COMMON ABBREVIATIONS
USED IN WRITING PRESCRIPTIONS

Abbreviation	Derivation	Meaning	Abbreviation	Derivation	Meaning
a̅a̅	ana	of each	o.m.	omni mane	every morning
a.c.	ante cibum	before meals	o.n.	omni nocte	every night
ad	ad	to, up to	os	os	mouth
ad lib.	ad libitum	freely as desired (at pleasure)	oz	uncia	ounce
			p.c.	post cibum	after meals
agit. ante sum.	agita ante sumendum	shake before taking	per	per	through or by
alt. dieb.	alternis diebus	every other day	pil.	pilula	pill
alt. hor.	alternis horis	alternate hours	p.o.	per os	orally
alt. noct.	alternis noctibus	alternate nights	p.r.n.	pro re nata	as required
aq.	aqua	water	PR		per rectum
aq. dest.	aqua destillata	distilled water	PTA		prior to appointment
b.i.d.	bis in die	two times a day	ptd		prior to discharge
b.i.n.	bis in nocte	two times a night	q	quaque	every
c., c̅	cum	with	q.h.	quaque hora	every hour
Cap.	capiat	let him take	q. 2 h.		every two hours
caps.	capsula	capsule	q. 3 h.		every three hours
comp.	compositus	compound	q. 4 h.		every four hours
Det.	detur	let it be given	q.i.d.	quater in die	four times a day
Dieb. tert.	diebus tertiis	every third day	q.l.	quantum libet	as much as desired
dil.	dilutus	dilute	q.n.	quaque nocte	every night
DS		double strength	q.p.	quantum placeat	as much as desired
D/W		distilled water	q.v.	quantum vis	as much as you please
EOD; eod		every other day	q.s.	quantum sufficit	as much as is required
elix.	elixir	elixir	R	recipe	take
ext.	extractum	extract	Rep.	repetatur	let it be repeated
fld.	fluidus	fluid	s, s̅	sine	without
Ft.	fiat	make	seq. luce.	sequenti luce	the following day
g	gramme	gram	Sig. or S.	signa	write on label
gr	granum	grain	s.o.s.	si opus sit	if necessary
gt	gutta	a drop	sp.	spiritus	spirits
gtt	guttae	drops	ss	semis	a half
h.	hora	hour	stat.	statim	immediately
h.d.	hora decubitus	at bedtime	supp		suppository
h.s.	hora somni	hour of sleep (bedtime)	syr.	syrupus	syrup
M.	misce	mix	t.d.s.	ter die sumendum	to be taken three times daily
m.	minimum	a minim			
mist.	mistura	mixture	t.i.d.	ter in die	three times a day
non rep.	non repetatur	not to be repeated	t.i.n.	ter in nocte	three times a night
noct.	nocte	in the night	tr. or tinct.	tinctura	tincture
O	octarius	pint	ung.	unguentum	ointment
ol.	oleum	oil	ut. dict.	ut dictum	as directed
o.d.	omni die	every day	vin.	vini	of wine
o.h.	omni hora	every hour	W/O		without

SPANISH-FRENCH-ENGLISH EQUIVALENTS OF COMMONLY USED MEDICAL TERMS AND PHRASES

English	Spanish	French
What is your name?	¿Cómo se llama usted? (¿Cuál es su nombre?)	Comment vous appelez-vous?
Where do you work?	¿Dónde trabaja? (¿Cuál es su profesión o trabajo?) (¿Qué hace usted?)	Où travaillez-vous?
You will need blood and urine tests.	Usted va a necesitar pruebas de sangre y de orina.	Vous avez besoin d'une analyse de sang et d'urine.
You will be admitted to a hospital.	Usted será ingresado al hospital.	Vous allez être admis à un hôpital.
May I help you?	¿Puedo ayudarle?	Puis-je vous aider?
How are you feeling? Where does it hurt?	¿Cómo se siente? ¿Dónde le duele?	Comment vous sentez-vous? Où avez vous mal?
Do you feel better today?	¿Se siente mejor hoy?	Vous sentez-vous mieux aujourd'hui?
Are you sleepy?	¿Tiene usted sueño?	Avez-vous sommeil?
The doctor will examine you now.	El doctor le examinará ahora.	Le médecin va vous examiner maintenant.
You should remain in bed today.	Usted debe quedarse en su cama hoy.	Vous devriez rester au lit aujourd'hui.
We want you to get up now.	Queremos que se levante ahora.	Nous voulons que vous vous leviez maintenant.
You may take a bath.	Puede bañarse.	Vous pouvez prendre un bain.
You may take a shower.	Puede darse una ducha.	Vous pouvez prendre une douche.
Have you noticed any bleeding?	¿Ha notado algún sangrado?	Avez-vous remarqué un saignement?
Do you still have any numbness?	¿Todavía siente adormecimiento?	Ressentez-vous encore un engourdissement?
Do you have any drug allergies?	¿Es usted alérgico(a) a algún medicamento?	Souffrez-vous d'allergie à n'importe quel médicaments?
I need to change your dressing.	Necesito cambiar su vendaje.	Je dois changer votre pansement.
What medications are you taking now?	¿Qué medicamentos está tomando ahora?	Quels médicaments prenez-vous actuellement?
Do you take any medications?	¿Toma usted algunas medicinas?	Prenez-vous des médicaments?
Do you have a history of	¿Padece	Avez-vous déjà souffert de
a. heart disease?	a. del corazón?	a. maladie du coeur?
b. diabetes?	b. de diabetes?	b. diabète?
c. epilepsy?	c. de epilepsia?	c. épilepsie?
d. bronchitis?	d. de bronquitis?	d. bronchite?
e. emphysema?	e. de enfisema?	e. emphysème?
f. asthma?	f. de asma?	f. asthme?
Do you need a sleeping pill?	¿Necesita una pastilla para dormir?	Avez-vous besoin d'un somnifère?
Do you need a laxative?	¿Necesita un laxante/purgante?	Avez-vous besoin d'un laxatif?
Relax. Try to sleep.	Relájese. Trate de dormir.	Détendez-vous. Essayez de dormir.
Please turn on your side.	Favor de ponerse/virarse de lado.	Veuillez vous tourner sur le côté.
Do you need to urinate?	¿Tiene que orinar?	Avez-vous besoin d'uriner?
Have you had any sickness from any medicine?	¿Le ha caído mal alguna medicina?	Avez-vous déjà eu des réactions à n'importe quel médicament?
Are you allergic to anything? Medicines, drugs, foods, insect bites?	¿Es usted alérgico(a) a algo? ¿Medicinas, drogas, alimentos, picaduras de insectos?	Êtes-vous allergique à quelque chose? Médicaments, drogues, aliments, piqûres d'insectes?
Do you use contact lenses, dentures? Do you have any loose teeth, removable bridges, or any prosthesis?	¿Usa usted lentes de contacto, dentadura postiza? ¿Tiene dientes flojos, dientes postizos, o cualquier próstesis?	Utilisez-vous des verres de contact, des prothèses dentaires? Avez-vous des dents qui se déchaussent, des ponts amovibles ou une prothèse?
Press the button when you want a nurse.	Apriete el botón cuando quiera llamar a una enfermera.	Appuyez sur le bouton pour appeler une infirmière.

Spanish adapted from Lister S. Wilber CJ: *Medical Spanish: the instant survival guide,* ed 4, London, Butterworth. French translations provided by Catherine Moor, translator, Montreal, Quebec, Canada.

MOSBY'S®
MEDICAL
DICTIONARY

ELEVENTH EDITION

MOSBY'S®
MEDICAL
DICTIONARY

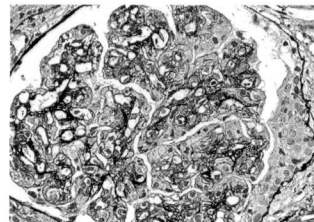 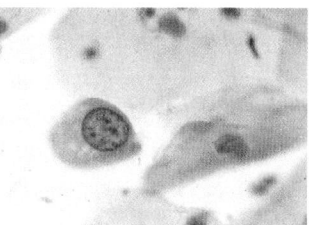 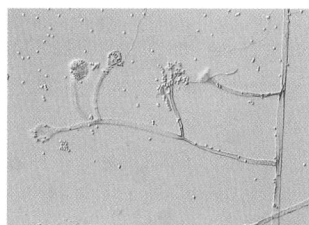

Illustrated in full color throughout

With over 2450 Illustrations

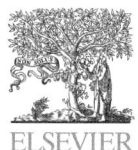

ELSEVIER

Elsevier
3251 Riverport Lane
St. Louis, Missouri 63043

MOSBY'S® MEDICAL DICTIONARY,
ELEVENTH EDITION

ISBN: 978-0-323-63915-6

Library of Congress Control Number: 2021933790

Executive Content Strategist: Sonya Seigafuse
Senior Content Development Manager: Luke Held
Senior Content Development Specialist: Sarah Vora
Publishing Services Manager: Julie Eddy
Senior Project Manager: Jodi Willard
Design Direction: Margaret Reid
Cover Illustrations:
Chromatin: (McKee, 1997)
Diabetic retinopathy: (Goldman and Shafer, 2012)
Lichtheimia: (Mahon, Lehman, and Manuselis, 2011)
Membranoproliferative glomerulonephritis: (Schena et al, 2015)

Printed in Canada

Last digit is the print number: 9 8 7 6 5 4 3 2

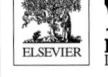

CONTENTS

EDITOR'S FOREWORD

Health care is complex, nuanced, and evolutionary in nature. The changes in health care can often be dramatic and rapid. Language is a tool of communication, and the language of health care is also complex, nuanced, evolving, and informed by words no longer in common use. The overarching goal of this edition of *Mosby's Medical Dictionary* is to assist the user to understand how words and phrases commonly encountered in the health care literature and clinical practice are used, have been used in the past, how they are spelled and pronounced and, in many instances, see examples of the words and phrases by utilizing full-color illustrations. Mastering the body of knowledge essential to professional practice requires access to definitions that enhance the understanding of the language of health care. All of the entries in this edition of *Mosby's Medical Dictionary* have been developed and reviewed to provide a single source of authoritative, up-to-date definitions for a wide variety of health care professionals and individuals who wish to better understand health care information and communicate it effectively.

The characteristics that have made the previous 10 editions of *Mosby's Medical Dictionary* an invaluable resource for the past 30 years have been retained. These include the use of a large and easy-to-read typeface, encyclopedic definitions for commonly referenced key terms, and a commonsense, strictly alphabetical organization of definitions. To assist readers in recognizing alternative spellings, selected British spellings are included where appropriate. Students, educators, and practitioners have praised the comprehensive and reliable nature of previous editions, and great care has been taken to ensure that tradition is continued in this 11th edition.

One of the most distinct features of *Mosby's Medical Dictionary* is the inclusion of high-quality, full-color illustrations and photographs throughout the book to enhance and clarify definitions of terms with a visual representation of many diseases, conditions, and equipment. *Mosby's Medical Dictionary* was the first English-language medical, nursing or health professional's dictionary to use full-color images. In addition, a Color Atlas of Human Anatomy contains clearly labeled helpful illustrations and is placed at the front of the dictionary for easy access.

It is impossible to adequately thank and acknowledge all of the many individuals who have contributed to the 11th edition of *Mosby's Medical Dictionary*. As an editor, I have been informed by innumerable students over the years, as well as colleagues in many professions and at many institutions, and inspired by the many patients that I, my students, and my colleagues have cared for and about. An interdisciplinary Editorial Board and numerous consultants and experts reviewed every entry in *Mosby's Medical Dictionary*. I am deeply indebted to all of them for the care and wisdom they shared in providing suggestions for revision and for additional entries.

It is an honor to work with professionals as dedicated to meeting the needs of readers as those of Elsevier. Tamara Myers provided expert guidance and was instrumental in gaining access to the considerable resources of Elsevier-Mosby, Saunders, Churchill-Livingstone, and Butterworth-Heinemann. The database used to facilitate the review and collaboration of multiple individuals in the construction of this edition was invaluable. Sarah Vora was an inspirational partner who was sensitive to the need to keep the work moving forward while at the same time sensitive to the need to allow time to properly research and refine the entries. Babette Morgan and Jodi Willard were extraordinary in their helpful and constructive input on entries and the labeling of images. The research associated with compiling a dictionary requires examining the literature, consulting with experts and verifying the accuracy of an entry. The availability of resources from Elsevier and the ability to consult with colleagues regarding a words meaning and use were critical to the completion of this and every previous edition of *Mosby's Medical Dictionary*.

In addition, my colleagues and students at Rutgers University, School of Nursing—Camden patiently reviewed materials, answered questions, and always provided just the right suggestion to assist me in making each and every definition and image maximally useful. I appreciate their contributions and trust they will all be proud to be associated with the 11th edition of *Mosby's Medical Dictionary*. Dr. Tyshaneka Saffold assisted with images and Dr. Staci Pacetti served on the Editorial Board.

It is impossible to not conclude without a thank you to my family. My niece, Olivia Felicia, is a talented photographer who enthusiastically assisted with images. My son, Kevin P. O'Toole, OTR, is an Occupational Therapist who was generous with his time and expertise, and critiques. I am fortunate to have children familiar with Latin and Greek for consultation on the etymology of many entries. My family has always been willing to indulge my passion for words and serve as the definition of love.

My thanks also go to the readers for using this work to learn or update their ability to communicate with others and improve patient care.

This edition was largely completed during a pandemic. In March 2020 the world changed and health, and the words used to describe health and health practices, became more important to many individuals. The vocabulary of health care was featured daily in news outlets. As editor, I was reminded of the importance of a reference that helped all users of the dictionary to understand and accurately express concepts related to health care.

Marie T. O'Toole, EdD, RN, FAAN, ANEF

EDITOR

Danny McGuire, BS, MEd, PhD
Professor and Chair
Department of Chemistry, Physics, and
    Engineering
Cameron University
Lawton, Oklahoma

Marc S. Micozzi, MD, PhD
Adjunct Professor
Department of Medicine
University of Pennsylvania School of
    Medicine
Philadelphia, Pennsylvania;
Department of Pharmacology
Georgetown University School of Medicine
Washington, DC

Linda Mollino, MSN, RN
Director of Career and Technical Programs
Health and Human Services
Oregon Coast Community College
Newport, Oregon

Quanza E. Mooring, PhD RN
Assistant Professor of Nursing
Department of Nursing
Texas Lutheran University
Seguin, Texas

Anne M. Moscony, OTD, CHT
Occupational Therapist, Certified Hand
    Therapist
Occupational Therapy
University of St. Augustine for Health Science
St. Augustine, Florida

Krishan K. Pandey, PhD
Associate Research Professor
Molecular Microbiology and Immunology
Saint Louis University
St. Louis, Missouri

Joseph William Robertson, DDS, BS
Department of Nursing and Health Professions
Oakland Community College
Royal Oak, Michigan

Bhupinder Singh, MD
Head Faculty of Health Sciences
Health Sciences
Biztech College
Canadian All Care College
University Health Network
Jammu Medical College
Ontario, Canada

Paul St. Jacques, MD
Professor of Anesthesiology
Anesthesiology
Vanderbilt University Medical Center
Nashville, Tennessee

Tim Randolph, PhD, MT(ASCP)
Associate Professor
Saint Louis University
St. Louis, Missouri

Paula Denise Silver, BS, PharmD
Medical Instructor
School of Health Science
ECPI University
Newport News, Virginia

Jennifer M. Stevenson, MHS, CCC-SLP, EdS
Speech-Language Pathologist
Great Beginnings Early Education Center
Lee's Summit R-7 School District
Therapy Relief at Hope
Lee's Summit, Missouri

Gary Thibodeau, PhD
Chancellor Emeritus and Professor Emeritus
    of Biology
University of Wisconsin—River Falls
River Falls, Wisconsin

Kajal Vora, FNP-C, MSN
Family Nurse Practitioner
Anesthesia Services
Emory University Hospital
Atlanta, Georgia

Patti Ward, PhD, RT(R)
Professor of Radiologic Technology
Health Sciences
Colorado Mesa University
Grand Junction, Colorado

Bradley M. Wright, PharmD, BCPS, FASHP
Associate Clinical Professor
Pharmacy Practice
Auburn University Harrison School of
    Pharmacy
Huntsville, Alabama

Nancy H. Wright, RN, BS, CNOR(R)
Wright Solutions
Curriculum Development
Health Care Education Compliance
Helena, Alabama

Wm. Kendall Wyatt, MD, RN, EMTP
Chief Resident Physician
Charleston Area Medical Center
Charleston, West Virginia

Jean Yockey, RN, PhD, MSN, FNP, ANA
Assistant Professor
Nursing
University of South Dakota
Vermillion, South Dakota

Nicole B. Zeller, MSN, RN
Nursing Faculty
Nursing
Lake Land College
Mattoon, Illinois

GUIDE TO THE DICTIONARY

A. ALPHABETICAL ORDER

The entries are alphabetized in dictionary style, that is, letter by letter, disregarding spaces or hyphens between words:

analgesic	**artificial lung**
anal membrane	**artificially acquired immunity**
analog	**artificial menopause**

(Alphabetized in telephone-book style, that is, word by word, the order would be different: **anal membrane / analgesic / analog; artificial lung / artificial menopause / artificially acquired immunity.**)

The alphabetization is alphanumeric; that is, words and numbers form a single list, numbers being positioned as though they were spelled-out numerals: **Nilstat / 90-90 traction / ninth nerve.** (An example of the few exceptions to this rule is the sequence **17-hydroxycorticosteroid / 11-hydroxyetiocholanolone / 5-hydroxyindoleacetic acid,** which can be found between the entries **hydroxychloroquine sulfate** and **hydroxyl,** not, as may be expected, **17-. . .** in letter "S," **11-. . .** in letter "E," and **5-. . .** in letter "F.").

Small subscript and superscript numbers are disregarded in alphabetizing: **No / N_2O / nobelium**

For the alphabetization of prefixes and suffixes, see F.

B. COMPOUND HEADWORDS

Compound headwords are given in their natural word order: **abdominal surgery,** not **surgery, abdominal; achondroplastic dwarf**, not **dwarf, achondroplastic**.

When appropriate, a reference is made elsewhere to the nonalphabetized element; the entry **dwarf,** for example, shows this indirect cross-reference: ". . . Kinds of dwarfs include **achondroplastic dwarf, . . .**" (followed by additional terms ending in "dwarf").

(NOTE: In this guide, the term "headword" is used to refer to any alphabetized and nonindented definiendum, be it a single-word term or a compound term.)

C. MULTIPLE DEFINITIONS

If a headword has more than one meaning, the meanings are numbered and are often accompanied by an indication of the field in which a sense applies: "**fractionation, 1.** (in neurology) . . . **2.** (in chemistry) . . . **3.** (in bacteriology) . . . **4.** (in histology) . . . **5.** (in radiology) . . ."

Smaller differences in meaning are occasionally separated by semicolons: "**enervation, 1.** the reduction or lack of nervous energy; weakness; lassitude, languor. **2.** removal of a complete nerve or of a section of nerve."

Words that are spelled alike but have entirely different meanings and origins are usually given as separate entries, with superscript numbers: "**aural^1,** pertaining to the ear or hearing . . ." followed by "**aural^2,** pertaining to an aura."

For reference entries that appear in the form of numbered senses, see the example of **balsam** at E.

D. THE ELEMENTS OF AN ENTRY

The entry headword has a large boldface type. For the most part, boldface terms indicate a corresponding headword or entry. The following elements may occur in boldface or italics in this order.

■ HEADWORD ABBREVIATIONS: **central nervous system (CNS)**

A corresponding abbreviation entry is listed: "**CNS,** abbreviation for **central nervous system.**" (For abbreviation entries, see F.)

Occasionally the order is reversed: "**DDT (dichlorodiphenyltrichloroethane),**" with a corresponding reference entry: "**dichlorodiphenyltrichloroethane.** See **DDT.**" (For reference entries, see E below.)

■ PLURAL OR SINGULAR FORMS that are not obvious. The first form shown is the more common except when plurals are of more or less equal frequency: "**carcinoma,** *pl. carcinomas, carcinomata*"; "**cortex,** *pl.* **cortices**"; "**data,** *sing.* **datum**"

A reference entry is listed only when the terms are alphabetically separated; for example, there are several entries between **data** and "**datum.** See **data.**"

■ HIDDEN ENTRIES, that is, terms that can best be defined in the context of a more general entry. For example, the definition of the entry **equine encephalitis** continues as follows: ". . . **Eastern equine encephalitis (EEE)** is a severe form of the infection . . . **western equine encephalitis (WEE),** which occurs . . . **Venezuelan equine encephalitis (VEE),** which is common in . . ." The corresponding reference entries are "**eastern equine encephalitis.** See **equine encephalitis.**"; "**western equine encephalitis.** See **equine . . .**"; and so forth. For further reference, from the abbreviations **EEE, WEE,** and **VEE,** see F.

■ INDIRECT CROSS-REFERENCES to other defined entries, shown as part of the definition and usually introduced by "Kinds of": "**dwarf,** . . . Kinds of dwarfs include **achondroplastic dwarf, asexual dwarf,** . . . and **thanatophoric dwarf.**"

The entry referred to may or may not show a reciprocal reference, depending on the information value.

■ SYNONYMOUS TERMS, preceded by "Also called," "Also spelled," or, for verbs and adjectives, "Also": "**abducens nerve,** . . . Also called **sixth cranial nerve.**"

A corresponding reference entry is usually given: "**sixth cranial nerve.** See **abducens nerve.**"

Occasionally the synonymous term is accompanied by a usage label: "**abdomen,** . . . Also called *(informal)* **belly.**"

If a synonymous term applies to only one numbered sense, it precedes rather than follows the definition, to avoid ambiguity: "**algology, 1.** the branch of medicine that is concerned with the study of pain. **2.** also called **phycology,** the branch of science that is concerned with algae." (Whenever a synonymous term *follows* the last numbered sense, it applies to all senses of the entry.)

■ (DIRECT) CROSS-REFERENCES, preceded by "See also" or "Compare," referring to another defined entry for additional information: "**abdominal aorta,** . . . See also **descending aorta.**"

The cross-reference may or may not be reciprocal.

Cross-references are also made to illustrations, tables, the color atlas, and the appendixes.

For cross-references from an abbreviation entry (with "See"), see F.

■ PARTS OF SPEECH related to the entry headword, shown as run-on entries that do not require a separate definition: "**abalienation, . . . —abalienate,** *v.,* **abalienated,** *adj.*"

E. REFERENCE ENTRIES

Reference entries are undefined entries referring to a defined entry. There, they usually correspond to the boldface terms for which reference entries are mentioned at D above.

However, many of the less frequently used synonymous terms are listed as a reference only; at the entry referred to, the reader's attention is not drawn to them with "Also called."

Some reference entries appear in the form of a numbered sense of a defined entry: "**balsam, 1.** any of a variety of resinous saps, generally from evergreens, usually containing benzoic or cinnamic acid. Balsam is sometimes used in rectal suppositories and dermatological agents as a counterirritant. **2.** See **balm.**"

If two or more alphabetically adjacent terms refer to the same entry or entries, they are styled as one reference entry: "**coxa adducta, coxa flexa.** See **coxa vara.**"

A reference entry that would be derived from a boldface term in an immediately adjacent entry is not listed again as a headword; it becomes a "hidden reference entry": "**acardius amorphus,** . . . Also called *acardius anceps.*" But *acardius anceps* is not listed again as a reference entry because it would immediately *follow* the entry, the next entry being **acariasis.** Likewise: "**acoustic neuroma,** . . . Also called **acoustic neurilemmoma, acoustic neurinoma, acoustic neurofibroma.**" But the three synonymous terms are not listed again as reference entries because they would immediately *precede* the entry, the entry ahead being **acoustic nerve.** Therefore:

> **If a term is not listed at the expected place, the reader might find it among the boldface or italicized terms of the immediately preceding or the immediately following entry.**

Selected British spellings are included where appropriate. These are included as reference entries, which refer the reader to the American spelling containing the definition. After the definition, the British spelling is given as an alternate spelling. For example: "**haematology.** See **hematology.**" The end of the definition for **hematology** says "Also spelled **haematology.**" As with other reference entries, when the reference entry would immediately precede or follow the main entry, it is not included as a separate entry, such as "**hyperkalemia** . . . Also spelled *hyperkalaemia.*"

F. OTHER KINDS OF ENTRIES

■ ABBREVIATION ENTRIES: Most abbreviation entries, including symbol entries, show the full form of the term in boldface: "**ABC,** abbreviation for **aspiration biopsy cytology.**" "**H,** symbol for the element **hydrogen.**" Implied reference is made to the entries **aspiration biopsy cytology** and **hydrogen** respectively.

Abbreviation entries for which there is no corresponding entry show the full form in italics: "**CBF,** abbreviation for *cerebral blood flow.*" "**f,** symbol for *respiratory frequency.*"

A combination of abbreviation entry and reference entry occurs when the abbreviation is that of a boldface or lightface term appearing under another headword. For example, the hidden entries at D (in addition to the reference entries shown there) are also referred to in the following manner: "**EEE,** abbreviation for **eastern equine encephalitis.** See **equine encephalitis.**" An example with a lightface term: "**HLA-A,** abbreviation for *human leukocyte antigen A.* See **human leukocyte antigen.**" The latter entry says ". . They are HLA-A, HLA-B, HLA-C . . ."

■ PREFIXES AND SUFFIXES: The large amount and the nature of prefix and suffix entries are an important feature of this dictionary. Through these entries the reader has additional access to the meanings of headwords and the words used in defining them. But such entries also give access to thousands of terms that are not included in this dictionary (and, to a large extent, are not found in any other reference work). For example, the entries **xylo-** and **-phage** (plus **-phagia, phago-,** and **-phagy**) may lead to the meaning of "xylophagous," namely, "wood-eating."

Prefix and suffix headwords consisting of variants are alphabetized by the first variant only. For example, "**epi-, ep-,** a prefix meaning 'on, upon' . . ." is followed by **epiblast** (notwithstanding "**ep-**"). The other variant or variants are listed in their own alphabetical place as reference entries referring to the first variant: "**ep-.** See **epi-.**"

■ ENTRIES WITH SPECIAL PARAGRAPHS: Among the entries on diseases, drugs, and procedures, at least 1100 feature special paragraphs, with headings such as:

observations, interventions, and *nursing considerations* (for disease entries),

indications, contraindications, and *adverse effects* (for drug entries),

method, nursing interventions, and *outcome criteria* (for procedure entries).

G. FURTHER COMMENTS

■ EPONYMOUS TERMS THAT END IN "SYNDROME" OR "DISEASE" are given with an apostrophe (and "s" where appropriate) if they are based on the name of one person: **Adie's syndrome; Symmers' disease.** If they are based on the names of several people, they are without apostrophe: **Bernard-Soulier syndrome; Brill-Symmers disease.**

■ ABBREVIATIONS AND LABELS IN ITALIC TYPE: The abbreviations are *pl.* (plural), *npl.* (noun plural), *sing.* (singular); *n.* (noun), *adj.* (adjective), *v.* (verb). The recurring labels are *slang, informal, nontechnical, obsolete, archaic; chiefly British, Canada, U.S.*

■ DICTIONARY OF FIRST REFERENCE for general spelling preferences is *Webster's New Collegiate Dictionary;* thereafter: *Webster's Third New International Dictionary.*

H. PRONUNCIATION

■ SYSTEM: See the Pronunciation Key on p. xiii. The pronunciation system of this dictionary is basically a system that most readers know from their use of popular English dictionaries, especially the major college or desk dictionaries. All symbols for English sounds are ordinary letters of the alphabet with few adaptations, and with the exception of the schwa, / <reve> / (the neutral vowel).

■ ACCENTS: Pronunciation, given between slants, is shown with primary and secondary accents, and a raised dot shows that two vowels or, occasionally, two consonants, between the slants are pronounced separately:

anoopsia /an′ō·op′sē·ə /
cecoileostomy /il′ē·os′t ə mē/
methemoglobin /met′hēm ə glō′bin, met·hē′ m ə glōbin/

Without the raised dot, the second /th/ in the last example would be pronounced as in "thin." (The pronunciation key lists the following paired consonant symbols as representing a single sound: /ch/, /ng/, /sh/, /th/, /th/, /zh/, and the foreign sounds /kh/ and /kh/–if no raised dot intervenes.)

■ TRUNCATION: Pronunciation may be given in truncated form, especially for alternative or derived words:

defibrillate /difī′brilāt, difib′-/
bacteriophage /baktir′ē· ə f ā j′, . . .—**bacteriophagy** /-of′ ə jē/, *n.*

In the last example, the reader is asked to make the commonsense assumption that the primary accent of the headword becomes a secondary accent in the run-on term: /baktir'ē·of'·əjē/.

■ LOCATION: Pronunciation may be given for any boldface term and may occur anywhere in an entry:

> **aura** /ôr 'e /, **1.** *pl.* **aurae** /ôr 'ē/, a sensation . . .
> **2.** *pl.* auras, an emanation of light . . .
> **micrometer, 1.** /mīkrom 'ə t ə r/, an instrument used for. . .
> **2.** /mī 'krōmē 't ə r/, a unit of measurement . . .

Occasionally it is given for a lightface term:

> **b.i.d.,** (in prescriptions) abbreviation for *bis in die* /dē 'ā/, a Latin phrase meaning . . .
> **boutonneuse fever. . . ,** an infectious disease . . . a tache noire /täshnô·är ' / or black spot . . .

■ LETTERWORD VERSUS ACRONYM: Letterwords are abbreviations that are pronounced by sounding the names of each letter, whereas acronyms are pronounced as words. If the pronunciation of an abbreviation is not given, the abbreviation is usually a letterword:

> **ABO blood groups** [read / ā 'b ē 'ō '/, not/ā 'bō/]

If the pronunciation is an acronym, this is indicated by pronunciation:

> **AWOL** / ā 'wôl/

Some abbreviations are used as both:

> *JAMA* /jä 'mä, jam 'ə, j ā 'ā 'em 'ā '/

■ FOREIGN SOUNDS: Non-English sounds do not occur often in this dictionary. They are represented by the following symbols:

/œ/	as in (French) **feu** /fœ/, **Europe** /œrôp'/; (German) **schön** /shœn/, **Goethe** /gœ't ə /
/Y/	as in (French) **tu** /tY/, **déjà vu** /d ā zhävY'/; (German) **grün** /grYn/, **Walküre** /vulkY'r ə /
/kh/	as in (Scottish) **loch** /lokh/; (German) **Rorschach** / rôr ' -shokh/, **Bach** /bokh, bäkh/
/kh/	as in (German) **ich** /ikh /, **Reich** /rīkh/ (or, approximated, as in English **fish:** /ish/, /rīsh/)
/N/	This symbol does not represent a sound but indicates that the preceding vowel is a nasal, as in French **bon** /bôN/, **en face** /äNfäs'/, or **international** /aNternäsyōnäl'/.
/nyə/	Occurring at the end of French words, this symbol is not truly a separate syllable but an /n/ with a slight /y/ (similar to the sound in ''onion'') plus a near-silent / ə /, as in **Bois de Boulogne** / b̄oo lō'nyə /, **Malgaigne** /mälg ā'nyə /.

Because this work is a subject dictionary rather than a language dictionary, certain foreign words and proper names are rendered by English approximations. Examples are **Müller** /mil'ə r/ (which is closer to German than /mY'l ə r/), **Niemann** /nē'mon/ (which is closer than /nē'män/), **Friedreich** /frēd'rīsh/ (which is close enough for anyone not used to pronouncing /*kh/), or **jamais vu,** for which three acceptable pronunciations are given: /zhäm ā vY'/ (near-French) and the approximations /zhäm ā vē ' / and /zhäm ā v ōo ' / (/-vē'/ being much closer to French than /-v ōo ' /). Depending on usage, a foreign word or name may be given with near-native pronunciation, with entirely assimilated English pronunciation (as **de Quervain's**

fracture /de k ə rv ā nz'/), or with both (as **Dupuytren's contracture** /dYpYitraNs', dēpē·itranz'/ or **Klippel-Feil syndrome** /klipel 'f ə l', klip'ə lfīl'/).

At any rate, the English speaker should not hesitate to follow whatever is usage in his or her working or social environment.

Many of the numerous *Latin* terms in this dictionary are not given with pronunciation, mainly because there are different ways (all of them understood) in which Latin is pronounced by the English speaker and may be pronounced by speakers elsewhere. However, guidance is given in many cases, often to reflect common usage.

LATIN AND GREEK PLURALS: The spelling of Latin and Greek plurals is shown in most instances. However, when the plural formation is regular according to Latin and Greek rules, the pronunciation is usually not included. Therefore, the following list shows the suggested pronunciation of selected plural endings that are frequently encountered in the field of medicine:

PLURAL ENDINGS	EXAMPLES
-a /-ə/	**inoculum,** *pl.***inocula** /inok'y ōolə/
-ae /-ē/	**vertebra,** *pl.***vertebrae** /vur'təbrē/
-ces /-sēz/	**thorax,** *pl.***thoraces** /thôr'əsēz/
	apex, *pl.***apices** /ā'pisēz/
-era /-ərə/	**genus,** *pl.***genera** /jen'ərə/
-ges /-jēz/	**meninx,** *pl.***meninges** /minin'jēz/
-i /-ī/	**calculus,** *pl.***calculi** /kal'kyəlsī /
	coccus, *pl.***cocci** /kok'sī /
-ia /-ē·ə /	**criterion,** *pl.***criteria** /krītir'ē·ə/
-ides /-idēz/	**epulis,** *pl.***epulides** /ipyoo'lidēz/
-ina /-ənə/	**foramen,** *pl.***foramina** /f ə ram'ənə/
-ines /-ənēz/	**lentigo,** *pl.***lentigines** /lentij ' ənēz/
-omata /-ō'm ətə/	**hematoma,** *pl.***hematomata** /hē'mə tō'mətə/
-ones /-ō ' nēz/	**comedo,** *pl.***comedones** /kom'ə dō'nēz/
-ora /-ərə/	**corpus,** *pl.***corpora** /kôr'pərə/
	femur, *pl.***femora** /fem'ərə/
-ses /-sēz/	**analysis,** *pl.***analyses** / ənal'əsēz/
-udes /- ōo ' dēz/	**incus,** *pl.***incudes** /ink ōo'dēz/
-us /- ōos/	**ductus** (/duk ' təs/), *pl.***ductus** /duk't ōos/

NOTE: Notwithstanding the listing of Latin and Greek plurals in this dictionary, and notwithstanding the foregoing examples, in most instances it is acceptable or even preferable to pluralize Latin and Greek words according to the rules of English words. (For certain kinds of entries, both the English and the foreign plurals are given in this dictionary, usually showing the English form first, as, for example, in nearly all **-oma** nouns: **hematoma,** *pl.***hematomas, hematomata.**)

W.D.G.

I. ETYMOLOGIES AND EPONYMS

The word roots, or etymologies, of the headwords in this dictionary are shown in square brackets following the pronunciations of the headwords. Meanings are given in roman typeface and represent the original connotation of the word from which the medical term is derived. In compound medical terms formed from two or more elements, a plus sign (+) is used to indicate an element has been translated in a previous head-word, as in [L *acidus* + Gk *philein* to love]. A semicolon (;) is used to separate word elements having more than one origin, as in [L *abdomen;* Gk *skopein* to view]. Word fragments representing etymologic elements, such as prefixes, are separated from the rest of the word root by a comma (,), as in [Gk *a, basis* not step]. A comma is also used to separate the abbreviation for the language of origin and its translation when the English-language equivalent for the word is the same, as in the term **ala** [L, wing].

The following abbreviations are used to identify language sources:

Afr	African	L	Latin
Ar	Arabic	ME	Middle
AS	Anglo-Saxon		English
Dan	Danish	OFr	Old French
D	Dutch	ONorse	Old Norse
Fr	French	Port	Portuguese
Ger	German	Scand	Scandinavian
Gk	Greek	Sp	Spanish
Heb	Hebrew	Swe	Swedish
It	Italian	Turk	Turkish
Jpn	Japanese		

Some other languages sources, such as Singhalese or Welsh, may be indicated without abbreviations.

Eponymous entries, in which the surname of an individual is incorporated in the headword, are also treated in square brackets with brief biographic details, as in **Alcock's canal** [Benjamin Alcock, Irish anatomist, b. 1801]. When an eponym contains two or more surnames, a semicolon (;) is used to separate the identities of the individuals. Medical terms derived from other proper nouns, such as geographic sites, are presented in a similar manner, as **Calabar swelling** [Calabar, a Nigerian seaport], or **ytterbium (Yb)** [Ytterby, Sweden].

K.N.A.

PRONUNCIATION KEY

Vowels

SYMBOLS	KEY WORDS
/a/	hat
/ä/	father
/ā/	fate
/e/	flesh
/ē/	she
/er/	air, ferry
/i/	sit
/ī/	eye
/ir/	ear
/o/	proper
/ō/	nose
/ô/	saw
/oi/	boy
/o͞o/	move
/o͝o/	book
/ou/	out
/u/	cup, love
/ur/	fur, first
/ə/	(the neutral vowel, always unstressed, as in) ago, focus
/ər/	teacher, doctor

Consonants

SYMBOLS	KEY WORDS
/b/	book
/ch/	chew
/d/	day
/f/	fast
/g/	good
/h/	happy
/j/	gem
/k/	keep
/l/	late
/m/	make
/n/	no
/ng/	sing, drink
/ng·g/	finger
/p/	pair
/r/	ring
/s/	set
/sh/	shoe, lotion
/t/	tone
/th/	thin
/*th*/	than
/v/	very
/w/	work
/y/	yes
/z/	zeal
/zh/	azure, vision

For /oe/, /Y/, /kh/, /*kh*/, /N/, and /nyə/, see FOREIGN SOUNDS , p. xiii.

COLOR ATLAS OF HUMAN ANATOMY

SKELETAL SYSTEM

ANTERIOR VIEW OF SKELETON

POSTERIOR VIEW OF SKELETON

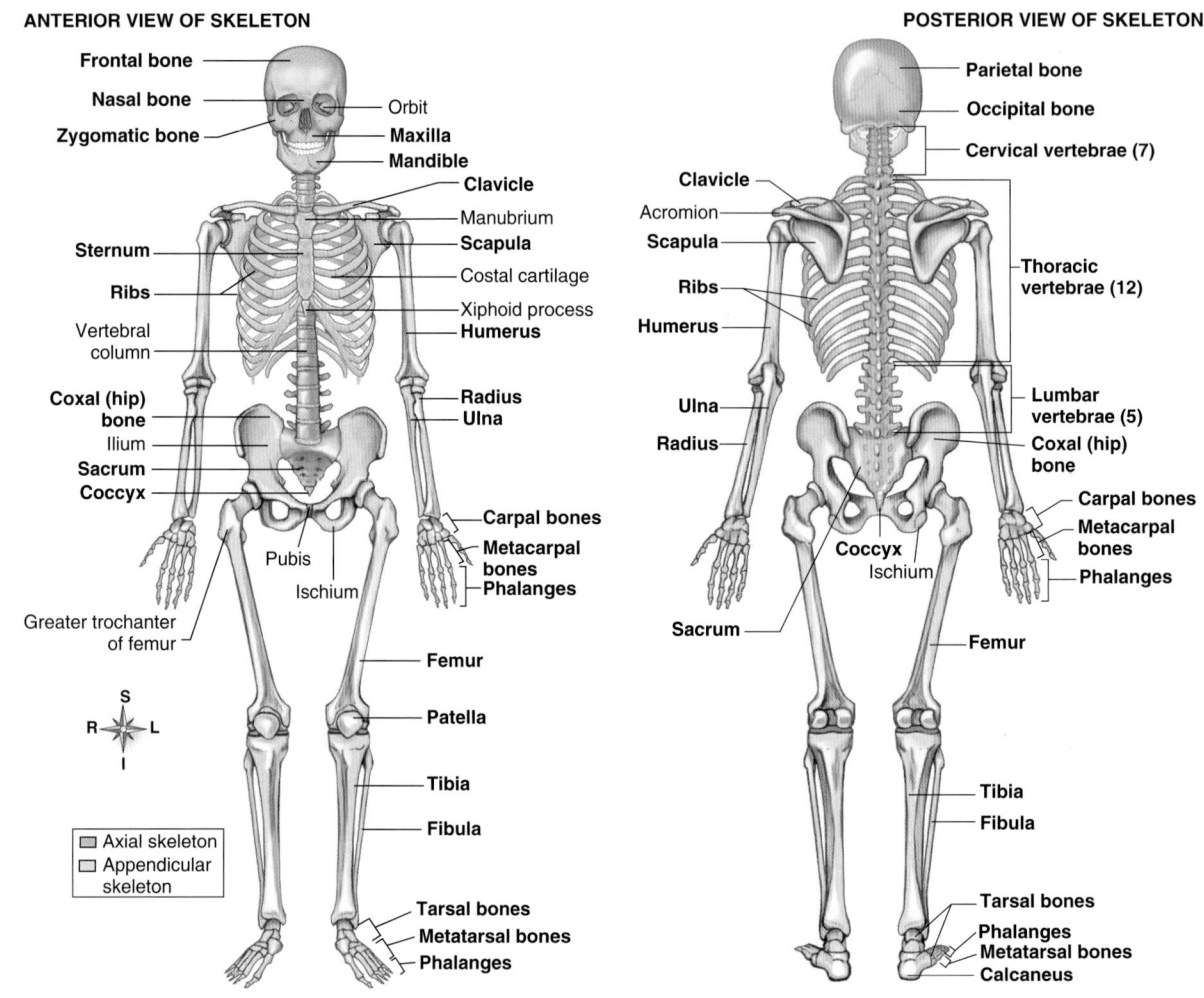

Anterior view labels:
Frontal bone
Nasal bone
Zygomatic bone
Orbit
Maxilla
Mandible
Clavicle
Manubrium
Scapula
Sternum
Ribs
Costal cartilage
Xiphoid process
Humerus
Vertebral column
Radius
Ulna
Coxal (hip) bone
Ilium
Sacrum
Coccyx
Pubis
Ischium
Carpal bones
Metacarpal bones
Phalanges
Greater trochanter of femur
Femur
Patella
Tibia
Fibula
Tarsal bones
Metatarsal bones
Phalanges

☐ Axial skeleton
☐ Appendicular skeleton

S
R — L
I

Posterior view labels:
Parietal bone
Occipital bone
Cervical vertebrae (7)
Clavicle
Acromion
Scapula
Ribs
Humerus
Thoracic vertebrae (12)
Ulna
Radius
Lumbar vertebrae (5)
Coxal (hip) bone
Carpal bones
Metacarpal bones
Phalanges
Coccyx
Ischium
Sacrum
Femur
Tibia
Fibula
Tarsal bones
Phalanges
Metatarsal bones
Calcaneus

ANTERIOR VIEW OF SKULL

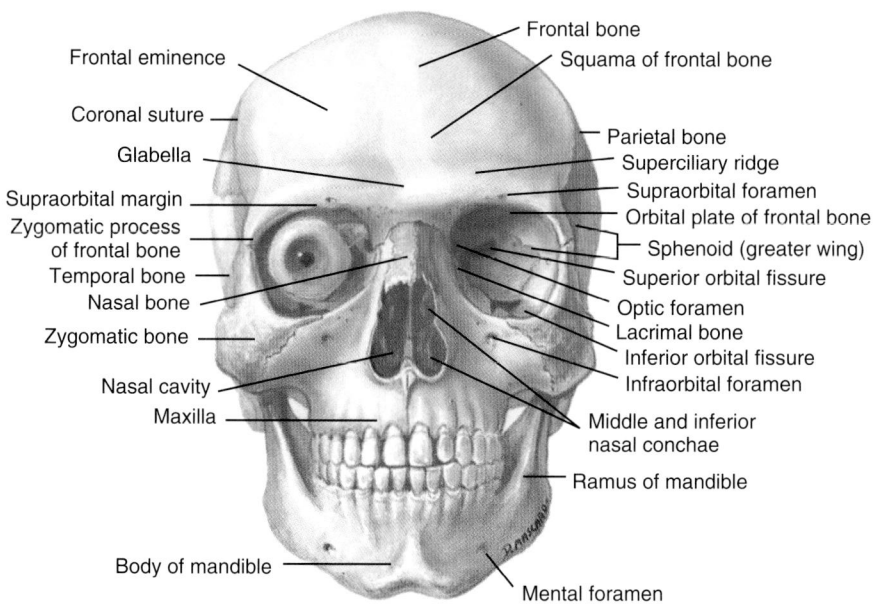

Frontal bone
Squama of frontal bone
Frontal eminence
Coronal suture
Glabella
Parietal bone
Superciliary ridge
Supraorbital foramen
Orbital plate of frontal bone
Supraorbital margin
Zygomatic process
of frontal bone
Sphenoid (greater wing)
Temporal bone
Superior orbital fissure
Nasal bone
Optic foramen
Zygomatic bone
Lacrimal bone
Inferior orbital fissure
Nasal cavity
Infraorbital foramen
Maxilla
Middle and inferior
nasal conchae
Ramus of mandible
Body of mandible
Mental foramen

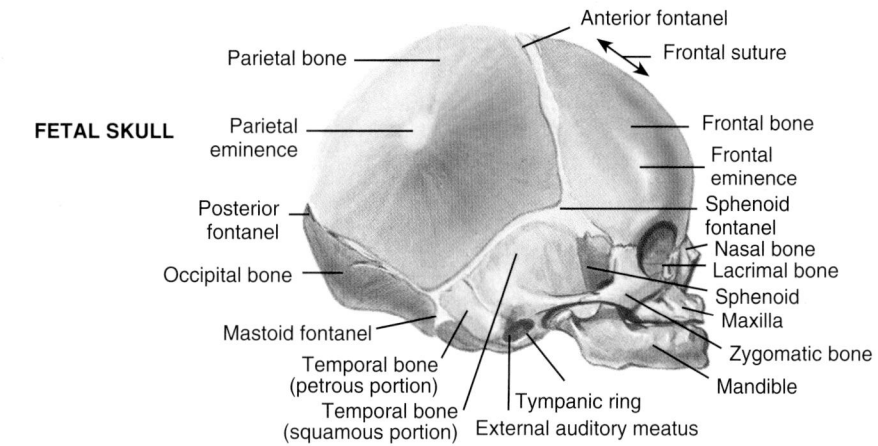

FETAL SKULL

Anterior fontanel
Frontal suture
Parietal bone
Frontal bone
Parietal
eminence
Frontal
eminence
Sphenoid
fontanel
Posterior
fontanel
Nasal bone
Lacrimal bone
Sphenoid
Occipital bone
Maxilla
Zygomatic bone
Mastoid fontanel
Mandible
Temporal bone
(petrous portion)
Tympanic ring
Temporal bone
(squamous portion)
External auditory meatus

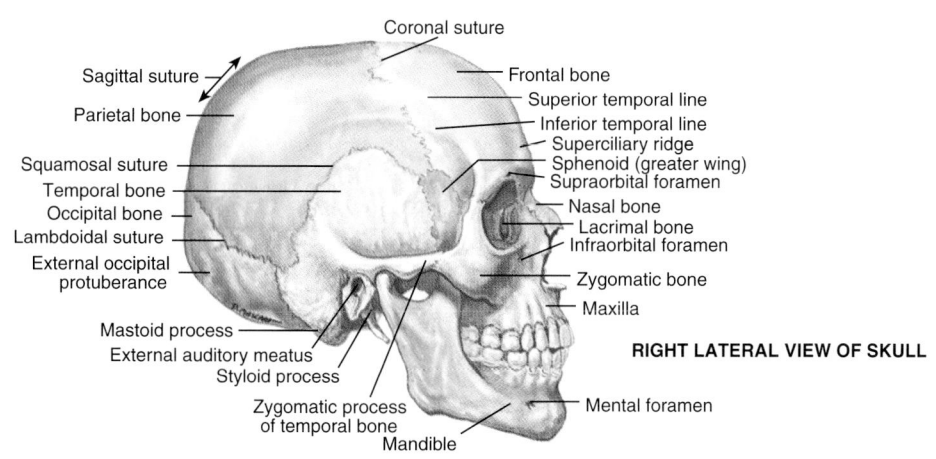

Coronal suture
Sagittal suture
Frontal bone
Superior temporal line
Parietal bone
Inferior temporal line
Superciliary ridge
Squamosal suture
Sphenoid (greater wing)
Supraorbital foramen
Temporal bone
Nasal bone
Occipital bone
Lacrimal bone
Lambdoidal suture
Infraorbital foramen
External occipital
protuberance
Zygomatic bone
Maxilla
Mastoid process
External auditory meatus
RIGHT LATERAL VIEW OF SKULL
Styloid process
Mental foramen
Zygomatic process
of temporal bone
Mandible

THORAX AND RIBS

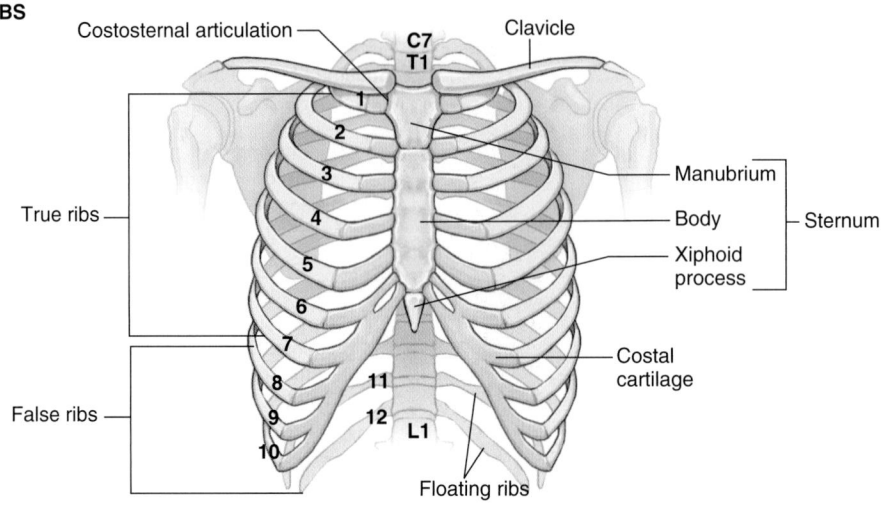

Costosternal articulation

Clavicle

C7
T1

1
2
3
4
5
6
7
8
9
10
11
12
L1

True ribs

False ribs

Floating ribs

Manubrium

Body

Xiphoid process

Sternum

Costal cartilage

PELVIS

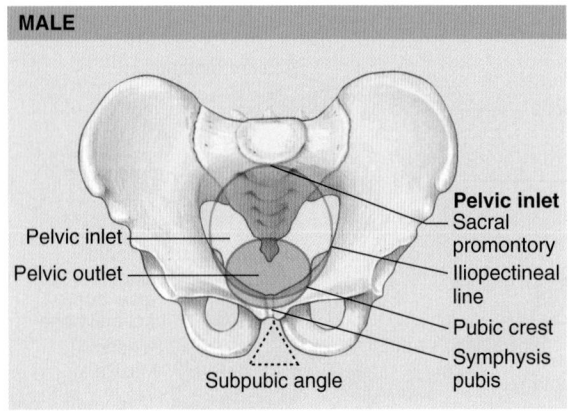

MALE

Pelvic inlet

Pelvic outlet

Subpubic angle

Pelvic inlet
Sacral promontory

Iliopectineal line

Pubic crest

Symphysis pubis

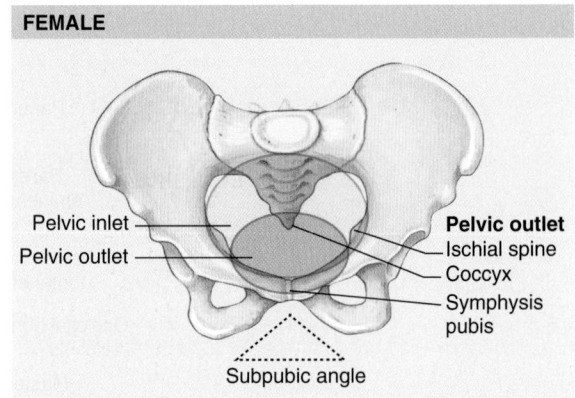

FEMALE

Pelvic inlet

Pelvic outlet

Subpubic angle

Pelvic outlet
Ischial spine
Coccyx
Symphysis pubis

INDIVIDUAL VERTEBRA

RIB

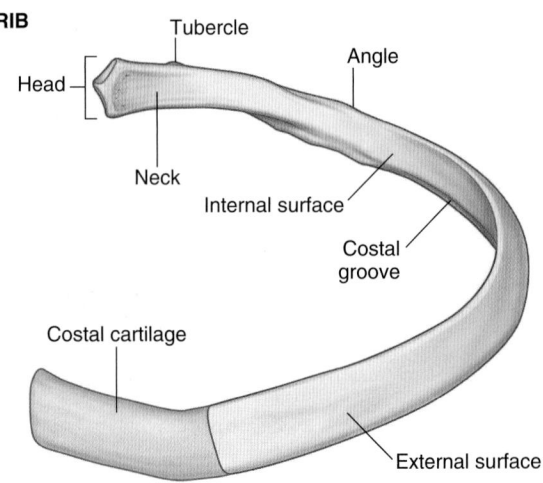

Head

Tubercle

Angle

Neck

Internal surface

Costal groove

Costal cartilage

External surface

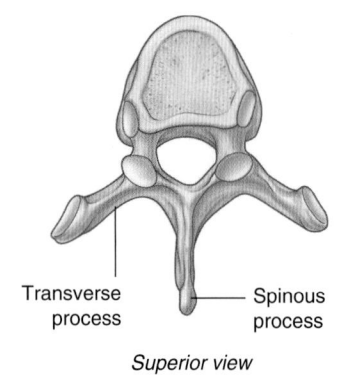

Transverse process

Spinous process

Superior view

VERTEBRAL COLUMN

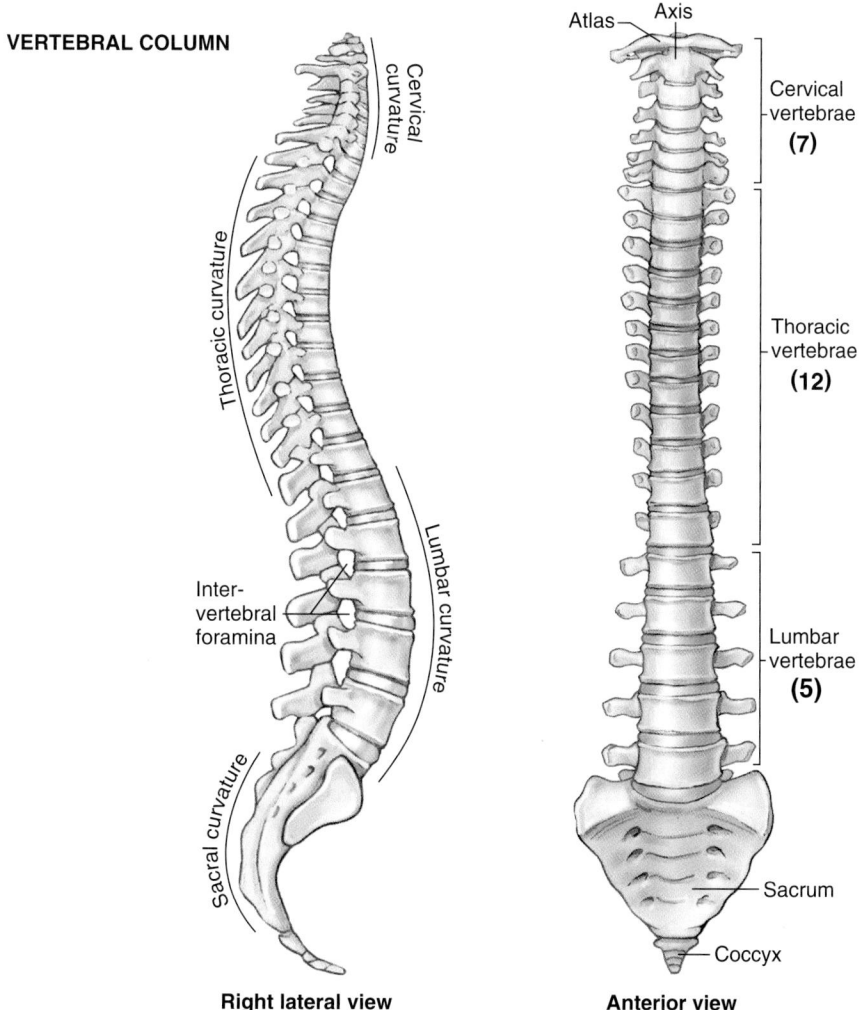

Cervical curvature

Thoracic curvature

Inter-vertebral foramina

Lumbar curvature

Sacral curvature

Right lateral view

Atlas

Axis

Cervical vertebrae **(7)**

Thoracic vertebrae **(12)**

Lumbar vertebrae **(5)**

Sacrum

Coccyx

Anterior view

FIRST CERVICAL VERTEBRA (ATLAS)

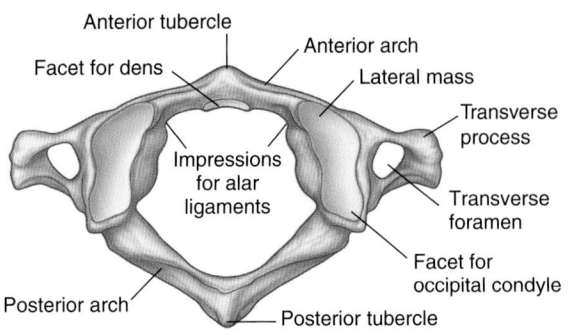

Anterior tubercle

Facet for dens

Anterior arch

Lateral mass

Transverse process

Impressions for alar ligaments

Transverse foramen

Facet for occipital condyle

Posterior arch

Posterior tubercle

SECOND CERVICAL VERTEBRA (AXIS)

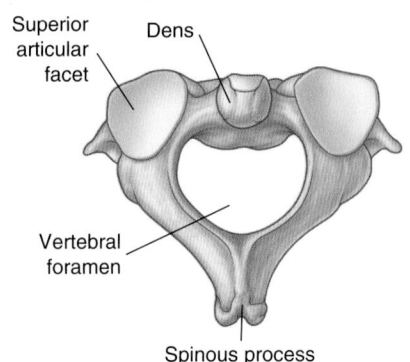

Superior articular facet

Dens

Vertebral foramen

Spinous process

FIFTH CERVICAL VERTEBRA

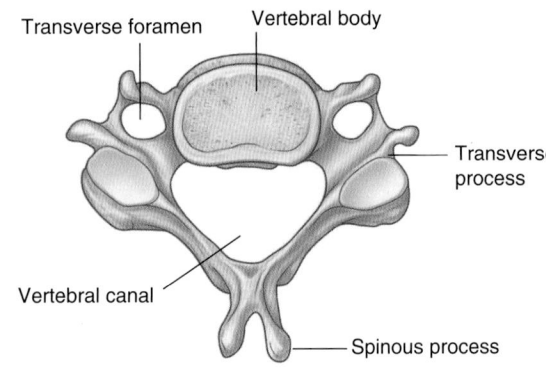

Transverse foramen

Vertebral body

Transverse process

Vertebral canal

Spinous process

THORACIC VERTEBRA

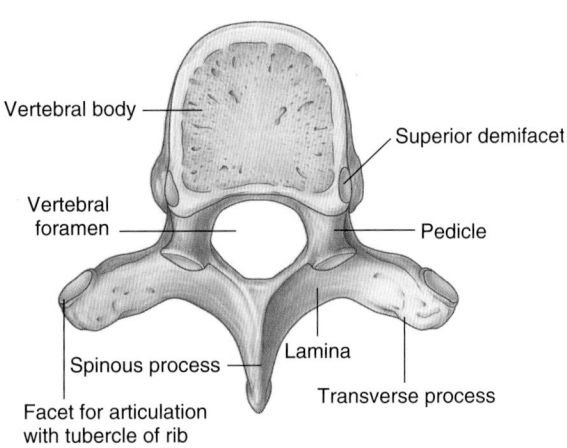

Vertebral body

Superior demifacet

Vertebral foramen

Pedicle

Spinous process

Lamina

Transverse process

Facet for articulation with tubercle of rib

LUMBAR VERTEBRA

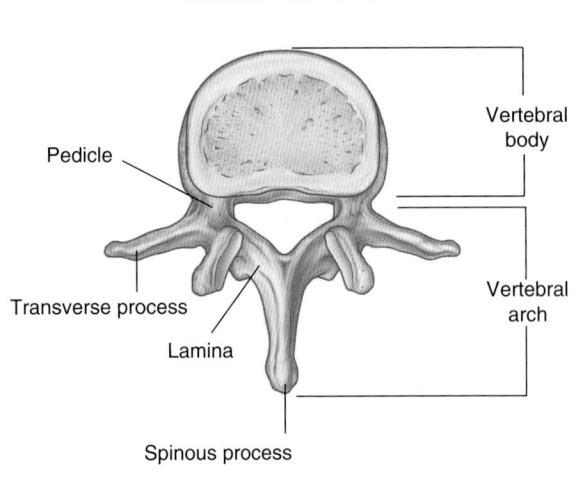

Pedicle

Vertebral body

Transverse process

Lamina

Vertebral arch

Spinous process

SACRUM AND COCCYX

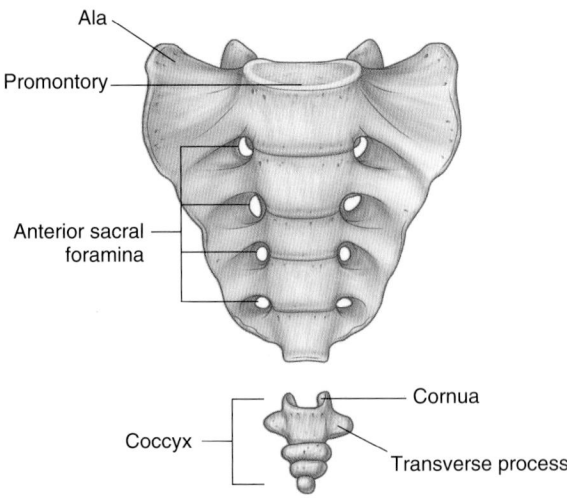

Ala

Promontory

Anterior sacral foramina

Cornua

Coccyx

Transverse process

MICROSCOPIC STRUCTURE OF BONE

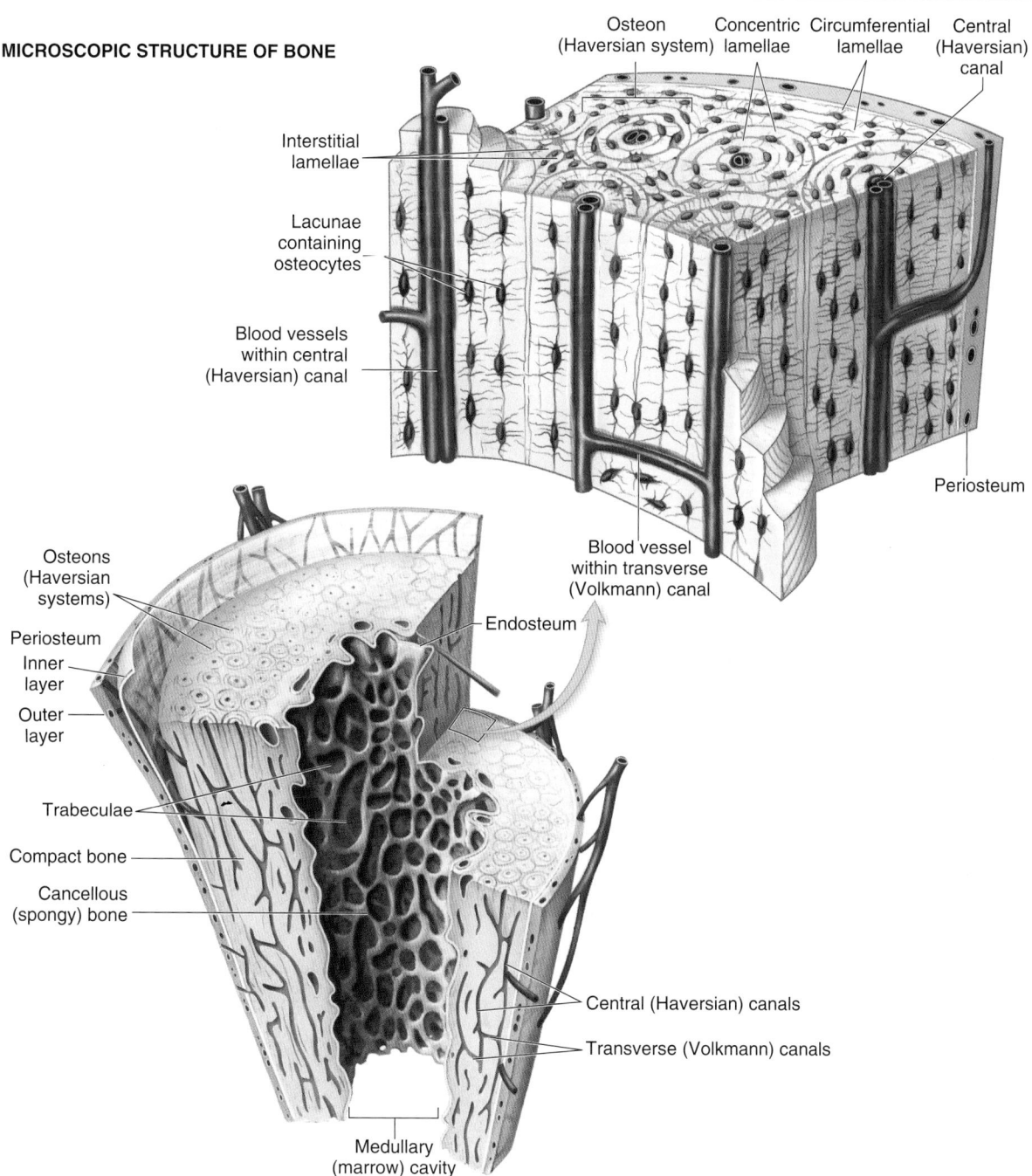

Osteon (Haversian system)   Concentric lamellae   Circumferential lamellae   Central (Haversian) canal

Interstitial lamellae

Lacunae containing osteocytes

Blood vessels within central (Haversian) canal

Periosteum

Blood vessel within transverse (Volkmann) canal

Osteons (Haversian systems)

Periosteum
Inner layer
Outer layer

Endosteum

Trabeculae

Compact bone

Cancellous (spongy) bone

Central (Haversian) canals

Transverse (Volkmann) canals

Medullary (marrow) cavity

MUSCULAR SYSTEM

ANTERIOR VIEW

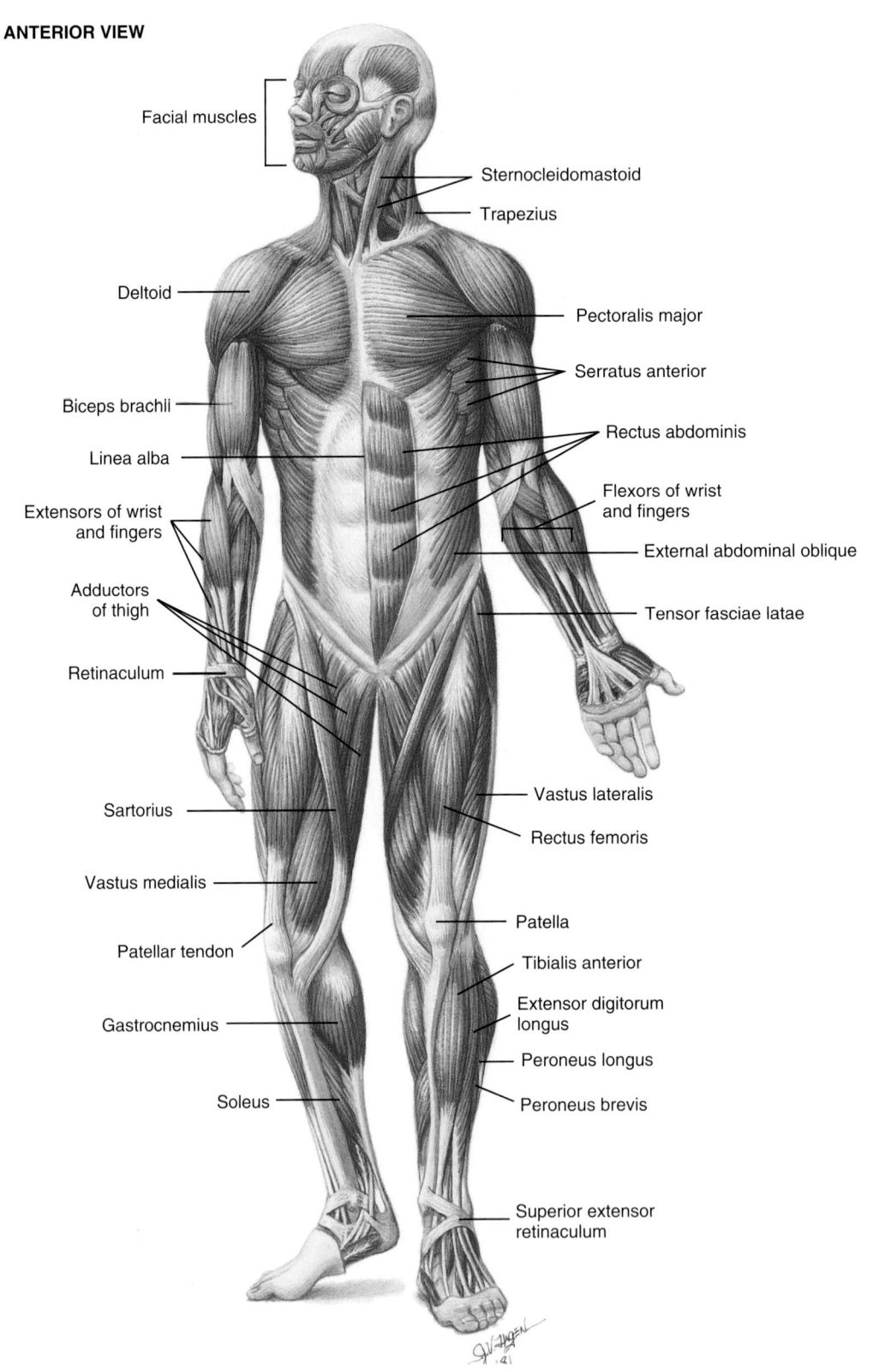

Facial muscles

Sternocleidomastoid

Trapezius

Deltoid

Pectoralis major

Serratus anterior

Biceps brachli

Rectus abdominis

Linea alba

Flexors of wrist
and fingers

Extensors of wrist
and fingers

External abdominal oblique

Adductors
of thigh

Tensor fasciae latae

Retinaculum

Vastus lateralis

Sartorius

Rectus femoris

Vastus medialis

Patella

Patellar tendon

Tibialis anterior

Extensor digitorum
longus

Gastrocnemius

Peroneus longus

Peroneus brevis

Soleus

Superior extensor
retinaculum

POSTERIOR VIEW

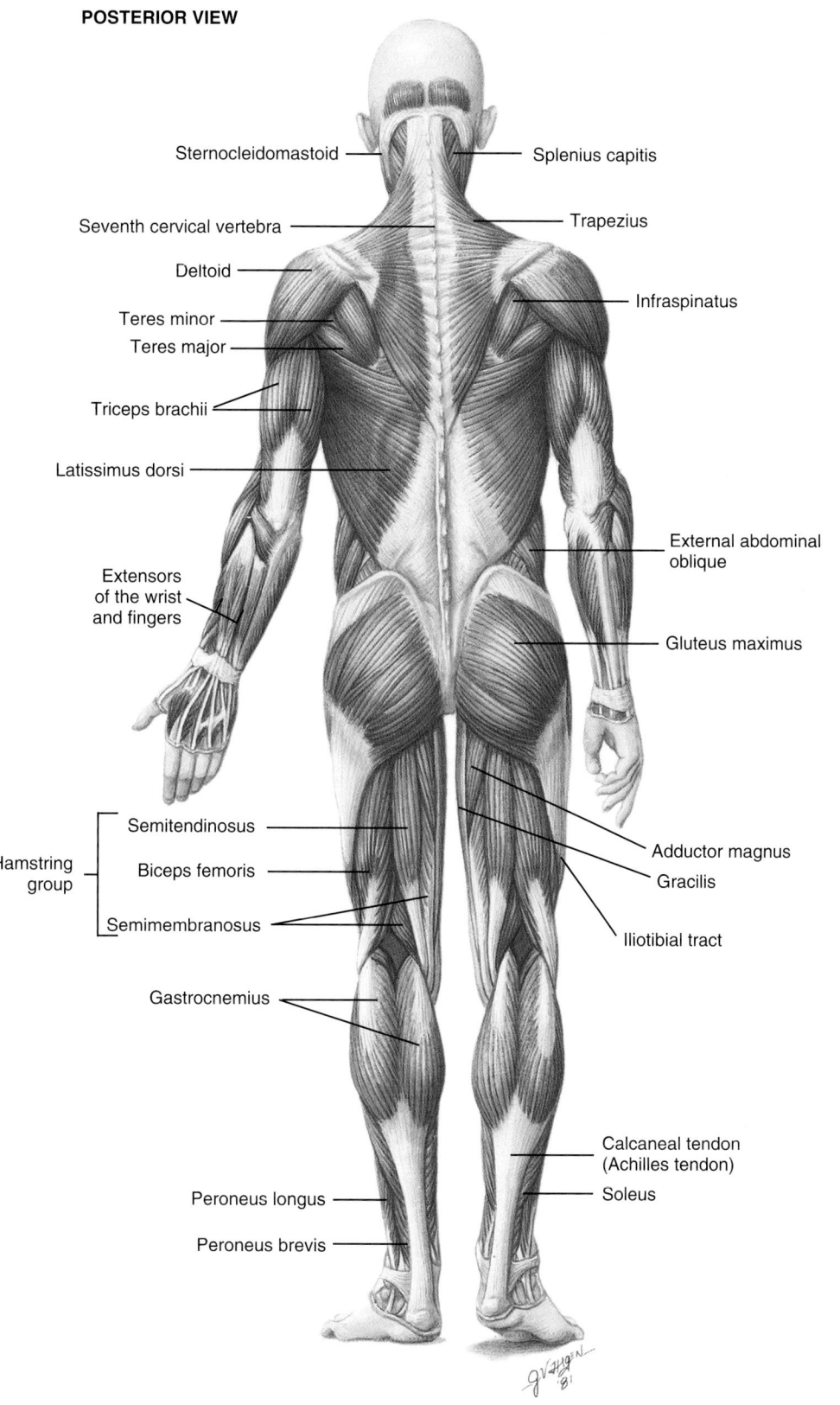

Sternocleidomastoid

Seventh cervical vertebra

Deltoid

Teres minor

Teres major

Triceps brachii

Latissimus dorsi

Extensors
of the wrist
and fingers

Hamstring
group

Semitendinosus

Biceps femoris

Semimembranosus

Gastrocnemius

Peroneus longus

Peroneus brevis

Splenius capitis

Trapezius

Infraspinatus

External abdominal
oblique

Gluteus maximus

Adductor magnus

Gracilis

Iliotibial tract

Calcaneal tendon
(Achilles tendon)

Soleus

**LATERAL AND ANTERIOR VIEWS OF
MUSCLES OF THE FACE AND ANTERIOR CRANIUM
AND SEVERAL MUSCLES OF MASTICATION**

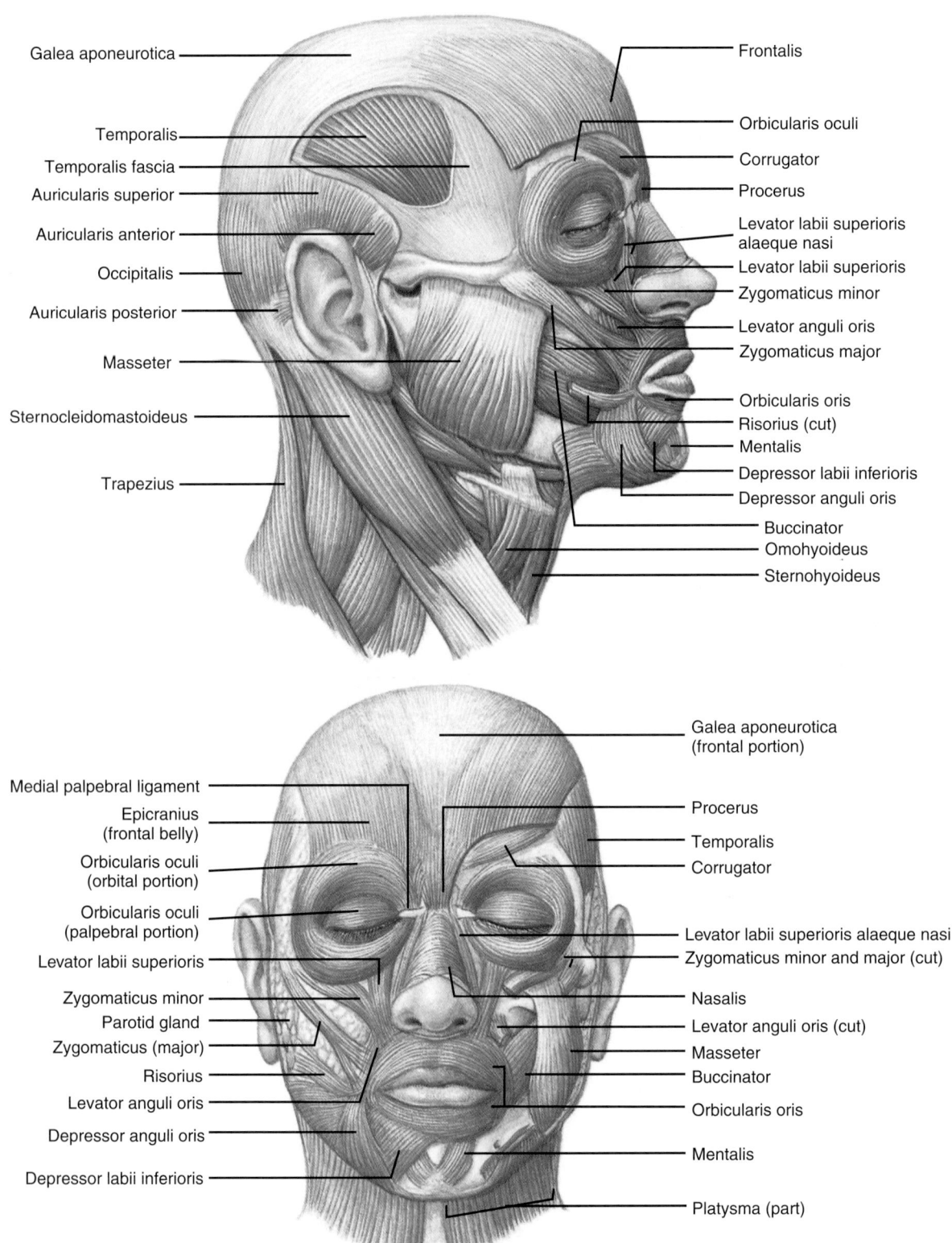

Galea aponeurotica

Frontalis

Temporalis

Orbicularis oculi

Temporalis fascia

Corrugator

Auricularis superior

Procerus

Auricularis anterior

Levator labii superioris
alaeque nasi

Occipitalis

Levator labii superioris

Auricularis posterior

Zygomaticus minor

Masseter

Levator anguli oris

Zygomaticus major

Sternocleidomastoideus

Orbicularis oris

Risorius (cut)

Mentalis

Trapezius

Depressor labii inferioris

Depressor anguli oris

Buccinator
Omohyoideus
Sternohyoideus

Galea aponeurotica
(frontal portion)

Medial palpebral ligament

Epicranius
(frontal belly)

Procerus

Temporalis

Orbicularis oculi
(orbital portion)

Corrugator

Orbicularis oculi
(palpebral portion)

Levator labii superioris

Levator labii superioris alaeque nasi

Zygomaticus minor and major (cut)

Zygomaticus minor

Nasalis

Parotid gland

Levator anguli oris (cut)

Zygomaticus (major)

Masseter

Risorius

Buccinator

Levator anguli oris

Orbicularis oris

Depressor anguli oris

Mentalis

Depressor labii inferioris

Platysma (part)

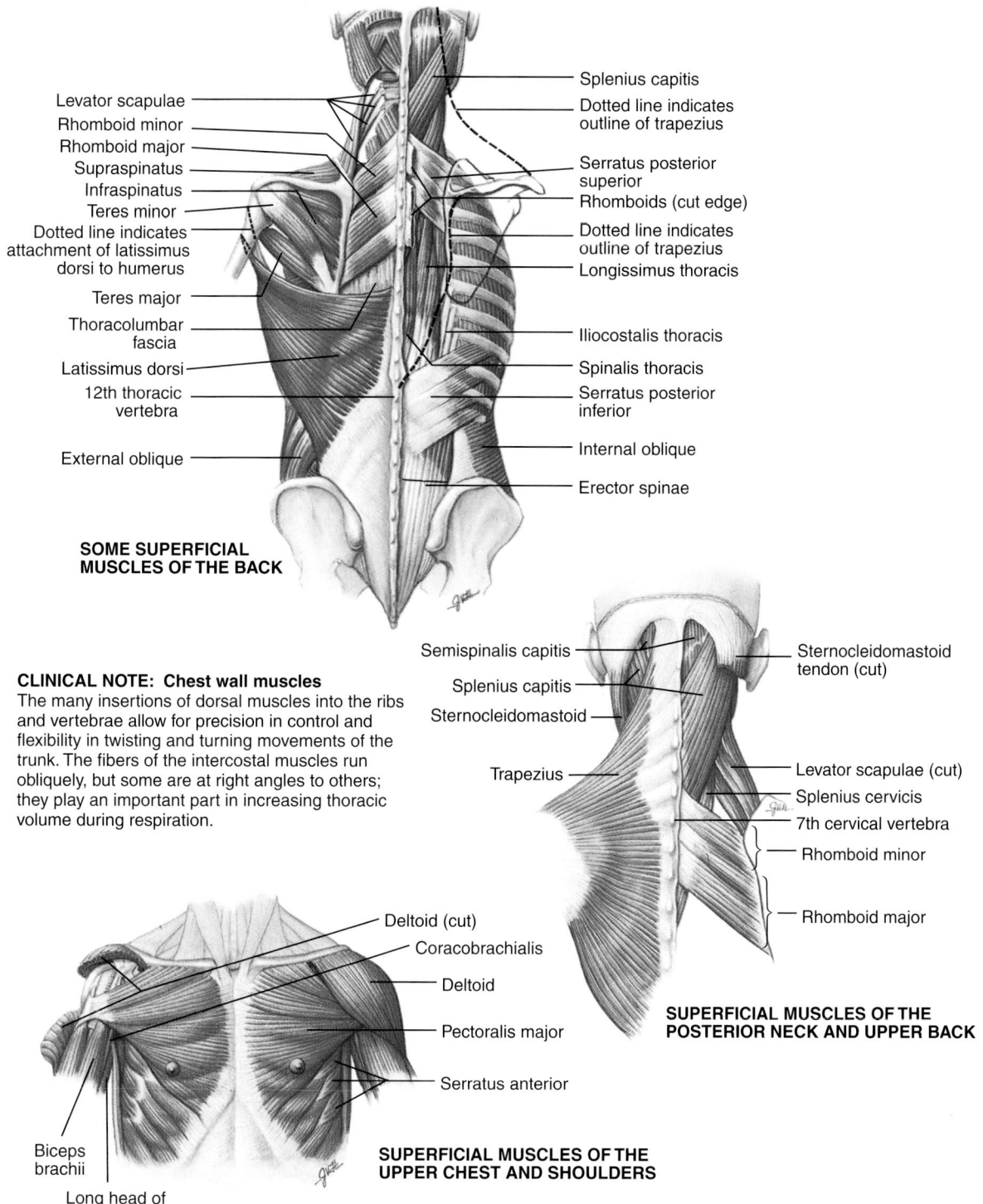

Levator scapulae
Rhomboid minor
Rhomboid major
Supraspinatus
Infraspinatus
Teres minor
Dotted line indicates attachment of latissimus dorsi to humerus
Teres major
Thoracolumbar fascia
Latissimus dorsi
12th thoracic vertebra
External oblique

Splenius capitis
Dotted line indicates outline of trapezius
Serratus posterior superior
Rhomboids (cut edge)
Dotted line indicates outline of trapezius
Longissimus thoracis
Iliocostalis thoracis
Spinalis thoracis
Serratus posterior inferior
Internal oblique
Erector spinae

SOME SUPERFICIAL MUSCLES OF THE BACK

CLINICAL NOTE: Chest wall muscles
The many insertions of dorsal muscles into the ribs and vertebrae allow for precision in control and flexibility in twisting and turning movements of the trunk. The fibers of the intercostal muscles run obliquely, but some are at right angles to others; they play an important part in increasing thoracic volume during respiration.

Semispinalis capitis
Splenius capitis
Sternocleidomastoid
Trapezius

Sternocleidomastoid tendon (cut)
Levator scapulae (cut)
Splenius cervicis
7th cervical vertebra
Rhomboid minor
Rhomboid major

SUPERFICIAL MUSCLES OF THE POSTERIOR NECK AND UPPER BACK

Deltoid (cut)
Coracobrachialis
Deltoid
Pectoralis major
Serratus anterior

Biceps brachii
Long head of the triceps

SUPERFICIAL MUSCLES OF THE UPPER CHEST AND SHOULDERS

CIRCULATORY SYSTEM

PRINCIPAL ARTERIES

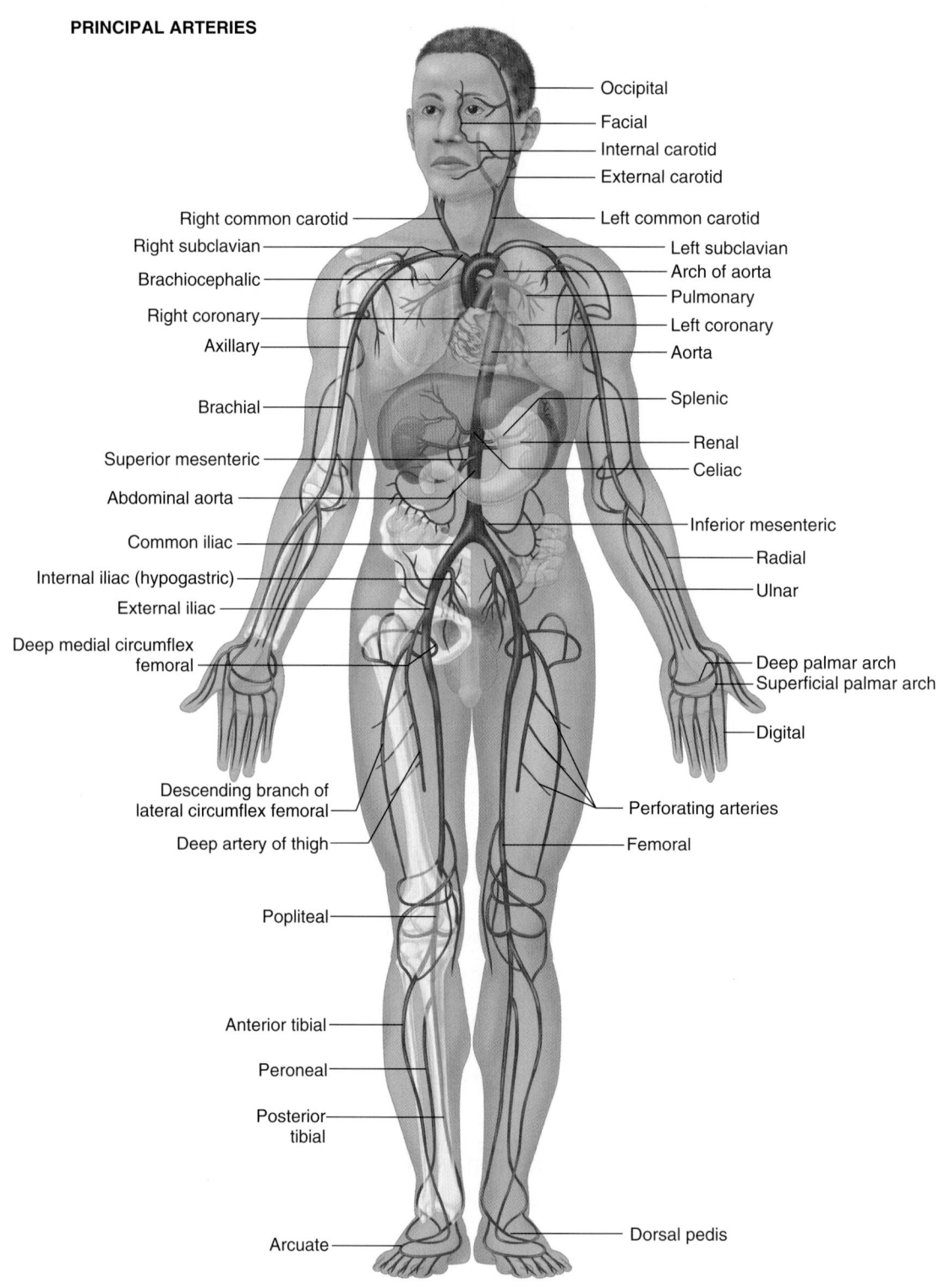

Occipital
Facial
Internal carotid
External carotid
Right common carotid — Left common carotid
Right subclavian — Left subclavian
Brachiocephalic — Arch of aorta
Right coronary — Pulmonary
Axillary — Left coronary
Aorta
Brachial — Splenic
Superior mesenteric — Renal
Abdominal aorta — Celiac
Common iliac — Inferior mesenteric
Internal iliac (hypogastric) — Radial
External iliac — Ulnar
Deep medial circumflex femoral
Deep palmar arch
Superficial palmar arch
Digital
Descending branch of lateral circumflex femoral
Deep artery of thigh — Perforating arteries
Popliteal — Femoral
Anterior tibial
Peroneal
Posterior tibial
Arcuate — Dorsal pedis

PRINCIPAL VEINS

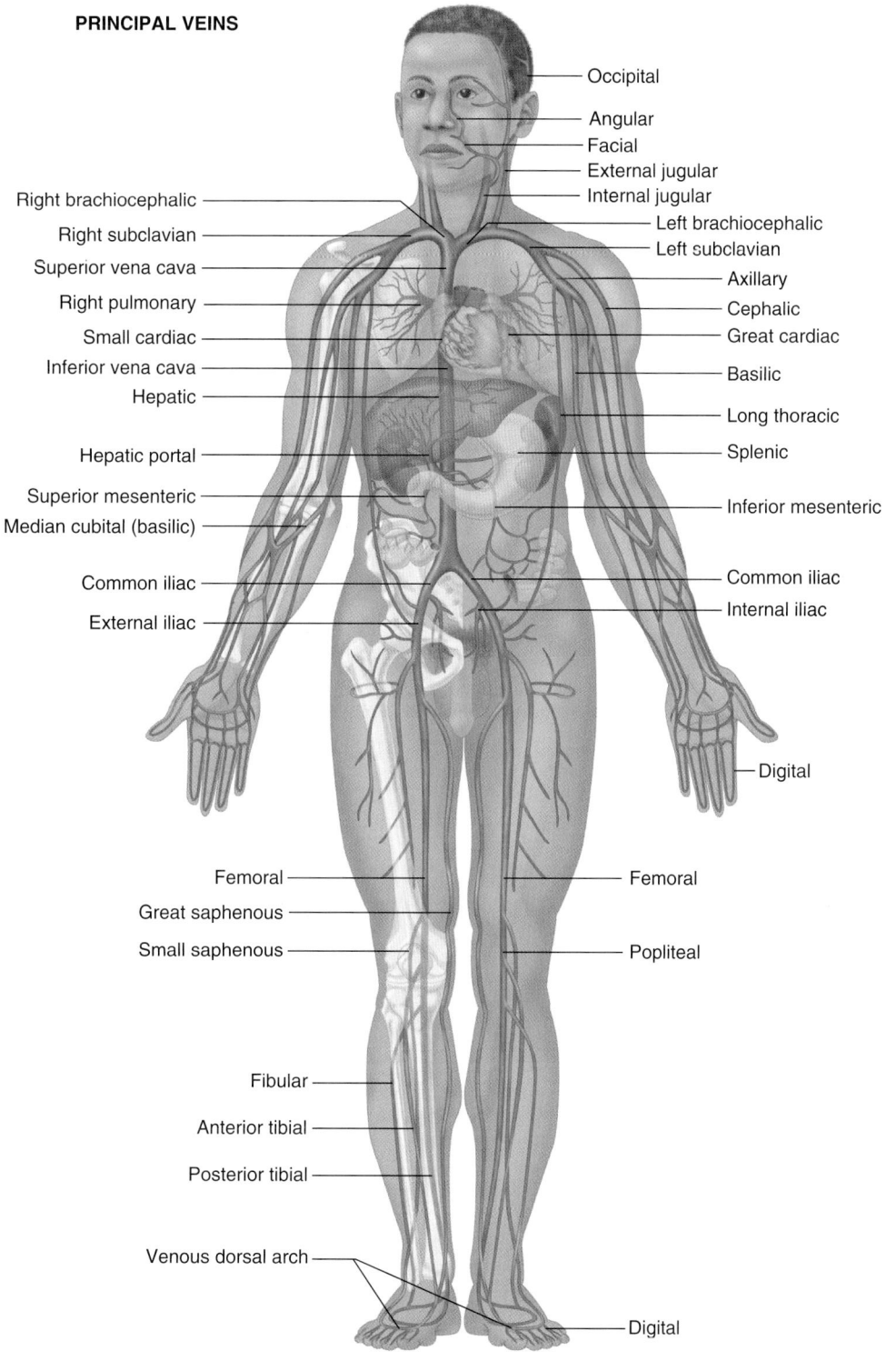

Occipital
Angular
Facial
External jugular
Internal jugular
Left brachiocephalic
Left subclavian
Axillary
Cephalic
Great cardiac
Basilic
Long thoracic
Splenic
Inferior mesenteric
Common iliac
Internal iliac
Digital
Femoral
Popliteal
Digital

Right brachiocephalic
Right subclavian
Superior vena cava
Right pulmonary
Small cardiac
Inferior vena cava
Hepatic
Hepatic portal
Superior mesenteric
Median cubital (basilic)
Common iliac
External iliac
Femoral
Great saphenous
Small saphenous
Fibular
Anterior tibial
Posterior tibial
Venous dorsal arch

MAJOR ARTERIES OF THE HEAD AND NECK

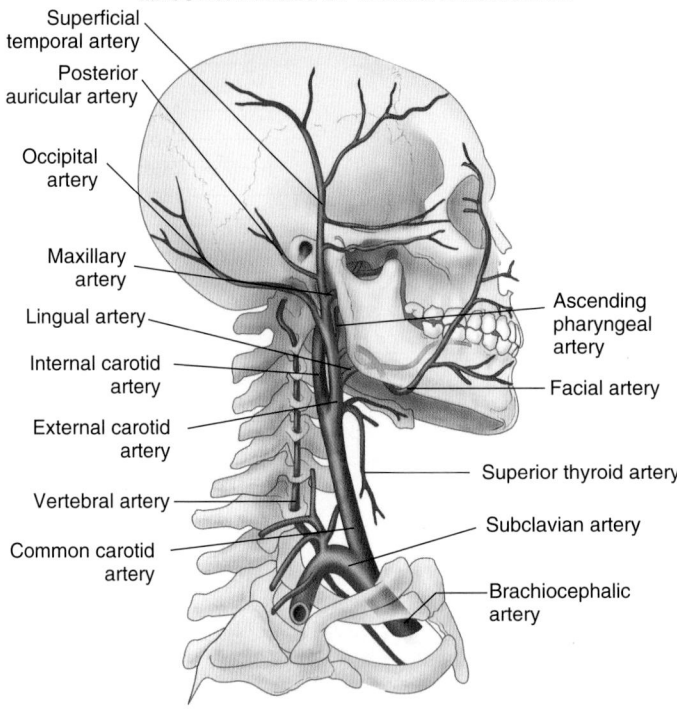

Superficial temporal artery

Posterior auricular artery

Occipital artery

Maxillary artery

Lingual artery

Internal carotid artery

External carotid artery

Vertebral artery

Common carotid artery

Ascending pharyngeal artery

Facial artery

Superior thyroid artery

Subclavian artery

Brachiocephalic artery

VEINS FORMING THE SUPERIOR VENA CAVA

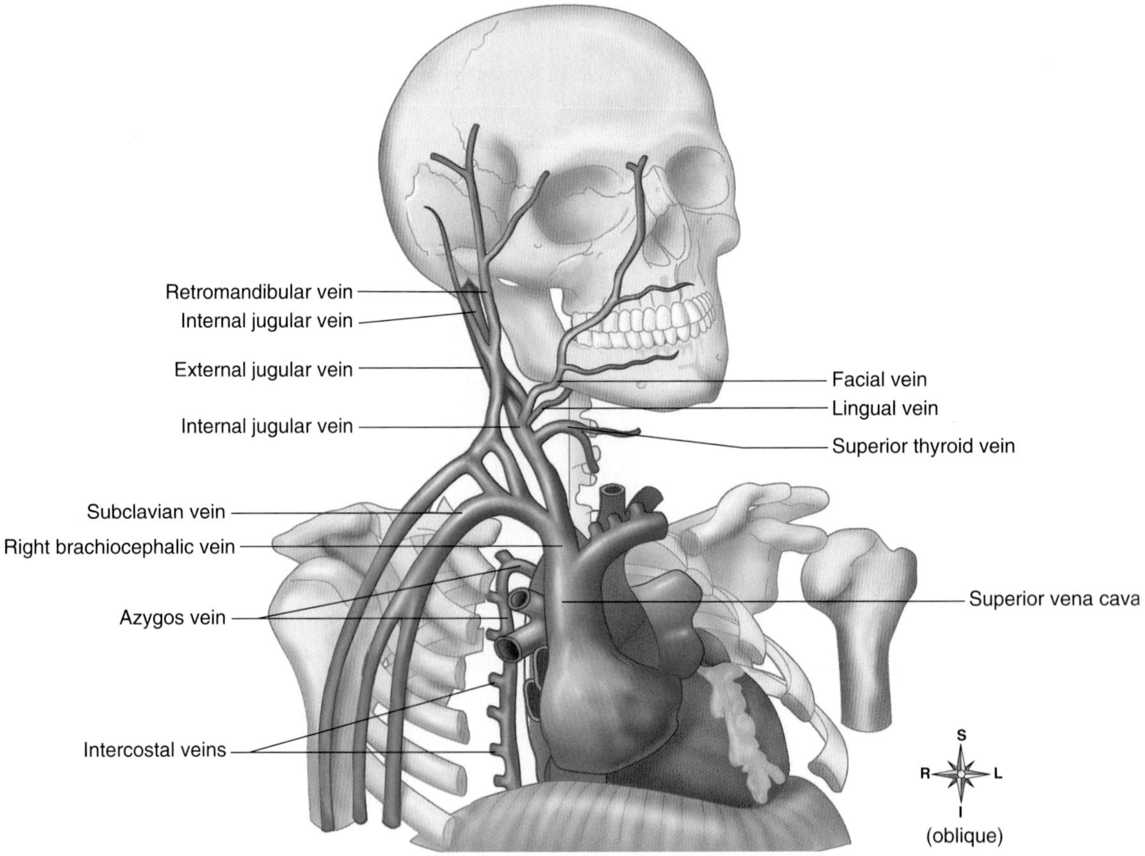

Retromandibular vein

Internal jugular vein

External jugular vein

Internal jugular vein

Subclavian vein

Right brachiocephalic vein

Azygos vein

Intercostal veins

Facial vein

Lingual vein

Superior thyroid vein

Superior vena cava

S
R — L
I
(oblique)

ANTERIOR VIEW OF THE HEART

Left common carotid artery

Brachiocephalic trunk

Superior vena cava

Ascending aorta

Pulmonary trunk

Conus arteriosus

Right pulmonary veins

Auricle of right atrium

Right coronary artery and cardiac vein

Right ventricle

Left subclavian artery

Arch of aorta

Ligamentum arteriosum

Auricle of left atrium

Left pulmonary veins

Great cardiac vein

Circumflex artery

Anterior interventricular branches of left coronary artery and cardiac vein

Left ventricle

Apex

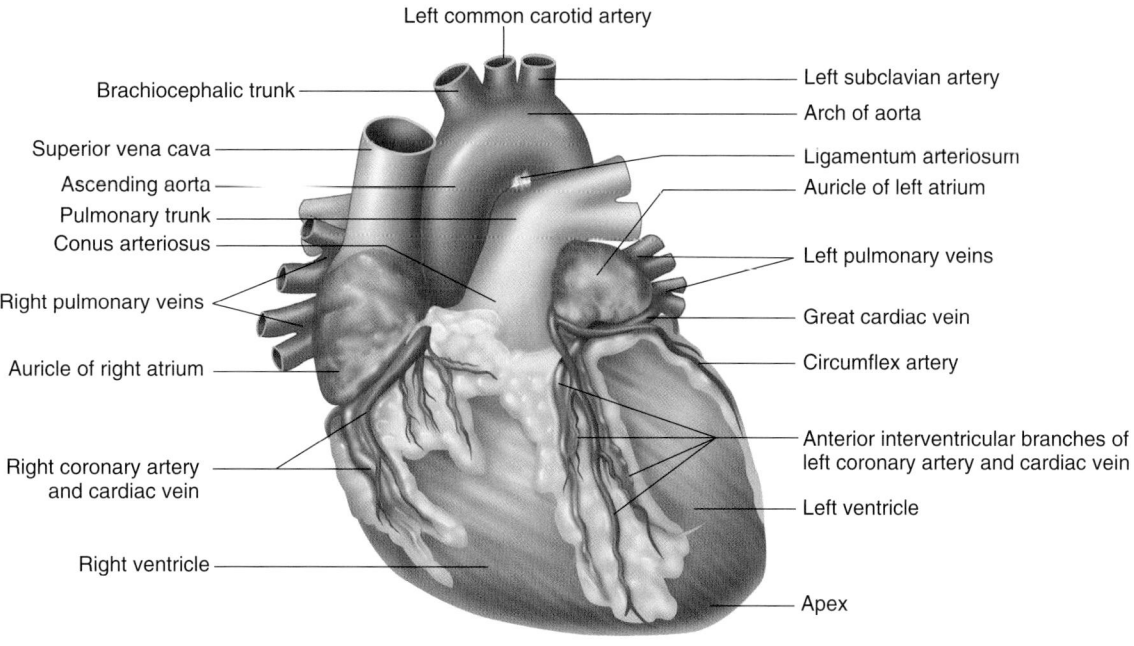

POSTERIOR VIEW OF THE HEART

Left common carotid artery

Left subclavian artery

Left pulmonary artery

Left pulmonary veins

Auricle of left atrium

Left atrium

Great cardiac vein

Posterior artery and vein of left ventricle

Left ventricle

Posterior interventricular sulcus

Apex

Brachiocephalic trunk

Aortic arch

Superior vena cava

Right pulmonary artery

Right pulmonary veins

Right atrium

Inferior vena cava

Coronary sinus

Posterior interventricular branch of right coronary artery

Middle cardiac vein

Right ventricle

MAJOR ARTERIES OF THE UPPER EXTREMITY

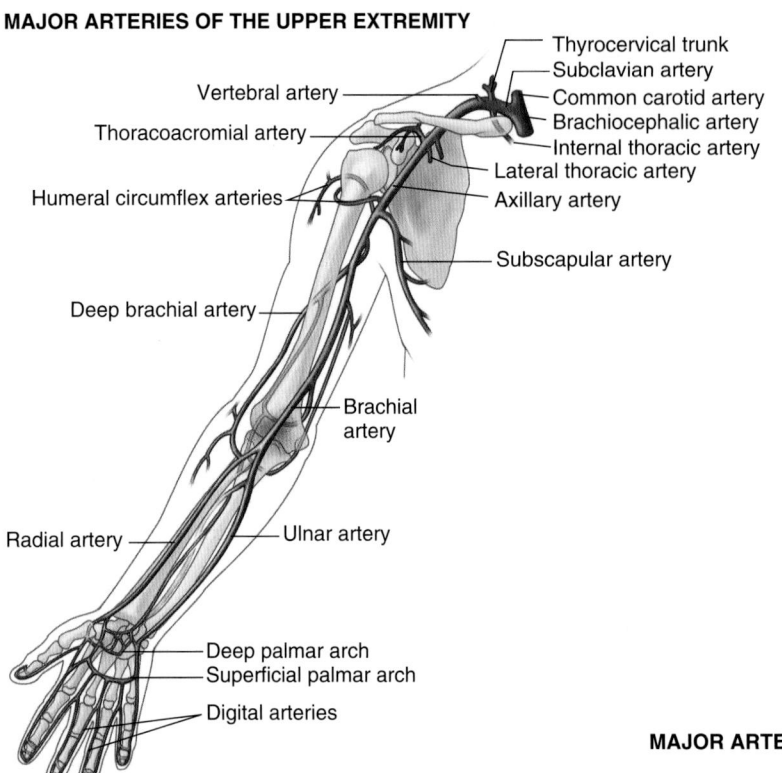

Thyrocervical trunk
Subclavian artery
Common carotid artery
Brachiocephalic artery
Internal thoracic artery
Lateral thoracic artery
Axillary artery

Vertebral artery
Thoracoacromial artery
Humeral circumflex arteries

Subscapular artery

Deep brachial artery

Brachial artery

Radial artery
Ulnar artery

Deep palmar arch
Superficial palmar arch

Digital arteries

MAJOR ARTERIES OF THE LOWER EXTREMITY

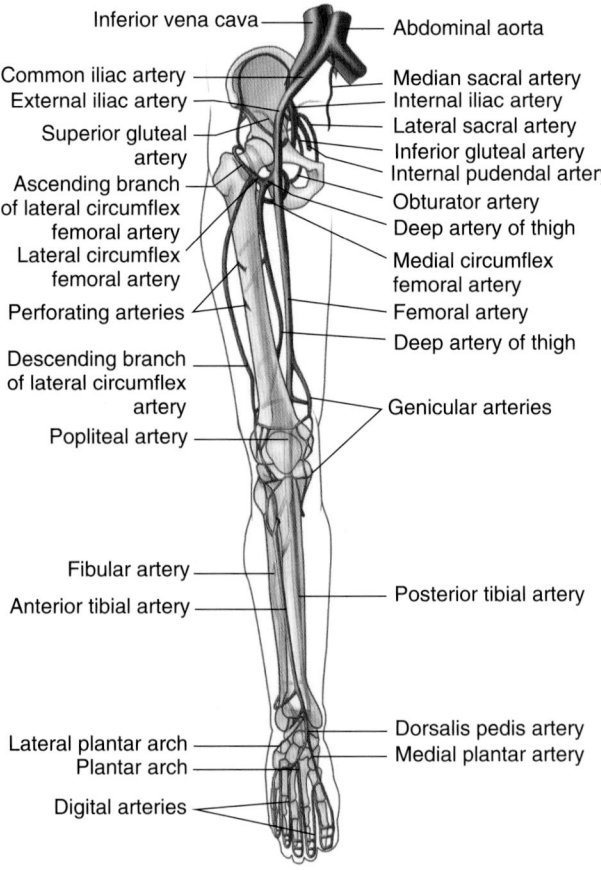

Inferior vena cava
Abdominal aorta

Common iliac artery
External iliac artery
Superior gluteal artery
Ascending branch of lateral circumflex femoral artery
Lateral circumflex femoral artery
Perforating arteries

Descending branch of lateral circumflex artery
Popliteal artery

Median sacral artery
Internal iliac artery
Lateral sacral artery
Inferior gluteal artery
Internal pudendal artery
Obturator artery
Deep artery of thigh
Medial circumflex femoral artery
Femoral artery
Deep artery of thigh

Genicular arteries

Fibular artery
Anterior tibial artery

Posterior tibial artery

Lateral plantar arch
Plantar arch

Dorsalis pedis artery
Medial plantar artery

Digital arteries

MAJOR VEINS OF THE UPPER EXTREMITY

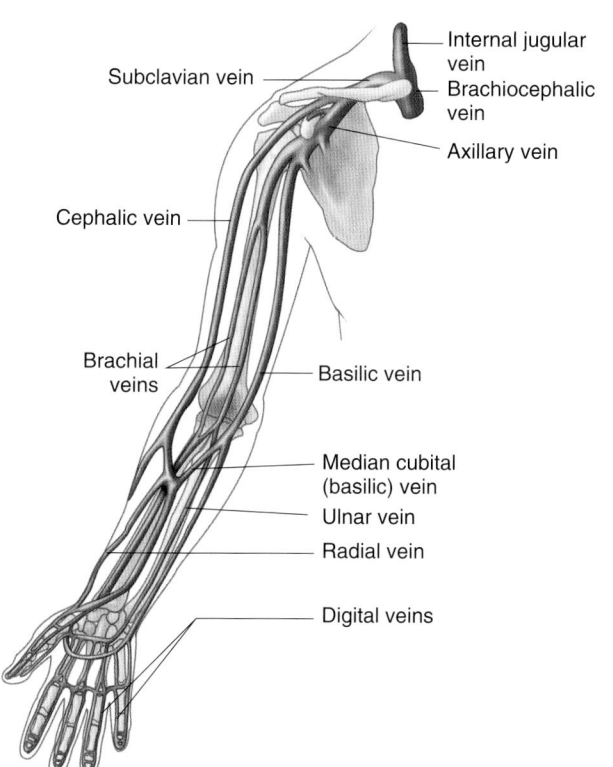

Internal jugular vein
Subclavian vein
Brachiocephalic vein
Axillary vein
Cephalic vein
Brachial veins
Basilic vein
Median cubital (basilic) vein
Ulnar vein
Radial vein
Digital veins

MAJOR VEINS OF THE LOWER EXTREMITY

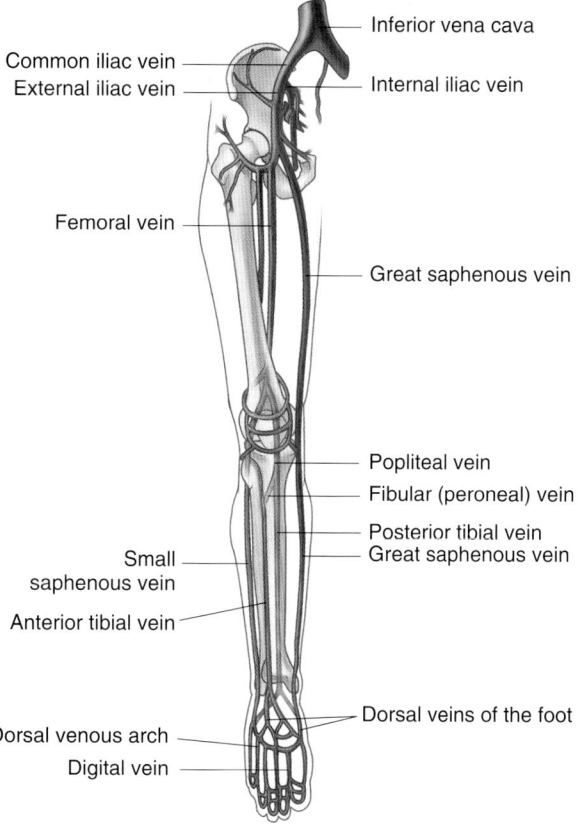

Inferior vena cava
Common iliac vein
External iliac vein
Internal iliac vein
Femoral vein
Great saphenous vein
Popliteal vein
Fibular (peroneal) vein
Posterior tibial vein
Great saphenous vein
Small saphenous vein
Anterior tibial vein
Dorsal veins of the foot
Dorsal venous arch
Digital vein

ENDOCRINE SYSTEM

GLANDS OF THE ENDOCRINE SYSTEM

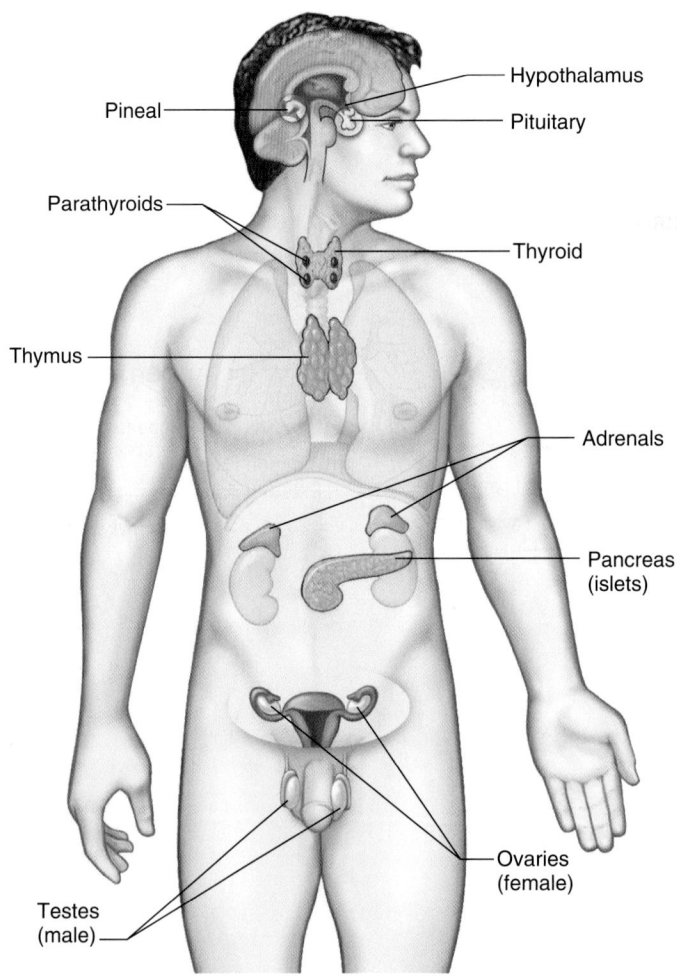

Pineal

Parathyroids

Thymus

Testes
(male)

Hypothalamus

Pituitary

Thyroid

Adrenals

Pancreas
(islets)

Ovaries
(female)

LOCATION OF THE PITUITARY AND PINEAL GLANDS

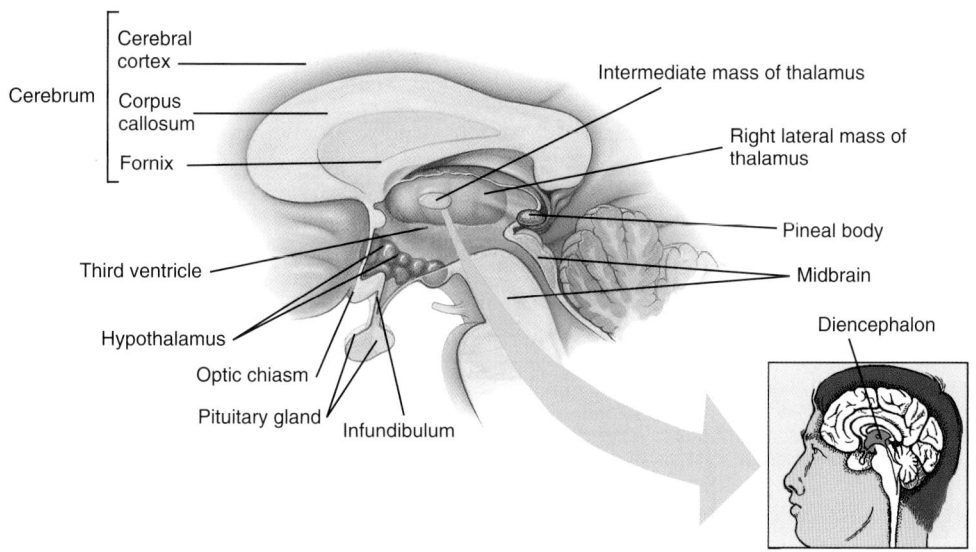

Cerebrum
- Cerebral cortex
- Corpus callosum
- Fornix

Intermediate mass of thalamus

Right lateral mass of thalamus

Pineal body

Midbrain

Third ventricle

Hypothalamus

Optic chiasm

Pituitary gland

Infundibulum

Diencephalon

GROSS ANATOMY OF THE THYROID GLAND

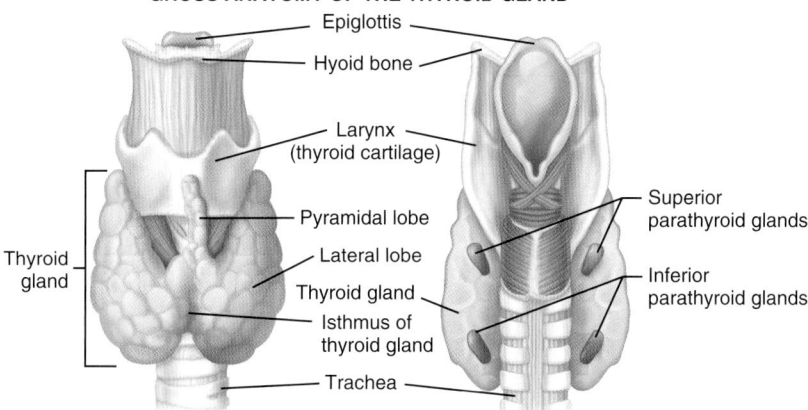

Epiglottis

Hyoid bone

Larynx (thyroid cartilage)

Pyramidal lobe

Lateral lobe

Thyroid gland

Isthmus of thyroid gland

Trachea

Thyroid gland

Superior parathyroid glands

Inferior parathyroid glands

PANCREAS

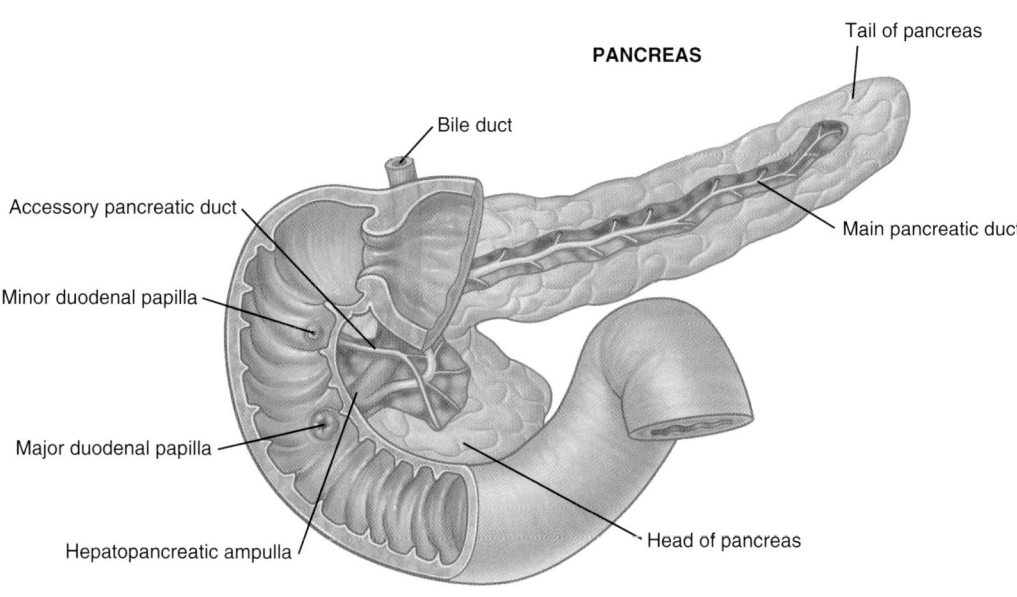

Tail of pancreas

Bile duct

Accessory pancreatic duct

Main pancreatic duct

Minor duodenal papilla

Major duodenal papilla

Hepatopancreatic ampulla

Head of pancreas

LYMPHATIC SYSTEM

ORGANS OF THE LYMPHATIC SYSTEM

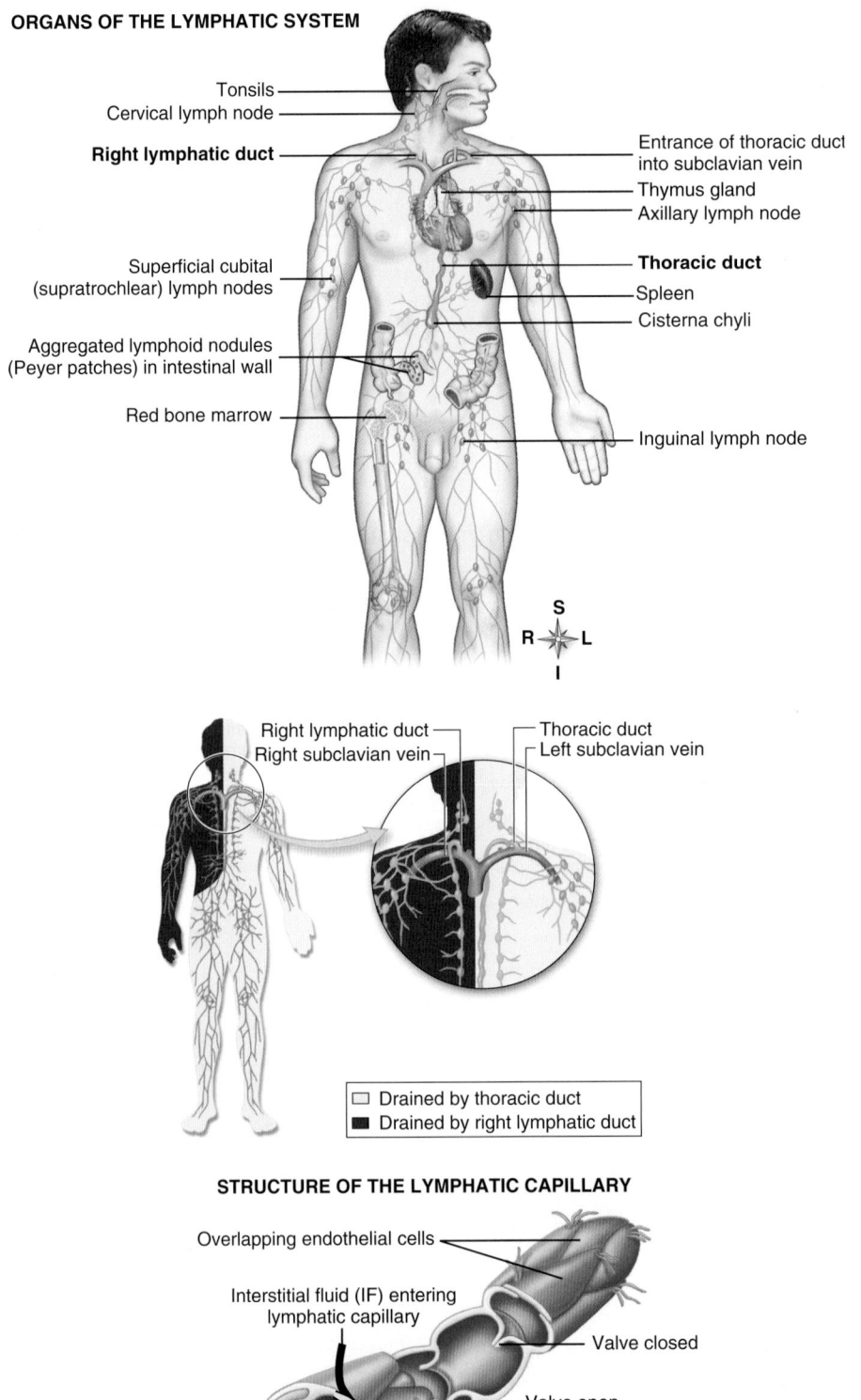

Tonsils

Cervical lymph node

Right lymphatic duct

Entrance of thoracic duct into subclavian vein

Thymus gland

Axillary lymph node

Superficial cubital (supratrochlear) lymph nodes

Thoracic duct

Spleen

Cisterna chyli

Aggregated lymphoid nodules (Peyer patches) in intestinal wall

Red bone marrow

Inguinal lymph node

S
R L
I

Right lymphatic duct

Right subclavian vein

Thoracic duct

Left subclavian vein

☐ Drained by thoracic duct
■ Drained by right lymphatic duct

STRUCTURE OF THE LYMPHATIC CAPILLARY

Overlapping endothelial cells

Interstitial fluid (IF) entering lymphatic capillary

Valve closed

Valve open

Direction of flow

Anchoring fibers

STRUCTURE OF THE SPLEEN

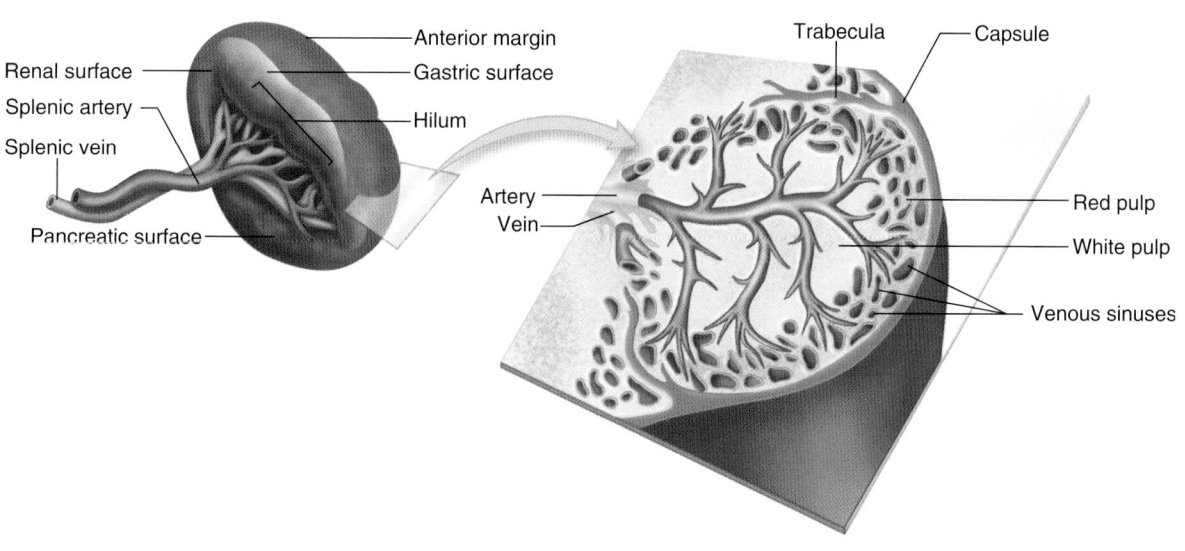

Anterior margin

Renal surface

Gastric surface

Splenic artery

Hilum

Splenic vein

Pancreatic surface

Trabecula

Capsule

Artery

Vein

Red pulp

White pulp

Venous sinuses

GROSS ANATOMY OF THE THYMUS

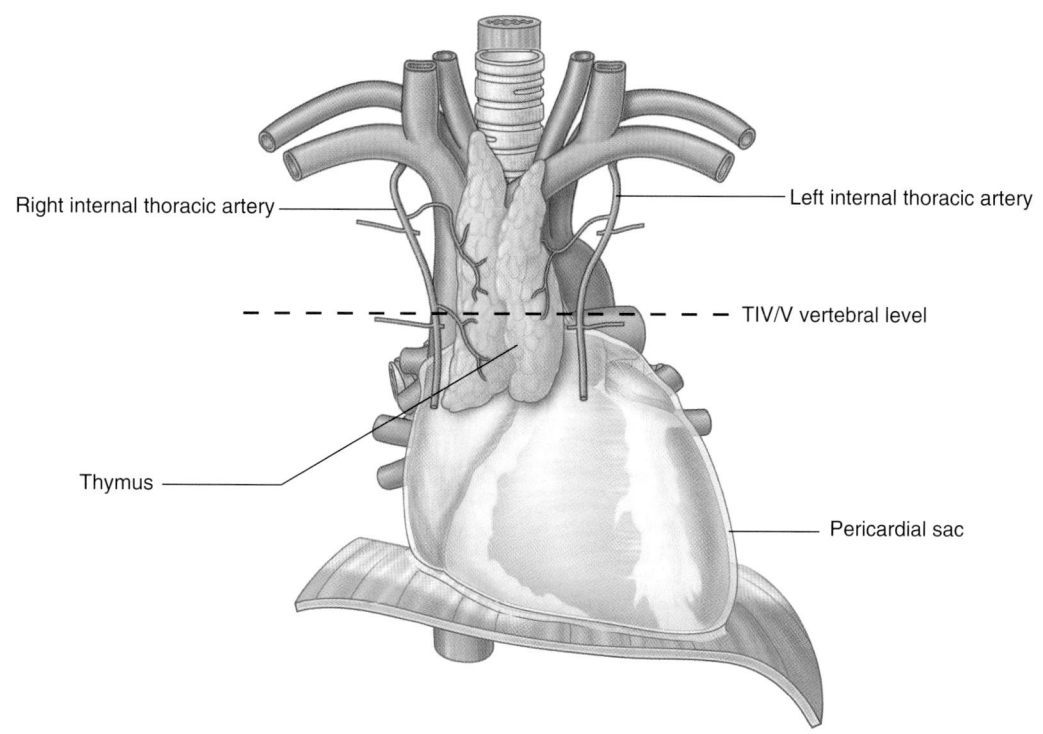

Right internal thoracic artery

Left internal thoracic artery

TIV/V vertebral level

Thymus

Pericardial sac

LYMPHATIC DRAINAGE SYSTEM
OF THE HEAD AND NECK

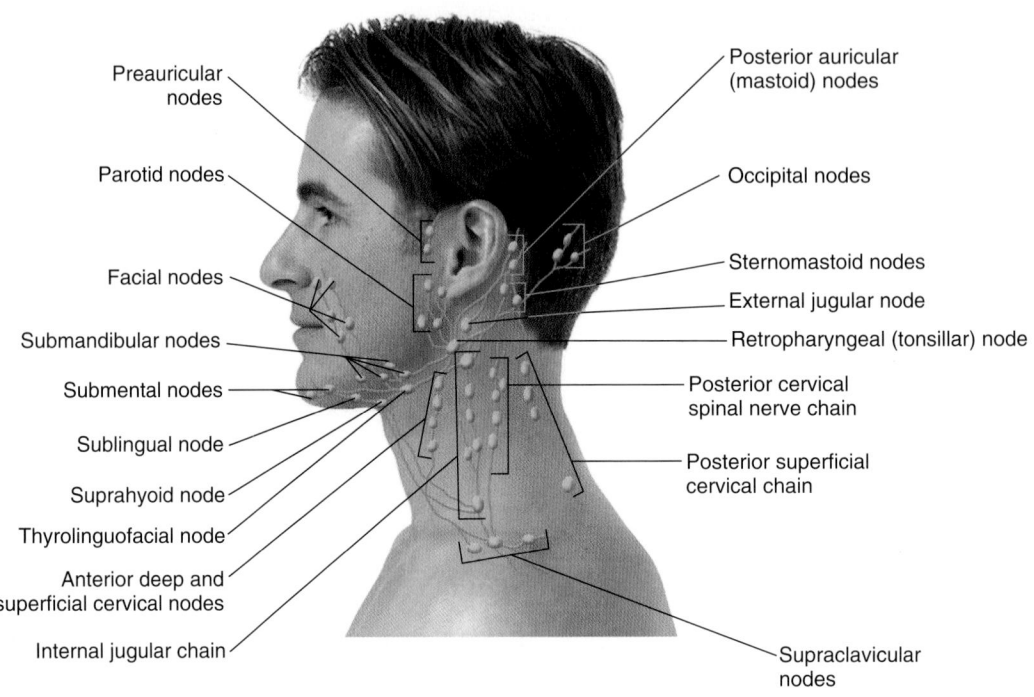

Preauricular nodes

Parotid nodes

Facial nodes

Submandibular nodes

Submental nodes

Sublingual node

Suprahyoid node

Thyrolinguofacial node

Anterior deep and superficial cervical nodes

Internal jugular chain

Posterior auricular (mastoid) nodes

Occipital nodes

Sternomastoid nodes

External jugular node

Retropharyngeal (tonsillar) node

Posterior cervical spinal nerve chain

Posterior superficial cervical chain

Supraclavicular nodes

SCHEMATIC SECTION OF A LYMPH NODE

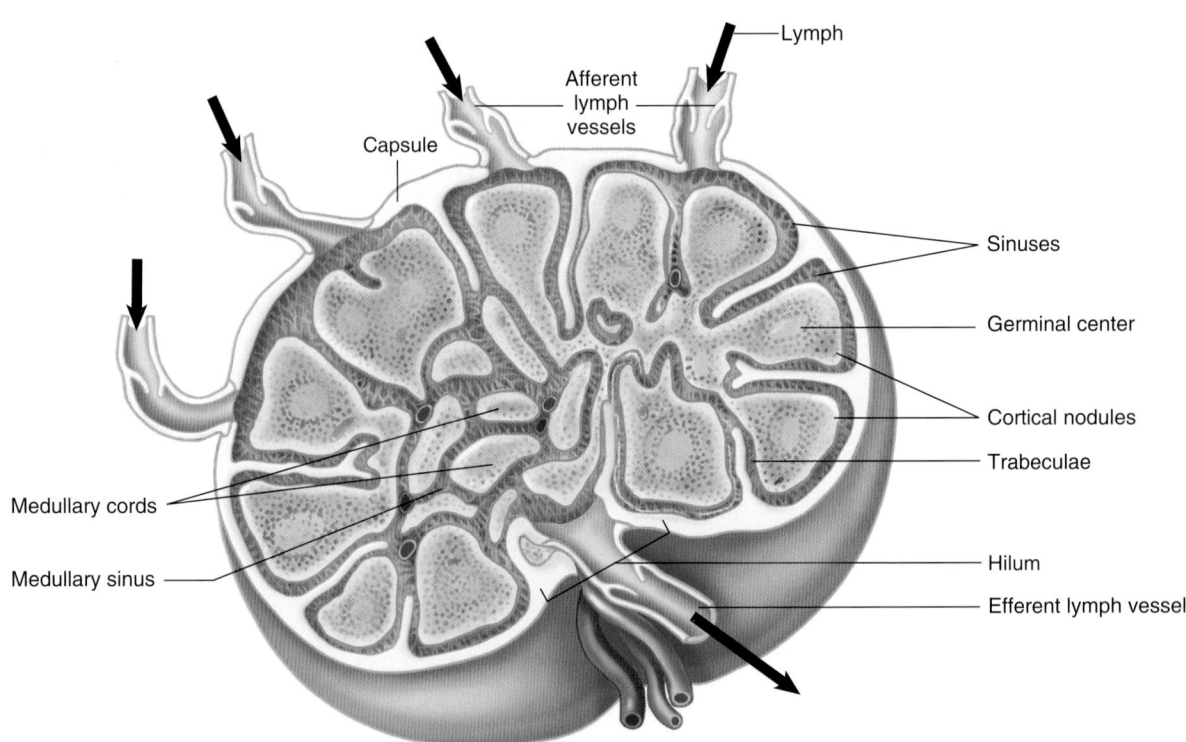

Lymph

Afferent lymph vessels

Capsule

Sinuses

Germinal center

Cortical nodules

Trabeculae

Medullary cords

Medullary sinus

Hilum

Efferent lymph vessel

NERVOUS SYSTEM

SIMPLIFIED VIEW OF THE NERVOUS SYSTEM

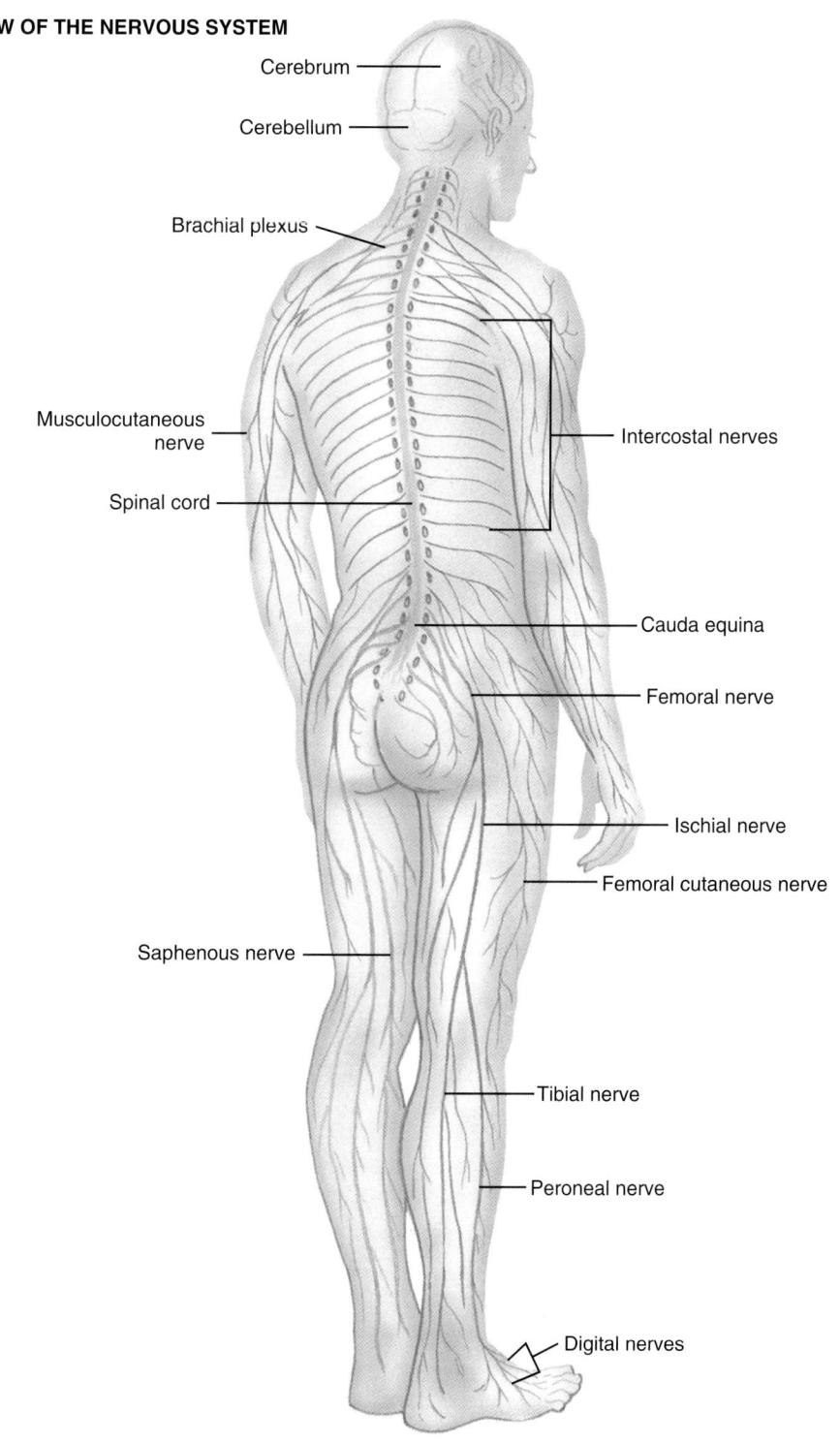

Cerebrum

Cerebellum

Brachial plexus

Musculocutaneous nerve

Spinal cord

Intercostal nerves

Cauda equina

Femoral nerve

Ischial nerve

Femoral cutaneous nerve

Saphenous nerve

Tibial nerve

Peroneal nerve

Digital nerves

GROSS ANATOMY OF THE SPINAL CORD

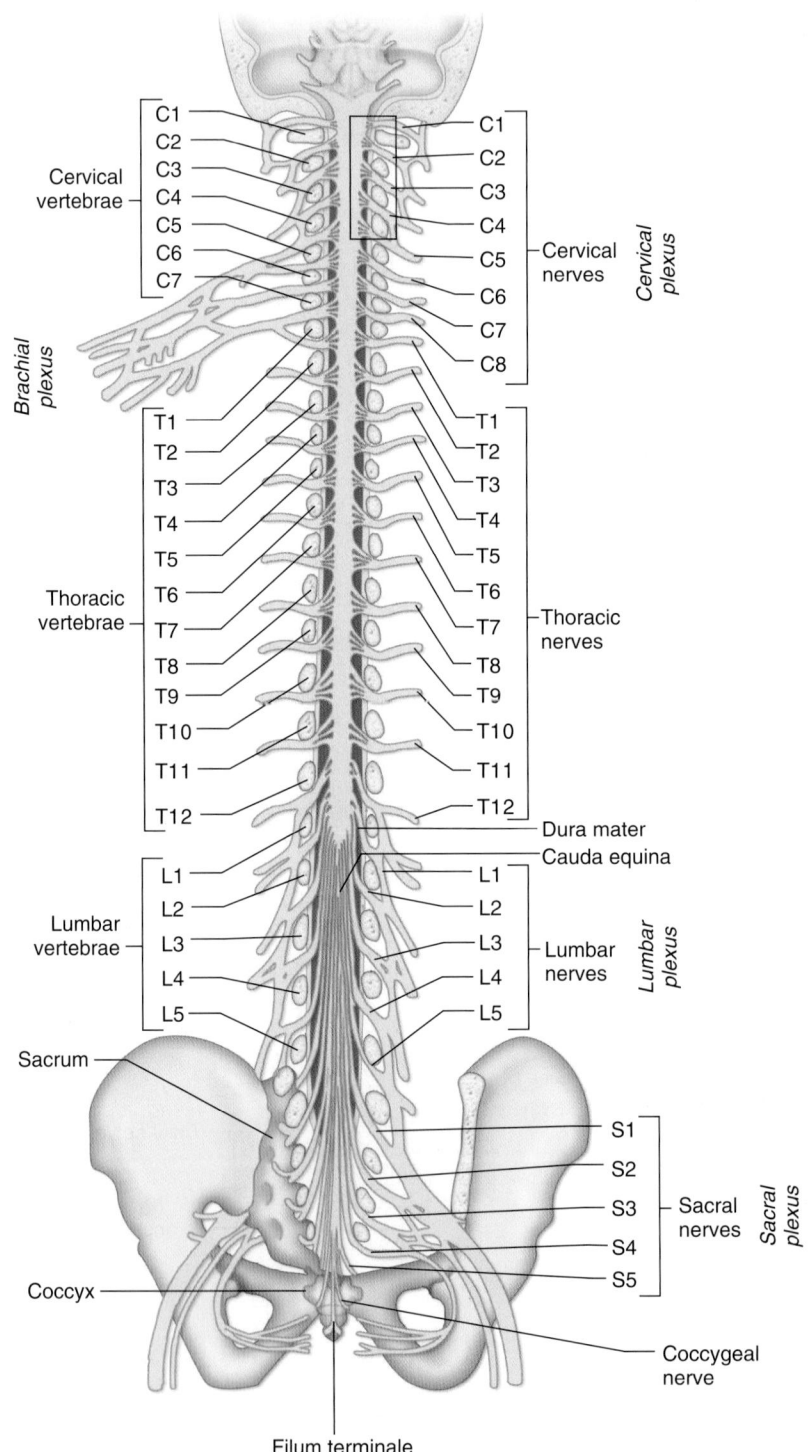

Cervical vertebrae — C1 C2 C3 C4 C5 C6 C7

Brachial plexus

Thoracic vertebrae — T1 T2 T3 T4 T5 T6 T7 T8 T9 T10 T11 T12

Lumbar vertebrae — L1 L2 L3 L4 L5

Sacrum

Coccyx

Filum terminale

C1 C2 C3 C4 C5 C6 C7 C8 — Cervical nerves — Cervical plexus

T1 T2 T3 T4 T5 T6 T7 T8 T9 T10 T11 T12 — Thoracic nerves

Dura mater
Cauda equina

L1 L2 L3 L4 L5 — Lumbar nerves — Lumbar plexus

S1 S2 S3 S4 S5 — Sacral nerves — Sacral plexus

Coccygeal nerve

CEREBRAL NUCLEI

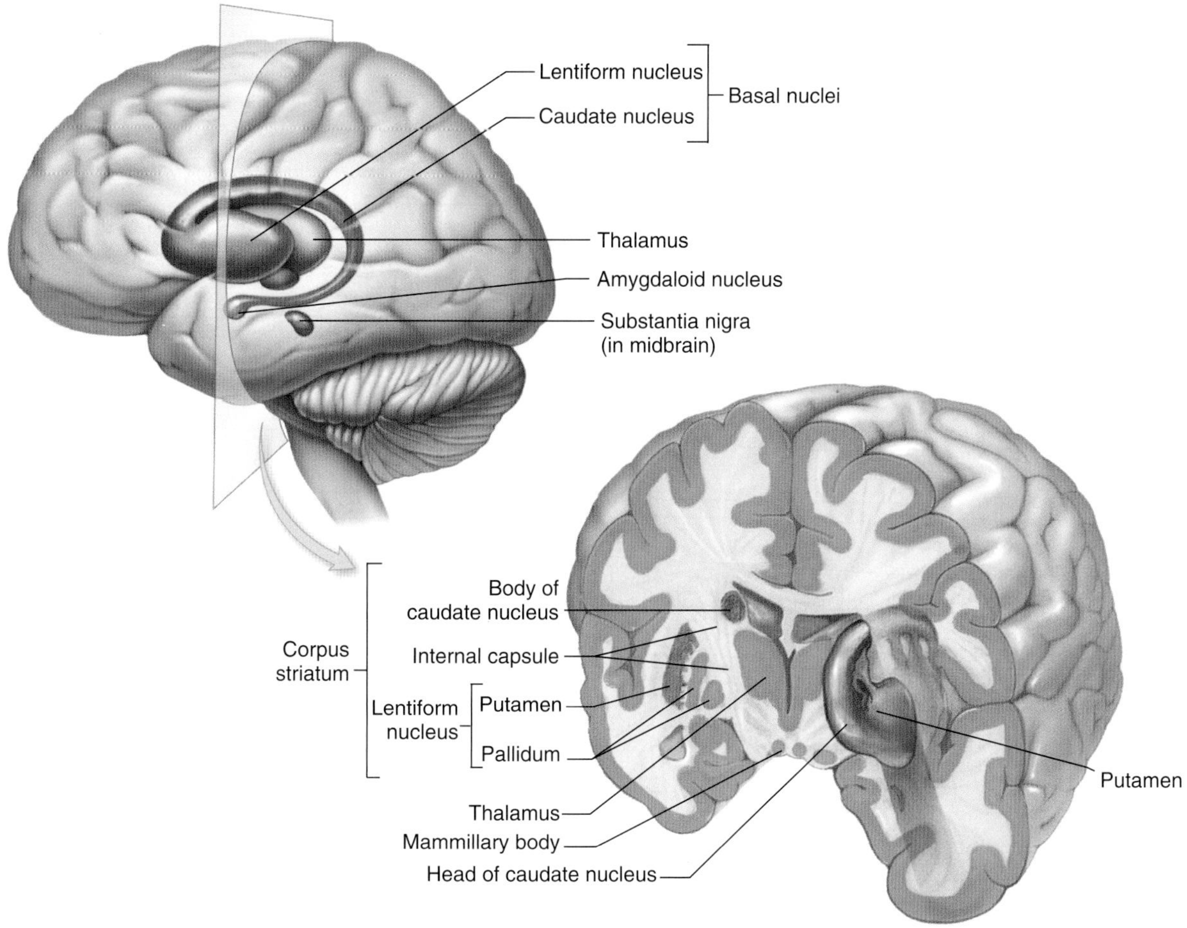

Lentiform nucleus — Basal nuclei
Caudate nucleus

Thalamus
Amygdaloid nucleus
Substantia nigra
(in midbrain)

Corpus
striatum

Body of
caudate nucleus

Internal capsule

Lentiform
nucleus

Putamen

Pallidum

Thalamus
Mammillary body
Head of caudate nucleus

Putamen

FUNCTIONAL AREAS OF THE CEREBRAL CORTEX

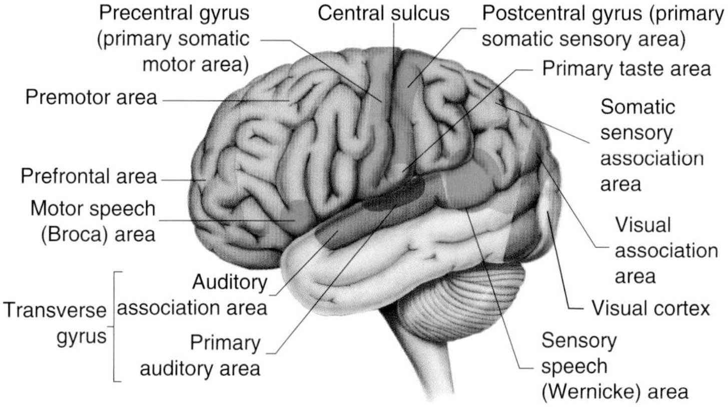

Precentral gyrus
(primary somatic
motor area)

Central sulcus

Postcentral gyrus (primary
somatic sensory area)

Premotor area

Primary taste area

Somatic
sensory
association
area

Prefrontal area

Motor speech
(Broca) area

Visual
association
area

Transverse
gyrus

Auditory
association area

Primary
auditory area

Visual cortex

Sensory
speech
(Wernicke) area

RETICULAR ACTIVATING SYSTEM

Radiations to cortex

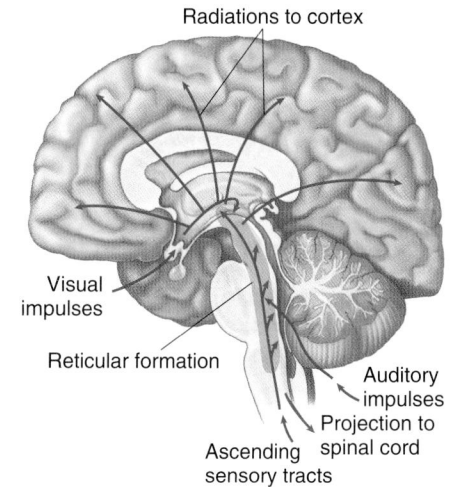

Visual
impulses

Reticular formation

Auditory
impulses

Projection to
spinal cord

Ascending
sensory tracts

BASE OF THE BRAIN

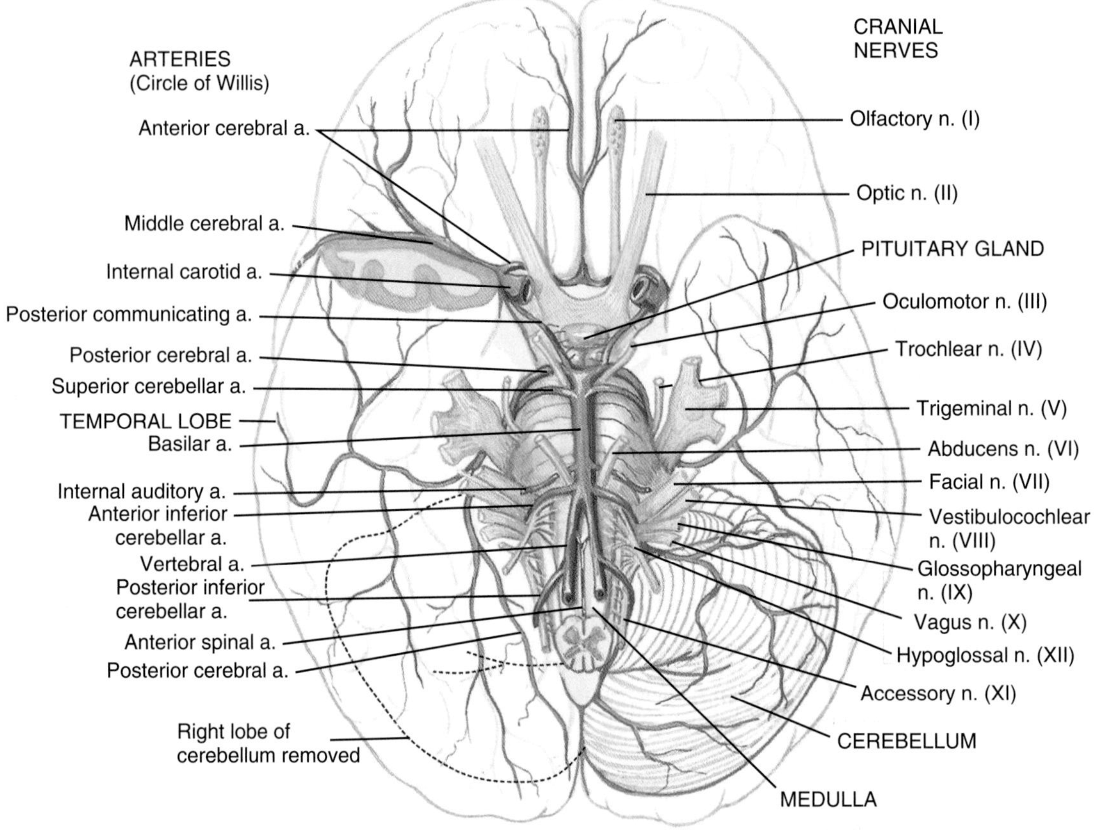

ARTERIES
(Circle of Willis)

Anterior cerebral a.

Middle cerebral a.

Internal carotid a.

Posterior communicating a.

Posterior cerebral a.

Superior cerebellar a.

TEMPORAL LOBE

Basilar a.

Internal auditory a.

Anterior inferior
cerebellar a.

Vertebral a.

Posterior inferior
cerebellar a.

Anterior spinal a.

Posterior cerebral a.

Right lobe of
cerebellum removed

CRANIAL
NERVES

Olfactory n. (I)

Optic n. (II)

PITUITARY GLAND

Oculomotor n. (III)

Trochlear n. (IV)

Trigeminal n. (V)

Abducens n. (VI)

Facial n. (VII)

Vestibulocochlear
n. (VIII)

Glossopharyngeal
n. (IX)

Vagus n. (X)

Hypoglossal n. (XII)

Accessory n. (XI)

CEREBELLUM

MEDULLA

BRAINSTEM AND DIENCEPHALON

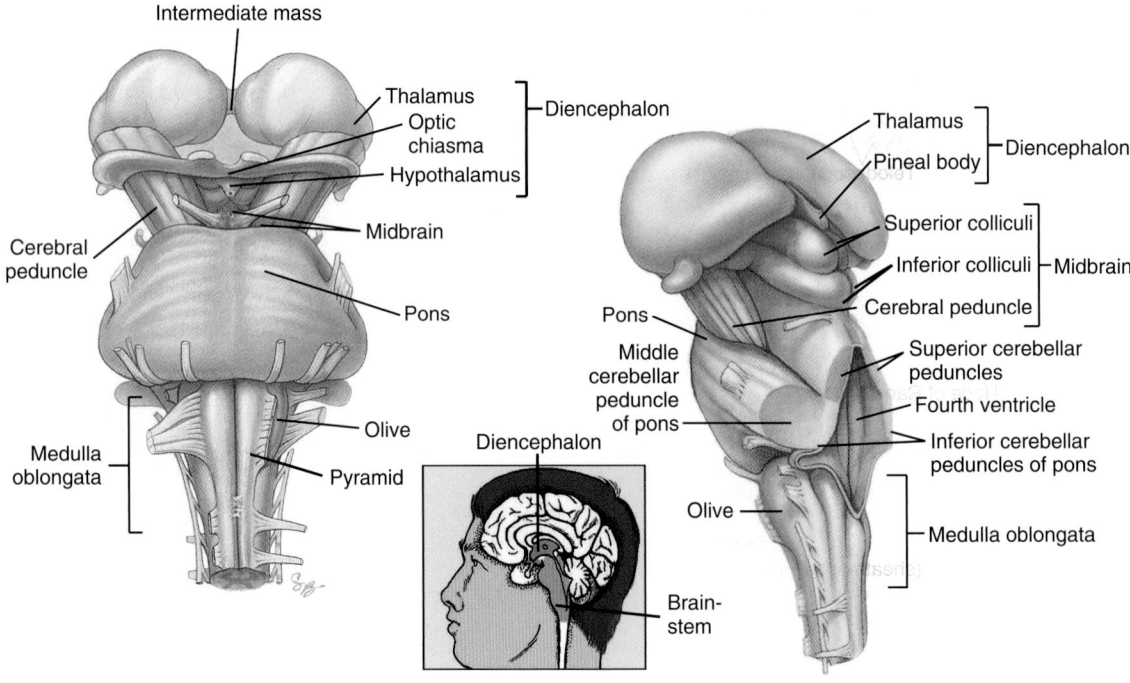

Intermediate mass

Thalamus
Optic chiasma
Hypothalamus
— Diencephalon

Cerebral peduncle

Midbrain

Pons

Medulla oblongata

Olive

Pyramid

Diencephalon

Brain-stem

Thalamus
Pineal body
— Diencephalon

Superior colliculi
Inferior colliculi
Cerebral peduncle
— Midbrain

Pons

Middle cerebellar peduncle of pons

Superior cerebellar peduncles

Fourth ventricle

Inferior cerebellar peduncles of pons

Olive

Medulla oblongata

BASIC STRUCTURE OF THE NEURON

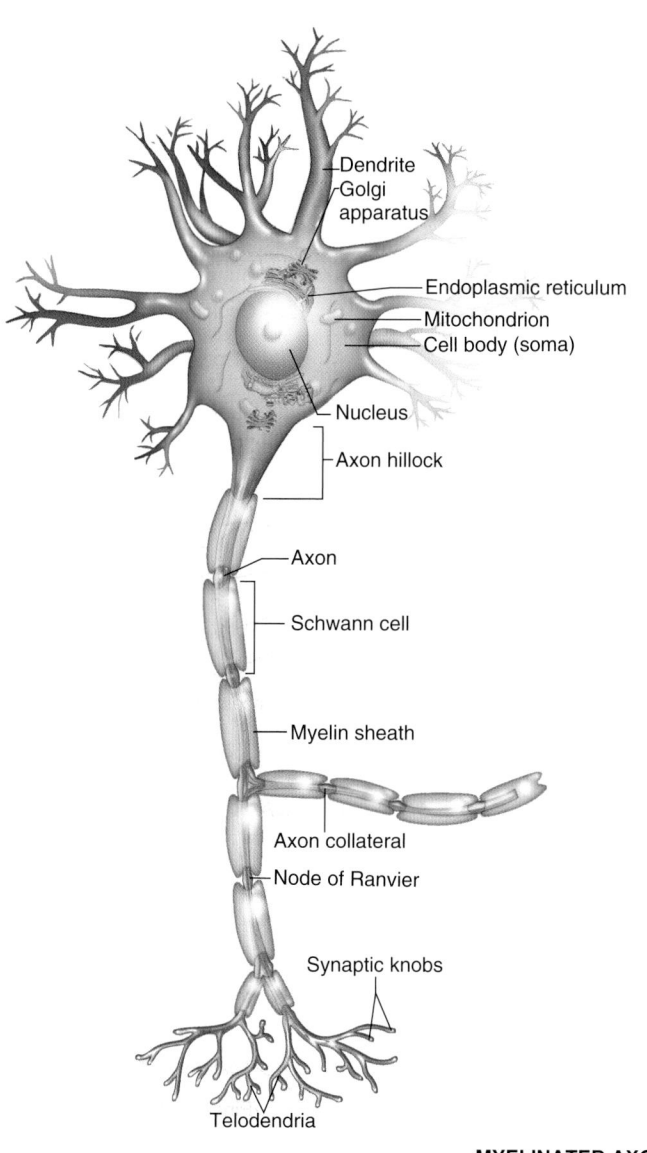

Dendrite
Golgi apparatus
Endoplasmic reticulum
Mitochondrion
Cell body (soma)
Nucleus
Axon hillock
Axon
Schwann cell
Myelin sheath
Axon collateral
Node of Ranvier
Synaptic knobs
Telodendria

MYELINATED AXON

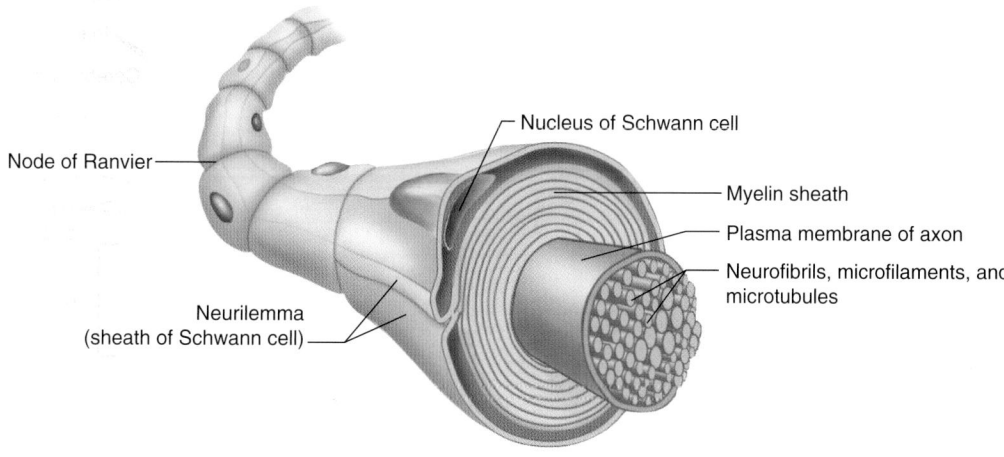

Node of Ranvier
Nucleus of Schwann cell
Myelin sheath
Plasma membrane of axon
Neurofibrils, microfilaments, and microtubules
Neurilemma (sheath of Schwann cell)

RESPIRATORY SYSTEM

ORGANS OF THE RESPIRATORY SYSTEM

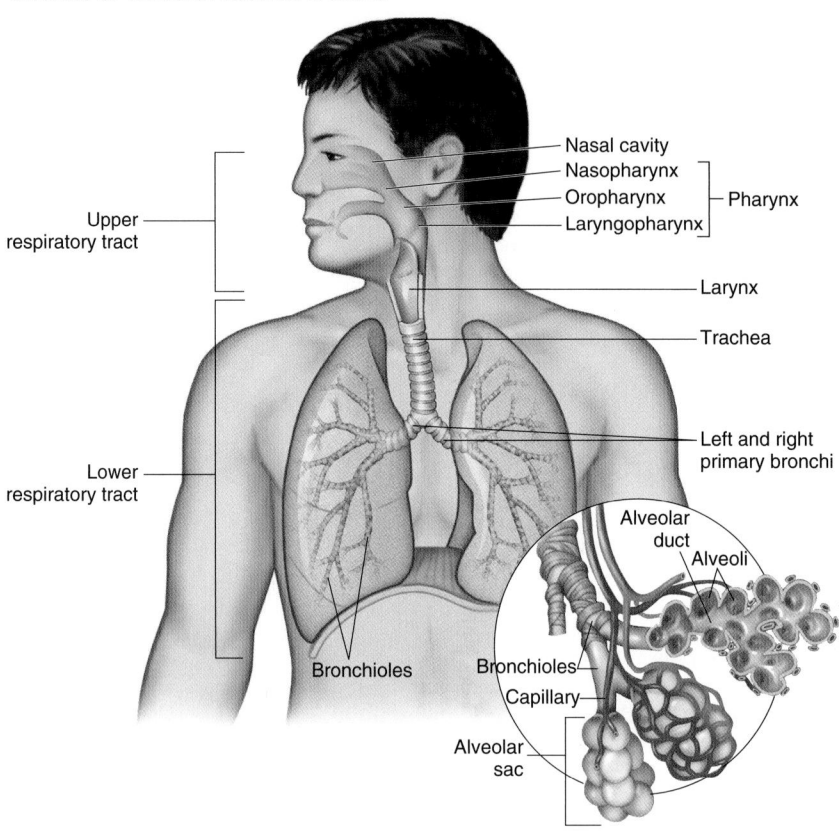

NASAL PASSAGES AND THROAT

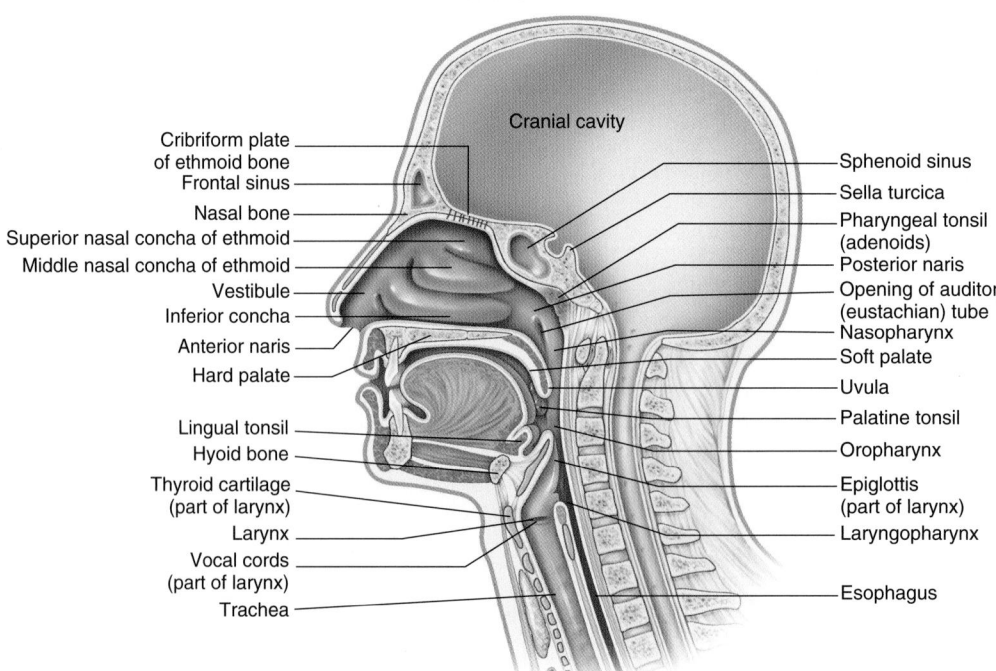

NASAL SEPTUM

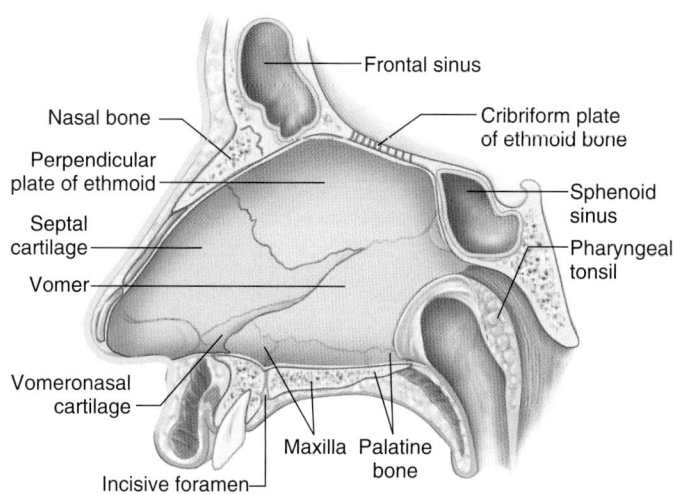

Frontal sinus

Nasal bone

Cribriform plate
of ethmoid bone

Perpendicular
plate of ethmoid

Sphenoid
sinus

Septal
cartilage

Pharyngeal
tonsil

Vomer

Vomeronasal
cartilage

Maxilla Palatine
bone

Incisive foramen

NASAL CAVITY

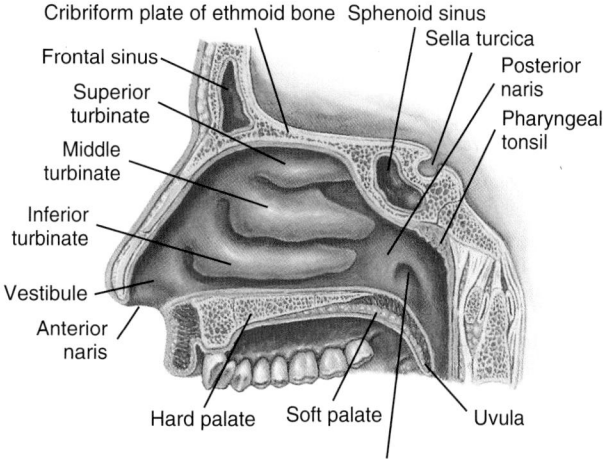

Cribriform plate of ethmoid bone Sphenoid sinus

Sella turcica

Frontal sinus

Posterior
naris

Superior
turbinate

Pharyngeal
tonsil

Middle
turbinate

Inferior
turbinate

Vestibule

Anterior
naris

Hard palate Soft palate Uvula

Opening of auditory (eustachian) tube

BONES OF THE NASAL CAVITY

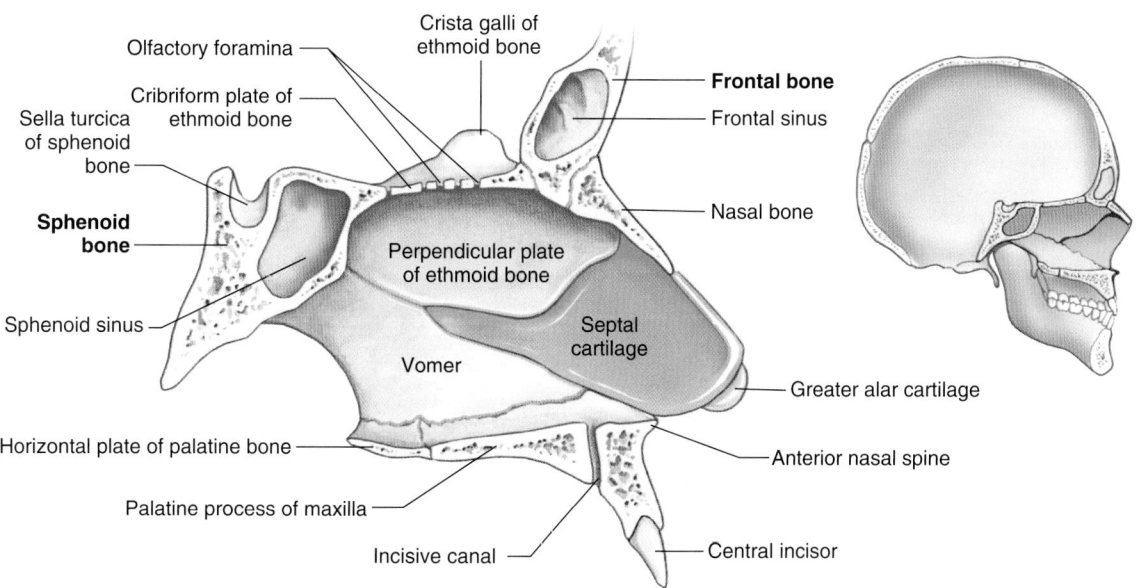

Crista galli of
ethmoid bone

Olfactory foramina

Frontal bone

Cribriform plate of
ethmoid bone

Frontal sinus

Sella turcica
of sphenoid
bone

Nasal bone

**Sphenoid
bone**

Perpendicular plate
of ethmoid bone

Sphenoid sinus

Septal
cartilage

Vomer

Horizontal plate of palatine bone

Greater alar cartilage

Palatine process of maxilla

Anterior nasal spine

Incisive canal

Central incisor

LUNGS

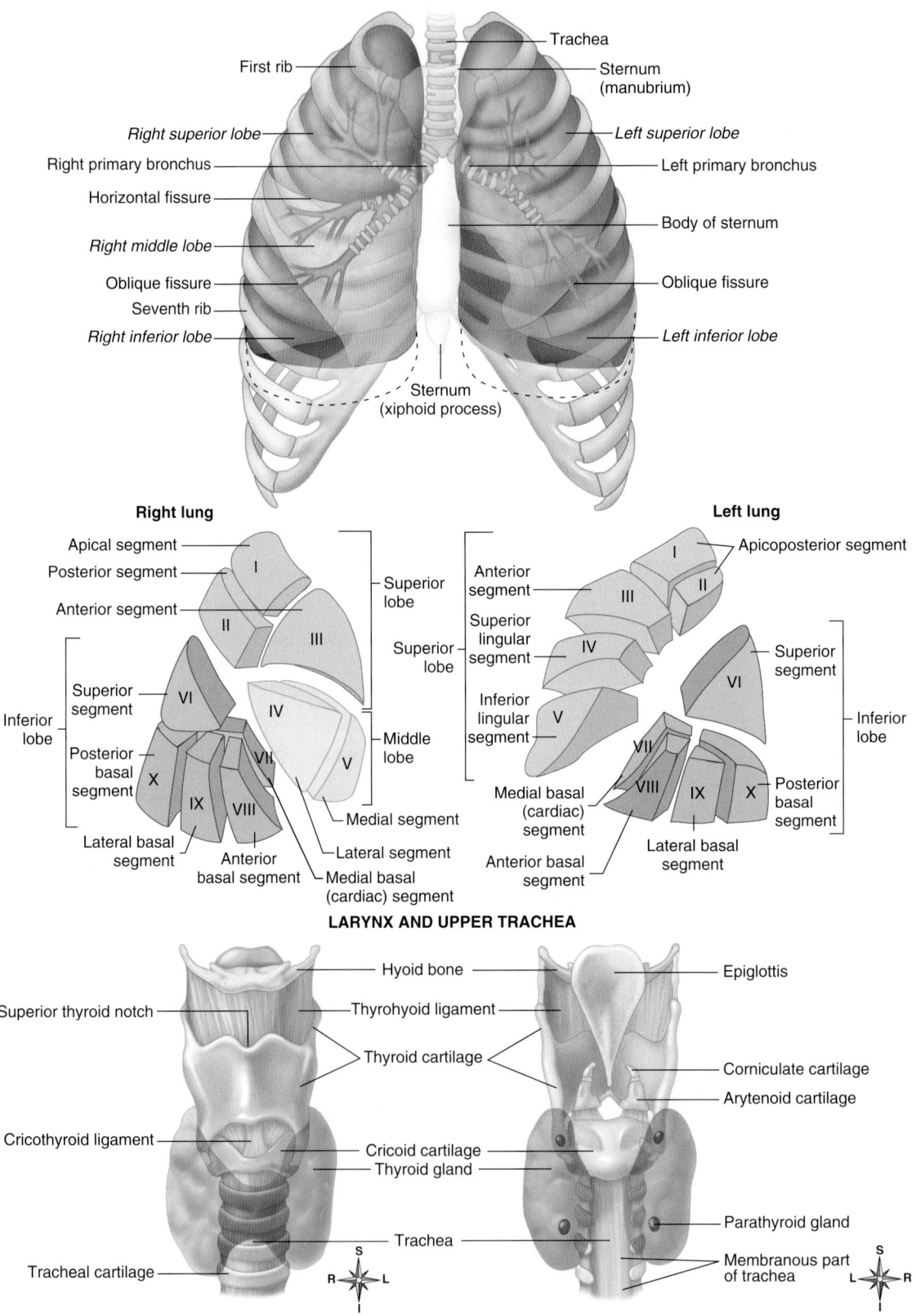

Trachea

First rib

Sternum (manubrium)

Right superior lobe

Left superior lobe

Right primary bronchus

Left primary bronchus

Horizontal fissure

Body of sternum

Right middle lobe

Oblique fissure

Oblique fissure

Seventh rib

Right inferior lobe

Left inferior lobe

Sternum (xiphoid process)

Right lung

Left lung

Apical segment — I

Apicoposterior segment

Posterior segment

Superior lobe

Anterior segment

Anterior segment — II

Superior lobe

Superior lingular segment — IV

Superior segment

III

Inferior lobe

Superior segment — VI

Inferior lingular segment — V

Inferior lobe

Posterior basal segment — X

IV

Middle lobe

VII

V

Medial basal (cardiac) segment

Posterior basal segment

IX — VIII

Medial segment

Lateral basal segment

Anterior basal segment

Lateral segment

Medial basal (cardiac) segment

Anterior basal segment

Lateral basal segment

LARYNX AND UPPER TRACHEA

Hyoid bone

Epiglottis

Superior thyroid notch

Thyrohyoid ligament

Thyroid cartilage

Corniculate cartilage

Arytenoid cartilage

Cricothyroid ligament

Cricoid cartilage

Thyroid gland

Parathyroid gland

Trachea

Tracheal cartilage

Membranous part of trachea

A-30

GAS-EXCHANGE STRUCTURES OF THE LUNG

Surfactant-producing (type II) cell

Fluid containing surfactant layer

Basement membranes

Red blood cell

Macrophage

Alveolus

Alveolar epithelium

Capillary

Interstitial space

Fluid containing surfactant

Capillary endothelium

Alveolar epithelium

RBC

O_2 O_2 O_2

CO_2 CO_2

CO_2

Basement membrane

Basement membrane

Alveolus

Capillary

Respiratory membrane

LARYNX

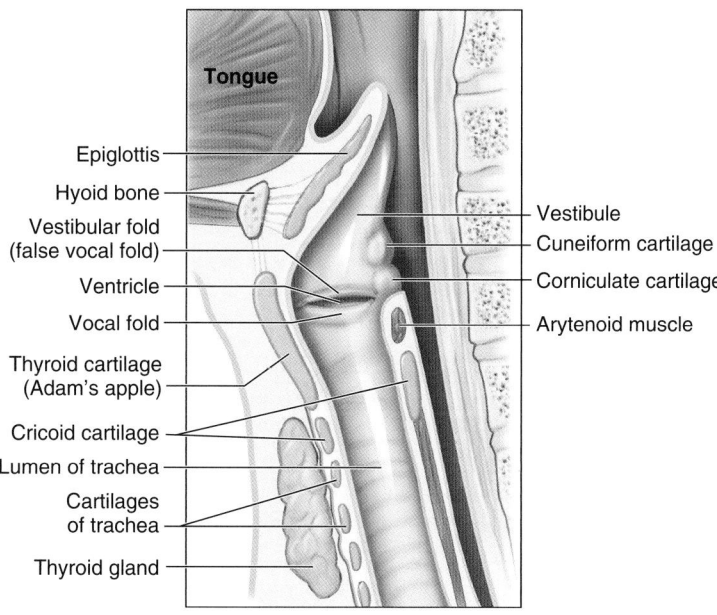

Tongue

Epiglottis

Hyoid bone

Vestibular fold (false vocal fold)

Ventricle

Vocal fold

Thyroid cartilage (Adam's apple)

Cricoid cartilage

Lumen of trachea

Cartilages of trachea

Thyroid gland

Vestibule

Cuneiform cartilage

Corniculate cartilage

Arytenoid muscle

DIGESTIVE SYSTEM

ORGANS OF THE DIGESTIVE SYSTEM AND SOME ASSOCIATED STRUCTURES

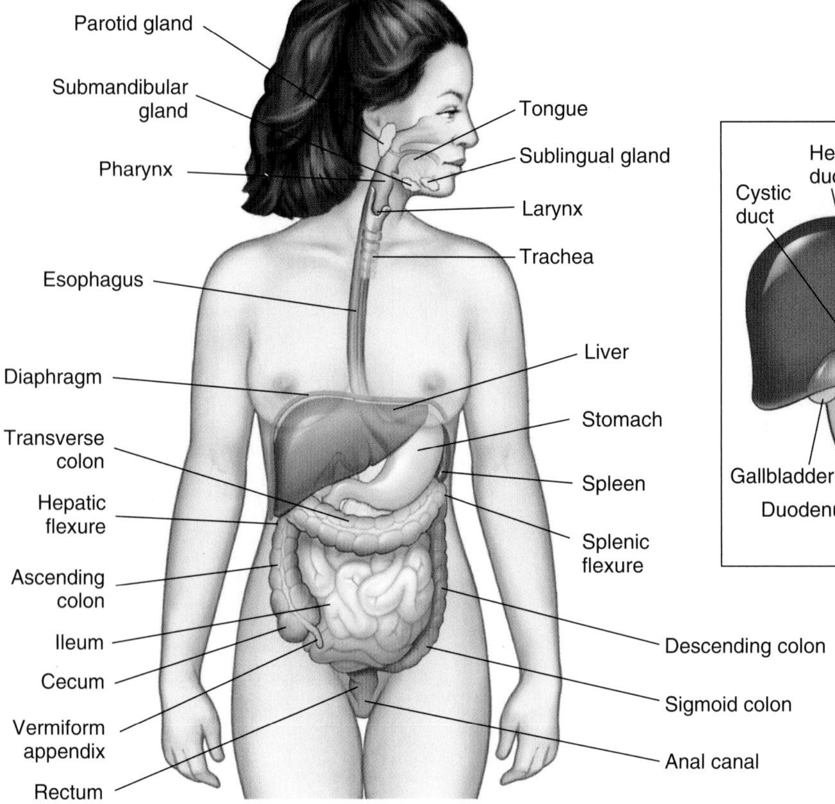

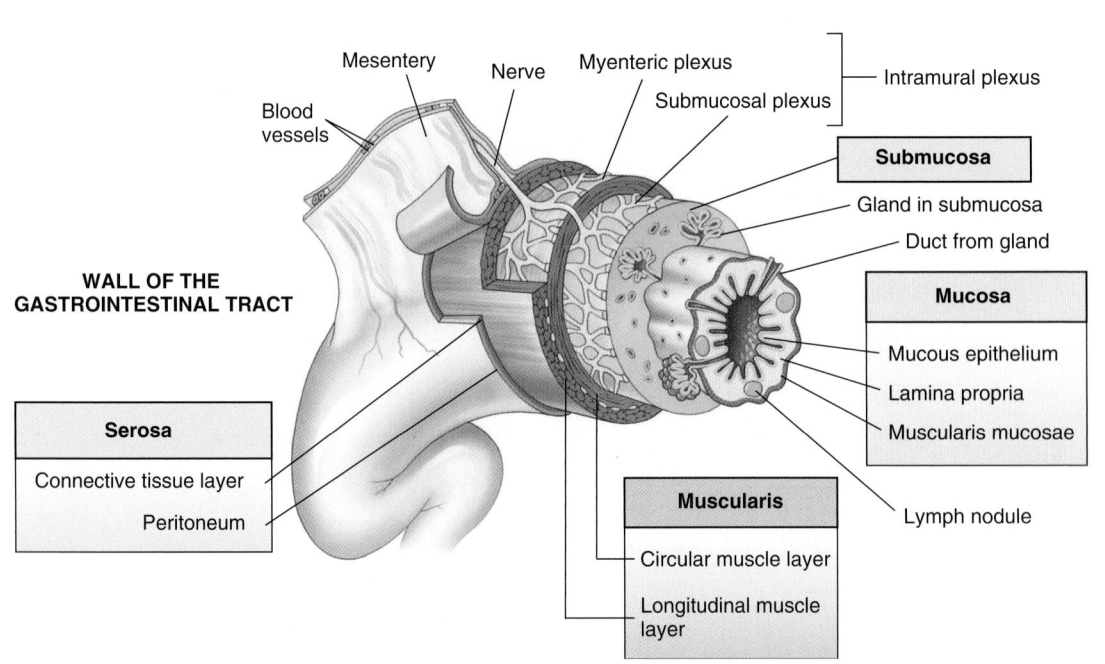

Parotid gland
Submandibular gland
Pharynx
Tongue
Sublingual gland
Larynx
Trachea
Esophagus
Diaphragm
Transverse colon
Hepatic flexure
Ascending colon
Ileum
Cecum
Vermiform appendix
Rectum
Liver
Stomach
Spleen
Splenic flexure
Descending colon
Sigmoid colon
Anal canal

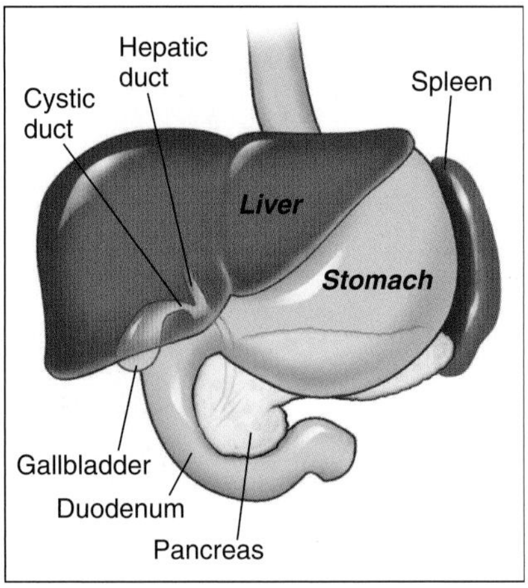

Hepatic duct
Cystic duct
Spleen
Liver
Stomach
Gallbladder
Duodenum
Pancreas

WALL OF THE GASTROINTESTINAL TRACT

Mesentery
Nerve
Myenteric plexus
Submucosal plexus
Intramural plexus
Blood vessels
Submucosa
Gland in submucosa
Duct from gland
Mucosa
Mucous epithelium
Lamina propria
Muscularis mucosae
Lymph nodule
Serosa
Connective tissue layer
Peritoneum
Muscularis
Circular muscle layer
Longitudinal muscle layer

LOCATION OF THE SALIVARY GLANDS

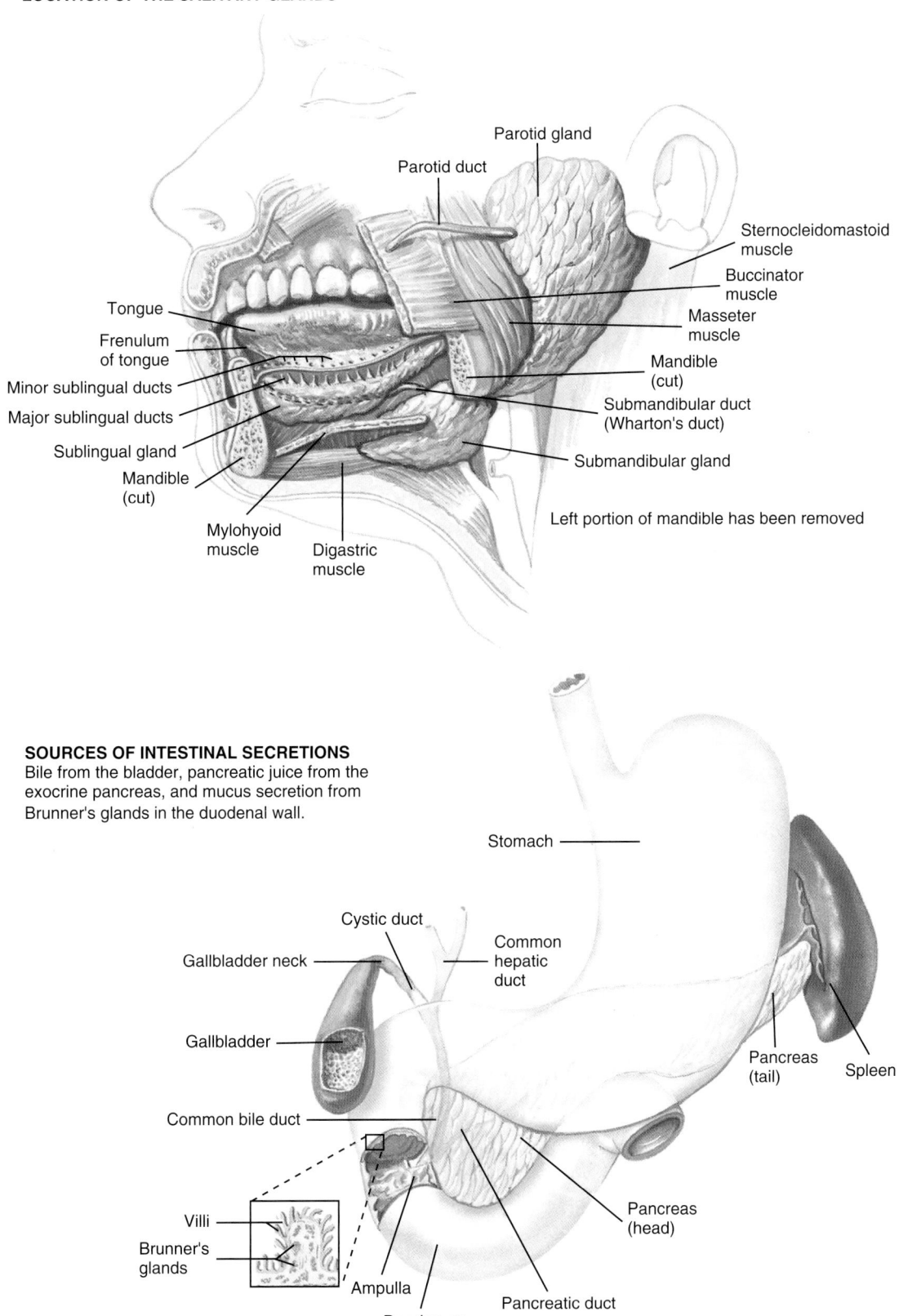

Parotid gland

Parotid duct

Sternocleidomastoid
muscle

Buccinator
muscle

Masseter
muscle

Mandible
(cut)

Submandibular duct
(Wharton's duct)

Submandibular gland

Tongue

Frenulum
of tongue

Minor sublingual ducts

Major sublingual ducts

Sublingual gland

Mandible
(cut)

Mylohyoid
muscle

Digastric
muscle

Left portion of mandible has been removed

SOURCES OF INTESTINAL SECRETIONS
Bile from the bladder, pancreatic juice from the
exocrine pancreas, and mucus secretion from
Brunner's glands in the duodenal wall.

Stomach

Cystic duct

Gallbladder neck

Common
hepatic
duct

Gallbladder

Pancreas
(tail)

Spleen

Common bile duct

Villi

Brunner's
glands

Pancreas
(head)

Ampulla

Pancreatic duct

Duodenum

LARGE INTESTINE

Enlarged detail of the large intestine, rectum, and anus shows the junction between the large and small intestines and the valvelike entry of the ileum into the cecum.

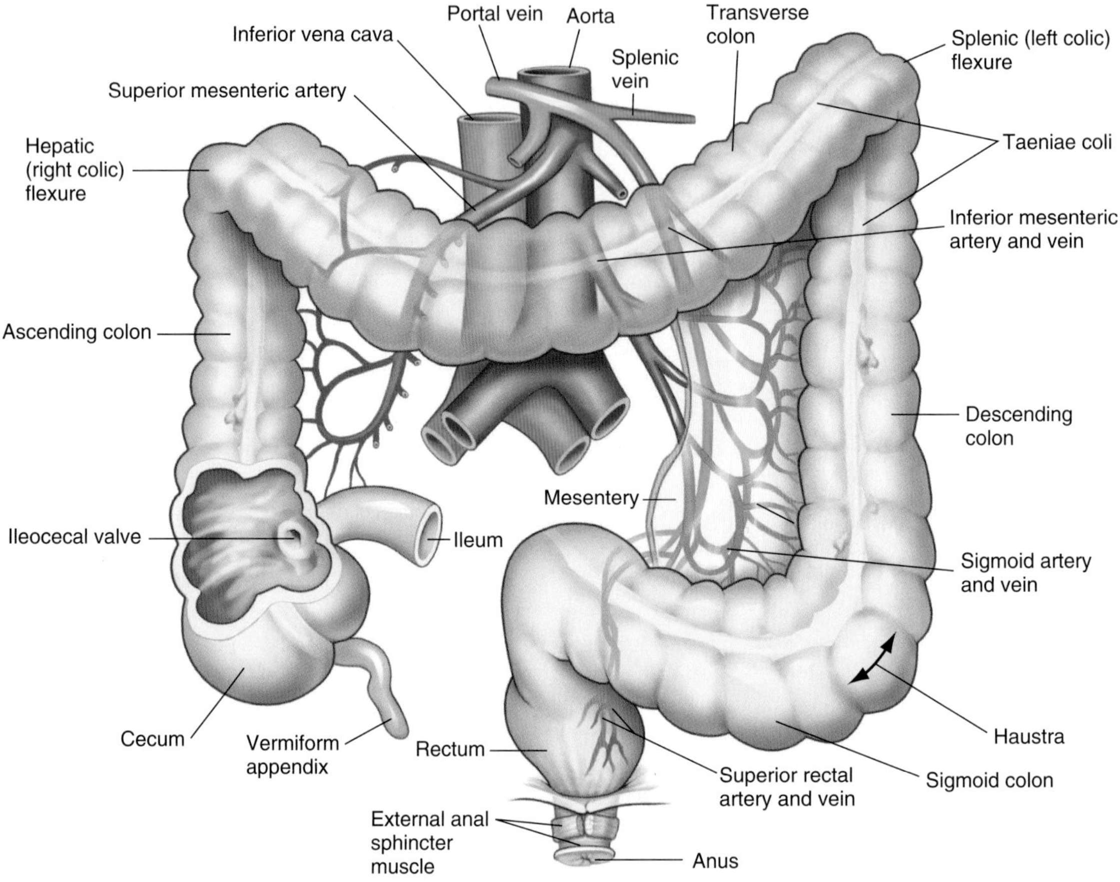

Portal vein
Aorta
Inferior vena cava
Superior mesenteric artery
Transverse colon
Splenic vein
Splenic (left colic) flexure
Hepatic (right colic) flexure
Taeniae coli
Inferior mesenteric artery and vein
Ascending colon
Descending colon
Mesentery
Ileocecal valve
Ileum
Sigmoid artery and vein
Cecum
Vermiform appendix
Rectum
Haustra
Superior rectal artery and vein
Sigmoid colon
External anal sphincter muscle
Anus

CECUM AND TERMINAL ILEUM

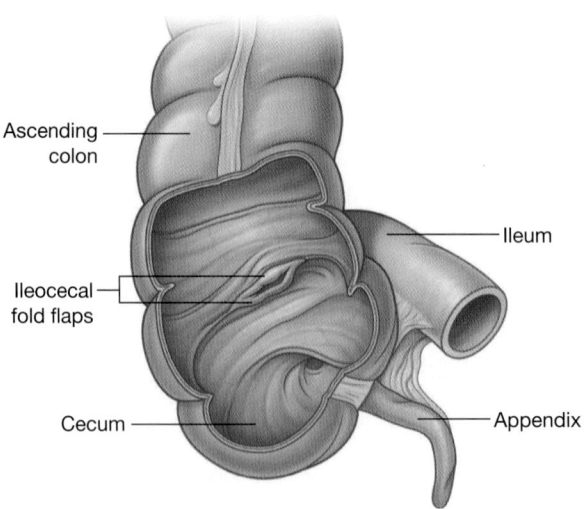

Ascending colon
Ileum
Ileocecal fold flaps
Cecum
Appendix

REPRODUCTIVE SYSTEM

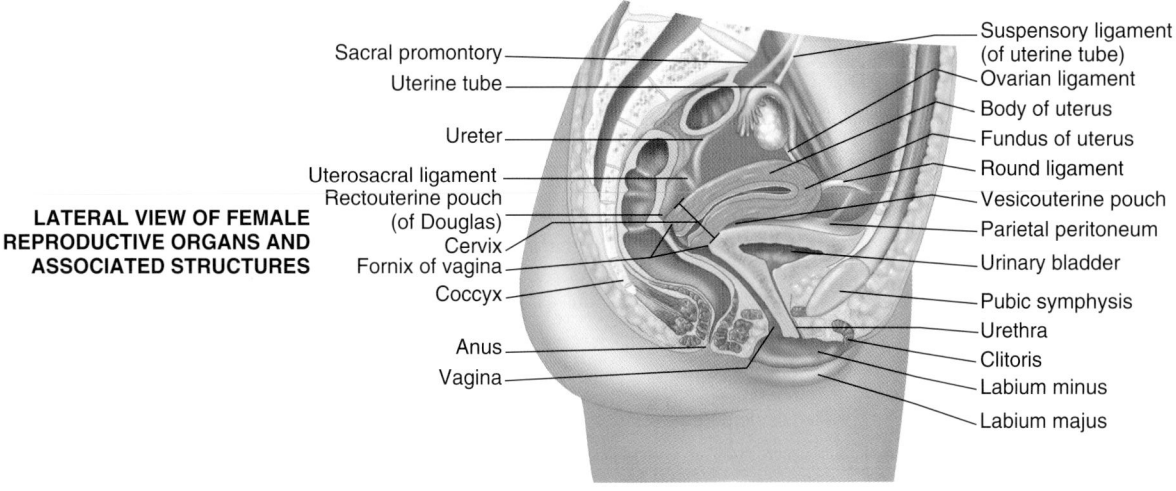

LATERAL VIEW OF FEMALE REPRODUCTIVE ORGANS AND ASSOCIATED STRUCTURES

Sacral promontory
Uterine tube
Ureter
Uterosacral ligament
Rectouterine pouch (of Douglas)
Cervix
Fornix of vagina
Coccyx
Anus
Vagina

Suspensory ligament (of uterine tube)
Ovarian ligament
Body of uterus
Fundus of uterus
Round ligament
Vesicouterine pouch
Parietal peritoneum
Urinary bladder
Pubic symphysis
Urethra
Clitoris
Labium minus
Labium majus

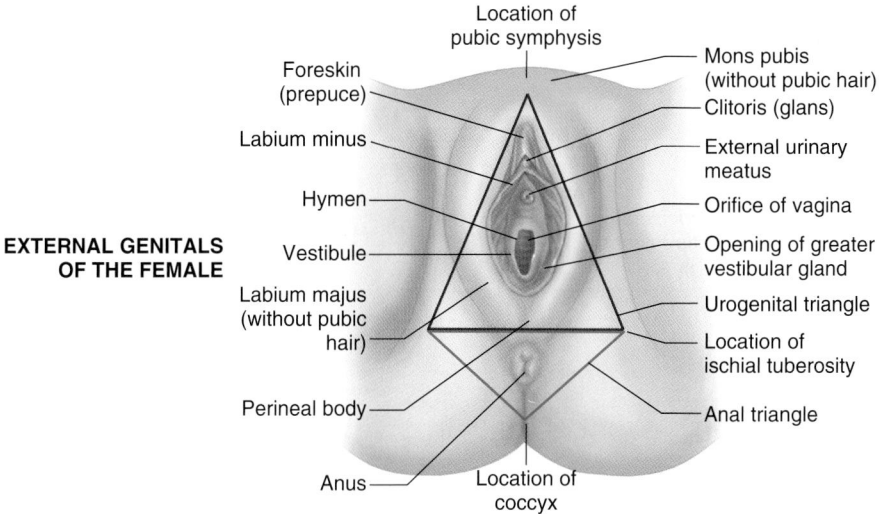

EXTERNAL GENITALS OF THE FEMALE

Location of pubic symphysis
Foreskin (prepuce)
Labium minus
Hymen
Vestibule
Labium majus (without pubic hair)
Perineal body
Anus
Location of coccyx

Mons pubis (without pubic hair)
Clitoris (glans)
External urinary meatus
Orifice of vagina
Opening of greater vestibular gland
Urogenital triangle
Location of ischial tuberosity
Anal triangle

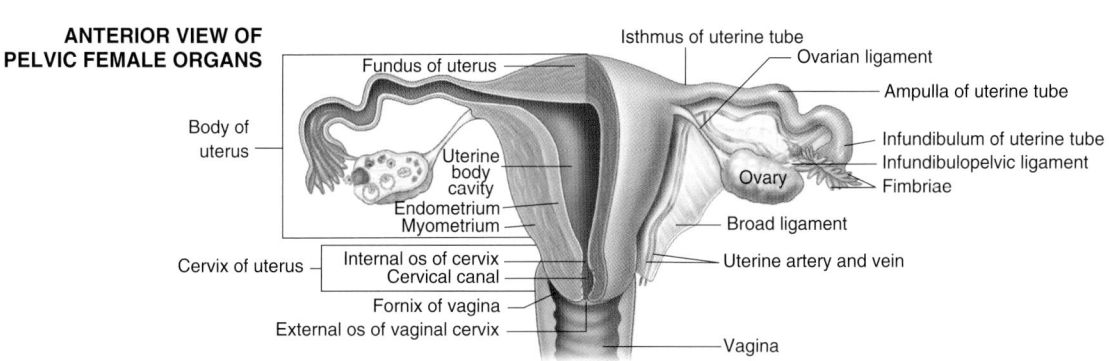

ANTERIOR VIEW OF PELVIC FEMALE ORGANS

Fundus of uterus
Body of uterus
Uterine body cavity
Endometrium
Myometrium
Cervix of uterus
Internal os of cervix
Cervical canal
Fornix of vagina
External os of vaginal cervix

Isthmus of uterine tube
Ovarian ligament
Ampulla of uterine tube
Infundibulum of uterine tube
Infundibulopelvic ligament
Fimbriae
Ovary
Broad ligament
Uterine artery and vein
Vagina

FEMALE BREAST

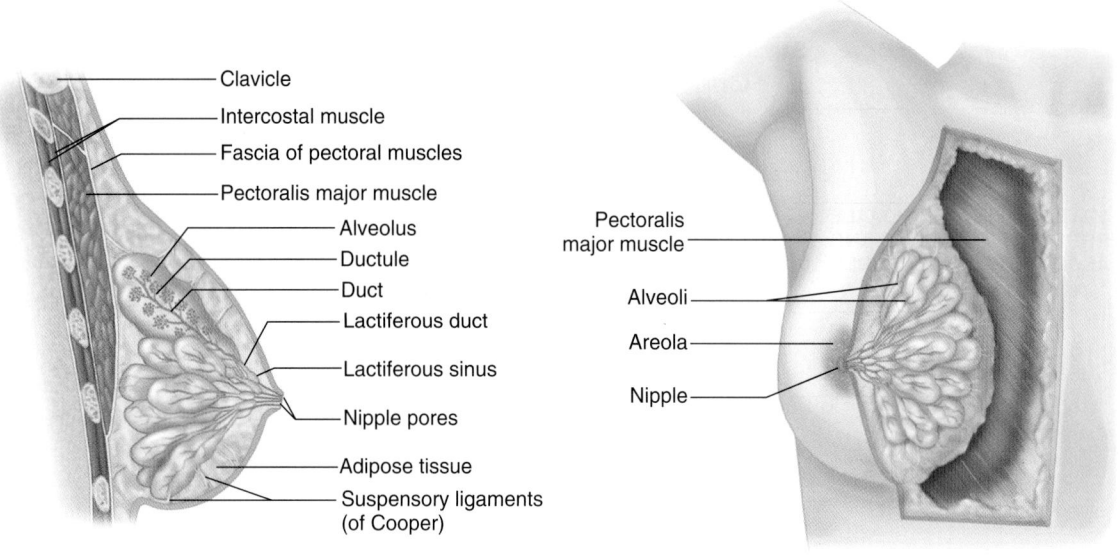

Clavicle
Intercostal muscle
Fascia of pectoral muscles
Pectoralis major muscle
Alveolus
Ductule
Duct
Lactiferous duct
Lactiferous sinus
Nipple pores
Adipose tissue
Suspensory ligaments
(of Cooper)

Pectoralis
major muscle
Alveoli
Areola
Nipple

LYMPHATIC SYSTEM AND THE FEMALE BREAST

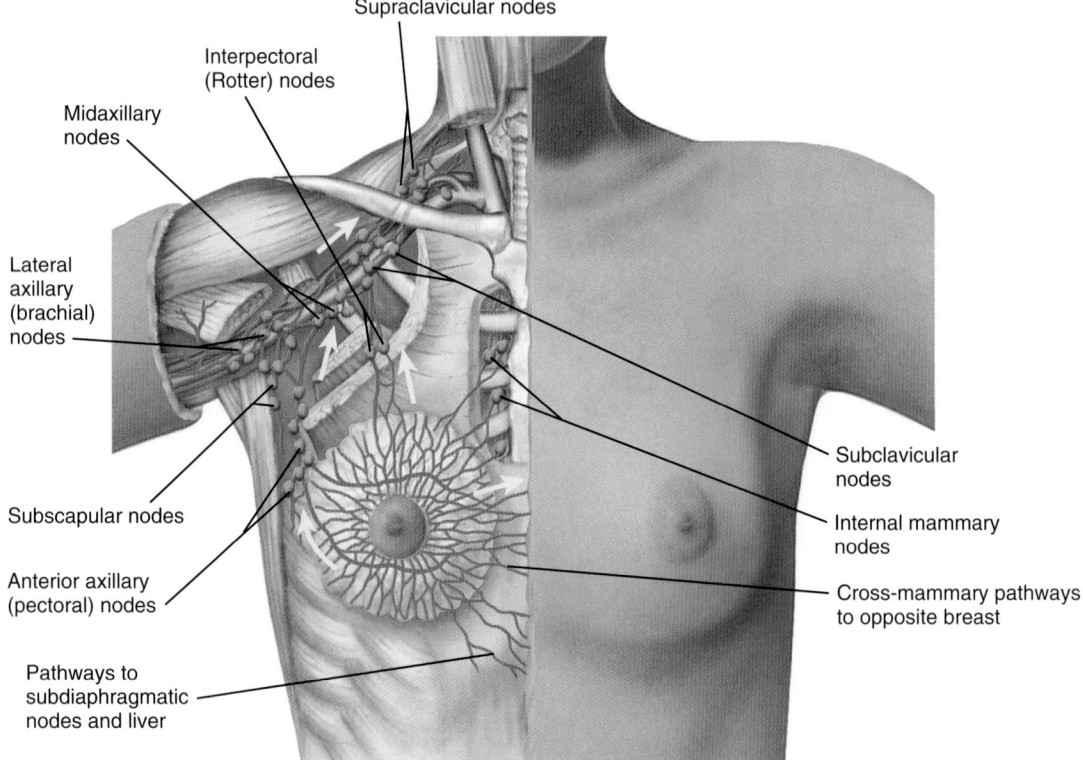

Supraclavicular nodes
Interpectoral
(Rotter) nodes
Midaxillary
nodes
Lateral
axillary
(brachial)
nodes
Subscapular nodes
Anterior axillary
(pectoral) nodes
Pathways to
subdiaphragmatic
nodes and liver

Subclavicular
nodes
Internal mammary
nodes
Cross-mammary pathways
to opposite breast

MALE REPRODUCTIVE ORGANS AND ASSOCIATED STRUCTURES

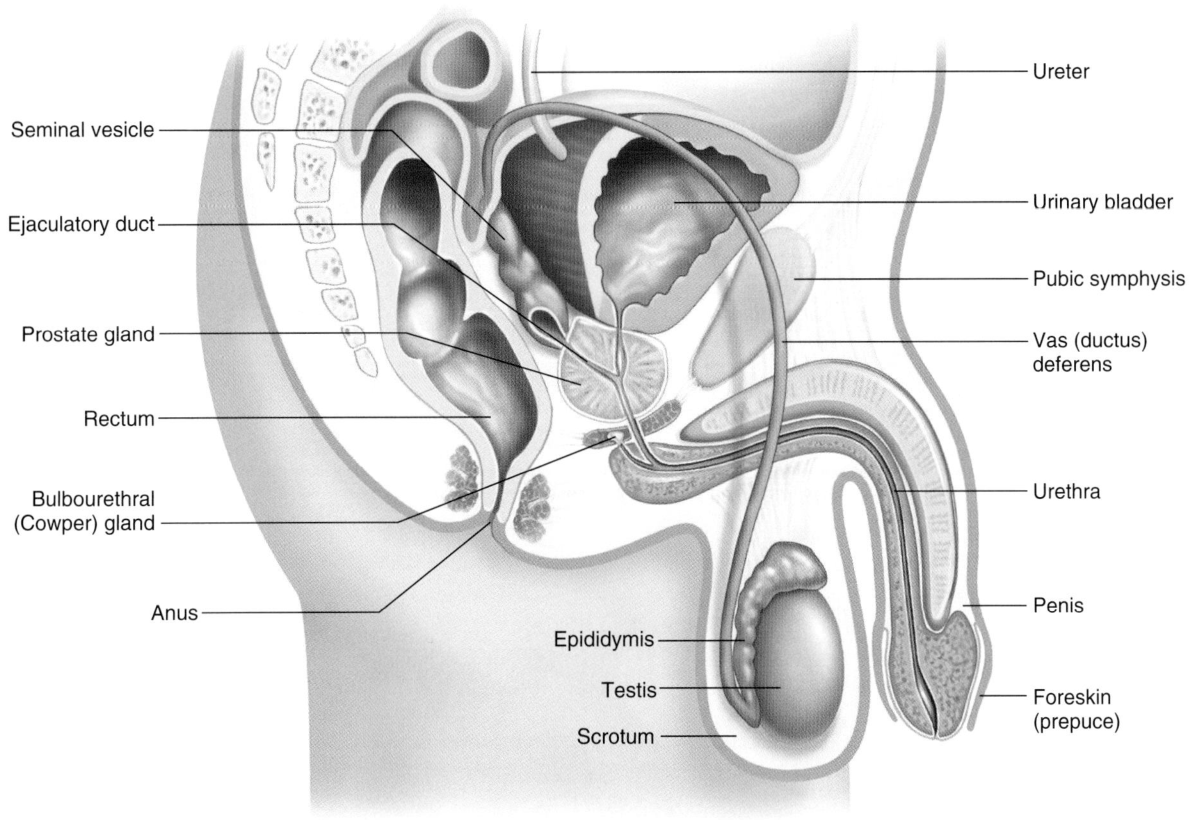

Seminal vesicle

Ejaculatory duct

Prostate gland

Rectum

Bulbourethral
(Cowper) gland

Anus

Epididymis

Testis

Scrotum

Ureter

Urinary bladder

Pubic symphysis

Vas (ductus)
deferens

Urethra

Penis

Foreskin
(prepuce)

EXTERNAL GENITALS OF THE MALE

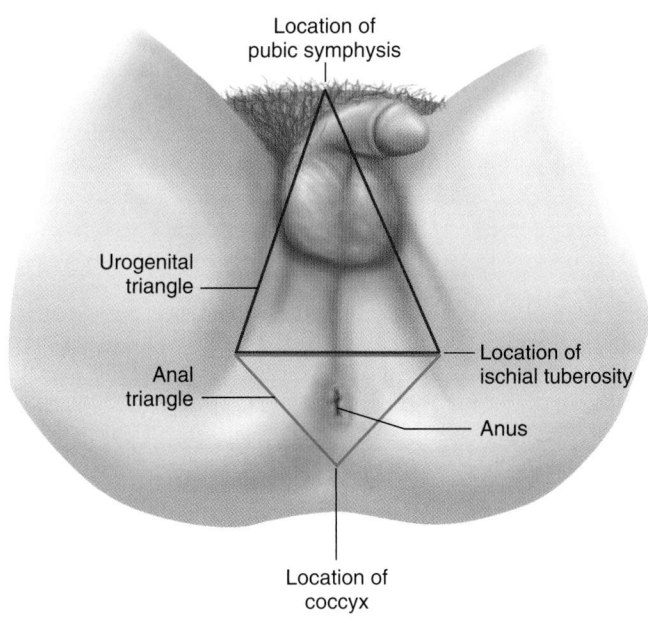

Location of
pubic symphysis

Urogenital
triangle

Anal
triangle

Location of
ischial tuberosity

Anus

Location of
coccyx

TUBULES OF THE TESTIS AND EPIDIDYMIS

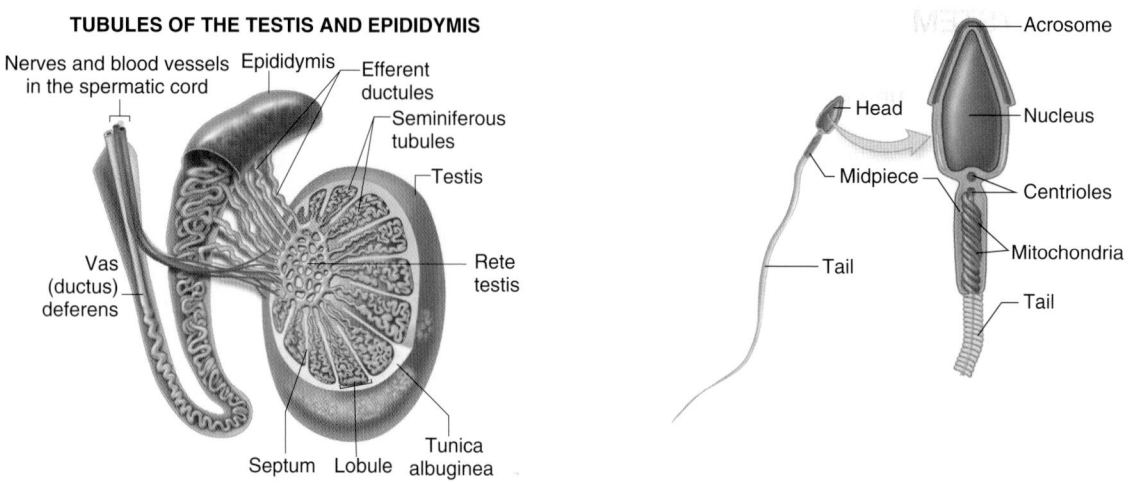

Nerves and blood vessels in the spermatic cord
Epididymis
Efferent ductules
Seminiferous tubules
Testis
Vas (ductus) deferens
Rete testis
Septum   Lobule   Tunica albuginea

Acrosome
Head
Nucleus
Midpiece
Centrioles
Mitochondria
Tail
Tail

ANTERIOR VIEW OF MALE REPRODUCTIVE STRUCTURES

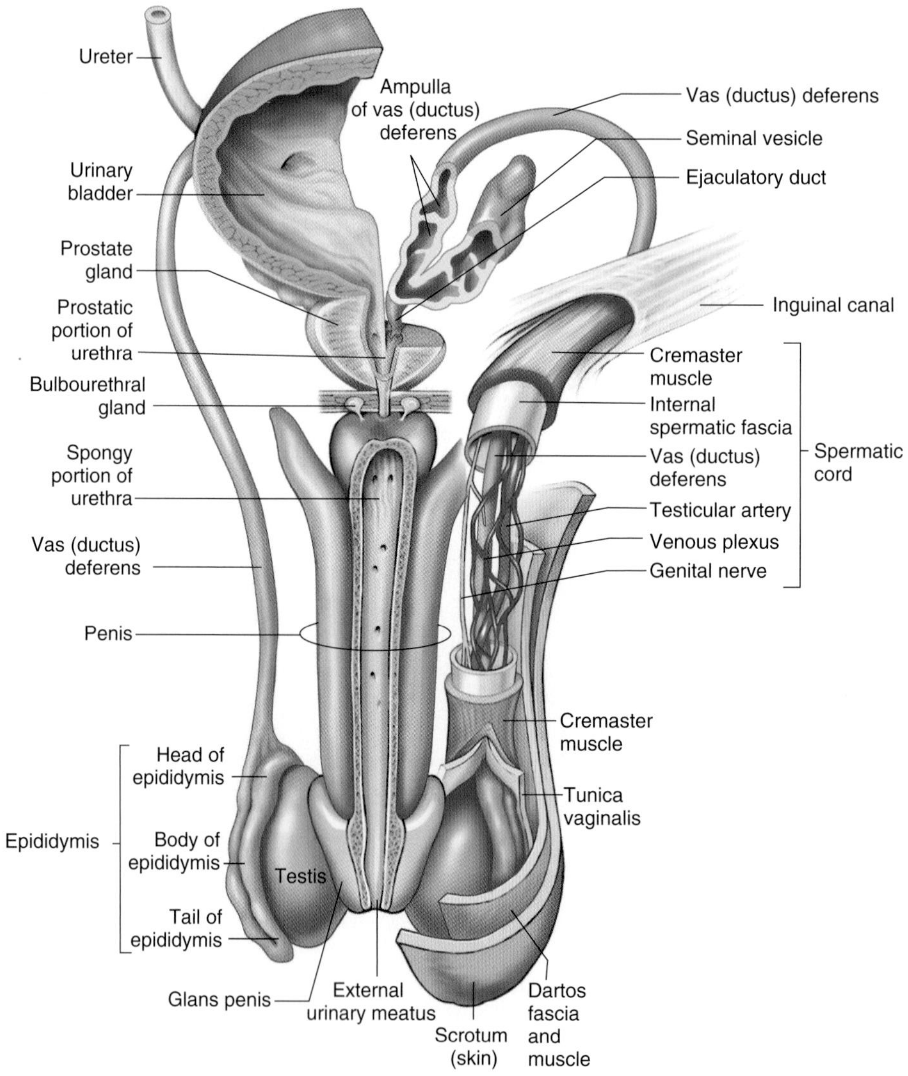

Ureter
Ampulla of vas (ductus) deferens
Vas (ductus) deferens
Seminal vesicle
Ejaculatory duct
Urinary bladder
Inguinal canal
Prostate gland
Cremaster muscle
Prostatic portion of urethra
Internal spermatic fascia
Bulbourethral gland
Vas (ductus) deferens
Spermatic cord
Spongy portion of urethra
Testicular artery
Venous plexus
Vas (ductus) deferens
Genital nerve
Penis
Cremaster muscle
Head of epididymis
Tunica vaginalis
Epididymis
Body of epididymis
Testis
Tail of epididymis
Glans penis
External urinary meatus
Scrotum (skin)
Dartos fascia and muscle

URINARY SYSTEM

URINARY SYSTEM AND SOME ASSOCIATED STRUCTURES

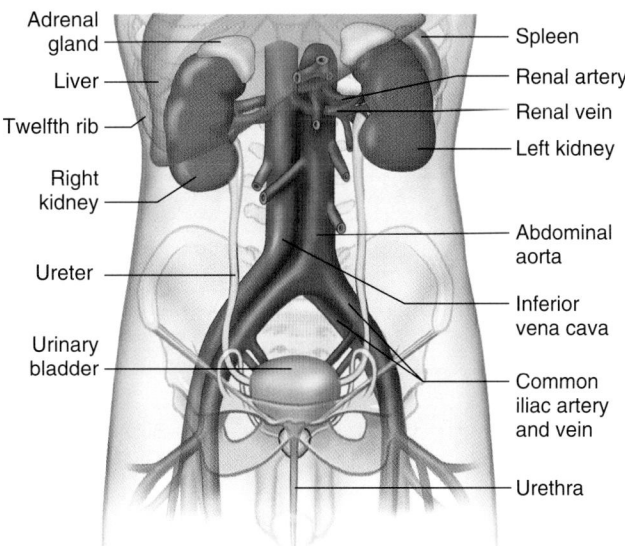

Adrenal gland — Spleen — Renal artery — Liver — Renal vein — Twelfth rib — Left kidney — Right kidney — Ureter — Abdominal aorta — Urinary bladder — Inferior vena cava — Common iliac artery and vein — Urethra

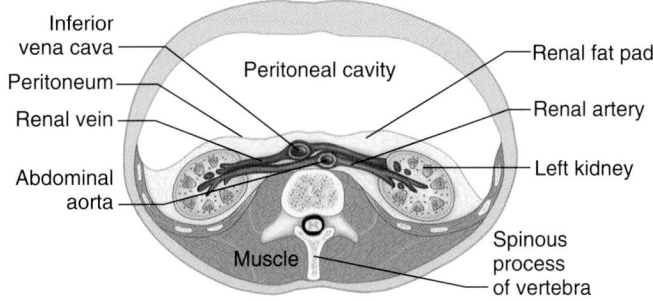

Inferior vena cava — Peritoneal cavity — Renal fat pad — Peritoneum — Renal artery — Renal vein — Left kidney — Abdominal aorta — Muscle — Spinous process of vertebra

BLADDER

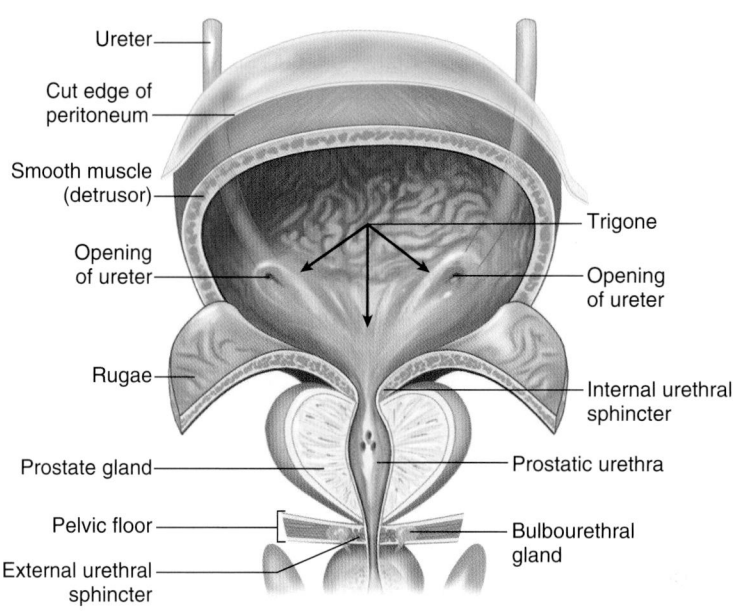

Ureter

Cut edge of peritoneum

Smooth muscle (detrusor)

Opening of ureter

Rugae

Prostate gland

Pelvic floor

External urethral sphincter

Trigone

Opening of ureter

Internal urethral sphincter

Prostatic urethra

Bulbourethral gland

INTERNAL STRUCTURE OF THE KIDNEY

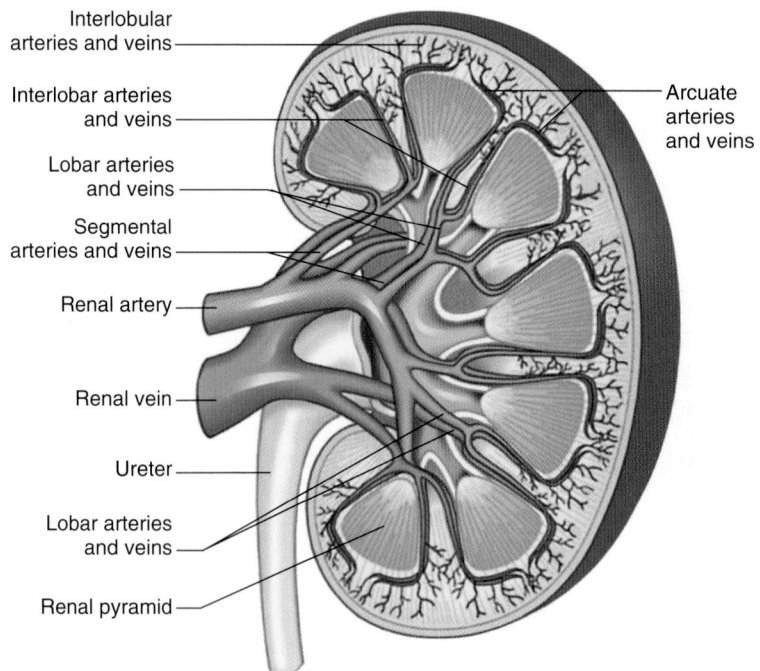

Interlobular arteries and veins

Interlobar arteries and veins

Lobar arteries and veins

Segmental arteries and veins

Renal artery

Renal vein

Ureter

Lobar arteries and veins

Renal pyramid

Arcuate arteries and veins

NEPHRON

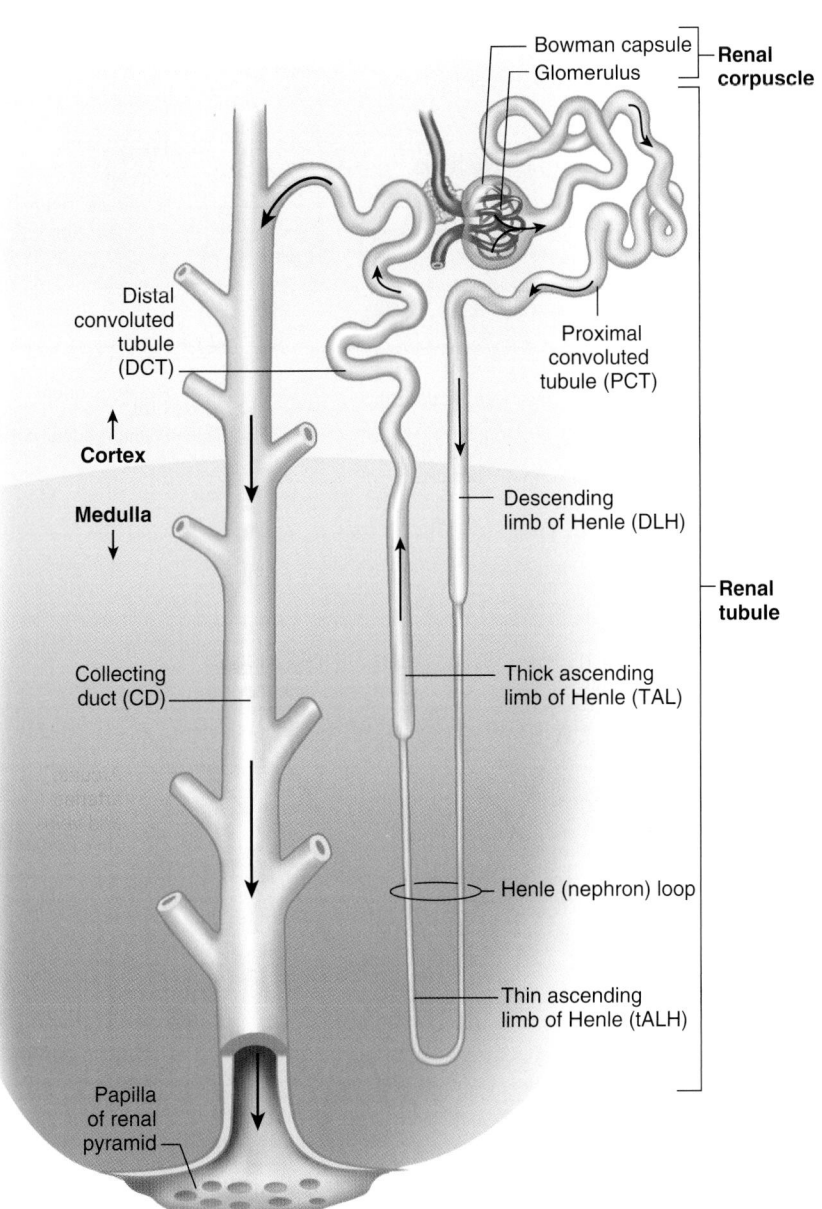

SPECIAL SENSES

GROSS ANATOMY OF THE EAR

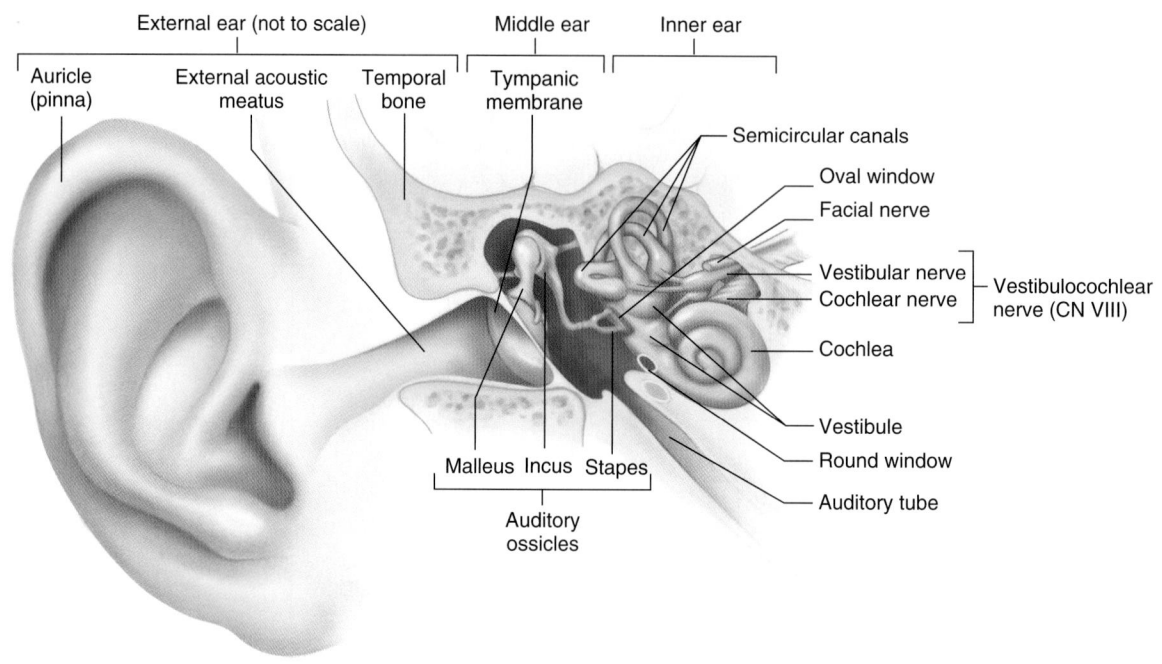

External ear (not to scale) | Middle ear | Inner ear

Auricle (pinna)
External acoustic meatus
Temporal bone
Tympanic membrane
Semicircular canals
Oval window
Facial nerve
Vestibular nerve
Cochlear nerve
Vestibulocochlear nerve (CN VIII)
Cochlea
Vestibule
Round window
Auditory tube
Malleus   Incus   Stapes
Auditory ossicles

STRUCTURE OF THE SKIN

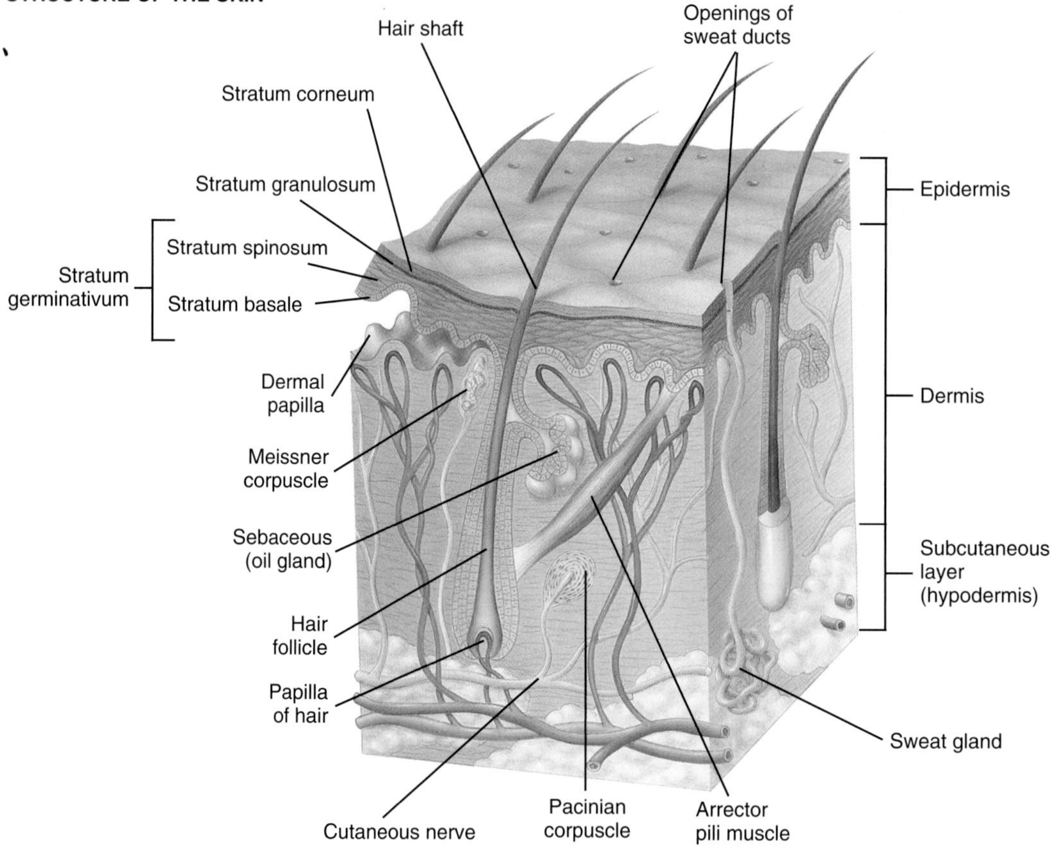

Hair shaft
Openings of sweat ducts
Stratum corneum
Stratum granulosum
Epidermis
Stratum spinosum
Stratum germinativum
Stratum basale
Dermal papilla
Dermis
Meissner corpuscle
Sebaceous (oil gland)
Hair follicle
Subcutaneous layer (hypodermis)
Papilla of hair
Sweat gland
Cutaneous nerve
Pacinian corpuscle
Arrector pili muscle

CROSS-SECTIONAL VIEW OF THE EYE

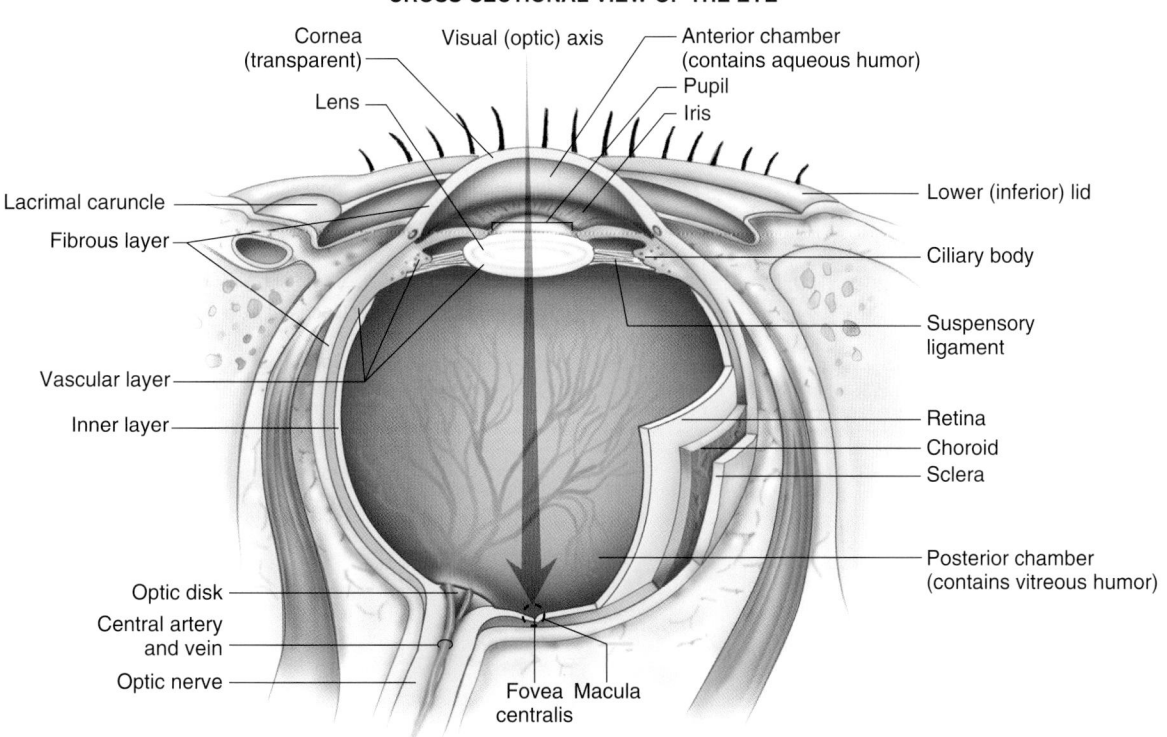

Cornea (transparent)
Visual (optic) axis
Anterior chamber (contains aqueous humor)
Lens
Pupil
Iris
Lacrimal caruncle
Lower (inferior) lid
Fibrous layer
Ciliary body
Suspensory ligament
Vascular layer
Inner layer
Retina
Choroid
Sclera
Posterior chamber (contains vitreous humor)
Optic disk
Central artery and vein
Optic nerve
Fovea Macula centralis

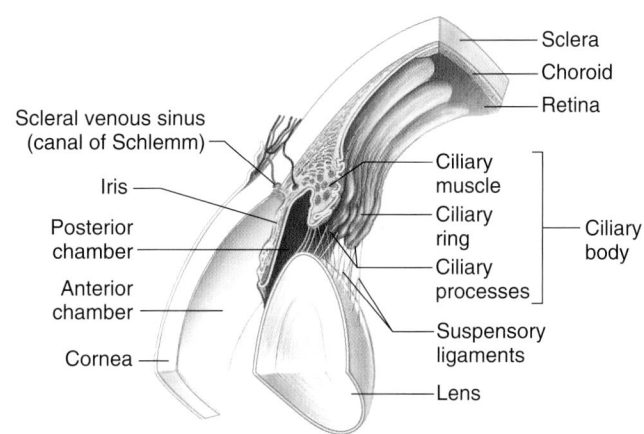

Sclera
Choroid
Retina
Scleral venous sinus (canal of Schlemm)
Iris
Ciliary muscle
Ciliary ring
Ciliary body
Posterior chamber
Ciliary processes
Anterior chamber
Suspensory ligaments
Cornea
Lens

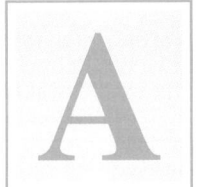

A

Å, symbol for **angstrom**.

a-, a Greek prefix meaning "without," "lack of," "not": *aphasia*.

A, α. See **alpha**.

A68, symbol for a protein found in the brain tissue of patients with Alzheimer disease. It is also found in the developing normal brains of fetuses and infants but begins to disappear by the age of 2 years. It is a major subunit of paired helical filaments and derivatized forms of tau protein, which is generally hyperphosphorylated. See also **tau protein**.

AA, **1.** abbreviation for **achievement age. 2.** abbreviation for **Alcoholics Anonymous. 3.** abbreviation for **amplitude of accommodation. 4.** abbreviation for **anesthesiologist assistant. 5.** abbreviation for **amino acid. 6.** abbreviation for **anterior apical. 7.** abbreviation for **arch of the aorta. 8.** abbreviation for *arm-ankle (pulse rate)*.

AAA, **1.** abbreviation for *American Association of Anatomists*. **2.** abbreviation for *acquired aplastic anemia*. **3.** abbreviation for **abdominal aortic aneurysm**.

āa, āa, ĀĀ, (in prescriptions) indicating an equal amount of each ingredient to be compounded. Abbreviation for **ana**.

AAAAI, abbreviation for **American Academy of Allergy, Asthma, and Immunology**.

AACE, **1.** abbreviation for *American Association of Clinical Endocrinologists*. **2.** abbreviation for *Association for the Advancement of Computing in Education*.

AACN, **1.** abbreviation for **American Association of Colleges of Nursing. 2.** abbreviation for **American Association of Critical Care Nurses**.

AAFP, abbreviation for *American Academy of Family Physicians*.

AAI, abbreviation for **ankle-arm index**. See **ankle-brachial index**.

AAL, abbreviation for **anterior axillary line**.

AAMC, abbreviation for **American Association of Medical Colleges**.

AAMI, **1.** abbreviation for **Association for the Advancement of Medical Instrumentation. 2.** abbreviation for *acute anterior myocardial infarction*. **3.** abbreviation for *age-associated memory impairment*.

AAN, abbreviation for **American Academy of Nursing**.

AANA, abbreviation for **American Association of Nurse Anesthetists**.

AANN, abbreviation for **American Association of Neuroscience Nurses**.

AAO–HNSF, abbreviation for *American Academy of Otolaryngology–Head and Neck Surgery*.

AAOMS, abbreviation for *American Association of Oral and Maxillofacial Surgeons*.

AAPA, **1.** abbreviation for **American Academy of Physician Assistants. 2.** abbreviation for *American Association of Psychiatric Administrators*.

Aaron sign /ˈa-rən ˈsīn/ [Charles D. Aaron, American physician, 1866–1951], a clinical sign in acute appendicitis indicated by referred pain or feeling of distress in the epigastric or precordial region when continuous firm pressure is applied over McBurney's point. See also **McBurney's point**.

AARP, Inc., a nonprofit U.S. organization of older persons, who may or may not be retired, with the goal of improving the welfare of persons over 50 years of age. Among other actions, the group seeks out health and wellness benefits for its members. The AARP advocates for older individuals on legislative, consumer, education, and legal issues. Formerly called **American Association of Retired Persons**.

Aarskog syndrome /ärsˈkog/ [Dagfinn Charles Aarskog, Norwegian pediatrician, 1928–2014], an X-linked syndrome characterized by wide-set eyes, nostrils that are tipped upward, a broad upper lip, a scrotal shawl, and small hands. Also called *Aarskog-Scott syndrome,* **faciodigitogenital syndrome, faciogenital dysplasia**.

Aase syndrome /äz/ [Jon Morton Aase, American pediatrician, b. 1936], a rare familial syndrome characterized by mild delayed growth, hypoplastic anemia, heart defects, variable leukocytopenia, triphalangeal thumbs, narrow shoulders, and late closure of fontanels, and occasionally by cleft lip, cleft palate, retinopathy, and web neck. Autosomal-dominant transmission has been suggested. Also called *Aase-Smith syndrome*.

AAUP, abbreviation for **American Association of University Professors**.

AAV, abbreviation for **adeno-associated virus**.

Ab, abbreviation for **antibody**.

ab-, abs-, prefixes meaning "from, off, away from": *abstract, abnormality*.

Abadie sign /äbˈə-dēʹ/ [Jean Marie Charles Abadie, French physician, 1842–1932], **1.** spasm of the muscle that raises the upper eyelid, seen in patients with exophthalmic goiter. **2.** loss of feeling in the Achilles tendon associated with the progressive loss of deep tendon reflexes, as seen in diabetes mellitus or syphilis.

abacavir /a-BAK-a-vir/, an antiviral that is a nucleoside reverse transcriptase inhibitor.

■ INDICATIONS: It is prescribed in combination with other antiretroviral agents for HIV-1 infection.

■ CONTRAINDICATIONS: Known hypersensitivity to this drug or moderate to severe hepatic impairment prohibits its use.

■ ADVERSE EFFECTS: Hypersensitivity reactions occur in approximately 5% of patients and can be fatal. Other life-threatening adverse effects include granulocytopenia, anemia, and lactic acidosis. Common side effects include fever, headache, malaise, insomnia, nausea, vomiting, diarrhea, anorexia, and rash.

abacterial /abˈaktirʺē·əl/, any atmosphere or condition free of bacteria; literally, without bacteria.

abaissement /äʹbäsmäNʺ/ [Fr, a lowering], a falling or depressing.

amyloid beta (amyloid β), an abnormal peptide, varying from 40 to 43 amino acids in length and found in aggregates in the cerebrovascular walls and the cores of the plaques in Alzheimer disease. The accumulation of certain forms of this substance is neurotoxic and plays a role in the initiation of the cognitive deficits that define Alzheimer disease. The exact mechanism is unknown.

A band, a muscle fiber contractile unit that contains both actin (thin filament) and myosin (thick filament). It is marked by partial overlapping of the actin and myosin filaments and extends the entire length of the myosin filaments as the dark area between two I bands of a sarcomere. There is no change in the length of the A band with muscle contraction. Compare **I band.**

abandonment of care /əban″dənment/, unilateral termination of care without the patient's consent or knowledge, or without adequate notice, while the patient is still in need of care. Also called **medical abandonment.**

abapical /abap″əkəl/, opposite the apex.

abarognosis /aber″agnō″sis/ [Gk, *a,* not, *baros,* weight, *gnosis,* knowledge], an inability to judge or compare the weight of objects, particularly those held in the hand.

abarthrosis, a form of articulation that allows considerable change in position and spatial relationship between the articulated parts and in which bones move freely upon one another. See **synovial joint**.

abarticular /ab″ärtik″yo͞olər/ [L, *ab,* away from, *articulus,* joint], **1.** pertaining to a condition that does not affect a joint. **2.** pertaining to a site or structure remote from a joint.

abarticular gout, extraarticular gout that affects structures other than joints, such as ligaments or other soft tissues. See also **tophaceous gout.**

abarticulation /ab′ärtik′yəlā″shən/, **1.** dislocation of a joint. **2.** a synovial joint.

abasia /əbā″zhə/ [Gk, *a, basis,* not step], the inability to walk caused by a lack of motor coordination. –*abasic,* **abatic,** *adj.*

abasia-astasia, the inability or refusal to walk or stand upright. Also called **astasia-abasia.**

abatacept, a monoclonal antibody agent.

■ INDICATIONS: This drug is used to treat acute or chronic rheumatoid arthritis that has not responded to other disease-modifying agents. It may be used in combination with other disease-modifying antirheumatic agents. It may not be used with tumor necrosis factor antagonists or anakinra.

■ CONTRAINDICATIONS: Tuberculosis and known hypersensitivity to this drug prohibit its use.

■ ADVERSE EFFECTS: Adverse effects of this drug include headache, asthenia, dizziness, abdominal pain, dyspepsia, nausea, rash, flushing, urticaria, pruritus, and wheezing. Life-threatening side effects include anaphylaxis, malignancies, and angioedema. Common side effects include hypertension, hypotension, injection site reaction, pharyngitis, cough, rhinitis, and upper respiratory tract infection.

abate /əbāt″/ [ME, *abaten,* to beat down], to decrease, become less intense, or reduce in severity or degree.

abatement /əbāt″mənt/, a decrease or lessening in severity of symptoms. –**abate,** *v.*

abatic, pertaining to an inability to walk. See **abasia.**

abaxial /abak″sē·əl/ [L, *ab, axis,* from axle], pertaining to a position outside the axis of a body or structure. In anatomical position, farther away from the midsagittal plane, or midline of the body.

Abbe-Estlander flap /ab″ē·est″landər/ [Robert Abbe, American surgeon, 1851–1928; Jakob A. Estlander, Finnish surgeon, 1831–1881], a surgical procedure that transfers a full-thickness section of one lip of the oral cavity to the other lip, using an arterial pedicle for ensuring survival of a graft.

Abbokinase, a plasminogen activator. Brand name for **urokinase.**

Abbott-Miller tube. See **Miller-Abbott tube.**

ABC, abbreviation for **aspiration biopsy cytology.**

abciximab /ab-sik″si-mab/, a human-murine monoclonal antibody Fab fragment that inhibits the aggregation of platelets; used in the prevention of thrombosis in percutaneous transluminal coronary angioplasty and administered by intravenous infusion.

■ INDICATIONS: It is prescribed as an adjunct to percutaneous transluminal coronary angioplasty or atherectomy.

■ CONTRAINDICATIONS: The drug should not be given to patients with active internal bleeding, recent GI or urinary bleeding of significance, history of stroke, thrombocytopenia, or recent major surgery.

■ ADVERSE EFFECTS: The side effects most often reported include bleeding, thrombocytopenia, pulmonary edema, atrioventricular block, and atrial fibrillation.

Abdellah, Faye Glenn [1919–2017], a nursing theorist who introduced a typology of 21 nursing problems in 1960 in Patient-Centered Approaches to Nursing. The concepts of nursing, nursing problems, and the problem-solving process are central to Abdellah's work. The typology is divided into three areas: (1) the physical, sociological, and emotional needs of the patient; (2) the types of interpersonal relationships between the nurse and the patient; and (3) the common elements of patient care. It was formulated in terms of nursing-centered services that can be used to determine the patient's needs and to teach and evaluate nursing students. It was based on systematic research studies. The typology provided a scientific body of knowledge unique to nursing, making it possible to move away from a disease-oriented model of educating nurses.

abdomen /ab″dəmən, abdō″mən/ [L, *abdominis,* belly], the portion of the body between the thorax and the pelvis. The abdominal cavity is lined by the peritoneum; contains the inferior portion of the esophagus, the stomach, the intestines, the liver, the spleen, the pancreas, and other organs; and is bounded by the diaphragm and the pelvic cavity. See also **abdominal regions.** –*abdominal, adj.*

abdominal actinomycosis /abdom″inəl/, a chronic bacterial disease caused by *Actinomyces,* gram-positive bacilli, and characterized by abdominal masses or abscesses. See **actinomycosis.**

abdominal adhesion /abdom″inəl/, the binding together of tissue surfaces of abdominal organs, usually involving the intestines and causing obstruction. The condition may be a response to surgery or result from trauma or chronic inflammation. The patient experiences abdominal distension, pain, nausea, vomiting, and increased pulse rate. Surgery may be required.

abdominal aorta, the portion of the descending aorta that passes through the diaphragm into the abdomen, descending anterior to the vertebral column and ending at the fourth lumbar vertebra, where it divides into the two common iliac arteries. It supplies blood to abdominal structures, such as the testes, ovaries, kidneys, and stomach. Its branches are the celiac, superior mesenteric, inferior mesenteric, middle suprarenal, renal, testicular, ovarian, inferior phrenic, lumbar, middle sacral, and common iliac arteries. Compare **thoracic aorta.** See also **descending aorta.**

abdominal aortic aneurysm (AAA), abnormal dilation of the abdominal aorta, usually in an area of severe atherosclerosis.

■ OBSERVATIONS: Occasionally the patient may experience abdominal, scrotal or back pain; however the majority of patients are asymtomatic until a rupture of the aneurysm occurs.

■ INTERVENTIONS: Ultrasound screening is recommended for men between the ages of 65 and 75 who have a history of smoking. Smoking cessation is imperative when an aneurysm is identified. Onetime ultrasonography screening for AAA in men age 55 years or older with a family history of AAA is also recommended.

■ PATIENT CARE CONSIDERATIONS: There is a very high mortality rate associated with a rupture of an AAA. Monitoring is important to ascertain the growth of the aneurysms before rupture.

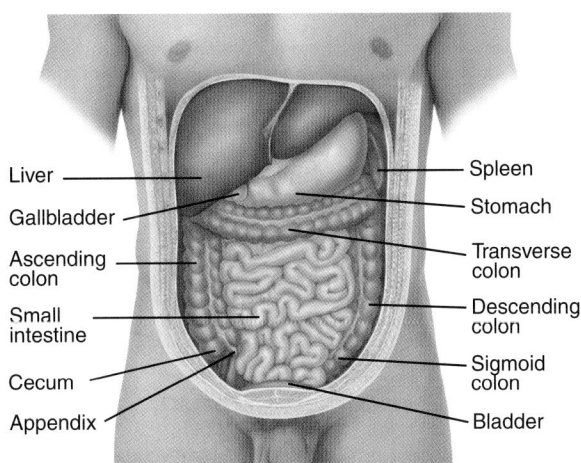

Abdominal cavity (Ball et al, 2015)

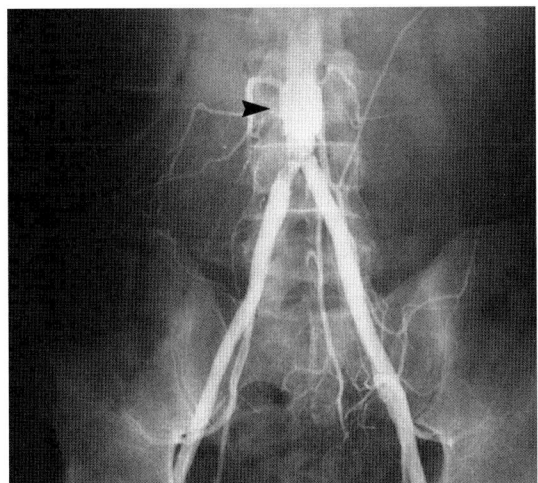

Abdominal aortic aneurysm (arrowhead) (Courtesy Riverside Methodist Hospital)

abdominal aortography, a radiographic study of the abdominal aorta after the introduction of a radiopaque contrast medium through a catheter. The catheter is usually inserted in the aorta through the femoral artery.

abdominal aponeurosis, the conjoined sheetlike tendons of the oblique and transverse muscles of the abdomen.

abdominal arteries, the arteries that branch from the anterior surface of the abdominal aorta to supply the gastrointestinal tract, as well as the liver, pancreas, and gallbladder. The celiac artery supplies the foregut, the superior mesenteric artery supplies the midgut, and the inferior mesenteric artery supplies the hindgut.

abdominal binder, a bandage or elasticized wrap that is applied around the lower part of the torso to support the abdominal musculature or to hold dressings in place.

abdominal breathing, a pattern of inspiration and expiration in which most of the ventilatory work is done with the abdominal muscles. The contractile force of the abdomen is used to elevate the diaphragm. Compare **diaphragmatic breathing.**

abdominal cavity, the space within the abdominal walls lying anterior to the vertebrae, between the diaphragm and the pelvic area, containing the liver, stomach, small intestine, colon, spleen, gallbladder, kidneys, associated tissues, and blood and lymphatic vessels surrounded by the abdominal fascia.

abdominal compartment syndrome, a rare, potentially lethal condition characterized by increased intraabdominal pressure and hypoperfusion of the intestines and other peritoneal and retroperitoneal structures. It is most commonly caused by blunt trauma.

abdominal decompression, 1. paracentesis or laparotomy to relieve the intraabdominal pressure associated with abdominal compartment syndrome. **2.** an obsolete obstetric technique in which the abdomen was enclosed in a chamber that permitted surrounding pressure to be controlled during the first stage of labor.

abdominal examination, the physical assessment of a patient's abdomen by visual inspection, auscultation, percussion, and palpation. Visual inspection of the normally oval shape of the abdominal surface while the patient is supine may reveal abnormal surface features indicating the effects of disease, surgery, or injury. Subsurface tumors, fluid accumulation, or hypertrophy of the liver or spleen may be observed as an abnormal surface feature. Auscultation may reveal vascular sounds that provide information about arterial disorders such as aortic aneurysms and bowel sounds that indicate intestinal function. In pregnancy, auscultation can detect fetal heartbeat and blood circulation in the placenta. Percussion helps detect the condition of internal organs. Palpation is used to detect areas of tenderness or rigidity, muscle tone and skin condition, and shapes and sizes of subsurface organs or masses.

abdominal fascia, an inclusive term for the fascia that forms part of the general layer lining the walls of the abdominal cavity and surrounding the abdominal organs; it is subdivided into visceral abdominal fascia, parietal abdominal fascia, and extraperitoneal fascia.

abdominal fistula, an abnormal passage or tract, usually from the gastrointestinal tract to the external surface of the abdomen.

abdominal gestation, (Obsolete) the implantation of a fertilized ovum outside the uterus but within the peritoneal cavity. Now called **abdominal pregnancy.** See also **ectopic pregnancy.**

abdominal girth, the circumference of the abdomen, usually measured at the umbilicus. Primarily used to evaluate and monitor fluid accumulation in the abdominal cavity, obesity, or accumulation of gas associated with bowel obstruction.

abdominal hernia,   a protrusion of bowel through a defect in or weakened portion of the abdominal musculature, often through the site of an old surgical scar or abdominal trauma. Also called **ventral hernia.** See also **hernia.**

abdominal hysterectomy,   a surgical procedure in which the uterus is removed through an incision in the abdominal wall. Formerly called **abdominohysterectomy.**

abdominal inguinal ring,   an opening of the inguinal canal on the abdominal wall through which the male spermatic cord or the female round ligament pass. The deep abdominal inguinal ring is marked by an oval depression on the deep aspect of the anterior abdominal wall, just above the inguinal ligament. The superficial abdominal inguinal ring is an oval opening in the aponeurosis of the external abdominal oblique muscle.

abdominal muscles,   the muscles between the thorax and the pelvis supporting the abdominal wall. The lateral parts of the wall are formed by the transverse abdominis, the internal oblique, and the external oblique. Anteriorly, on each side, a segmented muscle, the rectus abdominis, spans the distance between the inferior thoracic wall and the pelvis. Other muscles supporting the posterior aspect of the wall are the quadratus lumborum, the psoas major, and the iliacus.

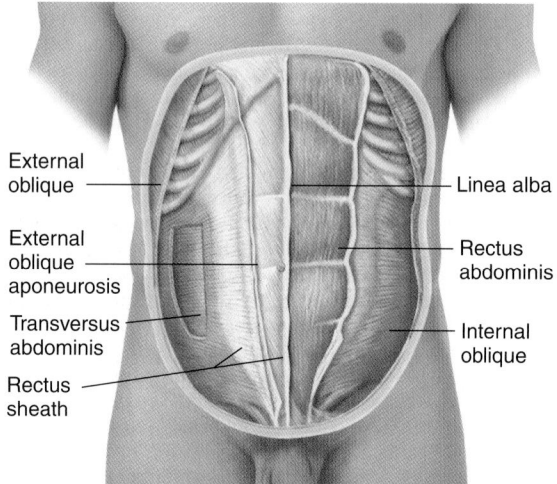

External oblique

External oblique aponeurosis

Transversus abdominis

Rectus sheath

Linea alba

Rectus abdominis

Internal oblique

Abdominal muscles *(Ball et al, 2015)*

abdominal nephrectomy [L, *abdominis,* belly; Gk, *nephr,* kidney, *ektomē,* cutting out],   the surgical removal of a kidney or kidneys through an abdominal incision.

abdominal nerves,   the network of nerve fibers passing through the posterior abdominal region anterolateral to the lumbar vertebral bodies, including the sympathetic trunks and associated splanchnic nerves, the abdominal prevertebral plexus and ganglia, and the lumbar plexus.

abdominal pain,   acute or chronic, localized or diffuse pain in the abdominal cavity. Abdominal pain is a significant symptom because its cause may require immediate surgical or medical intervention. The most common causes of severe abdominal pain are inflammation, perforation of an intraabdominal structure, circulatory obstruction, intestinal or ureteral obstruction, intestinal cramping, or rupture of an organ located within the abdomen. Specific conditions include appendicitis, perforated peptic ulcer, strangulated hernia, superior mesenteric arterial thrombosis, diverticulitis, and small and large bowel obstruction. Differential diagnosis of the cause of acute abdominal pain requires its localization and characterization by means of light and deep palpation; auscultation; percussion; and abdominal, rectal, or pelvic examination. Direct physical examination may be supplemented by various laboratory and radiological examinations. Aspiration of peritoneal fluid (paracentesis) for bacteriological and chemical evaluation is sometimes indicated. Conditions producing acute abdominal pain that may require surgery include appendicitis, acute or severe and chronic diverticulitis, acute and chronic cholecystitis, cholelithiasis, acute pancreatitis, perforation of a peptic ulcer, intestinal obstructions, abdominal aortic aneurysms, and trauma affecting any of the abdominal organs. Gynecological causes that may require surgery include pelvic inflammatory disease, ruptured ovarian cyst, and ectopic pregnancy. Abdominal pain associated with pregnancy may be caused by the weight of the enlarged uterus; rotation, stretching, or compression of the round ligament; or squeezing or displacement of the bowel. In addition, uterine contractions associated with preterm labor may produce severe abdominal pain. Chronic abdominal pain may be functional or may result from overeating or aerophagy. When symptoms are recurrent, an organic cause is considered. Organic sources include peptic ulcer, hiatal hernia, gastritis, chronic cholecystitis and cholelithiasis, chronic pancreatitis, pancreatic carcinoma, chronic diverticulitis, intermittent low-grade intestinal obstruction, and functional indigestion. Some systemic conditions may cause abdominal pain. Examples include systemic lupus erythematosus, lead poisoning, hypercalcemia, sickle cell anemia, diabetic acidosis, porphyria, tabes dorsalis, and black widow spider poisoning.

abdominal paracentesis [L, *abdominis,* belly; Gk, *para,* near, *kentesis,* puncturing],   a surgical procedure in which there is an external puncture of the abdominal cavity for the removal of fluid for diagnosis or treatment.

abdominal pregnancy,   extrauterine pregnancy implanted outside the uterus exclusive of implantation on or in the fallopian tube or ovary. Uncommon, with diagnosis by exclusion and confirmation by ultrasound or MRI. Depending on gestational age and location of implantation, therapy ranges from medical (methotrexate) to surgical, the latter often difficult, depending on the implantation site and the degree of vascularity in the implantation. Often the gestation is removed at surgery, but the placenta is left in situ to be treated by methotrexate. It is one of the rare causes of maternal death, almost always due to delayed diagnosis and hemorrhage. Formerly called **abdominocyesis.**

abdominal pressure,   a sensation or application of force surrounding structures within the abdomen.

abdominal prevertebral plexus,   the network of nerve fibers surrounding the abdominal aorta. It extends from the aortic hiatus of the diaphragm to the bifurcation of the aorta into the right and left common iliac arteries. Along its route, it is subdivided into the celiac plexus, the abdominal aortic plexus, and the superior hypogastric plexus.

abdominal pulse,   the rhythmic transmission of blood turbulence in the abdominal aorta.

abdominal quadrant,   any of four topographic areas of the abdomen divided by two imaginary lines, one vertical and one horizontal, intersecting at the umbilicus. The divisions are the left upper quadrant (LUQ), the left lower quadrant (LLQ), the right upper quadrant (RUQ), and the right lower quadrant (RLQ). Quadrants are most commonly utilized in clinical examination and practice. Compare **abdominal regions.**

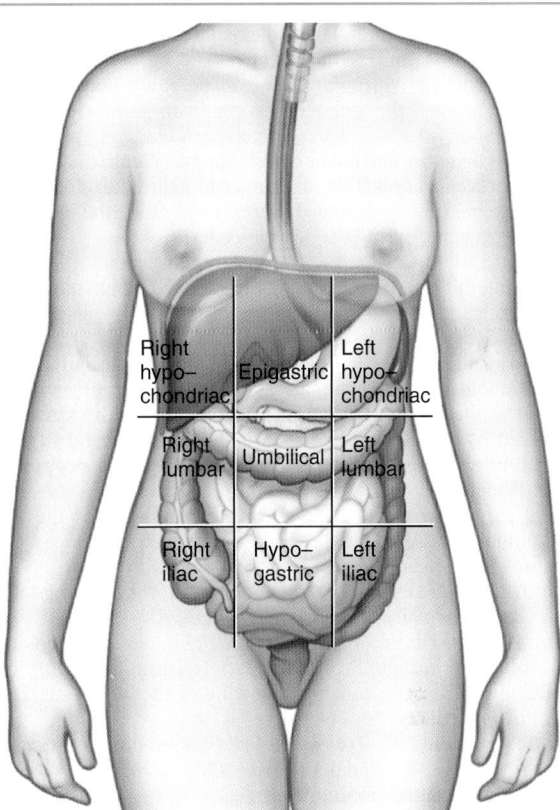

Abdominal regions (Herlihy, 2014)

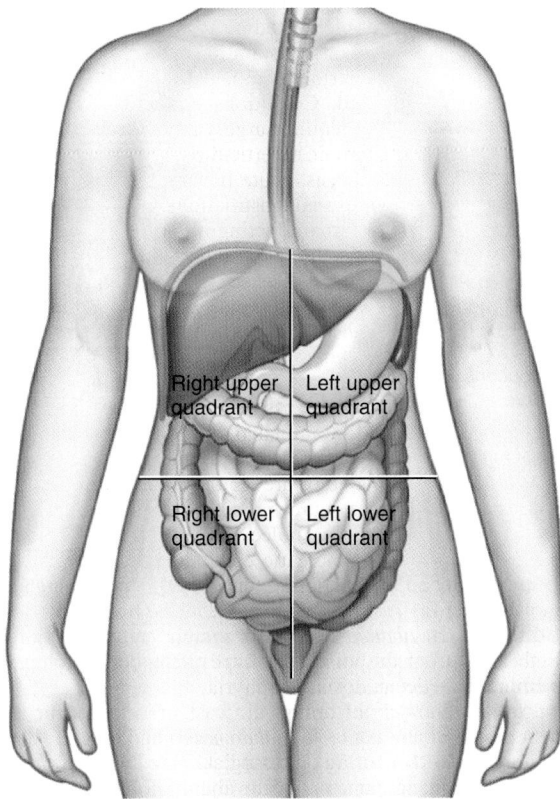

Abdominal quadrants (Herlihy, 2014)

abdominal reflex, a superficial neurological reflex obtained by firmly stroking the skin of the abdomen around the umbilicus. It normally results in a brisk contraction of abdominal muscles in which the umbilicus moves toward the site of the stimulus. This reflex is often lost in diseases of the pyramidal tract and can also be lost with age or abdominal surgery. See also **superficial reflex.**

abdominal regions, the nine topographic subdivisions of the abdomen, determined by four imaginary lines imposed over the anterior surface in a tic-tac-toe pattern. The upper horizontal line passes along the level of the cartilages of the ninth rib, the lower along the iliac crests. The two vertical lines extend on each side of the body from the cartilage of the eighth rib to the center of the inguinal ligament. The lines divide the abdomen into three upper, three middle, and three lower zones: right hypochondriac, epigastric, and left hypochondriac regions (upper zones); right lateral (lumbar), umbilical, and left lateral (lumbar) regions (middle zones); right inguinal (iliac), pubic (hypogastric), and left inguinal (iliac) regions (lower zones). Compare **abdominal quadrant.**

abdominal salpingectomy, removal of the fallopian tube or tubes through a surgical incision in the abdomen. Also called *celiosalpingectomy, laparosalpingectomy.*

abdominal splinting, a tensing or tightening of the abdominal wall muscles, usually occurring as an involuntary reaction to the pain of a visceral disease or disorder or to postoperative discomfort. Abdominal splinting, in turn, may result in hypoventilation and respiratory complications.

abdominal sponge, a special type of gauze pad used as an absorbent and sterile covering for the viscera. See also **sponge.**

abdominal surgery, any one of a number of procedures that involve the surgical management of the abdomen or abdominal organs. An open procedure requires a surgical incision that is closed with staples or sutures. Laparoscopic and robotic procedures require small incisions in which instruments are placed through long, hollow tubes attached to a camera. Laparoscopic incisions are also meticulously closed following the procedure. Kinds include **appendectomy, cholecystectomy, laparotomy.** See also **acute abdomen.**

abdominal tenaculum, a clip or clamp to hold abdominal tissue. See **tenaculum.**

abdominal testis, an undescended testicle in the retroperitoneal or abdominal region.

abdominal thrust, quick, hard movement with both arms encircling the patient's abdomen and using the fists to make a thrusting motion directed inward and upward toward the diaphragm to assist an adult to expel a foreign object in the airway. See **Heimlich maneuver.**

abdominal ultrasound, a diagnostic study that provides visualization of the abdominal aorta, liver, gallbladder, pancreas, biliary ducts, kidneys, ureters, and bladder. This test is used to diagnose and locate cysts, tumors, calculi, or abdominal aortic aneurysms or other malformations; to document the progression of various diseases; or to guide the insertion of instruments during surgical procedures.

abdominal viscera, the internal organs enclosed within the abdominal cavity, including the stomach, liver, intestines, spleen, pancreas, and components of the urinary and reproductive tracts.

abdominal wall, the boundaries of the abdominal cavity that enclose the abdominal cavity and the viscera within. It is multilayered, beginning superficially with skin, followed by subcutaneous tissue and fat, superficial fascia, abdominal musculature and fascia, and most deep, the peritoneum.

abdominal wound, a break in the continuity of the abdominal wall. A wound that exposes or penetrates the viscera raises the danger of infection or peritonitis.

abdomino- /abdom″inō-/, a combining form meaning "abdomen": *abdominoscopy, abdominogenital.*

abdominocardiac reflex /-kär″dē·ək/, an immediate, involuntary response of the heart to stimulation of the abdominal viscera, causing a slowing of the heart rate. The reflex is mediated through the vagus nerve.

abdominocentesis, *(Obsolete)* now called **paracentesis.**

abdominocyesis /abdom′inōsī·ē″sis/, *(Obsolete)* now called **abdominal pregnancy.**

abdominocystic, pertaining to the abdomen and gallbladder. Also called **abdominovesical.**

abdominogenital /-jen″itəl/, pertaining to the abdomen and reproductive system.

abdominohysterectomy, now called **abdominal hysterectomy.**

abdominohysterotomy /-his′tərot″əmē/, *(Obsolete)* now called **hysterotomy.**

abdominopelvic cavity /-pel″vik/, the space between the diaphragm and the pelvis. There is no structurally distinct separation between the abdominal and pelvic regions.

abdominoperineal /-per′inē″əl/, pertaining to the abdomen and the perineum, including the pelvic area, female vulva and anus, and male scrotum and anus.

abdominoplasty, a surgical procedure that removes excess fat and skin and tightens the abdominal muscles to create a smoother abdominal profile. Also called **tummy tuck.**

abdominoscopy /abdom′inos″kəpē/ [L, abdomen; Gk, *skopein,* to view], a procedure for examining the contents of the peritoneum in which an electrically illuminated tubular device is passed through a trocar into the abdominal cavity. Also called **peritoneoscopy.** See also **endoscopy, laparoscopy.**

abdominoscrotal /-skrō″təl/, pertaining to the abdomen and scrotum.

abdominothoracic arch /-thôras″ik/, the boundary between the thorax and the abdomen.

abdominovaginal /-vaj″inəl/, pertaining to the abdomen and vagina.

abdominovesical /-ves″ikəl/, pertaining to the abdomen and bladder. Also called **abdominocystic.**

ABD pad, a gauze pad, ranging in size from 5 × 9 to 12 × 16, with a filler for absorbency of wound drainage.

abducens muscle, the extraocular lateral rectus muscle that moves the eyeball outward. See also **extraocular muscles.**

abducens nerve [L, *abducere,* to take away], either of the paired sixth cranial nerves. It arises in the pons near the fourth ventricle, leaves the brainstem between the medulla oblongata and pons, and passes through the cavernous sinus and the superior orbital fissure. It controls the lateral rectus muscle, turning the eye outward. Also called *abducent,* **nervus abducens, sixth cranial nerve.**

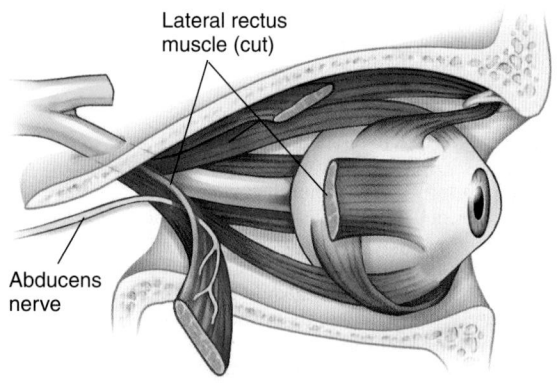

Lateral rectus muscle (cut)

Abducens nerve

Abducens nerve

abducent /abdoo″sənt/ [L, drawing away], pertaining to a movement away from the median line of the body.

abduction [L, *abducere,* to take away], movement of a limb away from the midline or axis of the body. Compare **adduction.** −*abduct, v.*

abduction boots, an orthopedic cast or orthotic for the lower extremities, available in both short- and long-leg configurations, with a bar incorporated at ankle level to provide hip abduction. Abduction boots are used for postoperative positioning and immobilization after certain surgical procedures. They also promote proper positioning during healing after surgical repair of the lower extremities. Compare *abduction pillow.*

abduction pillow, *n.,* a soft foam wedge placed between the thighs and secured with velcro straps; used to position the lower extremities and hold the hip in the correct position following hip replacement surgery.

abductor /abduk″tər/ [L, *abducere*], a muscle that draws a body part away from the midline or axis of the body, or one part from another. Compare **adductor.**

abductor digiti minimi of the foot, a muscle on the lateral side of the foot that abducts the little toe at the metatarsophalangeal joint. It is innervated by the lateral plantar branch of the tibial nerve.

abductor digiti minimi of the hand, a muscle that is the principal abductor of the little finger.

abductor hallucis, a muscle that forms the medial margin of the foot and contributes to a soft tissue bulge on the medial side of the sole. It abducts and flexes the great toe at the metatarsophalangeal joint and is innervated by the medial plantar branch of the tibial nerve.

abductor pollicis brevis, one of the three thenar muscles. It abducts the thumb, principally at the metacarpophalangeal joints. See **thenar muscles.**

abductor pollicis longus, a muscle that originates from the proximal posterior surfaces of the radius and ulna and from the related interosseous membrane. It forms a tendon that passes into the thumb and inserts on the lateral side of the base of the first metacarpal. Its major function is to abduct the thumb at the joint between the first metacarpal and trapezium bones.

abembryonic /ab′embrē·on″ik/, the area of a blastocyst opposite the early embryo.

aberrancy. See **aberrant ventricular conduction.**

aberrant, moving away from the usual standard, deviating from the natural type. See **aberration.**

aberrant conduction. See **aberrant ventricular conduction.**

aberrant goiter, an enlargement of a supernumerary or ectopic thyroid gland.

aberrant ventricular conduction (AVC), the temporary abnormal intraventricular conduction of a supraventricular impulse. It is usually associated with an increase in the duration of the QRS complex to more than 120 msec. This conduction pattern is fairly common after a very premature atrial beat and during the paroxysmal supraventricular tachycardia that is caused by antidromic circus movement tachycardia, also known as Wolff-Parkinson-White syndrome (using the atrioventricular node retrogradely and an accessory pathway antegradely). Also called **aberrancy, aberrant conduction, ventricular aberration.**

aberration /ab′ərā″shən/ [L, *aberrare*, to wander], **1.** any departure from the usual course or normal condition. **2.** abnormal growth or development. **3.** (in psychology) an illogical and unreasonable thought or belief, often leading to an unsound mental state. **4.** (in genetics) any change in the number or structure of the chromosomes. See also **chromosomal aberration. 5.** (in optics) any imperfect image formation or blurring caused by unequal refraction or focalization of light rays through a lens. **6.** (in botany and zoology) pertaining to an abnormal individual, such as certain atypical members of a species. −**aberrant,** *adj.*

abetalipoproteinemia (ABL) /əbā′təlip′ōprō′tinē″mē·ə/ [Gk, *a* + *beta*, not beta, *lipos*, fat, *proteios*, first rank, *haima*, blood], a group of rare inherited disorders of fat metabolism, characterized by the absence of apoprotein β-100 and manifested by acanthocytosis, low or absent serum beta-lipoprotein levels, and hypocholesterolemia. In severe cases, steatorrhea, ataxia, nystagmus, motor incoordination, and retinitis pigmentosa occur. Also called **Bassen-Kornzweig syndrome.**

abeyance /əbā″əns/ [Fr], a temporary state of inaction or temporary interruption of function.

abfraction, a pathological loss of tooth structure owing to biomechanical pressure and stress, forming V-shaped notches in the cervical area of the tooth. Compare **attrition, abrasion, erosion.**

ABG, abbreviation for **arterial blood gas.**

ABI, abbreviation for **ankle-brachial index.**

abient /ab′ē·ont/ [L, *abire*, to go away], characterized by a tendency to move away from stimuli. Compare **adient.** −**abience,** *n.*

ability /əbil″itē/, the capacity to act in a specific way because of the possession of appropriate sensory, motor, and life skills coupled with the mental and/or physical fitness necessary to become proficient.

AbioCor, an implantable artificial heart device for patients with end-stage heart failure. It is normally powered by an external console or battery packs, but also has an internal battery to power the pump for approximately 20 minutes when the external power supply is disconnected.

abiogenesis /ab′ē·ōjen″əsis/ [Gk, *a* + *bios*, not life, *genein,* to produce], the theory that life can originate from inorganic, inanimate matter. Compare **biogenesis.** −*abiogenetic, adj.*

abiosis /ab′ē·ō″sis/ [Gk, *a* + *bios,* not life], a nonviable condition or a situation incompatible with life. −*abiotic, adj.*

abiotrophy /ab′ē·ot″rəfē/ [Gk, *a* + *bios* + *trophe,* nutrition, growth], progressive degeneration or loss of function that is not due to any apparent injury. Usually applied to degenerative hereditary diseases of late onset. See also **atrophy.** −*abiotrophic, adj.*

ablastemic /ab′lastem″ik/, nongerminal or not germinating.

ablation /ablā″shən/ [L, *ab* + *latus,* carried away], **1.** vaporization or an excision of any part of the body, or removal of a growth or harmful substance. **2.** (in cardiology) a procedure used in the management of rapid or irregular rhythms in which cardiac tissue is destroyed. Kinds include **Cox Maze Procedure.** −*ablate, v.*

ablatio placentae, *(Obsolete)* now called **abruptio placentae.**

ABLB test, abbreviation for **alternate binaural loudness balance (ABLB) test.**

-able, -ible, suffixes meaning "able to" or "capable of": *durable, edible.*

ablepharia /ab′ləfer″ē·ə/, a defect or congenital absence of the eyelids (partial or total).

ABLS, abbreviation for **advanced burn life support.**

ablution /abloo″shən/ [L, *abluere,* wash away], **1.** the act of washing or bathing. −*ablutent, adj.* **2.** the act of cleaning the body.

ABMS, abbreviation for *American Board of Medical Specialties.*

abnerval current /abnur″vəl/ [L, *ab,* from; Gk, *neuron,* nerve], an electrical current that passes from a nerve to and through muscle.

abneural /abnoor″əl/, away from the central nervous system or the neural axis.

abnormal behavior /abnôr″məl/ [L, *ab* + *norma,* away from rule], behavior that deviates from what is commonly accepted by a group or society. See also **behavior disorder.**

abnormality /ab′nôrmal″itē/ [L, *ab* + *norma,* away from rule], a condition that differs from the usual cultural or scientifically accepted standards.

abnormal psychology, the study of emotional/behavioral, mental, or neuropsychological disorders.

abnormal tooth mobility, excessive movement of a tooth within its alveolus (socket) as a result of injury or disease in the supporting peridontium.

ABO blood group, a system for classifying human blood on the basis of antigenic components of red blood cells and their corresponding antibodies. The ABO blood group is identified by the presence or absence of two different antigens, A and B, on the surface of the red blood cell. The four blood types in this grouping, A, B, AB, and O, are determined by and named for these antigens. Each ABO blood group also contains naturally occurring antibodies to the antigens it lacks. Group A has A antigens on the red cells, with anti-B antibodies in the plasma. Group B has B antigens on the red cells and anti-A antibodies in the plasma. Group O has neither A nor B antigens, and both anti-A and anti-B in the plasma. AB has both A and B antigens on the red cells, and no anti-A or anti-B in the plasma. In addition to its significant role in transfusion therapy and transplantation, ABO blood grouping contributes to forensic medicine, to genetics, and to anthropology. See also **blood group, Rh factor, transfusion.**

A

aboiement /ä′bô·ämäN″/, an involuntary making of abnormal, animal-like sounds, such as barking. Aboiement may be a clinical sign of Gilles de la Tourette syndrome.

abort /əbôrt′/ [L, *ab,* away from, *oriri,* to be born], **1.** *(Nontechnical)* to deliver a nonviable fetus; to miscarry. Now called **miscarriage.** See also **spontaneous abortion. 2.** to terminate a pregnancy before the fetus has developed enough to be viable. See also **induced abortion. 3.** to terminate in the early stages or to discontinue before completion, as to arrest the usual course of a disease, to stop growth and development, or to halt a project.

abortifacient /əbôr′tifā″shənt/, **1.** causing abortion. **2.** an agent or medication that causes abortion.

abortion /əbor″shən/ [L, *ab* + *oriri*], the spontaneous or induced termination of pregnancy. Kinds include **habitual abortion, infected abortion, septic abortion, voluntary abortion.** See also **complete abortion, elective abortion, incomplete abortion, induced abortion, medical abortion, missed abortion, spontaneous abortion, therapeutic abortion.**

abortionist, a person performing elective and/or therapeutic terminations of pregnancy by surgical or medical means.

abortion on demand, removal by medical or surgical methods of a normally implanted intrauterine pregnancy at maternal request regardless of reason when no restrictive legal statutes prohibit the request. In general, refers to a normally implanted intrauterine gestation weighing less than 500 g. See also **elective abortion.**

abortion pill, *(Informal)* See **mifepristone.**

abortive infection /əbôr″tiv/, an infection in which some or all viral components have been synthesized but no infective virus is produced. The situation may result from an infection with defective viruses or because the host cell is nonpermissive and prohibits replication of the particular virus. Also called **nonproductive infection.**

abortus /əbôr″təs/, a fetus weighing less than 500 g. See also **abortion, miscarriage,** *products of conception.*

abortus fever, a form of brucellosis caused by *Brucella abortus,* an organism so named because it causes abortion in cows. Humans can become infected through broken skin by direct contact with tissue, blood, urine, vaginal secretions, aborted fetuses, or placentas of infected animals or by ingestion of infected raw dairy products. Symptoms include fever, sweats, arthralgia, and myalgia. Administration of doxycycline and gentamicin is the recommended treatment. Also called **Rio Grande fever.** See also **brucellosis.**

abouchement /ä′bōoshmäN′/ [Fr, a tube connection], the junction of a small blood vessel with a large blood vessel.

aboulia. See **abulia.**

above-elbow (AE) amputation, an amputation of the upper limb between the elbow and the shoulder. Also called **transhumeral amputation.**

above-knee amputation, amputation of the lower leg between the knee and the hip. Also called **transfemoral amputation.**

ABP, abbreviation for **arterial blood pressure.**

ABR, **1.** abbreviation for **auditory brainstem response. 2.** abbreviation for **absolute bed rest.**

abrachia /əbrä″kē·ə/ [Gk, *a* + *brachion,* without arm], the absence of arms. −*abrachial, adj.*

abrachiocephalia, congenital absence of the arms and head. See **acephalobrachia.**

abrasion /əbrā″zhən/ [L, *abradere,* to scrape off], a scraping or rubbing away of a surface, such as skin or teeth, by a substance or surface with a hardness greater than that of the tissue being scraped or rubbed away. Abrasion may be the result of trauma, such as a skinned knee; of therapy, as in dermabrasion for the removal of scar tissue; or of normal function, such as the wearing down of a tooth by improper tooth brushing. Compare **laceration.** See also **friction burn.** −**abrasive,** *adj.,* −*abrade, v.*

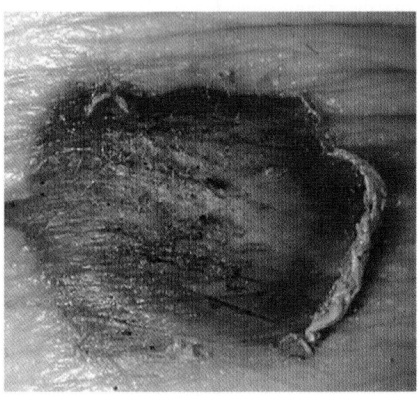

Skin abrasion *(Lynch, 2011)*

abrasion arthroplasty, reshaping of a joint by using a small tool or burr to grind down the surface inducing bleeding and fibrocartilaginous repair tissue to form a new articular surface that serves as a better joint covering.

abrasive, a substance used for grinding or polishing a surface. See **abrasion.**

abreact, the expression of repressed feelings by revisiting the situation in a way that relieves anxiety. See **abreaction.**

abreaction /ab′rē·ak″shən/ [L, *ab,* from, *re,* again, *agere,* to act], an emotional release resulting from mentally reliving or bringing into consciousness, through the process of catharsis, a long-repressed, painful experience. See also **catharsis.** −*abreact, v.*

abruption [L, *ab,* away from, *rumpere,* rupture], a sudden breaking off or tearing apart.

abruptio placentae [L, *ab,* away from, *rumpere,* to rupture], abnormal separation of a normally implanted intrauterine pregnancy. There are three types: complete (entire placenta separates), partial (part of placenta separates), marginal (separation limited to placental edge). This complication occurs in approximately 0.4%–1% of viable pregnancies. Risk factors include hypertension including preeclampsia and eclampsia, multiple gestation, smoking, cocaine use, trauma. Previous abruptio placentae increases the risk by fifteenfold to twentyfold. It is the most common cause of coagulopathy in pregnancy. Fetal survival depends on gestational age, degree of placental separation, and timeliness of delivery if required (vaginal or cesarean section). Also called **ablatio placentae, placenta abruptio, placental abruption.** Compare **placenta previa.** See also **Couvelaire uterus, fetal distress, placenta accreta, postpartum hemorrhage.**

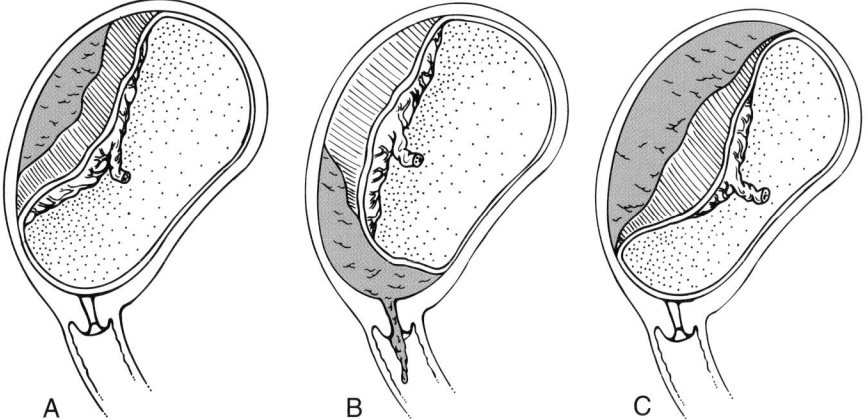

Abruptio placentae. A, Mild abruption with concealed hemorrhage. B, Severe abruption with external hemorrhage. C, Complete separation with concealed hemorrhage. *(McKinney et al, 2013)*

■ OBSERVATIONS: Bleeding from the site of separation causes abdominal pain, uterine tenderness, and tetanic uterine contraction. Bleeding may be concealed within the uterus or may be evident externally, sometimes as sudden massive hemorrhage. In severe cases, shock and death can result in minutes. Partial separation may cause little bleeding and may not interfere with fetal oxygenation.

■ INTERVENTIONS: If the pregnancy is near term, labor may be permitted or induced by amniotomy. A premature pregnancy may be allowed to continue under close observation of the mother on bed rest. In severe cases, cesarean section must be performed immediately and rapidly. Extensive extravasation of blood within the uterine wall may deplete fibrinogen, prolong clotting time, cause intractable bleeding, lead to disseminated intravascular coagulation, and by damaging the uterine musculature, prevent the uterus from contracting well after delivery. Uterine artery ligation or hysterectomy may be necessary to prevent exsanguination.

■ PATIENT CARE CONSIDERATIONS: The health care provider must be alert to the possibility that bleeding is present but concealed internally and that if all the blood can escape, there may be little pain.

abscess /ab″səs/ [L, *abscedere*, to go away], **1.** a cavity containing pus and surrounded by inflamed tissue, formed as a result of suppuration in a localized infection. Healing usually occurs when an abscess drains, is incised, or is permanently removed from the body. If an abscess is deep in tissue, drainage is accomplished by means of a sinus tract that connects it to the surface. Abscesses are able to form in almost any location on or within the body. Abscess formation can cause redness, pain, warmth, and swelling. **2.** an abscess that develops anywhere along the root length of a tooth. An acute abscess is usually characterized by pain caused by the pressure of pus against the nerve tissue within the tooth or within the periodontal tissues, redness caused by blood accumulation, and swelling caused by the suppuration. Chronic periodontal abscesses are frequently asymptomatic, and the patient is unaware of any draining pus. The source of the bacteria that causes the infection is the normal oral flora. See also **periapical abscess, acute abscess, chronic abscess.**

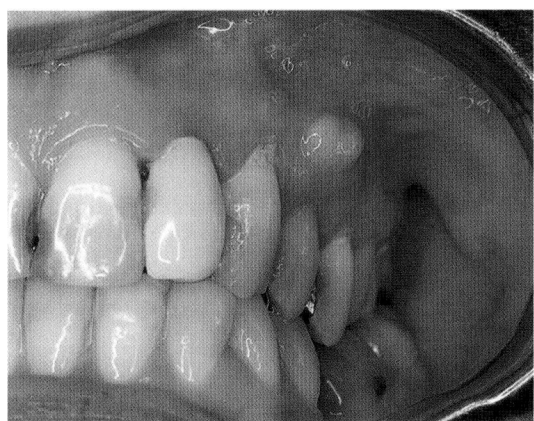

Abscess *(Regezi et al, 2012)*

abscissa /absis″ə/ [L, *ab,* away, *scindere,* to cut], the horizontal coordinate in a graph, along which are plotted the units of one of the variables considered in the study, as time in a time-temperature study. Compare **ordinate.**

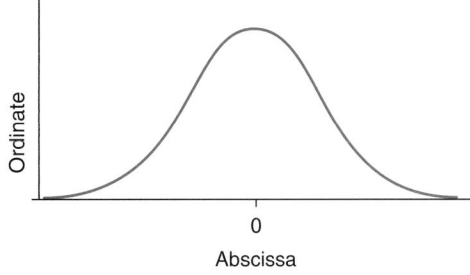

Abscissa *(Miller-Keane and O'Toole, 2005)*

abscission /absish″ən/ [L, *abscinere,* to cut away], the process of cutting away, as in corneal abscission, removal of the prominence of the cornea.

absconsio /abskon″shō/ [L, *ab,* away from, *condo,* hidden], a cavity or fossa.

abscopal /abskō″pəl/, pertaining to a systemic antitumor immune response in which nonirradiated lesions at a distance from the primary site of irradiation regress.

absence seizure, an epileptic seizure characterized by a sudden, momentary loss of consciousness. Occasionally it is accompanied by minor myoclonus of the neck or upper extremities, frequent blinking, slight symmetric twitching of the face, or loss of tonus. Seizures usually occur many times a day without a warning aura and are most frequent in children and adolescents, especially at puberty. Children often outgrow them. The patient experiencing a typical seizure has a vacant facial expression and ceases all voluntary motor activity; with the rapid return of consciousness, the patient may resume conversation at the point of interruption without realizing what occurred. During and between seizures, the patient's electroencephalogram shows 3-Hz spike-and-wave discharges. Anticonvulsant drugs used to prevent absence seizures include ethosuximide and valproic acid. Also called **absentia epileptica, petit mal seizure.** See also **epilepsy.**

absenteeism /ab′səntē″izəm/, (for health or related reasons) absence from work, a location, or a place where one is expected. The most common causes of absenteeism in health care professionals include influenza and musculoskeletal injuries. Causes of absenteeism also include illnesses (communicable and occupational), as well as psychological stress, burnout, family or child care issues, and disengagement.

absentia epileptica. See **absence seizure.**

absent without leave (AWOL) /ā″wôl/ [L, *absentia*], a military term that is also used in the medical field to describe a patient who departs from a psychiatric, day care, or medical facility without authorization.

Absidia /absid″ē·ə/, now called *Lichtheimia* sp.

absolute /ab″səloot/, unconditional, unrestricted, or independent of arbitrary standards.

absolute agraphia [L, *absolutus,* set loose; Gk, *a,* not, *graphein,* to write], a complete inability to write caused by a central nervous system lesion. The person is unable to write even the letters of the alphabet. See also **agraphia.**

absolute alcohol, a clear, colorless, highly hygroscopic liquid with a burning taste, containing at least 99.5% ethyl alcohol by volume. Sometimes called anhydrous alcohol. Also called **dehydrated alcohol.**

absolute (A) temperature, temperature that is measured from a base of absolute zero on the Kelvin scale or the Rankine scale.

absolute bed rest (ABR), restriction of a patient's activities. A person on absolute or strict bed rest must remain in bed at all times. Bed rest may be prescribed to maintain a pregnancy, in cases of severe pain associated with movement, or with orthopedic conditions in which it would be unsafe to be out of bed. It is associated with many hazards of immobility. Numerous research studies have demonstrated that bed rest is a greater stressor to the patient in many conditions than a less restrictive activity prescription would be. Compare **partial bed rest.**

■ PATIENT CARE CONSIDERATIONS: The cardiovascular, pulmonary, gastrointestinal, and musculoskeletal systems all suffer from inactivity and the recumbent position. Cardiac output and capacity, depth of respiration, and peristalsis decrease, while the risk of orthostatic hypotension, thromboembolism, and pulmonary disorders increases. Muscle tone, strength, and endurance decrease. Losses of muscle strength of as much as 10% to 15% have been demonstrated after only 1 week of bed rest. Over extended periods of immobility, collagen components of soft tissues begin to rearrange, resulting in joint capsule tightening and muscle contracture and atrophy. Osteoporotic changes with loss of bone density result from lack of weight bearing and reduction of muscular forces on the bones. Measures to offset the deleterious effects of immobility are indicated for those confined to bed rest, specifically bed mobility and exercise.

■ OUTCOME CRITERIA: Activities and exercises condition not only the musculoskeletal system, but also other body systems stressed by bed rest. Frequent range-of-motion exercises prevent stiffness in muscles and joints and provide sensory and proprioceptive stimulation. Conditioning exercises enhance cardiac, pulmonary, and gastrointestinal function. A coordinated effort by the health care team to provide instruction and assistance with an appropriate program to maintain mental and physical health can do much to promote the well-being of a patient immobilized by bed rest.

absolute discharge [L, *absolutus,* set free], a final and complete termination of the patient's relationship with a caregiving agency, indicating that the individual will no longer receive any level of care and/or assistance.

absolute glaucoma /ab′səloot/ [L, *absolutus* + Gk, *cataract*], complete blindness in which a glaucoma-induced increase in intraocular pressure results in permanent vision loss. The optic disc is white and deeply excavated, and the pupil is usually widely dilated and immobile. Also called *absolutum glaucoma,* **glaucoma consummatum.**

absolute growth, the total percentage increase in size of an organism or a particular organ or part, such as the limbs, head, or trunk.

absolute humidity, the actual mass or content of water in a measured volume of air regardless of temperature. It is usually expressed in grams per cubic meter or pounds per cubic foot or cubic yard.

absolute neutrophil count (ANC), the number of neutrophils in a milliliter of blood. The ANC is a measure of a person's immune status. Generally, if the count is above 1000, the person may safely mingle with other people or undergo chemotherapy, but a count below 500 indicates that a person is at high risk for infection and should be kept away from those with infectious diseases. Neutropenia by definition is an ANC below 1500/mm³. It is calculated by adding the number of segmented neutrophils and the number of basal neutrophils and multiplying the sum by the total white blood cell (WBC) count. The formula is ANC = Total WBC count × (% neutrophils + % bands)/100. Also called *absolute granulocyte count (AGC).*

absolute threshold [L, *absolutus,* set loose, AS, *therscold*], **1.** the lowest point at which a stimulus can be perceived. **2.** pertaining to millivolts of electrical charge determined by ion fluctuations or movement across plasma membranes that result in nerve or muscle stimulation.

absolute zero, the temperature at which all molecular activity except vibration ceases. It is a theoretical value derived by calculations and projections from experiments with the behavior of gases at extremely low temperatures. Absolute zero is estimated to be equal to −273.15° C or −459.67° F.

absorb, **1.** incorporating matter, energy, or liquids through a chemical or physical process. **2.** to receive, take in, or blend together spaces, situations, people's emotions, or circumstances.

absorbable gauze /əbsôr″bəbəl/, a material produced from oxidized cellulose that can be absorbed. It is applied or sutured directly to tissue to stop bleeding. After a clot forms, the gauze turns into a gel. Also called *absorbable cotton.*

absorbable surgical suture [L, *absorbere,* to suck up; Gk, *cheirourgos,* surgery; L, *sutura*], a suture made from material that can be completely incorporated by the body. Originally used for internal tissues, this type of suture is now also used for percutaneous tissue, facilitating healing but eliminating the need for suture removal.

absorbance /əbsôr″bəns/, the degree of absorption of light or other radiant energy by a medium exposed to the energy. It is expressed as the logarithm of the ratio of energy transmitted through a vacuum to the energy transmitted through the medium. For solutions, it is the logarithm of the ratio of energy transmitted through pure solvent to the energy transmitted through the solution. Absorbance varies with factors such as wavelength, solution concentration, and path length.

absorbed dose, the energy imparted by ionizing radiation per unit mass of irradiated material at a location of interest. The SI unit of absorbed dose is the gray (Gy); the non-SI (traditional) unit is referred to as rad, or radiation absorbed dose. 1 Gy equals 1 J/kg, and 1 Gy equals 100 rad.

absorbefacient /absôr″bifā″shənt/ [L, *absorbere,* to suck up + *facere,* to make], **1.** any agent that promotes or enhances the quality and ability to soak liquids more readily. **2.** causing or enhancing absorption.

absorbent /absôr″bənt/ [L, *absorbere,* to suck up], **1.** capable of attracting and incorporating substances into itself. **2.** a product or substance that can absorb liquids or gases.

absorbent dressing, a clean or sterile covering applied to a wound or incision to draw secretions into itself. Kinds of absorbent dressings are Teflon-coated gauze squares, fluffed gauze, and abdominal bandages.

absorbent gauze, a fabric or pad with various forms, weights, and uses, primarily designed to absorb fluid and/or excretions. It may be a rolled, single-layered fine fabric for spiral bandages, or it may be a thick, multilayered pad for a sterile pressure dressing. There may also be an adhesive backing.

absorbent point. See **paper point.**

absorption /absôrp″shən/ [L, *absorptio*], **1.** the incorporation of matter by other matter through chemical, molecular, or physical action, such as the dissolution of a gas in a liquid or the taking up of a liquid by a porous solid. **2.** (in physiology) the passage of nutrients and substances across and into tissues, such as the passage of digested food molecules into intestinal cells or the passage of liquids into kidney tubules. Kinds include **agglutinin absorption, cutaneous absorption, external absorption, intestinal absorption, parenteral absorption, pathological absorption. 3.** (in radiology) the process by which the energy of an electromagnetic photon is taken up by matter. **–absorb,** *v.*

absorption coefficient, the factor by which the intensity of electromagnetic energy decreases as it interacts with a unit thickness of an absorbing material. It is usually expressed per unit thickness.

absorption rate constant, a value describing how much drug is absorbed per unit of time.

absorption spectrum, a plot of percent transmittance, absorbance, logarithm of absorbance, or absorptivity of a compound as a function of wavelength, wave number, or frequency of radiation.

absorptivity /ab′sôrptiv″itē/, absorbance at a particular wavelength divided by the product of the concentration of a substance and the sample path length. Also called **absorption coefficient.**

abstinence /ab″stinəns/, voluntarily avoiding a substance, such as food or alcohol, or refraining from the performance of an act, such as sexual intercourse.

abstinence syndrome [L, *abstinere,* to hold back; Gk, *syn,* together, *dromos,* course]. **1.** See **withdrawal syndrome. 2.** See **neonatal abstinence syndrome.**

abstract /ab″strakt, abstrakt″/ [L, *abstrahere,* to drag away], **1.** a condensed summary of a scientific article, literary piece, or address. **2.** to collect data and extract files, including coding and billing information, from a medical record. **3.** (in pharmacology) the base in which other components are mixed and dissolved. **4.** difficult to understand because of lack of practicality. **5.** the process of gathering theoretical information to develop ideas with reference to the main idea.

abstraction /abstrak″shən/ [L, *abstrahere,* to drag away], (in dentistry) a condition in which teeth or other maxillary and mandibular structures are inferior to their normal position, away from the occlusal plane. Also called **infraclusion,** *infraocclusion.*

abstract thinking, the final, most complex stage in the development of cognitive thinking, in which thought is characterized by adaptability, flexibility, and the use of concepts and generalizations. Problem solving is accomplished by drawing logical conclusions from a set of observations, for example, making hypotheses and testing them. This type of thinking is generally developed by 12 to 15 years of age, usually after some degree of education. In psychiatry, many disorders are characterized by the inability to think abstractly. Compare **concrete thinking, syncretic thinking.**

abulia /əboo̅″lyə/ [Gk, *a + boule,* without will], a loss of the ability or a reduced capacity to exhibit initiative or to make decisions. Also spelled **aboulia.**

abuse /abyoo̅s″/ [L, *abuti,* to waste, *abusus,* using up], **1.** improper use of equipment, a substance, or a service, such as a drug or program, either intentionally or unintentionally. See also **substance abuse. 2.** Using words and/or physical action to hurt, attack, and do harm.

abused person [Fr, *abuser,* to disuse; L, *persona,* a role played], an individual who has been harmed or maltreated emotionally, verbally, sexually, or physically by another person or by a situation; a victim.

abutment /əbut″mənt/ [Fr, *abouter,* to place end to end], a tooth, root, or implant that supports and provides retention for a fixed or removable dental prosthesis. Compare **retainer.**

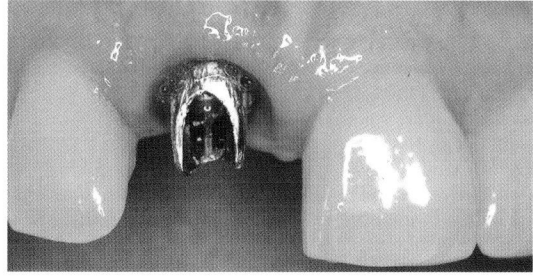

Frontal view of abutment *(Block, 2015)*

abutment tooth, a tooth selected to support a fixed or removable prosthesis. Compare **retainer.**

ABVD, an anticancer drug combination of *A*driamycin (doxorubicin), *b*leomycin, *v*inblastine, and *d*acarbazine.

Ac, 1. symbol for the element **actinium. 2.** abbreviation for **acetyl.**

AC, 1. abbreviation for **alternating current. 2.** abbreviation for *accommodative convergence.* See **AC/A ratio.**

a.c., (in prescriptions) denoting a Latin phrase meaning "before meals." Abbreviation for *ante cibum.*

A-C, abbreviation for *alveolar-capillary.*

acacia gum /ə-'kā-shə gəm/, a dried, gummy exudate of the acacia tree *(Acacia senegal)* used as a binding, suspending, or emulsifying agent in medicines. Also called **gum arabic.**

academic health center, an educational unit that includes a teaching hospital, a medical school, and at least one other school related to a health care profession; such centers deliver patient care services and degree-granting educational programs.

academic ladder /ak'ədem″ik/ [Gk, *akademeia,* school], the hierarchy of faculty appointments in an academic setting (university, college, or community college) through which a faculty member advances from the rank of instructor to assistant professor to associate professor to professor.

Academy of Nutrition and Dietetics, an organization that advances the nutritional well-being of the American public. Membership is primarily registered dietitians. Formerly called *American Dietetic Association (ADA).*

acai /ä·sä·ē/, an antioxidant extract from the berry of the acai palm tree *(Euterpe oleracea);* used in skin products and juices.

acalculia /a′kalkoo″lyə/ [Gk, *a,* not; L, *calculare,* to reckon], the inability to perform simple mathematic calculations the patient previously knew. Commonly seen in neurological disorders, it is assessed by having a patient count forward or backward or do mental addition or subtraction. See also **agraphia, constructional apraxia, dementia, finger agnosia, Gerstmann syndrome.**

acamprosate, an antialcoholic agent.

■ INDICATIONS: This drug is used for maintenance of abstinence from alcohol in alcohol dependence in combination with counseling.

■ CONTRAINDICATIONS: Severe renal disease, creatinine clearance of less than 30 mL/hr, and known hypersensitivity to this drug prohibit its use.

acampsia /əkamp″sē-ə/ [Gk, *a + kampsein,* not to bend], a condition in which a joint is rigid. See also **ankylosis.**

acanth-, acantho-, acantha /əkan″thə/ [Gk, *akantha,* thorn], combining forms meaning "thorny" or "spiny": *acanthesia, acanthocytosis.*

acanthamoebiasis /əkan′thəməbī″əsis/, a potentially fatal meningoencephalitis infection caused by *Acanthamoeba castellani,* a free-living ameboflagellate. It is commonly acquired by swimming in water contaminated by the microorganism. Cleaning contact lenses in contaminated solution can cause keratitis.

Acanthamoeba /əkan′thəmē″bə/, a genus of free-living ameboid protozoa typically found in moist soil and water. The organisms may enter the body through a break in the skin or even through the nasal mucosa, olfactory nerve, and mucous membranes of the eye. It may cause severe infections, such as keratitis (eye infection that can lead to blindness, especially with contact lens wearers), or systemic infections of the lung, genitourinary system, brain, and central nervous system. It is most common in persons with a compromised immune system. Disseminated cutaneous lesions caused by this organism are seen particularly in patients with AIDS. Although an infection may be fatal, cases are more commonly chronic and can persist for months.

acanthesia /ak′anthē″zhə/, pinprick paresthesia; an abnormality of cutaneous sensory perception that causes a simple touch to be felt as a painful pinprick.

acanthiomeatal line /əkan′thē·ō′mē·ā″təl/, a hypothetical line extending from the external acoustic (auditory) meatus to the acanthion (located at the base of the anterior nasal spine). In dentistry, a full maxillary denture is constructed so that its occlusal plane is parallel with this line. The line is used for radiographic positioning of the skull. See **acanthion.**

acanthion, a craniometric point at the center of the base of the anterior nasal spine.

acanthocheilonemiasis. See **mansonellosis.**

acanthocyte /əkan″thəsīt′/ [Gk, *akantha + kytos,* cell], an abnormal peripheral blood film erythrocyte with irregular spurlike projections. Predominant in abetalipoproteinemia; fewer occur in liver disease Compare **burr cell, elliptocyte.** See also **abetalipoproteinemia, acanthocytosis.**

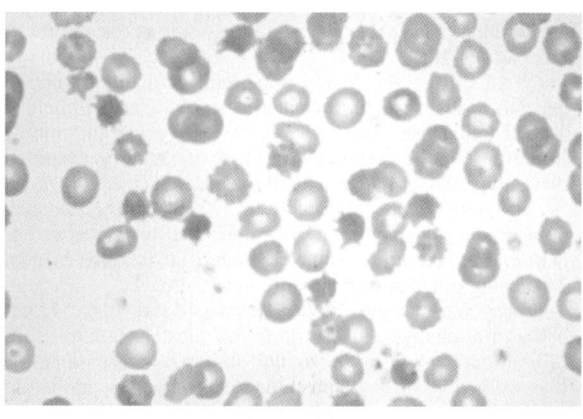

Acanthocyte *(Jaffe et al, 2011)*

acanthocytosis /akan′thōsītō″sis/ [Gk, *akantha + kytos + osis,* condition], the presence of acanthocytes on a peripheral blood film, most commonly associated with abetalipoproteinemia, in which as many as 80% of the erythrocytes are acanthocytes. Compare **crenated erythrocytes, elliptocytosis.** See also **abetalipoproteinemia.**

acanthoid, resembling a spinous process. See also **spinous process.**

acanthoma /ak′anthō″mə/ [Gk, *akantha + oma,* tumor], a localized skin hypertrophy that arises from the stratum spinosum. It may be benign or malignant.

acanthoma adenoides cysticum. See **trichoepithelioma.**

acanthoma fissuratum, a benign, firm, skin-colored, or erythematous nodule, grossly resembling basal cell carcinoma, occurring on the bridge of the nose or behind the ear, resulting from constant minor mechanical trauma. A common cause is poorly fitting glasses. Also called **granuloma fissuratum.**

acanthoma verrucosa seborrheica. See **seborrheic keratosis.**

acanthorrhexis /əkan′thôrek″sis/, the rupture of intercellular bridges of the stratum spinosum, as in eczema or allergic contact dermatitis.

acanthosis /ak′anthō″sis/ [Gk, *akantha + osis,* condition], an abnormal, diffuse hypertrophy of the stratum spinosum, as in eczema and psoriasis. See also **acanthosis nigricans.** *−acanthotic, adj.*

acanthosis nigricans /nē″grikanz′/, a skin disease characterized by dark, velvety thickening of the skin, common in the neck, axilla, and groin, and frequently associated with obesity and endocrine disorders. There are benign and malignant forms; the latter is most often associated with cancers of the GI tract. See also **acanthosis.**

A

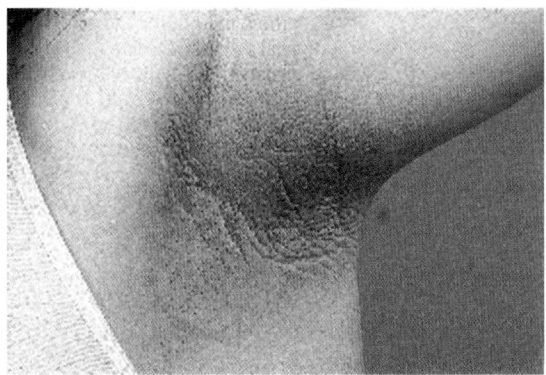

Acanthosis nigricans *(Glynn and Drake, 2012)*

acapnia /akap″nē·ə/, deficiency of carbon dioxide in the blood.

AC/A ratio, (in ophthalmology) the proportion between accommodative convergence (AC) and accommodation (A), or the amount of convergence automatically resulting from the dioptric focusing of the eyes at a specified distance. The ratio of accommodative convergence to accommodation is usually expressed as the quotient of accommodative convergence in prism diopters divided by the accommodative response in diopters.

acarbia /akär″bē·ə/ [Gk, *a,* not; L, *carbo,* coal], a decrease in the bicarbonate level in the blood.

acarbose, an oral alpha-glucosidase inhibitor.

■ INDICATIONS: It is prescribed in the treatment of type 2 diabetes mellitus; it slows the digestion of complex carbohydrates and reduces the demand for insulin. The drug is indicated for use with dietary modifications or other medications that treat diabetes in patients whose hyperglycemia is not sufficiently controlled by diet alone.

■ CONTRAINDICATIONS: It should not be used by patients with diabetic ketoacidosis or intestinal diseases that may impair digestion or absorption. Caution is advised for use in patients with renal dysfunction. It is contraindicated in patients with a serum creatinine >2.0 mg/dL

■ ADVERSE EFFECTS: The side effects most often reported include flatulence, diarrhea, and abdominal pain. Increased transaminase levels have been reported in patients taking high doses.

acardia /akär″dē·ə/ [Gk, *a* + *kardia,* without heart], a rare congenital anomaly in which the heart is absent. It is almost exclusively seen in a monozygous twin whose survival depends on the circulatory system of its twin. It is considered the most extreme form of twin-twin transfusion. *–acardiac, adj.*

acardius acephalus, a fetus that lacks a head, heart, and most of the upper part of the body.

acardius acormus, a fetus that lacks a heart and has a defective trunk, a severe complication in monozygotic twinning.

acardius amorphus, a nonviable fetus with no heart and a rudimentary body that does not resemble the normal form. Also called *acardius anceps.*

acariasis /ak′ərī″əsis/ [Gk, *akari,* mite, *osis,* condition], a disease, usually of the skin, caused by infestation with a wide variety of parasitic mites or worms. The gastrointestinal, genitourinary, and pulmonary systems may also be affected. Compare **scabies.** See also **acarid.**

acarid /ak″ərid/, one of the many mites and ticks that are members of the order Acarina, which includes a great number of parasitic and free-living organisms. Adults have four pairs of legs and round bodies, living as ectoparasites. Most are not yet described, but several types are of medical interest because they infect humans. Those associated with disease act as intermediate hosts of pathogenic agents, directly cause skin or tissue damage, and cause loss of blood or tissue fluids. Important as vectors of scrub typhus and other rickettsial diseases are the six-legged larvae of mites from the family Trombiculidae, which are parasites of humans, many other mammals, and birds. See also **chigger, scabies.**

acaro-, a combining form meaning "mites": *acariasis, acarodermatitis.*

acarodermatitis /ak′ərōdur″mətī″tis/ [Gk, *akari,* mite, *derma,* skin, *itis,* inflammation], a skin inflammation caused by mites or ticks.

acarophobia /-fō″bē·ə/, **1.** a morbid dread of tiny parasites or the delusion that tiny insects such as mites have invaded the skin. **2.** a fear of itching, particularly from parasites.

acaudal /ākô″dəl/ [Gk, *a,* without; L, *cauda,* tail], without a tail.

acc, ACC, abbreviation for **accommodation.**

accelerated hypertension, *(Obsolete)* See **malignant hypertension.**

accelerated idiojunctional rhythm, an automatic junctional rhythm with a rate greater than 59 beats/min but less than 100 beats/min.

accelerated idioventricular rhythm (AIVR), an automatic ectopic ventricular rhythm with a rate greater than 49 beats/min but less than 100 beats/min, without retrograde conduction to the atria. In acute myocardial infarction an AIVR can be a sign of spontaneous reperfusion or a result of thrombolytic therapy.

accelerated junctional rhythm, an ectopic junctional heart rhythm with a rate that exceeds the normal firing rate of junctional tissue, with or without retrograde atrial conduction. See also **junctional rhythm.**

accelerated respiration, an abnormally rapid rate of breathing, usually more than 25 breaths/min. See also **tachypnea.**

acceleration /aksel′ərā″shən/ [L, *accelerare,* to quicken], a change in the speed or direction of a moving object. Increasing speed is positive acceleration; decreasing speed is negative acceleration. Compare **deceleration.** *–accelerate, v.*

acceleration-deceleration injury, injury resulting from a collision between a body part and another object or body part while both are in motion; for example, a coup-contrecoup injury to the brain.

acceleration phase, **1.** *(Obsolete)* the first period of active labor. Now called **active phase of labor. 2.** (in bacteriology) a period of increased growth occuring prior to the lag phase in a culture of microbes.

accelerator /aksel″ərā″tər/ [L, *accelerare,* to quicken], **1.** a nerve or muscle that increases the rate of performance of some function. **2.** a slender nerve fiber passing through the sympathetic ganglion to the heart, causing an increase in heart rate. **3.** an agent or apparatus used to increase the rate at which a substance acts or a function proceeds.

accentuation /aksen′choo·ā″shən/ [L, *accentus,* accent], an increase in distinctness or loudness, as in heart sounds.

acceptable daily intake (ADI), the maximum amount of any substance in food or water that can be safely ingested by a human. Ingestion that exceeds this amount may cause toxic effects. This term is usually applied to additives, residues, or chemicals not normally found in foods.

acceptance of individuality, (in psychiatry) an index of family health in which differentiation or individuation is a valued goal.

acceptance of separation, an indicator of mental well-being in which a loss is dealt with in a healthy manner, indicating productive adaptability.

acceptor /aksep″tər/ [L, *accipere,* to receive], **1.** a compatible organism that receives living tissue, such as transfused blood or a transplanted organ, from another organism. Compare **donor. 2.** a substance or compound that combines with, or accepts, a part of another substance or compound, such as an atom, an ion, an electron, or an electron pair.

access /ak″ses/, a means of approach, such as the space needed for the manipulation of dental or surgical instruments. An example is vascular access in hemodialysis.

accessibility /ak″ses ǎ bil ity/, "the ability to access and benefit from products, devices, services, or environments that have been designed to be usable by people with disabilities."

access cavity [L, *accedere,* to approach], a coronal opening made to the center (pulp chamber) of a tooth, required for effective cleaning, shaping, and obturation of the pulp canals and pulp chamber during endodontic or root canal therapy.

accessory /akses″ərē/ [L, *accessonis,* appendage], **1.** a supplementary item, desirable but not necessary, used chiefly for convenience or for safety, such as the electric elevator mechanisms for hospital beds. **2.** a structure that contributes to the function of one of the main anatomical systems, such as the accessory sex organs in men and women or the accessory organs of the skin, including the hair, the nails, and the skin glands.

accessory chromosome. See **monosome.**

accessory diaphragm, a rare congenital anomaly in which a second diaphragm or portion of a diaphragm develops in the chest. It is usually found on the right side and is oriented upward and backward to the posterior chest wall. It may be separated from the true diaphragm by a lobe of a lung. It is often associated with cardiac anomalies.

accessory gland, glandular tissue that contributes in a secondary way to the function of a similar gland, which may be nearby or some distance away.

accessory ligament [L, *accessus,* extra, *ligare,* to bind], a ligament that helps strengthen a union between two bones, even though it is not part of a joint capsule.

accessory movement, movement that occurs between adjacent joint surfaces that is necessary for a full range of motion but is not under direct voluntary control. Examples include rolling of the humeral head in the glenoid fossa during shoulder flexion, and sliding of the distal carpus on the proximal carpus during wrist ulnar deviation.

accessory muscle, a relatively rare anatomical duplication of a muscle that may appear anywhere in the muscular system. The most common sign associated with an accessory muscle is the appearance of a soft tissue mass. Differential diagnosis without an exploratory operation is difficult because of the similar appearance of some tumors or soft tissue masses, such as ganglia. The appearance of the soft tissue mass associated with an accessory muscle may be transient, or it may be constant, depending on the location of the accessory muscle in relation to motion. In many individuals with accessory muscles, specific treatment is not indicated unless the accessory muscle interferes with normal function.

accessory muscle of respiration, any of the muscles of the neck, back, and abdomen that may assist the diaphragm and the internal and external intercostal muscles in respiration, especially in some breathing disorders or during exercise. Often elevated effort of breathing contributes to increased anterior-posterior diameter of the chest (barrel chest) over time.

accessory nasal sinuses [L, *accessus,* extra, *nasus,* nose, *sinus,* hollow], the paranasal sinuses that occur as hollows within the skull but open into the nasal cavity and are lined with a mucous membrane continuous with the nasal mucous membrane. See also **paranasal sinus.**

accessory nerve, either of a pair of cranial nerves essential for speech, swallowing, and certain movements of the head and shoulders. Each nerve has a cranial and a spinal portion, communicates with certain cervical nerves, and connects to the nucleus ambiguus of the brain. Also called **eleventh cranial nerve, nervus accessorius, spinal accessory nerve.**

Internal carotid artery Internal jugular vein

Accessory nerve [XI]

Sternocleidomastoid muscle Trapezius muscle

Accessory nerve *(Cronenwett and Johnston, 2014)*

accessory organ, an organ or other distinct collection of tissues that contributes to the function of another similar organ, such as the ocular muscles and eyelids, which contribute to the function of the eye.

accessory organs of the eye, the accessory organs of the eye: the eyelids, eyelashes, eyebrows, conjunctival sac, lacrimal apparatus, and extrinsic muscles of the eye. Also called **adnexa oculi.**

accessory pancreas [L, *accessus,* extra; Gk, *pan,* all, *kreas,* flesh], small clusters of pancreatic cells detached from the pancreas and sometimes found in the wall of the stomach or intestines.

accessory pancreatic duct, the small duct that branches from the pancreatic duct and opens into the duodenum near the mouth of the common bile duct. Compare **pancreatic duct.**

accessory pathway, an abnormal conduction pathway between an atrium and a ventricle. Ventricular activation via an accessory pathway slows initial ventricular contraction, producing preexcitation and the delta wave of Wolff-Parkinson-White syndrome. The delta wave shortens the P-R interval, and broadens the QRS complex. The most common associated arrhythmias are paroxysmal supraventricular tachycardia and atrial fibrillation. Patients may be cured by transvenous radiofrequency ablation of the accessory pathway or may be treated pharmacologically.

accessory phrenic nerve, the nerve that joins the phrenic nerve at the root of the neck or in the thorax, forming a loop around the subclavian vein. It may arise from the nerve to the subclavius muscle or from the trigeminal nerve. Compare **phrenic nerve.**

accessory placenta [L, *accessionis,* a thing added, *placenta,* flat cake], a small secondary placental unit attached only by placental vessels. Also called **succenturiate placenta.**

accessory root canal, an anatomical lateral branching of the pulp canal in a tooth, usually occurring in the apical third of the root.

accessory sign, an unusual sign that is not typical or characteristic of a particular disease.

accessory spleen [L, *accessus,* extra; Gk, *splen*], small nodules of splenic tissue that may occur in the gastrosplenic ligament, greater omentum, or other visceral sites.

accessory thymus [L, *accessus,* extra; Gk, *thymos,* thymelike], a nodule of thymic tissue that is isolated from the gland.

accessory tooth, a supernumerary, or extra, tooth. Also called **hyperdontia.**

access time, the amount of time required for a computer to retrieve data from its disk drive.

accident /ak″sidənt/ [L, *accidere,* to happen], any unexpected or unplanned event that may result in death, injury, property damage, or a combination of serious effects. The victim may or may not be directly involved in the cause of the accident. Accidents frequently are the result of both physical and mental factors that can result in unsafe operating systems at work, home, or other sites.

accident-prone, describing a person who experiences accidents and accompanying injuries at a much greater than average rate.

acclimate /əklī″mit, ak″limāt/ [L, *ad,* toward; Gk, *klima,* region], to adjust physiologically to a different climate or environment or to changes in altitude or temperature. Also called *acclimatize.* −*acclimatization, acclimation, n.*

accommodation (A, acc, ACC) /əkom′ədā″shən/ [L, *accommodatio,* adjustment], **1.** the state or process of adapting or adjusting one thing or set of things to another. See **reasonable accommodation. 2.** the continuous process or effort of the individual to adapt or adjust to surroundings to maintain a state of homeostasis, both physiologically and psychologically. **3.** adjustment, especially adjustment of the eye for seeing objects at various distances. This is accomplished by the ciliary muscle, which controls the lens of the eye, allowing it to flatten or thicken as is needed for distant or near vision.. See also **accommodation reflex. 4.** (in sociology) the reciprocal reconciliation of conflicts between individuals or groups concerning habits and customs, usually through a process of compromise, arbitration, or negotiation. Also called **adjustment.** Compare **adaptation.**

accommodation reflex, an adjustment of the eyes for near vision, consisting of pupillary constriction, convergence of the eyes, and increased convexity of the lens. Also called **ciliary reflex.** See also **light reflex.**

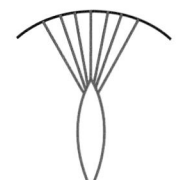 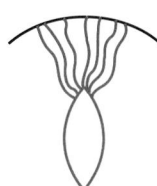

Ligaments tight—lens flattened   Ligaments relaxed—lens more rounded

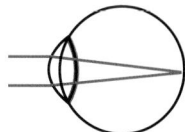 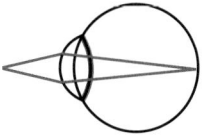

Rays from a *distant* object are focused on the retina by a flattened lens   Rays from a *nearby* object are focused on the retina by a more rounded lens

Accommodation reflex *(Marsh, 2003)*

accommodative strabismus /əkom″ədā′tiv/ [L, *accommodatio,* adjustment; Gk, *strabismos,* squint], **1.** strabismus resulting from abnormal demand on accommodation, such as esotropia resulting from uncorrected hyperopia or exotropia resulting from uncorrected myopia. **2.** strabismus resulting from the act of accommodation in association with a high AC/A ratio.

accountability /əkoun′təbil″itē/, responsibility for the moral and legal requirements of proper patient care.

accreditation /əkred′itā″shən/, a process whereby a professional association or nongovernmental agency grants recognition to a school or health care institution for demonstrated ability to meet predetermined criteria for established standards, such as the accreditation of hospitals by The Joint Commission in the United States or Accreditation Canada in Canada. Compare **certification.**

Accreditation Council for Occupational Therapy Education (ACOTE), the national body that accredits educational programs for occupational therapy and occupational therapy assistant programs.

Accreditation Review Council on Education in Surgical Technology and Surgical Assisting (ARC-STSA), a monitoring organization created in 1972 to establish, maintain, and promote standards of quality for the training, curriculum, and content of instruction in surgical technology and surgical assisting recognized through programmatic accreditation in cooperation with the Commission on Accreditation of Allied Health Education Programs (CAAHEP), the American College of Surgeons (ACS), and the Association of Surgical Technologists (AST).

accrementition /ak′rəmentish″ən/, a growth or an increase in size by the addition of similar tissue or material, as in cell division, binary fission, budding, or gemmation.

accretio cordis /əkrē″shē·ō/ [L, *accrescere,* to increase, *cordis,* heart], an abnormal condition in which the pericardium adheres to the plurae, diaphragm, or chest wall.

accretion /əkrē″shən/ [L, *accrescere,* to increase], **1.** growth by the addition of material similar to that already present. **2.** the adherence or growing together of parts that are normally separated. **3.** an accumulation of foreign material, especially within a cavity. −*accretive, adj.,* −*accrete, v.*

acculturation /əkul′chərā″shən/, **1.** accepting the norms, traditions, and history of a group different from one's own background. **2.** the modification of the culture of a group resulting from association with another group.

accumulated dose equivalent /əkyoo″myəlā′tid/, an estimate of an individual's absorbed dose of radiation over a lifetime, expressed in rem. Occupationally exposed persons are allowed no more than 5 rem/year, or 1 rem multiplied by age at any time during the person's lifetime. Also called **allowable dose.** See also **rem.**

accuracy /ak″yərəsē′/, the extent to which a measurement is close to the true value.

accurate empathy /ak″yərit/, an appropriate understanding of another person's feelings and experiences.

Accurbron, a bronchodilator. Brand name for **theophylline.**

Accutane, an antiacne agent. Brand name for **isotretinoin.**

ACDF, abbreviation for **anterior cervical decompression and fusion.**

ACE, abbreviation for **angiotensin-converting enzyme.**

ACE bandage, a trademark for a woven elastic bandage wrapped firmly around a joint or extremity to compress and support the area. It may also be used to secure dressings and in skin traction.

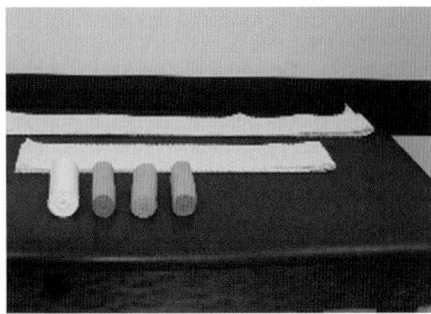

ACE bandage *(Browner and Fuller, 2012)*

acebutolol /as′əbo͞o″təlol/, a beta-adrenoreceptor blocking agent that inhibits the stimulation of the central nervous system alpha-adrenergic receptors and decreases sympathetic stimulation to the blood vessels and the heart.
- INDICATIONS: It is prescribed in the treatment of hypertension, angina pectoris, ventricular arrhythmias, and other cardiovascular disorders.
- CONTRAINDICATIONS: The drug should not be given to patients with asthma, persistent severe bradycardia, second- and third-degree heart block, overt heart failure, cardiogenic shock, and peripheral vascular disease. It is generally not recommended during pregnancy.
- ADVERSE EFFECTS: The most common side effects include fatigue, bradycardia, bronchospasm, flatulence, hypotension, muscle and joint pains, nausea, constipation, diarrhea, headache, rash, dizziness, and insomnia.

acedia /əsē′dē·ə/ [Gk, *akedia,* apathy], a condition of listlessness and a form of deep sadness marked by indifference and sluggish mental processes, making it difficult if not impossible to perform normal daily functions.

acellular /āsel″yələr/, without cells.

acentric /āsen″trik/ [Gk, *a* + *kentron,* not center], 1. having no center; lacking a middle point of reference. 2. (in genetics) describing a chromosome fragment that lacks the center for attachment.

-aceous /-ā″shəs/, a suffix meaning "having the appearance of" or "like" something specified: *papyraceous, sebaceous.*

ACEP, abbreviation for **American College of Emergency Physicians.**

acephal-, acephalo-, combining forms meaning "having no head": *acephalobrachia, acephaly.*

acephalia, absence of a head. See also **acephaly.**

acephalism. See **acephaly.**

acephalobrachia /asef′əlōbrā″kē·ə/ [Gk, *a* + *kephale,* without head, *brachion,* arm], a congenital anomaly in which a fetus lacks both arms and the head. Also called **abrachiocephalia.**

acephalocardia /-kär″dē·ə/ [Gk, *a,* not, *kephale,* head, *cardia,* heart], the congenital absence of both the head and the heart, as in a parasitic twin.

acephalus /əsef″ələs/ [Gk, *a* + *kephale,* without head], 1. headless. 2. a headless fetus.

acephaly /əsef″əlē/ [Gk, *a* + *kephale,* without head], a congenital defect in which the head is absent or not properly developed. Also called **acephalia, acephalism.** *–acephalic, adj.*

acerola /as′ərō″lə/, a small, cherrylike fruit of the genus *Malpighia* that grows in tropical climates. It is a richer source of vitamin C than any other known fruit. Also called **Barbados cherry.**

acesulfame-K /as′əsul″fām/, a synthetic noncaloric sweetener marketed under the trademark Sweet One®. It is approximately 200 times sweeter than sucrose. Heat does not affect its sweetening ability, an advantage over aspartame. Also called *acesulfame potassium.*

acet, abbreviation for *acetate carboxylate anion.*

acervuline /ah ser′ vu lin/, occurring in clusters; aggregated.

acet-, 1. a combining form meaning "vinegar": *acetyl.* 2. a prefix used for carboxylic acid derivatives and related compounds that have two carbons in the carbonyl-containing part of the structure. It is synonymous with *ethano-.* An example is acetic acid, or ethanoic acid, CH_3CO_2H.

acetabula. See **acetabulum.**

acetabular /as′ətab″yələr/ [L, *acetabulum,* little saucer], pertaining to the acetabulum; a concave surface where the femur articulates to form the hip joint.

acetabular angle, the angle between the acetabular line and Hilgenreiner's line, normally between 27 and 30 degrees in the neonatal hip. It is used in the radiographic assessment of developmental dysplasia of the hip. Also called *acetabular index.*

acetabular labrum, a fibrocartilaginous collar on the rim of the acetabulum that crosses the acetabular notch as the transverse acetabular ligament and converts the notch into a foramen.

acetabular line, a line following the slope of the acetabulum that is used in radiographic assessment of the hip joint. With Hilgenreiner's line it forms the acetabular angle.

acetabular notch, an indentation in the margin of the acetabulum.

acetabuloplasty /as″ətab″yəlōplas′tē/, a surgical procedure performed to reshape or remodel the acetabulum.

acetabulum /as′ətab″yələm/ *pl. acetabula* [L, vinegar cup], the large, cup-shaped cavity at the juncture and lateral surface of the ilium, the ischium, and the pubis, in which the ball-shaped head of the femur articulates.

acetal, 1. a colorless, volatile liquid used as a solvent and sometimes as a hypnotic. Also called *diethyl acetal.* 2. any compound with the general formula $R_2C(OR)_2$ or $RCH(OR)_2$, in which R indicates an alkyl or aryl group.

acetaldehyde (CH_3CHO) /as′ətəldē″hīd/, 1. a colorless, volatile liquid aldehyde with a pungent odor produced by the oxidation of ethyl alcohol. It is used in the manufacture of acetic acid, perfumes, and flavors. It is irritating to membranes and has a general narcotic action. 2. an intermediate in the metabolism of alcohol.

acetaminophen /əset′əmin″əfin/, an analgesic and antipyretic drug used in many nonprescription pain relievers. It has no antiinflammatory properties. It may be used with other products that do not contain additional acetaminophen.
- INDICATIONS: It is often recommended for the treatment of mild to moderate pain and fever. The dose should not exceed 4000 mg/24 hours.
- CONTRAINDICATIONS: Known hypersensitivity to acetaminophen prohibits its use. It should not be used in persons with liver disease.
- ADVERSE EFFECTS: Among the most serious adverse reactions are anaphylaxis, hepatotoxicity, and hemolytic anemia. Overdosing can result in fatal cyanosis and hepatic necrosis.

acetaminophen poisoning, a toxic reaction to the ingestion of excessive doses of acetaminophen. Many over-the-counter and prescription medications contain acetaminophen. Individuals may ingest an overdose accidentally when taking multiple products containing acetaminophen. Dosages exceeding 140 mg/kg can produce liver failure, and larger doses can be fatal. Large amounts of acetaminophen metabolites can overwhelm the glutathione-detoxifying mechanism of the liver, resulting in progressive necrosis of the liver within 5 days. The onset of symptoms may be marked by nausea and vomiting, profuse sweating, pallor, and oliguria.

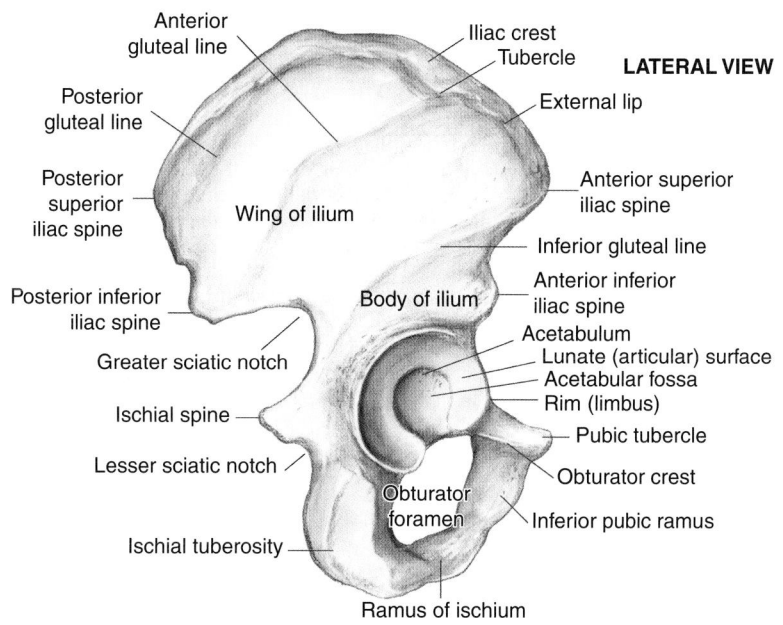

Acetabulum *(Chhabra and Browne, 2008)*

The incidence of nausea and vomiting increases, accompanied by jaundice and pain in the upper abdomen, hypoglycemia, encephalopathy, and kidney failure. Treatment requires inducing vomiting or performing gastric lavage, depending on the length of time since the ingestion. Acetylcysteine may prevent extensive liver damage if given via nasogastric tube soon after ingestion.

acetate ($CH_3CO_2^-$) /as″itāt/, an anion of the molecular formula $C_2H_3O_2$. It is the conjugate base of acetic acid.

acetate kinase, an enzyme that catalyzes the transfer of a phosphate group from adenosine triphosphate to acetate. Also called **acetokinase.**

acetaZOLAMIDE /as′ətəzō″ləmīd/, a carbonic anhydrase inhibitor diuretic agent.

■ INDICATIONS: It is prescribed for the treatment for glaucoma and edema and as an adjunctive agent for the treatment of refractory epilepsy and altitude sickness.

■ CONTRAINDICATIONS: Hyponatremia, hypokalemia, severe liver or kidney disease or dysfunction, Addison's disease, and known hypersensitivity to this drug or other sulfonamides prohibit its use.

■ ADVERSE EFFECTS: Among the most serious adverse reactions are anorexia and depression, particularly in the elderly; acidosis; hyperuricemia; and crystalluria. Paresthesias, GI disturbances, and lethargy are common.

Acetest®, a trademark for a product used to test for the presence of elevated quantities of ketone in the urine of patients with diabetes mellitus or other metabolic disorders. A large quantity of ketone causes a rapid change in the color of the Acetest tablet. See also **acetone in urine test, ketone bodies.**

acetic /əsē″tik, əset″ik/ [L, *acetum,* vinegar], pertaining to substances having the sour properties of vinegar or acetic acid or to chemical compounds possessing the radical CH_3CO^-.

acetic acid ($HC_2H_3O_2$), a clear, colorless, pungent liquid that is miscible with water, alcohol, glycerin, and ether and that constitutes 3% to 5% of vinegar. Acetic acid is produced commercially by the reaction of methanol with carbon monoxide in the presence of a catalyst, or it may be obtained from ethyl alcohol by the action of many aerobic bacteria. Various concentrations are used in the manufacture of plastics, dyes, insecticides, cellulose acetate, photographic chemicals, and pharmaceutic preparations, including vaginal jellies and antimicrobial solutions for the treatment of superficial infections of the external acoustic meatus. Also called **ethanoic acid.**

acetic fermentation, the production of acetic acid or vinegar from a weak alcoholic solution.

acetoacetic acid /as′ətō·əsē″tik, əsē′tō-/, a colorless, oily keto acid produced by the metabolism of lipids and pyruvates. It is excreted in trace amounts in normal urine and in elevated levels in diabetes mellitus, especially in ketoacidosis. Acetoacetic acid levels are also increased during starvation as a result of the incomplete oxidation of fatty acids. Soluble in water, alcohol, and ether, acetoacetic acid decomposes at temperatures below 100° C to acetone and carbon dioxide. Also called **acetone carboxylic acid, acetylacetic acid,** *beta-ketobutyric acid,* **diacetic acid.**

acetohydroxamic acid /as′ĕ-to-hi″droks-am′ik/, an inhibitor of bacterial urease used in the prophylaxis and treatment of struvite renal calculi, whose formation is favored by urease-producing bacteria, and as an adjunct in the treatment of urinary tract infections caused by urease-producing bacteria. It is administered orally.

acetokinase. See **acetate kinase.**

acetol kinase, an enzyme that catalyzes the transfer of a phosphate group from adenosine triphosphate to hydroxyacetone.

acetonaemia. See **ketonemia.**

acetone /as″ətōn/, **1.** a colorless, fragrant, volatile liquid ketone body found in small amounts in normal urine and in larger quantities in the urine of diabetics experiencing ketoacidosis or individuals experiencing starvation. It is one of the group of compounds called ketones. **2.** a commercial preparation used to clean the skin of fats and oils before some dermatological procedures; prolonged exposure to the compound can be irritating. It also has many varied industrial uses. Also called **2-propanone.**

acetone bodies. See **ketone bodies.**

acetone carboxylic acid. See **acetoacetic acid.**

acetone in urine test, a test for the presence of dimethyl-ketone in the urine of patients, used as a laboratory indication of ketosis and the severity of diabetes mellitus. Chemically treated test paper strips or sticks are exposed to urine. If acetone is present in the urine as the result of the incomplete breakdown of fatty and amino acids in the body, the test strips change color. The color may be visualized or analyzed by a spectrophotometer.

acetonide grouping, an acetone-based ketal, or a ketone-alcohol derivative present in some corticosteroid drugs, such as fluocinolone acetonide.

acetonuria /as′ətōnoo͞r′ē·ə/, the presence of acetone, diacetic acid, and beta-hydroxybutyric acid in the urine. Excretion in the urine of large amounts of acetone, an indication of incomplete oxidation of large amounts of lipids, commonly occurs in diabetic acidosis. See also **ketoaciduria.**

acetophenetidin. See **phenacetin.**

acetylacetic acid. See **acetoacetic acid.**

acetyl (CH₃CO, Ac), a monovalent radical associated with derivatives of acetic acid.

acetylcholine (ACh) /as′ətilkō′lēn, əsē′til-/, a direct-acting cholinergic neurotransmitter agent widely distributed in body tissues, with a primary function of mediating the synaptic activity of the nervous system and skeletal muscles. Its half-life and duration of activity are short because it is rapidly destroyed by acetylcholinesterase. Its activity also can be blocked by atropine at the junctions of nerve fibers with glands and smooth muscle tissue. It is a stimulant of the vagus and autonomic nervous system and functions as a vasodilator and cardiac depressant. It also has an effect at the neuromuscular junction that causes muscle contraction. Acetylcholine is used therapeutically as an adjunct to eye surgery and has limited benefits in certain circulatory disorders because of its short half-life.

acetylcholine receptor (AChR) antibody test, one of three blood tests for AChR to diagnose myasthenia gravis, the most sensitive of which is the AChR-modulating antibody test and the least sensitive of which is the AChR-blocking antibody test. The test used most often is the AChR-binding antibody test.

acetylcholinesterase (AChE) /-kō′lines″tərās/, an enzyme produced and released by the somatic nerves controlled by sympathetic and parasympathetic nerve ganglia. It inactivates and prevents the accumulation of the neurotransmitter acetylcholine, released during nerve impulse transmission, by hydrolyzing the substance to choline and acetate. The action reduces or prevents excessive firing of neurons at neuromuscular junctions. AChE is also present in hematopoietic cells. AChE is one of the fastest-acting enzymes in the body, with high catalytic activity and turnover.

acetylcoenzyme A /əsē′til·kō·en″zīm, as′ətil-/, a biomolecule that carries an activated form of the 2-carbon acetyl unit found in the course of several important metabolic processes. The formation of acetylcoenzyme A is the critical intermediate step between anaerobic glycolysis and the citric acid cycle. Also called *acetyl-CoA.*

acetylcysteine /-sis″tēn/, a mucolytic and acetaminophen antidote.

■ INDICATIONS: It is prescribed in nebulized or oral form for the treatment of chronic pulmonary disease, acute bronchopulmonary disease, atelectasis resulting from mucous obstruction, and acetaminophen poisoning.

■ CONTRAINDICATIONS: Known sensitivity to this drug prohibits its use.

■ ADVERSE EFFECTS: Among the most serious adverse reactions are stomatitis, nausea, rhinorrhea, and bronchospasm.

acetylene /aset′əlēn/, a colorless, highly flammable gas that is the simplest of the alkynes. Also called **ethyne.**

acetylsalicylic acid (ASA). See **aspirin.**

acetylsalicylic acid poisoning /əsē′təlsal′isil″ik, as′itəl-/, the toxic effects of overdosage of the commonly used antipyretic and analgesic drug, aspirin. Early symptoms include dizziness, ringing in the ears, changes in body temperature, GI discomfort, and hyperventilation. Severe poisoning is marked by respiratory alkalosis, which may lead to metabolic acidosis. Children and the elderly are particularly vulnerable to the potential toxic effects of salicylates. See also **Reye's syndrome, salicylate poisoning.**

acetyltransferase /-trans″fərās/, any of several enzymes that transfer acetyl groups from one compound to another.

ACG, **1.** abbreviation for *apexcardiography.* **2.** abbreviation for *apexcardiogram.*

ACh, abbreviation for **acetylcholine.**

ACH, abbreviation for **adrenocortical hormone.**

achalasia /ak′əlā″zhə/ [Gk, *a + chalasis,* without relaxation], a disorder characterized by the constriction of the lower portion of the esophagus, preventing normal swallowing. See also **dysphagia.**

Achard-Thiers syndrome /äsh″är terz″/ [Emile C. Achard, French physician, 1860–1941; Joseph Thiers, French physician, 20th century], a hormonal disorder generally seen in postmenopausal women with type 2, insulin-resistant diabetes mellitus, characterized by the growth of body hair in a masculine distribution. The exact cause of the disease is unknown. Treatment includes mechanical removal or bleaching of excess hair and hormonal therapy to correct endocrine imbalances related to systemic disease. See also **hirsutism.**

ache /āk/ [OE, *acan,* to hurt], **1.** a pain or discomfort characterized by persistence, dullness, and usually moderate intensity. An ache may be localized, such as a stomachache, headache, or bone ache, or a general ache, as in the myalgia that accompanies a viral infection or a persistent fever. **2.** to suffer from a dull, persistent pain of moderate intensity.

AChE, abbreviation for **acetylcholinesterase.**

acheiria /əkī′rē·ə/ [Gk, *a,* not, *cheir,* hand], **1.** a congenital absence of one or both hands. **2.** a lack of sensation of the hands or a feeling of their absence.

acheiropody /ak′ī·rop″ədē/ [Gk, *a,* not, *cheir,* hand, *pous,* foot], an autosomal-recessive disorder resulting in congenital absence of the hands and feet.

achievement age (AA) /əchēv″mənt/, the level of a person's educational development as measured by an achievement test and compared with the normal score for chronological age. Compare **mental age.** See also **developmental age.**

achievement quotient (AQ), a numeric expression of a person's achievement age, determined by various achievement tests, divided by the chronological age and expressed as a multiple of 100. Compare **intelligence quotient.**

achievement test, a standardized test for the measurement and comparison of knowledge or proficiency in various fields of vocational or academic study. Compare **aptitude test, intelligence test, personality test, psychological test.**

Achilles tendon /əkil″ēz/ [*Achilles,* Greek mythological hero], the common distal tendon of the soleus and gastrocnemius muscles of the leg. It is the thickest and strongest tendon in the body and connects the triceps surae to the heel bone. In an adult, it is about 15 cm long. The tendon becomes contracted about 4 cm above the heel and flares out again to insert into the calcaneus. Also called **tendo calcaneus.**

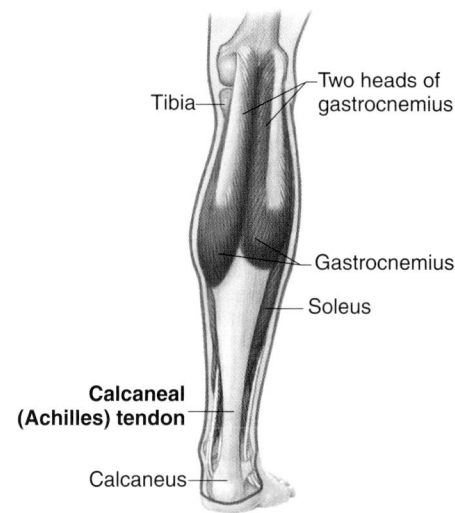

Achilles tendon *(Patton and Thibodeau, 2010)*

Achilles tendon reflex,   a deep tendon reflex consisting of plantar flexion of the foot when a sharp tap is given directly to the tendon of the gastrocnemius muscle at the back of the ankle. This reflex is often absent in people with peripheral neuropathies or diabetes. A sluggish return of the flexed foot may occur in patients with hypothyroidism and lower motor neuron diseases. A hyperactive reflex may be caused by hyperthyroidism or by pyramidal tract disease, as well as by any upper motor neuron disease. Also called **ankle reflex.** See also **deep tendon reflex.**

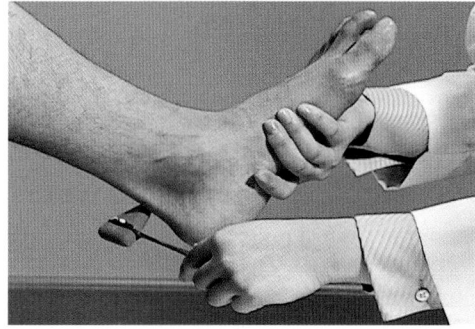

Elicitation of the Achilles tendon reflex *(Ball et al, 2015)*

achiral,   pertaining to the absence of chirality in a compound, as in stereochemical isomers.

achlorhydria /ā′klôrhī″drē·ə/   [Gk, *a + chloros,* not green, *hydor,* water],   an abnormal condition characterized by the absence of hydrochloric acid in gastric secretions. Achlorhydria occurs most commonly in atrophy of the gastric mucosa, gastric carcinoma, and pernicious anemia. It is also found in severe iron-deficiency anemia. Malignancy is expected when achlorhydria is seen in combination with peptic ulcers. Protein digestion is severely impaired in patients with achlorhydria, but overall digestion in the digestive tract is relatively normal because trypsin and other enzymes of the pancreas and small intestine are not affected. See also **achylia.** −*achlorhydric, adj.*

achloropsia /ā′klôrop″sē·ə/   [Gk, *a,* not, *chloros,* green, *opsis,* vision],   an inability to see green; green blindness.

acholia /akō″lē·ə/   [Gk, *a + chole,* without bile],   **1.** the absence of or a decrease in bile secretions. **2.** any condition that suppresses the flow of bile into the small intestine. −*acholic, adj.*

acholuria /ak′əloŏr″ē·ə/   [Gk, *a + chole,* without bile, *ouron,* urine],   the absence of bilirubin (bile pigment) from urine; it occurs in prehepatic jaundice, in which plasma bilirubin, attached to albumin, remains insoluble and is not excreted by the kidneys.

achondrogenesis /ākon′drōjen″əsis/,   the most severe form of chondrodysplasia; typically lethal before or soon after birth. Type 1A, called the Houston-Harris type, is characterized by infants with extremely short limbs, a narrow chest, short ribs that fracture easily, and soft skull bones. These infants also lack normal bone formation (ossification) in the spine and pelvis. In Type 1B, Parenti-Fraccaro type, affected infants have extremely short limbs, a narrow chest, and a prominent, rounded abdomen. The fingers and toes are short, and the feet may be rotated inward. Affected infants frequently have a soft outpouching around the umbilicus. Infants with Type 2, Langer-Saldino type, have short arms and legs, a narrow chest with short ribs, and underdeveloped lungs. This condition is also associated with a lack of ossification in the spine and pelvis. Distinctive facial features include a prominent forehead, a small chin, and in some cases an opening in the roof of the mouth (a cleft palate).

achondroplasia /ākon′drōplā″zhə/   [Gk, *a + chondros,* without cartilage, *plassein,* to form],   a rare disorder of the growth of cartilage in the epiphyses of the long bones and skull. It results in premature ossification, permanent limitation of skeletal development, and dwarfism typified by a protruding forehead and short, thick arms and legs on a normal trunk. Onset is in fetal life and the diagnosis can be made on prenatal ultrasound. It is inherited as an autosomal-dominant gene with most cases occurring as a sporadic mutation (affecting a fibroblast growth factor receptor). The majority of affected individuals die during gestation or the first year of life. Those who survive have relatively normal longevity. Also called **chondrodystrophy, fetal rickets.**

achondroplastic dwarf /-plas″tik/,   the most common type of dwarf, characterized by disproportionately short limbs, a normal-sized trunk, a large head with a depressed nasal bridge and small face, stubby hands, and lordosis. The condition results from an inherited defect in bone-forming tissue and is often associated with other defects or abnormalities, although there is usually no involvement of the central nervous system and intelligence is normal. See also **achondroplasia.**

AChR,   abbreviation for *acetylcholine receptor.*

achroma /akrō″mə/   [Gk, *a,* without, *chroma,* color],   **1.** the absence or lack of color. **2.** loss of normal pigmentation (hypopigmentation), as in albinism or leukoderma.

achromatic,   **1.** colorless. **2.** color-blind. **3.** a substance not colored by common staining agents. **4.** a lens that refracts white light without separating it into component colors.

achromatic lens /ak′rəmat″ik/   [Gk, *a,* without, *chroma,* color; L, *lentis,* lens],   a lens in which the focal lengths for red and blue colors of the spectrum are the same, refracting light without decomposing it into its component colors.

achromatic vision.   See **coloproctitis.**

achromatocyte.   See **achromocyte.**

achromatopsia.   See **color blindness.**

achromia /akrō″mēə/   [Gk, *a + chroma,* without color],   **1.** depigmentation. **2.** the absence or loss of natural pigmentation of the skin and iris. It may be congenital or acquired.

Achromobacter /akrō′mōbak″tər/,   a genus of gram-negative, rod-shaped, flagellated bacteria that do not form pigment on agar. Most species in the genus are saprophytic, nonpathogenic organisms found in water, soil, or the human digestive tract, but they may cause infection in the compromised host.

achromocyte /ākrō″məsīt/, a red cell artifact that stains more faintly than intact red cells.

Achromycin V, an antibiotic. Brand name for **tetracycline hydrochloride.**

achylia /ākī″lē·ə/ [Gk, *a,chylos,* not juice], an absence or severe deficiency of hydrochloric acid and pepsinogen (pepsin) in the stomach. This condition may also occur in the pancreas when the exocrine portion of that gland fails to produce digestive enzymes. Also called *achylosis.* See also **achlorhydria.**

achylous /əkī″ləs/, **1.** pertaining to a lack or loss of gastric juice or other digestive secretions. **2.** pertaining to a lack of chyle.

acicular /əsik″yələr/ [L, *aciculus,* little needle], long, straight, and pointed in appearance, as seen in certain leaves and crystals.

acid /as″id/ [L, *acidus,* sour], **1.** a compound that yields hydrogen ions when dissociated in aqueous solution (Arrhenius definition), acts as a hydrogen ion donor (Brønsted definition), or acts as an electron pair acceptor (Lewis definition). Acids turn blue litmus red, have a sour taste, and react with bases to form salts. Acids have chemical properties essentially opposite to those of bases. See also **alkali, base.** **2.** *(Slang)* LSD. **3.** sour or bitter to the taste. −*acidic, adj.*

acid-, a prefix meaning "sour, bitter, acid": *acidemia, acidophil.*

acidaemia, British spelling for acidemia. See **acidemia.** See also **propionic acidemia.**

acidalbumin, a substance formed by the action of mild acid solutions on albumin. Also called **metaprotein.**

acidaminuria, now called **aminoaciduria.**

acid-base balance, a condition existing when the net rate at which the body produces acids or bases equals the net rate at which acids or bases are excreted. The result of acid-base balance is a stable concentration of hydrogen ions in body fluids. See also **acid, base.**

acid-base metabolism, the metabolic processes that maintain the balance of acids and bases essential in regulating the composition of body fluids. Acids release hydrogen ions, and bases accept them; the concentration of hydrogen ions present in a solution governs whether it is acid, alkali, or neutral. Hydrogen ions in water are measured on a pH scale of 0.0 to 14.0, with a reading of 7.0 indicating neutral at 25° C. Above 7.0, the solution is alkaline; below, it is acidic. Blood is slightly alkaline, ranging from 7.35 to 7.45. Metabolic buffer systems within the body maintain this ratio, and when the ratio is upset, acidosis or alkalosis results. Acidosis may be caused by diarrhea, vomiting, uremia, diabetes mellitus, and the action of certain drugs. Alkalosis may be caused by overingestion of alkaline drugs, loss of chloride in gastric vomitus, and the action of certain diuretic drugs. See also **acid-base balance, acidosis, alkalosis, pH.**

acid burn, damage to tissue caused by exposure to an acid. The severity of the burn is determined by the strength of the acid and the duration and extent of exposure. Initial emergency treatment includes irrigating the affected area with large amounts of cool or room-temperature water. Compare **alkali burn.**

acid dust, an accumulation of highly acidic particles of dust. Such substances accumulate in the atmosphere and account for much of the smog hanging over large metropolitan areas. Many respiratory illnesses, such as lung cancer and

asthma, may be aggravated or caused by such dust. See also **acid rain.**

acidemia /as′idē″mē·ə/, decreased pH status of the blood or abnormal acidity in the blood. Specific types are denoted by prefixes: *lactacidemia, lipacidemia.*

acid etching, microscopic roughening of dental enamel with an acid (usually phosphoric acid) to promote mechanical retention of resin sealant by increasing the surface area available for bonding.

acid-fast bacillus (AFB), a type of bacillus that resists decolorizing by acid after accepting a stain. Examples include *Mycobacterium tuberculosis* and *M. leprae.*

acid-fast stain, a method of staining used in bacteriology in which a smear on a slide is treated with carbol-fuchsin stain or auramine-rhodamine stain, decolorized with acid alcohol, and counterstained with methylene blue or potassium permanganate to identify acid-fast bacteria. Acid-fast organisms resist decolorization and appear red or yellow against a dark background when viewed under a microscope. The stain may be performed on any clinical specimen but is most commonly used in examining sputum for *Mycobacterium tuberculosis,* an acid-fast bacillus. See also **Ziehl-Neelsen test.**

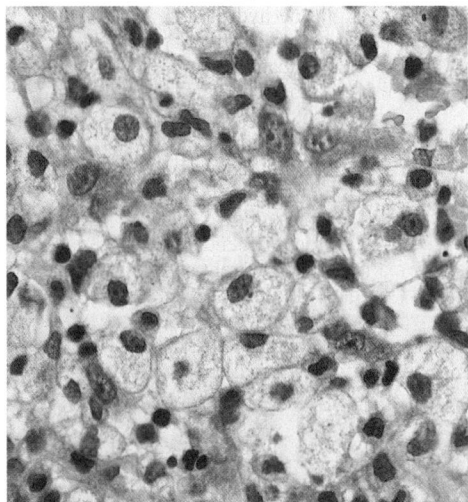

Acid-fast stain of mycobacterium *(Simon, 2013)*

acid flush, a runoff of precipitation with a high acid content, as may occur during thaws. Acid flushes may pollute rivers and reservoirs, killing fish and endangering the natural balance of the ecosystem. See also **acid rain.**

acidify. See **acid.**

acidity /asid″itē/ [L, *acidus,* sour], **1.** the degree of sourness, sharpness of taste, or ability of a chemical to yield hydrogen ions in an aqueous solution. **2.** the degree of gastric acid in the stomach. The acidity varies during any 24-hour period, but the pH averages 0.9 to 1.5. The main source of stomach acidity is hydrochloric acid secreted by the gastric glands of the stomach.

acid mist, a mist containing a high concentration of acid or particles of any toxic chemical, such as carbon tetrachloride or silicon tetrachloride. Such chemicals are often used by industry and stored in tanks that may leak their contents into residential areas, becoming especially dangerous if the toxic substance mixes with fog. Inhalation of acid mists may irritate the mucous membranes, the eyes, and the respiratory tract and seriously upset the chemical balances of the body. See also **acid rain.**

acid mucopolysaccharide,   **1.** long chains of molecules found in the ground substance of collagen, joint fluid, and mucoid material. **2.** a 24-hour urine diagnostic test used in the evaluation of genetic disorders known as mucopolysaccharidoses (MPS).

acidophil /as″idō̄fil, əsid″əfil/ [L, *acidus,* acid + Gk, *philein,* to love],   **1.** a particular staining pattern of cells and tissues when using haematoxylin and eosin stains. Specifically, a cell or cell constituent with an affinity for acid dyes. The most common such dye is eosin, which stains acidophilic organisms red and is the source of the related term eosinophilic. See also **eosinophilic. 2.** an organism that thrives in an acid medium. *−acidophilic, adj.*

acidophilic adenoma,   a tumor of the pituitary gland characterized by cells that can be stained red with an acid dye. Gigantism and acromegaly can result from the hypersecretion of growth hormone caused by an acidophilic adenoma. Also called **eosinophilic adenoma.**

acidophilus milk /as″idof″ələs/,   milk inoculated with cultures of *Lactobacillus acidophilus,* used in various enteric disorders to change the bacterial flora of the GI tract.

acidosis /as″idō″sis/ [L, *acidus* + Gk, *osis,* condition],   an abnormal increase in the hydrogen ion concentration in the blood, resulting from an accumulation of an acid or the loss of a base. It is indicated by a blood pH below the normal range (7.35 to 7.45). The various forms of acidosis are named for their cause; for example, renal tubular acidosis results from failure of the kidney to secrete hydrogen ions or reabsorb bicarbonate ions, respiratory acidosis results from respiratory retention of carbon dioxide, and diabetic acidosis results from an accumulation of ketones associated with a lack of insulin. Treatment depends on diagnosis of the underlying abnormality and concurrent correction of the acid-base imbalance. Compare **alkalosis.** *−acidotic, adj.*

acid phosphatase,   an enzyme found in the kidneys, serum, semen, and prostate gland. It is elevated in serum in prostate cancer and in trauma. Normal concentrations in serum are 0 to 1.1 Bodansky units/mL. See also **alkaline phosphatase.**

acid phosphatase test,   **1.** a presumptive test for the presence of semen in suspected rape cases. Also called *acid phosphatase assay.* **2.** a diagnostic tool used to monitor the response to treatment for prostatic cancer, particularly in regard to bony metastasis.

acid poisoning,   a toxic condition caused by the ingestion of a toxic acid agent such as hydrochloric, nitric, phosphoric, or sulfuric acid, some of which are ingredients in common household cleaning compounds. Compare **alkali poisoning.**

acid rain,   the precipitation of moisture, as rain, with high acidity caused by release into the atmosphere of pollutants from industry, motor vehicle exhaust, and other sources. Acid precipitation with a pH of 5.6 or lower is assigned responsibility by various authorities for numerous human health problems, fish kills, and the destruction of timber. Also called *acid precipitation,* **acid snow.** See also **acid dust, acid flush, acid mist.**

acid rebound,   the hypersecretion of gastric acid that may occur after the initial buffering effect of an antacid. It occurs most noticeably when antacids containing calcium carbonate are used.

acid salt,   a salt formed from an acid with two or more bases by only partial replacement of hydrogen ions from the related acid, leaving some degree of acidity. An example is sodium bicarbonate, which is also identified as sodium acid carbonate or sodium hydrogen carbonate.

acid snow.   See **acid rain.**

acidulous /əsid″yələs/,   slightly acidic or sour.

aciduria [L, *acidus* + Gk, *ouron,* urine],   the excretion of an acid in the urine. The condition may be caused by a diet rich in meat proteins or certain fruits, a medication used to treat a urinary tract disorder, an inborn error of metabolism, or ketoacidosis.

acinar adenocarcinoma.   See **acinic cell adenocarcinoma.**

acinar cell /as″inər/ [L, *acinus,* grape],   a cell of the tiny lobules of a compound gland or similar saclike structure, such as an alveolus.

Acinetobacter /as″inē″təbak″tər/,   a genus of nonmotile, aerobic bacteria of the family Neisseriaceae that often occurs in clinical specimens. The bacterium contains gram-negative or gram-variable cocci and does not produce spores. It grows on regular medium without serum and is oxidase negative and catalase positive. It is mainly found in water, and its disease activity is opportunistic. Most human disease is caused by *A. baumannii.* The bacterium can cause various infections, including pneumonia, wound infections, bacteremia, and meningitis. Most infections are nosocomial and occur in immunocompromised individuals, rarely occurring outside of intensive care units and other health care settings. The organism can also colonize patients without causing symptoms or infection, particularly in open wounds or tracheostomy sites. *Acinetobacter* is often resistant to those antibiotics used regularly.

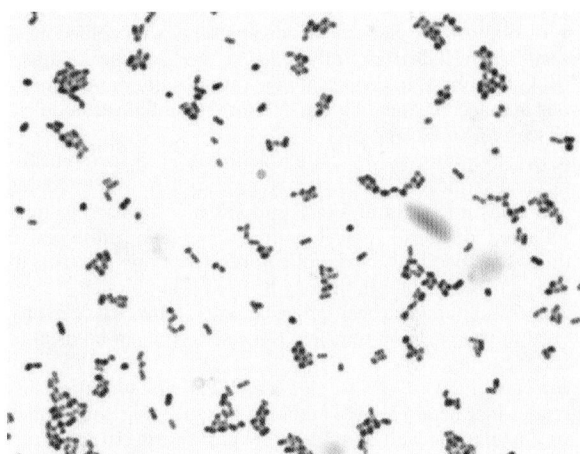

Acinetobacter *(Murray, Rosenthal, and Pfaller, 2005)*

acini,   plural form of acinus. See **acinus.**

acinic cell adenocarcinoma /asin″ik/ [L, *acinus,* grape],   an uncommon low-grade malignant neoplasm that develops in the secreting cells of racemose glands, especially the salivary glands. The tumor consists of cells with clear or slightly granular cytoplasm and small eccentric dark nuclei. Also called **acinar adenocarcinoma, acinous adenocarcinoma.**

aciniform /asin″ifôrm/ [L, *acinus,* grape, *forma,* shape],   shaped like a cluster of grapes. The term refers particularly to glandular tissue.

acinitis /as″inī″tis/,   any inflammation of the tiny, grape-shaped portions of certain glands. Compare **adenitis.**

acinotubular gland /as″inōt(y)o͞ob″yələr/ [grape-shaped],   a gland in which the acini are elongated or tube shaped.

acinous adenocarcinoma.   See **acinic cell adenocarcinoma.**

A

acinus /as″inəs/ *pl.* *acini* [L, grape], any small saclike structure, particularly one found in a gland. See **alveolus.**

acitretin /as″e-tret′in/, a second-generation retinoid used in the treatment of severe psoriasis. It is administered orally.

A.C. joint, abbreviation for *acromioclavicular joint.* See **acromioclavicular articulation.**

acknowledgment /ək΄nӓl əj mənt/, a therapeutic technique characterized by providing feedback to individuals, assuring them that they have been heard.

ACL, abbreviation for **anterior cruciate ligament.**

Aclovate, a topical corticosteroid. Brand name for **alclometasone dipropionate.**

ACLS, abbreviation for **advanced cardiac life support.**

acme /ak″mē/ [Gk, *akme,* point], the peak or highest point, such as the peak of intensity of a uterine contraction during labor or the peak of perfection.

acne /ak″nē/, a chronic disorder of the hair follicles and sebaceous glands characterized by pimple outbreaks, cysts, infected abscesses, and sometimes scarring. Characteristic lesions include open (blackhead) and closed (whitehead) comedones, inflammatory papules, pustules, and nodules. It seems to result from a combination of factors, such as thickening of the follicular opening, increased sebum production, the presence of bacteria, and the host's inflammatory response. Also called **acne vulgaris.** Kinds include **acne conglobata, acne fulminans, chloracne.** See also **comedo.**

■ OBSERVATIONS: Superficial acne presents with comedones, scattered pustules, and oily skin on the face, neck, upper back, and chest. In deep acne, the pustules are more numerous and accompanied by pus-filled cysts, inflamed nodules, abscesses, and scarring.

■ INTERVENTIONS: Manual extraction is used for comedones and surgical excision may be used for persistent nodules and sinus tracts. Intralesional steroids may be used to treat inflamed nodules. Topical antimicrobial and antiinfective drugs, comedolytics, and oral antiinfective drugs are used to treat pustules. Isotretinoin may be used if antibiotics are unsuccessful. Oral estrogen-progesterone is often successfully used to treat acne in females. Dermabrasion can be used to treat scarring.

■ PATIENT CARE CONSIDERATIONS: Patient education includes instruction to avoid picking or squeezing comedones or pustules, as well as to avoid exposure to coal tar products, cocoa butter, greasy cosmetics, or hair gels. Excessive cleansing is counterproductive. Patients should know that diet has been shown to have little or no influence on acne. Most over-the-counter preparations have no proven efficacy and may aggravate acne outbreaks. Therapy often includes a combination of a topical antibiotic combined with an antiinflammatory agent, such as the combination of clindamycin with benzoyl peroxide, and a topical retinoid. Patients started on oral isotretinoin should have baseline liver and lipid panels and a pregnancy test before use. Females should be counseled on the serious risks of this medication to a fetus should pregnancy occur. Females should be placed on two forms of birth control for 1 month before starting therapy, during therapy, and at least 1 month after therapy. All patients on this medication should avoid vitamin A supplements and prolonged exposure to the sun. Sunscreen and protective clothing should be used when exposed to sunlight.

acne atrophica /atrof″ikə/, a skin disorder characterized by small scars or pits left by an earlier occurrence of acne vulgaris.

acne cachecticorum, an eruption or irritation of the skin that may occur in patients who are very weak and debilitated. It is characterized by soft, mildly infiltrated pustular lesions.

acne conglobata /kon′glōbā″tə/, a severe form of acne with abscess, cyst, scar, and keloid formation. It may affect the lower back, buttocks, and thighs, as well as the face and chest. It affects more males than females, often beginning in young adulthood and persisting for many years. Also called **cystic acne.**

acneform /ak″nifôrm/. See **acneiform.**

acneform drug eruption, any of various skin reactions to a drug, characterized by papules and pustules resembling acne.

acne fulminans, severe scarring acne in teenage males, which may be accompanied by fever, polyarthralgia, crusted ulcerative lesions, weight loss, anemia, arthritis, and blood disorders.

acnegenic /ak′nijen″ik/ [Gk, *akme* + *genein,* to produce], causing or producing acne.

acneiform, resembling acne. Also spelled **acneform.**

acne keloid [Gk, *akme,* point, *kelis,* spot, *eidos,* form], an acneform disorder in which secondary pyogenic infection in and around pilosebaceous structures results in keloidal scarring. It is manifested as persistent folliculitis of the back of the neck associated with occlusion of the follicular orifices. It is most often encountered in black and Asian men.

acne medicamentosa, any type of acne resulting from a reaction to medication, such as to a steroid or the salt of a halogen. Also called **drug-induced acne.**

acne necrotica miliaris, a rare, chronic type of pruritic, pustular folliculitis of the scalp, forehead, and temples occurring mostly in adults and characterized by tiny pustules, probably a pyoderma or tuberculid. Also called **acne varioliformis.**

acne neonatorum, a skin condition of newborns caused by sebaceous gland hyperplasia and characterized by the localized formation of grouped comedones or papules on the nose, cheeks, and forehead.

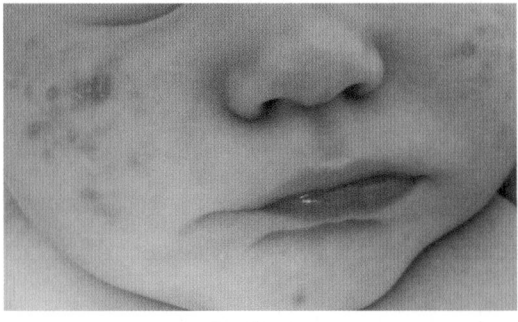

Acne neonatorum *(Maroñas-Jiménez and Krakowski, 2016)*

acne papulosa, a common skin condition in which comedones develop moderately inflamed papules. It is considered a papular form of acne vulgaris.

acne pustulosa, a form of acne in which the predominant lesions are pustular and may result in scarring.

acne rosacea. See **rosacea.**

acne urticaria /ur′tiker″ē·ə/, a form of acne marked by papules that are predominantly edematous and wheal-like and that have been aggravated by scratching.

acne varioliformis. See **acne necrotica miliaris.**

acne vulgaris. See **acne.**

A

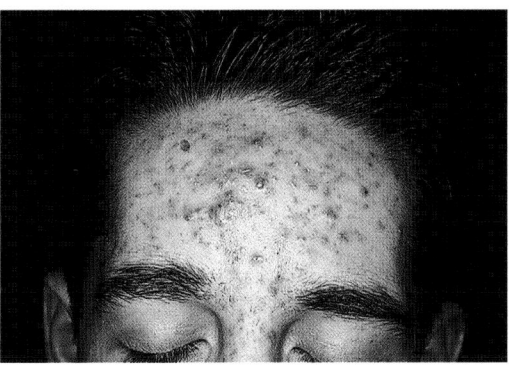

Acne vulgaris on the forehead *(Callen et al, 2000)*

ACNM, abbreviation for *American College of Nurse-Midwives.*

ACOEM, abbreviation for **American College of Occupational and Environmental Medicine.**

ACOG, abbreviation for **American College of Obstetricians and Gynecologists.**

acognosia /ak′og·nō″zhə/ [Gk, *ako(s),* remedy, *gnos(is),* knowledge], the knowledge or the study of remedies.

acorea /ā′kôrē″ə/ [Gk, *a,* without, *kore,* pupil], an absence of the pupil of the eye.

acoria /akôr″ē·ə/ [Gk, *a,* without, *koros,* satiety], a condition characterized by constant hunger and excessive ingestion of food, not from hunger but because of loss of the sensation of satiety.

acorn-tipped catheter, a flexible catheter with a bulbous, triangular-shaped tip used in various diagnostic procedures to occlude an orifice and prevent backflow of dyes used during the procedure.

ACOTE, abbreviation for **Accreditation Council for Occupational Therapy Education.**

acous-, acus-, acust-, acousto-, combining forms meaning "hearing": *acousma, acoustic.*

-acousia, -acusia, -acusis, -akusis, suffixes meaning a "(specified) condition of the hearing": *anacusis.*

acousma /əkooz″mə/ *pl. acousmas, acousmata* [Gk, *akousma,* something heard], a hallucinatory impression of strange sounds.

acoustic /əkoos′tik/ [Gk, *akouein,* to hear], pertaining to sound or hearing. Also **acoustical.**

-acoustic, -acoustical, **1.** suffixes meaning "the hearing organs." **2.** suffixes meaning "amplified sound waves": *otoacoustic emissions.* **3.** suffixes meaning pertaining to sound: *psychoacoustics.*

acoustic apparatus, the various components of the sense of hearing. See also **cochlea, inner ear, organ of Corti.**

acoustic cavitation, a potential biological effect of ultrasonography, marked by the growth and collapse of preexisting microbubbles under the influence of large-amplitude oscillations. As normally used, ultrasound pulses are too short to cause acoustic cavitation in human tissues.

acoustic center, the portion of the brain, in the temporal lobe of the cerebrum, in which the sense of hearing is located. Also called **auditory cortex.**

acoustic hair cell. See **auditory hair.**

acoustic-immittance audiometry, audiological testing used to evaluate the status of the external and middle ears and of the acoustic reflex arc. Kinds include **tympanometry, static compliance testing, acoustic reflex measures.**

acoustic impedance, interference with the passage of sound waves by objects in the path of those waves. It equals the velocity of sound in a medium multiplied by the density of the medium. The acoustic impedance of bone may be nearly five times as great as that of blood. Testing middle ear acoustic impedance is part of audiological evaluation used to detect middle ear problems.

acoustic meatus [Gk, *akoustikos,* hearing; L, *meatus,* a passage], the external or internal canal of the ear.

acoustic microscope, a microscope in which the object being viewed is scanned with sound waves and its image reconstructed with light waves. Acoustic microscopes produce excellent resolution of the objects being studied and allow close examination of cells and tissues without staining or damaging the specimen.

acoustic nerve. See **vestibulocochlear nerve.**

acoustic neuroma, a benign unilateral or bilateral vestibular schwannoma that develops from the vestibulocochlear nerve and grows within the auditory canal, occurring rarely with the vestibular or cochlear apparatus of the inner ear. Depending on the location and size of the lesion, tinnitus, progressive hearing loss, headache, facial numbness, papilledema, dizziness, and an unsteady gait may result. Paresis and difficulty in speaking and swallowing may occur in the later stage. Also called *acoustic neurilemmoma, acoustic neurinoma, acoustic neurofibroma schwannoma.*

acoustic reflex, a paired reaction with bilateral contraction following unilateral sound exposure. The muscle contractions pull the stapes out of the oval window and thus protect the internal ear from damage caused by loud noise. The acoustic reflex threshold is the lowest level of sound that will elicit an acoustic reflex and is in the range of 85 to 90 dB hearing level in individuals with normal hearing. Acoustic reflexes are usually elevated or absent in cases of conductive or sensorineural hearing loss and present at normal or lower levels in the case of cochlear hearing loss.

acoustic reflex measures, measurement of the acoustic reflex in response to intense sound, a component of the evaluation of middle ear function.

acoustics /əkoos″tiks/ [Gk, *akoustikos,* hearing], the science of sound.

acoustic shadow, in an ultrasound image, the absence of echoes produced by the presence of dense material, such as calculi, which impede the transmission of sound waves. It is often used to detect biliary calculi.

acoustic trauma, a sudden loss of hearing, partial or complete, caused by an extremely loud noise, a severe blow to the head, or other trauma. The greatest loss of hearing occurs at 4000 Hz. It may be temporary or permanent. Compare **noise-induced hearing loss.**

acoustooptics /əkoos′tō·op″tiks/, a field of physics that studies the generation of light waves by ultra–high-frequency sound waves. Knowledge gained by such study is applied chiefly in the transmission of information by acoustooptic devices.

ACP, **1.** abbreviation for **American College of Physicians.** **2.** abbreviation for **American College of Prosthodontists.** **3.** abbreviation for *advanced care planning.*

acquired /əkwī″ərd/ [L, *acquirere,* to obtain], pertaining to a characteristic, condition, or disease gained and/or obtained as a result of external conditions after birth. An example is acquired immunity. Compare **congenital, familial, hereditary.**

acquired cystic kidney disease, the development of cysts in a formerly noncystic kidney during end-stage renal disease.

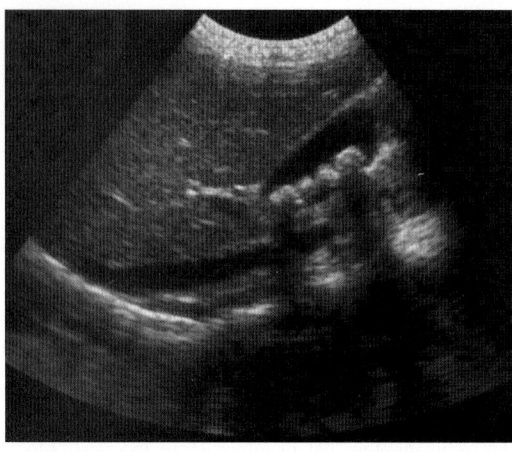
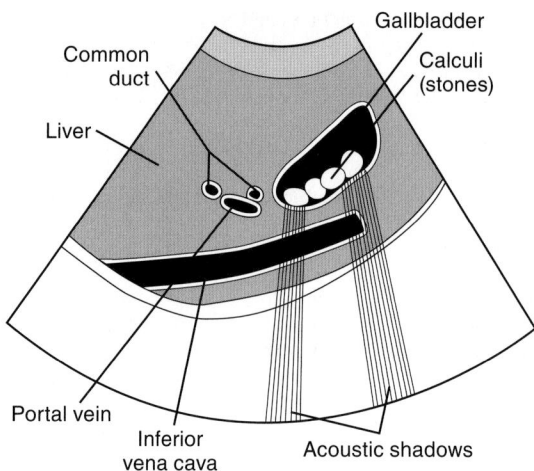

Calculi. Typically, calculi, or "stones," are distinguished by the fact that they impede (reflect, absorb, stop, decrease) sound waves. This creates a bright anterior surface and dark to anechoic posterior shadow. Note the sharp, well-defined edges of the shadows. (Tempkin, 2015)

acquired epileptic aphasia. See **Landau-Kleffner syndrome.**

acquired hypogammaglobulinemia [L, *acquirere*, to obtain; Gk, *hypo*, a deficiency, *gamma*, third letter of Greek alphabet; L, *globulus*, small globe; Gk, *haima*, blood], an acquired deficiency of the gamma globulin blood fraction. See also **hypogammaglobulinemia.**

acquired immunity, any form of immunity that is not innate and that is obtained during life as a result of exposure to an antigen, resulting in the formation of antibodies. It may be naturally or artificially acquired and actively or passively induced. Naturally acquired immunity is obtained by the development of antibodies resulting from an attack of infectious disease or by the transmission of antibodies from the mother through the placenta to the fetus or to the infant through colostrum and breast milk. Artificially acquired immunity is obtained by vaccination or by the injection of immune gamma globulin. Acquired immunity can be divided into cell-mediated immunity (T cells) and humoral immunity (B cells). Compare **natural immunity.** See also **active immunity, passive immunity.**

acquired immunodeficiency syndrome (AIDS), a syndrome involving a defect in cell-mediated immunity, characterized by a susceptibility to infection with opportunistic pathogens. The U.S. Centers for Disease Control and Prevention has defined AIDS as beginning when a person with HIV infection has a CD4 cell count below 200. See also **AIDS-dementia complex, AIDS-wasting syndrome.**

■ OBSERVATIONS: An individual may be diagnosed as having AIDS if he or she is infected with HIV, has a CD4+ count below 200, and exhibits one or more illnesses associated with impaired immune function. Symptoms often include extreme fatigue, intermittent fever, night sweats, chills, lymphadenopathy, enlarged spleen, anorexia and consequent weight loss, severe diarrhea, apathy, and depression. As the disease progresses, characteristics are a general failure to thrive, anergy, and any of a variety of recurring infections.

■ INTERVENTIONS: Treatment consists primarily of chronic symptom management and combined chemotherapy to counteract the opportunistic infections. There is no known cure. Drugs used to treat AIDS include antiretroviral therapies targeting HIV. These include reverse transcriptase inhibitors, which interfere with the virus's ability to synthesize DNA within host cells, and HIV protease inhibitors, which cause the production of noninfectious HIV particles. HIV integrase inhibitors are now part of the first line in the recommended treatment regimen. HIV integrase is responsible for integration of the viral genome into cellular DNA. These drugs are given in combinations (often called cocktails), with several options available that require just a single pill a day.

■ PATIENT CARE CONSIDERATIONS: Care of the patient with AIDS is complex and mandates a coordinated team approach that varies with the patient's symptoms. Intervention is directed at providing education to prevent the spread of disease and infection, promoting self-care and optimal nutrition, and providing emotional support for patients and their families. Prevention of opportunistic infections—such as candidiasis, Kaposi's sarcoma, tuberculosis, viral hepatitis, or pneumonia—is a priority. Patients with tumors, hematologic abnormalities, and infections require treatment for these disorders, along with care for their HIV-related symptoms.

acquired pellicle, an acellular film composed of salivary glycoproteins that firmly adheres to all surface structures of the oral cavity, including tooth surfaces, dental restorations and prostheses, and soft tissues. It is clear, translucent, insoluble, and not readily visible until a disclosing agent has been applied. Acquired pellicle can mineralize into dental calculus. The significance of the pellicle is that it appears to provide a barrier against acids. Acquired pellicle can be mechanically removed with toothbrushing, flossing, and mechanical dental hygiene prophylaxis. Compare **bacterial plaque.**

acquired reflex. See **conditioned reflex.**

acquired sterility [L, *acquirere*, to obtain, *sterilis*, barren], the failure to conceive after once bearing a child. Also called **one-child sterility, secondary infertility.**

acquired trait [L, *acquirere*, to obtain + *trahere*, to draw], a physical characteristic that is not inherited but may be an effect of the environment or of a somatic mutation.

ACR, 1. abbreviation for **American College of Radiology.** 2. abbreviation for **albumin/creatinine ratio.**

acral /ak″rəl/ [Gk, *akron*, extremity], pertaining to an extremity or apex.

acral erythema, erythema localized to the palms and soles, as in hand-foot syndrome.

Acremonium /ak″rĕ-mo′ne-um/, a genus of Fungi imperfecti of the former class Hyphomycetes. Some species produce cephalosporin antibiotics. Formerly called *Cephalosporium*.

acrid /ak″rid/ [L, *acris*, sharp], sharp or pungent, bitter, and unpleasant to the smell or taste.

acridine /ak″ridēn/, a dibenzopyridine compound used in the synthesis of dyes and drugs. Its derivatives include fluorescent yellow dyes and the antiseptic agents acriflavine hydrochloride, acriflavine base, and proflavine.

acrimony /akʺrəmōʹnē/ [L, *acrimonia,* pungency], **1.** a quality of bitterness, harshness, or sharpness. **2.** feelings of anger and negativity.

acrivastine /akʺri-vasʹtēn/, a nonsedating antihistamine used in the treatment of hay fever. It is administered orally.

■ INDICATIONS: When combined with the decongestant pseudoephedrine hydrochloride, it is prescribed in the treatment of allergic rhinitis.

■ CONTRAINDICATIONS: The drug should not be given to patients with known sensitivity to this drug or other alkylamine antihistamines or any components of the formulation. Since pseudoephedrine is a sympathomimetic, the use of this combination is contraindicated in patients using monoamine oxidase inhibitors or in those with severe coronary artery disease or severe hypertension. It is also contraindicated in those with renal insufficiency.

■ ADVERSE EFFECTS: The side effects most often reported include somnolence, headache, dizziness, nervousness, insomnia, tachycardia, palpitations, xerostomia, nausea, and muscle weakness.

acro-, a prefix meaning "extremities": *acrocentric, acrocyanosis.*

acrocentric /akʹrōsenʺtrik/ [Gk, *akron,* extremity, *kentron,* center], pertaining to a chromosome in which the centromere is located near one of the ends so that the arms of the chromosome are extremely uneven in length. Compare **metacentric, submetacentric, telocentric.**

acrocephalosyndactyly /akʹrō-sefʹə-lō-sin-dakʹti-lē/ [L, *acrocephaly + syndactyly*], any of a group of autosomaldominant disorders in which premature fusion of the cranium results in a conical deformity of the skull. Webbed fingers or toes are also present. The term is often used alone to denote Apert syndrome. See also **Apert syndrome.**

acrocephaly. See **oxycephaly.**

acrochordon /akʹrōkôrʺdon/, a benign, pedunculated growth of skin, commonly occurring on the eyelids, neck, axillae, or groin. Also called **skin tag.**

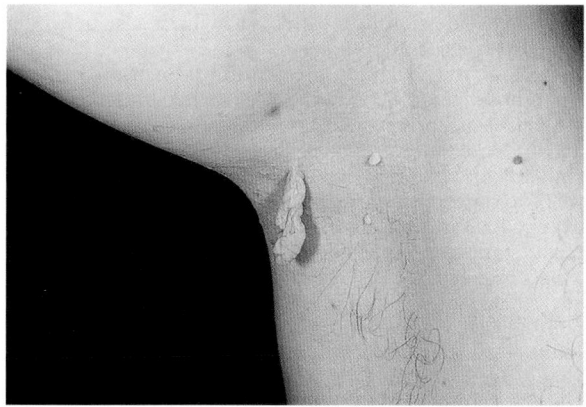

Acrochordon *(Callen et al, 2000)*

acrocyanosis, symmetrical cyanosis of the extremities, with persistent, uneven blue or red discoloration of the skin of the fingers, toes, wrists, or ankles accompanied by sweating or profuse coldness of the digits. Also called **Raynaud sign.**

acrodermatitis /-durʹmətīʹtis/ [Gk, *akron + derma,* skin, *itis,* inflammation], chronic inflammation of the skin of the hands and feet caused by a parasitic mite belonging to the order Acarina.

acrodermatitis enteropathica /enʹtərōpathʺikə/, a rare, chronic disease of infants characterized by vesicles and bullae of the skin and mucous membranes, alopecia, diarrhea, and failure to thrive. An autosomal-recessive disorder of zinc malabsorption, the disease may be lethal if not treated. Zinc sulfate is usually prescribed.

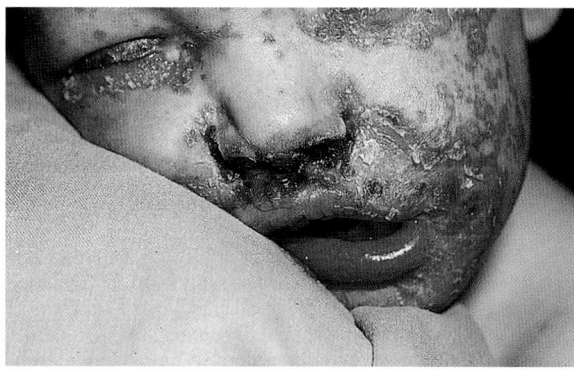

Acrodermatitis enteropathica *(Callen et al, 2000)*

acrodermatitis papulosa infantum. See **Gianotti-Crosti syndrome.**

acrodynia /akʹrōdinʺē·ə/ [Gk, *akron + odyne,* pain], a rare disease occurring in infants and young children caused by heavy metals poisoning, especially mercury poisoning. Symptoms include edema, pruritus, generalized rash, pink coloration of the extremities, scarlet coloration of the cheeks and nose, swollen and painful extremities, cold and clammy skin, profuse sweating, digestive disturbances, photophobia, polyneuritis, extreme irritability alternating with periods of listlessness and apathy, and failure to thrive. Children who have experienced this disorder may have residual health problems as adults. Also called **erythroderma polyneuropathy, Feer disease, Swift disease, pink disease.**

acroesthesia /akʹrō·esthēʺzhə/ [Gk, *akron,* extremity, *aisthesis,* sensation], a condition of increased sensitivity or pain in the hands or feet.

acrokeratosis verruciformis /akʹrōkerʹətōʺsis/, a skin disorder characterized by the appearance of flat, wartlike lesions on the dorsum of the hands and feet and occasionally on the wrists, forearms, and knees. It is an inherited disease, transmitted as a dominant trait. Lesions may transform into squamous cell carcinoma.

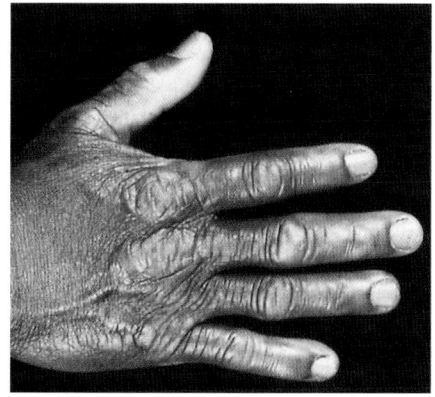

Acrokeratosis verruciformis *(du Vivier, 1993)*

acrokinesis /-kīnēʺsis/ [Gk, *akron,* extremity, *kinesis,* motion], a state in which the limbs possess an abnormally wide range of motion or unusual extension of movement.

acromegalia. See **acromegaly.**

acromegalic eunuchoidism /-məgal″ik/, a rare disorder characterized by genital atrophy and development of female secondary sex characteristics occurring in men with advanced acromegaly caused by a tumor in the anterior pituitary gland. Initially the gonadal function of the anterior lobe may be stimulated, but with the growth of the tumor the patient may become impotent; lose facial, axillary, and pubic hair; and acquire soft skin and a feminine distribution of fat. Also called **retrograde infantilism.**

acromegaly /ak′rəmeg″əlē/ [Gk, *akron* + *megas,* great], a chronic metabolic condition in adults caused by oversecretion of growth hormones by the pituitary gland. It is characterized by gradual, permanent, marked soft tissue enlargement and widening and thickening of skeletal bones in the face, jaw, hands, and feet. Hypertrophy of the vocal cords leads to deepening of the voice. Complications from increased growth hormone levels include atherosclerosis, peripheral neuropathy, hypertension, hyperglycemia, airway obstruction, cardiomyopathy, and visceromegaly involving the salivary glands, liver, spleen, and kidneys. Treatment normally includes radiation, pharmacological agents, or surgery, often involving partial resection of the pituitary gland. Also called **acromegalia.** Compare **gigantism.** *–acromegalic, adj.*

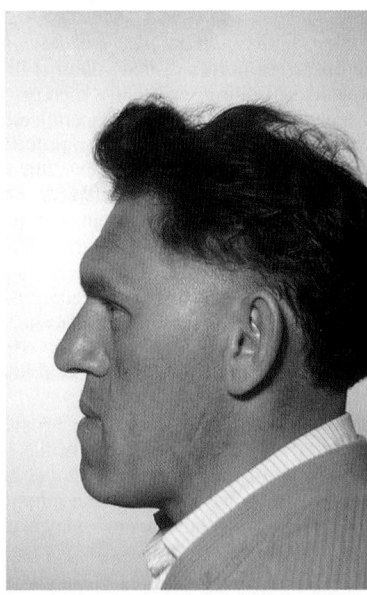

Individual with acromegaly *(Scully, 2014)*

acromial. See **acromion.**

acromicria /ak′rəmik″rē-ə/, an anomaly characterized by abnormally small hands and feet. The person may also possess unusually small facial features, such as the nose and ears, due to a deficiency in pituitary function after puberty.

acromioclavicular articulation /-mī′ōklavik″yələr/, the gliding joint between the acromial end of the clavicle and the medial margin of the acromion of the scapula. It forms the most superior portion of the shoulder. The joint has six ligaments.

acromiocoracoid /-kôr″əkoid/, pertaining to the acromion and coracoid process.

acromiohumeral /-hyoo″mərəl/, pertaining to the acromion and the humerus.

acromion /əkrō″mē·ən/ [Gk, *akron* + *omos,* shoulder], the lateral extension of the spine of the scapula, forming the highest point of the shoulder and connecting with the clavicle at a small oval surface in the middle of the spine. It gives attachment to the deltoid and trapezius muscles. Also called

acromion process. Compare **coracoid process.** *–acromial, adj.*

acromioscapular /-skap″yələr/, pertaining to the acromion and the scapula.

acro-osteolysis /ak′rō·os′tē·ol″isis/, destruction of the digit tips, including the bone, usually caused by vasospasm. It is characterized by loss of bone tissue in the hands, Raynaud's phenomenon, and sensitivity to cold temperatures. Causes include congenital conditions, scleroderma, Raynaud's disease, Buerger's disease, frostbite, and exposure to vinyl chloride.

acroparesthesia /ak′rōpar′isthē″zhə/ [Gk, *akron* + *para,* near, *aisthesis,* feeling], **1.** an extreme sensitivity at the tips of the extremities of the body, caused by nerve compression in the affected area or by polyneuritis. **2.** a disease characterized by tingling, numbness, and stiffness in the extremities, especially in the fingers, hands, and forearms. It sometimes produces pain, pallor, or mild cyanosis. The disease occurs in a simple form, which may produce acrocyanosis, and in an angiospastic form, which may produce gangrene.

acrophobia [Gk, *akron* + *phobos,* fear], a pathological fear or dread of high places that results in extreme anxiety. Psychotherapy attempts to overcome or eliminate the phobic response. See also **obsession, phobia, flooding.**

acrosomal cap, acrosomal head cap. See **acrosome.**

acrosomal reaction /ak″rəsō′məl/, the pattern of various chemical changes that occurs in the anterior of the head of the spermatozoon in response to contact with the ovum and that leads to the sperm's penetration and fertilization of the ovum.

acrosome /ak″rəsōm′/ [Gk, *akron* + *soma,* body], the cap-like structure surrounding the anterior end of the head of a spermatozoon. It is derived from the Golgi apparatus within the cytoplasm and contains degradative enzymes that function in the penetration of the ovum during fertilization. Also called **acrosomal cap, acrosomal head cap.** See also **acrosomal reaction.** *–acrosomal, adj.*

acrotic /əkrot″ik/ [Gk, *a* + *krotos,* not beating], **1.** pertaining to the surface of the body or to the skin glands. **2.** pertaining to an absent or weak pulse.

acryl-, acrylo-, prefixes meaning "acrylic compound."

acrylate, an anion, salt, ester, or conjugate base of acrylic acid. Also called *2-propenoate.*

acrylic acid (CH_2COOH) /əkril″ik/, a corrosive liquid used in the production of the plastic materials used in medical and dental procedures. Also called *2-propenoic acid.*

acrylic resin base, a cold- or heat-cured plastic polymer molded to conform to the tissues of the alveolar process; used to support prosthetic teeth.

acrylic resin dental cement, a free-flowing substance used for restoring or repairing damaged teeth. In powder form it contains polymethyl methacrylate, which acts as a filler, plasticizer, and polymerization initiator. In liquid form it contains methyl methacrylate with an inhibitor and an activator.

ACS, 1. abbreviation for *American Cancer Society.* **2.** abbreviation for *American Chemical Society.* **3.** abbreviation for **American College of Surgeons. 4.** abbreviation for **acute confusional state. 5.** abbreviation for *Association of Clinical Scientists.* **6.** abbreviation for **abdominal compartment syndrome.**

ACSM, abbreviation for *American College of Sports Medicine.*

act-, a prefix meaning "to do, drive, act": *action, activate.*

ACTH, abbreviation for **adrenocorticotropic hormone.**

Acthar, an adrenocorticotropic hormone injection. Brand name for **ACTH, corticotropin.**

-actide, a combining form designating a synthetic corticotropin.

actigraph /ak″tigraf′/, any instrument that records changes in the activity of a substance or an organism and produces a graphic record of the process, such as an electrocardiograph.

actin, a protein forming the thin filaments in muscle fibers that are pulled on by myosin cross-bridges to cause a muscle contraction. See also **myosin.**

actin-. See **actino-, actin-.**

acting out, the expression of intrapsychic conflict or painful emotion through overt behavior that is usually pathological, defensive, and unconscious and that may be destructive or dangerous. In controlled situations such as psychodrama, Gestalt therapy, or play therapy, this behavior may be therapeutic in that it may serve to reveal to the patient the underlying conflict governing the behavior. See also **transference.**

actinic /aktin″ik/ [Gk, *aktis,* ray], pertaining to radiation, such as sunlight or x-rays.

actinic burn, a burn caused by exposure to sunlight or another source of ultraviolet radiation.

actinic conjunctivitis [Gk, *aktis,* ray, + L, *conjunctivus,* connecting; Gk, *itis,* inflammation], an inflammation of the conjunctiva caused by exposure to the ultraviolet radiation of sunlight or other sources, such as acetylene torches, therapeutic lamps (sunlamps), and klieg lights. Also called **actinic ophthalmia.**

actinic dermatitis, a skin inflammation or rash resulting from exposure to sunlight, x-ray, or radiation. Chronic or recurrent actinic dermatitis can predispose to skin cancer. See also **actinic keratosis.**

actinic keratosis, a slowly developing, localized thickening and scaling of the outer layers of the skin as a result of chronic, prolonged exposure to the sun. It is more common in the fair skinned and elderly. It usually is a discrete, slightly raised, red-on-pink lesion located on a sun-exposed surface. Treatment of this premalignant lesion includes surgical excision, cryotherapy, and topical chemotherapy. Also called **senile keratosis, senile wart, solar keratosis.**

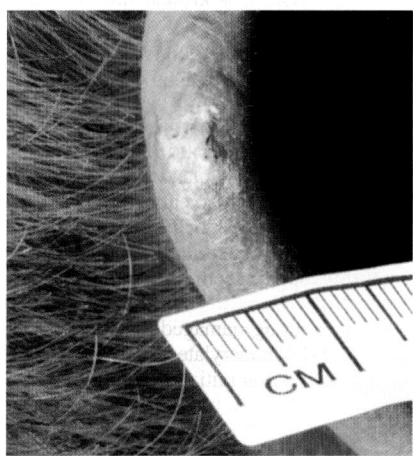

Actinic keratosis *(Walker and Colledge, 2015)*

actinic ophthalmia. See **actinic conjunctivitis.**

actinism, the ability of sunlight or similar forms of radiation to produce chemical changes.

actinium (Ac), a rare, radioactive metallic element. Its atomic number is 89; its atomic mass is 227. It occurs in some ores of uranium.

actino-, actin-, prefixes meaning "ray" or "radiation": *actinic, actinotherapy.*

Actinobacillus /ak″tinōbasil″əs/, a genus of small gram-negative bacillus, with members that are pathogenic for humans

and other animals. The species *Actinobacillus actinomycetemcomitans* is the cause of actinomycosis in humans.

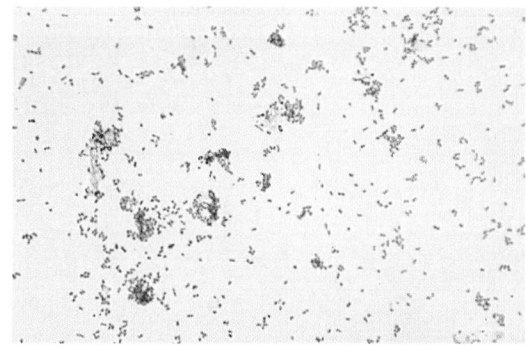

Actinobacillus *(Mahon, Lehman, and Manuselis, 2007)*

Actinomyces /ak″tinōmī″sēz/ [Gk, *aktis,* ray, *mykes,* fungus], a genus of anaerobic or facultative anaerobic, gram-positive bacteria. Species that may cause disease in humans, such as *Actinomyces israelii* (which causes actinomycosis), are normally present in the mouth and throat. Disease activity is normally limited to periodontal disease.

actinomycin A, the first of a group of chromopeptide antibiotic agents derived from soil bacteria. Most are derivatives of phenoxazine and contain actinocin. They are generally active against gram-positive and gram-negative bacteria and some fungi. Because of their cytotoxic properties, they are effective for certain types of neoplasms. See also **dactinomycin.**

actinomycin B, an antibiotic antineoplastic agent derived from *Actinomyces antibioticus.*

actinomycin D. See **dactinomycin.**

actinomycosis /ak″tinōmīkō″sis/, a chronic bacterial disease most frequently located in the jaw, thorax, or abdomen. It is characterized by deep, lumpy abscesses that extrude a thin, granular pus through multiple sinuses. The disease occurs worldwide but is seen most frequently in those who live in rural areas. It is not spread from person to person or from animals to humans. The most common causative organism in humans is *Actinomyces israelii,* a normal inhabitant of the bowel and mouth. Disease occurs after tissue damage, usually in the presence of another infectious organism. It can be diagnosed by microscopic identification of sulfur granules, pathognomonic of *Actinomyces,* in the exudate. There are several forms of actinomycosis. Orocervicofacial actinomycosis occurs with the spread of the bacterium into the subcutaneous tissues of the mouth, throat, and neck as a result of dental or tonsillar infection. Thoracic actinomycosis may represent proliferation of the organism from cervicofacial abscesses into the esophagus, or it may result from inhalation of the bacterium into the bronchi. Abdominal actinomycosis usually follows an acute inflammatory process in the stomach or intestines, such as appendicitis, diverticulum of the large bowel, or a perforation found in the groin or another area that drains exudate into the stomach. A large mass may be palpated, and sinus tracts from abscesses deep in the abdomen may form. Pelvic actinomycosis is most commonly associated with intrauterine devices. Central nervous system actinomycosis is a rare cause of brain abscess. Bacterial endocarditis is very rarely caused by actinobacillus infection. Musculoskeletal actinomycosis involves subcutaneous tissue, muscle, and bone. Disseminated *Actinomycosis* follows hematogenous spread of the infection and may involve the skin, brain, liver, and urogenital system. All forms of actinomycosis are treated with at least 6 weeks of daily injections of penicillin in large doses. Abdominal actinomycosis can be cured in 40% of cases, thoracic actinomycosis in 80%, and orocervicofacial actinomycosis in 90%.

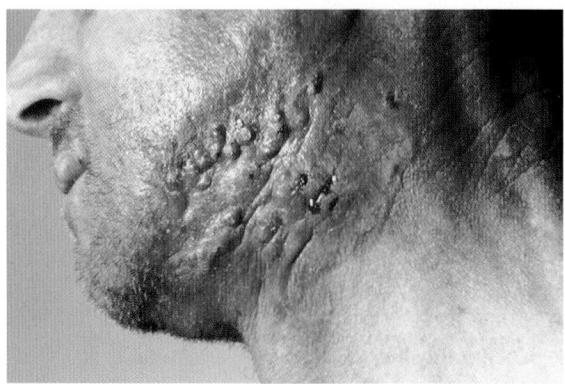

Actinomycosis *(Courtesy Professor I. Brook)*

actinomyosin, the complex consisting of parallel threads of actin and myosin proteins that constitutes muscle fibers. It is responsible for the contraction and relaxation of muscle. When a muscle fiber contracts, the two proteins slide past each other, shortening the fiber while increasing its apparent thickness. Also called **actomyosin.** See also **sliding filaments.**

actinotherapy, the use of ultraviolet light, other parts of the spectrum of the sun's rays, or x-rays to treat various disorders, particularly skin diseases.

action, **1.** an activity or exertion of power used to carry out a function or produce an effect. **2.** movement that is produced when a muscle contracts. For example, the action of the flexor carpi ulnaris (FCU) muscle is to flex and ulnarly deviate the wrist.

action current. See **action potential.**

action level, the level of concentration at which an undesirable or toxic component of a food or beverage is considered dangerous enough to public health to warrant government prohibition of the sale of that food. The U.S. Food and Drug Administration tests foods for action levels.

action potential, an electric impulse consisting of a self-propagating series of polarizations and depolarizations, transmitted across the plasma membranes of a nerve fiber during the transmission of a nerve impulse and across the plasma membranes of a muscle cell during contraction or another activity. In the absence of an impulse, the inside is electrically negative and the outside is positive (the resting potential). During the passage of an impulse at any point on the nerve fiber, the inside becomes positive and the outside, negative. Also called **action current.**

action therapies, treatments that stress change in inappropriate behavior by taking a specific action. Also called *action-oriented therapy.* Compare **talk therapy.**

action tremor [L, *agere,* to do, *tremor,* shaking], a slight shaking that occurs or is evident during voluntary movements of the upper extremities. Also called **intention tremor.**

Activase, a commercial form of tissue plasminogen activator. Brand name for **alteplase.**

activate, to begin a process or procedure that initiates an action. See **activation.**

activated charcoal, a general-purpose emergency antidote and a powerful pharmaceutic adsorbent.

■ INDICATIONS: It is prescribed in the treatment of acute poisoning and the control of flatulence.

■ CONTRAINDICATIONS: There are no known contraindications, but activated charcoal is ineffective in poisoning caused by a strong acid or an alkali, cyanide, organic solvents, ethanol, methanol, iron, and lithium. It should not be administered by mouth to unconscious persons.

■ ADVERSE EFFECTS: There are no known adverse effects.

activated clotting time (ACT) test, a blood test primarily used to monitor high doses of unfractionated (standard) heparin as an anticoagulant during cardiac angioplasty, hemodialysis, and cardiopulmonary bypass. It can also be used to monitor the dose of protamine sulfate required to reverse the effect of heparin. The test measures the time required for whole blood to clot after the addition of particulate activators.

activated 7-dehydrocholesterol. See **vitamin D$_3$.**

activated partial thromboplastin time (APTT). See **partial thromboplastin time.**

activated prothrombin complex concentrate (APCC), a therapeutic concentrate of activated coagulation factors II, VII, IX, and X, used to treat patients with hemophilia who have developed coagulation factor inhibitors, usually anticoagulation factor VIII or IX.

activated resin. See **self-curing resin.**

activated sludge process, the treatment of sewage using a combination of bacteria and air.

activating enzyme, an enzyme that promotes or sustains an activity, such as catalyzing the combination of amino acids to form peptides or proteins.

activation /ak′tivā″shən/, the promotion or production of an activity or process.

activation energy [L, *activus,* active], the energy required to convert reactants to transition-state species or an activated complex that will spontaneously proceed to products.

activation factor. See **factor XII.**

activator /ak″tivā′tər/, **1.** a substance, force, or device that stimulates activity in another substance or structure, especially a substance that activates an enzyme. **2.** a substance that stimulates the development of an anatomical structure in the embryo. **3.** an internal secretion of the pancreas. **4.** an apparatus for making substances radioactive, such as a cyclotron or neutron generator. **5.** (in dentistry) a removable orthodontic appliance that functions as a passive transmitter and stimulator of the perioral muscles.

active algolagnia. See **sadism.**

active anaphylaxis [Gk, *ana,* up, *phylaxis,* protection], hypersensitivity caused by the reaction of the immune system to the injection of a foreign protein. Compare **anaphylaxis.**

active assisted exercise [L, *activus*], the movement of the body or any of its parts primarily through the individual's own efforts but accompanied by the aid of a member of the health care team or some device, such as an exercise machine. See also **active exercise, passive exercise.**

active carrier [OFr, *carier*], a person without signs or symptoms of an infectious disease who carries the causal microorganisms and can transmit the disease to others.

active electrode [Gk, *elektron,* amber, *hodos,* way], an electrode that is applied at a specific point to produce stimulation in a concentrated area in electrotherapy or electrocautery.

active euthanasia, the ending of life by the deliberate administration of lethal agents by an individual other than the patient.

active exercise, an unassisted effort by an individual to engage in activity, exercise, or repetitive motion that causes voluntary contraction and relaxation of the muscles and movement of the body. Compare **passive exercise.** See also **aerobic exercise, anaerobic exercise.**

active expiration [L, *expirare,* to breathe out], a forced exhalation using the abdominal wall, internal intercostal muscles, and diaphragm.

active hyperemia [L, *activus* + Gk, *hyper,* excessive, *haima,* blood], the increased flow of blood into a particular body part, caused by an increase in vasoactive metabolites. It is associated with increased metabolism.

active immunity, a form of long-term acquired immunity. It protects the body against a new infection as the result of antibodies or T-cell mediated immunity that develops naturally after exposure to an infectious agent or artificially after a vaccination. Over time antibody counts may wane, resulting in the need for repeat vaccination or a "booster shot." Compare **passive immunity.** See also **acquired immunity, immune response, natural immunity.**

active labor [L, *activus,* active, *labor,* work], the second portion of the first stage of labor, characterized by rapid dilation and effacement, usually between 4 cm and near complete (10 cm) dilation. The progress of dilation is traditionally approximately 1 cm/hr in nulliparae and 1 to 2 cm/hr in multiparae in unfacilitated labor. See also **Friedman curve, labor.**

active listening, the act of alert and intentional hearing, interpretation, and demonstration of an interest in what a person has to say through verbal signal, nonverbal gestures, and body language.

active matrix array (AMA), a large-area integrated circuit that consists of millions of identical semiconductor elements and acts as the flat-panel image receptor in digital radiographic and fluoroscopic systems.

active movement, the movement of parts of the body as a result of voluntary muscle effort. Compare **passive movement.**

active-passive, (in psychiatry) a concept that characterizes persons as either actively involved in shaping events, such as being proactive, or passively reacting to them, such as being reactive.

active phase of labor, the stage of labor in which the cervix will dilate from 4 to 7 cm. Contractions during this phase will last about 45 to 60 seconds, with 3 to 5 minutes of rest between contractions.

active play, any activity from which one derives amusement, entertainment, enjoyment, or satisfaction by taking a participatory rather than a passive role. Children of all age groups engage in various forms of active play, from the exploration of objects and toys by the infant and toddler to the formal games, sports, and hobbies of the older child. Compare **passive play.**

active range of motion (AROM), the range of movement through which a patient can actively (without assistance) move a joint. Movement occurs because of the contraction of skeletal muscle(s). Movement may be measured in degrees using a goniometer. Compare **passive range of motion.**

active resistance exercise, the movement or exertion of the body or any of its parts performed totally through the individual's own efforts against a resisting force. See also **progressive resistance exercise.**

active resistance training (ART), a conditioning or rehabilitation program designed to enhance a patient's muscular strength, power, and endurance through progressive active resistance exercises and muscle overloading. Examples of this type of conditioning include push-ups and squats.

active sensitization [L, *agere,* to do, *sentire,* to feel], an immune response that is antibody-mediated and occurs as a result of a specific antigen being injected, ingested, or inhaled into the individual. This sensitizes the individual so that subsequent exposure to the same antigen elicits an immune response. See also **sensitization.**

active site, the place on the surface of an enzyme where its catalytic action occurs.

active specific immunotherapy, a therapy that attempts to stimulate specific antitumor responses with tumor-associated antigens as the immunizing materials.

active transport, the movement of materials across the membranes and epithelial layers of a cell by means of chemical activity that allows the cell to admit otherwise impermeable molecules against a concentration gradient. Expediting active transport are carrier molecules within the cell that bind and enclose themselves to incoming molecules. Active transport is the means by which the cell absorbs glucose and other substances needed to sustain life and health. Certain enzymes play a role in active transport, providing a chemical "pump" that typically uses adenosine triphosphate (ATP) to help move substances through the plasma membrane. Compare **osmosis, passive transport.**

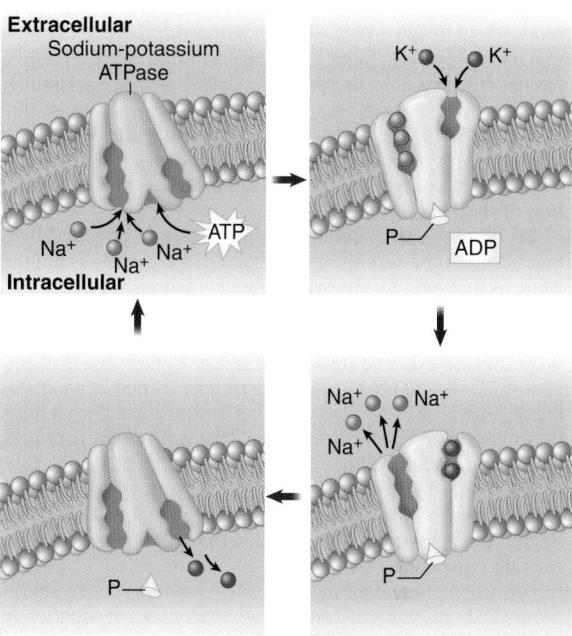

Active transport: the sodium-potassium pump
(Thibodeau and Patton, 2010)

activities of daily living (ADL) /aktiv″itēz/, activities oriented toward taking care of one's own body, such as bathing or showering, toileting and toilet hygiene, dressing, swallowing/eating, feeding, functional mobility, personal device care, personal hygiene and grooming, and sexual activity. Also referred to as basic activities of daily living (BADLs) and personal activities of daily living (PADLs).

activity, **1.** movements and or behaviors, as in something accomplished or planned. **2.** (in chemistry) the action of an enzyme on an amount of substrate that is converted to product per unit of time under defined conditions. **3.** (in occupational therapy) a pursuit and/or class of actions that is culturally recognized and defined, as the activity of shopping or the activity of playing cards.

activity analysis, the systematic process of identifying the subparts and/or steps needed to complete an activity and examining these components to determine the performance skills needed to complete the activity. This process includes identifying the physical, perceptual, cognitive, psychological, social, and cultural factors inherent in completing a specific activity or occupation. It is an essential skill of the occupational therapist, used to identify areas where the activity (or the environment within which the activity occurs) can be modified or adapted to enhance performance.

activity coefficient, a proportionality constant, γ, relating activity, α, to concentration, *c,* expressed in the equation, $\alpha = \gamma c$.

activity demands, the features of a task that influence the type and nature of effort required to successfully carry out the task (activity). Identifying the physical, cognitive, perceptual, and/or psychosocial requirements inherent in task completion is a necessary precursor to developing strategies that can enhance task or activity performance.

activity theory, (in aging) a concept proposed by Robert J. Havighurst [1900–1990] that continuing activities from middle age promotes well-being and satisfaction in aging. Thus older adults who are actively involved in a variety of situations and who establish new roles and relationships are more likely to age with a sense of satisfaction.

activity tolerance, the type and amount of exercise a patient may be able to perform without undue exertion or possible injury.

actomyosin /ak′təmī″əsin/. See **actinomyosin.**

actual cautery /ak″chŏŏ·əl/ [L, *actus,* act], the application of heat, rather than a chemical substance, in the destruction of tissue or to stop bleeding.

actual charge, the amount actually charged or billed by a practitioner for a service. The actual charge usually is not the same as that paid for the service by an insurance plan.

actualization, **1.** the fulfillment of a potential, as by a person who may develop capabilities through experience and education. **2.** the fulfillment of the highest level of human needs based on Maslow's hierarchy of needs. *−actualize, v.*

acu-, a combining form meaning "sharp," "clear," or "needle": *acuity, acupuncture.*

acuity /əkyŏŏ′itē/ [L, *acuere,* to sharpen], **1.** the clearness or sharpness of perception, such as visual acuity. **2.** the degree of illness, often used to determine staffing levels for nursing personnel.

acuminate /ə·kyŏŏ′mi·nāt/ [L, *acuminatus*], **1.** sharp-pointed. **2.** to sharpen something or to make it smaller in diameter with an increased length.

acuminate wart. See **genital wart.**

acupressure /ak″yəpresh″ər/ [L, *acus,* needle, *pressura,* pressure], a therapeutic technique of applying pressure with the fingers, beads, bracelets, or pellets in a specified way on designated points on the body to relieve pain, produce anesthesia, or regulate a body function.

acupressure needle, **1.** a slender pointed device used for insertion and manipulation at acupressure points to improve health and well-being. **2.** any of several needles inserted near a source of bleeding to help control blood loss. The needles exert pressure on tissues adjacent to the damaged vessel.

acupuncture /ak″yəpunk″chər/ [L, *acus* + *punctura,* puncture], a method of producing analgesia or altering the function of a body system by inserting fine, wire-thin needles into the skin at specific body sites along a series of lines, or channels, called meridians. Acupuncture is highly effective in treating both acute and chronic pain associated with multiple causes. It is effective for nausea associated with chemotherapy, or postoperatively. The efficacy and safety of acupuncture for the treatment of a wide variety of physical and psychological disorders are being explored by researchers in the health care community. *−acupuncturist, n.*

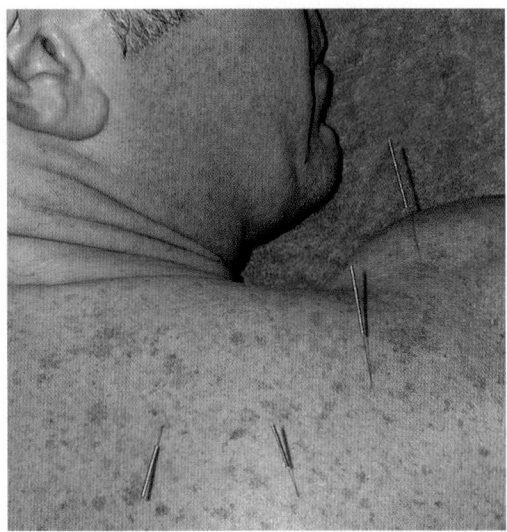

Individual receiving acupuncture *(Walker et al, 2014)*

acupuncture point, one of many discrete points on the skin along the several meridians (channels), or chains of points of the body. Stimulation of any of the various points affects the nervous system in a variety of ways. Also called *acupoints.*

acute /əkyŏŏt″/ [L, *acutus,* sharp], **1.** (of a disease or disease symptoms) beginning abruptly with marked intensity or sharpness, then subsiding after a relatively short period. **2.** sharp or severe. Compare **chronic.**

acute abdomen, an abnormal condition characterized by the acute onset of severe pain within the abdominal cavity. An acute abdomen requires immediate evaluation and diagnosis because it may indicate a condition that calls for surgical intervention. Information about the onset, duration, character, location, and symptoms associated with the pain is critical in making an accurate diagnosis. The patient is asked what decreases or increases the pain; constant, increasing pain is generally associated with appendicitis and diverticulitis, whereas intermittent pain more likely indicates an intestinal obstruction, ureteral calculi, or biliary calculi. Appendicitis may often be differentiated from a perforating ulcer by the slower onset or development of pain. Although the patient's report of the location of the pain is sometimes misleading because of referral, radiation, or reflection of pain, it may serve to identify a specific organ or system. Factors in the patient's history that are useful in the diagnosis and management of an acute abdomen include changes in bowel habits, weight loss, bloody stool, diarrhea, menses, vomiting, clay-colored stool, and previous abdominal surgery. Also called **surgical abdomen.** See also **abdominal pain.**

acute articular rheumatism. See **rheumatic fever.**

acute abscess, a recently formed collection of pus with little or no fibrosis in the wall of the cavity. It is accompanied by localized inflammation, pain, fever, and swelling. See also **abscess.**

acute ascending myelitis [L, *ascendere,* to go up; Gk, *myelos,* marrow, *itis,* inflammation], a severe inflammation of the spinal cord that extends progressively upward with corresponding interference in nerve functions. See also **myelitis.**

acute ascending spinal paralysis, a severe progressive spinal paralysis that spreads upward toward the brain.

acute air trapping, a condition of bronchiolar obstruction that results in early airway closure and trapping of air distal to the affected bronchiole. Air trapping can occur in persons with chronic obstructive pulmonary disease or asthma. Persons prone to episodes of acute air trapping learn to control expirations through pursed-lip breathing.

acute alcoholism, intoxication resulting from excessive consumption of alcoholic beverages. The syndrome is temporary and is characterized by depression of the higher nerve centers, causing impaired motor control, stupor, lack of coordination, and often nausea, dehydration, headache, and other physical symptoms. Compare **chronic alcoholism.** See also **alcoholism.**

acute atrophic paralysis [Gk, *a, trophe,* without nourishment, *paralyein,* to be palsied], a severe poliomyelitis involving the anterior horns of the spinal cord. It results first in flaccid paralysis of involved muscle groups and later in atrophy of those muscles.

acute angle [L, *acutus + angulus*], any angle of less than 90 degrees.

acute bacterial arthritis. See **septic arthritis.**

acute bronchitis. See **bronchitis.**

acute anicteric hepatitis [Gk, *a,* without, *ikteros,* jaundice, *hēpar,* liver, *itis,* inflammation], an acute hepatitis not accompanied by jaundice.

acute anterior poliomyelitis, an acute viral disease marked by inflammation of the anterior cornu (horn) of the spinal cord caused by poliomyelitis. Signs and symptoms include fever, pain, gastrointestinal disturbance, flaccid paralysis, and atrophy of muscular groups. See also **acute infectious paralysis.**

acute care, a pattern of health care in which a patient is treated for a brief but severe episode of illness, for the sequelae of an accident or other trauma, or during recovery from surgery. Acute care is usually given in a hospital by specialized personnel using complex and sophisticated technical equipment and materials, and it may involve intensive or emergency care. This pattern of care is often necessary for only a short time, unlike chronic care.

acute catarrhal sinusitis [Gk, *kata + rhoia,* flow; L, *sinus,* hollow], an inflammation that involves the nose and sinuses.

acute cervicitis, infection of the cervix marked by redness, edema, and bleeding on contact. Symptoms do not always occur but may include any or all of the following: copious, foul-smelling discharge from the vagina; pelvic pressure or pain; scant bleeding with intercourse; and itching or burning of the external genitalia. The principal causative organisms are *Trichomonas vaginalis*; *Candida albicans*; gonococcus, *Staphylococcus,* and *Streptococcus* species; and *Haemophilus vaginalis*. Diagnosis is by microscopic examination, confirmed in some cases by culture and Papanicolaou (Pap) smear. Specific antimicrobial medication may be effective. Acute cervicitis tends to be a recurrent problem because of reexposure to the germ, undertreatment, or predisposing factors such as human immunodeficiency virus infection, multiple sexual partners, or poor nutrition. See **cervicitis.**

acute childhood leukemia, a progressive, malignant disease of the blood-forming tissues. It is characterized by the uncontrolled proliferation of immature leukocytes and their precursors, particularly in the bone marrow, spleen, and lymph nodes. It is the most frequent cancer in children, with a peak onset occurring between 2 and 5 years of age. Cure rates are high. See also **acute lymphocytic leukemia, acute myeloid leukemia, leukemia.**

acute cholecystitis. See **cholecystitis.**

acute circulatory failure /sur″kyələtôr′ē/, a decrease in cardiac output resulting from cardiac or noncardiac causes and leading to tissue hypoxia. Acute circulatory failure usually happens so rapidly that the body does not have time to adjust to the changes. If not controlled immediately, the condition usually progresses to shock.

acute circumscribed edema [L, *circum,* around, *scribere,* to draw; Gk, *oidema,* swelling], a localized area of swelling or fluid retention, often associated with an inflammatory lesion or process.

acute compression syndrome. See **Beck's triad.**

acute confusional state (ACS), a form of delirium caused by interference with the metabolic or other biochemical processes essential for normal brain functioning. Symptoms may include disturbances in cognition and levels of awareness, short-term memory deficit, retrograde and anterograde amnesia, and disturbances in orientation, accompanied by restlessness, apprehension, irritability, and apathy. The condition may be associated with an acute physiological state, delirium, toxic psychosis, or acute brain syndrome which constitutes a medical emergency.

acute coronary syndrome, a term encompassing clinical presentations ranging from unstable angina through myocardial infarctions in which there is an interruption in the blood supply to the heart muscle.

acute delirium, an episode of acute organic reaction that is sudden, severe, and transient. Constitutes a medical emergency. See also **delirium.**

acute diarrhea [Gk, *dia + rhein,* to flow], a sudden severe attack of loose stools.

acute diffuse peritonitis [L, *diffundere,* to pour out; Gk, *peri,* near, *tenein,* to stretch, *itis,* inflammation], an acute widespread attack of peritonitis affecting most of the peritoneum and usually caused by infection or by a perforation of an abdominal organ (e.g., stomach or appendix). It is also a complication of peritoneal dialysis. Also called **generalized peritonitis.**

acute disease, a disease characterized by a relatively sudden onset of symptoms that are usually severe. An episode of acute disease results in recovery to a state comparable to the patient's condition of health and activity before the disease, in passage into a chronic phase, or in death. Examples are pneumonia and appendicitis. See also **chronic disease.**

acute disseminated encephalitis. See **acute disseminated encephalomyelitis.**

acute disseminated encephalomyelitis (ADEM), an acute disease of the brain and spinal cord with variable symptoms. It is thought to be an allergic reaction or immune attack resulting in inflammation that damages myelin tissue. Early symptoms may include fever, headache, vomiting, and drowsiness and progress to seizures, coma, and paralysis. It may be misdiagnosed as a severe attack of multiple sclerosis. Frequently patients who recover experience neurological disorders. Also called **acute disseminated encephalitis.**

acute diverticulitis, a sudden, severe, and painful disorder of the large intestine resulting from inflammation of one or more diverticula, or small pouches, in the wall of the bowel. The condition is typically diagnosed through x-rays and treated with antibiotics and/or surgically. If left untreated, the inflamed pouches may rupture, spilling fecal matter into the abdominal cavity and causing peritonitis.

acute endarteritis. See **endarteritis.**

acute epiglottitis, a severe, rapidly progressing bacterial infection of the epiglottis that can occur at any age but primarily occurring in young children between 2 and 7 years of age. It is characterized by sore throat, croupy stridor, and an inflamed epiglottis, which may cause sudden respiratory obstruction and possibly death. Symptoms also include fever and difficulty swallowing and breathing. The infection is generally caused by *Haemophilus influenzae,* type B, although streptococci may occasionally be the causative agents. Transmission occurs via infection with airborne particles or contact with infected secretions. Compare **croup.**

■ OBSERVATIONS: The diagnosis is made by bacteriological identification of *H. influenzae,* type B, in a specimen taken from the upper respiratory tract or in the blood. A lateral x-ray film of the neck shows an enlarged epiglottis and distension of the hypopharynx, which distinguishes the condition from croup. Direct visualization of the inflamed, cherry-red epiglottis by depression of the tongue or indirect laryngoscopy is also diagnostic but may produce total acute obstruction and should be attempted only by trained personnel with equipment to establish an airway or to provide respiratory resuscitation, if necessary.

■ INTERVENTIONS: Establishment of an airway is urgent, either by endotracheal intubation or by tracheostomy. Humidity and oxygen are provided, and airway secretions are drained or suctioned. IV fluids are usually required, and antibiotic therapy is initiated immediately. Steroids are useful.

■ PATIENT CARE CONSIDERATIONS: Intensive nursing care is required for a child with acute epiglottitis. The most acute phase of the condition passes within 24 to 48 hours, and intubation is rarely needed beyond 3 to 4 days. As the child responds to therapy, breathing becomes easier; rapid recovery usually occurs, so bed rest and quiet activity to relieve boredom become primary concerns for the health care team.

acute erosive gastritis. See **erosive gastritis.**

acute febrile neutrophilic dermatosis. See **Sweet syndrome.**

acute febrile polyneuritis. See **Guillain-Barré syndrome.**

acute fibrinous pericarditis [L, *fibra,* fibrous; Gk, *peri,* near, *kardia,* heart, *itis,* inflammation], an acute inflammation of the endothelial cells of the pericardium with fibers extending into the pericardial sac.

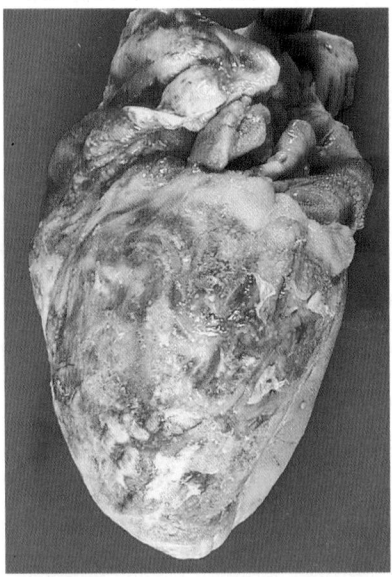

Acute fibrinous pericarditis *(Damjanov, 2012)*

acute focal bacterial nephritis. See **pyelonephritis.**

acute gastritis. See **gastritis.**

acute glaucoma, a serious eye condition that causes an increase in intraocular pressure. See **glaucoma.**

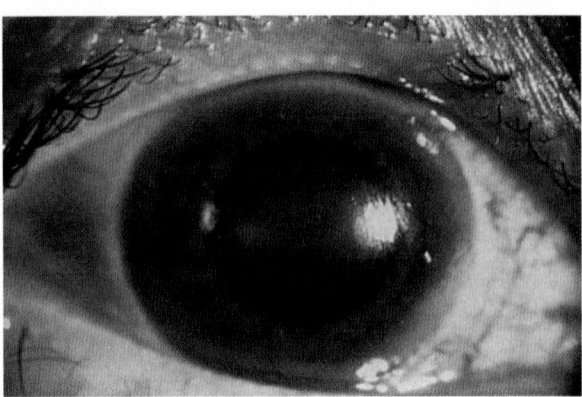

Acute glaucoma (primary closed-angle) *(Bertolini and Pelucio, 1995)*

acute glomerulonephritis. See **postinfectious glomerulonephritis.**

acute goiter [L, *guttur,* throat], a sudden enlargement of the thyroid gland. Clinical manifestations may include visible or palpable swelling at the base of the anterior neck, a tight feeling in the throat, cough, hoarseness, or difficulty swallowing or breathing.

acute granulocytic leukemia (AGL). See **acute myeloid leukemia.**

acute hallucinatory paranoia, a form of psychosis in which hallucinations are combined with the delusions of paranoia.

acute hallucinosis. See **alcoholic hallucinosis.**

acute hemorrhagic conjunctivitis, a highly contagious eye disease usually caused by enterovirus type 70 but also by coxsackie virus AZA. The disease is found primarily in densely populated humid areas, particularly developing countries or places with large immigrant populations. Clinical features include a sudden onset of severe ocular pain, blurred vision, photophobia, subconjunctival hemorrhage, chemosis, swelling of the eyelid, and a profuse watery discharge from the eye. Symptoms are caused by neutralizing antibodies to infection. A polymerase chain reaction analysis of conjunctival swab specimens from patients is a rapid method of identification of the infectious agent. Spontaneous improvement occurs within 2 to 4 days and is complete by 7 to 10 days. Management consists of hygienic measures and ophthalmic preparations.

acute hemorrhagic leukoencephalitis. See **acute necrotizing hemorrhagic encephalopathy.**

acute hemorrhagic pancreatitis [Gk, *haima,* blood, *rhegnynei,* to gush, *pan,* all, *kreas,* flesh], a potentially fatal inflammation of the pancreas characterized by bleeding, necrosis, and paralysis of the digestive tract.

acute hypoxia, a sudden or rapid depletion in available oxygen at the tissue level. The condition may result from asphyxia, airway obstruction, acute hemorrhage, blockage of alveoli by edema or infectious exudate, or abrupt cardiorespiratory failure. Clinical signs may include hypoventilation or hyperventilation to the point of air hunger and neurological deficits ranging from headache and confusion to loss of consciousness. Compare **chronic hypoxia.**

acute idiopathic polyneuritis. See **Guillain-Barré syndrome.**

acute illness, any illness characterized by signs and symptoms of rapid onset and short duration. It may be severe and impair normal functioning.

acute infectious paralysis [L, *inficere,* to stain; Gk, *paralyein,* to be palsied], acute disease caused by a poliovirus. Symptoms of minor disease include fever, headache, vomiting, sore throat, and frequently stiff back and neck. Major disease includes central nervous system involvement, pleocytosis in spinal fluid, and paralysis. Also called **acute anterior poliomyelitis.**

acute infective hepatitis.   See **hepatitis A.**

acute intermittent porphyria (AIP), an autosomal-dominant, genetically transmitted metabolic hepatic disorder caused by a deficiency of hydroxymethylbilane synthase. It is characterized by acute attacks of neurological dysfunction that can be started by environmental or endogenous factors. Women are affected more frequently than men, and attacks often are precipitated by starvation or severe dieting, alcohol ingestion, bacterial or viral infections, and a wide range of pharmaceutical products. Any part of the nervous system can be affected, and an initial common effect is mild to severe abdominal pain. Other effects can include tachycardia, hypertension, hyponatremia, peripheral neuropathy, and organic brain dysfunction marked by seizures, coma, hallucinations, and respiratory paralysis. A frequent diagnostic factor is a high level of porphyrin precursors in the urine, which usually increases during periods of acute attacks. Treatment is generally symptomatic, with emphasis on respiratory support, beta-blockers, and pain control. Education of the patient focuses on environmental factors, particularly medications such as barbiturates, that are known to cause an onset of symptoms, as well as avoidance of alcohol, sunlight, and skin trauma. A high-carbohydrate diet is reported to reduce the risk of acute attacks because glucose tends to block the induction of hepatic gamma-aminolevulinic acid synthetase, an enzyme involved in the porphyrias. Also called **intermittent acute porphyria.** See also **porphyria.**

acute laryngotracheobronchitis.   See **croup.**

acute lichenoid pityriasis.   See **Mucha-Habermann disease.**

acute lobar pneumonia, a form of pneumonia that can involve one or more lobes of the lung, characterized by a sudden onset, chills, fever, difficulty breathing, pleuritic chest pain, dry cough, rust-colored (blood-stained) sputum, and consolidation of the serofibrous fluid exuded by the alveoli. Most commonly, the condition results from infection by a virulent type of *Streptococcus pneumoniae.*

acute lymphoblastic leukemia (ALL), a hematologic, malignant disease characterized by large numbers of lymphoblasts in the bone marrow, circulating blood, lymph nodes, spleen, liver, and other organs. The number of normal blood cells is usually reduced. More than three fourths of cases in the United States occur in children, with the greatest number diagnosed between 2 and 5 years of age. The risk of the disease is increased for people with Down syndrome and for siblings of leukemia patients. Also called **acute lymphocytic leukemia.**

■ OBSERVATIONS: The disease has a sudden onset and rapid progression marked by fever, pallor, anorexia, fatigue, anemia, hemorrhage, bone pain, splenomegaly, and recurrent infection. Blood and bone marrow studies are used for diagnosis and for determination of the type of proliferating lymphocyte, which may be B cells, T cells (which usually respond poorly to therapy), or null cells that lack T or B cell characteristics.

■ INTERVENTIONS: Treatment includes intensive combination chemotherapy, therapy for secondary infections and hyperuricemia, and intrathecal methotrexate.

■ PATIENT CARE CONSIDERATIONS: The diagnosis of leukemia usually causes fear and anxiety. The coordinated support of the health care team is essential. When the patient is a child, it is important to determine the child's stage of development and relationships with parents, caregivers, or grandparents, in addition to preventing infection and monitoring the impact of medications and the the effect of the disease itself. Establishing a plan that includes age-appropriate activities, as well as including the patient and family in planning, will facilitate adjustment and maintenance of the quality of life for patients of all ages.

acute lymphocytic leukemia (ALL).   Also called **acute lymphoblastic leukemia.** See also **chronic lymphocytic leukemia.**

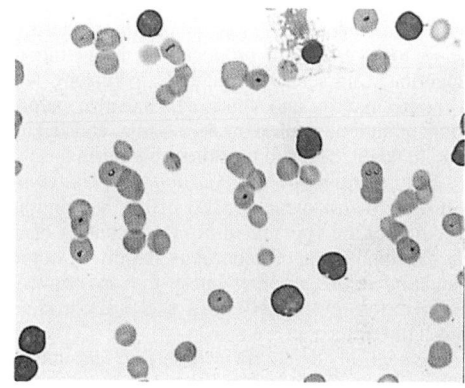

Acute lymphocytic leukemia *(Zitelli and Davis, 2012)*

acute lymphoid leukemia (ALL).   See **acute childhood leukemia.**

acute mountain sickness.   See **altitude sickness.**

acute myelitis, a sudden, severe inflammation of the spinal cord with a risk of permanent disability. See also **myelitis.**

acute myeloid leukemia (AML), a malignant neoplasm of blood-forming tissues characterized by the uncontrolled proliferation of immature granular leukocytes that usually have azurophilic Auer rods. Typical symptoms are spongy and bleeding gums, anemia, fatigue, fever, dyspnea, moderate splenomegaly, joint and bone pain, and repeated infections. The median age of diagnosis is 65, and incidence increases with age. The risk of the disease is increased among people who have been exposed to massive doses of radiation and who have certain blood dyscrasias, such as polycythemia, primary thrombocytopenia, and refractory anemia. Hispanics are also at greater risk. Variants of AML, in which only one cell line proliferates, are erythroid, eosinophilic, basophilic, monocytic, and megakaryocytic leukemias. The diagnosis is based on blood counts and bone marrow biopsies. Cytogenic analysis and immunophenotyping are also done for diagnosis. Chemotherapy, biotherapy, and bone marrow transplantation are used, but long remissions resulting from any form of treatment are rare. Also called **acute granulocytic leukemia,** *acute myelogenous leukemia,* **acute nonlymphocytic leukemia, myeloid leukemia, splenomedullary leukemia, splenomyelogenous leukemia.** See also **acute childhood leukemia, chronic myelocytic leukemia.**

acute myocardial infarction (AMI) [L, *acutus* + Gk, *mys,* muscle, *kardia,* heart; L, *infarcire,* to stuff], the early critical stage of necrosis of heart muscle tissue caused by blockage of a coronary artery. It is characterized by elevated S-T segments in the reflecting leads and elevated levels of cardiac enzymes. See also **myocardial infarction.**

acute necrotizing hemorrhagic encephalopathy, a degenerative brain disease, characterized by marked edema, numerous minute hemorrhages, necrosis of blood vessel walls, demyelination of nerve fibers, and infiltration of the meninges with neutrophils, lymphocytes, and histiocytes. Typical signs are severe headache, fever, and vomiting; seizures may occur, and the patient may rapidly lose consciousness. Treatment consists of decompression via withdrawal of cerebrospinal fluid. Also called **acute hemorrhagic leukoencephalitis.**

acute nephritis, a sudden inflammation of the kidney characterized by albuminuria and hematuria but without edema or urine retention. It affects children most commonly and usually involves only a few glomeruli. See also **nephritis.**

acute nicotine poisoning [L, *Nicotiana,* herb, *potio,* drink], a toxic condition produced by acute intoxication with nicotine. Characteristics include a burning sensation in the mouth, nausea and vomiting, diarrhea, palpitations, salivation, agitation, respiratory depression, and seizures that may lead to death. See also **nicotine poisoning.**

acute nongonorrheal vulvitis [L, *non,* not; Gk, *gone,* seed, *rhoia,* flow; L, *vulva,* wrapper; Gk, *itis,* inflammation], an inflammation of the vulva resulting from chafing of the vulvar lips, accumulation of sebaceous material, atopic reactions, local infections, or other causes that are nonvenereal.

acute nonlymphocytic leukemia (ANLL). See **acute myeloid leukemia.**

acute nonspecific pericarditis [Gk, *peri,* around, *kardia,* heart, *itis,* inflammation], an inflammation of the pericardium, with or without effusion. It often is associated with myocarditis but usually resolves without complications. See also **pericarditis.**

acute pain, severe pain, as may follow surgery or trauma or accompany myocardial infarction or other conditions and diseases. Acute pain occurring in the first 24 to 48 hours after surgery is often difficult to relieve, even with medications. Acute pain in individuals with orthopedic problems originates from the periosteum, the joint surfaces, and the arterial walls. Muscle pain associated with bone surgery results from muscle ischemia rather than muscle tension. Acute abdominal pain often causes the individual to lie on one side and draw up the legs in the fetal position. Compare **chronic pain.** See also **pain, pain intervention, pain mechanism.**

acute pancreatitis [Gk, *pan,* all, *kreas,* flesh, *itis,* inflammation], a sudden inflammation of the pancreas caused by autodigestion and marked by symptoms of acute abdomen and escape of pancreatic enzymes into the pancreatic tissues. The condition is associated with trauma, biliary disease, or alcoholism. The autodigestion is caused by premature activation of the digestive enzymes. Acute pancreatitis can also be of unknown cause. See also **pancreatitis.**

acute parapsoriasis. See **Mucha-Habermann disease.**

acute pharyngitis. See **pharyngitis.**

acute pleurisy, an inflammation of the pleura, often as a result of lung disease. It is characterized by irritation without recognizable pleural effusion and is localized. See also **pleurisy.**

acute primary myocarditis, **1.** an inflammation of the heart muscle, most commonly caused by a bacterial infection initiated locally or carried through the bloodstream. **2.** a severe inflammation of the heart muscle associated with degeneration of the muscle fibers and release of leukocytes into the interstitial tissues. See also **myocarditis.**

acute promyelocytic leukemia (AProL, APL), a malignancy of the blood-forming tissues, characterized by the proliferation of promyelocytes and blast cells with distinctive Auer rods. Symptoms include severe bleeding and bruises. The patient may also have a low fibrinogen level and platelet count. Management of the disease typically requires replacement of coagulation factors and administration of cytotoxic drugs. See also **leukemia.**

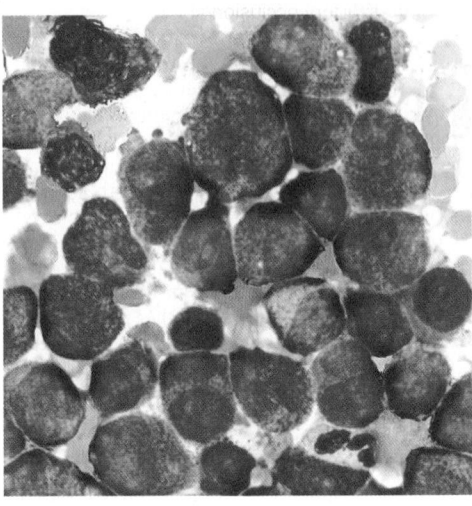

Acute promyelocytic leukemia *(Carr and Rodak, 2008)*

acute psychosis, one of a group of disorders in which ego functioning is either impaired or inhibited. The ability to process reality-based information is diminished and disordered. The cause may be a known psychological abnormality. In situations in which a physiological abnormality is not recognized, the functional impairment is still clearly present.

acute pyogenic arthritis, an acute bacterial infection of one or more joints, caused by trauma or a penetrating wound and occurring most frequently in children. Typical signs are pain, redness, and swelling in the affected joint; muscular spasms in the area; chills; fever; sweating; and leukocytosis. Treatment consists of immobilization of the joint, analgesia, sedation, and IV administration of an antibiotic. If required, the joint may be irrigated with normal saline solution and an antibiotic. Hospitalization is usually required. Also called **acute septic arthritis.**

acute radiation exposure, exposure of short duration to intense ionizing radiation, usually occurring as the result of an accidental spill of radioactive material. See **radiation exposure.** See also **chronic radiation exposure.**

acute rejection [L, *rejicere,* to throw back], after organ transplantation, the rapid reaction against allograft or xenograft tissue that is incompatible. It often occurs within a week of treatment, during which time the immune response increases in intensity.

acute renal failure (ARF), renal failure of sudden onset, such as from physical trauma, infection, inflammation, or toxicity. Symptoms include uremia and usually oliguria or anuria, with hyperkalemia and pulmonary edema. Three types are distinguished: prerenal, associated with poor systemic perfusion and decreased renal blood flow, such as with hypovolemic shock or congestive heart failure; intrarenal, associated with disease of the renal parenchyma, such as tubulointerstitial nephritis, acute interstitial nephritis, or nephrotoxicity; and postrenal, resulting from obstruction of urine flow out of the kidneys. See also **renal failure.**

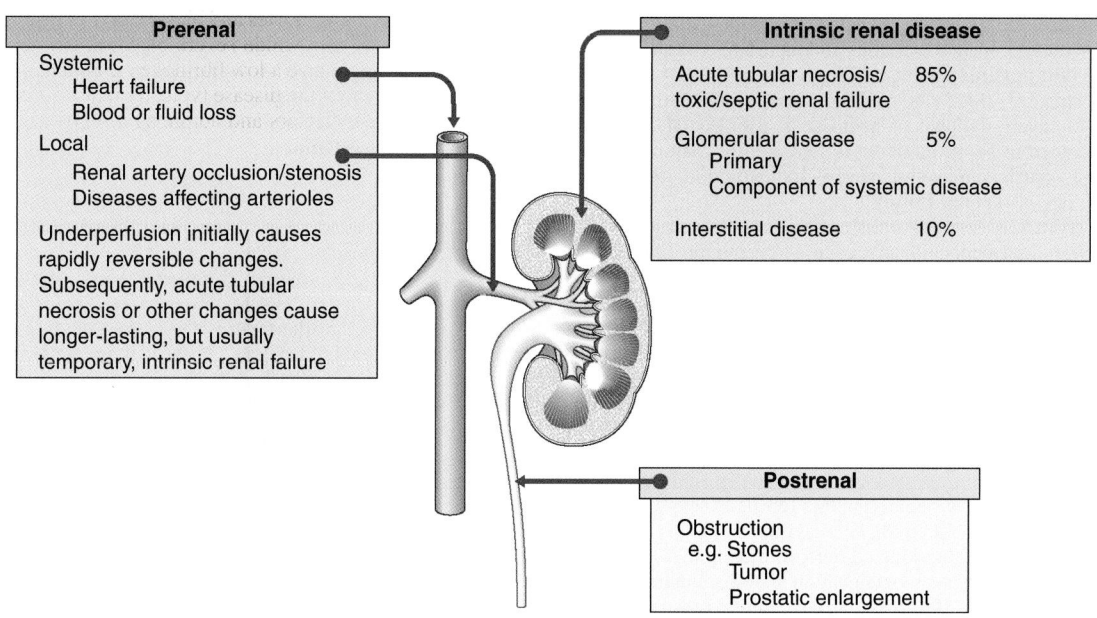

Prerenal

Systemic
    Heart failure
    Blood or fluid loss
Local
    Renal artery occlusion/stenosis
    Diseases affecting arterioles

Underperfusion initially causes
rapidly reversible changes.
Subsequently, acute tubular
necrosis or other changes cause
longer-lasting, but usually
temporary, intrinsic renal failure

Intrinsic renal disease

Acute tubular necrosis/ toxic/septic renal failure	85%
Glomerular disease Primary Component of systemic disease	5%
Interstitial disease	10%

Postrenal

Obstruction
    e.g. Stones
    Tumor
    Prostatic enlargement

Acute renal failure *(Colledge et al, 2010)*

acute respiratory distress syndrome.   See **adult respiratory distress syndrome.**

acute respiratory failure (ARF) [L, *acutus + respirare,* respiratory, *fallere,* to deceive], a sudden inability of the lungs to maintain normal respiratory function. The condition may be caused by an obstruction in the airways or by failure of the lungs to exchange gases in the alveoli. See **respiratory failure.**

acute rheumatic arthritis, joint inflammation that occurs during the acute phase of rheumatic fever.

acute schizophrenia, a disorder consisting of various degrees of psychosis, characterized by the sudden onset of personality disorganization. Symptoms include disturbances in thought, mood, and behavior. Positive symptoms include delusions, which may be bizarre in nature; hallucinations, especially auditory; disorganized speech; inappropriate affect; and disorganized behavior. Negative symptoms include flat affect, lack of volition, alogia, and anhedonia. Episodes appear suddenly in persons whose previous behavior has been relatively normal and are usually of short duration. Recurrent episodes are common, and in some instances a more chronic type of the disorder may develop. See also **schizoaffective disorder, schizophrenia, schizophreniform disorder.**

acute secondary myocarditis, a sudden, severe inflammation of the heart muscle, resulting from a disease of the endocardium or pericardium or a generalized infection. See also **myocarditis.**

acute septic arthritis.   See **acute pyogenic arthritis.**

acute septic myocarditis [Gk, *septikos,* putrid, *mys,* muscle, *kardia,* heart, *itis,* inflammation], a severe inflammation of the myocardium associated with pus formation, necrosis, and abscess formation. See also **myocarditis.**

acute suppurative arthritis [L, *suppurare,* to form pus], a form of arthritis characterized by invasion of the joint space by pyogenic organisms and the formation of pus in the joint cavity. Failure to recognize and treat septic arthritis can result in morbidity and, sometimes, death. Duration of the illness is usually 4 to 6 days. It most commonly affects children from 5 to 10 years of age. See also **septic arthritis, acute pyogenic arthritis.**

acute suppurative sinusitis [L, *acutus,* sharp, *suppurare,* to form pus, *sinus,* hollow; Gk, *itis,* inflammation], a purulent infection of the nasal sinuses. Symptoms are pain over the inflamed area, headache, chills, and fever.
■ DISEASE: The infection is treated with antibiotics, decongestants, and analgesics. If medical management fails, surgery is necessary.

acute tonsillitis [L, *acutus,* sharp, *tonsilla*; Gk, *itis,* inflammation], an inflammation of one or both tonsils associated with a catarrhal exudate over the tonsil or the discharge of caseous or suppurative material from the tonsillar crypts.

acute toxicity, the harmful effect of a toxic agent that manifests itself in seconds, minutes, hours, or days after ingestion or exposure.

acute transverse myelitis, an inflammation of the entire thickness of the spinal cord, affecting both the sensory and motor nerves. It can develop rapidly and is accompanied by necrosis and neurological deficit that commonly persist after recovery. Patients in whom spastic reflexes develop soon after the onset of this disease are more likely to recover. This disorder may result from a variety of causes, such as multiple sclerosis, measles, pneumonia, viral infections, and the ingestion of certain toxic agents such as carbon monoxide, lead, and arsenic. Such poisonous substances can destroy the entire circumference of the spinal cord, including the myelin sheaths, axons, and neurons, and can cause hemorrhage and necrosis.
■ INTERVENTIONS: Initial medical treatments are designed to reduce spinal cord inflammation and to manage and alleviate symptoms. Antiinflammatory corticosteroid therapy is prescribed soon after the diagnosis is made to decrease inflammation and to improve the chance for and speed of neurological recovery. Many forms of long-term rehabilitative therapy are available for people who have permanent disabilities resulting from transverse myelitis.
■ PATIENT CARE CONSIDERATIONS: There is no cure, and the prognosis for complete recovery is poor. Immediate patient care includes frequent assessment of vital signs, vigilance for signs of spinal shock, maintenance of a urinary catheter, and proper skin care. Strategies for carrying out activities in new ways to overcome, circumvent, or compensate for permanent

disabilities are essential. Functional independence is possible with appropriate therapies and facilitates the attainment of the best possible quality of life.

acute tubular necrosis (ATN), acute renal failure with mild to severe damage or necrosis of tubule cells, usually resulting from nephrotoxicity, ischemia after major surgery, trauma (crush syndrome), severe hypovolemia, sepsis, or burns. See also **renal failure.**

acute tubulointerstitial nephritis, an early stage of tubulointerstitial nephritis similar to acute pyelonephritis but with involvement farther into the renal medulla to involve the tubules, resulting in decreased renal function.

acute urethral syndrome [Gk, *ourethra,* urethra, *syn,* together, *dromos,* course], new, rapid-onset painful urination, urinary frequency, and suprapubic pain, most commonly associated with recent vigorous coitus and/or infection with gonorrhea or *Chlamydia.* Urethral discharge may be present.

acute vulvar ulcer, a nonvenereal, usually shallow lesion of the vulva, often associated with a febrile illness.

acyanotic /ā'sī·ənot″ik/ [Gk, *a,* not, *kyanos,* blue], lacking a blue appearance of the skin and mucous membranes. The lack is suggestive of adequate oxygenation. Compare **cyanosis.**

acyanotic congenital defect, a heart defect present at birth that does not produce blue discoloration of the skin and mucous membranes under normal circumstances. However, the condition does increase the load on the pulmonary circulation and may lead to cyanosis, right ventricular failure, or other complications during physical exertion. Kinds include **atrial septal defect.**

acyclovir /əsī″klōvir/, an antiviral agent with activity against herpesvirus types 1 and 2 and varicella zoster virus. Acyclovir is converted by a herpesvirus enzyme into a molecule (acyclovir triphosphate) that inhibits the synthesis of deoxyribonucleic acid (DNA) molecules in the virally infected cells, thereby inhibiting viral replication. ■ INDICATIONS: It is prescribed topically in an ointment for the treatment of herpes simplex lesions (cold sores) and both orally and systemically (oral and IV) in other types of herpes infections, including genital herpes, herpes encephalitis, chickenpox (varicella zoster), and shingles (herpes zoster). ■ CONTRAINDICATIONS: Known sensitivity to this drug prohibits its use. ■ ADVERSE EFFECTS: After topical use, irritation or pruritus may occur; after systemic use, diaphoresis, headache, and nausea may occur. When it is administered intravenously in the treatment of immunosuppressed patients, there may be pain at the site of the injection, and 1% to 10% of such patients experience acute renal failure.

acyesis /ā'sī·ē″sis/, **1.** (*Obsolete*) the absence of pregnancy. **2.** sterility in women.

acyl /ā'sil/, an organic radical derived from an organic acid via removal of the hydroxyl group from the carboxyl group. It is represented as R—CO—.

acylation /as'ilā″shən/, the incorporation into a molecule of an organic compound of an acyl group, —C(O)R.

-ad, a suffix meaning "toward (a specified terminus)": *cephalad.*

AD, 1. abbreviation for *Associate Degree.* **2.** abbreviation for **Alzheimer disease.**

ad-, a prefix meaning "to, toward, addition to, intensification": *adneural, adrenal.*

a.d., 1. abbreviation for **auris dextra. 2.** (in pharmacology) an abbreviation identified by the Institute for Safe Medication Practices as an error-prone abbreviation. Now written in full as *right ear.*

A/D, 1. See **analog-to-digital (A/D) converter. 2.** abbreviation for *anodal duration.* **3.** abbreviation for *average deviation.*

ADA, 1. abbreviation for *American Dental Association.* **2.** abbreviation for *American Diabetes Association.* **3.** abbreviation for **adenosine deaminase. 4.** abbreviation for **Americans With Disabilities Act.**

ADAA, 1. abbreviation for *American Dental Assistants Association.* **2.** abbreviation for *Anxiety Disorders Association of America.*

adactyly /ādak″tilē/ [Gk, *a,* without + *daktylos,* finger or toe], a congenital defect in which one or more digits of the hand or foot are missing.

Adalat, a calcium channel blocker. Brand name for **NIFEdipine.**

adalimumab, an antirheumatic immunomodulating agent used to treat patients older than 18 years of age with moderate to severe rheumatoid arthritis.

Adam, Evelyn, [b. 1929] a Canadian nursing theorist who applied the structure of a conceptual model for nursing in her book, *"Être Infirmière"* in 1979 ("To Be a Nurse," 1980). Adam believes that a theory is useful to more than one discipline, but that a conceptual model for a discipline is useful only to that discipline. A conceptual model consists of assumptions, beliefs and values, and major units. Adam developed Virginia Henderson's concepts within Dorothy E. Johnson's structure of a conceptual model. She describes the goal of nursing as maintaining or restoring the client's independence in the satisfaction of 14 fundamental needs. Each need has biological, physiological, and psychosocial aspects. The nurse complements and supplements the client's strength, knowledge, and will.

Adam's apple, (*Informal*) See **laryngeal prominence.**

Adams-Stokes syndrome [Robert Adams, Irish surgeon, 1791–1875; William Stokes, Irish physician, 1804–1878], a condition characterized by sudden, recurrent episodes of loss of consciousness caused by incomplete heart block. Seizures may accompany the episodes. Also called **Stokes-Adams syndrome.** See also **infranodal block.**

adapalene /ah-dap'ah-lēn/, a synthetic analog of retinoic acid used topically in the treatment of acne vulgaris.

adaptation /ad'aptā″shon/ [L, *adaptatio,* act of adapting], **1.** a change or response to stress of any kind, such as inflammation of the nasal mucosa in infectious rhinitis or increased crying in a frightened child. Adaptation may be normal, self-protective, and developmental, as when a child learns to talk; it may be all-encompassing, creating further stress, as in polycythemia, which occurs naturally at high altitudes to provide more oxygen-carrying erythrocytes but may also lead to thrombosis, venous congestion, or edema. The degree and nature of adaptation shown by a patient are evaluated regularly by the members of the health care team. They constitute a measure of the effectiveness of care, the course of the disease, and the ability of the patient to cope with stress. Compare **accommodation. 2.** (in occupational therapy) an outcome associated with a client's experience of relative mastery in occupational adaptation.

adaptation model, (in nursing) a conceptual framework that focuses on the patient as an adaptive system, one in which nursing intervention is required when a deficit develops in the patient's ability to cope with the internal and external demands of the environment. These demands are classified into four groups: physiological needs, the need for a positive self-concept, the need to perform social roles, and the need to balance dependence and independence. The nurse assesses the patient's maladaptive response and identifies the kind of demand that is causing the problem. Nursing care is planned to promote adaptive responses for coping successfully with the current stress on the patient's well-being. This model, first proposed by Sister Callista Roy, is frequently used as a conceptual framework for programs of nursing education.

adaptation syndrome. See **general adaptation syndrome.**

adapted clothing, clothing that has been modified, such as with taped hook and loop or Velcro fasteners, to permit individuals with disabilities to dress themselves with minimal difficulty.

adapter [L, *adaptatio,* the process of adjusting], a device for joining or connecting two or more parts of a system to enable it to function properly.

adaptive device /adap″tiv/ [L, *adaptatio,* process of adapting; OFr, *devise,* plan or design], any structure, design, instrument, contrivance, or equipment that enables a person with a disability to function more independently or with greater satisfaction. Examples include plate guards and grab bars. Also called **self-help device,** *assistive device.*

adaptive hypertrophy [L, *adaptatio,* process of adapting; Gk, *hyper,* excessive, *trophe,* nourishment], a reactive extension, growth, or expansion in the amount of tissue that compensates for a loss of the same or similar tissue so that function is not impaired.

adaptive response, **1.** an appropriate reaction to an environmental demand. **2.** the ability to adjust and respond to changes in a nondisruptive manner.

ADA Seal of Acceptance, an approval granted by the American Dental Association Council on Scientific Affairs to oral care products that are supported by adequate research evidence as to their safety and efficacy.

ADC, abbreviation for **AIDS-dementia complex.**

ADCC, abbreviation for *antibody-dependent cell-mediated cytotoxicity.*

ADC Van Disal /ā″dē′sē″vandī″səl/, *(Informal)* a term used as a mnemonic device for recalling the protocol of hospital admission orders. The letters stand for admission authorization, diagnosis, condition, vital signs, activity, nursing requirements, drugs, instructions, special studies, allergies, laboratory tests. Variations include ADC VAN DISMAL, ADC VANDALISM.

ADD, abbreviation for **attention deficit disorder.**

Addams, Jane [1860–1935], an American social reformer. In Chicago in 1889 she founded Hull House, one of the first social settlements in the United States, where volunteers from many disciplines lived and worked in their professions. She played a central role in most of the social reforms of her time and provided inspiration to professionals who were striving to establish high educational standards and better working conditions. She is often referred to as the "Mother of Social Work" and made numerous contributions to the professionalization of social work. She was co-recipient of the Nobel Peace Prize in 1931.

adder, any of numerous venomous elapid and viperine snakes. The death adder is found in Australia and New Guinea, and the puff adder is found in Africa and Arabia. See also **snakebite.**

addict /ad″ikt/ [L, *addicere,* to devote], a person who has become physiologically and psychologically dependent on a chemical such as alcohol or other drugs to the extent that normal social, occupational, and other responsible life functions are disrupted.

addiction /ədik″shən/, a compulsive, uncontrollable dependence on a chemical substance, habit, or practice to such a degree that either the means of obtaining or ceasing use may cause severe emotional, mental, or physiological reactions. Compare **habituation.**

addictive personality /ədik″tiv/, a personality marked by traits of compulsive and habitual use of a substance or practice in an attempt to cope with psychic pain engendered by conflict and anxiety.

addisonian crisis. See **adrenal crisis.**

addisonism [Thomas Addison, London physician, 1793–1860], a condition characterized by the physical signs of Addison disease, although loss of adrenocortical functions is not involved. The signs include an increase in the bronze pigmentation of the skin and mucous membranes caused by increased levels of melanocyte-stimulating hormone, as well as general debility.

Addison crisis. See **adrenal crisis.**

Addison disease [Thomas Addison, British physician, 1793–1860], a life-threatening condition caused by partial or complete failure of adrenocortical function, often resulting from autoimmune processes, infection (especially tubercular or fungal), neoplasm, or hemorrhage in the gland. All three general functions of the adrenal cortex (glucocorticoid, mineralocorticoid, and androgenic) are lost. Also called **Addison syndrome.** See also **adrenal crisis.**

■ OBSERVATIONS: The disease is characterized by increased bronze pigmentation of the skin and mucous membranes; weakness; decreased endurance; anorexia; dehydration; weight loss; GI disturbances; salt cravings; anxiety, depression, and other emotional distress; and decreased tolerance to physical and emotional stress. The person's requirements for glucocorticoid, mineralocorticoid, and salt are increased by stress, as in infection, trauma, and surgical procedures. The onset is usually gradual, over a period of weeks or months. Laboratory tests reveal abnormally low blood concentrations of sodium and glucose, a greater than normal level of serum potassium, and a decreased urinary output of certain steroids. The diagnosis is established if the amount of cortisol in the plasma and steroid in the urine does not increase after stimulation with adrenocorticotropic hormone.

■ INTERVENTIONS: Treatment includes replacement therapy with glucocorticoid and mineralocorticoid drugs, an adequate fluid intake, control of sodium and potassium balance, and a diet high in complex carbohydrates and protein. Follow-up care includes continued administration of glucocorticoid drugs.

■ PATIENT CARE CONSIDERATIONS: Complications include high fever, confused behavior, and adrenal crisis. With careful management, the patient's resistance to infection, capacity for work, and general well-being can be maintained. Nursing care includes administering corticosteroids and other drugs, observing the patient for signs of abnormal sodium and potassium levels, monitoring body weight and fluid intake and output, and encouraging adequate intake of nutrients. The patient also needs protection against stress while in the hospital and instruction in the importance of avoiding stress at home. The significance of emotional distress, the value of wearing a Medic Alert bracelet or tag, the signs of impending crisis, the use of a prepared kit for emergencies, and the importance of scrupulous attention to drug and diet regimens are emphasized before discharge. Discharge teaching also emphasizes the need to take cortisone after meals or with milk to prevent gastric irritation and the development of ulcers.

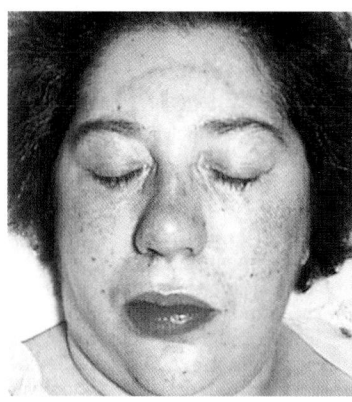

Patient with Addison disease *(Moll, 1997)*

Addison keloid.   See **morphea.**

Addison syndrome.   See **Addison disease.**

addition [L, *additio,* something added],   a chemical reaction in which two complete molecules combine to form a new product, usually by attachment to carbon atoms at a double or triple bond of one of the molecules.

additive /ad″itiv/,   any substance added intentionally or indirectly that becomes a part of the food, pharmaceutical, or other product. Additives may be introduced in growing, processing, packaging, storage, or cooking or other final preparation for consumption.

additive effect [L, *additio,* something added, *effectus*],   the combined effect of drugs that, when used together, produce an effect that is greater than the sum of their separately measured individual effects.

adducent /ədoō″sənt/,   an agent or other stimulus that causes a limb to be drawn toward the midline or axis of the body or causes the fingers or toes to move together.

adduction /əduk″shən/ [L, *adducere,* to bring to],   the movement of a limb toward the midline or axis of the body. Compare **abduction.** −*adduct, v.*

adductor /əduk″tər/,   a muscle that draws a part toward the midline or axis of the body. Compare **abductor, tensor.**

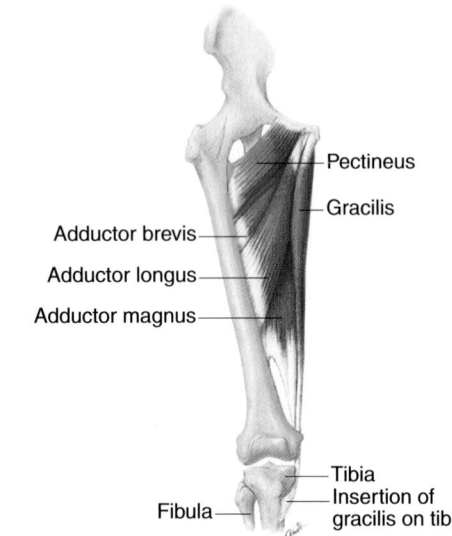

Pectineus
Gracilis
Adductor brevis
Adductor longus
Adductor magnus
Tibia
Insertion of gracilis on tibia
Fibula

Adductor brevis, adductor longus, and adductor magnus muscles of the anterior thigh *(Patton and Thibodeau, 2016)*

adductor brevis,   a somewhat triangular muscle in the thigh and one of the five medial femoral muscles. It acts to adduct and rotate the thigh laterally and to flex the leg. Compare **adductor longus, adductor magnus, gracilis, pectineus.**

adductor canal,   a triangular channel beneath the sartorius muscle and between the adductor longus and vastus medialis through which the femoral vessels and the saphenous nerve pass. Also called **Hunter's canal,** *subsartorial canal.*

adductor hiatus,   the opening in the tendon of insertion of the adductor magnus through which the femoral artery and vein pass into the popliteal space.

adductor longus,   the most superficial of the three adductor muscles of the thigh and one of five medial femoral muscles. It functions to adduct and flex the thigh. Compare **adductor brevis, adductor magnus, gracilis, pectineus.**

adductor magnus,   the long, heavy triangular muscle of the medial aspect of the thigh. The adductor magnus acts to adduct the thigh. The proximal portion acts to rotate the thigh medially and flex it on the hip; the distal portion acts to extend the thigh and rotate it laterally. Compare **adductor brevis, adductor longus, gracilis, pectineus.**

adductor pollicis,   a large triangular muscle that is a powerful adductor of the thumb and opposes the thumb to the rest of the digits in gripping. See **thenar muscles.**

adefovir dipivoxil,   an antiviral agent used to treat chronic hepatitis B.

ADEM,   abbreviation for **acute disseminated encephalomyelitis.**

aden-.   See **adeno-, aden-.**

adenalgia /ad″ənal″jə/   [Gk, *aden,* gland, *algos,* pain],   pain in any of the glands. Also called **adenodynia.**

adenectomy /ad″ənek″təmē/   [Gk, *aden* + *ektomē,* excision],   the surgical removal of any gland.

Aden fever,   now called **dengue fever.**

-adenia,   a suffix meaning "(condition of the) glands": *anadenia.*

adenine /ad″ənin/,   a purine base that is a component of DNA, RNA, adenosine monophosphate (AMP), cyclic AMP, adenosine diphosphate(ADP), and adenosine triphosphate (ATP).

adenine arabinoside.   See **vidarabine.**

adenine-D-ribose.   See **adenosine.**

adenitis /ad″ənī″tis/,   an inflammation of a lymph node causing swelling, enlargement, and/or pain. Acute adenitis of the cervical lymph nodes may accompany a sore throat and stiff neck, simulating mumps if severe. It is most often related to an oral, a pharyngeal, or an ear infection. Scarlet fever may cause acute suppurative cervical adenitis. Inflammation of the lymph nodes of the mesenteric portion of the peritoneum often produces pain and other symptoms similar to those of appendicitis, but characteristically mesenteric adenitis is preceded by respiratory infection, the pain is less localized and less constant than in appendicitis, and the pain does not increase in severity. Generalized adenitis is a secondary symptom of syphilis. Therapy requires treatment of the primary infection by the administration of antimicrobial agents, application of warm compresses, and occasionally, incision and drainage. Also called **lymphadenitis.** Compare **acinitis.**

adeno-, aden- /ad″ənō-/,   prefix meaning "gland": *adenocarcinoma, adenectomy.*

adenoacanthoma /ad″ənō·ak″anthō″mə/   [Gk, *aden* + *akantha,* thorn, *oma,* tumor],   a neoplasm that may be malignant or benign, derived from epithelial cells with squamous differentiation shown by some of the cells.

adenoameloblastoma /ad″ənō·amel″ōblastō″mə/ *pl. adenoameloblastomas, adenoameloblastomata,*   a benign tumor of the maxilla or mandible composed of ducts lined with columnar or cuboidal epithelial cells. It develops in tissue that normally gives rise to the teeth, and it most often occurs in young people.

adenoassociated virus (AAV),   a defective virus belonging to a group of DNA viruses of the Parvoviridae family that can reproduce only in the presence of adenoviruses. It is not yet known what role, if any, these organisms have in causing disease. No specific antiviral is available. When not replicating, it is integrated into the host genome and has been proposed as a vector for gene transfer.

adenocarcinoma /ad″ənōkärsinō″mə/ *pl. adenocarcinomas, adenocarcinomata* [Gk, *aden* + *karkinos,* crab, *oma*], *adj,* any one of a large group of malignant epithelial cell tumors of the glandular tissue. Specific tumors are diagnosed and named by cytological identification of the tissue affected; for example, an adenocarcinoma of the uterine cervix is characterized by tumor cells resembling the glandular epithelium of the cervix. −*adenocarcinomatous, adj.*

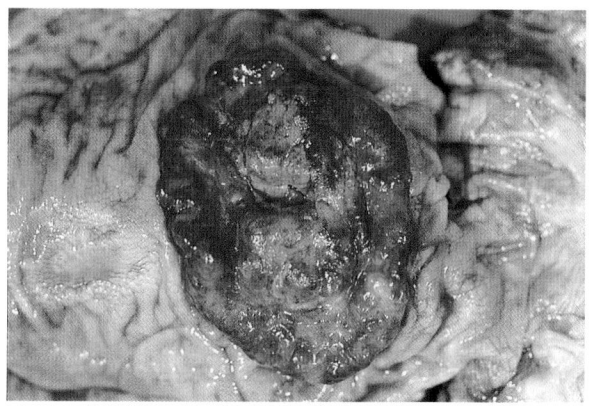

Adenocarcinoma *(Damjanov, 2012)*

adenocarcinoma in situ, a localized growth of abnormal glandular tissue that may become malignant. However, the abnormal cells do not extend beyond the basement membrane. It is most common in the endometrium and in the large intestine.

adenocarcinoma of the lung, a type of bronchogenic carcinoma made up of a discrete mass of cuboidal or columnar epithelial cells, generally at the lung periphery. Most of these tumors form glandular structures that contain mucin, although a few lack mucin and are solid. Growth is slow, but there may be early invasion of blood and lymph vessels by metastases while the primary lesion is still asymptomatic. Kinds include **bronchogenic adenocarcinoma.**

adenocele /ad″ənōsēl′/, a cystic, glandular tumor.

adenochondroma /ad′ənōkondrō″mə/ *pl. adenochondromas, adenochondromata* [Gk, *aden* + *chondros,* cartilage, *oma,* tumor], a neoplasm of cells derived from glandular and cartilaginous tissues, as a mixed tumor of the salivary glands. Also called **chondroadenoma.**

adenocyst /ad″ənōsist′/ [Gk, *aden* + *kytis,* bag], a benign tumor in which the cells form cysts. Also called **adenocystoma.**

adenocystic carcinoma, an uncommon malignant neoplasm composed of cords of uniform small epithelial cells arranged in a sievelike pattern around cystic spaces that often contain mucus. The tumor occurs most frequently in the salivary glands, breast, mucous glands of the upper and lower respiratory tract, and, occasionally, in vestibular glands of the vulva. The malignant slow growth tends to spread along nerves, causing neurological damage. Facial paralysis often results from adenocystic carcinoma of the salivary gland. Blood-borne metastases to lungs and liver have been reported. Standard treatment involves surgery followed by radiation. Also called **adenoid cystic carcinoma, adenomyoepithelioma, cribriform carcinoma, cylindroma.**

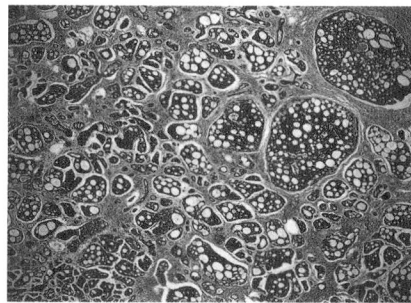

Adenocystic carcinoma *(Silverberg et al, 2006)*

adenocystoma. See **adenocyst.**

adenodynia /ad′ənōdin′ē·ə/, glandular pain. See **adenalgia.**

adenoepithelioma /ad′ənō·ep′ithē′lē·ō″mə/ *pl. adenoepitheliomas, adenoepitheliomata* [Gk, *aden* + *epi,* on, *thele,* nipple, *oma*], a neoplasm consisting of glandular and epithelial components.

adenofibroma /ad′ənōfībrō″mə/ *pl. adenofibromas, adenofibromata* [Gk, *aden* + L, *fibra,* fiber, *oma*], a tumor of the connective tissues that contains glandular elements.

adenofibroma edematodes, a neoplasm consisting of glandular elements and connective tissue in which marked edema is present.

adenohypophysis /ad′ənō′hīpof″isis/ [Gk, *aden* + *hypo,* beneath, *phyein,* to grow], the anterior lobe of the pituitary gland. It secretes growth hormone, thyroid-stimulating hormone, adrenocorticotropic hormone, melanocyte-stimulating hormone, follicle-stimulating hormone, luteinizing hormone, prolactin, beta-lipotropin molecules, and endorphins. The release of hormones from the hypothalamus regulates these secretions. Also called **anterior pituitary.**

adenoid /ad″ənoid/ [Gk, *aden* + *eidos,* form], **1.** having a glandular, particularly lymphoid, appearance. **2.** See **adenoids.**

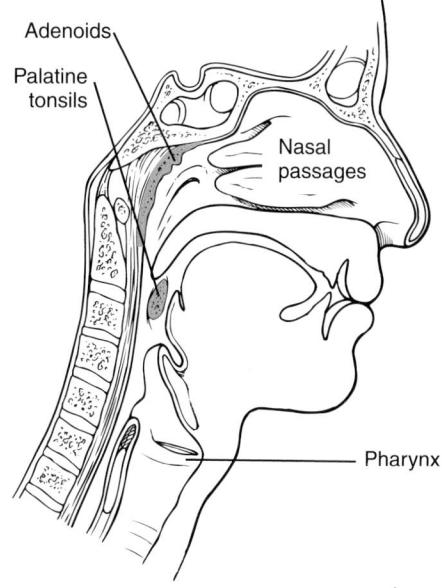

Adenoids *(Mosby, 2003)*

adenoidal speech, an abnormal manner of speaking caused by hypertrophy of the adenoidal tissue that normally exists in the nasopharynx of children. It is often characterized by hyponasality, with the consonants /m/, /n/, and /ng/ most affected. It may be self-limited with age-related growth of the craniofacial skeleton or corrected by a natural reduction of the swollen tissues or by surgical excision of the adenoids.

adenoid cystic carcinoma. See **adenocystic carcinoma.**

adenoidectomy /ad′ənoidek″təmē/ [Gk, *aden* + *eidos,* form, *ektomē,* excision], the removal of lymphoid tissue in the nasopharynx. This surgical procedure may be performed because the adenoids are enlarged, chronically infected, or causing obstruction. Normal adenoids may be excised as a prophylactic measure during tonsillectomy. The operation is performed with general anesthesia in children, but local anesthesia may be used in adults. After removal of the adenoids, bleeding is stemmed with pressure, or vessels may be ligated with sutures or electrocoagulation current may be used. After surgery, the patient is observed for signs of bleeding, and the pulse, blood pressure, and respiration rate are monitored. Discharge is usually the same day after recovery from anesthesia. Compare **adenotonsillectomy, tonsillectomy.**

adenoid facies, a long face and open-mouth posture, sometimes seen in children with hypertrophy of the pharyngeal tonsils ("adenoids"). Chronic nasal airway obstruction is believed to affect facial growth characteristics.

adenoid hyperplasia, enlarged adenoid glands, especially in children. Enlarged adenoids, often in association with enlarged tonsils, are a frequent cause of recurrent otitis media, sinusitis, conductive hearing loss, and partial respiratory obstruction. Severe obstruction can result in alveolar hypoventilation and pulmonary hypertension with congestive heart failure. Adenotonsillar hypertrophy is frequently seen in children with sickle cell disease. Treatment usually consists of an adenoidectomy.

adenoid hypertrophy [Gk, *aden,* gland, *eidos,* form, *hyper,* excessive, *trophe,* nourishment], the unusual growth of the pharyngeal tonsil.

adenoiditis /ad′ənoidī″tis/, an inflammation of the adenoids.

adenoids, one of two masses of lymphatic tissue situated on the posterior wall of the nasopharynx behind the posterior nares. During childhood these masses often swell and block the passage of air from the nasal cavity into the pharynx, preventing the child from breathing through the nose. Also called **pharyngeal tonsil.** –*adenoidal, adj.*

adenoleiomyofibroma /ad′ənōlī′ōmī′ōfibrō″mə/ [Gk, *aden* + *leios,* smooth, *mys,* muscle; L, *fibra,* fiber; Gk, *oma*], a glandular tumor with smooth muscle, connective tissue, and epithelial elements.

adenolipoma /ad′ənōlipō″mə/ *pl. adenolipomas, adenolipomata* [Gk, *aden* + *lipos,* fat, *oma*], a benign neoplasm consisting of elements of glandular and adipose tissue.

adenolipomatosis /ad′ənōlip′ōmətō″sis/, a condition characterized by the growth of adenolipomas in the groin, axilla, and neck.

adenolymphoma. See **papillary adenocystoma lymphomatosum.**

-adenoma, a suffix meaning a "tumor composed of glandular tissue or glandlike in structure": *sarcoadenoma, cystadenoma.*

adenoma /ad′ənō″mə/ *pl. adenomas, adenomata* [Gk, *aden* + *oma*], a benign tumor of glandular epithelium in which the cells of the tumor are arranged in a recognizable glandular structure. An adenoma may cause excess secretion by the affected gland, such as an acidophilic adenoma resulting in an excess of growth hormone. Kinds include **acidophilic adenoma, basophilic adenoma, insulinoma, fibroadenoma.** –*adenomatous, adenomatoid, adj.*

adenoma sebaceum /sebā″sē·əm/, firm skin-colored or red papules, often occurring in clusters on the cheeks, around the nose, and on the chin. They appear in childhood, from 5 years onward. The lesions are composed chiefly of fibrovascular tissue and are usually benign. Also called **angiofibroma.** See also **tuberous sclerosis.**

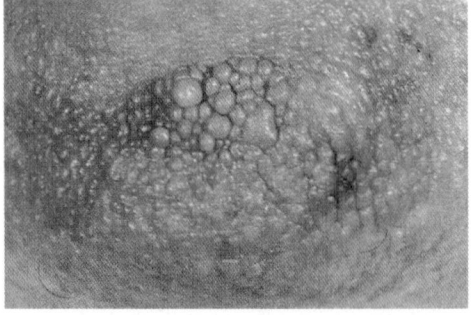

Adenoma sebaceum *(du Vivier, 1993)*

adenomatoid. See **adenoma.**

adenomatosis /ad′ənōmətō″sis/, an abnormal condition in which hyperplasia or tumor development affects two or more glands, usually the thyroid, adrenals, or pituitary.

adenomatous. See **adenoma.**

adenomatous goiter /ad′ənō″mətəs/, an enlargement of the thyroid gland caused by an adenoma or numerous colloid nodules.

adenomatous polyp [Gk, *aden,* gland, *oma,* tumor, *polys,* many, *pous,* foot], a tumor that develops in glandular tissue or epithelium. It is characterized by benign neoplastic changes in epithelium.

adenomatous polyposis coli (APC), a gene associated with familial adenomatous polyposis (FAP), an inherited disorder characterized by the development of myriad polyps in the colon, often occurring in adolescents and young adults ages 15 to 25. Untreated, the condition nearly always leads to colon cancer. The gene is located on chromosome 5.

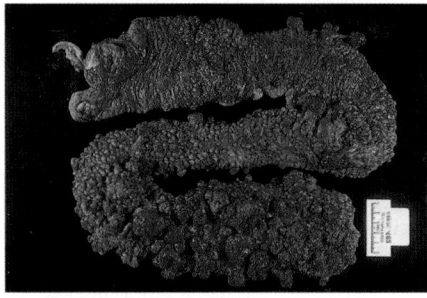

Adenomatous polyposis coli (APC) *(Skarin, 2010)*

adenomyoepithelioma. See **adenocystic carcinoma.**

adenomyofibroma /ad′ənōmī′ōfibrō″mə/ *pl. adenomyofibromas, adenomyofibromata* [Gk, *aden* + *mys,* muscle; L, *fibra,* fiber; Gk, *oma*], a fibrous tumor that contains glandular and muscular components.

adenomyoma /ad′ənōmī·ō″mə/ *pl. adenomyomas, adenomyomata,* a tumor of the endometrium of the uterus characterized by a mass of smooth muscle containing endometrial tissue and glands.

adenomyomatosis /ad′ənōmī′ōmətō″sis/, an abnormal condition characterized by the formation of benign nodules resembling adenomyomas, found in the uterus or in parauterine tissue.

adenomyosarcoma ad′ənōmī′ōsärkō″mə/, *pl. adenomyosarcomas, adenomyosarcomata* See **Wilms tumor.**

adenomyosis /ad′ənōmī·ō″sis/, **1.** a benign neoplastic condition characterized by tumors composed of glandular tissue and smooth muscle cells. **2.** a neoplastic condition characterized by the invasive growth of uterine mucosa in the uterus, pelvis, colon, or oviducts.

adenopathy /ad′ənop″əthē/ [Gk, *aden* + *pathos,* suffering], an enlargement of a lymph node anywhere in the body. Also called **lymphadenopathy.** –*adenopathic, adj.*

adenopharyngitis /ad′ənōfer′injī″tis/, an inflammation of the adenoids, pharynx, and pharyngeal lymphoid tissue.

adenosarcoma /ad′ənōsärkō″mə/*pl. adenosarcomas, adenosarcomata,* [Gk, *aden* + *sarx,* flesh, *oma*], a mixed malignant glandular tumor of connective tissue. It contains both glandular and sarcomatous elements.

adenosarcorhabdomyoma /ad′ənōsär′kōrab′dōmīō″mə/ *pl. adenosarcorhabdomyomas, adenosarcorhabdomyomata,* a tumor composed of glandular and connective tissue and striated muscle elements.

adenosine /əden″əsin, -sēn/, a compound derived from nucleic acid composed of adenine and a sugar, d-ribose.

Adenosine is the major molecular component of the nucleotides adenosine diphosphate, adenosine monophosphate, and adenosine triphosphate and of the nucleic acids DNA and RNA. Also called **adenine-d-ribose.** See also **adenosine phosphate.**

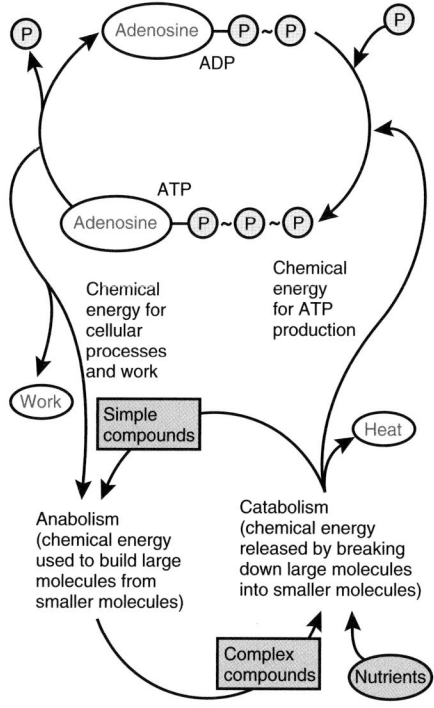

Adenosine *(Mosby, 2003)*

adenosine deaminase (ADA) /dē·am″inās/, an enzyme that catalyzes the conversion of adenosine to the nucleoside inosine through the removal of an amino group. A deficiency of ADA can lead to severe combined immunodeficiency syndrome. See also **adenosine.**

adenosine diphosphate (ADP), a product of the hydrolysis of adenosine triphosphate.

adenosine hydrolase, an enzyme that catalyzes the conversion of adenosine into adenine and ribose.

adenosine kinase, an enzyme in the liver and kidney that catalyzes the transfer of a phosphate group from adenosine triphosphate to produce adenosine diphosphate.

adenosine monophosphate (AMP), an ester, composed of adenine-d-ribose and phosphoric acid, that participates in energy released by working muscle. Also called **adenylic acid.**

adenosine phosphate, a compound consisting of the nucleotide adenosine attached through its ribose group to one, two, or three phosphate units, or phosphoric acid molecules. Kinds include **adenosine diphosphate, adenosine monophosphate, adenosine triphosphate.**

adenosine 3′,5′-cyclic monophosphate. See **cyclic adenosine monophosphate.**

adenosine triphosphatase (ATPase), an enzyme in skeletal muscle and other tissues that catalyzes the hydrolysis of adenosine triphosphate to adenosine diphosphate and inorganic phosphate. Among various enzymes in this group, mitochondrial ATPase is involved in obtaining energy for cellular metabolism, and myosin ATPase is involved in muscle contraction.

adenosine triphosphate (ATP), a compound consisting of the nucleotide adenosine (A) attached through its ribose

group to three phosphoric acid molecules (P). Hydrolysis of ATP to adenosine diphosphate (D) releases energy. By coupling a less favorable reaction in the cell with this hydrolysis, the less favorable reaction may proceed, allowing one to think of ATP as the cellular energy currency, especially in muscle.

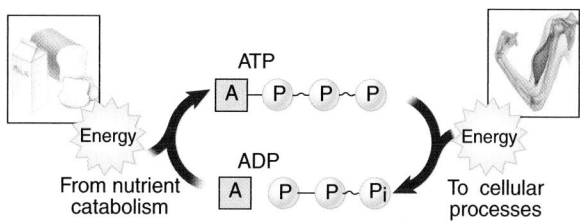

Adenosine triphosphate (ATP) *(Patton and Thibodeau, 2010)*

adenosis /ad′ənō″sis/, **1.** any disease of the glands, especially a lymphatic gland. **2.** excessive or proliferative development or enlargement of glandular tissue.

adenotomy /ad′ənot″əmē/ [Gk, *aden,* gland, *tomé,* a cutting], a dissection of or an incision into a gland.

adenotonsillectomy /ad′ənōton′silek″təmē/, the surgical removal of the adenoids and tonsils. Compare **adenoidectomy, tonsillectomy.**

adenovirus /ad′ənōvī″rəs/ [Gk, *aden* + L, *virus,* poison], any one of more than 55 medium-sized viruses of the Adenoviridae family, pathogenic to humans, that cause conjunctivitis, upper respiratory tract infection, cystitis, or GI infection. The viral genome is linear, double-stranded DNA of varying sizes (26-48 kb). After the acute and symptomatic period of illness, the virus may persist in a latent stage in the tonsils, adenoids, and other lymphoid tissue. Compare **rhinovirus.** *−adenoviral, adj.*

adenylate /əden″ilāt/, a salt or ester of adenylic acid.

adenylate cyclase, an enzyme that initiates the conversion of adenosine triphosphate to cyclic adenosine monophosphate, a mediator of many physiological activities.

adenylate kinase, an enzyme in skeletal muscle that makes possible the reaction ATP + AMP = 2ADP. Also called **myokinase.**

adenylic acid. See **adenosine monophosphate.**

adequate and well-controlled studies, the clinical and laboratory studies that the sponsors of a new drug are required by law to conduct to demonstrate the truth of the claims made for its effectiveness.

adermatoglyphia, the absence of fingerprints from birth. A rare mutation of a gene (SMARCAD1) expressed in the skin. The palms, fingers, toes, and soles of an affected person are also smooth and devoid of normal subtle ridges.

adermia /ədur″mē·ə/ [Gk, *a* + *derma,* without skin], a congenital or acquired skin defect or the absence of skin.

ADH, abbreviation for **antidiuretic hormone.**

ADHA, abbreviation for **American Dental Hygienists' Association.**

adherence /adhir″əns/, **1.** the quality of clinging or being closely attached. **2.** the process in which a person follows rules, guidelines, or standards, especially as a patient follows a prescription and recommendations for a regimen of care. *−adherent, adj., −adhere, v.*

adherent pericardium. See **pericardial adhesion.**

adherent placenta [L, *adhaerens,* sticking to, *placenta,* flat cake], a placenta that remains attached to the uterine wall beyond the normal time after birth of the fetus. See also **placenta accreta.**

adhesin /adhē″sin/, any one of a number of bacterial products that enables bacteria to adhere to and colonize a host.

Adherence is often an essential step in pathogenesis. Adhesins are attractive candidates for vaccines and/or components of accellular vaccines, such as those for pertussis.

adhesion /adhē″zhən/ [L, *adhaerens,* sticking to], a band of scar tissue that binds anatomical surfaces that normally are separate from each other. Adhesions most commonly form in the abdomen after abdominal surgery, inflammation, or injury. A loop of intestine may adhere to unhealed areas. Scar tissue constricting the bowel's lumen may cause intestinal obstruction, blocking intestinal flow and causing abdominal pain, nausea and vomiting, and distention. Nasogastric intubation and suction may relieve symptoms. If the intestinal obstruction does not resolve spontaneously, surgery to lyse adhesions may be necessary. See also **adhesiotomy.**

adhesiotomy /adhē″sē·ot″əmē/ [L, *adhaerens* + Gk, *temnein,* to cut], the surgical division or separation of adhesions, usually performed to relieve an intestinal obstruction. Also called **lysis.** See also **abdominal surgery.**

adhesive /adhē″siv/ [L, *adhaerens,* sticking to], the quality of a substance that enables it to become attached to another substance.

adhesive capsulitis, a shoulder condition characterized by stiffness, pain, and limited passive and active shoulder motion. It most often occurs in midlife, and may be idiopathic or associated with shoulder surgery or injury. Also called *frozen shoulder.* See also **capsulitis.**

adhesive pericarditis. See **pericardial adhesion.**

adhesive peritonitis, an inflammation of the peritoneum characterized by a fibrinous exudate that mats together the intestines and various other organs. This condition may be marked by an exudate of serum, fibrin, cells, and pus, accompanied by abdominal pain and tenderness, vomiting, constipation, and fever.

adhesive phlebitis. See **obliterative phlebitis.**

adhesive pleurisy, an inflammation of the pleura with exudation. It causes obliteration of the pleural space through the fusion of the visceral pleura covering the lungs and the parietal pleura lining the walls of the thoracic cavity.

adhesive skin traction, a type of skin traction in which the therapeutic pull of traction weights is applied with adhesive straps that stick to the skin over the body structure involved, especially a fractured bone. Adhesive skin traction is a short-term treatment used only when continuous traction is desired and skin care for the affected area is easily maintained. It is not suitable for clients with fragile skin. Compare **nonadhesive skin traction.**

adhesive tape, a strong fabric covered on one side with an adhesive. Often water repellent, it may be used to hold bandages and dressings in place, to immobilize a part, or to exert pressure.

ADI, abbreviation for **acceptable daily intake.**

adiadochokinesia /ā′dē·ad′əkō′kinē″zhə, ədī′ədō′kō-/, an inability to perform rapidly alternating movements, such as pronation and supination or flexion and extension. The activity is commonly included in a neurological examination.

adiaphoresis /ā′dē·əfôrē″sis/, an absence or deficiency of perspiration.

adiastole /ā′dī·as″təlē/ [Gk, *a,* not, *dia,* across, *stellein,* to set], the absence or imperceptibility of the diastolic stage of the cardiac cycle. See also **diastole.**

adiathermance /a′dī·əthur″məns/ [Gk, *a* + *dia,* not across, *therme,* heat], the quality of being unaffected by radiated heat.

adient /ad″ē·ənt/ [L, *adire,* moving toward], *n,* characterized by a tendency to move toward rather than away from stimuli. Compare **abient.** –*adience, n.*

Adie pupil /ā″dē/ [William J. Adie, English physician, 1886–1935], an abnormal condition of the eyes marked by one pupil that reacts much more slowly to light changes or to accommodation or convergence than the pupil of the other eye. It is considered a pupillary muscle problem. There is no specific treatment. Also called **tonic pupil.**

Adie syndrome [William J. Adie], Adie pupil accompanied by depressed or absent tendon reflexes, particularly the Achilles tendon and patellar reflexes.

adip-. See **adipo-, adip-.**

adipectomy. See **lipectomy.**

adipic /ədip″ik/ [L, *adeps,* fat], pertaining to fatty tissue.

adipo-, adip-, combining forms meaning "fat": *adipocele, adiponecrosis.*

adipocele /ad″ipōsēl″/ [L, *adeps* + Gk, *kele,* hernia], a hernia containing fat or fatty tissue. Also called **lipocele.**

adipocyte /ad″ipōsīt″/, a fat (adipose) cell, potentially containing a large fat vacuole consisting mainly of triglycerides.

adipofibroma /ad′ipōfībrō″mə/ *pl.* adipofibromas, adipofibromata [L, *adeps* + *fibra,* fiber; Gk, *oma*], a fibrous neoplasm of the connective tissue with fatty components.

adipokinesis /ad′ipō′kinē″sis/, the mobilization of fat or fatty acids in lipid metabolism.

adipokinin /ad′ipōkī″nin/, a hormone of the adenohypophysis that causes mobilization of fat from adipose tissues.

adipometer /ad′ipom″ətər/, an instrument for measuring the thickness of a skin area as a guide for calculating the amount of subcutaneous fat.

adiponecrosis /ad′ipōnikrō″sis/ [L, *adeps* + Gk, *nekros,* dead, *osis* condition], a rarely used term referring to necrosis of fatty tissue in the body. The condition may be associated with hemorrhagic pancreatitis. –*adiponecrotic, adj.*

adiponecrosis subcutanea neonatorum, an abnormal dermatological condition of the newborn characterized by patchy areas of hardened subcutaneous fatty tissue and a bluish-red discoloration of the overlying skin. The lesions, often a result of manipulation during delivery, spontaneously resolve from days to several weeks without scarring. Also called **pseudosclerema, subcutaneous fat necrosis.**

adipose /ad″ipōs/, tissue composed of fat-containing cells arranged in lobules. See also **fat.**

adipose capsule [L, *adeps,* fat, *capsula,* little box], a capsule of fatty tissue surrounding the kidney. Also called **renal fat.**

adipose degeneration. See **fatty degeneration.**

adipose tissue [L, *adeps,* fat; OFr, *tissu*], a collection of fat cells, or adipocytes. See also **fatty tissue.**

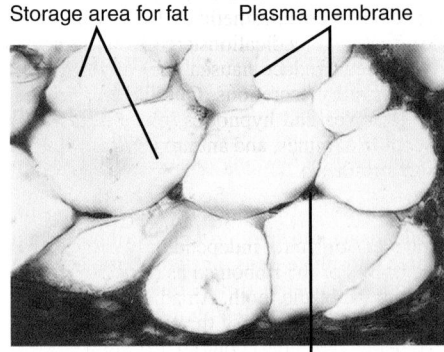

Storage area for fat Plasma membrane

Nucleus of adipose cell

Adipose tissue (© Ed Reschke; used with permission)

adipose tumor. See **lipoma.**

adiposis dolorosa. See **Dercum's disease.**

adiposis edematosa, a dimpling of the skin caused by subcutaneous fat. Also called **cellulite.**

adiposogenital dystrophy /ad′ipō′sōjen″itəl/ [L, *adeps* + *genitalis,* generation], a disorder occurring in males, characterized by genital hypoplasia and feminine secondary sex characteristics, including female distribution of fat. It is caused by hypothalamic malfunction or by a tumor in the adenohypophysis. Hypothermia, hypotension, and hypoglycemia are frequently associated with the disorder. Diabetes insipidus also results from hyposecretion of antidiuretic hormone, which causes increased output of diluted urine, electrolyte imbalances, and thirst. In addition, involvement of the satiety center may induce overeating and result in pronounced obesity. If a tumor is present, there may be drowsiness and symptoms of increased intracranial pressure (for example, subtle locus of control changes and headache). Treatment may include the administration of testosterone and a weight-reduction program, excision or radiological ablation of a tumor, and replacement of hormones, as necessary. Also called **Fröhlich syndrome.**

adipsia /ādip″sē·ə/ [Gk, *a* + *dipsa,* not thirst], an absence of thirst.

aditus /ad″itəs/ [L, *ad,* going to], an approach or an entry.

adjunct /ad″jungkt/ [L, *adjungere,* to join], (in health care) an additional substance, treatment, or procedure used for increasing the efficacy or safety of the primary substance, treatment, or procedure or for facilitating its performance. −*adjunctive, adj.*

adjunctive group /adjungk″tiv/, a group with specific activities and focuses, such as socialization, perceptual stimulation, sensory stimulation, or reality orientation, developing a common understanding.

adjunctive modalities, **1.** *(in occupational therapy)* methods that are complementary to purposeful activity, as well as supportive, but not the end goal of an occupational therapy intervention. See also **purposeful activity. 2.** *(in medicine and nursing)* additional methods used to add to or maximize the effects of primary treatments.

adjunctive psychotherapy, treatments that work together with other forms of therapy and concentrate on improving general mental and physical well-being without trying to resolve basic emotional problems. Kinds include **music therapy, recreational therapy.**

adjunct to anesthesia, one of a number of drugs or techniques used to enhance anesthesia but that are not classified as anesthetics. Adjuncts to anesthesia are used before an anesthetic is administered as premedications and during anesthesia to augment anesthetic effects or diminish undesirable side effects. Premedications are given to reduce anxiety, sedate the patient, reduce nausea and vomiting, and reduce oral and respiratory secretions. Opioid analgesics, benzodiazepines, sedatives and hypnotics, phenothiazines, anticholinergics, antihistamines, and antianxiety agents are common adjuncts to anesthesia.

adjustable axis face-bow. See **kinematic face-bow.**

adjustable orthodontic band /adjus″təbəl/, a soft-metal ribbon and mechanism for independently stretching the upper and lower halves of the ribbon so as to better conform to the anatomical shape of the tooth. An adjustable band automatically conforms to the shape of the tooth when it is tightened above and below the widest contour and allows attachment of an orthodontic appliance. See also **orthodontic band.**

adjusted age, the age of an infant based on due date or gestational age. For example, if a child is 8 months old but was born prematurely by 2 months, the adjusted age is 6 months.

adjusted death rate, a rate that controls for the effects of differences, such as age, in a population. See also **standardized death rate.**

adjustment, the changing of something to modify its relationship to something else. See also **accommodation.**

adjustment disorder [L, *adjuxtare,* to bring together], a temporary disorder of varying severity that occurs as an acute reaction to overwhelming stress in persons of any age who have no apparent underlying mental disorders. Symptoms include anxiety, withdrawal, depression, impulsive outbursts, crying spells, attention-seeking behavior, enuresis, loss of appetite, aches, pains, and muscle spasms. It can be persistent if symptoms continue for six months or more. It can develop in response to an identifiable stressor and result from situations such as separation of an infant from its mother, the birth of a sibling, loss or change of job, death of a loved one, or forced retirement. Symptoms usually recede and eventually disappear as stress diminishes. See also **anxiety disorder.**

adjuvant /ad″jəvənt/ [L, *ad* + *juvare,* to help], **1.** a pharmacological or immunological agent added to a therapeutic regimen to enhance the action of the main agent. These agents/drugs by themselves may have no therapeutic action. **2.** (in immunology) a substance added to an antigen that enhances or modifies the antibody response to the antigen. **3.** an additional treatment or therapy.

adjuvant chemotherapy, the use of additive or supplemental therapies in patients whose known disease has received local therapy, such as surgery, but who are at risk for recurrence or relapse based on protein expression, size of tumor, and characteristics of the tumor environment.

adjuvant radiotherapy, radiotherapy used in addition to surgical resection or chemotherapy in the treatment of cancer; typically used after initial treatment. The goal is to lower the risk that the cancer will return.

adjuvant therapy, the treatment of a disease with modalities or medications that are in addition to the main therapy.

ADL, abbreviation for **activities of daily living.**

adlerian psychology [Alfred Adler, Viennese psychiatrist, 1870–1937], a branch of psychoanalysis that focuses on physical security, sexual satisfaction, and social integration. See also **individual psychology.**

ad lib, a shortened form of a Latin phrase meaning "to be taken as desired." Abbreviation for *ad libitum.*

ADME, denoting the time course of drug distribution. Abbreviation for *absorption, distribution, metabolism, and elimination.*

Administration on Aging (AOA), the principal U.S. agency designated to carry out the provisions of the Older Americans Act of 1965. The AOA advises the U.S. Secretary of the Department of Health and Human Services and other federal departments and agencies on the characteristics and needs of older people and develops programs designed to promote their welfare. The federal government gives funds to states to create and maintain supportive services for older adults. The money is for programs that lead to the well-being of older adults and to their ability to live independently in their homes and communities. Some of these programs offer nutrition, transportation, guidance on elder rights, caregiving support, adult day care, and more. The administration has been in operation for over 35 years.

admission, **1.** the act of being received into a place or class of things. **2.** a patient accepted for service in a hospital, facility, or home health agency. **3.** a concession or acknowledgment.

ADN, abbreviation for **Associate Degree in Nursing.**

adneural /adnoo″əl/, **1.** located near or toward a nerve or nerve ending. **2.** pertaining to the stage of a nervous disorder in which the symptoms are apparent. Also called *adnerval.*

adnexa /adnek″sa/*sing.* **adnexus** [L, *adnectere,* to tie together], tissue or structures in the body adjacent to or near another, related structure. The ovaries and the fallopian tubes are adnexa of the uterus. Also called **annexa.** −*adnexal, adj.*

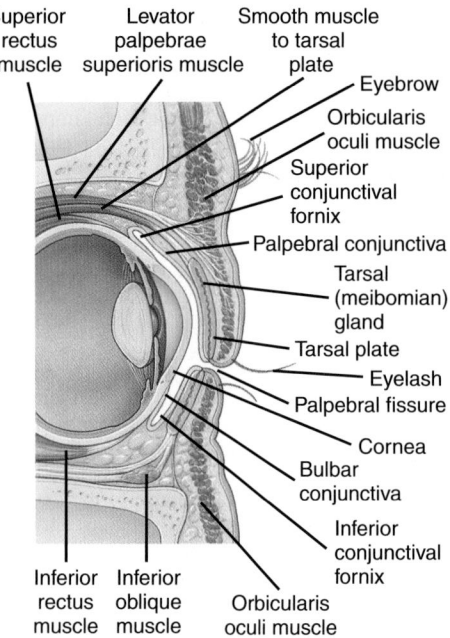

Adnexa oculi *(Thibodeau and Patton, 2007)*

adnexa oculi. See **accessory organs of the eye.**

adnexa uteri. See **uterine appendages.**

adnexectomy /ad′neksek″təmē/ [Gk, *ektomē,* excision], the surgical removal of accessory structures or appendages of an organ.

adnexitis /ad′neksī″tis/, inflammation or infection of the ovaries, fallopian tubes, and/or their supportive ligaments and membranes. See **pelvic inflammatory disease, gonorrhea,** *Chlamydia.*

adnexus. See **adnexa.**

-adol, a combining form designating an analgesic: *Panadol, Toradol.*

adolescence /ad′əles″əns/ [L, *adolescere,* to grow up], **1.** the period in development between the onset of puberty and adulthood. It usually begins between 10 and 14 years of age with the appearance of secondary sex characteristics and spans the teenage years, terminating at 18 to 20 years of age with the completion of the development of the adult form. During this period, the individual undergoes extensive physical, psychological, emotional, and personality changes. **2.** the state or quality of being adolescent or youthful. See also **postpuberty, prepuberty, psychosexual development, psychosocial development, pubarche.**

adolescent, 1. a young person in the process of developing from a child into an adult. **2.** one in the state or process of adolescence; a teenager.

adolescent vertebral epiphysitis. See **Scheuermann disease.**

adoption /ədop″shən/ [L, *adoptere,* to choose], **1.** a selection and inclusion in an established relationship or a choice of treatment protocol. **2.** the legal assumption of responsibility for an infant or child by an adult who is not the biologic parent.

ADP, abbreviation for **adenosine diphosphate.**

ADPKD, abbreviation for *autosomal-dominant polycystic kidney disease.*

adrenal /ədrē″nəl/ [L, *ad,* to, *ren,* kidney], pertaining to the adrenal glands, which are located atop the kidneys. Also called **suprarenal.**

adrenal cortex [L, *ad,* to, *ren,* kidney], the outer and greater portion of the adrenal gland, fused with the gland's medulla. In response to adrenocorticotropic hormone secreted by the adenohypophysis, it secretes mineralocorticoids (primary aldosterone), glucocorticoids (cortisol), and androgens. Adrenal androgens serve as precursors that are converted by the liver to testosterone and estrogens. Renin from the kidney controls adrenal cortical production of aldosterone. Compare **adrenal medulla. –adrenocortical,** *adj.*

adrenal cortical carcinoma, a malignant neoplasm of the adrenal cortex that may cause adrenal virilism or Cushing's syndrome. Such tumors vary in size and may occur at any age. Metastases frequently occur in the lungs, liver, and other organs.

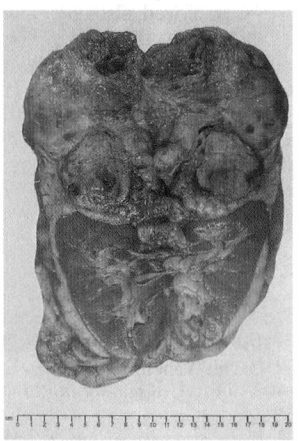

Adrenal cortical carcinoma *(Silverberg et al, 2006)*

adrenal crisis, an acute, life-threatening state of profound adrenocortical insufficiency in which immediate therapy is required. It is characterized by glucocorticoid deficiency, a drop in extracellular fluid volume, and hyperkalemia. Also called **addisonian crisis.** See also **Addison disease, adrenal cortex.**

■ OBSERVATIONS: Typically, the patient appears to be in shock or coma with a low blood pressure, weakness, and loss of vasomotor tone. The person's medical history may include abrupt discontinuation of exogenous steroids or Addison disease or reveal symptoms indicating its presence. Results of laboratory tests show hyperkalemia and hyponatremia.

■ INTERVENTIONS: An IV isotonic solution of sodium chloride containing a water-soluble glucocorticoid is administered rapidly. Vasopressor agents may be necessary to control hypotension. If the patient is vomiting, a nasogastric tube is inserted to prevent aspiration and relieve hyperemesis. Total bed rest and monitoring of blood pressure, temperature, and other vital signs are essential. After the first critical hours, the patient is followed as for Addison disease, and corticosteroid dosage is tapered to maintenance levels. Infection and a failure to increase the maintenance glucocorticoid (steroid) dose are common causes of crisis in people who have Addison disease.

■ PATIENT CARE CONSIDERATIONS: Nursing care during adrenal crisis includes eliminating all forms of stimuli, especially loud noises or bright lights. The patient is not moved unless absolutely necessary and is not allowed to perform self-care activities. If the condition is identified and treated promptly, the prognosis is good. Discharge instructions include a reminder to the patient to seek medical attention in any stressful situation, whether physiological or psychological, to prevent a recurrence of the crisis.

adrenalectomy /ədrē″nəlek″təmē/ [L, *ad + ren;* Gk, *ektomē,* excision], the total or partial surgical resection of one or both adrenal glands. It is performed to reduce the excessive secretion of adrenal hormones caused by an adrenal tumor or a malignancy. See also **Addison disease, Cushing syndrome.**

■ METHOD: Preoperative laboratory tests include electrolytes, fasting blood glucose, glucose tolerance, and an electrocardiogram. The optimization of blood pressure and intravascular volume are important measures to avoid hemodynamic complications. Preoperative preparation includes the use of alpha-adrenergic antagonists, beta-adrenergic antagonists with or without other antihypertensive agents, and fluid therapy. Insulin therapy for hyperglycemia may be necessary. The incision for an open adrenalectomy is made under the twelfth rib in the rear flank area with the patient under general anesthesia. Laparascopic adrenelectomy through a small incision in the abdominal wall may also be employed, also under general anesthesia

■ PATIENT CARE CONSIDERATIONS: Hemodynamic monitoring and preoperative steroid replacement are needed. Before surgery a nasogastric tube may be inserted. Careful intraoperative positioning is necessary for the patient with Cushing syndrome because of osteoporosis, fragile bones, and muscle wasting. In patients with pheochromocytoma, intraoperative manipulation of an adrenal tumor can cause a surge of catecholamines, resulting in a blood pressure increase. Postoperative care focuses on maintaining blood pressure with vasoconstrictors or vasodilators as needed, giving replacement doses of corticosteroids, and monitoring fluid and electrolyte status.

■ OUTCOME CRITERIA: With appropriate medications, resolution of symptoms is achieved in nearly all cases related to excessive secretions. When both glands are removed, the maintenance dosage of steroids continues for life. The prognosis for malignancies is usually poor.

adrenal gland, a small, triangular endocrine gland located on the superior portions of the kidneys and surrounded by the protective fat capsule of the kidneys. It is the result of the fusion of two organs, one forming the inner core, or medulla, and the other forming an outer shell, or cortex, each with independent functions. Also called **suprarenal gland.** See also **adrenal cortex, adrenal medulla.**

Adrenalin, an adrenergic. Brand name for **epinephrine.**

adrenaline. See **epinephrine.**

adrenal insufficiency [L, *ad,* to, *ren,* kidney, *in,* not, *sufficere,* to suffice], a condition in which the adrenal gland is unable to produce adequate amounts of cortical hormones. See also **Addison's disease.**

adrenalism /ah-dren′al-izm/, any disorder of adrenal function, whether of decreased or of heightened function.

adrenalize /ədrē″nəlīz/, to stimulate or excite.

adrenal medulla, the inner portion of the adrenal gland. Its cells secrete the catecholamines epinephrine and norepinephrine when stimulated by the sympathetic division of the autonomic nervous system. Compare **adrenal cortex.**

adrenal virilism, a condition characterized by hypersecretion of adrenal androgens, resulting in somatic masculinization. Excessive production of the hormone may be caused by a virilizing adrenal tumor, congenital adrenal hyperplasia, or an inborn deficiency of enzymes required to transform endogenous androgenic steroids to glucocorticoids. Girls born with adrenogenitalism may be pseudohermaphroditic with clitoral enlargement and labial fusion in infancy and later have low vocal pitch, acne, amenorrhea, and masculine distribution of hair and muscle development. Boys with congenital adrenogenitalism show precocious development of the penis, the prostate, and pubic and axillary hair, but their testes remain small and immature because negative feedback from the high level of adrenal androgens prevents the normal pubertal increase in pituitary gonadotropin levels. Children with the disorder are unusually tall, but their epiphyses close prematurely, and as adults they are abnormally short. Virilizing tumors are more common or more frequently diagnosed in women; they usually occur between 30 and 40 years of age but may arise later, after menopause. Signs of the tumor in women include hirsutism, amenorrhea, oily skin, ovarian changes, muscular hypertrophy, and atrophy of the uterus and breasts. Treatment may involve tumor resection, cortisol administration, and cosmetic surgery. Electrolytic hair removal may be indicated. Also called **adrenogenital syndrome.**

adrenarche /ad′rinär″kē/ [L, *ad + ren;* Gk, *arche,* beginning], the intensified activity in the adrenal cortex that occurs at about 8 years of age and increases the release of various hormones, especially androgens.

adrenergic /ad′rinur″jik/ [L, *ad + ren;* Gk, *ergon,* work], pertaining to sympathetic nerve fibers of the autonomic nervous system that liberate norepinephrine at a synapse where a nerve impulse passes. Compare **antiadrenergic, cholinergic.** See also **sympathomimetic.**

adrenergic blocking agent, a drug that blocks the secretion of epinephrine and norepinephrine at the postganglionic nerve endings of the sympathetic nervous system. See **antiadrenergic.**

adrenergic bronchodilator, a drug that acts on the beta$_2$ sympathetic nervous system of the receptors to relax bronchial

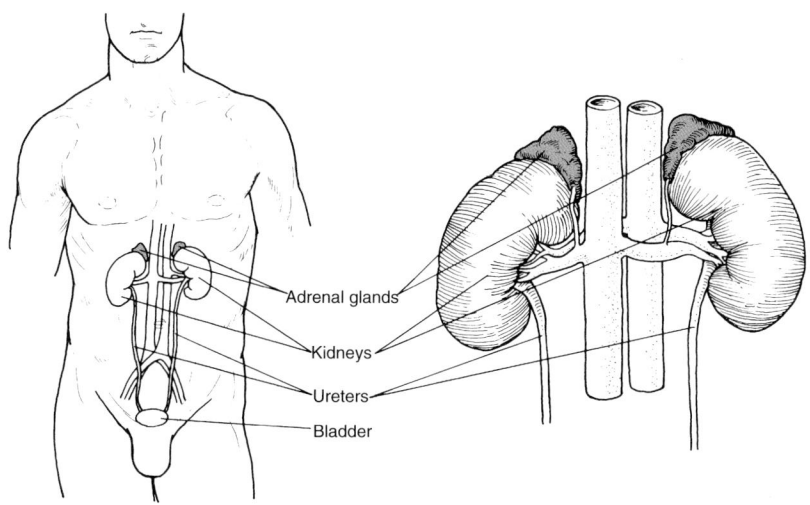

Adrenal gland *(Black and Hawks, 2009)*

smooth muscle cells. Examples include drugs that contain epinephrine, ephedrine, isoproterenol hydrochloride, or albuterol.

adrenergic fiber, a ganglionic nerve fiber of the autonomic nervous system that releases the neurotransmitter norepinephrine and, in some areas, dopamine. Most postganglionic sympathetic nerve fibers are of this type.

adrenergic receptor [L, *ad* + *ren,* kidney; Gk, *ergon,* work; L, *recipere,* to receive], a protein site in an organ, muscle, or gland that mediates the effects of neurotransmitters of the sympathetic nervous system, norepinephrine and epinephrine. Two types of adrenergic receptors are recognized: alpha-adrenergic and beta-adrenergic.

-adrenia, a combining form meaning "(degree or condition of) adrenal activity."

adrenocortical, referring to the structure and function of the adrenal cortex. See **adrenal cortex.**

adrenocortical cytomegaly, an abnormal enlargement of cells in the outer layer of the adrenal cortex.

adrenocortical hormone (ACH) [L, *ad,* to, *ren,* kidney, *cortex,* bark; Gk, *hormaein,* to set in motion], any of the hormones secreted by the cortex of the adrenal gland, including glucocorticoids, mineralocorticoids, and androgens.

adrenocorticotropic /ədrē′nōkôr′tikōtrop″ik/ [L, *ad* + *ren* + *cortex,* bark; Gk, *trope,* a turning], pertaining to stimulation of the adrenal cortex. Also spelled *adrenocorticotrophic.*

adrenocorticotropic hormone (ACTH), a hormone of the adenohypophysis that stimulates growth of the adrenal cortex and the synthesis and secretion of corticosteroids. ACTH secretion, regulated by corticotropin-releasing hormone from the hypothalamus, increases in response to a low level of circulating cortisol and to stress, fever, acute hypoglycemia, and major surgery. Under normal conditions a diurnal rhythm occurs in ACTH secretion, with an increase beginning after the first few hours of sleep and reaching a peak at the time a person awakens and a low in the evening. Normal ranges are from 15 to 100 pg/mL (10 to 80 ng/L) in the morning to less than 50 pg/mL (50 ng/L) in the evening. Normal values vary by laboratory. ACTH may be used in the treatment of rheumatoid arthritis, multiple sclerosis, and myasthenia. Also spelled *adrenocorticotrophic hormone.*

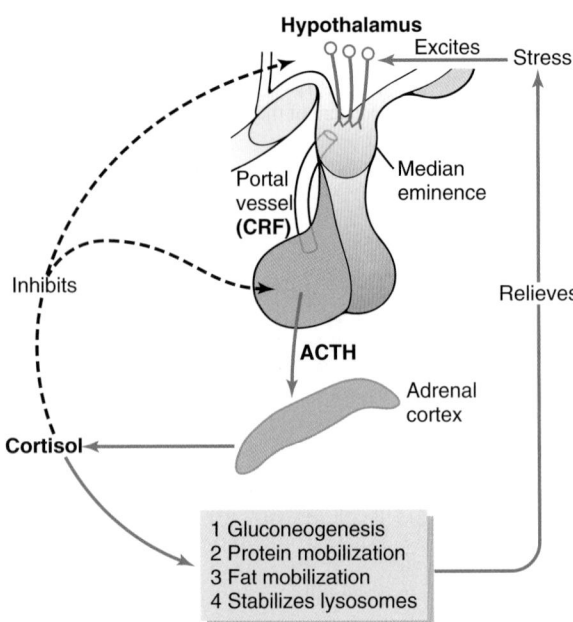

Hypothalamus

Excites — Stress

Portal vessel **(CRF)**

Median eminence

Inhibits

Relieves

ACTH

Adrenal cortex

Cortisol

1 Gluconeogenesis
2 Protein mobilization
3 Fat mobilization
4 Stabilizes lysosomes

Feedback mechanism of ACTH *(Hall and Guyton, 2011)*

adrenocorticotropic hormone test, a blood test used to study the functioning of the adenohypophysis by measuring cortisol levels. The test is used to diagnose Cushing syndrome and Addison disease, which are characterized by overproduction and underproduction of cortisol, respectively.

adrenocorticotropic hormone (ACTH) stimulation test with cosyntropin, a blood test performed on patients with adrenal insufficiency to indicate whether the adrenal gland is normal and capable of functioning if stimulated or if the patient has Addison disease or Cushing syndrome.

adrenocorticotropic hormone (ACTH) stimulation test with metyrapone, a blood or urine test similar to the ACTH stimulation test with cosyntropin. The test can confirm adrenal hyperplasia or adrenal adenoma or carcinoma. It can document that adrenal insufficiency exists as a result of pituitary disease rather than primary adrenal pathology. Metyrapone has been associated with life-threatening adrenal crisis in patients with primary insufficiency and should not be used on such patients.

adrenocorticotropin /-trop″in/, the adrenocorticotropic hormone secreted by the adenohypophysis that stimulates secretion of corticosteroid hormones by the adrenal cortex.

adrenodoxin /ədrē′nōdok″sin/, a nonheme iron protein, produced by the adrenal glands, that participates in the transfer of electrons.

adrenogenital syndrome (AGS), now called **congenital adrenal hyperplasia.**

adrenoleukodystrophy (ALD), a rare hereditary neonatal-childhood metabolic disorder that is transmitted as a recessive sex-linked trait and affects mainly males. It is characterized by adrenal atrophy and widespread cerebral demyelination, producing progressive mental deterioration, aphasia, apraxia, eventual blindness, and paralysis. In the neonate form the prognosis is poor, with death occurring usually in 1 to 5 years. The childhood form may be chronic and treatable for a few years with a special diet. Formerly called **Schilder disease.**

adrenomegaly /-meg″əlē/ [L, *ad* + *ren;* Gk, *megaly,* large], an abnormal enlargement of one or both adrenal glands.

adrenomimetic /-mimet″ik/, mimicking the functions of the adrenal hormones.

adrenotropic /-trop′ik/, having a stimulating effect on the adrenal glands.

Adriamycin RDF, an anthracycline antibiotic antineoplastic agent. Brand name for **DOXOrubicin hydrochloride.**

Adrucil, an antineoplastic. Brand name for **fluorouracil.**

ADRV, abbreviation for **adult rotavirus.**

Adson-Brown forceps [Alfred W. Adson, American neurosurgeon, 1887–1951; James B. Brown, American plastic surgeon, 1899–1971], a thumb forceps similar to the Adson forceps, having fine teeth at the tip, used for grasping delicate tissue. Also called **Brown-Adson forceps.**

Adson forceps [Alfred W. Adson, American neurosurgeon, 1887–1951], a small thumb forceps having a fine tip, with or without teeth.

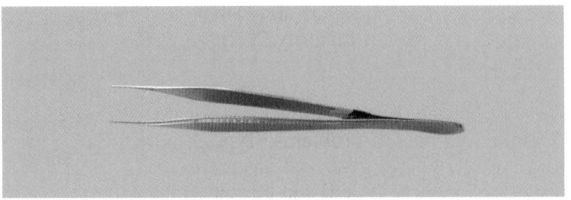

Adson tissue forceps *(Tighe, 2016)*

Adson's maneuver [Alfred W. Adson], a test for thoracic outlet syndrome. It is performed with the patient sitting with hands on the thighs. The examiner palpates both radial pulses as the patient takes a deep breath and holds it while extending the neck and turning the head toward the affected side. If the radial pulse on the affected side is significantly diminished or there is numbness or tingling in the hand, the result is regarded as positive. Also called *Adson's test*.

adsorbent /adsôr″bənt/, a substance, such as activated charcoal, that takes up another by the process of adsorption, as by the attachment of one substance to the surface of the other.

adsorption /adsôrp″shən/ [L, *ad* + *sorbere,* to suck in], *n,* a natural process whereby molecules of a gas or liquid adhere to the surface of a solid. The phenomenon depends on an assortment of factors such as surface tension and electrical charges. Many biological reactions involve adsorption. Adsorption is the principle on which chromatography is based and which allows for the separation of a mixture into component fractions for qualitative analysis. See also **chromatography**. −*adsorb, v.*

adtorsion /ad-tor′shun/, a turning inward of both eyes.

adult /ədult″, ad″ult/ [L, *adultus,* grown up], **1.** one who is fully grown and developed in mind, body, and spirit who has demonstrated the intellectual capacity and emotional and psychological stability to function independently. **2.** a person who has reached full legal age. Compare **child. 3.** any fully grown and mature organism.

adult celiac disease. See **celiac disease.**

adult ceroid lipofuscinosis, a nervous system disorder. Unlike other forms of neuronal ceroid lipofuscinosis, the adult form does not cause blindness. Type A is caused by mutations in the CLN6 gene and is inherited in an autosomal-recessive pattern. Type B can be caused by mutations in the DNAJC5 gene and is inherited in an autosomal-dominant pattern. Symptoms include movement disorders, seizures, dementia, and speech problems. Now called **adult neuronal ceroid lipofuscinosis.** See **Kufs disease.**

adult day-care center, a nonresidential facility for the supervised care of older adults, providing activities such as meals and socialization one or more days a week during specified daytime hours. The participants, primarily persons with physical and/or mental limitations who require socialization, physical assistance, and/or psychological assistance, return to their homes each evening. The program is often used as respite by family members caring for an older person who cannot be left alone safely in the home.

adult ego state, (in psychiatry) a part of the self that analyzes and solves problems, using information received from the parent ego and child ego states. It is assumed to be fully developed in a normal individual at the age of 12. The term is used in transactional analysis.

adulteration /ədul′tərā″shən/ [L, *adulterare,* to defile], an infusion and/or mixing with anything less than clear and clean, resulting in a preparation that is diluted or contaminated.

adult hemoglobin. See **hemoglobin A.**

adulthood, the phase of development characterized by physical and mental maturity. May be specified by law or culture.

adult neuronal ceroid lipofuscinosis, a disorder of the nervous system causing movement disorders, seizures, dementia, and speech problems. Type A is caused by mutations in the CLN6 gene and is inherited in an autosomal-recessive pattern. Type B can be caused by mutations in the DNAJC5 gene and is inherited in an autosomal-dominant pattern.

adult nurse practitioner, a registered nurse who has received additional education in the primary health care of adults. The additional education may be obtained through graduate-level education. The last examination for certification as an adult nurse practitioner was administered in 2016.

adult-onset diabetes, *(Obsolete)* now called **type 2 diabetes mellitus.**

adult polycystic disease (APD), *(Obsolete)* See **polycystic kidney disease.**

adult respiratory distress syndrome (ARDS), severe pulmonary congestion characterized by diffuse injury to alveolar-capillary membranes. Fulminating sepsis, especially when gram-negative bacteria are involved, is the most common cause. ARDS may occur after trauma; near-drowning; aspiration of gastric acid; paraquat ingestion; inhalation of corrosive chemicals, such as chlorine, ammonia, or phosgene; or the use of certain drugs, including barbiturates, chlordiazepoxide, heroin, methadone hydrochloride, propoxyphene hydrochloride, and salicylates. Other causes include diabetic ketoacidosis, fungal infections, high altitude, pancreatitis, tuberculosis, and uremia. Also called **acute respiratory distress syndrome, congestive atelectasis, hemorrhagic lung, noncardiogenic pulmonary edema, pump lung, shock lung, stiff lung, wet lung, chronic obstructive pulmonary disease.**

■ OBSERVATIONS: Signs and symptoms include dyspnea, tachypnea, adventitious breath sounds, hypoxemia, and decreased lung compliance. Changes occurring within the lung include damage to the alveolar-capillary membranes, leakage of plasma proteins into the alveoli, dilution of surfactant, cessation of surfactant production, hemorrhage, interstitial edema, impaired gas exchange, and ventilation-perfusion defects.

■ INTERVENTIONS: Treatment includes establishing an airway, administering oxygen, improving the underlying condition, removing the cause of ARDS, suctioning the respiratory passages as necessary, and reducing oxygen consumption. When ventilation cannot be maintained and there is evidence of a rising partial pressure of carbon dioxide in arterial blood, mechanical ventilation is necessary. Positive end-expiratory pressure (PEEP) is widely used in the treatment of ARDS. All interventions for ARDS are supportive; there is no cure.

■ PATIENT CARE CONSIDERATIONS: The patient with ARDS requires constant and meticulous care, reassurance, and observation for changes in respiratory function and adequacy, including signs of hypercapnia, hypoxemia (especially confusion), skin flushing, and behavior changes such as agitation and restlessness. Increasing hypoxia may be signaled by tachycardia, elevated blood pressure, increased peripheral resistance, and fulminating respiratory failure. If PEEP is being used, the patient is carefully observed for a sudden disappearance of breath sounds accompanied by signs of respiratory distress—an indication that pneumothorax may be present. Respiratory therapy, sterile suction techniques, and position changes are continued as necessary. The patient's weight is measured frequently, chest x-ray films are evaluated, and bacteriological cultures of secretions are analyzed for the causative organism. Throughout treatment, ventilation is carefully monitored through analysis of arterial blood gases. ARDS has a 50% mortality rate.

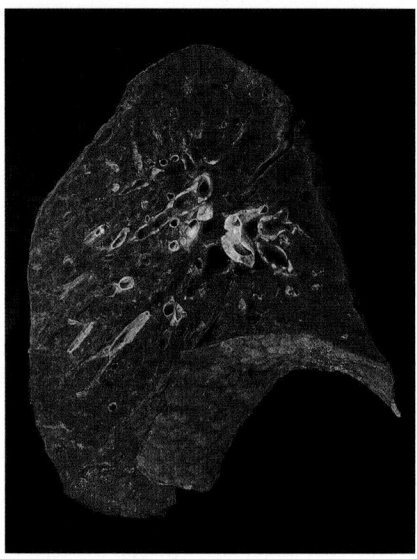

Diffuse alveolar damage in adult respiratory distress syndrome *(Finkbeiner, Ursell, and Davis, 2009)*

adult rickets. See **osteomalacia.**

adult rotavirus (ADRV), a form of rotavirus that causes severe diarrhea in adults. The virus resembles the usual rotavirus and its genome, but it is not antigenically related and does not react against rotavirus antibodies.

advanced burn life support (ABLS), assessment and management of burn patients provided by emergency care personnel from the scene of injury through the first 24 hours following injury. It includes evaluation of the patient, airway management and ventilatory support, fluid resuscitation, and determination of whether the patient should be transferred to a burn center.

advanced cardiac life support (ACLS), emergency medical procedures in which basic life support efforts of cardiopulmonary resuscitation are augmented by establishment of an IV fluid line, possible defibrillation, drug administration, control of cardiac arrhythmias, endotracheal intubation, and use of ventilation equipment.

advance directive [Fr, *avancer,* to move forward; L, *dirigere,* to direct], a legal written document with instructions related to medical care and end-of-life choices if the individual is unable to speak for himself or herself. See **durable power of attorney for health care, living will.**

advanced life support (ALS), a higher level of emergency medical care, usually provided by EMT-intermediates or paramedics. Typically ALS includes invasive techniques such as IV therapy, intubation, and/or drug administration.

advanced practice nurse (APN), a registered nurse having education beyond the basic nursing education and certified by a nationally recognized professional organization in a nursing specialty, or meeting other criteria established by a Board of Nursing in the United States or the Canadian Nurses Association (CNA) in Canada. The Board of Nursing or CNA establishes rules specifying which professional nursing organization certifications can be recognized for advanced practice nurses and sets requirements of education, training, and experience. Kinds include **certified nurse-midwife, nurse anesthetist, clinical nurse specialist, nurse practitioner.**

Advanced Trauma Life Support® (ATLS), an educational program developed by the American College of Surgeons, used worldwide, emphasizing a standardized approach to the care of patients in trauma emergency situations.

advancement /advans″/ [Fr, *avancer,* to move forward], a surgical technique in which a muscle or tendon is detached and then reattached at an advanced point.

adventitia /ad′ventish″ə/ [L, *adventitius,* coming from abroad], the outermost layer, composed of connective tissue with elastic and collagenous fibers, of an artery or another structure. Also called **tunica adventitia.**

adventitious, 1. pertaining to an accidental condition or an arbitrary action. 2. the absence of a genetic relationship or family association. 3. occurring at an inappropriate place, such as a coating on an artery.

adventitious bursa, an abnormal fluid-filled sac that develops as a response to friction or pressure.

adventitious crisis, a rare accidental and unexpected tragedy that may affect an entire community or population, such as an earthquake, flood, or airplane crash. In addition to injuries, loss of life, and property damage, an adventitious crisis often results in long-term psychological effects.

adventitious cyst, 1. an accumulation of fluid in a cystlike loculus but without an epithelial or other membranous lining. See also **pseudocyst. 2.** a cyst with a wall formed by a host cell and not by a parasite.

Abnormal (adventitious) lung sounds

Type	Physiology	Auscultation	Sound	Possible condition
Crackles	Air passing through fluid in small airways, or sudden opening of deflated, weakened airways	More commonly heard during inspiration	Fine high-pitched or coarse low-pitched popping sounds that are short and discontinuous	Pneumonia, heart failure, atelectasis, emphysema
Rhonchi	Large airway obstructed by fluid	Heard commonly during expiration	Low-pitched, continuous snoring sound	Chronic obstructive pulmonary disease (COPD), bronchospasm, pneumonia
Wheezes	Air passing through narrowed airways	Can be heard throughout inspiration and expiration	High-pitched, whistling sound	Airway obstruction, bronchospasm as in asthma, COPD
Pleural friction rub	Rubbing of inflamed pleura	May occur throughout respiratory cycle; heard best at base of lung at end of expiration	Scratching, grating, rubbing, creaking	Inflamed pleura, pulmonary infarction

From Monahan FD et al: *Phipps' medical-surgical nursing: health and illness perspectives,* ed 8, St Louis, 2007, Mosby.

adventitious sound, a breath sound that is not normally heard, such as a crackle, gurgle, rhonchus, or wheeze. It may be superimposed on normal breath sounds.

adverse childhood experiences (ACEs), traumatic events occuring before the age of 18, including but not limited to experiencing violence, abuse, or neglect; witnessing violence in the home; or having a family member attempt or die by suicide. ACEs are associated with risky health behaviors, chronic health problems, and a variety of negative outcomes as an adult. Understanding the impact of ACEs can lead to more trauma-informed interventions that help to mitigate negative outcomes.

adverse drug effect /advurs″, ad″vers/, an unintended reaction to a drug administered at normal dosage.

adverse drug reaction, any unwanted or unintended effect on the body as a result of the use of medications at normal therapeutic doses. Also called **drug reaction.**

adverse reaction, any harmful, unintended effect of a medication, diagnostic test, or therapeutic intervention.

advocacy /ad″vəkas′ē/, **1.** a process whereby a health care professional provides a patient with the information to make certain decisions, usually related to some aspect of the patient's health care. **2.** a method by which patients, their families, attorneys, health professionals, and citizen groups can work together to develop programs that ensure the availability of high-quality health care for a community. **3.** supporting a cause on behalf of another, such as a nurse advising a colleague on better care of a patient, a physical or occupational therapist lobbying for appropriate professional services, or any health care professional urging others that the patient's desires be honored.

adynamia /ad′inā″mē·ə/ [Gk, *a + dynamis,* not strength], a lack of physical strength resulting from a pathological condition. See also **asthenia.** *–adynamic, adj.*

adynamia episodica hereditaria, a condition of infancy, characterized by periodic muscle weakness and episodes of flaccid paralysis. It is inherited as an autosomal-dominant trait. Also called **hyperkalemic periodic paralysis.**

adynamic fever, a high temperature accompanied by muscular debility. Also called *asthenic fever.*

adynamic ileus. See **paralytic ileus.**

AEC syndrome, abbreviation for **ankyloblepharon–ectodermal dysplasia–clefting syndrome.** See **Hay-Wells syndrome.**

AED, abbreviation for **automated external defibrillator.**

Aedes /ā·ē′dēz/ [Gk, *aedes,* unpleasant], a genus of mosquito prevalent in tropical and subtropical regions. Several species are capable of transmitting pathogenic organisms to humans, including dengue fever, equine encephalitis, St. Louis encephalitis, tularemia, and yellow fever.

aer-. See **aero-, aer-.**

aeration [Gk, *aer,* air], **1.** the exchange of carbon dioxide for oxygen by blood in the lungs. **2.** the process of exposing a tissue or fluid to air or artificially charging it with oxygen or another gas, such as carbon dioxide. *–aerate, v.*

aero-, aer-, combining forms meaning "air" or "gas": *aerobe, aeration.*

Aerobacter aerogenes, a species of gram-negative aerobic bacteria that produces gas and acid from sugar and that is sometimes involved in souring milk. Also called *Enterobacter aerogenes.*

aerobe /er″ōb/ *pl.* aerobia [Gk, *aer + bios,* life], a microorganism able to live and grow in the presence of free oxygen. Compare **anaerobe, microaerophile.** Kinds include **facultative aerobe, obligate aerobe. –aerobic,** *adj.*

aerobic /erō″bik/, **1.** pertaining to the presence of air or oxygen. **2.** able to live and function in the presence of free oxygen. **3.** requiring oxygen for the maintenance of life. **4.** a chemical requiring the presence of oxygen.

aerobic capacity, the maximal amount of physiological work that an individual can do as measured by oxygen consumption. It is determined by a combination of aging and cardiovascular conditioning and is associated with the efficiency of oxygen extraction from the tissue.

aerobic exercise, any physical exercise that requires additional effort by the heart and lungs to meet the striated muscles' increased demand for oxygen. Aerobic exercise increases the breathing rate and ultimately raises heart and lung efficiency. Prolonged aerobic exercise (at least 20 minutes five times a week) is recommended for the maintenance of a healthy cardiovascular system. Examples of aerobic exercise include running, jogging, swimming, and vigorous dancing or cycling. Compare **anaerobic exercise.** See also **active exercise, passive exercise.**

aerobic glycolysis. See **glycolysis.**

aerobics. See **aerobic exercise.**

AeroBid /ār′ō-bid″/, an oral inhalation preparation. Brand name for **flunisolide.**

aerodontalgia /er′ōdontal″jə/ [Gk, *aer + odous,* tooth, *algos,* pain], a painful sensation in the teeth caused by a lowering of atmospheric pressure, as may occur at high altitudes.

aerodynamics, the study of air or other gases in motion or of bodies moving in air.

aerodynamic size, pertaining to the behavior of various aerosol particle sizes and densities.

aeroembolism. See **air embolism.**

Aeromonas /er′ōmō″nəs/, a genus of pathogenic, rod-shaped, gram-negative bacteria (schizomycetes) found in freshwater and saltwater, soil, and sewage. Various species affect fish, amphibians, reptiles, and animals, as well as humans, causing wound infections and gastroenteritis.

aerophagy /erof″əjē/ [Gk, *aer + phagein,* to eat], the excessive swallowing of air, usually an unconscious process associated with anxiety, resulting in abdominal distension or belching, gastric distress, and flatulence. It is often interpreted by the patient as signs of a physical disorder.

aerosinusitis /er′ōsī′nəsī″tis/ [Gk, *aer + L, sinus,* curve; Gk, *itis*], inflammation, edema, or hemorrhage of the frontal sinuses, caused by an expansion of air within the sinuses when the barometric pressure is decreased, as in an aircraft at high altitudes. Also called **barosinusitis.**

aerosol /er″əsol′/ [Gk, *aer;* L, *solutus,* in dissolved], **1.** nebulized particles suspended in a gas or in air. **2.** a pressurized gas containing a finely nebulized medication for inhalation therapy. **3.** a pressurized gas containing a nebulized chemical agent for sterilizing the air of a room.

aerosol bronchodilator therapy, the use of drugs that relax the respiratory tract smooth muscle tissue when administered as tiny droplets or a mist to be inhaled.

aerosol therapy, the use of an aerosol for respiratory care in the treatment of bronchopulmonary disease. Aerosol therapy allows the delivery of medications, humidity, or both to the mucosa of the respiratory tract and pulmonary alveoli. Agents delivered by aerosol therapy may relieve spasm of the bronchial muscles and reduce edema of the mucous membranes, liquefy bronchial secretions so that they are more easily removed, humidify the respiratory tract, and administer antibiotics locally by depositing them in the respiratory tract.

aerospace medicine /er″ōspās′/, a subspecialty of occupational medicine concerned with the physiological and psychological effects of air and space travel, safety in flight, and adaptation to environments associated with flight. See also **aviation medicine.**

aerotherapy /er′ōther″əpē/, the use of fresh air or air of differing pressures in treating disease, as in hyperbaric oxygenation.

aerotitis /er′ətī′tis/ [Gk, *aer* + *otikos,* ear, *itis*], an inflammation of the ear caused by changes in atmospheric pressure. Also called **barotitis.**

aerotitis media, inflammation or bleeding in the middle ear caused by a difference between the air pressure in the middle ear and that of the atmosphere, as occurs in sudden altitude changes, scuba diving, and hyperbaric chambers. Symptoms are pain, tinnitus, diminished hearing, and vertigo. Also called **barotitis media.**

Aesculapius /es′kyo̅o̅lā″pē·əs/, the ancient Greek god of medicine. According to legend, Aesculapius, the son of Apollo, was trained by the centaur Chiron in the art of healing; he became so proficient that he not only cured sick patients but also restored the dead to life. Because Zeus feared that Aesculapius could help humans escape death altogether, he killed the healer with a bolt of lightning. Later, Aesculapius was raised to the stature of a god and was worshipped also by the Romans, who believed he could prevent pestilence. Serpents were regarded as sacred by Aesculapius, and he is symbolized in modern medicine by a staff with a serpent entwined about it. See also **staff of Aesculapius.**

-aesthesia, -esthesia, suffixes meaning "(condition of) feeling, perception, or sensation": *kinesthesia, allesthesia.*

aesthetics. See **esthetics.**

aesthetic surgery. See **cosmetic surgery.**

-aesthetic. See **-esthetic, -esthetical, -esthes, -aesthetic, -aesthetical.**

AF, 1. abbreviation for **atrial fibrillation.** 2. abbreviation for **atrial flutter.**

af-. See **ad-.**

AFB, abbreviation for **acid-fast bacillus.**

afebrile /āfē″bril, āfeb′ril/ [Gk, *a* + *febris,* not fever], without fever. Also called **apyretic.** Compare **febrile.**

affect /əfekt′/ [L, *affectus,* influence], an outward, observable manifestation of a person's expressed feelings or emotions, such as flat, blunted, bland, or bright. –*affective, adj.*

affection /əfek″shən/ [L, influence], 1. an emotional state expressed by a warm or caring feeling toward another individual. 2. a disease process affecting all or a part of the human body.

affective disorder. See **mood disorder.**

affective intimacy, a measure of well-being in a family group that focuses on whether members feel close to one another yet do not lose their individuality.

affective learning, the acquisition of behaviors involved in expressing feelings in attitudes, appreciations, and values.

affective psychosis, a psychological reaction, such as psychotic depression or mania, in which the ego's functioning is impaired and there is loss of reality orientation. The primary clinical feature is a severe disorder of mood or emotions.

affect memory, a particular emotionally expressed feeling that recurs whenever a significant experience is recalled.

afferent /af″ərənt/ [L, *ad* + *ferre,* to carry], proceeding toward a center from the periphery, as applied to arteries, veins, lymphatic vessels, and nerves. Compare **efferent.**

afferent glomerular arteriole. See **vas afferens.**

afferent nerve [L, *ad* + *ferre,* to bear, *nervus*], a nerve fiber that transmits impulses from the periphery toward the central nervous system.

afferent pathway [L, *ad* + *ferre,* to bear; AS, *paeth* + *weg*], the course or route taken, usually by a linkage of neurons, from the periphery of the body toward the central nervous system.

afferent tract [L, *ad* + *ferre,* to bear, *tractus*], a pathway for nerve impulses traveling inward or toward the brain, the center of an organ, or another body structure. Also called **ascending tract.**

affidavit /af′idā″vit/ [L, he has pledged], a written statement that is sworn to before a notary public or an officer of the court.

affiliated hospital /əfil′ē·ā′tid/ [L, *ad* + *filius,* to son], a hospital that is associated to some degree with a medical school, a health profession, a health program, or another health care institution.

affinity /əfin″itē/ [L, *affinis,* related], 1. the measure of the binding strength of the antigen-antibody reaction. 2. the energy released or absorbed by an electron being added to a neutral atom in the gas phase.

affirmation [L, *affirmare,* to make firm], 1. (in psychology) autosuggestion; the point at which a tendency toward positive reaction or belief is observed by the therapist. 2. a positive thought or statement intended to reinforce desired behaviors or actions.

affirmative defense /əfur″mətiv/ [L, *affirmare,* to make firm], (in civil law) a denial of guilt or wrongdoing by a health care provider in a civil action in which one asserts that one adhered to the local standards of care. The defendant bears the burden of proof in an affirmative defense.

affusion /afyoo″zhən/ [L, *affundere,* to pour out], a culturally based form of therapy in which water is sprinkled or poured over the body or a particular body part. Although most often associated with baptism rituals, it is also used in facial and anti-anxiety treatments, especially in a spa environment.

afibrinogenemia /afī′brinō′jenē″mē·ə/ [Gk, *a,* not; L, *fibra,* fiber; Gk, *genein,* to produce, *haima,* blood], congenital absence of fibrinogen from the plasma associated with moderate to severe bleeding. Also spelled *afibrinogenaemia.*

aflatoxins /af′lātok″sins/ [Gk, *a,* not; L, *flavus,* yellow; Gk, *toxikon,* poison], a group of carcinogenic and toxic factors produced by *Aspergillus flavus* food molds. The degree of contamination will vary with geographic location and practices. Occurrence is influenced by environmental factors, especially those that encourage fungal growth. Aflatoxins are associated with potent carcinogenic effect in susceptible animals and acute toxicological effects in humans.

aflatoxicosis, an acute, subacute, or chronic syndrome associated with the consumption of foods contaminated with aflatoxins. The syndrome is most prevalent in developing countries. It is characterized by vomiting and abdominal pain. Pulmonary edema, convulsions, coma, and death, with cerebral edema and fatty involvement of the liver, kidneys, and heart, may also occur. Chronic exposure to aflatoxins is associated with changes in nutrition and immunity. Treatment involves the use of antimicrobials and supportive care related to symptomology.

AFMC, abbreviation for **Association of Faculties of Medicine of Canada.**

AFO, abbreviation for **ankle-foot orthosis.**

AFP, abbreviation for **alpha-fetoprotein.**

African hemorrhagic fever, any one of the hemorrhagic fevers that are known to occur in Africa, associated with morphologically similar but antigenically distinct viruses. Kinds include **Ebola virus disease, Lassa fever, yellow fever, Rift Valley fever, Marburg virus disease, Crimean-Congo hemorrhagic fever.**

African lymphoma, (*Obsolete*) now called **Burkitt lymphoma.**

African relapsing fever, now called **Borrelia duttoni.**

African sleeping sickness, now called **African trypanosomiasis.**

African tick fever, a tickborne or spotted fever caused by *Rickettsia africae* that develops into a diffuse rash.

Symptoms appear 2 weeks after the bite and often include fever, headache, muscle soreness, and rash. Multiple eschars, lymphangitis, lymphadenopathy, and edema are common. At the site of the tick bite the skin will be red and sore with a dark center. See also **relapsing fever.**

African tick typhus,   **1.** a rickettsial infection transmitted by ixodid (hard) ticks and characterized by fever, chills, maculopapular rash, headache, myalgia, arthralgias, and swollen lymph nodes. At the onset of the infection, a local lesion called tache noire appears at the site of the tick bite. The rash usually begins on the forearms and spreads over the rest of the body. The fever may persist into the second week, but death or complications are rare. **2.** tickborne rickettsial disease of the eastern hemisphere similar to Rocky Mountain spotted fever but less severe.

African trypanosomiasis,   a disease caused by the parasite *Trypanosoma brucei gambiense* (West African or Gambian trypanosomiasis) or *T. brucei rhodesiense* (East African or Rhodesian trypanosomiasis), transmitted to humans by the bite of the tsetse fly. African trypanosomiasis occurs only in the savannahs and woodlands of central and east Africa, where tsetse flies are found. The disease progresses through two phases: Stage 1 is marked by fever, lymphadenopathy, splenomegaly, and myocarditis. Stage 2 is marked by symptoms of central nervous system involvement, including lethargy, sleepiness, headache, convulsions, and coma. The disease is fatal unless treated, though it may be years before the patient reaches the neurological phase. Antimicrobial medications specific for the treatment of trypanosomiasis include suramin sodium, pentamidine isothionate, organic arsenicals, difluoromethylornithine, and eflornithine. Also called **African sleeping sickness, sleeping sickness.** Kinds include **Gambian trypanosomiasis, Rhodesian trypanosomiasis.** See also **trypanosomiasis.**

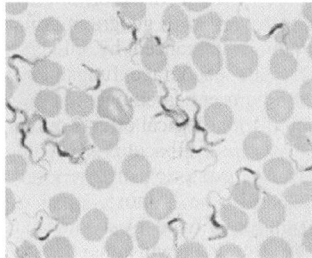

African trypanosomiasis: parasites in blood *(Kumar et al, 2010)*

Afrin,   an adrenergic vasoconstrictor. Brand name for **oxymetazoline hydrochloride.**

after-action report,   an analysis conducted after a disaster response or a disaster drill that includes all responders and agencies involved to evaluate actions taken and make recommendations for improvement.

afterbirth [AS, *aefter* + ME, *burth*],   the placenta, the amnion, the chorion, and some amniotic fluid, blood, and blood clots expelled from the uterus after childbirth.

aftercare [AS, *aefter* + *caru*],   health care offered a patient after discharge from a hospital or another health care facility. Patients frequently require professional services to manage health problems and conditions that no longer require inpatient status. Examples of aftercare include outpatient rehabilitation or home care services.

afterdepolarization /-dēpō′lərizā″shən/,   a membrane potential depolarization that follows an action potential. In cardiac muscles, it may be early (during phases 2 and 3 of the action potential) or delayed (during phase 4), and it is thought to cause atrial and ventricular tachycardia, especially in the setting of a long Q-T interval or digitalis poisoning. Also called **afterpotential.**

aftereffect,   a physical or psychological effect that continues after the stimulus is removed.

afterimage,   a visual sensation that continues after the stimulus ends. The image may appear in colors complementary to those of the stimulus.

afterload [AS, *aefter* + ME *lod*],   the load, or resistance, against which the left ventricle must eject its volume of blood during contraction. The resistance is produced by the volume of blood already in the vascular system and by the constriction of the vessel walls.

afterloading,   a technique for the administration of brachytherapy. Local catheters are surgically placed in the patient and subsequently loaded, under controlled conditions to protect health care personnel, with a radioactive source. See also **remote afterloading.**

afterpain [AS, *aefter* + Gk, *poine*, penalty],   one of many contractions of the uterus common during the first days after childbirth. Afterpains tend to be strongest during breastfeeding, in multiparas, after the birth of large babies, and after overdistension of the uterus. They usually resolve spontaneously but may require analgesia. Afterpains are normal and are an indication that the uterus is contracting as it should.

afterperception,   the apparent perception of a stimulus that continues after the stimulus is removed.

afterpotential,   an electrical event that follows and that is caused by preceding action potentials. See **afterdepolarization.**

afterpotential wave /-pəten″shəl/,   either of two smaller waves, positive or negative, that follow the main spike potential wave of a nerve impulse, as recorded on an oscillograph tracing of an action potential that propagates along a nerve fiber.

aftertaste /af′ter tāst/,   the sensation of taste following the ingestion of a food or medicine after the substance has been swallowed.

Ag,   symbol for the element **silver.**

ag-.   See **ad-.**

AGA,   abbreviation for **appropriate for gestational age (AGA) infant.**

against medical advice (AMA),   the decision of a client to stop a therapy or treatment despite the recommendation of medical professionals. See also **discharge against medical advice.**

agalactia /ā′gəlak″shə/   [Gk *a* + *gala,* not milk],   absence of or faulty secretion of milk following childbirth.

agalsidase beta,   a miscellaneous agent used intravenously to treat Fabry's disease. It lowers the amount of globotriaosylceramide (GL-3), which builds up in cells lining the blood vessels of the kidney and certain other cells in patients with Fabry's disease. See **Fabry's disease.**

■ CONTRAINDICATIONS: Known hypersensitivity to this drug prohibits its use.

■ PATIENT CARE CONSIDERATIONS: Infusion reactions are not uncommon and can be severe.

agamete /āgam′ēt/   [Gk, *a* + *gamos,* not marriage],   **1.** any of the unicellular organisms, such as bacteria and protozoa, that reproduce asexually by multiple fission instead of by the production of gametes. **2.** any asexual reproductive cell, such as a spore or merozoite, that forms a new organism without fusion with another gamete. See also **fungus.** −**agamic, -agamous,** *agametic, adj.*

agamic /āgam″ik/,   reproducing asexually, without the union of gametes; asexual.

agammaglobulinemia /agam′əglob′yo͞olinē″mē·ə/ [Gk, *a* + *gamma,* not gamma (third letter of Greek alphabet); L, *globulus,* small sphere; Gk, *haima,* blood], the absence of gamma globulin from the serum, associated with an increased susceptibility to infection. The condition may be transient, congenital, or acquired. The transient form is common in infancy before 6 weeks of age, when the infant becomes able to synthesize the immunoglobulin. The congenital form is rare and sex-linked, affecting male children; it results in decreased production of antibodies. The acquired form usually occurs in malignant diseases such as leukemia, myeloma, or lymphoma. Also spelled *agammaglobulinaemia.* See also **Bruton agammaglobulinemia, immune gamma globulin.**

■ OBSERVATIONS: Symptoms are related to a wide variety of bacterial infections, including but not limited to bronchitis, diarrhea, conjunctivitis, and pneumonia. Blood tests indicating low levels of immunoglobulins confirm the diagnosis.

■ INTERVENTIONS: Replacement therapy with human gamma globulin is effective in preventing severe infections. The aim is to maintain the gamma globulin level above 150 mg/100 mL of blood. Antibiotics are administered and are continued until all signs of infection are eliminated.

■ PATIENT CARE CONSIDERATIONS: Recurrent infections are not uncommon. The condition is also complicated by local damage to tissues related to scarring from the frequent infections. Genetic counseling should be considered for prospective parents with a family history of the disorder.

agamogenesis /əgam′ōjen″əsis/ [Gk, *a* + *gamos,* not marriage, *genein,* to produce], asexual reproduction, as by budding, binary fission of cells, or parthenogenesis. −*agamogonic, agamogenetic, agamogenic, agamocytogenic, adj.*

agamont, now called **schizont.**

agamous. See **agamete.**

aganglionic megacolon. See **Hirschsprung disease.**

aganglionosis /əgang′lē·ənō″sis/ [Gk, *a,* not, *gagglion,* knot, *osis,* condition], an absence of parasympathetic ganglion cells in the myenteric plexus; a diagnostic sign of congenital megacolon.

agar-agar /a″gära″gär/ [Malay], a dried hydrophilic, colloidal product obtained from certain species of red algae. Because it is unaffected by bacterial enzymes, it is widely used as the basic ingredient in solid culture media in bacteriology. Agar-agar is also used as a suspending medium, as an emulsifying agent, and as a bulk laxative. Also called *agar.*

agarose /ag″ärōs/, an essentially neutral fraction of agar used as a medium in electrophoresis, particularly for separation of serum proteins, hemoglobin variants, and lipoprotein fractions.

agastria /əgas″trē·ə/ [Gk, *a* + *gaster,* without stomach], the absence of a stomach. −*agastric, adj.*

AGC, abbreviation for *absolute granulocyte count (AGC).* Also called **absolute neutrophil count.**

age [L, *aetus,* lifetime], **1.** a stage of development at which the body has arrived, as measured by physical and laboratory standards, at what is normal for a male or female of the same chronological age. See also **developmental age. 2.** to undergo change as both the mind and body experience life and environmental influences. **3.** to grow old. The measure of time elapsed since a person's birth. See also **chronological age.**

age-associated cognitive impairment, a progressive decline in cognitive function that occurs as a result of the normal aging process. It can be caused by a number of factors, including nutrient deficiencies, the damaging effect of free radicals, adverse effects of medication, altered hormone balance, and decreased oxygen supply to brain cells. Its near-universality causes it to be confused with mild cognitive impairment or the very early stages of some dementias; careful testing and analysis are required.

aged /ājd/, **1.** people of advanced age. Chronological definitions of age may vary among countries and nationalities. Also called **elderly. 2.** a state of having grown older or more mature than others in a population group.

ageism /ā″jizəm/ [L, *aetas,* lifetime], an attitude that discriminates, separates, stigmatizes, or otherwise disadvantages people on the basis of chronological age.

agency [L, *agere,* to do], **1.** (in law) a relationship between two parties in which one authorizes the other to act on his or her behalf as agent. It usually implies a contractual arrangement between two parties managed by a third party, the agent. **2.** the business of any power or firm empowered to act for another. **3.** an organization that performs actions for others, particularly of a service nature.

Agency for Healthcare Research and Quality (AHRQ), a governmental agency of the U.S. Department of Health and Human Services. Its mission is to support research "to improve the outcomes and quality of health care, reduce its costs, address patient safety and medical errors, and broaden access to effective service." The agency systematically develops statements and recommendations to help individuals, institutions, and agencies make better decisions about health care based on research that provides evidence-based information. It publishes scientific information for other agencies and organizations on which to base clinical guidelines, performance measures, and other quality-improvement tools through its evidence-based practice centers, outcomes research findings for clinicians, and technology reviews. It provides access to scientific evidence, recommendations on clinical preventive services, and information on how to implement recommended preventive services in clinical practice. Formerly called *Agency for Health Care Policy and Research.*

Agency for Toxic Substances and Disease Registry (ATSDR), an agency of the U.S. Department of Health and Human Services, charged with performing specific functions concerning the effect on public health of hazardous substances in the environment. These functions include public health assessments of waste sites, health consultations concerning specific hazardous substances, health surveillance and registries, emergency responses to release of hazardous substances, applied research in support of public health assessments, information development and dissemination, and education and training concerning hazardous substances.

agender, an individual who does not identify as male or female.

agenesia. See **agenesis.**

agenesia corticalis /ā′jenē″zhə/ [Gk, *a* + *genein,* not to produce; L, cortex], the failure of the cortical cells of the brain, especially the pyramidal cells, to develop in the embryo, resulting in infantile cerebral paralysis and severe cognitive impairment.

agenesis /ājen″əsis/ [Gk, *a* + *genein,* not to produce], **1.** congenital absence of an organ or part, usually caused by a lack of primordial tissue and failure of development in the embryo. **2.** impotence or sterility. Also called **agenesia.** Compare **dysgenesis.** −*agenic, adj.*

agenetic fracture /ā′jenet″ik/, a spontaneous fracture caused by a defect or imperfection in bone development.

ageniocephaly /əjen′ē·ōsef″əlē/ [Gk, *a* + *genein,* not to produce, *kephale,* head], a form of otocephaly in which the brain, cranial vault, and sense organs are intact but the lower jaw is malformed. Also called *ageniocephalia.* −*ageniocephalic, ageniocephalous, adj.*

agenitalism /ājen″itəliz″əm/, **1.** any condition caused by the lack of sex hormones and the absence or malfunction of the ovaries or testes. **2.** congenital absence of genitalia.

agenosomia /ājen′əsō″mē·ə/, a congenital malformation characterized by the absence or defective formation of the genitals and protrusion of the intestines through an incompletely developed abdominal wall.

agent [L, *agere,* to do], **1.** (in law) a party authorized to act on behalf of another and to give the other an account of such actions. **2.** a substance capable of producing an effect.

Agent Orange, a U.S. military code name for a mixture of two herbicides, 2,4-D and 2,4,5-T, used as a defoliant during the Vietnam War between 1961 and 1971. The herbicides were unintentionally contaminated with the highly toxic chemical dioxin, which is believed to cause cancer and birth defects in animals and has been established as a cause of numerous health and environmental problems in those exposed to it. See also **dioxin.**

age of consent, (in medical jurisprudence) the age at which an individual is legally free to act as an adult, without parental permission for activities such as marrying, having sexual intercourse, or giving permission for medical treatment or surgery. The specific age of consent varies from 13 to 21 years, according to local laws.

age of majority, the age at which a person is considered to be an adult in the eyes of the law. It varies by activity from state to state.

age-related macular degeneration (AMD), a leading cause of blindness in individuals over the age of 50 due to damage to the macula, the part of the retina responsible for sharp, central vision.
- OBSERVATIONS: The early and intermediate stages of AMD usually start without symptoms. A comprehensive dilated eye exam can detect AMD; the exam usually includes an Amsler grid test. A blurred area near the center of vision is a common symptom as the disease progresses. A slow, progressive loss in central vision may become a significant disability.
- INTERVENTIONS: Lifestyle changes such as improvements to diet, control of blood pressure, and cessation of smoking may slow the progression of the disease. Currently, no curative treatment exists for AMD, and it is important to determine, with yearly dilated eye examinations, whether the condition is advancing. Researchers at the National Eye Institute have identified certain high-dose vitamins and minerals that can slow progression of the disease in people who have intermediate AMD. Advanced (or neovascular) AMD typically results in severe vision loss. However, therapies exist to stop further vision loss. They include the injection of medications to block the growth of new vessels in the eye, photodynamic therapy, and laser therapy.
- PATIENT CARE CONSIDERATIONS: Low-vision services and visual rehabilitation services will assist individuals in coping with the loss of vision and in maintaining independence.

age-specific, a description of data in which the age of the individual is significant for epidemiological or statistical purposes.

age 30 transition, (in psychiatry) a period between 28 and 33 years of age when an individual may reevaluate the choices made in his or her twenties. See also **midlife transition.**

ageusia /əgyoo̅′sē·ə/ [Gk, *a* + *geusis,* without taste], a loss or impairment of the sense of taste. Also called *gustatory anesthesia.*

agger /ag′ər, aj′ər/, a small protuberance or eminence of tissue, such as the curved elevation above the atrium of the nose.

agglomeration [L, *agglomerare,* to gather into a ball], a mass or cluster of individual units. −*agglomerate, v.*

agglutinant /əgloo̅′tənənt/ [L, *agglutinare,* to glue], **1.** something that causes adhesion, such as a circulating antibody adhering to an antigen. **2.** a substance that holds parts together during healing.

agglutination /əgloo̅′tinā″shən/ [L, *agglutinare,* to glue], the clumping of cells or particulate antigens as a result of interaction and cross-linking with agglutinins. −*agglutinate, v.*

agglutination reaction, the formation of an aggregate after the mixing of a soluble antibody with particulate antigen molecules in an aqueous medium. The visible aggregates are formed when specific antibody cross-links the antigens.

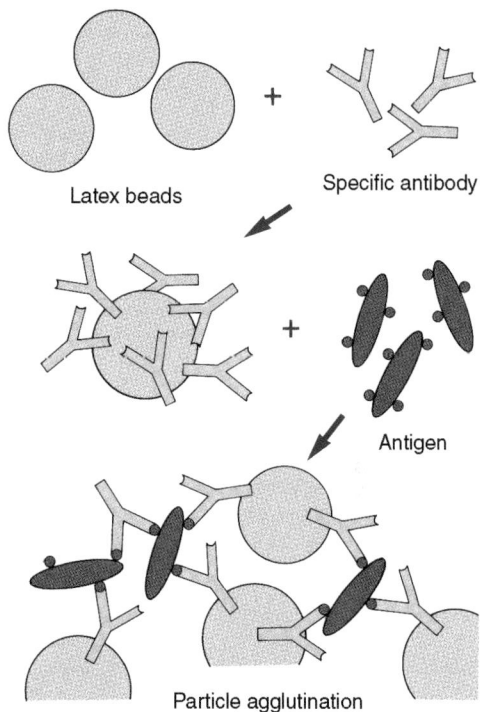

Agglutination reaction *(Tille, 2014)*

agglutination titer, the highest dilution of a serum that will produce clumping of cells or particulate antigens. It is a measure of the concentration of specific antibodies in the serum.

agglutinin /əgloo̅′tinin/, an antibody that interacts with antigens, resulting in agglutination. Usually multivalent, agglutinins react with insoluble antigens in stable suspension to form a cross-linking lattice that may clump or precipitate. Agglutinins are used in blood typing and in identifying or estimating the strength of immunoglobulins or immune sera. Compare **precipitin.** See also **blood typing, hemagglutination.**

agglutinin absorption, the removal of an antibody from immune serum via treatment with homologous antigen. The antibody attaches to the antigen, followed by centrifugation and separation of the antigen-antibody complex from the serum.

agglutinogen /ag′loo̅tin′əjin/ [L, *agglutinare* + Gk, *genein,* to produce], any antigenic substance that causes agglutination by the production of agglutinin.

aggravate /ag′ rah vāt″/ [L, *ad,* increase, *gravis,* heavy], to cause a health condition to deteriorate or increase in intensity.

aggregate /ag′rəgāt/ [L, *ad* + *gregare,* to gather together], **1.** the total of a group of substances or components making up a mass or complex. **2.** individuals, families, or other groupings who are associated because of similar social, personal, health care, or other needs or interests. Data on individual patients can be aggregated to allow conclusions about the patient population to be drawn. See also **aggregation.**

aggregate anaphylaxis, a hypersensitive immune response that produces an immediate, exaggerated reaction induced by an antigen that forms a soluble antigen-antibody complex.

aggregation /ag'rəgā″shən/ [L, *ad* + *gregare,* to gather together], an accumulation of substances, objects, or individuals, as in the clumping of blood cells or the clustering of clients with the same disorder. –**aggregate,** *v.*

aggression /əgresh′ən/ [L, *aggressio,* to attack], a forceful behavior, action, or attitude that is expressed physically, verbally, or symbolically. It may arise from innate drives or occur as a defense mechanism, often resulting from a threatened ego. It is manifested by either constructive or destructive acts directed toward oneself or against others. Kinds include **constructive aggression, destructive aggression, inward aggression.**

aggressive infantile fibromatosis, an uncommon condition, present at birth or developed during infancy or childhood, characterized by fast-growing, firm, painless, single or multiple nodules involving subcutaneous tissue, muscle, fascia, and tendons and seen anywhere on the body. Tumors are locally invasive but do not metastasize and have a high tendency to recur after excision.

aggressive periodontitis, *(Obsolete)* all periodontitis is now considered to be chronic.

aggressive personality, a personality with behavior patterns characterized by irritability, impulsivity, destructiveness, or violence in response to frustration.

aging [L, *aetas,* lifetime], the process of growing old. Biological aging results in part from a failure of body cells to function normally or to produce new body cells to replace those that are dead or malfunctioning. Normal cell function may be lost through infectious disease, malnutrition, exposure to environmental hazards, or genetic influences. Among body cells that exhibit early signs of aging are those that normally cease dividing after reaching maturity. Sociological and psychological theories of aging seek to explain the other influences on aging caused by the environment, engagement, personality, and nonbiological influences. Promoting health through attention to exercise, nutrition, and stress management is a key factor in maintaining body systems and mental health. See also **assessment of the aging patient.**

aging in place, an approach to living arrangements for the older adult that facilitates remaining in one's own home. An occupational therapist often suggests modifications to make the home safe. Community health nurses may provide support to manage chronic health problems. Other members of the health care team are involved as necessary.

agitated depression, *(Informal)* a combination of anxiety and depression. See **depression.**

agitation, a state of chronic restlessness and increased psychomotor activity generally observed as an expression of emotional tension and characterized by purposeless, restless activity. Pacing, talking, crying, and laughing sometimes are characteristic and may serve to release nervous tension associated with anxiety, fear, or other mental stress. –**agitate,** *v.*

agitographia /aj′itōgraf″ē·ə/ [L, *agitare* + Gk, *graphein,* to write], a condition characterized by abnormally rapid writing in which words or parts of words are unconsciously omitted. The condition is commonly associated with agitophasia.

agitophasia /aj′itōfā″zhə/ [L, *agitare* + Gk, *phasis,* speech], a condition characterized by abnormally rapid speech in which words, sounds, or syllables are unconsciously omitted, slurred, or distorted. The condition is commonly associated with agitographia. Also called *agitolalia.*

Agkistrodon /ag·kis′trōdon/, a genus of venomous pit vipers. *A. contortrix* is the copperhead, and *A. piscivorus* is the cottonmouth. See also **snakebite.**

aglossia /əglos″ē·ə/ [Gk, *a* + *glossa,* without tongue], congenital absence of the tongue; frequently associated with other craniofacial and limb defects.

aglutition /ag″ loo-tish′un/, inability to swallow.

agnathia /ag-nath″ē·ə/ [Gk, *a, gnathos,* not jaw], a rare and lethal developmental defect characterized by total or partial absence of the lower jaw. The maxilla, tongue, and the position of the ears may also be affected. Also called **agnathy, synotia.** See also **otocephaly.** –*agnathous, adj.*

agnathocephaly /ag-nath′əsef″əlē/ [Gk, *a* + *gnathos* + *kephale,* head], a congenital malformation characterized by the absence of the lower jaw, defective formation of the mouth, and placement of the eyes low on the face with fusion or approximation of the zygomas and the ears. Also called *agnathocephalia.* See also **otocephaly.** –*agnathocephalous, agnathocephalic, adj.*

agnathus /ag-nath″əs/ [Gk, *a* + *gnathos,* without jaw], a fetus with an absent or underdeveloped jaw.

agnathy. See **agnathia.**

agnogenic /ag″no-jen′ik/, of unknown origin.

agnogenic myeloid metaplasia. See **myeloid metaplasia.**

agnosia /ag·nō″zhə/ [Gk, *a* + *gnosis,* not knowledge], total or partial loss of the ability to recognize familiar objects or persons through sensory stimuli as a result of organic brain damage or dementia. The condition may affect any of the senses and is classified accordingly as auditory, visual, olfactory, gustatory, or tactile agnosia. Also called **agnosis.**

-agnosia, -agnosis, suffixes meaning "(condition of the) loss of the faculty to perceive": *autotopagnosia, paragnosia.*

-agogue, -agog, suffixes meaning an "agent promoting the expulsion of a (specified) substance": *lymphagogue, uragogue.*

agonal /ag″ənəl/ [Gk, *agon,* struggle], pertaining to death and dying.

agonal breathing, a gasping, labored respiratory pattern associated with cardiac arrest or the end of life.

agonal respiration, **1.** an abnormal breathing pattern. See **Cheyne-Stokes respiration, air hunger. 2.** the gasping breaths associated with the end of life.

agonal thrombus, a mass of blood platelets, fibrin, clotting factors, and cellular elements that forms in the heart of a dying patient with heart failure.

agonist /ag″ənist/ [Gk, *agon,* struggle], **1.** a contracting muscle whose contraction is opposed by another muscle (an antagonist). Also a muscle that works in support of another muscle, creating the same motion. The brachialis and biceps brachii are agonistic muscles. **2.** a drug or other substance having a specific cellular affinity that produces a predictable response.

agony /ag′ənē/ [Gk, *agon*], severe physical or emotional anguish or distress, as in pain.

agoraphobia /ag′orə-/ [Gk, *agora,* marketplace, *phobos,* fear], an anxiety disorder characterized by a fear of being in an open, crowded, or public place, such as a field, tunnel, bridge, congested street, or busy marketplace, where escape is perceived as difficult or help is not available in case of sudden incapacitation.

-agra, a suffix meaning a "pain or painful seizure": *cardiagra, trachelagra.*

agranular endoplasmic reticulum, the absence of ribosomes in endoplasmic retriculum. See **endoplasmic reticulum.** Compare **granular endoplasmic reticulum.**

agranulocyte /āgran″yoolōsīt′/ [Gk, *a,* not; L, *granulum,* small grain; Gk, *kytos,* cell], a leukocyte category characterized by the absence of cytoplasmic granules. Lymphocytes and plasma cells are agranulocytic. Compare **granulocyte.**

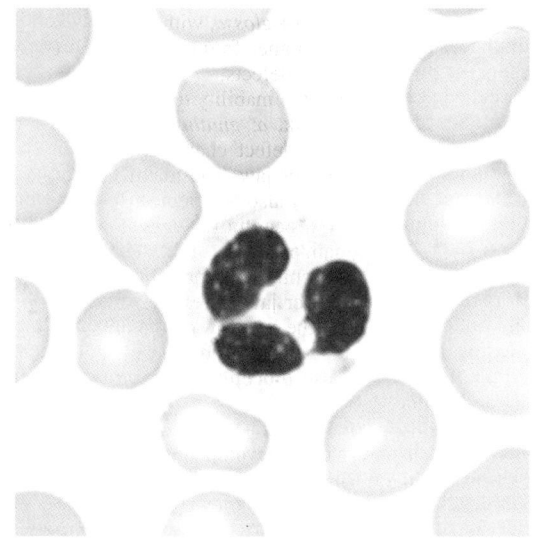

Agranulocyte *(Carr and Rodak, 2013)*

agranulocytosis /āgran′yo͞olō′sītō″sis/, severe reduction in the number of granulocytic leukocytes (basophils, eosinophils, and neutrophils). Reduction in polymorphonuclear neutrophils is neutrophilia, whereby the body is severely depleted in its ability to defend itself from bacterial infection. The acute disease may be an adverse reaction to a medication or the result of the effect of radiation therapy or chemotherapy on bone marrow

agraphesthesia. See **graphanesthesia.**

agraphia /āgraf″ē·ə/ [Gk, *a + graphein,* not to write], a loss of the ability to write, resulting from injury to the language center in the cerebral cortex. Compare **dysgraphia.** See also **absolute agraphia.** −*agraphic, adj.*

A:G ratio, the ratio of albumin to globulin in the blood serum. On the basis of differential solubility with a neutral salt solution, the normal values are 3.5 to 5 g/dL for albumin and 2.5 to 4 g/dL for globulin.

agrimony, an herb found in Asia, Europe, and the United States. Also called *agrimonia.*

■ INDICATIONS: Agrimony is used for mild diarrhea, gastroenteritis, intestinal secretion of mucus, inflammation of the mouth and throat, cuts and scrapes, postmenopausal symptoms, and amenorrhea. There is insufficient reliable information to assess its effectiveness.

■ CONTRAINDICATIONS: Agrimony is not recommended during pregnancy and lactation, in children, or in those with known hypersensitivity to it or to roses.

Agrobacterium, an environmental gram-negative, aerobic, rod-shaped bacillus. *A. tumefaciens* has been implicated in health care–associated urinary tract infections, peritonitis, wound infections, prosthetic valve endocarditis, and sepsis.

agrypnotic /ag′ripnot″ik/, **1.** a person who is unable to sleep. Also called **insomniac. 2.** a medication or psychostimulant causing wakefulness, such as caffeine, amphetamines, methylphenidate, and related drugs.

AGS, 1. abbreviation for *American Geriatrics Society.* **2.** abbreviation for **adrenogenital syndrome.**

agyria /əjī″rē·ə/, a congenital lack or underdevelopment of the convolutional pattern of the cerebral cortex. The cortical tissue is reduced, leading to severe cognitive impairment. Also called **lissencephalia, lissencephaly.**

AHA, 1. abbreviation for **American Hospital Association. 2.** abbreviation for **acetohydroxamic acid.**

"aha" reaction /ähä″/, *(Informal)* a sudden realization or inspiration, experienced especially during creative thinking or when an unexpected change in mental perspective reveals the solution to a problem.

AHF, abbreviation for **antihemophilic factor.**

AHH, abbreviation for **aryl hydrocarbon hydroxylase.**

AHIMA, abbreviation for *American Health Information Management Association.*

AHRQ, abbreviation for **Agency for Healthcare Research and Quality.** Formerly called **AHCPR.**

Ahumada-del Castillo syndrome /ä′ho͞omä″dädel′käs tē″- yō/ [Juan Carlos Ahumada, 1890–1976, Argentine gynecologist; Enrique B. del Castillo, 1897–1969, Argentine physician and endocrinologist], a form of secondary amenorrhea that may be associated with a pituitary gland tumor. It is characterized by both galactorrhea and amenorrhea, with low gonadotropin secretion, in the absence of a pregnancy.

AI, 1. abbreviation for **artificial intelligence. 2.** abbreviation for **artificial insemination. 3.** abbreviation for **apical impulse.**

AICC, abbreviation for **antiinhibitor coagulant complex.**

AICD, abbreviation for **automatic implanted cardioverter defibrillator.**

aid, assistance given a person who is ill, injured, or otherwise unable to cope with the normal demands of life.

aide /ād/, a worker who is an assistant to another. Kinds include **nurse's aide, occupational therapy aide,** *physical therapist aide, social and human services aide.*

AID, abbreviation for **artificial insemination—donor.**

AIDS /ādz/, abbreviation for **acquired immunodeficiency syndrome.**

AIDS-associated retinopathy. See **HIV-associated retinopathy.**

AIDS cholangiopathy, biliary duct disease that is a complication of acquired immunodeficiency syndrome. The most common effect is primary sclerosing cholangitis; some patients also have dysfunction of the sphincter of Oddi. This syndrome is most commonly caused by *Cryptosporidium parvum,* but it can also be caused by *Microsporidium,* cytomegalovirus, and *Cyclospora cayetanensis.* Its occurrence has been reduced by the advent of highly active antiretroviral therapy.

AIDS-dementia complex (ADC), type of dementia that occurs in 10% to 15% of patients with acquired immunodeficiency syndrome (AIDS). The condition is characterized by memory loss and by varying levels and forms of dementia. It may be caused by the destruction of brain neurons by the human immunodeficiency virus as autopsies indicate that the density of the neurons may be 40% lower in patients with AIDS than in healthy persons. Also called *AIDS-related dementia.*

AIDS nephropathy, 1. now called **HIV-associated nephropathy. 2.** any kidney disease that is associated with HIV.

AIDS-related complex (ARC), *(Obsolete)* a term used in the early years of the AIDS epidemic to identify the transition from asymptomatic HIV infection to the occurrence of symptoms.

AIDS serology test (AIDS screen, HIV antibody test), a test used to detect the antibody to the human immunodeficiency virus. Home testing kits are now available in addition to the tests performed by health care providers.

AIDS-wasting syndrome, a syndrome associated with acquired immunodeficiency syndrome (AIDS) in which patients have lost at least 10% of their body weight. Can be accompanied by at least 30 days of diarrhea or extreme weakness and fever not related to an infection.

AIH, abbreviation for **artificial insemination—husband/male partner.**

AILD, abbreviation for **angioimmunoblastic lymphadenopathy with dysproteinemia.** Now called **angioimmunoblastic T-cell lymphoma.**

AILD-type (lymphogranulomatosis X) T-cell lymphoma. See **angioimmunoblastic T-cell lymphoma.**

ailment [OE, *eglan*], any disease, physical disorder, or complaint, generally of a chronic, acute, or mild nature.

ainhum /ān′ hum or i′num/, a condition of unknown origin, seen chiefly in dark-skinned individuals, consisting of a linear constriction that causes spontaneous amputation of the fourth or fifth toe. See **autoamputation.**

air [Gk, *aer*], the colorless, odorless gaseous mixture constituting the earth's atmosphere. It consists of 78% nitrogen; 20% oxygen; almost 1% argon; small amounts of carbon dioxide, hydrogen, and ozone; traces of helium, krypton, neon, and xenon; and varying amounts of water vapor.

air abrasion, (in dentistry) a type of microabrasion in which a jet of air blows tiny particles against the tooth or cavity surface. Air abrasion systems use air, water, and specially formulated powders, usually of aluminum oxide, to deliver a controlled microabrasion spray for the mechanical removal of stain and biofilm attached to the tooth or cavity surface.

air bath, **1.** a tub that utilizes jets under the water surface to mix air into the solution. See **balneotherapy. 2.** an open-air treatment used in naturopathic medicine.

airborne contaminant, a material in the atmosphere that can affect the health of persons in the same or nearby environments. Particularly vulnerable are the tissues of the upper respiratory tract and lungs, including the terminal bronchioles and alveoli. The effects depend in part on the solubility of the inhaled matter. Inhaled contaminants may cause tissue damage, tissue reaction, disease, or physical obstruction. Some airborne contaminants, such as carbon monoxide, may have little or no direct effect on the lungs but can be absorbed into the bloodstream and carried to other organs or damage the blood itself. Biologically inert gases may dilute the atmospheric oxygen below the normal blood saturation value, thereby disturbing cellular respiration.

Airborne Precautions, guidelines recommended by the U.S. Centers for Disease Control and Prevention for reducing the risk of airborne transmission of infectious agents. Airborne droplet nuclei consist of small-particle residue (5 μm or smaller in size) of evaporated droplets that may remain suspended in the air for a long time. Airborne transmission occurs by dissemination of either airborne droplet nuclei or dust particles containing the infectious agent. Microorganisms carried in this manner can be widely dispersed by air currents and may be inhaled or deposited on a susceptible host from the source patient. Special air handling and ventilation are required to prevent airborne transmission. Airborne precautions apply to patients known or suspected to be infected with epidemiologically important pathogens that can be transmitted by the airborne route. Examples include measles (rubeola), varicella zoster virus infections, Legionella infection, disseminated zoster, and tuberculosis. Compare **Contact Precautions, Droplet Precautions.** See also **Standard Precautions, Transmission-Based Precautions.**

aircast splint, an inflatable device for temporarily immobilizing fractured or otherwise injured extremities. See **air splint.**

air compressor, a mechanical device that compresses air for storage and is used in handpieces and other air-driven medical and dental tools.

air embolism, the abnormal presence of air in the cardiovascular system, resulting in obstruction of blood flow. Air embolism may occur if a large quantity of air is inadvertently introduced by injection (for example, during IV therapy or surgery) or by trauma (for example, with a puncture wound). Also called **aeroembolism.** Compare **fat embolism, gas embolism.** See also **decompression sickness, embolus.**

air entrainment, the movement of room air into the chamber of a jet nebulizer used to treat respiratory diseases. Air entrainment increases the rate of nebulization and the amount of liquid administered per unit of time.

airflow pattern, the pattern of movement of respiratory gases through the respiratory tract. The pattern is affected by factors such as gas density and viscosity.

air fluidization, the process of blowing temperature-controlled air through a collection of microspheres to create a fluidlike movement. The technique is used in special mattresses designed to reduce pressure against a patient's skin. See also **air-fluidized bed.**

air-fluidized bed, a bed with body support provided by thousands of tiny soda-lime glass beads suspended by pressurized, temperature-controlled air. The patient rests on a polyester filter sheet that covers the beads. The special bed is designed for use by patients with or at risk for posterior pressure ulcers or with posterior burns, grafts, or donor areas. The pressure against the patient's skin surface is less than the capillary refilling. The improved capillary blood flow to the skin speeds the growth of granulation tissue.

air hunger, a form of respiratory distress characterized by gasping, labored breathing, or dyspnea.

airplane splint, an orthotic device used to immobilize a shoulder during healing from injury or surgery. The device maintains the shoulder at or about 90 degrees of glenohumeral abduction, with the elbow flexed. It extends to the waist and may be made of thermoplastic, plaster, or wire, and it may be supported by a trunk harness.

air pollution [L, *polluere,* to defile], contamination of the air by noxious fumes, aromas, or toxic chemicals.

air pump, a device that forces air into or out of a cavity or chamber.

air sac, a small, terminal cavity in the lung, consisting of the alveoli connected to one terminal bronchiole.

air sickness, *(Informal)* an inner ear and sensory system imbalance leading to feelings of nausea and uncomfortable sensations caused by air travel or, in some cases, by traveling on land at high elevations. Also called **motion sickness.** Compare **car sickness, seasickness.**

air splint, a device for temporarily immobilizing fractured or otherwise injured extremities. It consists of an inflatable cylinder that can be closed at either end and becomes rigid when filled with air under pressure. Also called **aircast splint.**

air swallowing, the intake of air into the digestive system, usually involuntarily, during eating, drinking, or chewing of gum. Air swallowing may also be an effect of anxious behavior. The problem occurs commonly in infants as a result of faulty feeding methods.

air thermometer, a device that measures the temperature of the atmosphere in degrees. See also **thermometer.**

airway [Gk, *aer* + AS, *weg,* way], **1.** a tubular passage for movement of air into and out of the lung. An airway with a diameter greater than 2 mm is defined as a large, or central, airway such as a mainstream bronchus; one smaller than 2 mm is considered a small, or peripheral, airway such as a terminal bronchus. **2.** a respiratory anesthesia device. **3.** an oropharyngeal tube used for mouth-to-mouth resuscitation.

airway conductance (Gaw), the instantaneous rate of gas flow in the airway per unit of pressure difference between the mouth, nose, or other airway opening and the alveoli. It is the reciprocal of airway resistance.

airway division, one of the 18 segments of the bronchopulmonary system. The segments are usually numbered from 1 to 10 for the right lung, which has three lobes, and from 1 to 8 for the left lung, which has two lobes.

airway obstruction, a mechanical impediment to the delivery of air to the lungs or to the absorption of oxygen in the lungs.

■ OBSERVATIONS: If the obstruction is minor, as in sinusitis or pharyngitis, the person is able to breathe, but not normally. If the obstruction is acute, the person may grasp the neck, gasp, become cyanotic, and lose consciousness.

■ INTERVENTIONS: Acute airway obstruction requires rapid intervention to save the person's life. In cases of obstruction caused by a bolus of food, a collection of mucus, or a foreign body in adults and children older than 1 year of age, the object may be removed manually, by suction, or with abdominal thrusts that create an artificial cough forceful enough to clear the obstruction. Obstruction caused by an inflammatory or allergic reaction may be treated with bronchodilating drugs, corticosteroids, intubation, and administration of oxygen. An emergency tracheotomy may be required if the obstruction cannot be mechanically or pharmacologically relieved within a few minutes.

■ PATIENT CARE CONSIDERATIONS: The patient is usually very apprehensive and may physically resist assistance. A rapid-response team should be summoned for inpatients or emergency dispatch for individuals in the community. Emergency care is begun and includes removing the obstruction, administering oxygen, and performing cardiopulmonary resuscitation, if necessary. See also **aspiration.**

airway resistance (Raw), a measure of the impedance to airflow through the bronchopulmonary system. It is the reciprocal of airway conductance.

AIUM, abbreviation for *American Institute of Ultrasound in Medicine.*

AK amputation, *(Informal)* abbreviation for **above-knee amputation.** See **transfemoral amputation.**

akaryocyte /āker″ē·əsīt′/ [Gk, *a,* not, *karyon,* kernel], a cell without a nucleus, such as an erthyrocyte.

akathisia /ak′əthē″zhə/ [Gk, *a + kathizein,* not to sit], a pathological condition characterized by restlessness and agitation, such as an inability to sit still. *−akathisiac, adj.*

akinesia /ā′kinē″zhə, ā′kīnē″zhə/ [Gk, *a, kinesis,* without movement], an abnormal state of motor and psychic hypoactivity. Also called **akinesis.** *−akinetic, adj.*

akinesis /a″ki·ne′sis/, the absence or impairment of the ability to initiate voluntary movement. It is a common symptom associated with Parkinson disease.

akinesthesia /ākin′esthē″zhə/, a loss of the sense of movement.

akinetic apraxia, the inability to perform a spontaneous movement. See also **apraxia.**

akinetic mutism, a state of apparent alertness in which a person is unable or refuses to move or to make sounds, resulting from a neurological or psychological disturbance.

akinetic seizure, a type of seizure disorder observed in children. It is a brief, generalized seizure in which the child suddenly falls to the ground.

Akineton, a peripheral anticholinergic. Brand name for **biperiden hydrochloride.**

Al, symbol for the element **aluminum.**

-al, a suffix designating a compound containing a member of the aldehyde group: *chloral, ethanal.*

-al, -ale, suffixes meaning "characterized by" or "pertaining to": *appendiceal, meningeal.*

ala /ā′lə/ *pl. alae* [L, wing], **1.** any winglike structure. **2.** the axilla. *−alar, adj.*

Ala, abbreviation for **alanine.**

ALA, abbreviation for **aminolevulinic acid.**

ala auris, *(Obsolete)* See **auricle.**

ala cerebelli /ser′əbel″ī/, a winglike structure of the central lobule of the cerebellum.

ala cinerea /sinir″ē·ə/, the triangular area on the floor of the brain's fourth ventricle from which the autonomic fibers of the vagus nerve arise.

alactasia. See **lactase deficiency.**

Alagille's syndrome /ä-lä·zhēl′/ [Daniel Alagille, French pediatrician, 1925–2005], an autosomal-dominant syndrome that affects the liver, heart, kidney, and other systems of the body. Can be associated with neonatal jaundice, cholestasis with peripheral pulmonary stenosis, and occasionally septal defects or patent ductus arteriosus, resulting from a low number or an absence of intrahepatic bile ducts. It is characterized by unusual facies and ocular, vertebral, and nervous system abnormalities.

ala nasi /nā″sī/, the outer flaring cartilaginous wall of the outer side of each nostril.

alanine (Ala or A) /al″ənin/, a nonessential, nonpolar (neutral) amino acid found in many food protein sources as well as in the body. It is degraded in the liver to produce important biomolecules such as pyruvate and glutamate. Its carbon skeleton also can be used as an energy source.

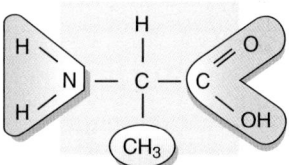

Chemical structure of alanine

alanine aminotransferase (ALT), an enzyme normally present in the serum and tissues of the body, especially the tissues of the liver. This enzyme catalyzes the transfer of an amino group from alanine to alpha-ketoglutarate, forming pyruvate and glutamate. The reaction is reversible. The enzyme is released into the serum as a result of tissue injury and increases in persons with acute liver damage. Normal findings are 5 to 35 IU/L. Also called **alanine transferase.** Compare **aspartate aminotransferase.**

alanine aminotransferase (ALT) test, a serum test that aids in the diagnosis of liver disease. Also called *alanine transaminase (ALT) test.* Formerly called *glutamate pyruvate transaminase (SGPT* or *GPT) test.*

alanine transferase, an intracellular enzyme in amino acid and carbohydrate metabolism found in high concentration in brain, liver, and muscle. An increased level indicates necrosis or disease in these tissues. See also **alanine aminotransferase.**

Al-Anon, an international organization that offers guidance, counseling, and support for the relatives, friends, and associates of alcoholics. See **Al-Anon Family Group.** See also **Alateen, Alcoholics Anonymous.**

Al-Anon Family Group, a fellowship and support group for individuals and families affected by alcohol abuse. See **Al-Anon.**

ala of the ethmoid, a small projection on each side of the crista galli of the ethmoid bone. Each ala fits into a corresponding depression of the frontal bone.

ala of the ilium, the upper flaring portion of the ilium.

ala of the sacrum, the flat extension of bone on each side of the sacrum.

A

alar, pertaining to a single wing; winglike. See **ala.**

ALARA, *(Informal)* acronym for *as low as reasonably achievable.* It refers to the principle that all radiation exposure, both to patients and to personnel, should be minimized as much as possible.

alar fold, 1. a fringed margin on either side of an infrapatellar fat pad in the knee joint formed by the synovial membrane. The synovial membrane covering the lower part of the infrapatellar fat pad is raised into a sharp midline fold directed posteriorly, the infrapateller synovial fold, which attaches to the margin of the intercondylar fossa of the femur. **2.** a fold extending from the nostril to the ventral nasal concha.

alar lamina [L, *ala,* wing, *lamina,* thin plate], the posterolateral area of the embryonic neural tube through which sensory nerves enter.

alar ligament, one of a pair of ligaments that connect the axis to the occipital bone and limit rotation of the cranium. Also called **check ligament, odontoid ligament.** Compare **membrana tectoria.**

alarm reaction, the first stage of the general adaptation syndrome. It is characterized by the release of adrenocorticotropic hormone (ACTH) by the pituitary gland and of epinephrine by the adrenal medulla, which cause increased blood glucose levels and a faster respiration rate, increasing the oxygen level of the blood. These actions provide the body with increased energy for dealing with stress.

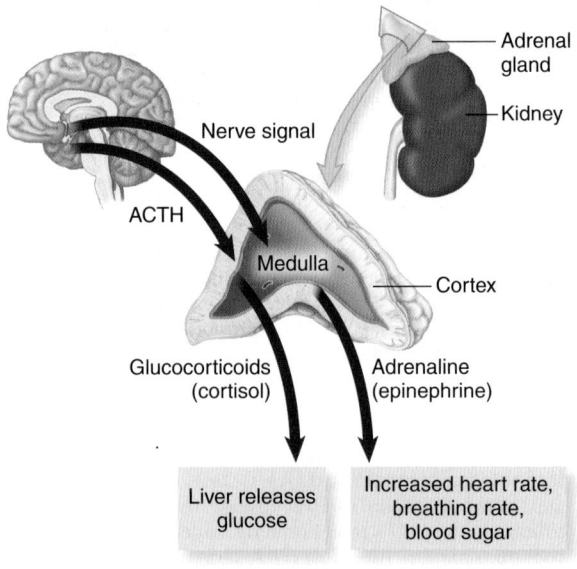

Alarm reaction *(Patton and Thibodeau, 2016)*

alar process [L, *ala,* wing, *processus*], a projection of the cribriform plate of the ethmoid bone articulating with the frontal bone.

alaryngeal speech /ā′lä·rin′je·əl spēch/ [Gk, *a,* without + *larynx*; ME, *speche*], methods of speech communication used after laryngectomy, including communication with an electrolarynx, a tracheoesophageal voice prosthesis, and use of esophageal speech.

alastrim /al″əstrim/ [Port, *alastrar,* to spread], a mild form of smallpox, with little rash. It is thought to be caused by a weak strain of the poxvirus that causes smallpox. Unlike smallpox, however, alastrim is rarely fatal. Also called **Cuban itch, Kaffir pox, milkpox, pseudosmallpox, pseudovariola, variola minor, West Indian smallpox, whitepox.** See also **smallpox.**

Alateen, an international organization that offers guidance, counseling, and support for the children of alcoholics. See also **Al-Anon, Alcoholics Anonymous.**

alatrofloxacin/trovafloxacin, a broad-spectrum quinolone antibiotic.

■ INDICATIONS: This drug is used to treat nosocomial pneumonia, community-acquired pneumonia, chronic bronchitis, acute sinusitis, complicated intraabdominal infections, infections of the skin and skin structure, urinary tract infections, chronic bacterial prostatitis, urethral gonorrhea in males, pelvic inflammatory disease, and cervicitis caused by susceptible organisms.

■ CONTRAINDICATIONS: Known hypersensitivity to quinolones, seizure disorders, cerebral atherosclerosis, and photosensitivity prohibit the use of this drug.

■ ADVERSE EFFECTS: Life-threatening side effects include pseudomembranous colitis and thrombocytopenia. Other adverse effects include headache, dizziness, insomnia, anxiety, nausea, flatulence, vomiting, diarrhea, abdominal pain, vaginitis, crystalluria, rash, pruritus, and photosensitivity.

ala vomeris /vō″məris/, an extension of bone on each side of the upper border of one of the unpaired facial bones in the skull.

alb-, a prefix meaning "white": *albinism, albumin.*

alba /al″bə/, literally, "white," as in *linea alba.*

albedo /albē″dō/ *pl. albedos* [L, *albus,* white], the fraction of solar energy (shortwave radiation) reflected from the earth back into space. It is a measure of the reflectivity of the earth's surface

albendazole /al-ben′dah-zōl/, a broad-spectrum anthelmintic used against many parasites, including those that cause echinococcosis and cysticercosis.

Albers-Schönberg disease /-shœn″burg, -shōn″-/ [Heinrich E. Albers-Schönberg, German radiologist and surgeon, 1865–1921], a rare condition transmitted as an autosomal-dominant trait in which there are bandlike areas of condensed bone at the epiphyseal lines of long bones and condensation of the edges of smaller bones. See also **osteopetrosis.**

■ OBSERVATIONS: Fractures are frequent, and recovery is slow. Deformities of the head, chest, or spine may occur. Anemia may also be present as the bone mass encroaches on bone marrow spaces. The cranial nerves may also be affected as bone is deposited in the skull.

■ INTERVENTIONS: Management is supportive and not curative. Bone marrow transplantation may be employed to provide cells that can be converted to osteoclasts. Other treatments include the administration of gamma interferon, a protein that delays progression of the disease, or calcitriol, a vitamin D compound that stimulates osteoclasts to dissolve and absorb bone.

■ PATIENT CARE CONSIDERATIONS: Health care professionals should offer surveillance, symptomatic treatment, and the prevention of complications. Measures to promote quality of life are important. Genetic counseling should be offered to families.

Albert disease [Eduard Albert, Austrian surgeon, 1841–1900], an inflammation of the bursa that lies between the Achilles tendon and the calcaneus. It is most frequently caused by injury but may also result from the wearing of poorly fitted shoes, increased strain on the tendon, excessive strenuous exercise, improper exercise techniques, or rheumatoid arthritis. Treatment includes an intrabursal injection of corticosteroid with lidocaine hydrochloride and warm compresses. If treatment is delayed, the inflammation may cause erosion of the calcaneus. Also called **anterior Achilles bursitis.**

albicans /al″bikənz/ [L, *albus,* white], white or whitish. See also **corpus albicans.**

albinism /al″biniz′əm/, a rare inherited disorder characterized by a lack of melanin in the skin. Pale skin that does not tan, white hair, pink eyes, nystagmus, astigmatism, and photophobia are associated with total albinism. Individuals with albinism are prone to severe sunburn, actinic dermatitis, and skin cancer. Compare **piebald, vitiligo.**

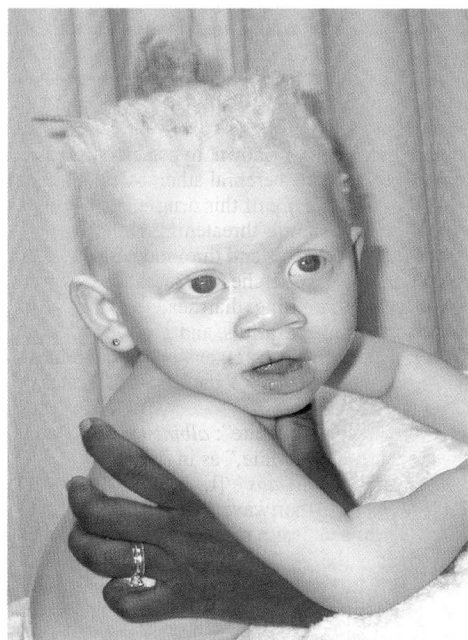

Child with albinism (Saadeh, 2007)

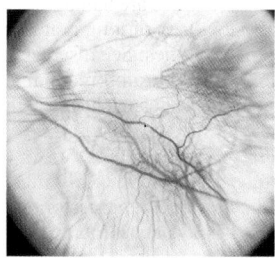

Pale fundus in albinism (Zitelli and Davis, 2012)

Albini nodules /äl·be′nēz/ [Giuseppe Albini, Italian physiologist, 1827–1911], gray nodules the size of a small grain, sometimes seen on the free edges of the atrioventricular valves of infants. Albini nodules are the remains of fetal structures.

albino /albī′nō/ [L, albus, white], (Obsolete) now called a person with albinism.

albinuria /al′binoor″ē·ə/, white cloudy urine.

Albright hereditary osteodystrophy (AHO), a rare disorder with a wide range of signs and symptoms, including short stature, obesity, round face, subcutaneous ossifications (formation of bone under the skin), and short fingers and toes. See also **pseudohypoparathyroidism.**

Albright syndrome /ôl″brīts/ [Fuller Albright, American physician and endocrinologist, 1900–1969], a disorder characterized by fibrous dysplasia of bone, isolated brown macules on the skin, and endocrine dysfunction. It causes precocious puberty in girls but not in boys. The bone lesions

are reddish gray, gritty fibromas containing areas of coarse fiber that may be confined to one bone or that occur in several areas, frequently causing deformities, pain, and pathological fractures. Treatment may involve osteotomy, curettage, and bone grafts. Also called **McCune-Albright syndrome.**

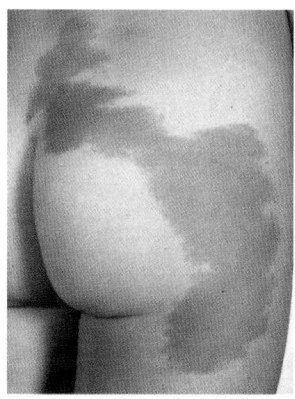

Albright syndrome (Courtesy Dr. David Atherton)

albumin /albyoo″min/ [L, albus, white], a water-soluble, heat-coagulable protein; the most abundant protein in blood plasma. Various albumins are found in practically all animal tissues and in many plant tissues. Determination of the levels and kinds of albumin in urine, blood, and other body tissues is the basis of a number of laboratory diagnostic tests.

albuminaturia, urine that contains a high level of albumin salts and has a low specific gravity.

albumin/creatinine ratio, the ratio of albumin to creatinine in the urine, calculated as a measure of albuminuria; used as a screening test for individuals at risk for the development of renal disease.

albumin (human), a plasma-volume expander.
■ INDICATIONS: It is prescribed in the treatment of hypoproteinemia, hyperbilirubinemia, and hypovolemic shock.
■ CONTRAINDICATIONS: Severe anemia, heart failure, and allergic reaction to albumin prohibit its use.
■ ADVERSE EFFECTS: Among the most serious adverse reactions are chills, hypertension, fever, and urticaria.

albumin microsphere sonicated, a microbubble, mean size 2 to 4.5 mm, created by heat treatment and sonication of diluted human albumin in the presence of octafluoropropane gas; sonicated albumin microspheres are injected intravenously as a diagnostic adjunct in echocardiography.

albuminous liver, (Obsolete) See **amyloid liver.**

albumin test [L, albus, white], any of several tests for the presence of albumin in the urine or blood. The test may be obtained to evaluate liver or renal function and/or nutritional status.

albuminuria, the presence of albumin in the urine, a common sign of renal or chronic disease. See also **proteinuria.**

-albuminuria, a suffix meaning a "(specified) condition characterized by excess serum proteins in the urine": noctalbuminuria, pseudalbuminuria.

albuterol, a beta$_2$ receptor adrenergic agent.
■ INDICATIONS: It is prescribed in the treatment of bronchospasm in patients with reversible obstructive airway disease, including asthma.
■ CONTRAINDICATIONS: Known sensitivity to this drug prohibits its use.
■ ADVERSE EFFECTS: Among the most serious adverse reactions are tachycardia, insomnia, dizziness, and hypertension.

alcalase, an protein-digesting enzyme found in certain laundry detergents. It may cause enzymatic detergent asthma.

Alcaligenes, an environmental gram-negative bacillus that can be found in the GI tract of humans and that can cause nosocomial infections in the compromised host.

alclometasone /al-klo-met′ah-sōn″/, a synthetic corticosteroid used topically for the relief of inflammation and pruritus.

alclometasone dipropionate, a topical corticosteroid.

■ INDICATIONS: It is prescribed for the relief of symptoms of inflammation and pruritus of corticosteroid-responsive dermatoses.

■ CONTRAINDICATIONS: It is contraindicated in patients with hypersensitivity to the drug. Children may absorb proportionally greater amounts of the drug per area of skin surface and should be treated with the smallest amount of the drug needed.

■ ADVERSE EFFECTS: Among adverse reactions are burning, stinging, and itching.

Alcock's canal [Benjamin Alcock, Irish anatomist, 19th century], a canal formed by the obturator internus muscle and the obturator fascia through which the pudendal nerve and vessels pass. Also called **pudendal canal.**

alcohol /al″kəhôl/ [Ar, *alkohl,* subtle essence], 1. a preparation containing at least 92.3% and not more than 93.8% by weight of ethyl alcohol, used as a topical antiseptic and solvent. 2. a clear, colorless, volatile liquid that is miscible with water, chloroform, or ether, obtained by the fermentation of carbohydrates with yeast. 3. a compound derived from a hydrocarbon by replacing one or more hydrogen atoms with an equal number of hydroxyl groups. Depending on the number of hydroxyl groups, alcohols are classified as monohydric alcohol, dihydric alcohol, and trihydric alcohol. –**alcoholic,** *adj., n.*

alcohol bath, an obsolete procedure for decreasing an elevated body temperature. It is no longer used because of the danger of inhaled fumes and absorption through the skin, causing toxicity.

alcoholic, 1. pertaining to alcohol or its effects on other substances. 2. a person who has developed a dependency on alcohol through abuse of the substance. It is less stigmatizing for health care professionals to refer to an individual as a person with an alcohol addiction rather than an alcoholic.

alcoholic ataxia [Ar, *alkohl,* essence; Gk, *ataxia,* disorder], a loss of coordination in performing voluntary movements associated with peripheral neuritis as a result of alcoholism. A similar form of ataxia may occur with neuritis resulting from other toxic agents. See also **Wernicke encephalopathy.**

alcoholic blackout, a form of amnesia in which a person has no memory of what occurred during a period of alcohol abuse and intoxication.

alcoholic cardiomyopathy [Ar, *alkohl,* essence; Gk, *kardia,* heart, *mys,* muscle, *pathos,* disease], a cardiac disease associated with alcohol abuse and characterized by an enlarged heart and low cardiac output. Treatment consists of abstinence from alcohol and results in marked reduction in heart size in over half of patients.

alcoholic cirrhosis. See **Laënnec cirrhosis.**

alcoholic coma [Ar, *alkohl* + Gk, *koma,* deep sleep], a state of unconsciousness that results from ingesting very high quantities of alcohol within short periods of time, causing severe alcohol intoxication.

alcoholic dementia [Ar, *alkohl* + L, *de,* away, *mens,* mind], a deterioration of normal cognitive and intellectual functions associated with long-term alcohol abuse.

alcoholic fermentation, the conversion of carbohydrates to ethyl alcohol.

alcoholic hallucinosis, a form of alcoholic psychosis characterized primarily by auditory hallucinations occurring in a clear sensorium, abject fear, and delusions of persecution. The condition develops in acute alcoholism as withdrawal symptoms shortly after prolonged and heavy alcohol intake is stopped or reduced, usually within 48 hours. Constitutes a medical emergency. Also called **acute hallucinosis.** See also **hallucinosis.**

alcoholic hepatitis, an acute toxic liver injury associated with excess ethanol consumption. It is characterized by necrosis, inflammation caused by the accumulation of polymorphonuclear leukocytes, and in many instances Mallory bodies.

alcoholic hepatopathy, a liver disease resulting from alcoholism, progressing in time to fibrosis and cirrhosis.

alcoholic ketoacidosis, the fall in blood pH (acidosis) sometimes seen in alcoholics and associated with a rise in the levels of serum ketone bodies.

alcoholic neuropathy, damage to the peripheral nerves as a result of nutritional deficiencies associated with alcohol consumption.

alcoholic-nutritional cerebellar degeneration, a sudden, severe incoordination in the lower extremities characteristic of poorly nourished alcoholics. The patient walks, if at all, with an ataxic or a wide-based gait. Treatment consists of improved nutrition, abstinence from alcohol, and physical therapy. See also **alcoholism.**

alcoholic paralysis [Ar, *alkohl,* essence; Gk, *paralyein,* to be palsied]. *(Obsolete)* See **alcoholic neuropathy.**

alcoholic psychosis, any of a group of severe mental disorders in which the ego's functioning is impaired, including pathological intoxication, delirium tremens, Korsakoff's psychosis, and acute hallucinosis. It is characterized by brain damage or dysfunction that results from excessive alcohol use.

Alcoholics Anonymous (AA), an international nonprofit organization, founded in 1935, consisting of abstinent alcoholics whose purpose is to stay sober and help others recover from the disease of alcoholism through a 12-step program, including group support, shared experiences, and faith in a higher power. The AA program, which emphasizes both medical and religious resources for help in overcoming alcoholism, consists of attending meetings and coping with abstinence "one day at a time." Meetings are held at convenient times in public locations such as factories, schools, churches, hospitals, and other community buildings. Similar groups who work with the children, relatives, friends, and associates of alcoholics are **Al-Anon** and **Alateen.**

alcoholic trance, *(Obsolete)* a state of automatism resulting from ethanol intoxication.

alcoholism /al″kəhôliz′əm/, the dependence on excessive amounts of alcohol, associated with a cumulative pattern of deviant behaviors. Alcoholism is a chronic illness with a slow, insidious onset, which may occur at any age. The cause is unknown, but genetic, cultural, and psychosocial factors are suspect, and families of individuals with alcoholism have a higher incidence of the disease. See also **acute alcoholism, chronic alcoholism.**

■ OBSERVATIONS: The most frequent health consequences of alcoholism are central nervous system depression and cirrhosis. The severity of each may be greater in the absence of food intake. Alcoholic patients also may suffer from alcoholic gastritis, peripheral neuropathies, auditory hallucinations, and cardiac problems. Abrupt withdrawal of alcohol in addiction causes weakness, sweating, and hyperreflexia. The severe form of alcohol withdrawal is delirium tremens.

■ INTERVENTIONS: Extreme caution should be used in administering drugs to alcoholic patients because of the possibility of additive central nervous system depression and toxicity caused by inability of the liver to metabolize the drugs. Treatment consists of psychotherapy (especially group therapy by organizations such as Alcoholics Anonymous) or administration of drugs, such as disulfiram, that cause an aversion to alcohol.

alcohol poisoning, poisoning caused by the ingestion of any of several alcohols, of which ethyl, isopropyl, and methyl are the most common. Ethyl alcohol (ethanol) is found in beverages, hairspray, and mouthwashes; ordinarily, it is lethal only if large quantities are ingested in a brief period. Isopropyl (rubbing) alcohol is more toxic. Methyl alcohol (methanol) is extremely poisonous: In addition to nausea, vomiting, and abdominal pain, it may cause blindness; death may follow the consumption of only 2 oz. Treatment for alcohol poisoning may include gastric lavage and other supportive interventions.

alcohol withdrawal syndrome, the clinical symptoms associated with cessation of alcohol consumption. These may include tremor, hallucinations, autonomic nervous system dysfunction, and seizures. See also **delirium tremens.**

ALD, abbreviation for **adrenoleukodystrophy.**

Aldactazide, a fixed-combination drug containing a thiazide diuretic and a potassium-sparing diuretic. Brand name for **hydrochlorothiazide, spironolactone.**

Aldactone, a potassium-sparing diuretic. Brand name for **spironolactone.**

aldehyde /al″dəhīd′/ [Ar, *alkohl* + L, *dehydrogenatum,* dehydrogenated], any of a large category of organic compounds derived from the oxidation of a corresponding primary alcohol, as in the conversion of ethyl alcohol to acetaldehyde, also known as ethanal. Each aldehyde is characterized by a carbonyl group (–CO–) attached directly to a hydrogen (–CHO) in its formula and can be converted into a corresponding acid by oxidation, as in the conversion of acetaldehyde to acetic acid.

aldesleukin, an antineoplastic agent.

■ INDICATIONS: This drug is used to treat metastatic renal cell carcinoma in adults and metastatic melanoma.

■ CONTRAINDICATIONS: Known hypersensitivity to this drug and abnormal thallium stress or pulmonary function tests prohibit this drug's use. This drug also must not be used in patients with organ allografts.

■ ADVERSE EFFECTS: Adverse effects of this drug include mental status changes, dizziness, sensory dysfunction, syncope, motor dysfunction, headache, impaired memory, depression, sleep disturbances, hallucinations, rigors, neuropathy, sinus tachycardia, dysrhythmias, bradycardia, PVCs, PACs, myocardial ischemia, reversible visual changes, stomatitis, anorexia, GI bleeding, dyspepsia, constipation, jaundice, ascites, dysuria, dry skin, purpura, petechiae, urticaria, arthralgia, myalgia, pulmonary congestion, tachypnea, pleural effusion, wheezing, and infection. Common side effects include fever, chills, hypotension, nausea, vomiting, diarrhea, pruritus, erythema, rash, and dyspnea. Life-threatening side effects include myocardial infarction, cardiac arrest, capillary leak syndrome, cerebrovascular accident, intestinal perforation, oliguria, anuria, proteinuria, hematuria, renal failure, thrombocytopenia, leukopenia, coagulation disorders, leukocytosis, eosinophilia, exfoliative dermatitis, pulmonary edema, respiratory failure, and apnea.

Aldoclor, a fixed-combination antihypertensive drug containing a diuretic and an antihypertensive agent. Brand name for **chlorothiazide, methyldopa.**

aldolase /al″dəlās/, enzyme found in muscle tissue that catalyzes the step in anaerobic glycolysis involving the breakdown of fructose 1,6-biphosphate to glyceraldehyde 3-phosphate. The enzyme can also catalyze the reverse reaction. Normal adult findings are 3 to 8.2 Sibley-Lehninger units/dL or 22 to 59 mU at 37° C. See also **glycolysis.**

aldolase test, a blood test that may be used in the assessment of muscular dystrophy and genetic disorders of the skeletal muscles.

Aldomet, an antihypertensive agent. Brand name for **methyldopa.**

Aldoril, a fixed-combination drug containing a thiazine diuretic and an antihypertensive agent. Brand name for **hydrochlorothiazide, methyldopa.**

aldose /al″dōs/, a monosaccharide (a simple sugar) that contains only one aldehyde (-CH=O) group per molecule. The chemical formula takes the form $Cn(H_2O)n$. The simplest possible aldose is the diose glycolaldehyde, which contains only three carbon atoms.

aldosterone /al″dōstərōn′, aldos″tərōn/, a mineralocorticoid steroid hormone produced by the adrenal cortex with action in the renal tubule to retain sodium, conserve water by reabsorption, and increase urinary excretion of potassium.

aldosterone test, a blood or 24-hour urine test used to measure the level of aldosterone; used as a screening test for Conn syndrome.

aldosteronism /al″dōstərō″nizəm, aldos″-/, a condition characterized by the hypersecretion of aldosterone, occurring as a primary disease of the adrenal cortex or, more often, as a secondary disorder in response to various extraadrenal pathological processes. Primary aldosteronism may be caused by adrenal hyperplasia or by an aldosterone-secreting adenoma. Secondary aldosteronism is associated with increased plasma renin activity and may be induced by nephrotic syndrome, cirrhosis, idiopathic edema, congestive heart failure, trauma, burns, or other kinds of stress. It is frequently noted in resistant hypertension. Also called **Conn syndrome, hyperaldosteronism.**

■ OBSERVATIONS: In many cases the only manifestation of aldosteronism is mild to moderate hypertension. Other signs and symptoms include episodic weakness, fatigue, paresthesia, polyuria, polydipsia, and nocturia. Glycosuria, hyperglycemia, and personality disturbances are occasionally manifested. Laboratory tests may show decreased plasma renin activity (measured after restricted sodium and/or diuretic therapy), increased aldosterone levels (measured after sodium loading), normal blood chemistry values, or hypernatremia and hypokalemia. A CT scan may be used to detect the presence of an adenoma.

■ INTERVENTIONS: Treatment includes regular monitoring and control of blood pressure and electrolytes. Aldosterone antagonists would be the first-line medications and may include spironolactone or eplerenone. A low-sodium diet, cessation of tobacco use, weight reduction (if indicated), and regular exercise are also advised. A unilateral adrenalectomy is performed if an adenoma or a carcinoma is present, and chemotherapy with mitotane may be an option.

■ PATIENT CARE CONSIDERATIONS: Nurses should focus on blood pressure monitoring and education. Instruction is needed in the use and expected side effects of medications, including gynecomastia, menstrual irregularities, and reduced libido with spironolactone. Dietary management (low sodium) should be addressed and a regular exercise regimen established and monitored. Counseling or referrals should be made for those who use tobacco products. The patient and a family member should be taught to monitor blood pressure on a regular basis. The importance of medical follow-up should be emphasized. Ongoing monitoring of electrolytes is also required, especially for those on medications to treat the disorder.

aldosteronoma al″dōstir′ənō″mə/*pl.* aldosteronomas, aldosteronomata/, an aldosterone-secreting adenoma of the adrenal cortex that is usually small and occurs more frequently in the left than the right adrenal gland. Aldosteronism with sodium retention, expansion of the extracellular fluid volume, potassium loss, and hypertension may occur.

-aldrate, a suffix designating an antacid aluminum salt.

Aldurazyme, brand name for **laronidase.**

alefacept, an immunosuppressive agent.

■ INDICATIONS: This drug is used to treat adults with moderate to severe plaque psoriasis.

■ CONTRAINDICATIONS: Known hypersensitivity to this drug prohibits its use.

alemtuzumab /al″em-tuz′u-mab″/, a recombinant, DNA–derived, humanized monoclonal antibody directed against the CD antigen CD52; it is administered intravenously as an antineoplastic drug in the treatment of B cell chronic lymphocytic leukemia.

alendronate, a bone-resorption inhibitor.

■ INDICATIONS: This drug is used to treat osteoporosis in postmenopausal women and Paget's disease.

■ CONTRAINDICATIONS: Known hypersensitivity to biphosphonates prohibits the use of this drug.

■ ADVERSE EFFECTS: Side effects include anemia, hypokalemia, hypomagnesemia, hypophosphatemia, osteonecrosis of the jaw, abdominal pain, anorexia, constipation, nausea, vomiting, bone pain, hypertension, urinary tract infection, and fluid overload.

Aleppo boil /əlep′ō/. See **cutaneous leishmaniasis.**

alertness [Fr, *alerte*], a measure of being mentally quick, active, and keenly aware of the environment.

aleukemia, an acute form of leukemia characterized by a diminished total white blood cell count in the peripheral blood, accompanied by a loss of normal bone marrow function. Also spelled *aleukaemia.*

aleukemic leukemia /ā′lo̅o̅kē″mik/, a type of leukemia in which the total leukocyte count remains within normal limits or is low and few abnormal forms appear in the peripheral blood. Diagnosis requires bone marrow biopsy. It occurs in 30% of all patients with leukemia, regardless of the specific type. Also called **aleukocythemic leukemia, subleukemic leukemia.**

aleukemic myelosis. See **myeloid metaplasia.**

aleukia /ālo̅o̅′kē·ə/ [Gk, *a + leukos*, not white], a marked reduction in or complete absence of leukocytes or platelets. Compare **leukopenia, thrombocytopenia.** See also **aplastic anemia.**

aleukocythemic leukemia. See **aleukemic leukemia.**

aleukocytosis /ālo̅o̅′kōsītō″sis/, absence of leukocytes from the blood.

Alexander's deafness [Gustav Alexander, Austrian otologist, 1873–1932], congenital deafness caused by cochlear aplasia involving chiefly the organ of Corti and adjacent ganglion cells of the basal coil of the cochlea; high-frequency hearing loss results. Also called *Alexander aplasia.*

Alexander disease /al′eg-zan′dər/ [W. Stewart Alexander, English pathologist, 20th century], an infantile form of leukodystrophy, characterized by a collection of eosinophilic material at the surface of the brain and around its blood vessels, resulting in brain enlargement. It also causes macrocephaly, seizures, and spasticity.

Alexander technique [Frederick Matthias Alexander, Australian actor, 1869–1955, who developed and taught the technique], a bodywork technique that uses psychophysical reeducation to correct dysfunctional habits of posture and movement. It is based on the principle that human movement is most fluid when the head leads and the spine follows to improve postural balance, coordination, and breathing; relieve stress and chronic pain; and improve general well-being.

alexandrite laser, a laser whose active medium is alexandrite doped with chromium, emitting light in the mid-infrared spectrum, tunable between 701 and 826 nm, and used usually at 755 nm. It is used for hair removal and other dermatological procedures.

alexia. See **word blindness.** *−alexic, adj.*

alexithymia /əlek′sithī″mē·ə, -thim″ē·ə/, an inability to experience and verbalize one's emotions.

alfa. See **alpha.**

alfacalcidol /al″fah-kal′si-dol/, a synthetic analog of calcitriol, to which it is converted in the liver. It is used in the treatment of hypocalcemia, hypophosphatemia, rickets, and osteodystrophy associated with various medical conditions, including chronic renal failure and hypoparathyroidism. Alfacalcidol is administered orally or intravenously.

alfalfa, an herb that is grown throughout the world.

■ INDICATIONS: This herb is used for poor appetite, hay fever and asthma, and high cholesterol. It may also be used as a nutrient source.

■ CONTRAINDICATIONS: Alfalfa is not recommended during pregnancy and lactation, in children, in persons using blood thinners, or in those with known hypersensitivity to it.

alfuzosin, an antiadrenergic agent.

■ INDICATIONS: This drug is used to treat symptoms of benign prostatic hyperplasia.

■ CONTRAINDICATIONS: Known hypersensitivity to this drug and moderate to severe hepatic impairment prohibit its use.

■ ADVERSE EFFECTS: Adverse effects of this drug include postural hypotension within a few hours of administration, chest pain, tachycardia, fatigue, nausea, abdominal pain, dyspepsia, constipation, impotence, priapism, general body pain, rash, upper respiratory infection, bronchitis, and sinusitis. Common side effects include dizziness and headache.

ALG, abbreviation for **antilymphocyte globulin.**

alg-. See **algesi-, alg-, alge-, algo-.**

alga /al″gə/ *pl.* algae [L, seaweed], any of a large group of mostly photosynthetic protists found worldwide in freshwater, in saltwater, and on land. *−algal, adj.*

algesi-, alg-, alge-, algo-, prefixes meaning "pain": *algesia, algophobia.*

-algesia, a suffix meaning "(condition of) sensitivity to pain": *asphalgesia, hyperthermalgesia.*

-algesic, a suffix meaning "sensitivity to pain": *analgesic, paralgesic.*

-algia, -algy, suffixes meaning "pain, painful condition": *epigastralgia, metrralgia.*

-algic, a suffix meaning "pain": *cardialgic, tibialgic.*

algid /al″jid/ [L, *algere*, to be cold], chilly or cold.

algid malaria [L, *algere*, to be cold], a rare complication of tropical malaria (occurring in 0.37% of cases) caused by the protozoan *Plasmodium falciparum.* It is characterized by cold skin, profound weakness, and severe diarrhea. See also **falciparum malaria, malaria.**

alginate /al′ji-nāt/, a salt of alginic acid, extracted from marine kelp. The calcium, sodium, and ammonium alginates have been used in foam, cloth, a thickening agent for foods, pharmaceutical preparations, and gauze for absorbent surgical dressings. Soluble alginates, such as those of sodium, potassium, or magnesium, form a viscous sol that can be changed into a gel by a chemical reaction with compounds such as calcium sulfate; this makes them useful as materials for taking dental impressions.

algo-. See **algesi-, alg-, alge-, algo-.**

algodystrophy /al′gōdis″trəfē/, a painful wasting of the muscles of the hands, often accompanied by tenderness and a loss of bone calcium. The condition may begin in the hand or in the shoulder and spread over the entire limb, causing contractures, edema, and cyanosis of the skin. It may also occur in the feet or legs. It may be associated with injury, heart disease, stroke, or a viral infection. Also called **complex regional pain syndrome.** See also **reflex sympathetic dystrophy.**

algolagnia /al′gōlag″nē·ə/ [Gk, *algos,* pain, *lagneia,* lust], a form of sexual perversion characterized by sadism or masochism. See also **sadomasochism.**

algologist /algol′əjist/, **1.** a person who specializes in the study of or the treatment of pain. **2.** a person who specializes in the science and research of the algae plant. Also called **phycologist.**

algology, **1.** the branch of medicine concerned with the study of pain. **2.** the branch of science concerned with the study of algae. Also called **phycologist.**

algophobia [Gk, *algos,* pain, *phobos,* fear], an anxiety disorder characterized by an abnormal, pervasive fear of experiencing pain or of witnessing pain in others.

algor [L, cold], the sensation of cold or a chill, particularly in the first stage of a fever.

algorithm /al″gərith′əm/, **1.** a step-by-step procedure for the solution to a problem by a computer, using specific mathematical or logical operations. **2.** an explicit protocol with well-defined rules to be followed in solving a health care problem.

algor mortis, the reduction in body temperature and accompanying loss of skin elasticity that occur after death. Also called **death chill.**

algospasm /al″gōspaz′əm/, an acute, painful spasm of the muscles. Now called **muscle cramp.**

aliasing, an artifact that is caused by undersampling of signal data in diagnostic imaging.

Alice in Wonderland syndrome, perceptual distortions of space and size, as experienced by the character Alice in the Lewis Carroll story. Similar hallucinogenic experiences have been reported by individuals using drugs of abuse and by patients with certain neurological diseases.

alienation /āl′yənā″shən/ [L, *alienare,* to estrange], the act or state of being estranged or isolated. See also **depersonalization.** −*alien, adj.,* −*alienate, v.*

alignment /əlīn′mənt/ [Fr, to put in a straight line], **1.** the arrangement of a group of points or objects along a line. **2.** the placement or maintenance of body structures in their proper anatomical positions, such as straightening of the teeth or repair of a fractured bone.

aliment [L, *alimentum,* to nourish], something that nourishes or feeds. −*alimentary, adj.*

alimentary bolus, a small, rounded mass of chewed food mixed with salivary enzymes that is ready to be swallowed. See **bolus.**

alimentary canal. See **digestive tract.**

alimentary duct. Also called **thoracic duct.**

alimentary system. Also called **digestive system.**

alimentary tract. Also called **digestive tract.**

alimentation, nourishment. See also **feeding.**

Alimta, brand name for **pemetrexed.**

aliphatic /al′ifat″ik/ [Gk, *aleiphar,* oil], pertaining to fat or oil, specifically hydrocarbon compounds that are open chains of carbon atoms, such as the fatty acids, rather than aromatic ring structures. Aliphatic compounds do not have conjugated unsaturated cyclic structures as are found in aromatic compounds such as benzene and naphthalene.

aliphatic acid, an acid containing a hydrocarbon fragment derived from a nonaromatic hydrocarbon.

aliphatic alcohol, an alcohol containing a hydrocarbon fragment derived from a fatty, nonaromatic hydrocarbon.

Examples include ethyl alcohol and isopropyl alcohol, both of which have fat-solvent properties as well as bactericidal effects.

-alis, a suffix meaning "pertaining to" something specified: *brachioradialis.*

aliskiren, a renin inhibitor used as an antihypertensive agent.

■ INDICATIONS: This drug is used to treat essential hypertension, alone or in combination with other antihypertensive agents.

■ CONTRAINDICATIONS: Use with angiotensin receptor blockers (ARBs) or angiotensin-converting enzyme inhibitors (ACEIs) in patients with diabetes and renal failure. Second- and third-trimester pregnancy and known hypersensitivity to this drug prohibit its use.

■ ADVERSE EFFECTS: Adverse effects of this drug include orthostatic hypotension, hypotension, headache, dizziness, renal stones, increased uric acid, rash, and hyperkalemia. Life-threatening side effects include angioedema. Patients with diabetes and renal failure are at significantly increased risk for complications.

alitretinoin, a second-generation retinoid, a class of chemical compounds that are related chemically to vitamin A.

■ INDICATIONS: It is a topical gel used to treat the cutaneous lesions of Kaposi's sarcoma.

■ CONTRAINDICATIONS: Known hypersensitivity and pregnancy prohibit this drug's use.

■ ADVERSE EFFECTS: Side effects include rash, stinging, warmth, redness, erythema, blistering, crusting, peeling, contact dermatitis, and pain at the site of application.

alkalemia [Ar, *al + galiy,* wood ash; Gk, *haima,* blood], increased pH of the blood, above the normal range of 7.35 to 7.45. Also spelled *alkalaemia.*

alkali /al″kəlī/ [Ar, *al + galiy,* wood ash], a compound with the chemical characteristics of a base. Usually used with reference to hydroxides of Group I metals and ammonium, alkalis combine with fatty acids to form soaps, turn red litmus blue, and enter into reactions with carbon dioxide that form water-soluble carbonates. See also **acid, base.** −*alkaline, adj.,* −**alkalinity,** *n.,* −**alkalize,** *v.*

alkali burn, damage to tissue caused by exposure to an alkaline compound such as lye. Treatment includes washing the area with copious amounts of water to remove the chemical. The victim should be immediately taken to a medical facility for assessment of tissue damage. Compare **acid burn.**

-alkaline, a suffix meaning "alkali": *subalkaline.*

alkaline ash /al″kəlīn/, residue in urine having a pH higher than 7.0.

alkali-ash diet, a diet designed to increase the blood and urinary pH in which the ingestion of specific fruits (avocados, tomatoes, and lemons) and vegetables (e.g., asparagus, cabbage, peas, and spinach) is encouraged. Restricted foods include meat, poultry, and cheese. Research suggests that the most rational approach should be based on the cumulative effects of foods because the maintenance of pH is a complex process in which the body adjusts to maintain equilibrium. However, a diet rich in fruit and vegetables promotes overall health.

alkaline bath, a bath taken in water containing sodium bicarbonate, used especially for skin disorders.

alkaline phosphatase, an enzyme present in all tissues and in high concentration in bone, liver, kidneys, intestines, biliary ducts, plasma, and teeth. It may be elevated in serum in some diseases of the bone and liver and some other illnesses. The function of alkaline phosphatase is the hydrolysis of organic phosphate esters present in the extracellular space.

Normal serum concentrations in adults are 1.5 to 4.5 Bodansky units; in children, 5 to 14 Bodansky units. See also **acid phosphatase.**

alkaline phosphatase test (ALP), a blood test used to determine a variety of liver and bone disorders such as extrahepatic and intrahepatic obstructive biliary disease, cirrhosis, hepatic tumors, hepatotoxic drugs, hepatitis, osteoblastic metastatic tumors, Paget's disease, rheumatoid arthritis, and hyperparathyroidism.

alkaline reflux gastritis, chronic gastritis caused by the reflux of alkaline intestinal contents after a partial gastrectomy.

alkaline reserve, the additional amount of sodium bicarbonate that the body produces to maintain a normal arterial pH (7.35 to 7.45) when the carbon dioxide level increases as a result of hypoventilation. The alkaline reserve is maintained by the kidneys, which control the excretion of bicarbonate ions in urine.

alkalinity /al′kəlin″itē/, the acid-base relationship of any solution that has a lower concentration of hydrogen ions or a higher concentration of hydroxide ions than pure water, which is an arbitrarily neutral standard with a pH of 7.0 at 25° C.

alkalinization /al′kəlinəzāshən/, **1.** the act of making a substance alkaline, as through the addition of a base. **2.** the state of becoming alkaline.

alkali poisoning, a toxic condition caused by the ingestion of an alkaline agent such as liquid ammonia, lye, and some detergent powders. Compare **acid poisoning.**

alkali reserves [Ar, *al + galiy,* wood ash + L, *reservare,* to save], the volume of carbon dioxide or carbonates at standard temperature and pressure in 100 mL of blood plasma. The principal buffer in blood is bicarbonate, which represents most of the alkali reserve. Hemoglobin phosphates and additional bases also act as buffers. If the alkali reserve is low, acidosis exists; if it is high, alkalosis exists.

alkalize. See **alkalinization,** def. 1.

alkaloid /al″kəloid/ [Ar, *al +* galiy; Gk, *eidos,* form], any of a large group of nitrogen-containing organic compounds produced by plants, including many pharmacologically active substances, such as atropine, caffeine, cocaine, morphine, nicotine, and quinine.

alkalosis /al′kəlō″sis/ [Ar, *al + galiy +* Gk, *osis,* condition], an abnormal condition of body fluids, characterized by a tendency toward a blood pH level greater than 7.45 caused by an excess of alkaline bicarbonate or a deficiency of acid. The treatment of uncompensated alkalosis involves the correction of dehydration and various ionic deficits to restore the normal acid-base balance in which the ratio of carbonic acid to bicarbonate is 20:1. When a buffer system, such as carbon dioxide retention or bicarbonate excretion, prevents a shift in pH, it is labeled compensated alkalosis. Compare **acidosis.** Kinds include **respiratory alkalosis, metabolic alkalosis.** See also **compensated alkalosis.**

alkane, a saturated aliphatic hydrocarbon containing no double or triple bonds in the carbon chain, such as propane.

alkaptonuria /alkap′tōnoor″ē·ə/ [Ar, *al + galiy +* Gk, *haptein,* to possess, *ouron,* urine], a rare inherited disorder marked by the excretion of large amounts of homogentisic acid in the urine, which is the result of the incomplete metabolism of the amino acids tyrosine and phenylalanine. The presence of the acid is indicated by darkening of urine when exposed to air or by brown or blue discoloration of the ears or eyes. Other indications are restricted joint mobility, kidney stones, and vascular hypertension. See also **ochronosis.** *−alkaptonuric, adj.*

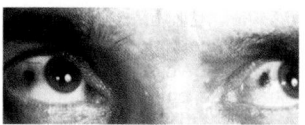

Alkaptonuria *(Moll, 1997)*

alkene /al″kēn/, an unsaturated aliphatic hydrocarbon containing at least one double bond in the carbon chain, such as ethylene or 1,3-butadiene. Also called **olefin.**

Alkeran, an alkylating antineoplastic agent. Brand name for **melphalan.**

alkyl /al″kil/, a hydrocarbon fragment derived from an alkane by the removal of one of the hydrogen atoms.

alkylamine /al″kiləmīn″/, an amine in which an alkyl group replaces one to three of the hydrogen atoms that are attached to the nitrogen atom of ammonia, such as methylamine (amino-methane).

alkylating agent /al″kilā′ting/, any substance that contains an alkyl radical and is capable of replacing a free hydrogen atom in an organic compound, or one that acts by a similar mechanism. This type of chemical reaction results in interference with DNA synthesis and RNA transcription, which in turn results in interference with mitosis and cell division, especially in rapidly proliferating tissue, causing cell death. Alkylating agents are radiometric in that their action is similar to that of irradiation. The agents are useful in the treatment of cancer and are a common class of chemotherapy agents. Agents include cyclophosphamide, mechlorethamine, thiotepa, busulfan, carmustine, lomustine, streptozocin altretamine, and procarbazine. Adverse effects include myleosuppression, particularly anemia and nausea, vomiting, and alopecia.

alkylation, a chemical reaction in which an alkyl group is transferred from an alkylating agent. When such organic reactions occur with a biologically significant cellular constituent such as deoxyribonucleic acid, they result in interference with mitosis and cell division.

alkyne /al″kīn/, an unsaturated aliphatic hydrocarbon containing at least one triple bond in the carbon chain, such as acetylene.

ALL, 1. abbreviation for **acute lymphoblastic leukemia. 2.** abbreviation for **acute lymphoid leukemia. 3.** abbreviation for **acute lymphocytic leukemia.**

allachesthesia /al′əkesthē″zhə/ [Gk, *allache,* elsewhere], an abnormality of touch sensation in which a stimulus is perceived to be at a point distant from where it is actually applied.

allanto-, a combining form meaning "allantois": *allantoidoangiopagus, allantotoxicon.*

allantoic. See **allantois.**

allantoidoangiopagus /al′əntoi′dō·an′jē·op″əgəs/ [Gk, *allantoeides,* sausagelike, *angeion,* vessel, *pagos,* fixed], conjoined monozygotic twin fetuses of unequal size that are united by the vessels of the umbilical cord. Also called **omphaloangiopagus.** See also **omphalosite.** *−allantoidoangiopagous, adj.*

allantoin /əlan′tō·in/, a chemical compound (5-ureidohydantoin), C4H6N4O3, that occurs as a white crystallizable substance found in many plants and in the allantoic and amniotic fluids and fetal urine of primates. It is also present in the urine of mammals other than primates as a product of purine metabolism. The substance, which can be produced synthetically by the oxidation of uric acid, was once used to promote tissue growth in the treatment of suppurating wounds and ulcers.

allantois /əlan″tois/ [Gk, *allas,* sausage, *eidos,* form], a tubular extension of the endoderm of the yolk sac that extends with the allantoic vessels into the connecting stalk of the embryo. In human embryos, allantoic vessels become the umbilical vessels and the chorionic villi. See also **body stalk, umbilical cord.** –**allantoic,** *adj.*

allele /əlēl″/, **1.** one of two or more alternative forms of a gene that occupy corresponding loci on homologous chromosomes. Each allele encodes a phenotypic feature or a certain inherited characteristic. An individual normally has two alleles for each gene, one contributed by the mother and one by the father. If both alleles are the same, the individual is homozygous; if the alleles are different, the individual is heterozygous. In heterozygous individuals, one of the alleles is usually dominant, and the other is recessive. In humans, for example, the allele for brown eyes is dominant, and the allele for blue eyes is recessive. **2.** one of two or more contrasting characteristics transmitted by alternative forms of a gene. Also called **allelomorph.** –**allelic,** *adj.*

allelo-, combining form meaning "another": *allelocatalysis, allelomorph.*

allelomorph. See **allele.**

Allen-Doisy test [Edgar Allen, U.S. endocrinologist, 1892–1943; Edward Doisy, U.S. biochemist and Nobel laureate, 1893–1986], a once-common bioassay test for estrogen and gonadotropins in which ovariectomized mice or rats were injected with an estrogenic substance. The appearance of cornified cells on vaginal smears and the disappearance of leukocytes constituted a positive reaction.

Allen test, a test for the patency of the radial artery after insertion of an indwelling monitoring catheter. It may also be used before obtaining arterial blood gases to assure adequate collateral blood flow. The patient's hand is formed into a fist while the nurse compresses the ulnar artery. Compression continues while the fist is opened. If blood perfusion through the radial artery is adequate, the hand should flush and resume its normal pinkish coloration. The accuracy and utility of the Allen test has been questioned in the research literature.

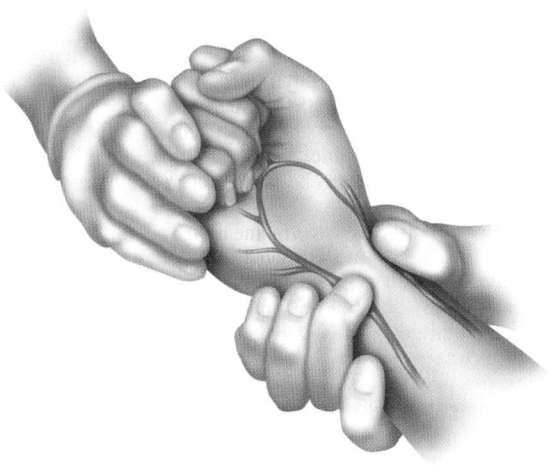

Allen test *(Custalow, 2005)*

allergen /al″ərjin/ [Gk, *allos,* other, *ergein,* to work, *genein,* to produce], an environmental substance that can produce a hypersensitive reaction in the body but may not be intrinsically harmful. Common allergens include pollen, animal dander, house dust, feathers, and various foods. Studies indicate that one of six Americans is hypersensitive to one or more allergens. Methods of identifying specific allergens affecting individuals include the patch test, the scratch test, the radioallergosorbent test, and the Prausnitz-Küstner test. See also **allergic reaction, allergy.** –**allergenic,** *adj.*

allergenic /al″ərjen″ik/, a substance capable of inducing hypersensitivity and provoking physical symptoms.

allergenic extract, a protein-containing extract purified from a substance to which a person may be sensitive. The extract may be used for diagnosis or for hyposensitization therapy.

allergic /əlur″jik/. See **allergy.**

allergic alveolitis. See **diffuse hypersensitivity pneumonia.**

allergic asthma, a form of asthma caused by exposure of the bronchial mucosa to an inhaled airborne antigen. The antigen causes the production of antibodies that bind to mast cells in the bronchial tree. The mast cells then release histamine, which stimulates contraction of bronchial smooth muscle and causes mucosal edema. Hyposensitization treatments are more effective for pollen sensitivity than for allergies to house dust, animal dander, mold, and insects. Psychological factors may provoke asthma attacks in bronchi already sensitized by antigens. Medication, including immunotherapy, can help relieve allergy symptoms. Often a diurnal pattern of histamine release occurs, causing variable degrees of bronchospasm at different times of the day. Also called **atopic asthma, extrinsic asthma.** See also **asthma, asthmatic eosinophilia, status asthmaticus.**

allergic bronchopulmonary aspergillosis, a form of aspergillosis that occurs in asthmatics when the fungus *Aspergillus fumigatus,* growing within the bronchial lumen, causes a type I or type III hypersensitivity reaction. The characteristics of the condition are similar to those of asthma, including dyspnea and wheezing. Chest examination and pulmonary function tests may reveal airway obstruction. Serological tests usually reveal precipitating antibodies to *A. fumigatus.* Bacteriological and microscopic examination of sputum may reveal *A. fumigatus* in addition to Charcot-Leyden crystals. Eosinophilia is usually also present. Compare **aspergillosis.**

allergic conjunctivitis, an inflammation of the conjunctiva caused by an allergy. Common allergens that cause this condition are pollen, grass, topical medications, air pollutants, occupational irritants, and smoke. This condition is bilateral, usually starts before puberty, and commonly recurs in a seasonal pattern. Also called **red eye.** See also **conjunctivitis.**

■ OBSERVATIONS: Common signs include itching, burning, and swelling around the eyes and excessive tearing. Eosinophils predominate in stained blood smears. The diagnosis is usually based on the results of cultures and sensitivity tests to identify the causative allergen.

■ INTERVENTIONS: Oral antihistamines and vasoconstrictor and corticosteroid eyedrops, such as predniSONE are typically prescribed.

■ PATIENT CARE CONSIDERATIONS: Cold compresses may be administered for comfort.

allergic contact dermatitis. See **allergic dermatitis.**

allergic coryza, acute rhinitis caused by exposure to any allergen to which the person is hypersensitive.

allergic dermatitis [Ger, *allergie,* reaction; Gk, *derma,* skin, *itis,* inflammation], a delayed type of hypersensitivity of the skin resulting from cutaneous contact with a specific allergen, with varying degrees of erythema, edema, and vesiculation. Such allergens include dyes, perfumes, poison ivy, certain chemicals, and metals. Also called **allergic contact dermatitis.**

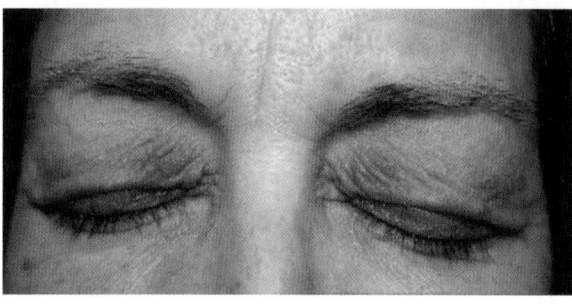

Allergic dermatitis *(Bolognia et al, 2012)*

allergic granulomatosis. See **Churg-Strauss syndrome.**

allergic interstitial nephritis, acute interstitial nephritis that is part of an allergic reaction, such as to medication. See also **interstitial nephritis.**

allergic interstitial pneumonitis. See **diffuse hypersensitivity pneumonia.**

allergic proctitis, in children, allergic gastroenteropathy having its focus in the rectum; in adults, rectal irritation possibly caused by chemicals in the rectum, such as after medical procedures, or inflammation caused by anal intercourse.

allergic purpura [Gk, *allos,* other, *ergein,* to work; L, *purpura,* purple], a chronic disorder of the skin associated with urticaria, erythema, asthma, and rheumatic joint swellings. Unlike in other forms of purpura, the platelet count, the bleeding time, and blood clotting are normal. Sensitization to foods, drugs, and insect bites is a factor.

allergic reaction, an unfavorable physiological response to an allergen to which a person has previously been exposed and to which the person has developed antibodies. The response may be characterized by a variety of symptoms, including urticaria, eczema, dyspnea, bronchospasm, diarrhea, rhinitis, sinusitis, laryngospasm, and anaphylaxis. Allergic reactions may be immediate or delayed. Eosinophilia is usually present and is revealed in the differential white blood cell count.

allergic rhinitis, inflammation of the nasal passages, usually associated with watery nasal discharge and itching of the nose and eyes, caused by a localized sensitivity reaction to an allergen, such as house dust, animal dander, or pollen. The condition may be seasonal, as in hay fever, or perennial, as in allergy to dust or animals. Treatment may include the local, systemic, or topical administration of antihistamines or steroids, avoidance of the antigen, and hyposensitization by injections of diluted antigen in gradually increasing amounts.

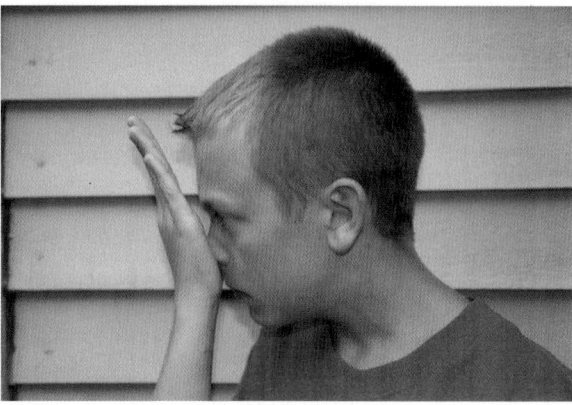

Allergic salute

allergic vasculitis, an inflammatory condition of the blood vessels that is induced by allergens such as iodides, penicillin, sulfonamides, and thioureas. It is characterized by itching, malaise, and a slight fever and by the presence of papules, vesicles, urticarial wheals, or small ulcers on the skin.

allergist /al′ərjist/, a physician who specializes in the diagnosis and treatment of allergic disorders and allergic reactions.

allergy /al″ərjē/ [Gk, *allos,* other, *ergein,* to work], a hypersensitive reaction to common, often intrinsically harmless substances, most of which are environmental. More than 50 million Americans have allergic reactions to airborne or inhaled allergens, such as cigarette smoke, house dust, and pollens. Symptoms of mild allergies, such as those associated with rhinitis, conjunctivitis, and urticaria, can be suppressed by antihistamines, with glucocorticoids administered as supplements to primary therapy. Severe allergic reactions, such as anaphylaxis and angioedema of the glottis, can cause systemic shock and death and commonly require immediate therapy with subcutaneous epinephrine or IV steroids, such as dexamethasone. See also **allergic reaction, allergy testing.**

allergy blood test, a blood test used to measure serum immunoglobulin E, which is an effective method of diagnosing allergy and of specifically identifying the allergen. This test can be helpful when the results of an allergy skin test are questionable, when the allergen is not available in a form for dermal injection, when the allergen may incite an anaphylactic reaction if injected into the patient, or when skin testing is particularly difficult (for example, in infants or patients with dermographia or widespread skin disease).

allergy immunotherapy, a specific series of treatments used to decrease an allergic immune response over time; the treatment often includes weekly injections of small doses of the allergen to decrease sensitivity.

allergy skin test, a skin test used to detect allergic reactions. Properly performed, it is considered the most convenient and least expensive test for detecting such reactions. The test involves injecting or topically scratching an allergen into the skin and then evaluating the wheal (swelling) and flare (redness) responses that follow. Positive reactions usually occur within 20 minutes.

allergy testing, any one of the various procedures used in identifying the specific allergens. Such tests are helpful in prescribing treatment to prevent allergic reactions or to reduce their severity. The most common is allergy skin testing, which exposes the patient to small quantities of the suspected allergens. Factors considered in performing allergy tests include the medical history of the patient, the allergy history, the environment, and the diet. Individuals to be tested are usually instructed to discontinue the use of any antihistamines at least 24 hours before the test because these drugs can interfere with normal test responses. Kinds include **intradermal test, scratch test, patch test, enzyme-linked immunosorbent assay, radioallergosorbent test.**

allesthesia /al′esthē″zha/, a referred pain or other sensation that is perceived at a remote site on the same or opposite side of the body stimulated. Also called **alloesthesia.**

all fours position, **1.** the sixth stage in the Rood system of ontogenetic motor patterns. In this stage, the lower trunk and lower extremities are brought into a co-contraction pattern while stretching of the trunk and limb girdles develops co-contractions of the trunk flexors and extensors. See **Rood System. 2.** (in obstetrics) a position in which the body rests on the arms and the knees with the knees held wide to open the pelvis.

allicin /al′i·sin/ [*Allium,* the genus of garlic], an oily substance extracted from garlic, having antibacterial activity.

allied health personnel, a distinct group of health professionals who apply their expertise to prevent disease transmission, diagnose, treat, and rehabilitate people of all ages and all specialties. Together with a range of technical and support staff they may deliver direct patient care, rehabilitation, treatment, diagnostics, and health improvement interventions to restore and maintain optimal physical, sensory, psychological, cognitive, and social functions.

alligator forceps, a device with long, thin angular handles and interlocking teeth; used in a variety of surgeries, primarily ear, nose, and throat procedures. Also called *alligator clamp.*

Allis forceps, a curved device with a scissorlike, atraumatic action. The device has serrated edges and is used for grasping biologic tissues. Also called *Allis clamp.*

allo-, all-, combining forms meaning "differing from the normal, reversal, or referring to another": *allopathy, allergic.*

alloantigen, proteins that vary from individual to individual that stimulate the production of antibodies. Graft rejection in human transplantation may be caused by immune responses to alloantigens on the graft, perceived as foreign by the recipient.

allochiria [Gk, *allos,* other, *chiria,* hand] a condition in which stimuli applied to one side of the body are erroneously perceived on the opposite side.

allodiploid /al′ōdip″loid/ [Gk, *allos,* other, *diploos,* double, *eidos,* form], **1.** an individual, an organism, a strain, or a cell that has two genetically distinct sets of chromosomes derived from different ancestral species, as occurs in hybridization. Compare **allopolyploid, autodiploid. 2.** also pertaining to such an individual, an organism, a strain, or a cell. −*allodiploidy, n.*

alloeroticism, alloerotism. See **heteroeroticism.**

alloesthesia. See **allesthesia.**

allogamy. See **cross-fertilization.**

allogenic /al′ōjen″ik/ [Gk, *allos* + *genein,* to produce], **1.** (in genetics) denoting an individual or cell type that is from the same species but genetically distinct. **2.** (in transplantation biology) denoting tissues, particularly stem cells from either bone marrow or peripheral blood, that are from the same species but antigenically distinct; homologous. Also spelled *allogeneic.* Compare **syngeneic, xenogeneic.** See also **alloantigen.**

allogenic graft. See **allograft.**

allograft /al′əgraft/ [Gk, *allos,* other + *graphion,* stylus], surgical transplantation of tissue between two genetically dissimilar individuals of the same species, such as between two humans who are not monozygotic twins. Tissues commonly used for allografts include cornea, cartilage, bone, artery, and cadaver skin stored in a skin-tissue bank. Also called **allogenic graft, homogenous graft, homograft, homologous graft.** Compare **autograft, isograft, xenograft.** See also **graft.**

allohexaploid. See **allopolyploid.**

allokeratoplasty /al′ōker″ətoplas′tē/, the repair of a cornea with synthetic transparent material.

allometric. See **allometry.**

allometric growth, the increase in size of different organs or parts of an organism at various rates. Also called **heterauxesis.** Compare **isometric growth.** See also **allometry.**

allometron /əlom″itron/, a quantitative change in the proportional relationship of the parts of an organism as a result of evolution.

allometry /əlom″itrē/ [Gk, *allos* + *metron,* measure], the measurement and study of the changes in proportions of the various parts of an organism in relation to the growth of the whole or of such changes within a series of related organisms. See also **allometric growth.** −*allometric, adj.*

allomorphism /al′ōmôr″fizəm/ [Gk, *allos,* other, *morphe,* form], **1.** a change in crystalline form without a change in chemical composition. **2.** a change in the shape of a group of cells caused by pressure or other physical factors.

allopathic physician /al′ōpath″ik/, a medical doctor (M.D.) who is educated in the principles of evidence-based practice and a biologically based approach to health and healing. Compare **chiropractic, homeopathy.** See also **Doctor of Medicine, Doctor of Osteopathy.**

allopathy /əlop″əthē/ [Gk, *allos* + *pathos,* suffering], a system of medical therapy in which a disease or an abnormal condition is treated by creating an environment that is antagonistic to the disease or condition; for example, an antibiotic toxic to a pathogenic organism is administered to treat an infection. Compare **chiropractic, homeopathy, osteopathy.** −*allopathic, adj.*

alloplast /al′ōplast/ [Gk, *allos,* other, *plassein,* to mold], a graft made of plastic, metal, or other synthetic material foreign to the human body. −*alloplastic, adj.*

alloplastic maneuver [Gk, *allos* + *plassein,* to mold], (in psychology) a process that is part of adaptation, involving an adjustment or a change in the external environment. Compare **autoplastic maneuver.**

alloplasty /al′ōplas′tē/ [Gk, *allos,* other, *plassein,* to mold], plastic surgery in which synthetic materials foreign to the human body are implanted. −*alloplastic, adj.*

allopolyploid /al′əpol″iploid/ [Gk, *allos* + *polyplous,* many times, *eidos,* form], **1.** an individual, an organism, a strain, or a cell that has more than two genetically distinct sets of chromosomes derived from two or more different ancestral species, as occurs in hybridization. Such individuals are referred to as allotriploid, allotetraploid, allopentaploid, allohexaploid, and so on, depending on the number of haploid sets of chromosomes they contain. Compare **allodiploid,** def. 1, **autodiploid.** See also **mosaic. 2.** *n,* also pertaining to such an individual, organism, strain, or cell. Also called **autopolyploid.**

allopurinol /al′əpyoor″ənôl/, a xanthine oxidase inhibitor uricosuric agent. Uricosuric medications (drugs) are substances that increase the excretion of uric acid in the urine, thus reducing the concentration of uric acid in blood plasma. In general, this effect is achieved by action on the proximal tubule of the kidney.

■ INDICATIONS: It is prescribed in the treatment of gout and other hyperuricemic conditions.

■ CONTRAINDICATIONS: It is not prescribed for children (except those with hyperuricemia resulting from malignancy), lactating mothers, or people suffering an acute attack of gout. Known hypersensitivity to this drug prohibits its use.

■ ADVERSE EFFECTS: Among the most serious adverse reactions are blood dyscrasias, severe rashes, and other allergic reactions. GI and ophthalmological disturbances also may occur.

allorhythmia /al′ōrith″mē′ə/, an irregular heart rhythm that occurs repeatedly.

all-or-none law, 1. the principle in neurophysiology stating that a stimulus must be strong enough to reach threshold to trigger a nerve impulse. Once threshold is achieved, the entire impulse is discharged. A weak stimulus will not produce a weak reaction. **2.** the principle that the heart muscle or nerve, under any stimulus above a threshold level, will respond either with a maximal strength response or with none at all. Also called **Bowditch effect.**

allostatic load, a term coined as a more precise alternative to the term *stress,* used to refer to environmental challenges that cause an organism to begin efforts to maintain stability (allostasis).

allosteric sites /al′ōster″ik/ [Gk, *allos* + *stereos,* solid], the sites, other than the active site or sites, of an enzyme that bind regulatory molecules.

allotetraploid. See **allopolyploid.**

allotransplantation, the transplantation of organs from a donor to a recipient of the same species but with a different genotype (an allograft).

allotrio-, a prefix meaning "strange or foreign": *allotriodontia, allotriogeustia.*

allotriodontia /əlot′rē·ōdon″shə/, **1.** the development of a tooth in an abnormal location, such as in a dermoid tumor. **2.** the transplantation of teeth from one individual to another.

allotriploid. See **allopolyploid.**

allotropic, 1. pertaining to a substance that is changed by digestion to retain some of its nutritive value. **2.** pertaining to an element that may exist in two or more forms at the atomic level, such as carbon, which exists as diamonds, graphite, and buckminsterfullerene (buckyballs, a crystalline form).

allowable charge /əlou″əbəl/, in the United States, the maximum dollar amount that a third party, usually an insurance company, will reimburse a provider for a specific service.

allowable costs, charges for health care services and/or supplies for which insurance benefits are available. Allowable costs vary across insurance companies.

allowable dose, permissible amount of radiation an individual or individual body part can receive in a specified period of time. See **accumulated dose equivalent.**

allowable error, a numerical interval assigned to each laboratory assay that provides limits for test imprecision. Often computed from the coefficient of variation at each of a series of decision levels and modified to meet consensus levels of clinical significance.

alloxan /əlok′san/, an oxidation product of uric acid that is found in the human intestine in diarrhea. Alloxan has been used to produce diabetes in experimental animals by destroying the insulin-secreting islet cells of the pancreas.

alloy /al″oi/ [Fr, *aloyer,* to combine metals], a mixture of two or more metals or of substances with metallic properties. Most alloys are formed by mixing molten metals that dissolve in each other. A number of alloys have medical applications, such as those used for prostheses and in dental amalgams.

almond oil, a viscous fluid expressed from the kernels of the fruit of almond trees. The sweet almond tree, *Prunus amygdalus,* which is native to the Mediterranean region, produces an oil that is used as a demulcent and a mild laxative. Bitter almond oil comes from a different tree *(Prunus amygdalus* var. *amara)* and contains toxic chemicals. Bitter almond oil is not recommended for ingestion.

almotriptan /al″mo-trip′tan/, an oral selective serotonin receptor agonist used in the acute treatment of a migraine.

aloe, a succulent found throughout the world.

■ INDICATIONS: Aloe vera gel is used externally for minor burns, skin irritations, minor wounds, frostbite, and radiation-induced injuries. Internally, it is used to heal intestinal inflammation and ulcers and to stimulate bile secretion as a digestive aid.

■ CONTRAINDICATIONS: Hypersensitivity to this plant, garlic, onions, or tulips prohibits the topical use of aloe. Aloe also should not be used on deep wounds. Internal use of the dried juice is contraindicated during pregnancy and lactation, in children younger than 12 years of age, and in those with kidney or cardiac disease or bowel obstruction. This product should not be used long term.

alopecia /al′əpē″shə/ [Gk, *alopex,* fox mange], a partial or complete lack of hair resulting from normal aging, an endocrine disorder, a drug reaction, an anticancer medication, or a skin disease. It can occur in both women and men and may be scarring (cicatricial), with permanent damage to the hair follicle, or nonscarring, in which the hair may regrow. Kinds include **alopecia areata, alopecia totalis, alopecia universalis, androgenetic alopecia, cicatricial alopecia, male pattern alopecia, premature alopecia.**

alopecia areata /er′ē-ā″tə/, a disease of unknown cause in which sudden well-defined bald patches occur. The bald areas are usually round or oval and located on the head and other hairy parts of the body. Hairs that look like exclamation points can sometime occur at a bald patch's edges. The condition is usually self-limited and often clears completely within 6 to 12 months without treatment. Recurrences are common. Anxiety and stress are common precipitating factors. Compare **alopecia totalis, alopecia universalis.**

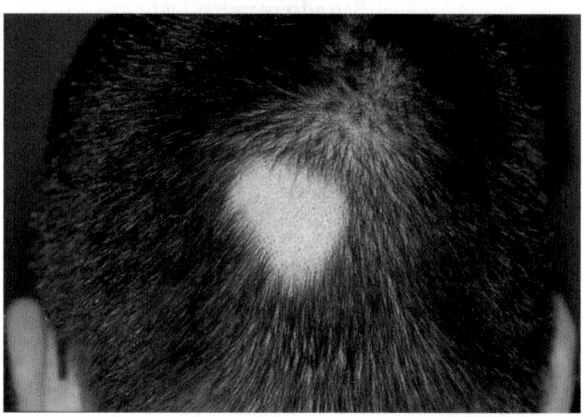

Alopecia areata *(Marks and Miller, 2013)*

alopecia congenitalis, congenital baldness in which there may be partial or complete absence of hair at birth.

alopecia neurotica, a loss of hair, usually occurring at one site, after a disease or an injury involving the nervous system.

alopecia prematura, baldness that occurs early in life, beginning as early as late adolescence.

alopecia senilis, natural hair loss that affects older persons.

alopecia totalis, an uncommon condition characterized by the loss of all hair on the scalp. The cause is unknown, and the baldness is usually permanent. No treatment is known. Compare **alopecia areata, alopecia universalis.**

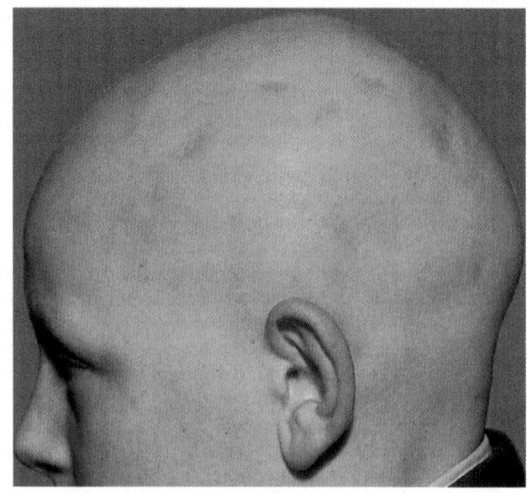

Alopecia totalis *(Bork et al, 1999)*

alopecia toxica, a form of hair loss attributed to a febrile illness.

alopecia universalis, a total loss of hair on all parts of the body. The condition is occasionally an extension of alopecia areata. Compare **alopecia areata, alopecia totalis.**

Aloxi, an antinausea medication. Brand name for **palonosetron.**

alpha /al″fə/, **1.** A, α, the first letter of the Greek alphabet. It is commonly used as a scientific notation, denoting the position of an atom in a molecule, identifying a nuclear particle, or designating a particular physiological rhythm. For example, it is used in chemical nomenclature to distinguish one variation in a chemical compound from others. **2.** referring to something for the first time.

alpha-adrenergic. See **adrenergic receptor.**

alpha-adrenergic blocking agent. See **antiadrenergic.**

alpha-adrenergic receptor. See **alpha receptor.**

alpha alcoholism, a mild form of alcoholism in which the dependence is psychological rather than physical. The person may consume alcohol in excessive amounts to relieve physical pain or psychological distress but is usually able to retain control when the distress subsides and can cease use of alcohol voluntarily.

alpha-aminoisovaleric acid, an essential amino acid needed for optimal growth in infants and for nitrogen equilibrium in adults. Also called **valine.**

alpha$_1$-antitrypsin [Gk, _anti,_ against, _trypsin_], a plasma protein produced in the liver that inhibits the action of proteolytic enzymes such as trypsin. Deficiencies are associated with liver disease in children and panacinar emphysema in adults. In the latter, the basic lesion is believed to result from effects of proteolytic enzymes on the walls of the alveoli. Also called **antitrypsin, alpha$_1$-proteinase inhibitor.**

alpha$_1$-antitrypsin test, a blood test performed on serum or plasma. Alpha$_1$-antitrypsin deficiency is a genetic disorder that may cause lung and liver disease.

alpha biofeedback, a procedure in which a person is presented with continuous information, usually auditory, on the state of his or her brain-wave pattern, with the intent of increasing the percentage of alpha activity; this is done with the expectation that it will be associated with a state of relaxation and peaceful wakefulness.

alpha cell [Gk, _alpha,_ first letter of the Greek alphabet; L, _cella,_ storeroom], one of a class of cells located in the adenohypophysis or in the pancreatic islets. Alpha cells in the pancreas produce glucagon, which raises the level of glucose in the blood.

alpha chain disease, the most prevalent form of heavy chain diseases; a rare family of syndromes associated with or representing a B cell malignancy variant. See also **immunoproliferative small intestine disease.**

alpha error, the probability of rejecting the null hypothesis given that it is true. It is denoted by the Greek letter α (alpha). Also called _alpha level._ Now called **type I error.**

Alpha Eta (ASAHP) /al″ fah a′tah/, the national honor society for allied health professions, founded in 1973.

alpha-fetoprotein (AFP), a protein that is normally synthesized by the liver, yolk sac, and GI tract of a human fetus, but may also be found at an elevated level in the sera of adults having certain malignancies. AFP measurements in amniotic fluid are used for the early diagnosis of fetal neural tube defects, such as spina bifida and anencephaly. Elevated serum levels may be present in ataxia-telangiectasia syndrome, hereditary tyrosinemia, cirrhosis, alcoholic hepatitis, hepatocellular carcinoma, and viral hepatitis. Although not a specific genetic marker for malignancies, AFP may be used to monitor the effectiveness of surgical and chemotherapeutic management of hepatomas and germ cell neoplasms.

alpha-fetoprotein (AFP) test, a blood test used to assist in diagnosing certain neoplastic conditions, such as hepatoma, some tumors and teratomas, Hodgkin disease, lymphoma, and renal cell carcinoma. Increased AFP concentrations also may indicate cirrhosis, active chronic hepatitis, and neural tube defects in the fetus.

alpha-galactosidase, a glycoside hydrolase enzyme that hydrolyzes the terminal alpha-galactosyl moieties (a part or functional group of a molecule) from glycolipids and glycoproteins. It predominantly hydrolyzes ceramide trihexoside, and it can catalyze the hydrolysis of melibiose into galactose and glucose.

alpha-globulins, one of a group of serum proteins classified as alpha, beta, or gamma on the basis of their electrophoretic mobility. Alpha-globulins have the greatest negative charge.

alpha-glucosidase inhibitor, any of a group of oral antihyperglycemic agents that act by competitive inhibition of alpha-glucosidase, delaying intestinal carbohydrate absorption and lessening postprandial increases in glucose levels. See **acarbose.**

alpha hemolysis, the development of a greenish zone around a bacterial colony growing on blood agar, characteristic of pneumococci and certain streptococci and caused by the partial decomposition of hemoglobin. Compare **beta hemolysis.**

alpha-hydroxypropionic acid, a hydroxybutyric acid with the hydroxyl group on the carbon adjacent to the carboxyl. The IUPAC name is 2-hydroxypropanoic acid. See also **lactic acid.**

alpha$_2$-interferon /in′tərfir″on/, a protein molecule effective in controlling the spread of common colds caused by rhinoviruses. It is administered as a nasal spray.

alpha-L-fucosidase, a lysosomal enzyme that catalyzes the hydrolysis of fucosides. A deficiency of this enzyme is a cause of fucosidosis.

alpha-methyldopa. See **methyldopa.**

alphanumeric, (in computer technology) data in the form of letters A to Z and numerals 0 to 9. The characters, which also may include punctuation marks, are used to facilitate the input of information to a computer as the interface between a keyboard and the computer processor.

alpha particle, a positively charged (+2) particle emitted from an atom during one kind of radioactive decay. It consists of two protons and two neutrons, the equivalent of a helium nucleus. Ordinarily, alpha particles are a weak form of radiation with a short range and are not considered hazardous unless inhaled or ingested.

alpha$_1$-proteinase inhibitor. See **alpha$_1$-antitrypsin.**

alpha receptor, any of the postulated adrenergic components of receptor tissues that respond to norepinephrine and to various blocking agents. The activation of alpha receptors causes physiologic responses such as increased peripheral vascular resistance, pupil dilation, and contraction of arrector muscles. Also called **alpha-adrenergic receptor.** Compare **beta receptor.**

alpha redistribution phase, a period after IV administration of a drug when the blood level of the drug begins to fall from its peak. It is caused primarily by redistribution of the drug throughout the body.

alpha rhythm. See **alpha wave.**

alpha state, a condition of relaxed, peaceful wakefulness devoid of concentration and sensory stimulation. It is characterized by alpha waves at a frequency of 8 to 13 Hz as recorded by an electroencephalograph and is accompanied by feelings of tranquility and a lack of tension and anxiety. Biofeedback training and meditation techniques are used to achieve this state.

Alpha Tau Delta /al″fə tou″ del″tə/, a national fraternity of professional nurses founded in 1921.

alpha-thalassemia [Gk, *thalassa,* sea + *haema,* blood], an anemia caused by a decreased rate of synthesis of the alpha chains of hemoglobin. The homozygous form is incompatible with life, the stillborn infant displaying severe hydrops fetalis; the heterozygous form may be asymptomatic or marked by mild anemia.

alpha-tocopherol. See **vitamin E.**

alphavirus /al′favī″rəs/, any of a group of very small Toga viruses consisting of a single molecule of single-stranded ribonucleic acid within a lipoprotein capsule. Many alphaviruses multiply in the cytoplasm of cells of arthropods and are transmitted to humans from mosquitoes, such as those causing equine encephalitis and Semiliki Forest virus. See also **encephalitis, Toga virus.**

alpha wave, one of several types of brain waves, characterized by a relatively high voltage or amplitude and a frequency of 8 to 13 Hz. Alpha waves are the "relaxed waves" of the brain and constitute the majority of waves recorded by electroencephalograms, registering the activity of the parietal and the occipital lobes and the posterior parts of the temporal lobes when the individual is awake but nonattentive and relaxed with the eyes closed. Opening and closing the eyes affect the patterns of the alpha waves and the beta waves. Also called **alpha rhythm, Berger wave.** Compare **beta wave, delta wave, theta wave.**

Alport syndrome [A.C. Alport, South African physician, 1880–1959], a form of hereditary nephritis (autosomal-dominant, autosomal-recessive, and X-linked). The trait is transmitted most often through females, who are often asymptomatic. In males, kidney impairment tends to develop in the third decade; death from renal complications occurs in middle age. Should not be confused with **Apert syndrome.**

■ OBSERVATIONS: The syndrome is associated with symptoms of glomerulonephritis, hematuria, progressive sensorineural hearing loss, and occasionally, vision problems.

■ INTERVENTIONS: Treatment is directed toward the relief of uremia or other kidney disorders. The use of ACE inhibitors may delay renal failure. Kidney transplantation and dialysis are sometimes successful treatments.

■ PATIENT CARE CONSIDERATIONS: The potential loss of renal function, hearing, and sight requires anticipatory guidance from the health care team. Testing for proteinuria should be initiated early. Genetic counseling should be offered to the family of individuals with Alport syndrome. The Alport Syndrome Foundation sponsors meetings and conferences to educate those affected by Alport syndrome.

alprazolam /alpraz″ələm/, a benzodiazepine antianxiety agent.

■ INDICATIONS: It is prescribed in the treatment of anxiety disorders or the short-term relief of the symptoms of anxiety.

■ CONTRAINDICATIONS: Acute narrow-angle glaucoma or known sensitivity to this drug or other benzodiazepines prohibits its use. It is contraindicated with ketoconazole and itraconazole. Pregnancy is also a contraindication.

■ ADVERSE EFFECTS: Among the most serious adverse reactions are drowsiness, light-headedness, and tolerance or physical dependence.

alprostadil, a proprietary form of prostaglandin E1 used to treat impotence and (temporarily) to maintain the patency of the ductus arteriosus in certain neonates.

■ INDICATIONS: It is recommended as palliative therapy for neonates awaiting surgery to correct congenital cardiac anomalies, such as tetralogy of Fallot and tricuspid atresia.

■ CONTRAINDICATIONS: It is contraindicated in respiratory distress syndrome and in cases of known hypersensitivity. This drug is contraindicated in pregnant patients.

■ ADVERSE EFFECTS: The most common adverse effects are apnea, fever, seizures, cerebral bleeding, flushing, bradycardia, and hypertension.

ALS, **1.** abbreviation for **advanced life support. 2.** abbreviation for **amyotrophic lateral sclerosis.**

Alström's syndrome [Carl Henry Alström, Swedish geneticist, 1907–1993], an inherited disease characterized by multiple system resistance to hormones. Clinical features include retinal degeneration leading to childhood blindness, type 2 diabetes mellitus, infantile obesity, nerve deafness, baldness, hyperuricemia, and hypertriglyceridemia. Males may also have high plasma gonadotropin levels and hypogonadism. The condition is transmitted through an autosomal-recessive gene.

ALT, abbreviation for **alanine aminotransferase.**

alteplase, a tissue plasminogen activator.

■ INDICATIONS: This drug is used for lysis of obstructing thrombi associated with acute MI and for other ischemic conditions requiring thrombolysis.

■ CONTRAINDICATIONS: Known hypersensitivity to this drug, active internal bleeding, recent cerebrovascular accident, severe uncontrolled hypertension, intracranial trauma or surgery, intraspinal trauma or surgery, aneurysm, and brain tumor prohibit the use of this drug.

■ ADVERSE EFFECTS: Adverse effects of this drug include urticaria and rash. Surface bleeding is a common side effect. Life-threatening side effects include sinus bradycardia, ventricular tachycardia, accelerated idioventricular rhythm, bradycardia, GI bleeding, genitourinary bleeding, intracranial bleeding, retroperitoneal bleeding, and anaphylaxis.

alteration, change.

altered state of consciousness (ASC) [L, *alter,* other], any state of awareness that differs from the normal awareness of a conscious person. Altered states of consciousness have been achieved, especially in Eastern cultures, by many individuals using various techniques, such as prolonged fasting, deep breathing, whirling, and chanting. Researchers now recognize that such practices can affect body chemistry and help induce the desired state. Experiments suggest that telepathy, mystical experiences, clairvoyance, and other altered states of consciousness may be subconscious capabilities in most individuals and can be used to improve health and help fight disease.

alteregoism /ôl′tərē″gō·iz′əm/, an altruistic feeling for an individual who is similar to or in a similar situation as oneself.

alternate binaural loudness balance (ABLB) test, a comparison of the intensity levels at which a given pure tone sounds equally loud to the normal ear and to the ear with hearing loss. The ABLB test is performed to determine the degree of sound distortion with unilateral sensorineural hearing loss.

alternate generation /ôl″tərnit/ [L, *alter,* other of two], a type of reproduction in which a sexual generation alternates with one or more asexual generations, as in many plants and simple animals. Also called **alternation of generations.**

alternating current (AC) /ôl″tərnā′ting/, an electrical current that reverses directions in a repetitive sinusoidal pattern. The frequency of repetition is 60 Hz. This means the direction of the current changes 60 times every second. Compare **direct current.** See also **current.**

alternating mydriasis, a visual disorder in which there is abnormal dilation of the pupils that affects the left and right eyes alternately. See also **mydriasis.**

alternating pulse, beating at regular intervals, but strength varies between strong and weak, without being consistent. Also called **pulsus alternans.**

alternation, the recurrent, successive occurrence of two functions or phases, such as when a nerve fiber responds to every other stimulus or when a heart produces an irregular beat with every other cardiac cycle.

alternation of generations. See **alternate generation.**

alternation rules, (in psychology) the sociolinguistic rules that establish options available to a person when he or she is speaking to someone else. The rules are influenced by social categories, such as kinship, gender, status, age, and type of interpersonal relationship.

alternative inheritance /ôltur″nətiv/, the acquisition of all genetic traits and conditions from one parent, as in self-pollinating plants and self-fertilizing animals.

alternative medicine, any of the systems of diagnosis and treatment differing in technique from that of the allopathic practitioner's use of medical therapies (alternatives to conventional medicine such as drugs and surgery) to treat disease and injury. Kinds include **acupuncture, aromatherapy, ayurveda, therapeutic touch (TT).** See also **complementary and alternative medicine.**

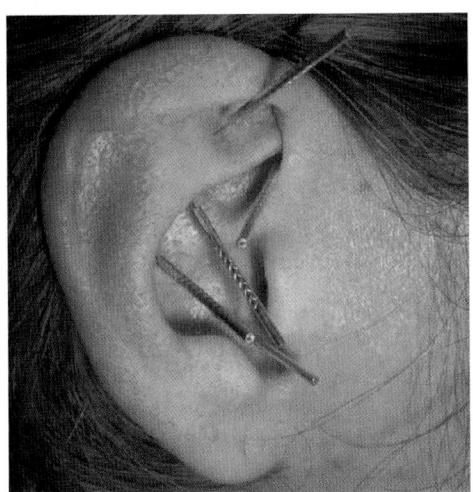

Alternative medicine: acupuncture for acute pain
(Walker et al, 2007)

alternative pathway of complement activation, a process of antigen-antibody interaction in which activation of the C3 step occurs without prior activation of C1, C4, and C2. The initiating substance may be endotoxin, yeast cell wall, bacterial capsule, or immunoglobulin A. See also *properdin system.*

alternator, a device for generating an electric current that changes polarity a specified number of times per second.

alternobaric vertigo, a condition of dysequilibrium caused by unequalized pressure differences in the middle ear, as may be experienced by divers during ascent. The pressure difference exerts its effect on the oval window of the inner ear.

alt hor, *(Obsolete)* (in prescriptions) a shortened Latin phrase meaning "every other hour." Abbreviation for *alternis horis.*

altitude /al″titood/ [L, *altitudo,* height], the level of elevation of any location on earth with reference to a fixed surface point, which is usually sea level. Several types of health effects are associated with altitude extremes, including a greater intensity of ultraviolet radiation that results from a thinner atmosphere. Barometric pressure decreases as altitude increases, so there are fewer molecules of oxygen. Thus breathing becomes faster and deeper, although demands of physical effort and cellular respiration are the same as at a lower altitude. High-altitude cardiac intolerance is usually worse in people with blood or pulmonary disorders. See also **altitude sickness.**

altitude anoxia [L, *altus,* high; Gk, *a,* without, *oxys,* sharp, *genein,* to produce], oxygen deprivation in a high-altitude atmosphere.

altitude sickness, a syndrome associated with the relatively lower amount of oxygen in the atmosphere at altitudes encountered during mountain climbing or travel in unpressurized aircraft or inner ear imbalance. Symptoms of mild altitude illness include headache, difficulty sleeping, loss of appetite, nausea and vomiting, fatigue, dizziness, rapid heart rate, and shortness of breath, especially on exertion. In severe cases, high-altitude pulmonary or cerebral edema may result, requiring emergency treatment and removal to lower altitudes. Also called **acute mountain sickness, bends, Monge disease.**

altretamine, an antineoplastic agent.
■ INDICATIONS: It is used for the palliative treatment of recurrent, persistent ovarian cancer after induction therapy agent.
■ CONTRAINDICATIONS: Known hypersensitivity to this drug, severe bone marrow depression, severe neurological toxicity, and pregnancy prohibit its use.
■ ADVERSE EFFECTS: Among the more serious adverse reactions are hepatic toxicity, leukopenia, thrombocytopenia, and anemia.

altruism /al″troo·iz′əm/, a sense of unconditional concern for the welfare of others. It may be expressed at the level of the individual, the group, or the larger social system. It is one of the curative factors of participating in group therapy. –*altruistic, adj.*

alum /al″əm/ [L, *alumen*], a topical astringent, used primarily in lotions and douches.

alumina /ah-loo′mi-nah/, **1.** a synthetically produced aluminum oxide, Al_2O_3, a white or nearly colorless crystalline substance that is used as a starting material for the smelting of aluminum metal. It also serves as the raw material for a broad range of advanced ceramic products and as an active agent in chemical processing. See **aluminum oxide. 2.** (in pharmaceuticals) aluminum hydroxide.

aluminum (Al) /əloo″minəm/ [L, *alumen,* alum], a widely used metallic element and the third most abundant of all the elements. Its atomic number is 13; its atomic mass is 26.97. Aluminum is commonly obtained by purifying bauxite to produce alumina, which is reduced to aluminum. It is light and durable and used extensively in the manufacture of aircraft components, prostheses, and dental appliances. Its compounds are components of many antacids, antiseptics, and astringents. Aluminum salts, such as aluminum hydroxychloride, can cause allergic reactions in susceptible individuals. Aluminum hydroxychloride is the most commonly used agent in antiperspirants and is also effective as a deodorant.

aluminum acetate solution. See **Burow's solution.**

aluminum attenuator, an aluminum filter used to control the hardness of an x-ray beam. The attenuator is inherent and/or added to the x-ray machine to remove low-energy x-ray photons from the primary beam. See **total filtration.**

aluminum hydroxide [L, *alumen,* alum; Gk, *hydor,* water, *oxys,* sharp], an antacid that works by chemical neutralization of hydrochloric acid in the stomach.

aluminum oxide, (Al_2O_3), a compound occurring naturally as various minerals. It is used in the production of abrasives, refractories, ceramics, and catalysts and in chromatography. It is also used to strengthen dental ceramics.

Alupent, a beta-adrenergic bronchodilator. Brand name for **metaproterenol sulfate.**

Alu sequences, a family of repeated DNA sequences found in large numbers in the human genome.

alve-, alveolo-, a prefix meaning "trough, channel, cavity": *alveolectomy, alveolus.*

alveobronchitis [L, *alveolus,* little hollow; Gk, *brongchos,* windpipe, *itis,* inflammation], an inflammation of the alveoli and bronchioles. Also called *alveobronchiolitis.* See also **bronchopneumonia.**

alveolar /alvē″ələr/ [L, *alveolus,* little hollow], pertaining to an alveolus.

alveolar air, the respiratory gases in an alveolus of the lung. Alveolar air can be analyzed for its content of oxygen, carbon dioxide, or other gases by collecting the last portion of air expelled by maximum exhalation. Also called **alveolar gas.**

alveolar air equation, a mathematical expression relating the approximate alveolar oxygen tension to the arterial partial pressure of carbon dioxide ($PaCO_2$), the fraction of inspired oxygen, and the ratio of carbon dioxide production to oxygen consumption.

alveolar arch, the arch of the upper or lower jaw from which the teeth project, formed by the alveolar processes.

alveolar-arterial end-capillary gas pressure difference, the gas pressure difference between the partial pressure of a gas, such as CO_2, in alveolar air and that in pulmonary capillary blood as the blood leaves the alveoli. It is measured in torr or millimeters of mercury (mm Hg).

alveolar-arterial gas pressure difference, the difference between the partial pressure of a gas, such as CO_2, in the alveoli and that in systemic arterial blood. The difference may indicate ventilation-perfusion mismatching. A negative difference indicates that the partial pressure of the gas is higher in systemic arterial blood than it is in alveolar air. It is measured in torr or millimeters of mercury (mm Hg).

alveolar artery, one of two arteries, the posterior and the anterior, that supply the maxillary (upper) teeth. There is also an inferior alveolar artery, which enters posteriorly and progresses into the mandible.

alveolar canal, any of the canals of the maxilla through which blood vessels and the nerves to the maxillary upper teeth pass. Also called *dental canal.*

alveolar-capillary membrane, a lung tissue structure, varying in thickness from 0.4 to 2 μm, through which diffusion of oxygen and carbon dioxide molecules occurs during respiration. It consists of an alveolar cell separated from a capillary cell by an interstitium and is essentially a fluid barrier.

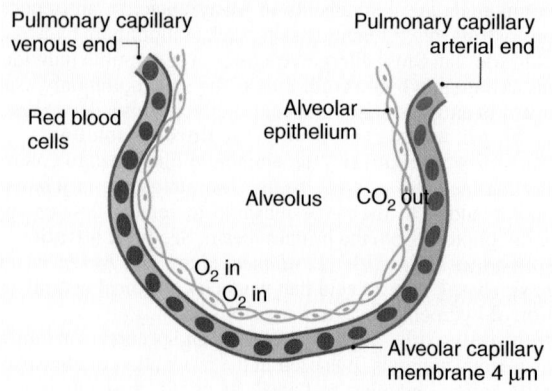

Alveolar-capillary membrane *(Qureshi, 2008)*

alveolar carcinoma. See **bronchioloalveolar carcinoma.**

alveolar cell carcinoma. See **bronchioloalveolar carcinoma.**

alveolar cleft, a break or gap in the continuity of the alveolar process, usually congenital. It typically occurs with a cleft lip and/or a cleft palate.

alveolar crestal fiber, any of the many white collagenous fibers of the periodontal ligament that extend diagonally from the cervical cementum to the alveolar crest. Alveolar fibers surround the tooth and assist in resisting horizontal tooth movements.

alveolar cyst, an air-filled cavity in a lung or in visceral tissues caused by rupture of an alveolus.

alveolar dead space. See **dead space.**

alveolar distending pressure, the pressure difference between the alveoli and the intrapleural space.

alveolar duct, any of the air passages in the lung that branch out from the bronchioles. The alveolar sacs arise from the alveolar ducts.

alveolar edema, an accumulation of fluid within the alveoli. The cause is usually the movement of blood components through the pulmonary capillary walls as a result of a change in osmotic pressure, an increased permeability of the walls, or related factors.

alveolar fistula. See **dental fistula.**

alveolar gas. See **alveolar air.**

alveolar gas volume (VA), the aggregate volume of gas in the alveoli of the lungs.

alveolar macrophage, a cell of the reticuloendothelial system in the lungs that engulfs and digests foreign substances inhaled into the alveoli.

alveolar microlithiasis, a rare disease characterized by the presence of calcium phosphate deposits in the alveoli and other parts of the bronchopulmonary system. The disease is familial in about half of cases.

■ OBSERVATIONS: Most individuals are asymptomatic for years. The diagnosis is detected at a late stage, when restrictive lung disease, hypoxia, and pulmonary hypertension are present. Fine, sandlike deposits may cause the entire lung to appear radiopaque on a radiograph. Serum levels of surfactant proteins A and D are also elevated.

■ INTERVENTIONS: Disodium etidronate has a benefical effect in some patients in regard to tissue calcification. Lung transplantation may be employed in the late stage of the disease.

■ PATIENT CARE CONSIDERATIONS: Other family members should be screened for the disease. The patient should be monitored carefully as calcium deposits may be found in other organs.

alveolar period, the period or phase in lung development beginning in utero after the terminal saccular period (about 32 to 36 weeks) and lasting until about 8 years of age. The terminal alveolar saccules subdivide several more times and mature alveoli form. Also called *alveolar phase.*

alveolar periosteum [L, *alveolus,* little hollow; Gk, *peri,* near, *osteon,* bone], a dense layer of connective tissue that lines the alveolar cavities of the upper and lower jaws, joining the bones to the horizontal fibers on the cementum of the teeth. See also **periosteum.**

alveolar pressure (PA), the pressure in the alveoli of the lungs.

alveolar process, the portion of the maxilla or the mandible that forms the dental arch and serves as a bony investment for the teeth. Its cortical covering is continuous with the compact bone of the body of the maxilla or the mandible and with the cancellous bone of the body of the jaws. Also called *alveolar bone.* See also **alveolar ridge.**

alveolar proteinosis, a very rare disease marked by the accumulation of plasma proteins, lipoproteins, and other blood components in the alveoli of the lungs, impairing the ability of the lungs to exchange oxygen and carbon dioxide. The disease tends to affect previously healthy young adults, with a higher incidence among males than females. The cause is unknown.

■ OBSERVATIONS: Clinical signs vary, although only the lungs are affected. Some patients are asymptomatic, whereas others experience dyspnea and an unproductive cough.

■ INTERVENTIONS: The condition may be treated with bronchopulmonary lavage. Correction of granulocyte-macrophage colony–stimulating factor (GM-CSF) deficiency with exogenous GM-CSF is an alternative therapy.

■ PATIENT CARE CONSIDERATIONS: The care of patients with minimal symptoms is conservatively managed. Patients with hypoxemia require a more aggressive approach. There is a risk of secondary infections.

alveolar ridge, the bony elevation of the maxilla or the mandible that contains the alveolar sockets (tooth sockets) of the teeth. See also **alveolar process.**

alveolar sac [L, *alveolus,* little hollow; Gk, *sakkos*], an air sac at one of the terminal cavities of lung tissue containing alveoli.

alveolar septum. Also called **interalveolar septum.**

alveolar sinus. See **dental fistula.**

alveolar socket [L, *alveolus,* little hollow; OFr, *soket*], the space in the alveolar process of the maxilla and mandible that accommodates a tooth.

alveolar soft part sarcoma, a tumor in subcutaneous or fibromuscular tissue, consisting of numerous large round or polygonal cells in a netlike matrix of connective tissue.

alveolar ventilation, the volume of air that ventilates all the perfused alveoli, equal to total ventilation minus dead space ventilation. The normal average is between 4 and 5 L/min.

alveolectomy /al′vē·ə·lek″tə·mē/ [L, *alveolus,* little hollow; Gk, *ektomē,* excision], the excision of a portion of the alveolar process performed to aid in the extraction of a tooth or teeth, modify the alveolar contour after tooth extraction, or prepare the mouth for dentures.

alveoli /al·vē′ō·lī/, pl. of alveolus. See **alveolus.**

alveolitis /al′vē·əlī″tis/, an inflammation of the alveoli of the lungs caused by the inhalation of an allergen. It is characterized by acute episodes of dyspnea, cough, diaphoresis, fever, weakness, and pain in the joints and muscles lasting from 12 to 18 hours. Recurrent episodes may lead to chronic obstructive pulmonary disease with weight loss, increasing exertional dyspnea, and interstitial fibrosis. X-ray images of the lungs may show cellular thickening of alveolar septa and ill-defined generalized infiltrates. Kinds include **bagassosis, farmer's lung, pigeon breeder's lung.**

alveoloplasty /alvē′əlōplas′tē/, surgical reconstruction and smoothing of the alveolar process or dental ridge. Also called **alveoplasty.**

alveoplasty. See **alveoloplasty.**

alveolotomy /al′vē·əlot′əmē/, an incision of a dental alveolus performed to drain pus from a dental infection.

alveolus /alvē′ələs/ *pl. alveoli* [L, *alveolus,* little hollow], **1.** a small outpouching along the walls of the alveolar sacs through which gas exchange between alveolar air and pulmonary capillary blood occurs. Also called **acinus, pulmonary alveolus. 2.** a tooth socket. See also **dental alveolus. –alveolar,** *adj.*

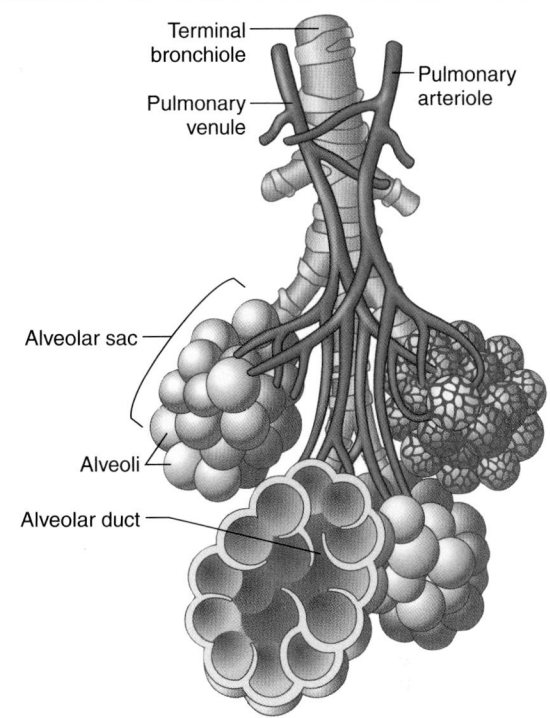

Alveoli *(Patton and Thibodeau, 2016)*

alymphocytosis /alim′fōsītō″sis/ [Gk, *a,* not; L, *lympha,* water; Gk, *kytos,* cell, *osis,* condition], absence of lymphocytes from the blood. Compare **lymphocytopenia.**

Alzheimer disease (AD) /ôl″zīmərz/ [Alois Alzheimer, German neurologist, 1864–1915], a condition characterized by progressive mental deterioration, often with confusion, memory failure, disorientation, restlessness, agnosia, speech disturbances, inability to carry out purposeful movement, and hallucinosis. There are three phases of disease progression over time: (1) preclinical Alzheimer characterized by changes that indicate the very earliest signs of disease; (2) mild cognitive impairment (MCI) or mild changes in memory and thinking abilities, enough to be noticed and measured, but not impairment that compromises everyday activities; (3) dementia due to Alzheimer disease. The patient may become hypomanic, refuse food, and lose sphincter control without focal impairment. The disease sometimes begins in middle life with slight defects in behavior and memory, usually an inability to incorporate new knowledge with old knowledge, but the symptoms can worsen dramatically with age. When the symptoms are severe, patients are unable to perform activities of daily living or orient to surroundings and do not recognize loved ones. Typical pathological features are miliary amyloid plaques in the cortex and fibrillary degeneration (tangles) in layers containing pyramidal ganglion cells. The cerebral cortex atrophies with widening of the cerebral sulci, especially in the frontal and temporal regions. Diagnostic criteria consist of a failure in at least three cognitive functions, including memory, use of language, visuospatial skills, personality, and calculating skills. Measurement of biomarkers in blood and cerebrospinal fluid, as well as neuroimaging tests to characterize brain changes, are assessments recommended by the Alzheimer's Association. Treatment may involve medications that are thought to decrease the rate of decline. Also called **senile dementia–Alzheimer type.**

■ PATIENT CARE CONSIDERATIONS: Care is initially concerned primarily with promoting activity and sleep and preventing agitation, violence, and injury. Death usually occurs 8 to 12 years after the first symptoms appear. Late-stage care is focused on palliative measures.

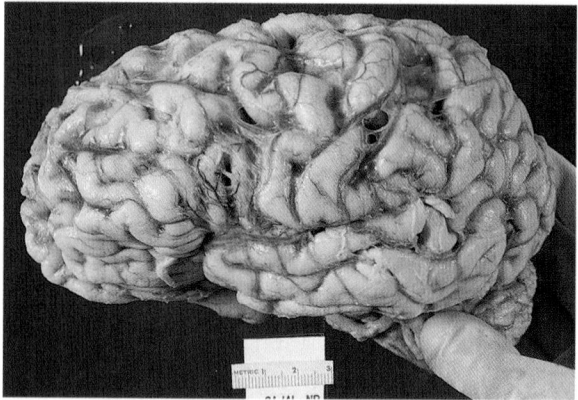

Brain in Alzheimer disease *(Finkbeiner, Ursell, and Davis, 2009)*

Alzheimer sclerosis [Alois Alzheimer; Gk, *sklerosis*, hardening], the degeneration of small cerebral blood vessels, resulting in mental changes.

Am, symbol for the element **americium.**

AMA, **1.** abbreviation for **American Medical Association. 2.** abbreviation for **antimitochondrial antibody. 3.** abbreviation for **active matrix array. 4.** abbreviation for **antimyocardial antibody (AMA) test. 5.** abbreviation for **against medical advice.**

amalgam /əmal″gəm/ [Gk, *malagma*, soft mass], **1.** a mixture or combination. **2.** an alloy of mercury, silver, and other metals commonly used in dentistry. **3.** See **dental amalgam.**

amalgam carrier, a dental instrument used to pick up a quantity of amalgam and transfer it into a prepared tooth cavity or a mold.

amalgam carver, a dental instrument for anatomically shaping dental amalgam while in a pliable state to restore natural contours, used in certain tooth cavity fillings or restorations.

amalgam condenser, a dental instrument used for compacting dental amalgam while in a pliable state, used for restoring teeth to a natural contour.

amalgam core, a rigid base or structure of dental amalgam that restores supragingival tooth structure and that is used for retaining a cast crown or bridge restoration. The core may be held in place by undercuts, slots, pins, or the pulp chamber of an endodontically treated tooth. Compare **cast core, composite core.** See also **core.**

amalgam tattoo, a discoloration of the gingiva or buccal membrane caused by particles of dental amalgam that migrate from an amalgam filling and become embedded within the tissue surface. The condition causes no symptoms and is usually left untreated.

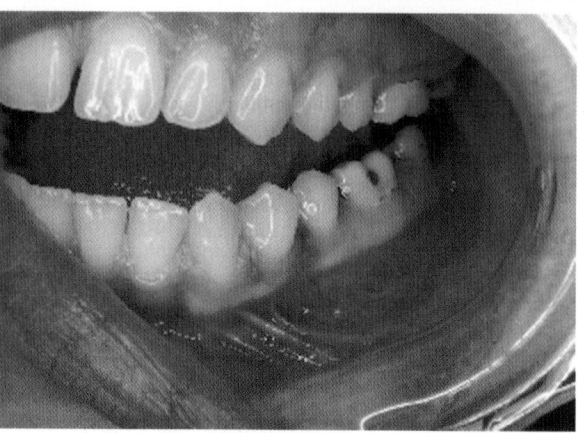

Amalgam tattoo *(Ibsen, 2014)*

Amanita [Gk, *amanitai*, fungus], a genus of mushrooms. Some species, such as *Amanita phalloides*, are poisonous, causing hallucinations, GI upset, and pain that may be followed by liver, kidney, and central nervous system damage. Also called *death cap*.

amantadine hydrochloride /əman″tədēn/, an antiviral and antiparkinsonian agent.

■ INDICATIONS: It is prescribed in the prophylaxis and early treatment of influenza virus A and in the treatment of parkinsonian symptoms and drug-induced extrapyramidal reactions.

■ CONTRAINDICATIONS: It is used with caution in patients with congestive heart failure and in women who are pregnant and lactating. Known hypersensitivity to this drug prohibits its use.

■ ADVERSE EFFECTS: Among the most serious adverse reactions are central nervous system effects and livedo reticularis. Nausea, dizziness, insomnia, nervousness, blurred vision, and slurred speech also may occur.

amastia /əmas″tē·ə/ [Gk, *a, mastos*, not breast], the absence of the breasts in women caused by a congenital defect, an endocrine disorder resulting in faulty development, a lack of development of secondary sex characteristics, or a bilateral mastectomy. Also called **amazia.**

amaurosis /am′ôrō″sis/ [Gk, *amauroein*, to darken], blindness, especially lack of vision resulting from a systemic cause such as disease of the optic nerve or brain, diabetes, renal disease, acute gastritis, or systemic poisoning produced by excessive use of alcohol or tobacco, rather than from damage to the eye itself. Unilateral or, more rarely, bilateral amaurosis may follow an emotional shock and may continue for days or months. One kind of congenital amaurosis is transmitted as an autosomal-recessive trait. –**amaurotic,** *adj.*

amaurosis fugax /foo″gaks/, a transient episodic blindness caused by decreased blood flow to the retina. Compare **amaurosis.**

amaurosis partialis fugax, a transitory partial blindness, usually caused by vascular insufficiency of the retina or the optic nerve as a result of carotid artery disease. Other related symptoms include dizziness, nausea, and vomiting.

amaurotic. See **amaurosis.**

amazia. See **amastia.**

amb-. See **ambi-, ambo-, amb-.**

amber [Ar, *anbar*], a hard fossilized resin derived from pine trees. An oil of amber, *Oleum succini,* has been used in some pharmaceutical preparations.

amber mutation [Ar, *anbar,* ambergris], a genetic alteration that causes the synthesis of a polypeptide chain to terminate prematurely because the triplet of nucleotides that normally codes for the next amino acid in the chain becomes uracil-adenine-guanine, the sequence that signals the end of the chain. See also **ochre mutation, opal mutation.**

ambi-, ambo-, amb-, prefixes meaning "on both sides" or "both": *ambidextrous, ambomalleal.*

ambidextrous /am′bēdek″strəs/ [L, *ambo,* both, *dexter,* right], able to use either the left or right hand to perform a task and write.

ambient /am′bē·ənt/ [L, *ambire,* on both sides], pertaining to the surrounding area or atmosphere, usually a defined area such as a room or another large enclosed space.

ambient air standard, the maximum tolerable concentration of any outdoor air pollutant as set by the Environmental Protection Agency (EPA) to protect public health and the environment. The EPA considers lead, the nitrogen oxides, particulate matter, sulfur dioxide, carbon monoxide, and ozone "criteria" pollutants. Research and medical evidence show a strong correlation between many diseases and toxic chemicals, but little is known about the precise effects and movement of airborne pollutants.

ambient noise [L, *ambiens,* around; ME, clamor], audible sounds in the environment.

ambient pressure, the atmospheric pressure, or pressure in the environment or surrounding area. It is given a reference value of zero (0) cm H_2O.

ambient temperature [L, *ambi,* around, *temperatura*], the amount of heat in the environment.

ambiguous /ambig″yoo·əs/ [L, *ambiguus,* to wander], having more than one direction, development, or interpretation or meaning.

ambiguous genitalia [L, *ambigere,* to go around], an atypical anatomy of the externally visible sex organs, making it difficult to determine the genetic sex.

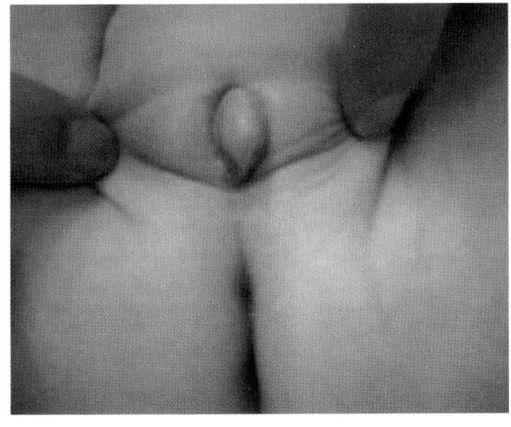

Ambiguous genitalia *(Murphy, Allen, and Jamieson, 2011)*

ambilateral, pertaining to or affecting both the right and the left side.

ambiopia. See **diplopia.**

ambivalence /ambiv″ələns/ [L, *ambo,* both, *valentia,* strength], **1.** a state in which a person concomitantly experiences conflicting feelings, attitudes, drives, desires, or emotions, such as love and hate, tenderness and cruelty, pleasure and pain toward the same person, place, object, or situation. In some situations, ambivalence is normal. Treatment in severe, debilitating cases consists of psychotherapy appropriate to the underlying cause. **2.** uncertainty and fluctuation caused by an inability to make a choice between opposites. **3.** a continuous oscillation or fluctuation. –*ambivalent, adj.*

ambivert /am″bivurt′/ [L, *ambo,* both, *vertere,* to turn], a person who possesses characteristics of both introversion and extroversion.

amblyopia /am′blē·ō″pē·ə/ [Gk, *amblys,* dull, *ops,* eye], impairment of vision not due to refractive errors, usually without an organic cause. Corrective lenses do not improve visual acuity. See also **toxic amblyopia.**

amblyopia cruciata. See **crossed amblyopia.**

ambo-. See **ambi-, ambo-, amb-.**

ambrisentan, an antihypertensive.
■ INDICATIONS: This drug is used to treat pulmonary arterial hypertension alone or in combination with other antihypertensives.
■ CONTRAINDICATIONS: Pregnancy, breastfeeding, and known hypersensitivity to this drug prohibits its use.
■ ADVERSE EFFECTS: Adverse effects of this drug include headache, fever, flushing, orthostatic hypotension, hypotension, peripheral edema, sinusitis, rhinitis, abdominal pain, constipation, anemia, rash, pharyngitis, and dyspnea.

Ambu bag, a brand name for a resuscitator bag used to assist ventilation. See also **bag-valve-mask resuscitator.**

ambulance /am″byələns/, a vehicle designed to transport ill or injured patients. It may be used under emergency or nonemergency conditions and is equipped with supplies and personnel to provide patient care en route.

ambulatory /am″byələtôr′ē/ [L, *ambulare,* to walk about], **1.** able to walk. The ability to get up and move about using the legs and feet for motion. **2.** pertaining to a patient who is not confined to bed. **3.** pertaining to a health service for people who are not hospitalized.

ambulatory anesthesia, the administration of anesthesia when the intent is to admit and discharge the patient on the day of the surgical procedure (same-day surgery). Also called **outpatient anesthesia.**

ambulatory automatism, aimless wandering or moving about or performance of mechanical acts without conscious awareness of the behavior. See also **fugue, poriomania.**

ambulatory blood pressure monitoring (ABPM), the recording of a patient's blood pressure at regular intervals under normal living and working conditions.

ambulatory care, health services provided on an outpatient basis to those who visit a hospital or another health care facility and depart after treatment on the same day.

ambulatory electrocardiograph. See **Holter monitor.**

ambulatory schizophrenia, *(Obsolete)* a mild form of psychosis, characterized mainly by a tendency to respond to questions with vague and irrelevant answers. The person also may seem somewhat eccentric and wander aimlessly.

ambulatory splint. *(Informal)* See **functional splint.**

ambulatory surgery center (ACS), a medical facility designed and equipped to handle surgery, pain management, and certain diagnostic procedures that do not require overnight hospitalization. Most patients who are in relatively good

A

health may receive treatment at ambulatory surgery centers. The centers may be associated with a general hospital or a specialty hospital or may function as independent medical facilities with prearranged emergency support. The centers are staffed with health professionals, as in conventional surgery departments. Also called *ambulatory surgical center.*

Ambu simulator, a brand name for a manikin used to teach cardiopulmonary resuscitation.

AM care /ā·em″/, routine hygienic care that is given before breakfast or early in the morning.

amcinonide /amsin″ōnīd/, a topical corticosteroid.
- INDICATIONS: It is used to treat inflammatory skin conditions.
- CONTRAINDICATIONS: Impaired circulation and known hypersensitivity to steroids prohibit its use.
- ADVERSE EFFECTS: Among the most common adverse reactions are itching, stinging, burning, and less frequently, various skin eruptions. Systemic side effects may result from prolonged or excessive application.

amdinocillin pivoxil, an ester of amdinocillin, administered orally in the treatment of urinary tract infections.

ameba /əmē″bə/ *pl.* *amebae, amebas* [Gk, *amoibe,* change], a microscopic single-celled parasitic organism. Several species may be parasitic in humans, including *Entamoeba histolytica* and *E. coli,* a nonpathogenic species of *Entamoeba* often confused with *E. histolytica.* Also spelled **amoeba.**

-ameba, -amoeba, suffixes meaning a "(specified) protozoan": *caudameba, Entamoeba.*

amebiasis /am′ēbī″əsis/, an infection of the intestine or liver by pathogenic amebae, particularly *Entamoeba histolytica,* acquired by ingesting fecally contaminated food or water. Infected carriers can be asymptomatic (luminal ambiasis); they may develop invasive intestinal disease with dysentery, colitis, or appendicitis or invasive extraintestinal disease with peritonitis and liver or lung abscess. Infection is most serious in infants, the elderly, and debilitated people. Amebiasis may require treatment with luminal amebicides (iodoquinol, paromomycin) to eradicate cysts and/or systemic treatment with metronidazole. Also spelled **amoebiasis.** See also **amebic abscess, amebic dysentery, hepatic amebiasis.**

amebic. See **ameba.**

amebic abscess /əmē″bik/, a collection of pus formed by disintegrated tissue in a cavity, usually in the liver, caused by *Entamoeba histolytica.* Cysts of the organism, ingested in fecally contaminated food or water, pass into the intestine, where active trophozoites are released. The trophozoites enter the intestinal mucosa, causing ulceration, nausea, vomiting, abdominal pain, and severe diarrhea, and they may invade the liver and produce an abscess. Oral metronidazole and oral or intramuscular chloroquine hydrochloride are used to treat hepatic amebic abscesses. See also **amebiasis.**

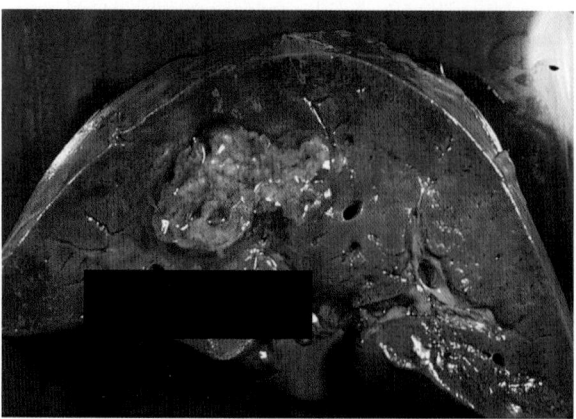

Amebic abscess *(Damjanov, 2006)*

amebic carrier state, a condition in which a patient may be a carrier of amebae without showing signs or symptoms of an amebic infection. A precocious carrier may appear healthy but may subsequently develop the amebic infection.

amebic dysentery, an inflammation of the intestine caused by infestation with *Entamoeba histolytica.* It is characterized by frequent, loose stools flecked with blood and mucus. Intestinal amebiasis may be accompanied by symptoms of liver involvement. Also called **intestinal amebiasis.** See also **amebiasis, hepatic amebiasis.**

amebic hepatitis, an inflammation of the liver caused by an infection with any of the various amebae, usually after an attack of amebic dysentery.

amebicide /əmē″bəsīd/, a drug or another agent that is destructive to amebae.

amebic liver abscess, the abscess formed in hepatic amebiasis, resulting from liquefaction necrosis caused by entrance of *Entamoeba histolytica* into the portal circulation.

ameboid movement /əmē″boid/ [Gk, *amoibe,* ameba, *eidos,* form; L, *movere,* to move], the ameba-like movement of certain types of body cells that can migrate through tissues, such as leukocytes. The movement generally consists of extension of a portion of the plasma membrane, probably caused by internal rearrangement or movement of the cytoskeleton. See also **diapedesis.**

amelanotic /am′ilənot″ik/ [Gk, *a, melas,* not black], pertaining to tissue that is unpigmented because it lacks melanin.

amelanotic melanoma, a melanoma that lacks melanin. See also **melanoma.**

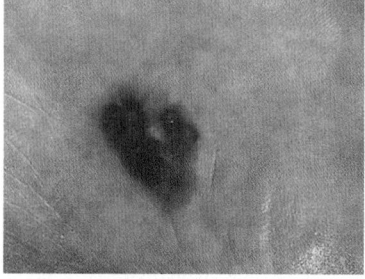

Amelanotic malignant melanoma *(du Vivier, 1993)*

amelia /əmē″lyə/ [Gk, *a, melos,* not limb], a congenital anomaly marked by the absence of one or more limbs. The term may be modified to indicate the number of legs or arms missing at birth, such as tetramelia for the absence of all four limbs.

amelification /əmel′ifikā″shən/ [OFr, *amel,* enamel; L, *facere,* to make], the differentiation of ameloblasts into the enamel of the teeth.

amelioration [L, *ad,* to, *melior,* better], an improvement in conditions.

ameloblast /am″ilōblast′/ [OFr, *amel* + Gk, *blastos,* germ], a specific epithelial cell from which tooth enamel is produced and deposited. Also called **enamel cell.** *−ameloblastic, adj.*

ameloblastic fibroma, a nonencapsulated odontogenic tumor composed of strands and small islands of mesenchymal and ameloblast-like epithelial cells that resembles the dental papilla without any formation of dentin or enamel.

ameloblastic fibro-odontoma, a tumor of the jaw that forms dentin and enamel. See also **composite odontoma.**

ameloblastic hemangioma, a highly vascular tumor of cells covering the dental papillae. See also **hemangioma.**

ameloblastic sarcoma, a malignant odontogenic tumor characterized by the proliferation of epithelial tissue and malignant mesenchymal tissue.

ameloblastoma /amˈəlōblastōˈˈmə/ [OFr, *amel* + Gk, *blastos,* germ, *oma*], a rare, highly destructive, benign, rapidly growing tumor of the jaw. Also called *adamantinoma, adamantoblastoma,* **epithelioma adamantinum.**

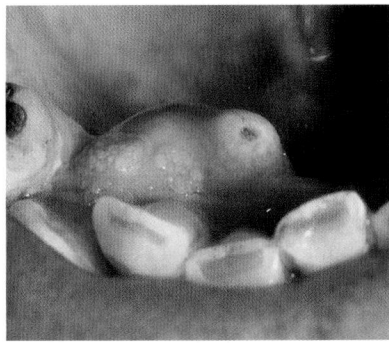

Ameloblastoma *(Regezi, Sciubba, and Jordan, 2008)*

amelodentinal /amˈəlōdenˈˈtinəl/[OFr, *amel* + L, *dens,* tooth], pertaining to both the enamel and the dentin of the teeth.

amelogenesis /amˈəlōjenˈˈəsis/ [OFr, *amel* + Gk, *genein,* to produce], the formation of the enamel of the teeth. −*amelogenic, adj.*

amelogenesis imperfecta, a condition characterized by brown or white chalky discoloration of the teeth and resulting from either severe enamel hypocalcification or enamel hypoplasia. The condition can be inherited as an autosomal-dominant, autosomal recessive, X-linked dominant, or X-linked recessive trait. With at least 14 different hereditary subtypes, the condition has numerous patterns of inheritance and a wide variety of clinical manifestations. The condition is classified according to severity: in agenesis, there is a complete lack of enamel; in enamel hypoplasia, defective matrix formation causes the enamel to be normal in hardness but deficient in quantity; and in enamel hypocalcification, defective maturation of ameloblasts results in enamel that is normal in quantity but soft and undercalcified. An ideal classification system for amelogenesis imperfecta has not been established yet. Also called **hereditary brown enamel, hereditary enamel hypoplasia.** Compare **dentinogenesis imperfecta.**

amenorrhea /āˈmenərēˈˈə/ [Gk, *a, men,* not month, *rhoia,* to flow], the absence of menstruation. Amenorrhea is normal before sexual maturity, during pregnancy, after menopause, and during the intermenstrual phase of the monthly hormonal cycle; it is otherwise caused by dysfunction of the hypothalamus, pituitary gland, ovary, or uterus; by the congenital absence or surgical removal of both ovaries or the uterus; or by medication. It may also occur in women who are underweight or who exercise extensively. Primary amenorrhea is the failure of menstrual cycles to begin. Secondary amenorrhea is the cessation of menstrual cycles once established. Also spelled *amenorrhoea.* See also **dietary amenorrhea, hypothalamic amenorrhea, postpill amenorrhea.** −*amenorrheic, adj.*

amentia /āmenˈˈshə/ [Gk, *a,* not; L, *mens,* mind], **1.** impaired development of intellectual capacity as a result of inadequate brain tissue. See **intellectual disability. 2.** a congenital mental deficiency.

American Academy of Allergy, Asthma, and Immunology (AAAAI), a professional organization with members in the United States, Canada, and 72 other countries. This membership includes allergists/immunologists, other medical specialists, and health care professionals who have a special interest in the research and treatment of allergic and immunologic diseases.

American Academy of Audiology, a professional association for audiologists, dedicated to providing quality hearing care services through professional development, education, research, and increased public awareness of hearing and balance disorders.

American Academy of Nursing (AAN), the honorary organization of the American Nurses Association, created to recognize superior achievement in nursing in order to promote advances and excellence in nursing practice, education, and research. A person elected to membership is given the title of Fellow of the American Academy of Nursing and may use the abbreviation FAAN as an honorific.

American Academy of Physical Medicine and Rehabilitation (AAPMR), a medical society for the specialty of physical medicine and rehabilitation concerned with advancing the specialty, promoting excellence in physiatric practice, and advocating on public policy issues related to persons with disabling conditions.

American Academy of Physician Assistants (AAPA), a national professional organization of physician assistants committed to transforming health through patient-centered, team-based medical practice.

American Association for Respiratory Care (AARC), an association for credentialed practitioners involved in the respiratory care profession or for student members enrolled in an educational program recognized or accredited by the AARC.

American Association of Colleges of Nursing (AACN), a national organization of baccalaureate and higher degree programs in nursing that was established to address issues in nursing education. AACN works to establish quality standards for nursing education; assists schools in implementing those standards; influences the nursing profession to improve health care; and promotes public support for professional nursing education, research, and practice.

American Association of Critical Care Nurses (AACN), a nursing specialty organization representing the interests of nurses with the responsibility of caring for acutely and critically ill patients.

American Association of Medical Colleges (AAMC), a national organization of faculty members and deans of medical schools and colleges that was established to monitor, develop, and administer rules, regulations, and standards for medical colleges.

American Association of Neuroscience Nurses (AANN), a national organization of nurses with the mission of advancement of neuroscience nursing as a specialty through the development and support of nurses to promote excellence in patient care.

American Association of Nurse Anesthetists (AANA), a professional association of certified registered nurse anesthetists and student registered nurse anesthetists. It promulgates education and practice standards and guidelines and affords consultation to both private and governmental entities regarding nurse anesthetists and their practice.

American Association of Occupational Health Nurses, a professional association dedicated to advancing the health, safety, and productivity of domestic and global workforces by providing education, research, public policy, and practice resources for occupational and environmental health nurses.

American Association of Retired Persons. See **AARP.**

American Association of University Professors (AAUP), a national organization of faculty members of institutions of higher learning. The AAUP represents faculty in matters of academic freedom, appointment policies, and procedures and serves as the bargaining agent for the faculties of some universities.

A

American College of Emergency Physicians (ACEP), a professional organization of physicians focused on support of quality emergency care and the physicians who provide such care.

American College of Obstetricians and Gynecologists (ACOG), a national organization for obstetricians and gynecologists.

American College of Occupational and Environmental Medicine (ACOEM), a professional organization whose members are concerned with the identification, prevention, diagnosis, and treatment of disorders associated with technology and industry.

American College of Physicians (ACP), a national professional organization for internal medicine specialists focused on scientific knowledge across the spectrum from health to complex illness.

American College of Prosthodontists (ACP), an organization of dentists who specialize in the diagnosis, treatment planning, rehabilitation, and maintenance of the oral function, comfort, appearance, and health of patients with clinical conditions associated with missing or deficient teeth or oral and maxillofacial tissues using biocompatible substitutes.

American College of Radiology (ACR), a national professional organization whose stated mission is to serve patients and society by empowering members to advance the practice, science, and professions of radiological care.

American College of Surgeons (ACS), a national professional organization of physicians who specialize in surgery. See also **Accreditation Review Committee on Education in Surgical Technology.**

American Dental Hygienists' Association (ADHA), an organization of dental hygienists committed to improving oral health; promoting dental hygiene education, licensure, practice, and research; and representing the legislative interests of dental hygienists.

American Hospital Association (AHA), a national organization that represents and serves individuals, institutions, and organizations that work to improve health services for all people. The AHA publishes several journals and newsletters.

American Joint Committee on Cancer (AJCC), a nonprofit organization that creates and publishes systems of classification for cancer staging, such as the TNM staging system and Collaborative Stage Data collection systems.

American Journal of Nursing, a professional journal containing articles of general and specialized clinical interest to nurses. It is the oldest nursing journal in the world.

American leishmaniasis, a group of infections caused by various species of the parasitic protozoa *Leishmania* of Central and South America characterized by cutaneous lesions at the site of the sandfly bite and transmitting infection and causing disfiguring ulcerative lesions of the nose, mouth, and throat or visceral disease. Illness may be prolonged, rendering patients susceptible to serious secondary infections. Also called **mucocutaneous leishmaniasis, New World leishmaniasis.** Kinds include **chiclero ulcer, espundia, forest yaws, uta.** See also **leishmaniasis.**

American Medical Association (AMA), a professional association whose membership is made up of the largest group of physicians and medical students in the United States, including practitioners in all recognized medical specialties, as well as general primary care physicians. The AMA is governed by a board of trustees and house of delegates who represent various state and local medical associations and U.S. government agencies such as the Public Health Service and medical departments of the army, navy, and air force. The AMA maintains directories of all U.S. licensed physicians (including nonmembers) in the United

States, including graduates of foreign medical colleges; researches prescription and nonprescription drugs; advises congressional and state legislators regarding proposed health care laws; and publishes a variety of journals that report on scientific and socioeconomic developments in the field of medicine. See also **British Medical Association, Canadian Medical Association Journal.**

American Medical Technologists (AMT), a nationally and internationally recognized certification agency and membership society for multiple allied health professionals, including laboratory, medical and dental office, and health education personnel. AMT is involved with the mission of public advocacy, working toward the cause of quality health care.

American mountain fever. See **Colorado tick fever.**

American National Standards Institute (ANSI), a private nonprofit organization that coordinates developments of standards for medical and other devices, services, and personnel in the United States and represents the United States in matters related to international standardization.

American Nephrology Nurses' Association (ANNA), a professional association that represents nurses who work in all areas of nephrology.

American Nurses Association (ANA), the national professional association of registered nurses in the United States. It was founded in 1896 to improve standards of health and the availability of health care. ANA advances the nursing profession by fostering high standards of nursing practice, promoting the rights of nurses in the workplace, projecting a positive and realistic view of nursing, and lobbying the Congress and regulatory agencies on health care issues affecting nurses and the public. The ANA is made up of 54 constituent associations from the 50 states, the District of Columbia, Guam, the Virgin Islands, and the Federal Nurses Association (FedNA), representing more than 900 district associations. National conventions are held biennially in even-numbered years. Members may join one or more of the five divisions of nursing practice: These divisions are coordinated by the Congress for Nursing Practice. The Congress evaluates changes in the scope of practice, monitors scientific and educational developments, encourages research, and develops statements that describe ANA policies regarding legislation affecting nursing practice. In addition, the ANA is politically active on the federal level in all issues relevant to nursing and the public. Statistical services enable the association to fulfill its role as the most authoritative source of data on nursing in the United States.

American Nurses Association—Political Action Committee (ANA-PAC), a committee established to promote the improvement of the health care system in the United States by raising money from constituent and state nursing association members and contributing to candidates for federal office who have demonstrated their belief in the legislative and regulatory agenda of the American Nurses Association.

American Occupational Therapy Association (AOTA), a national professional association established in 1917 to represent the interests and concerns of occupational therapy practitioners and students of occupational therapy and to improve the quality of occupational therapy services. Its major programs and activities are directed toward assuring the quality of occupational therapy services, improving consumer access to health care services, and promoting the professional development of members. AOTA educates the public and advances the profession by providing resources, setting standards, and serving as an advocate to improve health care.

American Psychiatric Association (APA), a national professional association for physicians who specialize in psychiatry. It is concerned with the development of standards for psychiatric facilities, the formulation of mental health programs, the dissemination of data, and the promotion of psychiatric education and research. It publishes the Diagnostic and Statistical Manual of Mental Disorders (DSM).

American Psychological Association (APA), a scientific and professional organization for psychologists.

American Red Cross, one of more than 192 national organizations that seek to reduce human suffering through various health, safety, and disaster-relief programs in affiliation with the International Red Cross and Red Crescent Societies. Clara Barton founded the American Red Cross in 1881, at age 59, and led it for the next 23 years. The president of the United States is honorary chairman of the organization, for which a 50-member board of governors, all volunteers, develops policy. The American Red Cross is a nongovernmental organization (NGO), relying on donations of time, money, and blood to do its work. Ninety percent of the Red Cross staff is made up of volunteers. The symbol of the American Red Cross is a red cross on a field of white.

American Registry of Radiologic Technologists (ARRT), an organization that offers credentials in medical imaging, interventional procedures, and radiation therapy. The group certifies and registers technologists in a range of disciplines by overseeing and administering education, ethics, and examination requirements.

American Sign Language (ASL), a method of manual communication used by some individuals with hearing disorders. Messages are conveyed by manipulation of the hands and fingers. ASL is a distinct language with its own grammar and syntax. Formerly called **Ameslan.**

American Society for Investigative Pathology (ASIP), a national professional organization of specialists in pathology and bacteriology engaged in research, investigation, and discovery of the cause of disease. Members include representatives of academic, clinical, governmental, hospital, and pharmaceutical communities.

American Society of Parenteral and Enteral Nutrition (ASPEN), an organization that provides education, support, and accreditation to persons who specialize in nutrition that is provided through IV, enteral, or related types of feeding.

American Society of Radiologic Technologists (ASRT), a national professional organization of people working in medical imaging and radiation therapy. The organization's stated mission is to advance and elevate the medical imaging and radiation therapy profession and to enhance the quality and safety of patient care.

American Speech-Language-Hearing Association (ASHA), the national professional, scientific, and credentialing association for members and affiliates who are audiologists; speech-language pathologists; speech, language, and hearing scientists; audiology and speech-language pathology support personnel; and students.

American Standard Safety System, a connection system for gas cylinders with a volume exceeding 25 cubic feet. The connections differ in thread type and size, right-handed and left-handed threading, internal and external threading, and nipple-seat design. This variability reduces the risk of errors, such as administering the wrong gas to a patient or utilizing equipment calibrated for one gas with another.

Americans With Disabilities Act, legislation approved by the U.S. Congress in July 1990 that would bar discrimination against persons with physical or mental disabilities in the areas of employment, state and local government services, public accommodations, transportation, and telecommunication. The Act defines disability as a condition that "substantially limits" such activities as walking, seeing,

caring for oneself, hearing, speaking, breathing, learning, and working. It applies to persons with acquired immunodeficiency syndrome (AIDS), diabetes, and cancer, as well as to alcoholics and substance abusers undergoing treatment. The law requires employers to make "reasonable accommodations" for workers who are otherwise qualified to carry out their job duties. Other entities affected include educational institutions, which are required to make "reasonable accommodations" for students with disabilities.

American trypanosomiasis. See **Chagas' disease.**

American Type Culture Collection (ATCC), a global nonprofit, nongovernmental organization that provides biological products and technical and educational services to research centers and laboratories in the academic, scientific, and medical communities.

americium (Am) /am′ərish″ē·əm/, a synthetic radioactive element of the actinide group. Its atomic number is 95; its atomic mass is 243.

Ameslan /am″islan/, now called **American Sign Language.**

Ames test /āmz/ [Bruce Nathan Ames, American molecular geneticist, b. 1928], a method of testing substances for possible carcinogenicity by exposing a strain of *Salmonella* to a sample of the substance. The rate of mutations observed is interpreted as an indication of the carcinogenic potential of the substance tested. Also called *mutagenicity test.*

amethopterin. See **methotrexate.**

ametropia /am′itrō″pē·ə/ [Gk, *ametros,* irregular, *opsis,* sight], a condition characterized by an optic defect involving an error of refraction, such as astigmatism, hyperopia, or myopia. –*ametropic, adj.*

Amevive, brand name for **alefacept.**

AMI, abbreviation for **acute myocardial infarction.**

Amicar, a hemostatic. Brand name for **aminocaproic acid.**

amicrobic /am′īkrob″ik/, not caused by or related to microbes.

amidase /am′i·dās/, **1.** an enzyme that catalyzes the formation of a monocarboxylic acid and ammonia by hydrolytic cleavage of the C–N bond of a monocarboxylic acid amide. **2.** a term used in the recommended and trivial names of some hydrolases acting on amides, particularly those acting on linear amides.

amide, **1.** a chemical compound formed from an organic acid by the substitution of an amino (NH_2, NHR, or NR_2) group for the hydroxyl (COOH) group. **2.** a chemical compound formed by the deprotonation of ammonia (NH_3) or a primary (RNH_2) or secondary (R_2NH) amine.

amide local anesthetic, any of the numerous compounds containing an amide chemical structure that blocks nerve transmission. A sodium channel blocker. Amides are metabolized by microsomal P-450 enzymes in the liver. Kinds include **bupivacaine hydrochloride, lidocaine hydrochloride, ropivacaine, articaine, mepivacaine, prilocaine hydrochloride.** See also **ester local anesthetic.**

amido-, a prefix meaning "the presence of the radical NH_2 along with the radical CO": *amidoacetal, amidobenzene.*

amifostine, a cytoprotective agent for cisplatin.

■ INDICATIONS: This drug is used to reduce renal toxicity when cisplatin is given to treat ovarian carcinoma. It also reduces xerostomia in radiotherapy for head and neck cancer.

■ CONTRAINDICATIONS: Known hypersensitivity to mannitol or aminothiol, hypotension, dehydration, and lactation prohibit the use of this drug.

■ ADVERSE EFFECTS: Dizziness, somnolence, sneezing, flushing, hiccups, hypocalcemia, rash, and chills are among this drug's side effects. Common side effects include hypotension, nausea, and vomiting.

A

Amigo, a trademark for a battery-operated, scooterlike vehicle that gives mobility to some patients who cannot walk.

amikacin sulfate /am′ikā″sin/, an aminoglycoside antibiotic.

■ INDICATIONS: It is prescribed in the treatment of various severe infections caused by susceptible strains of gram-negative bacteria.

■ CONTRAINDICATIONS: Concurrent use of certain diuretics or known hypersensitivity to this or other aminoglycosides prohibits its use. The drug is used with caution in patients who have impaired renal function or myasthenia gravis and those under the influence of neuromuscular blocking agents or other nephrotoxins.

■ ADVERSE EFFECTS: Among the most serious adverse reactions are nephrotoxicity, auditory and vestibular ototoxicity, and neuromuscular blockade. GI disturbances, pain at the site of injection, and hypersensitivity reactions may occur.

Amikin, an aminoglycoside antibiotic. Brand name for **amikacin sulfate.**

amiloride hydrochloride /am′ilôr″īd/, a potassium-sparing diuretic with antihypertensive activity. Its prototype is spironolactone.

■ INDICATIONS: It is prescribed as an adjunct in the treatment of congestive heart failure or hypertension. It is often given with a thiazide medication.

■ CONTRAINDICATIONS: Concurrent use of potassium-conserving agents, hyperkalemia, impaired renal function, or known hypersensitivity to this drug prohibit its use.

■ ADVERSE EFFECTS: Among the most serious adverse reactions are headache, diarrhea, nausea and vomiting, anorexia, hyperkalemia, dizziness, encephalopathy, impotence, muscle cramps, photosensitivity, irregular heart rhythm, confusion, and paresthesia.

amiloxate /am″il-ok′sāt/, an absorber of ultraviolet B radiation, used topically as a sunscreen.

amine /am′in, əmēn′/ [L, *ammonia*], (in chemistry) an organic derivative of ammonia in which one or more hydrogen atoms are replaced by alkyl or aryl groups.

amine pump, *(Informal)* an active transport system in the presynaptic nerve endings that takes up released amine neurotransmitters. Adverse reactions to some drugs, notably tricyclic antidepressants, block this function, resulting in a high concentration of norepinephrine in cardiac tissue and resultant tachycardia and arrhythmia. See also **monoamine oxidase inhibitor.**

amino-, a prefix for a chemical name indicated by the monovalent radical NH_2: *aminoacidopathy, aminotransferase.*

aminoacetic acid. See **glycine.**

amino acid (AA) /əmē′nō/, an organic chemical compound composed of one or more basic amino groups and one or more acidic carboxyl groups. A total of 20 of the more than 100 amino acids that occur in nature are the building blocks of proteins. The eight essential amino acids are isoleucine, leucine, lysine, methionine, phenylalanine, threonine, tryptophan, and valine. Arginine and histidine are essential in infants. Cysteine and tyrosine are semiessential because they may be synthesized from methionine and phenylalanine, respectively. The main nonessential amino acids are alanine, asparagine, aspartic acid, glutamine, glutamic acid, glycine, proline, and serine. From their structures, the amino acids can be classified as basic (arginine, histidine, lysine), acidic (aspartic acid, glumatic acid), or neutral (the remainder); each group is transported across cell membranes by different carrier methods. Individual amino acids represent the monomeric units that can be connected via peptide linkages (amide bonds) to produce polymeric structures called proteins according to the scheme below.

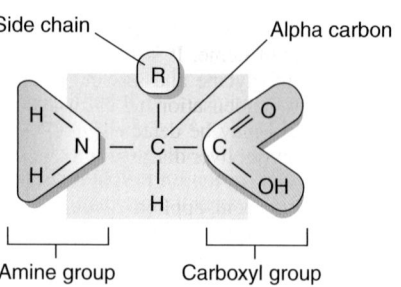

Basic chemical structure of an amino acid

amino acid group, a category of organic chemicals containing an amino group (NH_2), a carboxylic acid group (COOH), and a variable R group on the carbon separating the amino and carboxyl groups (often referred to as the alpha carbon). The R group may be comprised of nonpolar, polar, acidic, or basic side chains. The presence of the R group creates defined three-dimensionality, which is conserved in all naturally occurring amino acids.

aminoacidopathy /ə·mē′nō·as′id·op′ə·thē/, any of various disorders caused by a defect in an enzymatic step in the metabolic pathway of one or more amino acids or in a protein mediator necessary for transport of an amino acid into or out of a cell.

amino acid profiles, a series of blood or urine tests used to detect congenital amino acid metabolism defects.

amino acid residue, an amino acid molecule that has lost a water molecule by becoming joined to a molecule of another amino acid.

aminoaciduria /amē′nō·as′ido͞or″ē·ə/, the abnormal presence of amino acids in the urine that usually indicates an inborn error of metabolism, as in cystinuria. Formerly called **acidaminuria.**

aminobenzene. See **aniline.**

p-aminobenzoate /amē″no-ben′zo·āt/, any salt or ester of paraaminobenzoic acid. The potassium salt is administered orally as an antifibrotic in some dermatological disorders; various substituted esters, such as padimate O, are used as topical sunscreens.

aminobenzoic acid /-benzō″ik/, a metabolic product of the catabolism of the amino acid tryptophan. Also called **anthranilic acid.** See also **paraaminobenzoic acid** ($H_2NC_6H_4COOH$) (PABA).

aminocaproic acid /amē′nōkəprō″ik, am′inō-/, a hemostatic agent.

■ INDICATIONS: It is prescribed to stop excessive bleeding that results from hyperfibrinolysis.

■ CONTRAINDICATIONS: Active intravascular coagulation prohibits its use.

■ ADVERSE EFFECTS: Among the most serious adverse reactions are thrombosis and hypotension. Inhibition of ejaculation, nasal congestion, diarrhea, and allergic reactions also may occur.

aminoglycoside antibiotic. See **antibiotic.**

aminohydrolase. See **deaminase.**

aminolevulinic acid, a photochemotherapeutic agent. It is metabolized to protoporphyrin IX, a photosensitizer, which accumulates in the skin at the sites of application. On exposure of the sites to light of appropriate energy and wavelength together with oxygen, a photodynamic reaction occurs with cytotoxic effects.

■ INDICATIONS: It is used to treat nonhyperkeratotic actinic keratosis of the face and scalp.

■ CONTRAINDICATIONS: Known hypersensitivity to porphyrins contraindicates this drug's use.

■ ADVERSE EFFECTS: Side effects include crusts, hypopigmentation or hyperpigmentation, ulceration, pain, itching, bleeding, and pustules at the site of application.

aminolevulinic acid (ALA) /am′inōlev͞oolin″ik/, the aliphatic precursor of heme. It is formed in the body from the condensation of glycine and succinyl coenzyme A and undergoes further condensation to form porphobilinogen. Aminolevulinic acid may be detected in the urine of some patients with porphyria, liver disease, and lead poisoning.

aminolevulinic acid hydrochloride, the hydrochloride salt of aminolevulinic acid, applied topically in the treatment of nonhyperkeratotic actinic keratosis of the face and scalp.

aminophylline /am′ənōfil″in, əmē′nō-/, a bronchodilator.

■ INDICATIONS: It is prescribed in the treatment of bronchospasm associated with asthma, emphysema, and bronchitis.

■ CONTRAINDICATIONS: Known hypersensitivity to this drug or other xanthine medication prohibits its use. It is used with caution in patients who have peptic ulcers and those in whom cardiac stimulation would be harmful.

■ ADVERSE EFFECTS: Among the more serious adverse reactions are GI disturbances, central nervous system stimulation, palpitations, tachycardia, nervousness, and seizures.

aminophylline poisoning, an adverse reaction to an excessive intake of a methylxanthine drug such as caffeine or theophylline. The patient appears alternately restless, excited, and lethargic. Symptoms may include nausea, diarrhea, vomiting, abdominal pain, GI bleeding, headache, tinnitus, thirst, delirium, seizures, tachycardia, cardiac arrhythmias, and blood pressure changes.

aminopyrine /-pī′rin/, a white chemical compound with analgesic and antipyretic effects. Its continued or excessive use may lead to agranulocytosis.

aminosalicylic acid. See **paraaminosalicylic acid.**

5-aminosalicylic acid /ah-mē″nō-sal″əsil′ik/. See **mesalamine.**

aminosuccinic acid. See **aspartic acid.**

aminotransferase /-trans″fərās/, enzymes that catalyze the transfer of an amino group from an amino acid to an alpha-keto acid, with pyridoxal phosphate and pyridoxamine phosphate acting as coenzymes. Aspartate aminotransferase (AST), normally present in serum and various tissues, especially in the heart and liver, is released by damaged cells, and as a result, a high serum level may be diagnostic of myocardial infarction or hepatic disease. Alanine aminotransferase, a normal constituent of serum, especially in the liver, is released by injured tissue and may be present in high concentrations in the sera of patients with acute liver disease. Formerly called **transaminase.**

amiodarone hydrochloride, an oral antiarrhythmic drug.

■ INDICATIONS: It is prescribed for the treatment of life-threatening recurrent ventricular fibrillation and recurrent, hemodynamically unstable ventricular tachycardia refractory to other drugs; it is not considered induction therapy because of toxicities.

■ CONTRAINDICATIONS: This drug should not be given when patients have severe sinus-node dysfunction or second- or third-degree atrioventricular block or when episodes of bradycardia have resulted in syncope, except when used with a pacemaker. It also should not be used during pregnancy or in combination with certain other drugs such as ritonavir or certain quinolone antibiotics (e.g., sparfloxacin, moxifloxacin, gatifloxacin).

■ ADVERSE EFFECTS: Among the most serious adverse effects are pulmonary toxicity, liver dysfunction, nausea, vomiting, constipation, anorexia, malaise, fatigue, tremor, involuntary movements, visual disorders, bradycardia, cyanosis, and congestive heart failure.

Amipaque, a nonionic radiopaque contrast agent. Brand name for *metrizamide.*

Amitiza, brand name for **lubiprostone.**

amitosis /am′ətō″sis/ [Gk, *a, mitos,* not thread], cell division in which there is binary fission of the nucleus and cytoplasm (as in bacteria) without the complex stages of chromosome separation that occur in mitosis. −*amitotic, adj.*

amitriptyline /am′itrip″tilin/, a tricyclic antidepressant.

■ INDICATIONS: It is prescribed in the treatment of depression and has unlabeled uses for treating neuropathic pain and headaches.

■ CONTRAINDICATIONS: Concomitant administration of monoamine oxidase inhibitors, recent myocardial infarction, or known hypersensitivity to this drug or to other tricyclic medications prohibits its use. It is used with caution in patients who have a seizure disorder or cardiovascular disease or who are at risk for suicide.

■ ADVERSE EFFECTS: Among the more common adverse reactions are sedation and anticholinergic effects. A variety of cardiovascular and central nervous system effects may occur. This agent interacts with many other drugs.

AML, abbreviation for **acute myeloid leukemia.**

amlexanox /am-lek′sah-noks/, a topical antiulcerative agent used in the treatment of recurrent aphthous stomatitis.

amlodipine /amlō′dipēn/, a calcium channel blocker administered orally in the form of the besylate salt in the treatment of hypertension and chronic stable and vasospastic angina.

ammoni-, ammono-, a combining form meaning "ammonium": *ammoniemia, ammonolysis.*

ammonia (NH₃) /amō′nē·a/ [Gk, *ammoniakos,* salt of Ammon, Egyptian god], a colorless pungent gas produced by the decomposition of nitrogenous organic matter. Some of its many uses are as a fertilizer, an aromatic stimulant, a detergent, and an emulsifier.

ammoniacal fermentation /am′ənī″əkəl/, the production of ammonia and carbon dioxide from urea by the enzyme urease.

ammonia exposure, contact with ammonia, a chemical agent that is commonly available in both industry and commerce. Exposure to low concentrations of ammonia in air or solution may produce rapid skin or eye irritation. Exposure to high vapor concentrations can result in burning of the respiratory tract. See also **ammonia toxicity.**

ammonia level test, a blood test used to help diagnose severe liver diseases such as fulminant hepatitis, cirrhosis, and hepatic encephalopathy.

ammonia toxicity, exposure to ammonia at high levels. Ammonia acts on contact with moisture in the eyes, skin, and respiratory tract and any mucous surfaces to form caustic ammonium hydroxide. Ammonium hydroxide causes the necrosis of tissues through disruption of cell membrane lipids and leads to cellular destruction. As cell proteins break down, water is extracted, resulting in an inflammatory response that causes further damage. There is no antidote to ammonia toxicity. However, immediate decontamination of skin and eyes with copious amounts of water will hasten recovery. The individual should be removed from the area when ammonia vapors are high. A poison control center should be contacted immediately if ammonia is ingested.

ammonium (NH₄⁺), an ion formed by the reaction of ammonia (NH₃) with a hydrogen ion (H⁺). The ammonium ion is highly soluble in water but does not pass easily through cell membranes, as does the ammonia molecule, and its rate of excretion is influenced in part by the acidity of urine. The lower the pH, the greater the proportion of ammonium ions present, assuming a constant level of ammonia production from amino acid metabolism.

Ammon's horn. Also called **hippocampus.**

ammonuria /am′ōnŏ͞or″ē·ə/, urine that contains an excessive amount of ammonia.

amnesia /amnē″zhə/ [Gk, *a, mnasthai,* to forget], a loss of memory caused by brain damage or by severe emotional trauma. Kinds include **anterograde amnesia, posttraumatic amnesia, retrograde amnesia.** −*amnestic, amnesic, adj.*

amnesic aphasia [Gk, *a, mnasthai* + *a, phasis,* without speech], an inability to remember spoken words or to use words for names of objects, circumstances, or characteristics.

amnestic apraxia /amnes″tik/, the inability to carry out a movement in response to a request because of a lack of ability to remember the request. Often associated with dementia. See also **apraxia.**

amnio-, a prefix meaning "amnion": *amniocentesis, amnioscopy.*

amniocentesis /am′nē-ōsentē″sis/ [Gk, *amnos,* lamb's caul, *kentesis,* pricking], an obstetric procedure in which a small amount of amniotic fluid is removed for laboratory analysis.

■ METHOD: With the use of ultrasound imaging techniques, the position of the fetus and the location of the placenta are determined. The skin on the mother's abdomen is aseptically prepared, and a local anesthetic is usually injected. A needle attached to a syringe is introduced into a part of the uterus where there is the least chance of perforating the placenta or scratching the fetus. Between 20 and 25 mL of amniotic fluid is aspirated. Amniocentesis is performed to diagnose various inherited disorders, including chromosomal aberrations, neural tube defects, and Tay-Sachs disease. It is also performed to discover the sex of the fetus if certain sex-linked disorders are suspected. Later in pregnancy, amniocentesis may be performed to assess fetal lung maturity by testing the lecithin/sphingomyelin ratio and the presence of phosphatidyl-glycerol in the laboratory before elective delivery or for evidence of infection (chorioamnionitis).

■ PATIENT CARE CONSIDERATIONS: A woman must sign an informed consent form before amniocentesis. Specifically stated in the consent form are the reasons for performing the procedure and the facts that fluid is to be removed after needle puncture of the uterus, that ultrasound imaging techniques are usual adjuncts, that the procedure may fail to give the results intended, and that spontaneous abortion, nausea, abdominal pain, or fetal injury may occur. The woman is reassured that complications and failure are rare; she is given emotional support before, during, and after the procedure. In testing for inherited disorders, 10 days to 2 weeks is usually necessary for tissue culture before a diagnosis may be made; this waiting period may be extremely stressful for the mother. The woman is warned to report any signs of infection or of the onset of labor. $Rh_o(D)$ immunoglobulin should be given to pregnant women who are Rh negative.

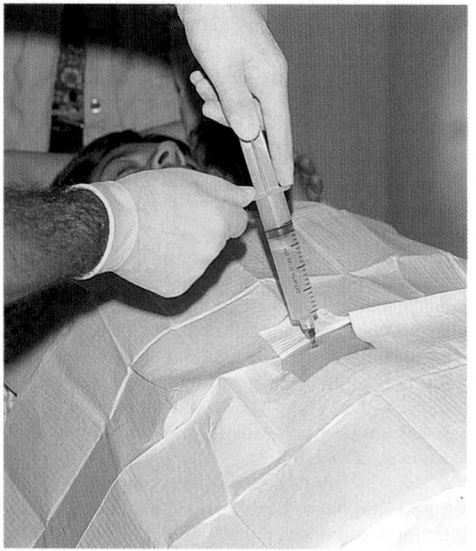

Amniocentesis: placement of needle *(Courtesy of Marjorie Pyle, RNC, LifeCircle, Costa Mesa, CA)*

amniography /am′nē-og″rəfē/, a procedure used to detect placement of the placenta by x-ray examination with injection of a radiopaque contrast medium into the amniotic fluid. It is seldom used, having been largely supplanted by ultrasonography.

amnioinfusion, infusion of a solution to increase intraamniotic fluid in cases of oligohydramnios or rupture of the membranes; the procedure may reduce the number and severity of variable decelerations due to cord compression during labor.

amnion /am″nē-on/ [Gk, *amnos,* lamb's caul], a membrane, continuous with and covering the fetal side of the placenta, that forms the outer surface of the umbilical cord. Compare **chorion. −amniotic,** *adj.*

amnionitis /am′nē-ōnī″tis/, an inflammation of the amnion. The condition may develop as a result of infection after early rupture of the fetal membranes.

amnion nodosum, a nodular condition of the fetal surface of the amnion and a manifestation of an intrauterine infection. It is frequently associated with prolonged membrane rupture.

amnioscopy /am′nē-os″kəpē/, a direct visual examination of the fetus and amniotic fluid with an endoscope that is inserted into the amniotic cavity through the uterine cervix or an incision in the abdominal wall.

amniotic. See **amnion.**

amniotic band disruption sequence syndrome, an abnormal condition of fetal development characterized by the development of fibrous bands within the uterus that entangle the fetus, leading to deformities in structure and function. The syndrome is associated with a variety of congenital anomalies, including clubfoot, missing limbs, simian creases, and skull and visceral defects. It can be detected in the uterus. Interventions are specific to the varied symptoms, and genetic counseling is suggested. Also called *amniotic band syndrome (ABS).*

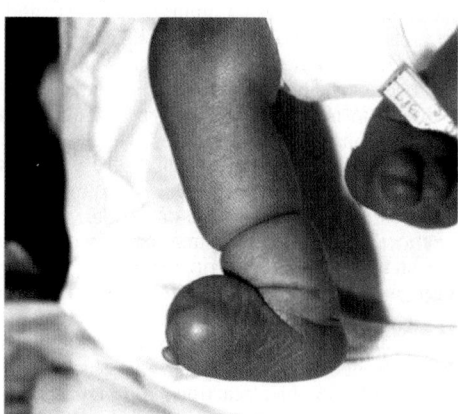

Amniotic bands *(Graham and Smith, 2007)*

amniotic cavity [Gk, *amnion,* fetal membrane; L, *cavum*], the fluid-filled space of the amniotic sac surrounding the fetus.

amniotic fluid, the fluid mixture surrounding the fetus. Its volume in a normal pregnancy increases from 250 to 800 mL between 16 and 32 weeks of gestation, remaining stable through 39 weeks and then declining to about 500 mL at 42 weeks. The origin of amniotic fluid in the first trimester is uncertain but probably includes transudation through the chorioamnion and fetal skin before its keratinization. Its volume thereafter is maintained by a balance of resorption by fetal swallowing and flow across the membranes into the fetus and uterus and production from the fetal lungs and kidneys (fetal urine). It provides a physical barrier to trauma and a medium for active chemical exchanges, as well as facilitating fetal movement, including fetal breathing (and thereby fetal lung growth) and swallowing. The cloudy appearance of the fluid is mainly due to desquamated fetal cells and lipids. See also **polyhydramnios, oligohydramnios.**

amniotic fluid embolism [Gk, *amnion;* L, *fluere,* to flow; Gk, *embolos,* plug],   entry of amniotic fluid into the maternal vascular system, usually during labor and delivery. When lodged in a pulmonary vessel, it causes rapid respiratory distress, cyanosis, cardiovascular collapse, hemorrhage associated with severe coagulopathy, and coma. Maternal death is not uncommon and is prevented by rapid total cardiovascular support and treatment of coagulopathy (disseminated intravascular coagulopathy, DIC). Now called **anaphylactoid syndrome of pregnancy.**

amniotic fold,   an embryonic growth feature observed in many vertebrates, particularly birds and reptiles. It consists of flaps of ectoderm and mesoderm that grow over the back of an embryo, fuse, and subsequently separate to form the amnion.

amniotic sac,   a thin-walled bag that contains the fetus and amniotic fluid during pregnancy. It has a capacity of 4 to 5 L at term. The wall of the sac extends from the margin of the placenta. The amnion, chorion, and decidua that make up the wall are each a few cell layers thick. They are closely applied—though not fused—to one another and to the wall of the uterus. The intact sac and its fluid provide for the equilibration of hydrostatic pressure within the uterus. During labor, the sac effects the uniform transmission of the force of uterine contractions to the cervix for dilation.

amniotome /am′ ne-o-tōm/,   an instrument for puncturing the fetal membranes.

amniotomy /am′nē-ot″əmē/,   artificial rupture of the fetal sac (membranes) using an amniotic hook (aminotome), usually with the intention of stimulating labor or allowing the introduction of intrauterine force pressure sensors and/or ECG electrodes applied to the fetal scalp to evaluate fetal well-being. Risks include prolapse of the umbilical cord and intrauterine infection.

amobarbital /am′ōbär″bətal/,   a barbiturate sedative-hypnotic. Also called **amylobarbitone.**
■ INDICATIONS: It is prescribed as an anticonvulsant and a preanesthetic and for short-term treatment of insomnia.
■ CONTRAINDICATIONS: Porphyria or known hypersensitivity to barbiturates prohibits its use. It is also contraindicated in patients with marked liver impairment or respiratory disease.
■ ADVERSE EFFECTS: Among the most serious adverse reactions are respiratory and circulatory depression, drug hangover, and various allergic reactions. It also interacts with many other drugs.

A-mode,   amplitude modulation in diagnostic ultrasonography. It represents the time required for the ultrasound beam to strike a tissue interface and return its signal to the transducer. The greater the reflection at the tissue interface, the larger the signal amplitude on the A-mode screen. See also **B-mode, M-mode.**

A-mode ultrasound [L, *ultra,* beyond, *sonus,* sound],   a display of ultrasonic echoes in which the horizontal axis of the visual display represents the time required for the return of the echo and the vertical axis represents the strength of the echo. The mode is used in echoencephalography. See also **A-mode.**

amoeba.   See **ameba.**

amoebiasis.   See **amebiasis.**

amok [Malay, *amoq,* furious],   a psychotic frenzy with a desire to kill anybody encountered. The murderous episodes may follow periods of severe depression.

amoric /ah-mo′rik/,   without particles.

amorph /ā″môrf, əmôrf″/   [Gk, *a, morphef,* not shape],   **1.** a mutant allele that has little or no effect on the expression of a trait. Compare **antimorph, hypermorph, hypomorph.** –*amorphic, adj.* **2.** abbreviation for **amorphous.**

amorphous /əmôr″fəs/   [Gk, *a,* not, *morphe,* form],   **1.** describing an object that lacks definite visible shape or form. **2.** (in chemistry) a substance that is not crystalline.

amorphous crystal,   a shapeless, poorly defined crystal or granule, e.g., phosphate salts that can be found in urine under basic conditions.

amoxapine /əmok″sepin/,   a tetracylic antidepressant (sometimes classified as a secondary amine tricylic).
■ INDICATIONS: It is prescribed in the treatment of mental depression.
■ CONTRAINDICATIONS: It is used with caution in conditions in which anticholinergics are contraindicated, in seizure disorders, and in cardiovascular disorders. Concomitant administration of monoamine oxidase inhibitors, recent myocardial infarction, or known hypersensitivity to this drug prohibits its use.
■ ADVERSE EFFECTS: Among the most serious adverse reactions are sedation and anticholinergic side effects. A variety of GI, cardiovascular, and neurological reactions may also occur. It is involved in many drug interactions.

amoxicillin /əmok′səsil″in/,   a beta-lactam semisynthetic oral penicillin antibiotic.
■ INDICATIONS: It is prescribed in the treatment of infections caused by a susceptible gram-negative or gram-positive bacteria.
■ CONTRAINDICATIONS: Known hypersensitivity to any penicillin prohibits its use.
■ ADVERSE EFFECTS: Among the most serious adverse reactions are anaphylaxis, nausea, and diarrhea. Allergic reactions and rashes are common.

Amoxil,   a beta-lactam antibiotic. Brand name for **amoxicillin.**

AMP,   abbreviation for **adenosine monophosphate.**

ampere (A) /am″pēr/   [André-Marie Ampère, French physicist, 1775–1836],   a unit of measurement of the amount of electric current. An ampere, according to the meter-kilogram-second (MKS) system, is the amount of current passed through a resistance of 1 ohm by an electric potential of 1 volt; in the International System (SI) of Units, an ampere is a unit of electric current that carries a charge of 1 coulomb through a conductor in 1 second. The standard international ampere is the amount of current that deposits 0.001118 g of silver per second when passed, according to certain specifications, through a silver nitrate solution. See also **ohm, volt, watt.**

amperometry /am′parom″ətrē/,   the measurement of current at a single applied potential.

amph-.   See **amphi-, amph-, ampho-.**

amphetamine poisoning,   the toxic effects of overdosage of drugs classified as amphetamines, including overdose or abuse of prescription medications and those manufactured synthetically in illegal laboratories.
■ OBSERVATIONS: Symptoms vary based on the amount, purity, and potency of the drug. They may include excitement, hyperthermia, tremors, tachycardia, hallucinations, delirium, seizures, and circulatory collapse.
■ INTERVENTIONS: Treatment is symptomatic and ranges from observation and sedation to management of circulatory collapse. Orogastric lavage with activated charcoal may

be performed. Patients with severe hyperthermia associated with psychomotor agitation require immediate measures to rapidly decrease temperature to prevent multiorgan failure and death. Great care must be taken with the administration and titration of medications to manage symptoms. Physical restraint should be avoided if possible.

■ PATIENT CARE CONSIDERATIONS: There is a high potential for abuse with amphetamines. Each member of the health care team should recognize the importance of behavioral counseling and therapy for individuals with an amphetamine addiction.

amphetamines /amfet″əmēnz/, a group of nervous system stimulants, including amphetamine and its chemical congeners dextroamphetamine and methamphetamine, that are subject to abuse because of their ability to produce wakefulness, euphoria, and weight loss. Abuse leads to compulsive behavior, paranoia, hallucinations, and suicidal tendencies. Amphetamines have many street names, such as **blackbeauties, lidpoppers, peppills, speed** (an injectable form), and **ice** (a crystalline form of methamphetamine that is smoked). See also **crack, dextroamphetamine sulfate, methamphetamine hydrochloride.**

amphetamine sulfate, a colorless water-soluble salt of amphetamine that stimulates the central nervous system. It has been used to treat certain respiratory complaints, fatigue, and narcolepsy and to effect weight loss. It formerly was used to treat obesity.

amphi-, amph-, ampho-, prefixes meaning "on both sides, around, double": *amphiarthrosis, amphoterism.*

amphiarthrosis. Also called **cartilaginous joint.**

amphidiarthrodial joint /am′fēdī″ärthrō″dē·əl/ [Gk, *amphi,* both kinds], a classification for joints that permit slight movement in more than one direction, as the symphysis pubis. Compare **diarthroidial joints.**

amphigenesis. See **amphigony.**

amphigenetic /am′fijənet″ik/ [Gk, *genein,* to produce], **1.** produced by the union of gametes from both sexes. **2.** bisexual; having both testicular and ovarian tissue.

amphigenous inheritance /amfij″ənəs/, the acquisition of genetic traits and conditions from both parents. Also called **biparental inheritance, duplex inheritance.**

amphigonadism /am′figō″nədiz′əm/, true hermaphroditism; the presence of both testicular and ovarian tissue in the same individual organism. –*amphigonadic, adj.*

amphigony /amfig″ənē/ [Gk, *amphi* + *gonos,* generation], sexual reproduction. Also called **amphigenesis.** –*amphigonic, adj.*

amphikaryon /am′fiker″ē·on/ [Gk, *amphi* + *karyon,* nucleus], a nucleus containing the diploid number of chromosomes. –*amphikaryotic, adj.*

amphimixis /am′fimik″sis/ [Gk, *amphi* + *mixis,* mingling], **1.** the union of germ cells in sexual reproduction. **2.** the union and integration of oral, anal, and genital libidinal impulses in the development of heterosexuality.

amphipathic /-path″ik/ [Gk, *amphi* + *pathos,* suffering], pertaining to a molecule having two sides with characteristically different properties, such as a detergent, which has both a polar (hydrophilic) end and a nonpolar (hydrophobic) end but is long enough so that each end demonstrates its own solubility characteristics.

ampho-. See **amphi-, amph-, ampho-.**

Amphojel, an antacid. Brand name for *aluminum hydroxide gel.*

amphoric breath sound /amfôr″ik/ [Gk, *amphoreus,* jug], an abnormal, resonant, hollow, blowing sound heard with a stethoscope over the thorax. It indicates a cavity opening into a bronchus or a pneumothorax.

amphoteric /am″fo-ter′ik/, **1.** capable of acting as both an acid and a base. **2.** capable of neutralizing either acids or bases.

amphotericin B /am′fəter″əsin/, an antifungal medication.

■ INDICATIONS: It is prescribed for topical or systemic use in the treatment of serious fungal infections.

■ CONTRAINDICATIONS: Known hypersensitivity prohibits its use.

■ ADVERSE EFFECTS: When it is used systemically, the most serious effects are nephrotoxicity and infusion-related reactions. Nausea, fever, chills, and shaking may occur on administration. With topical use, local hypersensitivity reactions are the most common adverse reactions.

amphotericin B cholesteryl complex, amphotericin B complexed with cholesteryl sulfate in a 1:1 ratio; it is administered by IV infusion in the treatment of disseminated aspergillosis in patients refractory to or intolerant of conventional amphotericin B therapy.

amphotericin B lipid complex, amphotericin B complexed with two phospholipids in a 1:1 drug-to-lipid ratio; it is administered by IV infusion in the treatment of invasive fungal infections in patients who are refractory to or intolerant of conventional amphotericin B therapy.

amphotericin B liposomal complex, amphotericin B intercalated into a single bilayer liposome; it is administered by IV infusion in the treatment of severe systemic fungal infections and kala-azars in patients refractory to or intolerant of conventional amphotericin B therapy.

amphoterism /-ter″izəm/ [Gk, *amphoteros,* pertaining to both], a quality of a chemical compound that permits it to act as an acid or a base. –**amphoteric,** *adj., n.*

ampicillin /am′pəsil″in/, a semisynthetic penicillin.

■ INDICATIONS: It is prescribed in the treatment of infections caused by a broad spectrum of sensitive gram-negative and gram-positive organisms.

■ CONTRAINDICATIONS: Known hypersensitivity to any penicillin prohibits its use.

■ ADVERSE EFFECTS: Among the most serious adverse reactions are anaphylaxis, nausea, and diarrhea. Fever, rashes, allergic reactions, and suprainfection also may occur.

ampicillin sodium, the sodium salt of ampicillin, prescribed as an antibiotic to treat gram-positive organisms and some gram-negative organisms.

amplification /am′plifikā″shən/ [L, *amplificare,* to make wider], **1.** (genetic) a process whereby certain targeted sequences of DNA are replicated by the polymerase chain reaction (PCR) in order to produce multiple copies of a single or limited number of genes. Often this refers to increasing the proportion of plasmid DNA relative to the amount of bacterial DNA. **2.** the replication in bulk of an entire DNA library. See also **polymerase chain reaction.** –*amplify, v.*

amplifier, a device that controls power from a mechanical, electrical, hydraulic, or other source so that the output is greater than the input.

amplitude /am″plityо̄od/ [L, *amplus,* wide], the width or breadth of range or displacement from equilibrium, e.g., maximum height of a sinusoidal wave from the mean or average position.

amplitude of accommodation (AA), the total accommodative power of the eye, determined by the difference between the refractive power for farthest vision and that for nearest vision.

amplitude of convergence, the difference in the power needed to turn the eyes from their far point to their near point of convergence. Also called **fusional amplitude, vergence ability.**

amprenavir, an antiviral (protease inhibitor).

■ INDICATIONS: It is used to treat HIV in combination with other antiretroviral agents.

■ CONTRAINDICATIONS: Known hypersensitivity prohibits its use.

■ ADVERSE EFFECTS: Life-threatening side effects include Stevens-Johnson syndrome and acute hemolytic anemia. Other serious adverse effects include new-onset diabetes, hyperglycemia, and exacerbation of preexisting diabetes mellitus. Common side effects include diarrhea, abdominal pain, nausea, paresthesia, and rash.

ampule /am″pyool/ [Fr, *ampoule,* phial], a small, sterile glass or plastic container that usually contains a single dose of a solution. Also spelled *ampoule.*

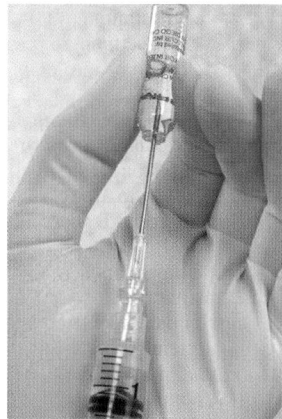

Withdrawal of medication from an ampule *(Lilley et al, 2014)*

ampulla /ampool″ə/ *pl.* **ampullae** [L, flasklike bottle], a rounded, saclike dilation of a duct, canal, or any tubular structure, such as the lacrimal duct, semicircular canal, fallopian tube, rectum, or vas deferens.

ampulla of the bile duct. Also called **hepatopancreatic ampulla.**

ampulla of the rectum, a flask-shaped dilation near the end of the rectum.

ampulla of Vater. See **hepatopancreatic ampulla.**

ampullar crest, the most prominent part of a localized thickening of the membrane that lines the ampullae of the semicircular ducts, covered with neuroepithelium, including hair cells, containing endings of the vestibular nerve. It is the site of sensory transduction of rotational motion.

ampullary aneurysm. See **saccular aneurysm.**

ampullary tubal pregnancy /ampool″lərē, am″pəler′ē/, implantation of an ectopic pregnancy in the ampulla of a fallopian tube; 80% of such extrauterine pregnancies happen with normal conception and 93% with assisted reproductive technology (ART).

ampullula /ampool″yələ/, a minute ampulla, such as a small lymph or blood vessel.

amputation /am″pyootā″shən/ [L, *amputare,* to excise], the surgical removal of a part of the body, a limb, or part of a limb to treat recurrent infection or gangrene in peripheral vascular disease; to remove malignant tumors; and to treat severe trauma. Kinds include **mastectomy, open amputation, closed amputation.**

amputation care, care for a patient who has undergone an amputation; the goal is physical and psychosocial adaptation to the loss. The body part removed will dictate the type of physical care required. Psychosocial recovery can be complex. Interventions require a team approach for successful recovery and rehabilitation.

■ METHOD: Patients and their families should be fully involved in the plans for rehabilitation, understand what is expected of them, and know the regimen of exercise and skills necessary for full functional recovery.

■ PATIENT CARE CONSIDERATIONS: Patients undergoing amputation will need assistance in dealing with changes in body image as they adjust to the loss. They should be encouraged and given the opportunity to express feelings of anxiety, grief, anger, and depression.

■ OUTCOME CRITERIA: A prosthesis may be delayed or immediate, depending on the condition of the patient and the reason for the amputation. Residual limbs are usually wrapped with elastic bandages. Early exercise is encouraged to facilitate full function with a prosthesis.

amputation flap, a fold of skin used to cover the end of a residual limb. See **closed amputation.**

amputation neuroma, a form of traumatic neuroma that may develop at the proximal end of a severed or injured nerve.

amputation-stump bandage, *(Informal)* an elastic bandage applied to cover the residual limb (stump) after an amputation. It helps to control edema and to shape the remaining portion of the limb (stump).

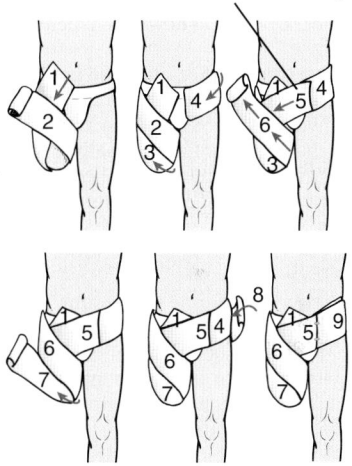

Start of second bandage

Amputation-stump bandaging for above-the-knee residual limb *(Mosby, 2003)*

amputee /am′pyootē″/, a person who has had all or a portion of an extremity traumatically or surgically removed.

amrinone lactate /am″rinōn/. See **inamrinone lactate.**

Amsler grid [Marc Amsler, Swiss ophthalmologist, 1891–1968], a checkerboard grid of intersecting dark horizontal and vertical lines with one dark spot in the middle. To discover a visual field defect, the person simply covers or closes one eye and looks at the spot with the other. A visual field defect is perceived as a defect, distortion, blank, or other fault in the grid. The person may record the defects directly on a paper copy of the grid that may be kept as a permanent record. The Amsler grid is used in testing for macular degeneration and is used to monitor an individual's central visual field. See **age-related macular degeneration.**

AMT, abbreviation for **American Medical Technologists.**

amu, abbreviation for **atomic mass unit.**

amusia /ə·myōo′zē·ə/ [Gk, *amousia,* want of harmony], an inability to recognize the significance of sounds, manifested as loss of the ability to recognize or produce music.

amyelia /am′ī-ēl″yə/ [Gk, *myelos,* marrow], the absence of a spinal cord; a rare congenital condition in which segments of the spinal cord are missing.

amyelinic neuroma /amī′əlin″ik/ [Gk, *a, myelos,* without marrow, *neuron,* nerve, *oma*], a tumor that contains only nonmyelinated nerve fibers.

amygdala /amig″dələ/ [Gk, *amygdale,* almond]. See **amygdaloid nucleus.**

amygdalin. See **Laetrile.**

amygdaloid /-dəloid/, resembling a small oval structure; shaped like an almond.

amygdaloid fossa [Gk, *amylon, eidos,* starchlike; L, *fossa,* ditch], a space in the wall of the oropharynx, between the pillars of the fauces, that is occupied by the palatine tonsil. Also called **tonsillar fossa.**

amygdaloid nucleus [Gk, *amygdale,* almond, *eidos,* form; L, *nucleus,* nut], one of the basal nuclei, found near the inferior horn of the lateral ventricle in the medial temporal lobe. It is considered part of the limbic system and is involved in memory and emotion. Also called **amygdala.**

amyl-. See **amylo-, amyl-.**

amyl alcohol /am″il/ [Gk, *amylon,* starch], a colorless, oily liquid with the formula $C_5H_{11}OH$ that is only slightly soluble in water but can be mixed with ethyl alcohol, chloroform, or ether. It is also known as 1-pentanol or normal pentanol.

amyl alcohol, tertiary. See **amylene hydrate.**

amylase /am′ilās/ [Gk, *amylon,* starch], an enzyme that catalyzes the hydrolysis of starch into smaller carbohydrate molecules. Alpha-amylase, found in saliva, pancreatic juice, malt, certain bacteria, and molds, catalyzes the hydrolysis of starches to dextrins, maltose, and maltotriose. Beta-amylase, found in grains, vegetables, malt, and bacteria, is involved in the hydrolysis of starch to maltose. Normal blood findings are 56 to 190 IU/L.

amylase test, a test performed on serum, plasma, or urine that is used to diagnose chronic or acute pancreatitis and other pancreatic disorders, such as pancreatic cancer. Increased amylase activity may also indicate nonpancreatic disorders, such as bowel perforation, penetrating peptic ulcer, duodenal obstruction, and other conditions.

amylene hydrate /am″əlēn/, a clear, colorless liquid, $(CH_3)_2C(OH)CH_2CH_3$ with a camphorlike odor, miscible with alcohol, chloroform, ether, or glycerin and used as a solvent and a hypnotic.

amylic fermentation /əmil″ik/, the formation of amyl alcohol from sugar.

amyl nitrite, a vasodilator.
- INDICATIONS: It is prescribed to relieve the angiospasm of angina pectoris and as an adjunct in the treatment of cyanide poisoning.
- CONTRAINDICATIONS: Known hypersensitivity to this drug or to other nitrites prohibits its use, as does head injury and narrow-angle glaucoma.
- ADVERSE EFFECTS: Among the serious adverse reactions are hypotension, allergic reactions, nausea, headache, and dizziness.

amylo-, amyl-, combining forms meaning "starch": *amylophagia, amylase.*

amylobarbitone. See **amobarbital.**

amyloid /am″iloid/ [Gk, *amylon,* starch, *eidos,* form], **1.** insoluble protein aggregates pertaining to or resembling starch. **2.** a starchlike protein-carbohydrate complex deposited abnormally in some tissues during certain chronic disease states, such as amyloidosis, rheumatoid arthritis, tuberculosis, and Alzheimer disease.

amyloid degeneration, degeneration of tissue resulting from deposition of amyloid complexes.

amyloid liver [Gk, *amylon,* starch, *eidos,* form; AS, *lifer*], *(Informal)* a liver in which the cells have been infiltrated with amyloid (glycoprotein) deposits. Also called **albuminous liver.**

amyloidosis /am′iloidō″sis/ [Gk, *amylon + eidos,* form, *osis,* condition], a progressive, incurable metabolic disease in which a waxy, starchlike glycoprotein (amyloid) accumulates in tissues and organs, impairing their function. The condition may be hereditary or acquired and may be systemic or organ specific. There is no known cure for amyloidosis, and treatment in the secondary type is aimed at alleviating the underlying chronic disease.
- OBSERVATIONS: Primary amyloidosis refers to light chain amyloidosis seen in multiple myeloma. Patients with secondary amyloidosis usually suffer from another chronic infectious or inflammatory disease, such as tuberculosis, osteomyelitis, rheumatoid arthritis, or Crohn's disease. Almost all organs can be affected, most often the heart, lungs, tongue, and intestines in primary amyloidosis, and the kidneys, liver, and spleen in the secondary type. Elderly patients tend to experience cardiac effects of the disease. Diagnosis is made through biopsy of the suspected organ or abdominal fat aspiration.
- INTERVENTIONS: There is no known cure for amyloidosis, and treatment in the secondary type is aimed at alleviating the underlying chronic disease.
- PATIENT CARE CONSIDERATIONS: Patients with renal amyloidosis are frequently candidates for kidney dialysis and transplantation.

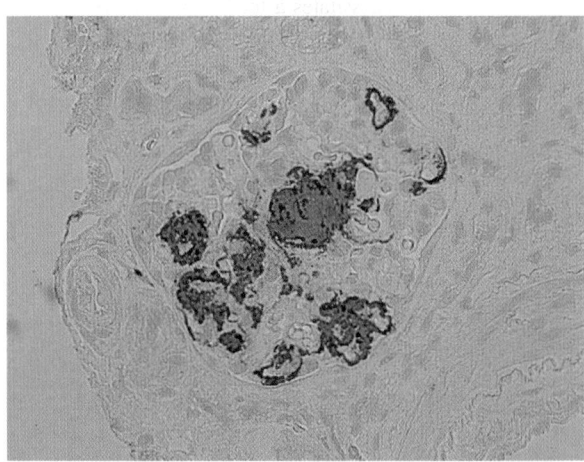

Amyloidosis of the kidney *(Rich et al, 2013)*

amyloid osteopathy, local osteoarticular lytic lesions often found in patients with hemodialysis-associated amyloidosis.

amyloid precursor protein (APP), a large transmembrane glycoprotein expressed on the cell surface and of uncertain function; it may be cleaved on the cell surface to a soluble form. Alternatively, cleavage may follow endocytosis and in some cases then yields 40 to 43 abnormal amino acid peptides, which aggregate to form amyloid β, associated with Alzheimer disease.

amylolysis /am′ēlol″isis/ [Gk, *amylon,* starch, *lysis,* loosening], the digestive process whereby starch is converted into sugars and dextrins by hydrolysis or by enzymatic activity.

amylopectinosis. See **Andersen's disease.**

amylophagia /am″əlo-f′jah/, the habit of eating starch, such as laundry starch or the compulsive consumption of purified starch. See also **pica.**

amylopsin, pancreatic amylase.

amylose, a minor constituent of starch (20%–30%) consisting of a linear chain of glucose molecules connected by linkages; it stains blue with iodine.

amyoplasia congenita. Also called **arthrogryposis multiplex congenita.**

amyotonia /ā′mī-ōtō″nē-ə/ [Gk, *a, mys,* not muscle, *tonos,* tone], an abnormal condition of skeletal muscle, characterized by a lack of tonus, weakness, and wasting, usually the result of motor neuron disease. Compare **myotonia.** –*amyotonic, adj.*

amyotrophic lateral sclerosis (ALS) /ā′mī-ōtrof″ik/ [Gk, *a,mys + trophe,* nourishment], a degenerative disease characterized by loss of the motor neurons, with progressive weakness and atrophy of the muscles of the hands, forearms, and legs, spreading to involve most of the body and face. It results from degeneration of the motor neurons of the anterior horns and corticospinal tracts, beginning in middle age and progressing rapidly, usually causing death within 2 to 5 years. Also called **Lou Gehrig disease,** *wasting palsy.* See also **Aran-Duchenne muscular atrophy.**

■ OBSERVATIONS: The initial symptom is weakness of the skeletal muscles, especially those of the extremities. As the disease progresses, the patient experiences difficulty in swallowing and talking, and dyspnea as the accessory muscles of respiration are affected. Mentation is not affected; the patient remains alert of the functional losses.

■ INTERVENTIONS: There is no known cure. For the most part, patients are cared for at home and are hospitalized when severe dysphagia necessitates a feeding tube or when treatment is necessary for acute respiratory problems.

■ PATIENT CARE CONSIDERATIONS: Interventions are planned and implemented by the health care team based on the patient's and family's needs during the course of the illness. In general, the major problems encountered are those related to dysphagia and the need to meet nutritional requirements and avoid aspiration; dyspnea and the promotion of patient comfort; aphasia and impaired verbal communication; weakness and impaired mobility and activity intolerance; constipation; pain and discomfort due to muscle cramps; and alteration in self-concept and body image. The patient and family will also need assistance in maintaining home care, coping with the effects of the illness, and maintaining optimal functioning. A variety of services including. but not limited to, community health nursing, physical therapy, occupational therapy, social services, mental health care, and medical care are essential to the adjustment of the patient and family to the disease process.

Amytal Sodium, a barbiturate. Brand name for *sodium amobarbital.*

an-, ana-, prefixes meaning "not, without": *anoxia, analgesia.*

-an, -ian, suffixes meaning "belonging to, characteristic of, similar to": *protozoan, salpingian.*

ANA, **1.** abbreviation for **American Nurses Association.** **2.** abbreviation for **antinuclear antibody.**

ana (āa, ā̄ā, AA). See **ā̄a, ā̄ā, AA.**

anabolic steroid /an′əbol″ik/ [Gk, *anaballein,* to build up], any of several compounds derived from testosterone or prepared synthetically to promote general body growth, to oppose the effects of endogenous estrogen, or to promote masculinizing effects. All such compounds cause a mixed androgenic-anabolic effect.

■ INDICATIONS: It is prescribed in the treatment of aplastic anemia, red-cell aplasia, and hemolytic anemia and in anemias associated with renal failure, myeloid metaplasia, and leukemia.

■ CONTRAINDICATIONS: It is contraindicated for the palliation of carcinoma of the breast; in pregnancy and serious cardiac, renal, and hepatic diseases; and with known hypersensitivity.

■ ADVERSE EFFECTS: Among the most serious adverse effects are acne, growth of facial hair, and hoarsening or deepening of the voice; other masculinizing features are common. Continued use of these compounds in women may also produce prominent musculature, hirsutism, and hypertrophy of the clitoris.

anabolism /ənab″əliz″əm/ [Gk, *anaballein,* to build up], the constructive phase of metabolism characterized by the conversion of simple substances into the more complex compounds of living matter. Compare **catabolism.** –*anabolic, adj.*

anabolite /ənab″ōlīt/ [Gk, *anaballein,* to build up], a product of the process of anabolism.

anacatadidymus /an′əkat′ədid″iməs/ [Gk, *ana,* up, *kata,* down, *didymos,* twin], conjoined twins that are fused in the middle but separated above and below.

anaclisis /an′əklī″sis/ [Gk, *ana + klisis,* leaning], **1.** a condition, normal in childhood but pathological in adulthood, in which a person is emotionally dependent on other people. **2.** a condition in which a person consciously or unconsciously chooses a love object because of a resemblance to the mother, father, or another person who was an important source of comfort and protection in infancy. –*anaclitic, adj.*

anaclitic depression /an′əklit″ik/, a syndrome occurring in infants, usually after sudden separation from the mothering person. Symptoms include apprehension, withdrawal, detachment, incessant crying, refusal to eat, sleep disturbances, and, eventually, stupor leading to severe impairment of the infant's physical, social, and intellectual development. If the mothering figure or a substitute is made available within 1 to 3 months, the infant recovers quickly with no long-term effects. See also **hospitalism.**

anacrotic pulse [Gk, *ana + krotos,* stroke], a pulse characterized by a transient drop in amplitude of the primary elevation on a sphygmographic tracing. It is seen in valvular aortic stenosis.

anacrotism /ənak″rətiz″əm/ [Gk, *ana, krotos,* stroke], a condition characterized by two arterial expansions per heartbeat and observed as a notch on the ascending limb of an arterial pulse pressure tracing. –*anacrotic, adj.*

anacusis /an′əko͞o″sis/ [Gk, *a, akouein,* not to hear], a total loss of hearing.

anadenia /an′ā-dē′nē-ə/ [Gk, *aden,* gland], *(Obsolete)* the absence of a gland.

anadicrotic pulse /an′ədīkrot″ik/ [Gk, *ana + dis,* twice, *krotos,* stroke], (on a sphygmographic tracing) a pulse characterized by two transient drops in amplitude on the curve of primary elevation.

anadidymus /an′ədid″iməs/ [Gk, *ana + didymos,* twin], conjoined twins that are united at the pelvis and lower extremities but are separated in the upper half. Also called **duplicatus anterior.**

anadipsia /an′ədip″sē-ə/ [Gk, *ana + dipsa,* thirst], extreme thirst, often occurring in the manic phase of bipolar disorder. The condition is the result of dehydration caused by the excessive perspiration, electrolyte imbalance, continuous urination, and relentless physical activity produced by the intense excitement characteristic of the manic phase. See also **polydipsia.**

Anadrol-50, an anabolic steroid. Brand name for **oxymetholone.**

anaemia. See **anemia.**

anaerobe /aner″ōb/ [Gk, *a* + *aer,* not air, *bios,* life], a microorganism that grows and lives in the complete or almost complete absence of oxygen. Anaerobes are widely distributed in nature and in the body. Compare **aerobe, microaerophile.** Kinds include **facultative anaerobe, obligate anaerobe.** See also **anaerobic infection.** −**anaerobic,** *adj.*

anaerobic /an′ərō″bik/, pertaining to the absence of air or oxygen.

anaerobic catabolism, the breakdown of complex chemical substances into simpler compounds, with the release of energy, in the absence of oxygen.

anaerobic exercise, any short-duration exercise that is powered primarily by metabolic pathways that do not use oxygen. Such pathways produce lactic acid, resulting in metabolic acidosis. Examples of anaerobic exercise include sprinting and heavy weight lifting. Compare **aerobic exercise.** See also **active exercise, passive exercise.**

anaerobic infection, an infection caused by an anaerobic organism such as *Clostridium,* usually occurring in deep puncture wounds that exclude air or in tissue that has diminished oxygen-reduction potential as a result of trauma, necrosis, or overgrowth of bacteria. This type of infection is characterized by abscess formation, foul-smelling pustular materials, and tissue destruction. Kinds include **gangrene, tetanus.**

anaerobic myositis. See **gas gangrene.**

anaesthesia. See **anesthesia.**

anaesthetic. See **anesthetic.**

anaesthetist. See **anesthetist.**

anagen, the first phase of the hair cycle, during which synthesis of the hair takes place.

anagrelide, an antiplatelet agent.

■ INDICATIONS: This drug is prescribed for essential thrombocythemia.

■ CONTRAINDICATIONS: Known hypersensitivity and hypotension prohibit its use.

■ ADVERSE EFFECTS: Life-threatening effects include congestive heart failure, myocardial infarction, myocardiopathy, cardiomegaly, complete heart block, atrial fibrillation, anemia, thrombocytopenia, ecchymosis, and lymphadenoma. Other serious effects include tachycardia, palpitations, arrhythmia, and seizures. Common side effects include orthostatic hypotension and rash.

anakhré /ah-nah-krā′/ [Fr, from native West African name]. See **goundou.**

anakinra, an antirheumatic agent and immunomodulator used to reduce the signs and symptoms of moderate to severe active rheumatoid arthritis in adults.

anal, pertaining to the anus.

anal agenesis, (*Obsolete*) now called **imperforate anus.**

anal canal, the final portion of the digestive tract, about 4 cm long, between the rectum and the anus.

anal character, (in psychoanalysis) a type of personality exhibiting patterns of behavior originating in the anal stage of childhood. It is characterized by extreme orderliness, obstinacy, perfectionism, cleanliness, punctuality, and miserliness, or their extreme opposites. Also called **anal personality.**

anal column, the highly vascular longitudinal folds of the anal canal in which the hemorrhoidal blood vessels are found.

anal crypt, the depression between rectal columns that encloses networks of veins that, when inflamed, are called hemorrhoids.

anal cryptitis, an inflammation of the mucous membrane of the anal crypts.

analeptic. See **central nervous system stimulant.**

anal eroticism, (in psychoanalysis) a libidinal fixation at or a regression to the anal stage of psychosexual development, often reflected as an anal character. Also called **anal eroticism.** Compare **oral eroticism.**

anal fissure, a painful linear ulceration or laceration of the skin at the margin of the anus. Also called **fissure-in-ano.**

anal fistula, an abnormal opening on the cutaneous surface near the anus, usually resulting from a local abscess of the crypt and common in Crohn's disease. A perianal fistula may or may not communicate with the rectum. Also called **fistula-in-ano.**

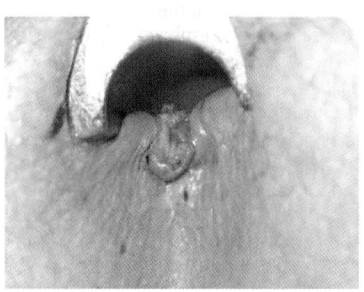

Anal fistula *(Herzig and Lu, 2010)*

anal fold, a slight elevation flanking the cloacal membrane and derived from a cloacal fold; anal folds form the border of the anus.

analgesia /an′əljē″zē·ə/ [Gk, *a, algos,* without pain], a decreased or absent sensation of pain.

analgesic /an′əljē″zik/, **1.** relieving pain. **2.** a drug that relieves pain. The opioid analgesics act on the central nervous system and alter the patient's perception; they are more often used for severe pain. The nonopioid analgesics act primarily at the periphery, do not produce tolerance or dependence, and do not alter the patient's perception; they are used for mild to moderate pain. Compare **anodyne.** See also **pain intervention.**

analgesic nephropathy [Gk, *a, algos,* without pain, *nephros,* kidney, *pathos,* disease], toxic damage to one or both kidneys resulting from the consumption of excessive amounts of nonsteroidal antiinflammatory drugs (NSAIDs) or similar analgesic medications.

analgia [Gk, *ana,* without, *algos,* pain], an absence of pain.

anal incontinence [L, *anus, incontinentia,* an inability to retain], the lack of voluntary control over fecal discharge.

anal membrane. See **cloacal membrane.**

anal membrane atresia, now called **imperforate anus.**

analog /an″əlog/ [Gk, *analogos,* proportionate], **1.** a substance, tissue, or organ that is similar in appearance or function to another but differs in origin or development, such as the eye of a fly and the eye of a human. **2.** a drug or other chemical compound that resembles another in structure or constituents but has different effects. Also spelled **analogue.** Compare **homolog.** −**analogous,** *adj.* **3.** (in computer processing) a continuous waveform that has varying amplitude to transmit electrical signals. Compare **digital.**

analogous /ənal″əgəs/ [Gk, *analogos*], something that is similar to a degree in function or form but different in structure or origin.

analog signal, a continuous electric waveform representing a specific condition, such as temperature, electrocardiogram waveforms, telephones, or computer modems.

analog-to-digital (A/D) converter, a device for converting analog information, such as temperature or electrocardiographic waveforms, into digital form for processing by a digital computer.

analogue, British spelling for analog. See **analog.**

anal orifice [L, *orificium,* an opening], **1.** the external opening at the end of the anal canal. **2.** the anus, surrounded by the anal sphincter muscle.

anal pecten, the corrugated epithelium within the anal transitional zone between the pectinate line and the anocutaneous line.

anal personality. See **anal character.**

anal phase. See **anal stage.**

anal plug, a mass of epithelial cells that temporarily occludes the anal canal in the embryo.

anal reflex, a superficial neurological reflex obtained by stroking the skin or mucosa of the region around the anus, which normally results in a contraction of the external anal sphincter. This reflex may be lost in disease of the pyramidal tract above the upper lumbar spine level (S3-S4). See also **superficial reflex.**

anal sadism, (in psychoanalysis) a sadistic form of anal eroticism, manifested by such behavior as aggressiveness and selfishness. Compare **oral sadism.**

anal sphincter, either of two sphincters (the internal and external anal sphincters) that open and close to control the evacuation of feces from the anus.

anal stage, (in psychoanalysis) the period in psychosexual development, occurring between 1 and 3 years of age, when preoccupation with the function of the bowel and the sensations associated with the anus are the predominant source of pleasurable stimulation. Adult patterns of behavior associated with fixation on this stage include extreme neatness, orderliness, cleanliness, perfectionism, and punctuality or their extreme opposites. Also called **anal phase.** See also **anal character, psychosexual development.**

anal stenosis, a rare complication associated with anorectal surgery in which the lumen of the bowel is narrowed. Mild stenosis can be managed with stool softeners and/or fiber supplements. Severe stenosis may require additional surgery.

anal verge [L, *anus* + *vergere,* to bend], the area between the anal canal and the perianal skin.

analysand /ənal″isand′/, a person undergoing psychoanalysis.

analysis /ənal″əsis/ [Gk, *ana* + *lyein,* to loosen], **1.** the separation into component parts. **2.** the separation of substances into their constituent parts and the determination of the nature, properties, and composition of compounds. See also **qualitative analysis, quantitative analysis. 3.** *(Informal)* psychoanalysis. **4.** (in occupational therapy) the process of determining the components or underlying parts that interact to allow individuals to complete daily activities; analysis includes a description of person, occupation, and environmental factors influencing one's ability to complete a desired activity. **5.** (in medical laboratory science) the determination of the composition, properties, activity, and quantity of selected substances. In most cases the substances are whole blood, plasma, or serum compounds named analytes. Analytes are assayed in an effort to predict, diagnose, and monitor the treatment of disorders. Analysis is usually quantitative, yielding binary (present versus absent) or continuous variables. −*analytic, adj.,* −**analyze,** *v.*

analysis of variance (ANOVA). See **ANOVA.**

analyst /an″əlist/, **1.** *(Informal)* a psychoanalyst. **2.** a person who analyzes the chemical, physical, or other properties of a substance or product.

analyte /an″əlīt/, a substance whose chemical constituents are being identified and measured. The term is usually applied to a component of blood or another body fluid.

analytic chemistry, a branch of chemistry that deals with identifying (qualitative chemistry) and measuring (quantitative chemistry) the components of chemical compounds or mixtures of compounds.

analytic psychology /an″əlit″ik/, **1.** the system in which phenomena such as sensations and feelings are analyzed and classified by introspective rather than by experimental methods. Compare **experimental psychology. 2.** a system of analyzing the psyche according to the concepts developed by Carl Gustav Jung. It differs from the psychoanalysis of Sigmund Freud in stressing a collective unconscious and a mystic, religious factor in the development of the personal unconscious while minimizing the role of sexual influence on early emotional and psychological development. Also called **Jungian psychology.**

analyze. See **analysis.**

analyzing /an″əlī″zing/, (in five-step nursing process) a category of nursing behavior in which the health care needs of the client are identified and the goals of care are defined. The nurse interprets data; identifies problems (nursing diagnoses) involving the patient, the patient's family, and significant others; defines goals and establishes priorities; integrates the information; and projects the expected outcomes of nursing interventions. Although analyzing follows assessing and precedes planning in the five steps of the nursing process, it is integral to effective nursing practice at all steps of the process. See also **assessing, evaluating, implementing, nursing process, planning.**

anamnesis /an″amnē″sis/ [Gk, *anamimneskein,* to recall], **1.** remembrance of the past. **2.** the accumulated data concerning a medical or psychiatric patient and the patient's background, including family, previous environment, experiences, and particularly, recollections, for use in analyzing his or her condition. Compare **catamnesis.**

anamnestic /an″amnes″tik/, **1.** pertaining to amnesia or memory. **2.** pertaining to the immunological memory and the immune response to an antigen to which immune cells have been exposed.

ANA-PAC, abbreviation for **American Nurses Association—Political Action Committee.**

anaphase /an″əfāz/ [Gk, *ana* + *phainein,* to appear], the third of four stages of division of the nucleus in mitosis and in each of the two divisions of meiosis. In anaphase of mitosis and of the second meiotic division, the centromeres divide, and the two chromatids, which are arranged along the equatorial plane of the spindle, separate and move to the opposite poles of the cell, forming daughter chromosomes. In anaphase of the first meiotic division, the pairs of homologous chromosomes separate from each other and move intact to the opposite poles of the cell. See also **cytokinesis, interphase, meiosis, metaphase, mitosis, prophase, telophase.**

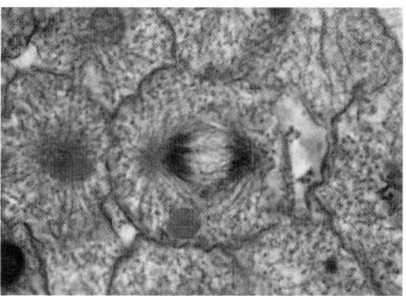

Anaphase *(© Ed Reschke; used with permission)*

anaphia /ənā″fē·ə/, an inability to perceive tactile stimuli.

anaphoresis, (in electrophoresis) the movement of anions in a solution or suspension toward the anode.

anaphylactic. See **anaphylaxis.**

anaphylactic hypersensitivity /an′əfilak″tik/ [Gk, *ana,* up, *phylaxis,* protection], an immediate, systemic hypersensitivity reaction to an exogenous antigen mediated by immunoglobulin E or G. It can be triggered by many substances, including drugs, especially penicillin and other antibiotics; foreign proteins used as therapeutic agents such as insulin, vaccines, allergen extracts, and muscle relaxants; insect venom, especially from bees, wasps, hornets, and fire ants; and certain foods such as shellfish, berries, chocolate, eggs, and nuts. Also called **type I hypersensitivity.** Compare **cytotoxic anaphylaxis, immunocomplex hypersensitivity.** See also **anaphylactic shock.**

anaphylactic reaction [Gk, *ana, phylaxis,* protection; L, *re, agere,* to act], an acute allergic response involving IgE-mediated, antigen-stimulated mast cell activation, resulting in histamine release. Exposure to the antigen may result in dyspnea, airway obstruction, shock, urticaria, and in some cases, death. Anaphylactic reactions may be caused by bee stings, foods, allergen extract, medications, or exercise. Rapid administration of subcutaneous epinephrine is the treatment of choice for severe reactions. Those with known allergies should wear a medical alert wristband. See also **anaphylactic shock.**

anaphylactic shock, a severe and sometimes fatal systemic allergic reaction to an allergen, such as a drug, vaccine, specific food, serum, allergen extract, insect venom, or chemical. This condition may occur within seconds to minutes from the time of exposure to the allergen and is commonly marked by respiratory distress and vascular collapse. The quicker the systemic atopic reaction in the individual after exposure, the more severe the associated shock is likely to be.

■ OBSERVATIONS: The first symptoms are intense anxiety, weakness, and a feeling of impending doom. Sweating and dyspnea may occur. These are followed, often quickly, by pruritus and urticaria. Other symptoms include hypotension, shock, arrhythmia, respiratory congestion, edema of the glottis, nausea, and diarrhea.

■ INTERVENTIONS: Treatment requires the immediate intramuscular or subcutaneous injection of epinephrine, The airway is maintained, and the patient is carefully monitored for signs of edema of the glottis, which may require the insertion of an endotracheal tube. The signs of edema of the glottis include stridor, hoarseness, and dyspnea. Cardiopulmonary resuscitation is indicated in cardiac arrest.

■ PATIENT CARE CONSIDERATIONS: Care requires appropriate emergency treatment and close monitoring for respiratory distress, hypotension, and decreased circulatory volume. Patients with a history of severe allergic reactions are instructed to avoid offending allergens; some patients must carry emergency anaphylaxis kits, such as an EpiPen Auto-Injector containing injectable epinephrine. Those with known allergies should wear a medical alert wristband.

anaphylactoid purpura. See **Henoch-Schönlein purpura.**

anaphylactoid syndrome of pregnancy, a quantity of amniotic fluid that enters the maternal blood system during labor and/or delivery, resulting in a systemic inflammatory response syndrome, causing vasospasm, pulmonary hypertension, myocardial damage, acute respiratory distress syndrome, and disseminated intravascular coagulation. It is estimated to occur in anywhere from 1 in 20,000 to 1 in 80,000 pregnancies, but it is a leading cause of maternal mortality. Formerly called **amniotic fluid embolism.**

anaphylatoxin /an′əfi′lətok″sin/, a fragment (C3a, C4a, or C5a) that is produced during the pathways of the complement system. Along with other mechanisms, it mediates changes in mast cells leading to the release of histamine and other immunoreactive or inflammatory reactive substances. If the degranulation of mast cells is too strong, it can cause allergic reactions.

anaphylaxis /an′əfilak″sis/ [Gk, *ana + phylaxis,* protection], an exaggerated, life-threatening hypersensitivity reaction to a previously encountered antigen. It is mediated by antibodies of the E or G class of immunoglobulins and results in the release of chemical mediators from mast cells. The reaction may consist of a localized wheal-and-flare reaction or generalized itching, hyperemia, angioedema, and in severe cases vascular collapse, bronchospasm, and shock. The severity of symptoms depends on the original sensitizing dose of the antigen, the number and distribution of antibodies, and the route of entry and dose of subsequently encountered antigen. Penicillin injection is the most common cause of anaphylactic shock. Insect stings, radiopaque contrast media containing iodide, aspirin, antitoxins prepared with animal sera, and allergens used in testing and desensitizing patients who are hypersensitive also produce anaphylaxis in some individuals. Kinds include **aggregate anaphylaxis, antiserum anaphylaxis, cutaneous anaphylaxis, cytotoxic anaphylaxis,** *indirect anaphylaxis, inverse anaphylaxis.* See also **anaphylactic reaction, anaphylactic shock.** –**anaphylactic,** *adj.*

■ OBSERVATIONS: Manifestations can range from mild to severe. Mild symptoms include mild nausea, anxiety, urticaria, itching, flushing, sneezing, nasal congestion, runny nose, cough, conjunctivitis, abdominal cramps, and tachycardia. Moderate reactions include a range of symptoms, including malaise; urticaria; pulmonary congestion, dyspnea, wheezing, and bronchospasm; hoarseness; edema of the periorbital tissue and/or tongue, larynx, and pharynx; dysphagia; nausea; vomiting; diarrhea; hypotension; syncope; and confusion. Severe anaphylaxis presents with pallor and cyanosis, stridor, airway obstruction, and hypoxia. If not treated immediately, respiratory arrest, cardiac arrhythmia, circulatory collapse, seizures, coma, and death rapidly ensue.

■ INTERVENTIONS: Treatment centers on immediate and aggressive management of emerging symptoms. Maintaining the airway and blood pressure is critical. Epinephrine and other drugs are used to counteract effects of mediator release and to block further mediator release. Vasoconstrictors are used to maintain blood pressure. Intubation or tracheostomy may be necessary to maintain an airway.

■ PATIENT CARE CONSIDERATIONS: The patient suffering an allergic reaction needs careful monitoring for signs of respiratory distress, hypotension, and decreased circulatory volume. Nursing interventions for anaphylactic shock center on the promotion of adequate ventilation and tissue perfusion. Airway needs are maintained, vital signs are monitored for hypotension, blood gases are monitored for acidosis, ECG is monitored for dysrhythmias, and fluid volume is replaced with IV solutions. Education about prevention of future attacks should include instruction in prophylaxis, such as avoiding known allergens, wearing a Medic Alert bracelet or necklace that identifies allergies, and ensuring that all medical records have allergies highlighted in a prominent place. Those with severe allergic reactions should consider carrying an anaphylaxis kit with preloaded epinephrine syringes.

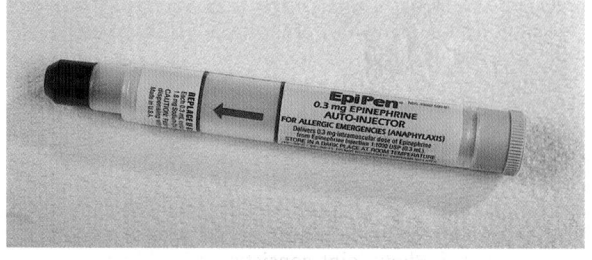

EpiPen used for anaphylaxis *(Bonewit-West, 2012)*

anaplasia /an′əplā″zhə/ [Gk, *ana* + *plassein,* to shape], a change in the structure and orientation of cells characterized by a loss of differentiation and reversion to a more primitive form. Anaplasia is characteristic of malignancy. Compare **aplasia.** −*anaplastic, adj.*

anaplastic astrocytoma. See **glioblastoma multiforme.**

anapnea /anap′nē·ə/ [Gk, *ana, pnoia,* breath], *(Obsolete)* restoration of breathing after a period of halted respiration.

anapophysis /an′ə·pof″i·sis/ [Gk, *an,* not, without + *apophysis,* a growing away], a small accessory vertebral process, especially one on a thoracic or lumbar vertebra.

Anaprox, a nonsteroidal antiinflammatory drug. Brand name for *naproxen sodium.*

anarthria /anär″thrē·ə/ [Gk, *a, arthron,* not joint], a loss of control of the muscles of speech, resulting in the inability to articulate words. The condition is usually caused by damage to a central or peripheral motor nerve. Damage can occur as a result of stroke.

anasarca /an′əsär″kə/ [Gk, *ana* + *sarx,* flesh], severe generalized, massive edema. Anasarca often occurs in congestive heart failure, liver failure, or renal disease. See also **edema.** −*anasarcous, adj.*

anastomosis /ənas′tōmō″sis/ [Gk, *anastomoien,* to provide a mouth], **1.** a connection between two vessels. **2.** a surgical joining of two ducts, blood vessels, or bowel segments to allow flow from one to the other. A vascular anastomosis may be performed to bypass an aneurysm or a vascular or arterial occlusion. With the patient under anesthesia, a section of the greater saphenous vein or a synthetic prosthesis is grafted to the prepared vessels. Postoperative nursing care includes preventing tissue injury and wound infection. Lack of blood flow may allow the graft to close. Pulses distal to the anastomosis are evaluated frequently. Capillary refilling time and the color and temperature of the skin are checked. Prophylactic antibiotic therapy may be started within hours. Urinary output is monitored. Kinds include **end-to-end anastomosis, end-to-side anastomosis, side-to-side anastomosis.** See also **bypass.** −*anastomotic, adj.,* −*anastomose, v.*

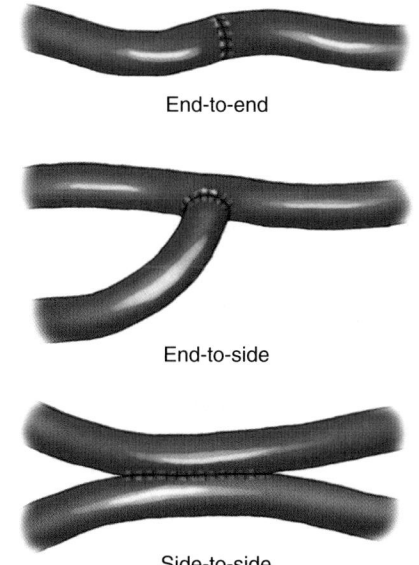

End-to-end

End-to-side

Side-to-side

Anastomosis *(LaFleur Brooks and LaFleur Brooks, 2014)*

anastomosis at elbow joint, a convergence of blood vessels at the elbow joint consisting of various veins and portions of the brachial and deep brachial arteries and their branches.

anastomotic, pertaining to a connection. See **anastomosis.**

anastrozole, a nonsteroidal aromatase inhibitor.
- INDICATIONS: It is prescribed in the treatment of advanced breast cancer for postmenopausal women whose disease has not responded to treatment with tamoxifen.
- CONTRAINDICATIONS: The drug is usually effective only in patients with estrogen-dependent tumors.
- ADVERSE EFFECTS: The side effects most often reported include hot flashes, diarrhea, fatigue, nausea, headache, and back pain.

anatomical, pertaining to anatomy or the structure of an organism. See **anatomy.**

anatomical age, the estimated age of an individual based on the stage of development or deterioration of the body as compared with that of other persons of the same chronological age.

anatomical crown, the portion of the dentin of a tooth that is covered by enamel. Compare **clinical crown.**

anatomical curve, the curvature of the different segments of the vertebral column. In the lateral contour of the back, the cervical and lumbar curves appear concave, and the thoracic and sacral curves appear convex.

anatomical dead space. See **dead space.**

anatomical height of contour, an imaginary line that encircles a tooth at the level of greatest circumference. Also called **surveyed height of contour.** See also **height of contour.**

anatomical incontinence, urinary incontinence associated with instability or excessive mobility of the bladder neck and adjacent urethra.

anatomical neck of the humerus [Gk, *ana,* up, *temnein,* to cut; AS, *hnecca;* L, *humerus,* shoulder], the portion of the humerus where there is a slight constriction adjoining the head.

anatomical pathology [Gk, *ana,* up, *temnein,* to cut, *pathos,* disease, *logos,* science], a medical specialty responsible for the examination of tissues and organs to assist in diagnosis of disease.

anatomical position, a standard position of the body: standing erect, facing directly forward, feet pointed forward and slightly apart, and arms hanging down at the sides with palms facing forward. This position is used as a reference to describe sites or motions of various parts of the body.

anatomical snuffbox, a small, cuplike depression on the back of the hand near the wrist formed by the three tendons reaching toward the thumb and index finger as the thumb is abducted and extended.

anatomical topography [Gk, *ana* + *temnein,* to cut, *topos,* place, *graphein,* to write], a system of identification of a body part in terms of the region in which it is located and its nearby structures.

anatomical zero joint position, the starting point of a joint range of motion.

anatomy /ənat″əmē/ [Gk, *ana* + *temnein,* to cut], **1.** the study, classification, and description of structures and organs of the body. **2.** the structure of an organism. Compare **physiology.** See also **applied anatomy, comparative anatomy, gross anatomy, microscopic anatomy, surface anatomy.** −*anatomical, adj.*

anatripsis /an′ətrip″sis/, a therapy that involves friction, usually neck, shoulder, and back therapeutic massage, with or without a simultaneous application of a medicine.

ANC, **1.** abbreviation for **absolute neutrophil count. 2.** abbreviation for **Army Nurse Corps.**

ANCA, abbreviation for *antineutrophil cytoplasmic antibody.*

-ance, a suffix changing a verb to a noun, as in *discontinuance.*

Ancef, a semisynthetic cephalosporin antibiotic. Brand name for **cefazolin sodium.**

ancestor [L, *antecessorem*], one from whom a person is descended, through the mother or the father. The term assumes a direct line of descent, excluding collateral family members of previous generations.

anchorage [Gk, *agkyra,* anchor], surgical fixation of a movable body part.

ancillary /an″səler′ē/ [L, *ancillaris,* handmaid], pertaining to something that is subordinate, auxiliary, or supplementary.

Ancobon, an antifungal. Brand name for **flucytosine.**

anconeus /angkō″nē-əs/ [Gk, *agkon,* elbow], one of seven superficial muscles of the posterior forearm. A small triangular muscle, it originates on the dorsal surface of the lateral condyle of the humerus and inserts in the olecranon. It functions to extend the forearm and abduct the ulna in pronation.

ancrod /ang″krod/, the venom of the Malayan pit viper, used to remove fibrinogen from the circulation to prevent or treat blood clotting.

-ancy, a suffix used to form nouns describing a quality: *buoyancy.*

ancylo-, ancyl-, anchyl-, anchylo-, ankylo-, ankyl-, combining forms meaning "bent or crooked, curved, stiff, fixed": *ancylostomiasis, ankylosis.*

Ancylostoma /ang′kilos″təmə/ [Gk, *angkylos,* crooked, *stoma,* mouth], a genus of nematode that is an intestinal parasite and causes hookworm disease. See also *Necator americanus.*

ancylostomiasis /an′səlos′təmī″əsis/, hookworm disease, more specifically that caused by *Ancylostoma duodenale, A. braziliense,* or *A. caninum.* Infection by *A. duodenale* is generally more harmful and less responsive to treatment than that by *Necator americanus,* which is the hookworm most often found in the southern United States. Larvae enter the host via the skin; the adult worm lives in the intestine. The adult worms abrade the intestinal wall, eventually causing severe anemia and debilitation. Heavy infection can cause serious health complications for pregnant women, neonates, children, and the malnourished. Clinical manifestations and treatment are similar for all types of hookworms. Infection may be prevented by eliminating fecal pollution of soil and by wearing shoes. See also **hookworm.**

Andersen disease [Dorothy Hansine Andersen, American pediatrician and pathologist, 1901–1963], a rare glycogen storage disease characterized by a genetic deficiency of branching enzyme (alpha-1:4, alpha-1:6 transglucosidase), causing the deposition in tissues of abnormal glycogen with long inner and outer chains. Also called **amylopectinosis, brancher glycogen storage disease, glycogen storage disease, type IV.**
■ OBSERVATIONS: Infants with the disease are not affected at birth but fail to thrive and soon show hepatomegaly, splenomegaly, and hypotonia of muscle associated with the progressive development of cirrhosis or heart failure of unknown mechanisms. Diagnosis is by enzyme assays of leukocytes and fibroblasts.
■ INTERVENTIONS: There is no specific therapy for the disease; treatment is directed toward control of symptoms. Liver transplantation may be an option for some individuals. Dietary measures to maintain normal blood sugar levels and to improve liver function and general overall nutrition should be employed.

■ PATIENT CARE CONSIDERATIONS: The coordinated effort of a team of health professionals, based on symptoms, is important to assist the patient and family to cope with the progressive nature of the disease. Genetic counseling should be considered.

Anderson Long Weighted Sump Tube, a weighted, mercury-free device for intestinal intubation and aspiration of gastrointestinal contents in patients with ileus and/or bowel obstructions.

Andersen-Tawil syndrome, a rare genetic disorder causing muscle weakness, arrhythmias, and developmental abnormalities.

Anderson-Hynes pyeloplasty, a surgical technique used in the management of pelvi-ureteric junction obstruction. See **dismembered pyeloplasty.**

Anderson triad syndrome, the presence of cystic fibrosis, celiac disease, and vitamin A deficiency.

-andr-, a combining form designating an androgen (steroid hormone) or characteristic of a male.

andreioma, androblastoma, now called **arrhenoblastoma.**

andro-, andr-, prefixes meaning "man or male": *androgen, androsterone.*

androgamone /an′drōgam″ōn/ [Gk, *andros,* man, *gamos,* marriage], a chemical secreted by male gametes that is believed to attract female gametes.

androgen /an″drəjin/ [Gk, *andros* + *genein,* to produce], any steroid hormone that increases male characteristics. Natural hormones, such as testosterone and its esters and analogs, are primarily used as substitution therapy. *—androgenic, adj.*

androgenetic alopecia, a common progressive, diffuse, symmetric loss of scalp hair. In men it begins in the 20s or early 30s with hair loss from the crown and the frontal and temple regions, ultimately leaving only a sparse peripheral rim of scalp hair (male pattern alopecia, often called male pattern baldness). In females it begins later, with less severe hair loss in the frontal area of the scalp. In affected areas, the follicles produce finer and lighter terminal hairs until terminal hair production ceases, with lengthening of the anagen phase and shortening of telogen of the hair cycle. The cause is unknown but is believed to be a combination of genetic factors and increased response of hair follicles to androgens. Additional medical conditions may be involved with hair loss. See also **male pattern alopecia.**

androgynous /androj″inəs/, **1.** (of a man or woman) having some characteristics of both sexes. Social role, behavior, personality, and appearance are reflections of individuality and are not determined by gender. **2.** hermaphroditic. Compare **gynandrous.** *—androgyny, n.*

android [Gk, *andros* + *eidos,* form], pertaining to something that is typically masculine, or manlike, such as an android pelvis.

android obesity, obesity in which fat is localized around the waist and in the upper body, most frequently seen in men and having a poorer prognosis for morbidity and mortality than the gynecoid type. Compare **gynecoid obesity.**

android pelvis, a type of pelvis with a structure characteristic of the male but not uncommon in women. The bones are thick and heavy, and the pelvic inlet is heart-shaped. The sacrum inclines anteriorly, the side walls are convergent, and the pubic arch is small. The diameters of the midplane and the pelvic outlet are smaller than in the normal gynecoid pelvis. Vaginal delivery is likely to be difficult unless the overall pelvis is large and the fetus is small. Compare **gynecoid pelvis.** See also **pelvis.**

andrology /androl″əjē/ [Gk, *andros,* man, *logos,* science], the study of the health of males; a medical specialty dealing with abnormalities associated with male reproductive and urological organs. Compare **gynecology.**

androma, *(Obsolete)* now called **arrhenoblastoma.**

andropause /an″drəpôs/, a change of life for males that may be expressed in terms of a career change, divorce, or reordering of life. It is associated with a decline in androgen levels that occurs in men during their late 40s or early 50s. Compare **menopause.**

androstenedione test, a blood test used to identify the presence of androstenedione, a precursor of testosterone; used for screening athletes to rule out the use of performance-enhancing drugs. It is also used to monitor ovarian and testicular malignancies and conditions associated with adrenocortical abnormalities.

androsterone /andros″tərōn/ [Gk, *andros + stereos,* solid], a byproduct of the breakdown of androgens excreted in the urine of both men and women but in higher amounts in men.

-ane, a suffix designating a saturated hydrocarbon of the methane series: *butane, propane.*

anecdotal /an″əkdot″əl/ [Gk, *anekdotos,* unpublished], pertaining to knowledge based on isolated observations and not yet verified by controlled scientific studies.

anecdotal record, a medical finding usually based on one or a few observed episodes of patient care, as distinguished from results compiled in a large-scale scientific or systematic study.

anechoic /an″ekō″ik/, (in ultrasonography) free of echoes; examples include a fluid-filled cyst.

Anectine, a depolarizing neuromuscular blocking agent. Brand name for **succinylcholine chloride.**

anejaculation, a failure of ejaculation of semen when the penis is stimulated by coitus or masturbation.

anemia /ənē″mē·ə/ [Gk, *a + haima,* without blood], inadequate tissue oxygenation. Usually caused by inadequate blood oxygen-carrying capacity. Anemia may be secondary to a decreased erythrocyte count, a decrease in quality hemoglobin to below the reference interval of 12 to 16 g/dL for women and 13.5 to 18 g/dL for men. Anemia may be caused by a decrease in erythrocyte production, an increase in erythrocyte destruction, or a loss of blood. A morphological classification system describes anemia by the hemoglobin content of the erythrocytes (normochromic or hypochromic) and by differences in erythrocyte size (macrocytic, normocytic, or microcytic). Any one of three tests (hemoglobin, hematocrit, or red blood cell count) can be used to diagnose anemia. See also **hemolytic anemia, hypoplastic anemia, iron-deficiency anemia, iron metabolism.**

■ OBSERVATIONS: Signs and symptoms include fatigue, exertional dyspnea, dizziness, headache, insomnia, pallor, confusion, or disorientation. Anorexia, dyspepsia, palpitations, tachycardia, cardiac dilation, and systolic murmurs also may occur. Iron deficiency is the most common cause. Additional laboratory studies may be required to establish the less common forms of anemia.

■ INTERVENTIONS: The therapeutic response to anemia is variable and depends on the causative factors. Moderate to severe anemia, with hemoglobin levels that are below 7 to 8 g/dL, may require transfusion of one or more units of packed red blood cells, especially if the condition is acute and specific clinical signs are present. Depending on the kind of anemia, treatment includes providing supplements of the deficient component, eliminating the cause of the blood loss, or alleviating the hemolytic component. The latter may involve administration of adrenal corticosteroids or splenectomy.

Appropriate laboratory tests are repeated at intervals to monitor the response and need for continued therapy. Erythropoietin injections may be used to stimulate erythrocyte production when anemia is secondary to chronic renal failure, the anemia of chronic disease, or chemotherapy.

-anemia, -anaemia, -nemia, suffixes meaning "(condition of) erythrocyte deficiency": *achlyanemia, melanemia.*

anemia of chronic disease, a decrease in the erythrocyte count as a result of a chronic inflammatory state.

anemia of pregnancy, an Hct <30% or Hgb <10g/dL. Physiologic anemia of pregnancy results from dilution because on average there is a 1000-mL increase in plasma volume and a 300-mL increase in red blood cell (RBC) volume. Iron-deficiency anemia is the most common nonphysiologic anemia of pregnancy because endogenous iron stores are insufficient to meet the increased iron requirements of pregnancy. Treatment is exogenous iron supplementation, generally 60 to 180 mg of elemental iron per day. Associated with anemia of pregnancy is a folate deficiency, which increases the risk of neural tube defects (NTDs). Treatment is exogenous folate of 0.4 to 1.0 mg/day.

anemic. See **anemia. −anemic,** *adj.*

anemic anoxia, a condition characterized by an oxygen deficiency in body tissues, resulting from a decrease in the number of erythrocytes or in the amount of hemoglobin in the blood.

anemic infarct, tissue necrosis from arterial occlusion. Also called **pale infarct, white infarct.**

anemo-, a prefix meaning "airflow" or "wind": *anemophobia.*

anencephalus /an″ən·sef′ə·ləs/, a fetus whose embryonic development proceeds with the lethal defect of an absence of a major portion of the brain and skull.

anencephaly /an″ensef″əlē/ [Gk, *a + encephalos,* without brain], a lethal neural tube defect in which absence of major portions of the brain and malformation of the brainstem occur. The cranium does not close, and the vertebral canal remains a groove. It is thought to be caused by a combination of genetic and environmental factors. It can be detected early in gestation by amniocentesis and analysis or by ultrasonography. See also **neural tube defect. −anencephalous,** *adj.*

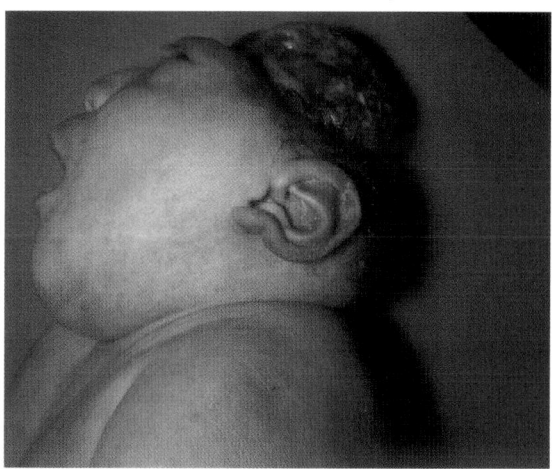

Infant with anencephaly *(Gilbert-Barness et al, 2007)*

anephric /ā·nef′rik/ [Gk, *a, nephros,* without kidney], without kidneys.

anephrogenesis /anef′rōjen″əsis/ [Gk, *a,* without, *nephros,* kidney, *genein,* to produce], the condition of being born without kidneys.

American Society of Anesthesiologists (ASA) physical status classification system

Classification	Definition	Adult examples
ASA I	A normal healthy patient.	Healthy, nonsmoking, no or minimal alcohol use.
ASA II	A patient with mild systemic disease.	Mild diseases only without substantive functional limitations. Examples include (but not limited to): current smoker, social alcohol drinker, pregnancy, obesity (30 < body mass index (BMI) < 40), well-controlled diabetes mellitus/hypertension, mild lung disease.
ASA III	A patient with severe systemic disease.	Substantive functional limitations; one or more moderate to severe diseases. Examples include (but not limited to): poorly controlled diabetes mellitus or hypertension, COPD, morbid obesity (BMI ≥40), active hepatitis, alcohol dependence or abuse, implanted pacemaker, moderate reduction of ejection fraction, end-stage renal disease (ESRD), undergoing regularly scheduled dialysis, premature infant postconceptional age <60 weeks, history (>3 months) of myocardial infarction (MI), cerebrovascular accident (CVA), transient ischemic attacks (TIA), or coronary artery disease (CAD)/stents.
ASA IV	A patient with severe systemic disease that is a constant threat to life.	Examples include (but not limited to): recent (<3 months) MI, CVA, TIA, or CAD/stents, ongoing cardiac ischemia or severe valve dysfunction, severe reduction of ejection fraction, sepsis, disseminated intravascular coagulation, acute respiratory distress, or ESRD not undergoing regularly scheduled dialysis.
ASA V	A moribund patient who is not expected to survive without the operation.	Examples include (but not limited to): ruptured abdominal/thoracic aneurysm, massive trauma, intracranial bleed with mass effect, ischemic bowel in the face of significant cardiac pathology or multiple organ/system dysfunction.
ASA VI	A declared brain-dead patient whose organs are being removed for donor purposes.	

Excerpted from *American Society of Anesthesiologists (ASA) physical status classification system* (Copyright © 2021) of the American Society of Anesthesiologists. A copy of the full text can be obtained from ASA, 1061 American Lane, Schaumburg, IL 60173-4973 or online at http://www.asahq.org.

anergia /ənur″jə/, **1.** a condition of lethargy or lack of physical activity. **2.** a diminished or absent sensitivity to commonly used test antigens.

aneroid /an″əroid/, relating to or denoting a barometer that measures air pressure by the action of the air in deforming the elastic lid of an evacuated box or chamber.

aneroid barometer, a device consisting of a flexible spring in a sealed, evacuated metal box that is used to measure atmospheric pressure. It is less accurate than a mercury barometer and is generally used for nonscientific work.

Anestacon, a local anesthetic jelly indicated for prevention and control of pain in procedures involving the male and female urethra, for topical treatment of painful urethritis, and as an anesthetic lubricant for endotracheal intubation (oral and nasal). Brand name for **lidocaine hydrochloride.**

anesthesia /an′esthē″zhə/ [Gk, *anaisthesia,* lack of feeling], the absence of all sensation, especially sensitivity to pain, as induced by an anesthetic substance, by hypnosis, or as occurs with traumatic or pathological damage to nerve tissue. Anesthesia induced for medical or surgical purposes may be topical, local, regional, sedation, or general and is named for the anesthetic technique or method. Also spelled **anaesthesia. −anesthetize,** *v.*

anesthesia machine, an apparatus for administering inhalation anesthetic gases and vapors and for controlling ventilation. Although there are many different models, all have the following features: a delivery system for medical gases, a flowmeter to measure fresh gas flow (such as medical air, oxygen, nitrous oxide), vaporizers for volatilizing and combining the anesthetic agents with oxygen and other carrier gases such as medical air and nitrous oxide, a circuit for delivering the gas to and from the patient, monitoring equipment or gauges, a ventilator, and a scavenging system to collect and discharge excess waste gas. It has multiple systems for detecting and alerting clinicians to potentially dangerous conditions.

anesthesia patients, classification of, a system developed by the American Society of Anesthesiologists (ASA) used to classify patients within six categories defined by physical health status, regardless of whether the health problems are related to the condition requiring anesthesia.

anesthesia screen, a metal frame on upright poles that is used to suspend a sterile barrier separating the surgical field from the anesthetist's access to the patient. Also called **ether screen.**

anesthesia technician, an operating-area employee who is skilled and knowledgeable in the supply and maintenance of anesthesiology-related materials and equipment.

anesthesiologist /an′əsthē′zē·ol″əjist/, a physician with an M.D., D.O., or equivalent degree from an accredited school of medicine who completes an accredited residency program in anesthesiology. Anesthesiologists may administer anesthesia directly or as part of an anesthesia team with certified registered nurse anesthetists and/or anesthesiologist assistants. Compare **nurse anesthetist.**

anesthesiologist assistant (AA), physician extenders who perform under the oversight of physician anesthesiologists to provide safe anesthesia care. Certification is granted by the National Commission for Certification of Anesthesiologist Assistants following the completion of an accredited graduate-level program and successful completion of the certification examination. Duties include the delivery and maintenance of quality anesthesia care, as well as advanced patient monitoring techniques. The exact details regarding delegation and licensing of anesthesiologist assistants differ from state to state and are regulated by the Board of Medicine and state statutes or regulations. Anesthesiologist assistants are defined as nonphysician anesthetists within the Centers for Medicare & Medicaid Services section of the Code of Federal Regulations. They may practice at any Veterans Affairs facility in the United States.

anesthesiology /-ol″əjē/, the branch of medicine that is concerned with the study and practice of anesthesia. It is a specialty requiring competency in general medicine, a broad understanding of surgical procedures, and a comprehensive knowledge of clinical obstetrics, chest medicine, neurology, pediatrics, pharmacology, biochemistry, cardiology, cardiovascular physiology, and respiratory physiology. See also **anesthesiologist, certified registered nurse anesthetist.**

anesthetic, a drug, gas, or other agent used to abolish the sensation of pain, to achieve adequate muscle relaxation during

A

Types of anesthesia

Type	Expected result	Method of administration	Risks
Local	Blocked sensation from peripheral nerves Blocked conduction of pain impulses in peripheral nerves	Administration of anesthetic agent to specific area of body by topical application or local infiltration	Allergic reaction Toxicity Cardiac or respiratory arrest Anxiety resulting from patient's "awake" state Infection
Regional			
■ Spinal	Analgesia Anesthesia Muscle relaxation	Anesthetic agent injected into cerebrospinal fluid (CSF) in subarachnoid space	Hypotension Total spinal anesthesia (inadvertent high level of spinal anesthesia, causing respiratory arrest and complete paralysis) Neurologic complications (tinnitus, arachnoiditis, meningitis, hematoma, paresthesias, bowel/bladder dysfunction, paralysis) Headache Infection
■ Epidural	Analgesia Anesthesia Muscle relaxation	Anesthetic agent injected into epidural space	Dural puncture Intravascular injection with possible convulsions, hypotension, cardiac arrest Hypotension Total spinal anesthesia Neurologic complications Hematoma Infection
■ Nerve block	Anesthesia of selected nerve	Local anesthetic injected around peripheral nerve	Inadvertent intravascular injection Nerve damage
■ Bier block	Anesthesia of extremity (usually used on upper extremity)	Anesthetic agent injected into veins of arm or leg while using pneumatic tourniquet	Infection Pain from tourniquet Overdose or toxicity of anesthetic agent
Minimal sedation	Sedation Anxiolysis Respiratory and cardiac function unaffected	Intravenous	Potential for impaired cognitive function and coordination
Moderate sedation and analgesia	Ability to maintain independent cardiorespiratory function Decreased level of consciousness Ability for purposeful responses to verbal and tactile stimuli Sedation Analgesia Amnesia Anxiolysis Rapid, safe return to activities of daily living	Intravenous May or may not have anesthesia provider in attendance Registered nurse often responsible for patient monitoring	Oversedation Respiratory depression, apnea Airway obstruction Hypotension Aspiration
Deep sedation and analgesia	Depressed consciousness Ability to respond purposefully after repeated or painful stimulation	Intravenous	Airway obstruction Inability to maintain spontaneous ventilation May require ventilatory support
General	Reversible unconsciousness Analgesia Anesthesia Amnesia Muscle relaxation (immobility) Depression of reflexes	Inhalation Intravenous	Oral or dental injury Cardiac or respiratory arrest Residual muscle paralysis Hypertension Hypotension Hypothermia Hyperthermia Renal dysfunction Neurologic dysfunction

Adapted from Monahan FD et al: *Phipps' medical-surgical nursing: health and illness perspectives,* ed 8, St Louis, 2007, Mosby.

surgery, to calm fear and allay anxiety, and to produce amnesia for the event.

anesthetist /ənes″thətist/, a general term used to describe a health care professional trained to administer anesthesia. Also spelled **anaesthetist.** See **anesthesiologist assistant, anesthesiologist, certified registered nurse anesthetist.**

anesthetize, to induce a lack of feeling or sensation. See **anesthesia.**

anetoderma /an′ətōdur″mə/ [Gk, *anetos,* relaxed, *derma,* skin], an idiopathic clinical change produced by focal damage to elastin fibers that results in loose/lax skin. Can occur as a primary defect or can be related to an underlying skin condition. There is no known effective treatment.

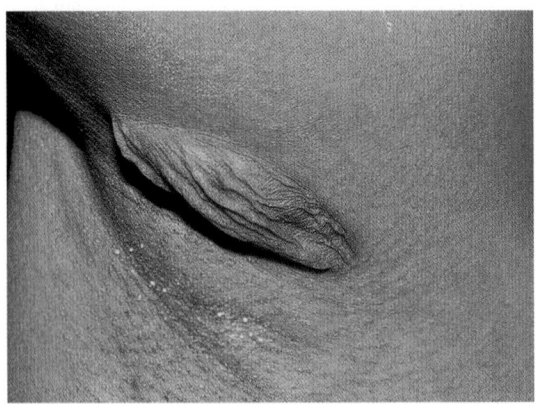

Anetoderma *(White and Cox, 2006)*

aneuploid /an″yo͞oploid/ [Gk, *a, eu,* not good, *ploos,* fold, *eidos,* form], **1.** an individual, organism, strain, or cell that has a chromosome number that is not an exact multiple of the haploid number characteristic of the species. **2.** also aneuploidic, pertaining to such an individual, organism, strain, or cell. Compare **euploid.** See also **monosomy, trisomy.**

aneuploidy /an″yo͞oploi′dē/, **1.** any variation in chromosome number that involves individual chromosomes rather than entire sets of chromosomes. There may be fewer chromosomes, as in Turner's syndrome (one X chromosome in females), or more chromosomes, as in Down syndrome (three copies of chromosome 21). Such individuals have various abnormal physiological and morphological traits. Compare **euploidy.** See also **chromosomal aberration, monosomy, trisomy. 2.** a phenomenon when the number of chromosomes in an individual, cell, or strain is not an exact multiple of haploid number characteristic of the species.

aneurysm /an″yo͞oriz′əm/ [Gk, *aneurysma,* widening], a localized dilation of the wall of a blood vessel. It may be caused by atherosclerosis and hypertension, or less frequently, by trauma, infection, or a congenital weakness in the vessel wall. Aneurysms are common in the aorta but also occur in peripheral vessels, especially in the popliteal arteries of older people. A sign of a large arterial aneurysm is a pulsating swelling that produces a blowing murmur on auscultation. Small aneurysms may produce no sound at all. An aneurysm may rupture, causing hemorrhage, or thrombi may form in the dilation and give rise to emboli that may obstruct smaller vessels. Aneurysms are usually named by the area in which they occur. Also called **vascular tumor.** Kinds include **abdominal aortic aneurysm, berry aneurysm, racemose aneurysm, compound aneurysm, fusiform aneurysm.** See also **pseudoaneurysm.** –*aneurysmal, adj.*

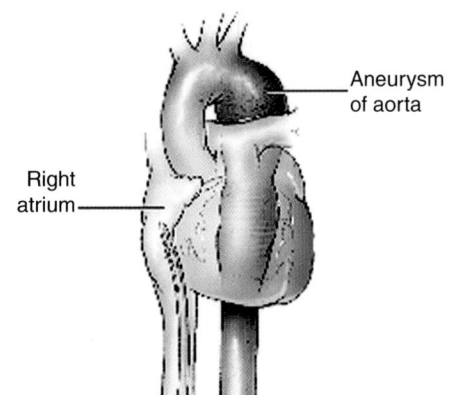

Aneurysm *(Doty, 2012)*

aneurysmal bone cyst, a cystic lesion that tends to develop in the metaphyseal region of long bones but may occur in any bone, including a vertebra. It may produce pain and swelling and generally increases in size gradually. Skin temperature around the bone may increase. It is usually removed surgically, but radiation may be used in cases when the tumor is not readily accessible.

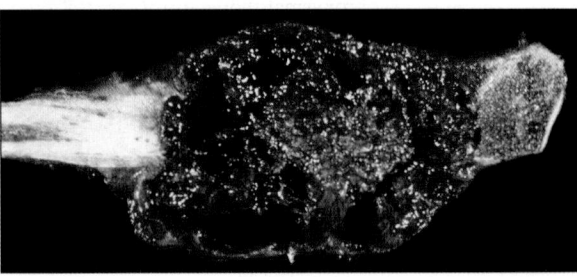

Aneurysmal bone cyst involving the proximal fibula
(Silverberg et al, 2006)

aneurysmal thrill, a vibration that can be felt over an aneurysm. In arterial aneurysms, the vibration is felt only in systole, but in arteriovenous aneurysms, it is felt during both systole and diastole.

aneurysmal varix [Gk, *aneurysma,* a widening; L, *varix,* a dilated vein], a varicose vein in which the enlargement is due to an acquired communication with an adjacent artery. Also called *aneurysmoid varix.*

aneurysmectomy, the surgical removal of an aneurysm.

aneurysm needle, a curved surgical apparatus equipped with a handle and eye at the point, used to ligate aneurysms.

ANF, abbreviation for *American Nurses Foundation.*

angel dust, *(Slang)* See **phencyclidine hydrochloride.**

angelica, an herb that belongs to the parsley family and is grown in cool northern climates.

■ INDICATIONS: Angelica is possibly safe and effective when prepared as a tea for the treatment of heartburn, colic, poor blood flow to the extremities, bronchitis, poor appetite, psoriasis, and vitiligo. It is also used to flavor alcoholic liqueurs and as an antiseptic.

■ CONTRAINDICATIONS: It contains furocoumarin derivatives, which make it unsafe for oral use or in extracts. Angelica should not be used during pregnancy and lactation or in children; it should be used only with caution in people with diabetes or bleeding disorders.

A

Angelman syndrome /ān′jəl·mən/, [Harry Angelman, English physician, 1915–1996], an autosomal-recessive syndrome characterized by jerky puppetlike movements, frequent laughter, cognitive impairment and delayed motor development, a peculiar open-mouthed facial expression, and seizures. It can be caused by a deletion on chromosome 15 inherited from the mother; the same deletion inherited from the father causes Prader-Willi syndrome.

anger [L, *angere,* to hurt], an emotional reaction characterized by extreme displeasure, rage, indignation, or hostility. It is considered to be of pathological origin when such a response does not realistically reflect a person's actual circumstances. However, expressions of anger vary widely in different individuals and cultures and may be considered functional under certain controlled circumstances.

angi-, a prefix meaning "blood."

angiitis /anjē·ī′tis/ [Gk, *angeion,* vessel, *itis*], an inflammation of a vessel, chiefly a blood or lymph vessel. See also **vasculitis.**

angina /anjī″nə, an″jinə/ [L, *angor, quinsy* (strangling)], **1.** a spasmodic, cramplike choking feeling resulting from insufficient oxygen supply to the myocardium, commonly caused by coronary artery disease. See **angina pectoris. 2.** characterized by a feeling of choking, suffocation, or crushing pressure and pain. Kinds include **decubitus angina, preinfarction angina, intestinal angina.**

angina pectoris, a paroxysmal thoracic pain caused most often by myocardial anoxia as a result of atherosclerosis or spasm of the coronary arteries. The pain usually radiates along the neck, jaw, and shoulder and down the inner aspect of the left arm. It is frequently accompanied by a feeling of suffocation and impending death. Attacks of angina pectoris are often related to exertion, emotional stress, eating, and exposure to intense cold, but unstable angina can occur in the absence of a stimulus or exertion. The pain may be relieved by rest and vasodilation of the coronary arteries by medication, such as nitroglycerin. Also called **cardiac pain.**

■ OBSERVATIONS: The chief symptom of stable angina is a highly variable, transient, substernal pain that typically starts with physical or emotional exertion and subsides with rest. It may range from a vague ache to an intense crushing sensation. Radiation to the left shoulder, arm, or jaw or to the back is common but does not occur in all cases. Attacks are exacerbated by cold. The most severe class of angina is a constant pain even at rest. Symptom patterns tend to be consistent and stable for a given individual. Any change in symptom patterns, such as an increase in attack frequency or intensity, should be viewed as serious. Such changes are known as unstable angina and are associated with the deterioration of atherosclerotic plaque. The pain in unstable angina is frequently not fully relieved by rest. Unstable angina is often a precursor to myocardial infarction. Tests include a stress test to deliberately induce an angina attack and check for electrocardiographic (ECG) changes. A test dose of nitroglycerin is administered to evaluate the degree of pain relief. Serum lipid and cardiac enzyme levels are evaluated to screen for cardiac risk factors. Nuclear scanning, angiography, and PET may be indicated to check myocardial perfusion and determine the presence of underlying coronary artery disease (CAD).
■ INTERVENTIONS: The first line of treatment is aggressive modification of risk factors, such as smoking, obesity, physical inactivity, elevated lipid levels, and elevated blood pressure. Drug therapy focuses on the prevention of myocardial insufficiency and pain relief and includes nitrates, beta-blockers, and calcium channel blockers. Prophylactic aspirin and statins are given for individuals with known CAD, and aspirin and heparin are used to treat intracoronary

blood clotting in unstable angina and to prevent progression to myocardial infarction. Coronary artery bypass is used for selected individuals with severe angina, localized CAD, no history of MI, and good ventricular function. Percutaneous coronary intervention may be emergently performed to compress plaque, and a stent may be placed to keep the coronary artery open. Angioplasty may be used to remove obstructive atherosclerotic lesions. Unstable angina necessitates immediate hospitalization, bed rest, and ECG monitoring for possible MI.
■ PATIENT CARE CONSIDERATIONS: The individual should be able to recognize and report symptoms of unstable angina. Nursing intervention during an acute attack is aimed at maintaining adequate tissue perfusion and relieving pain, including assessment and monitoring of vital signs and ECG patterns, auscultation of heart and lung sounds, administration of oxygen, and prompt administration of nitrates and narcotic analgesics as needed. Rest and cessation of all activity should occur until pain subsides. The nurse should provide comfortable positioning, and supportive calm reassurance to reduce anxiety. Patient education is tailored to the individual's symptom set and includes identification of precipitating factors and education to prevent or control those factors. The health care team plays a large role in reducing risk behaviors through smoking-cessation protocols, dietary modification (low-fat, low-sodium diet with complex carbohydrates and fruits), consistent aerobic exercise routines (three to four times weekly for at least 30 minutes), and stress-reduction activities. Education about medication effects and side effects is essential.

angina sine dolore /sē″nə dolôr″ə, sī″nē/, (*Obsolete*) a painless episode of coronary insufficiency. It is associated with diabetes mellitus. Now called **silent ischemia.**

angina trachealis. See **croup.**

angio-, angei-, angi-, combining forms meaning "a vessel, usually a blood vessel": *angioblastic, angiitis.*

angioblast /an′jēō·blast′/ [Gk, *angeion,* vessel + *blastos,* germ], **1.** the mesenchymal tissue of the embryo from which the blood cells and blood vessels differentiate. **2.** an individual vessel-forming cell.

angioblastic cord /an′jē·ōblas″tik/, any of the cordlike masses of splanchnic mesenchymal cells ventral to the primordial coelom. Angioblastic cords arrange themselves side by side to form the primordia of the endocardial tubes. Also called **angiogenic cell cluster.**

angioblastic meningioma, a tumor of the blood vessels of the meninges covering the spinal cord or the brain.

angioblastoma /an″jē·ōblastō″mə/ *pl.* angioblastomas, angioblastomata [Gk, *angeion,* vessel, *blastos,* germ, *oma*], a tumor of blood vessels in the brain. Kinds include **angioblastic meningioma, cerebellar angioblastoma.**

angiocardiogram /an′jē·ōkär″dē·ōgram′/, a radiographic image made during cardiac catheterization or coronary arteriography.

angiocardiography /-kär′dē·og″rəfē/ [Gk, *angeion* + *kardia,* heart, *graphein,* to record], the process of producing a series of radiographic images of the heart and its great vessels. A radiopaque contrast medium is injected through a catheter that is introduced through the femoral or radial artery. X-ray images are taken as the contrast medium passes through the heart and great vessels. Also called **cardiac angiography, angiography, cardiac catheterization.**

angiocatheter /an′jē·ōkath″ətər/, a hollow, flexible tube inserted into a blood vessel to withdraw or instill fluids.

angiochondroma /an′jē·ōkondrō″mə/ *pl.* angiochondromas, angiochondromata [Gk, *angeion* + *chondros,* cartilage, *oma*], a cartilaginous tumor characterized by an excessive formation of blood vessels.

angioedema /anˊjē·ō′idēʺmə/, a dermal, subcutaneous, or submucosal swelling that is acute, painless, and of short duration. It may involve the face, neck, lips, larynx, hands, feet, genitalia, or viscera. Angioedema may be hereditary or the result of a food or drug allergy, an infection, emotional stress, or a reaction to blood products. Treatment depends on the cause. Severe angioedema may require subcutaneous injections of epinephrine, intubation, or tracheotomy to prevent respiratory obstruction. Prevention depends on the identification and avoidance of causative factors. Also called **angioneurotic edema**. See also **anaphylaxis, serum sickness, urticaria.**

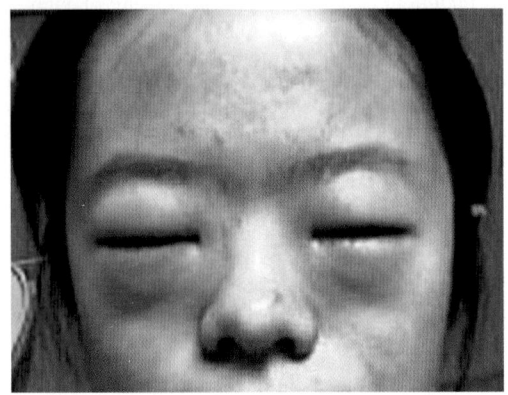

Individual with angioedema *(Limsuwan and Demoly, 2010)*

angioendothelioma, *(Obsolete)* now called **hemangioendothelioma.**

angiofibroma /anˊjē·ōfîbrō″mə/ *pl.* *angiofibromas, angiofibromata* [Gk, *angeion* + L, *fibra,* fiber; Gk, *oma*], an angioma containing fibrous tissue. Also called **fibroangioma, telangiectatic fibroma.**

angiogenesis /anˊjē·ōjen″əsis/ [Gk, *angeion* + *genesis,* origin], the formation of new blood vessels, a process controlled by chemicals produced in the body that stimulate blood vessels or form new ones. Angiogenesis plays an important role in the growth and spread of cancer. Angiogenesis also occurs in the healthy body for healing of wounds and restoring blood flow to tissues after injury.

angiogenesis inhibitor, a substance that blocks the formation of new blood vessels; particular useful in cancer.

angiogenic cell cluster. See **angioblastic cord.**

angiogenin /anˊjē·ōjen″in/, a protein that mediates the formation of blood vessels. A single-chain basic protein cloned from molecules of the tumor angiogenesis factor (TAF) in human colon cancer cells, angiogenin is used experimentally to stimulate the development of new blood vessels.

angioglioma /anˊjē·ōglē·ō″mə/ *pl.* *angiogliomas, angiogliomata* [Gk, *angeion* + *glia,* glue, *oma,* tumor], a highly vascular tumor composed of neuroglia.

angiogram /anʺjē·əgram/ [Gk, *angeion,* vessel, *gramma,* writing], the detailed radiographic images that highlight blood flow through a blood vessel after injection of a radiopaque contrast medium to demonstrate abnormalities such as blood clots or aneurysms. See also **arteriogram, phlebogram.**

angiograph /anʺjē·əgraf/ [Gk, *angeion,* vessel, *graphein,* to record], an instrument that records the patterns of pulse waves inside blood vessels. See also **sphygmograph.**

angiography /anˊjē·og″rəfē/ [Gk, *angeion* + *graphein,* to record], the x-ray visualization of the internal anatomy of the heart and blood vessels after the intravascular introduction of radiopaque contrast medium. The procedure is used as a diagnostic aid. The contrast medium may be injected into an artery or vein or introduced into a catheter inserted in a central or peripheral artery and threaded through the vessel to a visceral site. Because iodinated contrast agents are nephrotoxic, renal function also must be determined before angiography. After the procedure the patient is monitored for signs of bleeding at the puncture site, and bed rest for a number of hours is indicated. *–angiographic, adj.*

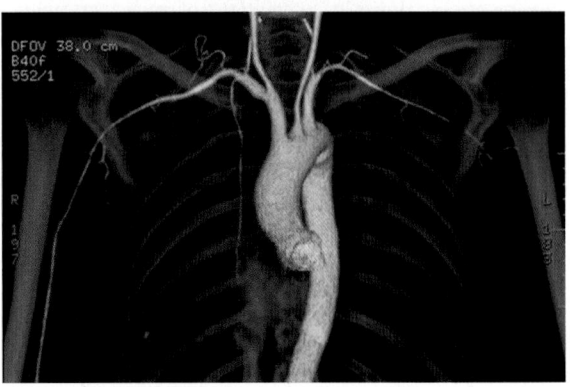

Angiography *(Cronenwett and Johnston, 2014)*

angiohemophilia. See **von Willebrand disease.**

angioimmunoblastic lymphadenopathy with dysproteinemia (AILD), now called **angioimmunoblastic T-cell lymphoma.**

angioimmunoblastic T-cell lymphoma (AITL), a rare, but aggressive systemic lymphoma of mature T cells involving deregulation of B cells and endothelial cells. Symptoms of angioimmunoblastic T-cell lymphoma (AITL) include fever, night sweats, and skin rash. As the disorder progresses, hepatosplenomegaly, hemolytic anemia, polyclonal hypergammaglobulinemia, and autoimmune disorders may develop. AITL accounts for 1% to 2% of all non-Hodgkins lymphoma cases in the United States.The Epstein-Barr virus (EBV) is observed in the majority of cases. Also called **immunoblastic lymphadenopathy, angioimmunoblastic lymphadenopathy with dysproteinemia.**

angiokeratoma /anʹjē·ōker′ətō″mə/ *pl.* *angiokeratomas, angiokeratomata* [Gk, *angeion* + *keras,* horn, *oma*], a benign, vascular neoplasm on the skin, characterized by clumps of dilated blood vessels and thickening of the epidermis, especially the scrotum and the dorsal aspect of the fingers and toes. Can occur as single or as multiple lesions of the vulva and scrotum.

angiokeratoma circumscriptum, a rare skin disorder characterized by discrete papules and nodules in small patches on the legs or on the trunk.

angiokeratoma corporis diffusum, a rare familial disease in which glycolipids are stored in many parts of the body, especially in the venous and cardiovascular systems, causing vasomotor, urinary, and cutaneous disorders and, in some cases, muscular abnormalities. Characteristic signs are dilation of blood vessels in the bathing suit areas; edema; hypertension; cardiomegaly, especially enlargement of the left ventricle; diffuse nodularity of the skin; albumin, erythrocytes, leukocytes, and casts in the urine; and vacuoles in muscle bundles. Also called **diffuse angiokeratoma, Fabry syndrome, Fabry disease.**

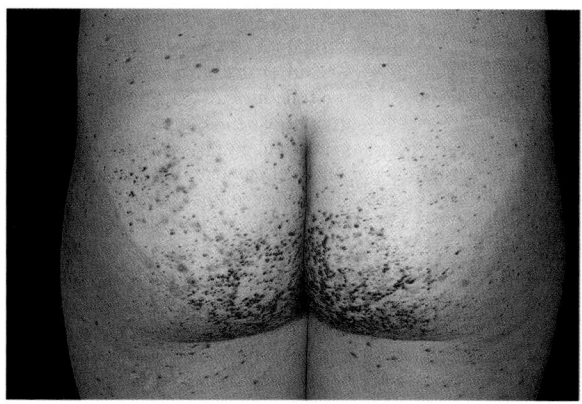

Angiokeratoma corporis diffusum *(Habif et al, 2011)*

angiokeratomas, angiokeratomata.   See **angiokeratoma.**

angiolipoma /an′jē·ōlipō″mə/ *pl.* *angiolipomas, angiolipomata* [Gk, *angeion* + *lipos,* fat, *oma*], a benign neoplasm containing blood vessels and tissue. Also called **lipoma cavernosum, telangiectatic lipoma.**

-angioma, suffix meaning a "tumor composed chiefly of blood and lymph vessels": *fibroangioma, glomangioma.*

angioma /an′jē·ō″mə/ *pl.* *angiomas, angiomata* [Gk, *angeion,* vessel + *oma,* tumor], any benign tumor with blood vessels (hemangioma) or lymph vessels (lymphangioma). Most angiomas are congenital; some, such as cavernous hemangiomas, may disappear spontaneously. Compare **angiosarcoma.**

angioma cavernosum.   See **cavernous hemangioma.**

angioma cutis, a nevus composed of a network of dilated blood vessels.

angioma lymphaticum.   See **lymphangioma.**

angioma serpiginosum /sərpij′inō″səm/ [Gk, *angeion* + *oma* + L, *serpere,* to creep], a cutaneous disease characterized by tiny vascular points, appearing as red dots in a serpentine or ring pattern.

angiomatosis /an′jē·ōmətō″sis/, a condition characterized by numerous vascular tumors.

angiomyoma /-mī·ō″mə/ *pl.* *angiomyomas, angiomyomata* [Gk, *angeion* + *mys,* muscle, *oma*], a tumor composed of vascular and muscular tissue elements.

angiomyoneuroma.   See **glomangioma.**

angiomyosarcoma /mī′ōsärkō″mə/ *pl.* *angiomyosarcomas, angiomyosarcomata* [Gk, *angeion* + *mys,* muscle, *sarx,* flesh, *oma*], a tumor containing vascular, muscular, and connective tissue elements.

angioneuroma.   See **glomangioma.**

angioneurotic anuria /-nŏŏrot″ik ənyŏŏr″ē·ə/ [Gk, *angeion* + *neuron,* nerve, *a* + *ouron,* not urine], an abnormal condition characterized by an almost complete absence of urine caused by destruction of tissue in the renal cortex.

angioneurotic edema, *(Obsolete)* now called **angioedema.**

angioneurotic gangrene [Gk, *angeion* + *neuron,* nerve, *gaggraina*], the death and putrefaction of tissue caused by an interruption of the blood supply resulting from thrombotic arteries or veins.

angiopathy /an′jē·op″əthē/ [Gk, *angeion,* vessel, *pathos,* disease], a disease of the blood vessels.

angioplasty /an″jēōplas′tē/ [Gk, *angeion,* vessel, *plassein,* to mold], the opening and restoration of blood vessels performed by inflating a balloon within the vessel lumen at the site of narrowing to reconstitute flow. See also **balloon angioplasty.**

angiopoiesis /-poi·ē″sis/ [Gk, *angeion,* vessel, *poien,* to make], the process of blood vessel formation.

angiorrhaphy /an′jē·ôr″əfē/ [Gk, *angeion,* vessel, *rhaphe,* suture], the repair by suture of any blood vessel.

angiosarcoma /-särkō″mə/, a rare, malignant tumor consisting of endothelial and fibroblastic tissue that proliferates and eventually surrounds vascular channels. It begins in the lining of the blood vessels. The condition usually occurs in older persons. Angiosarcoma has been associated with exposure to many foreign materials in the body, such as steel, shrapnel, and plastic. This tumor tends to be aggressive and recurs locally as well as metastasizing. Also called **hemangiosarcoma, malignant hemangioendothelioma.** Compare **angioma.**

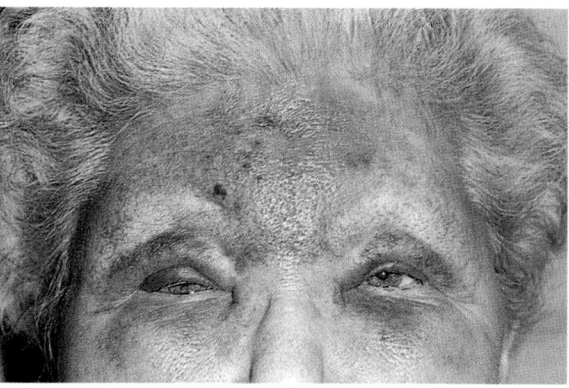

Individual with angiosarcoma *(Callen et al, 2000)*

angiosclerosis /-sklerō″sis/ [Gk, *angeion,* vessel, *skleros,* hard, *osis,* condition], a thickening and hardening of the walls of the blood vessels. See also **athetoid.**

angioscope /an″jē·əskōp/, a type of microscope attached to a small, flexible catheter that permits inspection of blood vessels.

angiospasm /an″jē·ōspaz′əm/, a sudden, transient constriction of a blood vessel. Also called **vasomotor spasm, vasospasm.** See also **vasoconstriction.**

angiostrongyliasis /an′jē·ō·stron′ji·lī′ə·sis/, infection by a species of *Angiostrongylus.* Infection comes after eating contaminated raw or insufficiently cooked hosts such as snails, slugs, prawns, or crabs. Most cases occur in Southeast Asia and the Pacific Basin. *A. costaricensis* causes abdominal or intestinal angiostrongyliasis. Abdominal cases have been reported in Costa Rica and occur most commonly in young children. *A. cantonensis* larvae migrate to the central nervous system and cause eosinophilic meningitis.

Angiostrongylus [Gk, *angeion,* vessel + *strongylos,* round], a genus of parasitic nematodes. Species *A. cantonensis* and *A. costaricensis* normally infect other animals but can cause angiostrongyliasis in humans.

angiotensin /-ten″sin/ [Gk, *angeion* + L, *tendere,* to stretch], a polypeptide in the blood that causes vasoconstriction, increased blood pressure, and the release of aldosterone from the adrenal cortex. Angiotensin is formed by the action of renin on angiotensinogen, an alpha$_2$-glycoprotein that is produced in the liver and that constantly circulates in the blood. Renin, stimulated by juxtaglomerular cells in the kidney in response to decreased blood volume and serum sodium levels, acts as an enzyme in the conversion of angiotensinogen to angiotensin I, which is rapidly hydrolyzed to form the active compound, angiotensin II. The vasoconstrictive action of angiotensin II decreases the glomerular filtration rate, and the concomitant action of aldosterone promotes sodium retention, with the result that blood volume and sodium reabsorption increase. Plasma angiotensin II increases during the luteal phase of the menstrual cycle and is probably responsible for an elevated level of aldosterone during that period. Angiotensin is inactivated by peptidases, called angiotensinases, in plasma and tissues.

angiotensin-converting enzyme (ACE), a glycoprotein (dipeptidyl carboxypeptidase) that catalyzes the conversion of angiotensin I to angiotensin II by splitting two terminal amino acids.

angiotensin-converting enzyme (ACE) inhibitor, a protease inhibitor found in serum that promotes vasodilation by blocking the formation of angiotensin II and slowing the degradation of bradykinin and other kinins. It decreases sodium retention, water retention, blood pressure, and heart size, treating heart failure by slowing changes to the ventricle.

angiotensin-converting enzyme (ACE) test, a serum or plasma test used to measure the activity of the enzyme that converts angiotensinogen into angiotensin. The test is primarily used to diagnose and monitor sarcoidosis.

angiotensinogen /-tensin″əjən/, a serum glycoprotein produced in the liver that is the precursor of angiotensin.

angle /ang″gəl/ [L, *angulus*], **1.** the space or the shape formed at the intersection of two lines, planes, or borders. The divergence of the lines, planes, or borders may be measured in degrees of a circle. **2.** (in anatomy and physiology) the geometric relationships between the surfaces of body structures and the positions affected by movement.

angle board, a device used in dentistry to establish reproducible angular relationships between a patient's head, the x-ray beam, the image receptor, and the x-ray film during dental imaging radiography.

angle-closure glaucoma. See **glaucoma.**

angle former, a hoe-shaped, paired dental instrument whose cutting edges are at an oblique angle to the axis of the blade. It is used to access angles and shape the dental restoration for a class III dental cavity preparation. Also called **bayonet angle former.**

angle of convergence, an angle formed between the visual axis of an eye focused on an object and a median line.

angle of incidence, 1. the measure of the deviation of the approach of a ray from the line perpendicular to the surface at the point of incidence. **2.** the angle at which an ultrasound beam hits the interface between two different types of tissues, such as the facing surfaces of bone and muscle. The angle is also affected by the difference in acoustic impedance of the different tissues.

angle of iris, the angle formed between the cornea and the iris at the periphery of the anterior chamber of the eye. The aqueous fluid normally drains through this angle, which may be blocked in glaucoma. Also called **filtration angle.**

angle of Louis [Pierre Charles Alexandre Louis, French physician, 1787–1872], the sternal angle between the manubrium and the body of the sternum.

angle of mandible, 1. anatomically, the region of the mandible where the inferior border of the mandible joins the posterior border of the ascending ramus. Also called **gonial angle. 2.** (in orthodontics) the measure in degrees of the relationship between the body and the ramus of the mandible. It is used in cephalometric measurements of skull radiographs.

angle of refraction [L, *refringere,* to break apart], the angle that a refracted ray of light makes with a line perpendicular to the refracting surface at the point of refraction. Also called **refracting angle.**

angle of Treitz /trīts/ [Wenzel Treitz, Czech physician, 1819–1872], a sharp curve or flexure at the junction of the duodenum and jejunum.

Angle's classification of malocclusion [Edward Hartley Angle, American orthodontist, 1855–1930], a classification of the various types of malocclusion. The classification is based on where the buccal groove of the mandibular first molar contacts the mesiobuccal cusp of the maxillary first molar: on the cusp (Class I, neutroclusion, or normal occlusion); distal to the cusp by at least the width of a premolar (Class II, distocclusion); or mesial to the cusp (Class III, mesioclusion). Each class contains two or more types or divisions. Also called **classification of malocclusion.**

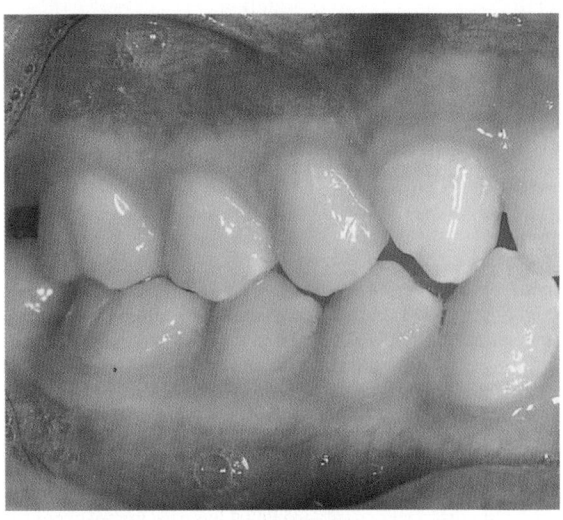

Angle's classification of malocclusion: Class I normal occlusion *(Courtesy Dr. Dona M. Seely, DDS, MSD, Orthodontics, Bellevue and Seattle, WA)*

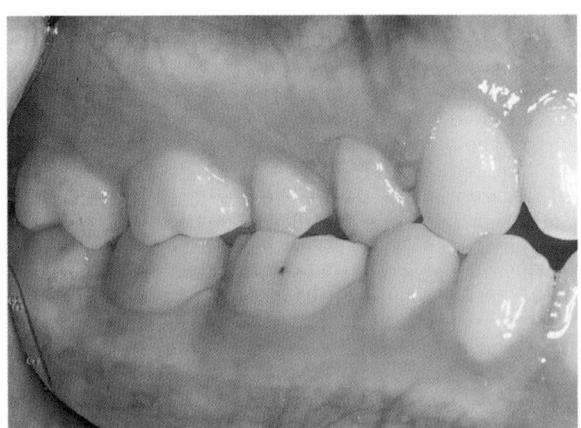

Angle's classification of malocclusion: Class III malocclusion *(Courtesy Dr. Dona M. Seely, DDS, MSD, Orthodontics, Bellevue and Seattle, WA)*

angor /ang″gôr/, a condition of extreme distress, usually occurring in intestinal or pectoral angina.

angstrom (Å) /ang″strəm/ [Anders Jonas Angström, Swedish physicist, 1814–1874], a unit of measure of length equal to 0.1 nanometer (1/10,000,000,000 meter), or 10^{-10} meter. Typically used to measure distances between atoms within molecules. Also called *angstrom unit.*

angular artery /ang′gu·lər är′tə·re/, a branch of the facial artery to the medial angle of the eye that supplies the lacrimal sac, lower eyelid, and nose.

angular cheilitis, angular cheilosis. See **perlèche.**

angular gyrus /ang″gyələr/ [L, *angulus* + Gk, *gyros*], a folded convolution in the inferior parietal lobe where it unites with the temporal lobe of the cerebral cortex.

angular movement [L, *angularis,* sharply bent], one of the four basic movements allowed by the various joints of the skeleton. It is a movement in which the angle between two adjoining bones is decreased, as in flexion, or increased, as in extension. Compare **circumduction, gliding, rotation.**

angular spinal curvature [L, *angulus* + *spina,* backbone, *curvatura,* bend], a sharp bending or sloping of the vertebral column. See also **gibbus deformity.**

angular stomatitis, superficial erosions and fissuring at the angles of the mouth. Also called **perlèche.**

angular vein, one of a pair of veins of the face, formed by the junction of the frontal and the supraorbital veins. At the root of the nose, each angular vein receives the flow of venous blood from the infraorbital, superior and inferior palpebral, and external nasal veins, becoming the first part of one of the two facial veins.

angulated fracture /ang″gyələ′tid/, a fracture in which the fragments of bone are at angles to one another.

angulation [L, *angulatus,* bent], **1.** an angular shape or formation. **2.** the discipline of precisely measuring angles, as in mechanical drafting and surveying. **3.** (in radiography) the direction of the useful beam of radiation in relation to the object being radiographed and the receptor used to record its image. See also **horizontal angulation, vertical angulation. 4.** the formation of a sharp obstructive angle, as in the intestines or ureters.

anhedonia /an′hēdō″nē·ə/ [Gk, *a* + *hedone,* not pleasure], the inability to feel pleasure or happiness in response to experiences that are ordinarily pleasurable. It is often a characteristic of major depression and schizophrenia. −**anhedonic,** *adj.*

anhidrosis /an′hidrō″sis, an′hī-/ [Gk, + without sweat], an abnormal condition characterized by inadequate perspiration.

anhidrotic /an′hidrot″ik, an′hī-/, **1.** pertaining to anhidrosis. **2.** an agent that reduces or suppresses perspiration.

anhidrotic ectodermal dysplasia, a congenital X-linked disorder fully expressed in males, or rarely an autosomal-recessive trait with full expression in both sexes, characterized by ectodermal dysplasia associated with aplasia or hypoplasia of the sudoriferous glands, hypothermia, alopecia, anodontia, conical teeth, and typical facies with frontal bossing, midfacial hypoplasia, saddle nose, large chin, and thick lips. Also called **Christ-Siemens-Touraine syndrome, congenital ectodermal defect, hypohidrotic ectodermal dysplasia, antihidrotic.**

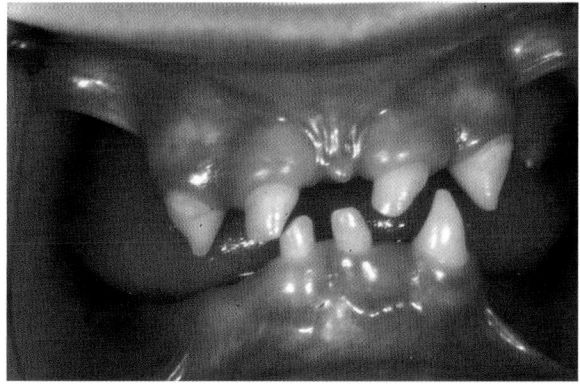

Anhidrotic ectodermal dysplasia *(Dean et al, 2011)*

anhydrase /anhī″drās/ [Gk, *a,* not + *hydor,* water], an enzyme that catalyzes the elimination of water molecules from certain compounds, as carbonic anhydrase dehydrates carbonic acid, thereby controlling the amount of carbon dioxide in the blood and lungs.

anhydride /anhī″drīd/ [Gk, *a* + *hydor,* without water], a chemical compound derived by the removal of water from one or more substances, especially an acid.

anhydrous /anhī″drəs/ [Gk, *a* + *hydor,* without water], an absence of water.

anicteric /an′ikter″ik/ [Gk, *a* + *icterus,* not jaundice], pertaining to the absence of jaundice (icterus).

anicteric hepatitis, a mild form of hepatitis in which there is no jaundice (icterus). Symptoms include anorexia, GI disturbances, and slight fever. Levels of aspartate aminotransferase and alanine aminotransferase are elevated. The infection may be mistaken for influenza or may be undetected. Compare **hepatitis.** See also **acute anicteric hepatitis.**

anideus /anid″ē·əs/, an anomalous, rudimentary embryo consisting of a simple rounded mass with little indication of the body parts. Also called **fetus anideus.** Kinds include **embryonic anideus.** −**anidian, anidous, anidean,** *adj.*

anidulafungin, a systemic antifungal agent.

■ INDICATIONS: This drug is used to treat *Candida albicans, C. glabrata, C. parapsilosis,* and *C. tropicalis.*

■ CONTRAINDICATIONS: Known hypersensitivity to this drug or other echinocandins prohibits its use.

■ ADVERSE EFFECTS: Common side effects include headache, nausea, anorexia, vomiting, diarrhea, rash, back pain, rigors, and increased aspartate aminotransferase and alanine aminotransferase. Adverse effects of this drug include dizziness, deep vein thrombosis, hypotension, hypokalemia, hypocalcemia, hyperglycemia, hyperkalemia, hypernatremia, and (rarely) hypomagnesemia. Life-threatening side effects include seizures, atrial fibrillation, right bundle branch block, sinus arrhythmia, thrombophlebitis, (rarely) superficial ventricular extra systoles, hepatic necrosis, neutropenia, thrombocytopenia, leukopenia, and coagulopathy.

aniline ($C_6H_5NH_2$) /an″ilēn/ [Ar, *alnil,* indigo], a toxic organic made synthetically. Its main use is in the manufacture of precursors to polyurethane and other industrial chemicals. Like most volatile amines, it has a characteristic foul odor. Industrial workers exposed to aniline are at risk of developing methemoglobinemia and bone marrow suppression. Also called **aminobenzene, benzenamine.**

aniline dye, a chemical used to color fabrics, wood, and leather. It may also be present in household items such as shoe polish. Aniline can be toxic if absorbed or ingested in large amounts. See **aniline.**

anilingus /ā′niling″gəs/, sexual stimulation of the anus by the tongue or lips.

anilism [Ar, *alnil,* indigo; Gk, *ismos,* state], a condition of poisoning resulting from exposure to aniline compounds. Symptoms generally include cyanosis, weakness, cold sweats, irregular pulse, breathing difficulty, coma, seizures, and possible sudden heart failure. See also **aniline.**

anima /an″imə/ [L, soul], **1.** the soul or life. **2.** the active ingredient in a drug. **3.** (in analytic psychology) a person's true inner unconscious being or personality. Compare **persona. 4.** (in analytic psychology) the female component of the male personality. Compare **animus.**

animal, a living organism that subsists on oxygen and the breakdown of organic substances taken into the body, usually by ingestion. Most animals are capable of voluntary movement.

animal-assisted therapy, 1. a therapeutic activity facilitated by occupational therapists with professionally trained animals in which the client interacts with the animal and the animal with the client to achieve identified goals. See also **sensory modulation. 2.** a goal-directed intervention provided by a health professional with specialized education in human interactions in which an animal is incorporated as a component of the treatment process.

animal control, actions safeguarding public health and safety related to the enforcement of animal-related local and national laws, statutes, and ordinances.

animal pole [L, *anima*], the active, formative part of an ovum. It contains the nucleus and the bulk of the cytoplasm and is the site where the polar bodies form. In mammals, the animal pole is also the site where the inner cell mass develops and gives rise to germ layers. Also called **germinal pole.** Compare **vegetal pole.**

animation, 1. the state of being alive. **2.** an ability to put into action a vivid appearance of life.

animus /an″iməs/ [L, spirit], **1.** the active or rational soul; the animating principle of life. **2.** (in analytic psychology) the male component of the female personality. Compare **anima. 3.** (in psychiatry) a deep-seated antagonism that is usually controlled but may erupt with virulence under stress.

anion /an″ī·ən/ [Gk, *ana + ion*, backward going], a negatively charged ion that is attracted to the positive electrode (anode) at which oxidation takes place in electrolysis. Compare **cation.** –*anionic, adj.*

anion-exchange resin, any one of the simple organic polymers with high molecular weights that exchange the resin anions with other anions in solution. Compare **cation-exchange resin.**

anion gap, the difference between the concentrations of serum or plasma cations and anions, determined by measuring the concentrations of sodium cations and chloride and bicarbonate anions. It is helpful in the diagnosis and treatment of acidosis, and it is estimated by subtracting the sum of chloride and bicarbonate concentrations in the plasma from that of sodium. It is normally about 8 to 14 mEq/L and represents the negative charges contributed to plasma by unmeasured ions or ions other than those of chloride and bicarbonate, mainly phosphate, sulfate, organic acids, and plasma proteins. Anions other than chloride and bicarbonate normally constitute about 12 mEq/L of the total anion concentration in plasma. Acidosis can develop with or without an associated anion increase. An increase in the anion gap often suggests diabetic ketoacidosis, drug poisoning, renal failure, or lactic acidosis and usually warrants further laboratory tests.

anion gap test, a calculation used to help identify the causes of metabolic acidosis, most of which are associated with an increased anion gap. The most commonly used formula is Anion Gap (AG) = Sodium – (Chloride + Bicarbonate [total CO_2]). See also **anion gap.**

aniridia /an″ī·rid′ē·ə/ [Gk, *a*, without + *iris*], an absence of the iris, a usually bilateral, hereditary anomaly.

anisakiasis /an″ī·sə·kī′ə·sis/, infection of humans or other animals with a nematode of the family Anisakidae, usually *Anisakis marina*. Human infection is usually caused by third-stage larvae eaten in sushi and undercooked infected marine fish such as herring. The larvae then burrow into the stomach wall, producing an eosinophilic granulomatous mass. Also called **eosinophilic granuloma.**

Anisakis /an″ī·sə′kis/ [Gk, *an*, not, without + *isos*, equal + *akis*, point], a genus of nematodes of the superfamily Ascaridoidea; species *A. marina* is the usual cause of human anisakiasis. Its organisms are found in the stomachs of marine animals and birds. Human infection occurs by ingestion of raw fish that contain larvae.

anise /an″is/, the fruit of the *Pimpinella anisum* plant. Extract of anise is used in the preparation of carminatives and expectorants.

aniseikonia /an″ī·sīkō″nē·ə/ [Gk, *anisos,* unequal, *eikon,* image], an abnormal ocular condition in which each eye perceives the same image as being of a different form and size.

anismus /ānis″məs/, an extreme contraction of the external anal sphincter. Clinical signs include constipation, perineal pain, and defecatory dysfunction.

aniso-, anis- /anī′sō-/, prefixes meaning "unequal, asymmetric, or dissimilar": *aniseikonia, anisognathy.*

anisocoria /-kôr″ē·ə/ [Gk, *anisos,* unequal, *kore,* pupil], an inequality of the diameter of the pupils of the two eyes.

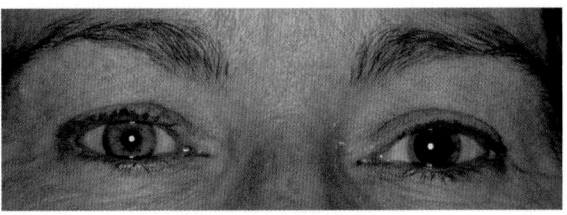

Anisocoria *(Lemmi and Lemmi, 2000)*

anisocytosis /anī′sōsītō″sis/ [Gk, *anisos + kytos,* cell], an abnormal condition of the erythrocytes characterized by variable diameter on a blood film and associated with increased red cell distribution width (RDW). Compare **poikilocytosis.** See also **macrocytosis, microcytosis.**

anisogamete /-gam″ēt/ [Gk, *anisos + gamos,* marriage], a gamete that differs considerably in size and structure from the one with which it unites, such as the macrogamete and microgamete of certain sporozoa. Also called **heterogamete.** Compare **isogamete.** –*anisogametic, adj.*

anisogamy /an″īsog″əmē/, sexual conjugation of gametes of unequal size and structure, as in certain thallophytes and sporozoa. Compare **heterogamy, isogamy.** –*anisogamous, adj.*

anisognathous /an″īsōnath″əs/ [Gk, *anisos + gnathos,* jaw], an abnormal condition in which the maxillary and mandibular arches or jaws are of significantly different sizes. –*anisognathic, adj.*

anisokaryosis /anī′sōker′ē·ō″sis/, a significant variation in nuclear size among cells of the same general type. –*anisokaryotic, adj.*

anisomastia /anī′sōmas″tē·ə/, a condition in which one female breast is much larger than the other.

anisometropia /anī′sōmetrō″pē·ə/ [Gk, *anisos + metron,* measure, *ops,* eye], an abnormal ocular condition characterized by a difference in the refractive powers of the eyes.

anisopia /an″īsō″pē·ə/, a condition in which the visual power of one eye is greater than that of the other.

anisopiesis /an″īsōpī·ē″sis/ [Gk, *anisos,* unequal, *piesis,* pressure], a condition of unequal arterial blood pressure on the left and right sides of the body.

anistreplase, a plasminogen activator.

■ INDICATIONS: This drug is used in acute MI for lysis of coronary artery thrombi. This drug is also used in acute S-T segment elevation MI and acute ischemic stroke.

■ CONTRAINDICATIONS: Known hypersensitivity to this drug or streptokinase; active internal bleeding; intraspinal or intracranial surgery; central nervous system neoplasms; severe, uncontrolled hypertension; cerebral embolism; thrombosis; hemorrhage; recent trauma; or history of cerebrovascular accident all prohibit the use of this drug.

■ ADVERSE EFFECTS: Life-threatening side effects include intracranial hemorrhage, dysrhythmias, GI bleeding, genitourinary bleeding, intracranial bleeding, retroperitoneal bleeding, thrombocytopenia, bronchospasm, lung edema, and anaphylaxis. Adverse effects of this drug include headache, fever, sweating, agitation, dizziness, paresthesia, tremor, vertigo, hypotension, conduction disorders, nausea, vomiting, decreased hematocrit, surface bleeding, rash, urticaria, phlebitis at the injection site, itching, flushing, low back pain, arthralgia, altered respirations, and dyspnea.

ankle [AS, *ancleow*], **1.** the joint of the tibia and fibula of the leg with the talus of the foot. **2.** the part of the lower limb where this joint is located.

ankle-arm index (AAI). See **ankle-brachial index.**

ankle bandage, a figure-eight bandage looped under the sole of the foot and around the ankle. The heel may be covered or left exposed, although covering is preferable because it prevents "window edema." See also **figure-eight bandage.**

ankle bone, *(Informal)* See **talus.**

ankle-brachial index (ABI), the ratio of ankle systolic pressure to the arm systolic pressure, used in assessing the status of lower extremity arteries. It is calculated by dividing the higher of the left and right ankle pressures by the higher of the two brachial artery pressures. Also called **ankle-arm index.**

ankle clonus, an involuntary tendon reflex that causes repeated flexion and extension of the foot. It may be caused by pressure on the foot or corticospinal disease. More than four beats of clonus is pathological.

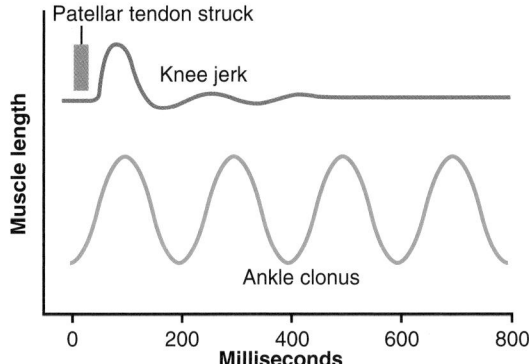

Graphic representation of ankle clonus *(Hall and Guyton, 2011)*

ankle-foot orthosis (AFO), any of a variety of protective external devices that can be applied to the ankle area to prevent injury in a high-risk athletic activity, to protect a previous injury such as a sprain, or to assist patients with chronic joint instability with walking. An AFO is often used by patients unable to dorsiflex the ankle during gait. It may be used to maintain anatomical position in a person that has a footdrop.

ankle joint [AS, *ancleow* + L, *jungere,* to join], a synovial hinge joint between the leg and the foot. The ankle joint is

composed of three bones: the tibia, which forms the inside portion; the fibula, which forms the outside portion; and the talus underneath. The ankle joint is responsible for the up-and-down motion of the foot.

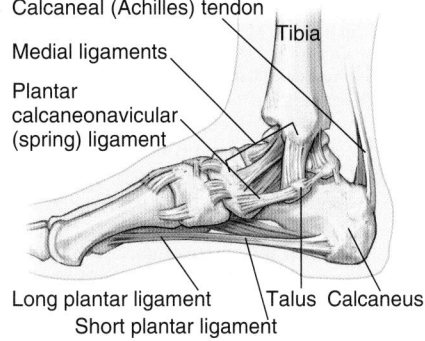

Ankle joint of the right foot: medial view

ankle reflex. See **Achilles tendon reflex.**

ankyl-, ankylo-. See **ancylo-, ancyl, anchyl-, anchylo-, ankylo-, ankyl-.**

ankyloblepharon /ang′kə·lō·blef′ə·ron/ [Gk, *agkylos,* crooked + *blepharon,* eyelid], the adhesion of the ciliary edges of the eyelid to each other.

ankyloblepharon–ectodermal dysplasia–clefting syndrome. See **Hay-Wells syndrome.**

ankyloglossia /ang′kilōglos″ē·ə/ [Gk, *agkylos,* crooked, *glossa,* tongue], a restriction of tongue movement as a result of fusion or adherence of the tongue to the floor of the mouth. Partial ankyloglossia is caused by a frenum of the tongue that is abnormally short or is attached too close to the tip of the tongue. Also called **tongue-tie.**

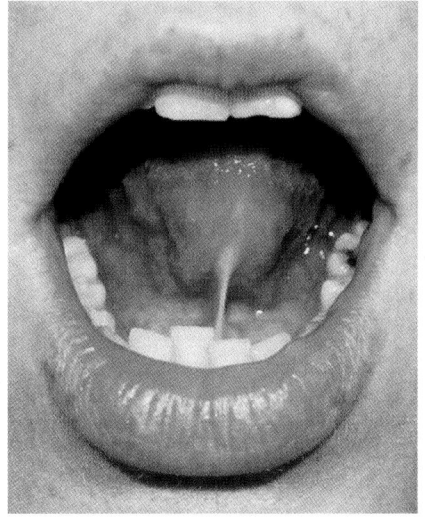

Ankyloglossia *(Cohen, 2013)*

ankylosed /ang″kilōst/, pertaining to the immobility or fusion of a joint resulting from pathological changes in the joint or in the adjacent tissues. It may be the result of injury or disease and may be partial or complete. Complete fusion of two bone ends at a joint means that no motion can occur at that joint.

ankylosing spondylitis /ang′kilō″sing/, a chronic inflammatory disease associated with human leukocyte antigen B27, first affecting the spine and adjacent structures and commonly progressing to eventual fusion (ankylosis) of the involved joints. In extreme cases a forward flexion of the spine, called a "poker spine" or "bamboo spine," develops. Also called **Marie-Strümpell arthritis, Marie-Strümpell disease.** See also **ankylosis, rheumatoid arthritis.**

■ OBSERVATIONS: The disease primarily affects males under 30 years of age and generally follows a course of 20 years. There is a strong hereditary tendency. In addition to the spine, the joints of the hip, shoulder, neck, ribs, and jaw are often involved. When the costovertebral joints are involved, the patient may have difficulty in expanding the rib cage while breathing. Ankylosing spondylitis is a systemic disease, often affecting the eyes and heart. Many patients also have inflammatory bowel disease.

■ INTERVENTIONS: The chronic nature of the disease requires a coordinated team approach. The medical aim of treatment is to reduce pain and inflammation in the involved joints, usually with nonsteroidal antiinflammatory drugs and tumor necrosis factor drugs. Physical therapy helps keep the spine as erect as possible to prevent flexion contractures. The occupational therapist examines surroundings (home, school, work environment) to determine the impact of the disease on everyday functions and responsibilities. Nursing care must focus on management of the medication regimen and coping with the chronic nature of the disease. In advanced cases, surgery may be performed to straighten a badly deformed spine.

■ PATIENT CARE CONSIDERATIONS: Care is complex and the patient should be encouraged to take an active role in management. Support groups are an important resource.

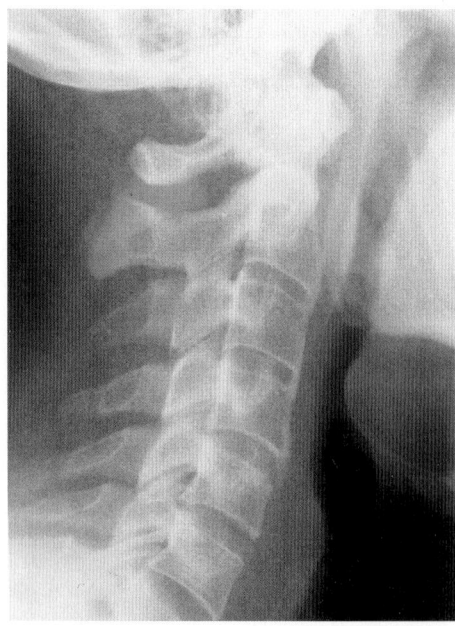

Ankylosing spondylitis (Goldman and Schafer, 2016)

ankylosis /ang′kilō″sis/ [Gk, *ankylosis,* bent condition], **1.** the fusion of a joint, often in an abnormal

position, usually resulting from destruction of articular cartilage and subchondral bone, as occurs in rheumatoid arthritis. It may also occur in immobilized patients when active or passive range of motion is not provided. Also called **acampsia.** Compare **pseudoankylosis. 2.** the surgically induced fusion of a joint to relieve pain or provide support. Also called **arthrodesis, fusion. −ankylosed,** *adj.*

anlage /ahn′lah-ge/, the beginnings of an organ or part in the developing embryo. See **primordium.**

ANLL, abbreviation for **acute nonlymphocytic leukemia.**

ANNA, abbreviation for **American Nephrology Nurses' Association.**

ANNA-1, abbreviation for **type 1 antineuronal antibody.**

ANNA-2, abbreviation for **type 2 antineuronal antibody.**

anneal [AS, *aelan,* to burn], **1.** to temper metals, glass, or other materials by controlled heating and cooling to make them more malleable and ductile. **2.** to cause the interaction of two separate strands of nucleic acid to form a duplex molecule, often by using a related technique of controlled heating and cooling.

annexa. See **adnexa.**

annihilation /ənī′əlā″shən/, the total transformation of matter into energy, as when an antimatter positron collides with an electron. Two photons are created, each with an energy equaling the mass of the individual particles at rest.

annular, describing a ring-shaped lesion surrounding a clear, normal, unaffected disk of skin.

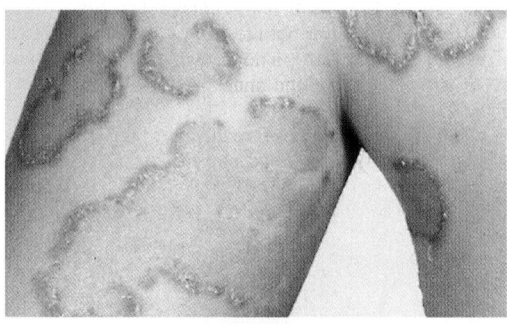

Annular psoriasis (du Vivier, 2013)

annular ligament. See **anular ligament.**

annulus. See **anulus.**

annulus conjunctivae. See **conjunctival ring.**

anode, the electrode at which oxidation occurs. −*anodal, adj.*

anodic stripping voltammetry /ənō′dik, anod″ik/, a process of electroanalytic chemistry used to detect trace metals. It involves the use of a metal-exchange reagent that releases lead or other metals from macromolecular binding sites.

anodontia /an′ōdon″tē·ə/ [Gk, *a,* not, *odous,* tooth], a congenital anomaly in which all of the teeth are missing. The term is generally applied to cases in which all teeth are missing and no tooth follicles are present. Compare **partial anodontia.**

anodyne /an″ədīn/ [Gk *a* + *odyne,* not pain], a medication or intervention that relieves or lessens pain. Compare **analgesic.**

anomalo-, anomal-, combining forms meaning "uneven, deviation from normal, or irregular": *anomalopia, anomalous.*

anomalous.   See **anomaly.**

anomalous trichromatism, anomalous trichromatic vision.

anomaly /ənom′əlē/ [Gk, *anomalos,* irregular], **1.** a deviation from what is regarded as normal. **2.** a congenital malformation, such as the absence of a limb or the presence of an extra finger. **−anomalous,** *adj.*

anomia /ənō″mē·ə/ [Gk, *a + onoma,* without name], a form of aphasia characterized by the inability to name objects. Comprehension and repetition are unaffected.

anomie /an″əmē/, a state of apathy, alienation, anxiety, personal disorientation, and distress resulting from the loss of social norms and goals previously valued.

anonychia /an″ō-nik′e·ə/ [Gk, *a + onyx,* without nail], an absence of a nail or nails.

anoopsia /an′ō-op″sē·ə/ [Gk, *ana,* up, *ops,* eye], a strabismus in which one or both eyes are deviated upward. Also called **hypertropia.**

Anopheles /ənof′əlēz/ [Gk, *anopheles,* harmful], a genus of mosquito containing over 90 species, many of which are vectors of malaria. See also *Plasmodium.*

anopia /anō″pē·ə/ [Gk, *a + ops,* not eye], a blindness resulting from a defect in or the absence of one or both eyes.

-anopia, -anopsia, **1.** suffixes meaning "(condition involving) nonuse or arrested development of the eye": *hemianopia, quadrantanopsia.* **2.** suffixes meaning "(condition of) defective color vision": *cyanopia, tritanopia.*

anoplasty /an″ōplas′tē/ [L, *anus* + Gk, *plassein,* to shape], a surgical repair or correction of a malformation of the anus.

anorchia /anôr″kē·ə/ [Gk, *a + orchis,* not testis], the congenital absence of one or both testes.

anorectal /ān′ōrek″təl, ā′nō-/ [L, *anus* + *rectus,* straight], pertaining to the anal and rectal portions of the large intestine.

anorectal abscess [L, *anus + rectus,* straight, *abscedere,* to go away], a tender, pus-filled mass in the area of the anus and rectum.

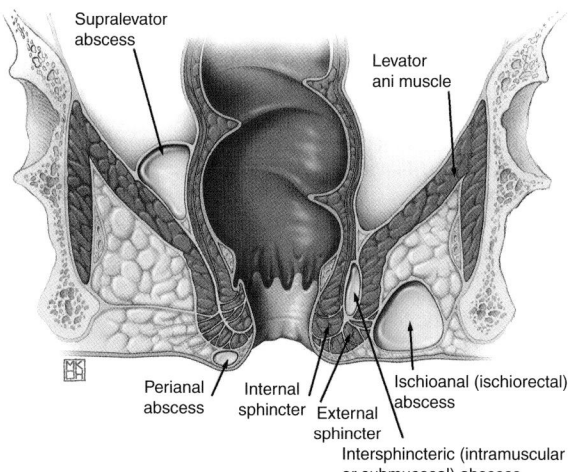

Common sites of anorectal abscess *(Pfenninger and Zainea, 2001)*

Supralevator abscess / Levator ani muscle / Perianal abscess / Internal sphincter / External sphincter / Ischioanal (ischiorectal) abscess / Intersphincteric (intramuscular or submucosal) abscess

anorectal stricture [L, *anus + rectus,* straight, *strictura,* compression], a narrowing of the anorectal canal. It is

sometimes congenital but also may result from surgery to correct an anal fissure or to remove hemorrhoids.

anorectic /an′ōrek″tik/, **1.** pertaining to anorexia. **2.** causing a loss of appetite, as an anorexiant drug. Also called *anorectous.*

anorectoperineal muscle, any of the bands of smooth muscle fibers extending from the perineal flexure of the rectum to the membranous urethra in the male.

anorexia /an′ōrek″sē·ə/ [Gk, *a + orexis,* not appetite], a lack or loss of appetite, resulting in the inability to eat. The condition may result from poorly prepared or unattractive food or surroundings, unfavorable company, or various physical and psychological causes. Compare **pseudoanorexia.** See also **anorexia nervosa.**

anorexia nervosa, a disorder characterized by a prolonged refusal to eat, resulting in emaciation, amenorrhea, emotional disturbance concerning body image, and fear of becoming obese. The condition is seen primarily in adolescents, predominantly in girls, and is usually associated with emotional stress or conflict, such as anxiety, irritation, anger, and fear, which may accompany a major change in the person's life. Treatment consists of measures to improve nourishment, followed by therapy to overcome the underlying emotional conflicts.

anorexiant /an′ôrek″sē·ənt/, a drug or other agent that suppresses the appetite, such as amphetamine.

anorexic.   See **anorectic,** def. 1.

anorgasmy /an′ôrgaz″mē/, inability to achieve orgasm during coitus or masturbation.

anorthopia /an′ôrthō″pē·ə/, a visual disorder in which straight lines appear to be curved or angular. The person also may have a diminished perception of symmetry and an inability to view objects in proper alignment.

anosmia /anoz″mē·ə/ [Gk, *a + osme,* without smell], a loss or an impairment of the sense of smell. It can occur as a temporary condition when a person has a head cold or respiratory infection or when intranasal swelling or other obstruction prevents odors from reaching the olfactory region. It becomes permanent when the olfactory neuroepithelium or any part of the olfactory nerve is destroyed as a result of intracranial trauma, neoplasms, or disease, such as atrophic rhinitis or the chronic rhinitis associated with the granulomatous diseases. In some instances, the condition may be caused by psychological factors, such as a phobia or fear associated with a particular smell. Also called *anosphresia, olfactory anesthesia.* Kinds include **anosmia gustatoria, preferential anosmia.** **−anosmic, anosmatic,** *adj.*

anosognosia /an′əsog·nō″zhə/ [Gk, *a + nosos,* not disease, *gnosis,* knowing], a lack of awareness or a denial of a neurological defect or illness in general, especially paralysis, on one side of the body. It may be attributable to a lesion in the right parietal lobe.

anotia /anō″tē·ə/ [Gk, *a + ous,* without ear], a congenital absence of one or both ears. Compare **microtia.**

ANOVA, a series of statistical procedures for comparing differences among three or more groups, rather than testing each pair of means separately, to determine if differences are due to chance. It is accomplished by examining the differences within the groups as well. Abbreviation for **analysis of variance.**

anovaginal /ā′nōvaj″inəl/ [L, *anus + vagina,* sheath], pertaining to the perineal region of the anus and vagina.

anovarism /an·ō′vər·iz·əm/ [Gk, *a,* without; L, *ovum,* egg], an absence of the ovaries. Also called *anovarianism.*

anovesical /-ves″ikəl/ [L, *anus + vesicula,* small bladder], pertaining to the anus and bladder.

anovular menstruation [Gk, *a + ovulum,* not egg], vaginal bleeding unassociated with a normal ovulatory cycle.

anovulation /an′ovyəlā″shən/, a failure of the ovaries to produce, mature, or release ova. The condition may result from ovarian immaturity or postmaturity; altered ovarian function, as in pregnancy and lactation; primary ovarian dysfunction, as in ovarian dysgenesis; or disturbed interaction of the hypothalamus, pituitary gland, and ovary caused by stress or disease. Oral contraceptives suppress ovulation. Anovulation may also be an adverse side effect of medications prescribed in the treatment of other disorders. —*anovular, anovulatory, adj.*

anoxemia /an′oksē″mē·ə/, a deficiency of oxygen in the blood. Also spelled *anoxaemia.* See also **hypoxia.**

anoxia /anok″sē·ə/ [Gk, *a + oxys,* not sharp], an abnormal condition characterized by a local or systemic lack of oxygen in body tissues. It may result from an inadequate supply of oxygen to the respiratory system, an inability of the blood to carry oxygen to the tissues, or a failure of the tissues to absorb the oxygen from the blood. Kinds include **anemic anoxia, stagnant anoxia.** See also **hypoxemia, hypoxia.** —*anoxic, adj.*

-ans, a suffix meaning "-ing": *penetrans, proliferans.*

ansa /an″sə/ *pl. ansae* [L, handle], (in anatomy) a looplike structure resembling a curved handle of a vase.

ansa cervicalis, one of three loops of nerves in the cervical plexus, branches of which innervate the infrahyoid muscles. Also called *ansa hypoglossi.*

-anserin, a suffix designating a serotonin antagonist.

ANSI, abbreviation for **American National Standards Institute.**

ant-. See **anti-, ant-.**

Antabuse, an alcohol-use deterrent agent. Brand name for **disulfiram.**

antacid /antas″id/ [Gk, *anti,* against, *acidus,* sour], **1.** opposing acidity. **2.** a drug or dietary substance that buffers, neutralizes, or absorbs hydrochloric acid in the stomach. Nonsystemic antacids containing aluminum and calcium are constipating; those containing magnesium have a laxative effect. Systemic antacids such as sodium bicarbonate are rarely used.

antagonism /antag″əniz′əm/ [Gk, *antagonisma,* struggle], **1.** an inhibiting action between physiological processes, such as muscle or hormone actions. **2.** the opposing actions of drugs.

antagonist /antagə″nist/ [Gk, *antagonisma,* struggle], **1.** one who contends with or is opposed to another. **2.** (in physiology) any agent, such as a drug or muscle, that exerts an opposite action to that of another or competes for the same receptor sites. Compare **agonist.** Kinds include **antimetabolite, associated antagonist, direct antagonist, opioid antagonist. 3.** (in dentistry) a tooth in the upper jaw that articulates during mastication or occlusion with a tooth in the lower jaw. —*antagonistic, adj.,* —*antagonize, v.*

antagonistic reflexes [Gk, *antagonisma* + L, *reflectere,* to bend back], spinal reflexes simultaneously activated to relax antagonistic muscle (muscle[s] opposing a movement) when the central nervous system sends a message to the agonist muscle (muscle causing movement) to contract. For example, when the biceps brachii muscle is activated to flex or bend the elbow, the triceps brachii muscle (that straightens the elbow) is inhibited from contracting. This allows smooth motion and prevents injury to either muscle. This process is called reciprocal inhibition.

antazoline /an-taz′o-lēn/, a derivative of ethylenediamine, used as an antihistamine. The phosphate salt is applied topically to the eyes in treatment of allergic conjunctivitis.

ante-, a prefix meaning "before in time or in place": *anteflexion, antepartal.*

antebrachial region /an′tə·brā′kē·əl/ [L. *ante,* before + *brachium,* arm], an anatomical term denoting the forearm, divided into the anterior or palmar antebrachial region and the posterior or dorsal antebrachial region.

antebrachium, (Obsolete) now called **forearm.**

antecardium, (Obsolete) now called the **epigastric region.**

antecedent /an′ti-sē″dənt/ [L, *antecedentem*], a thing or period that precedes others in time or order.

antecubital /-kyōo″bitəl/ [L, *ante,* before, *cubitum,* elbow], the surface of the arm in front of the elbow; at the bend of the elbow.

antecubital fossa [L, *ante,* before, *cubitum,* elbow, *fossa,* ditch], a depression at the bend of the elbow.

antecurvature /-kur″vəchər/, a slight degree of anteflexion or forward curvature.

antefebrile, the time preceding the development of a fever. During this period, the actual fever has not started, but there are other signs and symptoms, such as irritability and agitation, that may indicate the approaching fever.

anteflexion /-flek″shən/ [L, *ante + flectare,* bend], an abnormal position in which an organ is tilted acutely forward and/or folded over on itself.

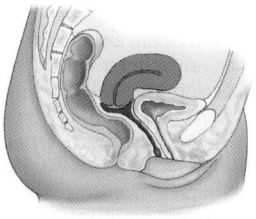

Anteflexion of the uterus *(Leonard, 2015)*

antegonial notch /-gō″nē·əl/ [L, *ante + gonia,* angle], a depression or concavity commonly present on the inferior border of the mandible on each side, immediately in front of the angle, or corner of the jaw, near the anterior margin of the masseter muscle attachment.

antegrade /an″təgrād/ [L, *ante,* before, *gredi,* to go], moving forward, or proceeding toward the front. Also called **anterograde.**

antegrade colonic enema, the creation of a continent stoma in the right colon through which an irrigation fluid may be infused. It is used in the management of chronic evacuation disorders when other methods to control constipation or fecal incontinence have not been successful. Also called *antegrade colonic irrigation.*

-antel, a combining form designating an anthelmintic.

ante mortem [L, *ante,* before, *mors,* death], before death.

antenatal, time of pregnancy prior to delivery. See **prenatal.**

antenatal care, the assessment, monitoring, and instruction in the time of pregnancy prior to labor and delivery. See **antepartal care.**

antenatal diagnosis. See **prenatal diagnosis.**

antepartal /an′təpär″təl/ [L, *ante + parturire,* to have labor pains], pertaining to the period spanning conception and labor.

antepartal care, care during the time of pregnancy prior to labor and delivery. A medical, surgical, gynecological, obstetric, psychosocial, and family history is taken, with particular emphasis on the discovery of familial or transmissible diseases. A physical examination is performed, including observation and evaluation of all body systems and pelvic organs. The vaginal part of the pelvic examination may include estimation of the size of the pelvis; a Papanicolaou

(Pap) smear; and tests for *Neisseria gonorrhoeae, Candida albicans, Chlamydia* species, *Trichomonas vaginalis,* herpes genitalis, and other infections. Blood pressure, weight, urinalysis (primarily for glucose and protein levels), measurement of fundal height, and auscultation of the fetal heart are routinely performed at monthly intervals or even more frequently in the second and third trimesters. Serum laboratory tests are performed to determine blood type and Rh factor, rubella titers, syphilis, hepatitis B, hematocrit, and hemoglobin or complete blood count. Ultrasound and/or amniocentesis may be performed if certain fetal abnormalities are suspected. Also called **antenatal care, prenatal care.** See also **intrapartal care, postpartal care.**

antepartum hemorrhage [Gk, *ante,* before; L, *parturire,* to have labor pains; Gk, *haima,* blood, *rhegnynai,* to burst forth], bleeding from the uterus during a pregnancy in which the placenta appears to be normally situated, particularly after the 28th week.

antepyretic /-pīret″ik/ [L, *ante,* before; Gk, *pyretos,* fever], before the onset of fever. Also called **antefebrile.**

anterior (A) /antir″ē·ər/ [L, *ante + prior,* foremost], **1.** the front of a structure. **2.** pertaining to a surface or part situated toward the front or facing forward. Compare **posterior.** See also **ventral.**

anterior Achilles bursitis. See **Albert's disease.**

anterior apical /antir″·ər ′ā·pi·kəl/, portion of the myocardium with blood supply from the left anterior descending coronary artery.

anterior asynclitism, the head of a fetus that is turned to the anterior side during labor. See **asyntaxia.**

anterior atlantoaxial ligament /atlan′tō·ak″sē·əl/, one of five ligaments connecting the atlas (C1) to the axis (C2). It is fixed to the inferior border of the anterior arch of the atlas and to the ventral surface of the body of the axis. Compare **posterior atlantoaxial ligament.**

anterior atlantooccipital membrane, one of two broad, densely woven fibrous sheets that form part of the atlantooccipital joint between the atlas and the occipital bone. Also called *anterior atlantooccipital ligament.* Compare **posterior atlantooccipital membrane.**

anterior axillary line (AAL), an imaginary vertical line on the body wall continuing the line of the anterior axillary fold with the upper arm.

anterior cardiac vein, one of several small vessels that return deoxygenated blood from the ventral portion of the myocardium of the right ventricle to the right atrium. See also **coronary sinus.**

anterior central gyrus. See **precentral gyrus.**

anterior cerebral commissure [L, *ante + prior,* foremost, *cerebrum,* brain, *commissura,* ajoining], a bundle of fibers in the anterior wall of the prosencephalon connecting the olfactory bulb and olfactory cortex on one side with the similar structures on the other side.

anterior cervical decompression and fusion (ACDF), a surgical procedure to treat cervical disk herniation or degeneration in the spine. A diskectomy is performed on the patient, who is under general anesthesia and supine, with the neck extended by a small shoulder roll placed horizontally. Fusion of a bone graft, either an autograft from the patient's iliac crest or an allograft from a bone bank, preserves the disk space and provides spinal stability. A spinal plate and screws are secured to the vertebral bodies above and below the graft. Patients should be observed postoperatively for dysphagia, hematoma, and recurrent laryngeal nerve palsy.

anterior chamber [L, *ante + prior,* foremost; Gk, *kamara,* an arched cover], the part of the anterior cavity of the eye in front of the iris. It contains the aqueous humor.

anterior column. See **anterior horn.**

anterior common ligament. See **anterior tibial node.**

anterior corticospinal tract, a group of nerve fibers in the anterior funiculus of the spinal cord, originating in the cerebral cortex.

anterior cruciate ligament (ACL), a strong band that arises from the posterior middle part of the lateral condyle of the femur, passes anteriorly and inferiorly between the condyles, and is attached to the depression in front of the intercondylar eminence of the tibia. The ACL is often injured in athletic activity and is the main control for stability during rotation of the knee.

anterior crural nerve, now called **femoral nerve.**

anterior cutaneous nerve, one of a pair of cutaneous branches of the cervical plexus. It arises from the second and the third cervical nerves and divides into the ascending and the descending branches. The ascending branches are distributed to the cranial, ventral, and lateral parts of the neck. The descending branches are distributed to the skin of the ventral and the lateral parts of the neck as far down as the sternum.

anterior drawer sign or test, a test for rupture of the anterior cruciate ligament. The result is positive if there is increased anterior gliding of the tibia when the knee is flexed at a 90-degree angle. See also **drawer sign.**

anterior elastic lamina, now called **Bowman's lamina.**

anterior ethmoidal artery, an artery that supplies the nasal septum and lateral wall and ends as the dorsal nasal artery.

anterior ethmoidal nerve, a nerve that innervates the anterior cranial fossa, the nasal cavity, and the skin of the lower half of the nose.

anterior fontanel, a diamond-shaped unossified area between the frontal and two parietal bones just above an infant's forehead at the junction of the coronal and sagittal sutures. Often called "soft spot" by non–health care professionals. See also **fontanel.**

anterior guide, (in dentistry) the portion of a dental articulator that is contacted by the incisal guide pin to maintain the selected separation of the upper and lower members of the articulator. The anterior guide influences the changing relationships of mounted casts in eccentric movements. Also called **incisal guide.** Compare **condylar guide.**

anterior horn [L, *ante + prior,* foremost, *cornu,* horn, *spina,* spine; Gk, *chorde,* string], one of the hornlike projections of gray matter into the white matter of the spinal cord. The anterior horn contains efferent fibers innervating skeletal muscle tissue and carrying motor commands. Also called **anterior column, ventral column, ventral horn.**

anterior horn cell, motor neuron in the anterior horn.

anterior longitudinal ligament, the broad, strong ligament attached to the ventral surfaces of the vertebral bodies. It extends from the occipital bone and the anterior tubercle of the atlas to the sacrum. Also called **anterior common ligament.** Compare **posterior longitudinal ligament.**

anterior malleolar artery, one of two arteries, the medial and the lateral, that arise from the anterior tibial artery and connect with vessels from the posterior tibial and fibular arteries to form an anastomotic network around the ankle.

anterior mediastinal node, a node in one of the three groups of thoracic visceral nodes of the lymphatic system that drains lymph from the nodes of the thymus, pericardium, and sternum. The nodes are located ventral to the brachiocephalic vein and to the arterial trunks from the aortic arch. See also **thoracic visceral node.**

anterior mediastinum, a caudal portion of the mediastinum in the middle of the thorax, bounded ventrally by the body of the sternum and parts of the fourth through the seventh ribs and dorsally by the parietal pericardium, extending downward as far as the diaphragm. Compare **middle mediastinum, posterior mediastinum, superior mediastinum.**

anterior nares, the ends of the nares, which open anteriorly into the nasal cavity and allow the inhalation and exhalation of air. Each is an oval opening that measures about 1.5 cm anteroposteriorly and about 1 cm in diameter. The anterior nares connect with the nasal fossae. Also called **nostrils.** Compare **posterior nares.**

anterior nasal spine, the sharp anterosuperior projection at the anterior extremity of the line of union of the two maxillae.

anterior neuropore, the opening of the embryonic neural tube in the anterior portion of the prosencephalon. It closes on day 25. Compare **posterior neuropore.** See also **horizon.**

anterior pituitary, glandular portion of the pituitary gland. See **adenohypophysis.**

anterior ramus, a branch of each spinal nerve as it exits the vertebral canal. The anterior rami form the major somatic plexuses of the body. Major visceral components of the peripheral nervous system are also associated mainly with the anterior rami of spinal nerves.

anterior rhizotomy [L, *ante + prior,* foremost; Gk, *rhiza,* root, *temnein,* to cut], the surgical cutting of the ventral root of a spinal nerve, usually to relieve persistent spasm, involuntary movement, or intractable pain.

anterior spinal artery, an artery that originates within the cranial cavity and passes inferiorly along the surface of the spinal cord. It is reinforced along its length by 8 to 10 segmental medullary arteries, the largest of which is the artery of Adamkiewicz.

anterior temporal artery, the anterior temporal branch of the middle cerebral artery. Its origin is the middle cerebral artery, and it supplies blood to the cortex of the anterior temporal lobe.

anterior tibial artery, one of two divisions of the popliteal artery, arising in back of the knee, dividing into six branches, and supplying various muscles of the leg and foot. Branches are the posterior tibial recurrent, anterior tibial recurrent, lateral anterior malleolar artery, medial anterior malleolar artery, lateral malleolar rete, and medial malleolar rete. Compare **posterior tibial artery.**

anterior tibial node, one of the small lymph glands of the lower limb, lying on the interosseous membrane of the leg near the proximal portion of the anterior tibial vessels. Compare **inguinal node, popliteal node.**

anterior tooth, a central incisor, lateral incisor, or cuspid of the maxillary or mandibular teeth. Compare **posterior tooth.**

anterior triangle of the neck, a triangular area bounded by the median line of the neck in front, the lower border of the mandible, and a line extending back to the sternocleidomastoid muscle.

antero-, anter- /an'tərō-/, prefixes denoting "front": *anterocclusion, anterolateral.*

anterocclusion /an'tərōkloo″shən/ [L, *ante + occludere,* to shut], a malocclusion in which the mandibular teeth are anterior to their normal position relative to the maxillary teeth. Compare **anteversion, def. 2.** See also **Angle's classification of malocclusion, mesiocclusion.**

anterograde, occurring in the normal direction or path of blood circulation; forward-moving. See **antegrade.**

anterograde amnesia [L, *ante + prior,* foremost, *gredi,* to go], **1.** the inability to form new memories. **2.** the inability to recall events that occur after the onset of amnesia, usually with an inability to form new memories, which can be temporary. Compare **anterograde memory, retrograde amnesia.**

anterograde memory, the ability to recall events in the distant past but not recent occurrences. Compare **anterograde amnesia.**

anteroinferior /an'tərō-infir″ē·ər/, situated in front of but at a lower level.

anterolateral /-lat″ərəl/, in front and on each side of another structure or object. Also called *anteroexternal.*

anterolateral thoracotomy, a surgical technique in which entry to the chest is made with an incision below the breast but above the costal margins. The incision involves the pectoralis, serratus anterior, and intercostal muscles. Compare **median sternotomy, posterolateral thoracotomy.**

anteromedial /an'tər·ō·mē′dē·əl/, located anteriorly and to the medial side.

anteromedial central artery, any of the branches of the anterior communicating artery that supply the corpus callosum, septum pellucidum, lentiform nucleus, and caudate nucleus.

anteroposterior (AP) /an'tərōpostir″ē·ər/ [L, *ante + prior,* foremost, *posterus,* coming after], from the front to the back of the body.

anteroposterior diameter of the pelvic outlet, the distance between the middle of the pubic symphysis and the upper border of the third sacral vertebra.

anteroposterior vaginal repair, a surgical procedure in which the upper and lower walls of the vagina are reconstructed to correct relaxed tissue. Relaxed vaginal tissue may result from aging changes, childbirth, or surgical trauma, or it may be inherited.

anterosuperior, situated in front of but at a higher level.

anteversion /-vur″shən/ [L, *ante + versio,* turning], **1.** an abnormal position of an organ in which it is tilted or bent forward on its axis, away from the midline. **2.** (in dentistry) the tipping or tilting of teeth or other mandibular structures more anteriorly than normal. Compare **anterocclusion. 3.** the angulation created in the transverse plane between the neck of the femur and shaft of the femur. The normal angle is between 15 and 20 degrees.

anthelmintic /ant'helmin″tik/ [Gk, *anti + helmins,* against worms], **1.** pertaining to a substance that destroys or prevents the development of parasitic worms, such as filariae, flukes, hookworms, pinworms, roundworms, schistosomes, tapeworms, trichinae, and whipworms. **2.** an anthelmintic drug. An anthelmintic may interfere with the parasites' carbohydrate metabolism, inhibit their respiratory enzymes, block their neuromuscular action, or render them susceptible to destruction by the host's macrophages. Drugs used in treating specific helmintic infections include piperazine, pyrantel pamoate, pyrvinium pamoate, mebendazole, niclosamide, hexylresorcinol, diethylcarbamazine, and thiabendazole.

-anthema, a suffix meaning a "(specified) type of skin eruption or rash": *enanthema, exanthema.*

anthraco-, a combining form meaning "carbuncle or coal": *anthraconecrosis, anthracosis.*

anthracosis /an'thrəkō″sis/ [Gk, *anthrax,* coal, *osis,* condition], a chronic lung disease characterized by the deposit of coal dust in the lungs and by the formation of black nodules on the bronchioles, resulting in focal emphysema. The condition occurs in coal miners and is aggravated by cigarette smoking. There is no specific treatment; most cases are asymptomatic, and preventing further exposure to coal dust may halt progress of the condition. Also called **black lung disease, coal worker's pneumoconiosis, miner's pneumoconiosis.** See also **inorganic dust.**

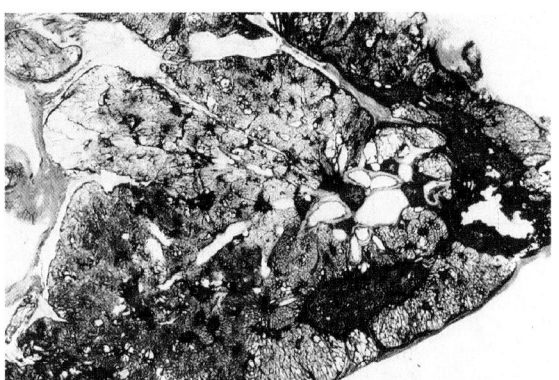

Anthracosis *(Lovaasen and Schwerdtfeger, 2015)*

anthralin /an″thrəlin/, a topical antipsoriatic.

■ INDICATIONS: It is prescribed in the treatment of psoriasis and chronic dermatitis, slowing the growth of skin cells.

■ CONTRAINDICATIONS: Known hypersensitivity to this drug prohibits its use. It is not applied to acute psoriatic eruptions or near the eyes.

anthranilic acid. See **aminobenzoic acid.**

anthrax /an″thraks/ [Gk, *anthrax,* coal, carbuncle], an acute infectious disease (reportable to public health officials) caused by the spore-forming bacterium *Bacillus anthracis* and occurring most frequently in herbivores (cattle, goats, sheep). Humans can become infected through skin contact, ingestion, or inspiration of spores from infected animals or animal products. Person-to-person transmission of inhalational disease does not occur. Anthrax in animals is usually fatal. Inspiration causes the most serious form in humans and is usually fatal, but in 95% of the cases it is acquired when a break in the skin has direct contact with infected animals and their hides. The cutaneous form begins with itching and then a 1- to 3-cm reddish-brown lesion that ulcerates and then forms dark eschar surrounded by brawny edema; the signs and symptoms that follow include internal hemorrhage, muscle pain, headache, fever, nausea, and vomiting. The pulmonary form, called woolsorter's disease, is often fatal unless treated early. Early symptoms include low-grade fever, nonproductive cough, malaise, fatigue, myalgia, profound sweating, and chest discomfort. Later symptoms include an abrupt onset of a high fever and severe respiratory distress (cyanosis, dyspnea, stridor). Treatment is a course of antibiotics, such as penicillin, doxycycline, ciprofloxacin, and/or ofloxacin. Contaminated surfaces should be cleaned with a 5% hypochlorite solution. A vaccine is available for veterinarians and for others for whom anthrax is an occupational hazard. The incubation period for anthrax is 7 to 42 days. Anthrax is an important potential bioterrorism agent. Also called **malignant edema, malignant pustule, ragpicker disease.**

■ OBSERVATIONS: Cutaneous anthrax begins as an itchy, raised, red-brown skin bump that develops into a vesicle and then a painless ulcer with a depressed black necrotic center. Lymph nodes in the adjacent area may be swollen, and there may be fever, fatigue, and headache. Eschar from the ulcer dries and drops off with little or no scarring after 1 to 2 weeks. Cutaneous forms respond readily to treatment, but 20% of untreated cases result in death. Inhalation anthrax starts with a brief prodrome that resembles a viral respiratory illness, followed by hypoxia, dyspnea, fever, muscle aches, headaches, and fatigue. Once the spores travel to the lymphatic system, respiratory failure and shock occur and death usually ensues regardless of treatment. Gastrointestinal anthrax presents with severe abdominal pain, fever, fatigue, anorexia, hematemesis, and bloody diarrhea. In some cases there may be lesions in the nose, mouth, and throat. The disease spreads systemically and is fatal in 30% to 60% of cases if not treated immediately. Diagnosis in all forms is made by history of possible exposure, by physical exam for presenting symptomatology, and by isolation of *Bacillus anthracis* in blood, skin lesions, or respiratory secretions. Serological testing with enzyme-linked immunosorbent assay can confirm diagnosis. An anthracis test (available in specialized labs) can be used to detect anthrax cell-mediated immunity. Chest x-rays may detect mediastinal widening, pleural effusion, and infiltrates in inhalation anthrax.

■ INTERVENTIONS: Antiinfectives, such as penicillin, doxycycline, ciprofloxacin, and/or ofloxacin are commonly used for cutaneous anthrax. IV hydration and ventilator support are used for the inhalation form. Local and state authorities need to be notified in all suspected cases. Use of the anthrax vaccine is recommended in limited use for those at risk (e.g., military personnel, veterinarians, and livestock handlers). Side effects are high, and the schedule is six doses over an 18-month period. Treatment for exposure is usually a postexposure anthrax vaccine and a 60-day course of antibiotics.

■ PATIENT CARE CONSIDERATIONS: Care for inhalation anthrax is largely supportive and centers on management of airway and mechanical ventilation, fluid management, and comfort measures. Every member of the health care team should be prepared for an effective response should anthrax be used in a bioterrorism event. This includes familiarization with workplace policies, procedures, and protocols, and maintenance of current knowledge regarding bioterrorism threats.

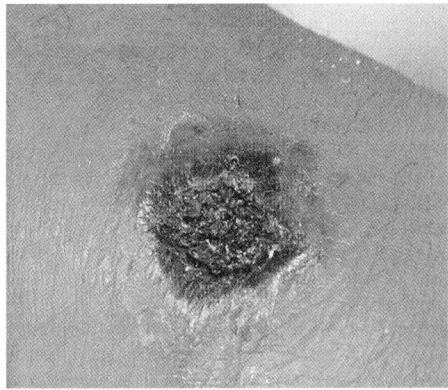

Cutaneous anthrax *(Courtesy of the Centers for Disease Control and Prevention)*

anthrax vaccine, a cell-free protein extract of cultures of *Bacillus anthracis,* used for immunization against anthrax.

anthropo-, a prefix meaning "man or human": *anthropoid, anthropology.*

anthropoid /an″thrəpoid/ [Gk, *anthropos,* human, *eidos,* form], resembling a man or human.

anthropoid pelvis [Gk, *anthropos,* human, *eidos,* form], a type of pelvis in which the pelvic inlet is oval and the anteroposterior diameter of the pelvic inlet is much greater than the transverse. The posterior portion of the space in the true pelvis is much greater than the anterior portion. If a woman's pelvis is large, vaginal delivery is not compromised, but the occiput posterior position of the fetus is favored. See also **pelvis.**

anthropology [Gk, *anthropos,* human, *logos,* science], the science of human beings, including physical characteristics, social structure, behavior, and environmental aspects.

anthropometry /an′thrəpom″ətrē/ [Gk, *anthropos + metron,* measure], the science of measuring the human body as to height, weight, and size of component parts, including skinfold thickness, to study and compare the relative proportions under normal and abnormal conditions. Also called *anthropometric measurement.* −*anthropometric, adj.*

anthropomorphism /an′thrəpōmôr″fizəm/ [Gk, *anthropos,* human, *morphe,* form], the assignment of human characteristics, motivations, and qualities to animals or inanimate objects.

anti-, ant-, prefixes meaning "against": *antibody, antacid.*

antiadrenergic /an′ti·ad′rənur″jik, an′tī-/ [Gk, *anti* + L, *ad + ren,* to kidney], **1.** pertaining to the blockage of the effects of impulses transmitted by the adrenergic postganglionic fibers of the sympathetic nervous system, blocking the response to norepinephrine at both alpha and beta receptors. **2.** an antiadrenergic agent. These drugs block the response to norepinephrine bound to alpha receptors and reduce the tonus of smooth muscle in peripheral blood vessels, causing increased peripheral circulation and decreased blood pressure. Alpha$_1$-blocking agents include ergotamine derivatives, phenoxybenzamine, phentolamine, and tolazoline hydrochloride; they are used to treat conditions such as migraines, Raynaud disease, pheochromocytoma, diabetic gangrene, and spastic vascular disease. Beta$_1$-blocking agents decrease the rate and force of heart contractions and are administered for hypertension, angina, and arrhythmias; propranolol hydrochloride and its congeners are examples. Also called **sympatholytic, sympatholytic agent.** Compare **adrenergic, anticholinergic.**

antiagglutinin /-əgl$\overline{oo}$″tinin/ [Gk, *anti,* against; L, *agglutinare,* to glue], a specific antibody that counteracts the effects of an agglutinin.

antiamebic /an′ti·əmē″bik/, pertaining to a medication that suppresses the growth of amebae or protozoa. Also spelled *antiamoebic.*

antianabolic /-an′əbol″ik/, pertaining to drugs or other agents that inhibit or retard anabolic processes, such as cell division and the creation of new tissue by protein synthesis.

antianaphylaxis /-an′əfilak″sis/ [Gk, *anti,* against, *ana,* back, *phylaxis,* protection], a procedure to prevent anaphylactic reactions by injecting a patient with small desensitizing doses of the antigen. Also called **allergy immunotherapy.**

antianemic /-ənē″mik/ [Gk, *anti + a + haima,* without blood], **1.** pertaining to a substance or procedure that counteracts or prevents a deficiency of erythrocytes, or red blood cells. **2.** an agent used to treat or prevent anemia. Whole blood or packed red blood cells are transfused in the treatment of anemia resulting from acute blood loss. Transfusions of blood components are used in the treatment of aplastic anemia. Iron-deficiency anemia is usually treated with oral preparations of ferrous sulfate, fumarate, or gluconate, but a parenteral preparation is indicated for people who are unable to absorb iron from the GI tract or for those who respond with nausea and diarrhea to the oral administration of iron. Cyanocobalamin is administered parenterally in the treatment of pernicious anemia. Folic acid is prescribed to correct a deficiency of that vitamin in the anemias accompanying general malnutrition or Laënnec's cirrhosis and to treat the anemia of infants on an exclusive milk diet. A combination of folic acid and vitamin B$_{12}$ is prescribed for people who are anemic as a result of an inadequate dietary intake of both vitamins.

antianginal /-anji″nəl/, **1.** pertaining to the reduction of myocardial oxygen consumption or the increase of oxygen supply to the myocardium to prevent symptoms of angina pectoris. **2.** an antianginal agent.

antiantibody /an′ti·an″tibod′ē/ [Gk, *anti* + *anti* + AS, *bodig*], an immunoglobulin formed as the result of the administration of an antibody that acts as an immunogen. The antiantibody then interacts with the antibody. See also **immune gamma globulin.**

antiantitoxin /-tok″sin/ [Gk, *anti* + *anti* + *toxikon,* poison], an antiantibody that may form in the body during immunization, inhibiting or counteracting the effect of the antitoxin administered.

antianxiety agent, a drug that reduces feelings of fear and apprehension. The group includes the benzodiazepine derivatives and a few less widely used nonbenzodiazepines such as meprobamate and hydroxyzine hydrochloride. Also called **anxiolytic.**

antiarrhythmic /-ərith″mik/ [Gk, *anti* + *rhythmos,* rhythm], **1.** pertaining to a procedure or substance that prevents, alleviates, or corrects an abnormal cardiac rhythm. Kinds include **defibrillator, pacemaker. 2.** an antiarrhythmic agent. The major antiarrhythmic drugs are lidocaine hydrochloride, amiodarone, beta-blockers, and calcium channel blockers. The antiadrenergic blocking agent propranolol hydrochloride may also be used in treating arrhythmias. In addition to their use in supportive care, lidocaine or amiodarone may be used to treat complete heart block and ventricular arrhythmias requiring an increased force of cardiac contractions to establish a normal rhythm. Atropine may be used in the treatment of bradycardia, a sedative in the treatment of tachycardia, and digitalis in the treatment of atrial fibrillation. Nondihydropyridine calcium channel blockers control arrhythmias by inhibiting calcium ion influx across the plasma membrane of cardiac muscle, thus slowing atrioventricular conduction and prolonging the effective refractory period within the AV node. See also **arrhythmia.**

antiarthritic /-ärthrit″ik/ [Gk, *anti,* against, *arthron,* joint, *itis,* inflammation], **1.** pertaining to a therapy that relieves symptoms of arthritis. **2.** an antiarthritic agent.

antibacterial /-baktir″ē·əl/ [Gk, *anti* + *bakterion,* small staff], **1.** pertaining to a substance that kills bacteria or inhibits their growth or replication. **2.** an antibacterial agent. Antibiotics synthesized chemically or derived from various microorganisms exert their bactericidal or bacteriostatic effect by interfering with the production of the bacterial plasma wall; by interfering with protein synthesis, nucleic acid synthesis, or plasma membrane integrity; or by inhibiting critical biosynthetic pathways in the bacteria.

antiberiberi factor. See **thiamine.**

antibiotic /-bī·ot″ik/ [Gk, *anti* + *bios,* life], **1.** pertaining to the ability to destroy or interfere with the development of a living organism. **2.** a chemical substance that has the capacity to kill or inhibit the growth of microorganisms.

antibiotic anticancer agent, a drug that blocks mammalian cell proliferation in addition to microbial proliferation, making them too dangerous for treating bacterial infections but useful for treating cancer. Kinds include **bleomycin sulfate, dactinomycin, DAUNOrubicin citrate liposomal, mitomycin.**

antibiotic resistant, 1. pertaining to strains of microorganisms that have developed a resistance to a particular antibiotic. **2.** pertaining to strains of microorganisms that are not sensitive to antibiotics.

antibiotic sensitivity test, a laboratory method for determining the susceptibility of organisms to therapy with antibiotics.

After the infecting organism has been recovered from a clinical specimen, it is cultured and tested against a panel of antibiotic drugs (the specific panel is determined by whether the organism is gram-positive or gram-negative). If the growth of the organism is inhibited by the action of the drug, it is reported as sensitive to that antibiotic. If the organism is not susceptible to the antibiotic, it is reported as resistant to that drug. See also **sensitivity test.**

antibody (Ab) /an″tibod′ē/ [Gk, *anti* + AS, *bodig*], a protein produced by plasma cells that can identify and neutralize pathogens, also known as immunoglobulin (Ig). Monomeric immunoglobulins consist of two heavy chains and two light chains, both having a constant region and a variable region. The variable region binds the antigen and needs to be highly variable in order to be able to recognize as many different antigens as possible. Different types of heavy chains characterize the five structurally distinct classes: IgA, IgD, IgE, IgG, and IgM. Also called **immunoglobulin.** See also **immune response.**

antibody absorption, the process of removing or tying up undesired antibodies in an antiserum reagent by allowing them to react with their antigens.

antibody therapy, the administration of parenteral immunoglobulins as a treatment for patients with immunodeficiency diseases.

antibody titer, the concentration of a serum or plasma antibody. Antibodies are individual immune responses to a variety of antigens, often pathogenic. A rising titer over a period of time indicates the active presence of an antigen, such as a bacterial infection.

antibromic, a deodorizing agent. See **deodorant.**

anticancer diet /-kan″sər/, a diet, based on recommendations of the American Cancer Society, National Cancer Institute, and National Academy of Sciences, to reduce cancer risk factors associated with eating habits.

anticarcinogenic /-kär′sinəjen″ik/ [Gk, *anti,* against, *karkinos,* crab, *oma,* tumor, *genein,* to produce], pertaining to a substance or device that neutralizes or moderates the effects of a cancer-causing substance.

anticardiolipin antibodies test, a serum or plasma test performed to detect antibodies to cardiolipin-bound proteins. Chronically elevated anticardiolipin antibodies are associated with antiphospholipid syndrome, a disorder characterized by arterial and venous thrombosis, low birth weights, and fetal loss.

anticentromere antibody test, a serum or plasma test that is used to diagnose the connective tissue disorder limited systemic sclerosis, which is sometimes named CREST syndrome for its clinical manifestations.

anticholinergic /-kō′lənur″jik/ [Gk, *anti* + *chole,* bile, *ergein,* to work], **1.** pertaining to a blockade of acetylcholine receptors that results in the inhibition of the transmission of parasympathetic nerve impulses. **2.** an anticholinergic agent that functions by competing with the neurotransmitter acetylcholine for its receptor sites at synaptic junctions. Anticholinergics are used to treat spastic disorders of the GI tract, to reduce salivary and bronchial secretions before surgery, or to dilate the pupil. Some are used to reduce parkinsonian symptoms and are often used as adjuvant therapy. Atropine in large doses stimulates the central nervous system and in small doses acts as a depressant. Among numerous agents are ipratropium, tiotropium, and benztropine. Also called **cholinergic blocking agent, parasympatholytic.** See also **antiadrenergic.**

anticholinergic poisoning, poisoning caused by overdosing with an anticholinergic or by ingesting of plants such as jimsonweed that contain belladonna alkaloids. It is characterized by dry mouth; hot, dry, flushed skin; fixed, dilated pupils; sinus tachycardia; urinary retention; disorientation; agitation; impairment of short-term memory; slurred speech; hallucinations; respiratory depression; seizures; and coma. In rare cases, death may occur. Treatment is by induced vomiting and administration of activated charcoal; physostigmine salicylate may be used in severe cases to reverse the anticholinergic effects. A poison control center should be contacted if poisoning is suspected.

anticholinesterase /an′tikol′ənes″tərās/, a drug that inhibits or inactivates the action of acetylcholinesterase. Drugs of this class cause acetylcholine to accumulate at the junctions of various cholinergic nerve fibers and their effector sites or organs, allowing potentially continuous stimulation of cholinergic fibers throughout the central and peripheral nervous systems. Anticholinesterases include physostigmine salicylate, neostigmine, edrophonium, and pyridostigmine. Neostigmine and pyridostigmine are prescribed in the treatment of myasthenia gravis; edrophonium is used in the diagnosis of myasthenia gravis and the treatment of overdose of curariform drugs. Anticholinesterases are also useful in the treatment of Alzheimer disease, with agents such as donepezil and rivastigmine. Many agricultural insecticides have been developed from anticholinesterases; these are the highly toxic chemicals called organophosphates. Nerve gases developed as potential chemical warfare agents contain potent, irreversible forms of anticholinesterase. Also called *acetylcholinesterase inhibitor.*

anticipation /antis′ipā″shən/, **1.** an appearance before the expected time of a periodic sign or symptom. **2.** expectation of standard symptoms or sequelae related to health and disease.

anticipatory adaptation /antis″əpətôr′ē/ [L, *anticipare,* to receive before], the act of adapting to a potentially distressing situation before actually confronting the problem. An example is when a person tries to relax before learning the results of a health examination.

anticipatory grief, feelings of grief that develop before, rather than after, a loss.

anticipatory guidance, the psychological preparation of a person to help relieve the fear and anxiety of an event expected to be stressful. An example is the preparation of a child for surgery by explaining what will happen and what it will feel like and showing equipment or the area of the hospital where the child will be. It is also used to prepare parents for the normal growth and development of their child.

anticipatory nausea and vomiting, nausea and/or vomiting occurring before a new cycle of chemotherapy in response to conditioned stimuli, such as the smells, sights, and sound of the treatment room. It usually occurs after the person has experienced acute nausea and vomiting.

anticoagulant /-kō·ag″yələnt/ [Gk, *anti* + *coagulare,* curdle], **1.** pertaining to a substance that prevents or delays coagulation of the blood. **2.** an anticoagulant drug. Heparin is a potent anticoagulant that interferes with the formation of thromboplastin, with the conversion of prothrombin to thrombin, and with the formation of fibrin from fibrinogen. Phenindione derivatives administered orally are vitamin K antagonists that prevent coagulation by inhibiting the formation of vitamin K–dependent clotting factors. See also **antithrombotic.**

anticoagulant citrate phosphate dextrose adenine solution, citrate phosphate dextrose adenine.

anticoagulant citrate phosphate dextrose solution, citrate phosphate dextrose.

anticoagulant therapy [Gk, *anti* + L, *coagulare,* to curdle; Gk, *therapeia*], the use of drugs that retard the formation and propagation of blood clots (thrombosis). In patients who have experienced thrombotic events, anticoagulant therapy is used to prevent secondary thrombosis, cerebrovascular occlusion, thrombophlebitis, deep venous thrombosis, and pulmonary embolism. Anticoagulants may be administered prophylactically subsequent to various types of surgery and in atrial fibrillation.

anticodon /anʹtikōʺdon/ [Gk, *anti* + *caudex,* book], a sequence of three nucleotides found in transfer RNA. Each anticodon pairs complementarily with a specific codon of messenger RNA during protein synthesis and specifies a particular amino acid in the protein. See also **genetic code, transcription, translation.**

anticomplement, a substance that combines with and neutralizes complement by preventing its union with an antibody.

anticonvulsant /-kənvulʺsənt/ [Gk, *anti* + L, *convellere,* to shake], **1.** pertaining to a substance or procedure that prevents or reduces the severity of epileptic or other convulsive seizures. **2.** an anticonvulsant drug. Hydantoin derivatives, especially phenytoin, apparently exert their anticonvulsant effect by stabilizing the plasma membrane and decreasing intracellular sodium levels; as a result, the excitability of the epileptogenic focus is reduced. Phenytoin prevents the spread of excessive discharges in motor areas and suppresses arrhythmias originating in the thalamus, frontal lobes, and other brain areas. Succinic acid derivatives, valproic acid, and various barbiturates are among the drugs prescribed to limit or prevent absence seizures. Gabapentin, topiramate, levetiracetam, and some benzodiazepines are also useful as anticonvulsants. Many of these agents can produce fetal malformations when administered to pregnant women. Also called **antiepileptic.**

anticyclic citrullinated peptide antibody test, a serum or plasma test among the studies used to diagnose rheumatoid arthritis, to differentiate rheumatoid arthritis from other forms of arthritis, and to assist in establishing a prognosis.

antideformity positioning and splinting /-dəforʺmi tē/, the use of splints, orthoses, braces, or similar devices to prevent or control contractures or other musculoskeletal deformities that may result from disuse, burns, or other injuries. Examples include the application of an axillary or airplane splint to prevent adduction contracture of the shoulder and a neck conformer splint to prevent flexion contractures of the neck.

anti-DNase B, a blood test used to diagnose acute rheumatic fever and poststreptococcal glomerulonephritis. Its results are variable and for accuracy should be done in conjunction with the antistreptolysin O titer test. Formerly called *antideoxyribonuclease-B titer test.*

antidepressant /-dəpresʺənt/, **1.** pertaining to a substance or a measure that prevents or relieves depression. **2.** a medication affecting neurotransmitters in the brain, such as dopamine, serotonin, and norepinephrine.

antidiabetic /-dīʹəbetʺik/, pertaining to an agent that prevents or relieves symptoms of diabetes by maintaining a normal blood sugar level.

antidiarrheal /-dīʹərēʺəl/, a drug or dietary fiber–forming agent that relieves the symptoms of diarrhea. The most effective antidiarrheal drugs are opioid derivatives, which slow intestinal motility to permit greater time for the absorption of water and electrolytes. Dietary fiber–forming agents improve stool consistency but may not decrease fluid and electrolyte loss. Infectious diarrhea (for example, traveler's diarrhea) may require antibiotics if severe.

antidiuretic /-dīʹəretʺik/ [Gk, *anti* + *dia,* through, *ourein,* to urinate], **1.** pertaining to the suppression of urine formation and/or excretion. **2.** an antidiuretic hormone, produced in hypothalamic nuclei and stored in the posterior lobe of the pituitary gland, that suppresses urine formation by permitting the resorption of water-collecting ducts in the kidneys. –*antidiuresis, n.*

antidiuretic hormone (ADH), a hormone that decreases the production of urine by increasing the reabsorption of water by the renal tubules. It is secreted by cells of the hypothalamus and stored in the neurohypophysis. ADH is released in response to a decrease in blood volume, an increased concentration of sodium or other substances in plasma, pain, stress, or the action of certain drugs. ADH causes contraction of smooth muscle in the digestive tract and blood vessels, especially capillaries, arterioles, and venules. Acetylcholine, methacholine, nicotine, large doses of barbiturates, anesthetics, epinephrine, and norepinephrine stimulate ADH release; ethanol and phenytoin inhibit production of the hormone. Increased intracranial pressure promotes inappropriate increases and decreases in ADH. Synthetic ADH is used in the treatment of diabetes insipidus. Normal values are 1 to 5 pg/mL or less than 1.5 ng/L. Also called **vasopressin.**

antidiuretic hormone (ADH) test, a serum or plasma test that may be used to diagnose diabetes insipidus (both the neurogenic and nephrogenic forms) and the syndrome of inappropriate ADH secretion (SIADH), which is associated with tumors, pulmonary diseases, infection, trauma, Addison disease, and myxedema.

anti-DNA antibody test, a blood test that is useful for the diagnosis and follow-up of systemic lupus erythematosus (SLE). The test uses double-stranded deoxyribonucleic acid (DNA) as antigen to detect anti-DNA antibodies. High titers characterize SLE, and low to moderate levels may indicate other rheumatic diseases as well as chronic hepatitis, infectious mononucleosis, and biliary cirrhosis.

antidote /anʺtidōt/ [Gk, *anti* + *dotos,* that which is given], a drug or other substance that opposes the action of a poison or a drug consumed in excess. An antidote may be mechanical, such as activated charcoal, which absorbs poisons in the GI tract and prevents their absorption; chemical, acting to neutralize the toxin or bind excess amounts of the agent; or physiological, acting to oppose the action of the poison, as when a sedative is given to a person who has ingested a large amount of a stimulant or when a receptor blocker is administered to a person who has taken a large dose of a receptor agonist.

antidromic conduction /anʹtidromʺik/ [Gk, *anti* + *dromos,* course], the conduction of a neural impulse backward from a receptor in the midportion of an axon. It is an unnatural phenomenon and may be produced experimentally. Because synaptic junctions allow conduction in one direction only, backward, antidromic impulses fail to pass the synapse, dying at that point. Compare **orthodromic conduction.**

antidyskinetic /anʹte-, anʹti-disʺki-netʹik/, **1.** pertaining to the relief or prevention of dyskinesia. **2.** an antidyskinetic agent.

antiembolism (AE) hose /-emʺbəlizʹəm/ [Gk, *anti* + *embolos,* plug], elasticized stockings worn to prevent the formation of emboli and thrombi, especially in patients who have had surgery or who have been restricted to bed. Return flow of the venous circulation is promoted, preventing venous stasis and dilation of the veins, conditions that predispose individuals to varicosities and thromboembolic disorders. Also called **thromboembolic disorder (TED) hose.**

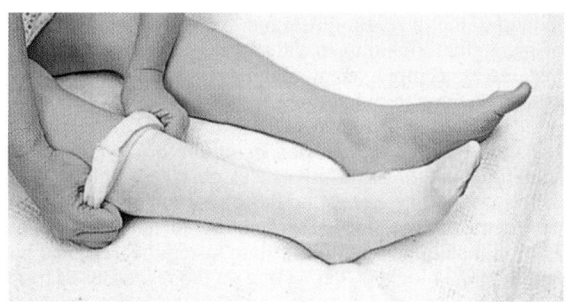

Antiembolism hose *(Elkin, Perry, and Potter, 2007)*

antiemetic /-imet″ik/ [Gk, *anti* + *emesis,* vomiting], pertaining to a substance or procedure that prevents or alleviates nausea and vomiting.

antiepileptic. See **anticonvulsant.**

antiestrogen /-es″trəjən/, a hormone-based product used predominantly in cancer chemotherapy. The group of antiestrogen drugs includes tamoxifen, fulvestrant, and anastrozole. They are used mainly in treating estrogen-dependent tumors, such as breast cancer.

antiextractable nuclear antigens test, a blood test used to help diagnose systemic lupus erythematosus and mixed connective tissue disease and to rule out other rheumatoid diseases.

antifebrile. See **antipyretic.**

antifibrillatory /-fibril″ətôr′ē/, pertaining to a medication or other agent that suppresses atrial or ventricular fibrillation.

antifilarial, pertaining to a substance or agent destructive to filariae. See **antimalarial.**

antiflux /an′ti·fluks/ [Gk, *anti,* against + L, *fluere,* to flow], a substance that prevents the attachment of solder.

antifungal /-fung″gəl/, **1.** pertaining to a substance that kills fungi or inhibits their growth or reproduction. **2.** an antifungal, antibiotic drug. Amphotericin B and fluconazole, both effective against a broad spectrum of fungi, probably act by binding to sterols in the fungal plasma membrane and changing the membrane's permeability. Amphotericin B has the broadest spectrum of action among antifungals. Miconazole and nystatin are both used topically. Amphotericin B and fluconazole, along with the echinocandins, are used systemically. Griseofulvin, another broad-spectrum antifungal agent, binds to the host's new keratin and renders it resistant to further fungal invasion. Miconazole nitrate inhibits the growth of common dermatophytes, including yeastlike *Candida albicans;* nystatin is effective against yeast and yeastlike fungi. Also called **antimycotic.**

antigalactic /-gəlak″tik/, pertaining to a drug or other agent that prevents or reduces milk secretion in mothers of newborns.

anti-GBM disease, a rare autoimmune disease; kidney or pulmonary disorder in which the glomerular basement membrane is damaged by an antigen-antibody reaction. The kidney itself may serve as the antigenic target in the reaction. Also called **Goodpasture syndrome.**

antigen /an″tijən/ [Gk, *anti* + *genein,* to produce], a substance that the immune system recognizes as foreign and mounts an immune response against. The immune response may be either production of an antibody, a cell-mediated response, or both.

antigen-antibody reaction, a process in which antibodies bind to antigens to form antigen-antibody complexes. These complexes may render toxic antigens harmless (neutralization), agglutinize antigens on the surface of microorganisms, or activate the complement system by exposing the complement binding sites on antibodies. Certain complement protein molecules immediately bind to these sites and trigger the activity of the other complement protein molecules, which cause antigen-bearing cells to lyse. Antigen-antibody reactions may start immediately with antigen contact or as much as 48 hours later. They normally produce immunity but may also be responsible for allergy, autoimmunity, and fetomaternal hematologic incompatibility. In the immediate allergic response, the antigen-antibody reaction activates certain enzymes and causes an imbalance between those enzymes and their inhibitors. Simultaneously released into the circulation are several pharmacologically active substances, including acetylcholine, bradykinin, histamine, immunoglobulin G, and leukotaxine. See also **allergen, allergic reaction, humoral immunity, serum sickness.**

antigenic. See **antigen.**

antigenic determinant, a site on an antigen molecule to which an antibody molecule binds. Also called **epitope.**

antigenic drift [Gk, *anti,* against, *genein,* to produce; AS, *drifan,* drift], a gradual, relatively minor change in the antigenicity of a virus, periodically producing a mutant antigen requiring new antibodies and vaccines to combat its effects. Compare **antigenic shift.**

antigenicity /an′tijənis″ətē/, the ability of an antigen to induce an immune response by binding specifically to a T cell receptor or antibody (B cell receptor). The degree of antigenicity of a substance depends on the kind and amount of that substance and on the degree to which the host is sensitive. Also called **immunogenicity.** See also **antigen-antibody reaction.**

antigenic shift, a sudden, major change in the antigenicity of a virus, seen especially in influenza viruses, resulting from the recombination of the genomes of two different strains; it is associated with pandemics because hosts do not have immunity to the new strain. Compare **antigenic drift.**

antigen presentation, biological assemblage of antigen molecules (peptides) presented to T cells on the surface of cells. Exogenous antigens are taken up by macrophages and dendritic cells and are digested in the lysosome, and the peptides are displayed within the class II major histocompatibility complex on the cell surface. Endogenous antigen peptides can be presented by any cell and are presented by a type I major histocompatibility complex. See also **antigen processing.**

antigen-presenting cell, a cell that can break down protein antigens into peptides and present the peptides, in conjunction with major histocompatibility complex class II molecules (HLA in humans), on the cell surface, where they can interact with T cell receptors. Dendritic cells and macrophages are types of antigen-presenting cells.

antigen processing, the process that prepares antigens for presentation to T cells. Exogenous antigens are endocytosed by antigen-presenting cells and degraded in endosomes/lysosomes. The peptides that have formed due to this process bind to major histocompatibility complex class II molecules and are then transported to the cell surface for presentation to CD4+ T cells. Endogenous proteins, including viral proteins in virus-infected cells, are degraded in the proteasome, and the resulting peptides are loaded on major histocompatibility complex class I molecules. The complex will be transported to the cell surface for presentation to CD8+ T cells.

antigenuria /an″ti-jĕ-nu′re-ah/, the presence of a specific antigen in the urine.

antigerminal pole. See **vegetal pole.**

antiglobulin /an′tiglob″yo͞olin/ [Gk, *anti* + L, *globulus,* small globe], an antibody against gamma globulin. See also **antiglobulin test, precipitin.**

antiglobulin test, a test for the presence of antibodies that coat and damage erythrocytes as a result of any of several diseases or conditions. The test can detect Rh antibodies in maternal blood and is used to anticipate hemolytic disease in the newborn. It is also used to diagnose and screen for autoimmune hemolytic anemias and to determine the compatibility of blood types. When exposed to a sample of the patient's serum, the antiglobulin serum causes agglutination if human globulin antibody or its complement is present. Also called **Coombs test.**

antiglomerular basement membrane antibodies test, a blood or tissue test used to diagnose Goodpasture's syndrome, which is associated with the presence of circulating glomerular basement membrane antibodies.

antigravity muscle /-grav″itē/, any of the muscle groups involved in the stabilization of joints or other body parts by opposing the effects of gravity. Examples include the muscles of the jaw that automatically keep the mandible raised and the mouth closed.

anti-G suit, a rarely used garment designed to produce pressure on the lower part of the body to shunt blood to the torso. See **military antishock trousers.**

antihelix, the semicircular ridge of the ear anterior and parallel to the helix.

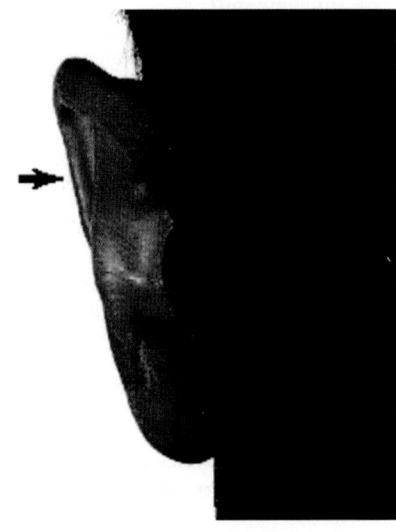

Antihelix of the ear *(Niamtu, 2011)*

antihemophilic C factor. See **factor XI.**

antihemophilic factor (recombinant), a sterile, purified, coagulation factor VIII concentrate produced by recombinant technology that possesses biological activity comparable with that of human plasma-derived coagulation factor VIII. It is used to prevent or stop hemorrhage during surgery or other procedures in patients with hemophilia A. It is administered intravenously.

antihemophilic factor VII concentrate (AHF) /-hē′mōfil″ik/, plasma derivative used to treat bleeding in patients with hemophilia A. It may be prepared by fractionation of human plasma or affinity column purification. A recombinant DNA product is also available.
■ CONTRAINDICATIONS: There are no known contraindications.
■ ADVERSE EFFECTS: The most serious adverse reaction is hepatitis, which occurs because the factor is obtained from pools of human plasma. Allergic reactions may also occur.

antihemorrhagic /-hē′môraj″ik/, any drug or agent used to prevent or control bleeding, such as thromboplastin or thrombin, either of which mediates the blood-clotting process. Antihemorrhagics may also include antifibrinolytics such as aminocaproic acid and tranexamic acid.

antihidrotic. See **anhidrotic.**

antihistamine /-his″təmin/ [Gk, *anti* + *histos,* tissue, amine (ammonia compound)], any substance capable of reducing the physiological and pharmacological effects of histamine, including a wide variety of drugs that block histamine receptors. Many such drugs are readily available as over-the-counter medicines for the management of allergies. Toxicity resulting from the overuse of antihistamines and their accidental ingestion by children is common and sometimes fatal. These substances do not completely stop the release of histamine, and the ways in which they act on the central nervous system are not completely understood. The antihistamines are divided into histamine$_1$ (H$_1$) and histamine$_2$ (H$_2$) blockers, depending on the responses to histamine they prevent. The most common H$_1$ blocking agent is diphenhydramine. H$_1$-blocking drugs, such as alkylamines, ethanolamines, ethylenediamines, and piperazines, are effective in the symptomatic treatment of acute allergies. Second-generation H$_1$ blockers, such as cetirizine, fexofenadine, and loratadine, cause less sedation. H$_2$-blocking agents include famotidine and nizatidine, and are used in the treatment of heartburn, peptic ulcer disease, and gastroesophageal reflux. Antihistamines can both stimulate and depress the central nervous system. −*antihistaminic, adj.*

antihistamine poisoning, an adverse reaction to an excessive intake of antihistamines. Symptoms include fatigue, lethargy, delirium, hallucinations, loss of striated muscle control, hyperreflexia, tachycardia, dilated pupils, and in severe cases, coma.

anti-Hu antibody, any of the polyclonal immunoglobulin G autoantibodies directed against the proteins of the Hu antigen family; they are associated with paraneoplastic sensory neuronopathy and, encephalomyelitis in oat cell carcinoma of the lung and more rarely, sarcoma and neuroblastoma. Also called **type 1 antineuronal antibody.**

antihypercholesterolemic /-hī′pərkō′les′tərōlē″mik/, a drug that prevents or controls an increase of cholesterol in the blood. Also called *dyslipidemic agent.* See also **antilipidemic.**

antihyperglycemic /an″te-, an″ti-hi″per-gli-se′mik/, **1.** pertaining to a substance or therapy that prevents or reduces high levels of glucose in the blood. **2.** an antihyperglycemic agent.

antihyperglycemic agent. Also called *antidiabetic agent.* See **hypoglycemic agent.**

antihyperkalemic /an″te-, an″ti-hi″per-kah-le′mik/, **1.** pertaining to a substance or procedure effective in decreasing or preventing increases in serum potassium levels. **2.** an antihyperkalemic agent.

antihyperlipidemic /an″te-, an″ti-hi″per-lipi″de′mik/, **1.** pertaining to a substance or procedure that promotes a reduction of lipid levels in the blood. **2.** an antihyperlipidemic agent. Also called *dyslipidemic.*

antihypertensive /-hī′pərten″siv/, **1.** pertaining to a substance or procedure that reduces high blood pressure. **2.** an antihypertensive agent. Various drugs achieve their antihypertensive effect by depleting tissue stores of catecholamines in peripheral sites, by blocking pressor receptors in the carotid sinus and heart, by blocking autonomic nerve impulses that constrict blood vessels, by stimulating central inhibitory alpha$_2$ receptors, or by causing vasodilation. Thiazides and other diuretic agents inhibit the reabsorption of sodium in the renal tubules, increasing urinary excretion of sodium and decreasing plasma and extracellular fluid volume, decreasing blood volume. Drugs that act on adrenergic control of blood pressure include beta-adrenergic blocking agents, which act at beta-adrenergic receptors in the heart and kidneys to reduce cardiac output and renin secretion, and others that act on alpha-adrenergic mechanisms in the central or sympathetic nervous system to reduce peripheral vascular resistance.

Vasodilators act directly on the arterioles to produce the same effect. Other drugs used to treat hypertension are hydrochlorothiazide (a diuretic agent), angiotensin-converting enzyme inhibitors, nonnitrate vasodilators, calcium channel blockers, and angiotensin receptor blockers. Most cases of hypertension can be controlled by one of these drugs or a combination of them. The proper combination is determined by the response of the individual and may be affected by patient factors. In some cases, several drugs must be tried before the right combination is identified. Compare **antihypotensive.**

antihypoglycemic /an″te-, an″ti-hi″po-gli-se″mik/, pertaining to a substance or therapy, such as dextrose or glucagon, that counteracts low blood sugar.

antihypotensive /-hī′pōten″siv/, **1.** pertaining to a substance or other agent that tends to increase blood pressure. **2.** an antihypotensive drug. Compare **antihypertensive.**

antiimmune /an′ti·imyo͞on″/ [Gk, *anti* + L, *immunis,* free from], pertaining to the prevention or inhibition of immunity. See also **immune response.**

antiinfective /-infek″tiv/ [Gk, *anti* + L, *inficere,* to stain], **1.** pertaining to an agent that prevents or treats infection. **2.** an antiinfective drug.

antiinflammatory /-inflam″ətor″ē/ [Gk, *anti* + L, *inflammare,* to set afire], **1.** pertaining to a substance or procedure that counteracts or reduces inflammation. **2.** an antiinflammatory drug.

antiinhibitor coagulant complex (AICC), a concentrated fraction from pooled human plasma, which includes vitamin K–dependent coagulation factors (factors II, VII, IX, and X), factors of the kinin-generating system, and factor VIII coagulant antigen. It is administered intravenously as an antihemorrhagic in hemophilic patients with factor VIII inhibitors. Its mechanism of action has not been elucidated but may result at least from part to its factor Xa content.

antiinitiator /-inish″ē-ātər/, a substance that is a potential cocarcinogen but that may protect cells against cancer development if given before exposure to an initiator. An example is the food additive butylated hydroxytoluene (BHT). An antiinitiator given after exposure to an initiator may also act as a promoter and encourage rather than block cancer development.

antileprotic /-leprot″ik/, **1.** a substance or other agent that is effective in treating leprosy. **2.** an antileprotic drug.

antilipidemic /an″tilip′idē″mik/ [Gk, *anti* + *lipos,* fat, *haima,* blood], **1.** pertaining to a regimen, diet, or agent that reduces the level of lipids in the serum. Antilipidemic diets and drugs are prescribed to reduce the risk of atherosclerosis for two reasons: atheromatous plaques contain free cholesterol, and lower serum cholesterol levels and a lower incidence of coronary artery disease are found more frequently in populations consuming a low-fat diet than in those on a high-fat diet. **2.** an antilipidemic drug, also known as a dyslipidemic agent. A number of pharmacological agents, including bile acid sequestrants and HMG-CoA reductase inhibitors, are used to reduce serum lipid levels. Cholestyramine and colestipol exert their antilipidemic action by combining with bile acids in the intestine to form an insoluble complex that is excreted in the feces; they may reduce serum cholesterol levels but prevent the absorption of essential fat-soluble vitamins and may be associated with several serious side effects. A newer class of agents interferes with the absorption of cholesterol from dietary and biliary sources. See also **hyperlipidemia.**

Antilirium, an acetylcholinesterase inhibitor. Brand name for **physostigmine salicylate.**

antiluetic, *(Obsolete)* an agent used to treat syphilis.

antilymphocyte globulin. See **antithymocyte globulin.**

antimalarial /-məler″ē-əl/, **1.** pertaining to a substance that destroys or suppresses the development of malaria plasmodia or to a procedure that exterminates the mosquito vectors of the disease, such as spraying insecticides or draining swamps. **2.** an antimalarial drug. Chloroquine and hydroxychloroquine sulfate are effective against *Plasmodium vivax, P. malariae,* and certain strains of *P. falciparum.* Patients with drug-resistant *P. falciparum* are often treated with a combination of quinine, pyrimethamine, and sulfadoxine.

antimessage, a strand of viral RNA that cannot act as messenger RNA because of its negative coding sequence. It must be converted to a positive-strand sequence by a viral transcriptase (RNA-dependent RNA polymerase) before its message can be translated in a host cell.

antimetabolite /-mətab″əlīt/ [Gk, *anti* + *metabole,* change], a drug or other substance that is an antagonist to or resembles a normal human metabolite and interferes with its function in the body, usually by competing for its receptors or enzymes. Among the antimetabolites used as antineoplastic agents are the folic acid analog methotrexate and the pyrimidine analog fluorouracil. The antineoplastic mercaptopurine, an analog of the nucleotide adenine and the purine base hypoxanthine, is a metabolic antagonist of both compounds. Thioguanine, another member of a large series of purine analogs, interferes with nucleic acid synthesis. Cytarabine, used in the treatment of acute myelocytic leukemia, is a synthetic nucleoside that resembles cytidine and kills cells that actively synthesize deoxyribonucleic acid (DNA), apparently by inhibiting the enzyme DNA polymerase.

antimicrobial /-mīkrō″bē-əl/ [Gk, *anti* + *mikros,* small, *bios,* life], **1.** pertaining to a substance that kills microorganisms or inhibits their growth or replication. **2.** an antimicrobial agent.

Antiminth, an anthelmintic. Brand name for **pyrantel pamoate.**

antimitochondrial antibody (AMA) /-mī′tōkon″drē-·əl/, an antibody that acts specifically against mitochondria. These antibodies are not normally present in the blood of healthy people.

antimitochondrial antibody (AMA) test, a blood test that is used to determine the presence of antimicrobial antibody in the blood. Low titers may occur in chronic hepatitis, drug-induced hepatotoxicity, and various other diseases. High titers are often diagnostic of primary biliary cirrhosis. Patients with autoimmune hepatitis, extrahepatic obstruction, or acute infection may also test positive for AMA.

antimitotic /-mītot″ik/, inhibiting cell division.

antimony (Sb) /an″təmō′nē/ [L, *antimonium*], a bluish, crystalline metallic substance occurring in nature which is listed as element number 51 on the Periodic Table of the Elements. Various antimony compounds are used in the treatment of filariasis, leishmaniasis, lymphogranuloma, schistosomiasis, and trypanosomiasis. They are also used as emetics.

antimony poisoning, a toxic effect caused by the ingestion or inhalation of antimony or antimony compounds. It is characterized by vomiting, diaphoresis, diarrhea, and a metallic taste in the mouth. Irritation of the skin or mucous membranes may result from external exposure. Severe poisoning resembles arsenic poisoning. Antimony and antimony compounds are common ingredients of many substances used in medicine and industry.

antimorph /an″təmôrf/ [Gk, *anti* + *morphe,* form], a mutant allele that inhibits or antagonizes the influence of the normal allele in the expression of a trait. Compare **amorph, hypermorph, hypomorph.**

antimuscarinic /-mus′kərin″ik/ [Gk, *anti* + L, *musca,* fly], effective against the poisonous activity of muscarine. Compare **muscarinic.**

antimutagen /-myoo″təjən/ [Gk, *anti* + L, *mutare,* to change; Gk, *genein,* to produce], **1.** any substance that reduces the rate of spontaneous mutations or counteracts or reverses the action of a mutagen. **2.** any technique that protects cells against the effects of mutagens. −*antimutagenic, adj.*

antimyasthenic /an″te-, an″ti-mi″as-then′ik/, **1.** counteracting or relieving muscular weakness in myasthenia gravis. **2.** an antimyasthenic.

antimycotic. See **antifungal.**

antimyocardial antibody (AMA) test, a blood test used to detect an autoimmune source of myocardial injury and disease, such as rheumatic heart disease, myocardiopathy, postthoracotomy syndrome, and myocardial infarction. This test may also be used to monitor the effect of treatment on these conditions.

antineoplastic /-nē′ōplas″tik/ [Gk, *anti* + *neos,* new, *plasma,* something formed], **1.** pertaining to a substance, procedure, or measure that prevents the proliferation of cells. **2.** a chemotherapeutic agent that controls or kills cancer cells. Drugs used in the treatment of cancer are cytotoxic but are generally more damaging to dividing cells than to resting cells. Cycle-specific antineoplastic agents are more effective in killing proliferating cells than resting cells, and phase-specific agents are most active during a specific phase of the cell cycle. Most anticancer drugs prevent the proliferation of cells by inhibiting the synthesis of deoxyribonucleic acid (DNA) by various mechanisms. Alkylating agents, such as mechlorethamine HCl derivatives, ethylenimine derivatives, and alkyl sulfonates, interfere with DNA replication by causing cross-linking of DNA strands and abnormal pairing of nucleotides. **Antimetabolites** exert their action by interfering with the formation of compounds required for cell division. Methotrexate, folic acid analog, and 5-fluorouracil, a pyrimidine analog, inhibit enzymes required for the formation of the essential DNA constituent thymidine. 6-Mercaptopurine, a hypoxanthine analog, and 6-thioguanine, an analog of guanine, interfere with the biosynthesis of purines. VinBLAStine sulfate and vinCRIStine sulfate, **alkaloids** derived from the periwinkle plant, disrupt cell division by interfering with the formation of the mitotic spindle. Antineoplastic antibiotics, such as DOXOrubicin HCl, daunomycin, and mitomycin, block or inhibit DNA synthesis; dactinomycin and plicamycin interfere with ribonucleic acid synthesis. Cytotoxic chemotherapeutic agents may be administered via the oral or intravenous route or by infusion. All have untoward and unpleasant side effects and are potentially immunosuppressive and dangerous. Estrogens and androgens, although not considered antineoplastic agents, frequently cause tumor regression when administered in high doses to patients with hormone-dependent cancers.

antineoplastic antibiotic, a chemical substance derived from a microorganism or a synthetic analog of the substance, used in cancer chemotherapy. Dactinomycin, used in the treatment of Wilms' tumor, testicular carcinoma, choriocarcinoma, rhabdomyosarcoma, and some other sarcomas, exerts its antineoplastic effect by interfering with ribonucleic acid (RNA) synthesis. Plicamycin, with a similar mechanism of action, is also administered for testicular cancer and for trophoblastic cancer. DOXOrubicin HCl, a broad-spectrum agent that is especially useful in treating breast carcinoma, lymphomas, sarcomas, and acute leukemia, and closely related daunomycin, which is also effective in acute leukemias, block the biosynthesis of RNA. Mitomycin C, prescribed for gastric, breast, cervical, and

head and neck carcinomas, cross-links strands of deoxyribonucleic acid (DNA). Bleomycin sulfate, used in the treatment of squamous cell carcinomas of the head and neck, testicular carcinoma, and lymphomas, damages DNA and prevents its repair. Antineoplastic antibiotics cause bone marrow depression and usually cause nausea and vomiting; several cause alopecia.

antineoplastic hormone, a chemically synthesized or a synthetic analog of the naturally occurring compound used to control certain disseminated cancers. Hormonal therapy is designed to counteract the effect of an endogenous hormone required for tumor growth. The estrogens diethylstilbestrol (DES) and ethinyl estradiol may be used in the palliative treatment of a prostatic carcinoma that is nonresectable or unresponsive to radiotherapy. An androgen, such as testosterone propionate, testolactone, or fluoxymesterone, may be administered after surgery to control disseminated breast cancer in women whose tumor is estrogen dependent. The antiestrogen tamoxifen produces responses in many patients with advanced estrogen-dependent breast cancer. Paradoxically, large doses of estrogen, frequently used to control disseminated breast cancer in postmenopausal women, apparently checks the growth of tumors by inhibiting the secretion of estrogen by the adrenal gland. Some progestins produce a favorable response in women with disseminated endometrial carcinoma and, occasionally, in patients with prostate or renal cancers. These progestins include megestrol acetate, medroxyprogesterone acetate, and 17-alpha-hydroxyprogesterone caproate.

antineoplaston, a peptide, amino acid derivative, or carboxylic acid proposed to control neoplastic cell growth using the patient's own biochemical defense system, which works jointly with the immune system. Antineoplaston therapy is not approved for general use due to lack of clinical evidence.

antineutrophil cytoplasmic antibody (ANCA) test, a serum or plasma test used to diagnose granulomatosis with polyangiitis (formerly called Wegener's granulomatosis) and systemic vasculitis. It is also used to monitor therapeutic response and to detect early relapse.

antinuclear antibody (ANA) /-noo″klē-ər/, an autoantibody directed against nuclear antigens. Antinuclear antibodies are found in the blood serum of patients with rheumatoid arthritis, systemic lupus erythematosus, Sjögren's syndrome, polymyositis, scleroderma, Raynaud's disease, mixed connective tissue disease, and a number of nonrheumatic disorders ranging from lymphomas, leukemias, primary biliary cirrhosis, thyroiditis, chronic active hepatitis, and adverse drug reactions. The antibodies are often detected with an immunofluorescent assay technique.

antinuclear antibody (ANA) test, a serum or plasma test used to detect antinuclear antibodies associated with systemic lupus erythematosis. ANAs bind the nuclei of fixed leukocytes in vitro. Their presence is confirmed through fluorescence-labeled antibodies that are detected microscopically.

antioncogene /an″ti-on″kəjēn/, a tumor-suppressing gene that may act by controlling cellular growth. When an antioncogene is inactivated, tumor cellular proliferation begins, and tumor activity accelerates.

antioxidant /-ok″sidənt/, a chemical or other agent that inhibits or retards oxidation of a substance to which it is added. Examples include butylated hydroxyanisole and butylated hydroxytoluene, which are added to foods or the packaging of foods containing fats or oils to prevent oxygen from combining with the fatty molecules, thereby causing them to become rancid.

antioxidation /-ok′sidā″shən/, the prevention of oxidation.

antiparallel /-per″ələl/ [Gk, *anti + parallelos,* side-by-side], pertaining to molecules, such as strands of DNA, that are parallel but are oriented in opposite directions.

antiparasitic /-per′əsit″ik/ [Gk, *anti + parasitos,* guest], **1.** pertaining to a substance or procedure that kills parasites or inhibits their growth or reproduction. **2.** an antiparasitic drug such as an amebicide, an antihelminthic, an antimalarial, a schistosomicide, a trichomonacide, or a trypanocide.

antiparietal cell antibodies, antibodies against the cells of the stomach that make and release intrinsic factor and stomach acid.

antiparietal cell antibody (APCA) test, a serum or plasma test employed to support the diagnosis of pernicious anemia–related vitamin B$_{12}$ deficiency. The APCA test is used in combination with assays of vitamin B$_{12}$, antiintrinsic factor antibodies, methylmalonic acid, and homocysteine to distinguish pernicious anemia from other causes of megaloblastic anemia.

antiparkinsonian /-pär″kənsōnē·ən/, pertaining to a substance or procedure used to treat parkinsonism. Drugs for this neurological disorder are of two kinds: those that compensate for the lack of dopamine in the corpus striatum and anticholinergic agents that counteract the activity of the abundant acetylcholine in the corpus striatum. Synthetic levodopa, a dopamine precursor that crosses the blood-brain barrier, reduces the rigidity, sluggishness, dysphagia, drooling, and instability characteristic of the disease but does not alter its relentless course. Centrally active cholinergic blockers, notably benztropine mesylate, biperiden hydrochloride, procyclidine hydrochloride, and trihexyphenidyl hydrochloride, may relieve tremors and rigidity and improve mobility. The antiviral agent amantadine hydrochloride is often effective in the treatment of parkinsonism; its mechanism of action is not established, but it apparently increases release of dopamine in the brain. Therapeutic approaches to the relief of the symptoms of parkinsonism include alcohol injection, cautery, cryosurgery, and surgical excision performed to destroy the globus pallidus (reducing rigidity) and parts of the thalamus (reducing tremor). Extrapyramidal symptoms similar to those of idiopathic parkinsonism are frequently induced by antipsychotic drugs.

antipathy /antip″əthē/ [Gk, *anti + pathos,* suffering], a strong feeling of aversion or antagonism to particular objects, situations, or individuals.

antiperistalsis /-per′əstal″sis/, a wave of contractions in the digestive tract that moves toward the oral end of the tract. In the duodenum, stomach, or esophagus it results in regurgitation. Also called **reverse peristalsis.**

antiperistaltic /-per′əstal″tik/ [Gk, *anti + peristellein,* to wrap around], **1.** pertaining to a substance that inhibits or diminishes peristalsis. **2.** an antiperistaltic agent. Opioids, such as paregoric, diphenoxylate hydrochloride, and loperamide hydrochloride, provide symptomatic relief of diarrhea. Anticholinergics reduce spasms of intestinal smooth muscle and are frequently prescribed to decrease excessive GI motility.

antiplatelet agent /-plāt″lit/, therapeutic agent that inhibits platelet function. Often employed to prevent clot propagation or secondary thrombosis in patients who have had a primary arterial thrombolytic event such as acute myocardial infarction, peripheral artery disease, or cerebrovascular accident.

antipode /an″tipōd/, something that is diametrically opposite.

antipraxia /-prak″sē·ə/, a condition in which functions or symptoms appear to oppose each other.

antiprogestin /-prōjes″tin/, a substance that interferes with the production, uptake, or effects of progesterone. The most common example is mifepristone.

antiprotease, a substance that can prevent the digestion of proteins. Also called **protease inhibitor.**

antiprothrombin /-prōthrom″bin/, a substance that inhibits the conversion of prothrombin to thrombin.

antiprotoplasmatic /-prō″təplasmat″ik/, pertaining to an agent that damages the protoplasm of cells.

antiprotozoal /an″te-, an″ti-pro-to-zo′al/, **1.** destroying protozoa or checking their growth or reproduction. **2.** an antiprotozoal agent. Kinds include **pentamidine isethionate, metronidazole.**

antipruritic /-pro͞orit″ik/ [Gk, *anti + L, prurire,* to itch], **1.** pertaining to a substance or procedure that tends to relieve or prevent itching. **2.** an antipruritic drug. Topical anesthetics, corticosteroids, and antihistamines are used as antipruritic agents.

antipsoriatic /an″tisôr″ē·at″ik/ [Gk, *anti + psora,* itch], pertaining to an agent that relieves the symptoms of psoriasis.

antipsychotic /-sīkot″ik/ [Gk, *anti + psyche,* mind, *osis,* condition], **1.** pertaining to a substance or procedure that counteracts or diminishes symptoms of a psychosis. **2.** an antipsychotic drug. Categories include typical antipyschotics, such as phenothiazines (prochlorperazine) and butyrophenones (haloperidol), and atypical agents. Atypical agents include olanzapine, aripiprazole, and clozapine. Atypical agents differ from typical agents with regard to their affinity for dopamine blockade and their side effect profiles. Formerly called *major tranquilizer.*

anti-Purkinje cell antibody (APCA). See **anti-Yo antibody.**

antipyresis /-pīrē″sis/ [Gk, *anti + pyretos,* fever], the condition or state of being free from fever.

antipyretic /-pīret″ik/ [Gk, *anti + pyretos,* fever], **1.** pertaining to a substance or procedure that reduces fever. −**antipyresis,** *n.* **2.** an antipyretic agent. Such drugs usually lower the thermodetection set point of the hypothalamic heat regulatory center, with resulting vasodilation and diaphoresis. Widely used antipyretic agents are acetaminophen, aspirin, and NSAIDs. Also called **antifebrile, antithermic.**

antipyretic bath, a bath in which tepid water (85° to 90° F; 29° to 32° C) is used to reduce body temperature.

antipyrotic /-pīrot″ik/ [Gk, *anti + pyr,* fire], *(Archaic)* pertaining to the treatment of burns or scalds.

antirabies serum, an antiserum obtained from the blood serum or plasma of animals immunized with rabies vaccine; it is used for postexposure prophylaxis against rabies if rabies immune globulin is unavailable.

antirachitic /-rəkit″ik/, pertaining to an agent used to treat rickets.

antiretroviral /an″te-, an″ti-ret′ro-vi″ral/, **1.** effective against retroviruses. **2.** a substance or drug that stops or suppresses the activity of retroviruses such as HIV.

anti-Rh agglutinin, an antibody to an Rh antigen on Rh+ erythrocytes that causes these cells to agglutinate. Appears in Rh− persons after exposure to Rh+ erythrocytes, as when an Rh− mother is pregnant with an Rh+ fetus. See also **Rh factor.**

antirheumatic /-ro͞omat″ik/ [Gk, *anti + rheumatismos,* that which flows], pertaining to the relief of symptoms of any painful or immobilizing disorder of the musculoskeletal system.

anti-Ri antibody, an autoantibody having neuronal binding characteristics similar to those of anti-Hu antibody but directed against a different RNA binding site; it is associated with paraneoplastic opsoclonus-myoclonus in small cell lung carcinoma and in cancer of the breast and fallopian tube. Also called **type 2 antineuronal antibody.**

antiseborrheic /-seb′ərē′ik/, pertaining to a drug or agent applied to the skin to control seborrhea or seborrheic dermatitis.

antisense /an″tēsens/, pertaining to a ribonucleic acid (RNA) molecule that is complementary to the messenger RNA (mRNA) produced by transcription of a given gene. Antisense RNA synthesized in the laboratory hybridizes with the complementary mRNA molecules, thereby blocking the synthesis of specific proteins. DNA sequence could also be used to hybridize with complementary mRNA and block protein synthesis. Antisense drugs have a potential to be used for therapy. Compare **sense.**

antisense strand, the strand of a double-stranded nucleic acid that is complementary to the sense strand in DNA, being the template strand on which the mRNA is synthesized. Compare **sense strand.**

antisepsis /-sep′sis/ [Gk, *anti* + *sepein,* putrefaction], processes, procedures, or chemical treatments that kill or inhibit microorganisms to prevent infection.

antiseptic /-sep″tik/, **1.** tending to inhibit the growth and reproduction of microorganisms. **2.** a substance that tends to inhibit the growth and reproduction of microorganisms when applied to living tissue. See also **disinfectant.**

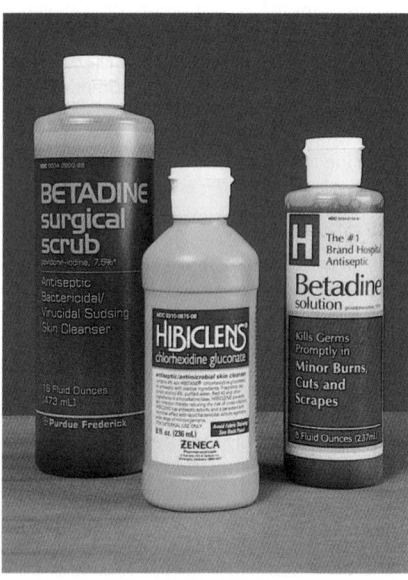

Antiseptic solutions *(Bonewit-West, 2012)*

antiseptic dressing, a fabric, gauze, or pad treated with an antiseptic, a germicidal, or a bacteriostatic solution and applied to a wound or an incision to prevent or treat infection.

antiserum /an″tisir′əm/ *pl.* **antisera, antiserums** [Gk, *anti* + L, whey], the serum of an animal or human containing antibodies against a specific disease, used to confer passive immunity to that disease. Antisera do not provoke the production of antibodies. There are two types of antisera: antitoxin neutralizes the toxin produced by specific bacteria but does not kill the bacteria, and antimicrobial serum acts to destroy bacteria by making them more susceptible to leukocytic action. Polyvalent antiserum acts on more than one antigenic determinant; monovalent antiserum acts on only one. Antibiotic drugs have largely replaced antimicrobial antisera. Caution must always be used in the administration of all antisera, since hepatitis or hypersensitivity reactions can result. Also called **immune serum.** Compare **vaccine.**

antiserum anaphylaxis, exaggerated hypersensitivity in a nonsensitized person after the injection of serum from a sensitized individual. Also called **passive anaphylaxis.** Compare **active anaphylaxis.**

antishock garment, a garment used to improve blood pressure. Kinds include **Non-Pneumatic Antishock Garment, military antishock trousers.**

antisialogog /-sī·al′əgōg′/ [Gk, *anti* + *sialon,* saliva, *agogos,* leading], a drug that reduces saliva secretion.

anti–smooth muscle antibody test, a blood test used primarily to help diagnose active autoimmune chronic hepatitis, although a low-level positive result may be associated with viral infections, malignancy, multiple sclerosis, primary biliary cirrhosis, and *Mycoplasma* infections.

antisocial personality /-sō″shəl/ [Gk, *anti* + L, *socius,* companion], a person who exhibits attitudes and overt behavior contrary to the customs, standards, and moral principles accepted by society. The individual appears to lack a sense of moral conscience. Also called **psychopathic personality, sociopathic personality.** See also **antisocial personality disorder.**

antisocial personality disorder, a condition characterized by repetitive behavioral patterns that are contrary to usual moral and ethical standards and cause a person to experience continuous conflict with society. Symptoms include aggression, callousness, impulsiveness, irresponsibility, hostility, a low frustration level, marked emotional immaturity, and poor judgment. A person who has this disorder overlooks the rights of others, is incapable of loyalty to others or to social values, is unable to experience guilt or to learn from past behaviors, is impervious to punishment, and tends to rationalize his or her behavior or to blame it on others.

antispasmodic /-spazmod″ik/, a drug or other agent that prevents smooth muscle spasms, as in the uterus, digestive system, or urinary tract. Belladonna and dicyclomine hydrochloride are among drugs used in antispasmodic preparations; Oxybutynin and tolterodine are examples of antispasmotic medications. See also **anticholinergic, cholinergic blocking agent.**

antispastic /an″te-, an″ti-spas′tik/, an antispasmodic with specific reference to striated muscle.

antisperm antibody (ASA), any of the various surface-bound antibodies found on spermatozoa after infection, trauma to the testes, or vasectomy; they interfere with fertilization or result in nonviable zygotes.

antispermatozoal antibody test, a fluid analysis or blood test used as a screening test for infertility. The test may be performed on men and women to detect the presence of sperm antibodies that may diminish fertility.

anti-SS-A (ro), anti-SS-B (La), and anti-SS-C antibody test, a blood test to measure the presence of antinuclear antibodies, which indicates Sjögren's syndrome.

antistreptolysin-O test (ASOT, ASO, ASLT) /an″tistrep′təlī″sinō′/, a serum test to identify and measure antibodies to streptolysin-O, an exotoxin produced by most group A and some group C or G streptococci. Elevated or rising titers indicate a current or recent strep infection. Often used to diagnose and monitor rheumatic fever or glomerulonephritis.

antithermic, *(Obsolete)* See **antipyretic.**

antithrombin /-throm″bin/, a plasma serine protease inhibitor that neutralizes thrombin. Antithrombin is a major coagulation control protein.

antithrombin (AT) test, an assay that determines the concentration and activity of antithrombin, a plasma serine protease that inhibits several coagulation enzymes, particularly thrombin (coagulation factor II) and coagulation factor X. Antithrombin is upregulated by therapeutic anticoagulant heparin in an effort to prevent or control thrombosis. Antithrombin deficiency is rare and is associated with thrombophilia, the tendency to form pathological blood clots. In heparin therapy, patients with acquired or congenital antithrombin deficiency respond only partially to heparin therapy, a condition named "heparin resistance." Formerly called *antithrombin III (ATT-III) test.*

antithrombotic /-thrombot″ik/, preventing or interfering with the formation of a thrombus or blood clotting. See also **anticoagulant.**

antithymocyte globulin (ATG) /an′tithī′məsīt/, the gamma globulin fraction of antiserum derived from animals that have been immunized against human thymocytes; an example is an immunosuppressive agent that causes specific destruction of T cells, used in treatment of allograft rejection. Also called **antilymphocyte globulin.**

antithymocyte globulin (ATG), a purified gamma globulin obtained from horses or rabbits immunized with human thymocytes; it is administered intravenously in the treatment of acute rejection occurring after renal transplantation.

antithyroglobulin antibody test, a serum or plasma test to identify and measure antithyroglobulin antibody, an autoantibody that may attack the thyroid gland. Antithyroglobulin antibody may reduce thyroid function in conditions such as Hashimoto thyroiditis or Graves disease. The antithyroglobulin test is performed in a profile of thyroid tests that may include free T_3, free T_4, and thyroid-stimulating hormone.

antithyroid drug /-thī′roid/, a preparation that inhibits the synthesis of thyroid hormones and is commonly used in the treatment of hyperthyroidism. The major antithyroid drugs are thioamide derivatives, such as propylthiouracil, and methimazole. Such substances interfere with the incorporation of iodine into the tyrosyl residues of thyroglobulin required for the production of the hormones thyroxine and triiodothyronine. They are often used to control hyperthyroidism during an anticipated remission and before a thyroidectomy.

antithyroid microsomal antibody test, a blood test used primarily in the differential diagnosis of thyroid diseases such as Hashimoto disease. This test is usually performed in conjunction with the antithyroglobulin antibody test. Also called **antithyroid peroxidase antibody (anti-TPO) test.**

antithyroid peroxidase (anti-TPO) antibodies, the main antigen of the thyroid microsomal fraction. It is elevated in the majority of the patients with thyroiditis.

antithyroid peroxidase (anti-TPO) antibody test, a serum or plasma test to identify and measure one of several autoantibodies that may reduce thyroid function as in Hashimoto thyroiditis or Graves disease.

antitoxin /-tok″sin/ [Gk, *anti* + *toxikon,* poison], a subgroup of antisera usually prepared from the serum of horses immunized against a particular toxin-producing organism, such as botulism antitoxin given therapeutically in botulism and tetanus and diphtheria antitoxins given prophylactically to prevent those infections.

anti-TPO, abbreviation for *antithyroid peroxidase.*

antitragus, an elevation of the auricle of the ear opposite the tragus and above the fleshy lobule.

antitrismus /-tris″məs/, a tonic muscular spasm that forces the mouth to open.

antitrust /-trust″/, (in law) against the operation, establishment, or maintenance of a monopoly in the manufacture, production, or sale of a commodity, provision of a service, or practice of a profession.

antitrypsin. See **alpha₁-antitrypsin.**

antitubercular /-tōōbur″kyələr/, any agent or group of drugs used to treat tuberculosis. At least two drugs, and usually three, are required in various combinations in active pulmonary tuberculosis infection. These medications include isoniazid, ethambutol hydrochloride, streptomycin sulfate, pyrazinamide, and rifampin. Supplements of pyridoxine (vitamin B_6) also may be needed to relieve the symptoms of peripheral neuritis that can occur as a side effect of isoniazid.

antitumor antibodies, a natural product that interferes with deoxyribonucleic acid in such a way as to prevent its further replication and the transcription of ribonucleic acid. They are known as antibiotics because they are produced from natural products in a manner similar to the production of antibiotics.

antitussive /an′titus″iv/ [Gk, *anti* + L, *tussive,* cough], **1.** against a cough. **2.** any of a large group of opioid and nonopioid drugs that act on the central and peripheral nervous systems to suppress the cough reflex. Because the cough reflex is necessary for clearing the upper respiratory tract of obstructive secretions, antitussives should not be used with a productive cough. Codeine phosphate and hydrocodone bitartrate are potent opioid antitussives. Dextromethorphan hydrobromide is an effective antitussive with minimal risk of dependence. Antitussives are administered orally, usually in a syrup with a mucolytic or expectorant and alcohol, but sometimes in a capsule with an antihistaminic and a mild analgesic.

antiurolithic /an″ti-u′ro-lith′ik/, **1.** preventing the formation of urinary calculi. **2.** an antiurolithic agent.

antivenin /an′tiven″in/ [Gk, *anti* + L, *venenum,* poison], a suspension of venom-neutralizing antibodies prepared from the serum of immunized horses. Antivenin confers passive immunity and is given as a part of emergency first aid for various snake and insect bites. Also spelled *antivenom.*

Antivert, an antihistaminic antivertigo agent. Brand name for **meclizine hydrochloride.**

antiviral, effective against viruses.

antivirus software, a software program written so that on execution (usually automatic when a computer is started) it scans the hard drive and related processors to identify, isolate, and eradicate viruses and other harmful malware and spyware. Modern antivirus software requests updates automatically on a schedule set either by default or by the user. See **malware.**

antivitamin factor [Gk, *anti* + L, *vita,* life, amine], a substance that inactivates a vitamin.

antixerophthalmic vitamin. See **vitamin A.**

anti-Yo antibody, polyclonal IgG autoantibody directed against Purkinje's cells and associated with paraneoplastic cerebellar degeneration in small cell carcinoma of the lung and cancer of the breast or ovary. Also called **anti-Purkinje cell antibody.**

Anton syndrome [Gabriel Anton, German neuropsychiatrist, 1858–1933], a form of anosognosia in which a person with partial or total blindness denies being visually impaired, despite medical evidence to the contrary. The patient typically contrives excuses for the inability to see, such as suggesting that the light is inadequate.

Antopol-Goldman lesion. See **subepithelial hematoma of renal pelvis.**

antr-. See **antro-, antr-.**

antra, pleural of antrum. See **antrum.**

antral gastritis [Gk, *antron,* cave], an abnormal narrowing of the antrum of the stomach. The narrowing is not a true gastritis but a radiographic finding that may represent a peptic ulcer or a tumor.

antrectomy /antrek″təmē/, a surgical procedure in which the portion of the stomach distal to the antrum is excised.

antro-, antr-, prefix meaning "antrum or sinus": *antrocele, antrodynia.*

antrum *pl.* **antra** [Gk, *antron,* cave], a cavity or chamber that is nearly closed and usually surrounded by bone. The antrum cardiacum is a dilation of the esophagus. The fluid-filled cavity in a mature graafian follicle of the ovary is also termed an antrum.

antrum of Highmore. See **maxillary sinus.**

Anturane, a uricosuric drug. Brand name for **sulfinpyrazone.**

anular /an′yələr/ [L, *annulus,* ring], also spelled **annular.**

anular ligament, a ligament that encircles the head of the radius and holds it in the radial notch of the ulna. Distal to the notch, the anular ligament forms a complete fibrous ring. Also spelled **annular ligament.**

anulus /an″yələs/, a ring of circular tissue, such as the whitish tympanic anulus around the perimeter of the tympanic membrane. Also spelled **annulus. –anular, annular,** *adj.*

anulus fibrosus, an outer ring of collagen in an intervertebral disk arranged in a lamellar configuration that surrounds a wider zone of fibrocartilage.

anuresis, the retention of urine in the bladder. Compare **anuria.**

anuria /ənoor′ē·ə/ [Gk, *a, ouron,* not urine], the absence of urine production or a urinary output of less than 100 mL/day. Anuria may be caused by a failure or kidney dysfunction, a decline in blood pressure below that required to maintain filtration pressure in the kidney, or an obstruction in the urinary passages. A rapid decline in urinary output, leading ultimately to anuria and uremia, occurs in acute renal failure. Also called **anuresis, prerenal anuria.** Compare **oliguria.** Kinds include **angioneurotic anuria, obstructive anuria, postrenal anuria, renal anuria.** *–anuric, anuretic, adj.*

anus /ā″nəs/, the opening of the rectum lying in the fold between the buttocks. It is surrounded by two sphincters that control the discharge of fecal material. **–anal,** *adj.*

anxietas /angzī″ətas/ [L, anxiety], a state of anxiety, nervous restlessness, or apprehension, often accompanied by a feeling of oppression in the epigastric region. Kinds include **anxietas presenilis, restless legs syndrome.**

anxietas presenilis [L, *anxietas* + *prae,* before, *senex,* aged], a state of extreme anxiety associated with the climacteric.

anxietas tibiarum, *(Obsolete)* now called **restless legs syndrome.**

anxiety /angzī″ətē/ [L, *anxietas*], anticipation of impending danger and dread accompanied by restlessness, tension, tachycardia, and breathing difficulty not necessarily associated with a specific or known stimulus. Kinds include **castration anxiety, free-floating anxiety, generalized anxiety disorder, separation anxiety, situational anxiety, panic disorder.**

anxiety attack, an acute, psychobiological reaction manifested by intense anxiety and panic. Symptoms include palpitations, shortness of breath, dizziness, faintness, profuse diaphoresis, pallor of the face and extremities, GI discomfort, and an intense feeling of imminent doom or death. Attacks usually occur suddenly, last from a few seconds to an hour or longer, and vary in frequency from several times a day to once a month. Treatment consists of reassurance, desensitization statement, separation of the individual from anxiety-producing situations, administration of a sedative if necessary, and appropriate psychotherapy to identify the stresses perceived as threatening.

anxiety disorder, a disorder in which anxiety is the most prominent feature. The symptoms range from mild, chronic tenseness, with feelings of timidity, fatigue, apprehension, and indecisiveness, to more intense states of restlessness and irritability that may lead to aggressive acts, persistent helplessness, or withdrawal. In extreme cases, the overwhelming emotional discomfort is accompanied by physical responses, including tremor, sustained muscle tension, tachycardia, dyspnea, hypertension, increased respiration, and profuse diaphoresis. Other physical signs include changes in skin color, nausea, vomiting, diarrhea, restlessness, immobilization, insomnia, and changes in appetite, all occurring without identification of a known underlying organic cause. See also **anxiety, anxiety attack, anxiety reaction, anxiety state, obsessive-compulsive disorder, phobia, posttraumatic stress disorder.**

Physiological, behavioral, cognitive, and affective responses to anxiety

Physiological	Physiological—cont'd	Behavioral	Cognitive—cont'd
Cardiovascular	*Neuromuscular*	Restlessness	Loss of objectivity
Palpitations	Increased reflexes	Physical tension	Fear of losing control
Racing heart	Startle reaction	Tremors	Frightening visual images
Increased blood pressure	Eyelid twitching	Startle reaction	Fear of injury or death
Faintness*	Insomnia	Hypervigilance	Flashbacks
Actual fainting*	Tremors	Rapid speech	Nightmares
Decreased blood pressure*	Rigidity	Lack of coordination	
Decreased pulse rate*	Fidgeting	Accident proneness	**Affective**
	Pacing	Interpersonal withdrawal	Edginess
Respiratory	Strained face	Inhibition	Impatience
Rapid breathing	Generalized weakness	Flight	Uneasiness
Shortness of breath	Wobbly legs	Avoidance	Tension
Pressure on chest	Clumsy movement	Hyperventilation	Nervousness
Shallow breathing			Fear
Lump in throat	*Urinary tract*	**Cognitive**	Fright
Choking sensation	Pressure to urinate*	Impaired attention	Frustration
Gasping	Frequent urination*	Poor concentration	Helplessness
		Forgetfulness	Alarm
Gastrointestinal	*Skin*	Errors in judgment	Terror
Loss of appetite	Flushed face	Preoccupation	Jitteriness
Revulsion toward food	Localized sweating (e.g.,	Blocking of thoughts	Jumpiness
Abdominal discomfort	palms)	Decreased perceptual field	Numbing
Abdominal pain*	Itching	Reduced creativity	Guilt
Nausea*	Hot and cold spells	Diminished productivity	Shame
Heartburn*	Pale face	Confusion	Frustration
Diarrhea*	Generalized sweating	Self-consciousness	Helplessness

*Parasympathetic response.

From Stuart GW: *Principles and practice of psychiatric nursing,* ed 10, St Louis, 2013, Mosby.

anxiety dream, a dream that is accompanied by restlessness and a gradual increase in pulse rate. Anxiety dreams tend to occur in children, who usually recall the content clearly.

anxiety reaction [L, *anxietas* + *re, agere,* to act], a clinical characteristic in which anxiety is the predominant feature or is experienced by a person facing a dreaded situation to the extent that his or her functioning is impaired. The reaction may be expressed as an anxiety attack, a phobia, or a compulsion.

anxiety state [L, *anxietas* + *ity,* state], a mental or emotional reaction characterized by apprehension, uncertainty, and irrational fear. Anxiety states may be accompanied by physiological changes such as diaphoresis, tremors, rapid heartbeat, dilated pupils, and xerostomia.

anxiolytic. See **antianxiety agent.**

AOA, abbreviation for **Administration on Aging.**

AORN, abbreviation for **Association of periOperative Registered Nurses.**

aorta /ā·ôr″tə/ [Gk, *aerein,* to raise], the main trunk of the systemic arterial circulation, comprising four parts: the ascending aorta, the arch of the aorta, the thoracic portion of the descending aorta, and the abdominal portion of the descending aorta. It starts at the aortic opening of the left ventricle, rises a short distance, bends over the root of the left lung, descends within the thorax on the left side of the vertebral column, and passes through the aortic hiatus of the diaphragm into the abdominal cavity. It branches into the two common iliac arteries. –*aortic, adj.*

aortic aneurysm, a localized dilation of the wall of the aorta caused by atherosclerosis, hypertension, connective tissue disease such as Marfan's, or less frequently, syphilis. The lesion may be a saccular distension or a fusiform or cylindrical swelling of a length of the vessel. Syphilitic aneurysms almost always occur in the thoracic aorta and usually involve the arch of the aorta. The more common atherosclerotic aneurysms are usually in the abdominal aorta below the renal arteries and above the bifurcation of the aorta. These lesions often contain atheromatous ulcers covered by thrombi that may discharge emboli, causing obstruction of smaller vessels. See also **dissecting aneurysm.**

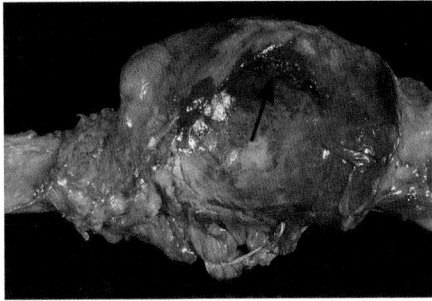

Ruptured abdominal aortic aneurysm *(Kumar et al, 2010)*

aortic angiogram. See **aortogram.**

aortic arch (AA). See **arch of the aorta.**

aortic arch syndrome, any of a group of occlusive conditions of the arch of the aorta, producing a variety of symptoms related to obstruction of the large branch arteries, including the brachiocephalic, left common carotid, and left subclavian. It may be caused by atherosclerosis, Takayasu's arteritis, syphilis, and other conditions. Symptoms include syncope, temporary blindness, hemiplegia, aphasia, and memory loss.

aortic atresia [Gk, *aeirein* + *a, tresis,* a boring], a congenital anomaly in which the aortic valve is blocked or missing, preventing normal blood flow.

■ OBSERVATIONS: Symptoms appear shortly after birth and include cyanosis, difficulty breathing, and irritability. The severity of symptoms is related to the degree of the defect, as well as the presence of other cardiac defects.

■ INTERVENTIONS: Prostaglandin (IV) may be prescribed to keep the ductus arteriosis open to permit blood flow. Multiple surgical procedures may be required to correct the deformity.

■ PATIENT CARE CONSIDERATIONS: Infants with congenital heart disease and their families require support. Long-term follow-up with regular evaluations is important.

aortic balloon pump. See **intraaortic balloon pump.**

aortic body, one of several small structures on the arch of the aorta that contain neural tissue sensitive to the chemical composition of arterial blood. The aortic bodies respond primarily to large reductions in blood oxygen content and trigger an increase in respiratory rate. See also **aortic-body reflex, carotid body.**

aortic-body reflex, a neural reflex in which a decrease in the oxygen content of arterial blood is sensed by the aortic bodies, which signal the medullary respiratory center to increase respiratory rate. See also **carotid-body reflex.**

aortic hiatus, an opening behind the diaphragm for the aorta and thoracic duct.

aortic insufficiency. See **aortic regurgitation.**

aortic notch [Gk, *aeirein,* to raise; OFr, *enochier*], the indentation on the descending limb of an arterial pulse sphygmogram. It marks the closure of the aortic valve. Also called **dicrotic notch.**

aortic obstruction [L, *obstruere,* to build against], a blockage or impediment that interrupts the flow of blood in the aorta.

aorticopulmonary septum, a septum, formed by fusion of the bulbar ridges during heart development, that divides the bulbus cordis into aortic and pulmonary trunks.

aortopulmonary window. Also called **aortopulmonary fenestration.**

aortic reconstruction, a surgical restoration of function to a damaged or obstructed aorta as by bypass or aortoplasty.

aortic regurgitant murmur [Gk, *aeirein,* to raise; L, *re,* again, *gurgitare,* to flow, *murmur,* humming], a high-pitched, soft, blowing, decrescendo, early diastolic heart murmur that is a sign of aortic regurgitation.

aortic regurgitation, the flow of blood from the aorta back into the left ventricle during diastole, resulting from a failure of the aortic valve to close completely. Also called **aortic insufficiency.**

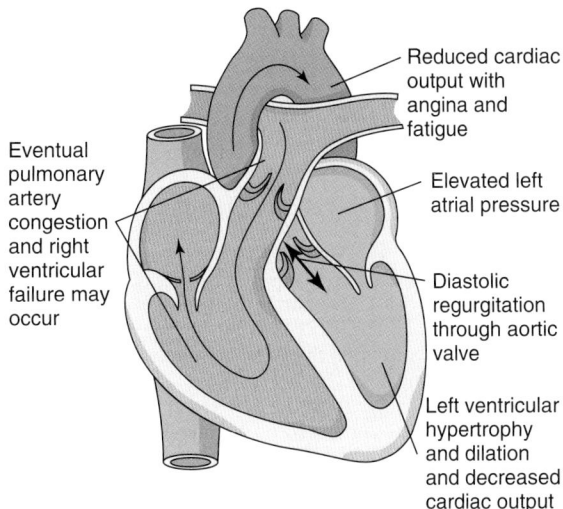

Effects of aortic regurgitation *(Beare and Myers, 1998)*

Reduced cardiac output with angina and fatigue

Elevated left atrial pressure

Diastolic regurgitation through aortic valve

Left ventricular hypertrophy and dilation and decreased cardiac output

Eventual pulmonary artery congestion and right ventricular failure may occur

aortic sinus [Gk, *aeirein,* to raise; L, *sinus,* little hollow], any of three dilations, one anterior and two posterior, between the aortic wall and the semilunar cusps of the aortic valve. Also called **Petit's sinus, sinus of Morgagni, sinus of Valsalva.**

aortic stenosis (AS) [Gk, *aeirein + stenos,* narrow, *osis,* condition], a narrowing or stricture of the aortic valve. Common causes include calcification of the valve because of age, congenital malformations such as bicuspid or unicuspid valves, or direct damage to the valve from rheumatic fever, which leads to fusion of the cusps. Surgical repair may be indicated. Surgery is followed by frequent examinations because prosthetic valve dysfunction and bacterial endocarditis are relatively common sequelae. See also **congenital cardiac anomaly, valvular heart disease.**

■ OBSERVATIONS: Aortic stenosis obstructs the flow of blood from the left ventricle into the aorta, causing decreased cardiac output and pulmonary vascular congestion. It may lead to congestive heart failure. Clinical manifestations include faint peripheral pulses, exercise intolerance, angina-type pain, syncope, and a harsh midsystolic murmur often introduced by an ejection sound. Diagnosis is confirmed by cardiac catheterization or echocardiography.

■ INTERVENTIONS: Surgical repair may be indicated. Surgery is followed by frequent examinations because prosthetic valve dysfunction and bacterial endocarditis are relatively common sequelae.

■ PATIENT CARE CONSIDERATIONS: Monitoring health and maintaining a heart-healthy lifestyle are important. Children with aortic stenosis are usually restricted from strenuous activities, but should be encouraged to be active.

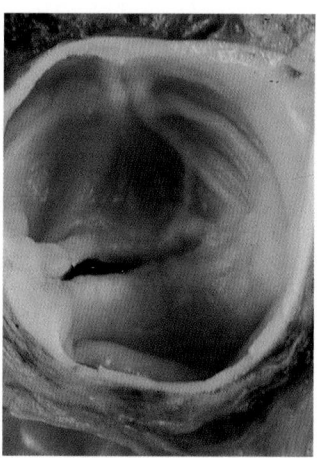

Aortic stenosis *(Damjanov and Linder, 2000)*

aortic thrill [Gk, *aeirein,* to raise; AS, *thyrlian*], a palpable chest vibration caused by aortic stenosis or an aortic aneurysm. It is usually felt in systole by placing the flat of the hand or the fingertips on the second intercostal space to the right of the sternum.

aortic valve, a valve in the heart between the left ventricle and the aorta. It is composed of three semilunar cusps that close in diastole to prevent blood from flowing back into the left ventricle from the aorta. The three cusps are separated by sinuses that resemble tiny buckets when they are filled with blood. These cup-shaped flaps grow from the lining of the aorta and, in systole, open to allow oxygenated blood to flow from the left ventricle into the aorta and on to the peripheral circulation. Compare **mitral valve, pulmonary valve, tricuspid valve.**

aortic valvular stenosis. See **subaortic stenosis.**

aortitis /ā′ôrtī′tis/, an inflammation of the aorta. It occurs most frequently in tertiary syphilis and occasionally in rheumatic fever.

aortocoronary /ā·ôr′tōkôr″əner′ē/ [Gk, *aeirein + L, corona,* crown], pertaining to the aorta and coronary arteries.

aortacoronary bypass [AS, *bi,* alongside; Fr, *passer*], *(Obsolete)* now called **coronary artery bypass graft (CABG).**

aortogram /ā·ôr′təgram/ [Gk, *aerein + gramma,* record], a radiographic image or set of images of the aorta made after the injection of a radiopaque contrast medium. Also called **aortic angiogram.**

aortography /ā·ôrtog″rəfē/ [Gk, *aerein + graphein,* to record], a diagnostic tool that uses a radiographic process to study the aorta and its branches after the patient is injected with any of various contrast media. −*aortographic, adj.*

aortopulmonary fenestration /ā·ôr′tōpul″məner′ē/ [Gk, *aerein + L, pulmoneus,* lung, *fenestra,* window], a congenital anomaly characterized by an abnormal fenestration in the ascending aorta and the pulmonary artery cephalad to the semilunar valve, allowing oxygenated and unoxygenated blood to mix, resulting in a decrease in the oxygen available in the peripheral circulation. Also called *aortic septal defect,* **aortopulmonary window.**

AOTA, abbreviation for **American Occupational Therapy Association.**

AOTF, abbreviation for *American Occupational Therapy Foundation.*

AP, abbreviation for **anteroposterior.**

ap-, apo-, prefixes meaning "separation or derivation from; away from": *apeidosis, aponeurosis.*

APA, **1.** abbreviation for **American Psychiatric Association. 2.** abbreviation for **American Psychological Association.**

APA Style, an editorial style used in many of the social and behaviorial sciences, with rules and guidelines published by the American Psychological Association.

APACHE IV /əpach″ē/, a system for classifying the severity of illness in patients in the intensive care unit. Abbreviation for *Acute Physiology and Chronic Health Evaluation.* See also **SAPS III.**

apareunia /ā′pəroo̅″nē·ə/, an inability to perform coitus caused by a physical or psychological sexual dysfunction.

apathetic hyperthyroidism /ap′əthet″ik/, a form of Graves disease mainly affecting older adults that causes a placid, aged facial appearance, apathetic behavior, and inactivity rather than the symptoms usually associated with hyperthyroidism. Medical treatment not only restores normal behavioral activity but also results in a more youthful physical appearance. Untreated, the patient is likely to succumb to the effects of stress or acute illness.

apathy /ap′əthē/ [Gk, *a, pathos,* not suffering], an absence or suppression of emotion, feeling, concern, or passion; an indifference to stimuli found generally to be exciting or moving. The condition is common in patients with neurasthenia, depressive disorders, and schizophrenia. −*apathetic, adj.*

apatite /ap′ətīt/ [Gk, *apate,* deceit], an inorganic mineral composed of calcium and phosphate. Apatite appears chemically as hydroxyapatite and fluorapatite in the bones and teeth.

APC,   **1.** abbreviation for **atrial premature complex. 2.** abbreviation for **adenomatous polyposis coli.**

APCA,   **1.** abbreviation for **antiparietal cell antibodies. 2.** abbreviation for **anti-Purkinje cell antibody.**

APCC,   abbreviation for **activated prothrombin complex concentrate.**

apepsia /āpep″sē·ə/   [Gk, *a,* without, *pepsis,* digestion], a condition involving a failure of the digestive functions.

aperient /əpir″ē·ənt/   [L, *aperire,* to open], a mild laxative.

aperistalsis /āper′istal″sis/   [Gk, *a,* without, *peristellein,* to clasp], a failure of the normal waves of contraction and relaxation that move contents through the digestive tract. Compare **peristalsis.**

aperitive /əper″itiv/   [L, *aperere,* to open], a stimulant of the appetite. Also called *aperitif.*

Apert syndrome /äper″/   [Eugène Charles Apert, French pediatrician, 1868–1940], a rare genetic condition characterized by an abnormal craniofacial appearance in combination with partial or complete fusion (webbing) of the fingers and toes. Also called **acrocephalosyndactyly.** Should not be confused with **Alport syndrome.**

■ OBSERVATIONS: Signs of Apert syndrome include a peaked and vertically elongated head, widespread and bulging eyes, and a high, arched posterior palate with bony defects of the maxilla and the mandible, including cleft palate or uvula and extreme malocclusion. The degree of fusion varies greatly and may be complete.

■ INTERVENTIONS: There is no known cure for Apert syndrome. Treatment is supportive; surgery to correct abnormalities may be performed.

■ PATIENT CARE CONSIDERATIONS: A characteristic feature is the premature joining of cranial bones, with resultant growth disturbances.

aperture /ap″ərchər/   [L, *apertura,* an opening], an opening or hole in an object or anatomical structure.

aperture of the frontal sinus,   an external opening of the frontal sinus into the nasal cavity.

aperture of the glottis,   an opening between the true vocal cords and the arytenoid cartilages.

aperture of the larynx,   an opening between the pharynx and larynx.

aperture of the sphenoid sinus,   a round opening between the sphenoid sinus and the nasal cavity, situated just above the superior nasal concha.

apex /ā″peks/ *pl.* **apices**   [L, tip], **1.** the top, the end, the summit, or the extremity of a structure, such as the apex cordis or the apices of the teeth. **–apical,** *adj.* **2.** pertaining to the end of the root of a tooth.

apex beat,   a pulsation of the left ventricle of the heart, palpable and sometimes visible at the fifth intercostal space in healthy adults, approximately 9 cm to the left of the midline. Also called **apical beat.**

apex cordis   [L, *apex + cordis,* of the heart], the pointed lower border of the heart. It is directed downward, forward, and to the left and is usually located at the level of the fifth intercostal space.

apexification /-if′ikā″shən/   [L, *apex + facere,* to make], a process of promoting apical closure of the root in an endodontically treated tooth by placement of mineral trioxide aggregate (MTA), calcium hydroxide paste, or other tissue-tolerant material in the root canal.

apexigraph /āpek″sigraf′/,   a device used for determining the position of the apex of a tooth root. Also called *electronic apex locator.*

apex murmur   [L, *apex,* summit, *murmur,* humming], a heart sound heard best at the apex of the heart, which in most individuals is at the level of the fifth intercostal space. Also called **apical murmur.**

apex of the heart,   the lowest superficial part of the heart, formed by the inferolateral part of the left ventricle.

apex of the urinary bladder,   the superior area of the urinary bladder, opposite the fundus. It is located at the junction of the superior and inferolateral surfaces of the bladder, and from it the middle umbilical ligament (urachus) extends to the umbilicus. Also called **vertex** or *summit of urinary bladder.*

apex pneumonia   [L, *apex,* summit; Gk, *pnemon,* lung], pneumonia in which consolidation is limited to the upper lobe of one lung. Also called **apical pneumonia.**

apex pulmonis /pəlmō″nis/   [L, *apex + pulmoneus,* lung], the rounded upper border of each lung, projecting above the clavicle.

APF,   a preparation of sodium fluoride acidulated to a lower, more acidic pH with phosphoric acid for topical application to the teeth for the prevention of dental caries. Abbreviation for *acidulated phosphate fluoride.*

Apgar score /ap″gär/   [Virginia Apgar, American anesthesiologist, 1909–1974], an evaluation of a newborn's physical condition, usually performed 1 minute and again 5 minutes after birth, based on a rating of five factors that reflect the infant's ability to adjust to extrauterine life. The system rapidly identifies infants requiring immediate intervention or transfer to a neonatal intensive care unit.

■ METHOD: The infant's heart rate, respiratory effort, muscle tone, reflex irritability, and color are scored from a low value of 0 to a normal value of 2. The five scores are combined, and the totals at 1 minute and 5 minutes are noted; for example, Apgar 9/10 is a score of 9 at 1 minute and 10 at 5 minutes.

■ PATIENT CARE CONSIDERATIONS: A low 1-minute score requires immediate intervention, including administration of oxygen, clearing of the nasopharynx, and usually transfer to a neonatal intensive care unit. A baby with a low score that persists at 5 minutes requires expert care, which may include assisted ventilation, umbilical catheterization, cardiac massage, blood gas analysis, correction of acid-base deficit, or medication to reverse the effects of maternal medication.

■ OUTCOME CRITERIA: A score of 0 to 3 represents severe distress, a score of 4 to 7 indicates moderate distress, and a score of 7 to 10 indicates an absence of difficulty in adjusting to extrauterine life. The 5-minute total score is normally higher than the 1-minute score. Because a normal, vigorous, healthy newborn almost always has bluish hands and feet at 1 minute, the first score for color will include a 1 rather than a perfect 2; however, at 5 minutes the blueness may have passed, and a score of 2 may be given. A 5-minute overall score of 0 to 1 correlates with a 50% neonatal mortality rate; infants who survive

Infant evaluation at birth—Apgar scoring system

Sign	0	1	2
Heart rate	Absent	Slow, <100	>100
Respiratory effort	Absent	Irregular, slow, weak cry	Good, strong cry
Muscle tone	Limp	Some flexion of extremities	Well-flexed
Reflex irritability	No response	Grimace	Cry, sneeze
Color	Blue, pale	Body pink, extremities blue	Completely pink

exhibit three times as many neurological abnormalities at 1 year of age as do children with a 5-minute score of 7 or more.

APhA, abbreviation for *American Pharmacists Association.*

APHA, abbreviation for *American Public Health Assoc iation.*

aphagia /əfā″jē·ə/ [Gk, *a* + *phagein,* not to eat], a condition characterized by the loss of the ability to swallow as a result of organic disease or psychological causes such as cerebrovascular accident and anxiety. See also **dysphagia.**

aphagia algera, a condition characterized by the refusal to eat or swallow because doing so causes pain.

aphakia /əfā″kē·ə/ [Gk, *a, phakos,* not lens], (in ophthalmology) a condition in which the crystalline lens of the eye is absent, usually because it has been surgically removed, as in the treatment of cataracts. Also called *aphacia.* –*aphakic, aphacic, adj.*

aphasia /əfā″zhə/ [Gk, *a* + *phasis,* not speech], a neurological condition in which language function is disordered or absent because of an injury to certain areas of the cerebral cortex. The deficiency may be sensory aphasia, in which language is not understood, or motor aphasia, in which words cannot be formed or expressed. Aphasia may be complete or partial, affecting specific language functions. Most commonly, the condition is a mixture of incomplete sensory and motor aphasia. It may occur after severe head trauma, prolonged hypoxia, or cerebrovascular accident. It is sometimes transient, as when the swelling in the brain following injury subsides and language returns. Compare **anomia, aphrasia.** Kinds include **Broca aphasia, Wernicke aphasia.** –*aphasic, adj.*

aphemia /əfē″mē·ə/, a loss of the ability to speak. The term is applied to emotional disorders as well as neurological causes. A person may suffer aphemia because a fear of speaking or a refusal to participate in verbal communication. –*aphemic, adj.*

apheresis /əfer″əsis, af′ərē″sis/ [Gk, *aphairesis,* removal], a procedure in which blood is temporarily withdrawn, one or more components are selectively removed, and the rest of the blood is reinfused into the donor. The process is used in treating various disease conditions in the donor and for obtaining blood elements for the treatment of other patients or for research. Also called **pheresis.** See also **leukapheresis, plasmapheresis, plateletpheresis.**

-aphia, -haphia, suffixes meaning a "condition of the sense of touch": *hyperaphia, paraphia.*

aphonia /āfō″nē·ə/ [Gk, *a, phone,* without voice], a condition characterized by loss of the ability to produce normal speech sounds that results from overuse of the vocal cords, organic disease, or psychological causes, such as anxiety. Kinds include **aphonia paralytica, spastic aphonia.** See also **speech dysfunction.** –*aphonous, aphonic, adj.*

aphonia paralytica /par′əlit″ikə/, a condition characterized by a loss of the voice caused by paralysis or disease of the laryngeal nerves. See also **aphonia.**

aphonic pectoriloquy /āfon″ik/, the abnormal transmission of voice sounds through a cavity or a serous pleural effusion, detected during auscultation of a lung.

aphonic speech, abnormal speech in which vocalizations are whispered.

aphonous. See **aphonia.**

aphoria /əfôr″ē·ə/, a condition in which physical weakness is not compromised as a result of exercise.

aphrasia /əfrā″zhə/, a form of aphasia in which a person may be able to speak single words or understand single words but is not able to communicate with words that are arranged in meaningful phrases or sentences.

-aphrodisia, a suffix meaning a "(specified) condition of sexual arousal": *anaphrodisia, hypoaphrodisia.*

aphronia /əfrō″nē·ə/ [Gk, *a, phronein,* not to understand], (in psychiatry) a condition characterized by an impaired ability to make commonsense decisions. –*aphronic, adj.*

aphtha /af″thē/ [Gk, *aphtha,* eruption], a small, shallow, painful ulceration that usually affects the oral mucosa but not underlying bone. Aphthae occasionally may affect other body tissues, including those of the GI tract and the external genitals. They do not appear to be infectious, contagious, or sexually transmitted. See also **aphthous stomatitis, foot-and-mouth disease.** –*aphthous, adj.*

aphthous fever. See **foot-and-mouth disease.**

aphthous stomatitis /af″thəs/ [Gk, *aphtha,* eruption, *stoma,* mouth, *itis,* inflammation], a recurring condition characterized by the eruption of painful ulcers (commonly called canker sores) on the mucous membranes of the mouth. Evidence suggests that the condition is an immune response. Heredity, some foods, emotional stress, cancer, and fever are also possible causes.

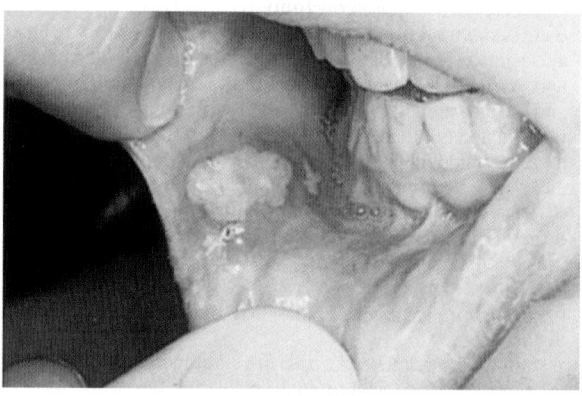

Aphthous stomatitis *(Feldman, Friedman, and Brandt, 2010)*

APIC, abbreviation for **Association for Professionals in Infection Control and Epidemiology.**

apical, **1.** pertaining to the tip or top of a structure, such as the heart, the lungs, or the tongue. See **apex. 2.** (in dentistry) the tip of the root portion of a tooth.

apical beat, the pulsation of the heart felt or auscultated over the apex of the heart at the point of maximal impulse. Also called **apex beat.**

apical curettage [L, *apex;* Fr, scraping], the debridement of the apical surface of a tooth and the removal of diseased soft tissues in the surrounding bony crypt. Compare **apicoectomy, root curettage, subgingival curettage.**

apical fiber, one of the many fibers of the periodontal ligament. These fibers radiate around the apex of the tooth at approximately right angles to their cementum attachment, extending into the bone at the bottom of the alveolus. Apical fibers resist forces that tend to lift the tooth from its socket and, with the other fibers of the periodontal ligament, stabilize the tooth against tilting movements.

apical impulse. See **precordial movement.**

apical lordotic view /lôrdot″ik/, a radiograph made with the patient leaning backward to the image receptor at an angle of 15 to 45 degrees to project the clavicles above the apices of the lungs for the purpose of better visibility. The view can also be generated through a 15- to 45-degree cephalic angle of the central ray.

apical membrane, the layer of plasma membrane on the apical side (the side toward the lumen) of the epithelial cells in a body tube or cavity, separated from the basolateral membrane by the zonula occludens.

apical murmur. See **apex murmur.**

apical odontoid ligament /ōdon″toid/, an upper cervical spine ligament connecting the axis (C2) to the occipital bone. It extends from the odontoid process of the axis (dens) to the anterior margin of the foramen magnum and lies between the two alar ligaments, blending with the anterior atlantooccipital membrane.

apical perforation, a mechanically induced channel running from the pulp canal into the periodontal space at or near the apex of the root.

apical periodontitis [L, *apex,* summit; Gk, *peri,* near, *odous,* tooth, *itis,* inflammation], an inflammation of the tissues around the apex of a tooth root.

apical pneumonia. See **apex pneumonia.**

apical pulse, the heartbeat as felt by palpation or heard with a stethoscope on the chest wall adjacent to the lowest and leftmost point of the heart.

apicectomy. See **apicoectomy.**

apices, pleural of apex. See **apex.**

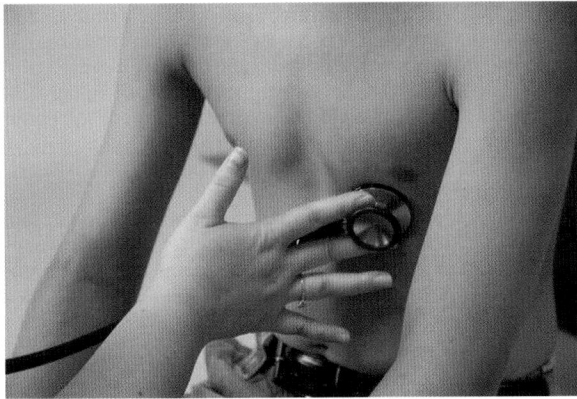

Palpation of the apical pulse

apicitis /ap′isī″tis/, an inflammation of the apex of a body structure, such as the apex pulmonis (lung) or the end of the root of a tooth.

apicoectomy /ap′ikō•ek″təmē/ [L, *apex* + Gk, *ektomē,* excision], (in dentistry) surgical removal of the apex or the apical portion of an infected or damaged tooth root, which is then usually sealed with MTA (mineral trioxide aggregate) and other biocompatible proprietary compounds, usually in conjunction with apical curettage or root canal therapy. The goal of the procedure is to prolong the useful life of the tooth. Also called **apicectomy, partial root amputation, root resection, root-end resection.**

apicotomy /ā′pikot″əmē/, a surgical incision into the highest point of a body structure.

apituitarism /ā′pityoo″itəriz′əm/ [Gk, *a,* without; L, *pituita,* phlegm; Gk, *ismos,* a state], an absence or loss of function of the pituitary gland.

APKD, abbreviation for **adult polycystic kidney disease.**

aplasia /əplā″zhə/ [Gk, *a, plassein,* not to form], **1.** a developmental failure resulting in the absence of an organ or tissue. **2.** (in hematology) a failure of the normal process of cell generation and development in the bone marrow. Compare **hyperplasia, hypoplasia.** See also **aplastic anemia. –aplastic,** *adj.*

aplasia cutis congenita [Gk, *a, plassein*; L, *cutis,* skin, *congenitus,* born with], the congenital absence of a localized area of skin. The defect occurs predominantly on the scalp, less frequently on the limbs and trunk. It is usually covered by a thin, translucent membrane or scar tissue, or it may be raw and ulcerated. The condition is genetically transmitted, although the mode of inheritance is not known.

aplastic. See **aplasia.**

aplastic anemia, a deficiency of all of the formed elements of blood (specifically erythrocytes, leukocytes, and platelets), representing a failure of the cell-generating capacity of bone marrow. Aplastic anemia is often of unknown origin and may involve destruction of bone marrow by exposure to toxic chemicals, ionizing radiation, or some antibiotics. Also spelled *aplastic anaemia.* Compare **alymphocytosis, hemolytic anemia, hypoplastic anemia.** See also **aleukia, leukopenia.**

Apley's scratch test, a method for assessing the general range of motion of the shoulders. The patient is asked to scratch the back of his or her head and then to scratch behind the back at the small of the back with the same hand. The

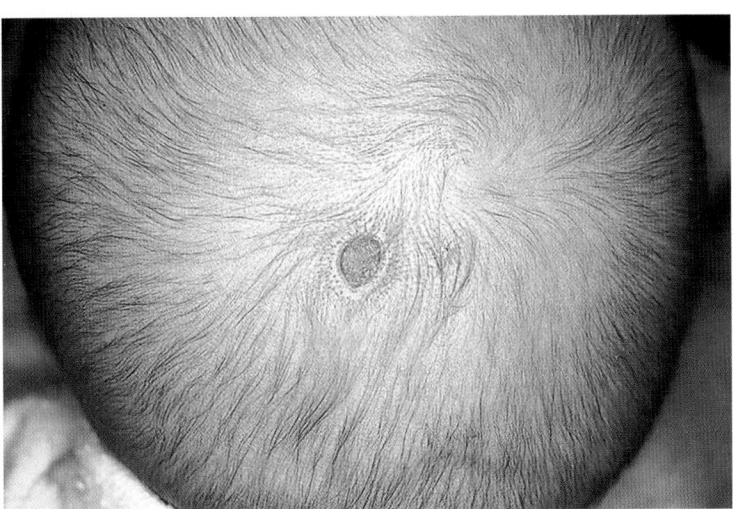

Aplasia cutis congenita *(Callen et al, 2000)*

test requires abduction and lateral rotation and adduction and medial rotation, thus giving a general impression of the available range of the shoulder.

Aplisol, brand name for a tuberculin purified protein derivative used for tuberculin tests.

APMA, abbreviation for *American Podiatric Medical Association.*

APN, abbreviation for **advanced practice nurse.**

apnea /apnē″ə, ap″nē·ə/ [Gk, *a + pnein,* not to breathe], an absence of spontaneous respiration. Kinds include **central sleep apnea, mixed sleep apnea, obstructive sleep apnea.** –*apneic, adj.*

apnea monitor [Gk, *a + pnein,* not to breathe], a device designed to sound an alarm if an individual stops breathing for a given period of time. It may be a bed pad (alarm mattress), chest electrode, chest belt, or nasal flow sensor.

apnea monitoring, the act of closely observing the respiration of individuals, particularly infants. The procedure may involve the use of electronic devices that detect changes in thoracic or abdominal movements and in heart rate. Such devices may include an alarm that sounds if breathing stops. See also **apnea monitor.**

apneumia /ap·noo″mē·ə/ [Gk, *a, pneumon,* without lung], a congenital absence of the lungs.

apneustic breathing /apnoo″stik/ [Gk, *a, pneusis,* not breathing], a pattern of breathing characterized by a prolonged inspiratory phase followed by expiration apnea. The rate of apneustic breathing is usually around 1.5 breaths per minute. This breathing pattern is often associated with head injury.

apneustic center, an area in the lower portion of the pons that controls the inspiratory phase of respiration. Disorders involving abnormal stimulation of the apneustic center can produce a gasping type of ventilation with maximum inspirations. Also called **pontine respiratory center.**

apnoea. See **apnea.**

apocrine gland /ap″əkrīn, -krin/ [Gk, *apo + krinein;* L, *secernere,* to separate], a gland whose secretion contains part of the secreting cell. Compare **holocrine gland, merocrine gland.**

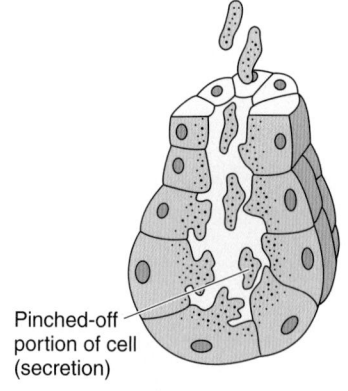

Pinched-off portion of cell (secretion)

Apocrine gland *(Gartner and Hiatt, 2007)*

apocrine miliaria. See **Fox-Fordyce disease.**

apocrine sweat gland [Gk, *apo,* from, *krinein,* to separate], one of the large dermal sudoriferous glands located in the axillary, anal, genital, and mammary areas of the body. Apocrine sweat glands open into the upper portion of a hair follicle instead of onto the skin's surface. Becoming functional only after puberty, they secrete perspiration containing nutrients consumed by skin bacteria. The bacterial waste products produce a characteristic odor. Compare **eccrine gland.** See also **sudoriferous gland.**

apodal /ə·pō″dəl/ [Gk, *a, pous,* without foot], having no feet. See also **symmelia.**

apodial symmelia. See **sirenomelia.**

apoenzyme /ap′ō·en″zīm/ [Gk, *apo + en,* into, *zyme,* ferment], the protein part of a holoenzyme. The nonprotein part is the prosthetic group, which is usually permanently attached to the apoenzyme.

apogee /ap″əjē/ [Gk, *apo + ge,* earth], the climax of a disease or the period of greatest severity of signs and symptoms, usually followed by a crisis.

Apokyn, a nonselective dopamine agonist. Brand name for **apomorphine.**

apolipoprotein /ap′ōlip′ōprō″tēn/ [Gk, *apo + lipos,* fat, *protos,* first], proteins that bind lipids (oil-soluble substances such as fat and cholesterol) to form lipoproteins. They transport the lipids through the lymphatic and circulatory systems.

apolipoprotein A-I, a protein component of lipoprotein complexes found in high-density lipoprotein (HDL) and chylomicrons. It is an activator of lecithin-cholesterol acyltransferase, which forms cholesteryl esters in HDL. All apoproteins of plasma lipoproteins bind and transport lipid in the blood. A deficiency of apolipoprotein A-I is associated with low HDL levels and Tangier disease.

apolipoprotein A-II, a protein component of lipoprotein complexes found in high-density lipoprotein and chlyomicrons, which activates hepatic lipase.

apolipoprotein A-III, a protein component of high-density lipoproteins. Also called **apolipoprotein D.**

apolipoprotein B-100, a protein component of lipoprotein involved in the hepatic transport of lipid as very–low-density lipoprotein and low-density lipoprotein (LDL). Apoprotein B-100 links to cellulose LDL receptors. It is elevated in the plasma of patients with familial hyperlipoproteinemia.

apolipoprotein C-I, a protein component of lipid that activates lecithin-cholesterol acyltransferase.

apolipoprotein C-II, a protein component of chylomicrons and very–low-density lipoprotein that activates lipoprotein lipase.

apolipoprotein D. See **apolipoprotein A-III.**

apolipoprotein E, a protein component of lipoprotein complexes found in very–low-density lipoprotein (VLDL), high-density lipoprotein, chylomicrons, and chylomicron remnants. It facilitates hepatic uptake of chylomicron and VLDL remnants and is elevated in patients with type III hyperlipoproteinemia. One form of apolipoprotein E has been linked to Alzheimer disease.

apolipoprotein A, a blood test used to evaluate the risks of atherogenic disease of the heart and peripheral arteries.

apomorphine, an antiparkinson agent.

■ INDICATIONS: This drug is used for acute, intermittent treatment of hypomobility episodes in advanced parkinsonism.

■ CONTRAINDICATIONS: Known hypersensitivity to this drug prohibits its use.

■ ADVERSE EFFECTS: Adverse effects of this drug include psychosis, hallucination, depression, dizziness, headache, confusion, yawning, dyskinesias, drowsiness, somnolence, edema, syncope, tachycardia, blurred vision, rhinorrhea, sweating, vomiting, constipation, dysphagia, dry mouth, impotence, and urinary frequency. Life-threatening side effects include sleep attacks, hemolytic anemia, leukopenia, and agranulocytosis. Common side effects include agitation, orthostatic hypotension, nausea, and anorexia.

aponeurosis /ap′ōno͞oro͞o″sis/ *pl.* **aponeuroses** [Gk, *apo* + *neuron,* nerve, sinew], a broad, flat sheet of fibrous connective tissue that serves as a tendon to attach muscles to bone or as fascia to bind muscles together or to other tissues at their origin or insertion. *–aponeurotic, adj.*

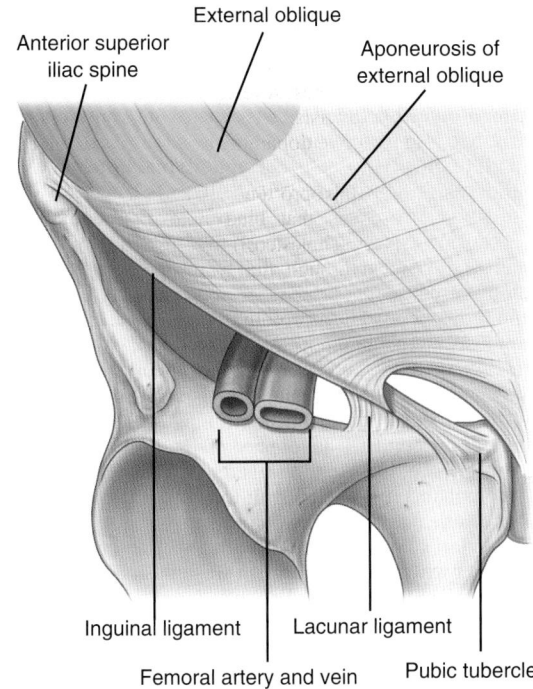

External oblique

Anterior superior iliac spine

Aponeurosis of external oblique

Inguinal ligament

Lacunar ligament

Femoral artery and vein

Pubic tubercle

Aponeurosis *(Drake, Vogl, and Mitchell, 2015)*

aponeurosis of the external abdominal oblique, the broad, flat membrane that covers the entire ventral surface of the abdomen and lies superficial to the rectus abdominis muscles. Fibers from both sides of the aponeurosis interlace in the midline to form the linea alba. The upper part of the aponeurosis serves as the inferior origin of the pectoralis major muscle; the lower part ends in the inguinal ligament.

aponeurotic fascia /-no͞orot″ik/ [Gk, *apo,* from, *neuron,* tendon], a thickened layer of connective tissue that provides attachment to a muscle.

aponeurotic fibroma, a firm, fixed nodule composed of fibroblastic tissue with finely stippled calcifications, not attached to the overlying skin and infiltrating into surrounding soft tissue. This recurrent benign tumor is seen mainly in people under 20 years of age, most often on the hand. Also called **juvenile aponeurotic fibroma.**

apophyseal. See **apophysis.**

apophyseal fracture, a fracture occurring in preadolescent individuals that separates the growth plate (apophysis) of a bone from the main osseous tissue at a point of strong tendinous or ligamentous attachment.

apophysis /əpof″isis/ [Gk, a growing away], any small projection, process, or outgrowth, usually on a bone without an independent center of ossification. Examples include the zy-gomatic apophysis of the temporal bone and the basilar apophysis of the occipital bone. *–apophysial,* **apophyseal,** *adj.*

apophysitis /əpof′əsī′tis/, an inflammation of an outgrowth, projection, or swelling, especially a bony outgrowth that is still attached to the rest of the bone. Apophysitis occurs due to excessive traction or stress most frequently affecting the calcaneus **(Sever's disease),** the knee **(Osgood-Schlatter),** the shoulder **(Little Leaguer shoulder),** or elbow **(Little Leaguer elbow).**

apoprotein /ap′ōprō′tēn/, a polypeptide chain not yet complexed to its specific prosthetic group.

apoprotein B-48, a protein component of lipoprotein found in chylomicrons. It is involved in the intestinal absorption of lipids.

apoptosis /ā′pōtō″sis, ā′poptō″sis/ [Gk, *apo,* away, *ptosis,* falling], necrosis of keratinocytes in which the nuclei of the necrotic cells dissolve and the cytoplasm shrinks, rounds up, and is subsequently phagocytized. The term generally refers to "programmed" cell death.

aposia /āpō″shə/ [Gk, *a,* not, *posis,* thirst], a complete lack of thirst.

apothecaries' measure /əpoth″əker′ēz/ [Gk, *apotheke,* store], a system of graduated liquid volumes originally based on the minim, formerly equal to one drop of water but now standardized to 0.06 mL; 60 minims equals 1 fluid dram, 8 fluid drams equals 1 fluid ounce, 16 fluid ounces equals 1 pint, 2 pints equals 1 quart, 4 quarts equals 1 gallon. See also **apothecaries' weight, metric system.**

apothecaries' weight, a system of graduated amounts arranged in order of heaviness and based on the grain, formerly equal to the weight of a plump grain of wheat but now standardized to 65 mg; 20 grains equals 1 scruple, 3 scruples equals 1 dram, 8 drams equals 1 ounce, 12 ounces equals 1 pound. Compare **avoirdupois weight.** See also **apothecaries' measure, metric system.**

apothecary /əpoth″əker′ē/ [Gk, *apotheke,* store], historic term used to denote a compounding pharmacist. See **pharmacist.**

apparatus /ap′ərat″əs/ [L, *ad,* toward, *parare,* to make ready], a device or a system composed of different parts that act together to perform some special function.

apparent leukonychia, a white discoloration of the nail that fades when pressure is applied and with maintenance of transparency of the nail plate.

appendage, 1. a less important portion of an organ. 2. an outgrowth, such as a tail. 3. a limb or limblike structure.

appendectomy /ap′əndek″təmē/ [L, *appendere* + Gk, *ektomē,* excision], the surgical removal of the vermiform appendix. This procedure can be performed via laparoscopy or open surgery. See also **abdominal surgery.**

appendical. See **appendix.**

appendical reflex /əpen″dikəl/, extreme tenderness at McBurney point, a diagnostic finding in appendicitis. Also called *McBurney reflex,* **McBurney sign.**

appendiceal, pertaining to the appendix, such as appendiceal cancer. See **appendix.**

appendiceal abscess. See **appendicular abscess.**

appendices. See **appendix.**

appendices epiploicae, now called **epiploic appendix.**

appendicial, now called **appendical.** See **appendix.**

appendicitis /əpen′disī″tis/ [L, *appendere* + Gk, *itis*], an inflammation of the vermiform appendix, usually acute, that, if undiagnosed, leads rapidly to perforation and peritonitis. The inflammation is caused by an obstruction such as a hard mass of feces or a foreign body in the lumen of the appendix, lymphoid hyperplasia, fibrous disease of the intestinal wall, an adhesion, or a parasitic infestation. Appendicitis is most likely to occur in teenagers and young adults and is more prevalent in male patients. Kinds include **chronic appendicitis.**

■ OBSERVATIONS: The most common symptom is constant pain in the right lower quadrant of the abdomen around McBurney's point, which the patient describes as having begun as intermittent pain in midabdomen. Rebound tenderness occurs at McBurney's point as well. Pain may also occur on the left side. Extreme tenderness occurs over the right rectus abdominis muscle. To decrease the pain, the patient keeps the knees bent to prevent tension of the abdominal muscles. Appendicitis is characterized by vomiting, a low-grade fever of 99° to 102° F, an elevated white blood cell count, rebound tenderness, a rigid abdomen, and decreased or absent bowel sounds. Other indications of peritonitis include increasing abdominal distension, acute abdomen, tachycardia, rapid and shallow breathing, and restlessness. If peritonitis is suspected, IV antibiotic therapy, fluids, and electrolytes are given.

■ PATIENT CARE CONSIDERATIONS: The nurse is alert to the signs and symptoms of rupture and peritonitis and provides education about the diagnosis, treatment, and recovery.

■ PATIENT CARE CONSIDERATIONS: Treatment is appendectomy within 24 to 48 hours of the first symptoms because delay usually results in rupture and peritonitis as fecal matter is released into the peritoneal cavity. The fever rises sharply once peritonitis begins. The patient may have sudden relief from pain immediately after rupture, followed by increased, diffuse pain.

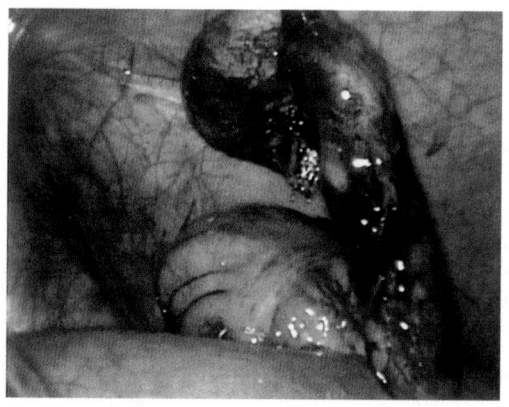

Appendicitis: laparoscopic view *(Zitelli and Davis, 2012)*

appendicitis pain [L, *appendere,* to hang upon, *poena,* penalty], severe general abdominal pain that develops rapidly and usually becomes localized in the lower right abdominal quadrant. It is accompanied by extreme tenderness over the right rectus abdominis muscle with rebound pain at McBurney's point. Occasionally, the pain is on the left side.

appendicular. See **appendix.**

appendicular abscess, **1.** an abscess on a limb. **2.** an abscess of the vermiform appendix. Also called **appendiceal abscess.**

appendicular artery, one of the four branches of the ileocolic artery, supplying the mesoappendix and the appendix.

appendicular skeleton, the bones of the limbs and their girdles, attached to the axial skeleton. Compare **axial skeleton.**

appendix /əpen″diks/ *pl. appendices, appendixes,* **1.** an accessory part attached to a main structure. Also called **appendage. 2.** See **vermiform appendix.** −**appendicular, appendiceal, appendicial, appendical,** *adj.*

appendix dyspepsia [L, *appendere* + Gk, *dys,* difficult, *peptein,* to digest], an abnormal condition characterized by impaired digestive function associated with chronic appendicitis. See also **dyspepsia.**

appendix epididymidis. See **epididymal appendix.**

appendixes. See **appendix.**

appendix vermiformis. See **vermiform appendix.**

apperception /ap′ərsep″shən/ [L, *ad,* toward, *percipere,* to perceive], **1.** mental perception or recognition. **2.** (in psychology) a conscious process of understanding or perceiving in terms of a person's previous knowledge, experiences, emotions, and memories. −**apperceptive,** *adj.*

appestat /ap″əstat/, the area of the hypothalamus of the brain that controls the appetite.

appetite /ap″ətīt/ [L, *appetere,* to long for], a natural or instinctive desire, such as for food.

apple picker's disease, an allergic reaction with respiratory complaints, associated with the handling of apples that have been treated with a fungicide.

apple sorter's disease, a form of contact dermatitis caused by contact with chemicals used in washing apples.

appliance /əplī″əns/ [L, *applicare,* to apply], **1.** a device used to perform a specific medical function or to have a specific therapeutic effect. **2.** (in dentistry) generally a device to correct a malocclusion, to correct an oral habit, or to stabilize an occlusion.

application /ap′likā″shən/, a computer program used to process a particular type of data, such as payroll, inventory, data about patients, scheduling of procedures and activities, pharmacy requisition and control, documentation of professional services, care planning, word processing, or spreadsheets. Also called *app.*

applicator /ap′likā″tər/, a rodlike instrument with a piece of cotton on the end, used for the local application of medication or probing of wound pockets or crevices. Also called *cotton swab.*

applied anatomy /əplīd″/, the study of the structure of the organs of the body as it relates to the diagnosis and treatment of disease. Also called **practical anatomy.** Compare **comparative anatomy.** See also **pathological anatomy, radiological anatomy, surgical anatomy.**

applied chemistry, the application of the study of chemical elements and compounds to industry and the arts.

applied psychology, **1.** the interpretation of historical, literary, medical, or other data according to psychological principles. **2.** any branch of psychology that emphasizes practical rather than theoretic approaches and objectives, such as child psychology, clinical psychology, educational psychology, and industrial psychology.

applied science, the use of existing knowledge and scientific techniques to advance understanding. See **science.**

apposition /ap′əsish″ən/ [L, *apponere,* to put to], the placement or position of adjacent structures or parts so that they can come into contact.

appositional growth, an increase in size by the addition of new tissue or similar material at the periphery of a particular part or structure, as in the addition of new layers in bone and tooth formation. Compare **interstitial growth.**

apposition suture, a stitch or series of stitches that holds the margins of an incision close together.

approach, the steps in a particular surgical procedure from division of the most superficial parts of the anatomy through exposure of the operation site.

approach-approach conflict [L, *ad + propiare,* to draw near], a conflict resulting from the simultaneous presence of two or more incompatible impulses, desires, or goals, each of which is desirable. Also called **double-approach conflict.** See also **conflict.**

approach-avoidance conflict, a conflict resulting from the presence of a single goal or desire that is both desirable and undesirable. See also **conflict.**

appropriate for gestational age (AGA) infant /əprō″prē·it/ [L, *ad,* toward, *proprius,* ownership], a newborn whose size, growth, and maturation are normal for gestational age, whether delivered prematurely, at term, or later than term. Such infants, if born at term, fall within the average range of size and weight on intrauterine growth curves, measuring from 48 to 53 cm in length and weighing between 2700 and 4000 g. Compare **small for gestational age (SGA) infant, large for gestational age (LGA) infant.** See also **gestational age.**

approximal /əprok″siməl/ [L, *approximare,* to approach], close or very near.

approximate /əprok″simāt/ [L, *ad + proximare,* to come near], **1.** to draw two tissue surfaces close together, as in the repair of a wound, or to draw the bones of a joint together as in physical therapy. **2.** almost correct.

approximator /əprok″səmā′tər/, a medical instrument used to draw together the edges of divided tissues, as in closing a wound or in repairing a fractured rib.

apraxia /əprak″sē·ə/ [Gk, *a + pressein,* not to act], an impairment in the ability to perform purposeful acts or to manipulate objects without any loss of strength, sensation, or coordination. Apraxia of speech is an inability to program the position of speech muscles and the sequence of muscle movements necessary to produce understandable speech, although understanding of speech remains intact. See also **amnestic apraxia, ideational apraxia, motor apraxia, developmental apraxia.** —*apraxic, adj.*

aprepitant, an antiemetic agent.

■ INDICATIONS: This drug is used to prevent nausea and vomiting associated with cancer chemotherapy (including high-dose cisplatin). It is used in combination with other antiemetics.

■ CONTRAINDICATIONS: Known hypersensitivity to this drug prohibits its use.

■ ADVERSE EFFECTS: Adverse effects of this drug include insomnia, anxiety, depression, confusion, peripheral neuropathy, bradycardia, deep vein thrombosis, hypertension, abdominal pain, anorexia, gastritis, vomiting, heartburn, serum creatine, proteinuria, dysuria, anemia, asthenia, fatigue, dehydration, fever, hiccups, tinnitus, and increased aspartate aminotransferase, alanine aminotransferase, and blood urea nitrogen. Life-threatening side effects include thrombocytopenia and neutropenia. Common side effects include headache, dizziness, diarrhea, constipation, and nausea.

Apresoline, a nonnitrate arteriolar vasodilator antihypertensive agent. Brand name for **hydrALAZINE hydrochloride.**

aprosody /āpros′odē/ [Gk, *a + prosodia,* not modulated voice], a speech disorder characterized by the absence of the normal variations in pitch, loudness, intonation, and rhythm of word formation.

aprosopia /ā′prəsō″pē·ə/ [Gk, *aprosopos,* faceless], a congenital absence of part or all of the facial structures. The condition is usually associated with other malformations.

aprotinin /ap′ro-ti′nin/, an inhibitor of proteolytic enzymes, used as an antihemorrhagic agent to reduce perioperative blood loss in patients undergoing cardiopulmonary bypass during coronary artery bypass graft; administered intravenously.

apselaphesia /ap-sel-ə-′fē-zē-ə/, *(Obsolete)* a loss of tactile sensations.

APTA, abbreviation for *American Physical Therapy Association.*

aptitude /ap″tətyo͞od/ [L, *aptitudo,* ability], a natural ability, tendency, talent, or capability to learn, understand, or acquire a particular skill; mental alertness or physical ability.

aptitude test, any of a variety of standardized tests for measuring an individual's ability to learn certain skills. Compare **achievement test, intelligence test, personality test, psychological test.**

Aptivus /AP-tih-vus/, a protease inhibitor. Brand name for **tipranavir.**

Apt test, a test for blood in the stool of a newborn. The test differentiates between maternal and newborn blood. The presence of newborn blood indicates active GI bleeding or necrotizing enterocolitis. Also called *alkali denaturation test.*

apyretic, **1.** See **afebrile. 2.** the absence of fever.

apyrexia /ā′pīrek″sē·ə/ [Gk, *a + pyrexis,* without fever], an absence or remission of fever.

aq. See **aqua.**

aqua (aq) /ä″kwə/, the Latin word for water.

AquaMEPHYTON, a vitamin K compound. Brand name for **phytonadione.**

aquaphobia /ä′kwəfō″bē·ə/ [L, *aqua,* water; Gk, *phobos,* fear], an irrational fear of water.

aquaporin /ak″wah-po′rin/, any of a family of proteins found in plasma membranes and forming a functional component of water channels.

aquapuncture /-pungk″chər/ [L, *aqua,* water, *punctura,* puncture], the injection of water under the skin or spraying of a fine jet of water onto the skin surface to relieve mild irritation. Most often associated with veterinary medicine.

aquatherapy. See **underwater exercise.**

aquathermia pad /-thur′mē·ə/, a waterproof plastic or rubber pad that can be applied to areas of muscle sprain, edema, or mild inflammation. The pad contains channels through which heated or cooled water flows. The device is connected by hoses to a bedside control unit that contains a temperature regulator, a motor for circulating the water, and a reservoir of distilled water. Although generally safer than a conventional heating pad, the aquathermia pad must be checked periodically to avoid the risk of acc idental burns. Also called *water flow pad.*

aquatic exercise. See **underwater exercise.**

aqueduct /-dukt/ [L, *aqua,* water, *ductus,* act of leading], any canal, channel, or passage through or between body parts, such as the cerebral aqueduct.

aqueduct of Sylvius. See **cerebral aqueduct.**

aqueous /ā″kwē·əs, ak″wē·əs/ [L, *aqua*], **1.** watery or waterlike. **2.** a medication prepared with water. **3.** a solution containing water.

aqueous chamber [L, *aqua,* water; Gk, *kamara,* something with an arched cover], either the anterior or the posterior chamber of the eye. The aqueous chambers contain the aqueous humor.

aqueous extract, a water-based preparation of a plant or an animal substance containing the biologically active portion of the plant or substance without its cellular residue.

aqueous humor, the clear, watery fluid circulating in the anterior and posterior chambers of the eye. It is produced by the ciliary body and is reabsorbed into the venous system primarily at the iridocorneal angle by means of the canal of Schlemm.

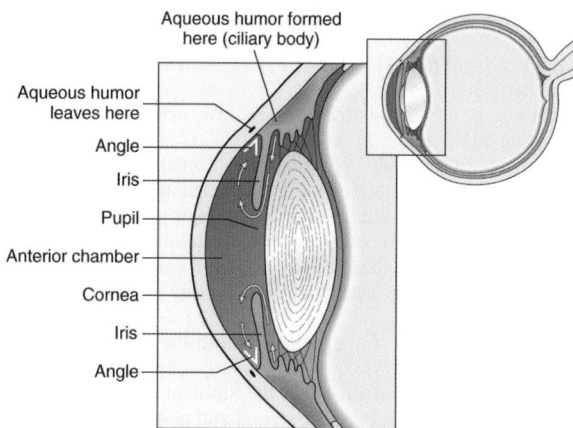

Aqueous humor formed here (ciliary body)

Aqueous humor leaves here

Angle

Iris

Pupil

Anterior chamber

Cornea

Iris

Angle

Aqueous humor *(Lovaasen and Schwerdtfeger, 2015)*

aqueous phase, a solution in a liquid state made up of a substance dissolved in water; distinguished from an organic phase.
aqueous solution [L, *aqua,* water + *solutus,* dissolved], a homogenous liquid preparation of any substance dissolved in water.
Ar, 1. symbol for the element **argon. 2.** abbreviation for *aromatic group.*
arabinosylcytosine. See **cytarabine.**
arachidonic acid /ar′əkidon″ik/ [L, *arachos,* a legume], a long-chain (20-carbon chain) polyunsaturated fatty acid that is a component of lecithin and serves as a starting material in the biosynthesis of prostaglandins and leukotrienes. In mammals, arachidonic acid is synthesized from linoleic acid.
arachnid [Gk, *arachne,* spider], a member of the phylum Arthropoda, class Arachnida, which includes spiders, scorpions, mites, and ticks.
arachnidism. See **arachnoidism.**
arachnitis /ar′əknī″tis/, an inflammation of the arachnoid membrane, characterized by pain, stinging, and neurological problems. Also called **arachnoiditis.**
arachno-, arachn-, combining forms meaning "arachnoid membrane" or "spider": *arachnoidal, arachnoidism.*
arachnodactyly /ərak′nōdak″tilē/ [Gk, *arachne,* spider, *dactylos,* finger], a congenital anomaly in which the fingers and toes are long, thin, and spiderlike. It is seen in Marfan syndrome.

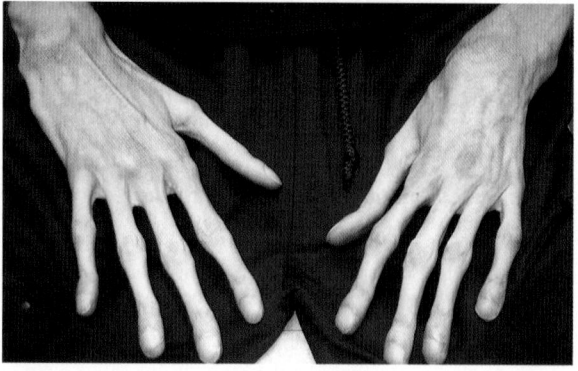

Arachnodactyly in Marfan syndrome *(Zitelli and Davis, 2012)*

arachnoid /ərak″noid/ [Gk, *arachne,* spider, *eidos,* form], resembling a cobweb or spiderweb, such as the arachnoid membrane. *−arachnoidal, adj.*
arachnoid cyst, a fluid-filled cyst between the layers of the leptomeninges, lined with arachnoid membrane, most commonly occurring in the sylvian fissure. Also called **leptomeningeal cyst.**
arachnoid granulations, clumps of arachnoid villi that project into the superior sagittal sinus.
arachnoidism /ərak″noidiz′əm/ [Gk, *arachne,* spider, *eidos,* form], the condition produced by the bite of a venomous spider.
arachnoiditis. See **arachnitis.**
arachnoid membrane, a thin, delicate membrane enclosing the brain and the spinal cord, interposed between the pia mater and the dura mater. The subarachnoid space lies between the arachnoid membrane and the pia mater, and the subdural space lies between the arachnoid membrane and the dura mater. Also called *arachnoid sheath.*
arachnoid trabeculae, fine filaments that pass from the arachnoid to the pia mater. They are embryological remnants.
arachnoid villi [Gk, *arachne,* spider, *villus,* shaggy hair], one of the many projections of fibrous tissue from the arachnoid membrane.
arachnophobia /ərak′nōfō″bē·ə/, a morbid fear of spiders.
Aramine, a mixed-adrenergic agonist. Brand name for **metaraminol bitartrate.**
Aran-Duchenne muscular atrophy /aran″dōōshen″/ [François A. Aran, French physician, 1817–1861; Guillaume B.A. Duchenne, French neurologist, 1806–1875], a form of amyotrophic lateral sclerosis affecting the hands, arms, shoulders, and legs at the onset before becoming more generalized.
arbitrary inference /är″bitrer′ē in″fərəns/, a form of cognitive distortion in which a judgment based on insufficient evidence leads to an erroneous conclusion.
arbitrator /är″bətrā′tər/ [L, *arbiter,* umpire], an impartial person appointed to resolve a dispute between parties. The arbitrator listens to the evidence presented by the parties in an informal hearing and attempts to arrive at a resolution acceptable to both parties. *−arbitration, n.*
arborization test. See **ferning test.**
arbovirus /är″bōvī″rəs/, any one of more than 300 viruses transmitted by the saliva of insects. The majority of human infections are asymptomatic, but symptomatic infections can be characterized by fever, rash, and bleeding into the viscera or skin. Some lead to encephalitis with fatality or permanent neurological damage. Vertebrate infection occurs when a contaminated arthropod takes a blood meal. Dengue, yellow fever, and equine encephalitis are three common arboviral infections. Treatment is symptomatic for all arbovirus infections. Vaccines have been developed to prevent infection from some arboviruses. Also called **arthropod-borne virus.**
arbutamine /ahr-bu′tah-mēn″/, a synthetic catecholamine with positive chronotropic and inotropic properties, used in echocardiography and diagnostic coronary angiography. It binds to and activates beta$_1$-adrenergic receptors in the myocardium, thereby increasing heart rate and increasing force of myocardial contraction.

arc [L, *arcus,* bow], a part of the circumference of a circle.

ARC, *(Obsolete)* abbreviation for **AIDS-related complex.**

arcade [L, *arcus,* bow], an arch or series of arches.

arch, any anatomical structure that is curved or has a bowlike appearance. Also called *arcus.*

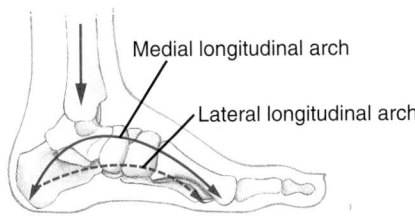

Arches of the foot *(Patton, 2016)*

arch-. See **archi-, arch-, arche-.**

arch bar, any one of various types of wires, bars, or splints that conform to the curvature of the teeth in the jaws, and are used in the treatment of fractures of the jaws and their supporting structures and in the stabilization of injured teeth.

arche-. See **archi-, arch-, arche-.**

-arche, a suffix meaning "beginning": *menarche.*

archenteric canal. See **neurenteric canal.**

archenteron /arken″təron/ *pl.* **archentera** [Gk, *arche,* beginning, *enteron,* intestine], the primitive digestive cavity formed by invagination into the gastrula, which is lined with endoderm during the embryonic development of many animals. It corresponds to the tubular cavity in the vertebrates that connects the amniotic cavity with the yolk sac. Also called **archigaster, coelenteron, gastrocoele, primitive gut.** See also **gastrula.** −*archenteric, adj.*

archeocortex. See **olfactory cortex.**

arches of the foot [L, *arcus,* bow; AS, *fot*], the bony curves of the instep, including the longitudinal (anteroposterior) and the transverse arches.

archetype /är″kətīp′/ [Gk, *arche* + *typos,* type], **1.** an original model or pattern from which a thing or group of things is made or evolves. **2.** (in analytic psychology) an inherited primordial idea or mode of thought derived from the experiences of the human race and present in the subconscious of the individual in the form of drives, moods, and concepts. See also **anima.** −*archetypic, archetypical, archetypal, adj.*

archi-, arch-, arche-, prefixes meaning "first, beginning, or original": *archiblastoma, archetype.*

archiblastoma /är″kiblastō″mə/ *pl.* **archiblastomas, archiblastomata** [Gk, *arche* + *blastos,* germ, *oma*], a tumor composed of cells derived from the layer of tissue surrounding the germinal vesicle.

archigaster. See **archenteron.**

archinephric canal, archinephric duct. See **pronephric duct.**

archinephron. See **pronephros.**

architectural barrier /är″kətek″chərəl/, a physical feature that limits or prevents people with disabilities from obtaining the goods or services that are offered. A common example would be parking spaces that are too narrow or that lack an adjacent access aisle for people who use wheelchairs and other mobility devices.

architecture /är″kitek′chər/ [Gk, *architekton,* master builder], **1.** (in computer technology) the basic design of a computer, including the memory, central processing unit, and input/output devices. **2.** the structuring of patient records in a format that facilitates their creation and exchange of information in an electronic health record. **3.** the compositions and arrangement of tissue, as in wound architecture or muscle architecture.

architis /ärkī″tis/ [Gk, *archos,* anus, *itis,* inflammation], *(Obsolete)* an inflammation of the anus. Now called **proctitis.**

arch length /ärch/, the distance from the distal point of the most posterior tooth on one side of the upper or lower jaw to the same point on the opposite side, usually measured through the points of contact between adjoining teeth. See also **available arch length.**

arch length deficiency, the difference in any dental arch between the length required to accommodate all the natural teeth and the actual length. The deficiency is determined by subtracting the sum of the widths of the teeth in millimeters from the existing arch length in millimeters. The negative value is the arch length deficiency.

arch of the aorta, the proximal one of the four portions of the aorta, giving rise to three arterial branches, called the brachiocephalic, left common carotid, and left subclavian arteries. The arch rises at the level of the border of the second sternocostal articulation of the right side, passes to the left in front of the trachea, bends dorsally, and becomes the descending aorta. Also called **aortic arch.**

arch width, (in dentistry) the distance between the left and right opposites in the upper or lower jaw, usually expressed in millimeters. The intercanine, interpremolar, or intermolar distance may be cited as the arch width.

arch wire, an orthodontic wire fastened to two or more teeth through attachments fixed to the teeth (fixed attachments), used to cause or guide tooth movement. See also **full-arch wire, sectional arch wire.**

arcing spring contraceptive diaphragm /är″king/, a kind of contraceptive diaphragm in which the flexible metal spring that forms the rim is a combination of a flexible coil spring and a flat band spring made of stainless steel. The silicone rubber dome is approximately 4 cm deep, and the diameter of the rubber-covered rim is between 65 and 80 mm. This kind of diaphragm is prescribed for a woman whose vaginal musculature is relaxed and does not afford strong support, as in first-degree cystocele, rectocele, or uterine prolapse. Compare **coil spring contraceptive diaphragm, flat spring contraceptive diaphragm.** See also **contraceptive diaphragm fitting.**

ARC-STSA, abbreviation for **Accreditation Review Council on Education in Surgical Technology and Surgical Assisting.**

arctation. See **stenosis.**

arcuate /är″kyoo·at/ [L, *arcuatus,* bowed], an arch or bow shape.

arcuate artery of the foot, a branch of the dorsalis pedis artery. Also called **metatarsal artery.**

arcuate ligament of the diaphragm, one of the three arc-shaped ligaments of the diaphragm that attach to the vertebral column.

arcuate scotoma [L, *arcuatus* bowed; Gk, *skotoma,* darkness], an arc-shaped blind area that may develop in the field of vision of a person with glaucoma. It is caused by damage to nerve fibers in the retina.

arcus senilis /senē″lis/ [L, bow, aged], an opaque ring, gray to white in color, that surrounds the periphery of the cornea. It is caused by deposits of cholesterol in the cornea or hyaline degeneration and occurs primarily in older persons. See also **gerontotoxon.**

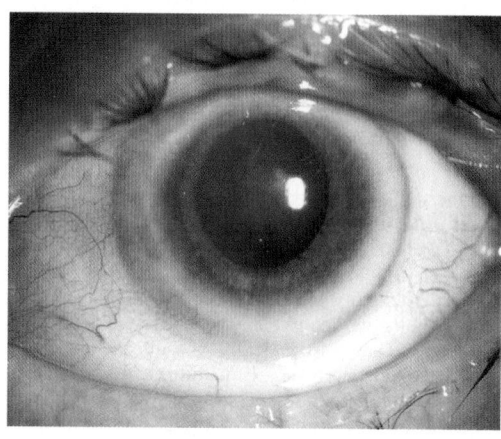

Arcus senilis *(Spalton et al, 2005)*

Arden's powder, a commercial preparation containing boric acid powder, alum powder, eucalyptus oil, thyme oil, menthol crystals and methyl salicylate, used in solution as an astringent douche.

ARDS, abbreviation for **adult respiratory distress syndrome.**

area /er″ē·ə/ [L, space], (in anatomy) a limited anatomical space that contains a specific structure of the body or within which certain physiological functions predominate, such as the aortic area and the association areas of the cerebral cortex.

Areas of Occupation, daily activities in which people engage, including activities of daily living (ADLs), instrumental activities of daily living (IADLs), education, work, play, leisure, and social participation.

areata /erē·ā″tə/, occurring in patches or circumscribed areas, such as hair loss. See **alopecia areata.**

area under the concentration curve (AUC), **1.** (in pharmacology) a method of measurement of the bioavailability of a drug based on a plot of blood concentrations sampled at frequent intervals. It is directly proportional to the total amount of unaltered drug in the patient's blood. **2.** (in laboratory science) a calculus derivation that helps analyze the efficacy of a laboratory assay. The area under the curve is computed from the shape of a plot of a continuous variable. One application is the analysis of a "receiver-operating characteristic curve"

that plots assay sensitivity against 1–specificity. An area under the curve value of 0.5 indicates a useless assay; a value of 1.0, usually unobtainable, reflects a "perfect" assay.

areflexia /ā′rēflek″sē·ə/, the absence of the reflexes.

Arenavirus /er′inəvī″rəs/, a genus of viruses usually transmitted to humans by contact with or inhalation of aerosolized excreta of wild, infected rodents. Individual arenaviruses are identified with specific geographic areas, such as Bolivian hemorrhagic fever in one river valley in Bolivia; Lassa fever in Nigeria, Liberia, and Sierra Leone; and Argentine hemorrhagic fever in two agricultural provinces in Argentina. Arenavirus infections are characterized by a slow onset of fever, sweats, malaise, headache, retro-orbital pain, muscle pain, rash, petechiae, hemorrhage, delirium, hypotension, and ulcers of the mouth. In rare cases in health care and family settings, some arenaviruses are associated with secondary person-to-person infection. Treatment is supportive, such as fluid and electrolyte balance, rest, and adequate nutrition. Preventative measures include rodent control. To date, there are no FDA-approved arenavirus vaccines, and current antiarenaviral therapy is limited to an off-label use of ribavirin that is only partially effective.

areola /erē″ōlə/ *pl. areolae,* **1.** a small space or a cavity within a tissue. **2.** a circular area of a different color surrounding a central feature, such as the discoloration about a pustule or the darkened area surrounding the nipple of the mammary gland. **3.** the part of the iris around the pupil.

areola of breast, the pigmented, circular area surrounding the nipple of each breast. Also called *areola mammae, areola papillaris.*

areolar /erē″ələr/ [L, *areola,* little space], pertaining to an areola.

areolar gland, one of the large modified sebaceous glands in the areolae encircling the nipples of the breasts of women. The areolar glands secrete a lipoid fluid that lubricates and protects the nipple during nursing and contain smooth muscle bundles that cause the nipples to become erect when stimulated. Also called **gland of Montgomery.**

areolar tissue, a kind of connective tissue having little tensile strength and consisting of loosely woven fibers and areolae. It occupies the interspaces of the body. Also called **fibroareolar tissue.** Compare **fibrous tissue.**

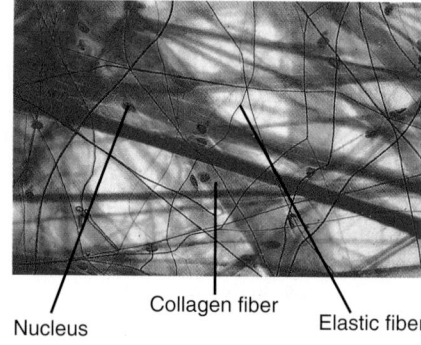

Nucleus   Collagen fiber   Elastic fiber

Areolar tissue *(© Ed Reschke; used with permission)*

areolitis /er′ē·əlī″tis/, an inflammation of the areolae of the breasts.

ARF, **1.** abbreviation for **acute respiratory failure. 2.** abbreviation for **acute renal failure.**

arformoterol, a long-acting adrenergic beta$_2$-agonist, sympathomimetic, and bronchodilator.

■ INDICATIONS: This drug is used to treat chronic obstructive pulmonary disease, including chronic bronchitis and emphysema.

■ CONTRAINDICATIONS: Tachydysrhythmias, severe cardiac disease, heart block, actively deteriorating chronic obstructive pulmonary disease, and known hypersensitivity to this drug, sympathomimetics, or racemic formoterol prohibit its use.

■ ADVERSE EFFECTS: Adverse effects of this drug include insomnia, headache, dizziness, stimulation, hallucinations, flushing, irritability, palpitations, tachycardia, hypertension or hypotension, angina, dysrhythmias, dry nose, irritation of nose and throat, heartburn, nausea, vomiting, flushing, sweating, anorexia, bad taste/smell changes, hypokalemia, muscle cramps, cough, wheezing, dyspnea, and dry throat. Life-threatening side effects include anaphylaxis and bronchospasm. Common side effects include tremors, anxiety, and restlessness.

Arg, abbreviation for **arginine.**

argatroban /ahr-gat′ro-ban″/, a non–heparin-based anticoagulant and direct thrombin inhibitor used to treat thrombosis when heparin-induced thrombocytopenia prevents continued heparin use; administered intravenously.

argentaffin cell /är′jentaf″in/ [L, *argentum,* gleaming, *affinitas,* affinity], a cell containing granules that stain readily with silver and chromium. Such cells occur in most regions of the GI tract and are especially abundant in the crypts of Lieberkühn. Also called **enterochromaffin cell, Kulchitsky cell.**

argentaffinoma /är′jentaf″inō″mə/ *pl. argentaffinomas, argentaffinomata,* a tumor that secretes large amounts of the hormone serotonin. It usually arises in the GI tract anywhere between the stomach and rectum and can metastasize to the liver. In the liver the tumor produces and releases large quantities of serotonin into the systemic bloodstream, resulting in carcinoid syndrome, which is characterized by flushing, swelling of the face, flat angioma on the skin, diarrhea, bronchial spasm, rapid pulse, low blood pressure, and tricuspid and pulmonary stenosis, often with regurgitation. Treatment is with surgery, radiation therapy, chemotherapy, or biotherapy. Carcinoid tumors are considered a type of endocrine tumor. Also called *carcinoid tumor.*

argentaffinoma syndrome. See **carcinoid syndrome.**

argentaffinomata. See **argentaffinoma.**

Argentine hemorrhagic fever, an acute febrile viral illness caused by an arenavirus transmitted to humans by contact with or inhalation of aerosolized excreta of infected rodents. Initially, it is characterized by chills, fever, headache, myalgia, anorexia, nausea, vomiting, and a general feeling of malaise. As the disease progresses, the victim may develop a high fever, dehydration, hypotension, flushed skin, abnormally slow heartbeat, bleeding from the gums and internal tissues, hematuria, and hematemesis. There may be involvement of the central nervous system, shock, and pulmonary edema. There is no specific treatment for the disease other than hydration, rest, warmth, and adequate nutrition. Rarely, IV fluids and dialysis are necessary. Usually, the prognosis is complete recovery. See also *Arenavirus,* **Bolivian hemorrhagic fever, Lassa fever.**

arginase /är″jinās/, an enzyme that catalyzes the hydrolysis of arginine during the urea cycle, producing urea and ornithine. The enzyme is found primarily in the liver but also occurs in the mammary gland, testes, and kidney.

arginase deficiency, an autosomal-recessive aminoacidopathy involving the biosynthesis of urea; arginine is elevated in blood and urine and may cause secondary cystinuria; orotic aciduria is common, but hyperammonemia is rare. Clinical signs include psychomotor retardation, hepatomegaly, and scalp discoloration. Also called **argininemia.**

arginine (Arg) /är″jinin/, an amino acid formed during the urea cycle by the transfer of a nitrogen atom from aspartate to citrulline. It can also be prepared synthetically. Certain compounds made from arginine, especially arginine glutamate and

arginine hydrochloride, are used intravenously in the management of conditions in which there is an excess of ammonia in the blood caused by liver dysfunction. See also **urea cycle.**

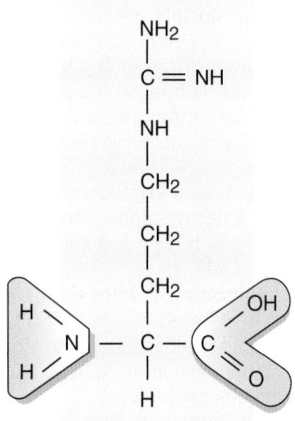

Chemical structure of arginine

argininemia /är′jininē″mē·ə/, arginase deficiency; arginine deficiency syndromes involve either T-cell dysfunction or endothelial dysfunction.

arginine vasopressin, vasopressin containing arginine, as that from humans and most other mammals; for medicinal uses. Also called **argipressin.**

argininosuccinic acidemia /ärjin′inō′suksin″ik/, an inherited amino acid metabolism disorder in which the lack of an enzyme, argininosuccinase, results in an excess of argininosuccinic acid in the blood. The condition is characterized by seizures and cognitive impairment. Treatment mainly involves a low-protein diet containing essential amino acids or amino acid analogs.

argipressin /ahr″gi-pres′in/, arginine vasopressin.

argon (Ar) /är″gon/ [Gk, *argos,* inactive], a colorless, odorless, chemically inactive gas making up approximately 1% of the atmosphere. Its atomic mass is 39.95; its atomic number is 18. It forms no known compounds.

Argyll Robertson pupil [Douglas M.C.L. Argyll Robertson, Scottish ophthalmologist, 1837–1909], a pupil that constricts on accommodation but not in response to light. It is most often seen in advanced neurosyphilis.

argyria /ärjī″rē·ə/ [Gk, *argyros,* silver], a permanent dull blue or gray to bronze discoloration of the skin, conjunctiva, and internal organs caused by excessive oral intake of silver salts.

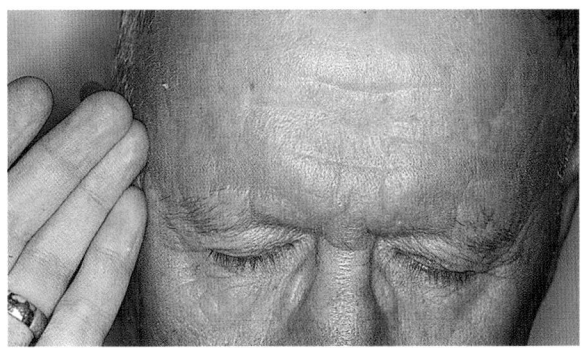

Individual with argyria *(Callen et al, 2000)*

argyrophil /ärjĭ″rəfil/ [Gk, *argyros,* silver, *philein,* to love], a cell or other object that is easily stained or impregnated with silver.

arhythmia. See **arrhythmia.**

ariboflavinosis /ārī′bōflā′vĭnō″sis/ [Gk, *a,* not, *ribose*; L, *flavus,* yellow; Gk, *osis*], a condition caused by deficiency of riboflavin (vitamin B$_2$) in the diet. It is characterized by bilateral lesions at the corners of the mouth, on the lips, and around the nose and eyes; by seborrheic dermatitis; and by various visual disorders. See also **riboflavin.**

aril, a botanical term used to denote an accessory seed coating that may form a fleshy, cuplike structure around the immature seed (ovule), as in yew and nutmeg. The aril is often brightly colored and edible.

Arimidex, an aromatase inhibitor used for treating estrogen-receptor–positive breast cancer, primarily in postmenopausal women. Brand name for **anastrozole.**

aripiprazole, an atypical antipsychotic agent used to treat schizophrenia and other disorders.

Aristocort, a glucocorticoid. Brand name for **triamcinolone.**

-arit, combining form designating an antirheumatic drug.

arithmetic mean. See **mean.**

Arkansas stone /är″kənsô/, a fine-grained stone of novaculite used to sharpen surgical instruments.

Arlidin, a beta-adrenergic agonist peripheral vasodilator. Brand name for *nylidrin hydrochloride.*

arm [L, *armus*], 1. the portion of the upper limb of the body between the shoulder and the elbow. The bone of the arm is the humerus. The muscles of the arm are the coracobrachialis, the biceps brachii, the brachialis, and the triceps brachii. 2. the arm and the forearm. See also **shoulder joint.**

ARM, abbreviation for **artificial rupture of membranes.** See **amniotomy.**

armamentarium /är′məmenter″ē·əm/ [L, *armamentum,* implement], the total therapeutic assets of a health care provider or medical facility, including medicines and equipment and collective resources available to provide care and treatment.

arm board, 1. a wheelchair component supporting a flaccid arm in the correct position to prevent or decrease subluxation of the shoulder joint and to prevent edema. 2. a board used to keep the arm still to permit the drawing of blood or starting of an IV needle. 3. a rigid board covered in a soft material used to immobilize the arm when a peripheral intravenous line is near an area of flexion and/or requires stability.

arm bone, (*Nontechnical*) layman's term for the humerus. See also **humerus.**

arm cylinder cast, an orthopedic device of plaster of paris, fiberglass, or thermoplastics used for immobilizing the upper limb from the wrist to the upper arm. It is most often applied to aid the healing of a dislocated elbow, for postoperative immobilization or positioning of the elbow, or in the correction of an elbow deformity, and treatment of forearm and humerus fractures.

armpit, (*Nontechnical*) layman's term for axilla. See also **axilla.**

Army Nurse Corps (ANC), a branch of the U.S. Army founded on February 2, 1901, with headquarters in Falls Church, Virginia.

Arnold-Chiari malformation /är″nəldkē·är″ē/ [Julius Arnold, German pathologist, 1835–1915; Hans Chiari, French pathologist, 1851–1916], a congenital herniation of the brainstem and lower cerebellum through the foramen magnum into the cervical vertebral canal. It is often associated with meningocele and spina bifida. See also **neural tube defect.**

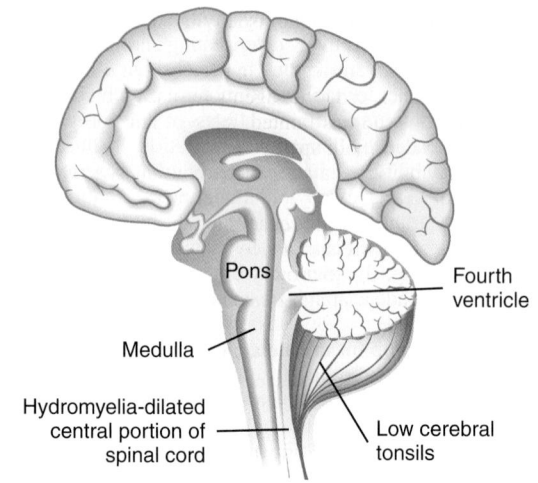

Arnold-Chiari malformation (*Huether and McCance, 2008*)

-arol, combining form designating a dicoumarol-type anticoagulant.

AROM, 1. abbreviation for **active range of motion. 2.** abbreviation for *artificial rupture of (fetal) membranes.*

aroma [Gk, spice], any agreeable odor or pleasing fragrance, especially of food, drink, spices, or medication.

aromatase /ah-ro′mah-tās/, an enzyme activity occurring in the endoplasmic reticulum and catalyzing the conversion of testosterone to the aromatic compound estradiol.

aromatase inhibitors, a class of drugs that inhibits aromatase activity and thus blocks production of estrogens. Such drugs are used to treat breast cancer and endometriosis.

aromatherapy, a form of herbal medicine that uses various oils from plants. The route of administration can be absorption through the skin or through inhalation. The aromatic biochemical structures of certain herbs are thought to act in areas of the brain related to past experiences and emotions (e.g., limbic system).

aromatic /er′ōmat″ik/ [Gk, *aroma,* spice], 1. pertaining to a strong but agreeable odor such as a pleasant spicy odor. 2. a stimulant or medicinal plant. 3. pertaining to organic chemical structures including a 6-carbon ring, such as benzol. 4. an essential oil, usually with a strong smell, that is derived from plants and used in cooking, perfumes, or aromatherapy.

aromatic alcohol, a fatty alcohol in which one or more of the hydrogen atoms of the hydrocarbon portion of the alcohol is replaced by an aromatic ring.

aromatic ammonia spirit [Gk, *aroma,* Ammon temple, ancient source of ammonium chloride salt, *spiritus,* breath], a strongly fragrant solution of ammonium carbonate in dilute liquid ammonia, oils, alcohol, and water for use as an inhalant to revive a person who has fainted. Also called **aromatic spirit of ammonia.**

aromatic bath, a medicated bath in which aromatic substances or essential oils are added to the water.

aromatic compounds, organic compounds that contain a benzene, naphthalene, or analogous ring. Many of these compounds have agreeable odors, which accounts for the use of this term for such compounds.

aromatic elixir [Gk, *aroma* + Ar, *al-iksir,* philosophers' stone], a pleasant-smelling flavoring agent added to some medications.

aromatic hydrocarbon [Gk, *aroma,* spice, *hydor,* water; L, *carbo,* coal], an organic compound that has a benzene or other aromatic ring, as distinguished from an open-chain aliphatic compound.

aromatic spirit of ammonia, a mixture of ammonia, ammonium carbonate, and other agents for use as an inhalant to revive a person who has fainted. Also called **smelling salt.** See **aromatic ammonia spirit.**

arousal [OE, to rise], a state of responsiveness to sensory stimulation.

arousal level, the state of sensory stimulation needed to induce active wakefulness in a sleeping infant. Arousal levels range from deep sleep to drowsy state.

ARPKD, abbreviation for *autosomal-recessive polycystic kidney disease.*

Arranon, brand name for **nelarabine.**

array [ME, *aray,* preparation], an arrangement or order of components or other objects, usually according to a predetermined system or plan.

arrector pili /ä·rek′tor pī′lī/ *pl. arrectores pilorum* [L, raisers of the hair], minute smooth muscles of the skin attached to the connective tissue sheath of the hair follicles; when they contract, they cause the hair to stand erect, producing cutis anserina (goose flesh).

arrest [L, *ad, restare,* to withstand], to inhibit, restrain, or stop, as to arrest the course of a disease. See also **cardiac arrest.**

arrested dental caries, tooth decay in which the area of decay has stopped progressing and infection is not present but in which the demineralized area in the tooth remains as a cavity.

arrested development, **1.** the cessation of one or more phases of the developmental process in utero before normal completion, resulting in congenital anomalies. **2.** a form of intellectual disability that develops in some children after they have progressed normally for the first 3 to 4 years of life. Can be classified as cognitive impairments, learning disorders, motor skills disorders, communication disorders, or pervasive developmental disorders. Also called **developmental arrest.**

arrest disorders, the cessation of progress during labor. Arrest disorders include secondary arrest of dilation (no progress in cervical dilation in more than 2 hours), arrest of descent (fetal head does not descend for more than 1 hour in primipara women and more than 0.5 hours in multipara women), and failure of descent of the fetus.

arrested labor [L, *ad + restare,* to withstand, *labor,* work], abnormality of the active (but not latent) phase of labor characterized by cessation of progress of labor.

arrheno-, prefix meaning "male": *arrhenoblastoma, arrhenogenic.*

arrhenoblastoma /erē′nōblastō″mə/ [Gk, *arrhen,* male, *blastos,* germ, *oma,* tumor], an ovarian neoplasm whose cells mimic those in testicular tubules and secrete male sex hormone, causing virilization in females. Also called **andreioma, androblastoma, androma, arrhenoma, Sertoli-Leydig cell tumor.**

arrhenogenic /erē′nōjen″ik/, producing only male offspring.

arrhenokaryon /erē′nōker″ē·on/ [Gk, *arrhen,* male, *karyon,* nucleus], an organism that is produced from an egg that has only paternal chromosomes.

arrhenoma. See **arrhenoblastoma.**

arrhinia /ə-rinxe-ə/ [Gk, *rhin,* nose], a rare congenital abnormality characterized by partial or complete absence of the nose. Also called *nasal agenesis.*

arrhythmia /ərith″mē·ə/ [Gk, *a + rhythmos,* without rhythm], any deviation from the normal pattern of the heartbeat. Compare **dysrhythmia.** −*arrhythmical,* **arrhythmic,** *adj.*

arrhythmic [Gk, without rhythm], pertaining to an absence or irregularity of normal rhythm of the heartbeat.

ARRT, abbreviation for **American Registry of Radiologic Technologists.**

arsenic (As) /är″sənik/ [Gk, *arsen,* strong], an element that occurs throughout the earth's crust in metal arsenides, arsenious sulfides, and arsenious oxides. Its atomic number is 33; its atomic mass is 74.92. This element has been used for centuries as a therapeutic agent and as a poison and continues to have limited use in some trypanocidal drugs. The introduction of nonarsenic trypanocidals with less dangerous side effects in the treatment of trypanosomiasis has greatly reduced its use. Exposure to arsenic can occur occupationally in mining, in the pesticide and pharmaceutical industries, and in glass and microelectronics manufacturing, as well as environmentally from both industrial and natural sources. The average concentration in the human adult is about 20 mg, which is stored mainly in the liver, kidney, GI tract, and lungs. The mechanisms for the biotransformation of arsenics in humans are not well understood. Most arsenics are slowly excreted in the urine and feces, which accounts for the toxicity of the element. Arsenic is a carcinogen. −*arsenic, adj.*

arsenic poisoning, toxic effect caused by the ingestion or inhalation of arsenic or a substance containing arsenic, an ingredient in some pesticides, herbicides, dyes, and medicinal solutions. Small amounts absorbed over a period of time may result in chronic poisoning, producing nausea, headache, coloration and scaling of the skin, hyperkeratoses, anorexia, and white lines across the fingernails. Ingestion of large amounts of arsenic results in severe GI pain, diarrhea, vomiting, and swelling of the extremities. Renal failure and shock may occur, and death may result. Determination of the presence of arsenic in the urine, hair, or fingernails is diagnostic.

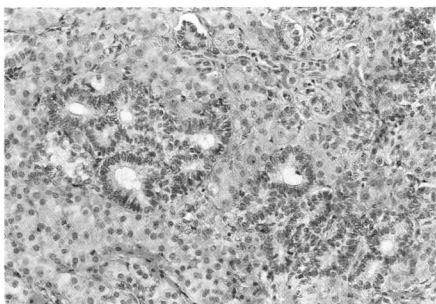

Arrhenoblastoma *(Fletcher, 2007)*

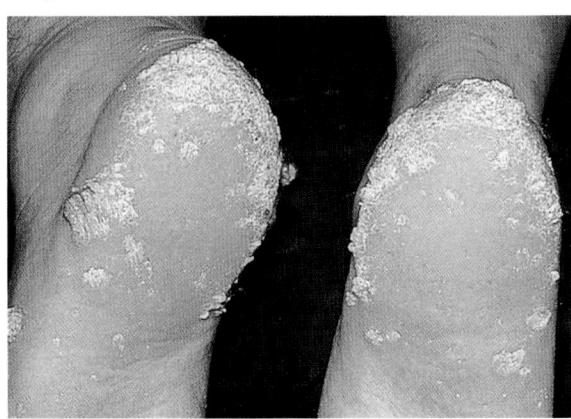

Arsenic keratoses *(Lawrence and Cox, 2002)*

arsenic stomatitis [Gk, *arsen,* strong; *stoma,* mouth, *itis,* inflammation], an abnormal oral condition associated with arsenic poisoning, characterized by dry, red, painful oral mucosa; ulceration; bleeding beneath the mucosa; and mobility of teeth. Compare **atabrine stomatitis, bismuth stomatitis.** See also **arsenic poisoning.**

arsenic trihydride. See **arsine.**

arsenic trioxide, an oxidized form of arsenic, used in weed killers and rodenticides. It is also administered intravenously as an antineoplastic in the treatment of acute promyelocytic leukemia.

arsenism /ahr′sĕ-nizm/, chronic arsenic poisoning.

arsine /ahr′sēn/, any of several colorless, volatile arsenical bases that are highly toxic and carcinogenic; the most common one is AsH_3, arsenous trihydride. Some of these compounds have been used in warfare, and a major industrial use is in the production of microelectronic components, as well as in metal refining. Inhalation leads to massive red blood cell hemolysis with secondary renal failure and jaundice. A garliclike odor may be noted with high concentrations. Initial symptoms include headache, vertigo, and nausea.

ART, abbreviation for **active resistance training.**

Artane, a synthetic antispasmodic, anticholinergic drug. Brand name for **trihexyphenidyl hydrochloride.**

artefact. See **artifact.**

arterectomy /är′tərek″təmē/, the surgical removal of a segment of an artery.

arteri-. See **arterio-, arteri-.**

arterial (A) /ärtir″ē·əl/ [Gk, *arteria,* airpipe], pertaining to an artery.

arterial bleeding. See **arterial hemorrhage.**

arterial blood gas (ABG), the oxygen and carbon dioxide content of arterial blood, measured by various methods to assess the adequacy of ventilation and oxygenation and the acid-base status of the body. Oxygen saturation of hemoglobin is normally 95% or higher. The partial pressure of arterial oxygen, normally 80 to 100 mm Hg, is increased in hyperventilation and decreased in cardiac decompensation, chronic obstructive pulmonary disease, and certain neuromuscular disorders. The partial pressure of carbon dioxide, normally 35 to 45 mm Hg, may be higher in emphysema, chronic obstructive pulmonary disease, and reduced respiratory center function; it may be lower in pregnancy and in the presence of pulmonary emboli and anxiety.

arterial blood gases (ABG) test, a profile performed on fresh whole arterial or capillary blood that reports pH, CO_2 saturation, bicarbonate, and O_2 saturation. The assays detect and define respiratory and metabolic acidosis and alkalosis, kidney function, and oxygenation.

arterial blood pressure (ABP), the pressure of the blood in the arterial system, which depends on the heart's pumping pressure, the resistance of the arterial walls, elasticity of vessels, the blood volume, and its viscosity.

arterial capillaries, microscopic blood vessels (capillaries) extending beyond the terminal ends of arterioles.

arterial catheter [Gk, *arteria,* airpipe, *katheter,* a thing lowered into], a tubular instrument that can be inserted into an artery either to draw blood or to measure blood pressure directly. More commonly referred to as an arterial line. Also called **Art-line.**

arterial circulation [Gk, *arteria* + L, *circulare,* to go around], the movement of blood through the arteries directed away from the heart to the tissues.

arterial hemorrhage, the loss of blood from an artery, often associated with vessel trauma or the removal of a large-bore arterial catheter. Also called **arterial bleeding.**

arterial insufficiency, inadequate blood flow in arteries. It may be caused by occlusive atherosclerotic plaques or emboli; damaged, diseased, or intrinsically weak vessels; arteriovenous fistulas; aneurysms; hypercoagulability states; or heavy use of tobacco. Signs of arterial insufficiency include pale, cyanotic, or mottled skin over the affected area, absent or decreased sensations, tingling, diminished sense of temperature, muscle pains, reduced or absent peripheral pulses, and, in advanced disease, arterial ulcers and atrophy of muscles in the involved extremity. Diagnosis includes checking and comparing peripheral pulses in contralateral extremities, angiography, ultrasound using a Doppler device, and skin temperature tests. Treatment may include a diet low in saturated fats, moderate exercise, sleeping on a firm mattress, use of a vasodilator, and, if indicated, surgical repair of an aneurysm or arteriovenous fistula. Use of tobacco products, prolonged standing, and sitting with the knees bent are discouraged.

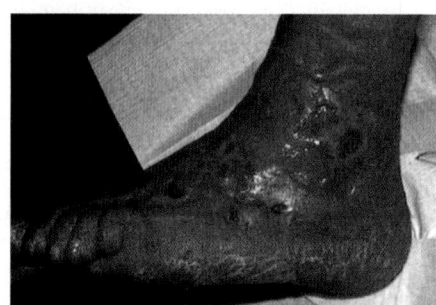

Ulcers in a patient with arterial insufficiency *(Graham-Brown and Bourke, 2007)*

arterial insufficiency of lower extremities, a condition characterized by hardening, thickening, and loss of elasticity of the walls of arteries in the legs. It causes decreased cir-

Arterial blood gases

Parameter	Measurement	Value
Acid-base balance	pH: hydrogen ion concentration	Normal: 7.35-7.45 Alkalemia: >7.45 Acidemia: <7.35
Oxygenation	Pao_2: partial pressure of dissolved O_2 in blood	Normal: 80-100 mm Hg Hyperoxia: >100 mm Hg Hypoxemia: <80 mm Hg, 95%-98%
Ventilation	Sao_2: percentage of O_2 bound to hemoglobin $Paco_2$: partial pressure of CO_2 dissolved in blood	Normal: 35-45 mm Hg Hypercapnia: >45 mm Hg Hypocapnia: <35 mm Hg

From Monahan FD et al: *Phipps' medical-surgical nursing: health and illness perspectives,* ed 8, St Louis, 2007, Mosby.

culation, sensation, and function. Symptoms include sharp, cramping pain during exercise or rest at night; numbness; skin changes ranging from pallor to ulceration; thickened toenails; and loss of hair on the legs. Dorsalis pedis, posterior tibial, and popliteal pulses may be diminished or absent. The ankle-brachial index is used as the initial screening test, and laboratory studies usually show elevated plasma lipid levels. See also **claudication.**

arterialized flap, a skin graft used in reconstructive surgery whose blood supply in the new site is maintained by a vein that is grafted to an artery.

arterial ligament, a small nonfunctional ligament attached to the superior surface of the pulmonary trunk and the inferior surface of the aortic arch. It is a vestige of the ductus arteriosus.

arterial line (A-line, Art-line), an arterial blood monitoring system consisting of a catheter inserted into an artery and connected to pressure tubing, a transducer, and a monitor. The device permits continuous direct blood pressure readings as well as access to the arterial blood supply when samples are needed for analysis.

arterial murmur, a sound produced by blood moving through a narrowed artery.

arterial nephrosclerosis [Gk, *arteria,* airpipe, *nephros,* kidney, *sklera,* hard, *osis,* condition], patchy atrophic scarring of the kidneys caused by arteriosclerotic narrowing of the lumens of the large branches of the renal artery, occurring in elderly or hypertensive persons and occasionally causing hypertension.

arterial network [Gk, *arteria* + L, *rete,* net], an anastomotic network of small arteries at a point before they branch into arterioles and capillaries. Also called **rete arteriosum.**

arterial palpitation [Gk, *arteria,* airpipe; L, *palpitare,* to flutter], a pulsation felt in an artery.

arterial pH, the hydrogen ion concentration of arterial blood. Normal range is 7.35 to 7.45.

arterial plethysmography, a manometric test that is usually performed to rule out occlusive disease of the lower extremities. It can also be used to identify arteriosclerotic disease in the upper extremity.

arterial port, the self-sealing diaphragm in a synthetic access device that allows repeated access to the vascular system for the delivery of medications and other fluids needed on an intermittent basis.

arterial pressure, the stress exerted by circulating blood on the artery walls. It is the product of the cardiac output and the systemic vascular resistance. A number of extrinsic and intrinsic factors regulate and maintain a reasonably constant arterial pressure. Extrinsic factors include neurological stimulation and hormones such as catecholamines and prostaglandins. Intrinsic factors include chemoreceptors and baroreceptors in the arterial walls that cause vasoconstriction or vasodilation. Arterial pressure is commonly measured with a sphygmomanometer and a stethoscope. Stress, hypervolemia, hypovolemia, and various drugs may alter the arterial pressure. Also called **arterial tension.** See also **blood pressure.**

arterial rete /rē"tē/ [Gk, *arteria,* airpipe; L, *rete,* net], a network of arteries and arterioles.

arterial sclerosis [Gk, *arteria,* airpipe, *sklerosis,* hardening], a thickening and hardening of the arteries caused by fibrosis or calcium deposition. See also **arteriosclerosis, atherosclerosis.**

arterial tension. See **arterial pressure.**

arterial thrill, a vibration that can be felt over an artery. It is usually associated with turbulent blood flow within the artery.

arterial wall, the fibrous and muscular wall of vessels that carry oxygenated blood from the heart to structures throughout the body, and of the pulmonary arteries that carry deoxygenated blood from the heart to the lungs. The wall of an artery has three layers: the tunica intima, the inner layer; the tunica media, the middle layer; and the tunica adventitia, the outer layer. Nerves from the autonomic nervous system constrict or dilate the vessel and thus control the flow of blood into the areas served by the artery. The middle layer in smaller arteries is almost entirely muscular and in larger arteries is more elastic. The thickness of the outer layer varies with the location of the artery. In protected areas, such as the abdominal and cranial cavities, the outer layer of associated arteries is very thin, but in more exposed locations, as in the limbs, it is much thicker. See also **tunica intima, tunica adventitia, tunica media.**

arteriectomy /ärtir'ē·ek"təmē/ [Gk, *arteria* + *ektomē,* excision], the surgical removal of a portion of an artery.

arteries, vessels through which the oxygenated blood passes away from the heart to various parts of the body. The wall of an artery consists typically of an outer layer (tunica adventitia), a middle layer (tunica media), and an inner layer (tunica intima). See **blood vessel.**

arterio-, arteri-, prefix meaning "artery": *arteriosclerosis, arteritis.*

arteriocapillary /är·tir'ē·ō·kap'i·lar'ē/ [Gk, *arteria* + L, *capillaris,* hairlike], pertaining to the arteries and the capillaries.

arteriofibrosis /ärtir'ē·ōfībrō"sis/, an inflammatory, fibrous thickening of the walls of the arteries and arterioles, resulting in a narrowing of the lumen of the vessels.

arteriogenic impotence, vasculogenic impotence caused by a disorder in the arteries supplying the penis, such as atherosclerosis or stenosis.

arteriogram /ärtir"ē·əgram'/, a series of radiographic images used to observe blood flow within an artery injected with a radiopaque contrast medium. See also **arteriography.**

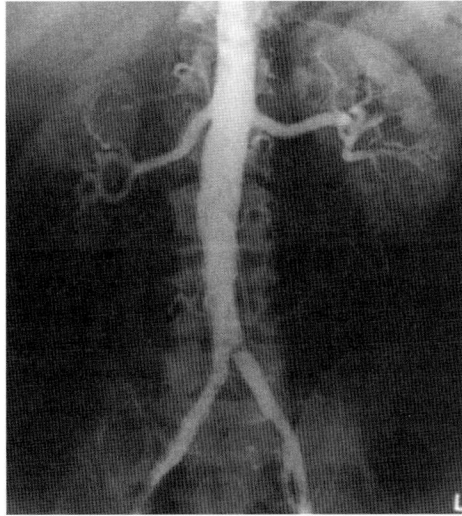

Renal arteriogram *(Gurley and Callaway, 2011)*

arteriography /ärtir'ē·og"rəfē/ [Gk, *arteria,* airpipe, *graphein,* to record], a diagnostic imaging test used to observe blood flow within arteries; the test consists of the production of images of vessels after a radiopaque contrast medium is introduced into the bloodstream or into a specific vessel by injection or through a catheter. See also **angiography.** *—arteriographic, adj.*

arteriole /ärtir″ē·ōl/ [L, little artery], the smallest of the arteries. Blood flowing from the heart is pumped through the arteries, to the arterioles, to the capillaries, into the veins, and returned to the heart. The muscular walls of the arterioles constrict and dilate in response to both local factors and neurochemical stimuli; thus, arterioles play a significant role in peripheral vascular resistance and in regulation of blood pressure. Also called *arteriola.* See also **artery.**

arteriolosclerosis /ärtir″ē·ō′ləskləro″sis/, pathological thickening, hardening, and loss of elasticity of arteriolar walls.

arteriopathy /ärtir″ē·op″əthē/ [Gk, *arteria + pathos,* suffering], a disease of an artery.

arterioplasty /ärtir″ē·əplas″tē/ [Gk, *arteria + plassein,* to mold], surgical repair or reconstruction of an artery. The procedure is often performed to correct an aneurysm.

arteriosclerosis /ärtir″ē·ō′sklərō″sis/ [Gk, *arteria + sklerosis,* hardening], a common disorder characterized by thickening, loss of elasticity, and calcification of arterial walls. It results in a decreased blood supply, especially to the cerebrum and lower extremities. The condition often develops with aging and in hypertension, nephrosclerosis, scleroderma, diabetes, and hyperlipidemia. Typical signs and symptoms include intermittent claudication, changes in skin temperature and color, altered peripheral pulses, bruits over an involved artery, headache, dizziness, and memory defects. Vasodilators and exercise may relieve symptoms, but there is no specific treatment. Preventive measures include therapy for predisposing diseases, adequate rest and exercise, avoidance of stress, and discontinuation of tobacco use. Also called **arterial sclerosis, hardening of the arteries.** Kinds include **atherosclerosis, Mönckeberg's arteriosclerosis. —arteriosclerotic,** *adj.*

arteriosclerosis obliterans [Gk, *arteria + skleros +* L, *obliterare,* efface], a gradual narrowing of the arteries with thrombosis and degeneration of the intima. The condition may lead to complete occlusion of an artery and subsequent gangrene.

arteriosclerotic /-sklərot″ik/ [Gk, *arteria + skleros,* hard], pertaining to a thickening, hardening, and calcification of the arterial wall.

arteriosclerotic aneurysm, an aneurysm arising in a large artery, most commonly the abdominal aorta, as a result of weakening of the wall in severe atherosclerosis. Also called **atherosclerotic aneurysm.**

arteriosclerotic heart disease (ASHD), a thickening and hardening of the walls of the coronary arteries.

arteriosclerotic retinopathy [Gk, *arteria,* airpipe, *sklerosis,* hardening; L, *rete,* net; Gk, *pathos,* disease], a disorder of the retina associated with hardening and thickening of the arteries supplying that part of the eye. It often accompanies hypertension.

arteriospasm /ärtir″ē·ōspaz′əm/ [Gk, *arteria + spasmos,* spasm], a sudden, abnormal contraction of an artery.

arteriostenosis /-stənō″sis/, a narrowing of an artery.

arteriotomy /ärtir″ē·ot″əmē/, a surgical incision in an artery.

arteriovenous (AV) /-vē″nəs/ [Gk, *arteria +* L, *vena,* vein], pertaining to arteries and veins.

arteriovenous anastomosis [Gk, *arteria +* L, *vena;* Gk, *anastomoein,* to form a mouth], a communication between an artery and a vein, either as a congenital anomaly or as a surgically produced link between vessels. See also **arteriovenous fistula.**

arteriovenous aneurysm, a dilation affecting both an artery and a vein, often as an abnormal linkage of the two.

arteriovenous angioma of the brain, a congenital tumor consisting of a tangle of coiled, usually dilated arteries and veins, islets of sclerosed brain tissue, and, occasionally, cartilaginous cells. The lesion, which may be distinguished by an intracranial bruit, generally arises in the vascular system of the pia mater and may grow to project deeply into the brain, causing seizures and progressive hemiparesis.

arteriovenous fistula, **1.** an abnormal communication between an artery and vein. It may occur congenitally or result from trauma, infection, arterial aneurysm, or a malignancy. A continuous murmur and palpable thrill may be detected over the fistula and may be obliterated by compressing the feeding artery; this maneuver may slow the heartbeat (Branham's sign). Chronic arteriovenous fistulas may cause varicosities, cutaneous ulcers, and cardiac enlargement resulting from high-output heart failure. A congenital fistula may result in a cavernous hemangioma. If an arteriovenous fistula is limited in size and is accessible, it can be treated by surgical excision. **2.** an anastomosis between an artery and vein created surgically to provide vascular access for hemodialysis.

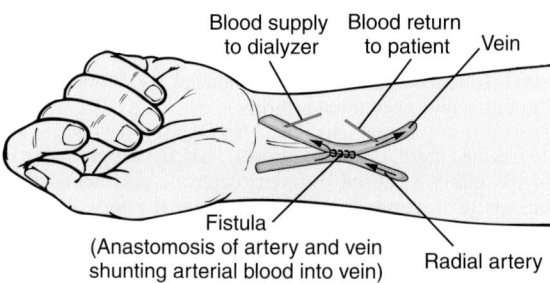

Arteriovenous fistula *(Lewis et al, 2011)*

arteriovenous oxygen (a-vo₂) difference, the arterial oxygen content minus the central venous oxygen content.

arteriovenous shunt (AV shunt), a passageway, artificial or natural, that allows blood to flow from an artery to a vein without going through a capillary network.

arteritis /är″tərī″tis/ [Gk, *arteria + itis*], inflammation of the inner layers or the outer coat of one or more arteries. It may occur as a clinical entity or accompany another disorder, such as rheumatoid arthritis, rheumatic fever, polymyositis, or systemic lupus erythematosus. Kinds include **infantile arteritis, rheumatic arteritis, Takayasu's arteritis, temporal arteritis.** See also **endarteritis, periarteritis.**

arteritis obliterans. See **endarteritis obliterans.**

arteritis umbilicalis, septic inflammation of the umbilical artery in newborns, usually caused by the bacterium *Clostridium tetani.*

artery /är″tərē/ [Gk, *arteria,* airpipe], one of the large blood vessels carrying blood in a direction away from the heart to the tissues. Compare **vein.** See also **arterial wall, arteriole.**

artery forceps, any forceps used for grasping, compressing, and holding the end of an artery during ligation. Generally self-locking, its handles are scissorlike. Artery forceps are atraumatic to prevent tissue damage. Also called **hemostatic forceps.**

arthral. See **articular.**

arthralgia /ärthral″jə/ [Gk, *arthron,* joint, *algos,* pain], joint pain. *—arthralgic, adj.*

-arthria, suffix meaning a "(specified) condition involving the ability to articulate": *anarthria, dysarthria.*

-arthritic, -arthritical, suffix meaning "arthritis": *antiarthritic, postarthritic.*

arthritis /ärthrī″tis/ [Gk, *arthron,* joint, *itis*], a complex family of musculoskeletal disorders consisting of more than 100 different diseases or conditions that can affect people of all ages, races, and genders. The most common type of arthritis is osteo-arthritis. See also **osteoarthritis, rheumatoid arthritis.**

arthritis deformans, *(Obsolete)* now called **rheumatoid arthritis.**

arthro-, arthr-, combining form meaning "joints, articulations": *arthralgia, arthrocentesis.*

arthrocentesis /är″thrōsintē″sis/ [Gk, *arthron + kentesis,* pricking], the puncture of a joint with a needle and the withdrawal of fluid, performed to obtain samples of synovial fluid for diagnostic purposes. It may also be used to instill medications and to remove fluid from joints to simply relieve pain. A local anesthetic is usually administered; surgical asepsis is observed in the procedure. Normal synovial fluid is a clear, straw-colored, slightly viscous liquid that forms a white, viscous clot when mixed with glacial acetic acid; if inflammation is present, as in rheumatoid arthritis, the fluid is watery and turbid, and its mixture with glacial acetic acid results in a flocculent, easily broken clot. The number of leukocytes, especially polymorphonuclear cells, and the protein content are increased, and the glucose level is decreased if inflammation is present. Synovial fluid samples are also cultured and examined microscopically to diagnose a septic process, such as bacterial arthritis.

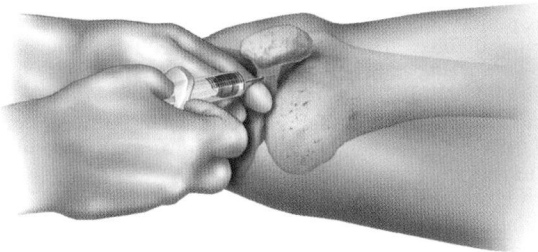

Arthrocentesis *(Custalow, 2005)*

arthrodiastasis, the application of an external fixator to stretch the joint capsule as an alternative to joint fusion or joint replacement.

arthrodesis, surgical fusion of a joint. See **ankylosis.**

arthrogram /är″thrəgram/, **1.** a radiographic image after introduction of contrast material. **2.** a nuclear medicine study used to detect the loosening of a prosthetic device.

arthrography [Gk, *arthron,* joint, *graphein,* to record], a diagnostic imaging procedure used to observe the inside of a joint following the introduction of radiolucent or radiopaque contrast medium.

arthrogryposis multiplex congenita [Gk, *arthron + gryposis,* joint curve; L, *multus,* many, *plica,* fold, *congenitus,* born with], fibrous stiffness of one or more joints, present at birth. It is often associated with incomplete development of the muscles that move the involved joints and degenerative changes of the motor neurons that innervate those muscles. The cause of the condition, which is uncommon, is unknown, although possible causes are fetal crowding and maternal neuromuscular disease. Physiotherapy to loosen the joints is the only treatment. Also called **amyoplasia congenita.**

arthrokinematic /är″thrəkin′əmat″ik/, pertaining to the movement of bone surfaces within a joint.

arthron /är″thron/ [Gk], a joint or articulation, including its various components of bones, cartilaginous inserts, all soft tissue structures intervening between the rigid skeletal parts, and the adjacent muscular elements.

arthropathy /ärthrop″əthē/ [Gk, *arthron + pathos,* suffering], any disease or abnormal condition affecting a joint. *−arthropathic, adj.*

arthroplasty /är″thrəplast′ē/ [Gk, *arthron + plassein,* to mold], the surgical reconstruction or replacement of a painful, degenerated joint to restore mobility in osteoarthritis or rheumatoid arthritis or to correct a congenital deformity. Also called **joint replacement.** See also **osteoarthritis.**

■ METHOD: Either the bones of the joint are reshaped and soft tissue or a metal disk is placed between the reshaped ends, or all or part of the joint is replaced with a metal or plastic prosthesis.

■ PATIENT CARE CONSIDERATIONS: Preoperative care may include the typing and crossmatching of blood. After surgery the patient may be placed in traction to immobilize the affected limb. Physical therapy to increase muscle strength and range of motion is allowed on a slow, progressive schedule. When a lower extremity is involved, weight-bearing activity may or may not be allowed. Frequent checks of distal circulation are made, and the nurse watches for bleeding, thrombophlebitis, pulmonary embolism, or fat embolism. Antibiotics are usually given to prevent infection, which is the most common cause of failure of the surgery.

■ OUTCOME CRITERIA: The goal of the procedure is the relief of pain and restoration of full range of motion.

arthropod /är″thrəpod′/ [Gk, *arthron + pous,* foot], a member of the Arthropoda, a large phylum of animal life that includes crabs and lobsters as well as mites, ticks, spiders, and insects. Arthropods generally are distinguished by a jointed exoskeleton (shell) and paired, jointed legs. They bite, sting, cause allergic reactions, and may serve as vectors for viruses and other disease-causing agents.

arthropod-borne virus. See **arbovirus.**

arthroscope /-skōp′/ [Gk, *arthron + skopein,* to watch], a fiberoptic instrument connected to a light source that is surgically inserted to examine joints. It is used primarily in knee and hand surgeries.

arthroscopic anterior cruciate ligament reconstruction, reconstruction of the anterior cruciate ligament (ACL), performed on individuals whose activities are compromised by instability of the knee and who have failed to respond to nonsurgical treatment options. Repair of the anterior cruciate ligament usually involves replacement of the ligament by either an autograft, allograft, or synthetic ligament. Autografts are the method of choice; synthetic devices may contribute to the development of chronic synovitis. The procedure is usually performed using an arthroscope.

arthroscopy /ärthros″kəpē/ [Gk, *arthron + skopein,* to watch], the examination of the interior of a joint, performed by inserting a specially designed endoscope through a small incision. The procedure, used chiefly in knee problems, permits biopsy of cartilage or synovium, diagnosis of a torn meniscus, and, in some instances, removal of loose bodies in the joint space. *−arthroscopic, adj.*

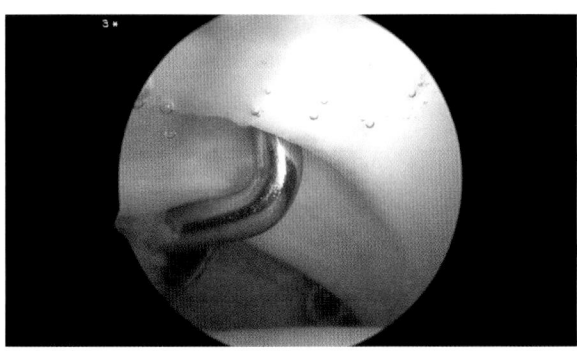

Arthroscopy *(Alwattar and Bharam, 2011)*

arthrous /är″thrəs/ [Gk,], **1.** pertaining to joints or the articulation of bones. **2.** pertaining to a disease of a joint.

Arthus reaction /ärtoōs″/ [Nicholas M. Arthus, French physiologist, 1862–1945], a rare, severe, immediate nonatopic hypersensitivity reaction to the injection of a foreign substance, that usually is not irritating but in certain individuals is antigenic. The reaction is thought to involve the formation of an antigen-antibody complex that activates complement. Acute local inflammation, usually in the skin and marked by edema, hemorrhage, and necrosis, occurs at the site of injection. Also called *Arthus phenomenon.* See also **serum sickness.**

articaine, an amide local anesthetic agent used in dentistry. The half-life is 20 minutes; it hydrolyzes quickly in the blood. It is commonly available as a 4% (40 mg/mL) solution in combination with epinephrine 1:100,000 or 1:200,000 to prolong its efficacy. See also **amide local anesthetic.**

articul-, combining form meaning "joint, structure, and function": *articular, articulatio.*

articular. See **articulate,** def. 1.

articular capsule [L, *articulare,* to divide into joints], an envelope of tissue that surrounds a freely moving joint, composed of an external layer of white fibrous tissue and an internal synovial membrane. See also **fibrous capsule.**

articular cartilage [L, *articulare + cartilago*], a type of hyaline connective tissue that covers the articulating surfaces of bones within synovial joints. See also **cartilage.**

articular disk, **1.** a small oval plate between the condyle of the mandible and the mandibular fossa. Displacement of or injury to the plate may be a cause of temporomandibular joint (TMJ) pain. **2.** the platelike cartilaginous end of certain bones in movable joints, sometimes closely associated with surrounding muscles or with cartilage.

articular fracture, a fracture involving the articulating surfaces of a joint.

articular head, a projection on a bone that forms a joint with another bone.

articular muscle, a muscle that is attached to the capsule of a joint.

articular process of vertebra, a bony outgrowth on a vertebra that forms a joint with an adjoining vertebra.

articulate /ärtik″yəlāt/ [L, *articulare,* to divide into joints], **1.** to form a joint. **2.** to configure the supraglottal airway to produce consonants and vowels, resulting in speech that is distinct and connected. See also **phonation, resonance, articulation,** def. 1. **–articulation,** *n.*

articulated /ärtik″yəlā′tid/, united by a movable joint.

articulated partial denture. See **partial denture.**

articulation, **1.** the process by which the supraglottal airway is shaped to form consonants and vowels into meaningful, understandable speech. **2.** the place of union or junction between two or more bones of the skeleton. See **joint. 3.** (in a university) the seamless transfer of credits from one institution of higher learning to another, usually the result of a partnership between a community college and a four-year college.

articulation of the pelvis /ärtik′yəlā″shən/, any one of the connections between the bones of the pelvis, involving four groups of ligaments. The first group connects the sacrum and the ilium; the second, the sacrum and the ischium; the third, the sacrum and the coccyx; and the fourth, the two pubic bones.

articulator /ärtik″yəlā′tər/ [L, *articulare,* to divide into joints], a mechanical device used in the fabrication and testing of dental prostheses. It simulates the temporomandibular joints and jaw members to which maxillary and mandibular plaster casts may be attached. Some articulators are adjustable, allowing movement of attached casts into various eccentric relationships.

artifact /är″təfakt/ [L, *ars,* skill, *facere,* to make], **1.** anything artificially made; may be extraneous, irrelevant, or unwanted, such as a substance, structure, or piece of data or information. **2.** (in radiography) storage, handling, or processing irregularities resulting in unwanted images or alterations in the appearance of the subject. **3.** (in ethology) an object constructed by individuals of a group that provides information about cultural practices.

artifactual modification /är′təfak″choo·əl/, a change in protein structure caused by in vitro manipulation.

artificial /är′tifish″əl/ [L, *artificium,* not natural], **1.** made by human work as a substitute for something that is natural. **2.** simulated; resulting from art in imitation of nature.

artificial abortion, *(Obsolete)* an abortion that is produced deliberately. Also called **induced abortion.** Now called **therapeutic abortion.**

artificial airway [L, *artificiosum,* skillfully made], a plastic or rubber device that can be inserted into the upper or lower respiratory tract to facilitate ventilation and/or the removal of secretions.

artificial ankylosis, *(Informal)* a surgical procedure in which there is artificial induction of joint ossification so that the joint becomes immovable. Now called **arthrodesis.**

artificial anus, *(Informal)* a surgical opening into the bowel, as in a colostomy.

artificial blood. See **perfluorocarbon.**

artificial crown, a dental prosthesis that restores part or all of the crown of a natural tooth. Compare **anatomical crown, clinical crown, partial crown.**

artificial dentition, replacements for natural teeth. Kinds include **full denture, partial denture, fixed bridge, endosseous implant.**

artificial eye, *(Informal)* a prosthetic device resembling the anterior surface of a normal eyeball. It is fitted under the upper and lower eyelid of an eye that has been removed.

artificial urinary sphincter, an implantable prosthetic device for treating urinary incontinence caused by an incompetent or absent sphincter; an artificial sphincter is created with an inflatable cuff around the bladder neck or bulbar urethra.

artificial heart, a mechanical device consisting of a pump and artificial ventricles capable of fully sustaining an individual's circulatory system. It is used to keep the patient alive until transplantation is possible. The first artificial heart to be successfully implanted was the Jarvik-7 in 1982. Kinds include **AbioCor, Berlin heart.**

artificial homologous insemination. Also called **artificial insemination—husband.** See **artificial insemination.**

artificial impregnation, artificial insemination with husband's or partner's sperm. Also called **artificial insemination—husband.** See **artificial insemination.**

artificial insemination (AI), the introduction of semen into the vagina or uterus by mechanical or instrumental means rather than by sexual intercourse. The procedure is planned to coincide with the expected time of ovulation so that fertilization can occur. Also called **artificial impregnation.** Kinds include **artificial insemination—husband, artificial insemination—donor.** See also **menstrual cycle.**

artificial insemination—donor (AID), artificial insemination in which the semen specimen is provided by an anonymous donor. The procedure is used primarily in cases where the partner is unable to provide a viable sperm sample. Also called **heterologous insemination.** Compare **artificial insemination—husband.**

Circulatory and ventricular assist devices (artificial hearts)

Pump type	Pump method	Ventricular support	Power and controller	Uses	Pump, console placement
Abiomed's BVS 5000™	• A pneumatic drive console • Can operate one or two blood pumps independently	• Right ventricle/ left ventricle/ biventricular	• External power and control console	• First FDA-approved device for all patients with potentially reversible heart failure ≤10 days • Bridge to transplant • Possible weaning from device as heart recovers	• External
Abiomed™ Impella	• Catheter pump • Inserted via femoral artery • Up to 2.5 L of blood delivered per minute	• Blood delivered by pump from left ventricle into ascending aorta	• Inserted percutaneously in the cardiac catheterization laboratory	• Active support in critical situations • Short-term circulatory support	• Minimally invasive catheter-based
Berlin Heart™	• One or two air-driven pumps (dependent on need for single or double ventricle support) • Air pulses drive rhythm of pumps	• Left and/or right ventricle	• Works with patient's heart to support ventricles	• Bridge to transplant • Special permission needed to use in the U.S. • For pediatric patients from newborn to adolescent	• Plastic pump chamber external to the body
BioMedicus™	• Centrifugal device—impeller inside cone that creates vortex • Can rotate to 5000 rpm • Maximum pump flow rate 10 L/min	• Right ventricle/ left ventricle/ biventricular ECMO (extracorporeal membrane oxygenation)	• External motor and power console • Internal battery, 45 min	• Cardiopulmonary bypass short term (≤5 days of circulatory support) • Postcardiotomy cardiogenic shock • Bridge to transplant • Transport of patient from hospital to hospital with transplant center	• External
CardioWest™ temporary Total Artificial Heart (TAH-t)	• Modern version of Jarvic-7	• Biventricular	• Only temporary artificial heart designed to beat in chest	• Bridge to transplant	• Internal
Thoratec VAD System	• Blood flows to the venous access device (VAD) through an atrial or ventricular cannula • Sensor detects the VAD is full of blood and ejects blood from pump into the aorta (left side) or pulmonary artery (right side)	• Right ventricle/ left ventricle/ biventricular	*Dual Drive Console:* • Two independent and identical modules that provide alternating pulses of air pressure and vacuum to provide pulsatile flow *TLC-II Mobility Cart:* • Single driver unit: Univentricular Biventricular • 4 rechargeable batteries *TLC Docking Station:* • Serves as a home base for portable driver • Downloads data • Allows for pump parameters to be changed • Battery charger	• Used to support total or partial circulatory assistance • Possible wean from Thoratec to a less invasive device (i.e., intra-aortic balloon pump [IABP]) • Bridge to transplant	• External
Novacor, Heartmate	• Passive filling of the pump • Aortic valve does not open • Pump output depends on flow from the right side • Can track the natural heart rhythm	• Left ventricular device only	• External microprocessor-based electronic controller powered by an AC external home unit as well as primary and secondary batteries • Life-threatening alarm systems cannot be muted • Can run in either auto or fixed rate mode • Battery charger	• Bridge to transplant • Bridge to recovery • Chronic or "end-stage" alternative therapy	• Pump inside body with percutaneous lead cable tunneled to exit site (usually above the right iliac crest)

Data Courtesy Colleen Becker RN, MSN, CCRN and Kathy Sue Rowland, RN, BS Educ.

artificial insemination—husband/male partner (AIH), artificial insemination in which the semen specimen is provided by the husband or male partner. The procedure is used primarily in cases of impotency, low sperm count, when the husband or male partner is incapable of sexual intercourse because of some physical disability or a vaginal disorder. Also called **artificial homologous insemination.** Compare **artificial insemination—donor.**

artificial intelligence (AI), a system that attempts to make it possible for a machine to perform functions similar to those performed by human intelligence, such as learning, reasoning, self-correcting, and adapting.

artificial kidney, *(Informal)* a device used to remove body waste, commonly excreted in urine, from circulating blood. It usually consists of a set of tubes or catheters that pass the blood through a dialysate solution, where wastes are removed by osmosis and diffusion. Also called **dialyzer, hemodialyzer, kidney machine.** See also **hemodialysis, peritoneal dialysis.**

artificial limb, *(Informal)* now called **prosthesis.**

artificial lung. See **extracorporeal membrane oxygenator.**

artificially acquired immunity. See **acquired immunity.**

artificial menopause [L, *artificiosus,* artificial, *men,* month; Gk, *pauein,* to cease], the termination of menstrual periods by surgery, radiation, or other methods. See also **menopause.**

artificial pacemaker. *(Nontechnical)* See **pacemaker.**

artificial respiration, now called **artificial ventilation.**

artificial rupture of membranes. See **amniotomy.**

artificial saliva [L, *artificiosum,* artifice, *saliva,* spittle], a mixture of carboxymethylcellulose, sorbitol, sodium, and potassium chloride in an aqueous solution. It is available in a spray container for the treatment of xerostomia (dry mouth).

artificial selection, the process by which the genotypes of successive plant and animal generations are determined through controlled breeding. Compare **natural selection.** See also **eugenics.**

artificial stone. See **dental stone.**

artificial tears, a pharmaceutical preparation of various polymers that can be instilled in the eyes of patients suffering from dry eye or keratoconjunctivitis sicca.

artificial ventilation, the process of supporting respiration by manual or mechanical means when normal breathing is inefficient or has stopped. If artificial ventilation is unsuccessful, the patient is repositioned and the airway is tested for the presence of an obstruction. Also called **artificial respiration.** See also **cardiopulmonary resuscitation, resuscitation, ventilator.**

Art-line. *(Informal)* See **arterial line.**

art therapist. a human service professional who uses art media and images, the creative process, and client responses to artwork in order to assess, treat, and rehabilitate patients with mental, emotional, physical, or developmental disorders. Through art, the therapist attempts to help the client access and express memories, trauma, and psychic conflict often not easily reached with words.

art therapy, the use of art media to reconcile emotional conflicts, foster self-awareness, and express unspoken and frequently unconscious concerns. Art therapy is often used when traditional forms of verbal psychotherapy have failed or have been rejected by an individual and when individuals have difficulty expressing feelings or use verbalization as a defense mechanism.

aryepiglottic fold /er′ē·ep′iglot″ik/, a mucosal fold on each of the lateral borders of the larynx. Together the folds enclose the superior margins of the quadrangular membranes and adjacent soft tissues. They function as a sphincter during swallowing.

aryl-, prefix designating an alkyl monovalent radical derived from an aromatic hydrocarbon and used to denote aromatic groups.

aryl hydrocarbon hydroxylase (AHH), an enzyme that converts carcinogenic chemicals in tobacco smoke and in polluted air into active carcinogens within the lungs.

arytenoid cartilage /ä·rit′ənoid kär′ti·ləj/ [Gk, *arytaina,* ladle + *eidos,* form; L, *cartilago*], one of the paired, pitcher-shaped cartilages of the back of the larynx at the upper border of the cricoid cartilage with attachments to the vocal chords.

As, symbol for the element **arsenic.**

AS, abbreviation for **aortic stenosis.**

as-. See **ad-.**

a.s., **1.** abbreviation for **auris sinistra. 2.** (in pharmacology) an abbreviation identified by the Institute for Safe Medication Practices as an error-prone abbreviation. Now written in full as *left ear.*

5-ASA, abbreviation for **5-aminosalicylic acid.** See **mesalamine.**

ASA, **1.** abbreviation for *American Society of Anesthesiologists.* **2.** abbreviation for **aspirin. 3.** abbreviation for **antisperm antibody. 4.** abbreviation for *American Statistical Association.*

ASAHP, abbreviation for **Association of Schools of Allied Health Professions (ASAHP).**

ASAP, abbreviation for *as soon as possible.*

asbestos /asbes″təs/ [Gk, *asbestos,* inextinguishable], a group of fibrous impure magnesium silicate minerals. Inhalation of the fibers can lead to pulmonary fibrosis if the fibers accumulate in terminal bronchioles. Continued exposure to asbestos fibers can result in lung cancer.

asbestos body, a structure found in the lungs of patients with asbestosis, consisting of an asbestos fiber engulfed by a macrophage or of a mass of asbestos spicules coated with calcium, iron salts, and other substances.

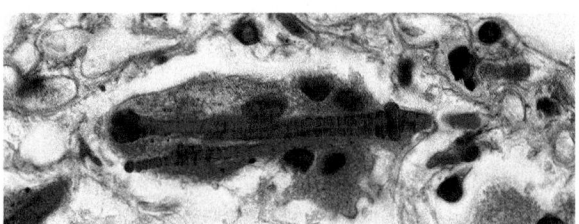

Asbestos body *(Silverberg et al, 2006)*

asbestosis /as-bes′-to′sis/ [Gk, *asbestos,* inextinguishable, *osis,* condition], a chronic lung disease caused by the inhalation of asbestos fibers that results in the development of alveolar, interstitial, and pleural fibrosis. See also **chronic obstructive pulmonary disease, inorganic dust.**

■ OBSERVATIONS: A comprehensive occupational and environmental history is important when asbestosis is being considered. Occupational exposure in construction, demolition, remodeling, mining, and shipbuilding increases risk, and exposure may have occurred 15 years or more before symptoms occur. Chest x-ray films show characteristic small linear opacities distributed throughout the lungs. The disease is progressive. Shortness of breath develops eventually into respiratory failure.

■ INTERVENTIONS: Asbestosis is an irreversible condition, but treatment options do exist to increase comfort, to slow the course of the disease, and to assist the patient to breathe more comfortably.

■ PATIENT CARE CONSIDERATIONS: Cigarette smoking and continuous exposure to asbestos aggravate the condition. The risk of developing lung cancer is significantly increased. Fatal mesothelial tumors sometimes occur.

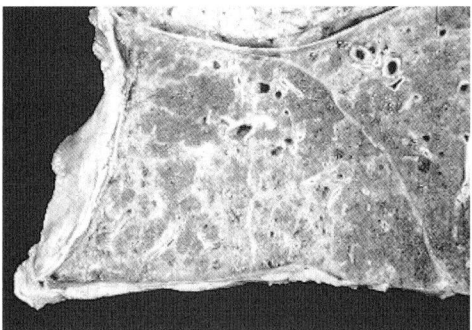

Asbestosis (Kumar et al, 2007)

ASC, **1.** abbreviation for **altered state of consciousness. 2.** abbreviation for **ambulatory surgery center.**

ascariasis /as′kərī″əsis/ [Gk, *askaris,* intestinal worm, *osis,* condition], the most common parasitic infection in the world, caused by a parasitic worm, *Ascaris lumbricoides,* that migrates through the lungs in its larval stage. The eggs are passed in human feces, contaminating the soil and allowing transmission to the mouths of others through hands, water, or food. After hatching in the small intestine, the larvae travel through the wall of the intestine and are carried by the lymphatics and blood to the lungs. The larvae are swallowed; they mature in the jejunum, where they release eggs; and the cycle is repeated.

■ OBSERVATIONS: Some individuals have no symptoms. Heavy intestinal infection may result in abdominal cramps and obstruction. In children infection may cause stunted growth. Early respiratory symptoms of coughing, wheezing, hemoptysis, and fever are caused by the migration of worms through the respiratory tract. The infective eggs are readily identified in the feces.

■ INTERVENTIONS: Piperazine citrate, pyrantel pamoate, mebendazole, and albendazole are effective treatments.

■ PATIENT CARE CONSIDERATIONS: The disease can be prevented by educating people, especially children, about good hygiene, such as handwashing, especially before preparing food. Washing fruits and vegetables before consumption is also important.

Ascaris /as″kəris/, **1.** a genus of nematode worms. **2.** large parasitic intestinal roundworms, such as *Ascaris lumbricoides,* a cause of ascariasis, found throughout temperate and tropic regions. They can infect the intestines of humans and swine.

ascaris, a nematode of the genus *Ascaris*; an intestinal worm.

ascending aorta /asen″ding/ [L, *ascendere,* to climb], one of the four main sections of the aorta, giving rise to the right and left coronary arteries, continuing as the arch of the aorta. See also **arch of the aorta.**

ascending colon, the segment of the colon that extends up from the first region of the large intestine known as the cecum, which is located in the lower right side of the colic fissure. It extends upward into the abdomen, where it joins with the transverse colon at the hepatic flexure on the right side.

ascending neuritis [L, *ascendere,* to rise; Gk, *neuron,* nerve, *itis,* inflammation], a nerve inflammation that begins on the periphery and moves upward along a nerve trunk.

ascending neuropathy, a disease of the nervous system that begins at a lower location and spreads upward. Kinds include **Guillain-Barré syndrome.**

ascending paralysis, a condition in which there is successive flaccid paralysis of the legs, then the trunk and arms, and finally the muscles of respiration. Causes include poliomyelitis, Guillain-Barré syndrome, and exposure to toxic chemicals, for example, botulinum toxin.

ascending pharyngeal artery, one of the smallest arteries that branch from the external carotid artery, deep in the neck. It supplies various organs and muscles of the head, such as the tympanic cavity, the longus capitis, and the longus colli. It divides into five branches: the pharyngeal, palatine, prevertebral, inferior tympanic, and posterior meningeal.

ascending poliomyelitis [L, *ascendere,* to rise; Gk, *polios,* gray, *myelos,* marrow, *itis,* inflammation], poliomyelitis that begins in the legs and spreads upward to involve the trunk and respiratory muscles. See also **ascending paralysis.**

ascending pyelonephritis, pyelonephritis caused by a urinary tract infection that has spread up the ureter and into the kidney.

ascending testis, a previously documented scrotal testicle that later ascends into an extrascrotal position.

ascending tract. See **afferent tract.**

ascending urography. See **urography.**

asceticism /aset″isiz′əm/ [Gk, *askein,* to exercise], (in psychiatry) a defense mechanism that involves repudiation of all instinctual impulses. The concept is derived from the religious doctrine that material things are evil and that only spiritual things are good.

Ascher syndrome /äsh′ər/ [Karl Wolfgang Ascher, Czech-born American ophthalmologist, 1887–1971], relaxation of the skin of the eyelid and redundancy of the mucous membrane and submucous tissue of the upper lip. In some patients nontoxic thyroid enlargement also occurs. The cause of the syndrome is unknown.

Aschoff bodies [Karl A.L. Aschoff, German pathologist, 1866–1942], tiny rounded or spindle-shaped nodules containing multinucleated giant cells, fibroblasts, and basophilic cells. They are found in joints, tendons, the pleura, and the cardiovascular system of patients who have or have had rheumatic fever.

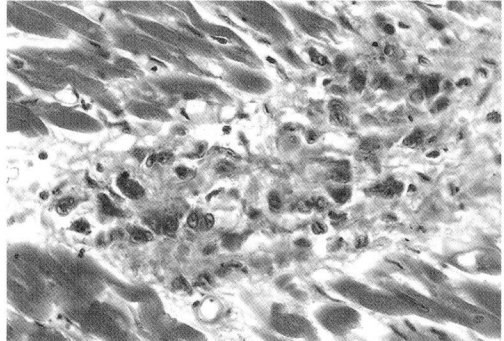

Aschoff bodies (Kumar et al, 2007)

ascites /əsī″tēz/ [Gk, *askos,* bag], an abnormal intraperitoneal accumulation of a fluid containing large amounts of protein and electrolytes. Ascites is a complication, for example, of cirrhosis, congestive heart failure, nephrosis, malignant neoplastic disease, peritonitis, or various fungal and parasitic diseases. See also **paracentesis.** −*ascitic, adj.*

■ OBSERVATIONS: Ascites may be observed when more than 500 mL of fluid has accumulated. Ultrasound examination can detect much smaller amounts. The condition may be accompanied by general abdominal swelling, hemodilution, edema, or a decrease in urinary output. Identification of ascites is made through palpation, percussion, and auscultation.

■ INTERVENTIONS: Ascites is treated with dietary therapy and diuretic drugs; abdominal paracentesis may be performed to relieve pain and improve respiratory and visceral function by relieving the pressure of the accumulated fluid. A peritoneovenous shunt may be surgically inserted to drain the ascites via a tube from the peritoneal cavity to the superior vena cava.

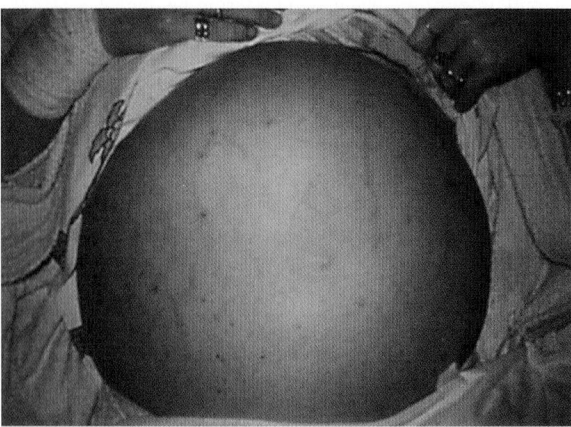

Ascites *(Butcher, 2004)*

ascites praecox /prē″koks/ [Gk, *askos* + L, *praematurus,* premature], an abnormal accumulation of fluid within the peritoneal cavity before the generalized edema associated with pericarditis. See also **ascites.**

ascitic fluid /əsit″ik/ [Gk, *askos,* bag], a watery fluid containing albumin, glucose, and electrolytes that accumulates in the peritoneal cavity in association with certain diseases, such as liver disease or congestive heart failure. The fluid occurs as leakage from the veins and lymphatics into extravascular spaces.

ASCO, abbreviation for *American Society of Clinical Oncology.*

ascorbemia /as′kôrbē″mē·ə/ [Gk, *a,* not; AS, *scurf,* scurvy; Gk, *haima,* blood], the presence of ascorbic acid in the blood in amounts greater than normal, usually reflecting only an excess of ascorbic acid intake. The condition is usually due to the use of ascorbic acid (vitamin C) supplements.

ascorbic acid /əskôr″bik/ [Gk, *a,* not; AS, *scurf,* scurvy], a water-soluble, white crystalline vitamin present in citrus fruits, tomatoes, berries, potatoes, and fresh green and leafy vegetables, including broccoli, brussels sprouts, collards, turnip greens, parsley, sweet bell peppers, and cabbage. It is essential for the formation of collagen and fibrous tissue for normal intercellular matrices in teeth, bone, cartilage, connective tissue, and skin, and for the structural integrity of capillary walls. It also aids in fighting bacterial infections and interacts with other nutrients. Signs of deficiency are bleeding gums, tendency to bruise, swollen or painful joints, nosebleeds, anemia, lowered resistance to infections, and slow healing of wounds and fractures. Severe deficiency

results in scurvy. A large excess of ascorbic acid may cause a burning sensation during urination, diarrhea, skin rash, and nausea and may disturb the absorption and metabolism of cyanocobalamin. Results of tests for glycosuria, uric acid, and iron may be inaccurate when the patient is receiving large amounts of the vitamin. Also called *antiscorbutic vitamin,* **vitamin C.** See also **ascorbemia, infantile scurvy, scurvy.**

ascorburia /as′kôrbyoŏr″ē·ə/ [Gk, *a,* not; AS, *scurf,* scurvy; Gk, *ouron,* urine], the presence of ascorbic acid in the urine in amounts greater than normal. It usually reflects only an excess intake, generally caused by the use of vitamin C supplements.

ascribed role /əskrībd″/, an assigned function in society, based on age, sex, or other factors, that is neither earned nor chosen by the person. See also **assumed role.**

ASD, abbreviation for **atrial septal defect.**

-ase, suffix used in naming enzymes; acts on the substance named in the word root (that precedes the suffix): *lipase, protease.*

Asendin, a tricyclic antidepressant. Brand name for **amoxapine.**

asepsis /āsep″sis/ [Gk, *a, sepsis,* not decay], **1.** the absence of germs. **2.** medical asepsis, procedures used to reduce the number of microorganisms and prevent their spread. Examples include handwashing and "no touch" dressing technique. **3.** procedures used to eliminate any microorganisms; sterile technique. An example is sterilization of surgical instruments. −**aseptic,** *adj.*

aseptic. See also **asepsis.**

aseptic-antiseptic, a combination of techniques to eliminate microorganisms and to reduce infection.

aseptic bone necrosis, a bone condition that results from poor blood supply to an area of bone, causing localized bone death. The dead areas of bone are weakened and can collapse. It may occur in patients taking corticosteroids. Typical bones affected by steroids include the femur bone of the hip, the humerus bone of the shoulder, and the tibia bone of the knee, sometimes in combinations and frequently affecting both sides of the body (bilateral). The condition may be asymptomatic or, if joint surfaces are involved, marked by severe pain and joint collapse. It may also be associated with an injury to the joint. Also called **avascular necrosis, osteonecrosis.**

aseptic fever, a fever not associated with infection. Mechanical trauma, as in a crushing injury, can cause fever even when no pathogenic microorganism is present. Although the exact mechanism is not understood, fever in such cases is believed to result from the breakdown of leukocytes or the absorption of avascular tissue.

aseptic gauze, any gauze that is free of microorganisms (sterile).

aseptic meningitis, an inflammation of the meninges that is caused by one of a number of viruses, including coxsackie viruses and echoviruses (which account for about half the cases), nonparalytic polioviruses, and mumps, or may be drug induced, such as with high-dose IV immunoglobulin. See also **viral meningitis.**

■ OBSERVATIONS: Viral meningitis is especially common in children during the late summer and early fall. In about one third of the cases no pathogen can be demonstrated, but analysis of cerebrospinal fluid reveals increased numbers of white blood cells, usually lymphocytes; normal glucose concentration; slightly elevated protein levels; and no bacteria. Symptoms vary, depending on the causative agent, and may include fever, headache, stiff neck and back, nausea, and skin rash.

■ INTERVENTIONS: No specific treatment is available. Supportive therapy is directed to maintaining hydration and controlling fever.

■ PATIENT CARE CONSIDERATIONS: Complete recovery, without complication or residual effect, is usual.

aseptic necrosis [Gk, *a, sepsis,* without decay, *nekros,* dead, *osis,* condition], cystic and sclerotic degenerative changes in tissues. A condition in which poor blood supply to an area of bone leads to bone death. It may follow an injury in the absence of infection. See also **avascular necrosis, osteonecrosis.**

aseptic peritonitis [Gk, *a, sepsis,* without decay, *peri,* near, *teinein,* to stretch, *itis,* inflammation], peritonitis in which inflammation of the peritoneum is caused by chemicals, radiation, or injury, rather than by an infectious agent.

aseptic technique, any health care procedure in which added precautions, such as the use of sterile gloves and instruments, are used to prevent contamination of a person, object, or area by microorganisms.

Asepto syringe, a brand name for a large bulb-fitted, blunt-tipped syringe used primarily for irrigating wounds.

asexual /āsek″shoo·əl/ [Gk, *a,* not; L, *sexus,* male or female], **1.** not sexual. **2.** pertaining to an organism that has no sexual organs. **3.** pertaining to a process that is not sexual. —**asexuality,** *n.*

asexual generation. See **asexual reproduction.**

asexuality. See **asexual.**

asexualization /āsek′shoo·əlīzā″shən/, the process of making one incapable of reproduction. Sterilization of an individual or animal by castration, vasectomy, removal of the ovaries, or use of chemicals.

asexual reproduction, any type of reproduction that occurs without the union of male and female gametes, such as fission, budding, sporulation, or parthenogenesis. Also called **asexual generation, direct generation, nonsexual generation.** Compare **sexual reproduction.**

ASHA, abbreviation for **American Speech-Language-Hearing Association.**

ASHD, abbreviation for **arteriosclerotic heart disease.**

Asherman's syndrome, secondary amenorrhea in a hormonally normal woman, caused by obliteration of the endometrial cavity by adhesions that form as a result of curettage, infection, or uterine ablation.

asialorrhea. See **hyposalivation.**

Asian flu. See **influenza.**

asiderosis /ā′sidərō″sis/, an iron deficiency and a cause of anemia.

ASIP, abbreviation for **American Society for Investigative Pathology.**

-asis, suffix meaning an "action, process, or result of": *metabasis, oxydasis.*

asitia, a sensation of revulsion associated with food or food odors.

Ask-Upmark kidney, a hypoplastic kidney with fewer lobules than usual and fissures on its surface; most affected persons have severe hypertension, sometimes with hypertensive encephalopathy and retinopathy. The condition may be either congenital or a result of vesicoureteral reflux with pyelonephritis.

ASL, abbreviation for **American Sign Language.**

ASCLS, abbreviation for *The American Society for Clinical Laboratory Science.*

Asn, abbreviation for **asparagine.**

ASO, abbreviation for **antistreptolysin-O test.**

asocial /āsō″shəl/ [Gk, *a,* without; L, *socius,* companion], withdrawn or disengaged from normal contacts with other individuals.

asoma /āsō″mə/ [Gk, *a,* not, *soma,* body], a fetus with an incomplete trunk and head.

ASO, abbreviation for **antistreptolysin-O test.**

ASPAN, abbreviation for *American Society of PeriAnesthesia Nurses.*

asparaginase /aspar″əjinās/ [Gk, *asparagos,* asparagus], an enzyme that catalyzes the hydrolysis of asparagine to asparaginic acid and ammonia. Asparaginase is used as a chemotherapeutic agent in the treatment of acute lymphoblastic leukemia and lymphosarcoma.

asparagine (Asn) /aspar″əjin/, a nonessential amino acid found in many food and body proteins. It is easily hydrolyzed to aspartic acid and has diuretic properties. See also **amino acid, protein.**

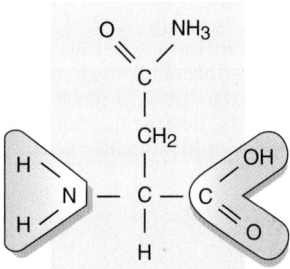

Chemical structure of asparagine

aspartame /aspär″tām, as″pərtām/, a white, almost odorless crystalline powder that is used as an artificial sweetener. It is formed by binding the amino acids of phenylalanine and aspartic acid. Approximately 180 times as sweet as the same amount of sucrose, it is used mostly to sweeten cold or uncooked foods. Unprotected aspartame tends to lose its sweetness in the presence of heat, moisture, and alkaline media. Use of this nonnutritive sweetener should be avoided by patients with phenylketonuria (PKU) because the substance hydrolyzes to form aspartate and phenylalanine.

aspartate aminotransferase (AST) /aspär″tāt/, an enzyme normally present in body serum and in certain body tissues, especially those of the heart and liver. This enzyme affects the intermolecular transfer of an amino group from aspartic acid to alpha-ketoglutaric acid, forming glutamic acid and oxaloacetic acid. The reaction is reversible. The enzyme is released into the serum because of tissue injury and thus may increase as a result of myocardial infarction and liver damage. Normal findings for adults are 8 to 20 U/L or 5 to 40 IU/L. Compare **alanine aminotransferase.** Formerly called **glutamic oxaloacetic transaminase, serum glutamic-oxaloacetic transaminase.**

aspartate aminotransferase (AST) test, a blood test usually used to detect the enzyme aspartate aminotransferase in the systemic circulation. It is often ordered in conjunction with another liver enzyme, alanine aminotransferase (ALT), or as part of a liver panel or comprehensive metabolic panel (CMP) to screen for or help diagnose liver disorders. AST and ALT are considered to be two of the most important tests to detect liver injury, although ALT is more specific for the liver than is AST and is more commonly increased than is AST. At times, AST is compared directly to ALT and an AST/ALT ratio is calculated. This ratio may be used to distinguish between different causes of liver damage and to distinguish liver injury from damage to heart or muscle. AST levels are often compared with results of other tests such as alkaline phosphatase (ALP), total protein, and bilirubin to help determine which form of liver disease is present. AST may be used to monitor the treatment of persons with liver disease and may be ordered either by itself or with other tests for this purpose. Sometimes AST is used to monitor persons who are taking medications potentially toxic to the liver. If AST levels increase, then the person may be switched to another medication. Formerly called **serum glutamic-oxaloacetic transaminase.** See **aspartate aminotransferase.**

aspartate kinase, an enzyme that catalyzes the transfer of a phosphate group from adenosine triphosphate to aspartate to produce phosphoaspartate.

aspartate transaminase. See **aspartate aminotransferase.**

aspartic acid (Asp) /aspär″tik/, a nonessential amino acid present in sugar cane, beet molasses, and breakdown products of many proteins. Pure aspartic acid is a water-soluble, colorless crystalline substance. Aspartic acid is interconvertible with oxaloacetic acid from the citric acid cycle. Aspartic acid is used in culture media, dietary supplements, detergents, fungicides, and germicides. Also called **aminosuccinic acid.** See also **amino acid, protein.**

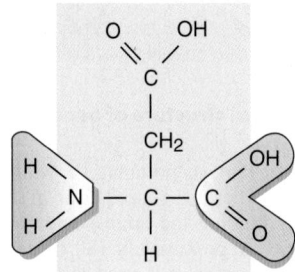

Chemical structure of aspartic acid

aspastic /āspas″tik/, not characterized by spasms.

aspect [L, *aspectus,* a look], the appearance, look, presentation, facing, or fronting of a person or object.

Asperger syndrome /äs′pər·gər/ [Hans Asperger, Austrian psychiatrist, 20th century], a developmental disorder characterized by severe impairment of social interactions and impairment in language and communication skills.

■ OBSERVATIONS: An obsessive interest in an object or topic is a characteristic of the disorder. Repetitive routines or rituals are also common, along with unusual patterns in speech and language. Uncoordinated movements are frequently observed.

■ INTERVENTIONS: Early treatment is important. It should be provided by a coordinated team attentive to the symptoms experienced by the patient and the support needed by the family.

■ PATIENT CARE CONSIDERATIONS: A predictable schedule that engages attention in structured activities will assist in coping with Asperger syndrome.

aspergillic acid /as′pərjil″ik/, an antibiotic substance derived from *Aspergillus flavus,* an aflatoxin-producing mold found on corn, grain, and peanuts. See also **aflatoxins.**

aspergillosis /as′pərjilō″sis/ [L, *aspergere,* to sprinkle; Gk, *osis,* condition], a relatively uncommon infection, growth, or allergic response caused by inhalation of a fungus of the genus *Aspergillus* that can cause inflammatory, granulomatous lesions on or in any organ. There are several forms of aspergillosis. Pulmonary aspergillosis is divided into two types: allergic bronchopulmonary aspergillosis (an allergic reaction to the fungus that develops with asthma)

and invasive aspergillosis (a serious infection with pneumonia, most often seen in immunosuppressed people already weakened by some other disorder). Topical fungicides can be used on the skin; amphotericin B is used to treat systemic aspergillosis, especially if it has spread to the lungs. Surgery may be required to remove an aspergilloma, a fungus ball that develops if bleeding occurs in an area of the lung previously diseased. The prognosis, as for most systemic fungal infections, is poor. Compare **allergic bronchopulmonary aspergillosis.**

Aspergillus /as′pərjil″əs/ [L, *aspergere,* to sprinkle], a genus of fungi that is a common contaminant in the laboratory and a cause of nosocomial infection. The fungus has hyphae and spores, lives in the soil, is ubiquitous, and proliferates rapidly. Inhalation of the spores of the two pathogenic species, *A. fumigatus* and *A. flavus,* is common, but infection is rare. However, allergic reaction to the spores can also occur.

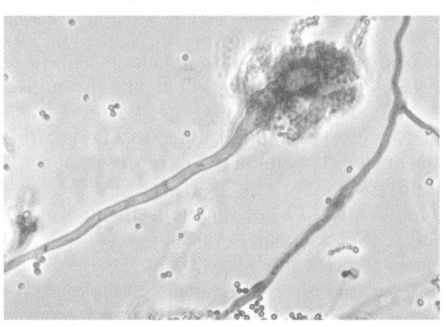

Aspergillus fumigatus *(Centers for Disease Control and Prevention Public Health Image Library ID#4297, Dr. Libero Ajello, 1963)*

aspermatic /ā′spurmat″ik/, unable to secrete or ejaculate semen.

aspermatogenesis /āspur′mətōjen″əsis/, failure of the testes to produce spermatozoa.

aspermia /āspur″mē·ə/ [Gk, *a, sperma,* without seed], lack of formation or ejaculation of semen.

asphyxia /asfik″sē·ə/ [Gk, *a* + *sphyxis,* without pulse], severe hypoxia leading to hypoxemia and hypercapnia, loss of consciousness, and, if not corrected, death. Some of the more common causes of asphyxia are drowning, electrical shock, aspiration of vomitus, lodging of a foreign body in the respiratory tract, inhalation of toxic gas or smoke, and poisoning. Oxygen and artificial ventilation are promptly administered to prevent damage to the brain. The underlying cause is then treated. See also **artificial ventilation. –asphyxiated,** *adj.,* **–asphyxiate,** *v.*

asphyxia neonatorum, a condition in which a newborn does not breathe spontaneously. The asphyxia may develop before or during labor or immediately after delivery. The condition may involve placental or neonatal pulmonary dysfunction with underlying causes that can include abruptio placentae, umbilical compression, or uterine tetany. Other factors include congenital defects, such as a diaphragmatic hernia, or adverse effects of anesthetics or analgesics administered to the mother. Immediate resuscitation is required to prevent death or brain damage. Also called **perinatal asphyxia.** See also **asphyxia pallida.**

asphyxia pallida /pal″ədə/, an abnormal condition in which a newborn appears pale and limp, shows signs of apnea, and suffers from bradycardia as marked by a heartbeat of 80 beats/min or less.

asphyxiate /asfik″sē·āt/ [Gk, *a + sphyxis,* without pulse], to induce an inability to breathe. Causes may include circulatory congestion, chemical poisoning, electrical shock, or physical suffocation.

asphyxiated. See **asphyxia.**

asphyxiating thoracic dysplasia. See **Jeune syndrome.**

asphyxiation [Gk, *a + sphyxis,* without pulse], a state of asphyxia or inability to breathe.

aspirant /as″pirənt/, the fluid, gas, or solid particles that are withdrawn from the body by aspiration methods.

aspirant maneuver, a procedure used in making radiographic images of the laryngopharyngeal area. The patient exhales completely, then slowly inhales while making a harsh, high-pitched sound. The maneuver adducts the vocal cords so that the ventricle of the larynx is clearly visible in the image.

aspirate /-rāt/ [L, *aspirare,* to breathe upon], **1.** to withdraw fluid or air from a cavity. The process is usually aided by use of a syringe or a suction device. See **paracentesis. 2.** when all or part of a food/liquid bolus enters the airway. **3.** (in phonetics) a release of air.

aspirating needle /-rā′ting/, a long, hollow needle used to remove fluid from a cavity, vessel, or structure of the body.

aspirating syringe, **1.** (in dentistry) a hypodermic syringe used to inject local anesthetics. Before administration of a local anesthetic at the desired location, the operator applies negative pressure checking for blood in the syringe. This ensures that the anesthetic solution will not be deposited in a blood vessel. **2.** a large-volume syringe with a tapered tip for insertion into tubes, allowing withdrawal of fluids when the piston is pulled back.

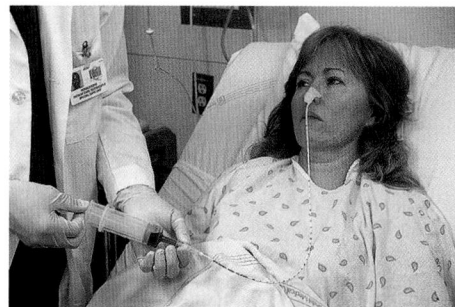

Aspirating nasogastric tube with aspirating syringe
(Perry and Potter, 2011)

aspiration /as′pirā′shən/, **1.** drawing in or out by suction. **2.** the act of withdrawing a fluid, such as mucus or serum, from the body by a suction device. **–aspirate,** *n.* **3.** the misdirection of food or liquid during swallowing or breathing, as in aspiration of saliva. May be related to mass effects of tumors or loss or diminished sensation, including loss of cough reflex. See also **aspiration pneumonia.**

aspiration biopsy, the removal of living tissue, for microscopic examination, by suction through a fine needle attached to a syringe. The procedure is used primarily to obtain cells from a lesion containing fluid or when fluid is formed in a serous cavity. See also **cytology, needle biopsy.**

aspiration biopsy cytology (ABC), a microscopic examination of cells obtained directly from living body tissue by aspiration through a fine needle. It is used primarily as a diagnostic procedure, generally as a technique for detecting nuclear and cytoplasmic changes in cancerous tissue. Compare **exfoliative cytology.**

aspiration drug abuse, the inhalation of a liquid, solid, or gaseous chemical into the respiratory system for nontherapeutic purposes. Examples include glue and solvent sniffing and cocaine snorting.

aspiration of vomitus, the inhalation of regurgitated gastric contents into the pulmonary system. See also **aspiration pneumonia.**

aspiration pneumonia, an inflammatory condition of the lungs and bronchi caused by inhaling foreign material or acidic vomitus. Aspiration pneumonia most commonly occurs in the right middle lobe and lower lobe due to the more vertical position of the right main bronchus. Compare **bronchopneumonia.** See also **pneumonia.**

■ OBSERVATIONS: Aspiration pneumonia may occur during anesthesia or recovery from anesthesia. At-risk patients include those with a decreased level of consciousness related to drugs and/or alcohol and those with swallowing difficulties or an impaired gag reflex.

■ INTERVENTIONS: Treatment depends on severity. Usual measures consist of prompt suctioning of the bronchi and administration of supplemental oxygen. Continued artificial ventilation may be required. Close monitoring of oxygenation status is imperative. The Infectious Diseases Society of America/American Thoracic Society Consensus Guidelines provide evidence-based recommendations for treatment.

■ PATIENT CARE CONSIDERATIONS: The patient's pulse rate, quality of respirations, level of consciousness, and skin color are carefully monitored. Secretions are removed by suction as necessary. Infection and respiratory failure are frequent complications. Aspiration pneumonia may be prevented by positioning unconscious patients with the head elevated 15 to 30 degrees and turned to the side and by paying careful attention to the maintenance of enteral feeding therapy and an adequate airway. A comprehensive swallowing evaluation in patients with risk factors for aspiration pneumonia may prevent further episodes.

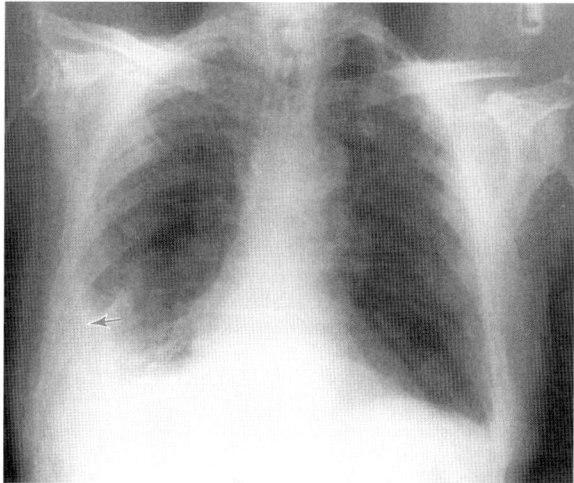

Aspiration pneumonia *(arrow) (Courtesy Dr. T. Scott Johnson)*

aspiration precautions, recommended practices to decrease the risk of aspiration of oropharyngeal secretions and regurgitated gastric contents. Recommendations include elevation of the head of the bed, appropriate sedative use, and assessment of placements of feeding tubes at 4-hour intervals, along with assessment for tolerance of the feeding and avoidance of bolus feedings. Proper care of endotracheal tube cuffs and swallowing assessments for at-risk patients are also recommended. The American Association of Critical Care Nurses has published evidence-based guidelines on the prevention of aspiration.

aspirator /as″pirā′tər/ [L, *aspirare,* to breathe upon], any instrument that removes a substance from a body cavity by suction, such as a bulb syringe, piston pump, or hypodermic syringe.

aspirin (ASA) /as″pirin/, an analgesic, antipyretic, and antiinflammatory agent; also used as an antithrombotic agent in low doses. Also called **acetylsalicylic acid.**

■ INDICATIONS: It is prescribed to reduce fever and relieve pain and inflammation. Low-dose aspirin therapy may be prescribed to reduce the risk of a heart attack in individuals at risk.

■ CONTRAINDICATIONS: Bleeding disorders, peptic ulcer, pregnancy, concomitant use of anticoagulants, or known hypersensitivity to salicylates prohibits its use.

■ ADVERSE EFFECTS: Among the most serious adverse reactions are ulcers, occult bleeding, clotting defects, renal toxicities, tinnitus, dyspepsia, and allergic reactions. Reye syndrome has been associated with aspirin use in children.

aspirin poisoning, now called **salicylate poisoning.**

asplenia /āsplē″nē·ə/ [Gk, *a,* without, *spleen*], absence of a spleen. The condition may be congenital or result from surgical removal.

ASRT, abbreviation for **American Society of Radiologic Technologists.**

assault /əsôlt″/ [L, *assilirere,* to leap upon], **1.** an unlawful act that places another person, without that person's consent, in fear of immediate bodily harm or battery. **2.** attack with intent to hurt. **3.** to threaten a person with bodily harm or injury. See **battery.**

assay /asā″, as″ā/ [Fr, *essayer,* to try], a laboratory measurement to determine the presence, the concentration, or the activity of a drug or other biological substances.

assertiveness /əsur″tivnes/, behavior directed toward claiming one's rights without denying those of others.

assertive training /əsur″tiv/ [L, *asserere,* to join to oneself], a therapeutic technique to help individuals become more self-assertive and self-confident in interpersonal relationships. It focuses on the direct, honest statement of feelings and beliefs, both positive and negative. The technique is learned by role playing in a therapeutic setting, usually in a group, followed by practice in actual situations. Also called *assertion training.*

assess, to examine for the purpose of evaluation and/or quality improvement. See **assessment.**

assessing /əses″ing/ [L, *assidere,* to sit beside], (in five-step nursing process) a category of nursing behavior that includes the gathering, verifying, and communicating of information related to the client. The nurse collects information from verbal interactions with the patient, the patient's family, and significant others; examines standard data sources for information; systematically checks for symptoms and signs; determines the patient's ability to perform self-care activities; examines the patient's environment; and identifies reactions of the staff (including the nurse who is performing the assessment) to the patient and to the patient's family and significant others. To verify the data, the nurse confirms the observations and perceptions by gathering additional information; discusses the decisions made by other members of the staff, when indicated; and personally evaluates and checks the patient's condition. The nurse reports the information that has been gathered and verified. Although assessing is the first of the five steps of the nursing process, preceding analyzing, it is integral to effective nursing practice at all steps of the process. See also **analyzing, evaluating, implementing, nursing process, planning.**

assessment /əses″mənt/ [L, *assidere,* to sit beside], **1.** (in a health care facility) an evaluation or appraisal of a condition.

2. the process of making such an evaluation. **3.** (in a problem-oriented medical record) an examiner's evaluation of the disease or condition based on the patient's subjective report of the symptoms and course of the illness or condition and the examiner's objective findings, including data obtained through laboratory tests, physical examination, medical history, and information reported by family members and other health care team members. See also **nursing assessment, problem-oriented medical record. –assess,** *v.*

assessment of the aging patient, an evaluation of the changes characteristic of advancing years exhibited by an elderly person.

■ METHOD: a comprehensive multidisciplinary approach provides the most useful information related to the health, psychosocial, and functional capabilities of the older adult.

■ PATIENT CARE CONSIDERATIONS: The health care provider faces the patient during the evaluation, establishes eye contact, repeats questions if necessary, avoids shouting, and addresses the person by name.

■ OUTCOME CRITERIA: Aging does not progress at a uniform rate, and its effects may vary widely from one individual to the next, but, in many cases, changes once considered normal in elderly patients are disease processes that may respond to treatment. A thorough assessment distinguishes the effects of pathological disorders from those of aging and provides the basis for care needed by the patient.

assimilate /əsim″əlāt/ [L, *assimilare,* to make alike], **1.** to convert food in the digestive tract to substances suitable for incorporation into the body and its tissues; anabolism. **2.** to incorporate components of a new culture into existing values.

assimilation [L, *assimulare,* to make alike], **1.** the process of incorporating nutritive material into living tissue, occurring after digestion and absorption or simultaneous with absorption. **2.** (in psychology) the incorporation of new experiences into a person's pattern of consciousness. Compare **apperception. 3.** (in sociology and anthropology) the process in which a person or a group of people of a different ethnic background becomes absorbed into a new culture. **–assimilate,** *v.*

assist-control mode, a system of mechanical ventilation in which the patient is allowed to initiate breathing, although the ventilator delivers a set volume with each breath. The ventilator can also be programmed to initiate breathing if the patient's breathing slows beyond a certain point or stops altogether.

assisted breech [L, *assistere,* to stand by], an obstetric operation in which a baby being born feet or buttocks first is permitted to deliver spontaneously as far as its umbilicus and is then extracted. Also called **partial breech extraction.** Compare **breech extraction.**

assisted circulation [L, *assistere,* to stand, *circulare,* to go around], a method of treating patients with severe circulatory deficiencies by introducing a mechanical pumping system to aid the blood flow.

assisted conception, now called **assisted reproductive technology.**

assisted death, a form of euthanasia in which an individual expressing a wish to die prematurely is helped to accomplish that goal by another person, either by counseling and/or by providing a poison or other lethal instrument. The assisted death may be regarded as a homicide or suicide by local authorities, and the person giving assistance may be held responsible for the death. See also **assisted suicide.**

assisted reproductive technology, the manipulation of egg and sperm in treating infertility. The processes include the administration of drugs to induce ovulation, fertilization, gamete intrafallopian transfer, zygote intrafallopian transfer, and cryopreservation of gametes. See also **in vitro fertilization.**

assisted respiration, the use of mechanical devices to facilitate a normal breathing pattern. Also called **mechanical ventilation.**

assisted suicide, a form of euthanasia in which a person wishes to commit suicide but feels unable to perform the act alone because of a physical disability or lack of knowledge about the most effective means. An individual who assists a suicide victim in accomplishing that goal may or may not be held responsible for the death, depending on local laws. The participation of health professionals in assisted suicide is controversial. Also called *physician-assisted suicide.* See also **euthanasia, suicide.**

assisted ventilation, the use of mechanical or other devices to help maintain respiration, usually by delivering air or oxygen under positive pressure. See also **IPPB, respiration.**

assistive listening device (ALD), a device other than a hearing aid that provides auditory assistance to those with hearing impairment or a central auditory processing disorder. See also **hearing aid, cochlear implant.**

assistive technology, educational or rehabilitative devices and equipment used to adapt (as to an environment) or to promote function. Examples are cognitive rehabilitative software, pressure systems for reducing edema, computer games to develop fine and gross motor coordination, limb prostheses, and wheelchairs.

assistive technology device, equipment that assists individuals with disabilities in performing occupations and/or daily activities. Kinds of assistive devices include hearing aids, adapted pencil grips, computer voice-recognition programs, and mobility aids, such as wheelchairs or canes.

assistive technology service (AT service), any service that directly assists an individual with disabilities in the selection, acquisition, and/or use of an assistive technology device.

assistive technology team (AT team), a group of professionals who make recommendations and carry out the training of an individual with a disability using an assistive technology device.

associated antagonist, one of a pair of muscles or group of muscles that pull in opposite directions but whose combined action results in moving a part in one direction.

Associate Degree in Nursing (ADN) /əsō′shē·āt/ [L, *associare,* to unite], an academic degree awarded on satisfactory completion of a 2-year course of study, usually at a community or junior college. The recipient is eligible to take the national licensing examination to become a registered nurse. An associate degree in nursing is not available in Canada or countries in the European Union.

associated movement, a movement of parts that act together, as of the eyes. See also **contralateral reflexes, synkinesis.**

associate nurse, a nurse with an Associate Degree in Nursing who can fulfill the functions and skills necessary to provide patient care. Articulation programs provide the opportunity for the nurse with an associate degree to earn a baccalaureate degree.

association /əsō′shē·ā″shən/ [L, *associare,* to unite], **1.** a connection, union, joining, or combination of things. **2.** (in psychology) the connection of remembered feelings, emotions, sensations, thoughts, or perceptions with particular persons, things, or ideas. Kinds include **association of ideas, clang association, controlled association, dream association, free association.**

association area, any part of the cerebral cortex involved in the integration of sensory information. Also called *association cortex.*

Association for Professionals in Infection Control and Epidemiology (APIC), a multidisciplinary international professional organization of infection preventionists.

Association for the Advancement of Medical Instrumentation (AAMI), a nonprofit organization involved in advancing understanding, safety, and efficacy of medical instrumentation and technology.

Association for the Education of Children with Medical Needs (AECMN), an interdisciplinary organization that provides professional support to individuals involved in the education of children with chronic illnesses and medical challenges.

associationist model of learning /əsō′shē·ā″shənist/, a theory that defines learning as behavioral change that is a result of reinforced practice. If the response has not been reinforced repeatedly, an alternative behavior may be substituted.

Association of Faculties of Medicine of Canada (AFMC), a Canadian organization of the deans and faculty members of the nation's 17 faculties of medicine. It is concerned with all aspects of the education of physicians and acts as the liaison between the member schools and other professional organizations and governmental agencies. The official languages of the AFMC are English and French.

association of ideas, a mental connection established between similar or simultaneously occurring ideas, feelings, or perceptions.

Association of periOperative Registered Nurses (AORN), the professional organization of perioperative nurses, which supports registered nurses in achieving optimal outcomes for patients undergoing operative or other invasive procedures. Formerly called *Association of Operating Room Nurses.*

Association of Schools of Advancing Health Professions (ASAHP), an organization of health care institutions and professionals with the goal of increasing public awareness of the unique contributions of allied health professionals in improving health and health care outcomes.

Association of Surgical Technologists (AST), established in 1969 as the national professional organization for surgical technologists and surgical assistants. See also **Accreditation Review Council on Education in Surgical Technology and Surgical Assisting.**

Association of Women's Health, Obstetric, and Neonatal Nurses (AWHONN), an organization of nurses working in obstetrics and gynecology in the United States. Formerly called **Nurses' Association of the American College of Obstetrics and Gynecology (NAACOG).**

association paralysis, a motor neuron disease in which atrophy, weakness, and fasciculation of the tongue, facial muscles, pharynx, and larynx occur. Also called **progressive bulbar paralysis.**

association test, a technique used in psychiatric diagnosis and in educational and psychological evaluation in which a person is asked to respond to a stimulus word with the first word that comes to mind. The time taken to respond and the associations offered are compared with pretested responses and are classified and enumerated for diagnostic significance. Also called **word association test.** See also **free association.**

associative play, a form of play in which a group of children participate in similar or identical activities without formal organization, group direction, group interaction, or a definite goal. The children may borrow or lend toys or pieces of play equipment, and they may imitate others in the group, but each child acts independently, as on a playground or among a group riding tricycles or bicycles. Compare **cooperative play.** See also **parallel play, solitary play.**

assortive mating, the matching of males and females for reproduction in a manner that avoids random selection.

assumed role /əsoomd″/, a role in life that an individual usually selects or achieves by choice, such as one's role in marriage or employment. See also **ascribed role.**

Normal physiologic changes associated with aging

- Thinning hair
- Loss of elasticity in skin
- Loss of height (due to changes in posture and joint compression)
- Difficulty in hearing high frequency sounds
- Lens changes resulting in presbyopia
- Decreased muscle mass
- Decrease in brain weight and blood flow
- Changes in sleep patterns

AST, **1.** abbreviation for **aspartate aminotransferase. 2.** abbreviation for **Association of Surgical Technologists.**

-ast, combining form designating an antiasthmatic or antiallergic drug not acting primarily as an antihistamine.

astasia /astā″zhə/ [Gk, *a, stasis,* not stand, *a, basis,* not step], a lack of motor coordination marked by an inability to stand or sit without assistance.

astasia-abasia, a form of ataxia in which the patient is unable to stand or walk because of lack of motor coordination but is able to carry out natural leg movements when sitting or lying down. This term is often used to describe psychogenic gait disturbances. Also called **abasia-astasia.**

astatine (At) [Gk, *astasis,* unsteady], a very unstable, radioactive element that occurs naturally in minute amounts. Its atomic number is 85; the atomic mass of its longest lived isotope is 210.

asteatosis /as′tē·ətō″sis/ [Gk, *a, stear,* without tallow, *osis,* condition], a dry skin condition caused by a deficiency of sebaceous gland secretions. Scales and fissures may result from the dryness. The condition is treated with creams and ointments that replace the missing skin oils.

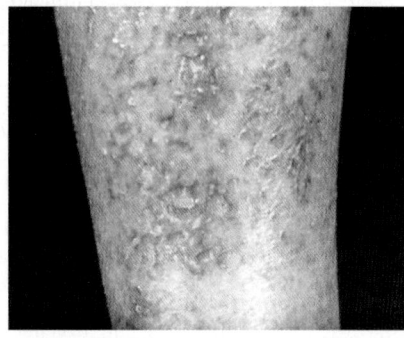

Asteatotic eczema *(du Vivier, 2013)*

-aster, suffix meaning "star-shaped": *diaster, oleaster.*

astereognosis /əstir′ē·og·nō″sis/ [Gk, *a, stereos,* not solid, *gnosis,* knowledge], an inability to identify objects or shapes by touch.

asterixis /as′tərik″sis/ [Gk, *a, sterixis,* not fixed position], a hand-flapping tremor, often accompanying metabolic disorders. The tremor is usually induced by extending the arm and dorsiflexing the wrist. Asterixis is seen frequently in hepatic encephalopathy. Also called **flapping tremor, liver flap.**

asteroid body [Gk, *aster,* star, *eidos,* form], a rare irregular star-shaped structure that develops in the giant cells in certain diseases, including sarcoidosis, actinomycosis, and nocardiosis, as well as in fibrin-rich exudates.

asthenia /asthē″nē·ə/ [Gk, *a + sthenos,* without strength], **1.** the lack or loss of strength or energy; weakness; debility. **2.** (in psychiatry) lack of dynamic force in the personality. Kinds include **myalgic asthenia,**

neurocirculatory asthenia. See also **adynamia.** –**asthenic,** *adj.*

-asthenia, suffix meaning "(condition of) debility, loss of strength and energy, depleted vitality": *neurasthenia, phlebasthenia.*

asthenic /asthen″ik/ [Gk, *a + sthenos,* without strength], pertaining to a condition of weakness, feebleness, or loss of vitality.

asthenic habitus [Gk, *a + sthenos,* without strength; L, *habere,* to have], a body structure characterized by a slender build with long limbs, an angular profile, and prominent muscles or bones. Compare **athletic habitus, pyknic.** See also **ectomorph.**

asthenic personality, now called **dependent personality disorder.**

asthenopia /as′thənō″pē·ə/ [Gk, *a, sthenos + ops,* eye], a condition in which the eyes tire easily because of weakness of the ocular or ciliary muscles. Symptoms include pain in or around the eyes, headache, dimness of vision, dizziness, and slight nausea.

asthma /az″mə/ [Gk, panting], a respiratory disorder causing narrowing of the airway that may be due to allergy or hypersentivity reactions. It is a complex disorder involving biochemical, immunological, infectious, endocrinological, and psychological factors. Also called **bronchial asthma.** See also **allergic asthma, childhood asthma, exercise-induced asthma, intrinsic asthma, organic dust, status asthmaticus.**

■ OBSERVATIONS: Asthma is characterized by recurring episodes of paroxysmal dyspnea, wheezing on expiration and/or inspiration caused by constriction of the bronchi, coughing, and viscous mucoid bronchial secretions.

■ INTERVENTIONS: Treatment may include elimination of the causative agent, hyposensitization, aerosol or oral bronchodilators, beta-adrenergic drugs, methylxanthines, cromolyn, leukotriene inhibitors, and short- or long-term use of corticosteroids. Sedatives and cough suppressants may be contraindicated. The goal of treatment is the control of symptoms and elmination of complications.

■ PATIENT CARE CONSIDERATIONS: The episodes may be precipitated by inhalation of allergens or pollutants, infection, cold air, vigorous exercise, or emotional stress.

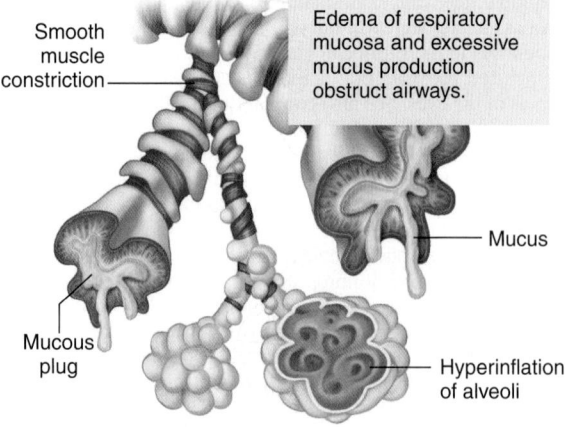

Smooth muscle constriction

Edema of respiratory mucosa and excessive mucus production obstruct airways.

Mucus

Mucous plug

Hyperinflation of alveoli

Asthma *(Patton and Thibodeau, 2016)*

-asthma, suffix meaning "(condition of) labored breathing."

asthma crystal, now called **Charcot-Leyden crystal.**

-asthmatic, suffix meaning "asthma, its symptoms, or its treatment."

asthmatic breathing /azmat″ik/ [Gk, *asthma,* panting; AS, *braeth*], breathing marked by prolonged wheezing on exhalation caused by spasmodic contractions of the bronchi.

asthmatic bronchitis, inflammation and swelling of the mucous membrane of the bronchi in a patient with asthma.

asthmatic cough [Gk, *asthma* + AS, *cohhetan*], a wheezing cough accompanied by signs of breathing difficulty.

asthmatic eosinophilia, a form of eosinophilic pneumonia, characterized by allergic bronchospasm, cough, fever, and expectoration of bronchial casts containing eosinophils and fungal mycelia. It is a result of hypersensitivity to the fungus *Aspergillus fumigatus* or *Candida albicans.* The condition usually occurs in the fourth or fifth decade of life and is twice as common in women as in men. Untreated, it may result in pleural effusion, pericarditis, ascites, encephalitis, hepatomegaly, and respiratory failure. Treatment is similar to that for asthma and includes administration of corticosteroids and antibiotics. Desensitization to the allergen is not usually effective. See also **allergic asthma, eosinophilic pneumonia.**

astigmatic /as′tigmat″ik/ [Gk, *a, stigma,* without point], pertaining to astigmatism, or an error of refraction in which a ray of light is not sharply focused on the retinal tissue but is spread over a more diffuse area. Astigmatism is due to differences in curvature in the various meridians of the cornea and lens of the eye.

astigmatic keratotomy, an operation in which the cornea is relaxed by a series of transverse incisions to flatten the meridian in which the incisions are made and increase the curvature in the meridian 90 degrees away. It is done for the correction of astigmatism.

astigmatism /əstig″mətiz′əm/ [Gk, *a, stigma,* without point], an abnormal condition of the eye in which the light rays cannot be focused clearly in a point on the retina because the spheric curve of the cornea or lens is not equal in all meridians. Vision is typically blurred; if uncorrected, it often results in visual discomfort or asthenopia. The person cannot accommodate to correct the problem. The condition usually may be corrected with contact lenses or with eyeglasses ground to neutralize the condition.

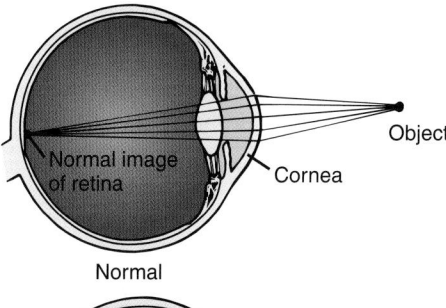

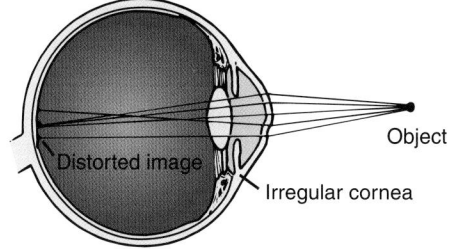

Astigmatism

-astine, combining form designating an antihistaminic.

Aston-Patterning [Judith Aston, American massage therapist], a bodywork technique to accommodate asymmetry and individual uniqueness of the human body to match human function to the environment. Movement patterns are taught to include the asymmetric pattern rather than allowing a tension pattern to develop. This technique has been applied to fitness training and ergonomic product design.

astragalus, **1.** See **talus. 2.** an herb that is grown throughout the world, most commonly in China, Japan, and Korea.
■ INDICATIONS: This herb is used as an immune stimulant; for viral infections, HIV/AIDS, cancer, and vascular disorders; to improve circulation; and to lower blood pressure. In most instances, there is insufficient reliable information regarding its effectiveness.
■ CONTRAINDICATIONS: Astragalus should not be used during pregnancy and lactation, in children, or during acute infections.

astringent /əstrin″jənt/ [Gk, *astringere,* to tighten], **1.** a substance that causes contraction of tissues on application, usually used locally. **2.** having the quality of an astringent. −*astringency, n.*

astringent douche, a cleansing stream containing substances such as alum that cause the mucous membrane of the vagina to constrict. See **Arden's powder™.**

astro-, prefix meaning "star" or "star-shaped": *astroblastoma, astrocytoma.*

astroblastoma /as′trōblastō″mə/ *pl. astroblastomas, astroblastomata* [Gk, *aster,* star, *blastos,* germ, *oma,* tumor], a malignant neoplasm of the brain and spinal cord. Cells of an astroblastoma lie around blood vessels or around connective tissue septa.

astrocyte /as″trōsīt′/ [Gk, *aster* + *kytos,* cell], a large star-shaped neuroglial cell with many branches, found in certain tissues of the nervous system.

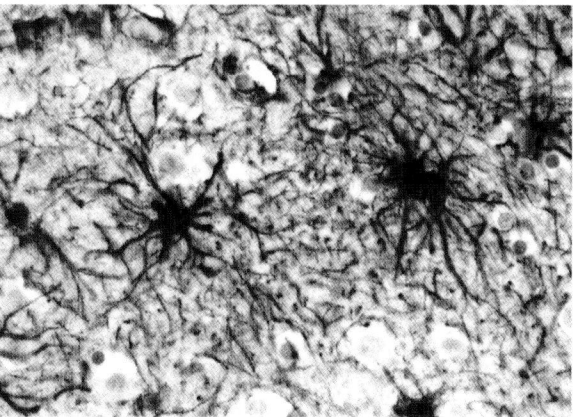

Astrocyte (Courtesy Dr. J. Corbo, Brigham and Women's Hospital)

astrocytoma /as′trōsītō″mə/ *pl. astrocytomas, astrocytomata* [Gk, *aster* + *kytos* + *oma*], a primary tumor of the brain composed of astrocytes and characterized by slow growth, cyst formation, invasion of surrounding structures, and often development of a highly malignant glioblastoma within the tumor mass. Complete surgical resection of an astrocytoma may be possible early in the development of the tumor. It may also be treated with radiation therapy postoperatively or if surgery is not possible. Also called *astrocytic glioma.*

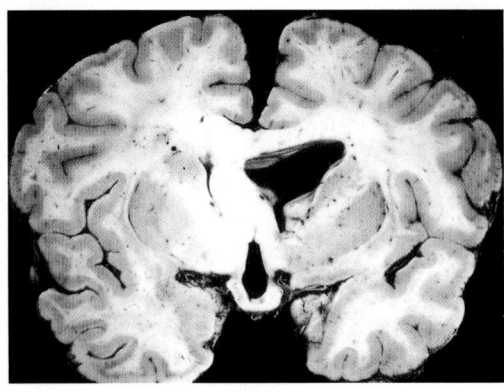

Astrocytoma *(Kumar et al, 2013)*

astrocytosis /as′trōsītō″sis/ [Gk, *aster* + *kytos* + *osis,* condition], an increase in the number of neuroglial cells with fibrous or protoplasmic processes frequently observed in an irregular area adjacent to degenerative lesions, such as abscesses, certain brain neoplasms, and encephalomalacia. Astrocytosis represents a reparative process and in some cases may be diffuse in a large region.

astrophobia, a fear of stars and the solar system.

asymbolia /ă-sim-boxle-ə/, the inability to recognize previously familiar sensations.

asymmetric /ā′simet″rik, as′imet″rik/ [Gk, *a* + *symmetria,* without proportion], 1. (of the body or parts of the body) unequal in size or shape. 2. different in placement or arrangement about an axis. Also called *asymmetrical.* Compare symmetric. −asymmetry, *n.*

asymmetric tonic neck reflex. See tonic neck reflex.

asymmetry. See asymmetric.

asymphytous /ə·sim′fə·təs/ [Gk, *a, symphysis,* not a growing together], separate or distinct; not grown together.

asymptomatic /āsimp′təmat″ik/ [Gk, *a,* without, *symptoma,* that which happens], without symptoms or signs of disease.

asymptomatic neurosyphilis [Gk, *a,* without, *symptoma, neuron,* nerve; Fr, *syphilide*], a form of neurosyphilis characterized by pathological changes in the cerebrospinal fluid, although there are no symptoms of nervous system damage. Asymptomatic neurosyphilis may occur many years before actual nervous system damage is noticeable.

asynchronous /āsing″krənəs/ [Gk, *a* + *synchronos,* not simultaneous], 1. (of an event or device) a computer operation in which a command is performed in response to a signal that the previous command has been completed. Data and messages can be transferred and paused, then started again, resulting in intermittent transmission. 2. a form of communication that does not occur simultaneously. Multiple individuals can participate in a conversation, but can do so at different times via messaging or communication boards.

asynclitism /āsing″klitiz′əm/ [Gk, *a* + *syn,* not together, *kleisis,* to lean], presentation of a parietal aspect of the fetal head to the maternal pelvic inlet in labor. The sagittal suture is parallel to the transverse diameter of the pelvis but anterior or posterior to it. In normal labor, the fetal head usually engages with some degree of asynclitism. Anterior asynclitism, in which the anterior part presents, is called Nägele obliquity. Posterior asynclitism is called Litzmann obliquity. See also cardinal movements of labor, engagement.

asyndesis /əsin′dəsis/, a mental disorder marked by an inability to assemble related ideas or thoughts into one coherent concept.

asynergy /āsin″ərjē/ [Gk, *a* + *syn* + *ergein,* to work], 1. a condition characterized by faulty coordination among groups of organs or muscles that normally function harmoniously. 2. the state of muscle antagonism found in cerebellar disease. See also ataxia, cerebellum.

asyntaxia /ā′sintak″sē·ə/ [Gk, *a* + *syn* + *taxis,* arrangement], any interference with the orderly sequence of growth and differentiation of the fetus during embryonic development, resulting in one or more congenital anomalies. Kinds include asyntaxia dorsalis. See also developmental anomaly.

asyntaxia dorsalis, failure of the neural tube to close during embryonic development. See also neural tube defect.

asystole /āsis″təlē/ [Gk, *a* + *systole,* not contraction], a life-threatening cardiac condition characterized by the absence of electrical and mechanical activity in the heart. Clinical signs include apnea and lack of pulse. Without cardiac monitoring, asystole cannot be distinguished from ventricular fibrillation. −asystolic, *adj.*

asystolic cardiac rhythm /ā′sistol″ik/, an electrocardiographic recording that appears as a flat line, indicating cardiac arrest.

At, symbol for the element astatine.

at-. See ad-.

atabrine stomatitis, an abnormal oral condition characterized by skin changes that resemble those of lichen planus. It may be associated with the use of atabrine hydrochloride (a preparation of the antimalarial drug quinacrine). Compare arsenic stomatitis, bismuth stomatitis.

ataractic /at′ərak″tik/ [Gk, *ataraktos,* quiet], pertaining to a drug or other agent that has a tranquilizing or sedating effect.

Atarax, an antianxiety, antiemetic, antipruritic, and anticholinergic drug. Brand name for hydrOXYzine hydrochloride.

ataraxia /at′ərak″sē′ə/ [Gk, *a,* not, *tarakos,* disturbed], a vague state of mental tranquility.

atavism /at″əviz′əm/ [L, *atavus,* ancestor], the appearance in an individual of traits or characteristics more like those of a grandparent or earlier ancestor than of the parents. Atavistic data may offer clues to a health care provider of genetic or familial health factors. −atavistic, *adj.*

atavistic [L, *atavus,* ancestor], pertaining to the tendency for a genetic trait of a remote ancestor to be expressed in an individual as a result of a chance recombination of genes.

ataxia /ətak″sē·ə/ [Gk, without order], an impaired ability to coordinate movement, often characterized by a staggering gait and postural imbalance. It can have many causes, including lesions in the spinal cord or cerebellum that may be the sequelae of birth trauma, congenital disorder, infection, degenerative disorder, neoplasm, toxic substance stroke, or head injury. See also hereditary ataxia. −ataxic, *ataxial, adj.*

ataxiaphasia /-fā″zhə/ [Gk, without order], a state in which a person is unable to connect words properly as needed to form a sentence.

ataxia-telangiectasia syndrome /tɒlan″jē·ektā″zhə/ [Gk, *ataxia* + *telos,* end, *angeion,* vessel, *ektasis,* expansion], a rare genetic disorder involving deficits in immunoglobulin metabolism that is transmitted as an autosomal-recessive trait. It usually begins in infancy with impaired motor control (ataxia) and progresses slowly with increasing cerebellar degeneration to severe disability. Permanent dilation of superficial blood vessels (telangiectasias) are most prominent on skin surfaces exposed to the sun: ears, face, and bulbar conjunctiva. Intellectual ability seems to stop at the level of 10 years of age in many cases. Affected individuals are susceptible to upper and lower respiratory infections and have an increased risk of malignancy, especially lymphoma. Also called Louis-Bar syndrome.

ataxic. See ataxia.

ataxic aphasia, now called nonfluent aphasia.

ataxic breathing, a type of breathing associated with a lesion in the medullary respiratory center and characterized by a series of inspirations and expirations. See also **Biot's respiration.**

ataxic dysarthria, abnormal speech characterized by slurring and discoordination of sounds because of neuromuscular dysfunction of the cerebellum. Timing range, force, and direction of speech motor movements are affected. See also **cerebellar speech.**

ataxic gait, an unsteady, staggering, and uncoordinated pattern when walking. See **cerebellar gait.**

ataxic speech. See **cerebellar speech.**

atazanavir, a protease inhibitor
■ INDICATIONS: Used in combination with other antiretroviral agents to treat HIV.
■ CONTRAINDICATIONS: Known hypersensitivity to this drug prohibits its use.
■ ADVERSE EFFECTS: Adverse effects of this drug include headache, depression, dizziness, insomnia, peripheral neurological symptoms, fatigue, fever, arthralgia, back pain, cough, lipodystrophy, and pain. Life-threatening side effects include hepatotoxicity and Stevens-Johnson syndrome. Common side effects include diarrhea, abdominal pain, nausea, rash, and photosensitivity.

ATCC, abbreviation for **American Type Culture Collection.**

-ate, **1.** suffix meaning "acted upon or being in a (specified) state": *degenerate, enucleate.* **2.** suffix meaning "possessing": *caudate, longipedate.* **3.** suffix meaning a "chemical compound derived from a (specified) source": *silicate, opiate.* **4.** suffix meaning an "acid compound": *oxalate, phosphate.*

atelectasis /at'ilek″təsis/ [Gk, *ateles,* incomplete, *ektasis,* expansion], an abnormal condition characterized by the collapse of alveoli, preventing the respiratory exchange of carbon dioxide and oxygen in a part of the lungs. Symptoms may include diminished breath sounds or aspiratory crackles, a mediastinal shift toward the side of the collapse, fever, and increasing dyspnea. As the remaining portions of the lungs eventually hyperinflate, oxygen saturation of the blood is often nearly normal. The condition may be caused by obstruction of the major airways and bronchioles, by compression of the lung as a result of fluid or air in the pleural space, or by pressure from a tumor outside the lung. Loss of functional lung tissue may secondarily cause increased heart rate, blood pressure, and respiratory rate. Secretions retained in the collapsed alveoli are rich in nutrients for bacterial growth, a condition often leading to stasis pneumonia in critically ill patients. See also **postoperative atelectasis, primary atelectasis.**

ateliosis /ətē′lē·ō″sis/ [Gk, *ateles,* incomplete, *osis,* condition], a form of dwarfism caused by the absence or destruction of eosinophil cells of the adenohypophysis. Affected individuals may appear childlike and have poorly developed muscles.

ateliotic dwarf /at′əlē·ot″ik/, a normally proportioned individual of unusually short stature whose skeleton is incompletely formed as a result of the nonunion of the epiphyses and diaphyses during bone development.

atelo-, prefix meaning "imperfect" or "incomplete": *atelorachidia.*

atelorachidia /at′əlôr′əkid″ē·ə/ [Gk, *ateles,* incomplete, *rhachis,* spine], a defective, incomplete formation of the spinal column. Also spelled *atelorhachidia.*

atenolol /aten″əlôl/, a beta$_1$ selective blocker.
■ INDICATIONS: It is prescribed for the treatment of hypertension and arrhythmias and for control of the ventricular rate in atrial fibrillation.
■ CONTRAINDICATIONS: Sinus bradycardia, second- or third-degree atrioventricular block, cardiogenic shock, or cardiac failure prohibits its use.
■ ADVERSE EFFECTS: Among the more serious adverse reactions are bradycardia, dizziness, and nausea.

ATG, abbreviation for **antithymocyte globulin.**

athelia /āthē″lē·ə/ [Gk, *a,* not, *thele,* nipple], an absence of nipples. The condition is rare but consistently associated with Poland's syndrome and some types of ectodermal dysplasia.

atherectomy /ath′ərek″təmē/, a minimally invasive surgical removal of an atheroma (plaque) in a major artery, utilizing an atherectomy catheter.

atherectomy catheter, a specially designed catheter for cutting away atheromatous plaque from the lining of an artery. A tiny metal cone at the tip of the catheter has cutting edges for loosening the plaque and has openings through which the plaque fragments can be aspirated. The catheter is positioned and monitored by fluoroscopy.

atheroembolic renal disease /ath′ərō·embol″ik/, a condition of gradual or rapid kidney failure resulting from obstruction of the renal arteries by atheromas and emboli. It is associated with atherosclerosis and hypertension and occurs most frequently in persons over 60 years of age. The patient is usually azotemic and also experiences emboli in other body areas.

atheroembolism /ath′ərō·em″bəliz′əm/, obstruction of a blood vessel by an atherosclerotic embolism originating from an atheroma in a major artery.

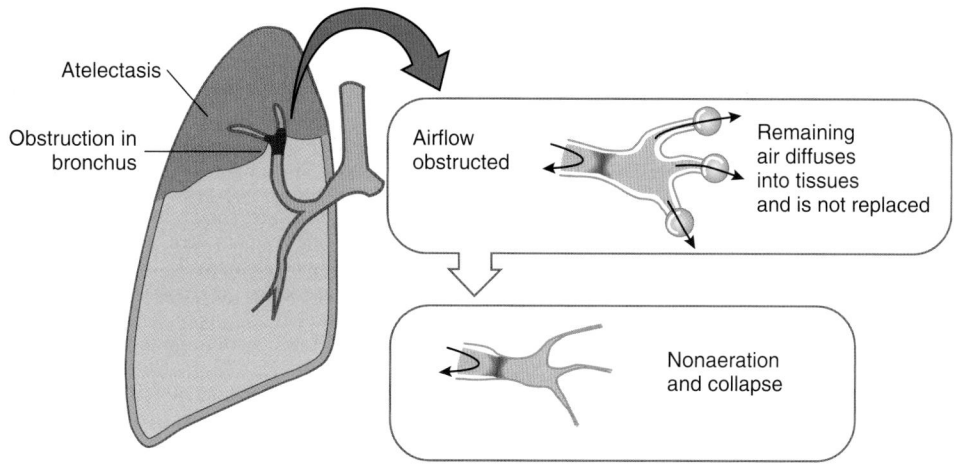

Atelectasis *(Gould, 2014)*

atherogenesis [Gk, *athere,* porridge, *oma,* tumor, *genein,* to produce], the formation of subintimal plaques in the lining of arteries. −*atherogenic, adj.*

atheroma /ath′ərō′mə/ [Gk, *athere,* meal, *oma,* tumor], an abnormal mass of fat or lipids, as in a sebaceous cyst or in deposits in an arterial wall. −**atheromatous,** *adj.*

atheromatosis /ath′ərōmətō″sis/, the development of many atheromas.

atheromatous [Gk, *athere,* meal, *oma,* tumor], pertaining to atheroma.

atheromatous plaque, a yellowish raised area on the lining of an artery formed by fatty deposits; indicative of atherosclerosis.

atherosclerosis /ath′ərō′sklərō″sis/ [Gk, *athere,* meal, *sklerosis,* hardening], a common disorder characterized by yellowish plaques of cholesterol, other lipids, and cellular debris in the inner layers of the walls of arteries. Atherosclerosis may be induced by injury to the arterial endothelium, proliferation of smooth muscle in vessel walls, or accumulation of lipids in hyperlipidemia. The condition begins as a fatty streak and gradually builds to a fibrous plaque or atheromatous lesion. The vessel walls become thick, fibrotic, and calcified, and the lumen narrows, resulting in reduced blood flow to organs normally supplied by the artery. The plaque eventually creates a risk for thrombosis and is one of the major causes of coronary heart disease, angina pectoris, myocardial infarction, and other cardiac disorders. Plaque rupture is usually provoked by activation of the sympathetic nervous system, such as sudden awakening, heavy physical exertion, or anger. See also **arteriosclerosis.** −*atherosclerotic, adj.*

■ OBSERVATIONS: Atherosclerosis usually occurs with aging and is often associated with tobacco use, obesity, high homocysteine levels from eating red meat, hypertension, elevated low-density lipoprotein and depressed high-density lipoprotein levels, and diabetes mellitus.

■ INTERVENTIONS: Antilipemic agents do not reverse atherosclerosis. Segments of arteries obstructed or severely damaged by atheromatous lesions may be replaced by patch grafts or bypassed, as in coronary bypass surgery; the lesion may be removed from the vessel via endarterectomy; or obstructed arteries may be opened by balloon angioplasty or by the insertion of stents.

■ PATIENT CARE CONSIDERATIONS: A diet low in cholesterol, calories, and saturated fats, together with avoidance of smoking, stress, and a sedentary lifestyle, may help prevent the disorder.

atherosclerotic aneurysm /-ot″ik/ [Gk, *athere* + *skleros,* hard, *aneurysma,* an arterial widening]. See **arteriosclerotic aneurysm.**

atherothrombosis /ath′ərō′thrombō″sis/, a condition in which a thrombus originates in an atheromatous blood vessel.

athetoid /ath″ətoid/, pertaining to athetosis, as in the involuntary, purposeless weaving motions of the body or its extremities.

athetosis /ath′ətō″sis/ [Gk, *athetos,* not fixed], slow, writhing, continuous, and involuntary movement of the extremities, as seen in some forms of cerebral palsy and in motor disorders resulting from lesions in the basal ganglia, tabes dorsalis, or other conditions.

athiaminosis /əthī′əminō″sis/, a condition resulting from lack of thiamine in the diet. See also **beriberi, thiamine.**

athlete's foot. *(Informal)* See **tinea pedis.**

athlete's heart /ath″lēts/, an enlarged but otherwise normal heart of an athlete trained for endurance. It is characterized by a low heart rate, an increased pumping capacity, and a greater ability to deliver oxygen to skeletal muscles. It may sometimes be confused with left ventricular hypertrophy. Also called **athletic heart syndrome.**

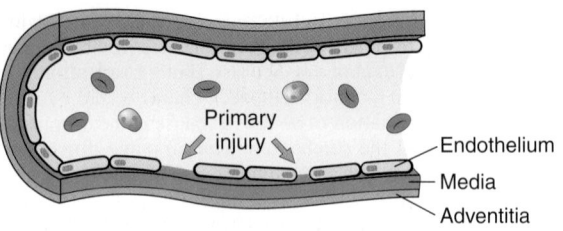

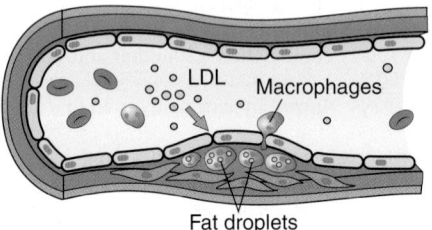

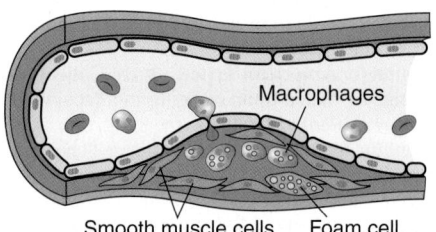

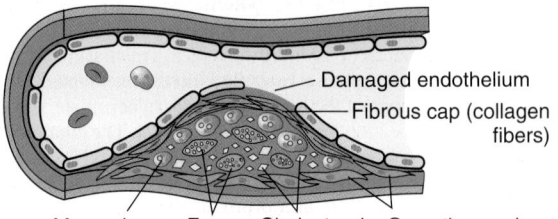

Pathogenesis of atherosclerosis *(Damjanov, 2012)*

athletic habitus /athlet″ik/, a physique characterized by a well-proportioned, muscular body with broad shoulders, thick neck, deep chest, and flat abdomen. Compare **asthenic habitus, pyknic.** See also **mesomorph.**

athletic heart syndrome. See **athlete's heart.**

athletic trainer, (in health care) an allied health professional who is an integral part of the health care system associated with sports. Through both academic preparation and practical experience, the athletic trainer provides a variety of services, including injury prevention and recognition and immediate care, treatment, and rehabilitation of athletic trauma. Certified athletic trainers earn a degree from an accredited athletic training curriculum.

Ativan, a benzodiazepine antianxiety agent. Brand name for **lorazepam.**

atlantal /ətlan″təl/, pertaining to the atlas, the first cervical vertebra.

atlantoaxial /ətlan′tō-ak″sē-əl/ [Gk, *atlas,* to bear, *axis,* pivot], pertaining to the first two cervical vertebrae.

atlantooccipital joint /-oksip″itəl/ [Gk, *atlas,* to bear; L, *ob,* against, *caput,* head], one of a pair of condyloid joints formed by the articulation of the atlas of the vertebral column with the occipital bone of the skull. It includes two articular capsules, two membranes, and two lateral ligaments. The atlantooccipital joint permits nodding and lateral movements of the head.

atlas [Gk, *atlas*, to bear, a mythical giant, compelled to uphold the world], the first cervical vertebra, articulating with the occipital bone and the axis.

ATLS, a course developed by the American College of Surgeons designed to teach a systematic, concise approach to the care of a trauma patient. Abbreviation for **Advanced Trauma Life Support®.**

atm, abbreviation for **atmosphere.**

atman /ät″män/, (in psychiatry) a concept derived from Eastern Indian philosophy that the highest value is knowledge of one's true self. The atman represents the most inward reality, the innermost spirit, and the highest controlling power of a person.

atmo-, prefix meaning "steam" or "vapor": atomizer.

atmosphere (atm) /at″məsfir/ [Gk, *atmos,* vapor, *sphaira,* sphere], **1.** the natural body of air that covers the surface of the earth. It is composed of approximately 21% oxygen, 78% nitrogen, and 1% argon and other gases, including small amounts of carbon dioxide, hydrogen, and ozone, as well as traces of helium, krypton, neon, and xenon and varying amounts of water vapor. **2.** an envelope of gas, which may or may not duplicate the natural atmosphere in chemical components. **3.** a unit of gas pressure that is usually defined as being equivalent to the average pressure of the earth's atmosphere at sea level, or about 14.7 pounds per square inch or 760 mm Hg. –*atmospheric, adj.*

atmospheric pressure /-fer″ik/, the pressure exerted by the weight of the atmosphere. The average atmospheric pressure at sea level is approximately 14.7 pounds per square inch. With increasing altitude the pressure decreases. At 30,000 feet, approximately the height of Mount Everest, the air pressure is 4.3 pounds per square inch. Also called **barometric pressure.**

ATN, abbreviation for **acute tubular necrosis.**

atom /at″əm/ [Gk, *atmos,* indivisible], **1.** (in chemistry and physics) the smallest division of an element that exhibits all the properties and characteristics of the element. It comprises neutrons, electrons, and protons. The number of protons in the nucleus of every atom of any given element is the same and is called its atomic number. **2.** *(Nontechnical)* the amount of any substance that is so small that further division is not possible. –*atomic, adj.*

atomic mass (A), the average mass, relative to the carbon-12 isotope, of an element is based on the average masses of the naturally occurring isotopes of that element. Also called **atomic weight.** See also **atomic mass unit.**

atomic mass unit (amu) /ətom″ik/, a mass exactly equal to one-twelfth the mass of one carbon-12 atom. The energy equivalent of 1 amu is 931.2 MeV. The mass equivalent of 1 amu is 1.66 X 10^{-24} g.

atomic number, the number of protons in the nucleus of an atom of a particular element. In a neutral atom, the atomic number equals the number of electrons. See also **atom, electron, proton.**

atomic theory [Gk, *atmos,* indivisible, *theoria,* speculation], the concept that all matter is composed of atoms that are in turn composed of protons, electrons, and neutrons. A chemical element is identified by the number of protons (atomic number) it contains.

atomic weight. See **atomic mass.**

atomize. See **nebulize.**

atomizer /at″əmī″zər/, a device used to reduce a liquid and eject it as a fine spray or vapor.

atomoxetine, a nonstimulant psychotherapeutic agent used to treat attention deficit–hyperactivity disorder.

atonia /ātō″nē·ə/ [Gk, *a* + *tonos,* without tone], decreased or absent muscle tone. See also **atonic.**

atonic /əton″ik/, **1.** weak. **2.** lacking normal tone, as in the case of a muscle that is flaccid. **3.** lacking vigor, such as an atonic ulcer, which heals slowly. –**atony,** *n.*

atonic bladder. See **flaccid bladder.**

atonic constipation, constipation caused by failure of the colon to respond to the normal stimuli for evacuation, caused by loss of muscle tone. It may occur in elderly or bedridden patients or after prolonged dependence on laxatives. Also called **colon stasis, lazy colon.** See also **fecal impaction, fecalith, inactive colon, constipation.**

atonic impotence. See **impotence.**

atonicity. See **atonia.**

atony, loss of muscular tone. See **atonic,** def. 2.

atopic /ātop″ik/ [Gk, *a* + *topos,* not place], pertaining to a hereditary tendency to experience immediate allergic reactions such as asthma or vasomotor rhinitis because of the presence of an antibody (atopic reagin) in the skin and sometimes the bloodstream. Although it may have a hereditary component, contact with the allergen must occur before the hypersensitivity reaction can develop. –**atopy,** *n.*

atopic allergy [Gk, *a,* not, *topos,* place], a form of allergy that afflicts persons with a genetic predisposition to hypersensitivity to certain allergens. Examples include asthma, hay fever, and food allergies.

atopic asthma. See **allergic asthma.**

atopic dermatitis, an intensely pruritic, often excoriated inflammation commonly found on the face and antecubital and popliteal areas of allergy-prone (atopic) individuals. In infancy and early childhood it is called infantile eczema. Also called *atopic eczema.* Compare **contact dermatitis.** See also **atopic.**

■ OBSERVATIONS: There are no specific cutaneous signs of atopic dermatitis. The lesions seen are a result of scratching from intense itching. The constant and severe itching sets up an itch-scratch-rash-itch cycle that produces red, scaly papules, which coalesce into plaques that ooze and crust. Common sites include the hands, face, upper trunk, and flexural areas, such as bends in knees and elbows. Lesions tend to be symmetric on extremities. Diagnosis is made primarily through clinical evaluation and evidence of personal or family history. Immunofluorescence may show that elevated IgE levels and serum eosinophilia is present as cases worsen.

■ INTERVENTIONS: Primary treatment for acute outbreaks includes emollient lotions to decrease dry skin; topical steroids or pimecrolimus cream (Elidel) or tacrolimus ointment to decrease inflammation; oral antihistamines or other antipruritics to control itching. Outbreak prevention is aimed at avoiding triggering factors, such as sudden temperature shifts, contact with irritants, foods that provoke exacerbations, stressful situations, allergens, or excessive hand washing.

■ PATIENT CARE CONSIDERATIONS: Nursing care is aimed at helping the individual break the itch-scratch cycle and reduce outbreaks. This includes proper use of topical medications, and instruction in ways to prevent or reduce outbreaks. Adequate rest can reduce the threshold for itching. Modest exercise in a controlled temperature environment can increase circulation. A balanced diet that avoids food triggers can strengthen skin protective functions. Hygiene is aimed at cleanliness, avoidance of drying, and maintenance of acidic pH on skin. Nails should be kept clipped to decrease abrasion from scratching. Affected individuals need to know that this is a genetically determined chronic disease with cycles of exacerbation and remission.

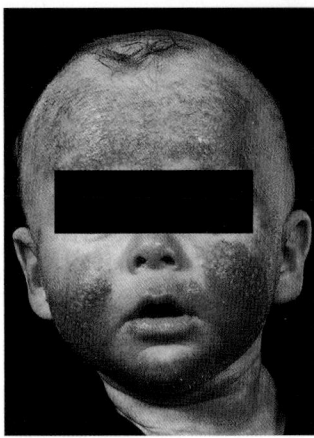

Toddler with atopic dermatitis *(Chan and Burrows, 2009)*

atopic reagin,   **1.** a plasma or cerebrospinal fluid antibody that generates allergic (atopic) reactions by causing histamine release. **2.** the antibody that is detected in the rapid plasma reagin test for syphilis. See also **reagin.**

atopognosia /ātop′əgnō″zhə/   [Gk, *a, topos,* not place, *gnosis,* knowledge],   a form of agnosia in which a person is unable to locate a tactile sensation correctly.

atopy,   a genetic predisposition toward the development of immediate hypersensitivity reactions.

atorvastatin,   an antihyperlipidemic, classified as an HMG-CoA reductase inhibitor.

■ INDICATIONS: This drug is used to lower the levels of both cholesterol and triglycerides in the plasma.

■ CONTRAINDICATIONS: Known hypersensitivity, pregnancy, lactation, and active liver disease prohibit the use of this drug.

■ ADVERSE EFFECTS: Myalgias, myopathy and rhabdomyolysis are dose-related effects. Liver dysfunction is rare and usually transient. Other adverse effects include rash, pruritus, alopecia, dyspepsia, flatus, pancreatitis, lens opacities, and headache.

atovaquone /ah-to′vah-kwōn/,   an antibiotic/antiparasitic used in the treatment of mild to moderate *Pneumocystis* pneumonia and in the prevention and treatment of falciparum malaria. It is administered orally.

atoxic,   not poisonous.

ATP,   abbreviation for **adenosine triphosphate.**

ATPase,   abbreviation for **adenosine triphosphatase.**

ATPD,   abbreviation for ambient temperature and pressure, dry.

ATPS,   abbreviation for ambient temperature and pressure, saturated. See **volume ATPS.**

atracurium,   an intermediate-duration nondepolarizing skeletal muscle relaxant used as an adjunct in anesthesia to create an ideal surgical field; it induces muscle paralysis, thereby reducing muscle tension in the surrounding surgical field. See also **cisatracurium.**

atransferrinemic anemia /ā′transfer′inē″mik/,   an iron-transport deficiency disease characterized by a failure of iron to move from the liver or other storage sites to tissues in which erythrocytes develop. The condition may be caused by a molecular defect in transferrin, an iron-binding protein. In addition to anemia, the patient usually suffers from hemosiderosis.

atraumatic /ā′trômat″ik/   [Gk, *a,* without, *trauma*],   pertaining to therapies or therapeutic instruments and devices that are unlikely to cause tissue damage.

atresia /ətrē″zhə/   [Gk, *a, tresis,* not perforation],   the absence of a normal body opening, duct, or canal, such as of the anus, vagina, or external ear canal. **–atretic,** *atresic, adj.*

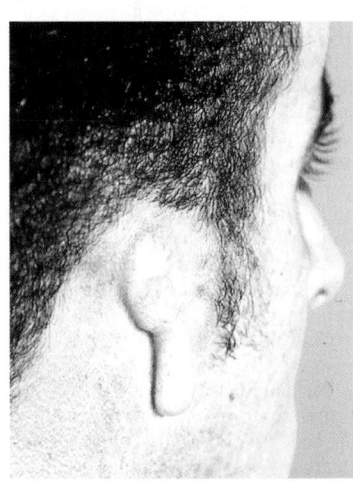

Atresia of the right external ear *(Myers, 2008)*

atresic teratism /ətrē″sik/   [Gk, *a, tresis* + *tera,* monster],   a congenital anomaly in which any of the normal openings of the body, such as the mouth, nares, anus, or vagina, fails to form.

atretic,   closed or missing. See **atresia.**

atria,   pleural of atrium. See **atrium.**

atrial complex,   the P wave of the electrocardiogram, representing electrical activity of the atria.

atrial extrasystole.   See **premature atrial complex.**

atrial fibrillation (AF) /ā″trē·əl/,   an abnormality of cardiac rhythm characterized by disorganized electrical activity in the atria and accompanied by an irregular ventricular response that is usually rapid. The atria quiver instead of pumping in an organized fashion, resulting in compromised ventricular filling and reduced stroke volume. Blood clots can form and travel to the lungs, forming a life-threatening pulmonary embolism, or to the brain, causing a life-threatening stroke.

atrial flutter (AF),   **1.** a type of atrial tachycardia characterized by contraction rates between 230/min and 380/min. Two kinds, typical and atypical, have been identified and are distinguished from each other by their rates and electrocardiographic (ECG) patterns. During typical atrial flutter the atrial rate is between 290/min and 310/min and produces "fence post" or "sawtooth" ECG waves. During atypical atrial flutter the atrial rate is higher, and the ECG waves lack the sawtooth appearance, and are often sinusoidal. For both types, ventricular contractions usually follow atrial contractions in a 1:2, 1:3, 1:4, or variable ratio. It may be cured with electrophysiological radiofrequency ablation. Compare **atrial fibrillation. 2.** a type of atrial tachycardia characterized by contraction rates between 230/min and 380/min. Two kinds, typical and atypical, have been identified and are distinguished from each other by their rates and electrocardiographic (ECG) patterns. During typical atrial flutter the atrial rate is between 290/min and 310/min and produces "fence post" or "sawtooth" ECG waves. During atypical atrial flutter the atrial rate is higher, and the ECG waves lack the sawtooth appearance, and are often sinusoidal. For both types, ventricular contractions usually follow atrial

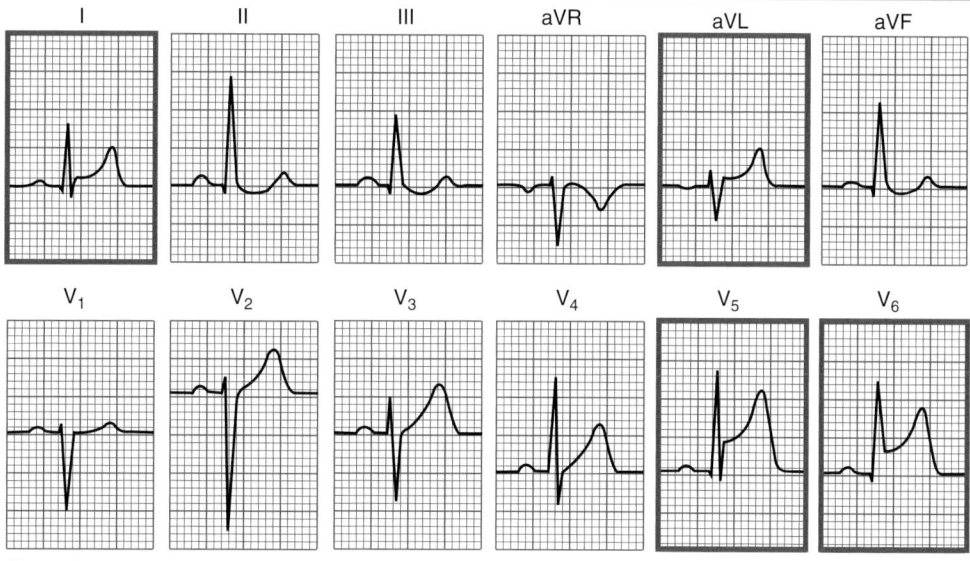

Phase 1

ECG strip showing atrial flutter *(Wesley, 2012)*

contractions in a 1:2, 1:3, 1:4, or variable ratio. It may be cured with electrophysiological radiofrequency ablation.

atrial gallop. See **S₄.**

atrial myxoma, a benign, pedunculated, gelatinous tumor that originates in the interatrial septum of the heart. The tumor is characterized by palpitations, disseminated neuritis, nausea, weight loss, fatigue, dyspnea, fever, and occasional sudden loss of consciousness. It is treated by surgical removal of the tumor.

atrial natriuretic peptide (ANP), a hormone involved in natriuresis and the regulation of renal and cardiovascular homeostasis. It is synthesized as a prohormone in the granules of the myocytes of the atrium and is released into the circulation in response to atrial dilation or increased intravascular fluid volume. It causes natriuresis, diuresis, and renal vasodilation; reduces circulating concentrations of renin, aldosterone, and antidiuretic hormone; and thereby normalizes circulating blood pressure and volume. Also called *atrial natriuretic factor.*

atrial pacing. See **pacing.**

atrial premature complex (APC). See **premature atrial complex.**

atrial septal defect (ASD), a congenital cardiac anomaly characterized by an abnormal opening between the atria. The severity of the condition depends on the size and location of the opening, which are related to the stage at which embryonic development of the septum was arrested. ASDs are classified as ostium primum defect, in which there is inadequate development of the endocardial cushions of the first septum of the fetal heart; ostium secundum defect, in which the aperture in the second septum of the fetal heart fails to close; and sinus venosus defect, in which the superior portion of the atrium fails to develop. ASDs increase the flow of oxygenated blood into the right side of the heart, which is usually well tolerated, since the blood is delivered under much lower pressure than in ventricular septal defect. Clinical manifestations include a characteristic harsh, scratchy systolic murmur and a fixed splitting of the second heart sound, which does not vary with respiration. X-ray films and electrocardiograms generally show right atrial and right ventricular enlargement,

although definitive diagnosis is made by cardiac catheterization or echocardiogram. Closure is indicated in most cases but is usually postponed until later childhood, unless the defect is severe. Closure may be done surgically or via a percutaneous approach. See also **endocardial cushion defect.**

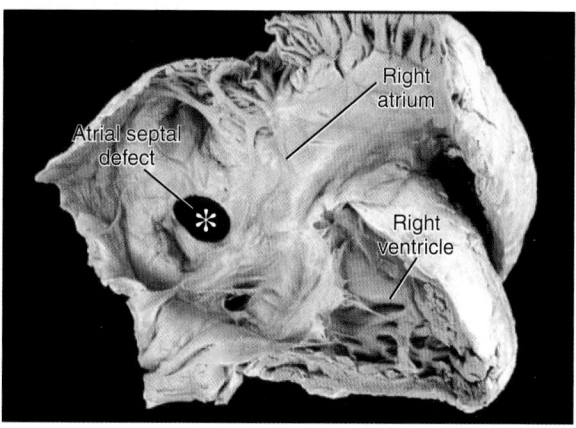

Atrial septal defect *(Damjanov and Linder, 2000)*

atrial septum [L, *atrium,* hall, *saeptum,* fence], the partition between the left and right atria of the heart.

atrial standstill, a condition of complete failure of the atria to contract. P waves are absent in all electrocardiogram surface leads, and A waves are absent in the jugular venous pulse and right atrial pressure tracings. Generally, a junctional escape pacemaker maintains ventricular activity during atrial standstill.

atrial systole, the contraction of the atria of the heart, which precedes ventricular contraction by a fraction of a second.

atrial tachycardia [L, *atrium,* hall; Gk, *tachys,* quick, *kardia,* heart], rapid beating of the atria caused by abnormal automaticity, triggered activity, or intraatrial reentry. The atrial rate is usually less than 200/min; however, in cases of digitalis excess, the rate increases gradually to 130/min to 250/min as the digitalis is continued. When there is 2:1 conduction, the atrial rhythm is irregular in 50% of cases. The contour of the P waves is different from that of the sinus P wave except in cases of digitalis-induced atrial tachycardia, when the P wave is almost identical to the sinus P wave. Vagal maneuvers have no effect on atrial tachycardia, although they do cause atrioventricular block. Atrial tachycardia may be either nonparoxysmal (common) or paroxysmal (uncommon). Also called **auricular tachycardia.**

atrichia /ātrik″ē·ə/ [Gk, *a,* not, *thrix,* hair], **1.** pertaining to a group of bacteria that lack flagella. **2.** the congenital or acquired absence of hair.

atrichosis /ā′trikō″sis/ [Gk, *a + trichia,* without hair, *osis,* condition], a congenital or acquired absence of hair.

atrio-, prefix meaning "atrium of the heart" or "entrance chamber."

atrioventricular (AV) /ā′trē·ōventrik″yələr/ [L, *atrium,* hall, *ventriculus*], pertaining to a connecting conduction event or anatomical structure between the atria and ventricles.

atrioventricular block (AVB) [L, *atrium + ventriculus,* little belly], a disorder of cardiac impulse transmission that reflects prolonged, intermittent, or absent conduction of impulses between the atria and ventricles. It commonly occurs at the AV node or within the bundle branch system. Treatment depends on where the block is located and whether it is transient or permanent. Heart rate–supporting drugs or pacemaker insertion are common options. See also **heart block, intraatrial block, intraventricular block, sinoatrial (SA) block.**

atrioventricular (AV) bundle, a band of atypical cardiac muscle fibers with few contractile units. It arises from the distal portion of the AV node and extends across the AV groove to the top of the interventricular septum, where it divides into the bundle branches. Also called **bundle of His.**

atrioventricular (AV) dissociation, a breakdown in the normal conduction of excitation through the heart, allowing the atria and ventricles to beat independently under the control of their own pacemakers.

atrioventricular (AV) junction [L, *jungere,* to join], the region of the heart that separates the atria from the ventricles. It includes the AV bundle (bundle of His) and surrounds the AV node. See also **junctional extrasystole.**

atrioventricular (AV) node, an area of specialized cardiac muscle that receives the cardiac impulse from the sinoatrial (SA) node and conducts it to the bundle of His and thence to the Purkinje fibers and walls of the ventricles. The AV node is located in the septal wall between the left and right atria.

atrioventricular (AV) septum, a small portion of membrane that separates the atria from the ventricles of the heart.

atrioventricular (AV) valve, a valve in the heart through which blood flows from the atria to the ventricles. The valve between the left atrium and left ventricle is the mitral (bicuspid) valve; the right AV valve is the tricuspid valve.

at risk, the state of an individual or population being vulnerable to a particular disease or event. The factors determining risk may be environmental, psychosocial, psychological, or physiological. An example of an environmental factor is exposure to harmful substances or organisms. An example of a physiological factor is genetic predisposition to a disease.

atrium /ā″trē·əm/ *pl. atria* [L, hall], a chamber or cavity, such as the right and left atria of the heart or the nasal cavity.

atrium of the ear, the external part of the ear, including the auricle and the tubular portion of the external auditory meatus.

atrium of the heart, one of the two upper chambers of the heart. The right atrium receives deoxygenated blood from the superior vena cava, the inferior vena cava, and the coronary sinus. The left atrium receives oxygenated blood from the pulmonary veins. Blood is emptied into the ventricles from the atria during diastole.

atrium proper, the space anterior to the crista terminalis of the right atrium of the heart.

Atromid-S, a fibric acid derivative used to lower plasma triglyceride (VLDL) levels. Brand name for **clofibrate.**

atrophia, a wasting or dimunition of size due to poor nutrition.

atrophic /ātrof″ik/ [Gk, *a,* without, *trophe,* nourishment], characterized by a wasting of tissues, usually associated with general malnutrition or a specific disease state. See also **dystrophic.**

atrophic acne, acne vulgaris in which, after the disappearance of small papular lesions, a stippling of tiny atrophic pits and scars remains.

atrophic catarrh [Gk, *a, trophe,* without nourishment, *kata,* down, *rhoia,* flow], an abnormal condition characterized by inflammation and discharge from the mucous membranes of the nose, accompanied by the loss of mucosal and submucosal tissue. Compare **hypertrophic catarrh.** See also **catarrh.**

atrophic cirrhosis [Gk, *a + trophe,* without nourishment, *kirrhos,* yellow-orange], a form of advanced portal cirrhosis with massive shrinking of the liver.

atrophic fracture, a spontaneous fracture caused by bone atrophy, as in the bones of a person with osteoporosis. Also called **pathological fracture.**

atrophic gastritis, a chronic inflammation of the stomach, associated with degeneration of the gastric mucosa. There are two types: a type associated with *Helicobacter pylori* and autoimmune, which is characterized by antiparietal and antiintrinsic factor antibodies. Autoimmune atrophic gastritis is seen in elderly patients and in persons with pernicious anemia; it rarely causes epigastric pain. See also **pernicious anemia.**

atrophic glossitis, a pathological condition in which the various papillae are lost from the dorsum of the tongue, which may result in a sensitive surface that makes eating difficult. See also **glossitis.**

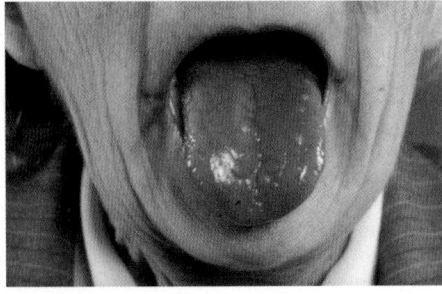

Atrophic glossitis *(Mangold, Torgerson, and Rogers, 2016)*

atrophic rhinitis [Gk, *a + trophe,* without nourishment, *rhis,* nose, *itis,* inflammation], a nasal condition, a form of chronic rhinitis, in which there is inflammation and atrophy of the mucous membrane of the nose, resulting in failure of the ciliary function and drying and crusting of the lining of the nasal passages. This may reduce the sense of smell. It commonly occurs as a result of viral infection such as the common cold but can also be caused by allergies.

atrophic vaginitis [Gk, *a* + *trophe,* without nourishment; L, *vagina,* sheath; Gk, *itis,* inflammation], degeneration, thinning, and dryness of the vaginal mucous membranes due to decreased estrogen, usually associated with menopause. See also **vaginitis.**

atrophied /at″rŏfēd/ [Gk, *a* + *trophe,* without nourishment], decreased in size because of disuse or disease, as an organ, tissue, or body part.

atrophoderma /at″rŏfədur″mə/ [Gk, *a* + *trophe* + *derma,* skin], the wasting away or decrease in thickness of the skin. The atrophy may affect the entire body surface or only localized areas. The condition is often associated with aging and may occur as a primary or secondary symptom of various diseases.

atrophy /at″rəfē/ [Gk, *a* + *trophe,* without nourishment], a wasting or decrease in size or physiological activity of a part of the body because of disease or other influences. A skeletal muscle may undergo atrophy as a result of lack of physical exercise or neurological or musculoskeletal disease. Cells of the brain and central nervous system may atrophy in old age because of restricted blood flow to those areas. See also **abiotrophy, aging. –atrophic,** *adj.,* **–atrophy,** *v.*

atrophy of aging, a decrease in function of various bodily systems and organs, including the brain.

atrophy of disuse [Gk, *a, trophe* + L, *dis,* opposite of, *usus*], a shrinkage or wasting away of tissues resulting from immobility or lack of exercise.

atropine /at″rŏpin/ [Gk, *Atropos,* one of the three Fates], an alkaloid from *Atropa belladonna* and *Datura stramonium* plants. It is a classic anticholinergic agent and is used to treat symptomatic bradycardia and topically to dilate pupils before eye examinations. Atropine is related to other drugs, such as scopolamine and hyoscyamine, and has a similar action of blocking parasympathetic stimuli by raising the threshold of response of effector cells to acetylcholine.

atropine sulfate, an antispasmodic and anticholinergic.

■ INDICATIONS: It may be prescribed in the treatment of GI hypermotility to decrease the tone of the detrusor muscle of the urinary bladder in urinary tract disorders, for cycloplegic refraction and dilation of the pupil in inflammation of the iris or the uvea, cardiac arrhythmias, and certain kinds of poisoning and as an adjunct to anesthesia.

■ CONTRAINDICATIONS: GI obstruction, glaucoma, hepatitis, liver or kidney dysfunction, porphyria, or known hypersensitivity to this drug or other anticholinergics prohibit its use.

■ ADVERSE EFFECTS: Among the more serious adverse reactions are tachycardia, angina, loss of taste, nausea, diarrhea, skin rash, blurred vision, and eye pain. Dry mouth and constipation are common effects.

atropine sulfate poisoning [Gk, *Atropos,* fate; L, *sulphur* + *potio,* drink], toxic effects of an overdose of a drug sometimes used as an adjunct to general anesthesia and to treat bradycardia. Symptoms include tachycardia, hot and dry flushed skin, dry mouth with thirst, restlessness and excitement, urinary retention, constipation, and a burning pain in the throat. Treatment may include the administration of physostigmine.

attached epithelial cuff. See **junctional epithelium.**

attached gingiva, gingival mucosal tissue that covers and is firmly attached to the alveolar process in the maxilla and mandible. Also called **alveolar gingiva.**

attachment [Fr, *attachement*], **1.** the state or quality of being affixed or attached. **2.** (in psychiatry) a mode of behavior in which one individual relates in an affiliative or dependent manner to another; a feeling of affection or loyalty that binds one person to another. See also **bonding. 3.** (in dentistry) any device, such as a retainer or artificial crown, used

to secure a partial denture to a natural tooth in the mouth, or that secures an artificial dental prosthesis to an implant. **4.** (in periodontology) the fixation of periodontal tissues to alveolar bone and tooth structure.

attachment apparatus, the various tissues that surround and support the teeth, including the cementum, the periodontal ligament, and the alveolar process. See also **masticatory system.**

attack, **1.** an episode in the course of an illness, usually characterized by acute and distressing symptoms. **2.** a rapid response to a condition.

attapulgite /at″ah-pul′jīt/, a clay mineral that contains aluminum silicate and is the main ingredient of Fuller's earth.

attending [L, *attendo,* to notice], (in psychology) pertaining to an enhanced readiness to perceive, with an adjustment of the brain and sense organs to focus on a situation.

attending physician [L, *attendere,* to stretch], the physician (who is on the medical staff of a hospital or health care facility) who is legally responsible for the health care given to a particular patient. In a university hospital setting, an attending physician often also has teaching responsibilities, holds a faculty appointment, and supervises residents and medical students.

attention [L, *attendere,* to stretch], the element of cognitive functioning in which the mental focus is maintained on a specific issue, object, or activity.

attention deficit disorder (ADD), a syndrome affecting children, adolescents, and adults characterized by short attention span, hyperactivity, and poor concentration. The symptoms may be mild or severe and are associated with functional deviations of the central nervous system without signs of major neurological or psychiatric disturbance. The people affected are usually of normal intelligence but often trail their peers in academic achievement. Other symptoms may include impairment in perception, conceptualization, language, memory, and motor skills; decreased attention span; increased impulsivity; and emotional lability. The condition is more prevalent in boys than in girls and may result from genetic factors, biochemical irregularities, perinatal or postnatal injury, or disease. There is no known cure, and symptoms may subside or disappear with time. Medications are frequently prescribed for children with hyperactive symptoms, and some form of psychotherapeutic counseling is recommended. Treatment of children is most effective with family and behaviorally oriented programs. Adult counseling tends to focus on specific issues such as time management and goal setting. Also called **hyperactivity, hyperkinesis, minimal brain dysfunction.** See also **learning disability.**

attention deficit–hyperactivity disorder (ADHD), a childhood mental disorder with onset before 7 years of age and involving impaired or diminished attention, impulsivity, and hyperactivity. Also called **hyperactive child syndrome.** See **attention deficit disorder.**

attenuated /əten″yoo·ā·tid/ [L, *attenuare,* to make thin], pertaining to the dilution of a solution or the reduction in virulence or toxicity of a microorganism or a drug by weakening it.

attenuated virus [L, *attenuare,* to make thin, *virus,* poison], a strain of virus whose virulence has been lowered by physical or chemical processes, or by repeated passage through the cells of another species. Vaccines made by attenuated strains are used to prevent smallpox, measles, mumps, rubella, polio, yellow fever, and other viruses.

attenuation /əten′yoo·ā″shən/ [L, *attenuare,* to make thin], **1.** the process of reduction. **2.** (in radiology) the reduction in intensity of an x-ray beam as it passes through matter. **3.** (in infectious diseases) taking an infectious agent and altering it so that it becomes harmless or less virulent. Attenuated viruses are often used as vaccine agents.

attenuation coefficient, a quantitative measure that characterizes how easily a material can be penetrated by a beam of light, sound, or energy. In radiography or ultrasound, the difference between the energy that enters a body part and the energy that is not detected. The difference is caused by the absorption and scattering of energy within the body tissues.

attenuator /əten″yoo-ā′tər/ [L, *attenuare,* to make thin], an agent that weakens the toxicity of a poisonous substance or the virulence of a microorganism.

Attenuvax, an active immunizing agent. Brand name for *live measles virus vaccine.*

attic. See **epitympanic recess.**

attitude /at′ətyo͞od, -to͞od/ [L, *aptitude,* fitness], **1.** a body position or posture, particularly the fetal position in the uterus, as determined by the degree of flexion of the head and extremities. **2.** (in psychiatry) any of the major integrative forces in the development of personality that gives consistency to an individual's behavior. Attitudes are cognitive in nature, formed through interactions with the environment. They reflect the person's innermost convictions about situations good or bad, right or wrong, desirable or undesirable.

attitudinal isolation /at′ətyo͞o″dənəl/ [L, *attitudo,* posture], a type of social isolation that results from a person's own cultural or personal values.

attitudinal reflex, any reflex initiated by a change in position of the head or by a change in position of the head with respect to the position of the body. Also called **statotonic reflex.** Kinds include **tonic labyrinthine reflex, tonic neck reflex.**

atto-, a prefix in the metric system indicating a value of one quintillionth, or 10^{-18}.

ATTR amyloidosis, the most common form of familial amyloidosis, in which any of numerous mutations of the gene encoding transthyretin cause systemic autosomal-dominant disorders characterized by polyneuropathies, cardiomyopathies, and variable organ involvement.

attrition /ətrish″ən/ [L, *atterere,* to wear away], **1.** the process of wearing away or wearing down by friction. **2.** the physiological wearing away of the teeth such as from normal mastication, grinding, bruxism, premature contacts, or abnormal tooth structures. See **abrasion, abfraction, erosion. 3.** a reduction in the number of participants in a study or program of study that happens when individuals withdraw or are dismissed.

-ature, combining form indicating "to join": *ligature.*

at. wt., abbreviation for **atomic weight.**

atypia /ātip″ēə/ [Gk, *a + typos,* without type], a condition of being irregular, not the same, or nonstandard.

atypical /ātip″əkəl/ [Gk, *a + typos,* without type], a condition or object that is not of a usual or standard type and that does not look or appear the same in character.

atypical measles syndrome (AMS), a form of measles (rubeola) reported in persons immunized with a killed measles vaccine used in the United States from 1962 to 1967 and in Canada until 1970. Immunization with inactivated measles virus does not provide immunity and can sensitize the patient to the virus, resulting in an alteration of the disease. Symptoms differ from those of typical measles, beginning with a sudden high fever, headache, abdominal pain, and coughing. The measles rash may appear only 1 or 2 days later, usually starting on the hands and feet, rather than the head and neck. The infection may be complicated by edema of the extremities and pneumonia and may persist for up to 3 months.

atypical Mycobacterium [Gk, *a + typos,* without type, *mykes,* fungus, *bakterion,* small staff], a group of mycobacteria, including pathogenic and nonpathogenic forms, that are classified according to their ability to produce pigments, growth characteristics, and reactions to chemical tests. Mycobacteria, nontuberculosis (atypical) does not require isolation precautions.

atypical pneumonia [Gk, *a + typos,* without type, *pneumon,* lung, *ia,* condition], a group of relatively mild symptoms of chills, headache, muscular pains, moderate fever, and coughing, but without substantive evidence of a bacterial infection. Chest radiographs may show mottling at the bases of the lungs. Eaton agent, or *Mycoplasma pneumoniae,* may be the cause of the symptoms. Also called **walking pneumonia.**

atypical polypoid adenomyoma, a rare and benign tumor that may be clinically and histologically mistaken for malignance.

atypical somatoform disorder, an abnormal condition marked by physical symptoms and complaints that appear related to a preoccupation with an imagined defect in one's personal appearance or ability.

Au, symbol for the element **gold.**

audible /ô″dəbəl/ [L, *audire,* to hear], capable of being heard. Some animals are able to hear sounds of higher or lower frequencies and different intensities than those audible to most humans.

audio-, combining form meaning "hearing": *audiology.*

audioanalgesia /ô·dē·ō·an′əljē″sē·a/ [L, *audire,* to hear; Gk, *a, algos,* not pain], the use of music or sounds to produce a level of minimal sedation along the continuum of sedation spectrum to enhance relaxation and to distract a patient's mind from pain, anxiety, or discomfort, as during dentistry, during labor and childbirth, or during procedures with sedation or regional anesthetic techniques. When used along with anesthetics, it is termed a co-sedation technique.

audiogenic epilepsy. See **auditory epilepsy.**

audiogram /ô″dē·ə·gram′/ [Gk, *audire + gramma,* record], a chart showing the faintest level at which an individual is able to detect sounds of various frequencies, usually in octaves from 125 Hz to 8000 Hz. See also **audiometry, speech banana.**

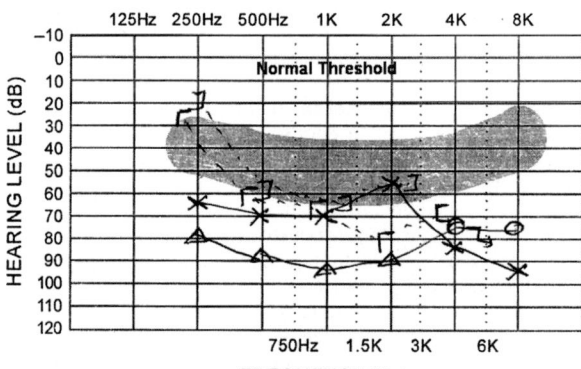

Audiogram *(Jacob et al, 2007)*

audiologist, a health professional with graduate education in normal hearing processes and hearing loss, who detects and evaluates hearing loss, and who determines how a client can best make use of remaining hearing. If a client can benefit from assistive listening devices such as hearing aids, the audiologist assists with the selection, fitting, and training in their use. See also **speech-language pathologist.**

audiology /-ol″əjē/ [L, *audire + Gk, logos,* science], a field of research and clinical practice devoted to the study of hearing disorders, assessment of hearing, hearing conservation, and aural rehabilitation. *—audiologic, audiological, adj.*

audiometer /ô′dē·om″ətər/ [L, *audire* + Gk, *metron,* measure], an electronic device for testing hearing. Earphones are placed over the ears (air-conduction testing), or a bone vibrator is placed on the mastoid (bone conduction testing). Hearing is tested by using tones from very low to very high frequencies at various decibels of intensity. The patient signals when a tone is heard, and the lowest level at which the patient hears is noted on an audiogram.

audiometrist /ô′dē·om″ətrist/, a technician who has received special training in the use of pure-tone audiometry equipment. An audiometrist conducts the hearing tests selected and interpreted by an audiologist, who supervises the process.

audiometry /ô′dē·om″ətrē/, the testing of the sensitivity of the sense of hearing. Various audiometric tests determine the lowest intensity of sound at which an individual can perceive auditory stimuli (hearing threshold) and distinguish different speech sounds. Pure tone audiometry assesses the person's ability to hear frequencies, usually ranging from 125 to 8000 Hz, and can indicate whether a hearing loss is caused by an outer ear, a middle ear, an inner ear, or an acoustic nerve problem. Speech audiometry tests the ability to understand selected words. Impedance audiometry is an objective method of assessing the resistance or compliance of the conducting mechanism of the middle ear with a probe inserted into the ear canal. −*audiometric, adj.*

audiovisual /ô′dē·ōvizh″əl/, pertaining to communication that uses both sight and sound messages.

audit /ô″dit/, **1.** a final statement of account. **2.** a review and evaluation of health care procedures and documentation for the purpose of comparing the quality of care provided with accepted standards; an examination of records or accounts to check accuracy

auditory /ô″dətôr′ē/ [L, *auditorius,* hearing], pertaining to the sense of hearing and the hearing organs involved.

auditory amnesia [L, *auditorius,* hearing; Gk, *amnesia,* forgetfulness], a loss of memory for the meaning of sounds. Also called **word deafness.**

auditory area [L, *auditorium,* hearing], the sound perception area of the cerebral cortex. It is located in the floor of the lateral fissure and on the dorsal surface of the superior temporal gyrus.

auditory brainstem response (ABR), an electrophysiological test used to measure hearing sensitivity and evaluate the integrity of ear structures from the auditory nerve through the brainstem. It is also used to screen hearing of newborns.

auditory canal. See **auditory meatus.**

auditory cortex. See **acoustic center.**

auditory epilepsy, a reflex form of epilepsy provoked by sounds. Also called **audiogenic epilepsy.**

auditory figure-ground, an auditory process that denotes the ability to focus on a particular sound, such as a voice, without being distracted by background sounds in the environment.

auditory hair [L, *audire,* to hear; AS, *haer*], one of the cells with hairlike processes in the spiral organ of Corti. The hairs, or cilia, function as sensory receptors. Also called **acoustic hair cell, cell of Corti.**

auditory hallucination [L, *audire,* to hear, *alucinari,* a wandering mind], commonly seen in schizophrenia. It is a subjective experience of hearing voices or other sounds despite the absence of an actual reality-based external stimulus to account for the phenomenon.

auditory meatus [L, *audire,* to hear, *meatus,* passage], **1.** the external auditory meatus, a tubelike channel of the external ear extending from the auricle to the tympanum of the middle ear. **2.** the internal auditory meatus, a short channel extending from the petrous part of the temporal

bone to the fundus near the vestibule. It contains the eighth cranial nerve. Also called **auditory canal.**

auditory nerve. See **vestibulocochlear nerve.**

auditory ossicles [L, *audire* + *ossiculum,* little bone], the malleus, the incus, and the stapes, three small bones in the middle ear that articulate with each other. As the tympanic membrane vibrates, it transmits sound waves through the ossicles to the cochlea.

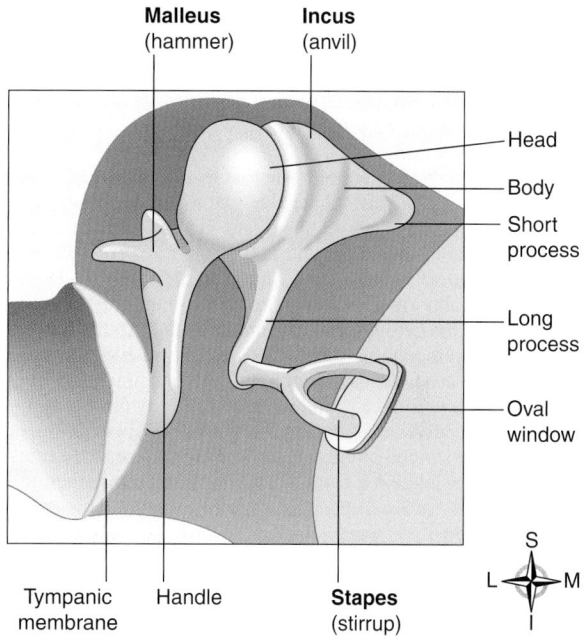

Auditory ossicles *(Waugh and Grant, 2014)*

auditory system assessment, an evaluation of the patient's ears and hearing and an investigation of present and past diseases or conditions that may be responsible for an auditory impairment.

■ METHOD: The client is questioned in verbal or written form regarding previous ear problems, especially childhood problems of otitis media, perforations of the eardrum, and drainage, and history of measles, mumps, or scarlet fever. Information is obtained about past or present ototoxic medications, such as aspirin, chemotherapeutic drugs, NSAIDs. streptomycin, aminoglycerides, or diuretics. Previous ear surgeries as well as tonsillectomy and adenoidectomy or head injury are also documented. Use of a hearing aid and problems with compacted cerumin are noted. Symptoms of dizziness, ringing in the ears, and hearing loss are recorded. Information regarding allergies, prematurity, and family members with hearing loss is documented. Chronic medical conditions such as diabetes or cancer as well as occupational exposures to high-noise environments, with or without protection, are also important. Recreational ear hazards, such as swimming or chronic exposure to loud music, are noted. Physical examination includes inspection and palpation of the external ear including the mastoid area for tenderness, swelling, redness, nodules, or lesions. Otoscopic examination is then performed to assess the ear canal and tympanic membrane. Diagnostic procedures indicated by the history may include audiometry, a mastoid x-ray film, Rinne and Weber tuning-fork tests, and microbiological studies for potential pathogens in smears of ear drainage.

■ PATIENT CARE CONSIDERATIONS: The health care provider conducts the interview, makes the observations, and collects the pertinent background information and the results of the diagnostic procedures.

■ OUTCOME CRITERIA: A thorough assessment of the patient's auditory system is essential in establishing the diagnosis of an ear disorder.

auditory threshold [L, *audire,* to hear; AS, *threscold*], the lowest intensity at which a sound may be heard. An audiologist typically determines a patient's threshold for pure tones and speech.

auditory verbal therapy, a rehabilitation method for children with hearing impairments that employs the use of residual hearing and amplification with hearing aids or cochlear implants.

auditory vertigo [L, *audire,* to hear, *vertigo,* dizziness], vertigo associated with ear disease. It is characterized by sensations of gyration and, when severe, with prostration and vomiting.

Auerbach plexus [Leopold Auerbach, German anatomist, 1828–1897; L, *plexus,* plaited], the myenteric plexus, a group of autonomic nerve fibers and ganglia located in the muscle tissue of the intestinal tract.

Auer rod /ou″ər/ [John Auer, American physiologist, 1875–1948], an abnormal, needle-shaped or round, pink-staining inclusion in the cytoplasm of myeloblasts and promyelocytes in acute myelogenous, promyelocytic, or myelomonocytic leukemia. These inclusions contain enzymes such as acid phosphatase, peroxidase, and esterase and may represent abnormal derivatives of cytoplasmic granules. The finding of Auer rods in stained blood smears helps to differentiate acute myelogenous leukemia from acute lymphoblastic leukemia.

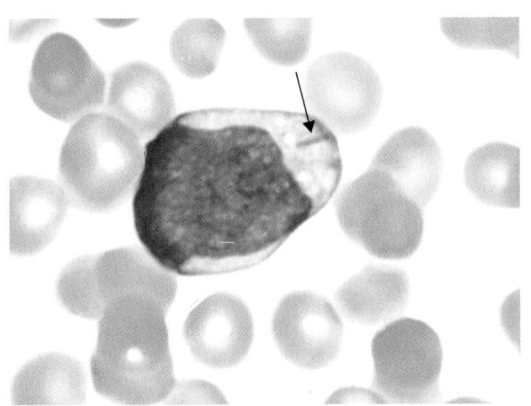

Auer rod *(Carr and Rodak, 2009)*

augmentation /ôg′məntā″shən/ [L, *augmentare,* to increase], **1.** stimulation of an increased rate of biological activity, such as faster cell division or heartbeat. **2.** breast enlargement through mammoplasty.

augmentation mammoplasty, a surgical procedure to increase the size of the breasts.

aur-, auri-, prefix meaning "ear": *auricle, aural.*

aura /ôr′ə/ [L, breath], **1.** a sensation, as of light, warmth, or emotion (such as fear) that may precede an attack of migraine or an epileptic seizure. **2.** an emanation of light or color surrounding a person as seen in Kirlian photography and studied in nursing research in healing techniques.

aural /ôr″əl/, **1.** pertaining to the ear or hearing. −**aurally,** *adv.* **2.** pertaining to an aura.

aural forceps, a dressing forceps with fine, bent tips used in surgery.

aurally. See **aural.**

aural rehabilitation, a form of therapy in which hearing-impaired individuals are taught to improve their ability to communicate. Methods taught include, but are not limited to, speech-reading, auditory training, use of hearing aids, and use of assistive listening devices such as telephone amplifiers. See **auditory verbal therapy.**

auramine /ôr″əmēn/, **1.** a yellow aniline dye used in the manufacture of paints, textiles, and rubber products. Auramine is possibly carcinogenic to humans. Also called **dimethylaniline. 2.** auramine O is a fluorescent stain used to identify acid-fast organisms.

auramine O, a fluorescent, yellow aniline dye used as a stain for the tubercle bacillus and for deoxyribonucleic acid (DNA).

auramine-rhodamine stain, a fluorescent dye consisting of auramine O, rhodamine B, and phenol that is used in the fluorochrome acid-fast staining method. The dye binds to mycolic acids in the cell wall of bacteria and resists decolorization with acid alcohol.

auranofin /ôr′ənof″in/, an oral gold disease-modifying antirheumatoid drug.

■ INDICATIONS: It can be prescribed for the treatment of rheumatoid arthritis, but is generally not first-line therapy.

■ CONTRAINDICATIONS: Auranofin is contraindicated for patients who have disorders that are caused by or aggravated by medicines containing gold or who have impaired kidney function.

■ ADVERSE EFFECTS: Among the most severe adverse effects are diarrhea, loose stools, abdominal pain, nausea, vomiting, rash, pruritus, stomatitis, anemia, leukopenia, granulocytopenia, thrombocytopenia, eosinophilia, proteinemia, hematuria, and elevated liver enzyme levels.

aurantiasis cutis /ôr′əntī″əsis/ [L, *aurantium,* orange; Gk, *osis,* condition; L, *cutis,* skin], a yellowish skin pigmentation that results from eating excessive amounts of foods containing carotene, such as carrots.

auras. See **aura.**

auriasis, skin discoloration resulting from treatment using gold salts. See **chrysiasis.**

auricle /ôr″ikəl/ [L, *auricula,* little ear], **1.** the external ear. Also called **pinna, ala auris. 2.** a small, cone-shaped pouch that extends from the upper and front part of the left or right cardiac atrium, so named because of its earlike shape. Also called *atrial appendix.*

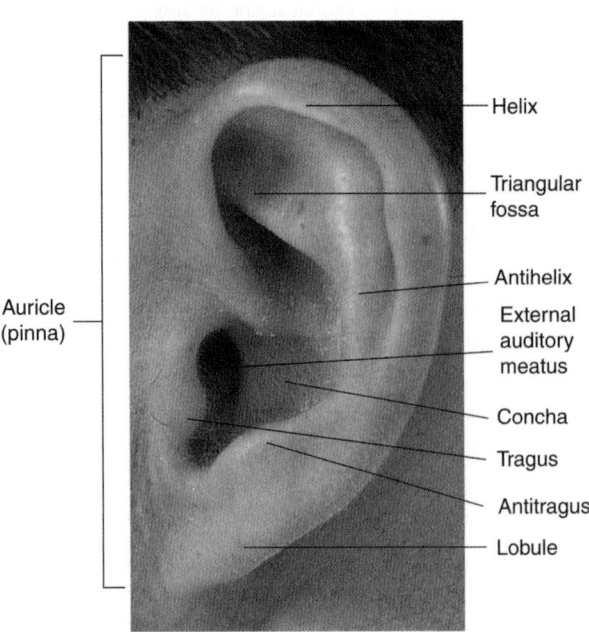

Auricle *(Wilson and Giddens, 2013)*

auricular /ôrik″yələr/, **1.** pertaining to the auricle of the ear. **2.** See **otic.**

auricular acupuncture, acupuncture performed using points on the ear that have been mapped to specific anatomical areas of the body.

auricular cervical nerve reflex. See **Snellen's reflex.**

auricularis anterior, one of three extrinsic muscles of the ear. It functions to move the auricula forward and upward. Some people can voluntarily contract the auricularis anterior to move the ears. Compare **auricularis posterior, auricularis superior.**

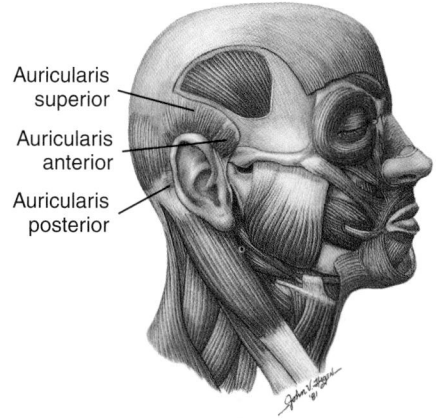

Auricularis
superior

Auricularis
anterior

Auricularis
posterior

Auricularis anterior, auricularis posterior, and auricularis superior *(Thibodeau and Patton, 2003)*

auricularis posterior, one of three extrinsic muscles of the ear. It serves to draw the auricula backward. Compare **auricularis anterior, auricularis superior.**

auricularis superior, a thin, fan-shaped muscle that is one of three extrinsic muscles of the ear. It acts to draw the auricula upward. Compare **auricularis anterior, auricularis posterior.**

auricular line, a hypothetical line passing through the external auditory meatuses and perpendicular to the Frankfort horizontal plane.

auricular point, the center of the external auditory meatus.

auricular tachycardia. See **atrial tachycardia.**

auricular tubercle, a small projection sometimes found on the edge of the helix of the ear. Also called *darwinian tubercle,* **Darwin's tubercle.**

auriculin /ôrik″yəlin/, a hormonelike substance with diuretic activity produced in the atria of the heart.

auriculocranial /-krā″nē·əl/, pertaining to the auricle of the ear and the cranium.

auriculotemporal /-tem″pərəl/, pertaining to the auricle of the ear and the temporal area of the skull.

auriculoventriculostomy /ôrik′yəlōventrik″yəlos″təmē/ [L, *auricula + ventriculus,* little belly; Gk, *stoma,* opening], a surgical procedure that directs cerebrospinal fluid into the general circulation in the treatment of hydrocephalus, usually in the newborn. In this procedure a polyethylene tube is passed from the lateral ventricle through a burr hole in the parietal skull area under the scalp and into the jugular vein, right atrium, superior vena cava, or abdomen for the discharge of cerebrospinal fluid. The tube, which has valves, is inserted to prevent reflux of the blood into the ventricles and to maintain the draining of excess cerebrospinal fluid when ventricular pressure increases. This procedure is performed to correct the communicating and the obstructive forms of hydrocephalus. Also called **ventriculoatrial shunt, ventriculoatriostomy.**

auris dextra (a.d.), the Latin term for right ear.

auris sinistra (a.s.), the Latin term for left ear.

aurothioglucose /ôr′ōthī′ōgloo″kōs/, an organic gold compound used as a disease-modifying antirheumatoid drug.

■ INDICATIONS: It is prescribed for adjunctive treatment of adult and juvenile rheumatoid arthritis, but generally no longer considered first-line therapy.

■ CONTRAINDICATIONS: Severe uncontrolled diabetes, renal or hepatic dysfunction, a history of infectious hepatitis, hypertension, heart failure, systemic lupus erythematosus, agranulocytosis, hemorrhagic diathesis, pregnancy, urticaria, eczema, colitis, or known hypersensitivity to this drug prohibit its use.

■ ADVERSE EFFECTS: Among the most serious adverse effects are kidney and liver damage and allergic reactions. Dermatitis and lesions of mucous membranes are common.

auscultate /ôs″kəltāt/ [L, *auscultare,* to listen], to practice auscultation, or to listen and interpret sounds produced within the body.

auscultation /ôs′kəltā″shən/ [L, *auscultare,* to listen], the act of listening for sounds within the body to evaluate the condition of the heart, blood vessels, lungs, pleura, intestines, or other organs or to detect the fetal heart sound. Auscultation may be performed directly with the unaided ear, but most commonly a stethoscope is used to determine the frequency, intensity, duration, and quality of the sounds. *—auscultatory, adj.,* **—auscultate,** *v.*

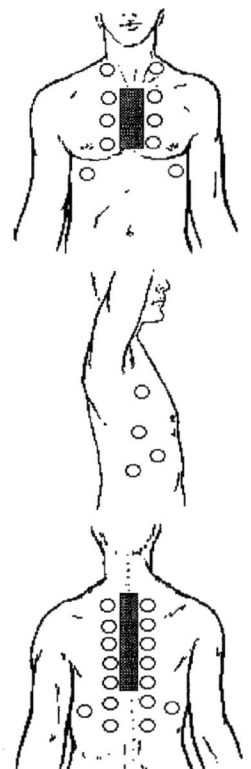

Normal location for auscultation of bronchovesicular breath sounds *(Magione, 2008)*

auscultatory gap, time in which sound is not heard in the auscultatory method of measuring blood pressure with a sphygmomanometer, occurring particularly in hypertension and in aortic stenosis.

Austin Flint murmur [Austin Flint, American physiologist, 1812–1886], a low-pitched sound characteristic of severe aortic regurgitation without mitral valve disease. It is typically heard during ventricular middiastole at the mitral valve area. It is caused by premature closure of the mitral valve by the jet of aortic regurgitation. Amyl nitrate may help differentiate this murmur from that of mitral valve stenosis.

Australia antigen, **1.** an envelope antigen known as hepatitis B surface antigen (HBsAg), found in acute or chronic hepatitis B. See also **hepatitis. 2.** a serological marker on the surface of the hepatitis B virus.

Australian lift, a type of shoulder lift used to move a patient who is unable to assume a sitting position on a bed or other surface. The lift is executed by two persons, one on each side of the patient, who place their shoulders near the patient under the patient's axillae. At the same time, the two lifters grasp each other's hands under the patient's thighs and make coordinated movements needed to lift the patient onto or from a bed or wheelchair.

Australian Q fever, a variety of Q fever occurring in Australia. It is enzootic in Australian animals, especially bandicoots (large rats). See also **Q fever.**

autacoid /ô″təkoid/, any one of the substances produced locally by one group of cells that acts locally near its site of synthesis.

authenticity /ô″thəntis″itē/, (in psychiatry) emotional and behavioral openness; a quality of being genuine and trustworthy.

authoritarian personality, a group of behavioral traits characteristic of one who advocates obedience and strict adherence to rules.

authority /ôthôr″ətē/, a relationship between two or more persons or groups characterized by the influence one may exercise over the other through ideas, commands, suggestions, or instructions.

authority figure, a person who by virtue of status, strength, knowledge, or other recognized superiority exerts influence over others.

autism spectrum disorders, a group of disorders characterized by impairment of development in multiple areas, including the acquisition of reciprocal social interaction, verbal and nonverbal communication skills, and imaginative activity, and by stereotyped interests and behaviors. Also called **pervasive developmental disorders.** Kinds include **autistic disorder, Rett's syndrome, childhood disintegrative disorder.**

autistic disorder /ôtis″tik/ [Gk, *autos,* self], a pervasive developmental disorder with onset in infancy or childhood, characterized by impaired social interaction, impaired communication, and a remarkably restricted repertoire of activities and interests. See also **infantile autism.** *–autistic, adj.*

autistic phase, a period of preoedipal development, according to Mahler's system of personality stages. It lasts from birth to around 1 month and is considered normal. Children then become aware that they cannot satisfy their body needs by themselves.

autistic thought, a form of thinking that is internally stimulated in which the ideas have a private meaning to the individual. Autistic thinking is a symptom in patients with schizophrenia. Fantasy life may be interpreted as reality.

auto-, aut-, prefix meaning "self": *autistic thought.*

autoactivation /-ak″tivā″shən/ [Gk, *autos,* self, *activus,* active], self-activation, as when a gland is stimulated by its own secretions.

autoagglutination /-əgloo″tənā″shən/ [Gk, *autos,* self; L, *agglutinare,* to glue], **1.** The clumping of red blood cells caused by an individual's own serum. Also called **autohemagglutination. 2.** the clumping of certain antigens or antigen-bearing cells, such as bacteria.

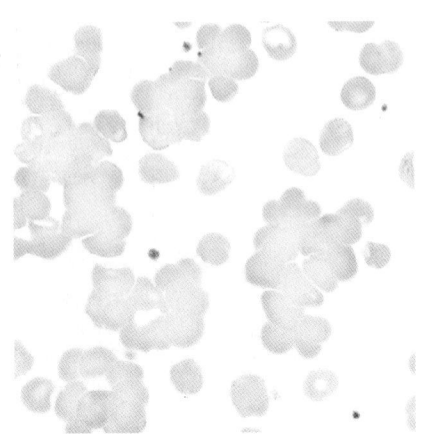

Autoagglutination *(Rodak and Carr, 2013)*

autoamputation /-amp″yŏŏtā″shən/, the spontaneous detachment of a body part, usually the fourth or fifth toe, as occurs among the males of some African peoples. A depression develops across the digitoplantar fold of the toe and gradually progresses until the toe falls off. The condition is usually painless and has no other symptoms. Also called **ainhum.**

autoantibody /ô″tō·an″tibod′ē/ [Gk, *autos + anti,* against; AS, *bodig,* body], an immunoglobulin produced by a person that recognizes an antigen on that person's own tissues. Several mechanisms may trigger the production of autoantibodies: an antigen, formed during fetal development and then sequestered, may be released as a result of infection, chemical exposure, or trauma, as occurs in autoimmune thyroiditis, sympathetic uveitis, and aspermia; there may be disorders of immune regulatory or surveillance function; antibodies produced against certain streptococcal antigens during infection may cross-react with myocardial tissue, causing rheumatic heart disease, or with glomerular basement membrane, causing glomerulonephritis; and normal body proteins may be converted to autoantigens by chemicals, infectious organisms, or therapeutic drugs. Some examples of autoantibodies are those found against gastric parietal cells in pernicious anemia, against platelets in autoimmune thrombocytopenia, and against antigens on the surface of erythrocytes in autoimmune hemolytic anemia. There is growing evidence that genetic factors increase the incidence and severity of autoimmune diseases.

autoantigen /ô″tō·an″tijin/ [Gk, *autos + anti,* against, *genein,* to produce], an endogenous body constituent that stimulates an autoimmune reaction. An autoantigen associated with Addison's disease has been identified as the enzyme 17 α-hydroxylase. Also called **self-antigen.** See also **autoantibody, autoimmune disease.**

autoaugmentation /-ôg″məntā″shən/, a surgical procedure in which the detrusor muscle of the bladder is removed, leaving the bladder epithelium otherwise intact.

autoblast /ô″təblast/, **1.** a free-living unicellular microorganism. **2.** an independent cell.

autocatalytic, acceleration of a chemical reaction by one of the products formed during the reaction.

autocatheterization /-kath″ərizā″shən/, the insertion of a catheter by the patient, usually referring to urinary catheterization. See also **self-catheterization.**

autochthonous /ôtok″thənəs/ [Gk, *autos,* self, *chthon,* earth], relating to a disease or other condition that appears to have originated in the part of the body in which it was discovered.

autochthonous idea [Gk, *autos* + *chthon,* earth], an idea that originates in the unconscious and arises spontaneously in the mind, independent of the conscious train of thought.

autoclassis /ôtok″ləsis/ [Gk, *autos,* self, *klassis,* breaking], the rupturing or breaking of a part of the body caused by a force or agent arising from within the body itself.

autoclave /ô″təklāv/, an appliance used to sterilize medical instruments or other objects with steam under pressure.

autocrine /ô″təkrin/, denoting the effect of a hormone on cells that produce it.

autodermic graft. See **autogenous graft.**

autodigestion, a condition in which gastric juices in the pancreas or stomach digest the organ's own tissues.

autodiploid /ô″tōdip″loid/ [Gk, *autos* + *diploos,* double, *eidos,* form], **1.** an individual, organism, strain, or cell containing two genetically identical or nearly identical chromosome sets that are derived from the same ancestral species and result from the duplication of the haploid set. **2.** also pertaining to such an individual, organism, strain, or cell. Compare **allodiploid, allopolyploid, autopolyploid.** –*autodiploidy, n.*

autoeroticism /-irot″əsiz′əm/ [Gk, *autos* + *eros,* self-love], **1.** sensual, sexual gratification of the self, usually obtained through the stimulus of one's own body without the participation of another person. It is derived from such acts as stroking, masturbation, and fantasy or from other oral, anal, or visual sources of stimulation. **2.** sexual feeling or desire occurring without any external stimulus. **3.** (in Freudian psychoanalytic theory) an early phase of psychosexual development, occurring in the oral and the anal stages. Compare **heteroeroticism.** –*autoerotic, adj.*

autoerythrocyte sensitization /ô′tō-ərith″rəsīt/ [Gk, *autos* + *erythros,* red, *kytos,* cell], a disorder characterized by recurrent spontaneous, painful bruising in patients with underlying psychosis and neurosis. Autoimmune hemolytic anemia, an extreme example of the condition, may cause fulminant hemolysis, fever, abdominal pain, hyperbilirubinemia, thrombosis, and shock.

autoerythrocyte sensitization syndrome. See **Gardner-Diamond syndrome.**

autogamy. /aw-togxə-me-/ [auto- + Gr. gamos marriage], a form of self-fertilization seen in some ciliate protozoa and plants.

autogenesis /ô″tōjen″əsis/ [Gk, *autos* + *genein,* to produce], **1.** abiogenesis. **2.** a self-produced condition; a condition originating from within the organism. Also called **autogeny.** Compare **heterogenesis, homogenesis.** –*autogenic, autogenetic, adj.*

autogenic therapy /-jen″ik/, a mental health therapy introduced by Wolfgang Luthe. It is based on the concept that natural forces in the brain are able to remove disturbing influences so that functional harmony can be restored in the mind and body. It was developed from research on sleep and hypnosis and involves biofeedback exercises.

autogenous /ôtoj″ənəs/, **1.** self-generating. **2.** originating from within the organism, as a toxin or vaccine.

autogenous graft [Gk, *autos,* self, *genein,* to produce, *graphion,* stylus], a skin graft transplanted from one site to another in the same individual.

autogenous vaccine [Gk, *autos,* self, *genein,* to produce; L, *vacca,* cow], a vaccine prepared from cultures of an infectious agent taken from the patient to be treated.

autogeny. See **autogenesis.**

autograft /ô″təgraft′/ [Gk, *autos* + *graphion,* stylus], surgical transplantation of any tissue from one part of the body to another location in the same individual. Autografts are used in several kinds of plastic surgery, most commonly to replace skin lost in severe burns. Compare **allograft, isograft, xenograft.** See also **graft.**

autographism, a skin condition characterized by wheals that develop from tracing on the skin with the fingernail or a blunted instrument. This condition makes the patient itch and may be associated with urticaria. Also called **dermatographia, Ebbecke's reaction.**

autohemagglutination. See **autoagglutination.**

autohemolysis /-hēmol″isis/ [Gk, *autos,* self, *haima,* blood, *lysein,* to loosen], the destruction of erythrocytes by hemolytic agents found in an individual's own blood.

autohexaploid, autohexaploidic. See **autopolyploid.**

autohypnosis [Gk, *autos, hypnos,* sleep], the self-induction of hypnosis by an individual who concentrates on one subject to attain an altered state of consciousness. It may also occur in a person who has become habituated to the process by undergoing hypnosis a number of times.

autoimmune /-imyo͞on″/ [Gk, *autos* + L, *immunus,* exempt], pertaining to an immune response to one's own tissues. See also **autoimmune disease.**

autoimmune disease, one of a large group of diseases characterized by altered function of the immune system of the body, resulting in an immune response against the body's own cells. Antigens normally present on the body's cells stimulate the development of autoantibodies which, unable to distinguish those antigens from external antigens, act against the body's cells to cause localized and systemic reactions. These reactions can affect almost any cell or tissue and cause a variety of diseases, including systemic lupus erythematosus (SLE) and autoimmune thyroiditis. Some autoimmune disorders, such as Hashimoto's disease, are tissue specific, whereas others, such as SLE, affect multiple organs and systems. Both genetic and environmental triggers may contribute to autoimmune disease. About 5% to 8% of the U.S. population is affected by an autoimmune disease. Most autoimmune diseases occur in women.

■ OBSERVATIONS: The manifestations and clinical characteristics depend on the specific disease and on the organ or organ systems affected. See specific diseases.

■ INTERVENTIONS: Therapy includes corticosteroid, antiinflammatory, and immunosuppressive drugs. Symptoms are treated specifically.

■ PATIENT CARE CONSIDERATIONS: Many autoimmune diseases are characterized by periods of crisis interrupted by periods of remission. During a crisis, the patient may be hospitalized and require extensive nursing care, with relief from pain, applications of heat or cold, range of motion exercises, or assistance in movement and ambulation. It is important also to teach the patient and the family the side effects of the drugs being prescribed and how the drugs are to be taken.

autoimmune polyglandular syndromes. See **polyglandular autoimmune syndromes.**

autoimmune response, an immune response of an organism against its own cells and tissues.

autoimmune theory of aging, a theory of aging that ascribes aging and cell death to preprogrammed decline in T cell function with age. T cells are white blood cells important for immunity. Their decline causes decreased self/nonself recognition, a weakened ability to produce antibodies or to fight infections, and an increased development of infections, tumors, and autoimmune disorders. See also **theories of aging.**

autoimmunity /-imyo͞o″nitē/, an abnormal condition in which the body reacts against constituents of its own tissues. Autoimmunity may result in hypersensitivity and autoimmune disease. See also autoantibody, autoantigen, autoimmune disease.

autoimmunization /-im′yənizā″shən/, the process whereby a person's immune system develops antibodies against one or more of the person's own tissues. See also **autoantibody, autoantigen, autoimmune disease.**

autoinfection, **1.** an infection by disease organisms already present in the body but developing in a different body part. **2.** a reinfection by microbes or parasitic organisms.

autoinfusion /-infyoo″zhən/, a technique for forcing blood from the extremities to the body core by applying bandages or a pressure device. It may be used to control bleeding, increase blood pressure, and, in surgery, to create a relatively bloodless surgical field.

autoinoculation /-inok′yəlā″shən/ [Gk, *autos* + L, *inoculare,* to graft], a secondary infection originating from a focus of infection already present in the body.

autointoxication /-intok′sikā″shən/ [Gk, *autos* + L, *in*; Gk, *toxikon,* poison], a condition of poisoning by substances generated by one's own body, as by toxins resulting from a metabolic disorder.

autokeratoplasty /-ker″ətōplas′tē/, the surgical transfer of corneal tissue from one eye of a patient to repair the cornea of the other.

autokinesia /-kinē″zhə/, voluntary movement.

autolesion /-lē″zhən/, a self-inflicted injury.

Autolet /ô″tōlet/, a trademark for a small, sharp instrument, as a lancet, that is used to obtain a capillary blood specimen.

autologous graft [Gk, *autos, logos, graphion,* stylus], the transfer of tissue from one site to another on the same body.

autologous stem cell transplantation (ASCT), a treatment for advanced or refractory solid tumors, such as neuroblastomas, lymphomas, and Ewing's sarcoma. Stem cells from the bone marrow or blood are withdrawn before high-dose irradiation or chemotherapy that destroys many of the remaining cells; afterwards the removed cells are reinfused to form a new population of blood cells.

autologous transfusion, a procedure in which blood is removed from a donor and stored for a variable period before it is returned to the donor's circulation. It is indicated for surgical procedures in which the likelihood of the need for a transfusion is high.

autolysis /ôtol″isis/, the spontaneous destruction of tissues by intracellular enzymes. It generally occurs in dying or dead cells.

automated external defibrillator (AED), a portable apparatus used in sudden cardiac arrest. It is programmed to provide step-by-step instructions, to analyze cardiac rhythms automatically, and to indicate with a voice prompt when to deliver a defibrillating shock.

automated reagin test (ART), a modification of the rapid plasma reagin (RPR) test for use with automated analyzers. It is used in clinical chemistry.

automatic behavior. See **automatism.**

automatic bladder, involuntary detrusor muscle contraction and urinary sphincter relaxation, resulting in spontaneous voiding, as in infants and children before toilet training. It can also be caused by spinal cord damage. See **reflex bladder.**

automatic implanted cardioverter defibrillator (AICD), a surgically implanted device that automatically detects and corrects potentially fatal arrhythmias.

automatic infiltration detector /ô′təmat″ik/ [Gk, *automatismos,* self-action], a temperature-sensitive device that activates an alarm and automatically stops an IV infusion when the IV fluid passes into tissue. The device detects any cooling of the skin at the IV site, a common sign of infiltration. The detector is usually secured to the skin with tape and attaches by a small cable to the fluid-monitoring circuit of an IV pump.

automaticity /ô′tōmətis″itē/, a property of specialized excitable tissue that allows self-activation through spontaneous development of an action potential, as in the pacemaker cells of the heart.

automatic mallet condenser. See **mechanical condenser.**

automatic speech, speech composed of or containing words or phrases, such as numbers, the alphabet, or greetings, that are overlearned and spoken rotely.

automation /ô′təmā″shən/, use of a machine designed to follow a predetermined sequence of individual operations repeatedly and automatically.

automatism /ôtom″ətiz′əm/ [Gk, *automatismos,* self-action], **1.** (in physiology) involuntary function of an organ system independent of apparent external stimuli, such as the beating of the heart, or dependent on external stimuli but not consciously controlled, such as the dilation of the pupil of the eye. **2.** (in philosophy) the theory that the body acts as a machine and that the mind, whose processes depend solely on brain activity, is a noncontrolling adjunct of the body. **3.** (in psychology) mechanical, repetitive, and undirected behavior that is not consciously controlled, as seen in psychomotor epilepsy, hysterical states, and such acts as sleepwalking.

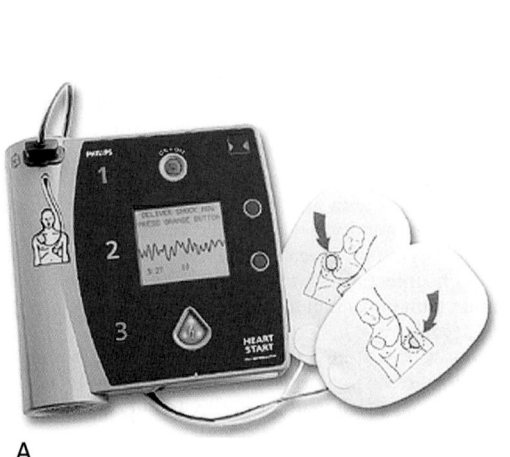
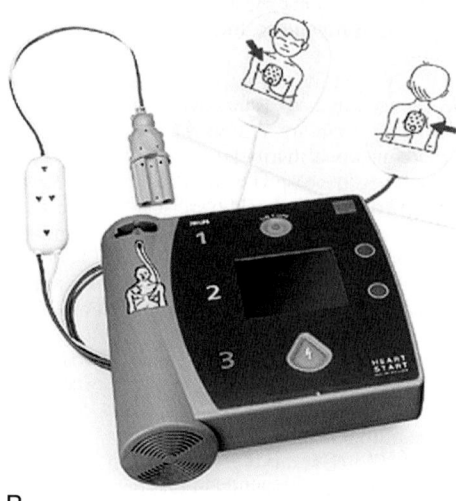

A B

Automated external defibrillator. A, Adult. B, Pediatric. *(Aehlert, 2012)*

Also called **automatic behavior.** Kinds include **ambulatory automatism, command automatism, immediate posttraumatic automatism.**

automnesia /ô′tōmnē″zhə/, the recollection of a previous experience.

autonomic /ô′tənom″ik/ [Gk, *autos + nomos,* law], **1.** having the ability to function independently without outside influence. **2.** pertaining to the autonomic nervous system.

autonomic bronchodilators, a category of drugs with actions that dilate bronchiolar smooth muscle tissue by acting on the autonomic nervous system. Examples include adrenergic drugs, such as albuterol, epinephrine, and salmeterol, and anticholinergic products, such as ipratropium and tiotropium.

autonomic drug, any of a large group of drugs acting in either the sympathetic or parasympathetic nervous system.

autonomic dysreflexia, a syndrome affecting persons with a spinal cord lesion above the midthoracic level (tetraplegics and some paraplegics) that is characterized by hypertension, bradycardia, severe headaches, pallor below and flushing above the cord lesions, and convulsions. It is the result of impaired function of the autonomic nervous system caused by simultaneous sympathetic and parasympathetic activity, such as may occur with bowel or bladder distension pain or a pressure ulcer. It is usually a medical emergency requiring care in an intensive care unit. A cerebrovascular accident and death may occur during an attack. Also called **autonomic hyperreflexia.**

autonomic epilepsy. See **vasomotor epilepsy.**

autonomic ganglion [Gk, *autos,* self, *nomos,* law, *ganglion,* knot], a physical grouping of autonomic neuron cell bodies. It can be near the target organ, as in the parasympathetic division, or more distant, as in the sympathetic division. See also **sympathetic ganglion.**

autonomic hyperreflexia. Also called **autonomic dysreflexia.**

autonomic imbalance [Gk, *autos,* self, *nomos,* law; L, *in,* not, *bilanx,* having two scales], a disruption of a segment of the autonomic nervous system, as in autonomic ataxia.

autonomic nerve [Gk, *autos,* self, *nomos,* law, *neuron,* nerve], a nerve of the autonomic nervous system, which includes both the sympathetic and parasympathetic nervous systems. It possesses the ability to function independently and spontaneously as needed to maintain optimal status of body activities.

autonomic nervous system, the part of the nervous system that regulates involuntary body functions, including the activity of the cardiac muscle, smooth muscles, and glands. It has two divisions, the sympathetic nervous system and the parasympathetic nervous system. The sympathetic component, which is often referred to as the "fight or flight" system, accelerates heart rate, constricts blood vessels, and raises blood pressure. The parasympathetic component, often called the "rest and digest" system, slows heart rate, increases intestinal peristalsis and gland activity, and relaxes sphincters.

autonomic reflex, any of a large number of normal reflexes governing and regulating the functions of the viscera. Autonomic reflexes control such activities of the body as blood pressure, heart rate, peristalsis, sweating, and urination.

autonomous /ôton″əməs/ [Gk, *autos,* self, *nomos,* law], being functionally independent.

autonomous bladder. See **flaccid bladder.**

autonomy /ôton″əmē/ [Gk, *autos + nomos,* law], the quality of having the ability or tendency to function independently. –**autonomous,** *adj.*

autonomy drive, a behavioral trait characterized by the attempt of an individual to master the environment and to impose his or her purposes on it.

auto-PEEP /aw′to-pēp″/. See **intrinsic positive end-expiratory pressure.**

autopentaploid, autopentaploidic. See **autopolyploid.**

autophagia /-fā″jə/, **1.** a mental disorder characterized by the biting or eating of one's own flesh, as may occur in Lesch-Nyan syndrome. **2.** the automatic consumption of one's own tissues by fasting or dieting. **3.** the metabolic action of catabolism.

autoplastic maneuver /-plas″tik/, (in psychology) a process that is part of adaptation, involving an adjustment within the self.

autoplasty /ô″təplas′tē/ [Gk, *autos + plassein,* to mold], a plastic surgery procedure in which autografts, or parts of the patient's own tissues, are used to replace or repair body areas damaged by disease or injury.

autoploid /ô″təploid/, having homologous chromosome sets, or two or more copies of a single haploid set.

autopodium /-pō″dē·əm/, the distal major subdivision of a hand or foot.

autopolymerizing resin. See **self-curing resin.**

autopolyploid /ô′tōpol″iploid/ [Gk, *autos + polyploos,* many times, *eidos* form], **1.** an individual, organism, strain, or cell that has more than two genetically identical or nearly identical sets of chromosomes that are derived from the same ancestral species. They result from the duplication of the haploid chromosome set and are referred to as autotriploid, autotetraploid, autopentaploid, autohexaploid, and so on, depending on the number of multiples of the haploid chromosomes they contain. –**autopolyploidy,** *n. autopolyploidic adj.* **2.** pertaining to such an individual, organism, strain, or cell. Compare **allopolyploid.** See also **allodiploid.**

autopolyploidy /ô′tōpol″iploi′dē/, the state or condition of having more than two identical or nearly identical sets of chromosomes. Compare **allopolyploid.**

autopsy /ô″topsē/ [Gk, *autos + opsis,* view], a postmortem examination performed to confirm or determine the cause of death. Also called **necropsy, necroscopy.** –*autopsical, autopsic, adj.,* –*autopsist, n.*

autopsy pathology, the study of disease by the examination of the body after death by a pathologist. The organs and tissues are first described by their appearance at the time of dissection, then by their appearance in the microscopic examination or laboratory analysis of small representative samples of tissue taken for their diagnostic value.

autoregulation [Gk, *autos,* self; L, *regula,* rule], an intrinsic capacity of organs to regulate their own blood flow or metabolic activity. The former process results from the contraction or relaxation of self-excitable smooth muscle, which causes the constriction or dilation of vessels. It allows organs to maintain constant blood flow and meet their metabolic needs despite variations in systemic arterial pressure.

autosensitization /-sen′sətīzā″shən/ [Gk, *autos,* self; L, *sentire,* to feel], the sensitization of an individual by humoral antibodies or by a delayed cellular reaction to substances in his or her own body tissues.

autosepticemia /-sep′tisē″mē·ə/, a systemic infection in which pathogens (microorganisms) are present in the circulating bloodstream, developing from an infection within the body and not introduced from outside the body.

autoserous treatment /ô′təsir″əs/ [Gk, *autos* + L, *serum,* whey], therapy of an infectious disease by inoculating the patient with the patient's own serum.

autosite /ô″təsīt/ [Gk, *autos* + *sitos,* food], the larger, more normally formed member of unequal or asymmetric conjoined twins on whom the other smaller fetus depends for various physiological functions and for nutrition and growth. Compare **parasitic fetus.** –*autositic, adj.*

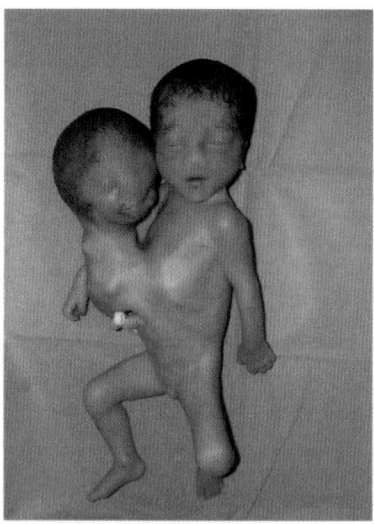

Conjoined fetuses with autosite on right *(Fujimori et al, 2004)*

autosmia /ôtoz″mē·ə/ [Gk, *autos,* self, *osme,* smell], awareness of one's own body odor.

autosomal /ô′təsō″məl/ [Gk, *autos* + *soma,* body], **1.** pertaining to or characteristic of an autosome. **2.** pertaining to any condition transmitted by an autosome.

autosomal-dominant inheritance, a pattern of inheritance in which the transmission of a dominant allele on an autosome causes a trait to be expressed. Males and females are usually affected with equal frequency. If both parents are heterozygous *(Aa),* each of their children has a 50% chance of being heterozygous, a 25% chance of being homozygous for the dominant allele *(AA),* and a 25% chance of being homozygous for the recessive allele *(aa);* children with either of the first two genotypes will express the trait of the dominant allele. If one parent is homozygous for the dominant allele, all of the children will express the trait. Achondroplasia, osteogenesis imperfecta, polydactyly, Marfan syndrome, and some neuromuscular disorders are transmitted through autosomal-dominant inheritance. Compare **autosomal-recessive inheritance.** See also **dominance.**

autosomal inheritance, a pattern of inheritance in which the transmission of traits depends on the presence or absence of certain alleles on the autosomes. The pattern may be dominant or recessive, and males and females are usually affected with equal frequency. The majority of hereditary disorders are the result of a defective gene on an autosome. Kinds include **autosomal-dominant inheritance, autosomal-recessive inheritance.** See also **inheritance.**

autosomal-recessive inheritance, a pattern of inheritance resulting from the transmission of a recessive allele on an autosome. Males and females are usually affected with equal frequency. If both parents are heterozygous *(Aa),* each of their children has a 25% chance of expressing the trait of the recessive allele. If both parents are homozygous recessive (aa), all of the children will express the trait. If one parent is homozygous recessive and the other is homozygous dominant *(AA),* none of the children will express the trait, but all will be carriers *(Aa).* There may be no family history of the trait; it becomes manifest when two carriers have a child who is homozygous recessive. Cystic fibrosis, phenylketonuria, and galactosemia are examples of traits that result from autosomal-recessive inheritance. Compare **autosomal-dominant inheritance.** See also **recessive.**

autosomatognosis /-sō′mətognō″sis/, a phantom sensation that an amputated part of the body is still attached.

autosome /ô″təsōm/, any chromosome that is not a sex chromosome and that appears as a homologous pair in a somatic cell. Humans have 22 pairs of autosomes, which transmit all genetic traits and conditions other than those that are sex-linked. Also called **euchromosome.** Compare **sex chromosome.** –*autosomal, adj.*

autosplenectomy /ô′tōsplinek″təmē/ [Gk, *autos* + *splen,* spleen, *ektomē,* excision], a progressive shrinking of the spleen that may occur in sickle cell anemia. The spleen is replaced by fibrous tissue and becomes nonfunctional.

autosuggestion [Gk, *autos* + L, *suggerere,* to suggest], an idea, thought, attitude, or belief suggested to oneself, often as a formula or incantation, as a means of controlling one's behavior. Compare **suggestion.**

autotetraploid, autotetraploidic. See **autopolyploid.**

autotopagnosia /ô′tōtop′əg·nō″zhə/ [Gk, *autos* + *topos,* place, *a* + *gnosis,* without knowledge], the inability to recognize or localize the various body parts because of organic brain damage. It is associated generally with lesions of the dominant hemisphere and may be an effect of some cases of cerebrovascular accident. It is also characterized by a loss of ability to distinguish left from right, manifested during a neurological examination when the patient is unable to perform a task such as touching the right ear with the left thumb. Retraining involves touching various parts of the patient's body and asking the patient to identify the area touched and by having the patient assemble human figure puzzles. Also called **body image agnosia, body-scheme disorder.** See also **agnosia, proprioception.**

autotoxemia /-toksē″mē·ə/, a form of poisoning caused by substances generated within the body as a result of the pathological alteration of the person's own tissues.

autotoxic, pertaining to autotoxins.

autotransfusion /-transfyoo″zhən/, the collection, anticoagulation, filtration, and reinfusion of blood from an active bleeding site, most commonly a hemothorax. It may be used in cases of major trauma or in major surgery when blood can be collected from a sterile site. Various techniques are used to perform autotransfusion, but the goal is the same—to maintain a sterile field, to prevent clotting of the collected blood, and to safely administer needed blood to the patient.

autotransplantation. See **autograft, autoplasty.**

autotriploid, autotriploidic. See **autopolyploid.**

autovaccination, the use of materials derived from an invading organism or the diseased tissue of an individual.

autozygous /-zī″gəs/, pertaining to genes in a homozygote that are copies of the same ancestral gene as a result of a mating between related individuals.

autumn fever, Now called **leptospirosis.**

aux-. See **auxo-, aux-.**

auxanology /ôks′ənol″əjē/ [Gk, *auxein,* to grow, *logos,* science], the scientific study of growth and development. —*auxanological, adj.*

auxesis, growth from increase in cell size without cell division. See also **hypertrophy.**

auxiliary /ôksil″yərē/ [L, *auxilium,* aid], an individual or group serving in assistive, supporting, or complementary tasks in a clinical setting.

auxiliary enzyme [L, *auxilium,* assist], an enzyme that links the enzyme being measured with an indicator enzyme. It is a component of the coupled assay system.

auxiliary storage, a storage device for adding to the main storage of the computer, using such media as external hard drives, compact disks, USB flash drives, DVDs, or tapes.

auxo-, aux-, prefix meaning "growth," "acceleration," or "stimulation": *auxesis.*

auxotonic /ôk′sōton″ik/, pertaining to muscle contractions that increase in force as the muscle shortens.

auxotox [Gk, *auxein,* increase, *toxikon,* poison], a chemical with a particular atomic grouping that, if added to a relatively benign substance, increases the toxic characteristics of the mixture.

AV, **1.** abbreviation for **arteriovenous. 2.** abbreviation for **atrioventricular.**

available arch length /əvā″ləbəl/ [ME, *availen,* to be of use], the length or space in a dental arch that is accessible for all of the natural teeth of an individual. See also **arch length, arch length deficiency, arch width.**

avalvular /āvalv″yələr/ [Gk, *a,* without; L, *valva,* valve], pertaining to an absence of one or more valves.

Avandia, an oral antidiabetic medication. Brand name for **rosiglitazone.**

avascular /āvas″kyələr/ [Gk, *a,* without; L, *vasculum,* vessel], **1.** pertaining to a tissue area that is not receiving a sufficient supply of blood. The reduced supply may be the result of blockage by a blood clot or of the deliberate stoppage of flow during surgery or during control of a hemorrhage. **2.** pertaining to a kind of tissue that does not have blood vessels.

avascular graft [Gk, *a,* without; L, *vasculum,* vessel; Gk, *graphion,* stylus], a tissue graft in which there is no infiltration of blood vessels.

avascularization [Gk, *a,* without; L, *vasculum,* vessel], a diversion of blood flow away from tissues.

avascular necrosis, the deterioration and death of tissue due to the absence of a blood supply. See **coagulation necrosis.**

Avastin, an angiogenesis inhibitor. Brand name for **bevacizumab.**

AVB, abbreviation for **atrioventricular block.**

average, (in mathematics) a value established by dividing the sum of a series by the number of its units.

aversion therapy /əvur″zhən/ [L, *aversus,* a turning away], a form of behavior therapy in which punishment or unpleasant or painful stimuli, such as electric shock or drugs that induce nausea, are used to suppress undesirable behavior. The procedure is used in treating such conditions as drug abuse, alcoholism, gambling, overeating, smoking, and various sexual deviations. Also called **aversive stimulus.** See also **behavior therapy.**

aversive stimulus /əvur″siv/, an undesirable stimulus, such as electric shock, that causes psychic or physical pain. See also **aversion therapy.**

avian influenza /ā″vē·ən/, a highly contagious viral disease of birds caused by an influenza A virus; it occurs in both mild and severe forms. The severe form is highly pathogenic and can result in a mortality rate for birds that can reach 90% to 100% within 48 hours. It may be transmitted to humans through contact with bird droppings or surfaces contaminated by them or through intermediate hosts such as pigs. Person-to-person transmission appears to be rare. Symptoms of avian influenza in humans range from typical influenza-like symptoms to eye infections, pneumonia, acute respiratory distress, and other severe and life-threatening complications. The only means of control when avian influenza has been observed in a flock of domestic fowl is destruction of infected birds and disinfection of the farm. Also called **bird flu.**

avian tuberculosis, a strain of tuberculosis in birds, caused by *Mycobacterium avium.* Birds consistently shed large amounts of the bacteria into the environment via feces. The organism is also pathogenic in humans and is especially problematic in the immunocompromised.

aviation medicine /āv′ē·ā″shən/, a branch of medicine that is concerned with the health effects of travel by aircraft, including such aspects as jet lag, restricted body movement for long periods, and reaction to violent aircraft movement in turbulent weather. See also **aerospace medicine, aviation physiology.**

aviation physiology, a branch of physiology that is concerned with the effects on humans and animals exposed for long periods to pressurized cabins, weightlessness, disturbances of biological rhythms, acceleration, and mental functions under stressful flying conditions.

avidin, a glycoprotein used in biotin function studies.

avidity /avid″itē/ [L, *avidus,* eager], an inexact measure of the binding strength of antibodies to multiple antigenic determinants on natural antigens.

A-V interval [L, *intervallum,* space between ramparts], the time between an atrial polarization and the next ventricular polarization. In a surface electrocardiogram, the A-V interval is the time between the beginning of the P wave and the beginning of the QRS complex. A normal interval is less than 200 msec. In His bundle electrograms (HBEs), the A-V interval is the time between the A wave and the V deflection. The A wave is the first deflection on the HBE and represents low right atrial activation. The V deflection is the last deflection on the HBE and represents ventricular activation; it is concurrent with the QRS complex on a surface electrocardiogram. Prolongation of this interval is known as first-degree heart block.

avirulent /āvir″yələnt/ [Gk, *a,* not; L, *virus,* poison], the inability of an agent to produce pathologic effects; not pathogenic.

avitaminosis /āvī′təminō″sis/ [Gk, *a,* not; L, *vita,* life, *amine,* chemical, *osis,* condition], a condition resulting from a deficiency of or lack of absorption or use of one or more dietary vitamins. Also called **hypovitaminosis.** Compare **hypervitaminosis.** See also *specific vitamins.*

AV nicking, a vascular abnormality in the retina of the eye, visible on ophthalmological examination, in which a vein is compressed by an arteriovenous crossing. The vein appears "nicked" as a result of constriction or spasm. It is a sign of hypertension, arteriosclerosis, or other vascular conditions.

avobenzone /av″o-ben′zōn/, a sunscreen that absorbs light in the UVA range.

Avogadro's constant /av′ogad″rōz/ [Amedeo Avogadro, Italian physicist, 1776–1856]. See **Avogadro's number.**

Avogadro's law [Amedeo Avogardo, Italian scientist 1776–1856], a natural law stating that equal volumes of all gases at a given temperature and pressure contain the same number of molecules.

Avogadro's number *(N$_A$)*, the number of atoms in exactly 12 g of the isotope of carbon ^{12}C, or 6.02×10^{23}. One mole of any monoatomic element contains this number of atoms and one mole of any polyatomic element or molecule contains this number of molecules.

avoidance [ME, *avoiden,* to empty], (in psychiatry) a conscious or unconscious defense mechanism, physical or psychological, by which an individual tries to avoid or escape from unpleasant stimuli, conflicts, or feelings, such as anxiety, fear, pain, or danger.

avoidance-avoidance conflict, a conflict resulting from the confrontation of two or more alternative goals or desires that are equally aversive and undesirable. Also called **double-avoidance conflict.** See also **conflict.**

avoidance conditioning, the establishment of certain patterns of behavior to avoid unpleasant or painful stimuli.

avoidant personality, a personality disorder characterized by hypersensitivity to rejection and a reluctance to start a relationship because of a fear of not being accepted uncritically. The person has a strong desire for affection and acceptance and may be distressed by an inability to relate comfortably with others.

avoirdupois weight /av′ərdəpoiz″/ [OF, *avoir de pois,* to have weight], the English system of weights in which there are 7000 grains, 256 drams, or 16 ounces to 1 pound. One ounce in this system equals 28.35 g, and 1 pound equals 453.59 g. Compare **apothecaries' weight.** See also **metric system.**

Avonex, an agent with antiviral and immunomodulatory properties used to treat multiple sclerosis. Brand name for **interferon beta-1a.**

avulse. See **avulsion.**

avulsed tooth /əvulst/ [L, *avulsio,* a pulling away], a tooth that has been forcibly and traumatically displaced from its normal position, usually completely forced from its alveolus. In some cases, if attended to early, it can be surgically reimplanted. Also spelled **evulsed tooth.** See also **avulsion.**

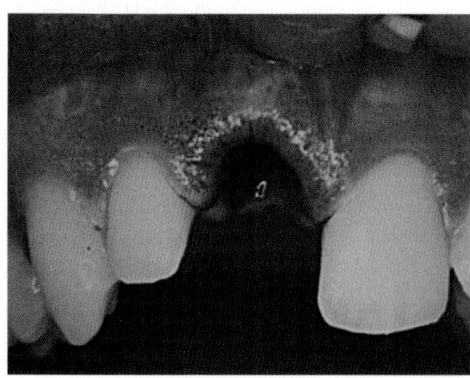

Avulsed tooth *(Adams, 2008)*

avulsion /əvul″shən/ [L, *avulsio,* a pulling away], the separation, by tearing, of any part of the body from the whole. **–avulse,** *v.*

avulsion fracture, a fracture caused by the tearing away of a fragment of bone where a strong ligamentous or tendinous attachment forcibly pulls the fragment away from osseous tissue.

AWHONN, a group focused on the health of women and newborns, which includes delivery of advocacy, research, information, and publications to improve the quality and delivery of health. Abbreviation for **Association of Women's Health, Obstetric, and Neonatal Nurses.**

axenic culture, a pure culture of microorganisms; one free from contaminating microorganisms or, in the case of parasites, without the presence of the host.

axetil, contraction for L-*acetoxyethyl.*

axi-, axio-, axo-, prefix meaning "axis": *axial, axolysis.*

axial (A) /ak″sē·əl/ [Gk, *axon,* axle], **1.** pertaining to or situated on the axis of a body structure or part. **2.** (in dentistry) relating to the long principal structure of a tooth.

axial current, the central part of the bloodstream in an artery.

axial gradient, **1.** the variation in metabolic rate in different parts of the body. **2.** the development toward the body axis or its parts in relation to the metabolic rate in the various parts.

axial illumination, standard light transmission path in a compound light microscope. The operator focuses light from the substage source onto the specimen using the field diaphragm and movable condenser. The light then enters the objective lens and the image is magnified. See also **illumination.**

axial neuritis. See **parenchymatous neuritis.**

axial resolution, the ability of an ultrasound system to discern and display two objects lying along the axis of an ultrasound beam.

axial skeleton [L, *axis,* axle; Gk, *skeletos,* dried up], the bones forming the axis of the skeleton, including the skull, vertebrae, ribs, and sternum. Compare **appendicular skeleton.**

axial spillway, a groove that crosses a cusp ridge or a marginal ridge and extends onto a long surface of a tooth. Compare **interdental spillway, occlusal spillway.**

axifugal /aksif″yəgəl/ [L, *axis,* axle, *fugere,* to flee], extending away from an axis or axion. Also called **axofugal.** Compare **centrifugal.**

axilla /aksil″ə/ *pl.* **axillae** [L, wing], a pyramid-shaped space forming the underside of the shoulder between the upper arm and the side of the chest. Also called **armpit.** –*axillary, adj.*

axillary artery [L, *axilla,* wing], one of a pair of continuations of the subclavian arteries that starts at the outer border of the first rib and ends at the distal border of the teres major, where it becomes the brachial artery. It has three parts and six branches, supplying various chest and arm muscles.

axillary block anesthesia. See **brachial plexus anesthesia.**

axillary dissection. See **axillary node dissection.**

axillary line, an imaginary vertical line on the body wall passing through a point midway between the anterior and posterior folds of the axilla.

axillary nerve, one of the last two branches of the posterior cord of the brachial plexus before the posterior cord becomes the radial nerve. It divides into a posterior branch and an anterior branch. The posterior branch innervates the teres minor, part of the deltoideus, and part of the skin overlying the deltoideus; the anterior branch innervates the deltoideus. Some fibers of the nerve also supply the capsule of the shoulder joint.

axillary node, one of the lymph glands of the axilla that help fight infections in the chest, armpit, neck, and arm and drain lymph from those areas. The 20 to 30 axillary nodes are divided into the lateral group, the anterior group, the posterior group, the central group, and the medial group. See also **lymphatic system, lymph node.**

axillary node dissection, surgical removal of axillary lymph nodes through an incision in the axilla. It is often a component of a modified radical mastectomy for women with invasive breast cancer. It may be done at the same time or after a lumpectomy. Also called **axillary dissection.**

axillary region, the area of the upper chest surrounding the axilla, lateral to the pectoral region.

axillary temperature [L, *axilla,* wing, *temperatura*], the body temperature as recorded by a thermometer placed in the axilla. The reading is generally 0.5° to 1° F less than the oral temperature.

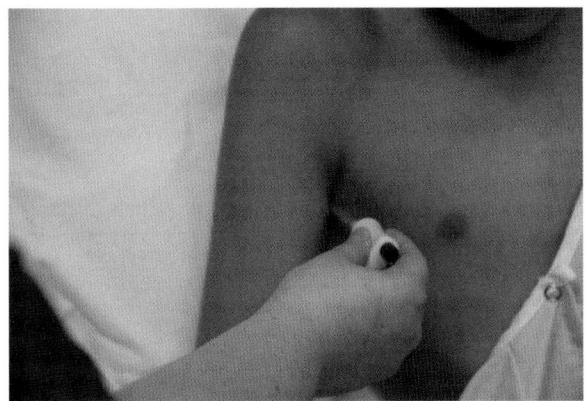

Monitoring axillary temperature

axillary vein, one of a pair of veins of the upper limb that becomes the subclavian vein at the outer border of the first rib. It receives deoxygenated blood from the venous tributaries. Compare **subclavian vein.**

axillary walls, the four walls of the axilla. The anterior wall is formed by the lateral part of the pectoralis major muscle, the pectoralis minor and subclavius muscles, and the clavipectoral fascia. The medial wall is formed by the upper thoracic wall and the serratus anterior muscle. The lateral wall is formed entirely by the intertubercular sulcus of the humerus. The posterior wall is formed by the costal surface of the scapula, the subscapularis muscle, the distal parts of the latissimus dorsi and teres major muscles, and the proximal part of the long head of the triceps brachii muscle.

axillofemoral bypass graft /ak′silōfem″ərəl/, a procedure in which a synthetic artery or a vein is surgically anastomosed between the axillary and common femoral arteries in cases of peripheral arterial insufficiency. The graft shunts blood between those arteries, increasing blood flow to the lower extremities.

axio-. See **axi-, axio-, axo-.**

axion /ak″sē·on/, **1.** the brain and spinal cord. **2.** the cerebrospinal axis.

axioplasm. See **axoplasm.**

axis /ak″sēz/ *pl.* **axes** [Gk, *axon,* axle], **1.** (in anatomy) a line that passes through the center of the body, or a part of the body, such as the frontal axis, binauricular axis, and basifacial axis. **2.** the second cervical vertebra, about which the atlas rotates, allowing the head to be turned, extended, and flexed. Also called **epistropheus, odontoid vertebra.**

axis artery, one of a pair of extensions of the subclavian arteries running into and supplying the upper limb, continuing into the forearm as the palmar interosseous artery.

axis cylinder. See **axon.**

axis deviation, an electrocardiogram trace in which the QRS axis of the heart in the frontal plane lies outside the usual range of −30–110 degrees. It represents an abnormal direction of ventricular depolarization.

axis traction, the process of assisting labor by applying traction to the fetal head with obstetrical forceps following the curve of Carus through the mother's birth canal. See also **forceps.**

axo-, a combining term referring to *axis* or *axion.*

axoaxonic synapse /ak′sō-akson″ik/ [Gk, *axon,* axle (to), *axon,* axle], a synapse in which the axon of one neuron comes into contact with the axon of another neuron.

axodendritic synapse /-dendrit″ik/ [Gk, *axon* + *dendron,* tree], a synapse in which the axon of one neuron comes into contact with the dendrites of another neuron.

axodendrosomatic synapse /-den′drōsōmat″ik/, a synapse in which the axon of one neuron comes into contact with both the dendrites and the cell body of another neuron.

axofugal. See **axifugal.**

axolysis /aksol″isis/, the degeneration of the axon of a nerve cell.

axon /ak″son/ [Gk, axle], an extension, usually long and slender, of a neuron capable of conducting action potentials or self-propagating nervous impulses. Axons can conduct impulses over great distances away from the cell body. Only ends of axons (terminals) can release neurotransmitters and stimulate other neurons/effectors. Compare **dendrite.** See also **action potential, neurotransmitter.**

axon flare, vasodilation, reddening, and increased sensitivity of the skin surrounding an injured area, caused by an axon reflex. It is considered part of a triple response in which injury or stroking of the skin results in local reddening, the release of histamine or a histamine-like substance, a surrounding flare, and wheal formation. A pinprick in the involved area causes more intense pain than a similar stimulus before injury.

axonography /ak′sonog″rəfē/, the recording of electrical activity in the axon of a nerve cell. Also called **electroaxonography.**

axonotmesis /ak′sənotmē″sis/ [Gk, *axon* + *temnein,* to cut], an interruption of the axon from nerve injury, with subsequent wallerian degeneration of the distal nerve segment. Connective tissue of the nerve, including the Schwann cell basement membranes, may remain intact.

axon reflex [Gk, *axon,* axle], a neuron reflex in which an afferent impulse travels along a nerve fiber away from the cell body until it reaches a branching, where it is diverted to an end organ without entering the cell body. It does not involve a complete reflex arc, and therefore it is not a true reflex.

axon sheath [Gk, *axon* + AS, *scaeth*], a laminated myelin sheath that is interrupted at intervals by nodes of Ranvier.

axoplasm /ak″sōplaz″əm/, cytoplasm of an axon that encloses the neurofibrils.

axoplasmic flow /ak′sōplaz″mik/ [Gk, *axon* + *plassein,* to shape], the continuous pulsing, undulating movement of the cytoplasm between the cell body of a neuron, where protein synthesis occurs, and the axon fiber to supply it with the substances vital for the maintenance of activity and for repair. The nerve fiber depends totally on the cell body for metabolites, and any interruption in the axoplasmic flow caused by disease or trauma results in the degeneration of the unsupplied areas of the axon.

axosomatic synapse /ak′sōsōmat″ik/ [Gk, *axon* + *soma,* body], a synapse in which the axon of one neuron comes into contact with the cell body of another neuron.

axotomy /ak″sot″əmē/, a nerve fiber procedure in which there is a surgical transection or severing of an axon.

Ayres, A. Jean [American occupational therapist and developmental psychologist, 1920–1989], developed the original theory and intervention techniques of sensory integration based on neuroscience and occupational therapy. Ayres Sensory Integration therapy (ASI) is used by occupational therapy practitioners to treat children and adults who experience difficulty in integrating information from the senses. ASI encompasses the theory, assessment methods, patterns of sensory integration and praxis problems, and intervention concepts, principles, and techniques developed by Ayres. Ayres is credited with expanding on the terms *just-right challenge, adaptive response,* and *praxis* in relation to a child's occupational performance. See also **Ayres Sensory Integration (ASI).**

Ayres Sensory Integration (ASI) [Jean Ayres, contemporary occupational therapist], (in occupational therapy) the theory, assessment methods, intervention concepts, principles, and techniques enhancing the capacity to perceive and organize sensory information to produce a meaningful adaptive response.

Aygestin, an oral progestin. Brand name for *norethindrone acetate.*

ayurveda /ĭ″yər-vaxdə/ [Sanskrit, *ayur,* life, *veda,* science], a form of alternative medicine with Hindu Indian origins, widely used in the Indian health system and increasingly in the Americas. The focus is on promoting health and well-being through traditional ancient cultural methods of health care for the body and mind. Dietary and herbal medicine products are integral to care. Colon cleansing to rid the body of toxins is also a method of care. Lifestyle analysis and change are the cornerstones of the healing process.

azacitidine, an antineoplastic hormone.
- INDICATIONS: This drug is used to treat myelodysplastic syndrome.
- CONTRAINDICATIONS: Pregnancy, advanced malignant hepatic tumors, and known hypersensitivity to this drug or mannitol prohibit its use.
- ADVERSE-EFFECTS: Adverse effects of this drug include anxiety, depression, dizziness, fatigue, headache, cardiac murmur, hypotension, tachycardia, nausea, vomiting, anorexia, constipation, abdominal pain, abdominal distension or tenderness, hemorrhoids, mouth hemorrhage, tongue ulceration, stomatitis, dyspepsia, dysuria, urinary tract infection, ecchymosis, irritation at injection site, rash, sweating, pyrexia, and hypokalemia. Life-threatening side effects include diarrhea, hepatotoxicity, hepatic coma, renal failure, renal tubular acidosis, leukopenia, anemia, thrombocytopenia, and neutropenia.

azatadine maleate /azat″ədēn/, a first-generation antihistamine used topically to treat allergic rhinitis.

azathioprine /az′əthī′ōprēn/, an immunosuppressive.
- INDICATIONS: It is prescribed to prevent organ rejection after transplantation and to treat lupus erythematosus and other systemic inflammatory diseases, such as rheumatoid arthritis, that are unresponsive to other agents.
- CONTRAINDICATIONS: Known hypersensitivity to this drug prohibits its use. It is contraindicated in rheumatoid arthritis and in pregnant women.
- ADVERSE EFFECTS: Among the most serious adverse reactions are bone marrow suppression and hepatotoxicity. Nausea and fever are common.

azelaic acid /az″ĕ-la′ik/, a dicarboxylic acid occurring in whole grains and animal products. It has antibacterial effects on both aerobic and anaerobic organisms, particularly *Propionibacterium acnes* and *Staphylococcus epidermidis*; normalizes keratinization; and has a cytotoxic effect on malignant or hyperactive melanocytes. It is applied topically in the treatment of acne vulgaris.

azelastine, an H1-selective antihistamine that also inhibits leukotriene and platelet-activating factor (PAF) synthesis and release.
- INDICATIONS: This drug is used to treat seasonal allergic rhinitis and seasonal allergic conjunctivitis.
- CONTRAINDICATIONS: Known hypersensitivity, acute asthma attacks, and lower respiratory tract disease prohibit this drug's use.
- ADVERSE EFFECTS: Side effects include sedation (more common with increased doses), increased drowsiness, weight increase, and myalgia.

Azelex /az·ĕ-leks/, a preparation used for treating acne. Brand name for **azelaic acid.**

-azepam, combining form designating a diazepam-type antianxiety agent.

azidothymidine. See **zidovudine.**

Azilect, a monoamine oxidase inhibitor. Brand name for **rasagiline.**

azithromycin, a macrolide antibiotic that suppresses the formation of protein by bacteria, retards bacterial growth, or causes death of the microorganisms. It does not suppress hepatic metabolism of other drugs like the macrolide prototype erythromycin and has a very long half-life, which makes it an appealing therapy against susceptible microorganisms.
- INDICATIONS: It is prescribed in the treatment of mild to moderate infections by certain bacteria in adults, including respiratory tract infections, skin disorders, and sexually transmitted diseases.
- CONTRAINDICATIONS: The drug should not be given to patients with allergies to erythromycin or any macrolide antibiotics or with kidney diseases. Azithromycin should be used with caution in patients with active liver disease.
- ADVERSE EFFECTS: The side effects most often reported include diarrhea, loose stools, nausea, stomach pains, or vomiting.

azo-, az-, prefix meaning "containing nitrogen": *azotemia.*

-azocine, combining form designating a narcotic agonist or antagonist.

azo compounds /ā″zō/ [Fr, *azote,* nitrogen], one of many organic aromatic compounds containing the divalent chromophore, –N═N–. They are produced by the alkaline reduction of nitro compounds among other methods.

azo dye, a type of nitrogen-containing compound used in commercial coloring materials. Some forms of the chemical are potential carcinogens.

azoic /āzō″ik/ [Gk, *a,* not, *zoe,* life], devoid of life.

azole antifungal, any of a group of antifungals characterized by the presence of an azole ring structure, which includes the triazoles and the imidazoles (qq.v.). They are usually fungistatic but can be fungicidal at higher concentrations and act by interfering with the enzyme activity of cytochrome P-450, decreasing the production of ergosterol and so damaging the cell membrane by altering its permeability and functions. Examples include fluconazole and miconazole.

-azoline, combining form designating an antihistaminic or local vasoconstrictor.

azoospermia /āzō′əspur″mē·ə/ [Gk, *a, zoon,* not animal, *sperma,* seed], lack of spermatozoa in the semen. It may be caused by testicular dysfunction, cancer chemotherapy, or blockage of the tubules of the epididymis, or it may be induced by vasectomy. Infertility, but not impotence, is associated with azoospermia. Compare **oligospermia.**

azoprotein /ā′zōpro″tēn/, a protein coupled to another substance through a diazo (–N═N–) linkage. Azoproteins are often used in immunochemical procedures.

Azorean disease, now called **Machado-Joseph disease.**

-azosin, combining form designating a prazosin-type anti-hypertensive agent.

azotemia /az′ōtē″mē·ə/ [Fr, *azote,* nitrogen; Gk, *haima,* blood], retention of excessive amounts of nitrogenous compounds in the blood. This toxic condition is caused by failure of the kidneys to remove urea from the blood and is characteristic of uremia. Also spelled *azotaemia.* See also **uremia.** *−azotemic, adj.*

azoturia /az′ōtŏŏr″ē·ə/ [Fr, *azote,* nitrogen; Gk, *ouron,* urine], an excess of nitrogenous compounds including urea in the urine.

AZT, a nucleoside reverse transcriptase inhibitor for HIV. Also called **azidothymidine, zidovudine.**

Azulfidine /ā zulf œdine/, a sulfonamide antibacterial agent used to treat ulcerative colitis and rheumatoid arthritis. Brand name for **sulfasalazine.**

azure /āz″hər/, one of a group of basic blue methylthionine or phenothiazine dyes used in staining blood and cell nuclei.

azurophil, any substance that is readily stained by an azure blue aniline dye. In laboratory hematology, azurophilic granules appear in certain white blood cells. *−azurophilic, adj.*

azurophilia /āzh′ŏŏrəfil″yə/, a condition in which the blood contains some cells that have granules that stain readily with azure (blue) dye.

azygography /az′īgog″rəfē/, the radiographic imaging of the azygos venous system after injection of a radiopaque contrast medium.

azygos. See **azygous.**

azygospore /az′igəspôr/ [Gk, *a + zygon,* not yoke, *sporos,* seed], a spore that is produced directly from a gamete that has not undergone conjugation, as in certain algae and fungi.

azygous /az″əgəs/ [Gk, *a + zygon,* not yoke], occurring as a single entity or part, such as any unpaired anatomical structure; not part of a pair. Also spelled **azygos.**

azygous lobe, a congenital malformation of the lung caused by a fold of pleural tissue carried by the azygous vein during descent into the thorax during embryonic development. It produces an extra lobe in the right upper lung and may appear on x-ray film as a fissure in the shape of an upside-down comma.

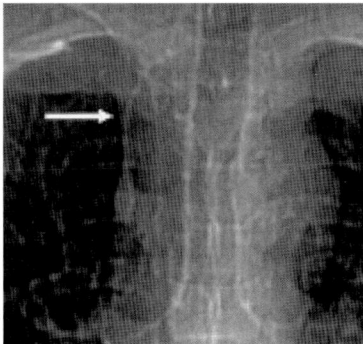

Azygous lobe *(González et al, 2009)*

azygous vein, one of the seven veins of the thorax. Beginning opposite the first or second lumbar vertebra, it rises through the aortic hiatus in the diaphragm and passes to the right of the vertebral column to the fourth thoracic vertebra, then arches ventrally over the root of the right lung, and ends in the superior vena cava. It receives numerous veins, such as the hemiazygous veins, several esophageal veins, and the right bronchial vein. In cases of obstruction to the inferior vena cava it is the principal vein that returns blood to the heart. Compare **internal thoracic vein, left brachiocephalic vein, right brachiocephalic vein.**

A

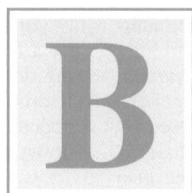

B, symbol for the element **boron.**

B, β. See **beta.**

B6 bronchus sign, an artifact in a lung radiographic image in which an air bronchogram appears in the superior segment of the lower lobe as a result of consolidation, atelectasis, or mass lesion.

B19 virus, a strain of human parvovirus associated with a number of diseases, including hemolytic anemia, erythema infectiosum, fifth disease, and symptoms of arthritis and arthralgia. B19 infects only humans. Approximately 50% of adults have been infected some time during childhood or adolescence. Children infected with erythema infectiosum, the most common illness caused by B19, develop a mild rash, usually across the face, which usually resolves in 7 to 10 days. Postinfection children develop lasting immunity. Infection in adults not previously infected with B19 is usually more severe, involving joint aches and swelling, most often resolving in 2 to 3 weeks.

Ba, symbol for the element **barium.**

BA, **1.** a degree in liberal arts or sciences with specialization in a major. Initialism for *Bachelor of Arts.* **2.** initialism for *blood alcohol.*

babbling, a stage in speech development characterized by the production of strings of speech sounds in vocal play, such as "ba-ba-ba." Kinds include **canonical babbling, integrative babbling.**

Babcock operation [William W. Babcock, American surgeon, 1872–1963], a snarelike surgical procedure for the removal of a varicosed saphenous vein by insertion of an acorn-tipped sound, tying the vein to the sound and drawing it out.

babesiosis /bəbē′sē·ō″sis/ [Victor Babés, Romanian bacteriologist, 1854–1926], a potentially severe and sometimes fatal disease caused by infection with protozoa of the genus *Babesia.* The parasite is introduced into the host through the bite of ticks and infects red blood cells. In the United States, incidence of the disease is highest in the Northeast and North Central regions. Symptoms include headache, fever, chills, vomiting, hepatosplenomegaly, hemolytic anemia, fatigue, myalgia, and hemolysis. Treatment is clindamycin or quinone. Most patients with babesiosis are asymptomatic. Approximately 25% of patients with babesiosis are also infected with Lyme disease. Also called *babesiasis.*

Babinski reflex /bəbin″skē/ [Joseph F.F. Babinski, French neurologist, 1857–1932], dorsiflexion of the big toe with extension and fanning of the other toes elicited by firmly stroking the lateral aspect of the sole of the foot. The reflex is normal in newborns and abnormal in children and adults, in whom it may indicate a lesion in the pyramidal tract or other neurological insult.

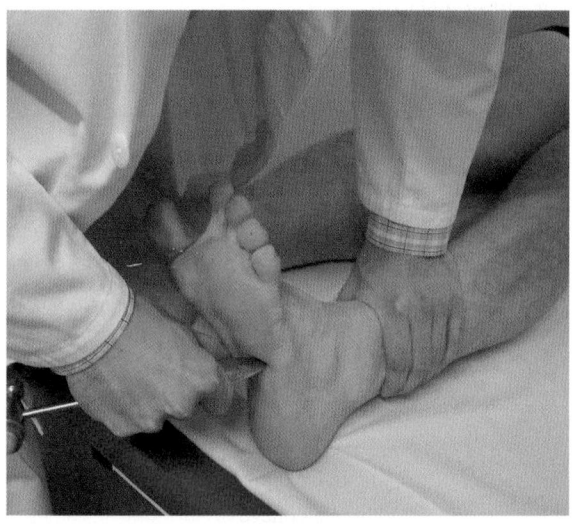

Babinski reflex *(Lehmeyer and Stumpfe, 2009)*

Babinski sign [Joseph Babinski], a series of partial responses that are pathognomonic of different degrees of upper motor neuron disease, including (1) absence of an ankle jerk in sciatica; (2) an extensor plantar response, with an extension of the great toe and adduction of the other toes; (3) a more pronounced concentration of the platysma muscle on the unaffected side during blowing or whistling; (4) pronation that occurs when an arm affected by paralysis is placed in supination; and (5) when a patient in a supine position with arms crossed over the chest attempts to assume a sitting position, the thigh on the affected side is flexed, and the heel is raised, while the leg on the unaffected side remains flat.

Babkin reflex /bab′ kin/, a reflex elicited in many newborn infants in which the infant's mouth opens in response to pressure by the examiner's thumbs on the palms of both hands of the infant. The persistence of the reflex beyond the fifth month of age is generally regarded as abnormal.

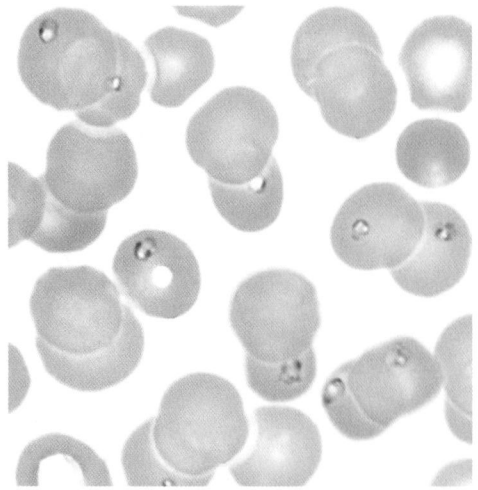

Babesiosis *(Carr and Rodak, 2009)*

baby [ME, *babe*], **1.** *n.*, an infant or young child, especially one who is not yet able to walk or talk. **2.** *v.*, *(Slang)* to treat gently or with special care.

baby bottle caries. See **early childhood caries.**

baby bottle tooth decay. See **early childhood caries**. Formerly called **nursing bottle caries.**

Baby-Friendly Hospital, an international initiative launched by the World Health Organization (WHO) and United Nations Children's Fund (UNICEF) in 1991 designed to support practices that protect, promote, and support breastfeeding in hospitals.

Baby Jane Doe regulations, rules established in 1984 by the U.S. Health and Human Services Department requiring state governments to investigate complaints about parental decisions involving the treatment of handicapped infants. The rules also allowed the federal government to have access to children's medical records and required hospitals to post notices urging physicians and nurses to report any suspected cases of denial of proper medical care to infants. The controversial regulations were found unlawful by a federal court. Nevertheless, regulations still exist that require health care providers to provide treatment for severely handicapped newborns except when death appears inevitable, when treatment merely prolongs inevitable death, or when treatment is considered so futile as to be inhumane. For the most part responsibility for enforcement has been transferred to hospital ethics boards and state child protective services agencies. Also called *Baby Doe rules.*

baby talk, **1.** *(Informal)* the speech patterns and sounds of young children learning to talk, characterized by mispronunciation, imperfect syntax, repetition, and phonetic modifications, such as lisping or stuttering. See also **lallation. 2.** the intentionally oversimplified manner of speech, imitative of young children learning to talk, used by adults in addressing children or pets. **3.** the speech patterns characteristic of regressive stages of various mental disorders, especially schizophrenia.

bacampicillin hydrochloride, a semisynthetic penicillin.
■ INDICATIONS: It is prescribed in the treatment of respiratory tract, urinary tract, skin, and gonococcal infections.
■ CONTRAINDICATIONS: Known sensitivity to this drug or other penicillins prohibits its use.
■ ADVERSE EFFECTS: Among the most serious adverse reactions are hypersensitivity reactions, gastritis, enterocolitis, and transient blood disorders.

Bachelor of Science in Nursing (BSN) /bach″ələr/, an academic degree awarded on satisfactory completion of a 4-year course of study in a college or university. The recipient is eligible to take the national certifying examination to become a registered nurse. A baccalaureate degree is a prerequisite to advancement in nursing education and advancement in many systems and institutions that employ nurses. Compare **Associate Degree in Nursing, diploma program in nursing.**

Bach remedies [Edward Bach, British physician 1886–1936], a set of 38 flower essences formulated to enhance mental or emotional well-being.

bacill-, combining form meaning "rod-shaped bacterium": *bacillemia, bacillosis.*

Bacillaceae /bas′əlā″si·ē/ [L, *bacillum*, small rod], a family of Bacilli of the order Bacillales consisting of gram-positive, rod-shaped cells that can produce cylindric, ellipsoid, or spheric endospores situated terminally, subterminally, or centrally. These cells are chemoheterotrophic and mostly saprophytic, commonly appearing in soil. Some are parasitic on insects and animals and are pathogenic. The family includes the genus *Bacillus,* which is aerobic, and the genus *Clostridium,* which is facultatively anaerobic.

bacillary angiomatosis /bas″əler′ē/, condition of multiple angiomata caused by an infection of Bartonella. The infectious agent is associated with contact with young cats infected with fleas and is also the cause of cat-scratch fever. It is manifested in persons with cellular immunodeficiency, such as human immunodeficiency virus (HIV)–infected patients, as small hemangioma-like lesions of the skin but may also involve the lymph nodes and viscera. The skin lesions are often mistaken for Kaposi's sarcoma. Infection is curable but can be fatal if untreated. Treatments include oral erythromycin, tetracycline, trimethoprim, and rifampicin.

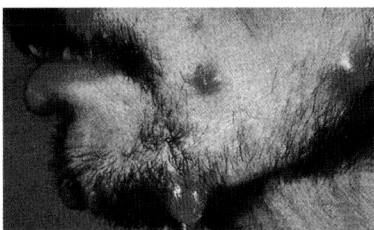

Bacillary angiomatosis *(Stone and Gorbach, 2000)*

bacillary dysentery, *(Obsolete)* now called **shigellosis.**

bacille Calmette-Guérin (BCG) /kalmet″gāran″/ [Léon C.A. Calmette, French bacteriologist, 1863–1933; Camille Guérin, French bacteriologist, 1872–1961], an attenuated strain of the *Mycobacterium bovis* bacillus that is given as a live bacterial vaccine to prevent the development of tuberculosis. It is most often administered intradermally with a multiple-puncture disk. When administered to infants in high-prevalence areas, there is some evidence that it prevents the more serious forms of tuberculosis. It may have some efficacy against leprosy. BCG is also instilled into the bladder as a treatment for bladder cancer to stimulate the immune response in people who have certain kinds of malignancy. It induces a positive tuberculin reaction and may mask early, active infection by removing the diagnostic sign of conversion from the negative to the positive skin reaction. See also **tuberculin test, tuberculosis.**

bacille Calmette-Guérin vaccine, an active immunizing agent prepared from an attenuated bacille Calmette-Guérin strain of *Mycobacterium bovis.*
■ INDICATIONS: It is prescribed most commonly for immunization against tuberculosis. It is instilled intravesically to treat carcinoma in situ of the urinary bladder in certain situations. It is seldom administered in the United States as an immunizing agent but is often given in many countries to infants, caregivers, etc., who are at high risk for intimate and prolonged exposure to people with active tuberculosis.
■ CONTRAINDICATIONS: Hypogammaglobulinemia, immunosuppression, or concomitant use of corticosteroids or isoniazid prohibits its use. It is not given after a vaccination for smallpox, nor is it given to patients with a positive tuberculin reaction or a burn.
■ ADVERSE EFFECTS: Among the most serious adverse reactions are anaphylaxis and disseminated pulmonary tuberculosis. Pain, inflammation, and granuloma may develop at the site of injection.

bacillemia /bas′əlē″mē·ə/, a condition in which bacilli are circulating in the blood. See also **bacteremia, sepsis, septicemia.**

bacilli /bəsil″ī/*sing.* bacillum [L, *bacillum,* small rod], any rod-shaped bacteria. See *Bacillus.*

bacilliform /bəsil″ifôrm/, rod-shaped, like a bacillus.

bacillosis /bas′əlō″sis/, a condition in which bacilli have invaded tissues, inducing symptoms of an infection.

bacillum. See **bacilli.**

bacilluria /bas′əloor″ē·ə/ [L, *bacillum* + Gk, *ouron,* urine], the presence of bacilli in the urine.

Bacillus /bəsil″əs/, **1.** a genus of aerobic, gram-positive, or facultatively anaerobic, spore-forming, rod-shaped microorganism of the family Bacillaceae, order Eubacteriales. The genus includes numerous species and is found in the environment in soil, water, dust, and air. Most species are nonpathogenic but may be pathogenic in immunosuppressed individuals and patients with indwelling devices. Two species, *B. anthracis* and *B. cereus,* are important as agents of disease in humans. Many microorganisms formerly classified as *Bacillus* are now classified in other genera. See also **acid-fast bacillus, Bacillaceae. 2.** any rod-shaped bacteria.

Bacillus anthracis, a species of gram-positive, facultative anaerobe that causes anthrax, a disease primarily of cattle and sheep. The spores of this organism, if inhaled, can cause a pulmonary form of anthrax in humans. When in contact with skin, it causes inflammatory lesions. It can also cause disease when ingested. Spores can live for many years in animal products, such as hides and wool, and in soil. In powdered and aerosol form it has been used as a biological weapon. If detected early enough, *B. anthracis* infections can be stopped by using antibiotics such as ciprofloxacin. See also **anthrax, woolsorter's disease.**

Bacillus cereus, a species of bacilli found in the soil. It causes food poisoning (an emetic type and a diarrheal type) by the formation of an enterotoxin in contaminated foods. The symptoms are similar to those of *Staphylococcus* food poisoning. It can also cause infections, such as ocular infections, and septicemia.

bacitracin /bas′itrā″sin/ [L, *bacillum* + *Tracy,* surname of patient in whom toxin-producing bacillus species was isolated], an antibacterial.
■ INDICATIONS: A common component of topical antibiotic ointments used for treating skin infections.
■ CONTRAINDICATIONS: Known hypersensitivity to this drug prohibits its use.
■ ADVERSE EFFECTS: Skin rash.

back [AS, *baec*], the posterior or dorsal portion of the trunk of the body between the neck and the pelvis. The back is divided by a middle furrow that lies over the tips of the spinous processes of the vertebrae. The skeletal portion of the back includes the thoracic and the lumbar vertebrae and both scapulae. The nerves that innervate the various muscles of the back arise from the segmental spinal nerves.

backache /bak″āk/ [AS, *baec* + ME, *aken*], a pain in the lumbar, lumbosacral, or cervical region of the back, varying in sharpness and intensity. Causes may include muscle strain or other muscular disorders or pressure on the root of a nerve, such as the sciatic nerve, caused in turn by a variety of factors, including a herniated vertebral disk. Treatment may include heat, ultrasound, and devices to provide support for the affected area. Additionally, it may require surgical intervention and medications to relieve pain and relax spasm of the muscle of the affected area.

back-action condenser, an instrument for compacting dental amalgams and other dental materials that has a U-shaped shank, which develops the condensing force from a pulling motion rather than from the more common pushing motions.

backboard, a long, flat, rigid piece of wood or other material that is placed under an accident victim with possible spinal injury. It is used to transport the patient to a hospital or as a firm surface for CPR.

backbone, *(Informal)* the vertebral column.

backcross [AS, *baec* + *cruc,* cross], **1.** a mating (cross) between a heterozygote and a homozygote. **2.** an organism or strain produced by such a cross. See also **testcross.**

backflow /bak′ flō″/, **1.** the flow of liquids in the opposite of the expected direction. **2.** pressure in a vein causing blood to enter an intravenous line. See also **back pressure.**

background level, the usual intensity of a chemical or other stimulus in the environment.

background radiation [AS, *baec* + OE, *grund,* ground], naturally occurring radiation emitted by soil, groundwater, building materials, radioactive substances in the body (especially potassium 40), and cosmic rays from outer space. Each year the average person is exposed to 2.28 millisieverts (mSv) of radon and thoron radiation, 0.21 mSv of external terrestrial radiation, 0.29 mSv of naturally occurring internal radiation, and 0.33 mSv of cosmic radiation. Background radiation levels may vary in different locales.

backing /bak′ing/ [AS, *baec*], **1.** (in dentistry) the piece of metal that supports a porcelain or resin facing on a fixed or removable partial denture. Also called *diatoric.* **2.** the peelable paper on an adhesive dressing that is removed before application.

back pressure [AS, *baec* + L, *premere,* to press], pressure that builds in a vessel or a cavity as fluid accumulates. The pressure increases and extends backward if the normal mechanism for egress or passage of the fluid is not restored. See also **backflow,** def. 2.

backscatter radiation. See **scattered radiation.**

backup, 1. *(Informal)* a duplicate computer, data file, equipment, or procedure for use in the event of equipment failure. **2.** the act of creating another copy of a file, group of files, or an entire computer hard drive.

baclofen, an antispastic agent.
■ INDICATIONS: It is prescribed to reduce the spasticity associated with multiple sclerosis, cerebral palsy, and spinal cord injury; not effective against spasticity caused by stroke.
■ CONTRAINDICATIONS: Known hypersensitivity to this drug prohibits its use.
■ ADVERSE EFFECTS: Among the more serious adverse reactions are confusion, hypotension, dyspnea, impotence, nausea, and transient drowsiness.

-bactam, combining form designating a beta-lactamase inhibitor.

bacter-. See **bacterio-, bacter-, bacteri-.**

bacteremia /bak′tirē″mē·ə/ [Gk, *bakterion,* small staff, *haima,* blood], the presence of bacteria in the blood. Undocumented bacteremias occur frequently and usually abate spontaneously. Bacteremia is demonstrated by blood culture. Antibiotic treatment, if given, is specific for the organism found and appropriate to the locus of infection. If untreated, bacteremia can be fatal. Compare **septicemia.** See also **septic shock.** −*bacteremic, adj.*

bacteremic shock, septic shock caused by the release of toxins by bacteria, usually gram-negative bacteria, in the blood. This causes dangerously low blood pressure, which deprives organs of an adequate blood supply. Bacteremic or septic shock is life-threatening. See **septic shock.**

bacteria /baktir″ē·ə/*sing. bacterium* [Gk, *bakterion,* small staff], a domain of life existing as small unicellular microorganisms. The genera vary morphologically, being spheric (cocci), rod-shaped (bacilli), spiral (spirochetes), or comma-shaped (vibrios). The nature, severity, and outcome of any infection caused by a bacterium are characteristic of that species.

-bacteria, suffix meaning "genus of microscopic plants forming the class Schizomycetes."

bacterial adherence /baktir″ēəl/, the process whereby bacteria attach themselves to cells or other surfaces before proliferating.

bacterial aneurysm, a localized dilation in the wall of a blood vessel caused by the growth of bacteria. It often follows septicemia or bacteremia and usually occurs in peripheral vessels. See also **mycotic aneurysm.**

bacterial cholangitis, the most common type of infection of the biliary tract, caused by bacterial infection. If bacteria invade the liver, they can enter the bloodstream and cause septicemia, which can be fatal.

bacterial count, a quantitive analysis of microbes. See **count.**

bacterial endocarditis, an acute or subacute bacterial infection of the endocardium or the heart valves or both. See also **endocarditis, subacute bacterial endocarditis.**

■ OBSERVATIONS: The condition is characterized by heart murmur, prolonged fever, bacteremia, splenomegaly, and embolic phenomena.

■ INTERVENTIONS: Prompt treatment of both types with antibiotics, such as penicillin, cephalosporin, or gentamicin given intravenously, is essential to prevent destruction of the valves and cardiac failure.

■ PATIENT CARE CONSIDERATIONS: The acute variety progresses rapidly and is usually caused by staphylococci. The subacute variety is usually caused by the lodging of *Streptococcus viridans* in heart valves damaged by rheumatic fever.

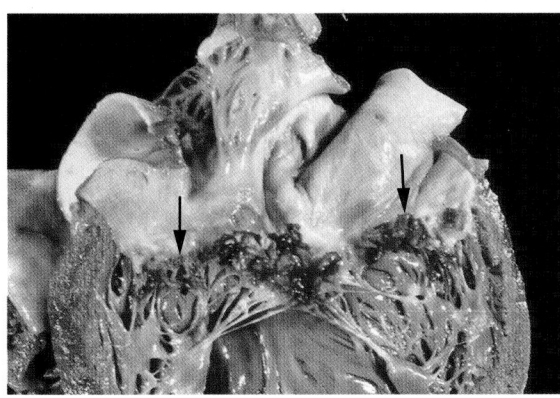

Bacterial endocarditis *(Kumar et al, 2007)*

bacterial enteritis, inflammation of the intestine caused by bacterial infection; the most common types in humans are *Campylobacter* enteritis, *Salmonella* enteritis, *Shigella* enteritis, and *Yersinia* enteritis.

bacterial enzyme, an enzyme produced by a bacterium.

bacterial food poisoning, a toxic condition resulting from the ingestion of food contaminated by certain bacteria. Acute infectious gastroenteritis caused by various species of *Salmonella* is characterized by fever, chills, nausea, vomiting, diarrhea, and general discomfort beginning 8 to 48 hours after ingestion and continuing for several days. Similar symptoms caused by *Staphylococcus,* usually *S. aureus,* appear much sooner and rarely last more than a few hours. Food poisoning caused by the neurotoxin of *Clostridium botulinum* is characterized by GI symptoms, disturbances of vision, weakness or paralysis of muscles, and, in severe cases, respiratory failure. See also **botulism.**

bacterial inflammation [L, *bacterium* + *inflammare,* to set afire], any inflammation that is part of a body's response to a bacterial infection.

bacterial kinase, **1.** a kinase of bacterial origin. **2.** a bacterial enzyme that activates plasminogen, the precursor of plasmin.

bacterial laryngitis, an inflammation of the larynx caused by a bacterial infection and usually associated with rhinosinusitis or laryngotracheal bronchitis. Signs of a bacterial infection are a cough and purulent rhinorrhea. Mild to moderate infections do not usually require treatment; more severe infections are treated with antibiotics. See also **laryngitis.**

bacterial meningitis, infection of the meninges by bacteria. If left untreated, it could be fatal or have significant sequelae. See **meningitis.**

bacterial overgrowth syndrome, a dramatic increase in the number of microorganisms in the small intestine. See **stasis syndrome.**

bacterial plaque, a dense, nonmineralized complex composed primarily of colonies of bacteria embedded in a gelatinous matrix. It contains amino acids, carbohydrates, proteins, lipids, and salts from saliva and gingival fluid; soluble food substances; shed leukocytes and epithelial cells; and products of bacterial metabolism. Plaque and the response of the host are the major causative factors in most dental diseases, including dental caries and inflammatory periodontal diseases. Also called **biofilm, dental plaque.**

bacterial pneumonia, pneumonia caused by bacteria, such as *Klebsiella pneumoniae, Mycoplasma pneumoniae, Staphylococcus aureus, Streptococcus pneumoniae, Streptococcus pyogenes,* and others.

bacterial prostatitis, a bacterial infection of the prostate. Acute bacterial infections usually involve gram-negative bacilli, such as *Escherichia coli.* Most cases are treated with a prolonged course (greater than 1 month) of broad-spectrum antimicrobial drugs. Abscesses may be associated with anaerobic bacteria. Chronic bacterial prostatitis is usually caused by gram-negative bacilli. It is less common and characterized by low back pain, dysuria, and perineal discomfort. See also **prostatitis.**

bacterial protein, a protein produced by a bacterium. Antibiotics frequently target bacterial protein synthesis, and some antibiotics inhibit bacterial protein synthesis.

bacterial resistance, the ability of certain strains of bacteria to develop a tolerance to specific antibiotics to which they once were susceptible.

bacterial toxin [Gk, *bakterion,* small staff, *toxikon,* poison], any poisonous substance produced by a bacterium. Kinds include **endotoxin, exotoxin.**

bacterial vaccine, a saline solution suspension of a strain of attenuated or killed bacteria prepared for injection into a patient to stimulate development of active immunity to that strain and against similar bacteria.

bacterial vaginosis [Gk, *bakterion,* small staff; L, *vagina,* sheath; Gk, *osis,* condition], a chronic inflammation of the vagina caused by bacterial imbalance (e.g., an overgrowth of the normal bacterial flora of the vagina). Vaginal flora commonly includes lactobacilli, streptococci, *Gardnerellavaginalis,* strains of Enterobacteriaceae, and anaerobes. Also called **vulvovaginitis.**

bacterial virus, a virus with the ability to infect and/or destroy bacteria. It is usually species-specific. See also **bacteriophage.**

bactericidal antibiotic [Gk, *bakterion* + *caedere,* to kill; Gk, *anti,* against, *bios,* life], an antibiotic drug that kills bacteria.

bactericide /baktir″əsīd/ [Gk, *bakterion* + L, *caedere,* to kill], any drug or other agent that kills bacteria. −*bactericidal, adj.*

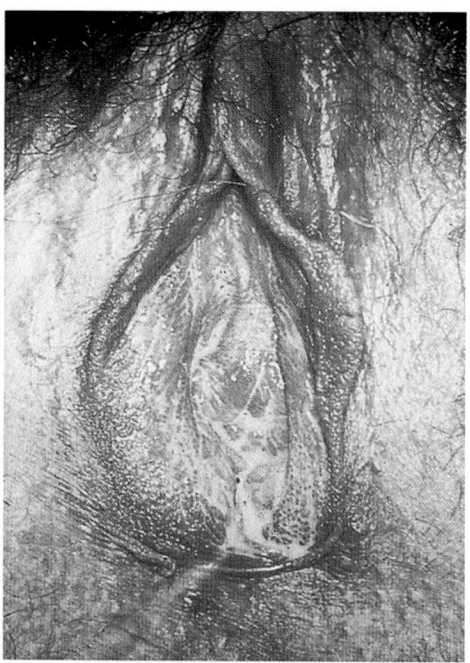

Bacterial vaginosis (Andrews, 2005)

bactericidin [Gk, *bakterion* + L, *caedere*, to kill], an antibody that kills bacteria in the presence of complement. Also called **bacteriocidin.**

bacterid /bak′ter-id/, a skin eruption due to bacterial infection elsewhere in the body.

bacteriemia. See **bacteremia.**

bacterio-, bacter-, bacteri-, combining form meaning "bacterial microorganism": *bacteriogenic, bactericide.*

bacteriocidal. See **bactericide.**

bacteriocidal antibiotic. See **bactericidal antibiotic.**

bacteriocidin. See **bactericidin.**

bacteriocin /baktir′ē-ɔsin/, a protein produced by certain species of bacteria that, by inducing metabolic block, are toxic to related strains of those bacteria. Also called **protein antibiotic.**

bacteriocinogenic /baktir′ē-ɔsin′ɔjen″ik/, pertaining to an organism capable of producing proteins with bactericidal activity.

bacteriogenic /baktir′ē-ɔjen″ik/, **1.** capable of producing bacteria. **2.** derived from or originating in bacteria. **3.** caused by bacteria.

bacterioidal. See **bacteroid.**

bacteriological /baktir′ē-ɔloj″ik/ [Gk, *bakterion*], pertaining to **bacteriology.** Also **bacteriologic.**

bacteriological sputum examination, a laboratory procedure to determine the presence or absence of bacteria in a sputum specimen. Part of the specimen is stained and examined microscopically on a glass slide, and part is inoculated on a culture medium and allowed to incubate for more specific examination later. Also called **smear, sputum culture and sensitivity test.**

bacteriologist /baktir′ē-ol″ɔjist/, a specialist in the scientific study of bacteria, viruses, and microorganisms.

bacteriology /-ol″ɔjē/ [Gk, *bakterion* + *logos*, science], the scientific study of bacteria.

bacteriolysin /baktir′ē-ɔlī″sin/ [Gk, *bakterion* + *lyein*, to loosen], an antibody that causes the breakdown of a particular species of bacterial cell. Complement usually also is necessary for this reaction. See also **bacteriolysis.**

bacteriolysis /baktir′ē-ol″ɔsis/, the intracellular or extracellular breakdown of bacteria, resulting in the release of the cell's contents. See also **bacteriolysin.** −*bacteriolytic, adj.*

bacteriophage /baktir″ē-ɔfāj′/ [Gk, *bakterion* + *phagein,* to eat], any virus that infects host bacteria, including the blue-green algae. Bacteriophages resemble other viruses in that each is composed of either ribonucleic acid (RNA) or deoxyribonucleic acid (DNA). They vary in structure from simple fibrous bodies to complex forms with contractile "tails." Bacteriophages associated with temperate bacteria may be genetically intimate with the host and are named for the bacterial strain for which they are specific, such as coliphage and corynebacteriophage. −*bacteriophagic, adj.,* −*bacteriophagy, n.*

bacteriophage typing, the process of identifying a species of bacterium according to the type of virus that attacks it.

bacteriophagic, bacteriphagy. See **bacteriophage.**

bacteriospermia /baktir′ēɔspur″mē-ɔ/, the presence of bacteria in semen or ejaculate.

bacteriostasis /baktir′ē-os″tɔsis/ [Gk, *bakterion* + Gk, *stasis,* standing still], a state of suspended growth and/or reproduction of bacteria. Compare **bactericide.** −*bacteriostatic, adj.*

bacteriostat, a chemical or biological agent that inhibits the growth of bacteria.

bacterium. See **bacteria.**

bacteriuria /baktir′ēyo͞or″ē-ɔ/, the presence of bacteria in the urine. The presence of more than 100,000 pathogenic bacteria per milliliter of urine is usually considered significant and diagnostic of urinary tract infection. Bacteriuria may be asymptomatic. See also **urinary tract infection.**

bacteroid /bak″tɔroid/, **1.** pertaining to or resembling bacteria. **2.** a structure that resembles a bacterium. Also spelled *bacterioid.* −*bacteroidal,* **bacterioidal,** *adj.*

Bacteroides /bak′tɔroi″dēz/ [Gk, *bakterion,* small staff, *eidos,* form], a genus of obligate anaerobic bacilli normally found in the colon, mouth, genital tract, and upper respiratory system. Severe infection may result from the invasion of the bacillus through a break in the mucous membrane into the venous circulation, where thrombosis and bacteremia may occur. Foul-smelling abscesses, gas, and putrefaction are characteristic of infection with this organism. Of the 30 species, *Bacteroides fragilis* is the most common and most virulent.

Bactrim, a fixed-combination drug containing two antibiotics, commonly prescribed to treat urinary tract infection. Brand name for **sulfamethoxazole and trimethoprim.**

BAER, abbreviation for **brainstem auditory evoked response.**

baffling, the process of removing large water particles from suspension in a jet nebulizer so that the particles entering the patient's airways are of a uniform therapeutic size. The function may be performed in part by a perforated plate against which liquid particles impinge and fracture and are reflected into the vapor chamber of the nebulizer.

bag [AS, *baelg*], a flexible or dilatable sac or pouch designed to contain gas, fluid, or semisolid material such as crushed ice. An Ambu bag or breathing bag is used to control the flow of respiratory gases entering the lungs of a patient. Several types of bags are used in medical or surgical procedures to dilate the anus, vagina, or other body openings.

bagasse /bɔgas″/ [Fr, cane trash], the crushed fibers or the residue of sugarcane, a source of the thermophilic actinomycetes antigen that is a cause of bagassosis hypersensitivity pneumonitis.

bagassosis /bag′ɔsō″sis/, a self-limited lung disease caused by an allergic response to bagasse, the fungi-laden, dusty debris left after the syrup has been extracted from sugarcane. It is characterized by fever, dyspnea, and malaise.

bagging, *(Informal)* the artificial ventilation performed with a respirator bag, such as a bag-valve-mask resuscitator (Ambu bag) or the reservoir bag on an anesthesia machine. The bag is squeezed to deliver positive pressure gases to the patient's lungs through a mask, an endotracheal tube, a laryngeal mask, or another breathing device. During general anesthesia, the anesthetist may use this technique to assist or control the respiration of an unconscious patient. Bagging may also be employed in the emergency response for basic and advanced life support.

bag-valve-mask resuscitator, a device consisting of a manually compressible container with a plastic bag of oxygen at one end and a one-way valve and mask that fit over the mouth and nose of the person to be resuscitated at the other end. Kinds include **Ambu bag™.**

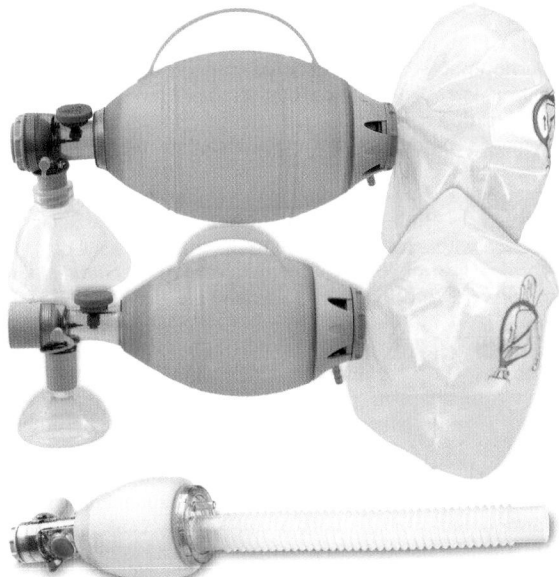

Bag-valve-mask resuscitators *(© 2015 Ambu)*

Bainbridge reflex [Francis A. Bainbridge, English physiologist, 1874–1921], a cardiac reflex in which stimulation of stretch receptors in the wall of the left atrium causes an increased pulse rate. It may be triggered by the infusion of large amounts of IV fluids or by backflow of blood in congestive heart failure.

Baker cyst [William M. Baker, British surgeon, 1839–1896], a synovial cyst that forms at the back of the knee. It is often associated with rheumatoid arthritis and may appear only when the leg is straightened. Also called *popliteal cyst.*

baker's itch [AS, *giccan,* to bake], a rash that may develop on the hands and forearms of bakery workers, probably as an allergic reaction to flours, flour mites, or other ingredients in bakery products.

BAL, 1. abbreviation for **British antilewisite. See dimercaprol. 2.** abbreviation for **bronchoalveolar lavage.**

balance [L, *bilanx,* having two scales], **1.** an instrument for weighing. **2.** a normal state of physiological equilibrium. **3.** a state of mental or emotional equilibrium. **4.** to bring into equilibrium.

balance billing, the difference between the charge a provider bills and the allowed amount by the government.

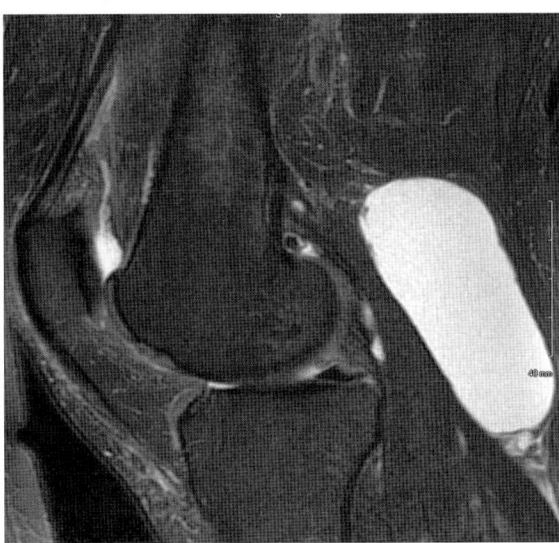

Baker cyst of the knee *(Miller et al, 2010)*

balanced anesthesia, a technique of general anesthesia utilizing the properties of various medications, narcotic analgesics, muscle relaxation, and inhalation agents and/or nitrous oxide to render the patient unconscious. This technique of combining individual drugs produces the desired effect to the optimum degree and minimizes undesirable effects. It provides both patient comfort and an appropriate surgical field.

balanced articulation, simultaneous contact between the upper and lower teeth as they glide over each other when the mandible is moved laterally. See also **balanced occlusion.**

balanced diet, a diet containing adequate energy and all of the essential nutrients that cannot be synthesized in adequate quantities by the body in amounts adequate for growth, energy needs, nitrogen equilibrium, repair, and maintenance of normal health.

balanced forearm orthosis (BFO), forearm orthosis for persons with severe weakness or paralysis of the elbow or forearm; it consists of a trough to support the forearm and a mechanism such as a Bowden cable linking it to the shoulder region so that small movements of the shoulder girdle or trunk produce motion at the elbow. See **mobile arm support.**

balanced occlusion, simultaneous contact between the upper and lower teeth on both sides and in the anterior and posterior occlusal areas of the jaws. An appropriate dental prosthesis is constructed with such an occlusion to stabilize the denture base and prevent the denture base from tipping or rotating in relation to the supporting structures. This term is primarily associated with intraoral assessment of occlusal harmony but may also be used in the process of pretesting the occlusion while the dentures are mounted on casts attached to an anatomical articulator. See also **balanced articulation.**

balanced polymorphism, in a population, the occurrence of a certain proportion of homozygotes and heterozygotes for specific genetic traits, which is maintained from generation to generation by the forces of natural selection. Compare **genetic polymorphism.**

balanced suspension, a system of splints, ropes, slings, pulleys, and weights for suspending extremities of the body, used as an aid to realignment and healing from fractures or from surgical intervention. See also **lower extremity suspension, upper extremity suspension.**

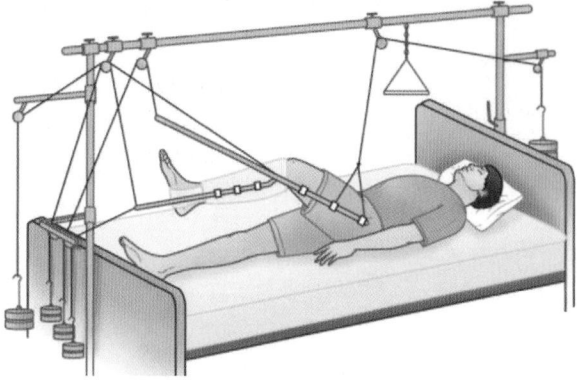

Balanced suspension *(Rothrock, 2007)*

balanced traction, a system of balanced suspension that supplements traction in the treatment of fractures of the lower extremities or after various operations affecting the lower parts of the body that require traction.

balanced translocation, the transfer of segments between nonhomologous chromosomes in such a way that the configuration and total number of chromosomes change, but each cell contains the normal amount of diploid or haploid genetic material. Usually the long arm of an acrocentric chromosome is transferred to another chromosome, and the small fragment containing the centromere is lost, leaving only 45 chromosomes. A person with a balanced translocation is phenotypically normal but may produce children with trisomies. Compare **reciprocal translocation, robertsonian translocation.**

balancing side, the side of the mouth opposite the working side (predominant chewing side) of dentition or a denture.

balanic /bəlan″ik/ [Gk, *balanos,* acorn], pertaining to the glans penis or the glans clitoridis.

balanic hypospadias. See **glandular hypospadias.**

balanitis /bal′ənī″tis/ [Gk, *balanos + itis*], inflammation of the glans penis.

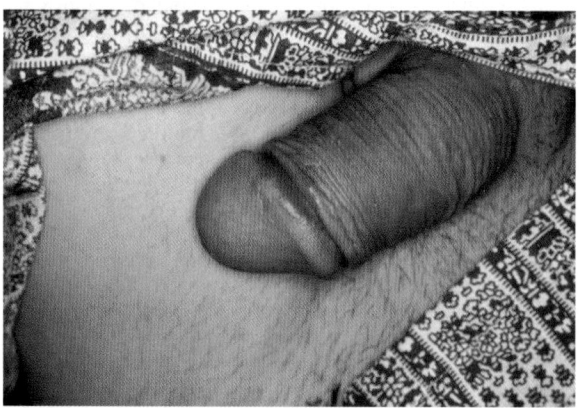

Balanitis *(Rakel and Rakel, 2016)*

balanitis circumscripta plasmacellularis, a benign lesion involving the inner surface of the prepuce and glans associated with shiny, moist lesions. The condition usually manifests in middle-aged or elderly uncircumcised males. The etiology is unknown but is thought to be due to local infections, poor hygiene, heat, friction, or constant rubbing. Also called **Zoon balanitis.**

balanitis diabetica, an inflammation of the glans penis or glans clitoridis caused by glucose content of the urine and commonly seen in persons with diabetes.

balanitis xerotica obliterans /zirot″ikə oblit″ərans/ [Gk, *balanos + itis + xeros,* dry, *tokos,* labor; L, *obliterare,* to efface], a chronic skin disease (lichen sclerosis et atrophicus) of the glans penis, characterized by a white indurated area surrounding the meatus, that may result in urethral stenosis. Treatment is with local antibacterial and antiinflammatory agents.

balano-, balan-, combining form meaning "the head of the penis" in males or the "glans clitoris" in females: *balanoplasty, balanitis.*

balanoplasty /bal″ənōplas′tē/ [Gk, *balanos + plassein,* to mold], an operation involving plastic surgery of the glans penis to correct a congenital defect or to serve an aesthetic purpose.

balanoposthitis /bal′ənōposthī″tis/ [Gk, *balanos + posthe,* penis, foreskin, *itis*], a generalized inflammation of the glans penis and prepuce in uncircumcised males, usually caused by poorly retractile foreskin and poor hygiene. It is characterized by soreness, irritation, and discharge, which occur as a complication of bacterial or fungal infection. A culture of the discharge can determine the causative agent—often a common venereal disease—so that specific antimicrobial therapy can then be instituted. Circumcision may be considered in severe cases. To relieve discomfort, the inflamed area can be irrigated with a warm saline solution several times a day.

balanopreputial /bal′ənōpripyoo″shəl/ [Gk, *balanos + L, praeputium,* foreskin], pertaining to the glans penis and the prepuce.

balanorrhagia /bal′ənōrā″jē·ə/ [Gk, *balanos + rhegnynai,* to burst forth], balanitis in which pus is discharged copiously from the penis.

balantidiasis /bal′əntidī″əsis/, an infection caused by ingestion of cysts of the protozoan *Balantidium coli,* the largest human protozoan. Pigs are the animal reservoir. In some cases, the organism is a harmless inhabitant of the large intestine, but infection with *B. coli* usually causes diarrhea. Infrequently the infection progresses, and the protozoan invades the intestinal wall and produces ulcers or abscesses, which may cause dysentery and death. Human infections, a rare event in industrialized countries, are usually acquired by ingestion of food or water contaminated by mammal feces. Diagnosis is made by identification of trophozoites in the stool or in sampled colonic tissue. Tetracycline, iodoquinol, or metronidazole is usually prescribed to treat the infection.

Balantidium coli /bal′əntid″ē·əm/ [Gk, *balantidion,* little bag, *kolon,* colon], the largest and the only ciliated protozoan species that is pathogenic to humans, causing balantidiasis. It is a normal inhabitant of the domestic hog and is transmitted to humans by the ingestion of cysts excreted in hog feces, occurring either during direct contact with pigs, handling of fertilizer that contains pig excrement, or contact with a water supply contaminated with excrement.

baldness [ME, *balled*], *(Informal)* absence of hair, especially from the scalp. See also **alopecia.**

BAL in Oil, a heavy metal antagonist. Brand name for **dimercaprol.**

Balint syndrome [Rudolph Balint, Hungarian neurologist, 1874–1929], a group of visual symptoms characterized by simultaneous anosognosia and optic ataxia. The patient experiences nystagmus, or loss of control of eye movements, and the inability to perceive all parts of a scene simultaneously. The patient may begin to follow a moving object but lose it. The cause is bilateral disease of the parietotemporal areas of the brain.

Balkan traction frame, an overhead, rectangular frame attached to the bed and used for attaching splints, suspending or changing the position of immobilized limbs, or providing continuous traction with weights and pulleys.

Balkan tubulointerstitial nephritis /tōō′byəlō·in′tər-stish″-əl/, a chronic kidney disorder marked by renal insufficiency, proteinuria, tubulointerstitial nephritis, and anemia. The onset is gradual, but end-stage disease occurs within 5 years after the first signs. About one third of the patients also suffer from urinary tract cancers. The disease is endemic in the Balkans but is not hereditary.

ball [ME, *bal*], **1.** *n.,* spherical object, such as one of the collagen balls embedded in hyaline cartilage. **2.** *v.,* placing together in a fitted, rounded connection. **−ball,** *v.*

Ballance's sign [Charles A. Ballance, English surgeon, 1856–1936], a dull percussion resonance sound heard on the right flank of a patient lying in the left decubitus position, an indication of a ruptured spleen. The sound is caused by an accumulation of liquid blood on the right side and coagulated blood on the left.

ball-and-socket joint, a synovial or multiaxial joint in which the globular (ball-shaped) head of an articulating bone is received into a cuplike cavity, allowing the distal bone to move around an indefinite number of axes with a common center, such as in hip and shoulder joints. Also called **enarthrosis, spheroidea.** Compare **condyloid joint, pivot joint, saddle joint.** See also **joint.**

ball-bearing feeder, *(Informal)* a balanced forearm suspension used for patients confined to a wheelchair with paralysis of the upper extremity. It is designed to improve performance in feeding, grooming, and desk skills. Components include a proximal ball-bearing and swivel arm; a distal ball-bearing and swivel arm; and a rocker arm and trough. See also **mobile arm support (MAS).**

ball-catcher position, a position of the hands used in making a radiograph to diagnose rheumatoid arthritis. The hands are held with the palms upward and the fingers cupped, as if to catch a ball.

Baller-Gerold syndrome /bä′lər ga′rōlt/ [Friedrich Baller, German physician, 20th century; M. Gerold, German physician, 20th century], an autosomal-recessive syndrome characterized by premature fusion of cranial bones (craniosynostosis) and partial or complete absence of the radius. Missing and/or malformed fingers may also occur.

ballism. See **ballismus.**

ballismus /bôl′iz′məs/ [Gk, *ballismo,* dancing], an abnormal neuromuscular condition characterized by uncoordinated swinging of the limbs and jerky movements. Ballism is associated with extrapyramidal disorders such as Sydenham chorea. The condition may occur in a unilateral form as hemiballismus. Also called **ballism.**

ballistic movement /bəlis″tik/, a high-velocity musculoskeletal movement, such as a tennis serve or boxing punch, requiring reciprocal coordination of agonistic and antagonistic muscles. These movements are characterized by high firing rates, high force production, and very brief contraction times.

ballistics /bəlis″tiks/ [Gk, *ballein,* to throw], the study of the motion, trajectory, and impact of projectiles, including bullets and rockets.

ballistocardiograph [Gk, *ballein,* to throw, *kardia,* heart, *graphein,* to record], an apparatus for recording body movements caused by the thrust of the heart during systolic ejection of the blood into the aorta and the pulmonary arteries. It has been used in measuring cardiac output and the force of contraction of the heart.

ballistocardiography /balis′tōkär′dē·og″rəfē/, the recording and monitoring of physical activity matched to the beating of the heart and the circulation of the blood.

ball of the foot, the part of the foot composed of the distal heads of the metatarsals and their surrounding fatty fibrous tissue pad.

balloon angioplasty /bəlōōn″/, a method of dilating or opening an obstructed blood vessel by threading a small, balloon-tipped catheter into the vessel. The balloon is inflated to compress arteriosclerotic lesions against the walls of the vessel, leaving a larger lumen, through which blood can pass. It is used in treating arteriosclerotic heart disease.

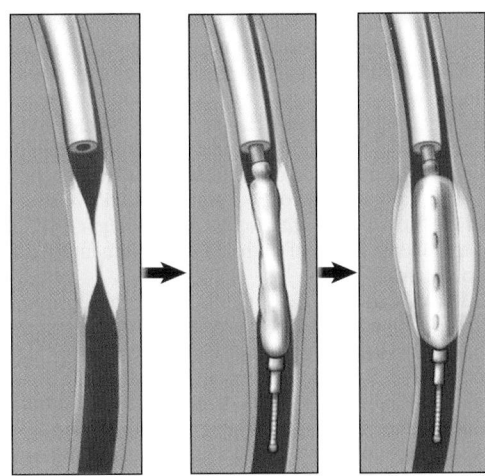

Balloon angioplasty *(Patton, 2016)*

balloon catheter radiation, a method for delivering internal radiation therapy to patients with breast cancer following lumpectomy. The goal is to destroy remaining cancer cells and to minimize damage to surrounding healthy tissue. Treatment usually lasts 5 to 7 days, after which time the catheter is removed. See also **MammoSite.**

balloon compression, a percutaneous therapy for trigeminal neuralgia. A balloon is inflated to compress the gasserian ganglion and produce trigeminal injury.

ballooning degeneration hydropic degeneration, a severe hepatocellular change. See **granular degeneration.**

balloon septostomy. See **Rashkind procedure.**

balloon tamponade [Fr, *tamponnade*], a procedure in which a device consisting of a flexible tube and two balloons is inserted into a passageway and the balloons are expanded to restrict the flow of blood or to force open a stenosis. See also **balloon angioplasty.**

balloon-tip catheter, a catheter bearing a nonporous inflatable sac around its far end. After insertion of the catheter, the sac can be inflated with air or sterile water, introduced via injection into a special port at the near end of the catheter. The inflated sac secures the catheter in the correct position. See also **Foley catheter, Swan-Ganz catheter.**

ballottable /bəlot″əbəl/ [Fr, *balloter,* a shaking about], pertaining to a use of palpation to detect movement of objects suspended in fluid, such as a fetus in amniotic fluid, or the patella bumping against the femur. See also **ballottement.**

ballottable head [Fr, *ballotage,* shaking up], during labor, a fetal head that has not descended and become fixed in the maternal bony pelvis. See also **engagement, cardinal movements of labor.**

ballottement /bä′lôtmäN″, bəlot″ment/ [Fr, tossing], a technique for palpating an organ or floating structure by bouncing it gently and feeling it rebound. In late pregnancy, a fetal head that can be ballotted is unengaged.

ball thrombus, a relatively round, coagulated mass of blood containing platelets, fibrin, and cellular fragments that may obstruct a blood vessel or an orifice, usually the mitral valve of the heart.

ball-valve action, the intermittent opening and closing of an orifice by a buoyant, ball-shaped mass, which acts as a valve. Some kinds of objects that may act in this manner are kidney stones, gallstones, and blood clots.

balm /bäm/ [Gk, *balsamon,* balsam], **1.** a healing or a soothing substance, such as any of various medicinal ointments. **2.** an aromatic plant of the genus *Melissa* that relieves pain. Also called **balsam. 3.** an herb used as a natural topical treatment.

balneology /bal′nē·ol″əjē/ [L, *balneum,* bath; Gk, *logos,* science], a field of study that deals with the chemical compositions of various mineral waters and their healing characteristics, especially in therapeutic bathing. –*balneological, adj.*

balneotherapy /bal′nē·ōther″əpē/ [L, *balneum* + Gk, *therapeia,* treatment], use of baths in the treatment of diseases and conditions.

balsalazide /bal-sal′ah-zīd/, a prodrug of the antiinflammatory mesalamine to which it is converted in the colon; administered orally in the treatment of ulcerative colitis.

balsam /bôl″səm/ [Gk, *balsamon*], **1.** any of a variety of resinous saps, generally from evergreens, usually containing benzoic or cinnamic acid. Balsam is sometimes used in rectal suppositories and dermatological agents as a counterirritant. Kinds include **balsam of peru. 2.** See **balm.**

balsam of peru, an oily resin that acts as a local protectant, used in perfumes, toiletries, and many medicines. It is an ingredient in hemorrhoid suppositories and ointment (e.g., Anusol™), tincture of benzoin, calamine lotion, and dental cement. It is frequently identified as an allergen.

Baltimore Longitudinal Study of Aging (BLSA), a long-range examination of interrelations between multiple correlates of aging. Although men of varied backgrounds were selected for the original study (1955) in order to explore uncontrolled factors that might lead to new knowledge regarding aging, the BLSA now includes both men and women. This is the longest-running study on aging in America. The study has provided scientific evidence as to what happens as men and women age. It is identifying normal aging patterns from patterns of disease, illness, and other causes, such as genetics and heredity. What has been learned from the studies has made a significant contribution to research supporting healthy aging. The awareness provided in areas such as exercise, diet, and physical activities, as well as all activities of daily living and lifestyle habits, equates to a significant contribution in terms of how aging can be managed today.

-bamate, combining form designating a propanediol or pentanediol derivative.

Bamberger's sign, dullness at the level of the scapula that disappears when the patient leans forward; a symptom associated with pericardial effusion.

bamboo spine /bamboo″/ [Malay, *bambu*], (in radiology) the appearance of the thoracic or lumbar spine with rigid characteristics of advanced ankylosing spondylitis. Also called **poker spine.** See also **ankylosing spondylitis.**

band [ME, *bande,* strip], **1.** (in anatomy) a bundle of fibers, as seen in tendon or striated muscle, that encircles a structure or binds one part of the body to another. **2.** (in dentistry) a strip of metal that fits around a tooth and serves as an attachment for orthodontic components. **3.** *(Informal)* the immature form of a segmented neutrophil characterized by a sausage-shaped nucleus. It is the only immature leukocyte

normally found in the peripheral circulation. Bands represent 3% to 5% of the total white cell number. An increase in the relative number of bands indicates bacterial infection or acute stress to the bone marrow.

band adapter, an instrument for aiding in the fitting of a circumferential orthodontic band to a tooth.

bandage /ban″dij/ [ME, *bande,* strip], **1.** *n,* a strip or roll of cloth or other material that may be wound around a part of the body in a variety of ways to secure a dressing, maintain pressure over a compress, or immobilize a limb or other part of the body. See also **cravat bandage. 2.** to apply a bandage.

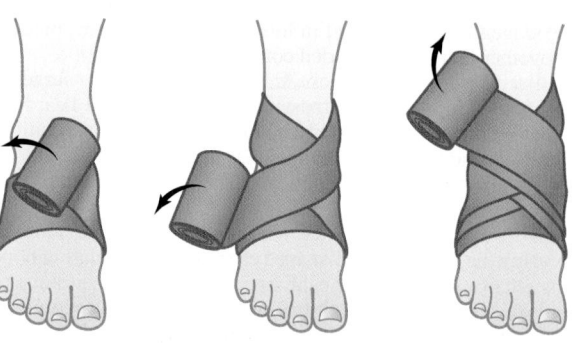

Figure-of-eight bandage for the ankle *(Proctor and Adams, 2014)*

bandage shears, a sturdy pair of scissors used to cut through bandages. The blades of most bandage shears are angled to the shaft of the instrument, and the lower blade is rounded and blunt to facilitate insertion under the bandage without harming the patient's skin. Also called *bandage scissors.*

band cell, a developing granular (immature) leukocyte in circulating blood, characterized by a curved or indented nucleus. Band cells are intermediate leukocytic forms between metamyelocytes and adult leukocytes with segmented nuclei.

band heterotopia, an anomaly of the cerebral cortex in which a heterotopic band of gray matter is found between the lateral ventricles and the cortex; affected patients may have cognitive impairment or epilepsy.

banding [ME, *bande,* strip], any of several techniques of staining chromosomes with fluorescent stains or chemical dyes that produce a series of transverse light and dark areas whose intensity and position are characteristic of each chromosome. Banding patterns are identified as C-banding, G-banding, Q-banding, or R-banding according to the staining technique used. Also called **chromosome banding.**

Bandl's ring, a thickened ring of myometrium in the lower uterine segment, associated with sustained obstructed labor. See **pathological retraction ring.**

bandpass, (in radiology) a measure of the number of times per second an electron beam can be modulated, expressed as Hertz (Hz). It is a factor that influences horizontal resolution on a cathode-ray tube. The higher the bandpass, the greater the horizontal resolution. Also called **bandwidth.**

band pusher, an instrument used for seating metal circumferential orthodontic bands into correct position on a tooth.

band remover, an instrument used to help take circumferential orthodontic bands off teeth.

bandwidth, **1.** the range of frequencies that can be satisfactorily transmitted or processed by a system. **2.** See **bandpass.**

bang. See **bhang.**

Bangkok hemorrhagic fever, *(Obsolete)* now called **dengue fever.**

bank, (for health or related reasons) a stored supply of human materials or tissues for future use by other individuals. Kinds include **blood bank, eye bank, tissue bank.**

Banting, Sir Frederick G. [Canadian physician, 1891–1941], co-winner, with John J. Macleod, of the 1923 Nobel prize for medicine and physiology for their research with the Canadian physiologist Charles H. Best showing the link between the pancreas and insulin in the control of diabetes. See also **Macleod, John J.**

Banti syndrome /ban″tēz/ [Guido Banti, Italian pathologist, 1852–1925], a chronic, progressive disorder secondary to portal hypertension. Obstruction of the blood vessels that lie between the intestines and the liver leads to venous congestion, enlargement of the spleen, and abnormal destruction of red and white blood cells. See also **congestive splenomegalia, cirrhosis, portacaval shunt, portal hypertension.**

■ OBSERVATIONS: Early symptoms are weakness, fatigue, and anemia. It is associated with splenomegaly, anemia, leukopenia, GI tract bleeding, and cirrhosis of the liver.

■ INTERVENTIONS: Surgical removal of the spleen and creation of a portacaval shunt to improve portal circulation are sometimes necessary. Because the syndrome is often a complication of alcoholic cirrhosis of the liver, medical treatment includes prescriptions for improved nutrition, vitamins, abstinence from alcohol, and rest.

■ PATIENT CARE CONSIDERATIONS: The patient requires physical and emotional support to deal with the disease trajectory associated with portal hypertension. If alcohol abuse is an underlying cause, the patient and family must learn to deal with abstinence.

BAO, abbreviation for **basal acid output.**

bar, **1.** (in physical science) a measure of air pressure. It is equal to 1000 millibars, or 10^6 dyne/cm2, or approximately 1 standard atmosphere (1 atm). Also called **barye. 2.** a long, narrow rigid structure that a patient can grasp to assist in stabilization. Kinds include **grab bar, parallel bar.**

bar-. See **baro-, bar-, bari-.**

Baraclude, antiviral agent for hepatitis B. Brand name for **entecavir.**

baragnosis /bar″ag-no′sis/, impairment of the ability to perceive differences in weight or pressure.

baralyme /ber″əlīm/ [Gk, *barys*, heavy; AS, *lim*, lime], a mixture of calcium and barium compounds used to absorb exhaled carbon dioxide in an anesthesia rebreathing system, a process that reduces the need for large amounts of fresh gas. See also **soda lime.**

Bárány's test. See **caloric test.**

-barb, combining form designating a barbituric acid derivative.

Barbados cherry. See **acerola.**

barber's itch. See **sycosis barbae.**

barbiturate /bärbich″ŏŏrāt, -ərit/ [Saint Barbara, drug discovered on day of the saint, 1864], a derivative of barbituric acid that acts as a sedative-hypnotic. These derivatives act by depressing the respiratory rate, blood pressure, temperature, and central nervous system. They have great addiction potential. Some barbiturates are used in anesthesia and in the treatment of refractory seizures.

barbiturate coma [Ger, Saint Barbara's Day; Gk, *koma*, deep sleep], an effect of barbituric acid or its derivatives, which may be rapid-acting sedatives, hypnotics, and respiratory depressants. Barbiturate coma may be intentionally induced for the treatment of some neurological conditions.

barbiturate poisoning. See **barbiturism.**

-barbituric, combining form used to designate compounds derived from barbituric acid.

barbiturism /bärbich″əriz′əm/, **1.** acute or chronic poisoning by any of the derivatives of barbituric acid. Ingestion of such preparations in excess of therapeutic quantities may be fatal or may produce physiological, pathological, and psychological changes, such as depressed respiration, cyanosis, disorientation, and coma. Immediate medical care should be promptly initiated. Also called **barbiturate poisoning. 2.** addiction to a barbiturate.

barbotage /bahr″bo-tahzh′/, repeated alternate injection and withdrawal of fluid with a syringe, as in gastric lavage or administration of an anesthetic agent into the subarachnoid space.

bar clasp arm, (in prosthetic dentistry) a clasp arm that originates from a denture base and serves as an extracoronal retainer to an abutment tooth.

Bard-Pic syndrome /bärd″pik″/ [Louis Bard, 19th century French physician, 1857–1930; Adrian Pic, French physician, b. 1863], *(Obsolete)* a condition characterized by progressive jaundice, enlarged gallbladder, and cachexia; associated with advanced pancreatic cancer.

Bard sign [Jean Louis Marius Bard, French physician, 1857–1930], the increased oscillations of the eyeball in organic nystagmus when the patient tries to visually follow a target moved from side to side across the line of sight. Such oscillations usually cease during the same test if the patient has congenital nystagmus.

bare lymphocyte syndrome, an immune deficiency condition caused by mutations in genes affecting expression or function of major histocompatibility complexes. It is inherited as an autosomal-recessive trait. The deficiency causes a severe combined immunodeficiency resulting from the lack of antigen presentation by type I and/or type II major histocompatibility complex.

baresthesia /bär′esthē″zhə/, sensitivity to weight or pressure.

bar graph [OF, *barre*], a graph in which frequencies are represented by bars extending from the ordinate or the abscissa, allowing the distribution of the entire sample to be seen at once.

bariatrics /ber′ē-at″riks/ [Gk, *baros,* weight, *iatros,* physician], the field of medicine that focuses on the treatment and control of obesity and diseases associated with obesity.

bariatric surgery, surgical procedures that cause weight loss by restricting the amount of food the stomach can hold, causing malabsorption of nutrients, or by a combination of both gastric restriction and malabsorption. Kinds include **gastric bypass, biliopancreatic diversion, gastric sleeve.**

baritosis /ber′ətō″sis/, a benign form of pneumoconiosis caused by an accumulation of barium dust in the lungs. Barium does not cause fibrosis and is not a common cause of functional impairment. The condition is most likely to affect persons involved in the mining and processing of barite, a barium-containing compound used in the manufacture of paints.

barium (Ba) /ber″ē-əm/ [Gk, *barys,* heavy], a pale yellow, metallic element classified with the alkaline earths. Its atomic number is 56; its atomic mass is 137.36. The acid-soluble salts of barium are poisonous. Fine, milky barium sulfate is used as a radiopaque contrast medium in radiographic imaging of the digestive tract.

barium enema, a rectal infusion of barium sulfate, a radiopaque contrast medium that is retained in the lower intestinal tract during radiographic studies for diagnosis of obstruction, tumors, or other abnormalities. The procedure may be used therapeutically in children to reduce nonstrangulated intussusception. Also called **contrast enema.**

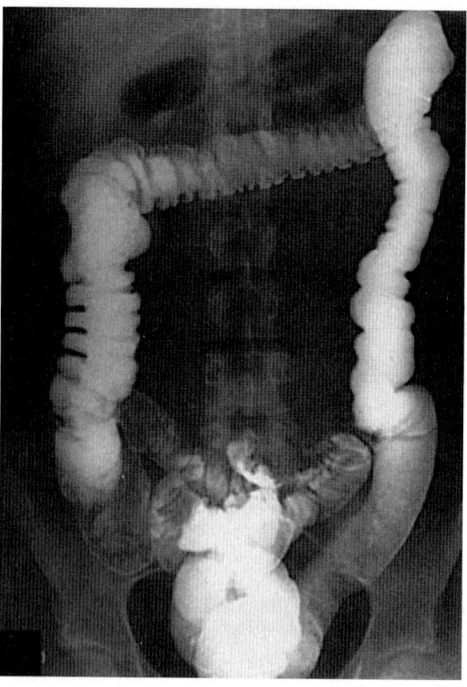

Barium enema *(Ehrlich, 2013)*

barium enema with air contrast. See **double-contrast barium enema.**

barium meal. See **gastrointestinal series.**

barium poisoning, a condition characterized by a severe, rapid decrease in plasma potassium levels and a shift of potassium into cells caused by the ingestion of soluble barium salts. The patient may experience nausea, vomiting, abdominal cramps, bloody diarrhea, dizziness, arrhythmias, ringing in the ears, cardiac arrest, and respiratory failure.

barium sulfate, a radiopaque medium used as a diagnostic aid in radiology.
- INDICATIONS: It is prescribed for radiographic examination of the GI tract.
- CONTRAINDICATIONS: Known hypersensitivity to this drug prohibits its use.
- ADVERSE EFFECTS: Among the more serious complications is severe constipation.

barium swallow [Gk, *barys*, heavy; AS, *swelgan*, to swallow], a medical imaging procedure in which a radiopaque barium sulfate suspension is administered orally and is used to examine the upper GI (gastrointestinal) tract. Also called **esophagography.** See also **barium meal.**

Barker, Phil, a nursing theorist who developed the Tidal Model of Health Recovery for psychiatric and mental health nursing. Psychiatric patients often feel that they are drowning in the flux of constant change and need rescue. Their life stories, or experiences, must be carefully evaluated to determine what resources they have for recovery and what kind of support is needed from and for the nurses who are caring for the patients.

Barlow syndrome [John B. Barlow, South African cardiologist, 1924–2008], an abnormal cardiac condition characterized by an apical systolic murmur, a systolic click, and an electrocardiogram indicating inferior ischemia. These signs are associated with mitral regurgitation caused by prolapse of the mitral valve. Also called **floppy-valve syndrome.** See also **mitral valve prolapse (MVP) syndrome.**

Barnard, Kathryn E. [1938–2020], a nursing theorist who developed the Child Health Assessment Interaction Model. Her model and theory were the outcome of the Nursing Child Assessment Project (1976–1979). Barnard believes that the parent-infant system is influenced by individual characteristics of each member. Those characteristics are modified to meet the needs of the system by adaptive behavior. The interaction between parent (or caregiver) and child is shown in Barnard's model to take place with five cues and activities: (1) the infant's clarity in sending cues; (2) the infant's responsiveness to the parent; (3) the parent's sensitivity to the child's cues; (4) the parent's ability to recognize and alleviate the infant's distress; and (5) the parent's social, emotional, and cognitive growth-fostering activities. A major issue in Barnard's theoretic assertions is that the nurse gives support to the mother's sensitivity and response to her infant's cues rather than trying to change her characteristics or mothering style.

baro-, bar-, bari-, combining form meaning "pressure, heaviness, weight": *baresthesia, barognosis, bariatrics.*

barognosis /ber′əgnō″sis/ *pl.* **barognoses** [Gk, *baros,* weight, *gnosis,* knowledge], the ability to perceive and evaluate weight, especially that held in the hand.

barograph /ber″əgraf′/ [Gk, *baros* + *graphein,* to record], an instrument that continually monitors barometric pressure and records pressure changes on paper.

barometer /bərom″ətər/ [Gk, *baros* + *metron,* measure], an instrument for measuring atmospheric pressure, commonly consisting of a slender tube filled with mercury, sealed at one end, and inverted into a reservoir of mercury. At sea level the normal height of mercury in the tube is 760 mm. At higher elevations the mercury column height (barometric pressure) is less. Fluctuations in barometric pressure may precede major changes in weather. –**barometric,** *adj.*

barometric pressure. See **atmospheric pressure.**

baroreceptor /ber′ōrisep″tər/ [Gk, *baros* + L, *recipere,* to receive], one of the pressure-sensitive nerve endings in the walls of the atria of the heart, the aortic arch, and the carotid sinuses. Baroreceptors stimulate central reflex mechanisms that allow physiological adjustment and adaptation to changes in blood pressure via changes in heart rate, vasodilation, or vasoconstriction. Baroreceptors are essential for homeostasis. Also called **pressoreceptor.**

barosinusitis. See **aerosinusitis.**

Barosperse, a radiopaque medium. Brand name for **barium sulfate.**

barotitis. See **aerotitis.**

barotitis media. See **aerotitis media.**

barotrauma /ber′ōtrô″mə, -trou″mə/ [Gk, *baros* + *trauma,* wound], physical injury sustained as a result of exposure to changing air pressure, or rupture of the tympanic membranes, as may occur among scuba divers or caisson workers or anyone near dynamite or gas explosions. Barotrauma may be iatrogenic as in the case of excessive ventilator pressures leading to lung injury. Compare **decompression sickness.**

Barr body. See **sex chromatin.**

barrel chest, a large, rounded thorax, as in the inspiratory phase, considered normal in some stocky individuals and certain others who live in high-altitude areas and consequently have increased vital capacity. Barrel chest may also be a sign of chronic obstructive pulmonary disease. Also called **emphysematous chest.**

barrel distortion, outward bowing of gridded straight lines in an image, resulting from lens distortion such that the lateral magnification at the center of the image is greater than that at the edges.

Barr-Epstein virus. See **Epstein-Barr virus.**

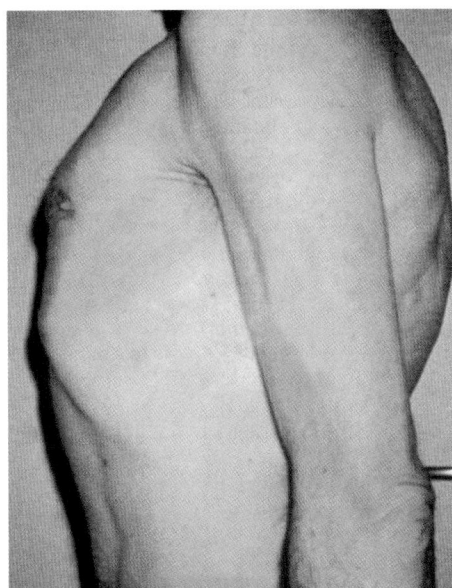

Barrel chest *(From Mc Donald FS, ed. Mayo Clinic images in internal medicine, with permission. © Mayo Clinic Scientific Press and CRC Press.)*

Barré pyramidal sign /bärä″/ [Jean A. Barré, French neurologist, 1880–1971], a diagnostic sign indicating a disease of the pyramidal tracts. The patient lies facedown and the legs are flexed at the knee. The patient is unable to maintain this position. Also called *pyramidal drift, Barré test.*

Barrett esophagus [Norman R. Barrett, English surgeon, 1903–1979], a disorder of the lower esophagus marked by a benign ulcerlike lesion in columnar epithelium, resulting most often from chronic irritation of the esophagus by gastric reflux of acidic digestive juices. Major symptoms include dysphagia, decreased lower esophageal (LES) pressure, frequent heartburn and, less commonly, chest pain. Symptoms may be relieved by eating frequent small meals, avoiding foods that produce gas, taking antacid medication, and elevating the head of the bed to prevent passive reflux when lying down. Treatment consists of proton pump inhibitors and H$_2$ blockers. The lesion is considered premalignant, and surveillance endoscopy is performed to screen for esophageal cancer. Also called **Barrett syndrome.**

Barrett syndrome [Norman R. Barrett, English surgeon, 1903–1979]. See **Barrett esophagus.**

barrier /ber″ē·ər/ [ME, *barrere*], **1.** a wall or other obstacle that can restrain or block the passage of substances. Barrier methods of contraception, such as the condom or cervical diaphragm, prevent the passage of spermatozoa into the uterus. Membranes and cell walls of body tissues function as screenlike barriers to permit the movement of water or certain other molecules from one side to the other while preventing the passage of other substances. Skin is an important barrier that protects against the entry of microorganisms and the exit of body fluids. Barriers in kidney tissues adjust automatically to regulate the retention or excretion of water and other substances according to the needs of organ systems elsewhere in the body. **2.** something nonphysical that obstructs or separates, such as barriers to communication or compliance. **3.** (in radiography) any device that intercepts beams of x-rays. A primary barrier is one that blocks the passage of the useful x-ray beam, such as the walls and floor. A secondary barrier is one that intercepts only leakage and scattered x-ray emissions. An example is the ceiling.

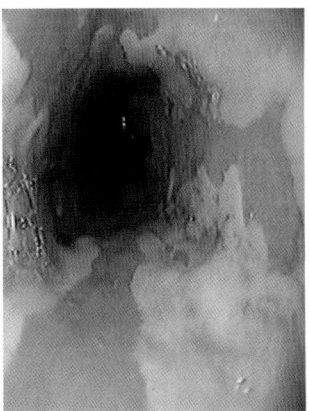

Barrett syndrome *(Goldman et al, 2008)*

barrier creams, ointments, lotions, and similar preparations applied to exposed areas of the skin to protect skin cells from exposure to various allergens, irritants, and carcinogens, including sunlight.

barrier-free design [AS, *freo,barreres;* L, *designare,* to mark out], the design of homes, workplaces, and public buildings that allows individuals with physical disabilities or other disabilities to access and participate in the use of such structures to complete everyday activities. It typically refers to eliminating architectural barriers.

barrier methods, contraceptive methods, such as condoms and diaphragms, in which a plastic or rubber barrier blocks passage of spermatozoa through the vagina or cervix. See also **contraception.**

Barsony-Koppenstein method, a technique for creating radiographic images of the cervical intervertebral foramina.

Barthel Index (BI) [D.W. Barthel, 20th century American psychiatrist], a disability profile scale developed by D.W. Barthel in 1965 to evaluate a patient's self-care abilities in 10 areas, including bowel and bladder control. The patient is scored from 0 to 15 points in various categories, depending on his or her need for help, such as in feeding, bathing, dressing, and walking. This measurement tool is most commonly used with patients with neuromuscular and musculoskeletal conditions who are in an inpatient rehabilitation setting. It has been used with rehabilitation patients to predict length of stay and to indicate the amount of care needed.

bartholinitis /bär″təlinī″tis/ [Caspar T. Bartholin, Danish anatomist, 1655–1738; Gk, *itis*], an inflammatory condition of one or both Bartholin glands, caused by bacterial infection. Usually the causative microorganism is a species of *Streptococcus, Staphylococcus,* or *Escherichia coli,* or a strain of gonococcus. The condition is characterized by swelling of one or both glands, pain, and development of an abscess in the infected gland. A fistula may develop from the gland to the vagina, anus, or perineum. Treatment includes local application of heat, often by soaking in hot water; antibiotics; or, if necessary, incision of the gland and drainage of the purulent material or excision of the entire gland and its duct.

Bartholin abscess /bär″təlinz/ [Caspar T. Bartholin; L, *abscedere,* to go away], an abscess of the greater vestibular gland (also called Bartholin gland) of the vulva.

Bartholin cyst [Caspar T. Bartholin], a cyst that arises from one of the vestibular or Bartholin glands or from its ducts and fills with clear fluid that replaces the suppurative exudate characteristic of chronic inflammation.

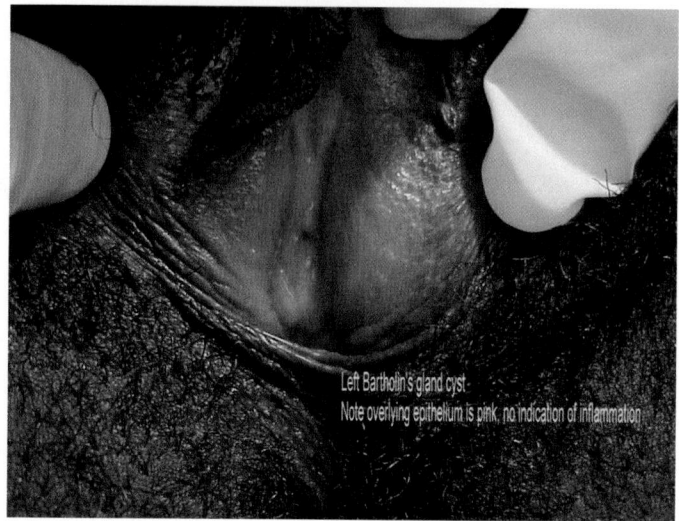

Left Bartholin's gland cyst:
Note overlying epithelium is pink, no indication of inflammation

Bartholin cyst *(Bieber, Horowitz, and Sanfilippo, 2006)*

Bartholin duct [Caspar T. Bartholin], the major channel for drainage of the sublingual salivary gland.

Bartholin gland [Caspar T. Bartholin], one of two small mucous-secreting glands located on the posterior and lateral aspect of the vestibule of the vagina. Also called **greater vestibular gland.**

Bartholin gland carcinoma [Caspar T. Bartholin], a rare malignancy comprising 1% to 2% of vulvar carcinomas that occurs deep in the labia majora. Treatment is radical vulvectomy and bilateral lymphadenectomy. Recurrence is common, but the 5-year survival rate is 85%.

Barton, Clara, (1821–1912), an American philanthropist, humanitarian, and founder of the American National Red Cross. During the U.S. Civil War, she was a volunteer nurse, often on the battlefield, and at its end she organized a bureau of records to help in the search for missing men. When the Franco-Prussian War erupted, she assisted in the organization of military hospitals in Europe in association with the International Red Cross. This experience led to her advocacy of the establishment of an American Red Cross organization of which she became the first president.

Bartonella /bär'tənel″ə/ [Alberto Barton, Peruvian bacteriologist, 1871–1950], a genus of small gram-negative flagellated pleomorphic coccobacilli, some of which are opportunistic pathogens. Members of the genus infect red blood cells and the epithelial cells of the lymph nodes, liver, and spleen. They are transmitted at night by the bite of a sandfly of the genus *Phlebotomus*. Three species are considered important in human disease. *B. bacilliformis* causes bartonellosis. Because of its distinctive appearance, it is easily identified on microscopic examination of a smear of blood stained with Wright's stain. *B. henselae* is the causative agent of cat-scratch fever and bacillary angiomatosis. *B. quintana* causes trench fever and may cause peliosis of the liver.

Barton, George [1871–1923], an architect who in 1917 organized a group of individuals interested in the advancement of occupational therapy and served as president of the group, the National Society for the Promotion of Occupational Therapy. Barton became interested in occupational therapy during a long convalescence, when he recognized the importance of activity in assisting him to cope with his illness and deal with his disabilities. The National Society for the Promotion of Occupational Therapy became the American Occupational Therapy

Association in 1921. See also **American Occupational Therapy Association.**

Bartonella henselae, the etiological agent of cat-scratch fever. Feline infection results in chronic asymptomatic bacteremia, which may last up to 17 months. Approximately 40% of cats are infected with the organism. Most human infections occur between September and February and follow a cat bite or scratch.

bartonellosis /bär'tənəlō″sis/, an acute infection caused by *Bartonella bacilliformis,* transmitted by the bite of a sandfly. It is characterized by fever, severe anemia, bone pain, and, several weeks after the first symptoms are observed, multiple nodular or verrucous skin lesions. The disease is endemic in the valleys of the Andes in Peru, Colombia, and Ecuador. The treatment usually includes chloramphenicol, penicillin, streptomycin, or tetracycline. Untreated, the infection is often fatal. Also called **Carrión disease, Oroya fever, verruga peruana.**

Barton forceps. See **obstetric forceps.**

Barton fracture [John R. Barton, American surgeon, 1794–1871], a distal radius fracture with dislocation of the radiocarpal joint; it is the most common fracture dislocation of the wrist joint.

Bartter syndrome /bär'tərz/ [Frederick C. Bartter, American physiologist, 1914–1983], autosomal-recessive renal tubular disorders characterized by hypokalemia, hypochloremia, metabolic alkalosis, and hyperreninemia with normal blood pressure. There are excessive urinary losses of sodium, chloride, and potassium. The syndrome is traditionally classified into three main clinical variants: neonatal (or antenatal) Bartter syndrome, classic Bartter syndrome, and Gitelman syndrome. Early signs in childhood are abnormal physical growth (dwarfism) and cognitive impairment, often accompanied by chronic hypokalemia and alkalosis.

bary-, combining form meaning "heavy" or "difficult."

barye. See **bar,** def. 1.

basal /bā″səl/ [Gk, *basis,* foundation], pertaining to the fundamental, basic, or lowest level, as basal anesthesia, which produces the first stage of unconsciousness, and the basal metabolic rate, which indicates the lowest metabolic rate.

basal acid output (BAO), the minimum amount of gastric hydrochloric acid produced by an individual after fasting for 8 hours. The normal adult volume is 2 to 5 mEq/hr. It is used in the diagnosis of various diseases of the stomach and intestines, such as gastric ulcers and Zollinger-Ellison syndrome. It is most useful in the evaluation of the effectiveness of acid suppression with medications or surgical vagotomy and to evaluate patients for hyperacidity.

basal body temperature method of family planning, a natural method of family planning that relies on identification of the fertile period of the menstrual cycle by noting the rise in basal body temperature that occurs with ovulation. The progesterone-mediated rise is 0.5° to 1° F; rate and pattern vary greatly from woman to woman, and to some extent from cycle to cycle in any one woman. The woman keeps careful records over several cycles, taking her temperature at the same time every morning before getting out of bed or doing anything else. She may take her temperature orally or rectally in the same way every day. Talking, getting up, smoking a cigarette, eating, or even moving about in bed may change the temperature. Many other factors may also affect the reading, including infection, stress, a bad night's sleep, medication, or environmental temperature. If any of these factors is present, the woman notes them on her record. Abstinence is required to avoid pregnancy from 6 days before the earliest day that ovulation was noted to occur during the preceding 6 months until the third day after the rise in temperature in the current cycle. The days after that period are considered "safe" infertile days. Another way of calculating the possible beginning of the fertile days is to subtract 19 days from the shortest complete menstrual cycle of the preceding 6 months. The basal body temperature method is more effective when used with the ovulation method than is either method used alone. The combination of these methods is called the symptothermal method of family planning. Compare **ovulation method of family planning.**

basal body temperature (BBT), the temperature of the body under conditions of absolute rest, taken orally or rectally, after sleep, and before the patient does anything, including getting out of bed, smoking a cigarette, moving around, talking, eating, or drinking.

basal bone,   **1.** (in prosthodontics) the osseous tissue of the mandible and the maxilla, which provides support for artificial dentures. **2.** (in orthodontics) the fixed osseous structure that limits the movement of teeth in the creation of a stable occlusion.

basal cell, any one of the cells in the deepest layer of stratified epithelium; the base.

basal cell acanthoma.   See **basal cell papilloma.**

basal cell carcinoma [Gk, *basis* + L, *cella,* storeroom; Gk, *karkinos,* crab, *oma,* tumor], a malignant epithelial cell tumor that begins as a pearly-appearing papule and enlarges peripherally, developing a central crater that erodes, crusts, and bleeds. Metastasis is rare, but local invasion destroys

underlying and adjacent tissue. It occurs most frequently in sun-exposed areas of the body, such as the face, ears, neck, scalp, shoulders, and back. The primary known cause of the cancer is excessive exposure to the sun or to radiation. Treatment is eradication of the lesion, often by electrodesiccation, laser, or cryotherapy. Lesions may also be treated with topical or injection chemotherapy or radiation. Also called *basal cell epithelioma,* **basaloma, basiloma, carcinoma basocellulare, hair matrix carcinoma.** See also **rodent ulcer.**

basal cell papilloma,   now called **seborrheic keratosis.**

basal energy expenditure (BEE),   now called **basal metabolic rate.**

basal ganglia [Gk, *basis* + *ganglion,* knot],   areas of gray matter, largely composed of cell bodies, within each cerebral hemisphere. The most important are the caudate nucleus, the putamen, the substantia nigra, the subthalamic nucleus, and the pallidum. The basal ganglia are surrounded by the rings of the limbic system and lie between the thalamus of the diencephalon and the white matter of the hemisphere.

Basaljel,   an antacid. Brand name for *aluminum carbonate gel.*

basal lamina [Gk, *basis* + L, *lamina,* plate],   a thin, noncellular layer of ground substance lying just under epithelial tissue surfaces. Constituting the amorphous portion of the basement membrane, it can be examined with an electron microscope. Also called **basement lamina.**

basal layer.   See **stratum basale.**

basal layer of endometrium,   the deepest layer of the endometrium, which contains the blind ends of the uterine glands; the cells of this layer undergo minimal change during the sexual cycle.

basal layer of epidermis.   See **stratum basale.**

basal membrane,   the innermost layer of the epidermis.

basal metabolic rate (BMR),   the amount of energy used in a unit of time by a fasting, resting subject to maintain vital functions. The rate, determined by the amount of oxygen used, is expressed in Calories consumed per hour per square meter of body surface area or per kilogram of body weight. Also called **basal energy expenditure.** See also **Calorie.**

basal metabolism [Gk, *basis* + *metabole,* change],   the amount of energy needed to maintain essential body functions, such as respiration, circulation, temperature, peristalsis, and muscle tone. Basal metabolism is measured when the subject is awake and at complete rest, has not eaten for 14 to 18 hours, and is in a comfortable, warm environment. It is expressed as a basal metabolic rate, according to calories per hour per square meter of body surface. See also **Calorie.**

basaloid carcinoma /bā″səloid/   [Gk, *basis* + *eidos,* form, *karkinos,* crab, *oma,* tumor],   a rare transitional malignant neoplasm of the anal canal containing areas that resemble basal cell carcinoma of the skin. Basaloid carcinoma is rapidly invasive. Tumor may spread to the skin of the perineum.

basaloma.   See **basal cell carcinoma.**

basal seat,   (in dentistry) the oral structures that support a denture. See also **basal seat outline.**

basal seat area.   See **stress-bearing area.**

basal seat outline,   a profile on the oral mucous membrane or on a plaster cast model of the entire oral area to be covered by a denture. See also **basal seat.**

basal temperature.   See **basal body temperature.**

basal temperature chart [Gk, *basis,* foundation; L, *temperatura* + *charta,* paper],   a daily temperature chart, usually including the temperature on awakening. A basal temperature chart is sometimes used by women to establish a date of ovulation, when the temperature may show a sudden increase, or as a means of natural family planning to determine "safe days" for coitus.

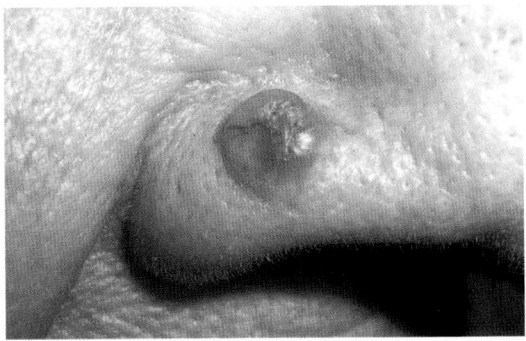

Basal cell carcinoma *(Rakel and Rakel, 2016)*

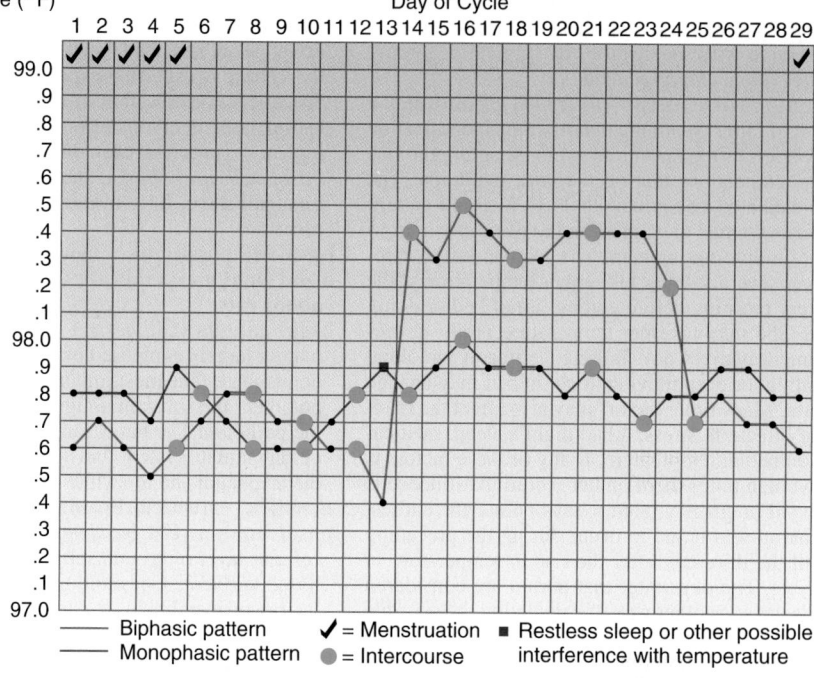

Temperature (°F) Day of Cycle

Basal temperature rise during ovulation (McKinney et al, 2009)

basal tidal volume, the amount of air inhaled and exhaled by a healthy person at complete rest, with all bodily functions at a minimal level of activity, adjusted for age, weight, and sex. See also **tidal volume.**

base [Gk, *basis,* foundation], **1.** a chemical compound that increases the concentration of hydroxide ions in aqueous solution. See also **acid, alkali. 2.** a molecule or radical that takes up or accepts hydrogen ions. **3.** an electron pair donor. **4.** the major ingredient of a compounded material, particularly one that is used as a medication. Petroleum jelly is frequently used as a base for ointments.

base analog [Gk, *basis + analogos,* proportionate], a chemical analog of one of the purine or the pyrimidine bases normally found in RNA or DNA. Modified base analogs have been used in therapy to block polymerization and replication of a pathogen's genome.

Basedow goiter /bä″sədōz/ [Karl A. von Basedow, German physician, 1799–1854], a name for a colloid goiter. A colloid goiter occurs when there is insufficient iodine to produce adequate levels of thyroid hormones. The thyroid gland compensates by enlarging, causing an increase in hormone production.

base excess, a measure of metabolic alkalosis or metabolic acidosis (negative value of base excess) expressed as the amount of acid or alkali needed to titrate 1 L of fully oxygenated blood to a pH of 7.40, the temperature being held at a constant 37° C and the PCO_2 at 40 mm Hg.

base-forming food, a food that increases the pH of the urine. Base-forming foods mainly are fruits, vegetables, and dairy products, which are sources of sodium and potassium. Some foods that are acidic in their natural state may be converted to alkaline metabolites.

baseline /bās″līn/ [Gk, *basis* + L, *linea*], **1.** a known value or quantity with which an unknown is compared when measured or assessed (e.g., baseline vital signs). **2.** the patient's initial information at diagnosis or assessment against which later tests will be compared; level of performance or aggregate findings before therapy. **3.** (in radiology) any of several basic anatomical planes or locations used for positioning purposes. They include the orbitomeatal, infraorbitomeatal, acanthomeatal, and glabellomeatal lines.

baseline behavior, a specified frequency and form of a particular behavior during preexperimental or pretherapeutic conditions.

baseline condition, an environmental condition during which a particular behavior reflects a stable rate of response before the introduction of experimental or therapeutic conditions.

baseline fetal heart rate, the mean fetal heart rate pattern, assessed between uterine contractions. An electronic fetal monitor is used to detect abnormally rapid or slow rates (less than 110 or more than 160 beats/min) at term.

baseline pain, the highest, most consistent level of pain over a period of time.

Basel Nomina Anatomica, an international system of anatomical terminology adopted at a meeting in Basel, Switzerland, in 1895.

basement lamina, now called **basal lamina.**

basement membrane [Fr, *soubassement,* under base], the fragile noncellular layer that secures the overlying epithelium to the underlying tissue. It is the deepest layer, may contain reticular fibers, and can be selectively stained with silver stains. Also called **basal lamina, basement lamina.**

base of gastric gland, a component of the basic secretory unit of the stomach. The isthmus and neck of the gland lead down to the lowest portion, the base.

base of renal pyramid, the part of a renal pyramid that is directed away from the renal sinus.

base of the heart, the portion of the heart opposite the apex. It is superior and medially located. It forms the upper border of the heart, lies just below the second rib, and primarily involves the left atrium, part of the right atrium, and the proximal portions of the great vessels.

base of the skull, the floor of the skull containing the anterior, middle, and posterior cranial fossae and numerous foramina, such as the optic foramen, foramen ovale, foramen lacerum, and foramen magnum.

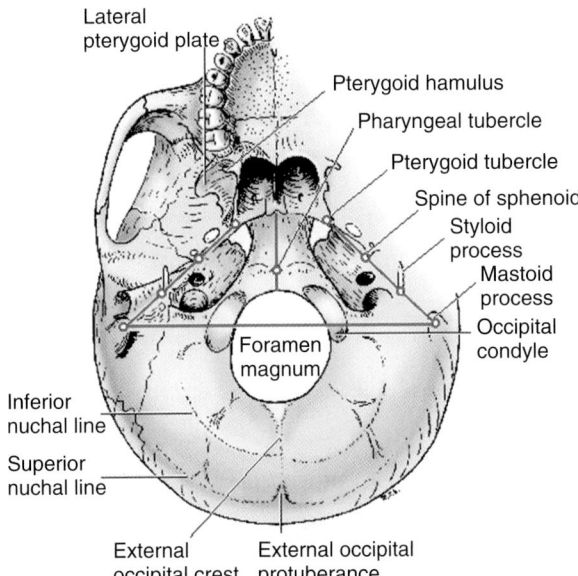

Lateral pterygoid plate
Pteygoid hamulus
Pharyngeal tubercle
Pterygoid tubercle
Spine of sphenoid
Styloid process
Mastoid process
Occipital condyle
Foramen magnum
Inferior nuchal line
Superior nuchal line
External occipital crest
External occipital protuberance

Base of the skull *(Sinnatamby, 2011)*

base pair, a pair of nucleotides in the complementary strands of a DNA molecule that interact through hydrogen bonding across the axis of the helix. One of the nucleotides in each pair is a purine (either adenine or guanine), and the other is a pyrimidine (either thymine or cytosine). Because of distinct hydrogen bonding capacity, adenine always pairs with thymine, and guanine always pairs with cytosine.

base pairing, the formation of base pairs in DNA.

baseplate [Gk, *basis* + ME, *plate*], a temporary prosthetic structure that represents the base of a denture, used for making records of maxillomandibular relationships, for evaluating lip line and lip fullness, for arranging artificial denture teeth, or for ensuring a precise fit of a denture by trial placement in the mouth. Also called *record base,* **temporary base.**

baseplate wax, a pink-colored dental wax containing about 75% paraffin or ceresin with additions of beeswax and other waxes and resins; used chiefly to establish the initial arch form in making trial dentures for the arrangement of artificial denture teeth, and for the construction of complete dentures.

base ratio, the ratio of the molar quantities of purine and pyrimidine bases in DNA and RNA.

bas-fond /bäfôN′/ [Fr, bottom], the bottom or fundus of any structure, especially the fundus of the urinary bladder.

basi-, basio-, bas-, baso-, prefix meaning "a foundation or base": *basal, basophil.*

-basia /bā″zhə/, suffix meaning "ability to walk": *brachybasia, dysbasia.*

-basic, suffix meaning "relating to or containing alkaline compounds": *tetrabasic.*

basic aluminum carbonate gel, an aluminum hydroxide–aluminum carbonate gel, used as an antacid, for treatment of hyperphosphatemia in renal insufficiency, and to prevent phosphate urinary calculi.

basic amino acid, an amino acid that has a positive electric charge in solution at a pH of 7. The basic amino acids are arginine, histidine, and lysine.

Basic Cardiac Life Support, *(Informal)* now called **basic life support.**

basic group identity, (in psychiatry) the shared social characteristics, such as world view, language, values, and ideological system, that evolve from membership in an ethnic group.

basic health services, the minimum degree of health care considered to be necessary to maintain adequate health and protection from disease.

basic human needs, (in psychology) fundamental requirements that must be satisfied before higher level needs are met. Physiological requirements include air, water, food, clothing, shelter, and procreation. See **Maslow's hierarchy of needs.**

basic life support (BLS) [Gk, *basis,* foundation; AS, *lif* + L, *supportare,* to bring up to], the care that health care providers and public safety professionals provide to patients who are experiencing respiratory arrest, cardiac arrest, or airway obstruction. BLS includes psychomotor skills for performing high-quality cardiopulmonary resuscitation (CPR), using an automated external defibrillator (AED), and relieving an obstructed airway for patients of all ages.

basic salt, a salt that contains an unreplaced hydroxide ion from the base generating it, such as Ca(OH)Cl.

Basidiobolus /bəsid′ē·ob′ələs/ [Gk, *basis,* foundation + *bolos,* a throw], a mainly saprobic genus of fungi of the family Basidiobolaceae. The species *B. ranarum* causes a mycotic infection called entomophthoromycosis in humans.

basifacial /bā″sifā″shəl/ [Gk, *basis* + L, *facies,* face], pertaining to the lower portion of the face.

basilar /bas″ilər/ [Gk, *basis,* foundation], pertaining to a base or a basal area.

basilar artery, the single posterior arterial trunk formed by the junction of the two vertebral arteries at the base of the skull. It extends from the inferior to the superior border of the pons before dividing into the left and right posterior cerebral arteries. It supplies the internal ear and parts of the brain. Its branches are the pontine, labyrinthine, anterior inferior cerebellar, superior cerebellar, and posterior cerebral.

basilar artery insufficiency syndrome, the composite of clinical indicators associated with insufficient blood flow through the basilar artery; a condition that may be caused by arterial occlusion. Common signs of this syndrome include dizziness, blindness, numbness, depression, dysarthria, dysphagia, and weakness on one side of the body.

basilar artery occlusion, an obstruction of the basilar artery, resulting in dysfunction involving cranial nerves III through XII, cerebellar dysfunction, hemiplegia or tetraplegia, and loss of proprioception.

basilar membrane, the cellular structure that forms the floor of the cochlear duct and is supported by bony and fibrous projections from the cochlear wall. It provides a fibrous base for the spiral organ of Corti.

basilar plexus [Gk, *basis* + L, braided], the venous network interlaced between the layers of the dura mater over the basilar portion of the occipital bone. It connects the two petrosal sinuses and communicates with the anterior vertebral venous plexus.

basilar sulcus [Gk, *basis* + L, furrow], the grove of the brina that cradles the basilar artery in the midline of the pons.

basilar vertebra, the lowest or last of the lumbar vertebrae.

basilic vein /bəsil″ik/, one of the four superficial veins of the arm, beginning in the ulnar part of the dorsal venous network and running proximally on the posterior surface of the ulnar side of the forearm. It is often chosen for blood testing. Compare **dorsal digital vein, median antebrachial vein.**

basiliximab, a monoclonal antibody used for immunosuppression.

■ INDICATIONS: This drug is used in combination with cyclosporine and corticosteroids to treat acute allograft rejection in renal transplant patients.

■ CONTRAINDICATIONS: Known hypersensitivity to this drug contraindicates its use.

■ ADVERSE EFFECTS: Life-threatening effects of this drug include pulmonary edema and cardiac failure. Other adverse effects include hypotension, headache, constipation, abdominal pain, infection, and moniliasis. Common side effects include pyrexia, chills, tremors, dyspnea, wheezing, chest pain, vomiting, nausea, and diarrhea.

basiloma, now called **basal cell carcinoma.**

basiloma terebrans /ter″əbrənz/ [Gk, *basis* + *oma* + L, *terebare,* to bore], an invasive basal cell epithelioma.

basin, a receptacle for collecting or holding fluids. A kidney-shaped basin is commonly used as an emesis receptacle.

basio-. See **basi-, basio-, bas-, baso-.**

basioccipital /bā′si·oksip′ətəl/ [Gk, *basis* + L, *occiput,* back of the head], pertaining to the basilar process of the occipital bone.

basion /bā′sē·on/ [Gk, *basis,* foundation], the midpoint on the anterior margin of the foramen magnum of the occipital bone.

basis, the lowest anatomical part of an organ or other structure.

basis pedunculi cerebri. See **crus cerebri.**

basket /bas′ket/, **1.** a small mesh receptacle inserted through a ureteroscope to retrieve renal stones. **2.** a stainless steel wire receptacle used for cleaning surgical instruments.

basket cell [L, *bascauda,* dishpan], **1.** deep stellate cells (neurons) of the cerebral cortex with a horizontal axon that sends out branches. Each axon branch or collateral breaks up into a basketlike mesh that surrounds a Purkinje cell. **2.** myoepithelial cells of mammary glands stimulated by oxytocin.

basket extraction, an endoscopic surgical procedure in which a basket catheter is used to entrap and fragment calculi.

basolateral membrane, the layer of plasma membrane of epithelial cells that is adjacent to the basement membrane and separated from the apical membrane by the zonula occludens.

basophil /bā′səfil/ [Gk, *basis* + *philein,* to love], a granulocytic white blood cell characterized by cytoplasmic granules that stain blue when exposed to a basic dye. Basophils represent 1% or less of the total white blood cell count. The relative number of basophils increases in myeloproliferative diseases and decreases in severe allergic reactions. An increase in number is seen during the healing phase of inflammation. Basophils produce histamine during inflammatory reactions. Also called **basophilic erythrocyte.** Compare **eosinophil, neutrophil.** See also **agranulocyte,** differential white blood cell count, granulocyte, leukocyte. —*basophilic, adj.*

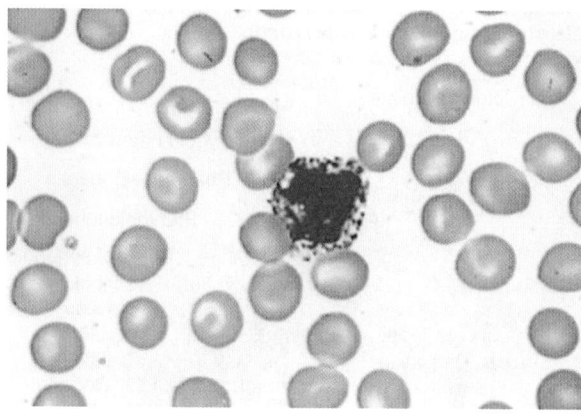

Basophil *(Ramé and Thérond, 2011)*

basophilic adenoma [Gk, *basis* + *philein,* to love, *aden,* gland, *oma*], a tumor of the pituitary gland composed of cells that can be stained with basic dyes. Compare **acidophilic adenoma, chromophobic adenoma.**

basophilic erythrocyte. See **basophil.**

basophilic leukemia [Gk, *basis* + *philein,* to love, *leukos,* white, *haima,* blood], an acute or chronic malignant neoplasm of blood-forming tissues, characterized by large numbers of immature basophilic granulocytes in peripheral circulation and in tissues. See also **acute myeloid leukemia.**

basophilic stippling [Gk, *basis* + *philein,* to love; D, *stippen,* to prick], the presence of punctate blue nucleic acid remnants in red blood cells, observed under the microscope on a Wright-Giemsa–stained blood film. Stippling is characteristic of lead poisoning. See also **basophil, lead poisoning.**

basosquamous cell carcinoma /bā′sōskwā″məs/ [Gk, *basis* + L, *squamosus,* scaly], a malignant epidermal tumor composed of basal and squamous cells.

Bassen-Kornzweig syndrome. See **abetalipoproteinemia.**

batch processing [ME, *baten,* to bake], a processing mode used with computers in which accumulated similar programs or input data are processed simultaneously.

bath [AS, *baeth*], (in the hospital) a cleansing procedure performed by or for patients, as needed for hygienic or therapeutic purposes, to help prevent infection, preserve the unbroken condition of the skin, stimulate circulation,

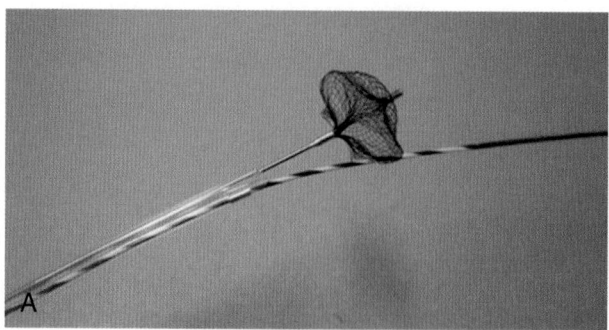
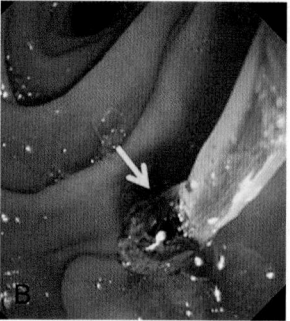

Basket extraction *(Onda et al, 2015)*

promote oxygen intake, maintain muscle tone and joint mobility, and provide comfort. The bath may be a bed bath, a shower, or a partial bath, depending on the patient's condition and preference. The bath period may be used to instruct the patient on hygienic measures, range-of-motion exercises, and general measures to promote skin health.

bath blanket, a thin, lightweight cloth used to cover a patient during a bath. It absorbs moisture while keeping the patient warm. See also *blanket bath.*

bathesthesia /bath″əsthē″zhə/ [Gk, *bathys,* deep, *aisthesia,* feeling], sensitivity to deep structures in the body. Also called **bathyesthesia.**

bathmic evolution, now called **orthogenic evolution.**

bathy-, batho-, prefix meaning "depth, deep": *bathyanesthesia.*

bathyanesthesia /bath′ēan′esthē″zhə/ [Gk, *bathys,* deep, *anaisthesia,* loss of feeling], a loss of deep feeling, such as that associated with organs or structures beneath the body surface, or muscles and joints; a loss of sensitivity to deep structures in the body.

bathycardia /bath′ēkär″dē·ə/ [Gk, *bathys,* deep, *kardia,* heart], a condition in which the heart is located at an abnormally low site in the thorax.

bathyesthesia. See **bathesthesia.**

Batten disease /bat′en/, **1.** also called **Vogt-Spielmeyer disease. 2.** more generally, any or all of the group of disorders constituting neuronal ceroid lipofuscinosis.

battered baby syndrome, an infant who has experienced physical abuse. Also called **shaken baby syndrome.** See **child abuse.**

battered woman syndrome (BWS), a subcategory of posttraumatic stress disorder (PTSD) in which a woman who has experienced physical and emotional abuse continues to reexperience the abuse after it ceases; avoids activities; is in a state of hyperarousal and/or hypervigilance; has difficulty with interpersonal relationships, sexuality, and intimacy issues; and has a distorted body image.

battery [Fr, *batterie*], **1.** a device of two or more electrolytic cells connected to form a single source providing direct current or voltage. **2.** a series or a combination of tests to determine the cause of a particular illness or the degree of proficiency in a particular skill or discipline. **3.** (in law) the unlawful use of force on a person. See **assault.**

Battey bacillus /bat′ē/ [Battey Hospital, in Rome, Georgia, where bacteria strain was first isolated], a bacillus, later renamed *Mycobacterium intracellulare,* that causes a chronic pulmonary disease resembling tuberculosis. It is considered an opportunistic pathogen and does not commonly infect healthy individuals. The organism is resistant to most of the common bacteriostatic and antibiotic medications but may be treated with multiple drug regimens. Surgical resection of involved lung tissue may be necessary and may improve the outcome in serious cases. Rest, good nutrition, and general supportive care are usually recommended. Compare **tuberculosis.**

battledore placenta /bat″əldôr′/ [ME, *batyldoure,* a beating instrument; L, *placenta,* flat cake], a condition in which the umbilical cord is attached at the margin of the placenta. It rarely occurs and does not affect placental functioning. Also called **placenta battledore.**

Battle sign [William H. Battle, English surgeon, 1855–1936], bruising and palpable bogginess of the area behind the ear that may indicate a fracture of a bone of the lower skull.

baud /bôd/ [J.M.E. Baudot, French inventor, b. 1845], a measure of data flow or the speed with which a computer device transmits information.

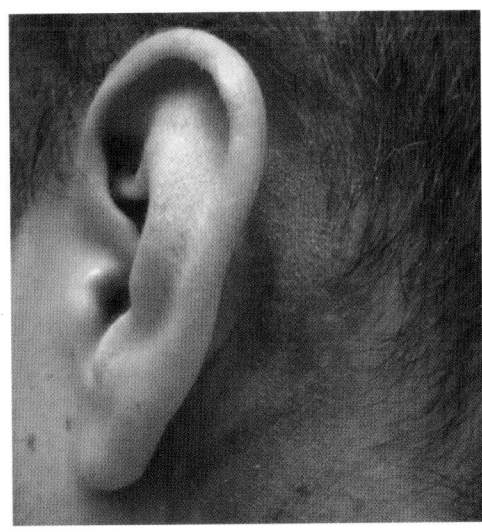

Battle sign *(Parillo and Dellinger, 2014)*

bavituximab, an IgG monoclonal antibody that binds to the surface of certain tumor cells and viruses. The body's immune system detects the antibody and may destroy the cell or virus.

bay, an anatomical depression or recess, usually containing fluid, such as the lacrimal bay of the eye.

Bayes' theorem /bāz″/ [Thomas Bayes, British mathematician, 1702–1761], a mathematic statement that describes an assay's clinical sensitivity and specificity based on its true positive and true negative rates. A true positive assay is one in which the result correctly predicts a condition. A true negative assay is one in which the result correctly predicts the absence of a condition. A false positive occurs when the assay predicts a condition that does not exist, and a false negative occurs when the assay predicts the absence of a condition that is in fact present. The positive predictive value of an assay is computed as the proportion of individuals with a disease and a positive laboratory result compared with all individuals who have a positive result. The clinician considers all clinical effectiveness data when interpreting a laboratory assay result.

Bayley Scales of Infant Development [Nancy Bayley, 20th century American psychologist], a three-part scale for assessing the development of children between the ages of 2 months and 2½ years. Infants are tested for perception, memory, and vocalization on the mental scale; sitting, stair climbing, and manual manipulation on the motor scale; and attention span, social behavior, and persistence on the behavioral scale.

Baylisascaris /bā′lis·as′kä·ris/, a genus of ascarid nematodes found in the intestines of mammals, particularly raccoons. *B. columnaris* infests the central nervous system of dogs. *B. procyonis* is usually found in raccoons and rodents, but fecal contamination from those animals can cause spread to domestic animals and humans, resulting in larva migrans or eosinophilic encephalitis, which is often fatal.

bayonet angle former. See **angle former.**

bayonet condenser [Fr, *baionette*], an instrument used in dentistry for compacting restorative material. It has an off-set nib and a shank with right-angle bends, used primarily for varying the line of force in the compaction of gold. There are many variations in angle, length, and diameter of the nib.

BBB, 1. abbreviation for **bundle branch block. 2.** abbreviation for **blood-brain barrier.**

BBT, abbreviation for **basal body temperature.**

BCAA, abbreviation for **branched-chain amino acids.**

B cell, a category of lymphocyte that originates in the bone marrow and produces antibodies. A precursor of the plasma cell, it is one of the two lymphocytes that play a major role in the body's immune response. Also called **B lymphocyte.** Compare **T cell.** See also **plasma cell.**

B-cell growth/differentiation factor, substances that are necessary for the differentiation, growth, and maturation of plasma cells and B memory cells.

B cell lymphoma, any in a large group of non-Hodgkin lymphomas characterized by malignant transformation of the B cells. See also **non-Hodgkin lymphoma.**

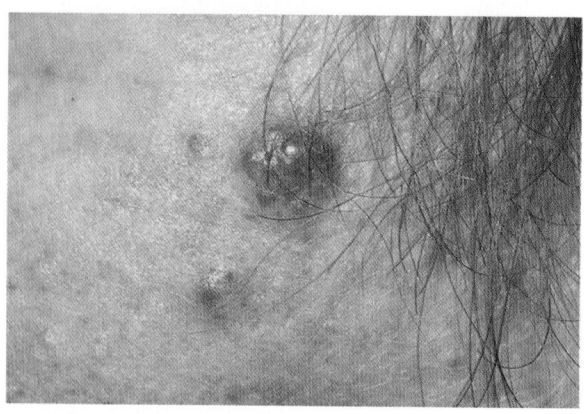

B cell lymphoma *(White and Cox, 2006/Courtesy Dr. L. Barco)*

B cell–mediated immunity, the ability to produce an immune response induced by B lymphocytes. Contact with a foreign antigen stimulates B cells to differentiate into plasma cells, which release antibodies. Plasma cells also generate memory cells, which provide a rapid response if the same antigen is encountered again. T cells play a crucial role in the differentiation of B cells into plasma cells.

B cell stimulating factor-1. See **interleukin-4.**

BCG, abbreviation for **bacille Calmette-Guérin.**

BCG solution, an aqueous suspension of bacille Calmette-Guérin for instillation into the bladder to activate the immune system in treatment of superficial bladder cancers. It reduces the risk of a subsequent bladder cancer developing, although the exact mechanism of action is unknown.

BCG vaccine. See **bacille Calmette-Guérin vaccine.**

BCHC diet, initialism for *Bristol Cancer Help Center (BCHC) diet.*

BCLS, abbreviation for **Basic Cardiac Life Support.**

BCNU. See **carmustine.**

B complex vitamins, a large group of water-soluble nutrients that includes thiamine (vitamin B_1), cyanocobalamin (vitamin B_{12}), niacin (vitamin B_3), pyridoxine (vitamin B_6), riboflavin (vitamin B_2), biotin, folic acid, and pantothenic acid. The B complex vitamins are essential, for example, for the conversion of simple carbohydrates like glucose and the carbon skeletons of amino acids into energy, and for the metabolism of fats and proteins. Good sources include brewer's yeast, liver, whole grain cereals, nuts, eggs, meats, fish, and vegetables. Because some B complex vitamins are produced by intestinal bacteria, taking antibiotics may destroy these bacteria. Symptoms of vitamin B deficiency include nervousness, depression, insomnia, neuritis, anemia, alopecia, acne or other skin disorders, and hypercholesterolemia.

b.d. See **b.i.d.**

BDI, abbreviation for **Beck's depression inventory.**

B-DNA, a long, thin form of deoxyribonucleic acid in which the helix is right-handed.

Be, symbol for the element **beryllium.**

beaded /bē″did/ [ME, *bede*], **1.** having a resemblance to a row of beads. **2.** pertaining to bacterial colonies that develop along the inoculation line in various stab cultures. **3.** bacteria that stand out due to colored stain, appearing in a rounded, beaded shape.

beak, **1.** any pointed anatomical structure, such as the beak of the sphenoid bone. **2.** a pair of dental pliers used in shaping prostheses. **3.** a radiographic image of a bony protuberance adjacent to a degenerative intervertebral disk.

beaker /bēk′er/, a round laboratory vessel of various materials, usually with parallel sides and often with a pouring spout.

beaker cell, now called **goblet cell.**

beak sign, a descriptive appearance for the abnormal structures on radiographic images of the GI tract. A barium swallow is used to facilitate the visibility of the distal esophagus in achalasia as it narrows and makes a right angle, appearing as a bird's beak, before entering the stomach.

Beals syndrome /bēlz/ [Rodney Kenneth Beals, American orthopedic surgeon, 1931–2008], an autosomal-dominant syndrome characterized by long, thin extremities with abnormally long fingers and toes, multiple joint contractures, kyphoscoliosis, and malformed ears; it is a form of hereditary bone dysplasia. Also called **congenital arachnodactyly.** Should not be confused with **Marfan syndrome.**

■ OBSERVATIONS: Individuals with Beals' syndrome are unable to fully extend joints. As a result, muscles can become tight and short, restricting movement. When contractures are present at birth, they can delay motor development.

■ INTERVENTIONS: The treatment varies, depending on presentation. A treatment team, usually composed of pediatricians, orthopedists, nurses, and occupational and physical therapists, is important to achieve normal life expectancy. Physical therapy will improve mobility of joints and strengthen muscles. Surgical procedures may be necessary to release joints and other parts of the body that are permanently contracted. Orthotic devices may be necessary. Occupational therapy will help individuals use assistive technology or compensate for limited movement to complete desired occupations.

■ PATIENT CARE CONSIDERATIONS: Individuals with Beals syndrome should be monitored for cardiovascular complications.

beam [ME, *beem*, tree], **1.** a bedframe fitting for pulleys and weights, used in the treatment of patients requiring weight traction. See **Balkan traction frame. 2.** (in radiology) the primary radiation emitted from an x-ray tube.

BEAM /bēm, bē″ā′em″/, abbreviation for **brain electric activity map.**

beam alignment, (in radiography) the process of positioning the radiographic tube head so that it is aligned properly with the image receptor.

beam collimation, **1.** the restriction of the size and shape of the x-ray beam to the area being examined or treated by confining the beam with metal diaphragms or shutters with high radiation-absorption power. See **beam restrictor. 2.** (in dentistry) a beam-restricting device with either a round or rectangular opening. According to federal regulations, the round collimator reduces the diameter of the x-ray beam to no more than 2.75 inches as it exits the tubehead.

beam hardening, the process of increasing the average energy level of an x-ray beam by filtering out the low-energy photons.

BE amputation, abbreviation for **below-elbow (BE) amputation.**

beam quality, the energy of an x-ray beam. The penetrating power of the x-ray beam is controlled by the kilovoltage.

beam restrictor, a device that reduces the size of the beam of radiation emitted from x-ray equipment.

beam splitter, a device that reflects light from the output phosphor of an image intensifier to a recording device.

beam therapy. See **chromotherapy, external beam radiotherapy.**

bean [ME, *bene*], the pod-enclosed flattened seed of numerous legumes; an important source of incomplete proteins in a balanced diet.

bearing down /ber″ing/ [OE, *beran*, to bear, *adune*, down], a voluntary effort by a woman in the second stage of labor to aid in the expulsion of a fetus. By applying the Valsalva maneuver, the mother increases intraabdominal pressure.

bearing down pains [OE, *beran*, to bear, *adune*, down; L, *poena*, penalty], the extreme discomfort experienced by a woman during the second stage of labor while performing the Valsalva maneuver to help expel the fetus.

beat, **1.** the mechanical contraction or electrical activity of the heart muscle, which may be detected and recorded as the pulse or on the electrocardiogram, respectively. **2.** a throb or pulsation.

Beau's lines /bōz″/ [Joseph H.S. Beau, French physician, 1806–1865], transverse depressions that appear as white lines across the fingernails as a sign of an acute severe illness such as malnutrition, systemic disease, thyroid dysfunction, trauma, or coronary occlusion.

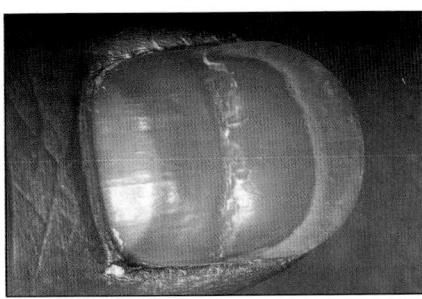

Beau's lines *(Graham-Brown and Bourke, 2007)*

becaplermin /bĕ-kap′ler-min/, a recombinant platelet-derived growth factor used in treatment of chronic severe dermal ulcers of the lower limbs in diabetes mellitus.

Beck, Cheryl Tatano, a nursing theorist whose Postpartum Depression Theory asserts that postpartum depression results from a feeling of loss of control due to a combination of physiological, psychological, and environmental stressors and that symptoms are varied and likely to be multiple. Beck describes four stages of postpartum depression (encountering terror, dying of self, struggling to survive, and regaining control) and identifies 22 key propositions related to postpartum depression.

Becker muscular dystrophy (BMD) [Peter E. Becker, German geneticist, 1908–2000], a chronic degenerative disease of the muscles, characterized by progressive weakness. It occurs in childhood, more frequently in boys between 8 and 20 years of age. It occurs less frequently, progresses more slowly, and has a better prognosis than the more common pseudohypertrophic form of muscular dystrophy. The pathophysiological characteristics of the disease are not understood; it is transmitted genetically as an autosomal-recessive trait. Also called **benign pseudohypertrophic muscular dystrophy.** Compare **Duchenne muscular dystrophy.**

■ OBSERVATIONS: Muscle weakness in the lower extremities that progressively worsens; eventually the individual may be unable to walk. Muscle weakness in the upper body is not as severe as in the lower body. Respiratory compromise is sometimes present.

■ INTERVENTIONS: There is no known cure; treatment is symptomatic. The goal of treatment is to maximize the person's quality of life. This goal is best achieved with a coordinated interprofessional team that focuses on keeping the individual active and engaged in self-care.

■ PATIENT CARE CONSIDERATIONS: Support groups may assist the patient and family in dealing with the chronic, progressive nature of the disease.

Beck's depression inventory (BDI) [Aaron T. Beck, American psychiatrist, b. 1921], a system of classifying a total of 18 criteria of depressive illness. It was developed by Aaron T. Beck in the 1960s as a diagnostic and therapeutic tool for the treatment of childhood affective disorders. The BDI is similar to the 21-criteria DSM-IV diagnostic system of the 1980s except that the DSM-IV scale includes loss of interest, restlessness, and sulkiness, which are missing from the BDI; the Beck inventory lists somatic complaints and loneliness, which are criteria not included in the DSM-III inventory. See also *DSM.*

Beck triad [Claude Schaeffer Beck, American surgeon, 1894–1971], a combination of three symptoms that characterize cardiac tamponade: high central venous pressure as evidenced, for example, by jugular venous distension; low arterial pressure; and muffled heart sounds.

Beckwith-Wiedemann syndrome [John B. Beckwith, American pathologist, b. 1933], a hereditary disorder of unknown cause associated with neonatal hypoglycemia and hyperinsulinism. Formerly called **EMG syndrome.**

■ OBSERVATIONS: Clinical manifestations include unusual growth in both height and weight until approximately the age of 8, a large tongue, and an umbilical hernia. There is enlargement of internal organs, with hyperplasia of the kidney and pancreas and extreme enlargement of the cells of the adrenal cortex.

■ INTERVENTIONS: The management of blood sugar levels is critical. Subtotal pancreatectomy is often necessary in cases of beta cell hyperplasia, nesidioblastosis, or beta cell tumor of the pancreas. Surgical repair of abdominal defects is often necessary.

■ PATIENT CARE CONSIDERATIONS: Children who survive infancy generally do well. Monitoring for signs of tumors is important.

beclomethasone dipropionate, a glucocorticoid.

■ INDICATIONS: It is prescribed in a metered-dose inhaler in the maintenance treatment of bronchial asthma, as prophylactic therapy, and as an aerosol for nasal inhalation to treat chronic allergic rhinitis.

■ CONTRAINDICATIONS: Status asthmaticus, acute asthma, or known hypersensitivity to this drug prohibits its use.

■ ADVERSE EFFECTS: Among the more serious adverse reactions of systemic administration are the symptoms of adrenal insufficiency. Hoarseness, sore throat, and fungal infections of the oropharynx and larynx may occur. Good oral and dental hygiene after each use is requisite.

becquerel (Bq) /bekrel″, bek′ərel″/ [Antoine H. Becquerel, French physicist, 1852–1908], the SI unit of radioactivity, equal to one radioactive decay per second. See also **curie.**

bed [AS, *bedd*], **1.** (in anatomy) a supporting matrix of tissue, such as the nailbeds of modified epidermis over which the fingernails and the toenails move as they grow. **2.** an elevated support for the body during sleep.

bed board, a rigid, slender surface that is placed under a mattress to give added support to a patient with back problems.

bedbug [AS, *bedd* + ME, *bugge,* hobgoblin], a blood-sucking wingless arthropod of the species *Cimex lectularius* or the species *C. hemipterus* that feeds on humans and other animals. Bedbugs are most active at night. The bite, which causes itching, pain, swelling, and redness, can be treated with a lotion or cream containing a corticosteroid or other topical antiinflammatory or analgesic preparation. Infestations of the areas harboring the bedbugs must be treated.

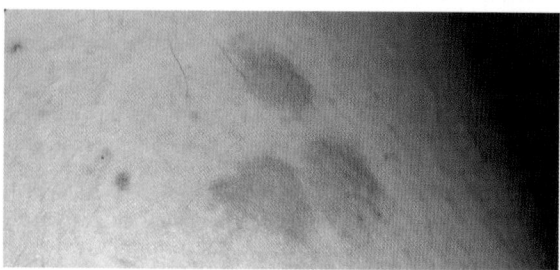

Bedbug bite *(Kliegman et al, 2016)*

bed cradle, a frame placed over a bed to prevent sheets or blankets from touching the patient. See also **footboard.**

Bedford finger stall, a removable finger orthotic that holds the injured and an adjacent finger in a static position, usually extension. It can be worn for prolonged periods.

Bednar aphthae /bed″när/ [Alois Bednar, Austrian pediatrician, 1816–1888], the small yellowish, slightly elevated ulcerated patches that occur on the posterior portion of the hard palate of infants who place infected objects in their mouths. It is also associated with malnutrition. Compare **Epstein pearls, thrush.**

bed pan, a vessel, made of metal or plastic, used to collect feces and urine of bedridden patients.

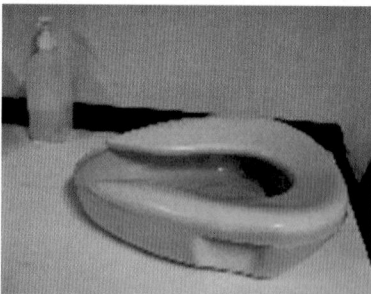

Bed pan *(Nicol et al, 2012)*

bed rest, the restriction of a patient to bed for therapeutic reasons for a prescribed period.

bedridden, describing a person who is unable or unwilling to leave the bed due to physical or emotional conditions.

bed sharing, the practice of having an infant or child sleep on the same surface as an adult. Compare **co-sleeping.**

bedside manner, the behavior of a health care provider as perceived by a patient or peers.

bedsore, *(Informal)* now called **pressure ulcer.**

bedwetting. *(Nontechnical)* See **enuresis.**

BEE, abbreviation for **basal energy expenditure.**

bee cell pessary. See **pessary.**

beef tapeworm. See *Taenia saginata.*

beef tapeworm infection [OF, *buef,* cow; AS, *taeppe, wyrm*], an infection caused by the tapeworm *Taenia saginata,* transmitted to humans when they eat contaminated beef. The adult worm can live for years in the intestine of humans without causing any symptoms. The infection is rarely found in North America and Western Europe, where beef is carefully inspected before being made available and is often thoroughly cooked before eating, but it is common in other parts of the world. Infection can be prevented by cooking beef until it is no longer pink inside. A public health measure is to prevent cattle from eating vegetation contaminated with human feces. See **tapeworm infection.**

bee sting [AS, *beo* + *stingan*], an injury caused by the venom of bees or wasps (vespids), usually accompanied by pain and swelling. The stinger of the honeybee usually remains implanted and should be removed. Pain may be alleviated by application of an ice pack or a paste of sodium bicarbonate and water. Serious reactions may result from multiple stings, stings on some areas of the head, or the injection of venom directly into the circulatory system. In a hypersensitive person, a single bee sting may result in death through anaphylactic shock and airway obstruction. Hypersensitive individuals are encouraged to carry emergency treatment supplies, including epinephrine, with them when the possibility of bee sting exists. Compare **wasp, yellow jacket venom.**

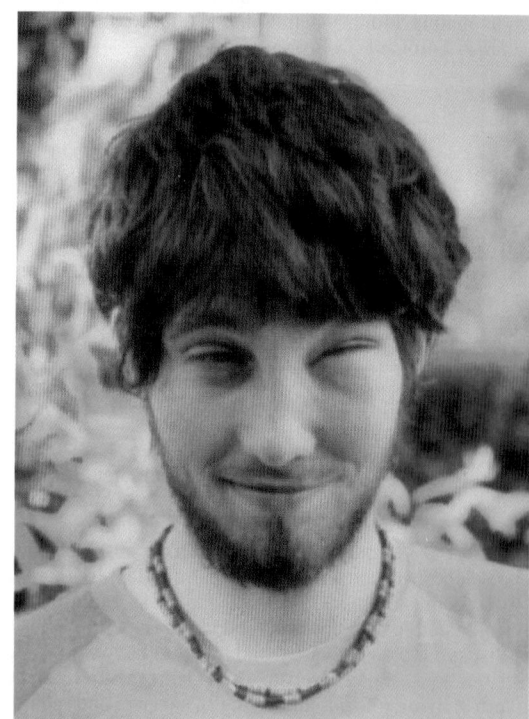

Eye swelling from bee sting *(de Graaf et al, 2009)*

beet sugar, sucrose from sugar beets.

behavior /bihā″vyər/ [ME, *behaven*], **1.** the manner in which a person acts or performs. **2.** any or all of the activities of a person, including physical actions, which are observed directly, and mental activity, which is inferred and interpreted. Kinds include **abnormal behavior, automatic behavior, invariable behavior, variable behavior.**

behavioral health professional services and treatments designed to address mental health and substance abuse disorders.

behavioral isolation /behā″vyərəl/, social isolation that results from a person's socially unacceptable behavior.

behavioral marital therapy, a form of marital therapy using principles and techniques from behavior therapy; it attempts to alleviate marital distress by increasing positive, pleasant interactions between the couple.

behavioral medicine, a multidisciplinary field focused on the study of the interactions of behavior, physiology, and biochemical states to maintain and improve health through changes in behavior.

behavioral objective, the description of an outcome for therapy or health education that identifies a specific behavior or pattern of behavior.

behavioral science, any of the various interrelated disciplines, such as psychiatry, psychology, sociology, nursing, and anthropology, that observe and study human activity, including psychological and emotional development, interpersonal relationships, values, and mores.

behavioral systems model, a framework originating in psychology as behavioral systems theory (BST) extended by Dorothy E. Johnson to describe factors that may affect the stability of a person's behavior. The model examines systems of behavior, not the behavior of an individual at any particular time. In one model, behavior is defined as an integrated response to stimuli. Several subsystems of behavior form the eight human microsystems, which are ingestion, elimination, dependency, sex, achievement, affiliation, aggression, and restoration. Each subsystem comprises several structural components called *imperatives,* which are goal, set, choice, action, and support. The goal of nursing care is to attain, maintain, or restore balance of the subsystems of behavior for the stability of the patient.

behavior disorder, any of a group of antisocial behavior patterns occurring primarily in children and adolescents, such as overaggressiveness, overactivity, destructiveness, cruelty, truancy, lying, disobedience, perverse sexual activity, criminality, alcoholism, and drug addiction. It includes oppositional defiance disorder and autism spectrum disorders. Treatment may include psychotherapy, milieu therapy, medication, and family counseling. See also **antisocial personality disorder.**

behaviorism, a school of psychology founded by John B. Watson that studies and interprets behavior by observing measurable responses to stimuli without reference to consciousness, mental states, or subjective phenomena, such as ideas and emotions. See also **neobehaviorism.**

behaviorist, an individual with the belief that behavior is based on a stimulus-response reaction.

behavioristic psychology. See **behaviorism.**

behavior modification, purposeful, conscious change in behavior based on an identified need to do so. May be accomplished individually or with the help of professionals, particularly those trained in behavior-modification therapy. See **behavior therapy.**

behavior reflex, now called **conditioned response.**

behavior therapy, a kind of psychotherapy that attempts to modify observable maladjusted patterns of behavior by substituting a new response or set of responses to a given stimulus. The treatment techniques involve the methods, concepts, and procedures derived from experimental psychology; they

include assertiveness training, aversion therapy, contingency management, flooding, modeling, operant conditioning, and systemic desensitization. Also called **behavior modification.** See also **biofeedback.**

behaviour, also spelled **behavior.**

Behçet disease /bā″set/ [Hulusi Behçet, Turkish dermatologist, 1889–1948], a rare syndrome that includes a severe, chronic multisystem inflammatory illness of unknown cause. Also called *Behçet syndrome.*

■ OBSERVATIONS: The disease mostly affects young males and is characterized by severe uveitis and retinal vasculitis. Other signs may include optic atrophy and small, shallow, painful, white or gray lesions of the mouth and the genitals, indicating diffuse vasculitis. It may involve all organs and affect the central nervous system.

■ INTERVENTIONS: Corticosteroids and immunosuppressive therapy may be considered. Treatment is symptomatic and focuses on reducing discomfort and preventing serious complications.

■ PATIENT CARE CONSIDERATIONS: The disease is most common in Japan, Turkey, and Israel, but rare in the United States. The variability of symptoms makes the coordination of care an important consideration.

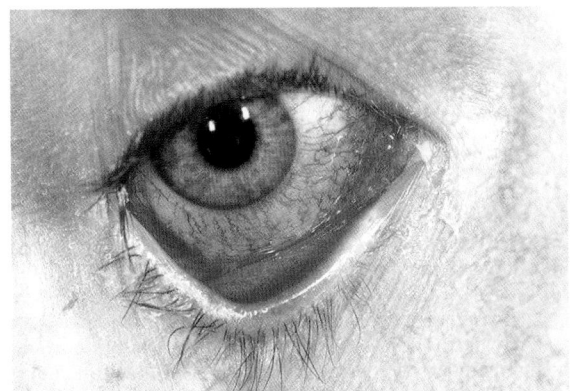

Behçet disease conjunctivitis *(Regezi, Sciubba, and Jordan, 2008)*

bejel /bej″əl/ [Ar, *bajal*], a nonvenereal form of endemic syphilis prevalent among children in the Middle East and North Africa, caused by the spirochete *Treponema pallidum* subsp. *endemicum.* It is transmitted by person-to-person contact and by the sharing of drinking and eating utensils. Also called **dichuchwa, endemic syphilis, frenga, siti.**

■ OBSERVATIONS: The primary lesion is usually on or near the mouth, appearing as a mucus patch, followed by the development of pimplelike sores on the trunk, arms, and legs. Chronic ulceration of the nose and soft palate occurs in the advanced stages of the infection. Destructive changes in the tissues of the heart, central nervous system, and mouth, often associated with the venereal form of syphilis, rarely develop.

■ INTERVENTIONS: Intramuscular injection of penicillin is effective in curing the infection, but if extensive tissue destruction has occurred, scar tissue forms and may be permanently disfiguring.

■ PATIENT CARE CONSIDERATIONS: Transmission is by close contact. Public health measures related to case finding and control of the spread of the disease are important.

Békésy audiometry /bek″əsē/ [George von Békésy, Hungarian-American physicist and Nobel laureate, 1899–1972], a type of hearing test in which the subject controls the intensity of the stimulus by pressing a button while listening to a pure tone whose frequency slowly moves through the entire audible range. The intensity diminishes as long as the button is pressed. When the intensity is too low for the subject to hear the tone, the button is released and the intensity begins to increase. When the subject again hears the tone, the button is again pressed, yielding a zigzag tracing. Continuous and interrupted tones are used, and the tracings of the two are compared. The test may be used to differentiate between hearing losses of cochlear and neural origins.

Bekhterev-Mendel reflex. See **Mendel's reflex.**

bel [Alexander G. Bell, Canadian inventor, 1847–1922], a unit that expresses intensity of sound. It is the logarithm (to the base 10) of the ratio of the power of any specific sound to the power of a reference sound. The most common reference sound has a power of 10^{-16} watts per square centimeter, or the approximate minimum intensity of sound at 1000 cycles per second that is perceptible to the human ear. An increase of 1 bel approximately doubles the intensity or loudness of most sounds. See also **decibel.**

belching. (Informal) See **eructation.**

belladonna /bel′ədon″ə, belädôn″ä/ [It, fair lady], the dried leaves, roots, and flowering or fruiting tops of *Atropabelladonna,* a common perennial called deadly nightshade, containing the alkaloids hyoscine and hyoscyamine. Hyoscyamine has anticholinergic and antispasmodic properties.

belladonna alkaloids, a group of anticholinergic alkaloids occurring in belladonna *(Atropa belladonna).*

Bell-Magendie law, a finding in neurophysiology that states that the anterior roots of the spinal cord are mainly motor, while the posterior roots are mainly sensory. See **Bell's law.**

bellows murmur /bel″ooz/ [AS, *belg,* bag; L, humming], a hollow, blowing sound, such as that of air moving in and out of a bellows.

bellows ventilator, a respiratory care device in which oxygen and other gases are mixed in a mechanism that contracts and expands. The system pressure is increased or decreased in the chamber surrounding the bellows. The gases are moved into the patient circuit when the system pressure increases. As the patient exhales, the bellows contracts and fills again with gases from air and oxygen intakes.

bell-shaped curve, the curve of the probability density function of the normal distribution, resembling the outline of a bell. Also called **normal curve.**

Bell's law [Charles Bell, Scottish surgeon, 1774–1842], an axiom stating that the anterior spinal nerve roots (and spinal cord and medulla) contain only motor and posterior spinal nerve roots (and spinal cord and medulla) are sensory. Also called **Bell-Magendie law, Magendie's law.**

Bell palsy [Charles Bell, Scottish surgeon, 1774–1842], a unilateral paralysis of the facial nerve, thought to result from trauma to the nerve, compression of the nerve, or infection, of which herpes simplex virus is thought to be the most common. Any or all branches of the nerve may be affected. The person may not be able to close an eye or control salivation on the affected side. It usually resolves over weeks but can leave some permanent damage, including decreased taste and hypersensitivity to noise on the affected side. Also called *Bell paralysis, idiopathic facial paralysis (IFP).*

Bell phenomenon [Charles Bell], a sign of peripheral facial paralysis, manifested by the upward and outward rolling of the eyeball when the affected individual tries to close the eyelid. It occurs on the affected side in peripheral facial paralysis.

belly [AS, *beig,* bag], the fleshy central bulging portion of a muscle.

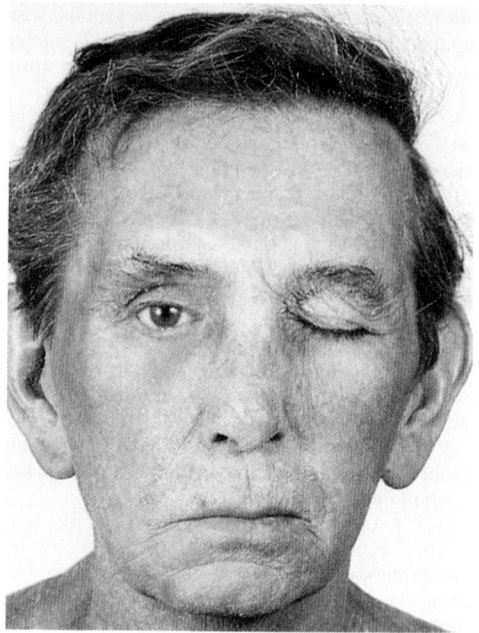

Patient with Bell palsy *(Perkin et al, 1986)*

belly button. (Informal) See **umbilicus.**

belonephobia /bel′ənəfō″bē·ə/ [Gk, *belone,* needle, *phobos,* fear], a morbid fear of sharp-pointed objects, especially needles and pins.

below-elbow (BE) amputation, an amputation of the arm below the elbow; the most common indication is severe trauma.

below-knee (BK) amputation. See **long below-knee (BK) amputation, short below-knee (BK) amputation.**

belt restraint, a device used around the waist to secure a patient on a stretcher or in a chair.

Benadryl, a first-generation antihistamine. Brand name for **diphenhydrAMINE hydrochloride.**

Bence Jones protein /bens/ [Henry Bence Jones, English physician, 1814–1873], a protein found almost exclusively in the urine of patients with multiple myeloma. The protein constitutes the light chain component of myeloma globulin; it coagulates at temperatures of 45° to 55° C and redissolves completely or partially on boiling. See also **multiple myeloma, protein.**

Bence Jones protein test, a urine test whose positive result most commonly indicates multiple myeloma. The test is used to detect and monitor the presence of monoclonal free immunoglobulin light chains (FLCs), important tumor markers in the treatment and clinical course of multiple myeloma and similar diseases. More recently, immunochemical assays for FLCs have been developed for both urine and blood.

bench research, (Informal) any research done in a controlled laboratory setting using nonhuman subjects. The focus is on understanding cellular and molecular mechanisms that underlie a disease or disease process.

-bendazole, combining form designating a tibendazole-type anthelmintic.

Bender's Visual Motor Gestalt test [L, *visus,* vision, *movere,* to move; Ger, *Gestalt,* form; L, *testum,* crucible; Lauretta Bender, American psychiatrist, 1897–1987], a standard psychological test in which the subject copies a series of patterns.

bending fracture, **1.** a fracture indirectly caused by the bending of an extremity, such as the foot or the great toe. **2.** a deformity of a long bone caused by multiple small fractures.

bendrofluazide. See **bendroflumethiazide.**

bendroflumethiazide /ben′drōfloo̅′məthī″əzīd/, a diuretic and antihypertensive.

■ INDICATIONS: It is prescribed in the treatment of hypertension and edema.

■ CONTRAINDICATIONS: Anuria or known hypersensitivity to this drug, to other thiazide medication, or to sulfonamide derivatives prohibits its use.

■ ADVERSE EFFECTS: Among the more serious are hypokalemia, hyperglycemia, hyperuricemia, and hypersensitivity reactions.

bends, *(Informal)* now called **decompression sickness.**

beneficence /bĕ nef′ĭ–sens/, the doing of active goodness, kindness, or charity, including all actions to benefit others. In bioethics, the principle of beneficence refers to a moral obligation to act for the benefit of others.

beneficiary /ben′əfish″ərē/, a person or group designated to receive certain profits, benefits, or advantages, as the recipient of a will or insurance policy.

beneficiary member. See **enrollee.**

benefit. See **covered benefit.**

benefit year, benefits coverage that ends on December 31, regardless of the initial date of enrollment.

Benemid, a uricosuric agent. Brand name for **probenecid.**

benign /binīn″/ [L, *benignus,* kind], **1.** (of a tumor) noncancerous and therefore not a direct threat to life, even though treatment eventually may be required for health or cosmetic reasons. Compare **malignant.** See also **benign neoplasm. 2.** description of a biopsy from a tumor that identifies tissue as nonmalignant and not a direct threat to life, based on cellular characteristics and a lack of invasive properties.

benign congenital hypotonia, a condition marked by signs of weakness and a loss of muscle tone in babies, resulting from nonprogressive weakness of skeletal muscles from birth.

benign cystic nephroma, multilocular cyst of kidney.

benign essential tremor. See **essential tremor.**

benign familial chronic pemphigus [L, *benedicere,* to bless, *familia,* household; Gk, *pemphix,* bubble], a hereditary condition of the skin characterized in the early stages by blisters that break, leaving red, eroded areas followed by crusts. It most commonly occurs on the neck, groin, and axillary regions. It presents in late adolescence or early adulthood. Also called **Hailey-Hailey disease.**

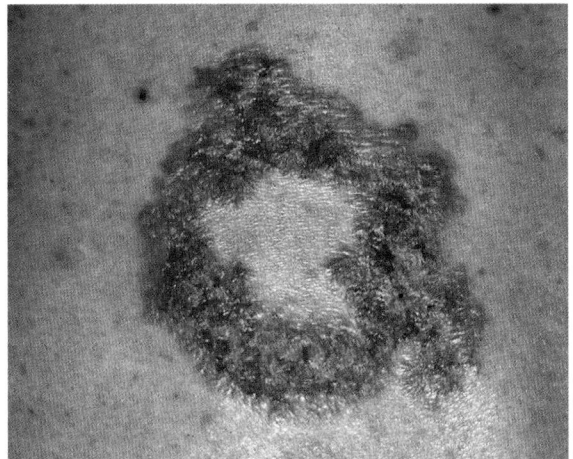

Benign familial chronic pemphigus *(Habif, 2016)*

benign familial hematuria, a rare, usually benign disorder characterized by abnormally thin basement membranes of the glomerular capillaries and persistent hematuria. Autosomal-dominant inheritance is suspected.

benign forgetfulness, a temporary memory block in which some fact from the recent or remote past is forgotten but later recalled.

benign giant lymph node hyperplasia, a condition resembling lymphoma but without recognizable malignant cells, characterized by isolated masses of lymphoid tissue and lymph node hyperplasia, usually in the abdominal or mediastinal area. One variety has numerous small germinal centers near blood vessels with vascular proliferation; a second type consists of sheets of plasma cells and fewer but larger germinal centers. The disease may be either benign or premalignant and overlap with autoimmune diseases. Also called **Castleman disease.**

benign hypertension, a misnomer implying a harmless elevation of blood pressure. Because any sustained elevation of blood pressure may adversely affect health, it is incorrect to refer to the condition as "benign." See also **essential hypertension.**

benign intracranial hypertension, formerly called **pseudotumor cerebri.** Now called **idiopathic intracranial hypertension.**

benign juvenile melanoma, a noncancerous pink or fuchsia raised papule with a scaly surface, usually on a cheek. Occurring most commonly in children between 9 and 13 years of age, it may be mistaken for a malignant melanoma. Also called **compound melanocytoma, spindle cell nevus, Spitz nevus.**

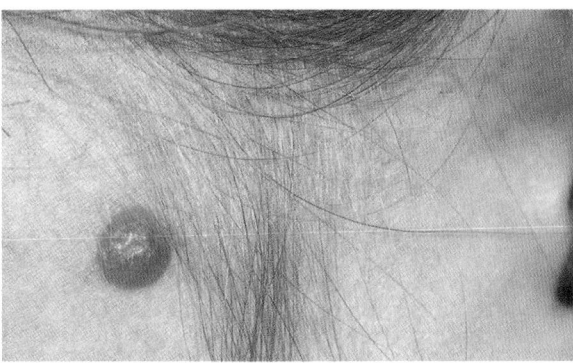

Benign juvenile melanoma *(Habif, 2010)*

benign lymphocytic meningitis, also called **sterile meningitis.** Now called **aseptic meningitis.**

benign lymphoreticulosis. See **cat-scratch fever.**

benign mesenchymoma [L, *benignare* + Gk, *meso,* middle, *egchyma,* infusion, *oma,* tumor], a benign neoplasm that has two or more definitely recognizable mesenchymal elements in addition to fibrous tissue.

benign migratory glossitis, now called **geographic tongue.**

benign mucosal pemphigoid. See **cicatricial pemphigoid.**

benign myalgic encephalomyelitis, chronic muscle fatigue, visual and hearing difficulties, low-grade fever, stiff neck, urinary frequency, and insomnia unrelieved by rest. Also called **Iceland disease, Royal free disease.** See **postviral fatigue syndrome.**

benign neoplasm [L, *benignare* + Gk, *neos,* new, *plasma,* formation], a localized tumor that has a fibrous capsule, limited potential for growth, a regular shape, and cells that are well differentiated. A benign neoplasm does not invade surrounding tissue or metastasize to distant sites. Also called **benign tumor.** Compare **malignant neoplasm.** Kinds include **adenoma, fibroma, hemangioma, lipoma.**

benign nephrosclerosis, a renal disorder marked by arteriolosclerotic (arteriosclerosis affecting mainly the arterioles) lesions in the kidney. It is associated with hypertension.

benign paroxysmal peritonitis. See **familial Mediterranean fever.**

benign paroxysmal positional vertigo, recurrent vertigo and nystagmus occurring when the head is placed in certain positions. It can be debilitating and can cause difficulty in walking straight. It is usually not associated with central nervous system lesions.

■ OBSERVATIONS: Patients may experience the sensation of disorientation in space combined with a sensation of motion accompanied by nystagmus, nausea and/or vomiting, perspiration, pallor, increased salivation, and general malaise. Diagnosis is made by history and clinical exam in conjunction with ENG and positional testing. Audiology, ABR, CT, or MRI may be used to rule out other causes of vertigo.

■ INTERVENTIONS: Treatment is focused on a series of vestibular exercises, including gait training, sets of visual vestibular head and eye movements, and Epley maneuvers. If exercises provoke nausea, premedication with antiemetics may be necessary. Surgical plugging of the posterior semicircular canal may be done in individuals with an intractable recurrent pattern of vertigo attacks that are unresponsive to exercise therapy.

■ PATIENT CARE CONSIDERATIONS: Care focuses on demonstration and return demonstration of prescribed exercises.

benign prostatic hyperplasia (BPH), a histological diagnosis associated with nonmalignant, noninflammatory enlargement of the prostate, most common among men over 50 years of age. Also called **benign prostatic hypertrophy.** Compare **prostatitis.**

■ OBSERVATIONS: BPH diagnosis can only be made after biopsy or resection; otherwise the diagnosis is benign prostatic enlargement. BPH is usually progressive and may lead to urethral obstruction and to interference with urine flow, urinary frequency, nocturia, dysuria, and urinary tract infections.

■ INTERVENTIONS: Treatment may include medication, localized application of heat, balloon dilation, laser vaporization, and microwave hyperthermia. Surgical resection of the enlarged prostate is sometimes necessary.

■ PATIENT CARE CONSIDERATIONS: Some men may experience temporary problems with sexual function after benign prostatic hyperplasia surgery.

benign prostatic hypertrophy. See **benign prostatic hyperplasia.**

benign pseudohypertrophic muscular dystrophy. See **Becker muscular dystrophy.**

benign stupor, a state of apathy or lethargy, such as occurs in severe depression.

benign thrombocytosis. See **thrombocytosis.**

benign tumor. (Informal) See **benign neoplasm.**

benne oil, a nutrient-rich oil used in cooking and for medicinal purposes derived from an ancestor of the sesame seed. See **sesame oil.**

Benner, Patricia [b. 1942], a nursing theorist who confirmed the levels of skill acquisition in nursing practice in *From Novice to Expert*: *Excellence and Power in ClinicalNursing Practice* (1984). Benner used systematic descriptions of five stages: novice, advanced beginner, competent, proficient, and expert. Thirty-one competencies emerged from an analysis of actual patient care episodes. From this work seven areas

of nursing practice having a number of competencies with similar intents, functions, and meanings developed. They are identified as (1) the helping role, (2) the teaching-coaching function, (3) the diagnostic and patient-monitoring function, (4) effective management of rapidly changing situations, (5) administering and monitoring therapeutic interventions and regimens, (6) monitoring and ensuring the quality of health care practices, and (7) organizational work-role competencies. Benner's work describes nursing practice in the context of what nursing actually is and does rather than from context-free theoretic descriptions.

Bennett angle [Norman G. Bennett, English dentist, 1870–1947], the angle formed by the sagittal plane of the working side condyle and the path of the advancing balancing side condyle during lateral mandibular movement, as viewed in the horizontal plane.

Bennett hand tool test, a test used in occupational therapy and prevocational testing to measure hand function, coordination, and speed of performance while using common hand tools, such as a wrench and screwdriver.

Bennett fracture [Edward H. Bennett, Irish surgeon, 1837–1907], a fracture that runs obliquely through the base of the first metacarpal bone and into the carpometacarpal joint, detaching the greater part of the articular facet. A Bennett fracture may be associated with dorsal subluxation or with dislocation of the first metacarpal.

Benoquin, a depigmenting agent. Brand name for **monobenzone.**

benserazide /ben-ser'ah-zīd/, an inhibitor of the decarboxylation of peripheral levodopa to dopamine, having actions similar to those of carbidopa. When given with levodopa, benserazide produces higher brain concentrations of dopamine with lower doses of levodopa, thus lessening the side effects seen with higher doses. It is used orally in conjunction with levodopa as an antiparkinsonian agent.

bent fracture, (Informal) now called **greenstick fracture.**

bentonite [Fort Benton, Montana], colloidal, hydrated aluminum silicate that, when added to water, swells to approximately 12 times its dry size. It is used as a bulk laxative and as a base for skin care preparations. Also called **mineral soap.**

bentoquatam /ben'to-kwah"tam/, a topical skin protectant used to prevent or reduce allergic contact dermatitis from contact with poison ivy, oak, and sumac.

Bentyl, an anticholinergic antispasmodic. Brand name for **dicyclomine hydrochloride.**

benzalkonium chloride, a disinfectant and fungicide prepared in an aqueous solution in various strengths.

benzathine penicillin G. See **penicillin G benzathine.**

benzenamine. Also called **aniline.**

benzene /ben"zēn/, a colorless, highly flammable liquid hydrocarbon (C_6H_6) derived by catalytic reforming during petroleum refining. The prototypical aromatic compound, it is used in the production of various organic compounds, including pharmaceuticals and as an industrial solvent. It is a known carcinogen.

benzene poisoning, a toxic condition caused by ingestion of benzene, inhalation of benzene fumes, or exposure to benzene-related products such as toluene or xylene, characterized by blurred vision, nausea, headache, dizziness, and incoordination. In acute cases, respiratory failure, convulsions, or ventricular fibrillation may cause death. Chronic exposure may result in aplastic anemia (a form of leukemia). See also **nitrobenzene poisoning.**

benzethonium chloride /ben'zəthō"nē·əm/, a topical anti-infective used for disinfecting the skin and for treating some infections of the eye, nose, and throat. It is also used as a preservative in some pharmaceutical preparations.

benzhexol hydrochloride. See **trihexyphenidyl hydrochloride.**

benzo[a]pyrene dihydrodiol epoxide (BPDE-I), a carcinogenic derivative of benzo[a]pyrene associated with tobacco smoke.

benzocaine /ben″zəkān/, an ester-type, local anesthetic agent derived from aminobenzoic acid that is most useful when applied topically. It is used as an adjunct in sedation for passage of the fiberoptic scope for esophagogastroduodenoscopy (EGD) and in many over-the-counter compounds for pruritus and pain. In dentistry it is applied topically to oral tissues before the administration of local anesthesia. Benzocaine has a low incidence of toxicity, but sensitization to it may result from prolonged or frequent use. Topical application of benzocaine may cause methemoglobinemia in infants and small children. A minimum of 5% benzocaine is required in a compound to be effective.

benzodiazepine derivative /ben″zōdī·az″əpin/, one of a group of psychotropic agents, including the tranquilizers chlordiazepoxide, diazepam, oxazepam, lorazepam, and chlorazepate, prescribed to alleviate anxiety, and the hypnotics flurazepam, clonazepam, temazepam, and triazolam, prescribed in the treatment of insomnia. Tolerance and physical dependence occur with prolonged high dosage. Withdrawal symptoms, including seizures, may follow abrupt discontinuation. Adverse reactions to the benzodiazepines include drowsiness, ataxia, and a paradoxical increase in aggression and hostility. These reactions are not common with the usual recommended dosage.

benzoic acid /benzō″ik/, a keratolytic agent, usually used with salicylic acid as an ointment in the treatment of athlete's foot and ringworm of the scalp. It has little antifungal action but makes deep infections accessible to more potent preparation. Mild irritation may occur at the site of application.

benzonatate /benzō″nətāt/, a nonopiate antitussive.

■ INDICATIONS: It is prescribed to suppress the cough reflex.

■ CONTRAINDICATIONS: Known hypersensitivity to this drug prohibits its use.

■ ADVERSE EFFECTS: Hypersensitivity reactions, such as bronchospasm, laryngospasm, and cardiovascular collapse, may occur and may be serious. Vertigo, sedation, headache, and constipation may sometimes occur. The pill should be swallowed whole; a choking feeling and oral numbness may occur if the capsule is chewed or sucked.

benzoyl peroxide /benzō″il/, an antibacterial, keratolytic drying agent.

■ INDICATIONS: It is prescribed in the treatment of acne.

■ CONTRAINDICATIONS: Known hypersensitivity to this drug prohibits its use. It is not used in the eye, on inflamed skin, or on mucous membranes.

■ ADVERSE EFFECTS: Among the more serious adverse reactions are excessive drying and allergic contact sensitization.

benzthiazide /benzthī″əzid/, a diuretic and antihypertensive.

■ INDICATIONS: It is prescribed in the treatment of hypertension and edema.

■ CONTRAINDICATIONS: Anuria or known hypersensitivity to this drug, to other thiazide medication, or to sulfonamide derivatives prohibits its use.

■ ADVERSE EFFECTS: Among the more serious adverse effects are hypokalemia, hyperglycemia, hyperuricemia, and hypersensitivity reactions.

benztropine mesylate /benztrō″pēn/, an anticholinergic and antihistaminic agent.

■ INDICATIONS: It may be prescribed as adjunctive therapy in the treatment of drug-induced extrapyramidal symptoms and all forms of parkinsonism.

■ CONTRAINDICATIONS: Known sensitivity to this drug prohibits its use, and it is not administered to children less than 3 years of age.

■ ADVERSE EFFECTS: Among the most serious adverse reactions are blurred vision, nausea and vomiting, depression, and skin rash. Other adverse effects include urinary retention, constipation, and dry mouth.

benzyl alcohol /ben″zil/, a clear, colorless, oily liquid, derived from certain balsams, used as a topical anesthetic and as a bacteriostatic agent in solutions for injection. Also called **phenyl carbinol, phenyl methanol.**

benzyl benzoate /benzō″āt/, a clear, oily liquid with a pleasant, pervasive fragrance. It is used as an agent to destroy lice and scabies, as a solvent, and as a flavor for gum.

benzyl carbinol. See **phenylethyl alcohol.**

beractant /ber-ak″tant/, a substance obtained from bovine lungs containing mostly phospholipids. It mimics the action of human pulmonary surfactant and is used in prevention and treatment of respiratory distress syndrome of the newborn. Administered by endotracheal intubation.

Berdon syndrome, also called **megacystis-microcolon-intestinal hypoperistalsis.**

bereavement /bərēv″mənt/ [ME, bereven, to rob], a form of grief with anxiety symptoms that is a common reaction to the loss of a loved one. It may be accompanied by insomnia, hyperactivity, and other effects. Although bereavement does not necessarily lead to depressive illness, it may be a triggering factor in a person who is otherwise vulnerable to depression. See also **grief, mourning.**

Berger disease [Jean Berger, 20th-century French nephrologist], a disorder characterized by the deposition of immunoglobulin A (IgA) in the kidneys. Also called **mesangial IgA nephropathy.**

■ OBSERVATIONS: The onset of disease is usually in childhood or early adulthood, and males are affected twice as often as females. Recurrent episodes of macroscopic hematuria and proteinuria are present when renal function is impaired.

■ INTERVENTIONS: Controlling blood pressure and cholesterol levels can slow the progression of the disease.

■ PATIENT CARE CONSIDERATIONS: The condition may or may not progress to renal failure over a period of many years. A spontaneous remission occurs in some cases.

Berger's paresthesia [Oskar Berger, 19th-century German neurologist; Gk, para, near, aisthesia, sensation], chronic paresthesia. See **paresthesia.**

Berger wave. See **alpha wave.**

Bergonié-Tribondeau law /ber′gônē″tribôdō′/ [Jean A. Bergonié, French radiologist, 1857–1925; Louis F.A. Tribondeau, French physician, 1872–1918], a rule of radiobiology stating that the radiosensitivity of a tissue depends on the number of undifferentiated cells in the tissue, their mitotic activity, and the length of time they are actively proliferating.

beriberi /ber′ēber″ē/ [Sinhalese, beri, weakness], a disease of the peripheral nerves caused by a deficiency of or an inability to assimilate thiamine. It frequently results from a diet limited to polished white rice, and it occurs in endemic form in eastern and southern Asia. Rare cases in the United States are associated with stressful conditions, such as hypothyroidism, infections, pregnancy, lactation, and chronic alcoholism. Also called **athiaminosis.** See also **thiamine.**

■ OBSERVATIONS: Symptoms are fatigue, diarrhea, appetite and weight loss, disturbed nerve function causing paralysis and wasting of limbs, edema, and heart failure.

■ INTERVENTIONS: Administration of thiamine prevents and cures most cases of the disease.

■ PATIENT CARE CONSIDERATIONS: Beriberi is usually fatal if left untreated. With treatment, symptoms usually improve rapidly.

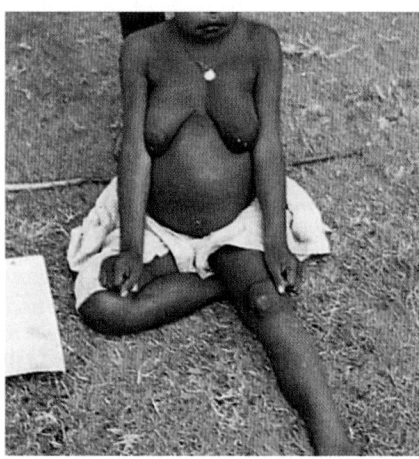

Woman with cardiac beriberi (McLaren, 1992)

berkelium (Bk) /burk″lē·əm/ [Berkeley, California], an artificial radioactive transuranic element. Its atomic number is 97.

Berlin heart, a small artificial heart used in infants and children with severe heart failure.

berlock dermatitis [Fr, *breloque,* bracelet charm], a temporary skin condition, characterized by hyperpigmentation and skin lesions. It is caused by a unique reaction to psoralen-type photosynthesizers, commonly used in perfumes, colognes, and pomades, such as oil of bergamot. Also spelled *berloque dermatitis.*
■ OBSERVATIONS: Berlock dermatitis commonly produces an acute erythematous reaction, similar to that associated with sunburn. The area affected becomes hyperpigmented and surrounded by darker pigmentation. Areas of the neck where perfume containing oil of bergamot is applied often become affected by pendantlike lesions. Diagnosis is based on the appearance of such signs and on patient history, which may include recent exposure to psoralens.
■ INTERVENTIONS: Treatment seeks to identify and eliminate the cause of the condition. Topical steroids may be administered to relieve discomfort.
■ PATIENT CARE CONSIDERATIONS: Patients benefit from advice about the complications of prolonged exposure to sunlight and ultraviolet light. They also appreciate the reassurance that the lesions will vanish within a few months.

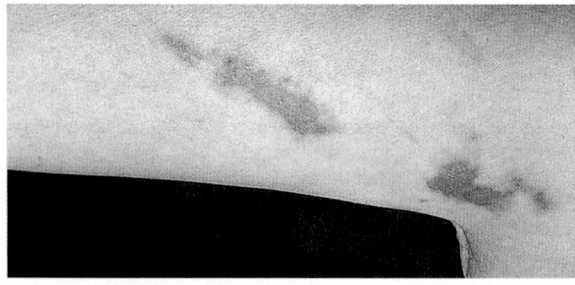

Berlock dermatitis (Callen et al, 2000)

Bernard-Soulier syndrome /bernär″soolyā″/ [Jean A. Bernard, French hematologist, 1907–2006; Jean-Pierre Soulier, French hematologist, 1915–2003], an autosomal-recessive bleeding disorder characterized by an absence of or a deficiency in the ability of the platelets to adhere to von Willebrand factor because of the relative lack of membrane glycoprotein Ib/V/IX. On microscopic examination the platelets appear large and gray. The use of aspirin may provoke hemorrhage. After trauma or surgery, loss of blood may be greater than normal and a transfusion may be required.

Bernoulli's principle /bərnoo″lēz/ [Daniel Bernoulli, Swiss scientist, 1700–1782], (in physics) the principle stating that the sum of the velocity and the kinetic energy of a fluid flowing through a tube is constant. The greater the velocity, the less the lateral pressure on the wall of the tube. Thus, if an artery is narrowed by atherosclerotic plaque, the flow of blood through the constriction increases in velocity and decreases in lateral pressure. Also called *Bernoulli's law.*

Bernoulli theorem /bər·noo″lē/, in an experiment involving probability, the larger the number of trials, the closer the observed probability of an event approaches its theoretical probability.

berry aneurysm [ME, *berye* + Gk, *aneurysma,* widening], a small, saccular dilation of the wall of a cerebral artery. It occurs most frequently at the junctures of vessels in the circle of Willis. A berry aneurysm may be the result of a congenital developmental defect and may rupture without warning, causing intracranial hemorrhage. Smoking and hypertension increase the likelihood of rupture.

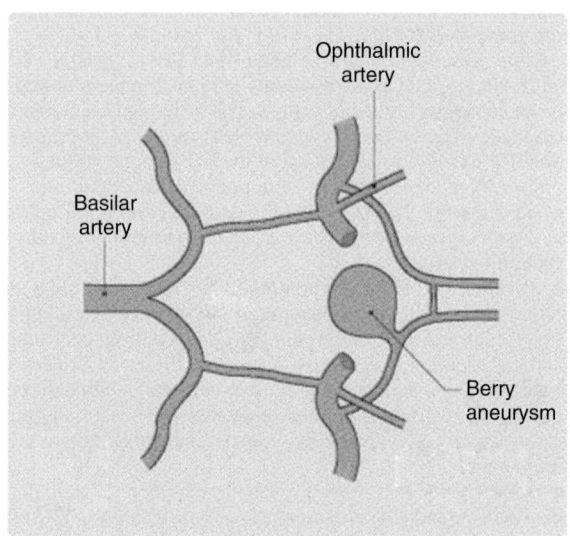

Common sites of berry aneurysms (Russ, 2006)

Bertin column hypertrophy, congenital enlargement of renal columns (columns of Bertin), a benign condition sometimes mistaken for a renal tumor. Also called *renal column hypertrophy.*

berylliosis /bəril′ē·ō″sis/, poisoning that results from the inhalation of dusts or vapors containing beryllium or beryllium compounds. The substance also may enter the body through or under the skin. Also called *chronic beryllium disease (CBD).* See also **inorganic dust.**
■ OBSERVATIONS: Characterized by granulomas throughout the body and by diffuse pulmonary fibrosis, resulting in a dry cough, shortness of breath, and chest pain.
■ INTERVENTIONS: Symptoms may be treated with corticosteroids or methotrexate. In severe cases, lung transplantation may be considered.

■ PATIENT CARE CONSIDERATIONS: Symptoms may not appear for several years after exposure. A team approach including public and occupational health professionals, as well as pulmonary specialists, should be employed.

beryllium (Be), a steel-gray, lightweight metallic element. Its atomic number is 4; its atomic mass is 9.012. Beryllium occurs naturally as beryl and is used in metallic alloys and in fluorescent powders. Inhalation of beryllium fumes or particles may cause the formation of granulomas in the lungs, skin, and subcutaneous tissues. See also **berylliosis.**

best practice /prə·nən·sē·ā″·shən/ [L, *pro,* unamateurishly, *nuntio,* I declare], *n., v., adj.,* the use of scientific evidence, regulations, and expert opinion to determine the most appropriate course of action when addressing a health care problem.

bestiality /bes′chē·al′itē/ [L, *bestia,* beast], **1.** sexual relations between a human being and an animal. Also called **zooerastia. 2.** conduct or behavior characterized by beastlike appetites or instincts.

besylate, a contraction for benzenesulfonate.

beta /bē″tə, bā″tə/, B, β, the second letter of the Greek alphabet, used in scientific notation to denote position of a carbon atom in a molecule, a type of protein configuration, or identification of a type of activity such as beta-blocker, beta particle, or beta rhythm. It is used in statistics to represent a type II error in the interpretation of study results.

beta-adrenergic antagonist, a substance or drug that can inhibit the binding of norepinephrine to the beta receptors (in the heart and bronchial smooth muscle). Binding of norepinephrine to the beta receptors initiates physiological responses such as increasing the rate and force of contraction of the heart, as well as relaxing bronchial and vascular smooth muscle. Beta-adrenergic antagonists can be used to lower blood pressure and heart rate and relieve bronchospasm.

beta-adrenergic blocking agent. See **antiadrenergic.**

beta-adrenergic receptor. See **beta receptor.**

beta-adrenergic stimulating agent. See **adrenergic.** See also **sympathomimetic.**

beta-alaninemia /-al′əninē″mē·ə/, an inherited metabolic disorder marked by a deficiency of an enzyme, beta-alanine-alpha-ketoglutarate aminotransferase. The clinical signs include seizures, drowsiness, and, if uncorrected, death. The condition is sometimes treated with vitamin B₆ (pyridoxine).

beta-blocker, *(Informal)* a popular term for a beta-adrenergic blocking (or beta receptor antagonist) agent. See **antiadrenergic.**

beta-carotene [Gk, beta; L, *carota,* carrot], a vitamin A precursor and ultraviolet screening agent.

■ INDICATIONS: It is prescribed to ameliorate photosensitivity in patients with erythropoietic protoporphyria.

■ CONTRAINDICATIONS: It is used with caution in patients with impaired renal or hepatic function. Known hypersensitivity to this drug prohibits its use.

■ ADVERSE EFFECTS: No serious adverse reactions have been observed. Diarrhea may occur.

beta cells, 1. insulin-producing cells situated in the islets of Langerhans. Their insulin-producing function tends to accelerate the movement of glucose, amino acids, and fatty acids out of the blood and into the cellular cytoplasm, countering glucagon function of alpha cells. **2.** the basophilic cells of the anterior lobe of the pituitary gland.

beta decay, a type of radioactivity that results in the emission of beta particles, either electrons or positrons. See also **beta particle.**

Betadine, a topical antiinfective agent. Brand name for **povidone-iodine.**

beta error, now called **type II error.**

beta-fetoprotein, a protein found in fetal liver and in some adults with liver disease. Compare **alpha-fetoprotein.** See also **ferritin, fetoprotein.**

beta-galactosidase. See **lactase.**

Betagan, a topical glaucoma drug. Brand name for **levobunolol hydrochloride.**

beta-glucan (β-glucan), a soluble form of dietary fiber found in oats and barley.

beta hemolysis, the development of a clear zone around a bacterial colony growing on blood agar, characteristic of certain pathogenic bacteria. Compare **alpha hemolysis.**

beta-hemolytic streptococci, the pyogenic streptococci of groups A, B, C, E, F, G, H, K, L, M, and O that cause hemolysis of red blood cells in blood agar in the laboratory. These organisms cause most of the acute streptococcal infections seen in humans, including scarlet fever, many cases of pneumonia and sepsis syndrome, and streptococcal sore throat. Penicillin is usually prescribed to treat these infections when they are suspected, even before the results of the bacteriological culture are available, because it is known that these organisms as a group are usually sensitive to the effects of penicillin and because the sequelae of untreated streptococcal infection may include glomerulonephritis and rheumatic fever.

betahistine /ba″tah-his′tēn/, a histamine analogue used as the hydrochloride salt and as a vasodilator to reduce the frequency of attacks of vertigo in Ménière's disease, especially in patients having a high frequency of such attacks; administered orally.

17β-hydroxycorticosterone, cortisol. See **hydrocortisone.**

beta-hydroxyisovaleric aciduria, an inherited metabolic disease caused by a deficiency of an enzyme needed to metabolize the amino acid leucine. The condition results in an accumulation of leucine in the tissues, causing maple sugar odor in the urine, ketoacidosis, intellectual disabilities, and muscle atrophy. See **maple syrup urine disease.**

beta₂-interferon. See **interleukin-6.**

beta-lactam antibiotic, any of a group of antibiotics, including the cephalosporins, carbapenems, and penicillins, whose chemical structure contains a beta-lactam ring.

beta-lactamase /-lak″təmāz/ [*lactam,* a cyclic amide, *ase,* enzyme], an enzyme produced by various types of bacteria that catalyzes the hydrolysis of the beta-lactam ring of some penicillins, cephalosporins, and carbapenems, producing penicilloic acid and rendering the antibiotic ineffective. Also called **cephalosporinase, penicillinase.**

betamethasone, a glucocorticoid.

■ INDICATIONS: It is prescribed for topical corticosteroid-responsive dermatoses and injected directly into lesions (bursitis or rheumatoid arthritis, for example) to help control pain and inflammation.

■ CONTRAINDICATIONS: Systemic fungal infections, dermatological viral and fungal infections, impaired circulation, or known hypersensitivity to this drug prohibits its use.

■ ADVERSE EFFECTS: Prolonged use has been associated with hyperglycemia, glaucoma, osteoporosis, and peptic ulcer disease.

beta₂-microglobulin (B₂M) test, a test that analyzes blood, urine, or fluid for increased levels of B₂M, a protein found on the surface of all cells. Increased levels in the urine indicate renal tubule disease; drug-induced renal toxicity; heavy metal–induced renal disease; lymphomas, leukemia, or myeloma; or AIDS. Increased serum levels indicate lymphomas, leukemia, or myeloma; glomerular renal disease; renal transplant rejection; viral infections, especially HIV and cytomegalovirus; or chronic inflammatory processes.

beta-naphthylamine /-nafthil″əmēn/, an aromatic amine used in aniline dyes and linked to the development of bladder cancer in humans.

beta-oxidation, a catabolic process in which fatty acids are used by the body as a source of energy. The fatty acid molecules are converted through a series of intermediates into acetylcoenzyme A molecules, which then enter the tricarboxylic acid (TCA) cycle along with metabolites of carbohydrates and proteins.

beta particle, an electron emitted from the nucleus of an atom during radioactive decay of the atom. Beta particles have a range of 10 m in air and 1 mm in soft tissue. Also called **beta rays.**

Betapen-VK, an antibiotic. Brand name for *penicillin V potassium.*

beta phase, the period immediately following the alpha, or redistribution, phase of drug administration. During the beta phase the blood level of the drug falls more slowly as it is metabolized and excreted from the body.

beta rays, a stream of beta particles, as emitted from atoms of disintegrating radioactive elements. Normally, the element is a nuclide with a high ratio of neutrons to protons.

beta receptor, any one of the postulated adrenergic (sympathetic fibers of autonomic nervous system) components of receptor tissues that respond to epinephrine and such blocking agents as propranolol. Activation of beta receptors causes various physiological reactions such as relaxation of the bronchial muscles and an increase in the rate and force of cardiac contraction. Also called **beta-adrenergic receptor.** Compare **alpha receptor.**

beta rhythm. See **beta wave.**

beta-thalassemia, an anemia that is caused by diminished synthesis of beta chains of hemoglobin due to mutations in the HBB gene. The homozygous form is known as thalassemia major, and the heterozygous form is known as thalassemia minor. See **thalassemia.**

betatron /bā″tətron/, a cyclic accelerator that produces high-energy electrons for radiotherapy. The magnetic field of the betatron deflects electrons into a circular orbit, and an increasing magnetic orbital flux produces an induced circumferential electric field that accelerates them.

beta wave, one of several types of brain waves, characterized by relatively low voltage and a frequency of more than 13 Hz. Beta waves are the "busy waves" of the brain, recorded by electroencephalograph from the frontal and the central areas of the cerebrum when the patient is awake and alert with eyes open. Also called **beta rhythm.** Compare **alpha wave, delta wave, theta wave.**

betaxolol hydrochloride /betak″səlol/, a topical drug for open-angle glaucoma (Betoptic). An oral preparation (Kerlone) is indicated for the management of hypertension.
- INDICATIONS: It is prescribed for the relief of ocular hypertension and chronic open-angle glaucoma (ophthalmic) and for the management of hypertension (oral).
- CONTRAINDICATIONS: Betaxolol hydrochloride is contraindicated in patients with sinus bradycardia, greater than first-degree atrioventricular (AV) block, cardiogenic shock, and overt heart failure. The ophthalmic preparation is used with caution by patients who are also receiving oral beta-adrenergic blocking drugs.
- ADVERSE EFFECTS: Adverse reactions include stinging and tearing of the eyes. Systemic effects are rare. Adverse effects of the oral preparation are bradycardia, fatigue, dyspnea, and lethargy.

bethanechol chloride /bethan″əkol/, a cholinergic agonist.
- INDICATIONS: It is prescribed in the treatment of fecal and urinary retention and neurogenic atony of the bladder.

- CONTRAINDICATIONS: Uncertain strength of the bladder, obstruction of the GI or urinary tract, hyperthyroidism, peptic ulcer, bronchial asthma, cardiovascular disease, epilepsy, Parkinson's disease, hypotension, or known hypersensitivity to this drug prohibits its use. It is not given during pregnancy. It is never given intramuscularly or intravenously.
- ADVERSE EFFECTS: Among the more serious adverse reactions are flushing, headache, GI distress, diarrhea, excessive salivation, sweating, and hypotension.

Betopic, a topical glaucoma medication. Brand name for **betaxolol hydrochloride.**

Betz cells [L, *cella,* storeroom; Vladimir A. Betz, Russian anatomist, 1834–1894], **1.** large pyramidal neurons of the motor cortex with axons that form part of the pyramidal tract associated with voluntary movements. **2.** upper motor neurons.

bevacizumab, a DNA-derived monoclonal antibody that selectively binds to and inhibits activity of human vascular endothelial growth factor to reduce microvascular growth and inhibition of metastatic disease progression.
- INDICATIONS: This drug is used to treat metastatic carcinoma of the colon or rectum in combination with 5-FU IV. It is also being investigated for use as an adjunctive in breast and renal cancer.
- CONTRAINDICATIONS: Known hypersensitivity to this drug prohibits its use.
- ADVERSE EFFECTS: Adverse effects of this drug include hypertension, hypotension, nausea, vomiting, anorexia, diarrhea, constipation, abdominal pain, anorexia, colitis, stomatitis, proteinuria, urinary frequency and urgency, bilirubinemia, hypokalemia, dyspnea, and upper respiratory tract infection. Life-threatening side effects include deep vein thrombosis, hypertensive crisis, GI hemorrhage, nephritic syndrome, leukopenia, neutropenia, thrombocytopenia, exfoliative dermatitis, and hemorrhage. Common side effects include asthenia and dizziness.

bevel /bev″əl/ [OFr, *baif,* open mouth angle], **1.** any angle, other than a right angle, between two planes or surfaces. **2.** (in dentistry) any angle other than 90 degrees between a tooth cut and a cavity wall in the preparation of a tooth cavity. Compare **cavosurface bevel, contra bevel. 3.** the slanted portion of a needle tip that facilitates nontraumatic entry into a vein.

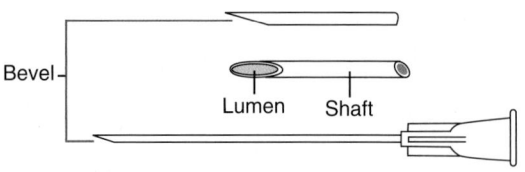

Beveled needle tip *(Mosby, 2003)*

bexarotene, a second-generation retinoid.
- INDICATIONS: This drug is prescribed for cutaneous T cell lymphoma. Investigational uses include treatment of breast cancer.
- CONTRAINDICATIONS: Pregnancy and known hypersensitivity to retinoids prohibit bexarotene's use.
- ADVERSE EFFECTS: Life-threatening adverse reactions include acute pancreatitis, leukopenia, and neutropenia. Other serious side effects include asthenia, infection, anemia, and hypothyroidism. Among the drug's common side effects are headache, nausea, abdominal pain, and diarrhea.

bezoar /bē″zôr/ [Ar, *bazahr,* protection against poison], a hard ball of hair or vegetable fiber that may develop within the stomach of humans. More often it is found in the stomachs of ruminants. Bezoars were once thought to have magical properties.

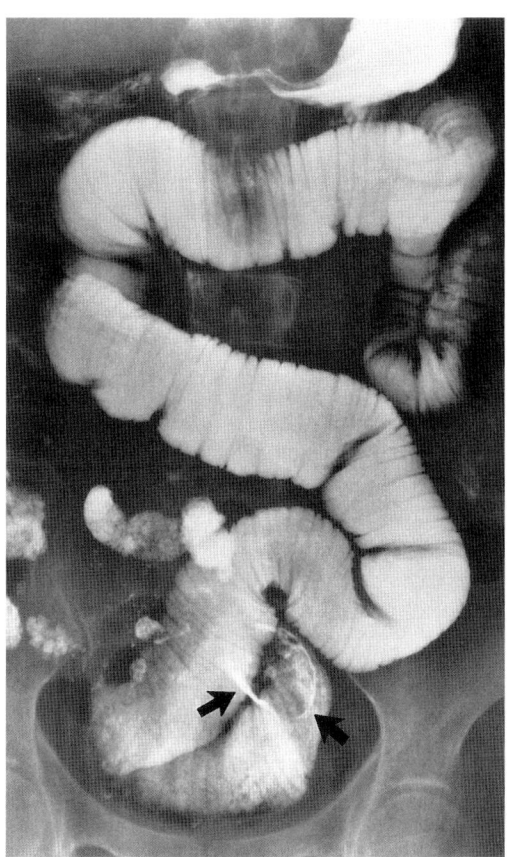

Radiographic image of bezoar *(Eisenberg and Johnson, 2012)*

Bg Bennett-Goodspeed antigens, HLA Class I antigens that may be expressed on mature red blood cells: HLA-B7 (Bga), HLA-B17 (B57 or B58) (Bgb), and HLA-A28 (A68 or A69) (Bgc).

Bh, symbol for the element **bohrium.**

bhang /bang/ [Hindi, *bag*], an Asian Indian hallucinogenic composed of dried leaves and the young stems of uncultivated *Cannabis sativa.* It is usually ingested as a boiled mixture with milk, sugar, or water. It produces euphoria. It also may be smoked or chewed. Also spelled **bang.** See also **cannabis.**

BHC, abbreviation for *benzene hexachloride.*

Bi, symbol for the element **bismuth.**

bi-, prefix meaning "twice, two": *biarticular, bicuspid.*

BIA, abbreviation for **bioelectric impedance analysis.**

-bia, suffix meaning "creature possessing a mode of life": *aerobia.*

biarticular, having or affecting two joints. Also called **diarticular.**

bias /bī″əs/ [MFr, *biais*], **1.** an oblique or a diagonal line. **2.** a prejudiced or subjective attitude. **3.** (in statistics) the distortion of statistical findings from the true value. There can be many kinds of bias; some may be caused by the sampling process, but bias can be caused by other factors. **4.** (in electronics) a voltage applied to an electronic device, such as a vacuum tube or a transistor, to control operating limits. See also **detection bias.**

biased sample /bī″əst/ [OFr, *biais,* slant; L, *exemplum,* sample], (in research) a sample of a group in which all factors or participants are not equally balanced or objectively represented.

biasing /bī″əsing/, a method of treating neuromuscular dysfunction by contracting a muscle against resistance, causing the muscle spindles to readjust to the shorter length and the muscle tissue to be more responsive and sensitive to stretching.

biauricular /bī·aw·rik′yo͞o·lər/ [L, *bis,* twice + *auriculus,* little ear], pertaining to the two auricles of the ears. Also called **binauricular.**

Biavax, brand name for **rubella and mumps virus vaccine.**

bibliotherapy, a type of group therapy in which books, poems, and newspaper articles are read in the group to help stimulate thinking about events in the real world and to foster relations among group members.

bicalutamide, an anticancer chemotherapy agent.

■ INDICATIONS: It is prescribed in the treatment of metastatic prostate cancer. The drug acts by binding to androgen receptors within target cells, preventing androgens from binding to them.

■ CONTRAINDICATIONS: The drug should not be given to patients who have an allergic reaction to it. Bicalutamide should be used with caution in patients with moderate to severe liver dysfunction.

■ ADVERSE EFFECTS: The side effects most often reported include hot flashes, general body pain, asthenia, constipation, nausea, and diarrhea.

bicameral /bī·kam′ər·əl/ [L, *bis,* twice + *camera,* vaulted chamber], having two chambers.

bicameral abscess /bīkam″ərəl/, an abscess with two separate cavities or chambers divided by a thin membrane or septum.

bicapsular /bī·kap′syo͞o·lər/ [L, *bis,* twice + *capsula,* little box], having two capsules, as an articular capsule.

bicarbonate (HCO₃⁻) /bīkär″bənāt/ [L, *bis,* twice, *carbo,* coal], an anion of carbonic acid in which only one of the hydrogen atoms has been removed, as in sodium bicarbonate ($NaHCO_3$). Also called **hydrogen carbonate.**

bicarbonate of soda. Also called **sodium bicarbonate.**

bicarbonate precursor, an injection of sodium lactate used in the treatment of metabolic acidosis. It is metabolized in the body to sodium bicarbonate.

bicarbonate therapy, a procedure to increase a patient's stores of bicarbonate when there are signs of severe acidosis. It is usually performed only in certain cases, and with extreme caution, as a stopgap measure to neutralize acidosis partially when the patient's blood pH has fallen to levels that may be hazardous to the survival of vital tissues.

bicarbonate transport, the route by which most of the carbon dioxide is carried in the bloodstream. Once dissolved in the blood plasma, carbon dioxide combines with water to form carbonic acid, which immediately ionizes into hydrogen and bicarbonate ions. The bicarbonate ions serve as part of the alkaline reserve.

bicellular /bī·sel′yo͞o·lər/ [L, *bis,* twice + *cella,* storeroom], made up of two cells, or having two cells.

biceps, (*Informal*) a muscle having two heads; frequently used to refer to the muscles that flex and supinate the forearm.

biceps brachii /bī″seps brā″kē·ī/ [L, *bis,* twice, *caput,* head, *bracchii,* arm], the long fusiform muscle of the upper arm on the anterior surface of the humerus, arising in two heads from the scapula. It flexes the arm and the forearm and supinates the hand. Also called **biceps, biceps flexor cubiti.** Compare **brachialis, triceps brachii.**

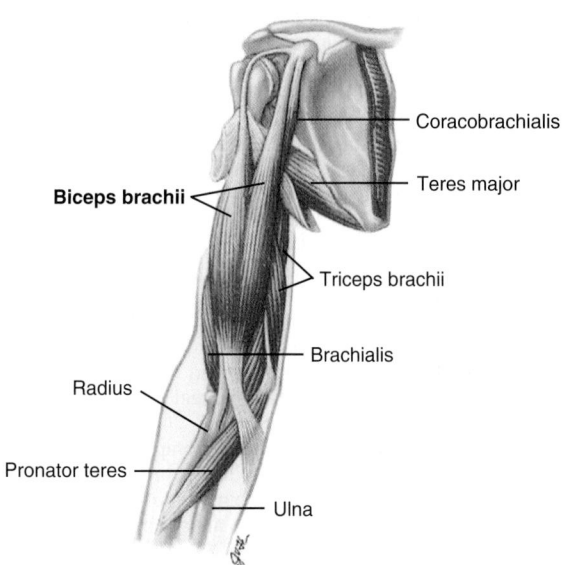

Biceps brachii *(Patton, 2016)*

biceps femoris [L, *bis*, twice, *caput*, head, *femoris*, thigh], one of the posterior femoral muscles. It has two heads at its origin. The biceps femoris flexes the leg and rotates it laterally and extends the thigh, rotating it laterally. It is one of the hamstring muscle group and lies on the posterior, lateral side of the thigh.

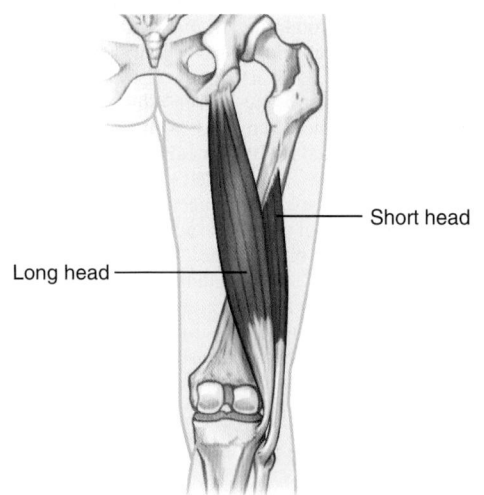

Biceps femoris

biceps flexor cubiti. See **biceps brachii.**

biceps reflex, a contraction of a biceps muscle produced when the tendon is tapped with a percussor in testing deep tendon reflexes. See also **deep tendon reflex.**

Bichat's membrane /bishäz/ [Marie F.X. Bichat, French anatomist, 1771–1802], an elastic lining beneath the endothelium of an arterial wall.

bichromatic analysis /-krōmat″ik/ [Gk, *bios* + *chroma*, color], the spectrophotometric monitoring of a reaction at two wavelengths. It is used to correct for background color.

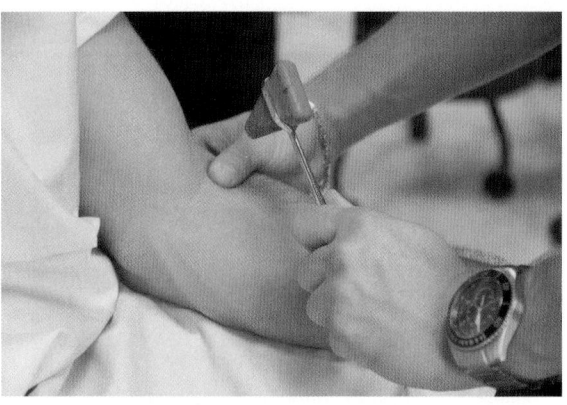

Biceps reflex testing *(Seidel et al, 2011)*

Bicillin C-R /bi-sil′in/, combination preparation of two antibiotics. Brand name for *penicillin G benzathine and penicillin G procaine.*

bicipital aponeurosis, a flat sheet of connective tissue that fans out from the medial side of the tendon to blend with deep fascia covering the anterior compartment of the forearm.

bicipital groove /bīsip″ətəl/ [L, *bis*, twice, *caput*, head; D, *groeve*], a groove between the greater and lesser tubercles of the humerus for passage of the tendon of the long head of the biceps muscle.

biclor /bī″klôr/, abbreviation for *two chloride anions in a salt.*

biconcave /bīkon″kāv/ [L, *bis*, twice, *concavare*, to make hollow], concave on both sides, especially as applied to a lens. −*biconcavity, n.*

biconvex /bīkon″veks/ [L, *bis* + *convexus*, vaulted], convex on both sides, especially such as applied to a lens. −*biconvexity, n.*

bicornate /bīkôr″nāt/ [L, *bis* + *cornu*, horn], having two horns or processes.

bicornate uterus, a uterus with two bodies and cervices sharing a common vagina, the result of incomplete fusion of the müllerian ducts. See **uterus bicornis, müllerian duct.**

bicornuate, also spelled **bicornate.**

bicuspid /bīkus″pid/ [L, *bis* + *cuspis*, point], **1.** having two cusps or points. **2.** a premolar tooth; a first premolar and a second premolar are found in each quadrant of the adult dentition.

bicuspid valve, a valve with two cusps. See **mitral valve.**

bicycle ergometer [L, *bis*, twice; Gk, *kyklos*, circle, *ergon*, work, *metron*, measure], a stationary bicycle used in fitness testing to estimate the exercise intensity (power output) from the rpm and the resistance to pedaling, which can be adjusted to vary the intensity.

b.i.d., (in prescriptions) a Latin phrase meaning "twice a day." Abbreviation for **bis in die.**

bidactyly /bīdak″tilē/ [L, *bis* + Gk, *daktylos*, finger], an abnormal condition in which the second, third, and fourth digits on a hand are missing and only the first and fifth are present. Formerly called **lobster claw deformity.** −*bidactylous, adj.*

bidermoma /bī′dərmō″mə/ [L, *bis* + Gk, *derma*, skin, *oma*, tumor], a neoplasm composed of cells and tissues originating in two germ layers.

bidet /bidā″/ [Fr, pony], a fixture resembling a toilet bowl, with a rim to sit on and usually equipped with plumbing implements for cleaning the genital and rectal areas.

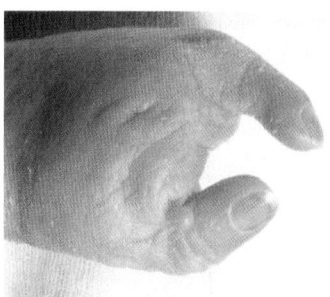

Bidactyly *(Courtesy Dr. Christine L. Williams, New York Medical College)*

biduotertian fever /bī′dōō·ətur″shən/ [L, *bis* + *dies,* day, *tertius,* three], a form of malaria characterized by overlapping paroxysms of chills, fever, and other symptoms. It is caused by infection with two strains of *Plasmodium,* each having its own cycle of symptoms, such as in quartan and tertian malaria. Compare **double quartan fever.** See also **malaria.**

Bier block /bēr blok/ [August Karl Gustav Bier, German surgeon, 1861–1949], regional anesthesia accomplished after intravenous injection of an exsanguinated extremity with a preservative-free local anesthetic such as 0.5% lidocaine. Used for surgical procedures on the arm below the elbow or the leg below the knee. A Bier block is performed by first inserting an intravenous catheter and then connecting a saline-flushed port, such as a hep-lock. The affected extremity is then sequentially and tightly wrapped with an Esmarch's bandage to exsanguinate the extremity. A pneumatic double tourniquet, placed proximal to the elbow or knee is then inflated to a pressure that is 100 torr (mm Hg) greater than the systolic blood pressure. The local anesthetic is then injected intravenously, while the double tourniquet prevents the local anesthetic from entering the systemic circulation. A Bier block is limited to procedures of short duration (less than 1 hour). See also **anesthesia, regional anesthesia.**

bifid /bī″fid/ [L, *bis* + *findere* to cleave], cleft, or split into two parts, as in the spinous processes of the cervical vertebrae.

bifid scrotum, separation of the two halves of the scrotum, as in penoscrotal transposition.

bifid tongue [L, *bis* + *findere,* to cleave; AS, *tunge*], a tongue divided by a longitudinal furrow. Also called **cleft tongue.**

bifid ureter, one in which proximal segments come from two different collecting systems but join to form one ureter before reaching the bladder.

bifid uvula, bifurcation of the uvula, a minor anomaly seen more commonly in Native Americans than in other population groups. Considered an incomplete form of cleft palate.

bifocal /bīfō″kəl/ [L, *bis* + *focus,* hearth], **1.** pertaining to the characteristic of having two foci. **2.** (of a lens) having two areas of different focal lengths.

bifocal contact lens, a small, thin corrective lens placed directly on the cornea that contains corrections for both near and far vision. See also **contact lens.**

bifocal glasses [L, *bis,* twice, *focus,* hearth; AS, *glaes*], corrective eyeglasses in which each lens is made up of two segments of different refractive powers or strengths. Generally, the upper part of the lens is used for ordinary or distant vision, and the smaller, lower section for near vision for close work, such as reading or sewing.

biforate /bīfôr″āt/ [L, *bis* + *forare,* to pierce twice], having two perforations or foramina.

bifrontal suture /bīfron″təl/ [L, *bis* + *frons,* front, *sutura*], the interlocking lines of fusion between the frontal and parietal bones of the skull.

bifurcate /bīfur″kāt/ [L, *bis,* twice, *furca,* fork], pertaining to the division or branching of an object into two branches, such as the branching of blood vessels or bronchi. −*bifurcated, adj.*

bifurcate ligament, a V-shaped ligament in the foot that connects the anterior process of the calcaneus to the cuboid and navicular bones.

bifurcation /bī′fərkā″shən/ [L, *bis* + *furca,* fork], a splitting into two branches, such as the trachea, which branches into the two bronchi.

bigeminal /bījem″inəl/ [L, *bis,* twice, *geminus,* twin], pertaining to pairs, twins, or dual events, such as a bigeminal pulse, which is characterized by two beats in rapid succession. See also **bigeminy.**

bigeminal pulse, an abnormal pulse in which two beats in close succession are followed by a pause during which no pulse is felt. Compare **trigeminal pulse.** See also **trigeminy.**

bigeminal rhythm [L, *bis* + *geminus,* twin; Gk, *rhythmos*], an abnormal heartbeat in which ectopic ventricular or atrial beats alternate with and are precisely coupled to sinus beats, or in which ventricular ectopic beats occur in pairs, as in ventricular tachycardia with 3:2 exit block. Also called **bigeminy, coupled rhythm.**

bigeminy /bījem″inē/ [L, *bis* + *geminus,* twin], an association in pairs. See **bigeminal rhythm.**

bilabial /bī-lā′bē-əl/, a consonantal speech sound produced by using the two lips, such as *b, p,* or *m.*

bilaminar /bīlam″ənər/ [L, *bis* + *lamina,* plate], pertaining to or having two layers, such as the ectoderm and endoderm of the blastula, and the basal lamina interspersed with reticular fibers to form the basement membrane of the epithelium.

bilaminar blastoderm, the stage of embryonic development before mesoderm formation in which only the ectoderm and endoderm primary germ layers have formed. Compare **trilaminar blastoderm.**

bilateral /bilat″ərəl/ [L, *bis* + *lateralis,* side], **1.** having two sides. **2.** occurring or appearing on two sides; for example, a patient with bilateral hearing loss may have partial or total hearing loss in both ears. **3.** having two layers.

bilateral carotid artery [L, *bis,* twice, *latus,* side; Gk, *karos,* heavy sleep], a main artery to the head and neck that divides into left and right branches and again into external and internal branches.

bilateral coordination, the ability to use both sides of the body in a synchronized fashion to accomplish both fine and gross motor activities.

bilateral integration, the ability of an individual to use both sides of the body together in a coordinated fashion.

bilateral long-leg spica cast, an orthopedic device of plaster of paris, fiberglass, or other casting material that encases and immobilizes the trunk cranially as far as the nipple line and both legs caudally as far as the toes. A horizontal crossbar to improve immobilization connects the parts of the cast encasing both legs at ankle level. It is used to aid the healing of fractures of the hip, the femur, the acetabulum, and the pelvis and to correct hip deformities. Compare **one-and-a-half spica cast, unilateral long-leg spica cast.**

bilateral symmetry [L, *bis* + *latus,* side; Gk, *syn,* together, *metron,* measure], similar structure of the halves of an organism.

Bilbao tube /bilbō″ə/, a long, thin, flexible tube that is used to inject barium into the small intestine. The tube is guided with a stiff wire from the mouth to the end of the duodenum under fluoroscopic control.

bilberry, an herb found in the central, Northern, and Southeastern regions of Europe.

■ INDICATIONS: This herb is used for diabetic retinopathy, macular degeneration, glaucoma, cataract, capillary fragility, varicose veins, hemorrhoids, and mild diarrhea; possibly effective for some indications but controlled clinical trials do not support its use for improving vision.

■ CONTRAINDICATIONS: Bilberry should not be used during pregnancy and lactation or in children until more research is available.

bile /bīl/ [L, *bilis*], a bitter, yellow-green, viscid alkaline fluid secreted by the liver. Stored in the gallbladder, bile receives its color from the presence of bile pigments such as bilirubin. Bile passes from the gallbladder through the common bile duct in response to the cholecystokinin (CCK) produced in the duodenum in the presence of a fatty meal. Bile emulsifies these fats (breaks them into smaller particles and lowers the surface tension), preparing them for further digestion and absorption in the small intestine. Any interference in the flow of bile will result in the presence of unabsorbed fat in the feces and in jaundice. Also called **gall.** See also **biliary obstruction, jaundice.** –**biliary,** *adj.*

bile acid, a steroid acid of the bile, produced during the metabolism of cholesterol. On hydrolysis, bile acid yields glycine and choleic acid.

bile duct. See **biliary duct.**

bile duct abscess, a cavity containing pus and surrounded by inflamed tissue in the bile duct.

bile pigments, a group of substances that contribute to the colors of bile, which may range from a yellowish green to brown. A common bile pigment is bilirubin, which contains a reddish iron pigment derived from the breakdown of old red blood cells.

bile salts [L, *bilis*, bile; AS, *sealt*], a mixture of sodium salts of the bile acids and cholic and chenodeoxycholic acids synthesized in the liver as a derivative of cholesterol. Their low surface tension contributes to the emulsification of fats in the intestine and their absorption from the GI tract.

bile solubility test, a bacteriological test used in the differential diagnosis of pneumococcal and streptococcal infection.

Bilharzia, now called *Schistosoma.*

bilharziasis, now called **schistosomiasis.**

bili-, prefix meaning "bile": *biliary, biligenesis.*

biliary /bil′ē-er′ē/, pertaining to bile or to the gallbladder and bile ducts, which transport bile. These are often called the biliary system and biliary tract. See also **bile, biliary calculus.**

biliary abscess, an abscess of the gallbladder or liver.

biliary atresia, congenital absence or underdevelopment of one or more of the biliary structures, causing jaundice and early liver damage. As the condition worsens, the child's growth may be delayed, and portal hypertension may develop. Surgery can correct the defective ducts in only a small percentage of cases. Liver transplantation is an option. Most infants die in early childhood from biliary cirrhosis. It is essential to distinguish between this condition and neonatal hepatitis, which is treatable. See also **biliary cirrhosis.**

biliary calculus [L, *bilis*, bile, *calculus*, pebble], a stone formed in the biliary tract, consisting of cholesterol or bile pigments and calcium salts. Also called **choledocholithiasis, gallstone.** See also **cholangitis, cholecystitis, cholelithiasis.**

■ OBSERVATIONS: Biliary calculi may cause jaundice, right upper quadrant pain, obstruction, and inflammation of the gallbladder.

■ INTERVENTIONS: If stones cannot pass spontaneously into the duodenum, cholangiography or similar processes will reveal their location, and they can be removed surgically.

■ PATIENT CARE CONSIDERATIONS: The pain associated with biliary calculi can be severe.

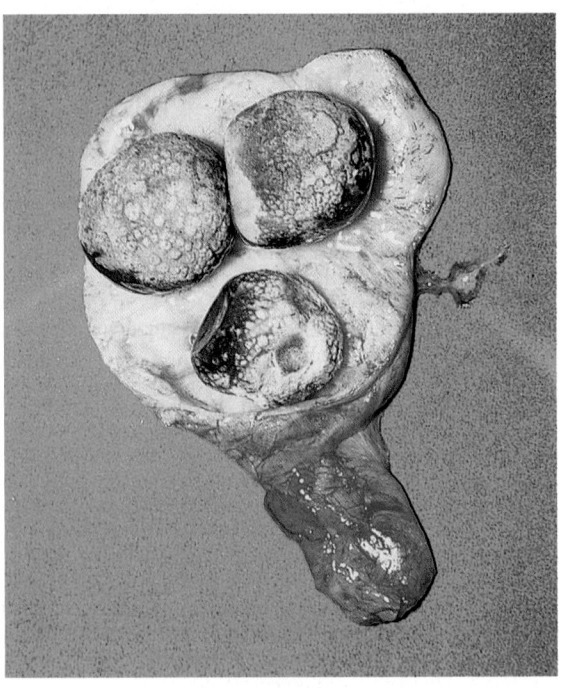

Biliary calculi *(Cross, 2013)*

biliary cirrhosis [L, *bilis* + *kirrhos,* yellow-orange, *osis,* condition], now called **primary biliary cholangitis.**

biliary colic [L, *bilis* + *kolikos,* colon pain], a type of smooth muscle or visceral pain specifically associated with the passing of stones through the bile ducts. Also called **cholecystalgia.** See also **biliary calculus.**

biliary duct, one of the muscular ducts through which bile passes from the liver and gallbladder to the duodenum. See also **common bile duct.**

biliary dyskinesia, pain or discomfort in the epigastric region resulting from spasm, especially of the sphincter of Oddi, following cholecystectomy. It interferes with bile drainage.

biliary dyspepsia, *(Obsolete)* a digestive upset caused by an inadequate flow of bile into the duodenum.

biliary fistula, an abnormal passage from the gallbladder, a bile duct, or the liver to an internal organ or the surface of the body. Biliary fistulae into the duodenum may complicate cholelithiasis; a gallstone may become impacted, usually in the ileocecal valve, and cause intestinal obstruction.

biliary glands. See **glands of bile duct.**

biliary obstruction, blockage of the common or cystic bile duct, usually caused by one or more gallstones. It impedes bile drainage and produces an inflammatory reaction. Less common causes of biliary obstruction include choledochal cysts, pancreatic and duodenal tumors, Crohn's disease, pancreatitis, echinococcosis, ascariasis, and sclerosing cholangitis. Stones, consisting chiefly of cholesterol, bile pigment, and calcium, may form in the gallbladder and in the hepatic duct in persons of either sex at any age but are more common in middle-aged women. Increased amounts of serum cholesterol in the blood, such as occurs in obesity, diabetes, hypothyroidism, biliary stasis, and inflammation of the biliary system, promote gallstone formation. Cholelithiasis may be asymptomatic until a stone lodges in a biliary duct, but the patient usually has a history of indigestion and discomfort after eating fatty foods. A calculus biliary obstruction should be considered cancerous until proven otherwise.

■ OBSERVATIONS: Biliary obstruction is characterized by severe epigastric pain, often radiating to the back and shoulder, nausea, vomiting, and profuse diaphoresis. The dehydrated patient may have chills; fever; jaundice; clay-colored stools; dark, concentrated urine; an electrolyte imbalance; and a tendency to bleed because the absence of bile prevents the synthesis and absorption of fat-soluble vitamin K.

■ INTERVENTIONS: The patient in the acute care setting is placed in semi-Fowler's position and is usually administered intermittent nasogastric suctioning, parenteral fluids with electrolytes and fat-soluble vitamins, and medication for pain. Antibiotics, anticholinergic and antispasmodic drugs, and a cholecystogram or ultrasound scan may be ordered. The blood pressure, temperature, pulse, and respirations are monitored, and the patient is helped to turn, cough, and deep breathe every 2 to 4 hours. Fluid intake and output are measured, and the color and character of urine and stools are noted. When the nasogastric tube is removed, the patient initially receives a low-fat liquid diet and progresses to a soft or normal diet, as tolerated; up to 2500 mL of fluids a day are encouraged or administered intravenously, unless contraindicated. Cholecystectomy is usually the definitive treatment, but in most cases surgery is delayed until the patient's condition is stabilized and any prothrombin deficiency (caused by vitamin K malabsorption) is corrected.

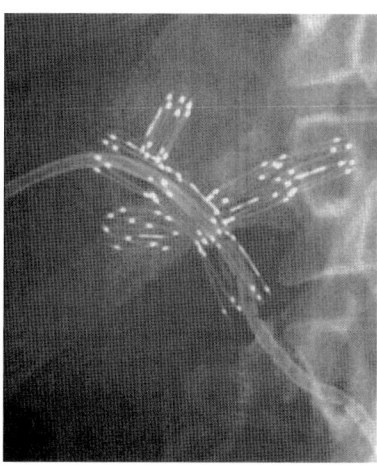

Stents in place to correct biliary obstruction (Feldman, Friedman, and Brandt, 2006)

biliary pseudolithiasis, pain in the bile ducts with symptoms resembling those of cholelithiasis but in the absence of gallstones.

biliary system, the gallbladder, bile ducts, some cells within the liver, and bile ducts outside the liver. See **biliary.**

biliary tract [L, *bilis,* bile, *tractus*], the pathway for bile flow from the canaliculi in the liver to the opening of the bile duct into the duodenum.

biliary tract cancer, a rare adenocarcinoma in a bile duct, often causing jaundice, pruritus, and weight loss. The lesion may be papillary or flat and ulcerated. The tumor is often unresectable at diagnosis. See also **cholangiocarcinoma.**

biligenesis /bil′ijen″əsis/, the process by which bile is produced.

bilingulate /bīling″gyəlit/ [L, *bis,* twice, *lingula,* little tongue], having two tongues or two tonguelike structures or processes.

biliopancreatic diversion, a surgical treatment for obesity consisting of resection of the distal two thirds of the stomach and attachment of the ileum to the proximal stomach. The duodenum and jejunum are bypassed and empty their secretions into the distal ileum through a new anastomosis. Also called *biliopancreatic bypass.*

bilious /bil″yəs/ [L, *bilis,* bile], **1.** pertaining to bile. **2.** characterized or affected by disordered liver function and especially excessive secretion of bile.

bilious vomiting, the vomiting of bile. Also called *cholemesis.*

bilirubin /bil′iroo″bin/ [L, *bilis* + *ruber,* red], the orange-yellow pigment of bile, formed principally by the breakdown of hemoglobin in red blood cells after termination of their normal lifespan. Water-insoluble unconjugated bilirubin normally travels in the bloodstream to the liver, where it is converted to a water-soluble, conjugated form and excreted into the bile. In a healthy person, about 250 mg of bilirubin is produced daily. The majority of bilirubin is excreted in the stool. The characteristic yellow pallor of jaundice is caused by the accumulation of bilirubin in the blood and in the tissues of the skin. Testing for bilirubin in the blood provides information for diagnosis and evaluation of liver disease, biliary obstruction, and hemolytic anemia. Normal levels of total bilirubin are 0.1 to 1.2 mg/dL or 2 to 21 μmol/L. See also **jaundice.**

bilirubin blood test, a blood test performed in cases of jaundice to help determine whether the jaundice is caused by hepatocellular dysfunction (as in hepatitis) or extrahepatic obstruction of the bile ducts (as with gallstones or tumor blocking the bile ducts). Total serum bilirubin is made up of conjugated (direct) and unconjugated (indirect) bilirubin, with varying ratios of each characterizing different diseases.

bilirubin cast, a tubular structure in a histological examination containing bilirubin, giving it a yellow-brown color, as seen with obstructive jaundice.

bilirubin diglucuronide, a conjugated water-soluble form of bilirubin, formed in the liver by esterification of two molecules of glucuronide to the bilirubin molecule; this is the usual form in which bilirubin is found in the bile.

bilirubinemia /-ē″mē·ə/ [L, *bilis,* bile, *ruber,* red; Gk, *haima,* blood], the presence of bilirubin in the blood.

bilirubinuria /-ōōr″ē·ə/, the presence of bilirubin, a yellow-gold pigment that is a product of bile catabolism, in urine. Bilurubinuria may indicate liver disease, bile duct obstruction, or hemolytic anemia.

biliuria /bil′iyoor″ē·ə/ [L, *bilis* + Gk, *ouron,* urine], the presence of bile pigments in the urine.

biliverdin /bil′ivur″din/ [L, *bilis* + *virdis,* green], a greenish bile pigment formed in the breakdown of hemoglobin and converted to bilirubin. See also **bile, bilirubin.**

billing limit. See **limiting charge.**

Billings method [Evelyn (1918–2013) and John (1918–2007) Billings, Australian physicians], a way of estimating ovulation time by changes in the cervical mucus that occur during the menstrual cycle. See also **ovulation method of family planning.**

Billroth operation I [Christian A. Billroth, Austrian surgeon, 1829–1894], the surgical removal of the pylorus in the treatment of gastric cancer or peptic ulcer disease. The proximal end of the duodenum is anastomosed to the stomach.

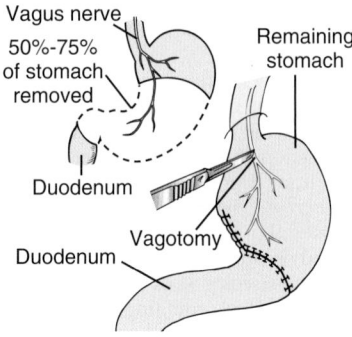

Billroth operation I *(Lewis et al, 2011)*

Billroth operation II [Christian A. Billroth], the surgical removal of the pylorus and the first part of the duodenum. The cut end of the stomach is anastomosed to the jejunum, which is pulled through the transverse mesocolon from the lower abdomen. The remaining duodenum carrying biliary and pancreatic secretions drains into the ileum through a new anastomosis in the lower abdomen. Also called **gastrojejunostomy.**

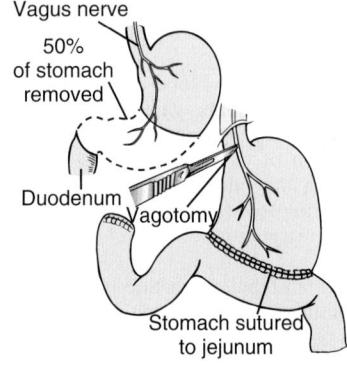

Billroth operation II *(Lewis et al, 2011)*

Bill's maneuver [Arthur H. Bill, American obstetrician, 1877–1961], an obstetric procedure in which a forceps is used to rotate the fetal head at midpelvis before extraction of the head during birth.

bilobate /bīlōʺbāt/ [L, *bis,* twice, *lobus,* lobe], having two lobes.

bilobate placenta [L, *bis,* twice, *lobus,* lobe, *placenta,* flat cake], a placenta with two connected lobes. Also called **placenta bipartitia.**

bilobulate /bīlobʺyəlāt/, having two lobules. Also called *bilobular.*

bilocular /bīlokʺyələr/ [L, *bis + loculus,* compartment], **1.** divided into two cells. **2.** containing two cells. Also called *biloculate.*

Biltricide, an anthelmintic agent. Brand name for *praziquantel.*

bimanual /bīmanʺyoo·əl/ [L, *bis + manus,* hand], with both hands.

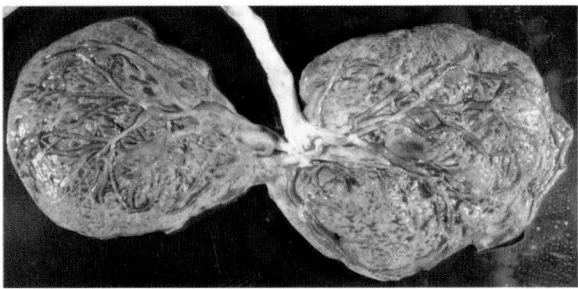

Bilobate placenta *(Crum et al, 2018)*

bimanual examination [L, *bis + manos,* hand], an examination, usually vaginal, that requires the use of both of the examiner's hands.

bimanual palpation, the examination of a woman's pelvic organs in which the examiner places one hand on the abdomen and one or two fingers of the other hand in the vagina. The size, shape, and consistency of the cervix, uterus, and adnexa are then assessed and noted.

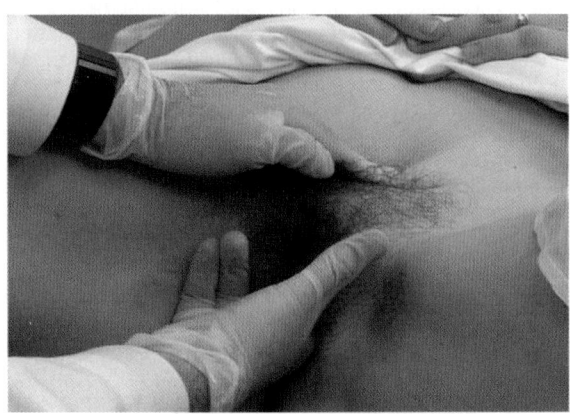

Bimanual palpation *(Swartz, 2014)*

bimanual percussion [L, *bis,* twice, *manus,* hand, *percutere,* to strike through], a diagnostic technique of producing sound vibrations in body cavities by the use of two hands, one serving as the plexor, or "hammer," and the other as the pleximeter, or striking plate. See also **percussion.**

bimastoid /bīmasʺtoid/, pertaining to the two mastoid processes of the temporal bone.

bimatoprost /b-matʹo-prost/, a synthetic prostaglandin analogue that acts as an ocular hypotensive; applied topically to the conjunctiva in the treatment of open-angle glaucoma and ocular hypertension.

bimaxillary /bīmakʺsilerʹē/ [L, *bis + maxilla,* jawbone], **1.** pertaining to both the upper and lower jaws. **2.** of or relating to the two halves of the maxilla.

bimodal distribution /bīmoʺdəl/ [L, *bis + modus,* measure], the distribution of quantitative data into two clusters. It is suggestive of two separate normally distributed populations from which the data are drawn.

bimolecular reaction $(E_2, S_N 2)$ /bīʹmolekʺyələr/, an elementary reaction in which more than one molecule is involved in the slow step of a biochemical mechanism. It may follow second-order reaction rate or second-order kinetics.

bin-, prefix meaning "twice, two": *binocular, binovular.*

binangle /bin″ang·gəl/ [L, *bini,* twofold, *angulus,* angle], a double-ended surgical or operative instrument that has a shank with two offsetting angles.

binary fission /bī″nərē/ [L, *bini,* twofold, *fissionis,* splitting], the division of a cell or nucleus into two equal parts. It is the common form of asexual reproduction among bacteria, protozoa, and other unicellular organisms. Also called **simple fission.** Compare **multiple fission.**

binary number, a number in base 2 represented by 0s and 1s. For example, the number 2 in the decimal form is written as 10 in the binary form, the decimal number 3 is written as 11, the decimal number 4 is written as 100 in the binary form, and so on.

binaural /bī·naw′rəl/ [L, *bis,* twice + *auris,* ear], pertaining to both ears.

binaural stethoscope, *(Obsolete)* now called **diaphragm stethoscope.**

binauricular. See **biauricular.**

bind [AS, *binden*], **1.** to bandage or wrap in a band. **2.** to join together with a band or with a ligature. **3.** (in chemistry) to combine or unite molecules by using reactive groups within the molecules or by using a binding chemical. Binding is especially associated with chemical bonds that are fairly easily broken, such as in the bonds between toxins and antitoxins.

binder, a bandage made of a large piece of material to fit and support a specific body part.

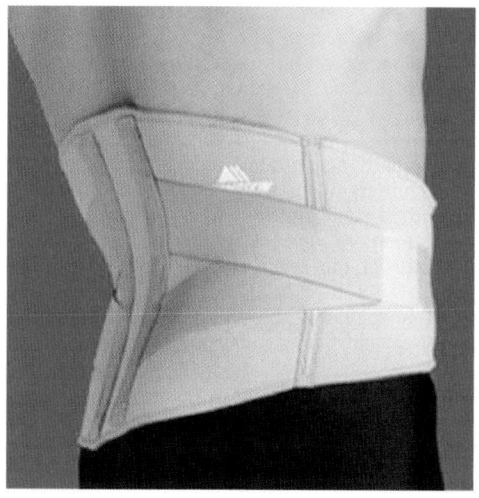

Abdominal binder *(Cameron and Monroe, 2011)*

binding energy, **1.** the amount of energy required to separate a nucleus into its individual nucleons. **2.** the energy released as the nucleus forms from nucleons.

binding site [ME, *binden* + L, *situs*], the location on the surface of a cell or a molecule where other cell fragments or molecules attach to initiate a chemical or physiological action.

binding sites, **1.** concave features on antibody molecules that serve as locations for binding antigens. Because of possible variations in antibody amino acid sequences and molecule configurations, each kind of antibody can provide combining sites for a specific antigen. **2.** locations on protein molecules where drugs or other substances may become bound by intermolecular forces or electrochemical attraction.

Binet age /binā′/ [Alfred Binet, French psychologist, 1857–1911], the mental age of an individual, especially a child, as determined by the Binet-Simon tests, which are evaluated on the basis of tested intelligence of the "normal" individual at any given age.

binge eating. See **bulimia.**

binocular /bīnok″yələr, bin-/ [L, *bini* + *oculus,* eye], **1.** pertaining to both eyes, especially regarding vision. **2.** a microscope, telescope, or field glass that can accommodate viewing by both eyes.

binocular fixation, the process of having both eyes directed at the same object at the same time, which is essential for good depth perception.

binocular ophthalmoscope, an ophthalmoscope having two eyepieces used for stereoscopic examination of the eye.

binocular parallax /per″əlaks/ [L, *bini* + *oculus* + Gk, *parallax,* in turn], the difference in the angles formed by the sight lines to two objects situated at different distances from the eyes. Binocular parallax is a major factor in depth perception. Also called **stereoscopic parallax.**

binocular perception, the visual ability to judge depth or distance by virtue of having both eyes functioning normally.

binocular vision, the simultaneous use of both eyes so that the images perceived by each eye are combined to appear as a single image. Compare **diplopia.**

binocularity, the ability to focus on an object with both eyes and perceive a single image.

binomial /bīnō″mē·əl/, **1.** containing two names or terms. **2.** the unique, two-part scientific name used to identify a plant. The first name is the genus; the second, the species. A designation of the variety may also follow to further differentiate the plant. Use of the binomial is the only reliable way to accurately specify a particular herb, since common names differ from region to region and a single common name may often denote several herbs that differ widely from one another.

binomial nomenclature [L, *bis,* twice; Gk, *nomos,* law; L, *nomenclatio,* calling by name], a system of classification of animals, plants, and other life forms (developed by Carl Linné, an 18th-century Swedish naturalist) that assigns a two-part Latinized name referring respectively to the organism's genus and species, such as *Homo sapiens* for humans.

binovular /bīnov″yələr/ [L, *bini* + *ovum,* egg], developing from two distinct ova, as in dizygotic twins. Also **diovular.**

binovular twins. See **dizygotic twins.**

Binswanger disease /bin′swäng·ər/ [Otto Binswanger, German neurologist, 1852–1929], a degenerative dementia of presenile onset caused by thinning of the subcortical white matter of the brain caused by arteriosclerosis and thromboembolism affecting the blood vessels that supply the white matter and deep structures of the brain. Associated with multiple subcortical strokes.

binuclear /bīnōō″klē·ər/ [L, *bis,* twice, *nucleus,* nut kernel], having two nuclei, as in the example of a heterokaryon or binucleate hybrid cell. Also called *binucleate.*

bio- /bī′ō-/, prefix meaning "life": *bioassay, biopsy.*

bioactive [Gk, *bios,* life; L, *activus,* with energy], having an effect on or causing a reaction in living tissue.

bioactive compound, a chemical substance found in fruits, nuts, and vegetables that may play a role in the prevention of cancer and other chronic diseases. Kinds include **lycopene, lignan.**

bioactivity /-aktiv″itē/, any response from or reaction in living tissue. **–bioactive,** *adj.*

bioassay /bī′ō·as″ā, -əsā′/ [Gk, *bios* + Fr, *assayer,* to try], the laboratory determination of the concentration of a drug or other substance in a specimen by comparing its effect on an organism, an animal, or an isolated tissue with that of a standard preparation. Also called **biological assay.**

bioastronautics /-as'trōnôt″iks/, the science dealing with the biological aspects of space travel.

bioavailability /-əvā'libil″itē/ [Gk, *bios* + ME, *availen,* to serve], the degree of activity or amount of an administered drug or other substance that becomes available for activity in the target tissue.

bioburden, the number of organisms on a surface before sterilization.

biocenosis /-sənō″sis/ [Fk, *bios,* life, *koinos,* common], an ecological community.

biochemical genetics. See **molecular genetics.**

biochemical marker /-kem″ikəl/ [Gk, *bios* + *chemeia,* alchemy], any hormone, enzyme, antibody, or other substance that is detected in the urine, blood, or other body fluids or tissues that may serve as a sign of a disease or other abnormality. An example is markedly elevated C-reactive protein in acute inflammation.

biochemical recurrence. See **biochemical relapse**.

biochemical relapse, a rise in the level of prostate-specific antigen (PSA) following treatment that may provide evidence of an early recurrence but does not equal a clinical relapse. Also called **biochemical recurrence, PSA failure.**

biochemistry /-kem″istrē/, the chemistry of organisms and life processes. Also called **biological chemistry, physiological chemistry.** −*biochemical, adj.*

biochemorphics /-kemôr″fiks/, the study of the relationship between chemical structure and biological function.

bioclimatology /-klī'mətol″əjē/, the study of the relationship and interactions between climate and organisms.

biocybernetics /-sī'bərnet″iks/, the science of communication and control within and among organisms and of the interaction between organisms and mechanical or electronic systems.

biodegradable /-digrā″dəbəl/ [Gk, *bios,* life; L, *de,* away, *gradus,* step], the natural ability of a chemical substance to be broken down into less complex compounds or compounds having fewer carbon atoms by bacteria or other microorganisms.

biodynamics /-dīnam″iks/, the study of the effects of dynamic physical processes, such as radiation, on organisms.

bioelectric impedance analysis (BIA) /-ilek″trik/, a method of measuring the fat composition of the body, compared to other tissues, by its resistance to electricity. Fat tissue does not conduct electricity. Muscle and bone are poor conductors. The method is reported to be 95% accurate, depending on body water content, which may fluctuate with exercise, diet, sweating, and use of alcohol or drugs. See also **total body electric conductivity.**

bioelectricity /-ilektris″itē/ [Gk, *bios* + *elektron,* amber], electrical current that is generated by living tissues, such as nerves and muscles. The electrical potentials of human tissues, recorded by electrocardiograph, electroencephalograph, and similar sensitive devices, are used in diagnosing the condition of various vital organs.

bioenergetics /-en'ərjet″iks/ [Gk, *bios* + *energein,* to be active], a system of exercises based on the concept that natural healing will be enhanced by bringing the patient's body rhythms and the natural environment into harmony.

bioequivalent /bī'ō·ikwiv″ələnt/ [Gk, *bios* + L, *aequus,* equal, *valere,* to be strong], (in pharmacology) pertaining to two drugs with identical active ingredients possessing similar bioavailability and producing the same effect at the site of physiological activity. It often pertains to brand and generic versions of the same drug entity.

bioethics /bī'ō·eth′iks/ [Gk, *bios,* life + *ethos,* the habits of humans or animals], values and rules involved in the study and investigation of living organisms.

biofeedback /-fēd″bak/ [Gk, *bios* + AS, *faedan,* food, *baec,* back], a process providing a person with visual or auditory information about the autonomic physiological functions of his or her body, such as blood pressure, muscle tension, and brain wave activity, usually through use of instruments. By trial and error, the person learns consciously to control these processes, which were previously regarded as involuntary. Biofeedback may be used clinically to treat many conditions, such as pain, anxiety, hypertension, insomnia, and migraine headache.

biofilm /bi′o-film″/, **1.** well-organized colonies of bacteria clustered together to form microcolonies. These colonies of bacteria attach to surfaces, where they assume different characteristics from planktonic bacteria. **2.** (in dentistry) bacterial plaque that adheres tenaciously to tooth surfaces, restorations, and prosthetic appliances. See **bacterial plaque.**

bioflavonoid /bī′ōflā″vənoid/ [Gk, *bios* + L, *flavus,* yellow; Gk, *eidos,* form], a generic term for any of a group of colored flavones found in many fruits. Once believed to reduce capillary bleeding, bioflavonoids are now considered nonessential nutrients. Bioflavonoids are frequently used in herbal preparations, but there is insufficient evidence to support efficacy.

biogenesis /bī′ōjen″əsis/ [Gk, *bios* + *genein,* to produce], **1.** the doctrine that living material can originate only from preexisting life and not from inanimate matter. Also called **biogeny. 2.** the origin of life; ontogeny and phylogeny. Compare **abiogenesis.** −*biogenetic, adj.*

biogenetic law, a biologically discredited hypothesis. See **recapitulation concept.**

biogenic /bī′ōjen″ik/, **1.** produced by the action of a living organism, such as fermentation. **2.** essential to life and the maintenance of health, such as food, water, and proper rest.

biogenic amine, one of a large group of naturally occurring biologically active compounds, most of which act as neurotransmitters. The most dominant, norepinephrine, is involved in such physiological functions as emotional reactions, memory, sleep, and arousal from sleep. Other biochemicals of the group include three catecholamines: histamine, serotonin, and dopamine. These substances are active in regulating blood pressure, elimination, body temperature, and many other centrally mediated body functions.

biogeny. See **biogenesis,** def. 1.

biogravics /-grav″iks/, the study of the effects of gravity, including reduced and increased gravitational forces, on organisms.

biohazard /-haz′ərd/ [Gk, *bios,* life; OFr, *hasard*], anything that is a risk to organisms, such as ionizing radiation or harmful bacteria or viruses.

bioimpedance analysis, a method for analyzing the water content of the body through variations in bioimpedance among different types of tissue. It is often used to estimate the percentage of body fat by measuring fat to lean body mass.

bioinstrument, a sensor or other device implanted into or attached to a living organism for the purpose of recording physiological data, such as brain activity or heart function.

biokinetics /-kinet″iks/ [Gk, *bios,* life, *kinetikos,* moving], the study of the movements within developing organisms.

biological /-loj″ik/ [Gk, *bios* + *logos,* science], **1.** pertaining to organisms and their products. **2.** any preparation made from organisms or their products and used as a diagnostic, preventive, or therapeutic agent. Also spelled *biologic.* Kinds include **antigen, antitoxin, sera, vaccine, monoclonal antibody.**

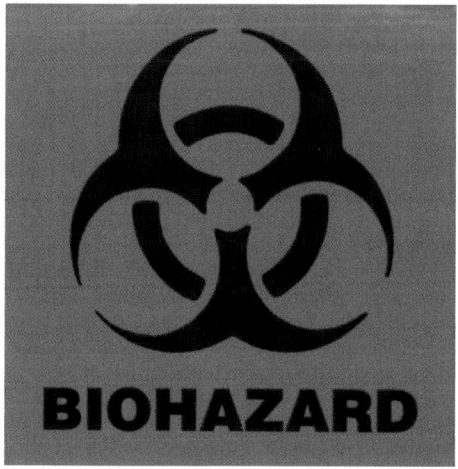

Biohazard label *(Bonewit-West, 2013)*

biological activity, the inherent capacity of a substance, such as a drug or toxin, to alter one or more chemical or physiological functions of a cell, tissue, organ, or organism. The biological activity of a substance is determined not only by the substance's physical and chemical nature but also by its concentration and the duration of cellular exposure to it. Biological activity may reflect a "domino effect," in which the alteration of one function disrupts the normal activity of one or more other functions.

biological armature, the connective tissue-rich aggregate of larger ducts, vessels, and autonomic nerves that in many mammalian exocrine glands serves as an internal framework whose function of support, and often anchorage, resembles that of the armature within a clay sculpture.

biological assay. See **bioassay.**

biological chemistry, an interdisciplinary combination of biology and chemistry. See **biochemistry.**

biological death, death attributed to natural causes. Biological death refers to permanent cellular damage, resulting from lack of oxygen, that is not reversible.

biological dressing, a dressing for burn injuries that is made from pigskin or synthetic materials with characteristics like those of human skin. The dressing is most effective in treating burns that are of uniform depth and of superficial partial thickness. It should be applied as soon as possible after the injury and should adhere to the wound during healing.

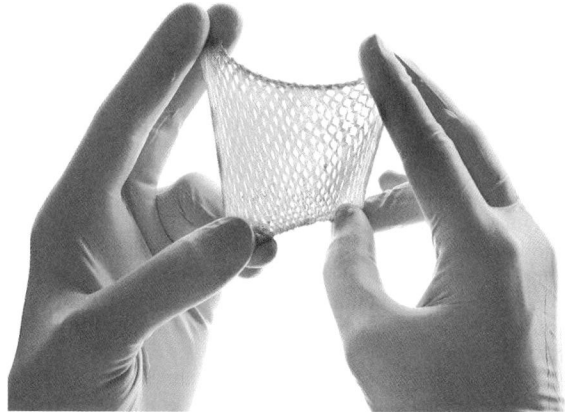

Biological dressing *(©2014 Soluble Solutions, LLC: TherasSkin®)*

biological half-life, the time required for the body to eliminate half of an administered dose of any substance by regular physiological processes. The biological half-life is approximately the same for stable and radioactive isotopes of a specific element. Also called *metabolic half-life.* See also **effective half-life, half-life.**

biological monitoring, **1.** a process of measuring the levels of various physiological substances, drugs, or metabolites within a patient during diagnosis or therapy. **2.** the measurement of toxic substances in the environment and the identification of health risks to the population. Biological monitoring often uses indirect methods of identifying and measuring substances, such as analyses of samples of blood, urine, feces, hair, nails, sweat, saliva, or exhaled air and extrapolation from metabolic effects.

biological plausibility, a method of reasoning used to establish a cause-and-effect relationship between a biological factor and a particular disease.

biological psychiatry, a school of psychiatric thought that stresses the physical, chemical, and neurological causes of and treatments for mental and emotional disorders.

biological rhythm [Gk, *bios,* life, *logos,* science, *rhythmos*], the periodic recurrence of a biological phenomenon, such as the respiratory cycle, the sleep cycle, or the menstrual cycle. Also called **biorhythm.**

biological vector, an animal carrier. See **vector.**

biologist /bī·ol″əjist/ [Gk, *bios,* life, *logos,* science], a person who studies life sciences.

biology /bī·ol″əje/, the scientific study of life. Scientists may specialize in one or more branches of study. Kinds include **biometry, cytology, ecology, evolution, genetics, molecular biology, paleontology, physiology.**

biolysis /bī·ol″isis/ [Gk, *bios,* life, *lysis,* loosening], the disintegration or dissolution of organic matter resulting from the activity of organisms, such as bacterial action on living tissue.

biome /bī″ōm/ [Gk, *bios* + *oma,* tumor, mass], the collection of biological communities existing in and characteristic of a broad geographic region, such as desert, tropical forest, or savanna. A biome includes all organisms of a particular region.

biomechanical frame of reference, a framework in which the evaluation and intervention focuses on range of motion, strength, endurance, and preventing contractures and deformities; used primarily with orthopedic disorders.

biomechanics [Gk, *bios* + *mechane,* machine], the study of mechanical laws and their application to living organisms, especially the human body and its locomotor system. −*biomechanic, biomechanical, adj.*

biomedical, pertaining to the biological aspects of medicine.

biomedical engineering /-med″ikəl/ [Gk, *bios* + L, *medicare,* to heal], a system of scientific techniques that is applied to biological processes to solve practical medical problems or answer questions in biomedical research.

biometry /bī·om″ətrē/, the application of statistical methods in analyzing data obtained in biological or anthropological research. See also **biology.**

biomicroscopy /-mīkros″kəpē/, **1.** microscopic examination of living tissue in the body. **2.** ophthalmic examination of the eye by use of a slit lamp and a magnifying lens. See also **slit lamp, slit-lamp microscope.**

bionics /bī·on″iks/, the science of applying electronic principles and devices, such as computers and solid-state miniaturized circuitry, to medical problems. An example of the application of bionics is the development of artificial pacemakers to correct abnormal heart rhythms. −*bionic, adj.*

biopharmaceutics /-fär′məsoo̅′tiks/, the study of the chemical and physical properties of drugs, their components, and their activities in living organisms. See also **pharmacokinetics, pharmacodynamics.**

biophysics, the application of physical laws to life processes of organisms.

biopotentials /-pəten″shəls/, a voltage produced by a tissue of the body, particularly muscle tissue during a contraction. Electrocardiography depends on measurement of changing potentials in contracting heart muscle. Electromyography and electroencephalography function similarly in the diagnosis of neuromuscular and brain disorders, respectively.

biopsy /bī′opsē/ [Gk, bios + opsis, view], **1.** the removal of a small piece of living tissue from an organ or other part of the body for microscopic examination to confirm or establish a diagnosis, estimate prognosis, or follow the course of a disease. **2.** the tissue excised for examination. **3.** (Informal) to excise tissue for examination. Kinds include **aspiration biopsy, needle biopsy, punch biopsy, surface biopsy.**

biopsychic /bī′ōsī′kik/ [Gk, bios + psyche, mind], pertaining to mental factors as they relate to living organisms.

biopsychology. See **psychobiology.**

biopsychosocial /bī′ōsī′kōsō″shəl/ [Gk, bios + psyche, mind; L, socius, companion], pertaining to the complex of biological, psychological, and social aspects of life.

biopsychosocial diagnosis, a holistic approach to diagnosis that takes into consideration the medical, developmental, psychological, spiritual, and social conditions and symptoms that are present and how they interact to produce a particular patient's condition.

bioptic, a vision-enhancement lens for individuals with low vision.

bioptome tip catheter /bī·op″tōm/, a catheter with a special end designed for obtaining endomyocardial biopsy samples. It is threaded through a guiding catheter to the right ventricle, where it snips small tissue samples from the septal wall for pathological examination. The bioptome tip device is used to monitor heart transplantation patients for early signs of tissue rejection.

biorhythm. See **biological rhythm.**

biosafety, a system for the safe handling of toxic and dangerous biological and chemical substances. Guidance in biosafety is offered by the U.S. Centers for Disease Control and Prevention, Occupational Safety and Health Administration, and National Institute for Occupational Safety and Health. In Canada, the Public Health Agency of Canada offers guidance.

biosimilar, a drug, vaccine, or other complex biological product that is highly similar to a product that has been approved by the U.S. Food and Drug Administration or Health Canada, with only minor differences in inert components of the product.

-biosis, suffix meaning "a specific way of living": macrobiosis, symbiosis.

biostatistics /-stətis″tiks/, numeric data on births, deaths, diseases, injuries, and other factors affecting the general health and condition of human populations. Also called **vital statistics.**

biosynthesis /-sin″thəsis/ [Gk, bios + synthesis, putting together], any one of thousands of chemical processes continually occurring throughout the body in which less complex molecules form more complex biomolecules, especially the carbohydrates, lipids, proteins, nucleotides, and nucleic acids. Biosynthetic reactions constitute the anabolism of the body. −biosynthetic, adj.

biosystem, any organism or complex system of organisms.

biotaxis /bī′ōtak″sis/ [Gk, bios + taxis, arrangement], the ability of cells to develop into certain forms and arrangements. See also **cytoclesis.** −biotactic, adj.

biotaxy /bī′ōtak′sē/, **1.** biotaxis. **2.** the systematic classification of organisms according to their phenotypic characteristics; taxonomy.

biotechnology /-teknol″əjē/ [Gk, bios + techne, art, logos, science], **1.** the study of the relationships between humans or other living organisms and machinery, such as the health effects of computer equipment on office workers or the ability of airplane pilots to perform tasks when traveling at supersonic speeds. **2.** the industrial application of the results of biological research, particularly in fields such as recombinant deoxyribonucleic acids (DNA) or gene splicing, which permits the production of synthetic hormones or enzymes by combining genetic material from different species. See also **recombinant DNA.**

biotelemetry /-təlem″ətrē/, the transmission of physiological data, such as electrocardiographic (ECG) and electroencephalographic (EEG) recordings, heart rate, and body temperature by radio or telephone systems. Transmission of such data uses sophisticated electronic devices developed for the study of the effects of space travel on animals and humans; it has progressed to the use of communication satellites for relaying such data from one part of the world to another.

bioterrorism, the calculated use, or threatened use, of biological agents or chemicals that can cause harm or catastrophic risk if used inappropriately as a strategic method of control against civilian populations. The goal is to attain political or ideological objectives by intimidation or coercion.

bioterrorism infectious agents testing, microbiological tests for infectious agents feloniously employed to sicken or kill, including botulism, anthrax, Yersinia pestis, Francisella tularensis, and other bacteria, fungi, and toxins. Testing may include blood tests, urine tests, stool tests, tissue cultures, sputum cultures, lymph node biopsies, and skin tests.

bioterrorism preparedness, the development of plans and strategies in anticipation of a bioterrorism attack. Planning should include measures to take before, during, and after the attack.

biotherapy, a type of therapy that uses substances obtained from living organisms to treat a disease (such as cancer). Kinds include **antibody therapy, gene therapy, hematopoietic growth factor, interferon, interleukin, vaccine.** See also **immunotherapy.**

-biotic, suffix meaning "life": antibiotic; also, meaning "possessing a (specified) mode of life": gnotobiotic.

biotic factor /bī·ot″ik/, an environmental influence on living things, as distinguished from climatic or geological factors.

biotic potential, the possible growth rate of a population of organisms under ideal conditions, which include an absence of predators and an unlimited availability of nutrients and space for expansion.

biotin /bī″ətin/ [Gk, bios, life], a colorless, crystalline, water-soluble B complex vitamin that acts as a coenzyme in fatty acid production and in the oxidation of fatty acids and carbohydrates. It also aids in the use of protein, folic acid, pantothenic acid, and vitamin B_{12}. Rich sources are egg yolk, beef liver, kidney, unpolished rice, brewer's yeast, peanuts, cauliflower, and mushrooms. Formerly called **vitamin H.** See also **avidin.**

biotin deficiency syndrome, an abnormal condition caused by a deficiency of biotin, a B complex vitamin. It is characterized by dermatitis, hyperesthesia, muscle pain, anorexia, slight anemia, and changes in electrocardiographic activity of the heart. The average daily requirement of biotin for an adult is 100 to 200 mcg; the average American diet provides 100 to 300 mcg of the vitamin. Because biotin is synthesized by intestinal bacteria, naturally occurring deficiency in adults is unknown, although it can be induced by large quantities of raw egg whites in the diet. Symptoms include scaly dermatitis, grayish pallor, extreme lassitude, anorexia, muscle pains, insomnia, some precordial distress, and slight anemia. Some authorities consider seborrheic dermatitis in infants a form of biotin deficiency.

biotope /bī″ətōp/ [Gk, *bios* + *topos,* place], a specific biological habitat or site.

biotoxin /bī″ətoks″in/, poison produced by and derived from plants and animals. Biotoxins can be absorbed by ingesting or inhaling the toxin. There are different types of toxins, depending upon the mode of toxicity or biological target, including hcmotoxins, mycotoxins, necrotoxins, cytotoxins, and neurotoxins. Examples of biotoxins include abrin, from the jequirity bean or rosary pea *(Abrus precatorius)*; ricin, from castor beans; and strychnine, from *Strychnos nux-vomica.*

biotransformation /-trans′fôrmā″shən/ [Gk, *bios* + L, *trans,* across, *formare,* to form], the chemical changes a substance undergoes in the body, such as by the action of enzymes. See also **metabolic.**

Biot respiration /bē·ō″/ [Camille Biot, French physician, 1878–1918], an abnormal respiratory pattern, characterized by short episodes of rapid, uniformly deep inspirations followed by 10 to 30 seconds of apnea. Biot respiration is symptomatic of meningitis or increased intracranial pressure.

bipalatinoid /bī′palat″inoid, -pal″-/, describing a two-compartment capsule with different medications in each side. It is designed so that the two substances become mixed and activated as the gelatin capsule dissolves.

biparental inheritance. See **amphigenous inheritance.**

biparietal /bīpərī″ətəl/ [L, *bis,* twice, *paries,* wall], pertaining to the two parietal bones of the head, such as the biparietal diameter.

biparietal diameter (BPD), the transverse distance between the protuberances of the two parietal bones of the skull.

biparietal suture [L, *bis + paries,* wall, *sutura*], the interlocking lines of fusion between the two parietal bones of the skull.

bipartite /bīpär″tīt/, having two parts.

biped /bī″ped/, **1.** having two feet; moving with two feet. **2.** any animal with only two feet.

bipedal /bīpē″dəl, -ped″əl/ [L, *bis,* twice, *pes,* foot], capable of locomotion on two feet.

bipenniform /bīpen″ifôrm′/ [L, *bis + penna,* feather, *forma,* form], (of body structure) having the bilateral symmetry of a feather, such as the pattern formed by the fasciculi that converge on both sides of a muscle tendon in the rectus femoris. Compare **multipenniform, penniform, radiate.**

biperforate /bī·pər′fə·rāt/ [L, *bis,* twice + *perforatus,* bored through], having two perforations.

biperiden hydrochloride /bīper″idən/, a synthetic anticholinergic agent.

■ INDICATIONS: It may be prescribed in the treatment of Parkinson's disease and drug-induced extrapyramidal disorders. Biperiden hydrochloride is administered orally, and biperiden lactate is administered intramuscularly or intravenously.

■ CONTRAINDICATIONS: Narrow-angle glaucoma, asthma, obstruction of the genitourinary or GI tract, or known hypersensitivity to this drug prohibits its use.

■ ADVERSE EFFECTS: Among the more serious adverse reactions are blurred vision, central nervous system effects, urinary

retention, postural hypotension, tachycardia, dry mouth, decreased sweating, and hypersensitivity reactions.

biphasic /bīfā″zik/ [L, *bis* + Gk, *phasis,* appearance], having two phases, parts, aspects, or stages.

bipolar /bīpō″lər/ [L, *bis* + *polus,* pole], **1.** having two poles, such as in certain electrotherapeutic treatments using two poles or in certain types of bacterial staining that affects only the two poles of the microorganism under study. **2.** (of a nerve cell) having an afferent and an efferent process.

bipolar cell, a cell, such as a retinal neuron, with two main processes arising from the cell body.

bipolar disorder, a major mood disorder characterized by episodes of mania, depression, or mixed mood. One or the other phase may be predominant at any given time, one phase may appear alternately with the other, or elements of both phases may be present simultaneously. Characteristics of the manic phase are excessive emotional displays, such as excitement, elation, euphoria, or in some cases irritability accompanied by hyperactivity, boisterousness, impaired ability to concentrate, decreased need for sleep, and seemingly unbounded energy. In extreme mania, a sense of omnipotence and delusions of grandeur may occur. In the depressive phase, marked apathy and underactivity are accompanied by feelings of profound sadness, loneliness, guilt, and lowered self-esteem. Causes of the disorder are multiple and complex, often involving biological, psychological, interpersonal, and social and cultural factors. The disorder is a biological illness that can be precipitated or exacerbated by psychosocial stressors. See also **major depressive disorder.**

bipolar electrocautery, an electrocautery in which both active and return electrodes are incorporated into a single handheld instrument so that the current passes between the tips of the two electrodes and affects only a small amount of tissue.

bipolar lead /lēd/, *(Informal)* a tracing produced by such a lead on an electrocardiograph.

bipolar version, a method for changing the position of a fetus in which one hand is placed on the abdomen of the mother and two fingers of the other hand are inserted into the uterus.

bipotentiality /bī′pəten′shē·al″itē/ [L, *bis* + *potentia,* power], the characteristic of acting or reacting according to either of two possible states.

bird breeder's lung. See **pigeon breeder's lung.**

bird face retrognathism, a classification of malocclusion (class II distoocclusion). See **retrognathism.**

bird flu. See **avian influenza.**

birth [ME, *burth*], **1.** the event of being born, the entry of a new person from its mother into the world. Kinds include **breech birth, live birth, stillbirth.** See also **effacement, labor. 2.** the childbearing event, the bringing forth by a mother of a baby. **3.** a medical event; the delivery of a fetus by an obstetric attendant.

birth canal, *(Informal)* the passage that extends from the inlet of the true pelvis to the vaginal orifice through which an infant passes during vaginal birth. See also **clinical pelvimetry.**

birth center, a health facility with services limited to maternity care for women judged to be at minimum risk for obstetric complications that would require hospitalization.

birth certificate, a legal document recording information about a birth, including, among other details, the date, time, and location of the event; identity of the mother and father; and identity of the attending physician or licensed midwife.

birth control. See **contraception.**

birth defect. See **congenital anomaly.**

birthing chair, a special seat used in labor and delivery to promote the comfort of the mother and facilitate the birthing process. The chair may be specially designed, having many technical features, or it may be a simple three-legged stool with a high, slanted back and a circular seat with a large central hole in it. The newer birthing chairs allow women to sit straight up or to recline. The chair has a lower section that may be removed or folded out of the way. Lights, mirrors, and basins may be attached. The upright position appears to shorten the time in labor, particularly the second or expulsive stage of labor, probably because of gravity and increased participation of the mother. The chair is not suitable for use with anesthesia.

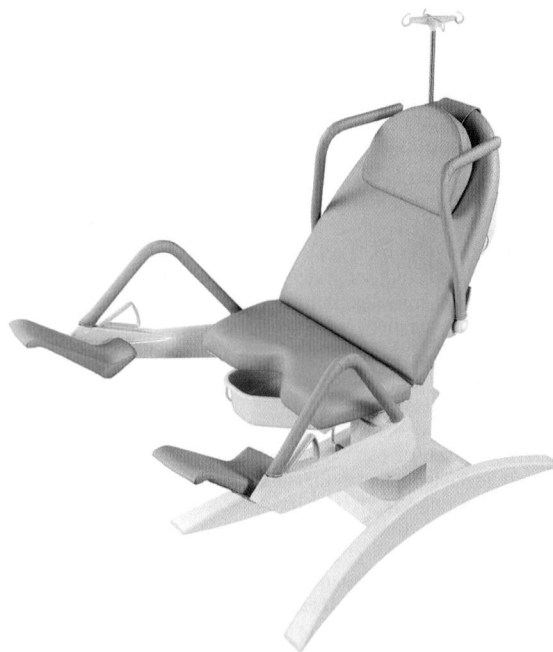

Birthing chair (© 2015 BORCAD cz.)

birthing pool, a receptacle holding more than 100 gallons of water, with a filtering system and heater, for use during labor and delivery in water births. It may be inflatable or permanent.

birth injury, trauma suffered by a baby while being born. Kinds include **cerebral palsy, Erb's palsy.**

birthmark, a benign marking that usually appears as skin pigmentation. See **nevus.**

birth mother, the biological mother whose egg contributed to conception of a child. The child may be borne by that woman, or the child may have been conceived in a surrogate mother.

birth palsy [ME, *burth* + Gk, *paralyein,* to be palsied], a loss of motor or sensory nerve function in some body part caused by a nerve injury during the birth process. Also called **birth paralysis.**

birth paralysis. See **birth palsy.**

birth parent, one of an individual's two biological parents.

birth rate, the proportion of the number of live births in a specific area during a given period to the total population of that area, usually expressed as the number of births per 1000 of population. Compare **crude birth rate, refined birth rate, true birth rate.**

birth trauma, 1. any physical injury suffered by an infant during the process of delivery. **2.** the supposed psychic shock, according to some psychiatric theories, that an infant suffers during delivery.

birth weight, the measured heaviness of a baby when born, usually about 3500 g (7.5 lbs). In the United States, 97% of newborns weigh between 2500 g (5.5 lbs) and 4500 g (10 lbs). Babies weighing less than 2500 g at term are considered small for gestational age. Babies weighing more than 4500 g are considered large for gestational age and are often infants of mothers with diabetes mellitus.

bis-, prefix meaning "twice, two": *bisacromial, bisferious.*

bisacodyl /bisak″ōdil/, a cathartic.

■ INDICATIONS: It is prescribed in the treatment of acute or chronic constipation or for emptying of the bowel before or after surgery or before diagnostic radiographic procedures.

■ CONTRAINDICATIONS: Abdominal pain, nausea, vomiting, rectal fissures, ulcerated hemorrhoids, or known hypersensitivity to this drug prohibits its use.

■ ADVERSE EFFECTS: Among the more serious adverse reactions are colic, abdominal pain, and diarrhea.

bisacromial /bīsəkrō″mē·əl/, pertaining to both acromions, the triangular, flat, bony plates at the end of the scapula.

bisalbuminemia /bis′albyo͞om′inē″mē·ə/, a condition in which two types of albumin exist in an individual. The two types are expressed by heterozygous alleles of the albumin gene and are detected by differences in the mobility of the types on electrophoretic gels.

bisect /bīsekt″/ [L, *bis* + *secare,* to cut], to divide into two equal lengths or parts.

bisexual /bīsek″sho͞o·əl/ [L, *bis* + *sexus,* male or female], **1.** hermaphroditic; having gonads of both sexes. **2.** possessing physical or psychological characteristics of both sexes. **3.** engaging in both heterosexual and homosexual activity. **4.** desiring sexual contact with persons of both sexes.

bisexual libido, (in psychoanalysis) the tendency in a person to seek sexual gratification with people of either sex.

bisferious pulse /bisfer″ē·əs/ [L, *bis* + *ferire,* to beat], an arterial pulse that has two palpable peaks, the second of which is slightly weaker than the first. It may be detected in cases of aortic regurgitation and obstructive cardiomyopathy. Compare **dicrotic pulse.**

bishydroxycoumarin. See **dicumarol.**

bis in die (b.i.d.) /dē″ā/, a Latin phrase, used in prescriptions, meaning "twice a day." It is more commonly used in its abbreviated form.

bismuth (Bi) /biz″məth, bis″-/ [Ger, *wismut,* white mass], a reddish, crystalline, trivalent metallic element. Its atomic number is 83. Its atomic mass is 208.98. It is combined with various other elements, such as oxygen, to produce numerous salts used in the manufacture of many pharmaceutic substances.

bismuth gingivitis, a dark bluish line along the gingival margin caused by bismuth used in the treatment of gastrointestinal disorders or by industrial exposure. See also **bismuth stomatitis, gingivitis.**

bismuth stomatitis, an abnormal oral condition caused by the systemic use of bismuth compounds over prolonged periods. It is characterized by a blue-black line on the inner aspect of the gingival sulcus or dark pigmentation of the buccal mucosa, sore tongue, metallic taste, and burning sensation in the mouth. Compare **arsenic stomatitis, atabrine stomatitis.**

bismuth subsalicylate, a bismuth salt of salicylic acid, administered orally in the treatment of diarrhea and gastric distress, including nausea, indigestion, and heartburn. Also used in the treatment of peptic ulcer disease associated with *Helicobacter pylori* infection.

bisoprolol /bis″o-pro′lol/, a synthetic beta-adrenergic blocking agent, used as the fumarate salt; administered orally as an antihypertensive agent. Also used in the treatment of systolic heart failure.

bisphosphonate /bis-fos′fo-nāt/, a class of drugs that prevent the loss of bone mass; used to treat osteoporosis and similar diseases. Also called **diphosphonate.**

bit /bit/, the smallest unit of information in a computer. Bits are the building blocks for all information processing in digital electronics and computers. Eight bits equals one byte. Abbreviation for *binary digit.* See also **byte.**

bitart, abbreviation for **bitartrate carboxylate anion.**

bitartrate /bītär″trāt/, a salt or monoester of tartaric acid; the monoanion of tartaric acid, $C_4H_5O_6$.

bite [AS, *bitan*], **1.** the act of cutting, tearing, holding, grinding, crushing, or gripping with the teeth. **2.** the lingual portion of an artificial tooth between its shoulder and its incisal edge. **3.** an occlusal record or relationship between the upper and lower teeth or jaws. Compare **closed bite, open bite.**

bite block, **1.** a wedge-shaped device used to protect the teeth and tongue and to hold the mouth open during medical or dental procedures and some emergency situations. Caution is required to ensure that the device does not fall into the unprotected airway. **2.** (in dentistry) an artificial dental structure. See **occlusion rim.**

bitegauge /bīt″gāj′/ [AS, *bitan* + OFr, *gauge,* measure], a prosthetic dental device that helps attain proper occlusion of the upper and lower teeth.

biteguard [AS, *bitan* + OFr, *garder,* to defend], a resin plastic or rubber appliance that covers the occlusal and incisal surfaces of the teeth. It is used to stabilize the teeth, to provide a platform for the excursive glides of the mandible, and to eliminate the effects of nocturnal grinding (bruxism) of the teeth. Also called **biteplane, night guard.** Compare **mouth guard.**

biteguard splint, a device, usually made of resin or rubber, for covering the occlusal and incisal surfaces of the teeth and for protecting them from traumatic occlusal forces during immobilization and stabilization processes. See also **Gunning's splint.**

bitelock /bīt″lok′/, a dental device for retaining occlusion rims in the same relation outside and inside the mouth.

bitemporal /bītem″pərəl/ [L, *bis,* twice, *tempora,* temples], pertaining to both temples or both temporal bones.

bitemporal hemianopia [L, *bis,* twice, *tempora,* temples; Gk, *hemi,* half, *opsis,* vision], a loss of the temporal half of the vision in each eye, usually resulting from a lesion in the chiasmal area, such as a pituitary tumor.

biteplane /bīt″plān/, **1.** See **occlusal plane. 2.** a metal sheet laid across the biting surfaces of the upper or lower teeth to determine the relationship of the teeth to the occlusal plane. **3.** an orthodontic appliance of heat-cured acrylic resin worn over the maxillary occlusal surfaces and used to treat pain of the temporomandibular joint and adjacent muscles. **4.** See **biteguard.**

biteplate /bīt″plāt/, a device used in dentistry as a diagnostic or therapeutic aid for prosthodontics or orthodontics. It is made of wire and plastic and is constructed to be worn within the right and left maxillary arches. It may also be used in the correction of temporomandibular joint problems or as a splint in restoring the full mouth.

bite reflex, a swift, involuntary biting action that may be triggered by stimulation of the oral cavity. The bite can be difficult to release in some cases, such as when a spoon or tongue depressor is placed in a patient's mouth.

bite wing film image [AS, *bitan* + ME, *winge*], a dental radiographic image or film onto which a horizontal or vertical projection plane or tab presents so that the teeth can hold the image sensor or film in position during exposure; used to view the interproximal area of posterior teeth and bone. Also called **interproximal film image.** See also **bite wing radiograph.**

bite wing radiograph, a dental radiographic image that reveals the coronal portions of maxillary and mandibular teeth and portions of the alveolar bone and the interdental septa. See also **bite wing film image.**

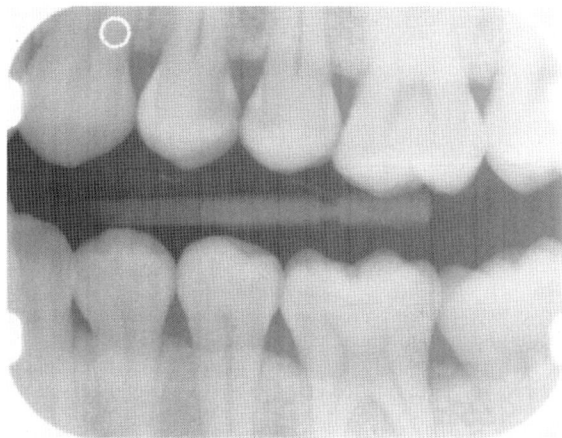

Bite wing radiograph *(Daniel et al, 2008)*

Bithynia /bəthin′ē·ə/, a genus of snails, species of which act as intermediate hosts to *Opisthorchis,* which can cause cancer and infection in humans. Found in Thailand and Laos.

biting in childhood, a natural behavior trait and reflex action in infants, acquired at about 5 to 6 months of age in response to the introduction of solid foods in the diet and the beginning of the teething process. The activity represents a significant modality in the psychosocial development of the child, because it is the first aggressive action the infant learns, and through it the infant learns to control the environment. The behavior also confronts the infant with one of the first inner conflicts, because biting can produce both pleasing and displeasing results. Biting during breastfeeding causes withdrawal of the nipple and anxiety in the mother, yet it also serves as a means of soothing teething discomfort. Infants continue to use biting as a mechanism for exploring their surroundings. Toddlers and older children often use biting for expressing aggression toward their parents and other children, especially during play or as a means of gaining attention. Most children normally outgrow the tendency unless they have severe maladaptive or emotional problems. See also **psychosexual development, psychosocial development.**

Bitot's spots /bitōz″/ [Pierre Bitot, French surgeon, 1822–1888], white or gray triangular deposits on the bulbar conjunctiva adjacent to the lateral margin of the cornea, a clinical sign of vitamin A deficiency. Also called *Bitot's patches.*

bitrochanteric lipodystrophy /bī′trōkənter″ik/ [L, *bis* + Gk, *trochanter,* runner; *lipos,* fat, *dys,* bad, *trophe,* nourishment], an abnormal and excessive deposition of fat on the buttocks and the outer aspect of the upper thighs, occurring most commonly in women. See also **lipodystrophy.**

bivalent /bīvā″lənt/ [L, *bis* + *valere,* to be powerful], (in genetics) a pair of synapsed homologous chromosomes that are attached to each other by chiasmata during the early first meiotic prophase of gametogenesis. The structure serves as the basis for the tetrads from which gametes are produced during the two meiotic divisions. Also called **divalent.** *–bivalence, n.*

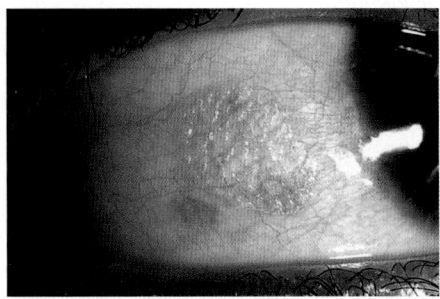

Bitot's spots *(Spalton et al, 2005)*

bivalent antibody, an antibody that has two binding sites that can cross-link one antigen to another. IgG antibodies have two antigen-binding sites (bivalent), while IgM antibodies have 10 identical binding sites (polyvalent).

bivalent chromosome, a pair of synapsed homologous chromosomes during the early stages of gametogenesis. See also **bivalent.**

bivalirudin /bi-val′roo-din/, a direct thrombin inhibitor used intravenously along with other agents in patients undergoing transluminal coronary angioplasty.

bivalved cast [L, *bis* + *valva,* valve], a cast that is cut in half to detect or relieve pressure underneath, especially when a patient has decreased or no sensation in the portion of the body surrounded by the cast. "Windows" are often cut out of the cast over the pressure areas to assess circulation or open wounds under the cast.

bivalve speculum, a medical tool used for direct visualization of a body orifice; it has two blades, which are adjustable. See also **speculum.**

biventricular pacing, a procedure during which a lead is used to deliver current directly to the left ventricle, in addition to those used to deliver current to the right atrium and ventricle so that the ventricles can be induced to pump in synchrony. See also **pacing.**

bizarre leiomyoma. See **epithelioid leiomyoma.**

Björnstad's syndrome /byôrn′städz/ [R. Björnstad, Swedish dermatologist, 20th century], a rare autosomal-recessive disorder characterized by congenital sensorineural deafness and tightly curled hair.

Bk, symbol for the element **berkelium.**

BK, Abbreviation for below-knee; most commonly used in reference to amputations. Abbreviation for *below-knee.*

BK amputation, abbreviation for **below-knee (BK) amputation.** See **long below-knee (BK) amputation, short below-knee (BK) amputation.**

B-K mole syndrome. See **dysplastic nevus syndrome.**

black beauties, *(Slang)* a street name for drugs. See **amphetamines.**

black cohosh, a perennial herb that grows throughout the United States and in parts of Canada.

■ INDICATIONS: This herb is used to treat the symptoms of menopause (hot flashes and nervous conditions associated with menopause) and dysmenorrhea (menstrual cramps, pain, inflammation); generally considered to be effective against mild symptoms but not a substitute for estrogen-containing prescriptions needed to control more severe vasomotor symptoms.

■ CONTRAINDICATIONS: Black cohosh should not be used during pregnancy, since uterine stimulation can occur. It also should not be used during lactation or in children.

Black Creek Canal virus, a virus of the genus *Hantavirus* that causes pulmonary syndrome. Named for the Black Creek Canal area in Florida, where it was first isolated from cotton rats.

black damp, a gas found in mines. See **damp.**

black death, a historic medieval epidemic. See **bubonic plague.**

Blackett-Healy method, a positioning procedure for producing x-ray images of the subscapularis area. The patient is placed in a supine position with the affected shoulder joint centered on the midline of the image, the arm abducted, and the elbow flexed. The opposite shoulder is raised about 15 degrees and supported with a sandbag.

black eye, *(Informal)* contusion around the eye with bruising, discoloration, and swelling. It is usually treated for the first 24 hours with ice packs to reduce swelling, then with hot compresses to aid in resorption of blood from the hematoma. Also called **periorbital ecchymosis.**

Blackfan-Diamond anemia. See **Diamond-Blackfan syndrome.**

black fever. See **kala-azar.**

black hairy tongue. See **parasitic glossitis.**

black haw, an herb found in the eastern United States and across southeastern Canada.

■ INDICATIONS: This herb is used for dysmenorrhea, menstrual cramps and pain, menopausal metrorrhagia, hysteria, asthma, and heart palpitations. It is also used to lower blood pressure. It is possibly effective at relieving uterine spasms, but effectiveness in other instances has not been verified.

■ CONTRAINDICATIONS: Black haw should be used with caution in people with kidney stones since it contains oxalic acid.

blackhead. *(Informal)* See **comedo.**

black light. See **Wood's light.**

black lung disease. See **anthracosis.**

black measles [AS, *blac* + OHG, *masala*], **1.** *(Informal)* See **hemorrhagic measles. 2.** historical name for **Rocky Mountain spotted fever.**

blackout, *(Informal)* a temporary loss of vision or consciousness.

black plague. See **bubonic plague.**

Black's Classification of Caries [G.V. Black, 1836–1915, American dentist]. See **classification of caries.**

blackwater fever, a rare, serious complication of chronic falciparum malaria, characterized by jaundice, hemoglobinuria, acute renal failure, and passage of bloody, dark red or black urine caused by massive intravascular hemolysis. Death occurs in 20% to 30% of all cases. See also **falciparum malaria, malaria,** *Plasmodium.*

Blackwell, Elizabeth, (1821–1910), a British-born American physician; the first woman to be awarded a medical degree in the United States. She established the New York Infirmary, a 40-bed hospital staffed entirely by women, in which she advanced the role of women in medicine and educated nurses in a 4-month course. She was an abolitionist and worked with Dorothea Dix during the U.S. Civil War.

black widow spider [AS, *blac* + *widewe;* ME, *spithre*], *Latrodectus mactans,* a species of spider found in the United States, whose bite causes pain and sometimes death. Spider bites release a neurotoxin called latrotoxin.

black widow spider antivenin, a passive immunizing agent.

■ INDICATIONS: It is prescribed in the treatment of black widow spider bite.

■ CONTRAINDICATIONS: Known hypersensitivity to this drug or to horse serum prohibits its use.

■ ADVERSE EFFECTS: Among the more serious adverse effects are allergic reactions.

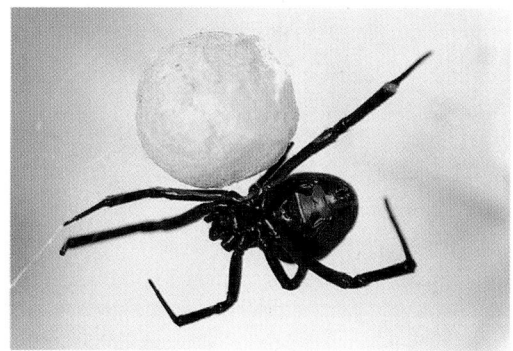

Black widow spider with fresh egg case *(Courtesy Michael Cardwell & Associates)*

black widow spider bite [AS, *blac* + *widewe*; ME, *spithre* + AS, *bitan*], the bite of the spider species *Latrodectus mactans,* a poisonous arachnid found in many parts of the world. Black widow venom contains some enzymatic proteins, including a peptide that affects neuromuscular transmission. The bite is perceived as a sharp pinprick pain, followed by a dull pain in the area of the bite; restlessness; anxiety; sweating; weakness; and drooping eyelids. Muscular rigidity starts at the location of the bite and moves peripherally to the chest. Small children, elderly adults, or persons with heart disorders are most severely affected and may require hospitalization and the administration of an antivenin. Immediate treatment includes keeping the victim quiet and immobilizing the bite area at the level of the heart.

bladder [AS, *blaedre*], a hollow, muscular, expandable sac that collects and stores urine before excretion. Also called **urinary bladder.**

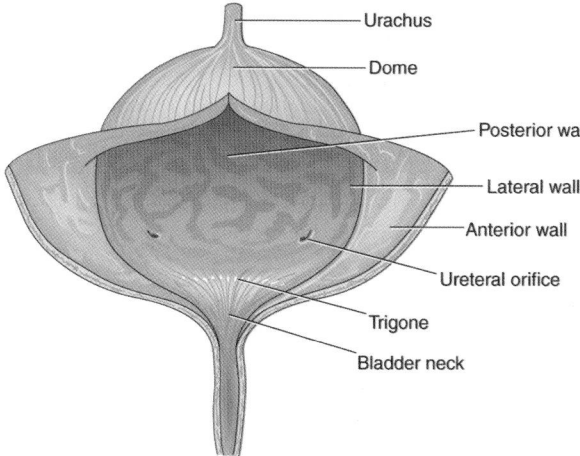

Urachus
Dome
Posterior wall
Lateral wall
Anterior wall
Ureteral orifice
Trigone
Bladder neck

Bladder *(Buck, 2015)*

bladder augmentation, augmentation cystoplasty, often achieved with the addition of a flap of bowel or stomach to the bladder to increase bladder volume.

bladder calculus. See **vesical calculus.**

bladder cancer, the most common malignancy of the urinary tract, characterized by multiple growths that tend to recur in a more aggressive form. Bladder cancer occurs more often in men than in women and is more prevalent in urban than in rural areas. The risk of bladder cancer increases with cigarette smoking and exposure to aniline dyes, beta-naphthylamine, mixtures of aromatic hydrocarbons, or benzidine and its salts, used in chemical, paint, plastics, rubber, textile, petroleum, and wood industries and in medical laboratories. Other predisposing factors are chronic urinary tract infections, calculous disease, and schistosomiasis. The majority of bladder malignancies are transitional cell carcinomas; a small percentage are squamous cell carcinomas or adenocarcinomas. See also **cystectomy.**

■ OBSERVATIONS: Symptoms of bladder cancer include painless hematuria, frequent urination, and dysuria. Irritation from the tumor may mimic cystitis. Urinalysis, excretory urography, cystoscopy, or transurethral biopsy is performed for diagnosis.

■ INTERVENTIONS: Superficial or multiple lesions may be treated by fulguration or open loop resection. A segmental resection is usually performed if the tumor is at the dome or in a lateral wall of the bladder. Total cystectomy may be performed for an invasive lesion of the trigone and necessitates the creation of a urinary diversion. Radiation therapy and/or chemotherapy may be valuable under certain circumstances, such as unresectable tumor growth. Internal irradiation, the introduction of radioisotopes via a balloon of a catheter, or the implantation of radon seeds may be used in treating small localized tumors on the bladder wall. Medications that are often used as palliatives are BCG, 5-fluorouracil, thiotepa, and doxorubicin.

■ PATIENT CARE CONSIDERATIONS: Patients may have a recurrence up to 10 years after successful treatment.

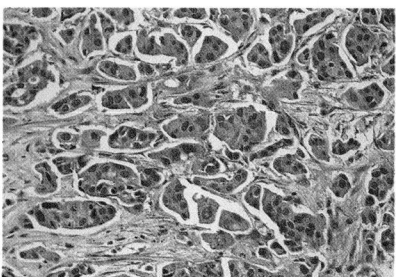

Transitional cell carcinoma of bladder cancer *(Fletcher, 2007)*

bladder cancer markers test, a urine test used for the detection and surveillance of carcinoma. Currently, there is a high incidence of false-positive and false-negative results; new assays are under development.

bladder flap, *(Informal)* the vesicouterine fold of peritoneum incised during low cervical cesarean section so that the bladder can be separated from the uterus to expose the lower uterine segment for incision. The flap is reapproximated with sutures during closure to cover the uterine incision. See also **cesarean section.**

bladder hernia, a protrusion of the urinary bladder through an opening in the inguinal area.

bladder irrigation [AS, *blaedre* + L, *irrigare,* to conduct water], the washing out of the bladder by a continuous or intermittent flow of saline or a medicated solution. The bladder also may be irrigated by an oral intake of fluid.

bladder neck dyssynergia, incomplete opening of the bladder neck during urination, resulting in partial obstruction of urinary flow. Also called **smooth sphincter dyssynergia.**

bladder neck incision, surgical incision of the bladder neck to facilitate the passage of urine and a stronger urinary stream. The operation is similar to but less extensive than bladder neck resection.

bladder neck resection, surgical removal of tissue from the bladder neck to treat obstruction.

bladder neck suspension, any of various methods of surgical fixation of the urethrovesical junction area and the bladder neck to restore the neck to a high retropubic position for relief of stress incontinence. The group includes the Marshall-Marchetti-Krantz operation and the Burch, Pereyra, and Stamey procedures. Also called **colposuspension.**

bladder outlet obstruction (BOO), obstruction of the outflow of urine from the bladder resulting from various etiologies; causes include benign prostatic hyperplasia, prostate cancer, bladder neck contracture, stricture, and a variety of other conditions.

bladder retraining [AS, *blaedre* + L, *trahere,* to draw], a system of therapy for urinary incontinence in which a patient practices withholding urine while maintaining a normal intake of fluid. The interval between urination is increased from about 1 hour to 3 to 4 hours over a period of 10 days. The patient also learns to recognize and react to the urge to urinate.

bladder sphincter [AS, *blaedre* + Gk, *sphingein,* to bind], a circular muscle surrounding the opening of the urinary bladder into the urethra.

bladder wall, the surrounding structure of the urinary bladder, consisting of the serous coat, subserous layer, muscular coat, submucous layer, and mucous coat.

Blakemore-Sengstaken tube. See **Sengstaken-Blakemore tube.**

Blalock-Taussig procedure /blā″loktô″sig/ [Alfred Blalock, American surgeon, 1899–1964; Helen B. Taussig, American physician, 1898–1986], surgical construction of a shunt between the right subclavian artery and the right pulmonary artery as a temporary measure to overcome congenital heart malformations, such as tetralogy of Fallot, in which there is insufficient pulmonary blood flow. Echocardiography is used to assess the malformation. General anesthesia and a cardiac bypass machine are used for the operation. The subclavian artery is joined end to side with the pulmonary artery, directing blood from the systemic circulation to the lungs. Thrombosis of the shunt is the major postoperative complication. Permanent surgical correction is performed in early childhood. See also **heart surgery.**

blame placing, the process of placing responsibility for one's behavior on others.

blanch /blanch, blänch/ [Fr, *blanchir,* to become white], **1.** to cause to become pale, as a nailbed may be blanched by using digital pressure. **2.** to press blood away and wait for return, such as blanching of fingernails and return of blood. **3.** to become white or pale, as from vasoconstriction accompanying fear or anger.

blanch test [Fr, *blanchir,* to become white; L, *testum,* crucible], a test of blood circulation in the fingers or toes. Pressure is applied to a fingernail or toenail until normal color is lost. The pressure is then removed, and, if the circulation is normal, color should return almost immediately, within about 2 seconds. The time may be prolonged by dehydration; a compromise of circulation, such as arterial occlusion; hypovolemic shock; or hypothermia. See also **capillary refill.**

bland [L, *blandus*], mild or having a soothing effect.

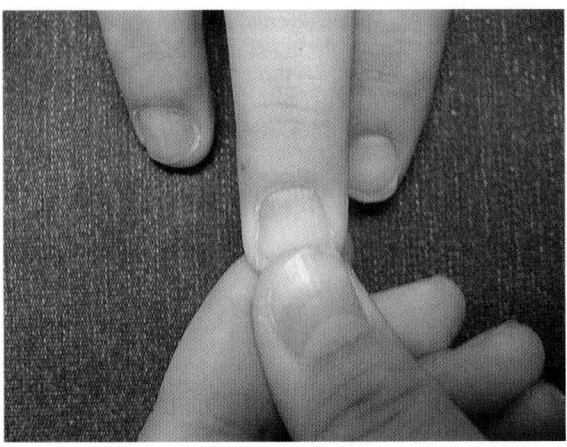

Blanch test *(Cummings et al, 2008)*

bland aerosols, aerosols that consist of water, saline solutions, or similar substances that do not have important pharmacological action. They are primarily used for humidification and liquefaction of secretions.

bland diet, a diet that is mechanically, chemically, physiologically, and sometimes thermally nonirritating to the GI tract. It is often prescribed in the treatment of ulcerative colitis, gallbladder disease, diverticulitis, gastritis, idiopathic spastic constipation, and mucous colitis and after abdominal surgery. Historically, it was first called the "white diet" (or Sippy diet, after Dr. Sippy, who developed it). This allowed the use of only white foods, such as milk, cream, mashed potatoes, and hot cereal (e.g., Cream of Wheat). It has progressed to what has been called the "liberal bland diet," which allows all foods except caffeine, alcohol, black pepper, spices, or any other food that could be considered irritating. The clinical value of the traditional bland diet has never been proven, and thus its use as a treatment for GI problems is questionable.

blank, a solution containing all of the reagents needed for analysis of a substance except the substance tested; typically used for the calibration of an instrument for chemical analysis.

blast, **1.** a primitive cell, such as an embryonic germ cell. **2.** a cell capable of building tissue, such as an osteoblast in growing bone.

-blast, suffix meaning an "embryonic state of development": *megaloblast, osteoblast.*

blast cell [Gk, *blastos,* germ], any immature cell, such as an erythroblast, lymphoblast, or neuroblast.

blastema /blastē″mə/ *pl. blastemas, blastemata* [Gk, bud], **1.** any mass of cells capable of growth and differentiation, specifically the primordial, undifferentiated cellular material from which a particular organ or tissue develops. **2.** in certain animals, a group of cells capable of regenerating a lost or damaged part or creating a complete organism in asexual reproduction. **3.** the budding or sprouting area of a plant. See also **primordium.** *–blastemic, blastemal, blastematic, adj.*

-blastema /-blas′təmə/, suffix meaning a "beginning substance or foundation for new growth": *blastema.*

blastemata, blastemal, blastematic, blastemic. See **blastema.**

blastic transformation, a late stage in the progress of chronic granulocytic leukemia. The leukemic cells become more undifferentiated and morphologically and genetically more abnormal, with more aggressive growth patterns. Signs of anemia and blood platelet deficiency are present, and half of the blood cells in the bone marrow are immature forms. Blastic transformation indicates that resistance to therapy has developed in the patient who has entered a terminal stage of leukemia.

blastid /blas′tid/ [Gk, *blastos,* germ], the site in the fertilized ovum where the pronuclei fuse and the nucleus forms. Also spelled *blastide.*

blastin /blas″tin/ [Gk, *blastanein,* to grow], any substance that provides nourishment for or stimulates the growth or proliferation of cells, such as allantoin.

blasto-, blast-, combining form meaning "an early embryonic or developing stage": *blastocoele, blastema.*

blastocoele /blas″təsēl′/ [Gk, *blastos,* germ, *koilos,* hollow], the fluid-filled cavity of the blastocyst in mammals and the blastula or discoblastula of lower animals. The cavity increases the surface area of the developing embryo to allow better absorption of nutrients and oxygen. Also called **cleavage cavity, segmentation cavity, subgerminal cavity.** Also spelled *blastocoel, blastocele.*

blastocyst /blas″təsist/ [Gk, *blastos* + *kystis,* bag], the embryonic form that follows the morula in human development. Implantation in the wall of the uterus usually occurs during this stage, approximately 8 to 13 days after fertilization. The blastocyst consists of an outer layer (trophoblast) that is attached to the inner cell mast.

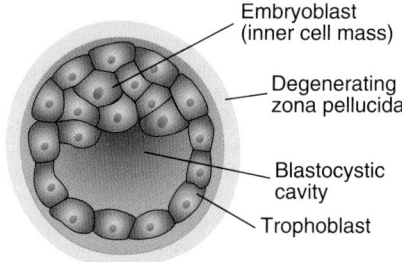

Early blastocyst *(Moore and Persaud, 2012)*

blastocyst cavity, the fluid-filled cavity developing in the morula as it becomes a blastocyst.

blastocyte /blas″təsīt/ [Gk, *blastos* + *kytos,* cell], an undifferentiated embryonic cell that precedes germ layer formation. −*blastocytic, adj.*

blastocytoma. See **blastoma.**

blastoderm /blas″tədurm′/ [Gk, *blastos* + *derma,* skin], the layer of cells forming the wall of the blastocyst in mammals and the blastula in lower animals during the early stages of embryonic development. It is produced by the cleavage of the fertilized ovum and gives rise to the primary germ layers, the ectoderm, mesoderm, and endoderm, from which the embryo and all of its membranes are derived. Also called **germinal membrane.** Kinds include **bilaminar blastoderm, embryonic blastoderm, extraembryonic blastoderm, trilaminar blastoderm.** −*blastodermal, blastodermic, adj.*

blastodisk /blas″tədisk/, the disklike, yolk-free area of cytoplasm surrounding the animal pole in a yolk-rich ovum, such as that of birds and reptiles. The blastodisk is the site where cleavage occurs after fertilization. As cleavage continues, the blastodisk develops into the embryo. Also spelled **blastodisc.**

blastogenesis /blas″tōjen″əsis/ [Gk, *blastos* + *genein,* to produce], **1.** asexual reproduction by budding. **2.** the transmission of hereditary characteristics by the germ plasm. Compare **pangenesis. 3.** the early development of an embryo during cleavage and formation of the germ layers. **4.** the process of transforming small lymphocytes in tissue culture into large, blastlike cells by exposure to phytohemagglutinin or other substances, often for the purpose of inducing mitosis. −*blastogenetic, adj.*

blastogenic /-jen″ik/, **1.** originating in the germ plasm. **2.** initiating tissue proliferation. **3.** relating to or characterized by blastogenesis.

blastogenic factor, lymphocyte-transforming factor.

blastogeny /blastoj″ənē/, **1.** the early stages in ontogeny. **2.** the germ plasm history of an organism or species, which traces the history of inherited characteristics.

blastokinin /blas″təkī″nin/ [Gk, *blastos* + *kinein,* to move], a globulin, secreted by the uterus in many mammals, that may stimulate and regulate the implantation process of the blastocyst in the uterine wall. Also called **uteroglobulin.**

blastolysis /blastol″isis/ [Gk, *blastos* + *lysis,* loosening], destruction of a germ cell or blastoderm. −*blastolytic, adj.*

blastoma /blastō″mə/ [Gk, + tumor], a neoplasm of embryonic tissue that develops from the blastema of an organ or tissue. A blastoma derived from a number of scattered cells is pluricentric; one arising from a single cell or group of cells is unicentric. Also called **blastocytoma.** −**blastomatous,** *adj.*

blastomatosis /blast″tōmətō″sis/ [Gk, *blastos* + *oma,* tumor, *osis,* condition], the development of many tumors from embryonic tissue.

blastomatous. See **blastoma.**

blastomere /blas″təmēr/ [Gk, *blastos* + *meros,* part], any of the cells formed from the first mitotic division of a fertilized ovum (zygote). The blastomeres further divide and subdivide to form a multicellular morula in the first several days of pregnancy. Also called **segmentation cell.** See also **blastula.** −*blastomeric, adj.*

blastomere biopsy, a technique for preimplantation genetic diagnosis, in which a blastomere is removed from a 6- or 8-cell embryo and tested for genetic abnormalities.

blastomerotomy /-merot″əmē/ [Gk, *blastos* + *meros,* part, *tome,* cut], destruction of a blastomere. Also called **blastotomy.** −*blastomerotomic, adj.*

Blastomyces /blas′tōmī″sēz/ [Gk, *blastos* + *mykes,* fungus], a genus of yeastlike fungi, usually including the species *Blastomyces dermatitidis,* which causes North American blastomycosis, and *Paracoccidioides brasiliensis,* which causes South American blastomycosis.

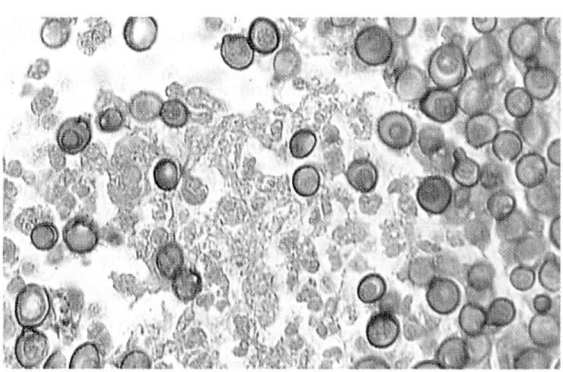

Blastomyces *(Forbes, Sahm, and Weissfeld, 2007)*

blastomycosis /blas′tōmīkō″sis/ [Gk, *blastos* + *mykes,* fungus, *osis,* condition], an infectious disease caused by a yeastlike fungus, *Blastomyces dermatitidis.* It usually affects only the skin but may cause acute pneumonitis or disseminated disease and invade the lungs, kidneys, central nervous system, and bones. Also called **Gilchrist disease.** See also **fungus, mycosis, North American blastomycosis.**

■ OBSERVATIONS: Skin infections are almost always a result of hematogeneous seeding from a primary infection and often begin as small papules on the hand, face, neck, or other exposed areas where there has been a cut, bruise, or other injury. The infection may spread gradually and irregularly into surrounding areas. Lung infection is caused by inhalation of airborne conidia. When the lungs are involved, mucous membrane lesions resemble squamous cell carcinoma. The person usually has a cough, dyspnea, chest pain, chills, and a fever with heavy sweating. Diagnosis is made by identification of the disease organism in a culture of specimens from lesions.

■ INTERVENTIONS: Treatment usually involves the administration of amphotericin B in pulmonary disease or itraconazole or ketoconazole in systemic disease. Recovery usually begins within the first week of treatment.

■ PATIENT CARE CONSIDERATIONS: The disease is most common in river valleys of North America, particularly in the southeastern United States, but outbreaks have occurred in Africa and Latin America. The mortality rate is approximately 5%.

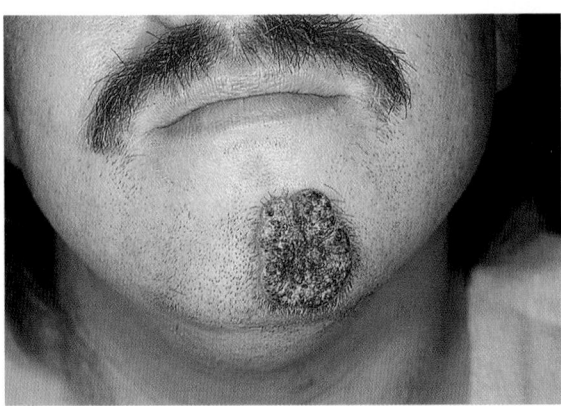

Blastomycosis *(Callen et al, 2000)*

blastopore /blas″təpôr/ [Gk, *blastos* + *poros,* opening], (in embryology) the opening into the archenteron made by invagination of the blastula.

blastoporic canal. See **neurenteric canal.**

blastosphere. See **blastula.**

blastotomy. See **blastomerotomy.**

blastula /blas″tyələ/ [Gk, *blastos,* germ], an early stage of the process through which a zygote develops into an embryo, characterized by a fluid-filled sphere formed by a single layer of cells. The spheric layer of cells is called a blastoderm; the fluid-filled cavity is the blastocoele. The blastula develops from the morula stage and is usually the form in which the embryo becomes implanted in the wall of the uterus. Also called **blastosphere.**

-blastula, suffix meaning an early embryonic stage in the development of a fertilized egg: *discoblastula.*

blastulation, the transformation of the morula into a blastocyst or blastula by the development of a central cavity, the blastocoele.

BLB mask, abbreviation for **Boothby-Lovelace-Bulbulian (BLB) mask.**

bleaching /blēch′ing/ [ME, *blechen*], the act or process of removing stains or color by chemical means.

bleaching agents, medications and over-the-counter preparations used to depigment the skin. The products may be used by persons whose skin has become hyperpigmented through exposure to sunlight and particularly for melasma associated with pregnancy, the use of oral contraceptives, or hormone replacement therapy. Most agents are sold as creams or lotions and contain hydroquinone.

bleach poisoning, an adverse reaction to ingestion of hypochlorite salts commonly found in household and commercial bleaches. Symptoms include pain and inflammation of the mouth, throat, and esophagus; vomiting; shock; and circulatory collapse. A poison control center should be contacted immediately if bleach poisoning is suspected.

bleb /bleb/ [ME, blob], **1.** an accumulation of fluid under the skin. **2.** an anatomical structure with a blisterlike appearance.

bleed [AS, *blod,* blood], **1.** to lose blood from the blood vessels of the body. The blood may flow externally through an orifice or a break in the skin or flow internally into a cavity, into an organ, or between tissues. **2.** to cause blood to flow from a vein or an artery.

bleeder, **1.** (*Slang*) a person who has hemophilia or any other vascular or hematological condition associated with a tendency to hemorrhage. **2.** (*Slang*) a blood vessel that bleeds, especially one cut during a surgical procedure.

bleeding, the release of blood from the vascular system as a result of damage to a blood vessel. See also **blood clotting.**

bleeding diathesis, a predisposition to abnormal blood clotting.

bleeding precautions, modifications in activities of daily living that minimize the risk of bleeding, such as avoiding contact sports, wearing gloves when gardening, avoiding sharp objects (i.e., razors), avoiding aspirin and medications containing aspirin, using care when brushing teeth, and avoiding injections when possible.

bleeding time, (*Obsolete*) the time required for blood to stop flowing from a forearm incision of specific dimensions under controlled blood pressure. The test, also called the Duke or Ivy bleeding time, uses a specially designed lancet and is meant to measure platelet function. The bleeding time has no ability to predict bleeding risk and is obsolete. Medical laboratory scientists discourage the use of the bleeding time. See also **hemostasis.**

blemish [OFr, *bleme,* to deface], a skin stain, alteration, defect, or flaw.

blended family [ME, *blenden,* to mix], a family formed when parents and/or partners bring together children from previous marriages and relationships.

blending inheritance, the apparent fusion in offspring of distinct, dissimilar characteristics of the parents. Blended characteristics are usually of a quantitative nature, such as height, and fail to segregate in successive generations. The phenomenon is the result of multiple pairs of genes that have a cumulative effect. See also **polygene.**

blenno-, blenn-, combining form meaning "mucus": *blennorrhea.*

blennorrhea /blen′ərē″ə/ [Gk, *blennos,* mucus, *rhoia,* flow], excessive discharge of mucus. Also called *blennorrhagia.* Also spelled *blennorrhoea.*

Blenoxane, an antineoplastic. Brand name for **bleomycin sulfate.**

bleomycin sulfate /blē·əmī″sin/, an antineoplastic antibiotic.

■ INDICATIONS: It is prescribed in the treatment of a variety of neoplasms.

■ CONTRAINDICATIONS: Hypersensitivity to this drug prohibits its use.

- ADVERSE EFFECTS: Among the most serious adverse reactions are pneumonitis, pulmonary fibrosis, and a syndrome of hyperpyrexia and circulatory collapse. Rashes and skin reactions commonly occur.

blephar-. See **blepharo-, blephar-.**

blepharal /blef′ərəl/ [Gk, *blepharon,* eyelid], pertaining to the eyelids.

blepharedema /blef′əridē″mə/, a fluid accumulation in the eyelid, causing a swollen appearance.

-blepharia, suffix meaning "(condition of the) eyelid": *macroblepharia.*

blepharitis /blef′ərī″tis/ [Gk, *blepharon + itis*], an inflammatory condition of the lash follicles and meibomian glands of the eyelids, characterized by swelling, redness, and crusts of dried mucus on the lids. Ulcerative blepharitis is caused by bacterial infection. Nonulcerative blepharitis may be caused by psoriasis, seborrhea, or an allergic response.

- OBSERVATIONS: Individuals report a foreign-body sensation of the eye. There are red eyelid margins, flaking and scaling around lashes, an itching and burning sensation, and loss of lashes. Light sensitivity, conjunctivitis, and possible corneal inflammation may also occur. In ulcerative blepharitis there are crusts on the eyelids that bleed when removed. Small pustules develop in lash follicles, and eyelids become "glued" together by dried drainage during sleep. Lid margins thicken over time with misdirected growth and/or loss of eyelashes. Corneal pannus, ulcerative keratitis, and lid ectropion can occur in severe cases. Diagnosis is made by clinical examination, and lab tests may be run to isolate the causative agent. Individuals with chronic diseases such as diabetes, gout, anemia, and rosacea or a history of sties, chalazia, or chronic infections of the mouth and/or throat are at greater risk.

- INTERVENTIONS: Blepharitis is often resistant to various therapies. Topical antiinfective ointments and drops are used, but the mainstay of treatment is the use of eyelid scrubs. Resistant cases may require oral antibiotic treatment.

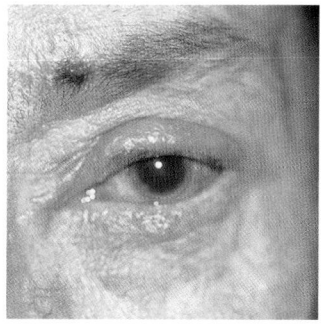

Blepharitis *(Kanski, 2002)*

blepharo-, blephar-, combining form meaning "eyelid" or "eyelash": *blepharochalasis, blepharoplasty.*

blepharoadenoma /-ad′inō″mə/ pl. *blepharoadenomas, blepharoadenomata,* a glandular epithelial tumor of the eyelid.

blepharoatheroma /-ath′ərō″mə/ pl. *blepharoatheromas, blepharoatheromata,* a tumor of the eyelid.

blepharochalasis /blef′ə·rō·kal′ə·sis/ [Gk, *blepharon,* eyelid + *chalasis,* relaxation], relaxation of the skin of the eyelid because of atrophy of the intercellular tissue.

blepharoclonus /blef′ərok″lōnəs/, a condition characterized by muscle spasms of the eyelid, appearing as increased winking.

blepharoncus /blef′əron″kəs/ [Gk, *blepharon + onkos,* swelling], a tumor of the eyelid.

blepharophimosis /blef′ə·rō·fi·mō′sis/ [Gk, *blepharon,* eyelid + *phimōsis,* a muzzling], abnormal narrowness of the palpebral fissure in the horizontal direction, caused by lateral displacement of the medial canthus.

blepharoplasty /blef′əroplas′tē/ [Gk, *blepharon,* eyelid, *plassein,* to mold], plastic surgery to restore or repair the eyelid and eyebrow by removing excess skin, muscle, or fat. Also called **brow lift.**

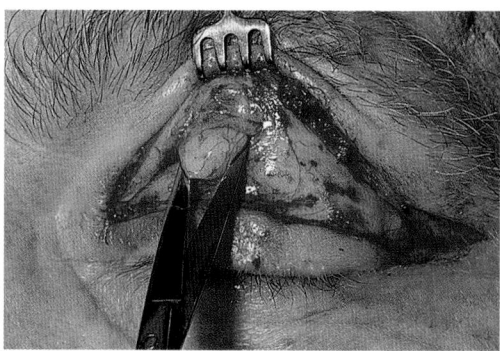

Excision of fat during a blepharoplasty *(Tyers and Collin, 2008)*

blepharoplegia /-plē″jē·ə/ [Gk, *blepharon + plege,* stroke], paralysis of muscles of the eyelid.

blepharospasm /blef″ərōspaz′əm/ [Gk, *blepharon,* eyelid, *spasmos,* spasm], the involuntary contraction of eyelid muscles. The condition may be caused by a local lesion of the eye, a neurological irritation, or psychological stress.

blessed thistle, an annual herb found in Europe and Asia.

- INDICATIONS: This herb is used for loss of appetite, indigestion, and intestinal gas. It is probably safe when used as recommended, but evidence of effectiveness is lacking.

- CONTRAINDICATIONS: Blessed thistle should not be used during pregnancy, in children, or in those with known hypersensitivity to the herb.

Bleuler, Eugen /bloi″lər/ [Swiss psychiatrist, 1857–1939], a pioneer investigator in the fields of autism and schizophrenia. Bleuler introduced the term schizophrenia to replace dementia praecox and identified four primary symptoms of schizophrenia, known as Bleuler's "4 A's": ambivalence, associative disturbance, autistic thinking, and affective incongruity.

blighted ovum /blī″tid/, a fertilized ovum that fails to develop. On x-ray or ultrasonic visualization it appears to be a fluid-filled cyst attached to the wall of the uterus. It may be empty, or it may contain amorphous parts. Many first-trimester spontaneous abortions represent the expulsion of a blighted ovum. Suction curettage may be necessary if the blighted ovum is retained.

blind, 1. to withhold intervention information from a researcher or participant in a scientific study. See also **double-blind study. 2.** See **blindness.**

blind fistula [AS, *blind* + L, pipe], an abnormal passage with only one open end; the opening may be on the body surface or on or within an internal organ or structure. Also called **incomplete fistula.**

blindgut, digestive cavity with one opening. See **cecum.**

blind intubation, insertion of an endotracheal tube without direct visualization of the glottis. See **intubation.**

blind loop [AS, *blind* + ME, *loupe*], a redundant segment of intestine. Bacterial overgrowth occurs and may lead to malabsorption, obstruction, and necrosis. Blind loops may be created inadvertently by surgical procedures, such as side-to-side ileotransverse colostomy.

blind loop syndrome. See **stasis syndrome.**

blindness [AS, *blind*], the absence of sight. The term may indicate a total loss of vision or may be applied in a modified manner to describe certain visual limitations, as in yellow color blindness (tritanopia) or word blindness (dyslexia). Legal blindness is defined as best corrected visual acuity less than 20/200 in the better eye or marked constriction of the visual fields.

blind spot, 1. a normal gap in the visual field occurring when an image is focused on the space in the retina occupied by the optic disc. 2. an abnormal gap in the visual field caused by a lesion on the retina or in the optic pathways or resulting from hemorrhage or choroiditis, often perceived as light spots or flashes.

blink reflex [ME, *blenken* + L, *reflectere,* to bend back], the automatic closure of the eyelid when an object is perceived to be rapidly approaching the eye.

blister, a vesicle or bulla of the skin containing watery matter or serum.

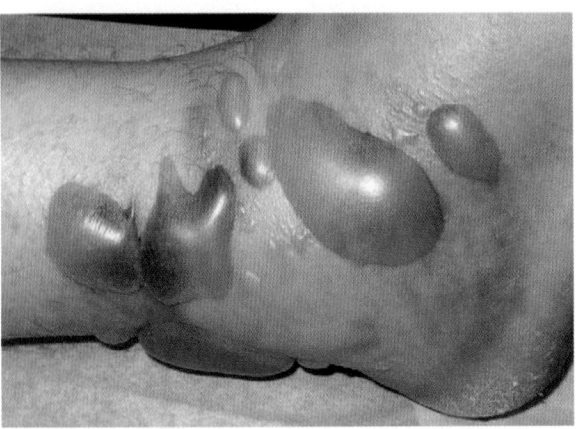

Blister *(Coughlin and Saltzman, 2014)*

blister agents/vesicants, chemicals that cause blistering of the skin or mucous membranes on contact. These agents include phosgene oxime, lewisite, distilled mustard, mustard gas, nitrogen mustard, sesqui mustard, and sulfur mustard. Exposure is mainly by inhalation or by contact with the skin or eyes. Inhalation causes shortness of breath, tachypnea, and hemoptysis, and death may result from the accumulation of fluid in the lungs; contact with the skin causes blistering and necrosis; and ocular contact causes swelling of the eyelids and corneal damage and can lead to blindness. Exposure to high doses affects the cardiovascular and nervous systems and may lead to cardiac arrest, convulsions, and coma. If these agents are ingested, nausea, vomiting, hematemesis, and diarrhea result. No antidote exists for most blister agents, and treatment consists of removal of clothing, washing the exposed areas, and supportive care. Lewisite can be neutralized by the application of British antilewisite (dimercaprol) if it is done soon after exposure.

bloat [ME, *blout*], a swelling or filling with gas, such as distension of the abdomen that results from swallowed air or from intestinal gas. The stomach on percussion will have a tympanic sound.

Blocadren, a beta-adrenergic receptor blocking agent. Brand name for **timolol maleate.**

Bloch-Sulzberger incontinentia pigmenti, Bloch-Sulzberger syndrome. See **incontinentia pigmenti.**

block [OFr, *bloc*], 1. a disruption in the conduction of a nerve impulse. The term may apply to stoppage of nerve conduction as produced by local anesthetics, inhibition of beta receptors by beta-blocker drugs, inhibition of calcium channels by calcium channel blocker drugs, or prevention of neuromuscular transmission by blockade of nicotinic receptors by muscle-relaxant drugs. 2. a device to maintain separation of the teeth, such as a bite block.

blockade /blokād″/, an agent that interferes with or prevents a specific action in an organ or tissue, such as a cholinergic blockade that inhibits transmission of acetylcholine-stimulated nerve impulses along fibers of the autonomic nervous system.

blockage. See **obstruction.**

block anesthesia, 1. See **conduction anesthesia.** 2. the loss of feeling or sensation induced by injecting a local anesthetic agent close to a nerve trunk. Examples in dentistry include Gow-Gates block anesthesia and inferior alveolar block anesthesia. Differs from local infiltration of anesthesia. Compare **regional anesthesia.**

blocked pleurisy. See **encysted pleurisy.**

blocker. See **blocking agent.**

blocking [ME, *blok*], 1. preventing the transmission of an impulse, such as by an antiadrenergic agent or by the injection of an anesthetic. 2. interrupting an intracellular biosynthetic process, such as by the injection of actinomycin D or the action of an antivitamin. 3. an interruption in the spontaneous flow of speech or thought. 4. repressing an idea or emotion to prevent it from obtruding into the consciousness.

blocking agent, 1. an agent that inhibits a biological action, such as movement of an ion across the cell membrane, passage of a neural impulse, or interaction with a specific receptor. 2. an agent used in hybridization experiments (Southern, Northern, and Western blotting) to avoid nonspecific binding of probe to the membrane.

blocking antibody, an antibody that reacts with an antigen but fails to cross-link with other antigens and cause agglutination. When such antibodies are present in high concentration, they interfere with the action of other antibodies by occupying all the antigenic sites. See also **antigen-antibody reaction, hapten.**

blockout /blok′out/ [OFr, *bloc* + AS, *ūt*], (in dentistry) elimination of undesirable undercut areas in a plaster cast, filling them in with a suitable material, usually a hard blockout wax; this includes all areas that would offer interference to placement or removal of the denture framework and those not crossed by a rigid part of the denture. A blockout creates a common path of insertion.

blood [AS, *blod*], the liquid pumped by the heart through all the arteries, veins, and capillaries. The blood is composed of a clear yellow fluid, called plasma, and the formed elements, which are red cells, white cells, and platelets. The major function of the blood is to transport oxygen and nutrients to the cells and to remove carbon dioxide and other waste products. Adults normally have a total blood volume of 7% to 8% of body weight, or 70 mL/kg of body weight for men and about 65 mL/kg for women. Compare **lymph.** See also **blood cell, erythrocyte, leukocyte, plasma, platelets.**

blood agar, a culture medium consisting of blood (usually sheep's blood) and nutrient agar, used in bacteriology to cultivate certain microorganisms, including *Staphylococcus epidermidis, Streptococcus pneumoniae,* and *Clostridium perfringens.*

blood agents, poisons that affect the body by being absorbed into the blood. Blood agents include arsine and cyanide. Exposure to both may occur by inhalation, and cyanide exposure may also occur by ingestion and absorption through the skin and eyes. Arsine causes hemolysis, resulting in generalized weakness, jaundice, delirium, and renal failure; high doses may result in death. There is no antidote and treatment is supportive. Cyanide prevents cells from using oxygen, leading to cell death, and poisoning especially affects the cardiovascular and nervous systems and can lead to heart and brain damage and death from respiratory failure. Treatment consists of the administration of an antidote and supportive care.

blood albumin [AS, *blod* + L, *albus*], the plasma protein circulating in blood serum. Also called **serum albumin.**

blood and urine cortisol, a blood or urine test that assists in the evaluation of adrenal activity. Adrenal hyperfunction may indicate Cushing disease, adrenal adenoma or carcinoma, ectopic ACTH-producing tumors, or hyperthyroidism, whereas hypofunction may indicate congenital adrenal hyperplasia, Addison disease, hypopituitarism, hypothyroidism, or liver disease.

blood uric acid, a blood plasma or serum test that measures uric acid concentration. Hyperuricemia (elevated blood uric acid) is related to gout, kidney stones, kidney failure, leukemia, myeloma, lead poisoning, and dehydration.

blood bank, an organizational unit responsible for collecting, processing, and storing blood and components for transfusion and other purposes. The blood bank is usually a subdivision of a laboratory in a hospital and is often charged with the responsibility for pretransfusion compatibility testing and other serological tests. See also *bank blood,* **component therapy, transfusion.**

blood bank technology specialist, a medical laboratory scientist with a specialty certification in immunohematology and transfusion medicine as a specialist in blood banking (SBB) from the American Society for Clinical Pathology. These specialists are responsible for the operations of blood banks and transfusion services, from routine testing to the most advanced procedures. Most are technical supervisors and laboratory managers and oversee reference laboratories, but they may also work in other areas, such as education and research.

blood bilirubin test, a quantitative blood plasma or serum assay of the bile pigment, bilirubin. Total bilirubin consists of bilirubin diglucuronide (conjugated, water soluble, direct) and unconjugated (albumin-bound, water insoluble, indirect). Prehepatic disease such as hemolytic anemia is associated with unconjugated bilirubin; hepatocellular disease or posthepatic bile duct obstruction, such as gallstones, is associated with conjugated bilirubin.

blood blister, a blister containing blood. It may be caused by a pinch, a bruise, or persistent friction.

blood-borne pathogens, pathogenic microorganisms that are transmitted via human blood and cause disease in humans. They include, but are not limited to, hepatitis B virus (HBV) and human immunodeficiency virus (HIV). A number of pathogens can be transmitted percutaneously, often by needlestick injuries.

blood-brain barrier (BBB) [AS, *blod* + *bragen* + ME, *barrere*], an anatomical-physiological feature of the brain thought to consist of walls of capillaries in the central nervous system and surrounding astrocytic glial membranes. The barrier separates the parenchyma of the central nervous system from blood. The blood-brain barrier prevents or slows the passage of some drugs and other chemical compounds, radioactive ions, and disease-causing organisms such as viruses from the blood into the central nervous system.

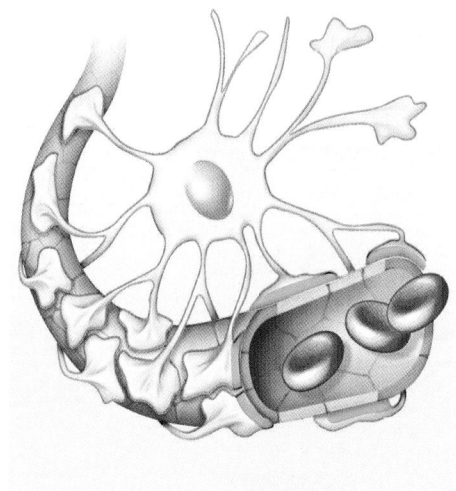

Blood-brain barrier

blood buffers [AS, *blod* + ME, *buffe,* to cushion], whole blood, carbon dioxide, and bicarbonate ions that maintain the proper pH. See also **buffer, arterial pH.**

blood capillaries [AS, *blod* + L, *capillaris,* hairlike], the minute vessels connecting arterioles and venules, the walls of which act as a semipermeable membrane for exchanges of various substances between the blood and tissue fluid. A capillary wall generally has a thickness of one simple squamous epithelial cell, permitting easy diffusion of gas molecules and other dissolved substances. Occasional small openings permit diapedesis of leukocytes, distribution of nutrients to the tissues supplied by the capillary network, and collection of waste products released by the cells.

blood cell, any of the formed elements of the blood, including red cells (erythrocytes), white cells (leukocytes) and platelets (thrombocytes). Blood cells constitute about 50% of the total volume of the blood. See also **erythrocyte, leukocyte, platelets.**

blood cell casts [AS, *blod* + L, *cella,* storeroom; ONorse, *kasta*], urinary sediment containing blood cells, typically red or white blood cells.

blood chloride test, a blood test performed as part of a panel of electrolyte testing. It is performed along with other electrolyte tests to indicate the patient's acid-base balance and hydration status.

blood circulation [AS, *blod* + L, *circulare,* to go around], the circuit of blood through the body, from the heart through the arteries, arterioles, capillaries, venules, and veins and back to the heart.

blood clot [AS, *blod* + *clott,* lump], a semisolid, gelatinous mass, the final result of the clotting process in blood. Red cells, white cells, and platelets are enmeshed in an insoluble fibrin network of the blood clot. Compare **embolus, thrombus.** See also **blood clotting, fibrinogen.**

blood clotting, the conversion of blood from a free-flowing liquid to a semisolid gel. Although clotting can occur within an intact blood vessel, the process usually starts with tissue damage. Within seconds of injury to the vessel wall, platelets adhere to the site. If normal amounts of calcium, platelets, and tissue factors are present, prothrombin is converted to thrombin. Thrombin acts as a catalyst for the conversion of fibrinogen to a mesh of insoluble fibrin, in which all the formed elements are immobilized. Also called *blood coagulation.* Compare **hemostasis.** See also **anticoagulant, coagulation.**

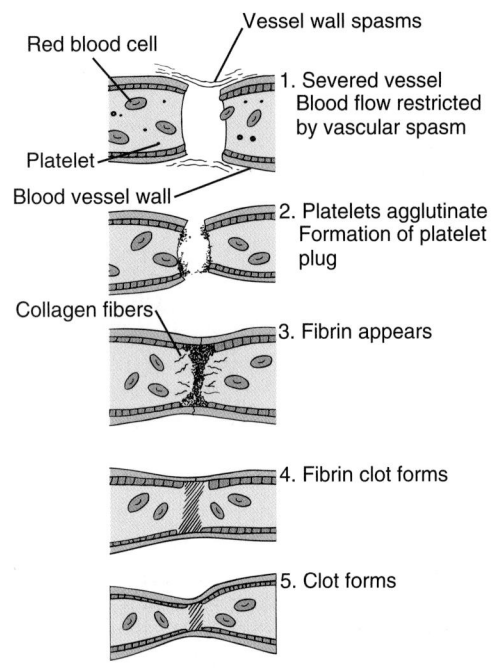

Red blood cell

Vessel wall spasms

Platelet

Blood vessel wall

Collagen fibers

1. Severed vessel
Blood flow restricted
by vascular spasm

2. Platelets agglutinate
Formation of platelet
plug

3. Fibrin appears

4. Fibrin clot forms

5. Clot forms

Blood clotting *(Mosby, 2003)*

blood component therapy, transfusion of one or more of the components of whole blood to treat a specific deficiency.

blood corpuscle [AS, *blod* + L, *corpusculum,* little body], *(Obsolete)* an archaic term for a blood cell, an erythrocyte, a leukocyte, or sometimes a thrombocyte.

blood count. See **complete blood count.**

blood creatinine test, a quantitative measure of plasma or serum creatinine that is elevated in impaired renal function or renal failure. The creatinine level is used in estimating the glomerular filtration rate. The creatinine assay is sometimes paired with the blood urea nitrogen assay.

blood crossmatching, the direct matching of donor and recipient blood to prevent the transfusion of incompatible blood types. Crossmatching tests for agglutination of (1) donor red blood cells (RBCs) by recipient serum and (2) recipient RBCs by donor serum.

blood culture and sensitivity test, a blood culture obtained to detect the presence of bacteria in the blood (bacteremia). Bacteria present are identified and tested for resistance to antibiotics.

blood culture medium, a liquid enrichment medium for the growth of bacteria in the diagnosis of blood infections (bacteremia and septicemia). It contains a suspension of brain tissue in meat broth with dextrose, peptone, and citrate and has a pH of 7.4.

blood donor, an individual who gives blood or blood components. See also **blood bank, transfusion.**

blood doping, *(Slang)* the administration of blood, red blood cells, or related blood products to an athlete to enhance performance, often preceded by the withdrawal of blood so that training continues in a blood-depleted state.

blood dyscrasia [AS, *blod* + Gk, *dys,* bad, *krasis,* mingling], a pathological condition in which any of the constituents of the blood are abnormal in structure, function, or quality, as in leukemia or hemophilia.

blood fluke, a parasitic flatworm of the class Trematoda, genus *Schistosoma,* including the species *S. haematobium, S. japonicum,* and *S. mansoni.*

blood gas, **1.** gas dissolved in the liquid part of the blood. Blood gases include oxygen, carbon dioxide, and nitrogen. **2.** a laboratory test to determine oxygen, carbon dioxide, bicarbonate, and hydrogen ion (pH) concentrations in whole blood.

blood gas analysis (BGA), the determination of oxygen and carbon dioxide concentrations and pressures with the pH of the blood by laboratory tests; the following measurements may be made: PO_2, partial pressure of oxygen in arterial blood; PCO_2, partial pressure of carbon dioxide in arterial blood; SO_2, percent saturation of hemoglobin with oxygen in arterial blood; total CO_2 content of (venous) plasma; and pH.

blood gas determination, an analysis of the pH of the blood and the concentration and pressure of oxygen and carbon dioxide in the blood. It can be performed as an emergency procedure to assess acid-base balance and ventilatory status. Blood gas determination is often important in the evaluation of cardiac failure, hemorrhage, kidney failure, drug overdose, shock, uncontrolled diabetes mellitus, or any other condition of severe stress. The blood for examination is drawn from an artery, as ordered in a heparinized syringe, sealed from air, placed on ice, and immediately transported for analysis. Normal adult arterial blood gas values are pH 7.35 to 7.45; PCO_2 35 to 45 mm Hg; HCO_3^- 21 to 28 mEq/L; PO_2 80 to 100 mm Hg; O_2 saturation 95% to 100%. See also **acid-base balance, acidosis, alkalosis, oxygenation, $PaCO_2$, pH, PO_2.**

blood gas tension, the partial pressure of a gas in the blood.

blood glucose [AS, *blod* + OFr, *livel* + Gk, *glykys,* sweet], **1.** referring to the glucose in the bloodstream. Glucose is a simple monosaccharide sugar that is circulated throughout the body via the blood. It provides energy. The presence and function of insulin are essential, facilitating the entry of glucose into the cells. **2.** a laboratory measure performed on serum or plasma specific for the monosaccharide glucose. The assay is usually performed after a fasting period, typically 8 hours.

blood glucose level, the concentration of glucose in the blood, represented in milligrams of glucose per deciliter of blood. Normal adult blood glucose levels range from 70 to 115 mg/dL (4 to 6 mmol/L) with generally higher levels after 50 years of age. A fasting serum glucose of 126 mg/dL on two or more occasions signifies diabetes mellitus. A fasting serum glucose of 100 to 125 mg/dL is considered an impaired fasting glucose, a type of prediabetes that increases the risk of developing type 2 diabetes. If a random blood glucose test is done, a level of 200 mg/dL or higher is usually an indicator of diabetes mellitus. See glucose tolerance test. See also **hypoglycemia, hyperglycemia, glycosylated hemoglobin.**

blood glucose test, a blood test used to detect hyperglycemia or hypoglycemia. This test must be performed frequently in patients with newly diagnosed diabetes mellitus to assist in monitoring and adjusting the insulin dose. See also **fasting plasma glucose.**

blood group, the classification of blood based on the presence or absence of genetically determined antigens on the surface of the red cell. Many blood group systems have been described, including ABO, Rh, MNS, P, Kell, Duffy, Kidd, Lutheran, Kx, H, Xg, and others, as well as collections of high- and low-frequency antigens. Their relative importance depends on their clinical significance in transfusion therapy, organ transplantation, maternal-fetal compatibility, and genetic studies. See also **ABO blood group.**

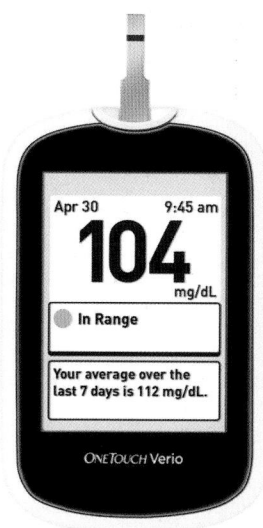

Blood glucose test *(©Lifescan Inc.)*

blood island, one of the clusters of mesodermal cells that proliferate on the outer surface of the embryonic yolk sac and give it a lumpy appearance.

blood lactate, lactic acid that appears in the blood as a result of anaerobic metabolism when oxygen delivery to the tissues is insufficient to support normal metabolic demands.

bloodless, 1. any organ or body part that lacks blood or appears to lack blood. **2.** a surgical field in which the normal local blood supply has been redirected to other areas.

bloodless phlebotomy [AS, *blod* + ME, *les* + Gk, *phleps,* vein, *tomos,* cutting], a technique of trapping blood in a body region by the application of tourniquet pressure that is less than the pressure needed to interrupt arterial blood flow.

bloodletting, *(Informal)* the therapeutic opening of an artery or vein to withdraw blood from a particular area. It is sometimes performed to treat polycythemia and congestive heart failure. Now called **phlebotomy.**

blood level, the concentration or activity level of a serum, plasma, or whole blood analyte. Analytes may include metabolic materials and external materials such as drugs.

blood osmolality [AS, *blod* + Gk, *ōsmos,* impulsion], the osmotic pressure of blood. It measures the amount of solute concentration per unit of total volume of a particular solution. The normal values in serum are 280 to 295 mOsm/L. See also **osmolality.**

blood osmolality test, a blood test that measures the concentration of solutes. Osmolality identifies patients with fluid and electrolyte imbalance, seizures, coma, and ascites. The test also detects and monitors hydration status, acid-base balance, and antidiuretic hormone (ADH) levels.

blood patch. See **epidural blood patch.**

blood pH, the hydrogen ion concentration of the blood, a measure of blood acidity or alkalinity. The normal pH values for arterial whole blood are 7.35 to 7.454; for venous whole blood, 7.36 to 7.41; and for venous serum or plasma, 7.35 to 7.45.

blood plasma [AS, *blod* + Gk, *plassein,* to mold], the liquid portion of the blood, free of its formed elements and particles. Plasma represents approximately 50% of the total volume of blood and contains glucose, proteins, amino acids, and other nutritive materials; urea and other excretory products; and hormones, enzymes, vitamins, and minerals. Compare **serum.** See also **blood, plasma protein, pooled plasma.**

blood platelet. See **platelets, thrombocyte.**

blood poisoning, *(Informal)* now called **septicemia.**

blood potassium (K+) test, a blood test that detects the serum concentration of potassium, the major cation within cells. Potassium levels are followed carefully in patients with uremia, renal insufficiency, Addison's disease, or vomiting and diarrhea; in those on steroid therapy; in those taking potassium-depleting diuretics; and in those taking digitalis-like drugs.

blood pressure (BP) [AS, *blod* + L, *premere,* to press], the pressure exerted by the circulating volume of blood on the walls of the arteries and veins and on the chambers of the heart. Blood pressure is regulated by the homeostatic mechanisms of the body by the volume of the blood, the lumen of the arteries and arterioles, and the force of cardiac contraction. In the aorta and large arteries of a healthy young adult, blood pressure is approximately 120 mm Hg during systole and 70 mm Hg during diastole. See also **hypertension, hypotension.**

■ METHOD: The indirect blood pressure is most often measured by auscultation using an aneroid or pressure sensor sphygmomanometer, a stethoscope, and a blood pressure cuff.

■ INTERVENTIONS: The intervals at which the patient's blood pressure is to be taken are determined by the patient's condition. The pressure should be taken in both arms the first time the procedure is performed; persistent major differences between the two readings are indicative of a vascular occlusion. The width of the cuff should be one-third to one-half the circumference of the limb used. Thus, a larger cuff is required for a large patient or for any patient if the pressure is taken at the thigh.

■ OUTCOME CRITERIA: Any factor that increases peripheral resistance or cardiac output increases the blood pressure. Therefore, it is important to obtain a blood pressure reading when the patient is at rest. Increased peripheral resistance usually increases the diastolic pressure, and increased cardiac output tends to increase the systolic pressure. Blood pressure increases with age, primarily as a result of the decreased distensibility of the veins. As a person grows older, an increase in systolic pressure precedes an increase in diastolic pressure.

blood pressure monitor [AS, *blod* + L, *premere,* to press, *monere,* to warn], a device that automatically measures blood pressure and records the information continuously. Automatic monitoring of blood pressure is often used in surgery or in an intensive care unit, where frequent monitoring is required. Automated blood pressure monitors can also be used for self-monitoring of blood pressure.

blood protein [AS, *blod* + Gk, *proteios,* of first rank], any of the large variety of proteins normally found in the blood, such as albumin, globulin, hemoglobin, and proteins bound to hormones or other compounds. See also **plasma protein, serum protein.**

blood protein test (blood albumin), a serum chemistry test that measures albumin, a protein that makes up 55%-60% of total serum protein and that helps maintain colloidal osmotic pressure. Albumin is elevated in dehydration and multiple myeloma and becomes reduced in acute or chronic inflammation, liver disease, renal dysfunction, increased protein catabolism, and plasma volume expansion. Albumin is often measured as part of serum protein electrophoresis, which also provides serum globulin levels.

blood pump, 1. a device for regulating the flow of blood into a blood vessel during transfusion. **2.** a component of a heart-lung machine that pumps the blood through the machine for oxygenation and then through the peripheral circulatory system of the body. Also called **mechanical**

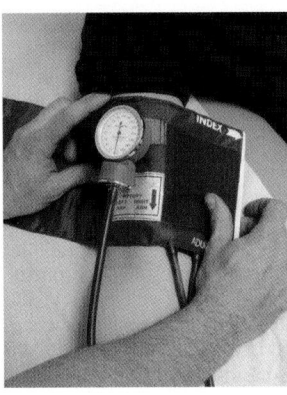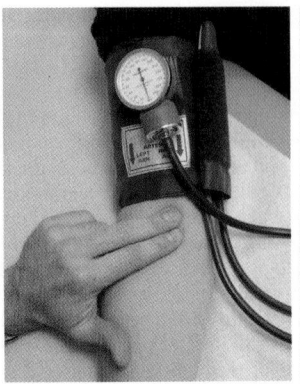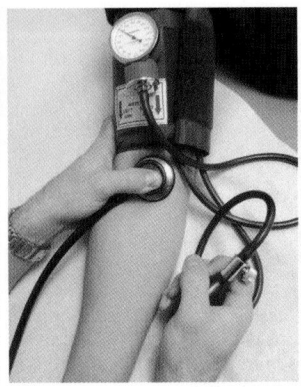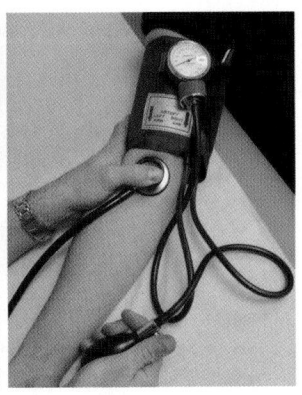

Measurement of blood pressure (Bonewit-West, 2013)

heart-lung, heart-lung machine. See also **cardiopulmonary bypass, oxygenation.**

blood relative, (Informal) a related person who shares some of the same genetic material through a common ancestry.

blood serum. See **serum.**

bloodshot, (Informal) a redness of the conjunctiva or sclera of the eye caused by dilation of blood vessels in the tissues.

blood film, a whole blood monolayer skillfully prepared on a microscopic slide and stained with a polychrome dye such as Wright stain. The film is examined visually or by pattern-recognition instruments to characterize the distribution and morphology of erythrocytes, leukocytes, and platelets. The blood film is part of a complete blood count and is used to support the diagnosis of viral and bacterial infections and hematological and metabolical diseases.

blood sodium test (Na⁺), a plasma or serum test that is a member of an electrolyte panel that also includes measurements of levels of potassium, chloride, and carbon dioxide. An elevated sodium level, hypernatremia, is associated with dehydration or adrenal or renal disorders. A reduced sodium level, hyponatremia, is associated with renal insufficiency, the use of diuretics, and endocrine disorders.

bloodstream, the blood that flows freely through the circulatory system.

blood substitute, a substance used for a replacement or volume expansion for circulating blood. Plasma, human serum albumin, packed red cells, platelets, leukocytes, and concentrates of clotting factors are often administered in place of whole blood transfusions in the treatment of various disorders. Substances that are sometimes used to expand blood volume include dextran, hetastarch, albumin solutions, or plasma protein fraction. Perfluorocarbon emulsions, although potentially toxic, have been used as blood substitutes.

blood sugar, one of a group of closely related substances, such as glucose, fructose, and galactose, that are normal constituents of the blood and are essential for cellular metabolism. Also called **blood glucose.**

blood test, a laboratory test performed on whole blood, plasma, or serum that is used to predict or diagnose disorders and to monitor their treatment. Over 70% of clinical diagnoses rely on blood tests.

blood transfusion [AS, blod + L transfundere, to pour through], the administration of whole blood or a component, such as packed red cells, to replace blood lost through trauma, surgery, or disease. See also **transfusion reaction.**

■ METHOD: Needed equipment is gathered; orders are reviewed; transfusion consent is completed; and blood component is obtained, verified, and inspected per institution protocol. It is extremely important that the blood component to be transfused is compatible with the individual receiving the transfusion and that the correct individual is receiving the transfusion. Once verification of product and individual is confirmed, the blood component is hung using the appropriate tubing and setup and is infused. A piggybacked 0.9% normal saline solution is set up to follow the infusion or to flush the line in the event of a transfusion reaction. Infusion must be completed in under 4 hours to prevent bacterial growth. Individuals must be carefully monitored for a transfusion reaction during infusion. Vital signs should be checked every 5 minutes for at least the first 15 minutes of infusion, and regularly thereafter. In addition, the patient should be monitored for signs and symptoms of transfusion reaction, such as fever; facial flushing; rapid, thready pulse; cold, clammy skin; itching; swelling at infusion site; dizziness; dyspnea; or low back or chest pain. (Stop an infusion immediately at any sign of transfusion reaction.) The blood infusion rate is slow upon initiation of the transfusion to decrease harm if an early transfusion reaction occurs. After infusion, IV tubing is cleared with saline solution and the blood bag is discarded according to institutional policy.

■ OUTCOME CRITERIA: No signs of transfusion reaction. Laboratory values show positive response to administration of blood component.

blood typing, a blood test used to determine the character of the blood of prospective blood donors and of expectant mothers and newborns on the basis of agglutinogens in the erythrocytes. The test detects the presence of ABO antigens as well as the Rh factor. See also **blood group.**

blood urea nitrogen (BUN) [AS, blod + Gk, ouron, urine, nitron, soda, genein, to produce], a measure of the amount of urea in the blood. Urea forms in the liver as the end product of protein metabolism, circulates in the blood, and is excreted through the kidney in urine. The BUN, determined by a blood test, is directly related to the metabolic function of the liver and the excretory function of the kidney. Normal findings (in mg/dL) are 10 to 20 for adults, 5 to 18 for children and infants, 3 to 12 for newborns, and 21 to 40 for cord blood. In the elderly, the BUN may be slightly higher than the normal adult range. A critical value of 100 mg/dL indicates serious impairment of renal function. Also called **urea nitrogen, serum urea nitrogen.** Compare **creatinine.** See also **azotemia.**

blood vessel, any one of the network of muscular tubes that carry blood. Kinds include **artery, arteriole, capillary, vein, venule.**

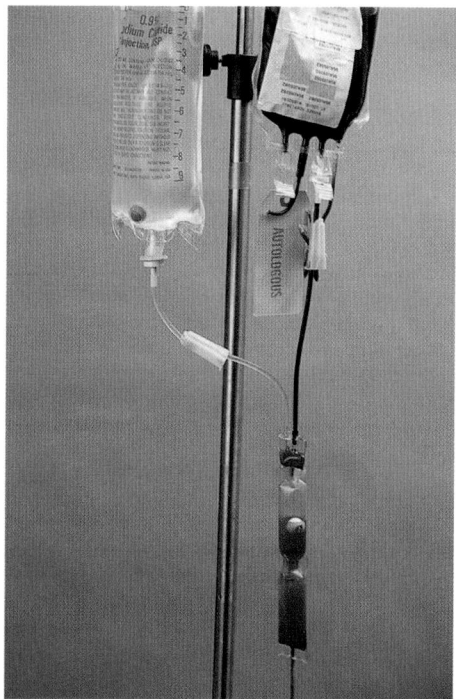

Setup for blood transfusion *(Cooper and Gosnell, 2015)*

blood warming coil, a device constructed of coiled plastic tubing immersed in a warm water bath and used for the warming of blood before massive transfusions, such as those often required for patients who experience extensive bleeding. Administration of cold blood in such transfusions may cause hypothermia and/or shock. The blood warming coil is a prepackaged sterile single-use device. Compare **electric blood warmer.**

bloody show, the passage of blood-tinged mucus late in pregnancy. Bloody show results from the thinning (effacement) of the cervix and the simultaneous extrusion of the mucous plug, with a small amount of bleeding from vessels in the area. Usually considered to appear at the start of the latent phase of labor, although active labor may not follow for many days. See also **effacement.**

bloody sputum [AS, *blod* + L, *sputum,* spittle], blood-tinged material expelled from the respiratory passages. The amount and color of blood in sputum expelled by coughing or clearing the throat may indicate the cause and location of the bleeding. Swallowed blood regurgitated from the stomach most often loses its vital coloring, however, thus eliminating the opportunity to judge the origin.

blooming, an increase in x-ray focal spot size at increased tube current and/or decreased tube potential.

Bloom syndrome [David Bloom, American physician, 1892–1980], a rare genetic disease occurring mainly in Ashkenazi Jews. It is transmitted as an autosomal-recessive trait and is characterized by growth delay, dilated capillaries of the face and arms, sensitivity to sunlight, and an increased risk of malignancy.

blot, **1.** a technique for transferring electrophoretically separated components from a gel onto a nitrocellulose membrane, chemically treated paper, or filter for analysis. It is frequently used to analyze genetic material. **2.** the substrate containing the transferred material. See also **Northern blot test, Southern blot test, Western blot test.**

blotch, *(Informal)* a skin discoloration that may vary in severity from an area of pigmentation to large pustules or blisters.

blow-out fracture, a break in the floor of the orbit caused by a blow that suddenly increases the intraocular pressure.

blowpipe /blō′pīp/ [AS, *blāwan* + *pīpe*], a tube through which a current of air or other gas is forced on a flame to concentrate and intensify the heat.

BLS, abbreviation for **basic life support.**

blue baby [OFr, *blou* + ME, *babe*], *(Informal)* an infant born with cyanosis caused by a congenital heart lesion that results in a right-to-left shunt, most commonly tetralogy of Fallot. Other causative lesions include transposition of the great vessels and incomplete expansion of the lungs (congenital atelectasis). Congenital cyanotic heart lesions are diagnosed by cardiac catheterization, angiography, or echocardiography and are corrected surgically, preferably in early childhood. See also **congenital cardiac anomaly, tetralogy of Fallot, transposition of the great vessels.**

blue cohosh, a perennial herb found in the Midwest and Eastern regions of the United States. Serious toxicities are associated with the use of blue cohosh for menstrual irregularities, and there is insufficient evidence of its efficacy.

Blue Cross, an independent nonprofit U.S. corporation that functions as a health insurance agency, providing protection for an enrolled patient by covering all or part of the person's hospital expenses. Blue Cross programs vary in different communities because of state laws regulating them. See also **Blue Shield.**

blue diaper syndrome [OFr, *blou*; ME, *diapre,* patterned fabric], a defect of tryptophan absorption in which, because of intestinal bacterial action on the tryptophan, the urine contains abnormal indoles, giving it a blue color. Compare **Hartnup's disease.**

blue dome cyst, a spherical dilation of a mammary duct in which bleeding has occurred.

blue dot sign, a tender blue or black spot beneath the skin of the testis or epididymis; a sign of testicular torsion of the appendix testis or, less commonly, appendix epididymis.

blue fever, *(Informal)* Rocky Mountain spotted fever, so named for the dark cyanotic discoloration of the skin after the initial rickettsial infection. The disease is characterized by headache, chills, and fever, as well as a rash. See also **rickettsiosis, Rocky Mountain spotted fever, typhus.**

blue-green algae, *(Nontechnical)* now called **cyanobacteria.**

blue-green algae poisoning. *(Nontechnical)* See **cyanobacteria poisoning.**

blue line, a bluish discoloration sometimes observed along the marginal gingiva in cases of gingivitis. It is a sign of chronic lead or bismuth poisoning.

blue nevus [OFr, *blou* + L, *naevus,* mole], a sharply circumscribed, usually benign, steel blue skin nodule with a diameter between 2 and 7 mm. It is found on the face or upper extremities, grows very slowly, and persists throughout life. The dark color is caused by large, densely packed melanocytes deep in the dermis of the nevus. Nodular blue nevi found on the buttocks or in the sacrococcygeal region occasionally become malignant. Any sudden change in the size of such a lesion demands surgical attention and biopsy. Compare **melanoma.**

blue phlebitis, a severe form of thrombosis of a deep vein, usually the femoral vein. The condition is acute and fulminating and is usually accompanied by vast edema and cyanosis of the limb distal to the occluding thrombus. It can lead to venous gangrene. Also called **phlegmasia cerulea dolens.**

blue rubber bleb nevus [OFr, *blou,* blue; + ME, *rubben,* to scrape; + ME, *bleb,* blob; + L, *naevus,* mole],　a type of congenital nevus, transmitted as an autosomal-dominant trait, characterized by blue hemangiomas with soft elevated nipple-like centers, found on the skin surface, in the GI tract, and sometimes on mucous membranes. It may be accompanied by pain, regional hyperhidrosis, or GI bleeding.

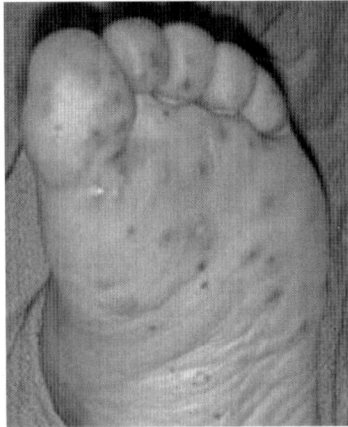

Blue rubber bleb nevus syndrome *(Coran, 2012, 2006)*

blues,　**1.** *(Informal)* a designation for Blue Cross and Blue Shield health insurance systems. **2.** *(Informal)* a common term for a temporary, transient feeling of low mood or mild depression (not yet diagnosed).

Blue Shield,　an independent nonprofit U.S. corporation that offers patient protection for costs of surgery and other medical services. Although Blue Cross and Blue Shield are technically separate organizations, they generally coordinate their functions in providing benefits covering both hospital costs and physician fees. See also **Blue Cross.**

blue spot,　**1.** *(Informal)* one of a number of small grayish blue spots that may appear near the armpits or around the groins of individuals infested with lice, such as in pediculosis corporis and pediculosis pubis. These spots are usually less than 1 cm in diameter and are caused by a substance in the saliva of lice that converts bilirubin to biliverdin. Also called **macula cerulea. 2.** *(Informal)* one of a number of dark blue round or oval spots that may appear as a congenital condition in the sacral regions of certain children less than 4 or 5 years of age. They usually disappear spontaneously as the affected individual matures. Also called **Mongolian spot.**

Blumberg sign /blum′ berg/,　pain on abrupt release of steady pressure (rebound tenderness) over the site of a suspected abdominal lesion, as seen in peritonitis.

blunt dissection [ME, *blunt* + L, *dissecare,* to cut apart],　a dissection performed by separating tissues along natural lines of cleavage without cutting.

blunt-ended DNA,　a segment of DNA in which the ends of both strands are even with each other.

blunting,　a decrease in the intensity of emotional expression from the level one would normally expect as a reaction to a specific situation. It is the opposite of overreaction and may be marked by apathy, minimal response, or indifference.

blush [ME, *blusshen,* to redden],　a brief, diffuse erythema of the face and neck, commonly the result of dilation of superficial small blood vessels in response to heat or sudden emotion.

BLV-HTLV retroviruses,　a genus similar in morphology and replication to the type C retroviruses. Organisms have a

long latency and cause B and T cell leukemia and lymphoma and neurological disease. Included in this genus are human T-lymphotropic viruses 1 and 2.

B lymphocyte.　See **B cell.**

BM,　abbreviation for **bowel movement.**

β₂m,　abbreviation for *beta₂-microglobulin.*

BMA,　abbreviation for **British Medical Association.**

BMD,　abbreviation for **Bureau of Medical Devices.** Now called **National Center for Devices and Radiological Health.**

BMI,　abbreviation for **body mass index.**

B-mode,　brightness modulation in diagnostic ultrasonography. Bright dots on an oscilloscope screen represent echoes, and the intensity of the brightness indicates the strength of the echo. See also **A-mode, M-mode.**

BMR,　abbreviation for **basal metabolic rate.**

BNA,　abbreviation for *Basel Nomina Anatomica.*

BNP,　abbreviation for **brain natriuretic peptide.**

BOA,　abbreviation for **born out of asepsis.**

board,　a service in which an individual in a residential home provides living accommodations to another, usually an older adult. Persons providing this service do not necessarily have to be skilled and/or licensed health care personnel. See also **custodial care, board and care.**

board and care,　nonmedical, community-based residential care for individuals who can care for themselves; meals and supervision are provided. Assistance with activities of daily living may be provided, but not skilled nursing assistance. Most states, provinces, and territories require licensing for board and care homes.　Also called *adult foster care homes.*

board certification,　**1.** the process by which physicians are certified in a given medical specialty or subspecialty. Certification is awarded by the 23-member boards of the American Board of Medical Specialties on completion of accredited training and examinations and fulfillment of individual requirements of the board. **2.** the process by which health care professionals demonstrate competency in their areas of practice through examination, length of supervised practice, and/or educational attainment. National boards and professional associations establish the standards for certification.

board certified,　denoting a health care professional who has completed the certification requirements established by a specialty board and has been certified as a specialist in a particular field of medicine, nursing, occupational therapy, physical therapy, radiological technology, or other health profession.

board eligible,　denoting a health care professional who has completed all of the requirements for certification but has not completed the process.

boarder baby,　**1.** *(Informal)* an infant abandoned to a hospital because the mother is unable to care for him or her. **2.** in some hospitals, any infant still in the nursery after the mother's discharge for any reason (even if only temporarily).

board of health,　an administrative body acting on a municipal, county, state, provincial, or national level. The functions, powers, and responsibilities of boards of health vary with the locales. Each board is generally concerned with the recognition of the health needs of the people and the coordination of projects and resources to meet and identify these needs. Among the tasks of most boards of health are disease prevention, health education, and implementation of laws pertaining to health.

Bobath, Karel and Berta,　Karel Bobath, a psychiatrist and neurophysiologist, and Berta Bobath, a physical therapist, developed the original neurodevelopmental treatment (NDT) theory and intervention techniques to address abnormal tone and movement patterns in persons with neurological conditions such as cerebral palsy and cerebral vascular accident. See also **neurodevelopmental treatment.**

bobbing, the act of moving up and down, usually with a jerking motion.

Bochdalek hernia [Vincent Bochdalek, 1801–1883, Czech anatomist], a hernia through the defect in the left posterior pleuroperitoneal canal of the diaphragm.

Bodansky unit /bōdăn″skē/ [Aaron Bodansky, American biochemist, 1887–1961], the quantity of alkaline phosphatase that liberates 1 mg of phosphate ion from glycerol 2-phosphate in 1 hour at 37° C and under other standardized conditions.

body [AS, *bodig*], **1.** the whole structure of an individual with all the organs. **2.** a cadaver (corpse). **3.** the largest or the main part of any structure, such as the body of the stomach. Also called **corpus, soma.**

body awareness, internal sense of body structures and their relationships to each other.

body burden, **1.** the state of activity of a radioactive chemical in the body at a specified time after administration. **2.** chemicals stored in the body that may be detected by analysis.

body cast [AS, *bodig,* body; ONorse, *kasta*], a molded orthotic device that may extend from the chest to the groin to immobilize the spine.

body cavity, any of the spaces in the human body that contain organs. One major cavity, the thoracic cavity, is subdivided into a pericardial and two pleural cavities.

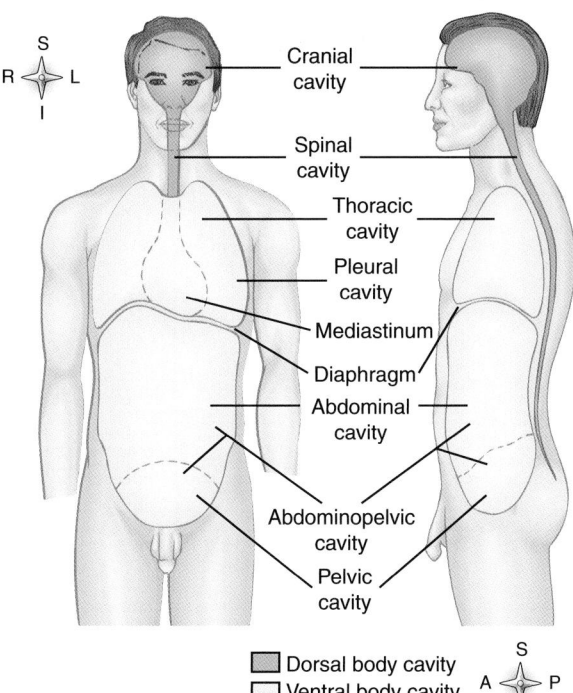

Major body cavities *(Patton and Thibodeau, 2010)*

body composition, the relative proportions of protein, fat, water, and mineral components in the body. It varies among individuals as a result of differences in body density and degree of obesity.

body fluid [AS, *bodig* + L, *fluere,* to flow], fluid contained in the three fluid compartments of the body: the plasma of the circulating blood, the interstitial fluid between the cells, and the cell fluid within the cells. See also **blood plasma, interstitial fluid, extracellular fluid, intracellular fluid.**

body image [AS, *bodig* + L, *imago,* likeness], a person's concept of his or her physical appearance. The mental representation, which may be realistic or unrealistic, is constructed from self-observation, the reactions of others, and a complex interaction of attitudes, emotions, memories, fantasies, and experiences, both conscious and unconscious. A marked inability to conceptualize one's personal body characteristics may be caused by organic brain damage, as in autotopagnosia; by a physical disability, such as the loss of a limb; or by psychological and emotional disturbances, as in anorexia nervosa.

body image agnosia. See **autotopagnosia.**

body jacket, an orthopedic cast that encases the trunk of the body but does not extend over the cervical area; it may be equipped with shoulder straps. The cast is used to help position and immobilize the trunk for the healing of spinal injuries and scoliosis and after spinal surgery. Compare **Risser cast.** See also **thoracolumbosacral orthosis.**

body language [AS, *bodig* + L, *lingua,* tongue], a set of nonverbal signals, including body movements, postures, gestures, spatial positions, facial expressions, and body adornment, that give expression to various physical, mental, and emotional states. See also **kinesics.**

body louse, *Pediculushumanuscorporis.*

body mass index, a formula for determining obesity. It is calculated by dividing a person's weight in kilograms by the square of the person's height in meters. An adult with a BMI of 25 to 29.9 is considered overweight. A BMI of 30 or greater indicates obesity.

International classification of adult underweight, overweight, and obesity according to body mass index (BMI)

	BMI (kg/m²)	
Classification	*Principal cut-off points*	*Additional cut-off points*
Underweight	**<18.50**	**<18.50**
Severe thinness	<16.00	<16.00
Moderate thinness	16.00–16.99	16.00–16.99
Mild thinness	17.00–18.49	17.00–18.49
Normal range	**18.50–24.99**	**18.50–22.99**
		23.00–24.99
Overweight	**≥25.00**	**≥25.00**
Pre-obese	25.00–29.99	25.00–27.49
		27.50–29.99
Obese	**≥30.00**	**≥30.00**
Obese class I	30.00–34.99	30.00–32.49
		32.50–34.99
Obese class II	35.00–39.99	35.00–37.49
		37.50–39.99
Obese class III	≥40.00	≥40.00

Data from World Health Organization, 2015. Retrieved from http://apps.who.int/bmi/index.jsp?introPage=intro_3.html.

body mechanics, **1.** the field of physiology that studies muscular actions and the function of muscles in maintaining body posture. Knowledge gained from such studies is especially important in the prevention of injury during the performance of tasks that require the body to lift and move. **2.** the application of kinesiology to the use of proper body movement when engaged in daily activities. The goal of proper body mechanics is the prevention and/or correction of problems associated with posture and with the performance of tasks that require the body to lift and move.

body movement, motion of all or part of the body, especially at a joint or joints. Kinds include **adduction, abduction, extension, flexion, rotation, circumduction.**

body odor, an unpleasant scent associated with stale perspiration. Freshly secreted perspiration is odorless, but after exposure to the atmosphere and bacterial activity at the surface of the skin, chemical changes occur to produce the odor. Common body odor usually can be eliminated by washing and cleansing. Body odors can also be the result of illness or environmental changes, discharges from a variety of skin conditions, cancer, fungal infections, hemorrhoids, leukemia, and ulcers. See also **bromhidrosis.**

body of Retzius /ret″sē-əs/ [Magnus G. Retzius, Swedish anatomist, 1842–1919], any one of the masses of protoplasm containing pigment granules at the lower end of a hair cell of the organ of Corti in the internal ear.

body plethysmograph [AS, *bodig* + Gk, *plethynein,* to increase, *graphein,* to record], a device for studying alveolar pressures, lung volumes, and airway resistance. The patient sits or reclines in an airtight compartment and breathes normally. The pressure changes in the alveoli are reciprocated in the compartment and are recorded automatically.

body position, attitude or posture of the body. See also **anatomical position, decubitus position, Fowler's position, prone, supine, Trendelenburg position.**

body righting reflex. See **righting reflex.**

body scheme, a piagetian term for a cognitive structure that develops in infants in the sensorimotor period during the first 2 years of life as they learn to differentiate between themselves and the world around them. See also **Piaget, Jean.**

body-scheme disorder. See **autotopagnosia.**

body-section radiography, a radiographic technique in which the image receptor and x-ray tube are synchronously moved in opposite directions to produce a more distinct image of a selected body plane. The process has the effect of blurring adjacent body structures during exposure. Also called **tomography.**

body stalk, the elongated part of the embryo that is connected to the chorion. See also **allantois.**

body surface area, the outer aspects of the human body, a calculation of which is sometimes used in the determination of medication doses. The height and the weight of the patient must be known to determine body surface area. See **surface area.**

body systems model, a conceptual framework in which illness is studied in relation to the functional systems of the body, such as the circulatory, nervous, GI, and reproductive. In this model, care is directed to manipulating the patient's environment in such a way that the signs and symptoms of the health problem are alleviated. As the body systems model traditionally focuses on the disease rather than the patient, current educational programs tend to integrate it with other concepts that allow the practitioner to approach the patient in a more holistic framework. Also called **medical model.**

body temperature, the level of heat produced and sustained by the body processes. Variations and changes in body temperature are major indicators of disease and other abnormalities. Heat is generated within the body

through metabolism of nutrients and lost from the body surface through radiation, convection, and evaporation of perspiration. Heat production and loss are regulated and controlled in the hypothalamus and brainstem. Fever is usually a function of an increase in heat generation; however, some abnormal conditions, such as congestive heart failure, produce slight elevations of body temperature through impairment of the heat loss function. Contributing to the failure to dissipate heat are reduced activity of the heart, lower rate of blood flow to the skin, and the insulating effect of edema. Diseases of the hypothalamus or interference with the other regulatory centers may produce abnormally low body temperatures. Normal adult body temperature, as measured orally, is 98.6° F (37° C). Oral temperatures ranging from 96.5° F to 99° F are consistent with good health, depending on the person's physical activity, the environmental temperature, and that person's usual body temperature. Axillary temperature is usually from 0.5° F to 1° F lower than the oral temperature. Rectal temperatures may be 0.5° F to 1° F higher than oral readings. Body temperature appears to vary 1° F to 2° F throughout the day, with lows recorded early in the morning and peaks between 6 pm and 10 pm. This diurnal variation may increase in range during a fever. Whereas adult body temperature, normal and abnormal, tends to vary within a relatively narrow range, children's temperatures respond more dramatically and rapidly to disease, changes in environmental temperature, and levels of physical activity.

body type, the general physical appearance of an individual human body. Three commonly used terms for body types are ectomorph, describing a thin, fragile physique; endomorph, denoting a round, soft body; and mesomorph, indicating a muscular, athletic body of average size. See also **asthenic habitus, athletic habitus, ectomorph, endomorph, mesomorph, pyknic.**

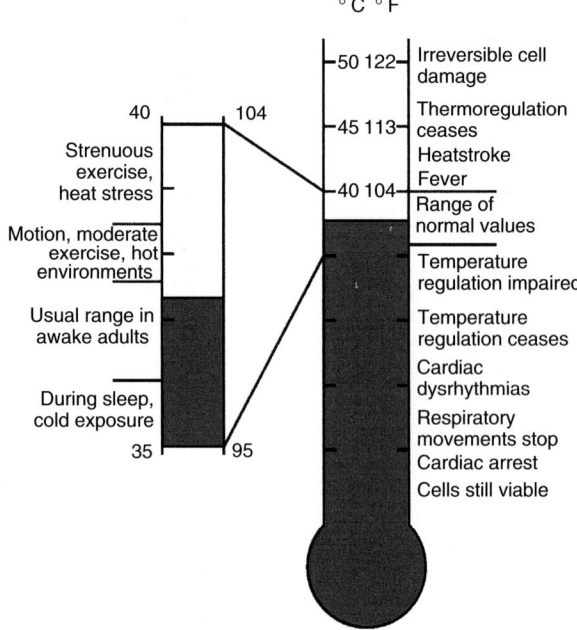

Normal and abnormal body temperatures *(Thibodeau and Patton, 2003)*

body-weight ratio, a relation expressed by dividing the body weight in grams by the height in centimeters.

Boeck's disease, Boeck's sarcoid [C. Boeck, Swedish histologist, 1845–1917]. See **sarcoidosis.**

Boerhaave syndrome /bôr″häv/ [Hermann Boerhaave, Dutch physician, 1668–1738], a condition marked by spontaneous rupture of the esophagus, usually preceded by severe vomiting, leading to mediastinitis and pleural effusion. Clinical manifestations are violent retching or vomiting. Emergency care with surgery and drainage is needed to save the life of the patient.

Bohn nodules [H. Bohn, German physician, 1832–1888], benign palatal cysts of the newborn. Compare **Epstein pearls.**

Bohr effect [Christian Bohr, Danish physiologist, 1855–1911], the effect of CO_2 and H^+ on the affinity of hemoglobin for molecular O_2. Increasing PCO_2 and H^+ decreases oxyhemoglobin saturation, whereas decreasing concentrations have the opposite effect. In humans a decrease of pH from 7.4 to 7.3 at 40 mm Hg PO_2 decreases oxyhemoglobin saturation by 6%. The Bohr effect is particularly significant in the capillaries of working muscles and the myocardium and in maternal and fetal exchange vessels of the placenta.

bohrium (Bh), a chemical element with the atomic number 107. Named after Neils Bohr and first synthesized by a Russian research team in 1976. See **element 107.** Should not be confused with **boron.**

boil [AS, *byle,* sore], a skin abscess. A tender, swollen area that forms around a hair follicle. See also **furuncle.**

boiling point [ME, *boilen,* to make bubbles; L, *pungere,* to prick], **1.** the temperature at which a substance passes from the liquid to the gaseous state at a particular atmospheric pressure. **2.** the temperature at which the vapor pressure of a liquid equals the external pressure. See also **evaporation.**

-bol, combining form designating an anabolic steroid.

bole /bōl/, any of a variety of soft, friable clays of various colors, although usually red from iron oxide. They consist of hydrous silicate of aluminum, are used as pigments, and were once commonly used as absorbents and astringents.

Bolivian hemorrhagic fever /bəliv″ē·ən/, a febrile illness caused by the Machupo virus generally transmitted by contact with or inhalation of aerosolized rodent urine and droppings or by eating food that is contaminated with infected rodent feces. Person-to-person infection has been documented, but it is very rare. After an incubation period of 1 to 2 weeks, the patient experiences chills, fever, weakness, headache, muscle ache, anorexia, nausea, and vomiting. As the disease progresses, hypotension, dehydration, bradycardia, pulmonary edema, and internal hemorrhage may occur. The mortality rate may reach 30%; pulmonary edema is the most common cause of death. There is no specific therapy. Peritoneal dialysis is sometimes performed. Also called **Machupo.** See also *Arenavirus,* **Argentine hemorrhagic fever, Lassa fever.**

bolus /bō″ləs/ [Gk, *bolos,* lump], **1.** a round mass, specifically a mass of solids and semisolids that have been chewed (masticated) and mixed with saliva during the oral preparation to swallow prior to being digested. Also called **alimentary bolus. 2.** a large round preparation of medicinal material for oral ingestion, usually soft and not prepackaged. **3.** a dose of a medication or a contrast material, radioactive isotope, or other pharmaceutic preparation injected rapidly by the intravenous route. **4.** (in radiotherapy) material used to fill in irregular body surfaces to improve dose distribution for hyperthermia or to increase the dose to the skin when high-energy photon beams are used. **5.** a clumping in the stomach of ingested foreign material, often the result of habitual behavior.

bolus dose, an amount of IV medication administered rapidly to decrease the response time or to be used as a loading dose before an infusion, quickly raising the concentration of the medication in blood. See also **bolus.**

bombard /bombärd″/, **1.** to shower a drug or tissue sample with radioactive particles from a nuclear isotope source. **2.** to overload or overstimulate with sound, information, or attention.

Bombay phenotype /bombā″/ [Bombay, India, where first reported], a rare genetic trait in which there is no expression of the A, B, or H antigens on the red blood cells. Bombay phenotypes (genetically hh) lack the H gene, which normally produces the H antigen, a precursor for A and B antigens. Since H is not expressed, A or B cannot be expressed. The serum contains anti-A, anti-B, and anti-H. See also **ABO blood group.**

bombesin /bom′bə·sin/, a neurohormone and pressor substance found in small amounts in brain and intestinal tissue under normal conditions and in increased amounts in certain pulmonary and thyroid tumors. It is a potent mitogen (stimulator of mitosis) and its effects on gastrin and other hormones are attributed to increased cell numbers.

bond, **1.** a strong coulombic force between atoms in a substance due to attraction of ions of opposite charge for each other or of the nuclei for shared electrons. See also **coulomb, Coulomb's law. 2.** a strong, meaningful interpersonal relationship between people and/or their pets, work, or other things they care deeply about. **3.** to join together securely with an adhesive substance.

bonding [ME, *band,* to bind], **1.** (in dentistry) a technique of joining orthodontic brackets or other attachments directly to the enamel surface of a tooth, using orthodontic adhesives. **2.** The restoration of anterior teeth with a tooth-colored composite resin material. **3.** the reciprocal attachment process that occurs between an infant and the parents, especially the mother. Bonding is significant in the formation of affectionate ties that later influence both the physical and psychological development of the child. It is usually initiated immediately after birth by placing the nude infant on the mother's abdomen so that both the parent and the child can see and touch one another and begin to interact. The newborn is in an alert, reactive state for about 30 minutes to 1 hour after birth and displays such behaviors as crying, sucking, clinging, grasping, and following with the eyes, which in turn stimulate the expression of parenting instincts. Also called **maternal-child attachment.** See also **maternal deprivation syndrome, maternal-infant bonding.**

bond specificity, the nature of enzyme action that causes the disruption of only certain bonds between atoms.

bone [AS, *ban*], **1.** the dense, hard, and somewhat flexible connective tissue constituting the framework of the human skeleton. It is composed of compact osseous tissue surrounding spongy cancellous tissue permeated by many blood vessels and nerves and enclosed in membranous periosteum. **2.** any single element of the skeleton, such as a rib, the sternum, or the femur. Also called **os.** See also **connective tissue.**

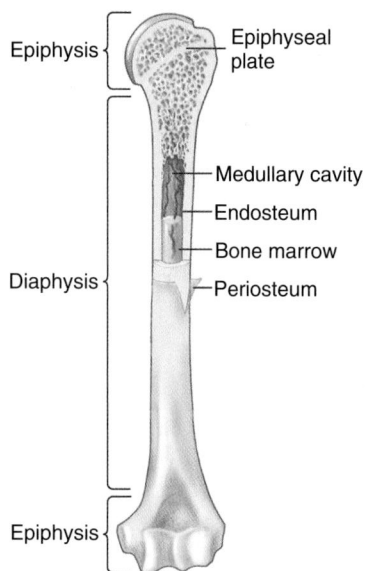

Structure of a long bone *(Muscolino, 2011)*

Epiphysis

Epiphyseal plate

Medullary cavity

Endosteum

Bone marrow

Periosteum

Diaphysis

Epiphysis

bone age [AS, *ban* + L, *aetas*], the stage of development or decline of the skeleton or its segments, as seen in radiographic examination, when compared with x-ray views of the bone structures of other individuals of the same chronological age (usually seen on x-rays of the hand and wrist).

bone-anchored hearing aid, a hearing aid that allows direct bone conduction of sound to the cochlea by means of a sound-processing device attached to an osseointegrated titanium fixture implanted posterior to the ear.

bone cancer [AS, *ban* + Gk, *karkinos,* crab], a skeletal malignancy occurring as a sarcoma or in an area of rapid growth or as metastasis from cancer elsewhere in the body. Primary bone tumors are rare; the incidence peaks during adolescence, decreases, and then rises slowly after 35 years of age. In adults, bone cancer is linked to exposure to ionizing radiation. Paget's disease, hyperparathyroidism, chronic osteomyelitis, old bone infarcts, and fracture callosities increase the risk of many bone tumors. Most osseous malignancies are metastatic lesions found most often in the spine or pelvis and less often in sites away from the trunk. These are referred to as cancers of the primary site and not bone cancer. See also **chondrosarcoma, Ewing's sarcoma, fibrosarcoma, multiple myeloma, osteosarcoma.**
■ OBSERVATIONS: Bone cancers progress rapidly but are often difficult to detect. Alkaline phosphatase levels are elevated in osteoblastic tumors, and serum calcium and urinary calcium levels are increased in highly destructive lesions. X-ray films, radioisotopic scanning, arteriography, and biopsy are diagnostic.
■ INTERVENTIONS: Surgical treatment consists of local resection of slow-growing tumors or amputation, including the joint above the tumor, if the lesion is aggressive. Radiotherapy may be given preoperatively or as the primary form of treatment.
■ PATIENT CARE CONSIDERATIONS: As with any malignancy a coordinated team approach is imperative to provide the best quality of life possible. Nursing care will often focus on the management of the medication regimen and the control of pain. There is evidence that maintaining a healthy weight and being physically active reduces the risk of developing other cancers and complications. Physical and occupational

therapists should determine a safe exercise program based on the patient's condition. Prosthetic and orthotic devices are often prescribed.

bone cell [AS, *ban* + L, *cella,* storeroom], an osteocyte, osteoblast, or osteoclast; a cell with myriad spidery processes embedded in the matrix of bone. See also **osteoblast.**

bone-cutting forceps, a type of forceps that has long handles, single or double joints, and heavy blades for cutting bone.

bone cyst [AS, *ban* + Gk, *kytis,* cyst], **1.** a dilation in the wall of a blood vessel in a bone, usually eccentrically placed. **2.** a sac in bone tissue in the parathyroid disorder osteitis fibrosa.

bone densitometry, any of several methods of determining bone mass by measuring radiation absorption by the skeleton. Common techniques include single-photon absorptiometry (SPA) of the forearm and heel, dual-photon absorptiometry (DPA) and dual-energy x-ray absorptiometry (DXA) of the spine and hip, quantitative computed tomography (QCT) of the spine and forearm, radiographic absorptiometry (RA) of the hand, and quantitative ultrasound (QU).

bone graft, the transplantation of a piece of bone from one part of the body to another to repair a skeletal defect.

bone lamella [AS, *ban,* bone, *lamella,* plate], a thin plate of bone matrix; a basic structural unit of mature bone.

bone loss. See **bone recession.**

bone marrow [AS, *ban* + ME, *marowe*], the soft, organic, spongelike material in the cavities of bones; also called medulla ossium. It is a network of blood vessels and special connective tissue fibers that hold together a composite of fat- and blood-producing cells. Its chief function is to manufacture erythrocytes, leukocytes, and platelets. These blood cells normally do not enter the bloodstream until they are fully developed, so the marrow contains cells in all stages of growth. If the body's demand for leukocytes is increased because of infection, the marrow responds immediately by increasing production. The same is true if more erythrocytes are necessary, as in hemorrhage or anemia. Red marrow is found in many bones of infants and children and in the spongy (cancellous) bone of the proximal epiphyses of the humerus and femur and the sternum, ribs, and vertebral bodies of adults. Fatty yellow marrow is found in the medullary cavity of most adult long bones.

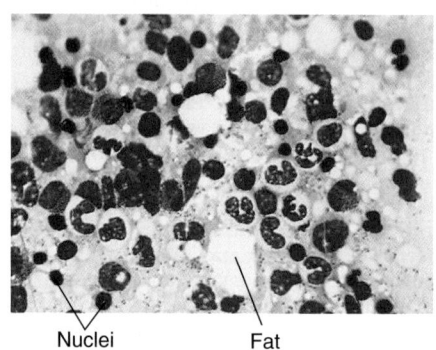

Nuclei   Fat

Bone marrow *(© Ed Reschke; used with permission)*

bone marrow aspiration, removal of bone marrow fluid via a needle to diagnose a number of conditions, including leukemia, lymphoma, and multiple myeloma. Bone marrow aspiration is also used for bone marrow transplantation. See also **bone marrow transplantation.**

bone marrow biopsy, a tissue section taken from the hematopoietic portion of iliac crest or sternal bone marrow using a coring device. A stained bone marrow biopsy is examined microscopically to characterize bone marrow histology (architecture). Histology supports the diagnosis of anemia, polycythemia, leukemia, myeloma, thrombocytopenia, thrombocytosis, tumor infiltrates, or inadequate or excessive iron stores. The bone marrow biopsy is employed in combination with a bone marrow aspirate, flow cytometry, and molecular analysis for the diagnosis and monitoring of hematological disorders.

bone marrow failure, failure of the hematopoietic function of the bone marrow. See also **hematopoietic system.**

bone marrow infusion, *(Nontechnical)* a method of injecting a fluid substance through an aspiration needle directly into the marrow cavity of a long bone when intravenous access is not possible. The substance is absorbed into the general circulation almost immediately. Also called **intraosseous infusion.**

bone marrow reserve, a storage pool of mature neutrophils in the bone marrow that can be released as necessary.

bone marrow suppression, ineffective bone marrow activity, resulting in reduction in the number of platelets, red cells, and white cells, such as in aplastic anemia. Also called **myelosuppression.**

bone marrow transplantation, the transplantation of bone marrow from a healthy donor to stimulate production of normal blood cells. The marrow may be autologous (from a previously harvested and stored self-donation) or allogeneic (from a living related donor or a living unrelated donor). The bone marrow is removed from the donor by aspiration and infused intravenously into the recipient. Used to treat malignancies, such as leukemia, lymphoma, myeloma, and selected solid tumors; and nonmalignant conditions, such as aplastic anemia, immunological deficiencies, and inborn errors of metabolism. Transplantation is usually preceded by chemotherapy and total body radiation of the recipient.

bone plate [AS, *ban,* bone; OFr, *plate*], a metal plate used to reconstruct a bone that has been fractured. The plate is designed to hold bone fragments in apposition.

bone recession [AS, *ban* + L, *recedere,* to recede], (in dentistry) apical progression of the level of the alveolar crest, resulting in decreased bone support for the teeth. The condition, which may be horizontal or vertical, is associated with inflammatory periodontal disease. Also called **bone resorption, bone loss.**

bone resorption, the healing and remodeling process of bone. See also **bone recession.**

bone scan, the injection of a radioactive substance to enable visualization of a bone via the image produced by a nuclear medicine camera's capture of the emission of radioactive particles.

bone tissue [AS, *ban* + OFr, *tissu*], a hard form of connective tissue composed of osteocytes and a calcified collagenous intercellular substance arranged in thin plates. Also called **bony tissue.** See also **connective tissue.**

bone turnover biochemical markers test, a serum, plasma, or urine test to monitor the treatment of osteoporosis, hyperparathyroidism, bone tumors, or Paget disease. Examples of markers include N-telopeptide (NTx), C-telopeptide (CTx), deoxypyridinoline (DPD), tartrate-resistant acid phosphatase (TRAP), bone-specific alkaline phosphatase, and osteocalcin. Also called *bone resorption markers test, bone formation markers test.*

bone x-ray, radiographic studies to detect abnormalities of the bones or joints.

Bonine, an antiemetic. Brand name for **meclizine hydrochloride.**

Bonnevie-Ullrich syndrome. See **Turner syndrome.**

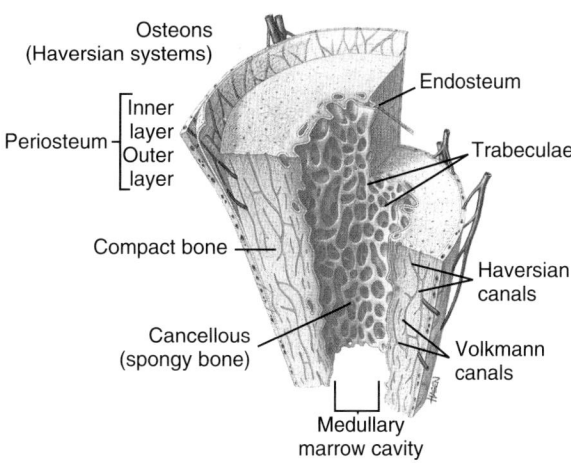

Bone tissue *(Thibodeau and Patton, 2007)*

Bonnie Pruden myotherapy, a relaxation technique that uses the application of touch to certain points and spots in, on, and near the muscles of the body, which creates responses in associated areas.

Bonwill triangle [William G.A. Bonwill, American dentist, 1833–1899], an equilateral triangle formed by lines from the contact points of the lower central incisors (or the median line of the residual ridge of the mandible) to the mandibular condyle on each side and from one condyle to the other.

bony labyrinth, a series of bony cavities in the inner ear. See **membranous labyrinth.**

bony landmark [AS, *ban* + AS, *land, mearc*], any distinct groove or prominence on a bone that serves as a guide to the location of other body structures. An example is the posterior superior iliac crest.

bony palate. See **hard palate.**

bony thorax [AS, *ban* + Gk, *thorax,* chest], the skeletal part of the chest, including the thoracic vertebrae, ribs, and sternum.

bony tissue. See **bone tissue.**

BOO, abbreviation for **bladder outlet obstruction.**

book retinoscopy, a measure of accommodation in which retinoscopy is performed while the patient focuses on reading a book. It is commonly used with children.

booster injection, the administration of an additional dose of antigen within a defined period of time, such as a vaccine or toxoid, usually in a smaller amount than the original immunization. It is given to maintain the immune response at an appropriate level.

booster phenomenon /bōōs′ter/, on a tuberculin test, an initial false-negative result caused by a diminished response that becomes positive on subsequent testing.

booster response, response of the immune system to a subsequent encounter with the same antigen. This includes antibody production and/or cell-mediated immunity. See **secondary antibody response, immunological memory.**

boot, **1.** a shoelike prosthetic device for holding a leg or arm during treatment. **2.** a basketweave bandage that covers the foot and lower leg. **3.** an airtight device in which the arm or leg can be inserted and the air pumped out, creating a partial vacuum to divert blood flow from the surrounding area.

Boothby-Lovelace-Bulbulian (BLB) mask, an apparatus for the administration of oxygen consisting of a mask fitted with an inspiratory-expiratory valve and a rebreathing bag.

boracic acid. See **boric acid.**

borage, an annual herb found in North America and Europe. Its safety when used in amounts ingested for medicinal purpose has not been established.

borage oil, the oil extracted from the seeds of borage (*Borago officinalis*). It is an herbal supplement used for the treatment of neurodermatitis. It is also a food supplement.

borate /bôr″āt/, any salt of boric acid. Borate salts and boric acid, although formerly used as mild antiseptic irrigant solutions, especially for ophthalmic conditions, are highly poisonous when taken internally or absorbed through a cut, abrasion, or other wound in the skin. Because of the potential for fatal poisoning, such solutions are rarely used now. See also **boric acid.**

borborygmos /bôr″bərig″məs/ *pl.* borborygmi [Gk, *borborygmos*, bowel rumbling], an audible abdominal sound produced by hyperactive intestinal peristalsis. Borborygmi are audible abdominal sounds produced by hyperactive intestinal peristalsis. Borborygmi are very loud rumbling, gurgling, and tinkling noises heard in auscultation, often without a stethoscope. The increased intestinal activity noted at times in cases of gastroenteritis and diarrhea result in borborygmi that do not have the intensity or the episodic character of "normal borborygmi." Borborygmi that are high-pitched and accompanied by vomiting, distension, and intestinal cramps suggest a mechanical obstruction of the small intestine and often precede complete bowel obstruction.

border [OFr, *bordure*], an edge or boundary of a body structure.

borderline [OFr, *bordure* + L, *linea*], pertaining to a state of health in which the patient has some of the signs and symptoms of a disease but not enough to justify a definite diagnosis.

borderline personality [OFr, *bordure* + L, *linea* + *personalis*], a personality disorder in which there are impairments in personality. The impairments can refer to self or interpersonal relationships. There is also the presence of pathological personality traits related to either empathy or intimacy.

Bordetella /bôr″ditel″ə/ [Jules J.B.V. Bordet, Belgian bacteriologist, 1870–1961], a genus of gram-negative coccobacilli, some species of which are pathogens of the respiratory tract of humans, including *Bordetella bronchiseptica*; *B. parapertussis*, which causes mild pharyngitis; and *B. pertussis*, the causative agent of pertussis. See also **parapertussis, pertussis.**

boric acid /bôr″ik/, **1.** a white odorless powder or crystalline substance used as a buffer (H_3BO_3). The powder is highly poisonous when taken internally. Also called **boracic acid, orthoboric acid. 2.** (in ophthalmology) an eyewash solution with weak antiseptic properties used to cleanse or irrigate the eyes.

boric acid poisoning, an adverse reaction to the ingestion or absorption through the skin of boric acid, a mild but potentially lethal antiseptic. Symptoms include nausea, vomiting, diarrhea, rash, convulsions, and shock. A poison control center should be contacted immediately if boric acid poisoning is suspected.

Bornholm disease [named for the Danish island of Bornholm], formerly called **epidemic pleurodynia.** Now called **epidemic myalgia.**

born out of asepsis (BOA), (in a hospital) denoting a newborn who was not delivered in the usual place in an obstetric unit. Depending on the policy of the institution, a BOA-designated infant may have been born on the way to the hospital, in the hospital, on the way to the delivery suite, or in a labor room.

■ OBSERVATIONS: Initial assessment in the admitting unit includes evaluation of respiration, quality of cry, skin color, apical pulse rate, muscle tone, reflexes, temperature, condition of umbilical cord or cord stump, ability to suck, presence of meconium, congenital defect, skin eruption, or signs of sepsis, including jaundice, anorexia, vomiting, diarrhea, irritability or lethargy, high-pitched cry, and hypothermia or hyperthermia.

■ INTERVENTIONS: The usual steps in caring for a newborn are performed. Head and chest circumferences are measured, weight is taken, and the baby is placed in a warmer until the axillary temperature is 36.5° C. Vitamin K and silver nitrate are usually given. In many hospitals, BOA infants are placed in a special nursery and isolated from other infants to prevent contagion if they are infected.

■ PATIENT CARE CONSIDERATIONS: Daily care for the BOA infant is the same as that given to other newborns, but, in addition, the BOA baby is closely observed for signs of sepsis. The parents are involved in the care of the infant as soon as possible, and the usual instructions are given at discharge for home care of the baby.

boron (B) /bôr″on/, a nonmetallic element whose atomic number is 5; its atomic mass is 10.81. Elemental boron occurs in the form of dark crystals and as a greenish yellow amorphous mass. Certain concentrations of this element are toxic to plant and animal life, but plants need traces of boron for normal growth. It is the characteristic element of boric acid, which is used chiefly as a dusting powder and ointment for minor skin disorders. Boric acid in solution was formerly extensively used as an antiinfective and eyewash, but the high incidence of toxic reactions and fatalities associated with these preparations has greatly reduced their use.

Borrelia /bərel″ē·ə/ [Amédée Borrel, French bacteriologist, 1867–1936], a genus of coarse, unevenly coiled helical spirochetes, several species of which cause tick-borne and louse-borne diseases. Many animals serve as reservoirs and hosts for *Borrelia*. The spirochete may be identified by microscopic examination of a smear of blood stained with Wright stain; it is also easily inoculated onto culture media for bacterial culture and identification.

Borrelia burgdorferi /burg′dôrfer″ī/, the causative agent in Lyme disease. The organism is transmitted to humans by tick vectors, primarily *Ixodes dammini*. The disease is most common in the Northeastern, North-Central, and Northwestern regions of the United States and Canada.

bortezomib, a miscellaneous antineoplastic.

■ INDICATIONS: This drug is used to treat multiple myeloma when at least two other treatments have failed.

■ CONTRAINDICATIONS: Pregnancy and known hypersensitivity to this drug, boron, or mannitol prohibit its use.

■ ADVERSE EFFECTS: Adverse effects of this drug include hypotension, edema, anemia, fatigue, malaise, weakness, arthralgia, bone pain, muscle cramps, myalgia, back pain, abdominal pain, constipation, diarrhea, dyspepsia, nausea, vomiting, anorexia, anxiety, insomnia, dizziness, headache, peripheral neuropathy, rigors, paresthesia, cough, pneumonia, dyspnea, upper respiratory infection, dehydration, weight loss, herpes zoster, rash, pruritus, and blurred vision. Life-threatening side effects include neutropenia and thrombocytopenia.

bosentan, an endothelial receptor antagonist used to treat pulmonary arterial hypertension.

boss [ME, *boce*], a swelling, eminence, or protuberance on an organ, such as a tumor or overgrowth that is raised and stands out on a bone surface or a tooth. For example, on the forehead it is often a sign of rickets.

Boston exanthema [Boston; Gk, *ex*, out, *anthema*, blossoming], an epidemic disease characterized by scattered, pale red maculopapules on the face, chest, and back, occasionally accompanied by small ulcerations on the tonsils and soft palate. There is little or no adenopathy, and the rash disappears spontaneously in 2 or 3 weeks. It is caused by echovirus 16 and requires no treatment. Compare **herpangina.**

Botox, a neurotoxin produced by the bacterium *Clostridium botulinum.* Current uses include cosmetic procedures as it paralyzes the underlying muscles, reducing wrinkling. It may also be used to treat excessive sweating, migraine headaches, selected muscular disorders, and some bladder and bowel disorders.

Botryoid odontogenic cyst, a multicystic and multilocular odontogenic cyst closely related to the lateral periodontal cyst. See also **lateral periodontal cyst.**

bottle feeding [OFr, *bouteille* + AS, *faeden*], feeding an infant or young child from a bottle with a rubber nipple on the end as a substitute for or supplement to breastfeeding.

bottle mouth caries. See **early childhood caries.**

botulinum toxin /boch′əlī″nəm/ [L, *botulus,* sausage; Gk, *toxikon,* poison], any of a group of potent bacterial toxins produced by different strains of *Clostridium botulinum.* It may be used therapeutically for blepharospasm or cosmetically to relax facial wrinkles. It is also used in the management of overactive bladder and migraine headaches. The strains are sometimes identified by letters of the alphabet, such as A, B, or C. Also called **Botox,** *botulinus toxin.*

botulism /boch′əliz′əm/ [L, *botulus,* sausage], an often fatal form of food poisoning caused by an endotoxin produced by the bacillus *Clostridium botulinum.* In the United States, approximately 25% of cases are food-borne botulism, 72% are infant botulism, and the rest are wound botulism. In food-borne botulism, the toxin is ingested in food contaminated by *C. botulinum,* although it is not necessary for the live bacillus to be present if the toxin has been produced. In infant botulism, which is associated with eating unpasteurized honey, infants may consume pores that produce the toxin. In wound botulism, the toxin may be introduced into the human body through a wound contaminated by the organism. Botulism differs from most other types of food poisoning in that it develops without gastric distress and occurs 18 hours up to 1 week after the contaminated food has been ingested. Botulism is characterized by lassitude, fatigue, and visual disturbances, such as double vision, difficulty in focusing the eyes, and loss of ability of the pupil to accommodate to light. Muscles may become weak, and dysphagia often develops. Nausea and vomiting occur in fewer than half the cases. Affected infants are lethargic, feed poorly, are constipated, and have a weak cry and poor muscle tone. Hospitalization is required, and antitoxins are administered. Sedatives are given, mainly to relieve anxiety. Approximately 8% of the cases of botulism are fatal, usually as a result of delayed diagnosis and respiratory complications. Most botulism occurs after eating improperly canned or cooked foods. Reporting botulism to public health authorities is mandatory. See also *Clostridium.*

■ OBSERVATIONS: Symptoms usually appear 18 to 36 hours after ingestion of a contaminated food substance. Severity of symptoms is related to the quantity of the botulinum toxin that was ingested and include dry mouth, diplopia, loss of pupillary light reflex; nausea, vomiting, cramps, and diarrhea. Dysphagia, dysarthria, and progressive descending muscular paralysis may follow. Botulism is fatal in about 8% of cases, usually because of respiratory paralysis or circulatory failure. Serum may be positive for botulinal toxins, and cultures may be taken of stomach contents, feces, or suspected food to confirm the causative organism.

■ INTERVENTIONS: The trivalent botulinal antitoxin is administered as soon as possible after onset and clinical diagnosis.

The GI tract is purged using laxatives, gastric lavage, and high colonic enemas to dilute and decrease absorption of the toxin. Tracheostomy and mechanical ventilation may be instituted if necessary. Care is supportive with a long recovery period and the need for rehabilitation to regain muscle tone, strength, and function.

■ PATIENT CARE CONSIDERATIONS: Health care providers should be alert to signs and symptoms of serum sickness that frequently occur after the administration of the antitoxin, including fever, arthralgia, lymphadenopathy, skin eruption, pain, pruritus, and erythematous swelling at the injection site. Individuals may also report joint and muscle aches, chest pain, and difficulty breathing. The care of the health care team for acute illness is largely supportive and involves airway management, prevention of aspiration, fluid and electrolyte management, pain management, nutrition management, prevention of skin breakdown and contractures during paralysis, minimization of stimuli, precise communication because of altered vision and loss of speech, and allaying anxiety about paralysis and treatment. Primary prevention targets education of consumers in the safe handling, storage, and preparation of food. Health professionals should also be prepared for an effective response should botulinum toxin be used in a bioterrorism event. This includes familiarization with institution policies, procedures, and protocols and maintenance of current knowledge regarding bioterrorism threats.

bouba, **1.** See **yaws. 2.** the association of sounds with certain shapes.

Bouchard node /bŌŌshär″/ [Charles J. Bouchard, French physician, 1837–1915], an abnormal cartilaginous or bony enlargement of a proximal interphalangeal joint of a finger, usually occurring in diseases of the joints, such as rheumatoid arthritis. Compare **Heberden node.**

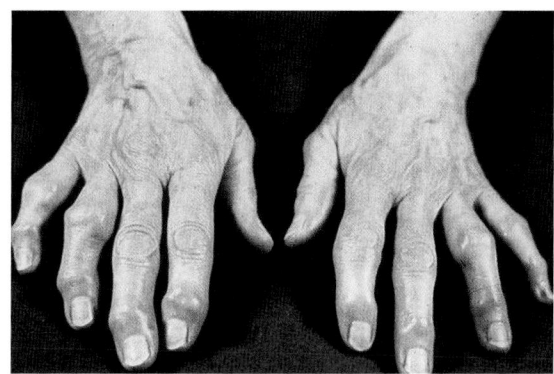

Bouchard nodes *(Monahan, 2007)*

bougie /bŌŌ″zhē, bŌŌzhē″/ [Fr, candle], a thin cylindric instrument made of rubber, waxed silk, or other flexible material for insertion into canals of the body in order to dilate, examine, or measure them.

-boulia. See **-bulia, -boulia.**

boundary /boun″dərē/, **1.** (in psychology) an ability to separate the self from others, setting personal boundaries that help maintain one's self-image and self-concept. **2.** in social psychology, the ability to separate self from others in interpersonal relationships in a way in which all parties share but are uniquely individual and respectful. **3.** a professional boundary in which a professional is able to maintain a professional self that is separate from the client, patient, or the patient's significant others.

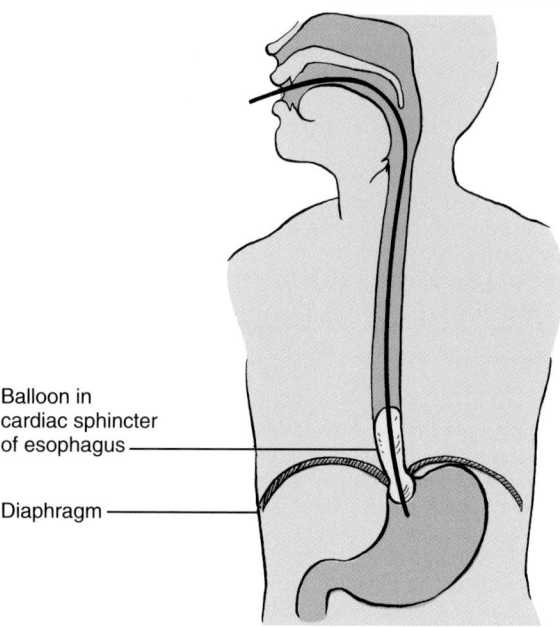

Balloon in
cardiac sphincter
of esophagus

Diaphragm

Passage of a bougie *(Black and Hawks, 2005)*

boundary lubrication, a coating of a thin layer of molecules on each weight-bearing surface of a joint to facilitate a sliding action by the opposing bone surfaces.

boundary maintenance mechanisms, (in psychology) behavior and practices that exclude members of some groups from the customs and values of another group.

bound carbon dioxide, carbon dioxide that is transported in the bloodstream as part of a sodium bicarbonate molecule, as distinguished from dissolved carbon dioxide or bicarbonate ion.

bounding pulse [OFr, *bondir,* to leap; L, *pulsare,* to beat], a pulse that feels full and springlike on palpation as a result of an increased thrust of cardiac contraction or an increased volume of circulating blood within the elastic structures of the vascular system.

bound water, water in the tissue of the body bound to macromolecules or organelles.

bouquet fever, *(Obsolete)* now called **dengue fever.**

Bourdon regulator, a commonly used adjustable device with an attached pressure gauge for controlling the flow of oxygen or other gases from cylinders in medical applications.

Bourneville disease, now called **tuberous sclerosis.** Should not be confused with **tuberculosis.**

bouton /boōtôN″, boō″ton/ [Fr, button], **1.** a button, pustule, or knoblike swelling, such as the expanded end of an axon at a synapse (terminaux) that comes into contact with cell bodies of other neurons. **2.** a lesion associated with cutaneous leishmaniasis. **3.** a small abscess of the intestinal mucosa in amebic dysentery.

boutonneuse fever /boō″tənoōz′/ [Fr, *bouton,* button; L, *febris*], a febrile disease of the Mediterranean area, the Crimea, Africa, and India caused by infection with *Rickettsia conorii,* transmitted to humans through the bite of a tick. The onset of the disease is characterized by a lesion called a *tache noire,* or black spot, at the site of the infection; fever lasting from a few days to 2 weeks; and a papular erythematous rash that spreads over the body to include the skin of the palms and soles. The disease is usually a mild form of rickettsial disease, but severe complications occur in approximately 10% of patients. Usually, mild forms only are observed in children. Treatment usually involves administration of antibiotics. There is no prophylactic medication available, and prevention depends primarily on avoiding ticks. See also **rickettsiosis, Rocky Mountain spotted fever.**

boutonnière deformity /boō′tônyer″/ [Fr, buttonhole], an abnormality of a finger marked by fixed flexion of the proximal interphalangeal joint and hyperextension of the distal interphalangeal joint. The central slip of the digit extensor tendon mechanism attenuates or ruptures over the PIP joint, and the associated lateral bands slip below the axis of the joint, thus pulling the PIP into a flexed posture. The condition occurs in rheumatoid arthritis and can occur following trauma to a finger.

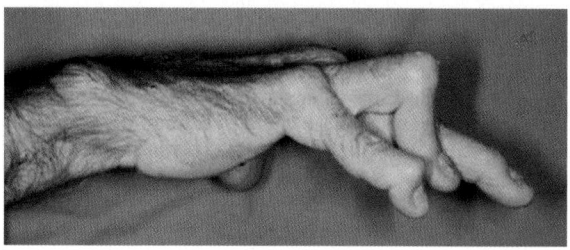

Boutonnière deformity *(Townsend et al, 2012)*

bovine spongiform encephalopathy (BSE), an infection of cattle characterized by degenerative, clumsy, apprehensive behavior, and death. The BSE brain tissue is perforated and spongy in appearance. The disease was first observed in cattle by veterinarians in 1883. It has been associated with other spongiform encephalopathies such as scrapie in sheep and goats and Creutzfeldt-Jakob disease (CJD) in humans. In European "mad cow" disease, it is believed the disease was transmitted to cattle through livestock feed that contained remains of scrapie-infected sheep. The disease was then transmitted to humans who ate BSE-infected beef.

bovine tuberculosis /bō″vīn/ [L, *bos,* ox, *tuber,* swelling; Gk, *osis,* condition], a form of tuberculosis caused by *Mycobacterium tuberculosis* that primarily affects cattle but is occasionally found in other mammals and, rarely, humans. Mastitis and pulmonary symptoms can occur.

Bowditch effect [H.P. Bowditch, American physiologist, 1840–1911]. See **all-or-none law.**

bowel. See **intestine.**

bowel bypass syndrome, a series of adverse effects that may follow bowel bypass surgery and include chills, fever, joint pain, and skin inflammation on the arms, legs, and thorax.

bowel continence, the ability to control the discharge of fecal material. In children, bowel control is largely a maturational process. A variety of neurological problems can interfere with bowel continence in the adult. Achieving bowel continence is a priority in rehabilitation settings. See also **bowel training, toilet training.**

bowel elimination, the discharge of fecal material from the intestinal tract.

bowel incontinence, an inability to control the discharge of fecal material. This can range from leaking a small amount of stool and flatus to a total inability to anticipate defecation, with resultant soiling. See **incontinence.** See also **encopresis.**

bowel irrigation, the installation of fluids into the lower gastrointestinal tract for the purpose of lavage.

bowel management, a regimen for individuals who are unable to anticipate or control the discharge of fecal material. It is an important component of the care of a patient with a spinal cord injury. See also **toilet training.**

bowel movement, the evacuation of fecal material from the intestinal tract.

bowel resection, an excision of a diseased or injured section of the small or large intestine through a laparoscope or an abdominal incision to treat obstruction, inflammatory bowel disease, cancer, ruptured diverticulum, ischemia, or traumatic injury. After excision, the bowel is reanastomosed.

bowel training [OFr, *boel*], a method of establishing regular evacuation by reflex conditioning used in the treatment of fecal incontinence, impaction, chronic diarrhea, and autonomic hyperreflexia. In patients with autonomic hyperreflexia, distension of the rectum and bladder causes paroxysmal hypertension, restlessness, chills, diaphoresis, headache, elevated temperature, and bradycardia.

■ METHOD: The patient's previous bowel habits are assessed, and the necessity of developing a program to induce an evacuation at the same time each day or every other day is explained. Exercises to strengthen abdominal muscles, such as pushing up, bearing down, and contracting the musculature, are demonstrated. The patient is instructed to recognize and respond promptly to signals indicating a full bowel and to develop cues to stimulate the urge to defecate, such as drinking coffee or massaging the abdomen. Fluids to 3000 mL daily are encouraged, exercise is increased as able, and the importance of eating well-balanced meals that include bulk and roughage is discussed. Depending on the patient and the problem, the training program may involve drinking warm fluid, ensuring privacy, and inserting a lubricated glycerin suppository before the set time. The possibility that emotional stress or illness may cause accidental incontinence after the program has been established is discussed. Many clients require weeks or months of training to achieve success.

■ INTERVENTIONS: It is important that patients fully participate in the planning of the program as the activities become a part of the patient's daily routine. As the program is implemented, revisions may be necessary. Regular exercise and physical activity, when possible, are interventions that contribute to the success of the program.

■ OUTCOME CRITERIA: Reflex conditioning is often an effective method of developing regular bowel habits for incontinent patients, especially those who are highly motivated and are given good instruction and understanding support.

bowel urgency, the sudden, almost uncontrollable need to defecate.

bowenoid papulosis. See **Bowen's disease.**

Bowen disease [John T. Bowen, American dermatologist, 1857–1941], a form of intraepidermal carcinoma (squamous cell). It is characterized by red-brown scaly or crusted lesions that resemble a patch of psoriasis or dermatitis. Treatment includes curettage and electrodesiccation. A corresponding lesion found on the glans penis is called erythroplasia of Queyrat. Also called *Bowen precancerous dermatosis.*

Bowen technique, a system of gentle but powerful soft tissue mobilizations using the thumbs and fingers over muscles, tendons, nerves, and fascia to restore the self-healing mechanism of the body. This technique has been used for

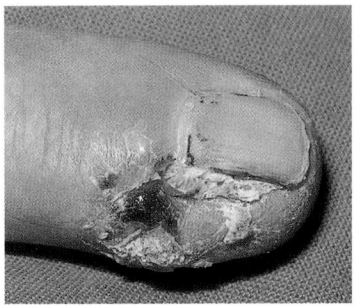

Bowen disease *(White and Cox, 2006)*

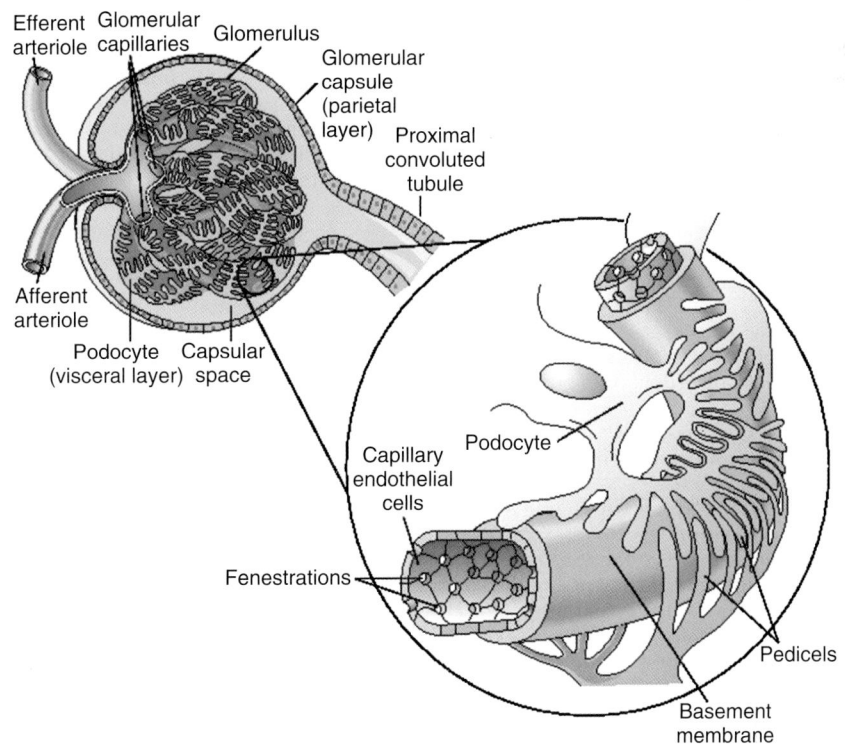

Bowman's capsule *(Copstead-Kirkhorn and Banasik, 2014)*

conditions affecting the musculoskeletal system, including back, neck, hip, and shoulder pain.

bowleg, *(Informal)* See **genu varum.**

Bowman's capsule /bōʹmanz/ [William Bowman, English anatomist, 1816–1892], the cup-shaped end of a renal tubule or nephron enclosing a glomerulus. With the glomerulus, it is the site of filtration in the kidney. Also called **glomerular capsule.**

Bowman's glands [William Bowman; L, *glans,* acorn], branched tubuloalveolar glands in mucous membranes of the mouth. They keep the mouth surfaces moist.

Bowman's lamina [William Bowman; L, *lamina,* plate], a tough membrane beneath the corneal epithelium. Also called **anterior elastic lamina,** *Bowman's layer, Bowman's membrane.*

bowtie filter /bōʹtī/, a filter shaped like a bowtie that may be used in computed tomography to compensate for the shape of the patient's head or body. It is used with fan-shaped x-ray beams to equalize the amount of radiation reaching the image receptor.

boxer's ear. *(Informal)* See **pachyotia.**

boxer's fracture [Dan, *bask,* a blow; L, *fractura,* break], a break in one or more metacarpal bones, usually the fourth or the fifth, caused by punching a hard object. The distal fracture fragment is typically angulated and/or impacted.

boxing, the forming of vertical walls, most commonly made of wax, to produce the desired shape and size of the base of a dental plaster cast.

boxing wax [L, *buxis,* box; AS, *weax*], (in dentistry) a thin sheet of flexible wax used for forming walls around an impression to be poured with dental plaster to form a cast model.

Boyd amputation [H.B. Boyd, American surgeon], amputation at the ankle with removal of the talus and fusion of the tibia and calcaneus.

Boykin, Anne, a nursing theorist who, with Savina O. Schoenhofer, wrote *Nursing as Caring: A Model for Transforming Practice,* which postulates that caring is the end, not the means, of nursing. The authors describe caring in nursing as a mutual process between caring for persons in which the nurse artistically responds with authentic presence to calls for nursing. It is a concept not unique *to* nursing but *in* nursing. All activities of nursing emanate from a commitment to caring and engender a respect for the specialness of each person.

Boyle's law /boilz/ [Robert Boyle, English scientist, 1627–1691], (in physics) the law stating that the product of the volume and pressure of a gas contained at a constant temperature remains constant.

BP, abbreviation for **blood pressure.**

BPD, **1.** abbreviation for **bronchopulmonary dysplasia. 2.** abbreviation for **bipolar disorder. 3.** abbreviation for **biparietal diameter.**

BPDE-I, acronym for *benzopyrene dihydrodiol epoxide.*

BPH, abbreviation for **benign prostatic hyperplasia.**

bpm, initialism for *beats per minute.*

BPRS, abbreviation for **Brief Psychiatric Rating Scale.**

Br, symbol for the element **bromine.**

brace [OFr, *bracier,* to embrace], an orthotic device, sometimes jointed, used to support and hold any part of the body in the correct position to allow function and healing, such as a leg brace that permits walking and standing. Compare **splint.** See also **durable medical equipment.**

brachi- /brāʹkē-/, prefix meaning "arm": *brachialgia, brachiocephalic.*

-brachia /-brāʹkē-ə/, suffix meaning an "anatomical condition involving an arm": *acephalobrachia, microbrachia.*

brachial /brāʹkē-əl/ [Gk, *brachion,* arm], pertaining to the arm.

brachial artery, the principal artery of the upper arm that is the continuation of the axillary artery. It has three branches and terminates at the bifurcation of its main trunk into the radial artery and the ulnar artery.

brachialgia /-alʹjē-ə/ [L, *brachium,* arm; Gk, *algos,* pain], a severe pain in the arm, often related to a disorder involving the brachial plexus.

brachialis /brāʹkē-əlʹis/ [Gk, *brachion,* arm], a muscle of the upper arm covering the distal half of the humerus and the anterior part of the elbow joint. It functions to flex the forearm. Compare **biceps brachii, triceps brachii.**

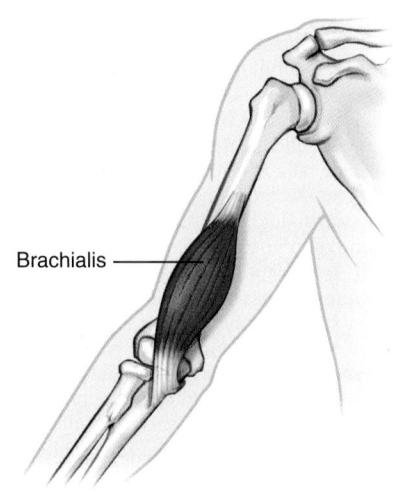

Brachialis

Brachialis

brachial paralysis [L, *brachium,* arm; Gk, *paralyein,* to be palsied], paralysis of an arm or a hand as a result of a lesion of the brachial plexus. See also **Erb's palsy.**

brachial plexus [Gk, *brachion* + L, braided], the plexus that innervates the upper limb, formed by the anterior rami of cervical spinal nerves C5 to C8 and T1. It is initially formed in the neck and continues through the axillary inlet into the axilla. See also **plexus.**

brachial plexus anesthesia, an anesthetic block of the upper extremity, performed by injecting local anesthetic near the plexus formed by the last four cervical and first two thoracic spinal nerves. The plexus extends from the transverse processes of the spine to the apex of the axilla, where the terminal nerves are formed. Because of the anatomy of this area, many approaches are possible. Approaches include the axillary (in the armpit), supraclavicular and infraclavicular (above and below the collarbone), and interscalene (between the anterior and middle scalene muscles of the neck) areas. Also called **brachial plexus block.** See also **regional anesthesia.**

brachial plexus block. See **brachial plexus anesthesia.**

brachial plexus paralysis. See **Erb's palsy.**

brachial pulse [Gk, *brachion* + L, *pulsare,* to beat], the pulse of the brachial artery, palpated in the antecubital space. See also **pulse.**

Brachial plexus

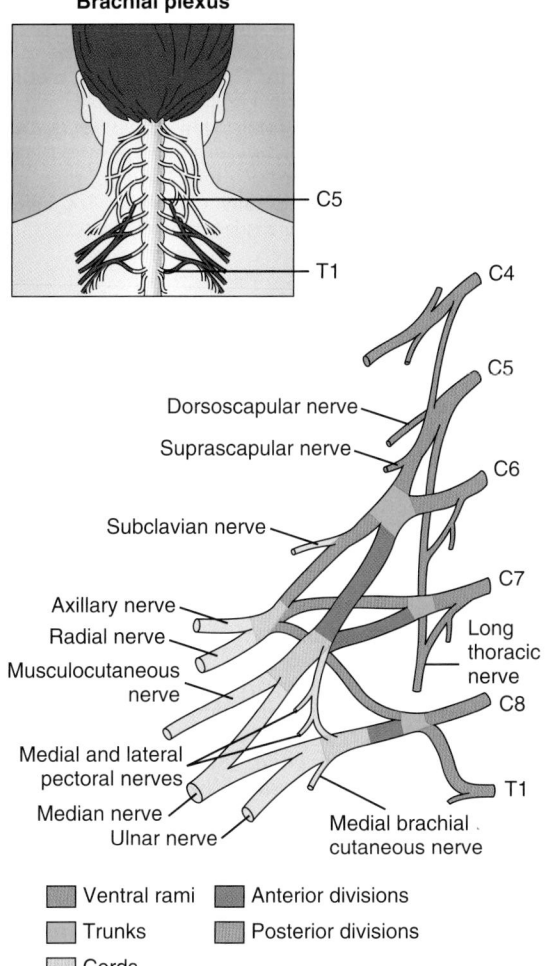

Ventral rami — Anterior divisions

Trunks — Posterior divisions

Cords

Brachial plexus *(Thibodeau and Patton, 2007)*

brachial region, an anatomical term used to refer to the arm (shoulder to elbow), divided into anterior and posterior brachial regions.

brachial vein, a vein in the arm that accompanies the brachial artery and drains into the axillary vein.

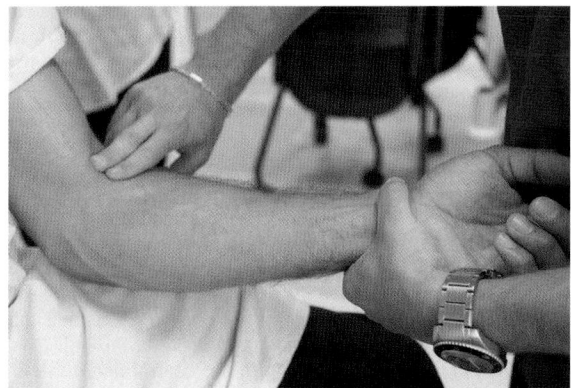

Assessment of brachial pulse *(Courtesy Rutgers School of Nursing—Camden. All rights reserved.)*

brachiocephalic, relating to the arm and head.

brachiocephalic arteritis. See **Takayasu's arteritis.**

brachiocephalic artery, first branch of the aortic arch. See also **innominate artery.**

brachiocephalic trunk. See **innominate artery.**

brachiocephalic vein, the vein feeding the superior vena cava, collecting blood from the subclavian and jugular veins. See also **innominate vein.**

brachiocubital /-kyoo″bitəl/ [Gk, *brachion* + L, *cubitus,* elbow], pertaining to the arm and forearm.

brachioplasty, a surgical procedure to shape, lift, and tighten sagging skin of the upper arm related to excess skin or fat.

brachioradialis /-rā′dē·al″is/, the most superficial muscle on the radial side of the forearm. It functions to flex the forearm.

brachioradialis reflex [Gk, *brachion* + L, *radial, reflectare,* to bend backward], a deep tendon reflex elicited by striking the lateral surface of the forearm proximal to the distal head of the radius, characterized by normal slight elbow flexion and forearm supination. It is accentuated by disease of the

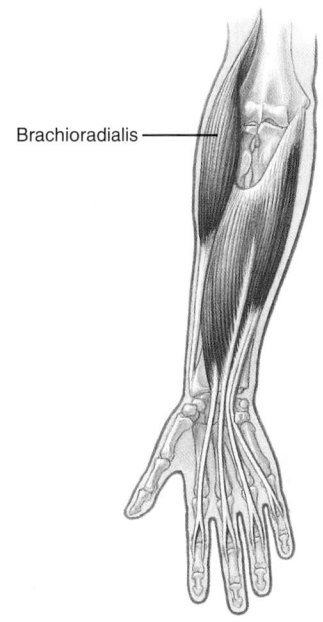

Brachioradialis *(Patton and Thibodeau, 2010)*

pyramidal tract above the level of the fifth cervical vertebra. See also **deep tendon reflex.**

-brachium /-brā″kē·əm/, **1.** suffix meaning "the upper arm from shoulder to elbow." **2.** suffix meaning "an arm or arm-like growth": *antebrachium.*

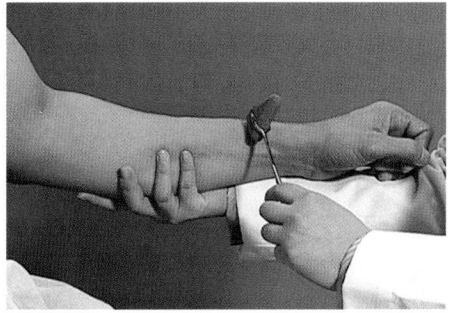

Brachioradialis reflex testing *(Ball et al, 2015)*

brachy- /brak′ē-/, prefix meaning "short": *brachybasia, brachydactyly.*

brachybasia /-bā″zhə/, abnormally slow walking, with a short, shuffling gait. The condition is associated with cerebral hemorrhage pyramidal tract disease, or Parkinson's disease.

brachycephaly /-sef′əlē/ [Gk, *brachys,* short, *kephale,* head], a congenital malformation of the skull in which premature closure of the coronal suture results in excessive lateral growth of the head, giving it a short, broad appearance. Also called *brachycephalia, brachycephalism.* See also **craniostenosis.** −*brachycephalous, brachycephalic, adj.*

brachydactyly /-dak″təlē/, an inherited condition in which fingers or toes are abnormally short due to unusually short bones.

brachygnathia. See **micrognathia.**

brachytherapy [Gk, *brachys,* short, *therapeia,* treatment], the placement of radioactive sources, such as seeds, needles, or catheters, in contact with or implanted into the tumor tissues to be treated for a specific period. Sources can be temporary or permanent. The rationale for this treatment is to provide a high absorbed dose of radiation in the tumor tissues and a very limited absorbed low dose in the surrounding normal tissues. Traditional brachytherapy implants deliver low doses of radiation; the newest variations deliver high doses. Compare **teletherapy.**

bracket /brak′ət/ [Fr, *braguette,* codpiece], a support projecting from the main structure. An orthodontic bracket is a small metal attachment soldered or welded to an orthodontic band or cemented directly to the teeth, serving to fasten the arch wire to the band or tooth. Also called **orthodontic attachment.** See also **orthodontic appliance, orthodontic band.**

bracketing /brak′ et-ing/, a technique used in qualitative research in which the researcher's knowledge about an experience is suspended or set aside.

Bradford solid frame [Edward H. Bradford, American surgeon, 1848–1926], a rectangular metal orthopedic device that provides support for the entire body and is especially appropriate for patients who are less than 5 years of age, hyperactive, or mentally challenged. The main purpose of the device is to assist in maintaining proper immobilization, positioning, and alignment by controlling movement. To facilitate care, the Bradford solid frame is not placed directly on a bed but is elevated at both ends by plywood blocks or other suitable devices. It is most often used with Bryant traction but never with balanced suspension traction, cervical traction, cervical tongs, or certain other kinds of traction.

Bradford split frame [Edward H. Bradford, American surgeon, 1848–1926], a rectangular metal orthopedic device covered with two separate pieces of canvas fastened at both ends of the frame. Used especially in pediatrics to aid in the immobilization of children in traction, it is divided in the middle by a large opening designed to accommodate the excretory functions of an incontinent patient in a hip spica cast. The division also allows the upper and lower extremities of the patient to be elevated separately and the cast to be kept clean and dry.

Bradley method [Robert Bradley, 20th-century American physician], a method of psychophysical preparation for childbirth, comprising education about the physiological characteristics of childbirth, exercise, and nutrition during pregnancy, and techniques of breathing and relaxation for control and comfort during labor and delivery. The father is extensively involved in the classes and acts as the mother's "coach" during labor. Among the advantages of the method are its simplicity, the father's involvement, and the realistic approach to the efforts and discomfort of labor. Also called **husband-coached childbirth.** Compare **Lamaze method, Read method.**

brady- /brad′ē-/, prefix meaning "slow, dull": *bradycardia, bradykinesia, bradyphagia.*

bradyarrhythmia /-ərith″mē·ə/ [Gk, *bradys,* slow, *a* + *rhythmos,* without rhythm], any disturbance of cardiac rhythm in which the heart rate is less than 60 beats/min.

bradycardia /-kär″dē·ə/ [Gk, *bradys,* slow, *kardia,* heart], a condition in which the heart rate is less than 60 beats/min. Bradycardia takes the form of sinus bradycardia, sinus arrhythmia, and second- or third-degree atrioventricular block. Sinus bradycardia may be caused by excessive vagal tone, decreased sympathetic tone, or anatomical changes. It is common in athletes and is relatively benign. It may even be beneficial in acute myocardial infarction (especially inferior). Pathological bradycardia may be symptomatic of a brain tumor, digitalis toxicity, heart block, or vagotonus. Cardiac output is decreased, causing faintness, dizziness, chest pain, and eventually syncope and circulatory collapse. Treatment may include administration of atropine, implantation of a pacemaker, or change in medical treatment.

bradycardia-tachycardia syndrome [Gk, *bradys* + *kardia,* + *tachys,* fast, *kardia* + *syn,* together, *dromos,* course], a disorder characterized by a heart rate that alternates between being abnormally low (less than 60 beats/min) and abnormally high (greater than 100 beats/min). Also called *bradytachycardia,* **tachycardia-bradycardia syndrome.** See also **sick sinus syndrome, sinus node dysfunction.**

bradyecoia, *(Obsolete)* mild hearing loss.

bradyesthesia /-esthē″zhə/ [Gk, *bradys,* slow, *aisthesis,* feeling], a slowness in perception.

bradykinesia /-kinē″zhə, -kīnē″zhə/ [Gk, *bradys* + *kinesis,* motion], an abnormal condition characterized by slowness of all voluntary movement and speech, such as caused by parkinsonism, other extrapyramidal disorders, and certain tranquilizers.

bradykinin /-kī″nin/ [Gk, *bradys* + *kinein,* to move], a peptide containing nine amino acid residues produced from α_2-globulin by the enzyme kallikrein. Bradykinin is a potent vasodilator.

bradylalia. See **bradyphasia.**

bradyphagia /-fā″jə/, a habit of eating very slowly.

bradyphasia /-fā″zhə/, an abnormally slow manner of speech, often associated with mental illness. Also called **bradylalia.**

bradypnea /-pnē″ə/ [Gk, *bradys* + *pnein,* to breath], an abnormally low rate of breathing (lower than 12 breaths/min). Compare **hypopnea.** See also **respiration rate.**

Bragg curve [William H. Bragg, English physicist, 1862–1942], the path followed by ionizing particles used in a radiation treatment. Because certain particles reach a peak of potential near the end of their path, the Bragg curve can be used to direct the radiation to deep-seated tumors while significantly sparing normal overlying tissues.

Braille /brāl, brä″yə/ [Louis Braille, French teacher of the visually impaired, 1809–1852], a system of printing for the visually impaired consisting of raised dots or points that can be read by touch.

brain [AS, *bragen*], the portion of the central nervous system contained within the cranium. It consists principally of the cerebrum, thalamus, hypothalamus, cerebellum, midbrain, pons, and medulla. Specialized cells in its mass of convoluted, soft gray or white tissue coordinate and regulate the functions of the central nervous system, integrating the functions of the body as a whole.

brain abscess [AS, *bragen* + L, *abscedere,* to go away], a pocket of infection in a part of the brain. It is usually a result of the spread of an infection from another source, such as the skull, sinuses, or other structures in the head. The infection also may be secondary to a disease in the bones, the nervous system outside the brain, or the heart. Also called **cerebral abscess, intracranial abscess.**

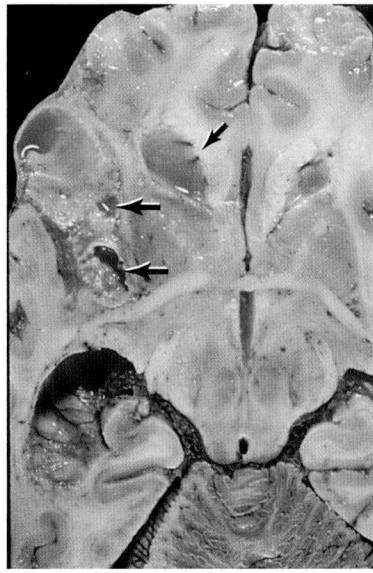

Brain abscess *(Damjanov and Linder, 2000)*

brain attack, a term signifying that a stroke is in progress and an emergency situation exists. So called by the American Stroke Association to draw attention to the situation, as in heart attack. See **cerebrovascular accident.**

brain compression. See **cerebral compression.**

brain concussion [AS, *bragen* + L, *concussus,* a shaking], a bruising to cerebral tissues caused by a violent jarring or shaking or other blunt, nonpenetrating injury to the brain resulting in a sudden change in momentum of the head. Characteristically, after a mild concussion there may be a transient loss of consciousness followed, on awakening, by a headache. Severe concussion may cause prolonged unconsciousness and disruption of certain vital functions of the brainstem, such as respiration and vasomotor stability. The treatment for a person recovering from a concussion consists principally of observation for signs of intracranial bleeding and increased intracranial pressure. Also called **concussion.**

brain death [AS, *bragen* + *death*], an irreversible form of unconsciousness characterized by a complete loss of brain function while the heart continues to beat. The legal definition of this condition varies from state to state. The usual clinical criteria for brain death include the absence of reflex activity, movements, and spontaneous respiration requiring mechanical ventilation or life support to continue any cardiac function. The pupils are dilated and fixed. Because hypothermia, anesthesia, poisoning, or drug intoxication may cause deep physiological depression that resembles brain death, these parameters must be within normal limits prior to testing. Diagnosis of brain death may require evaluating and demonstrating that electrical activity of the brain is absent on

two electroencephalograms performed 12 to 24 hours apart. Brain death can be confirmed with electroencephalograms showing a complete lack of electrical activity (a flat line) or vascular perfusion studies showing a lack of blood flow to the brain. Also called **irreversible coma.** Compare **coma, sleep, stupor.**

brain edema. See **cerebral edema.**

brain electric activity map (BEAM), a topographic map of the brain created by a computer that is able to respond to the electric potentials evoked in the brain by a flash of light. Potentials recorded at 4-msec intervals are converted into a many-colored map of the brain, showing them to be positive or negative. The waves may be observed traveling through the brain. If the wave is disordered, blocked, too small, or too large, a tumor or other lesion may be causing the abnormal pattern.

brain fever, *(Obsolete)* any inflammation of the brain or meninges. See also **encephalitis.**

brain natriuretic peptide (BNP), a hormone, originally isolated from porcine brain tissue, having biological effects similar to those of atrial natriuretic peptide and stored mainly in the myocardium of the cardiac ventricles. Blood levels of BNP are elevated in hypervolemic states, such as congestive heart failure and hypertension.

brain scan [AS, *bragen* + L, *scandere,* to climb], a diagnostic procedure used to image the brain. Common modalities include CT, MRI, and PET. Imaging can be done with or without a contrast medium used to localize and identify intracranial masses, lesions, tumors, or infarcts. In nuclear medicine modalities intravenously injected radioisotopes accumulate in abnormal brain tissue and are traced and photographed by a scintillator or scanner. The nature and rate of accumulation of radioisotopes in pathological tissue are diagnostic of some lesions. Compare **computed tomography.** See also **isotope, radioisotope.**

Brain's reflex [Walter R. Brain, English physician, 1895–1966; L, *reflectere,* to bend back], the reflexive extension of the flexed paralyzed arm of a hemiplegia patient when assuming a quadrupedal posture. Also called **quadripedal extensor reflex.**

brainstem [AS, *bragen* + *stemm*], the portion of the brain comprising the medulla oblongata, the pons, and the mesencephalon. It performs motor, sensory, and reflex functions and contains the corticospinal and reticulospinal tracts. The 12 pairs of cranial nerves from the brain arise mostly from the brainstem. Compare **medulla oblongata, mesencephalon, pons.**

brainstem auditory evoked response (BAER), the electric activity that may be recorded from the brainstem in the first 10 msec after presentation of an auditory stimulus. In a subject with normal brainstem functioning, seven peaks are observed. A delayed, normally shaped waveform may indicate a hearing loss caused by pathology such as an inner ear canal tumor; one or more missing peaks may indicate a neural disorder.

brain swelling. *(Informal)* See **cerebral edema.**

brain syndrome, a group of symptoms resulting from impaired function of the brain. It may be acute and reversible, or chronic and irreversible. An organic mental disorder is a specific organic mental syndrome in which the cause is known or presumed. An organic mental syndrome is a temporary or permanent brain dysfunction of any cause.

brain tumor, an invasive neoplasm of the intracranial portion of the central nervous system. Brain tumors cause significant rates of morbidity and mortality but are occasionally treated successfully. In adults 20% to 40% of malignancies in the brain are metastatic lesions from cancers in the breast,

B

lung, GI tract, or kidney or a malignant melanoma. These are referred to as secondary tumors. The origin of primary brain tumors is not known, but the risk is increased in individuals exposed to vinyl chloride, in the siblings of cancer patients, and in recipients of renal transplantation being treated with immunosuppressant medication. Causes under investigation are genetic changes, heredity, ionizing radiation, environmental hazards, viruses, and injury. Gliomas, chiefly astrocytomas, are the most common malignancies. Medulloblastomas occur often in children. Surgery is the initial treatment for most primary tumors of the brain. Postoperative nursing care includes assessment of the patient to detect elevation in intracranial pressure.

■ OBSERVATIONS: Symptoms of a brain tumor are often those of increased intracranial pressure, such as headache, nausea, vomiting, papilledema, lethargy, and disorientation, but vary depending on the site of a tumor. Localizing signs, such as loss of vision on the side of an occipital neoplasm, may occur. Diagnostic measures include visual field and funduscopic examinations, skull x-ray examinations, electroencephalography, brain scanning, magnetic resonance imaging, computed tomography, and spinal fluid studies. Cerebral angiography is used for information about vascular supply.

■ INTERVENTIONS: Radiotherapy is indicated for inoperable lesions, medulloblastomas, and tumors with multiple foci and is used in postoperative treatment of residual tumor tissue. The blood-brain barrier impedes the effect of some antineoplastic agents, but the administration of disk-shaped drug wafers is an emerging practice. A coordinated team approach to care will be dictated by the patient's symptoms.

■ PATIENT CARE CONSIDERATIONS: A brain tumor can have a profound effect on activities of daily living. Symptoms are dependent on location and size.

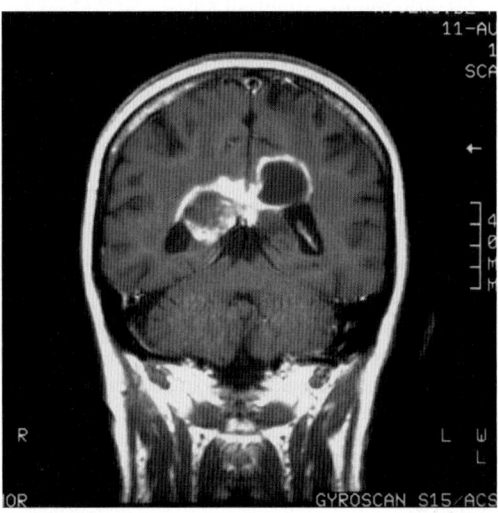

Brain tumor *(Courtesy Riverside Methodist Hospitals)*

brainwashing, intensive indoctrination, usually of a political or religious nature, applied to individuals to develop in their minds a specific belief and motivation.

brain wave [AS, *bragen* + *wafian*], any of a number of patterns of rhythmic electric impulses produced in different parts of the brain. Most patterns, identified by the Greek letters alpha, beta, delta, gamma, kappa, and theta, are similar for all normal persons and are relatively stable for each individual. Brain waves help in the diagnosis of certain neurological disorders, such as epilepsy or brain tumors. See also **alpha wave, beta wave, delta wave, theta wave.**

bran, a coarse outer covering or coat (seed husk) of cereal grain, such as wheat or rye. Bran provides a source of dietary fiber, B vitamins, iron, magnesium, and zinc. When separated from the meal or flour portion of a grain, it is less nutritious.

branch, (in anatomy) an offshoot arising from the main trunk of a nerve or blood vessel.

branched-chain amino acids (BCAA), leucine, isoleucine, and valine; they are incorporated into proteins or catabolized for energy.

branched-chain ketoaciduria. See **maple syrup urine disease.**

branched tubular gland [OFr, *branche*], one of the many multicellular glands with one excretory duct from two or more tube-shaped secretory branches, such as some of the gastric glands.

brancher glycogen storage disease. See **Andersen's disease.**

branchial /brang″kē·əl/ [Gk, *branchia*, gills], pertaining to body structures of the face, neck, and throat area, particularly the muscles.

branchial arches [Gk, *branchia*, gills; L, *arcus*, bow], arched structures in the embryonic pharynx.

branchial cleft [Gk, *branchia*, gills; ME, *clift*], a linear depression in the pharynx of the early embryo opposite a branchial or pharyngeal pouch.

branchial cyst [Gk, *branchia*, gills, *kystis*, bag], a lump of tissue derived from a branchial remnant in the neck.

branchial fistula, a congenital abnormal passage from the pharynx to the external surface of the neck, resulting from the failure of a branchial cleft to close during fetal development. Also called **cervical fistula.**

branching canal. See **collateral pulp canal.**

branchiogenic /brang′kē·ōjen″ik/ [Gk, *branchia*, gills, *genein*, to produce], pertaining to any tissues originating in the branchial cleft or arch. Also called **branchiogenous.**

branchio-oto-renal syndrome /brang′kē·ō·ō′tō·rē′nəl/ [Gk, *branchia*, gills + *ous*, ear + L, *ren*, kidney], branchial arch anomalies (preauricular pits, branchial fistulas or pits) associated with congenital deafness resulting from dysgenesis of the organ of Corti, and with renal dysplasia. It is inherited as an autosomal-dominant trait with high penetrance and variable expression.

brand name, a product with a unique name or trademark protected by a patent. See **trademark.**

Brandt-Andrews maneuver [Thure Brandt, Swedish obstetrician, 1819–1895; Henry R. Andrews, English obstetrician, 1871–1942], a method of expressing the placenta from the uterus in the third stage of labor. One hand grasps the umbilical cord while the other is placed on the mother's abdomen with the fingers over the anterior surface of the uterus. While the hand on the abdomen is pressed backward and slightly upward, the other applies gentle traction on the cord.

Braschi valve, a one-way valve put into the inspiratory limb of a ventilator circuit to measure the intrinsic positive end-expiratory pressure.

brass founder's ague, now called **metal fume fever.**

brassy cough [AS, *brase*, brassy, *cohhetan*, to cough], a high-pitched cough caused by irritation of the recurrent pharyngeal nerve or by pressure on the trachea.

brassy eye, an eye inflammation. See **chalkitis.**

Braun's canal. See **neurenteric canal.**

brawny arm, a swollen arm caused by lymphedema, usually after a mastectomy.

Braxton Hicks contractions, irregular uterine contractions unassociated with cervical effacement and dilation.

These contractions are initially painless, but in the third trimester Braxton Hicks contractions may intermittently become rhythmic, relatively close together, and painful. They often resolve with hydration and ambulation. It may be difficult to distinguish Braxton Hicks contractions from true labor pains by history alone. See **preterm contractions, false labor.**

Braxton Hicks version /brak″stən hiks″/ [John Braxton Hicks, English physician, 1823–1897], *(Obsolete)* one of several types of maneuvers formerly used to turn the fetus from an undesirable position to one that is more likely to facilitate delivery. See also **version.**

Brazelton assessment. See **Neonatal Behavioral Assessment Scale.**

Brazilian trypanosomiasis. See **Chagas' disease.**

BRCA1, symbol for a breast cancer gene. BRCA1 is a tumor suppressor gene. A healthy BRCA1 gene produces a protein that protects against unwanted cell growth. The protein is packaged by the cell's Golgi apparatus into secretory vesicles, which release their contents on the cell's surface. The protein circulates in the intracellular space, attaching itself to neighboring cell receptors. The receptors signal the cell nuclei to stop growing. When the gene is defective, it produces a faulty protein that is unable to prevent proliferation of abnormal cells as they evolve into potentially deadly breast cancer. BRCA1 may also normally inhibit ovarian cancer.

BRCA2, symbol for a breast cancer gene with activity similar to that of BRCA1.

breach of contract, (in law) the failure to perform as promised or agreed to in a contract. The breach may be complete or partial and may entail repudiation, failure to recognize the contract, or prevention or hindrance of performance. The health care industry is highly regulated to protect patients. The accidental release of confidential protected health information is an example of a breach of contract.

breach of duty, **1.** (in law) the failure to perform an act required by law. **2.** the performance of an act in an unlawful manner and/or in a manner that is not appropriate to the profession.

breakbone fever. *(Obsolete)* See **dengue fever.**

break test, a test of a person's muscle strength by application of resistance after the person has reached the end of a range of motion following completion of activity. Resistance is applied gradually in a direction opposite to the line of pull of the muscle or muscle group being tested. The resistance is released immediately if there is any sign of pain or discomfort.

braking radiation. See **bremsstrahlung radiation.**

breakthrough, (in psychiatry) a sudden new insight into a problem and its solution after a period of little or no progress.

breakthrough analgesia, analgesia administered for the relief of pain perceived while already anesthetized with a local or regional anesthetic. Breakthrough analgesia could be performed by reanesthetizing the area surrounding the surgical area or by administration of an intravenous analgesic.

breakthrough bleeding, the escape of uterine blood between menstrual periods; a possible side effect of fibroids or oral contraceptive use.

breakthrough dose, the dose of an analgesic required for the relief of breakthrough pain. Also called **rescue dose.**

breakthrough pain, a transient increase in pain intensity that occurs in patients with stable, baseline persistent pain.

breast [AS, *breast*], **1.** the anterior aspect of the surface of the chest. **2.** a mammary gland.

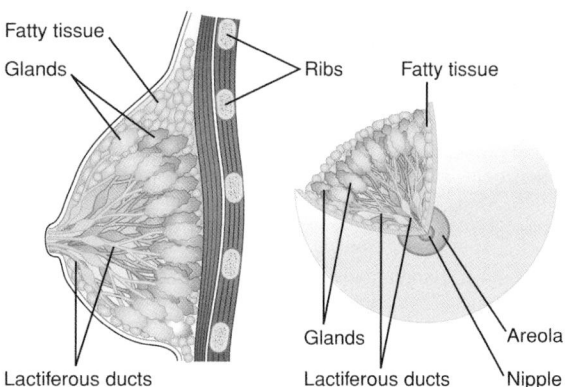

Breast *(Buck, 2015)*

breast abscess, a true abscess following unresolved postpartum breast infection (mastitis). Treatment is surgical drainage of the abscess and antibiotic therapy, the most common pathogens being *Staphylococcus aureus,* group A or B streptococcus, *Beta haemophilus,* and *Escherichia coli.*

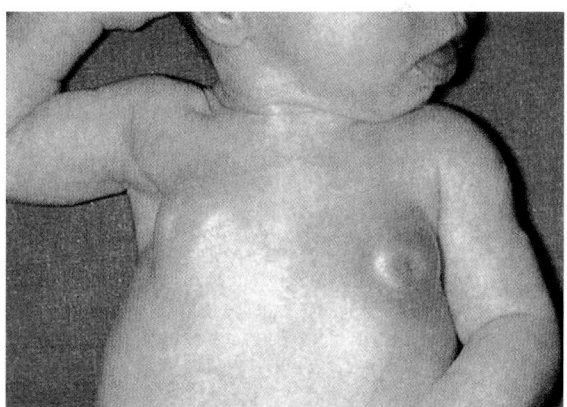

Breast abscess *(Mansel et al, 2009)*

breast augmentation, *(Informal)* common name for augmentation mammoplasty.

breast cancer, a malignant neoplastic disease of breast tissue, a common malignancy in women and very rarely in men. The incidence increases with age from the third to the fifth decade and reaches a second peak at age 65. Known risk factors include age, certain genetic abnormalities, a family history of breast cancer, nulliparity or late parity (over age 30 years), exposure to ionizing radiation, early menarche, and late menopause. Women who take postmenopausal estrogen therapy are also at increased risk. The diagnosis may be established by a careful physical examination, mammography, and cytological examination of tumor cells obtained by biopsy. Infiltrating ductal carcinomas are found in about 75% of cases, and infiltrating lobular, infiltrating medullary, colloid, comedo, or papillary carcinomas in the others. Inflammatory carcinomas account for approximately 1% of cases. Metastasis through the lymphatic system to axillary lymph nodes and to bone, lung, brain, and liver is common, but there is evidence that primary carcinomas of the breast may exist in multiple sites and that tumor cells may enter the bloodstream directly without passing through lymph nodes. See also **lumpectomy, mastectomy, scirrhous carcinoma.**

■ OBSERVATIONS: A mass detected by breast self-examination, clinical breast examination, or mammogram requires follow-up. Increasing numbers of breast cancers are found on mammogram. Definitive diagnosis is made by incisional, excisional, fine needle, or stereotactic core biopsy of the mass. Pain, tenderness, changes in breast shape, dimpling, and nipple retraction rarely occur until the disease reaches an advanced stage. Prognosis dims markedly as the number of involved lymph nodes increases. Pleural effusion, ascites, pathological fracture, and spinal compression can occur with advanced disease.

■ INTERVENTIONS: Surgical treatment may consist of a mastectomy or a lumpectomy, with dissection of axillary nodes, or sentinel lymph node biopsy for women without palpable lymph nodes. Postoperative radiotherapy, chemotherapy, or both are often prescribed. Chemotherapeutic agents frequently administered in various combinations are cyclophosphamide, methotrexate, 5-fluorouracil, phenylalanine mustard (L-PAM), thiotepa, DOXOrubicin, vinCRIStine, paclitaxel, and predniSONE. The presence of estrogen receptors in breast tumors is considered an indication for hormonal manipulation such as the administration of antiestrogens. Implantation of a prosthesis after mastectomy is optional and does not appear to decrease survival probability. Reconstructive surgery is common, with few complications. Adjunct systemic multidrug chemotherapy is used primarily for premenopausal node-positive women. Adjunct hormone therapy (estrogens, androgens, and progestins) is used primarily for postmenopausal node-positive or receptor-positive women. Antiestrogen therapy (Tamoxifen and aromatase inhibitors) is used as first-line therapy; biological therapy with trastuzumab (Herceptin) is used in select patients for treatment of metastatic disease. Emotional needs, such as fear over a cancer diagnosis, grieving over loss of a breast, and altered body image, must be addressed. Counseling may be needed. Referrals can be made for age-specific recovery support groups. Referral may also be made for fitting and construction of a breast prosthesis or surgical reconstruction of the breast. The need for long-term follow-up of physical and emotional sequelae is stressed.

■ PATIENT CARE CONSIDERATIONS: Nurses, physicians, and primary health care providers have responsibilities for patient care at all levels of the care continuum, from primary care and screening to acute and long-term follow-through after diagnosis and medical treatment for breast cancer. Health professionals play a major role in early detection and should educate and instruct women age 50 and older to get a biannual mammogram and clinical breast exam. Women

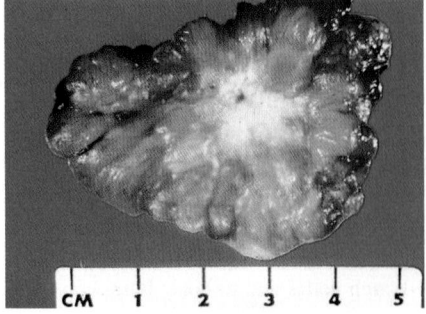

Breast cancer: invasive ductal carcinoma *(Kumar et al, 2013)*

at increased risk (i.e., family history, known genetic mutation, prior thoracic radiation) should talk with their health care provider about more frequent and earlier screening. All women should practice breast awareness (know how their breasts normally look and feel) and report any breast change promptly to their health care provider.

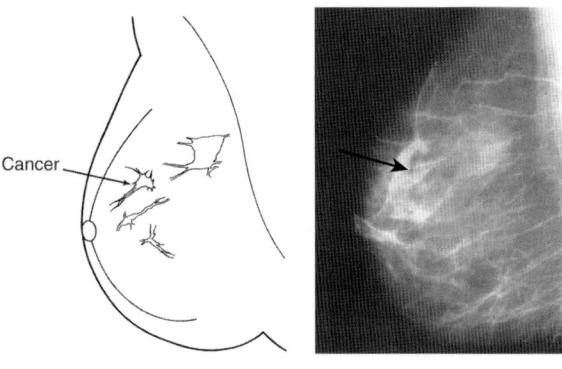

Breast cancer *(Leonard, 2011)*

breast cancer genetic screening test (BRCA genetic testing), a molecular test performed on whole blood to detect germ-line mutations in the BRCA1 or BRCA2 genes. The presence of BRCA1 or BRCA2 mutations confers a congenital predisposition for breast or ovarian cancer, and BRCA2 variations include a relationship to breast cancer in males. Hereditary breast cancer accounts for 5%-10% of all breast cancer cases.

breast cancer tumor analysis, a microscopic examination of breast cancer tissue to predict the probability of cancer recurrence.

breast ductal lavage, a fluid analysis of exfoliated cells from breast ducts to assess breast cancer risk.

breast examination, a process in which the breasts and their accessory structures are observed and palpated in assessing the presence of changes or abnormalities. There are benefits and limitations to self-breast examination, but in general women should be familiar with how their breasts normally look and feel. A clinical breast examination is performed by a health professional; a breast examination performed by the patient is known as a self-breast examination. See also **self-breast examination, clinical breast examination.**

■ METHOD: The breasts are observed with the patient sitting with her arms at her sides; sitting with her arms over her head, back straight, then leaning forward; and, finally, sitting upright as she contracts the pectoral muscles by placing hands on hips. The breasts are observed for symmetry of shape and size and for surface characteristics, including moles or nevi, hyperpigmentation, retraction or dimpling, edema, abnormal distribution of hair, focal vascularity, or lesions. With the patient still sitting, the axillary nodes and the supraclavicular and subclavicular areas are palpated. With the patient lying on her back, each breast is shifted medially, and the glandular area in each is palpated with the flat of the fingers of a hand in concentric circles or in a pattern like the spokes of a wheel, from the periphery inward. The areolar areas, the nipples, and the axillary tail of Spence in the upper outer quadrant extending toward the axilla are then palpated. The nipple is squeezed to check for discharge.

■ INTERVENTIONS: The breasts should be examined when they are not tender or swollen. Research has not shown a clear benefit of regular physical breast exams done by either a health professional or by women themselves. Most often when breast cancer is detected because of symptoms (such as a lump), a woman discovers the symptom during usual activities such as bathing or dressing.

■ OUTCOME CRITERIA: Early diagnosis greatly improves the rate of cure in cancer of the breast.

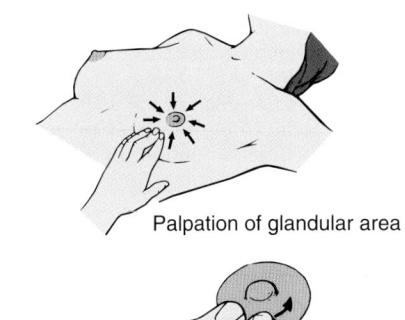

Palpation of glandular area

Palpation of areolar area

Compression of nipple

Breast examination

breastfeeding [AS, *braest* + ME, *feden*], **1.** suckling or nursing, giving a baby milk from the breast. Breastfeeding encourages postpartum uterine involution and slows the natural return of the menses. The World Health Organization recommends continued breastfeeding up to 2 years of age or beyond. Also called **nursing. 2.** taking milk from the breast. See also **breast milk, lactation.**

breast implant, the surgical placement of prosthetic material in a breast, either to increase the breast's size or for reconstruction after a mastectomy.

breast milk [AS, *braest* + *meoluc*], human milk. The composition is mostly water, protein, fat, carbohydrates, amino acids, vitamins, minerals, enzymes, white cells, and long-chain fatty acids. The exact composition of breast milk changes as the infant ages and suckles. The World Health Organization (WHO) recommends that a child breastfeed for at least 2 years. Compare **colostrum.** See also **breastfeeding.**

breast milk jaundice, jaundice and hyperbilirubinemia in breastfed infants that occur in the first weeks of life as a result of a metabolite in the mother's milk that inhibits the infant's ability to conjugate bilirubin to glucuronide for excretion. See also **hyperbilirubinemia of the newborn.**

■ OBSERVATIONS: Breast milk jaundice usually peaks around the tenth day of life. Serum bilirubin levels usually exceed 5 mg/100 mL but rarely reach dangerous levels of 20 mg/100 mL, at which point kernicterus may develop. The infant seems normal and healthy, but the skin, the whites of the eyes, and the serum are jaundiced (yellow).

■ INTERVENTIONS: If serum bilirubin exceeds acceptable levels, breastfeeding should continue frequently to enhance stooling and decrease the chance for enterohepatic circulation. Phototherapy may be used to accelerate excretion of bilirubin through the skin. The use of oral supplementation with glucose water or water alone is not recommended.

■ PATIENT CARE CONSIDERATIONS: The primary concerns of the nurse are to observe for signs of increasing jaundice, to monitor serum bilirubin levels, and usually to reassure the mother that her child is well and that the jaundice resolves slowly but completely in time.

breast pump, a mechanical or electronic device for withdrawing milk from the breast.

breast scintigraphy, a nuclear scan used to identify breast cancer in patients whose dense breast tissue precludes accurate evaluation by conventional mammography. It is also used as a second-line imaging modality in patients with an indeterminate mammogram and in women with lumpy breasts.

breast self-examination (BSE). See **self-breast examination.**

breast shadows, artifacts caused by breast tissue that appear on chest radiographs of women. The shadows accentuate the underlying tissue and may cause the appearance of an interstitial disease process. Breast nipples may also appear on the radiograph as "coin lesions," requiring that a second radiograph with special markers attached to the nipples be made so that the two films can be compared.

breast sonogram, an ultrasound test that is used primarily to determine if a mammographic abnormality or a palpable lump is a cyst (fluid-filled) or a solid tumor (benign or malignant). It is also used to examine symptomatic women who should not be exposed to mammographic radiation, such as pregnant women or women under the age of 25 with dense breast tissue.

breast transillumination [AS, *braest* + L, *trans,* through, *illuminare,* to light up], a method of examining the inner structures of the breast by directing light through the outer wall. Evidence suggests mammography is superior to this procedure for the detection of breast cancer. See also **diaphanography.**

breath, the air inhaled and exhaled during ventilation of the lungs.

Breathalyzer® /breth″əlī′zər/, a trademark for a device that analyzes exhaled air. It is commonly used to test for blood alcohol levels; the test is based on the relationship between alcohol in the breath and alcohol in the blood circulating through the lungs. Also spelled *Breathalyser.*

breath-holding /breth-/ [AS, *braeth* + ME, *holden*], a form of voluntary apnea that is usually but not necessarily performed with a closed glottis. Although breath-holding may be prolonged for several minutes, it is invariably terminated either voluntarily or when the person or child loses consciousness.

breathing, the alternate inspiration and expiration of air into and out of the lungs to support life. See **respiration.**

breathing biofeedback, the monitoring of breathing rate, volume, rhythm, and location by sensors placed on the chest and abdomen, used in the treatment of asthma, hyperventilation, and anxiety. The feedback is displayed to the patient visually and is used by the patient to learn to breathe more slowly, deeply, and rhythmically using the abdominal muscles.

breathing cycle /brē″thing/, a ventilatory cycle consisting of an inspiration followed by the expiration of a volume of gas called the tidal volume. The duration or total cycle time of a breathing cycle is the breathing or ventilatory period. Also called **respiratory cycle.**

breathing frequency (f). See **respiration rate.**

breathing nomogram [AS, *braeth* + Gk, *nomos,* law, *gramma,* a record], a chart that presents scales of data for body weight, breathing frequency, and predicted basal tidal volume arranged so that one can find an unknown value on one scale by drawing a line that connects known values on the other two scales.

breathing-related sleep disorder, any of several disorders characterized by sleep disruption caused by some breathing problem, resulting in excessive sleepiness or insomnia. Kinds include **central sleep apnea, obstructive sleep apnea, primary alveolar hypoventilation.**

breathing tube. *(Nontechnical)* See **endotracheal tube, nasotracheal tube.**

breathing work, the energy required for breathing movements. It is the cumulative product of the instantaneous pressure developed by the respiratory muscles and the volume of air moved during a breathing cycle.

breathlessness. *(Nontechnical)* See **dyspnea.**

breath odor, an odor usually produced by substances or diseases in the lungs or mouth. Certain specific odors are associated with some diseases, such as diabetes, liver failure, uremia, or a lung abscess.

breath sound [AS, *braeth* + L, *sonus*], the sound of air passing in and out of the lungs, as heard with a stethoscope. Vesicular, bronchovesicular, and bronchial breath sounds are normal. Decreased breath sounds may indicate an obstruction of an airway, collapse of a portion or all of a lung, thickening of the pleurae of the lungs, emphysema, or other chronic obstructive pulmonary disease.

breath test, any of various tests in which a person's breath is analyzed for presence of something abnormal. Subgroups called the ^{13}C breath tests and ^{14}C breath tests involve administration of organic compounds labeled with carbon 13 (heavy carbon) or carbon 14 (radioactive carbon), respectively, and measuring the subsequent levels of labeled carbon dioxide in the patient's breath; the labeled compound may be found to be metabolized in the GI tract normally, too fast, or too slow.

breath tests, diagnostic tests for intestinal disorders such as bacterial overgrowth, ileal disease, lactase deficiency, and steatorrhea. Lactose malabsorption is treated by giving the patient 12.5 to 25.0 g of lactose and measuring the amount of hydrogen excreted in the breath. If lactose absorption is impaired in the small intestine, colonic bacteria ferment the lactose, releasing hydrogen, which is excreted in the breath. Bacterial overgrowth is tested with ^{14}C-cholylglycine, which is normally absorbed by the ileum and recycled via the enterohepatic circulation. In cases of bacterial overgrowth the labeled glycine is removed by conjugation in the small intestine, absorbed, and metabolized, resulting in an increase of ^{14}CO$_2$ in the breath. Breath tests are also used to test for the presence of *Helicobacter pylori*.

Breckinridge, Mary, (1881–1965), the American nurse who founded the Frontier Nursing Service in Kentucky to improve the obstetric care of women living in remote mountainous areas. The nurses in the service had training in midwifery and reached their patients on horseback and on foot, often encountering personal danger. The service began training midwives and stimulated the establishment of other midwifery schools.

Breda disease. See **espundia.**

breech birth [ME, *brech* + *burth*], a delivery that is bottom first rather than head first, occurring in about 2% of singleton deliveries at term. There are three breech presentations: frank breech (both feet near head), complete breech (legs are crossed and feet are not near the head), and incomplete or footling breech (one or both feet are extended). Breech presentation is more common in a multiple pregnancy or in women with polyhydramnios, uterine anomalies, or uterine fibroid tumors. Fetal conditions associated with breech birth include hydrocephalus and anencephaly. The risks of vaginal delivery include entrapment of the "aftercoming head" and umbilical cord prolapse. Facilitating delivery of the aftercoming fetal head may be done using Piper forceps. Because of these serious risks, many prefer cesarean section rather than a trial of breech delivery. Also because of these risks, manual version to a cephalic presentation (external cephalic

version, ECV) may be considered, generally between 36 and 38 weeks gestational age, when there is a lesser incidence of reversion to the breech. See also **assisted breech, breech presentation, complete breech, footling breech, frank breech, version and extraction.**

breech extraction [ME, *brech* + L, *ex,* out, *trahere,* to pull], an obstetric operation in which an infant being born feet or buttocks first is grasped before any part of the trunk is born and delivered by traction. Compare **assisted breech.**

breech presentation [ME, *brech* + L, *praesentare,* to show], intrauterine position of the fetus in which the buttocks or feet present. Compare **vertex presentation.** Kinds include **complete breech, footling breech, frank breech.** See also **breech birth.**

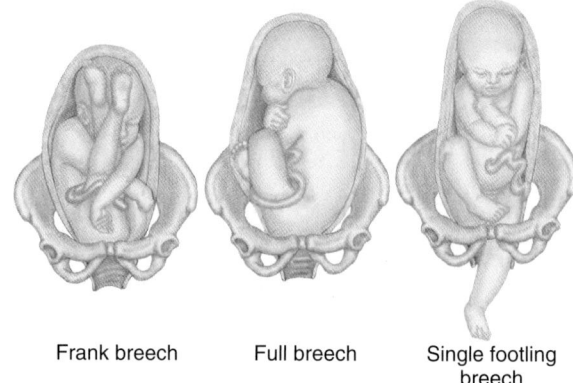

Frank breech   Full breech   Single footling breech

Breech presentation *(McKinney et al, 2013)*

bregma /breg″mə/ [Gk, the front of the head], the junction of the coronal and sagittal sutures on the top of the skull. −**bregmatic,** *adj.*

bremsstrahlung radiation /brems″shträ″lōong/ [Ger, braking radiation], a type of radiation produced by the interaction between projectile electrons and the nuclei of target atoms. Also called **braking radiation, deceleration radiation.**

Brenner tumor [Fritz Brenner, German pathologist, 1877–1969], an uncommon benign ovarian neoplasm consisting of nests or cords of epithelial cells containing glycogen that are enclosed in fibrous connective tissue. The tumor may be solid or cystic and is sometimes difficult to distinguish from certain granulosa-theca cell neoplasms.

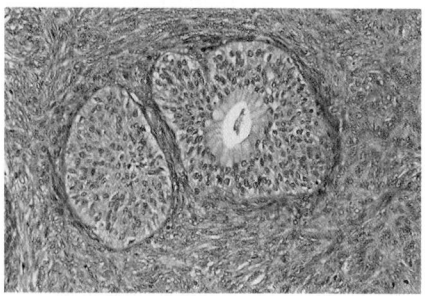

Brenner tumor *(Fletcher, 2007)*

Breslow thickness, the greatest thickness of a primary cutaneous melanoma, measured in millimeters in a biopsy specimen from the granular layer of the epidermis down to the deepest point of invasion. Thickness is one of many prognostic factors identified by the American Joint Committee on Cancer in its cancer staging system. See also **cancer staging.**

Brethine, a beta₂-receptor agonist agent. Brand name for **terbutaline sulfate.**

bretylium tosylate /britil″ē·əm/, an antiarrhythmic agent.

■ INDICATIONS: It is prescribed in the treatment of selected life-threatening ventricular arrhythmias when other measures have not been effective.

■ CONTRAINDICATIONS: Known hypersensitivity to this drug prohibits its use.

■ ADVERSE EFFECTS: Among the more serious adverse reactions are hypotension, nausea and vomiting, anginal pain, and nasal stuffiness.

brevi- /brev′ē-/, prefix meaning "short": *brevicollis.*

brevicollis, shortness of the neck.

Brevicon, a drug combination used as an oral contraceptive. Brand name for **norethindrone, ethinyl estradiol.**

Brevital Sodium, short-acting barbiturate anesthetic. Brand name for **methohexital sodium.**

brewer's yeast /broo″ərz/ [ME, *brewen,* to boil, *yest,* foam], a preparation containing the dried pulverized cells of a yeast, such as *Saccharomyces cerevisiae,* that is used as a leavening agent and as a dietary supplement. It is one of the best sources of the B complex vitamins and a rich source of many minerals and a high grade of protein.

Bricanyl, a beta₂-receptor agonist agent administered via inhalation. Brand name for **terbutaline sulfate.**

brick dust urine, a reddish discoloration signaling precipitated urates in acidic urine.

bridge. See **bridgework.**

bridge of Varolius. See **pons.**

bridgework, a fixed partial denture that is cemented to abutment teeth with a pontic or pontics in between. Also called **bridge.** See also **abutment, pontic, retainer.**

bridging [AS, *brycg*], **1.** a physical rehabilitation technique that strengthens abdominal and leg muscles. Reclining with knees bent, the patient plants the feet on a firm surface and lifts the buttocks off the surface. **2.** (in nursing) a technique for supporting a part of the body, such as the testicles in treating orchitis, using a Bellevue bridge made of a towel or other material. **3.** positioning a patient so that bony prominences are free of pressure on the mattress by using pads, bolsters of foam rubber, or pillows to distribute body weight over a larger surface.

Brief Psychiatric Rating Scale (BPRS), a rating scale for assessing psychopathology on the basis of a small number of items, usually 16 to 24, encompassing psychosis, depression, and anxiety symptoms.

brief psychotherapy, (in psychiatry) treatment directed to the active resolution of personality or behavioral problems rather than to the speculative analysis of the unconscious. It usually concentrates on a specific problem or symptom and is limited to a specified number of sessions with the therapist.

brief psychotic disorder, an episode of psychotic symptoms (incoherence, loosening of associations, delusions, hallucinations, disorganized or catatonic behavior) with sudden onset, lasting less than 1 month. If it occurs in response to a stressful life event, it may be called brief reactive psychosis.

brief reactive psychosis, a short episode, usually less than 2 weeks, of psychotic behavior that occurs in response to a significant psychosocial stressor.

brightness gain /brīt″nes/, the increase in illumination level of a radiograph produced by an image intensifier. It is calculated as the minification gain multiplied by the flux gain. The product is the ratio of the number of photons at the output phosphor to the number at the input phosphor.

Brill-Symmers disease. See **giant follicular lymphoma.**

Brill-Zinsser disease /bril″zin″sər/ [Nathan E. Brill, American physician, 1860–1925; Hans Zinsser, American bacteriologist, 1878–1940], a mild form of epidemic typhus that recurs in a person who appears to have completely recovered from a severe case of the disease years earlier. Some rickettsiae remain in the body after the symptoms of the disease abate, causing the recurrence of symptoms, especially when stress, illness, or malnutrition weakens the person. Treatment with antibiotics may eradicate the organism. See also **epidemic typhus, murine typhus, rickettsiosis, typhus.**

brim, **1.** edge or margin. **2.** the edge of the upper border of the true pelvis, or the pelvic inlet. See also **pelvis.**

brim of true pelvic cavity. See **iliopectineal line.**

brimonidine /bri-mō′ni-dēn/, an alpha-adrenergic receptor agonist used as the tartrate salt in treatment of open-angle glaucoma and ocular hypertension. It is administered topically to the conjunctiva.

Brinnell hardness test [Johann A. Brinnell, Swedish engineer, 1849–1925], a means of determining the surface hardness of a material by measuring the resistance the material offers to the impact of a steel ball. The test result is recorded as the Brinnell hardness number (BHN); harder materials have higher BHNs. The Brinnell hardness test is commonly used to measure abrasion resistance of materials used in dental restorations, such as amalgam, composite, cements, and porcelains. Compare **Knoop hardness test.**

brinzolamide /brin-zo′lah-mīd/, a carbonic anhydrase inhibitor used topically in the treatment of open-angle glaucoma and ocular hypertension.

Briquet syndrome. See **somatization disorder.**

British antilewisite. See **dimercaprol.**

British Medical Association (BMA), a voluntary professional organization of physicians and medical students in the United Kingdom.

British Pharmacopoeia, the official British reference work setting forth standards of strength and purity of medications and containing directions for their preparation to ensure that the same prescription written by different doctors and filled by different pharmacists will contain exactly the same ingredients in the same proportions. The first *British Pharmacopoeia* was published in 1864 by the General Medical Council; it superseded the *London Pharmacopoeia,* which had been published since 1618. See also **British Medical Association,** *United States Pharmacopeia.*

British thermal unit (BTU), a unit of heat energy. The amount of thermal energy that must be absorbed by 1 lb of water to raise its temperature by 1° at 39.2° F. It is also equivalent to 1055 joules or 252 calories.

brittle diabetes, poorly controlled diabetes mellitus in which blood glucose levels are unstable. See also **type 1 diabetes mellitus.**

broach, (in dentistry) an elongated, tapering dental instrument that contains multiple projecting sharp barbs, used in removing pulpal material and cotton or paper points from the pulp canal.

broad beta disease, type III familial hyperlipoproteinemia in which a lipoprotein, high in cholesterol and triglycerides, accumulates in the blood. The condition, which affects males in their twenties and females in their thirties and forties, is characterized by yellowish nodules (xanthomas) on the elbows and knees, peripheral vascular disease, and elevated serum cholesterol levels. Persons with this disease are at risk of development of early coronary disease. Therapy includes dietary measures to reduce weight and levels of serum lipids. Also called **dysbetalipoproteinemia, hyperlipidemia type III.** See also **hyperlipidemia, hyperlipoproteinemia.**

broad ligament [ME, *brood* + L, *ligare,* to tie], a folded sheet of peritoneum draped over the uterine tubes, the uterus, and the ovaries. It extends from the sides of the uterus to the sidewalls of the pelvis, dividing the pelvis from side to side and creating the vesicouterine fossa and pouch in front of the uterus and the rectouterine fossa and pouch behind it. See also **cardinal ligament.**

broad ligament of the liver [ME, *brod* + L, *ligare,* to bind; AS, *lifer*], a crescent-shaped fold of peritoneum attached to the lower surface of the diaphragm, connecting with the liver and the anterior abdominal wall. Also called **falciform ligament of liver.**

broad-spectrum antibiotic, an antibiotic that is effective against a wide range of infectious microorganisms.

Broca aphasia /brō″kə/ [Pierre P. Broca, French neurologist, 1824–1880], a type of aphasia consisting of nonfluent speech, with a laconic and hesitant, telegraphic quality caused by a large dominant hemisphere frontal lesion extending to the central sulcus. The patient's agrammatic speech is characterized by abundant nouns and verbs but few articles and prepositions; the resulting speech is economical but lacking in syntax. Compare **Wernicke aphasia.**

Broca's area [Pierre P. Broca], an area involved in speech production situated on the inferior frontal gyrus of the brain. See also **aphasia, Broca's aphasia, motor speech areas, speech centers.**

Broca's fissure [Pierre P. Broca], a cleft or groove encircling Broca's area in the left frontal area of the brain.

Broca's plane [Pierre P. Broca], a plane that includes the tip of the interalveolar septum between the upper central incisors and the lowest point of the left and right occipital condyles.

Brödel bloodless line, a longitudinal light-colored zone on the anterior surface of the kidney near the convex border, considered to be less vascularized than other areas because it is the border between two areas of arterial distribution.

Brodie abscess [Benjamin Brodie, English surgeon, 1783–1862], **1.** a subacute form of osteomyelitis consisting of a painless staphylococcal infection of bone, usually in the metaphysis of a long bone of a child, characterized by a necrotic cavity surrounded by dense granulation tissue. Also called **circumscribed abscess of bone.** See also **osteomyelitis. 2.** a chronic abscess of bone surrounded by dense fibrous tissue and sclerotic bone.

Brodmann's areas /brod″manz, brōt″mons/ [Korbinian Brodmann, German anatomist, 1868–1918], the 47 different areas of the cerebral cortex that are associated with specific neurological functions and distinguished by different cellular components. They control movements of the lips and vocal cords as well as motor speech. Compare **motor area.** See also **cerebral cortex.**

broken cell preparation. See **homogenate.**

broker, a licensed and regulated person or business assisting individuals in applying for coverage and enrolling in a Qualified Health Plan (QHP) through the Health Care Marketplace in the United Sates. Also called **agent.**

brom, abbreviation for *bromide anion.*

bromazepam /bro-maz′ĕ-pam/, a benzodiazepine used as an antianxiety agent and as a sedative and hypnotic. It is administered orally.

brom-, bromo-, combining form meaning a compound containing bromine or meaning "odor, stench": *bromhidrosis.*

bromelain /brō′məlān/, any of several enzymes that catalyze cleavage of proteins on the carboxyl side of alanine, glycine, lysine, and tyrosine bonds. Differing forms are derived from the fruit (fruit bromelain) and stem (stem bromelain) of the pineapple plant. The enzyme is administered orally as an antiinflammatory agent (especially to relieve swelling in the nasal and paranasal sinuses) and is also used in immunology to render red cells agglutinable by incomplete antibody.

Bromfed, a fixed combination of an antihistamine and a decongestant. Brand name for **brompheniramine maleate,** *pseudoephedrine maleate.*

bromhidrosis /brō′midrō″sis/ [Gk, *bromos,* stench, *hidros,* sweat], an abnormal condition in which the apocrine sweat has an unpleasant odor. The odor is usually caused by bacterial decomposition of perspiration on the skin. Treatment includes frequent bathing, changing of socks and underclothes, and the use of deodorants, antibacterial soaps, and foot powders. Also called **body odor.**

bromide /brō′mīd/ [Gk, *bromos,* stench], an anion of bromine. Bromide salts, once widely prescribed as sedatives, are now seldom used for that purpose because they may cause serious mental disturbances as side effects.

bromide poisoning, an adverse reaction to ingested bromide. Symptoms include nausea, vomiting, an acnelike rash, slurred speech, ataxia, psychotic behavior, and coma.

bromine (Br) /brō″mēn/, a corrosive, toxic red-brown liquid element of the halogen group. Its atomic number is 35; its atomic mass is 79.904. It exists naturally as a diatomic molecule, Br_2. Bromine is used in industry, in photography, in the manufacture of organic chemicals and fuels, and in medications. Bromine gives off a red vapor that is extremely irritating to the eyes and the respiratory tract. Liquid bromine causes serious skin burns. Compounds of bromine have been used as sedatives, hypnotics, and analgesics and are still used in some nonprescription, over-the-counter preparations. Prolonged use of these products may cause brominism, a toxic condition characterized by acneiform eruptions, headache, loss of libido, drowsiness, and fatigue. See also **bromide.**

bromo-. See **brom-, bromo-.**

bromocriptine mesylate /brō′mōkrip″tēn/, a dopamine receptor agonist.

■ INDICATIONS: It is prescribed for the treatment of amenorrhea and galactorrhea associated with hyperprolactinemia, female infertility, and Parkinson's disease.

■ CONTRAINDICATIONS: Sensitivity to any ergot alkaloid prohibits its use. The drug was disqualified for use in suppressing postpartum lactation by the FDA in 1994 because of a previously unrecognized increase in intracranial hemorrhages.

■ ADVERSE EFFECTS: Among the more severe adverse reactions are palpitations, hypotension, bradycardia, hallucinations, syncope, nausea, ataxia, dyspnea, dysphagia, and confusion.

bromoderma /brō′mōdur″mə/ [Gk, *bromos,* stench, *derma,* skin], an acneiform, bullous, or nodular skin rash occurring as a hypersensitivity reaction to ingested bromides.

brompheniramine maleate /brom′fənir″əmin/, an antihistamine.

■ INDICATIONS: It is prescribed in the treatment of allergic reactions, including rhinitis, skin reactions, and itching.

■ CONTRAINDICATIONS: Asthma or known hypersensitivity to this drug prohibits its use. It is not given to newborns, lactating mothers, or other people for whom anticholinergic medications are contraindicated.

■ ADVERSE EFFECTS: Drowsiness, skin rash, hypersensitivity reactions, dry mouth, and tachycardia commonly occur.

Brompton's cocktail [Developed at the Royal Brompton Hospital in England.], *(Obsolete)* an analgesic solution that contained alcohol, morphine or heroin, and, in some cases, a phenothiazine. Formulations varied; it is no longer in use. The cocktail was administered in the control of pain in the terminally ill patient. Also called *Brompton's mixture.*

bronch-, broncho-, combining form meaning "bronchus": *bronchiectasis, bronchodilation.*

bronchi(o)-, prefix meaning relationship to a bronchus. See also **bronch(o)-.**

bronchial /brong′kē·əl/ [Gk, *bronchos,* windpipe], pertaining to the bronchi or bronchioles.

bronchial artery, the nutritive vascular system of the pulmonary tissues, originating from the thoracic aorta or one of its branches. The vascular system interconnects within the lung with branches of the pulmonary arteries and veins.

bronchial asthma. See **asthma.**

bronchial atresia, occlusion or obstruction of a lobar or segmental bronchus, usually in the left upper lobe; the affected lung segment is often hyperinflated because of leakage of air through the alveolar pores.

bronchial breath sound [Gk, *bronchos,* windpipe], a normal sound heard with a stethoscope over the main airways of the lungs, especially the trachea. Expiration and inspiration produce noise of equal loudness and duration, sounding like blowing through a hollow tube. The expiratory sound is heard during the greater part of expiration, whereas the inspiratory sound stops abruptly at the height of inspiration, with a pause before the sound of expiration is heard. Also called **tracheal breath sound.**

bronchial cast, a cylindrical solid or semisolid plug that blocks a bronchus and is sometimes expectorated.

bronchial challenge, bronchial challenge test, a challenge test in which a nonspecific agent such as histamine or methacholine is applied to the bronchi and the bronchi are assessed for a bronchoconstriction reaction. Also called **bronchial provocation.** See **inhalational challenge test.**

bronchial cough, a cough associated with bronchiectasis and heard in its early stages as hacking and irritating, becoming looser in later stages.

bronchial drainage. See **postural drainage.**

bronchial fremitus, a vibration that can be palpated on the chest wall (usually the posterior thorax) over a bronchus. It results from congestion by secretions that rattle as air passes during respiration. See also **fremitus.**

bronchial hyperreactivity [Gk, *bronchos* + *hyper,* excess; L, *re,* again, *agere,* to act], an abnormal respiratory condition characterized by reflex bronchospasm in response to histamine or a cholinergic drug, such as methacholine. It is a universal feature of asthma and is used in the differential diagnosis of asthma and heart disease.

bronchial murmur, a murmur heard as a blowing sound, caused by air flowing in and out of the bronchial tubes.

bronchial pneumonia. See **bronchopneumonia.**

bronchial provocation. See **bronchial challenge, bronchial challenge test.**

bronchial secretion, a substance produced in the bronchial tree that consists of mucus secreted by the goblet cells and mucous glands of the bronchi, protein salts released from disintegrating cells, plasma fluid, and proteins, including fibrinogen, that have escaped from pulmonary capillaries.

bronchial spasm. *(Informal)* See **bronchospasm.**

bronchial toilet, special care that is given to patients with tracheostomies and respiratory disorders, including stimulation of coughing, deep breathing, and suctioning of the respiratory tract with a tracheobronchial aspiration pump.

bronchial tree, an anatomical complex of the trachea and bronchi. The bronchi branch from the trachea. The right bronchus is wider and shorter than the left bronchus and branches into three secondary bronchi, one passing to each of the three lobes of the right lung. The left bronchus is smaller in diameter and about twice as long as the right bronchus. It is also more horizontal and more susceptible to obstruction.

It branches into the secondary bronchi for the inferior and the superior lobes of the left lung. The bronchus is sometimes described as a bronchial tube.

bronchial tube. See **bronchus.**

bronchial washing [Gk, *bronchos,* windpipe; ME, *was-shen,* to wash], irrigation of the bronchi and bronchioles performed during bronchoscopy to cleanse the tubes and to collect specimens for laboratory examination.

bronchiectasis /brong′kē·ek″tə·sis/ [Gk, *bronchos* + *ektasis,* stretching], an abnormal condition of the bronchial tree characterized by irreversible dilation and destruction of the bronchial walls. The condition is sometimes congenital but is more often a result of bronchial infection or of obstruction by a tumor or an aspirated foreign body. Symptoms include a constant cough producing copious purulent sputum; hemoptysis; chronic sinusitis; clubbing of fingers; and persistent moist, coarse crackles. Some of the complications of bronchiectasis are pneumonia, lung abscess, empyema, brain abscess, and amyloidosis. Treatment includes frequent postural drainage, expectorants, antibiotics, and, rarely, surgical resection of the affected part of the lungs.

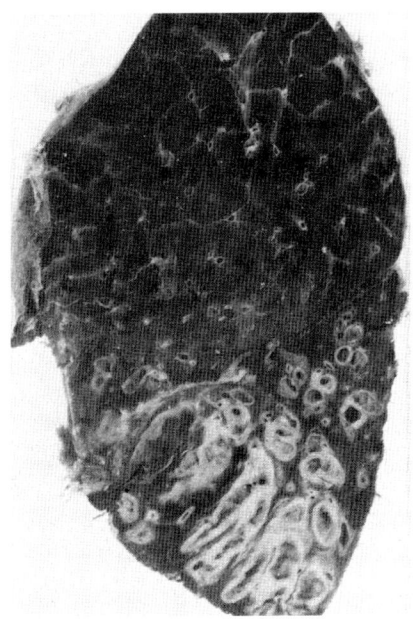

Bronchiectasis *(Irwin and Tecklin, 2004)*

■ OBSERVATIONS: The individual is often asymptomatic early in the disease. A chronic cough with sputum production is the most common presenting sign. Hemoptysis, recurrent pneumonia, dyspnea, wheezing, and fatigue are also frequently seen. Fever, night sweats, weight loss, fetid breath, and hemoptysis may also be present. Moist crackles in lung bases may be heard on auscultation. Sputum appears purulent and foamy with sediment and has a large number of WBCs. Sputum cultures and Gram's stain are used to identify microorganisms. Chest x-rays reveal increased markings, honeycombing, and tram tracking. Pulmonary function studies show a decrease in vital capacity and expiratory flow. CT scans are used to detect cystic lesions and rule out neoplastic obstruction. Bronchography may be used when surgery is contemplated to visualize bronchiectatic areas. Clubbed fingers, pulmonary hypertension, right ventricular failure, and cor pulmonale are complications associated with long-standing disease.

■ INTERVENTIONS: Acute treatment includes medications, such as mucolytics to clear secretions; antibiotics to treat bacterial infection; and bronchodilators to reduce dyspnea. Chest physiotherapy, with postural drainage, is used to clear secretions. Adequate hydration and a vaporizer help liquefy secretions. Supplemental oxygen is administered for hypoxemia. Bronchial resection is used to treat confined disease, which is unresponsive to conservative therapy.

■ PATIENT CARE CONSIDERATIONS: The focus of nursing, medical, and respiratory therapy care during acute episodes is to promote airway clearance and effective breathing patterns through respiratory monitoring, cough enhancement, anxiety reduction, and rest. Preventive and chronic care focuses on avoidance of air pollution and contact with individuals with respiratory infections; prompt identification and treatment of respiratory infection; maintenance of adequate nutrition and hydration; smoking cessation as applicable; and use of influenza and pneumonia vaccines for prophylaxis.

bronchiolar. See **bronchiole.**

bronchiolar collapse /brong″kyələr/ [L, *bronchiolus,* little windpipe, *conlabi,* to fall], a condition in which bronchioles, which are pliable and lack cartilaginous support, become compressed by surrounding structures in the absence of inflowing air needed to keep them inflated. The condition occurs in disorders such as emphysema, cystic fibrosis, and bronchiectasis.

bronchiole /brong″kē·ōl/ [L, *bronchiolus,* little windpipe], a small airway of the respiratory system extending from the bronchi into the lobes of the lung. There are two divisions of bronchioles: The terminal bronchioles passively conduct inspired air from the bronchi to the respiratory bronchioles and expired air from the respiratory bronchioles to the bronchi. The respiratory bronchioles function similarly, allowing the exchange of air and waste gases between the alveolar ducts and the terminal bronchioles. –**bronchiolar,** *adj.*

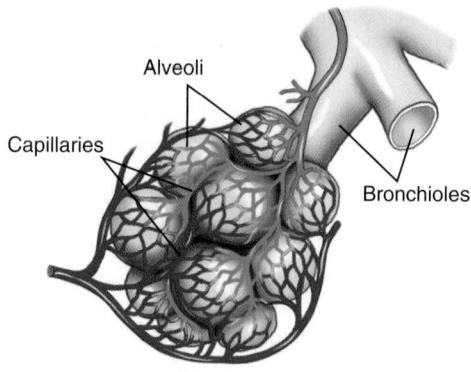

Bronchioles *(LaFleur Brooks, 2014)*

bronchiolitis /brong″kē·ōlī″tis/ [L, *bronchiolus,* little windpipe; Gk, *itis,* inflammation], an acute viral infection of the lower respiratory tract that occurs primarily in infants less than 12 months of age. It begins as a mild upper respiratory tract infection and over a period of 2 to 3 days develops into more severe respiratory distress. It is characterized by expiratory wheezing, inflammation, and obstruction at the level of the bronchioles. The most common causative agents are the respiratory syncytial viruses (RSVs) and the parainfluenza viruses. Mycoplasma pneumoniae, rhinoviruses, enteroviruses, and measles virus are less common causative agents. Transmission occurs by infection with airborne particles or by contact with infected secretions. The diagnosis consists of

evidence of hyperinflation of the lungs through percussion or chest x-ray.

■ OBSERVATIONS: The condition typically begins as an upper respiratory tract infection with serious nasal discharge and often with low-grade fever. Increasing respiratory distress follows, characterized by tachypnea, tachycardia, intercostal and subcostal retractions, a paroxysmal cough, an expiratory wheeze, and often an elevated temperature. The chest may appear barrel-shaped; x-ray films show hyperinflated lungs and a depressed diaphragm. Respiration becomes more shallow, causing increased alveolar oxygen tension and leading to respiratory acidosis. Complete obstruction and absorption of trapped air may lead to atelectasis and respiratory failure. Blood gas determinations indicate the degree of carbon dioxide retention.

■ INTERVENTIONS: Routine treatment includes administering humidity and mist, generally combined with oxygen; ensuring an adequate fluid intake, usually given intravenously because of tachypnea, weakness, and fatigue; suctioning the airways to remove secretions; and promoting rest. Endotracheal intubation is indicated when carbon dioxide retention occurs, when bronchial secretions do not loosen and clear, or when oxygen therapy does not alleviate hypoxia. Such medications as antibiotics, bronchodilators, corticosteroids, cough suppressants, and expectorants are not routinely used. Ribavirin may be used when RSV is the causative agent but is generally used only in the high-risk population. Sedatives are contraindicated because of their suppressant effect on the respiratory tract. The infection typically runs its course in 7 to 10 days, with good prognosis. The disorder is often confused with asthma. A family history of allergy, the presence of other allergic manifestations, and improvement with epinephrine injection are usually indicative of asthma, not bronchiolitis. Cystic fibrosis, pertussis, the bronchopneumonias, and foreign body obstruction of the trachea are other disorders that may be confused with bronchiolitis.

■ PATIENT CARE CONSIDERATIONS: The focus of care is to promote rest and to conserve the child's energy by reducing anxiety and apprehension; to increase the ease of breathing with humidity and oxygen as needed; to aid in changing position for comfort; and to induce drainage of secretions or to suction when necessary. Vital signs and chest and breath sounds are continuously monitored to detect early signs of respiratory distress.

bronchiolitis obliterans, a form of bronchiolitis in which the exudate is not expectorated but becomes organized and obliterates the bronchial tubes, causing collapse of the affected part of the lungs.

bronchiospasm. See **bronchospasm.**

bronchitis /brongkī″tis/ [Gk, *bronchos,* windpipe, *itis,* inflammation], acute or chronic inflammation of the mucous membranes of the tracheobronchial tree. Caused by the spread of upper respiratory viral or sometimes bacterial infections to the bronchi, it is often observed with or after childhood infections, such as measles, whooping cough, diphtheria, and typhoid fever. See also **chronic bronchitis, chronic obstructive pulmonary disease, respiratory syncytial virus.**

■ OBSERVATIONS: Acute bronchitis is frequently preceded by an upper respiratory infection. The most common presenting sign is a dry, hacking cough that increasingly produces viscous mucus. Other symptoms include low-grade fever, substernal pain, and fatigue. Rhonchi and occasional wheezing may be heard when auscultating lungs. Diagnosis is usually made from the type of cough and sputum. Chest x-rays are taken to rule out other disorders. Arterial blood gases are monitored when the underlying chronic disease is present, and sputum is cultured for evidence of superimposed infection. Pneumonia is the most common complication. Acute respiratory failure occurs in some individuals with underlying pulmonary disease. Chronic bronchitis may be asymptomatic for years. A productive cough with copious mucopurulent sputum, peripheral cyanosis, and variable dyspnea are typical presenting signs. The cough becomes increasingly progressive and the sputum production more copious. Wheezing, tachypnea, and tachycardia may also be present. Several attacks per year are common. Chest x-rays reveal cardiac enlargement, congested lung fields, and thickened bronchial markings. Pulmonary function studies show increased residual volume and decreases in forced vital capacity and forced expiratory volume. PaO_2 is decreased and $PaCO_2$ increased on arterial blood gas results. Sputum cultures show presence of multiple microorganisms and neutrophils. Cor pulmonale, pulmonary hypertension, right ventricular hypertrophy, and respiratory failure are common complications seen in chronic bronchitis.

■ INTERVENTIONS: Treatment for acute episodes include medications, such as inhaled bronchodilators for wheezing, expectorants for cough, and antipyretics for fever. Antiinfective drugs are used only with concomitant chronic obstructive pulmonary disease (COPD) or a superimposed infection. Adequate hydration and a vaporizer help liquefy secretions. Treatment for chronic bronchitis includes antiinfective drugs for infection, bronchodilators to reduce dyspnea, and corticosteroids to reduce inflammation. Chest physiotherapy is used to loosen secretions. Oxygenation is used for hypoxia. Health promotion in individuals with chronic disease include a consistent exercise program to improve ventilatory and cardiac function; smoking cessation programs and use of flu and pneumonia vaccines for prophylaxis.

■ PATIENT CARE CONSIDERATIONS: The focus of care during acute episodes is supportive and includes rest, increased fluids, and use of a steam vaporizer. Education plays a large role for those suffering from chronic bronchitis and includes information on the disease process; instruction on medication administration (schedule and use of spacer), home use of oxygen, chest physiotherapy program, effective coughing, exercise program, nutrition plan to decrease weight if indicated, smoking cessation if indicated, and proper use of respirators in workplace if exposed to respiratory irritants. Importance of long-term and consistent follow-up should be stressed.

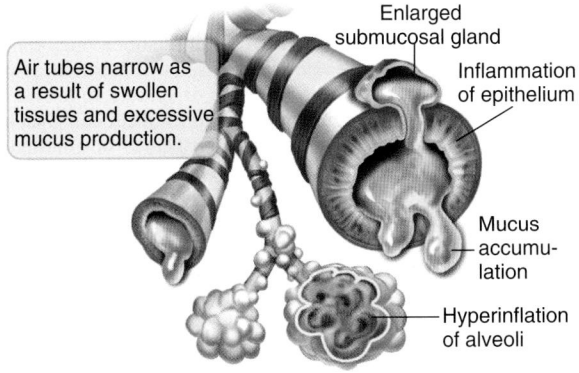

Chronic bronchitis (Patton, 2016)

bronch(o)-, combining form meaning relationship to a bronchus. See also **bronchi(o)-.**

bronchoalveolar /-alvē″ələr/ [Gk, *bronchos,* windpipe; L, *alveolus,* little hollow], pertaining to the terminal air sacs at the ends of the bronchioles.

bronchoalveolar lavage (BAL), a diagnostic procedure in which small amounts of physiological solution are injected through a fiberoptic bronchoscope into a specific area of the lung, while the rest of the lung is sequestered by an inflated balloon. The fluid is then aspirated and inspected for pathogens, malignant cells, and mineral bodies.

bronchoaortic constriction, thoracic constriction of esophagus.

bronchoconstriction [Gk, *bronchos,* windpipe; L, *constringere,* to draw tight], a narrowing of the lumen of the bronchi, restricting airflow to and from the lungs.

bronchodilation /-di′lā″shən/ [Gk, *bronchos,* windpipe; L, *dilatare,* to widen], a widening of the lumen of the bronchi, allowing increased airflow to and from the lungs.

bronchodilator /-dilā″tər/, a substance, especially a drug, that relaxes contractions of the smooth muscle of the bronchioles to improve ventilation to the lungs. Pharmacological bronchodilators are prescribed to improve aeration in asthma, bronchiectasis, bronchitis, and emphysema. Commonly used bronchodilators include albuterol, ipratropium, and combinations of these drugs. The adverse effects vary, depending on the particular class of the bronchodilating drug. In general, bronchodilators are given with caution to people with impaired cardiac function. Nervousness, irritability, gastritis, or palpitations of the heart may occur.

bronchofibroscopy, the visual examination of the tracheobronchial tree through a fiberoptic bronchoscope. It can be used for the collection of sputum or tissue samples in the diagnosis of pneumonia or cancer. It is also used for diagnosing/treating hemoptysis. See also **fiberoptic bronchoscopy.**

bronchogenic /-jen″ik/ [Gk, *bronchos* + *genein,* to produce], originating in the bronchi.

bronchogenic adenocarcinoma, the more common type of adenocarcinoma of the lung. See also **adenocarcinoma of the lung.**

bronchogenic carcinoma, one of the more than 90% of malignant lung tumors that originate in bronchi. Lesions, usually resulting from cigarette smoking, may cause coughing and wheezing, fatigue, chest tightness, and aching joints. In the late stages, bloody sputum, clubbing of the fingers, weight loss, and pleural effusion may be present. Diagnosis is made by bronchoscopy, sputum cytological examination, lymph node biopsy, radioisotope scanning procedures, or exploratory surgery. Surgery is the most effective treatment, but well over 50% of cases are unresectable when first detected. Palliative treatment includes radiotherapy and chemotherapy.

bronchogenic cyst, a cyst that develops in the lungs or mediastinum. It may be asymptomatic or cause cough, stridor, wheezing, or dyspnea. It may also become infected or malignant, requiring surgical removal.

bronchography /brongkog″rəfē/, an x-ray visualization of the bronchi after they have been coated with a radiopaque substance.

broncholithiasis /-lithī″əsis/, inflammation of the bronchi caused by an accumulation of hard concretions or stones on their lining.

bronchomediastinal trunk, one of the two lymphatic vessels, right and left, that drain the lung and bronchi, mediastinal structures, and thoracic wall.

bronchomotor tone, the state of contraction or relaxation of the smooth muscle in the bronchial walls that regulates the caliber of the airways.

Air tubes narrow as a result of swollen tissues and excessive mucus production.

Enlarged submucosal gland

Inflammation of epithelium

Mucus accumulation

Hyperinflation of alveoli

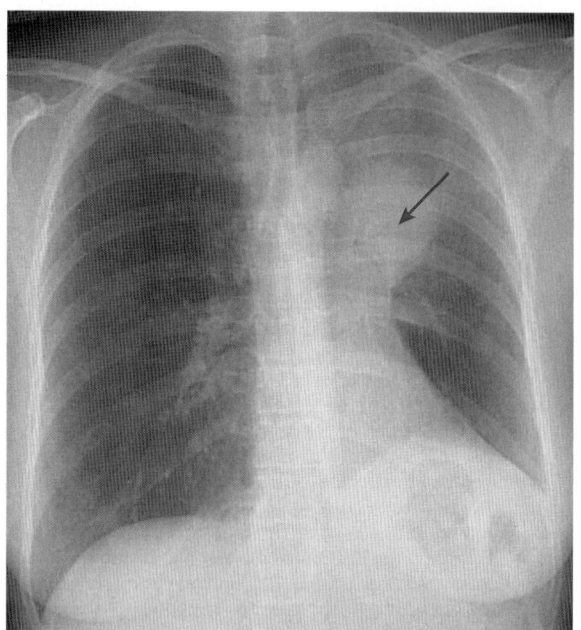

Bronchogenic carcinoma—in a radiograph *(Klatt, 2015)*

bronchophony /brongkof″ənē/ [Gk, *bronchos* + *phone,* voice], an increase in the intensity and clarity of vocal resonance that may result from an increase in lung tissue density, such as in the consolidation of pneumonia. It is assessed by having the patient repeat a word such as "ninety-nine" during auscultation.

bronchopleural fistula /-ploor″əl/, an abnormal passageway between a bronchus and the pleural cavity.

bronchopneumonia [Gk, *bronchos* + *pneumon,* lung], an acute inflammation of the lungs and bronchioles, characterized by chills, fever, high pulse and respiratory rates, bronchial breathing, cough with purulent bloody sputum, severe chest pain, and abdominal distension. The disease is usually a result of the spread of infection from the upper to the lower respiratory tract, most commonly caused by the bacterium *Mycoplasma pneumoniae, Staphylococcus pyogenes,* or *Streptococcus pneumoniae.* Atypical forms of bronchopneumonia may occur in viral and rickettsial infections. The most common cause in infancy is the respiratory syncytial virus. Bronchopneumonia may lead to pleural effusion, empyema, lung abscess, peripheral thrombophlebitis, respiratory failure, congestive heart failure, and jaundice. Treatment includes administration of an antibiotic, oxygen therapy, supportive measures to keep the bronchi clear of secretions, and relief of pleural pain. Also called **bronchial pneumonia, catarrhal pneumonia.** Compare **aspiration pneumonia, eosinophilic pneumonia, interstitial pneumonia.** See also **lobar pneumonia, respiratory syncytial virus.**

bronchoprovocation inhalation test, a pulmonary function test performed on patients with a history of asthma who have normal pulmonary function at rest. In a specific test, the patient inhales a particular antigen while the forced expiratory volume (FEV) is measured. In a nonspecific test, the patient inhales a substance such as histamine periodically at increasing concentrations while the FEV is measured.

bronchopulmonary /-pul″mōner′ē/ [Gk, *bronchos* + L, *pulmonis,* lung], pertaining to the bronchi and the lungs.

bronchopulmonary dysplasia (BPD) /-pool″məner′ē/, a chronic respiratory disorder characterized by scarring of lung tissue, thickened pulmonary arterial walls, and mismatch between lung ventilation and perfusion. It often occurs in infants who have been dependent on long-term artificial ventilation.

bronchopulmonary hygiene, the care and cleanliness of the respiratory tract and of ventilatory/respiratory therapy equipment. Hygienic care may include providing assistance with postural drainage and controlled coughing techniques, percussion, vibration, and nasotracheal or endotracheal suctioning. Respiratory care equipment is a potential source and reservoir of infectious organisms and must be cleaned and sterilized periodically.

bronchopulmonary lavage [Gk, *bronchos,* windpipe; L, *pulmonis,* lung; Fr, *lavage,* washing out], the irrigation or washing out of the bronchi and bronchioles to remove pulmonary secretions.

bronchopulmonary segment, the area of lung supplied by a segmental bronchus and its accompanying pulmonary artery branch. Each segment is shaped like an irregular cone with the apex at the origin of the segmental bronchus and the base projected peripherally onto the surface of the lung.

bronchoscope /brong″kəskōp′/, a curved, flexible tube for visual examination of the bronchi. It contains fibers that carry light down the tube and project an enlarged image up the tube to the viewer. The bronchoscope is used to examine the bronchi, to secure a specimen for biopsy or culture, or to aspirate secretions or a foreign body from the respiratory tract. See also **fiberoptic bronchoscopy.** *–bronchoscopic, adj.*

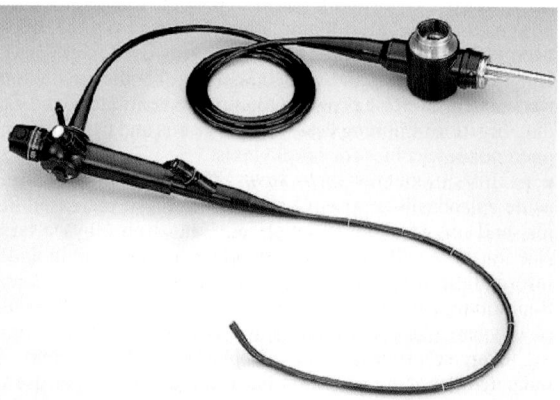

Fiberoptic bronchoscope *(Courtesy Olympus America, Inc.)*

bronchoscopy /brongkos″kəpē/, the visual examination of the tracheobronchial tree, using the standard rigid, tubular metal bronchoscope or the narrower, flexible fiberoptic bronchoscope. The procedure also may be used for suctioning, for obtaining a biopsy specimen and fluid or sputum for examination, for removing foreign bodies, and for diagnosing such conditions as localized atelectasis, bronchial obstruction, lung abscess, and tracheal extubation. See also **bronchial washing, bronchoscope.**

bronchospasm /-spaz′əm/, an excessive and prolonged contraction of the smooth muscle of the bronchi and bronchioles, resulting in an acute narrowing and obstruction of the respiratory airway. The contractions may be localized or general and may be caused by irritation or injury to the respiratory mucosa, infections, or allergies. A cough with generalized wheezing usually indicates the condition. Bronchospasm is a chief characteristic of asthma. Treatment includes the use of active bronchodilators, catecholamines, corticosteroids, or methylxanthines and preventive drugs such as cromolyn sodium. Also called **bronchial spasm, bronchiospasm.** See also **asthma, bronchitis.**

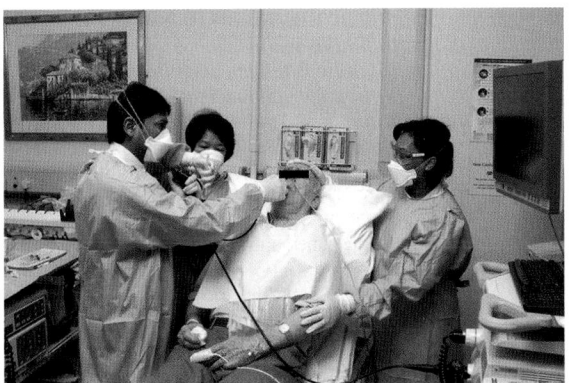

Bronchoscopy *(Shah, 2007)*

bronchospirometry /-spīrom″ətrē/, a technique for the study of the ventilation and gas exchange of each lung separately by the introduction of a catheter into either the left or the right mainstem bronchus. A double-lumen tube permits simultaneous but separate sampling of the gas from both lungs.

bronchotracheal. See **tracheobronchial.**

bronchovesicular /-vesik″yələr/, pertaining to the bronchi, bronchioles, and alveoli.

bronchovesicular sounds [Gk, *bronchos,* windpipe; L, *vesicula,* small bladder, *sonus,* sound], one of three normal breath sounds that occurs between the sounds of the bronchial tubes and those of the alveoli, or a combination of the two sounds.

bronchus /brong′kəs/ *pl. bronchi* [L; Gk, *bronchos,* windpipe], any one of several large air passages in the lungs through which pass inhaled air and exhaled air. Each bronchus has a wall consisting of three layers. The outermost is made of dense fibrous tissue and reinforced with cartilage. The middle layer is a network of smooth muscle. The innermost layer consists of ciliated mucous membrane. Also called **bronchial tube.** Kinds include **lobar bronchus, primary bronchus, segmental bronchus.** See also **bronchiole.** –**bronchial,** *adj.*

Bronkodyl, a bronchial smooth muscle relaxant. Brand name for **theophylline.**

Brønsted acid [Johannes N. Brønsted, Danish physical chemist, 1879–1947], a molecule or an ion that acts as a hydrogen ion donor.

Brønsted base [Johannes N. Brønsted], a molecule or an ion that acts as a hydrogen ion acceptor.

brontophobia, fear of thunder. Also called **tonitrophobia.**

bronze diabetes, *(Nontechnical)* iron overload. Now called **hereditary hemochromatosis.**

broth, **1.** a fluid culture medium, such as a solution of lactose or thioglycollate, used to support the growth of bacteria for laboratory analysis. **2.** a beverage or other clear fluid made with meat extract and water, such as chicken bouillon.

Brovana, long-acting beta₂ agonist. Brand name for **arformoterol.**

brow, the forehead, particularly the eyebrow or ridge above the eye.

brow lift, forehead lift. It is the removal or alteration of muscles and tissues of forehead to raise the eyebrows and minimize frown lines. Compare **blepharoplasty.**

Brown-Adson forceps [James B. Brown, American plastic surgeon, 1899–1971; Alfred W. Adson, American neurosurgeon, 1887–1951]. See **Adson-Brown forceps.**

brown fat [ME, *broun* + AS, *faett,* filled], a type of fat present in newborns and rarely found in adults. Brown fat is a unique source of heat energy for the infant because it has greater thermogenic activity than ordinary fat. Brown fat deposits occur around the kidneys, neck, and upper chest.

Brownian motion /brou″nyən/ [Robert Brown, Scottish botanist, 1773–1858], a random movement of microscopic particles suspended in a liquid or gas, such as the continuing erratic behavior of dust particles in still water. The movement is produced by the natural kinetic activity of molecules of the fluid that strike the foreign particles. Also called *Brownian movement.*

brown recluse spider, a small poisonous arachnid, *Loxosceles reclusa,* also known as the brown or violin spider, found in both North and South America. The bite produces a characteristic necrotic lesion. The venom from its bite usually creates a blister surrounded by concentric white and red circles. This so-called bull's-eye appearance is helpful in distinguishing it from other spider bites. There is little or no initial pain, but localized pain develops in about an hour. The patient may experience systemic symptoms; nausea, fever, and chills are common, but the reaction is usually self-limited. Immediate treatment includes keeping the victim quiet and immobilizing the bite area at the level of the heart. A bleb forms, sometimes in a target or bull's-eye pattern. The blood-filled bleb increases in size and eventually ruptures, leaving a black scar. Antivenin is not available in the United States or Canada.

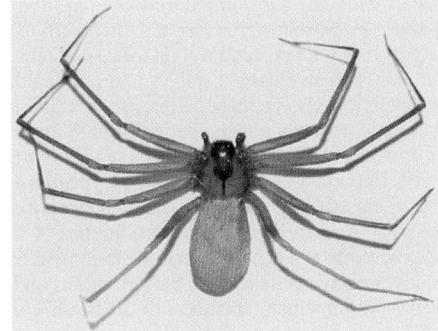

Brown recluse spider *(Courtesy Indiana University Medical Center)*

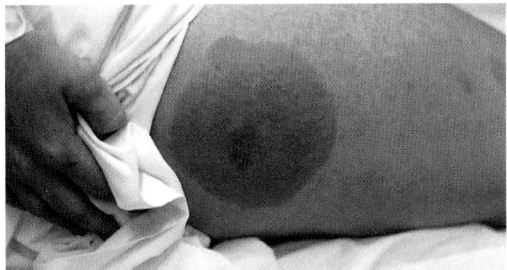

Brown recluse spider bite after 48 hours *(Auerbach, 2012)*

Brown-Séquard's syndrome /broun″sākärz″/ [Charles E. Brown-Séquard, French physiologist, 1817–1894], a traumatic neurological disorder resulting from compression or transection of one side of the spinal cord above the tenth thoracic vertebrae, characterized by spastic paralysis and loss of postural sense (proprioception) on the body's injured side, and loss of the senses of pain and heat on the other side of the body.

brown spider. See **brown recluse spider.**

brow presentation, presentation in which the brow, or forehead, of the fetus is the first part of the body to enter the birth canal. Because the diameter of the fetal head at this angle may be greater than that of the mother's pelvic outlet, a cesarean section may be recommended. However, the fetus usually converts to a vertex presentation. If not and labor is obstructed, alternatives for delivery include rotation of the fetal head using forceps or cesarean section.

Brucella abortus. See **abortus fever.**

brucellosis /broo′səlō′sis/ [David Bruce, English pathologist, 1855–1931], a disease caused by any of several species of the gram-negative coccobacillus *Brucella*: *Brucella melitensis, B. abortus, B. suis,* and *B. canis,* the latter of which is very rare and causes only mild illness. It is primarily a disease of animals (including cattle, pigs, sheep, camels, goats, and dogs); humans usually acquire it by ingestion of contaminated milk or milk products or raw meat or marrow, through a break in the skin, through contact with an infected animal, or through inhalation of dust from contaminated soil. Brucellosis is most prevalent in rural areas among farmers, veterinarians, meat-packers, slaughterhouse workers, and livestock producers. Laboratory workers are also at risk. Also called **Cyprus fever,** *dust fever,* **Gibraltar fever, Malta fever, Mediterranean fever, rock fever, undulant fever.** See also **abortus fever.**

■ OBSERVATIONS: It is characterized by fever, chills, sweating, malaise, and weakness. The fever often occurs in waves, rising in the evening and subsiding during the day, and at intervals separated by periods of remission. Other signs and symptoms may include anorexia and weight loss, headache, muscle and joint pain, and an enlarged spleen, and orchiepididymitis in young men. In some victims the disease is acute; more often it is chronic, recurring over a period of months or years.

■ INTERVENTIONS: Although brucellosis itself is rarely fatal, treatment is important because serious complications such as pneumonia, endocarditis, meningitis, and encephalitis can occur. Additionally, brucellosis can be debilitating. A combination of doxycycline and gentamycin is the treatment of choice. Additonally, treatments depend on the symptoms and will require intervention by many members of the health care team.

■ PATIENT CARE CONSIDERATIONS: This organism is considered a potential agent of bioterrorism due to its low infectious dose (10–100 organisms) and method of infection by way of aerosol, allowing distribution over a large area.

Brudzinski sign /broodzin″skē/ [Josef Brudzinski, Polish physician, 1874–1917], an involuntary flexion of the hip and knee when the neck is passively flexed. It can occur in patients with meningitis. Compare **Kernig sign.**

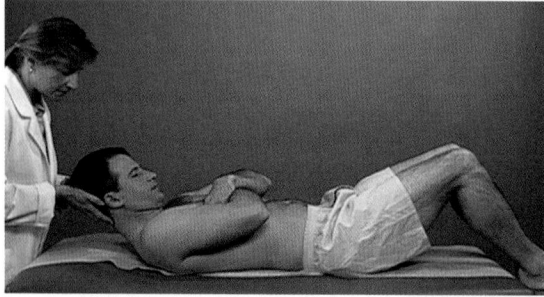

Brudzinski sign (Ball et al, 2015)

Brueghel syndrome. See **Meige disease.**

Brugia /bruj′ə/ [S.L. Brug, Dutch parasitologist in Indonesia, 1879–1946], a genus of nematodes of the superfamily Filarioidea that parasitize humans and other mammals. See also **filariasis.**

bruise. *(Informal)* See **contusion, ecchymosis.**

bruit /broo′ē/ [Fr, noise], an abnormal blowing or swishing sound or murmur heard while auscultating a carotid artery, the aorta, an organ, or a gland, such as the liver or thyroid, and resulting from blood flowing through a narrow or partially occluded artery. The specific character of the bruit, its location, and the time of its occurrence in a cycle of other sounds are all of diagnostic importance. Bruits are usually of low frequency and are heard best with the bell of a stethoscope.

Brunnstrom hemiplegia classification [Signe Brunnstrom, Swedish physical therapist], a poststroke evaluation to measure the degree of recovery; it assesses muscle tone and voluntary control of movement patterns. Results indicate the patient's progress through stages of recovery.

brush biopsy, the use of a catheter with bristles that is inserted into the body to collect cells from tissues.

brush border, microvilli on the free surfaces of certain epithelial cells, particularly the absorptive surfaces of the intestine and the proximal convoluted tubules of the kidney.

Brushfield spots [Thomas Brushfield, English physician, 1858–1937; ME, *spotte,* stain], pinpoint white or light yellow spots on the iris of a child with Down syndrome. Occasionally, they are seen in infants without the syndrome.

Bruton agammaglobulinemia [Ogden C. Bruton, American physician, 1908–2003], a sex-linked, inherited condition characterized by the absence of gamma globulin in the blood. Those (usually children) affected by the syndrome are deficient in antibodies and susceptible to repeated infections. Compare **agammaglobulinemia.**

bruxism /bruk′sizəm/ [Gk, *brychein,* to gnash the teeth], the compulsive, conscious or unconscious grinding or clenching of the teeth, especially during sleep or as a mechanism for releasing tension during periods of extreme stress in the waking hours. Also called **bruxomania, attrition.**

bruxomania. See **bruxism.**

Bryant's traction [Thomas Bryant, English physician, 1828–1914; L, *trahere,* to pull], an orthopedic mechanism used to immobilize both lower extremities in the treatment of a fractured femur or in the correction of a congenital hip dislocation. The mechanism consists of a traction frame supporting weights, which are connected by ropes that run through pulleys to traction foot plates. The traction pull elevates the lower extremities to a vertical position with the patient supine, the trunk and the lower extremities forming a right angle. The weight applied to the traction mechanism is usually less than 35 lbs. Compare **Buck's traction.**

BSA, abbreviation for **body surface area.**

BSE, abbreviation for **self-breast examination, bovine spongiform encephalopathy.**

BSN, initialism used informally in the United States and most of Canada to denote a Bachelor of Science in Nursing degree as well as other bachelor's degrees with a major in nursing, such as BSc, BscN, BS, and BA. See **Bachelor of Science in Nursing.**

BT, abbreviation for **bleeding time.**

BTPD, initialism for *body temperature, ambient pressure, dry.*

BTPS, abbreviation for *body temperature, ambient pressure, saturated (with water vapor).* See **volume BTPS.**

BTU, abbreviation for **British thermal unit.**

buba, a single primary lesion caused by a spirochete. See **yaws.**

bubble-diffusion humidifier, a device that provides humidified oxygen or other therapeutic gases by allowing the gas to bubble through a reservoir of water.

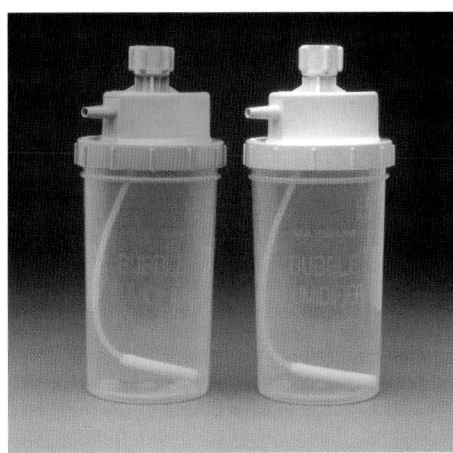

Bubble-diffusion humidifiers *(Courtesy Allied Health Care)*

bubble goniometer, a device used for measuring joint angles, consisting of a spirit level and a pendulum. Compare **gravity goniometer.** See also **goniometry.**

bubble oxygenator, a heart-lung device that oxygenates the blood while it is diverted outside the patient's body.

bubo /byoo″bo/ *pl. buboes* [Gk, *boubon,* groin], a greatly enlarged, tender, inflamed lymph node usually in the groin that is associated with diseases such as chancroid, lymphogranuloma venereum, and syphilis. Treatment includes specific antibiotic therapy, application of moist heat, and sometimes incision and drainage.

bubonic plague /byoobon″ik/ [Gk, *boubon,* groin; L, *plaga,* stroke], the most common form of plague. The symptoms are caused by an endotoxin released by a bacillus, *Yersinia pestis,* usually introduced into the body by the bite of a rat flea that has bitten an infected rat. Inoculation with plague vaccine confers partial immunity; infection provides lifetime immunity. Also called **black death, black plague.** Compare **pneumonic plague, septicemic plague.** See also **bubo, plague,** *Yersinia pestis.*

■ OBSERVATIONS: It is characterized by painful buboes in the axilla, groin, or neck; fever often rising to 106° F (41.11° C); prostration with a rapid, thready pulse; hypotension; delirium; and bleeding into the skin from the superficial blood vessels.

■ INTERVENTIONS: Treatment includes antibiotics, supportive nursing care, surgical drainage of buboes, isolation, and stringent precautions against spread of the disease.

■ PATIENT CARE CONSIDERATIONS: Conditions favor a plague epidemic when a large infected rodent population lives with a large nonimmune human population in a damp, warm climate. Improved sanitary conditions and eradication of rats and other rodent reservoirs of *Y. pestis* may prevent outbreaks of the disease. Killing the infected rodents, which may include ground squirrels and rabbits, and not the fleas allows a continued threat of human infection. It is a possible agent of bioterrorism if the bacilli are aerosolized and has the highest potential for negative public health consequences.

bucardia /bookär″dē·ə/, *(Obsolete)* extreme enlargement of the heart.

bucca-. See **bucco-, bucc-, bucca-, bucci-.**

buccal /buk″əl/ *pl. bucca* [L, *bucca,* cheek], pertaining to the inside of the cheek, the surface of a tooth, or the gum beside the cheek.

buccal administration of medication, oral administration of a drug, usually in the form of a tablet, by placing it between the cheek and the teeth or gum until it dissolves.

buccal artery, a branch of the maxillary artery that supplies the buccinator muscle, the skin, and mucous membrane of the cheek. See also **buccinator.**

buccal bar, a portion of an orthodontic appliance consisting of a rigid metal wire that extends anteriorly from the buccal side of a molar band. See also **arch bar, labial bar, lingual bar.**

buccal cavity, the vestibule of the mouth, specifically the area lying between the teeth and cheeks.

buccal contour [L, *bucca* + *cum,* together with, *tornare,* to turn], the shape of the buccal side of a posterior tooth. It is usually characterized by a slight occlusocervical convexity that has its largest prominence at the gingival third of the clinical buccal surface.

buccal exotosis, a nonmalignant surface growth occurring on the outer or facial surface of the maxilla and/or mandible, usually found in the premolar and molar region.

buccal fat pad, a fat pad in the cheek under the subcutaneous layer of the skin and over the buccinator muscle. It is particularly prominent in infants and is often called a sucking pad.

buccal fentanyl, an opioid analgesic. The tablet formulation is placed in the mouth to dissolve.

■ INDICATIONS: This drug is used to treat breakthrough pain in cancer patients who are taking regularly scheduled doses of another opiate pain medication and who are tolerant to opiates.

■ CONTRAINDICATIONS: Known intolerance or hypersensitivity to this drug or its components prohibits its use. This drug must not be used in the management of acute or postoperative pain.

■ ADVERSE EFFECTS: Adverse effects include sedation, euphoria, constipation, miosis, decreased respirations, and pruritus. Bradycardia and hypotension are rare but may occur in overdose.

buccal flange [L, *bucca* + OFr, *flanche,* flank], the portion of a denture base that occupies the cheek side of the mouth and extends distally from the buccal notch. Compare **labial flange, lingual flange.** See also **flange.**

buccal frenum, a fold or band of mucous membrane connecting the alveolar ridge to the cheek and separating the labial vestibule from the buccal vestibule.

buccal glands [L, *bucca,* cheek, *glans,* acorn], small salivary glands located between the buccinator muscle and the mucous membranes in the vestibule of the mouth.

buccal mucosa, the mucous membranes lining the inside of the mouth.

buccal nerve, a branch of the anterior trunk of the mandibular nerve that supplies general sensory nerves to the skin of the cheek, oral mucosa, and buccal gingivae of the lower molars. It may also carry the motor innervations to the lateral pterygoid muscle and to part of the temporalis muscle.

buccal notch, a depression in a denture flange that accommodates the buccal frenum. See also **labial notch.**

buccal smear, a sample of cells removed from the buccal mucosa to obtain a specimen for chromosome or DNA analysis for genetic testing, or for a sex chromatin test to determine the genetic sex of an individual. See also **sex chromatin.**

buccal splint, material that is placed on the buccal surfaces of fixed partial denture units to hold the units in position for assembly.

B

buccal vestibule, that portion of the gutter or vestibule of the mouth that lies between the cheeks and the teeth and gingivae or residual alveolar ridges extending distally from the labial vestibule.

bucci-. See **bucco-, bucc-, bucca-, bucci-.**

buccinator /buk″sinā′tər/ [L, *buccina,* trumpet], the main muscle of the cheek and one of the 12 muscles of the mouth. It is pierced by the duct of the parotid gland opposite the second molar tooth. The buccinator, innervated by buccal branches of the facial nerve, compresses the cheek, acting as an important accessory muscle of mastication by holding food under the teeth. It also plays a role in other oral functions, such as sucking, smiling, whistling, and speech.

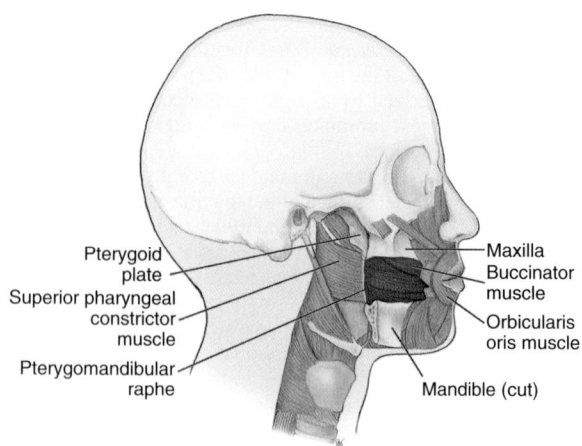

Buccinator *(Fehrenbach and Herring, 2012)*

bucco-, bucc-, bucca-, bucci-, combining form meaning "cheek": *buccal, buccinator.*

buccocclusion /buk′ə·kloo͞′zhən/ [L, *bucca,* cheek + *occludere,* to close up], a malocclusion in which the dental arch or the quadrant of a dental arch or group of teeth is positioned closer to the cheek than normal. Compare **linguoocclusion.**

buccogingival /buk′ōjinjī″vəl/, pertaining to the internal mouth structures, particularly the cheeks and gums.

buccolinguomasticatory triad /buk′ōling′wōmas″təkə-tôr′e/ [L, *bucca,* cheek, *lingua,* tongue, *masticare,* to gnash the teeth], a complex of involuntary lip, tongue, jaw, and head movements seen in tardive dyskinesia.

buccopharyngeal /buk′ōfərin″jē·əl/, pertaining to the cheek and the pharynx or to the mouth and the pharynx.

buccopharyngeal fascia, a thin layer of fascia that coats the outside of the muscular part of the pharyngeal wall.

buccopharyngeal membrane. See **pharyngeal membrane.**

buccula /buk″yələ/ [L, *bucca,* cheek], a fold of fatty tissue, literally a "little cheek" beneath the chin. Also called **double chin.**

bucket handle fracture [OFr, *buket,* tub; ME, *handel,* part grasped; L, *fractura,* break], a fracture of the wider end of a long bone along the growth plate forming an arc along the proximal margin. New bone formation leads to a thickened appearance and simulates the appearance of a handle; often indicative of child abuse–related injury.

bucking, 1. (*Informal*) gagging, coughing. **2.** involuntary resistance to positive pressure ventilation in a patient with an endotracheal tube in place.

buck knife, a periodontal surgical knife with a spear-shaped cutting point, used to make an interdental incision associated with a gingivectomy.

Buck's fascia [Gurdon Buck, American surgeon, 1807–1877], the deep fascia encasing the erectile tissue of the penis.

Buck's skin traction [Gurdon Buck, American physician, 1807–1877), an orthopedic procedure that applies traction to the lower extremity with the hips and the knees extended. It is used in the treatment of hip and knee contractures, in postoperative positioning and immobilization, and in disease processes of the hip and the knee. It is also used to maintain alignment of the hip and leg in patients with hip fractures until reduction of the hip can be performed. This type of traction may be unilateral, involving one leg, or bilateral, involving both legs. Also called **Buck's traction.**

Buck's traction [Gurdon Buck, American physician; L, *trahere,* to pull], one of the most common orthopedic mechanisms by which pull is exerted on the lower extremity with a system of ropes, weights, and pulleys. Buck's traction, which may be unilateral or bilateral, is used to immobilize, position, and align the lower extremity in the treatment of contractures and diseases of the hip and knee. The mechanism commonly consists of a metal bar extending from a frame at the foot of the patient's bed, supporting traction weights connected by a rope passing through a pulley to a cast or a splint around the affected body structure. Also called **Buck's skin traction.** Compare **Bryant's traction.**

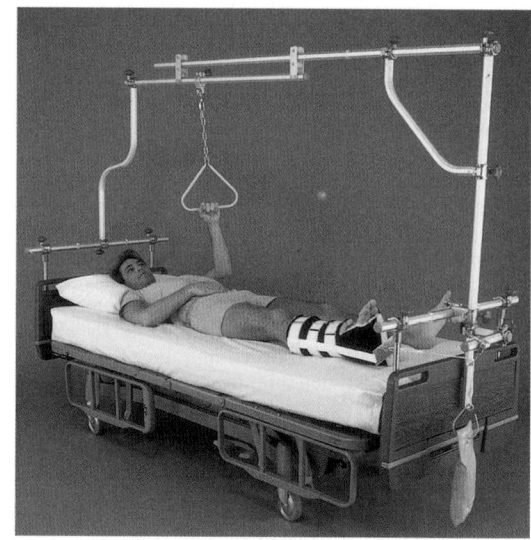

Buck's traction *(Christensen, 2010)*

Bucky diaphragm [Gustav P. Bucky, American radiologist, 1880–1963; Gk, *diaphragma,* partition], a moving grid that limits the amount of scattered radiation reaching a radiographic image receptor, thereby increasing the contrast. Also called *Bucky grid.*

buclizine hydrochloride /boo͞′kləzēn/, an antiemetic/antivertigo drug derived from piperazine that has anticholinergic and antihistaminic properties. It is used to treat nausea, vomiting, and dizziness from motion sickness.

bud [ME, *budde*], any small outgrowth that is the beginning stage of a living structure, such as a limb bud from which an upper or lower limb develops.

Budd-Chiari syndrome /bud″kē·är″ē/ [George Budd, English physician, 1808–1882; Hans Chiari, Czech-French pathologist, 1851–1916], a disorder of hepatic circulation, marked by occlusion of the hepatic veins, that leads to liver enlargement, ascites, extensive development of collateral vessels, and severe portal hypertension. It may be congenital. Also called **Chiari syndrome, Rokitansky disease.**

budding [ME, *budde*], a type of asexual reproduction in which an organism produces a budlike projection containing chromatin that eventually detaches and develops into an independent organism. It is common in simple organisms, such as sponges, yeasts, and molds.

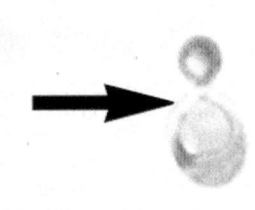

Budding *(Tille, 2014)*

buddy splint, a splinting or taping technique commonly used after a finger or toe injury requiring immobilization. The injured and an adjacent digit are typically splinted or taped together to limit or encourage the range of motion of the affected digit. Also called **buddy tape.**

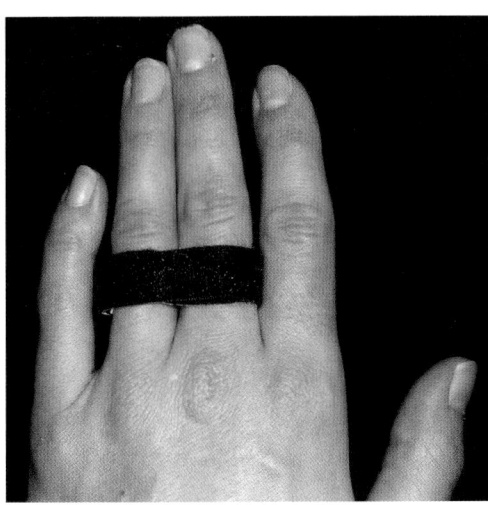

Buddy splint *(Tang et al, 2012)*

buddy tape. See **buddy splint.**

budesonide, a nasal and oral corticosteroid antiinflammatory agent, available under the brand name Pulmicort for use in a nebulizer or Turbuhaler.

■ INDICATIONS: It is prescribed in the management of symptoms of seasonal or perennial allergic rhinitis or perennial nonallergic rhinitis. Nebulizer solutions are used for the treatment of asthma in children.

■ CONTRAINDICATIONS: The drug should not be given to patients who have an allergic reaction to the drug or to any of its components or to patients with an untreated infection of the mucous membranes.

■ ADVERSE EFFECTS: Side effects include nasal or throat irritation, dysphonia, and oral candidiasis.

Buerger disease. See **thromboangiitis obliterans.**

Buerger's postural exercises [Leo Buerger, American physician, 1879–1943; L, *ponere,* to place, *exercere,* to continue working], exercises designed to maintain circulation in a limb.

buffalo hump, an accumulation of fat on the back of the neck associated with the prolonged use of large doses of glucocorticoids or the hypersecretion of cortisol caused by Cushing syndrome.

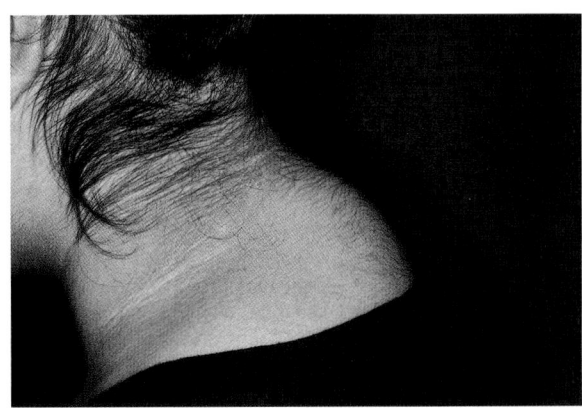

Buffalo hump *(Paller and Mancini, 2016)*

buffer [ME, *buffe,* to cushion], a substance or group of substances that tends to control the hydrogen ion concentration in a solution by reacting with hydrogen ions of an acid added to the system or releasing hydrogen ions to a base added to the system. Buffers minimize significant changes of pH in a chemical system. Among the functions carried out by buffer systems in the body is maintenance of the acid-base balance of the blood and of the proper pH in kidney tubules. See also **blood buffers, pH.**

buffer anions, the negatively charged bicarbonate, protein, and phosphate ions that comprise the buffer systems of the body.

buffer cations, the positively charged ions associated with the buffering anions of the body's electrolytes, mainly protein cations.

buffered insulin human, human regular insulin buffered with phosphate. It is used particularly in continuous infusion pumps but is also administered subcutaneously, intramuscularly, or intravenously.

buffer solution [ME, *buffet* + L, *solutus,* dissolved], a solution that will minimize changes in pH value despite dilution or addition of a small amount of base or acid.

buffy coat [ME, *buffet* + Fr, *cote*], a grayish white layer of white blood cells and platelets that accumulates on the surface of sedimented erythrocytes when blood is allowed to stand or is centrifuged.

bug, **1.** an error in a computer program (software bug) or a flaw in computer hardware (hardware bug), usually resulting in an inability to process data correctly. **2.** *(Nontechnical)* a common term for germs, microorganisms, viruses, or bacteria.

bulb [L, *bulbus,* swollen root], any rounded structure, such as the eyeball, hair roots, and certain sensory nerve endings.

bulbar /bul″bər/ [L, *bulbus*], **1.** pertaining to a bulb. **2.** pertaining to the medulla oblongata of the brain and the cranial nerves.

bulbar ataxia [L, *bulbus*, swollen root; Gk, *ataxia*, without order], a loss of motor coordination caused by a lesion in the medulla oblongata or pons.

bulbar conjunctiva, the thin, clear membrane that is part of the conjunctiva covering the eyeball. See **conjunctiva.**

bulbar myelitis [L, *bulbus*, swollen root; Gk, *myelos*, marrow, *itis*, inflammation], an inflammation of the central nervous system involving the medulla oblongata.

bulbar palsy [L, *bulbus*, swollen root; Gk, *paralyein*, to be palsied], a form of paralysis resulting from a defect in the motor centers of the medulla oblongata. See also **bulbar poliomyelitis.**

bulbar paralysis, a degenerative neurological condition characterized by progressive paralysis of cranial nerves and involving the lips, tongue, mouth, pharynx, and larynx. The condition occurs most commonly in people over 50 years of age, in multiple sclerosis, and in amyotrophic lateral sclerosis.

bulbar poliomyelitis [L, *bulbus*, swollen root; Gk, *polios*, gray, *myelos*, marrow, *itis*, inflammation], a form of poliomyelitis that involves the medulla oblongata and gradually progresses to bulbar paralysis with respiratory and circulatory failure.

bulbiform /bul″bifôrm/, shaped like a bulb.

bulbocavernosus reflex, bulbospongiosus reflex, the contraction of the bulbospongiosus muscle when the dorsum of the penis is tapped or the glans penis is compressed. The response can be elicited in women by applying pressure to the clitoris. This reflex is useful in the evaluation of patients with spinal shock.

bulbospongiosus, a muscle that covers the bulb of the penis in the male and the bulbus vestibuli in the female. Also called *accelerator urinae*, **ejaculator urinae.** Formerly called **bulbocavernosus.**

bulbourethral gland /-yoōrē″thrəl/, one of two small glands located on each side of the prostate, draining to the wall of the urethra. Bulbourethral glands secrete a fluid component of the seminal fluid. Also called **Cowper's gland.**

bulbous [L, *bulbus*, swollen root], pertaining to a structure that resembles a bulb or that originates in a bulb.

bulb syringe, a device with a flexible bulb that replaces the plunger for instillation or aspiration. Bulb syringes can be used to irrigate an external orifice, such as the auditory canal. See also **syringe.**

-bulia, -boulia, suffix meaning "(condition of the) will": *abulia.*

bulimia /boōlim″ē·ə/ [Gk, *bous*, ox, *limos*, hunger], a disorder characterized by an insatiable craving for food, often resulting in episodes of continuous eating and often followed by purging, depression, and self-deprivation. Also called **binge eating.** See also **anorexia nervosa.**

bulimic /boōlim″ik/, pertaining to bulimia.

bulk. See **dietary fiber.**

bulk cathartic [ME, *bulke,* heap; Gk, *kathartikos,* evacuation of bowels], a cathartic (laxative) that acts by softening and increasing the mass of fecal material in the bowel. Bulk cathartics contain a hydrophilic agent such as methylcellulose or psyllium seed.

bulla /boōl″ə, bul″ə/ *pl. bullae* [L, bubble], a thin-walled blister of the skin or mucous membranes greater than 1 cm in diameter containing clear, serous fluid. Compare **vesicle.** —**bullous,** *adj.*

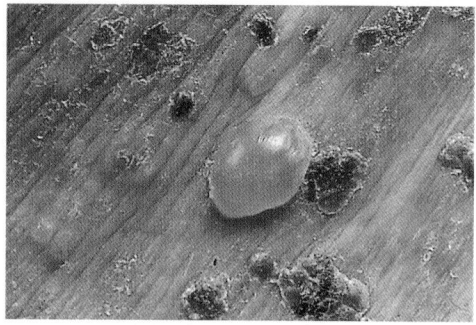

Bulla *(du Vivier, 1993)*

bulldog forceps, short spring forceps for clamping an artery or vein for hemostasis. The jaws may be padded to prevent injury to vascular tissue.

bullet forceps, a kind of forceps that has thin, curved, serrated blades that are designed for extracting a foreign object, such as a bullet, from the base of a puncture wound.

bullous. See **bulla.**

bullous congenital ichthyosiform erythroderma. See **epidermolytic hyperkeratosis.**

bullous disease /boōl″əs/, any disease marked by eruptions of blisters, or bullae, filled with fluid on the skin or mucous membranes. Kinds include **pemphigus.**

bullous emphysema, single or multiple large cystic alveolar dilations of lung tissue. Also called **cystic emphysema.**

bullous impetigo, a form of impetigo in which the skin lesions are bullae instead of vesicles. The crusts are thin and greenish yellow. Infection is treated with oral anti-staphylococcal antibiotics.

bullous myringitis [L, *bulla* + *myringa,* eardrum], an inflammatory condition of the eardrum, characterized by painful fluid-filled vesicles on the tympanic membrane and the sudden onset of severe pain in the ear. The condition often occurs with bacterial otitis media. Treatment includes administration of antibiotics and analgesics and surgical draining of the vesicles. See also **otitis media.**

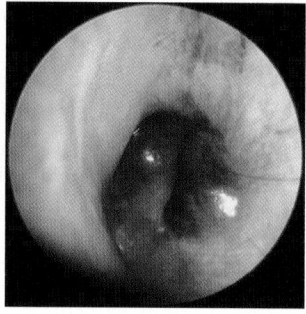

Bullous myringitis *(Swartz, 2014)*

bullous pemphigoid [L, *bulla,* bubble; Gk, *pemphix,* bubble, *eidos,* form], a rare autoimmune disease causing blisters. It presents with tense bullae filled with serous fluids. The origin is unknown, but it is associated with antihypertensive medications, such as furosemide, some antibiotics, and NSAIDs (nonsteroidal antiinflammatory drugs). Treatment includes oral steroids and other immunosuppressive medications.

bullous urticaria. See **urticaria bullosa.**

bullseye rash, a characteristic skin lesion associated with Lyme disease. See **erythema migrans.**

bumetanide /boōmet′ənīd/, a loop (high ceiling) diuretic related to furosemide.

■ INDICATIONS: It is prescribed for edema caused by cardiac, hepatic, or renal disease.

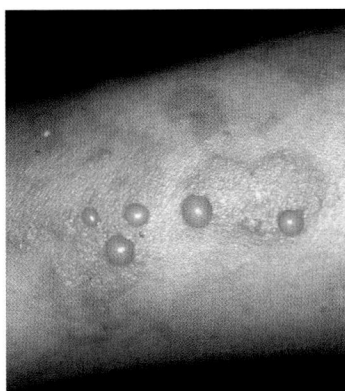

Bullous pemphigoid *(Habif, 2016)*

■ CONTRAINDICATIONS: Anuria, electrolyte depletion, or known sensitivity to this drug prohibits its use.

■ ADVERSE EFFECTS: Among the most serious adverse reactions are hypokalemia, hyperuricemia, and azotemia.

Bumex, a loop diuretic. Brand name for **bumetanide.**

Buminate, a blood volume expander. Brand name for **albumin (human).**

BUN, abbreviation for **blood urea nitrogen.**

-bund, suffix meaning "prone to" something specified: *moribund.*

bundle, a group of nerve fibers or other threadlike structures running in the same direction. See also **fasciculus.**

bundle branch [Dan, *bondel* + Fr, *branche*], a segment of the network of specialized conducting fibers that transmits electrical impulses within the ventricles of the heart. Bundle branches are a continuation of the atrioventricular (AV) bundle, which extends from the upper part of the intraventricular septum. The AV bundle divides into a left and a right branch, each going to its respective ventricle by passing down the septum and beneath the endocardium. Within the ventricles the bundle branches subdivide and terminate in the Purkinje fibers.

bundle branch block (BBB), an inability of cardiac impulses to be conducted down the bundle branches, causing a broad and abnormally shaped QRS complex. BBB is commonly seen in high-risk, acute, anterior wall myocardial infarction. It may be caused by ischemia or necrosis of the bundle branches, trauma (as in surgical manipulation), or mechanical compression of the branches by a tumor. A pacemaker may be inserted if further deterioration of conduction is anticipated. See also **left bundle branch block, right bundle branch block.**

bundle of His, specialized heart muscle cells for conduction. See **atrioventricular (AV) bundle.**

bunion /bun′yən/ [Gk, *bounion,* turnip], an abnormal, medial enlargement of the joint at the base of the great toe. It is caused by inflammation of the bursa, usually as a result of heredity, degenerative joint disease, or chronic irritation and pressure from poorly fitted shoes. It is characterized by soreness, swelling, thickening of the skin, and lateral displacement of the great toe.

bunionectomy /bun′yənek″təmē/, surgical removal of a bunion.

bunionette /bun′yənet″/, an abnormal enlargement and inflammation of the joint at the base of the small toe. Also called **tailor's bunion.**

Bunnell block, a small wooden block used in exercise of the fingers after surgery. The exercises with the block allow each joint to be exercised individually with full tendon excursion while the other joints are held extended.

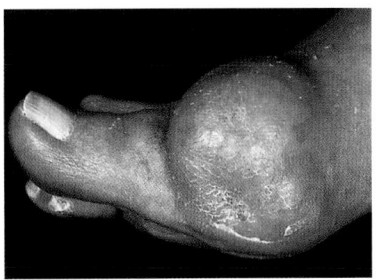

Bunion *(du Vivier, 1993)*

Bunsen burner /bōōn″sən, bun″sən/ [Robert E.W. Bunsen, German chemist, 1811–1899], a standard laboratory gas burner designed to produce nearly complete combustion in a smokeless flame.

Bunyamwera virus infection /bun′yəmwir″ə/ [Bunyamwera, town in Uganda where the type of species was isolated], one of a group of arthropod-borne viruses of the genus *Bunyavirus,* composed of over 150 virus types in the family Bunyaviridae, that infect humans and are carried by mosquitoes from rodent hosts. Related viruses cause California encephalitis, Rift Valley fever, and other diseases characterized by headache, weakness, low-grade fever, myalgia, and a rash. Convalescence is prolonged. Outbreaks have occurred in North America, South America, Africa, and Europe.

buoyant density, the thickness or compactness of a substance that allows it to float in a standard fluid.

buphthalmos. See **congenital glaucoma.**

bupivacaine hydrochloride /byōōpiv″əkān/, a local anesthetic.

■ INDICATIONS: It is prescribed for caudal, epidural, peripheral, or sympathetic anesthetic block.

■ CONTRAINDICATIONS: Known hypersensitivity to this drug or to any of the amide class of local anesthetics prohibits its use.

■ ADVERSE EFFECTS: Among the more serious adverse reactions are central nervous system disturbances, cardiovascular depression, respiratory arrest, cardiac arrest, and hypersensitivity reactions.

Buprenex, a parenteral opioid analgesic. Brand name for *buprenorphine hydrochloride.*

buprenorphine /bu″prĕ-nor′fēn/, a synthetic opioid agonist-antagonist derived from thebaine, used in the form of the hydrochloride salt as an analgesic for moderate to severe pain and as an anesthesia adjunct. Administered sublingually or by intramuscular or IV injection.

■ INDICATIONS: It is administered parenterally for the relief of moderate to severe pain and is used in tablet form to treat opioid dependence.

■ CONTRAINDICATIONS: This controlled substance is contraindicated for patients who may be opioid dependent.

■ ADVERSE EFFECTS: Among the reported adverse effects are respiratory depression, sedation, nausea, dizziness, vertigo, headache, vomiting, miosis, diaphoresis, and hypotension.

buPROPion /bōōprō″pē·on/, a heterocyclic mood-elevating drug used to treat some types of depression (brand name: Wellbutrin) and to promote smoking cessation (brand name: Zyban).

bur. See **burr.**

Burch procedure /berch/, a type of bladder neck suspension for stress incontinence, consisting of fixation of the lateral vaginal fornices to the iliopectineal ligaments.

burden, **1.** load. **2.** a heavy, oppressive load, as in an overwhelming task.

burdock root, a perennial herb found in the United States, China, and Europe.

■ INDICATIONS: This herb is used for skin diseases, inflammation, rashes, colds and fever, cancer, gout, and arthritis; there are insufficient data to know if it is effective.

■ CONTRAINDICATIONS: Burdock is probably safe except in those who are hypersensitive to this plant. Burdock also should be used cautiously in people with diabetes or cardiac disorders.

Bureau of Medical Devices (BMD), now called **National Center for Devices and Radiological Health.**

buret /byo͞oret′/ [Fr, small jug], a laboratory utensil used to deliver a wide range of volumes accurately. Also spelled *burette.*

buried penis, a concealed penis of normal size that is hidden under the skin of the abdomen or scrotum. It can occur at any age but is most common in children.

buried suture [L, *sutura*], *(Informal)* an absorbable running suture placed in the dermis below the skin edges. This technique brings the skin edges together and the suture material is not visible, hence the term "buried suture."

Burke, Mary Lermann, a nursing theorist who, with Georgene Gaskill Eakes and Margaret A. Hainsworth, developed the Theory of Chronic Sorrow to describe the ongoing feelings of loss that arise from illness, debilitation, or death. See also **Theory of Chronic Sorrow.**

Burkholderia /bərk′holdēr″ēə/, a genus of gram-negative, aerobic, rod-shaped bacteria that includes several species formerly classified in the genus *Pseudomonas,* including the agents of glanders and melioidosis. The bacteria are both human and plant pathogens. Their role in the biodegradation of polychlorinated biphenols also makes them important environmental bacteria.

Burkholderia cepacia, formerly *Pseudomonas cepacia.* A group of bacteria found in the environment that are often resistant to common antibiotics. Immunocompromised persons or those with chronic lung disease, especially cystic fibrosis, are susceptible to infection. In patients without cystic fibrosis, *B. cepacia* infections are almost all nosocomial or related to IV drug abuse. Outbreaks have been related to intraaortic balloon pumps, contaminated water sources, respiratory therapy equipment such as reusable electronic ventilator probes, or contaminated disinfectants. A variety of approaches including strict segregation of cystic fibrosis patients based on the presence of this organism have been tried in order to reduce nosocomial transmission. Even a single significant nosocomial infection with *B. cepacia* may warrant investigation.

Burkholderia mallei, a nonmotile species that causes glanders. It is primarily a disease of horses, mules, and donkeys but may also infect humans and other animals. It is a potential agent for bioterrorism.

Burkholderia pickettii, formerly called *Pseudomonas pickettii. B. pickettii* has been responsible for epidemics of bloodstream infections associated with contaminated distilled or sterile water.

Burkholderia pseudomallei, a species that inhabits water and soil and causes melioidosis. Infection is spread via contact with a contaminated source and is a predominant disease of tropical climates. The species is a potential agent for bioterrorism. See also **melioidosis.**

Burkitt lymphoma /bur″kit/ [Denis P. Burkitt, English surgeon in Africa, b. 1911], a malignant neoplasm composed of undifferentiated lymphoreticular cells that form a large osteolytic lesion in the jaw or, in children, an abdominal mass. The tumor, which is seen chiefly in Central Africa, is characteristically a gray-white mass, sometimes containing areas of hemorrhage and necrosis. Central nervous system involvement often occurs, and other organs may be affected. The Epstein-Barr virus (EBV), a herpesvirus, is associated with this lymphoma; however, most non-African cases are EBV negative. Chemotherapy can often cure the disease. Also called **African lymphoma,** *Burkitt tumor.*

burn [AS, *baernan*], any injury to tissues of the body caused by hot objects or flames, electricity, chemicals, radiation, or gases in which the extent of the injury is determined by the nature of the agent, length of time exposed, body part involved, and depth of burn. The treatment of burns includes pain relief, careful asepsis, prevention of infection, regulation of body temperature, maintenance of the balance in the body of fluids and electrolytes, and good nutrition. First priority with burns of the airway is airway control. Severe burns of any origin may cause shock, which is treated before the wound. Burns are sometimes classified as first-, second-, third-, and fourth- degree. First-degree burns involve only a superficial layer of epidermal cells. Second-degree burns may be divided into superficial partial-thickness and deep partial-thickness wounds. Damage in second-degree burns extends through the epidermis to the dermis but is usually not sufficient to prevent skin regeneration. In third-degree burns the entire thickness of the epidermis and dermis is destroyed. Fourth-degree burns are full-thickness injuries that penetrate the subcutaneous tissue, muscle, and periosteum or bone. See also **chemical burn, electrocution, thermal burn.**

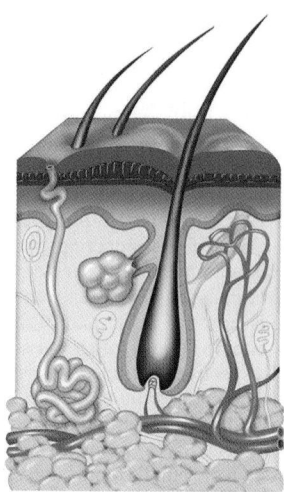

First-degree burn: damaged epidermis and edema

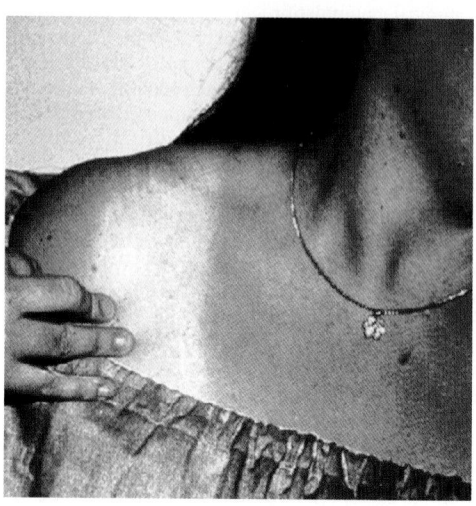

First-degree burn *(AACN, 2008)*

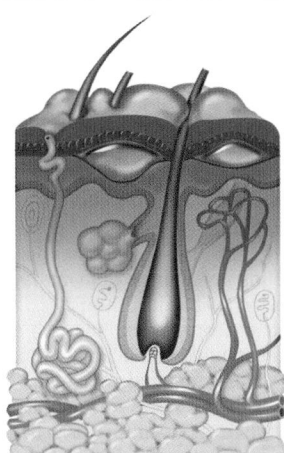

Superficial partial-thickness second-degree burn

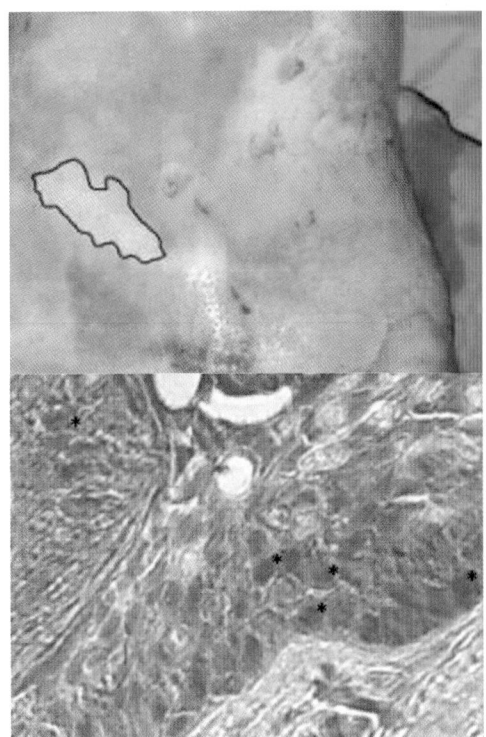

Deep partial-thickness second-degree burn *(Gravante et al, 2006)*

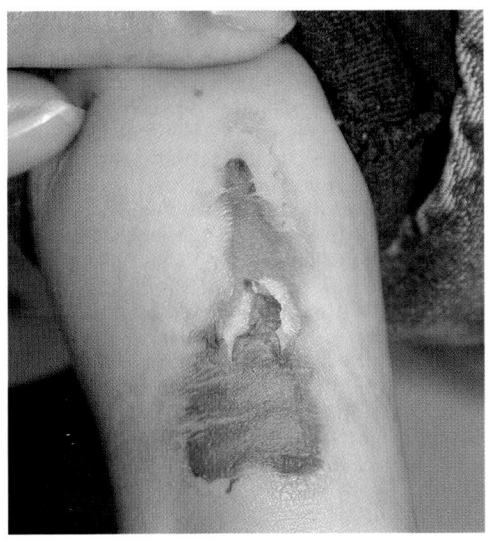

Superficial partial-thickness second-degree burn
(Chiang et al, 2011)

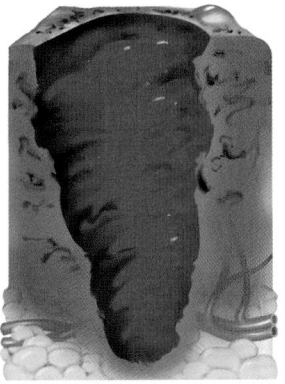

Third-degree burn

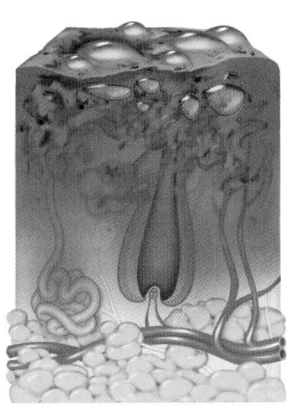

Deep partial-thickness second-degree burn

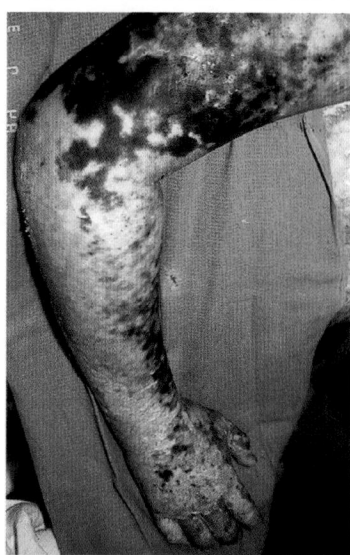

Third-degree burn *(Frazier, 2013)*

burn center, a health care facility that is designed to care for patients who have been severely burned. A number of burn centers has been established throughout the United States and Canada to provide sophisticated advanced techniques of care for burn victims.

burn recovery, the successful rehabilitation of a patient following a major burn injury, with reintegration into the home and community.

burner syndrome, a condition of burning pain, especially in the upper extremities, and sometimes accompanied by shoulder girdle weakness. It may be experienced during contact sports, such as football, as a result of a blow to the head or shoulder. It is attributed to an upper trunk neuropathy of the brachial plexus.

Burnett syndrome. See **milk-alkali syndrome.**

burning drops sign, a sensation of hot liquid dripping into the abdominal cavity caused by a perforated stomach ulcer.

burning feet syndrome, a neurological disorder characterized by symptoms of a burning sensation in the sole of the foot. The burning tends to be more intense at night and may also involve the hands. Possible causes include causalgia from injury to the sciatic nerve, degeneration of the spinal cord, and polyneuropathy. The condition is also associated with diabetes mellitus, kidney disease, and a B vitamin deficiency. Also called **Gopalan's syndrome.**

burning mouth syndrome, a burning sensation of the oral mucous membranes and tongue that is often associated with aging in terms of menopause and hormonal changes, although it can also suggest other conditions or infections, such as yeast infections.

burning pain [AS, *baernan,* to burn; L, *poena,* penalty], a descriptor used to communicate the sensation patients are experiencing. It may be related to neurological problems or excruciating pain experienced associated with an injury or thermal burn. The term is also used sometimes to describe heartburn or myocardial pain.

burnisher /bur′nishər/ [ME, *burnischen,* to make brown], a dental instrument shaped with rounded smooth edges of the nib, used to closely adapt, polish, or work-harden a metallic material to an underlying object, usually the margin of a gold restoration.

burnishing /bur′nish·ing/ [ME, *burnischen,* to make brown], **1.** (in dentistry) the process of adapting, polishing, and/or work-hardening a metal restoration under the sliding pressure of a smooth hard instrument, as in finishing the surface of a gold restoration. **2.** (in dentistry) smoothing and adapting the margins of a thin, annealed sheet of platinum to form a band about a tooth as a matrix for a restoration.

burnout, a popular term for a mental or physical energy depletion after a period of chronic, unrelieved job-related stress characterized sometimes by physical illness. The person suffering from burnout may lose concern or respect for other people and often has cynical, dehumanized perceptions of people, labeling them in a derogatory manner. Causes of burnout peculiar to the health professions often include stressful, even dangerous, work environments; lack of support; lack of respectful relationships within the health care team; low pay scales compared with other professions; shift changes and long work hours; understaffing of hospitals; pressure from the responsibility of providing continuous high levels of care over long periods; and frustration and disillusionment resulting from the difference between job realities and job expectations.

burn therapy, the management of a patient burned by flames, hot liquids, explosives, chemicals, or electric current or who has suffered skin damage from extreme cold. Partial-thickness burns may be first-degree, involving only the epidermis, or second-degree, involving the epidermis and dermis, whereas full-thickness or third-degree burns involve all skin layers. Second-degree burns covering more than 30% of the body and third-degree burns on the face and extremities or on more than 10% of the body surface are critical. In the first 48 hours of a severe burn, vascular fluid, sodium chloride, and protein rapidly pass into the affected area, causing local edema, blister formation, hypovolemia, hypoproteinemia, hyponatremia, hyperkalemia, hypotension, and oliguria. The initial hypovolemic stage is followed by a shift of fluid in the opposite direction, resulting in diuresis, increased blood volume, and decreased serum electrolyte level. Potential complications in serious burns include circulatory collapse, renal damage, gastric atony, paralytic ileus, infections, septic shock, pneumonia, and stress ulcer (Curling's ulcer), characterized by hematemesis and peritonitis.

■ METHOD: The extent of the burn, its cause, its time of occurrence, and the patient's age, weight, allergies, and any preexisting illness are all critical elements for the burn team to consider when providing care. If respiratory distress is present, endotracheal intubation or tracheostomy may be performed. Fluid intake and output are measured hourly; if a child excretes less than 1 mL/kg of urine or an adult less than 0.5 mL/kg, a diuretic or an increase in IV infusion of fluid may be necessary. Blood transfusions, steroid therapy, and antipyretics may be ordered; aspirin is contraindicated. Burned extremities are elevated, and contractures are prevented by using orthotics to keep affected areas properly aligned. The patient is weighed daily at the same time on the same scale, and, after the initial acute period, an adequate intake of a high-calorie, high-protein diet is encouraged. Tranquilizers may be given before wound care, but narcotics for pain usually are not needed after the acute phase. The patient is encouraged to stand for a few minutes every hour or every second hour and is generally able to walk in 7 to 10 days, but convalescence may be prolonged. Burn patients often are frightened, withdrawn, and disoriented initially, but after a few days they may become angry, depressed, or rebellious and need emotional support to help them cooperate with their treatment and rehabilitation. Extensive plastic surgery and repeated skin grafts may be required to restore function and the physical appearance of burn patients.

■ INTERVENTIONS: The burn patient requires intensive, prolonged care to prevent complications and disfiguring contractures. A team approach to the complex care of this patient is imperative. For example, the nurse administers parenteral fluids and medication, implements wound care, closely monitors the patient's condition, limits physical discomfort, provides emotional support and diversion, and encourages the family to visit regularly and become involved in the patient's care. Physical therapists will initiate an aggressive therapy program; most burn patients need therapy at least twice daily. During the rehabilitation phase, physical therapy is critical to overcome the long-standing catabolic state and disuse atrophy. Occupational therapists can fabricate an orthosis to preserve range of motion and prevent or correct scar contractures. The burn team will meet regularly to ensure that the needs of the patient are met and that the treatment plan is coordinated in a way in which all disciplines can contribute their expertise to recovery.

■ OUTCOME CRITERIA: The outcome for the severely burned patient depends greatly on the detailed, near-constant care required during the acute phase of treatment. Scarring may cause residual dysfunction and discouragement. Encouragement to participate fully in ongoing therapy and to continue treatments is essential.

Burow's solution /byoor″ōz/ [Karl A. Burow, German physician, 1809–1874], a liquid preparation containing aluminum sulfate, acetic acid, precipitated calcium carbonate, and water, used as a topical astringent, antiseptic, and antipyretic for a wide variety of skin disorders. Also called **aluminum acetate solution.**

burp, **1.** *(Informal)* to belch, or eructate; to expel gas from the stomach through the mouth. **2.** a belch, or eructation.

burr, a rotary instrument fitted into a handpiece and used to cut teeth or bone. Also spelled **bur.**

burr cell [ME, *burre* + L, *cella,* storeroom], a form of mature erythrocyte in which the cells or cell fragments have spicules, or tiny projections, on the surface.

burr holes, holes drilled in the skull during surgery to drain and irrigate an abscess and/or to release increasing intracranial pressure.

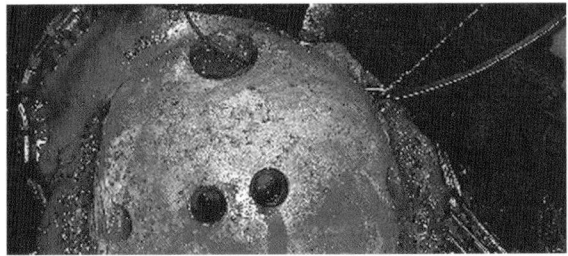

Burr holes for craniotomy *(Shah et al, 2012)*

burrowing flea. See **chigoe.**

bursa /bur″sə/ *pl.* **bursae** [Gk, *byrsa,* wineskin], **1.** a fibrous sac between certain tendons and the bones beneath them. Lined with a synovial membrane that secretes synovial fluid, the bursa acts as a small cushion that allows the tendon to move over the bone as it contracts and relaxes. Bursae may enlarge if subject to excessive forces, causing bursitis. See also **adventitious bursa, bursa of Achilles, olecranon bursa, prepatellar bursa. 2.** a sac or closed cavity. See also **omental bursa, pharyngeal bursa.**

bursa-equivalent tissue, bursal equivalent tissue, a hypothesized lymphoid tissue in nonavian vertebrates, including human beings, equivalent to the bursa of Fabricius

in birds: the site of B lymphocyte maturation. It now appears that B lymphocyte maturation occurs primarily in the bone marrow.

bursal abscess /bur″səl/, a collection of pus in the cavity of a bursa.

bursa of Achilles, bursa separating the tendon of Achilles and the calcaneus.

bursectomy /bərsek″təmē/ [Gk, *byrsa,* wineskin, *ektomē,* cutting out], the excision of a bursa.

bursitis /bərsī″tis/, inflammation of the bursa, the connective tissue structure surrounding a joint. Bursitis may be precipitated by arthritis, infection, injury, or excessive or traumatic exercise or effort. Kinds include **housemaid's knee, miner's elbow, weaver's bottom.** See also **rheumatism.**

■ OBSERVATIONS: The chief symptom is severe pain of the affected joint, particularly on movement.

■ INTERVENTIONS: Treatment goals include the control of pain and the maintenance of joint motion. Acute pain is often treated with an intrabursal injection of an adrenocorticosteroid. Other common treatments are analgesics and antiinflammatory agents. Additional measures may include a combination of rest, splints, and heat and cold application, as well as physical or occupational therapy.

■ PATIENT CARE CONSIDERATIONS: After the inflammation has subsided, heat may be helpful. In chronic cases, surgery may be required to remove calcium deposits.

burst, to break suddenly while under tension or expansion.

burst fracture [ME, *bersten* + L, *fractura,* break], any fracture that disperses multiple bone fragments, usually at or near the end of a bone. It frequently occurs in a vertebra.

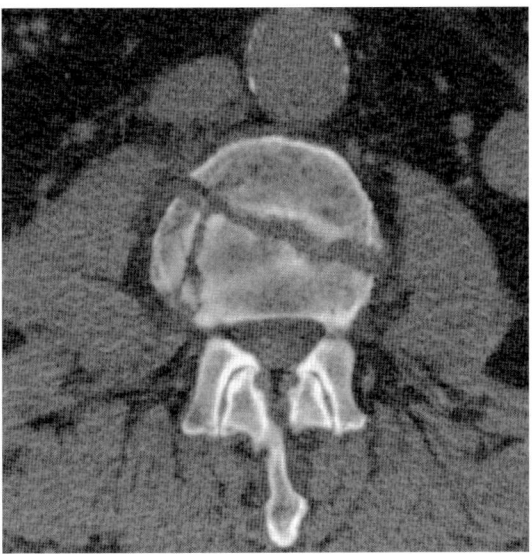

Burst fracture of the third lumbar vertebra *(Courtesy Ohio State University Medical Center)*

Burton's line [Henry Burton, English physician, 1799–1849], a dark blue stippled line along the gingival margin, which is a sign of lead poisoning. See also **blue line.**

Buruli ulcer /boo̅o̅′rə·le/ [Buruli, district in Uganda], an ulcer of the skin with widespread necrosis of subcutaneous fat. It is caused by a species of *Mycobacterium ulcerans* and manifested by a small, firm, painless, movable subcutaneous nodule that enlarges and ulcerates. It occurs principally in Central Africa (the Nile river banks) but has also been seen in other tropical areas.

bus, a set of parallel wires in a computer to which the central processing unit and all input-output units are connected. Each separate wire carries the electric current representing 1 bit. Buses interconnect the parts of the computer that communicate with each other, such as a video card or modem.

Busse-Buschke disease, now called **cryptococcosis.** Should not be confused with **Buschke disease.**

Buschke-Löwenstein tumor. See **giant condyloma.**

Buschke disease, also called **scleredema.** Should not be confused with **Busse-Buschke disease.**

bushy chorion, the region of the chorion that bears villi.

BuSpar, an oral antianxiety drug. Brand name for **buspirone hydrochloride.**

buspirone hydrochloride /bŏospir″ōn/, an antianxiety agent not related chemically to others. Administered orally as the hydrochloride salt. Unlike benzodiazepines, it has low abuse potential, takes several days to weeks to exert its effect, does not intensify the effects of other CNS depressants, and is less sedating.

■ INDICATIONS: It is prescribed for generalized anxiety disorders.

■ CONTRAINDICATIONS: This drug is contraindicated in patients with severe hepatic or renal impairment. Patients taking a benzodiazepine drug should be gradually withdrawn from that medication before starting therapy with buspirone.

■ ADVERSE EFFECTS: Among adverse reactions reported are dizziness, headache, light-headedness, excitement, and nausea.

busulfan /bŏosul″fən/, an alkylating agent.

■ INDICATIONS: It is prescribed in the treatment of chronic myelocytic leukemia.

■ CONTRAINDICATIONS: Radiation therapy, depressed neutrophil or platelet counts, concurrent administration of neoplastic medication, or known hypersensitivity to this drug prohibits its use.

■ ADVERSE EFFECTS: Among the more serious adverse reactions are alveolar hyperplasia (busulfan lung), depression of the bone marrow, and severe nausea and diarrhea. Amenorrhea commonly occurs.

butabarbital sodium /byŏo′təbär″bitôl/, a sedative; intermediate-acting barbiturate.

■ INDICATIONS: It is prescribed for the relief of anxiety, nervous tension, and insomnia.

■ CONTRAINDICATIONS: Porphyria, seizure disorders, or known hypersensitivity to this drug prohibits its use.

■ ADVERSE EFFECTS: Among the more serious adverse reactions are jaundice, skin rash, and paradoxical excitement.

butamben picrate /byŏotam″bən pik″rāt/, a topical local anesthetic for the temporary relief of pain from minor burns.

butane (C_4H_{10}), a colorless petroleum-based gas. It is the fourth member of the paraffin series of hydrocarbons.

butanoic acid. See **butyric acid.**

butanol. See **butyl alcohol.**

Butazolidin, an NSAID drug. Brand name for *phenylbutazone.*

butenafine /bu-ten′ah-fēn/, a topical antifungal agent used as the hydrochloride salt in the treatment of athlete's foot, jock itch, and ringworm.

Butisol Sodium, a barbiturate sedative-hypnotic. Brand name for **butabarbital sodium.**

Butler-Albright syndrome, a type of distal renal tubular acidosis occurring later than infancy and having autosomal-dominant inheritance. Also called *Lightwood-Butler-Albright syndrome.*

butoconazole nitrate /byŏo′təkō″nəzōl/, an intravaginal antifungal cream.

■ INDICATIONS: It is prescribed for the treatment of vulvovaginal fungal infections caused by *Candida* species.

■ CONTRAINDICATIONS: Its use is contraindicated during the first trimester of a pregnancy.

■ ADVERSE EFFECTS: Adverse reactions include vulvar and vaginal burning and itching.

butorphanol tartrate /byŏotôr″fənôl/, an agonist/antagonist opioid of the phenanthrene family.

■ INDICATIONS: It is administered parentally for surgical premedication, as an analgesic component of balanced anesthesia, for prompt relief of moderate to severe pain associated with surgical procedures, and as a nasal spray for the relief of migraine pain.

■ CONTRAINDICATIONS: Butorphanol tartrate is not given to patients known to be sensitive to phenanthrenes or to persons dependent on opioids because it may provoke withdrawal symptoms.

■ ADVERSE EFFECTS: Toxicity may result from the use of butorphanol with other opioids.

butt, **1.** to place two flat surfaces together to form a joint. **2.** (in dentistry) to place directly against the tissues covering the residual alveolar ridge. **3.** (in dentistry) to place a dental restoration directly against a flat surface of a prepared tooth.

butter, a soft, solid substance, such as the dairy produced by churning cream.

butterfly bandage [AS, *buttorfleoge*], a narrow adhesive strip with broader winglike ends used to approximate the edges of a superficial wound and to hold the edges together as they heal. It is used in place of a suture in certain cases.

butterfly fracture, a bone break in which the center fragment contained by two fracture lines forms a triangle resembling a butterfly's wing.

butterfly needle, a short needle attached to plastic stabilizers at 90 degrees. It is used for IV access to small veins of adults and children.

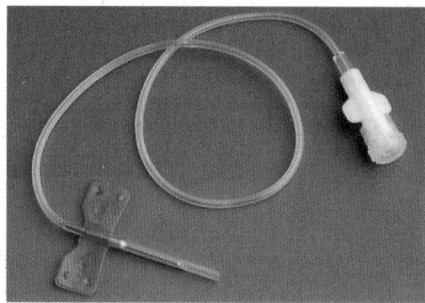

Butterfly needle *(Courtesy Medline Industries)*

butterfly rash, an erythematous eruption of both cheeks joined by a narrow band of rash across the nose. It may be seen in lupus erythematosus, rosacea, and seborrheic dermatitis.

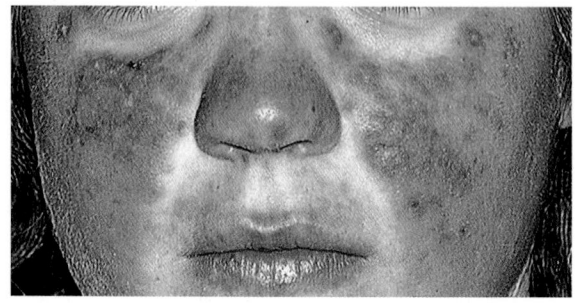

Butterfly rash *(Habif, 2016)*

buttermilk [Gk, *boutyron,* butter; AS, *meoluc*], **1.** the slightly sour-tasting liquid remaining after the solids in cream have been churned into butter. It is nearly fat free and is nutritionally comparable to whole milk. **2.** cultured milk made by the addition of certain organisms to fat-free milk.

butter stools, (Informal) a fatty fecal discharge from the bowels, as may occur in steatorrhea.

buttock augmentation, a reconstructive cosmetic surgery for reshaping or enhancing the buttocks.

buttocks, the fleshy hillocks at the lower posterior part of the torso comprising fat and the gluteal muscles. Also called **nates.**

button /but′ən/ [OFr, *boton*], a knoblike elevation or structure.

buttonhole [OFr, *boton* + AS, *hol*], a small slitlike hole in the wall of a structure or a cavity of the body.

buttonhole fracture, a fracture caused by a straight perforation of a bone, such as by a bullet.

buttonhole stenosis, an extreme narrowing of a vessel. The term usually refers to the mitral valve, in which the valve cusps are contracted to form an opening shaped like a buttonhole.

buttonhook, an adaptive device designed to help patients who have limited finger range of motion, dexterity, or weakness with fastening buttons on clothing. It consists of a small, usually metal hook for pulling buttons through buttonholes, as on gloves, dresses, or shirts.

button suture, a technique in suturing in which the ends of the suture material are passed through buttons on the surface of the skin and tied. It is used to prevent the suture from cutting through the skin.

buttressing, a phenomenon of osteoarthritis in which osteophytes at the hip joint extend across the femoral neck inferior to the femoral head and combine, with a proliferation along the medial aspect of the femoral neck.

buttress plate, a thin, flat metal plate used as an internal fixation apparatus to provide support in the surgical repair of a fracture, especially long bones.

butyl /byoo′til/ [Gk, *boutyron,* butter, *hyle,* matter], a hydrocarbon radical (C_4H_9), most compounds of which are obtained from petroleum. It exists as four isomers: n-butyl, isobutyl, secondary butyl, and tertiary butyl. Butyl compounds, some of which are toxic and irritating, are used in a variety of industrial and medical applications, including anesthesia.

butyl alcohol (C_4H_9OH), a clear, toxic liquid used as an organic solvent. It exists as four isomers, n-butyl, isobutyl, secondary butyl, and tertiary butyl alcohol. Also called **butanol.**

butyr-, combining form meaning "butter": *butyric.*

butyric acid (C_3H_7OOH) /byootir′ik/, a clear, colorless liquid with an odor of rancid butter or vomit that is miscible with water, alcohol, glycerin, and ether. Butyric acid is obtained commercially from 1-butanol by oxidation and can be obtained from carbohydrates by butyric fermentation. It is used in the production of artificial flavors. In the human body, high-fiber foods are transformed by colonic bacteria into short-chain fatty acids (SCFA) that include butyrate. Also called **butanoic acid, propylformic acid.**

butyric fermentation, the conversion of carbohydrates to butyric acid.

butyrophenone /byoo′tərōfē′nōn/, one of a group of structurally related antipsychotics. They are used in treating psychosis, to decrease the choreic symptoms of Huntington's disease and the tics and coprolalia of Gilles de la Tourette's syndrome, and are used as an adjunct in neuroleptanesthesia. Principal butyrophenones are haloperidol and droperidol. Butyrophenones are pharmacologically and clinically similar to phenothiazines.

BWS, abbreviation for **battered woman syndrome.**

Byetta, injectable antidiabetic agent. Brand name for **exenatide.**

Byler disease, progressive familial intrahepatic cholestasis; an autosomal-recessive disorder caused by an error in conjugated bile salt metabolism, with early onset of loose, foul-smelling stools; jaundice; hepatosplenomegaly; and dwarfism.

bypass [AS, *bi,* alongside; Fr, *passer*], **1.** any one of various surgical procedures to divert or shunt the flow of blood or other natural fluids from normal anatomical courses. A bypass may be temporary or permanent. Bypass surgery is commonly performed in the treatment of cardiac and GI disorders. **2.** a term used by some hospitals to signal that its emergency department lacks the personnel and equipment to handle additional patients, thereby advising that ambulances transporting new patients be diverted to other hospitals.

by-product material, **1.** the radioactive waste of nuclear reactors. **2.** something produced in the making of something else.

byssinosis /bis′inō″sis/ [Gk, *byssos,* flax, *osis,* condition], an occupational respiratory disease characterized by shortness of breath, cough, and wheezing. The condition is an allergic reaction to dust or fungi in cotton, flax, and hemp fibers. Compare **pneumoconiosis.** See also **organic dust.**

■ OBSERVATIONS: The symptoms are typically more pronounced on Mondays, when workers return after a weekend break. They are reversible in the early stages, but prolonged exposure results in chronic airway obstruction, bronchitis, and emphysema with fibrosis, leading to respiratory failure, pulmonary hypertension, and cor pulmonale.

■ INTERVENTIONS: Treatment is symptomatic for the irreversible changes of emphysema and chronic bronchitis.

■ PATIENT CARE CONSIDERATIONS: In the United States, the disease is most common in North Carolina, South Carolina, and Georgia in individuals working in the textile industry.

byte /bīt/, the amount of memory required to encode one character of information (letter, number, or symbol) in a computer system; it is normally 8 bits. See also **bit.**

Borrelia duttoni, an infection caused by the spirochete *Borrelia duttonii,* which is transmitted by the soft tick *Ornithodoros moubata,* found in human dwellings in tropical Africa. Also called **African relapsing fever, tick-borne relapsing fever,** *Dutton relapsing fever.* See also **relapsing fever.**

■ OBSERVATIONS: The spirochete enters the lesion through a tick bite, characteristically producing a high fever, chills, rapid heartbeat, headache, joint and muscle pain, vomiting, and neurological disorders. The symptoms recur in a pattern of remissions and peaks of fever and other effects.

■ INTERVENTIONS: Treatment with tetracycline is usually effective in curing the infection.

■ PATIENT CARE CONSIDERATIONS: The infection is spread through the community as ticks bite infected people, thereby acquiring the spirochete for inoculation in others.

Byzantine arch palate /biz″əntēn/, a congenital anomaly of the roof of the mouth marked by incomplete fusion of the palatal process and the nasal spine.

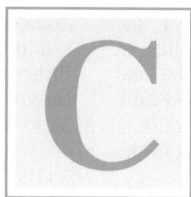

C, 1. symbol for **capacitance. 2.** symbol for **clearance.** (Subscripts denote the substance [e.g., C_I or C_{In} denote inulin clearance]). **3.** symbol for *heat capacity.*

c, 1. symbol for **small calorie. 2.** symbol for **centi-. 3.** symbol for *capillary blood.*

C, 1. symbol for **canine tooth. 2.** symbol for the element **carbon. 3.** symbol for **large calorie. 4.** symbol for **compliance. 5.** symbol for **cathode. 6.** symbol for **Celsius. 7.** symbol for **clonus. 8.** symbol for **complement. 9.** symbol for **contraction. 10.** symbol for **coulomb. 11.** abbreviation for **cytosine. 12.** symbol for **cervical vertebra.**

C1, C2, ..., 1. symbol for **cervical nerves. 2.** symbol for **cervical vertebra.**

C1 INH, abbreviation for *C1 inhibitor.*

C1q nephropathy, a type of immune complex glomerulonephritis with deposits of complement component C1q in the kidneys. Primarily found in children and young adults. Symptoms include loss of protein and/or blood in urine resulting from damage to the kidneys. It may ultimately cause kidney failure.

C3 NeF, abbreviation for **C3 nephritic factor.**

C3 nephritic factor (C3 NeF), an autoantibody that recognizes complement factors important for regulation of the complement system. Binding of the C3 NeF induces overactive complement that may be deposited in glomerular capillary walls and mesangial tissues, precipitating or contributing to local inflammation and kidney damage.

Ca, symbol for the element **calcium.**

CA 125, a blood tumor marker for ovarian or other glandular cell carcinomas. Although an elevated level does not necessarily indicate the presence of cancer, increases in the level of the antigen may signal continuing tumor growth, which may indicate a poor prognosis. Abbreviation for *cancer antigen 125.*

CA 19-9, a blood tumor marker for pancreatic, hepatobiliary, and colorectal cancer. This tumor marker is used in diagnosis, but is more useful in the evaluation of a patient's response to treatment and in surveillance of the disease. Abbreviation for *cancer antigen 19-9.*

CA 15-3 tumor marker test, a blood test used to determine the presence of the cancer antigen 15-3 tumor-associated serum marker. This serum marker is used for staging breast cancer and monitoring its treatment.

CA 27.29, a blood tumor marker used for staging breast cancer and monitoring its treatment. Abbreviation for *cancer antigen 27.29.*

CA 125 tumor marker test, a blood test used to determine the presence of CA 125 serum tumor marker, which has a high degree of sensitivity and specificity for ovarian cancer. It is also used to determine a patient's response to therapy and for posttreatment surveillance.

cabergoline /cah-ber′go-lēn/, a dopamine receptor agonist used in treatment of hyperprolactinemia, administered orally.

CABG, See **coronary artery bypass graft.** Abbreviation for **coronary artery bypass graft.**

Cabot rings /kab″ot/ [Richard C. Cabot, American physician, 1868–1939], threadlike figures, often appearing as loops or rings, in red blood cells of patients with severe anemia. The inclusions are seen in Wright stain blood films. Also called *Cabot bodies.*

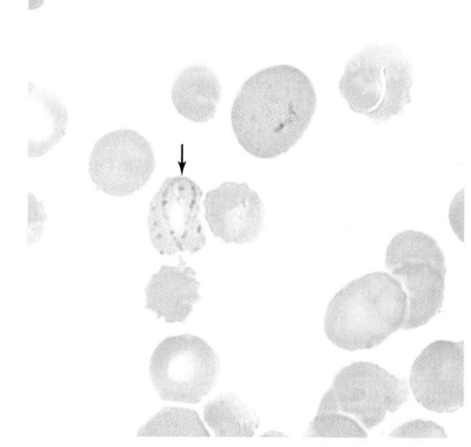

Cabot rings *(Carr and Rodak, 2013)*

cac-. See **caco-, cac-.**

CaC₂, chemical formula for **calcium carbide.**

CaC₂O₄, chemical formula for **calcium oxalate.**

cacao /kəkā′ō/, **1.** cocoa. **2.** the seeds of *Theobroma cacao* from which cocoa solids and butter are extracted. See also **cocoa butter.**

cache /kash/, (in computer technology) a fast storage buffer in the central processing unit or hard drive used to increase the amount and speed of data processing. Also called *cache memory.*

cachectic /kəkek″tik/ [Gk, *kakos,* bad, *hexis,* state], pertaining to a state of generally poor health, malnutrition, and weight loss.

cachet /käshā″/ [Fr, tablet], an edible disk-shaped wafer or capsule that encloses a dose of medicine.

cachexia /kəkek″sē·ə/ [Gk, *kakos,* bad, *hexis,* state], general ill health and malnutrition, marked by weakness and emaciation, usually associated with severe disease, such as advanced malignancy or AIDS. Also called *cachexy.* **–cachectic,** *adj.*

cachinnation /kak′ənā″shən/ [L, *cachinnare,* to laugh aloud], excessive laughter with no apparent cause, often part of the behavioral pattern in individuals with schizophrenia. **–cachinnate,** *v.*

caco-, cac-, prefix meaning "ill, unpleasant, or bad": *cachexia, cacophony.*

cacodemonomania /kak′ōdē′mənōmā″nē·ə/ [Gk, *kakos* + *daimon,* spirit, *mania,* madness], a condition in which an individual claims to be possessed by an evil spirit.

cacophony /kəkof″ənē/ *pl. cacophonies* [Gk, *kakos* + *phone,* voice], a harsh or discordant sound or a mixture of confused, different sounds. **–cacophonic, cacophonous,** *adj.*

cacoplastic /kak′əplas″tik/, **1.** pertaining to a low or inferior grade of structure or organization. **2.** pertaining to a state of abnormal growth.

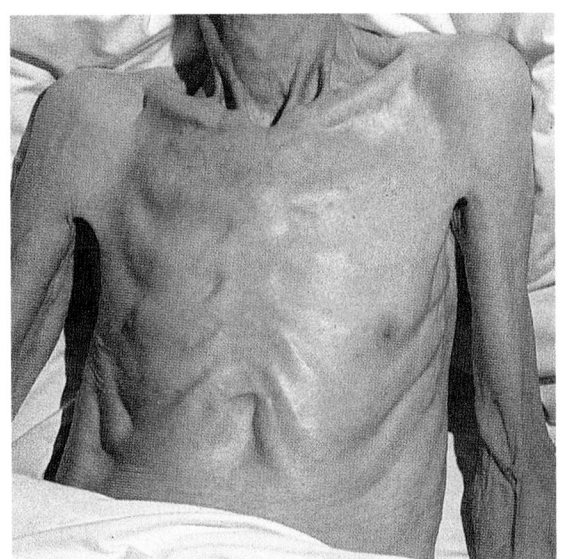

Adult male with cachexia *(Forbes and Jackson, 2003)*

of acidic foods prepared and stored in cadmium-lined containers, as lemonade in certain metal cans. The effects may include vomiting, dyspnea, headache, prostration, pulmonary edema, and possibly, years later, cancer. Maternal cadmium exposure can affect fetal development.

caduceus /kədoo″sē·əs/ [L; Gk, *karykeion*, herald], the wand of the god Hermes or Mercury, used as the symbol for the U.S. Army Medical Corps. It is represented as a staff with two serpents coiled around it and is often confused with the staff of Æsculapius, a rod with one snake entwined about it.

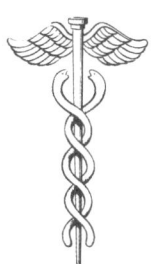

Caduceus *(Mosby, 2003)*

caec-, caeco-. See **cec-, ceco-.**
caecal, also spelled **cecal.**
caecostomy, also spelled **cecostomy.**
caenogenesis, also spelled **cenogenesis.**
Caesarean hysterectomy. See **cesarean hysterectomy.**
Caesarean section. See **cesarean section.**
caesium. See **cesium.**
café-au-lait spot /kaf″ā·ōlā″/ [Fr, coffee with milk], an oval-shaped, pale tan macule. Simultaneous development of several café-au-lait spots is associated with neurofibromatosis, but occasional café-au-lait spots occur normally. See also **neurofibromatosis.**

cacosmia /kakoz″mē·ə/ [Gk, *kakos* + *osme*, odor], the perception of foul odor or stench when none exists. In most instances the condition results from psychological factors, as in olfactory hallucinations that occur during certain psychoses, although it may be caused by a brain lesion. Also spelled **kakosmia.**

CAD, **1.** abbreviation for **coronary artery disease. 2.** abbreviation for *computer-assisted design.*

cadaver /kədä″vər/ [L, dead body], a corpse used for dissection and anatomic study.

cadaver graft, the transfer of tissue from the body of a dead individual to repair a defect in a living person. The tissue is treated to prevent disease transmission and rejection. Also called **postmortem graft.** See also **allograft.**

cadaveric donor, an organ or tissue donor who has died and donated his or her body for study, research, and examination after death or for the removal of tissue and anatomical parts. See also **cadaveric donor transplantation.**

cadaveric donor transplantation, allogeneic transplantation of an organ or tissue from a cadaver.

cadaveric renal transplant (CRT), a kidney transplant from a deceased donor.

cadence /kā″dəns/ [L, *cadere,* to fall], a rhythm, as in voice, music, or movement.

cade oil. See **juniper tar.**

cadmium (Cd) /kad″mē·əm/, a metallic, bluish-white element that resembles tin. Its atomic number is 48; its atomic mass is 112.40. Cadmium has many uses in industry and is found in cigarette smoke. See also **cadmium poisoning.**

cadmium nephropathy, chronic tubulointerstitial nephritis caused by prolonged low-level cadmium poisoning. Elevated levels of urinary beta$_2$ microglobulin are associated with renal dysfunction in persons chronically exposed to low but cumulative cadmium in the environment or work setting.

cadmium poisoning, poisoning resulting from excessive exposure to cadmium. The inhalation of cadmium in fumes created by welding, smelting, or other industrial processes involving solder is one of many sources of exposure. Cadmium bromide, used in engraving, lithography, and photography, can cause severe GI symptoms if swallowed. Cadmium may also cause poisoning by the ingestion

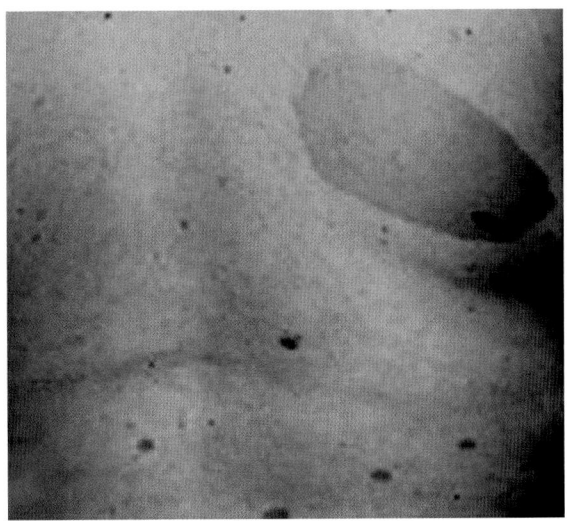

Café-au-lait spot *(King and Zamora, 2006)*

café coronary /kəfā″/, (*Informal*) a collapse of a person who is eating, caused by asphyxiation resulting from obstruction of the glottis by a food bolus. Because the signs are similar to those of a heart attack, such episodes are frequently mistaken for coronary occlusions. Also called **foreign body obstruction.**

Cafergot, a fixed-combination drug commonly administered in the treatment of migraine headaches. Brand name for **caffeine, ergotamine tartrate.**

caffeine /kafēn″, kaf″ē·in/ [Ar, *qahwah,* coffee], a central nervous system stimulant.

■ INDICATIONS: It is prescribed to treat migraine, as well as to counteract drowsiness and mental fatigue.

■ CONTRAINDICATIONS: It is used with caution in patients with heart disease and peptic ulcer. Known hypersensitivity to this drug prohibits its use.

■ ADVERSE EFFECTS: Among the most serious adverse reactions are tachycardia and diuresis. GI distress, restlessness, and insomnia are common.

caffeine breath test, a breath test for liver function in which the patient is given a dose of caffeine labeled with carbon 13. Excessively low levels of labeled carbon dioxide in the patient's breath indicate inadequate metabolism of it by the liver, as in patients who have cirrhosis or who smoke.

caffeinism /kaf-ēn-izm/, an agitated state induced by chronic, excessive ingestion of caffeine.

caffeine poisoning [Ar, *qahwah,* coffee; L, *potio,* drink], a toxic condition caused by the chronic ingestion of excessive amounts of caffeine, which is found in coffee, tea, cola beverages, and certain stimulant drugs. Symptoms include restlessness, anxiety, general depression, tachycardia, dysrhythmias (premature atrial contractions), tremors, nausea, diuresis, and insomnia. In cases of caffeine poisoning, death may result from cardiovascular and respiratory collapse. A poison control center should be called whenever poisoning is suspected.

Caffey disease. See **infantile cortical hyperostosis.**

Caffey syndrome [John Caffey, American pediatrician, 1895–1978], the battered baby syndrome, first described by John Caffey in 1946. Now called **shaken baby syndrome.** Should not be confused with **Caffey disease.**

CAGE /kāj/, a mnemonic abbreviation formed by the letters contained in four questions designed to screen alcoholic patients: *C*ut down, *A*nnoyed by criticism, *G*uilt about drinking, and *E*ye-opener drinks.

CAH, **1.** abbreviation for **chronic active hepatitis. 2.** abbreviation for **congenital adrenal hyperplasia.**

CAAHEP, abbreviation for *Commission on Accreditation of Allied Health Education Programs.*

CAI, abbreviation for **computer-assisted instruction.**

-caine, suffix usually indicating a synthetic alkaloid anesthetic: *cocaine.*

caisson disease. Also called **decompression sickness.**

cajeputol [Indonesian, *kayu,* wood, *putih,* white], a volatile oil used in topical treatments for muscle aches.

caked /kākt/ [ONorse, *kaka*], *(Informal)* formed into a compact mass or crust, as the scab of coagulated blood on a healing wound.

caked breast, *(Informal)* an accumulation of milk in the secreting ducts of the breast after childbirth, causing all or a part of the breast to become hardened and the tissues to become engorged. Now called **lactation mastitis.**

CAL, abbreviation for **chronic airflow limitation.**

cal, abbreviation for **calorie.**

Cal, abbreviation for **Calorie.**

Calabar swelling /kal″əbär/ [Calabar, a Nigerian seaport], a localized angioedema and erythema usually on the extremities, characterized by migratory, swollen lumps of subcutaneous tissue caused by a parasitic filarial worm (Loa) endemic to Central and West Africa. The swollen areas move with the worm through the body at a speed of about 1 cm/min and may become as large as a small egg. Kinds include *Loa loa.* See also **loiasis.**

Caladryl, a topical fixed-combination drug containing a skin protective substance and an antihistamine. Brand name for **calamine, diphenhydrAMINE hydrochloride.**

calamine /kal″əmīn/ [Gk, *kadmeia,* zinc ore], a pink, odorless powder used as a protectant or as an astringent and sometimes prepared as a lotion. It is composed of zinc oxide with 0.5% ferric oxide.

Calan, a calcium channel blocker. Brand name for *verapamil hydrochloride.*

calc-, calci-, prefix meaning "lime or calcium": *calciuria, calcification.*

calcane-, calcaneo-, prefix meaning "heel": *calcaneodynia, calcaneum.*

calcaneal, **1.** toward the heel. **2.** See **calcaneum, calcaneus.**

calcaneal epiphysitis, a painful disorder involving the calcaneus at its epiphysis. The condition tends mainly to affect children who are physically active and whose heel bones are still divided by a layer of cartilage. The stress of jumping and other athletic activities may break the union of the bone segments at the cartilage layer. Treatment may require immobilization of the foot in a cast. Also called **Sever disease.**

calcaneal spur, abnormal, often painful bony outgrowth on the lower surface of the calcaneus, resulting from chronic traumatic pressure on the heel. Also called **heel spur.**

calcaneal tendon. See **Achilles tendon.**

calcaneal tuberosity, a transverse elevation on the plantar surface of the calcaneus to which are attached the abductor digiti minimi, the long plantar ligament, and various other muscles, including the abductor hallucis and the flexor digitorum brevis.

calcanean. See **calcaneum, calcaneus.**

calcaneodynia /kalkā′nē·ōdin″ē·ə/ [L, *calcaneum* + Gk, *odyne,* pain], a painful condition of the heel.

calcaneovalgus, calcaneovarus. See **clubfoot.**

calcaneum, calcaneus /kalkā″nē·əs/ [L, *calcaneum,* heel], the heel bone. The largest of the tarsal bones, it articulates proximally with the talus and distally with the cuboid. Also called **os calcis.** **–calcaneal, calcanean,** *adj.*

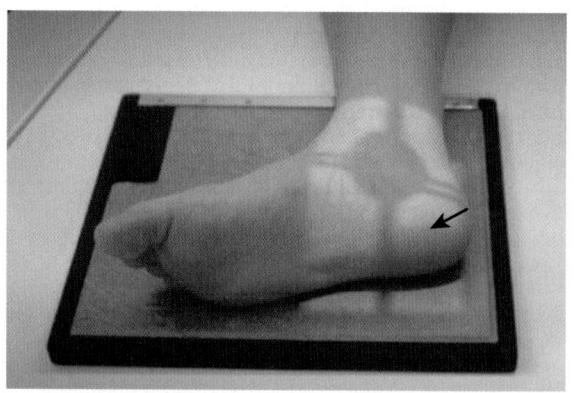

Calcaneus (Bontrager and Lampignano, 2005)

calcar /kal″kär/, a spur or a structure that resembles a spur, as in the calcar femorale of the femur.

calcar avis /ā″vis/ [L, *calcar,* spur, *avis,* bird], a projection on the medial wall of the posterior horn of the lateral ventricle of the brain. It is associated with the lateral extension of the calcarine fissure. Also called **hippocampus minor.**

calcareous /kalker″ē·əs/ [L, *calcar,* spur], **1.** pertaining to calcium or lime; hard and chalky **2.** containing calcium or lime.

calcareous metastasis, the deposition of calcium salts in visceral organs as a result of hyperparathyroidism, absorptive diseases of the bone, or any cause of hypercalcemia, particularly when associated with hyperphosphatemia. Also called **metastatic calcification.**

calcar femorale /kal′kär fem′ə·rā′lē/ [L], the plate of strong tissue that strengthens the neck of the femur.

calcaria. See **calcar.**

calcarine /kal″kərīn/, **1.** having the shape of a spur. **2.** pertaining to the calcar.

calcarine fissure, a groove between the cuneus and the lingual gyrus on the medial surface of the occipital lobe of the brain. Also called *calcarine sulcus.*

calcemia, excess calcium in the blood. Also called **hypercalcemia.** Compare **hypocalcemia.**

calcergy /kal″sərjē/, local calcification of soft tissues at the site of injection of certain types of medications.

calci-. See **calc-, calci-.**

calcifediol /kal′sife″dē·ol/, a major transport form of vitamin D.
- ■ INDICATIONS: It is prescribed in the treatment of metabolic bone disease associated with chronic renal failure.
- ■ CONTRAINDICATIONS: Hypercalcemia, vitamin D toxicity, malabsorption syndrome, decreased renal function, or known hypersensitivity to this drug prohibits its use.
- ■ ADVERSE EFFECTS: Among the most serious adverse effects are renal toxicity and those reactions associated with hypercalcemia, such as soft tissue calcification and GI and central nervous system disturbances.

calciferol /kalsif″ərôl/ [L, *calx,* lime, *ferre,* to bear], a fat-soluble, crystalline unsaturated alcohol produced by ultraviolet irradiation of ergosterol in plants. It is used as a dietary supplement in the prophylaxis and treatment of rickets, osteomalacia, and other hypocalcemic disorders. Also called **ergocalciferol, oleovitamin D₂, vitamin D₂.** See also **rickets, viosterol.**

calcific aortic disease [L, *calx,* lime], an abnormal condition characterized by small deposits of calcium in the aorta.

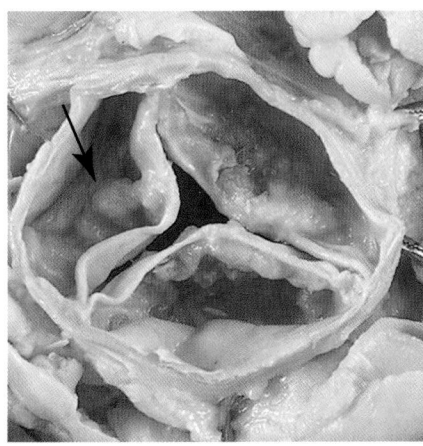

Calcific aortic stenosis *(Kumar et al, 2007)*

calcification [L, *calx* + *facere,* to make], the accumulation of calcium salts in tissues. Normally, about 99% of all the calcium entering the human body is deposited in the bones and teeth; the remaining 1% is dissolved in body fluids such as blood. Disorders affecting the delicate balance between calcium and other minerals, parathyroid hormone, and vitamin D can result in calcium deposits in arteries, kidneys, lung alveoli, and other tissues, interfering with normal organ function. See also **calcitonin, calcium, calculus.**

calcific tendinitis [L, *calx,* lime, *facere,* to make, *tendo,* tendon; Gk, *itis,* inflammation], a chronic inflammation of a tendon resulting from an accumulation of calcium deposits in the tissue.

calcified fetus. See **lithopedion.**

Calcimar, brand name for **calcitonin.**

calcination /kal′sinā″shən/ [L, *calcinare,* to burn lime], the heating of inorganic materials to drive off water. It is used in dentistry to manufacture plaster and stone from gypsum. Compare **calcification.**

calcinosis /kal′sənō″sis/, a condition characterized by abnormal deposits of calcium salts in various tissues. The deposits appear as nodules or plaques and may occur in the skin, connective tissue, muscles, or intervertebral disks. Usually the nodules occur secondary to dermatomyositis or to a preexisting inflammatory degenerative or neoplastic dermatosis, primarily scleroderma.

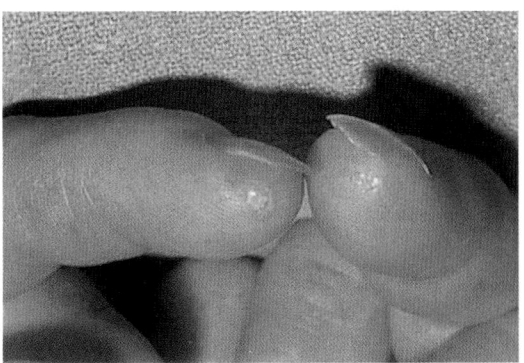

Calcinosis cutis *(Moll, 1997)*

calcipenia /kal′sipē″nē·ə/, a deficiency of calcium in the body tissues and fluids.

calcipotriene /kal′sĭpotri′ēn/, a synthetic derivative of cholecalciferol (vitamin D₃), applied to the skin to treat psoriasis.

calcitonin /kal′sitō″nin/ [L, *calx* + Gk, *tonos,* tone], a hormone produced in parafollicular cells of the thyroid that participates in regulating the blood level of calcium and stimulates bone mineralization. A synthetic preparation of the hormone is used in the treatment of certain bone disorders. Calcitonin acts to reduce the blood level of calcium and to inhibit bone resorption, whereas parathyroid hormone acts to increase blood calcium level and bone resorption. Vitamin D also contributes to the regulation of calcium homeostasis. Also called **salmon calcitonin, thyrocalcitonin.**

calcitonin test, a blood test used to evaluate patients who have or are suspected of having medullary carcinoma of the thyroid. It is also used to monitor response to therapy, to predict recurrence of the cancer, and to screen those with a family history of the disease.

calcitriol /kalsit″rē·ôl/, the active form of vitamin D; a regulator of calcium metabolism.
- ■ INDICATIONS: It is prescribed in the management of hypocalcemia in patients undergoing chronic renal dialysis and in patients with hypoparathyroidism.
- ■ CONTRAINDICATIONS: Hypercalcemia, evidence of vitamin D toxicity, malabsorption syndrome, decreased renal function, or known sensitivity to this drug prohibits its use.
- ■ ADVERSE EFFECTS: Among the more serious adverse reactions are renal toxicity and those associated with hypercalcemia, such as soft tissue calcification.

calcium (Ca) /kal″sē·əm/ [L, *calx,* lime], **1.** calcium is the fifth most abundant element in the human body and is mainly present in the bone. The body requires calcium ions for the transmission of nerve impulses, muscle contraction, blood coagulation, cardiac functions, and other processes. It is a component of extracellular fluid and of soft tissue cells. The average daily human intake of calcium varies from 200 to 2500 mg. In North America, dairy products are the major dietary sources of this element. The daily dietary allowances recommended by the Food and Nutrition Board vary from 360 mg for infants to 1200 mg for women 15 to 18 years of age. More than 90% of the calcium in the body is stored in the skeleton, which constantly exchanges its supplies with the calcium of the interstitial fluids. The endocrine system controls the concentration of ionized calcium in the plasma. Only a fraction of this amount is ionized and diffusible; the rest is bound to proteins, especially albumin. It is the ionized, diffusible portion of calcium that participates in the physiological changes associated with hypocalcemia. About one third of the calcium ingested by humans is absorbed, primarily in the small bowel. Vitamin D, calcitonin, and parathyroid hormone are essential in the metabolism of calcium. The degree of cell permeability varies inversely with calcium ion concentration. Abnormally high levels of ionized calcium in the extracellular fluid can produce muscle weakness, lethargy, and coma. A relatively small decrease from the normal level of this element can produce seizures. Normal adult blood levels of calcium are 9 to 10.5 mg/dL or 2.25 to 2.75 nmol/L. **2.** an alkaline earth metal element. Its atomic number is 20; its atomic mass is 40.08. Its metallic form is a white flammable solid, brittle and somewhat harder than lead. Calcium is commonly produced by the electrolysis or thermal dissociation of calcium chloride. Calcium carbonate is the most common calcium compound. Calcium also occurs as a component of the natural compound gypsum, which forms plaster of paris when heated. It is also a component of calcium cyanamid, a fertilizer and progenitor of other nitrogen compounds.

calcium carbonate (CaCO$_3$), precipitated chalk; a white powder sometimes used in antacids.

calcium channel, a slow voltage-gated channel very permeable to calcium ions and slightly permeable to sodium ions, existing in three subtypes designated *L, M,* and *N* and located throughout the body. In excitable cells the action potential results from the transmembrane fluxes of Na$^+$, Ca^{2+}, and K$^+$. Calcium channels are the main cause of action potentials in certain smooth muscles, and the N channels regulate neurotransmitter release. Also called **calcium-sodium channel.**

calcium channel blocker, a drug that inhibits the flow of calcium ions across the membranes of smooth muscle cells. By reduction of the calcium flow, smooth muscle tone is relaxed and the risk of muscle spasms is diminished. Calcium channel blockers are used primarily in the treatment of heart diseases marked by coronary artery spasms (e.g., variant angina).

calcium chloride (CaCl$_2$), a granular white chemical with an unpleasant taste. It is used in a concentrated solution of the chloride salt of calcium to replenish calcium in the blood and also has uses in cardiac resuscitation.

■ INDICATIONS: It is prescribed for the treatment of hypocalcemic tetany and as an antidote for lead or magnesium poisoning or magnesium sulfate overdose.

■ CONTRAINDICATIONS: Renal insufficiency, ventricular fibrillation, hypercalcemia, or known hypersensitivity to this drug prohibits its use. Calcium chloride is never injected into tissue.

■ ADVERSE EFFECTS: Among the more serious adverse reactions is hypercalcemia.

calcium citrate, a salt used as a calcium supplement and in the treatment of hyperphosphatemia in renal osteodystrophy.

calcium gluconate (C$_{12}$H$_{22}$CaO$_{14}$), an odorless, tasteless white powder or granules administered orally or intravenously to treat hypocalcemia caused by disease or medications.

calcium glycerophosphate, a calcium salt administered intramuscularly or intravenously in conjunction with calcium lactate in the treatment and prophylaxis of hypocalcemia.

calcium hydroxide (Ca[OH]$_2$), a white powder that is used widely in the food industry to fortify beverages with calcium. Also called **slaked lime.**

calcium oxalate (CaC$_2$O$_4$), a small, colorless crystal that may be present in urine or may be a component of renal calculi.

calcium oxide (CaO), a compound formed by the calcination of chalk or marble. It is very caustic when it comes into contact with moist skin and mucous membranes. Also called *calx, quicklime.*

calcium phosphate (Ca$_3$[PO$_4$]$_2$), an odorless, tasteless white powder used as a calcium supplement, laxative, and antacid.

calcium pump, a theorized, energy-requiring mechanism for transmitting calcium ions across a plasma membrane from a region of low calcium ion concentration to one of higher concentration. Compare **sodium-potassium pump.**

calcium-sodium channel. See **calcium channel.**

calcium sulfate (CaSO$_4$), a moisture-absorbing white powder used for making plaster casts. Also called **plaster of paris.**

calcium (Ca) test, *(Informal)* a blood or urine test used to evaluate parathyroid function and calcium metabolism by directly measuring the total amount of calcium in the blood. It is used to monitor patients with renal failure, renal transplantation, hyperparathyroidism, and various malignancies, as well as to monitor calcium levels during and after large-volume blood transfusions.

calcium urate, the calcium salt of uric acid; a less common type of renal calculus. Compare **calcium oxalate.**

calciuria /kal′siŏŏr″ē-ə/ [L, *calx,* lime; Gk, *ouron,* urine], the presence of calcium in the urine.

calcofluor white stain, a nonspecific fluorochrome stain that binds to cellulose and chitin in cell walls of fungi, *Pneumocystis jiroveci* cysts, and parasites. It is used to detect these organisms in clinical specimens.

calcospherite /kal′kəsfir″īt/, a spherical mass of calcium salts and organic matter found in an area of calcification.

calculogenesis /kal′kyəlōjen″əsis/, the formation of calculi.

calculous /kal″kyələs/, **1.** describing a substance that has the hardness of stone. **2.** an abnormal concretion, usually composed of mineral salts, occuring within the body, chiefly in hollow organs or their passages. Kinds include **gallstone, kidney stone.**

calculous pyelonephritis, infection of the kidney in association with urinary calculi, which may be obstructive.

calculous pyonephrosis, pus and calculi in the kidney.

calculus /kal″kyələs/ *pl. calculi* [L, little stone], **1.** an abnormal stone formed in body tissues by an accumulation of mineral salts. Calculi are usually found in biliary and urinary tracts. Also called **stone.** Kinds include **biliary calculus, renal calculus. 2.** (in dentistry) a deposit of mineralized bacterial plaque biofilm, calcium phosphate, calcium carbonate, and organic matter that accumulates on the teeth or a dental prosthesis. Calculus that forms coronal to the gingival crest, called supragingival calculus, is chalky and cream-colored but may be stained by drinks such as tea or coffee, tobacco, and food. Calculus that forms in the gingival pocket, or the periodontal pocket, called serumal calculus, subgingival calculus, or veneer, is usually denser and darker than supragingival calculus; slight deposits may be invisible until dried with air, lending a chalky appearance. It harbors bacteria, Also called **tartar.** See also **serumal calculus, subgingival calculus, veneer,** def. 2.

Calderol, a transport form of vitamin D. Brand name for **calcifediol.**

Caldwell-Luc procedure [George Caldwell, American physician, 1834–1918; Henri Luc, French physician, 1855–1925], surgical drainage of the sinus into the nose following opening of the maxillary sinus. Now largely replaced by endoscopic sinus surgery for sinusitis. It is still employed for large tumors within or adjacent to the maxillary sinus and removal of odontic tumors or cysts. See also **sinus surgery.**

Caldwell-Moloy pelvic classification /kôl″dwelməloi″/ [William E. Caldwell, American obstetrician, 1880–1943; Howard C. Moloy, American gynecologist, 1903–1953], a system for classifying the structure of the bony pelvis of the female. The types in this system are android, anthropoid, gynecoid, and platypelloid. The sacrum, coccyx, sidewalls, sacrosciatic notch, ischial spines, pubic arch, and ischial tuberosities are the anatomical points of reference used to determine pelvic type. The classification system requires that a mixed pelvis be named for the character of its posterior section with the name of the type characterized by the anterior portion after a hyphen, as in a gynecoid-android pelvis. See also **pelvic classification.**

calefacient /kal′əfā″shənt/ [L, *calare*, to be warm, *facere*, to make], **1.** *adj.,* making or tending to make anything warm or hot. **2.** *n,* an agent that imparts a sense of warmth when applied, such as a hot-water bottle or a hot compress.

calf *pl.* **calves** [ONorse, *kalfi*], the fleshy mass at the back of the leg below the knee, composed chiefly of the gastrocnemius muscle.

calfactant, a natural lung surfactant extract.

■ INDICATIONS: It is used in the prevention and treatment (rescue) of respiratory distress syndrome in premature infants.

■ CONTRAINDICATIONS: No contraindications are known at present.

■ ADVERSE EFFECTS: Concurrent illnesses that have occurred during treatment with this drug include pulmonary air leaks, pulmonary interstitial emphysema, apnea, pulmonary hemorrhage, patent ductus arteriosus, intracranial hemorrhage, severe intracranial hemorrhage, necrotizing enterocolitis, posttreatment sepsis, and posttreatment infection. Other serious adverse effects include bradycardia, oxygen desaturation, vasoconstriction, hypotension, and hypertension.

calf muscle pump, an action of the calf (soleus) muscles in which the muscles contract and squeeze the popliteal and tibial veins, forcing the blood in those veins to move upward toward the heart. Also called **soleus pump.**

caliber /kal″ibər/ [Fr, *calibre,* bore of a gun], **1.** the inside diameter of a tube or a canal, such as a blood vessel. Also spelled **calibre. 2.** measure of quality.

calibration /kal′ibrā″shən/ [Fr, *calibre,* the bore of a gun], the process of adjusting a device by comparing it to established standards and making adjustments to ensure accuracy.

calibrator, **1.** an instrument used to measure the size of an opening. **2.** instruments of gradually increasing size used to increase the diameter of an opening, such as a dilator of a urethral stricture.

calibre, the diameter of a tube or tube-like structure.

Caliciviridae /kalis′ivir″idē/, a family of plus-stranded ribonucleic acid viruses that have a nonenveloped virion 35 to 40 nm in diameter. It is associated with episodes of gastroenteritis and upper respiratory infection in humans and animals, including exanthema in swine.

caliculus /kalik″yələs/, a cup-shaped structure.

California encephalitis, arthropod-borne encephalitis or encephalomeningitis, induced by an arbovirus. Infection usually is caused by a mosquito bite. Epidemics occur mainly in the Midwest, on the eastern seaboard, and in Texas and Louisiana. The virus was first isolated in California. See also **arbovirus, encephalitis.**

■ OBSERVATIONS: The infection generally follows one of two clinical courses. The mild form is characterized by headache, malaise, gastrointestinal symptoms, and a fever that may reach 104° F. The more severe form may be marked by a sudden onset of fever, vomiting, headaches, lethargy, and signs of neurological involvement such as loss of reflexes, disorientation, seizure, loss of consciousness, and flaccid paralysis.

■ INTERVENTIONS: Treatment usually involves administration of anticonvulsant and sedative medications.

■ PATIENT CARE CONSIDERATIONS: Recovery usually begins in 1 week. Mortality rate is very low, but a significant number of patients have neurological sequelae for 1 year or more.

californium (Cf) [state of California], an artificial element in the actinide group. Its atomic number is 98; the atomic mass of its longest-lived isotope is 251. Californium-252 is a potent source of neutrons.

caliorraphy /kal′ə·ôr″əfē/, surgical repair of the calyces of the kidney, usually performed to improve urinary drainage into the ureters.

calipers /kal″ipərz/ [Fr, *calibre,* bore of a gun], an instrument with two hinged, adjustable, curved legs, used to measure the thickness or the diameter of a convex or solid body. It is also used to measure space on a graph and in measuring ECG patterns.

calisthenics /kal′isthen″iks/, a system of exercise in which emphasis is on movements of muscle groups rather than on power and effort. An objective is usually to elevate the heart rate for prolonged periods of time.

calix-. See **calyx-, calix-.**

Calliphoridae /kal′əfôr″ədē/ [Gk, *kallos,* beauty, *pherein,* to bear], a family of medium-sized to large, usually hairy, metallic blue or green flies that belong to the order Diptera. The flies serve as pathogenic vectors and may cause intestinal or nasopharyngeal infection with fly larvae in humans. These flies include the genera *Auchmeromyia, Calliphora, Chrysomyia, Cochliomyia, Cordylobia, Lucilia, Phaenicia, Phormia,* and *Sarcophaga.*

callomania /kal′ōmā″nē·ə/ [Gk, *kallos,* beauty, *mania,* madness], a psychological condition characterized by delusions of personal beauty.

callosal /kəlō″səl/ [L, *callosus,* hard], pertaining to the corpus callosum.

callosal agenesis, defect of the callosal structures of the brain; congenital absence of corpus callosum.

callosal fissure /kəlōs″əl/ [L, *callosus,* hard, *fissura,* cleft], a groove following the convex aspect of the corpus callosum.

callosity, a thick, hardened area of skin, usually caused by friction. See also **callus,** def. 1. **–callosity,** *n.*

callosomarginal fissure /kəlō″sōmär″jənəl/, a long, irregular groove on the medial surface of a cerebral hemisphere. It divides the cingulate gyrus from the medial frontal gyrus and from the paracentral lobule. Also called **cingulate sulcus.**

callosum. See **corpus callosum.**

callous. See **callus.**

callous ulcer /kal″əs/ [L, *callosus,* hard, *ulcus,* ulcer], an ulcer with a hard indurated base and thick inelastic margins.

It lacks a blood supply and is frequently associated with edema of the legs.

callus /kal″əs/ [L, hard skin], **1.** a common, usually painless thickening of the stratum corneum at locations of external pressure or friction. Also called **callosity.** Compare **corn.** **2.** an unorganized network of woven bone formed about the ends of a broken bone; it is absorbed as repair is completed (provisional callus) and ultimately replaced by true bone (definitive callus). Also called **keratoma.** –**callous,** *adj.*

calmative /kä″mətiv/, a medication or herbal remedy having a calming or quieting effect.

calmodulin /kalmod″yəlin/, a calcium-binding protein that mediates a variety of biochemical and physiological processes, including the contraction of smooth muscles and the release of norepinephrine. Calmodulin may act independently of, in concert with, or antagonistically to reactions involving cyclic adenosine monophosphate.

calor /kal″ôr/ [L, warmth], heat, such as that generated by inflammation of tissues or from the body's normal metabolic processes. Compare **dolor, rubor, tumor.** See also **loss of function, cardinal signs of inflammation.**

calor-, calori-, combining form meaning "heat": *caloric, calorie.*

caloric /kalôr″ik/, pertaining to heat or calories.

caloric test, a procedure in which the ear canal is alternately irrigated with warm water or air and cold water or air. The warm irrigation produces a rotatory nystagmus toward the irrigated side. Cold irrigation produces a rotatory nystagmus away from the irrigated side. If the vestibular portion of the ear is normal, all irrigations will produce nystagmus that is approximately equal in intensity. If the vestibular portion of the ear is diseased, irrigation may produce less nystagmus than would occur in the normal ear. Also called **Bárány's test.** See also **electronystagmography.**

calorie (cal) /kal″ôrē/ [L, *calor,* warmth], (in biochemistry) the amount of heat required to raise the temperature of 1 g of water 1° C at a pressure of 1 atmosphere. Also called **small calorie.** Compare **Calorie.** –**caloric,** *adj.*

Calorie (Cal, kcal), (in nutrition) a unit, equal to the large calorie, used to denote the heat expenditure of an organism and the fuel or energy value of food. Digestive processes reduce food to usable "fuel," which the body "burns" in the complex chemical reactions that sustain life. Also called **great calorie, kilocalorie, kilogram calorie, kcalorie, large calorie.** Compare **calorie.**

calorific /kal″ərif″ik/, (in biochemistry) pertaining to the production of heat.

calorigenic /kəlôr″ijen″ik/ [L, *calor,* warmth; Gk, *genein,* to produce], pertaining to a substance or process that produces heat or energy or that increases the consumption of oxygen.

calorimeter /kal″ərim″ətər/, a device used for measuring quantities of heat generated by friction, chemical reaction, or the human body. –*calorimetric, adj.*

calorimetry /kal″ərim″ətrē/ [L, warmth; Gk, measure], the measurement of the amount of heat released or heat absorbed, typically determined by the use of a bomb calorimeter. Compare **direct calorimetry, indirect calorimetry.** –*calorimetric, adj.*

calvaria /kalver″ē·ə/, the skullcap or superior portion of the skull, which varies greatly in shape from individual to individual. In some persons the calvaria is relatively oval, in others it is more circular. The fontanels, or soft spots, in the skull of an infant are situated on the surface of the calvaria at the junction of the sagittal and coronal sutures and at the junction of the sagittal and lambdoid sutures. Also called *calva.* See also **bregma.**

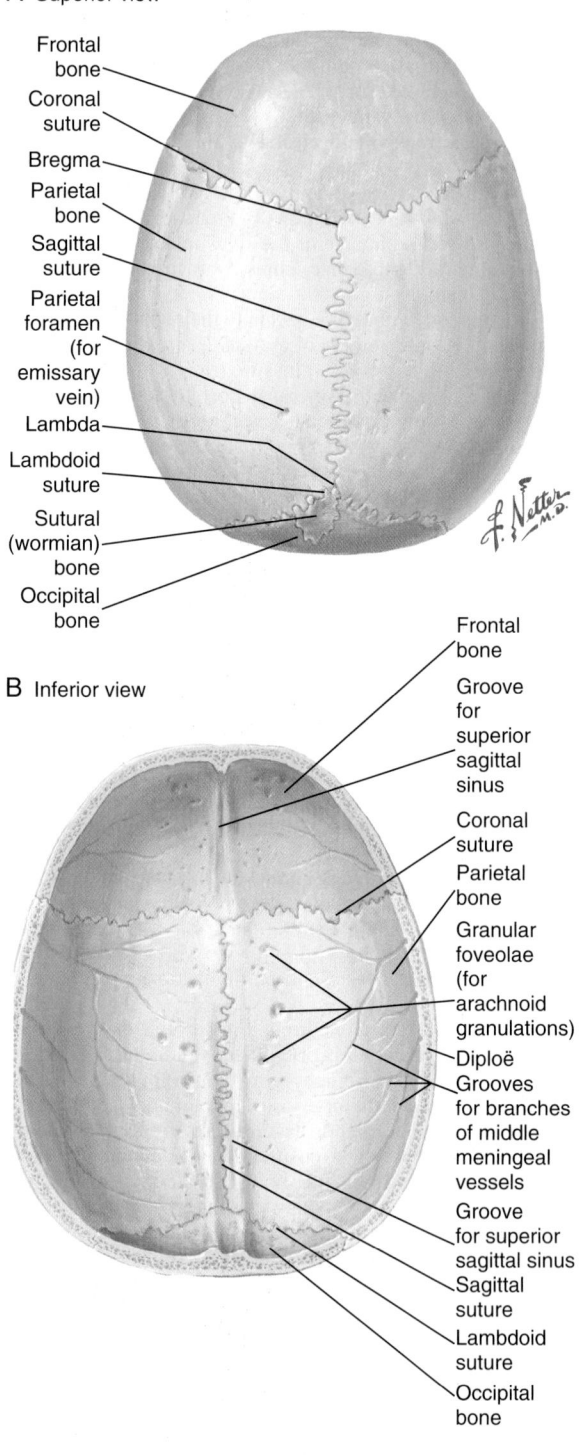

A Superior view

Frontal bone
Coronal suture
Bregma
Parietal bone
Sagittal suture
Parietal foramen (for emissary vein)
Lambda
Lambdoid suture
Sutural (wormian) bone
Occipital bone

B Inferior view

Frontal bone
Groove for superior sagittal sinus
Coronal suture
Parietal bone
Granular foveolae (for arachnoid granulations)
Diploë
Grooves for branches of middle meningeal vessels
Groove for superior sagittal sinus
Sagittal suture
Lambdoid suture
Occipital bone

Calvaria *(Netter, 2011)*

Calvé-Perthes disease, now called **Legg-Calvé-Perthes disease.**

calvities /kalvish″i·ēz/ [L, *calvus,* without hair], *(Obsolete)* baldness. Now called **alopecia.** –*calvous, adj.*

calyceal fornix, the inner border of a renal calyx where it touches a papilla or papillae.

calyces, plural of calyx. See **calyx.**

calyx /kal″isēz/ *pl.* **calyces** [Gk, *kalyx,* shell], **1.** a cup-shaped structure within an organ. **2.** a renal calyx. **3.** the wall of an ovarian follicle after expulsion of the ovum at ovulation.

calyx-, calix-, prefix meaning "cuplike": *calyces.*

CAM, abbreviation for **complementary and alternative medicine.**

cambium layer [L, *cambire,* to exchange], **1.** (in anatomy and physiology) the loose inner cellular layer of the periosteum that develops during ossification. **2.** (in botany) a cellular layer of formative tissue that lies between the wood and the bark in plants.

camera /kam″ərə/ [L, vaulted chamber], (in anatomy) any compartment, cavity, or chamber, as those of the eye, tooth, or heart.

Cameron ulcer, a peptic ulcer within a sliding hiatal hernia. It may be accompanied by chronic bleeding or be clinically silent.

Camey neobladder [M. Camey, French physician], a type of artificial urinary bladder using segments of the intestine to create a U-shaped (Camey I and II) or Z-shaped (modified Camey II) urinary reservoir.

camisole restraint, a type of restrictive device to immobilize patients at risk of harming themselves or others; used in mental health facilities. Also called **straitjacket.**

cAMP, abbreviation for **cyclic adenosine monophosphate.**

Camper's fascia [Petrus Camper, Dutch anatomist, 1722–1789], the superficial fatty layer of the superficial fascia of the abdominal wall.

camphor /kam″fər/ [L, *camphora*], a colorless or white crystalline substance with a penetrating odor and pungent taste, occurring naturally in certain plants, especially *Cinnamomum camphora.* It is present in some over-the-counter topical pain relievers, as well as in ointments applied to the chest. Its use is common in ayurveda practices. Also called **camphor, gum camphor.**

camphorated oil /kam″fərā′tid/ [Malay, *kapur,* chalk; L, *oleum,* oil], a colorless to yellowish liquid with the penetrating, pungent odor of camphor. It is derived from a combination of a dozen organic chemicals, including terpenes, safrole, and acetaldehyde obtained from the camphor laurel plant. It is used mainly as a liniment, as a counterirritant, and to increase local blood flow. In the 1980s, all solutions that contain 20% camphorated oil were removed from the U.S. market because of safety concerns. It continues to be available without a prescription in lower concentrations and in Canada.

camphor liniment, a pharmaceutic preparation of 12.5% camphor, with alcohol, lavender oil, and ammonia, used to increase blood flow to an area in the relief of rheumatic symptoms. See also **camphorated oil.**

camphor poisoning, a severe toxic condition resulting from the accidental ingestion of camphorated oils. Symptoms may include headache, hallucinations, nausea, vomiting, diarrhea, convulsions, and kidney failure. A poison control center should be contacted immediately if poisoning is suspected.

campimeter /kampim″ətər/, (in ophthalmology) an instrument for determining the integrity of the central field of vision.

Campral, a medication used in the management of alcohol dependence. Brand name for **acamprosate.**

camptocormia /kamp′tōkôr″mē·ə/, a condition in which the back is habitually tilted forward although the spinal column remains flexible. It is frequently diagnosed as a psychological conversion, and there is often a history of trauma.

camptodactyly /kamp′tədak″təlē/ [Gk, *kamptos,* bent, *daktylos,* finger], congenital digital flexion deformity that usually occurs in the proximal interphalangeal joint of the small finger(s) but may occur in multiple digits. –*camptodactylic, adj.*

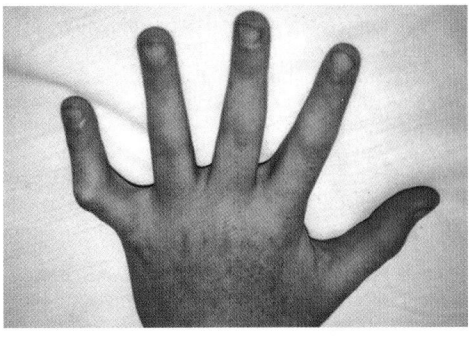

Camptodactyly *(Canale and Beaty, 2013)*

camptomelia /kamp′təmē″lyə/ [Gk, *kamptos,* bent, *melos,* arm], a congenital anomaly characterized by bending of one or more limbs, causing permanent bowing or curving of the affected area. –*camptomelic, adj.*

Campylobacter [Gk, *campylos,* curved, *bakterion,* small staff], a genus of bacteria found in the family Spirillaceae. The organisms consist of gram-negative, non–spore-forming, spirally curved motile rods that have a single polar flagellum at either or both ends of the cell. They move in a characteristic coillike motion. The organisms are microaerophiles, requiring little or no oxygen for growth. *C. jejuni* is a common cause of food poisoning. *C. fetus* consists of several subspecies that cause human infections, as well as abortion and infertility in cattle. Also called *Vibrio fetus.*

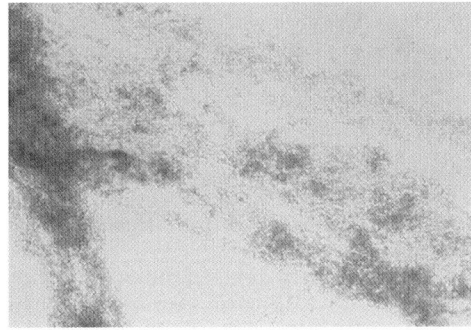

Campylobacter *(Mahon, Lehman, and Manuselis, 2011)*

Campylobacter enteritis, intestinal infection of humans or other mammals by a species of *Campylobacter,* characterized by diarrhea that may be bloody, abdominal pain with cramps, and fever. The cause is usually ingestion of contaminated food or water. Also called *enteric campylobacteriosis.*

Campylobacter gastroenteritis, bacterial gastroenteritis in humans or other mammals, caused by infection with *Campylobacter jejuni,* most commonly acquired from contact with infected individuals; from consumption of contaminated food, water, or other beverages; or from exposure to contaminated objects or environmental surfaces. Infection is usually characterized by diarrhea that may be bloody, abdominal pain with cramps, and fever. The cause is usually ingestion of contaminated food or water. Generally, adherence to good personal hygiene by personnel before and after all contacts with patients and their food, and standard precautions will minimize the risk of transmission of enteric pathogens.

■ PATIENT CARE CONSIDERATIONS: Most infections are self-limited. Patients should drink extra fluids as long as the diarrhea lasts. Antimicrobial therapy is needed only for patients with severe disease or those at high risk for severe disease, such as people with immune systems that are severely weakened from medications or other illnesses. Azithromycin and fluoroquinolones are commonly used for treatment, but resistance to fluoroquinolones is common.

campylobacteriosis /kam′pəlōbaktēr′ē-ō′sis/, infection with organisms of the genus *Campylobacter*.

Campylobacter pylori, *(Obsolete)* now called *Helicobacter pylori*.

camsylate, shortened word form for camphorsulfonate.

Camurati-Engelmann disease [Mario Camurati, Italian physician, 1896–1948; Guido Engelmann, 20th-century Czechoslovakian surgeon], an inherited disorder of bone development marked by an onset of symptoms of muscular pain, weakness, and wasting, mainly in the legs, during childhood. The symptoms vary individually from mild to disabling. Radiographic examination usually reveals thickening of the periosteal and medullary surfaces of the diaphyseal edges of the long bones. In some cases compression of nerve tissue may occur. The symptoms usually subside during early adulthood. Also called **progressive diaphyseal dysplasia.**

Canadian Association of Occupational Therapists (CAOT), The Canadian Association of Occupational Therapists (CAOT) is the national organization that supports the more than 17,000 occupational therapists (OTs) and occupational therapy assistants (OTAs) who work or study in Canada. Additionally, CAOT provides leadership in the development and promotion of the occupational therapy profession in Canada and internationally.

Canadian Association of Practical Nurse Educators (CAPNE), a Canadian national association representing the interest of practical nurses that includes educators and regulatory bodies from each province/territory except Quebec.

Canadian Association of Schools of Nursing (CASN), the Canadian Association of Schools of Nursing/Association *(canadienne des écoles de sciences infirmières)* is the national voice for nursing education, research, and scholarship and represents baccalaureate and graduate nursing programs in Canada.

Canadian Association of University Teachers (CAUT), a Canadian national organization representing the interests of all who teach in the universities of the provinces and territories of Canada. The official languages of the CAUT are English and French.

Canadian Dental Association, a federation of Canadian provincial and territorial dental associations dedicated to the promotion of optimal oral health and the advancement of a unified profession.

Canadian crutch, a crutch designed to provide support around the forearm rather than the axilla. A cuff fits around the lower arm. Also called **forearm crutch, lofstrand crutch.**

Canadian Journal of Public Health (CJPH), the official publication of the Canadian Public Health Association.

Canadian Medical Association Journal (CMAJ), the official publication of the Canadian Medical Association.

Canadian Nurses Association (CNA), the official national organization for the professional registered nurses of Canada who are members of the nine provincial nurses'

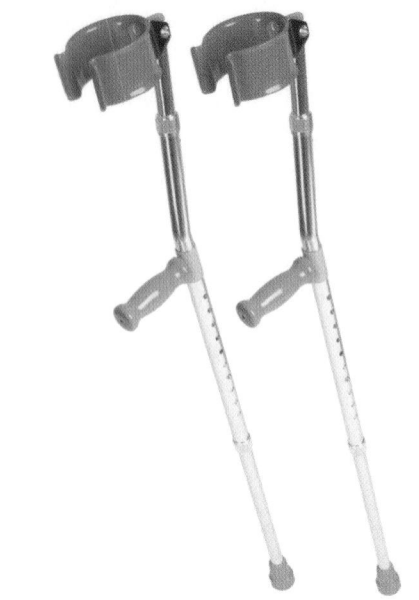

Canadian crutch *(©2015 Medline Industries, Inc.)*

associations, the Northwest Territories Registered Nurses Association, and the Yukon Registered Nurses Association. The CNA, a federation of these 11 associations, is supported by membership fees from the association members. The chief objective of the CNA is to promote high standards of nursing practice, education, research, and administration in order to achieve high quality of nursing care in the interest of the people of Canada. It is concerned with the standards of education for nurses, social and economic welfare of nurses, advancement of competence and expertise within the profession, promotion of unity and understanding among the members, and national and international representation of the organized profession of nurses. A board of elected directors and a permanent staff working at CNA House in Ottawa manage the affairs of the organization. Among the services provided are a research and advisory unit that studies trends in nursing and health and prepares briefs when necessary; a national library containing reference works, the national and international archives of nursing, and up-to-date lists of educational programs in nursing; an information service that collects and disseminates information about nursing and publishes The Canadian Nurse and L'infirmière Canadienne; a labor relations service; a certification program; a testing service; a governmental liaison service; and an international service that facilitates a working relationship with various organizations such as the World Health Organization and the Pan American Health Organization. All services are provided in the two official languages of Canada, English and French. The CNA is a member of the International Council of Nursing.

Canadian Nurses Foundation (CNF), a national Canadian foundation organized to support scholarship in nursing. The CNF awards financial support to nurses undertaking baccalaureate and graduate studies in nursing and to nurses conducting research in nursing.

Canadian Model of Occupational Performance and Engagement (CMOP-E), a conceptual model for occupational therapy developed by Polatajko, Townsend, and Craik in 2007. This model represents an expansion of the Canadian Model of Occupational Performance (CMOP), which was developed by the Canadian Association of Occupational Therapists (CAOT) in 1997. The model identifies and emphasizes the dynamic interplay among the components of the model, which are the person, the occupation, and the environment. *Engagement* was added as a conceptual advancement on the original model, as it was identified as an important aspect of human occupation. This advancement was necessitated by developments and improvements in knowledge of occupation-based, client-centered, and evidence-based occupational therapy practice.

Canadian Occupational Performance Measure (COPM), a tool to enable personalized health care. Designed for use by occupational therapists, the measure serves to identify issues of personal importance to the client and to detect changes in a client's self-perception of occupational performance over time. The COPM, which initiates the conversation with clients about performance issues in everyday living, provides the basis for setting intervention goals. Multidisciplinary health care teams have also used the COPM extensively as an initial client-centered assessment. The COPM is intended for use as an outcome measure; as such, it should be administered at the beginning of services and at appropriate intervals thereafter, as determined by the client and therapist.

Canadian Orthopedic Nurses Association (CONA), a national Canadian organization concerned with the nursing care of orthopedic patients and the continuing education of nurses working in orthopedics. Membership includes orthopedic nurses and other professionals concerned with orthopedics.

Canadian Public Health Association (CPHA), a national Canadian organization concerned with issues in public health and epidemiology. Membership is open to professionals and to others interested in these issues.

Canadian Red Cross, a charity that is part of the largest humanitarian network in the world, the International Red Cross and Red Crescent Movement. This network includes the International Committee of the Red Cross, the International Federation of Red Cross and Red Crescent Societies (Federation), and 192 national Red Cross and Red Crescent Societies. The mission of the Canadian Red Cross is to improve the lives of vulnerable people by mobilizing the power of humanity in Canada and around the world.

canal /kənal′/ [L, *canalis,* channel], **1.** (in anatomy) a narrow tube or channel. Kinds include **adductor canal, Alcock's canal, alimentary canal. 2.** (in dentistry) one of the accessory root canals and collateral pulp canals in the teeth.

canal debridement, the removal of infected skin and debris from the external auditory canal.

canalicular /kan′əlik″yələr/, pertaining to a small tubelike structure.

canalicular period, the period or phase of prenatal lung development lasting in different parts of the lungs from the sixteenth or seventeenth week to the twenty-sixth week or later and followed by the terminal saccular period. Basic structures of the gas-exchanging parts of the lungs form and become vascular, and primordial alveoli called the terminal saccules begin to form, enabling respiration to begin. Fetuses delivered after respiration begins may be viable. Also called *canalicular phase.*

canalicular testis, an undescended testis located between the internal and external inguinal rings.

canaliculus /kan′əlik″yələs/ *pl. canaliculi* [L, little channel], a very small tube or channel, such as the microscopic haversian canaliculi throughout bone tissue.

canaliculus of chorda tympani, a small canal that opens off the facial canal just before its termination, transmitting the chorda tympani nerve into the tympanic cavity. Also called *canal of chorda tympani, Civinini canal.*

canalization /kan′əlīzā″shən/, the formation of tubelike openings or passages through any tissue.

canal obturation, the filling of the pulp canal, or root canal, completely and densely with a nonirritating hermetic sealing agent. Also called **root canal filling.** See also **root canal therapy.**

canal of Corti [Alfonso Corti, Italian anatomist, 1822–1888], a space between the inner and outer rods and the basilar membrane of the cochlea in the organ of Corti. Also called **Corti's tunnel.**

canal of Schlemm /shlem/ [Friedrich Schlemm, German anatomist, 1795–1858], a tiny vein at the angle of the anterior chamber of the eye that connects with the pectinate villi, draining the aqueous humor and funneling it into the bloodstream. Also called **Schlemm's canal.**

canavanine /kan′əvan″in/, an amino acid antagonist present in alfalfa sprouts in concentrations of about 15,000 ppm, or 1.5% by weight. Canavanine can displace arginine in cellular proteins, thereby rendering them inactive. Consumption may disrupt proteins associated with autoimmune disease.

cancellous /kan″siləs/ [L, *cancellus,* lattice], (of tissue) latticelike, porous, spongy. Cancellous tissue is normally present in the interior of many bones, where the spaces are usually filled with marrow.

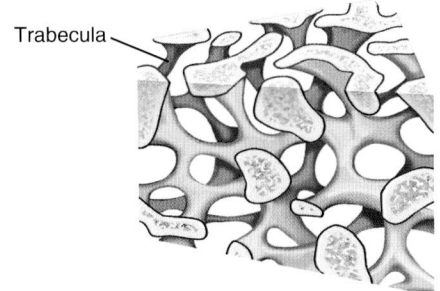

Trabecula

Cancellous bone

cancellous bone, a reticular latticelike arrangement of bony plates and trabeculae occurring at the ends of the long bones and in the interior of some irregular bones, such as the vertebrae containing red bone marrow. Also called **spongy bone.**

cancer /kan″sər/ [L, crab], **1.** a neoplasm characterized by the uncontrolled growth of cells that tend to invade surrounding tissue and to metastasize to distant body sites. **2.** any of a large group of malignant neoplastic diseases characterized by the presence of malignant cells. Each cancer is distinguished by the nature, site, or clinical course of the lesion. The basis of cancer is believed to reside in alterations in deoxyribonucleic acid (DNA), usually at several loci in the genes, but many potential causes are recognized. In men, the most common types of newly diagnosed cancer are the prostate, lung, and colorectal. In women, the most common cancer is breast cancer. Many viruses induce malignant tumors in animals; an infectious cause is likely in some human cancers. An excessive rate of malignant tumors in organ transplantation recipients after immunosuppressive therapy indicates that the immune system plays a major role in controlling the proliferation of anaplastic cells.

■ OBSERVATIONS: The incidence of different kinds of cancer varies markedly with gender, age, ethnic group, and geographic location. Cancer is second only to heart disease as a cause of mortality in the United States and Canada and is a leading cause of death in children between 3 and 14 years of age. In the United States and Canada, common sites for the development of malignant tumors are the skin, lung, prostate, breast, and colon.

■ INTERVENTIONS: Surgery remains a major form of treatment, but irradiation is widely used as preoperative, postoperative, or primary therapy; chemotherapy, with single or multiple antineoplastic agents, is often highly effective.

■ PATIENT CARE CONSIDERATIONS: Many malignant lesions are curable if detected in the early stage. Patients with a diagnosis of cancer need a coordinated plan of care to ensure the best possible outcome.

TNM staging system

T: Primary tumor

TX	Primary tumor is not assessable
T0	No evidence of primary tumor
Tis	Carcinoma in situ
T1, T2, T3, T4	Progressive increase in tumor size and involvement locally

N: Regional lymph nodes

NX	Nodes are not assessable
N0	No metastasis to regional lymph nodes
N1, N2, N3	Increasing degrees of involvement of regional lymph nodes

Note: Extension of primary tumor directly into lymph nodes is considered metastasis to lymph nodes. Metastasis to a lymph node beyond the regional ones is considered to be a distant metastasis.

M: Distant metastasis

MX	Presence of distant metastasis is not assessable
M0	No distant metastasis
MI	Presence of distant metastasis

From *Miller-Keane Encyclopedia & dictionary of medicine, nursing, & allied health,* ed. 6, St. Louis, 1997, Saunders.

Cancer incidence by site and gender in 2015*

Male		Female	
Type	%	Type	%
Prostate	26	Breast	29
Lung	14	Lung	13
Colon/rectum	8	Colon/rectum	8
Urinary bladder	7	Uterus	7
Melanoma (skin)	5	Non-Hodgkin's lymphoma	4
Non-Hodgkin's lymphoma	5	Melanoma (skin)	4

*Estimates exclude basal and squamous cell skin cancers and in situ carcinomas except urinary bladder.
Data from *Cancer facts and figures,* Atlanta, 2015, American Cancer Society.

Seven warning signs of cancer

C	hange in bowel or bladder habits
A	sore that does not heal
U	nusual bleeding or discharge from any body orifice
T	hickening or a lump in the breast or elsewhere
I	ndigestion or difficulty in swallowing
O	bvious change in a wart or mole
N	agging cough or hoarseness

From Lewis SL et al: *Medical-surgical nursing: assessment and management of clinical problems,* ed 8, St. Louis, 2011, Mosby.

cancericidal /kanˈsərisĭ″dəl/ [L, *cancer,* crab, *caedere,* to kill], pertaining to a substance or procedure capable of destroying cancer cells.

cancer immunotherapy, treatments that target the immune system, causing it to attack malignant cells. The treatments are designed to either stimulate the body's own immune response, or immune system components may be administered. The immune response may be general, or it may be specific to the cancerous cells.

cancer in situ, *(Nontechnical)* now called **carcinoma in situ.**

cancer of the small intestine, a neoplastic disease of the duodenum, jejunum, or ileum. Adenocarcinomas, the most common tumors, occur more frequently in the duodenum or upper jejunum and form polypoid or constricting napkin-ring growths. Lymphomas, found most often in the lower small intestine, may impair bowel motility by invading nerves and in some cases are associated with a malabsorption syndrome. Less common tumors of the small intestine are carcinoids, usually found in the ileum, and sarcomas, including Kaposi's sarcoma, usually seen in the jejunum and ileum. A leiomyosarcoma may sometimes form a large extraluminal mass.

■ OBSERVATIONS: Characteristics vary, depending on the kind of tumor and the site, but may include abdominal pain, vomiting, weight loss, diarrhea, intermittent bowel obstruction, GI bleeding, or a mass in the right abdomen. Diagnosis typically is made with barium radiographic examination, but results of such studies may be inconclusive until lesions are large. CT scans of the abdomen or an abdominal ultrasound are utilized to visualize bulky tumors and to evaluate metastasis.

■ INTERVENTIONS: Surgery, including a wide resection of mesenteric lymph nodes, is typically indicated for adenocarcinomas and carcinoids. Irradiation occasionally is indicated. Chemotherapy is often useful, particularly for lymphoma.

■ PATIENT CARE CONSIDERATIONS: The prognosis for 5-year survival is poor. Factors affecting the prognosis include tumor stage and the presence of metastases at diagnosis.

cancerous /kanˈsərəs/ [L, crab, *oma,* tumor], pertaining to or resembling a malignancy.

cancer staging, a system for describing the exact location, size, and extent of spread of a malignant tumor, used to plan treatment and predict prognosis. Staging may involve a physical examination, diagnostic procedures, surgical exploration, and histological examination. The system developed by the American Joint Committee for Cancer Staging and End Results Reporting uses the letter *T* to represent the tumor, *N* for the regional lymph node involvement, *M* for distant metastases, and numeric subscripts in each category to indicate the degree of dissemination. According to this

American Cancer Society guidelines for the early detection of cancer

Screening for	*Recommendation*

The American Cancer Society recommends these screening guidelines for most adults.

Breast cancer
- Yearly mammograms are recommended starting at age 40 and continuing for as long as a woman is in good health
- Clinical breast exam and breast self-exam: Research does not show a clear benefit of physical breast exams done by a health professional or self-exams by women for breast cancer screening. Due to this lack of evidence, regular clinical breast exams and breast self-exams are not recommended. However, all women should be familiar with how their breasts normally look and feel and report any changes to a health care provider right away.

The American Cancer Society recommends that some women because of their family history, a genetic tendency, or certain other factors be screened with MRI in addition to mammograms. (The number of women who fall into this category is small: less than 2% of all the women in the U.S.) Talk with your doctor about your history and whether you should have additional tests at an earlier age.

Colorectal cancer and polyps

Beginning at age 50, both men and women should follow one of these testing schedules:

Tests that find polyps and cancer
- Flexible sigmoidoscopy every 5 years*, or
- Colonoscopy every 10 years, or
- Double-contrast barium enema every 5 years*, or
- CT colonography (virtual colonoscopy) every 5 years*

Tests that primarily find cancer
- Yearly fecal occult blood test (gFOBT)**, or
- Yearly fecal immunochemical test (FIT) every year**, or
- Stool DNA test (sDNA), interval uncertain**

The tests that are designed to find both early cancer and polyps are preferred if these tests are available to you and you are willing to have one of these more invasive tests. Talk to your doctor about which test is best for you.

The American Cancer Society recommends that some people be screened using a different schedule because of their personal history or family history. Talk with your doctor about your history and what colorectal cancer screening schedule is best for you.

Cervical cancer
- **Cervical cancer testing should start at age 21. Women under age 21 should not be tested**
- **Women between the ages of 30 and 65** should have a Pap test plus an HPV test (called "co-testing") done every 5 years. This is the preferred approach, but it's OK to have a Pap test alone every 3 years.
- **Women over age 65** who have had regular cervical cancer testing with normal results should not be tested for cervical cancer. Once testing is stopped, it should not be started again. Women with a history of a serious cervical precancer should continue to be tested for at least 20 years after that diagnosis, even if testing continues past age 65.
- **A woman who has had her uterus removed (and also her cervix)** for reasons not related to cervical cancer and who has no history of cervical cancer or serious precancer should not be tested.
- **A woman who has been vaccinated against HPV** should still follow the screening recommendations for her age group.

Some women because of their history may need to have a different screening schedule for cervical cancer.

Endometrial (uterine) cancer

The American Cancer Society recommends that at the time of menopause, all women should be informed about the risks and symptoms of endometrial cancer. Women should report any unexpected bleeding or spotting to their doctors.

Some women because of their history may need to consider having a yearly endometrial biopsy. Please talk with your doctor about your history.

Prostate cancer

The American Cancer Society recommends that men make an informed decision with their doctor about whether to be tested for prostate cancer. Research has not yet proven that the potential benefits of testing outweigh the harms of testing and treatment. The American Cancer Society believes that men should not be tested without learning about what we know and don't know about the risks and possible benefits of testing and treatment.

Starting at age 50, talk to your doctor about the pros and cons of testing so you can decide if testing is the right choice for you. If you are African American or have a father or brother who had prostate cancer before age 65, you should have this talk with your doctor starting at age 45. If you decide to be tested, you should have the PSA blood test with or without a rectal exam. How often you are tested will depend on your PSA level.

*If the test is positive, a colonoscopy should be done.
**The multiple stool take-home test should be used. One test done by the doctor in the office is not adequate for testing. A colonoscopy should be done if the test is positive.
Data from the American Cancer Society: American Cancer Society Guidelines for the Early Detection of Cancer. Retrieved from: http://www.cancer.org/Healthy/FindCancerEarly/CancerScreeningGuidelines/american-cancer-society-guidelines-for-the-early-detection-of-cancer.

system, $T_1N_0M_0$ designates a small localized tumor; $T_2N_1M_0$ is a larger primary tumor that has extended to regional nodes; and $T_{43}NM_3$ is a very large lesion involving regional nodes and distant sites. PTNM is a TNM confirmed by pathology. CTNM is a clinical assessment of TNM. Tx is used when the tumor is unevaluated.

cancr-, cancri-, cancro-, prefix meaning "cancer": *cancriform, cancroid.*

cancriform /kang″krifôrm′/ [L, crab, *forma,* form], pertaining to a lesion resembling a cancer.

cancroid [L, crab; Gk, *eidos,* form], pertaining to a lesion resembling a cancer.

cancrum /kang″krəm/, a gangrenous, ulcerative, inflammatory lesion. Cancrum nasi is a gangrenous, ulcerative condition often associated with rhinitis in children.

candela, formerly called **candle power.** See **candle.**

candesartan, an antihypertensive in the angiotensin II receptor antagonist class.

■ INDICATIONS: It is used to treat hypertension, either alone or in combination with other drugs.

■ CONTRAINDICATIONS: Known hypersensitivity to this drug prohibits its use.

■ ADVERSE EFFECTS: Angioedema is a potentially life-threatening side effect. Dizziness, diarrhea, cough, and upper respiratory infection are common side effects. Other side effects include fatigue, headache, nausea, arthralgia, and pain.

Candida /kan″didə/ [L, *candidus,* white], a genus of yeast, including the common pathogen *Candida albicans,* which is an agent of opportunistic oral and genital infections in humans. Formerly called ***Monilia.***

Candida albicans /al″bəkanz/, a common budding yeast; a microscopic fungal organism normally present in the mucous membranes of the mouth, intestinal tract, and vagina of healthy people. Under certain circumstances, it may cause superficial infections of the skin, mouth, or vagina. Infection of the esophagus and severe invasive systemic infections may occur in persons who are immunocompromised. See also **candidiasis.**

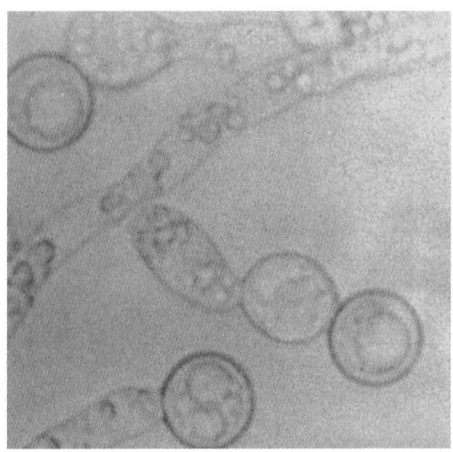

Candida albicans *(Courtesy Dr. Ellen Wald, University of Wisconsin Children's Hospital)*

Candida endocarditis, mycotic endocarditis caused by a species of *Candida.*

Candida glabrata. See ***Torulopsis glabrata.***

Candida guilliermondii, a species of *Candida* that sometimes causes cutaneous candidiasis, fungal infections of the nails. Rare systemic infections include meningitis and endocarditis, particularly in individuals using addictive drugs intravenously.

Candida kefyr, an opportunistic species that occasionally causes human disease and has been isolated from nails and pulmonary specimens. Formerly called ***Candida pseudotropicalis.***

Candida krusei, an extremely rare non-albicans species of *Candida* occasionally associated with candidiasis, esophagitis, endocarditis, and vaginitis.

Candida lusitaniae, an extremely rare species that causes opportunistic infections in humans. This species often demonstrates resistance to amphotericin B, the major antifungal antimicrobial used to treat invasive infections and mycoses.

candidal vaginitis, candidal vulvovaginitis, now called **vulvovaginal candidiasis.**

Candida peritonitis, peritonitis caused by a species of *Candida,* usually as a complication of peritoneal dialysis, with symptoms that include abdominal pain with or without mild fever, nausea, and vomiting.

Candida pneumonia. See **pulmonary candidiasis.**

Candida pseudotropicalis. See *Candida kefyr.*

Candida stellatoidea, a species that sometimes causes *Candida* vaginitis or endocarditis. It is closely related to *Candida albicans.*

Candida vaginitis, *Candida* vulvovaginitis. See **vulvovaginal candidiasis.**

candidiasis /kan′didī″əsis/ [L, *candidus* + Gk, *osis,* condition], any infection caused by a species of *Candida,* usually *Candida albicans.* The nails, rectum, and skin folds are sites of infection. Diaper rash, intertrigo, vaginitis, conjunctivitis, and thrush are common topical manifestations of candidiasis. Oral candidiasis without a history of recent antibiotic therapy, cytotoxic therapy, corticosteroid therapy, radiation therapy to the head and neck, or immunosuppressive disorder may indicate the possibility of human immunodeficiency virus infection. The most common source for candidemia is the GI tract and intravascular catheters. Also called *candidosis, moniliasis.*

■ OBSERVATIONS: This common form of vaginitis presents with a thick, cheesy white or yellow discharge, intense itching, and redness and swelling of labia and vulva. Symptoms exacerbate in the week that precedes menses, and menstruation provides some relief of the itching. Diagnosis is based on symptomatology and positive wet mount or culture.

■ INTERVENTIONS: Treatment targets the infective agent with the use of topical and/or oral antifungal agents.

■ PATIENT CARE CONSIDERATIONS: Instruction in correct use of vaginal applications of medications is needed. Stress should be placed on the need to complete the full course of antifungal treatment. Education should include the importance of vaginal hygiene/cleanliness to prevent an environment for pathogen growth. Douching should be avoided because it destroys the protective vaginal environment. Tight, nonporous, nonabsorbent underclothing should be avoided.

Candiru fever /kan″diroo′/, an arbovirus infection transmitted to humans by the bite of a sandfly, characterized by an acute fever, headache, and muscle aches. Recovery occurs, without treatment, within a few days. The infection occurs mainly in the forests of Brazil. See also **arbovirus, phlebotomus fever.**

candle [L, *candela,* light], (in optics) the basic unit of measurement for luminous intensity, equal to ⅟₆₀ of the luminous intensity of a square centimeter of a black body heated to 1773.5° C or the solidification temperature of platinum, adopted in 1948 as the international standard of luminous intensity. Also called **candela.**

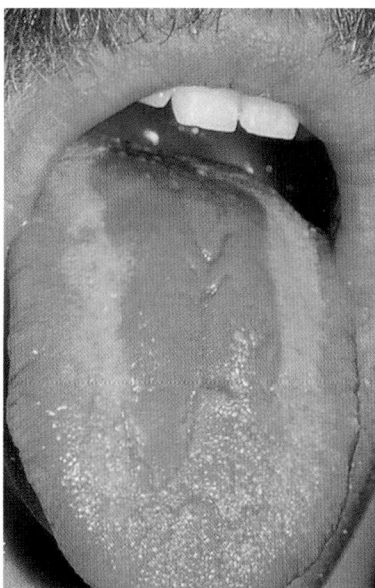

Oral candidiasis *(Friedman-Kien and Cockerell, 1996)*

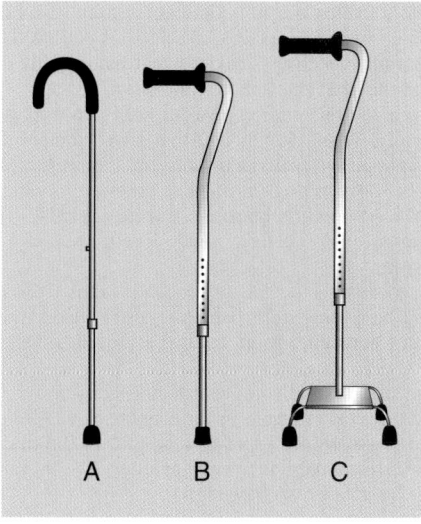

Single- and quad-foot canes *(Mosby, 2003)*

candle power (CP), *(Obsolete)* now called **candela.** See **candle.**

candy-striper, *(Informal)* a hospital volunteer, named for the striped pink-and-white uniforms worn by the young women who originated the role in the 1940s; typically, candy-stripers are junior high or high school students. Although the tradition of the uniform has changed, young men and women continue to serve as volunteers.

cane [Ar, *qanah,* reed], a sturdy wooden or metal shaft or walking stick used to give support and mobility during walking to a person with impaired mobility. A cane should be of an appropriate length to allow a person with an injured leg to walk with it held on the side of the noninjured leg. In walking, the person may rest his or her weight on the cane and the injured leg while moving the unaffected leg forward. To take the next step, the weight is placed on the sound leg while the injured leg and cane are moved forward. The cane should allow 25 degrees of elbow flexion.

cane sugar, sucrose from sugarcane.

canine fossa /kā″nīn/ [L, *canis,* dog; L, ditch], (in dentistry) either of the wide depressions on the external surface of each maxilla, superolateral to the canine tooth socket. It is the origin of the levator anguli oris muscle. Also called **maxillary fossa.**

canine tooth, any of the four teeth, one on each side of the upper and lower jaws, situated between the lateral incisor and the first premolar. The canine teeth are larger and stronger than the incisors and have characteristics of both anterior and posterior teeth. Canines are the longest rooted teeth in the dentition, and serve as a turning point and transition between anterior and posterior teeth. They project beyond the occlusal level of the other teeth in both arches. Their roots sink deeply into the bones, causing marked prominences on the alveolar arch. The upper (maxillary) canine teeth, or eyeteeth, are larger and longer than the mandibular canines and have a distinct basal ridge. The lower (mandibular) canine teeth, or stomach teeth, are situated nearer the midline than the maxillary canines, and their summits (cuspal edges) correspond to the intervals between the upper canines and incisors. The crowns of the canines are very large and conic and taper to blunted points or cusps. The primary canines lie between the primary lateral incisors and primary first molars and erupt about 16 to 20 months after birth, whereas the adult permanent canines erupt during the eleventh or twelfth year of life. The canines serve to powerfully grasp, tear, and cut food in preparation for further mastication.

canities /kanish″i·ēz/, loss of pigment, as in the graying of hair or the appearance of white streaks in the nails.

canker /kang″kər/ [L, *cancer,* crab], an ulcer or sore in the mouth or genitals. Also called **aphthous stomatitis, chancre.**

canker sore, an ulcerous lesion of the mouth, characteristic of aphthous stomatitis. It is hereditary and not contagious. Most often the sores heal without treatment. Sodium lauryl sulfate, which is present in most toothpastes, may worsen the symptoms. Antimicrobial mouthwashes or corticosteroid topical treatment are sometimes prescribed. See also **aphthous stomatitis.**

cannabis /kan″əbis/ [Gk, *kannabis,* hemp], a psychoactive herb (marijuana) derived from the flowering tops of hemp plants. Prescription use of cannabis for medical purposes is now legal in many states and Canadian provinces. However, the use and possession of marijuana continues to be considered a federal offense. All parts of the plant contain psychoactive substances. Cannabinoids, or psychoactive substances synthesized by the hemp plant, include cannabinol, cannabidiol, cannabinolic acid, cannabigerol, cannabicyclol, and several isomers of tetrahydrocannabinol (THC). THC is believed to cause the most characteristic psychological effects, which include alterations of mood, memory, motor coordination, cognitive ability, and self-perception. Low doses of cannabis commonly hinder complex actions, such as driving and flying, which involve complex sensory perception, concentration, and information processing. Cannabis may also enhance the nondominant senses of touch, taste, and smell. Higher doses in some persons can produce delusions, paranoid feelings, anxiety, and panic. This drug also increases the heart rate and systolic blood pressure. Cannabis is about three times more powerful when smoked than when taken orally. Research indicates that some cannabinoids may be therapeutic as anticonvulsants or antiemetics and may be helpful in reducing intraocular pressure associated with glaucoma. Also called **bhang, ganja, grass, hashish, marijuana,** *pot,* **reefer, tea, weed.** See also **medical marijuana.**

cannon A wave [L, *cane,* tube; AS, *wafian*], a powerful atrial wave in the jugular venous pulse caused by the contraction of the right atrium against a closed tricuspid valve. Rapid, regular cannon A waves (the "frog sign") are diagnostic of paroxysmal supraventricular tachycardia. Irregular cannon A waves are seen in atrioventricular (AV) dissociation and are therefore especially helpful in the diagnosis of ventricular tachycardia, which includes AV dissociation in 50% of cases. See also **frog sign.**

cannula /kan′yələ/ *pl. cannulas, cannulae* [L, small tube], a flexible tube that may be inserted into a duct or cavity to deliver medication or drain fluid. It may be guided by a sharp, pointed instrument (trocar). A body fluid may be passed through the cannula to the outside. See also **nasal cannula.** *−cannular, cannulate, adj.*

cannulation /kan′yələ″shən/, the insertion of a cannula into a body duct or cavity, as into the trachea, bladder, or a blood vessel. Also called *cannulization. −cannulate, cannulize, v.*

canonical babbling, a pattern of speech that begins at approximately 6 to 7 months of age. The child's oral musculature and voice are coordinated and capable of producing sounds that are recognized as real syllables. The primary feature of this period of development is the emergence of sequences of consonant-vowel syllables with adultlike timing. Babies sound as if they are trying to produce real words. There is no evidence, however, that these sounds are linked to a specific referent. Compare **integrative babbling.**

CANS, abbreviation for *Council for the Advancement of Nursing Science.*

cantering rhythm [Canterbury gallop; Gk, *rhythmos,* beat], a pattern of three heart sounds in each cardiac cycle, resembling the canter of a horse. See also **gallop.**

cantharis /kan′thäris/ *pl. cantharides* [Gk, *kantharis,* beetle], the dried insect *Cantharis vesicatoria,* which contains cantharidin, used in dilute amounts in homeopathic preparations. Its best-known traditional use has been as an aphrodisiac. There is insufficient evidence to support its use or efficacy. Also called **Spanish fly.**

cantho-, prefix meaning "canthus (the corner of the eye)": *canthoplasty.*

canthoplasty /kan′thōplas′tē/, a form of plastic surgery used to lengthen the palpebral fissure through the lateral canthus or to restore a defective canthus (the junction of eyelids) to help create an upward slant in the outer corner of the eyelid or to correct a droopy appearance.

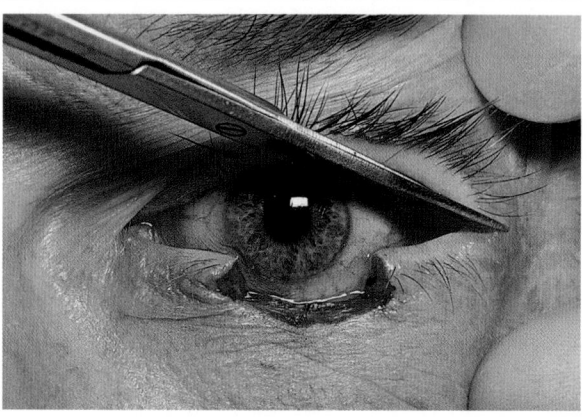

Canthoplasty *(Tyers and Collin, 2008)*

canthorraphy /kanthôr″əfē/, a surgical procedure to suture the eyelids at either canthus.

canthus /kan′thəs/ *pl. canthi* [Gk, *kanthus,* corner of the eye], the angle at the medial and the lateral margins of the eyelids. The medial canthus opens into a small space containing the opening to a lacrimal duct. Also called **palpebral commissure.** *−canthical, adj.*

Cantil, an anticholinergic antispasmodic. Brand name for **mepenzolate bromide.**

Cantor tube [Meyer O. Cantor, American physician, b. 1907], a long, single-lumen nasoenteric tube with a small, sealed, mercury-filled, rubber bag at the distal end, used to relieve obstructions in the small intestine. The tube also contains drainage holes to allow for aspiration of intestinal contents. Now largely replaced by the Andersen long weighted sump tube due to concerns related to potential failure of the mercury weighted bag.

CaO, chemical formula for **calcium oxide.**

Ca(OH)$_2$, chemical formula for **calcium hydroxide.**

CAOT, abbreviation for **Canadian Association of Occupational Therapists.**

cap, 1. the maximum dollar amount a health insurance company would pay in lifetime benefits for care. The Affordable Care Act of 2010 banned lifetime limits in the United States for essential health benefits; however some insurance plans were grandfathered and exempt from this cap. Services that are not considered essential benefits are often subject to a cap. 2. *(Informal)* in dentistry, an artificial crown.

CAP, 1. abbreviation for **College of American Pathologists.** 2. abbreviation for **catabolic activator protein.**

capacitance (C) /kəpas″ətəns/, 1. a measure of electrostatic capacity or the amount of stored electrical charge per unit of electrical potential. 2. the ability of a body to store an electrical charge. Any object that can be electrically charged exhibits capacitance.

capacitance vessels [L, *capacitas,* capacity], 1. the blood vessels that hold the major portion of the intravascular blood volume. 2. the veins.

capacitation /kəpas′itā″shən/, the process in which the spermatozoon, after it reaches the ampulla of the fallopian tube, undergoes a series of changes that lead to its ability to fertilize an ovum. Capacitation accomplishes three changes in sperm requisite to their fertilizing an ovum. First is the ability to undergo the acrosome reaction. In the acrosome reaction the seminal plasma factors that coat the sperm are removed, and receptor mobility is restricted, all associated with decreased stability of the acrosomal membrane. As the sperm approaches the ovum, a rapid breakdown of the outer acrosomal membrane occurs, completing the acrosomal reaction. The second changes involve the egress of the enzyme contents of the acrosome, including hyaluronidase, corona-disposing enzyme, and the protease acrosin, all of which facilitate sperm penetration and fusion with the ovarian membrane. Third, the sperm become hypermotile, and this increased velocity is thought to be crucial in zona penetration by the sperm.

capacity /kəpas′i·tē/ [L, *capacitas*], **1.** the power or ability to hold, retain, or contain or the ability to absorb. **2.** mental ability to receive, accomplish, endure, or understand. **3.** the volume or potential volume of material (solid, liquid, or gas) that can be held or contained.

capacity factor /kəpas″itē/ [L, *capacitas + factum,* to make], the ratio of the elution volume of a substance to the void volume in the column.

Capastat, an antibiotic. Brand name for **capreomycin.**

CAPD, abbreviation for **continuous ambulatory peritoneal dialysis.**

capecitabine, an antineoplastic and antimetabolite.

- INDICATIONS: It is used to treat metastatic colorectal and breast cancers.
- CONTRAINDICATIONS: Pregnancy and known hypersensitivity to 5-fluorouracil prohibit its use. It also should not be used in infants.
- ADVERSE EFFECTS: Life-threatening effects include neutropenia, lymphopenia, thrombocytopenia, and myelosuppression. Other serious adverse effects include anemia, hyperbilirubinemia, and edema. Common side effects include nausea, vomiting, anorexia, diarrhea, and stomatitis.

capeline bandage /kap″əlin/ [Fr, hooded cape], a covering applied like a cap. It is used for protecting the head, the shoulder, or a residual limb. Also called **Hippocrates' bandage.**

Capgras syndrome /käpgrä′/ [Jean Marie Joseph Capgras, French psychiatrist, 1873–1950], a form of delusional misidentification in which the patient believes that other persons in the environment are not their real selves but doubles.

Capillaria /kap′ilar′ē·ə/ [L, *capillaris,* hairlike], a genus of nematodes of the family Trichuridae. *C. philippinensis* is a parasite of the human intestine in the Philippines. See also **capillariasis.**

capillariasis /kap′ilərī′əsis/, infection with nematodes of the genus *Capillaria,* species of which attack various different animals. Human infection is usually by *C. philippinensis,* which infests the intestines and causes severe diarrhea, malabsorption, and often death. More rarely, infection with *C. hepatica* can cause human hepatic capillariasis, and infection with *C. aerophila* can cause human pulmonary capillariasis.

capillaries. See **blood vessel.**

capillaritis /kap′ilərī″tis/ [L, *capillaris,* hairlike; Gk, *itis,* inflammation], inflammation of a capillary or capillaries characterized by a progressive pigmentary disorder of the skin and capillaries. It does not involve any systemic problems and runs a benign self-limiting course.

capillarity. See **capillary action.**

capillary /kap″iler′ē/ [L, *capillaris,* hairlike], one of the microscopic blood vessels (about 0.008 mm in diameter) joining arterioles and venules. The wall consists of a single

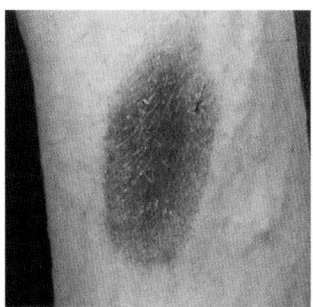

Capillaritis *(du Vivier, 1993)*

layer of endothelial cells, which are specialized squamous epithelial cells. Blood and tissue fluids exchange various substances across these walls.

capillary action, the process involving molecular adhesion by which the surface of a liquid in a tube is either elevated or depressed, depending on the cohesiveness of the liquid molecules. The more cohesive the molecules, the more depressed will be the surface of the liquid. Less cohesive liquid molecules will adhere to the surfaces of the tube in which they are contained and elevate the surface of the liquid. The ability of a liquid to flow against gravity in a narrow space such as a thin tube is an example of capillary action. Also called **capillary attraction, capillarity.**

capillary angioma. See **cherry angioma.**

capillary attraction. See **capillary action.**

capillary bed, a capillary network.

capillary blood sample, a small amount of blood obtained by pricking the skin of the heel, finger, or earlobe with a lancet or needle so that it can be used for examination and/or analysis. Individuals can be taught to obtain this sample at home when frequent monitoring is necessary, as in blood glucose monitoring.

capillary flames. *(Nontechnical)* See **telangiectatic nevus.**

capillary fracture, any thin, hairlike break in a bone.

capillary fragility, a condition in which weakened capillaries rupture easily when stressed, observed as bleeding under the skin.

capillary hemangioma, a blood-filled birthmark or benign tumor consisting of closely packed small blood vessels. Commonly found during infancy, it first grows, then may spontaneously disappear in early childhood without treatment. Surgical removal is not usually attempted unless frequent trauma and bleeding are present. However, surgery may be performed later for cosmetic reasons. Also called **hemangioma simplex, strawberry hemangioma, strawberry mark, nevus vascularis.** Compare **cavernous hemangioma, nevus flammeus.**

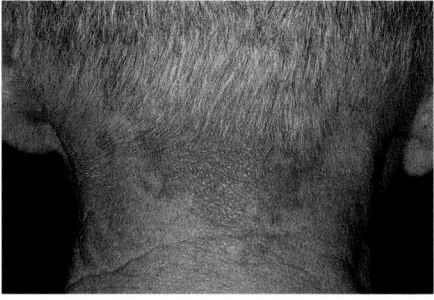

Capillary hemangioma *(Habif, 2011)*

capillary hemorrhage, an oozing of blood from the capillaries.

capillary permeability [L, *capillaris,* hairlike, *permeare,* to pass through], a condition of the capillary wall structure that allows blood elements and waste products to pass through the capillary wall to tissue spaces. Capillaries are selectively permeable, preventing passage of some molecules and permitting others. A balance is normally present between the amount of plasma entering the tissues from the capillaries and the amount reentering the circulatory system. The lining of the capillary may be affected by inflammation or injury, resulting in increased capillary permeability. The increased permeability allows more fluid to enter the tissues, resulting in swelling and/or edema.

capillary pressure [L, *capillaris,* hairlike, *premere,* to press], **1.** the pressure within capillary walls due to the force of blood. **2.** a difference in force between fluids (e.g., oil and water) in contact with each other in small tubelike structures.

capillary pulse. See **Quincke pulse.**

capillary refill. See **blanch test.**

capillary refilling, the process whereby blood returns to a portion of the capillary system after its blood supply has been interrupted briefly. Capillary refilling is tested by pressing firmly on a fingernail and estimating the time required for blood to return after pressure is released. In a normal person with good cardiac output and digital perfusion, capillary refilling should take less than 3 seconds. A time of more than 3 seconds is considered a sign of sluggish digital circulation, and a time of 5 seconds is regarded as abnormal.

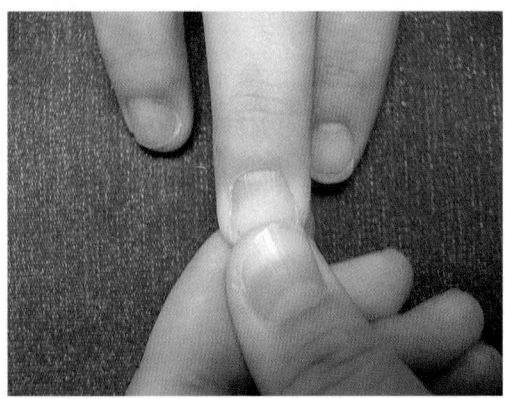

Assessing capillary refill *(Cummings et al, 2009)*

capillary tufting, an abnormal condition in which pulmonary capillaries project as tufts, or small masses, into the alveoli.

capillus /kəpil″əs/ *pl. capilli* [L, filament], one of the hairs of the body, specifically one of the hairs of the scalp.

capit-, capito-, combining form meaning "head": *capital, capitate.*

capita. See **caput.**

capital /kap′itəl/ [L, *caput,* head], **1.** of the highest importance; involving danger to life. **2.** of or pertaining to the head of the femur. Often referred to as the capital femoral epiphysis.

capitate /kap′itāt/, having the shape of a head.

capitate bone [L, *caput,* head; AS, *ban*], one of the largest carpal bones, located at the center of the wrist and having a rounded head that fits the concavity of the scaphoid and the lunate bones. Also called **os capitatum, os magnum.**

capitation, a payment method for health care services. The physician, hospital, or other health care provider is paid a contracted rate for each member assigned, referred to as "per-member-per-month" rate, regardless of the number or nature of services provided. The contractual rates are usually adjusted for age, gender, illness, and regional differences.

capitulum /kəpich″ələm/ *pl. capitula* [L, small head], **1.** a small, rounded prominence on a bone where it articulates with another bone. **2.** the lateral humeral condyle.

capitulum of the humerus, a rounded eminence at the distal, lateral end of the humerus that articulates with the radius.

Caplan syndrome [Anthony Caplan, English physician, 1907–1976], a condition of pneumoconiosis with symptoms of rheumatoid arthritis and radiographic evidence of intrapulmonary nodules. It is caused by inhalation of coal dust and results in inflammation and scarring of the lungs. Although there is no treatment for Caplan syndrome, it is important to treat the rheumatoid arthritis. Also called **rheumatoid pneumoconiosis.**

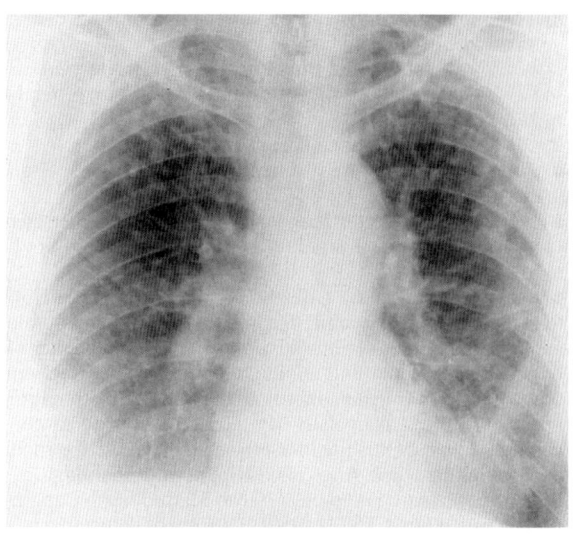

Caplan syndrome *(Hochberg et al, 2015)*

-capnia, suffix meaning "(condition of) carbon dioxide content in the blood": *acapnia, hypocapnia.*

capnogram, measurement of carbon dioxide. See **capnograph, end-tidal CO$_2$.**

capnograph /kap″nəgraf′/ [Gk, *kapnos,* smoke, *graphein,* to record], an instrument used in anesthesia, intensive care, and respiratory therapy to produce a capnogram, a tracing that shows the concentration of carbon dioxide in each exhaled breath. It is used to monitor the adequacy of spontaneous and mechanical ventilation. Also called **capnogram.**

capnometry /kapnom″ətrē/, the measurement of carbon dioxide in a volume of gas. The most common monitoring units are based on the selective absorption of infrared light by carbon dioxide and water vapor. Capnometry may also be performed by using mass spectrometry. See also **end-tidal CO$_2$.**

capotement /käpōtmäN″, kəpōt″mənt/, an irregular vibration causing a splashing sound, made by fluid movements in a dilated stomach containing air and fluid.

Capoten, an angiotensin-converting enzyme inhibitor. Brand name for **captopril.**

capping, **1.** a process by which cell-surface molecules aggregate on a plasma membrane. **2.** *(Informal)* the practice of replacing the covering on a syringe needle. A "sharps" container should be used for the disposal of used syringes. If an appropriate container is unavailable, the Occupational Safety and Health Administration (OSHA) mandates that a mechanical device be used to recap needles.

cap polyposis, a rare type of polyposis coli in which inflammatory polyps have elongated crypts and caps of purulent, fibrinous exudate.

capreomycin /kap′rē·ōmī′sin/, an antibiotic and antitubercular agent.

■ INDICATIONS: It is prescribed in the treatment of pulmonary infections caused by capreomycin-susceptible strains of *Mycobacterium tuberculosis* when the primary agents are ineffective or cannot be used.

■ CONTRAINDICATIONS: Known sensitivity to this drug prohibits its use. It must be used with caution in patients with preexisting renal or auditory impairment.

■ ADVERSE EFFECTS: Among the most serious adverse reactions are nephrotoxicity, hearing loss, tinnitus, vertigo, leukocytosis, leukopenia, urticaria, and skin rash.

capric acid $(CH_3[CH_2]_8COOH)$ /kap′rik/ [L, *caper,* goat], a white crystalline carboxylic acid with a rancid odor, occurring as a glyceride in natural oils. Capric acid is used in the production of perfumes, flavors, wetting agents, and food additives. Also called **decanoic acid.**

caprizant /kap′rizant/, *(Obsolete)* describing an irregular leaping or bounding pulse.

caproic acid $(CH_3[CH_2]_4COOH)$ /kaprō′ik/, a carboxylic acid present in milk fat and some plant oils. It is used in the production of artificial flavors. Also called **hexanoic acid.**

caps-, kaps-, capsul-, capsulo-, prefix meaning "capsule" or "container": *capsulation, capsuloplasty.*

capsaicin /kapsa′isin/, an alkaloid irritating to the skin and mucous membranes; the pungent active principle in capsicum. It is used in a cream that is a counterirritant and topical analgesic and also in pepper spray. See also **capsicum.**

capsicum, an herbal product derived from peppers native to tropical areas of the Americas.

■ INDICATIONS: It is used for muscle spasms, the pain of inflammation, neuromas, psoriasis, and dry mouth. It is also used as a food antioxidant and as a food seasoning.

■ CONTRAINDICATIONS: It is contraindicated in those with known hypersensitivity, in women who are pregnant or lactating, and in children until more research is available. It should not be used in open wounds or abrasions or near the eyes. It can cause extreme burns and blisters in its undiluted form.

capsid /kap′sid/ [L, *capsa,* box], the layer of protein enveloping the genome of a virion. A capsid is composed of structural units called capsomeres. Its symmetry may be cubic (icosahedral) or helical.

capsomere /kap′səmir/, one of the building blocks of a viral capsid. It consists of groups of identical protein molecules and is visible in an electron microscope.

capsul-, capsulo-. See **caps-, kaps-, capsul-, capsulo-.**

capsula, an anatomic structure. See **capsule,** def. 3.

capsular /kap′sələr/ [L, *capsula,* little box], pertaining to or resembling a small container (capsule).

capsular pattern, a series of limitations of joint movement when the joint capsule is a limiting structure. An example is the range in glenohumeral joints, from flexion as the least limited movement to external rotation as the most limited movement. It occurs only in synovial joints that are controlled by muscles and not in joints that depend primarily on ligamentous stability, such as the sacroiliac.

capsular swelling test, the swelling of capsules of bacteria when they are mixed with their specific antigen. See also **quellung reaction.**

capsular vascular plexus, the network of veins and arteries adjacent to and within the renal capsule.

capsulation /kap′syo͞o·lā′shən/ [L, *capsula,* little box], the enclosure of a medicine in a capsule.

capsule /kap′syəl, kap″səl/ *pl. capsuli* [L, *capsula,* little box], **1.** a small soluble container, usually made of gelatin, used for enclosing a dose of medication for swallowing. Compare **tablet. 2.** a membranous shell surrounding certain microorganisms, such as the pneumococcus bacterium. **3.** a well-defined anatomical structure that encloses an organ or part, such as the capsule of the adrenal gland. Also called **capsula.**

capsule endoscopy, an orally administered, disposable capsule containing video chips and a transmitter that moves passively through the gastrointestinal tract via peristalsis, recording images in the esophagus, stomach, small bowel, and colon. The images are examined for pathology, and the capsule is expelled with feces. Preparation for the procedure is similar to that required for a colonoscopy.

capsulectomy /kap′sələk′təmē/, the surgical excision of a capsule, usually the capsule of a joint or of the lens of the eye.

capsule of the kidney, the fibrous connective tissue enclosure of the kidney. Fatty tissue covers the fibrous capsule and helps protect the organ from bumps and shocks. Compare **Bowman's capsule.**

capsule of the lens. See **lens capsule.**

capsuli, a curved vessel or container. See also **capsule.**

capsulitis /-ī′tis/ [L, *capsula,* little box; Gk, *itis,* inflammation], inflammation of an anatomical capsule (e.g., adhesive capsulitis of the shoulder).

capsuloma /kap′sələ″mə/ *pl. capsulomas, capsulomata* [L, *capsula* + Gk, *oma,* tumor], a neoplasm of the capsule or the subcapsular area of the kidney.

capsuloplasty /kap′sələ̄plas′tē/, plastic surgery performed on the capsule of a joint for repair or reconstruction.

capsulorrhaphy /kap′sələ̄r′əfē/, surgical repair of a tear in a capsule, most often of a joint, to prevent further deterioration.

capsulorrhexis /kap′sələ̄rek″sis/, a surgical technique in which a continuous circular tear in the anterior capsule is made in the crystalline lens to allow phacoemulsification of the lens nucleus during cataract surgery.

capsulotomy /kap′sələt″əmē/ [L, *capsula* + Gk, *temnein,* to cut], an incision into a capsule, such as in an operation to remove a cataract.

captain-of-the-ship doctrine, *(Obsolete)* the historical medicolegal principle that the physician is ultimately responsible for all patient-care activities and that he or she thus may be held accountable and may be sued for negligence or malpractice when the act at issue is performed by an employee or other person under the physician's control, even if not ordered by the physician.

captive reinsurance company, a reinsurance company organized to serve only one client (e.g., one company or a related group of industries).

captopril /kap″tōpril/, an angiotensin-converting enzyme inhibitor.

■ INDICATIONS: It is prescribed for the treatment of hypertension and congestive heart failure.

■ CONTRAINDICATIONS: Known sensitivity to this drug prohibits its use.

■ ADVERSE EFFECTS: Among the most serious adverse reactions are hypotension, proteinuria, renal failure, neutropenia, agranulocytosis, angioneurotic edema, angina, myocardial infarction, Raynaud's disease, cough, hyperkalemia, and congestive heart failure.

capture /kap″chər/, **1.** the catching and holding of a nuclear particle, as an electron, or an electrical impulse originating elsewhere. **2.** (in cardiology) the capture of control of the atria or ventricles after a period of independent beating caused by ectopic beats or an atrioventricular block. **3.** (in cardiology) the ability of a pacemaker to electrically stimulate a cardiac chamber.

capture beat, the return of atrial control over ventricular contraction, following a period of atrioventricular dissociation.

capture-recapture method, a plan for epidemiological studies of health problems such as acquired immunodeficiency syndrome, substance abuse, or prostitution. The method provides for comparative analysis of data from various independent sources and adjusting for missing cases.

caput /kā″pət, kap″ət/ *pl. capita* [L, head], **1.** the head. **2.** the enlarged or prominent extremity of an organ or part.

caput femoris /fem″əris/, the head of the femur. It articulates with the acetabulum; formed by the ilium, ischium, and pubis.

caput fibulae /fib″yəlē/, the head of the fibula. It articulates with the lateral condyle of the tibia.

caput humeri /hyoo̅″mərī/, the head of the humerus. It articulates with the glenoid cavity of the scapula.

caput mallei /mal″ē·ī/, the head of the malleus. It articulates with the incus.

caput mandibulae /mandib″yəlē/, the articular process of the ramus of the mandible.

caput medusae /mədoo̅″sē/ [L, head of Medusa, a mythical snake-haired Gorgon], a pattern of dilated cutaneous veins radiating from the umbilical area of a newborn. The feature is also observed in adults with cirrhosis of the liver with portal hypertension.

caput ossis metacarpalis, the metacarpal head. It articulates with the proximal phalanx of the same digit.

caput phalangis /falan″jis/, the articular head at the distal end of the proximal and middle phalanges.

caput radii /rā″dē·ī/, the head of the radius. It articulates with the capitulum of the humerus on its lateral side.

caput stapedis /stapē″dis/, the head of the stapes.

caput succedaneum /suk′sədənē″əm/ [L, *caput*, head, *succeder,* to replace], a localized pitting edema in the scalp of a fetus that may overlie sutures of the skull. It is usually formed during labor as a result of the circular pressure of the cervix on the fetal occiput. On vaginal examination the swelling may be mistaken for unruptured membranes. If the caput enlarges appreciably during labor, it may cause an erroneous impression of fetal descent on successive examinations. At birth the baby's head may appear markedly deformed, but the swelling begins to resolve immediately and is usually gone in a few days. Compare **cephalhematoma, molding.**

Carabelli cusp [Georg Carabelli, Austrian dentist, 1787–1842], an accessory cusp usually found on the mesiolingual cusp of a maxillary adult permanent first molar. It may be unilateral or bilateral and varies in size. It is commonly seen in persons of Caucasian ancestry but is rarely found in persons of Mongolian or Inuit heritage.

Carafate, an antiulcer drug that forms a protective layer over the ulcer site. Brand name for *sucralfate.*

caramiphen /käram′ifen/, an anticholinergic agent with actions similar to but weaker than those of atropine. The edisylate ester is administered orally as an antitussive, and the hydrochloride ester is administered orally in treatment of Parkinson's disease.

carapace /kar″əpās/ [Sp, *carapacho,* hard shell], a horny shield or shell covering the dorsal surface of an animal such as a turtle.

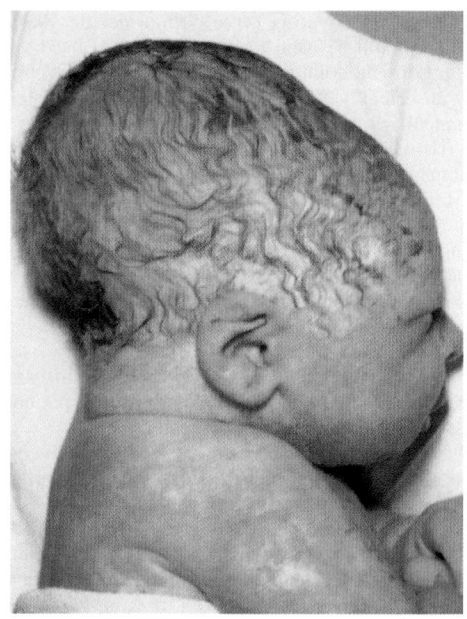

Caput succedaneum *(Beischer, Mackey, and Coblitz, 1997)*

carate, now called **pinta.**

carb, 1. abbreviation for **carbonate. 2.** abbreviation for **carbohydrate.**

carb-. See **carbo-, carbon-, carbono-, carb-, carbi-.**

carbamate /kär″bəmāt/, any of a group of anticholinesterase enzymes that cause reversible inhibition of cholinesterase. They are used in certain medications and insecticides. Some carbamates are toxic and may cause convulsions and death through ingestion or skin contact. Atropine, an anticholinergic medication, is a commonly recommended antidote.

carbamate kinase, a liver enzyme that catalyzes the transfer of a phosphate group from adenosine triphosphate, associated with ammonia and carbon dioxide, to form adenosine diphosphate and carbamoylphosphate.

carbamazepine /kär′bəmaz″əpin/, an anticonvulsant and specific analgesic for trigeminal neuralgia.

■ INDICATIONS: Often a drug of choice for treating partial seizures, generalized tonic-clonic seizures, and other mixed seizures. It is prescribed in the treatment of trigeminal and glossopharyngeal neuralgia and has unlabeled uses for certain affective disorders (e.g., bipolar disorder). It is also used in the treatment of intermittent explosive disorders and rage.

■ CONTRAINDICATIONS: Concomitant use of monoamine oxidase inhibitors, a history of bone marrow depression, pregnancy, or known hypersensitivity to this drug or to any of the tricyclic antidepressants prohibits its use.

■ ADVERSE EFFECTS: Among the more serious adverse reactions are life-threatening blood dyscrasias, drowsiness, dizziness, ataxia, nausea, syndrome of inappropriate diuretic hormone, and dermatological and hypersensitivity reactions. Routine blood tests are recommended.

carbamide peroxide /kär″bəmīd/, a topical antiinfective.

■ INDICATIONS: It is prescribed to treat canker sores and other minor inflammatory conditions of the gums and mouth and to soften impacted earwax.

■ CONTRAINDICATIONS: Perforated eardrum prohibits its use.

■ ADVERSE EFFECTS: The most serious adverse reaction is local irritation.

carbamino compound /kär′bam″inō/, a chemical complex formed by the binding of carbon dioxide molecules to plasma proteins. A small fraction of carbon dioxide binds with protein as it leaves a tissue cell.

carbaminohemoglobin, a chemical complex formed by carbon dioxide and hemoglobin after the release of oxygen by the hemoglobin to a tissue cell. The action is similar to that of the formation of a carbamino compound. It accounts for nearly 25% of the carbon dioxide released in the lung. Also spelled *carbaminohaemoglobin.*

carbenicillin disodium /kär′bənəsil″in/, a semisynthetic penicillin antibiotic with an extended spectrum that includes *Pseudomonas aeruginosa.*

■ INDICATIONS: It is prescribed in the treatment of certain infections caused by sensitive gram-negative aerobic bacilli.

■ CONTRAINDICATIONS: Known hypersensitivity to this drug or to other penicillins prohibits its use.

■ ADVERSE EFFECTS: Among the more serious adverse effects are hypersensitivity reactions, neurological disturbances, and clotting defects. The high sodium content (5.5 to 6.5 mEq/g) may aggravate fluid and electrolyte imbalance in people affected with kidney, heart, or liver disease.

carbetapentane /kärba′täpen′tān/, an antitussive agent with mild atropine-like antisecretory activity used as the tannate salt in treatment of cough associated with upper respiratory infections. It is administered orally.

carbi-. See **carbo-, carbon-, carbono-, carb-, carbi-.**

carbide, a binary compound of carbon. The various compounds range in stability from explosive copper or silver carbides to hard abrasive compounds, such as silicon carbide.

carbidopa /kär′bidō′pə/, a dopa decarboxylase inhibitor that cannot cross the blood-brain barrier. It is administered to people with Parkinson's disease to inhibit peripheral metabolism of levodopa. This property is significant in that it allows a greater proportion of peripheral levodopa to cross the blood-brain barrier for central nervous system effect.

■ INDICATIONS: It is prescribed in combination with levodopa in the treatment of idiopathic Parkinson's disease because it inhibits the degradation of levodopa in the periphery, thereby permitting a larger percentage of orally administered doses to enter the brain.

■ CONTRAINDICATIONS: Glaucoma, hypertension, use of a monoamine oxidase inhibitor within the past 14 days, or known hypersensitivity to this drug prohibits its use.

■ ADVERSE EFFECTS: Among the most serious adverse reactions are GI bleeding, cardiac irregularity, hemolytic anemia, tardive dyskinesia, mental depression, blurred vision, and activation of malignant melanoma.

carbinoxamine maleate /kär′bənok″səmēn/, an antihistamine found in some fixed-combination cold and allergy medications.

■ INDICATIONS: It is prescribed in the treatment of allergic reactions, including rhinitis, skin reactions, and itching.

■ CONTRAINDICATIONS: Asthma or known hypersensitivity to this drug prohibits its use. It should not be administered to infants or lactating mothers. It should be used with caution in patients with renal, cardiac, and liver disorders.

■ ADVERSE EFFECTS: Among the more serious adverse reactions are tachycardia and other side effects of anticholinergic medications. Drowsiness, skin rash, hypersensitivity reactions, and dry mouth commonly occur.

carbo-, carbon-, carbono-, carb-, carbi-, combining form meaning "carbon, carbonic acid, or charcoal": *carbohydrate, carbonate,*

Carbocaine hydrochloride, a local anesthetic. Brand name for *mepivacaine hydrochloride.*

carbocyclic, being or having an organic ring composed of carbon atoms. See **closed-chain.**

carbohydrate /kär′bōhī′drāt/ [L, *carbo,* coal; Gk, *hydor,* water], any of a group of organic compounds, the most important of which are the saccharides, starch, cellulose, and glycogen. Carbohydrates constitute the main source of energy for all body functions, particularly brain functions, and are necessary for the metabolism of other nutrients. They are synthesized by all green plants and in the body are either absorbed immediately or stored in the form of glycogen. Cereals, vegetables, fruits, rice, potatoes, legumes, and flour products are the major sources of carbohydrates. They can also be manufactured in the body from some amino acids and the glycerol component of fats. Symptoms of deficiency include fatigue, depression, breakdown of essential body protein, and electrolyte imbalance. Muscle protein-sparing amounts of food carbohydrates have been estimated to be 50 to 100 g/day for most people. Excessive consumption of simple carbohydrates is associated with tooth decay and is carefully monitored in persons with diabetes. The dietary reference intake for carbohydrates is 130 g/day.

carbohydrate intolerance, inability to properly metabolize one or more carbohydrates, as in fructose intolerance and glucose intolerance.

carbohydrate loading, a dietary practice of some endurance athletes, such as marathon runners, intended to increase glycogen stores in the muscle tissue. The original, or "classic," carbohydrate loading regimen began with a period of several days on a low-carbohydrate diet designed to deplete

Summary of carbohydrate classes

Chemical class n	Class members	Sources
Monosaccharides (single sugars, simple carbohydrates)	Glucose (dextrose)	Corn syrup (commonly used in processed foods)
	Fructose	Fruits, honey
	Galactose	Lactose (milk)
Disaccharides (double sugars, simple carbohydrates)	Sucrose	Table sugar (sugar cane, sugar beets)
	Lactose	Molasses
	Maltose	Milk
		Starch digestion, intermediate
		Sweetener in food products
		Starch digestion, final
Polysaccharides (multiple sugars, complex carbohydrates)	Starch	Grains and grain products (cereal, bread, crackers, baked goods)
	Glycogen	Rice, corn, bulgur
		Legumes
		Potatoes and other vegetables
		Storage form of carbohydrate in animal tissue (not a dietary source)

From Nix S: *Williams' basic nutrition and diet therapy,* ed 13, St. Louis, 2009, Mosby.

C

stored glycogen, followed by consumption of a diet high in complex carbohydrates for 3 days before the event. A more modern approach advocates that athletes routinely consume the high-carbohydrate diet recommended for the general population (55% to 60% of total calories) and eat extra carbohydrates (70%) for 3 days before an event. The practice is controversial and is not universally accepted.

carbohydrate metabolism, the sum of the anabolic and catabolic processes of the body involved in the synthesis and breakdown of carbohydrates, principally glucose, fructose, and galactose. Some of the processes are glycogenesis and glycolysis. Energy-rich phosphate bonds are produced in many metabolic reactions requiring carbohydrates.

carbohydrate utilization test, any of several tests for identification of yeasts and certain other organisms according to a profile of carbohydrate assimilation.

carbolated camphor /kär″bōlā′tid/ [L, *carbo,* coal, *camphora*], *(Obsolete)* a mixture of 1.5 parts camphor with 1 part each of alcohol and phenol; formerly used as an antiseptic dressing for wounds.

carbol-fuchsin solution /kär′bolfook″sin/ [L, *carbo,* coal; Leonard Fuchs, German botanist, 1501–1566], **1.** a preparation used in the treatment of superficial fungal infections. It contains boric acid, phenol, resorcinol, fuchsin, acetone, and alcohol in water. Also called *carbol-fuchsin,* **Castellani paint. 2.** a staining agent for use in acid-fast stains.

carbol-fuchsin stain [L, *carbo,* coal; Leonard Fuchs], a solution of dilute phenol and basic fuchsin used on microorganisms and cell nuclei for microscopic examination. Also called **Ziehl stain.** See also **acid-fast stain, Kinyoun stain.**

carbolic acid (C_6H_5OH) /kärbol″ik/ [L, *carbo,* coal, *acidus,* sour], a poisonous, colorless to pale pink crystalline compound obtained from coal tar distillation or oxidation of cumene and converted to a clear liquid with a strong odor and burning taste by the addition of 10% water. In solution it is a powerful disinfectant. Also called **hydroxybenzene, oxybenzene, phenic acid, phenol, phenylic acid, phenylic alcohol.**

carbolic acid poisoning. See **phenol poisoning.**

carbolism /kär″boliz′əm/, poisoning by phenol, also known as carbolic acid. See **phenol poisoning.**

carbon (C) /kärbən/ [L, *carbo,* coal], a nonmetallic, almost always tetravalent element. Its atomic number is 6; its atomic mass is 12.011. Carbon occurs in pure form in diamonds, graphite, and fullerenes and is a component of all living tissue. The study of organic chemistry focuses on the vast number of carbon compounds. Carbon occurs in impure form in charcoal, coke, and soot, and in the atmosphere as carbon dioxide. Carbon is essential to the chemical mechanisms of the body, participating in many metabolic processes and acting as a component of carbohydrates, amino acids, triglycerides, deoxyribonucleic and ribonucleic acids, and many other compounds. See also **carbon-11, carbon-14.**

carbon-11 (^{11}C), a radioactive isotope of carbon with a half-life equation number of 20.39 minutes. Carbon-11 is used as a device for visualizing and showing the internal outlines of body organs and parts in tomography. Compare **carbon-14.**

carbon-13 (^{13}C), a naturally occurring isotope of carbon, with an atomic mass of 13, occurring 1.11% of the time. It is used as a tracer in liver function tests and a few metabolic tests.

carbon-14 (^{14}C), a radioactive isotope of carbon with a half-life equation number of 5730 years. Carbon-14 is used as a chemical compound in the research of cancer. Compare **carbon-11.**

carbonate (CO_3^{2-}) /kär″bənāt/, a CO_3^{2-} anion. Carbonates are in equilibrium with bicarbonates in water and frequently occur in compounds as insoluble salts, such as calcium carbonate.

carbonate dehydratase. See **carbonic anhydrase.**

carbon cycle, the steps by which carbon in the form of carbon dioxide is extracted from and returned to the atmosphere by living organisms, especially human beings. The process starts with the photosynthetic production of carbohydrates by plants, progresses through the consumption of carbohydrates by animals and human beings, and ends with the exhalation of carbon dioxide by those same animals and human beings and with the release of carbon dioxide during the decomposition of dead plants and animals. Various chemical processes intervene between the ingestion of carbohydrates and the release of carbon dioxide. Carbohydrate metabolism starts with the movement of glucose through plasma membranes and subsequently involves glycolysis, the processes of the citric acid cycle, electron transport, and oxidative phosphorylation. See also **citric acid cycle.**

carbon damp, asphyxiation in an enclosed space. See **damp.**

carbon dioxide (CO_2) [L, *carbo* + Gk, *dis,* twice, *oxys,* sharp], a colorless, odorless gas produced by the oxidation of carbon; also a "greenhouse" gas. Carbon dioxide, as a product of cell respiration, is carried by the blood to the lungs and is exhaled. The acid-base balance of body fluids and tissues is affected by the level of carbon dioxide and its carbonate compounds. Solid carbon dioxide (dry ice) is used in the treatment of some skin conditions. Normal adult blood levels of carbon dioxide are 23 to 30 mEq/L or 23 to 30 mmol/L (SI units). See also **greenhouse effect.**

carbon dioxide acidosis, *(Obsolete)* now called **respiratory acidosis.**

carbon dioxide bath, a therapeutic treatment taken in water that is saturated with carbon dioxide. There is insufficient evidence to show that this type of activity is more effective than no treatment. See also **Nauheim bath, balneotherapy.**

carbon dioxide content (CO_2 content) **test,** a test performed on plasma or serum, often as part of an electrolyte profile that includes sodium, potassium, and chloride levels. It is used to assess pH status.

carbon dioxide inhalation, a carefully controlled procedure in which carbon dioxide gas is administered in the treatment of anxiety or following resuscitation to ameliorate hemorrhagic shock–induced lung injury.

carbon dioxide (CO_2) **narcosis,** a condition of confusion, tremors, convulsions, and possible coma that may occur if blood levels of carbon dioxide increase to 70 mm Hg or higher. Individuals with chronic obstructive pulmonary disease can have CO_2 narcosis without these symptoms because they develop a tolerance to elevated CO_2. When ventilation is sufficient to maintain a normal oxygen partial pressure in the arteries, the carbon dioxide partial pressure is generally near 40 mm Hg. See also **carbon dioxide poisoning.**

carbon dioxide poisoning, a condition of toxic effects caused by inhaling excessive amounts of carbon dioxide. Carbon dioxide is a respiratory stimulant, but it is also an asphyxiant. High concentrations can cause unconsciousness and death from ventilatory failure. Particularly vulnerable are persons who work in confined spaces with poor air circulation, such as mine shafts, silos, or holds of ships. Faulty home furnaces also have been implicated in many deaths. See also **carbon dioxide** (CO_2) **narcosis.**

carbon dioxide pressure. See **carbon dioxide tension.**

carbon dioxide response, the ventilatory reaction to increased concentrations of carbon dioxide in inhaled air. The respiration rate increases linearly up to a concentration of 8% to 10%, rises more gradually up to a concentration of about 20%, and decreases at higher concentrations. At concentrations of around 25%, the person is conscious but unable to perform simple tasks. At concentrations of 30%, carbon dioxide is an anesthetic.

carbon dioxide retention, any increased body stores of carbon dioxide resulting from impaired carbon dioxide elimination in conditions such as alveolar hypoventilation, strangulation, apnea, and ventilation-perfusion abnormalities. Respiratory acidosis may result from carbon dioxide retention.

carbon dioxide slush, solid carbon dioxide combined with a solvent, such as acetone, and sometimes also alcohol, used as an escharotic to treat skin lesions, such as warts and moles, and as a peeling agent in chemabrasion.

carbon dioxide stores, the amount of carbon dioxide contained in the body as a gas and in the form of carbonic acid, carbonate, bicarbonate, and carbaminohemoglobin. During a steady state of ventilation and aerobic respiration, the rate at which carbon dioxide leaves the body equals the rate at which it is produced, and carbon dioxide stores remain constant.

carbon dioxide tension (PCO_2), the partial pressure of carbon dioxide, a measure of the relative concentration of the gas in air or in a fluid, such as plasma. It is expressed quantitatively in millimeters of mercury (mm Hg). Alveolar PCO_2 directly reflects pulmonary gas exchange in relation to blood flow. Alveolar PCO_2 usually decreases as the respiration rate increases. Normal values for arterial and alveolar PCO_2 are between 35 and 45 mm Hg. Higher levels occur in conditions of slow blood flow and respiration. Below-normal values are caused by hyperventilation and lead to respiratory alkalosis. Also called **carbon dioxide pressure.** See also **carbon dioxide, hypercapnia, hyperventilation, hypoventilation.**

carbon dioxide therapy, the therapeutic inhalation of a low concentration of carbon dioxide gas. Such therapy may be used to dilate the blood vessels, stimulate the cardiovascular brain centers and central nervous system, overcome hyperventilation, assist in developing a productive cough needed to remove mucous secretions, and control hiccups.

carbonemia /kär″bənē′mē-ə/, excessive carbonic acid in the blood.

carbon fiber, a material consisting of graphite fibers in a plastic matrix. The properties of carbon fibers include high stiffness, high tensile strength, low weight, high chemical resistance, high temperature tolerance, and low thermal expansion. Carbon fibers are usually combined with other materials to form a composite. When combined with graphite to form carbon-carbon composites, it has a very high heat tolerance. It is used in radiological devices to reduce patient exposure to x-rays.

carbonic acid (H_2CO_3) /kärbon′ik/ [L, *carbo,* coal, *acidus,* acid], an unstable acid formed by dissolving carbon dioxide in water. It is the basis of carbonated beverages and is related to the carbonate group of compounds. Its production in the body is catalyzed by carbonic anhydrase.

carbonic anhydrase /anhī′drās/, an enzyme that assists rapid reciprocal or mutual conversion of carbon dioxide and water into carbonic acid, protons, and bicarbonate ions. It plays a key role in the regulation of pH and fluid balance in different parts of the body. Also called **carbonate dehydratase.**

carbonic anhydrase inhibitor, a substance that decreases the rate of carbonic acid and H^+ production in the kidney, thereby increasing the excretion of solutes and the rate of urinary output. An example of a carbonic anhydrase inhibitor is acetazolamide. Some carbonic anhydrase inhibitors are used as diuretics, others in the treatment of glaucoma.

carbon monoxide (CO) [L, *carbo* + Gk, *monos,* single, *oxys,* sharp], a colorless, odorless, poisonous gas produced by the combustion of carbon or organic fuels in a limited oxygen supply, as in the cylinders of an internal combustion engine or an improperly set oil or gas furnace. CO binds to hemoglobin approximately 210 times stronger than oxygen, preventing the formation of oxyhemoglobin and reducing the oxygen supply to the tissues. Prolonged exposure to high levels of CO results in asphyxiation.

carbon monoxide poisoning, a toxic condition in which carbon monoxide gas has been inhaled and binds to hemoglobin molecules, thus displacing oxygen from the red blood cells and decreasing the capacity of the blood to carry oxygen to the cells of the body. Characteristically, headache, dyspnea, drowsiness, confusion, cherry-pink skin, unconsciousness, and apnea occur in sequence as the level of carbon monoxide in the blood increases. Cherry-red skin is a late sign most commonly noted in fatalities. The most common source of carbon monoxide in cases of poisoning is exhaust fumes from an automobile.

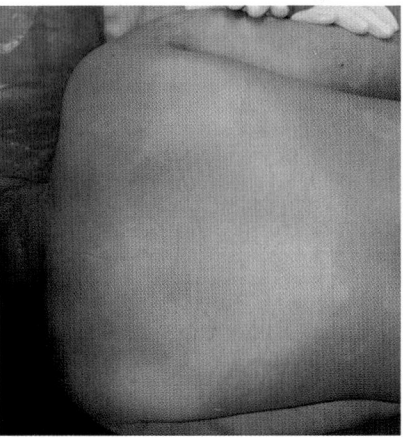

Cherry-pink skin associated with carbon monoxide poisoning *(Mohankumar et al, 2012)*

carbon tetrachloride (CCl_4) [L, *carbo* + Gk, *tetra,* four, *chloros,* greenish], a colorless, volatile toxic liquid used as a solvent. CCl_4 is particularly toxic to the kidneys and liver; permanent damage to these organs may result from exposure.

carbon tetrachloride poisoning [L, *carbo,* coal; Gk, *tetra,* four, *chloros,* greenish; L, *potio,* drink], toxic effects of exposure to carbon tetrachloride, a colorless commercial dry cleaning fluid also used in fire extinguishers and industrial solvents. It may attack both liver and kidneys. Symptoms include persistent headache, nausea, vomiting, diarrhea, uremia, lethargy, confusion resulting from central nervous system depression, and degeneration of the liver and kidneys. Ingestion of the liquid or inhalation of the fumes usually results in headaches, nausea, central nervous system depression, abdominal pain, and convulsions. In poisoning by inhalation, ventilatory assistance and oxygen may be necessary. A poison control center should be contacted if carbon tetrachloride poisoning is expected.

carboplatin /kär″bōplat′in/, one of a series of platinum analog drugs used in cancer therapy. It is commonly administered intravenously for the treatment of ovarian cancer.

carboprost, a synthetic analog of dinoprost used as an oxytocic for termination of pregnancy and missed abortion, administered intramuscularly.

carboxyfluoroquinolone /kärbok′sēfloo′ərōkwī′nəlōn/, any of a group of oral quinolone antibiotics that are generally effective against Enterobacteriaceae and show varying activity against *Pseudomonas* and other species. The drugs differ in their oral absorption.

carboxyhemoglobin /kärbok′sēhē″məglō′bin, -hem″-/ [L, *carbo* + Gk, *oxys,* sharp, *haima,* blood; L, *globus,* ball], a hemoglobin variant produced by the exposure of hemoglobin to carbon monoxide. Carbon monoxide from the environment is inhaled into the lungs, absorbed through the alveoli, and bound to hemoglobin in the blood, blocking the sites for oxygen transport. Oxygen levels decrease, and hypoxia and anoxia may result. Also spelled *carboxyhaemoglobin.* See also **carbon monoxide poisoning, oxyhemoglobin.**

carboxyhemoglobin test, a measurement of the carboxyhemoglobin level in whole blood. A level higher than 5% in a nonsmoker or 10% in a smoker confirms carbon monoxide poisoning.

carboxyl /kärbok″sil/, a monovalent radical (R–COOH) characteristic of organic acids. The hydrogen of the radical can be replaced by metals to form salts.

carboxylase /kärbok′səlās/, an enzyme that catalyzes the addition of a molecule of carbon dioxide to another compound to form a carboxyl group.

carboxylation /-lā″shən/, a chemical process in which a carboxylic acid group (COOH) is introduced into a substrate.

carboxylic acid /kär′bok·sil′ik as′id/, any of a group of organic acids containing the carboxyl radical R–COOH, including amino acids and fatty acids.

carboxymethylcellulose /kärbok″semeth″ilsel′ulōs/, a substituted cellulose polymer of variable size. The sodium or calcium salt is used as a pharmaceutical suspending agent, tablet excipient, and viscosity-increasing agent. The sodium salt is also used as a laxative.

carboxymethylcellulose calcium, the calcium salt of carboxymethylcellulose, used as a tablet disintegrant in pharmaceutical preparations. See also **carboxymethylcellulose.**

carbuncle /kär″bungkəl/ [L, *carbunculus,* little coal], a large site of staphylococcal or streptococcal infection containing purulent matter in deep, interconnecting subcutaneous pockets. Pus eventually discharges to the skin surface through openings. Common sites for carbuncles are the back of the neck and the buttocks. Treatment may include the use of antibiotics, hot compresses, and surgical drainage. Compare **furuncle.**

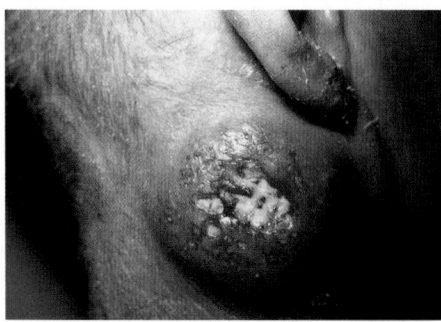

Carbuncle *(Conlon and Snydman, 2000)*

carbunculosis /karbung′kyəlō″sis/, an abnormal condition characterized by a cluster of deep, painful abscesses that drain through multiple openings onto the skin surface, usually around hair follicles. Carbunculosis is a form of folliculitis, most commonly caused by the bacterium *Staphylococcus aureus* and less frequently by *methicillin-resistant Staphylococcus aureus (MRSA).* The lesions caused by this condition may cause fever and malaise. Diabetics and the immunosuppressed are more susceptible to carbunculosis. Men are more susceptible to carbuncles than are women.

■ OBSERVATIONS: Carbunculosis commonly follows persistent *S. aureus* infection and furunculosis. Diagnosis is based on obvious skin lesions, a patient history of previous furunculosis, and *S. aureus* in wound culture.

■ INTERVENTIONS: Treatment of carbunculosis requires the administration of systemic antibiotics and surgical drainage. The prognosis depends on the severity of the infection and the physical condition of the patient.

■ PATIENT CARE CONSIDERATIONS: Health care for this disorder is mainly supportive and educative to impress the patient with the importance of meticulous personal and family hygiene. Patient teaching includes explaining the importance of reducing sugar and fat intake and cautioning the patient not to squeeze a carbuncle or furuncle because it may rupture into the surrounding area. The patient is also instructed not to share towels and washcloths with other family members because this practice may spread the bacteria. Also stressed are the importance of thoroughly laundering towels and washcloths before reusing them and the need for daily changes of laundered clothes and bedsheets. The patient is additionally encouraged to change dressings frequently and to discard them in paper bags. Because carbunculosis often follows furunculosis, a disorder associated with diabetes, the patient should have a thorough physical examination.

carcin-, carcino-, combining form meaning "cancer": *carcinogen.*

carcinoembryonic antigen (CEA) /kär′sənō·em′brē·on″ik/ [Gk, *karkinos,* crab, *en,* into, *bryein,* to grow, *anti,* against, *genein,* to produce], an antigen present in very small quantities in adult tissue. Changes in CEA values are used to monitor tumor response to treatment. The reference range for serum CEA is 0 to 3 ng/mL in nonsmokers and 0 to 5 ng/mL in smokers.

carcinogen /kärsin″əjin/ [Gk, *karkinos* + *genein,* to produce], a substance or agent that causes the development or increases the incidence of cancer. The U.S. Department of Health and Human Services publishes a biennial report that contains a list of all substances that either are known to be human carcinogens or may reasonably be anticipated to be human carcinogens. **–carcinogenic,** *adj.*

carcinogenesis /kär′sinəjen″əsis/, the process of initiating and promoting cancer. Compare **malignant transformation, oncogenesis, sarcomagenesis, tumorigenesis.**

carcinogenic /kär′sinəjen″ik/, pertaining to the ability to cause the development of a cancer. Also spelled *cancerigenic, cancerogenic.* **–carcinogenicity,** *n.*

carcinoid /kär″sinoid/ [Gk, *karkinos* + *eidos,* form], a small yellow tumor derived from argentaffin cells in the GI mucosa that secrete serotonin and other catecholamines. Carcinoid tumors spread slowly locally but may metastasize widely. There are typically no systemic symptoms until metastasis occurs. Also called **argentaffinoma, Kulchitsky cell carcinoma.** See also **argentaffin cell, carcinoid syndrome.**

carcinoid syndrome, the systemic effects of serotonin-secreting carcinoid tumors, which include flushing, diarrhea, cramps, skin lesions resembling pellagra, labored breathing, palpitations, and valvular heart disease, especially of the tricuspid and pulmonary valve. Treatment includes surgical excision of the tumor, if feasible. Chemotherapy and radiation treatment are occasionally used. Also called **argentaffinoma syndrome.** See also **carcinoid.**

carcinolysis /kär′sinol″isis/ [Gk, *karkinos* + *lysis,* loosening], the destruction of cancer cells. See also **cancericidal.** −*carcinolytic, adj.*

carcinoma /kär′sinō″mə/ [Gk, *karkinos* + *oma,* tumor], a malignant epithelial neoplasm that tends to invade surrounding tissue and to metastasize to distant regions of the body. Carcinomas develop most frequently in the skin, large intestine, lungs, stomach, prostate, cervix, or breast. The tumor is firm, irregular, and nodular, with a well-defined border. Microscopically, the cells are characterized by abnormal size and shape, disproportionately large nuclei, and clumps of nuclear chromatin. −**carcinomatous,** *adj.*

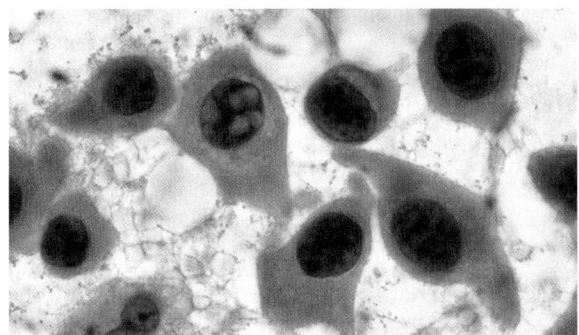

Carcinoma cells showing loss of cohesion *(McKee, 1997)*

carcinoma basocellulare, *(Obsolete)* now called **basal cell carcinoma.**

carcinoma cutaneum, *(Obsolete)* cancers of the skin. Now called **basal cell carcinoma, squamous cell carcinoma.**

carcinoma en cuirasse /äN″kēräs″/ [Gk, *karkinos* + *oma* + Fr, breastplate], a rare recurrence of breast cancer characterized by progressive extensive fibrosis and rigidity of the skin of the chest, neck, back, and abdomen.

carcinoma fibrosum. See **scirrhous carcinoma.**

carcinoma gigantocellulare. See **giant cell carcinoma.**

carcinoma in situ /insit″oo, insī″too/ [Gk, *karkinos* + *oma* + L, in position], a premalignant neoplasm that has not invaded the basement membrane but shows cytological characteristics of cancer. Such neoplastic changes in stratified squamous or glandular epithelium frequently occur on the uterine cervix and in the anus, bronchi, buccal mucosa, esophagus, eye, lip, penis, uterine endometrium, and vagina. Also called **cancer in situ, intraepithelial carcinoma, preinvasive carcinoma.** See also **erythroplasia of Queyrat.**

carcinoma lenticulare /len′tikoōlär′ə/ [Gk, *karkinos* + *oma* + L, lens], a form of tuberous carcinoma or scirrhous skin cancer characterized by the development of many small, flat nodules that coalesce to form larger areas resembling a fungus infection.

carcinoma medullare, carcinoma molle. See **medullary carcinoma.**

carcinoma mucocellulare. See **Krukenberg tumor.**

carcinoma scroti /skrō″tī/, an epithelial cell carcinoma of the scrotum.

carcinoma spongiosum /spon′jē·ō″səm/, a soft and spongy carcinoma with small and large cavities. See also **medullary carcinoma.**

carcinomata, *(Obsolete)* now called **carcinoma.**

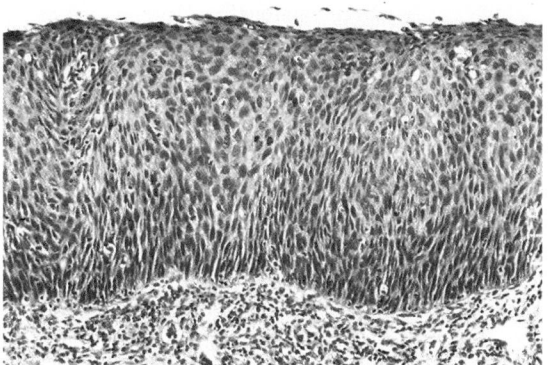

Carcinoma in situ *(Kumar et al, 2010)*

carcinoma telangiectaticum /telan′jē·ektat″ikəm/ [Gk, *karkinos* + *oma* + *telos,* end, *angeion,* vessel, *ektasis,* dilation], a neoplasm of the capillaries of the skin causing dilation of the vessels and red spots on the skin that blanch with pressure.

carcinomatoid /kär′sinō″mətoid/, resembling a carcinoma.

carcinomatosis. See **carcinosis.**

carcinomatous /-om″ətəs/, pertaining to carcinoma. See also **carcinous.**

carcinomatous pericarditis. See **neoplastic pericarditis.**

carcinoma tuberosum. See **tuberous carcinoma.**

carcinoma villosum. See **villous carcinoma.**

carcinophilia /kär′sinō″fil″yə/ [Gk, *karkinos* + *philein,* to love], the property in which there is an affinity for carcinomatous tissue. −*carcinophilic, adj.*

carcinosarcoma /kär′sinōsärkō″mə/ [Gk, *karkinos* + *sarx,* flesh, *oma,* tumor], a malignant neoplasm composed of carcinomatous and sarcomatous cells. Tumors of this type may occur in the esophagus, thyroid gland, and uterus.

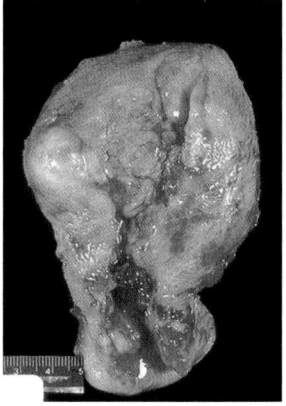

Carcinosarcoma *(Fletcher, 2007)*

carcinosis /kär′sinō″sis/ *pl. carcinoses,* a condition characterized by the development of many carcinomas throughout the body. Also called **carcinomatosis.** Kinds include **carcinosis pleurae, miliary carcinosis, pulmonary carcinosis.**

carcinosis pleurae /ploo″rē/, a secondary malignancy of the pleura in which nodules develop throughout the membranes.

carcinostatic /kär′sinōstat″ik/ [Gk, *karkinos* + *statikos,* causing to stand], pertaining to the tendency to slow or halt the growth of a carcinoma.

carcinous. See **carcinomatous.**

Cardarelli sign [Antonio Cardarelli, Italian physician, 1831–1927], an abnormal lateral pulsation of the trachea, particularly associated with aneurysm or dilation of the aortic arch.

cardia /kär″dē·ə/ [Gk, *kardia,* heart], **1.** the opening between the esophagus and the cardiac portion of the stomach. **2.** the portion of the stomach surrounding the esophagogastric connection, characterized by the absence of acid cells. –**cardiac,** *adj.*

cardia-, cardi-, cardio-, combining form meaning "heart": *cardiac, periocardiocentesis.*

-cardia, suffix meaning a "type of heart action or location": *bradycardia, dextrocardia.*

cardiac /kär″dē·ak/ [Gk, *kardia,* heart], **1.** pertaining to the heart. **2.** pertaining to the part of the stomach closest to the esophagus.

-cardiac, suffix meaning "to characterize types and locations of heart ailments": *intracardiac, pericardiac.*

cardiac action potential, the transmembrane potential in the heart consisting of five phases: 0, the upstroke or rapid depolarization, which initiates the heartbeat in response to an influx of Na^+; 1, early rapid repolarization; 2, plateau in response to an influx of Ca^{2+}; 3, final rapid repolarization in response to an influx of K^+; and 4, resting membrane potential and diastolic depolarization. Abnormalities of the heart or its conduction system that alter the cardiac action potential lead to the development of cardiac arrhythmias.

cardiac aneurysm, an enlargement of the cardiac tissue, which may include the aorta, atria, or ventricle. It is often associated with hypertension or myocardial infarction. See **ventricular aneurysm.**

cardiac angiography. See **angiocardiography.**

cardiac apex. See **apex cordis.**

cardiac apnea [Gk, *kardia + a + pnein,* not to breathe], an abnormal, temporary absence of respiration, such as occurs in Cheyne-Stokes respiration.

cardiac arrest [Gk, *kardia +* L, *ad + restare,* to withstand], a sudden cessation of cardiac output and effective circulation. It is usually precipitated by ventricular fibrillation or ventricular asystole. When cardiac arrest occurs, delivery of oxygen and removal of carbon dioxide stop, tissue cell metabolism becomes anaerobic, and metabolic and respiratory acidosis ensue. Immediate initiation of cardiopulmonary resuscitation is required to prevent heart, lung, kidney, and brain damage and death. Also called **cardiopulmonary arrest.** See also **cardiopulmonary resuscitation.**

cardiac arrhythmia [Gk, *kardia + a + rhythmos,* without rhythm], **1.** *(Nontechnical)* an abnormal cardiac rate or rhythm. The condition is caused by a failure of the sinus node to maintain its pacemaker function or by a defect in the electrical conduction system. Kinds include **bradycardia, ectopic beat, heart block, tachycardia. 2.** most accurately, the absence of a cardiac rhythm, as in asystole.

cardiac asthma, *(Nontechnical)* the wheezing that can occur in patients with left heart failure. Cardiac asthma is not true asthma. The wheezing is due to a decrease in airway diameter caused by pulmonary congestion, not bronchoconstriction.

cardiac atrophy, a wasting of heart muscle usually caused by cachexia, aging, or a mediastinal tumor.

cardiac care, comprehensive health care provided to individuals and families experiencing problems associated with cardiac disease, including the diagnosis, treatment, and rehabilitation services needed to improve physiological function, to maintain or improve quality of life, and to prevent complications.

cardiac catheter, a long, fine catheter designed to be passed into the heart through a blood vessel. Used for diagnosis, it allows the determination of blood pressure and the rate of blood flow in the vessels and chambers of the heart and the identification of abnormal anatomy. Medication may be instilled directly through the catheter into a coronary vessel, often seen by tomography.

cardiac catheterization, a diagnostic procedure in which a catheter is introduced through an incision into a large artery or vein, usually of an arm or a leg, and threaded through the circulatory system to the heart.

■ METHOD: The sterile radiopaque catheter 100 to 125 cm in length ultimately reaches the superior vena cava, and then enters into the right atrium (or through an artery leading to the left ventricle) and other structures to be studied. The course of the catheter is followed with fluoroscopy, and radiographs may be taken. An electrocardiogram is monitored on an oscilloscope. As the catheter tip passes through the chambers and vessels of the heart, blood pressure is monitored, and blood samples are taken to study the oxygen content.

■ PATIENT CARE CONSIDERATIONS: An antibiotic is often given the day before the procedure. Cardiac catheterization takes from 1 to 3 hours. The patient has to lie still but may be asked to cough or breathe deeply during the procedure. It is anxiety producing, and the patient needs explanation and emotional support. A young child may need a sedative. The pulse on the operative side and the blood pressure on the other side of the body are monitored at least every 15 minutes for 1 hour and every half hour thereafter. During left heart catheterization, peripheral pulses are also monitored. The temperature may be elevated for several hours, and there may be pain at the incision site. The patient is prevented from bending the hip on the operative side after the study. A sand bag or other counterpressure dressing is applied to the site to prevent bleeding at the insertion site. The nurse observes the site for bleeding and for signs of infection, thrombophlebitis, and cardiac arrhythmia. Cardiac catheterization is typically performed by a special team in a special laboratory. By offering information and counseling, a member of the team may be of great help to the patient before and after the procedure.

■ OUTCOME CRITERIA: Many conditions may be accurately identified and assessed by using cardiac catheterization, including congenital heart disease, coronary artery disease, tricuspid stenosis, and valvular incompetence. Among the risks of the procedure are local infection, cardiac arrhythmia, and thrombophlebitis.

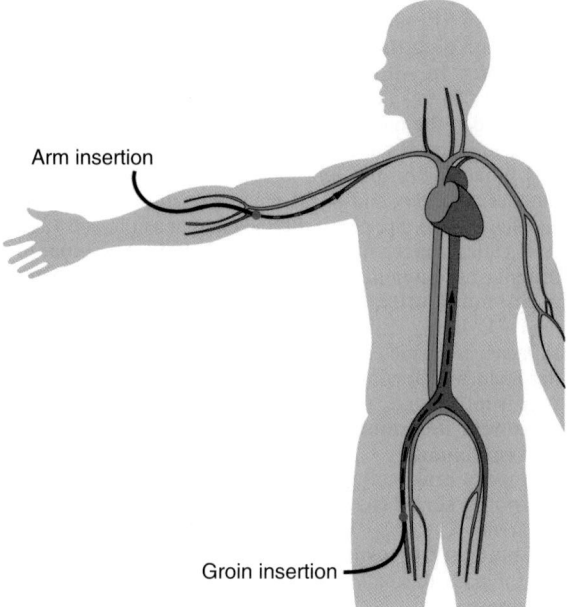

Arm insertion

Groin insertion

Insertion sites for cardiac catheterization *(Pagana and Pagana, 2006)*

Common cardiac arrhythmias

Description	Classic characteristics	Etiology and pathology	Clinical manifestations	Management
Sinus bradycardia Heart rate less than 60 beats/min (possibly normal in highly trained athletes and other healthy adults, particularly during sleep)	Pacemaker site: SA node Rhythm: regular Rate: <60 beats/min P waves: normal QRS complex: normal Intervals: normal Ectopic beats: possibly present	Inferior wall myocardial infarction Increased intracranial pressure Addison's disease Myxedema Hypothermia Anorexia nervosa Drugs: digitalis, beta-blockers (propranolol, nadolol) Vagal stimulation from severe pain, fear, vomiting, bearing down during defecation	This condition is usually asymptomatic but may cause dizziness, angina, disorientation, hypotension, syncope, or heart failure if cardiac output decreases.	This rhythm is treated only if it is symptomatic, and then treatment is directed at increasing heart rate. Causative factor should be removed if possible. Atropine should be administered intravenously. Pacemaker is used in refractory cases.

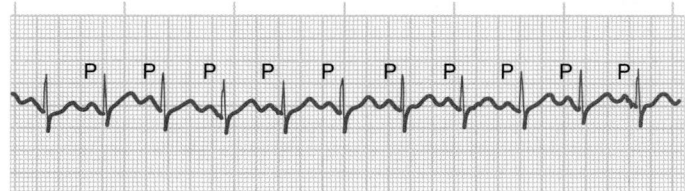

Description	Classic characteristics	Etiology and pathology	Clinical manifestations	Management
Sinus tachycardia Heart rate between 100 and 160 beats/min	Pacemaker site: SA node Rhythm: regular Rate: >100 beats/min P waves: normal but in rapid rhythms possibly more peaked or lost in T wave QRS complex: normal Intervals: possible shortening of PR and QT intervals as rate increases	Possible occurrence in normal individuals as a result of fear, anxiety, physical exertion Ingestion of alcohol and caffeine Use of nicotine, atropine, and catecholamines Accompaniment of pathological processes that raise metabolic rate, such as fever and thyrotoxicosis Short-term compensatory mechanism to maintain circulation of oxygenated blood to tissues during myocardial ischemia and infarction, pulmonary embolism, heart failure, anemia, hypoxemia, and hypovolemia	This condition is often asymptomatic, although it occasionally causes subjective feelings of palpitations. Patients with preexisting heart disease may experience light-headedness, angina, disorientation, and syncope.	Underlying cause is corrected or eliminated. As indicated, beta-adrenergic blocking agents, calcium channel blockers, digoxin, and adenosine are used to control arrhythmia.

Continued

Common cardiac arrhythmias—cont'd

Description	Classic characteristics	Etiology and pathology	Clinical manifestations	Management
Paroxysmal atrial tachycardia				
Very rapid, regular heart rate of 150-250 beats/min that occurs and stops suddenly	Pacemaker site: atrial tissue Rhythm: regular Rate: 150-250 beats/min P waves: usually hidden in previous T wave QRS complex: normal Intervals: immeasurable PR interval, regular R-R interval	Usual preceding rhythm: frequent premature atrial contractions Possible cause: sympathetic nervous system stimulation or hypermetabolic states Patients at risk: those with ischemic heart disease, rheumatic heart disease, and myocarditis	Patients may experience symptoms of decreased cardiac output. Patients may complain of palpitations, racing heartbeat, dizziness, dyspnea, angina, diaphoresis, and fatigue.	Vagal stimulation by means of Valsalva maneuver or carotid sinus pressure is used. Adenosine, 6-mg intravenous bolus over 1–2 sec, is rapidly administered, followed by 20-mL saline flush. Verapamil, propranolol, or digitalis is administered if adenosine is not effective. Synchronized cardioversion is used if patient not responsive to drug therapy or is hemodynamically unstable.

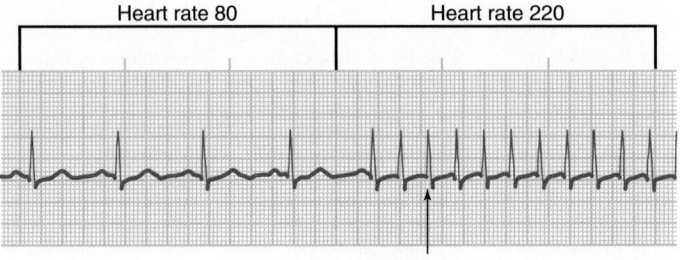

Heart rate 80 | Heart rate 220

Hidden P wave

Description	Classic characteristics	Etiology and pathology	Clinical manifestations	Management
Atrial flutter				
Atrial arrhythmia that occurs when an atrial ectopic pacemaker discharges impulses at 250-400 beats/min (less common than atrial fibrillation)	Pacemaker site: ectopic focus in atrial tissue Rhythm: usually regular but possibly irregular Rate: atrial rate—250-400 beats/min, ventricular rate—depends on AV conduction ratio P waves: presence of flutter waves QRS complex: normal Intervals: immeasurable PR interval, regular or irregular R-R interval	Occurrence in patients with cardiomyopathy, hypoxia, heart failure, pericarditis, myocarditis, hyperthyroidism, pulmonary disease, pulmonary emboli Trigger: reentry conduction Only some impulses from AV node are conducted through to ventricles.	This condition may be asymptomatic, or patient may complain of palpitations or fluttering feeling in chest or throat. Patient may become hypotensive and develop cool, clammy skin.	Digitalis, beta-blockers, and calcium channel blockers are administered to slow impulse conduction time. If AV conduction rate is 1:1, immediate synchronized cardioversion is done. Atrial overdrive pacing may be considered if time and patient's condition permit.

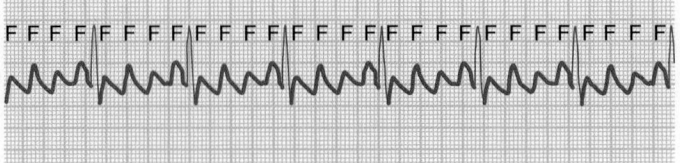

F F F F F F F F F F F F F F F F F F F F F F F F F F F F F F F

Common cardiac arrhythmias—cont'd

Description	Classic characteristics	Etiology and pathology	Clinical manifestations	Management
Atrial fibrillation				
Arrhythmia in which chaotic ectopic atrial foci cause the atria to quiver rather than contract Atrial rate >400 beats/min	Pacemaker site: many ectopic foci in atrial tissue Rhythm: irregular Rate: atrial rate—>400 beats/min P waves: presence of chaotic F waves QRS complex: normal Intervals: lack of P waves, irregular R-R interval	In healthy people, possible association with stress or excessive alcohol consumption Chronic atrial fibrillation in patients with heart failure, mitral valve disease, rheumatic heart disease, hypertension, and hyperthyroidism Relationship with atrial reentry mechanism Only a few impulses from AV node pass through to the ventricle	Signs and symptoms are related to rate of ventricular response. If ventricular response is rapid, patient experiences manifestations of decreased cardiac output and is at risk for heart failure and myocardial ischemia. Blood pooling in atria places patient at risk for thrombus formation and embolization to the brain and other organs.	Ventricular rate is controlled. Anticoagulation therapy is performed. Arrhythmia is converted to sinus rhythm.

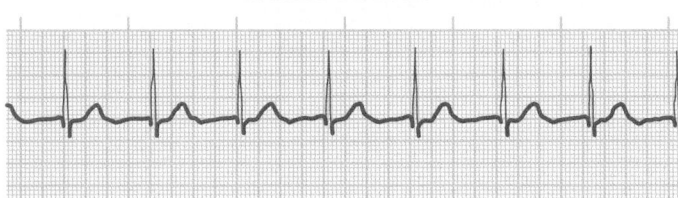

Description	Classic characteristics	Etiology and pathology	Clinical manifestations	Management
Junctional rhythm				
Rhythm that originates in or around the AV node	Pacemaker site: AV node Rhythm: regular Rate: 40-60 beats/min P waves: possibly present, possibly inverted and found before, in, or after QRS complex QRS complex: usually normal Intervals: shorter-than-normal PR interval, normal R-R interval	Occurrence only when dominant pacemaker of heart fails to function Cause: retrograde stimulation of atria, which do not contract simultaneously with ventricles, reducing cardiac output Possible cause: certain drugs or damage to the AV node secondary to acute myocardial infarction or ischemia	This rhythm is similar to other bradyarrhythmias. Symptoms include manifestations of decreased cardiac output.	Pharmacological management is used to increase heart rate. Temporary pacemaker may be inserted. Underlying cause is identified and treated.

Description	Classic characteristics	Etiology and pathology	Clinical manifestations	Management
Premature ventricular contractions				
	Pacemaker site: ventricular tissue (single or multiple foci) Rhythm: irregular Rate: normal 60 to 100 beats/min P waves: not present because impulses originate in the ventricles QRS complex: usually wide and bizarre, usually no longer than 0.10 sec, possibly with same focus in the ventricles or with variety of configurations if occurring from multiple foci in ventricles Intervals: absent PR intervals	Association with stimulants such as caffeine, alcohol, aminophylline, epinephrine, isoproterenol, and digoxin Associated diseases: acute myocardial infarction, mitral valve prolapse, heart failure, and coronary artery disease Possibly unifocal or multifocal	Most patients are asymptomatic, but some may complain of palpitations and skipped beats.	Treatment is indicated when six or more occur per minute, ventricular couplets or triplets appear, or multifocal premature ventricular contractions occur. Lidocaine is drug of choice; procainamide is second choice if lidocaine is ineffective.

Continued

Common cardiac arrhythmias—cont'd

Description	Classic characteristics	Etiology and pathology	Clinical manifestations	Management

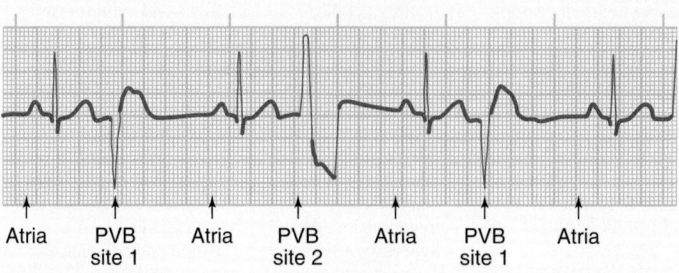

Atria   PVB   Atria   PVB   Atria   PVB   Atria
site 1   site 2   site 1

Ventricular tachycardia

Description	Classic characteristics	Etiology and pathology	Clinical manifestations	Management
Arrhythmia originating in an ectopic focus in the ventricles	Pacemaker site: ventricular (single or multiple foci) Rhythm: atrial—indeterminable, ventricular—typically regular but possibly slightly irregular Rate: ventricular—100 to 250 beats/min P waves: usually buried in QRS complex, possible presence of retrograde P waves QRS complex: wide, bizarre, and independent of P waves, possibly with same configuration as premature ventricular contractions Intervals: indeterminable	Occurrence when more than three premature ventricular contractions occur in succession with a heart rate of >100 beats/min Usual association: coronary artery disease, acute myocardial infarction, electrolyte imbalances, or cardiomyopathy	Patients may complain of palpitations, dizziness, chest pain, and shortness of breath. Signs and symptoms of decreased cardiac output are present. If this rhythm is rapid or sustained, loss of consciousness may occur.	If rate <100 beats/min and patient is hemodynamically stable, no treatment is necessary. Lidocaine is administered if patient is hemodynamically stable but rate is >100 beats/min. Procainamide is administered if lidocaine is ineffective. Bretylium is third drug of choice. If patient is hemodynamically unstable, immediate synchronized cardioversion is performed.

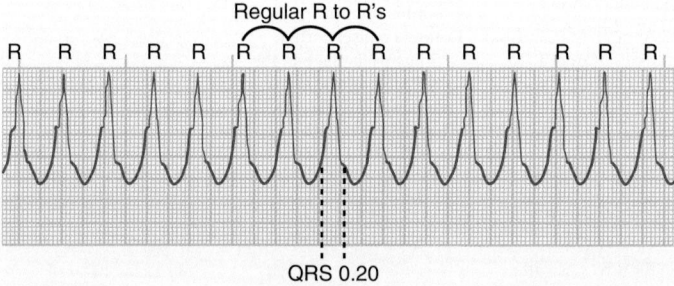

Regular R to R's

R R R R R R R R R R R R R R R R

QRS 0.20

Ventricular fibrillation

Description	Classic characteristics	Etiology and pathology	Clinical manifestations	Management
Rapid, ineffective, and disorganized depolarization of the ventricles	Pacemaker site: ventricular tissue (multiple foci) Rhythm: irregular, uncoordinated, without specific pattern Rate: rapid, uncoordinated, cannot be determined P waves: none QRS complex: rapid, irregular, not discernible Intervals: not discernible	Characteristics: disorganization of electrical impulses, conduction, and ventricular contraction Occurrence with coronary artery disease, acute myocardial infarction, myocardial ischemia, and cardiomyopathy Possible induction by procedures such as cardiac catheterization or cardiac pacing Possible occurrence with thrombolytic therapy, coronary reperfusion, accidental electrical shock, hyperkalemia, and hypoxia	Loss of consciousness may occur. Pulse, heart sounds, and blood pressure are absent. The patient's pupils are dilated, cyanosis develops rapidly, and seizures are possible.	Immediate CPR and defibrillation are performed after advanced cardiac life-support measures.

Common cardiac arrhythmias—cont'd

Description	Classic characteristics	Etiology and pathology	Clinical manifestations	Management

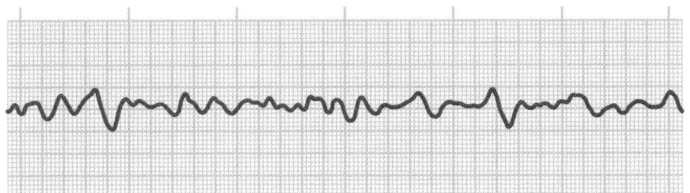

First-degree atrioventricular block

Block in which every impulse from the SA node is conducted to the ventricles, but a delay occurs at the AV node.	Pacemaker site: SA node Rhythm: regular Rate: 60–100 beats/min P waves: normal QRS complex: normal Intervals: P-R interval >0.20 sec	Association with organic heart diseases such as rheumatic fever, chronic ischemic heart disease, myocardial infarction, hyperthyroidism, and vagal stimulation Additional association with drugs such as digitalis, beta-blockers, and calcium channel blockers	A soft S_1 is heard. Patients may have asymptomatic bradycardia or be otherwise asymptomatic.	Underlying cause is treated. Usually, treatment is not required, but patients should be monitored closely.

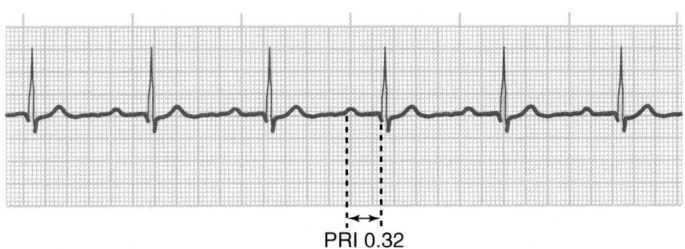

PRI 0.32

Second-degree atrioventricular block, type I (also called *Mobitz type I* or *Wenckebach*)

Failure of some of the SA impulses to be conducted to the ventricles	Pacemaker site: SA node Rhythm: atrial—regular, ventricular—irregular Rate: atrial—normal, ventricular—normal but possibly slower than atrial rate P waves: normal or prolonged QRS complex: normal width with pattern of one nonconducted QRS Intervals: normal	Usual cause: myocardial ischemia in an acute myocardial infarction of inferior wall Possible cause: digitalis toxicity, acute rheumatic fever, electrolyte imbalance, vagal stimulation, or quinidine or procainamide therapy	S_1 tends to become progressively softer with intermittent pauses. Otherwise, this rhythm is usually asymptomatic. If ventricular rate is slow, hypotension and syncope can occur.	Usually, no treatment is required if patient is asymptomatic. Underlying cause is treated when necessary. Atropine is administered, temporary pacemaker is inserted, or both treatments are used if patient is symptomatic.

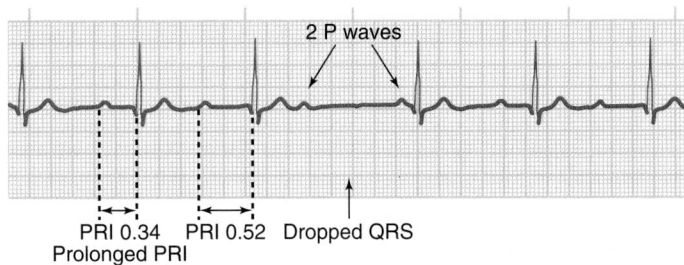

2 P waves

PRI 0.34   PRI 0.52   Dropped QRS
Prolonged PRI

Continued

Common cardiac arrhythmias—cont'd

Description	Classic characteristics	Etiology and pathology	Clinical manifestations	Management
Second-degree atrioventricular block, type II (also called *Mobitz type II*)				
Failure of some of the sinus impulses to be conducted to the ventricles	Pacemaker site: SA node Rhythm: atrial—regular, ventricular—irregular Rate: atrial—normal, ventricular—normal, but may be slower than atrial rate P waves: occur in multiples QRS complex: widening preceded by two or more P waves Intervals: normal	Association with myocardial infarction of acute anterior or anteroseptal wall, rheumatic and other silent heart diseases, or digitalis toxicity Occurrence lower in the AV node than type I block	This rhythm is more serious than type I second-degree block because a certain number of impulses from the sinus node are not conducted to the ventricles. This almost always occurs in the His-Purkinje system. Patients may be hypotensive, have bradycardia, and exhibit symptoms of decreased cardiac output.	Treatment is necessary even if patient is asymptomatic. If acute myocardial infarction has occurred, pacemaker is inserted. Isoproterenol is last resort in emergency situation.

3 P waves

P   P   P   P   P   P

3:1 block

Illustrations from Monahan FD et al: *Phipps' medical-surgical nursing: foundations for clinical practice,* ed 8, St. Louis, 2007, Mosby.
AV, Atrioventricular; *SA,* sinoatrial.

cardiac cirrhosis [Gk, *kardia,* heart, *kirrhos,* yellow-orange, *osis,* condition], an increase of fibrous tissue in the liver resulting from congestive heart failure, chronic myocarditis, or cardiac fibrosis.

cardiac compression. See **cardiac tamponade.** See also **chest compression.**

cardiac conduction defect, any impairment of the electrical pathways and specialized muscular fibers that conduct impulses through the heart and result in atrial and ventricular contraction. Conduction defects may develop between the sinus and atrioventricular (AV) nodes, between the sinus node and the AV bundle, or within the AV bundle or the left or right bundle branches. Defective transmission of cardiac impulses may be caused by ischemia, necrosis, drugs, electrolyte disturbances, or trauma. See also **heart block.**

cardiac cycle [Gk, *kardia + kyklos,* circle], the cycle of events in the heart during which an electrical impulse is conducted from the sinus node to the atrioventricular (AV) node, to the AV bundle, to the bundle branches, and to the Purkinje fibers, causing depolarization of the atria followed by depolarization of the ventricles. Depolarization leads to contraction. The contractions of the left and the right atria are nearly simultaneous; they precede the nearly simultaneous contractions of the ventricles. Structural, chemical, or electrical abnormalities may cause a large variety of anomalies in the cardiac cycle.

cardiac decompensation, a condition of congestive heart failure in which the heart is unable to ensure adequate cellular perfusion in all parts of the body without assistance. Causes may include myocardial infarction, increased workload, infection, toxins, or defective heart valves.

cardiac depressant [L, *deprimere,* to press down], an agent that decreases heart rate and contractility. See also **antiadrenergic, calcium channel blocker.**

cardiac dyspepsia, a digestive disorder associated with heart disease.

cardiac dyspnea [Gk, *dys,* difficult, *pnoia,* breath], breathing distress caused by heart disease. It is most commonly the result of pulmonary venous congestion.

cardiac edema [Gk, *oidema,* swelling], an accumulation of serum fluid from blood plasma in the interstitial tissues as a result of congestive heart failure. In severe cases, the fluid may also accumulate in serous cavities.

cardiac electric axis, the main direction of electrical current flow in the heart. It may be calculated in the frontal plane by using limb leads or in the horizontal plane by using precordial leads. See also **Einthoven's triangle.**

cardiac exercise stress test, a noninvasive electrodiagnostic and/or nuclear test used to evaluate chest pain in patients with suspected coronary disease, to determine the safe limits of exercise during a cardiac rehabilitation program, to detect labile or exercise-related hypertension, to detect intermittent claudication, to evaluate the effectiveness of antianginal or antiarrhythmic drugs, and to evaluate the effectiveness of cardiac surgical intervention.

cardiac failure. See **heart failure.**

cardiac hypertrophy, an abnormal enlargement of the heart muscle, often associated with increased afterload. It frequently accompanies long-standing hypertension and congestive heart failure.

cardiac impulse [Gk, *kardia + L, impellere,* to set in motion], **1.** the mechanical movement of the thorax caused by the beating of the heart. It is readily palpable and easily recorded. See also **point of maximum impulse. 2.** the electrical stimulus generated by the heart for pacing purposes.

cardiac index, a measure of the cardiac output of a patient per square meter of body surface area. Its normal range in a healthy adult is 2.8 to 4.2 L/min/m^2.

cardiac insufficiency, the inability of the heart to pump efficiently. See also **cardiac decompensation.**

cardiac massage, repeated, rhythmic compression of the heart applied directly, during surgery, or through the intact chest wall in an effort to maintain circulation after cardiac arrest or ventricular fibrillation. Also called **heart massage, chest compression.**

cardiac monitor, a device for the continuous observation of cardiac function. It may include electrocardiograph and oscilloscope readings, recording devices, and a visual and/or audible record of heart function and rhythm. An alarm system may be set to identify abnormal rhythms or heart rates.

cardiac monitoring, a continuous check on the functioning of the heart with an electronic instrument that provides an electrocardiographic reading on an oscilloscope. Each ventricular contraction of the heart is indicated by either a flashing light or an audible sound. The indicator is often integrated with an alarm system that is triggered by a pulse rate above or below predetermined limits. See also **electrocardiograph.**

cardiac murmur, an abnormal sound heard during auscultation of the heart, caused by altered blood flow into a chamber or through a valve. A murmur is classified by the quality of the sound, its time of occurrence during the cardiac cycle, its duration, and its intensity on a scale of I to VI. Also noted are the part of the heart over which the murmur is heard and any parts to which it radiates. In certain age groups, many systolic murmurs are benign and of no significance, whereas others signal a cardiac disorder. Diastolic murmurs are always pathological. Also called **heart murmur.**

cardiac muscle, a special striated muscle of the myocardium containing dark intercalated disks at the junctions of abutting fibers. Cardiac muscle is an exception among involuntary muscles, which are characteristically smooth. Its contractile fibers resemble those of skeletal muscle but are only one third as large in diameter, are richer in sarcoplasm, are abundant in mitochondria, and contain centrally located nuclei. Compare **smooth muscle, striated muscle.**

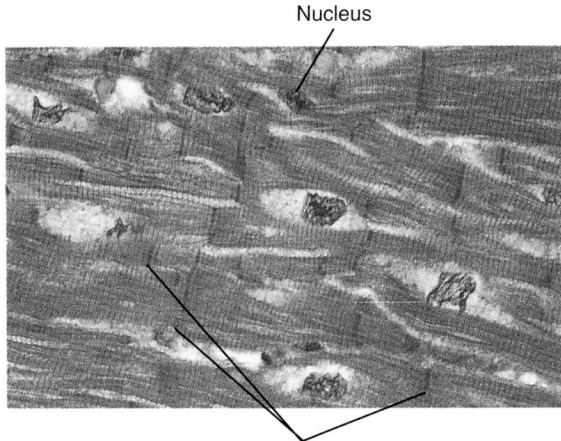

Nucleus

Intercalated disks

Cardiac muscle (© Ed Reschke; Used with permission)

cardiac nerves, the three autonomic nerves that supply the heart, including the inferior, superior, and middle (or great) cardiac nerves.

cardiac nuclear scanning, a nuclear scan used to detect myocardial ischemia, infarction, wall dysfunction, and decreased ejection fraction. It is commonly used as the imaging method portion of cardiac stress testing. Specific indications for this test include screening of adults for past and recent infarction, quantification and surveillance of myocardial infarction, and evaluation of the following: chest pain and ECG changes, myocardial perfusion before and after surgery, effectiveness of therapy for coronary artery perfusion, ventricular function in patients with myocardial disease, and status of patients receiving cardiotoxic drugs.

cardiac output (CO), the volume of blood expelled by the ventricles of the heart with each beat (the stroke volume) multiplied by the heart rate. Cardiac output is commonly measured by the thermodilution technique. A normal, resting adult has a cardiac output of 4 to 8 L per minute.

cardiac pacemaker. See **pacemaker.**

cardiac pain. See **angina pectoris.**

cardiac plexus [Gk, *kardia* + L, pleated], one of several nerve networks situated close to the arch of the aorta. The cardiac plexuses contain sympathetic and parasympathetic nerve fibers that follow the right and left coronary arteries into the heart. Some of these fibers terminate in the sinus node; others terminate in the atrioventricular node and in the atrial myocardium.

cardiac radionuclide imaging [Gk, *kardia* + L, *radiare,* to shine, *nucleus,* nut kernel, *imago,* image], the noninvasive examination of the heart using a radiopharmaceutical and a detection device, such as a gamma camera, positron camera, or rectilinear scanner. Clinical applications of cardiac radionuclide imaging are the gated cardiac blood pool scan, myocardial imaging, and detection of myocardial necrosis.

cardiac reflex [L, *reflectere,* to bend back], a neural mechanism that automatically increases or reduces the heart rate. Stimulation of stretch receptors in the right side of the heart by increased venous return increases the heart rate, whereas increased arterial blood pressure stimulates nerve endings in the carotid sinus and aortic arch to reduce the heart rate.

cardiac regurgitation [Gk, *kardia,* heart; L, *re + gurgitare,* to flow], a backward flow of blood through one or more defective heart valves.

cardiac rehabilitation [Gk, *kardia,* heart; L, *re + habilitas,* ability], a supervised program of progressive exercise, psychological support, education, and training to enable a patient to resume the activities of daily living on an independent basis following a myocardial infarction. The patient may require special training to adapt to a new occupation and lifestyle.

cardiac reserve, the potential capacity of the heart to function well beyond its basal level in response to alterations in physiological demands.

cardiac rhythm [Gk, *kardia,* heart, *rhythmos*], the recurring beat of the heart.

cardiac souffle /soo″fəl/ [Gk, *kardia,* heart; Fr, puff], a heart murmur having a soft, blowing sound.

cardiac sphincter [Gk, *kardia + sphingein,* to bind], a sphincter between the esophagus and the stomach opening at the approach of food that can then be swept into the stomach by rhythmic peristaltic waves.

cardiac standstill, the complete cessation of ventricular contractions and ejection of blood by the heart. Cardiac standstill requires immediate cardiopulmonary resuscitation and pacing. See also **cardiac arrest.**

cardiac stenosis [Gk, *kardia,* heart; Gk, *stenos,* narrow, *osis,* condition], a nonvalvular obstruction of blood flow through any heart chamber. The cause may be a thrombosis or tumor.

cardiac stimulant, a pharmacological agent that increases the action of the heart. Cardiac glycosides increase the force of myocardial contractions and decrease the heart rate and conduction velocity, allowing more time for the ventricles to relax and become filled with blood. These glycosides are used in the treatment of congestive heart failure, atrial flutter and fibrillation, paroxysmal atrial tachycardia, and cardiogenic shock. Toxic signs and symptoms that result from an overdose or the cumulative effect of slowly eliminated digitalis preparations include anorexia, nausea, vomiting, diarrhea, abdominal pain, headache, muscle weakness, confusion, drowsiness, irritability, visual disturbances, bradycardia or tachycardia, ectopic heartbeats, bigeminy, and a pulse deficit. Toxic effects may be attributed to an overdose or decreased growth hormone–releasing factor. Epinephrine, a potent vasopressor and cardiac stimulant, is sometimes used to restore heart rhythm in cardiac arrest but is not used in treating heart failure or cardiogenic shock. Isoproterenol hydrochloride, which is related to epinephrine, may be used in treating heart block. Inamrinone, dobutamine hydrochloride, and dopamine are used in the short-term treatment of cardiac decompensation resulting from depressed contractility.

cardiac syncope /sing″kəpē/ [Gk, *kardia,* heart, *syncope,* fainting], a temporary loss of consciousness caused by inadequate cerebral blood flow resulting from a sudden failure in cardiac output for any reason.

cardiac tamponade /tam′pənäd″/, compression of the heart produced by the accumulation of blood or other fluid in the pericardial sac. Also called **cardiac compression, pericardial tamponade.**

■ OBSERVATIONS: Signs of cardiac tamponade may include distended neck veins, hypotension, decreased heart sounds, tachypnea, peripheral pulses that are weak or absent or that fall sharply during inspiration (pulsus paradoxus), reduced left atrial pressure, and pericardial friction rub. The patient, who is usually anxious and restless, may sit upright or lean forward, and the skin may be pale, dusky, or cyanotic. The electrocardiogram generally shows decreased cardiac voltage and may show electrical alternans, and the chest x-ray film may reveal an enlarged heart shadow ("water bottle" heart).

■ INTERVENTIONS: The patient is maintained on bed rest; the head of the bed is elevated 45 degrees, and a defibrillator and emergency drugs are kept at the bedside. IV saline is the initial therapy of choice to maintain filling pressures in the heart. Blood pressure, respiration, apical pulse, and atrial and pulmonary wedge pressures are checked every 15 to 30 minutes. Auscultation for pulsus paradoxus is performed, and peripheral pulses are checked every 30 minutes. A 12-lead electrocardiogram is usually ordered, and the patient is placed on a cardiac monitor with the rhythm strip checked every hour. A Doppler echocardiogram is done initially and may be repeated a few days later. Cardiotonic and antiarrhythmic drugs are administered as ordered. Aspiration of the fluid in the pericardial sac (pericardiocentesis) is performed, and, if surgery is indicated, the patient is prepared for the procedure. In cases in which bleeding vessels are the cause of the tamponade, the vessels are ligated.

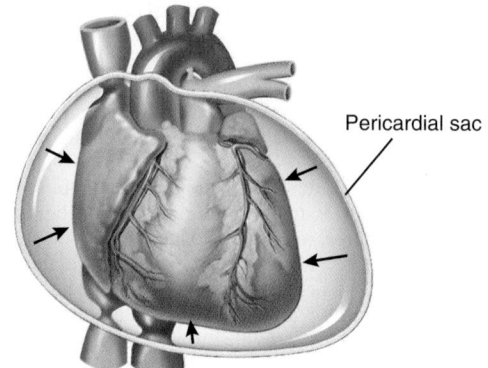

Cardiac tamponade

cardiac thrombosis [Gk, *kardia,* heart, *thrombos,* lump, *osis,* condition], a blood clot located at a heart valve or in one of the heart chambers. A left ventricular thrombosis may follow a large myocardial infarction.

cardiac valve. See **heart valve.**

cardial notch, the superior angle created when the esophagus enters the stomach.

cardiasthenia /kar′dē·asthē″nē·ə/ [Gk, *kardia,* heart, *a,* without, *sthenos,* strength], a form of neurasthenia in which cardiovascular symptoms are prominent.

cardiectomy /kär′dē·ek″təmē/, **1.** removal of the heart. **2.** removal of the cardiac portion of the stomach.

cardiectopia /kär′dē·ektō″pē·ə/, abnormal positioning of the heart in the thoracic cavity.

cardinal /kär′dənal/ [L, *cardo,* hinge], pertaining to something so fundamental that other things hinge on it, such as a cardinal trait that influences one's total behavior.

cardinal frontal plane [L, *cardo,* hinge, *frons,* forehead, *planum,* level ground], the plane that divides the body into front and back portions. Also called **vertical plane.**

cardinal horizontal plane. See **transverse plane.**

cardinal ligament [L, *cardo,* hinge, *ligare,* to bind], a sheet of subserous fascia extending across the female pelvic floor as a continuation of the broad ligament. See also **broad ligament.**

cardinal movements of labor, a group of overlapping rather than distinct movements of the fetus as it accommodates and moves progressively through the birth canal during normal labor. Disaccommodations in these movements are the causes of the protraction and arrest disorders comprising abnormal labor patterns. See **engagement, flexion, internal rotation, extension, external rotation, expulsive stage of labor.**

cardinal position of gaze, (in ophthalmology) one of six positions to which the normal eye may be turned. This test evaluates the functioning of the six extraocular muscles and cranial nerves III, IV, and VI. The positions and the corresponding muscles and nerves are as follows: (1) straight nasal: medial rectus and the third cranial nerve; (2) up nasal: inferior oblique and the third cranial nerve; (3) down nasal: superior oblique and the fourth cranial nerve; (4) straight temporal: lateral rectus and the sixth cranial nerve; (5) up temporal: superior rectus and the third cranial nerve; and (6) down temporal: inferior rectus and the third cranial nerve. Also called **extraocular movement.**

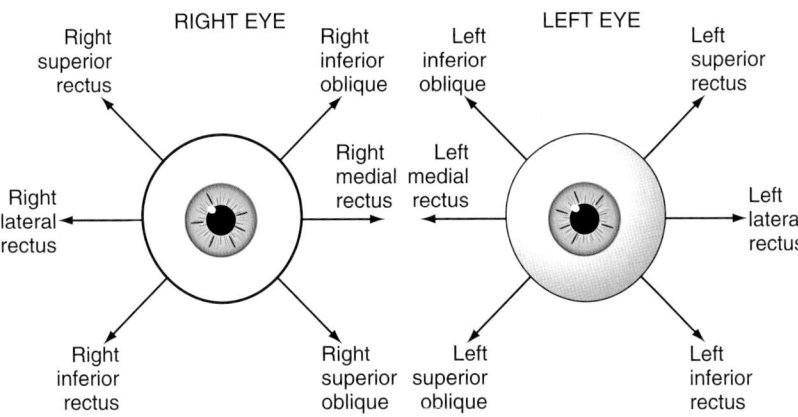

Ocular muscle movement in cardinal positions of gaze *(Rakel and Rakel, 2011)*

cardinal sagittal plane. See **median plane.**

cardinal symptom, a symptom fundamental or key to an illness or health condition; a component of the diagnostic criteria. Also called **primary symptoms.** Compare **sign.** See **symptom.**

cardinal signs of inflammation, symptoms associated with the body's complex response to irritants, infections, and/or cellular abnormalities. See **calor, rubor, dolor, loss of function, tumor.**

cardioangiography. See **angiocardiography.**

Cardiobacterium, a gram-negative genus of facultative anaerobic rod-shaped bacteria that is part of the normal flora of the human nasopharynx region. It is associated with endocarditis, causing 5% to 10% of cases.

cardiocatheterization. See **cardiac catheterization.**

cardiocele /kär′dē-ōsēl′/, protrusion of the heart through an opening in the diaphragm or the abdominal wall.

cardiocirculatory /kär′dē-ōsur″kyo͞olətôr′ē/ [Gk, *kardia* heart; L, *circulare,* to go around], pertaining to the heart and the circulation.

cardioesophageal reflux /-əsof′əjē″əl/ [Gk, *kardia,* heart, *oisophagos,* gullet; L, *refluere,* to flow back], a backward flow or regurgitation of stomach contents into the esophagus. Repeated episodes of reflux can lead to esophagitis. Among factors contributing to the condition are stomach pressure greater than esophageal pressure, hiatal hernia, and incompetence of the lower esophageal sphincter.

cardiogenic /-jen″ik/, originating in the heart muscle.

cardiogenic mesoderm, splanchnic mesoderm in the cardiogenic region where the embryonic heart develops that gives rise to the paired endocardial tubes.

cardiogenic shock [Gk, *kardia* + *genein,* to produce; Fr, *choc*], an abnormal condition often but not always characterized by a low cardiac output associated with acute myocardial infarction and congestive heart failure. Cardiogenic shock is fatal in about 80% of cases, and immediate therapy is necessary. Depending on the signs, therapy may include diuretics, vasoactive drugs, and the application of various devices. Compare **hypovolemic shock.** See also **electric shock, septic shock, shock.**

cardiogram. See **electrocardiogram.**

cardiograph. See **electrocardiograph.**

cardiography. See **electrocardiography.**

cardiohepatomegaly /-hep′ətōmeg″əlē/, enlargement of the heart and liver.

cardioinhibitory /kär′dē-ō′inhib″itôr′ē/, slowing or inhibiting the rate or strength of ventricular contractions.

cardiokinetic /kär′rdē-ōki·net′ik/ [Gk, *kardia,* heart + *kinesis,* motion], **1.** *adj.,* stimulating the action of the heart. **2.** *n.,* an agent that stimulates action of the heart.

cardiologist /-ol″əjist/, a physician who specializes in the diagnosis and treatment of disorders of the heart.

cardiology /-ol″əjē/ [Gk, *kardia* + *logos,* science], **1.** the study of the anatomy, normal functions, and disorders of the heart. **2.** the specialized field of health care concerned with cardiovascular health.

cardiomegaly /kär′dē-ōmeg″əlē/ [Gk, *kardia* + *megas,* large], enlargement of the heart.

cardiomyopathy, any disease of the myocardium causing enlargement. Also called **myocardiopathy.**

cardiomyopexy /kär′dē-omī″əpek′sē/ [Gk, *kardia* + *mys,* muscle, *pexis,* fixation], a surgical procedure in which a muscle, such as the pectoral, is fixated to the cardiac muscle and pericardium to improve myocardial blood supply.

cardiopathy /kär′dē-op″əthē/ [Gk, *kardia,* heart, *pathos,* disease], a disease of the heart.

cardiopericarditis /-per′ikärdī″tis/, inflammation of the heart and the pericardium.

cardioplasty /kär″dē-ōplas′tē/, a surgical repair to correct a defect in the cardiac sphincter of the esophagus that frequently leads to cardiospasm. Cardiospasm is caused by failure of the sphincter to relax so that food can enter the stomach. Also called *esophagogastroplasty.*

cardioplegia /-plē″jə/ [Gk, *kardia* + *plege,* stroke], **1.** paralysis of the heart. **2.** the arrest of myocardial contractions by hypothermia, electrical stimuli, or injection of chemicals for the purpose of performing surgery on the heart. See also **cardiac standstill.**

cardioprotectant /kär′dē-ōprōtek′tant/, **1.** *adj.,* counteracting cardiotoxic effects. **2.** *n.,* an agent, such as a beta-blocker, that so acts.

cardiopulmonary /-pul″məner′ē/ [Gk, *kardia* + L, *pulmo,* lung], pertaining to the heart and lungs.

cardiopulmonary arrest. See **cardiac arrest.**

cardiopulmonary bypass, a procedure used in heart surgery in which the blood is diverted from the right atrium or vena cava by means of a pump, which oxygenates the blood and then returns it directly to the aorta, bypassing the heart and lungs during the surgery.

cardiopulmonary murmur [Gk, *kardia,* heart; L, *pulmo,* lung, *murmur,* humming], a sound heard over the heart during breathing and synchronous with the heartbeat; caused by vibrations that result when the heart strikes the lung tissue with every beat. Also called **cardiorespiratory murmur.**

cardiopulmonary resuscitation (CPR), a basic emergency procedure for life support. It is used in cases of cardiac arrest to establish effective circulation and ventilation in order to prevent irreversible cerebral damage resulting from anoxia. External cardiac massage compresses the heart between the lower sternum and the thoracic vertebral column. During compressions, blood is forced into systemic and pulmonary circulation, and venous blood refills the heart when the compression is released. Current guidelines recommend restoring circulation with chest compressions and, when available, defibrillation to restart the heart. Compressions and defibrillation should take priority over airway and ventilation interventions by health care providers and trained rescuers. See also **hands-only CPR.**

cardiorespiratory. See **cardiopulmonary.**

cardiorespiratory murmur, movement of the air in the lungs that mimics a cardiac murmur. It disappears when the breath is held. Also called **cardiopulmonary murmur.**

cardiorrhaphy /kär′dē·ôr″əfē/ [Gk, *kardia* + *rhaphe,* suture], an operation in which the heart muscle is sutured.

cardioselectivity /-sel′əktiv″ītē/, selectivity of a drug, such as a beta-adrenergic agent, for heart tissue over other tissues of the body.

cardiospasm /kär″dē·əspaz′əm/ [Gk, *kardia* + *spasmos,* pull], a form of achalasia characterized by a failure of the cardiac sphincter at the distal end of the esophagus to relax. It causes dysphagia and regurgitation and sometimes requires surgical division of the muscle.

cardiotachometer /kär′dē·ō′təkom″ətər/ [Gk, *kardia* + *tachos,* speed, *metron,* measure], an instrument that continually monitors and records the heartbeat.

cardiotherapy, treatment of heart disease.

cardiothoracic ratio /-thôras″ik/, the ratio of the diameter of the heart at its widest point to the maximum width of the thoracic cavity, assessed by examining a chest x-ray. The normal ratio is less than 1:2.

cardiotomy /kär′dē·ot″əmē/ [Gk, *kardia* + *temnein,* to cut], **1.** an operation in which the heart is incised. **2.** an operation in which the cardiac end of the stomach or cardiac orifice is incised.

cardiotomy reservoir, in cardiopulmonary bypass, a collection chamber for blood suctioned from the heart chambers and pericardium.

cardiotonic /kär′dē·ōton″ik/ [Gk, *kardia* + *tonos,* tone], **1.** pertaining to a substance that tends to increase the efficiency of contractions of the heart muscle. **2.** a pharmacological agent that increases the force of myocardial contractions. Cardiac glycosides, derived from certain plant alkaloids, exert a tonic effect by altering the transport of electrolytes across the myocardial membrane, causing a decreased efflux of sodium and calcium and a decreased influx of potassium. Digitoxin and digoxin, widely used cardiac glycosides obtained from leaves of a species of foxglove, increase the force of myocardial contractions, extend the refractory period of the atrioventricular node, and, to a lesser degree, affect the sinoatrial node and the heart's conduction system.

cardiotoxic /-tok″sik/ [Gk, *kardia* + *toxikon,* poison], having a toxic or injurious effect on the heart.

cardiovascular /kär′dē·ōvas″kyələr/ [Gk, *kardia* + L, *vasculum,* small vessel], pertaining to the heart and blood vessels.

cardiovascular assessment, an evaluation of the condition, function, and abnormalities of the heart and circulatory system.

■ METHOD: The patient is asked to describe the onset, duration, location, and characteristics of any pain present and the occurrence of weakness, fatigue, shortness of breath, fever, coughing, wheezing, and palpitations. Questions are asked about episodes of fainting, indigestion, nausea, edema of extremities, cyanosis, and vision changes, and whether the hands and feet ever feel numb or cold. The person's general appearance, assumed position, rate and rhythm of all arterial pulses, presence of pulsus paradoxus or pulsus alternans, and the distension, pulsation, and pressure of neck veins are observed. Blood pressure, temperature, and rate and character of respirations are checked. The precordium is examined for the point of maximal impulse, symmetry, the cardiac border, pulsations, and evidence of lifts or bulges. Auscultation of the chest is performed to determine the intensity, pitch, duration, timbre, origin, and frequency of heart sounds and murmurs and to identify the location and character of breath sounds, including crackles, rhonchi, and rubs. Color, temperature, turgor, and dryness or sweating of the skin are noted, and the appearance of the extremities, capillary filling time, nails, and lesions are described. The patient's level of consciousness, reflexes, neurological signs, and responses to pain are recorded, along with data on concurrent hypertension, obesity, diabetes, and any pulmonary and renal conditions. Information is obtained about any previous cardiovascular surgery and illnesses, such as rheumatic fever, myocardial infarction, angina, congenital heart disease, occlusive vascular disease, and lung and kidney disorders. Pertinent background data include the patient's response to stress; coping methods; relationships; occupation; environment; sleep pattern and number of pillows used; exercise level, including number of blocks walked and flights of stairs climbed; leisure activities; and use of alcohol, tobacco, and other drugs. Other factors considered in the evaluation are the patient's history of medication with digitalis preparations, antihypertensives, diuretics, aspirin, sleeping pills, over-the-counter cold and influenza remedies; use of illegal drugs such as cocaine; and family history of heart disease, hypertension, diabetes, obesity, vascular disorders, stroke, and renal disease.

■ INTERVENTIONS: The health care professional usually obtains the patient's history, records the external observations, checks the vital signs, auscultates the chest, and assembles the pertinent background information and reports on diagnostic tests. In specialty areas such as a coronary care unit, the nurse may interpret electrocardiographic tracings, and the health care provider may adjust medications. Each member of the team will focus on the development of goals that enhance cardiovascular health.

■ OUTCOME CRITERIA: An accurate and complete assessment of cardiovascular function is an essential adjunct to a complete physical examination and is vital to the diagnosis and proper continuing care of a patient with cardiovascular disease.

cardiovascular disease, any abnormal condition characterized by dysfunction of the heart and blood vessels. In the United States, cardiovascular disease is the leading cause of death. Kinds include **atherosclerosis, myocardiopathy, rheumatic heart disease, syphilitic endocarditis, systemic venous hypertension.**

cardiovascular reflex, a reflex in which heart and circulatory functions are altered in response to changes in heart rate, vascular tone, blood volume, or other variables, usually involving bioreceptors.

cardiovascular shunt [Gk, *kardia,* heart; L, *vasculum,* small vessel; ME, *shunten*], any abnormal passage between chambers of the heart or between the systemic and pulmonary circulatory systems.

cardiovascular system, the network of anatomical structures, including the heart and blood vessels, that circulate blood throughout the body. The system includes thousands of kilometers of vessels that deliver nutrients and other essential materials to the fluids surrounding the cells and that remove waste products and convey them to excretory organs.

cardiovascular technologist, an allied health professional who performs diagnostic examinations at the request or direction of a physician in invasive cardiology, noninvasive cardiology, and/or peripheral vascular study. Through subjective data collection and/or recording, the technologist obtains information from which a correct anatomical and physiological diagnosis may be established for each patient.

cardioversion /-vur″zhən/ [Gk, *kardia* + L, *vertere,* to turn], the restoration of the heart's normal sinus rhythm through an electric shock delivered by a defibrillator. Application of the shock is synchronized to the QRS complex. Cardioversion is used to slow the heart or to restore the heart's normal sinus rhythm when drug therapy is ineffective at doing so. Cardioversion may also be done pharmacologically, with IV antiarrhythmic medication. Also called *cardiovert.*

cardioverter /-vur″tər/, a defibrillator or other instrument used to convert abnormal heart rhythms into normal rhythms.

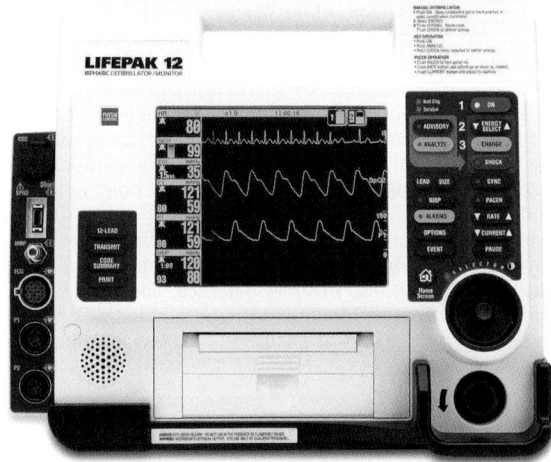

Cardioverter *(©2015 Physio-Control, Inc.)*

carditis /kärdī″tis/, inflammation of the heart muscle, usually resulting from infection. In most cases more than one layer of muscle is involved. Chest pain, cardiac arrhythmia, circulatory failure, and damage to the structures of the heart may occur. Kinds include **endocarditis, myocarditis, pericarditis.**

Cardizem, a calcium channel blocker. Brand name for **diltiazem.**

career ladder, **1.** (in health care education) a pathway for upward mobility that begins with earning a basic certification or degree and building on that expertise by adding additional certifications and advanced degrees. **2.** (in a field of study) a pathway for advancement in the professional role in an institution. Many facilities provide detailed advice to their staffs in regard to assuming more responsibilities within their scope of practice to allow for career advancement.

caregiver, **1.** one who contributes the benefits of medical, social, economic, or environmental resources to a dependent or partially dependent individual, such as a critically ill person. **2.** one who takes on the responsibility for functions of daily living when a person is unable to care for himself or herself, including their projects and causes.

care plan, a written strategy that begins with observations, assessments, and recognition of patient/client needs. With that information, a plan is set and followed to treat or intervene. The goal is to achieve healthy outcomes: restoration, maintenance, or rehabilitation of health. Goals and outcomes are evaluated at set times. Care plans are developed by members of the health care team and appear on the patient record. See also **nursing care plan.**

CARF, abbreviation for **Commission on Accreditation of Rehabilitation Facilities.**

caries /ker″ēz/ [L, decay]. See **dental caries.**

carina /kərē″nə/ *pl. carinae* [L, keel], any structure shaped like a ridge, cleft, or keel, such as the carina of the trachea, that projects from the lowest tracheal cartilage.

caring behaviors, actions characteristic of concern for the well-being of a patient, such as sensitivity, comforting, attentive listening, honesty, and nonjudgmental acceptance.

cariocas /kär′ē-ō″kəs/, a form of lateral movement in a gait cycle in which the side-stepping leg is moved successively behind and then in front of the stance leg. The resulting walking pattern is not in balance and alignment.

cariogenic /ker′ē-ōjen″ik/, tending to produce dental caries.

carious, having caries or decayed areas, especially of the teeth.

carisoprodol /ker′isōprō″dol/, a skeletal muscle relaxant.
■ INDICATIONS: It is prescribed for the relief of muscle spasm.
■ CONTRAINDICATIONS: Porphyria or known hypersensitivity to this drug or to chemically similar drugs, such as meprobamate, prohibits its use.
■ ADVERSE EFFECTS: Among the more serious adverse reactions are ataxia, drowsiness, pronounced weakness, visual disturbances, mental confusion, anaphylactic shock, erythema multiforme, and allergic reactions.

C-arm, an imaging scanner intensifier, so named because of its configuration. C-arms have radiographic capabilities, though they are used primarily for fluoroscopic imaging during surgical, orthopedic, critical care, and emergency care procedures.

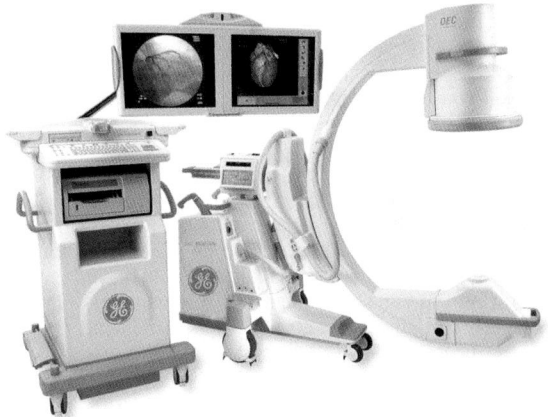

C-arm *(Frank, Long, and Smith, 2012)*

carmalum. See **carmine dye.**

carminative /kärmin″ətiv/ [L, *carminare,* to cleanse], **1.** *adj.,* pertaining to a substance that relieves flatulence and abdominal distension. **2.** *n.,* an agent that relieves gaseous distension and painful spasms, especially after meals.

carmine dye /kär″min/ [AR, *qirmize* + AS, *deag*], a dye formerly used in histological cell analysis that stains glycogen and mucin. Also called **carmalum.**

carmustine /kärmus″tin/, a lipid-soluble nitrosourea, 1, 3-bis (2-chloroethyl)-l-nitrosourea, used as a single antineoplastic agent or with other approved chemotherapeutic agents in the treatment of brain tumors, multiple myeloma, Hodgkin's disease, and non-Hodgkin's lymphomas. Also called **BCNU.**

carnal /kär″nəl/ [L, *caro,* flesh], pertaining to the flesh or body or worldly things, as distinguished from spiritual.

carneous /kär″nē-əs/, fleshlike.

carnitine /kär″nitin/, a substance found in skeletal and cardiac muscle and certain other tissues that functions as a carrier of fatty acids across the membranes of the mitochondria. It is used therapeutically in treating angina and certain deficiency diseases, particularly endocardial fibroelastosis, and as an antithyroid agent. It has actions that closely resemble those of amino acids and B vitamins.

carnitine palmitoyltransferase /kär′nitēn päl′mitō′əltrans′-fərās/, an enzyme that catalyzes the transfer between coenzyme A and carnitine of long-chain fatty acids. Deficiency is a cause of defective fatty acid oxidation. Also spelled *carnitine palmityltransferase.*

carnitine palmityltransferase deficiency /kär′ni·tēn päl′mitiltrans′fərās dēfish′ənsē/, an autosomal-recessive disorder of lipid metabolism, seen more often in men, in which the altered enzyme is abnormally regulated, resulting in muscle aches, fatigability, and myoglobinuria (but without lipid accumulation), occurring after prolonged exercise, particularly in the cold or after fasting.

Carnitor, an amino acid derivative. Brand name for **levocarnitine.**

carnivore /kär″nivôr/ [L, *caro,* flesh, *vorare,* to devour], an animal belonging to the order Carnivora, classified as a flesh eater, with appropriate teeth and a characteristically simple stomach and a short intestine for such a diet. −*carnivorous, adj.*

carnosine /kär′nōsēn/ [L, *caro*], a dipeptide composed of beta-alanine and histidine, found in humans in skeletal muscle and in the brain, particularly in the primary olfactory pathways. It may play a role as a neurotransmitter.

carnosinemia /kär′nōsinē′mē·ə/, accumulation of carnosine in the blood.

carob /kar′əb/ [Ar. *alkharrubah*], *Ceratonia siliqua,* a tree native to the Mediterranean basin. A powder from the fruit of the tree is sometimes used for digestive problems. See also **carob bean.**

carob bean, the fruit of the carob tree whose seed is leguminous. The finely pulverized meal of the dried ripe fruit contains albuminous proteins, carbohydrates, and small amounts of fat and crude fiber and has been used for centuries in pharmaceutic formulations as an adsorbent and demulcent in treatment of diarrhea. It is generally regarded as safe, but its effectiveness in treating diarrhea has not been rigorously assessed.

carotene /kar″ətin/ [L, *carota,* carrot], a red or orange organic compound found in carrots, sweet potatoes, egg yolk, fish oils, and leafy vegetables, such as beet greens, spinach, and broccoli. Beta-carotene, the most common form of carotene, is a provitamin and in the body is converted to vitamin A. See also **vitamin A.**

carotenemia /kar′ətinē″mē·ə/, the presence of high levels of carotene in the blood, resulting in an abnormal yellow appearance of the plasma and skin. It differs from jaundice in that the conjunctivae are not discolored. It may be caused either by excessive consumption of carotene-containing foods or drinks, such as carrots or carrot juice, or from a decreased ability to convert the carotenoids to vitamin A. It may also occur in diabetes mellitus and hypothyroidism. Also called **pseudojaundice,** *xanthemia.* Compare **jaundice.**

carotenoid /kərot″ənoid/, any of a group of red, yellow, or orange highly unsaturated pigments that are found in foods such as carrots, sweet potatoes, and leafy green vegetables. Many of these substances, such as carotene, are used in the formation of vitamin A in the body, whereas others, including lycopene and xanthophyll, show no vitamin A activity. Also spelled *carotinoid.*

carotenosis. See **carotenemia.**

caroticotympanic canaliculi, tiny passages in the temporal bone interconnecting the carotid canal and the tympanic cavity that carry communicating twigs between the internal carotid and tympanic plexuses. Also called *caroticotympanic foramina.*

caroticotympanic nerves, the plexus of nerves surrounding the internal carotid artery.

carotid /kərot″id/ [Gk, *karos,* heavy sleep], pertaining to the arteries that supply the head and neck. See also **carotid body, carotid sinus, common carotid artery.**

carotid arch [Gk, *karos,* heavy sleep; L, *arcus,* bow], the third arch of the aorta, the source of the common carotid arteries.

carotid body [Gk, *karos* + AS, *bodig*], a small structure containing neural tissue at the bifurcation of the carotid arteries. It monitors the pressure and oxygen content of the blood and therefore assists in regulating blood pressure and respiratory rate.

carotid-body reflex [Gk, *karos* + AS, *bodig* + L, *reflectere,* to bend back], a normal chemical reflex initiated by a decrease in oxygen concentration in the blood and, to a lesser degree, by increased carbon dioxide and hydrogen ion concentrations that act on chemoreceptors at the bifurcation of the common carotid arteries. The resulting nerve impulses cause the respiratory center in the medulla to increase respiratory activity. Compare **aortic-body reflex.**

carotid-body tumor, a benign round, firm growth that develops at the bifurcation of the common carotid artery. The tumor may cause dizziness, nausea, and vomiting if it impedes the flow of blood and pressure is increased in the vascular system. Surgical excision is the usual treatment in some cases.

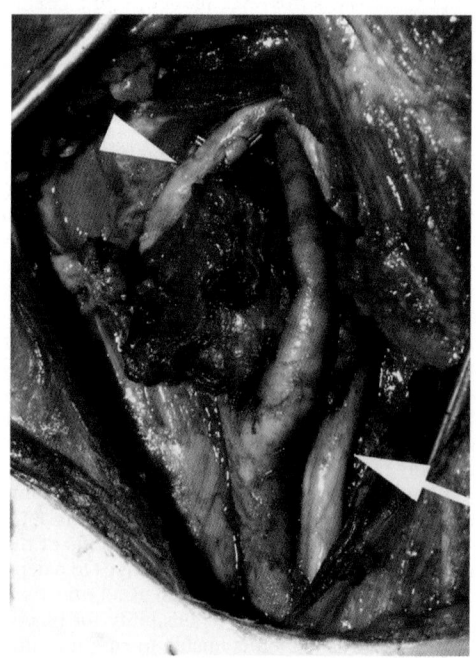

Carotid-body tumor *(Townsend et al, 2008)*

carotid bruit, a murmur heard over the carotid artery in the neck, suggesting arterial narrowing. It is usually secondary to atherosclerosis. Stroke is likely if the narrowing is severe and the condition is untreated.

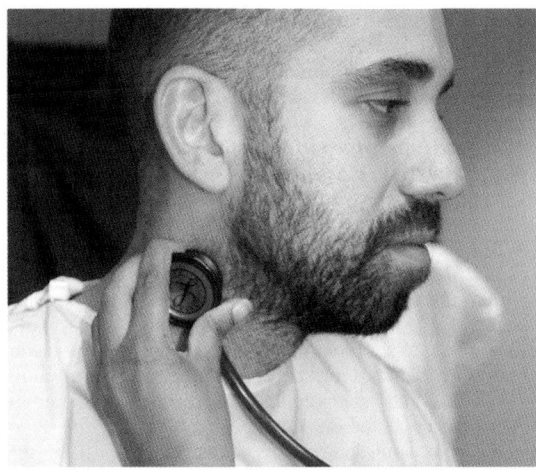

Ausculation for carotid bruits *(Courtesy Rutgers School of Nursing—Camden. All rights reserved.)*

carotid duplex scanning, a noninvasive ultrasound test used on the extracranial carotid artery to detect occlusive disease directly. It is often performed for patients with headaches and neurological symptoms such as transient ischemic attacks, hemiparesis, paresthesia, and acute speech or visual defects.

carotid endarterectomy (CEA), surgical excision of atheromatous segments of the endothelium and tunica media of the carotid artery, leaving a smooth tissue lining and facilitating blood flow through the vessel. The surgery is performed on vessels with stenosis to decrease the risk of stroke.

carotid plexus [Gk, *karos* + L, pleated], any one of three nerve plexuses associated with the carotid arteries. Compare **common carotid plexus, external carotid plexus, internal carotid plexus.**

carotid pulse, the pulse of the carotid artery, palpated by gently pressing a finger in the area between the larynx and the sternocleidomastoid muscle in the neck. See also **pulse.**

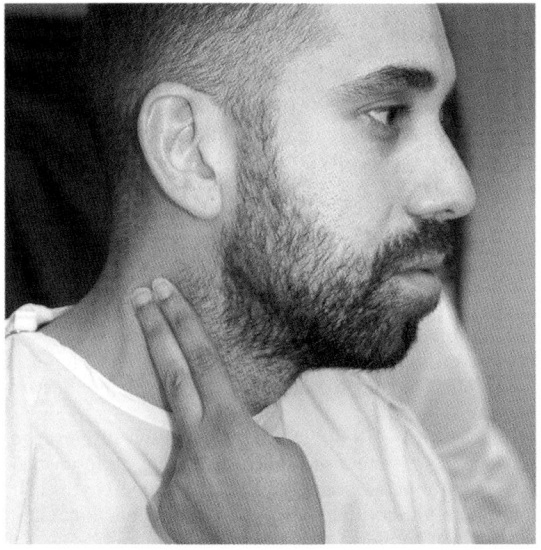

Assessment of the carotid pulse *(Courtesy Rutgers School of Nursing—Camden. All rights reserved.)*

carotid sheath, the fibrous tissue enclosing the carotid artery, jugular vein, and vagus nerve on each side of the neck.

carotid sinus [Gk, *karos* + L, curve], a dilation of the arterial wall at the bifurcation of the common carotid artery. It contains sensory nerve endings from the glossopharyngeal nerve that respond to changes in blood pressure.

carotid sinus massage, firm rubbing at the bifurcation of the carotid artery at the angle of the jaw. It creates an elevation of blood pressure in the carotid sinus that results in reflex slowing of atrioventricular conduction and sinus rate. The technique may be used to reduce the heart rate in tachyarrhythmia.

carotid sinus reflex, a neural mechanism in which an increase in blood pressure in the carotid artery at the level of its bifurcation triggers a decrease in heart rate. See also **carotid sinus syndrome.**

carotid sinus syndrome, a temporary loss of consciousness that sometimes results in provoked convulsive seizures as a result of the intensity of the carotid sinus reflex when pressure builds in one or both carotid sinuses. Also called *carotid sinus syncope.*

carotidynia /kərot′idin″ē·ə/ [Gk, *karos* + *odyne,* pain], a pain along the length of the common carotid artery, caused by pressure.

carp-, carpo-, combining form meaning "wrist": *carpal, carpometacarpal.*

-carp, suffix meaning "fruit": *monocarp, pericarp.*

carpal /kär′pəl/ [Gk, *karpos,* wrist], pertaining to the carpus, or wrist.

-carpal, combining form referring to the wrist: *metacarpal, radiocarpal.*

carpal arch, the arch formed by the carpal bones; the sides and roof of the carpal tunnel.

carpal bones, the eight bones of the wrist, which are arranged in two rows, a proximal and a distal row, each consisting of four bones. The proximal row consists of the scaphoid (navicular), the lunate, the triquetrum, and the pisiform bones. The distal row consists of the trapezium (greater multiangular), the trapezoid (lesser multiangular), the capitate, and the hamate bones. Also called **wrist.**

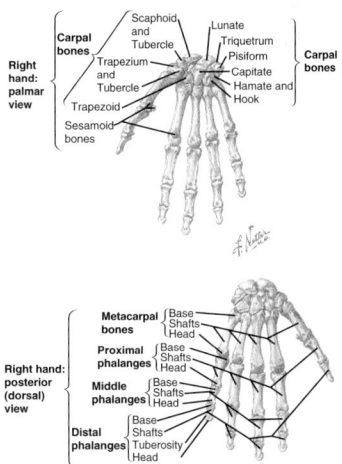

Carpal bones *(Copyright © 2015 Elsevier Inc. All rights reserved. www.netterimages.com)*

carpal ligaments, the four ligaments of the hand: the dorsal ligament, a thick band of white fibrous tissue on the dorsum of the wrist, attached to the lower end of the radius and to the styloid process of the ulna; the radiate ligament of the wrist, which projects from the head of the capitate bone to the volar aspects of other carpal bones; the broad, flat transverse ligament, which is attached to the tubercle of the scaphoid and the crest of the trapezium; and the volar ligament, a superficial part of the flexor retinaculum of wrist. See also **flexor retinaculum of wrist.**

carpal spasm, a sudden, powerful, involuntary contraction observed as a tetanic flexion of the hands and wrists.

carpal tunnel [Gk, *karpos* + Fr, *tonnel*], a tunnel formed by the carpal bones and the flexor retinaculum through which pass the median nerve and the tendons of the flexor digitorum profundus, the flexor digitorum superificialis, and the flexor pollicis longus.

carpal tunnel release, a surgical procedure for treating carpal tunnel syndrome in which the flexor retinaculum of the wrist is cut to release compression of the median nerve.

carpal tunnel syndrome, a common painful disorder of the wrist and hand, caused by compression on the median nerve between the inelastic carpal ligament and other structures within the carpal tunnel. It is often seen in cumulative trauma to the wrist. Symptoms may result from trauma, synovitis, or tumor or may develop with rheumatoid arthritis, amyloidosis, acromegaly, or diabetes. Symptomatic treatment usually relieves mild symptoms of recent onset, but if the pain becomes disabling, the injection of corticosteroids often yields dramatic relief. Surgical division of the transverse carpal ligament to relieve nerve pressure is usually curative. ■ OBSERVATIONS: The median nerve innervates the palm and the radial side of the hand; compression of the nerve causes weakness, pain with opposition of the thumb, and burning, tingling, or aching, sometimes radiating to the forearm and shoulder joint. Weakness and atrophy of muscles may increase from lack of use as a result of pain that impairs thumb and finger dexterity. Pain may be intermittent or constant and is often most intense at night. Diagnosis can be confirmed by electromyography. ■ INTERVENTIONS: Symptomatic treatment usually relieves mild symptoms of recent onset, but if the pain becomes disabling, the injection of corticosteroids often yields dramatic relief. Patients with both severe and mild-to-moderate carpal tunnel syndrome benefit from wearing wrist splints. Surgical division of the transverse carpal ligament to relieve nerve pressure is usually curative. ■ PATIENT CARE CONSIDERATIONS: There should be a thorough review of activities and the patient's functional level in performing these activities. An occupational therapist or physical therapist should identify repetitive and/or resistive motions involving the wrist, as well as digital flexion and extension during activity. It is also critical to identify poor body mechanics and posture and to provide instruction for correction.

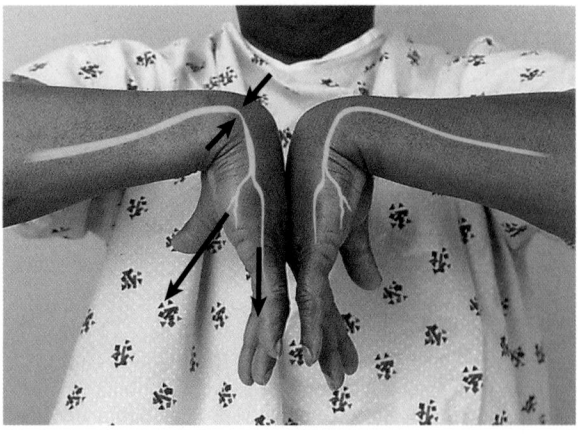

Procedure for assessing carpal tunnel syndrome *(Seidel et al, 2015)*

Carpenter syndrome /kär′pəntərz/ [George Carpenter, British physician, 1859–1910], an autosomal-recessive form of acrocephalopolysyndactyly characterized also by cognitive impairment and shortened digits. Also called *acrocephalopolysyndactyly.* See also **Noack syndrome, Sakati-Nyhan syndrome, Goodman syndrome.**

carpometacarpal (CMC) joint /-met′əkär″pəl/ [Gk, *karpos,* wrist, *meta,* next, *karpos*], any of the joints formed by the distal row of carpal bones and the bases of the metacarpals. The joints are essential for movements of the hand.

carpopedal /-ped″əl/ [Gk, *karpos,* wrist; L, *pes,* foot], pertaining to the wrist and foot.

carpopedal spasm [Gk, *karpos* + L, *pes,* foot], a spasm of the hand, thumbs, foot, or toes that sometimes accompanies tetany.

carrier /ker″ē·ər/ [OFr, *carier*], **1.** a person or animal who harbors and can potentially spread an organism that causes disease in others but does not become ill. **2.** one whose chromosomes carry a recessive gene. **3.** an immunogenic molecule or part of a molecule that is recognized by T cells in an antibody response.

carrier-free, **1.** relating to a radioisotope in pure form, free of dilution by stable isotope carriers. **2.** describing a substance in which every molecule is marked by a radioactive tracer or other tag.

Carrión disease. See **bartonellosis.**

Carroll Quantitative Test of Upper Extremity Function, a six-part assessment of a person's ability to grasp and lift objects of different shapes and sizes. It is designed to determine an individual's level of function in the arm and hand movements required for the activities of daily living.

carrying angle, the angle at which the humerus and radius articulate.

carry-over [L, *carrus,* wagon; AS, *ofer*], test system contamination when specimens or reagents from a prior or separate aliquot become mixed with a current test system, causing erroneous results.

car sickness [L, *carrus,* wagon; AS, *seoc*], *(Informal)* a form of kinesia caused by the motion of a vehicle. Compare **air sickness.** See also **kinesia.**

carteolol /kär′te·älol/, a beta-adrenergic blocking agent with intrinsic sympathetic activity, administered orally as an antihypertensive and applied topically to the conjunctiva in the treatment of glaucoma and ocular hypertension.

cartilage /kär′tilij/ [L, *cartilago*], a nonvascular dense supporting connective tissue composed of chondrocytes and various ratios of fibers to ground substance. It is found chiefly in the joints, the thorax, and various rigid tubes, such as the larynx, trachea, nose, and ear. Temporary cartilage, such as sesamoid bones (knee) and those that compose most of the fetal skeleton at an early stage, is later replaced by bone. Permanent cartilage remains unossified, except in certain diseases and, sometimes, in advanced age. Kinds include **elastic cartilage, hyaline cartilage, white fibrocartilage.** –**cartilaginous,** *adj.*

cartilage-capped exostosis, a small fragment of the growth plate separated from the rest of the bone. See **exostosis cartilaginea.**

cartilage graft, a surgical transplantation of cartilage to correct congenital ear and nose defects in children and to treat severe injuries in adults. Because chondrocytes can be allografted without the risk of an immune reaction, cadaver cartilage can be used for tissue grafts.

cartilage-hair hypoplasia [L, *cartilago* + AS, *haer* + Gk, *hypo,* under, *plasis,* forming], a genetic disorder characterized by dwarfism caused by hypoplasia of the cartilage; multiple skeletal abnormalities; and excessively sparse, short, fine, brittle hair that is usually light colored. It is inherited as an autosomal-recessive trait. The condition is found primarily among Amish people in the United States and Canada.

cartilage of auditory tube, the cartilage on the inferomedial surface of the temporal bone that supports the walls of the cartilaginous portion of the auditory tube.

cartilage tissue. See **connective tissue.**

cartilaginous. See **cartilage.**

cartilaginous bone, bone that develops by endochondral ossification in a preexisting cartilage. Also called **endochondral bone.**

cartilaginous joint [L, *cartilago* + *junger,* to join], a slightly movable joint in which cartilage unites bony surfaces. Two types of articulation involving cartilaginous joints are synchondrosis and symphysis. Also called **amphiarthrosis, junctura cartilaginea.** Compare **fibrous joint, synovial joint.**

cartilaginous septum of nose, the plate of cartilage forming the anterior part of the nasal septum.

cartilaginous skeleton [L, *cartilago* + Gk, *skeletos,* dried up], the parts of the skeleton that are formed by cartilage.

CARTOS II /kär″tos/, a technique in which serial copies of electron micrographs are programmed on a computer for display on a screen. The image can be manipulated for study of all dimensions of the structure. Abbreviation for *computer-aided reconstruction by tracing of serial sections.*

Cartrol, an antihypertensive agent. Brand name for *carteolol hydrochloride.*

caruncle /kär″ungkəl/ [L, *caruncula,* small piece of flesh], a small, fleshy projection, such as one of the lacrimal caruncles at the inner canthus of the eye or the hymenal caruncles that are the hymenal remnants.

carunculae hymenales [L, *caruncula* + Gk, *hymen,* membrane], *(Obsolete)* now called **hymenal tag.**

carvedilol, an alpha-/beta-adrenergic blocker.

■ INDICATIONS: It is used to treat congestive heart failure and essential hypertension, either alone or in combination with other antihypertensives.

■ CONTRAINDICATIONS: Known hypersensitivity to this drug, bronchial asthma, class IV decompensated cardiac failure, second- or third-degree heart block, cardiogenic shock, or severe bradycardia and pulmonary edema prohibit the use of carvedilol.

■ ADVERSE EFFECTS: Life-threatening effects of this drug include atrioventricular block, bradycardia, congestive heart failure, pulmonary edema, and thrombocytopenia. Other serious adverse effects include somnolence, depression, ataxia, diarrhea, dependent edema, peripheral edema, extrasystoles, hypertension, hypotension, palpitations, peripheral ischemia, urinary tract infection, viral infection, and hypertriglyceridemia.

carve-out, **1.** a service not covered in a health insurance contract. It is usually reimbursed according to a different arrangement or rate formula than those services specified under the contract umbrella. **2.** a population subgroup for whom separate health care arrangements are made.

CAS, abbreviation for **coronary artery scan.**

CASA, abbreviation for **computer-aided semen analysis.**

cascade /kaskād″/ [L, *cadere,* to fall], any process that develops in stages, with each stage dependent on the preceding one, often producing a cumulative effect.

cascade humidifier, a bubbling respiratory care device in which gases travel down a tower and pass through a grid into a chamber of heated water. The displaced water rises above the grid, forming a liquid film that is converted to a froth as the gas also rises from the chamber through the grid. The

process results in an airflow that can have a relative humidity of up to 100%.

cascara sagrada, an herbal product taken from the bark of a tree native to parts of the coast of the northwestern United States and southwestern Canada.

■ INDICATIONS: It is used for chronic constipation, hepatitis, and gallstones.

■ CONTRAINDICATIONS: Generally regarded as safe for short-term use, it should not be used by those who are hypersensitive to this product, by women who are pregnant or lactating, or by children younger than age 2 years until more research is available. Also, it is contraindicated where GI bleeding, obstruction, abdominal pain, nausea, vomiting, appendicitis, or Crohn disease is present.

case [L, *causus,* a happening], **1.** an episode of illness or injury. **2.** a container or receptacle.

caseation /kā′sē·ā″shən/ [L, *caseus,* cheese], a form of tissue necrosis in which the cellular outline is lost and the appearance is that of crumbly or liquefied cheese. It is typical of tuberculosis. See also **caseous.** −*caseate, v.*

caseation necrosis [L, *caseus,* cheese; Gk, *nekros,* dead, *osis,* condition]. See **caseous necrosis.**

case-control study, a nonexperimental research design using an epidemiological approach in which previous cases of the condition are used in lieu of new information gathered from a randomized population. A group of patients with a particular disease or disorder, such as myocardial infarction, is compared with a control group of persons who have not had that medical problem. The two groups, matched for age, sex, and other personal data, are examined to determine which possible factor (e.g., cigarette smoking, coffee drinking) may account for the increased disease incidence in the case group. See also **retrospective study.**

case fatality rate [L, *causus,* a happening, *fatum,* fate, L, *rata,* share], the number of registered deaths caused by any specific disease, expressed as a percentage of the total number of reported cases of a specific disease; the proportion of individuals contracting a disease who die of that disease.

case finding, the act of locating individuals with a disease.

case history [L, *causus* + *historia*], a patient's complete medical record before a current illness or injury. The history includes any infectious diseases experienced by the person; all immunizations, hospitalizations, and therapies; information relating to deaths or illnesses of parents and other close family members; allergies; and congenital or acquired physical defects, as well as a broad mental health history for the patient and patient's family.

casein, a white powder protein that occurs naturally in milk. It contains phosphorus and sulfur and is regarded as a "complete protein" because it contains all essential amino acids. Casein is precipitated when milk turns sour.

case management, **1.** a problem-solving process through which appropriate services to individuals and families are assured. **2.** a method of structuring acute care for all patients in three dimensions: work design, clinical management roles, and concurrent monitoring and feedback. **3.** a patient-centered, goal-oriented process of assessing the need of an individual for particular services and obtaining those services and monitoring care. See also **managed care.**

case nursing [L, *casus,* a happening, *nutrix,* nourish], an organizational mode for allocation of nursing staff in which one nurse is assigned to provide total nursing care to one or more patients. See also **primary nursing.**

caseous /kā″sē·əs/,   **1.** cottage cheese-like. Describing the mixture of fat and protein that appears in some body tissues undergoing necrosis. **2.** pertaining to the cheesy covering on fetuses that protects them during their prolonged presence in amniotic fluid. See also **vernix caseosa.**

caseous abscess,   an accumulation of pustular material with the consistency of viscous cheese. See **cheesy abscess.**

caseous fermentation [L, *caseus,* cheese, *fermentum,* yeast],   the coagulation of soluble casein to form insoluble calcium paracaseinate through the action of rennin.

caseous necrosis,   necrosis that transforms tissue into a dry cheeselike mass. It occurs primarily in tuberculosis. Also called **caseation necrosis.** See also **cheesy necrosis.**

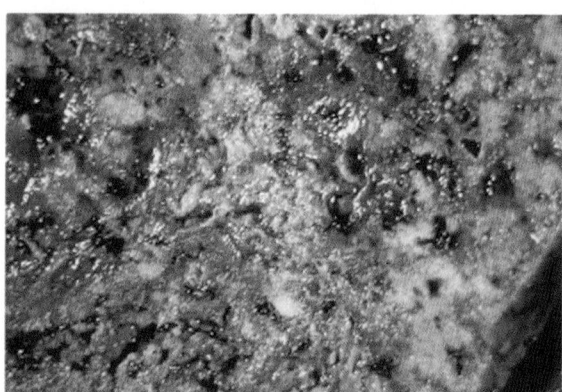

Caseous necrosis *(Kradin, 2010)*

case rate,   a pricing method in which a flat amount, often a per diem rate, covers a defined group of procedures and services. It is often used in services such as obstetrics and cardiovascular surgery for exceptions to a relative value scale or resource-based relative value scale. Also called *case price* or *bundled payment.*

case study,   a detailed analysis of a person or group with a particular disease or condition, noting characteristics of the disease or condition. Case studies are often used to call attention to new diseases or to diseases entering new populations.

$CaSO_4$,   chemical formula for **calcium sulfate.**

Casodex,   an anticancer chemotherapy agent. Brand name for **bicalutamide.**

cast [ONorse, *kasta*],   **1.** a stiff, solid dressing formed with plaster of paris or other material around a limb or other body part to immobilize it during healing. Kinds include **body jacket, long-arm cast, long-leg cast, short-arm cast, short-leg cast, spica cast. 2.** a mold of a part or all of a patient's teeth and internal jaw area for fitting prostheses or dentures. **3.** a tiny structure formed by deposits of mineral or other substances on the walls of renal tubules, bronchioles, or other organs. Casts often appear in samples of urine or blood collected for laboratory examination. **4.** the deviation of an eye from the normal parallel lines of vision, such as in strabismus.

cast brace,   a combination of a brace within a cast at a joint.

cast core [ONorse, *kasta* + L, *cor,* heart],   (in dentistry) a custom precise metal form, shaped like a tooth, prepared for an artificial crown. Its purpose is to replace the missing clinical crown of the tooth with a stable structure. The cast metal form incorporates a post and is cemented into the root canal for the retention of an artificial tooth crown. Compare **amalgam core, composite core.** See also **core.**

Castellani paint.   See **carbol-fuchsin solution.**

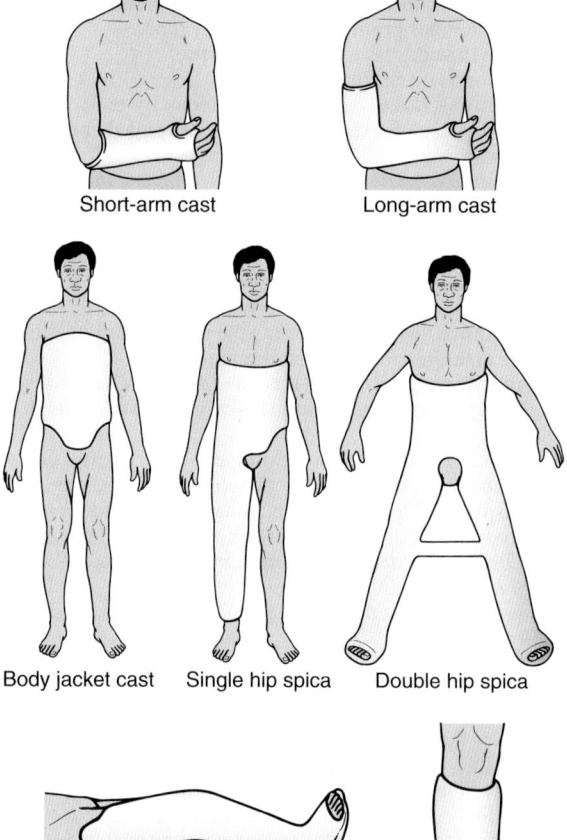

Short-arm cast   Long-arm cast

Body jacket cast   Single hip spica   Double hip spica

Long-leg cast

Short-leg cast

Casts *(Lewis et al, 2011)*

casting,   **1.** the act of encasing a body part in a cast. **2.** (in dentistry) the process by which crowns, inlays, and other metallic restorations are produced.

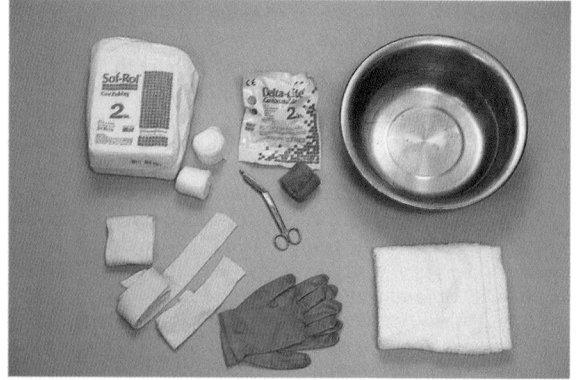

Casting materials *(Perry, Potter, and Elkin, 2012)*

casting tape, an adhesive or resin-impregnated mesh used for shaping lightweight casts.

Castleman disease /kas′əlmən/ [Benjamin Castleman, American pathologist, 1906–1982]. See **benign giant lymph node hyperplasia.**

castor oil /kas″tər/ [L, beaver, *oleum,* olive oil], an oil derived from *Ricinus communis,* used as a stimulant cathartic.

- INDICATIONS: It is prescribed as a cleansing preparation of the bowel or colon before examination and, rarely, for constipation.
- CONTRAINDICATIONS: Symptoms of appendicitis, intestinal obstruction or perforation, and fecal impaction prohibit its use. It is not to be used during menstruation or pregnancy.
- ADVERSE EFFECTS: Among the most serious adverse reactions are rectal bleeding and laxative dependence. Nausea, abdominal cramps, and dizziness also may occur.

cast post, (in dentistry) a custom fabricated insert within the root canal of a tooth being restored. Compare **cast core.**

castration /kastrā″shən/ [L, *castrare,* to castrate], the surgical excision of one or both testicles or ovaries, performed most frequently to reduce the production and secretion of certain hormones that may stimulate the proliferation of malignant cells in women with breast cancer or in men with prostate cancer. The patient must be informed that bilateral excision of the gonads causes sterility. See also **oophorectomy, orchidectomy.**

castration anxiety, **1.** (in Freudian psychoanalytic theory) the fantasized fear of injury or loss of the genital organs, often as the reaction to a repressed feeling of punishment for forbidden sexual desires. It may also be caused by some apparently threatening everyday occurrence, such as a humiliating experience, loss of a job, or loss of authority. **2.** a general threat to the masculinity or femininity of a person or an unrealistic fear of bodily injury or loss of power. Compare **penis envy.** See also **anxiety disorder.**

cast saw, a tool used to cut through a cast. It is used to split or remove the cast.

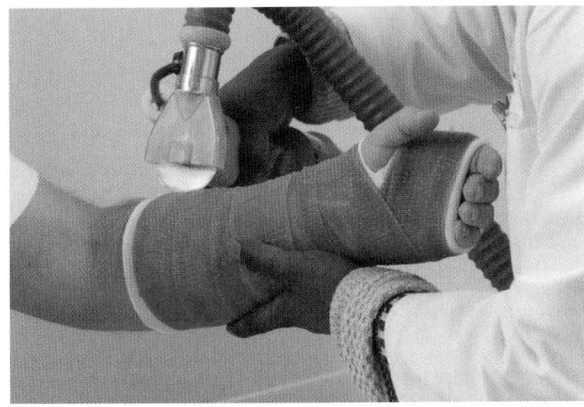

Cast saw cutting off a cast *(Bonewit-West, 2012)*

cast shoe, a shoe worn over a foot that is encased in a cast.

cast stabilization, the use of rods, pins, wooden shafts, or other devices to lend stability to a cast.

casualty /kazh″əltē/ [L, *casus,* chance], **1.** a serious or fatal accident or injury. **2.** the victim of a serious or fatal

accident or injury. **3.** a person killed, wounded, or otherwise disabled in war.

casuistics /kazh′əwis″tiks/ [L, *casus,* a happening], documentation of history of illness, treatment, and outcomes.

CAT /kat/, abbreviation for **computerized axial tomography.** See **computed tomography.**

cata-, cat-, prefix meaning "down, under, against, lower, with": *catabiosis, catabolism.*

catabasis /kətab″əsis/ *pl. catabases* [Gk, *kata,* down, *bainein,* to go], the phase in which a disease declines. −*catabatic, adj.*

catabiosis /kat′əbī-ō″sis/, the normal aging of cells. −*catabiotic, adj.*

catabolic. See **catabolism.**

catabolic activator protein, (in molecular genetics) a protein that participates in initiating the transcription of ribonucleic acid in organisms without a true nucleus, such as bacteria.

catabolic illness /kat′əbol″ik/, a disorder characterized by weight loss and diminished muscle mass and body fat. Underlying causes include infection, injury, organ system failure, chemotherapy, and uncontrolled diabetes mellitus, particularly type 1.

catabolism /kətab″əliz′əm/ [Gk, *kata + ballein,* to throw], a metabolic process in which complex substances are broken down by living cells into simple compounds. The process liberates energy for use in work, energy storage, or heat production. Carbon dioxide and water are produced, as well as energy. Compare **anabolism.** −**catabolic,** *adj.*

catabolite activator protein. See **CAP.**

catachronobiology /kat′əkrō′nōbī-ol″əjē/, the study of the harmful effects of time on living systems. See also **chronobiology.**

catacrotism /kətak″rətiz′əm/ [Gk, *kata + krotein,* to strike], an anomaly of the pulse, characterized by one or more small additional waves in the descending limb of the pulse tracing. −*catacrotic, adj.*

catagen, the brief portion of the hair cycle in which growth of the hair (anagen) stops and resting (telogen) begins.

catagenesis /kat′əjen″əsis/ [Gk, *kata,* down, *genein,* to produce], a form of evolution that is retrogressive.

catalase /kat″əlās/ [Gk, *katalein,* to dissolve], a heme enzyme, found in almost all biological cells, that catalyzes the decomposition of hydrogen peroxide to water and oxygen.

catalepsy /kat″əlep′sē/ [Gk, *kata + lambanein,* to seize], an abnormal state characterized by a trancelike level of consciousness and postural rigidity. It occurs in hypnosis and in certain organic and psychological disorders such as schizophrenia, epilepsy, and hysteria. −*cataleptic, adj.*

catalysis /kətal″əsis/ [Gk, *katalein,* to dissolve], an increase in the rate of a chemical reaction by the addition of a substance that is neither permanently altered nor consumed by the reaction. Compare **negative catalysis.** See also **catalyst.** −*catalytic, adj.,* −**catalyze,** *v.*

catalyst /kat″əlist/ [Gk, *katalein,* to dissolve], a substance that influences the rate of a chemical reaction without being permanently altered or consumed by the process. Most catalysts, including enzymes in living organisms, accelerate chemical reactions; negative catalysts slow such reactions. See also **enzyme, negative catalysis.**

-catalytic, -catalytical, suffix meaning "a chemical reaction caused by an agent unchanged by the reaction": *autocatalytic, photocatalytic.*

catalyze. See **catalysis.**

catamenia. See **menses.**

catamnesis /kat′amnē″sis/ [Gk, *kata* + *men,* month], the medical history of a patient from the onset of an illness. Compare **anamnesis,** def. 2.

cataphoria /kat′əfôr″ē·ə/, a tendency of the visual axes of both eyes to assume a low plane after the visual fusional stimuli have been eliminated.

cataphylaxis /kat′əfəlak″sis/ [Gk, *kata* + *phylax,* guard], **1.** the migration of leukocytes and antibodies to the site of an infection. **2.** the deterioration of the natural defense system of the body. –*cataphylactic, adj.*

cataplexy /kat″əplek″sē/ [Gk, *kata* + *plexis,* stroke], a condition characterized by sudden loss of muscle tone, usually resulting in a fall, caused by strong emotions, such as anger, fear, or surprise, often associated with narcolepsy. –*cataplectic, adj.*

Catapres, an antihypertensive drug. Brand name for **clonidine hydrochloride.**

cataract /kat″ərakt/ [Gk, *katarrhakies,* waterfall], an abnormal progressive condition of the lens of the eye, characterized by loss of transparency. A yellow, brown, or white opacity can be observed within the lens, behind the pupil. Most cataracts are caused by degenerative changes, often occurring after 50 years of age. The tendency to develop cataracts is inherited. Trauma, such as a puncture wound, may result in cataract formation. Less often, exposure to such poisons as dinitrophenol or naphthalene causes them. Congenital cataracts are usually hereditary but may be caused by viral infection during the first trimester of gestation. If cataracts are untreated, sight is eventually lost. At onset, vision is blurred; then bright lights glare diffusely, and distortion and double vision may develop. Uncomplicated cataracts of old age (senile cataracts) are usually treated with excision of the lens and either surgical insertion of an intraocular lens or prescription of special contact lenses or glasses. The soft cataracts of children and young adults may be either incised and drained or fragmented by ultrasound. See also **congenital cataract, senile cataract.**

■ OBSERVATIONS: Symptoms of cataracts include progressive, painless blurring and distortion of objects, glare from bright lights, and gradual loss of vision. Signs include a yellow, brown, or white coloring on the pupil and myopia. The crystalline lens of the eye becomes cloudy and opaque. Cataracts are identified by a complete ophthalmoscopic examination, including funduscopy and slit lamp examination. The primary complication is blindness.

■ INTERVENTIONS: Surgical removal of the lens is the primary treatment and is performed only after vision becomes compromised. Follow-up laser surgery is frequently needed to remove a secondary membrane that can form. Topical antiinfective drugs and mydriatic-cycloplegics are used preoperatively, and corticosteroids, antibiotics, and mydriatics are used postoperatively. Corrective lenses may be used to correct vision, and strong lighting may be used to enhance vision until surgery is performed.

■ PATIENT CARE CONSIDERATIONS: Before surgery, care is focused on assessment and attention to self-care deficits related to decreasing vision. Preoperative care includes education about the surgical experience and lens implants and reduction of anxiety about impending surgery. Postoperative education focuses on proper use and instillation of eyedrops, prevention of infection, and activity restrictions. Recovery is usually rapid, and most individuals are able to resume activities of daily living within a week.

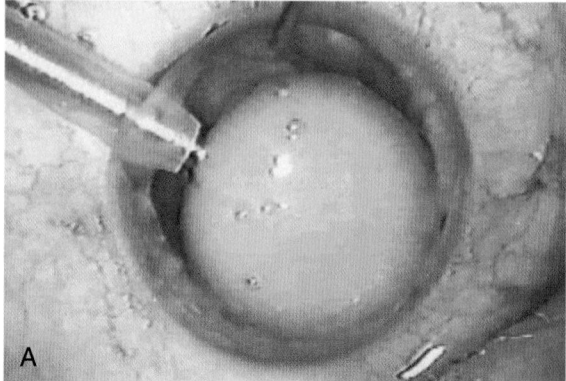

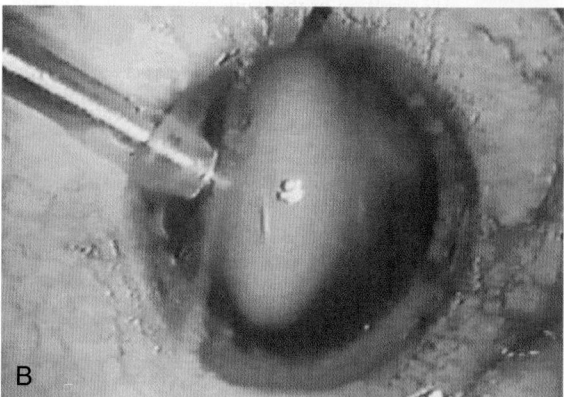

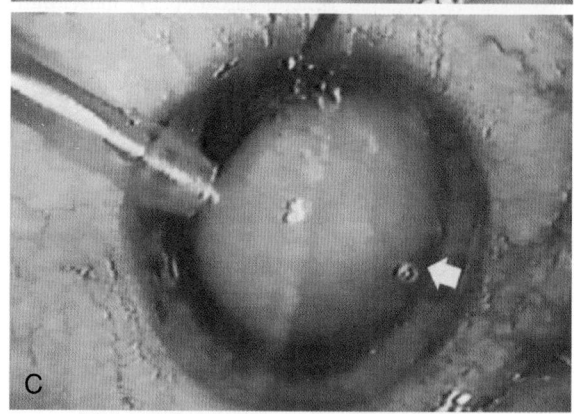

Cataract *(Brazitikos et al, 1999)*

cataractogenic /kat′ərak′tōjen″ik/, pertaining to agents that may cause cataracts.

cataract removal, removal of a cloudy lens from the interior of the eye. The most common method of removal is extracapsular in which the lens cortex and nucleus are expressed from the eye after the anterior portion of the capsule is removed, leaving the posterior capsule behind. An intraocular lens is usually implanted after lens removal for visual correction. In recent years, sutureless cataract techniques have increased in popularity because of the rapidity of rehabilitation. Clear cornea microincisions allow the use of topical anesthesia in place of retrobulbar anesthesia.

catarrh /kətär″/ [Gk, *kata + rhoia,* flow], inflammation of the mucous membranes with discharge, especially inflammation of the air passages of the nose and the trachea. See also **rhinitis.** −*catarrhal,* **catarrhous,** *adj.*

catarrhal conjunctivitis [Gk, *kata + rhoia* + L, *conjunctivus,* connecting; Gk, *itis,* inflammation], a simple form of inflammation of the conjunctiva, usually associated with an infection such as a cold, allergy, exposure to pollution, or physical irritation as by an eyelash in the eye. It is accompanied by discharge and can be acute or chronic.

catarrhal croup [Gk, *kata + rhoia* + Scot, to croak], severe laryngitis accompanied by a croupy cough. See also **croup.**

catarrhal dysentery, inflammation of the gastrointestinal tract with foul-smelling stools. See **sprue.**

catarrhal ophthalmia [Gk, *kata + rhoia + ophthalmos,* eye], an inflammation of the conjunctiva with a discharge. See also **catarrhal conjunctivitis.**

catarrhal pneumonia. See **bronchopneumonia.**

catarrhal stomatitis, inflammation of the mucous membranes of the mouth; characterized by edema and pain. See **simple stomatitis.**

catarrhous, inflamed. See **catarrh.**

catastrophic care /kat′əstrof″ik/ [Gk, *katastrophe,* sudden downturn; L, *garrire,* to babble], a pattern of health care that involves intensive, highly specialized life-support care of an acutely ill or severely traumatized patient.

catastrophic health insurance, **1.** health insurance that awards benefits to pay for the cost of severe or lengthy disability or illness. Benefits on some policies are not paid until a specified minimum amount paid by the insured is exceeded. Most policies have a limit in total benefits paid, and payment for certain kinds of services may be precluded or limited to a maximum indemnity. **2.** a marketplace insurance category with a low premium and a higher-than-average deductible. You must be under 30 or have a hardship exemption to purchase this insurance plan, which is designed to protect the buyer from the cost of a catastrophic illness.

catastrophic illness, any illness that requires lengthy hospitalization, extremely expensive therapies, or other care that would deplete a family's financial resources unless covered by special medical insurance policies. In Canada, catastrophic illness is covered by the Canada Health Care System.

catastrophic reaction [Gk, *katastrophe,* sudden downturn; L, *re,* again, *agere,* to act], **1.** the uncoordinated response to a drastic shock or a sudden threatening condition, as often occurs in the victims of car crashes and disasters. **2.** an intense, spontaneous, aggressive, and confused outburst from a patient with severe dementia in response to something that is perceived as immensely frustrating. Violence is a potential.

catatonia /kat′ətō′nē·ə/ [Gk, *kata + tonos,* tension], a state of psychologically induced immobility with muscular rigidity at times interrupted by agitation. It is manifested usually as immobility with extreme muscular rigidity or, less commonly, as excessive, impulsive activity. See also **catatonic schizophrenia.** −*catatonic, adj.*

catatonic excitement /kat′əton′ik/, a state of extreme agitation characterized by purposeless movement.

catatonic schizophrenia [Gk, *kata + tonos + schizein,* to split, *phren,* mind], a form of schizophrenia characterized by alternating periods of extreme withdrawal and extreme excitement. During the withdrawal stage, stupor, waxy flexibility, muscular rigidity, mutism, blocking, negativism, and catalepsy (cerea flexibilitas) may be seen. During the period of excitement, purposeless and impulsive activity may range from mild agitation to violence. See also **catatonia.**

catatonic stupor, a form of catatonia characterized by a marked decrease in response to the environment with a reduction in spontaneous movement. Patients with this disorder sometimes appear unaware of their environment.

cat-bite fever. See **cat-scratch fever.**

CAT-CAM, abbreviation for **contoured adducted trochanteric controlled alignment method.**

catchment /kach′ment/, the catching or collecting of water, especially the collection of rainwater.

catchment area [L, *capere,* to take, *area,* space], the specific geographic area for which a particular institution, especially a mental health center, is responsible.

catch-up growth [L, *capere* + As, *uf, gruowan*], an acceleration of the growth rate following a period of growth delay caused by a secondary deficiency, such as acute malnutrition or severe illness. The phenomenon, which routinely occurs in premature infants, involves rapid increase in weight, length, and head circumference and continues until the normal individual growth pattern is resumed. The severity, duration, and developmental timing at which the deficiency occurs may result in some growth inadequacy or permanent deficit, especially in such tissue as the brain.

cat-cry syndrome [L, *catta,* cat, *quiritare,* to cry out; Gk, *syndromos,* course], a rare congenital disorder characterized at birth by a kittenlike cry caused by a laryngeal anomaly. The condition is associated with a defect in chromosome 5. Other characteristics include low birth weight, microcephaly, "moon face," wide-set eyes, strabismus, and low-set misshapen ears. Infants are hypotonic; heart defects and mental and physical impairments are common. Also called **chromosome 5p-syndrome, cri-du-chat syndrome.**

catecholamine /kat′əkəlam″in/, any one of a group of sympathomimetic compounds composed of a catechol (1,2-dihydroxyphenyl) moiety carrying an alkyl side chain with an amine group on the side chain. Some catecholamines are produced naturally by the body and function as key neurological chemicals.

catechol-o-methyl transferase (COMT) /kat′əkol′ōmeth″il/, an enzyme that deactivates the catecholamines dopa, dopamine, epinephrine, and norepinephrine.

categoric data /kat′əgôr″ik/ [Gk, *kategorikos,* affirmation; L, *datus,* giving], (in research) any data that are classified by name rather than by number, such as race, religion, ethnicity, or marital status. Also called **nominal data.**

categoric variable, a characteristic in a research study that denotes placement of data into categories, such as gender.

Category A Diseases/Agents, a designation by the U.S. Centers for Disease Control and Prevention (CDC) for bioterrorism agents that includes dangerous illnesses, germs, or bacteria introduced to a population by simple methods with the intent to cause harm and alter well-being, physically and mentally. They create widespread public panic and disruption. See also **Category B Diseases/Agents, Category C Diseases/Agents.**

Category B Diseases/Agents, a designation by the U.S. Centers for Disease Control and Prevention (CDC) for bioterrorism agents that includes dangerous illnesses, germs, and/or bacteria that are moderately easy to disseminate, result in moderate morbidity rates and low mortality rates, and require specific enhancements of the diagnostic capacity and enhanced disease surveillance. See also **Category A Diseases/Agents, Category C Diseases/Agents.**

Category C Diseases/Agents, a designation by the U.S. Centers for Disease Control and Prevention (CDC) for bioterrorism agents that includes emerging pathogens that could be engineered for mass dissemination in the future because of availability, ease of production and dissemination, and potential for high morbidity and mortality rates and major health impact. See also **Category A Diseases/Agents, Category B Diseases/Agents.**

cat-eye syndrome [L, *catta* + AS, *eage* + Gk, *syndromos,* course], a rare congenital autosomal anomaly, marked by the presence of an extra, small chromosome 22 and pupils that resemble the vertical pupils of a cat. Anal atresia and heart abnormalities are common. Those with this syndrome may have normal intelligence or varying degrees of intellectual delay. Also called *Schmid–Fraccaro syndrome.*

catgut [L, *catta* + AS, *guttas*], an absorbable suture material, prepared from the intestines of mammals, used to close surgical wounds. It can be treated with chromic salts to delay absorption and enhance strength.

catharsis /kəthär″sis/, **1.** a cleansing or purging. **2.** the therapeutic release of pent-up feelings and emotions by open discussion of ideas and thoughts. **3.** the process of drawing repressed ideas and feelings into the consciousness by the technique of free association, often in conjunction with hypnosis and the use of hypnotic drugs. Also called **psychocatharsis.** See also **abreaction. −cathartic,** *n.*

cathartic /kəthär″tik/ [Gk, cleansing], **1.** *adj.,* pertaining to a substance that causes evacuation of the bowel. **2.** *n.,* an agent that promotes bowel evacuation by stimulating peristalsis, increasing the fluidity or bulk of intestinal contents, softening the feces, or lubricating the intestinal wall. The term *cathartic* implies a fluid evacuation, in contrast to *laxative,* which implies the elimination of a soft, formed stool. Cathartics that increase peristalsis, usually by irritating intestinal mucosa, include certain plant substances, such as aloe, colocynth, croton oil, podophyllum senna, phenolphthalein, bisacodyl, and dehydrocholic acid. Saline cathartics, such as sodium sulfate, magnesium sulfate, and magnesium hydroxide, dilute the intestinal contents by retaining water through osmotic forces. Suppositories containing sodium biphosphate, sodium acid pyrophosphate, and sodium bicarbonate induce defecation when the salts react to form carbon dioxide and the expanding gas stimulates peristalsis. Also called **coprogogue. −catharsis,** *n.*

cathectic. See **cathexis.**

catheter /kath″ətər/ [Gk, *katheter,* something lowered], a hollow flexible tube that can be inserted into a vessel or cavity of the body to withdraw or instill fluids, directly monitor various types of information, and visualize a vessel or cavity. Most catheters are made of soft plastic, rubber, or silicon. Kinds include **acorn-tipped catheter, angiocatheter, Foley catheter, intrauterine catheter.**

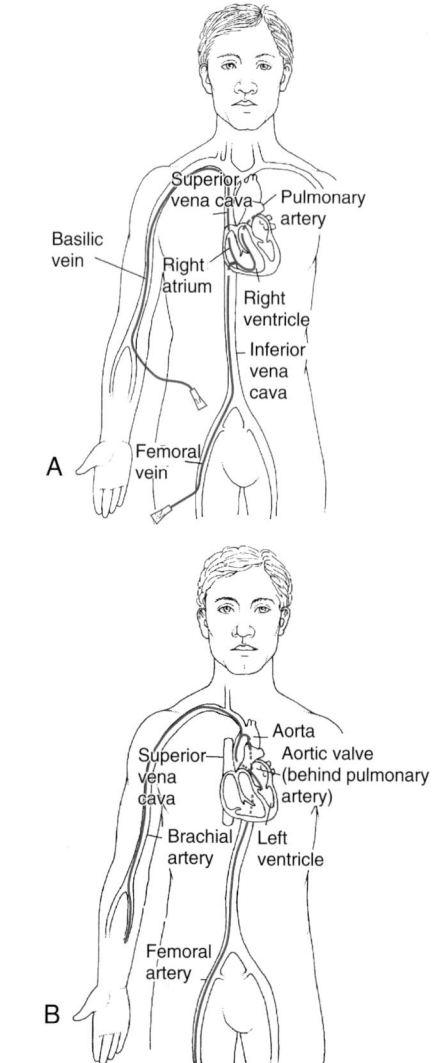

A, Right-sided heart catheterization. The catheter is inserted into the femoral vein and advanced through the inferior vena cava (or, if into an antecubital or basilic vein, through the superior vena cava), right atrium, and right ventricle and into the pulmonary artery. B, Left-sided heart catheterization. The catheter is inserted into the femoral artery or the antecubital artery. The catheter is passed through the ascending aorta, through the aortic valve, and into the left ventricle. *(Mosby, 2003)*

catheter ablation, use of a small, thin, flexible wire tubing to deliver energy frequency to destroy very small areas of tissue. See also **radiofrequency ablation.**

catheter hub, a threaded plastic connection at the end of an IV catheter.

catheterization /kath′ətur͞izā″shən/, the introduction of a catheter (a hollow flexible tube) into a body cavity or organ to inject or remove a fluid. See also **female catheterization, Foley catheter, male catheterization. −catheterize,** *v.*

cathexis /kəthek″sis/ [Gk, *kathexis,* retention], the conscious or unconscious attachment of emotional feeling and importance to a specific idea, person, or object. **–cathectic,** *adj.*

cathode (C) /kath″ōd/ [Gk, *kata,* down, *hodos,* way], **1.** the electrode at which reduction occurs. **2.** the negative side of the x-ray tube, which consists of the focusing cup and the filament.

cathode ray, an invisible stream of electrons emitted by a negative electrode and propelled at high velocity through a vacuum x-ray tube toward an anode.

cathode ray oscilloscope [Gk, *kata* + *hodos* + L, *radius* + *ocillare,* to swing; Gk, *skopein,* to view], an instrument that produces a visual representation of electrical variations by means of the fluorescent screen of a cathode ray tube. Oscilloscopes have many applications in medicine and in nursing, such as the displaying of patients' brain waves and heartbeats for monitoring and diagnostic purposes.

cathode ray tube (CRT), a vacuum tube that focuses a beam of electrons onto a spot on a screen coated with a phosphor, creating a visible image of information on the face of the tube. For the most part, CRT use has been replaced by newer display technologies.

cation /kat″ī·on/ [Gk, *kata,* down, *ion,* going], a positively charged ion. Compare **anion.**

cation-exchange resin, any one of various insoluble organic polymers with high molecular weights that exchange their cations for other cations in solution. Cation-exchange resins are used especially to restrict intestinal sodium absorption in patients with edema. Compare **anion-exchange resin.**

catling, a long, sharp, double-edged surgical knife used in amputation. Also called *catlin.*

catoptric /kətop″trik/ [Gk, *katoptron,* mirror], pertaining to a reflected image or reflected light, such as from a mirror.

cat pox. See **cowpox.**

cat's claw, an herb that belongs to the madder family, found in South America and Southeast Asia.

■ INDICATIONS: It is used for cancer, herpes, arthritis, gastritis, gout, wounds, and gastric ulcers. There may be short-term benefits when used for osteoarthritis, but effectiveness for other indications has not been proven.

■ CONTRAINDICATIONS: It is contraindicated during pregnancy and lactation and in children younger than 3 years of age until more research is available. It also should not be used in people with muscular sclerosis, tuberculosis, or hemophilia or in those who have had organ transplants.

cat-scratch fever, a disease that results from the scratch or bite of a healthy cat. It is caused by the bacterium Bartonella. Inflammation and pustules are found on the scratched skin and lymph nodes in the neck, head, groin, or axilla and swell 2 weeks later. There may be spontaneous remission of symptoms in about 2 weeks. Although patients are seldom seriously ill, fever, loss of appetite, headache, and malaise may occur and symptoms can persist for months. Antibiotics may be prescribed for persistent infection. Also called **benign lymphoreticulosis,** *cat scratch disease.*

cat's eye amaurosis [L, *catta* + AS, *aege* + Gk, *amauroin,* to darken], a monocular blindness, with a bright reflection from the pupil caused by a white mass in the vitreous humor resulting from inflammation or a malignant lesion. Also called **leukocoria.**

Caucasian [ancient geographic region of the Caucasus, in southeastern Europe], a reference to the Caucasus nationality, whose general physical type has the characteristic of lighter-colored skin. The term is common in the United States in demographic surveys.

caud-, prefix meaning "tail": *caudal, caudocephalad.*

caudad /kô″dad/ [L, *cauda,* tail], toward the tail or end of the body, away from the head. Compare **cephalad.**

cauda equina [L, *cauda* + *equus,* horse], the lower end of the spinal cord at the first lumbar vertebra and the bundle of lumbar, sacral, and coccygeal nerve roots that emerge from the spinal cord at the first lumbar vertebra. It descends from the lower spinal cord and occupies the vertebral canal below the cord.

caudal /kô″dəl/, toward the distal end of the body or an inferior position.

caudal anesthesia, the injection of a local anesthetic agent into the caudal (end) portion of the epidural space through the sacral hiatus to anesthetize sacral and lower lumbar nerve roots. Once popular in obstetrics, it is now rarely performed except in pediatric anesthesia. Complications of caudal anesthesia include infection, a high (5% to 10%) rate of failure, frequent neurological complications, dural puncture, and hypotension. See also **regional anesthesia.**

caudal eminence, a tail-like eminence produced by a proliferating mass of mesodermal cells at the caudal end of the early vertebrate embryo. It is the remnant of the primitive node and the precursor of hindgut, adjacent notochord and somites, and the caudal part of the spinal cord. Also called **tail bud.**

caudal ligaments, bands of fibrous tissue attaching the skin to the coccyx. Remnants of the embryonic notochord, they form a small cup-shaped depression. Also called **caudal retinaculum.**

caudal regression syndrome, failure of formation of part or all of the coccygeal, sacral, and occasionally lumbar vertebral units and the corresponding segments of the caudal spinal cord, with resulting neurogenic dysfunction of bowel and bladder. The syndrome is more common in infants born to mothers with diabetes. It is a complex condition that may have multiple etiologies. Also called **sacral agenesis.**

caudal retinaculum. See **caudal ligaments.**

caudate /kô″dāt/, having a tail.

caudate lobe of the liver [L, *cauda,* tail; Gk, *lobos,* lobe; AS, *lifer*], a part of the right lobe of the liver that lies near the inferior vena cava.

caudate nucleus [L, *cauda,* tail, *nucleus,* nut kernel], a crescent-shaped mass of gray matter lateral to the thalamus in the floor of the anterior horn and body of the lateral ventricle.

caudate process [L, *cauda* + *processus,* projection], a small elevation of tissue that extends obliquely from the lower extremity of the caudate lobe of the liver to the visceral surface of the right lobe. It separates the fossa for the gallbladder from the beginning of the fossa for the inferior vena cava.

caudocephalad /kô′dōsef″əlad/ [L, *cauda,* tail; Gk, *kephale,* head; L, *ad,* toward], movement from the tail toward the head.

caul /kôl/ [ME, *cawel,* basket], an intact amniotic sac surrounding the fetus at birth. The sac usually ruptures or is ruptured during the course of labor or delivery. When it remains intact, it must be torn or cut to allow the baby to breathe.

cauliflower ear [L, *caulis,* cabbage, *fiore,* flower; AS, *eare*], a thickened, deformed pinna and external ear (with an appearance like the vegetable cauliflower) that is caused by repeated trauma, such as that suffered by boxers. Plastic surgery may be a means of restoring the normal appearance of the ear.

caumesthesia /kô′məsthē″zhə/ [Gk, *kauma,* heat, *aisthesis,* feeling], an abnormal condition in which a patient has a low temperature but experiences a sense of intense heat. **–caumesthetic,** *adj.*

caus-, caut-, prefix meaning "burn": *causalgia, cautery.*

causalgia /kôzal″jə/ [Gk, *kausis,* burning, *algos,* pain], a severe sensation of burning pain, often in an extremity, sometimes accompanied by local erythema of the skin caused by peripheral nerve injury.

causal hypothesis /kô″səl/ [L, *causa,* cause; Gk, *hypotithenia,* foundation], (in research) a hypothesis that predicts a cause-and-effect relationship among the variables to be studied.

causal hypothesis testing study, (in research) an experimental design used in testing a hypothesis that predicts a cause-and-effect relationship within the data to be studied.

causality /kôsal″itē/, (in research) a relationship between one phenomenon or event (A) and another (B) in which A precedes and causes B. The direction of influence and the nature of the effect are predictable and reproducible and may be empirically observed. Causality is difficult to prove. Some social scientists contend that it is impossible to prove a causal relationship.

causal treatment, treatment directed against the cause of the disease. See **treatment.**

causation /kôsā″shən/ [L, *causa*], (in law) the existence of a reasonable connection between the misfeasance, malfeasance, or nonfeasance of the defendant and the injury or damage suffered by the plaintiff. In a lawsuit in which negligence is alleged, the harm suffered by the plaintiff must be proved to result directly from the negligence of the defendant; causation must be demonstrated.

cause [L, *causa*], any process, substance, or organism that produces an effect or condition.

CAUSN, abbreviation for *Canadian Association of University Schools of Nursing.*

caustic /kôs″tik/ [Gk, *kaustikos,* burning], **1.** *n.,* any substance that is destructive to living tissue, such as silver nitrate, nitric acid, or sulfuric acid. **2.** *adj.,* exerting a burning or corrosive effect.

caustic poisoning, the accidental ingestion of strong acids or alkalis, resulting in burns and tissue damage to the mouth, esophagus, and stomach. The victim experiences immediate pain, swelling, and edema. The pulse may be weak and rapid. Respirations become shallow, and edema may close the airway. Complications, which include circulatory shock, perforation of the esophagus, and pharyngeal edema leading to asphyxia, can be fatal. See also **acid burn, alkali burn.**

caustics, strong alkaline chemicals, such as hydrofluoric acid, that destroy soft body tissues, resulting in deep penetrating burns and corrosion of the skin, eyes, and mucous membranes on contact. Caustics are usually the hydroxides of light metals. Exposure may be by inhalation or ingestion. Treatment of exposure to these agents involves irrigation of exposed areas and neutralization of the substance.

CAUT, abbreviation for **Canadian Association of University Teachers.**

cauterization /kô′tərīzā″shən/ [Gk, *kauterion,* branding iron], the process of burning a part of the body by cautery.

cauterize /kô″tərīz/ [Gk, *kauterion,* branding iron], **1.** to burn tissues by thermal heat, including steam, hot metal, or solar radiation; electricity; or another agent such as laser or dry ice, usually with the objective of destroying damaged or diseased tissues, preventing infections, or coagulating blood vessels. See also **chemical cauterization. 2.** to apply a cautery; to perform cauterization.

cautery /kô″tərē/ [Gk, *kauterion,* branding iron], **1.** a device or agent used in the coagulation of tissue by heat or caustic substances. **2.** a destructive effect produced by a cauterizing agent.

cautery knife, a surgical knife that cuts tissue and seals it to prevent bleeding. The knife is connected to an electric source that generates the heat necessary for cauterization.

cav-, cavo-, prefix meaning "hollow": *cavity, cavogram.*

cava. See **cavum.**

cavalry bone. See **rider's bone.**

Cavell, Edith /kəvel″/, (1865–1915), an English nurse. Trained at London Hospital, in 1907 she was named head of a nurses training school in Brussels. After the Germans occupied Belgium in World War I, she nursed or sheltered more than 200 fleeing soldiers and helped them reach Holland. To her, this was an extension of her nursing: helping those in need. For this, she was arrested by the Germans, tried, and shot on October 12, 1915. Her execution, which she met with courage and fortitude, brought her widespread admiration.

caveola, *pl.* **caveolae,** a small pit, depression, or invagination, such as any of the minute pits or incuppings of the cell membrane formed during pinocytosis, which close and then pinch off to form small, free, fluid-filled vesicles in the cytoplasm.

Caverject, an injectable prostaglandin-derived drug for the treatment of male impotence. Brand name for **alprostadil.**

cavernoma. See **cavernous hemangioma.**

cavernous /kav″ərnəs/ [L, *caverna,* hollow place], containing cavities or hollow spaces. See also **cavernous hemangioma.**

cavernous angioma. See **cavernous hemangioma.**

cavernous body of the clitoris, cavernous body of the penis. See **corpus cavernosum.**

cavernous hemangioma [L, *caverna,* hollow place; Gk, *haima,* blood, *oma,* tumor], a benign, congenital, red or purple tumor consisting of enlarged blood vessels. The scalp, face, and neck are the most common sites, but these tumors have been found in the liver and other organs. Superficial cavernous hemangiomas are friable and easily infected if the skin is broken. Treatment includes observation, irradiation, sclerosing solutions, and laser surgery and excisional surgery. Also called **angioma cavernosum, cavernoma.** Compare **capillary hemangioma, nevus flammeus.**

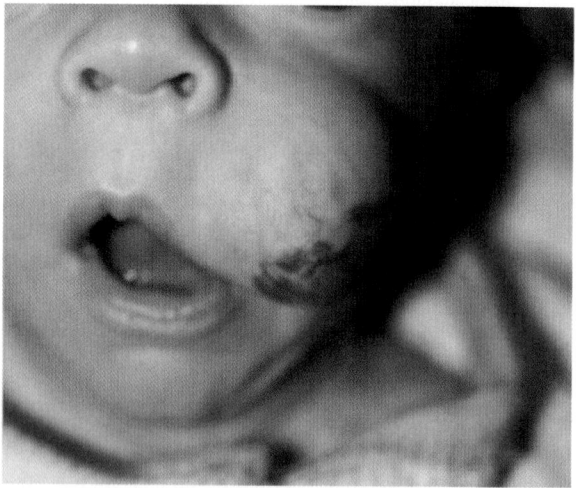

Infant with cavernous hemangioma *(Courtesy Department of Dermatology, School of Medicine, University of Utah)*

cavernous lymphangioma. See **lymphangioma cavernosum.**

cavernous nerve, one of the terminal branches of the inferior hypogastric plexuses that innervate the erectile tissues of the penis.

cavernous sinus [L, *caverna* + *sinus,* curve], one of a pair of irregularly shaped bilateral venous channels between the sphenoid bone of the skull and the dura mater. It is one of the five anterior inferior venous sinuses that drain the blood from the dura mater into the internal jugular vein.

Trochlear nerve [IV]

Abducent nerve [VI]

Internal carotid artery

Oculomotor nerve [III]

Pituitary gland

Dura mater

Diaphragma sellae

Sphenoid (paranasal) sinus

Cavernous (venous) sinus

Ophthalmic division of trigeminal nerve [V₁]

Maxillary division of trigeminal nerve [V₂]

Cavernous sinus *(Drake, Vogl, and Mitchell, 2015)*

cavernous sinus syndrome, an abnormal condition characterized by edema of the conjunctiva, the upper eyelid, and the root of the nose and by paralysis of the third, fourth, and sixth cranial nerves. It is caused by a thrombosis of the cavernous sinus.

cavernous sinus thrombosis, a syndrome, usually secondary to infections near the eye or nose, characterized by orbital edema, venous congestion of the eye, and palsy of the nerves supplying the extraocular muscles. The infection may spread to involve the cerebrospinal fluid and meninges. Treatment involves antibiotics and sometimes anticoagulants.

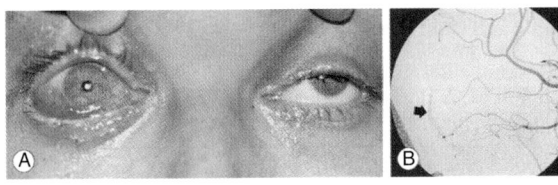

Cavernous sinus thrombosis *(Albert et al, 2008)*

CAVH, abbreviation for **continuous arteriovenous hemofiltration.**

cavitary /kav″iter′ē/ [L, *cavus,* hollow], **1.** *adj.,* denoting the presence of one or more cavities. **2.** *n.,* any parasite having a body cavity or an alimentary canal.

cavitate /kav″itāt/ [L, *cavus,* hollow], to rapidly form and collapse vapor pockets or bubbles in a flowing fluid with low-pressure areas, often causing damage to surrounding structures.

cavitation, **1.** the formation of deep open spaces within the body, such as those formed in the lung by tuberculosis. **2.** any cavity within the body, such as the pleural cavities.

cavity /kav″itē/ [L, *cavus*], **1.** a hollow space within a larger structure, such as the peritoneal cavity or the oral cavity. See also **body cavity. 2.** *(Nontechnical)* a space in a tooth formed by dental caries.

cavity classification, a method for describing dental caries based on the tooth surfaces on which they occur (labial, buccal, lingual, incisal, occlusal, or root), the type of surface on which they occur (pit and fissure or smooth), and their numeric designation according to the classification of caries. Also called **Black's Classification of Caries.** See also **classification of caries.**

cavity prep. See **prepared tooth cavity.**

cavity preparation, a procedure for the removal of diseased hard tissues of a tooth and the shaping of the surgical site to an acceptable form necessary to receive and retain a particular type of restoration.

cavogram /kav″əgram′/ [L, *cavus* + Gk, *gramma,* record], an angiogram of the inferior or superior vena cava.

cavosurface /kāv′ōsur′fəs/ [L, *cavus,* cavity + *superficies,* surface], the contact between a dental cavity preparation and natural tooth structure.

cavosurface angle /kāv′ōsur″fəs/, the angle formed by the junction of the wall of a prepared tooth cavity with the external natural tooth structure.

cavosurface bevel [L, *cavus* + *superficies,* surface; OFr, *baif,* open mouth], the incline of the angle of a prepared tooth cavity wall where it contacts the enamel wall. Compare **bevel, contra bevel.**

cavum /kā″vəm/ *pl. cava,* **1.** any hollow or cavity. **2.** the inferior or superior vena cava.

cavus /kā″vəs/ [L, *cavus,* cavity], an abnormally high or exaggerated arch of the foot. See also **clawfoot.**

cayenne pepper. See **capsicum.**

CBA, abbreviation for **cost-benefit analysis.**

CBC, abbreviation for **complete blood count.**

CBF, abbreviation for **cerebral blood flow.**

CBI, abbreviation for **continuous bladder irrigation.**

cc, 1. abbreviation for **cubic centimeter. 2.** (in pharmacology) an abbreviation identified by the Institute for Safe Medication Practices as an error-prone abbreviation. Now called **mL. 3.** a measurement of volume.

CC, 1. abbreviation for **chief complaint. 2.** abbreviation for **closing capacity.**

CCD, abbreviation for **charge-coupled device.**

CCK test, abbreviation for **cholecystokinin test.**

CCK-HIDA scan, cholecystokinin hepatobiliary (CCK-HIDA) scintigraphy used as a diagnostic measure in the evaluation of abdominal pain when gallbladder disease is suspected. To prepare for the scan, the patient fasts for 4 or more hours. Following the fast, technetium-99m-EHIDA is injected systemically via an intravenous site. Then 1½ hours later cholecystokinin (CCK) is infused over 45 minutes. Imaging begins 5 minutes before infusion, and the gallbladder ejection fraction is monitored.

CCNE, abbreviation for **Commission on Collegiate Nursing Education.**

CCP, abbreviation for **complement control protein.**

CCPD, abbreviation for **continuous cycling peritoneal dialysis.**

CCRN®, denoting certification as a critical-care registered nurse by the American Association of Critical-Care Nurses Certification Corporation.

CCU, **1.** abbreviation for **coronary care unit. 2.** abbreviation for **critical care unit.**

Cd, symbol for the element **cadmium.**

CD4, symbol for a glycoprotein expressed on the surface of helper T lymphocytes and other immune cells. CD4 serves as a receptor for human immunodeficiency virus envelope glycoprotein gp120. Binding of the viral glycoprotein gp120 to CD4 is the first step in viral entry, leading to the fusion of viral and cell membranes. CD4 count is used as an indicator of treatment timing in HIV patients. Abbreviation for *cluster of differentiation 4.*

CD4 cell, CD4+ cell, a major classification of T lymphocytes, referring to those that carry the CD4 antigen; most are helper cells. HIV infection causes a drastic decrease in CD4+ T cells.

CD4 cell count, a measure of the number of "helper" T cells that carry the CD4 glycoprotein on their cell surface and that help B cells produce certain antibodies. The human immunodeficiency virus (HIV) binds to CD4 and kills T cells bearing this glycoprotein. Thus the CD4 cell count is an indicator of the progress of an HIV infection and helps measure the effectiveness of anti-HIV drugs. CD4 T cells mainly produce interleukin 2, an autocrine and paracrine T cell growth factor; preactivated or memory CD4 T cells secrete a much larger array of lymphokines on restimulation. See also **CD4, CD8 cell, human immunodeficiency virus, T cell.**

CD4/CD8 ratio, the ratio of the number of CD4 T cells to the number of CD8 T cells. In healthy individuals the ratio must be greater than 1. The ratio is important in monitoring the function of the immune system in patients who have viral infections or who have undergone tissue transplantation, either of which may cause an increase in the number of CD8 T cells.

CD8 cell, a T lymphocyte that recognizes antigens presented by major histocompatibility complex (MHC) class I molecules present on infected or cancer cells. Binding of the T cell receptor with the MHC-I/antigen complex induces killing of the infected or cancer cell by the CD8 T cell. Antigen-presenting cells and CD4 T cells are essential for initial CD8 T cell activation. Activated CD8 T cells can secrete large amounts of gamma-interferon, a cytokine involved in the body's defense against viruses. Also called **cytotoxic T cell.** See also **cell-mediated cytotoxicity.**

CD8 cell, CD8+ cell, a major classification of T lymphocytes, referring to those that carry the CD8 antigen; the major subtypes are the cytotoxic T lymphocytes and the suppressor cells. See also **T lymphocyte, cytotoxic T lymphocytes.**

CD8 T lymphocytes, CD8+ T lymphocytes. See **CD8 cell, CD8+ cell.**

CDA, **1.** abbreviation for **certified dental assistant. 2.** abbreviation for **Canadian Dental Association.**

CD antigen, any of a number of cell-surface markers expressed by leukocytes and used to distinguish cell lineages, developmental stages, and functional subsets. Such markers can be identified by specific monoclonal antibodies and are numbered by their cluster of differentiation, as in CD1, CD2, etc.

cdc, abbreviation for **cell division cycle.**

CDC, abbreviation for **Centers for Disease Control and Prevention.**

CDE, **1.** the major symbols used in one system for the nomenclature of the Rh system in which D is the same as

Rh0, the major determining factor of Rh positivity. **2.** abbreviation for **certified diabetes educator.**

CDH, abbreviation for **congenital dislocation of the hip.**

C. difficile. Also called *C. diff.* See *Clostridium difficile.*

CDK, abbreviation for **cyclin-dependent kinase.**

CDR, abbreviation for **computed dental radiography.**

Ce, symbol for the element **cerium.**

CEA, **1.** abbreviation for **carcinoembryonic antigen. 2.** abbreviation for **carotid endarterectomy.**

ceasmic /sē·az″mik/ [Gk, *keazein,* to split], pertaining to or characterized by a persistent embryonic fissure or abnormal cleavage of parts.

ceasmic teratism [Gk, *keazein + teras,* monster], a congenital anomaly caused by developmental arrest, in which body parts that should be fused remain in their fissured embryonic state, such as in cleft palate.

cec-, ceco-, prefix meaning "cecum": *cecopexy.*

cecal /sē″kəl/ [L, *caecus,* blind, blind gut], **1.** pertaining to the cecum. **2.** pertaining to the optic disc or the blind spot in the retina. Also spelled **caecal.**

cecal appendix. See **vermiform appendix.**

cecal artery, one of the branches of the ileocolic artery that supply the cecum.

cecal volvulus, a type of colonic volvulus consisting of twisting or displacement and anomalous rotation of the cecum, such as in volvulus neonatorum or Ladd's syndrome. It can cause obstruction.

Ceclor, a cephalosporin antibiotic. Brand name for **cefaclor.**

cecocolostomy /sē″kōkəlos″təmē/ [L, *caecus,* blind, blind gut; Gk, *kolon,* colon, *stoma,* mouth], **1.** a surgical operation that creates an anastomosis between the cecum and the colon. **2.** the anastomosis produced by this operation.

cecofixation. See **cecopexy.**

cecoileostomy /-il′ē·os″təmē/ [L, *caecus + ilia,* intestine, *stoma,* mouth], a surgical operation that connects the ileum with the cecum. Also called **ileocecostomy.**

cecopexy /sē″kōpek′sē/ [L, *caecus + Gk, pexis,* fix], a surgical operation that fixes or suspends the cecum to stabilize its excessive mobility. Also called **cecofixation.**

cecostomy /sēkos″təmē/ [L, *caecus + Gk, stoma,* mouth], the surgical construction of an opening into the cecum, performed as a temporary measure to relieve intestinal obstruction in a patient who cannot tolerate major surgery. With the patient under local anesthesia, a tube is inserted into the cecum to allow drainage of feces. The procedure may also be done to decompress the large bowel and prevent distension until peristalsis is restored after intestinal surgery. Also spelled **caecostomy.** See also **abdominal surgery, intestinal obstruction.**

cecum /sē″kəm/ [L, *caecus,* blind, blind gut], a pouchlike structure or cul-de-sac constituting the first part of the large intestine. It is inferior to the junction of the ascending colon and joins the ileum, the last segment of the small intestine, at the ileocecal valve.

Cedax, an oral cephalosporin. Brand name for **ceftibuten.**

CeeNU, an antineoplastic. Brand name for **lomustine.**

cef-, prefix designating a cephalosporin.

cefaclor /sē″fəklôr/, a cephalosporin antibiotic.

■ INDICATIONS: It is prescribed in the treatment of selected infections caused by susceptible strains of bacteria.

■ CONTRAINDICATIONS: Known hypersensitivity to cephalosporins prohibits its use. It is used with caution in patients who are allergic to penicillin.

■ ADVERSE EFFECTS: Among the most serious adverse reactions are hypersensitivity reactions and diarrhea, nausea, and vomiting.

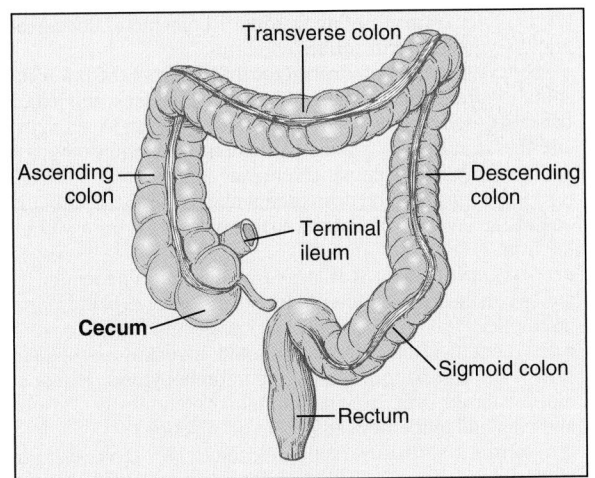

Cecum *(Levy et al, 2006)*

cefadroxil monohydrate /sē′fədrok″sil/, a cephalosporin antibiotic.
■ INDICATIONS: It is prescribed in the treatment of selected bacterial infections.
■ CONTRAINDICATIONS: Known hypersensitivity to cephalosporins prohibits its use. It is administered with caution to patients with a history of allergy to penicillins.
■ ADVERSE EFFECTS: Among the most serious adverse reactions are hypersensitivity reactions and severe diarrhea, nausea, and vomiting.

Cefadyl, an antibiotic. Brand name for **cephapirin.**

cefamandole nafate /sēfəman″dōl naf″āt/, a cephalosporin antibiotic.
■ INDICATIONS: It is prescribed in the treatment of infections caused by susceptible bacterial strains.
■ CONTRAINDICATIONS: Known hypersensitivity to cephalosporins prohibits its use. It is used with caution in patients who are allergic to penicillin.
■ ADVERSE EFFECTS: Among the most serious adverse reactions are hypersensitivity reactions, phlebitis, superinfection, and pain on intramuscular injection.

cefazolin sodium /sēfaz″ōlin/, a cephalosporin antibiotic.
■ INDICATIONS: It is prescribed in the treatment of infections caused by susceptible bacterial strains.
■ CONTRAINDICATIONS: Known hypersensitivity to this drug or to any cephalosporin medication prohibits its use, as does severely impaired renal function. It is used with caution in patients who are allergic to penicillin or other drugs.
■ ADVERSE EFFECTS: Among the more serious adverse reactions are pain at the site of injection and hypersensitivity reactions.

cefdinir, a broad-spectrum, third-generation cephalosporin antibiotic.
■ INDICATIONS: This drug is used to treat *Haemophilus influenzae, H. parainfluenzae, Morganella catarrhalis, Streptococcus pneumoniae, Staphylococcus pyogenes,* and S. *aureus.*
■ CONTRAINDICATIONS: Known hypersensitivity to cephalosporins prohibits its use. It also should not be used in infants less than 1 month old.
■ ADVERSE EFFECTS: Life-threatening effects include proteinuria, nephrotoxicity, renal failure, leukopenia, thrombocytopenia, agranulocytosis, neutropenia, lymphocytosis, eosinophilia, pancytopenia, hemolytic anemia (rare), and anaphylaxis. Other serious adverse effects include bleeding, anemia, thrombophlebitis; and increased aspartate aminotransferase (AST), alanine aminotransferase (ALT),

bilirubin, lactic dehydrogenase, alkaline phosphatase, and blood urea nitrogen. Common side effects include nausea, vomiting, diarrhea, and anorexia.

cefditoren pivoxil, an antiinfective agent used to treat acute bacterial exacerbation of chronic bronchitis, pharyngitis/tonsillitis, and uncomplicated skin and skin structure infections.

cefepime, a fourth-generation cephalosporin.
■ INDICATIONS: It is used to treat infections caused by gram-negative bacilli, including *Escherichiacoli, Proteus,* and *Klebsiella;* gram-positive organisms, including *Streptococcus pneumoniae, S. pyogenes,* and *Staphylococcus aureus;* and infections of the lower respiratory tract, urinary tract, skin, and bone.
■ CONTRAINDICATIONS: Known hypersensitivity to cephalosporins prohibits its use. It also should not be used in infants less than 1 month old.
■ ADVERSE EFFECTS: Life-threatening effects include nephrotoxicity, renal failure, leukopenia, thrombocytopenia, agranulocytosis, neutropenia, lymphocytosis, eosinophilia, pancytopenia, hemolytic anemia (rare), and anaphylaxis. Other serious effects include GI bleeding; increased aspartate aminotransferase (AST), alanine aminotransferase (ALT), bilirubin, lactic dehydrogenase, and alkaline phosphatase; proteinuria, candidiasis, increased blood urea nitrogen, and thrombophlebitis. Common side effects include nausea, vomiting, diarrhea, and anorexia.

cefepime hydrochloride, the hydrochloride salt of cefepime, used in treatment of infections of the skin and soft tissue and of the respiratory and urinary tracts, administered intramuscularly or intravenously.

Cefizox, a cephalosporin antibiotic. Brand name for **ceftizoxime sodium.**

Cefobid, a cephalosporin antibiotic. Brand name for **cefoperazone sodium.**

cefonicid sodium /sēfon″isid/, a parenteral cephalosporin-type antibiotic.
■ INDICATIONS: It is prescribed for bacterial infections of the lower respiratory or urinary tract, skin, bones, and joints; septicemia; and surgical prophylaxis.
■ CONTRAINDICATIONS: A history of allergy to cephalosporins or acute anaphylactic or urticarial reactions to penicillin prohibit its use.
■ ADVERSE EFFECTS: Among the more serious adverse reactions are pain and phlebitis at the injection site and occasionally allergic reactions and GI effects.

cefoperazone sodium /sē′fōper″əzōn/, a third-generation cephalosporin antibiotic.
■ INDICATIONS: It is prescribed in the treatment of respiratory tract, bone, joint, skin, and female genital tract infections and of bacterial septicemia.
■ CONTRAINDICATIONS: Hypersensitivity to the cephalosporins or known sensitivity to this drug prohibits its use.
■ ADVERSE EFFECTS: Among the most serious adverse reactions are pruritus, urticaria, transient eosinophilia, neutropenia, and injection site reactions.

Cefotan, a cephalosporin antibiotic. Brand name for **cefotetan disodium.**

cefotaxime sodium /sēfōtak″zēm/, a third-generation cephalosporin antibiotic.
■ INDICATIONS: It is prescribed for lower respiratory tract, genitourinary, gynecological, skin, bone and joint, and central nervous system infections and for bacterial septicemia caused by strains of susceptible microorganisms.
■ CONTRAINDICATIONS: Hypersensitivity to the cephalosporins or known hypersensitivity to this drug prohibits its use.

C

■ ADVERSE EFFECTS: The most serious adverse reactions are pruritus, colitis, fungal infections, and injection site reactions.

cefotetan disodium /sē′fōtet″ən/, a parenteral second-generation cephalosporin antibiotic with greater activity against anaerobes and gram-negative bacilli than first-generation cephalosporins.

■ INDICATIONS: It is prescribed for bacterial infections of the lower respiratory tract, urinary tract, skin, abdomen, bones or joints, or reproductive organs and for surgical prophylaxis.

■ CONTRAINDICATIONS: It is contraindicated for patients who are hypersensitive to cefotetan or to other cephalosporin antibiotics.

■ ADVERSE EFFECTS: Among adverse reactions reported are skin rash, diarrhea, eosinophilia, positive Coombs' test results, and elevated liver enzyme levels.

cefoxitin sodium /sēfok″sitin/, a parenteral second-generation cephalosporin antibiotic with greater activity against anaerobes and gram-negative bacilli than first-generation cephalosporins.

■ INDICATIONS: It is prescribed for bacterial infections of the lower respiratory tract, urinary tract, skin, abdomen, bones or joints, or reproductive organs and for surgical prophylaxis.

■ CONTRAINDICATIONS: Known hypersensitivity to cephalosporins prohibits its use. It is administered with caution to patients who are allergic to penicillin and related antibiotics or who have impaired renal function.

■ ADVERSE EFFECTS: Among the most serious adverse reactions are hypersensitivity reactions, phlebitis, superinfection, and pain on intramuscular injection.

ceftazidime /seftaz″idēm/, a parenteral third-generation cephalosporin-type antibiotic.

■ INDICATIONS: It is prescribed for treatment of documented *Pseudomonas aeruginosa* infection and other bacterial infections of the lower respiratory tract, urinary tract, skin, abdomen, blood, bones and joints, and central nervous system.

■ CONTRAINDICATIONS: It is contraindicated in patients who are hypersensitive to this product or to other cephalosporin antibiotics.

■ ADVERSE EFFECTS: Among adverse reactions reported are pruritus, fever, skin rash, diarrhea, eosinophilia, thrombocytosis, phlebitis, discomfort at the site of injection, and positive Coombs' test result.

ceftibuten, an oral third-generation cephalosporin.

■ INDICATIONS: It is prescribed in the treatment of chronic bronchitis, acute bacterial otitis media, pharyngitis, and tonsillitis.

■ CONTRAINDICATIONS: It should not be given to children with abdominal pain, vomiting, and diarrhea.

■ ADVERSE EFFECTS: The side effects most often reported include nausea, headache, diarrhea, dyspepsia, dizziness, and abdominal pain.

ceftizoxime sodium /sef′tizok″zēm/, a third-generation cephalosporin antibiotic.

■ INDICATIONS: It is prescribed in the treatment of infections caused by susceptible bacterial strains (does not include *Pseudomonas aeruginosa*), primarily in the respiratory system, genitourinary system, bone, joints, and skin.

■ CONTRAINDICATIONS: Known sensitivity to this drug prohibits its use. It is used with caution in patients who are allergic to penicillin.

■ ADVERSE EFFECTS: Among the most serious adverse reactions are hypersensitivity reactions, neutropenia, leukopenia, thrombocytopenia, and pain at the injection site.

ceftriaxone sodium /sef′trī-ak″sōn/, a parenteral third-generation cephalosporin antibiotic.

■ INDICATIONS: It is prescribed for infections of the lower respiratory tract, urinary tract, skin, abdomen, bones, and joints. It is also used to treat gonorrhea, septicemia, and meningitis and in surgical prophylaxis, particularly in coronary bypass operations. It has a comparatively long half-life and, although its dosage must still be decreased with renal impairment, it is one of the few cephalosporins that is eliminated primarily by the liver.

■ CONTRAINDICATIONS: It is contraindicated in patients who are hypersensitive to this product or to other cephalosporin antibiotics.

■ ADVERSE EFFECTS: Among reported adverse reactions are skin rash, diarrhea, eosinophilia, thrombocytosis, leukopenia, increased liver enzyme and blood urea nitrogen levels, and pain and tenderness at the site of injection.

cefuroxime sodium /sef′ōorok′zēm/, a cephalosporin antibiotic.

■ INDICATIONS: It is prescribed in the treatment of lower respiratory tract, urinary tract, skin, and gonococcal infections; bacterial septicemia; and meningitis and for the prevention of postoperative infections.

■ CONTRAINDICATIONS: Hypersensitivity to the cephalosporins or known sensitivity to this drug prohibits its use.

■ ADVERSE EFFECTS: Among the most serious adverse reactions are pruritus, urticaria, transient eosinophilia, neutropenia, leukopenia, and injection site reactions.

CEJ, abbreviation for **cementoenamel junction.**

cel-, coel-, 1. prefix meaning "a cavity of the body": *coelenteron.* 2. prefix meaning "a swelling or tumor, hernia": *celosomia.* 3. prefix meaning "belly" or "abdomen": *coelom.*

-cele, suffix meaning "relating to a hernia or swelling": *rectocele, cystocele.*

celecoxib /sel″ekok′sib/, a nonsteroidal antiinflammatory drug of the COX-2 inhibitors group, administered orally for symptomatic treatment of arthritis.

Celestone, a glucocorticoid. Brand name for **betamethasone.**

Celexa /sĕ-lek′sə/, an antidepressant. Brand name for **citalopram.**

celiac /sē′lē-ak/ [Gk, *koilia,* belly], pertaining to the abdominal cavity.

celiac artery [Gk, *koilia,* belly, *arteria,* airpipe], a thick visceral branch of the abdominal aorta, arising caudal to the diaphragm, usually dividing into the left gastric, common hepatic, and splenic arteries.

celiac disease [Gk, *koilia* + L, *dis,* opposite of; Fr, *aise,* ease], an inborn error of metabolism characterized by the inability to hydrolyze peptides contained in gluten. Gluten is found in wheat, oats, and barley. Also called **celiac sprue, gluten-induced enteropathy, nontropical sprue.** Compare **malabsorption syndrome.**

■ OBSERVATIONS: The disease affects adults and young children, who suffer from abdominal distension, vomiting, diarrhea, muscle wasting, and extreme lethargy. A characteristic sign is a pale, foul-smelling stool that floats on water because of its high fat content.

■ INTERVENTIONS: Most patients respond well to a high-protein, high-calorie, gluten-free diet. Rice and corn are good substitutes for wheat, and any vitamin or mineral deficiencies can be corrected with oral preparations.

■ PATIENT CARE CONSIDERATIONS: There may be a secondary lactose intolerance, and it may become necessary to eliminate all milk products from the diet. Prognosis for full recovery is excellent. Failure to respond generally indicates misdiagnosis.

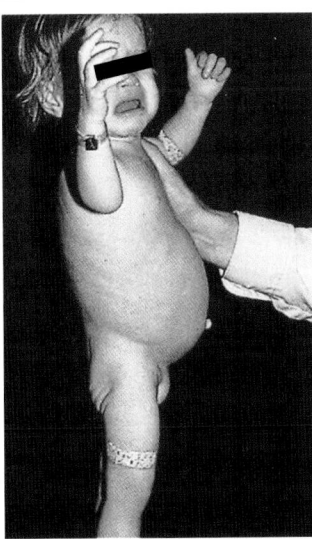

Child with celiac disease: abdominal distension *(Zitelli and Davis, 2012)*

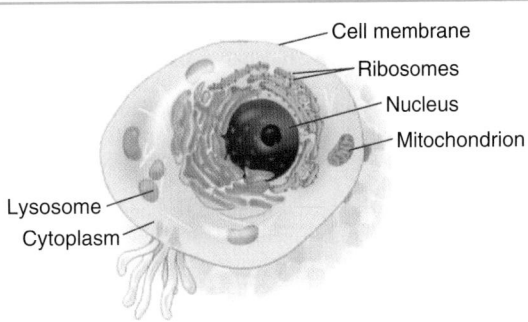

Cell *(Shiland, 2016)*

celiac ganglion, a group of nerve cells located on each side of the crura of the diaphragm. The cells are connected to the celiac plexus.

celiacoduodenal part of suspensory muscle of duodenum, a band of smooth muscle that passes from the terminal duodenum to join the phrenicoceliac part (pars phrenicocoeliaca) and end in connective tissue that attaches to the celiac trunk.

celiac plexus. See **solar plexus.**

celiac rickets [Gk, *koilia* + *rhachis,* spine, *itis,* inflammation], arrested growth and osseous deformities resulting from malabsorption of fat and calcium. See also **celiac disease, rickets.**

celiac sprue. See **celiac disease.**

celio-, prefix meaning "belly or abdomen": *celiocolpotomy*

celiocolpotomy /sē′lē·ōkəlpot″əmē/ [Gk, *koilia* + *kolpos,* vagina, *temnein,* to cut], an incision into the abdomen with a surgical approach through the vagina for oviduct sterilization or diagnostic inspection.

celioscope, *(Obsolete)* now called **laparoscope.**

cell [L, *cella,* storeroom], the fundamental unit of all living tissue. Eukaryotic cells consist of a nucleus, cytoplasm, and organelles surrounded by a plasma membrane. Within the nucleus are the nucleolus (containing ribonucleic acid) and the chromatin (containing protein and deoxyribonucleic acid), which form chromosomes, wherein are located the determinants of inherited characteristics. Organelles within the cytoplasm include the endoplasmic reticulum, ribosomes, Golgi apparatus, mitochondria, lysosomes, and centrosome. Prokaryotic cells are much smaller and simpler than eukaryotic cells, even lacking a nucleus. The specialized nature of body tissue reflects the specialized structure and function of its constituent cells. See also **cell theory. –cellular,** *adj.*

cella /sel″ə/ [L, storeroom], an enclosed space.

cell bank, a storage facility for frozen tissue samples held for research purposes and for surgical reconstruction of damaged body structures.

cell biology. See **cytology.**

cell body [L, *cella* + AS, *bodig*], the part of a cell that contains the nucleus and surrounding cytoplasm exclusive of any projections or processes, such as the axon and dendrites of a neuron or the tail of a spermatozoon.

cell culture [L, *cella,* storeroom, *colere,* to cultivate], living cells that are maintained in vitro in artificial media of serum and nutrients for the study and growth of certain strains of microorganisms or for experiments in controlling diseases, such as cancer. They are routinely used to culture viruses that cause infections.

cell death, 1. terminal failure of a cell to maintain essential life functions. See also **necrosis, apoptosis. 2.** the point in the process of dying at which vital functions have ceased at the cellular level. **3.** programmed cell death.

cell determination, the process by which an undifferentiated embryonic cell becomes committed to develop into a specific type of cell. Cell determination appears to involve the selective activation of certain sets of genes and the inactivation of others.

cell division, the continuous process by which a cell alternates between a long interphase period and mitosis. Mitosis involves four stages: prophase, metaphase, anaphase, and telophase. Cell division does not occur in discrete steps: each phase is part of a continuous process that may require hours for its completion. During the interphase period new deoxyribonucleic acid, ribonucleic acid, and protein molecules are synthesized before the start of the next prophase. Compare **meiosis.** See also **mitosis.**

cell division cycle (cdc), the sequence of events that occur during the growth and division of cells.

CELLector, a brand name for a device that modifies human blood cells by circulating them through a box containing a number of polystyrene plates. Genetically engineered monoclonal antibodies are permanently attached to the polystyrene plates, which capture specifically targeted cells while the rest of the cells are transfused back into the patient's body. The device is used in bone marrow transplantation.

cell inclusion [L, *cella,* storeroom, *in* + *claudere,* to shut], any foreign matter or residual elements of the cytoplasm that are enclosed within a cell. They are metabolic products of the cell (for example, granules or crystals). Also called **metaplasm.**

cell line [L, *cella* + *linea*], a colony of animal cells derived and developed as a subculture from a primary cell culture.

cell mass [L, *cella,* storeroom, *massa*]. See **inner cell mass.**

cell-mediated cytotoxicity, cytolysis of a target cell by effector lymphocytes, such as cytotoxic T lymphocytes or natural killer cells. It can also be antibody-dependent (antibody-dependent cell-mediated cytotoxicity) when antibodies coat target cells and are consequently recognized and killed by killer cells.

cell-mediated hypersensitivity, hypersensitivity initiated by antigen-specific T lymphocytes. Unlike forms of hypersensitivity mediated by antibodies, it takes one or more days to develop and can be transferred by lymphocytes but not by serum. The term is often equated with delayed hypersensitivity, or type IV hypersensitivity. Kinds include **rheumatoid arthritis, type 1 diabetes mellitus, multiple sclerosis.**

cell-mediated hypersensitivity reaction.   See **hypersensitivity reaction.**

cell-mediated immunity,   immune response that does not involve antibodies. Cell-mediated immune responses can involve the destruction of infected cells or cancer cells by CD8 T cells or natural killer cells. CD4 T cells also provide protection against different pathogens via activation of CD8 T cells and secretion of cytokines. Primarily directed at microorganisms that survive in phagocytes and microorganisms (viruses and bacteria) that infect nonphagocytic cells. Also called **cellular immunity.**

cell membrane.   See **plasma membrane.**

cell of Corti.   See **auditory hair.**

cell organelle [L, *cella,* storeroom; Gk, *organon,* instrument],   any of a number of membrane-bound structures within a cell that have specific functions, such as reproduction or metabolism. Kinds include **mitochondrion, Golgi apparatus.**

cell receptor,   a protein located either on a cell's surface, in its cytoplasm, or in its nucleus that binds to a specific ligand (typically an ion or a molecule), initiating signal transduction and a change in cellular activity.

cells of Paneth /pä″nət, pan″əth/   [Josef Paneth, Austrian physiologist, 1857–1890],   large granular epithelial cells found in intestinal glands. They secrete digestive enzymes and bactericidal lysozyme. Also called **Davidoff's cells.**

cell-surface marker,   an antigenic determinant found on the surface of a specific type of cell.

cell theory,   the proposition that cells are the basic units of all living tissues or organisms and that cellular function is the essential process of living things.

cellular /sel″yələr/   [L, *cella,* storeroom],   pertaining to or consisting of the smallest units of life (cells).

cellular hypersensitivity reaction.   See **cell-mediated hypersensitivity.**

cellular immunity [L, *cellula,* little cell, *immunis,* exempt],   the mechanism of acquired immunity characterized by the dominant role of T cell lymphocytes. Cellular immunity is involved in resistance to infectious diseases caused by viruses and some bacteria and in delayed hypersensitivity reactions, some aspects of resistance to cancer, certain autoimmune diseases, graft rejection, and certain allergies. It does not involve the production of humoral antibody but instead involves the activation of leukocytes and natural killer cells. Also called **cell-mediated immunity.** Compare **humoral immunity.**

cellular infiltration,   the migration and grouping of cells, especially blood cells, within tissues throughout the body.

cellular pathology.   See **pathology.**

cellulite /sel″yəlīt/,   *(Nontechnical)* fat and fibrous tissue deposits that result in dimpling of the skin. Also called **adiposis edematosa.**

cellulitis /sel′yəli″tis/   [L, *cellula,* little cell; Gk, *itis,* inflammation],   a diffuse acute bacterial infection of the skin and subcutaneous tissue characterized most commonly by local heat, redness, pain, and swelling and occasionally by fever, malaise, chills, and headache. Abscess and tissue destruction usually follow if antibiotics are not taken. The infection is more likely to develop in the presence of damaged skin, poor circulation, or diabetes mellitus. In addition to appropriate antibiotics, treatment includes warm soaks, elevation, and prevention of pressure to the affected areas.

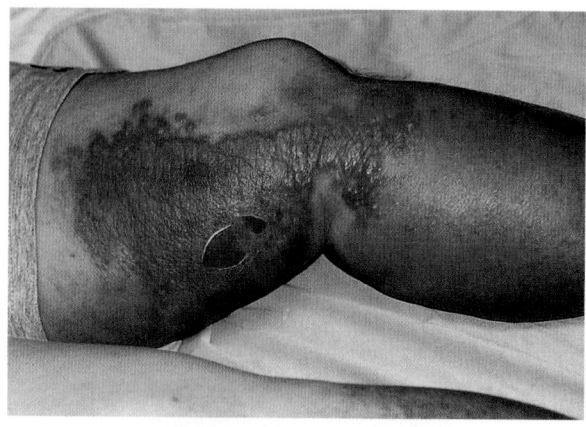

Cellulitis *(Black and Hawks, 2009)*

cellulose /sel″yo͞olōs/   [L, *cellula,* little cell],   a colorless, insoluble, indigestible, transparent, solid polysaccharide that is the primary constituent of the cell walls of plants. In the diet it provides the bulk necessary for proper digestive tract functioning. Rich sources are fruits, such as apples and bananas, and legumes, bran, and green vegetables, especially celery. See also **dietary fiber.**

cellulose sodium phosphate,   an insoluble, nonabsorbable cation-exchange resin prepared from cellulose. It binds calcium and is used to prevent formation of calcium-containing kidney stones.

cell wall,   the structure that covers and protects the plasma membrane in some kinds of cells, such as certain bacteria and all fungi and plant cells. The cell walls of plant cells are composed of cellulose.

celom, celomic.   See **coelom.**

Celontin,   an anticonvulsant. Brand name for **methsuximide.**

celosomia /sē′ləsō″mē·ə/   [Gk, *kele,* hernia, *soma,* body],   a congenital malformation characterized by a fissure or absence of the sternum and ribs and protrusion of the viscera.

celothelioma,   *(Obsolete)* now called **mesothelioma.**

Celsius (° C) /sel″sē·əs/   [Anders Celsius, Swedish scientist, 1701–1744],   a widely used international temperature scale in which 0° is the freezing point of water and 100° is the boiling point of water at sea level. To convert to Fahrenheit, multiply the Celsius temperature by 1.8, then add 32. Also called **centigrade.** Compare **Fahrenheit.**

Celsius thermometer,   a device for measuring temperature in Celsius degrees. See **Celsius.**

cement /siment″/   [L, *caementum,* rough stone],   **1.** a sticky or mucilaginous substance that hardens into a firm mass and helps neighboring tissue cells stick together. **2.** any of a variety of dental materials used to fill cavities or to hold bridgework or other dental prostheses in place. **3.** a material, such as methyl methacrylate, used in the fixation of a prosthetic joint in adjacent bone.

cemental fiber /simen″təl/   [L, *caementum,* rough stone, *fibra*],   any one of the many fibers of the periodontal membrane that extend from the cementum to the intermediate plexus, where their terminations are mixed with those of the alveolar fibers.

cementation /sē′məntā′shən/   [L, *caementum,* rough stone],   (in dentistry) the attachment of a restoration or bracket with an adhesive. For example, cementation may be used to attach an inlay, onlay, or crown to a natural tooth, or an orthodontic band or bracket.

cement base, (in dentistry) a layer of a stable dental restorative material, sometimes containing medication, that is applied to the bottom of a prepared tooth cavity to protect the pulp, reduce the bulk of metallic restoration, or eliminate undercuts in a tapered preparation.

cementifying fibroma /-ifī″ing/ [L, *caementum* + *facere,* to make, *fibra,* fiber; Gk, *oma,* tumor], **1.** an intraosseous lesion composed of fibrous connective tissue enclosing foci of calcified material resembling cancellous bone or cementum, which is thought to arise from the periodontal ligament. **2.** a rare odontogenic tumor composed of varying amounts of fibrous connective tissue resembling cementum.

cementoblast /simen′təblast/, one of the large cuboidal cells that is responsible for the formation of cementum, the outer covering of the root of the tooth. See also **cementum.**

cementoblastoma /simen′tōblastō″mə/ *pl.* cementoblastomas, cementoblastomata [L, *caementum* + Gk, *blastos,* germ, *oma,* tumor], a rare, benign odontogenic tumor representing a true neoplasm of cementum that primarily affects mandibular permanent first molars in children and young adults under the age of 30 years. Radiographically, it appears as a well-defined radiopaque mass surrounded by a thin radiolucent halo. Treatment consists of enucleation of the tumor and removal of the involved tooth or teeth. Should not be confused with **cementoma.**

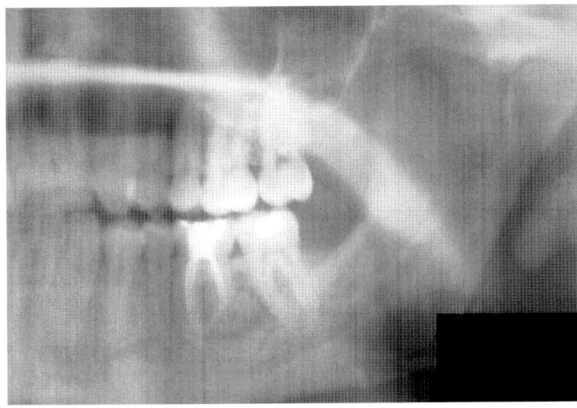

Cementoblastoma *(Regezi, Sciubba, and Jordan, 2008)*

cementocyte /simen″təsīt/, a cell found in the cementum of teeth. Its function is unknown, but it may respond to changes in normal and traumatic occlusal forces as well as endocrine signals actively directing local cementum metabolism.

cementoenamel junction (CEJ), the junction of the coronal border of the cementum and the apical border of the enamel.

cementoma /sē′mentō″mə/ *pl.* cementomas, cementomata [L, *caementum* + Gk, *oma,* tumor], a rare benign neoplasm of cementoblasts, microscopically resembling an osteoblastoma, that is fused to the root of a tooth. It occurs predominantly in the mandible and is typically seen within the second and third decades of life, with no gender predilection. It may be present as a mass of fibrous connective tissue, as fibrous connective tissue with spicules of cementum, or as a calcified mass resembling cementum. Radiographically, early cementomas appear as well-defined radiolucencies at the apex of mandibular anterior teeth that are often mistaken for periapical lesions. Older lesions may appear to calcify with time. An important diagnostic indication is that these teeth test vital to vitality testing. Kinds include **cementoblastoma, cementifying fibroma.**

cementum /simen″təm/, the bonelike calcified connective tissue that covers the roots of the teeth and helps to support them by providing a place of attachment for the periodontal ligament fibers and underlying dentin.

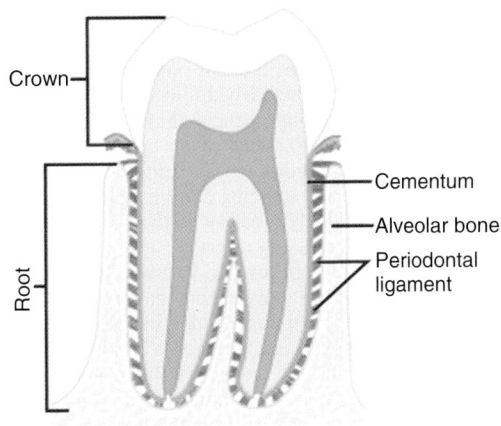

Cementum *(Bath-Balogh and Fehrenbach, 2011)*

cen, abbreviation for **centromere.**

CEN, abbreviation for **certified emergency nurse.**

cen-, prefix meaning "common": *cenesthesia.*

cenesthesia /sē′nesthē″zhə/ [Gk, *koinos,* shared in common, *aisthesis,* feeling], the general sense of existing, derived as the aggregate of all the various stimuli and reactions throughout the body at any specific moment to produce a feeling of health or of illness. Also called **coenesthesia, coenesthesis,** *cenesthesis.*

ceno-, prefix meaning "new, empty, or having a common feature": *cenogenesis.*

cenogenesis /sē′nōjen″əsis/ [Gk, *kenos,* empty, *genein,* to produce], the development of structural characteristics that are absent in earlier forms of a species, as an adaptive response to environmental conditions. Also spelled **caenogenesis, coenogenesis, kenogenesis.** Compare **palingenesis.** *−coenogenetic, caenogenetic, cenogenetic, adj.*

cenophobia, a morbid fear of open spaces. See **kenophobia.**

censor [L, *censere,* to assess], **1.** a person who monitors or evaluates books, newspapers, plays, works of art, speech, or other means of expression in order to suppress certain kinds of information. **2.** (in psychoanalysis) a psychic suppression that allows unconscious thoughts to rise to consciousness only if they are heavily disguised.

census [L, *censere,* to assess], **1.** an enumeration of the population, usually conducted periodically as a function of an official agency. In addition to counting heads, the census often collects information about members of a household, sources of income, types of dwellings, and matters relating to the health of the community. **2.** in the hospital setting, the number of patients in the hospital.

cente-, prefix meaning "puncture": *centesis.*

center [Gk, *kentron*], **1.** the middle point of the body or geometric entity, equidistant from points on the periphery. **2.** a group of neurons with a common function, such as the accelerating center in the brain that controls the heartbeat. **3.** a facility or concentration of researchers and/or clinicians where specialized activities are concentrated.

center-edge angle of Wiberg [G. Wilberg, Swedish orthopedic surgeon, 1902–1988], the angle formed by a line drawn perpendicular to a baseline that passes through the center of the femoral heads and a line connecting the center of the femoral head and the superior border of the acetabulum, used in radiographic evaluation of the hip joint. It is less than 20 degrees in developmental dysplasia of the hip.

center of excellence (COE), a tertiary or quaternary health care provider that is identified as the most expert and cost efficient and produces the best outcomes. There are no strict universal criteria established to be designated a COE; however, some accrediting agencies have established standards for specialties. Also called *center of quality.*

center of gravity, the midpoint or center of the weight of a body or object. In the standing adult human the center of gravity is in the midpelvic cavity, between the symphysis pubis and the umbilicus.

Centers for Disease Control and Prevention (CDC), a federal agency of the U.S. government that provides facilities and services for the investigation, identification, prevention, and control of disease. It is concerned with all of the epidemiological aspects and the laboratory diagnosis of disease. Immunization programs, quarantine regulations and programs, laboratory standards, and community surveillance for disease are among the activities of the CDC, which is located in Atlanta. Many state and local health workers and scientists receive training in specific techniques there. Originally the Communicable Disease Center, it was concerned only with communicable diseases; today its interests include environmental health, smoking, malnutrition, poisoning, and issues in occupational health. The name was changed again in 1992 to include its prevention function.

Centers for Medicare and Medicaid Services, an agency of the U.S. Department of Health and Human Services. It is responsible for oversight of the rules, regulations, and directives related to insurance benefits, coverage, payments to doctors, and standards for health care. Formerly called **Health Care Financing Administration.**

centesis /sentē″sis/ [Gk, *kentesis,* pricking], a perforation or a puncture of a cavity, such as paracentesis or thoracocentesis.

centi- (c), prefix meaning "a hundred or a hundredth": *centiliter, centipoise.*

centigrade, a scale. See **Celsius.**

centigram (cg), a mass equal to one hundredth of a gram, or 10 milligrams.

centigray (cGy) /sen′tigra/, a unit of absorbed radiation dose equal to one hundredth (10^{-2}) of a gray, or 1 rad.

centiliter (cL), a volume equal to one hundredth of a liter, or 10 milliliters.

centimeter (cm) /sen″timē′tər/ [L, *centum,* hundred; Gk, *metron,* measure], the metric unit of measurement equal to one hundredth of a meter, or 0.3937 inch.

centimeter-gram-second system (cgs, CGS), the internationally accepted scientific system of expressing length, mass, and time in basic units of centimeters, grams, and seconds. The CGS system is almost universally being replaced by the Système International d'Unités (SI, or the International System of Units), based on the meter, kilogram, and second.

centipede bite /sen″təpēd/ [L, *centum,* hundred, *pes,* foot], a wound produced by the poison claws and the first body segment of a centipede, an elongate arthropod with many pairs of legs. The bite of a few species, including *Scolopendra morsitans* in the southern United States, may cause painful local inflammation, fever, headache, vomiting, and dizziness.

centipoise /sen″təpois/ [Jean L.M. Poiseuille, French physiologist, 1797–1869], a measure of the viscosity of a liquid, equal to one hundredth of a poise. The viscosity of glycerin is 1490 centipoise, compared with 1.005 centipoise for water.

centrad [L, *centum,* hundred], **1.** pertaining to a central direction, toward the center. **2.** a unit of measure equal to one hundredth part of a radian. **3.** a measure of the refractive strength of a prism.

central [Gk, *kentron,* center], pertaining to or situated at a center or middle.

central amaurosis [Gk, *kentron + amauroein,* to darken], blindness caused by a disease of the central nervous system.

central anesthesia, a loss of feeling or sensation as a result of a lesion in the central nervous system.

central auditory processing disorder (CAPD), difficulty in processing and interpreting auditory stimuli in the absence of a peripheral hearing loss, usually resulting from a problem in the brainstem or cerebral cortex. Children with CAPD often have difficulty with written language tasks and may exhibit other learning disabilities as well.

central biasing /bī″əsing/, a theory of pain modulation in which higher centers such as the cerebral cortex influence the perception of and response to pain.

central canal of spinal cord [Gk, *kentron + L, canalis,* channel], the conduit that runs the entire length of the spinal cord and contains some of the 140 mL of cerebrospinal fluid (CSF) in the body of the average individual. The central canal of the spinal cord lies in the center of the cord between the ventral and the dorsal gray commissures and extends toward the cranium into the medulla oblongata, where it opens into the fourth ventricle of the brain. Lumbar puncture, often performed to obtain samples of CSF for diagnostic purposes, draws fluid from the subarachnoid space around the spinal cord and not from the central canal. See also **lumbar puncture.**

central catheter [Gk, *kentron,* central, *katheter,* a thing lowered into], a catheter inserted into either a central artery or a central vein for diagnostic or therapeutic procedures.

central chemoreceptor, any of the sensory nerve cells or chemical receptors that are located in the medulla of the brain. Also called **medullary chemoreceptor.**

central chondrosarcoma [Gk, *kentron + chondros,* cartilage, *sarx,* flesh, *oma,* tumor], a malignant cartilaginous tumor that forms inside a bone. Also called **enchondrosarcoma.**

central core disease, an autosomal-dominant muscle disorder characterized by dense, amorphous, hyaline changes in the central portion of the myofibrils, which lack organelles. Onset is in infancy and causes delayed motor development, especially in the lower limbs. Also called **Shy-Magee syndrome.**

central deafness. See **central auditory processing disorder.**

central electrode, a key part of a radiation detection instrument, consisting of a positively charged rigid wire in the center of a gas-filled cylinder. The electrode attracts electrons liberated by the ionization effects of radiation and converts them into an electric current.

central facilitation, (in chiropractic) a model based on neurophysiological findings that explains the symptoms of subluxogenic pain and discomfort that arise from nonspinal sites.

central fissure. See **central sulcus.**

central implantation. See **superficial implantation.**

central incisor, one of the two teeth located closest to the sagittal plane in the maxilla and mandible.

central line, *(Informal)* IV tubing inserted for continuous access to a central vein, either the jugular or subclavian, for administering fluids and medicines and for obtaining diagnostic information. Keeping the central line in place ensures accessibility to the venous system in case the peripheral veins collapse. It may also be used for kidney dialysis and long-term drug therapy. See also **central venous catheter.**

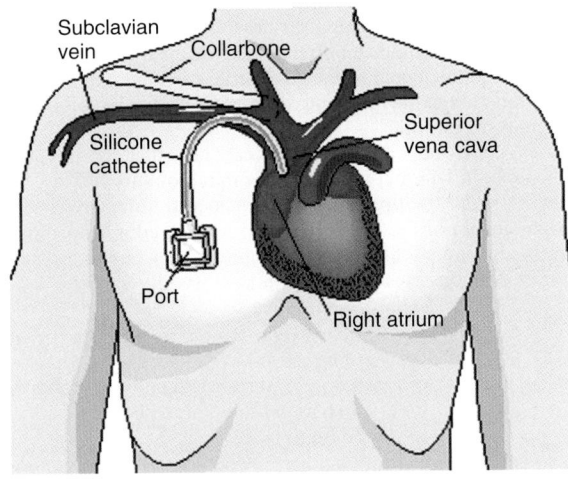

Central line with port access *(Perry and Potter, 2010)*

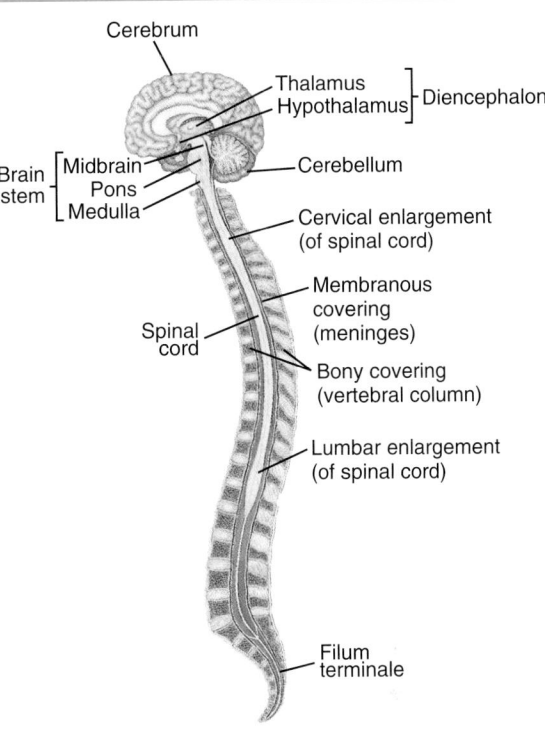

Central nervous system *(Patton and Thibodeau, 2010)*

central lobe, one of the lobes constituting each of the cerebral hemispheres, lying hidden in the depths of the lateral sulcus. The central lobe can be seen only if the lips of the sulcus are parted or cut away. Also called **island of Reil.** Compare **frontal lobe, occipital lobe, parietal lobe, temporal lobe.**

central necrosis [Gk, *kentron,* central, *nekros,* dead, *osis,* condition], death of the central part of a tissue or organ.

central nervous system (CNS) [Gk, *kentron* + L, *nervus,* nerve; Gk, *systema*], one of the two main divisions of the nervous system, consisting of the brain and the spinal cord. The central nervous system processes information to and from the peripheral nervous system and is the main network of coordination and control for the entire body. The brain controls many functions and sensations, such as sleep, sexual activity, muscular movement, hunger, thirst, memory, and emotions. The spinal cord extends various types of nerve fibers from the brain and acts as a switching and relay terminal for the peripheral nervous system. The 12 pairs of cranial nerves emerge directly from the brain. Sensory nerves and motor nerves of the peripheral system leave the spinal cord separately between the vertebrae but unite to form 31 pairs of spinal nerves containing sensory fibers and motor fibers. More than 10 billion neurons constitute but one tenth of the brain cells; the other cells consist of neuroglia that support the neurons. The neurons and the neuroglia form the soft, jellylike substance of the brain, which is supported and protected by the skull. The brain and the spinal cord are composed of gray matter and white matter. The gray matter primarily contains nerve cells and associated processes; the white matter consists predominantly of bundles of myelinated nerve fibers. Compare **peripheral nervous system.** See also **brain, spinal cord.**

central nervous system depressant, any drug that decreases the function of the central nervous system, such as alcohol, tranquilizers, barbiturates, and hypnotics. Such drugs can produce tolerance, physical dependence, and compulsive drug use. These substances depress excitable tissue throughout the central nervous system by stabilizing neuronal membranes, decreasing the amount of transmitter released by the nerve impulse, and generally depressing postsynaptic responsiveness and ion movement. Larger dosages cause anesthesia and potentially fatal respiratory and cardiovascular depression. Central nervous system depressants elevate the seizure threshold and can produce physical dependence in a relatively short period. After alcohol the most abused depressants are the short-acting barbiturates, especially pentobarbital, secobarbital, glutethimide, methyprylon, and methaqualone. These substances have popular street names on the illicit market, such as "reds" (secobarbital) and "yellows" (pentobarbital). Sudden withdrawal of general central nervous system depressants that have been used in high doses for prolonged periods can be fatal to some individuals.

central nervous system stimulant, a substance that quickens the activity of the central nervous system by increasing the rate of neuronal discharge or by blocking an inhibitory neurotransmitter. Many natural and synthetic compounds stimulate the central nervous system, but only a few are used therapeutically. Caffeine, a potent central nervous system stimulant, is used to help restore mental alertness and overcome respiratory depression, but it may cause nausea, nervousness, tinnitus, tremor, tachycardia, extrasystoles, diuresis, and visual disturbances. Amphetamines, sympathomimetic amines with central nervous system stimulating activity, are used in treating narcolepsy and obesity, but these drugs have a high potential for abuse and may cause dizziness, restlessness, tachycardia, increased blood pressure, headache, mouth dryness, an unpleasant taste, GI symptoms, and urticaria. Various amphetamines, especially deanol acetamidobenzoate, a precursor of acetylcholine, are prescribed for hyperkinetic child syndrome because central nervous system stimulants may act as depressants in children. Doxapram is used to stimulate the respiratory center and restore consciousness after anesthesia and to treat acute sedative-hypnotic intoxication. Also called **analeptic.**

central nervous system tumor, a neoplasm of the brain or spinal cord that characteristically does not spread beyond the cerebrospinal axis, although it may be highly invasive locally and have widespread effects on body functions. Intracranial neoplasms are about four times more common than those arising in the spinal cord. From 20% to 40% of brain tumors are metastatic lesions from primary cancer elsewhere, such as in the breast, lung, GI tract, kidney, or a site of melanoma. See also **brain tumor, spinal cord tumor.**

central neurogenic hyperventilation (CNHV) [Gk, *kentron* + *neuron,* nerve, *genein,* to produce], a pattern of breathing during coma marked by rapid, regular ventilations at a rate of about 25 per minute. Increasing regularity rather than rate indicates an increasing depth of coma.

central neuronal plasticity, (in chiropractic) the tendency for the neuronal responses to noxious stimuli to spread to other central pathways, producing the symptoms of referred pain.

central odontogenic fibroma, a rare, benign tumor of the maxilla or mandible composed of radiolucent odontogenic epithelium embedded in stroma. There is a 2:1 female predilection.

central pain [Gk, *kentron* + L, *poena,* penalty], pain caused by a lesion in the central nervous system.

central paralysis [Gk, *kentron* + *paralyein,* to be palsied], paralysis caused by a lesion in the central nervous system.

central pathway, a nerve tract in the brain or spinal cord.

central placenta previa [Gk, *kentron* + L, *placenta,* flat cake, *praevius,* preceding], placenta previa in which the placenta completely covers the internal os. Delivery by cesarean section is almost always required. Also called **complete previa.** See also **placenta previa.**

central processing unit (cpu, CPU), the component of a computer that controls the encoding and execution of instructions, consisting mainly of an arithmetic unit, which performs arithmetic functions, and an internal memory, which controls the sequencing of operations. Also called **processor.**

central ray (CR), the central portion of the x-ray beam with minimal divergence of the beam rays. It is directed toward the center of the image receptor or of the object being imaged. See also **elongation, image foreshortening, cone cutting.** ■ METHOD: In dentistry, when utilizing the paralleling technique of image acquisition, the central ray should be perpendicular to the long axes of both the tooth and the image receptor. If the central ray is positioned incorrectly, the resulting image is distorted or missing.

central scotoma [Gk, *kentron* + *skotos,* darkness, *oma,* tumor], an area of blindness or site of depressed vision involving the macula of the retina.

central sensitization, (in chiropractic) a state in which neurons activated by noxious mechanical and chemical stimuli are sensitized by such stimuli and become hyperresponsive to all subsequent stimuli delivered to the neurons' receptive fields.

central sleep apnea, a form of sleep apnea resulting from decreased respiratory center output. It may involve primary brainstem medullary depression resulting from a tumor of the posterior fossa, poliomyelitis, or idiopathic central hypoventilation.

central slip, the part of the extensor tendon of a finger that inserts into the middle phalanx.

central stimulant. See **central nervous system stimulant.**

central sulcus [Gk, *kentron* + L, furrow], a cleft separating the frontal from the parietal lobes of the brain. Also called **central fissure, fissure of Rolando.**

central tendon, a broad connective tissue sheet that forms the diaphragm. It is composed of interlacing fibers that arise from the lumbar vertebrae, the costal margin, and the xiphoid process of the sternum.

central venous blood pressure, the blood pressure in the superior vena cava, measured by inserting a catheter attached to a manometer directly outside the right atrium. It is approximately equal to the right atrial pressure. On physical examination, it may be approximated by evaluation of jugular venous distension.

central venous catheter, a catheter that is threaded through the internal jugular, antecubital, or subclavian vein, usually with the tip resting in the superior vena cava or the right atrium of the heart. It is also used to administer fluids or medications for hemodynamic monitoring and to measure central venous pressure.

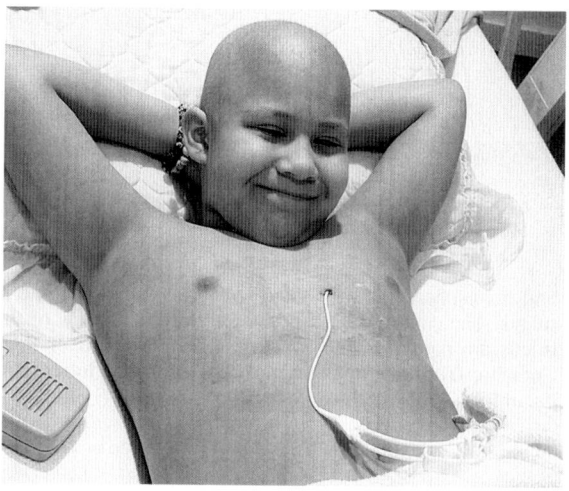

Child with central venous catheter for medication administration *(Hockenberry and Wilson, 2007)*

central venous oxygen saturation (CVSO$_2$), the oxygen saturation in the vena cava. The CVSO$_2$ is measured through a central venous catheter and is useful in measuring cardiac output. A reading of less than 55% usually indicates a falling cardiac output and probable cardiac failure.

central venous pressure (CVP), the blood pressure in the large veins of the body, as distinguished from peripheral venous pressure in an extremity. It is measured with a water manometer that may be attached to the head of a patient's bed and to a central venous catheter inserted into the vena cava or electronically with a transducer. The normal CVP values are 2 to 14 cm H$_2$O.

central venous pressure monitor (CVP monitor), a device for measuring and recording the venous blood pressure by means of an indwelling venous catheter and a pressure manometer. It is used to evaluate the right ventricular function, the right atrial filling pressure, and the circulating blood volume.

central venous return, the blood from the venous system that flows into the right atrium through the vena cava.

central vertigo [Gk, *kentron* + L, *vertigo,* dizziness], vertigo that is caused by a central nervous system disorder.

central vision, vision that results from images falling on the macula of the retina.

central zone, a cone-shaped area of the prostate composed mainly of stromal cells, found deep to the peripheral zone and extending from there to the base of the prostate.

Centrax, a benzodiazepine antianxiety agent. Brand name for **prazepam.**

centre. See **center.**

centrencephalic /sen′trensifal″ik/ [Gk, *kentron* + *enkephalos,* brain], pertaining to the center of the encephalon.

centri-. See **centro-, centri-.**

centriacinar emphysema /sentrē·əsin′ər/, one of the types of emphysema, characterized by enlargement of air spaces in the proximal part of the acinus, primarily at the level of the respiratory bronchioles. Also called **centrilobular emphysema, focal emphysema.**

centric /sen′trik/, **1.** See **central. 2.** *(Informal)* (in dentistry) a shorthand term referring to centric relation or centric occlusion.

centriciput /sentris″ipŏŏt/, the central part of the head, between the occiput and the sinciput.

centric occlusion, the position of the mandible in relation to the maxilla where the teeth of each jaw are intermeshed and bite forces are distributed equally.

centric relation, the position of the mandible in relation to the maxilla in which the mandible is positioned midline with the mandibular condyles as posterior and superior as possible within the mandibular fossa. This position is used to determine occlusal relations and positioning for the fabrication of denture prosthetics.

centrifugal /sentrif″yəgəl/, denoting a force that is directed outward, away from a central point or axis. The force does not actually exist but is a manifestation of inertia. See also **centripetal force.**

centrifugal current, an electrical current in the body with the positive pole near the nerve center and the negative pole at the periphery. Also called **descending current.**

centrifugal force, an inertial force in a rotating system, directed outward from the axis of rotation and inversely proportional to the distance from the axis of rotation. The force is the product of the mass of an object and its radial acceleration; thus in centrifugation, the heavier components of a mixture are separated from the other components by being thrown to the periphery of the orbit.

centrifuge /sen″trifyōōj′/ [Gk, *kentron* + L, *fugere,* to flee], a device for separating components of different densities contained in liquid by spinning them at high speeds. Centrifugal force causes the heavier components to move to one part of the container, leaving the lighter substances in another. −**centrifugal,** *adj.,* −**centrifuge,** *v.*

centrilobular /sen′trəlob″yələr/ [Gk, *kentron* + L, *lobulus,* small lobe], pertaining to the center of a lobule.

centrilobular emphysema. See **centriacinar emphysema.**

centriole /sen″trē·ōl′/ [Gk, *kentron*], an intracellular organelle, usually a component of the centrosome. Often occurring in pairs, centrioles are associated with cell division and can be closely studied only with an electron microscope. They are tiny cylinders positioned at right angles to each other, with walls consisting of nine bundles of fine tubules, three tubules to a bundle. Numerous centrioles occur in some large cells, such as the giant cells in bone marrow. The precise function of centrioles is still unknown, but they appear to aid in the formation of the spindle that develops during mitosis.

centripetal /sentrip″ətəl/ [Gk, *kentron* + L, *petere,* to seek], **1.** denoting an afferent direction, such as that of a sensory nerve impulse traveling toward the brain. **2.** denoting the direction of a force pulling an object toward an axis of rotation or constraining an object to a specific curved path.

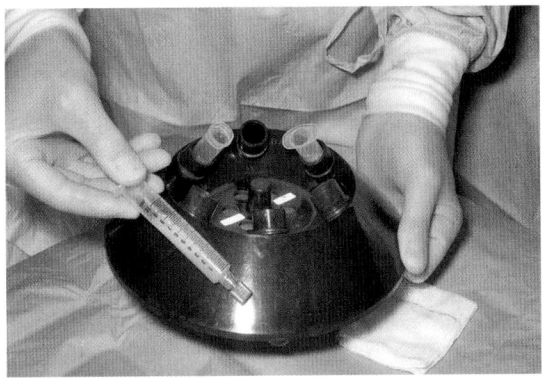

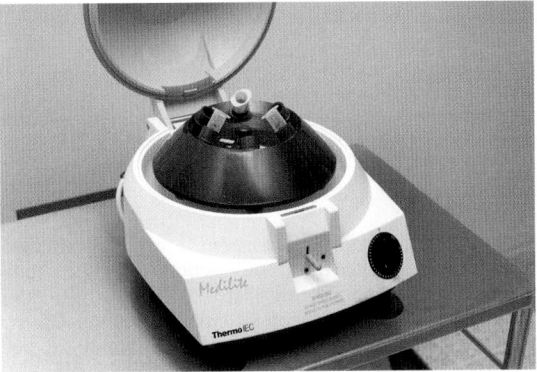

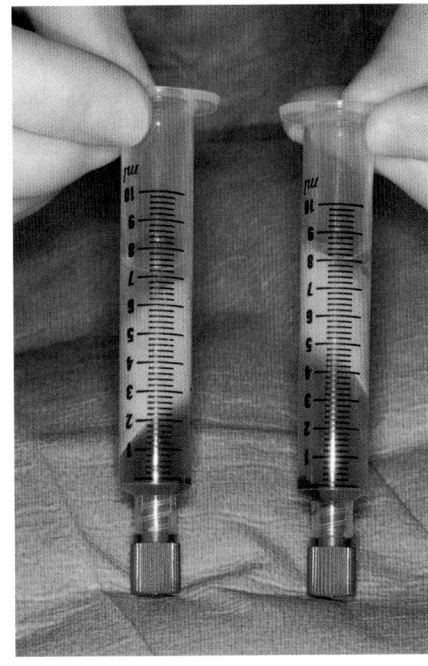

Capped syringes in centrifuge; centrifuge loaded; separation of layers by centrifugation *(Tyers and Collin, 2008)*

centripetal current, an electrical current passing through the body from a peripheral positive electrode to a negative pole near the nerve center. Also called *ascending current.*

centripetal force, the force, directed toward the axis of rotation, required to keep an object moving in a circular path.

centro-, centri-, combining form meaning "center, central, to the center": *centrosome, centriciput.*

centromere (cen) /sen″trəmir/ [Gk, *kentron* + *meros,* part], the constricted region of a chromosome that joins the two chromatids to each other and attaches to spindle fibers in mitosis and meiosis. During cell division the centromeres split longitudinally, half going to each of the new daughter chromosomes. The position of the centromere is constant for a specific chromosome and is identified as acrocentric, metacentric, submetacentric, or telocentric. Also called **kinetochore, kinomere, primary constriction.** –*centromeric, adj.*

centrosome [Gk, *kentron* + *soma,* body], a self-propagating cytoplasmic organelle present in animal cells and in the cells of some lower plants; it is important during cellular division. The structure, which consists of the centrosphere and the centrioles, is located near the nucleus of the cell center or attraction sphere and functions as the dynamic center of the cell, especially during mitosis. Also called **cytocentrum, microcentrum, paranuclear body.**

centrosphere [Gk, *kentron* + *sphaira,* ball], the condensed area of cytoplasm surrounding the centrioles in the centrosome of a cell.

centrostaltic /sen′trōstôl″tik/, pertaining to the center of movement.

centrum, *pl.* **centra** [Gk, *kentron*], any kind of center, especially one related to a body structure, as the centrum semiovale of a cerebral hemisphere.

CEO, C.E.O., abbreviation for **chief executive officer.**

CEP, abbreviation for **congenital erythropoietic porphyria.**

cephal-. See **cephalo-, cephal-.**

cephalad /sef″əlad/ [Gk, *kephale,* head], toward the head; away from the ends or tail. Compare **caudad.**

cephalalgia /sef′əlal″jə/ [Gk, *kephale,* head, *algos,* pain], headache, often combined with another word to indicate a specific type of headache, such as histamine cephalalgia. Also called **cephalgia.** See also **histamine headache.**

cephalea agitata, cephalea attonita /sef′əlē″ə/, a violent headache that is frequently an early symptom of an infection.

cephaledema /sef′əlidē″mə/, a swelling of the brain caused by fluid accumulation. See also **cerebral edema.**

cephalexin /sef′əlek″sin/, an oral first-generation cephalosporin antibiotic.

■ INDICATIONS: It is prescribed for oral treatment of selected infections caused by susceptible bacterial strains, especially lower respiratory tract, urinary tract, skin and soft tissue, and bone and joint infections. It is also used as a prophylaxis against bacterial endocarditis in high-risk patients undergoing surgical or dental procedures.

■ CONTRAINDICATIONS: Known hypersensitivity to this drug or to any cephalosporin medication prohibits its use, as does severely impaired renal function. It is used with caution in patients who are allergic to penicillin or other drugs.

■ ADVERSE EFFECTS: Nausea, diarrhea, and hypersensitivity reactions may occur.

cephalgia, headache. See **cephalalgia, headache.**

cephalhematoma /sef′əlhē″mətō″mə, -hem′ətō″mə/, swelling caused by subcutaneous bleeding and accumulation of blood. It may begin to form in the scalp of a fetus during labor and enlarge slowly in the first few days after birth. It is usually a result of trauma, often caused by forceps or vacuum-assisted births. Also spelled *cephalhaematoma.* Compare **caput succedaneum, molding.**

-cephalia, suffix meaning a specified "(condition of the) head": *hemicephalia, acephalia.*

cephalic /sifal″ik/, pertaining to the head.

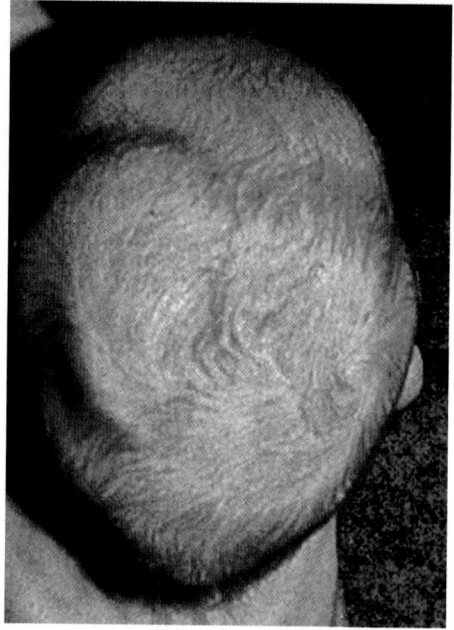

Cephalhematoma *(Paller and Mancini, 2011)*

-cephalic, suffix meaning "relating to the head": *holocephalic, ultrabrachycephalic.*

cephalic index [Gk, *kephale,* head, *index,* pointer], a ratio between the breadth and length of the head. It is calculated as 100 times the maximum breadth of the head, measured at the greatest diameter of the cranial vault above the supramastoid crest, divided by the maximum length measured from the most prominent point on the glabella to the opisthocranion. It is used primarily to estimate fetal age and head shape.

cephalic presentation, a classification of fetal position in which the head of the fetus is the presenting part. Cephalic presentation is usually further qualified by an indication of the part of the head presenting, such as the occiput, brow, or chin. See also **brow presentation.**

cephalic vein, one of the four superficial veins of the upper limb. It receives deoxygenated blood from the dorsal and palmar surfaces of the forearm. Compare **basilic vein, dorsal digital vein, median antebrachial vein.**

cephalo-, cephal-, prefix meaning "head": *cephalocaudal, cephalocentesis.*

cephalocaudal /sef′əlōkô″dəl/ [Gk, *kephale* + L, *cauda,* tail], **1.** pertaining to the long axis of the body, or the relationship between the head and the base of the spine. Also called **cephalocercal. 2.** denoting a pattern of motor development that occurs in widening circles and proceeds ventrally and caudally.

cephalocele /sef′əlōsēl′/, the protrusion of a part of the brain through an opening in the skull. The opening may be congenital or may result from an injury. Also called **cerebral hernia.**

cephalocentesis /-sentē″sis/, the puncture of the skull with a hollow needle, performed to allow drainage of fluid or an abscess.

cephalocercal, *(Obsolete)* now called **cephalocaudal.**

cephalogram. See **cephalometric radiograph projection.**

cephalometric radiograph projection /sef′əlōmet′rik rä′dē·ō·graf/, an extraoral imaging technique of the head, including the mandible, in full lateral view; used for making cranial measurements especially for use in orthodontic treatment planning. Also called **cephalogram.**

cephalometric tracing, a line drawing of structural outlines of craniofacial landmarks and facial bones made directly from a cephalometric radiogram.

cephalometry /-ətrē/, scientific measurement of the head, such as that performed in dentistry to determine appropriate orthodontic procedures for correcting malocclusions and other abnormal conditions. *–cephalometric, adj.*

cephalomotor /sef′əlōmō′tər/ [Gk, *kephale,* head, + L, *motare,* to move about], moving the head; pertaining to motions of the head.

cephalopagus. See **craniopagus.**

cephalopelvic /-pel′vik/, pertaining to a relationship between the fetal head and the maternal pelvis.

cephalopelvic disproportion (CPD) [Gk, *kephale* + L, *pelvis,* basin, *dis,* opposite of, *proportio,* similarity], an obstetrical condition in which a baby's head is too large or a mother's birth canal too small to permit normal labor or birth. In relative CPD, the size of the baby's head is within normal limits but larger than average or the size of the mother's birth canal is within normal limits but smaller than average, or both; relative CPD is often overcome by molding of the head, the forces of labor, or the use of forceps to effect delivery. In absolute CPD, the baby's head is markedly or abnormally enlarged or the mother's birth canal is markedly or abnormally contracted, making vaginal delivery impossible. See also **clinical pelvimetry, dystocia.**

cephalophlebitis, an inflammation of the vena cava.

Clinical Care Classification, a standardized nursing terminology developed by Dr. Virginia Saba; originally called the Home Heath Care Classification.

cephalosporinase. See **beta-lactamase.**

Cephalosporium /sef′əlōspo′re·um/. See *Acremonium.*

cephalothin sodium /sef′əlō′thin/, a parenteral first-generation cephalosporin antibiotic.

■ INDICATIONS: It is prescribed in the treatment of infections caused by susceptible bacterial strains causing respiratory, genitourinary, gastrointestinal, skin and soft tissue, and bone and joint infections, or septicemia. It is effective against many gram-positive bacilli and cocci (other than enterococcus) and some gram-negative bacilli.

■ CONTRAINDICATIONS: Known hypersensitivity to this drug or to any cephalosporin medication prohibits its use. It is prescribed with caution for patients who are allergic to penicillin.

■ ADVERSE EFFECTS: Among the more serious adverse reactions are pain at the site of injection and hypersensitivity reactions.

-cephalus [Gk, *kephale,* head], **1.** suffix meaning an abnormal condition of the head, as indicated by the stem to which the ending is attached, such as *hydrocephalus.* **2.** suffix indicating an individual having an abnormal condition of the head, especially a congenital anomaly of the fetus, such as *dicephalus.*

-cephaly [Gk, *kephale,* head], suffix meaning an abnormal condition of the head.

-cephaly, -cephalia, suffix meaning a "(specified) condition of the head": *macrencephaly.*

cephapirin /sef′əprin/, a parenteral first-generation cephalosporin antibiotic.

■ INDICATIONS: It is prescribed in the treatment of bacterial infections caused by cephapirin-susceptible strains of a wide variety of microorganisms that cause septicemia, endocarditis, osteomyelitis, and bacterial infections of the respiratory tract, urinary tract, and skin.

■ CONTRAINDICATIONS: Known sensitivity to cephalosporin antibiotics prohibits its use.

■ ADVERSE EFFECTS: Among the most serious adverse reactions are neutropenia, leukopenia, anemia, bone marrow depression, and allergic reactions.

cephradine /sef′rədēn/, an oral first-generation cephalosporin antibiotic.

■ INDICATIONS: It is prescribed in the treatment of certain infections caused by susceptible bacterial strains causing respiratory, genitourinary, gastrointestinal, skin and soft tissue, and bone and joint infections, or septicemia. It is effective against many gram-positive bacilli and cocci (other than enterococcus) and some gram-negative bacilli.

■ CONTRAINDICATIONS: Known hypersensitivity to this drug or to any cephalosporin medication prohibits its use. It is prescribed with caution for patients who are allergic to penicillin.

■ ADVERSE EFFECTS: Nausea, diarrhea, and hypersensitivity reactions may occur.

-ceptor [shortened from *receptor;* L, *recipere,* to receive], suffix denoting a receptor, with the root preceding it specifying the type.

cer-, prefix meaning "wax": *cerumen.*

cera, wax. Ordinary yellow beeswax is sometimes identified as cera flava; white beeswax, bleached by exposure to air and sunlight, is known as cera alba.

ceramics /səram′iks/, **1.** (in dentistry) the process of making dental restorations from fused porcelain and other glasses. **2.** a hard, heat-resistant inorganic material.

ceramidase /səram′idās/, an enzyme of the hydrolase class that catalyzes the cleavage of a ceramide to form sphingosine and a fatty acid anion, a step in the degradation of sphingolipids. See also **Farber's disease, Farber's lipogranulomatosis.**

ceramidase deficiency. See **Farber's disease, Farber's lipogranulomatosis.**

ceramide /ser′əmīd/, the basic unit of the sphingolipids, consisting of sphingosine or a related base attached by means of its amino group to a long-chain fatty acyl group.

cerato-, kerato-, prefix meaning "cornea" or "horny tissue": *keratomalacia.*

cercaria /sərker′ē·ə/ *pl.* cercariae [Gk, *kerkos,* tail], a minute, wormlike early developmental form of trematode. It develops in a freshwater snail, is released into the water, and swims toward the sun, rising to the surface of the water in the warmest part of the day. Cercariae enter the body of the next host by ingestion, by direct invasion through the skin, or through a cut or other break in the skin. Some cercariae of the genera *Schistosoma, Chlonorchis, Paragonimus, Fasciolopsis,* and *Fasciola* are known to infect humans. They encyst and complete their development in various organs of the body. Each species tends to migrate to one organ, such as *Fasciola hepatica,* which grows to become a liver fluke. See also **fluke, schistosomiasis.**

cerclage /serkläzh′/ [Fr, cask hooping], **1.** an orthopedic procedure in which the ends of an oblique bone fracture or the chips of a broken patella are bound together with a wire loop or a metal band to hold them in position until healed. **2.** a procedure in which a taut silicone band is applied around the sclera to restore contact between the retina and the choroid when the retina is detached. **3.** an obstetric procedure in which a nonabsorbable suture is used for holding the cervix closed to prevent spontaneous abortion in a woman who has an incompetent cervix. The suture is removed when the pregnancy is at full term to allow labor to begin. See also **incompetent cervix.**

cerea flexibilitas /sirē′ə flek′sibil′itas/ [L, waxlike flexibility], a cataleptic state, frequently observed in catatonic schizophrenia, in which the limbs maintain the positions in which they are placed for an indefinite period. Also called **flexibilitas cerea, waxy flexibility.** See also **catalepsy.**

cerebella. See **cerebellum.**

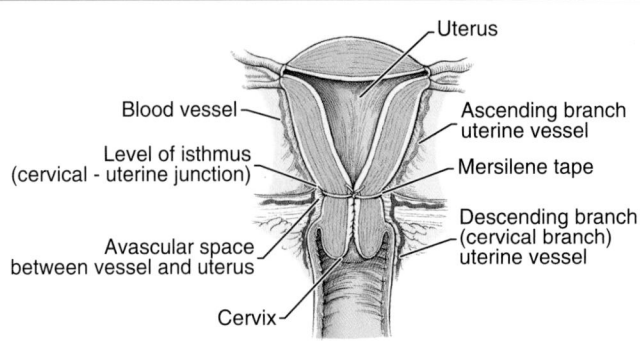

Cerclage *(Gabbe et al, 2012)*

cerebellar /ser′əbel″ər/ [L, *cerebellum,* small brain], pertaining to the cerebellum.

cerebellar angioblastoma [L, *cerebellum* + Gk, *angeion,* vessel, *blastos,* germ, *oma*], a cystic tumor in the cerebellum composed of a mass of blood vessels. It is frequently associated with von Hippel-Lindau disease. See also **von Hippel–Lindau disease.**

cerebellar artery, one of the three major arteries (superior, posterior inferior, and anterior inferior) on each side that supply the cerebellum.

cerebellar artery occlusion, an obstruction of one of the arteries supplying the cerebellum. It can result in ipsilateral ataxia, facial analgesia, contralateral hemiparesis, and loss of temperature and pain sensations.

cerebellar ataxia [L, *cerebellum,* small brain; Gk, *ataxia,* without order], a loss of muscle coordination caused by a lesion in the cerebellum.

cerebellar atrophy [L, *cerebellum* + Gk, *a* + *trophe,* without nourishment], deterioration and wasting of tissues of the cerebellum. Causes of the condition include nutritional and metabolic factors such as alcohol abuse and degenerative disease. See also **spinocerebellar disorder.**

cerebellar cortex, the superficial gray matter of the cerebellum covering the white substance in the medullary core. It consists of two layers, an external molecular layer and an internal granule cell layer. Also called **cortical substance of cerebellum.**

cerebellar cyst, a cyst that develops in the white matter of the cerebellum and that can be associated with an astrocytoma.

cerebellar falx, a small sickle-shaped process of the dura mater attached to the occipital bone above and projecting into the posterior cerebellar notch between the two cerebellar hemispheres. Also called **falx cerebelli.**

cerebellar gait [L, *cerebellum,* small brain; ONorse, *geta,* a way], a staggering gait in which the person walks with a wide base and has difficulty turning. The feet can be turned outward, and the person puts his or her weight first on the heel and then on the toes. The condition is caused by a lesion in the cerebellum or cerebellar pathways. Also called **ataxic gait.**

cerebellar hemangioblastoma, a hemangioblastoma of the cerebellum, often cystic. An autosomal-dominant form is associated with von Hippel-Lindau disease. See also **von Hippel–Lindau disease.**

cerebellar inferior peduncle [L, *cerebellum,* small brain, *inferior,* lower, *pes,* foot], a band of nerve fibers that forms the lateral boundary of the bottom part of the fourth ventricle and carries afferent fibers into the cerebellum.

cerebellar middle peduncle [L, *cerebellum,* small brain, *medius* + *pes,* foot], a lateral extension of the transverse nerve fibers of the pons. It consists mainly of fibers from the pontine nuclei to the neocerebellum.

cerebellar notch, **1.** anteriorly, a broad depression that lies dorsal to the midbrain and separates the cerebellar hemispheres. **2.** posteriorly, a deep depression adjacent to the falx cerebelli.

cerebellar rigidity, a stiffness of the trunk muscles caused by a midline (vermal) lesion in the cerebellum. In some cases, the limbs may also be rigid and the neck and back arched, as in opisthotonos.

cerebellar speech [L, *cerebellum* + AS, *spaec*], abnormal speech caused by diseases of the cerebellum, characterized by slow, jerky, and slurred articulation that may be intermittent and explosive or monotonous and unvaried in pitch. Also called **scanning speech.** See also **ataxic speech.**

cerebellar superior peduncle [L, *cerebellum,* small brain, *superior* + *pes,* foot], a band of nerve fibers that passes from the cerebellum on each side of the superior medullary velum. It includes nerve tracts linking the dentate nucleus to the red nucleus of the midbrain and to the thalamus.

cerebellar tentorium, a horizontal projection of the meningeal dura mater that covers and separates the cerebellum in the posterior cranial fossa from the posterior parts of the cerebral hemispheres. It is attached posteriorly to the occipital bone and laterally to the superior border of the petrous part of the temporal bone. The anterior and medial borders of the tentorium cerebelli are free, forming an oval opening into the midline through which the midbrain passes. Also called **tentorium cerebelli.** Compare **cerebellar falx, cerebral falx.**

cerebellar tremor [L, *cerebellum,* small brain, *tremor,* shaking], an intention tremor or trembling during voluntary movements, caused by lesions in the cerebellum.

cerebellomedullary cistern. Also called **cisterna magna.**

cerebellopontine /ser′əbel′ōpon″tīn/ [L, *cerebellum* + *pons,* bridge], leading from the cerebellum to the pons varolii.

cerebellospinal /ser′əbel′ōspī′nəl/ [L, *cerebellum* + *spina,* backbone], leading from the cerebellum to the spinal cord.

cerebellum /ser′əbel″əm/ *pl. cerebellums, cerebella* [L, small brain], the part of the brain located in the posterior cranial fossa behind the brainstem. It consists of two lateral cerebellar hemispheres, or lobes, and a middle section called the vermis. Three pairs of peduncles link it with the brainstem. The cerebellum is concerned primarily with coordinating voluntary muscular activity, such as posture, balance, coordination, and speech.

cerebr-, combining form meaning "cerebrum": *cerebroid.*

cerebra. See **cerebrum.**

cerebral /ser′əbrəl, sərē′brəl/, pertaining to the cerebrum.

-cerebral, suffix referring to the brain.

cerebral abscess. See **brain abscess.**

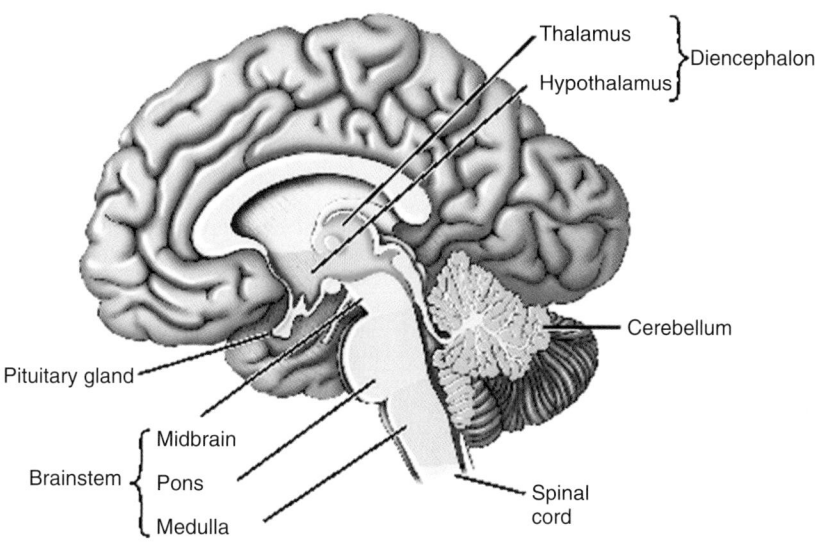

Cerebellum *(Herlihy, 2014)*

cerebral amyloid angiopathy, vascular amyloidosis affecting small- and medium-sized arteries of the leptomeninges and cerebral cortex, resulting in microinfarcts, microhemorrhages, or large hemorrhages. It may be asymptomatic or may result in hemorrhagic stroke or dementia. It usually occurs in the elderly, and most cases are sporadic. A hereditary form with autosomal-dominant inheritance also exists.

cerebral aneurysm [L, *cerebrum,* brain; Gk, *aneurysma,* a widening], an abnormal, localized dilation of a cerebral artery. It is most commonly the result of congenital weakness of the tunica media or muscle layer of the arterial wall. Cerebral aneurysms may also be caused by infection, such as occurs in subacute bacterial endocarditis or syphilis, and by neoplasms, arteriosclerosis, and trauma. The most frequent sites are the middle cerebral, internal carotid, basilar, and anterior cerebral arteries, especially at bifurcations of vessels. Cerebral aneurysms may occur in infancy or old age. They may be fusiform dilations of the entire circumference of an artery or saccular outcroppings of the side of a vessel. The outcroppings may be as small as a pinhead or as large as an orange but are usually the size of a pea. Cerebral aneurysms pose a danger of rupture and intracranial hemorrhage.

cerebral angiography [L, *cerebrum,* brain; Gk, *angeion,* vessel, *graphein,* to record], a radiographic imaging procedure used to visualize the vascular system of the brain after injection of a radiopaque contrast medium.

cerebral anoxia, a condition in which oxygen is deficient in brain tissue. This state, which is caused by circulatory failure, can exist for no more than 4 to 6 minutes before the onset of irreversible brain damage.

cerebral aqueduct [L, *cerebrum* + *aqueductus,* water canal], the narrow conduit in the midbrain, between the third and the fourth ventricles, that conveys the cerebrospinal fluid throughout the cerebrum, cerebellum, and brainstem. Also called **aqueduct of Sylvius.**

cerebral arteriovenous malformation. See **arteriovenous angioma of the brain.**

cerebral artery, one of the arteries that supply the brain. The middle cerebral artery is the largest of the cerebral arteries and the vessel most commonly affected by a cerebrovascular accident. See also **cerebrovascular accident.**

Anterior — Aneurysm

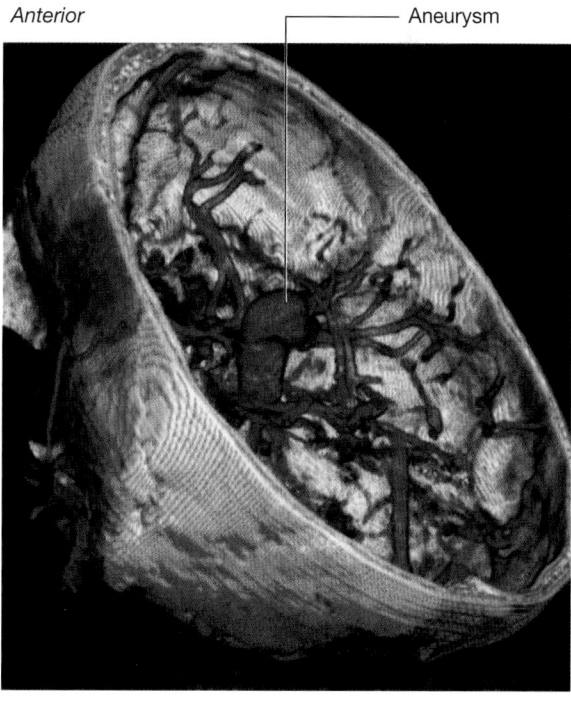

Posterior

Cerebral aneurysm *(Drake, Vogl, and Mitchell, 2015)*

cerebral blood flow (CBF), **1.** the blood supply to the brain in a given period of time. CBF is determined by blood viscosity, cerebral vascular resistance (CVR), and cerebral perfusion pressure (CPP). CBF = CPP/CVR. **2.** the circulation of blood through the vascular system of the brain.

cerebral cavity. See **cranial cavity.**

cerebral compression [L, *cerebrum,* brain, *comprimere,* to press together], any abnormal condition resulting from hemorrhage, abscess, or tumor that increases intracranial pressure. If untreated, the compression destroys the brain tissues and causes herniation of the brain. Also called **brain compression.**

cerebral cortex [L, *cerebrum* + *cortex,* bark], a layer of neurons and synapses (gray matter) on the surface of the cerebral hemispheres, folded into gyri with about two thirds of its area buried in fissures. It integrates higher mental functions, general movement, visceral functions, perception, and behavioral reactions. It has been classified in many different ways. More than 200 areas have been identified on the basis of differences in myelinated fiber patterns, as well as 47 separate function areas with different cell designs. For example, stimulation of the precentral cortex or motor area with electrodes causes contractions of voluntary muscles. Destruction of a motor speech area in the frontal operculum causes motor aphasia or speech defects despite healthy, intact vocal organs. Stimulation of the frontal area affects circulation, respiration, pupillary reaction, and other visceral activity. Also called **pallium.** See also **cerebrum.**

cerebral deafness. See **central auditory processing disorder.**

cerebral depressant [L, *cerebrum,* brain, *deprimere,* to press down], a drug or other agent that has a sedating effect on the brain, reducing activity and alertness and, in some instances, causing a loss of consciousness. See also **central nervous system depressant.**

cerebral dominance, the specialization of each of the two cerebral hemispheres in the integration and control of different functions. In 90% of the population, the left cerebral hemisphere specializes in or dominates the ability to speak and write and the capacity to understand spoken and written words. The areas that control these activities are situated in the frontal, parietal, and temporal lobes of the left hemisphere. In the other 10% of the population, either the right hemisphere or both hemispheres dominate the speech and writing abilities. The right cerebral hemisphere dominates the integration of certain sounds other than those associated with speaking, such as sounds of coughing, laughter, crying, and melodies. The right cerebral hemisphere perceives tactile stimuli and visual spatial relationships better than the left cerebral hemisphere does. See also **Brodmann's areas, Broca's area.**

cerebral edema [L, *cerebrum* + Gk, *oidema,* swelling], an accumulation of fluid in the brain tissues. Causes include infection, tumor, trauma, or exposure to certain toxins. Because the skull cannot expand to accommodate the fluid pressure, brain tissues are compressed. Early symptoms are changes in level of consciousness: sluggishness, then dilation of one or both pupils, and finally a gradual loss of consciousness. Cerebral edema can be fatal.

cerebral embolism [L, *cerebrum* + *embolos,* plug], a condition in which an embolus blocks blood flow through the vessels of the cerebrum, resulting in tissue ischemia distal to the occlusion. See also **cerebrovascular accident.**

cerebral falx, a sickle-shaped fold of dura mater membrane extending into and following along the longitudinal fissure and separating the two hemispheres of the cerebrum. It assists with anchoring the cerebrum in place in the skull. Also called **falx cerebri.**

cerebral fossa, the stem of the lateral sulcus of the cerebrum, which forms a furrow separating the orbital surface of the frontal lobe from the temporal lobe.

cerebral gigantism [L, *cerebrum* + Gk, *gigas,* giant], an abnormal condition characterized by excessive weight and size at birth, accelerated growth during the first 4 or 5 years after birth without any increase in the level of growth hormone, and then reversion to normal growth. Some typical signs of this condition are prognathism, downward-slanting

eyes, an elongated skull, moderate intellectual disability, and impaired coordination. Also called **Soto syndrome.**

cerebral gyrus. See **gyrus.**

cerebral hemiplegia [L, *cerebrum* + Gk, *hemi,* half, *plege,* stroke], paralysis of one side of the body caused by a brain lesion. See also **hemiplegia.**

cerebral hemisphere [L, *cerebrum* + Gk, *hemi,* half, *sphaira,* ball], one of the halves of the cerebrum. The two cerebral hemispheres are divided by a deep longitudinal fissure and are connected medially at the bottom of the fissure by the corpus callosum. Prominent grooves, subdividing each hemisphere into four major lobes, are the central sulcus, the lateral fissure, and the parietooccipital fissure. Each hemisphere also has a fifth major lobe deep in the brain. The hemispheres consist of an external gray layer and an internal white matter that surrounds islands of gray matter called nuclei (the basal ganglia).

cerebral hemorrhage [L, *cerebrum* + Gk, *haima,* blood, *rhegnynei,* to burst forth], a hemorrhage from a blood vessel in the brain. Three criteria used to classify cerebral hemorrhages are location (subarachnoid, extradural, subdural), kind of vessel involved (arterial, venous, capillary), and origin (traumatic, degenerative). Each kind of cerebral hemorrhage has distinctive clinical characteristics. Most cerebral hemorrhages occur in the region of the basal ganglia and are caused by the rupture of a sclerotic artery as a result of hypertension. Other causes of rupture include congenital aneurysm, cerebrovascular thrombosis, and head trauma.

■ OBSERVATIONS: Bleeding may lead to displacement or destruction of brain tissue. Extensive hemorrhage is usually fatal. Depending on the extent and the location of the damaged tissue, residual effects may include aphasia, diminished mental function, hemiplegia, or disturbance of the function of a special sense.

■ INTERVENTIONS: A computed tomography scan may be performed to locate the lesion and to differentiate the hemorrhage from an embolus or thrombus, or cerebral angiography may be used for these purposes. Lumbar puncture may be performed to reveal blood in the spinal fluid if subarachnoid bleeding is suspected, but computed tomography must be performed first because of the risk of brain herniation if high intracranial pressure is present. Surgery is sometimes necessary to stop the bleeding and to prevent death from greatly increased intracranial pressure, although it has not been shown to improve long-term outcome. Treatment is usually supportive.

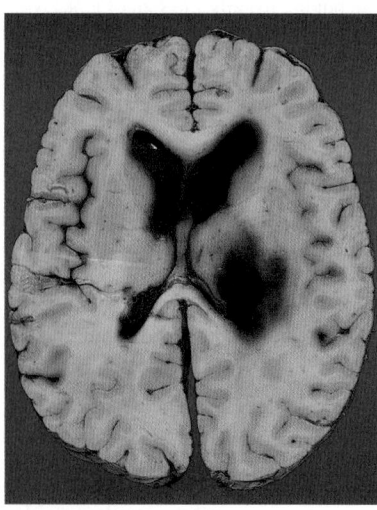

Cerebral hemorrhage *(Finkbeiner, Ursell, and Davis, 2009)*

cerebral hernia. See **cephalocele.**

cerebral infarction. See **cerebrovascular accident.**

cerebral lobes, the well-defined areas of the cerebral cortex, demarcated by fissures, sulci, and arbitrary lines, which include the frontal, temporal, parietal, and occipital lobes.

cerebral localization, 1. the determination of various areas in the cerebral cortex associated with specific functions, such as the 47 Brodmann's areas. **2.** the diagnosis of a cerebral condition, such as a brain lesion, by analyzing the signs manifested by the patient to determine the area of the brain affected.

cerebral nerves. See **cranial nerves.**

cerebral palsy (CP) [L, *cerebrum* + Gk, *para,* beyond, *lysis,* loosening], a motor function disorder caused by a permanent, nonprogressive brain defect or lesion present at birth or shortly thereafter. The disorder is usually associated with premature or abnormal birth and intrapartum asphyxia, causing damage to the nervous system. Also called **congenital cerebral diplegia, Little disease.**

■ OBSERVATIONS: The neurological deficit may result in a wide variety of symptoms, including spastic hemiplegia, monoplegia, diplegia, or tetraplegia; athetosis or ataxia; seizures; paresthesia; varying degrees of intellectual impairment; and impaired speech, vision, and hearing. Difficulties with breathing, sucking, swallowing, and responsiveness are usually apparent soon after birth, but the characteristic stiff, awkward movements of the infant's limbs may be missed for several months. Walking is usually delayed, and when it is attempted, the child manifests a typical scissors gait. The arms may be affected only slightly, but the fingers are often spastic. Deep-tendon reflexes are exaggerated, and there may be slurred speech, delay in development of sphincter control, and athetotic movements of the face and hands.

■ INTERVENTIONS: Early identification of the disorder facilitates the development of a comprehensive plan for infants with cerebral palsy and the initiation of an individualized therapeutic program. Treatment is individualized and may include the use of orthotics, braces, and supports; surgical correction of deformities; physical, occupational, and speech therapy; and various indicated drugs, such as muscle relaxants, oral antispasticity and antidystonic medications, injectable botulinum toxin, and anticonvulsants.

■ PATIENT CARE CONSIDERATIONS: Cerebral palsy includes a large group of childhood movement disorders. The pattern of symptoms and their severity vary widely, depending on the area of the central nervous system compromised. A multidisciplinary team approach is vital for all aspects of management to improve function and minimize disability.

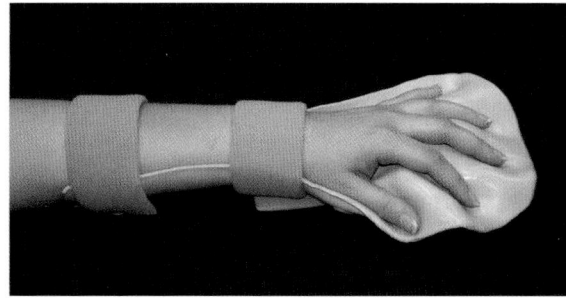

Splint for spastic hand due to cerebral palsy *(Canale and Beaty, 2008)*

cerebral peduncle [L, *cerebrum,* brain, *pes,* foot], a pair of ovoid masses of nerve fibers at the upper border of the pons that disappear into the left and right hemispheres of the cerebrum. It includes corticopontine and pyramidal-tract fibers and helps constitute the central portion of the midbrain.

cerebral perfusion pressure (CPP), a parameter that is related to the amount of blood flow to the brain. It is calculated by subtracting the intracranial pressure from the mean systemic arterial blood pressure.

cerebral sulci, the furrows on the surface of the brain between the gyri. See also **gyrus.**

cerebral thrombosis [L, *cerebrum* + Gk, *thrombos,* lump, *osis,* condition], an abnormal condition in which a blood clot forms in a cerebral blood vessel.

cerebral vertigo [L, *cerebrum,* brain, *vertigo,* dizziness], vertigo that is caused by organic brain disease. See also **central vertigo.**

cerebral vomiting, vomiting caused by a disorder of the central nervous system, especially stimulation of the vomiting center, usually without preceding nausea.

cerebriform carcinoma. See **medullary carcinoma.**

cerebroatrophic hyperammonemia. See **Rett's syndrome.**

cerebrocerebellar atrophy /ser″əbrōser′əbel″ər/ [L, *cerebrum,* brain, *cerebellum,* small brain; Gk, *a* + *trophe,* without nourishment], a deterioration of the cerebellum caused by certain abiotrophic diseases.

cerebrocostomandibular syndrome /ser″əbrōkos′tō·man dib′yŏŏlər/ [L, *cerebrum,* brain + *costa,* rib + *mandibula,* mandible], an extremely rare autosomal-recessive syndrome of severe micrognathia and costovertebral abnormalities, including small bell-shaped thorax, incompletely ossified aberrant rib structure, and abnormal rib attachment to vertebrae. There are also palatal defects, glossoptosis, prenatal and postnatal growth deficiencies, and in some cases moderate to severe intellectual disabilities, the latter sometimes related to neonatal respiratory distress.

cerebrohepatorenal syndrome /ser″əbrōhep′ətō·rē′nəl/, an autosomal-recessive disorder characterized by craniofacial abnormalities, hypotonia, hepatomegaly, polycystic kidneys, jaundice, and death in early infancy, and associated with absence of peroxisomes in the liver and kidneys. Also called **Zellweger syndrome.**

cerebroid /ser″əbroid/ [L, *cerebrum* + Gk, *eidos,* form], white matter in the brain transmitting signals from one location of the cerebrum to another.

cerebroma /ser′əbrō″mə/ *pl.* cerebromas, cerebromata, any unusual mass of brain tissue.

cerebromedullary tube. See **neural tube.**

cerebromeningitis /-men′inji″tis/. See **meningitis.**

cerebropathia psychia toxemia, *(Obsolete)* now called **Korsakoff psychosis.**

cerebroretinal angiomatosis. See **von Hippel–Lindau disease.**

cerebroside /ser″əbrōsīd′/, any of a group of glycolipids found in the brain and other tissues of the nervous system, especially the myelin sheath.

cerebroside sulfatase [L, *cerebrum,* brain, *sulfur,* brimstone, *ase,* enzyme], an enzyme of the hydrolase class that catalyzes the reaction of cerebroside 3-sulfate + H_2O. A deficiency of the enzyme, which is transmitted through an autosomal-recessive gene, is the cause of sulfatide lipidosis. See also **sulfatide lipidosis.**

cerebrospinal /ser″əbrōspī′nəl, sərē″brō-/, pertaining to or involving the brain and the spinal cord.

cerebrospinal axis [L, *cerebrum,* brain, *spina,* spine, *axle*], a line formed by the brain and spinal cord about which the body turns.

cerebrospinal fever, *(Obsolete)* now called **meningococcal meningitis.**

cerebrospinal fluid (CSF), the fluid that flows through and protects the four ventricles of the brain, the subarachnoid spaces, and the spinal canal. It is composed mainly of secretions of the choroid plexuses in the lateral ventricles and in the third and the fourth ventricles of the brain and is clear and colorless. Changes in the carbon dioxide content of CSF affect the respiratory center in the medulla, helping to control breathing. A brain tumor may press against the cerebral aqueduct and shut off the flow of the fluid from the third to the fourth ventricle, causing fluid accumulation in the lateral and third ventricles, called internal hydrocephalus. Other blockages of the flow of CSF, such as those caused by blood clots, result in serious complications. Certain illnesses and various diagnoses may require microscopic examination and chemical analysis of CSF. Samples of the fluid may be removed by lumbar puncture between the third and the fourth lumbar vertebrae or from the cisterna magna.

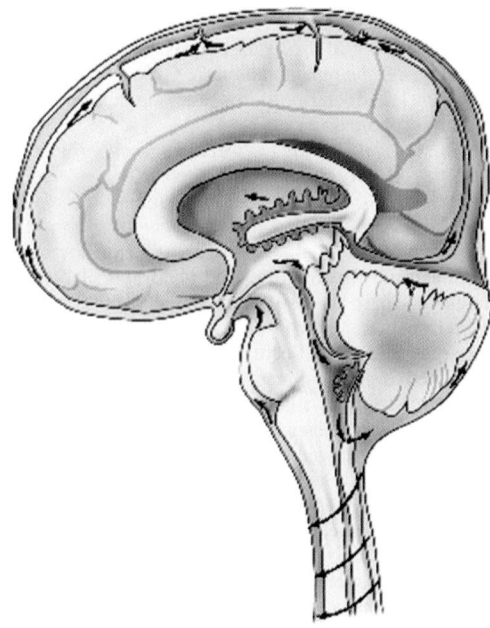

Cerebrospinal fluid (CSF) *(Winn, 2011)*

cerebrospinal ganglion, a cluster of sensory ganglia neurons on roots of cranial and spinal nerves. The neurons lack dendrites and have no synapses on their cell bodies. See also **autonomic ganglion, dorsal root ganglion, ganglion.**

cerebrospinal nerves, the 12 pairs of cranial nerves and 31 pairs of spinal nerves that originate in the brain and spinal cord.

cerebrospinal otorrhea, a discharge of cerebrospinal fluid (CSF) from the ear. Basal skull fractures can transverse the paranasal air sinuses of the middle ear within the temporal bone, resulting in a dural tear. CSF can then leak through the dural tear and drain from the ear. Compare **cerebrospinal rhinorrhea.**

cerebrospinal pressure [L, *cerebrum* + *spina* + *premere,* to press], the pressure of cerebrospinal fluid in the central nervous system. It usually measures between 100 and 150 mm of H_2O or 10 and 15 mm Hg and is measured by a manometer attached to the end of a needle after it has been inserted into the subarachnoid space via lumbar puncture (most commonly). See also **cerebrospinal fluid.**

cerebrospinal rhinorrhea [L, *cerebrum,* brain, *spina,* spine; Gk, *rhis,* nose, *rhoia,* flow], a discharge of cerebrospinal fluid (CSF) from the nose. Basal skull fractures can transverse the paranasal air sinuses of the frontal bone, resulting in a dural tear. CSF can then leak through the dural tear and drain from the nose. Compare **cerebrospinal otorrhea.**

cerebrotendinous xanthomatosis. See **van Bogaert's disease.**

cerebrovascular /ser′əbrōvas″kyələr, sərē′brō-/ [L, *cerebrum* + *vasculum,* little vessel], pertaining to the vascular system and blood supply of the brain.

cerebrovascular accident (CVA), an abnormal condition of the brain characterized by occlusion by an embolus, thrombus, or cerebrovascular hemorrhage or vasospasm, resulting in ischemia of the brain tissues normally perfused by the damaged vessels. The sequelae of a cerebrovascular insult depend on the location and extent of ischemia. Paralysis, weakness, sensory change, speech defect, aphasia, or death may occur. Symptoms remit somewhat after the first few days as brain swelling subsides. In the United States, 80% of cerebrovascular incidents are ischemic and 20% are hemorrhagic. Also called **brain attack,** *cerebrovascular insult,* **stroke.**

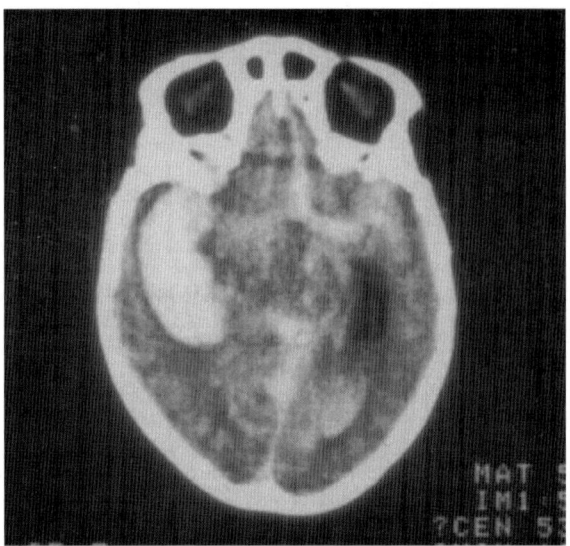

Radiographic image of cerebrovascular accident *(Little et al, 2013)*

cerebrum /ser″əbrəm, sərē″brəm/ *pl. cerebrums, cerebra* [L, brain], the largest and uppermost section of the brain, divided by a longitudinal fissure into the left and right cerebral hemispheres. At the bottom of the groove, the hemispheres are connected by the corpus callosum. The internal structures of the hemispheres merge with those of the diencephalon and further communicate with the brainstem through the cerebral peduncles. The surface of the cerebrum is called gyri. Each lobe bears the name of the bone under which it lies. The cerebrum performs sensory functions, motor functions, and less easily defined integration functions associated with various mental activities. It generates a variety of electrical waves that may be recorded as an electroencephalogram to localize areas of brain dysfunction, to identify altered states of consciousness, or to establish brain death. See also **cerebral cortex, cerebral hemisphere.** —**cerebral,** *adj.*

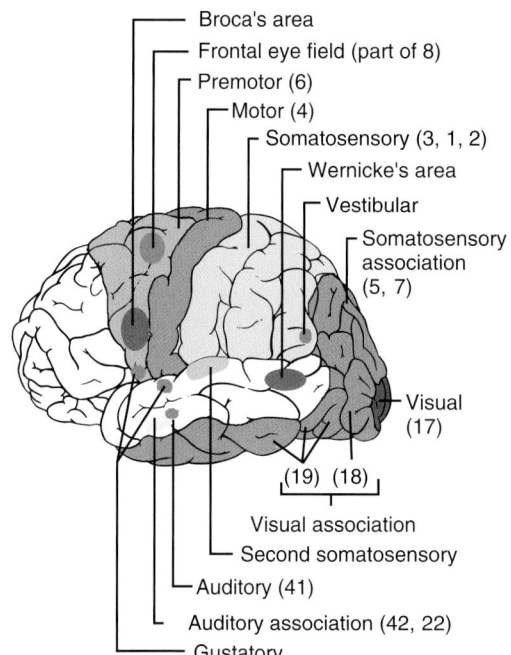

- Broca's area
- Frontal eye field (part of 8)
- Premotor (6)
- Motor (4)
- Somatosensory (3, 1, 2)
- Wernicke's area
- Vestibular
- Somatosensory association (5, 7)
- Visual (17)
- (19) (18)
- Visual association
- Second somatosensory
- Auditory (41)
- Auditory association (42, 22)
- Gustatory

Functional areas and lobes of the cerebrum *(Mosby, 2003)*

Cerezyme, an analog of the human enzyme beta-glucocerebrosiderase used for long-term therapy of Type 1 Gaucher's disease. Brand name for **imiglucerase.**

cerium (Ce) /sir″ē·əm/ [L, *Ceres,* Roman goddess of agriculture], a ductile gray rare earth element. Its atomic number is 58; its atomic mass is 140.13. A compound of cerium, cerium oxalate, is used as a sedative, an antiemetic, and an antitussive.

cerium nitrate, a topical antiseptic used in the treatment of burns to control bacterial and fungal infections.

cerivastatin, an HMG-CoA reductase inhibitor (Baycol) withdrawn from the market in August 2001 after several cases of fatal rhabdomyolysis.

ceroid /sir″oid/ [L, *cera,* wax; Gk, *eidos,* form], a golden, waxy pigment appearing in the cirrhotic livers of some individuals, in the GI tract, in the nervous system, and in the muscles. It is an insoluble, acid-fast, sudanophilic pigment.

ceroma /sirō″mə/ *pl. ceromas, ceromata* [L, *cera,* wax; Gk, *oma,* tumor], *(Obsolete)* a neoplasm that has undergone degeneration, causing it to have a waxy consistency.

certifiable /sur″tifī′əbəl/ [L, *certus,* certain, *facere,* to make], **1.** *(Informal)* a term now inappropriately used to refer to an individual with a mental illness. Originally, *certifiable* in a mental health context referred to the incontrovertible presence of mental illness in an individual deemed incompetent by experts. **2.** pertaining to infectious diseases or dangerous conditions that must be reported to local health authorities.

certificate of medical necessity, a prescription, form, or other formal document containing information to provide evidence that durable medical equipment is reasonable and necessary for the diagnosis or treatment of illness or injury or to improve function.

certificate-of-necessity, certificate-of-need (CON), a statement or certificate issued by a governmental agency for proposed construction or modification of a health facility that ensures that the facility will be needed at the time of its completion. The certificate is issued to the individual or group intending to build or modify the facility for additional services. The process is intended to prevent duplication of services in a community.

certification [L, *certus,* certain, *facere,* to make], **1.** a process in which an individual, an institution, or an educational program is evaluated and recognized as meeting certain predetermined standards. Certification is usually made by a nongovernmental agency. The purpose of certification is to ensure that the standards met are those necessary for safe and ethical practice of the profession or service. **2.** (in health care) (in nursing) a process in which the professional organization or association verifies that a person who is licensed has met the standards for specialty practice specified by the profession. The purpose of certification is to assure other professionals and the public that the person has mastered the skills necessary to practice a particular specialty and has acquired the standard body of knowledge common to that specialty. Compare **accreditation.**

certified diabetes educator (CDE), a credential administered by the National Certification Board for Diabetes Educators signifying that a health care professional possesses specialized knowledge and expertise in diabetes self-management education.

certification in nursing, one of two processes in which a professional organization formally recognizes the competence of a nurse to practice a subspecialty of nursing. One process, certification for excellence, bases recognition on professional achievement, advanced education, and superior performance. The second process, entry level certification, bases recognition on advanced education in a program approved by the certifying organization. Criteria vary according to the particular requirements of the professional organization but always require current licensure as a registered nurse and usually include an examination and certain educational or practice requirements. Submission and evaluation of documented clinical practice and a statement of a philosophy of practice may also be required by some professional organizations.

certified dental assistant (CDA) /sur″tifīd/, a person who has successfully completed the education, training, and testing requirements of the Dental Assisting National Board (DANB). See also **dental assistant.**

certified emergency nurse (CEN), a nurse who has had training in emergency nursing and successfully completed an examination given by the Board of Certification of Emergency Nursing based on emergency nursing practice in the United States. To remain certified, a CEN must be reexamined every 4 years (or 8 years if specified educational requirements are met within 4 years).

Certified First Assistant (CFA), **1.** a credential offered by the National Board of Surgical Technology and Surgical Assisting following rigorous training, education, and completion of a program with qualifications specific to the surgical suite. **2.** an individual who has earned the credential of CFA and performs the roles and duties of a surgical assistant. See also **surgical assistant.**

certified medical assistant (CMA [AAMA]), an allied health professional responsible for a variety of administrative and clinical tasks to support physicians, primarily in offices and clinics. Specific duties vary from office to office depending on location, size, specialty, and state law. Certification is provided by the American Association of Medical Assistants following successful completion of an accredited program and a certification examination.

certified medical transcriptionist. See **medical transcriptionist.**

certified milk, raw milk that is obtained, handled, and marketed in compliance with state health laws. The milk must be produced by disease-free cows that are regularly inspected by a veterinarian and are milked by sterilized equipment in hygienic surroundings. It must contain less than a specified low bacterial count. The sale of raw milk is illegal in some states.

certified nurse-midwife (CNM), (according to the American College of Nurse-Midwives) "an individual educated in the two disciplines of nursing and midwifery, who possesses evidence of certification according to the requirements of the American College of Nurse-Midwives. Nurse-midwifery practice is the independent management of care of essentially normal newborns and women, antepartally, intrapartally, postpartally, and/or gynecologically, occurring within a health care system which provides for medical consultation, collaborative management, or referral and is in accord with the qualifications, standards, and functions for the practice of nurse-midwifery as defined by the American College of Nurse-Midwives." See also **midwife.**

certified occupational therapy assistant (COTA), an allied health paraprofessional who supports occupational therapists in providing rehabilitative care to patients with mental, emotional, or physical impairments that prevent them from working or living independently. Occupational therapy assistants aim to help patients recover from, or compensate for, an ailment and resume a productive life. Almost all programs to become an occupational therapy assistant lead to associate's degrees. Certification, licensing, or registration is mandated to work in most states. Some states utilize the certification exam offered by the National Board for Certifying Occupational Therapy for licensure.

certified registered nurse anesthetist (CRNA), an advanced practice nurse who provides anesthesia care to patients in solo practice settings or as a member of the anesthesia team model for all types of surgeries and procedures. The certified registered nurse anesthetist (CRNA) has completed postgraduate education and passed a national certification examination. See also **nurse anesthetist.**

Certified Registered Nurse Infusion (CRNI®), a certification offered by the Infusion Nurses Certification Corporation (INCC) to indicate a registered nurse has attained a specialized level of practice in providing infusion therapy to patients, including collaboration in the safe administration of intravenous medications.

certified respiratory therapist (CRT), a health care professional who performs routine care, management, and treatment of patients with respiratory disorders. Certification requires completion of an approved training course and passing an examination by the National Board for Respiratory Care.

Certified Surgical Technologist (CST), 1. credential offered by the National Board of Surgical Technology and Surgical Assisting. **2.** an allied health professional who as a member of the surgical team is responsible for providing an optimal surgical environment by performing perioperative duties, including preparing the operating room; gathering necessary equipment and supplies; opening sterile supplies; preparing the sterile field including the back table and Mayo stand set-ups; performing counts; assisting in applying sterile drapes; anticipating the needs of the surgeon during the procedure; passing instrumentation and supplies to the surgeon; caring for specimens; applying sterile dressings; and preparing the O.R. for the next procedure. CSTs are experts in aseptic technique and constantly ensure that all members of the surgical team adhere to the principles of aseptic technique.

certify /sur″tifī/, **1.** to guarantee formally that certain requirements based on expert knowledge of significant, pertinent facts have been met. **2.** to attest, by a legal process, that someone is insane. **3.** to attest to the fact of someone's death in writing, usually on a form required by a local authority. **4.** to declare that a person has satisfied certain requirements for membership or acceptance into a professional or other group. See also **board certification. −certification,** *n.*

Cerubidine, an antineoplastic drug. Brand name for *DAUNOrubicin hydrochloride.*

cerulean /sirōō″lē·ən/ [L, *caelum,* sky], sky-blue in color.

ceruloplasmin /sirōō′lōplaz″min/ [L, *caelum,* sky; Gk, *plassein,* to shape], a blue glycoprotein in plasma that transports 96% of the plasma copper. A major decrease is seen in Wilson's disease.

cerumen /sirōō″mən/ [L, *cera,* wax], a yellowish or brownish waxy secretion produced by vestigial apocrine sweat glands in the external ear canal; it is a mixture of secretions and sloughed epithelial cells. It is typically expelled from the ear canal spontaneously. Also called **earwax.** See also **ceruminosis.**

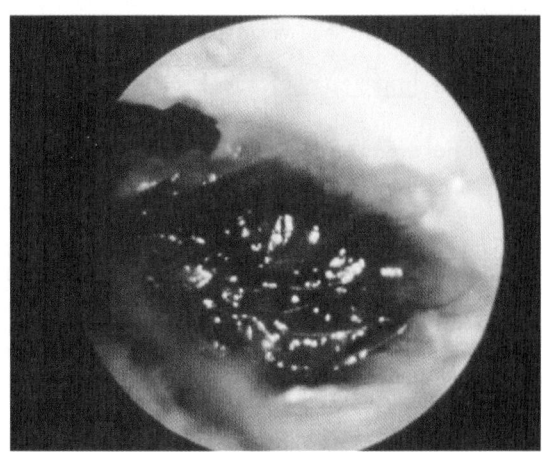

Cerumen *(Siglar, 1994)*

cerumen impaction. See **ceruminosis.**

ceruminolytic agent [L, *cera,* wax; Gk, *lysis,* a loosening; L, *agere,* to do], a medication that dissolves or loosens cerumen (earwax) to allow for its removal.

ceruminoma /serōō′minō″mə/, an adenocarcinoma in the external auditory meatus.

ceruminosis /sirōō′minō″sis/, excessive buildup of cerumen (earwax) in the external auditory canal. It can cause discomfort, symptoms of hearing loss, tinnitus, dizziness, or local irritation leading to the development of infection. Removal of excess cerumen is accomplished by the local use of a wax-softening agent by a health care professional, followed by careful flushing with an ear syringe if the tympanic membrane is intact. Impacted cerumen can occlude the canal or press against the tympanic membrane and is often seen in those who use cotton swabs, hearing aids, or earplugs, or in people with an ear canal anatomic abnormality. A cerumen spoon is sometimes used to scoop out hardened collections of wax. Also called **cerumen impaction.**

ceruminous /sirōō″minəs/, pertaining to earwax.

ceruminous gland, one of a number of tiny structures in the external ear canal, believed to be modified sweat glands. They secrete a waxy cerumen instead of watery sweat.

cervic-, prefix meaning "neck": *cervicitis, cervicodynia.*

cervical /sur″vikəl/ [L, *cervix,* neck], **1.** pertaining to the neck or the region of the neck. **2.** pertaining to the constricted area of a necklike structure, such as the neck of a tooth or the cervix of the uterus.

cervical abortion [L, *cervix* + *ab,* away from, *oriri,* to be born], spontaneous expulsion of an ectopic cervical pregnancy. See also **ectopic pregnancy.**

cervical adenitis [L, *cervix* + Gk, *aden,* gland, *itis,* inflammation], an abnormal condition characterized by enlarged, tender lymph nodes of the neck. It often occurs in association with acute infections of the throat. Most lymph nodes respond well to oral antibiotic treatment targeting the infectious agent. However, some may need to be opened and drained. Children often present with associated fever.

cervical amputation, the removal of the neck (cervix) of the uterus.

cervical artery, an artery that supplies the muscles of the neck.

cervical biopsy, the removal of cervical tissue for microscopic examination to diagnose chronic cervical infection or cervical cancer.

cervical canal, the canal within the uterine cervix, which protrudes into the vagina. The uterine end of the canal is closed at the internal os and, in the nullipara, at the distal end by the external os. The canal is a passageway through which the menstrual flow escapes and, vastly dilated and effaced by labor, through which the infant must pass to be delivered vaginally. Various diagnostic and therapeutic procedures require dilation of the muscular cervix surrounding the canal, including endometrial biopsy, suction and surgical curettage, and radium implantation. Pelvic inflammatory disease is the result of the entry of pathogenic bacteria into the uterus through the cervical canal. Sperm must travel upward through the canal to reach the uterus and fallopian tubes.

cervical cancer, a neoplasm of the uterine cervix that can be detected in the early, curable stage by the Papanicolaou (Pap) test. The exact cause is unknown, but factors that may be associated with the development of cervical cancer are coitus at an early age, relations with many sexual partners, genital herpesvirus infections (such as cytomegalovirus), human papillomavirus (HPV), multiparity, and poor obstetric and gynecological care. Cervical dysplasia may regress, persist, or progress to clinical disease, but carcinoma in situ is considered to be a precursor of invasive carcinoma. About 90% of cervical tumors are squamous cell carcinomas, fewer than 10% are adenocarcinomas, and others are mixtures of these kinds, or, in rare cases, sarcomas. Cervical cancer invades the tissues of adjacent organs and may metastasize through lymphatic channels to distant sites, including the lungs, bone, liver, brain, and paraaortic nodes.

■ OBSERVATIONS: Early cervical neoplasia is usually asymptomatic, but there may be a watery vaginal discharge or occasional spotting of blood; advanced lesions may cause a dark, foul-smelling vaginal discharge, leakage from bladder or rectal fistulas, anorexia, weight loss, and back and leg pains. Pap smears of cervical cells are highly important in screening, but definitive diagnoses are based on colposcopic examination and cytological study of specimens obtained by biopsy.

■ INTERVENTIONS: Treatment depends on the kind and the extent of the malignancy, the age of the woman, and her general health. Also considered are her wishes in regard to maintaining her reproductive function. Carcinoma in situ may be treated by excisional conization or cryosurgery. Invasive tumors may be treated with radiotherapy or hysterectomy. Chemotherapy has a mainly palliative role.

■ PATIENT CARE CONSIDERATIONS: Vaccination against HPV types 16 and 18, which are responsible for most cervical cancer cases, is now recommended for young women as a preventive measure.

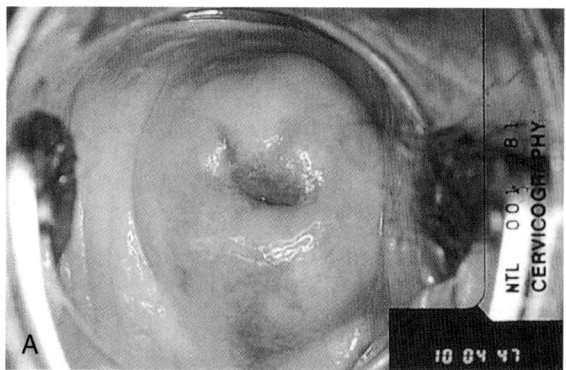
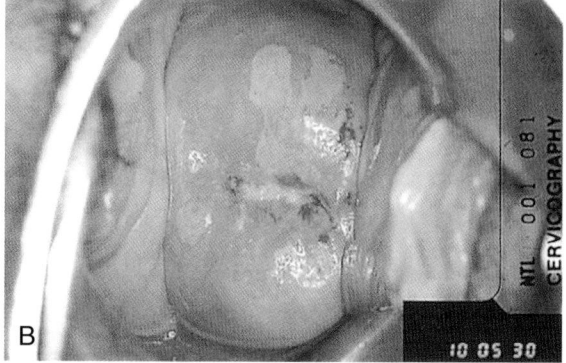
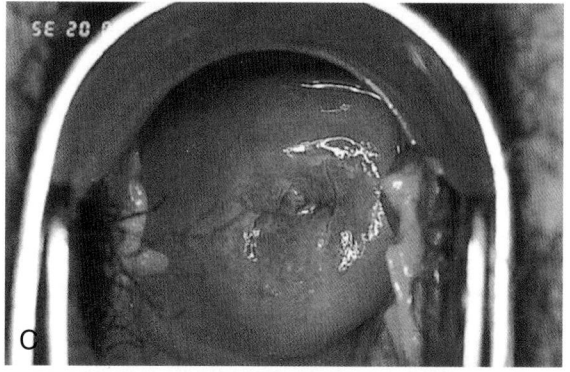
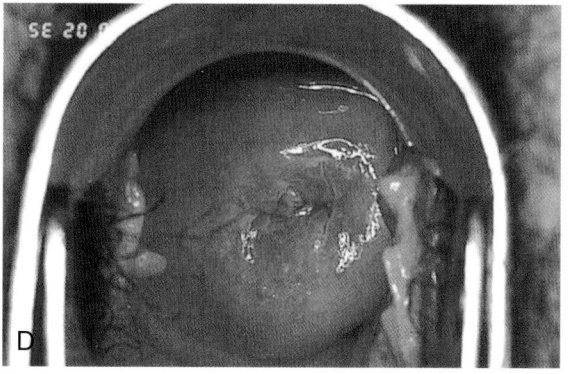

Cervical cancer *(Symonds and McPherson, 1994)*

cervical cap, a mechanical cap fitted over the cervix to provide barrier contraception, preventing sperm from entering the cervical canal. See also **barrier methods.**

cervical cauterization, the destruction of abnormal cervical tissues using heat, electricity, or freezing. Most commonly used for the treatment of cervical dysplasia and symptomatic benign cervical cysts.

cervical conization, the excision of a cone-shaped tissue section from the endocervix, performed to obtain a tissue sample to establish a precise diagnosis. It may be performed with a scalpel or laser ("cold knife" technique) or with a wire loop heated electrically (large loop excision). See also **cone biopsy.**

cervical cyst [L, *cervix,* neck; GK, *kystis,* bag], any benign cystic lesion on the endocervix or exocervix. See **nabothian cyst.**

cervical dilation /dil′ā″shən/ [L, *dilatare,* to widen], the diameter of the opening of the cervix in labor as measured on vaginal examination. It is expressed in centimeters or finger breadths; one finger breadth is approximately 2 cm. At full dilation the diameter of the cervical opening is 10 cm.

Primigravida

Before labor

Early effacement

Complete effacement

Complete dilation

Cervical dilation *(McKinney et al, 2009)*

cervical disk syndrome, an abnormal condition characterized by compression or irritation of the cervical nerve roots in or near the intervertebral foramina before the roots divide into the anterior and posterior rami. When it is caused by ruptured intervertebral disks, degenerative cervical disk disease, or cervical injuries, it may produce varying degrees of malalignment, causing nerve root compression. Most cervical disk syndromes are caused by injuries that involve hyperextension. Edema usually occurs in all cases of cervical disk syndrome. Nonsurgical intervention, which is usually

a successful treatment, may include immobilization of the cervical vertebrae to decrease irritation and to provide rest for the traumatized area. Other treatment may include special exercises, heat therapy, and intermittent traction. Mild analgesics are usually successful in controlling the pain associated with cervical disk syndrome, especially when used with immobilization. Surgery is recommended only when signs and symptoms persist despite nonsurgical treatment. The prognosis for this condition is usually good, but recurrence of symptoms is common. Also called **cervical root syndrome.** See also **herniated disk, whiplash injury.**

■ OBSERVATIONS: Pain, the most common symptom, usually emanates from the cervical area but may radiate down the arm to the fingers and increase with cervical motion. The pain may increase sharply with coughing, sneezing, or any radical movement. Other signs and symptoms may be paresthesia, headache, blurred vision, decreased skeletal function, and weakened hand grip. Physical examination may reveal varying degrees of muscular atrophy, sensory abnormalities, muscular weakness, and decreased reflexes. Radiographic examination may show a loss of normal lordosis associated with the cervical vertebrae and may also reveal some minor malalignment of the vertebrae.

■ INTERVENTIONS: Nonsurgical intervention, which is usually a successful treatment, may include immobilization of the cervical vertebrae to decrease irritation and to provide rest for the traumatized area. Other treatment may include special exercises, heat therapy, and intermittent traction. Mild analgesics are usually successful in controlling the pain associated with cervical disk syndrome, especially when used with immobilization. Surgery is recommended only when signs and symptoms persist despite nonsurgical treatment.

■ PATIENT CARE CONSIDERATIONS: The prognosis for this condition is usually good, but recurrence of symptoms is common.

cervical dysplasia, atypical squamous or columnar tissues of the cervix that may slowly progress to carcinoma; associated with HPV infection. See also **human papillomavirus, cervical cancer.**

cervical erosion [L, *cervix + erodere,* to consume], a condition in which the squamous epithelium of the cervix is abraded as a result of irritation caused by infection or trauma such as childbirth and replaced by columnar epithelium.

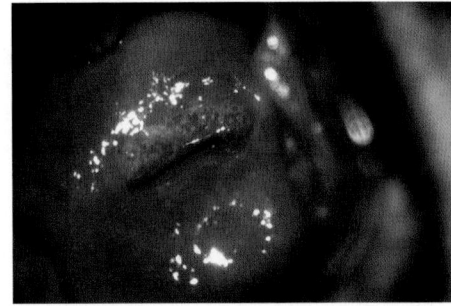

Cervical erosion *(Greer et al, 2001)*

cervical fistula, an abnormal passage from the cervix to the vagina or bladder. It may be caused by a malignant lesion, radiotherapy, surgical trauma, or injury during childbirth. A cervical fistula communicating with the bladder permits leakage of urine, causing irritation, odor, and embarrassment.

cervical infertility, female factor infertility caused by abnormal interaction between the sperm and the cervical mucus.

cervical intraepithelial neoplasia (CIN) /in′trə·ep′ithē
″lē·əl/, abnormal changes in the basal layers of the squamous epithelial tissues of the uterus. The disorder is graded according to its pathological progress, from CIN1 to CIN3; CIN3 represents carcinoma of the cervix. The disorder is associated with human papillomaviruses. See also **human papillomavirus.**

cervical lordosis, the dorsally concave curvature of the cervical spinal column when seen from the side.

cervical mucus, a secretion of the columnar epithelium lining the upper portion of the cervical canal of the uterus. The mucus that is secreted by endocervical glands changes in appearance and consistency throughout the menstrual cycle. For the first few days after menstruation, little mucus is secreted. As ovulation approaches, increasing amounts of sticky cloudy-white or yellowish secretions are seen. Around the time of ovulation, the volume of mucus increases, and it becomes clear, slippery, and elastic, resembling the uncooked white of an egg. After ovulation the mucus becomes cloudy, thick, sticky, and progressively less profuse until menstruation supervenes to begin the cycle again. It forms the endocervical "plug" in pregnancy, which when released causes "bloody show." See also **mucous plug, ovulation method of family planning.**

cervical mucus method of family planning, a type of natural family planning that relies on inspection of the cervical mucus. See also **contraception, ovulation method of family planning.**

cervical nerves [L, *cervix,* neck, *nervus,* nerve], the eight pairs of spinal nerves that arise from the cervical segments of the spinal cord, from above the atlas to below the seventh vertebra. The first four supply the head and neck, and the other four mainly innervate the upper limbs, scalp, and back. See also **cervical plexus.**

cervical os. See **external cervical os, internal cervical os.**

cervical pleura, the dome-shaped layer of parietal pleura lining the cervical extension of the pleural cavity. Also called **dome of pleura, pleural cupola.**

cervical plexus, the network of nerves formed by the ventral primary divisions of the first four cervical nerves. Each nerve, except the first, divides into the superior branch and the inferior branch, and both branches unite to form three loops. The plexus is located opposite the cranial aspect of the first four cervical vertebrae. It communicates with certain cranial nerves and numerous muscular and cutaneous branches.

cervical plexus block, anesthetic nerve block at any point below the mastoid process from the second cervical vertebra to the sixth cervical vertebra. This method is used for operations on the area between the jaw and clavicle, such as for carotid endarterectomy. Complications may include Horner's syndrome, inadvertent stellate ganglion or brachial plexus block, vertebral artery bleeding or infection, subarachnoid or peridural penetration, phrenic nerve block or palsy manifested by respiratory failure, or laryngeal nerve block, manifested by sudden hoarseness.

cervical polyp [L, *cervix* + Gk, *polys,* mean, *pous,* foot], an outgrowth of columnar epithelial tissue of the endocervical canal, usually attached to the canal wall by a slender pedicle. Often there are no symptoms, but multiple or abraded polyps may cause bleeding, especially with contact during coitus. Treatment of a symptomatic polyp is excision.

cervical radiculopathy, disease of the cervical nerve roots, often manifesting as neck or shoulder pain.

cervical regions, the various anatomical regions of the neck, including anterior, lateral, and posterior cervical regions and the region over the sternocleidomastoid muscle.

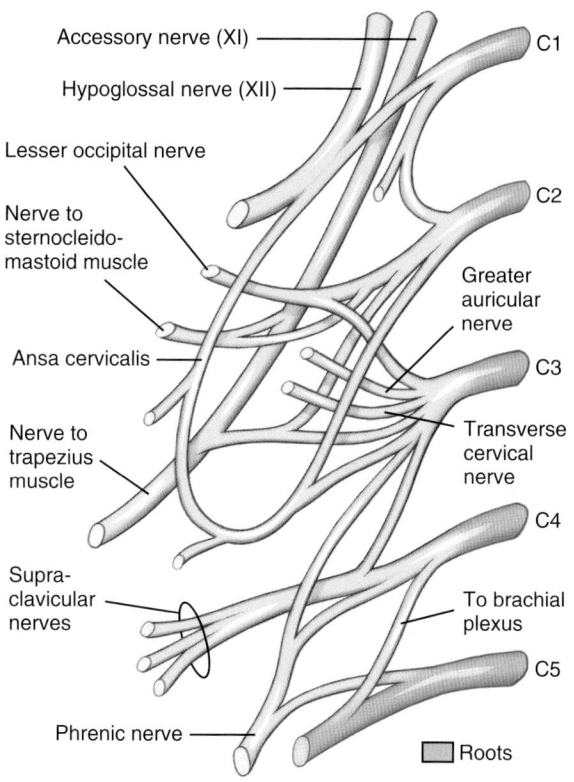

Accessory nerve (XI)　　C1
Hypoglossal nerve (XII)
Lesser occipital nerve
C2
Nerve to sternocleido-mastoid muscle
Greater auricular nerve
Ansa cervicalis
C3
Nerve to trapezius muscle
Transverse cervical nerve
C4
Supra-clavicular nerves
To brachial plexus
C5
Phrenic nerve
Roots

Cervical plexus

cervical rib, a supernumerary rib that articulates with a cervical vertebra, usually the seventh, but does not reach the sternum.

cervical root syndrome. See **cervical disk syndrome.**

cervical smear [L, *cervix* + AS, *smero,* grease], a small amount of the secretions and superficial cells of the cervix, secured from the external os of the cervix with a sterile applicator or special small wooden or plastic spatula. For a Papanicolaou's smear, it is obtained from the squamocolumnar junction of the uterine cervix and from the vaginal vault and endocervical canal. The specimen is spread on a labeled glass slide and sent for cytological examination. For bacteriological culture and identification, only the applicator is used; the specimen is spread on a glass slide and stained and examined under a microscope or placed in or on a culture medium and sent to a bacteriological laboratory for culture and identification.

cervical spinal fusion, surgery to relieve severe neck pain, as well as pain in shoulders, arms, and hands, caused by abnormal movement or adjustment of adjacent vertebrae, a pinched nerve, or spinal compression. The adjacent vertebrae are joined with metal devices and/or a bone graft made from human bone or a ceramic material. An anterior or posterior surgical approach may be used.

cervical spine (C-spine), that portion of the spine comprising the cervical vertebrae.

cervical spondylosis [L, *cervix* + Gk, *spondylos,* vertebra, *osis,* condition], a form of degenerative joint and disk disease affecting the cervical vertebrae and resulting in compression of the associated nerve roots. Symptoms include pain or loss of feeling in the affected arm and shoulder and stiffness of the cervical spine.

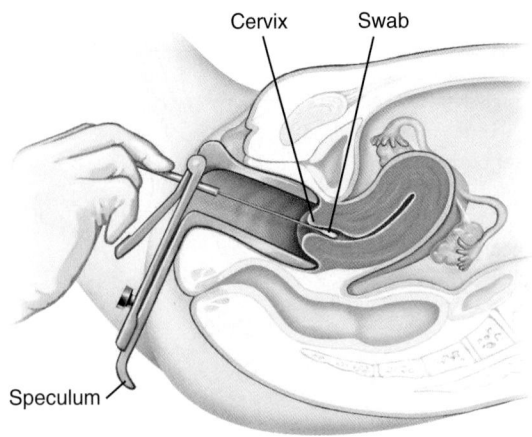

Cervix Swab

Speculum

Obtaining a cervical smear

cervical stenosis [L, *cervix* + Gk, *stenos,* narrow, *osis,* condition], a narrowing or complete closure of the canal between the body of the uterus and the cervical os (endocervical canal).

cervical tenaculum. See **tenaculum.**

cervical traction, a system of traction applied to the cervical spine by applying a force to lift the head.

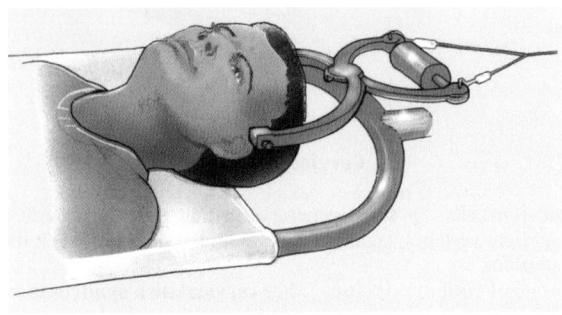

Cervical traction *(Bowden et al, 1998)*

cervical triangle, one of two triangular areas formed in the neck by the oblique course of the sternocleidomastoid muscle. The anterior triangle is bounded by the midline of the throat anteriorly, the sternocleidomastoid laterally, and the body of the mandible superiorly. The posterior triangle is bounded by the clavicle inferiorly and by the borders of the sternocleidomastoid and the trapezius superiorly.

cervical vertebra (C), one of the first seven segments of the vertebral column. They differ from the thoracic and lumbar vertebrae through the presence of a vertical costotransverse foramen in each transverse process. The first cervical vertebra (atlas) has no body, supports the head, and contains a smooth, oval facet for articulation with the dens of the second cervical vertebra. The dens extends from the cranial portion of the body of the second cervical vertebra (axis), which has a very large, strong spinous process with a bifid extremity. The seventh cervical vertebra has a very long, prominent spinous process that is nearly horizontal and is often used as a palpable reference for locating the other cervical vertebrae. The bodies of the four remaining cervical vertebrae are small, oval, and broader than the other three in transverse diameter and contain large, triangular foramina within their transverse processes. Their spinous processes are short

and bifid. Compare **coccygeal vertebra, lumbar vertebra, sacral vertebra, thoracic vertebra.** See also **vertebra.**

cervicitis /sur′visī″tis/, inflammation of the cervix, usually associated with bacterial vaginosis, trichomoniasis, or candidiasis. May be asymptomatic or associated with often foul-smelling, purulent discharge. Often recurrent due to reexposure. Diagnosis is by microscopic evaluation of the discharge and/or culture. Cervicitis is treated with an appropriate antibiotic or sometimes cautery. Kinds include **acute cervicitis, chronic cervicitis.**

cervico-, prefix meaning "neck": *cervicodynia, cervicolabial.*

cervicodynia /sur′vikōdin″ē·ə/, pain in the neck; discomfort in the upper cervical posterior area. Also called **trachelodynia.**

cervicogenic dorsalgia, upper back pain caused by a cervical spine disorder.

cervicogenic headache, (in chiropractic) a condition in which headaches, particularly those classified as muscle tension headaches involving referred pain, are the result of cervical subluxations.

cervicogenicity dysfunction /-jenis″itē/, (in chiropractic) a syndrome of hypomobility, tender points in soft tissues, reduced regional ranges of cervical motion, and static misalignment.

cervicogenic sympathetic syndrome, (in chiropractic) any of a large group of bodily disorders involving the cervical spine and the associated sympathetic trunk of nerve fibers. The effects usually include causalgia and reflex sympathetic dystrophy.

cervicolabial /sur′vikōlā″bē·əl/ [L, *cervix* + *labium,* lip], pertaining to or situated on the lip side of the neck of an incisor or a canine tooth.

cervicoplasty /sur″vikōplas′tē/, **1.** plastic surgery performed on either the uterine cervix or the neck. **2.** the removal of excess skin on the neck; also known as a neck lift.

cervicothoracic /-thôras″ik/, pertaining to the neck and thorax.

cervicothoracic ganglion. See **stellate ganglion.**

cervicouterine /sur′vikōyoo″tərin/, pertaining to or situated at the cervix of the uterus.

cervicovaginitis /-vaj′inītis/, an inflammation of the cervix and vagina.

cervicovesical /sur′vikōves″ikəl/ [L, *cervix* + *vesica,* bladder], pertaining to the cervix of the uterus and the bladder.

cervix /sur″viks/ *pl. cervices cervixes,* the part of the uterus that lies partly in the vagina and partly in the pelvic cavity, joining the body (corpus) of the uterus at a narrow junction termed the isthmus. The cervix in a healthy woman who has not had children is a cylinder 2 to 3 cm in length, while the corpus is 7 to 8 cm in length and 4 to 5 cm in width, roughly pear shaped. The outer part of the cervix (the exocervix) is composed of squamous cells, changing at the squamocolumnar junction into columnar glandular cells (the endocervix) leading into the corpus. During labor the cervix thins (effacement) and opens (dilates), allowing the fetus to be born. Also called **neck of uterus.** See also **effacement, endocervix.**

ceryl alcohol /sē″ril/ [L, *cera,* wax; Ar, *alkohl,* essence], a fatty alcohol present in many waxes. Also called **hexacosanol.**

Cesamet, a synthetic cannabinoid. Brand name for **nabilone.**

cesarean hysterectomy /sizer″ē·ən/ [L, *Caesarlex,* Caesar's law; Gk, *hystera,* womb, *ektomē,* excision], a surgical operation in which the uterus is removed at the time of cesarean section. It is performed most often for complications of cesarean section, usually intractable hemorrhage.

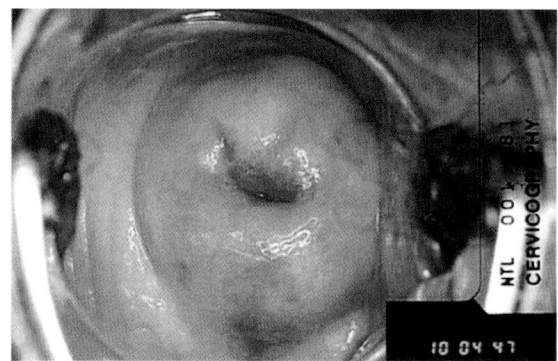

Cervix *(Symonds and Mcpherson, 1994)*

Less often it is done to treat preexisting gynecological disease, such as an intraepithelial cervical neoplasia or cancer.

cesarean section (CS) [L, *Caesarlex,* Caesar's law, *sectio*], a surgical procedure in which the uterus is opened by a transverse incision in the lower uterine segment (lower segment transverse cesarean section, LSTCS) or a vertical incision through the corpus of the uterus (classical cesarean section, vertical cesarean section) to deliver a baby. The abdomen may be opened by either a transverse or vertical incision. Maternal indications for a cesarean section include protraction and descent disorders (dysfunctional labor) and abnormal placental position (e.g., placenta previa) or premature separation of the placenta during labor (e.g., abruptio placenta). Fetal indications include breech, transverse, or other noncephalic presentations and evidence of a nonreassuring fetal status (formerly called fetal distress). After cesarean section a trial of labor is usually appropriate in a subsequent pregnancy. See also **classic cesarean section, extraperitoneal cesarean section, low cervical cesarean section.**

cesium (Cs) /sē′zē-əm/ [L, *caesius,* sky blue], an alkali metal element. Its atomic number is 55; its atomic mass is 132.9. Like other alkali metals, cesium emits electrons when exposed to visible light and is used in photoelectric cells and in television cameras. Also spelled **caesium.**

cesium-137 (^{137}Cs), a radioactive material with a half-life of 30.2 years that is used in radiotherapy as a sealed source of gamma rays intended for application to various malignancies that are treated by brachytherapy. Cesium has replaced radium for such applications. See also **brachytherapy.**

cesspool fever. *(Slang)* See **typhoid fever.**

cestode. See **tapeworm.**

cestode infection, cestodiasis. See **tapeworm infection.**

cestoid /ses″toid/ [Gk, *kestos,* girdle, *eidos,* form], **1.** cestodelike, or resembling a tapeworm. **2.** a class of platyhelminth flatworms of the Cestoda subclass, usually found in the small intestine.

Cetacaine, a fixed-combination anesthetic spray, containing several local anesthetics, applied to mucous membranes. Brand name for **benzocaine**, *butyl aminobenzoate,* **tetracaine hydrochloride.**

cetirizine, an H1-histamine antagonist.

■ INDICATIONS: It is used to treat allergy symptoms and rhinitis.

■ CONTRAINDICATIONS: Known hypersensitivity to this drug, lactation, and severe hepatic disease prohibit its use. It also should not be used in newborns or premature infants.

■ ADVERSE EFFECTS: Life-threatening effects include hemolytic anemia, thrombocytopenia, leukopenia, agranulocytosis, pancytopenia, and dysrhythmias (rare). Other serious adverse effects include urinary retention, impotence, diarrhea, vomiting, sedation, confusion, blurred vision, tremors, hypotension, palpitations, bradycardia, and tachycardia. Common side effects are thickening of bronchial secretions, nausea, drowsiness, and headache.

cetrorelix /set″rorel′iks/, a gonadotropin-releasing hormone antagonist used to inhibit premature luteinizing hormone surges in women undergoing controlled ovarian stimulation during infertility treatment, administered subcutaneously.

cetuximab, a miscellaneous, antineoplastic, monoclonal antibody that inhibits epidermal growth factor receptors.

■ INDICATIONS: This drug is used alone or in combination with irinotecan for epidermal growth factor receptors expressing metastatic colorectal carcinoma.

■ CONTRAINDICATIONS: Known hypersensitivity to this drug or murine proteins prohibits its use.

■ ADVERSE EFFECTS: Adverse effects of this drug include rash, pruritus, acne, and dry skin. Life-threatening side effects include leukopenia, anemia, toxic epidermal necrolysis, angioedema, renal failure, interstitial lung disease, pulmonary embolus, anaphylaxis, sepsis, and infection. Common side effects include headache, insomnia, depression, nausea, diarrhea, vomiting, anorexia, mouth ulceration, dehydration, constipation, abdominal pain, blepharitis, cheilitis, cellulitis, cysts, alopecia, skin or nail disorder, conjunctivitis, asthma, malaise, fever, back pain, cough, dyspnea, and peripheral edema.

cetyl alcohol ($C_{16}H_{33}OH$) /sē′til/ [L, *cetus,* whale; Ar, *alkohl,* essence], a fatty alcohol derived from spermaceti, used as an emulsifier and stiffening agent in creams and ointments. Also called **hexadecanol, palmityl alcohol.**

cetyl palmitate, esters of cetyl alcohol and saturated high–molecular-weight fatty acids, principally palmitic acid, used as an emulsifying and stiffening agent.

cetylpyridinium chloride /sē′təlpī′ridin″ē-əm/, an antiinfective used as a preservative in pharmaceutic preparations and as a topical cleanser and local anesthetic (Cepacol). It is inactivated by soap, serum, and tissue fluids; therefore, the surface of the skin must be clean and well rinsed.

■ INDICATIONS: It is prescribed prophylactically to prevent infection of the skin or mucous membranes.

■ CONTRAINDICATIONS: Known hypersensitivity to this drug is the only contraindication.

CEU, abbreviation for **continuing education unit.**

cevimeline /sevim′älēn/, a cholinergic agonist used as the hydrochloride salt in the treatment of xerostomia associated with Sjögren's syndrome; administered orally.

cevitamic acid. See **ascorbic acid.**

Cf, symbol for the element **californium.**

CF, abbreviation for **cystic fibrosis.**

CFA, abbreviation for **Certified First Assistant.**

cg, abbreviation for **centigram.**

CGD, abbreviation for **chronic granulomatous disease.**

cGMP, abbreviation for **cyclic guanosine monophosphate.**

cgs, CGS, abbreviation for **centimeter-gram-second system.**

cGy, abbreviation for **centigray.**

C_2H_2, chemical formula for **acetylene.**

C_2H_4, chemical formula for **ethylene.**

C_6H_6, chemical formula for **benzene.**

Ch1, symbol for **Christchurch chromosome.**

Chaddock reflex [Charles G. Chaddock, American neurologist, 1861–1936], an abnormal reflex, induced by firmly stroking the ulnar surface of the forearm, characterized by flexion of the wrist and extension of the fingers in fanlike position. It is seen on the affected side in hemiplegia.

Compare **Gordon's reflex, Oppenheim reflex.** See also **Babinski reflex.**

Chaddock sign [Charles G. Chaddock], a variation of Babinski reflex elicited by firmly stroking the side of the foot just distal to the lateral malleolus, characterized by extension of the great toe and fanning of the other toes. It is seen in pyramidal tract disease. See also **Babinski reflex.**

Chadwick's sign /chad″wiks/ [James R. Chadwick, American gynecologist, 1844–1905], a sign of pregnancy that develops after the sixth week and consists of a dark bluish or purplish-red vaginal or cervical mucosa as a result of increased blood supply to the area.

chafe [L, *calefacere,* to make warm], to irritate the skin by friction, such as when rough material rubs against an unprotected area of the body.

chafing, superficial irritation of the skin by friction.

Chagas disease /chag′əs/ [Carlos Chagas, Brazilian physician, 1879–1934], a protozoal infection caused by *Trypanosoma cruzi,* transmitted to humans by certain species of bloodsucking reduviid (triatomine) bugs, which are found only in the Americas and mainly in poorer areas of Latin America. Also called **American trypanosomiasis, Brazilian trypanosomiasis, South American trypanosomiasis, Cruz trypanosomiasis,** *Trypanosoma cruzi, Chagas-Cruz disease.* See also **trypanosomiasis.**

■ OBSERVATIONS: The most recognized sign of acute infection, which is common in children and rare in adults, is a swelling of the eyelids on the side of the face near the insect bite, known as Romaña's sign. The acute form is also marked by a lesion at the site of the bite, fever, weakness, enlarged spleen and lymph nodes, edema of the face and legs, and tachycardia. This form resolves within 4 months unless complications, such as encephalitis, develop. The chronic form may be manifested by cardiomyopathy or by dilation of the esophagus or colon. Often, infections are asymptomatic.

■ INTERVENTIONS: Treatment with nifurtimox and benznidazole is, at best, only partially effective.

■ PATIENT CARE CONSIDERATIONS: It may occur in acute or chronic form, both of which can be asymptomatic or life threatening. Natural reservoirs include dogs, armadillos, and rodents.

Chagres fever /chag′ris/ [Chagres River, Panama; L, *febris*], a phlebotomus arbovirus infection transmitted to humans through the bite of a sandfly. The disease is rarely fatal and is characterized by fever, headache, and muscle pains of the chest or abdomen. There may be nausea and vomiting, giddiness, weakness, photophobia, and pain on moving the eyes. The infection usually subsides within a week. Supportive treatment includes analgesics, bed rest, and adequate fluid intake. The disease is most common in Central America. Also called **Panama fever.**

chain [L, *catena*], **1.** a length of several units linked together in a linear pattern, such as a polypeptide chain of amino acids or a chain of atoms forming a chemical molecule. **2.** a group of individual bacteria linked together, such as streptococci formed by a chain of cocci. **3.** the serial relationship of certain structures essential to function, such as the chain of ossicles in the middle ear. Each of the small bones moves successively in response to vibration of the tympanic membrane, thus transmitting the auditory stimulus to the oval window. **4.** a connected series, such as a chain of events.

chaining, a system of learning behaviors in which each response is a stimulus for the next response.

chain reaction, **1.** (in chemistry) a reaction that proceeds through one or more reactive intermediates; one of the required reactive intermediates (usually free radicals) is formed in each step of the reaction. Examples include the polymerization of organic monomers into plastics or in the free radical halogenation of hydrocarbons. **2.** (in physics) a reaction that perpetuates itself by the proliferating fission of nuclei and the release of atomic particles that cause more nuclear fissions.

chain reflex, a series of reflexes, each stimulated by the preceding one.

chalasia /kəlā″zhə/ [Gk, *chalasis,* relaxation], abnormal relaxation or incompetence of the cardiac sphincter of the stomach, resulting in reflux of the gastric contents into the esophagus with subsequent regurgitation. Conservative treatment in infancy includes feeding several small meals a day to prevent distension of the stomach and holding the baby upright while giving the feeding. The symptoms and treatment are similar to those of a hiatal hernia. See also **gastroesophageal reflux.**

chalazion /kəlā″zion/ [Gk, hailstone], a small, nonmalignant, localized swelling of the eyelid resulting from obstruction and retained secretions of the meibomian glands. Treatment can include warm wet compresses, but the condition often requires surgery for correction. Compare **hordeolum, sty.**

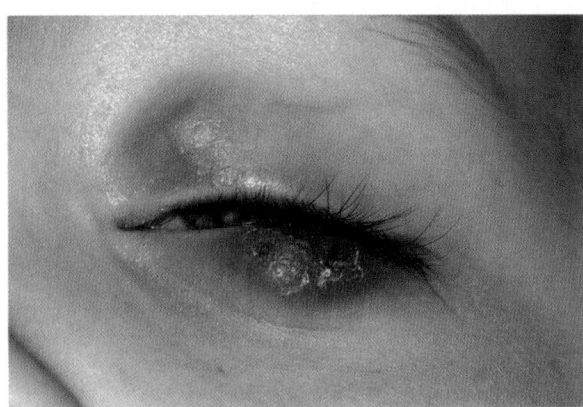

Chalazion *(Albert and Miller, 2008)*

chalice cell. See **goblet cell.**

chalicosis /kal′ikō″sis/, a type of fibrosis that results from the inhalation of impure calcium dusts. Pure calcium dusts are soluble and are absorbed. Calcium dusts from marble, limestone, or Portland cement usually do not cause fibrosis. Respiratory impairment is generally caused by the presence of free silica in the calcium dust.

chalkitis /kalkī″tis/ [Gk, *chalkos,* brass, *itis,* inflammation], deposits of copper in the ocular tissue that cause inflammation of the eyes and result from rubbing the eyes with the hands after touching or handling brass. Also called **brassy eye.**

challenge, **1.** a method of testing the sensitivity of an individual to a hormone, allergen, or other substance by administering a sample. A small amount may be injected to determine whether the immune system will react by producing appropriate antibodies. **2.** a term used to describe the rapid or concentrated infusion of a substance such as potassium or magnesium in the face of a life-threatening deficiency or rapid infusion of IV fluid to differentiate between fluid deficit or renal failure as the cause of severely decreased urine output. **3.** a physical or mental/emotional obstacle.

chalone /kā″lōn/ [Gk, *chalan,* to relax], any one of numerous polypeptide inhibitors that are elaborated by a tissue and function like hormones on specific target organs.

chamaeprosopy /kam′əpros″əpē/ [Gk, *chamai,* low, *prosopon,* face], a facial appearance characterized by a low brow and a broad face. *−chamaeprosopic, adj.*

chamber [Gk, *kamara,* vaulted enclosure], **1.** a hollow but not necessarily empty space or cavity in an organ, as in the anterior and posterior chambers of the eye or the atrial and ventricular chambers of the heart. **2.** a room or closed space used for research or therapeutic purposes, such as a decompression chamber or hyperbaric oxygen chamber.

Chamberlain's line [W.E. Chamberlain, American radiologist, 1891–1947], a line that extends from the posterior of the hard palate to the dorsum of the foramen magnum.

Chinese medicine, the diverse body of medical theory and practice that has evolved in China, comprising four branches: acupuncture and moxibustion, herbal medicine, qi gong, and tui na. Although Chinese medicine encompasses a variety of theory and practice, all of its forms share certain underlying characteristics. The body and mind are considered together as a dynamic system subject to cycles of change and affected by the environment, and emphasis is on supporting the body's self-healing ability. Fundamental to Chinese medicine are the yin-yang principle and the concept of basic substances that pervade the body: qi, jing (essence), and shen (spirit), collectively known as the three treasures, and the blood (a fluid and material manifestation of qi) and body fluids (which moisten and lubricate the body). Disease arises from a disturbance of qi within the body, the particular pathological process depending on the location of the disturbance; causes are classified into three groups, external (which are environmental), internal (emotions), and miscellaneous (such as diet, fatigue, or trauma). Diagnosis is by visual assessment, listening and smelling, questioning, and palpation; a single biomedical disease may be associated with a large number of Chinese medicine diagnoses, and one diagnosis in Chinese medicine may encompass a number of biomedical diseases. Once a diagnosis is established, therapy aims at restoring the body's homeostasis by treating the root cause of the disease.

Chamberlen forceps [Peter Chamberlen, English obstetrician, 1560–1631], *(Obsolete)* one of the earliest kinds of obstetric forceps, introduced in the 17th century.

chamfer /cham′fər/, the finish line on an extracoronal cavity preparation for a crown restoration in which the junction between the crown and the remaining tooth structure is formed to create a sloping shoulder at the apical terminus of the restoration. See **margin.**

chamomile /kam′əmēl/, an herb with both annual and perennial forms, native to Germany, Hungary, and other areas of Europe, now growing freely in the United States and Canada.
■ INDICATIONS: It is used externally as an antiseptic and soothing agent for inflamed skin and minor wounds. Internally, it is used as an antispasmodic, gas-relieving, and antiinflammatory agent for the treatment of digestive problems; as a light sleep aid and sedative for adults and children; and as a possible anticancer agent. It is likely safe when used in medicinal amounts for a short term.
■ CONTRAINDICATIONS: It should not be used during pregnancy (Chamaemelum nobile) and lactation; it may be used in children. Cross-hypersensitivity may result from allergy to sunflowers, ragweed, or members of the aster family (echinacea, feverfew, milk thistle). People with asthma should also avoid its use.

CHAMPUS, *(Obsolete)* abbreviation for **Civilian Health and Medical Programs for Uniformed Services.** Now called **TRICARE.**

chancr-. See **cancr-, cancri-, cancro-.**

chancre /shang″kər/ [Fr, canker], **1.** a skin lesion, usually of primary syphilis, that begins at the infection site as a papule 10 to 30 days after exposure to the spirochete and develops into a red, bloodless, painless ulcer with a scooped-out appearance. It heals without treatment and leaves no scar. Two or more chancres may develop at the same time, usually in the genital area but sometimes on the hands, face, or other body surface. The chancre teems with *Treponema pallidum* spirochetes and is highly contagious. Also called **venereal sore. 2.** a papular lesion or ulcerated area of the skin that marks the point of infection of a nonsyphilitic disease, such as tuberculosis. Compare **chancroid.** See also **syphilis.**

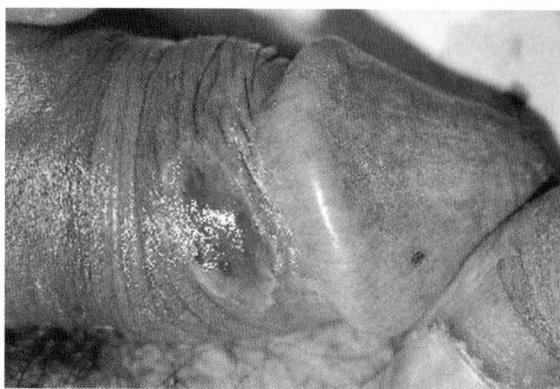

Chancre *(James et al, 2016)*

chancroid /shang″kroid/ [Fr, *chancre,* canker; Gk, *eidos,* form], a highly contagious sexually transmitted disease caused by infection with the bacillus *Haemophilus ducreyi.* It characteristically begins as a papule, usually on the skin of the external genitalia; it then grows and ulcerates, other papules form, and, if untreated, the bacillus spreads, causing buboes in the groin. It is often associated with tender and enlarged inguinal lymph nodes. An intradermal skin test is more reliable than smear and culture techniques in diagnosing this condition. Azithromycin or ceftriaxone are prescribed to treat chancroid. Because the lesion resembles syphilis and lymphogranuloma venereum, the diagnosis must be made before treatment to prevent obscuring simultaneous infections. Symptoms may not appear until 10 days after infection. Also called **venereal ulcer.** Compare **chancre.**

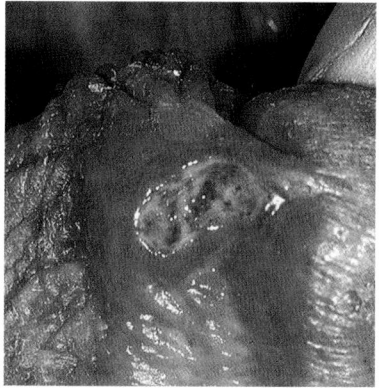

Chancroid *(Habif et al, 2010)*

chancrous /shang″krəs/, describing a condition of chancres or lesions resembling chancres.

change agent, 1. a role in which communication skills, education, and other resources are applied to help a client adjust to changes caused by illness or disability. **2.** a role to help members of an organization adapt to organizational change or to create organizational change.

change of life. *(Informal)* Also called **menopause.**

channel [L, *canalis,* pipe], **1.** a passageway or groove that conveys fluid, such as the central channels that connect the arterioles with the venules. **2.** membrane-bound globular proteins that allow diffusion of specific ions and molecules across a cell membrane along their concentration gradients.

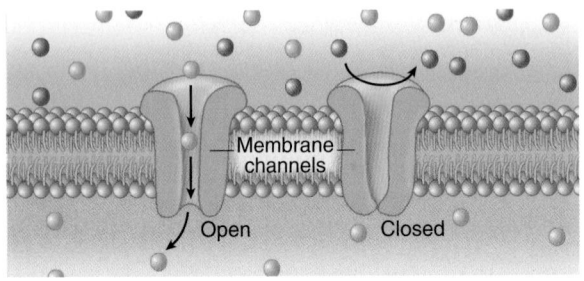

Membrane channel *(Patton, 2016)*

channeling, referral of increased numbers of patients in exchange for discounted prices. It does not apply in Canada.

channel ulcer [L, *canalis,* pipe, *ulcus,* sore], a rare type of peptic ulcer found in the pyloric canal between the stomach and the duodenum. See also **peptic ulcer.**

Chantix, a medication used for cessation of smoking. Brand name for **varenicline.**

chaos /kā″əs/, total disorganization with no causal relationships operating.

chaotic atrial tachycardia. See **multifocal atrial tachycardia.**

chaparral, an herbal product harvested from a shrub found in Mexico and the Southwestern United States.

■ INDICATIONS: Use of this herb is not recommended because it is potentially toxic to the liver and kidneys.

■ CONTRAINDICATIONS: Do not use it during pregnancy and lactation or in children until more research is completed. Persons with liver or renal disease should also avoid its use. The American Herbal Product Association has recommended that companies not sell chaparral products until the hepatoxicity question has been clarified, but it is still readily available.

Chapman lymphatic reflexes, (in chiropractic) a method of using body wall reflexes to influence the motion of fluids. After a surface locus has been contacted by the tip of the examiner's finger, a firm gentle contact is maintained and a rotary motion is imparted to the finger to express the fluid content of the locus into the surrounding tissues.

chapped /chapt/ [ME, *chappen,* cracked], pertaining to skin that is roughened, cracked, or reddened by exposure to cold or excessive moisture evaporation. Stinging or burning sensations often accompany the disorder. Prevention is achieved through protection against exposure to cold and wind and by maintaining a proper level of moisture. Treatment includes the avoidance of frequent washing, the replacement of soaps and detergents with superfatted soaps, and the application of emollients. Compare **frostbite.** −*chap, v.*

character [Gk, *charassein,* to engrave], **1.** the integrated composite of traits and behavioral tendencies that enables a person to react in a relatively consistent way to the customs and mores of society. Character, as

contrasted with personality, implies volition and morality. Compare **personality. 2.** any letter, number, symbol, or punctuation mark, usually composed of 8 bits or 1 byte, that can be transmitted as output by a computer. See also **bit.**

character analysis, a systematic investigation of the personality of an individual with special attention to psychological defenses and motivations, usually undertaken to improve behavior.

character disorder, a chronic, habitual, maladaptive, and socially unacceptable pattern of behavior and emotional response. See also **personality disorder.**

characteristic /kar′əktəris′tik/ [Gk, *charassein,* to engrave], **1.** *adj.,* typical of an individual or other entity. **2.** *n.,* a trait that distinguishes an individual or entity.

characteristic radiation, radiation produced when an outer-shell electron moves closer to the nucleus or "falls in" to replace an ejected inner-shell electron of a target atom. The energy of the radiation produced is equal to the difference in binding energies of the electron shells.

charcoal. See **activated charcoal.**

Charcot-Bouchard aneurysm /shärkō″bōōshär″/ [Jean M. Charcot, French neurologist, 1825–1893; Charles J. Bouchard, French physician, 1837–1886], a small, round dilation of a small artery in the cerebral cortex or basal ganglia. Charcot-Bouchard aneurysms often occur in individuals with very high blood pressure.

Charcot-Leyden crystal /shärkō″lī′dən/ [Jean M. Charcot; Ernst V. von Leyden, German physician, 1832–1910], any of the proteinaceous crystalline structures shaped like narrow, double pyramids found in the sputum of persons suffering from asthma and found in the feces of dysentery patients. Charcot-Leyden crystals occur in association with the fragmentation of eosinophils. Also called **asthma crystal, leukocytic crystal.**

Charcot-Marie-Tooth disease /shärkō″mərē″tooth″/ [Jean M. Charcot; Pierre Marie, French neurologist, 1853–1940; Howard H. Tooth, English neurologist, 1856–1925], a progressive hereditary disorder characterized by degeneration of the peroneal muscles of the fibula, resulting in clubfoot, foot drop, and ataxia. Progressive arm weakness can also be present as distal muscles atrophy. Compare **peripheral neuropathy.**

Charcot fever /shärkō″/ [Jean M. Charcot], a syndrome characterized by recurrent chills and fever, jaundice, and abdominal pain in the right upper quadrant that occurs with inflammation of the bile ducts. It is caused by the intermittent impaction of a stone in the ducts.

Charcot foot /shär·kō″/ [Jean M. Charcot], a hallmark symptom of the peripheral neurological disorder known as Charcot-Marie-Tooth disease; involves weakness of the foot and lower leg muscles, which may result in foot drop and a high-stepped gait with frequent tripping or falls. Foot deformities, such as high arches and hammertoes (a condition in which the middle joint of a toe bends upward) are also characteristic due to weakness of the small muscles in the feet.

Charcot joint. See **neuropathic joint disease.**

Charcot's triad [Jean M. Charcot; Gk, *trias,* three], a set of three signs of brainstem involvement in multiple sclerosis: intention tremor, nystagmus, and scanning speech. Also called *Charcot's neurological triad.*

CHARGE association, a syndrome of associated defects, including coloboma of the eye, heart anomaly, choanal atresia, intellectual disability, and genital and ear anomalies.

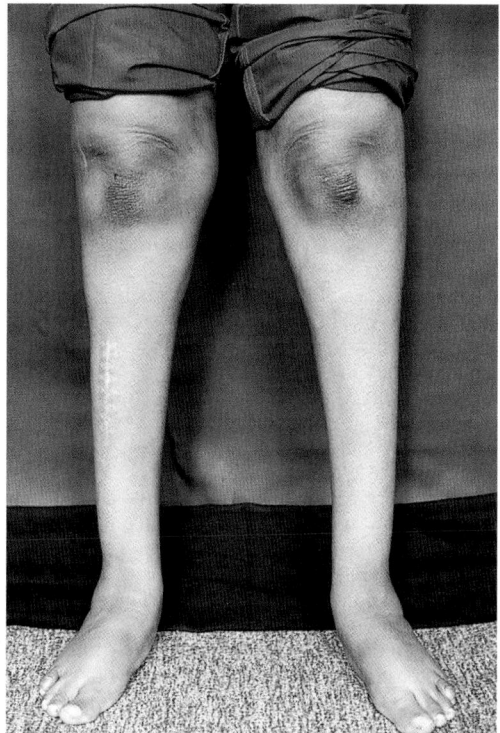

Child with Charcot-Marie-Tooth disease *(Zitelli and Davis, 2012)*

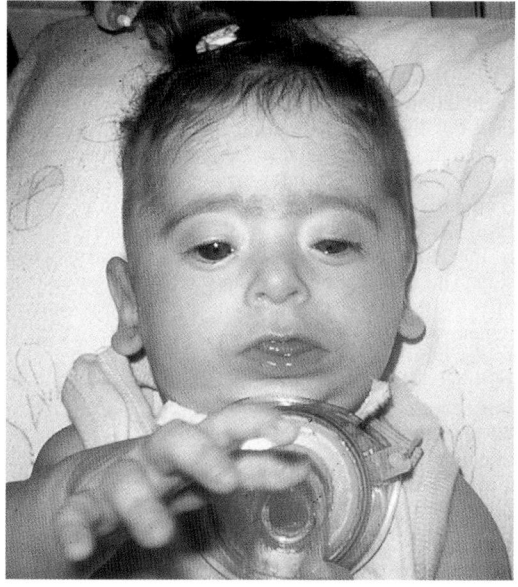

Infant with CHARGE association *(Zitelli and Davis, 2012/ Courtesy Dr. W. Tunnessen, Children's Hospital of Philadelphia.)*

charge-coupled device (CCD),   **1.** an array of semiconductors so arranged that the output of one serves as the input of the next. CCDs are often used to convert light patterns into electrical signals. See also **charge-coupled image sensor. 2.** in dental imaging, one type of image receptor found within an intraoral sensor.

charge-coupled image sensor,   two-dimensional electronic array for converting light patterns into electrical signals.

charge nurse,   the nurse assigned to manage the operations of the patient care area for the shift, in addition to patient care, if necessary. Responsibilities may include staffing, delegation of nursing assignments, admissions and discharge, and coordination of activities in the patient care area.

charlatan /shär″lətən/ [Fr, imposter],   a totally unqualified individual posing as an expert, especially an individual pretending to be a physician. Also called **quack.** −*charlatanical, adj.*

Charles' law,   (in physics) a law stating that, at constant pressure in a flexible container, the volume of an ideal gas is directly proportional to the temperature. When applying the gas laws, the unit of temperature must be in Kelvin. See also **Gay-Lussac's law.**

charley horse /chär″lē hôrs′/,   (*Informal*) a sudden painful condition in any muscle in the lower legs characterized by acute discomfort. It is the result of a strain, tear, or bruise of the muscle; is aggravated by movement; and is often associated with athletic activity. Treatment includes rest and massage. Compare **cramp.**

chart /chärt/ [L, *charta,* paper],   **1.** a patient record of data in tabular or graphic form. **2.** *v.,* to note data in a patient record (computerized or paper), usually at prescribed intervals. **3.** a group of symbols of graduated size for measuring visual acuity.

charta /kär″tə/ *pl. chartae* [L, paper],   a piece of paper, especially one treated with medicine, as for external application, or with a chemical for a special purpose, such as litmus paper.

charting,   the act of compiling data on clinical records or charts (computerized or paper). The charts are updated regularly to keep members of the health care team advised of changes in the patient's condition. The data usually include responses to treatment, interventions undertaken, care provided, fluctuations in temperature, pulse rates, respiration, other variable factors, and much more, including all nursing care. By law, charting is required by all health and allied health professionals directly involved with patient assessment and care. See also **documentation.**

chauffeur's fracture /shō″fərz/ [Fr, stoker; L, *fractura,* break],   any fracture of the radial styloid, produced by a twisting or a snapping type of injury. Historically, this fracture is so named as it was a common injury when chauffeurs experienced the backfire of a car while cranking the engine.

Chaussier's areola /shōsyāz″/ [François Chaussier, French anatomist, 1746–1828; L, little space],   an areola of indurated tissue surrounding a malignant pustule.

CHB,   abbreviation for **complete heart block.**

CHC,   abbreviation for **community health center.**

CHD,   **1.** abbreviation for **coronary heart disease.** See **coronary artery disease. 2.** abbreviation for **congenital heart disease.** See **congenital cardiac anomaly.**

checkup [Fr, *eschec,* acquire; AS, *uf*],   (*Informal*) a thorough study or examination of the health of an individual. See also **health assessment.**

Chédiak-Higashi syndrome /ched″ē·ak·higä″shē/ [Moises Chédiak, 20th-century Cuban physician; Ototaka Higashi, 20th-century Japanese physician],   a congenital autosomal-recessive disorder, characterized by partial albinism, photophobia, pale optic fundi, massive leukocytic inclusions, psychomotor abnormalities, recurrent infections, and early death. Antenatal diagnosis can be made by amniocentesis and tissue culture. Bone marrow transplantation from an HLA-matched sibling is the therapy of choice. Treatment includes acyclovir, high-dose intravenous gamma globulin, and microtubulytic drugs, such as vincristine, vinblastine, and colchicine.

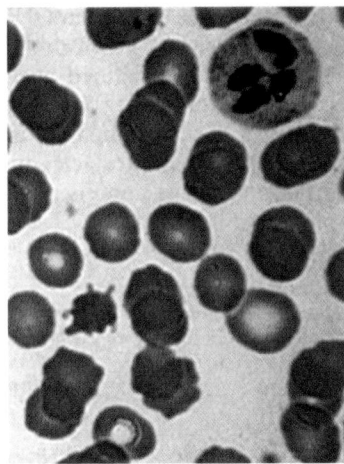

Chédiak-Higashi syndrome: peripheral blood smear
(Gahl, 2006)

cheek [AS, *ceace*], **1.** a fleshy prominence, especially the fleshy protuberances on both sides of the face between the eye and the jaw and between the ear and the nose and mouth. **2.** *(Informal)* a buttock.

cheekbone. See **zygomatic bone.**

cheesy abscess [AS, *cese* + L, *abscedere,* to go away], an abscess that contains a yellowish, semisolid, cheeselike material, such as a tuberculous abscess. Also called **caseous abscess.**

cheesy necrosis, tissue death in which the structures have degenerated into a white, cheesy mass. See also **caseous necrosis.**

cheil-. See **cheilo-, cheil-.**

cheilectomy /kīlek″təmē/, surgical removal of irregular surfaces, usually bone spurs, in the lining of a joint.

-cheilia, -chilia, suffix meaning "(condition of the) lips": pachycheilia.

cheilitis /kīlī″tis/ [Gk, *cheilos,* lip, *itis,* inflammation], an abnormal condition of the lips characterized by inflammation and cracking of the skin. There are several forms, including those caused by excessive exposure to sunlight, allergic sensitivity to cosmetics, and vitamin deficiency. Compare **cheilosis.**

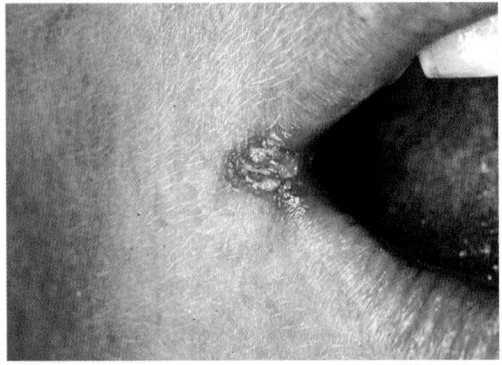

Cheilitis *(Mosca and Hathorn, 2006)*

cheilo-, cheil-, prefix meaning "lip": *cheilocarcinoma, cheiloplasty.*

cheilocarcinoma /kī′lōkär′sinō″mə/ *pl. cheilocarcinomas, cheilocarcinomata,* a malignant epithelial tumor of the lip.

cheiloplasty /kī″ləplas′tē/ [Gk, *cheilos,* lip, *plassein,* to mold], surgical correction of a defect of the lip.

cheilorrhaphy /kīlôr″əfē/ [Gk, *cheilos,* lip, *raphe,* suture], a surgical procedure that sutures the lip, such as in the repair of a congenitally cleft lip or a lacerated lip.

cheilosis /kīlō″sis/, a noninflammatory disorder of the lips and mouth characterized by bilateral scales and fissures, resulting from a deficiency of riboflavin in the diet.

cheir-. See **cheiro-, cheir-, chir-, chiro-.**

cheiralgia /kīral″jə/ [Gk, *cheir* + *algos,* pain], a pain or localized discomfort in the hand, especially that associated with arthritis. −*cheiralgic, adj.*

-cheiria. See **-chiria, -cheiria.**

cheiro-, cheir-, chir-, chiro-, prefix meaning "hand": *cheiromegaly, cheiroplasty.*

cheirognostic /kī′ragnos″tik/ [Gk, *cheir,* hand, *gnostikos,* knowing], pertaining to the ability to distinguish between the left and right hands and sides of the body.

cheiromegaly /kī′rōmeg″əlē/ [Gk, *cheir* + *megas,* large], an abnormal condition characterized by excessively large hands out of proportion to other parts of the body.

cheiroplasty /kī″rōplas′tē/, a surgical procedure to restore an injured or congenitally deformed hand to normal use. Also called **chiroplasty.** −*cheiroplastic, adj.*

chelate /kē″lāt/ [Gk, *chele,* claw], **1.** *n.,* a polydentate ligand, either ionic or neutral, that forms a chemical complex with metal ions in solution. An example is the interaction of a metal ion and two or more polar groups of a single molecule. **2.** *n.,* (in medicine) any coordination compound composed of a central metal ion and an organic molecule with multiple bonds arranged in ring formations, used especially in chemotherapeutic treatments for metal poisoning. **3.** *adj.,* pertaining to chelation.

chelating agent /kē″lāting/, a substance that promotes chelation. Chelating agents are used in the treatment of metal poisoning. They convert the metal to an inert substance that can be eliminated by the body. Kinds include **EDTA.** See also **chelation.**

chelation /kēlā″shən/, a chemical reaction in which there is a combination with a metal to form a ring-shaped molecular complex in which the metal is firmly bound and isolated. See also **chelating agent.**

chelation therapy, the use of a chelating agent to remove toxic metals from the body, the treatment of heavy metal poisoning. There is insufficient evidence that chelation therapy is effective in the management of disorders not associated with heavy metal poisoning.

cheloid, cheloidal. See **keloid.**

cheloidosis. See **keloidosis.**

chemabrasion /kem′əbrā″zhən/ [Gk, *chemeia,* alchemy; L, *ab* + *radere,* to scrape off], a method of treating scars, chromatosis, or other skin disorders by applying chemicals that remove the surface layers of skin cells. See also **chemical cauterization, chemosurgery.**

chemexfoliation. See **chemical peel.**

chemical /kem″əkəl/ [Gk, *chemeia,* alchemy], **1.** *n.,* a substance composed of chemical elements or a substance produced by or used in chemical processes. **2.** *adj.,* pertaining to chemistry.

chemical action, any process in which elements and/or compounds react with each other to produce a chemical change. For example, hydrogen and oxygen combine to produce water.

chemical affinity [Gk, *chemeia,* alchemy; L, *affinis,* related], **1.** an attraction that results in the formation of molecules from atoms. **2.** an attraction between chemicals caused by polarity, as used in affinity chromatography.

chemical agent, any chemical power, active principle, or substance that can produce an effect in the body by interacting with various body substances, such as aspirin, which produces an analgesic effect.

chemical antidote [Gk, *chemeia* + *anti,* against, *dotos,* that which is given], any substance that reacts chemically with a poison to form a compound that is harmless. There are few true antidotes, and treatment of poisoning depends largely on eliminating the toxic agent before it can be absorbed by the body.

chemical burn, tissue damage caused by exposure to a strong acid or alkali, such as phenol, creosol, mustard gas, or phosphorus. See also **acid burn, acid poisoning, alkali burn, alkali poisoning.**

chemical carcinogen [Gk, *chemeia,* alchemy, *karkinos,* crab, *oma,* tumor, *genein,* to produce], any chemical agent that can induce the development of cancer in living tissue.

chemical cauterization [Gk, *chemeia* + *kauterion,* branding iron], the corroding or burning of living tissue by a caustic chemical substance, such as potassium hydroxide. Also called **chemocautery,** *chemical cautery.*

chemical cystitis, allergic cystitis occurring in reaction to a chemical substance in the body. See also **drug-induced cystitis.**

chemical disaster, the accidental release of a quantity of toxic chemicals or harmful substances and compounds into the environment, resulting in death or injury to workers or members of nearby communities. Examples include the release of methyl isocyanate from a chemical plant in Bhopal, India, at a cost of 2000 lives; and a nuclear accident at Chernobyl, Ukraine, requiring the removal of 160,000 people from their homes.

chemical energy. See **energy.**

chemical equivalent, a drug or chemical containing similar amounts of the same ingredients as another drug or chemical.

chemical gastritis, inflammation of the stomach caused by the ingestion of a chemical compound. Treatment is determined by the substance ingested. Compare **corrosive gastritis, erosive gastritis.**

chemical indicator, **1.** a commercially prepared device that monitors all or part of the physical conditions of the sterilization cycle. It usually consists of a sensitive ink dye that changes color under certain conditions. **2.** a compound added to a reaction system to show, typically by a change in color, when the process is complete, as in an acid-base titration.

chemical mediator, a neurotransmitter chemical, such as acetylcholine.

chemical name, the exact designation of the chemical structure of a drug as determined by the rules of accepted systems of chemical nomenclature.

chemical peel, a cosmetic therapy to reduce or improve wrinkles, blemishes, pigment spots, and sun-damaged areas of the skin. Using a chemical solution of phenol, trichloroacetic acid, or alpha hydroxy fruit acid, the top skin layers are peeled away, allowing new, smoother skin with tighter cells to occupy the surface. Immediately after the peel, there may be considerable swelling, which subsides after 7 to 10 days as new skin begins to form. Other chemical solutions used include glycolic acid, retinol, Jessner's solution, beta hydroxy acid, and combinations thereof. Also called **chemexfoliation, chemoexfoliation.**

chemical peritonitis [Gk, *chemeia,* alchemy, *peri,* near, *teinein,* to stretch, *itis,* inflammation], an inflammation of the peritoneum resulting from chemicals, including digestive substances, in the peritoneum. See also **peritonitis.**

chemical restraint [Gk, *chemeia,* alchemy; *restringere,* to confine], the use of psychotropics, hypnotics, or anxiolytics to control a potentially violent patient.

chemical shift, (in nuclear magnetic resonance spectrometry) the spectral position of a resonance in the substance of interest relative to the spectral position of the resonance of a standard. Nonequivalent atoms of a molecule have different chemical shifts.

chemical shift artifacts, artifacts in magnetic resonance caused by small differences in resonance frequencies of different chemical compounds (e.g., water and fat).

chemical sympathectomy, the removal of a sympathetic nerve tract or ganglion by injection of a corrosive chemical such as phenol; used principally for the amelioration of neuropathic pain.

chemical warfare, the waging of war with poisonous chemicals and gases.

cheminosis /kem'ənō″sis/ [Gk, *chemeia* + *osis,* condition], any disease caused by a chemical substance.

chemist, **1.** a person with special education and training in the structures, characteristics, and actions of chemicals. **2.** in Great Britain, Australia, and New Zealand, a pharmacist.

chemistry /kem″istrē/ [Gk, *chemeia,* alchemy], the science dealing with the elements, their compounds, and the molecular structure and interactions of matter. Kinds include **inorganic chemistry, organic chemistry.**

chemistry, normal values, the amounts of various substances in the normal human body, determined by testing a large sample of people presumed to be healthy. Normal values are expressed in ranges of numbers, and ranges vary for different age groups and from laboratory to laboratory. For example, a normal concentration of a substance in the blood might be expressed as 5 to 20 mg/dL. Although variations from normal values may be highly significant tools in the diagnoses of certain diseases, in all cases an abnormal result must be cautiously interpreted. See **reference intervals.**

chemo- /kem′ō-, kē′mō-/, combining form meaning "by chemical reaction" or "a chemical or chemistry": *chemokinesis.*

chemoattractant /kē′mō·ətrak′tənt/ [Gk, *chemeia,* alchemy + L, *attrahere,* to draw to], a chemotactic factor that induces positive chemotaxis.

chemocautery. See **chemical cauterization.**

chemodifferentiation /-dif′əren′shē·ā″shən/, a stage in embryonic development that precedes and controls specialization and differentiation of the cells into rudimentary organs.

chemoexfoliation. See **chemical peel.**

chemokine /kē′mōkīn/ [Gk, *chemeia,* alchemy + *kinēsis,* movement], any of a group of low-molecular-weight chemoattractant proteins, identified on the basis of their ability to induce chemotaxis or chemokinesis in leukocytes (or in particular populations of leukocytes) during both homeostasis and inflammation. The group is divided into four subgroups on the basis of genetic, structural, and functional criteria. They function as regulators of the immune system and may also play roles in the circulatory and central nervous systems. See also **cytokine.**

chemokinesis /kē′mōki·nē′sis/ [Gk, *chemeia,* alchemy, *kinesis,* movement], increased nondirectional activity of cells caused by the presence of a chemical substance. Compare **chemotaxis.**

chemonucleolysis /-noo̅′klē·ol″isis-/ [Gk, *chemeia* + L, *nucleus,* nut kernel; Gk, *lysein,* to loosen], a method of dissolving the nucleus pulposus of an intervertebral disk by the injection of a chemolytic agent, such as the enzyme chymopapain. The procedure is used primarily in the treatment of a herniated disk and other intervertebral disk lesions.

chemoprevention, the use of natural, synthetic or biological substances to suppress or prevent a disease such as cancer. Also called **chemoprophylaxis.**

chemoprophylaxis /-prō'filak″sis/ [Gk, *chemeia* + *prophylax,* advance guard], administration of a medicine or chemical agent with the purpose of disease prevention, such as the use of antimicrobial drugs to prevent the acquisition of pathogens in an endemic area or to prevent their spread from one body area to another.

chemoprotectant, **1.** *adj.,* providing protection against the toxic effects of chemotherapy agents. **2.** *n.,* an agent that so acts.

chemoradiotherapy, combined modality therapy using chemotherapy and radiotherapy, designed to reduce the need for surgery by maximizing the interaction between the radiation and the therapeutic agent or agents.

chemoreceptor /-risep″tər/ [Gk, *chemeia* + L, *recipere,* to receive], a sensory nerve cell activated by chemical stimuli. For example, chemoreceptors in the carotid artery are sensitive to the partial pressure of carbon dioxide in the blood; they signal the respiratory center in the brain to increase or decrease the rate of breathing.

chemoreflex /-rē″fleks/, any reflex initiated by the stimulation of chemical receptors, such as those of the carotid and aortic bodies, which respond to changes in carbon dioxide, hydrogen ion, and oxygen concentrations in the blood. See also **chemoreceptor.**

chemoresistance, **1.** a specific resistance by components of a cell to chemical substances. **2.** the resistance of bacteria or a cancer cell to a chemical designed to treat the disorder.

chemosis /kimō″sis/ [Gk, *cheme,* cockle, *osis,* condition], an abnormal edematous swelling of the mucous membrane covering the eyeball and lining the eyelids. Usually the result of local trauma or infection, chemosis may also occur in acute conjunctivitis. Obstruction of normal lymph flow, such as might result from growth of a tumor within the eye socket, may less commonly cause chemosis. Systemic disorders, such as angioneurotic edema, anemia, and Bright's disease, may also cause the condition. Also called **conjunctival edema.**

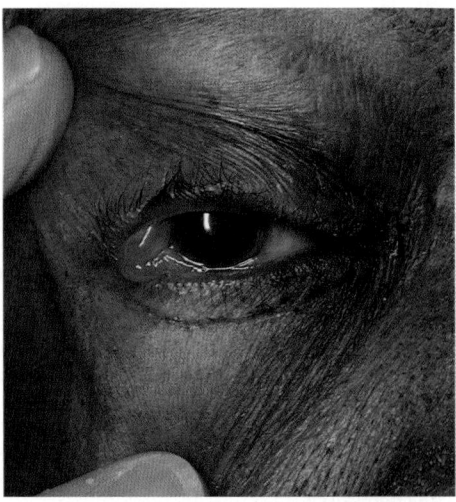

Chemosis *(Swartz, 2014)*

chemostat /kē″məstat′/, a device that assures a steady rate of cell division in bacterial populations by maintaining a constant environment.

chemosurgery /-sur″jərē/ [Gk, *chemeia* + *cheirourgos,* surgeon], the destruction of malignant, infected, or gangrenous tissue by the application of chemicals. The technique is used successfully to remove skin cancers.

chemotactic /-tak″tik/ [Gk, *chemeia,* alchemy, *taxis,* arrangement], pertaining to a tendency of cells to migrate toward or away from certain chemical stimuli.

chemotaxis /-tak″sis/ [Gk, *chemeia* + *taxis,* arrangement], movement toward or away from a chemical stimulus. Chemotaxis is a cellular function, particularly of neutrophils and monocytes, whose phagocytic activity is influenced by chemical factors released by invading microorganisms.

chemotherapeutic agent /-ther′əpyoo″tik/, any chemical used to treat cancer. It is usually used to refer to antineoplastic drugs.

chemotherapeutic index, a system for judging the safety and effectiveness of a drug as a ratio between the dose that is lethal to 50% of animals (LD_{50}) and the median effective (ED_{50}) or minimal curative dose.

chemotherapy /-ther″əpē/, the treatment of cancer, infections, and other diseases such as cancer with chemical agents. The term has been applied over the centuries to a variety of therapies, including malaria therapy with herbs and use of mercury for syphilis. In modern usage, chemotherapy usually entails the use of chemicals to destroy cancer cells on a selective basis. The cytotoxic agents used in cancer treatments generally function in the same manner as ionizing radiation; they do not kill the cancer cells directly but instead impair their ability to replicate. Most of the commonly used anticancer drugs act by interfering with deoxyribonucleic acid and ribonucleic acid activities associated with cell division. Chemotherapeutic agents are often used in combination to intercept cell replication at various points of the cell cycle. These agents are also often used in combination with other cancer treatments such as radiation therapy and targeted therapy for their synergistic effect. For example, a cytotoxic agent may be used to render a tumor cell more sensitive to the effects of ionizing radiation, thus allowing the cancer to be controlled with smaller doses of radiation. Chemotherapy is not selective; it kills healthy cells as well as cancer cells. *−chemotherapeutic, adj.*

chemotherapy (unsealed radioactive), the oral or parenteral administration of a radioisotope, such as iodine 131 (^{131}I) for the treatment of hyperthyroidism or thyroid cancer or phosphorus 32 (^{32}P) for leukemia, polycythemia vera, or peritoneal ascites resulting from widely disseminated carcinoma.

■ METHOD: The patient needs to be isolated during the half-life of the radioisotope (8.1 days for ^{131}I, 14 days for ^{32}P, and 2.7 days for ^{198}Au) to prevent radiation exposure to other persons.

■ INTERVENTIONS: Therapy with radioactive iodine is performed on an outpatient basis. The dose of the isotope is low, so radiation precautions are not needed. Disposal of urine, feces, and dressings follows a prespecified protocol.

■ OUTCOME CRITERIA: Radioactive iodine usually counteracts hyperthyroidism and is frequently used in conjunction with surgery in the treatment of thyroid cancer. Radioactive phosphorus often controls polycythemia vera, but other agents are generally more effective in leukemia therapy. Radioactive gold is usually administered as a last resort in advanced lung cancer or peritoneal ascites resulting from malignant disease.

chenodeoxycholic acid /kē′nōdē·ok′sikō″lik/, a secondary bile acid. It is used in vivo to dissolve small, noncalcified cholesterol gallstones in a small percentage of patients who cannot tolerate surgery or other methods to remove gallstones. Compare **endoscopic retrograde**

cholangiopancreatography, percutaneous transhepatic cholangiography. See also **ursodeoxycholic acid.**

cherophobia /kē′rō′fō′bē·ə/, **1.** a morbid aversion to cheerfulness. **2.** avoidance of events that normally cause happiness.

cherry angioma [L, *cerasus* + *angeion,* vessel, *oma,* tumor], a small, bright red, clearly circumscribed vascular tumor on the skin. It occurs most often on the trunk but may appear anywhere on the body. The lesion is common; more than 85% of people over 45 years of age have several cherry angiomas. Also called **capillary angioma, capillary hemangioma,** *Campbell de Morgan spots,* **senile angioma.**

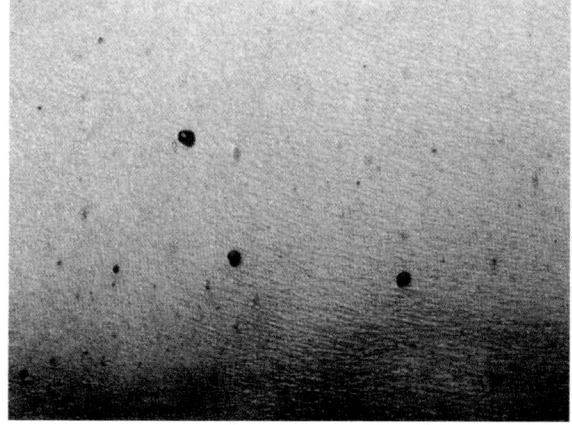

Cherry angioma *(Nanda, 1996)*

cherry red spot, an abnormal red circular area of the choroid, visible through the fovea centralis of the eye and surrounded by a contrasting white edema. It is associated with cases of infantile cerebral sphingolipidosis and sometimes appears in the late infantile form of Tay-Sachs disease. Also called **Tay's spot.**

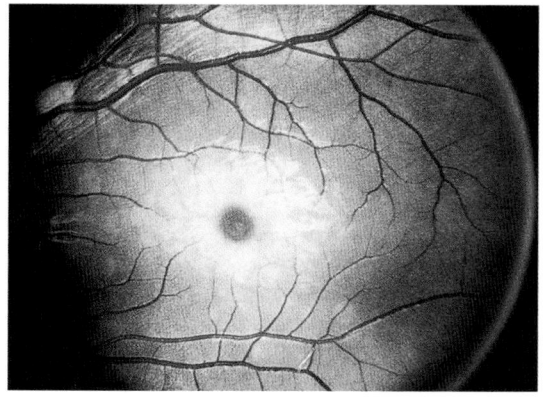

Cherry red spot at the macula *(Kanski and Bowling, 2011)*

cherubism /cher″əbiz′əm/ [Heb, *kerubh*], an abnormal hereditary condition characterized by progressive bilateral swelling at the angle of the mandible, especially in children. In some cases of cherubism, the entire jaw swells and the eyes turn up, enhancing the cherubic facial appearance. The condition tends to regress during adult life.

chest [AS, *box*], **1.** see **thorax. 2.** the outside front part of the basic thoracic structure. See also **thoracic cage, thoracic cavity.**

chest bandage, any of several types of fabric dressings for chest injuries, including a three-cornered open chest wrapping or a figure-eight roller bandage spica.

chest binder, a broad bandage or girdle, with or without shoulder straps, that encircles the chest and aids in supplying heat or other therapies. A chest binder also may be used to support the breasts.

chest compression, the act of depressing the chest at least 2 inches (5 cm) and at a rate of at least 100 per minute to maintain circulation in a pulseless individual. See also **cardiopulmonary resuscitation.**

chest cavity, the part of the body enclosed by the ribs and the sternum. See **body cavity.**

chest drainage, the withdrawal of air, blood, or fluids from the chest cavity through a tube commonly inserted into the pleural space. The tube may be connected to a suction device that helps establish the negative pressure necessary to reinflate a collapsed lung.

chest lead /lēd/, **1.** One of the six positive electrodes placed on the surface of the chest over different regions of the heart to record electrical activity. These six leads are named V1 to V6. **2.** *(Informal)* the tracing produced by such a lead on an electrocardiograph.

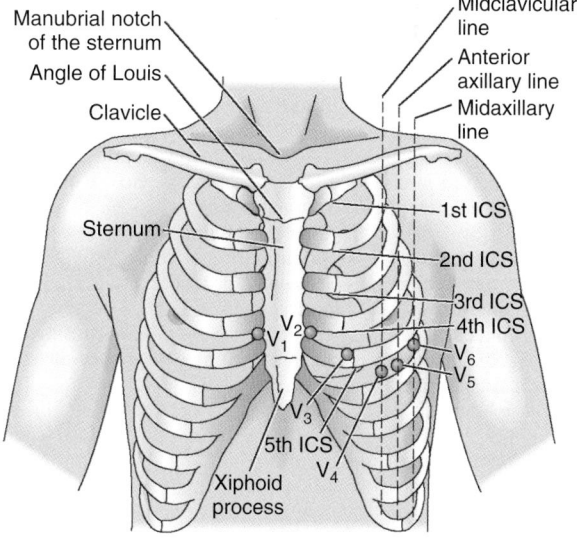

Chest leads *(Chester, 1999)*

chest pain [AS, *cest,* box; L, *poena,* punishment], a physical complaint that requires immediate diagnosis and evaluation. Chest pain may be symptomatic of cardiac disease, such as angina pectoris, myocardial infarction, aortic stenosis, or pericarditis, or of pulmonary disease, such as pleurisy, pneumonia, or pulmonary embolism or infarction. The source of chest pain may also be musculoskeletal, gastrointestinal, or psychogenic. The use of illegal drugs such as cocaine may also cause chest pain. Over 90% of severe chest pain in adults is caused by coronary disease, spinal root compression, or psychological disturbance.

■ OBSERVATIONS: Evaluation of chest pain requires determining the quality of the pain (dull, sharp, or crushing), locating the site of the pain (in the center or side of the chest), and determining how long the pain has persisted, how it has developed, and whether it has occurred in the past. The patient is asked to describe the spread of pain to other parts of the body and to identify such factors as exertion, emotional dis-

tress, movement, eating, or deep breathing that aggravate or relieve the pain. If the pain is reproducible by palpation during physical examination, it is unlikely to be cardiac in origin.
■ PATIENT CARE CONSIDERATIONS: Because of its association with life-threatening heart disease, chest pain causes extreme anxiety, which tends to mask other symptoms that would aid in diagnosis and treatment. Reassuring the person being examined assists in proper diagnosis. Other specific cardiovascular conditions associated with chest pain are myocardial infarction, angina pectoris, pericarditis, and a dissecting aneurysm of the thoracic aorta. Musculoskeletal conditions include rib fractures, swelling of the rib cartilage, and muscle strain. GI conditions associated with chest pain include esophagitis, peptic ulcers, hiatal hernia, gastritis, cholecystitis, and pancreatitis.

chest physiotherapy, **1.** see **cupping and vibrating, percussion. 2.** a technique designed to loosen and mobilize mucus so that it can be expectorated.

chest prominences and depressions, any unnatural surface features of the chest that may be caused by congenital defects, diseases such as emphysema, enlarged organs, tumors, traumas, or occupational hazards. See also **barrel chest, flail chest, funnel chest, pigeon breast.**

chest regions, the topographic parts or subdivisions of the chest: presternal, mammary, inframammary, and axillary.

chest thump [AS, *cest,* box], *(Informal)* a sharp blow delivered to the chest in the precordial area to restore a normal heartbeat after a witnessed cardiac arrest.

chest tube, a catheter inserted through the rib space of the thorax into the pleural space to remove air and/or fluid, thereby restoring negative pressure in the pleural space. It is attached to a water-seal chest drainage device. It is commonly used after chest surgery and lung collapse.

chest wall percussion. See **percussion.**

chest x-ray, the most commonly performed diagnostic x-ray examination. A chest x-ray produces images of the heart, lungs, airways, blood vessels, and the bones of the spine and chest. An x-ray (radiograph) is a noninvasive medical test that helps health care professionals diagnose and treat medical conditions.

chewing reflex, a pathological sign in adults with brain damage, characterized by repetitive chewing motions when the mouth is stimulated.

Cheyne nystagmus /shăn/ [John Cheyne, Scottish physician, 1777–1836], an involuntary eye movement with a rhythm that resembles that of Cheyne-Stokes respiration.

Cheyne-Stokes respiration (CSR) [John Cheyne; William Stokes, Irish physician, 1804–1878; L, *respirare* to breathe], an abnormal pattern of respiration, characterized by alternating periods of apnea and deep, rapid breathing. The respiratory cycle begins with slow, shallow breaths that gradually become abnormally rapid and deep. Breathing gradually becomes slower and shallower and is followed by 10 to 20 seconds of apnea before the cycle is repeated. Each episode may last from 45 seconds to 3 minutes. Underlying CSR is a complex alteration in the functioning of the respiratory center in the brain, caused by dysfunction of the diencephalon or by bilateral hemispheric lesions. The respiratory center may have a reduced sensitivity to the concentrations of blood gases, as is seen in cerebrovascular disease, in tumors of the brainstem, and in severe head injury. CSR may be triggered by changes in blood chemical processes, especially in elderly patients with degenerative arterial disease or respiratory diseases, such as bronchopneumonia. In an otherwise healthy person, CSR may be caused by hyperventilation, exposure to high altitudes, or an overdose of a narcotic or hypnotic drug. CSR occurs more frequently during

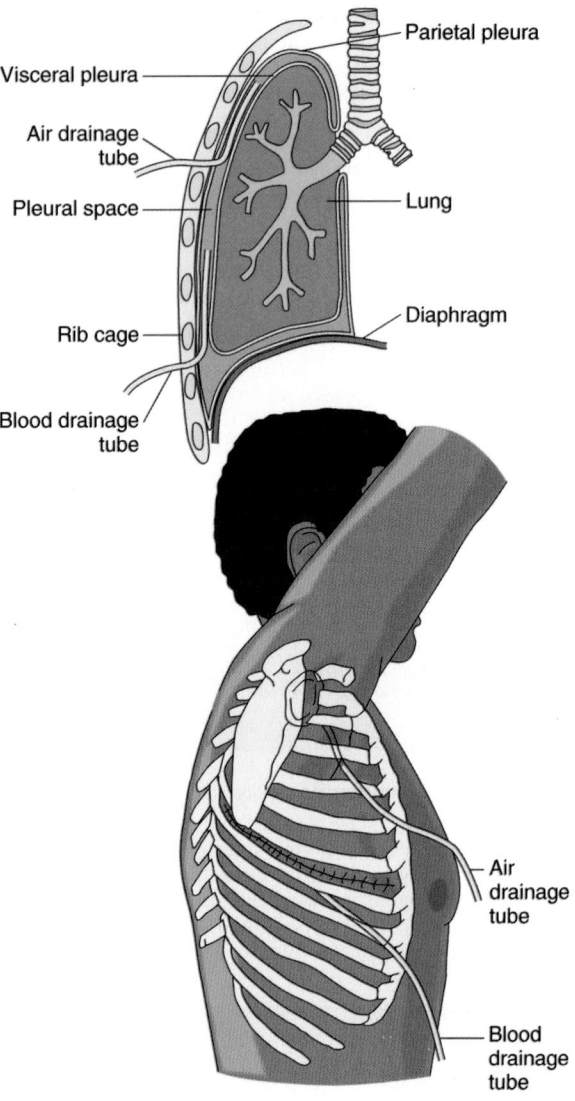

Placement of chest tubes *(Ignatavicius and Workman, 2016)*

sleep. Also called **agonal respiration, periodic breathing.** Compare **Biot's respiration.**

-chezia, -chesia, suffix meaning "(condition of) defecation, especially involving the discharge of foreign substances": *hematochezia.*

CHF, abbreviation for **congestive heart failure.**

chi /kī/, X, the 22nd letter of the Greek alphabet, sometimes used in scientific notation to designate the 22nd in a series.

ch'i, a Chinese concept of a fundamental life energy that flows in orderly ways along meridians, or channels, in the body. The energy can be either positive or negative. See also **acupuncture.**

CHI, abbreviation for **creatinine height index.**

Chiari-Frommel syndrome /kē·är″ēfrom″əl/ [Johann B. Chiari, German obstetrician, 1817–1854; Richard Frommel, German gynecologist, 1854–1912], a hormonal disorder that occurs after pregnancy in which weaning does not spontaneously end lactation. It is usually the result of a decrease in pituitary gonadotropins and an excess of pituitary prolactin and may be accompanied by amenorrhea. Treatment includes observation, hormonal therapy, and investigation to confirm or rule out pituitary tumor.

Chiari malformation /kē·ä′rē/ [Hans Chiari, Austrian pathologist, 1851–1916], a congenital anomaly in which the cerebellum and medulla oblongata, which is elongated and flattened, protrude into the spinal canal through the foramen magnum. It is classified into three types according to severity, ranging from prolapse of the cerebellar tonsils into the spinal canal without elongation of the brainstem (type I) to complete herniation of the cerebellum to form an occipital encephalocele (type III). It may be accompanied by hydrocephalus, spina bifida, syringomyelia, and mental defects. The classic form, type II, better known as Arnold-Chiari malformation, is tonsillar herniation with a myelomeningocele, a form of spina bifida. Also called *Chiari deformity*. See also **Arnold-Chiari malformation.**

Chiari syndrome. See **Budd-Chiari syndrome.**

chiasm /kī′azəm/ [Gk, *chiasma,* lines that cross], **1.** the crossing of two lines or tracts, as of the optic nerves at the optic chiasm. **2.** (in genetics) the crossing of two chromatids in the prophase of meiosis. −**chiasmal, chiasmic,** *adj.*

chiasma /kī·az′mə/ [Gk, lines that cross], a visible connection between homologous chromosomes during the first meiotic division in gametogenesis. Chiasmata appear as X-shaped configurations during the late prophase stage and provide the means by which homologous chromosomes exchange genetic material. See also **crossing over.** −*chiasmatic,* **chiasmic,** *adj.*

chiasmal. See **chiasm.**

chiasmapexy /kī·az″məpek″sē/, surgery involving the optic chiasm.

chiasmatypy. See **crossing over.**

chiasmic. See **chiasm, chiasma.**

chickenpox /chik″ənpoks′/ [AS, *cicen* + ME, *pokke*], an acute, highly contagious viral disease caused by a herpesvirus, varicella zoster virus. It occurs primarily in young children and is characterized by crops of pruritic vesicular eruptions on the skin. The disease is transmitted by direct contact with skin lesions or, more commonly, by droplets spread from the respiratory tract of infected persons, usually in the prodromal period or the early stages of the rash. The vesicular fluid and the scabs are infectious until entirely dry. Indirect transmission through uninfected persons or objects is rare. The diagnosis is usually made by physical examination and by the characteristic appearance of the disease. The virus may be identified by culture of the vesicle fluid. Also called **varicella.**

■ OBSERVATIONS: The incubation period averages 2 to 3 weeks, followed by slight fever, mild headache, malaise, and anorexia occurring about 24 to 36 hours before the rash begins. The prodromal period is usually mild in children but may be severe in adults. The rash, which is highly pruritic, begins as macules and progresses in 1 or 2 days to papules and, finally, to vesicles surrounding an erythematous base and containing clear fluid. Within 24 to 48 hours the vesicles turn cloudy and become umbilicated, are easily broken, and become encrusted. The lesions, which erupt in crops so that all three stages are present simultaneously, first appear on the back and chest and then spread to the face, neck, and limbs; they occur only rarely on the soles and palms. In severe cases, laryngeal or tracheal vesicles in the pharynx, larynx, and trachea may cause dyspnea and dysphagia. Prolonged fever, lymphadenopathy, and extreme irritability from pruritus are other symptoms. The symptoms last from a few days to 2 weeks.

■ INTERVENTIONS: Routine treatment consists of rest; medications to reduce fever; applications of topical antipruritics,

such as wet compresses, calamine lotion, or a paste made from baking soda and water; or oral antihistamines, given for the relief of itching. Infected vesicles may be treated with neomycin-bacitracin, and systemic antibiotics may be given if the secondary bacterial infection is extensive. People who are susceptible and at risk for severe disease when exposed to the infection may be passively protected with zoster immune globulin, varicella-zoster immune globulin, immune serum globulin, or zoster immune plasma. A vaccine for active immunization is available for individuals 12 months of age and older. Babies born to women in whom chickenpox develops within 5 days of delivery are especially likely to have a severe case of the disease. One attack of the disease usually confers permanent immunity, although recurring episodes of herpes zoster occur, especially in elderly or debilitated people, resulting from reactivation of the virus. Herpes zoster virus, like all herpesviruses, lies dormant in certain sensory nerve roots after primary infection.

■ PATIENT CARE CONSIDERATIONS: Chickenpox in childhood is usually benign. Few cases require hospitalization. It may be serious or fatal in immunocompromised people, such as those infected with human immunodeficiency virus, those receiving chemotherapy or radiotherapy for malignant disease, those who have undergone organ transplantation, those with congenital or acquired defects in cell-mediated immunity, or those receiving high doses of steroids. Common complications are secondary bacterial infections, such as abscesses, cellulitis, pneumonia, and sepsis, and hemorrhagic varicella (tiny hemorrhages that may occur in the vesicles or surrounding skin). Less common complications are encephalitis, Reye's syndrome (associated with the use of aspirin), thrombocytopenia, and hepatitis.

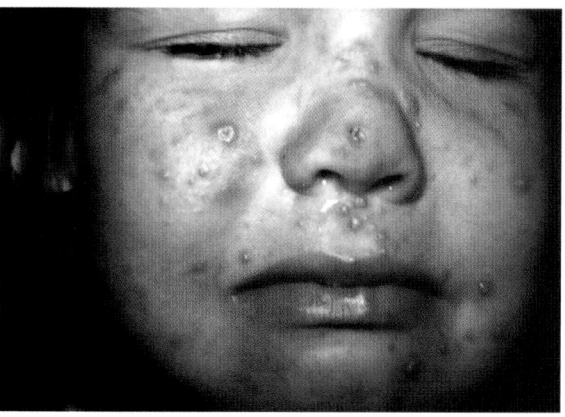

Child with chickenpox *(Kliegman and Stanton, 2016)*

chiclero ulcer /chikler″ō/ [Mex, *tzictli,* chicle; L, *ulcus*], a kind of American leishmaniasis caused by *Leishmania mexicana.* It is endemic among the workers in the Yucatan and Central America who harvest chicle from the forest. The disease is characterized by cutaneous ulcers on the head that usually heal spontaneously within 6 months, except for those on the pinna of the ear, which may last for years and cause scarring and deformities. See also **American leishmaniasis, leishmaniasis.**

chicory, a perennial herb native to Europe but now found in the United States, Canada, India, Egypt, and elsewhere.

■ INDICATIONS: It is used as a coffee substitute, as a source of fructooligosaccharides, as a mild laxative for children, and as a treatment for gout, rheumatism, loss of appetite, and digestive distress. It is generally recognized as safe in foods and may be effective as an appetite stimulant; there is insufficient reliable information for its other indications.

■ CONTRAINDICATIONS: It is contraindicated during pregnancy and lactation and in children. People who are hypersensitive to chicory or asteraceae/composit herbs also should avoid its use, and it is contraindicated for people with gallstones.

χ² distribution.   See **chi square distribution.**

Chido-Rodgers blood group /chē′dōroj′ərz/, a blood group consisting of nine antigens that are fragments of the C4 component of complement that attaches to the red cell from plasma.

chief cell [Fr, chef; L, *cella,* storeroom], **1.** any one of the simple columnar epithelial cells or the simple cuboidal epithelial cells that line the gastric glands and secrete pepsinogen and intrinsic factor, which are needed for the digestion and absorption of vitamin B_{12} and the normal development of red blood cells. Pernicious anemia may be caused by the absence of intrinsic factor. Also called **zymogenic cell. 2.** any one of the epithelioid cells with pale-staining cytoplasm and a large nucleus containing a prominent nucleolus. Cords of such cells form the main substance of the pineal body. **3.** any one of the polyhedral epithelial cells, within the parathyroid glands, which contain pale, clear cytoplasm and a vesicular nucleus.

chief complaint (CC), a subjective statement made by a patient describing the most significant or serious symptoms or signs of illness or dysfunction that caused him or her to seek health care. It is used most often in a health history. Also called **presenting symptom.**

chief executive officer (CEO, C.E.O.), the most senior official of an organization or institution.

chief resident, a senior resident physician who acts temporarily as the clinical and administrative director of the house staff in a department of the hospital. The period of duty varies depending on the size of the department, the length of the residency, and the number of house staff members.

chief surgeon, a surgeon appointed or elected head of the surgeons on the staff of a health care facility.

chigger /chig″ər/ [Fr, *chique*], the larva of *Trombicula* mites found in tall grass and weeds. It sticks to the skin and causes irritation and severe itching. Also called **harvest mite, red bug, red mite.** Compare **chigoe.**

chigoe /chig″ō/, a flea, *Tunga penetrans,* found in tropical and subtropical America and Africa. The pregnant female flea burrows into the skin of the feet, causing an inflammatory condition that may lead to spontaneous amputation of a toe. Also called **burrowing flea, sand flea, jigger.** Compare **chigger.**

chikungunya /chik′ungun′yə/ [Swahili, that which bends up], a self-limited disease resembling dengue, not transmissible among people. It was once seen mainly in Africa and Southeast Asia but is now also seen in the Americas. It is caused by an alphavirus transmitted chiefly by mosquitoes of the genus *Aedes.* Avoiding mosquito bites is important in prevention. Its most prominent symptoms are musculoskeletal, and it has occasionally been associated with hemorrhagic fever. It is a possible agent for bioterrorism, dispersed as an aerosol or via infected mosquitoes.

chikungunya encephalitis /chik′əngun″yə/ [Swahili, that which bends up; Gk, *enkephalos,* brain, *itis,* inflammation], a togavirus infection characterized by a high fever that begins abruptly, muscle aches, a rash, and pain in the joints. It is transmitted by the bite of a mosquito and occurs mainly in Africa, in Asia, and on some of the Pacific islands, including Guam. The fever may last for a week, then rise again after a remission of several days. Pain in the joints may

continue after other symptoms have ceased. Supportive nursing care and symptomatic relief are the only treatments. The disease is almost always self-limiting and rarely fatal.

chilblain /chil″blān/ [AS, *cele,* cold, *bleyn,* blister], redness and swelling of the skin caused by excessive exposure to cold. Burning, itching, blistering, and ulceration that are similar to those characteristic of a thermal burn may occur. Treatment includes protection against cold and injury, gentle warming, and avoidance of tobacco. Also called **pernio.** Compare **frostbite.**

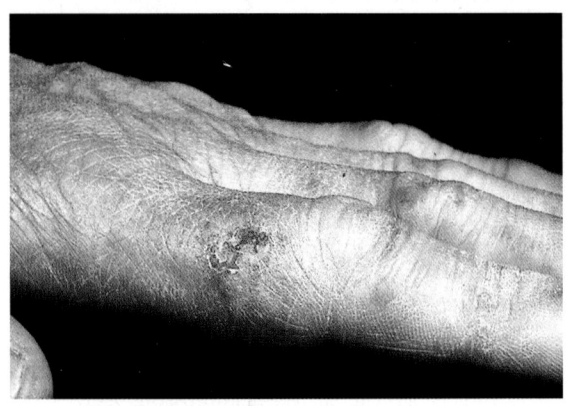

Chilblain *(du Vivier, 1993)*

chilblain lupus erythematosus, a form of discoid lupus erythematosus aggravated by cold, initially resembling chilblains, in which the lesions consist of small, hardened, reddened nodular areas on the exposed areas of the body, especially the finger knuckles.

child [AS, *cild*], **1.** a person of either sex between the time of birth and adolescence. **2.** an unborn or recently born human being; fetus; neonate; infant. **3.** an offspring or descendant; a son or daughter or a member of a particular tribe or clan.

child abuse, the physical, sexual, or emotional maltreatment of a child. Child abuse predominantly affects children less than 3 years of age and is the result of multiple and complex factors involving both the parents and the child, compounded by various stressful environmental circumstances, such as inadequate physical and emotional support within the family and any major life change or crisis, especially those crises arising from marital strife. Parents at high risk for abuse are characterized as having unsatisfied needs, difficulty in forming adequate interpersonal relationships, unrealistic expectations of the child, and a lack of nurturing experience, often involving neglect or abuse in their own childhoods. Predisposing factors among children include the temperament, personality, and activity level of the child; order of birth in the family; sensitivity to parental needs; and requirement for special physical or emotional care resulting from illness, premature birth, or congenital or genetic abnormalities. Identification of abused children or potential child abusers is a major concern for all health care workers. Obvious physical marks on a child's body, such as burns, welts, or bruises, and signs of emotional distress, including symptoms of failure to thrive, are common indications of some degree of neglect or abuse. Often, radiograph films to detect healed or new fractures of the extremities or diagnostic tests to identify sexual molestation are necessary. If abuse is suspected, the health care worker is required to make the necessary report. Special counseling services or support groups, such as Parents Anonymous, help families in which a child is abused. The nurse can play a significant role in preventing abuse by promoting a positive parent-child relationship, especially in the neonatal period, by teaching parents proper child care and disciplinary techniques, by explaining normal child development and behavior so that parents can formulate realistic guidelines for discipline, and by identifying parents at risk for child abuse. Compare **child neglect.**

■ OBSERVATIONS: Abuse may reveal itself through physical, sexual, and/or emotional manifestations. Physical signs include unexplained bruising on soft tissue areas, such as the face, back, neck, buttocks, upper arms, thighs, ankles, and back of legs; multiple bruises at different stages of healing; burns; bites; cuts; unexplained head or abdominal injuries; multiple fractures; or x-ray evidence of multiple old fractures. The child may exhibit a fear of being hit or hurt. The child may be wearing long-sleeve shirts or similar clothing to hide injuries. Patterns of sexual abuse are evidenced as torn, stained, or bloody underclothing; bruising, redness, swelling, or bleeding of the genitalia, vagina, or rectum; statements that it hurts to walk or sit; and complaints of pain or itching in the genital area. The child may play out abuse with dolls or playmates. Emotional abuse may be exhibited in the child as inappropriate behavior or developmental delays in speech or social interactions. This may be accompanied by facial tics, rocking motions, and odd reactions to persons in authority. Emotional abuse is often seen in combination with other forms of abuse or neglect. Patterns of neglect are evidenced through a lack of care and attention. The child may have to provide care for himself or herself that is inappropriate for his or her age or developmental level. The child may be unresponsive or withdrawn, or may not respond to the caregiver's coaxing. Nonorganic failure to thrive or malnutrition should be considered when a healthy baby appears to have lost weight or physical tone, especially when the infant is 25% below the expected growth curve. Diagnosis is typically made by social service, health care, and legal experts after history, investigation, and physical examination. A physical exam is conducted to show injuries or evidence of past injuries and general state of health and hygiene (height or weight parameters that are less than expected, malnourishment, and unkempt appearance). Information, drawing, or play behaviors from child that include evidence of abuse are also diagnostic tools, as are observation of child-parent interactions (eye contact, touching, verbal interaction, and/or parental concern). Severe injury, disability, developmental delay, mental impairment, and death are all complications of chronic and/or severe physical abuse. Abuse victims have an increased likelihood of becoming abusers.

■ INTERVENTIONS: Initial interventions are geared toward stabilizing injuries and preventing further abuse. If serious signs are obvious, the situation should be reported to the appropriate local sources for immediate investigation. If the child is perceived to be in immediate danger, child protection should be sought through the local child protection agency. If the signs are vague or inconsistent, observations need to be documented and reported to appropriate local sources for investigation. Long-term interventions include monitoring, therapy, and support for child and abuser(s).

■ PATIENT CARE CONSIDERATIONS: Nurses, physicians, and other primary health care providers serve as a front-line resource for the detection and prevention of child abuse. This includes the identification of high-risk dependent child relationships, such as lack of prenatal care; previous history of child abuse or neglect; prior removal of other children from the home; parents with a history of substance abuse, depression, or other psychiatric illness; parents with a history of

domestic violence; parents who were themselves abused as children; lack of adequate support networks or resources; and infants or children with high care demands. The provider needs to do a thorough assessment for signs of abuse or neglect, monitor parent-child interactions, and report any suspicions through appropriate channels. The nurse is also instrumental in the institution of actions, such as parenting classes, home visits, early intervention, support groups for parents, and counseling to prevent or halt abuse. Social agency referrals should be made for financial assistance, food, clothing, and shelter needs. Education centers on teaching about realistic expectations for child behavior at various stages of development, and about appropriate forms of discipline and on providing information on available community resources, such as Parents Anonymous or Parents United International.

childbearing period [AS, *cild + beran,* to bear; Gk, *peri,* around, *hodos,* way], the reproductive period in a woman's life from puberty to menopause. It is the time during which she is physiologically able to conceive children. The deferment of childbearing has prompted many women to turn to reproductive technology to extend the childbearing period.

childbed fever, historic term for progressive infection of the fetal membranes and amniotic fluid to the uterus and beyond, which was a common cause of postpartum maternal death. With modern antibiotic therapy maternal death is rare although there is considerable maternal morbidity. Its incidence is increased with premature spontaneous rupture of membranes (PSROM), prolonged labor, and preterm labor. Now called **puerperal fever.** See also **premature rupture of membranes, chorioamnionitis.**

childbirth. See **birth.**

childbirth center, a health facility where prenatal care and delivery services are made available to low-risk pregnant women by a team of nurse-midwives, obstetricians, pediatricians, and ancillary health professionals.

child development, the various stages of physical, social, and psychological growth that occur from birth through young adulthood. See also **adolescence, development, growth, infant, neonatal period, psychosexual development, psychosocial development, toddler.**

childhood, **1.** the period in human development that extends from birth until the onset of puberty. **2.** the state or quality of being a child. See also **development, growth.**

childhood aphasia, an inability to process language, caused by a brain dysfunction in childhood.

childhood asthma, a reversible obstructive lung disease. It is a chronic inflammatory disorder of the airways caused by increased airway reaction to various stimuli. Most children who have asthma develop symptoms before 5 years of age. Asthma in young children (less than 5 years old) is hard to diagnose. It can be a life-threatening disease if not properly managed. It is the third leading cause of hospitalization among children under the age of 15 and a leading cause of school absenteeism.

■ OBSERVATIONS: The symptoms of asthma vary widely in frequency, duration, and degree of symptoms. They may range from frequent coughing spells (which may occur during play, at night, or while laughing or crying), occasional periods of wheezing, and slight dyspnea to severe attacks that can lead to total airway obstruction (resulting in status asthmaticus) and respiratory failure. The child with acute asthma has shortness of breath, chest congestion or tightness; chest pain (particularly in younger children); inability to talk, eat, or play; vomiting; or excessive use of stomach muscles to breathe

■ INTERVENTIONS: Management of asthma in children is based on symptoms and prevention of attacks. In the long-

term management of asthma in children, an effort is made to control the symptoms with the minimum amount of medication, increasing the number and frequency of medications as symptoms increase and reducing the level as symptoms are brought under control. A written asthma action plan is an important tool to let patients and their caregivers know how well treatment is working. The plan outlines the steps needed to manage the child's asthma.
■ PATIENT CARE CONSIDERATIONS: Prognosis varies considerably; asthma symptoms that start in childhood can disappear for some teens and young adults. For others, symptoms go away only to return a few years later. But some children with asthma, particularly those with severe asthma, never outgrow it. The primary focus of care for children with asthma is to relieve symptoms of respiratory distress. The health care team implements measures to promote physical comfort, induce rest, and reduce fatigue and anxiety. An especially important role is to reassure the child and parents about procedures, equipment, and prognosis. Each member of the health care team plays a significant role in the long-term support of children with chronic asthma, primarily in teaching the child and parents about the disease, about how to avoid triggers, and how to cope with the condition.

childhood disintegrative disorder, pervasive developmental disorder characterized by marked regression in a variety of skills, including language, social skills or adaptive behavior, play, bowel or bladder control, and motor skills, after at least 2 years but less than 10 years of apparently normal development.

childhood myxedema [AS, *cildhad* + Gk, *myxa,* mucus, *oidema,* swelling], a juvenile form of hypothyroidism characterized by atrophy of the thyroid gland after a severe infection of the gland. Also called **juvenile myxedema.**

childhood-onset pervasive developmental disorders, disturbances in thought, affect, social relatedness, and behavior that emerge usually between the ages of 30 months and 12 years of age. An example is autism. See also **pervasive developmental disorders.**

childhood polyarteritis nodosa (CPAN), a rare and often fatal disease causing inflammation of small and medium arteries. Clinical signs are dependent on the systems involved and may include skin involvement, myalgia/muscle tenderness, hypertension, peripheral neuropathy, and/or renal involvement.

childhood polycystic disease. See **polycystic kidney disease.**

childhood triad, three types of behavior—fire setting, bed-wetting, and cruelty to animals—that may predict emerging sociopathy when they occur consistently or in combination. Also called **Macdonald triad.**

child life specialist, a professional who specializes in the use of developmental, educational, and therapeutic interventions that help children and their families cope with challenging life events and experiences, such as those related to health care and hospitalization.

child neglect, the failure by parents or guardians to provide for the basic human needs of a child by physical or emotional deprivation that interferes with normal growth and development or that places the child in jeopardy. Compare **child abuse.** See also **failure to thrive, maternal deprivation syndrome.**

Child Occupational Self-Assessment (COSA), a self-assessment tool and an outcome measure based on the Model of Human Occupation designed to capture the perceptions of children regarding their own sense of occupational competence and the importance of everyday activities and tasks related to school, home, and the community.

child psychology, the study of the mental, emotional, and behavioral development of infants and children. See also **applied psychology.**

Child-Pugh classification, a classification of severity of cirrhosis with five different parameters assigned scores of 1 to 3, with 3 being the most negative or severe finding, that are then added together. The parameters are hepatic encephalopathy, ascites, total bilirubin, serum albumin, and prothrombin time (PT), international normalized ratio (INR).

child welfare, a service agency sponsored by the community or special organizations that provide for the physical, social, or psychological care of children.

Children's Health Insurance (CHIP), low-cost health coverage for children in families that have no health insurance and do not qualify for Medicaid. There is no charge for well-care and dental visits. Also called *Children's Health Insurance Program.*

-chilia. See **-cheilia, -chilia.**

chill [AS, *cele*], **1.** the sensation of cold caused by exposure to a cold environment. **2.** an attack of shivering with pallor and a feeling of coldness, often occurring at the beginning of an infection and accompanied by a rapid rise in temperature.

chilo-, prefix for medical terms relating to the lips. See also **cheilo-, cheil-.**

Chilomastix /kī'lōmas″tiks/, a genus of flagellate protozoa, such as *Chilomastix mesnili,* a nonpathogenic intestinal parasite of humans. Infection with this organism may be the occasional cause of diarrhea in children. Transmission is through the oral-fecal route.

chimera /kimir″ə, kīmir″ə/ [Gk, *khimaros,* fire-breathing monster], an organism carrying cell populations derived from two or more different zygotes of the same or different species. Chimeras include recipients of tissue grafts from other individuals. Compare **mosaic.**

chimerism /kimir″izəm/, a state in bone marrow transplantation in which bone marrow and host cells exist compatibly without signs of graft-versus-host rejection disease.

chimney-sweeps' cancer, the first reported occupational disease, initially described in 1775. See **scrotal cancer.**

chin, the raised triangular portion of the mandible and the soft tissue over it below the lower lip. It is formed by the mental protuberance.

Chinese herbal medicine, a highly complex system of diagnosis and treatment using medicinal herbs, one of the branches of traditional Chinese medicine. Herbs used range from the nontoxic and rejuvenating, such as ginseng, which are used to support the body's healing system, to highly toxic ones, such as aconite, used in the treatment of disease.

Chinese restaurant syndrome, (*Informal*) a group of transient symptoms consisting of tingling and burning sensations of the skin, facial pressure, headache, and chest pain that occur immediately after eating food containing monosodium glutamate, frequently used in Chinese cooking. It is a pharmacological reaction and not an allergic reaction. See also **monosodium glutamate.**

Chinese rhubarb, an herb used in Western and traditional medicine. See *Rheum palmatum.*

chin reflex, chin-jerk reflex. See **jaw jerk.**

chinstick, a joystick (used to control a cursor or other movements on a computer screen) that is activated by the chin, without the use of hands. Different joysticks require more force than others. In addition, some joysticks have up to three programmable control buttons that perform various functions. Some, however, work only with software written specifically for use with them. See also **mouthstick.**

CHIP, abbreviation for **Children's Health Insurance Program.**

chip [AS, *kippen,* to slice], **1.** *n.,* a relatively small piece of a bone or tooth. **2.** *v.,* to break off or cut away a small piece. **3.** *n.,* a semiconductor in which an integrated circuit is embedded.

chip fracture, any small fragmental fracture, usually one involving a bony process near a joint. See also **avulsion fracture.**

chip graft, a transplant consisting of small pieces of cartilage or bone that are packed into defective bone structures.

chir-. See **cheiro-, cheir-, chir-, chiro-.**

chiral, (in physical science) describing a compound that cannot be superimposed on its mirror image.

chiralgia /kəral′jə/, a pain in the hand, particularly one that does not result from trauma, nerve injury, or physiological problems.

chirality, using the right or left hand. See **handedness.**

-chiria, -cheiria, suffix meaning a "(specified) condition involving stimulus and its perception": *allochiria.*

chiro-. See **cheiro-, cheir-, chir-, chiro-.**

chiroplasty, surgury specific to the hands. See **cheiroplasty.**

chiropodist, (*Obsolete*) now called **podiatrist.**

chiropody, (*Obsolete*) now called **podiatry.**

chiropractic /kī′rōprak″tik/ [Gk, *cheir,* hand, *practikos,* efficient], a system of therapy based on the theory that the state of a person's health is determined in general by the condition of his or her nervous system. In most cases, treatment provided by chiropractors involves the mechanical manipulation of the spinal column. Some practitioners employ radiology for diagnosis and use physiotherapy and diet in addition to spinal manipulation. Chiropractic care does not include drugs or surgery. A chiropractor is awarded the degree of Doctor of Chiropractic, or D.C., after completing at least 2 years of premedical studies followed by 4 years of training in an approved chiropractic school. Compare **allopathic physician, osteopath.**

chiropractor /-prak″tər/, health care professionals who focus on disorders of the musculoskeletal system and the nervous system, and the effects of these disorders on general health. Chiropractic care is used most often to treat neuromusculoskeletal complaints, including but not limited to back pain, neck pain, pain in the joints of the arms or legs, and headaches. Chiropractic physicians practice a drug-free, hands-on approach to health care that includes patient examination, diagnosis, and treatment. Chiropractors have broad diagnostic skills and are also trained to recommend therapeutic and rehabilitative exercises, as well as to provide nutritional, dietary, and lifestyle counseling.

chirospasm, (*Obsolete*) now called **writer's cramp.**

chisel fracture, an incomplete fracture in which there is oblique detachment of a bone fragment from the head of the radius.

chi square (χ^2) /kī/, (in statistics) a statistic test for an association between observed data and expected data represented by frequencies. The test yields a statement of the probability of the obtained distribution having occurred by chance alone.

chi square distribution /kī skwar/, a theoretical probability distribution of the sum of the squares of a number *(k)* of normally distributed variables whose mean is 0 and standard deviation is 1. The parameter *k* is the number of degrees of freedom. It is widely used for statistical significance in biology and medicine. Also written χ^2 *distribution.*

Chlamydia /kləmid″ē-ə/ [Gk, *chlamys,* cloak], **1.** a microorganism of the genus *Chlamydia.* **2.** a genus of microorganisms that live as intracellular parasites, have a number of properties in common with gram-negative bacteria, and are currently classified as specialized bacteria. Three species of *Chlamydia* have been recognized; all are pathogenic to humans. These are *Chlamydia trachomatis (C. trachomatis), Chlamydia psittaci (C. psittaci),* and *Chlamydia pneumoniae.* It is one of the most common sexually transmitted diseases. See also **psittacosis.** −*chlamydial, adj.*

■ OBSERVATIONS: There may be no symptoms. When present in women, symptoms may include abnormal vaginal discharge, painful intercourse, and itching or burning in the perineal area. In men, there may be a small amount of penile discharge, painful urination, and swelling of the scrotum.

■ INTERVENTIONS: Treatment consists of one of the following: doxycycline, azithromycin, erythromycin, levofloxacin, or ofloxacin. Another important measure includes encouraging patients to refer for testing any sexual partners of the past 60 days.

■ PATIENT CARE CONSIDERATIONS: The health care provider should educate the patient about condom use, medications, and avoidance of sexual intercourse until drug therapy is completed and symptoms are gone.

chlamydial perihepatitis, inflammation of the visceral or diaphragmatic surface of the liver caused by extension of a chlamydial infection.

Chlamydia pneumoniae pneumonia /klə·mid′ē·ə n$\overline{oo}$·mō′-nē·ē/, a mild form of primary atypical pneumonia caused by infection with *C. pneumoniae,* characterized by fever, rales, and infiltration of a middle or lower lobe; the recovery period is usually prolonged. Treatment is on a case-by-case basis. Macrolides are the typical antibiotics prescribed.

Chlamydia test, a microscopic examination or blood test used to determine the presence of the many *Chlamydia* species that cause human diseases such as respiratory tract infections, sexually transmitted disease, eye disease, genital and urethral infections, and pelvic inflammatory disease.

Chlamydia trachomatis pneumonia /klə·mid′ē·ə trəkom′ə·tis/, a mild type of bacterial pneumonia, usually seen in infants whose mothers are infected with *C. trachomatis.* Characteristics include coughing, tachypnea, and eosinophilia. Treatment consists of one of the following: doxycycline, azithromycin, erythromycin, levofloxacin, or ofloxacin.

chloasma /klō·az″mə/ [Gk, *chloazein,* to be green], tan or brown pigmentation, particularly of the forehead, cheeks, and nose, commonly associated with pregnancy, the use of oral contraceptives, or hormone replacement therapy. The hyperpigmentation may be permanent or may disappear, only to recur with subsequent pregnancies or use of oral contraceptives, and is frequently treated with bleaching agents such as hydroquinone. Also called **gravidarum chloasma, mask of pregnancy, melasma.**

chloasma traumaticum, a pigmentary discoloration that results from friction on the skin.

chloasma uterinum, a dark discoloration of the face in pregnancy associated with elevated estrogen and melanocyte-stimulating hormone levels. It may persist to some extent in some women postpartum. Also called **chloasma, mask of pregnancy.**

chlor-, prefix meaning "green": *hyperchloremia, chlorine.*

chloracne /klôrak″nē/ [Gk, *chloros,* green, *akme,* point], a skin condition characterized by small, black follicular plugs and papules on exposed surfaces, especially on the arms, face, and neck of workers in contact with chlorinated compounds, such as cutting oils, paints, varnishes, and lacquers. Avoidance of contact with chlorinated compounds or the use of protective garments prevents the condition.

chloral hydrate, a sedative and hypnotic.

■ INDICATIONS: It is prescribed for the short-term (less than 2 weeks) relief of insomnia, anxiety, or tension and as a sedative/hypnotic for diagnostic procedures.

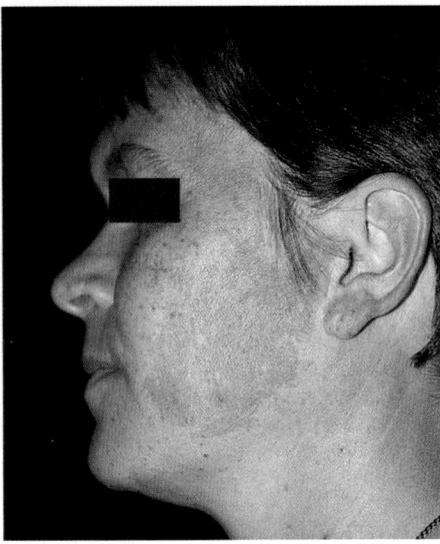

Chloasma *(Gruber and Hansch, 2007)*

■ CONTRAINDICATIONS: Liver or kidney dysfunction or known hypersensitivity to this drug prohibits its use.
■ ADVERSE EFFECTS: Among the more serious adverse reactions are GI disturbances, skin rash, paradoxic excitement, and hypotension.

chloral hydrate poisoning, an adverse reaction to ingestion of trichloroethylidine glycol, also known as chloral hydrate, which is sometimes used as a hypnotic because of its depressive effects on the central nervous system. Symptoms include irritation of the digestive tract, vomiting, depressed breathing, shock, confusion, and injury to the liver and kidneys.

chlorambucil /klôr′ambōō″sil/, an alkylating agent.
■ INDICATIONS: It is prescribed in the treatment of a variety of malignant neoplastic diseases, including chronic lymphocytic leukemia and Hodgkin's disease.
■ CONTRAINDICATIONS: Bone marrow depression or known hypersensitivity to this drug prohibits its use. It is not given during pregnancy or within 28 days of chemotherapy or radiation therapy. Pregnancy should be avoided for 1 month after discontinuing use.
■ ADVERSE EFFECTS: Among the more serious adverse reactions are bone marrow depression, GI disturbance, skin rash, and hepatotoxicity.

chloramphenicol /-amfē″nikol/, an antibacterial and antirickettsial.
■ INDICATIONS: It is used for the treatment of serious infections when the microorganism is resistant to less toxic antibiotics and also when its ability to penetrate to the site of the infection is superior to less toxic alternative antibiotics.
■ CONTRAINDICATIONS: It is used only when safer drugs are contraindicated; pregnancy, lactation, or known hypersensitivity to this drug also prohibits its use.
■ ADVERSE EFFECTS: Among the more serious adverse reactions are bone marrow depression, aplastic anemia, and gray syndrome (characterized by circulatory collapse, cyanosis, acidosis, abdominal distension, coma, and death).

chlordane poisoning. See **chlorinated organic insecticide poisoning.**

chlordiazepoxide /klôr′dī·az′əpok″sīd/, an antianxiety drug of the benzodiazepine type.
■ INDICATIONS: It is prescribed in the treatment of anxiety, nervous tension, and alcohol withdrawal symptoms.

■ CONTRAINDICATIONS: Acute narrow-angle glaucoma, pregnancy, or known hypersensitivity to this drug prohibits its use. It should be used with caution in patients who are depressed or have a history of drug dependence.
■ ADVERSE EFFECTS: Adverse effects include respiratory depression. Among the more serious adverse reactions are withdrawal symptoms that appear on discontinuation of treatment. Drowsiness and fatigue commonly occur.

chlorhexidine /-hek″sidēn/, an antimicrobial agent used as a surgical scrub, hand rinse, and topical antiseptic. It is effective against gram-positive organisms, gram-negative organisms, aerobes, facultative anaerobes, and yeast.

chlorhydria. See **hyperchlorhydria.**

-chloric, suffix meaning "referring to or containing chlorine": *hydrochloric acid.*

chloride /klôr″īd/ [Gk, *chloros,* green], an anion of chlorine. Metal chlorides are salts of hydrochloric acid; the most common is sodium chloride (table salt).

chloride blood test, a blood test performed as part of multiphasic testing of electrolytes. It is performed along with other electrolyte tests to indicate the patient's acid-base balance and hydrational status.

chloride shift, an exchange of chloride ions in red blood cells in peripheral tissues in response to PCO_2 of blood. The shift reverses in the lungs.

chloridometer /klôr′idom″ətər/, an instrument for measuring the level of chlorides in body fluids.

chloriduria, an excessive level of chlorides in the urine.

chlorinated /klôr″ənā′tid/ [Gk, *chloros,* greenish], pertaining to material that contains or has been treated with chlorine.

chlorinated organic insecticide poisoning, poisoning resulting from the inhalation, ingestion, or absorption of chlorophenothane (DDT) and other insecticides containing chlorophenothane, such as heptachlor, dieldrin, and chlordane. It is characterized by vomiting, weakness, malaise, convulsions, tremors, ventricular fibrillation, respiratory failure, and pulmonary edema. Also called **DDT poisoning.**

chlorination [Gk, *chloros,* green], the disinfection or treatment of water or other substances with free chlorine.

chlorine (Cl) /klôr″ēn/, a yellowish-green gaseous element of the halogen group. Its atomic number is 17; its atomic weight mass is 35.453. It has a strong, distinctive odor; is irritating to the respiratory tract; and is poisonous if ingested or inhaled. It occurs in nature chiefly as a component of sodium chloride in seawater and in salt deposits. It is used as a bleach and as a disinfectant to purify water for drinking or for use in swimming pools. Chlorine compounds in general use include many solvents, cleaning fluids, and chloroform. Most of the solvents and cleaning fluids containing chlorine are toxic when inhaled or ingested.

chloroacetophenone (CN) /klo″ro·as″etofe′nōn/, an organic chemistry component and compound commonly used in the production of tear gas and mace.

chloroform /klôr″əfôrm′/ [Gk, *chloros* + L, *formica,* ant], **1.** a nonflammable volatile liquid that was the first liquid inhalation anesthetic to be discovered. (Nitrous oxide was the first gaseous inhalation anesthetic agent discovered.) Chloroform has a low margin of safety and significant toxicity. It is no longer used as an anesthetic agent. **2.** a solvent that is hepatotoxic and nephrotoxic if ingested. Chloroform may also be released to the air as a result of its formation in the chlorination of drinking water, wastewater, and swimming pools. Other sources include pulp and paper mills, hazardous waste sites, and sanitary landfills. The major effect from short-term inhalation exposure to chloroform is central nervous system depression.

chloroleukemia /klôr′ōlo͞okē″mē·ə/ [GK, *chloros,* green, *leukos,* white, *haima,* blood], a kind of myelogenous leukemia in which specific tumor masses are not seen at autopsy, but body fluids and organs are green. See also **myelogenous.**

chlorolymphosarcoma /-lim′fōsärkō″mə/ *pl. chlorolymphosarcomas, chlorolymphosarcomata* [Gk, *chloros* + L, *lympha,* water; Gk, *sarx,* flesh, *oma,* tumor], a greenish neoplasm of myeloid tissue occurring in patients with myelogenous leukemia. The mononuclear cells in the peripheral blood are believed to be lymphocytes rather than myeloblasts, such as found with chloroma.

chloroma /klôrō″mə/ *pl. chloromas, chloromata,* a malignant greenish neoplasm of myeloid tissue that occurs anywhere in the body of patients who have myelogenous leukemia. The green pigment is primarily myeloperoxidase (verdoperoxidase). The tumor tissue fluoresces bright red under ultraviolet light. Also called **chloromyeloma, granulocytic sarcoma.**

Chloromycetin, an antibacterial and antirickettsial drug. Brand name for **chloramphenicol.**

chloromyeloma. See **chloroma.**

chlorophyll /klôr″əfil/ [Gk, *chloros* + *phyllon,* leaf], one of several pigments that absorb light energy and participate in the production of carbohydrates in photosynthetic organisms. Chlorophylls a and b are found in plants, chlorophyll c occurs in brown algae, and chlorophyll d occurs in red algae. Chlorophyll molecules contain a porphyrin ring system that binds a central magnesium ion. See also **photosynthesis.**

chloroprocaine /-prō″kān/, a local anesthetic with a chemical structure similar to that of procaine.

chloroquine /klôr″əkwīn′/, an antimalarial.

■ INDICATIONS: It is prescribed in the treatment of malaria, extraintestinal amebiasis, rheumatoid arthritis, discoid lupus erythematosus, scleroderma, pemphigus, and photoallergic reactions.

■ CONTRAINDICATIONS: Retinal or visual field changes, porphyria, or known hypersensitivity to this drug prohibits its use.

■ ADVERSE EFFECTS: Among the more serious adverse reactions are GI disturbances, headache, visual disturbances resulting from retinal damage, and pruritus. It can turn the skin blue/black and/or the urine brown/black, bleach the hair, and cause photosensitivity.

chlorosis /klôrō″sis/, *(Obsolete)* an iron-deficiency anemia of young women characterized by hypochromic, microcytic erythrocytes and a small reduction in the total number of erythrocytes. See also **anemia.**

chlorothiazide /-thī″əzīd/, a thiazide diuretic chemically related to sulfonamides; an antihypertensive.

■ INDICATIONS: It is prescribed in the treatment of hypertension and edema.

■ CONTRAINDICATIONS: Anuria or known hypersensitivity to thiazide medication or to sulfonamide derivatives prohibits its use.

■ ADVERSE EFFECTS: Among the more serious adverse reactions are hypokalemia, hyperglycemia, and hyperuricemia. Hypersensitivity reactions may occur.

chlorpheniramine maleate /-fenir″əmēn/, an antihistamine.

■ INDICATIONS: It is prescribed in the treatment of a variety of hypersensitivity reactions, including rhinitis, skin rash, and pruritus.

■ CONTRAINDICATIONS: Asthma or known hypersensitivity to this drug prohibits its use. It is not given to newborns or lactating mothers.

■ ADVERSE EFFECTS: Among the more serious adverse reactions are skin rash, hypersensitivity reactions, and tachycardia. Drowsiness and dry mouth commonly occur.

chlorpheniramine polistirex, sulfonated styrene-divinylbenzene copolymer complex with chlorpheniramine, having the same actions as the base, used in cough and cold preparations, administered orally.

chlorpheniramine tannate, the tannate salt of chlorpheniramine, having the same actions as the base, used in cough and cold preparations, administered orally.

chlorproMAZINE /-prō″məzēn/, a phenothiazine drug used as an antipsychotic and antiemetic.

■ INDICATIONS: It is prescribed in the treatment of psychotic disorders (mania, schizophrenia), severe nausea and vomiting, and intractable hiccups.

■ CONTRAINDICATIONS: Parkinson's disease, concurrent administration of central nervous system depressants, liver or renal dysfunction, severe hypotension, or known hypersensitivity to this drug or to other phenothiazine medication prohibits its use.

■ ADVERSE EFFECTS: Among the more serious adverse effects are hypotension, alteration in cardiac conduction, liver toxicity, a variety of extrapyramidal reactions, blood dyscrasias, and hypersensitivity reactions.

chlorproPAMIDE /-prō″pəmīd/, an oral antidiabetic of the sulfonylurea class.

■ INDICATIONS: It is prescribed in the treatment of non–insulin-dependent diabetes mellitus.

■ CONTRAINDICATIONS: Liver or kidney dysfunction or known hypersensitivity to this drug prohibits its use.

■ ADVERSE EFFECTS: Among the most serious adverse reactions are hematological derangements and jaundice. Hypoglycemia, GI distress, and rashes are common adverse effects.

chlortetracycline hydrochloride /-tet′rəsī″klēn/, a tetracycline antibiotic used as a topical antiinfective.

■ INDICATIONS: It is prescribed in the treatment of bacterial infections.

■ CONTRAINDICATIONS: It is available topically only and has little systemic effect. Known hypersensitivity to this drug or to other tetracycline medication prohibits its use.

■ ADVERSE EFFECTS: Burning, stinging, and yellowing of the skin may occur.

chlorthalidone /-thal″idōn/, a diuretic and antihypertensive; a sulfonamide derivative.

■ INDICATIONS: It is prescribed in the treatment of high blood pressure and edema.

■ CONTRAINDICATIONS: Anuria or known hypersensitivity to this drug, to other thiazide medication, or to sulfonamide derivatives prohibits its use.

■ ADVERSE EFFECTS: Among the more serious adverse reactions are hypokalemia, hyperglycemia, hyperuricemia, and hypersensitivity reactions.

Chlor-Trimeton, an antihistamine. Brand name for **chlorpheniramine maleate.**

chlorzoxazone /-zok″səzōn/, a skeletal muscle relaxant.

■ INDICATIONS: It is prescribed for the relief of muscle spasm.

■ CONTRAINDICATIONS: Impaired liver function and known hypersensitivity to this drug prohibit its use.

■ ADVERSE EFFECTS: Among the more serious adverse reactions are jaundice and GI bleeding.

CHN, a nursing specialty certification offered by the Board of Nephrology Examiners Nursing Technology (BONENT). Abbreviation for *certified hemodialysis nurse.*

choana /kō″ənə/ *pl. choanae,* **1.** a funnel-shaped channel. **2.** See **posterior nares.**

choanal atresia /kō″ənəl/ [Gk, *choane,* funnel, *a + tresis,* not hole], a congenital anomaly in which a bony or membranous occlusion blocks the passageway between the nose and pharynx. The condition, which is caused by the failure of the nasopharyngeal septum to rupture during embryonic development, can result in serious ventilation problems in the neonate; therefore providing an oral airway or endotracheal intubation may be necessary. The defect is usually repaired surgically shortly after birth.

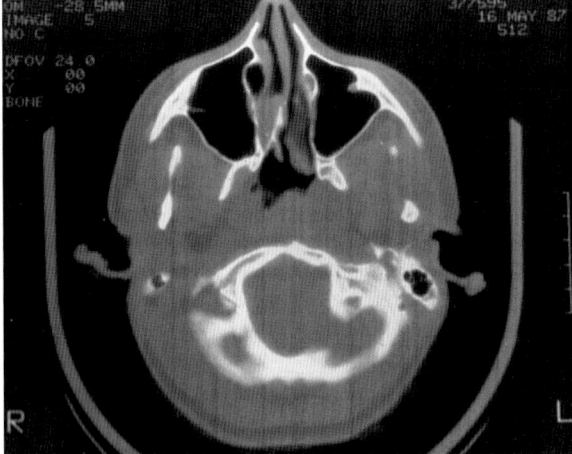

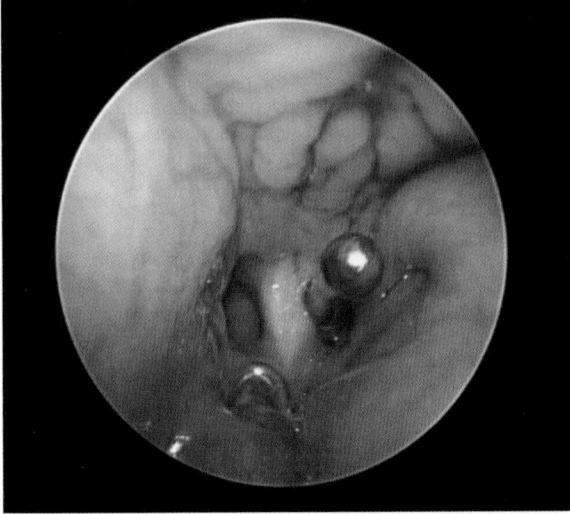

Unilateral choanal atresia *(Myers and Carrau, 2008)*

chocolate cyst [Mex, *chocolatl* + Gk, *kystis,* bag], an ovarian cyst seen in patients with endometriosis, filled with dark red or brown hemosiderin-laden fluid. See also **endometriosis, ovarian cyst.**

choke [ME, *choken*], to interrupt breathing by compression or obstruction of the larynx or trachea.

choke damp, nitrogen and carbon dioxide. See **damp.**

choked disc. See **papilledema.**

chokes, a respiratory condition, occurring in decompression sickness, characterized by shortness of breath, substernal pain, and a nonproductive paroxysmal cough caused by bubbles of gas in the blood vessels of the lungs.

choke-saver, **1.** a curved forceps that can be inserted into the throat of a person who is choking on a food bolus or similar swallowed object. The tweezerlike device can grasp and retrieve the object. See also **Magill forceps. 2.** a program that trains food service employees to recognize a choking victim and administer the Heimlich maneuver. See also **Heimlich maneuver.**

choking, the condition in which a respiratory passage is blocked by constriction of the neck, an obstruction in the trachea, or swelling of the larynx. It is characterized by decreased movement of air through the airways or sudden coughing and a red face that rapidly becomes cyanotic. The person cannot breathe and clutches his or her throat. Emergency treatment requires removal of the obstruction and resuscitation if necessary. See also **Heimlich maneuver.**

choking/lung/pulmonary agents, chemicals that cause severe irritation or swelling of the respiratory tract. Agents include ammonia, bromine, chlorine, osmium tetraoxide, phosgene, phosphine, and phosphorus. When inhaled, they cause damage to the lungs, either by their corrosive effects or by cytotoxicity, leading to respiratory distress and death from respiratory failure. Treatment consists of supportive care.

chol-. See **chole-, chol-, cholo-.**

cholagogue /kō″ləgog/ [Gk, *chole,* bile, *agogein,* to draw forth], a drug that stimulates the flow of bile.

cholangiectasis /kōlan′jē·ek″təsis/, dilation of the bile ducts, usually as a sequela to obstruction.

cholangi(o) [Gk, *choledochos,* bile duct], combining form for bile duct.

cholangiocarcinoma /kōlan′jē·ōkär′sinō″mə/, a cancer of the biliary epithelium. Risk factors include ulcerative colitis and infestation of liver flukes. Diagnosis is based on histological evaluation, and the prognosis is poor.

cholangiocellular carcinoma. See **cholangiohepatoma.**

cholangiogram /kōlan″jē·əgram′/, an x-ray image of the bile ducts produced after injection of a radiopaque contrast medium. A cholangiogram is routinely performed before, during, or after biliary tract surgery. A postoperative x-ray image may be made after injecting an iodinated contrast medium through an indwelling T-tube. The medium also may be introduced directly into the biliary system or intravenously. See also **cholangiography, cholecystography.**

cholangiography /kōlan′jē·og″rəfē/, a special roentgenographic test procedure for outlining the major bile ducts by the IV injection or direct instillation of a radiopaque contrast material. See also **cholecystography.**

■ METHOD: For IV cholangiography the contrast agent is given slowly by vein, and x-ray films are taken of the region of the gallbladder. Operative and postoperative cholangiography use the injection of contrast material into the common bile duct via a drainage T-tube inserted during surgery to reveal any small, residual gallstones that are present. In percutaneous transhepatic cholangiography the contrast material is injected through a long needle or needle catheter, which is introduced directly through the skin into the substance of the liver. Endoscopic retrograde cholangiography is accomplished by cannulating the ampulla of Vater through a flexible fiberoptic duodenoscope and instilling radiopaque material directly into the common bile duct.

■ INTERVENTIONS: IV cholangiography cannot be used in the presence of severe liver disease or jaundice because the dye will not be concentrated and excreted into the bile. The patient fasts, and fluids are restricted overnight. An early morning cleansing enema is given, usually followed by a sedative. The patient is warned about a brief burning sensation that occurs as the dye is injected. For percutaneous transhepatic cholangiography, sedative premedication is often ordered and a local anesthetic injected at the site of needle puncture. Appropriate evaluation for bleeding tendencies must be carried out before percutaneous transhepatic cholangiography. Bile peritonitis is occasionally a complication of T-tube or percutaneous cholangiography, and close nursing observation is essential after the test is completed. For endoscopic retrograde cholangiography, nothing is given by mouth after midnight, an explanation is given to the patient, dentures are removed, and, to permit administration of medications, IV infusion is begun. The endoscope is passed with the patient in the left lateral position; then the patient is turned to the prone position, the ampulla is cannulated, the dye is injected, and films are taken. Vital signs are observed and the patient is given a light meal 2 to 4 hours after the procedure.

■ OUTCOME CRITERIA: The resulting cholangiograms from any of these procedures are examined for unobstructed outlining of the biliary system. Calculi may be noted as shadows within the opaque medium.

cholangiohepatitis /kō·lan′jē·ō·hep′ə·tī′tis/ [Gk, *chole,* bile + *angeion,* vessel + *hepar,* liver + *-itis,* inflammation], severe inflammation of the bile passages, often associated with liver fluke infestation that causes obstruction of the bile ducts.

cholangiohepatoma /kōlan′jē·ō·hep′ətō″mə/ *pl. cholangiohepatomas, cholangiohepatomata,* a primary carcinoma of the liver that develops in the bile ducts in which an abnormal mixture of liver cord cells and bile duct cells exists. Also called **cholangiocarcinoma, cholangiocellular carcinoma.** See also **hepatoma.**

cholangiolitis /-lī″tis/, an abnormal condition characterized by inflammation of the fine tubules of the bile duct system (small bile radicles or cholangioles), which may cause cholangiolitic cirrhosis. −*cholangiolitic, adj.*

cholangioma /kōlan′jē·ō″mə/, a neoplasm of the bile ducts.

cholangiopancreatography /kōlan-jē·ə-paŋ-krē-ə-′tägrə-fē/ [Gk, *chole,* bile + *pan,* all, *kreas,* flesh, *graphein,* to record], the radiographic examination of the bile and pancreatic ducts after introduction of a radiopaque contrast medium.

cholangioscopy /kōlan′jē·os″kəpē/, direct examination of the bile ducts with a fiberoptic endoscope.

cholangiostomy /kōlan′jē·os″təmē/ [Gk, *chole,* bile, *angeion,* vessel, *stoma,* mouth], a surgical operation performed to form an opening in a bile duct.

cholangitis /kō′lanjī″tis/, inflammation of the bile ducts, caused either by bacterial invasion or by obstruction of the ducts by calculi or a tumor. The condition is characterized by severe right upper quadrant pain, jaundice (if an obstruction is present), and intermittent fever. Blood tests reveal an elevated level of serum bilirubin. Diagnosis is made by ultrasound evaluation and cholangiography. Treatment uses antibiotics for infection and surgery for acute obstruction. See also **biliary calculus.**

cholate, any salt or ester of cholic acid; an anion of cholic acid.

chole-, chol-, cholo-, prefix meaning "bile": *cholecystectomy, cholelithotomy, cholesterase.*

cholecalciferol. See **vitamin D₃.**

cholecystagogue /kō′ləsis″təgog′/, a drug that stimulates emptying of the gallbladder.

cholecystalgia, *(Obsolete)* now called **biliary colic.**

cholecystectomy /kō′lisistek″təmē/ [Gk, *chole* + *kystis,* bag, *ektomē,* excision], the surgical removal of the gallbladder, performed to treat cholelithiasis, cholecystitis, and gallbladder cancer. Surgery may be delayed while the acute inflammation is treated. Under general anesthesia, the gallbladder is excised and the cystic duct ligated, the common duct is explored, and any stones found are removed. The most common complication is disruption of the hepatic or other ducts of the biliary system, requiring surgical correction. Wound infection, hemorrhage, bile leakage, and jaundice may also occur. When possible, cholecystectomy is done as a laparoscopic procedure. See also **cholecystitis, cholelithiasis.**

cholecystic /kō′lisis″tik/, pertaining to the gallbladder.

cholecystitis /kō′lisistī″tis/ [Gk, *chole* + *kystis,* bag, *itis,* inflammation], acute or chronic inflammation of the gallbladder. Acute cholecystitis is usually caused by a gallstone that cannot pass through the cystic duct. Pain is felt in the right upper quadrant of the abdomen, accompanied by nausea, vomiting, eructation, and flatulence. The patient may exhibit a positive Murphy's sign. Diagnosis is usually made with ultrasound. Surgery is the preferred mode of treatment. Chronic cholecystitis, the more common type, has an insidious onset. Pain, often felt at night, may follow a fatty meal. Complications include biliary calculi, pancreatitis, and carcinoma of the gallbladder. Again surgery is the preferred treatment. See also **biliary calculus, cholecystectomy, cholelithiasis.**

■ OBSERVATIONS: Common manifestations for cholecystitis may range from indigestion to moderate to severe abdominal or shoulder pain accompanied by fever and jaundice. Symptoms for acute cholecystitis include colicky pain in right upper quadrant and right lower scapula, nausea and vomiting, and low-grade fever. Manifestations indicative of chronic cholecystitis include anorexia, flatulence, nausea, fat intolerance, episodic or diffuse abdominal pain, and heartburn. The gallbladder may be palpable, and palpation of right upper quadrant may elicit tenderness and stoppage of inspiration (Murphy's sign). History may show ingestion of a large fatty meal before onset of pain. Ultrasonography is often performed initially to visualize gallstones. A nuclear imaging (hepatobiliary iminodiacetic acid scan) is useful in diagnosing acute cholecystitis. Necrosis and perforation of the gallbladder with generalized peritonitis, cholangitis with or without septic shock, pancreatitis, biliary cirrhosis, and bowel obstruction with perforation and peritonitis are all complications of biliary disease.

■ INTERVENTIONS: Conservative treatment of a cholecystitis attack includes control of pain, prevention of infection, and maintenance of fluid and electrolyte balance. Gastric decompression to reduce stimulation of the gallbladder may be indicated for control of severe nausea and vomiting. Antiinfective drugs are used to prevent infection, analgesics to treat pain, anticholinergics to reduce secretions, and antispasmodics to reduce smooth muscle spasms. Fat soluble vitamins and bile salts may also be prescribed. Laparoscopic cholecystectomy may be indicated to remove the gallbladder in acute disease. Endoscopic balloon or basket procedures may be used to remove stones. An endoscope retrograde cholangiopancreatography with or without stent placements and sphincterotomy may be used to extract ductal stones. Pulverization of stones by lithotripsy or dissolution of stones by oral ursodiol or methyl terbutyl instilled into gallbladder may also be used.

■ PATIENT CARE CONSIDERATIONS: Acute care is directed toward pain relief and fluid and electrolyte management. Preoperative care includes education about the surgical experience and reduction of anxiety about impending surgery. Postoperative care focuses on pain management, adequate ventilation, and prevention of postsurgical complications, such as bleeding or infection of surgical site. Education for those with an intact gallbladder includes instruction in a low-fat diet, institution of a consistent exercise program, and maintenance of normal weight. Any weight loss needs to be done slowly (1 to 2 lb a week) to prevent sludgy bile. If stones have been removed, the individual needs to understand that stones can recur and that medical follow-up is necessary.

cholecyst(o) [Gk, *choledochos,* bile duct], a combining form meaning gallbladder.

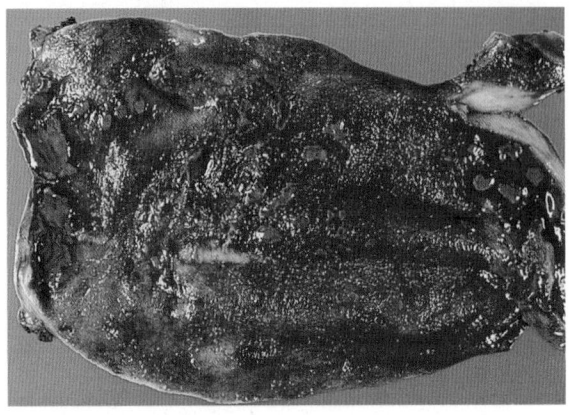

Acute cholecystitis *(Damjanov and Linder, 2000)*

cholecystoduodenostomy /kō'lēsis'tōdoo'ōdənos'təmē/ [Gk, *chole* + *kystis* + L, *duodeni,* twelve fingers], surgical anastomosis of the gallbladder and the duodenum to facilitate drainage of bile into the intestine when the bile duct is blocked.

cholecystogram /kō'lisis''təgram'/, *(Obsolete)* a diagnostic study replaced by ultrasound of the gallbladder.

cholecystoileostomy /kō'lisis'tō·il'ē·os''təmē/ [Gk, *chole,* bile, *kystis,* bag, *eilein,* to twist, *stoma,* mouth], a surgical procedure performed to connect the gallbladder to the ileum. The connection may occur spontaneously after cholecystitis.

cholecystojejunostomy /kō'lē·sis'tōjəjoonos''təmē/ [Gk, *chole* + *kystis* + L, *jejunus,* empty], surgical anastomosis of the gallbladder and the jejunum. The anastomosis may occur spontaneously after cholecystitis.

cholecystokinin /-kī''nin/ [Gk, *chole* + *kystis,* bag, *kinein,* to move], a hormone produced by the mucosa of the upper intestine that stimulates contraction of the gallbladder and secretion of pancreatic enzymes.

cholecystokinin test (CCK test), a test to assess gallbladder function. After IV administration of cholecystokinin, the resultant pancreatic secretion of amylase, trypsin, and lipase is measured by collection through a tube in the duodenum. Compare **CCK-HIDA scan.** See also **secretin-cholecystokinin test.**

cholecystolithiasis /kō'lisis'tōlithī''əsis/, the presence of gallstones in the gallbladder.

cholecystolithotomy /ko'lisis'tōlithot'ämē/, incision of the gallbladder for removal of gallstones.

cholecystolithotripsy /kō'lisis'tōlith''ətripsē/, a procedure for crushing gallstones in the gallbladder or common bile duct with a specialized instrument called a lithotrite.

cholecystosonography /kō'lisis'tōsōnog''rəfē/, a method of examining the gallbladder using ultrasound.

choledochal /-dok''əl/ [Gk, *chole,* bile, *dochus,* containing], pertaining to the common bile duct.

choledochal cysts, rare congenital dilations of the bile ducts.

choledochojejunostomy /kōled'ədok'ōjē'joonos''təmē/ [Gk, *chole,* bile, *dochus,* containing; L, *jejunus,* empty; Gk, *stoma,* mouth], a surgical procedure in which the bile duct is connected to the jejunum.

choledocholith /kōled''əkōlith'/, a gallstone in the common bile duct.

choledocholithiasis. See **biliary calculus.**

choledocholithotomy /-lithot''əmē/ [Gk, *chole* + *dochus,* containing, *lithos,* stone, *temnein,* to cut], a surgical operation to make an incision in the common bile duct to remove a gallstone.

choledocholithotripsy /-lith''ətrip'sē/, a procedure for crushing gallstones in the common bile duct with a specialized instrument called a lithotrite.

choledocholitis, an inflammation of the common bile duct.

Choledyl, a theophylline derivative. Brand name for **oxtriphylline.**

choleic /kōlē''ik/, pertaining to bile.

cholelithiasis /-lithī''əsis/ [Gk, *chole* + *lithos,* stone, *osis,* condition], the presence of gallstones in the gallbladder. The condition affects about 20% of the population above 40 years of age and is more prevalent in women and in persons with cirrhosis of the liver. Many patients complain of unlocalized abdominal discomfort, eructation, and intolerance to certain foods. Others have no symptoms. In patients with severe attacks of biliary pain associated with cholelithiasis, cholecystectomy is recommended to prevent such complications as cholecystitis, cholangitis, and pancreatitis. Also called **chololithiasis.** See also **biliary calculus, cholecystitis.**

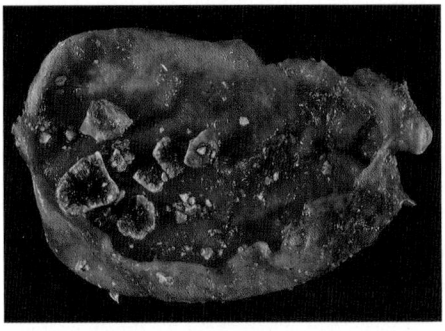

Cholelithiasis *(Kumar et al, 2007)*

cholelithic dyspepsia /kō'lilith''ik/ [Gk, *chole* + *lithos,* stone, *dys,* bad, *peptein,* to digest], an abnormal condition characterized by sudden attacks of indigestion associated with dysfunction of the gallbladder. See also **dyspepsia.**

cholelithotomy /-lithot''əmē/, a surgical operation to remove gallstones through an incision in the gallbladder.

cholera /kol''ərə/ [Gk, *chole* + *rhein,* to flow], an acute bacterial infection of the small intestine. The disease is spread by water and food that have been contaminated by feces of persons previously infected. The symptoms are caused by cholera toxin, which is produced by the infecting organism, *Vibrio cholerae.* The profuse, watery diarrhea, as much as a liter an hour, depletes the body of fluids and electrolytes. Complications include circulatory collapse, cyanosis, destruction of kidney tissue, and metabolic acidosis. The rate of mortality is as high as 50% if the infection remains untreated. See also *Vibrio cholerae,* **vibrio gastroenteritis.**

■ OBSERVATIONS: Symptoms include severe watery diarrhea and vomiting, muscular cramps, dehydration, and depletion of electrolytes.

■ INTERVENTIONS: Treatment includes, first and foremost, replacement of fluids and electrolytes (oral rehydration therapy) or IV fluids and, second, the administration of antibiotics.

■ PATIENT CARE CONSIDERATIONS: A cholera vaccine is available for people traveling to areas where the infection is endemic, but it provides incomplete protection. Preventive measures are critically important and include eating only cooked foods and, when unsure about the quality of the water supply, drinking only water that has been boiled or decontaminated by iodine or that has been commercially bottled.

choleragen /kol″ərəjin/,   an exotoxin produced by the bacterium *Vibrio cholerae* that stimulates the secretion of electrolytes and water into the small intestine in Asiatic cholera, causing diarrhea and loss of body fluids and weakening the patient.

cholera sicca,   *(Obsolete)* a rare malignant form of cholera. Also called **dry cholera.**   Now called **cholera siderans.**

cholera siderans,   a type of cholera seen during epidemics in which the patient experiences a massive outpouring of fluid and electrolytes into the digestive system and dies of toxemia before the usual symptoms of vomiting and diarrhea develop. Mortality is high with this condition, and it is often not recognized as cholera.

cholera vaccine,   an active immunizing agent against cholera.
■ INDICATIONS: It is prescribed as an immunization against cholera.
■ CONTRAINDICATIONS: Immunosuppression, acute infection, concomitant administration of corticosteroids, or known hypersensitivity to this drug prohibits its use.
■ ADVERSE EFFECTS: The most serious adverse reaction is anaphylaxis.

choleresis /kō′lərē″sis/,   the secretion of bile by the liver.

choleretic /kō′ləret″ik/   [Gk, *chole + eresis,* removal],   **1.** *adj.,* stimulating the production of bile in the liver either by cholepoiesis or by hydrocholeresis. **2.** *n.,* a choleretic agent.

choleric /kol″ərik, kəler″ik/,   having a volatile temper or an irritable nature.

choleriform /kōler″ifôrm/,   resembling cholera. Also called *choleroid.*

cholescintigraphy /kō′ləsintig″rəfē/,   a nuclear imaging procedure used to evaluate the function of the gallbladder and bile ducts. The procedure involves the injection of a radioactive tracer.

cholestasis /-stā″sis/   [Gk, *chole + stasis,* standing still],   interruption in the flow of bile through any part of the biliary system, from liver to duodenum. It is essential to determine whether the cause is within the liver (intrahepatic) or outside it (extrahepatic). Intrahepatic causes include hepatitis, drug and alcohol use, metastatic carcinoma, and pregnancy. Extrahepatic causes include presence of an obstructing calculus or tumor in the common bile duct and carcinoma of the pancreas. Symptoms of both types of cholestasis include jaundice, pale and fatty stools, dark urine, and intense itching over the skin. If liver disease is suspected, liver biopsy examination can confirm the suspicion, and attempts can be made to treat the underlying disorder. Extrahepatic cholestasis usually requires surgery. See also **cholestatic hepatitis.** −*cholestatic, adj.*

cholestatic hepatitis,   jaundice with bile stasis in inflamed intrahepatic bile ducts usually caused by the toxic effects of a drug. Signs are persistent jaundice, itching, and elevated alkaline phosphatase levels. These signs usually abate when the hepatitis remits. See also **cholestasis, hepatitis.** −*cholestatic, adj.*

cholestatic jaundice /-stat″ik/,   a yellowing of the skin caused by thickening of bile, obstruction of hepatic ducts, or changes in liver cell function.

cholesteatoma /kōles′tē·ətō″mə/   [Gk, *chole + stear,* fat, *oma,* tumor],   a cystic mass composed of epithelial cells and cholesterol that is found in the middle ear and occurs as a congenital defect or as a serious complication of chronic otitis media. The mass may occlude the middle ear, or enzymes produced by it may destroy the adjacent bones, including the ossicles. Surgery is required to remove a cholesteatoma. See also **otitis media.**

cholesterase /kəles″tərās′/   [Gk, *chole + aither,* air; Ger, *saure,* acid; *ase,* enzyme suffix],   an enzyme in the blood and other tissues that forms cholesterol and fatty acids by hydrolyzing cholesterol esters.

cholesteremia.   See **cholesterolemia.**

cholesterol /kəles″tərôl/   [Gk, *chole + steros,* solid],   a waxy lipid soluble compound found only in animal tissues. A member of a group of compounds called sterols, it is an integral component of every cell in the body. It facilitates the absorption and transport of fatty acids. Cholesterol acts as the precursor for the synthesis of various steroid hormones, including cortisol, cortisone, and aldosterone in the adrenal glands, and of the sex hormones progesterone, estrogen, and testosterone. It sometimes precipitates along with other compounds in the gallbladder to form gallstones. Cholesterol is found in foods of animal origin and is continuously synthesized in the body, primarily in the liver. Increased levels of low-density lipoprotein cholesterol may be associated with the pathogenesis of atherosclerosis, whereas higher levels of high-density lipoprotein cholesterol appear to lower the person's risk for heart disease. Normal adult levels of total blood cholesterol are 150 to 200 mg/dL or 3.9 to 5.2 mmol/L (SI units). Also called *cholesterin.* See also **high-density lipoprotein, low-density lipoprotein, sterol.**

Chemical structure of cholesterol *(Patton and Thibodeau, 2010)*

cholesterol embolism,   an embolism resulting from fracture of a plaque of atherosclerosis, most frequently caused by trauma to the aorta during cardiac catheterization.

Cholesterol and lipoprotein profile classification

Cholesterol reading	Classification
Total cholesterol (mg/dL)	
<200	Desirable
200–239	Borderline high risk
≥240	High risk
LDL cholesterol (mg/dL)	
<100	Optimal
100–129	Near optimal
130–159	Borderline high risk
160–189	High risk
≥190	Very high risk
HDL cholesterol (mg/dL)	
≥60	Optimal
<40	Low
Triglycerides (mg/dL)	
<150	Normal
150–199	Borderline high risk
200–499	High risk
≥500	Very high risk

cholesterolemia /-ē″mē·ə/, **1.** the presence of excessive amounts of cholesterol in the blood. **2.** Also called **cholesteremia.** See also **hypercholesterolemia.**

cholesteroleresis /kəles′tərôler″isis, -erē′sis/ [Gk, *chole, steros + eresis,* removal], the increased elimination of cholesterol in the bile.

cholesterol metabolism, the sum of the anabolic and catabolic processes in the synthesis and degradation of cholesterol in the body. Serum cholesterol level is increased when it is ingested and is quickly absorbed. Cholesterol is also synthesized in the liver and can be synthesized by most other body tissues. As more cholesterol is ingested, less is synthesized by the body. Cholesterol is removed from the body by degradation in the liver and excretion in the bile.

cholesterolopoiesis /kəles′tərō′lōpō·ē″sis/ [Gk, *chole + steros + poiesis,* producing], the elaboration of cholesterol by the liver.

cholesterolosis /kəles′tərəlō″sis/, an abnormal condition, found in about 5% of patients with chronic cholecystitis, in which deposits of cholesterol occur within large macrophages in the submucosa of the gallbladder. This produces a spotty appearance, sometimes referred to as a strawberry gallbladder. Cholesterolosis is often associated with gallstones and may be asymptomatic or accompanied by biliary colic. Also called *cholesterosis.* See also **cholecystitis.**

cholesterol-restricted diet. See **low-cholesterol diet.**

cholesterol test, a blood test used to identify patients who are at risk for arteriosclerotic heart disease. Because cholesterol alone is not a totally accurate predictor of heart disease, this test is usually done as a part of lipid profile testing, which also evaluates levels of lipoproteins and triglycerides.

cholesteryl ester storage disease /kōles″təril/, an inherited disorder in which there is an accumulation of neutral lipids, such as cholesterol esters and glycerides, in body tissues. The disease may be asymptomatic or be characterized by hepatosplenomegaly, fat in the stools (steatorrhea), and adrenal calcification. The cause is a deficiency of the enzyme cholesterol ester hydrolase. There is no specific treatment. A form of the disorder affecting infants, with symptoms in the first weeks after birth, is Wolman disease.

cholesteryl ester transfer protein (CETP), a plasma glycoprotein that plays a role in the movement of cholesterol from the peripheral tissue to the liver by mediating the transfer of cholesteryl esters from HDL cholesterol to apolipoprotein B–containing proteins, which are then metabolized to lipoproteins that are removed from the circulation by receptors in the liver. Deficiency of this protein, an autosomal-dominant trait, results in markedly higher plasma levels of HDL cholesterol and apolipoprotein A-I. Also called *plasma lipid transfer protein.*

cholestyramine /-tir″əmēn/, a drug used to treat hypercholesterolemia that acts on the liver's bile acids. It binds to bile acids and causes increased fecal elimination, which causes increased oxidation of cholesterol to bile acids, thereby lowering blood cholesterol levels.

cholestyramine resin, an ion-exchange resin and antihyperlipemic agent.

■ INDICATIONS: It is prescribed for oral administration to increase bile acid excretion in the stool, for the treatment of hyperlipoproteinemia, and for pruritus resulting from partial biliary obstruction.

■ CONTRAINDICATIONS: Complete biliary obstruction or known hypersensitivity to this drug prohibits its use.

■ ADVERSE EFFECTS: Among the more serious adverse reactions are fecal impaction, GI disturbances, and depletion of vitamins A, D, and K. Constipation is common. It interferes with the absorption of many other drugs, so other medicines should be given 1 hr before or 4-6 hr after cholestyramine.

-cholia, -choly, suffix meaning "(condition of the) bile": *dyscholia.*

cholic acid, a bile acid synthesized in the liver from cholesterol. Cholan-24-oic acid is stored in the liver bound to coenzyme A and converted to glycine and taurine bile salts before secretion into bile.

choline /kō″lēn/ [Gk, *chole,* bile], a lipotropic substance that can be synthesized by the body. Under certain circumstances it is considered by some to be essential. Found in most animal tissues, choline is a primary component of acetylcholine, the neurotransmitter, and functions with inositol as a basic constituent of lecithin. It prevents fat deposits in the liver and facilitates the movement of fats into the cells. The richest sources of choline are liver, kidneys, brains, wheat germ, brewer's yeast, and egg yolk. See also **inositol, lecithin.**

choline bitartrate, the bitartrate salt of choline, used as a dietary supplement.

choline chloride, the chloride salt of choline, used as a dietary supplement.

choline esters, a group of cholinergic drugs that acts at sites or organs where acetylcholine is the neurotransmitter. Kinds include **bethanechol chloride, methacholine,** *carbachol.*

choline magnesium trisalicylate, a combination of choline and magnesium salicylates, used as an analgesic, antipyretic, antiinflammatory, and antirheumatic and administered orally.

cholinergic /-ur″jik/ [Gk, *chole + ergon,* to work], **1.** pertaining to nerve fibers that liberate acetylcholine at the myoneural junctions. **2.** the tendency to transmit or to be stimulated by or to stimulate the elaboration of acetylcholine. Also called **cholinergic stimulant.** Compare **adrenergic, anticholinergic.**

cholinergic blocking agent, any agent that blocks the action of acetylcholine and substances similar to acetylcholine. Such agents, in effect, block the action of cholinergic nerves that transmit impulses by the release of acetylcholine at their synapses.

cholinergic crisis, a pronounced muscular weakness and respiratory paralysis caused by excessive acetylcholine, often apparent in patients suffering from myasthenia gravis as a result of overmedication with anticholinesterase drugs. Intubation and mechanical ventilation are necessary until the crisis resolves.

cholinergic fiber [Gk, *chole,* bile, *ergon,* work; L, *fibra*], a nerve fiber of the autonomic nervous system that releases the neurotransmitter acetylcholine. Cholinergic fibers include all preganglionic fibers, all postganglionic sympathetic fibers to sweat glands, and efferent fibers innervating skeletal muscle.

cholinergic nerve, a nerve that releases the neurotransmitter acetylcholine at its synapse. The cholinergic nerves include all the preganglionic sympathetic and preganglionic parasympathetic nerves, the postganglionic parasympathetic nerves, the somatic motor nerves to skeletal muscles, and some nerves to sweat glands and to certain blood vessels.

cholinergic receptor [Gk, *chole,* bile, *ergein,* to work; L, *recipere,* to receive], a specialized sensory nerve ending that responds to the stimulation of acetylcholine.

cholinergic stimulant. See **cholinergic.**

cholinergic urticaria [Gk, *chole + ergon,* to work; L, *urtica,* nettle], an abnormal and usually temporary vascular reaction of the skin, often associated with sweating, in susceptible individuals subjected to stress, strong exertion, or hot weather. The condition is characterized by small, pale, itchy papules surrounded by reddish areas. It is caused by the action of acetylcholine on mast cells. Compare **urticaria.**

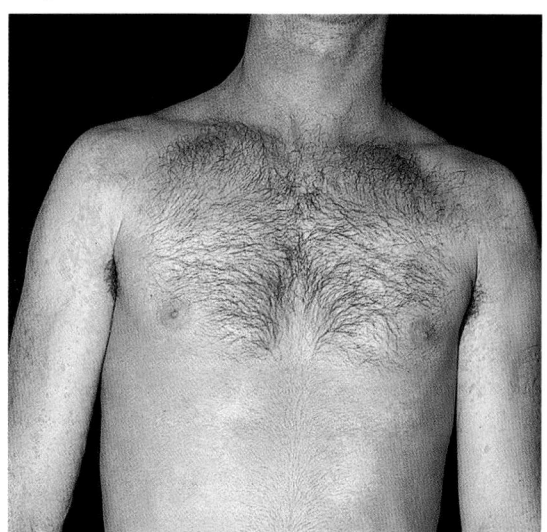

Adult male with cholinergic urticaria *(Callen et al, 2000)*

choline salicylate, the choline salt of salicylic acid, used as an analgesic, antipyretic, antiinflammatory, and antirheumatic, administered orally.

cholinesterase /kō′lines″tərās/, an enzyme that acts as a catalyst in the hydrolysis of acetylcholine to choline and acetate. It provides the off mechanism during cholinergic neurotransmission.

cholinesterase inhibitor. See **anticholinesterase.**

cholinesterase test, a blood test done to identify patients with pseudocholinesterase deficiency before anesthesia or to identify patients who may have been exposed to organophosphate poisoning.

cholo-. See **chole-, chol-, cholo-.**

Cholografin, a diagnostic contrast medium used in radiology. Brand name for *iodipamide.*

chololithiasis /kō′ləlithī′əsis/. See **cholelithiasis.**

Choloxin, an antihyperlipoproteinemic agent. Brand name for *dextrothyroxine sodium.*

-choly. See **-cholia, -choly.**

cholylglycine. See **glycocholic acid.**

cholyltaurine, a bile salt, the taurine conjugate of cholic acid. Also called *taurocholic acid.*

chondr-. See **chondro-, chondr-, chondri-.**

chondral /kon″drəl/, pertaining to cartilage.

chondralgia /kondral″jə/, pain that appears to originate in cartilage.

chondrectomy /kondrek″təmē/, the surgical excision of a cartilage.

chondri-. See **chondro-, chondr-, chondri-.**

-chondria, -chondrion, **1.** suffix meaning "a condition involving granules in cell composition": *mitochondrion.* **2.** suffix from Greek *hypochondrion* ("below the cartilage"). The hypochondriac region was regarded as the seat of emotion in ancient Greece.

chondrial bone [Gk, *chondros,* cartilage; AS, *ban,* bone], bone that forms under the periosteal membrane. Also called **perichondrial bone.**

chondriocont /kon″drē·ōkont′/, a threadlike or rod-shaped mitochondrion.

chondriome /kon″drē·ōm/ [Gk, *chondros,* cartilage], the total mitochondrial content of a cell, taken as a unit. Also called *chondrioma.*

chondriomite /kon″drē·ōmīt′/ [Gk, *chondros* + *mitos,* thread], a single, granular mitochondrion or a group of such mitochondria that appear in a chain formation.

chondriosome, *(Obsolete)* now called **mitochondrion.**

chondritis /kondrī″tis/, any inflammatory condition affecting the cartilage.

chondro-, chondr-, chondri-, prefix meaning "cartilage": *chondroblast, chondroclast, chondrocostal.*

chondroadenoma. See **adenochondroma.**

chondroangioma /kon′drō·an′jē·ō″mə/ *pl. chondroangiomas, chondroangiomata* [Gk, *chondros* + *angeion,* vessel, *oma,* tumor], a benign mesenchymal tumor containing vascular and cartilaginous elements.

chondroblast /kon″drōblast/ [Gk, *chondros* + *blastos,* germ], any one of the cells that develop from the mesenchyma and form cartilage. Chondroblasts secrete the extracellular matrix of cartilage and play an important role in endochondrial ossification and especially in longitudinal bone growth. Formerly called **chondroplast.**

chondroblastoma /kon′drōblastō″mə/ *pl. chondroblastomas, chondroblastomata,* a benign tumor, derived from precursors of cartilage cells, that develops most frequently in the epiphyses of the proximal humerus, distal femur, and the proximal tibia. It is more common in boys than girls, typically appearing during the teenage years. The lesions may contain scattered areas of calcification and necrosis. Also called **Codman tumor.**

chondrocalcinosis /kon′drōkal′sinō″sis/ [Gk, *chondros* + L, *calyx,* lime; Gk, *osis,* condition], an arthritic disease in which calcium deposits are present in the peripheral joints. It resembles gout and often occurs in patients over 50 years of age who have osteoarthritis or diabetes mellitus. It most commonly invades the knee joint. Aspiration of synovial fluid from the affected joints reveals crystals of calcium salts, especially calcium pyrophosphate dihydrate. Inflammation and pain may be relieved by intraarticular injections of hydrocortisone and by antiinflammatory medications. Also called **pseudogout.** Compare **gout.**

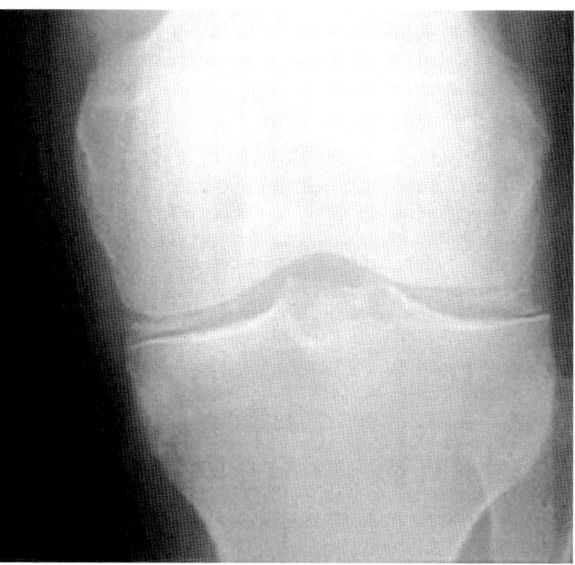

Chondrocalcinosis *(Browner and Fuller, 2012)*

chondrocarcinoma /kon′drōkär′sinō″mə/ *pl. chondrocarcinomas, chondrocarcinomata* [Gk, *chondros* + *karkinos*, crab, *oma*, tumor], a malignant epithelial tumor in which cartilaginous metaplasia is present.

chondroclast /kon″drōklast′/ [Gk, *chondros* + *klasis*, breaking], a giant multinucleated cell associated with the resorption of cartilage. −*chondroclastic, adj.*

chondrocostal /kon′drōkos″təl/ [Gk, *chondros* + L, *costa*, rib], pertaining to the ribs and the costal cartilages.

chondrocyte /kon″drəsīt/ [Gk, *chondros* + *kytos*, cell], any one of the polymorphic cells that reside in the cartilage of the body and maintain the extracellular matrix. Each contains a nucleus, a relatively large amount of clear cytoplasm, and the common organelles. −*chondrocytic, adj.*

chondrodysplasia /kon′drōdisplā″zhə/ [Gk, *chondros* + *dys*, bad, *plassein*, to form], an inherited bone dysplasia characterized by abnormal growth appearing as stippling at the ends of bones, particularly the long bones of the arms and legs. Bones of the hands and feet may be similarly affected.

chondrodysplasia punctata, an inherited form of dwarfism characterized by skin lesions, radiographic evidence of epiphyseal stippling, and a pug nose. There are two types of the anomaly: a benign Conradi-Hünermann form marked by mild asymmetric limb shortening and a lethal rhizomelic form with marked proximal limb shortening. The Conradi-Hunermann form of the disorder is transmitted by an autosomal-dominant gene and the rhizomelic form by an autosomal-recessive gene.

chondrodystrophia calcificans congenita /-distrō″fē·ə/ [Gk, *chondros* + *dys*, bad, *trophe*, nourishment; L, *calyx*, lime, *congenitus*, born with], an inherited defect characterized by many small opacities in the epiphyses of the long bones. This sign is present on x-ray images of the newborn. Dwarfism, contractures, cataracts, cognitive disability, and short, stubby fingers develop as the infant grows into childhood. Also called *chondrodystrophia fetalis calcificans.*

chondrodystrophic myotonia. See **Schwartz-Jampel syndrome.**

chondrodystrophy /kon′drōdis″trəfē/ [Gk, *chondros* + *dys*, bad, *trophe*, nourishment], a group of disorders in which there is abnormal conversion of cartilage to bone, particularly in the epiphyses of the long bones. Patients are dwarfed, with normal trunks and shortened extremities. See also **achondroplasia.**

chondroectodermal dysplasia /kon′drō·ek′tədur″məl/, an inherited form of dwarfism marked by distal limb shortening, an extra finger or toe next to the smallest finger or toe, and cardiovascular abnormalities. It is transmitted by an autosomal-recessive gene. Also called **Ellis−van Creveld syndrome.**

chondroendothelioma /kon′drō·en′dōthē′lē·ō″mə/ *pl. chondroendotheliomas, chondroendotheliomata* [Gk, *chondros* + *endon*, within, *thele*, nipple, *oma*, tumor], a benign mesenchymal tumor containing cartilaginous and endothelial components.

chondrofibroma /kon′drōfībrō″mə/ *pl. chondrofibromas, chondrofibromata*, a fibrous tumor that contains cartilaginous components.

chondrogenesis /kon′drōjen″əsis/, the development of cartilage. −*chondrogenetic, adj.*

chondroid /kon″droid/, resembling cartilage.

chondroid lipoma, an uncommon benign fatty neoplasm occurring as a well-circumscribed, yellow, sometimes encapsulated, slowly growing mass under the skin, typically affecting middle-aged adults, usually women, and most often involving the limb girdles or proximal extremities. It is

characterized by a lobular growth pattern and is composed of large vacuolated cells resembling lipoblasts.

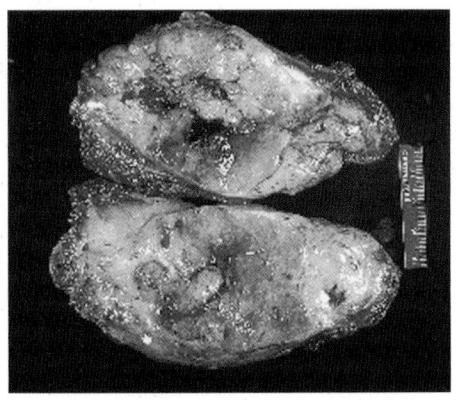

Chondroid lipoma *(Rosai, 2011)*

chondrolipoma /kon′drōlipō″mə/ *pl. chondrolipomas, chondrolipomata*, a benign mesenchymal tumor containing fatty and cartilaginous components.

chondroma /kondrō″mə/ *pl. chondromas, chondromata*, a benign, fairly common tumor of cartilage cells that grows slowly within cartilage (enchondroma) or on the surface (ecchondroma). Kinds include **joint chondroma, synovial chondroma.** See also **ecchondroma, enchondroma.** −*chondromatous, adj.*

-chondroma, suffix meaning a "benign cartilaginous tumor": *osteochondroma.*

chondromalacia /kon′drōməlā″shə/ [Gk, *chondros* + *malakia*, softness], a softening of cartilage. *Chondromalacia fetalis* is a lethal congenital form of the condition in which a stillborn infant has soft and pliable limbs. *Chondromalacia patellae* occurs in young adults after knee injury and is characterized by swelling, pain, and degenerative changes, which are revealed on x-ray examination.

chondroma sarcomatosum. See **chondrosarcoma.**

chondromatosis /kon′drōmətō″sis/, a condition characterized by the presence of many cartilaginous tumors. Kinds include **synovial chondroma.**

chondromatous. See **chondroma.**

chondromere /kon″drōmir/ [Gk, *chondros* + *meros*, part], a cartilaginous embryonic vertebra and its costal component.

chondromyoma /kon′drōmī·ō″mə/ *pl. chondromyomas, chondromyomata* [Gk, *chondros* + *mys*, muscle, *oma*, tumor], a benign mesenchymal tumor containing myomatous and cartilaginous tissue.

chondromyxofibroma /kon′drōmik′sōfībrō″mə/ [Gk, *chondros* + *myxa*, mucus; L, *fibra*, fiber, *oma*, tumor], a benign tumor that develops from cartilage-forming connective tissue. The lesion, typically a firm, grayish-white mass, tends to occur in the knee and small bones of the foot and may be confused with chondrosarcoma. Also called **chondromyxoid fibroma.**

chondromyxoid /kon′drōmik″soid/ [Gk, *chondros* + *myxa*, mucus, *eidos*, form], composed of cartilaginous and myxoid elements.

chondromyxoid fibroma. See **chondromyxofibroma.**

chondrophyte /kon″drōfīt/ [Gk, *chondros* + *phyton*, growth], an abnormal mass of cartilage. −*chondrophytic, adj.*

chondroplasia /-plā″zhə/ [Gk, *chondros,* cartilage, *plassein,* to form], the formation of cartilage.

chondroplast. See **chondroblast.**

chondroplasty /kon″drōplas′tē/ [Gk, *chondros* + *plassein,* to mold], the surgical repair of cartilage.

chondrosarcoma /kon′drōsärkō″mə/ *pl.* chondrosarcomas, chondrosarcomata [Gk, *chondros* + *sarx,* flesh, *oma,* tumor], a malignant neoplasm of cartilaginous cells or their precursors that occurs most frequently in long bones, the pelvic girdle, and the scapula. The tumor is a large, smooth, lobulated growth composed of nodules of hyaline cartilage that may show slight to marked calcification. Also called **chondroma sarcomatosum.** **–chondrosarcomatous,** *adj.*

chondrosarcomatosis /kon′drōsär′kōmətō″sis/, a condition characterized by multiple malignant cartilaginous tumors.

chondrosarcomatous. See **chondrosarcoma.**

chondrosis /kondrō″sis/, 1. the development of the cartilage of the body. 2. a cartilaginous tumor.

chondrosternal joint. See **sternocostal articulation.**

chondrotomy /kondrot″əmē/, a surgical procedure for dividing a cartilage.

CHOP /chop/, an anticancer drug combination that is typically used in non-Hodgkin lymphoma and will often be combined with a monoclonal antibody such as rituximab. Abbreviation for *cyclophosphamide, doxorubicin, vincristine, and prednisone.*

chopping, a therapeutic exercise to improve the strength and coordination of upper trunk nerves and muscles by lifting the arms overhead and lowering them in a chopping or slashing movement.

chord-, root/combining form meaning "string, cord": *chordoma, chordotomy.*

chorda /kôr″də/, a string filament such as a nerve or tendon.

chordae tendineae, the strands of tendon that anchor the cusps of the mitral and tricuspid valves to the papillary muscles of the ventricles of the heart, preventing prolapse of the valves into the atria during ventricular contraction. Also called **tendinous cords.**

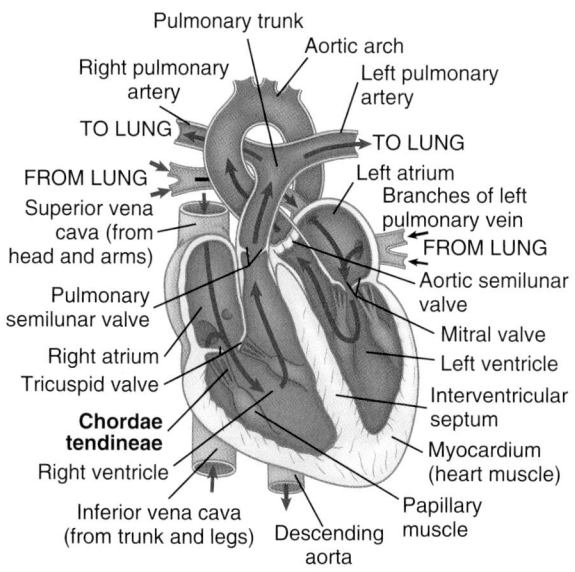

Chordae tendineae *(McCance and Huether, 2014)*

chordal canal. See **notochordal canal.**

chorda tympani, a branch of the facial nerve that carries taste from the anterior two thirds of the tongue and parasympathetic innervation to all salivary glands below the level of the oral fissure.

chordee /kôr″dē, kôr″dā/ [Gk, *chorde,* cord], a congenital defect of the genitourinary tract resulting in a ventral curvature of the penis, caused by presence of a fibrous band of tissue instead of normal skin along the corpus spongiosum. The condition is often associated with hypospadias and is surgically corrected in early childhood. The goals of surgery are to improve the appearance of the genitalia cosmetically for psychological reasons, to construct an organ that allows the boy to void in a standing position, and to produce a sexually adequate organ.

chorditis /kôrdī″tis/, 1. inflammation of a spermatic cord. 2. inflammation of the vocal cords or of the vocal folds.

chorditis nodosa, the formation of small white nodules on one or both vocal cords in persons who use their voices excessively. Also called *chorditis tuberosa.* See also **vocal cord nodule.**

chordoid /kôr″doid/ [Gk, *chorde* + *eidos,* form], resembling the notochord or notochordal tissue, cell-like material present in embryonic development.

chordoma /kôrdō″mə/ *pl.* chordomas, chordomata, a rare tumor that develops from the fetal notochord. It is usually located in the midline, behind the sella; it is slow growing but highly invasive. The most common chordomas are of the sacrum and cervical spine.

chordotomy /kôrdot″əmē/ [Gk, *chorde* + *temnein,* to cut], surgery in which the anterolateral tracts of the spinal cord are surgically divided to relieve pain.

chorea /kôrē″ə/ [Gk, *choreia,* dance], a condition characterized by involuntary rapid, purposeless motions, as flexing and extending of the fingers, raising and lowering of the shoulders, or grimacing. The movements often appear to be well coordinated. In some forms the person is also irritable, emotionally unstable, physically weak, and restless. See also **chorea gravidarum, Huntington disease, Sydenham chorea.** **–choreic,** *adj.*

chorea gravidarum /kôr″ē·əgrav′idär″əm/, a type of movement disorder that occurs during the early months of pregnancy. It may be a form of Sydenham chorea associated with a history of rheumatic fever. More commonly, it is triggered in some women taking oral contraceptives. Symptoms should recede within hours or days of delivery. See also **Sydenham chorea.**

chorea minor, *(Obsolete)* now called **Sydenham chorea.**

choreic. See **chorea.**

choreic ataxia /kôrē″ik/ [Gk, *choreia,* dance, *ataxia,* without order], a form of ataxia in which patients lack muscular coordination and movements are marked by involuntary twitching and abrupt jerking.

choreiform /kərē″əfôrm′/, resembling the rapid jerky, involuntary, and uncoordinated movements associated with chorea.

choreiform spasm [Gk, *choreia,* dance; L, *forma* + Gk, *spasmos*], a condition of involuntary muscle contractions that result in dancing motions. In one type, powerful contractions of the leg muscles cause a leaping, jumping action. It can also involve arm, shoulder, and neck muscles.

choreoacanthocytosis. See **neuroacanthocytosis.**

choreoathetoid cerebral palsy /kôr′ē·ō·ath″ətoid/, a form of cerebral palsy characterized by choreiform (jerky, ticlike twitching) and athetoid (slow, writhing) movements.

choreoathetosis /kôr′ē·ō·ath′ətō″sis/ [Gk, *choreia,* dance, *athetos,* not fixed], irregular involuntary movements that may involve the face, neck, trunk, extremities, or respiratory muscles, giving an appearance of restlessness. The writhing movements may vary from subtle to wild and ballistic and are commonly associated with administration of levodopa in parkinsonism. Levodopa-induced involuntary movement (dyskinesia) occurs most commonly 1 to 3 hours after administration of the drug.

chorio-, combining form meaning "protective fetal membrane": *choriocele, chorioamnionitis.*

chorioadenoma /kərē′ō·ad′inō″mə/ *pl. chorioadenomas, chorioadenomata* [Gk, *chorion,* skin, *aden,* gland, *oma,* tumor], an epithelial cell tumor of the outermost fetal membrane that is intermediate in the malignant development of a hydatid mole to invasive choriocarcinoma.

chorioadenoma destruens /-des″trōō·əns/ [Gk, *chorion + aden + oma +* L, *destruere,* to pull down], an invasive hydatidiform mole in which the chorionic villi of the mole penetrate into the myometrium and parametrium of the uterus and metastasize to distant parts of the body, most commonly to the lungs. Also called **metastasizing mole.**

chorioamnionic /-am′nē·ot″ik/, pertaining to the chorion and the amnion.

chorioamnionitis /-am′nē·ōnī″tis/ [Gk, *chorion + amnion,* fetal membrane, *itis,* inflammation], a progressive infection of the fetal membranes and amniotic fluid to the uterus and beyond. With modern antibiotic therapy maternal death is rare although there is considerable maternal morbidity. Its incidence is increased with premature spontaneous rupture of membranes (PSROM), prolonged labor, and preterm labor.

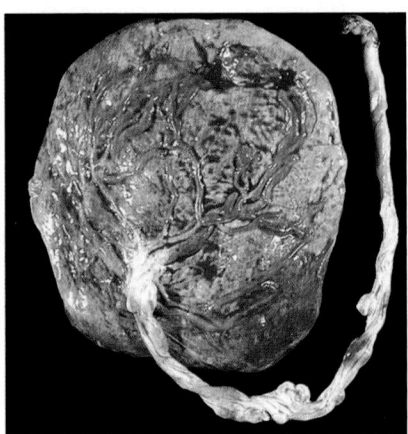

Chorioamnionitis *(Zitelli and Davis, 2007)*

choriocarcinoma /kôr′ē·ōkär′sinō″mə/ *pl. choriocarcinomas, choriocarcinomata,* an epithelial malignancy of fetal origin that develops from the chorionic portion of the products of conception. Also called **chorioepithelioma, chorionic carcinoma, chorionic epithelioma.**

■ OBSERVATIONS: The primary tumor usually appears in the uterus as a soft, dark red, crumbling mass, may invade and destroy the uterine wall, and may metastasize through lymph or blood vessels, forming secondary hemorrhagic and necrotic tumors in the vaginal wall, vulva, lymph nodes, lungs, liver, and brain. The urine often contains much more chorionic gonadotropin than is expected in pregnancy.

■ INTERVENTIONS: This form of cancer, which is more common in older women, responds to chemotherapy with cytotoxic drugs such as methotrexate. Rarely, a choriocarcinoma may arise in a teratoma of the testis, mediastinum, or pineal gland; chemotherapy is usually ineffective in treating these tumors.

■ PATIENT CARE CONSIDERATIONS: The cure rate for women is very high if the disease is diagnosed early.

choriocele /kôr″ē·əsēl′/ [Gk, *chorion + kele,* hernia], a hernia or protrusion of the tissue of the choroid layer of the eye.

chorioepithelioma. See **choriocarcinoma.**

choriogenesis /kôr′ē·ōjen″əsis/, the development of the chorion, which is first evident in the first month of pregnancy. The chorion continues to expand to accommodate the fetus and serves as the outer barrier between the fetus and the uterus. −*choriogenetic, adj.*

choriogonadotropin /ko″re·ōgon″ä-dotro″pin/. See **chorionic gonadotropin.**

choriogonadotropin alfa, human chorionic gonadotropin produced by recombinant technology, used to induce ovulation and pregnancy in certain infertile, anovulatory women and to increase the numbers of oocytes for patients attempting conception using assisted reproductive technologies, such as gamete intrafallopian transfer or in vitro fertilization. It is administered subcutaneously.

choriomeningitis. See **lymphocytic choriomeningitis.**

chorion /kôr″ē·on/ [Gk, *chorion,* skin], the outermost extraembryonic membrane composed of trophoblast lined with mesoderm. It develops villi about 2 weeks after fertilization and is vascularized by allantoic vessels 1 week later. It gives rise to the placenta and persists until birth as the outer of the two layers of membrane containing the amniotic fluid and the fetus. Compare **amnion.** See also **amniotic sac.**

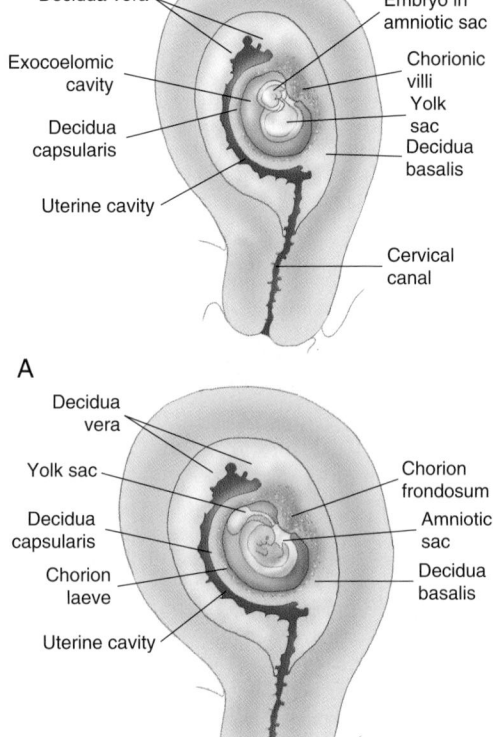

Chorion *(Hagen-Ansert, 2012)*

chorionic carcinoma, chorionic epithelioma. See **choriocarcinoma.**

chorionic cavity, extraembryonic coelom.

chorionic gonadotropin (CG) /kôr′ē·on″ik/ [Gk, *chorion* + *gone,* seed, *trophe,* nutrition], a chemical component of the urine of pregnant women and pregnant mares. This glycoprotein hormone is secreted by the placental trophoblastic cells. It is composed of two subunits, alpha and beta, and helps maintain the corpus luteum during pregnancy. The alpha subunit is nearly identical to follicle-stimulating, luteinizing, and thyroid-stimulating hormones. The specific hormonal effects of chorionic gonadotropin are activated by the beta portion. They include stimulation of the corpus luteum to secrete estrogen and progesterone and to decrease lymphocyte activation. Chorionic gonadotropin is also administered in the treatment of some cases of cryptorchidism and male hypogonadism and in the induction of ovulation in some infertile women. Also called **human chorionic gonadotropin.** See also **gonadotropin.**

chorionic plate [Gk, *chorion* + *platys,* flat], the part of the fetal placenta that gives rise to chorionic villi, which attach to the uterus during the early stage of formation of the placenta. It forms the fetal side of the placental disc, and its development is responsible for a normal placenta.

chorionic sac [Gk, *chorion,* skin, *sakkos,* sack], the saclike membrane that develops from the blastocyst wall to envelop the embryo.

chorionic villus [Gk, *chorion* + L, *villus,* shaggy hair], any of the tiny vascular fibrils on the surface of the chorion that infiltrate the maternal blood sinuses of the endometrium and help form the placenta.

chorionic villus sampling (CVS) [Gk, *chorion,* skin + L, *villos,* shaggy hair + L, *exemplum,* example], the sampling of placental tissues for prenatal diagnosis of potential genetic defects. The sample is obtained through a catheter inserted into the cervix. One of the main advantages of having this test instead of amniocentesis is that it can be done earlier in pregnancy. Also called *chorionic villus biopsy,* **CVB.** Compare **amniocentesis.**

chorioretinitis /kôr′ē·ōret′ini″tis/, an inflammatory condition of the choroid and retina of the eye, usually as a result of parasitic or bacterial infection. It is characterized by blurred vision, photophobia, and distorted images.

chorioretinopathy /kôr′ē·ōret′ənop″əthē/ [Gk, *chorion* + L, *rete,* net; Gk, *pathos,* disease], a noninflammatory process caused by disease that involves the choroid and the retina. Also called **choroidoretinitis.**

choroid /kôr″oid/ [Gk, *chorion* + *eidos,* form], a vascular layer of tissue between the retina and the sclera of the eye that supplies blood to the outer retina.

choroidal malignant melanoma /kôroi″dəl/ [Gk, *chorion* + *eidos* + L, *malignus,* ill-disposed; Gk, *melas,* black, *oma,* tumor], a tumor of the choroid coat of the eye that grows into the vitreous humor, causing detachment and degeneration of the overlying retina. Typically mound-shaped or mushroom-shaped, the neoplasm may break through the sclera and appear under the conjunctiva.

choroideremia /kôr′oidərē′mē·ə/ [Gk, *chorion,* skin + *eidos,* form + *erēmia,* destitution], hereditary primary degeneration of the retina, transmitted as an X-linked trait and beginning in the first decade of life. In males, the earliest symptom is usually night blindness, followed by constricted visual field and eventual blindness as the degeneration of the pigment epithelium of the retina progresses to complete atrophy. In females, it is nonprogressive; usually there is normal vision and often an atypical pigmentary retinopathy.

choroiditis /kôr′oidī″tis/, an inflammatory condition of the choroid membrane of the eye. Compare **chorioretinopathy.**

choroid membrane, a vascular layer of tissue between the retina and the sclera of the eye.

choroidocyclitis /kôroi′dōsiklī″tis/ [Gk, *chorion* + *eidos* + *kyklos,* circle, *itis,* inflammation], an abnormal condition characterized by inflammation of the choroid and the ciliary processes.

choroidopathy /kôr′oidop″əthē/, noninflammatory degeneration of the choroid.

choroidoretinitis. See **chorioretinopathy.**

choroid plexectomy /pleksek″təmē/ [Gk, *chorion* + *eidos* + L, *plexus,* pleated; Gk, *ektomē,* excision], a surgical procedure for the reduction of cerebrospinal fluid production in the ventricles of the brain in hydrocephalus, usually in the newborn. The procedure involves transcortical entry of the lateral ventricles to coagulate or to excise the choroid plexuses and seeks to correct a communicating type of hydrocephalus.

choroid plexus [Gk, *chorion* + *eidos* + L, pleated], any one of the tangled masses of small, specialized vessels contained within the lateral, the third, and the fourth ventricles of the brain, responsible for producing cerebrospinal fluid.

Chotzen syndrome. See **Saethre-Chotzen syndrome.**

Christchurch chromosome (Ch1) [Christchurch, city in New Zealand], an abnormally small, acrocentric chromosome (either chromosome 21 or chromosome 22) in which the short arm is missing or partially deleted. The aberration is associated with chronic lymphocytic leukemia but has also been found in patients with various other defects. See also **Philadelphia chromosome.**

Christian Science, a religious system founded in 1879 by Mary Baker Eddy based on the metaphysical teachings of Phineas P. Quimby. It holds that healing should be achieved through spiritual means, that sickness and death are illusions resulting from a false sense of separation from God. Members of the religion are called Christian Scientists.

Christian-Weber disease [Henry A. Christian, American physician, 1876–1951; Frederick Parkes Weber, English physician, 1863–1962], a rare form of panniculitis characterized by nodular formations in the subcutaneous tissues and prolonged intermittent relapsing fever.

Christmas disease. See **hemophilia B.**

Christmas factor. See **factor IX.**

Christ-Siemens-Touraine syndrome [Josef Christ, 1871–1949, German physician and dentist; Herman W. Siemens, 1861–1969, German dermatologist; Albert Touraine, 1883–1962, French dermatologist]. See **anhidrotic ectodermal dysplasia.**

chrom-. See **chromo-, chrom-, chromat-, chromato-.**

chromaffin /krō″məfin/ [Gk, *chroma,* color; L, *affin,* affinity], having an affinity for staining with chromium salts, especially brown staining of the cells of the adrenal, coccygeal, and carotid glands; certain cells of the adrenal medulla; and cells of the paraganglions. Also called **chromaphil.**

chromaffin body. See **paraganglion.**

chromaffin cell, any one of the special cells that compose the paraganglia and are connected to the ganglia of the celiac, renal, suprarenal, aortic, and hypogastric plexuses. The chromaffin cells of the adrenal medulla secrete two catecholamines, epinephrine and norepinephrine, which affect smooth muscle, cardiac muscle, and glands in the same way as sympathetic stimulation, by increasing and prolonging sympathetic effects.

chromaffinoma. See **pheochromocytoma.**

chromaphil. See **chromaffin.**

-chromasia, suffix meaning "(condition of the) stainability of tissues": *metachromasia.*

chromate (CrO_4^{2-}), any salt of chromic acid.

chromatic /krōmat″ik/ [Gk, *chroma,* color], **1.** pertaining to color. **2.** stainable by a dye. **3.** pertaining to chromatin. Also called **chromatinic.**

-chromatic. See **-chromic, -chromatic.**

chromatic dispersion [Gk, *chroma* + L, *dis,* apart, *spargere,* to scatter], the splitting of light into its various component wavelengths or frequencies, such as with a prism, to separate and study the different colors.

chromatid /krō″mətid/ [Gk, *chroma,* color], one of the two identical, threadlike filaments of a chromosome. Chromatids are produced by the self-replication of the chromosome during interphase and are held together by a common centromere. During anaphase of mitosis and meiosis II, the chromatids separate to become daughter chromosomes.

chromatid deletion, the breakage of a chromatid, sometimes caused by radiation. If the breakage occurs in the G_1 phase of the cell cycle, before DNA synthesis, subsequent replication will produce two sister chromatids with material missing and two acentromeric fragments called isochromatids.

chromatin /krō″mətin/ [Gk, *chroma,* color], the material within a cell nucleus from which the chromosomes are formed. It consists of fine, threadlike strands of DNA attached to proteins called histones and is readily stained with basic dyes. Chromatin occurs in two forms, euchromatin and heterochromatin, which are distinguishable during the phases of the cell cycle by their different degrees of staining, which in turn depends how tightly they are coiled. During cell division, portions of the chromatin condense and coil to form the chromosomes. Also called **chromoplasm, karyotin.** See also **chromatid, euchromatin, heterochromatin, sex chromatin. –chromatinic,** *adj.*

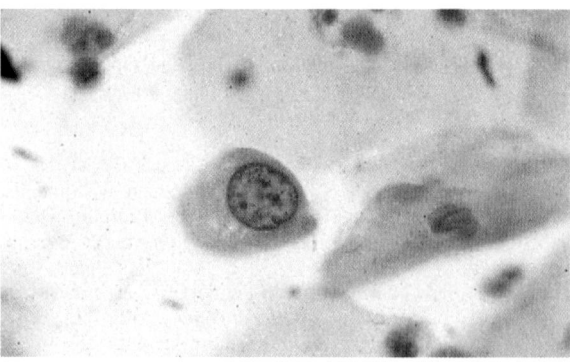

Rim of chromatin outlining the nuclear membrane
(McKee, 1997)

chromatinic. See **chromatic.**

chromatin-negative, lacking sex chromatin. The term applies to the nuclei of cells in normal males as well as those in individuals with certain chromosomal abnormalities.

chromatin nucleolus. See **karyosome.**

chromatin-positive, containing sex chromatin. The term applies to the nuclei of cells in normal females as well as those in individuals with certain chromosomal abnormalities.

chromatism /krō″mətiz″əm/, **1.** an abnormal condition characterized by hallucinations in which the affected individual sees colored lights. **2.** abnormal pigmentation or aberration.

chromatogram /krōmat″əgram′/, **1.** the record produced by the separation of gaseous substances or dissolved chemical substances moving through a column of absorbent material that filters out the various absorbates in different layers. **2.** any graphic record produced by any chromatographic method.

chromatography /krō′mətog″rəfē/, any one of several processes for separating and analyzing various gaseous or dissolved chemical materials. Kinds include **column chromatography, displacement chromatography, gas chromatography, ion exchange chromatography, paper chromatography. –***chromatographic, adj.*

chromatopsia /krō′mətop″sē·ə/ [Gk, *chroma* + *opsis,* vision], **1.** an abnormal visual condition that makes colorless objects appear tinged with color. **2.** a form of color blindness characterized by the imperfect perception of various colors. It may be caused by a deficiency in one or more of the retinal cones or by defective nerve circuits that convey color-associated impulses to the cerebral cortex. The most common defect in color sense is the inability to distinguish red from green, a defect evident in about 10% of men and 1% of women. Compare **chromesthesia.**

chromatosis /-ō″sis/, condition of abnormal skin pigmentation in any part of the body. See also **chloasma, vitiligo.**

chromaturia /-ōōr″ē·ə/ [Gk, *chroma,* color, *ouron,* urine], the production of urine that has an abnormal color.

chromesthesia /krō′misthē″zhə/ [Gk, *chroma* + *aisthesis,* feeling], **1.** the color sense that depends on the mixture of wavelengths in the light that enters the eye and the response of the different types of retinal cones associated with color vision. The human eye can distinguish hundreds of different colors that are combinations of the basic light wavelengths for red, green, and blue. Some of the retinal cones can be stimulated by the whole visual spectrum, and variable stimulation of all the cones can produce all the color sensations known to humans. Changes in the pigments within the cones affect color vision, and defects in the cones cause various kinds of color blindness. **2.** an abnormal condition characterized by the confusion of other senses, such as taste and smell, with imagined sensations of color. Compare **chromatopsia.**

chromhidrosis /krō′midrō″sis/ [Gk, *chroma* + *hidros,* sweat], a rare, functional disorder in which apocrine sweat glands secrete colored sweat. The sweat may be yellow, blue, green, or black and often also fluoresces. A known cause is occupational exposure to copper, catechols, or ferrous oxide.

-chromia, suffix meaning a "state or condition of pigmentation": *xanthochromia, erythrochromia.*

-chromic, -chromatic, suffix meaning color: *hypochromic.*

chromic catgut /krō″mik/ [Gk, *chroma,* color; L, *catta;* AS, *guttas*], surgical catgut that has been treated with chromium trioxide to strengthen it. It is an absorbable suture used as a ligature.

chromic myopia, a kind of color blindness characterized by the ability to distinguish colors only of those objects that are close to the eye.

chromium (Cr) /krō″mē·əm/ [Gk, *chroma,* color], a hard, brittle metallic element. Its atomic number is 24; its atomic mass is 51.99. It does not occur naturally in pure form but exists in combination with iron and oxygen in chromite, a mineral found chiefly in Africa, Albania, Russia, and Turkey. Chromium strongly resists corrosion and is used extensively to plate other metals, harden steel, and, in combination with other elements, form colored compounds. Stainless steels are more than 10% chromium and strongly resist rusting. Traces of chromium occur in plants and animals, and there is evidence that this element may be important in human nutrition, especially in carbohydrate metabolism. Some experts estimate that the safe and adequate daily intake of chromium ranges from 0.1 to 0.2 mg, depending on the age of the individual. Workers in chromite mines are susceptible to pneumoconiosis caused by the inhalation of chromite dust particles that lodge in the lung. Chromate salts have been identified as potential carcinogens. Chromium 51 isotope is used in blood studies.

chromium Cr 51 edetate, a complex of chromium 51 with edetic acid, used in the measurement of the glomerular filtration rate.

chromo-, chrom-, chromat-, chromato-, prefix meaning "color": *achromocyte, chromatopsia.*

chromobacteriosis /krō′məbaktir′ē·ō″sis/, an extremely rare, usually fatal systemic infection caused by a gram-negative bacillus *Chromobacterium violaceum.* It is found in fresh water in tropic and subtropic regions and enters the body through a break in the skin. The disease is characterized by sepsis, multiple liver abscesses, and severe prostration. Early diagnosis, surgical drainage of abscesses, and administration of chloramphenicol markedly improve the chance of survival.

chromoblastomycosis /krō′mōblas′tōmīkō″sis/ [Gk, *chroma* + *blastos,* germ, *mykes,* fungus, *osis,* condition], a chronic infectious skin disease caused by any multiple species to two genera of fungi Cladosporium and Phialophora found in the soil. Infection is characterized by the appearance of pruritic, warty nodules that develop in a cut or other break in the skin, occurring typically on the leg or foot. What may first appear as a small dull-red lesion gradually develops into a large ulcerated growth appearing like cauliflower tips in structure. Over a period of weeks or months additional warty growths may appear elsewhere on the skin along the path of lymphatic drainage. Common complications are secondary infection, lymphedema, and ulceration. Treatment includes surgical excision and, in some cases, topical application of systemic antibiotics. Flucytosine is the most commonly used antifungal agent. Also called **chromomycosis, verrucous dermatitis.** See also **mycosis,** *specific fungal infections.*

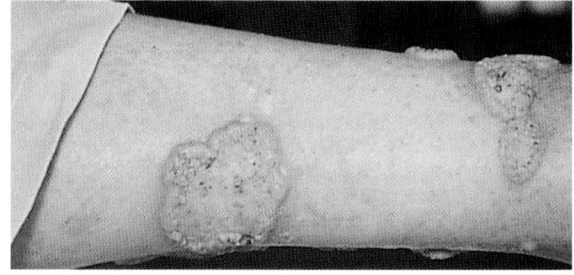

Chromoblastomycosis *(Murray et al, 2002)*

chromocenter. See **karyosome.**
chromocystoscopy. See **cystochromoscopy.**

chromogen /krō″mōjən/, a substance that absorbs light, producing color.

chromolipid, chromolipoid. See **lipochrome.**

chromomere /krō″məmir/ [Gk, *chroma* + *meros,* part], any of the series of beadlike structures that lie along the chromonema of a chromosome during the early stages of cell division. Chromomeres are most often seen in prophase II of meiosis. The position of each chromomere is relatively constant for each chromosome and probably reflects the chromosome's DNA coiling pattern. Also called **idiomere.** See also **karyomere.**

chromomycosis. See **chromoblastomycosis.**

chromonema /krō′mənē″mə/ *pl. chromonemata* [Gk, *chroma* + *nema,* thread], the part of a chromosome along which the chromomeres lie during cell division. See also **chromosome.** −*chromonemic, chromonemal, chromonematic, adj.*

chromophilic /krō′məfil″ik/ [Gk, *chroma* + *philein,* to love], denoting a cell, tissue, or microorganism that is easily stained, particularly certain leukocytes. Compare **chromophobic.**

chromophobe. See **chromophobia.**

chromophobe adenoma. See **chromophobic adenoma.**

chromophobia /krō′məfō″bē·ə/ [Gk, *chroma* + *phobos,* fear], **1.** the resistance of certain cells and tissues to stains. **2.** a morbid aversion to colors. −**chromophobe,** *n.*

chromophobic /krō′məfō″bik/, denoting a cell, tissue, or microorganism that is not easily stained, particularly certain cells of the anterior lobe of the pituitary gland. Compare **chromophilic.**

chromophobic adenoma, a tumor of the pituitary gland composed of cells that do not stain with acid or basic dyes. Diabetes insipidus and other conditions resulting from deficiency of one or more pituitary hormones are associated with this tumor. Also called **chromophobe adenoma.**

chromoplasm. See **chromatin.**

chromosensitive, descriptive of a substance that is affected by and responds to changes in chemical composition.

chromosomal. See **chromosome.**

chromosomal aberration /-sō″məl/ [Gk, *chroma* + *soma,* body; L, *aberrare,* to wander], any change in the structure or number of any of the chromosomes of a given species. In humans, a number of physical disabilities and disorders are directly associated with aberrations of both the autosomes and the sex chromosomes, including Down, Turner's, and Klinefelter's syndromes. The incidence of most chromosomal disorders is significantly higher than that of single-gene disorders. See also **trisomy.**

chromosomal nomenclature, a standard nomenclature system for identifying chromosomes in an individual as well as any deletions or additions of specific chromosomes or parts of chromosomes. The full complement of human chromosomes is represented as 46, XX for a normal female and 46, XY for a normal male. The pairs of autosomes are numbered from 1 to 22 according to decreasing length and are divided into seven groups: 1 through 3, group A; 4 and 5, group B; 6 through 12, group C; 13 through 15, group D; 16 through 18, group E; 19 and 20, group F; and 21 and 22, group G. Chromosomal aberrations are designated by indicating the total chromosomal number, sex complement, and group or specific chromosome in which the addition or deletion occurs. For example, 47, XY, G + indicates a male with an extra chromosome in the G group; 47, XX, 21 + indicates a female with an extra chromosome 21, a chromosomal aberration that results in Down syndrome. The short arm of a chromosome is designated by *p,* the long arm by *q,* and a translocation by *t.*

chromosomal sex [Gk, *chroma,* color, *soma,* body; L, *sexus,* male or female], the sex of an individual as determined, in mammals, by the presence or absence of a Y chromosome.

chromosome /krō″məsōm/ [Gk, *chroma* + *soma,* body], any of the threadlike structures in the nucleus of a cell that function in the transmission of genetic information. Each consists of a double strand of DNA attached to proteins called histones. The genes, which contain the genetic material that controls the inheritance of traits, are arranged in a linear pattern along the length of each DNA strand. Chromosomes are readily stainable with basic dyes and can be seen easily during cell division, when they are compactly coiled and in their most condensed state. During interphase the chromosomes disperse into chromatin and undergo self-replication, forming identical chromatids that separate during mitosis so that each new cell receives a full set of chromosomes. Each species has a characteristic number of chromosomes in each somatic cell. In humans, there are 46 chromosomes, including 22 homologous pairs of autosomes and 1 pair of sex chromosomes. One member of each pair is derived from each parent. Kinds include **Christchurch chromosome, daughter chromosome, gametic chromosome, giant chromosome, homologous chromosomes, monosome, Philadelphia chromosome, sex chromosome, somatic chromosome, W chromosome.** See also **centromere, chromatid, chromatin, Denver classification, gene, karyotype, mitosis.** –**chromosomal,** *adj.*

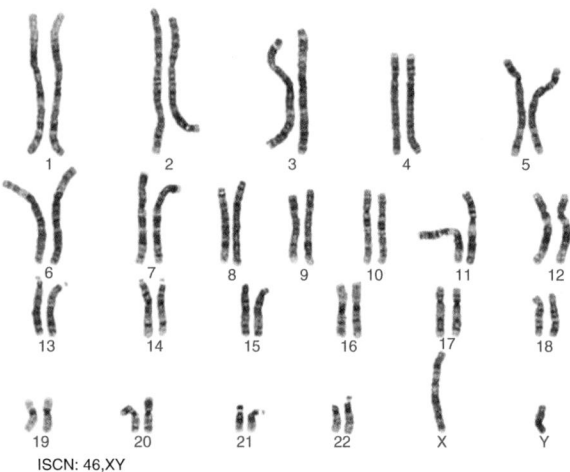

Chromosomes *(Courtesy National Institutes of Health)*

ISCN: 46,XY

chromosome 5p-syndrome. See **cat-cry syndrome.**

chromosome analysis, a laboratory procedure that isolates the chromosome pairs so that they may be visualized.

chromosome banding. See **banding.**

chromosome coil, the spiral formed by the coiling of two or more chromonemata in a chromosome.

chromosome complement, the normal number of chromosomes found in the somatic cells of a given species. In humans it is 46, consisting of 22 pairs of homologous autosomes and 1 pair of sex chromosomes.

chromosome karyotype test, a blood test used to study an individual's chromosome makeup to determine chromosomal defects associated with disease or the risk of developing disease. It is useful in evaluating congenital anomalies, cognitive impairment, and delayed puberty, as well as in the prenatal diagnosis of serious congenital diseases such as Klinefelter syndrome and Down syndrome and other suspected genetic disorders.

chromosome mapping. See **mapping.**

chromosome painting. See **fluorescent in situ hybridization.**

chromosome puff, a band of accumulated chromatin located at a specific site on a giant chromosome. It is indicative of gene activity, specifically DNA and RNA synthesis at that site. Such bands appear at certain chromosomal locations within a given tissue at specific developmental stages in insects and are significant in the study of the mode of genetic transmission.

chromosome walking, a molecular genetic technique by which overlapping molecular clones that span large chromosomal intervals are isolated.

chromotherapy /krō″məther″əpē/, a system of treating disease with colored lights chosen from specific regions of the spectrum.

chromotrope /krō″mətrōp/ [Gk, *chroma* + *trepein,* to turn], **1.** a component of tissue that stains metachromatically with metachromatic dyes. **2.** any one of several dyes differentiated by numeric suffixes. –*chromotropic, adj.*

chron-. See **chrono-, chron-.**

chronaxy /krō″naksē/ [Gk, *chronos,* time, *axia,* value], (in electroneuromyography) a measure of the shortest duration of an electrical stimulus needed to excite nerve or muscle tissue.

-chronia, -chrone, -chronic, 1. suffix meaning "correspondence of time between muscle and nerve": *isochronia.* **2.** suffix meaning the "time of formation of a part or tissue": *isochronic.*

chronic /kron″ik/ [Gk, *chronos,* time], (of a disease or disorder) persisting for a long period, often for the remainder of a person's lifetime. Compare **acute.**

Analysis of human chromosomes

Description of chromosomes		Group	Autosomes	Sex chromosomes	Number of chromosomes in all body (somatic) cells	
Size	Position of centromere				Male	Female
Large	Metacentric or submetacentric	A	1, 2, 3		6	6
Large	Submetacentric	B	4, 5		4	4
Medium	Metacentric and submetacentric	C	6, 7, 8, 9, 10, 11, 12	X	15	16
Medium	Acrocentric (subterminal)	D	13, 14, 15		6	6
Small	Metacentric and submetacentric	E	16, 17, 18		6	6
Smallest	Metacentric	F	19, 20		4	4
Small	Acrocentric (subterminal)	G	21, 22	Y	5	4
				TOTAL	**46**	**46**

chronic abscess, a persistent or recurrent accumulation of pus within a tissue. See **abscess.**

chronic active hepatitis (CAH), a potentially fatal form of hepatitis complicated by portal inflammation and extending into the parenchyma. There may be progressive destruction of the liver lobule with necrosis and fibrosis leading to scarring and cirrhosis. Possible causes include viral infections, drugs, and autoimmune reactions.

chronic airflow limitation. See **chronic obstructive pulmonary disease.**

chronic airway obstruction, a type of pulmonary disorder, such as emphysema or chronic bronchitis, in which the upper or lower airway is chronically obstructed. The patient, when at rest, breathes at a normal rate and may have prolongation of the expiratory phase with pursed-lip breathing. The patient may be barrel-chested and have large supraclavicular fossae. During inspiration, the intercostal spaces retract, and accessory muscles are used.

chronic alcoholic delirium. See **Korsakoff's psychosis.**

chronic alcoholism, a pathological condition resulting from the habitual use of alcohol in excessive amounts. The syndrome involves complex cultural, psychological, social, and physiological factors and usually impairs an individual's health and ability to function normally in society. Symptoms of the disease include anorexia, diarrhea, weight loss, neurological and psychiatric disturbances (most notably depression), and fatty deterioration of the liver, sometimes leading to cirrhosis. Treatment depends on the severity of the disease and its resulting complications; nutritional therapy, use of tranquilizers in the detoxification process, and hospitalization may be necessary. Alcoholism is not often detected in patients admitted to the hospital for care after an accident or for esophagitis, gastritis, peripheral neuropathy, anemia, or depression, all of which are secondary effects of alcoholism. If the patient is to undergo an operation, it is imperative that the anesthesiologist be notified of the condition, which can affect sensitivity to anesthetics. Alcoholism is a family disease, and the health professional can be instrumental in guiding the patient's family to seek treatment. Long-term support for alcoholics and their families is offered by such organizations as Alcoholics Anonymous, Al-Anon, Alateen, and rehabilitation facilities for alcoholism. Compare **acute alcoholism.** See also **alcoholism.**

chronic anterior poliomyelitis, an inflammation of the gray matter in the spinal cord, resulting in atrophy of muscles of the upper extremities and neck, with long periods of remission of symptoms. See also **poliomyelitis.**

chronic appendicitis, a type of appendicitis characterized by thickening or scarring of the vermiform appendix, caused by previous inflammation.

chronic bacterial prostatitis. See **prostatitis.**

chronic bronchitis, a very common, debilitating pulmonary disease, characterized by greatly increased production of mucus by the glands of the trachea and bronchi and resulting in a cough with expectoration for at least 3 months of the year for more than 2 consecutive years.

■ OBSERVATIONS: The condition has a strong association with smoking. Productive cough and chronic inflammation, often with wheezing or rhonchi, are universal features, followed by progressive dyspnea on exertion, repeated purulent respiratory infections, airway narrowing and obstruction, and often respiratory failure. Cor pulmonale with right ventricular heart failure is a common result. In some patients secondary polycythemia results from chronic hypoxemia. Prolonged expiratory phase, prominent cough, cyanosis, and acute attacks of respiratory distress with rapid, labored respirations may result. Common laboratory findings include elevated hematocrit, with or without respiratory acidosis; abnormal liver function caused by right-sided heart failure and hepatic congestion; pathogenic bacteria in the sputum; abnormal pulmonary function test results; and often chest x-ray signs of increased bronchial markings.

■ INTERVENTIONS: Patients with chronic bronchitis should be immunized against influenza and pneumococcal infections. Broad-spectrum antibiotics are usually prescribed during acute exacerbations of symptoms. Bronchodilators, such as albuterol, and sympathomimetic drugs, such as terbutaline and metaproterenol, are prescribed to prevent worsening of the condition. Adrenergics and anticholinergics, like albuterol and Atrovent, are used to maintain lung function. Heart failure is managed with appropriate medication.

■ PATIENT CARE CONSIDERATIONS: The patient should be encouraged to discontinue smoking and to avoid exposure to toxic inhalants, such as hair sprays, aerosol insecticides, and occupational irritants and poisons. The use of low-flow oxygen in the home requires patient/family education and monitoring. Exercise, especially walking, is often indicated.

chronic calcific pancreatitis, pancreatitis with calcification in the ducts, usually associated with exocrine insufficiency and diabetes mellitus.

chronic care, the provision of health care to individuals who have conditions lasting for a long period of time, usually longer than 3 months, with the primary goal of control of the disease. Compare **acute care.**

chronic carrier, an individual who acts as host to pathogenic organisms for an extended period without displaying any signs of disease.

chronic cervicitis, a persistent inflammation of the cervix that usually occurs among women in their reproductive years. Symptoms include a thick, irritating, malodorous discharge that may in severe cases be accompanied by significant pelvic pain. The cervix looks congested and enlarged, nabothian cysts are often present, and there are signs of eversion of the cervix and often old lacerations from childbirth. A Pap smear should be performed before treatment. The most effective treatments are hot and cold cautery. See **cervicitis.**

chronic cholecystitis. See **cholecystitis.**

chronic cystic mastitis. See **fibrocystic disease of the breast.**

chronic delirium [Gk, *chronos,* time; L, *delirare,* to rave], a form of delirium in which the patient shows signs of an altered level of awareness but is afebrile. The condition is sometimes associated with exhaustion, malnutrition, and wasting.

chronic dieting syndrome, the extreme practice of following fad diets, often leading to harmful physical and psychological effects. Also called **dieting syndrome.**

chronic disease, a disease that persists over a long period. The symptoms of chronic disease are sometimes less severe than those of the acute phase of the same disease. Chronic disease may be progressive, result in complete or partial disability, or even lead to death. Kinds include **diabetes mellitus, emphysema, arthritis.** See also **acute disease.**

chronic endoarteritis [Gk, *chronos,* time, *endon,* within, *arteria,* airpipe, *itis,* inflammation], persistent inflammation of the tunica intima of an arterial wall. It may be accompanied by fatty degeneration of arterial tissue and calcium deposits. Also called **endarteritis deformans.**

chronic endocarditis [Gk, *chronos,* time, *endon,* within, *kardia,* heart, *itis,* inflammation], persistent inflammation of the endocardium that usually follows an attack of acute endocarditis, syphilis, or an atheroma. It frequently involves the cardiac valves, making them incompetent. Also called **valvular endocarditis.**

chronic erosive gastritis.   See **erosive gastritis.**

chronic fatigue syndrome (CFS),   a condition characterized by disabling fatigue, accompanied by a constellation of symptoms, including muscle pain, multijoint pain without swelling, painful cervical or axillary adenopathy, sore throat, headache, impaired memory or concentration, unrefreshing sleep, and postexertional malaise. This diagnosis requires that a patient have four or more symptoms concurrently that persist for 6 or more months. The diagnosis is one of exclusion. Also called *immune dysfunction syndrome.*

chronic gastritis,   long-standing inflammation of the lining of the stomach. See **gastritis.**

chronic glaucoma,   primary open-angle glaucoma. See **glaucoma.**

chronic glomerulonephritis,   a noninfectious disease of the glomeruli of the kidney characterized by proteinuria, hematuria, edema, and decreased production of urine. Of unknown cause, it is asymptomatic for years. The symptoms develop slowly, and the disease progresses to kidney failure. Transplantation and dialysis are the only treatments available. See also **postinfectious glomerulonephritis, subacute glomerulonephritis, uremia.**

chronic gout [Gk, *chronos,* time; L, *gutta,* drop],   a persistent disorder of purine metabolism, characterized by abnormally high levels of serum uric acid and attacks of arthritis, with deposits of urates in the joints. The disorder may be familial and if untreated can lead to renal failure. See also **gout.**

chronic granulocytic leukemia.   See **chronic myelocytic leukemia.**

chronic granulomatous disease,   sex-linked recessive disorder in which myeloperoxidase is diminished in the primary granules of neutrophils, causing delayed intracellular killing of fungi and bacteria by neutrophils.

chronic hepatitis [Gk, *chronos,* time, *hēpar,* liver, *itis,* inflammation],   a state in which symptoms of hepatitis continue for several months and may increase in severity. In some cases of hepatitis B, the patient may become a lifelong carrier of the antigen and may show prolonged evidence of the infection. See also **alcoholic hepatitis, anicteric hepatitis, cholestatic hepatitis, hepatitis, hepatitis A, hepatitis B, hepatitis C, hepatitis D, hepatitis E.**

chronic hyperplastic rhinitis [Gk, *chronos,* time, *hyper,* excess, *plassein,* to form, *rhis,* nose, *itis,* inflammation],   chronic inflammation of the mucous membranes of the nose, with polyp formation.

chronic hyperplastic sinusitis [Gk, *chronos,* time, *hyper,* excess, *plassein,* to form; L, *sinus,* hollow; Gk, *itis,* inflammation],   chronic sinus inflammation, with polyp formation in the nose and sinuses.

chronic hypertrophic emphysema.   See **panacinar emphysema.**

chronic hypertrophic rhinitis [Gk, *chronos,* time, *hyper,* excess, *trophe,* nourishment, *rhis,* nose, *itis,* inflammation],   a condition of chronic inflammation of the nasal mucosa associated with enlargement of the mucous membrane.

chronic hypoxia,   a usually slow, insidious reduction in tissue oxygenation resulting from gradually destructive or fibrotic lung diseases, congenital or acquired heart disorders, or chronic blood loss. The patient experiences persistent mental and physical fatigue, shows sluggish mental responses, and complains of a loss of ability to perform physical tasks. Unless treated, the condition may lead to disability. There may be

some physiological adjustment to the lack of oxygen as occurs in individuals who move from sea level to mountainous areas, where oxygen pressures are reduced. Compare **acute hypoxia.**

chronic idiopathic xanthomatosis.   See **Hand-Schuller-Christian disease.**

chronic illness,   any disorder that persists over a long period and affects physical, emotional, intellectual, vocational, social, or spiritual functioning.

chronic immune thrombocytopenic purpura.   See **immune thrombocytopenic purpura.**

chronic inflammatory demyelinating polyneuropathy (CIDP),   a slowly progressive autoimmune neurological disorder with demyelination of the peripheral nerves and nerve roots, characterized by progressive weakness and impaired sensory function (loss of reflexes) in the limbs and enlargement of the peripheral nerves and usually by elevated protein in the cerebrospinal fluid. It occurs most commonly in young adults, particularly males. Presenting symptoms often include tingling or numbness of the digits, weakness of the limbs, hyporeflexia or areflexia, fatigue, and abnormal sensations. Compare **Guillain-Barré syndrome.**

chronic inflammatory demyelinating polyradiculoneuropathy,   a rare form of symmetrical motor neuron paralysis similar to Guillain-Barré syndrome but progressing more slowly or in a fluctuating pattern.

chronic interstitial nephritis.   See **interstitial nephritis.**

chronic intestinal ischemia.   See **intestinal angina.**

chronic intractable pain [Gk, *chronos,* time; L, *intractabilis* + *poena,* penalty],   excruciating, persistent pain that fails to respond to nonnarcotic analgesics and other treatment measures.

chronicity /krōnis″itē/,   having had a condition over a long period of time; a state of being chronic.

chronic leg ulcer [Gk, *chronos,* time; ONorse, *leggr* + L, *ulcus,* ulcer],   a wound of the lower extremity persisting for more than 6 weeks and showing no signs of healing after 3 or more months. It is typically associated with varicose veins, deep venous insufficiency, or a similar circulatory obstacle. Nonvenous causes of leg ulceration include arterial disease; ulcers may also be caused by trauma or have a bacterial, mycotic, hematological, neoplastic, neurological, or systemic origin.

■ OBSERVATIONS: Appearance will vary and can include complete loss of the epidermis and often portions of the dermis and even subcutaneous fat. The ulcer may be painful and have a foul odor.

■ INTERVENTIONS: Usually, treatment includes elevation of the leg two or three times daily, elastic support applied to the limb of the ambulatory patient, and avoidance of maceration of the wound. Because many factors lead to the development of the ulcer, it is important to have the input of the interdisciplinary team in the long-term management and treatment plan.

■ PATIENT CARE CONSIDERATIONS: Leg ulcers can be debilitating and greatly reduce patients' quality of life. A well-coordinated approach to delivering the correct treatment option for individual patients, based on accurate assessment of the underlying pathophysiology, is essential.

chronic lingual papillitis [Gk, *chronos* + L, *lingua,* tongue, *papilla,* nipple; Gk, *itis*],   an inflammatory disorder of the tongue, sometimes extending to the buccal mucosa and palate. It is characterized by irregularly scattered red patches, thinning of the lingual papillae, severe burning pain, and shedding of epidermal tissue. The disorder affects middle-aged individuals, especially women, and occurs in attacks alternating with remissions that last weeks or months. Also called **Moeller's glossitis.**

chronic low blood pressure,   a condition in which systolic and diastolic blood pressures are consistently below their normal values (approximately 120 and 70 mm Hg, respectively, in a young adult). Low blood pressure is not always suggestive of underlying disease; a careful assessment of accompanying symptoms, if present, should be undertaken.

chronic lymphocytic leukemia (CLL) [Gk, *chronos* + L, *lympha,* water; Gk, *kytos,* cell, *leukos,* white, *haima,* blood], a neoplasm of blood-forming tissues, characterized by a proliferation of small, long-lived lymphocytes, chiefly B cells, in bone marrow, blood, liver, and lymphoid organs. CLL is the most common leukemia in adults and the only leukemia to which there is a possible inheritable genetic predisposition. CLL is rare in persons less than 50 years of age, increases in frequency with age, and is more common in men than in women. The disease has an insidious onset and progresses to cause malaise, ready fatigability, anorexia, weight loss, nocturnal sweating, lymphadenopathy, and hepatosplenomegaly. Most patients can continue normal activities for years; 25% die of unrelated diseases. No treatment is curative, but remissions may be induced by chemotherapy or irradiation. Compare **acute lymphoblastic leukemia.**

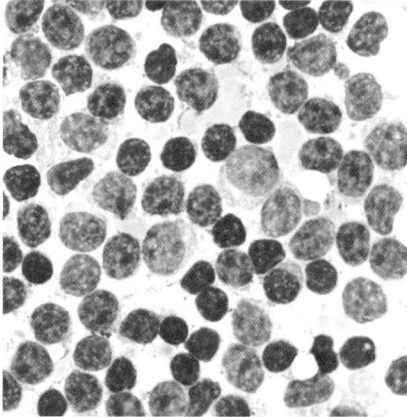

Chronic lymphocytic leukemia *(Carr and Rodak, 2009)*

chronic mastitis, *(Nontechnical)* an inflammation of breast tissue that can occur in the nonlactating woman. Now called *granulomatous mastitis.* See **mastitis.**

chronic mountain sickness [Gk, *chronos,* time; L, *montana;* AS, *soec*], a form of altitude sickness in which the increased production of red cells results in polycythemia. Some symptoms, such as headache, weakness, and limb aches, occasionally develop in indigenous mountain dwellers as well as in persons who have become acclimatized to the higher altitudes. See also **altitude sickness.**

chronic mucocutaneous candidiasis, a heterogeneous group of disorders, unified by impaired cell-mediated immunity against *Candida* species; a rare form of candidiasis characterized by candidal infection lesions of the skin, mucous membranes, GI tract, and respiratory tract. This disease usually occurs during the first year of life or with immune system dysfunction but can develop at any time. It affects both males and females and may be associated with an inherited defect of the cell-mediated immune system that allows autoantibodies to develop against target organs. The humoral immune system functions normally in this disease.

The onset of infections associated with the disease may precede endocrinopathy.

■ OBSERVATIONS: Diagnosis of this disease usually includes laboratory tests, which commonly show a normal T cell count and normal immunological responses to antigens other than *Candidaalbicans.* The endocrinopathy associated with this disease may include nonimmunological aberrations, such as hypocalcemia, abnormal hepatic function, hyperglycemia, iron deficiency, and abnormal vitamin B_{12} absorption. Required after diagnosis of chronic mucocutaneous candidiasis are evaluations of numerous physiological mechanisms, such as adrenal, gonadal, pancreatic, parathyroid, pituitary, and thyroid functions.

■ INTERVENTIONS: Chronic mucocutaneous candidiasis resists treatment with topical antifungal agents, miconazole, and nystatin. Endocrinopathies associated with the disease must be treated individually by hormone replacement; some success in this regard has been reported with experimental injections of thymosin and levamisole. Most success in treating severe cases has been achieved with transfer factor from a *Candida-positive* donor, with IV amphotericin B. Some success against systemic infection may also be possible with amphotericin B, but that agent is highly nephrotoxic. Some patients respond fairly well to fetal thymus transplantation. Plastic surgery may aid patients in coping with disfigurements caused by the disease. Treatment may also include oral or intramuscular iron replacement.

■ PATIENT CARE CONSIDERATIONS: Patients with chronic mucocutaneous candidiasis must be closely monitored for signs of other associated diseases, such as Addison's disease, diabetes, hepatitis, and pernicious anemia. Patients suffering psychologically from disfigurements associated with the disease often respond positively to encouragement and appropriate referrals for support or counseling. Amphotericin B, a nephrotoxin, is involved in the treatment. Therefore, the patient must be carefully monitored for renal function. Patients benefit from calm explanations of the progressive manifestations of the disease and the importance of regular endocrinological checkups.

chronic myelocytic leukemia (CML), a malignant neoplasm of blood-forming tissues, characterized by a proliferation of granular leukocytes and, often, of megakaryocytes. The disease occurs most frequently in adults older than 50 years of age and begins insidiously. Also called **chronic myelogenous leukemia.** See also **acute myeloid leukemia.**

■ OBSERVATIONS: Progress is marked by malaise, fatigue, heat intolerance, bleeding gums, purpura, skin lesions, weight loss, hyperuricemia, abdominal discomfort, and massive splenomegaly. Differential blood count and bone-marrow biopsies are performed to aid in the diagnosis. The alkaline phosphatase activity of the leukocytes is low, and the Philadelphia chromosome is present in myeloblasts in most patients with CML.

■ INTERVENTIONS: Therapy with an oral alkylating agent is usual, but advanced CML is refractory to chemotherapy. Appropriate support and educational programs that address the physical and emotional effects of CML are an important component of management.

■ PATIENT CARE CONSIDERATIONS: A highly collaborative environment involving patients and their families is important in the management of CML.

C

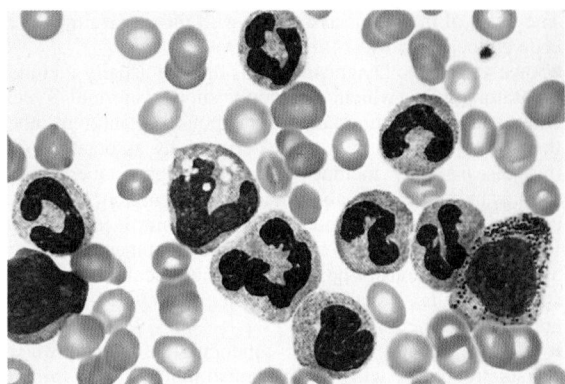

Chronic myelocytic leukemia *(Courtesy Dr. Robert W. McKenna, Department of Pathology, University of Texas Southwestern Medical School)*

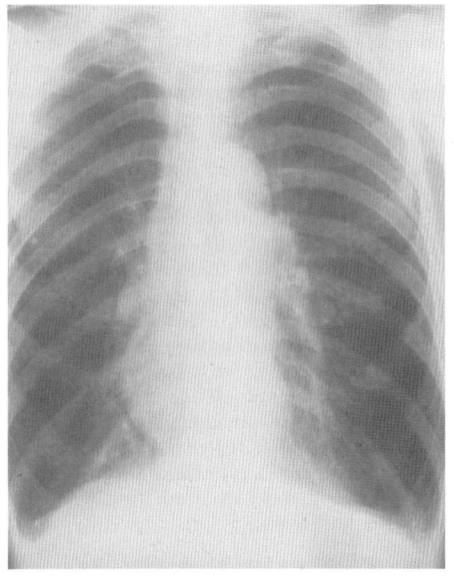

COPD radiograph with hyperinflation *(Mottram, 2013)*

chronic myelogenous leukemia /mī′əlōsit″ik/, myeloproliferative neoplasm characterized by the unregulated and excessive production of cells of the myelocytic maturation series and presence of the BCR/ABL 1 mutation. Also called **chronic myelocytic leukemia.** Compare **acute lymphocytic leukemia, chronic lymphocytic leukemia, leukemoid reaction.** See also **acute myeloid leukemia, leukocytosis.**

chronic myocarditis [Gk, *chronos,* time, *mys,* muscle, *kardia,* heart, *itis,* inflammation], inflammation of the myocardium that persists after an acute bacterial infection. Chronic myocarditis is characterized by degeneration of muscle tissue and fibrosis or infiltration of interstitial tissues. See also **myocarditis.**

chronic nephritis [Gk, *chronos,* time, *nephros,* kidney, *itis,* inflammation], a form of kidney inflammation usually secondary to another disease, such as chronic pyelonephritis. In chronic interstitial nephritis the kidney becomes small and granular with thickening of arteries and arterioles and proliferation of interstitial tissue. There may be functional abnormalities, such as urea retention, hematuria, and casts.

chronic nephropathy, a kidney disorder characterized by generalized or local damage to the tubulointerstitial areas of the kidney. The condition frequently results from more than a single cause, such as diabetes and a bacterial infection. Toxins, in the form of drugs or heavy metals, including cadmium or lead, are common causes, as are gout, cystinosis, and other metabolic disorders. Sickle cell disease is one of several inherited factors that may contribute to chronic nephropathy, but the condition can also develop from no known cause. Symptoms include polyuria, renal acidosis, edema, proteinuria, and blood in the urine. Treatment varies with correction of underlying causal factors. See also **kidney disease.**

chronic nonerosive gastritis, any type of chronic gastritis that does not involve deep penetration of the gastric mucosa.

chronic obstructive lung disease. See **chronic obstructive pulmonary disease.**

chronic obstructive pancreatitis, pancreatitis caused by dilation of one of the major ducts proximal to an obstruction, usually from a tumor or scarring, which may be the result of earlier acute pancreatitis. Removal of the obstruction may improve pancreatic function.

chronic obstructive pulmonary disease (COPD), a progressive and irreversible condition characterized by diminished inspiratory and expiratory capacity of the lungs. The condition is aggravated by cigarette smoking and air pollution. Also called **chronic obstructive lung disease.** Kinds include **asthma, chronic bronchitis, emphysema.**

chronic (open-angle) glaucoma. See **glaucoma.**

chronic pain, pain that continues or recurs over a prolonged period (usually longer than 12 weeks), caused by various diseases or abnormal conditions. Chronic pain may be less intense than acute pain. The person with chronic pain does not usually display increased pulse and rapid respiration because these autonomic reactions to pain cannot be sustained for long periods. Some factors that can complicate the treatment of persons with chronic pain are scarring, continuing psychological stress, and medication. Compare **acute pain.** See also **pain, pain intervention, pain mechanism.**

chronic pancreatitis [Gk, *chronos,* time, *pan,* all, *kreas,* flesh, *itis,* inflammation], chronic inflammation of the pancreas with fibrosis and calcification of the gland. It may follow repeated acute attacks and can lead to diabetes. Causes include alcohol abuse, genetic diseases such as cystic fibrosis, and conditions obstructing the pancreatic duct.

chronic peritonitis [Gk, *chronos,* time, *peri,* near, *tenein,* to stretch, *itis,* inflammation], a form of peritonitis in which the peritoneum thickens and ascites develops. The condition is usually associated with another disorder, such as pericarditis or polyserositis.

chronic pigmented purpura, any of a group of benign dermatoses of unknown cause, not associated with underlying systemic disease, consisting of minimal inflammation with tiny hemorrhages from capillaries in the upper dermis, visible as red dots on the skin. Kinds include **lichen aureus,** *pigmented purpuric lichenoid dermatitis, purpura annularis telangiectodes, Schamberg disease.*

chronic progressive myelopathy, gradually progressive spastic paraparesis associated with infection by human T-lymphotropic virus 1, characterized by progressive difficulty in walking and weakness of the lower extremity, sensory disturbances, and urinary incontinence, with no evidence of spinal compression or motor neuron involvement. Also called *HTLV-I–associated myelopathy,* **tropical spastic paraparesis.**

chronic prostatitis, inflammation of the prostate gland causing long-term pain. See **prostatitis.**

chronic purulent synovitis, **1.** inflammation of the lining of a joint with the presence of pus. **2.** See **chronic synovitis.**

chronic pyelonephritis. See **pyelonephritis.**

chronic radiation exposure, radiation contact that occurs and accumulates over a lifetime. It can be small, continuous amounts, as in the background radiation associated with radioactive materials in the soil, or radiation that is intermittent and associated with an occupation.

chronic regional pain syndrome. See **reflex sympathetic dystrophy.**

chronic rejection, immune rejection of transplanted tissue that may continue for several months.

chronic renal failure (CRF), gradual loss of kidney function, with progressively more severe renal insufficiency until the stage called chronic irreversible kidney failure or end-stage renal disease. Symptoms may include polyuria, anorexia or nausea, dehydration, and neurological symptoms.

chronic rheumatism [Gk, *chronos,* time, *rheumatismos,* that which flows], a term used to encompass more than 100 types of diseases, including many types of arthritis. Arthritic conditions are distinguished by red, swollen joints and inflamed connective tissues such as cartilage, synovial tissue, and tendons. Other rheumatic diseases are considered autoimmune diseases, meaning that the body's own immune system is turning on parts of the body. See also **rheumatism.**

chronic serous synovitis, inflammation of a synovial membrane associated with copious nonpurulent material, usually painful, particularly on motion, due to effusion in a synovial sac. It may be caused by rheumatic fever, rheumatoid arthritis, tuberculosis, trauma, gout, or other conditions. See also **chronic synovitis.**

chronic synovitis [Gk, *chronos,* time, *syn,* together; L, *ovum,* egg; Gk, *itis,* inflammation], persistent inflammation of the synovial membrane of a joint. Kinds include **chronic purulent synovitis, chronic serous synovitis.** See also **synovitis.**

chronic tetanus [Gk, *chronos,* time, *tetanos,* convulsive tension], **1.** a form of tetanus with a delayed onset, slow progression of the disease, and milder than usual symptoms. **2.** a reactivated tetanus infection in a healed wound.

chronic thromboembolic pulmonary hypertension, persistent pulmonary hypertension caused by obstruction of a major pulmonary artery by an unresolved embolus or multiple small pulmonary emboli.

chronic tuberculous mastitis, a rare infection of the breast resulting from extension of tuberculosis of underlying ribs. The condition is also characterized by multiple sinus tracts and the presence of tuberculosis elsewhere in the body.

chronic tubulointerstitial nephritis, tubulointerstitial nephritis that has progressed to the point at which there is interstitial fibrosis with shrunken kidneys, a lowered glomerular filtration rate, and danger of renal failure.

chronic undifferentiated schizophrenia, a condition marked by the symptoms of more than one of the classic types of schizophrenia—simple, paranoid, or catatonic. See also **acute schizophrenia.**

chrono-, chron-, prefix meaning "time": *chronotropism.*

chronobiologist /kron″o-bi-ol′ah-jist/, a specialist in biology with a focus on the rhythms of living organisms.

chronobiology, the study of the effects of time on living systems.

chronograph /kron″əgraf/ [Gk, *chronos + graphein,* to record], a device that records small intervals of time, such as a stopwatch. −*chronographic, adj.*

chronological /kron′əloj″ik/ [Gk, + reason], **1.** arranged in time sequence. **2.** pertaining to chronology. Also *chronologic.*

chronological age, the age of an individual expressed as time that has elapsed since birth. The age of an infant is expressed in hours, days, or months; the age of children and adults is expressed in years.

chronopsychophysiology /kron′ōsī′kofis′ē·ol″əjē/, the science of physiological cyclic processes in the body.

chronotherapeutics /kron′ōther′əpyoo″tiks/, a branch of medicine concerned with effects of circadian rhythms in human health, such as the hour of the day when asthma symptoms or heart attacks are most likely to occur, the best time of day for treating certain complaints, and the best times to administer medication or chemotherapy to enhance activity or lessen toxicity.

chronotropism /krənot″rəpiz′əm/ [Gk, *chronos + trepein,* to turn], the act or process of affecting the regularity of a periodic function, especially interference with the rate of the heartbeat. −*chronotropic, adj.*

chrys-, prefix meaning "gold": *chrysotherapy.*

Chrysanthemum /krisan′thəməm/, a genus of perennial flowering herbs of the family Compositae, native to the Balkans and the Middle East. They are a common cause of contact dermatitis, and their powdered flowers are insecticidal and scabicidal. *Chrysanthemum morifolium* is a common ingredient in Chinese herbal therapies.

chrysarobin /kris′ərō″bin/, a substance obtained from the wood of the *Andiraararoba* tree native to Brazil. It is used as an irritant in the treatment of parasitic skin diseases and psoriasis.

chrysiasis /krəsī″əsis/ [Gk, *chrysos,* gold, *osis,* condition], an abnormal condition that may develop after gold therapy, characterized by the deposition of gold in body tissues. Also called **auriasis.**

chrysotherapy /kris′ōther″əpē/ [Gk, *chrysos + therapeia,* treatment], the treatment of any disease with gold salts. −*chrysotherapeutic, adj.*

Chua K'a, a holistic counseling system of muscle tension release that emphasizes clarification and cleansing of the mind and emotions.

Churg-Strauss syndrome /churg″strous″/ [Jacob Churg, 20th-century American pathologist; Lotte Strauss, 20th-century American pathologist], a systemic autoimmune condition that causes inflammation of small and medium-sized blood vessels. The cause is unknown. See also **vasculitis.**

■ OBSERVATIONS: The syndrome develops in several stages: (1) airway inflammation (often asthma), (2) hypereosinophilia, and (3) vasculitis. If present, skin lesions consist of tender subcutaneous nodules and bruise-like spots. The eosinophil count is generally high. A biopsy of affected tissue will demonstrate a characteristic pattern with eosinophils present in the tissue.

■ INTERVENTIONS: Treatment goals are directed to reducing the inflammation and suppression of the immune system. Medications usually include high doses of corticosteroids and cyclophosphamide (Cytoxan).

■ PATIENT CARE CONSIDERATIONS: The disease can be fatal if untreated; with aggressive treatment, remission is possible.

Chvostek sign, Chvostek-Weiss sign /khvôsh″tek/ [Franz Chvostek, Austrian surgeon, 1835–1884], an abnormal spasm of the facial muscles elicited by light taps on the cheek to stimulate the facial nerve in patients who are hypocalcemic. It is a sign of tetany. Checking for this sign is especially important after thyroid or parathyroid surgery.

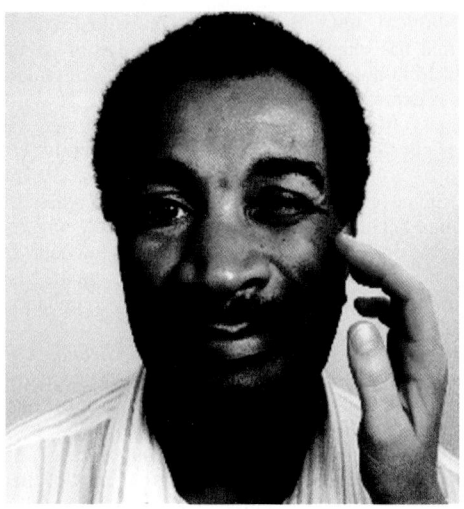

Chvostek sign *(Ignatavicius and Workman, 2016)*

chyl-.   See **chylo-, chyl-, chyli-.**

chyle /kīl/   [Gk, *chylos,* juice],   the cloudy or turbid, white or pale yellow liquid products of digestion taken up by the small intestine. Consisting mainly of emulsified fats, chyle passes through finger-like projections in the small intestine, called lacteals, and into the lymphatic system for transport to the venous circulation at the thoracic duct in the neck. Also called **chylus. –chylous,** *adj.*

chyle cistern,   a dilation at the beginning of the thoracic duct, situated ventrally to the body of the second lumbar vertebra, on the right side of and dorsally to the aorta. It receives the two lumbar lymphatic trunks and the intestinal lymphatic trunk. Also called **Pecquet's cistern.**

chyle leak,   a rare complication of trauma and/or surgery in which the milky, odorless fluid known as chyle moves from its normal location within the lymphatic system to the thoracic, pertioneal, or cardiac cavity. A fistula may also develop. Kinds include **chylous ascites, chylothorax.**

chyli-.   See **chylo-, chyl-, chyli-.**

-chylia,   suffix meaning "(condition of the) digestive juices, or chyle": *achylia.*

chyliform ascites.   See **chylous ascites.**

chylo-, chyl-, chyli-,   prefix meaning "chyle": *chylocele.*

chylocele /kī′ləsēl/,   a cystic lesion caused by an effusion of chylous fluid into the tunica vaginalis of the testes.

chyloid /kī′loid/,   resembling the chyle that fills the lacteals of the small intestine during the digestion of fatty foods.

chylomediastinum   /kī′lōmē′dē·astī″nəm/   [Gk, *chylos,* juice; L, *mediastinus,* midway],   the presence of chyle in the mediastinum.

chylomicron /kī′lōmī″kron/   [Gk, *chylos + mikros,* small],   minute lipoproteins measuring less than 0.5 µm in diameter. Chylomicrons consist of about 90 triglycerides with small amounts of cholesterol, phospholipids, fat-soluble vitamins, and protein. They are synthesized in the GI tract and carry dietary fat from the intestinal mucosa via the thoracic lymphatic duct into the plasma and ultimately to the liver and tissues. The remnant chylomicron particles are removed by the liver.

chylosus ascites.   See **chylous ascites.**

chylothorax /kī′lōthôr″aks/   [Gk, *chylos + thorax,* chest],   a condition marked by the effusion of chyle from the thoracic duct into the pleural space. The cause is usually a traumatic injury to the neck or a tumor that invades the thoracic duct. Treatment is directed at repairing damage to the duct.

chylous /kī′ləs/   [Gk, *chylos,* juice],   pertaining to or resembling chyle.

chylous ascites,   an abnormal condition characterized by an accumulation of chyle in the peritoneal cavity. Chylous ascites results from an obstruction in the thoracic duct that may be caused by a tumor or by a destructive lesion, resulting in rupture of a lymph vessel. Also called *ascites adiposus,* **chyliform ascites, chylosus ascites, fatty ascites, milky ascites.** See also **ascites.**

chyluria /kīloōr″ē·ə/   [Gk, *chylos + ouron,* urine],   a milky appearance of the urine caused by the presence of chyle.

chylus.   See **chyle.**

chymase /kī′mās/,   a serine protease present in human mast cells, most prominent in skin and connective tissue, where it can cleave angiotensin and stimulate mucous glands.

chyme /kīm/   [Gk, *chymos,* juice],   the viscous, semifluid contents of the stomach present during digestion of a meal. Chyme then passes through the pylorus into the duodenum, where further digestion occurs.

chymopapain   /kī′mōpəpā″ēn/   [Gk, *chymos* + Sp, *papaya*],   a proteolytic enzyme isolated from the fruit of *Carica papaya* and related to papain. It is used in the treatment of prolapsed intervertebral or herniated disks.

chymosin.   See **rennin.**

chymotrypsin /kī′mōtrip″sin/   [Gk, *chymos + tryein,* to rub, *pepsin,* digestion],   **1.** a proteolytic enzyme produced by the pancreas that catalyzes the hydrolysis of casein and gelatin. **2.** a yellow crystalline powder prepared from an extract of ox pancreas that is used in treating digestive disorders in which the enzyme is present in less than normal amounts or is totally lacking.

chymotrypsinogen /kī′mōtripsin″əjən/,   a substance produced in the pancreas that is the zymogen precursor to the enzyme chymotrypsin. It is converted to chymotrypsin by trypsin.

Ci,   abbreviation for **curie.**

CI,   abbreviation for *Colour Index.*

Cialis,   medication for erectile dysfunction. Brand name for **tadalafil.**

cibophobia /sē′bə-/   [L, *cibus,* food; Gk, *phobos,* fear],   an abnormal or morbid aversion to food or to eating.

cicatrices.   See **cicatrix.**

cicatricial alopecia /sisətrish″əl/,   a form of baldness produced by scar formation in dermatoses such as lupus erythematosus, usually progressing to permanent baldness.

cicatricial entropion.   See **cicatrix, entropion.**

cicatricial pemphigoid [L, *cicatrix,* scar; Gk, *pemphix,* blister or bubble + *eidos,* form],   a benign, chronic, usually bilateral, subepidermal blistering disease chiefly involving the mucous membranes, especially those of the mouth and eye. It heals by scarring and may lead to slow shrinkage of the affected tissues, and to blindness if untreated. Also called **benign mucosal pemphigoid.**

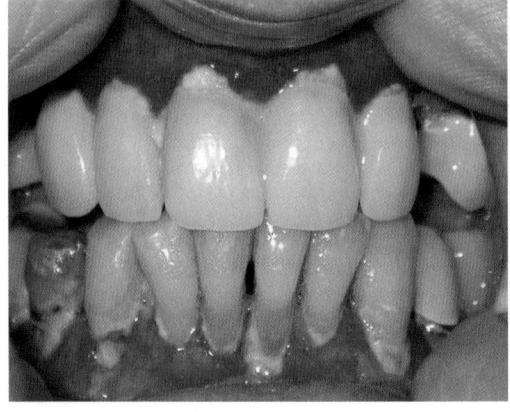

Cicatricial pemphigoid *(Marks and Miller, 2013)*

cicatricial scar [L, *cicatrix,* scar; Gk, *eschara,* scab], a fibrous scar that remains after a wound has healed.

cicatricial stenosis [L, *cicatrix,* scar; Gk, *stenos,* narrow, *osis,* condition], the narrowing of a duct or tube caused by the formation of scar tissue.

cicatrix /sik″ətriks, sikā″triks/ *pl. cicatrices* [L, scar], scar tissue that is avascular, pale, contracted, and firm after the earlier phase of skin healing characterized by redness and softness. Also called **scar.** −**cicatricial,** *adj.,* −**cicatrize,** *v.*

cicatrize /sik″ətrīz/ [L, scar], to heal so as to form a scar.

ciclopirox /sī″kləpī″roks/, a topical antifungal agent.

■ INDICATIONS: It is prescribed in the treatment of tinea and candidiasis.

■ CONTRAINDICATIONS: Known sensitivity to this drug prohibits its use.

■ ADVERSE EFFECTS: Among the most serious adverse reactions are local reactions of irritation, pruritus at the application site, burning, and worsening of clinical signs and symptoms.

ciclosporin. See **cyclosporin.**

cicutism /sik″yo͞otiz′əm/ [L, *Cicuta,* hemlock; Gk, *ismos,* process], poisoning caused by water hemlock, resulting in cyanosis, dilated pupils, convulsions, and coma. Treatment usually includes the use of activated charcoal and anticonvulsant drugs. Intubation and mechanical ventilation may be required. A poison control center should be contacted if cicutism is suspected.

CID, abbreviation for **cytomegalic inclusion disease.**

-cide, -cid, suffix meaning "killing": *amebicide, herbicide.*

-cidin, suffix designating an antibiotic: *bactericidin.*

cidofovir, an antiviral.

■ INDICATIONS: It is used to treat cytomegalovirus retinitis in patients with AIDS.

■ CONTRAINDICATIONS: Known hypersensitivity to acyclovir or this drug prohibits its use.

■ ADVERSE EFFECTS: Life-threatening effects include coma, hemorrhage, hematuria, granulocytopenia, thrombocytopenia, irreversible neutropenia, anemia, and eosinophilia. Other serious adverse effects include confusion, psychosis, tremors, somnolence, arrhythmias, hypertension/hypotension, retinal detachment in cytomegalovirus retinitis, abnormal liver function tests, increased creatinine, increased blood urea nitrogen, and phlebitis.

cigarette smoking, the inhalation of the gases and hydrocarbon vapors generated by slowly burning tobacco in cigarettes. The practice stems partly from the effect on the nervous system of the nicotine contained in the smoke. In addition to nicotine, nearly 1000 other chemicals have been identified in cigarette smoke, including carcinogenic polycyclic aromatic alcohols, cocarcinogenic phenols and fatty acids, carbon monoxide, hydrogen sulfide, hydrocyanic acid, nitrogen oxides, and various irritants that suppress protease inhibition and impair alveolar macrophage function. Cigarette smoke is addictive and is considered more dangerous than pipe or cigar smoke because it is less irritating and therefore more likely to be inhaled. See also **lung cancer, nicotine.**

ciguatera /se″gwätə′rəh/, a form of fish poisoning, marked by GI and neurological symptoms, caused by ingestion of tropical or subtropical marine fish, such as the barracuda, grouper, or snapper that have accumulated ciguatoxin in their tissues. Ciguatoxin is heat resistant and is not detoxified by cooking. This form of poisoning is often misdiagnosed as multiple sclerosis.

ciguatera poisoning /sē′gwəter″ə/ [Sp, *cigua,* sea snail; L, *potio,* drink], a nonbacterial food poisoning that results from eating fish contaminated with the ciguatoxin. Many of the over 300 varieties of fish from the Caribbean or South Pacific have been implicated; barracuda is a common source. The toxin is believed to block acetylcholinesterase activity. Characteristics of ciguatera poisoning are vomiting, diarrhea, tingling or numbness of extremities and the skin around the mouth, itching, muscle weakness, pain, and respiratory paralysis. Cold liquids feel hot to the surfaces of the mouth and throat. No specific treatment has been developed.

ciguatoxin /se′gwätok″sin/, a heat-stable toxin originating in a dinoflagellate as a pretoxin and concentrating in active form in the tissue of certain marine fish (usually tropical reef fish), causing ciguatera in humans who eat the fish.

cili-, **1.** prefix meaning "eyelid": *ciliary.* **2.** prefix meaning "eyelash": *cilia.* **3.** prefix meaning "minute vibratile": *ciliate.*

cilia /sil″ē-ə/*sing. cilium*[L, eyelids or eyelashes], **1.** eyelashes. **2.** small, hairlike processes projecting from epithelial cells on the outer surfaces of some tissues, aiding metabolism by producing motion, eddies, or current in a fluid. In the lung, cilia wave mucus, pus, and dust upward.

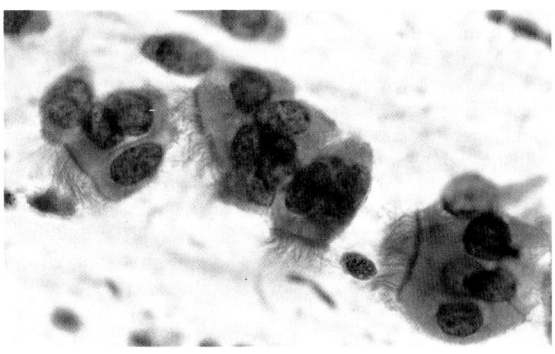

Cilia *(McKee, 1997)*

ciliary /sil″ē·er′ē/ [L, *cilia*], **1.** pertaining to the eyelashes or eyelids. **2.** referring to the filaments on cells that propel movement.

ciliary artery, any of the branches of the ophthalmic artery that, along with the retinal artery, supply the eye.

ciliary body [L, *cilia*], the thickened part of the vascular tunic of the eye that joins the iris with the anterior portion of the choroid. It is composed of the ciliary crown, ciliary processes and folds, ciliary orbiculus, ciliary muscle, and a basal lamina.

ciliary canal, the spaces of the iridocorneal angle.

ciliary disc, the thin part of the ciliary body extending between its crown and the ora serrata retinae.

ciliary ganglion, a small parasympathetic ganglion in the orbit of the eye, which controls pupillary and accommodative reflexes.

ciliary gland, one of the numerous tiny, modified sweat glands arranged in several rows near the free margins of the eyelids. The apertures of the glands lie near the attachments of the eyelashes. Acute localized bacterial infection of one or more of the ciliary glands causes external sties. Also called **glands of Moll Zeis. Compare tarsal gland.**

ciliary margin, the peripheral border of the iris, continuous with the ciliary body.

ciliary movement, the upward waving motion of the hairlike processes projecting from the epithelium of the respiratory tract and from certain microorganisms.

ciliary mucus transport, the movement of mucus-trapped particles from the upper respiratory tract to the lower pharynx, propelled by the motion of microscopic cilia lining the tract.

ciliary muscle, a semitransparent circular band of smooth muscle fibers attached to the choroid of the eye, the chief agent in glowing lens adjustment of the eye to assume a more spherical shape. It draws the ciliary process centripetally, relaxing the suspensory ligament of the crystalline lens and allowing the lens to become more convex.

ciliary process, any one of about 80 tiny, fleshy projections on the posterior surface of the iris, forming a frill around the margin of the crystalline lens of the eye. The processes compose one of the two zones of the ciliary body of the eye and are formed by infolding of the various layers of the choroid. They secrete nutrient fluids to nourish the lens, cornea, and vitreous body. See also **ciliary body.**

ciliary reflex. See **accommodation reflex.**

ciliary ring, a small grooved band of tissue, about 4 mm wide, that forms the posterior part of the ciliary body of the eye. It extends from the ora serrata of the retina to the ciliary processes and is thicker near the ciliary processes as a result of the thickness of the ciliary muscle.

ciliary zone, an outer circular area on the anterior surface of the iris, separated from the inner circular area by the angular line. The ciliary zone contains the stroma of the iris. Also called **zonule of Zinn.**

Ciliata /sil″ē·ā′tə/, a class of protozoa of the subphylum Ciliophora, characterized by cilia throughout the life cycle. The class includes the subclasses Euciliata and Protociliata. The only significant ciliate affecting humans is the intestinal parasite *Balantidium coli,* which causes dysentery.

ciliate /sil″ē·it/, of or having cilia, as certain epithelial cells of the body or protozoa of the class Ciliata.

ciliated epithelium /sil″ē·ā′tid/ [L, *cilia* + Gk, *epi,* upon, *thele,* nipple], any epithelial tissue that projects cilia from its surface, such as portions of the epithelium in the respiratory tract and the uterine tubes.

ciliopathies, a group of disorders caused by a defect in the assembly and disassembly of cilia during the cell cycle. Since nearly every cell in the body contains cilia, defects affect multiple organ systems.

Ciliophora, a phylum of protozoa whose members, called ciliates, use cilia for locomotion and feeding.

ciliospinal /sil″ē·ōspī′nəl/, pertaining to a relationship between the ciliary body of the eye and the spinal cord.

ciliospinal reflex [L, *cilia* + *spina,* backbone, *reflectere,* to bend back], a normal brainstem reflex initiated by scratching or pinching the skin of the neck or face, causing dilation of the pupil. Also called **pupillary skin reflex.**

cilium. See **cilia.**

-cillin, suffix designating a penicillin.

cilostazol, a platelet aggregation inhibitor.
- INDICATIONS: It is used to treat intermittent claudication.
- CONTRAINDICATIONS: Known hypersensitivity to this drug, congestive heart failure, active liver disease, blood dyscrasias, and active bleeding prohibit its use.
- ADVERSE EFFECTS: Life-threatening effects include atrial fibrillation/flutter, cerebral infarct, cerebral ischemia, congestive heart failure, cardiac arrest, myocardial infarction, nodal dysrhythmias, bleeding (epistaxis, hematuria, conjunctival hemorrhage, GI bleeding), agranulocytosis, neutropenia, and thrombocytopenia. Serious adverse effects include palpitations, tachycardia, vomiting, colitis, cholelithiasis, ulcer, and diabetes mellitus. Common side effects include vertigo, diarrhea, rash, back pain, headache, infection, myalgia, peripheral edema, cough, pharyngitis, and rhinitis.

cimbia /sim″bē·ə/, a girdlelike band of white fibers that extends across the surface of the cerebral peduncle.

cimetidine /simet″idēn/, an H2-receptor antagonist.
- INDICATIONS: It is prescribed to inhibit the production and secretion of acid in the stomach in the treatment of gastroesophageal reflux disease, pancreatitis, duodenal ulcers, and hypersecretory conditions. It is also used in the treatment of warts.
- CONTRAINDICATIONS: Known hypersensitivity to this drug prohibits its use. Not recommended with the use of tricyclic depressants.
- ADVERSE EFFECTS: Among the more serious adverse reactions are diarrhea, dizziness, rash, confusion (usually in elderly patients given large doses), and gynecomastia. Cimetidine inhibits several forms of cytochrome P450 and, therefore, has effects on many other drugs.

Cimex lectularius. See **bedbug.**

CIN, abbreviation for **cervical intraepithelial neoplasia.**

cinacalcet, a calcium receptor agonist that directly lowers parathyroid hormone levels by increasing sensitivity of calcium-sensing receptors to extracellular calcium.
- INDICATIONS: This drug is used to treat hypercalcemia in parathyroid carcinoma and secondary hyperparathyroidism in chronic kidney disease requiring dialysis.
- CONTRAINDICATIONS: Known hypersensitivity to this drug prohibits its use.
- ADVERSE EFFECTS: Adverse effects of this drug include dizziness, hypertension, nausea, diarrhea, vomiting, anorexia, access infection, noncardiac chest pain, asthenia, and myalgia.

cinchona /singkō″nə, chinchō″nə/ [countess of Chinchon, Peru], the dried bark of the stem or root of species of *Cinchona,* containing the alkaloids quinine and quinidine.

cinchonine, an alkaloid of cinchona used as an antimalarial agent, chiefly in the form of the sulfate salt, administered orally.

cinchonism /sin″kōniz′əm/, a condition resulting from excessive ingestion of cinchona bark or its alkaloid derivatives (quinine or quinidine). Cinchonism is characterized by hearing loss, headache, tinnitus, and signs of cerebral congestion. See also **quinine.**

cine-, kine-, kinesio-, prefix meaning "movement": *cineangiogram, cineradiography.*

cineangiocardiogram /sin″ē·an′jē·ōkär″dē·əgram′/, a radiographic image of the cardiovascular system produced by cineangiocardiography.

cineangiocardiography /sin″ē·an′jē·ōkär′dē·og″rəfē/ [Gk, *kinesis,* movement, *angeion,* vessel, *kardia,* heart, *graphein,* to record], the production of images of the cardiovascular system by a combination of fluoroscopic, radiographic, and motion-picture techniques. See also **cineradiography.**

cineangiogram /sin″ē·an′jē·əgram′/, a motion-picture recording of a portion of the cardiovascular system obtained after injection of radiopaque contrast medium.

cinefluorography. See **cineradiography.**

cinematics, recording of an anatomic structure in motion. See **kinematics.**

cineplastic amputation, amputation in which the stump is formed in a fashion to be usable for producing motion of a prosthesis. See **kineplasty.**

cineradiography /sin′irā′dē·og″rəfē/ [Gk, *kinesis,* movement; L, *radiere,* to shine; Gk, *graphein,* to record], the recording of images that appear on a fluorescent screen, especially images of body structures during and following the introduction of a contrast medium. Cineradiography incorporates the techniques of cinematography, fluoroscopy, and radiography as a diagnostic technique. Also called **cinefluorography.** See also **cineangiocardiography.**

cinesia, *(Obsolete)* now called **kinesia.**

-cinesis, -cinesia. See **-kinesis, -kinesia.**

cingulate /sing″gyəlit/ [L, *cingulum,* girdle], **1.** having a zone or a girdle, usually with transverse markings. **2.** pertaining to a cingulum.

cingulate sulcus. See **callosomarginal fissure.**

cingulectomy /sing′gyoŏolek″təmē/ [L, *cingulum* + Gk, *ektomē,* excision], the surgical excision of a portion of the cingulate gyrus in the frontal lobe of the brain and the immediately surrounding tissue.

cingulotomy /sing′gyoŏolot″əmē/ [L, *cingulum* + *temnein,* to cut], a procedure in brain surgery to alleviate intractable pain by producing lesions in the tissue of the cingulate gyrus of the frontal lobe. The operation interrupts the fibers of the white matter in the gyrus by the stereotactic application of heat or cold.

cinnamon /sin′əmən/ [Gk, *kinnamomon*], the aromatic inner bark of several species of a tree native to the East Indies and China. Saigon cinnamon is commonly used as a carminative, an aromatic stimulant, and a spice. −*cinnamic, adj.*

circa [L, *circa,* about], approximate, as an approximate date or number.

circadian dysrhythmia /sərkā″dē·ən, sur′kədē″ən/ [L, *circa,* about, *dies,* day; Gk, *dys,* bad, *rhythmos,* rhythm], the biological and psychological stress effects of jet lag, or rapid travel through several time zones. In addition to a shift in normal eating and sleeping patterns, disruption of medication schedules and other therapies may occur.

circadian rhythm [L, *circa,* about, *dies,* day; Gk, *rhythmos,* rhythm], a pattern over 24 hours of usual changes in behavior, sleep, eating, and waking patterns. Circadian rhythms can be unique to individuals, causing some to function better later in the day or at night rather than mornings or daytime. They often change temporarily during adolescence.

circinate /sur″sināt/ [L, *circinare,* to make round], having a ring-shaped outline or formation; annular.

circle [L, *circulus*], (in anatomy) a circular or nearly circular structure of the body, such as the circle of Willis and circle of Zinn. −*circular, adj.*

circle of Carus. See **curve of Carus.**

circle of least confusion, **1.** (in optics) a disc representing the image of a theoretical point made by a spherocylindrical lens. **2.** smallest cross-section of the blur circle between two focal lines formed by an astigmatic lens.

circle of Willis [Thomas Willis, English physician, 1621–1675], a vascular network at the base of the brain formed by the interconnection of the middle cerebral, anterior cerebral, posterior cerebral, basilar, anterior communicating, and posterior communicating arteries.

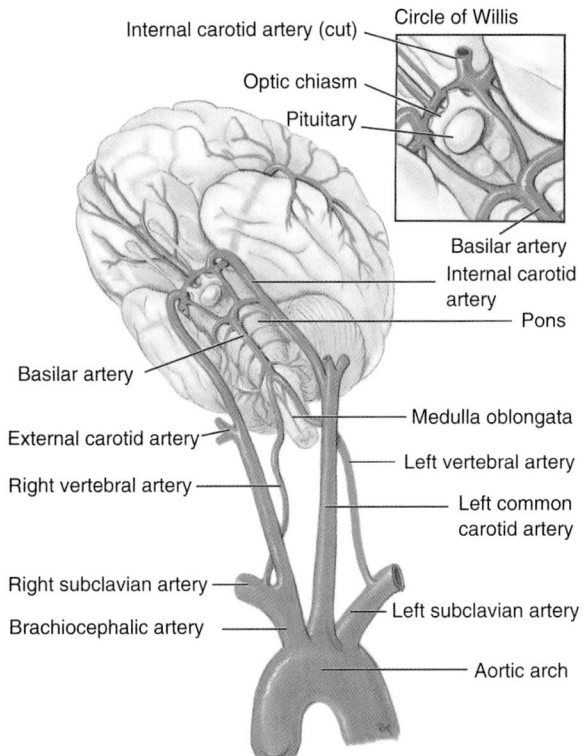

Circle of Willis

Internal carotid artery (cut)
Optic chiasm
Pituitary
Basilar artery
Internal carotid artery
Pons
Basilar artery
External carotid artery
Right vertebral artery
Medulla oblongata
Left vertebral artery
Left common carotid artery
Right subclavian artery
Left subclavian artery
Brachiocephalic artery
Aortic arch

View from below of arterial supply of the brain

Circle of Willis *(Applegate, 2011)*

CircOlectric (COL) bed, a brand name for an electronically controlled bed that can be vertically rotated 210 degrees, allowing a patient to move vertically from the prone to supine position. It is used especially in orthopedics and in the treatment of patients with severe burns and pressure ulcers. The bed consists of a strong aluminum circular frame supporting an anterior and a posterior straight frame within the exterior aluminum circle. The patient is "sandwiched" and secured between the two straight frames during rotation. Compare **Foster bed, hyperextension bed, Stryker wedge frame.**

circuit /sur″kit/ [L, *circuitus,* going around], a course or pathway, particularly one through which an electric current passes. Current passes through a closed or continuous circuit and stops if the circuit is open, interrupted, or broken. See also **volt.**

circuit training, a method of physical exercise in which activities are arranged in sets and the participant moves quickly from one activity to another with a minimum of rest between activities.

circular. See **circle.**

circular bandage /sur″kyələr/ [L, *circularis,* round], a bandage wrapped around an injured part, usually a limb or a digit.

circular fiber, any one of the many fibers in the free gingiva that encircle the teeth coronal to the alveolar crest; not attached to cementum. Compare **alveolar crestal fiber, apical fiber.**

circular fold, one of the numerous annular projections in the small intestine. They vary in size and frequency in the duodenum, the jejunum, and the ileum and are formed by mucous and submucous tissue. Also called **plica circularis, valve of Kerkring.**

circulation /sur″kyəlā″shən/ [L, *circulatio,* to go around], movement of an object or substance through a circular course so that it returns to its starting point, such as the circulation of blood through the circuitous network of arteries and veins.

circulation rate [L, *circulatio,* to go around, *ratum,* calculation], the rate of blood flow, usually expressed as the amount of blood pumped through the heart per minute. The rate varies with such factors as blood volume and cardiac contractility.

circulation time, the time required for blood to flow from one part of the body to another. Timing a particle of blood involves injecting a traceable dye or radioisotope into a vein and timing its reappearance in an artery at the point of injection. Alternatively, a substance that can be tasted, such as saccharin, can be injected and the time it takes to travel to the tongue noted. The resulting time helps determine problems with heart failure and decreased cardiac output.

circulatory failure [L, *circulatio + fallere,* to deceive], inability of the cardiovascular system to supply the cells of the body with enough oxygenated blood to meet their metabolic demands. The condition may result from abnormal cardiac function, as in myocardial infarction; from an inadequate circulating volume of blood, as occurs in hemorrhage; or from mass systemic vasodilation, as may occur in gram-negative septicemia. See also **shock.**

circulatory fluid. See **blood, lymph.**

circulatory overload [L, *circulatio,* to go around; AS, *ofer* + ME, *lod*], an elevation in blood pressure caused by an increased blood volume, as by transfusion. The condition can lead to heart failure or pulmonary edema.

circulatory system, the network of channels through which blood circulates.

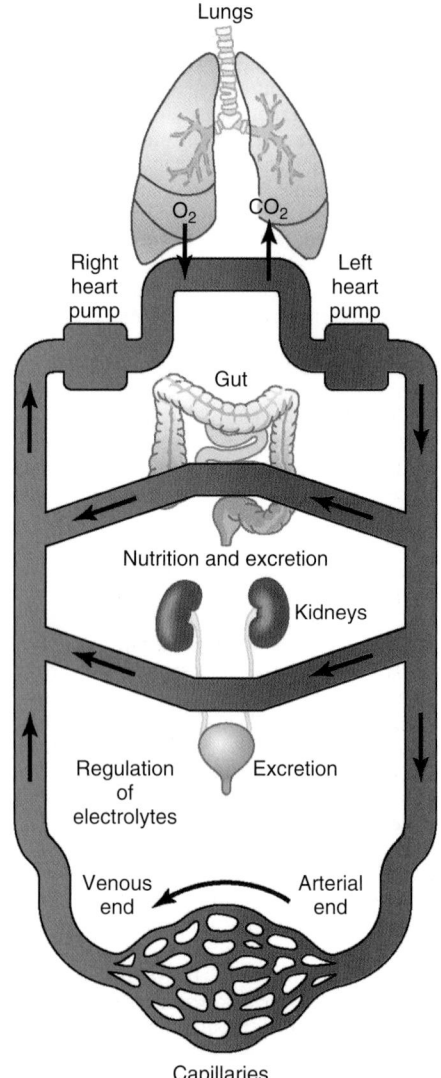

Circulatory system *(Hall, 2011)*

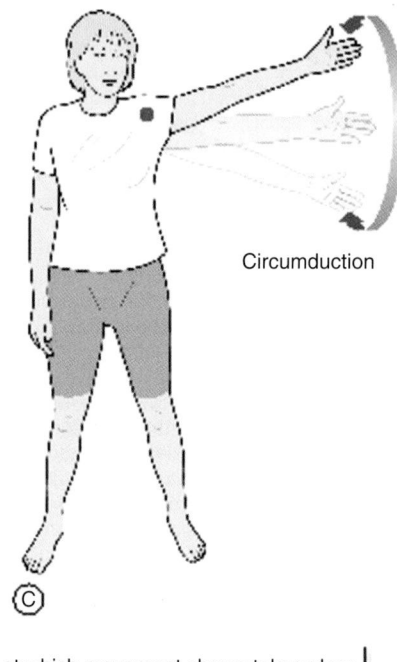

Circumduction

● joint at which movement shown takes place

Circumduction *(Waugh and Grant, 2014)*

circum-, prefix meaning "around": *circumanal, circumcision.*

circumanal /sur′kəmā″nəl/ [L, *circum,* around, *anus*], pertaining to the area surrounding the anus.

circumcision /-sizh″ən/ [L, *circum,* around, *cadere,* to cut], a surgical procedure in which the prepuce of the penis is excised. Circumcision is widely performed on newborn boys. The operation is performed on newborns with penile block anesthesia, using one of several kinds of clamps. It is sometimes performed on adult males in the treatment of phimosis and balanitis. Circumcision is a significant ritual in some religions.

circumcorneal /-kôr″nē·əl/, pertaining to the area of the eye surrounding the cornea.

circumduction /sur′kəmduk″shən/ [L, *circum + ducere,* to lead], **1.** one of the four basic movements allowed by the various joints of the skeleton. It is a combination of abduction, adduction, extension, and flexion. An example is the motion of a bone whose head articulates with a cavity, such as the femur with the acetabulum. The motion of the bone circumscribes a cone, the apex of which is in the cavity and the base of which is described by the distal end of the bone. **2.** the circular movement of a limb or of the eye. Compare **angular movement, gliding, rotation.**

circumference /surkum″fərens/ [L, *circum,* around, *ferre,* to bear], **1.** the perimeter or periphery of a circle. **2.** a circular plane surface of a joint.

circumferential /sərkum″fəren″shəl/, encircling; pertaining to a circumference or perimeter.

circumferential fibrocartilage [L, *circum + ferre,* to bring, *fibra,* fiber, *cartilago*], a structure made of fibrocartilage, in which fibrocartilaginous rims surround the margins of various articular cavities, such as the glenoid labra of the hip and the shoulder. The rims deepen such cavities and protect their edges. Compare **connecting fibrocartilage, interarticular fibrocartilage, stratiform fibrocartilage.**

circumferential implantation. See **superficial implantation.**

circumflex /sur″kəmfleks/ [L, *circum,* around, *flexcere,* to bend], winding around; pertaining to blood vessels or nerves that wind around other body structures, as in the circumflex coronary artery.

circumlocution /-lōkoo″shən/, the subconscious or learned use of pantomime, nonverbal communication, or word substitution by a patient because a word is difficult to retrieve or has been forgotten. See also **anomia, stuttering.**

circummarginate placenta, a placenta with a thinner ring of membranous tissue on the fetal surface than that of a circumvallate placenta. It is associated rarely with fetal malformation but usually has no clinical significance.

circumoral /sur′kəmôr″əl/ [L, *circum + os,* mouth], pertaining to the area of the face around the mouth.

circumoral pallor [L, *circum,* around, *os,* mouth, *pallor,* paleness], paleness of the skin area around the mouth, a possible sign of scarlet fever, pheochromocytoma, or shock.

circumscribed /-skrībd″/ [L, *circum,* around, *scribere,* to draw], within a well-defined area, or in one with definite boundaries or limits.

circumscribed abscess [L, *circum,* around, *scribere,* to draw, *abscedere,* to go away], an accumulation of pustular material separated from surrounding tissues by a wall of fibroblasts. Often difficult to treat, it may be drained or aspirated using the technique of needle aspiration. Antibiotic therapy is usually indicated. Kinds include **peritonsillar abscess, appendicular abscess, lung abscess, Brodie's abscess.**

circumscribed abscess of bone.   See **Brodie's abscess.**

circumscribed pleurisy.   See **encysted pleurisy.**

circumscribed scleroderma, *(Obsolete)*   now called **localized scleroderma.**

circumstantiality /-stan′shē·al″itē/   [L, *circum* + *stare,* to stand],   (in psychiatry) a speech pattern in which a patient has difficulty in separating relevant from irrelevant information while describing an event. The patient often includes all details and presents them in a sequential order, with the result that the main thread of thought becomes lost as one association leads to another. Frequently the person may need to have questions repeated because the main point of answers has become lost in the confusion of unnecessary detail. Compare **flight of ideas.**

circumvallate papilla.   See **papilla.**

circus movement,   **1.** an unusual and involuntary rolling or somersaulting caused by injured neural structures that control body posture, such as the cerebral pedicles or the vestibular apparatus. **2.** an unusual circular gait caused by injury to the brain or spinal cord. **3.** a mechanism associated with the excitatory wave of the atrium of the heart and atrial flutter or fibrillation. The wave travels a circular path characterized by a gap between the refractory and the excitatory tissue, usually resulting in conduction of only a fraction of the impulses to the ventricle.

cirrh-,   prefix meaning "yellow": *cirrhosis.*

cirrhosis /sirō″sis/   [Gk, *kirrhos,* yellow-orange, *osis,* condition],   a chronic degenerative disease of the liver in which the lobes are covered with fibrous tissue, the parenchyma degenerates, and the lobules are infiltrated with fat. Gluconeogenesis, detoxification of drugs and alcohol, bilirubin metabolism, vitamin absorption, GI function, hormonal metabolism, and other functions of the liver deteriorate. Blood flow through the liver is obstructed, causing back pressure and leading to portal hypertension and esophageal varices. Unless the cause of the disease is removed, hepatic coma, GI hemorrhage, and kidney failure may occur. Cirrhosis is most commonly the result of chronic alcohol abuse; other causes include nutritional deprivation, hepatitis, and cardiac problems.

■ OBSERVATIONS: Cirrhosis is often asymptomatic in early disease or may manifest as abdominal pain, diarrhea, nausea, vomiting, fatigue, and fever. As the disease progresses, manifestations such as chronic dyspepsia, constipation, anorexia, weight loss, pruritus, easy bruising, bleeding gums, nosebleeds, upper gastrointestinal bleeding, and enlarged liver are seen. Late disease is accompanied by telangiectasis, spider angiomas, enlarged breasts, testicular atrophy, jaundice, impotence, enlarged spleen, depression, abdominal vein distension, ascites, encephalopathy, and peripheral neuropathy. Diagnostic tests include abnormal liver function studies, including elevations in alkaline phosphatase, aminotransferase, and alanine aminotransferase. A CBC may show evidence of anemia, leukopenia, or thrombocytopenia. Protein metabolism tests show decreased total protein, decreased albumin, and increased globulin. Cholesterol levels are decreased as a result of abnormalities in fat metabolism. Prothrombin time is prolonged, and bilirubin metabolism is abnormal. Blood glucose may be reduced. Ultrasonography is used to reveal hepatosplenomegaly and enlarged portal veins. Liver scans show reduced liver uptake. Liver biopsy will show definitive histological changes in the liver cells and reveal altered structure in the lobes.

■ INTERVENTIONS: The first step is elimination of toxic agents, such as alcohol or drugs. Therapy is aimed at liver cell regeneration and the prevention or treatment of symptoms. This includes rest to reduce metabolic demands on the liver; a high-calorie, high-protein (unless hepatic encephalopathy is present), high-carbohydrate, and low-fat, low-sodium diet; diuretics to reduce edema; digestants to promote fat digestion; supplemental vitamins; and stool softeners. Ascites may be treated with abdominal paracentesis or peritoneovenous shunt. Esophageal varices may be treated by using blood and blood products, gastric lavage, or esophageal balloon to stem bleeding. Variceal sclerosis may be performed via endoscopy to eliminate the varicosities. A portal systemic shunt may be surgically placed to treat resistant esophageal varices. A transjugular intrahepatic portosystemic shunt may be used to divert portal blood from the liver to relieve portal hypertension. Renal dialysis is used to treat renal failure. Hepatic encephalopathy is managed by reducing ammonia formation through reduced protein intake, administering lactulose to decrease pH in the intestines, and administering antibiotics to reduce bacterial flora in the colon. Liver transplantation may be the only hope for those with advanced disease.

■ PATIENT CARE CONSIDERATIONS: Care for individuals with acute disease is multifaceted, complex, and dictated by the stage of the disease and presenting symptomatology. The focus is on strength conservation. This includes balancing rest and activity and correcting nutritional imbalances. Edema and ascites produce itching and impaired skin integrity. Skin care requires careful diligence to prevent excoriation and breakdown. Ascites can also produce shortness of breath from pressure placed on the diaphragm. Sensory perception may be decreased secondary to peripheral neuropathy. This places the individual at increased risk for injury and requires the implementation of injury prevention protocols. Infection control measures should also be in effect to reduce the possibility of infection from environmental pathogens in these susceptible individuals. Careful monitoring is needed to spot early signs of life-threatening complications, such as hepatic encephalopathy or esophageal bleeding. In the individual with hepatic encephalopathy, the focus is on monitoring systems affected by increased ammonia levels and assessing whether levels are effectively being reduced. Adequate hydration must be maintained with careful monitoring for fluid and electrolyte and acid-base imbalances, reduction of protein, prevention of constipation, and strict bed rest. Chronic care focuses on education. Individuals need to understand that this disease is chronic in nature and requires continuous care to reduce or prevent serious complications. Prompt treatment needs to be sought at any sign of complication. Instruction is needed about diet, medication use and restrictions, skin care, infection protection, and importance of complete alcohol abstinence. Referrals may be made to substance abuse programs and community or home health care agencies.

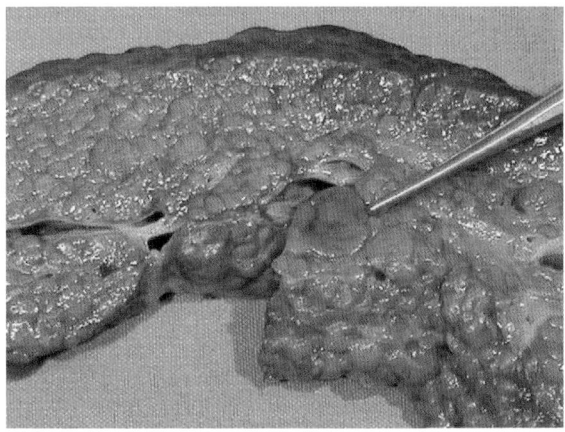

Cirrhosis *(Odze and Goldblum, 2009)*

cirsoid aneurysm, an enlarged tortuous vessel. Also called **racemose aneurysm.**

cis arrangement. See **cis configuration.**

cisatracurium, a nondepolarizing neuromuscular blocker.

- INDICATIONS: It is used to facilitate endotracheal intubation and skeletal muscle relaxation during mechanical ventilation, surgery, or general anesthesia.
- CONTRAINDICATIONS: Known hypersensitivity to this drug prohibits its use.
- ADVERSE EFFECTS: Life-threatening effects include prolonged apnea, bronchospasm, cyanosis, and respiratory depression. Other serious adverse effects include bradycardia, tachycardia, and increased/decreased blood pressure.

cis configuration /sis/, **1.** the presence of the dominant alleles of two or more pairs of genes on one chromosome and the recessive alleles on the homologous chromosome. **2.** the presence of the mutant genes of a pair of pseudoalleles on one chromosome and the wild-type genes on the homologous chromosome. Compare **coupling, trans configuration. 3.** (in chemistry) a form of geometric or stereoisomerism in which two substituent groups are on the same side of a double bond or aliphatic ring. Also known as Z (zusammen) configuration. Also called **cis arrangement, cis position.**

cisgender /sis-jen-der/, an individual with a match between gender identity and biological sex assigned at birth. Compare **transgender.**

cisplatin /sisplat″in/, an antineoplastic.

- INDICATIONS: It is prescribed in combination with vinblastine and bleomycin in the treatment of neoplasms such as metastatic testicular, prostatic, and ovarian tumors, and Hodgkin's lymphoma.
- CONTRAINDICATIONS: Preexisting renal dysfunction, myelosuppression, hearing impairment, or known hypersensitivity to this drug or other drugs containing platinum prohibits its use.
- ADVERSE EFFECTS: Among the most serious adverse reactions are nephrotoxicity, ototoxicity, myelosuppression, severe nausea, anorexia, vomiting, and allergic reactions.

cis position. See **cis configuration.**

cistern /sis″tərn/ [L, *cisterna,* vessel], a closed space serving as a reservoir for lymph or other body fluids, especially one of the enlarged subarachnoid spaces containing cerebrospinal fluid.

cisterna /sistur″nə/ *pl. cisternae* [L, vessel], a cavity that serves as a reservoir for lymph or other body fluids. Kinds include **cisterna chyli,** *cisterna subarachnoidea.*

cisterna chyli, the dilated portion of the thoracic duct at its origin in the lumbar region.

cisterna magna, the enlarged subarachnoid space between the undersurface of the cerebellum and the posterior surface of the medulla oblongata.

cisternal puncture /sistur″nəl/ [L, vessel, *punctura,* a piercing], the insertion of a needle into the cisterna magna to withdraw cerebrospinal fluid for examination, usually performed with fluoroscopic guidance. The puncture is made between the atlas and the occipital bone.

cistron /sis″tron/ [L, *cis,* this side, *trans,* across], a fragment or portion of DNA that codes for a specific polypeptide. It is the smallest unit functioning as a transmitter of genetic information. In modern molecular genetics the cistron is essentially synonymous with the gene. It can include regions preceding and following the coding DNA as well as introns.

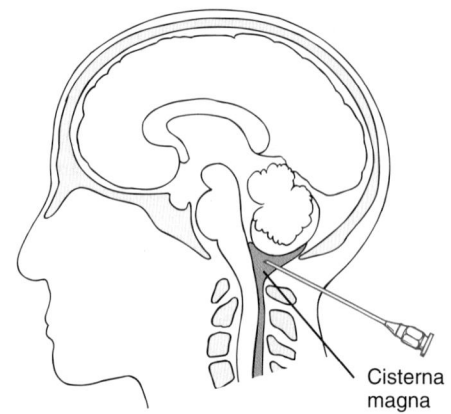

Cisternal puncture *(Mosby, 2003)*

cisvestitism /sisves″titiz′əm/ [L, *cis,* this side, *vestis,* garment], the practice of wearing attire appropriate to the sex of the individual involved but not suitable to the age, occupation, or status of the wearer, as when a male bookkeeper impersonates a male police officer by wearing a police uniform.

cit, abbreviation for **citrate.**

citalopram, an antidepressant in the selective serotonin-reuptake inhibitor class.

- INDICATIONS: It is used to treat major depressive disorder.
- CONTRAINDICATIONS: Known hypersensitivity to this drug prohibits its use. It should not be used with MAO inhibitors. It interacts with several forms of cytochrome P450 and therefore influences many other drugs.
- ADVERSE EFFECTS: Life-threatening effects include convulsions, hemorrhage, first-degree atrioventricular block, and myocardial infarction. Other serious adverse effects include hallucinations, delusions, psychosis, vomiting, asthma, hyperventilation, respiratory infection, dyspnea, bronchitis, pneumonia, angina pectoris, hypertension, palpitations, tachycardia, bradycardia, thrombophlebitis, arthritis, amenorrhea, cystitis, urine retention, and viral infection. Common side effects are numerous, affecting the GI, integumentary, respiratory, cardiovascular, genitourinary, and central nervous systems. Some are also systemic.

Citanest Hydrochloride, a local anesthetic. Brand name for **prilocaine hydrochloride.**

citicoline /sit′ikō″lin/, a natural substance that is a component of cell membranes. A pharmaceutic version is available in the United States as a supplement that is used to improve memory.

citrate (cit) /sit″rāt, sī″trāt/ [L, *kitron,* citron], **1.** an anion of citric acid. **2.** the act of treating with a citrate or citric acid. −*citration, n.*

citrated plasma, plasma from blood collected and mixed with sodium citrate, which prevents clotting. Citrated plasma is most often used for coagulation testing.

citric acid /sit″rik/ [Gk, *kitron,* citron; L, *acidus,* sour], a white, crystalline organic acid soluble in water and alcohol. It is extracted from citrus fruits, especially lemons and limes, or obtained by fermentation of sugars and is used as an acidulating agent, an antioxidant, and a flavoring agent in foods, carbonated beverages, and certain pharmaceutic products, especially laxatives. Compare **ascorbic acid.**

citric acid cycle [Gk, *kitron,* citron; L, *acidus,* sour; Gk, *kyklos,* circle], a sequence of enzymatic reactions involving the metabolism of carbon chains of sugars, fatty acids, and amino acids to yield carbon dioxide, water, and high-energy phosphate bonds. The cycle is initiated when pyruvate combines with coenzyme A (CoA) to form a two-carbon unit, acetyl-CoA, which enters the cycle by combining with four-carbon oxaloacetic acid to form six-carbon citric acid. In subsequent steps, isocitric acid, produced from citric acid, is oxidized to oxalosuccinic acid, which loses carbon dioxide to form alpha-ketoglutaric acid. Succinic acid, resulting from the oxidative decarboxylation of alpha-ketoglutaric acid, is oxidized to fumaric acid, and its oxidation regenerates oxaloacetic acid, which condenses with acetyl-CoA, closing the cycle. The citric acid cycle provides a major source of adenosine triphosphate energy and also produces intermediate molecules that are starting points for a number of vital metabolic pathways including amino acid synthesis. Also called **Krebs cycle, tricarboxylic acid cycle.** See also **acetylcoenzyme A.**

citrin /sit″rin/ [Gk, *kitron,* citron], a crystalline flavonoid concentrate that is used as a source of bioflavonoid.

citrovorum factor. See **folinic acid.**

citrulline /sitrul″ēn/ [L, *Citrullus,* watermelon], an amino acid produced from ornithine during the urea cycle. It is subsequently transformed to arginine by the transfer of a nitrogen atom from aspartate.

citrullinemia /-ē″mē·ə/, a disorder of amino acid metabolism caused by a deficiency of the enzyme argininosuccinic acid synthetase. The clinical features include vomiting, convulsions, and coma. It is treated with a low-protein diet that provides an essential amino acid mixture, ketoacid analogs of amino acids, and arginine.

Civilian Health and Medical Programs for Uniformed Services (CHAMPUS). *(Obsolete)* See **TRICARE.**

CJPH, abbreviation for **Canadian Journal of Public Health.**

C/kg, a unit of radiation exposure in the SI system, coulombs per kilogram of air. 1 roentgen = 2.58×10^{-4} C/kg.

CK isoenzyme fraction, one of several blood-borne enzymes that are released after myocardial necrosis. The isoenzyme of creatine kinase (CK) is identified as MB isomer, or MB-CK, and is a diagnostic clue to heart damage. Formerly called **creatine phosphokinase.** See also **aspartate aminotransferase, lactate dehydrogenase.**

cL, abbreviation for **centiliter.**

Cl, symbol for the element **chlorine.**

clade /klād/, (in biology) a grouping of organisms descended from one common ancestor.

Claforan, an antibiotic. Brand name for **cefotaxime sodium.**

claim, an itemized statement of services and costs from a health care provider or facility submitted to the insured for payment.

claims-made policy [L, *clamere,* to cry out; ME, *maken* + L, *politicus,* the state], a professional liability insurance policy that covers the holder for the period in which a claim of malpractice is made. The alleged act of malpractice may have occurred at some previous time, but the policy insures the holder when the claim is made. Compare **occurrence policy.**

clairvoyance /klervoi″əns/, the alleged power or ability to perceive or to be aware of objects or events without the use of the physical senses. See also **extrasensory perception, parapsychology, telepathy.**

clamp [AS, *clam,* to hold together], an instrument with serrated jaws and locking handles, used for gripping, holding, joining, supporting, or compressing an organ, vessel, or tissue. In surgery, clamps generally are used for hemostasis and clamping tissue.

clamp forceps. See **pedicle clamp.**

clam poisoning. See **shellfish poisoning.**

clang association /klang/ [L, *clangere,* to resound, *associare,* to unite], the mental connection between dissociated ideas made because of similarity in the sounds of the words used to describe the ideas. The phenomenon occurs frequently in schizophrenia. See also **looseness of association.**

clap. *(Slang)* See **gonorrhea.**

clapping [AS, *cloeppan,* to beat], **1.** (in massage) the procedure of making percussive movements on a patient's body, usually on the chest wall or back, by lowering the cupped palms alternately in a series of rapid, stimulating blows. In this procedure the movement of the hands is from the wrist. Clapping stimulates the circulation and refreshes the skin. It is often done to improve the comfort of bedridden patients, especially during administration of a bath. Also called **percussion. 2.** a therapeutic technique usually used in conjunction with postural drainage. The rhythmic motion of cupped hands gently tapping the chest loosens secretions in individuals with cystic fibrosis.

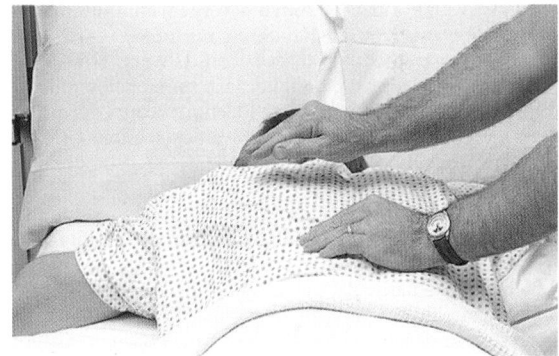

Clapping *(Potter et al, 2013)*

clapping and vibrating, a technique for dislodging and removing mucus and fluid from the lungs. Compare **high-frequency oscillation.** See also **clapping; postural drainage.**

Clapton line [Edward Clapton, English physician, 1830–1909], a greenish line at the base of the teeth, indicative of copper poisoning.

clarification /kler′ifikā″shən/ [L, *clarus,* clear, *facere,* to make], (in psychology) an intervention technique designed to guide the patient in focusing on and recognizing gaps and inconsistencies in his or her statements.

clarify /kler″əfī/, (in chemistry) to clear a turbid liquid by allowing any suspended matter to settle, by adding a substance that precipitates any suspended matter, or by heating. **–clarification,** *n.*

Clarks rule [Cecil Clark, 20th-century British physician; L, *regula,* model], *(Obsolete)* a method of calculating the approximate pediatric dosage of a drug for a child by using this formula: weight in pounds/150 × adult dose. See also **pediatric dosage.**

-clasia, suffix meaning a "(specified) condition involving crushing or breaking up": *osteoclasia.*

clasp [ME, *clippen,* to embrace], **1.** (in dentistry) a sleeve-like fitting that is fastened over a tooth to hold a partial denture in place. **2.** (in surgery) any device for holding together tissues, especially bones.

clasp arm, (in dentistry) an extension, usually from a minor connector, of the clasp of a removable partial denture, that provides retention, reciprocation, or stabilization to an abutment tooth.

clasp-knife reflex, an abnormal sign in which a spastic limb resists passive motion and then suddenly gives way, similarly to the motion of the blade of a jackknife. It is an indication of damage to the pyramidal tract.

clasp-knife spasticity, increased tension in the extensor of a joint when it is passively flexed, giving way suddenly on exertion of further pressure. See **clasp-knife reflex.**

clasp torsion, the twisting of a retentive clasp arm on a removable partial denture.

classical conditioning, a form of learning, based on the behaviorist theory of I. Pavlov, in which a previously neutral stimulus begins to elicit a given response through associative training. Also called **respondent conditioning.** See also **conditioned reflex.**

classical Western massage, methods of massage based on European concepts of anatomy and physiology and using five basic techniques: effleurage, pétrissage, friction, tapotement, and vibration.

classic cesarean section [L, *classicus,* first-class, *Caesar lex,* Caesar's law, *sectio,* a cutting], a method for surgically delivering a baby through a vertical midline incision of the upper segment of the uterus. For many practitioners this is the fastest method of cesarean delivery. However, it produces a weaker scar, and, because the upper segment is thicker and more vascular, more bleeding occurs during surgery than from the low cervical cesarean section. Compare **extraperitoneal cesarean section.** See also **cesarean section.**

classic tomography [L, *classicus* + Gk, *tome,* section, *graphein,* to record], a method that moves the x-ray source and the x-ray plate during an exposure to produce an image in which all but a particular plane is blurred out. This allows an approximate isolation of the image of a detail, which might otherwise be obscured by overlying or underlying structures. This technique is especially valuable in visualizing air-filled structures such as the lungs and paranasal sinuses. See also **computed tomography.**

classic typhus. See **epidemic typhus.**

classic visceral leishmaniasis, a form of leishmaniasis caused by *Leishmania donovani,* transmitted by the sandfly *Phlebotomus argentipes,* usually affecting older children or young adults. Humans are the only reservoir hosts. It occurs primarily in eastern India and Bangladesh.

classification /klas′ifikā″shən/ [L, *classis,* collection, *facere,* to make], **1.** (in research) a process in data analysis in which data are grouped according to previously determined characteristics. −*classify, v.* **2.** (in pharmacology) the categorization of drugs by type, purpose, or control (i.e., controlled substances).

classification of caries [L, *classis,* collection, *facere,* to make, *caries,* decay], a system for dividing dental caries into six possible classes based on the part of the tooth they affect. Class I caries are pits and fissures in the occlusal surfaces of posterior teeth or the lingual surfaces of maxillary incisors. Class II caries begin on the proximal surfaces of premolars and molars and can break through to the occlusal surfaces. Class III caries affect the proximal surfaces of incisors and canines, excluding the incisal angles. Class IV caries affect the proximal surfaces of incisors and canines, including the incisal angles. Class V pertains to caries that affect the gingival third of the labial, buccal, and lingual surfaces. A modification of this classification system (not included in Black's original Classification) adds another group, Class VI, consisting of caries on the incisal edges and cusp tips. Classification of caries provides dentists a basis for design of cavity preparations according to the type of restorative material used. Also called **Black's Classification of Caries.** See also **cavity classification.**

classification of malocclusion. See **Angle's classification of malocclusion.**

classification schemes, systems of organizing data or information, usually involving categories of items with similar characteristics. Kinds include *Nursing Interventions Classification,* **Diagnostic and Statistical Manual of Mental Disorders, International Classification of Diseases.**

class II biological safety cabinet, a container that recirculates air through a high-efficiency filter. It is usually located in a hospital pharmacy and is used to prepare chemotherapeutic agents in an environment that protects personnel from exposure.

-clast, suffix meaning "something that breaks": *osteoclast.*

-clastic, suffix meaning "causing disintegration": *osteoclastic.*

claudication /klô′dikā″shən/ [L, *claudicatio,* a limping], cramplike pains in the calves caused by poor circulation of the blood to the leg muscles. The condition is commonly associated with atherosclerosis. The disorder is usually manifested after walking and is relieved by rest. Claudication may require arterial bypass grafting, such as femoral popliteal bypass. Claudication must be differentiated from rest pain, a condition that requires surgical intervention and signals limb threat.

claustra. See **claustrum.**

claustrophobia /klôs′trə-/ [L, *claustrum,* a closing; Gk, *phobos,* fear], a morbid fear of being in or becoming trapped in enclosed or narrow places. The phenomenon is observed more often in women than in men and can generally be traced to some traumatic situation involving enclosed spaces, usually occurring in childhood. Treatment consists of psychotherapy to uncover the cause of the phobic reaction, followed by behavior therapy, specifically systematic desensitization or flooding technique.

claustrum /klôs″trəm/ *pl. claustra* [L, a closing], **1.** a barrier, as a membrane that partially closes an aperture. **2.** a thin sheet of gray matter composed chiefly of spindle cells, situated lateral to the external capsule of the brain and separating the internal capsule from white matter of the insula. Also called *claustrum of insula.*

clavicle /klav″ikəl/ [L, *clavicula,* little key], a long, curved, horizontal bone directly above the first rib, forming the ventral portion of the shoulder girdle. It articulates medially with the sternum and laterally with the acromion of the scapula and accommodates the attachment of numerous muscles. It is shorter, thinner, less curved, and smoother in the female than in the male and is thicker, more curved, and more prominently ridged for muscle attachment in persons performing consistent strenuous manual labor. Also called **collarbone.**

clavicle strap, strapping applied to immobilize the clavicle during fracture healing.

clavicular /kləvik″yələr/, pertaining to the clavicle (collarbone).

clavicular notch [L, *clavicula* + OFr, *enochier*], one of a pair of oval depressions at the superior end of the sternum. A clavicular notch is situated on each side of the sternum and articulates with the clavicle from the same side.

clavipectoral fascia, a thick sheet of connective tissue that connects the clavicle to the floor of the axilla.

clavipectoral triangle, an anatomical triangle formed by the clavicle, the deltoid, and the pectoralis major. It contains the cephalic vein. Also called **deltopectoral triangle.**

clavus, a thickening of the skin. See **corn.**

clawfoot, [AS, *clawu* + *foot*], a deformity of the foot characterized by an excessively high arch with hyperextension of the toes at the metatarsophalangeal joints, flexion at the interphalangeal joints, and shortening of the Achilles tendon. The condition may be present at birth or appear later as a result of contractures or an imbalance of the muscles of the foot, as in neuromuscular diseases such as Friedreich's ataxia and peroneal muscular atrophy. Surgical treatment is indicated in severe cases, especially in children. In milder forms, the pain from the excessive pressure under the metatarsal heads can be relieved by sponge, rubber, or leather insoles fitted into the shoes. Also called **gampsodactyly, griffe des orteils, pes cavus, talipes cavus.**

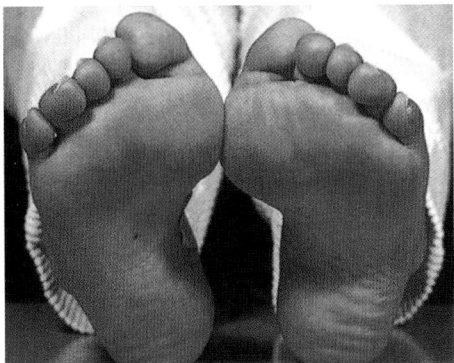

Clawfoot *(Perkin, 2002)*

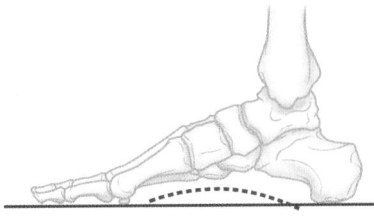

Expected arch

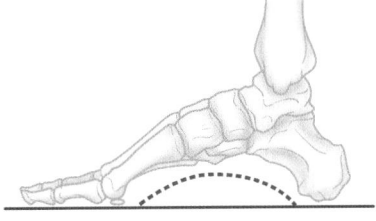

Clawfoot of pes cavus

Clawfoot *(Perkin, 2002)*

clawhand [AS, *clawu* + *hand*], refers to an abnormal posture of the hand, characterized by hyperextension of the metacarpal phalangeal joints and flexion (or ''clawing'') of the middle and distal interphalangeal joints. Indicative of a low-level or distal lesion of the ulnar nerve, with consequent paresis or paralysis of the ulnar innervated intrinsic muscles of the hand. There is a loss of the normal balance between the extrinsic digit extensors and the intrinsic digit flexors and flattening of the normal arches of the hand. Claw hand posture is typically less noticeable in the index and long digits because the lateral two lumbricals, which flex the MCP joints of the index and long digits, are innervated by the median nerve. Also called **main en griffe.**

claw-type traction frame, an orthopedic apparatus that holds various pieces of traction equipment, such as pulleys, ropes, and the weights that suspend or apply traction to various parts of the body. It consists of two metal uprights, one at the head of the bed and the other at the foot. Both uprights are secured to the bed by clawlike attachments and support an overhead metal bar secured to the uprights by metal clamps. Compare **Balkan traction frame, IV-type traction frame.**

clean-catch specimen, a urine specimen that is as free of bacterial contamination as possible without the use of a catheter. This type of specimen is needed to test urine for culture and sensitivity. After appropriate cleansing of the external genitalia, the client begins the urinary stream, allowing the initial portion to escape. The initial stream cleans or flushes the urethral orifice and meatus of resident bacteria. During the middle portion of voiding, the client collects the specimen. The procedure is easiest while using toilet facilities.

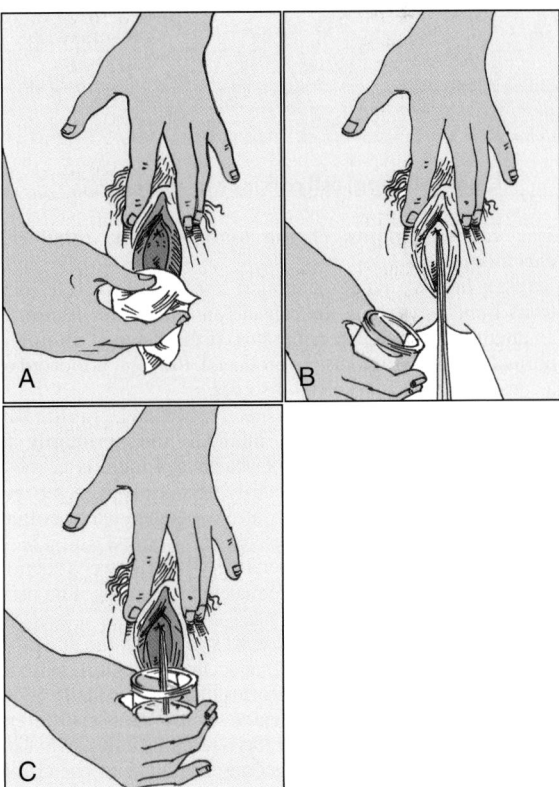

Clean-catch specimen *(Garrels, 2015)*

cleansing enema, an enema, usually composed of water and soapsuds, administered to remove all formed fecal material from the colon. See also **soapsuds enema.**

clearance (C) /klir″əns/ [L, *clarus,* clear], the removal of a substance from the blood via the kidneys. Kidney function can be tested by measuring the amount of a specific substance excreted in the urine in a given length of time.

clear cell [L, *clarus* + *cella,* storeroom], **1.** a type of cell found in the parathyroid gland that does not take on a color with the ordinary tissue stains used for microscopic examination. **2.** the principal cell of most renal cell carcinomas and occasionally of ovarian and parathyroid tumors. **3.** a specific type of epidermal cell, probably of neural origin, that has a dark-staining nucleus but clear cytoplasm with hematoxylin and eosin stain.

clear cell carcinoma, 1. a malignant tumor of the tubular epithelium of the kidney. Characteristically the malignant cells contain abundant clear cytoplasm. See also **renal cell carcinoma. 2.** an uncommon ovarian neoplasm characterized by cells with clear cytoplasm.

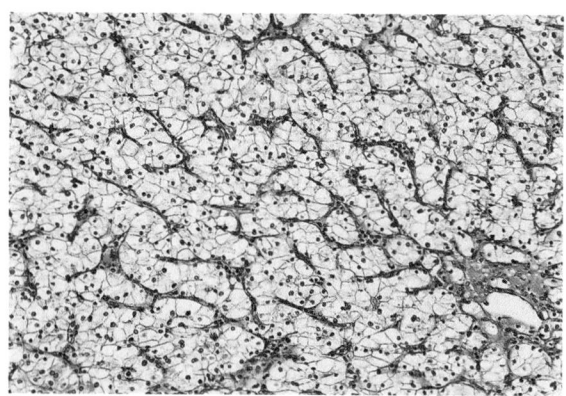

Clear cell renal cell carcinoma *(Fletcher, 2007)*

clear cell carcinoma of the kidney. See **renal cell carcinoma.**

clearing test, a range of motion test that moves the joint to its limits, stretching the capsule and other soft tissues in an attempt to reproduce symptoms. If the range of motion is normal and no symptoms are produced, the joint is cleared as a cause of a musculoskeletal disorder.

clear-liquid diet [L, *clarus* + *liquere,* to flow], a diet that supplies fluids and provides minimal fiber, primarily to relieve thirst and maintain water balance. Liquid is at room temperature and consists primarily of dissolved sugar and flavored liquids, such as ginger ale, sweetened tea or coffee, fat-free broth, plain gelatin desserts, and strained fruit juices. The diet is often used postoperatively until bowel function returns. It is nutritionally inadequate and should not be used for more than two days.

cleavage /klē″vij/ [AS, *cleofan,* to split], **1.** the series of repeated mitotic cell divisions that occur in an ovum immediately after fertilization. It transforms the single-celled zygote into a multicellular embryo capable of growth and differentiation. During cleavage, the embryo remains uniform in size as its cells, or blastomeres, become smaller with each division. Kinds include **determinate cleavage, equal cleavage, indeterminate cleavage, partial cleavage, total cleavage, unequal cleavage. 2.** the act or process of splitting, primarily a complex molecule into two or more simpler molecules. –**cleave′** *v.*

cleavage cavity. See **blastocoele.**

cleavage cell. See **blastomere.**

cleavage line, any one of a number of linear striations in the skin that delineate the general structural pattern, direction, and tension of the subcutaneous fibrous tissue. They correspond closely to the crease lines on the surface of the skin and are present in all areas of the body but are visible only in certain sites, such as the palms of the hands and soles of the feet. In general the lines run obliquely, lying in the direction in which the skin stretches the least, perpendicular to the direction of the greatest stretch. Incisions made parallel to these lines heal with much less scarring than those made perpendicular to them. To a certain degree, cleavage lines determine the direction and arrangement of lesions in skin diseases. Also called **Langer line.**

cleavage nucleus. See **segmentation nucleus.**

cleavage plane, 1. the area in a fertilized ovum where cleavage takes place; the axis along which any cell division occurs. **2.** any plane within the body where organs or structures can be separated with minimal damage to surrounding tissue.

cleave, to split. See **cleavage.**

cleft [ME, *clift*], **1.** division. **2.** a fissure, especially one that originates in the embryo, as the branchial cleft or the facial cleft.

cleft cheek, a transverse facial cleft, appearing as an abnormally large mouth. It is caused by the failure of the maxillary and mandibular processes to fuse during embryonic facial development.

cleft foot, a rare congenital anomaly in which a single cleft extends proximally into the foot, sometimes as far as the midfoot. Generally, one or more toes and parts of their metatarsals are absent, and often the tarsals are abnormal. Although the deformity varies in degree and type, the first and fifth rays usually are present.

cleft hand, a rare congenital disorder in which the hand develops in two parts because of the failure of a digit and metacarpal to form normally during embryonic development. There is a V-shaped gap in the hand due to the absence of central digits. Also called **ectrodactyly.**

cleft lip, a multifactorial congenital anomaly consisting of one or more clefts in the upper lip (with or without cleft palate) that result from a failure in the embryo of the maxillary and median nasal processes to close. Treatment is surgical repair, usually in infancy. Formerly called **harelip.** See also **cleft palate, multifactorial inheritance.**

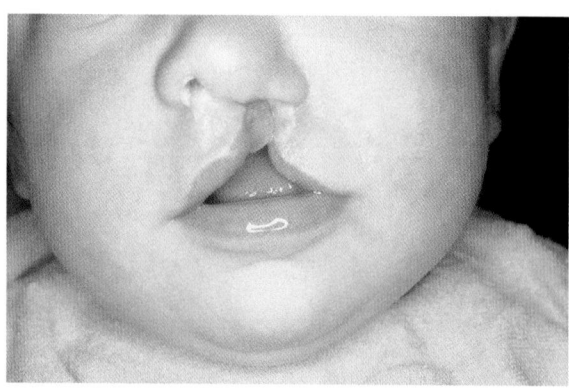

Infant with cleft lip *(Kanski, 2006)*

cleft-lip repair, the surgical correction of a unilateral or bilateral congenital interruption of the upper lip, usually resulting from the embryological failure of the median nasal and maxillary processes to unite.

■ METHOD: A cleft lip may sometimes be repaired during the infant's first 48 hours of life, but some surgeons follow a "rule of 10s" and perform the operation when the child is 10 weeks old, weighs 10 or more pounds, and has a hemoglobin level of at least 10 g/dL. Before surgery, elbow restraints, used to prevent the infant from touching the incision, are prepared in the proper size and are sent to the operating room with the patient. After surgery the infant is maintained with ventilatory support as necessary until respirations are normal. Essential observations include assessment for respiratory stridor or obstruction, excessive bleeding, separation of the incision, and redness under the elbow restraints used to keep the hands from the mouth. The infant is given clear liquids and juices through a syringe (Asepto) or special feeding unit. Parenteral fluids are administered until oral intake is adequate. Milk products, solids, and a nipple or pacifier are not allowed. The diet and manner of feeding may vary, but the infant is fed while held with the head up or is placed in a cardiac chair and burped after the intake of each ounce of food. The elbow restraints are worn at all times except when range-of-motion exercises are performed, one arm at a time, while skin care is administered to that limb.

■ INTERVENTIONS: Many members of the health care team are involved in the care of an infant undergoing this surgery. The nurse provides preoperative and postoperative care and prepares for the infant's discharge.

■ OUTCOME CRITERIA: Modern surgical techniques permit remarkable repair of cleft lips. In some cases a second operation is required to eliminate the scar.

cleft palate, a congenital defect characterized by a fissure in the midline of the palate, resulting from the failure of the two sides to fuse during embryonic development. The fissure may be complete, extending through both the hard and soft palates into the nasal cavities, or it may show any degree of incomplete or partial cleft. Together these abnormalities are the most common of the craniofacial malformations, accounting for half of the total number of defects. Feeding is best accomplished with special devices. Surgical repair of the defect is usually done in the first year of life. Care of the child requires a team approach that can include an oral and maxillofacial surgeon, a plastic surgeon, orthodontist, dentist, nurse, speech and hearing therapists, and social workers. Long-term postoperative problems, including speech impairment and hearing loss, improper tooth development and alignment, chronic respiratory and ear infections, and varying levels of emotional and social maladjustment, may be largely prevented by modern techniques and reconstructive surgery. See also **cleft lip.**

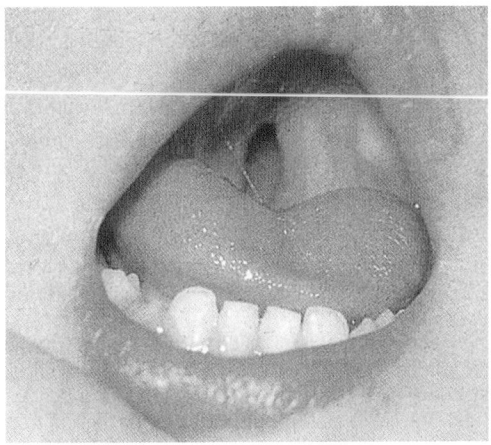

Cleft palate *(Greig and Garden, 1996)*

cleft-palate repair, the surgical correction of a congenital fissure in the midline of the partition separating the oral and nasal cavities. Palatal clefts range from a simple separation in the uvula to an extensive fissure involving the soft and hard palates and extending forward unilaterally or bilaterally through the alveolar ridge. A cleft lip often accompanies a cleft palate. Repair of a cleft palate is usually undertaken when a child is at least 6 months old and must be achieved before normal speech can be produced.

■ METHOD: Before surgery, properly sized elbow restraints to prevent the child from touching the mouth are prepared and sent to the operating room with the patient. Parenteral fluids are administered until the oral intake is adequate. Clear liquids and juices are given by cup only; straws, nipples, pacifiers, utensils, or toys may not be put into the mouth. Milk products and solids are contraindicated, but the kind of feeding ordered may vary. The child is fed in a high chair when possible, and a bib is used to accommodate drooling. Only circumoral mouth care is administered; the teeth are not brushed. The elbow restraints are worn continuously, except when daily range-of-motion exercises are performed and skin care is administered, to one arm at a time. With improvement the child is permitted to walk as tolerated.

■ INTERVENTIONS: Before discharge the nurse ensures that the parents understand the postoperative plan of care. Speech therapists should follow the child until it is clear that speech is normal.

■ OUTCOME CRITERIA: Depending on the extent and nature of a cleft palate, it may be repaired in one or in several operations. Some experts believe that early repair of a defect in the bony palate can lead to structural malrelations and advise delaying the operation until the child is between 5 and 7 years of age and has achieved more bone growth. Successful repair often greatly improves the child's oronasopharyngeal physiological function, speech, and appearance.

cleft-palate speech, faulty speech caused by a cleft palate, often characterized by hypernasality; difficulty with pressure consonants, voice, and articulation; and other problems resulting from the velopharyngeal insufficiency.

cleft sternum, a fissure in the sternum caused by a failure in embryonic development.

cleft tongue [ME, *clift* + AS, *tunge*], a tongue divided by a longitudinal fissure. Also called **bifid tongue.**

cleft uvula, an abnormal congenital condition in which the uvula is split into halves as a result of the failure of the posterior palatine folds to unite.

cleido-, cleid-, prefix meaning "clavicle," or collarbone: *cleidocranial dystocia.*

cleidocranial dysostosis /klī′dōkrā″nē·əl/ [Gk, *kleis,* key, *kranion,* skull, *dys,* bad, *osteon,* bone], a rare abnormal hereditary condition characterized by defective ossification of the cranial bones and by the complete or partial absence of the clavicles. It is transmitted as an autosomal-dominant trait. The defective ossification of the cranial bones delays the closing of the cranial sutures and produces large fontanels. The complete or partial absence of the clavicles allows the shoulders to be drawn together. This condition also involves dental and vertebral anomalies. Also called **cleidocranial dysplasia, dystrophia.** See also **dysostosis.**

cleidocranial dysplasia, an inherited disorder that affects the development of teeth and bones. The clavicles are usually either poorly developed or absent. It is often associated with delayed maturation of the skull, delayed closure of the fontanels, and extra pieces of bone in these spaces; failure of exfoliation and eruption of teeth; the presence of unerupted supernumerary teeth; gingival cysts; and an underdeveloped maxilla.

clemastine /klemas″tēn/, an antihistamine.

■ INDICATIONS: It is prescribed in the treatment of symptoms of allergic rhinitis, pruritus, or conjunctivitis.

■ CONTRAINDICATIONS: Use by lactating mothers or those undergoing monamine oxidase inhibitor therapy or having known sensitivity to this drug or other antihistamines is contraindicated. It is also contraindicated with narrow-angle glaucoma, asthma, symptomatic prostatic hypertrophy, and bladder-neck destruction.

■ ADVERSE EFFECTS: Among the most serious adverse reactions are hypersensitivity, skin rash, and tachycardia. Transient drowsiness commonly occurs.

clenching /klench′ing/ [ME, *clenchen*], the clamping and pressing of the jaws and teeth together in centric occlusion, frequently associated with acute nervous tension or physical effort, such as pushing or lifting a heavy object or performing a difficult task. See also **bruxism.**

Cleocin, an antibiotic. Brand name for **clindamycin hydrochloride.**

cleoid /klē′oid/ [ME, *cle,* claw + Gk, *eidos,* form], in dentistry a carving instrument with a blade shaped like a pointed spade or claw, with cutting edges on both sides used to contour dental amalgam while in its plastic state. Usually associated with a discoid, a round carving instrument on its opposite end.

cleptomania. See **kleptomania.**

clergyman's sore throat, loss of the voice from overuse, as by clergymen. Also called *dysphonia clericorum.*

click /klik′/ [Fr, *cliquer,* to clash], **1.** a single sound, such as the snapping, cracking, or crepitant noise during excursions of the mandibular condyle. The sound is associated with dysfunction of the temporomandibular joint. **2.** a sound associated with movement in a joint, suggesting structural or arthritic changes. **3.** an extra heart sound that occurs during systole. See also **ejection click, systolic click.**

click-murmur syndrome. See **Barlow's syndrome.**

client /klī″ənt/ [L, *clinare,* to lean], **1.** a person who is recipient of a professional service. **2.** a recipient of health care regardless of the state of health. **3.** a patient.

client-centered therapy, 1. a nondirective method of group or individual psychotherapy, originated by Carl Rogers, an American psychologist, in which the therapist's role is to listen to and then reflect or restate without judgment or interpretation the words of the client. The goal of the therapy is personal growth achieved by the client's increased awareness and understanding of his or her attitudes, feelings, and behavior. **2.** an approach to treatment whereby the health care provider includes the client in every part of the evaluation and intervention programs, including the decision about the plan of action.

client satisfaction, general approval of the organization and delivery of health care services by the patient.

client/server system, a computer configuration in which the workload is divided between a client computer and a server, as might be used in a health care management plan; often used to remotely store or access information, such as electronic health record (EHR) data.

climacteric, 1. See **menopause. 2.** See **andropause.**

climate /klī″mit/ [Gk, *klima,* inclination], **1.** a composite of the prevailing weather conditions that characterize any particular geographic region, including air pressure, temperature, precipitation, sunshine, and humidity. Because these factors affect health, they must be considered in the diagnosis and treatment of certain illnesses, especially those affecting respiration. **2.** the general condition surrounding something, as in a climate of goodwill. −*climatic, adj.*

climax /klī″maks/ [Gk, *klimax,* ladder], a peak of intensity, such as a sexual orgasm or the high point of a fever.

climbing fiber [ME, *climben* + L, *fibra*], a type of nerve fiber that carries impulses to the Purkinje cells of the cerebellar cortex.

clindamycin hydrochloride /klin′dəmī″sin/, an antibacterial drug.

■ INDICATIONS: It is prescribed in the treatment of certain serious bacterial infections (including anaerobic and some gram-positive organisms).

■ CONTRAINDICATIONS: Hypersensitivity to this drug or to lincomycin prohibits its use.

■ ADVERSE EFFECTS: Among the more serious adverse reactions are pseudomembranous colitis, severe GI disturbances, and hypersensitivity.

clinic [Gk, *kline,* bed], **1.** an ambulatory care site where persons who do not require hospitalization receive medical care. **2.** a group practice of doctors, such as the Mayo Clinic. **3.** a meeting place for doctors, nurses, medical students, and other health care providers involved in care where instruction can be given at the bedside of a patient or in a similar setting. **4.** a seminar or other scientific medical meeting. **5.** a detailed published report of the diagnosis and treatment of a health care problem.

-clinic, suffix meaning "places set aside for medical treatment": *polyclinic.*

clinical /klin″ikəl/ [Gk, *kline,* bed], **1.** pertaining to a clinic. **2.** pertaining to direct bedside medical or nursing care. **3.** pertaining to materials or equipment used in the care of a sick person. **4.** pertaining to experience of students in an educational program or experience.

clinical analysis, the use of laboratory data, including blood tests, urinalysis, and microscopic tissue studies, in determining a diagnosis and treatment regimen.

clinical assessment, an evaluation of a patient's physical condition and prognosis based on information gathered from physical and laboratory examinations and the patient's history and interview.

clinical assistant, a person who follows standard operating procedures to collect and prepare specimens and who performs appropriate laboratory tests. Clinical assistants complete a postsecondary clinical assistant program.

clinical breast examination (CBE), a breast examination performed by a health professional. It provides an opportunity to check for lumps and other abnormalities. It should be combined with a careful history to identify risk factors associated with breast cancer.

clinical crown, that portion of enamel visibly present in the oral cavity; the visible portion of the tooth that is coronal to the deepest part of the gingival crevice. Compare **anatomical crown.**

clinical-crown/clinical-root ratio, the length of the part of a tooth that is coronal to the junctional epithelium divided by the length of the tooth's root that is apical to the junctional epithelium. The ratio is useful in the diagnosis and prognosis of periodontal disease and treatment planning for fixed or removable prosthodontic restorations. Also called **crown/root ratio.**

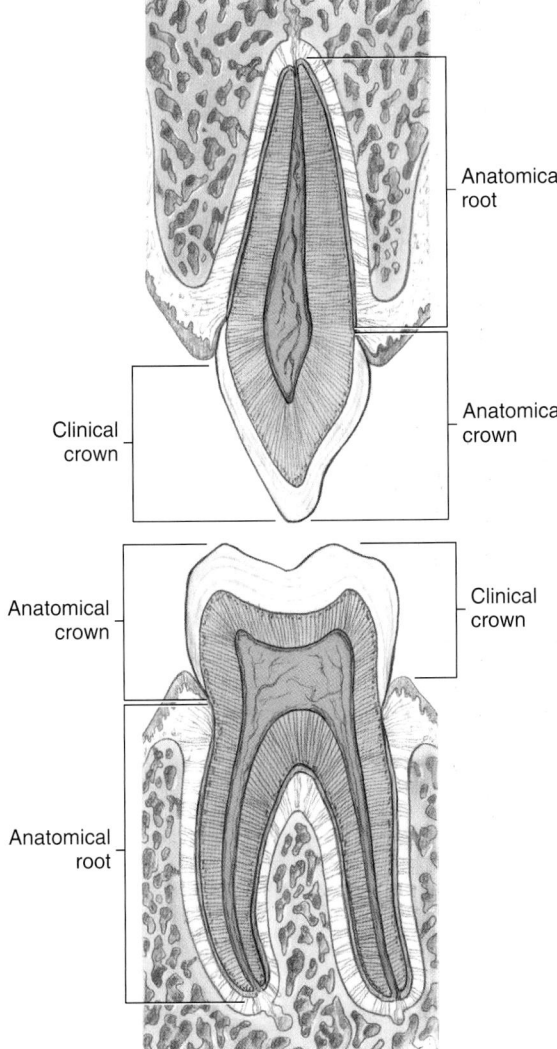

Clinical crown *(Fehrenbach and Popowics, 2016)*

clinical cytogenetics, the branch of genetics that studies the relationship between chromosomal aberrations and pathological conditions.

clinical diagnosis, a diagnosis made on the basis of knowledge obtained by medical history and physical examination alone, without benefit of laboratory tests or x-ray images.

clinical disease, a stage in the history of a pathological condition that begins with anatomical or physiological changes that are sufficient to produce recognizable signs and symptoms of a disease.

clinical epidemiology, the application of the science of epidemiology in a clinical setting. Emphasis is on a medically defined population, as opposed to statistically formulated disease trends derived from examination of larger population categories.

clinical genetics, a branch of genetics that studies inherited disorders and investigates the possible factors that may influence the occurrence of pathological conditions. Also called **medical genetics.**

clinical horizon, the time before an illness presents visible measurable causes, problems, and complications. Compare **subclinical.**

clinical humidity therapy, respiratory therapy in which water vapor is added to the therapeutic gases to make breathing them more comfortable.

clinical judgment, the application of information based on actual observation of a patient combined with subjective and objective data that lead to a conclusion. See also **clinical reasoning.**

clinical laboratory, a laboratory in which tests directly related to the care of patients are performed. Such laboratories use material obtained from patients for testing, as compared with research laboratories, where animal and other sources of test material are also used.

clinical laboratory scientist/medical technologist (CLS/ MT), an allied health professional who, in conjunction with pathologists or other physicians or medical scientists, performs specialized chemical, microscopic, and bacteriological tests of blood, tissue, and fluids. In addition to possessing the skills of clinical laboratory technicians/medical laboratory technicians, clinical laboratory scientists/medical technologists perform complex analyses, fine-line discrimination, and error correction. They have knowledge of physiological conditions affecting test results so they can develop data that may be used by a physician in determining the presence, extent, and, as far as possible, cause of a disease. They are held accountable for accurate results, establish and monitor quality assurance programs, and modify procedures as necessary. Preparation includes a baccalaureate degree and at least 1 year of professional/clinical education.

clinical laboratory technician/medical laboratory technician—associate degree, a clinical laboratory technician and allied health professional who, under the supervision of a pathologist or other physician, clinical laboratory scientist/medical technologist, or other medical scientist, performs specialized chemical, microscopic, and bacteriological tests of blood, tissue, and fluids. The technician can demonstrate discrimination between similar items and correction of errors by the use of preset strategies, is able to recognize factors that directly affect procedures and results, and monitors quality assurance procedures. Preparation is usually 2 academic years, with the graduate receiving an associate's degree.

clinical laboratory technician/medical laboratory technician—certificate, an allied health professional who, under the supervision of a pathologist or other physician, clinical laboratory scientist/medical technologist, or other medical scientist, performs routine, uncomplicated laboratory tests of blood, tissue, and fluids. Clinical education is usually 12 months, with the graduate receiving a certificate. This certificate is no longer being offered for new students.

clinical laboratory technician, kinds include **clinical laboratory technician/medical laboratory technician— associate degree, clinical laboratory technician/medical laboratory technician—certificate.** See also **medical laboratory technician.**

clinical medicine, a system of health maintenance based on direct observation of and communication with a patient.

clinical nurse leader, a registered nurse with a master's degree and certification who oversees the integration of care for patients using evidence-based practice. CNL® is a trademark of the American Association of Colleges of Nursing (AACN). In Canada, clinical nurse leaders include registered nurses and registered psychiatric nurses.

clinical nurse specialist (CNS), an advanced practice registered nurse who holds a minimum of a master's degree in nursing and certification by the American Nurses Credentialing Center (ANCC) or designated nursing specialty organization. The CNS, as a practitioner, assumes a leadership role in the distribution of clinical care to a specific patient population while interacting within the total health care system. The unique functions of the CNS are based on clinical expertise and judgment and include caring for patients, delegating responsibility, teaching other staff members, and influencing and effecting change with respect to the needs of the patient, family and the health care system through contributions to and utilization of evidence-based care.

clinical observations, 1. a requirement of many professional programs in which a student or potential student watches the activities associated with the patient care role in preparation for assumption of that role. Also called **shadowing. 2.** a record compiled by a health care professional that documents a patient's condition, the treatments provided to the patient, and the outcomes of those treatments. **3.** observations of a client's behavior that are used to create an intervention plan and determine progress toward goals.

clinical-pathological conference, a teaching conference in which a case is presented to a clinician, who then demonstrates the process of reasoning that leads to his or her diagnosis. A pathologist then presents an anatomical diagnosis, based on the study of tissue removed at surgery or obtained in autopsy. Often the students will have been asked to suggest a diagnosis based on the same information presented to the clinician. A discussion usually follows and serves to demonstrate the origin of errors present in any of the diagnoses offered.

clinical pathology, the laboratory study of disease by a pathologist using techniques appropriate to the specimen being studied. Kinds include **hematology, microbiology, immunology, toxicology.**

clinical pathway, a description of practices, usually in the form of an algorithm, likely to result in favorable outcomes for patients with a particular diagnosis that uses prospectively defined resources to minimize cost. It may be based on research, literature, or common practice. Also called **critical pathway.** See also **practice guideline.**

clinical pearl, a short, straightforward piece of clinical advice.

clinical pelvimetry, assessment of the bony pelvic portion of the birth canal by systematic pelvic and rectovaginal examination at the start of prenatal care and usually again in the first pelvic examinations in labor. Findings may be expressed in several ways: (1) clinical interpretations of adequate, borderline, or inadequate, (2) by Caldwell-Moloy type, (3) estimation of the length of the pelvic diameters associated with labor (including obstetric conjugate, interspinous diameter, transverse diameter, diagonal conjugate). Compare **x-ray pelvimetry.** See also **birth canal, cephalopelvic disproportion, dystocia.**

clinical practice guideline, systematically developed statements to assist practitioner and patient decisions about appropriate health care in specific clinical circumstances.

clinical psychology, the branch of psychology concerned with the diagnosis, treatment, and prevention of a wide range of personality and behavioral disorders, as well as mental health issues. See also **applied psychology,** def. 2.

clinical reasoning, higher order thinking in which the health care provider, guided by best evidence or theory, observes and relates concepts and phenomena to develop an understanding of their significance. See **clinical judgment.**

clinical research center, an organization, often associated with a medical school or a teaching hospital, that studies, analyzes, correlates, and describes medical cases. Such centers usually have extensive laboratory facilities and specialized staffs of physicians and medical technicians. Clinical research centers often offer free or very inexpensive medical care for patients participating in various research programs and often produce significant new medical information distributed through articles, journals, reports, seminars, and lectures. Funding for such facilities may be generated through minimal fees charged for various medical services and through grants.

clinical specialist, a health care provider who has advanced training in a particular field of practice. Many professional organizations provide certifications to assist the health care community and patients in identifying providers with advanced clinical knowledge, experience, and skills in special areas of practice within their disciplines.

clinical thermometer [Gk, *kline,* bed, *thermē,* heat, *metron,* measure], an electronic thermometer with disposable sheaths, designed for measuring body temperature. Measurement can be oral, rectal, axillary, or facial. Formerly called *bedside thermometer.*

clinical thermometry, a method for determining temperature in heated tissue.

clinical trial exemption (CTX), authorization to administer an investigational agent to patients or volunteer subjects under specified conditions of a particular research study in a clinical setting.

clinical trials, organized studies to provide large bodies of clinical data for statistically valid evaluation of treatment to determine safety and efficacy.

clinician /klinish″ən/, a health professional whose practice is based on direct observation and treatment of a patient, as distinguished from other types of health workers, such as laboratory technicians and those employed in research.

clinic without walls, a health care organization formed by the merger of selected functions, such as administrative, billing and collections, purchasing, personnel, and payroll, of various physician groups without the merger of any physical facilities.

Clinitest, reagent tablets used to test for the presence of reducing sugars, such as glucose, in the urine. The tablets contain copper sulfate, and the procedure is a modified version of Benedict's qualitative test. The tablets are rarely used in current practice.

Clinitron bed. See **fluidized air bed.**

clino-, prefix meaning "to bend or make lie down" or a "sloping shape": *clinodactyly.*

clinocephaly /klī′nōsef″əlē/ [Gk, *klinein,* to bend, *kephale,* head], a congenital anomaly of the head in which the upper surface of the skull is saddle shaped or concave. Also called *clinocephalism.* −*clinocephalic, clinocephalous, adj.*

clinodactyly /klī′nōdak″təlē/ [Gk, *klinein* + *dactylos,* finger], a congenital anomaly characterized by abnormal lateral or medial bending of one or more fingers or toes. Also called *clinodactylism.* −*clinodactylic, clinodactylous, adj.*

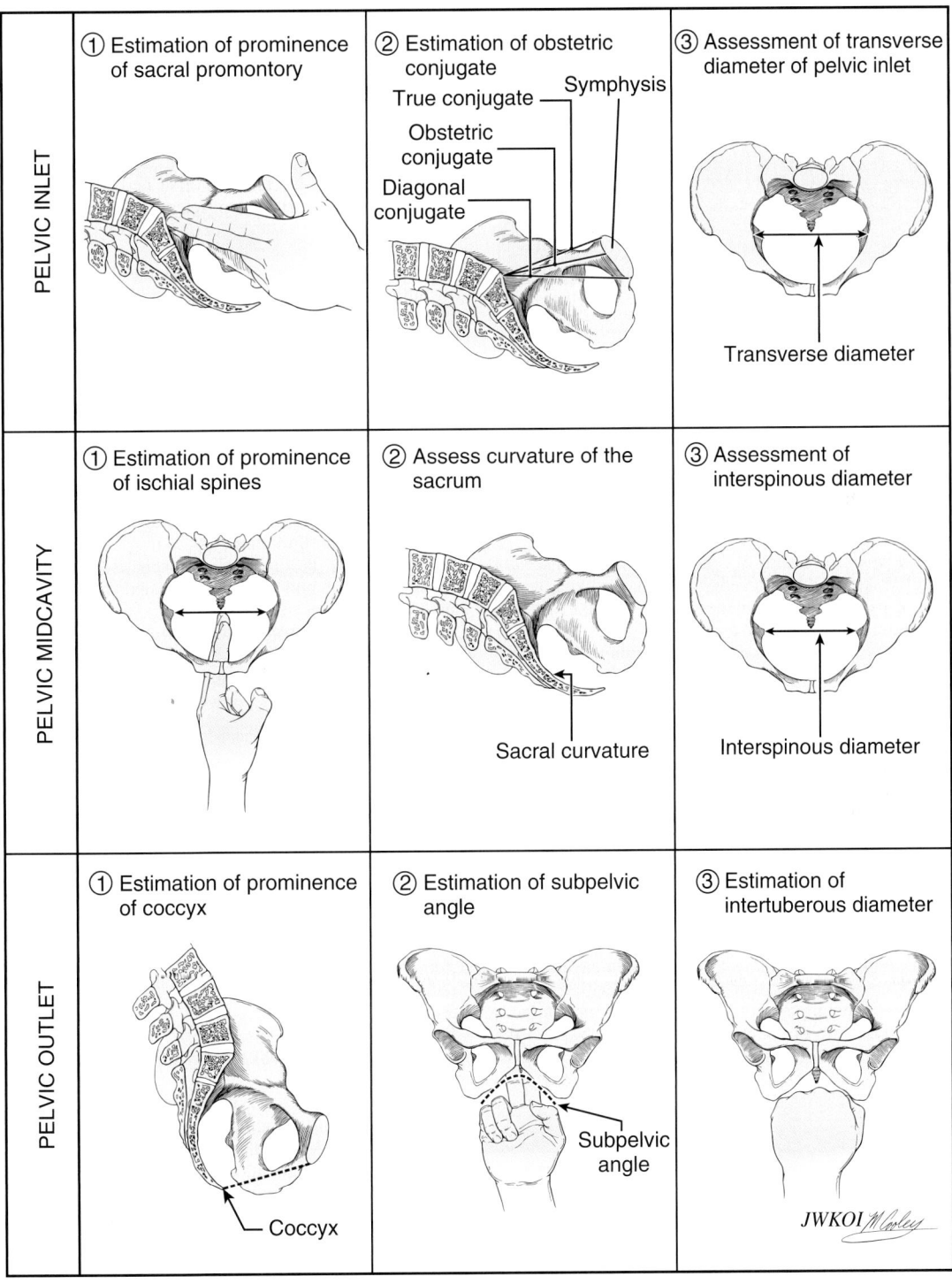

Clinical pelvimetry measurements *(Gabbe et al, 2012)*

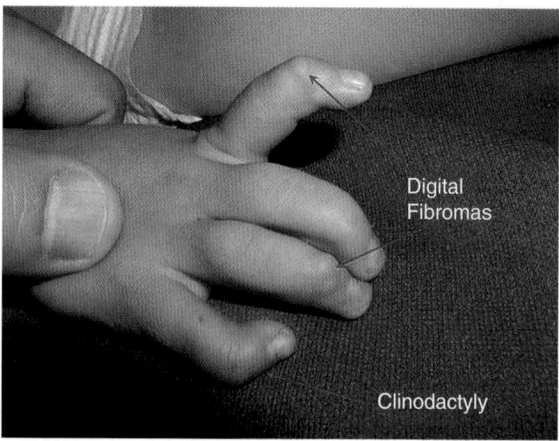

Digital Fibromas

Clinodactyly

Clinodactyly *(Izadpanah et al, 2007)*

clinoid processes /klī′noid/ [Gk, *kline*, bed, *eidos*, form; L, *processus*], the anterior, middle, and posterior processes of the sphenoid bone at the base of the skull.

clinometer /klīnom″ətər/, an instrument used to measure angular convergence of the eyes or the degree of paralysis of extraocular muscles. Also called **clinoscope.**

Clinoril, a nonsteroidal antiinflammatory drug. Brand name for **sulindac.**

clinoscope. See **clinometer.**

clip [AS, *clyppan*, to embrace], a surgical device used for grasping the skin to align the edges of a wound and to stop bleeding, especially of the smaller blood vessels. It is also used in radiography for localization.

clitoridectomy /klit′əridek″təmē/, the ancient ritual excising of all or part of the clitoris, and sometimes part of the labia, usually prior to puberty. It is a form of female genital mutilation and is considered a violation of the human rights of girls and women all over the world. The World Health Organization has repeatedly spoken out against the practice, and many nations have enacted laws criminalizing the practice. A deliberately misleading euphemism is female circumcision. See also **female genital mutilation.**

clitoridotomy, ritual removal or splitting of the clitoral hood, a form of female genital mutilation. Often inappropriately compared to male circumcision. See also **female genital mutilation.**

clitoris /klit″əris/ [Gk, *kleitoris*], the vaginal erectile structure of the female homologous to the corpora cavernosa of the penis. It consists of two corpora cavernosa within a dense layer of fibrous membrane, joined along their inner surfaces by an incomplete fibrous septum. It is situated beneath the anterior labia commissure, partially hidden between the anterior extremities of the labia minora and partly covered by a prepuce. –*clitoral, adj.*

clitoritis /klit′ôrī″tis/, inflammation of the clitoris.

clivus /klī″vəs/ [L, slope], **1.** an inclined surface. **2.** the bony surface of the posterior cranial fossa sloping upward from the foramen magnum to the dorsum sellae.

CLL, abbreviation for **chronic lymphocytic leukemia.**

cloaca /klō-ā″kə/ *pl. cloacae* [L, sewer], **1.** (in embryology) the end of the hindgut before the developmental division into the rectum, the bladder, and the primitive genital structures. **2.** (in pathology) an opening into the sheath of tissue around a necrotic bone.

cloacal fold, a slight elevation located just lateral to the cloacal membrane early in the fifth week of embryonic development. Cloacal folds later divide into urogenital folds and anal folds.

cloacal membrane /klō·ā″kəl/, a thin sheath that separates the internal and external portions of the cloaca in the developing embryo. It is formed from endoderm and ectoderm and closes the fetal anus during early prenatal development; it later ruptures and is absorbed so that the anal canal becomes continuous with the rectum. Also called **anal membrane.**

cloacal septum. See **urorectal septum.**

cloacal sphincter, the developing muscle surrounding the caudal end of the cloaca in the embryo. Its posterior part will become the external anal sphincter and its anterior part becomes the superficial transverse perineal, bulbospongiosus, and ischiocavernosus muscles.

clobetasol propionate /klōbet″əsol prō″pyōnāt/, a topical corticosteroid antiinflammatory.

■ INDICATIONS: It is prescribed for the short-term treatment of inflammation and pruritus associated with certain moderate to severe types of dermatitis.

■ CONTRAINDICATIONS: It is contraindicated for prolonged use, for applications to large areas of poor skin integrity, and with the use of occlusive dressing.

■ ADVERSE EFFECTS: Adverse reactions may include hyperglycemia, glycosuria, Cushing syndrome, and suppression of hypothalamic-pituitary-adrenal functions. Because of the greater ratio of skin surface to body weight in children, they are at risk of absorbing a greater proportion of topical steroid.

clocortolone pivalate /klōkôr″təlōn piv″əlāt/, a topical corticosteroid antiinflammatory.

■ INDICATIONS: It is prescribed for the short-term treatment of inflammation and pruritus associated with certain moderate to severe types of dermatitis.

■ CONTRAINDICATIONS: Viral and fungal diseases of the skin or local impairment of circulation prohibits its use.

■ ADVERSE EFFECTS: Among the more serious adverse reactions are systemic side effects that may result from prolonged or excessive application. Local irritation of the skin may occur.

clofibrate /klō″fəbrāt/, an antihyperlipidemic.

■ INDICATIONS: It is prescribed in the treatment of high blood levels of triglycerides occurring alone or in combination with high cholesterol levels.

■ CONTRAINDICATIONS: Liver or kidney dysfunction, pregnancy, lactation, biliary cirrhosis, or known hypersensitivity to this drug prohibits its use.

■ ADVERSE EFFECTS: Among the more serious adverse reactions are nausea, diarrhea, weight gain, and a syndrome resembling influenza. This drug interacts with many other drugs and should not be used together with the HMG-CoA reductase inhibitors (statins) used to lower plasma cholesterol levels because this combination has an increased risk for myositis and rhabdomyolysis.

Clomid, a nonsteroidal fertility drug. Brand name for **clomiPHENE citrate.**

clomiPHENE citrate /klō″məfēn/, a nonsteroidal drug that acts to stimulate ovulation by interacting with estrogen receptors in the hypothalamus in a manner that leads to the release of pituitary gonadotropins.

■ INDICATIONS: It is prescribed primarily for the treatment of anovulation and oligoovulation in women desiring pregnancy.

■ CONTRAINDICATIONS: Abnormal vaginal bleeding, liver dysfunction, or known hypersensitivity to this drug prohibits its use.

■ ADVERSE EFFECTS: Among the more serious adverse reactions are enlargement of the ovaries, hot flashes, blurred vision, gastric upset, rashes, and abdominal pain.

clomiPHENE stimulation test, a test used to evaluate gonadal function in males who show signs of abnormal pubertal development. Clomiphene, a nonsteroidal analog of estrogen, stimulates the hypothalamic-pituitary system to raise follicle-stimulating hormone and luteinizing hormone levels of the blood. Failure to respond to clomiphene indicates hypothalamic-pituitary disease, possibly a pituitary tumor. See also **clomiPHENE citrate, gonadotropin.**

clomiPRAMINE /klōmip′rämēn/, a tricyclic antidepressant of the dibenzazepine class, used in the form of the hydrochloride salt, also used as an antianxiety agent. Used in the treatment of obsessive-compulsive disorder, panic disorder, bulimia nervosa, cataplexy associated with narcolepsy, and chronic severe pain.

clonal /klō′nəl/, pertaining to a clone.

clonal marker, a defective or functionally unidentified DNA sequence in a clone of cancer cells. Such sequences are used to monitor the growth of cancer cells after chemical or other treatments.

clonal selection theory, (in immunology) a scientific model of the function of cells of the immune system in response to an antigen. Immunity to an antigen is the result of immunological memory related to the cloning of two types of lymphocytes. The first clone acts immediately to combat infection, and the second, longer-lasting clone remains in the immune system, resulting in immunity to that antigen.

clonazepam /klōnaz′′əpam/, a benzodiazepine anticonvulsant.
- ■ INDICATIONS: It is prescribed in the treatment of absence seizures in patients unresponsive to succinimides, of atonic and myotonic seizures, and of panic disorder.
- ■ CONTRAINDICATIONS: Liver disease, acute narrow-angle glaucoma, pregnancy, or known hypersensitivity to this drug or to other benzodiazepine drugs prohibits its use. It is not given during lactation. Interactions with alcohol may increase phenytoin levels. The herbs kava-kava and valerian may increase sedation.
- ■ ADVERSE EFFECTS: Among the more serious adverse reactions are thrombocytopenia, leukocytosis, eosinophilia, and respiratory depression. Abuse and addiction are serious problems and are not uncommon.

clone [Gk, *klon,* a plant cutting], a group of genetically identical cells or organisms derived from a single common cell or organism through mitosis. **–clonal,** *adj.*

-clonia, suffix meaning "(condition involving) spasms": eyelid myoclonia.

clonic /klon′ik/ [Gk, *klonos,* tumult], pertaining to increased reflex activity, as in upper motor neuron lesions when repetitive muscular contractions and relaxations in rapid succession are induced by stretching. See also **clonus.**

clonic convulsion [Gk, *klonos,* tumult; L, *convulsio,* cramp], a form of seizure characterized by rhythmic alternate involuntary contraction and relaxation of muscle groups.

clonic spasm [Gk, *klonos,* tumult, *spasmos*], involuntary alternating contractions and relaxations of muscles in rapid succession.

clonidine hydrochloride /klō′nədēn/, an alpha₂-agonist used as an antihypertensive. It stimulates alpha₂-adrenergic receptors in the brainstem to decrease sympathetic nervous system outflow. It is also administered epidurally to treat pain.
- ■ INDICATIONS: It is prescribed alone or in combination for the reduction of high blood pressure and is an adjunct for the treatment of cancer pain when pain persists during intraspinal opiate treatments. It may be used in the treatment of attention deficit hyperactivity disorder (ADHD) when a patient cannot tolerate or does not respond to stimulants or antidepressants.
- ■ CONTRAINDICATIONS: Known hypersensitivity to this drug prohibits its use.
- ■ ADVERSE EFFECTS: Among the more serious adverse reactions is a withdrawal syndrome that occurs on discontinuation of the medication characterized by tachycardia, a rapid increase in blood pressure, and anxiety. Drowsiness, sexual dysfunction, and dry mouth commonly occur.

cloning /klō′ning/, a procedure for producing multiple copies of genetically identical organisms or cells or of individual genes. Organisms may be cloned by transplanting blastocysts from one embryo into an empty zona pellucida, or nuclei from the cells of one individual into enucleated oocytes. Cells may be cloned by growing them in culture under conditions that promote cell reproduction. Genes may be cloned by isolating them from the genome of one organism and incorporating them into the genome of an asexually reproducing organism, such as a bacterium or a yeast.

clonorchiasis /klō′nôrkī′′əsis/, an infestation of the Chinese liver fluke, *Clonorchis sinensis.* It is a known risk factor for development of cholangiocarcinoma. See also *Clonorchis sinensis,* **schistosomiasis.**

Clonorchis sinensis /klōnôr′′kis sinen′′sis/, the Chinese or Oriental liver fluke, a trematode that is acquired by humans who eat raw, imperfectly cooked, pickled, salted, or smoked fish that is the intermediate host of the parasite. The fluke exists in a dormant stage as a cercaria, encysted in the skin of a fish and unable to continue its life cycle until ingested by a warm-blooded animal, in which the larvae mature and produce eggs. The eggs are excreted in the feces of the host to enter water, where the new generation evolves first in aquatic snails and then in fish. In human hosts the liver fluke lives in the bile ducts and gallbladder, causing chronic liver disease with enlargement of the liver, diarrhea, edema, and, eventually, death. Cholangitis, cholelithiasis, pancreatitis, and cholangiosarcoma are common complications and may be fatal. The adult fluke can survive in the biliary duct of its host for up to 50 years. Treatment is with praziquantel or albendazole. Also called *Opisthorchis sinensis.*

clonus (C) /klō′nəs/ [Gk, *klonos,* tumult], an abnormal pattern of neuromuscular activity, characterized by rapidly alternating involuntary contraction and relaxation of skeletal muscle. Compare **tonus. –clonic,** *adj.*

C-loop, a surgically formed loop of bowel with a C shape.

clopidogrel, a platelet aggregation inhibitor.
- ■ INDICATIONS: It is used to reduce the risk of stroke and myocardial infarction in high-risk patients.
- ■ CONTRAINDICATIONS: Known hypersensitivity, active bleeding, and increased risk for bleeding (e.g., peptic ulcers) prohibit its use.
- ■ ADVERSE EFFECTS: Intracranial hemorrhage is a potential life-threatening side effect. Other adverse effects include rash, pruritus, nausea, vomiting, diarrhea, epistaxis, purpura, edema, hypertension, chest pain, headache, dizziness, musculoskeletal pain, upper respiratory tract infection, bronchitis, urinary tract infection, and hypercholesterolemia.

Cloquet's hernia [J.G. Cloquet, German surgeon, 1790–1883], a femoral hernia. See **crural hernia.**

clor, abbreviation for *chloride anion.*

clorazepate dipotassium /klôraz′′əpāt dī-potassium/, a benzodiazepine antianxiety drug.
- ■ INDICATIONS: It is prescribed in the treatment of anxiety, nervous tension, and alcohol withdrawal.
- ■ CONTRAINDICATIONS: Psychosis, acute narrow-angle glaucoma, or known hypersensitivity to this drug prohibits its

use. Cross-addiction in alcohol withdrawal should be guarded against.

■ ADVERSE EFFECTS: Among the more serious adverse reactions are withdrawal symptoms that occur on discontinuation of treatment. Drowsiness and fatigue commonly occur. Addiction is possible.

closed amputation [L, *claudere,* to shut, *amputare,* to cut away], an amputation in which one or two broad flaps of muscular and cutaneous tissue are retained to form a cover over the end of the bone. It is performed only when no infection is present at the site of the stump. Compare **open amputation.**

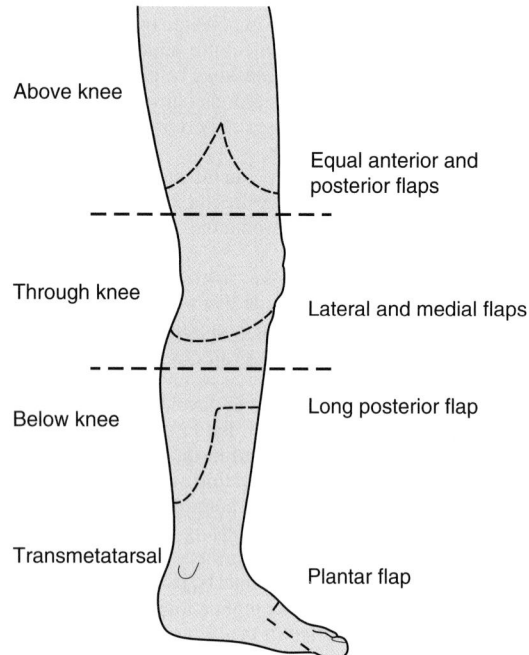

Locations for closed amputation *(Garden et al, 2012)*

closed-angle glaucoma, obstruction or damage to the trabecular network, interfering with aqueous humor drainage. See **glaucoma.**

closed bite [L, *claudere* + AS, *bitan*], an abnormal overbite; a decrease in the occlusal vertical dimension produced by various factors, such as tooth abrasion, tooth loss, and insufficient eruption of supportive posterior teeth. Compare **open bite.**

closed-cavity tympanomastoidectomy, tympanomastoidectomy with tympanoplasty and maintenance of an intact posterior wall of the ear canal.

closed-chain, (in organic chemistry) pertaining to a compound in which the carbon atoms are bonded to form a closed ring. Also called **carbocyclic.**

closed-chain exercise, *(Informal)* exercise in which the distal aspect of the extremity is in contact with a support surface such as the floor or a balance board. Also called **closed kinetic chain exercises.** Compare **open-chain exercise.**

closed-circuit breathing, rebreathing of a contained gas mixture, either directly or after recirculation of the gas through a water-absorbing or carbon dioxide–absorbing unit. An example is breathing through a spirometer.

closed-circuit helium dilution, a technique for measuring residual lung volume and functional residual capacity in which a patient breathes through a spirometer containing a known concentration of helium.

closed dislocation [L, *claudere,* to shut, *dis,* apart, *locare,* to place], a joint dislocation not accompanied by a break in the skin.

closed drainage, a system for wound care in which a small compression device is used to remove accumulated fluids and collect them in a reservoir. Accurate measurement of drainage is facilitated by use of a closed system. See **drainage.**

closed fracture [L, *claudere,* to shut, *fractura*], a fracture in which the bone does not break the skin. In otherwise healthy patients, closed fractures usually heal when treated appropriately, which may include a period of immobilization and non–weight-bearing or a surgical intervention. Compare **compound fracture.** Formerly called **simple fracture.**

closed group, (in psychotherapy) a group in which all members are admitted at the same time and vacancies that occur in the membership are not filled.

closed kinetic chain exercises, physical activity in which a portion of the body remains in contact with a floor or a board, as in push-ups or squats. Also called **closed-chain exercise.**

closed loop, a biological feedback system in which a substance produced in the body affects the mechanism that causes its own production.

closed loop obstruction, a type of small-bowel obstruction in which two areas of the bowel are obstructed at a single location, forming a closed loop.

closed-panel HMO, (in the United States) a health maintenance organization (HMO) in which physicians are either employees of the HMO or belong to a group of physicians that contracts with it. See also **health maintenance organization.**

closed physician-hospital organization (PHO), (in the United States) an organization of selected physicians on a hospital medical staff who have proved to be high-quality, cost-effective practitioners.

closed reduction of fractures [L, *claudere,* to shut, *reducere,* to lead back, *fractura*], the manual correction of the alignment, angulation, and rotation of fractures without incision.

closed system, a system that does not interact with its environment.

closed-system helium dilution method, a technique for measuring functional residual capacity and residual volume. It is based on the principle that if a known volume and concentration of helium are added to a patient's respiratory system, the helium will be diluted in proportion to the lung volume to which it is added. Helium, an inert gas, is not significantly absorbed from the lungs by the blood.

closed-wound suction, any one of several techniques for draining potentially harmful fluids, such as blood, pus, serosanguineous fluid, and tissue secretions, from surgical wounds. Such fluids interfere with wound healing and often promote infection. Postoperative drainage aids the healing process by removing dead spaces where extravascular fluids collect and helps draw healing tissues together. Closed-wound suction is often an important part of postoperative treatment and may be accomplished with a variety of reliable devices that create a gentle negative pressure to drain away undesirable exudates. The technique is used as an aid to many operations, such as mastectomies, breast augmentations, plastic and reconstructive procedures, and urological and urogenital procedures. It is generally used whenever the wound drainage is greater than 100 mL in 24 hours. Closed-wound suction devices usually consist of disposable transparent containers attached to suction tubes and portable suction pumps.

■ METHOD: After thoroughly irrigating the wound to remove blood clots and debris, the surgeon inserts the perforated tubing into the wound and draws it out through healthy tissue, approximately 5 cm from the incision line. When silicone tubing is used, the tube is passed through a stab wound made adjacent to the surgical wound. With the drainage tubing emerging away from the incision line, the suction system remains completely closed. Air cannot infiltrate the wound and cause contamination. When the suction tube has been inserted, the wound is closed, and a light dressing is applied. Because the tubing drains most fluids, the dressing usually does not require frequent changing. Closed-wound suction usually continues postoperatively for 2 or 3 days or until the wound stops exuding fluid. Suction is much longer after mastectomies. The surgeon then removes the suction tubing, and all drainage components of the suction device are discarded.

■ INTERVENTIONS: While the suction is functioning, the transparent tubing and reservoir are checked regularly as a precaution against clogging and for monitoring of the volume of exudate drawn from the wound. In some individuals, closed-wound suction systems can also accommodate antibiotic drips, which are connected to accessory tubing placed within the wound beside the suction tube. Closed-wound suction also allows irrigation of the wound with special flow controls to permit a periodic change in the flow direction of solutions.

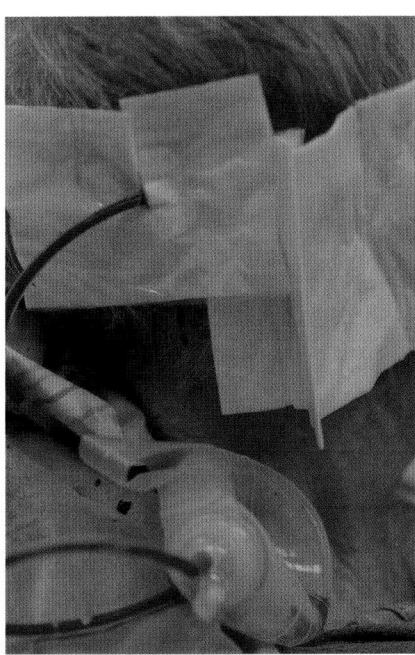

Closed-wound drainage system *(Nouri, 2008)*

closing capacity (CC), a measure of lung volume equal to the sum of closing volume and residual volume.

closing volume (CV), the volume of gas remaining in the lungs when the small airways begin to close during a controlled maximum exhalation. Closing volume normally increases with age and is also increased in obstructive airway disease.

clostridial /klostrid″ē·əl/ [Gk, *kloster,* spindle], pertaining to anaerobic spore-forming bacteria of the genus *Clostridium.*

clostridial myonecrosis. See **myonecrosis.**

clostridial toxin assay, a stool test to diagnose *Clostridium difficile* bacterial infection of the intestine.

Clostridium /-ē·əm/ [Gk, *kloster,* spindle], a genus of spore-forming anaerobic bacteria of the Bacillaceae family. *Clostridium novyi, C. septicum,* and *C. bifermentans* are involved in gas gangrene. *C. botulinum* causes botulism and produces the toxin used in the drug Botox for some cosmetic procedures. *C. perfringens* causes food poisoning, cellulitis, and wound infections. *C. tetani* is the cause of tetanus. *C. difficile* can cause a range of symptoms affecting the gastrointestinal tract, ranging from diarrhea to life-threatening inflammation.

Clostridium botulinum [Gk, *kloster,* spindle], a species of anaerobic bacteria that causes botulism in humans and botulism-like diseases in other animals. Botulinus food poisoning results from ingesting food containing preformed toxins produced by the species. It is a proteolytic pathogen commonly present in soil, where its endospores can survive for years. Their resistance to heat makes them an important source of poisoning in improperly cooked or canned foods.

Clostridium difficile /difis″ilē/, a common inhabitant of the colon flora in human infants and sometimes in adults. It produces a toxin that causes pseudomembranous enterocolitis in persons receiving antibiotic therapy, causing watery diarrhea. It is highly infectious and can affect all ages. Also called *C. difficile, C. diff.*

Clostridium perfringens [Gk, *kloster,* spindle], a species of anaerobic gram-positive bacteria capable of causing gas gangrene and food poisoning in humans and various digestive and urinary tract diseases in livestock. The oval spores of the bacteria are found in the soil and in the intestinal tracts of humans and animals. It is the third most common form of food poisoning in the United States, Canada, and the United Kingdom. Incubation time is 6 to 24 hours, usually 10 to 12 hours. Symptoms include abdominal cramps and diarrhea. Vomiting is rare. Also called *Clostridium welchii.* See also **gas gangrene.**

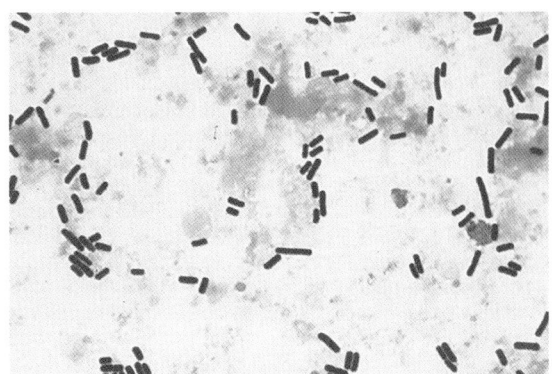

Clostridium perfringens *(Kumar et al, 2010)*

closure /klō″zhər/ [L, *claudere,* to shut], **1.** the surgical closing of a wound by suture or staple. **2.** a visual phenomenon in which the mind sees an entire figure when only a portion is actually visible. See also **flask closure. 3.** the ending of something, as in closure of the grieving process.

closylate /klos″ilāt/, USAN-approved contraction for *p*-chlorobenzenesulfonate.

clot, a semisolid mass, as of blood or lymph. See **blood clot.**

clothes lice. See *Pediculus humanus corporis.*

clot retraction, the shrinking of a semisolid mass formed by the coagulation of blood, lymph, or other fluid. A normal standing blood clot is completely retracted in about 24 hours, although the time depends on such factors as the number of platelets in the clot.

clot retraction test, *(Obsolete)* a blood test used to evaluate bleeding disorders. It measured the time required for blood in a test tube to form a clot and for the clot's edges to retract from the sides of the glass tube. This test is no longer used in most laboratories.

clotrimazole /klōtrim″əzōl/, a broad-spectrum antifungal agent of the imidazole group used in topical applications to treat fungal and yeast infections, including tinea pedis, tinea corporis, tinea versicolor, oral candidiasis, and vaginal candidiasis.

■ INDICATIONS: It is prescribed in the treatment of superficial fungal infections and candidal vulvovaginitis. Oral troches are used for prophylaxis against fungal infections in neutropenic patients.

■ CONTRAINDICATIONS: Known hypersensitivity to this drug prohibits its use. It is not prescribed for ophthalmic use; contact with eyes should be avoided.

■ ADVERSE EFFECTS: The most serious adverse reactions are severe hypersensitivity reactions of the skin. The use of oral troches often causes liver enzyme abnormalities.

clotting, the formation of a jellylike substance over the ends or within the walls of a blood vessel. See **blood clotting.**

clotting time [AS, *clott*], *(Obsolete)* the time required for blood to form a clot, tested by collecting a small sample of blood in a glass tube and examining it for clot formation. The first appearance of a clot is noted and timed. The normal coagulation time in glass tubes is 5 to 15 minutes. This simple test has been used to diagnose hemophilia, but it does not detect mild coagulation disorders. It is rarely used in clinical practice. Also called **prothrombin time.** Compare **bleeding time.**

cloud baby [AS, *clud + babe*], *(Obsolete)* a term of historic interest used to describe the spread of infections by a newborn who appears well and healthy but is a carrier of infectious organisms.

clouded sensorium. See **clouding of consciousness.**

clouding of consciousness, a mental state in which a patient is confused about or is not fully aware of the immediate surroundings. Also called **clouded sensorium.**

cloudy swelling. *(Informal)* See **granular degeneration.**

clove /klōv/ [L, *clavus,* nail], the dried flower bud of *Eugenia caryophyllata.* It contains the lactone caryophyllin and a volatile oil used as a dental analgesic, a germicide, and a salve. Clove is also used as a spice and a carminative against nausea, vomiting, and flatulence.

clove-hitch sling, a bandage that begins with a clove-hitch knot at the center. The loop made is fitted to the hand. The two loose ends are extended over and behind the shoulders and tied beside the neck. Longer ends may be drawn down the back of the shoulders and under each axilla to be tied over the chest. It provides support for an injured upper extremity.

cloverleaf nail /klō″vərlēf′/ [AS, *clafre + leaf + nagel*], a surgical nail shaped in cross section like a cloverleaf, used for internal fixation procedures.

cloverleaf skull deformity, a congenital defect characterized by a trilobed skull, resulting from the premature closure of multiple cranial sutures during embryonic development. The condition is associated with hydrocephalus, facial anomalies, and skeletal deformities.

cloxacillin sodium /klok′səsil″in/, a penicillinase-resistant penicillin used for bacterial infections.

■ INDICATIONS: It is prescribed in the treatment of serious bacterial infections, primarily those caused by penicillinase-producing strains of staphylococci.

■ CONTRAINDICATIONS: Known hypersensitivity to this drug or to any penicillin prohibits its use.

■ ADVERSE EFFECTS: Among the more serious adverse reactions are GI discomfort, rash, and hypersensitivity.

CLS/MT, an allied health professional usually with a bachelor's degree in clinical and/or biological science, working in hospitals and clinic-type settings, and educated to independently perform test procedures and complex analyses. Abbreviation for **clinical laboratory scientist/medical technologist.**

CLT/MLT, an allied health professional, with or without a degree in clinical and/or biological science, working in hospitals and clinic-type settings, performing test procedures unique to chemical, microscopic, and bacterial examination. May work supervised and/or unsupervised, depending on education, training, and degree. Abbreviation for **clinical laboratory technician/medical laboratory technician—associate degree, clinical laboratory technician/medical laboratory technician—certificate.**

clubbing [ME, *clubbe*], an abnormal enlargement of the distal phalanges with a flattening of the curvature of the nail margin at the cuticle, where the nail meets the cuticle. It usually is associated with cyanotic heart disease or advanced chronic pulmonary disease but sometimes occurs with biliary cirrhosis, colitis, chronic dysentery, thyrotoxicosis, and sickle cell anemia. Clubbing occurs in all the digits but is most easily seen in the fingers. Advanced clubbing is obvious, but early clubbing may be difficult to diagnose. Clubbing is present if the transverse diameter of the base of the fingernail is greater than the transverse diameter of the most distal joint of the digit. The nail base angle measures more than 160 degrees. See also **Schamroth window test.**

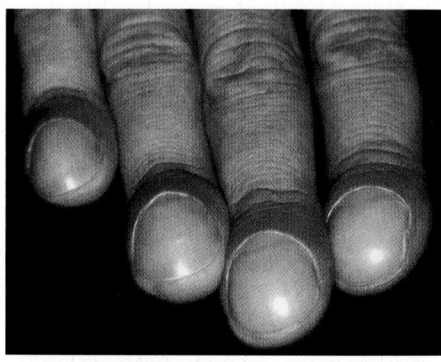

Clubbing *(Thiers, 2006)*

clubfoot [ME, *clubbe* + AS, *fot*], a congenital deformity of the foot, sometimes resulting from intrauterine constriction and characterized by unilateral or bilateral deviation of the metatarsal bones of the forefoot. Ninety-five percent of clubfoot deformities are equinovarus, characterized by medial deviation and plantar flexion of the forefoot, but a few are calcaneovalgus, or calcaneovarus, characterized by lateral deviation and dorsiflexion either outward from or inward toward the midline of the body. Treatment depends on the extent and rigidity of the deformity. Splints and casts in infancy may produce complete correction. Surgery in several steps may be necessary to achieve normal function. See also **Denis Browne splint, talipes.**

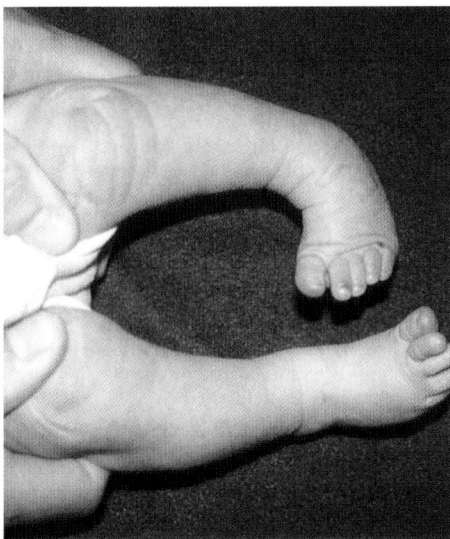

Clubfoot (James et al, 2013)

club hair, a hair in the resting, or final, stage of the growth cycle, before shedding, the bulb of which become a club-shaped mass. See also **hair.**

cluster analysis [AS, *clyster,* growing together; Gk, *analyein,* to loosen], (in statistics) a complex technique of data analysis of numeric scale scores that produces clusters of variables related to one another. The technique is performed with computer software or statistics programs.

cluster breathing, a breathing pattern in which a closely grouped series of respirations is followed by apnea. The activity is associated with a lesion in the lower pontine region of the brainstem. See also **Biot respiration, Cheyne-Stokes respiration.**

cluster headache, a condition characterized by attacks of intense unilateral pain, occurring most often over the eye and forehead. It is accompanied by flushing and watering of the eyes and nose. Cluster headaches are more common in males, occur in cycles, and are exacerbated with alcohol use. The attacks occur in groups with a duration of several hours. See also **histamine headache.**

clusterin /klus′terin/, a multifunctional glycoprotein with roles in the metabolism and transport of lipids and membrane fragments, secretion of hormones, reproductive biology, inhibition of assembly of the membrane attack complex of complement activation, programmed cell death, and modulation of intercell interactions. Its expression is enhanced in tissue injury and remodeling, and in degenerative diseases such as Alzheimer disease.

cluster-of-differentiation (CD) antigen, one of a group of cell-surface molecules that are used to classify leukocytes into subsets. Kinds include **CD4 cell, CD4+ cell, CD8 cell.**

cluttering [ME, *clotter*], a speech disorder of dysfluency characterized by a rapid delivery with uneven rhythmic patterns and omission or transposition of various speech sounds or syllables. The condition is commonly associated with other learning disabilities, such as difficulty in learning to speak, read, and spell.

clysis /klī′sis/ [Gk, *klyster,* washout], the nonoral insertion or injection of a fluid into tissue spaces, the rectum, or the abdominal cavity, such as the administration of an enema. It is used when IV access is not possible.

cm, abbreviation for **centimeter.**

Cm, symbol for the element **curium.**

cm², abbreviation for **square centimeter.**

cm³, abbreviation for **cubic centimeter.**

CMA, 1. abbreviation for Canadian Medical Association. **2.** abbreviation for **certified medical assistant.**

CMAJ, abbreviation for **Canadian Medical Association Journal.**

CMC, abbreviation for *carpometacarpal.* See **carpometacarpal (CMC) joint.**

CMF, an anticancer drug combination of cyclophosphamide, methotrexate, and fluorouracil.

CMHC, abbreviation for **community mental health center.**

CMI, abbreviation for **computer-managed instruction.**

CML, abbreviation for **chronic myelogenous leukemia.**

cmm, abbreviation for **cubic millimeter.**

CMRNG, abbreviation for *chromosomally mediated resistant Neisseria gonorrhoeae.*

CMS, abbreviation for **Centers for Medicare and Medicaid Services.** Formerly called **Health Care Financing Administration.**

CMT, abbreviation for **certified medical transcriptionist.** See **medical transcriptionist.**

CMV, abbreviation for *cytomegalovirus.*

CN, abbreviation for **chloroacetophenone.**

CNA, 1. abbreviation for **Canadian Nurses Association. 2.** abbreviation for certified nursing assistant. See also **nursing assistant.**

CNATS, abbreviation for *Canadian Nurses Association Testing Service.*

CNF, abbreviation for **Canadian Nurses Foundation.**

CNHV, abbreviation for **central neurogenic hyperventilation.**

Cnidaria, a phylum of invertebrate animals that includes jellyfish, sea anemones, hydroids, and corals. Formerly called **Coelenterata.**

CNM, abbreviation for **certified nurse-midwife.**

CNNT, abbreviation for **Council of Nephrology Nurses and Technicians.**

CNOR, a certification as a perioperative nurse, validating professional achievement of standards of practice by a registered nurse providing care for patients before, during, and after surgery.

CNRN, abbreviation for *certified neuroscience registered nurse.*

CNS, 1. abbreviation for **central nervous system. 2.** abbreviation for **clinical nurse specialist.**

CNSC, abbreviation for *certified nutrition support clinician.*

CNS sympathomimetic, a drug, such as cocaine or an amphetamine, whose effects mimic those of sympathomimetic nervous system stimulation.

Co, symbol for the element **cobalt.**

CO, 1. chemical formula for **carbon monoxide. 2.** abbreviation for **cardiac output.**

co-, col-, com-, con-, cor-, prefix meaning "together, with": *coagulate, coarctate.*

co-sleeping, the practice of sleeping in the same room with an infant or child. Compare **bed sharing.**

CO₂, chemical formula for **carbon dioxide.**

CoA, abbreviation for **coenzyme A.**

coaching, (in health care) interventions designed by a health care professional, in collaboration with individual patients, to assist in the successful self-management of patients' health and illness-related conditions and the achievement of optimal outcomes.

coaching model, (in occupational therapy) a framework used to enable occupational change and foster optimal health and well-being. In the coaching model occupational performance is the dynamic interaction of person, occupation, and environment. Coaching enables by beginning at the level of the person (affective, cognitive, spiritual). As a result of the client's action-reflection-learning cycle throughout the coaching process, changes can occur at all three levels (person/occupation/environment).

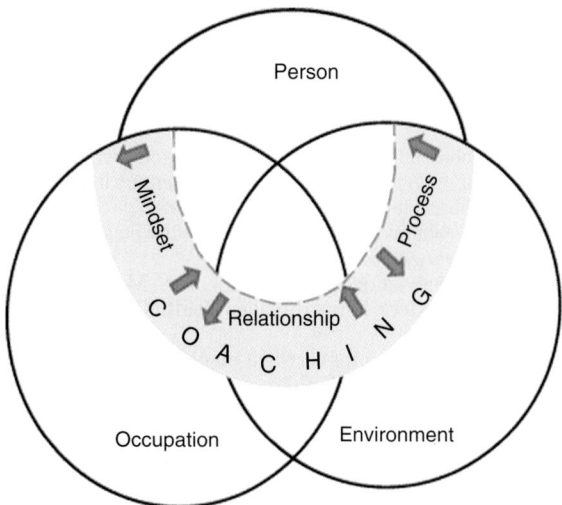

Coaching model *(Courtesy of Dr. Wendy Pentland)*

coagglutination /kō′əgloo′tənā″shən/ [L, *cum* + *agglutinare*, to glue], a clumping of red blood cells by mixtures of protein antigens and their antisera.

coagulability /kō·ag′yələbil″itē/ [L, *coagulare*, to curdle], the state of being able to coagulate or form blood clots.

coagulant /kō·ag″yələnt/ [L, *coagulare*, to curdle], an agent that causes a coagulum, or blood clot, to form.

coagulase /kō·ag″yəlās/ [L, *coagulare,* to curdle], an enzyme produced by bacteria, particularly *Staphylococcus aureus,* that promotes the formation of fibrin from fibrinogen to form thrombi.

coagulate /kō·ag″yəlāt/, to undergo or cause to undergo the chemical process whereby a fluid becomes curdled or clotted. –**coagulated,** *adj.*

coagulated /kō·ag″yəlā′tid/, curdled; changed to a clotted state.

coagulation /kō·ag′yəlā″shən/ [L, *coagulare,* to curdle], **1.** the process of transforming a liquid into a solid, especially of the blood. See also **blood clotting. 2.** (in colloid chemistry) the transforming of the liquid dispersion medium into a gelatinous mass. **3.** the hardening of tissue by some physical means, as by electrocoagulation or photocoagulation. –*coagulable, adj.*

coagulation cascade, the series of steps beginning with activation of the intrinsic or extrinsic pathways of coagulation and proceeding through the common pathway of coagulation to the formation of the fibrin clot. Each step involves activation of a proenzyme (zymogen), the activated form catalyzing activation of the following step. See also **common pathway of coagulation, extrinsic pathway of coagulation, intrinsic pathway of coagulation.**

coagulation current, an electric current delivered by a needle ball or variously shaped points to bind tissues together. See also **electrocautery, electrocoagulation.**

coagulation factor, plasma proteins in the coagulation system that circulate as inactive zymogens or cofactors. When activated by tissue damage, they form complexes that ultimately produce thrombin, an enzyme that cleaves fibrinogen to produce a fibrin clot and stops the bleeding. See also **blood clotting, coagulation, fibrinogen, hemophilia A, hemophilia B, hemophilia C.**

coagulation factor IX (human), a purified, sterile, dried concentrate of factor IX derived from pooled human plasma, used in the prophylaxis and treatment of bleeding in patients with hemophilia B, administered intravenously.

coagulation factor IX (recombinant), a sterile, dried concentrate of factor IX prepared by recombinant means, used in the prophylaxis and treatment of bleeding in patients with hemophilia B, administered intravenously.

coagulation factors concentration test, a set of blood tests used to measure the quantity of a number of specific factors suspected to be responsible for defects in hemostasis and to help the clinician determine the appropriate treatment. Deficiencies of these factors may result from inherited genetic defects, acquired diseases, or drug therapy.

coagulation factor VIIa, recombinant, an antihemophilic.

■ INDICATIONS: This drug is prescribed to prevent the bleeding associated with hemophilia A or B when inhibitors to Factor VIII or IX are present.

■ CONTRAINDICATIONS: Factors that prohibit its use include known hypersensitivity to this product or to mouse-, hamster-, or bovine-derived products.

■ ADVERSE EFFECTS: Life-threatening side effects include hemorrhage, hemarthrosis, decreased fibrinogen plasma, diffuse intravascular coagulation, coagulation disorder, and thrombosis. Other adverse effects include fever, headache, hypertension, bradycardia, pain, redness at the injection site, pruritus, purpura, and rash.

coagulation necrosis, necrosis in which tissue becomes a dry, opaque, eosinophilic mass containing outlines of anucleated cells. It results from the denaturation of proteins following hypoxic injury, such as that caused by ischemia in infarction. Also called **avascular necrosis, ischemic necrosis.**

coagulation pathways, processes by which blood changes from a liquidlike substance to a gel-like substance. See **common pathway of coagulation, extrinsic pathway of coagulation, intrinsic pathway of coagulation.**

coagulation time. See **clotting time.**

coagulative /kō·ag″yəlā′tiv/, **1.** *adj.,* causing blood clot formation. **2.** *n.,* an agent that assists in the formation of blood clots.

coagulopathy /kō·ag′yəlop″əthē/, a pathological condition that reduces the ability of the blood to coagulate, resulting in uncontrolled bleeding.

coalesce /kō·əles″/ [L, *coalescere,* to grow together], **1.** to grow together. **2.** to unite.

coal tar, a topical drug for treating eczema.

■ INDICATIONS: It is prescribed in the treatment of chronic skin conditions, such as dandruff, seborrheal dermatitis, and psoriasis.

■ CONTRAINDICATIONS: Known hypersensitivity to this drug prohibits its use.

■ ADVERSE EFFECTS: Among the most serious adverse effects are skin irritation and local hypersensitivity reactions.

coal tar creosote, creosote obtained by high temperature carbonization of bituminous coal. It is a brown-to-black, oily liquid, a mixture of aromatic hydrocarbons, tar acids, and tar bases, mainly used as a wood preservative. It is toxic to humans and other animals by contact, ingestion, or inhalation, and coal tar is a human carcinogen.

coal worker's pneumoconiosis. See **anthracosis.**

Coanda effect, a phenomenon of fluid movement similar to the Bernoulli effect in which passage of a stream of gas next to a wall results in a pocket of turbulence between the wall and the gas flow. The turbulence forms a low-pressure bubble that makes the gas stream adhere to the wall. The principle is used in fluidic ventilators.

coaptation splint /kō′aptā″shən/ [L, *coaptare,* to fit together; ME *splinte*], a small splint fitted to a fractured limb to prevent overriding of the fragments of bone during adjustment of the fracture. A longer splint usually covers the small one to provide more support and fixation of the entire limb. It is commonly used for fractures of the humeral shaft.

coarct /kō·ärkt″/ [L, *coarctare,* to press together], the act of narrowing or constricting, especially the lumen of a blood vessel.

coarctate retina /kō·ärk″tāt/ [L, *coarctare,* to press together, *rete,* net], a funnel-shaped retina caused by a leakage of fluid between the retina and the choroid.

coarctation /kō′ärktā″shən/, a compression, shriveling, or stricture of the walls of a vessel, such as the aorta.

coarctation of the aorta, a congenital cardiac anomaly characterized by a localized narrowing of the aorta. It results in increased pressure proximal to the defect and decreased pressure distal to it. The most common site of coarctation is just beyond the origin of the left subclavian artery from the aorta, resulting in high blood pressure in the upper extremities and head and low blood pressure in the lower extremities.
■ OBSERVATIONS: Symptoms are directly related to the pressure changes created by the constriction. Clinical manifestations include dizziness, headaches, fainting, epistaxis, reduced or absent femoral pulses, and muscle cramps in the legs from tissue anoxia during increased exercise. Diagnosis is based on characteristic pressure changes in the upper and lower body and specific radiological and echocardiographic findings, including notching of the lower ribs, left ventricular hypertrophy, and dilation of the aorta proximal to the stricture. A murmur may or may not be present.
■ INTERVENTIONS: Surgical repair is recommended for minor defects because of the high incidence of untreated complications, including aortic rupture, hypertension, infective endocarditis, subarachnoid hemorrhage, and congestive heart failure.
■ PATIENT CARE CONSIDERATIONS: Early detection and treatment usually lead to a successful outcome. The health care team should recognize that careful follow-up is necessary.

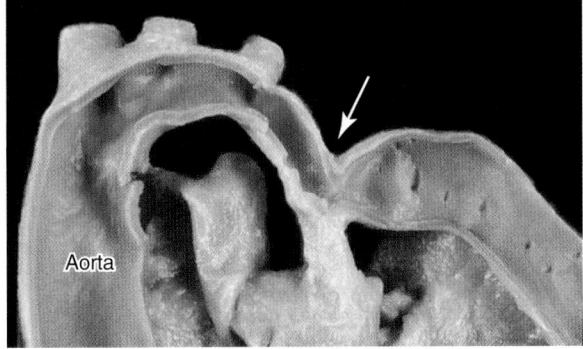

Coarctation of the aorta *(Damjanov and Linder, 2000)*

coarse /kôrs/ [ME, *cors,* common], (in physiology) involving a wide range of movements, such as those associated with tremors and other involuntary motions of the skeletal muscle.

coarse crackle [ME, *cors,* common, *krakelen*], an abnormal inspiratory breathing sound caused by air moving through an excessive amount of fluid in an airway, as in pulmonary edema.

coarse fremitus, a rough, loud, tremulous vibration of the chest wall noted on palpation of the chest during a physical examination as the person inhales and exhales. It is most common in pulmonary conditions characterized by consolidation. See also **fremitus.**

coarse tremor [ME, *cors,* common; L, *tremor,* shaking], a tremor in which the movements are relatively slow and may involve larger muscle groups.

coat [ME, *cote*], **1.** a membrane that covers the outside of an organ or part. **2.** one of the layers of a wall of an organ or part, especially a canal or a vessel.

coated tablet [ME, *cote* + Fr, *tablette*], a solid disc of one or more pharmaceutic agents that is (1) coated with sugar or a flavoring to mask the taste or (2) enteric-coated, meaning that it is coated with a substance that resists dissolution in the stomach but allows release of the medication in the intestine.

coated tongue [ME, *cote* + AS, *tunge*], a tongue with a white, yellow, or brown furred-appearing surface, representing a possible accumulation of mycelia, bacteria, food debris, or desquamated epithelial cells. There are many possible causes, ranging from a fungal infection, mouth breathing, dehydration, medications, certain foods, alcohol use, smoking, or fever. Also called **furred tongue.**

Coats disease, Coats retinitis. See **exudative retinopathy.**

cobalamin /kōbôl″əmin/ [Ger, *kobold,* mine goblin], a generic term for a chemical portion of the vitamin B_{12} molecule. See also **cyanocobalamin.**

cobalt (Co) /kō″bôlt/ [Ger, *kobold,* mine goblin], a metallic element that occurs in the minerals cobaltite, smaltite, and linnaeite. Its atomic number is 27. Its atomic mass is 58.93. Extensive deposits of cobalt minerals are found in Ontario, Canada. Pure cobalt is obtained by reducing the oxide with aluminum or carbon. It is used in special alloys, such as Alnico. Cobalt is a component of vitamin B_{12}, is found in most common foods, and is readily absorbed by the GI tract. This element is common in the human diet, but the precise daily intake requirement is not known, and cobalt deficiency in humans has not been seen. Cobaltous chloride has been given to some patients with certain types of anemia because of cobalt's capacity to produce polycythemia. Accidental intoxication by cobaltous chloride, especially by children, may produce cyanosis, coma, and death. Some amounts of cobalt stimulate the production of erythropoietin, by a process not yet understood, but large doses depress erythrocyte production. The only disease for which the use of cobalt is still advocated is normochromic, normocytic anemia associated with renal failure. The radioisotope ^{60}Co or cobalt-60 emits gamma rays and is often used as an encapsulated radiation source in the treatment of cancer.

cobalt-60 (^{60}Co), a radioactive isotope of the element cobalt with a mass of 60 and a half-life of 5.2 years. ^{60}Co emits high-energy gamma rays and is the most frequently used radioisotope in radiotherapy.

cobalt lung. See **hard metal disease.**

cobalt poisoning, poisoning from long-term excessive exposure to cobalt, seen in those who work with it. It was formerly seen in beer drinkers because cobalt was added to beer as a foam stabilizer. Symptoms include nausea, vomiting, tinnitus, nerve deafness, and cardiomyopathy.

Coban, a brand name for an elastic pressure wrap applied to reduce edema. It adheres to itself and may be used as a secondary dressing for patients allergic to tape. See also **cohesive bandage.**

Cobb collar, congenital stenosis of the bulbar urethra.

COBOL /kō″bol/, a high-level compiler computer language for programming, now used primarily to maintain legacy systems. Abbreviation for *common business oriented language.*

cobra /kō′brä/, any of numerous extremely poisonous elapid snakes commonly found in Africa, Asia, and India. They are capable of expanding the neck region to form a hood and have two comparatively short, erect, deep grooved fangs. A serum obtained from animals inoculated with cobra venom is used in counteracting the effects of the venom. Species include the Asian cobra and king cobra of Asia and the Egyptian cobra found throughout Africa and the Arabian peninsula. See also **snakebite.**

COBRA /kō′brə/, benefits that give a qualified worker the right to choose the right to continue group health benefits for limited periods of time at a cost available to other members in the group. Abbreviation for **Consolidated Omnibus Budget Reconciliation Act.**

Cobra head deformity, the appearance of a ureterocele in excretory urography, with the distal ureter slightly dilated and projecting into the bladder and an area of lesser density visible around it.

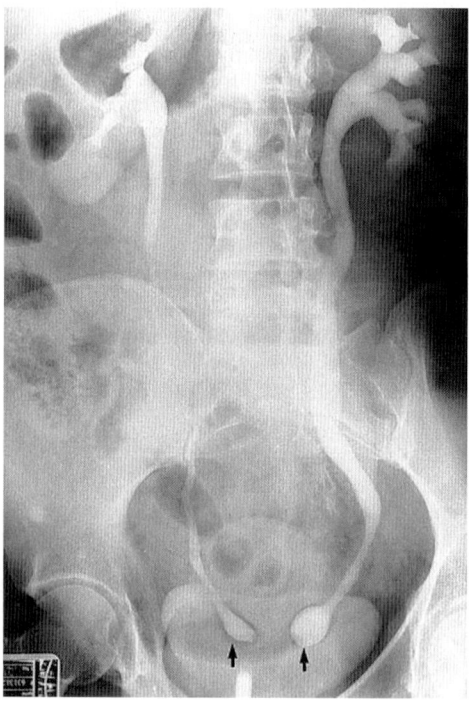

Cobra head deformity *(Mettler, 2014)*

cobra venom solution [L, *colubra,* snake, *venenum,* venom, *solutus,* dissolved], a sterile physiological salt solution containing minute amounts of cobralysin, the hemolytic substance in cobra venom.

coca, a species of South American shrubs native to Bolivia and Peru and cultivated in Indonesia. The leaves are dried and then chewed for their stimulant effect by some of the people of the region. It is a natural source of cocaine.

cocaine baby /kōkān″/, *(Slang)* a term for an infant with prenatal cocaine exposure. Now called **infant of chemically dependent mother.** See also **neonatal abstinence syndrome, prenatal cocaine exposure.**

cocaine hydrochloride, a white crystalline powder used as a local anesthetic. It was originally derived from coca leaves but can also be prepared synthetically. Cocaine is a Schedule I drug under the Controlled Substances Act of 1970. Cocaine hydrochloride solution should be freshly made; it deteriorates rapidly on standing and cannot be heat-sterilized.

■ INDICATIONS: Can be used to treat prolonged epistaxis in a 4% topical solution. It is sometimes used topically for its anesthetic properties. Cocaine use should be limited. It is highly addictive.

■ CONTRAINDICATIONS: It is incompatible with all alkaloid precipitants, mercurials, and silver nitrate. Central nervous system overstimulation may result from use with monoamine oxidase inhibitors, amphetamines, or guanethidine. Combination with epinephrine or norepinephrine can lead to cardiac arrhythmias or ventricular fibrillation. Persons with severe cardiovascular disease, thyrotoxicosis, hypotension, or hypertension should not take this drug.

■ ADVERSE EFFECTS: Among the most serious adverse effects are excitement, depression, euphoria, restlessness, tremors, vertigo, nausea, vomiting, hypotension, hypertension, abdominal cramps, exophthalmia, mydriasis, peripheral vascular collapse, tachypnea, tachycardia, chills, fever, coma, and death from respiratory failure.

cocaine hydrochloride poisoning [Sp, *coca* + *HCl* + L, *potio,* drink], toxic effects of exposure to the colorless crystalline alkaloid derived from coca leaves. Although used as a local analgesic for a century, cocaine is highly toxic with moderate vasoconstrictor activity and serious psychotropic effects. Symptoms include nervous excitement, restlessness, incoherent speech, fever, hypertension, stroke, and cardiac arrhythmias, leading to convulsions, collapse, respiratory arrest, and death. The euphoric effect of cocaine lasts about 30 minutes. A crystalline form of cocaine with the street names *crack* and *rock* is smoked.

cocarcinogen /kōkär″sənəjən/ [L, *cum,* together with; Gk, *karkinos,* crab, *genein,* to produce], an agent that alone does not transform a normal cell into a cancerous state but in concert with another agent can effect the transformation.

coccal. See **coccus.**

cocci-, cocco-, prefix meaning "seed, berry" or "spherical bacterial cell": *coccoid.*

Coccidia, a subclass of parasitic protozoa found in humans, other vertebrates, and some invertebrates. Among the species of coccidians pathogenic to humans is *Cyclospora cayetanensis.*

coccidian, **1.** *adj.,* pertaining to Coccidia. **2.** *n.,* a protozoan in the subclass Coccidia.

Coccidioides /kok·sid′ē·oi′dēz/, a pathogenic dimorphic genus of Fungi Imperfecti of the form-class Euascomycetes, form-family Onygenacaea. In soil it grows as a mycelium with infectious units called arthrospores; in tissue as a spherule with endospores. *C. immitis* causes coccidioidomycosis and fungal pneumonia.

coccidioidomycosis /koksid′ē·oi′dōmīkō″sis/ [Gk, *kokkos,* berry, *eidos,* form, *mykes,* fungus, *osis,* condition], an infectious fungal disease caused by the inhalation of spores of the protozoon *Coccidioides immitis* or *C. posadasii,* which is carried on windborne dust particles. The disease is endemic in hot, dry regions of the southwestern United States and Central and South America and is an opportunistic disease associated with human immunodeficiency virus infection and leukemia. Primary infection is characterized by symptoms resembling those of the common cold or pulmonary infection. Secondary infection, occurring after a period of remission and lasting from weeks to years, is marked by low-grade fever, anorexia and weight loss, cyanosis, dyspnea, hemoptysis, focal skin lesions resembling erythema nodosum, and arthritic pain in the bones and joints. The diagnosis is made by finding that the patient has been living in or visiting an endemic area and by identifying *C. immitis* in sputum, exudate, or tissue. Treatment usually consists of bed rest and the administration of antifungal agents, such as amphotericin B or fluconazole. Also called **desert fever, desert rheumatism, San Joaquin fever, valley fever.**

coccidiosis /kok′sidē·ō″sis/ [Gk, *kokkos* + *osis,* condition], a parasitic disease of tropical and subtropical regions caused by the ingestion of oocysts of the protozoon *Isospora belli* or *I. hominis.* Symptoms include fever, malaise, abdominal discomfort, and watery diarrhea. The infection is usually self-limited, lasting 1 to 2 weeks, but occasionally it persists, resulting in malabsorption syndrome and, rarely, death. No specific therapy has been found. Compare **coccidioidomycosis.**

cocco-. See **cocci-, cocco-.**

coccoid /kok″oid/ [Gk, *kokkos,* berry, *eidos,* form], having a spherical shape; resembling a micrococcus.

coccus /kok″əs/ *pl. cocci* [Gk, *kokkos,* berry], a bacterium that is round, spheric, or oval, such as gonococcus, pneumococcus, staphylococcus, and streptococcus. **–coccal,** *adj.*

-coccus, suffix meaning a "berry-shaped organism": *enterococcus, pneumococcus.*

coccyalgia /kok′si·al″jə/, a pain in or near the coccyx.

coccyg-, coccygo-, prefix meaning "coccyx": *coccygeal, coccygodynia.*

coccygeal. See **coccyx.**

coccygeal body. See **coccyx.**

coccygeal vertebra, one of the four segments of the vertebral column that fuse to form the adult coccyx. They are considered rudimentary vertebrae and have no pedicles, laminae, or spinous processes. Compare **cervical vertebra, lumbar vertebra, sacral vertebra, thoracic vertebra.** See also **coccyx, vertebra.**

coccygeus /koksij″ē·əs/ [Gk, *kokkyx,* cuckoo's beak], one of two muscles in the pelvic diaphragm. Stretching across the pelvic cavity like a hammock, it is a triangular sheet of muscle and tendinous fibers. It acts to draw the coccyx ventrally, helping to support the pelvic floor. Compare **levator ani.**

coccygodynia /kok′sigōdin″ē·ə/, pain or discomfort in the coccygeal area. Also called **coccyalgia,** *coccydynia.*

coccyx /kok″siks/ *pl. coccyges* [Gk, *kokkyx,* cuckoo's beak], the beaklike bone joined to the sacrum by a disk of fibrocartilage at the base of the vertebral column. It is formed by the union of three to five probably vestigial rudimentary

vertebrae. The pieces of the coccyx fuse together in males at an earlier period in life than in females. In both the coccyx becomes fused with the sacrum by the sixth decade of life. The coccyx is freely movable on the sacrum during pregnancy. **–coccygeal,** *adj.*

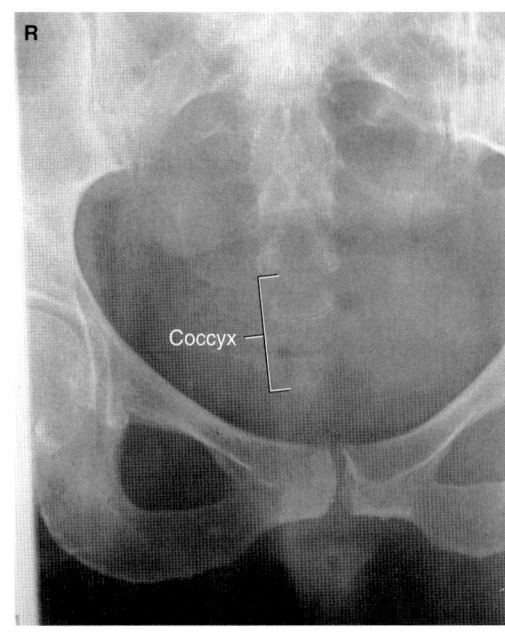

Coccyx *(Frank et al, 2012)*

cochineal /koch′inēl″/ [L, *coccineus,* bright red], a red dye prepared from the dried female insects of the species *Coccus cacti* containing young larvae. During the preparation of the dye the larvae are extracted with an aqueous solution of alum. The resulting dye has been used in coloring medicines.

cochlea /kok″lē·ə/ [L, snail shell], the auditory portion of the inner ear. It is a spiral tunnel about 30 mm long with two full and three quarter-turns, resembling a tiny snail shell and containing the sense organ for hearing. **–cochlear,** *adj.*

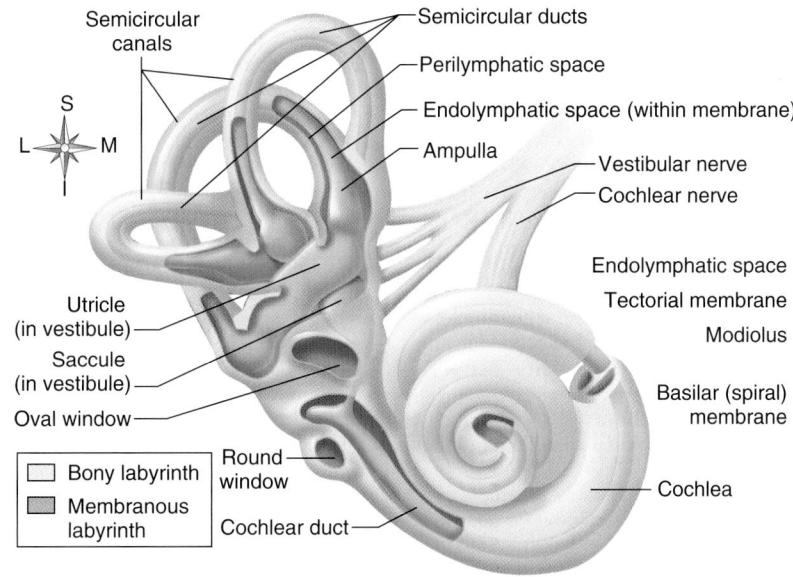

Cochlea *(Patton and Thibodeau, 2010)*

cochlear canal /kok′lē·ər/ [L, *cochlea* + *canalis,* channel], a bony spiral tunnel within the cochlea of the internal ear. It contains one opening that communicates with the tympanic cavity, a second that connects with the vestibule, and a third that leads to a tiny canal opening on the inferior surface of the temporal bone.

cochlear hearing loss, sensorineural hearing loss resulting from a defect in the receptor or transducing mechanisms of the cochlea.

cochlear implant, an electronic device that is surgically implanted into the cochlea of an individual with a severe to profound bilateral hearing loss. A transmitter placed outside the scalp sends signals to a receiver under the scalp, which in turn transmits an electrical code to the auditory nerve. A microphone is located behind the ear to collect the sound waves that are transmitted through a microprocessor. The microprocessor analyzes the sound waves and relays data back to electrodes in the implanted device. The patient receives electrical pulses that are translated into sound vibrations that can be distinguished as neural sensations. Although the implant does not transmit speech in the same manner as it would be perceived by a person with normal hearing, it allows the individual to perceive and distinguish sounds that would not otherwise be audible to him or her and to use those sounds along with other environmental cues to improve communication. Also called **cochlear prosthesis.**

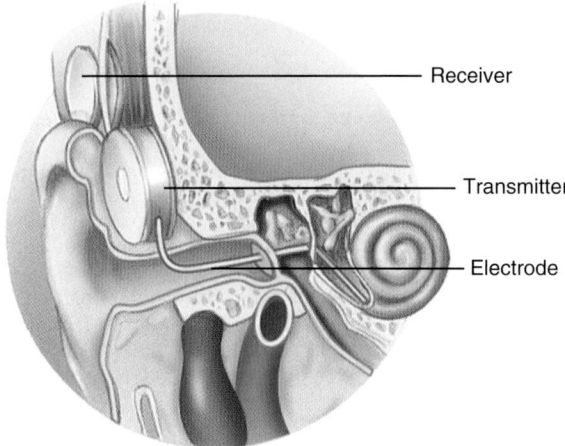

Receiver

Transmitter

Electrode

Cochlear implant *(Patton and Thibodeau, 2010)*

cochlear nerve [L, *cochlea,* snail shell, *nervus,* nerve], one of the main divisions of the eighth cranial nerve, with fibers that arise in spiral ganglion cells of the spiral organ and terminate in the dorsal and ventral cochlear nuclei of the brainstem. See also **vestibulocochlear nerve.**

cochlear prosthesis. See **cochlear implant.**

cochlear toxicity, poisonous effects of drugs that may result in hearing disorders, such as sensorineural hearing loss and tinnitus. Aminoglycoside antibiotics and vancomycin are examples of medications causing cochlear toxicity. See also **ototoxicity.**

cochlear window. See **round window.**

cochleovestibular /kok′lē·ō′vestib″yələr/, pertaining to the cochlea and vestibule of the ear.

Cochrane Reviews, a database providing access to abstracts and summaries to support evidence-based decision making.

Cockayne syndrome /kok·ān′/ [Edward Alfred Cockayne, English physician, 1880–1956], a rare autosomal-recessive syndrome of dwarfism with retinal atrophy and deafness, associated with progeria, prognathism, cognitive impairment, and photosensitivity. Features include a failure to thrive, microcephaly, and impaired development of the nervous system. The syndrome has three subtypes. Classical, or type I, Cockayne syndrome has an onset during early childhood. Type II has more severe symptoms and is apparent at birth. Type III has the mildest symptoms of the three types and appears later in childhood.

cockroach, the common name for members of the Blattidae family of insects, which infest homes, workplaces, and other areas inhabited by humans. Cockroaches transmit a number of disease agents, including bacteria, protozoa, and eggs of parasitic worms.

cocktail [AS, *cocc* + *toegel,*], *(Informal)* an unofficial mixture of drugs, usually in solution, combined to achieve a specific purpose. This term is frequently used when combining medications to treat patients who are HIV positive.

cockup splint, *(Obsolete)* a splint used to immobilize the wrist and leave the fingers free. Now called **wrist-hand orthotic.**

cocoa butter, a fatty extract of cocoa beans that is found in chocolate and moisturizers. It is traditionally used in the management of stretch marks, but randomized controlled trials do not support the efficacy of this use.

coconsciousness /kōkon″shəsnəs/, (in psychiatry) conscious states the patient is not aware of because they are not in the focus of attention but on the fringe of the content of consciousness. Thus something can be recalled and drawn into consciousness only when the conditions of consciousness are favorable.

cocontraction /kō′kəntrak″shən/, the simultaneous contraction of agonist and antagonist muscles around a joint. This is a normal neurological response when trying to increase the stability of the joint, such as when cocontracting hip and leg muscles to maintain posture when on a moving surface. Cocontraction of muscles around a joint occurs when learning a new motor skill, as riding a bike.

COD, abbreviation for *cause of death.*

code [L, *caudex,* book], **1.** (in law) a published body of statutes, such as a civil code. **2.** a collection of standards and rules of behavior, such as a dress code. **3.** a symbolic means of representing information for communication or transfer, such as a genetic code. **4.** a system of notation that allows information to be transmitted rapidly, such as Morse code, or in secrecy, such as a cryptographic code. **5.** *(Informal)* a discreet signal used to summon a special team to resuscitate a patient, as in "Code zero, 3 west" announced over a public address system to summon the team to the west wing of the third floor without alarming patients or visitors. "To code" means to cease respirations and/or heart function. See also **no code. 6.** to enter data by use of a given programming language into a computer. Compare **decode, encode.**

Code for Nurses, a set of guidelines for carrying out nursing responsibilities adopted by the American Nurses Association (ANA) in 1985. In 1994, the American Nurses Association determined that these guidelines were nonnegotiable and determined that each nurse had an obligation to adhere to the Code, and in 2001 a completely revised version of the Code of Ethics for Nurses was accepted by the ANA. The code was revised again in 2015.

codeine phosphate, an opioid analgesic and antitussive.

■ INDICATIONS: It is prescribed to suppress cough and to relieve mild to moderate pain.

■ CONTRAINDICATIONS: Known hypersensitivity to opiates is the only contraindication.

■ ADVERSE EFFECTS: Among the more serious adverse reactions are depression of the central nervous system, paradoxic excitement, and drug dependence.

codeine sulfate, a water-soluble salt of monomethylmorphine, an alkaloid derived from opium. It is used as a mild hypnotic, analgesic, and cough reflex suppressant. Dependency on the drug is possible, but is less likely to produce addiction than is morphine.

code of ethics, a statement encompassing the set of rules based on values and the standards of conduct to which practitioners of a profession are expected to conform. Kinds include **Code for Nurses, Hippocratic oath.**

codependent, a state of close association with a person who is dependent on or addicted to a potentially destructive behavior, such as substance abuse, gambling, or smoking. The codependent person facilitates the behavior of the dependent one.

code team, a specially trained and equipped team of physicians, nurses, and technicians that is available to provide advanced cardiac life support when summoned by an emergency code set by the institution. A code team usually includes a physician, registered nurse, respiratory therapist, and pharmacist.

coding [L, *caudex,* book], the process of organizing information into categories, which are assigned codes for the purposes of sorting, storing, and retrieving the data.

coding strand. See **sense strand.**

cod-liver oil, a pale-yellow, partially destearinated fatty oil extracted from the fresh livers of *Gadus morhua* and other fish of the family Gadidae. A rich source of fat-soluble vitamins A and D, it is useful in the treatment of nutritional deficiency of those vitamins. The oil must be stored in a cool, dark place, or it becomes rancid. See also **osteomalacia, rickets, tetany.**

Codman exercises [Ernest A. Codman, American surgeon, 1869–1940; L, *exercere,* to keep at work], mild exercises for restoring range of motion and function in the arms or shoulders after injury and immobilization of the limbs. The patient flexes the trunk and supports the upper body with the unaffected extremity. The injured extremity hangs free and can be moved in pendulum fashion through motion of the trunk without active contraction of the shoulder muscles. Also called **pendulum exercises.**

Codman tumor, *(Obsolete)* now called **chondroblastoma.**

codominance /kōdom″ənənts/ [L, *cum,* together with, *dominare,* to rule], the equal degree of dominance of two alleles or traits fully expressed in a phenotype, as when a person inherits both the I^A and I^B genes of the ABO blood group and has type AB blood. –*codominant, adj.*

codominant inheritance, the transmission of a trait or condition in which both alleles of a pair are given full expression in a heterozygote, as in the alleles for the AB or MNS blood group antigens and the leukocyte antigens.

codon /kō″don/, a unit of three adjacent nucleotides along a DNA or messenger RNA molecule that designates a specific amino acid to be incorporated into a polypeptide. The order of the codons along the DNA or messenger RNA determines the sequence of the amino acids in the polypeptide. Also called **trinucleotide.** See also **anticodon, genetic code.**

coefficient /kō′efish″ənt/ [L, *cum,* together with, *efficere,* to effect], a mathematic relationship between factors that can be used to measure or evaluate a characteristic under specified conditions. Examples include Henry's law, which measures solubility coefficient; Graham's law, which calculates diffusion coefficient; and the oxygen-utilization coefficient, which measures the amount of oxygen in a patient's venous blood in terms of the proportion of oxygen in his or her arterial blood.

coel-, prefix meaning "colon," denoting relationship to a cavity or space: *coelenteron.*

-coele, suffix form of *coel-.*

coelentera. See **coelenteron.**

Coelenterata. See **Cnidaria.**

coelenteron /sēlen″tərən/ *pl.* **coelentera** [Gk, *koilos,* hollow, *enteron,* intestine], the digestive cavity of animals in the phylum Cnidaria, such as the hydra and the jellyfish. See also **archenteron.**

coelom /sē″ləm/ [Gk, *koilos,* hollow], the body cavity of the developing embryo. It is situated between the layers of lateral mesoderm and in mammals gives rise to the pericardial, pleural, and peritoneal cavities. Also called **somatic cavity.** Kinds include **extraembryonic coelom.** –*celomic, coelomic, adj.*

coelosomy /sē″ləsō′mē/ [Gk, *koilos* + *soma,* body], a congenital anomaly characterized by protrusion of the viscera from the body cavity.

coenesthesia, coenesthesis, awareness of self through physiological stimuli. See **cenesthesia.**

coenogenesis. See **cenogenesis.**

coenzyme /kō·en″zīm/ [L, *cum,* together with, *en,* in, *zyme,* ferment], a nonprotein substance that combines with an apoenzyme to form a complete enzyme or holoenzyme. Coenzymes include some of the vitamins, such as B$_1$ and B$_2$, and have smaller molecules than enzymes. Coenzymes are dialyzable and heat-stable and usually dissociate readily from the protein portions of the enzymes with which they combine. See also **acetylcoenzyme A.**

coenzyme A (CoA) [L, *cum* + *en,* into, *zyme,* ferment], an important metabolite in the citric acid cycle. Although not a true enzyme, it plays a significant role in the transfer of acetyl groups and the metabolism of acids and amino acids.

coenzyme Q, any of several quinines that function as electron-carrying coenzymes involved in the electron transport chain or in aerobic cellular respiration. Also called **ubiquinone,** *coenzyme Q10.*

coffee [Ar, *qahwah*], the dried and roasted ripe seeds of *Coffea arabica, C. liberica,* and *C. robusta* trees, which may have originated in Africa and now grow in almost all tropical areas. Coffee contains the alkaloid caffeine and is the basis for a stimulating drink that has been used in treating the common headache, chronic asthma, and narcotic poisoning. The caffeine in coffee is potentially addictive; withdrawal symptoms include irritability and headache.

coffee-ground vomitus, dark brown vomitus the color and consistency of coffee grounds, composed of gastric juices and old blood and indicative of slow upper GI bleeding. Compare **hematemesis.**

Coffin-Lowry syndrome /kof′in lou′rē/ [Grange S. Coffin, American pediatrician, b. 1923; R. Brian Lowry, Irish-born Canadian physician, 20th century], a rare genetic disorder with onset in the postnatal period characterized by many parts of the body. Signs and symptoms are more severe in males than in females, and features can range from severe to very mild in women. Males typically have severe to profound intellectual disability and delayed development. Some experience stimulus-induced drop episodes (SIDEs) when startled with a loud noise. Characteristic facial features may include a prominent forehead, widely spaced and downward-slanting eyes, a short nose with a wide tip, and a wide mouth with full lips. It is transmitted with X-linked intermediate inheritance.

Coffin-Siris syndrome /kof′in sir′is/ [G.S. Coffin; Evelyn Siris, American radiologist, 1914–1987], hypoplasia or absence of the fifth fingers and toenails associated with growth and mental deficiencies; coarse facies; mild microcephaly; hypotonia; lax joints; mild hirsutism; and occasionally cardiac, vertebral, or GI anomalies.

C

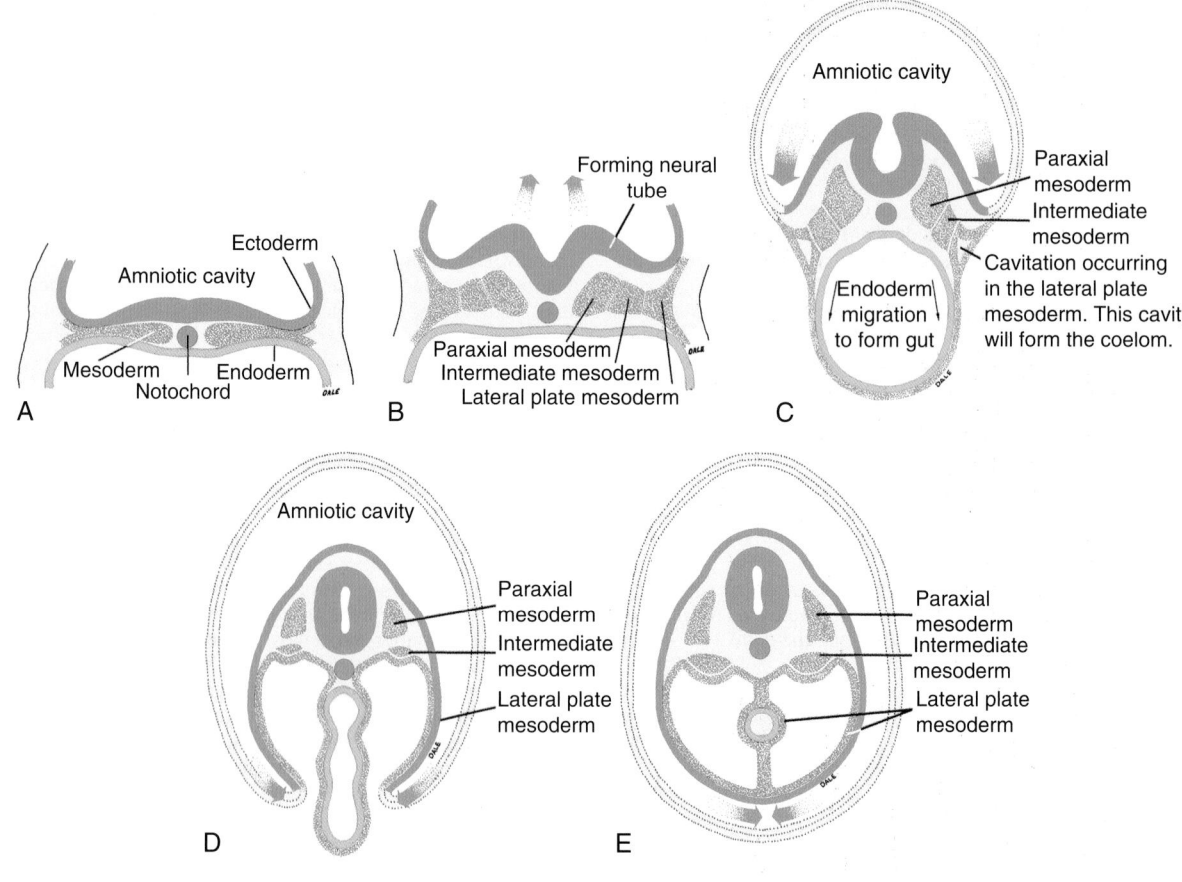

Coelom *(Nanci, 2013)*

Cogan syndrome /koʹgən/ [David Glendenning Cogan, American ophthalmologist, 1908–1993], a rare autoimmune disease usually affecting young Caucasian adults. Symptoms include a combination of nonsyphilitic interstitial keratitis and audiovestibular symptoms resembling Ménière's disease. Symptoms develop in a time span of less than two years.

Cogentin, an antiparkinson drug. Brand name for **benztropine mesylate.**

cognition /kognishʺən/ [L, *cognoscere,* to know], the mental process characterized by knowing, thinking, learning, understanding, and judging. Compare **conation. –cognitive,** *adj.*

cognitive /kogʺnitiv/, pertaining to the mental processes of comprehension, judgment, memory, and reasoning, as contrasted with emotional and volitional processes.

cognitive behavioral therapy (CBT), an approach to problem solving that helps persons understand their thoughts and develop strategies to change behaviors. Founded by Dr. Aaron Beck, an American psychiatrist (b. 1921), CBT is effective in the treatment of mood disorders as well as many other mental health conditions. CBT is accomplished in psychotherapy groups and/or in individual counseling. The goal is to identify how one's own thoughts and beliefs lead to certain behaviors and to make changes in thinking first, become aware of behaviors, and then move toward a positive change in both.

cognitive development, the developmental process by which an infant becomes an intelligent person, acquiring knowledge with growth and improving his or her ability to think, learn, reason, and abstract. Jean Piaget demonstrated the orderly sequence of this process from early infancy through childhood. See also **psychosexual development, psychosocial development.**

cognitive dissonance [L, *cognoscere,* to know, *dis,* opposite of, *sonare,* to sound], a state of tension resulting from a discrepancy in a person's emotional and intellectual frame of reference for interpreting and coping with his or her environment. It usually occurs when new information contradicts existing assumptions or knowledge.

cognitive distortion, errors in thinking that continue even when there is obvious contradictory evidence. Examples of cognitive distortions include all-or-nothing thinking, overgeneralization, labeling, mental filter, disqualifying the positive, jumping to conclusions (mind reading), magnification or minimization (catastrophizing), emotional reasoning ("should" and "must" statements), and personalization.

cognitive function, an intellectual process by which one becomes aware of, perceives, or comprehends ideas. It involves all aspects of perception, thinking, reasoning, and remembering. Compare **conation.**

cognitive learning, 1. learning that is concerned with acquisition of problem-solving abilities and with intelligence and conscious thought. **2.** a theory that defines learning as a behavioral change based on the acquisition of information about the environment.

cognitive psychology, 1. the study of the development of thought, language, and intelligence in humans. **2.** the field of psychology concerned with ways of knowing, mental processes, retention, decay or interference in thinking, learning, memory, and related areas of study.

cognitive restoration, an intervention technique, used primarily in rehabilitation medicine and educational psychology, designed to restore cognitive functioning.

cognitive restructuring, a change in attitudes, values, or beliefs that alters a person's self-expression. It occurs as a result of insight or behavioral achievement.

cognitive structuring, the process of reviewing with a patient the changes that have occurred in his or her thinking in order to instill a sense of those changes, and of his or her role in bringing about those changes.

cognitive therapy, any of the various methods of treating mental and emotional disorders that help a person change attitudes, perceptions, and patterns of thinking, from rational to realistic thoughts about self and situations. Kinds include **behavior therapy, existential therapy, Gestalt therapy, transactional analysis.**

cogwheel respiration, a breathing pattern characterized by a repeated series of brief interruptions of inhalation and exhalation.

cogwheel rigidity [ME, *cugge,* tooth on a gear; AS, *hweol* + L, *rigiditas,* unbending], an abnormal rigor in muscle tissue characterized by jerky movements when the muscle is passively stretched. The condition is often found in cases of Parkinson's disease and in the use of some first-generation antipsychotic medications.

cohabitate /kōhab′itāt/, to live together in a relationship when not married.

Cohen syndrome M. Michael Cohen, Jr., American pathologist (1937–2018), a rare autosomal-recessive genetic disorder with mutations in the VPS13B/COH1 gene. Symptoms are variable but are most often characterized by flaccid muscle tone; abnormalities of the head, face, hands, and feet; poor vision; neutropenia; and intellectual disability. Affected individuals usually have microcephaly. Also called **Pepper syndrome.**

Cohen technique, a type of ureteroneocystostomy in which the ureter is excised from the bladder and reimplanted in a new submucosal tunnel that is directed laterally across the trigone (transtrigonal) toward the contralateral side.

cohere /kōhir′/ [L, *cohaerere,* to cling together], to stick together, as similar molecules of a common substance.

coherence /kōhir′əns/, **1.** the property of sticking together, as the molecules within a common substance. **2.** (in psychology) the logical pattern of expression and thought evident in the speech of a normal, stable individual. −*coherent, adj.*

cohesive bandage /kōhē″siv/, a dressing material that will adhere to itself but not to other surfaces.

cohesiveness /kōhē″sivnəs/ [L, *cohaerere,* to cling together], **1.** (in psychiatry) a force that attracts members to a group and causes them to remain in it. **2.** (in dentistry) a property of annealed pure gold that allows it to fuse together under pressure and to closely adapt to the walls of a tooth preparation, making possible the use of 24–carat gold sheets or pellets as dental restorative material in single-tooth restorations. **3.** (in biochemistry) the property of the forces of attraction within an object that holds it together as compared to adhesion which is the forces of attraction existing between two different objects or surfaces that hold them together.

cohesive terminus, a single-stranded end projecting from a double-stranded DNA segment that can be joined by molecular genetic techniques to an introduced DNA fragment. Also called **sticky end.**

COHN, abbreviation for *certified occupational health nurse.*

cohort /kō″hôrt/ [L, *cohortem,* large group], (in statistics) a collection or sampling of individuals who share a common characteristic, such as members of the same age or the same sex.

cohort study, (in research) a study concerning a specific subpopulation, such as the children born between March and May in a given year or those born in the same months in a given year. See also **prospective study.**

coil, *(Slang)* a term used for some kinds of intrauterine contraceptive devices. See **intrauterine device.**

coiled tubular gland [L, *colligere,* to gather together, *tubulus,* small tube, *glans,* acorn], one of the many multicellular glands that contain a coiled, tube-shaped secretory portion, such as the sweat glands.

coil spring contraceptive diaphragm, a kind of contraceptive diaphragm in which the flexible metal spring that forms the rim is a coiled, circular spring. Seven sizes, in increments of 0.5 cm, allow fitting to a woman's pelvic anatomy, facilitating barrier contraception.

coincidence counting /kō·in″sidəns/ [L, *coincidere,* to occur together], the detection of two photons that arrive at separate counters simultaneously as the result of annihilation of a positron (created during a radioactive decay) and an electron. Coincidence counting greatly reduces the significance of any background radiation in radiography.

coinfection /ko′in-fek″shun/, simultaneous infection of a cell or organism by separate pathogens, as by hepatitis B and hepatitis D viruses.

coinsurance, an individual's share of the cost of a service provided by a health insurer or plan, calculated as a percent of the amount allowed for the service.

coital headache /kō″itəl/, an uncommon type of headache, mainly affecting men, that begins during or immediately after coitus. The complaint may last for several minutes to several hours.

coitus /kō″itəs/ [L, *coire,* to come together], intimacy-based physical interaction of any kind between two people, causing sexual excitation and/or orgasm in one or both partners. In the context of human reproduction, also called sexual intercourse, defined as a penis inserted into the vagina and ejaculation of semen containing sperm after sufficient sexual stimulation. Also called *coition.* See also **copulation, sexual intercourse.** −*coital, adj.*

coitus interruptus, withdrawal of the penis from the vagina during sexual intercourse before ejaculation as a form of contraception. The pregnancy rate associated with this practice is estimated to be as high as 27%. See **withdrawal method.**

COL, abbreviation for **CircOlectric (COL) bed™.**

col-, colo-, colon-, colonic-, prefix meaning "colon": *colonoscope.*

Colace, a stool softener. Brand name for *docusate sodium sulfosuccinate.*

colation /kōlā″shən/ [L, *colare,* to strain], the act of filtering or straining, as urine is often strained for medical examination.

ColBENEMID, a combination drug product used as an anti-gout medication. Brand name for **probenecid, colchicine.**

colchicine /kol″chəsēn/ [Gk, *kolchikon*], a gout suppressant that suppresses leukocyte mobility and phagocytosis in joints.

■ INDICATIONS: It may be prescribed in the treatment of acute gout and prophylaxis of recurrent gouty arthritis.

■ CONTRAINDICATIONS: Ulcer, ulcerative colitis, or known hypersensitivity to this drug prohibits its use. The drug is highly toxic and is not given to elderly, debilitated patients or to those who have chronic renal, hepatic, cardiovascular, or GI disease.

■ ADVERSE EFFECTS: Among the most serious adverse reactions are severe GI distress, including diarrhea with blood, bone marrow depression, peripheral neuritis, liver dysfunction, and alopecia. It is in pregnancy category D.

cold [AS, *kald*], **1.** *adj.,* the absence of heat. **2.** *n.,* a contagious viral infection of the upper respiratory tract, usually caused by a strain of rhinovirus. It is characterized by rhinitis, tearing, low-grade fever, and malaise and is treated symptomatically with rest, mild analgesia, decongestants, and increased fluid intake. Also called **common cold.** Compare **influenza. 3.** *adj.,* a distant method of relating; not friendly.

COLD /kōld/, abbreviation for **chronic obstructive lung disease.** See **chronic obstructive pulmonary disease.**

cold abscess, an abscess that does not show common signs of heat, redness, and swelling. See also **abscess,** def. 1.

cold agglutinin, a nonspecific antibody, found on the surface of red blood cells in certain diseases, that may cause clumping of the cells at temperatures below 36° C and may cause hemolysis. The phenomenon does not occur at body temperature. Mycoplasma pneumonia, infectious mononucleosis, and many lymphoproliferative disorders are associated with cold agglutinins.

cold agglutinin disease [AS, *kald* + L, *agglutinare,* to glue, *dis,* without; Fr, *aise,* ease], a disorder characterized by autoantibodies that agglutinate red blood cells at below-normal body temperatures. They occur in the sera of patients with mycoplasmal pneumonia.

cold-blooded, unable to regulate body heat. Fish, reptiles, and amphibians, which have internal temperatures that are close to the temperatures of the environments in which they live, are cold-blooded. Also called **poikilothermic.** Compare **warm-blooded.**

cold caloric irrigation, a procedure for testing the integrity of brainstem function. It is carried out by irrigating the external auditory canal of the patient with a cold saline solution while the head is flexed at approximately 30 degrees, after checking the patency of the ear canal. The stimulus results in jerky but regular eye movements (nystagmus) in a normal patient. Absence of the reaction may be a sign of a lesion at the pontine level of the brainstem. Also called **caloric test.**

cold cautery. See **cryocautery.**

cold compress [AS, *kald* + L, *comprimere,* to press together], a pad of damp, thickly folded, soft, absorbent cloth, dipped into cold water, wrung out, and applied to a body part for the relief of pain or reduction of inflammation or as a comfort measure.

cold-curing resin, (in dentistry) a plastic that hardens or chemically cures upon the mixing of a solid powder and a liquid polymer, producing an exothermic chemical reaction and forming a solid plastic substance. See **self-curing resin.**

cold environment, a human environment arbitrarily designated as one in which the temperature is below 10° C (50° F). Nearly two thirds of the world population, including most of North America, Europe, and Asia north of the Indian subcontinent, live in a naturally cold environment for at least a part of each year. The human body generally begins to experience some functional impairment when unprotected in temperatures below 15° C (59° F). The hands and fingers lose sensitivity, and the risk of errors and accidents increases. The body's hemostatic mechanism reacts with vasoconstriction, reducing heat loss to the environment but cooling the skin with a resultant chilling of the extremities. When vasoconstriction no longer eases the thermal strain between the skin and the environment, muscular hypertonus and shivering become mechanisms for maintaining body temperature.

cold hemoglobinuria. See **hemoglobinuria.**

cold injury, any of several abnormal and often serious physical conditions caused by exposure to cold temperatures. Kinds include **chilblain, frostbite, hypothermia, immersion foot.**

cold mist tent, a medical device for delivering humidified oxygen in an enclosed space. See **Croupette®.**

cold-pressor test, a diagnostic test in which one hand is immersed in ice water for approximately 60 seconds. In most cases, it triggers vascular sympathetic activation resulting in an increase in blood pressure and heart rate. It is used in the evaluation of hypertension and dysfunction of the autonomic nervous system.

cold-sensitive mutation, a genetic alteration resulting in a gene that functions only at high temperature.

cold sore. *(Informal)* See **herpes simplex.**

cold stress. See **hypothermia.**

cold ulcer, a small gangrenous ulceration on an extremity caused by poor circulation.

cold urticaria [AS, *kald* + L, *urtica,* nettle], wheals caused by exposure to cold temperatures. Compare **cholinergic urticaria.**

cold-wet-sheet pack, *(Obsolete)* a form of somatic therapy used indiscriminately and sometimes as a restraint in psychiatric hospitals of the past. While this type of therapy is rarely seen in clinical practice in North America today, it is still being used, particularly with the mentally ill or cognitively challenged in countries around the world, where it may be referred to as "packing." Today in North America, cold-wet-sheet pack therapy can be found in use in some spas or chosen by some as an alternative treatment to medications or other more invasive methods of treatment in the case of some chronic conditions or anxiety.

colectomy /kəlek″təmē/ [Gk, *kolon,* colon, *ektomē,* excision], surgical excision of part or all of the colon, performed to treat cancer of the colon, diverticulitis, or severe chronic ulcerative colitis. For several days before surgery a low-residue diet is prescribed. Antibiotics, bowel-cleansing enemas, or an oral bowel preparation solution are given to reduce the number of bacteria in the bowel. Parenteral fluids and electrolytes are given, and a nasogastric tube is passed. The nurse gives postoperative care as for any abdominal surgery. The nasogastric tube is connected to suction and remains in place until bowel sounds are heard. See also **abdominal surgery.**

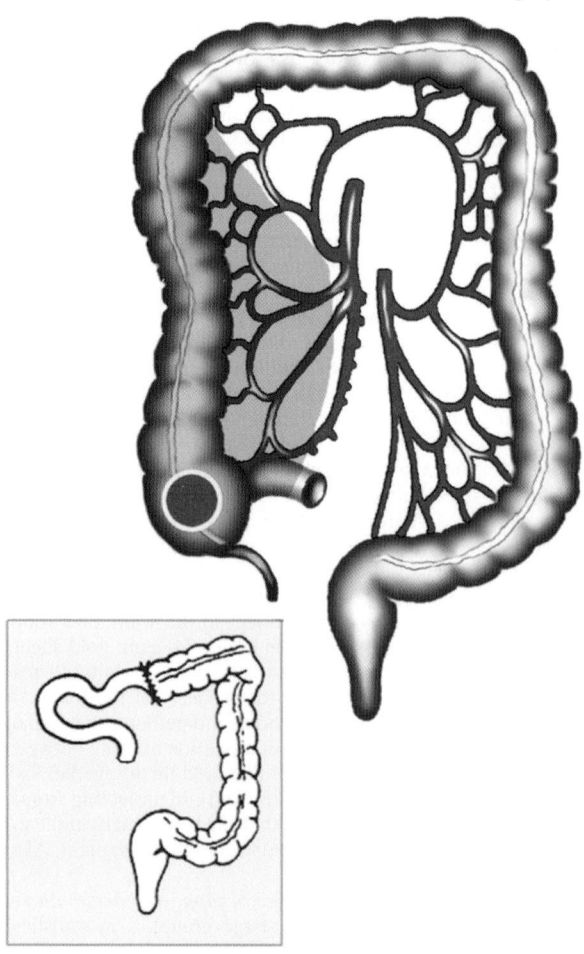

Colectomy *(Feldman et al, 2016)*

colesevelam /ko″lesev′elam/, a polymer that binds bile acids in the intestine and prevents them from being reabsorbed, resulting in decreased serum levels of total cholesterol, low-density lipoprotein cholesterol (LDL-C), and apolipoprotein B and increased levels of high-density lipoprotein cholesterol. It is administered orally as the hydrochloride salt. It is an adjunctive therapy to reduce elevated LDL-C levels in patients with primary hypercholesterolemia.

Colestid, an antihyperlipidemic. Brand name for **colestipol hydrochloride.**

colestipol hydrochloride /kōles″tipol/, an antihyperlipidemic that acts by sequestering bile acids in the intestine for excretion, thus reducing plasma levels of cholesterol when the liver removes cholesterol to synthesize new bile.

■ INDICATIONS: It is prescribed in the treatment of hypercholesterolemia and xanthoma.

■ CONTRAINDICATIONS: Biliary obstruction or known hypersensitivity to this drug prohibits its use.

■ ADVERSE EFFECTS: Among the more serious adverse reactions are skin rash; fecal impaction; and a deficiency of vitamins A, D, and K.

colfosceril /kolfos′eril/, a synthetic pulmonary surfactant used as the palmitate ester in combination with tyloxapol and as an alcohol in prophylaxis and treatment of neonatal respiratory distress syndrome, instilled into the endotracheal tube for intratracheal administration.

colic /kol″ik/ [Gk, *kolikos,* colon pain], **1.** *n.,* sharp visceral pain resulting from torsion, obstruction, or smooth muscle spasm of a hollow or tubular organ, such as a ureter or the intestines. Kinds include **biliary colic, infantile colic, renal colic. 2.** pertaining to the colon. **3.** unexplained crying in a healthy baby between 2 weeks and 5 months of age. Affects 10% to 20% of all infants and is more common in boys. Possible causes are digestive tract immaturity, food intolerances, hunger or overfeeding, lack of sleep, loneliness, tension, or overheated milk or formula. –**colicky,** *adj.*

colicinogen /kol′isin″əjən/ [*(E.) coli* + L, *caedere,* to kill; Gk, *genein,* to produce], an extrachromosomal segment of DNA in some strains of *Escherichia coli* that induces secretion of a colicin, a protein lethal to other strains of the bacterium. Colicins attach to specific receptors on the cell membrane and impair the synthesis of macromolecules or the production of energy. Also called *colicinogenic factor.*

colicky. See **colic.**

coliform /kol″ifôrm/ [*(E.) coli* + L, *forma,* form], **1.** pertaining to the colon-aerogenes group, or the *Escherichia coli* species of microorganisms, which comprises most of the intestinal flora in humans and other animals. Presence of coliforms is used as a standard indication of water pollution with fecal matter. **2.** having the characteristic of a sieve or cribriform structure, such as some of the porous bones of the skull.

colistimethate sodium /kō′listim″əthāt/, an antibiotic. Also called *colistin sulfomethate sodium.*

■ INDICATIONS: It is prescribed in the treatment of GI infections caused by certain gram-negative microorganisms and as a topical medication.

■ CONTRAINDICATIONS: Known hypersensitivity to this drug prohibits its use.

■ ADVERSE EFFECTS: Among the more serious adverse reactions are nephrotoxicity and neurotoxicity.

colistin sulfate /kōlis″tin/, an antibacterial and steroid agent.

■ INDICATIONS: It is prescribed topically in the treatment of infections of the outer ear and systemically for the treatment of serious gram-negative infections and gastroenteritis caused by *Escherichia coli.*

■ CONTRAINDICATIONS: Known hypersensitivity to this drug prohibits its use.

■ ADVERSE EFFECTS: Among the more serious systemic reactions are respiratory arrest, renal toxicity, and neuromuscular blockade.

colitis /kōlī″tis/, an inflammatory condition of the large intestine. Inflammatory bowel disease is characterized by severe diarrhea, bleeding, and ulceration of the mucosa of the intestine. Weight loss and pain are significant. Steroids, fluids, electrolytes, antibiotics, and careful attention to diet are the usual modes of therapy. Most of the diseases of this group are of unknown origin. Kinds include **Crohn disease, ulcerative colitis.** –*colitic, adj.*

collaborative power structure /kəlab″ərətiv′/, an arrangement whereby adult members of a functional family or organization make major decisions and are in agreement about power distribution.

collagen /kol″əjən/ [Gk, *kolla,* glue, *genein,* to produce], a fibrous insoluble protein consisting of bundles of tiny reticular fibrils that combine to form the white glistening inelastic fibers of the tendons, the ligaments, and the fascia. It is found in connective tissue, including skin, bone, ligaments, and cartilage. It represents 30% of total body protein. –**collagenous,** *adj.*

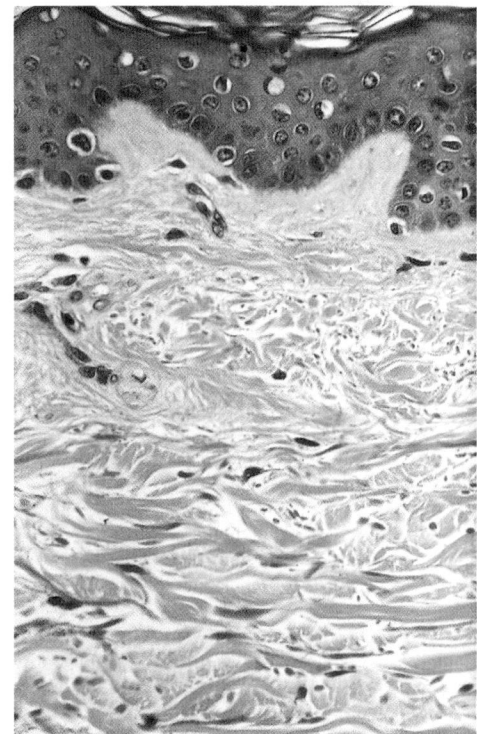

Collagen *(du Vivier, 2013)*

collagenase /kəlaj″ənās/, a medication applied as an ointment for debridement of decubitus ulcers, burns, and other epidermal lesions. It is also injected into the penis for treatment of Peyronie's disease and into the wrist, ankle, etc. for the treatment of Dupuytren's disease (restricted movement caused by thickening of the fascia). It is an enzyme preparation derived from the fermentation of *Clostridium histolyticum.*

collagen disease, an abnormal condition characterized by extensive disruption of the connective tissue, often involving inflammation and fibrinoid degeneration. Collagen diseases include polyarteritis nodosa, systemic lupus erythematosus, osteoarthritis, and rheumatoid arthritis. See also **collagen vascular disease.**

collagen injection, a reconstructive technique in cosmetic surgery to enhance the lips, to fatten sunken facial skin, or to remove the appearance of wrinkles in the forehead or around the mouth.

collagenoblast /kəlaj″ənōblast′/ [Gk, *kolla + genein + blastos,* germ], a cell that differentiates from a fibroblast and functions in the formation of collagen. It can also transform into cartilage and bone tissue by metaplasia.

collagenous. See **collagen.**

collagenous colitis /kəlajənəs kōlī′tis/, a type of colitis of unknown cause, characterized by deposits of collagenous material beneath the epithelium of the colon, with crampy abdominal pain; marked reduction in fluid and electrolyte absorption, leading to watery diarrhea; and no mucosal ulceration.

collagenous fiber /kəlaj″ənəs/, any one of the tough, white protein fibers that constitute much of the intercellular substance and the connective tissue of the body. Collagenous fibers contain collagen. They are often arranged in bundles that strengthen the tissues in which they are embedded.

collagen shield, a material derived from porcine scleral tissue, used in promotion of corneal healing. The shield enhances the penetration and effective time of subconjunctival antibiotics and corticosteroids. The collagen shield is designed to dissolve within 12 hours.

collagen vascular disease, any of a group of acquired disorders that have in common diffuse immunological and inflammatory changes in small blood vessels and connective tissue. Common features include arthritis, skin lesions, iritis and episcleritis, pericarditis, pleuritis, subcutaneous nodules, myocarditis, vasculitis, and nephritis. Also often associated are Coombs' test–positive hemolytic anemia, thrombocytopenia, leukopenia, B and T cell abnormalities, antinuclear antibodies, cryoglobulins, rheumatoid factors, false-positive serological test results for syphilis, alterations in serum complement, and immunological abnormalities. The diseases usually included in this category are mixed connective tissue disease, necrotizing vasculitis, and other vasculopathies; polymyositis; relapsing polychondritis; rheumatic fever; rheumatoid arthritis; scleroderma; and systemic lupus erythematosus. The cause of most of these diseases is unknown. Hereditary factors and deficiencies, autoimmunity, environmental antigens, infections, allergies, and antigen-antibody complexes in various combinations are probably involved. Also called **connective tissue disease.**

collapse /kəlaps″/ [L, *collabi,* to fall together], **1.** *(Nontechnical)* a state of extreme depression or a condition of complete exhaustion caused by physical or psychosomatic problems. **2.** an abnormal condition characterized by shock. **3.** the abnormal sagging of an organ or the obliteration of its cavity.

collapse of the lung [L, *collabi,* to fall together; AS, *lungen*], a reduction in the volume of a lung. The condition results from increased intrapleural pressure caused by accumulation of air or fluid in the pleural cavity or from a loss of internal pressure and elastic recoil of the lung. See also **atelectasis, hemothorax, pneumothorax.**

collapsing pulse. See **Corrigan pulse.**

collar [L, *collum,* neck], any structure that encircles another, usually around its neck, such as the periosteal bone collars that form around the diaphyses of young bones.

collarbone. *(Informal)* See **clavicle.**

collateral /kōlat″ərəl/ [L, *cum,* together with, *lateralis,* side], **1.** secondary or accessory. **2.** (in anatomy) a small branch, such as any one of the arterioles or venules in the body, as in collateral circulation.

collateral circulation [L, *cum + latus,* side, *circulare,* to go around], an accessory blood pathway developed through enlargement of secondary vessels after obstruction of a main channel.

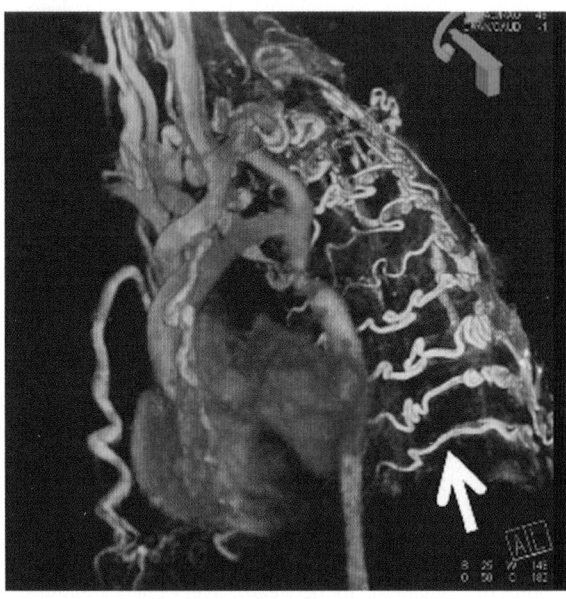

Image showing collateral circulation *(Lang, 2011)*

collateral fissure, a fissure separating the subcalcarine and subcollateral gyri of the cerebral hemisphere.

collateral innervation, reinnervation of denervated neurons caused by sprouting of uninjured axons in the vicinity.

collateral ligaments of interphalangeal joints of foot, fibrous bands, one on either side of each of the interphalangeal joints of the toes.

collateral ligaments of interphalangeal joints of hand, thick, fibrous bands on each side of the interphalangeal joints of the fingers. They prevent lateral or medial deviation of the joint.

collateral ligaments of the metacarpophalangeal joints, thick, fibrous bands on either side of each metacarpophalangeal joint, holding the two bones involved in each joint firmly together and preventing lateral or medial deviation during flexion of the joint.

collateral ligaments of the metatarsophalangeal joints, strong fibrous bands on either side of each metatarsophalangeal joint, holding the two bones involved in each joint firmly together.

collateral pulp canal, a branch of a tooth's pulp canal that emerges from the root at a place other than the apex. Also called **branching canal.** Compare **accessory root canal.**

collateral ventilation, the ventilation of alveoli in the lungs through indirect pathways, such as Kohn's pores in alveolar septa or anastomosing bronchioles.

collateral vessel [L, *cum + latus,* side, *vascellum,* small vase], a branch of an artery or vein used as an accessory to the blood vessel from which it arises.

collecting system, a group of renal calices and its pelvis considered as a unit.

collecting tubule [L, *colligere,* to gather, *tubulus,* small tube], any one of the many relatively straight tubules of the kidney that funnel urine into papillary ducts in the renal pelvis. The small collecting tubules play an important role in maintaining the fluid balance of the body by allowing water to osmose through their membranes into the interstitial fluid in the renal medulla. Antidiuretic hormone in the blood makes the collecting tubules permeable to water. If no antidiuretic hormone is present in the blood, membranes of the collecting tubules are practically impermeable to water. See also **Bowman's capsule, kidney.**

collective bargaining /kəlek″tiv/, the use of collective action by employees in negotiating working conditions and economic issues with their employer.

collective hysteria. See **mass hysteria.**

collective unconscious [L, *colligere,* to gather; AS, *un,* not; L, *conscious,* aware], (in analytic psychology) that portion of the unconscious common to all humans. Also called **racial unconscious.** See also **analytic psychology.**

collector, (in medicine) a device with various modifications, used for gathering secretions from the bronchi and esophagus for bacteriological and cytological examination.

college [L, *collegium,* society], **1.** an institution of higher learning. **2.** an organization of individuals with common professional training and interests, as the American College of Nurse-Midwives, the American College of Cardiology, or the American College of Surgeons. **3.** in Canada, referring to regulatory bodies overseeing professions such as the College of Registered Nurses of British Columbia, the College of Registered Psychiatric Nurses of British Columbia, and the College of Licensed Practical Nurses of British Columbia.

College of American Pathologists (CAP), a national professional organization of physicians who specialize in pathology.

Colles' fascia /kol″ēz/ [Abraham Colles, Irish surgeon, 1773–1843; L, band], the deep inner layer of the subcutaneous, superficial fascia of the perineum, constituting a distinctive structure in the urogenital region of the body. It is a strong, smooth sheet of tissue containing elastic fibers that give it a characteristic yellow tint.

Colles fracture [Abraham Colles], a break in or near the distal radius within 2.5 cm of the joint of the wrist, which causes displacement of the hand to a dorsal and lateral position. Colles fractures commonly occur when there is a fall with an outstretched hand. Also called **silver-fork fracture.**

colligative /kol″igā′tiv/ [L, *colligere,* to gather], (in physical chemistry) pertaining to those properties of matter (especially solutions) that depend on the numbers of particles, such as molecules and ions, rather than the chemical identity of any one particle. Colligative properties of solutions include boiling point, freezing point, vapor, pressure, and osmotic pressure.

collimate [L, *collineare,* to align], to make parallel.

collimator /kol″imā′tər/ [L, *collinare,* to bring into alignment], a device for limiting the size and shape of a radiation beam. It is used to reduce patient exposure to ionizing radiation, and the production of scatter radiation, thereby increasing radiographic quality.

colliquation /kol″ikwā″shən/ [L, *cum,* together with, *liquifacere,* to make liquid], **1.** the degeneration of a body tissue to a liquid state, usually associated with necrotic tissue. **2.** abnormal discharge of a body fluid.

colliquative /kol″ikwā′tiv/, characterized by a profuse fluid discharge, as in suppurating wounds and body structures that are infected.

collision tumor /kəlizh″ən/ [L, *cum,* together with, *laedere,* to strike], a tumor formed when two separate growths, developing close to each other, join. See also **carcinoma.**

collodion /kəlō″dē·ən/ [Gk, *kolla,* glue, *eidos,* form], a clear or slightly opaque, highly flammable liquid composed of pyroxylin, ether, and alcohol. It dries to a strong, transparent film that is used as a surgical dressing.

collodion baby, an infant whose skin at birth is covered with a scaly, parchmentlike membrane. The collodion baby is not a disease entity but is the first expression of some forms of ichthyosis. See also **harlequin fetus, lamellar exfoliation.**

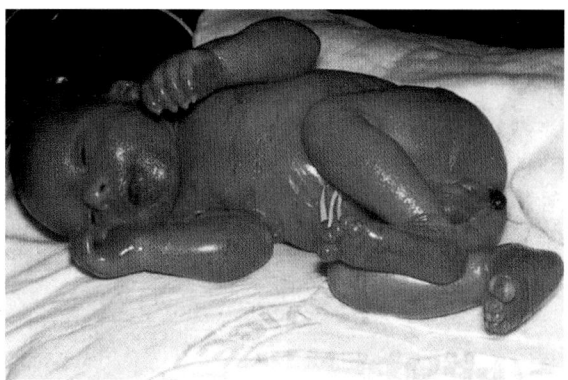

Collodion baby *(Courtesy Dr. D.A. Burns)*

colloid /kol″oid/ [Gk, *kolla,* glue, *eidos,* form], a state or division of matter in which large molecules or aggregates of molecules (1 to 100 nm in size) do not precipitate and are dispersed in another medium. In a suspension colloid the particles are insoluble and the medium may be solid, liquid, or gas. In an emulsion colloid the particles are usually water, and the medium is any of several complex hydrophilic, organic substances that become evenly dispersed among the particles of water. Compare **solution, suspension.**

colloidal solution /koloi″dəl/ [Gk, *kolla,* glue, *eidos,* form; L, *solutus,* dissolved], a solution in which small particles, such as large polymeric molecules, are homogenously dispersed through a liquid medium. See also **colloid.**

colloidal sulfur, a form of very finely divided sulfur that is used in the treatment of acne and other skin disorders.

colloid bath, a bath taken in water that contains such substances as bran, gelatin, and starch, used to relieve irritation and inflammation. See also **emollient bath.**

colloid chemistry, the science dealing with the composition and nature of chemical colloids.

colloid corpuscle, a starchlike body of little pathological significance found in the nervous tissue, prostate, and pulmonary alveoli. Also called **corpus amylaceum.** See also **amyloid.**

colloid cyst [Gk, *kolla,* glue, *eidos,* form, *kystis,* bag], **1.** a thyroid gland follicle distended with thyroid secretion. **2.** a cyst in the third ventricle, leading to hydrocephalus. **3.** a cyst with gelatinous contents.

colloid osmotic pressure. See **oncotic pressure.**

colloid substance, a jellylike substance formed in the deterioration of the protoplasm of tissues.

colloid suspension [Gk, *kolla,* glue, *eidos,* form; L, *suspendere,* to hang], a system of solids dispersed in a liquid medium, with particles generally smaller than 100 nm.

collum /kol″əm/, the anatomical necklike structure between the head and shoulders.

collyrium /kolir″ē·əm/, an eyewash or an ophthalmic liquid containing medications to be instilled into the eye.

coloboma /kol′əbō″mə/ *pl. colobomas, colobomata* [Gk, *koloboma,* defect], a congenital or pathological defect in the ocular tissue of the body, usually affecting the iris, ciliary body, or choroid by forming a cleft that extends inferiorly. Colobomas are usually the result of the failure of part of the fetal fissure to close. –*colobomatous, adj.*

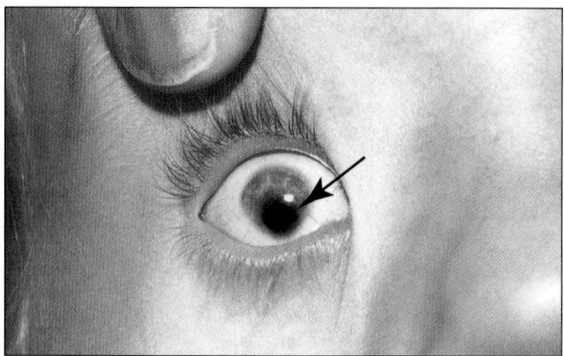

Coloboma *(David and Hoyt, 2005)*

coloenteritis, *(Obsolete)* now called **enterocolitis.**

colon /kō″lən/ [Gk, *kolon*], the portion of the large intestine extending from the cecum to the rectum. It has four segments: the ascending colon, transverse colon, descending colon, and sigmoid colon. –**colonic,** *adj.*

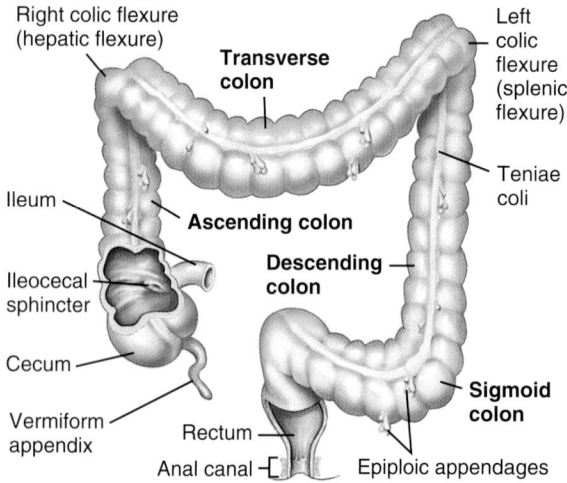

Colon

colon hydrotherapy, an extended and more complete form of an enema as well as a method of removing waste from the large intestine without using drugs. Colon hydrotherapy is used to treat constipation or impaction, as preparation for diagnostic studies of the large intestine (barium enema, sigmoidoscopy, or colonoscopy), and as preparation before or after surgery. The procedure is also used for bowel training for paraplegics or quadriplegics, those with arthritis, and patients who have suspected autointoxication or intestinal toxemia.

colonic. See **colon.**

-colonic /kōlon″ik/, suffix meaning "relating to the colon": *vesicocolonic.*

colonic fistula [Gk, *kolon* + L, pipe], an abnormal passage from the colon to the surface of the body or an internal organ or structure. In regional enteritis chronic inflammation may lead to the formation of a fistula between two adjacent loops of bowel.

An external opening from the colon to the surface of the abdomen may be created surgically after the removal of a malignant or severely ulcerated segment of the bowel. See also **colostomy.**

colonic intussusception, intussusception involving two segments of the colon; telescoping of the colon. One section of the colon tunnels over the adjacent section, resulting in bowel obstruction.

colonic irrigation, a procedure for washing the inner wall of the colon by filling it with water, then draining it. It is not considered an enema, but rather a technique for removing any material that may be present high in the colon.

colonic volvulus, volvulus or spasmodic contraction involving any portion of the colon, causing colic. Kinds include **cecal volvulus, sigmoid volvulus, transverse colon volvulus.**

colonization /kol′ənīzā″shən/, **1.** the invasion of a new habitat by a new species. **2.** the presence and multiplication of microorganisms without tissue invasion or damage. The colonies develop when a bacterial cell begins reproducing.

colono-, combining form meaning the "part of the large intestine between the cecum and rectum": *colonography, colonoscope.*

colonography /ko″lonog′rah-fe/, imaging of the colon, as by computed tomography or magnetic resonance imaging. Also called **virtual colonoscopy.**

colonoscope /kō″lənōskōp′/ [Gk, *kolon* + *skopein*, to watch], a long, flexible endoscope, usually fiberoptic, that permits examination of the interior of the entire colon. See also **endoscope.**

colonoscopy /kō′lənos″kəpē/, the examination of the mucosal lining of the colon by using a colonoscope, an elongated endoscope. It requires the cleansing of the client's large intestine, clear liquids the evening before the examination, and taking nothing by mouth for several hours before the exam. The client is usually sedated with IV medication.

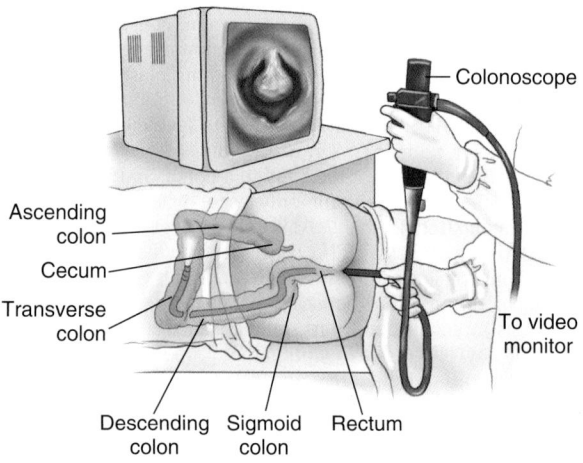

Extent of bowel examined

☐ Colonoscopy

☐ Sigmoidoscopy

Colonoscopy *(LaFleur Brooks and LaFleur Brooks, 2012)*

colon stasis. See **atonic constipation.**

colony /kol″ənē/ [L, *colonia*], **1.** (in bacteriology) a mass of microorganisms in a culture that originates from a single cell. Some kinds of colonies, according to different configurations, are smooth colonies, rough colonies, and dwarf colonies.

2. (in cell biology) a mass of cells in a culture or in certain experimental tissues, such as a spleen colony.

colony counter, a device used for counting colonies of bacteria growing in a culture. It usually consists of an illuminated, transparent plate divided into sections of known area. Petri dishes containing colonies of bacteria are placed over the plate, and the colonies are counted according to the number within the areas viewed.

colony-stimulating factor (CSF), secreted glycoproteins that cause hematopoietic stem cells to proliferate and differentiate into a specific kind of white blood cell.

coloproctectomy /kō′ləproktek″təmē/, surgical removal of the colon and rectum.

coloproctitis /kō′ləpraktī″tis/, an inflammation of both the colon and rectum. Also called **colorectitis, rectocolitis.**

coloptosis /kō′lōptō″sis/ [Gk, *kolon* + *ptosis,* fall], the prolapse or downward displacement of the colon, especially of the transverse portion.

-color, suffix meaning "hue or hues": *versicolor.*

Colorado tick fever, a relatively mild, self-limited arbovirus infection transmitted to humans by the bite of the wood tick *Dermacentor andersoni.* It is endemic in the mountainous regions above 5000 feet in the western United States and Canada and is most prevalent in the spring and summer months. The virus has been isolated from *D. andersoni* ticks in Alberta and British Columbia. It occurs most frequently in those with recreational or occupational exposure (hiking or fishing) in enzootic loci. Symptoms, which appear 3 to 6 days after the tick bite, occur in two phases separated by a period of remission and include chills, fever, and headache; pain in the eyes, legs, and back; and sensitivity to light. Treatment is supportive; analgesics can be given for headache and other pains. Also called **American mountain fever, mountain fever, mountain tick fever.** Compare **Rocky Mountain spotted fever.**

color blindness [L, color; AS *blint*], an abnormal condition characterized by an inability to distinguish colors of the spectrum clearly. In most cases it is not a blindness but a weakness in perceiving colors distinctly. There are two forms of color blindness: Daltonism, the more common form, is characterized by an inability to distinguish reds from greens. It is an inherited, sex-linked disorder. Total color blindness, or achromatic vision, is characterized by an inability to perceive any color at all. Only white, gray, and black are seen. It may be the result of a defect in or absence of the cones in the retina. Also spelled **colour blindness.**

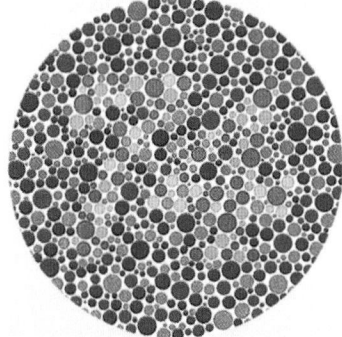

Color blindness chart *(Courtesy S. Ishihara, Washington University Department of Ophthalmology)*

color dysnomia /disnō″mē·ə/ [L, color; Gk, *dys,* difficult, *onoma,* name], an inability to name colors despite an ability to match and distinguish them. It may be caused by expressive dysphasia.

colorectal /kō′lōrek′təl/ [Gk, *kolon,* colon + L, *rectus,* straight], pertaining to or affecting the colon and rectum.

colorectal cancer /kō′lərek′təl/ [Gk, *kolon,* colon; L, *rectus,* straight], a malignant neoplastic disease of the large intestine, characterized by a change in bowel habits; the passing of blood (melena), which may be occult initially; and anemias. Malignant tumors of the large bowel usually occur after 50 years of age, are slightly more frequent in women than in men, and are common in the Western world. They are rare in children. Inherited syndromes (FAP, HNPCC) significantly increase the risk of colorectal cancer. The risk of large bowel cancer is also increased in patients with chronic ulcerative colitis, villous adenomas, and especially familial adenomatous polyposis of the colon. 75% of all colorectal cancers have no known predisposing factors, but people who have a high-fat diet and low activity levels may be more likely than others to have this cancer. In the vermiform appendix, carcinoid is the most common tumor. Most lesions of the large bowel are adenocarcinomas. These tumors have a long preinvasive stage, and, when they invade, they tend to grow slowly.

■ OBSERVATIONS: Rectal tumors may cause pain, bleeding, and a feeling of incomplete evacuation. They may metastasize slowly through lymphatic channels and veins and occasionally prolapse through the anus. Typical napkin ring tumors in the sigmoid and descending colon grow circumferentially and constrict the intestinal lumen, causing partial obstruction and production of flat or pencil-shaped stools. Manifestations include progressive abdominal distension, pain, vomiting, constipation, cramps, and bright red blood on the stool's surface. Malignant lesions in the ascending colon are usually large growths that may be palpable on physical examination; they generally cause severe anemia and nausea. There may be dark red or mahogany-colored blood mixed with the stool. The diagnosis of colorectal cancer is based on digital rectal examination, testing for blood in the stool, proctosigmoidoscopic examination of the sigmoid, and x-ray studies of the GI tract. Colonoscopy is the definitive test for colorectal cancer. Suspicious polyps may be removed for histological study, often through a sigmoidoscope or colonoscope or by laparotomy.

■ INTERVENTIONS: Surgical treatment of colorectal cancer may involve a wide resection of the lesion, the surrounding colon, and the attached tissues. Tumors of the rectum may require removal of the entire rectum by abdominoperineal resection and the creation of a permanent colostomy. Chemotherapy and irradiation may be administered as palliative therapy or adjuvant treatment.

■ PATIENT CARE CONSIDERATIONS: The care of the patient after a diagnosis of colorectal cancer focuses on coping with a possible loss of or alteration in body function, maintaining adequate nutrition, and preventing deterioration.

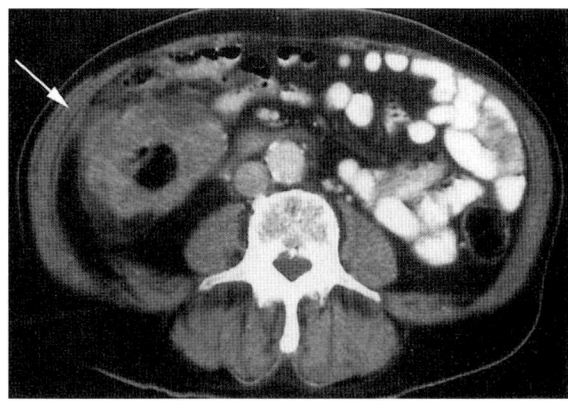

Colorectal cancer *(Garden et al, 2012)*

colorectitis. See **coloproctitis.**

colorimetry /kol′ərim″ətrē/, measurement of the intensity of color in a fluid or substance as compared with that in a standard solution. See also **spectrophotometry.**

color therapy, the therapeutic use of light of specific colors. It encompasses a number of methods used in complementary medicine, including the direction of light of specific colors at the chakras associated with the colors, the stimulation of acupoints, and the use of light of specific wavelengths to facilitate healing. Color therapy is often employed as a complementary treatment for seasonal affective disorder, depression, and stress.

color vision, a recognition of color as the result of changes in the pigments of the cones in the retina that react to varying intensities of red, green, and blue light. The exact mechanisms of color vision are not completely understood, but some experts believe they depend on three specialized types of cones, each type responding to red, green, or blue light. Some retinal cones respond to the entire visual spectrum. See also **color blindness.**

colosigmoidoscopy /kō′lōsig′moidos″kəpē/ [Gk, *kolon* + *sigma,* S-shaped, *eidos,* form, *skopein,* to look], the direct examination of the sigmoid portion of the colon with a sigmoidoscope.

colostomate /kəlos″təmāt/ [Gk, *kolon* + *stoma,* mouth; L, *atum,* one acted upon], a person who has undergone a colostomy.

colostomy /kəlos″təmē/ [Gk, *kolon* + *stoma,* mouth], surgical creation of an artificial anus on the abdominal wall by incising the colon and bringing it out to the surface, performed for cancer of the colon, benign obstructive tumors, and severe abdominal wounds. Immediate postoperative care is the same as for abdominal surgery. Compare **enterostomy.** Kinds include **loop colostomy, double-barrel colostomy.**

■ METHOD: A colostomy may be single-barreled, with one opening, or double-barreled, with distal and proximal loops opening onto the abdomen. The latter is performed for complete blockage of the lower bowel or in paraplegia to simplify daily management. A temporary colostomy may be done to divert feces after surgery, as in the repair of Hirschsprung's disease, or from an inflamed area; it is repaired when the colon has healed or the inflammation subsides.

■ PATIENT CARE CONSIDERATIONS: Preoperative care focuses on teaching the patient what to expect after surgery and preparation for the procedure. A high-calorie clear liquid diet is given. An antibiotic, usually neomycin, is prescribed to reduce the bacterial count in the bowel, and bowel-cleansing methods are used. Postoperatively, care of the stoma, management of the evacuation of feces, and protection of the skin surrounding the stoma must be addressed. Care must also focus on psychosocial issues; depression and poor self-image are common following this procedure.

■ OUTCOME CRITERIA: Recovery will vary, depending on the type of colostomy and the reason the colostomy is needed.

colostomy irrigation, a procedure used by colostomates to clear the bowel of fecal matter and to help establish an evacuation schedule. Many colostomates establish a regular schedule of evacuation with irrigation, but the procedure may be unsatisfactory for those who have a liquid or semisoft fecal stream, for patients who before the operation had a tendency to experience diarrhea under stress, or for patients with irregular bowel habits.

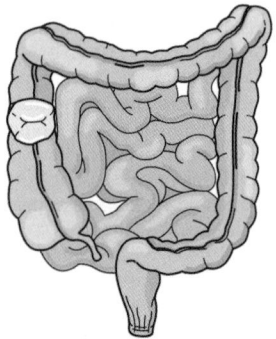

The **ascending colostomy** is done for right-sided tumors.

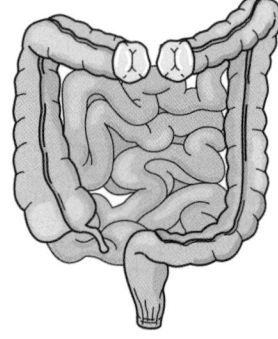

The **transverse (double-barreled) colostomy** is often used in such emergencies as intestinal obstruction or perforation because it can be created quickly. There are two stomas. The proximal one, closest to the small intestine, drains feces. The distal stoma drains mucus. Usually temporary.

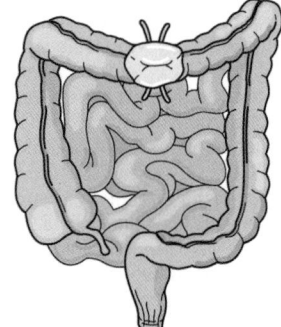

The **transverse loop colostomy** has two openings in the transverse colon, but one stoma. Usually temporary.

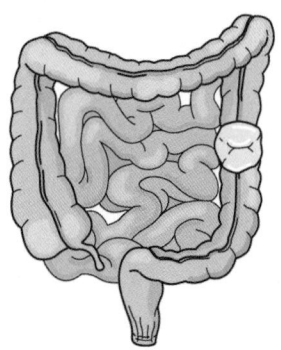

Descending colostomy

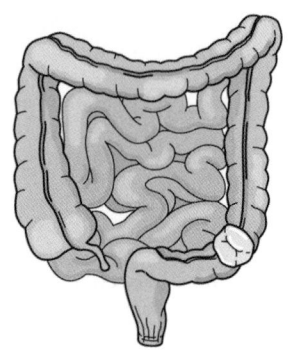

Sigmoid colostomy

Types of colostomies *(Monahan et al, 2007)*

colostrum /kəlos″trəm/ [L, first milk after birth], the fluid secreted by the breast during pregnancy and the first days after the delivery before lactation begins. It consists of immunologically active substances (maternal antibodies) and white blood cells, water, protein, fat, minerals, vitamins, and carbohydrate in a thin, yellow serous fluid. Compare **breast milk.**

colotomy /kōlot″əmē/, a surgical incision into the colon, usually performed through the abdominal wall.

colour blindness, also spelled **color blindness.**

Colour Index, a publication of dyers, colorists, and textile chemists that specifies all the standard industrial pigments and stains according to five-digit numbers associated with chemical coloring materials. For example, methylene blue is assigned number 52015.

colovaginal /kō′lōvaj″inəl/ [Gk, *kolon,* colon; L, *vagina,* sheath], pertaining to the colon and vagina, or to a communication between the two structures.

colovesical fistula, a fistula connecting the colon and the urinary bladder. Also called **vesicocolonic fistula.**

colp-. See **colpo-, colp-, kysth-, kystho-.**

colpalgia /kolpal″jə/, *(Obsolete)* a pain in the vagina.

colpectomy /kolpek″təmē/, the surgical excision of the vagina.

colpitis /kolpī″tis/, an inflammation of the vagina.

colpo-, colp-, kolpo-, kysth-, kystho-, combining form meaning "vagina": *colporrhaphy.*

colpocystocele /kol′pəsis″təsēl/, the prolapse of the urinary bladder into the vagina, usually through the anterior vaginal wall.

colpohysterectomy /-his′tərek″təmē/ [Gk, *kolpos,* vagina, *hystera,* womb, *ektomē,* excision], vaginal hysterectomy. See also **hysterectomy.**

colporrhaphy /kolpôr″əfē/ [Gk, *kolpos* + *raphe,* suture], a minimally invasive surgical procedure in which defects in the vagina are corrected by tightening muscles and returning stuctures to their usual anatomic position.

colposcope /kol″pəskōp/, a lighted instrument with lenses for direct examination of the surfaces of the vagina and cervix.

colposcopy /kolpos″kəpē/ [Gk, *kolpos* + *skopein,* to watch], a detailed examination of the vulva, vagina, and/or cervix with an optical magnifying instrument (colposcope). Its use facilitates directed biopsy of tissues suspicious for dysplasia or carcinoma rather than random biopsy sampling. Performed upon visualization of a lesion, because of an abnormal Pap smear or positive HPV test, or sometimes postcoital bleeding.

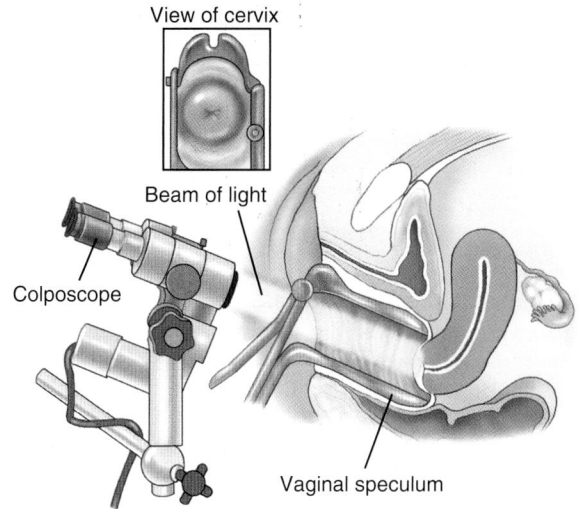

Colposcopy *(Leonard, 2015)*

colposuspension /kol″posuspen′shun/, bladder neck suspension.

colpotomy /kolpot″əmē/ [Gk, *kolpos* + *temnein,* to cut], any surgical incision into the wall of the vagina.

columbium. See **niobium.**

columella, **1.** a small column. **2.** the fleshy terminal portion of the nasal septum.

column, any elongated, cylindrical anatomical structure. It is usually oriented vertically and may provide structural support.

columna posterior. See **posterior horn.**

columnar cell /kəlum″nər/ [L, *columna,* column, *cella,* storeroom], an epithelial cell that appears long and narrow when sectioned along its long axis.

columnar epithelium [L, *columna,* column; Gk, *epi,* upon, *thele,* nipple], a type of epithelial cell that resembles a hexagonal prism.

column chromatography [L, *columna* + Gk, *chroma,* color, *graphein,* to record], the process of separating and analyzing a group of substances according to the differences in their absorption affinities for a given absorbent as evidenced by pigments deposited during filtration through the same absorbent contained in a glass cylinder or tube. The substances are dissolved in a liquid that is passed through the absorbent. The absorbates move down the column at different rates and leave behind a band of pigments that is subsequently washed with a pure solvent to develop discrete pigmented bands that constitute a chromatograph. The cylinder of absorbent is then pushed from the tube, and the individual bands are either separated with a knife or further diluted with the pure solvent and collected in the bottom of the tube for analysis. Effective column chromatography depends on the selection of the appropriate absorbent and solvent and a flow rate that is slow enough to allow complete diffusion of the absorbates from the solvent to the absorbent and the slowing of the absorbates according to their different affinities for the absorbent. Compare **gas chromatography, ion exchange chromatography.**

Coly-Mycin M, a parenteral antibacterial agent. Brand name for **colistimethate sodium.**

Coly-Mycin S, otic steroid and antibiotic combination. Brand name for **hydrocortisone, neomycin sulfate, colistin sulfate.**

com-. See **co-, col-, com-, con-, cor-.**

coma /kō″mə/ [Gk, *koma,* deep sleep], a state of profound unconsciousness, characterized by the absence of spontaneous eye openings, response to painful stimuli, and vocalization. The person cannot be aroused. Coma may be the result of trauma, space-occupying brain tumor, hematoma, cerebral edema, toxic metabolic condition, acute infectious disease with encephalitis, vascular disease, or brain ischemia. See also **Glasgow Coma Scale, unconscious.**

-coma, suffix meaning "(condition of) profound unconsciousness": *semicomatose.*

comatose /kō″mətōs/, pertaining to a state of coma, or abnormally deep sleep, caused by illness or injury.

combat fatigue [L, *com,* together, *battuere,* to beat, *fatigare,* to tire], any of a variety of psychological disorders, usually temporary but sometimes permanent, resulting from exhaustion, the stress of combat, or the cumulative emotions and psychological strain of warfare or other traumatic situations. It is characterized by anxiety, depression, irritability, memory and sleep disorders, and various related symptoms. Also called *combat neurosis,* **war neurosis.** See also **posttraumatic stress disorder, shell shock.**

combination chemotherapy /kom′binā″shən/, the simultaneous use of two or more anticancer drugs.

combined anesthesia. See **balanced anesthesia.**

combined carbon dioxide [L, *com,* together, *bini,* two-fold], the portion of the total carbon dioxide that is contained in blood carbonate, calculated as the difference between the total and dissolved carbon dioxide.

combined cycling ventilator, a mechanical ventilator that has more than one mechanism to recycle gases, such as equipment that may have time cycling or pressure cycling as a backup to a volume cycling control device.

combined oral contraceptive, an oral contraceptive pill that includes both an estrogen and a progestin.

combined oxygen, the oxygen that is physically bound to hemoglobin as oxyhemoglobin (HbO_2). One gram-molecular weight of oxygen can combine with 16,700 g of hemoglobin, and each gram of oxygen can bind with and carry 1.34 mL of oxygen.

combined patterns, a method of evaluating a patient's neuromuscular functions through tests that reveal the degree of coordination between movement patterns of the trunk and the extremities.

combined system disease, a disorder of the nervous system caused by a deficiency of vitamin B_{12} that results in pernicious anemia and degeneration of the spinal cord and peripheral nerves, marked by increased difficulty in walking, spasticity in lower extremities, a feeling of vibration in the legs, and a loss of sense of position. Also called **subacute combined degeneration of the spinal cord.** See also **cyanocobalamin, pernicious anemia.**

Combitube /kom′bit(y)oob/, a double-lumen tube with inflatable balloon cuffs that seal off the hypopharynx from the oropharynx and esophagus, used for airway management. It is inserted blindly, entering either the esophagus or trachea. If it enters the esophagus, one lumen, which has a blind distal end and side holes, functions as an esophageal obturator airway. If it enters the trachea, the other lumen, which has an open distal end, functions as a standard cuffed endotracheal tube.

Combivir /kom′bivir/, a combination preparation of the nucleoside analogs zidovudine and lamivudine, used in the treatment of HIV infection and AIDS. Brand name for **zidovudine, lamivudine.**

combustion /kəmbus″chen/, the process of burning or oxidation, which may be accompanied by light and heat. Oxygen itself does not burn, but it supports combustion. The rate of combustion is influenced by both oxygen concentration and its partial pressure.

comedo /kom″idō/ *pl. comedones* [L, *comedere,* to consume], blackhead (open comedo) or whitehead (closed comedo), the basic lesion of acne vulgaris, caused by an accumulation of keratin and sebum within the opening of a hair follicle. Compare **milium.**

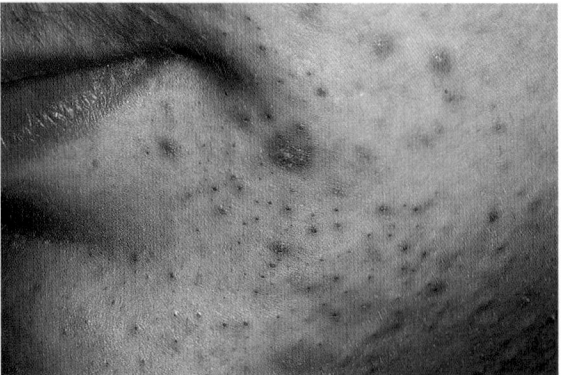

Comedos *(James et al, 2016)*

comedocarcinoma /kom′idōkär′sinō″mə/ *pl. comedocarcinomas, comedocarcinomata* [L, *comedere,* to consume; Gk, *karkinos,* crab, *oma,* tumor], a malignant intraductal neoplasm of the breast, in which the central cells degenerate and may be easily expressed from the cut surface of the tumor. Growth confined to the mammary ducts carries a better prognosis than do invasive breast lesions.

comedogenicity /kom′idōjənis″itē/, the ability of certain drugs or agents, such as anabolic steroids, to produce acne comedones.

comedomastitis, a dilated mammary duct.

comedones. See **comedo.**

comet assay. See **single-cell gel electrophoresis.**

comfort measure [L, *com,* together, *fortis,* strong], any action taken to promote the soothing of a patient, such as a back rub, a change in position, the prewarming of a stethoscope or bedpan, or administration of selected medications or treatments.

comfort zone [ME, *comforten* + Gk, *zone,* belt], **1.** the boundaries of temperature, humidity, wind velocity, and solar radiation within which a person dressed in a specified manner can perform certain tasks without discomfort. **2.** the psychological feeling of belonging or being comfortable in a specific area and/or role.

comfrey, a perennial herb found in the United States, Australia, and parts of Asia; also cultivated in Japan.

■ INDICATIONS: It is used for bruises, sprains, broken bones, acne, and boils. It is considered safe and possibly effective when used topically.

■ CONTRAINDICATIONS: Medicinal teas of comfrey are considered unsafe. Use of topical comfrey is not recommended during pregnancy and lactation, in children, and in those who are hypersensitive to this product. Internal use may cause fatal hepatotoxicity. It should not be used for more than 6 weeks or topically on broken skin.

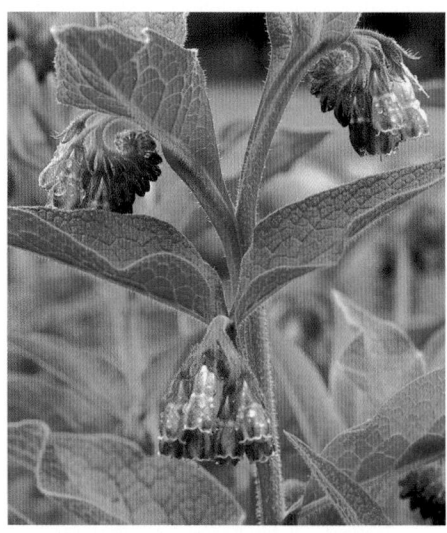

Comfrey plant *(Ulbricht, 2010)*

comitant strabismus. See **concomitant strabismus.**

Comité International des Poids et Mesures (CIPM) /kômitä″aNternäsyōnäl″dāpô·ä″āmesYr″/, a group of scientists who meet periodically to define the international (SI) units of physical quantities, such as the volume of a liter, the length of a meter, or the precise amount of time in a minute. See also **SI units.**

command [L, *commendare,* to protect], (in computer processing) an order given to the computer to execute a specific instruction, such as a code that evokes a particular program or performs a particular function.

command automatism, a condition characterized by an abnormal mechanical responsiveness to commands, usually followed without critical judgment, such as may be seen in hypnosis and certain psychotic states.

command hallucination, a condition in which individuals hear and sometimes obey voices that command them to perform certain acts. The hallucinations may influence them to engage in behavior that is dangerous to themselves or to others. Command hallucinations can be found in schizophrenia. On some occasions, only when the commands are powerful enough, violence, including murder, may occur. It is essential for health professionals to assess for this feature of the illness. See also **schizophrenia.**

commensal /kəmen″səl/ [L, *com,* together, *imensa,* table], (two different species) living together in an arrangement that is not harmful to either and that may be beneficial to both. Some bacteria in the digestive tract of humans aid in the processing of food and produce B vitamins needed for normal health while causing no harm (normal flora). Compare **parasite, synergist.**

commensalism /kəmen″səliz′əm/, a symbiosis in which one species benefits but the other species is neither helped nor harmed.

comminuted /kom″inyo͞o′tid/ [L, *comminuere,* to break into pieces], crushed or broken into a number of pieces.

comminuted fracture, a fracture in which the bone is broken in several places or is shattered, creating numerous fragments. Also called **fragmented fracture.**

Commission E, a German interdisciplinary regulatory committee whose function is to review herbal drugs and preparations from medicinal plants and evaluate and approve their safety and efficacy.

Commission on Accreditation of Rehabilitation Facilities, an independent accrediting agency covering and coordinating many human health services and disciplines in areas such as aging, behavioral health, children, vision services, employment, and more.

Commission on Collegiate Nursing Education (CCNE), an autonomous accrediting agency whose mission includes the assessment and identification of nursing programs that engage in effective educational practices, having a scope of the institutions of higher education in the United States offering nursing programs at the bachelor's, master's, and doctor of nursing practice level.

commissure /kom″iso͝or, -syo͝or/, **1.** a band of nerve fiber or other tissue that crosses from one side of the body to the other, usually connecting two structures or masses of tissue. **2.** a site of union of two anatomical parts, as the corner of the eye, lips, or labia.

commissurotomy /kom″isho͝orot″əme̅/ [L, *commissura,* a connection; Gk, *temnein,* to cut], the surgical division of a fibrous band or ring connecting corresponding parts of a body structure. A commissurotomy is commonly performed to separate the thickened, adherent leaves of a stenosed mitral valve.

commitment [L, *committere,* to entrust], **1.** the placement or confinement of an individual in a specialized hospital or other institutional facility. See also **institutionalize. 2.** the legal procedure of admitting a mentally ill person to an institution for psychiatric treatment. The process varies from state to state but usually involves

judicial or court action based on medical evidence certifying that the person is mentally ill. See also **certification. 3.** a pledge or contract to fulfill some obligation or agreement, used especially in some forms of psychotherapy or marriage counseling.

common baldness, androgenetic alopecia, in men called common male baldness and in women called common female baldness. Hair loss in women may be age-related or hormonal, or it may be associated with genetic predisposition; the hair thins all over the scalp, usually permanently, but the frontal hairline is maintained.

common bile duct [L, *communis,* common, *bilis,* bile, *ducere,* to lead], the duct formed by the juncture of the cystic and hepatic ducts.

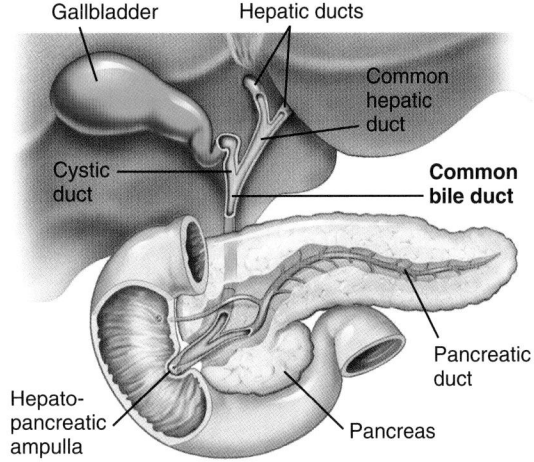

Common bile duct

common carotid artery [L, *communis* + Gk, *karos,* heavy sleep, *arteria,* airpipe], one of the two major arteries supplying blood to the head and neck. Each divides into an external carotid artery and an internal carotid artery.

common carotid plexus, a network of nerves on the common carotid artery, supplying sympathetic fibers to the head and the neck, with branches that accompany the cranial blood vessels. The common carotid plexus is formed by the internal and external carotid plexuses and by the cervical ganglia of the sympathetic system.

common cold. See **cold.**

common core standards (CCS), learning goals for English language arts and mathematical skills established for individual grade levels. Occupational and physical therapy goals, as well as the goals of the school nurse, must take the common core standards into consideration to establish educationally appropriate goals for a student requiring an individualized education program (IEP).

common fibular nerve, a nerve originating from the sciatic nerve that gives origin to two cutaneous branches, the sural communicating nerve, which contributes to the innervation of the skin over the lower posterolateral side of the leg, and the lateral sural cutaneous nerve, which innervates the skin over the upper lateral leg. It then continues around the neck of the fibula and enters the lateral compartment, where it divides into the superficial fibular nerve and the deep fibular nerve. The superficial fibular nerve innervates the fibularis longus and brevis and some of the dorsal areas of the foot and toes. The deep fibular nerve innervates the anterior compartment of the leg.

common hepatic artery, the visceral branch of the celiac trunk of the abdominal aorta, passing posterior to the pylorus and dividing into five branches: the gastroduodenal, right gastric, right hepatic, left hepatic, and middle hepatic.

common iliac artery, a division of the abdominal aorta, starting in front of the fourth lumbar vertebra, passing caudally about 5 cm, and dividing into external and internal iliac arteries. The right common iliac artery is somewhat longer than the left.

common iliac node, a node in one of the seven groups of parietal lymph nodes serving the abdomen and the pelvis. They drain the internal and external iliac nodes and pass their materials to the lateral aortic nodes. Compare **external iliac node, iliac circumflex node, internal iliac node.** See also **lymph, lymphatic system, lymph node.**

common iliac vein, one of the two veins that are the sources of the inferior vena cava, formed by the union of the internal and external iliac veins, ventral to the sacroiliac articulation. Each common iliac vein receives the iliolumbar and, in some individuals, the lateral sacral veins. The left common iliac vein also receives the middle sacral vein. Neither of the common iliacs contains valves. Compare **external iliac vein, internal iliac vein.**

common pathway of coagulation, the pathway common to both intrinsic and extrinsic coagulation pathways. Once activated, factor X forms a complex with its cofactor, factor V, to convert prothrombin to thrombin. Thrombin splits peptides from fibrinogen to produce a fibrin clot. See also **extrinsic pathway of coagulation, intrinsic pathway of coagulation.**

common tendinous ring, the thickening of the periorbita around the optic canal and the central part of the superior orbital fissure in the posterior part of the bony orbit. It is the point of origin of the four rectus muscles.

common variable immunodeficiency (CVID), a heterogeneous group of disorders characterized by hypogammaglobulinemia, decreased antibody production in response to antigenic challenge, and recurrent pyogenic infections, and often associated with hematological and autoimmune disorders. Most patients have normal numbers of circulating B cells that can identify antigens and proliferate, but they lack plasma cells and may have an intrinsic defect of B cell differentiation. Two less common forms are also recognized, one caused by a disorder of T lymphocyte regulation and one caused by production of autoantibodies against T and B lymphocytes.

commotio cordis, damage to the heart, frequently fatal, resulting from a sharp nonpenetrating blow to the adjacent body surface.

commune /kom″yoon/, **1.** a small community of people who share certain social and economic objectives. Members may also share property ownership and control local political leadership and are committed to the concept of holistic medicine. **2.** *v.,* to communicate in a deep, intimate way with another, with nature, or with the inner self.

communicability period /kəmyoo′nəkəbil″itē/, the time during which an infectious agent may be transferred directly or indirectly from an infected person to another person, from an infected animal to humans, or from an infected person to animals, including arthropods. For measles the communicability period ranges from 4 days before the appearance of a rash until 5 days after the onset of symptoms.

communicable /kəmyoo′nəkəbəl/ [L, *communis,* common], transmissible by direct or indirect means, as a communicable disease. See also **contagious.**

communicable disease, any disease transmitted from one person or animal to another directly, by contact with excreta or other discharges from the body; indirectly, by means of substances or inanimate objects, such as contaminated drinking glasses, toys, or water; or by means of vectors, such as flies, mosquitoes, ticks, or other insects. Communicable diseases may be caused by bacteria, chlamydia, fungi, parasites, rickettsiae, and viruses. To control a communicable disease, it is important to identify the organism, prevent its spread to the environment, protect others against contamination, and treat the infected person. Many communicable diseases, by law, must be reported to the local health department. Also called **contagious disease.**

Communicable Disease Center, *(Obsolete)* now called **Centers for Disease Control and Prevention (CDC).**

communicating hydrocephalus /kəmyoo′nikā″ting/ [L, *communicans* + Gk, *hydor,* water, *kephale,* head], a form of hydrocephalus in which there is an increase in cerebrospinal fluid that involves the entire ventricular system and the subarachnoid space. It is caused by an abnormality in the ability to absorb fluid in the subarachnoid space. No obstruction exists in the ventricular pathways.

communication /kəmyoo′nikā″shən/ [L, *communis,* common], any process in which a message containing information is transferred, especially from one person to another, by any of a number of media. Communication may be verbal or nonverbal; it may occur directly, such as in a face-to-face conversation or with the observation of a gesture; or it may occur remotely, spanning space and time, such as in writing and reading or in making or playing back of a recording. Communication is basic to all health care professions and contributes to the development of all therapeutic relationships. See also **kinesics, therapeutic communication.**

communication channels, (in communication theory) any gesture, action, sound, written word, or visual image used in transmitting messages.

communication disorders, 1. (in speech-language pathology) deficits resulting from genetic influences, injury, or disease. Communication disorders include cleft palate, oral-motor dysfunction, and laryngeal anomalies. People with speech problems may say sounds unclearly, have a hoarse or raspy voice, or repeat sounds or pause when speaking (stuttering). People with language disorders may have problems understanding, talking, reading, or writing. See also **speech language disorders. 2.** See **social (pragmatic) communication disorder.**

communication theme, (in psychiatry) a recurrent concept or idea that ties together components of communication. Kinds include **content theme, mood theme,** *interaction theme.*

communication theory, a hypothesis that describes a model for information transfer consisting of a source of information (the sender), a transmitter, a communication channel, a source of noise (interference), a receiver, and a purpose for the message.

community /kəmyoo′nitē/ [L, *communis,* common], **1.** a group of species who reside in a designated geographic area and who share common interests or bonds. **2.** a person's natural environment, where the person works, plays, and performs other daily activities. **3.** an area with geographic and often political boundaries demarcated as a district, country, metropolitan area, city, township, or neighborhood. **4.** a place whose members have a sense of identity and belonging, and shared values, norms, communication styles and patterns of behavior.

community-acquired infection, an infection contracted outside a health care setting or an infection present on admission. Community-acquired infections are often distinguished from nosocomial, or hospital-acquired, diseases by the types of organisms that affect patients who are recovering from a disease or injury. Community-acquired respiratory infections

Communicating with patients who have special needs

Patients with difficulty hearing
Avoid shouting.
Use simple sentences.
Punctuate speech with facial expression and gestures.

Patients with difficulty seeing
Communicate verbally before touching the patient.
Orient the patient to sounds in the environment.
Inform the patient when the conversation is over and when you are leaving the room.

Patients who are mute or cannot speak clearly
Place sign by unit call system to answer call light in person's room.
Listen attentively, be patient, and do not interrupt.
Do not finish patients' sentences for them.
Ask simple questions that require ''yes'' or ''no'' answers.
Allow time for understanding and responses.
Use visual cues (e.g., words, pictures, objects) when possible.
Allow only one person to speak at a time.
Do not shout or speak too loudly.
Encourage the client to converse.
Let the patient know if you do not understand.
Use communication aids as needed:
Pad and felt-tipped pen or Magic Slate
Flash cards
Communication board with words, letters, or pictures denoting basic needs
Computer toy (''speak and spell'' type)
Call bells or alarms
Sign language
Use of eye blinks or movement of fingers for simple responses (''yes'' or ''no'')

Patients who are cognitively impaired
Reduce environmental distractions while conversing.
Get the patient's attention before speaking.
Use simple sentences and avoid long explanations.
Avoid shifting from subject to subject.
Ask one question at a time.
Allow time for the client to respond.
Include family and friends to conversations, especially in subjects known to the patient.

Patients who are unresponsive
Call the patient by name during interactions.
Communicate both verbally and by touch.
Speak to the patient as though he or she could hear.
Explain all procedures and sensations.

Patients who do not speak English
Speak to the patient in a normal tone of voice (shouting may be interpreted as anger).
Establish a method for the client to signal the desire to communicate (call light or bell).
Provide a professional interpreter/translator as needed:
Use a person familiar with the patient's culture and with biomedicine if possible.
Allow plenty of time for the interpreter to transmit messages.
Communicate directly to the patient and family rather than the interpreter.
Ask one question at a time.
Avoid making comments to the interpreter about the patient or family (they may understand some English).
Develop a communication board, pictures, or cards using words translated into English for the patient to make basic requests (e.g., pain medication, water, elimination)
Have a dictionary (English/Spanish or appropriate) available if the patient can read.

From Potter PA et al: *Basic nursing: essentials for practice,* ed 7, St. Louis, 2009, Mosby.

commonly involve strains of *Haemophilus influenzae* or *Streptococcus pneumoniae* and are usually more antibiotic sensitive. Community-acquired infections are sometimes distinguished by the type of organism with the prefix CA. For example, the designation for an community-acquired infection with MRSA is CA-MRSA.

community dental health coordinator (CDHC), a person whose duties are to assist dentists in improving dental care for patients with limited or no care. A CDHC works with other dental team members under the remote supervision of a dentist. CDHCs increase access for underserved people by coordinating their dental needs, triaging care based on emergent or urgent needs, and organizing transportation and other logistical or social support as needed. A CDHC is not intended to substitute for a dentist in providing clinical care; performs no irreversible procedures; does not diagnose; screens patients for emergent, urgent, or routine dental care; and may places temporary restorations after consulting with the supervising dentist. CDHC duties can vary by state dental rules.

community health center, a site for providing primary health care designed to meet the unique needs of the people in its surrounding community. The emphasis on a local approach to health care, combined with comprehensive preventive care, is designed to provide more cost-effective health care.

community health nursing, a field of nursing that is a blend of primary health care and nursing practice with public health nursing. The community health nurse conducts a continuing and comprehensive practice that is preventive, curative, and rehabilitative. The philosophy of care is based on the belief

that care directed to the individual, the family, and the group contributes to the health care of the population as a whole. The community health nurse is not restricted to the care of a particular age or diagnostic group. Participation of all consumers of health care is encouraged in the development of community activities that contribute to the promotion of, education about, and maintenance of good health. These activities require comprehensive health programs that pay special attention to social and ecological influences and specific populations at risk.

community medicine, a branch of medicine that is concerned with the health of the members of a community, municipality, or region. The emphasis in community medicine is on the early diagnosis of disease, the recognition of environmental and occupational hazards to good health, and the prevention of disease in the community.

community mental health, a holistic, psychosocial treatment philosophy based on the social model of psychiatric care that advocates that a comprehensive range of mental health services be readily accessible to all members of the community.

community mental health center (CMHC), a community-based center that provides comprehensive mental health services, including ambulatory and inpatient care. The specific services to be provided are defined in an act of the U.S. Congress, the Community Mental Health Centers Act; these requirements have been updated periodically. The costs of consultation and educational services, instruction, development, and initial operation of the facility are paid for by the federal government. The organization, management, and operation of CMHCs are also specified by the act. Consumer representation in each of these areas is required. In Canada, a CMHC is a clinic much like a public health clinic, with a focus on mental health promotion and mental illness prevention. It does not include inpatient care. Assessments and outpatient and ongoing care are provided for those struggling with mental health issues, such as anxiety or grief and loss, and for those with mental illness.

community mobility, the ability to navigate the geographic, social, and physical environments outside the home environment. It includes the use of public and private transportation, walking, bicycling, driving, and other forms of transportation.

community psychiatry, the branch of psychiatry concerned with the development of an adequate and coordinated program of mental health care for residents of specified catchment areas. See also **community mental health center.**

community rating, a mechanism used by insurance companies in the United States to determine the percent of cost sharing for members of a group health insurance plan. Medical expenses are estimated based on a geographic region, with all members paying the same amount. Compare **experience rating.**

community reintegration, the return and acceptance of a person with a cognitive or physical disability as a participating member of the community.

Comolli sign /kōmō″lēs/ [Antonio Comolli, Italian pathologist, 1879–1975], a triangular swelling corresponding to the shape of the scapula after a fracture of that bone.

comorbidity, pertaining to a disease or other pathological process that occurs simultaneously with another.

compact bone /kom″pakt, kompakt″/ [L, *compingere,* to put together], hard, dense bone that is usually found at the periphery of skeletal structures, as distinguished from spongy cancellous bone.

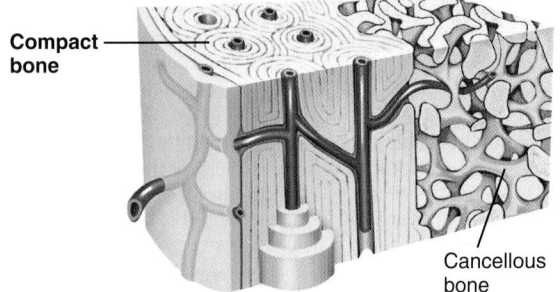

Compact bone

Cancellous bone

Compact bone

compact disc (CD), an optical disk on which computer data are encoded or on which sound is recorded in a digital format.

companion animal, a domesticated animal that provides health benefits to a person. Companion animals may help relieve stress or serve a more active role, as do guide dogs for persons with visual impairments, dogs trained to detect telephone or doorbell sounds for persons with hearing deficits, or dogs who can detect seizures in individuals with seizure disorders and then signal for help.

companionship /kəmpan″yənship′/ [L, *com,* together, *panis,* food], **1.** (in psychiatric nursing) the assignment of a staff member to stay with a disturbed patient to provide support and to protect the patient from self-harm or harm to others. In constant companionship the disturbed patient is accompanied in all activities until the staff member is convinced the patient has regained control. Also called *constant observation.* **2.** an inherent human social need for contact with another.

comparative anatomy /kəmper″ətiv/ [L, *com + par,* equal], the study of the morphological characteristics of all living animals. A comparison of the forms indicates a progression on a scale from the simplest to the most highly specialized animals. The adult stage of animals that are lower in the scale resembles the immature stages of many higher-level animals. See also **applied anatomy, ontogeny, phylogeny.**

comparative embryology, the study of the similarities and differences among various organisms during the embryological period of development.

comparative genomic hybridization, a cytogenetic technique in which reference DNA and the DNA to be studied, as from a tumor or an embryo, are labeled with green- and red-fluorescing fluorochromes, respectively. Genetic abnormalities are detected by changes in the green-to-red ratio.

comparative method, the analytic method in which the test method is compared to a standard, known reference method. It allows errors to be attributed to the test method because the accuracy of the reference method is known.

comparative physiology, the study of the similarities and differences of the vital processes found in various species of living organisms to determine fundamental physiological relationships between members of the animal and plant kingdoms.

comparative psychology, **1.** the study of human behavior as it relates to, or differs from, animal behavior. **2.** the study of the psychological and behavioral differences among various peoples.

compartment model /kəmpärt″mənt/, a mathematic representation of the body or an area of the body created to study physiological or pharmacological kinetic characteristics. A compartment model can simulate all of the biological processes involved in the kinetic behavior of a drug after it has been introduced into the body, leading to a better understanding of its pharmacodynamic effects. Studies most frequently use one- or two-compartment models. In a one-compartment model the body assumes the characteristics of a homogeneous unit in which an administered drug diffuses instantaneously in the volume of body fluid. In a two-compartment model the body is represented as two distinct compartments, a central and a peripheral compartment, with two separate fluid volumes.

compartment syndrome [L, *com + partiri,* to share], **1.** an acute pathological condition caused by elevation of tissue pressure within a closed space, resulting in the progressive development of compression and consequent reduction of blood supply. The compression may result from swelling within an overly restrictive dressing or cast or from nonexpansive muscle fascia. Clinical manifestations include swelling, restriction of movement, brown urine, myoglobinuria, vascular compromise, and severe pain or lack of sensation. Severe pain may appear out of proportion to the injury and is one of the earliest manifestations of this emergency situation. It can result in a permanent contracture deformity of the hand or foot, with or without a fracture. In severe cases, it can lead to necrosis and necessitate the amputation of an extremity. Treatment includes elevation, removal of restrictive dressings or casts, and potentially a surgical decompression or open fasciotomy. See also **Volkmann contracture.** **2.** a chronic pathological condition caused by elevation of tissue pressure within a closed space (compartment) during exercise. Clinical manifestations are pain in the affected extremity (usually the lower legs) and occasional numbness. Symptoms are relieved by rest and will recur with renewed exercising. This condition is not a medical emergency and is treated by eliminating the aggravating activities or limited fasciotomy.

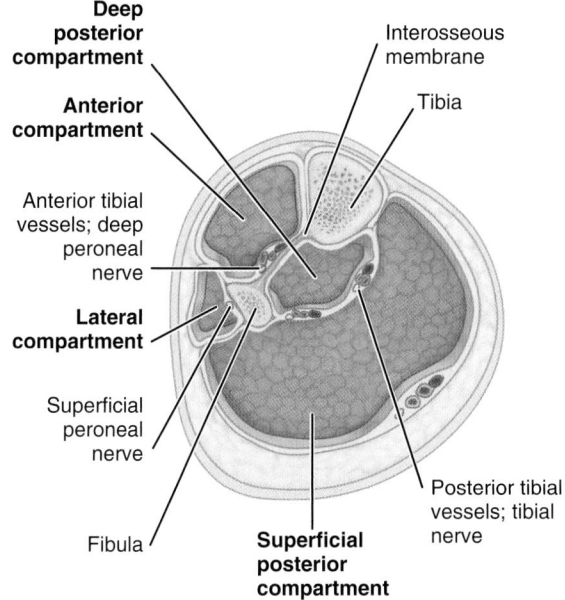

Deep posterior compartment

Anterior compartment

Anterior tibial vessels; deep peroneal nerve

Lateral compartment

Superficial peroneal nerve

Fibula

Interosseous membrane

Tibia

Posterior tibial vessels; tibial nerve

Superficial posterior compartment

NORMAL ANATOMY

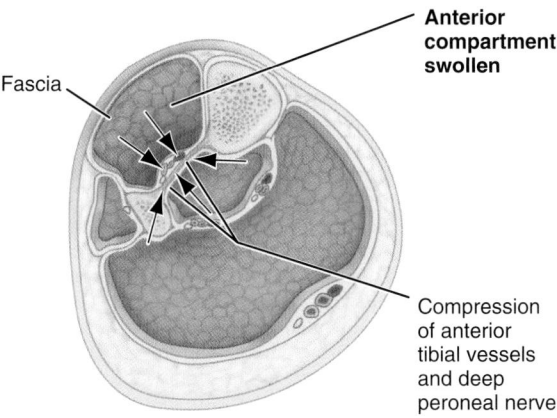

Fascia

Anterior compartment swollen

Compression of anterior tibial vessels and deep peroneal nerve

ANTERIOR COMPARTMENT SYNDROME

Anterior compartment syndrome (Black and Hawks, 2009)

compatibility /kəmpat′əbil″itē/ [L, *compatibilis,* agreeable], **1.** the quality or state of existing together in harmony; congruity. **2.** the orderly, efficient integration of the elements of one system with those of another. **3.** the formation of a stable chemical or biochemical system, specifically in medication, so that two or more drugs can be administered at the same time without producing undesired side effects or without canceling or affecting the therapeutic effects of the others. **4.** (in immunology) the degree to which the body's defense system tolerates the presence of foreign material, such as transfused blood, grafted tissue, or transplanted organs, without an immune reaction. Usually identical twins are completely compatible. **5.** (in blood grouping or crossmatching) the lack of reaction between blood groups so that there is no agglutination when the red blood cells of one

sample are mixed with the serum of another sample; no reaction from transfused blood. **−compatible,** *adj.*

compatible, **1.** capable of harmonious coexistence, said of two or more medications that are suitable for simultaneous administration without nullification or aggravation of their effects. **2.** denoting a donor and recipient of a blood transfusion in which there is no transfusion reaction. **3.** histocompatible.

Compazine, a phenothiazine. Brand name for **prochlorperazine.**

compendium /kəmpen″dē·əm/ *pl. compendia* [L, *compendere,* to weigh], a collected body of information on the standards of strength, purity, and quality of drugs. The official compendia in the United States are the *United States Pharmacopoeia,* the *Homeopathic Pharmacopoeia of the United States,* and their supplements. See also **formulary.**

compensated acidosis /kom″pənsā′tid/ [L, *compensare,* to balance, *acidus,* sour; Gk, *osis,* condition], a condition in which the pH of the blood is maintained within normal limits (adult/child: 7.35 to 7.45) although the blood bicarbonate level is below normal or the PCO_2 is above normal. This compensation is accomplished by the lungs and/or kidneys altering their functions.

compensated alkalosis, a condition in which the blood bicarbonate is increased or the PCO_2 is decreased but compensation by the lung and kidneys keeps the blood pH within the normal range.

compensated flowmeter [L, *compensare,* to balance], a gas therapy device with a scale that is calibrated against a constant pressure of 50 psi instead of the atmosphere. It is equipped with a valve distal to the gauge to record the output to the patient accurately.

compensated gluteal gait, one of the more common abnormal gaits associated with a weakness of the gluteus medius. It is a variation of the Trendelenburg gait. It involves the dropping of the pelvis on the unaffected side of the body during the walking cycle between the moment of heel strike on the affected side and before the moment of heel strike on the unaffected side. The compensated gluteal gait is also characterized by the dropping of the entire trunk downward and sideways over the affected hip and a short step on the unaffected side. In a compensated gait the trunk is forcibly thrown laterally during the weight-bearing or stance phase in the movement of the affected lower limb. This lateral movement is the result of an attempt to shift a significant portion of body weight above and outside the center of rotation of the affected hip. During this movement the erector spinae and the quadratus lumborum of the involved side function to lift the whole weight of the pelvis and the opposite lower extremity off the ground to allow the uninvolved leg to clear during its swing phase.

compensated heart failure, an abnormal cardiac condition in which heart failure is compensated for by such mechanisms as increased sympathetic stimulation of the heart, fluid retention with increased venous return, increased end-diastolic ventricular volume and fiber length, and ventricular hypertrophy. Progressive decline in cardiac function may be minimized by the administration of beta-blockers, digitalis glycosides, and angiotensin-converting enzyme inhibitors, to improve myocardial function and diuretics to relieve pulmonary and peripheral congestion. See also **heart failure.**

compensating current /kom″pənsā′ting/, an electric current that neutralizes the intensity of a muscle current.

compensating curve, the curvature of alignment of the occlusal surfaces of the teeth, developed to compensate for the paths of the condyles as the mandible moves from centric

C

to eccentric positions. For full dentures, it is used to maintain posterior tooth contacts to keep the dentures seated on the alveolar ridge on the molar teeth and to provide balancing contacts associated with a protruding mandible. The compensating curve corresponds to the curve of Spee in natural teeth.

compensating filter, a device used to absorb radiation during the radiographic process. The compensating filter is placed over a body area to compensate for body areas of various thicknesses and to even out the resulting radiographic densities. For example, a wedge may be placed over a foot with the thick portion over the toes and the thin edge toward the heel to compensate for the range of thickness of the foot. See also **bowtie filter.**

compensation /kom′pənsā″shən/ [L, *compensare,* to balance], **1.** the process of counterbalancing any defect in body structure or function. **2.** the process of maintaining an adequate blood flow through such cardiac and circulatory mechanisms as tachycardia, fluid retention with increased venous return, and ventricular hypertrophy. Lack of compensation indicates a diseased heart muscle. See also **compensated heart failure. 3.** a complex defense mechanism that allows one to avoid the unpleasant or painful emotional stimuli that result from a feeling of inferiority or inadequacy. Examples include making an extraordinary effort to overcome a disability, scorning a quality that one lacks ("sour grapes"), and substituting hard work and excellent performance in one field for a lack of ability in another. **4.** changes in structural relationships that accommodate foundation disturbances and maintain balance. See also **overcompensation.**

compensator /kom″pənsā′tər/, a device used in radiotherapy to correct for irregularities in body surfaces by providing a differential attenuation of the x-ray beam before it reaches the patient. The result is a more uniform distribution of radiation dose in the tumor. Compensators are generally mounted on the collimator system of a teletherapy unit.

compensatory hypertrophy /kəmpen″sətôr′ē/ [L, *compensare,* to balance], an increase in the size or the function of an organ or part to counteract a structural or functional defect. See also **compensated heart failure.**

compensatory movement patterns, movements of the body that an individual uses to achieve functional movement due to reduced voluntary muscle control or available range of motion. For example, an individual who elevates the scapula and performs trunk extension to substitute for reduced shoulder flexion during a reaching task.

compensatory pause, a pause noted on an electrocardiogram after a premature complex. It precedes the next normal complex.

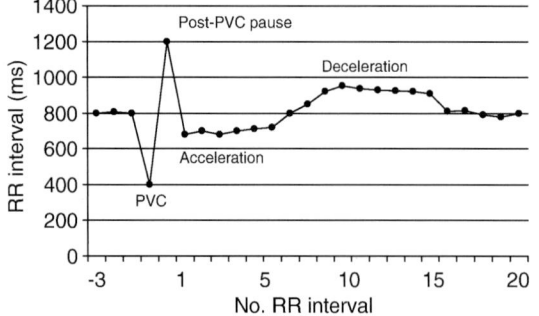

Compensatory pause: graph showing the physiological changes in sinus RR interval, which follow a PVC with a typical compensatory pause (HR turbulence) *(Lanza, 2007)*

competence /kom″pətəns/ [L, *competentia,* capable], **1.** (in embryology) the total capacity of an embryonic cell to react to determinative stimuli in various ways of differentiation. **2.** the ability of bacteria to take up donor deoxyribonucleic acid molecules. **3.** an expected standard of skill and knowledge by a health care professional. **4.** the ability of a patient to manage activities of daily living.

competent community /kom″pətənt/, a population that is aware of resources and alternatives, can make reasoned decisions about issues facing the group, and can cope adaptively with problems. It parallels the concept of positive mental health.

competitive antagonist, a substance that interferes with usual metabolic activity by competing for binding sites on a substrate (the substance on which an enzyme acts in a chemical reaction) or on an enzyme that ordinarily attacks the substrate. The antagonist is usually an analog of the substrate. See also **antimetabolite.**

competitive-binding assay /kompet″itiv/ [L, *competere,* to come together], an analytic procedure based on the reversible binding of a ligand to a binding protein. In proportion to its concentration, the ligand competes with a labeled derivative for binding to the limited number of available binding sites.

competitive displacement, the tendency of one drug to displace another at nonspecific protein-binding sites (e.g., plasma albumin) when both drugs are taken at the same time. Only free drug is able to bind to its specific target proteins. An example is phenylbutazone, which has a greater affinity for binding sites on plasma proteins than warfarin. As a result, if both drugs are taken at the same time, fewer binding sites are available for warfarin, thereby increasing its free concentration in the plasma and increasing its anticoagulant action in the liver to potentially undesirable levels.

competitive identification, the unconscious modeling of one's personality on that of another as a means of outdoing or bettering the other person. See also **identification.**

competitive inhibitor, an inhibitor of an enzyme reaction that competes with the substrate by binding at the active site.

complaint [L, *complangere,* to beat the breast], **1.** (in law) a pleading by a plaintiff made under oath to initiate a suit. It is a statement of the formal charge and the cause for action against the defendant. For a minor offense the defendant is tried on the basis of the complaint. A more serious felony prosecution requires an indictment with evidence presented by a state's attorney. **2.** *(Informal)* any ailment, problem, or symptom identified by a patient, a member of the patient's family, or other knowledgeable person. The chief complaint often causes the patient to seek health care.

complement (C) /kom″pləmənt/ [L, *complementum,* that which completes], a system of at least 20 complex enzymatic serum proteins. In an antigen-antibody reaction, activation of complement causes cell lysis. Complement is also involved in other physiological reactions, including inflammation, anaphylaxis, and phagocytosis. See also **antibody, antigen, antigen-antibody reaction, immune gamma globulin.**

complement abnormality, an unusual condition characterized by deficiencies or dysfunctions of any of the 11 serum proteins known as complement and designated C1-C11. The most common abnormalities are C2 and C3 deficiencies and C5 familial dysfunction. Patients with complement abnormalities may be more susceptible to infections and to collagen vascular diseases. Primary complement abnormalities may be inherited, whereas secondary complement abnormalities may stem from immunological reactions, such as drug-induced serum disease, which depletes complement.

Complement deficiencies may be associated with other illnesses, such as acute streptococcal glomerulonephritis, acute systemic lupus erythematosus, and dermatomyositis.

■ OBSERVATIONS: Increased susceptibility to systemic bacterial infection is associated with C2 and C3 deficiencies and with C5 familial dysfunction. Chronic renal failure and lupus erythematosus may also be associated with C2 deficiency. Signs of C5 dysfunction are malaise, diarrhea, and seborrheic dermatitis. Diagnosis of complement abnormalities is difficult and often expensive. Some indications are electrocardiographic conduction abnormalities; detection of complement and immunoglobulins in the walls of blood vessels in glomerulonephritis; cerebrospinal fluid pleocytosis; increased erythrocyte sedimentation rate; and presence in the urine of red blood cells (RBCs), RBC casts, and protein.

■ INTERVENTIONS: Replacement of complement-fixing antibodies and control of infection and associated illnesses are part of standard treatment for complement abnormalities. The patient commonly receives transfusion of fresh plasma to replace antibodies. Bone marrow transplantations and injection of gamma globulin may also be used, but the former carries the risk of a fatal graft-versus-host reaction. Complement abnormalities are usually corrected temporarily by replacement therapy, but no permanent cure is available.

■ PATIENT CARE CONSIDERATIONS: Patients should be carefully monitored, especially if they are receiving gamma globulin injections. Patients also should be instructed to exercise scrupulous hygiene, to seek prompt treatment of even the smallest wounds, and to avoid crowds or persons with active infections. Members of the health care team should be alert for early signs of ataxia or slight changes in mental activity that may signal neurological damage caused by infection.

complemental inheritance /kom′pləmen″təl/, the expression of a trait as a result of the presence of two independent pairs of nonallelic genes. Both of the genes must be present for the trait to appear in the phenotype.

complementary and alternative medicine (CAM), a large and diverse set of systems of diagnosis, treatment, and prevention based on philosophies and techniques other than those used in conventional Western medicine, often derived from traditions of medical practice used in other (non-Western) cultures. Such practices may be described as alternative, that is, existing as a body separate from and as a replacement for conventional Western medicine, or complementary, that is, used in addition to conventional Western practice. CAM is characterized by its focus on the whole person as a unique individual, on the energy of the body and its influence on health and disease, on the healing power of nature and the mobilization of the body's own resources to heal itself, and on the treatment of the underlying causes, rather than symptoms, of disease. Many of the techniques have not been validated by controlled studies.

complementary feeding /kom′pləmen″tərē/ [L, *complementum,* that which completes], a supplemental feeding given to an infant who is making the transition to solid foods while still breastfeeding. The World Health Organization identifies this an an important period for the infant. The transition from exclusive breastfeeding to family foods typically covers the period from 6 months through 18 to 24 months of age.

complementary gene, either member of two or more nonallelic gene pairs that interact to produce an effect not expressed in the absence of any of the pairs. Also called **reciprocal gene.**

complement assay, a blood test used primarily to measure serum complement in an effort to diagnose angioedema and to monitor the activity of disease in patients with systemic lupus erythematosus nephritis, membranoproliferative nephritis, or poststreptococcal nephritis.

complement cascade, a biochemical process involving the C1 to C9 complement proteins in which one protein interacts with another in a specific sequence called a complement pathway. C5b with C6, C7, C8, and C9 form the membrane attack complex that initiates cell lysis. Other molecules, such as C3a and C5a, act as cytokines, leading to inflammation.

complement control protein (CCP), any of a large family of proteins involved in complement regulation, encoded in a closely linked gene cluster, and having one or more stretches of a common short repeated sequence. See also **complement.**

complement fixation, an immunological reaction in which an antigen combines with an antibody and its complement, causing the complement factor to become inactive or fixed. The complement-fixation reaction can be tested in the laboratory by exposing the patient's serum to antigen, complement, and specially sensitized red blood cells. Complement-fixation tests can be used to detect antibodies for infectious diseases, especially syphilis and viral illnesses. They are rarely used in clinical practice today. See also **anticomplement, complement, immune system, immunity, Wassermann blood test.**

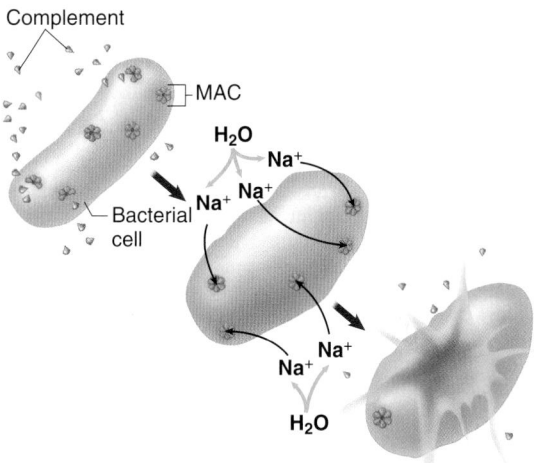

Complement fixation *(Patton and Thibodeau, 2010)*

complement-fixation test, any serological test in which complement fixation is detected, indicating the presence of a particular antigen. Specific C-F tests are used to aid in the diagnosis of amebiasis, Rocky Mountain spotted fever, trypanosomiasis, and typhus. They are rarely used in contemporary clinical practice.

complement inactivation [L, *in + activus, complere,* to complete], the loss of activity of complement proteins in blood, achieved by heating the serum to about 133° F (56° C).

complement protein molecule [L, *complementum + proteios,* first rank], any of the protein molecules that are chief humoral mediators of antigen-antibody reactions in the immune system. Complement proteins stimulate phagocytosis and inflammation. Nine are involved in the "classical pathway" cascade that results in the lysis of antibody-coated bacteria. They are designated C1 to C9. Overall, more than 30 complement proteins have been identified so far.

complete abortion [L, *complere,* to fill up], spontaneous expulsion of the entire contents of a documented pregnancy (fetus, placenta, membranes) before the time of extrauterine viability. Because no products of conception remain in the uterus, surgical evacuation is not needed. Compare **incomplete abortion, missed abortion.** See **miscarriage.**

complete bed bath, a bath in which the entire body of a patient is washed while he or she is in bed.

complete blood count (CBC), a standard hematological test profile performed on whole blood that measures erythrocyte, leukocyte, and thrombocyte parameters of volume and morphology, typically automated. A CBC is one of the most routinely performed tests in a clinical laboratory and one of the most valuable screening and diagnostic techniques. The normal red blood cell (RBC) count in adult males is 4.7 to 6.1 million/mm³. In adult females the normal RBC is 4.2 to 5.4 million/mm³. Each type of white blood cell can be represented as a percentage of the total number of white cells observed. This is called a differential count. The normal adult WBC count is 5000 to 10,000/mm³. Electronic blood counters also automatically determine hemoglobin or hematocrit and include this value in the CBC. See also **differential white blood cell count, erythrocyte, hematocrit, hemoglobin, leukocyte.**

complete breech, a buttocks-first fetal presentation with the legs folded on the thighs and the thighs on the abdomen. (The feet are next to the thighs and not the head as in frank breech presentation.) Compare **frank breech.** See also **breech birth.**

complete color blindness, monochromatic vision.

complete denture. See **full denture.**

complete dislocation [L, *complere,* to fill up, *dis,* apart, *locare,* to place], a dislocation in which the articular surfaces of the joint are completely separated.

complete fistula, an abnormal passage from an internal organ or structure to the surface of the body or to another internal organ or structure.

complete fracture, a bone break that completely disrupts the continuity of a bone across its entire width.

complete health history, a health history that includes a history of the chief complaint, present illness, past and present health, social history, occupational history, sexual history, psychological status, and family health history. See also **functional health history, health history.**

complete heart block (CHB) [L, *complere,* to fill up; Gk, *kardia,* heart; OFr, *bloc*], a total failure of impulses to be conducted from the atria to the ventricles. It causes the atria and ventricles to beat independently. It requires the use of a pacemaker to maintain a normal heart rate. Also called **third-degree AV heart block.**

complete hernia [L, *complere,* to fill up, *hernia,* rupture], a hernia characterized by protrusion of the hernial sac and abdominal contents through the abdominal wall.

complete paralysis [L, *complere,* to fill up; Gk, *paralyein,* to be palsied], paralysis characterized by a complete loss of motor function. Compare **paresis.**

complete previa. See **central placenta previa.**

complete protein, a protein that contains all the essential amino acids in appropriate amounts to allow normal growth and tissue maintenance when adequate energy is provided in the diet. Examples are casein (milk protein), eggs, fish, poultry, cheese, meat and some whole grains, such as quinoa.

complete rachischisis, a rare congenital fissure of the entire vertebral column and spinal cord, resulting from failure of the embryonic neural tube to close. The condition is characterized by flaccid paralysis and impaired sensations. It is often accompanied by other birth defects, such as cleft palate, cleft lip, and hydrocephalus, and is frequently fatal. Also called **holorachischisis, rachischisis totalis.** Compare **spina bifida.**

complete response (CR), (in oncology) the total disappearance of a tumor.

complex /kom″pleks, kəmpleks′/ [L, *complexus,* an embrace], **1.** a group of items, such as chemical molecules, that are related in structure or function as are the iron and protein portions of hemoglobin or the cobalt and protein portions of vitamin B₁₂. **2.** a combination of signs and symptoms of disease that forms a syndrome. **3.** (in psychology) a group of associated ideas with strong emotional overtones that affect a person's attitudes toward a specific subject.

complex carbohydrate, a polysaccharide, such as a carbohydrate, that is composed of a large number of glucose molecules, so called to distinguish it from a simple sugar. See also **carbohydrate.**

complex cavity, a cavity that involves more than one surface of a tooth. Compare **gingival cavity.**

complex fracture, a closed fracture in which the soft tissue surrounding the bone is severely damaged.

complex odontoma, a mixed odontogenic tumor consisting of both epithelial and mesenchymal dental hard tissues resembling enamel and dentin. It is an amorphous conglomeration of dental hard tissue consistent with a hamartoma, not a neoplasm. Compare **compound odontoma.**

complex protein, a protein that contains a simple protein and at least one molecule of another substance, as a glycoprotein, lipoprotein, nucleoprotein, proteoglycan, or hemoglobin.

complex regional pain syndrome, a neuromuscular condition characterized by pain and stiffness in the shoulder and arm, limited joint motion, swelling of the hand, muscle atrophy, and decalcification of the underlying bones. It is thought that a disturbance to the sympathetic nervous system is responsible for this condition. The condition occurs most commonly after myocardial infarction. Also called *RSD (reflex sympathetic dystrophy syndrome),* **causalgia, shoulder-hand syndrome.** See **reflex sympathetic dystrophy.**

complex spatial relations, the perceptual relationship of one figure or part of a figure to another.

complex sugars, sugar molecules that can be hydrolyzed or digested to yield two molecules of the same or different simple sugars, such as sucrose, lactose, and maltose. Also called **disaccharide, polysaccharide.**

compliance (C) /kəmplī″əns/ [L, *complere,* to complete], **1.** fulfillment by a patient of a caregiver's prescribed course of treatment. **2.** also called **pulmonary compliance.** (in respiratory physiology) a measure of distensibility of the lung volume produced by a unit pressure change. **3.** the quality of yielding to pressure or force without disruption, or an expression of the distensibility of an air- or fluid-filled organ, e.g., the lung or urinary bladder, in terms of volume per unit of pressure.

compliance factor, a measure of the expansion of the flexible tubing in a mechanical ventilating system when pressure is applied.

complicated dislocation [L, *complicare,* to fold together, *dis,* apart, *locare,* place], a joint dislocation accompanied by damage to the corresponding articular soft tissue.

complicated fracture, a fracture accompanied by injury to neighboring soft tissues, such as nerves and blood vessels.

complicated labor [L, *complicare,* to fold together, *labor, work*], **1.** any labor that does not follow an entirely normal course or that is facilitated in some manner. **2.** a labor resulting in untoward outcomes, fetal or maternal.

complication [L, *complicare,* to fold together], **1.** a disease or injury that develops during the treatment of a preexisting disorder. An example is a bacterial infection that is acquired by a person weakened by a viral infection. The complication frequently alters the prognosis. **2.** a problem that arises during labor that puts the neonate, mother, or both at risk.

component /kəmpō″nənt/ [L, *componere,* to assemble], a significant part of a larger unit.

component drip set, a device used for delivering IV fluids, especially whole blood. It includes plastic tubing and a combination drip chamber and filter. Compare **component syringe set, microaggregate recipient set, straight line blood set, Y-set.**

component syringe set, a device used for delivering IV fluids. It includes plastic tubing, two slide clamps, a Y-connector, and a syringe. The component syringe set may be used in various procedures, such as the transfusion of platelets and cryoprecipitates. In such transfusions the component syringe set is used primarily to prevent clogging the IV line. Compare **component drip set, microaggregate recipient set, straight line blood set, Y-set.**

component therapy, transfusion of an individual blood component rather than whole blood to treat a specific deficiency, avoid volume overload, and prevent reactions to unneeded blood products. Compare **plasmapheresis.** See also **packed cells, pooled plasma.**

composite core /kəmpos″it/ [L, *componere,* to assemble], a buildup of composite resin designed and placed in the pulp chamber and root canal of an endodontically treated tooth to allow the tooth to be used as a foundation for a crown or bridge. Compare **amalgam core, cast core.** See also **core.**

composite graft, a transplantation that involves more than one type of tissue, such as skin and cartilage. The term may also refer to an artificial vessel graft, an aortic valve prosthesis used to replace the ascending aorta valve.

compos mentis /kom″pōs men″tis/, having a sound mind. Compare **non compos mentis.**

compound /kom′pound/ [L, *componere,* to assemble], **1.** *n.,* (in chemistry) a substance composed of two or more different elements, chemically combined in definite proportions, that cannot be separated by physical means. **2.** *n.,* any substance composed of two or more different ingredients. **3.** *adj.,* denoting an injury characterized by multiple factors, such as a compound fracture. **4.** *v.,* to make a substance by combining ingredients, such as a pharmaceutic.

compound aneurysm, a localized dilation of an arterial wall in which some of the layers of the wall are distended and others are ruptured or dissected.

compound dislocation. See **open dislocation.**

compound fracture, a fracture in which the broken end or ends of the bone have torn through the skin. Also called **open fracture.**

compound joint [L, *componere,* to assemble, *jungere,* to join], a joint that involves more than two bones. Kinds include **elbow, knee.**

compound melanocytoma. See **benign juvenile melanoma.**

compound microscope [L, *componere,* to assemble; Gk, *mikros,* small, *skopein,* to view], a microscope with two or more simple or complex lens systems.

compound odontoma, an odontogenic tumor composed of mature enamel, dentin, cementum, and pulp tissue in the shape of miniature or rudimentary small teeth. See **composite odontoma, odontoma.**

compound tubuloalveolar gland /too″byəlō′alvē″ələr/, one of the many multicellular glands with more than one secretory duct that contains both tube-shaped and sac-shaped portions, such as the salivary glands.

comprehensive care, **1.** the provision of multiple services in a primary care setting. **2.** care that addresses social and psychological aspects of health in addition to physical care. See **holistic health care.**

Comprehensive Health Manpower Training Act of 1971, legislation passed by the U.S. Congress to provide educational funding for nurse-practitioner and physician-assistant programs.

Comprehensive Health Planning (CHP) and Public Health Services Amendments, legislation passed by the U.S. Congress in 1966 that emphasized regional planning and introduced the concept that each person has a "right to health care."

comprehensive medical care, a health care program that provides for preventive medical care and rehabilitative services in addition to traditional chronic and acute illness services.

compress /kom″pres/ [L, *comprimere,* to press together], a soft pad, usually made of cloth, used to apply heat, cold, or medication to the surface of a body area. A compress also may be applied over a wound to help control bleeding. Compare **dressing.**

compressed air hazards. See **decompression sickness.**

compressibility factor /kəmpres′ibil″itē/, a measure of the amount of tidal volume that may be trapped in a mechanical ventilator system in relation to the water pressure applied. It is expressed in milliliters of gas per centimeter of water pressure.

compressible volume /kəmpres″əbəl/, a part of the tidal volume of gas produced by a mechanical ventilator that is prevented from reaching a patient by compression of the gas and expansion of the flexible tubing in the equipment.

compression /kəmpresh″ən/ [L, *comprimere,* to press together], **1.** the act of pressing, squeezing, or otherwise applying pressure to an organ, tissue, or body area. An intracranial tumor or hemorrhage may cause compression of brain tissue. Kinds of pathological compression include compression fracture, in which bone surfaces are forced against each other, causing a break, and compression paralysis, marked by paralysis of a body area caused by pressure on a nerve. **2.** the pressing or squeezing of substances together so that they occupy a smaller volume of space (e.g., compressing gas into a pressurized aerosol can).

compression amplification. See **gray scale display.**

compression fracture, a bone break, especially in a short bone, that disrupts osseous tissue and collapses the affected bone. Axial loading is the usual mechanism of injury. The bodies of vertebrae are often sites of compression fractures.

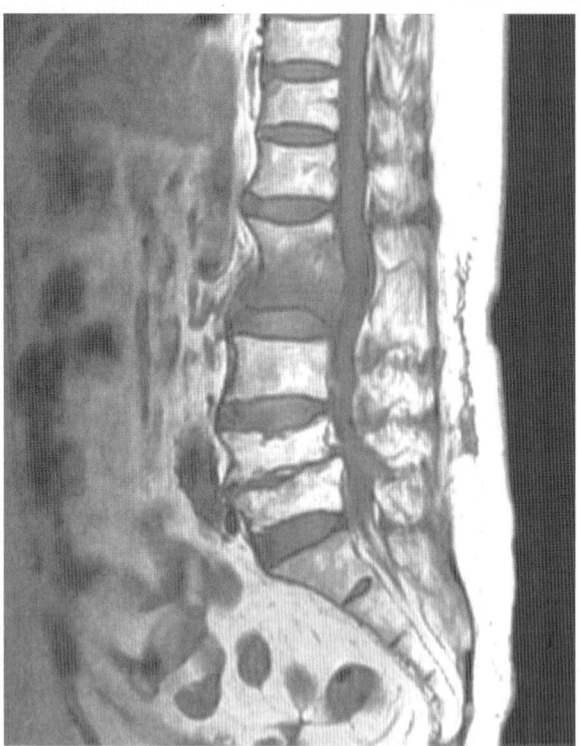

MRI showing compression fracture of L1-L2 *(Woo et al, 2015)*

compression neuropathy, any of several disorders involving damage to sensory nerve roots or peripheral nerves, caused by mechanical pressure or localized trauma. Compression neuropathy is characterized by paresthesia, weakness, or paralysis. The carpal, peroneal, radial, and ulnar nerves are most commonly involved. Compare **neuritis.** See also **paresthesia.**

compression paralysis [L, *comprimere,* to press together; Gk, *paralyein,* to be palsied], a paralysis caused by sustained pressure on a peripheral nerve. The condition may be temporary or permanent, depending on the duration and intensity of pressure.

compressions, (in physical science) regions of high molecular density, such as a great amount of ultrasound energy, within a longitudinal wave.

compressive atelectasis /kəmpres″iv/, a condition in which a region of the lung cannot be ventilated as a result of intrathoracic pressures that compress the alveoli in that region. The condition may result from a pulmonary embolism, which releases chemicals that cause vasoconstriction and bronchospasm, leading to alveolar compression.

compressor naris /kompres″ôr när″is/, the transverse part of the nasalis muscle that serves to depress the cartilage of the nose and to draw the ala toward the septum. Compare **dilator naris.**

compromise /kom″prəmīs/ [L, *com,* together, *promittere,* to promise], **1.** an action that may involve a change in a person's behavior, as in substituting goals or delaying satisfaction of needs in one area to reduce stress in another. **2.** an illness or condition that can affect another part of the body.

compromise body image, a new body image acquired by a patient as part of his or her adjustment to a physical dysfunction. It may harbor important emotional factors for the individual. A compromise body image incorporates and modifies unacceptable features of the condition through psychological defense mechanisms such as denial, sublimation, repression, and overcompensation.

compromised host, a person who is less than normally able to resist infection because of immunosuppressive therapy, immunological defect, severe anemia, or concurrent disease or condition, including human immunodeficiency virus infection, metastatic malignancy, cachexia, or severe malnutrition.

Compton scatter [Arthur H. Compton, American physicist, 1892–1962], an interaction process of photons with tissue in the diagnostic and therapeutic radiology energy range. In this process, the incoming photon transfers energy to an electron in the tissue and is deflected, or reemitted, with reduced energy in a different direction.

compulsion [L, *compellere,* to urge], an irresistible, repetitive irrational impulse to perform an act that is usually contrary to one's ordinary judgments or standards, yet results in overt anxiety if it is not completed. The compulsion also acts to decrease anxiety. The impulse is usually the result of an obsession. Compulsions are characteristic of an obsessive-compulsive disorder. Compare **phobia.** See also **compulsive ritual, obsession, obsessive-compulsive disorder.**

compulsion need [L, *compellere,* to urge; Gk, *neuron,* nerve, *osis,* condition], an irresistible, irrational urge to perform certain acts repeatedly in spite of conscious recognition that doing so is abnormal behavior.

compulsive /kəmpul″siv/ [L, *compellere,* to urge], pertaining to an act repeatedly performed under the stress of pathological, intense need.

compulsive eating, an eating disorder characterized by continuous or frequent excessive eating over which an individual does not feel he or she has control, and which usually leads to weight gain and obesity. Eating is not connected to hunger, and food intake may be rapid or secret. Compensatory behaviors like purging, laxative use, or excessive exercise do not occur. Generally the amount eaten at any one time is not large; when it is, the disorder is usually called binge eating.

compulsive idea [L, *compellere,* to urge], a recurring irrational idea that persists in the mind, usually generating an irresistible urge to perform an inappropriate act. Also called **imperative idea.**

compulsive personality, a type of character structure with a pattern of chronic and obsessive adherence to rigid standards of conduct. The person is usually excessively conscientious and inhibited, is extremely inflexible, has an extraordinary capacity for work, and lacks a normal ability to relax and to relate to other people. The compulsive person is likely to follow repetitive patterns of behavior, such as snapping the fingers, crossing the legs, tapping the foot, or refusing to walk on cracks in the sidewalk, and often leads an impoverished emotional life, being dominated by a need for order, cleanliness, punctuality, rules, and systems. See also **compulsive personality disorder.**

compulsive personality disorder, a mental condition in which an irrational preoccupation with order, rules, ritual, and detail interferes with everyday functioning and normal behavior. The disorder is characterized by an excessive devotion to work, a pathological adherence to a definite set of rules or system of behavior, and a persistent, compulsive following of specific rituals. The person cannot make decisions when faced with unexpected situations and cannot take pleasure in the normal activities of daily life. Psychotherapy is the usual treatment and may include behavior therapy with desensitization and flooding to reduce maladaptive anxiety.

See **obsessive-compulsive disorder.** See also **compulsive personality.**

compulsive polydipsia, a compelling urge to drink excessive amounts of liquid. The condition is psychogenic; it is not caused by any organic dysfunction or physical deprivation. Extreme cases can result in death from water intoxication and electrolyte imbalance. Also called **psychogenic polydipsia.** Should not be confused with **diabetes insipidus.**

compulsive ritual, a series of acts a person feels must be carried out even though he or she recognizes that the behavior is useless and inappropriate, commonly seen in obsessive-compulsive disorder. Failure to complete the acts causes extreme tension or anxiety. See also **obsessive-compulsive disorder.**

computed dental radiography (CDR), a computer-assisted technology for projecting and storing digital radiographic images of the teeth and jaws.

computed radiography (CR), imaging technology that records radiographic image data on photostimulable phosphor plates. The acquired image data are converted to a digital image by an external reader. Digitized images can be stored and manipulated by a computer and displayed on a high-resolution monitor or recorded on film by using a laser printer. See also **digital radiography.**

computed tomography (CT) /kəmpyo͞o″tid/, **1.** a computerized x-ray imaging technique in which a narrow beam of x-rays is aimed at a patient and quickly rotated around the body, producing signals that are processed by the machine's computer to generate an image of a detailed cross-section of tissue. Image slices can be displayed individually or stacked together by the computer to generate a 3-D image of the patient. The procedure, first used in 1972, is painless, noninvasive, and requires no special preparation. Formerly called **computerized axial tomography. 2.** (in dentistry) an imaging technique often used to view the temporomandibular joint area or a presurgical dental implant site. Also called *cone-beam imaging, cone-beam computed tomography (CBCT).*

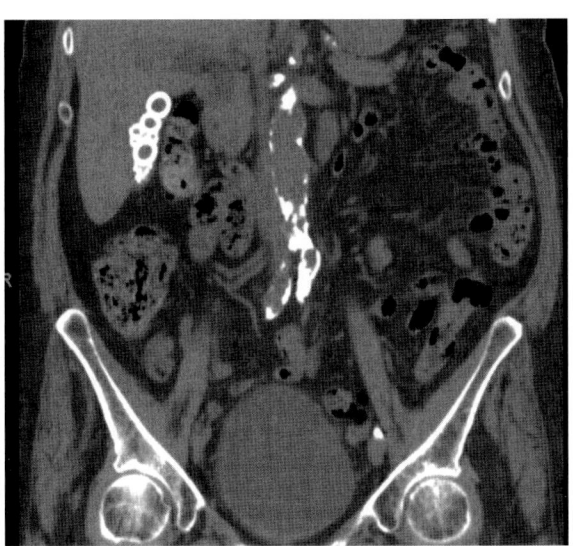

Computed tomography (Klein, 2010)

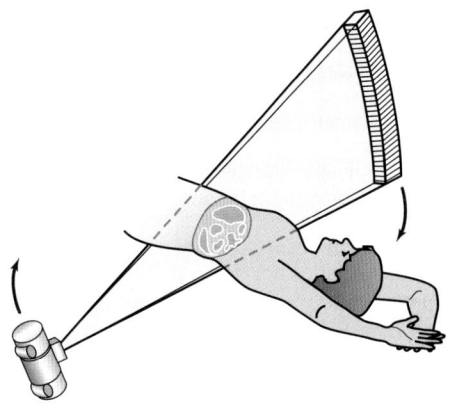

Computed tomography scan (Frank, Long, and Smith, 2012)

computed tomography angiography, the use of computed tomography to visualize blood vessels throughout the body after the injection of radiopaque contrast medium.

computed tomography of the abdomen, a noninvasive radiographic procedure performed with contrast dye to diagnose pathological conditions of the abdominal and retroperitoneal organs. See also **computed tomography.**

computed tomography of the brain, a radiographic procedure performed with contrast dye to diagnose pathological conditions of the brain. It can also identify multiple sclerosis and other degenerative abnormalities. See also **computed tomography,** def. 1.

computed tomography of the chest, a noninvasive radiographic procedure performed with contrast dye to diagnose and evaluate pathological conditions of the chest. Fractures can also be seen. See also **computed tomography,** def. 1.

computed tomography portogram, an x-ray test with contrast dye used to identify tumors of the liver smaller than 2 cm. The contrast medium is injected through a catheter in the splenic artery, rather than through a peripheral vein as in a routine CT scan.

computed tomography scanogram, a CT technique used especially to measure discrepancies in limb length. CT scout images of the joints of the upper or lower extremity are taken, followed by placement of the CT cursors over the joints to obtain measurements. The CT scanogram is more consistently reproduced and radiation doses are lower than in the conventional imaging technique (orthoroentgenography). See also **orthoroentgenography, scanography.**

computer [L *computare* to calculate], an electronic device that processes and stores large amounts of information very quickly. See also **mainframe computer, microcomputer, minicomputer.**

computer-aided semen analysis (CASA), any of various methods of automated, objective, standardized evaluation of sperm concentration and movement in a semen sample, to assess the individual's potential fertility or infertility. Most techniques use video recordings showing movements of multiple spermatozoa.

computer-assisted instruction (CAI), a teaching process that uses a computer in the presentation of instructional materials, often in a way that requires the student to interact with it.

computerized axial tomography (CAT). See **computed tomography.**

computer-managed instruction (CMI), a system in which a computer is used to manage several aspects of instruction, including learning assessment through administration of pretests and posttests; design and preparation of learning prescriptions; and calculation, analysis, and storage of student scores.

COMT, abbreviation for **catechol-o-methyl transferase.**

CON, abbreviation for **certificate-of-necessity, certificate-of-need.**

con-. See **co-, col-, com-, con-, cor-.**

CONA, abbreviation for **Canadian Orthopedic Nurses Association.**

conation /kōnā″shən/ [L, *conari,* to attempt], the mental process characterized by desire, impulse, volition, and striving. Compare **cognition.** –*conative, adj.*

-conazole, suffix designating a miconazole-type systemic antifungal agent.

concanavalin A /kon′kənav″əlin/, a protein isolated from the jack bean that reacts with polyglucosans in the blood of mammals and causes blood cells to agglutinate. It has been used in immunology to stimulate T cell production.

concatenates /kənkat″ənāts/, long molecules formed by continuous repeating of the same molecular subunit.

concave [L, *concavare,* to make hollow], curved like the interior of an arched circle. Compare **convex.**

concave-convex joint relationship /kon″kāv, konkāv″/, a relationship in which one of a joint's articulating surfaces is concave and the other is convex.

concave spherical lens [L, *concavare,* to make hollow; Gk, *sphaira,* ball; L, *lentil*], a lens with curved, depressed surfaces that cause light rays to diverge. It is used for the management of myopia (nearsightedness).

concavity /kən·kav″itē/, a deep depression or inward curving surface of an organ or body structure.

concealed accessory pathway /kənsēld/ [L, *con,* together, *celare,* to hide], a connection between the atria and ventricles that is capable of retrograde conduction only. The electrocardiogram is normal (no delta wave) during sinus rhythm and is not associated with preexcitation, but the patient is prone to paroxysmal supraventricular tachycardia caused by orthodromic circus movement tachycardia. Conduction into the ventricles is normal during atrial fibrillation because the accessory pathway does not conduct in that direction.

concealed hemorrhage, the escape of blood from a ruptured vessel into internal organs or cavities.

concealed junctional extrasystole, an impulse that arises in and discharges the atrioventricular (AV) node or the AV bundle but fails to reach either the atria or the ventricles. It is identified by its blocking or delaying effect on subsequent AV conduction.

concealed penis, a penis buried below the surface of the abdomen, thigh, or scrotum. Causes include poor skin fixation at the base of the penis, scarring after penile surgery, or excessive obesity. See also **buried penis.**

conceive /kənsēv″/ [L, *concipere,* to take together], to become pregnant.

concentrate /kon″səntrāt/ [L, *con + centrum,* center], **1.** *v.,* to decrease the bulk of a liquid mixture and increase the quantity of dissolved substances per unit of volume by the removal of solvent through evaporation or other means. **2.** *n.,* a substance, particularly a liquid, that has been strengthened and reduced in volume through such means.

concentration /kon′səntrā′shən/ [L, *concentratio*], **1.** increase in strength by evaporation. **2.** the ratio of the mass or volume of a solute to the mass or volume of the solution or solvent. See also **molality, molarity. 3.** to focus or direct one's thoughts or attention. **4.** a means of expressing the amount of herb and solvent used in formulating an herbal preparation. For example, a tincture with a 1:5 concentration contains 1 part of the herb in grams to 5 parts of the solvent in milliliters. Should not be confused with **potency.**

concentration gradient, a difference in the concentration of a substance on two sides of a permeable barrier.

concentric /kənsen″trik/ [L, *con + centrum,* center], describing two or more circles that have a common center.

concentric contraction, a muscle contraction that occurs when the muscle fibers shorten as tension develops. A concentric contraction of the biceps brachii occurs, for example, when an elbow is bent or flexed to raise a hand to the mouth. Compare **eccentric contraction.** See also **isotonic exercise.**

concentric fibroma, a fibrous tumor surrounding the uterine cavity.

concentric hypertrophy [L, *con + centrum,* center; Gk, *hyper,* excessive, *trophe,* nourishment], a type of tissue overgrowth in which the walls of an organ continue to increase but the exterior size remains the same and the internal size diminishes.

concept /′kän-ˌsept/ [L, *concipere,* to take together], a construct or abstract idea or thought that originates and remains within the mind. –**conceptual,** *adj.*

concept analysis, examination of the attributes of a concept as it occurs in ordinary usage in order to identify the meanings attached to the concept.

conception /kənsep″shən/ [L, *concipere,* to take together], **1.** the beginning of pregnancy, usually taken to be the instant that a spermatozoon enters an ovum and forms a viable zygote. **2.** the act or process of fertilization. **3.** the act or process of creating an idea or notion. **4.** the idea or notion created; a general impression resulting from the interpretation of a symbol or set of symbols.

conceptional age, in fetal development the number of weeks since conception. Because the exact time of conception is difficult to determine except in some cases of the use of artificial reproductive technology, conceptional age is assumed to be 2 weeks less than gestational age. Gestational age is in turn the number of weeks that have elapsed between the first day of the last normal menstrual period in an idealized 28-day menstrual cycle and the date of delivery. See also **estimated date of delivery, Naegele's rule.**

conception control. See **contraception, family planning.**

conceptive /kənsep″tiv/ [L, *concipere,* to take together], **1.** able to become pregnant; capable of fertility. **2.** pertaining to or characteristic of the mental process of forming ideas or impressions.

concept mapping, a method of visualizing relationships among various concepts. A branching, hierarchical diagram of concepts shows how they are connected using arrows and labels that identify interrelationships.

conceptual, an image of something held in the mind; an abstract notion or idea. See **concept.**

conceptual disorder /kənsep″choo·əl/ [L, *concipere,* to take together], a disturbance in thought processes, cognitive activities, or ability to formulate concepts.

conceptual framework, a group of concepts that are broadly defined and systematically organized to provide a focus, a rationale, and a tool for the integration and interpretation of information. Usually expressed abstractly through word models, a conceptual framework is the conceptual basis for many theories, such as communication theory and general systems theory. Conceptual frameworks also provide a foundation and organization for the educational plan in schools of nursing, occupational therapy, physical therapy, and other professional programs.

conceptus /kənsep″təs/ [L, *concipere,* to take together], the product of conception; the fertilized ovum and its enclosing membranes at all stages of intrauterine development, from implantation to birth. See also **embryo, fetus.**

concha /kong″kə/, a body structure that is shell shaped, as the cavity in the external ear that surrounds the external auditory canal meatus, patella, or vulva.

conchitis /kongkī″tis/, an inflammation of a concha of the ear or nose.

concoction /kənkok″shən/ [L, *con* + *coquere,* to cook], *(Informal)* a remedy prepared from a mixture of two or more drugs or substances that have been heated.

concomitant /konkom″itənt/ [L, *con* + *comitari,* to accompany], accompanying; designating one or more of two or more things, occurring simultaneously, that may or may not be interrelated or produced as a result of the others.

concomitant strabismus, a condition of crossed eyes in which the angle of squint is the same in all directions of gaze for a given testing distance. Also called **comitant strabismus.**

concomitant symptom, any symptom that accompanies a primary symptom.

concordance /kənkôr″dəns/ [L, *concordare,* to agree], the expression of one or more specific traits in both members of a pair of twins. Compare **discordance.** –*concordant, adj.*

concrescence /kənkres′əns/ [L, *concrescere,* to be formed], **1.** a growing together; a union of parts originally separate. **2.** (in embryology) the flowing together and piling up of cells. **3.** (in dentistry) the union of the roots of two adjacent teeth by a deposit of cementum.

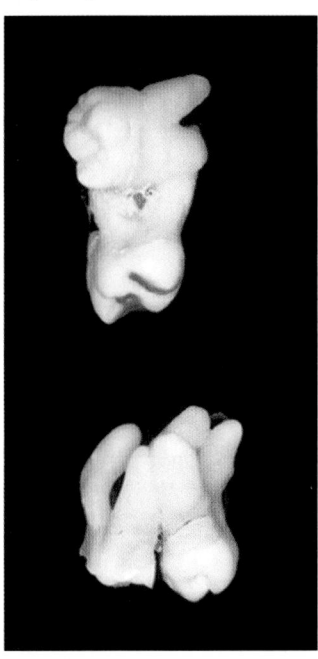

Concrescence *(Mosby, 2008)*

concreteness /kənkrēt″nes/ [L, *concrescere,* to be formed], communication in the here and now; simplicity; lack of abstraction.

concrete operation /kon″krēt, konkrēt″/, a thought process based on tangible rather than abstract points of reference.

concrete thinking, **1.** a stage in the development of the cognitive thought processes in the child. During this phase thought becomes increasingly logical and coherent so that the child is able to classify, sort, order, and organize facts while still being incapable of generalizing or dealing in abstractions. Problem solving is accomplished in a concrete, systematic fashion based on what is perceived, keeping to the literal meaning of words, as in applying the word *horse* to a particular animal and not to horses in general. In Piaget's classification this stage occurs between 7 and 11 years of age, is preceded by syncretic thinking, and is followed by abstract thinking. Compare **abstract thinking, syncretic thinking. 2.** the inability to abstract, to discern innuendo or hidden meaning, or to understand humor or concepts. This type of thinking is seen, for example, in some cases of schizophrenia, fetal alcohol syndrome, Asperger's syndrome, or brain injury. It is also seen in states of high anxiety.

concretion, **1.** an abnormal union of two adjacent parts. **2.** a hard inorganic mass in a natural cavity or in tissue. See also **calculus.**

concurrent infection [L, *concurrere,* to run together, *inficere,* to stain], a condition during which a person has two or more simultaneous infections.

concurrent nursing audit. See **nursing audit.**

concurrent review, part of a utilization management program in which health care is reviewed as it is provided (usually while the patient is still in the hospital). Reviewers, usually nurses, monitor appropriateness of the care, the setting, and the progress of discharge plans. The ongoing review is directed at keeping costs as low as possible and maintaining effectiveness of care.

concurrent sterilization, a method of preparing an infant-feeding formula in which all ingredients and equipment are sterilized before mixing.

concurrent validity, validity of a test or a measurement tool that is established by simultaneously applying a previously validated tool or test to the same phenomenon, or database, and comparing the results. Concurrent validity is achieved if the results are highly correlated (the same or similar) at a statistically significant level. See also **validity.**

concussion /konkush″ən/ [L, *concutere,* to shake violently], **1.** damage to the brain caused by a violent jarring or shaking, such as a blow, sports injury, or an explosion. **2.** *(Informal)* See **brain concussion.**

condensation /kon′dənsā″shən/ [L, *condensare,* to make thick], **1.** a reduction to a denser form, such as from water vapor to a liquid. **2.** (in psychology) a process, often present in dreams, in which two or more concepts are fused so that a single symbol represents the multiple components. In some cases of schizophrenia condensation, several thoughts and feelings fuse into a single verbal or nonverbal message and may be expressed in repetitive statements or gestures that can have a variety of meanings.

condensation nuclei, neutral particles, such as dust, in the atmosphere that are able to absorb or adsorb water and grow. At relatively high humidities they form fogs or hazes. Condensation nuclei consisting of sulfuric or nitric acid vapors or nitrogen oxides may be a source of respiratory irritants.

condensed milk, a thick liquid prepared by the evaporation of half of the water content of cow's milk.

condenser, an instrument for compacting dental restorative material into a prepared tooth cavity. It has a working end, or nib, with a flat or serrated face.

condition /kəndish″ən/ [L, *condicere,* to make arrangements], **1.** *n.,* a state of being, specifically in reference to physical and mental health or well-being. **2.** *n.,* anything that is essential to or restricts or modifies the appearance or occurrence of something else. **3.** *v.,* to train a person or an animal, usually through specific exercises and repeated exposure to a particular state or thing. **4.** *v.,* (in psychology) to subject a person or animal to conditioning or associative learning so that a specific stimulus always elicits a particular response. See also **classical conditioning.**

conditional discharge /kəndish″ənəl/, **1.** a specified leave of absence or liberty from a psychiatric hospital in which certain behaviors are expected from the patient and the original commitment order remains in effect. Also called **pass, temporary absence. 2.** an order entered into a patient's record in advance of the actual discharge date specifying criteria to be met prior to discharge.

conditionally essential nutrients, nutrients that must be supplied to the body only under special conditions, such as stress, illness, or aging.

conditioned avoidance response, a learned reaction that is performed either consciously or unconsciously to avoid an unpleasant or painful stimulus.

conditioned escape response, a learned reaction that is performed either consciously or unconsciously to stop or to escape from an aversive stimulus.

conditioned orientation reflex (COR), the response, in a child under the age of 2 years, of turning his or her head toward the source of a sound. When the child responds appropriately by turning toward the sound, he or she is rewarded by seeing a toy move or light up. See also **visual response audiometry.**

conditioned reflex, a reflex developed gradually by training in association with a specific repeated external stimulus. An example of a conditioned reflex is that in Pavlov's experiment in which a dog salivates at the ringing of a bell if, over a period of time, every feeding is preceded by the bell-ringing stimulus. Also called **acquired reflex.** See also **classical conditioning.**

conditioned response, an automatic reaction learned through training to a stimulus that does not normally elicit such response. Such responses can be physical or psychological and are produced by repeated association of some physiological function or behavioral pattern with an unrelated stimulus or event. In Pavlov's classic experiments, dogs learned to associate the sound of a ringing bell with feeding time so that they salivated at the sound of the bell, regardless of whether or not food was given to them. Also called **acquired reflex, behavior reflex, conditioned reflex, trained reflex.** Compare **unconditioned response.** See also **classical conditioning, operant conditioning.**

conditioned stimulus [L, *conditio + stimulus,* goad], any stimulus to which a reflex response has been conditioned by previous training or experience. See also **classical conditioning, operant conditioning.**

conditioning /kəndish″əning/ [L, *condicere,* to make arrangements], a form of learning based on the theories of early 20th-century scientists such as Ivan Pavlov, B.F. Skinner, John Watson, and Edward Thorndike in which there is the development of a response or set of responses to a stimulus or series of stimuli. Kinds include **classical conditioning, operant conditioning.**

condom /kon″dəm/, a soft, flexible sheath made of plastic, rubber, or lambskin that covers the penis. Condoms prevent the exchange of body fluids during sexual activity, thereby conception. With the exception of lambskin condoms, a condom also protects the users from sexually transmitted diseases. Also called **prophylactic, rubber.**

condom catheter, an external urinary collection device that fits over the penis like a condom, used in the management of urinary incontinence. Also called **Texas catheter.**

conduct disorder /kon″dukt/, (in psychiatry) an enduring set of behaviors that evolves over time, characterized by aggression and violations of the rights of others.

conducting zone, the portion of the respiratory system that provides a route for air, humidification of incoming air, and removal of debris and pathogens.

conduction /kənduk″shən/ [L, *conducere,* to lead], **1.** (in physics) a process in which heat is transferred from one substance to another because of a difference in temperature; a process (often electrical) in which energy is transmitted through a conductor. **2.** (in physiology) the process by which a nerve impulse is transmitted. *−conductive, adj.*

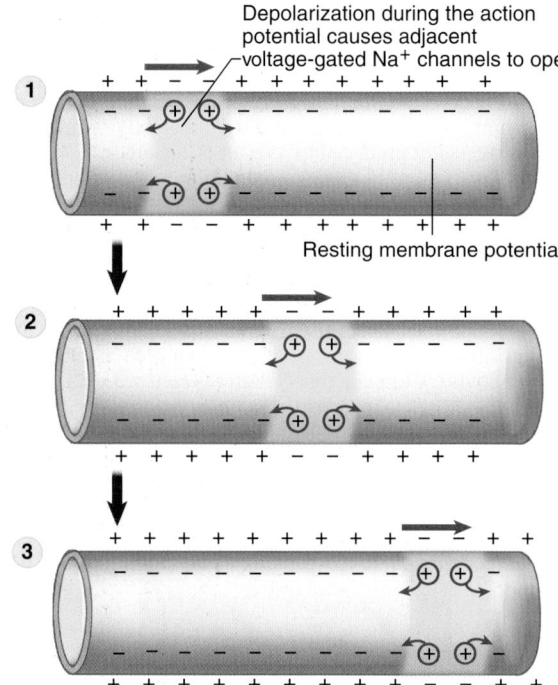

Depolarization during the action potential causes adjacent voltage-gated Na$^+$ channels to open

Resting membrane potential

Conduction of an action potential *(Patton, 2016)*

conduction anesthesia, a loss of sensation, especially pain, in a region of the body, produced by injecting a local anesthetic along the course of a nerve or nerves to inhibit the conduction of impulses to and from the area supplied by that nerve or nerves. Also called **block anesthesia, nerve block anesthesia.** See also **anesthesia, regional anesthesia.**

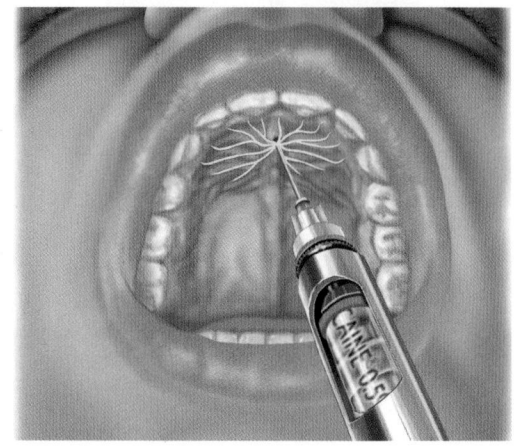

Conduction anesthesia *(Custalow, 2005)*

conduction aphasia, a dissociative speech phenomenon in which a patient has no difficulty in comprehending words seen or heard and no dysarthria, yet has problems in self-expression. The patient may substitute words similar in sound or meaning for the correct ones but is unable to repeat from dictation, to spell, or to read aloud. The patient is alert and aware of the deficit. A common cause is an embolus in a branch of the middle cerebral artery. The caregiver should try to reduce tension and frustration in the patient, encourage socialization, find alternate means of communication for the patient, use simple language and direct questions requiring simple answers, and help the family to understand the problem and effectively cope with it. See also **aphasia.**

conduction deafness. See **conductive hearing loss.**

conduction pathway, the route followed by nerve impulses propagated along synaptically connected neurons.

conduction system, specialized tissue that carries electrical impulses, such as bundle branches and Purkinje fibers in the heart.

conduction system of the heart, the network of highly specialized muscle tissue that transmits the electrical impulses needed for a heartbeat. It includes the sinus and atrioventricular (AV) nodes, the conducting fibers between the nodes, the AV bundle (bundle of His), the left and right bundle branches, and the Purkinje fibers. See also **cardiac cycle.**

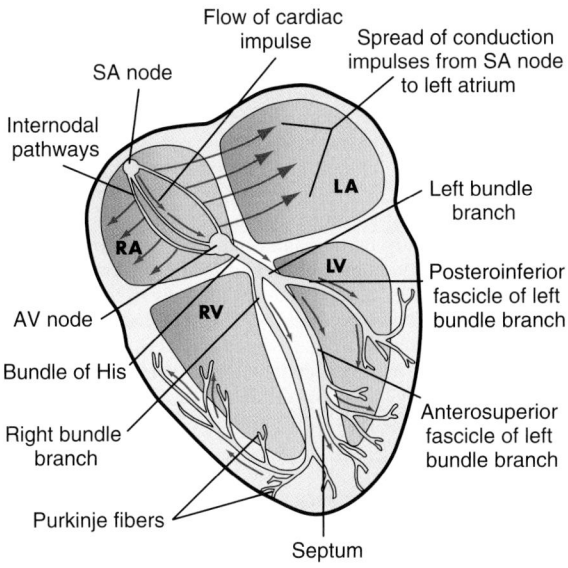

Conduction system of the heart *(Kinney, 1996)*

Labels on figure:
- Flow of cardiac impulse
- SA node
- Spread of conduction impulses from SA node to left atrium
- Internodal pathways
- LA
- Left bundle branch
- RA
- LV
- Posteroinferior fascicle of left bundle branch
- AV node
- RV
- Bundle of His
- Anterosuperior fascicle of left bundle branch
- Right bundle branch
- Purkinje fibers
- Septum

conduction velocity, the speed with which an electrical impulse can be transmitted through excitable tissue, as in the movement of an action potential through His-Purkinje fibers of the heart.

conductive hearing loss /kənduk″tiv/ [L, *conducere,* to lead], a form of hearing loss in which sound is inadequately conducted through the external or middle ear to the sensorineural apparatus of the inner ear. Sensitivity to sound is diminished, but clarity (interpretation of the sound) is not changed as long as the sound is sufficiently loud. This type of hearing loss can be caused by fluid in the middle ear, an ear infection, poor eustachian tube functioning, a hole in the eardrum, benign tumors, cerumen in the ear canal, an object stuck in the ear, or problems with how the outer or middle ear is formed. Also called **conduction deafness.** Compare **sensorineural hearing loss, mixed hearing loss.**

conductivity, the ability of an electric or other system to transmit sound, heat, light, or electromagnetic energy.

conductor, **1.** any substance through which electrons flow readily. **2.** (in psychiatry) a family therapist who uses his or her own personality to give direction to patients in therapy.

conduit /kon″dit, kon″doo·it/, **1.** an artificial channel or passage that connects two organs or different parts of the same organ. **2.** a tube or other device for conveying water or other fluids from one region to another.

condylar fracture /kon″dilər/ [Gk, *kondylos,* knuckle], any break in a condyle, a rounded projection on a bone at a hinge joint. Such fractures usually occur at the distal end of the humerus or the femur or at the end of a digit phalange, where the condylar fracture fragment may detach.

condylar guide, a mechanical device on a dental articulator, designed to guide articular movement similar to that produced by the condyles within the mandibular fossae of the temporomandibular joints. Compare **anterior guide.**

condyle /kon″dīl/ [Gk, *kondylos,* knuckle], a rounded projection at the end of a bone that anchors muscle ligaments and articulates with adjacent bones. *−condylar, adj.*

-condyle, -condylus, suffix meaning a "knucklelike projection on a bone": *epicondyle.*

condyloid /kon″diloid/ [Gk, *kondylos,* knuckle], resembling a knuckle.

condyloid joint [L, *kondylos* + *eidos,* form]. See **ellipsoid joint.**

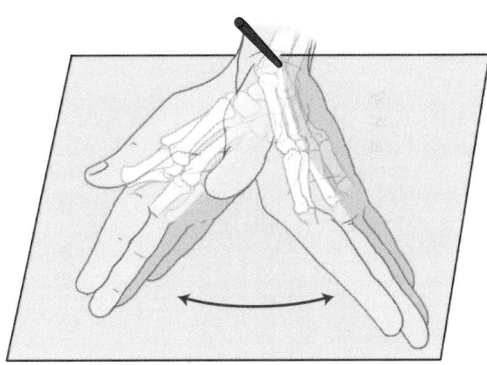

Condyloid joint *(Muscolino, 2011)*

condyloma /kon″dilō″mə/ *pl.* condylomas, condylomata [Gk, *kondyloma,* a knob], an elevated lesion. See **genital wart.**

condyloma acuminatum, soft, fleshy growths of the vulva, vagina, cervix, urethreal meatus, perineum, and anus resulting from human papillomavirus (HPV) infection. Lesions are often symmetric because of the viral transmission of the condition through direct skin-to-skin contact. See **genital wart.**

condyloma latum, a flat, moist papular growth that appears in secondary syphilis in the coronal sulcus of the perineum or on the glans penis. See also **syphilis.**

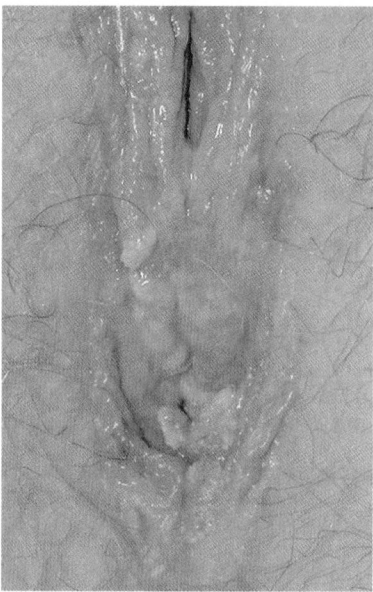

Condyloma latum *(Seidel et al, 2006)*

condylomatum acuminatum, *(Obsolete)* now called **condyloma acuminatum.**

-condylus. See **-condyle, -condylus.**

cone /kōn/ [Gk, *konos,* cone], **1.** a photoreceptor cell in the retina of the eye that enables a person to visualize colors. There are three kinds of retinal cones, one each for the colors blue, green, and red; other colors are seen by stimulation of more than one type of cone. **2.** a cone-shaped device attached to radiological equipment to focus x-rays on a small target of tissue. See also **cone biopsy.** *−conical, conic, adj.*

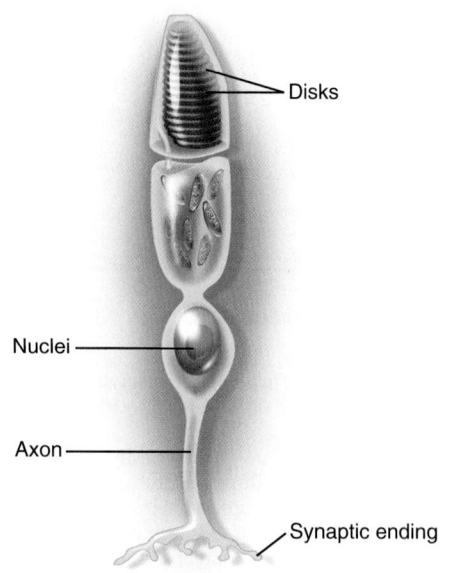

Cone cell of the retina

cone biopsy, surgical removal of a cone-shaped segment of the cervix, including both epithelial and endocervical tissue.

The cone of tissue is excised and examined microscopically to establish a precise diagnosis, usually to confirm or evaluate a positive Papanicolaou's test result. After surgery, hemorrhage sometimes occurs. If bleeding occurs 7 to 10 days later, suturing may be required. See also **biopsy, cone.**

cone cutting, a technical error resulting from a misalignment of the x-ray tube, cone, and/or image receptor. This results in the loss of one portion of the radiographic image.

confabulation /kənfab′yəlā″shən/ [L, *con + fabulari,* to speak], the fabrication of experiences or situations, often recounted in a detailed and plausible way to fill in and cover up cognitive impairment or memory loss, which may be caused by alcoholism, especially in people with Korsakoff's psychosis; head injuries; dementia; or lead poisoning. Also called **fabrication.**

confession /kənfesh″ən/, an act of seeking forgiveness through another for a real or imagined transgression.

confidence coefficient [L, *confidere,* to rely on; L, *coefficiens*], the probability that a confidence interval will contain the true value of the population parameter. For example, if the confidence coefficient is 0.95, 95% of the confidence intervals so calculated for each of a large number of random samples would contain the parameter.

confidence interval [L, *confidere,* to rely on, *intervallum,* area within ramparts], a type of statistical interval estimate for an unknown parameter: a range of values believed to contain the parameter, with a predetermined degree of confidence. Its endpoints are the confidence limits, and it has a stated probability (confidence coefficient) of containing the parameter.

confidence limits [L, *confidere,* to rely on, *limes,* limit], the endpoints or boundaries of a confidence interval, delineating the minimum and maximum values of the range expected to contain the parameter.

confidentiality /kon′fiden′shē·al″itē/, **1.** the nondisclosure of information except to another authorized person; in health care a professional and legal responsibility. **2.** (in research) protection of study participants such that an individual participant's identity cannot be linked to the information provided to the researcher and is never publicly divulged.

configuration /kənfig′yərā″shən/ [L, *configuare,* to form from], **1.** the hardware, software, and peripherals assembled to work as a computer unit for a specific situation or purpose. **2.** the general form, shape, or appearance of an object. **3.** (in chemistry) the arrangement in space of the atoms of a molecule.

configurationism. See **Gestalt psychology.**

confinement /kənfīn″mənt/ [L, *confinis,* common boundary], **1.** a state of being held or restrained within a specific place in order to hinder or minimize activity. **2.** *(Obsolete)* the final phase of pregnancy, during which labor and childbirth occur.

confinement deprivation, an emotional disorder that may result when an individual is separated from familiar surroundings or denied contact with familiar persons or objects. It may occur when one is confined to a single room.

conflict /kon″flikt/ [L, *conflictere,* to strike together], **1.** a mental struggle, either conscious or unconscious, resulting from the simultaneous presence of opposing or incompatible thoughts, ideas, goals, or emotional forces, such as impulses, desires, or drives. **2.** a painful state of consciousness caused by the arousal of such opposing forces and the inability to resolve them; a kind of stress found to a certain degree in every person. **3.** (in psychoanalysis) the unconscious emotional struggle between the demands of the id and those of the ego and superego or between the demands of the ego and the restrictions imposed by society. Kinds include

approach-approach conflict, approach-avoidance conflict, avoidance-avoidance conflict, extrapsychic conflict, intrapsychic conflict.

confluence of the sinuses /kon″floo·əns/ [L, *confluere,* to flow together], the wide union of the superior sagittal, the straight, and the occipital sinuses with the two large transverse sinuses of the dura mater. The right transverse sinus usually receives most of the blood from the superior sagittal sinus; the left transverse sinus receives the blood from the straight sinus. The confluence is one of six posterior superior sinuses of the dura mater, draining blood from the section and an inner bulging granular section.

confluent /kon″floo·ont/ [L, *confluere,* to flow together], running together, such as the sinuses of the dura mater, or some skin eruptions.

conformational disease, a general term for a number of disorders, such as Alzheimer disease and Pick's disease, caused by mutations in the structure of specific proteins, leading to the aggregation and deposition of abnormal proteins.

confounding /konfoun′ding/, **1.** interference by a third variable so as to distort the association being studied between two other variables, because of a strong relationship with both of the other variables. **2.** a relationship between two causal factors such that their individual contributions cannot be separated.

confrontational visual field testing /kon′frəntā″shənəl/ [L, *con* + *frons,* forehead], a method of assessing a patient's visual field by moving an object into the periphery of each of the visual quadrants. The test is conducted while one eye is covered and the vision of the other is fixed on a point straight ahead. The patient reports when the moving object, which may be the examiner's finger, is first detected at the edge of the visual field.

confusion /kənfyoo″shən/ [L, *confundere,* to mingle], a mental state characterized by disorientation regarding time, place, person, or situation. It causes bewilderment, perplexity, lack of orderly thought, and inability to choose or act decisively and perform the activities of daily living. It can be brief and temporary. It is usually, but not always, symptomatic of an organic mental disorder, but it may also accompany severe emotional stress, various psychological disorders, or appear as a side effect of some medications. −*confusional, adj.*

confusional state, a mild form of delirium. It may occur in any age group or may accompany preexisting brain disease. It may be triggered by a sudden or unexpected change in the person's environment. The confusion may be characterized by failure to perform activities of daily living, memory deficits, disruptive behavior, and inappropriate speech.

congener /kon″jənər/ [L, *con* + *genus,* origin], one of two or more things that are similar or closely related in structure, function, or origin. Examples of congeners are muscles that function identically, chemical compounds similar in composition and effect, and species of the same genus of plants or animals. −*congenerous, adj.*

congenital /kənjen″itəl/ [L, *congenitus,* born with], present at birth, as a congenital anomaly or defect. Compare **acquired, familial, hereditary.**

congenital absence of sacrum and lumbar vertebrae, an abnormal condition present at birth and characterized by varying degrees of deformity, ranging from the absence of the lower segment of the coccyx to the absence of the entire sacrum and all lumbar vertebrae. Congenital absence of the sacrum and the lumbar vertebrae is relatively rare. Lesser degrees of this anomaly may present so few signs that marked deformities are not present, and the condition may not be diagnosed unless accidentally found on radiographic examination. More severe forms display gross deformities and neurological deficits. Signs and symptoms of the more severe kinds include short stature, flattened buttocks, muscle paralysis to varying degrees, muscle atrophy in the lower extremities, foot deformities, contractures of the hips and knees, and varying degrees of loss of sensation, especially sensation distal to the knees. The treatment varies greatly for the congenital absence of the sacrum and lumbar vertebrae and depends on severity. Surgical intervention may be reconstructive or may involve disarticulation procedures at various spinal levels and subsequent fusion of the remaining vertebrae. Depending on the severity, many patients with this anomaly gain enough stability to sit and to walk with assistance through surgery. The most severe forms are usually fatal.

congenital adrenal hyperplasia (CAH), a group of disorders that have in common an enzyme defect resulting in low levels of cortisol and increased secretion of adrenocorticotropic hormone. The net effects are adrenal gland hyperplasia and increased production of cortisol precursors and androgens. During intrauterine life the disorder leads to pseudohermaphroditism in female infants and macrogenitosomia in male infants. Treatment involves hydrocortisone therapy and reconstructive surgery. See also **adrenal virilism, macrogenitosomia, pseudohermaphroditism.**

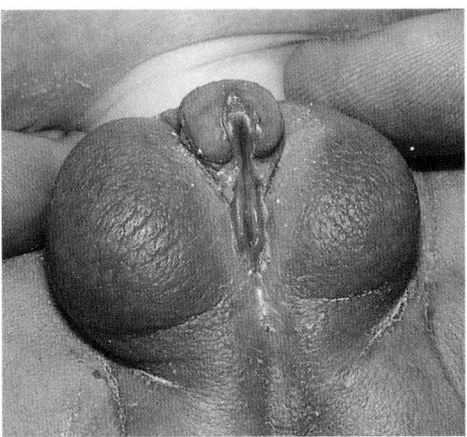

Pseudohermaphroditism associated with congenital adrenal hyperplasia *(Zitelli and Davis, 2012)*

congenital amputation, the absence of a fetal limb or part at birth. The condition previously was attributed to amputation by constricting bands in utero but now is regarded as a developmental defect.

congenital anomaly, any abnormality present at birth, particularly a structural one, that may be inherited genetically, acquired during gestation, or inflicted during parturition. Also called **birth defect.**

congenital arachnodactyly (CCA), also called **Beals syndrome.**

congenital cardiac anomaly, any structural or functional abnormality or defect of the heart or great vessels present at birth. Congenital heart anomalies are a major cause of neonatal distress and the most common cause of death in the newborn other than problems related to prematurity. Approximately 90% of all deaths from congenital heart anomalies occur during the first year of life. Congenital heart defects may be inherited or result from environmental factors, such as maternal infection or exposure to radiation or noxious substances during pregnancy. Most defects are

C

probably caused by an interaction between inherited and environmental factors that results in arrested embryonic development. Congenital heart anomalies are classified as broadly cyanotic, in which unoxygenated blood mixes with oxygenated blood in the systemic circulation, and acyanotic, in which such mixing does not occur. The general effects of cardiac malformations on cardiovascular functioning are increased cardiac workload, increased pulmonary vascular resistance, inadequate cardiac output, and, in the case of cyanotic anomalies, decreased oxygen saturation. The general physical symptoms of these pathophysiological alterations are growth delay, decreased exercise tolerance, recurrent respiratory infections, dyspnea, tachypnea, tachycardia, cyanosis, tissue hypoxia, and murmurs, all of which vary in severity, depending on the type and degree of the defect. Also called **congenital heart disease.** Kinds include **atrial septal defect, coarctation of the aorta, tetralogy of Fallot, transposition of the great vessels, tricuspid atresia, ventricular septal defect.** See also **aortic stenosis, patent ductus arteriosus, pulmonary stenosis, valvular stenosis.**

congenital cataract, an opaque eye lens present at birth. See **cataract.**

congenital central hypoventilation syndrome (CCHS), an extremely rare form of sleep apnea that causes an individual to stop breathing when falling asleep. A genetic mutation is thought to be the cause of the brainstem's failure to appropriately prompt breathing. Also called **Ondine curse syndrome.**

congenital cerebral diplegia, *(Obsolete)* now called **cerebral palsy.**

congenital cloaca. See **persistent cloaca.**

congenital cyanosis [L, *congenitus,* born with; Gk, *kyanos,* blue, *osis,* condition], cyanosis present at birth caused by a congenital heart disease or atelectasis of the lungs. See also **blue baby.**

congenital cyst [L, *congenitus,* born with; Gk, *kystis,* bag], a cyst present at birth, such as a dermoid cyst resulting from an embryonic defect in the skin or midline structures.

congenital cytomegalovirus disease. See **cytomegalic inclusion disease.**

congenital dermal sinus, a channel present at birth, extending from the surface of the body and passing between the bodies of two adjacent lumbar vertebrae to the spinal canal.

congenital dislocation of the hip (CDH), an orthopedic defect, present at birth, in which the head of the femur does not articulate with the acetabulum as a result of an abnormal shallowness of the acetabulum. Treatment consists of maintaining continuous abduction of the thigh so that the head of the femur presses into the center of the shallow cavity, causing it to deepen. Also called **congenital subluxation of the hip.** See also **Frejka splint.**

congenital ectodermal defect. See **anhidrotic ectodermal dysplasia.**

congenital erythropoietic porphyria (CEP) [L, *congenitus,* born with; Gk, *erythros,* red, *poein,* to make, *porphyros,* purple], a rare autosomal-recessive trait caused by a defect in hemoglobin synthesis in erythrocytes and release of porphyrin from normoblasts in the bone marrow. Symptoms may include mutilating lesions, hemolytic anemia, splenomegaly, excessive urinary excretion of uroporphyrin and coproporphyrin, and invariably erythrodontia and hypertrichosis. Skin photosensitivity may be extreme, and can lead to blistering, severe scarring, and increased hair growth. Also called *Gunther disease.*

congenital facial diplegia. See **Möbius syndrome.**

congenital generalized fibromatosis, the presence of small, hard, round fibromas of the subcutaneous and muscle tissues, the viscera, and the osseous systems, usually at birth. Visceral involvement may cause symptoms such as intestinal obstruction, diarrhea, and respiratory disturbances. Death is usually during the first few months of life. Also called **infantile fibromatosis.**

congenital glaucoma, a rare form of glaucoma affecting infants and young children, which results from a congenital closure of the iridocorneal angle by a membrane that obstructs the outflow of aqueous humor and increases the intraorbital pressure. The condition is progressive, is usually bilateral, and may damage the optic nerve. It may be corrected surgically. Symptoms include tearing, photophobia, and enlargement of the eye, known as buphthalmos or hydrophthalmos. See also **glaucoma.**

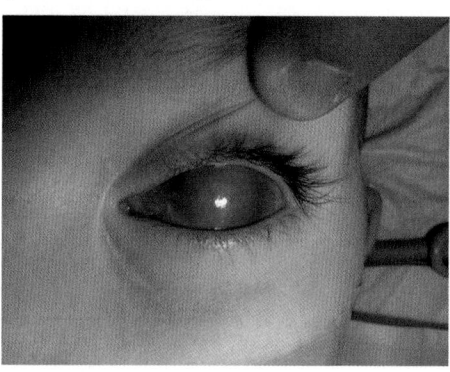

Child with congenital glaucoma *(Brightbill, 2009)*

congenital goiter, an enlargement of the thyroid gland at birth. It may be caused by a deficiency of enzymes or iodine required for the production of thyroxine.

congenital heart disease (CHD). See **congenital cardiac anomaly.**

congenital hernia [L, *congenitus,* born with, *hernia,* rupture], a hernia caused by a defect present at birth, as an umbilical hernia.

congenital hypogammaglobulinemia [L, *congenitus,* born with; Gk, *hypo,* deficiency, *gamma,* third letter of Greek alphabet; L, *globus,* small globe, *haima,* blood], a genetic disease characterized by a deficiency of gamma globulin and antibody in the serum. The cause may be a genetic defect leading to a failure of development of a normal beta-lymphocyte system and immune responses.

congenital hypoplastic anemia. See **Diamond-Blackfan syndrome.**

congenital immunity [L, *congenitus,* born with, *immunis,* free from], the immunity one has at birth that is acquired from the mother's antibodies as they pass through the placenta.

congenital jaundice [L, *congenitus,* born with; Fr, *jaune,* yellow], jaundice present at birth or during the first 24 hours of life.

congenital laryngeal stridor [L, *congenitus,* born with; Gk, *larynx* + L, *stridens,* a grating noise], a harsh respiratory sound that some infants make the first weeks after birth.

congenital leukemoid reaction. See **transient myeloproliferative disorder.**

congenital lobar emphysema [L, *congenitus,* born with; Gk, *lobos,* lobe; Gk, *en,* in, *physema,* a blowing], a respiratory disease that occurs in infants when air enters the lungs but cannot leave easily. The lungs become overinflated, causing respiratory function to decrease and air to leak out into the space around the lungs. Also called *congenital lobar overinflation.*

congenital lymphedema.   See **Milroy's disease.**

congenital megacolon.   See **Hirschsprung disease.**

congenital nonspherocytic hemolytic anemia, a group of blood disorders made up of a number of similar inherited diseases, each with a deficiency of one of the enzymes of red cell glycolysis. Most are associated with varying degrees of hemolysis, but all are less severe than, and are to be differentiated from, the more serious disorder associated with spherocytosis. Compare **hemolytic anemia, spherocytic anemia.** See also **elliptocytosis, glucose-6-phosphate dehydrogenase (G6PD) deficiency, heme, sickle cell anemia.**

congenital oculofacial paralysis.   See **Möbius syndrome.**

congenital pancytopenia.   See **Fanconi's anemia.**

congenital polycystic disease.   See **polycystic kidney disease.**

congenital pouch colon, a developmental anomaly of the colon in which part or all of it is replaced by a dilated pouch, accompanied by anorectal malformation and a fistula between the colon and the genitourinary tract.

congenital pulmonary arteriovenous fistula, a direct connection between the arterial and venous systems of the lung present at birth that results in a right-to-left shunt and permits unoxygenated blood to enter the systemic circulation. The anomaly is probably caused by faulty development of the network of vessels covering the embryonic lungs. It is often accompanied by hereditary hemorrhagic telangiectasis (Rendu-Osler-Weber disease). The fistula may be single or multiple and may occur in any part of the lung. If it is in an accessible site, surgical correction is the method of treatment.

congenital rubella syndrome, a collection of birth defects caused by transmission of the rubella virus from an infected mother to a fetus during the first trimester of pregnancy. Anomalies include cataracts, congenital heart disease, and sensorineural hearing loss. The infant may be small for gestational age and exhibit hyperbilirubinemia, thrombocytopenia, and hepatomegaly.

congenital scoliosis, an abnormal condition present at birth, characterized by a lateral curvature of the spine. It results from specific congenital rib and vertebral anomalies. The causative and pathological characteristics of congenital scoliosis are divided into six categories. Category I is associated with partial unilateral failure of the formation of a vertebra. Category II is associated with complete unilateral failure of the formation of a vertebra. Category III is associated with bilateral failure of segmentation with the absence of disk space. Category IV is associated with the unilateral failure of segmentation with the unsegmented bar. Category V is associated with the fusion of ribs. Category VI is associated with any condition not covered in the other categories. Category IV scoliosis seems to progress more rapidly and cause the greatest degree of deformity. The degree of obvious deformity caused by congenital scoliosis depends on the cause of the disease. The deformity increases with growth and age, usually progressing slowly during periods of slow growth of the trunk of the body. Treatment of congenital scoliosis may be surgical or nonsurgical. Some kinds of nonsurgical treatment techniques are exercise programs and use of orthotic devices, such as scoliosis splints or a Milwaukee brace. Surgical intervention in this disease may involve an anterior or a posterior spinal fusion. In a few individuals, additional procedures, such as spinal osteotomy, use of the Harrington rod, or halo traction, may be required. See also **scoliosis.**

congenital short neck syndrome, a rare congenital malformation of the cervical spine in which the cervical vertebrae are fused, usually in pairs, into one mass of bone, causing decreased neck motion and decreased cervical length, sometimes with neurological involvement. The posterior portion of the laminar arches in the cervical area is not fully developed; the result is spina bifida in the cervical region, usually involving the lower cervical vertebrae and, in some cases, one or more of the upper thoracic vertebrae. Congenital short neck syndrome is often associated with a cervical rib or with hemivertebrae. Neurological complications, such as nerve-root compression and peripheral nerve symptoms, are secondary to deformities of the vertebral bodies. The extreme shortness of the neck is the most common sign of this deformity, which allows only limited motion, lateral bending, and rotation. When the deformity involves nerve-root compression, symptoms of peripheral nerve involvement, such as pain or a burning sensation, may be evident, accompanied by paralysis, hyperesthesia, or paresthesia. Involvement of the spinal cord may present signs of abnormalities of lower extremities with associated signs of an upper motor lesion. Congenital short neck syndrome may require no treatment. Mild associated symptoms may be alleviated with traction, cast application, or cervical collars. Surgery may be required to relieve neurological manifestations. Also called **Klippel-Feil syndrome.**

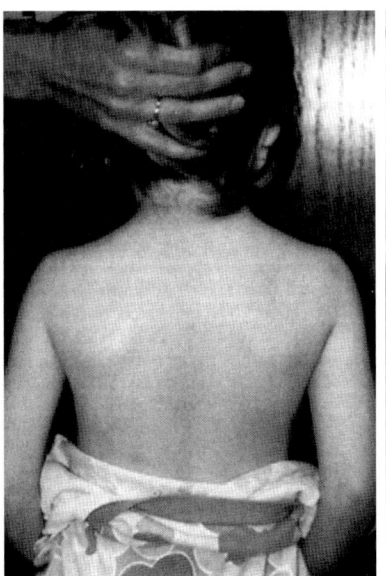 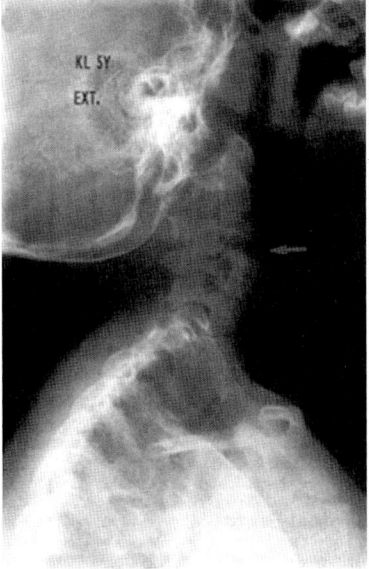

Congenital short neck syndrome *(Zitelli and Davis, 2007)*

congenital subluxation of the hip.   See **congenital dislocation of the hip.**

congenital syphilis [L, *congenitus,* born with; Gk, *syn,* together, *philein,* to love],   a form of syphilis acquired in utero, caused by the spirochete *Treponema pallidum.* Nearly 50% of infected infants die shortly before or after birth. It is generally characterized by osteitis, rashes, coryza, and wasting in the first months of life. Later childhood signs of the infection include interstitial keratitis, deafness, and notches in the incisor teeth (called Hutchinson's teeth). Some infected infants may appear disease-free at birth, but typical signs of the disease develop in adolescence. Infants are treated with penicillin; all infected infants require an ophthalmic examination. If untreated, the infection may cause deafness, blindness, disability, or death. See also **syphilis.**

congested /kənjes″tid/, **1.** having an excessive accumulation of a substance such as blood. The condition may be the result of increased production of the substance and/or outflow of the substance. It also can result from a decreased ability of the heart to pump, leading to lung congestion. **2.** having a blocked nasal or sinus passage. Mouth breathing may be necessary.

congestion /kənjes″chən/ [L, *congerere,* to accumulate],   an abnormal accumulation of fluid in an organ or body area. The fluid is often mucus, but it may be bile or blood.

congestive /kənjes″tiv/,   pertaining to congestion.

congestive atelectasis, *(Obsolete)* now called **adult respiratory distress syndrome.**

congestive cardiomyopathy [L, *congerere,* to accumulate; Gk, *kardia,* heart, *mys,* muscle, *pathos,* disease],   a heart muscle disease characterized by heart failure and enlargement.

congestive dysmenorrhea [L, *congerere,* to accumulate; Gk, *dys,* difficult, *men,* month, *rhein,* to flow], *(Obsolete)* a form of secondary dysmenorrhea caused by pelvic congestion, which arises from an increased blood supply in the area caused by pelvic disease.

congestive heart failure (CHF),   an abnormal condition that reflects impaired cardiac pumping and the inability to maintain the metabolic needs of the body. Its causes include myocardial infarction, ischemic heart disease, and cardiomyopathy. Failure of the ventricles to eject blood efficiently results in volume overload, ventricular dilation, and elevated intracardiac pressure. Increased pressure in the left side of the heart causes pulmonary congestion. Increased pressure in the right side causes systemic venous congestion and peripheral edema. See also **heart failure.**

congestive splenomegalia [L, *congerere,* to accumulate; Gk, *splen* + *megas,* large],   an enlarged spleen associated with gastric hemorrhage, anemia, portal hypertension, and cirrhosis of the liver. Also called **Banti syndrome,** *congestive splenomegaly,* **hepatolienal fibrosis.**

conglomerate silicosis /kənglom″ərit/ [L, *con* + *glomerare,* to wind into a ball],   a severe form of silicosis marked by conglomerate masses of mineral dust in the lungs, causing acute shortness of breath, coughing, and production of sputum. The conglomerates may encroach on the pulmonary circulation, causing pulmonary hypertension, right ventricular hypertrophy, pulmonary fibrosis, and complete disability. Cor pulmonale usually develops. See also **silicosis.**

congruent communication /kong″groo·ənt/,   a communication pattern in which the person sends the same message on both verbal and nonverbal levels.

-conia,   suffix meaning "small particles in the (specified) fluid or part of the body": *otoconia, statoconia.*

conic, conical.   See **cone.**

conic papilla,   any of numerous projections on the tongue. See **papilla.**

Conidiobolus /konid″e·ob′olus/,   a genus of perfect fungi. *C. coronatus* is usually a saprobe but sometimes causes entomophthoromycosis (a chronic granulomatous disease) in humans and horses.

coning,   the squeezing of the brain and brainstem through the foramen magnum as a result of swelling. It may lead to a loss of basic cardiorespiratory function.

conium.   See **hemlock.**

conivaptan,   a vasopressin receptor antagonist.

■ INDICATIONS: This drug is used to treat euvolemia hyponatremia in those hospitalized.

■ CONTRAINDICATIONS: Hypovolemia and known hypersensitivity to this drug prohibit its use.

■ ADVERSE EFFECTS: Adverse effects of this drug include headache, confusion, insomnia, hypotension, hypertension, orthostatic hypotension, phlebitis, nausea, vomiting, constipation, dry mouth, hematuria, polyuria, urinary tract infection, pollaklura, anemia, erythema, injection site reaction, dehydration, hyperglycemia, hypoglycemia, hypokalemia, hypomagnesia, hyponatremia, oral candidiasis, pain, peripheral edema, and pneumonia. Atrial fibrillation is a life-threatening side effect.

conization /kon′īzā″shən/,   the removal of a cone-shaped sample of tissue. See also **cone biopsy.**

conjoined manipulation /kənjoind″/ [L, *con* + *jungere,* to yoke together],   the use of both hands in obstetric and gynecological procedures, with one positioned in the vagina and the other on the abdomen.

conjoined tendon.   See **inguinal falx.**

conjoined twins,   two fetuses developed from the same ovum who are physically united at birth. The defect ranges from a superficial anatomical union of varying extent between equally or nearly equally formed fetuses to one in which only a part of the body is duplicated or in which a small, incompletely developed fetus, or parasite, is attached to a more fully formed one, the autosite. Conjoined twins result when separation of the blastomeres in early embryonic development does not occur until a late cleavage phase and is incomplete, causing the fused condition. Viability depends on the extent of the fusion and the degree of development of the fetuses. Formerly called **Siamese twins.**

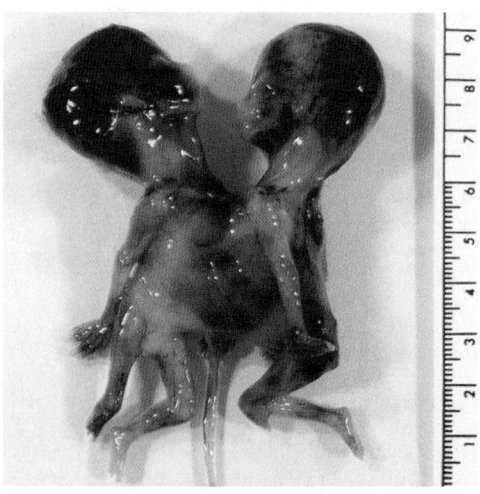

Conjoined twins at 12 weeks of development *(Courtesy Dr. D.K. Kalousek, Department of Pathology, University of British Columbia, Children's Hospital)*

conjoint family therapy /kənjoint″/, a form of psychotherapy in which a therapist sees a single nuclear family and addresses the issues and problems raised by family members.

conjugata /kon′jəgā″tə/ [L, *conjugere,* to yoke together], pertaining to the combined diameters of the pelvis, measured from the center of the promontory of sacrum to the back of the symphysis pubis.

conjugated bilirubin. See **bilirubin.**

conjugated estrogen /kon″jəgā′tid/, a mixture of sodium salts of estrogen sulfates, chiefly those of estrone, equilin, and 17-alpha-dihydroequilin. Conjugated estrogens may be prescribed to relieve postmenopausal vasomotor symptoms, such as hot flashes; to treat atrophic vaginitis, female hypogonadism, or primary ovarian failure; and to provide palliation in advanced prostatic carcinoma and metastatic breast cancer in selected patients. The drug is also used to treat and prevent osteoporosis. Continued use of estrogens can increase the risk of endometrial carcinoma, gallbladder disease, and thromboembolic disorders. Because of the danger of damage to the fetus, all female sex hormones are contraindicated during pregnancy. Among the adverse effects of conjugated estrogens are breakthrough bleeding, breast tenderness, nausea, headache, water retention, and skin eruptions. Current preliminary evidence suggests that there are no cardiovascular benefits to estrogen use during menopause, evidence that led to early discontinuation of the clinical study and changes in the product labeling. Coronary heart disease, the focus of the study, was actually increased in the treatment group, along with breast cancer, stroke, and thromboembolism. Topical agents rather than systemic estrogen should be used for treating vulvar or vaginal atrophy. Nonestrogen agents are recommended for the treatment and prevention of osteoporosis.

conjugate deviation [L, *conjugere,* to yoke together, *deviare,* to turn aside], pertaining to movements of the two eyes in which their visual axes function in parallel. The cause is a dysfunction of the ocular muscles, which allows the eyes to diverge to the same side when at rest.

conjugated hyperbilirubinemia, hyperbilirubinemia caused by defective excretion of conjugated bilirubin by the liver cells or by anatomical obstruction to bile flow within the liver or in the extrahepatic bile duct system. Kinds include **Dubin-Johnson syndrome, Rotor's syndrome.**

conjugated protein, a compound that contains a protein molecule united to a nonprotein substance, such as a carbohydrate or lipid.

conjugate paralysis [L, *conjugere,* to yoke together; Gk, *paralyein,* to be palsied], a condition of paralysis of the conjugate movements of the two eyes, up or down, or to the right or left. There is no diplopia. The cause is a cranial nerve lesion.

conjugation /kon′jəgā″shən/, **1.** (in biology) an exchange or transfer of genetic information between two individuals in certain types of unicellular organisms, including bacteria and some protozoa. In *Paramecium,* for example, both partners swap micronuclear material. The exchanged material is incorporated and passed on to progeny after replication. **2.** (in chemistry) a network of atoms connected together by alternating single and double bonds.

conjugon /kon″jo͞ogon/, an extrachromosomal segment of DNA that induces bacterial conjugation.

conjunctiva /kon′jungktī″və/ [L, *conjunctivus,* connecting], the mucous membrane lining the inner surfaces of the eyelids and anterior part of the sclera. The palpebral conjunctiva lines the inner surface of the eyelids and is thick, opaque, and highly vascular. The bulbar conjunctiva is loosely connected, thin, and transparent, covering the sclera of the anterior third of the eye. *−conjunctival, adj.*

conjunctival burn /-ī″vəl/, a chemical burn of the conjunctiva. Emergency treatment involves irrigating the eye with copious amounts of water until the chemical has been neutralized, as indicated by paper pH indicators. A topical ophthalmic anesthetic may be instilled to relieve pain. Emergency medical care should be sought.

conjunctival edema, swelling of the eye. See **chemosis.**

conjunctival fornix. See **inferior conjunctival fornix, superior conjunctival fornix.**

conjunctival reflex, a protective mechanism of the eye in which the eyelids close whenever the conjunctiva is touched. Compare **corneal reflex.**

conjunctival ring, a narrow ring at the junction of the conjunctiva and the periphery of the cornea. Also called **annulus conjunctivae, limbus.**

conjunctival sac [L, *conjunctivus,* connecting; Gk, *sakkos*], the potential space enclosed by the conjunctiva and the eyelids.

conjunctival test, a procedure used to identify offending allergens by instilling the eye with a dilute solution of the allergenic extract. A positive reaction in the allergic patient causes tearing and redness of the conjunctiva within 5 to 15 minutes. See also **allergy testing.**

conjunctivitis /kənjungk′tivī″tis/, inflammation of the conjunctiva, caused by bacterial or viral infection, allergy, or environmental factors. Red eyes, thick discharge, sticky eyelids in the morning, and inflammation without pain are characteristic results of the most common cause, bacteria. The cause may be found by microscopic examination or bacteriological culture of the discharge. Choice of treatment depends on the causative agent and may include antibacterial agents, antibiotics, or corticosteroids. Also called **pinkeye.** See also **choroiditis, uveitis.**

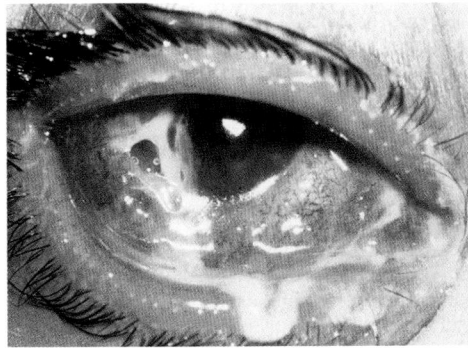

Adult with conjunctivitis (*Courtesy American Academy of Ophthalmology*)

conjunctivitis of newborn [L, *conjunctivus,* connecting, *itis,* inflammation; ME, *newe + borne*], a condition characterized by a purulent discharge from the eyes of an infant during the first 3 weeks of life. Frequent causes include gonococcal and chlamydial infections, which may lead to blindness if untreated. Also called **ophthalmia neonatorum.**

connecting fibrocartilage [L, *con + nectere,* to bind], a disk of fibrocartilage found between many joints, especially those with limited mobility, such as the spinal vertebrae. Each disk is composed of concentric rings of fibrous tissue separated by cartilaginous laminae. The disk swells outward if it is compressed by the vertebrae above or below. Compare **circumferential fibrocartilage, interarticular fibrocartilage, stratiform fibrocartilage.**

connective /kənek″tiv/ [L, *cum,* together with, *nectere,* to bind], pertaining to a binding or connection.

connective tissue, tissue that supports and binds other body tissue and parts. It derives from the mesoderm of the embryo and is dense, containing large numbers of cells and large amounts of intercellular material. The intercellular material is composed of fibers in a matrix or ground substance that may be liquid, gelatinous, or solid, such as in bone and cartilage. Connective tissue fibers may be collagenous or elastic. The matrix or ground material surrounding fibers and cells is a dynamic substance, susceptible to its own special diseases. Kinds include **bone tissue, dense connective tissue, fibrous tissue, loose connective tissue, cartilage tissue.**

connective tissue disease. See **collagen vascular disease.**

connector /kə·nek″tər/ [L, *con* + *nectere,* to bind], **1.** anything serving as a link between two separate objects or units. **2.** (in dentistry) the part of a fixed partial denture that unites a retainer of natural tooth/teeth or implant abutment and the pontic. It may be rigid or nonrigid.

connexin 26, a protein found on the GJB2 gene. Autosomal-recessive mutation of the gene encoding it is the most common cause of congenital sensorineuronal hearing loss.

connexon /kənek″son/ [L, *con* + *nectere,* to bind], the functional unit of a gap junction; the hexagonal array of membrane-spanning proteins around a central channel that connects with its counterpart in an adjacent cell to form the intercellular pore of the gap junction. See also **gap junction.**

Conn syndrome [Jerome W. Conn, American physician, 1907–1994; Gk, *syn,* together, *dromos,* course], primary aldosteronism, characterized by excessive secretion of aldosterone with symptoms of headache, fatigue, nocturia, and polyuria. The patient may also experience hypertension, hypokalemic alkalosis, potassium depletion, and hypervolemia. It may be caused by adrenal hyperplasia or an aldosterone-secreting adenoma. See also **aldosteronism.**

conoid tubercle, a tubercle on the inferior surface of the lateral third of the clavicle that gives attachment to the coracoclavicular ligament.

Conor disease, an infectious disease caused by a tick. See **Marseilles fever.**

Conradi-Hünermann syndrome /kon·rä′dē· hu′nər·män/ [Erich Conradi, German physician, 20th century; Carl Hünermann, German physician, 20th century], a rare genetic disorder characterized by skeletal malformations, skin abnormalities, cataracts, and short stature. The specific symptoms and severity of the disorder may vary greatly from one individual to another. Conradi-Hünermann syndrome is classified as a form of chondrodysplasia punctata, a group of disorders characterized by the formation of small, hardened spots of calcium on the "growing portion" or heads of the long bones (stippled epiphyses) or inside other areas of cartilage in the body. Conradi-Hünermann syndrome is inherited as an X-linked dominant trait that occurs almost exclusively in females.

consanguinity /kon′sang·gwin″itē/ [L, *con* + *sanguis,* blood], a hereditary or "blood" relationship between persons that results from having a common parent or ancestor.

conscience [L, *conscientia,* to be privy to information], **1.** the moral, self-critical sense of what is right and wrong. **2.** (in psychoanalysis) the part of the superego system that monitors thoughts, feelings, and actions and measures them against internalized values and standards.

conscientiousness /kon′she·en′shusnes/, **1.** a principled commitment to do something, such as to provide health care. **2.** acting in a way that is considered right or proper.

conscious /kon″shəs/ [L, *conscire,* to be aware], **1.** *adj.,* (in neurology) *capable* of responding to sensory stimuli; awake, alert; aware of one's external environment. **2.** *n.,* (in psychiatry) *that* part of the psyche or mental functioning in which thoughts, ideas, emotions, and other mental content are in complete awareness. Compare **preconscious, unconscious.**

consciousness /kon″shəsnes/, a clear state of awareness of self and the environment in which attention is focused on immediate matters, as distinguished from mental activity of an unconscious or subconscious nature.

conscious proprioception, the conscious awareness of body position and movement of body segments. It is regulated by the lemniscal system through pathways that begin in joint receptors and end in the parietal lobe of the cerebral cortex; it enables the cortex to refine voluntary movements.

conscious sedation, *(Obsolete)* now called **moderate sedation.**

consensual /konsen″shoo·əl/ [L, *con* + *sentire,* to feel], **1.** pertaining to a reflex action in which stimulation of one body part results in a response in another. **2.** agreeing or giving permission to an act.

consensual light reflex, a normally present crossed reflex in which light directed at one eye causes the opposite pupil to contract. In monocular blindness the pupil of the blind eye reacts consensually with stimulation of the seeing eye but does not cause constriction of the pupil of either eye. Also called **consensual reaction to light.** Compare **direct light reflex.** See also **light reflex.**

consensually validated symbols, symbols that are accepted as representing a common understanding.

consensual reaction, contraction of the pupil of one eye when the other retina is stimulated. It is a normal reflex and a test to evaluate the second and third cranial nerves.

consensual reaction to light. See **consensual light reflex.**

consensual reflex /konsen″shoo·əl/ [L, *con* + *sentire,* to feel], pertaining to a reflex action in which stimulation of one body part results in a response in another.

consensual validation, **1.** a mutual agreement by two or more persons about a particular meaning that is to be attributed to verbal or nonverbal behavior. **2.** the determination that a measuring tool (e.g., a test) measures what it is supposed to measure.

consensus sequence /kənsen″səs/, a sequence of nucleotides or amino acids similar or identical between regions of homology in different but related DNA, RNA, or protein sequence.

consensus statement, a document developed by an independent panel of experts, usually multidisciplinary, convened to review the research literature for the purpose of advancing the understanding of an issue, procedure, or method.

consent /kənsent″/ [L, *consentire,* to agree], to give approval, assent, or permission. A person must be of sufficient mental capacity and of the age at which he or she is legally recognized as competent to give consent (age of consent). See also **informed consent.**

consenting adult, an adult who willingly agrees to participate in an activity with one or more other adults. The term is usually applied to sexual activity.

consequences /kon″səkwen″səs/, stimulus events following a behavior that strengthen or weaken it. They may be either reinforcers or punishers, positive or negative.

conservation of energy /kon″sərvā″shən/ [L, *conservare,* to preserve], (in physics) a law stating that in any closed system the total amount of energy is constant; it may be transformed from one form into another, but the total amount of energy never changes.

conservation of matter, (in physics) a law stating that in any closed system the total amount of matter or mass is constant; it may be transformed from one chemical form or composition into another, but the total amount of matter never changes. See also **conservation of energy.**

conservation principles of nursing, a conceptual framework for nursing, created by Myra Estrine Levine, that is directed at maintaining the wholeness or integrity of the patient when the normal ability to cope is disturbed by stress. Nursing intervention is determined by the patient's need to conserve energy and to maintain structural, personal, and social integrity. The patient is perceived as a person whose wholeness is threatened by stress. Subjective and objective indicators of stress are assessed by the nurse, the stimuli for the stress are identified, and the level of integrity in each area is evaluated. The nurse acts as a "conservationist." The goal of the Four Conservation Principles of Nursing is to promote adaptation and maintain wholeness by using the principles of conservation. The model guides the nurse in focusing on the influences and responses at the organismic level.

conservative treatment, treatment designed to avoid radical medical therapeutic measures or operative procedures. See **treatment.**

Consolidated Omnibus Budget Reconciliation Act (COBRA), (for health or related reasons) legislation that provides for limited continuation of health coverage for individuals and families at the individual's own expense when the individual terminates employment from an organization that provides health insurance. The law applies only to organizations with a specified minimum number of employees.

consolidation /kənsol′idā″shən/ [L, *consolidare,* to make solid], **1.** the combining of separate parts into a single whole. **2.** a state of solidification. **3.** (in medicine) the process of becoming solid, as when the lungs become firm and inelastic in pneumonia.

consolidation of individuality and emotional constancy [per Hungarian-American physician/psychiatrist Margaret Mahler's (1897–1996)], (in psychiatry) the fourth and final subphase in Mahler's system of the separation-individuation phase of preoedipal development. It begins toward the end of the second year and is seen as open ended. A degree of object constancy is accomplished, and separation of self and object representations is established.

constancy /kon″stənsē/, an absence of variation in quality of distinctive features despite location, rotation, size, or color of an object.

constant /kon′stant/, a fact or principle that is not subject to change.

continuous arteriovenous hemofiltration (CAVH), a procedure to remove excess fluid and toxins that does not typically involve use of blood pumps but uses the patient's own mean arterial pressure to generate a driving force across a hemofilter membrane.

constant positive airway pressure. See **continuous positive airway pressure.**

constant positive pressure ventilation. See **continuous positive pressure ventilation.**

constant pressure generator, a machine that provides or generates a constant gas pressure throughout the inspiratory cycle of breathing. The pressure may range from a low value, such as 12 cm H_2O, to a high value of as much as 3500 cm H_2O, as required.

constant region, the part of an immunoglobulin or T cell receptor in which the amino acid sequence is relatively constant in all molecules of that class of immunoglobulin or T cell receptor. The constant region of an immunoglobulin determines its particular function. Compare **variable region.**

constant touch, a technique to diagnose the sensibility of an injured body part, such as a hand, by pressing the eraser end of a pencil or another object in various areas to determine the person's ability to detect the pressure.

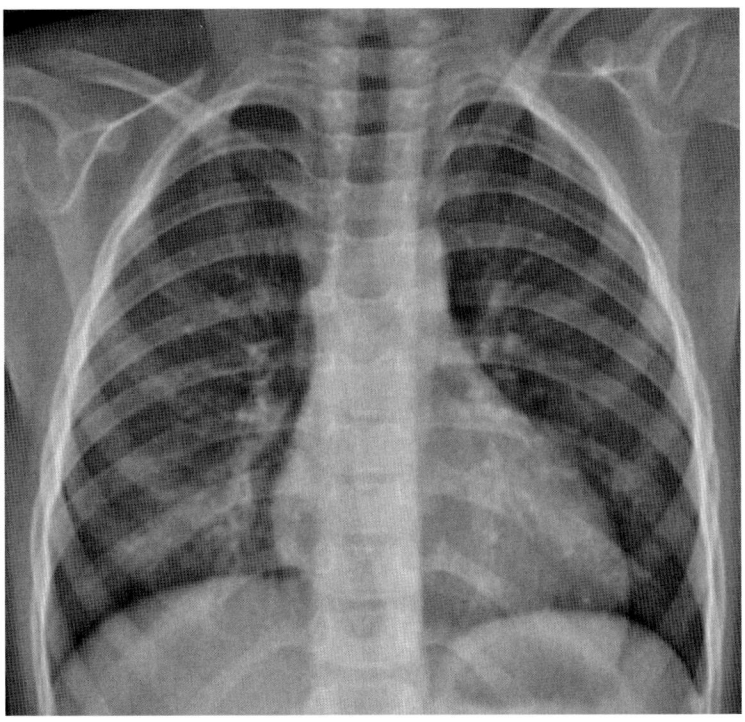

Lung consolidation in the inferior right region *(Giulio et al, 2018)*

constipation /kon'stipā″shən/ [L, *constipare,* to crowd together], difficulty in passing stools or incomplete or infrequent passage of hard stools. There are many causes, both organic and functional. Among the organic causes are intestinal obstruction, diverticulitis, and tumors. Functional impairment of the colon may occur in elderly or bedridden patients who fail to respond to the urge to defecate. For constipation that is not organically caused, the health care provider can encourage a liberal diet of fruits, vegetables, and plenty of water. The patient should be encouraged to exercise moderately, if possible, and to develop regular, unhurried bowel habits. See also **atonic constipation.** –*constipated, adj.*

■ OBSERVATIONS: Manifestations of constipation range from vague abdominal discomfort and a feeling of "fullness" to acute abdominal pain and nausea and vomiting. Decreased history of stools; hard, dry stools; small stools; bloody stools; increased flatulence; increased rectal pressure and pain; straining to evacuate; and decreased appetite are also common. A Valsalva maneuver during straining to pass stool can cause serious problems for individuals with cardiac disease or cerebral edema. Complications include fecal impaction and perforation of the colon. Chronic constipation can lead to diverticulosis and mucosal ulcers of the rectum, particularly in older adults. Most constipation is diagnosed on clinical exam, although abdominal x-rays or sigmoidoscopy may be helpful.

■ INTERVENTIONS: Most cases of constipation are managed with diet therapy, increased activity levels, stool softeners, bulk-forming agents, laxatives, and enemas. Constipation from slowed or absent GI motility requires a long-term bowel program.

■ PATIENT CARE CONSIDERATIONS: The overall goals of care are to relieve the constipated state, produce regular soft, well-formed stools, and prevent complications, such as mucosal tears or bleeding hemorrhoids. Laxatives and/ or enemas may be used for immediate relief. Assessment of elimination, nutrition, and activity patterns will assist the nurse in tailoring an educational approach aimed at preventing a pattern of chronic constipation. Emphasis on a high fiber diet, adequate fluid intake, and regular exercise is the cornerstone. Specific exercises to improve abdominal tone may be needed. Health professionals should discourage regular use of laxatives and enemas for fecal elimination because it may lead to constipation, electrolyte imbalances, and enlarged colon with chronic use.

constitution, the general bodily health of an individual, expressed by the person's physical and mental ability to function adequately in adverse circumstances.

constitutional delay /kon'stityoō″shənəl/ [L, *constituere,* to establish], a variation of normal growth in which there is slowed growth during the first 2 to 3 years of life, followed by normal or near-normal resumption of growth. The condition may relate to an inherited trait and/or a family history of short stature.

constitutional disease [L, *constituere,* to set up; Gk, *dis,* without; Fr, *aise,* ease], any disease associated with the inborn physical condition of the client, such as a hereditary susceptibility or inheritable illness.

constitutional symptom, a symptom that affects the general well-being or general status of a patient. Examples include weight loss, shaking, chills, fever, and vomiting.

constitutive resistance /kənstich″ootiv/, the bacterial resistance to antibiotics that is contained in the deoxyribonucleic acid molecules of the organism. The trait can be passed on to daughter cells through cell division, but it cannot be transmitted to other species of bacteria.

constriction /kənstrik″shən/ [L, *constringere,* to draw tight], an abnormal closing or reduction in the size of an opening or passage of the body, as in vasoconstriction of a blood vessel. See also **stenosis.**

constriction ring, in normal labor a ridge on the inner uterine surface forms between the passively thinning lower uterine segment and the actively thickening upper uterine segment (corpus). In cases of premature rupture of membranes and/or prolonged or protracted labor, a thicker, more prominent pathological structure forms, termed a pathological retraction ring (of Bandl) or a pathological construction ring. This may also occur between the births of twins. If labor is impeded, cesarean birth may be required. Compare **pathological retraction ring.**

constrictive cardiomyopathy /kənstrik″tiv kär'dē·omī·op″əthe/ [L, *constringere,* to draw tight; Gk, *kardia,* heart, *mys,* muscle, *pathos,* disease], a heart disorder characterized by decreased diastolic compliance of the ventricles, imitating constrictive pericarditis. Also called **restrictive cardiomyopathy.**

constrictive pericarditis, a fibrous thickening of the pericardium caused by gradual scarring or fibrosis. The pericardium may undergo calcification and gradually becomes rigid, resisting the normal dilation of the heart chambers during the blood-filling phases of the cardiac cycle.

constrictor /kənstrik″tər/, a muscle that binds or restricts an opening, such as the ciliary body fibers that control the size of the pupil.

constructional apraxia /kənstruk″shənəl/ [L, *construere,* to build], a form of apraxia characterized by the inability to copy drawings or to manipulate objects to form patterns or designs. It is caused by a right hemisphere lesion. The deficit is tested by asking the patient to copy two-dimensional geometric patterns, such as circles, squares, diamonds, and hexagons, and to copy three-dimensional structures constructed of 1-inch building blocks.

constructive aggression /kənstruk″tiv/, an act of self-assertiveness in response to a threatening action for purposes of self-protection and preservation. See also **aggression.**

constructive interference, (in ultrasonography) an increase in amplitude of sound waves that results when multiple waves of equal frequency are transmitted precisely in phase.

construct validity /kon″strəkt/, validity of a test or a measurement tool that is established by demonstrating its ability to identify or measure the variables or constructs that it proposes to identify or measure. The judgment is based on the accumulation of correlations from numerous studies using the instrument being evaluated. See also **validity.**

consultant /kənsul″tənt/ [L, *consultare,* to deliberate], a person who, by training and experience, has acquired a special knowledge in a subject area that has been recognized by a peer group and who is invited to guide, teach, or advise others in a professional capacity.

consultation /kon′səltā″shən/ [L, *consultare,* to deliberate], a process in which the help of a specialist is sought to identify ways to correct problems in patient management or in planning and implementation of health care programs.

consultee-centered communication /kon′sultē″/, expert advice or guidance that is given a consultee (health care provider) to improve the consultee's capacity to function more effectively in working with patients.

consumption coagulopathy, *(Obsolete)* now called **disseminated intravascular coagulation.**

contact [L, *contingere,* to touch], **1.** the touching or drawing together of two surfaces, as those of upper and lower teeth. The term is often used attributively, as in contact dermatitis and contact lens. **2.** the moving together, either directly or indirectly, of two individuals so as to allow the transmission of an infectious organism from one to the other. **3.** a person who has been exposed to an infectious disease. **4.** physical touch.

contact allergy, hypersensitivity to a substance that produced a reaction in a previous contact or that is structurally similar to another substance that produced such a reaction. Substances that can cause a contact allergy include poison ivy, metals, detergents, cosmetics, foods, and topical medicines.

contact dermatitis, a skin rash resulting from exposure to a primary irritant or to a sensitizing antigen. In the first, or nonallergic, type, a primary irritant, such as an alkaline detergent or an acid, causes a lesion similar to a thermal burn. Emergency treatment is to drench liberally and immediately with water. In the second, or allergic, type, sensitizing antigens cause an immunological change in certain lymphocytes. Subsequent exposure to the antigen causes the lymphocytes to release irritating chemicals, leading to inflammation, edema, and vesiculation. Poison ivy and nickel dermatitis are common examples of this type of delayed hypersensitivity reaction. The diagnosis can be aided by patch testing with suspected antigens. Treatment includes avoidance of the irritant or sensitizer, administration of topical corticosteroid preparations, and use of soothing or drying lotions. In severe cases, systemic corticosteroids may be used. Also called **dermatitis venenata.** Compare **atopic dermatitis.** See also **hypersensitivity reaction.**

■ OBSERVATIONS: Contact dermatitis is caused by contact with irritants and manifests as skin irritation at the site of contact. This irritation can vary from transient redness to bulla formation. Itching is common, and weeping and crusting may be present. Diagnosis is made through clinical evaluation, detailed history to locate possible source of contact rash, and patch testing to isolate allergens.

■ INTERVENTIONS: Removal of irritant from the skin with soap and water is the first line of treatment. Treatment then focuses on alleviating the itching and rash. Cool, wet cloths are effective for treating blistering. Oral antihistamines and colloidal oatmeal baths are used to control itching. Erythema may be treated with topical steroids. Oral corticosteroids are reserved for severe or widespread dermatitis.

■ PATIENT CARE CONSIDERATIONS: Subsequent exposure to the antigen causes the lymphocytes to release irritating chemicals, leading to inflammation, edema, and vesiculation. Poison ivy and nickel dermatitis are common examples of this type of delayed hypersensitivity reaction.

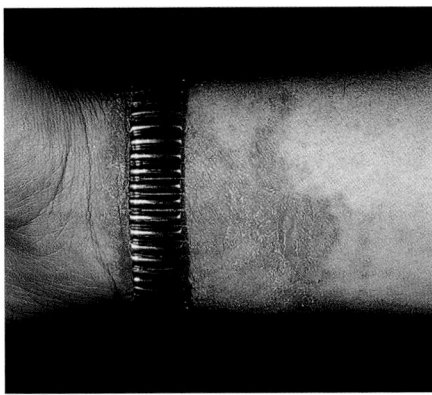

Contact dermatitis *(Habif et al, 2011)*

contact factor, a coagulation factor. Kinds include **prekallikrein, factor XII, factor VII.**

contact hour, **1.** a 50-minute "hour" used to measure time for continuing education programs. **2.** the actual amount of time in interacting with an instructor; class time.

contact lens, a small, curved lens, primarily plastic in composition, shaped to fit the person's eye either to correct refractive error or to enhance appearance. The two primary forms of contact lenses are (1) rigid gas-permeable lenses, which are small, are durable, and have little to no water absorption; and (2) soft lenses, which are larger, are more fragile, and have a 30% to 70% water content. Contact lenses float on the precorneal tear film.

contactor /kəntak″tər/, a switching device that is part of the timer for the control of voltage across an x-ray tube.

Contact Precautions, guidelines recommended by the Centers for Disease Control and Prevention for reducing the risk of transmission of epidemiologically important microorganisms by direct or indirect contact. Direct-contact transmission involves skin-to-skin contact and physical transfer of microorganisms to a susceptible host from an infected or colonized person. This can occur when health care personnel perform patient-care activities that require physical contact, such as turning or bathing the patient. Direct-contact transmission can also occur between two patients, such as by hand contact, with one patient serving as the source of infectious microorganisms and the other as a susceptible host. Indirect contact transmission involves contact of a susceptible host with a contaminated intermediate object, usually inanimate, in the patient's environment. Contact Precautions apply to specified patients known or suspected to be infected or colonized with epidemiologically important microorganisms that can be transmitted by direct or indirect contact. Compare **Airborne Precautions, Droplet Precautions.** See also **Standard Precautions, Transmission-Based Precautions.**

contact shield, a protective device constructed of lead or other material that is positioned directly on or over the eyes, gonads, or other radiosensitive areas of a patient to be exposed to an x-ray beam.

contagion /kəntā″jən/ [L, *contingere,* to touch], the transmission of an infection by direct contact, droplet spread, or contact with contaminated fomites, such as clothing, bedding, dishes, or other objects the infected person has used.

contagious /kəntā″jəs/ [L, *contingere,* to touch], infectious; transmitted from person to person by direct or indirect contact. See also **communicable. –contagion,** *n.*

contagious disease. See **communicable disease.**

contagious pustular dermatitis [L, *contingere,* to touch, *pustula,* pustules; Gk, *derma,* skin, *itis,* inflammation], a skin disease normally affecting sheep and goats but transmitted to humans who handle infected animals. It is caused by a pox virus and results in lesions on the hands, and occasionally on the face. The lesions resolve spontaneously, but slowly. Also called **ecthyma contagiosum, orf.**

containment, the keeping of something within limits.

contaminant /kəntam″inənt/ [L, *contaminare,* to bring in contact], an agent that causes contamination, pollution, or spoilage, such as a mold spore that makes food unsafe to eat.

contaminated culture /kəntam″inātid/, a bacterial culture that has acquired unwanted foreign microorganisms.

contamination /-ā″shən/ [L, *contaminare,* to pollute], a condition of being soiled, stained, touched, or otherwise exposed to harmful agents, making an object potentially unsafe for use as intended or without barrier techniques. An example is entry of infectious or toxic materials into a previously clean or sterile environment.

content analysis, a systematic procedure for the quantification and objective examination of qualitative data, such as observations and written or oral messages, by the classification and evaluation of terms, themes, or ideas; for example, the measurement of frequency, order, or intensity of occurrences in a communication to determine their meaning or effect.

content theme, a type of communication theme in which a single concept links varied topics of discussion. See **communication theme.**

content validity, **1.** validity of a test or a measurement as a result of the use of previously tested items or concepts within the tool. See also **validity. 2.** the degree to which the items within a research instrument or measurement tool represent the universe of content for the concept being measured or the domain of a given behavior.

context [L, *contextus,* to weave together], (in communications theory) the setting, meaning, and language of a message. If a message is interpreted without strict regard for these limits, it is taken out of context.

continence /kon″tinəns/ [L, *continere,* to contain], **1.** the ability to control bladder or bowel function. **2.** the use of self-restraint.

continent ileal reservoir, an intraabdominal pouch having a volume of at least 500 mL and a valve created from a portion of the ileum, pulled through the stoma, and lying flat against the abdominal wall. It maintains continence of feces and is emptied by a catheter when full. See also **continent ileostomy.**

continent ileostomy /kon″tinənt/, an ileostomy that drains into a surgically created pouch or reservoir in the abdomen. Involuntary discharge of intestinal contents is prevented by a nipple valve created from the ileum. This method eliminates the need for the patient to wear an external pouch over the stoma. Also called **Kock pouch.**

■ METHOD: After surgery the pouch is kept relatively empty by means of a catheter placed in it at surgery. The catheter is removed a week or two afterward, depending on the status of intestinal function and wound healing. Once the indwelling catheter is removed, the pouch is drained by periodically inserting a catheter through the stoma into the pouch through the valve. The time allowed to elapse between catheterizations is gradually lengthened as the capacity of the pouch increases to between 500 and 1000 mL. Six months after surgery drainage may be necessary only three or four times a day. The patient learns to recognize a feeling of fullness that indicates the need for drainage. When the patient is seated on the toilet, the dressing over the stoma is removed, and the tip of a French size 28 to 32 catheter is lubricated and inserted into the stoma. The distal end of the catheter is in a receptacle or in the toilet, at least 30 cm below the stoma. The lubricated tip of the catheter is advanced carefully through the stoma. Resistance is usually felt at a depth of about 5 cm where the valve covers the opening to the pouch. Flow usually begins when the tip of the catheter has passed the valve, at a distance of approximately 7.5 cm from the stoma. Complete drainage may require up to 15 minutes.

■ INTERVENTIONS: After surgery the patient is usually instructed to add foods one at a time. High-fiber foods and those that cause gas formation are particularly likely to be problematic. Thick secretions may be thinned by the injection of a little water into the pouch through the catheter. The stoma may be covered with a stoma cap or dressing. It is important to teach the patient to prevent irritation of the skin around the stoma. Nonallergenic tape may be used to hold the pad in place. After healing, if there is no danger of a blow to the abdomen, a pad is often not necessary. After surgery activity is resumed as the patient is able to tolerate it. There is no reason for activity to be curtailed once healing is complete and the person feels well.

■ OUTCOME CRITERIA: The patient may expect to be able to care for the stoma and to manage the drainage of the pouch. A continent ileostomy has several advantages, including the prevention of unpleasant odors and the convenience of eliminating the need for a colostomy or ileostomy bag.

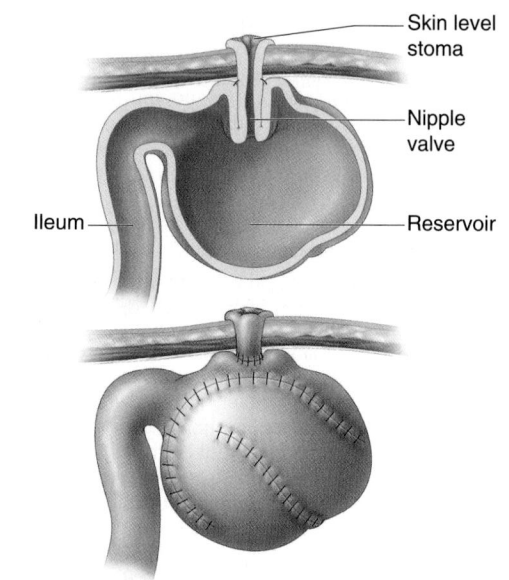

Continent ileostomy (Bailey et al, 2013)

continent urostomy. See **Indiana pouch.**

contingency contracting /kəntin″jənsē/ [L, *contingere,* to touch], a formal agreement between a psychotherapist and a patient undergoing behavior therapy regarding the consequences of certain actions by both parties.

contingency management, any of a group of techniques used in behavior therapy that attempts to modify a behavioral response by controlling the consequences of that response. Kinds include **contingency contracting, shaping, token economy.**

contingent nurse. See **float nurse.**

continua, ongoing. See **continuum,** def. 1.

continuing care nurse /kəntin″yo͞o·ing/ [L, *continuare,* to unite], a nurse who specializes in coordination of the overall needs of the patient with the potential health care resources of the community. Much of the emphasis is on discharge planning and assessment of the availability of participation in the patient's care after discharge by members of the family or other parties. Continuing care nursing responsibilities and discharge planning ideally begin at the time a patient is admitted to a hospital. Also called **nurse navigator.**

continuing education, formal educational programs designed to promote knowledge, skills, professional attitudes, and competency. The programs are usually short-term and specific. A certificate may be awarded for completion of a course, and a number of continuing education units or contact hours may be conferred. Continuing education is required for relicensure in many states. It is not to be confused with academic degree-granting programs, such as advanced education or graduate education. See also **contact hour.**

continuing education unit (CEU), a point awarded to a professional person by a professional organization for having attended an educational program relevant to the goals of the organization. A value is established for the course, and that number of points is given. Many states require professionals in the various fields of medicine, allied health, and nursing to obtain a specific number of CEUs annually for relicensure and to ensure continued competency. See also **contact hour.**

continuity theory /kon′tinyo͞o″itē/, a concept that an individual's personality does not change as the person ages, with the result that his or her behavior becomes more predictable.

continuous ambulatory peritoneal dialysis (CAPD) /kəntin″yoo·əs/ [L, *continuare,* to unite, *ambulare,* to walk about; Gk, *peri,* near, *tenein,* to stretch, *dia,* through, *lysis,* loosening], a maintenance system of peritoneal dialysis in which an indwelling catheter permits fluid to drain into and out of the peritoneal cavity by gravity.

continuous bladder irrigation (CBI), a continuous infusion of a sterile solution into the bladder, usually by using a three-way irrigation closed system with a triple-lumen catheter. One lumen is used to drain urine; another is used to inflate the catheter balloon, and the final lumen carries the irrigation solution. CBI is primarily used following genitourinary surgery to keep the bladder clear and free of blood clots or sediment. See also **drainage.**

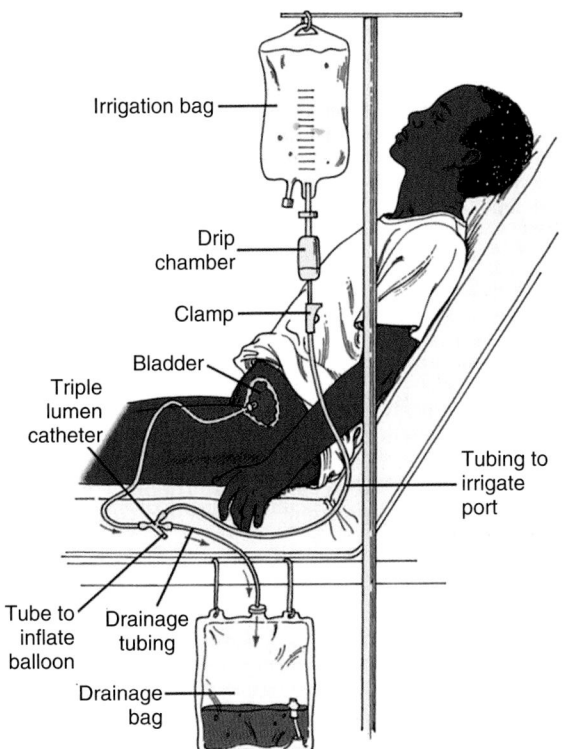

Irrigation bag
Drip chamber
Clamp
Bladder
Triple lumen catheter
Tubing to irrigate port
Tube to inflate balloon
Drainage tubing
Drainage bag

Continuous bladder irrigation *(Potter et al, 2013)*

continuous cycling peritoneal dialysis (CCPD), a type of dialysis in which the patient is attached to an automatic cycler for short exchanges while sleeping at night. Mobility is not feasible because of the cumbersome equipment. During waking hours the patient receives long dialysis exchanges but has ambulatory freedom.

continuous fever, a fever that persists steadily for a prolonged period. Compare **intermittent fever.**

continuous mandatory ventilation. See **assist-control mode.**

continuous murmur [L, *continuare,* to unite, *murmur,* humming], an uninterrupted heart murmur or cervical venous hum that characteristically begins in systole and persists through diastole. Cervical venous hum is a normal finding in children; other continuous murmurs are always pathological.

continuous negative chest wall pressure, a pressure below ambient pressure that is applied to the chest wall during the entire respiratory cycle, thus increasing transpulmonary pressure.

continuous passive motion (CPM), a technique for maintaining or increasing the amount of movement in a joint, using a mechanical device that applies force to produce joint motion without using active muscle contraction.

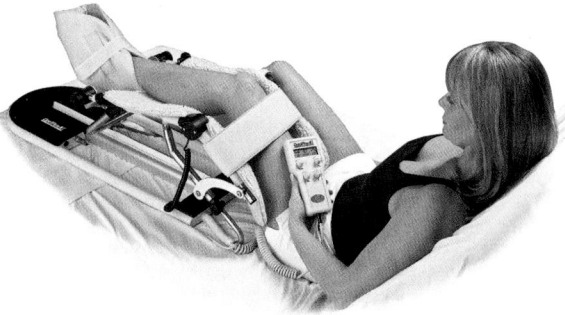

Continuous passive motion *(Courtesy The Chattanooga Group, Inc., Hixson, Tenn)*

continuous phase [L, *continuare,* to unite; Gk, *phasis,* appearance], the phase of a colloidal solution corresponding to that of the solvent of a true solution. Also called **external phase, dispersion medium.**

continuous positive airway pressure (CPAP), a method of noninvasive or invasive ventilation assisted by a flow of air delivered at a constant pressure throughout the respiratory cycle. It is performed for patients who can initiate their own respirations but who are not able to maintain adequate arterial oxygen levels without assistance. CPAP may be given through a ventilator and endotracheal tube, through a nasal cannula, or into a hood over the patient's head. Respiratory distress syndrome in the newborn and sleep apnea are often treated with CPAP. Portable CPAP machines are increasingly common in the home to deal with sleep apnea. Also called **constant positive airway pressure, CPPB.** Compare **positive end-expiratory pressure.**

continuous positive pressure ventilation (CPPV), a pressure above ambient pressure maintained in the upper airway throughout the breathing cycle. The term is usually applied to positive end-expiratory pressure and mechanical ventilation. Also called **constant positive pressure ventilation, CPPB.** See also **continuous positive airway pressure.**

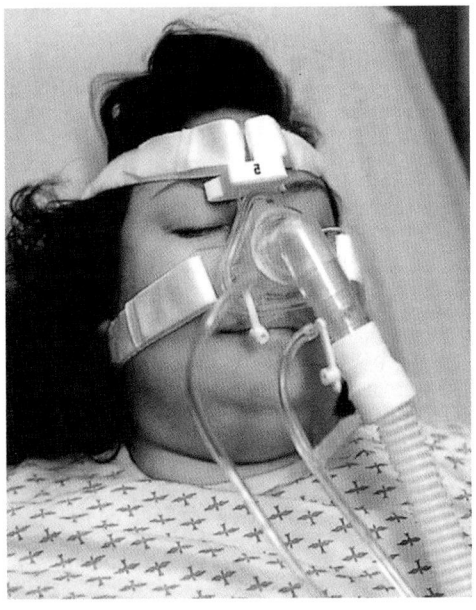

Continuous positive airway pressure *(Perry, Potter, and Elkin, 2012)*

continuous quality improvement (CQI), a system that seeks to improve the provision of services with an emphasis on future results. Like total quality management, CQI uses a set of statistical tools to understand subsystems and uncover problems, but its emphasis is on maintaining quality in the future, not just controlling a process. Once a process that needs improvement is identified, a team of knowledgeable individuals is gathered to research and document each step of that process. Once specific expectations and the means to measure them have been established, implementation aims at preventing future failures and involves the setting of goals, education, and the measurement of results. If necessary, the plan may be revised on the basis of the results, so that the improvement is ongoing.

continuous regional anesthesia [L, *continuare*, to unite], a method for maintaining regional nerve block. A local anesthetic solution is infused at intervals or at a slow rate to infiltrate epidural or spinal spaces, usually via an indwelling catheter.

continuous reinforcement, a schedule of strengthening or rewarding behavior in which omission of a response is followed by a reinforcing event or behavior. It is based on the principles of operant conditioning developed by B.F. Skinner.

continuous tremor, fine, rhythmic, purposeless movements that persist during rest but sometimes disappear briefly during voluntary movements. The pill-rolling movements and trembling of Parkinson's disease are typical of continuous tremors. Also called **resting tremor.** Compare **intention tremor.** See also **tremor.**

continuous tub bath, a therapeutic bath, usually prescribed in the treatment of some dermatological conditions, in which the patient lies supported in a medicated solution of tepid (38°C [100°F]) water. See also **hydrotherapy.**

continuous wave (CW), 1. an uninterrupted flow of energy, such as a beam of laser light. **2.** sound intensity that remains constant while ultrasound is being produced.

continuum /kəntin″yōo·əm/ *pl. continua,* **1.** a continuous series or whole. **2.** (in mathematics) a system of real numbers.

contour /kon′toor/ [Fr], **1.** *n.,* the normal outline or configuration of the body or of a part. **2.** *v.,* to shape a solid along certain desired lines.

contoured adducted trochanteric controlled alignment method (CAT-CAM) /kon′toord/, a design for an artificial lower limb that holds the femur in adduction, for persons who have undergone above-the-knee amputations.

contouring /kon′tooring/, the process of forming a curved shape.

contra-, prefix meaning "against": *contraception, contralateral.*

contra-angle /kon′trə·ang′gəl/ [L, *contra,* against + *angulus,* angle], a slant or divergence by which the working point of a surgical instrument is brought close to, but not aligned with, the long axis of its shaft. It may involve two, three, or four bends, or angles, in its shank.

contra-angle handpiece, a handpiece (dental drill) in which two or more angles or bends are used to set the shaft at a desired angle to access hard-to-reach areas of the oral cavity.

contra bevel [L, *contra,* against; OFr, *baif,* open mouth], **1.** the angle between a dental cutting blade and the base of the periodontal pocket when the blade is held

so that it separates the sulcular epithelium from the external epithelium of the gingiva. Also called **reverse bevel. 2.** an external bevel of a tooth preparation extending onto a buccal or lingual cusp from an intracoronal restoration.

contraception /kon′trəsep″shən/ [L, *contra + concipere,* to take in], a process or technique for preventing pregnancy by means of a medication, device, or method that blocks or alters one or more of the processes of reproduction in such a way that sexual union can occur without impregnation. Also called **birth control, conception control.** Kinds include **cervical cap, condom, contraceptive diaphragm, injectable contraceptive, intrauterine device, natural family planning method, oral contraceptive, spermatocide, sterilization,** *subdermal contraceptive implant.* See also **basal body temperature method of family planning, planned parenthood.**

contraceptive /kon′trəsep″tiv/ [L, *contra + concipere,* to take in], any device or technique that prevents pregnancy. See also **contraception.**

contraceptive diaphragm, a contraceptive device consisting of a hemisphere of thin rubber bonded to a flexible ring, inserted into the vagina together with spermicidal jelly or cream up to 2 hours before coitus. Fitted between the pubic symphysis and the posterior fornix of the vagina, the diaphragm cups the cervix in a pool of spermicide so that spermatozoa encounter a physical barrier, thus preventing conception. The rate of failure of the diaphragm method of contraception is approximately 2 unplanned pregnancies in 100 women using the method properly for 1 year. The principal advantage of the diaphragm is that it has no systemic effects. Diaphragms are manufactured in seven standard sizes from 55 to 100 mm in diameter. Also called **diaphragm.** Kinds include **arcing spring contraceptive diaphragm, coil spring contraceptive diaphragm, flat spring contraceptive diaphragm.**

contraceptive diaphragm fitting, a clinical procedure in which the pelvic dimensions of an individual woman are matched to the appropriate contraceptive diaphragm (diaphragm). Proper fitting depends on accurate clinical evaluation of the size of the vagina, position of the uterus, depth of the arch behind the symphysis pubis, and degree of support afforded by the muscles surrounding the vagina and selection thereby of the best type and size of diaphragm. See also **arcing spring contraceptive diaphragm, coil spring contraceptive diaphragm, flat spring contraceptive diaphragm.**

contraceptive effectiveness, the effectiveness of a method of contraception in preventing pregnancy. For clinical purposes it combines the theoretic effectiveness of the device, medication, or method and the use effectiveness. It is sometimes represented as a percentage but more accurately as the number of pregnancies per 100 woman-years. The average pregnancy rate for a couple who are sexually active and do not use contraceptives is equivalent to 85 pregnancies per 100 woman-years. A contraceptive method that results in a pregnancy rate of fewer than 10 pregnancies per 100 woman-years is considered highly effective. See also **pregnancy rate, woman-year.**

contraceptive jelly [L, *contra,* opposed, *concipere,* to take in, *gelare,* to congeal], a gelatinous preparation containing a spermicide to be introduced into the vagina to prevent conception.

Advantages and disadvantages of contraceptive methods

Method	Advantages	Disadvantages
Abstinence	100% effective in preventing sexually transmitted diseases (STDs) and pregnancy	Peer pressure to conform Relatively high failure rate from noncompliance
Withdrawal (coitus interruptus) Withdrawal of penis before ejaculation	No medical visit necessary	High failure rate Some seminal fluid often released before ejaculation Ejaculate at vaginal orifice may enter vagina No STD protection
Calendar method Refrain from intercourse during fertile period (time of ovulation)	Teaches girls about their menstrual cycle Encourages couple participation	High failure rate Requires a regular, predictable menstrual cycle (irregular menses are common for first 2 yr after menarche) No STD protection
Barrier methods *Condom*	Minimal side effects Easy to use Available without prescription Portable Provides protection against STDs Spermicidal condoms increase effectiveness for pregnancy and STD prevention Inexpensive in comparison to female condom Female participation Made of polyurethane; no latex sensitivities and can be used with oil-based lubricants Provides protection from STDs	Requires consistent use Requires premeditated intent for sexual union May decrease sensation
Male—Penile covering to trap sperm	Provides protection against STDs	Misuse results in failure Small percentage of people have latex sensitivity or allergies Decreased spontaneity
Female—Inserted into vagina with base covering part of perineum; may be inserted 8 hr before intercourse	Female participation Made of polyurethane; no latex sensitivities	Improper use may lead to pregnancy or development of STD May be difficult to insert Coital dependent Noisy
Diaphragm Cervical covering to prevent sperm from reaching egg Must be used in conjunction with spermicidal jelly May be inserted 4-6 hr before intercourse If inserted early, should be checked for placement before coitus	Can be fitted in virgins Low failure rate when used correctly Few contraindications May be reused	High failure rate in adolescents because of inconvenience of use Requires consistent use Requires fitting and instruction by medical personnel Requires premeditated intent for sexual union Requires body awareness and comfort with touching oneself for insertion Little STD protection May increase incidence of UTI
Cervical Cap Soft rubber dome with a firm but pliable rim; fits over base of the cervix close to the junction of the cervix and vaginal fornices	May be inserted hours before intercourse Insertion and removal similar to diaphragm	Available in only 4 sizes Must remain in place at least 6 hr after intercourse, but no more than 48 hr Not recommended for women with abnormal Pap test, history of toxic shock syndrome, or who have difficulty with proper fitting No STD protection

Continued

Advantages and disadvantages of contraceptive methods—cont'd

Method	Advantages	Disadvantages
Chemicals		
Spermicidal foam, jelly, cream, and suppositories	Available without prescription	High failure rate unless combined with condom
Substance inserted into vagina to kill sperm	Inexpensive	Possible for sperm to be ejaculated directly into uterine os, bypassing spermicide in vagina
	Easy to use	Must be used shortly before coitus; therefore requires interruption of sexual experience
	No major health concerns	Repeated sexual union requires repeated application
		Requires premeditated intent for sexual union
		Messy
		Nonoxynol-9 associated with increased transmission of human immunodeficiency virus to females; should not be used with anal sex in male partner sex for same reason
		No STD protection
Oral contraceptives		
Estrogen and progesterone-like compounds	99% effective if used correctly	Higher failure rate in adolescents than in older women
Inhibit ovulation by blocking release of gonadotropins from anterior pituitary gland	Safe for adolescents	Need to follow precise instructions; requires continued motivation, consistent use
	Method of choice for most adolescents	Requires prescription
	Administered by mouth	Price substantial for teenager
	Becomes a ritual not associated with sexual activity	No STD protection
	Regulates menses, decreases dysmenorrhea and acne, decreases menstrual flow	Possible side effects include headaches, missed or scanty periods, breakthrough bleeding, blood clot
	Prevents ovarian and endometrial cancers	Increased rates of chlamydia
	Prevents functional ovarian cysts	
Medroxyprogesterone acetate (DEPO-PROVERA)		
Progestin that suppresses hormonal cycle and prevents ovulation	No interruption of sex	No STD protection
Injection given every 3 mo	Invisible method	Possible side effects include significant weight gain, decreased high-density lipoproteins, irregular menses or amenorrhea, decreased libido, depression
		Fertility may be delayed after discontinuation
		Must return to care provider every 3 mo for injection
		Food and Drug Administration recommends discontinuation after 2 yr because of decreased bone density
Ortho evra transdermal system		
4.5-cm (1.75-in) square patch with norelgestromin and ethinyl estradiol	88.2% effective in perfect users	Not recommended for women >90 kg (198 lb)
Hormonal patch applied to skin weekly for 3 consecutive weeks (21 days)	Simple to use	Possible side effects include skin reaction at site, nausea, headache, dysmenorrhea, breast tenderness
Suppresses ovulation, thickens cervical mucus, and thins endometrium	Regular menstrual cycles	Slight increase risk of blood clot formation over combination oral contraceptive pill
	Not associated with sexual activity	Patch may be visible
	Avoids first-pass metabolism, resulting in more constant levels	No STD protection
NuvaRing		
Etonogestrel plus ethinyl estradiol	99.3% effective	Device may be felt by female or partner during sexual intercourse
Soft, flexible, transparent ring placed in vagina for 3 wk	Immediate return to ovulation at discontinuation	Device may fall out
Suppresses ovulation	May leave in place during sexual intercourse	Possible side effects include headache, vaginitis, leukorrhea, nausea, breakthrough bleeding
	Avoids first-pass metabolism, resulting in more constant levels	May have late withdrawal bleeding requiring placement of ring during menses
	No spermicide needed	No STD protection
	No vaginal erosion	
	No weight gain	

Advantages and disadvantages of contraceptive methods—cont'd

Method	Advantages	Disadvantages
Levonorgestrel intrauterine system (MIRENA)		
T-shape intrauterine device that releases 20 mcg/day of levonorgestrel	>99% effective	Risk of perforation at time of insertion
Inserted within 7 days of menses and remains in place for 5 yr	Effectively prevents fertilization, resulting in low rates of ectopic pregnancy	2%-12% expulsion rate
Thickens cervical mucus, inhibits sperm mobility and function	Reduced length and quantity of menstrual bleeding	Not recommended in nulliparous women or women not in monogamous relationships
	Reduced dysmenorrhea	Possible side effects include abdominal pain, headache, vaginal discharge, and breast pain
	No weight gain	No STD protection
Emergency or postcoital contraceptions		
Emergency contraception works in one of three ways: by suppressing or delaying ovulation, by preventing the meeting of sperm and egg, or by preventing implantation	Useful in unplanned sexual intercourse or contraceptive failure	No STD protection
Progestin-only pill given within 72 hours of intercourse	May be given to adolescent in advance in case of an emergency	May cause nausea if combination method used
or	Available without prescription for adults	May change timing of next menstrual cycle
Insertion of a copper-releasing intrauterine device up to 7 days after unprotected intercourse		

Modified from Hockenberry MJ, Wilson D: *Wong's nursing care of infants and children,* ed 10, St. Louis, 2015, Mosby.

contraceptive method, any act, device, or medication for avoiding conception or a viable pregnancy. See also **cervical cap, condom, contraceptive diaphragm, intrauterine device, natural family planning method, oral contraceptive, spermatocide, sterilization.**

contract [L, *con + trahere,* to draw], **1.** *n.,* an agreement or a promise that meets certain legal requirements, including competence of both or all parties to make the contract, proper lawful subject matter, mutuality of agreement, mutuality of obligation, and consideration (the exchange of something of value in payment for the obligation undertaken). **2.** *v.,* to make such an agreement or promise. –**contractual,** *adj.*

contracted kidney, a kidney that is greatly reduced in size and function as a result of an overgrowth of fibrous tissue and a diminished blood supply. The condition occurs in arteriolar nephrosclerosis and glomerulonephritis.

contractile /kəntrak″tīl/ [L, *con,* with, *trahere,* to draw], capable of becoming reduced in size or length or of being drawn together in response to some stimulus.

contractile ring dysphagia [L, *con + trahere,* to draw; AS, *hring*], an abnormal condition characterized by difficulty in swallowing caused by an overreactive interior esophageal sphincteric mechanism that induces painful sticking sensations under the lower sternum. Compare **dysphagia lusoria, vallecular dysphagia.**

contractility /kon′traktil″itē/, the ability of muscle tissue to contract when its thick (myosin) and thin (actin) filaments slide past each other.

contraction /kəntrak″shən/ [L, *con + trahere,* to draw], **1.** a reduction in size, especially of muscle fibers. **2.** an abnormal shrinkage. **3.** (in labor) a rhythmic tightening of the musculature of the upper uterine segment that begins as mild tightening and becomes very strong late in labor, occurring as frequently as every 2 minutes and lasting over 1 minute. Contractions decrease the size of the uterus and propel the fetus through the birth canal. **4.** abnormal smallness of the birth canal or part of it, a cause of dystocia. Inlet contraction exists if the anteroposterior diameter is 10 cm or less or if the transverse diameter is 11.5 cm or less. Midpelvic contraction exists if the sum of the measurements in centimeters of the interspinous diameter (normally 10.5 cm) and the posterior sagittal diameter (normally 5 cm) is 13.5 cm or less. Outlet contraction exists if the intertuberous diameter is 8 cm or less. See also **clinical pelvimetry, concentric contraction, dystocia, eccentric contraction, x-ray pelvimetry.**

contractions stress test (CST), ultrasound monitoring of fetal heart rate patterns during uterine contractions induced by exogenous oxytocin administration or endogenous oxytocin associated with nipple stimulation. Conceptually, decelerations (slowing) from the baseline fetal heart rate or fetal bradycardia are considered harbingers of placental insufficiency during the stress of labor. Management of such a "positive CST" depends on the nature of the altered fetal heart rate and the entire obstetric clinical situation. Indications for testing include maternal conditions (e.g., antiphospholipid syndrome, maternal cyanotic heart disease, systemic lupus erythematosus, chronic renal failure, insulin-treated diabetes, and hypertension) and pregnancy-related or fetal conditions (e.g., pregnancy-induced hypertension, preeclampsia, decreased fetal movement, oligohydramnios, polyhydramnios, intrauterine growth restriction [IUGR], postterm pregnancy, unexplained previous fetal demise, monochorionic diamniotic multiple gestation). See also **fetal nonstress test, oxytocin challenge test, fetal biophysical profile.**

contract-model HMO, a model in which the health maintenance organization (HMO) contracts with individual physicians rather than groups of providers for services not provided directly by the HMO.

contractual, pertaining to an agreement or arrangement. See **contract.**

contracture /kəntrak″chər/ [L, *contractura,* a pulling together], an abnormal condition of a joint, characterized by decreased motion and stiffness. It may be caused by atrophy and shortening of muscle fibers resulting from immobilization or by loss of the normal elasticity of connective tissues or the skin, as from the formation of extensive scar tissue over a joint. See also **Volkmann contracture.**
- OBSERVATIONS: A goniometer is used to determine the range of motion of a joint.
- INTERVENTIONS: The goals of the health care team are to prevent deformity and to preserve or enhance range of motion.

A coordinated approach will assist in the achievement of these goals. Physical and/or occupational therapy may be used to remediate deficits in range of motion and strength. The fabrication or provision of an orthotic device designed to maintain tissue length and prevent contracture may also be employed as a therapeutic tool. Surgery may be necessary to lengthen muscles. ■ PATIENT CARE CONSIDERATIONS: Prevention of contractures is a responsibility of every member of the health care team, including the patient. When contractures develop in a hospital setting, it is important to continue treatment when the patient is discharged. Follow-up by a home health nurse is often necessary to ensure that the patient and family understand the treatment plan.

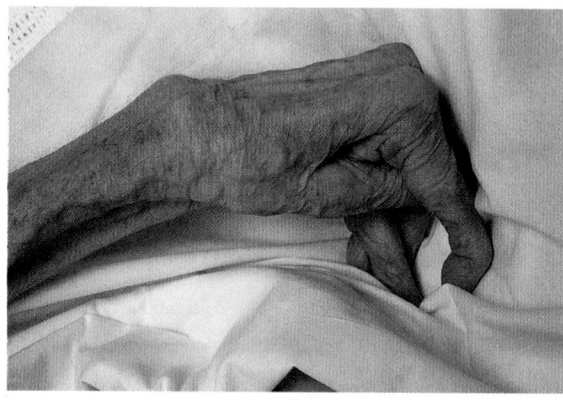

Contracture *(Sorrentino and Remmert, 2012)*

contraindicate /kon′trə·in″dikāt/ [L, *contra,* against, *indicare,* to make known], to report the presence of a disease or physical condition that makes it impossible or undesirable to treat a particular client in the usual manner or to prescribe medicines that might otherwise be suitable.

contraindication /-in′dikā″shən/ [L, *contra,* against, *indicare,* to make known], a factor that prohibits the administration of a drug or the performance of an act or procedure in the care of a specific patient. For example, pregnancy is a contraindication for the administration of tetracycline, immunosuppression may be a contraindication for vaccination, and complete placenta previa is a contraindication for vaginal delivery.

contralateral /-lat″ərəl/ [L, *contra* + *lateralis,* side], affecting or originating on the opposite side of a point of reference, such as a point on a body.

contralateral reflexes [L, *contra,* against, *latus,* side, *reflectere,* to bend back], an overflow phenomenon of the nervous system in which a reflex is elicited on one side of the body by a stimulus to the opposite side.

contrast /kon″trast/ [L, *contra,* against, *stare,* to stand], a measure of the difference in optic density, radiation transmission, pixel brightness, or other parameters between two adjacent areas in a radiographic image. Contrast plays an important role in the ability of a radiologist to perceive image detail.

contrast agent. See **contrast medium.**

contrast bath, a bath in which the patient alternately immerses a part of the body, usually the hands or feet, in hot and cold water for a specified period. The procedure is used to increase the blood flow to a particular area. The technique is used most often by physical therapists to reduce inflammation to restore mobility and function.

contrast examination, the use of radiopaque materials to make internal organs visible on an x-ray image. Because of their high atomic numbers, substances such as iodine and barium have an x-ray photoelectrical interaction that is nearly 400 times that of soft tissue. As a result, internal organs or cavities outlined by such substances are more visible.

contrast medium *pl.* **contrast media,** a substance that is swallowed or introduced via injection, catheter, or enema to facilitate radiographic imaging of internal structures that otherwise are difficult to visualize radiographically. A positive contrast medium absorbs more x-rays than the tissue or structure being examined, resulting in a more radiopaque appearance; a negative contrast medium absorbs fewer x-rays than the tissue or structure being examined, resulting in a more radiolucent appearance. Also called **contrast agent.**

contrast nephropathy, kidney damage by an iodinated contrast medium, usually seen in patients already weakened by some other condition, such as diabetes mellitus, proteinuria, hypovolemia, multiple myeloma, or preexisting renal insufficiency. There is usually a sharp decline in the glomerular filtration rate after administration of the agent, sometimes with acute renal failure, followed in a few days by return to the patient's previous level of function. Also called *contrast medium nephrotoxicity.*

contrecoup, a contusion of an area that occurs on the side opposite of impact. Compare **coup.**

contrecoup injury /kôtrekoo′/ [L, *contra,* against; Fr, *coup,* blow; L, *injuria*], an injury, usually involving the brain, in which the tissue damage is on the side opposite the trauma site, as when a blow to the left side of the head results in brain damage on the right side.

contributory negligence /kəntrib″yətôr′ē/, a legal term describing a situation in which both the plaintiff and the defendant share in the negligence that caused injury to the plaintiff.

control [Fr, *controler,* to register], **1.** *v.,* to exercise restraint or maintain influence over a situation, as in self-control, the conscious limitation or suppression of impulses. **2.** *n.,* a standard against which conclusions may be measured, as in a "control group."

control cable, a stainless steel wire, usually contained in a flexible stainless steel housing, used to move or lock a prosthesis into place.

control gene, a gene, such as an operator or a regulator, that controls the transcription of a structural gene by either inducing or repressing RNA synthesis.

control group, a set of items or people that serves as a standard or reference for comparison with an experimental group. A control group is similar to the experimental group in number and is identical in specified characteristics, such as sex, age, annual income, parity, or other factors, but does not receive the experimental treatment or intervention.

controlled area, a part of a hospital or other health facility that is occupied primarily by personnel who work with radioactive materials. It is designed with barrier shielding to confine the radiation exposure rate in the area to less than 100 milliroentgen per week.

controlled association, **1.** a direct connection of relevant ideas that results from a specific stimulus. **2.** a process of drawing repressed ideas into the consciousness in response to words spoken by a psychoanalyst. Also called **word association.**

controlled hypotension. See **deliberate hypotension.**

controlled ovarian hyperstimulation, a method of assisted reproductive technology consisting of carefully monitored administration of agents designed to induce ovulation by a greater number of ovarian follicles and thus increase the probability of an oocyte being fertilized. Also called *controlled ovarian stimulation.*

controlled oxygen therapy, the administration of oxygen to a patient on a dose-response basis in which oxygen is regarded as a drug and only the smallest amount of it is used to obtain a desired therapeutic effect.

controlled partial rebreathing anesthesia method (CPRAM), a technique to allow the reuse of exhaled anesthetic gases combined with some amount of fresh anesthetic gas.

controlled substance [Fr, *controle,* to register; L, *substantia,* essence], any drug defined in the five categories of the federal Controlled Substances Act of 1970. The categories, or schedules, cover opium and its derivatives, hallucinogens, depressants, and stimulants. Schedule I drugs have a high abuse potential and no approved medical uses. Drugs in Schedules II to V all have approved medical indications, with decreasing abuse and dependence liabilities as the schedule number increases. In Canada, categories are identified by Health Canada's Office of Controlled Substances (OCS).

Controlled Substances Act, a U.S. law enacted in 1970 that regulates the prescribing and dispensing of psychoactive drugs, including stimulants, depressants, and hallucinogens. The act lists five categories of restricted drugs, organized by their medical acceptance, abuse potential, and ability to produce dependence. A similar act exists in Canada.

controlled ventilation, the use of an intermittent positive pressure breathing unit or other respirator that has an automatic cycling device that replaces spontaneous respiration. Some units measure expired volume, nebulize medication or fluids in the air, exert negative pressure at the end of expiration, or have a variety of alarms.

control of hemorrhage, the limitation or cessation of the flow of blood from a break in the wall of a blood vessel. See also **Stop the Bleed.**

■ METHOD: Some of the methods for controlling hemorrhage are direct pressure, use of a tourniquet, and application of pressure on pressure points proximal to the wound. Direct pressure with a thick compress is applied in such a way that the edges of the wound are drawn together. A tourniquet is applied proximal to the site of bleeding only in the most extreme emergency, for the limb may then have to be removed as a result of tissue anoxia stemming from the use of the tourniquet. Firm manual pressure is applied to a pressure point over the main artery supplying the wound. Points used to obtain the pulse may be used as pressure points to stop hemorrhage.

■ INTERVENTIONS: Blood flow to an area is limited by restricting activity, elevating the part, and applying pressure. Specific treatment depends on the cause of the hemorrhage and the patient's condition. In addition to IV infusion equipment and fluids, the nurse may anticipate the need for vasopressor drugs, ventilatory assistance, central venous pressure monitoring equipment, and materials for obtaining and recording the blood pressure and urinary output. If signs of shock are present, the patient may be placed supine at a 45-degree angle to the pelvis, with the knees straight and the pelvis slightly higher than the chest. The head may be supported with a pillow. The person may be given oxygen, and the central venous pressure may be measured to determine the need for replacement of fluid volume. Sudden, severe hemorrhage with signs of shock usually is treated with IV infusion of fluids and transfusion of blood. The application of additional warmth to the skin is not recommended because heat increases the metabolism and the need for oxygen.

■ OUTCOME CRITERIA: Signs of continued bleeding—tachycardia, cold sweat, decreasing blood pressure, and patient anxiety—alert the health care provider to the probability that bleeding has begun again or that replacement fluids administered after the hemorrhage are inadequate. The person is kept calm and quiet. If the fluid balance is promptly restored, recovery is usual. Excessive loss of blood leads to hypoxia of all the tissues of the body, including the brain and vital organs, and causes death.

control process, a system of establishing standards, objectives, and methods and measuring actual performance, comparing results, reinforcing strengths, and taking necessary corrective action.

contuse /kontoōz″/, to injure a body part without breaking the skin.

contusion /kənt(y)oō″zhən/ [L, *contundere,* to bruise], an injury that does not disrupt the integrity of the skin, caused by a blow to the body and characterized by swelling, discoloration, and pain. The immediate application of cold may limit the development of a contusion. Also called **bruise.** Compare **ecchymosis.**

United States classification of controlled substances

Schedule	Dispensing restrictions	Examples
C-I	Only with approved protocol	Heroin, lysergic acid diethylamide (LSD), marijuana, mescaline, peyote, psilocybin, and methaqualone
C-II	• Written prescription only (if telephoned in, written prescription required within 72 hr) • No prescription refills • Container must have warning label	Codeine, cocaine, hydromorphone, meperidine, morphine, methadone, secobarbital, pentobarbital, oxycodone, amphetamine, methylphenidate, and others
C-III	• Written or oral prescription that expires in 6 mo • No more than five refills in 6-mo period • Container must have warning label	Codeine with selected other medications (e.g., acetaminophen), hydrocodone, pentobarbital rectal suppositories, and dihydrocodeine combination products
C-IV	• Written or oral prescription that expires in 6 mo • No more than five refills in 6-mo period • Container must have warning label	Phenobarbitol, chloral hydrate, meprobamate, the benzodiazepines (e.g. diazepam, temazepam, lorazepam), dextropropoxyphene, pentazocine, and others
C-V	Written prescription or over the counter (varies with state law)	Medications generally for relief of coughs or diarrhea containing limited quantities of certain opioid controlled substances

From Lilley et al: *Pharmacology and the nursing process,* ed 6, St. Louis, 2011, Mosby.

Canadian controlled substance chart

Drugs	Canada
LSD, mescaline (peyote), harmaline, psilocin and psilocybin (magic mushrooms)	**Part J of the Food and Drug Regulation (FDR)** • Considered "restricted drugs" • High misuse potential • No recognized medical use • New guidelines in effect April 1, 2014 for medical use of marihuana. Under the Marihuana for Medical Purposes Regulations, individuals, with medical documentation from their health care practitioner, can access marihuana for medical purposes from licensed producers.
Sedatives such as barbiturates and derivatives (secobarbital), thiobarbiturates (pentothal sodium); anabolic steroids (androstanolone), weight reduction drugs (anorexiants)	**Part G of the FDR** • Controlled drugs • Misuse potential • Only prescribed if required for medical condition • Specified number of refills (conditions apply) • Records must be kept • May be administered under emergency situations (conditions apply)
Amphetamines, benzphetamine, methamphetamine, phenmetrazine, phendimetrazine, testosterone	**Part G of the FDR** • Designated controlled drug • May be used for designated medical conditions outlined in FDR
Benzodiazepine tranquilizers such as diazepam, lorazepam, flunitrazepam, zolpidem	**Benzodiazepines and Other Targeted Substances Regulations** • Misuse potential • Only prescribed if required for medical condition • Specified number of refills (conditions apply) • Records must be kept • May be administered under emergency situations (conditions apply)
Opiates: heroin, morphine, codeine more than 8 mg, amidones (methadone), coca and derivatives (cocaine), phencyclidine (PCP), benzazocines (analgesics such as pentazocine), fentanyls	**Narcotic Control Regulation** • High misuse potential • Written prescriptions for specific medical conditions* • Records of opiate prescription file must be kept • No refills (limited amounts in a prescription) • Heroin and methadone are subject to specific controls **Schedule F of the FDR** (replaced by the **Prescription Drug List**) is a list of medicinal ingredients that, when found in a drug, require a prescription. It does not include medicinal ingredients that, when found in a drug, require a prescription if those ingredients are listed in *Controlled Drugs and Substances Act* Schedules. • Low misuse potential

From Skidmore-Roth L: Evolve Resources for *Mosby's 2016 nursing drug reference,* St. Louis, 2016, Mosby.
*Verbal prescriptions are permitted for certain opioid preparations (such as Tylenol No. 2 and No. 3), but not for opiate alone, or opiates with 1 other active nonopioid ingredient.

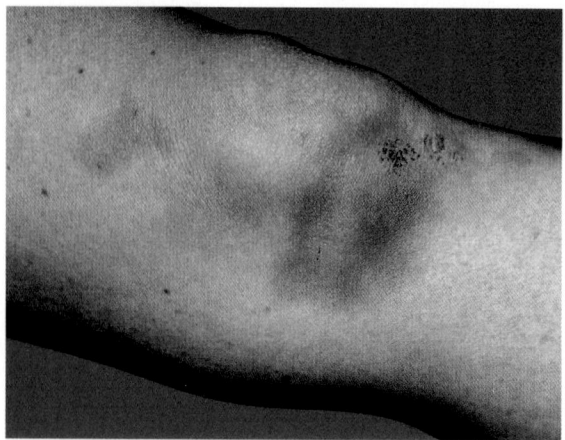

Contusion *(Cummings et al, 2009)*

conus medullaris, the terminal end of the spinal cord.

convalescence /kon′vəles″əns/ [L, *convalescere,* to grow strong], the period of recovery after an illness, injury, or surgery.

convalescent carrier, a person who has recovered from the symptoms of an infectious disease but is still capable of transmitting pathogens to others.

convalescent home. See **extended care facility.**

convection /kənvek″shən/ [L, *convehere,* to bring together], (in physics) the transfer of heat through a gas or liquid by the circulation of heated particles.

convergence /kənvur″jəns/ [L, *convergere,* to bend together], the movement of two objects toward a common point, such as the turning of the eyes inward to see an object close to the face. –*convergent, adj.*

convergent evolution, the evolution of nonhomologous organs in distantly related species in response to similar environmental conditions. Although of different origin, the organs appear similar in function, shape, or form.

convergent nystagmus, an intermittent spasmodic movement of the eyes in which they move rhythmically toward each other and slowly return to the original position. It is usually caused by a tumor of the anterior aqueduct of Silvius, third ventricle, or midbrain.

convergent squint, convergent strabismus. See **esotropia.**

conversion /kənvur″zhən/ [L, *convertere,* to turn around], **1.** changing from one form to another; transmutation. **2.** (in obstetrics) the correction of a fetal position during labor. **3.** (in psychiatry) an unconscious defense mechanism by which emotional conflicts that ordinarily cause anxiety are repressed and transformed into symbolic physical symptoms that have no organic basis. Loss of sensation, paralysis, pain, and other dysfunctions of the nervous system are the most common somatic expressions of conversion. **4.** (in traditional use) changing from one religion to another or a spiritual awakening from not having faith to acquiring it.

conversion disorder, a mental illness in which repressed emotional conflicts are changed into sensory, motor, or visceral symptoms with no underlying organic cause, such as blindness, anesthesia, hypesthesia, hyperesthesia, paresthesia, involuntary muscular movements (for example, tics or tremors), paralysis, aphonia, mutism, hallucinations, catalepsy, choking sensations, and respiratory difficulties. The person who has a conversion disorder may be indifferent to the symptoms yet firmly believes the condition exists. Causal factors include a conscious or unconscious desire to escape from or avoid some unpleasant situation or responsibility or to obtain sympathy or some other secondary gain. Treatment usually consists of psychotherapy. Also called **conversion hysteria, conversion reaction, somatoform disorder.**

conversion dysphonia, an inability to speak, usually psychogenic in nature. Conversion disorders have been reported to affect aspects of communication other than the voice. Formerly called **hysteric aphonia.**

conversion factor, a dollar value multiplied by a procedure's unit value, from the *Current Procedural Terminology* codes or a relative value scale, used to calculate the payment amount for contracted services or to set a price for a service.

conversion hysteria, *(Obsolete)* now called **conversion disorder.**

conversion reaction, an ego defense mechanism whereby intrapsychic conflict is expressed symbolically through physical symptoms. An example would be a person who becomes blind after seeing a sight that is so horrific that he or she is unable to cope with the image.

convex [L, *convextus,* vaulted], having a surface that curves outward. Compare **concave.**

convex spherical lens [L, *convehere,* to bring together; Gk, *sphaira,* ball; L, *lentil*], a lens that has sides that curve outward like a section of the exterior of a sphere and that brings light to a focus. It is used in the treatment of hyperopia (farsightedness).

convoluted /kon″vəloo′tid/ [L, *convolutus,* rolled together], twisted, rolled together, with one part over another in a scroll.

convoluted kidney tubules [L, *convolutus,* rolled together; ME, *kidenei;* L, *tubulus*], pertaining to the proximal convoluted tubule of the nephron that leads from the glomerulus to the connecting ducts, and between the Bowman's capsule and the loop of Henle. The proximal and distal sections are convoluted, whereas the ascending and descending limbs of Henle's loop are relatively straight.

convoluted seminiferous tubules, the long threadlike tubes in the areolar tissue of the testes. The testes also contain straight segments of seminiferous tubules.

convolution /kon′vəloo′shən/ [L, *convolutus,* rolled together], a tortuous irregularity or elevation caused by a structure being infolded on itself, such as the gyri of the cerebrum. See also **gyrus.**

convulsion, tonic and/or clonic movements. See **seizure.**

convulsive seizure /kənvul″siv/ [L, *convulsio,* cramp; OFr, *seisir*], a type of seizure in which there are shakes, twists, jerks, and generalized stiffening. This type of seizure may indicate an epileptic disorder or may be the result of high fever, meningitis, high levels of blood glucose or sodium, or other electrolyte disorders.

coordination of benefits (COB), the process of determination of payment responsibilities for a patient covered under multiple insurance policies, including Medicare.

convulsive syncope, a fainting episode. See **vasodepressor syncope.**

convulsive tic, a disorder of the facial nerve, causing involuntary spasmodic contractions of the facial muscles supplied by that nerve. Also called **hemifacial spasm.** See also **Gilles de la Tourette's syndrome.**

Cook catheter, a flexible catheter sometimes used in place of the Tenckhoff catheter in peritoneal dialysis.

Cooley anaemia, Cooley anemia. See **thalassemia.**

Coolidge tube [William D. Coolidge, American physician, 1873–1977], a basic type of hot-cathode x-ray tube that, with modern refinements, has been used in radiology since it was invented in 1913.

cooling [AS, *colian,* cool], reducing body temperature by the application of a hypothermia blanket; cold, moist dressings; or ice packs. Subnormal body temperature may be induced to reduce metabolic function before some kinds of surgery or after a cardiac arrest when a patient does not regain consciousness when spontaneous circulation returns. Very high fevers of any origin may be treated in part by reduction of the fever with cooling techniques. See also **hypothermia, hypothermia blanket.**

cooling rate, the rate at which temperature decreases with time (°C/min) immediately after the completion of hyperthermia treatment.

Coombs positive hemolytic anemia /koomz/ [Robin R.A. Coombs, British immunologist, 1921–2006], a form of anemia that results from premature destruction of circulating red blood cells. See also **antiglobulin test.**

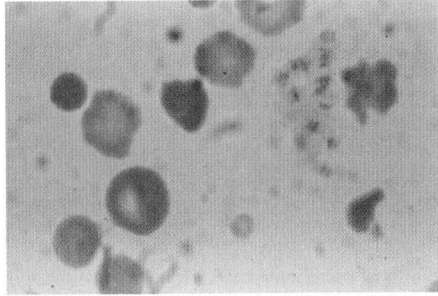

Coombs positive hemolytic anemia *(Zitelli and Davis, 2012)*

Coombs test. See **antiglobulin test.**

cooperative play /kō·op″erativ′/, **1.** any organized recreation among a group of children in which activities are planned for the purpose of achieving some goal. It usually occurs among older children. Compare **associative play, parallel play, solitary play. 2.** (in mental health and brain injury/brain rehabilitation) the ability to participate in play cooperatively and to plan next moves individually and together in the play.

Cooper's ligament. See **pectineal ligament.**

coordinated reflex /kō·ôr″dinā′tid/ [L, *coordinare,* to arrange], a sequence of muscular actions that occur in a purposeful, orderly progression, such as the act of swallowing.

CO-oximeter, a device that uses spectrophotometry to measure relative blood concentrations of oxyhemoglobin, carboxyhemoglobin, methemoglobin, and reduced hemoglobin.

copayment /kō″pāmənt/, (in the United States) an amount paid by a health insurance plan enrollee for each office or emergency department visit or purchase of prescription drugs in addition to the amount paid by the insurance company. See also **deductible.**

COPD, abbreviation for **chronic obstructive pulmonary disease.**

Cope loop catheter, a type of nephrostomy catheter with a loop at the end to hold it in place.

coping [Gk, *kolaphos,* buffet], a process by which a person deals with stress, solves problems, and makes decisions. The process has two components, cognitive and noncognitive. The cognitive component includes the thought and learning necessary to identify the source of the stress. The noncognitive components are automatic and focus on relieving the discomfort. Many defense mechanisms fall into this category. Although sometimes useful, noncognitive measures may fail to relieve the stress because the response may be inappropriate, may have the wrong effect, and, as it replaces cognitive coping measures, may prevent the person from learning more about the cause and finding a better solution for the problem.

coping mechanism, any effort directed to stress management, including task-oriented and ego defense mechanisms, the factors that enable an individual to regain emotional equilibrium after a stressful experience. It may be an unconscious process.

coping resources, the characteristics of a person, group, or environment that are helpful in assisting individuals in adapting to stress.

coping style, the commonly used cognitive, affective, or behavioral responses of a person to problematic or traumatic life events.

copolymer /kōpol′əmər/ [L, *co,* together or with; Gk, *polys,* many, *meros,* parts], a polymer containing monomers of more than one kind.

COPP, an anticancer drug combination of cyclophosphamide, procarbazine, prednisone, and vincristine.

copper (Cu) [L, *cuprum*], a malleable, reddish-brown metallic element. Its atomic number is 29; its atomic mass is 63.55. Copper occurs in a pure state in nature and in many ores. It is a component of several important enzymes in the body and is essential to good health. Copper deficiency is rare because only 2 to 5 mg daily, easily obtained from a variety of foods, is sufficient for a proper balance. Copper accumulates in individuals with Wilson's disease, primary biliary cirrhosis, and, occasionally, chronic extrahepatic biliary tract obstruction. It is an excellent conductor of heat and electricity and a valuable component of numerous alloys, and it may be compounded with arsenic to form insecticides. See also **ceruloplasmin, hepatolenticular degeneration.**

copper gluconate, a salt of copper used in the prophylaxis and treatment of copper deficiency.

copperhead /kop″ərhed′/ [L, *cuprum* + ME, *hed*], a poisonous pit viper (*Agkistrodon contortrix*) found mainly in the southeastern United States. The reddish brown, darkly banded snake is responsible for nearly 40% of the snakebites in the United States. Few bites are fatal. Pain, swelling, fang marks, and a bruise are usually present.

Immediate treatment includes keeping the victim quiet and immobilizing the bite area at the level of the heart while seeking medical attention. Antivenin is available but is rarely indicated. See also **coral snake, cottonmouth, rattlesnake.**

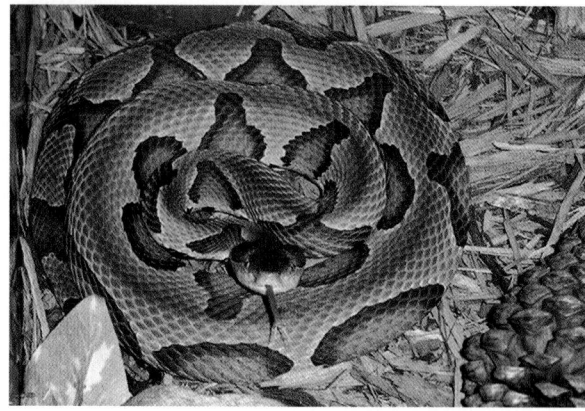

Copperhead *(Courtesy CDC/Edward J. Wozniak D.V.M., Ph.D)*

Copper T, a T-shaped intrauterine contraceptive device.

copro-, copr-, kopr-, kopra-, prefix meaning "feces": *coprolalia, coprolith.*

coprogogue, (*Obsolete*) now called **cathartic.**

coprolalia /kop′rōlā″lyə/ [Gk, *kopros,* dung, *lalein,* to babble], the excessive use of obscene language.

coprolith /kop″rōlith/, a hard mass of feces in the intestinal tract, usually caused by excessive absorption of water from the large intestine.

coprology, the study and analysis of fecal material. Also called **scatology.**

coproporphyria /kop′rōpôrfir″ē·ə/ [Gk, *kopros + porphyros,* purple], a rare autosomal-dominant metabolic disorder in which large quantities of nitrogenous substances, called porphyrins, are excreted in the feces. Attacks, with varying GI and neurological symptoms, may be precipitated by certain drugs, including barbiturates, sulfonamides, and steroids. Patients are often helped by a high-carbohydrate diet. Also called **hereditary coproporphyria.** See also **acute intermittent porphyria, coproporphyrin, porphyria.**

coproporphyrin /kop′rōpôr″firin/ [Gk, *kopros + porphyros,* purple], **1.** any of the nitrogenous organic substances normally excreted in the feces that are products of the breakdown of bilirubin from hemoglobin decomposition. **2.** a test used to measure red blood cell porphyrin levels.

copula /kop′ū·lə/ [L, *copulae,* link], **1.** any connecting part or structure. **2.** a median ventral elevation on the embryonic tongue, formed by union of the second pharyngeal arches, that represents the future root of the tongue. Also called *copula linguae.*

copulation, intercourse. See **coitus.**

CoQ, abbreviation for **coenzyme Q.**

cor /kôr/, **1.** the heart. **2.** relating to the heart.

cor-. See **co-, col-, com-, con-, cor-.**

coracoacromial /kôr′əkō·əkrō″mē·əl/, pertaining to the coracoid process and the acromion of the scapula.

coracobrachialis /kôr′əkōbrā′kē·al″is/, a muscle with its origin on the scapula and its insertion on the inner side of the humerus. It functions to adduct and flex the arm.

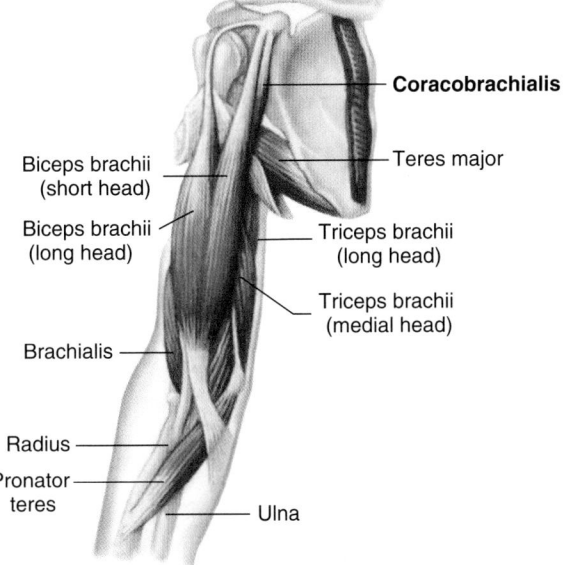

Biceps brachii (short head)

Biceps brachii (long head)

Brachialis

Radius

Pronator teres

Ulna

Coracobrachialis

Teres major

Triceps brachii (long head)

Triceps brachii (medial head)

Coracobrachialis muscle *(Patton and Thibodeau, 2010)*

coracoid process /kôr′əkoid/ [Gk, *korax,* crow, *eidos,* form; L, *processus*], the thick, curved extension of the superior border of the scapula, to which the pectoralis minor is attached. Compare **acromion.**

coral calculus, *(Obsolete)* now called **dendritic calculus.**

coral snake, a poisonous snake with transverse red, yellow, and black bands that is native to the southern United States. Bites are rare; pain does not always result, but neuromuscular and respiratory effects may be severe. Immediate treatment includes keeping the victim quiet and immobilizing the bite area at the level of the heart. Ventilatory support should be provided. Antivenin is available.

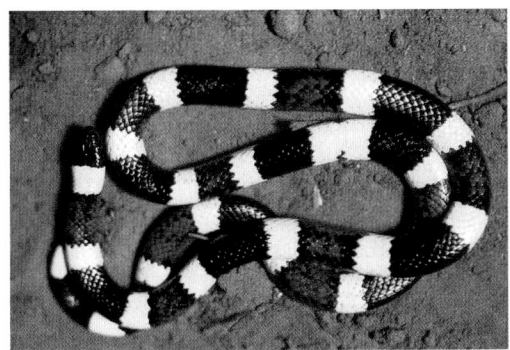

Coral snake *(Courtesy St. Louis Zoo)*

cord [Gk, *chorde,* string], any long, rounded, flexible structure. The body contains many different cords, such as the spermatic, vocal, spinal, neural, umbilical, and hepatic cords. Cords serve many different purposes, depending on location, kind of enclosed cells, and body parts or tissue involved.

cordal, pertaining to a cord, such as the umbilical cord.

Cordarone, an oral antiarrhythmic drug. Brand name for **amiodarone hydrochloride.**

cord blood, blood taken from the umbilical cord vein or artery of the fetus. Like bone marrow, cord blood is rich in stem cells. It can be frozen and stored for later transfusion, for example, in cord blood transplantation.

cord blood transplantation, the removal of blood from the umbilical cord of a fetus or its placenta for the treatment of blood diseases. Cord blood transplantation has been performed successfully in patients with leukemia, aplastic anemia, Fanconi's anemia, immunodeficiency, and genetic and metabolic disorders.

cordiform /kor′di-form/, heart shaped.

corditis /kôrdī′tis/ [Gk, *chorde* + *itis,* inflammation], an inflammation of the spermatic cord, accompanied by pain in the testis, often caused by an infection originating in the urethra or by a tumor, hydrocele, or varicocele. Inflammatory conditions of the testis may lead to swelling and tenderness.

cord presentation. See **funic presentation.**

Cordran, a topical glucocorticoid. Brand name for **flurandrenolide.**

core [L, *cor,* heart], **1.** a kind of main computer memory. **2.** main bank or repository for receiving all specimens and collections. Also called **laboratory core. 3.** (in dentistry) a section of a mold, usually of plaster, made over assembled parts of a dental restoration to record and maintain their relationships so that the parts can be reassembled in their original position; the retainer portion to which a dental restoration is attached. See **composite core, cast core, cast post. 4.** the center of a structure, as in core temperature of the body.

core-, coro-, prefix meaning "pupil of the eye": *corectopia.*

corectopia, displacement of the pupil from a central position.

core gender identity. See **gender identity.**

core temperature [L, *cor,* heart, *temperatura*], the temperature of deep structures of the body, such as the liver, as compared to that of peripheral tissues.

Corgard, a nonselective beta-adrenergic blocking agent. Brand name for **nadolol.**

-coria, suffix meaning "(condition of the) pupil": *anisocoria, platycoria.*

Cori cycle [Carl F. Cori, American physician, 1896–1984; Gerty T. Cori, American biochemist, 1896–1957; co-Nobel laureates in 1947], a physiological mechanism whereby lactate, produced by glycolysis of glucose in contracting muscle, is converted back to glucose in the liver and returned via the circulation to the muscles.

Cori disease /kôr′ē/ [Carl F. Cori; Gerty T. Cori], a rare type of glycogen storage disease in which the lack of an enzyme results in abnormally large deposits of glycogen in the liver, skeletal muscles, and heart. Signs are an enlarged liver, hypoglycemia, acidosis, and, occasionally, stunted growth. Symptoms can be controlled by giving the patient frequent small meals rich in carbohydrate and protein. Also called **Forbes disease; glycogen storage disease, type III;** *glycogenosis.*

corium. See **dermis.**

corkscrew esophagus /kôrk′skroō/ [ME *cork,* bark; L, *scrofa,* sow; Gk, *oisophagos,* gullet], a neurogenic disorder in which normal peristaltic contractions of the esophagus are replaced by spastic movements that occur spontaneously or with swallowing or gastric acid reflux. Difficulty in swallowing, weight loss, severe pain over the upper chest, and a characteristic corkscrew image on radiogram are the symptoms usually present. Management may include the use of antispasmodic drugs, avoidance of cold fluids, surgical dilation, or myotomy. Compare **achalasia.** See also **dysphagia.**

cork worker's lung, hypersensitivity pneumonitis seen in cork handlers, caused by inhalation of moldy cork dust containing spores of various species of *Penicillium.*

-cormia, -cormy, suffix meaning an "abnormal development of the trunk of the body": *camptocormia, nanocormia.*

corn [L, *cornu,* horn], a horny mass of condensed epithelial cells overlying a bony prominence. Corns result from chronic friction and pressure. The conic shape of the corn compresses the underlying dermis, making it thin and tender. Corns can become soft and macerated by perspiration. Treatment includes relief of the mechanical pressure and surgical paring or chemical peeling of the excess keratin. Also called **clavus.** Compare **callus,** def. 1.

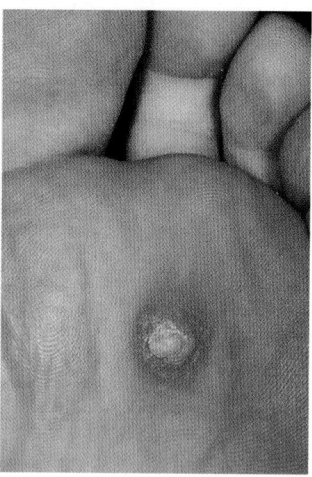

Corn *(Habif, 2004)*

cornea /kôr″nē·ə/ [L, *corneus,* horny], the convex, transparent anterior part of the eye, comprising one sixth of the outermost tunic of the eye bulb. It allows light to pass through it to the lens. The cornea is a fibrous structure with five layers: the anterior corneal epithelium, continuous with that of the conjunctiva; the anterior limiting layer (Bowman's membrane); the substantia propria; the posterior limiting layer (Descemet's membrane); and the endothelium of the anterior chamber (keratoderma). It is dense, uniform in thickness, and nonvascular, and it projects like a dome beyond the sclera, which forms the other five sixths of the eye's outermost tunic. The degree of corneal curvature varies among different individuals and in the same person at different ages; the curvature is more pronounced in youth than in advanced age. –*corneal, adj.*

corneal abrasion /kôr″nē·əl/ [L, *corneus,* horny, *abrasio,* scraping], the rubbing off of the outer layers of the cornea. A scratch or a small amount of dirt or sand trapped under the eyelid can cause a corneal abrasion.

corneal corpuscle, one of the fixed flattened connective tissue cells between the lamellae of the cornea. Also called **keratocyte.**

corneal grafting, transplantation of corneal tissue from one human eye to another, performed to improve vision in corneal scarring or distortion or to remove a perforating ulcer. Preoperative preparation includes constricting the pupil with a miotic drug, such as pilocarpine. With the patient under local anesthesia the affected area is excised, using an operating microscope; an identical section of clear cornea is cut from the donor eye and sutured in place, using an operating microscope. Cataract surgery may be performed at the same time. After surgery the eye is covered with a protective metal shield. The patient is cautioned against coughing, sneezing, vomiting, sudden movement, and lifting. The dressing is changed daily, and antibiotics are instilled. A complication that may occur after several weeks is a clouding over of the graft, a result of the rejection of foreign tissue. Corticosteroid

drugs administered immediately postoperatively may prevent the reaction. Healing is slow, and the sutures are usually left in place for 1 year. Also called **corneal transplantation, keratoplasty.**

corneal loupe, (in ophthalmology) a magnifying lens designed especially for examining the cornea.

corneal reflex, a protective mechanism for the eye in which the eyelids close when the cornea is touched. This reflex is mediated by the ophthalmic division of the fifth cranial nerve (sensory) and seventh cranial nerve (motor) and may be used as a test of integrity of those nerves. People who wear contact lenses may have a diminished or absent corneal reflex. Compare **conjunctival reflex.**

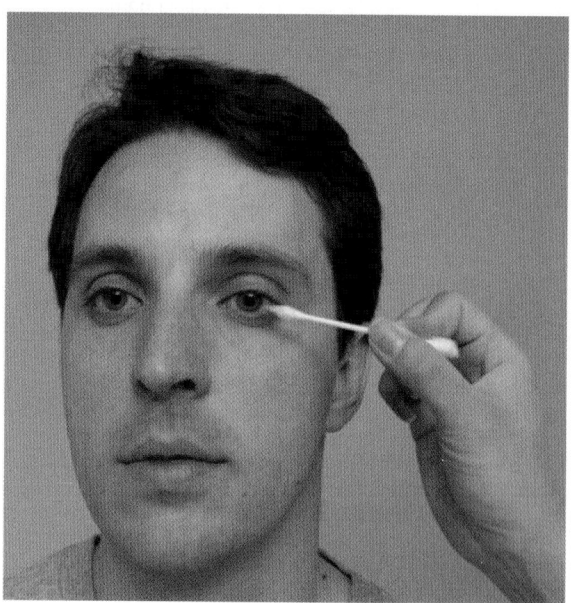

Assessment of corneal reflex *(Magee, 2014)*

corneal transplant. See **corneal grafting.**

corneal transplantation. See **corneal grafting.**

Cornelia de Lange syndrome (CdLS) /kôr·nā′lē·ä dā läng′/ [Cornelia de Lange, Dutch pediatrician, 1871–1950], a congenital syndrome of severe cognitive impairment with many other abnormalities, such as dwarfism, brachycephaly, low-set ears, webbed neck, carp mouth, peculiar shape of the nose, bushy eyebrows meeting at the midline, unruly coarse hair on the forehead and neck, and flat spadelike hands with short tapering fingers.

corneoblepharon /kôr′nē·ōblef″əron/. See **symblepharon.**

corneous. See **horny, keratic,** def. 1.

corneus layer. See **stratum corneum.**

cornification /kôr′nifikā″shən/, the conversion of cells into the horny layer of the skin. Also called **keratinization.** –*cornify, v.*

corn oil, a refined fixed oil obtained from the corn plant, *Zea mays,* used as a solvent and vehicle for medicinal agents and as a vehicle for injections. It has also been promoted as a source of polyunsaturated fatty acids in special diets.

corn pad, a device that helps relieve the pressure and pain of a corn on the toes by transferring the pressure to surrounding unaffected areas. Corn pads are constructed of pliable fabric and fashioned in various ways to accommodate different sites on the feet. See also **corn.**

cornua /kôr″noo·ə/, an anatomic structure that resembles a horn, as on the coccyx.

cornual pregnancy /kôr″nyoo·əl/ [L, *cornu,* horn, *praegnans,* childbearing], an ectopic pregnancy in one of the straight or curved extensions of the body of the uterus. The signs include a uterus that is asymmetric and tender, as well as cramping and spotting. The cornu of the uterus usually ruptures between 12 and 16 weeks of the pregnancy unless the condition is treated surgically to remove the products of conception. In most cases the uterus can be repaired. Also called **interstitial pregnancy.** See also **ectopic pregnancy.**

cornu posterioris. Also called **posterior horn.**

coro-. See **core-, coro-.**

corona /kərō″nə/ [L, crown], **1.** a crown. **2.** a crownlike projection or encircling structure, such as a process extending from a bone. —*coronal,* **coronoid,** *adj.*

coronal plane. See **frontal plane.**

coronal section [L, *corona,* crown, *sectio*], a section of the body cut in the plane of the coronal suture, or parallel to it.

coronal suture, the serrated transverse suture between the frontal bone and the parietal bone on each side of the skull.

corona radiata. See **radiate crown.**

coronary /kôr″əner′ē/ [L, *corona,* crown], **1.** *adj.,* pertaining to encircling structures, such as the coronary arteries. **2.** *adj.,* pertaining to the heart. **3.** *(Nontechnical) n.,* a myocardial infarction or occlusion.

coronary arteriovenous fistula, an unusual congenital abnormality characterized by a direct communication between a coronary artery, usually the right, and the right atrium or ventricle, the coronary sinus, or the vena cava. There may be a left-to-right shunt of small magnitude causing no symptoms, but a large shunt may result in growth failure, limited exercise tolerance, dyspnea, and anginal pain. Possible complications of a large shunt are bacterial endocarditis, rupture of an aneurysmal fistula, thrombus formation that causes occlusion or distal embolization, and in rare cases pulmonary hypertension and congestive heart failure. A loud continuous murmur heard at the lower or midsternal border of the heart suggests a coronary arteriovenous fistula; the diagnosis may be confirmed by coronary arteriography or aortography. Closure of the fistulous tract is a safe surgical procedure with excellent long-term results.

coronary artery, one of a pair of arteries that branch from the aorta, including the left and the right coronary arteries. Because these vessels and their branches supply the heart, any dysfunction or disease that affects them can cause serious, sometimes fatal complications. Coronary arterial anastomoses occur throughout the heart and are especially numerous within the interventricular and interatrial septa, at the apex of the heart, at the crux, over the anterior surface of the right ventricle, and between the sinus-node artery and the other atrial arteries. These anastomoses are more numerous and larger in the epicardium than in the endocardium, and they provide important collateral circulation in the recovery of patients who suffer coronary occlusions. The branches of the coronary arteries are affected by many different disorders, such as embolic, neoplastic, inflammatory, and noninflammatory diseases.

coronary artery bypass graft (CABG), open heart surgery in which a section of a vein or internal mammary artery is grafted from the aorta onto one of the coronary arteries, bypassing a narrowing or blockage in the coronary artery. The operation is performed in coronary artery disease to improve the blood supply to the heart muscle and to relieve anginal pain. Coronary arteriography pinpoints the areas of obstruction before surgery. Under general anesthesia and with the use of a cardiopulmonary bypass machine, one end of a 15- to 20-cm segment of saphenous vein from the patient's leg is grafted to the ascending aorta. The other end is sutured to the clogged coronary artery at a point distal to the stoppage. The internal mammary artery may also be used as graft tissue. Usually double or triple grafts are done for multiple areas of blockage. After surgery, close observation in an intensive care unit is essential to ensure adequate ventilation and cardiac output. The systolic blood pressure is not allowed to drop significantly below the preoperative baseline, nor is it allowed to rise significantly, because hypertension can rupture a graft site. Arrhythmias are treated with medications

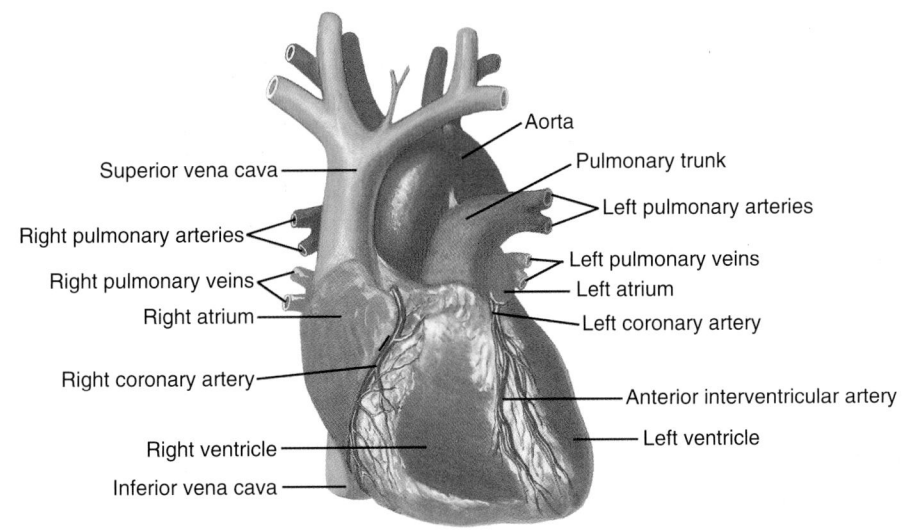

Coronary artery *(McCance and Huether, 2014)*

- Aorta
- Pulmonary trunk
- Left pulmonary arteries
- Left pulmonary veins
- Left atrium
- Left coronary artery
- Anterior interventricular artery
- Left ventricle
- Superior vena cava
- Right pulmonary arteries
- Right pulmonary veins
- Right atrium
- Right coronary artery
- Right ventricle
- Inferior vena cava

or by electrical cardioversion. The patient is usually discharged within 5 to 8 days, unless complications occur.

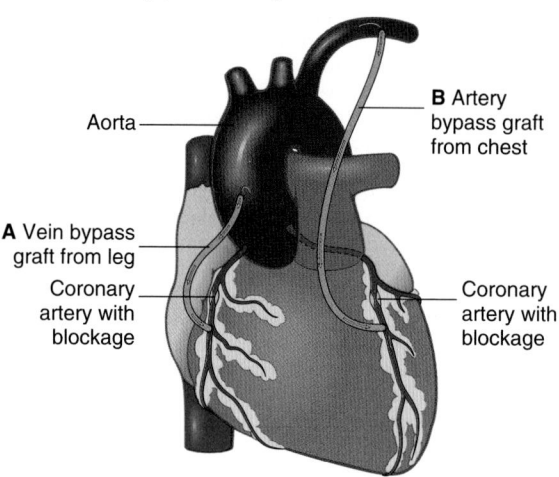

Coronary artery bypass graft *(Monahan et al, 2007)*

Image labels: Aorta; **B** Artery bypass graft from chest; **A** Vein bypass graft from leg; Coronary artery with blockage; Coronary artery with blockage

coronary artery disease (CAD), an abnormal condition that may affect the heart's arteries and produce various pathological effects, especially the reduced flow of oxygen and nutrients to the myocardium. The most common kind of coronary artery disease is coronary atherosclerosis, now the leading cause of death in the Western world. Other coronary artery diseases include coronary arteritis and fibromuscular hyperplasia of the coronary arteries. Also called **coronary heart disease.**
■ OBSERVATIONS: Angina pectoris, the classic symptom of coronary artery disease, results from myocardial ischemia. Diagnosis of coronary artery disease is usually based on patient history and tests such as exercise stress tests, electrocardiography, coronary angiography, and myocardial perfusion imaging.
■ INTERVENTIONS: Treatment concentrates on reducing myocardial oxygen demand or on increasing oxygen supply. Therapy commonly includes the administration of nitrates, such as nitroglycerin or isosorbide dinitrate; a beta-adrenergic blocker; or calcium channel blockers. Surgical interventions include coronary artery bypass surgery, angioplasty, insertion of cardiac stents, and atherectomy. The prevalence of coronary artery disease highlights the importance of preventive measures, such as reduced caloric intake by the obese patient; lowered salt, fats, and cholesterol consumption; regular exercise; abstention from the use of tobacco products; and reduction of stress.
■ PATIENT CARE CONSIDERATIONS: Many of the risk factors for heart disease can be modified to reduce mortality and health care costs. Improved models of care using a team-based approach provide the opportunity to cost effectively prevent complications related to chronic cardiovascular problems subsequent to coronary artery disease. Rehabilitation of the patients following acute exacerbation should stress the importance of following the prescribed regimens of diet, medication, exercise, and cessation of tobacco use.

coronary artery fistula, a congenital anomaly characterized by an abnormal connection between a coronary artery and a heart chamber or another blood vessel. The coronary artery abnormally attaches to one of the chambers of the heart (an atrium or ventricle) or another blood vessel (for example, the pulmonary artery).

coronary artery scan (CAS), a noninvasive method for the early detection of coronary atherosclerosis, using electron beam CT to detect and measure calcium, which is the marker for atherosclerosis, in the coronary arteries.

coronary bypass. See **coronary artery bypass graft.**

coronary care nursing, the nursing care provided to patients with cardiovascular disease. Nursing in this setting requires specialized technical knowledge, judgment, and skills, as well as the ability to give emotional support to patients and their families during the acute stage of cardiac dysfunction. Cardiac/Vascular Nurse Certification is offered through the American Nurses Credentialing Center, a subsidiary of the American Nurses Association.

coronary care unit (CCU), a critical care unit used for the treatment and monitoring of patients experiencing acute cardiac episodes.

coronary collateralization, the spontaneous development of new blood vessels in or around areas of restricted blood flow to the heart muscle.

coronary heart disease. *(Informal)* See **coronary artery disease.**

coronary ligament, one of the ligaments that connects the liver to the diaphragm.

coronary occlusion, an obstruction of an artery that supplies the heart muscle. When complete, it causes myocardial infarction; when incomplete, it may cause angina. The underlying pathophysiological characteristic is atherosclerotic plaque, which usually develops slowly by buildup of lipid and macrophage complexes. Rapid plaque accumulation is frequently caused by hemorrhage within a plaque. If the plaque ruptures, platelets aggregate, fibrin is deposited, spasm occurs, and a thrombus develops, resulting in acute myocardial infarction. Treatment includes prompt IV thrombolysis and administration of heparin. Primary percutaneous transvenous coronary angioplasty can achieve prompt reperfusion. See also **coronary artery disease.**

coronary plexus [L, *corona,* crown, *plexus,* plaited], a network of autonomic nerve fibers located near the base of the heart.

coronary sinus, the wide venous channel, about 2.25 cm long, situated in the coronary sulcus and covered by muscular fibers from the left atrium. Through a single semilunar valve it drains five coronary veins: the great cardiac vein, the small cardiac vein, the middle cardiac vein, the posterior vein of the left ventricle, and the oblique vein of the left atrium.

coronary sulcus, a surface groove encircling the heart that separates the atria from the ventricles. It contains the right coronary artery, the small cardiac vein, the coronary sinus, and the circumflex branch of the left coronary artery.

coronary thrombosis, development of a thrombus that blocks a coronary artery, often causing myocardial infarction and death. Coronary thromboses commonly develop in segments of arteries with atherosclerotic lesions.

coronary valve [L, *corona,* crown, *valva,* folding door], a semicircular fold of endocardium that may prevent the backflow of blood from the right atrium into the coronary sinus. Also called **thebesian valve.**

coronary vein, one of the veins of the heart that drains blood from the capillary beds of the myocardium through the coronary sinus into the right atrium. A few small coronary veins that collect blood from a small area in the right ventricle drain directly into the right atrium.

Coronaviridae /kôr′ənəvir″idē/, a family of four antigenic groups of single-stranded ribonucleic acid viruses. Some strains of the organism are associated with upper respiratory infections in humans. One example from this family is the virus that causes SARS (severe acute respiratory syndrome).

coronavirus /kôr′ənəvī″rəs/ [L, *corona* + *virus,* poison], a member of Coronaviridae, a family of viruses that includes several types capable of causing acute respiratory illnesses, including severe acute respiratory syndrome (SARS) and COVID-19. These viruses infect a wide variety of mammals (including humans) and birds. Along with rhinoviruses, coronaviruses are considered the primary causes of the common cold. Reinfection with the same genotype can occur. Other diseases caused by coronaviruses include hepatitis,

Decreasing risk factors for coronary artery disease

Hypertension	• Monitor home blood pressure (BP) and attend regular checkups. • Take prescribed medications for BP control. • Reduce salt intake. • Stop tobacco use. Avoid exposure to environmental tobacco (secondhand) smoke. • Control or reduce weight. • Perform physical activity daily.
Elevated serum lipids	• Reduce total fat intake. • Reduce animal (saturated) fat intake. • Take prescribed medications for lipid reduction. • Adjust total caloric intake to achieve and maintain ideal body weight. • Engage in daily physical activity. • Increase amount of complex carbohydrates, fiber, and vegetable proteins in diet.
Tobacco use	• Begin a smoking cessation program. • Change daily routines associated with smoking to reduce desire to smoke. • Substitute other activities for smoking. • Ask caregivers to support efforts to stop smoking. • Avoid exposure to environmental tobacco smoke.
Physical inactivity	• Develop and maintain at least 30 min of moderate physical activity daily (minimum 5 days a week). • Increase activities to a fitness level.
Psychological state	• Increase awareness of behaviors that are harmful to health. • Alter patterns that are conducive to stress (e.g., get up 30 min earlier so breakfast is not eaten on way to work). • Set realistic goals for self. • Reassess priorities in light of health needs. • Learn effective stress management strategies. • Seek professional help if feeling depressed, angry, anxious, etc. • Plan time for adequate rest and sleep.
Obesity	• Change eating patterns and habits. • Reduce caloric intake to achieve body mass index of 18.5–24.9 kg/m². • Increase physical activity to increase caloric expenditure. • Avoid fad and crash diets, which are not effective over time. • Avoid large, heavy meals. Consider smaller, more frequent meals.
Diabetes	• Follow the recommended diet. • Control or reduce weight. • Take prescribed antidiabetic medications. • Monitor blood glucose levels regularly.

From Lewis SL et al: *Medical-surgical nursing: assessment and management of clinical problems*, ed 9, St. Louis, 2014, Mosby.

neurological disease, infectious peritonitis, nephritis, and pancreatitis.

coroner /kôr″ənər/ [L, *corona*, crown], a public official who investigates the causes and circumstances of deaths that occur within a specific legal jurisdiction or territory, especially those that may have resulted from unnatural causes. See also **medical examiner.**

coronoid. See **corona.**

coronoid fossa /kô″rənoid/ [L, *corona* + Gk, *eidos*, form; L, *fossa*, ditch], a small depression in the distal dorsal surface of the humerus that receives the coronoid process of the ulna when the forearm is flexed.

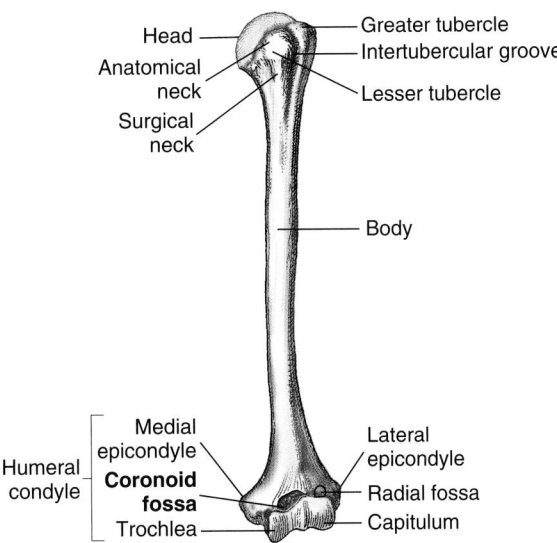

Coronoid fossa *(Frank, Long, and Smith, 2012)*

coronoid process of the mandible, a prominence on the anterior surface of the ramus of the mandible to which each temporal muscle attaches.

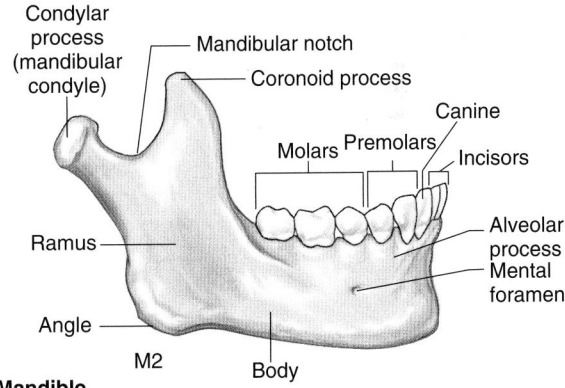

Coronoid process of the mandible *(Patton, 2016)*

coronoid process of the ulna, a wide, flaring projection of the proximal end of the ulna. The proximal surface of the process forms the lower part of the trochlear notch.

corpectomy, the removal of a vertebral body.

corpor-, prefix meaning "body": *corpora, corporis.*

corpora lutea. See **corpus luteum.**

corporate practice of medicine, (in the United States) the role of nonpracticing physicians or nonprofessional corporations in employment relationships with physicians engaged in providing health care. Laws governing corporate practice of medicine vary among different states, but generally they require practitioner control over diagnosis and treatment, practitioner setting of fees, a reasonable relationship between services provided by layperson or corporation and amounts charged to the practitioner, and an unaltered practitioner-patient relationship.

corpse /kôrps/ [L, *corpus,* body], the body of a dead human being.

corpulence /kôr″pyələns/ [L, *corpus,* body], obesity.

corpulent /kôr″pyələnt/, obese; of excessive weight.

cor pulmonale /kôr pŏŏl′mənal″ē/ [L, heart + *pulmoneus,* lungs], enlargement of the heart's right ventricle caused by primary lung disease. In some patients, the left ventricle also increases in size. Cor pulmonale eventually results in failure of the right ventricle, which cannot accommodate an increase in pressure as easily as the left ventricle. Pulmonary hypertension associated with this condition is caused by some disorder of the pulmonary parenchyma or of the pulmonary vascular system between the origin of the left pulmonary artery and the entry of the pulmonary veins into the left atrium.

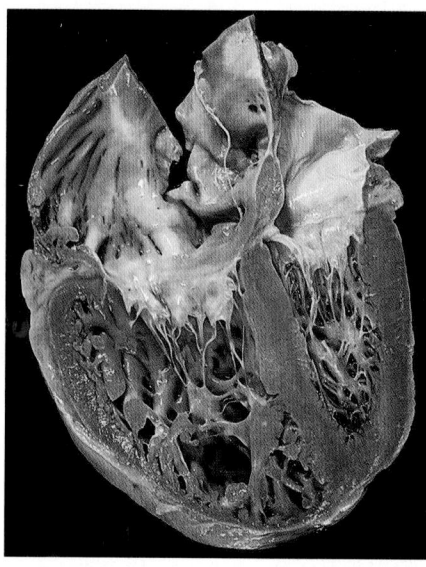

Cor pulmonale *(Kumar et al, 2010)*

corpus. See **body.**

corpus albicans /kôr″pəs/, a pale white spot on the surface of the ovary that arises from the corpus luteum if conception does not occur. Compare **corpus luteum.**

corpus amylaceum. See **colloid corpuscle.**

corpus callosum /kôr′pəs kalō′səm/, **1.** a transverse band of nerve fibers joining the cerebral hemispheres. It is located at the bottom of the longitudinal fissure between the two hemispheres and is covered by the cingulate gyrus. **2.** the largest commissure of the brain, connecting the cerebral hemispheres.

corpus cavernosum [L, body + *caverna,* hollow place], a type of spongy erectile tissue within the penis or clitoris. The tissue becomes engorged with blood during sexual excitement.

corpuscle /kôr″pəsəl/ [L, *corpusculum,* little body], **1.** any cell of the body. **2.** a red or white blood cell. Also called **corpuscule.** −*corpuscular, adj.*

corpuscular radiation /kôrpus″kyələr/ [L, *corpusculum* + *radiare,* to emit rays], the radiation associated with subatomic particles, such as electrons, protons, neutrons, or alpha particles, which travel in streams at various velocities. All such particles have definite masses and radiation properties that are very different from those of electromagnetic radiations, which have no mass and travel as waves at the speed of light. See also **background radiation, leakage radiation, scattered radiation.**

corpuscule. See **corpuscle.**

corpus femoris [L, *corpus,* body + *femur,* thigh], the main part or shaft of the femur.

corpus luteum /kôr″pəs lōō″tē·əm/ *pl. corpora lutea* [L, *corpus,* body, *luteus,* yellow], an anatomical structure on the ovary's surface, consisting of a spheroid of yellowish tissue 1 to 2 cm in diameter that grows within the ruptured ovarian follicle after ovulation. The pleated wall of the collapsed follicle is made up of several layers of granulosa cells that grow toward the center of the cavity to form the structure. During a woman's reproductive years, a corpus luteum forms after every ovulation. It acts as a short-lived endocrine organ that secretes progesterone, which serves to maintain the decidual layer of the uterine endometrium in the richly vascular state necessary for implantation and pregnancy. If conception occurs, the corpus luteum grows and secretes increasing amounts of progesterone. It reaches its maximum function and size (2 to 3 cm) at 10 to 12 weeks of gestation. It persists, slowly diminishing in size and function, until 6 months after

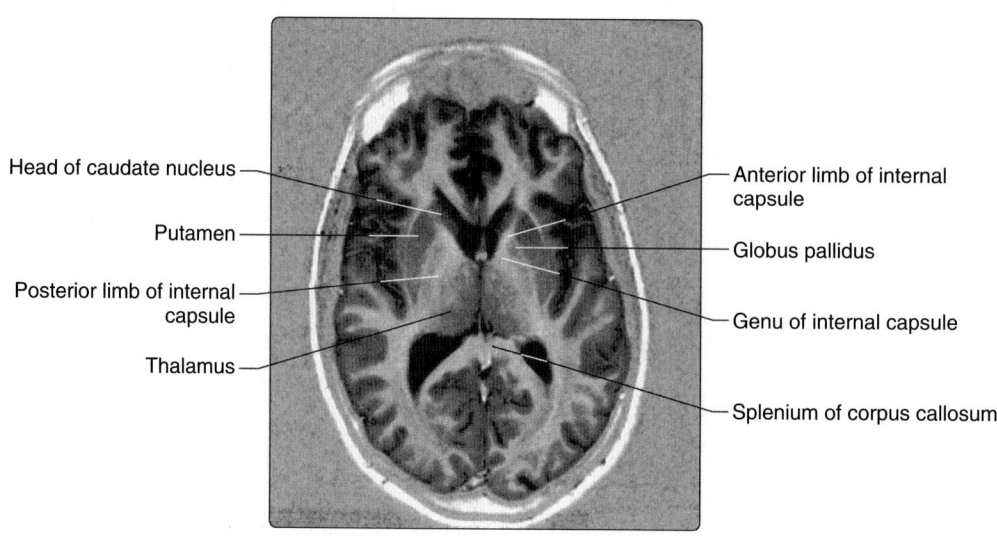

Corpus callosum *(Crossman and Neary, 2010)*

the onset of gestation. During the 2 weeks before menstruation, the corpus luteum secretes progesterone in decreasing amounts, atrophies, undergoes fibrotic degeneration, and becomes a pale spot on the surface of the ovary. Compare **corpus albicans.**

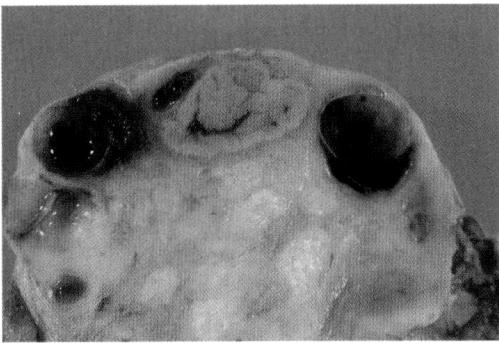

Corpus luteum *(Greer et al, 2001)*

corpus spongiosum /spon′jē·ō″səm/, one of the cylinders of spongy tissue, with the corpora cavernosa, on the dorsum of the penis from bulb to glans. It contains the urethra and erectile tissue.

corpus uteri, that part of the uterus above the isthmus and below the orifices of the fallopian tubes.

corrected pressure [L, *corrigere,* to make straight], a method of applying Boyle's law of gas pressures to adjust simultaneously for changes in both pressure and humidity.

corrective emotional experience /kərek″tiv/, a process by which a patient gives up old behavior patterns and learns or relearns new patterns by reexperiencing early unresolved feelings and needs.

corrective exercise. See **therapeutic exercise.**

corrective therapist. See **kinesiotherapist.**

correlation /kôr′əlā″shən/ [L, *com + relatio,* a carrying back], (in statistics) a relationship between variables that may be negative (inverse), positive, or curvilinear. Correlation is measured and expressed by using numeric scales.

correlative differentiation /kərel″ətiv/, (in embryology) specialization or diversification of cells or tissues caused by an inductor or other external factor. Also called **dependent differentiation.**

correspondence, (in ophthalmology) the relationship between corresponding points on each retina. The simultaneous stimulation of the points results in the sensation of viewing a single object.

Corrigan pulse [Dominic J. Corrigan, Irish physician, 1802–1880], a bounding pulse in which a great surge is felt, followed by a sudden and complete absence of force or fullness in the artery. This kind of pulse is associated with aortic regurgitation and occurs in excited emotional states; in various cardiac conditions, including patent ductus arteriosus; and as a result of systemic arteriosclerosis. Also called **collapsing pulse, water-hammer pulse.**

corrode. See **corrosive.**

corrosion /kərō″zhen/, a result of an oxidation-reduction reaction, or deterioration of a substance by a destructive agent. See also **corrosive.**

corrosion of surgical instruments [L, *corrodere,* to gnaw away], the rusting of surgical instruments or the gradual wearing away of their polished surfaces caused by oxidation and the action of contaminants. Though minimized by the use of stainless steel alloys in the fabrication of the instruments, corrosion persists as a problem, even when cleaning

procedures seem more than adequate. It usually results from inadequate cleaning and drying of surgical instruments after use, sterilization with solutions that eat into the surface, overexposure to such solutions, or a faulty autoclave. Cleanliness is the single most important factor in preventing corrosion. Any foreign material, either organic or inorganic, on the surface of stainless steel is likely to promote corrosion, and microscopic examinations often reveal foreign material and chlorides from cleaning solutions scattered over the surface of cleaned and sterilized instruments. The more chromium in the stainless steel alloys of which surgical instruments are made, the more resistant the instruments are to corrosion. Carbon, which hardens such alloys, also reduces their resistance to corrosion. Most corrosion of surgical instruments is superficial and may be removed by soaking in a solution of ammonia and alcohol or by repolishing by the manufacturer.

corrosive /kərō″siv/ [L, *corrodere,* to gnaw away], **1.** *adj.,* pertaining to the destruction or degradation of a substance or tissue, especially by chemical action. **2.** *n.,* an agent or substance that degrades a substance or tissue. For example, a corrosive can cause the formation of rust on metals. **−corrosion,** *n.,* **−corrode,** *v.*

corrosive gastritis, an acute inflammatory condition of the stomach caused by the ingestion of an acid, alkali, or other corrosive chemical in which the lining of the stomach is eaten away by the corrosive substance. The amount of tissue destruction and recommended treatment depend on the nature of the corrosive agent and the extent of exposure. Also called **toxic gastritis.** Compare **chemical gastritis, erosive gastritis.** See also **acid poisoning, alkali poisoning.**

corrugator supercilii /kôr′əgā″tər soo′pərsil″ē·ī/ [L, *corrugare,* to wrinkle; *super,* above, *cilium,* eyelash], one of the three muscles of the eyelid. Arising from the medial end of the superciliary arch and inserting into the skin above the orbital arch, it is innervated by the temporal and zygomatic branches of the facial nerve and functions to draw the eyebrow downward and inward, as if to frown. Also called *corrugator.* Compare **levator palpebrae superioris, orbicularis oculi.**

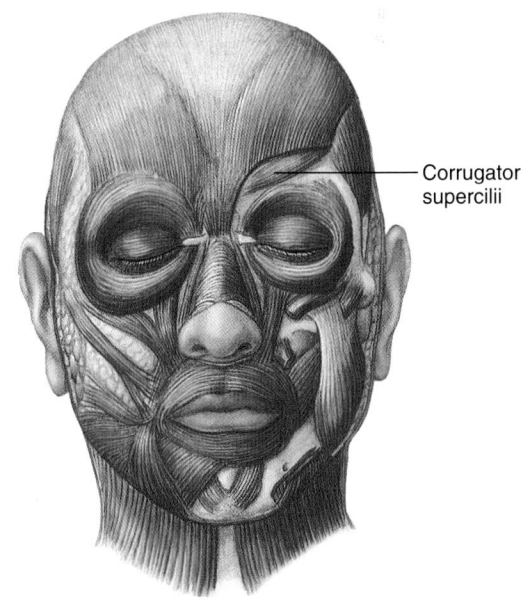

Corrugator supercilii

Corrugator supercilii *(Patton, 2016)*

-cort, suffix designating a cortisone derivative.

cortex /kôr'teks/ *pl.* **cortices** [L, bark], the outer layer of a body organ or other structure, as distinguished from the internal substance. –*cortical, adj.*

cortex corticis, part of the renal cortex, consisting of a narrow peripheral zone where the renal columns do not have visible renal corpuscles.

cortex of the lens, the softer, external part of the lens of the eye.

cortic-, prefix meaning "cortex" or "bark": *corticospinal, cortical, corticalization.*

cortical audiometry. See **audiometry.**

cortical blindness /kôr'tikəl/ [L, *cortex* + AS, *blind*], loss of vision that results from a lesion in the visual center of the cerebral cortex of the brain.

cortical bone, bone that contains layers of matrix arranged in parallel osteons. It is found as the outer covering of spongy bone and forms the walls of medullary canals of long bones. Cortical bone is 70% to 90% mineralized. Also called **compact bone.**

cortical evoked potential, a recording of electrical activity in the cerebral cortex in response to a stimuli.

cortical fracture [L, *cortex* + *fractura,* break], a fracture that involves the cortex of a bone.

corticalization, the increase of size and gyri of the cerebral cortex. See also **cerebral cortex.**

cortical labyrinth, a network of tubules and blood vessels in the renal cortex.

cortical march, the spread of abnormal electrical activity from one area of the cerebral cortex to adjacent areas, characteristic of jacksonian epilepsy. Also called **epileptic march, jacksonian march.**

cortical radiate arteries, arteries originating from the arcuate arteries of the kidney and distributed to the renal glomeruli. Also called **interlobular arteries of kidney.**

cortical rim sign, in computed tomography of the kidney, a thin rim of peripheral cortex that is perfused and visible when other parts of the cortex are not because of capsular collateral arteries. It indicates cortical necrosis, renal vein thrombosis, or infarction of the nonperfused parts. Also called *rim sign.*

cortical substance of cerebellum. See **cerebellar cortex.**

cortices. See **cortex.**

corticomedullary border, the area where the renal medulla and cortex come together.

corticopontocerebellar fibers, the corticopontine fibers and pontocerebellar fibers considered together.

corticospinal tract, any of two groups of nerve fibers (the anterior corticospinal tract and lateral corticospinal tract) that originate in the cerebral cortex and run through the spinal cord. They are responsible for carrying motor fibers.

corticosteroid /kôr'tikōstir″oid/ [L, *cortex* + *steros,* solid], any one of hormones elaborated by the adrenal cortex (excluding the sex hormones of adrenal origin) that influence or control key processes of the body. These processes include carbohydrate and protein metabolism, maintenance of serum glucose levels, electrolyte and water balance, and functions of the cardiovascular system, the skeletal muscle, the kidneys, and other organs. The corticosteroids synthesized by the adrenal glands include the glucocorticoids and the mineralocorticoids. The principal glucocorticoids are cortisol and corticosterone. The only physiologically important mineralocorticoid in humans is aldosterone. These hormones may be manufactured and administered exogenously. The glucocorticoids tend to cause the cells of the body to shift from carbohydrate

catabolism to fat catabolism, to accelerate the breakdown of proteins to amino acids, and to help maintain normal blood pressure. The secretion of these hormones increases during stress, especially that produced by anxiety and severe injury. Chronic overproduction of these substances is associated with various disorders, such as Cushing syndrome. A high blood level of glucocorticoids markedly increases the number of eosinophils and decreases the size of lymphatic tissues, especially the thymus and the lymph nodes. The decrease in lymphocytes slows antibody formation and affects the body's immune system. Aldosterone is the most powerful of the natural mineralocorticoids in the regulation of electrolyte balance, especially in the balance of sodium and potassium. Cortisol induces sodium retention and potassium excretion, but less effectively than aldosterone. The effects of the corticosteroids on the cardiovascular system, which are not precisely understood, are most evident in hypocortisolism, when the reduction in blood volume, accompanied by increased viscosity, may cause hypotension and cardiovascular collapse. The absence of corticosteroids decreases capillary permeability, decreases vasomotor response of small vessels, and reduces cardiac size and output. The skeletal muscles require adequate amounts of corticosteroids to function normally; excessive amounts cause them to function abnormally. Cortisol and its synthetic analogs can prevent or reduce inflammation by inhibiting edema, leukocytic migration, and disposition of collagen and by causing other complications associated with inflammatory processes. The antiinflammatory actions of synthetic hormones can be harmful, however, because they mask the disease process and prevent accurate observation of its progress. Hypoadrenalism may result from the too rapid withdrawal of such drugs after prolonged therapy. Toxic effects associated with prolonged large dose corticosteroid therapy include fluid and electrolyte imbalance, hyperglycemia and glycosuria, increased susceptibility to infections, myopathy, arrested growth, ecchymoses, Cushing syndrome, acne, and behavioral disturbances. Myopathy, characterized by weakness of the proximal musculature of the arms and the legs and associated shoulder and pelvic muscles, may also develop. Corticosteroid therapy may also produce behavioral changes, such as schizophrenia, suicidal tendencies, nervousness, and insomnia. See also **adrenal crisis.**

corticosteroid-binding globulin. See **transcortin.**

corticotroph /kor'tikōtrof″/, a small, irregularly stellate, acidophilic cell of the adenohypophysis, having small, sparsely distributed secretory granules and secreting adrenocorticotropic hormone and beta-endorphin. Also called *corticotrope,* **corticotropic cell.**

corticotroph adenoma. See **corticotropinoma.**

corticotropic cell. See **corticotroph.**

corticotropin. See **adrenocorticotropic hormone.**

corticotropinoma /kor'ti·kō·trō′pi·nō′mə/, a pituitary adenoma made up predominantly of corticotrophs. Excessive adrenocorticotropic hormone (corticotropin) secretion may cause Cushing disease or Nelson syndrome. See also **Cushing disease, Nelson syndrome.**

corticotropin-releasing hormone (CRH) /kôr'tikōtrop ″in/, a polypeptide hormone secreted by the hypothalamus into the pituitary portal system where it triggers the release of adrenocorticotropic hormone from the pituitary gland.

cortisol /kôr'təsôl/, a steroid hormone produced naturally by the adrenal gland, identical to chemically synthesized hydrocortisone.

■ INDICATIONS: It is prescribed for adrenocortical insufficiency, topically for inflammation, and as an adjunct for the treatment of ulcerative colitis.

■ CONTRAINDICATIONS: Fungal infections or known hypersensitivity to this drug prohibits its systemic use. Viral or fungal infections of the skin, impaired circulation, or known hypersensitivity to this drug prohibits its topical use.

■ ADVERSE EFFECTS: Among the more serious adverse reactions to this drug are GI, endocrine, neurological, fluid, and electrolyte disturbances. Hypersensitivity reactions may result from topical administration.

cortisone /kôr″təsōn/, a synthetic glucocorticoid.

■ INDICATIONS: It is prescribed for adrenocortical insufficiency inflammation.

■ CONTRAINDICATIONS: Fungal infections or known hypersensitivity to this drug prohibits its systemic use. Viral or fungal infections of the skin, impaired circulation, or known hypersensitivity to this drug prohibits its topical use.

■ ADVERSE EFFECTS: Among the more serious adverse reactions to the systemic administration of the drug are GI, endocrine, neurological, fluid, and electrolyte disturbances, so the drug must be used with caution when there are preexisting conditions. Skin reactions may result from topical administration. Therapy lasting longer than a few days can lead to hypothalamic-pituitary-adrenal suppression.

Corti's organ. See **organ of Corti.**

Cortisporin, a brand name for several topical fixed-combination drugs that contain a glucocorticoid (hydrocortisone) and two to three antibacterials (neomycin sulfate, polymyxin B sulfate, and/or bacitracin zinc). See also **hydrocortisone, neomycin sulfate, polymyxin B sulfate, bacitracin.**

Corti's tunnel. See **canal of Corti.**

cor triatriatum /kôr trī·ā′trē·ā′tum/, a congenital anomaly caused by failure of resorption of the embryonic common pulmonary vein, resulting in division of the left atrium by a fibromuscular diaphragm, the posterosuperior chamber receiving the pulmonary venous return and the anteroinferior chamber communicating with the left atrial appendage and mitral orifice. This results in a heart with three atrial chambers. The orifice between the two compartments may be reduced or absent, producing pulmonary venous obstruction.

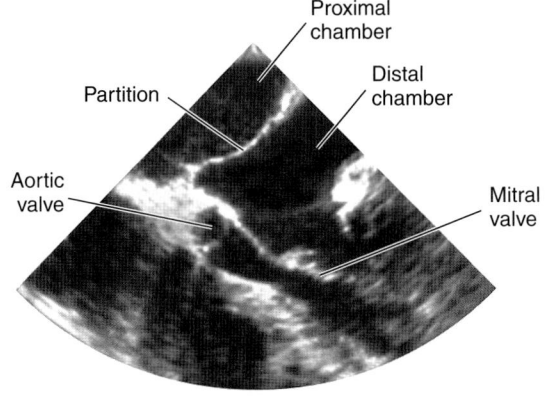

Cor triatriatum *(Kouchoukos et al, 2013)*

Corvert, a drug that controls atrial fibrillation and atrial flutter. Brand name for **ibutilide.**

Corynebacterium /kôr′inē′baktir′ē·əm/ [Gk, *koryne,* club, *bakterion,* small staff], a common genus of aerobic and facultative, anaerobic, gram-positive, nonmotile, rod-shaped curved bacilli that includes many species. The most common pathogenic species are *C. acnes,* commonly found in acne lesions, and *C. diphtheriae,* the cause of diphtheria. Nondiphtherial corynebacteria have been recognized as pathogenic, especially in immunocompromised patients. The most common infection with these organisms is bacteremia in association with infections involving devices such as heart valves, catheters, and neurological shunts. See also *Propionibacterium.*

coryza. See **rhinitis.**

coryza spasmodica. See **hay fever.**

coryza virus. See **rhinovirus.**

Corzide, a combination antihypertensive medication. Brand name for **nadolol, bendroflumethiazide.**

cosine law /kō″sīn/, a rule that optimal irradiation occurs when the source of radiation is at right angles to the center of the area being irradiated.

Cosmegen, an antineoplastic drug. Brand name for **dactinomycin.**

cosmesis /kosmē″sis/, the elective use of cosmetics or surgery for preserving or enhancing self-image.

cosmetic acne, a type of contact acne, usually of a low grade, seen on the chin and cheeks of persons habitually using facial cosmetics. The usual lesions are closed comedones or papular pustules.

cosmetic dermatitis /kosmet″ik/ [Gk, *kosmesis,* adornment], a form of irritant or allergic contact dermatitis caused by ingredients in cosmetic products. The meaning is commonly broadened to include soaps, shampoos, deodorants, and depilatories in addition to perfumes, coloring agents, and toiletries. This inflammatory skin disease can be manifested in a broad spectrum, ranging from erythema to eczema.

cosmetic surgery, reconstruction of cutaneous or underlying tissues, performed to improve, enhance, and correct a structural defect or to remove a scar, birthmark, or normal evidence of aging. Also called **aesthetic surgery.** Compare **plastic surgery.** Kinds include **blepharoplasty, rhinoplasty, rhytidoplasty.**

cosmic radiation /kos″mik/, high-energy particles with great penetrating power that originate in outer space and reach the earth as part of normal background radiation. The particles include high-energy atomic nuclei.

cost-, costi-, costo-, prefix meaning "rib": *costal, costalgia.*

costa /kos″tē/ *pl. costae,* a rib.

costal /kos″təl/ [L, *costa,* rib], **1.** pertaining to a rib. **2.** situated near a rib or on a side close to a rib.

costal arch [L, *costa + arcus,* bow], an arch formed by the shafts of the ribs.

costal cartilage, the cartilage at the anterior end of each rib.

costal facet, one of three sites on each side of a typical thoracic vertebra for articulation with ribs.

costalgia /kostal″jə·ə/ [L, *costa,* rib; Gk, *algos,* pain], a pain in the ribs.

costal groove, a groove along the inferior margin of the superior rib that accommodates the intercostal nerves and associated major arteries and veins.

costal notch, an indentation beside a costal cartilage on the side of the sternum.

cost analysis [L, *costare,* to stand firm; Gk, *ana,* again, *lyein,* to loosen], an analysis of the disbursements and expenses of an activity, agency, department, or program.

COSTAR /kō″stär/, a system that creates and stores electronic patient records, including medical history, physical examination information, laboratory reports, diagnosis, and treatments. Abbreviation for *COmputer STored Ambulatory Record system.*

cost-based value, a relative value scale used to determine the total units of services provided by a medical practice. The total cost of running the practice and the total units of service are then used to calculate the costs for each service provided.

cost-benefit analysis (CBA), a type of economic evaluation of medical care expense. It compares the expected monetary benefit derived from different health interventions with the expected cost of providing each of the interventions to determine the best or most profitable option.

cost-benefit ratio, a mathematic representation of the relationship of the cost of an activity to the benefit of its outcome or product.

cost cap, *(Informal)* a limit on the amount of money that an agency, department, or institution may spend.

cost center, a department, division, or other subunit of an institution established within its accounting system so that the income and expenses of the subunit can be separated from the income or expenses of other centers and monitored for cost and benefit.

cost control, the process of monitoring and regulating the expenditure of funds by an agency or institution. Budgets, reports, and cost-accounting procedures are performed to achieve cost control.

costectomy /kostek″təmē/, surgical removal of a rib or resection of rib.

cost-effectiveness, the extent to which an activity is thought to be as valuable as it is expensive. A public-assistance program that issued vouchers for nutritious foods in pregnancy might be considered cost-effective if it lowered the costly incidence of perinatal morbidity.

cost-effectiveness analysis (CEA), a type of economic evaluation used to determine the best use of money available for medical care. It compares different kinds of interventions with similar, but not identical, effects on the basis of the cost per unit achieved.

Costen syndrome. See **temporomandibular joint (TMJ) pain dysfunction syndrome.**

cost model, (in the United States) a managed care system in which all components of patient care are defined as costs as opposed to sources of revenue.

costocervical /kos′tōsur″vikəl/ [L, *costa,* rib, *cervix,* neck], pertaining to or involving the ribs and the neck.

costochondral /kos′təkon″drəl/ [L, *costa* + Gk, *chondros,* cartilage], pertaining to a rib and its cartilage.

costochondritis /kos′təkondrī″tis/, an inflammation of the costal cartilage of the anterior chest wall, characterized by pain and tenderness.

costoclavicular /-klavik″yələr/ [L, *costa* + *clavicula,* little key], pertaining to or involving the ribs and the clavicle.

costoclavicular line, an imaginary vertical line between the sternal and midclavicular lines. Also called **parasternal line.**

costophrenic (CP) angle /-fren″ik/ [L, *costa* + *phrenicus,* diaphragm], the angle between the diaphragm and the chest wall at the bottom of the lung.

costosternal /-stur″nəl/, pertaining to or involving the ribs and the sternum.

costotransverse articulation /-transvurs″/ [L, *costa* + *transversus,* a cross direction], any of the 20 gliding joints between the ribs and articulating vertebrae, except the eleventh and twelfth ribs. The five ligaments that associate with each costotransverse joint are the articular capsule, the superior costotransverse ligament, the posterior costotransverse ligament, the ligament of the neck of the rib, and the ligament of the tubercle of the rib.

costovertebral /-vur″təbrəl/, of or relating to a rib and the vertebral column.

costovertebral angle (CVA), one of two angles that outline a space over the kidneys. The angle is formed by the lateral and downward curve of the lowest rib and the vertical column of the spine itself. CVA tenderness to percussion is a common finding in pyelonephritis and other infections of the kidney and adjacent structures.

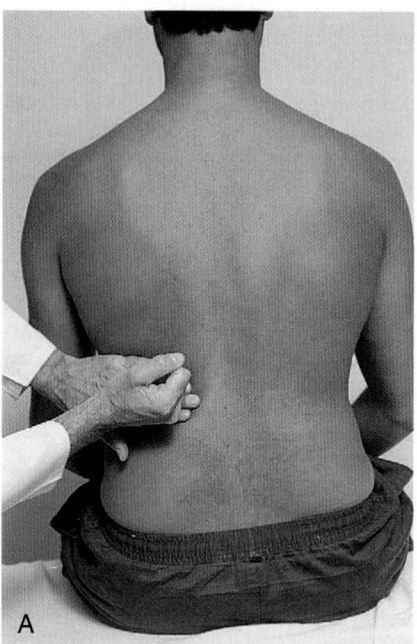

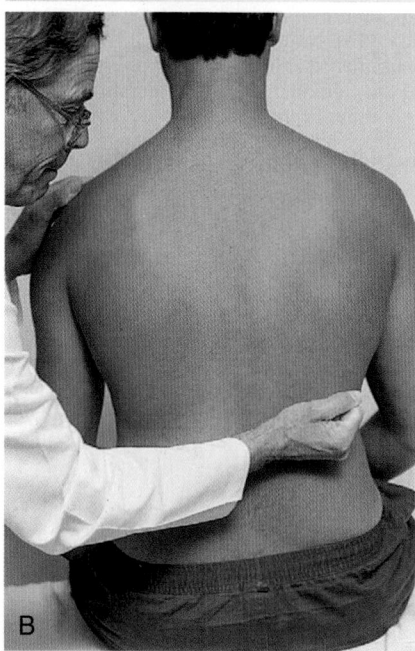

Percussion over the costovertebral angle *(Seidel et al, 2003)*

cost-sharing program, (in the United States) a financial risk-management strategy often used by insurance companies and self-insured employers in which employees share the cost of health services, such as through deductibles and coinsurance.

cost shifting, (in the United States) a mechanism for reducing inpatient costs by providing services in an outpatient setting. The inpatient cost per case is reduced, but the overall cost to the organization does not change.

cost-utility analysis (CUA), a type of economic evaluation of different approaches to managed health care costs. It compares the degree to which quality of life is improved per dollar spent. A quality-of-life index is used to compare interventions, including quality-adjusted life years.

cosyntropin /kō'sintrop″in/, a synthetic form of adrenocorticotropic hormone that is used in the diagnosis and treatment of adrenal hypofunction disorders such as Addison's disease to determine if the disorder is primary (adrenal dysfunction) or secondary (hypothalamic-pituitary axis dysfunction).

COTA, abbreviation for **certified occupational therapy assistant.**

Cotazym, a pancreatic enzyme preparation. Brand name for *pancrelipase.*

cot death. See **sudden infant death syndrome.**

cotton /kot′n/, **1.** a plant of the genus *Gossypium.* **2.** a textile material derived from the seeds of this plant.

cotton-mill fever. See **byssinosis.**

cottonmouth, a poisonous pit viper *(Agkistrodon piscivorus)* commonly found near water and swamps of the southeastern part of the United States. The symptoms of the bite of a cottonmouth are rapid swelling, severe pain, skin discoloration at bite marks, and weakness. Antivenin and ventilatory/circulatory support are the usual treatments. Also called **water moccasin.**

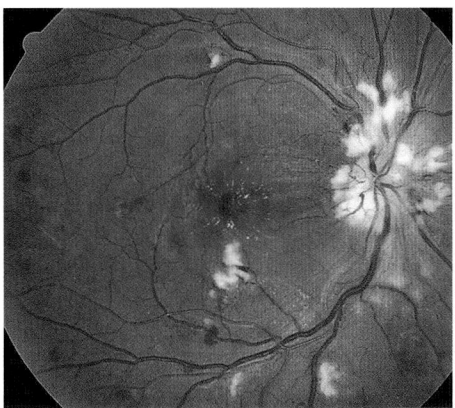
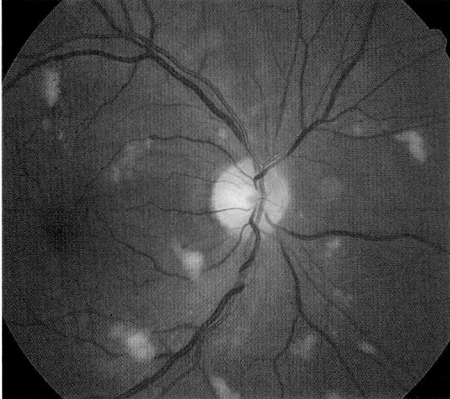

Cotton-wool exudate *(Zitelli and Davis, 2007)*

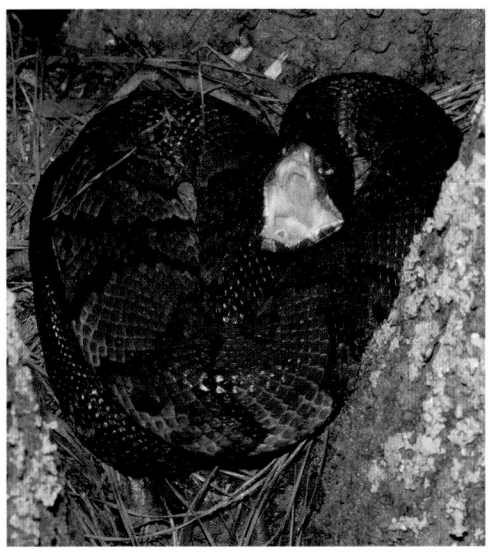

Cottonmouth *(Likens, 2009)*

Cotton fracture, a fracture involving the medial, lateral, and posterior malleoli of the ankle. Also called **trimalleolar fracture.**

cotton-wool exudate [Ar, *qutun* + AS, *wull* + ME, *spot*], a white fluffy-appearing lesion, an infarction of the nerve fiber layer, observed on the retina of patients with certain systemic conditions, such as diabetes, giant cell arteritis, acquired immunodeficiency syndrome, hypertension, and lupus. It can also be observed in retinal infections.

cotyledon /kot′ilē″don/ [Gk, *kotyledon,* cup shaped], one of the visible segments on the maternal surface of the placenta. A typical placenta may have 15 to 28 cotyledons, each consisting of fetal vessels, chorionic villi, and intervillous space.

cotyloid /kot″iloid/, cup shaped, as the acetabulum.

coudé catheter /ko͞odā′/ [Fr, *coude,* elbow], an elbowed catheter with an olive tip for a strictured urethra.

cough /kôf/ [AS, *cohhetan*], a sudden audible expulsion of air from the lungs. Coughing is preceded by inspiration, the glottis is partially closed, and the accessory muscles of expiration contract to expel the air forcibly from the respiratory passages. Coughing is an essential protective response that serves to clear the lungs, bronchi, and trachea of irritants and secretions or to prevent aspiration of foreign material into the lungs. It is a common symptom of diseases of the chest and larynx. Chronic coughing may be indicative of tuberculosis, lung cancer, bronchiectasis, asthma, or bronchitis. Otitis media, allergies, subdiaphragmatic irritation, congestive heart failure, and mitral valve disease may be associated with episodes of severe chronic coughing. Coughing is a reflex action that may be induced voluntarily and, to some extent, voluntarily inhibited. The cough-reflex center is located in the medulla of the brain. It responds to stimulation transmitted by the glossopharyngeal (CN9) or vagus (CN10) nerve. The reflex is initiated by chemical or mechanical irritation of the pharynx, larynx, or tracheobronchial tree. Because the function of coughing is to clear the respiratory tract of secretions, it is important that the cough expel accumulated debris. If it does not because of, for example, weakness or inhibition by pain, instruction in effective coughing and deep-breathing exercises is helpful. Persons with chronic coughs may obtain symptomatic relief through environmental controls that reduce irritants in and humidify air. Medication may help dilate the bronchi, liquefy secretions, and increase expectoration. Antitussive medications are sometimes prescribed even in the absence of mucus or congestion. When congestion is present and the patient is unable to cough up the mucus, an expectorant may be prescribed.

cough fracture, a break in a rib, usually the fourth to eighth rib, caused by violent coughing.

cough syncope [AS, *cohhetan* + Gk, *syncope,* fainting], a temporary loss of consciousness during coughing. The coughing increases the intrathoracic pressure enough to impede venous return, thereby interfering with normal blood flow to the brain.

cough variant asthma, asthma characterized by minimal wheezing and a nonproductive, often severe, cough lasting from a few hours to days.

coulomb (C) /kōō″lŏm/ [Charles A. de Coulomb, French physicist, 1736–1806], the SI unit of electricity equal to the quantity of charge transferred in 1 second across a conductor in which there is a constant current of 1 ampere, or 1 ampere-second.

Coulomb's law [Charles A. de Coulomb], (in physics) a law stating that the force of attraction or repulsion between two electrically charged bodies is directly proportional to the strength of the electrical charges and inversely proportional to the square of the distance between them.

coulometry /kōōlom″ətrē/, a type of electroanalytic chemistry in which a reagent generated at the surface of an electrode reacts with a substance to be measured. The substance, usually a metal ion, is measured in terms of the coulombs required for the reaction.

Coulter counter /kōl″tər/ [W.H. Coulter, 20th-century American engineer], an electric device that rapidly identifies and counts red and white blood cells present in a small specimen of human blood.

Coumadin, an anticoagulant. Brand name for **warfarin sodium.**

coumarin /kōō″mərin/, a class of orally active anticoagulant agents with warfarin as its prototype.

■ INDICATIONS: It is prescribed for prophylaxis and treatment of thrombosis and embolism.

■ CONTRAINDICATIONS: Known hypersensitivity to the drug prohibits its use. It is not prescribed to patients who are at risk for hemorrhage or who are pregnant.

■ ADVERSE EFFECTS: The most serious adverse reaction is hemorrhage. Many other drugs interact with this drug to increase or decrease its effect.

counseling [L, *consulere,* to consult], the act of providing advice and guidance to a patient or his or her family, a therapeutic technique that helps the patient recognize and manage stress and that facilitates interpersonal relationships between the patient and the family, significant others, or the health care team. Therapeutic counseling requires advanced practice skills for nurses and social workers, but is within the scope of practice for psychologists, psychiatrists, and certified or licensed counselors. See also **genetic counseling.**

counselor, a human services professional who deals with human development concerns through support, therapeutic approaches, consultation, evaluation, teaching, and research. Specializations include, but are not limited to, community counselor, gerontological counselor, spiritual counselor, grief counselor, marriage and family counselor/therapist, mental health counselor, school counselor, and student affairs practitioner. Kinds include **genetic counselor, rehabilitation counselor.**

count [L, *computere,* to calculate], a computation of the number of objects or elements present per unit of measurement. Kinds include *Addis count,* **bacterial count, complete blood count, platelet count.**

counterclaim [L, *contra,* against, *clamere,* to cry out], (in law) a claim made by a defendant establishing a cause for action in his or her favor against a plaintiff. The purpose of a counterclaim is to oppose or detract from a plaintiff's claim or complaint.

counterconditioning, a process used in behavioral therapy in which a learned response is replaced by an alternative response that is less disruptive.

countercurrent, a change in the direction of flow of a fluid. An example is the countercurrent in the ascending branch of a kidney tubule where osmolality undergoes a reversal after a gradual change in sodium chloride concentrations.

countercurrent multiplication, the mechanism in the loops of Henle of the renal tubules by which urine is concentrated. It is dependent on unique solute transport processes at different parts of the loops of Henle and the vasa recta.

counterinjunction /-injungk″shən/, (in transactional analysis) an overt message from the parent ego state of the mother or father that may be difficult to follow if it conflicts with earlier parental instructions. For example, the person may obey an earlier injunction to avoid close relationships, then be instructed later to "grow up and get married."

counterirritant, an agent used to produce an irritation in one part of the body, intended to relieve irritation in some other part.

counterphobic behavior /-fō″bik/, an expression of reaction to a phobia by a patient who actively seeks exposure to the type of situation that precipitates phobic symptoms. Examples are thrill-seeking and risk-taking activities.

counterpulsation /-pulsā″shən/ [L, *contra* + *pulsare,* to beat], **1.** the action of a circulatory-assist pumping device that is synchronized with cardiac systole and diastole to decrease the work of the heart. **2.** the process of increasing the intraaortic pressure in diastole by inflation of an intraaortic balloon and deflation of the balloon immediately before the next systole.

counterregulatory hormones, hormones that oppose the action of insulin by increasing blood glucose levels. They stimulate the release of glucose from the liver and decrease movement of glucose into cells. Kinds include **glucagon, epinephrine, growth hormone, cortisol.**

countershock [L, *contra* + Fr, *choc*], a high-intensity, short-duration electric shock applied to an area of the heart, resulting in total cardiac depolarization. See also **cardioversion, defibrillation.**

counterstain, a second stain added to a previously stained tissue sample to make cellular details more distinct.

countertraction /-trak″shən/ [L, *contra* + *trahere,* to pull], a force that counteracts the pull of traction, such as the force of body weight resulting from the pull of gravity. Orthopedic countertraction may be obtained by altering the angle of the body-weight force in relation to the pull of traction, such as by elevating the foot of the bed with blocks to attain the Trendelenburg position. The magnitude of countertraction is usually increased gradually by methodically changing the position of a patient and by adding or removing weights from weight hangers.

countertransference /-transfur″əns/, the conscious or unconscious emotional response of a psychotherapist or psychoanalyst to a patient. The response may be positive or negative but can provide useful data in the therapy.

countertransport /-trans″pôrt/ [L, *contra* + *trans,* across, *portare,* carry], the simultaneous transport of two different substances across the same membrane, each in the opposite direction.

counting cell hemocytometer [OFr, *conter* + L, *cella,* storeroom; Gk, *haima,* blood, *metron,* measure], a device for counting the number of cells in a volume of blood or other fluid. It consists of a microscope slide with a counting chamber. The chamber has a known volume and the slide has a ruled area to help count the cells.

counts per minute (cpm), a measure of the rate of ionizing emissions by radioactive substances.

coup /koo/ [Fr, blow], **1.** any blow or stroke or the effects of such a blow to the body, usually used with a French word identifying a type of stroke. **2.** a wound resembling a sword cut. Also called **en coup de sabre. 3.** also called *coup de soleil.* See also **sunstroke. 4.** administration of a drug in small amounts over a short period rather than in a single larger dose. Also called **coup sur coup. 5.** an injury most often associated with a blow to the skull in which the force of the impact is transmitted through the skull bones to the opposite side of the head, where the bruise, fracture, or other sign of injury appears. Also called **contrecoup.**

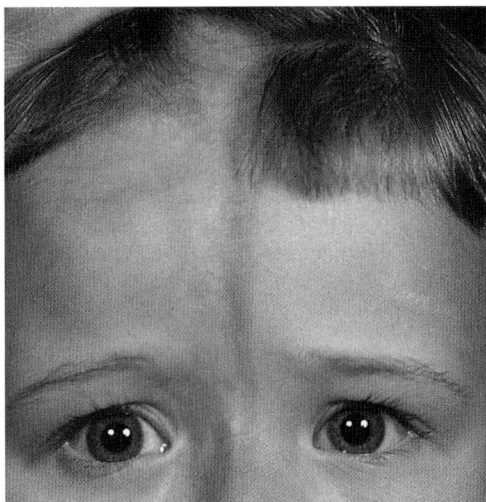

Coup de sabre (du Vivier, 1993)

coupled pacing, a pacemaker mode designed to apply electrical stimulation near the end of the T-wave to create a retrograde activation of the atrioventricular (AV) node and in turn to prevent rapid ventricular conduction during atrial fibrillation (AF). See **pacing.**

coupled rhythm, heartbeats occurring in pairs; the second beat is usually a premature ventricular contraction. See **bigeminal rhythm.**

couples' therapy, psychotherapy in which couples, who may be married or unmarried, undergo therapy together.

coupling /kup″ling/ [L, *copula,* bonding], **1.** the act of coming together, joining, or pairing. **2.** (in genetics) the situation in linked inheritance in which the nonalleles of two or more mutant genes are located on the same chromosome and are close enough that they are likely to be inherited together. **3.** (in radiation therapy) the efficiency of transfer of power from an applicator to the treatment site. Compare **repulsion.** See also **cis configuration. 4.** (in cardiology) the regular occurrence of a premature beat.

coupling interval, the interval between the dominant heartbeat and a linked ectopic beat. It is measured from the beginning of a normal QRS complex to the beginning of the ectopic QRS complex that follows it.

coup sur coup. See **coup.**

courseware /kôrs″wer/, software programs for use in instruction.

Courvoisier's law /koorvô·äzē·āz″/ [Ludwig Courvoisier, Swiss surgeon, 1843–1918], a statement that the gallbladder is smaller than usual if a gallstone blocks the common bile duct but is dilated if the common bile duct is blocked by something other than a gallstone, such as pancreatic cancer.

couvade /kooväd″/, a custom in some non-Western cultures whereby the husband goes through mock labor while his wife is giving birth.

Council of Nephrology Nurses and Technicians, a council of the National Kidney Foundation providing opportunities for collaboration and networking among colleagues to improve clinical practice and promote career advancement. The council advances the well-being of patients and works to effect changes in kidney health care legislation and public policies.

Couvelaire uterus /koovəler″/ [Alexandre Couvelaire, French obstetrician, 1873–1948], a hemorrhagic process in uterine musculature that may accompany severe abruptio placentae. Extravasated blood effuses between the muscle fibrils and under the uterine peritoneum. The uterus takes on a purplish color and does not contract well. Also called **uteroplacental apoplexy.** See also **abruptio placentae.**

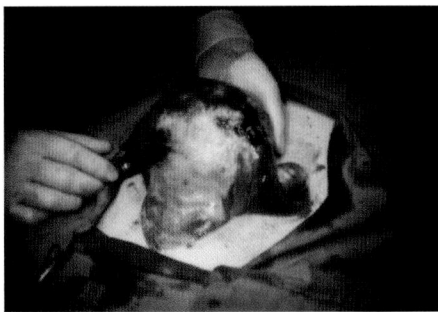

Couvelaire uterus (Greer et al, 2001)

covalent bond, a chemical bond that forms by the sharing of two electrons between atoms. A double bond is formed when four electrons are shared between two atoms; a triple bond is formed when six electrons are shared between two atoms.

coverage /kuv″ərij/, **1.** the extent to which services rendered by a health care program cover the potential need for them. **2.** *n.,* benefits available to an individual covered under a health plan.

covered benefit, a health service included in the premium of a policy paid by or on behalf of the enrolled patient. Also called **benefit,** *covered service.*

COVID-19, a pandemic associated with a variety of symptoms, including respiratory failure and death, caused by the coronavirus SARS-CoV-2. Older adults and people with severe underlying health conditions are at highest risk for developing serious complications. The mode of transmission is by respiratory droplets or by touching a surface or object that has the virus on it and then touching the mouth, nose, or eyes.

Cowden disease [Cowden, family name of the first recorded case], an autosomal-dominant disorder characterized by excessive hair growth, gingival fibromatosis, facial papules, hemangiomas, multiple noncancerous growths, and postpubertal fibroadenomatous breast enlargement. Also called **hamartoma syndrome.**

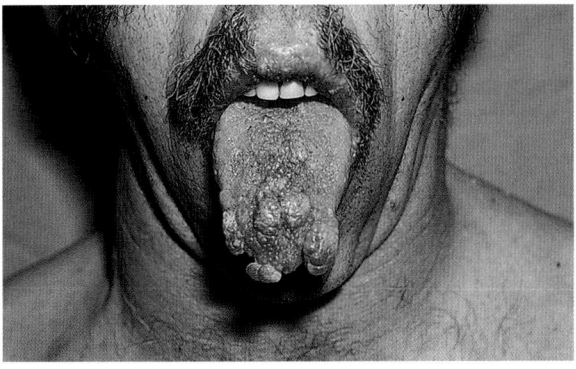

Adult with Cowden disease (Callen et al, 2000)

Cowper's gland /kou″pərz/ [William Cowper, English surgeon, 1666–1709], either of two round, pea-sized tubular glands embedded in the urethral sphincter of the male beneath the bulb of the male urethra. Normally yellow, they consist of several lobes with ducts that join and form a single excretory duct, emptying mucus into the urethra. Also called **bulbourethral gland.** Compare **Bartholin gland.**

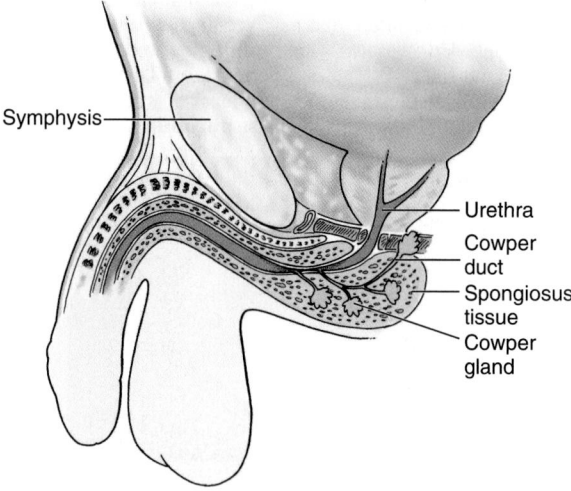

Cowper's gland (Gearhart et al, 2010)

Cowper's syringocele, a cystlike swelling of a bulbourethral gland (Cowper's gland) or one of its ducts, seen in infant boys or occasionally in older males. There are four types of syringocele, which are classified as either open or closed. Symptoms associated with an open syringocele are postvoid dribbling and hematuria. A closed syringocele is more likely to cause obstructive symptoms such as dysuria and urinary retention. Also called *Cowper's cyst.*

cowpox /kou″poks/ [AS, *cu* + ME, *pokkes*], a mild infectious disease characterized by a pustular rash, caused by the vaccinia virus. Animals that carry the vaccinia virus are cows, cats, and rodents. Human cases are usually rare. Transmission to humans can occur during the milking of a cow with active lesions on the udder and teats, but the disease is usually transmitted by domesticated cats. Cowpox infection usually confers immunity to smallpox, because of the similarity of the variola and vaccinia viruses. Also called **cat pox.** See also **smallpox, vaccinia.**

COX-2 inhibitors, cyclooxygenase-2 inhibitors, a group of nonsteroidal antiinflammatory drugs (NSAIDs) that act by inhibiting cyclooxygenase-2 activity. Many COX-2 inhibitors were taken off the market by the U.S. Food and Drug Administration (FDA), and others are the subject of class-action suits for cardiac and other toxicities. One of the members of this group is celecoxib.

coxa /kok″sə/ *pl. coxae* [L, hip], the hip joint; the head of the femur and the acetabulum of the innominate bone.

coxa adducta, coxa flexa. See **coxa vara.**

coxal articulation /kok″səl/ [L, *coxa* + *articularis,* relating to the joints], the ball-and-socket joint of the hip, formed by the articulation of the head of the femur into the cup-shaped cavity of the acetabulum. It involves seven ligaments and permits very extensive movements, such as flexion, extension, adduction, abduction, and medial and lateral rotation. Also called **hip joint.** Compare **shoulder joint.**

coxa magna, an abnormal widening of the head and neck of the femur.

Cox-Maze procedure /ka″ks meɪz/ [James Cox, American physician], a surgical ablation treatment for atrial fibrillation in which a "maze" of scar tissue is created to block aberrant cardiac impulses and restore a normal rhythm. The minimally invasive version uses radiofrequency waves to create the scar tissue. Also called **maze procedure.**

coxa plana. See **Perthes disease.**

coxa valga, a hip deformity in which the angle normally formed by the axis of the head and neck of the femur and the axis of its shaft is significantly increased.

coxa vara, a hip deformity in which the angle normally formed by the axis of the head and neck of the femur and the axis of its shaft is decreased. Also called **coxa adducta, coxa flexa.**

coxa vara luxans, a fissure or crack in the neck of the femur with dislocation of the head, caused by coxa vara.

Coxiella burnetii, a highly infectious, gram-negative bacterium that grows preferentially in the vacuoles of the host cell and causes Q fever. Also called *Rickettsia burnetii.*

coxsackie virus /koksak″ē-/ [Coxsackie, New York; L, *virus,* poison], any of 30 serologically different small RNA enteroviruses associated with a variety of symptoms and primarily affecting children during warm weather. The coxsackieviruses resemble the virus responsible for poliomyelitis, particularly in size. Both are picornaviruses. Coxsackie viruses can be divided into two groups. Group A is the milder form, causing herpangina and hand-foot-and-mouth disease. Group B causes epidemic pleurodynia. Both types can cause myocarditis, pericarditis, aseptic meningitis, and several exanthems. There is no known preventive measure except isolation of infected persons, and the treatment is generally directed to relief of symptoms. See also **viral infection.**

CP, abbreviation for **cerebral palsy.**

CPAN®, a professional certification designation for registered nurses caring for patients who have experienced sedation, analgesia, and anesthesia in a hospital or ambulatory care facility. Abbreviation for *certified postanesthesia nurse.*

CPAP, a technique to maintain the patency of an airway by the application of constant pressure during the entire respiratory cycle to prevent its collapse. Abbreviation for **continuous positive airway pressure.**

CPD, 1. abbreviation for **cephalopelvic disproportion.** 2. abbreviation for **childhood polycystic disease.**

CPDA-1, abbreviation for *citrate phosphate dextrose adenine.*

C peptide, a biologically inactive residue of insulin formation in the beta cells of the pancreas. When proinsulin is converted to insulin, an equal amount of C peptide, a chain of amino acids, is also secreted into the bloodstream. Beta cell secretory function can be determined by measuring the C peptide in a blood sample.

C-peptide test, a blood test used to evaluate levels of C-peptide, which correlate with insulin levels in the blood. Direct measurement of C-peptide measures the capacity of the pancreatic beta cells to secrete insulin. It is used to evaluate patients with suspected insulinoma, renal failure, pancreas transplant, factitious hypoglycemia, radical pancreatectomy, and diabetes mellitus.

CPHA, abbreviation for **Canadian Public Health Association.**

CPK, abbreviation for **creatine phosphokinase.**

CPM, abbreviation for **continuous passive motion.**

cpm, abbreviation for **counts per minute.**

CPPB, abbreviation for *continuous positive pressure breathing.* See **continuous positive airway pressure.**

CPPD, abbreviation for *calcium pyrophosphate dihydrate.* See **chondrocalcinosis.**

CPPV, abbreviation for **continuous positive pressure ventilation.**

CPR, abbreviation for **cardiopulmonary resuscitation.**

CPRAM, abbreviation for *controlled partial rebreathing anesthesia method.* See **controlled partial rebreathing anesthesia method.**

cps, abbreviation for **cycle per second.**

CPT codes, a coding system for medical procedures, defined in the publication *Current Procedural Terminology,* that allows for comparability in pricing, billing, and utilization review. CPT codes are used to bill for professional health-care services and time.

cpu, CPU, abbreviation for **central processing unit.**

CQI, abbreviation for **continuous quality improvement.**

CR, abbreviation for **computed radiography.**

Cr, symbol for the element **chromium.**

crab louse [AS, *crabba* + *lus*], a species of louse, *Pthirus pubis,* that infests the hairs of the genital area. It is often transmitted between persons by sexual contact but can also be spread by shared bedding. Pubic lice are usually easily killed with 1% permethrin or pyrethrin shampoo. Formerly called *Pediculus pubis.* See also **lice, pediculosis.**

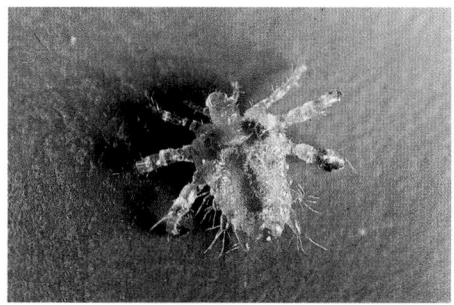

Crab louse *(Habif et al, 2011)*

crabs /krabz/, *(Informal)* popular name for *Pthirus pubis.*

crack [ME, *craken*], a street drug made by chemically converting cocaine hydrochloride to a form that can be smoked. Smoking crack is a faster, more direct way of getting cocaine molecules into the brain. Because larger amounts of the drug reach the brain more quickly, the effects are more intense than when cocaine, in the white-powder form, is injected, ingested, or inhaled. Also called **crack cocaine, freebase.**

crack baby, an unprofessional term referring to an infant who was exposed to the effects of cocaine in utero by a mother who used the "crack" form of the drug while pregnant. See also **cocaine baby, neonatal abstinence syndrome.**

crack cocaine, crack. See **cocaine hydrochloride, crack.**

cracked-pot sound [ME, *craken* + *pott* + L, *sonus,* sound], a sound sometimes heard on percussion over a cavity with an opening to a bronchus.

cracked tooth syndrome [ME, *craken*; AS, *toth*], a group of symptoms caused by the presence of a cracked tooth, including pain with applied pressure from biting or chewing, or application of cold; pulpitis can occur if left untreated.

crackle, a common, abnormal respiratory sound consisting of discontinuous bubbling noises heard on auscultation of the chest during inspiration. Fine crackles have a popping sound produced by air entering distal bronchioles or alveoli that contain serous secretions, as in congestive heart failure, pneumonia, or early tuberculosis. Coarse crackles may originate in the larger bronchi or trachea and have a lower pitch.

Crackles are not cleared by coughing. Compare **rhonchus, wheeze.** Formerly called **rale.** See also **coarse crackle.**

crackling rale. See **subcrepitant rale.**

cradle cap [AS, *cradel* + *caeppe*], a common seborrheic dermatitis of the scalp in infants. Also called **seborrhea capitis.**

■ OBSERVATIONS: Characterized by thick, yellow, greasy, or waxy scales that may be reddened. It may also involve the skin on the nose, eyebrows, ears, and trunk.

■ INTERVENTIONS: Treatment may include application of oil or ointment to soften the scales and frequent shampoos. A weak 0.5% hydrocortisone cream can be effective in controlling the problem but is usually not necessary.

■ PATIENT CARE CONSIDERATIONS: Cradle cap usually resolves on its own within a few months. Parents should be encouraged to wash the baby's scalp daily with a mild shampoo and to gently brush the scalp to remove scales.

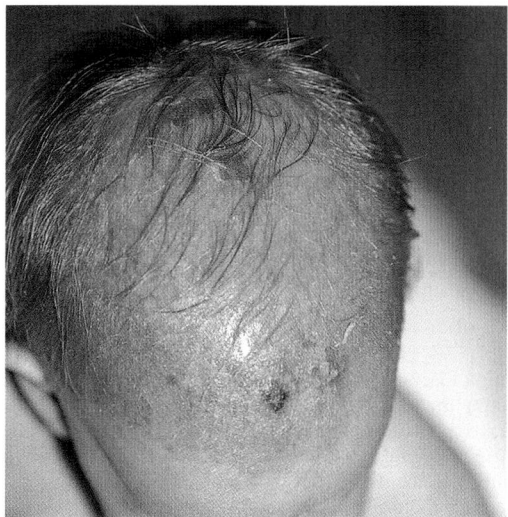

Cradle cap *(Callen et al, 2000)*

cramp [AS, *crammian,* to fill], **1.** a spasmodic and often painful contraction of one or more muscles. **2.** a pain resembling a muscular cramp. Kinds include **heat cramp, writer's cramp.** See also **charley horse, dysmenorrhea, wryneck, torticollis.**

cranberry, an herbal product whose edible berries are harvested from a small shrub found in the United States (from Alaska to Tennessee) and in Canada.

■ INDICATIONS: It is used for urinary tract infections (UTIs) and works by decreasing bacterial adherence to the walls of the bladder, urethra, and so on. Although likely effective to some degree, patients should not rely on cranberry juice for treating UTIs.

■ CONTRAINDICATIONS: Those with known hypersensitivity, oliguria, or anuria should not use cranberry.

-crania, suffix meaning "(condition of the) skull or head": *hemicrania.*

cranial. See **cranium.**

cranial arteritis, *(Obsolete)* now called **temporal arteritis.**

cranial bones /krā″nē-əl/ [Gk, *kranion,* cranium; AS, *ban*], the bones of the skull, particularly the part of the cranium that encloses the brain.

cranial cavity, the cavity of the skull containing the brain and other tissues. Also called **cerebral cavity.**

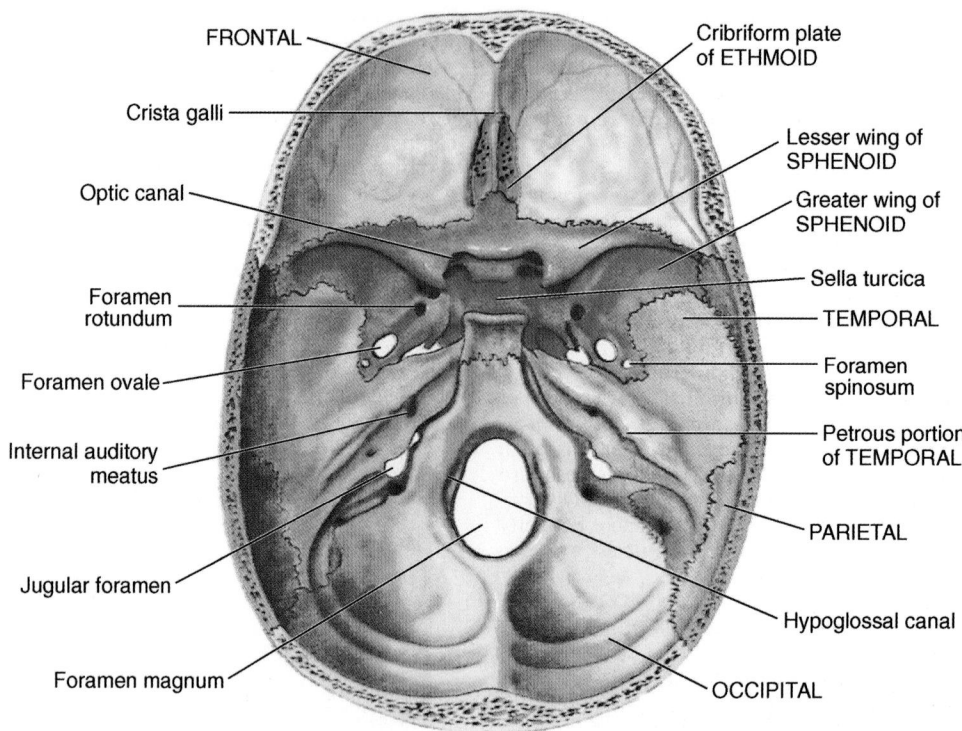

FRONTAL
Crista galli
Optic canal
Foramen rotundum
Foramen ovale
Internal auditory meatus
Jugular foramen
Foramen magnum

Cribriform plate of ETHMOID
Lesser wing of SPHENOID
Greater wing of SPHENOID
Sella turcica
TEMPORAL
Foramen spinosum
Petrous portion of TEMPORAL
PARIETAL
Hypoglossal canal
OCCIPITAL

Cranial cavity *(Solomon, 2009)*

cranial fibrous joints, **1.** the sutures and ligaments connecting the bones of the skull to each other. **2.** (in dentistry) the gomphoses holding the teeth in their sockets in the jaws.

cranial nerves [Gk, *kranion,* skull; L, *nervus*], the 12 pairs of nerves emerging from the cranial cavity through various openings in the skull. Beginning with the most anterior, they are designated by Roman numerals and named (I) olfactory, (II) optic, (III) oculomotor, (IV) trochlear, (V) trigeminal, (VI) abducens, (VII) facial, (VIII) vestibulocochlear (acoustic), (IX) glossopharyngeal, (X) vagal, (XI) accessory, and (XII) hypoglossal. The cranial nerves originate in the base of the brain and carry impulses for such functions as smell, vision, ocular movement, pupil contraction, muscular sensibility, general sensibility, mastication, facial expression, glandular secretion, taste, cutaneous sensibility, hearing, equilibrium, swallowing, phonation, tongue movement, head movement, and shoulder movement. Certain cranial nerves, particularly V, VII, and VIII, contain two or more distinct functional components considered as independent nerves by some authorities. Some anatomists also classify the terminal nerve as the first cranial. Also called **cerebral nerves.**

cranial sensory ganglion, the ganglion found on the root of each cranial nerve, containing the cell bodies of afferent (sensory) neurons.

cranial sutures, the interlocking lines of fusion (fibrous joints) of the bones forming the skull. The lines gradually become less prominent as a person matures. The gaps between the sutures form the fontanels in an infant. Also called **suturae cranii.**

cranial synchondroses, the cartilaginous junctions between the bones of the cranium.

craniectomy /krā′nē-ek″təmē/ [Gk, *kranion,* cranium, *ektomē,* excision], the surgical removal of a portion of the cranium.

cranio-, prefix meaning "skull" or "cranium": *craniopagus, craniosacral.*

craniocarpotarsal dystrophy. See **Freeman-Sheldon syndrome.**

craniocele. See **encephalocele.**

craniocervical /krā′nē-ōsur′vikəl/ [Gk, *kranion* + L, *cervix,* neck], pertaining to the junction of the skull and neck, particularly the area of the foramen magnum. Because of the complex of nerve fibers and blood vessels in the region and the flexibility of the cervical spine, craniocervical tissues are particularly vulnerable to a variety of compression and traction disorders.

craniodidymus /krā′nē-ōdid″iməs/ [Gk, *kranion* + *didymos,* twin], a two-headed fetus in which the bodies are fused.

craniofacial /-fā″shəl/ [Gk, *kranion,* cranium; L, *facies,* face], pertaining to the cranium and the face.

craniofacial dysostosis [Gk, *kranion* + L, *facies,* face; Gk, *dys,* bad, *osteon,* bone], an abnormal hereditary condition characterized by acrocephaly, exophthalmos, hypertelorism, strabismus, parrot-beaked nose, and hypoplastic maxilla with relative mandibular prognathism. This condition is transmitted as an autosomal-dominant trait. See also **dysostosis.**

craniohypophyseal xanthoma /krā′nē-ōhī′pōfiz″ē·əl/ [Gk, *kranion* + *hypo,* deficient, *phyein,* to grow, *xanthos,* yellow, *oma,* tumor], a condition in which cholesterol deposits are formed around the hypophyses of the bones, as in Hand-Schüller-Christian disease.

craniology /krā′nē-ol′əjē,/ the study of the shape, size, proportions, and other features of the human skull. It is now usually associated with anthropological research. A historically discredited theory was that the shape of the head determined a person's character and personality.

craniometaphyseal dysplasia /-met′əfiz″ē·əl/, an inherited bone disorder characterized by paranasal overgrowth, thickening of the skull and jaw, and entrapment of cranial nerves. The long bones have widened, club-shaped metaphyses. The patient may experience nasorespiratory infections, associated with bone overgrowth at the sinuses, and malocclusion of the jaws.

craniopagus /krā′nē·op″əgəs/ [Gk, *kranion* + *pagos,* fixed], conjoined twins united at the heads. Fusion can occur at the frontal, occipital, or parietal region. Also called **cephalopagus.**

craniopharyngeal /krā′nē·ōfərin″jē·əl/ [Gk, *kranion* + *pharynx,* throat], pertaining to the cranium and the pharynx.

craniopharyngioma, /krā′nē·ōfərin′jē·ō″mə/ *pl. craniopharyngiomas, craniopharyngiomata,* a congenital pituitary tumor, appearing most often in children and adolescents, that arises in cells derived from Rathke's pouch or the hypophyseal stalk. The lesion, a solid or cystic body ranging in size from 1 to 8 cm, may expand into the third ventricle or the temporal lobe and frequently becomes calcified. The tumor may interfere with pituitary function, damage the optic chiasm, disrupt hypothalamic control of the autonomic nervous system, and cause hydrocephalus. Increased intracranial pressure, severe headaches, vomiting, stunted growth, defective vision, irritability, somnolence, and infantile genitalia are often associated with the lesion in children. Development of the tumor after puberty usually results in amenorrhea in women and loss of libido and potency in men. Also called **ameloblastoma, pituitary adamantinoma, Rathke pouch tumor,** *craniopharyngeal duct tumor.*

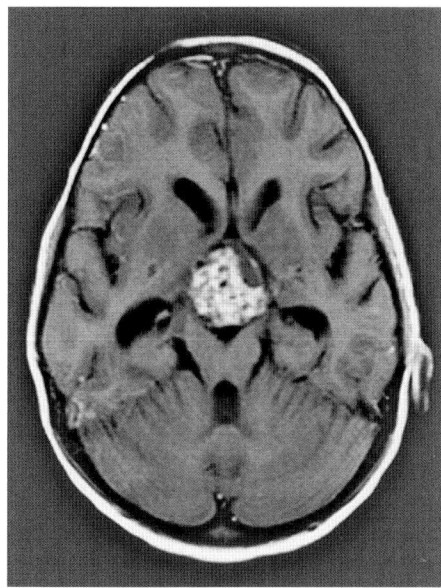

Craniopharyngioma *(Goetz et al, 2007)*

cranioplasty /krā″nē·ōplast′tē/, reconstruction surgery performed on the skull.

craniosacral therapy, a form of gentle manual manipulation used for diagnosis and for making corrections in a system made up of cerebrospinal fluid, cranial and dural membranes, cranial bones, and sacrum. This system is proposed to be dynamic with its own physiological frequency. Through touch and pressure, tension is supposed to be reduced and cranial rhythms normalized, leading to improvement in health.

craniospinal /krā′nē·ōspī′nəl/ [Gk, *kranion,* skull + L, *spina,* backbone or spine], pertaining to the cranium and the vertebral column.

craniostenosis /krā′nē·ō′stənō″sis/ [Gk, *kranion* + *stenos,* narrow, *osis,* condition], a congenital deformity of the skull that results from premature closure of the sutures between the cranial bones. The severity of the malformation depends on which sutures close, the point in the developmental process where the closure occurred, and the success or failure of the other sutures to compensate by expansion. Impaired brain growth may or may not be involved. The most common form of the condition is permanent closure of the sagittal suture with anteroposterior elongation of the skull. Surgery is generally indicated when multiple sutures are fused to relieve cerebral pressure and may be performed for cosmetic reasons. See also **brachycephaly, oxycephaly, plagiocephaly, scaphocephaly.** −*craniostenotic, adj.*

craniostosis /krā′nē·ostō″sis/ [Gk, *kranion* + *osteon,* bone, *osis,* condition], premature ossification of the sutures of the skull, often associated with other skeletal defects. The sutures close before or soon after birth. Without surgical correction the growth of the skull is inhibited, the head is deformed, and the eyes and brain are often damaged. Also called *craniosynostosis.*

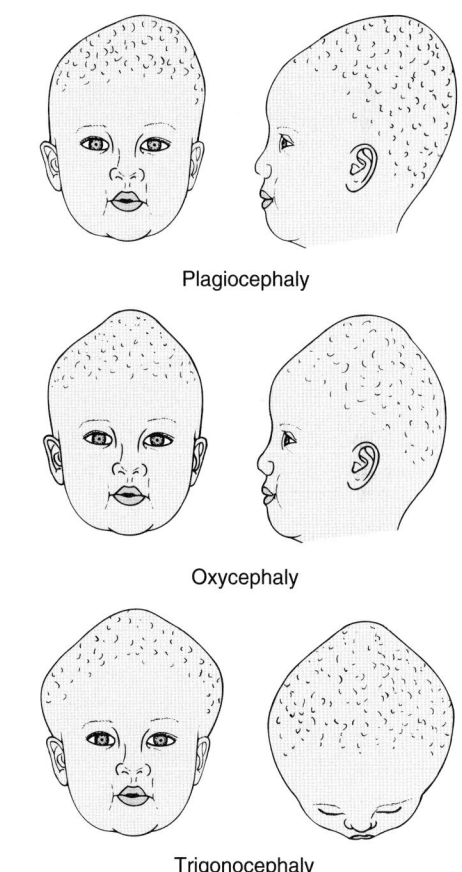

Plagiocephaly

Oxycephaly

Trigonocephaly

Craniostosis *(Mosby, 2003)*

craniotabes /krā′nē·ōtā″bēz/ [Gk, *kranion* + L, *tabes,* wasting], benign congenital thinness of the top and back of the skull of a newborn. The condition is common because the rate of brain growth exceeds the rate of calcification of the skull during the last month of gestation. The bones feel brittle when pressed by an examiner's fingers. Craniotabes disappears with normal nutrition and growth but may persist in infants in whom rickets develops.

craniotomy /krā″nē·ot″əmē/ [Gk, *kranion,* cranium, *temnein,* to cut], any surgical opening into the skull, performed to relieve intracranial pressure, to control bleeding, or to remove a tumor. X-ray images of the skull are taken before surgery, and a computed tomographic (CT) scan or an electroencephalogram is done to establish the diagnosis. The operative site is shaved and cleansed. A semicircular skin incision is made just above the hairline, a series of burr holes is made and connected with a cut, and the flap of bone is removed. The meninges are incised, and the brain is exposed. The flap may be replaced after surgery or left off temporarily to prevent the buildup of pressure from cerebral edema.

craniotubular /-toōb″yələr/, pertaining to a bossing, or overgrowth, of bone that produces an abnormal contour and increased bone density. Kinds include **craniometaphyseal dysplasia.**

cranium /krā″nē·əm/ [Gk, *kranion,* skull], the bony portion of skull that holds the brain. It is composed of eight bones: the frontal, occipital, sphenoid, ethmoid, and paired temporal and parietal bones. **–cranial,** *adj.*

-cranium, suffix meaning "skull": *epicranium, pericranium.*

crankcase-spool catheter /krangk″kās/, a special elastic catheter stored within a plastic spool to facilitate its insertion, especially for hyperalimentation. When fully inserted, the crankcase-spool catheter is usually lodged in the subclavian vein. The catheter is highly flexible, and each revolution of the spool feeds about 5 inches of the catheter into the vein involved. When the crankcase-spool catheter is fully inserted, a radiographic exposure is made of the insertion area to confirm its correct placement. The crankcase-spool catheter is less irritating than a regular catheter, allows greater limb movement, and minimizes the risk of thrombosis. It may, however, cause complications, such as occlusion, phlebitis, infection, and catheter sensitivity. Occlusion of the vein, a common risk, is usually countered by flushing the vein with dilute streptokinase.

crash [ME, *crasschen,* to break violently], a serious malfunction of computer hardware or software that generally results in the loss of function and any data that have not been saved to a file.

crash cart, a cart carrying emergency equipment and supplies, such as medications, suction devices, sutures, scalpels, surgical needles, sponges, swabs, retractors, hemostats, forceps, airways, O_2 supplies, IV supplies, tracheal tubes, and often a cardiac monitor with a defibrillator. Hospital emergency departments and intensive care units usually have several crash carts equipped according to prescribed specifications. Efficient, effective emergency care often depends on the careful provisioning of crash carts and the precise knowledge of their layouts.

-crasia, suffix meaning a "(specified) condition involving loss of control": *dyscrasia.*

crater, a pitlike depression, such as where an ulcer has been surgically removed.

cravat bandage /krəvat″/ [Fr, *cravate,* scarf, *bande,* strip], a triangular bandage, folded lengthwise. It may be

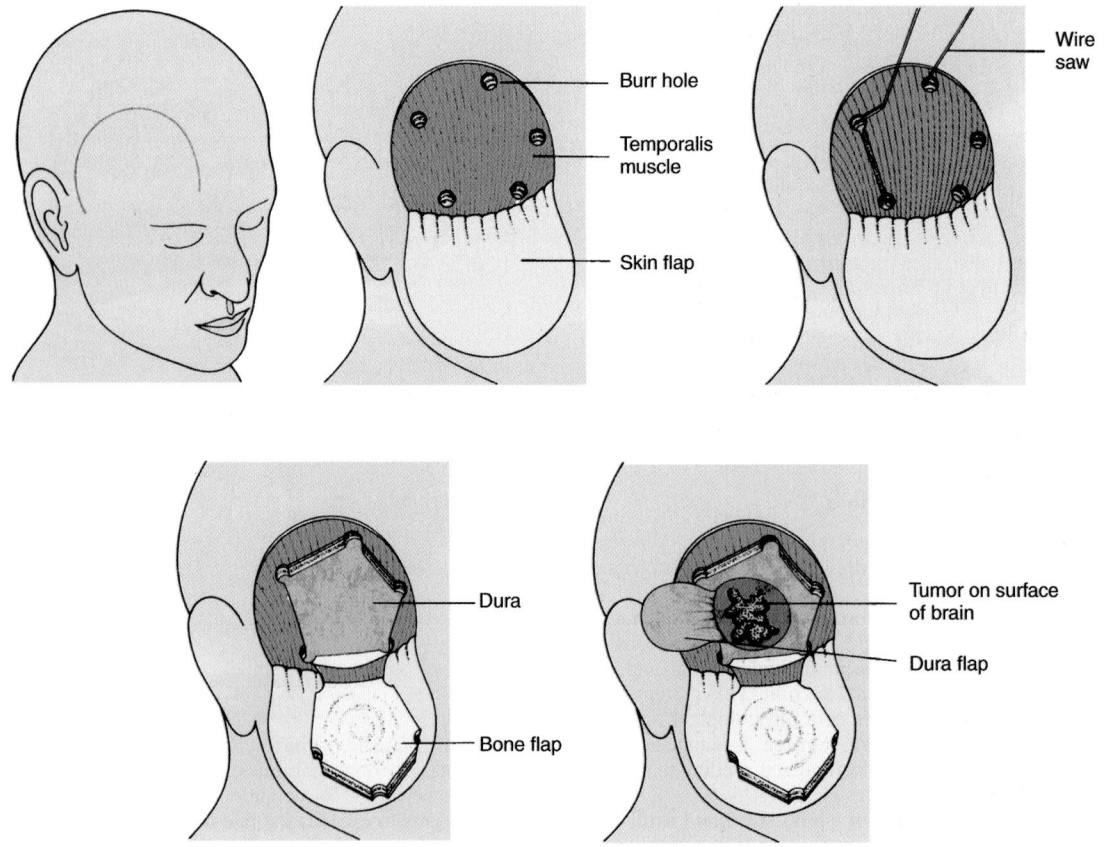

Craniotomy *(Urden et al, 2008)*

Burr hole

Temporalis muscle

Skin flap

Wire saw

Dura

Bone flap

Tumor on surface of brain

Dura flap

used as a circular, figure-eight, or spiral bandage to control bleeding or to tie splints in place.

cravat bandage for clenched fist, a pressure dressing made by folding the points of a triangular bandage to form a band about the fist.

cravat bandage for fracture of the clavicle, a sling dressing that includes a 2- to 4-inch soft pad in the armpit. The triangular bandage is placed with the center point on the affected shoulder. The hand and wrist are laid against it. The opposite ends are lifted to cover and support the arm. The bandage ends are drawn together and fastened at the back.

cravat elbow bandage, a triangular dressing that holds the elbow at a 45-degree angle, beginning with the center over the point of the elbow. The bandage is completed with one end around the forearm and the other around the upper arm.

cravat sling bandage, a support for a fractured arm prepared by laying the wrist on the center of the triangular bandage while the forearm is at a right angle. The two ends of the bandage are carried around the neck and tied.

crawling reflex. See **symmetric tonic neck reflex.**

C-reactive protein (CRP) /-rē·ak″tiv/, a protein not normally detected in the serum but present in many acute inflammatory conditions and with necrosis. CRP appears in the serum before the erythrocyte sedimentation rate begins to rise, often within 24 to 48 hours of the onset of inflammation. Acute rheumatic fever is monitored with serial estimations of CRP because the serum level of the protein is the most sensitive indicator of rheumatic activity. Bacterial infections and widespread neoplastic disease are also associated with C-reactive protein in the serum. CRP disappears when an inflammatory process is suppressed by salicylates, steroids, or both. Also called **serum C-reactive protein.**

C-reactive protein (CRP) test, a blood test used to detect and diagnose bacterial infectious disease, postsurgical wound infection, and inflammatory disorders such as acute rheumatic fever and rheumatoid arthritis. In addition, it is used as an adjunct in detecting acute bacterial meningitis in an acutely febrile child and a cardiovascular risk assessment marker when high sensitivity assays are used.

cream [Gk, *chrisma,* oil], **1.** the portion of milk rich in butterfat. **2.** any fluid mixture of thick consistency. Creams are often used as a method of applying medication to the surface of the body. Compare **ointment.**

crease [ME, *creste,* crest], an indentation or margin formed by a doubling back of tissue, such as the folds on the palm of the hand and sole of the foot.

creat-, prefix meaning "flesh": *creatorrhea.*

creatinase /krē·at′i·nās/ [Gk, *kreas,* flesh], an enzyme that catalyzes the conversion of creatine to sarcosine and urea.

creatine /krē″ətēn, -tin/ [Gk, *kreas,* flesh], an important nitrogenous compound produced by metabolic processes in the body. Combined with phosphorus, it forms a high-energy phosphate. In normal metabolic reactions the phosphorus is transferred to a molecule of adenosine diphosphate to produce a molecule of very high-energy adenosine triphosphate. See also **creatinine.**

creatine kinase (CK), an enzyme of the transferase class in muscle, brain, and other tissues. It catalyzes the transfer of a phosphate group from adenosine triphosphate to creatine, producing adenosine diphosphate and phosphocreatine. The reaction stores energy in muscle and brain tissue. Also called **creatine phosphokinase.** See also **Duchenne's muscular dystrophy.**

creatine kinase (CK) test, a blood test used to detect damage to the heart muscle, skeletal muscles, and brain. Serum

CK levels are elevated whenever such damage occurs. CK is the main cardiac enzyme studied in patients with heart disease.

creatine phosphate (CP) [Gk, *kreas,* flesh; Du, *potasschen*], an enzyme that increases in blood levels when muscle damage has occurred, as in pseudohypertrophic muscular dystrophy.

creatine phosphokinase. See **creatine kinase.**

creatinine /krē·at″inēn, -nin/, a substance formed from the metabolism of creatine, commonly found in blood, urine, and muscle tissue. It is measured in blood and urine tests as an indicator of kidney function. Normal adult blood levels of creatinine are 0.5 to 1.1 mg/dL for females and 0.6 to 1.2 mg/dL for males. While the creatinine levels may decrease in the elderly due to reduced muscle mass they may also increase due to a decrease in kidney function. Serum creatinine in the elderly will not increase until 50% of nephrons are no longer functional. See also **creatine.**

creatinine clearance test, a measure of plasma or serum creatinine concentration and creatinine concentration in a 24-hour urine collection specimen. The two values are used in a mathematical formula to derive creatinine clearance, a measure of kidney function.

creatinine height index (CHI), a value calculated from a 24-hour urinary excretion of creatinine compared with a healthy individual of the same height. It is an indicator of lean muscle mass and malnutrition, particularly in young males. See also **creatinine clearance test.**

creatinuria /krē′ətinoor′ē·ə/, increased concentration of creatine in the urine, as seen in muscular dystrophy, poliomyelitis, and various other conditions.

creatorrhea, the presence of undigested muscle fibers in the feces.

credentialing /kriden″shəling/, examination and review of the credentials of individuals meeting a set of educational or occupational criteria and therefore being licensed in their fields. Strict credentialing is required by both hospital and managed care accreditation bodies, as well as regulatory bodies for the health professions. The process is conducted periodically because of the responsibility of organizations for any claims of malpractice by their staffs but more importantly for the organizations' commitment to excellence in patient care. See also **certify.**

credentials /kriden″shelz/, a predetermined set of standards, such as licensure or certification, establishing that a person or institution has achieved professional recognition in a specific field of health care. See also **credentialing.**

Credé's maneuver /kredā″z/ [Karl S. Credé, German physician, 1819–1892], a technique for aiding the expulsion of the placenta. The uterus is pushed toward the birth canal by pressure exerted by the thumb of one hand on the posterior surface of the abdomen and the other hand on the anterior surface.

Credé method /kredā″/ [Karl S. Credé, German physician, 1819–1892], a technique for promoting the expulsion of urine by manual compression of the bladder through external pressure on the lower abdominal wall.

Credé's prophylaxis /kredā″z/ [Karl S. Credé], the instillation of a 1% silver nitrate solution into the conjunctiva of newborns to prevent ophthalmia neonatorum.

creep, a rheological effect of metals and other solid materials that may become elongated or deformed as a result of a load being applied for a long period. For example, creep can occur in silver amalgam fillings that have been in place for some time.

creeping eruption. See **cutaneous larva migrans.**

cremaster /krimas″tər/ [Gk, *kremastos,* hanging], a thin muscular layer that spreads out over the spermatic cord in a series of loops. It is a continuation of the obliquus internus. The muscle arises from the inguinal ligament and inserts into the crest of the pubis and into the sheath of the rectus abdominis. It is innervated by the genital branch of the genitofemoral nerve and functions to draw the testis up toward the superficial inguinal ring in response to cold or to stimulation of the nerve.

cremasteric arteries, the arteries that originate from the external iliac artery and accompany the spermatic cord into the scrotum in men or follow the round ligament of the uterus through the inguinal canal in women.

cremasteric fascia, a layer contributed by the internal oblique muscle to the coverings of the structures traversing the inguinal canal. This layer contains the cremasteric muscle.

cremasteric muscle. See **cremasteric fascia.**

cremasteric reflex /krē′məstər″ik/, a superficial neural reflex elicited by stroking the skin of the upper inner thigh in a male. This action normally results in a brisk retraction of the testis on the side of the stimulus. The reflex is lost in diseases of the pyramidal tract above the level of the first lumbar vertebra. See also **superficial reflex.**

crematorium /krē′mətôrē·əm/, a facility for the disposal of the deceased by burning at high temperatures.

crenated, scalloped or notched.

crenated erythrocytes, the formation of abnormal notching around the edge of a red blood cell.

crenation /krinā″shən/ [L, *crena,* notch], the formation of notches or leaflike scalloped edges on an object. Red blood cells exposed to a hypertonic saline solution acquire a notched, shriveled surface as a result of the osmotic effect of the solution. They are then called crenated red blood cells. −*crenate,* **crenated,** *adj.*

creosol /krē″əsol/, an oily liquid that is one of the active constituents (phenol) of creosote. Should not be confused with **cresol.**

creosote /krē″əsōt/, a flammable oily liquid with a smoky odor that is used primarily as a wood preservative. It can cause a wide variety of health problems, ranging from cancer and corneal damage to convulsions, dermatitis, and vertigo. Persons who work with treated wood are usually at the greatest risk of exposure.

crepitant /krep″itənt/ [L, *crepitans,* crackling], pertaining to the feel or sound of crackling or rattling, or of rough surfaces being rubbed together.

crepitant crackle [L, *crepitans,* crackling], an abnormal breathing sound produced at the end of inspiration and caused by air entering collapsed alveoli or just collapsed alveoli and atelectasis that contain fibrous exudate. It occurs in pneumonia, tuberculosis, and pulmonary edema.

crepitus /krep″itəs/ [L, crackling], **1.** flatulence or the noisy discharge of fetid gas from the intestine through the anus. **2.** a sound or feel that resembles the crackling noise heard when rubbing hair between the fingers or throwing salt on an open fire. Crepitus is associated with gas gangrene, rubbing of bone fragments, air in superficial tissues, or crackles of a consolidated area of the lung in pneumonia. Also called *crepitation.* **3.** a clicking sound often heard in movement of joints, for example, in temporomandibular joint resulting from joint irregularities.

cresc-, prefix meaning "to grow": *crescendo angina.*

crescendo angina /krishen″dō/ [L, *crescere,* to increase], a form of angina pectoris associated with ischemic electrocardiographic changes and marked by increased frequency, provocation, intensity, or character.

crescendo murmur [L, *crescere,* to increase, *murmur,* humming], a low-pitched sound of steadily increasing intensity to a sudden termination.

crescent /kres′ənt/ [L, *crescere,* to increase], **1.** *adj.,* shaped like a new moon or half moon; circular but open in appearance. **2.** *n.,* a structure that has this shape.

crescent bodies /kres′ənt/, **1.** (in a blood smear) large, pale, crescent-shaped cells produced from fragile erythrocytes as a blood film preparation is made. **2.** large, round bodies with pink crescentlike margins found in the blood of some anemia patients. Also called **achromocyte, selenoid cells.**

cresol /krē′sol/, a mixture of three isomers of an organic acid in a liquid with a phenolic odor. It is derived from coal tar and used in synthetic resins and disinfectants. Cresol is a potentially lethal protoplasmic poison that can be absorbed through the skin. Symptoms of chronic poisoning include skin eruptions, digestive disorders, uremia, jaundice, nervous disorders, vertigo, and mental changes. Acute poisoning by oral intake of 8 g or more can cause circulatory collapse and death. See also **phenol poisoning.**

crest, a narrow elongated elevation, as the iliac crest.

Crestor, brand name for **rosuvastatin.**

CREST syndrome /krest/, a disease of skin and blood vessels and, in severe cases, the lungs, digestive tract, or heart. Abbreviation for *calcinosis, Raynaud phenomenon, esophageal dysfunction, sclerodactyly, and telangiectasis.* Also called **limited scleroderma.**

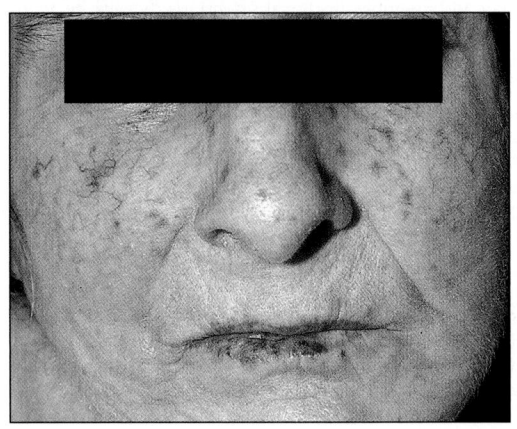

Woman with CREST syndrome *(White and Cox, 2006)*

cretin. See **cretinism.**

cretin dwarf /krē″tən/, a person in whom short stature is caused by infantile hypothyroidism and severe deficiency of thyroid hormone. Also called **hypothyroid dwarf.** See also **cretinism.**

cretinism /krē″təniz′əm/ [Fr, *cretin,* idiot], a congenital condition characterized by severe hypothyroidism and often associated with other endocrine abnormalities. Typical signs of cretinism include dwarfism, mental deficiency, puffy facial features, dry skin, large tongue, umbilical hernia, and muscular incoordination. The disorder occurs usually in areas where the diet is deficient in iodine and where goiter is common. Pregnant and breastfeeding women should take an iodine supplement and use iodized table salt to avoid an iodine deficiency. Early treatment with thyroid hormone generally promotes normal physical growth in infants but may not prevent cognitive impairment. The use of iodized salt has dramatically reduced the incidence of cretinism worldwide. The condition is increasingly rare, but in some geographic areas where iodine in the food is not sufficient, it remains a public health issue. See also **familial cretinism.** −*cretinous, adj.*

cretinoid, possessing physical characteristics associated with cretinism or being affected by cretinism. See also **cretinism.**

Creutzfeldt-Jakob disease /kroits″felt yä″kôp/ [Hans G. Creutzfeldt, German neurologist, 1885–1964; Alfons M. Jakob, German neurologist, 1884–1931], a rare fatal encephalopathy caused by infectious prion particles. The disease occurs in middle age. It is the human variant of mad cow disease. Also called **Jakob-Creutzfeldt disease, spastic pseudoparalysis, spastic pseudosclerosis, prion disease.**

■ OBSERVATIONS: Symptoms are progressive and include dementia, dysarthria, muscle wasting, and various involuntary movements such as myoclonus and athetosis. Deterioration is obvious week to week.

■ INTERVENTIONS: Transmission between humans is unusual, but the disease has been observed years after exposure to needles, instruments, and electrodes previously used in the treatment of a patient with the disease. Isolation is not necessary. Special care in disposal or sterilization of potentially infective items is always necessary. The goal of the health care team is to make the patient as comfortable as possible.

■ PATIENT CARE CONSIDERATIONS: There is no known cure. Most patients will die within a year.

crevice /krev″is/, a cleft or fissure, like that between the gum and the neck of a tooth.

CRH, abbreviation for **corticotropin-releasing hormone.**

CRHP, abbreviation for *Canadian Respiratory Health Professionals.*

crib /krib/ [L, *cribrum,* sieve], **1.** any racklike structure. **2.** a removable anchorage from an orthodontic appliance. **3.** a habit-breaking orthodontic appliance used for the treatment of tongue-thrust swallowing. **4.** a bed for an infant or small child, usually with slatted sides.

crib death. *(Informal)* See **sudden infant death syndrome.**

cribriform /krib″rifôrm′/ [L, *cribrum,* sieve], describing a structure with many perforations or punctures, as in the cribriform plate of the ethmoid bone.

cribriform carcinoma. See **adenocystic carcinoma.**

cribriform plate of the ethmoid bone, a sievelike structure that allows small olfactory nerve fibers to pass through its foramina from the nasal mucosa to the olfactory bulb.

crico-, prefix meaning "ring": *cricoid, cricoidectomy.*

cricoarytenoid muscles, one of the muscles that opens and closes the rima glottidis, innervated by the laryngeal branches of the vagus nerves.

cricoid /krī″koid/ [Gk, *krikos,* ring, *eidos,* form], *adj.,* having a ring shape. Kinds include **cricoid cartilage.**

cricoid cartilage, a ring-shaped cartilage of the larynx, consisting of a narrow anterior arch and a posterior wide quadrilateral lamina, connected to the thyroid cartilage by the cricothyroid ligament at the level of the sixth cervical vertebra.

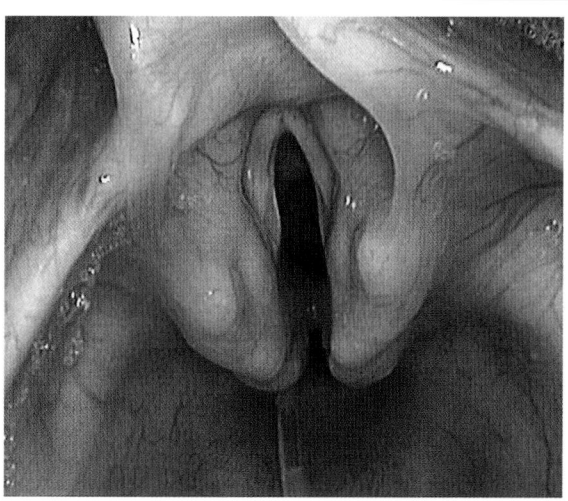

Cricoid cartilage *(Flint et al, 2010)*

cricoidectomy /-ek″təmē/ [Gk, *krikos + eidos + ektomē,* excision], a surgical procedure for removing the ring-shaped cricoid cartilage in the throat.

cricoid pressure, a technique to reduce the risk of the aspiration of stomach contents during induction of general anesthesia. The cricoid cartilage is pushed against the body of the sixth cervical vertebra, compressing the esophagus to prevent passive regurgitation. The technique cannot, however, and should not be used to stop active vomiting. Cricoid pressure is applied before intubation, immediately after injection of anesthetic drugs, and as a part of "rapid sequence" intubation. Once a mainstay of aspiration prevention, the effectiveness of this technique has recently been called into question. Cricoid pressure may also be used to move the larynx posteriorly and/or superiorly to facilitate visualization during laryngoscopy. Also called **Sellick's maneuver.**

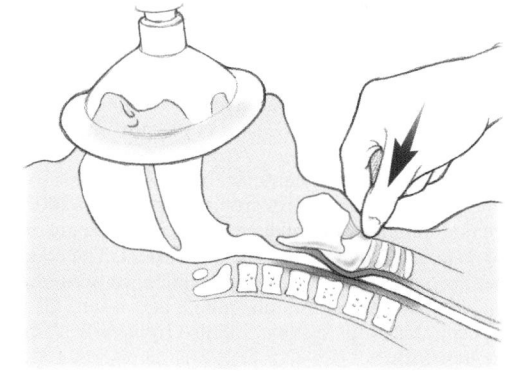

Cricoid pressure *(Aehlert, 2012)*

cricopharyngeal /krī′kōfərin″jē·əl/ [Gk, *krikos + pharynx,* throat], pertaining to the cricoid cartilage and the pharynx.

cricopharyngeal incoordination, a defect in the normal swallowing reflex. The cricopharyngeus muscle ordinarily serves as a sphincter to keep the top of the esophagus closed except when the person is swallowing, vomiting, or belching. The trachea remains open for breathing, but air normally does not enter the esophagus during respiration.

In swallowing the reverse effect occurs, and the larynx is closed while food slides past it into the esophagus, which is located immediately behind the larynx. When the somewhat complex series of neuromuscular actions is not properly coordinated as a result of disease or injury, the patient may choke, swallow air, regurgitate fluid into the nose, or experience discomfort in swallowing food. See also **dysphagia.**

cricothyroid membrane /-thī″roid/, a fibroelastic membrane including the cricothyroid ligament that connects the cricoid and thyroid cartilages. Also called **elastic membrane.**

cricothyrotomy /krī′kōthīrot″əmē/ [Gk, *krikos* + *thyreos,* shield, *eidos,* form, *temnein,* to cut], an emergency incision into the larynx, performed to open the airway in a person who is choking. A small vertical midline cut is made just below the thyroid cartilage and above the cricoid cartilage. The incision is opened farther with a transverse cut through the cricothyroid membrane, and the wound is spread open with a knife handle or other dilator. The new opening must be held open with a tracheostomy tube that is open at both ends to allow air to move in and out. Also called *cricothyroidotomy.* Compare **tracheostomy.**

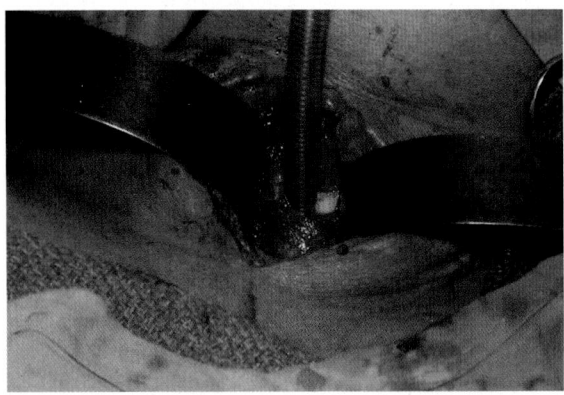

Cricothyrotomy *(Flint et al, 2015)*

cricotracheal ligament, the ligament that runs from the lower border of the cricoid cartilage to the adjacent upper border of the first tracheal cartilage.

cri-du-chat syndrome. See **cat-cry syndrome.**

Crigler-Najjar syndrome /krig″lər naj″är/ [John F. Crigler, Jr., American pediatrician, b. 1919; Victor A. Najjar, Lebanese-born American microbiologist, 1914–2002], a congenital familial autosomal anomaly, in which glucuronyl transferase, an enzyme, is deficient or absent. The condition is characterized by nonhemolytic jaundice, an accumulation of unconjugated bilirubin in the blood, and severe disorders of the central nervous system. See also **hyperbilirubinemia of the newborn.**

crime [L, *crimen*], any act that violates a law and may have criminal intent.

Crimean-Congo hemorrhagic fever /krīmē″ən/, an arbovirus infection caused by the virus *Nairovirus* of the family Bunyaviridae, transmitted to humans through the bite of a tick, characterized by fever, dizziness, muscle ache, vomiting, headache, and other neurological symptoms. After several days in severe cases, bleeding from the skin and mucous membranes, particularly from the mouth and nose; bloody sputum or vomit; and blood-tinged feces may be seen. Transfusion may be necessary to replace lost blood; otherwise treatment is symptomatic and supportive. The mortality rate is approximately 30%. Death occurs in the second week of infection. No specific medication or therapy is available for prevention or cure. It occurs mainly in Russia, Asia, and Africa; agricultural workers are most often afflicted. See also **hemorrhagic fever, Omsk hemorrhagic fever.**

criminal psychology, the study of the mental processes, motivational patterns, and behavior of criminals. Compare **forensic psychiatry.**

-crinat, suffix designating an ethacrynic acid–derived diuretic.

-crine, 1. suffix designating an acridine derivative. **2.** suffix meaning "to separate or secrete": *autocrine, endocrine, holocrine.*

crisis /krī″sis/ [Gk, *krisis,* turning point], **1.** a transition for better or worse in the course of a disease, usually indicated by a marked change in the intensity of signs and symptoms. **2.** a turning point in events affecting the emotional state of a person, such as death or divorce. A crisis can result in personality growth or personality disorganization. **3.** a characteristically self-limiting period of from 4 to 6 weeks that constitutes a transitional phase representing both the danger of increased psychological vulnerability and an opportunity for personal growth. See also **crisis intervention.**

crisis intervention, (in psychiatry) a short-term intense therapy that emphasizes identification of the event that triggered the emotional trauma. Focus is on neutralizing the trauma and mobilizing coping skills.

crisis-intervention unit, a group trained in emergency medical treatment and in various methods for rendering psychiatric therapeutic assistance to a person or group of persons during a period of crisis, especially instances involving suicide attempts or drug abuse. Such networks are found within community hospitals, in health care centers, or as specialized self-contained units, such as suicide-prevention centers, and operate 24 hours a day. The primary objectives of such crisis assistance are to help the person cope with the immediate problem and to offer guidance and support for long-term therapy.

crisis resolution, (in psychiatry) the development of effective adaptive and coping devices to resolve a crisis.

crisis theory, a conceptual framework for defining and explaining the phenomena that occur when a person faces a problem that appears to be unsolvable. The theory is the basis of crisis therapy.

crisscross inheritance [Christ cross; L, *in* + *hereditas,* in heredity], the inheritance of characteristics or conditions from the parent of the opposite sex.

crista. See **crest.**

crista ampullaris /kris′tə am′pəlar′is/ [L], the most prominent part of a localized thickening of the membrane that lines the ampullae of the semicircular ducts, covered with neuroepithelium containing endings of the vestibular nerve.

crista galli, a prominent wedge of bone projecting superiorly from the ethmoid.

crista obliqua, an elevated crest of variable prominence, consisting jointly of the triangular ridge of the distobuccal cusp and the distal ridge of the mesiolingual cusp. It courses obliquely across the occlusal surface of the maxillary molars to link the apices of the distobuccal and the mesiolingual cusps.

criterion /krītir″ē·ən/ *pl. criteria* [Gk, *kriterion,* a means for judging], a standard or rule by which something may be judged, such as a health condition, or a diagnosis established. Criteria are sets of rules or principles against which something may be measured, such as health care practices.

critical care. See **intensive care.**

critical care unit (CCU), a specially equipped hospital area designed for the treatment of patients with sudden life-threatening conditions. CCUs contain resuscitation and monitoring equipment and are staffed by personnel specially trained and skilled in recognizing and immediately responding to cardiac and other emergencies. See also **intensive care unit.**

critical organs /krit″ikəl/ [Gk, *krisis,* turning point, *organon,* instrument], tissues that are the most sensitive to irradiation, such as the gonads, lymphoid organs, and intestine. The skin, cornea, oral cavity, esophagus, vagina, cervix, and optic lens are the second-most sensitive organs to irradiation.

critical pathway. See **clinical pathway.**

critical period [Gk, *kritikos,* critical, *peri,* near, *hodos,* way], a period during a developmental or rehabilitation crisis. Examples include the brief period in which a zygote may be formed, the period in which a patient may survive a myocardial infarction, or the period in which an embryo is most vulnerable to the effects of medications used by the mother.

critical period of development, 1. a specific time during which the environment has its greatest impact on an individual's development. 2. the time during gestation when critical organ systems are formed.

critical point, the temperature and pressure at which, in a sealed system, the density of the liquid form of a substance is equal to the density of its gas form, and the two are not visibly separated, becoming a single fluid phase instead.

critical pressure, the pressure exerted by a fluid in a closed system at the critical temperature.

critical temperature, the highest temperature at which a substance can exist as a liquid.

Crixivan, an antiretroviral protease inhibitor. Brand name for **indinavir.**

CRNA, abbreviation for **certified registered nurse anesthetist.**

CRNI®, abbreviation for **Certified Registered Nurse Infusion.**

crocodile shagreen /shagrēn″/, a rare degenerative disorder involving either of two membranes of the cornea in which the cornea exhibits opacities separated by clear zones. The disorder may affect Descemet's deep membrane or Bowman's superficial membrane.

Crohn disease /krōnz/ [Burrill B. Crohn, American physician, 1884–1983], a chronic inflammatory bowel disease of unknown origin, usually affecting the ileum, the colon, or another part of the GI tract. Diseased segments may be separated by normal bowel segments, which give it the characteristic "skip lesions." Also called **regional enteritis.** Compare **ulcerative colitis.** See also **colitis, ileitis.**

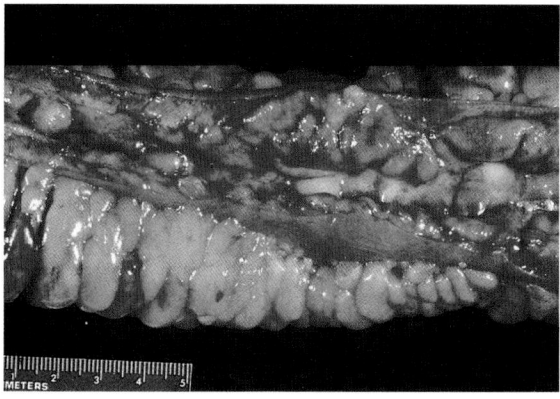

Crohn disease *(Kumar et al, 2007)*

Comparison of ulcerative colitis and Crohn disease

	Ulcerative colitis	*Crohn disease*
Usual area affected		
	Left colon, rectum	Distal ileum, right colon Can occur anywhere in gastrointestinal tract
Extent of involvement		
	Diffuse areas, contiguous	Segmental areas, noncontiguous
Inflammation		
	Mostly mucosal	Transmural
Mucosal appearance		
	Shallow mucosal ulcerations, edematous, superficial bleeding	Cobblestone effect, granulomas Thickened walls, narrowed lumen
Complications		
	Loss of absorption and elasticity	Fistulas
	Replacement of mucosa by scar tissue	Perianal disease Strictures
	Development of pseudopolyps that may become malignant	Abscesses Perforation
	Toxic megacolon	Anemia
	Hemorrhoids	Malabsorption of fat and fat-soluble vitamins
	Bleeding	

From Monahan FD et al: *Phipps' medical-surgical nursing: health and illness perspectives,* ed 8, St. Louis, 2007, Mosby.

Cromer blood group /krō′mər/, a blood group consisting of 12 red cell antigens located on the complement regulatory glycoprotein, decay-accelerating factor (DAF of CD55).

-cromil, suffix designating a cromoglycic acid-type antiallergic agent.

cromolyn sodium /krom″əlin/, a drug that blocks mast cell degranulation in response to antigen, which leads to decreased release of histamine, leukotrienes, and other inflammatory mast cell products. Also called *cromoglycic acid.*

■ INDICATIONS: It is prophylactically prescribed to prevent bronchial asthma.

■ CONTRAINDICATIONS: Known hypersensitivity to this drug prohibits its use; the drug is effective only for asthma prophylaxis, not treatment of an acute asthma attack.

■ ADVERSE EFFECTS: Bronchospasm, wheezing, nasal congestion, pharyngeal irritation, and other hypersensitivity reactions may occur.

Cronkhite-Canada syndrome /krong″kīt/ [Leonard W. Cronkhite, American physician, b. 1919; Wilma J. Canada, 20th-century American radiologist], an abnormal familial condition characterized by GI polyposis accompanied by ectodermal defects, such as nail atrophy, alopecia, and excessive skin pigmentation. In some individuals it is also accompanied by protein-losing enteropathy, malabsorption, and deficiency of blood calcium, potassium, and magnesium.

cross [L, *crux*], 1. (in genetics) a mating between individuals with different phenotypes. Kinds include **dihybrid cross, monohybrid cross, polyhybrid cross, trihybrid cross.** 2. any individual, organism, or strain produced from such a mating.

cross-bite [L, *crux* + AS, *bitan, toth*], a deviated tooth occlusion with the line of the mandibular teeth or a single tooth labial and/or buccal to the maxillary teeth.

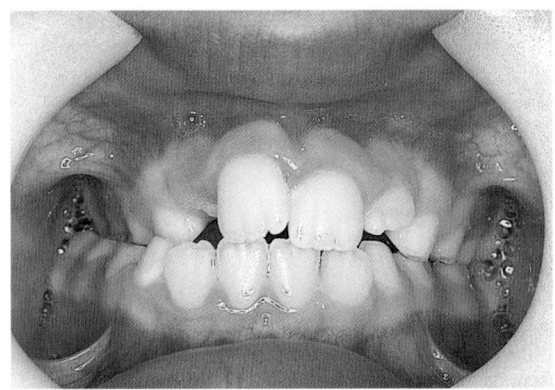

Cross-bite *(Millett and Welbury, 2000)*

crossbreeding [L, *crux* + *bredan*], the production of offspring by the mating of individuals of different varieties, strains, or species; hybridization. See also **inbreeding.** –*crossbred, adj.*

crossed amblyopia [L, *crux,* cross; Gk, *amblys,* dull, *ops,* eyes], a visual disorder in which the patient is unable to see on one side of the visual field, associated with hemianesthesia of the opposite side of the body. Also called **amblyopia cruciata.**

crossed extension reflex, one of the spinally mediated reflexes normally present in the first 2 months of life, demonstrated by the adduction and extension of one leg when the foot of the other leg is stimulated. When present in adults, it indicates hyperactive reflexes.

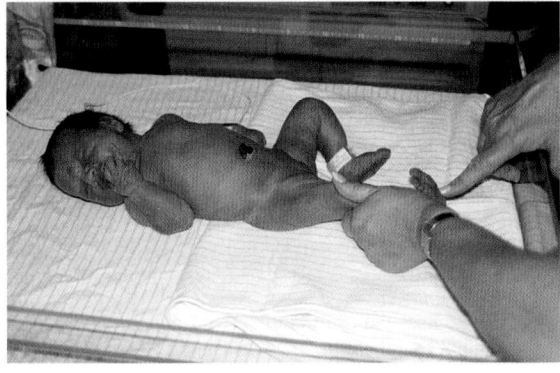

Crossed extension reflex *(Courtesy Marjorie Pyle, RNC, Lifecircle)*

crossed fused ectopic kidney, a rare congenital anomaly of the urinary system in which one kidney crosses over to the opposite side and the parenchyma of the two kidneys fuse.

crossed grid, an assembly of two parallel x-ray grids that are oriented at right angles to each other to eliminate scattered radiation from more than one direction during radiography. Also called **crosshatch grid.** See also **grid.**

crossed leg palsy, palsy of the fibular nerve, caused by sitting with one leg crossed over the other.

crossed reflex, any neural reflex in which stimulation of one side of the body results in a response on the other, such as the consensual light reflex.

cross-eye. *(Informal)* See **esophoria, esotropia.**

cross-fertilization, **1.** the union of gametes from different species or varieties to form hybrids. **2.** the fertilization of the flower of one plant by the pollen of a different plant. Also called **allogamy.**

crosshatch grid. See **crossed grid.**

cross infection [L, *crux,* cross, *inficere,* to stain], the transmittal of an infection from one patient to another patient or sometimes from one body system to another in the same patient, especially in patients whose immune system is depressed. The infection can be transmitted by contaminated objects or bodily secretions.

crossing over, the exchange of sections of chromatids between homologous pairs of chromosomes during the prophase stage of the first meiotic division. Crossing over occurs through the formation of chiasmata and results in the recombination of genes. Also called **chiasmatypy.**

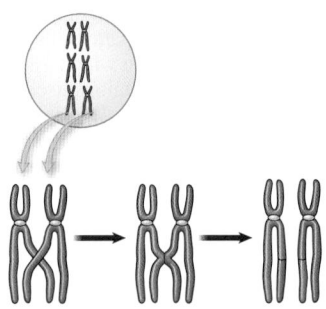

Crossing over *(Patton, 2016)*

cross-link /kros'link"/, a bond formed between polymer chains, either between different chains or between different parts of the same chain.

crossmatching [L, *crux* + AS, *gemaecca,* matching], a procedure in blood transfusions and organ transplantation. The recipient's erythrocytes or leukocytes are incubated with the donor's serum and vice versa. Various testing procedures are then performed to ensure that the donor and recipient have blood group compatibility or histocompatibility. Compare **blood typing.** See also **ABO blood group, Rh factor, transfusion, transfusion reaction.**

crossover /kros"ovər/ [L, *crux* + AS, *ofer*], the result of the recombination of genes on homologous pairs of chromosomes during meiosis. See also **crossing over.**

cross-reacting antibody [L, *crux,* cross, *re* + *agere,* to act; Gk, *anti* + AS, *bodig,* body], an antibody that reacts with antigens that are similar to, but different from, the specific antigens with which it originally reacted.

cross-resistance, resistance to a particular antibiotic that often results in resistance to other antibiotics, usually from a similar chemical class, to which the bacteria may not have been exposed. Cross-resistance can occur, for example, to both colistin and polymyxin B or to both clindamycin and lincomycin.

cross section, **1.** a transverse section cut through a structure. **2.** (in nuclear physics) of a specific atom or particle at a specific radiation, the area perpendicular to the direction of the radiation that one attributes to the atom or particle.

cross-sectional [L, *crux* + *secare,* to cut], (in statistics) pertaining to the sampling of a defined population at one point in time, performed in a nonexperimental research design. Compare **longitudinal.**

cross-sectional anatomy, the study of the relationship of the structures of the body by the examination of cross sections of the tissue or organ. Compare **surface anatomy.**

cross-sensitivity, a sensitivity to one substance that predisposes an individual to sensitivity to other substances that are related in chemical structure. Cross-sensitivity with allergic reactions may develop between antibiotics of similar chemical structures.

cross-sequential /-sikwen″shəl/ [L, *crux* + *sequi,* to follow], (in statistics) pertaining to data that compare several cohorts at different points in time.

cross-species transplant, a tissue or organ from an animal of one species that has been implanted into an animal of another species. Also called **xenotransplant.**

Cross syndrome. See **oculocerebral-hypopigmentation syndrome.**

cross-tolerance, a tolerance to other drugs that develops after exposure to a different agent. An example is the cross-tolerance that develops between alcohol and barbiturates.

crotalid /krot′älid/, pit viper.

Crotalus /krot′älus/, a large genus of venomous rattlesnakes with numerous species in North America and others in Central and South America. See also **snakebite.**

crotamiton /krōtam″iton/, a scabicide.

■ INDICATIONS: It is prescribed in the treatment of scabies and other pruritic skin diseases.

■ CONTRAINDICATIONS: Known hypersensitivity to this drug prohibits its use. It is not applied near the eyes or on the mouth or raw skin.

■ ADVERSE EFFECTS: Among the most serious adverse reactions are irritation and allergic reactions of the skin.

croup /krōōp/ [Scot, to croak], an acute infection of the upper and lower respiratory tract that occurs primarily in infants and young children 3 months to 3 years of age after an upper respiratory tract infection. It is characterized by hoarseness; irritability; fever; a distinctive harsh, brassy cough that sounds like a seal's bark; persistent stridor during inspiration; and dyspnea and tachypnea, resulting from obstruction of the larynx. Cyanosis or pallor occurs in severe cases. The most common causative agents are the parainfluenza viruses, especially type 1, followed by the respiratory syncytial viruses and influenza A and B viruses. Croup can also be caused by bacteria, allergies, and inhaled irritants. Also called **acute laryngotracheobronchitis, angina trachealis,** *exudative angina,* **laryngostasis.** Compare **acute epiglottitis.** *–croupous, croupy, adj.*

■ OBSERVATIONS: Transmission occurs through infection with airborne particles or with infected secretions. Leukocytosis with an increased proportion of polymorphonuclear cells may be present at first, followed by leukopenia and lymphocytosis. A lateral neck x-ray film shows subepiglottic narrowing and a normal-sized epiglottis, which differentiate the condition from acute epiglottitis. Onset of the acute stage is rapid, usually occurs at night, and may be precipitated by exposure to cold air. The child's condition often improves in the morning, but it may worsen at night.

■ INTERVENTIONS: Routine treatment consists of bed rest, adequate fluid intake, and alleviation of airway obstruction to ensure adequate respiratory exchange. Children with mild infections are usually managed at home with supportive measures, such as the use of acetaminophen to reduce fever and vaporizers, humidifiers, or steam from hot running water in an enclosed bathroom to reduce the spasm of the laryngeal muscles and to free secretions. Hospitalization is indicated for children with dehydration; progressive stridor and respiratory distress; and hypoxia, cyanosis, or pallor. Endotracheal intubation and tracheostomy may be necessary. Humidity and oxygen are usually prescribed. The vital signs are continuously monitored; changes in pulse and respiration may be early signs of hypoxia and impending airway obstruction. Fluids are often given intravenously to reduce physical exertion and the possibility of vomiting, with its attendant increased risk of aspiration. Corticosteroids and inhaled racemic epinephrine are often used. Other drugs, such as expectorants, bronchodilators, and antihistamines, are

rarely used, and sedatives are contraindicated because they exert a depressant effect on the respiratory tract.

■ PATIENT CARE CONSIDERATIONS: The primary focuses of care are to ease breathing by providing humidity and to monitor continuously for signs of respiratory distress and impending airway obstruction, with intubation and tracheostomy equipment kept readily available. To conserve the child's energy and to reduce apprehension, the health care provider encourages rest, disturbs the child as little as possible, remains in attendance, provides comfort with a familiar toy or other device, and encourages parental involvement whenever possible. Fever is usually reduced by the cool atmosphere of the mist tent; antipyretics are given as needed. To prevent chilling, frequent changes of clothing and bed linen are often necessary in the humid environment. The health care provider also explains the condition to the parents and discusses appropriate care after discharge, including continued use of humidity and ensuring of adequate hydration and proper nutrition. In most children the condition is relatively mild and runs its course in 3 to 7 days. The infection may spread to other areas of the respiratory tract and may cause complications, such as bronchiolitis, pneumonia, and otitis media. The most serious complication is laryngeal obstruction, which may cause death. If a tracheostomy is required, as may happen with a small percentage of children, other complications, such as infection, atelectasis, cannula occlusion, tracheal bleeding, granulation, stenosis, and delayed healing of the stoma, may develop.

Croupette /krōōpet″/, a brand name for a device that provides cool humidification with the administration of oxygen or of compressed air. The Croupette consists of a nebulizer with attached tubing that connects with a canopy to enclose the patient and contain the humidifying mist. The patient's environment may be cooled by using a Croupette with its own refrigeration unit. This device is most often used with pediatric patients to relieve hypoxia and liquefy secretions. Also called **cold mist tent.**

croupous, croupy. See **croup.**

Crouzon syndrome /krōōzonz″/ [Octave Crouzon, French neurologist, 1874–1938; L, *dis* + Fr, *aise,* ease], a genetic disorder caused by mutations in the FGFR2 gene, characterized by a malformed skull; various ocular disorders, including exophthalmos, strabismus, and optic atrophy; a beaked nose; and an underdeveloped upper jaw. In addition, individuals with Crouzon syndrome may have dental problems and hearing loss. Cleft lip and palate are sometimes present.

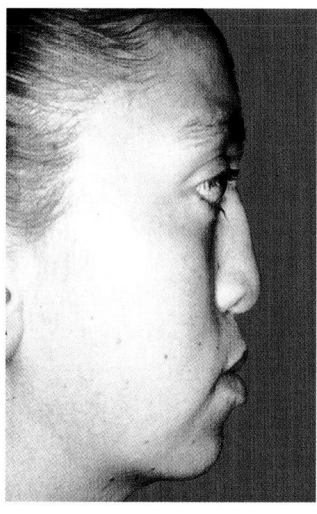

Woman with Crouzon syndrome *(Carlson, 2009/Courtesy A.R. Burdi)*

crowding /kroud′ing/ [ME, *crowden*], (in dentistry) the condition in which the teeth are too close together and have abnormal positions, such as overlapping, displacement in various directions, or a twist in position. See **arch length, arch length deficiency, arch width.**

Crow-Fukase syndrome, a multisystem disorder strongly associated with plasma cell dyscrasia. See **POEMS syndrome.**

crowing inspiration. See **laryngismus stridulus.**

crown [L, *corona*], **1.** the upper part of an organ or structure, such as the top of the head. **2.** the portion of a human tooth that is covered by enamel.

crown-heel length [L, *corona* + AS, *hela, lengthu*], the length of an embryo, fetus, or newborn as measured from the crown of the head to the heel. It is compared to the standing height of an older individual.

crowning [L, *corona*], (in obstetrics) time at the end of labor in which the fetal head is seen at the introitus of the vagina and "retracts" less and less with each subsequent contraction until birth.

crown/root ratio. See **clinical-crown/clinical-root ratio.**

crown-rump length, the length of an embryo, fetus, or newborn as measured from the crown of the head to the prominence of the buttocks.

CRP, abbreviation for **C-reactive protein.** See **C-reactive protein (CRP) test.**

CRRN, abbreviation for *certified rehabilitation registered nurse.*

CRST syndrome. See **CREST syndrome.**

CRT, 1. abbreviation for **cadaveric renal transplant. 2.** abbreviation for **cathode ray tube. 3.** abbreviation for **certified respiratory therapist.**

crucial /kroo′shəl/ [L. *crucialis*], most important; having an urgent priority.

cruciate /kroo′shē·āt/ [L, *crux*, cross], shaped like a cross.

cruciate anastomosis /kroo″shē·āt/ [L, *crux*, cross; Gk, *anastomoein*, to provide a mouth], an anastomosis in the upper part of the thigh, formed between the first perforating branch of the profunda femoris artery, the inferior gluteal artery, and the lateral and medial femoral circumflex arteries.

cruciate ligament of the atlas [L, *crux*, cross, *ligare*, to bind], a crosslike ligament attaching the atlas to the base of the occipital bone above and the posterior surface of the body of the axis below.

crucible /kroo″səbəl/, a cone-shaped vessel made of a refractory material, used in chemistry to melt or calcine materials at temperatures too high for other laboratory equipment to tolerate.

cruciform /kroo″sifôrm/ [L, *crux*, cross], in the shape of a cross.

cruciform ligament, any cross-shaped band of white fibrous tissue connecting bones and forming a joint capsule. Examples are the anterior and posterior cruciate ligaments of the knee and the cruciate ligament of the atlas.

crude birth rate [L, *crudus*, raw; ME, *burth* + L, *reri*, to reckon], the number of births per 1000 people in a population during 1 year. Compare **birth rate, refined birth rate, true birth rate.**

crude herb, a raw plant before it is processed or dried.

cruor /kroo″ôr/ [L, blood], a blood clot containing erythrocytes.

crur-, prefix meaning "leg" or "thigh": *crura, crural, crureus.*

crura. See **crus.**

crural /kroo″rəl/, pertaining to the leg between the knee and ankle.

crural hernia [L, *crus,* leg, *hernia,* rupture], **1.** a hernia that protrudes behind the posterior layer of the femoral sheath. Also called **Cloquet's hernia. 2.** a common type of groin hernia that occurs most often in obese females.

crural ligament. See **inguinal ligament.**

crura of anthelix, the two ridges on the external ear marking the superior termination of the anthelix and bounding the triangular fossa.

crureus. See **vastus intermedius.**

crus /krus/ *pl. crura* [L, leg], **1.** the leg from knee to foot. **2.** a structure resembling a leg, such as the crura of anthelix.

crus cerebri /ser″əbrī, -brē/ [L, *crus* + *cerebrum,* brain], either of the two cerebral peduncles, composed of the descending fiber tracts passing from the cerebral cortex to form the longitudinal fascicles of the pons. Also called **basis pedunculi cerebri.**

crushing wound /krush″ing/ [ME, *crushen* + AS, *wund*], a break in the external surface of the body caused by a severe force applied against the tissues. The body structures may be crushed without signs of external bleeding. An example is having the tip of the finger crushed in a door when it is suddenly closed. Also called *crush injury.*

crush syndrome [ME, *crushen*], a severe, life-threatening condition caused by extensive crushing trauma, characterized by destruction of muscle and bone tissue, hemorrhage, and fluid loss resulting in hypovolemic shock, hematuria, renal failure, and coma. Massive supportive therapy, including fluids, electrolytes, antibiotics, analgesia, oxygen, and intensive care with close monitoring of all vital functions, is usually necessary.

crust [L, *crusta,* shell], a solidified, hard outer layer formed by the drying of a body exudate, such as blood or pus, common in dermatological conditions such as eczema, impetigo, seborrhea, and favus and during the healing of burns and lesions; a scab. Also called *crusta.*

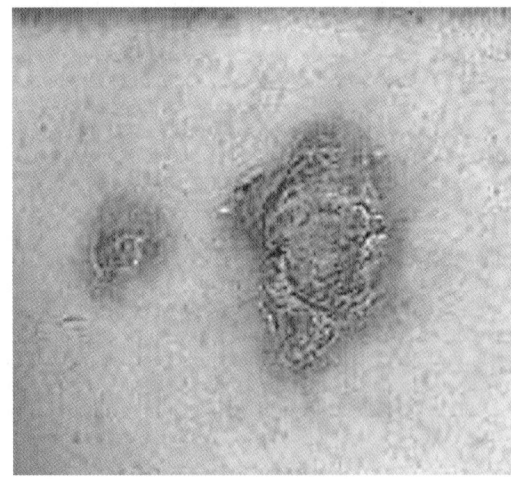

Crust (du Vivier, 1993)

crutch [AS, *cryce*], a wooden or metal staff that aids a person in walking. The most common kind of crutch is the axillary crutch, which reaches from the ground almost to the axilla. It has a padded, curved surface at the top that fits under the arm and a crossbar that is held in the hand at the level of the palms to support the body. It is important that the crutches be properly fitted and that the person be taught how to use them safely and how to achieve a stable and acceptable gait. See also **Canadian crutch.**

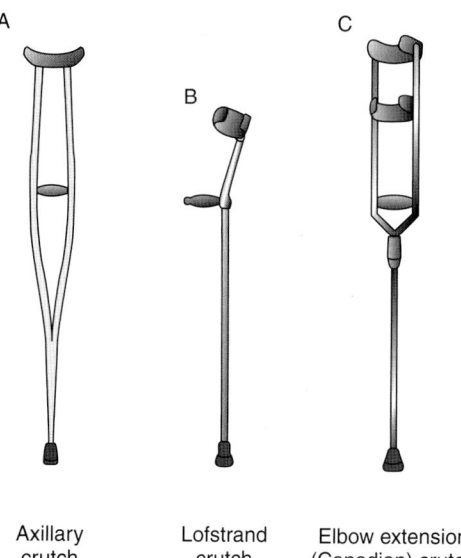

Types of crutches *(Mosby, 2003)*

Crutchfield tongs [William G. Crutchfield, American neurosurgeon, 1900–1972; ME, *tonges*], an instrument that is attached to the skull to hyperextend the head and neck of patients with fractured cervical vertebrae for the purpose of immobilizing and aligning the vertebrae.
■ METHOD: The tips of the tongs are inserted into small burr holes drilled in each parietal region of the skull; the surrounding skin is sutured and covered with a collodion dressing. A rope tied to the center of the tongs passes over a pulley at the head of the bed and is attached to a weight of 10 to 20 pounds, which hangs freely.
■ OUTCOME CRITERIA: A patient may be immobilized by Crutchfield tongs before surgery is performed. During an operation on the cervical spine and spinal cord, the tongs may be left in place for proper alignment.

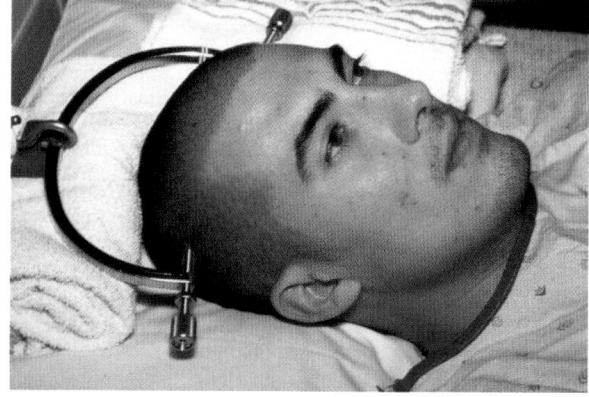

Crutchfield tongs *(Christensen and Kockrow, 2010)*

crutch gait, a gait achieved by a person using crutches. The gait selected and learned is determined by the physical and functional abilities of the patient and the diagnosis. In a two-point gait, the patient uses each crutch with the opposing leg. In a three-point gait, weight is borne on the noninvolved leg, then on both crutches, and then on the noninvolved leg again.

Weight-bearing on the involved leg initially is partial or prevented. A four-point gait gives stability but requires bearing weight on both legs. Each leg is used alternately with each crutch. The swing-to and swing-through gaits are often used by paraplegic patients with weight-supporting braces on the legs. Weight is borne on the supported legs. The crutches are placed one stride in front of the person, who then swings to that point or through the crutches to a spot in front of them.

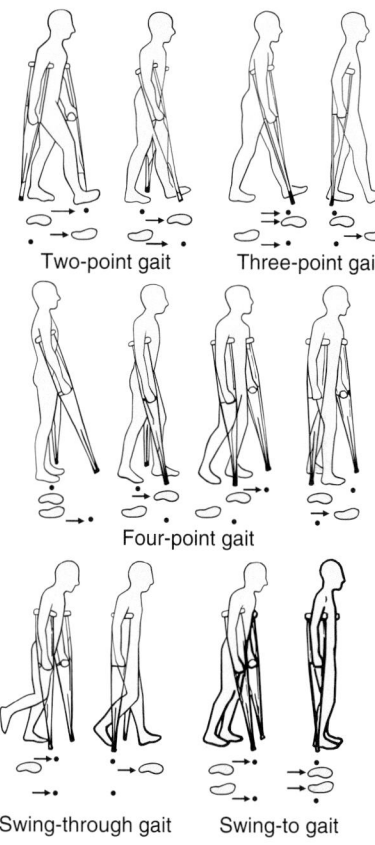

Two-point gait   Three-point gait

Four-point gait

Swing-through gait   Swing-to gait

Crutch gaits

crutch palsy, the temporary or permanent loss of sensation or muscle control resulting from pressure on the radial nerve by a crutch. The radial nerve passes under the axillary area superficially. Pressure, often caused by mismatching of the height of the patient and the crutch, can lead to paralysis of the elbow and wrist extensors.
Cruveilhier-Baumgarten syndrome /krYvāyā″boum″gä rtən/ [Jean Cruveilhier, French pathologist, 1791–1874; Paul Baumgarten, German pathologist, 1848–1928], recanalization of the paraumbilical veins with cirrhosis of the liver, portal hypertension, and splenomegaly.
crux /kruks, krŏŏks/ [L], **1.** formed by two lines, one vertical and the other horizontal. **2.** a difficult problem. **3.** a vital, basic, or decisive point.
Cruz trypanosomiasis. See **Chagas' disease.**
cry [OFr, *crier*], **1.** a sudden, loud, voluntary or automatic vocalization in response to pain, fear, or a startle reflex. **2.** weeping (the flowing of tears), as a reaction to pain or joy or as an emotional response to depression or grief. **3.** See **cat-cry syndrome.**
crying vital capacity (CVC), a measurement of the tidal volume while an infant is crying. The CVC may be valuable

in monitoring infants with lung diseases that cause changes in functional residual capacity.

cryo-, cry-, crymo-,   prefix meaning "cold": *cryocautery, cryonics, cryosurgery.*

cryoanesthesia /krī′ō·an′isthē″zhə/   [Gk, *kryos,* cold, *aisthesis,* feeling],   local anesthesia produced by applying a tourniquet and chilling an area to near-freezing temperature. It is used to diminish neural sensitivity to pain during brief minor surgical procedures.

cryocautery /krī′ōkô″tərē/   [Gk, *kryos + kauterion,* branding iron],   the application of any substance, such as solid carbon dioxide, that destroys tissue by freezing. Also called **cold cautery.**

cryogen /krī″əjən/   [Gk, *kryos + genein,* to produce],   **1.** a chemical that induces freezing, used to destroy diseased tissue without injury to adjacent structures. Cell death is caused by dehydration after cell membranes rupture. **2.** (in magnetic resonance imaging) a chemical used to cool the MRI electromagnet so that the magnet remains superconducting and higher magnified strengths can be achieved. Kinds include **carbon dioxide, liquid nitrogen,** *liquid helium,* **nitrous oxide.** *–cryogenic, adj.*

cryoglobulin /krī′ōglob″yoōlin/   [Gk, *kryos + L, globulus,* small sphere],   an abnormal plasma protein that precipitates and coalesces at low temperatures and dissolves and disperses at body temperature.

cryoglobulinemia /krī′ōglob′yoōlinē″mē·ə/   [Gk, *kryos + L, globulus,* small sphere; Gk, *haima,* blood],   the presence of cryoglobulins in the blood. Presence of cryoglobulins may be associated with a variety of clinical disorders including Waldenström's macroglobulinemia, hepatitis C, multiple myeloma, and leukemia.

cryoglobulin test,   a blood test to assess the presence of cryoglobulin, which is associated with lymphoid malignancies, connective tissue disease, acute and chronic infections, and liver disease.

cryonics /krī·on″iks/   [Gk, *kryos,* cold],   the techniques in which cold is applied for a variety of therapeutic goals, including brief local anesthesia, destruction of superficial skin lesions, and preservation of cells, tissue, organs, or the entire body. *–cryonic, adj.*

cryoprecipitate /-prisip″itāt/,   **1.** any precipitate formed on cooling of a solution. **2.** a preparation rich in factor VIII needed to restore normal coagulation in hemophilia. It is collected from fresh human plasma that has been frozen and thawed.

cryopreservation /krī′ōpres′ərvā″shən/,   a method of preserving tissues and organs in a viable state at extremely low temperatures.

cryostat /krī″ōstat/   [Gk, *kryos + statos,* standing],   a device used in surgical treatment of pathological disorders that consists of a special microtome used for freezing and slicing sections of tissue for study by a surgical pathologist. See also **microtome.**

cryosurgery /-sur″jərē/   [Gk, *kryos + cheirourgos*],   use of subfreezing temperature to destroy tissue. Cryosurgery is performed in the destruction of the ganglion of nerve cells in the thalamus in the treatment of Parkinson's disease, in the destruction of the pituitary gland to halt the progress of some kinds of metastatic cancer, and in the treatment of various cancers and lesions of the skin. The process is also used in ophthalmology to cause the edges of a detached retina to heal and to remove cataracts. The coolant is circulated through a metal probe, chilling it to as low as −160° C (−256° F), depending on the chemical used. The moist tissues adhere to the cold metal of the probe and freeze. Cells are dehydrated

as their membranes burst; eventually they are discarded or absorbed by the body.

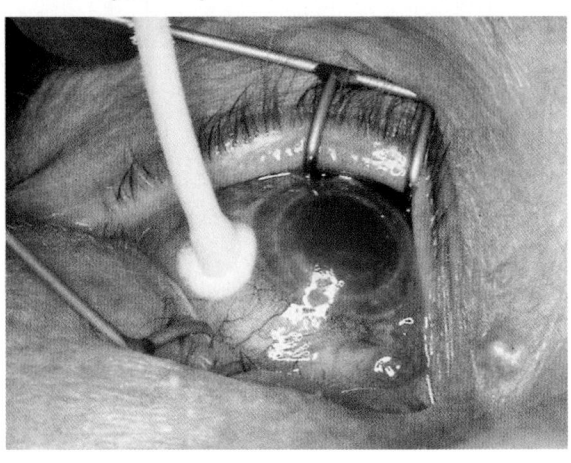

Cryosurgery (Jaffe, 1996)

cryotherapy /krī′ōther″əpē/   [Gk, *kryos + therapeia*],   a treatment using cold as a destructive medium. Cutaneous tags, warts, condyloma acuminatum, and actinic keratosis are some of the common skin disorders responsive to cryotherapy. Solid carbon dioxide or liquid nitrogen is applied briefly with a sterile cotton-tipped applicator or cryospray instrument. Blistering, followed by necrosis, results. The procedure may be repeated.

crypt /kript/   [Gk, *kryptos,* hidden],   a blind pit or tube on a free surface. Kinds include **anal crypt, dental crypt, synovial crypt.**

crypt-.   See **crypto-, crypt-, krypto-.**

cryptic /krip″tik/   [Gk, *kryptos,* hidden],   pertaining to something concealed or hidden.

crypto-, crypt-, krypto-,   combining form meaning "hidden": *cryptocephalus, cryptodidymus, cryptogenic.*

cryptocephalus /krip′tōsef″ələs/   [Gk, *kryptos + kephale,* head],   a malformed fetus that has a small, underdeveloped head. *–cryptocephalic, cryptocephalous, adj., –cryptocephaly, n.*

cryptococcosis /krip′tōkokō″sis/,   an infectious disease caused by the fungus *Cryptococcus neoformans,* which, after inhalation, spreads from the lungs to the brain and central nervous system, skin, skeletal system, and urinary tract. The disease occurs in all parts of the world, but 85% of the cases occur in North America, where it is most likely to afflict persons with immunodeficiencies such as human immunodeficiency virus (HIV) and middle-aged men in the southeastern United States. It is especially associated with breathing dust from pigeon droppings. Also called **Busse-Buschke disease, European blastomycosis, torulosis.** See also *Cryptococcus.*

■ OBSERVATIONS: It is characterized by the development of nodules or tumors filled with a gelatinous material in visceral and subcutaneous tissues. Initial symptoms may include coughing or other respiratory effects because the lungs are a primary site of infection. After the fungus spreads to the meninges, neurological symptoms, including headache, blurred vision, and difficulty in speaking, may develop. The diagnosis is made by isolation and identification of the fungus in sputum, pus, or tissue biopsy specimens.

■ INTERVENTIONS: Amphotericin B and fluconazole may be administered to control the infection. In patients with HIV, maintenance therapy with fluconazole may be indicated, but it does not affect survival and is not considered cost-effective.

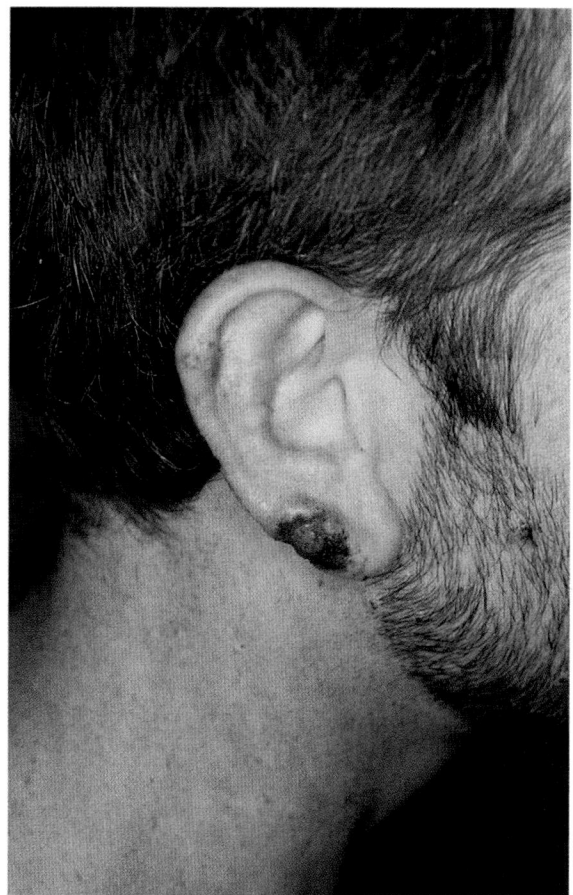

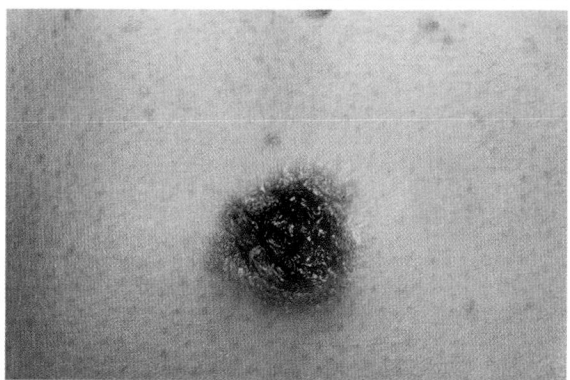

Cryptococcosis *(Callen, 1993)*

Cryptococcus /-kok″əs/, a genus of encapsulated yeasts that reproduce by budding rather than by producing spores. Many nonpathogenic species of *Cryptococcus* are commonly found in the soil and on the skin and mucous membranes of people who are well. Certain pathogenic species exist. *C. neoformans* is the most important. See also **fungus, yeast.**

Cryptococcus neoformans, a species of encapsulated yeasts that causes cryptococcosis, a potentially fatal infection that can affect the lungs, skin, and brain.

cryptodidymus /krip′tōdid″əməs/ [Gk, *kryptos + didymos,* twin], conjoined twins, one of which is a small, underdeveloped fetus concealed within the body of the other, more fully formed autosite.

crypt of iris, any one of the small pits in the iris along its free margin encircled by the circulus arteriosus minor. Also called *crypt of Fuchs.*

crypt of Lieberkühn, gland in the intestinal mucous membrane. See **Lieberkühn's glands.**

cryptogenic /-jen″ik/ [Gk, *kryptos,* hidden, *genein,* to produce], **1.** *adj.,* pertaining to a disease of unknown cause. **2.** *n.,* a parasitic organism living within another organism.

cryptogenic infection, a disease caused by pathogenic microorganisms of obscure or unknown origin.

cryptogenic septicemia, a systemic infection in which pathogens are present in the bloodstream but no primary focus of infection can be identified.

cryptomenorrhea /krip′tōmenôrē″ə/ [Gk, *kryptos* + L, *mens,* month; Gk, *rhoia,* flow], an abnormal condition in which the products of menstruation are retained within the vagina because of an imperforate hymen or, less often, within the uterus because of an occlusion of the cervical canal. Cryptomenorrhea is usually accompanied by subjective symptoms of menstruation with scant or absent flow and sometimes by severe pain. If the flow is completely obstructed, uterotubal reflux of menstrual flow into the pelvic cavity may cause peritonitis, pain, adhesions, and endometriosis. −*cryptomenorrheal, adj.*

cryptophthalmos /krip′təfthal″məs/ [Gk, *kryptos + ophthalmos,* eye], a rare congenital anomaly of the eye characterized by skin passing continuously from the forehead to the cheek over a malformed eye. It may be isolated but more commonly is seen as a part of Fraser's syndrome. Cryptophthalmos is classified into three types: complete, incomplete, and abortive. Treatment is by surgical reconstruction.

cryptophthalmos syndrome. See **Fraser syndrome.**

cryptorchidism /kriptôr″kidiz′əm/ [Gk, *kryptos,* hidden, *orchis,* testis], a developmental defect in which one or both testicles fail to descend into the scrotum and are retained in the abdomen or inguinal canal. The testes normally migrate into the scrotal sac at birth, but normal testicular descent depends on timely and synchronous development of other embryonic structures. Infants with undescended testicles diagnosed after 6 months of age should be referred to a specialist for evaluation. Also called *cryptorchid testis,* **undescended testis,** *cryptorchis.*

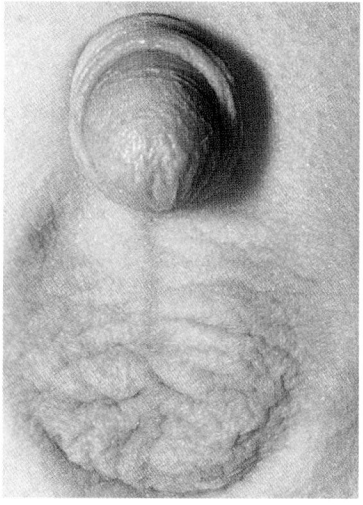

Cryptorchidism *(Courtesy Dr. Ellen Wald, Children's Hospital of Pittsburgh)*

cryptosporidiosis, an opportunistic infection caused by the intestinal parasites *Cryptosporidium parvum,* a very common parasite in animals, and *C. hominis.* The disease was relatively unknown as a human pathogen before a 1993 epidemic in the Milwaukee, Wisconsin, area, where 400,000 persons were stricken with diarrhea after drinking water contaminated with the parasite. Other sources of infection include raw or undercooked foods contaminated with *Cryptosporidium* oocysts, direct contact with infected humans or animals, and contact with recreational water. Symptoms of watery diarrhea, abdominal cramps, nausea, vomiting, and low-grade fever may appear 2 to 10 days after infection. They may lead to dehydration and weight loss. The symptoms may last 1 or 2 weeks and may be life-threatening to persons with suppressed immune systems. Treatment emphasizes rest, replenishment of body fluids and electrolytes, and medications to control diarrhea. Paromomycin may be partially effective in the treatment of cryptosporidiosis in persons with HIV infection. There is no known safe and effective cure for cryptosporidiosis. The drug nitzoxanide has been approved for the treatment of diarrhea caused by cryptosporidiosis, but it should be used only in patients with healthy immune systems. Fecal material from patients suffering from crytosporidiosis is infectious and should be handled accordingly. Care should be taken to avoid infection of immunocompromised patients by means of contact with symptomatic patients in a hospital environment.

cry reflex, a normal infantile reaction to pain, hunger, or need for attention. The reflex may be absent in an infant born prematurely or in poor health.

crystal /kris″təl/ [Gk, *krystallos*], a solid substance, either organic or inorganic, the atoms or molecules of which are arranged in a regular, repeating three-dimensional pattern known as a unit cell, which determines the shape of a crystal. −**crystalline,** *adj.*

crystal gold. See **mat gold.**

crystalline, describing material with a regular geometric shape. Crystalline substances have a very narrow melting point range.

crystalline lens /kris″təlin, -līn/ [Gk, *krystallos* + L, lentil], a transparent structure of the eye that is enclosed in a capsule between the iris and the vitreous humor and is slightly overlapped at its margin by the ciliary processes. It refracts light to focus images on the retina. The capsule of the lens is a transparent elastic membrane that touches the free border of the iris anteriorly and is secured by the suspensory ligament of the lens. The circumference of the capsule recedes from the iris to form the posterior chamber of the eye. The lens is biconvex in structure, with the posterior surface more convex than the anterior, derived from surface ectoderm. It is composed of a soft cortical material, a firm nucleus, and concentric laminae and is covered anteriorly by transparent epithelium. In the fetus the lens is very soft and has a slightly reddish tint; in the adult it is colorless and firm; in old age it becomes flattened, more dense, slightly opaque, and amber-tinted. See also **eye.**

crystallization /kris″təlīzā″shən/ [Gk, *krystallos,* rock crystal], *v.,* the production of crystals, either by cooling a liquid or gas to a solid state or by cooling a solution until the solute precipitates as a crystalline deposit; crystals can also be produced by evaporation of a liquid from a solution or slow vapor diffusion techniques.

crystalloid /kris″təloid/ [Gk, *krystallos* + *eidos,* form], a substance in a solution that can diffuse through a semipermeable membrane. Compare **colloid.**

crystalluria /kris″təloor″ē-ə/, the presence of crystals in the urine. The condition may be caused by metabolic disorders, inherited diseases, or medications.

Crystodigin, a cardiac glycoside. Brand name for **digitoxin.**

Cs, symbol for the element **cesium.**

CS, abbreviation for **cesarean section.**

c-section. (*Informal*) See **cesarean section.**

CSF, 1. abbreviation for **cerebrospinal fluid.** 2. abbreviation for **colony-stimulating factor.**

C-spine, abbreviation for **cervical spine.**

CSR, abbreviation for **Cheyne-Stokes respiration.**

c-src, a tyrosine kinase that participates in signal transduction pathways that regulate growth of cells. It hybridizes with oncogenes of the highly virulent Rous sarcoma virus. The human c-src gene is located at 20g12-13 on the long arm of chromosome 20.

CST, 1. abbreviation for **contractions stress test.** 2. abbreviation for **Certified Surgical Technologist.**

CT, abbreviation for **computed tomography.**

CT number. See **Hounsfield unit.**

CTX, abbreviation for **clinical trial exemption.**

Cu, symbol for the element **copper.**

CUA, abbreviation for **cost-utility analysis.**

Cuban itch, a mild form of smallpox. See also **alastrim.**

cubic centimeter (cc, cu cm, cm³) [Gk, *kybos* + L, *centum,* hundred; Gk, *metron,* measure], a theoretical cube or its equivalent, each edge of which is 1 centimeter long. One cubic centimeter is equivalent to 1 milliliter.

Cubicin, brand name for **daptomycin.**

cubic millimeter (cu mm, mm³), a unit of volume equal to 1 millionth of a liter. One cubic millimeter is equivalent to 1 microliter.

cubital /kyoo″bitəl/, pertaining to the elbow.

cubital fossa, a depression in the front of the elbow, immediately lateral to the tendon of the biceps brachii muscle.

cubitus /kyoo″bitəs/, 1. the elbow. 2. the forearm.

cuboidal epithelium /kyoōboi″dəl/ [Gk, *kybos,* cube, *eidos,* form, *epi,* above, *thele,* nipple], simple epithelial cells that are generally cube shaped and one layer thick. Stratified cuboidal cells are found in the mammary glands, the salivary glands, and in some sweat glands.

cuboid bone /kyoo″boid/ [Gk, *kybos,* cube, *eidos,* form], the outer cuboidal tarsal bone on the lateral side of the foot, proximal to the fourth and fifth metatarsal bones. It articulates with the calcaneus, lateral cuneiform, and fourth and fifth metatarsal bones and occasionally with the navicular. Also called **os cuboideum.**

cuboidodigital reflex. See **Mendel's reflex.**

cu cm, abbreviation for **cubic centimeter.**

cue /kyoo/, a stimulus that determines or may prompt the nature of a person's response.

cuff, (*Informal*) an inflatable elastic tube that is placed around a limb and inflated with air to restrict arterial circulation during blood pressure examination. See also **cuffed endotracheal tube, Dacron cuff.**

cuffed endotracheal tube, an endotracheal tube with a balloon at one end that may be inflated to tighten the fit in the lumen of the airway. The balloon forms a cuff that prevents gastric contents from passing into the lungs and gas from leaking back from the lungs. Both high-pressure and low-pressure cuffs are used. Overinflation of the cuff can cause contusion, hemorrhage, mucosal sloughing, or stenosis.

cuffing, a pathological condition in which cufflike borders of leukocytes form around small blood vessels, as in certain infections.

cuirass /kwiras″/ [Fr, *cuirasse*, breastplate], **1.** a negative-pressure full-body respirator. It consists of a rigid shell that conforms to the surfaces of the body from the neck to the hips. Ventilating pressure is delivered through a flexible hose attached to the top of the device. An electrically driven pump is adjusted to match the timing of the patient's spontaneous breathing. Also called *cuirass ventilator.* **2.** a tightly fitted chest bandage.

cul-de-sac /kul″dəsak, kYdesok″/ *pl. culs-de-sac, cul-de-sacs* [Fr, bottom of the bag], a blind pouch or cecum, such as the conjunctival cul-de-sac and the dural cul-de-sac.

cul-de-sac of Douglas [James Douglas, Scottish anatomist, 1675–1742], a pouch formed by the caudal portion of the parietal peritoneum. Also called **pouch of Douglas, rectouterine excavation, rectouterine pouch.**

culdocentesis /kul″dōsentē″sis/, the use of needle puncture or incision through the vagina to remove intraperitoneal fluid, including purulent material.

culdoplasty /kul″dōplas′tē/ [Fr, *cul-de-sac,* bottom of the bag; Gk, *plassein,* to mold], plastic surgery to correct a defect in the posterior fornix of the vagina.

culdoscope /kul″dəskōp′/, an endoscope with an attached light that can be inserted through the posterior wall of the vagina for examination of the pelvic viscera.

culdotomy /kuldot″əmē/, incision or needle puncture of cul-de-sac of Douglas by way of the vagina.

Culex /koo″leks/, a genus of humpbacked mosquitoes (Culicidae). It includes species that transmit viral encephalitis and filariasis. *Culex pipiens* is the most widely distributed mosquito globally.

Cullen sign [Thomas S. Cullen, American gynecologist, 1868–1953], the appearance of faint, irregularly formed hemorrhagic patches on the skin around the umbilicus. The discolored skin is usually blue-black and becomes greenish brown or yellow. A Cullen sign may appear 1 to 2 days after the onset of anorexia and the severe, poorly localized abdominal pains that are characteristic of acute hemorrhagic pancreatitis. It is also present in massive upper GI hemorrhage and ruptured ectopic pregnancy. Compare **Grey Turner sign.** See also **pancreatitis.**

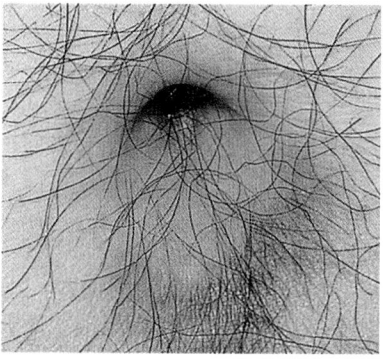

Cullen sign *(Greig and Garden, 1996)*

Culp-De Weerd pyeloplasty, pyeloplasty in which a spiral flap is turned down and incorporated into the adjacent ureter.

cult, a specific complex of beliefs, rites, and ceremonies associated with some particular person or object, which is maintained by a social group. A cult is often considered as having magical significance. Cults can be closed and exclusive to members only, secretive and protective of their beliefs. Cults indoctrinate their members in ways of being and doing.

cultural assimilation /kul″chərəl/, a process by which members of a minority group lose cultural characteristics that distinguish them from the dominant cultural group or take on the cultural characteristics of another group.

cultural event, a unique interaction of values, beliefs, ways, and mannerisms, celebrated and shared.

cultural healer, a member of an ethnic or cultural group who uses traditional methods of healing rather than conventional scientific methods to provide health care for other members of the group or members of another ethnic minority group.

culturally relativistic perspective, an ability to understand the behavior of transcultural patients (those who move from one culture to another) within the context of their own culture. See also **transcultural nursing.**

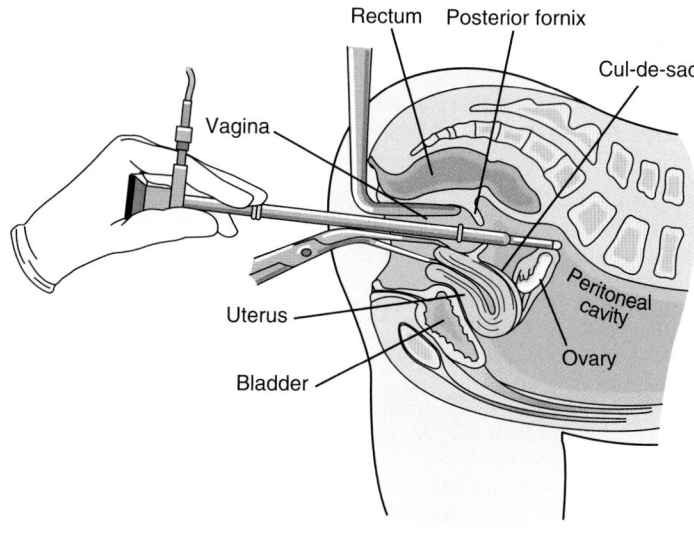

Culdoscope *(Phipps et al, 2003)*

cultural relativism, a belief that one's cultural norms, values, ethics, beliefs, and actions are influenced by that person's cultural background and cultural identity.

culture /kul′chər/ [L, *colere,* to cultivate], **1.** (in microbiology) a laboratory test involving the cultivation of microorganisms or cells in a special growth medium. See also **medium. 2.** (in psychology) a set of learned values, beliefs, customs, and behavior that is shared by a group of interacting individuals. **3.** in the humanities and social sciences, the beliefs of individuals in a group that contribute to their sense of identity, acceptance, and belonging.

culture-bound, (in anthropology) a term that connects the interpretation of an event to the beliefs of a particular culture. In health, examples of culture-bound conditions include diseases that are believed to be related to the "evil eye," illnesses that are attributed to spirits, or beliefs that prayer is necessary for healing.

culture medium. See **medium.**

culture procedure, (in bacteriology) any of several techniques for growing colonies of microorganisms to identify a pathogen and to determine its sensitivity to various antibiotics. Usually a specimen is secured by using sterile technique and a small amount is placed into or on one or more culture media, because different organisms are nourished by different nutrients and grow best at different specific pH levels. The environment in which the media are held during observation is maintained at body temperature, and the ambient oxygen level is adjusted to achieve an aerobic or anaerobic state. All procedures are aseptic, and all equipment is sterile to prevent accidental contamination of the media. As colonies appear in or on the media, small amounts of each (there are often several) are spread onto other media to allow examination of a pure specimen of the microorganisms.

culture shock, the psychological effect of a drastic change in the cultural environment of an individual. The person may exhibit feelings of helplessness, discomfort, and disorientation in attempting to adapt to a different cultural group with dissimilar practices, values, and beliefs.

cum /ko͞om/ [L], together with.

cu mm, abbreviation for **cubic millimeter.**

cumulative /kyo͞o′myəlā′tiv/ [L, *cumulare,* to pile on], increasing by incremental steps with an eventual total that may exceed the expected result.

cumulative action, 1. the increased activity of a therapeutic measure or agent when administered repeatedly, as the cumulative action of a regular exercise program. **2.** the increased activity demonstrated by a drug when repeated doses accumulate in the body and exert a greater biological effect than the initial dose.

cumulative dose, the total dose that accumulates as a result of repeated exposure to radiation or a radiopharmaceutical product.

cumulative gene. See **polygene.**

cumulus /kyo͞o′myo͞o·ləs/ *pl. cumuli* [L], a little mound, usually formed by a collection of cells.

cune-, prefix meaning "wedge": *cuneate, cuneiform, cuneus.*

cuneate /kyo͞o′nē·āt/ [L, *cuneus,* wedge], (of tissue) wedge shaped, especially in relation to cells of the nervous system.

cuneiform /kyo͞onē′əfôrm′/ [L, *cuneus,* wedge, *forma*], **1.** *adj.,* (of bone and cartilage) wedge shaped. **2.** *n.,* bone of the foot between the navicular and metatarsals.

cuneiform bone, one of the three small tarsal bones of the foot. Also called **triangular bone.**

cuneiform cartilage [L, *cuneus,* wedge, *forma + cartilago*], one of two small pieces of yellow, elongated, elastic, laryngeal cartilage at the edge of the aryepiglottic fold, above and anterior to the corniculate cartilage.

-cuneo, cuneo-, combining form meaning "wedge-shaped structures": *cuneiform bone.*

cuneus /kyo͞o′nē·əs/, a wedge-shaped region of the cerebral cortex lying between the parietooccipital and postcalcarine sulci on the mesial surface of the occipital lobe.

cunnilingus /kun′əling′gəs/, the oral stimulation of the female genitalia.

cup arthroplasty of the hip joint [L, *cupa,* cask; Gk, *arthron,* joint, *plassein,* to mold], the surgical replacement of the head of the femur by a metal or plastic mold to relieve pain and increase motion in arthritis or to correct a deformity. The damaged or diseased bone is removed, and the acetabulum and the head of the femur are reshaped. A cup is inserted between the two and becomes the articulating surface of the femur. After surgery the patient's legs are placed between an abduction pillow to hold them in a position of abduction extension and internal rotation to keep the cup in place in the acetabulum. Continued abduction may be necessary for 6 weeks. Possible complications include infection, thrombophlebitis, pulmonary embolism, and fat embolism. The patient receives extensive physical therapy. A walker or crutches are necessary to prevent full weight-bearing for 6 months, and an exercise program must be followed for several years. Compare **hip replacement.** See also **arthroplasty, knee replacement, osteoarthritis, plastic surgery.**

cup/disc ratio, (in ophthalmology) the mathematic relationship between the horizontal or vertical diameter of the optic nerve cup and the diameter of the optic disc.

cupola. See **cupula.**

cupping, 1. (in respiratory care) See **clapping. 2.** (in complementary medicine) a counterirritant technique from Eastern medicine of applying a suction device to the skin to draw blood to the surface of the body.

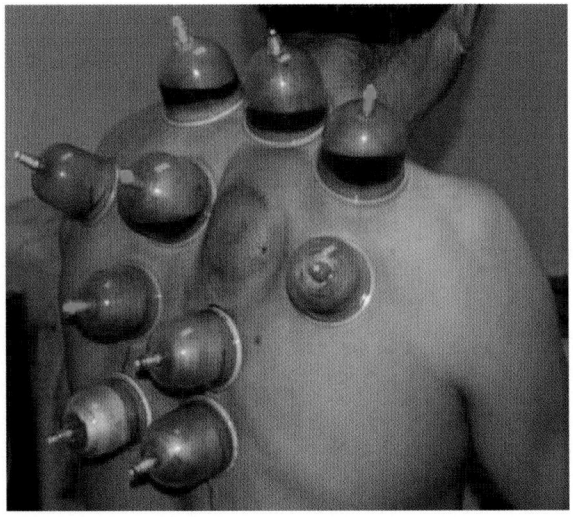

Cupping *(Yao et al, 2016)*

cupric /kyōō″prik/ [L, *cuprum,* copper], pertaining to copper in its divalent form, as cupric sulfate. Also called *copper (II),* as in copper (II) sulfate.

cupric sulfate, a crystalline salt of copper used as an emetic, astringent, and fungicide, as an oral antidote to phosphorus poisoning, as a topical treatment of cutaneous phosphorus burns, and as a catalyst in iron-deficiency anemia.

Cuprimine, a chelating agent used in the treatment of poisoning by heavy metals. Brand name for *D-penicillamine.*

cupula /kyōō″pələ/, any cup- or dome-shaped structure, such as the top of a lymphatic nodule in the small intestine. Also spelled **cupola.**

cupular caecum of cochlear duct, the closed blind apical end of the cochlear duct.

cupulolithiasis /kyōō′pyōōlōlithī″əsis/ [L, *cupula,* little cup; Gk, *lithos,* stone], a severe, long-lasting vertigo brought on by movement of the head to certain positions. Among the many possible causes are otitis media, ear surgery, and injury to the inner ear. In addition to extreme dizziness, signs are nausea, vomiting, and ataxia. There is no treatment except avoidance of the offending head positions. See also **positional vertigo.**

curanderismo [Spanish, *curandero,* healer], combination of beliefs, traditions, and cultural practices used to support both mental and physical healing and well-being. See **Latin American medical practices.**

curare /kyōōrä″rē/ [S. Am. Indian, *ourari*], a substance derived from tropical plants of the genus *Strychnos.* It is a potent neuromuscular blocker that acts by preventing transmission of neural impulses across the myoneural junctions. A large dose can cause complete paralysis, but action is usually reversible with acetylcholinesterase inhibitors (cholinergic agonists). Pharmacological preparations of the substance are used as adjuncts to general anesthesia. The use of curare or other neuromuscular blocking agents requires respiratory and ventilatory assistance by a qualified anesthetist or anesthesiologist. Also called **tubocurarine chloride.**

curariform /kyōōrä″rifôrm′/ [*curare*+L, *forma*], **1.** chemically similar to curare. **2.** having the effect of curare.

curative treatment, interventions, therapies, and medications designed to eliminate or correct a disease or condition. See **treatment.**

cure /kyōōr/ [L, *cura*], **1.** restoration to health of a person afflicted with a disease or other disorder. **2.** the favorable outcome of the treatment of a disease or other disorder. **3.** *(Informal)* a course of therapy, a medication, a therapeutic measure, or another remedy used in treatment of a medical problem, as faith healing, fasting, rest cure, or work cure.

curet /kyōōret″/ [Fr, *curette,* scoop], **1.** *n.,* a surgical instrument shaped like a spoon or scoop for scraping and removing material or tissue from an organ, cavity, or surface. A curet may be blunt or sharp and is designed in a shape and size appropriate to its use. Also spelled *curette.* **2.** *v.,* to remove tissue or debris with such a device. Kinds include **Hartmann's curet.**

curettage /kyōōr″ətäzh′/ [Fr, *curette,* scoop], scraping of material from the wall of a cavity or other surface, performed to remove tumors or other abnormal tissue or to obtain tissue for microscopic examination. Curettage also refers to clearing unwanted material from fistulas and areas of chronic infection. It may be performed with a blunt or a sharp curet or by suction.

curie (Ci) /kyōōr″ē/ [Marie Skladowska Curie, Polish-born chemist and physicist, 1867–1934; Pierre Curie, French

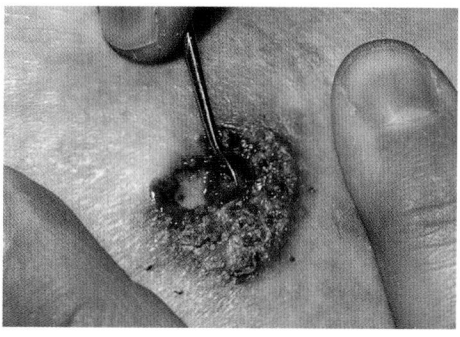

Curettage *(Habif, 1996)*

chemist and physicist, 1859–1906; both Nobel laureates], *(Obsolete)* the non-SI unit used to measure the intensity of radioactivity in a material; the term was used before adoption of the SI unit, becquerel (Bq). One curie is equal to 3.70×10^{10} Bq.

curing /kyōōr″ing/ [L, *curare,* to take care of or heal], (in dentistry) a method for promoting and accelerating hardening processes by using dampness, heat, cold, chemical agents, electromagnetic radiation, or other agents.

curium (Cm) /kyōō″rē·əm/ [Marie Skladowska Curie; Pierre Curie], a radioactive metallic element. Its atomic number is 96. Its atomic mass is 247. Curium is an artificial element produced by bombarding plutonium with helium ions in a cyclotron. Numerous isotopes of curium are produced by bombarding lighter transuranium elements. The radioactivity of curium causes it to glow in the dark.

-curium, suffix designating a neuromuscular blocking agent.

Curling ulcer [Thomas B. Curling, English surgeon, 1811–1888], a gastroduodenal ulcer that develops in people who have suffered severe stress, such as superficial burns, intracranial lesions, or severe bodily injury. Curling first diagnosed it in patients who had severe burns. The pathophysiological characteristics include hypotension from shock, which decreases the blood supply to gastric mucosa, which leads to ischemia. Also called *Curling stress ulcer.*

CURN®, a certification offered by the Certification Board for Urology Nurses and Associates. Abbreviation for *certified urological registered nurse.*

-curonium, suffix designating a neuromuscular blocking agent.

currant jelly clot /kur″ənt/ [ME, *corauns* + L, *gelare,* to congeal; AS, *clott*], a red, jellylike blood clot that is rich in hemoglobin from erythrocytes in the clot.

current /kur′ənt/ [L, *currere,* to run], **1.** a flowing or streaming movement. **2.** a flow of electrons along a conductor in a closed circuit; an electric current. **3.** certain physiological electrical activity and characteristics of blood circulation. Physiological currents include abnerval current, action current, axial current, centrifugal current, centripetal current, compensating current, demarcation current, and electrotonic current. See also **alternating current, direct current, volt, watt.**

-current, suffix meaning "running, flowing, happening": *countercurrent, recurrent.*

current of injury. See **demarcation current.**

Current Procedural Terminology, a system developed by the American Medical Association for standardizing the terminology and coding used to describe medical services and procedures. See also *CPT* **codes.**

C

current validity. See **validity.**

curriculum vitae (CV) /kərik″ələm wē″tī, -vē″tē/ *pl.* *curricula vitae* [L, *curriculum,* course, *vita,* life], a summary of educational and professional experiences, including activities and honors, to be used in applications for employment, for biographic citations on professional meeting programs, or for related purposes. Also called **resume, résumé.**

Curschmann's spiral /ko̅o̅rsh″monz/ [Heinrich Curschmann, German physician, 1846–1910; Gk, *speira,* coil], coiled fibrils of mucus occasionally found in the sputum of persons with bronchial asthma.

cursor /kur″sər/, a moving marker or pointer on a computer monitor that indicates a position.

curvature /kur″vəchər/, a bending or curving of a line from the course of a straight line.

curvature myopia, a type of nearsightedness caused by refractive errors associated with an excessive curvature of the cornea.

curve [L, *curvare,* to bend], (in statistics) a straight or curved line used as a graphic method of demonstrating the distribution of data collected in a study or survey.

curve of Carus [Karl G. Carus, German anatomist, 1789–1869], the normal axis of the pelvic outlet. Also called **circle of Carus.**

curve of occlusion, **1.** an imaginary curved surface that is described by the incisal and occlusal surfaces of the teeth. **2.** the curve of dentition on which lie the occlusal surfaces of the teeth. See also **reverse curve.**

curve of Spee /shpā, spē/ [Ferdinand Graf von Spee, German embryologist, 1855–1937], the anatomical curvature of the occlusal alignment of the teeth. It begins at the tip of the lower canine, follows the buccal cusps of the natural premolars and molars, and continues to the anterior border of the mandibular ramus. This compensation allows a smaller distance between the posterior teeth with an accompanying larger amount of opening of the anterior teeth. It is a useful landmark for arrangement of dental images or radiographs. Compare **compensating curve.**

curve of Wilson /wil″sən/ [Dr. George Wilson, American prosthodontist], the curvature of the cusps of the teeth as projected on the frontal plane. That of the mandibular dental arch is concave, and that of the maxillary dental arch is convex.

curvi-, prefix for terms relating to curvature: *curvilinear.*

curvilinear /cur″vilin″ē·ər/ [L, *curvus,* bent, *linea,* line], pertaining to a curved line.

curvilinear trend [L, *curvus,* bent, *linea,* line; AS, *trendan,* to turn], (in statistics) a trend in which a graphic representation of the data yields a curved line. The value of the independent variable may be expressed as a polynomial coefficient; by a more complete mathematic expression, such as a logistic curve; or by a smoothing process, such as a moving average.

Curvularia /ker″vular″eə/, a genus of imperfect fungi commonly found in soil and elsewhere. *C. lunata* is found in human mycetomas (chronic granulomatous disease).

cushingoid /ko̅o̅sh″ingoid/ [Harvey W. Cushing, American surgeon, 1869–1939; Gk, *eidos,* form], having the appearance and facial characteristic of Cushing disease: fat pads on the upper back and face, ruddy complexion, striae on trunk, thin legs, and excess facial hair.

Cushing disease /ko̅o̅sh″ing/ [Harvey W. Cushing, American neurosurgeon, 1869–1939], a metabolic disorder characterized by abnormally increased secretion of adrenocortical steroids, particularly cortisol, caused by increased amounts of adrenocorticotropic hormone

(ACTH) secreted by the pituitary, such as by a pituitary adenoma. Also called **hyperadrenalism.** Compare **Cushing syndrome.**

■ OBSERVATIONS: Excess adrenocortical hormones result in accumulations of fat on the abdomen, chest, upper back, and face and occurrence of edema, hyperglycemia, increased gluconeogenesis, muscle weakness, acne, purplish striae on the skin, decreased immunity to infection, osteoporosis with susceptibility to bone fractures, and facial hair growth in women. Diabetes mellitus may become a chronic condition.

■ INTERVENTIONS: Therapy is aimed at removal or destruction of ACTH-secreting tissue, most commonly by surgical or radiological procedures. The adrenal glands may be totally or subtotally removed and pharmacological preparations of adrenal steroids administered.

■ PATIENT CARE CONSIDERATIONS: Cushing disease affects many systems, and a team approach will assist the patient in coping with system changes. The chronic nature of the disease mandates education so that the patient is able to monitor symptoms and responses to medications. Changes in appearance and hormonal changes may affect the patient's emotional well-being. Assessment of the patient's level of activity and ability to carry out routine and self-care activities is important.

Cushing syndrome [Harvey W. Cushing], a metabolic disorder resulting from the chronic and excessive production of cortisol by the adrenal cortex or by the administration of glucocorticoids in large doses for several weeks or longer. When occurring spontaneously, the syndrome represents a failure in the body's ability to regulate the secretion of cortisol or adrenocorticotropic hormone (ACTH). (Normally cortisol is produced only in response to ACTH, and ACTH is not secreted in the presence of high levels of cortisol.) The most common cause of the syndrome is a pituitary tumor that increases secretion of ACTH. Also called **hyperadrenocorticism.** See also **Addison disease, Cushing disease, Nelson syndrome.**

■ OBSERVATIONS: Characteristically the patient with Cushing syndrome has a decreased glucose tolerance; central obesity; round "moon" face; supraclavicular fat pads; an overhanging, striae-covered pad of fat on the chest and abdomen; buffalo hump; scant menstrual periods or decreased testosterone levels; muscular atrophy; edema; hypokalemia; and some degree of emotional change. The skin may be abnormally pigmented and fragile; minor infections may become systemic and long-lasting. Children with the disorder may stop growing. Hypertension, kidney stones, and psychosis may also occur.

■ INTERVENTIONS: The objective of all treatment is decreased cortisol secretion. The source of the excess ACTH is discovered by a series of tests that challenge the function of the adrenal and pituitary glands. If the excess ACTH is caused by an adenoma of the anterior pituitary, irradiation or surgical excision of the tumor corrects the condition. If the condition is the result of medication, decreasing or changing the dosage may alleviate the symptoms.

■ PATIENT CARE CONSIDERATIONS: Care of the hospitalized patient with Cushing syndrome is similar to that of patients with Addison disease, Cushing disease, and other endocrinological disorders. Weight and electrolyte and fluid balance are monitored, an adequate balanced diet is urged, and emotional changes are observed with a goal of maintaining emotional equilibrium.

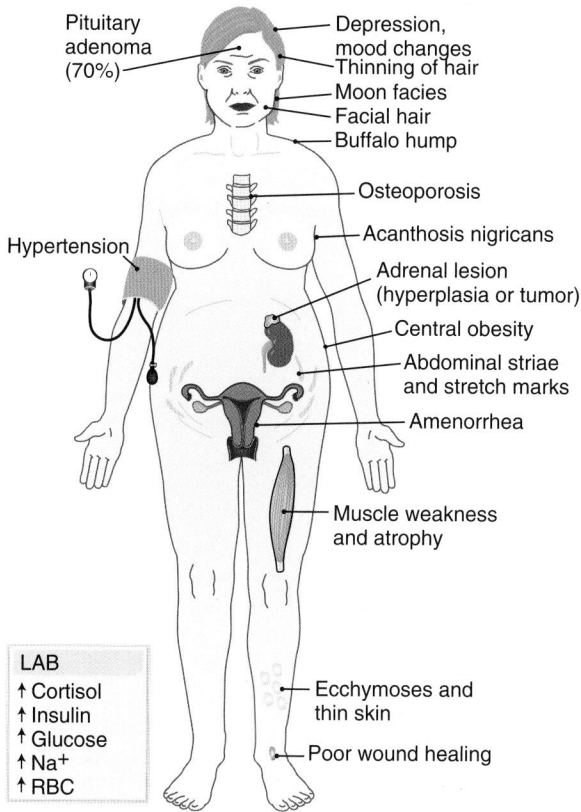

- Pituitary adenoma (70%)
- Depression, mood changes
- Thinning of hair
- Moon facies
- Facial hair
- Buffalo hump
- Osteoporosis
- Hypertension
- Acanthosis nigricans
- Adrenal lesion (hyperplasia or tumor)
- Central obesity
- Abdominal striae and stretch marks
- Amenorrhea
- Muscle weakness and atrophy
- Ecchymoses and thin skin
- Poor wound healing

LAB
↑ Cortisol
↑ Insulin
↑ Glucose
↑ Na⁺
↑ RBC

Cushing syndrome *(Damjanov, 2008)*

cushion [OFr, *coissin*], any anatomical structure that resembles a pad or pillow.

cusp [L, *cuspis,* point], **1.** a sharp projection or a rounded eminence that rises from the chewing surface of a tooth, such as the two pyramidal cusps that arise from the premolars. **2.** any one of the small flaps on the valves of the heart, as the ventral, dorsal, and medial cusps of the right atrioventricular valve.

cuspid /kus″pid/ [L, *cuspis,* point], a tooth with one cusp, or point; a canine tooth. Also called **unicuspid.**

cuspless tooth /kusp″les/, **1.** a tooth without cusps, or prominences, on its occlusal surface, possibly as a result of attrition. **2.** a posterior denture tooth that is purposefully manufactured without prominences to stabilize a denture during mastication.

custodial care /kəstō″dē·əl/ [L, *custodia,* guarding, *garrire,* to chatter], services and care of a nonmedical nature provided on a long-term basis, usually for convalescent and chronically ill individuals. Kinds include **board, personal assistance, board and care.**

customary and reasonable charge, (in the United States) a fee usually established by health insurance or government agencies that is considered to be the "usual" cost of a specific medical service. The fee is commonly based on the amount the company or agency will pay for that service and may vary with geographic area.

cut, a split in both strands of a DNA molecule. See also **nick.**

cut-, root/combining form meaning "skin": *subcutaneous, cuticle.*

cutaneous /kyo͞otā″nē·əs/ [L, *cutis,* skin], pertaining to the skin.

cutaneous absorption, the taking up of substances through the skin.

cutaneous anaphylaxis, a localized hypersensitivity reaction in the form of a wheal and flare. It occurs in sensitized individuals when, as a test of sensitivity to various allergens, an antigen is injected into the skin. See also **antiserum anaphylaxis.**

cutaneous anthrax, small blisters or ulcers on the skin after contact with anthrax spores. See **anthrax.**

cutaneous horn, a protruding keratotic growth of the skin, the base of which may show changes of actinic keratosis or carcinoma.

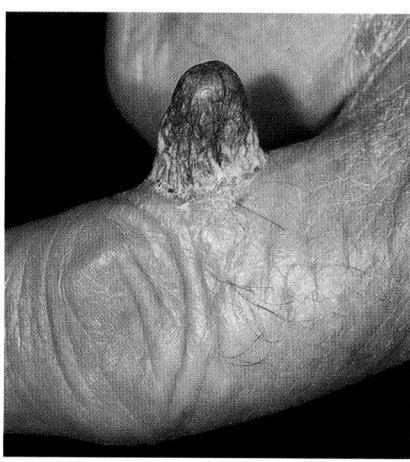

Cutaneous horn *(Habif, 2016)*

cutaneous immunofluorescence biopsy, a microscopic examination of skin tissue for evaluation and diagnosis of immunologically-mediated dermatitis.

cutaneous larva migrans, a skin condition caused by a hookworm, *Ancylostoma braziliense,* a parasite of cats and dogs. Its ova are deposited in the ground with the feces of infected animals, develop into larvae, and invade the skin of people, particularly bare feet, although any skin may be involved. The larvae rarely develop into adult hookworms in the human body, but as they migrate through the epidermis, a trail of inflammation follows the burrow, causing severe pruritus. Secondary infections often occur if the skin has been broken by scratching. It is the most commonly tropically acquired dermatosis. Beaches and other moist sandy areas are common locations of infection. Also called **creeping eruption.**

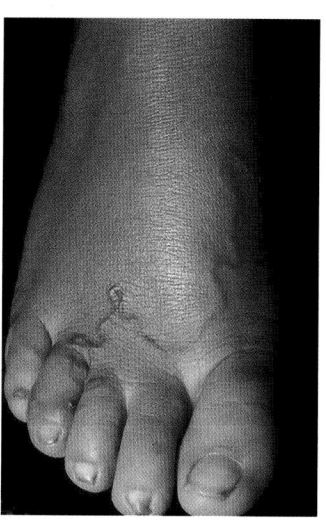

Cutaneous larva migrans *(Habif, 2016)*

cutaneous leishmaniasis, a dermatological disease caused by the parasite *Leishmania tropica*, transmitted to humans by the bite of the sand fly. This form of leishmaniasis, characterized by ulcerative lesions, occurs primarily in Africa, Asia, and some Mediterranean countries. The sore causes no systemic symptoms, but is susceptible to secondary infections. Treatment options include infrared therapy and injection of ulcers with sodium antimony gluconate. Also called **Aleppo boil, Delhi boil, Old World leishmaniasis, tropical sore.** Formerly called **oriental sore.** See also **leishmaniasis.**

cutaneous lupus erythematosus, one of the two main types of lupus erythematosus. It may involve only the skin or may precede involvement of other body systems. It may be chronic (discoid lupus erythematosus); subacute (systemic lupus erythematosus); or acute (characterized by an acute edematous, erythematous eruption, often with systemic exacerbations). The acute form may be the presenting symptom of systemic lupus erythematosus, such as after sun exposure.

cutaneous membrane. See **skin.**

cutaneous nerve, any mixed peripheral nerve that supplies a region of the skin.

cutaneous nevus [L, *cutis,* skin, *naevus,* birthmark], a discoloration of a skin area, such as a strawberry birthmark.

cutaneous papilloma, a small brown or flesh-colored outgrowth of skin, occurring most frequently on the neck of an older person. Also called **cutaneous tag, skin tag.**

cutaneous sensation [L, *cutis,* skin, *sentire,* to feel], a sensation experienced in or arising from receptors of the skin.

cutaneous tag. See **cutaneous papilloma.**

cutdown [ME, *cutten + doun*], a dissection to access a deep vein for puncture that is not accessible by venipuncture. The skin is cleansed before the procedure; the incision is sutured, and a sterile dressing is applied at its conclusion. See also **venipuncture.**

cuticle /kyo͞oʹtəkəl/ [L, *cuticula,* little skin], **1.** See **epidermis. 2.** the sheath of a hair follicle. **3.** the thin edge of cornified epithelium at the base of a nail.

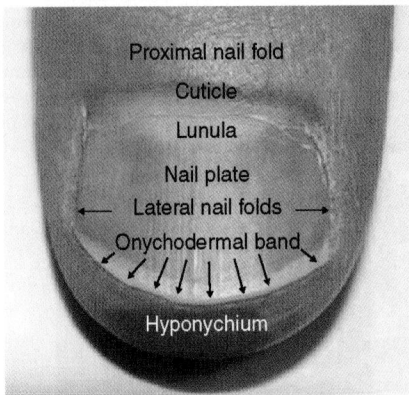

Cuticle *(McKee et al, 2005)*

cuticula /kyo͞otikʺyələ/, the cuticle; a narrow region of epidermis that covers the proximal surface of a fingernail or toenail.

cutis. See **skin.**

cutis laxa /kyo͞oʹtəs/ [L, skin, *laxus,* loose], abnormally loose, relaxed skin resulting from an absence of elastic fibers in the skin, usually a hereditary condition.

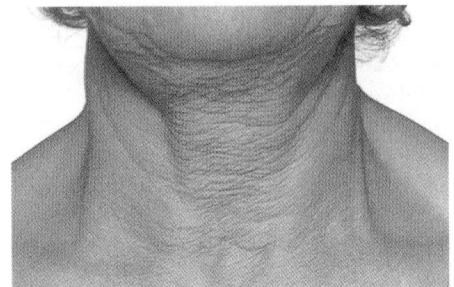

Cutis laxa *(Lawrence and Cox, 2002)*

cutis marmorata, skin that has a "marbled" appearance caused by conspicuous dilation of small vessels. See also **livedo.**

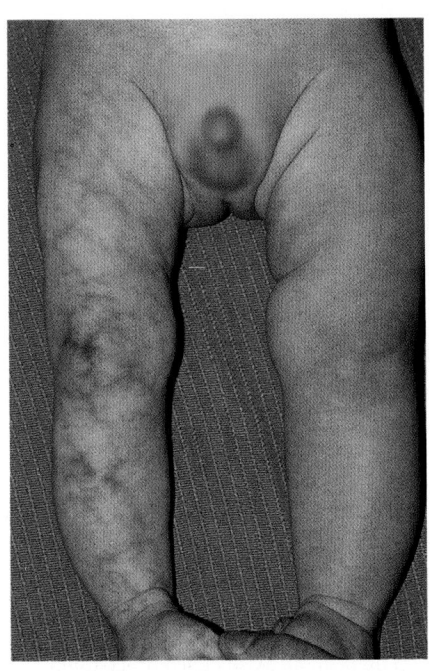

Infant with cutis marmorata *(Bolognia et al, 2014)*

cutting oil dermatitis, a skin disorder that affects machinists and others who use cutting oils as coolants and lubricants. Exposure to the oil obstructs hair follicles, sweat ducts, and sebaceous glands, leading to development of comedones and folliculitis. Sometimes there are secondary infections complicated by minute metal particles in the oil.

cuvette /kyo͞ovetʹ/ [Fr, *cuva,* tub], a small transparent tube or container with specific optical properties. The chemical composition of the container determines the vessel's use, such as Pyrex glass for examining materials in the visible spectrum or silica for those in the ultraviolet range. It is used in laboratory research and analyses, such as photometric evaluations, colorimetric determinations, and turbidity studies.

CV, 1. abbreviation for **closing volume. 2.** abbreviation for **curriculum vitae.**

CVA, 1. abbreviation for **cerebrovascular accident. 2.** abbreviation for **costovertebral angle.**

CVB, abbreviation for *chorionic villus biopsy.* See **chorionic villus sampling.**

CVC, abbreviation for **crying vital capacity.**

CVID, abbreviation for **common variable immunodeficiency.**

CVP, **1.** abbreviation for **central venous pressure. 2.** an anticancer drug combination of *c*yclophosphamide, *v*incristine, and *p*rednisone.

CVP monitor, abbreviation for **central venous pressure monitor.**

CW, abbreviation for **continuous wave.**

cyan-. See **cyano-, cyan-.**

cyanide poisoning /sī″ənid, -nīd/ [Gk, *kyanos,* blue], poisoning resulting from the ingestion or inhalation of cyanide from such substances as bitter almond oil, wild cherry syrup, prussic acid, hydrocyanic acid, or potassium or sodium cyanide. Characterized by impaired intracellular oxygenation, symptoms include tachycardia, drowsiness, seizures, headache, apnea, and cardiac arrest. Death may result within 1 to 15 minutes.

cyano-, cyan-, prefix meaning "blue": *cyanobacteria, cyanopsia, cyanosis.*

cyanobacteria /sī″ənōbaktir′ē·ə/ [Gk, *kyanos,* blue + *bacterion,* small staff], blue-green bacteria, unicellular or filamentous organisms that fix both carbon dioxide (in the presence of light) and nitrogen. Several species are common causes of water pollution and cause cyanobacteria poisoning. Formerly called **blue-green algae.**

cyanobacteria poisoning, poisoning by cyanobacteria, usually as a result of drinking contaminated water. In most cases it is a subacute condition characterized by liver damage with jaundice and sometimes bloody diarrhea and photosensitization. Drinking of heavily contaminated water may cause acute symptoms including muscle tremors, ataxia, dyspnea, cyanosis, and hyperesthesia so that a slight touch may cause convulsions and opisthotonos, which can be fatal. Also called **blue-green algae poisoning.**

cyanocobalamin /sī″ənōkōbal″əmin/ [Gk, *kyanos* + Ger, *kobald,* mine goblin], a red crystalline, water-soluble substance that is the common pharmaceutic form of vitamin B_{12}. It is involved in the metabolism of protein, fats, and carbohydrates; normal blood formation; and neural function. It is the first substance containing cobalt found to be vital to life. It cannot be produced synthetically but can be obtained from cultures of *Streptomyces griseus.* Rich dietary sources are liver, kidney, meats, fish, and dairy products. Deficiency can be caused by the absence of intrinsic factor (produced in the stomach), which is necessary for the absorption of cyanocobalamin from the GI tract. Deficiency can also occur in persons whose diet is strictly vegetarian, thereby excluding meat and dairy sources of the nutrient. Symptoms of deficiency include nervousness, neuritis, numbness and tingling in the hands and feet, poor muscular coordination, and menstrual disturbances. Cyanocobalamin (via injection) is used in the prophylaxis and treatment of pernicious anemia, tropical and nontropical sprue, and other macrocytic and megaloblastic anemias. It is relatively nontoxic, even when administered in amounts greater than those recommended for therapeutic purposes. Also called *antipernicious anemia factor,* **vitamin B_{12}, extrinsic factor.** See also **intrinsic factor, pernicious anemia.**

cyanomethemoglobin /sī″ənō′met·hē′məglō″bin/ [Gk, *kyanos* + *meta,* together with, *haima,* blood; L, *globus,* ball], product of an in vitro reaction in which hemoglobin from whole blood is reduced to methemoglobin and converted to a stable compound using potassium ferricyanide and potassium cyanide.

cyanopsia /sī″ənop″sē·ə/, a visual condition in which everything appears to have a blue tint.

cyanosed /sī″ənōst/, having a bluish discoloration of the skin, fingernails, and mucous membranes caused by a deficiency of oxygen in the blood. Also called **cyanotic.**

cyanosis /sī″ənō″sis/ [Gk, *kyanos,* blue, *osis,* condition], bluish discoloration of the skin and mucous membranes caused by an excess of deoxygenated hemoglobin in the blood or a structural defect in the hemoglobin molecule, such as in methemoglobin. **−cyanotic,** *adj.*

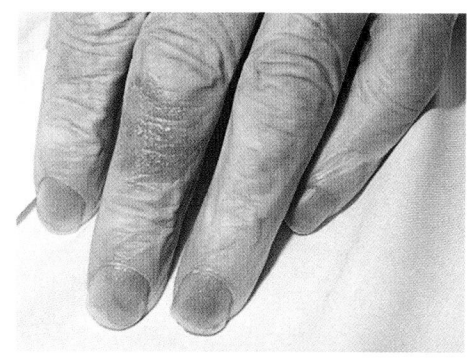

Cyanosis *(Henry and Stapleton, 2004)*

cyanotic, having a blue tinge to the skin, mucous membranes, or nailbeds. See also **cyanosed.**

cyanotic congenital heart defect /sī″ənot″ik/, an inborn heart defect that allows the mixing of unsaturated (venous) blood with saturated (arterial) blood to produce cyanosis.

cyberknife /sī″bərnīf/, a robotic radiosurgery system that delivers multiple beams of radiation, used to treat benign tumors and cancers and other medical conditions located anywhere in the body. It consists of a linear accelerator and a robotic arm.

cybernetics /sī″bərnet″iks/, the science of control and communication in living and nonliving systems, as in comparative study of electronic computers and the living brain.

cycl-. See **cyclo-, cycl-.**

cyclamate /sī″kləmāt/, an artificial nonnutritive sweetener formerly used in the form of calcium or sodium salt. It is banned in the United States.

cyclandelate /sīklan″dəlāt/, a peripheral vasodilator.
 ■ INDICATIONS: It is prescribed in the treatment of muscular ischemia and peripheral vascular obstruction or spasm.
 ■ CONTRAINDICATIONS: Pregnancy or known hypersensitivity to this drug prohibits its use.
 ■ ADVERSE EFFECTS: Tachycardia, weakness, GI distress, and flushing may occur.

cyclarthrosis /sī″klärthrō″sis, sik′-/, a pivot joint, capable of rotation.

cycle [Gk, *kyklos,* circle], a series of events that recurs at specified intervals. An example is influenza, which usually occurs in an annual cycle.

cyclencephaly /sīk″lənsef″əlē/ [Gk, *kyklos,* circle, *enkephalos,* brain], a developmental anomaly characterized by the fusion of the two cerebral hemispheres. **−cyclencephalic, cyclencephalous,** *adj.,* **−cyclencephalus,** *n.*

cycle per second. See **hertz.**

cyclic /sik″lik, sī″klik/ [Gk, *kyklos,* circle], pertaining to or occurring in a cycle or cycles, such as a chemical compound that contains a ring of atoms, as in cyclohexane (C_6H_{12}). See also **closed-chain.**

cyclic adenosine monophosphate (cAMP) /sik″lik, sī″klik/, a cyclic nucleotide formed from adenosine triphosphate by the action of adenyl cyclase. This cyclic compound, known as the "second messenger," participates in the action of catecholamines, vasopressin, adrenocorticotropic hormone, and many other hormones. Also called **adenosine 3′,5′-cyclic monophosphate.**

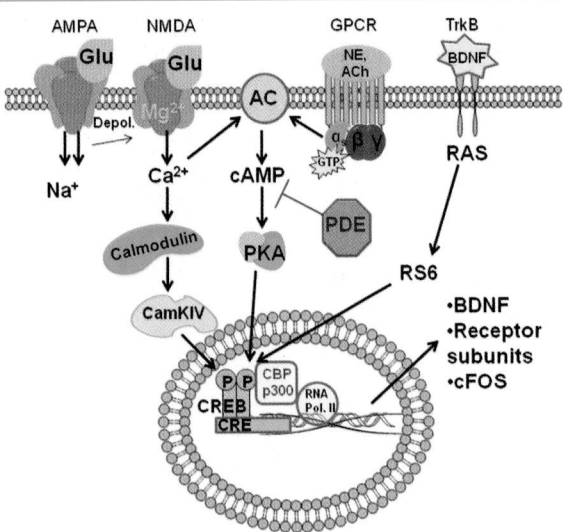

Cyclic adenosine monophosphate *(Hansen and Zhang, 2013)*

cyclic guanosine monophosphate (cGMP), a substance that mediates the action of certain hormones in a manner similar to that of cyclic adenosine monophosphate. In response to the stimulation of cholinergic receptors in a parasympathetic nerve, guanylate cyclase triggers the conversion of guanosine triphosphate to cGMP with the release of various enzymes. Atropine, an anticholinergic drug, can block cholinergic stimulation by means of this process.

cyclic neutropenia /sik′lik no͞o′trōpē′nē-ə/, a chronic type of neutropenia that abates and recurs, accompanied by malaise, fever, stomatitis, and various types of infections.

cyclic phosphate. *(Informal)* See **cyclic adenosine monophosphate.**

cyclic vomiting, periodic episodes of vomiting associated with migraine and usually accompanied by headaches and symptoms of ketosis. The episodes may begin in childhood.

cyclin /sī′klin/, one of a class of intracellular proteins that appear during the eukaryotic cell cycle. The cyclin concentration increases during the cycle until halfway to the mitosis stage, when it drops to zero. Cyclin may act as a molecular switch that activates mitosis when its concentration reaches a certain point.

cyclin-dependent kinase (CDK), a protein kinase that is activated by cyclin and involved in the regulation of the cell cycle.

-cycline, suffix designating a tetracycline-derivative antibiotic.

cycling /si′kling/, the ending of an inspiratory phase of mechanical ventilation.

cyclitis /siklī′tis/ [Gk, *kyklos* + *itis*], inflammation of the ciliary body that causes redness of the sclera adjacent to the cornea of the eye.

cyclizine hydrochloride /sī′klizēn/, an antihistamine and antiemetic/antivertigo agent.

■ INDICATIONS: It is prescribed in the treatment or prevention of motion sickness or vertigo.

■ CONTRAINDICATIONS: Known hypersensitivity to this drug prohibits its use. It is not given to newborns or lactating mothers.

■ ADVERSE EFFECTS: Among the more serious adverse reactions are skin rash, hypersensitivity reactions, and tachycardia. Drowsiness, dryness of the mouth, and worsening vision occur commonly.

cyclo-, cycl-, prefix meaning "round, recurring," often with reference to the eye: *cyclodialysis, cyclopia.*

cyclobenzaprine hydrochloride /sī′kləben″zəprēn/, a muscle relaxant.

■ INDICATIONS: It is prescribed in the short-term treatment of muscle spasm.

■ CONTRAINDICATIONS: Hyperthyroidism, cardiac arrhythmia, cardiac failure, concomitant use of a monoamine oxidase inhibitor, or known hypersensitivity to this drug prohibits its use. It is used with caution in conditions in which anticholinergics are contraindicated.

■ ADVERSE EFFECTS: The most serious adverse effects are hypersensitivity reactions. Drowsiness, dry mouth, and dizziness commonly occur.

cyclocephaly. See **cyclopia.**

Cyclocort, a glucocorticoid. Brand name for **amcinonide.**

cyclodestruction /sī′klədistruk″shən/, (in ophthalmology) a procedure to damage the ciliary body in order to diminish the production of aqueous fluid in the treatment of glaucoma; usually done by cryotherapy.

cyclodialysis /-dī·al″isis/, **1.** a surgical procedure performed on patients with glaucoma. A pathway is opened between the anterior chamber of the eye and the suprachoroidal space, allowing excess fluid to drain and reducing intraocular pressure. **2.** separation of the ciliary body from the sclera, usually as a result of trauma, causing decreased intraocular pressure, or hypotony.

cycloduction /-duk″shən/, (in ophthalmology) the range of rotation of an eye around its visual axis, which allows binocular single vision to be maintained when the head is tilted.

cyclooxygenase /si′klō·ok′səjĕnās/, an activity of the enzyme prostaglandin endoperoxide synthase.

cyclophosphamide /-fos″fəmīd/, an alkylating agent.

■ INDICATIONS: It is prescribed in the treatment of neoplasms and as an immunosuppressant in organ transplantation.

■ CONTRAINDICATIONS: It is teratogenic in animals. It is not used during pregnancy. Adequate methods of contraception should be considered for both males and females who are using it. It is used neither in patients with known hypersensitivity to the drug nor in patients with severely depressed bone marrow function. It is used with caution with impaired renal or hepatic function or with various blood disorders.

■ ADVERSE EFFECTS: Among the more serious adverse reactions are anorexia, vomiting, alopecia, leukopenia, cardiotoxicity, thrombocytopenia, and potentially serious hemorrhagic cystitis.

cyclopia /sīklō″pē-ə/ [Gk, *Cyclops,* mythic one-eyed giant], a developmental anomaly characterized by fusion of the orbits into a single cavity containing one eye. The condition is usually combined with various other head and facial defects. Also called **cyclocephaly, synophthalmia.**

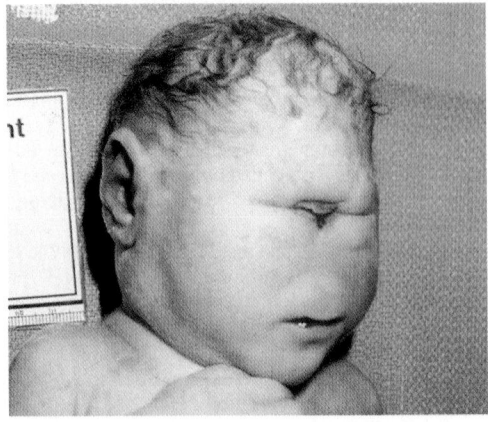

Fetus with cyclopia *(Courtesy Dr. A.E. Chudley, Department of Pediatrics and Child Health, University of Manitoba, Children's Hospital)*

cycloplegia /sī′kləplē″jə/ [Gk, *kyklos* + *plege*, stroke], paralysis of accommodation, as induced by certain ophthalmic drugs to allow examination of the eye. It causes pupillary dilation and relaxation of accommodation. See also **cycloplegic.**

cycloplegic /sī′kləplē″jik/, **1.** *adj.,* pertaining to a drug or treatment that causes paralysis of the ciliary muscles of the eye. **2.** *n.,* one of a group of anticholinergic drugs used to paralyze the ciliary muscles of the eye for ophthalmological examination or surgery. Any of the cycloplegics may cause adverse effects in persons sensitive to anticholinergics.

cycloplegic refraction, a type of static refraction, measured after lens accommodation is paralyzed by administration of cycloplegic eyedrops.

cyclopropane /sī′klōprō″pān/, an explosive anesthetic gas. It has been replaced by the nonflammable halogenated hydrocarbons.

cyclops. *(Obsolete)* See **cyclopia.**

cycloSERINE /sī′klōser″ēn/, an antibiotic.

■ INDICATIONS: It is prescribed in the treatment of active pulmonary and extrapulmonary tuberculosis.

■ CONTRAINDICATIONS: Epilepsy, depression, severe anxiety, psychosis, severe renal insufficiency, excessive concurrent use of alcohol, or known hypersensitivity to this drug prohibits its use.

■ ADVERSE EFFECTS: Among the most serious reactions are central nervous system toxic effects, including tremor, drowsiness, convulsions, and psychotic changes. Pyridoxine may be given concurrently to prevent these effects. Other side effects include arrhythmias and optic neuritis.

Cyclospora cayetanensis, a pathogenic protozoon that causes diarrhea, cramps, and fever in humans. The microorganism, a coccidian parasite about 0.01 mm in diameter, was identified in 1979, after the first known cases of the infection were diagnosed. Before 1996 only three outbreaks of *Cyclospora* infection had been reported in the United States and Canada. It is diagnosed much more frequently now, and is often referred to as "traveler's diarrhea." Although *Cyclospora* is transmitted by the fecal-oral route, person-to-person transmission is unlikely because oocytes require days to weeks under favorable conditions to become infectious after leaving an infected host.

cyclosporin, any of a group of biologically active metabolites of *Tolypocladium inflatum* Gams and certain other fungi. Nine have been identified and are designated cyclosporin A through I. The major forms are cyclosporin A and C, which are cyclic oligopeptides with immunosuppressive, antifungal, and antipyretic effects. As immunosuppressants, cyclosporines primarily affect T lymphocytes. They are widely used in organ transplantation to suppress rejection and are known to be a human carcinogen. Also spelled **ciclosporin.**

cyclothymic disorder /-thīm′ik/ [Gk, *kyklos* + *thymos,* mind], a disorder of mood, wherein the essential feature is a chronic mood disturbance of at least 2 years' duration, involving numerous periods of depression and hypomania, but not of sufficient severity and duration to meet the criteria for a major depressive or manic episode. See also **bipolar disorder, depression, dysthymic disorder.**

cyclothymic personality, a personality characterized by swings in mood from elation to depression.

cyclotomy /sīklot″əmē/, a surgical procedure for the correction of a defect in the ciliary muscle of the eye.

cyclotron /sī′klətron/ [Gk, *kyklos* + *electron,* amber], a device used to accelerate charged particles or ions along a spiral path within a magnetic field. The particles bombard targets, where they create radioactive species.

cyclotropia /sī′klōtrō″pe·ə/, (in ophthalmology) a condition in which the ocular position of one eye is rotated around its axis with respect to the other eye.

cylinder, a solid body having a circular transverse section. Exceptions include hollow gas cylinders, crossed cylinders used to measure astigmatism, and terminal cylinders of sensory nerve fibers.

cylindrical grasp /silin″drikəl/, the normal position of the hand and fingers when holding cylindrical objects, such as a glass tumbler, railing, or pot handle. The fingers and thumb close and flex around the object, which is stabilized against the palm of the hand. It occurs as a reflex action in infants and later develops into a voluntary gross grasp.

cylindrical lens, a lens with at least one nonspherical surface, used to correct astigmatism.

cylindroma /sil′indrō″mə/ *pl.* cylindromas, cylindromata [Gk, *kylindros,* cylinder], a tumor that appears to have cylinders of stroma surrounded by epithelial cells. See also **adenocystic carcinoma.**

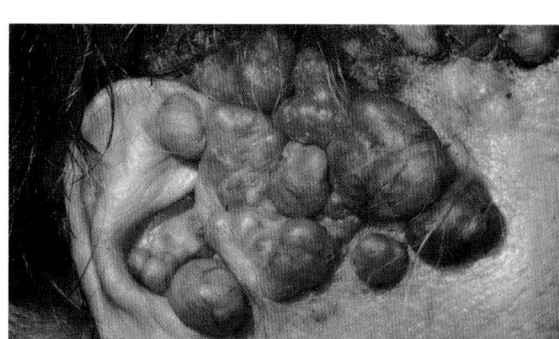

Cylindroma *(Hordinsky, Sawaya, and Scher, 2000)*

cyma line /sī″mə/, an S-shaped line seen on radiographs at the articulation of the talonavicular and calcaneocuboid bones of the foot. An abnormality in the joint, including pronation or supination of the talar head, appears as a broken cyma line on radiographs.

Cymbalta, brand name for **duloxetine.**

cyno-, cyn-, prefix meaning "dog, doglike": *cynophobia.*

cynophobia, a persistent, irrational fear of dogs.

cypionate /sī″pyōnāt/, contraction of *cyclopentanepropionate.*

cyproheptadine hydrochloride /sī′prōhep″tədēn/, an antihistamine.

■ INDICATIONS: It is prescribed in the treatment of hypersensitivity reactions, including rhinitis, skin rash, and pruritus.

■ CONTRAINDICATIONS: Asthma or known hypersensitivity to this drug prohibits its use. It is not given to newborns or lactating mothers.

■ ADVERSE EFFECTS: Among the more serious adverse reactions are skin rash, hypersensitivity, and tachycardia. Drowsiness and dry mouth commonly occur.

Cyprus fever. See **brucellosis.**

Cys, abbreviation for **cysteine.**

cyst /sist/ [Gk, *kystis,* bag], a closed sac lined with epithelium and containing fluid or semisolid material. It may or may not be infected. −**cystic,** *adj.*

cyst-. See **cysto-, cyst-, cysti-, cystido-.**

-cyst, -cystis, combining form meaning "pouch" or "bladder": *cystitis, enterocystoplasty, cystogram.*

cystadenocarcinoma /sis′tədē′nəkär′sinō″mə/, a type of pancreatic or liver tumor that evolves from a mucus cystadenoma. Clinical features include epigastric pain and a palpable abdominal mass that may also be seen by ultrasonography or computed tomographic scan. It is treated by surgical removal of the tumor or total pancreatectomy.

cystadenoma /sis′tədinō″mə/ *pl.* cystadenomas, cystadenomata [Gk, *kystis* + *aden,* gland, *oma,* tumor], **1.** an adenoma associated with a cystoma. **2.** an adenoma containing multiple cystic structures. The cysts may be serous, containing serum, or pseudomucinous, containing clear, serous fluid or thick, viscid fluid.

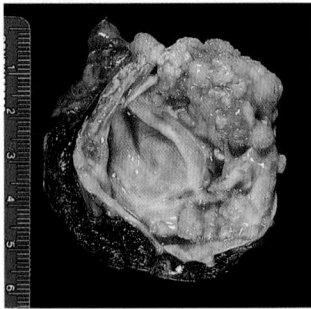

Serous cystadenoma *(Courtesy Dr. Christopher Crum, Brigham and Women's Hospital)*

Cystagon, a product used in the treatment of nephropathic cystinosis. Brand name for **cysteamine bitartrate.**

cystathioninemia /sis′təthī′əninē″mē-ə/, an inherited metabolic disorder, caused by a deficiency of the enzyme cystathionase, that causes an excess of the amino acid methionine. Some patients are asymptomatic, whereas others show signs of cognitive impairment, as well as thrombocytopenia and acidosis. It is treated with large doses of pyridoxine (vitamin B_6).

cysteamine /siste′ämēn″/, a sulfhydryl amine that is part of coenzyme A. It reduces intracellular cystine levels and is used in treatment of nephropathic cystinosis. It is administered orally.

cysteamine bitartrate, an anticysteine that reacts with cystine in the cell lysosomes to convert it to cysteine and a mixed disulfide compound, which can then exit the lysosome in patients with a metabolic defect causing cystinosis.

■ INDICATIONS: It is prescribed in the treatment of an inherited amino acid metabolic disease in which cysteine accumulates in the cells and can lead to the formation of crystals that can damage various organs, especially the kidneys (nephropathic cystinosis).

■ CONTRAINDICATIONS: It should not be given to patients with allergy to cysteamine or penicillamine, depression, drowsiness, lethargy, neurological disorders, or diseases of the liver or digestive tract.

■ ADVERSE EFFECTS: The side effects most often reported include vomiting, diarrhea, constipation, appetite loss, nausea, headaches, convulsions, and seizures.

cystectomy /sistek″təmē/ [Gk, *kystis* + *ektomē,* excision], a surgical procedure in which all or part of the urinary bladder is removed, as may be required in treating bladder cancer.

cysteine (Cys) /sis″tēn/, an amino acid containing a polar side chain found in many proteins in the body, including keratin. It is a metabolic precursor of cystine and an important source of sulfur for various body functions. Compare **cystine.**

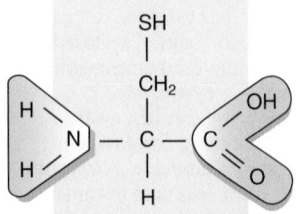

Chemical structure of cysteine

cysti-. See **cysto-, cyst-, cysti-, cystido-.**

cystic /sis″tik/ [Gk, *kystis,* bag], **1.** pertaining to a cyst. **2.** pertaining to a fluid-filled sac, such as the gallbladder or urinary bladder.

cystic acne. See **acne conglobata.**

cystic bile, concentrated bile stored in the gallbladder.

cystic carcinoma, a malignant neoplasm containing closed cavities or saclike spaces. These tumors may occur in the breast and ovary.

cystic diverticulum, a ventral outgrowth at the base of the hepatic diverticulum in the embryo. It gives rise to the gallbladder and cystic duct.

cystic duct, the duct through which bile from the gallbladder passes into the common bile duct.

cystic emphysema. See **bullous emphysema.**

cysticercosis /sis′tisərkō″sis/ [Gk, *kystis* + *kerkos,* tail, *osis,* condition], an infection and infestation by the larval stage of the pork tapeworm *Taenia solium* or the beef tapeworm *T. saginata.*

■ OBSERVATIONS: The invasive, early phase of the infection is characterized by fever, malaise, muscle pain, and eosinophilia.

■ INTERVENTIONS: Prophylaxis depends on eating only thoroughly cooked pork or beef. The antiparasitic drugs praziquantel or albendazole may be used to treat this infection on a case-by-case basis. In some cases, surgery may be necessary to remove the larvae, or cysticerci.

■ PATIENT CARE CONSIDERATIONS: The eggs are ingested and hatch in the intestine; the larvae invade the subcutaneous tissue, brain, eye, muscle, heart, liver, lung, and peritoneum. They attach themselves with two rows of hooklets, grow, mature, and become covered with a dense, fibrous capsule. Years later, seizures and personality change may appear if the brain is affected, and calcification and destruction of local structures are apparent in other infested areas of the body.

cysticercus /sis′tisur″kəs/ *pl. cysticercosis,* a larval form of tapeworm of the genus *Taenia.* It consists of a single scolex enclosed in a bladderlike cyst.

cystic fibroma, a fibrous tumor in which cystic degeneration has occurred.

cystic fibrosis (CF), an inherited autosomal-recessive disorder of the exocrine glands, causing those glands to produce abnormally thick secretions of mucus, elevation of sweat electrolytes, increased organic and enzymatic constituents of saliva, and overactivity of the autonomic nervous system. The glands most affected are those in the pancreas and respiratory system and the sweat glands. Also called **fibrocystic disease of the pancreas, mucoviscidosis.**

■ OBSERVATIONS: The earliest manifestation is meconium ileus, an obstruction of the small bowel by viscid stool. Other early signs are a chronic cough, persistent upper respiratory infections, and frequent, foul-smelling stools. The most reliable diagnostic tool is the sweat chloride test, which shows elevations of levels of chloride.

■ INTERVENTIONS: Because there is no known cure, treatment is directed at prevention of respiratory infections, which are the most frequent cause of death. Mucolytic agents and bronchodilators are used to help liquefy the thick, tenacious mucus. Physical therapy measures, such as postural drainage and breathing exercises, can also dislodge secretions. Broad-spectrum antibiotics may be used prophylactically. Surgery may be indicated for some cases that cannot be treated effectively with medications. Heart-lung and double-lung transplantations have been successful.

■ PATIENT CARE CONSIDERATIONS: Cystic fibrosis is usually recognized in infancy or early childhood, chiefly among Caucasians. Life expectancy in cystic fibrosis has improved markedly over the past several decades, and with early diagnosis and treatment most patients can be expected to reach adulthood.

cystic fibrosis transmembrane conductance regulator, a regulator of secretion in many exocrine tissues. Abnormalities in the gene cause cystic fibrosis, leading to abnormal chloride channels in cell membranes of the respiratory epithelium, pancreas, salivary glands, sweat glands, intestines, and reproductive tract. Also called *cystic fibrosis transmembrane regulator, cystic fibrosis transmembrane regulator protein.*

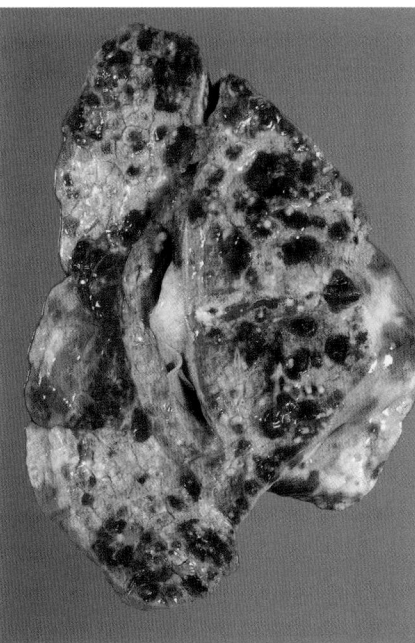

Cystic fibrosis *(Cooke and Stewart, 2004)*

cystic goiter, an enlargement of the thyroid gland, containing cysts resulting from mucoid or colloid degeneration or liquefaction.

cystic hygroma. See **cystic lymphangioma.**

cystic kidney [Gk, *kystis,* bag; ME, *kidenei*], pertaining to any of several kidney disorders in which cysts form, including congenital polycystic disease, solitary renal cysts, or cortical cysts associated with nephrosclerosis.

cystic kidney disease, cystic disease of kidney. See **acquired cystic kidney disease, polycystic kidney disease.**

cystic lymphangioma, a cystic growth formed by lymph vessels, usually congenital and occurring most frequently in the neck, axilla, or groin of children. Also called **cystic hygroma, lymphangioma cysticum.**

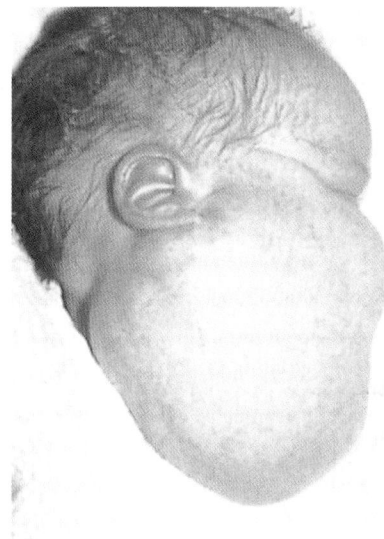

Infant with cystic lymphangioma *(Greig and Garden, 1996)*

cystic mastitis, a form of mammary dysplasia with inflammation and the formation of nodular cysts in the breast tissue. The cysts contain a turbid fluid. Symptoms may vary with individual breast changes that occur during the menstrual cycle.

cystic mole. See **hydatid mole.**

cystic myxoma, a tumor of connective tissue that has undergone cystic degeneration.

cystic nephroblastoma, multilocular cyst of kidney.

cystic neuroma, a neoplasm of nerve tissue that has degenerated and become cystic. Also called **false neuroma.**

cystic pyelitis, pyelitis with formation of submucosal cysts.

cystic pyeloureteritis, a type of ureteral inflammation in which there are subendothelial cysts projecting into the lumen of the ureter and renal pelvis.

cystic renal dysplasia, renal or kidney developmental abnormality in which there are cysts.

cystic tumor, a tumor with cavities or sacs containing a semisolid or a liquid material.

cystido-. See **cysto-, cyst-, cysti-, cystido-.**

cystine /sis″tin/, a compound consisting of two cysteine residues joined by a disulfide (S-S) linkage. Compare **cysteine.**

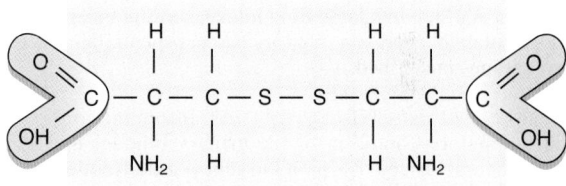

Chemical structure of cystine

cystinosis /sis′tinō″sis/ [*cystine* + Gk, *osis,* condition], a congenital disease characterized by glucosuria; proteinuria; cystine deposits in the liver, spleen, bone marrow, and cornea; rickets; excessive amounts of phosphates in the urine; and growth delay. Also called *cystine storage disease,* **Fanconi syndrome.** See also **cystine.**

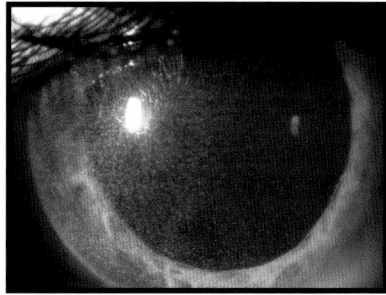

Cystinosis *(Freund et al, 2017)*

cystinuria /sis′tinŏŏr″ē·ə/ [*cystine* + Gk, *ouron,* urine], **1.** abnormal presence of the amino acid cystine in the urine collected in a 24-hour specimen. **2.** an inherited defect of the renal tubules, characterized by excessive urinary excretion of cystine and several other amino acids. The disorder is caused by an autosomal-recessive trait that impairs cystine reabsorption by the kidney tubules. In high concentration, cystine tends to precipitate in the urinary tract and form kidney or bladder stones. Treatment attempts to prevent the formation of stones or to dissolve

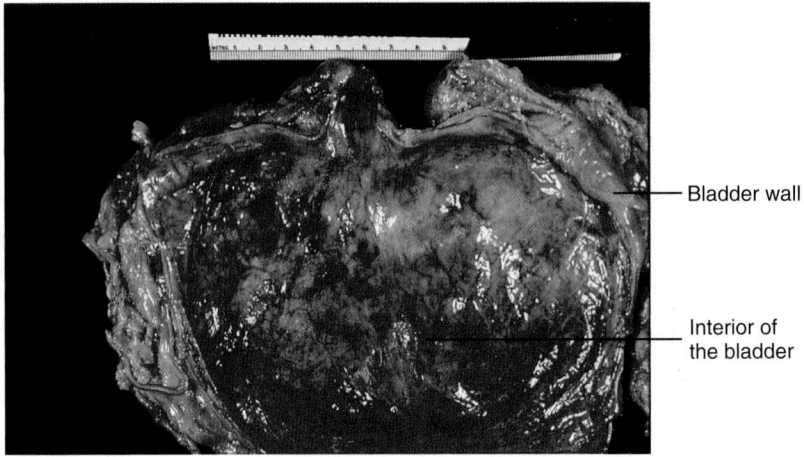

Bladder wall

Interior of
the bladder

Cystitis *(Damjanov, 2012)*

them by increasing the volume of urine flow, decreasing the pH of the urine, and increasing the solubility of cystine. In addition to a large fluid intake, sodium bicarbonate, acetazolamide, and, in refractory cases, D-penicillamine are sometimes prescribed.

-cystis. See **-cyst, -cystis.**

cystitis /sistī″tis/ [Gk, *kystis* + *itis,* inflammation], an inflammatory condition of the urinary bladder and ureters, characterized by pain, urgency and frequency of urination, and hematuria. It may be caused by a bacterial infection, calculus, or tumor. Increased sexual activity in women can cause cystitis, and certain venereal diseases such as gonorrhea and chlamydia may cause cystitis-like symptoms. Depending on the diagnosis, treatment may include antibiotics, increased fluid intake, medications to control bladder wall spasms, and, when necessary, surgery.

-cystitis, suffix meaning "inflammation of a bladder or cyst": *cholecystitis, dacryocystitis, paracystitis.*

cystitis colli, inflammation of the bladder and bladder neck.

cystitis cystica, cystitis with formation of multiple submucosal cysts in the bladder wall.

cysto-, cyst-, cysti-, cystido-, prefix meaning "bladder, cyst, or sac": *cystocele.*

cystocele /sis″təsēl′/ [Gk, *kystis* + *kele,* hernia], a herniation or protrusion of the urinary bladder through the wall of the vagina. Compare **rectocele, vesicocele.**

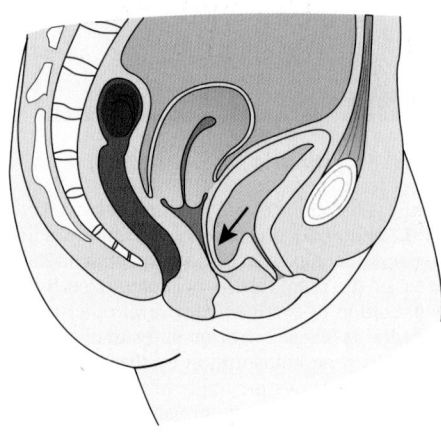

Cystocele *(Proctor and Adams, 2014)*

cystocerebral syndrome, encephalopathy caused by increased bladder wall tension. The condition is reversible, requiring immediate relief of bladder distension; if untreated, acute renal failure may result.

cystochromoscopy /sis″təkrōmos″kəpē/, examination of the bladder after administration of a colored dye, performed as an investigation of renal function and urinary system condition. Also called **chromocystoscopy.**

cystofibroma /-fībrō″mə/, a fibrous benign tumor that contains or is covered with cysts.

cystogram /sis″təgram′/ [Gk, *kystis* + *gramma,* record], a radiographic image of the bladder produced by cystography.

cystography /sistog″rəfē/, the radiographic examination of the urinary bladder after introduction of a radiopaque contrast medium.

cystoid /sis″toid/ [Gk, *kystis,* bag + *eidos,* form], pertaining to or resembling a cyst or bladder.

cystoid macular edema, thickening of the macula with cystic changes, increased fluid within the sensory retina of the macula, and disruption of the blood-retinal barrier and consequent leakage on fluorescein angiography, with leaking capillaries in the posterior pole and around the optic disc, often a result of cataract surgery.

cystojejunostomy /-ji′jōōnos″təmē/, drainage of a cyst, such as a pancreatic pseudocyst, into the jejunum.

cystolith, *(Obsolete)* now called **vesical calculus.**

cystolithalopaxy /-lith″əlōpek′sē/, removal of a kidney stone from the urinary bladder by crushing, followed by extraction of the particles by means of irrigation.

cystolithotomy /-lithot″əmē/, removal of a bladder stone from the urinary bladder following surgical opening of the bladder. Also called *cystolithectomy,* **vesical lithotomy.**

cystoma /sistō″mə/ *pl.* cystomas, cystomata [Gk, *kystis* + *oma,* tumor], any tumor or growth containing cysts, especially one in or near the ovary.

-cystoma, suffix meaning a "cystic tumor": *adenocystoma, osteocystoma, papilloadenocystoma.*

cystometer /sistom″ətər/, an instrument that measures bladder capacity in relation to changing urine pressure.

cystometrogram /sis′tōmet″rəgram′/, the graphic results of the measurements made during cystometrography. The term is also used to describe the test.

cystometrography (CMG) /sis′tōmətrog″rəfē/, a urological procedure that measures the amount of pressure exerted on the bladder at various bladder volumes. The test helps determine bladder capacity, bladder wall compliance, detrusor stability, and sensations of filling. It is often done in conjunction with electromyography and other urodynamic tests.

cystometry /sistom″ətrē/ [Gk, *kystis* + *metron*, measure], the study of bladder function by use of a device that provides data on the response to increased pressure.

cystoparesis /sis″tōpäre′sis/, paralysis of the urinary bladder. Also called **cystoplegia.**

cystoplasty, a surgical procedure to increase the size of the bladder.

cystoplegia. See **cystoparesis.**

cystoprostatectomy /-pros′tətek″təmē/, surgical removal of the bladder, prostate gland, and seminal vesicle.

cystosarcoma phyllodes /sis″tōsärkō″mə filō″dēs/, a malignant stromal breast tumor that grows rapidly and tends to recur if not adequately excised. The pattern of the cells resembles leaves.

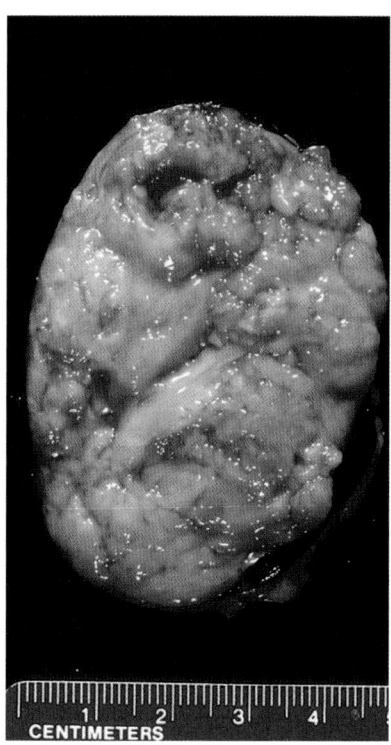

Cystosarcoma phyllodes *(Courtesy Dr. N. Weidner, Brigham and Women's Hospital)*

cystoscope /sis″təskōp′/ [Gk, *kystis* + *skopein,* to look], an instrument for examining and treating lesions of the urethra or bladder. There are both rigid and flexible types. The rigid instrument consists of an obturator for introduction, an outer sheath, a lighting system, a viewing lens, and ports for catheters and operative devices. The flexible cystoscope is a self-contained endoscope with ports for instrumentation and irrigation. Flexible

cystoscopes are more commonly used today and incorporate fiberoptics.

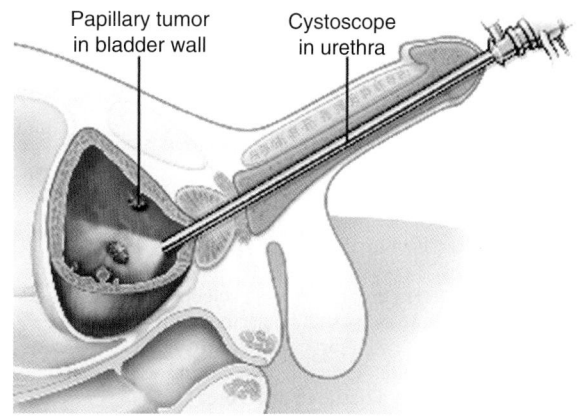

Cystoscope *(Thibodeau and Patton, 2010)*

cystoscopic. See **cystoscopy.**

cystoscopic urography. See **retrograde cystoscopy.**

cystoscopy /sistos″kəpē/, insertion of a rigid or flexible cystoscope into the urethra for visualization and instrumentation of the lower urinary tract. The procedure is often performed in urological offices with local anesthesia. The bladder is distended with water while the patient is supine or in the lithotomy position. After the examination the patient is observed for the common complications of local urethral trauma and signs of urinary infection. See also **cystoscope. –cystoscopic,** *adj.*

Cystospaz, an anticholinergic/antispasmodic agent. Brand name for *hyoscyamine.*

cystostomy /sistos″təmē/, an opening made in the bladder for drainage, usually through a catheter inserted through the abdominal wall.

cystotomy /sistot″əmē/, surgical incision of the urinary bladder.

cystoureterography /sis′təyoor′ətərog″rəfē/, the radiographic examination of the urinary bladder and ureters after introduction of a radiopaque contrast medium.

cystourethrogram /sis′təyoorē″thrəgram′/, a radiographic image of the urinary bladder and urethra produced by cystourethrography.

cystourethrography /sis′təyoor′ēthrog″rəfē/, the radiographic examination of the urethra and urinary bladder after introduction of a radiopaque contrast medium.

cysts of liver, small, single, simple, watery sacs in the liver, usually not associated with symptoms. The cause is unknown.

cyt-, cyto-, prefix meaning "cell" or "cytoplasm": *cytochrome, cytogenesis, cytosome.*

Cytadren, an inhibitor of adrenocorticosteroid biosynthesis. Brand name for *aminoglutethimide.*

cytapheresis /sī′tōfer″əsis/ [Gk, *kytos* + *aphairesis,* withdrawal], selective removal of a cellular component of blood by apheresis. Red cells, granulocytes, or platelets may be harvested. Cytapheresis is used to collect specific components from blood donors, or, in the case of therapeutic cytapheresis, to remove excess cellular components from patients with blood disorders.

cytarabine /siter″əbēn/, an antineoplastic agent. Also called **arabinosylcytosine,** *ARA-C,* **cytosine arabinoside.**

■ INDICATIONS: It is prescribed in the treatment of acute and chronic myelocytic leukemia, acute lymphocytic leukemia, and erythroleukemia.

■ CONTRAINDICATIONS: Known hypersensitivity to this drug prohibits its use.

■ ADVERSE EFFECTS: The most serious adverse reactions are bone marrow depression, stomatitis, phlebitis, liver toxicity, fever, and GI disturbances.

-cyte, suffix meaning a "cell" of a specified type: *astrocyte, hemocyte, plasmacyte.*

-cythemia, -cythaemia, suffix meaning a "condition involving cells in the blood": *erythrocythemia, rhestocythemia, thrombocythemia.*

cyto-. See **cyt-, cyto-.**

cytoanalyzer /sī′tō·an′əlī′zər/, an electronic device that screens samples of smears of suspected malignancies.

cytoarchitectonic /sī′tō-är″kitekton″ik/ [Gk, *kytos,* cell; L, *architectura,* architecture], pertaining to the cellular arrangement within a tissue or structure.

cytoarchitecture /-är′kitek″chər/, the typical pattern of cellular arrangement within a particular tissue or organ, as in the cerebral cortex. −*cytoarchitectural, adj.*

cytobiotactic, cytobiotaxis, influence exerted by one cell on the action of another. See **cytoclesis.**

cytoblast. See **nucleus.**

cytocentrum. See **centrosome.**

cytocerastic. See **cytokerastic.**

cytochemism /sī′tōkem″izəm/ [Gk, *kytos* + *chemeia,* alchemy], the chemical activity within the living cell, specifically the various reactions to and affinity for chemical substances.

cytochemistry /-kem″istrē/, the study of the various chemicals within a living cell and their actions and functions.

cytochrome /si″tōkrōm/ [Gk, *kytos,* cell, *chroma,* color], 1. a class of hemoproteins whose function is electron transport. These proteins have the ability to change the valence of the heme iron, alternating between ferrous and ferric states. 2. proteins involved in mitochondrial electron transport systems associated with adenosine triphosphate (ATP) production.

cytochrome c oxidase, an enzyme complex of the inner mitochondrial membrane that catalyzes the transfer of electrons from cytochrome *c* to oxygen, oxidizing cytochrome and reducing oxygen in the final step of the electron transport chain by which oxygen is used for fuel combustion.

cytochrome-c oxidase deficiency, a hereditary defect in the cytochrome-*c* oxidase complex that prevents the transfer of electrons from cytochrome *c* to molecular oxygen, ultimately halting adenosine triphosphate production. Manifestations are extremely variable and include myopathies, encephalopathies, ocular and cardiac defects, sensorineural deafness, Fanconi syndrome, diabetes mellitus, and short stature. Inheritance may be autosomal recessive, X-linked, or, possibly, maternal (mitochondrial), depending on the part of the cytochrome-*c* oxidase complex that is affected.

cytochrome P-450 [Gk, *kytos,* cell, *chroma,* color], a protein involved with extramitochondrial electron transport in the liver and in the metabolism or bioactivation of drugs.

cytocide [Gk, *kytos* + L, *caedere,* to kill], any substance that is destructive to cells. −*cytocidal, adj.*

cytoclesis /sī′tōklē″sis/ [Gk, *kytos* + *klesis,* calling for], the influence exerted by one cell on the action of other cells; the vital principle of all living tissue. Also called **cytobiotactic, cytobiotaxis.** −*cytobiotactic, cytocletic, adj.*

cytoctony /sītok′tənē/ [Gk, *kytos* + *ktonos,* killing], the destruction of cells in culture by viruses.

cytode /sī′tōd/ [Gk, *kytos* + *eidos,* form], the simplest type of cell, consisting of a protoplasmic mass without a nucleus, such as a bacterium.

cytodendrite /-den″drīt/. See **dendrite.**

cytodiagnosis /-dī′əgnō″sis/, diagnosis of a suspected pathological tissue by a microscopic examination of the cells in the sample.

cytodieresis /sī′tōdī·er″isis/ *pl. cytodiereses* [Gk, *kytos* + *diairesis,* separation], cell division, especially the phenomena involving the division of the cytoplasm. See also **cytokinesis, meiosis, mitosis.** −*cytodieretic, adj.*

cytodifferentiation /-dif′əren″shē·ā″shən/ [Gk, *kytos* + L, *differentia,* difference], 1. a process by which embryonic cells acquire biochemical and morphological properties essential for specialization and diversification. 2. the total and gradual transformation from an undifferentiated to a fully differentiated state.

cytofluorograph /-flôr″əgraf/, a diagnostic instrument used to measure the level of CD4 T lymphocytes in human immunodeficiency virus–positive patients.

cytogene /sī′təjēn/ [Gk, *kytos* + *genein,* to produce], a self-replicating particle within the cytoplasm of a cell that is derived from genes in the nucleus and is capable of transmitting hereditary information.

cytogenesis /sī′tōjen″əsis/ [Gk, *kytos* + *genein,* to produce], the origin, development, and differentiation of cells. −*cytogenic, adj.,* −*cytogenetics, n.*

cytogeneticist /sī′tōjənet″isist/, a scientist who specializes in the study of the origin, structure, differentiation, and function of cells, especially the chromosomes.

cytogenetics /sī′tōjənet″iks/, the branch of genetics that studies the cellular constituents concerned with heredity, primarily the structure, function, and origin of the chromosomes. Also called **cytogenics.** Kinds include **clinical cytogenetics.**

cytogenetic technologist, an allied health professional who studies chromosomes. The cytogenetic technologist determines how specimens will be collected, transported, and handled for cytogenetic analysis. After receiving a baccalaureate degree, cytogenetic technologists complete a 1-year certificate program.

cytogenic /-jen″ik/, pertaining to the formation of cells.

cytogenic gland, a glandular organ that secretes living cells, specifically the testes and ovaries.

cytogenic reproduction, the formation of a new organism from a germ cell, either sexually through the fusion of gametes to form a zygote or asexually by means of spores. Also called **cytogony.**

cytogenics. See **cytogenetics.**

cytogeny /sītoj″ənē/, 1. See **cytogenetics.** 2. the origin and development of cells. −*cytogenic, cytogenous, adj.*

cytogony /sītog″ənē/. See **cytogenic reproduction.**

cytohistogenesis /sī′tōhis′tōjen″əsis/ [Gk, *kytos* + *histos,* tissue, *genein,* to produce], the structural development and formation of cells. −*cytohistogenetic, adj.*

cytohyaloplasm, *(Obsolete)* now called **hyaloplasm.**

cytoid /sī′toid/ [Gk, *kytos* + *eidos,* form], like a cell.

cytoid body, a small white spot on the retina of each eye seen by using an ophthalmoscope to examine the eyes; often noted in patients affected with systemic lupus erythematosus.

cytokerastic /sī′tōkəras″tik/ [Gk, *kytos* + *kerastos,* mixed], pertaining to or characteristic of cellular development from a simple to a more complex arrangement.

cytokine /sī′təkīn/, one of a large group of low–molecular-weight proteins secreted by various cell types and involved in cell-to-cell communication, coordinating antibody and

Types and functions of cytokines

Type	Primary functions
Interleukins (ILs)	
IL-1	Augments the immune response; inflammatory mediator; promotes maturation and clonal expansion of B cells; enhances activity of NK cells; activates T cells, activates macrophages
IL-2	Induces proliferation and differentiation of T cells; activation of T cells, NK cells, and macrophages; stimulates release of other cytokines (α-IFN, TNF, IL-1, IL-6)
IL-3 (multicolony colony-stimulating factor)	Hematopoietic growth factor for hematopoietic precursor cells
IL-4	B-cell growth factor; stimulates proliferation and differentiation of B cells; induces differentiation into T_H2 cells; stimulates growth of mast cells
IL-5	B cell growth and differentiation; promotes growth and differentiation of eosinophils
IL-6	T- and B-cell growth factor; enhances the inflammatory response; promotes differentiation of B cells into plasma cells; stimulates antibody secretion; induces fever; synergistic effects with IL-1 and TNF
IL-7	Promotes growth of T and B cells
IL-8	Chemotaxis of neutrophils and T cells; stimulates superoxide and granule release
IL-9	Enhances T-cell survival; mast cell activation
IL-10	Inhibits cytokine production by T and NK cells; promotes B-cell proliferation and antibody responses; potent suppressor of macrophage function
IL-11	Synergistic action with IL-3 and IL-4 in hematopoiesis; is a multifunctional regulator of hematopoiesis and lymphopoiesis; osteoclast formation; elevates platelet count; inhibits proinflammatory cytokine production
IL-12	Promotes α-IFN production; induction of T helper cells; activates NK cells; stimulates proliferation of activated T and NK cells
IL-13	B cell growth and differentiation; inhibits proinflammatory cytokine production
IL-14	Stimulates proliferation of activated B cells
IL-15	Mimics IL-2 effects; stimulates proliferation of T cells and NK cells
IL-16	Proinflammatory cytokine; chemoattractant of T cells, eosinophils, and monocytes
IL-17	Promotes release of IL-6, IL-8, and G-CSF; enhances expression of adhesion molecules. Associated with the Th17 response.
IL-18	Induces α-IFN, IL-2, and GM-CSF production; important role in development of T helper cells; enhances NK activity; inhibits production of IL-10
IL-19	Similar to IL-10
IL-20	Similar to IL-10
IL-21	Similar to IL-2, IL-4, and IL-5
IL-22	Similar to IL-10
IL-23	Similar to IL-12; promotes memory T cell proliferation
IL-24	Similar to IL-10
IL-25	Promotes T_H2 cytokine production
IL-26	Similar to IL-10
IL-27	Similar to IL-12
Interferons (IFNs)	
α-Interferon (α-IFN)	Type 1 interferon. Inhibits viral replication; activates NK cells and macrophages; antiproliferative effects on tumor cells.
β-Interferon (β-IFN)	Type 1 interferon. Produced by fibroblasts and has antiviral activity. Used in treatment of multiple sclerosis.
γ-Interferon (γ-IFN)	Type 2 interferon. Activates macrophages, neutrophils, and NK cells; promotes B cell differentiation; inhibits viral replication. Hallmark cytokine of a Th1 reaction.
Tumor necrosis factor (TNF)	Activates macrophages and granulocytes; promotes the immune and inflammatory responses; kills tumor cells; is responsible for extensive weight loss associated with chronic inflammation and cancer
Colony-stimulating factors (CSFs)	
Granulocyte colony-stimulating factor (G-CSF)	Stimulates proliferation and differentiation of neutrophils; enhances functional activity of mature PMNs
Granulocyte-macrophage colony-stimulating factor (GM-CSF)	Stimulates proliferation and differentiation of PMNs and monocytes
Macrophage colony-stimulating factor (M-CSF)	Promotes proliferation, differentiation, and activation of monocytes and macrophages
Erythropoietin	Stimulates erythroid progenitor cells in bone marrow to produce red blood cells

NK, Natural killer; *PMN,* polymorphonuclear neutrophil.

Modified from Lewis SL et al: *Medical-surgical nursing: assessment and management of clinical problems,* ed 8, St. Louis, 2011, Mosby.

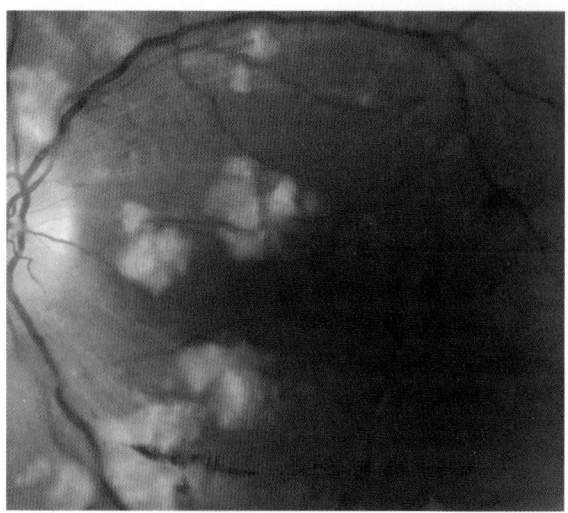

Cytoid body *(Kanski and Bowling, 2011)*

T-cell immune interactions and regulating immune reactivity. Kinds include **interferon, interleukin, lymphokine.**

cytokine assay, a blood test to detect interleukins, used predominantly for research. Clinically, cytokine assays may be used to measure the progression of inflammatory disease, AIDS, and various malignancies; determine disease risk; determine treatment of disease; and monitor patients receiving cytokine or anticytokine therapy.

cytokine network, a group of cytokines that modulate and regulate signaling between cells during an immune response.

cytokinesis /sī'tōkinē"sis, -kīnē"sis/ [Gk, *kytos + kinesis,* movement], the division of the cytoplasm, exclusive of nuclear division, that occurs during the final stages of mitosis and meiosis to form daughter cells. See also **karyokinesis.** *−cytokinetic, adj.*

cytological map [Gk, *kytos + logos,* science; L, *mappa,* table napkin], a graphic representation of the location of genes on a chromosome, based on correlating the genetic recombination results of testcrosses with the structural analysis of chromosomes that have undergone changes, such as deletions or translocations, as detected by banding techniques.

cytological sputum examination, a microscopic examination of a specimen of bronchial secretions, including a search for cells that may be cancerous or otherwise abnormal.

cytologic, cytological. See **cytology.**

cytologist /sītol"əjist/, a biologist who specializes in the study of cells, especially one who uses cytological techniques in the differential diagnosis of neoplasms.

cytology /sītol"əjē/ [Gk, *kytos + logos,* science], the study of cells, including their formation, origin, structure, function, biochemical activities, and pathological characteristics. Also called **cell biology.** Kinds include **aspiration biopsy cytology, exfoliative cytology.** *−cytologic, cytological, adj.*

cytolymph. See **hyaloplasm.**

cytolyses. See **cytolysis.**

cytolysin /sītol"isin/ [Gk, *kytos + lyein,* to loosen], an antibody that dissolves antigenic cells. Kinds include **bacteriolysin, hemolysin.**

cytolysis /sītol"isis/ *pl. cytolyses* [Gk, *kytos + lyein,* to loosen], the destruction or breakdown of cells, primarily by the disintegration of the plasma membrane. Kinds include **immune cytolysis.** *−cytolytic, adj.*

cytomegalic /sī'tōmegal"ik/, describing a condition characterized by abnormally large cells.

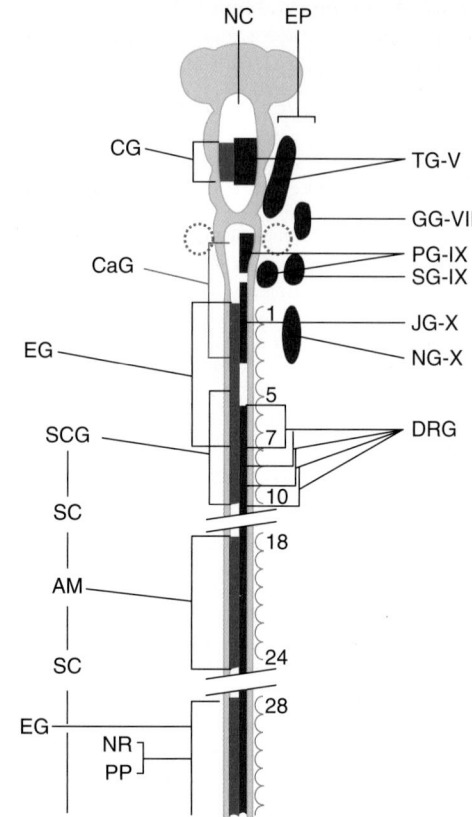

Cytological map *(Squire, 2009)*

cytomegalic inclusion disease (CID) [Gk, *kytos + megas,* large; L, *in, claudere,* in enclosure], a viral infection caused by cytomegalovirus (CMV), a member of the herpesvirus family. There are three forms: CMV inclusion disease of the newborn; acute acquired CMV infection, which is similar to infectious mononucleosis; and CMV in immunocompromised persons. See also **TORCH syndrome.**

■ OBSERVATIONS: Symptoms depend on the type of CID. When acquired in utero, results may range from spontaneous abortion or fatal neonatal illness to birth of a normal infant, depending on such factors as the virulence of the viral strain, fetal age when infected, and primary or recurrent nature of the mother's infection. About 10% of newborns with congenital CMV show clinical signs, such as microcephaly, delayed growth, hepatosplenomegaly, hemolytic anemia, and pathological fracture of long bones. In 5% to 25% of asymptomatic infections, infants develop significant psychomotor, hearing, ocular, or dental abnormalities. In adults, it is often characterized by malaise, fever, lymphadenopathy, pneumonia, hepatosplenomegaly, and superinfection with various bacteria and fungi as a result of the depression of immune response characteristic of herpesviruses.

■ INTERVENTIONS: Good hygiene is recommended to avoid transmission. Women who work with young children and are pregnant or planning to become pregnant are at high risk, especially if their first CMV infection is acquired during pregnancy. Antiviral drugs such as ganciclovir and acyclovir are used in immunocompromised patients to prevent infection or reduce viral load in infected patients.

■ PATIENT CARE CONSIDERATIONS: CMV infections associated with organ transplant are now treated with cytomegalovirus immune globulin intravenous (human) (CMV IGIV). It is now also used for prophylaxis.

Cytomegalovirus /sī'tōmeg'əlōvī'rəs/ [Gk, *kytos* + *megas,* large; L, *virus,* poison], a member of a group of large species–specific herpes–type viruses with a wide variety of disease effects. Infection results in characteristically enlarged cells with intranuclear inclusions. Opportunistic infection with this virus is common in immunocompromised individuals, causing clinical illnesses such as cytomegalovirus retinitis, pneumonia, esophagitis, colitis, adrenalitis, and hepatitis. It can also cause cytomegalic inclusion disease, a variety of gastrointestinal infections, and encephalitis. See also **cytomegalic inclusion disease, TORCH syndrome.**

cytomegalovirus disease. See **cytomegalic inclusion disease.**

cytomegalovirus (CMV) test, a blood test for CMV infection.

cytomegalovirus immune globulin, a purified immunoglobulin derived from pooled adult human plasma selected for high titers of antibody against cytomegalovirus. It is administered intravenously for treatment and prophylaxis of cytomegalovirus disease in transplant recipients.

cytomegaly /cītōmeg'älē/, abnormal enlargement of a cell or group of cells.

Cytomel, a thyroid hormone. Brand name for **liothyronine sodium.**

cytometer /sītom″ətər/ [Gk, *kytos* + *metron,* measure], a device for counting and measuring the number of cells within a specified amount of fluid, such as blood, urine, or cerebrospinal fluid.

cytometry /sītom″ətrē/, the counting and measuring of cells, specifically blood cells. −cytometric, *adj.*

cytomitome /sī'təmī″tōm/ [Gk, *kytos* + *mitos,* thread], the fibrillary network within the cytoplasm of a cell, as contrasted with that inside the nucleus. See also **karyomitome.**

cytomorphology /-môrfol″əjē/ [Gk, *kytos* + *morphe,* shape, *logos,* science], the study of the various forms of cells and the structures contained within cells. −cytomorphological, *cytomorphologic, adj.,* −cytomorphologist, *n.*

cytomorphosis /sī'tōmôr″fəsis/ [Gk, *kytos* + *morphosis,* shaping], the various changes that occur within a cell during the entire course of its life cycle.

cyton. See **perikaryon.**

cytopathic /-path″ik/, pertaining to the effect of disease or another disorder on a cell, such as damage from a virus or nuclear radiation.

cytopathogenic effect /-path′əjen″ik/, the degenerative or morphological changes in a cultured cell caused by cytopathic damage, including chromosomal aberrations, membrane permeability, and protein synthesis. The damage is especially associated with the multiplication of certain viruses.

cytopathological /sītōpath′olojikal/, relating to, or characterizing, cytopathology.

cytopathology /-pathol″əjē/, the study of changes at the cellular level caused by disease.

cytopenia /-pē″nē·ə/ [Gk, *kytos* + *penes,* poor], a deficiency in numbers of the blood cell elements.

cytophagy /sītof″əjē/, cell destruction by phagocytes.

cytophotometer /sī'tōfətom″ətər/ [Gk, *kytos* + *phos,* light, *metron,* measure], an instrument for measuring light density through stained portions of cytoplasm, used for locating and identifying chemical substances within cells.

cytophotometry /sī'tōfətom″ətrē/, the identification of chemical substances within cells by using a cytophotometer. Also called **microfluorometry.** −cytophotometric, *adj.*

cytophysiology /-fis′ē·ol′əjē/ [Gk, *kytos* + *physis,* nature, *logos,* science], the study of the biochemical processes involved in the functioning of individual cells. −cytophysiological, *cytophysiologic, adj.,* −cytophysiologist, *n.*

cytoplasm /sī″təplaz′əm/ [Gk, *kytos* + *plassein,* to mold], all of the substance of a cell other than the nucleus and the cell wall. See also **cell, nucleus.**

cytoplasmic bridge. See **intercellular bridge.**

cytoplasmic inheritance /sī'tōplaz″mik/, the acquisition of traits or conditions controlled by self-replicating substances within the cytoplasm, such as mitochondria or chloroplasts, rather than by genes on the chromosomes in the nucleus. The phenomenon occurs in plants and some animals but has not been demonstrated in humans.

Cytosar-U, an antineoplastic medication. Brand name for **cytarabine.**

cytoscopy /sītos″kəpē/ [Gk, *kytos* + *skopein,* to watch], the diagnostic study of cells obtained from patient specimens with the aid of microscopes and other laboratory equipment.

cytosine (C) /sī″təsin/, a pyrimidine base that is a component of DNA and RNA. In free or uncombined form it occurs in trace amounts in most cells, usually as a product of the enzymatic hydrolysis of nucleic acids and nucleotides. On hydrolysis, it is converted to urea and ammonia. See also **thymine, uracil.**

cytosine arabinoside. See **cytarabine.**

cytosis /sītō″sis/, a condition in which there is a greater than normal number of cells in a tissue or organ.

cytoskeleton /-skel″ətən/ [Gk, *kytos* + *skeletos,* dried body], the cytoplasmic elements that function as a supportive system within a cell, especially an epithelial cell. The cytoskeleton has three main components: microfilaments, microtubules, and intermediate filaments.

cytosol /sī′tōsôl/, the liquid medium of the cytoplasm (i.e., cytoplasm minus organelles and nonmembranous insoluble components).

cytosome /sī″təsōm/, a multilayered, membrane-bound, lamellar body found in type II pneumocytes. It is a precursor of pulmonary surfactant.

cytotechnologist, an allied health professional who works with a pathologist to detect changes in body cells that may be important in early diagnosis of cancer and other diseases. The cytotechnologist prepares cellular samples and examines them under a microscope to evaluate for abnormalities in structure.

cytotoxic. See **cytotoxin.**

cytotoxic anaphylaxis [Gk, *kytos* + *toxikon,* poison, *hyper,* above], complement-dependent hypersensitivity to foreign cells or to alterations of cell-surface antigens that is mediated by immunoglobulin G (IgG) or M (IgM). It causes immediate destruction of cells, as seen in hemolytic disease of the newborn and in severe transfusion reactions. Also called **cytotoxic hypersensitivity, type II hypersensitivity.** Compare **anaphylactic hypersensitivity, immunocomplex hypersensitivity.** See also **immune gamma globulin.**

cytotoxic drug, any pharmacological compound that inhibits the proliferation of cells within the body. Such compounds as the alkylating agents and the antimetabolites designed to destroy cells (with a high growth fraction) are commonly used in chemotherapy. Cytotoxic agents have a potential for producing teratogenesis, mutagenesis, and carcinogenesis.

cytotoxic hypersensitivity. See **cytotoxic anaphylaxis.**

cytotoxic hypersensitivity reaction. See **hypersensitivity reaction.**

cytotoxic killer T cell, an antigen-stimulated activated CD8 T cell. See also **CD4, CD8 cell.**

cytotoxic T cell, a T cell that has the capacity of killing other cells. Most cytotoxic T cells are major histocompatibility complex (MHC) molecules class I restricted CD8 T cells. In very particular cases, CD4 T cells can also kill. Formerly called **cytotoxic killer T cell.** See **CD8 cell.**

cytotoxic T lymphocytes [L, *natura* + ME, *kullen,* to kill, *cella,* storeroom], antigen-stimulated activated CD8 T cells.

cytotoxin /sī′tōtok″sin/ [Gk, *kytos* + *toxikon,* poison], a substance that has a toxic effect on certain cells. An antibody may act as a cytotoxin. −**cytotoxic,** *adj.*

cytotrophoblast /sī′tōtrof″əblast′/ [Gk, *kytos* + *trophe,* nutrition, *blastos,* germ], the inner layer of cells of the trophoblast of the early mammalian embryo that gives rise to the outer surface and villi of the chorion. Also called **Langhans layer.** Compare **syncytiotrophoblast.** −*cytotrophoblastic, adj.*

cytotropism /sī′tōtrop″izm/, a characteristic of some cells and agents that enables them to approach other cells or selectively bind to them.

Cytovene, an antiviral drug. Brand name for **ganciclovir.**

Cytoxan, an antineoplastic drug. Brand name for **cyclophosphamide.**

CYVADIC, an anticancer drug combination of cyclophosphamide, vinCRIStine, DOXOrubicin, and dacarbazine.

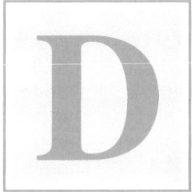

D

d, **1.** symbol for **deciduous dentition. 2.** abbreviation for **deuterium. 3.** abbreviation for **density. 4.** abbreviation for **death. 5.** abbreviation for **diopter. 6.** abbreviation for **dose. 7.** symbol for **deci-. 8.** abbreviation for **diameter. 9.** symbol for *one-tenth.*

D, **1.** symbol for *dead space gas.* **2.** symbol for **diffusing capacity. 3.** abbreviation for **diopter. 4.** abbreviation for **dexter. 5.** abbreviation for **vitamin D. 6.** symbol for **density. 7.** symbol for **diameter.**

d4T, symbol for *dideoxythymidine.*

Da, symbol for **dalton.**

DA, abbreviation for **developmental age.**

daboia /dəboi′ə/ [Hind, *dabna,* to lurk], a local name for Russell's viper, a large, very poisonous snake indigenous to India and Southeast Asia. Its venom is used in some laboratories to test the coagulation pathway.

dacarbazine /dekär″bəzēn/, an alkylating agent used as an antineoplastic drug.

■ INDICATIONS: It is prescribed primarily in the treatment of malignant melanoma and Hodgkin's disease.

■ ADVERSE EFFECTS: Among the more serious adverse reactions are bone marrow depression, GI symptoms, kidney and liver impairment, alopecia, and fever.

daclizumab, an immunosuppressant.

■ INDICATIONS: It is used to help prevent acute allograft rejection in renal transplant patients.

■ CONTRAINDICATIONS: Known hypersensitivity to this drug contraindicates its use.

■ ADVERSE EFFECTS: Life-threatening effects are pulmonary edema, tachycardia, thrombosis, renal tubular necrosis, and hydronephrosis. Other adverse effects include headache, prickly sensation, coughing, atelectasis, congestion, constipation, abdominal pain, pyrosis, hypertension, bleeding, oliguria, dysuria, renal damage, and impaired wound healing. Common side effects include chills, tremors, dyspnea, wheezing, vomiting, nausea, and diarrhea.

Dacogen, brand name for **decitabine.**

D/A converter. Also called *DAC, D2A* converter, *D-to-A* converter. See **digital-to-analog converter.**

dacrocystorhinotomy (DCR), the establishment of a new lacrimal duct for direct drainage into the nasal cavity to treat dacryocystitis resistant to antibiotic treatment.

Dacron cuff, a sheath of Dacron surrounding an atrial or venous catheter to prevent accidental displacement.

dacryadenitis. See **dacryoadenitis.**

dacryo-, dacry-, prefix meaning "tears": *dacryoadenitis, dacryocystectomy, dacryostenosis.*

dacryoadenitis /dak′rē·ō·ad′ənī″tis/, an inflammation of the lacrimal gland. The condition may be seen in a mumps infection that involves a lacrimal gland. Also called **dacryadenitis.**

dacryocyst /dak″re·ōsist′/ [Gk, *dakryon,* tear, *kytis,* bag], a lacrimal sac at the medial angle of the eye.

dacryocystectomy /dak′rē·ōsistek″təmē/ [Gk, *dakryon* + *kytis,* bag, *ektomē,* excision], partial or total excision of the lacrimal sac.

dacryocystitis /dak′rē·ōsistī″tis/, an infection of the lacrimal sac caused by obstruction of the nasolacrimal duct. It can be chronic or acute and is congenital in some cases. It is characterized by tearing and discharge from the eye. In the acute phase the sac becomes inflamed and painful. The disorder is nearly always unilateral and usually occurs in infants. It occurs on the left side more commonly than on the right because of the structure of the lacrimal sac. Systemic administration of antibiotics is usual; local topical treatment is seldom effective; rarely a dacryocystorhinostomy may be required. Compare **dacryostenosis.**

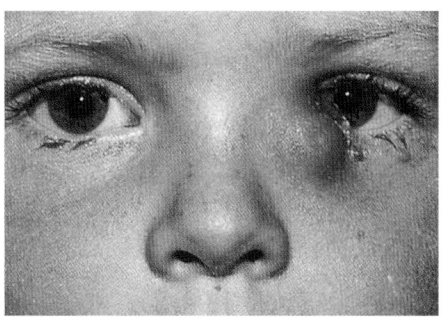

Child with dacryocystitis *(Zitelli et al, 2012)*

dacryocystorhinostomy /dak′rē·ōsis′tôrīnos″təmē/ [Gk, *dakryon* + *kytis,* bag, *rhis,* nose, *stoma,* mouth], a surgical procedure for restoring drainage into the nose from the lacrimal sac when the nasolacrimal duct is obstructed.

dacryon. See **tears.**

dacryostenosis /dak′rē·ōstinō″sis/ [Gk, *dakryon* + *stenos,* narrow, *osis,* condition], an abnormal stricture of the nasolacrimal duct, occurring either as a congenital condition or as a result of infection or trauma. Dacryocystorhinostomy may be required to correct this condition. Compare **dacryocystitis.**

dactinomycin /dak′tinōmī″sin/, an antibiotic used as an antineoplastic agent.

■ INDICATIONS: It is prescribed in the treatment of a variety of malignant neoplastic diseases, including testicular cancer, melanoma, Wilms' tumor, and rhabdomyosarcoma.

■ CONTRAINDICATIONS: Herpes zoster infection, chickenpox, or known hypersensitivity to this drug prohibits its use.

■ ADVERSE EFFECTS: Among the more serious adverse reactions are bone marrow depression, severe GI disturbances, proctitis, alopecia, and ulcers of the mouth.

dactyl /dak″til/ [Gk, *daktylos,* finger], a digit (finger or toe). **–dactylic,** *adj.*

dactyl-. See **dactylo-, dactyl-.**

-dactyly, suffix meaning "digit (finger or toe)": *arachnodactyly, pachydactyly.*

dactyledema /dak′tilidē″mə/, swelling of the fingers or toes.

-dactylia, suffix meaning "(condition of the) fingers or toes": *perodactylia, syndactylia.*

dactylic. See **dactyl.**

dactylion /daktil″ē·on/, a condition of complete or partial webbing of fingers.

dactylitis /dak′tilī″tis/, **1.** a painful inflammation of the fingers or toes, usually associated with sickle cell anemia or certain infectious diseases, particularly syphilis or tuberculosis. **2.** a sausage-shaped digit associated with psoriatic arthritis.

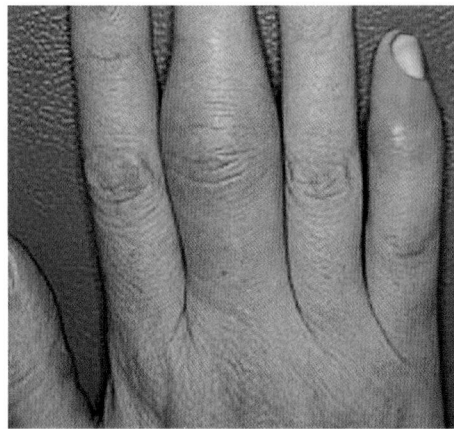

Dactylitis (Zitelli and Davis, 2007)

dactylo-, dactyl-, prefix meaning "finger" or "toe": *dactylion, dactyledema, dactylitis.*

DAF, abbreviation for *decay-accelerating factor.*

DAI, abbreviation for **diffuse axonal injury.**

daily adjusted progressive resistance exercise (DAPRE), a program of isotonic exercises that allows for individual differences in the rate at which a patient regains strength in an injured or diseased body part.

daily living skills, routine tasks and social skills required for care for one's self, usually acquired and developed from childhood into adulthood. See also **activities of daily living.**

Daily Reference Values (DRVs), a set of dietary standards applicable to adults and children over the age of 4 for eight nutrients and food compartments: total fat, saturated fat, cholesterol, total carbohydrates, dietary fiber, protein, potassium, and sodium. They are part of the U.S. Food and Drug Administration Daily Value label reference.

dairy food substitute, a group of foods that includes imitation cream; soy, almond, and rice milk; and dairy-free butter spreads. Although similar in taste and texture to genuine dairy products, nondairy products can differ markedly in composition from the products they resemble. They are consumed by individuals with allergies, as a component of a vegan diet, or for other health concerns.

Dakin's solution [Henry D. Dakin, American biochemist, 1880–1952; L, *solutus,* dissolved], an antiseptic solution containing boric acid and 0.4% to 0.5% of sodium hypochlorite, used in a dilute solution for wound irrigation and for treatment of athlete's foot.

dalfopristin /dalfo′pristin/, a semisynthetic antibacterial effective against a variety of gram-positive organisms. It is used in conjunction with quinupristin in the treatment of serious bacteremia caused by vancomycin-resistant *Enterococcus faecium* and complicated skin and skin structure infections caused by *Streptococcus pyogenes* or methicillin-sensitive *Staphylococcus aureus*; it is administered intravenously.

Dalmane, a benzodiazepine sedative-hypnotic drug. Brand name for **flurazepam hydrochloride.**

dalteparin sodium, a low-molecular-weight heparin.
■ INDICATIONS: It is prescribed to prevent deep vein thrombosis in adults undergoing abdominal surgery who are at risk for clotting. It is also used for the treatment of unstable angina and non–Q-wave myocardial infarction to prevent ischemic complications in patients with concurrent aspirin therapy.
■ CONTRAINDICATIONS: It should not be given to patients with allergy to dalteparin, heparin, or pork products or to patients with certain blood disorders.
■ ADVERSE EFFECTS: The side effects most often reported include heavy or unusual bleeding, black stools, or bruising or pain at the site of injection.

dalton [John Dalton, English chemist and mathematician, 1766–1844], **1.** an unofficial unit of atomic mass that was based on $\frac{1}{16}$ of the gram mass of oxygen until 1961; it is now based on $\frac{1}{12}$ the mass of carbon-12. Also called **atomic mass unit. 2.** (in biochemistry) unit (kilodaltons) that expresses the molecular weight (mass) of proteins and nucleic acids.

daltonism /dôl″təniz′əm/ [John Dalton], (*Informal*) a form of red-green color blindness. It is genetically transmitted as a sex-linked autosomal-recessive trait.

Dalton's law of partial pressures /dôl″tənz/ [John Dalton, English chemist and mathematician, 1766–1844], (in physics) a law stating that, in a mixture of nonreacting gases, the total pressure exerted is equal to the sum of the partial pressures of the individual gases in the same quantity at the same temperature. See also **Avogadro's law, Boyle's law, Gay-Lussac's law.**

dam, a barrier to the flow of fluid, as a dam placed around a tooth to protect it from saliva and bacteria during restoration. See also **rubber dam.**

damages /dam′ijəs/ [L, *damnum,* loss], (in law) a sum of money awarded to a plaintiff by a court as compensation for any loss, detriment, or injury to the plaintiff's person, property, or rights caused by the malfeasance or negligence of the defendant. Actual damages are awarded to reimburse the plaintiff for the loss or injury sustained. Nominal damages are awarded to show that a legal wrong has been committed although no recoverable loss can be determined. Punitive damages exceed the actual cost of injury or damage and are awarded when the defendant has acted with malice or reckless disregard of the plaintiff's rights.

damp [AS, vapor], a potentially lethal atmosphere in caves and mines. Kinds include **black damp, choke damp, fire damp, white damp.**

damping [AS, vapor], a gradual decrease in the amplitude of a series of waves or oscillations, such as an arterial pressure waveform.

danaparoid, an anticoagulant.
■ INDICATIONS: It is used to prevent vein thrombosis in hemodialysis, stroke, elective surgery for malignancy or total hip replacement, and hip fracture surgery.
■ CONTRAINDICATIONS: Hypersensitivity to this drug, sulfites, or pork products prohibits its use. Other factors that contraindicate its use include hemophilia, leukemia with bleeding, thrombocytopenia, purpura, cerebrovascular hemorrhage, cerebral aneurysm, severe hypertension, and other severe cardiac disease.
■ ADVERSE EFFECTS: Life-threatening side effects include hemorrhage and thrombocytopenia. Hypersensitivity reactions and rash are additional adverse effects.

danazol /dan″əzol/, a synthetic androgen that acts to suppress the output of gonadotropins from the pituitary, suppress ovarian hormone production, and directly block ovarian hormone receptors.
■ INDICATIONS: It is prescribed in the treatment of endometriosis, fibrocystic breast disease, and hereditary angioedema

when alternative hormonal therapy is ineffective, contraindicated, or intolerable.

■ CONTRAINDICATIONS: Genital bleeding; cardiac, liver, or kidney dysfunction; or known hypersensitivity to this drug prohibits its use. It is not prescribed during pregnancy or lactation.

■ ADVERSE EFFECTS: Among the most serious adverse reactions are muscle spasms, nausea, weight gain, acne, edema, oily skin, voice changes, and other androgenic effects.

dance/movement therapy (DMT), **1.** (in psychology), a movement-based therapeutic technique that aids in release of expressions or feelings and aids in promoting feeling and awareness. It is an intimate and powerful medium for therapy because it is a direct expression of the mind and body. **2.** (in occupational therapy) a creative art therapy that can be conducted individually or in groups to facilitate emotional, cognitive, and physical integration. Goals may include promotion of body awareness or improvements in self-control and in the communication of emotions.

dance reflex [ME, *dauncen* + L, *reflectere,* to bend back], a normal response in the neonate to simulate walking by a reciprocal flexion and extension of the legs when held in an erect position and inclined forward with the soles touching a hard surface. The reflex disappears by about 3 to 6 weeks of age and is replaced by controlled, deliberate movement. Also called **step reflex, stepping reflex.**

dander, dry scales shed from the scalp of humans or the skin of animals with fur. Allergies to animals are frequently the result of the animal's dander.

dandruff /dan″druf/, an excessive amount of scaly material composed of dead, keratinized epithelium shed from the scalp that may be a mild form of seborrheic dermatitis or psoriasis. Treatment with a keratolytic shampoo is usually recommended to soften and remove the scales.

dandy fever. See **dengue fever.**

Dandy-Walker cyst [Walter E. Dandy, American neurosurgeon, 1886–1946; Arthur E. Walker, American surgeon, 1907–1995], a cystic malformation of the fourth ventricle of the brain resulting from hydrocephalus. Diagnosis of the defect is made with computed tomographic scan, x-ray films, and less commonly a ventriculogram. Also called *Dandy-Walker malformation.* See also **hydrocephalus, shunt.**

Danocrine, an anterior pituitary suppressant. Brand name for **danazol.**

danthron /dan″thron/, a stimulant laxative. Products containing danthron are no longer available in the United States and Canada since it was found to be carcinogenic in animal models.

Dantrium, a skeletal muscle relaxant used in the treatment of malignant hyperthermia or malignant hyperpyrexia. Brand name for **dantrolene sodium.** See also **Ryanodex.**

dantrolene sodium /dan″trəlēn/, a skeletal muscle relaxant that acts directly on the skeletal muscle to prevent the release of calcium from the sarcoplasmic reticulum that is needed for muscle contraction.

■ INDICATIONS: It is prescribed in the treatment of muscle spasticity resulting from injury to the spinal cord or cerebrum when the person is immobile and flaccid limbs are preferable to spastic limbs. It is not indicated in treatment of spasm from rheumatic disorders. It is used intravenously for the management of malignant hyperthermia.

■ CONTRAINDICATIONS: Dantrolene should not be used when spastic muscles are needed to maintain posture or balance. Liver dysfunction or known hypersensitivity to this drug also prohibits its use.

■ ADVERSE EFFECTS: The most serious adverse reaction is potentially fatal hepatotoxicity. Common reactions include confusion, drowsiness, diarrhea, dizziness, fatigue, and

muscular weakness. Side effects may continue for several days.

DAP, **1.** abbreviation for **Draw-a-Person Test. 2.** abbreviation for **dose area product.**

dapiprazole /däpip′räzōl/, an alpha-adrenergic blocking agent used topically on the conjunctiva as the hydrochloride salt to reverse pharmacologically induced mydriasis.

DAPRE, abbreviation for **daily adjusted progressive resistance exercise.**

dapsone (DDS) /dap″sōn/, a bacteriostatic and bactericidal sulfone derivative.

■ INDICATIONS: It is prescribed in the treatment of leprosy and dermatitis herpetiformis and for prophylaxis against toxoplasmosis and *Pneumocystis carinii* in immunocompromised patients.

■ CONTRAINDICATIONS: Known hypersensitivity to this drug prohibits its use. It is not recommended for use during pregnancy or lactation.

■ ADVERSE EFFECTS: Among the more serious adverse reactions are hemolysis (particularly in people who have glucose-6-phosphate dehydrogenase deficiency), leprosy reactional state, methemoglobinemia, neuropathy, nausea, anorexia, toxic hepatic aplastic anemia, and skin rash. Dapsone was carcinogenic in animal models.

-dapsone, suffix designating a diaminodiphenylsulfone-derivative antimycobacterial agent.

daptomycin, a miscellaneous antiinfective agent.

■ INDICATIONS: This drug is used to treat complicated skin and skin structure infections caused by *Staphylococcus aureus* (including methicillin-resistant strains), *S. agalactiae, S. dysgalactiae,* and *Enterococcus faecalis* (vancomycin-susceptible strains only).

■ CONTRAINDICATIONS: Known hypersensitivity to this drug prohibits its use.

■ ADVERSE EFFECTS: Adverse effects of this drug include hypotension, hypertension, increased creatinine phosphokinase, nausea, constipation, diarrhea, vomiting, dyspepsia, headache, insomnia, dizziness, muscle pain or weakness, arthralgia, fungal infection, urinary tract infection, anemia, nephrotoxicity, rash, and pruritus. A life-threatening side effect is pseudomembranous colitis.

Daraprim, an antimalarial drug. Brand name for **pyrimethamine.**

darbepoetin alfa, a hematopoietic agent used to treat anemia associated with chronic renal failure or anemia in nonmyeloid malignancies.

Darbid, an anticholinergic drug. Brand name for *isopropamide iodide.*

Darier disease [Ferdinand-Jean Darier, French dermatologist, 1856–1938], an autosomal-dominant skin disorder. Also called **keratosis follicularis.**

Darier sign /däryā″/ [Ferdinand-Jean Darier, French dermatologist, 1856–1938], a burning or itching sensation induced by stroking skin lesions in cases of urticaria pigmentosa. The area may become raised and red due to mast cell degranulation.

dark adaptation, a normal increase in sensitivity of the retinal rod cells of the eye to detect any light that may be available for vision in a dimly lighted environment. The process is accompanied by an adjustment of the pupils to allow more light to enter the eyes.

darkfield microscopy [AS, *deorc,* hidden, *feld,* field; Gk, *mikros,* small, *skopein,* to look], examination of a microscopic specimen illuminated by a peripheral light source. The illumination causes the specimen to appear to glow against a dark background. In laboratory diagnosis, the technique is used primarily to identify the syphilis spirochete. Also called *darkfield illumination.* See also **ultramicroscopy.**

D

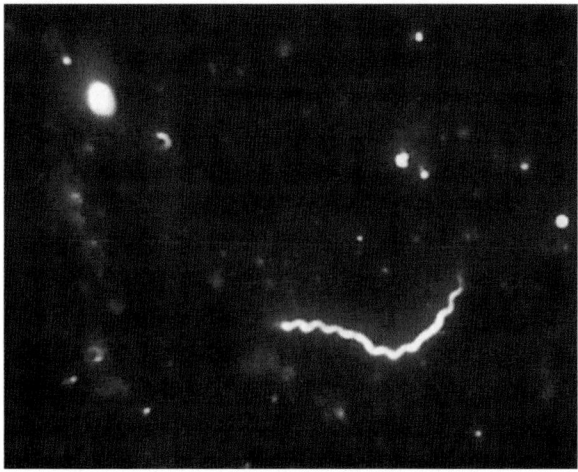

Darkfield microscopy: positive examination
(Morse et al, 2003)

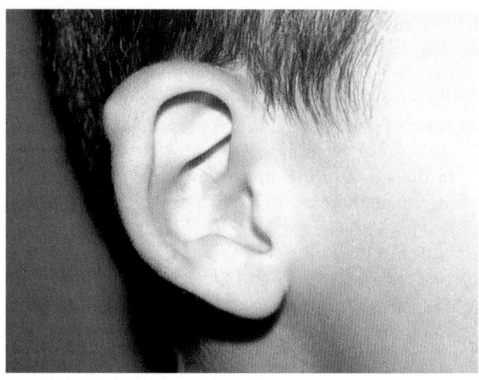

Darwinian ear *(Guyuron et al, 2009)*

Darwin's tubercle [Charles R. Darwin, English naturalist, 1809–1882]. See **auricular tubercle, darwinian ear.**

DAS, abbreviation for **data acquisition system.**

dasatinib, a miscellaneous antineoplastic drug.
- INDICATIONS: This drug is used to treat chronic myelogenous leukemia, accelerated blast crisis, and chronic phase and acute phase lymphoblastic leukemia.
- CONTRAINDICATIONS: Pregnancy and known hypersensitivity to this drug prohibit its use.
- ADVERSE EFFECTS: Adverse effects of this drug include headache, dizziness, insomnia, neuropathy, asthenia, arrhythmias, chest pain, congestive heart failure, pericardial effusion, constipation, diarrhea, GI bleeding, mucositis, stomatitis, fluid retention, edema, increased or decreased weight, pain, arthralgia, myalgia, cough, dyspnea, pulmonary edema and hypertension, pneumonia, and urinary tract infection. Life-threatening side effects include central nervous system hemorrhage, vomiting, neutropenia, thrombocytopenia, and bleeding. Common side effects include nausea, anorexia, abdominal pain, rash, and pruritus.

DASE, abbreviation for **Denver Articulation Screening Examination.**

DASH (Dietary Approach to Stop Hypertension) diet, a diet high in fruits, vegetables, and low-fat dairy products; low in saturated and total fats; low in cholesterol; and high in fiber. The diet is often described as the three plus five plan: three dairy, five fruits, and five vegetables per day. Research studies support the hypothesis that this diet reduces blood pressure and may play a role in the prevention of high blood pressure.

data /dā″tə, dat″ə, dä″tə/ *sing. datum* [L, *datum,* giving], **1.** pieces of information, especially those that are part of a collection to be used in an analysis of a problem, such as the diagnosis of a health problem. **2.** demographic details, clinical documentation, tests and test outcomes, and other information used in decision making and/or the development of models stored and processed by a computer.

data acquisition system (DAS), **1.** (in radiology) a radiation detection system that measures the amount of radiation passing through a patient and reaching the detector. The system converts analog signals to digital data that can be analyzed by a computer. **2.** (in computer processing) a collection of software and hardware that allows the measurement or control of physical characteristics of something in the real world. It involves the converting of samples into digital numeric values that can be manipulated by a computer.

data analysis, (in research) the phase of a study that includes classifying, coding, and tabulating information needed to perform quantitative or qualitative analyses according to the research design and appropriate to the data.

darkroom, a room in a hospital or similar facility for the storage and processing of light-sensitive materials.

Darling disease. See **histoplasmosis.**

dartoic tissue, tissue that resembles the tunica dartos, as in a tumor with muscular elements.

dartos fascia, the thin layer of subcutaneous tissue underlying the skin of the scrotum consisting mainly of nonstriated muscle fibers (the dartos muscle). Also called **tunica dartos,** *dartos.*

darunavir, an antiretroviral drug.
- INDICATIONS: This drug is used to inhibit HIV-1 protease by preventing maturation of the virus.
- CONTRAINDICATIONS: Known hypersensitivity to this drug prohibits its use.
- ADVERSE EFFECTS: Adverse effects of this drug include dizziness, somnolence, anorexia, dry mouth, nephrolithiasis, rash, pain, asthenia, hyperlipidemia, and lipodystrophy. Life-threatening side effects include insulin-resistant hyperglycemia and ketoacidosis. Common side effects include headache, insomnia, diarrhea, abdominal pain, nausea, and vomiting.

Darvocet-N, a fixed-combination drug containing an analgesic-antipyretic and an opioid analgesic. It was removed from the market worldwide because of serious adverse effects. Brand name for **acetaminophen,** *propoxyphene napsylate.*

Darvon, an opioid analgesic that was removed from the market worldwide because of serious adverse effects. Brand name for **propoxyphene hydrochloride.**

darwinian [Charles R. Darwin, English naturalist, 1809–1882], related to the theory of evolution and other theories of Charles Darwin.

darwinian ear /därwin″ē-ən/ [Charles R. Darwin, English naturalist, 1809–1882], an external ear with a thickening and/or point toward the top of the helix. It was first described by Charles Darwin as a vestigial structure retained through evolution. Also called **Darwin's tubercle, auricular tubercle.**

darwinian reflex [Charles R. Darwin, English naturalist, 1809–1882]. See **grasp reflex.**

darwinian theory [Charles R. Darwin, English naturalist, 1809–1882], a theory advanced by Charles Darwin that states that organic evolution results from the natural selection of those variants of organisms that are best suited to survive in their environments. Also called *darwinism.* Compare **lamarckism.** —**darwinian,** *adj.*

Data analysis follows collection of information and precedes its interpretation or application.

database, a store or bank of information in a form that can be processed by computer. It provides a mechanism for organizing large volumes of information, often categorically, to allow for more rapid retrieval and analysis.

data collection, (in research) the phase of a study that includes the gathering of information and identification of sampling units as directed by the research design. Data collection precedes data analysis.

data mining, the process of analyzing large, existing computerized data sets from different perspectives and summarizing them into useful information to gain new insights, discover new relationships, and identify patterns.

data processing, the techniques and practices involved in the manipulation of information by a computer.

data retrieval, the recovery of information from an organized filing system, such as a computer database or paper files.

dataset /dă″təset/, a collection of similar and related data for processing by computer.

data source, the origin of information relevant to a patient's level of wellness and health patterns.

data validation, the process of determining whether information gathered during the process of data collection is complete and accurate.

date/acquaintance rape, a sexual assault or rape by a person known to the victim, such as a date, employer, friend, or casual acquaintance. See also **rape.**

datum, a singular piece of information. See **data,** def. 1.

daughter cell [ME, *doughter,* female, child; L, *cella,* storeroom], one of the cells produced by the division of a parent cell.

daughter chromosome [ME, *doughter,* female, child; Gk, *chroma,* color, *soma,* body], either of the paired chromatids that separate and migrate to the opposite ends of the cell during the anaphase stage of mitosis. Each contains the complete genetic information of the original chromosome and is formed during interphase by the replication of the DNA in the chromosome.

daughter cyst, a small secondary parasitic cyst, usually a derivative of a hydatid cyst. See also **hydatid cyst.**

daughter element, an element that results from the radioactive decay of another element. For example, technetium-99 is the daughter element created by the decay of molybdenum-99.

daughter product. See **decay product.**

DAUNOrubicin citrate liposomal /dô′nōrōo″bisin/, an anthracycline antibiotic antineoplastic agent.
- INDICATIONS: It is prescribed in the treatment of advanced Kaposi's sarcoma in HIV patients.
- CONTRAINDICATIONS: Known hypersensitivity to this drug prohibits its use. It is also contraindicated in pregnancy, during lactations, and in patients with systemic infections or cardiac disease.
- ADVERSE EFFECTS: Serious adverse effects include chest pain and edema.

Davidoff's cells, epithelial cells. See **cells of Paneth.**

da Vinci Surgical System /də·vin′chē/, a proprietary robotic platform for minimally invasive surgery, consisting of a console, a patient-side cart to which a set of up to four electromechanical arms is attached, and a 3-D video display system. Instruments mounted on the robotic arms are introduced into the patient's body through minute incisions. The system translates the hand motions of the surgeon seated at the console into movements of the instruments inside the patient. The surgeon views the operative field through a 3-D camera attached to one of the arms. Cardiac, urological, gynecological, and colorectal surgeries are commonly performed using this system.

Davis ureterotomy [D.M. Davis, American urologist, 1887–1982], a procedure combining a ureteral incision with the placement of a stent, usually for long or multiple strictures below the ureteropelvic junction. The ureter heals to form a watertight closure over the stent, and the stent is then withdrawn.

DAWN /dôn/, abbreviation for **Drug Abuse Warning Network.**

dawn phenomenon [ME, *daunen* + Gk, *phainomenon,* anything seen], a tendency for persons with diabetes mellitus to experience hyperglycemia upon awakening in the morning because of increased cortisol and growth hormone secretion in the predawn hours. Compare **Somogyi effect.**

day blindness, vision difficulty in light. See **hemeralopia.**

day care [OE, *daeg* + *cearu*], a specialized program or facility that provides care for infants and preschool children, usually within a group framework. Day-care centers vary in size and function and range from neighborhood parent-supervised play groups to formal nursery schools or organized centers

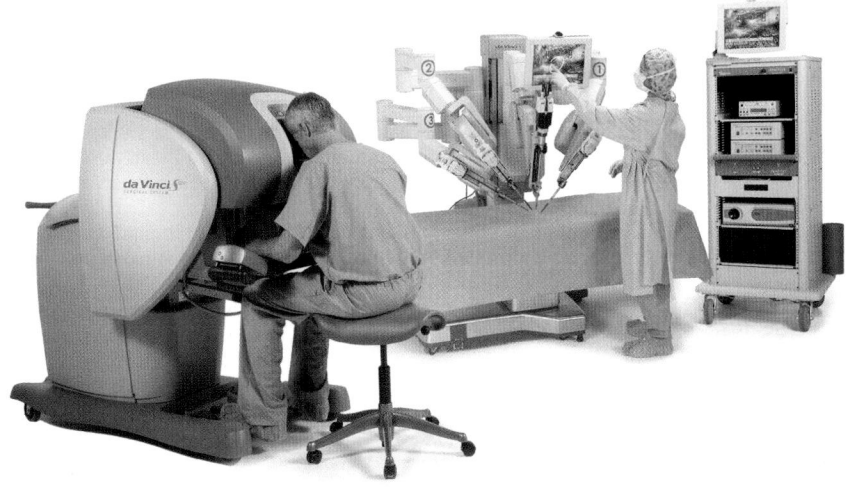

da Vinci Surgical System *(Copyright © 2015 Intuitive Surgical, Inc. All rights reserved.)*

run by trained personnel. Most day-care programs incorporate a daily schedule of play, outdoor activities, games and projects, creative or educational play, and snack and rest periods. Federal regulations require that states have policies in place for infection control, safety of the physical premises, and health and safety training appropriate to the setting. State policies in regard to these regulations vary.

daydream, a usually nonpathological reverie that occurs while a person is awake.

day health care services, the provision of hospitals, nursing homes, or other facilities for health-related services to adult patients who are ambulatory or can be transported and who regularly use such services for a certain number of daytime hours but do not require continuous inpatient care. See also **adult day-care center.**

day hospital [OE, *daeg* + L, *hospes,* guest], a psychiatric program that offers therapeutic activities during daytime hours for patients. See also **partial hospitalization program.**

day patient, a patient who does not require an overnight stay for treatment. Compare **inpatient.**

dB, abbreviation for **decibel.**

Db, symbol for the element **dubnium.**

D&C, abbreviation for **dilation and curettage.**

DC, abbreviation for **direct current.**

d/c, **1.** abbreviation for *discontinue.* **2.** abbreviation for **discharge.**

DCC gene, a gene normally expressed in the mucosa of the colon but reduced or absent in a small proportion of patients with colorectal cancer.

DCR, abbreviation for **dacrocystorhinotomy.**

DD, abbreviation for **developmental disability.**

DDAVP, an antidiuretic drug. Brand name for **desmopressin acetate.**

ddC, abbreviation for *2'3'-dideoxycytidine.* See **zalcitabine.**

DDD pacing, a specific type of electrical heart pacemaker mode. The letters indicate *D*ual pacing for both chambers, *D*ual chamber activity sensing, and *D*ual response (triggering and inhibition). Compare **VVI pacing.**

ddI, an antiretroviral medication. Abbreviation for *2',3'-dideoxyinosine.* See **dideoxyinosine.**

D-dimer test, a confirmatory test for disseminated intravascular coagulation that can also indicate when a clot is lysed by thrombolytic therapy. The fragment D-dimer assesses both thrombin and plasmin activity.

DDP, -DDP. See **cisplatin.**

D.D.S., abbreviation for *Doctor of Dental Surgery.* See also **dentist.**

DDST, abbreviation for **Denver Developmental Screening Test.**

DDT (dichlorodiphenyltrichloroethane), a nonbiodegradable water-insoluble chlorinated hydrocarbon once used worldwide as a major insecticide, especially in agriculture. In recent years knowledge of its adverse impact on the environment has led to restrictions in its use. In addition, because tolerance in formerly susceptible organisms develops rapidly, DDT has been largely replaced by organophosphate insecticides in the United States and Canada, where DDT was banned in the 1970s. It is still used as a pediculicide where epidemic-scale delousing is justified, as in barracks and refugee camps. Its value as a scabicide is marginal, because scabies and crab lice quickly become resistant to it. See also **scabicide.**

DDT poisoning. See **chlorinated organic insecticide poisoning.**

D&E, abbreviation for **dilation and evacuation.**

DE, abbreviation for **dose equivalent.**

de-, prefix meaning "to do the opposite," "away," "off," "to remove entirely," "down," or "from": *decapitation, decant, decay.*

DEA, abbreviation for **Drug Enforcement Agency.**

deactivation /dē·ak'tivā″shən/ [L, *de,* from, *activus,* active], the process of becoming or making something inactive or inoperable or removing it from use.

dead, pertaining to the absence of all vital functions in a previously living organism.

dead-end host [AS, *dead* + *ende* + L, *hospes,* guest], **1.** a host from which infectious agents are not transmitted to other susceptible hosts. **2.** any host organism from which a parasite cannot escape to continue its life cycle. Humans are dead-end hosts for trichinosis, because the larvae encysted in muscle and human flesh are unlikely to be a source of food for other animals susceptible to this parasite. Compare **definitive host, intermediate host, reservoir host.**

dead fetus syndrome, a condition in which the fetus has died but has remained in the uterus for some time. The condition leads to a blood coagulation disorder and disseminated intravascular coagulation, and the eventual delivery is usually accompanied by massive bleeding. See also **disseminated intravascular coagulation.**

deadly quartet, a combination of risk factors that includes upper body obesity, glucose intolerance, hypertriglyceridemia, and hypertension. Now called **metabolic syndrome.** See also **syndrome X.**

dead pulp. See **nonvital pulp.**

dead space [AS, dead; L, *spatium*], **1.** a cavity that remains after the incomplete closure of a surgical or traumatic wound, leaving an area in which blood can collect and delay healing. **2.** the amount of lung in contact with ventilating gases but not in contact with pulmonary blood flow. Alveolar dead space is characterized by alveoli that are ventilated by the pulmonary circulation but are not perfused. The condition may exist when pulmonary circulation is obstructed, as by a thromboembolus. Anatomical dead space is an area in the trachea, bronchi, and air passages containing air that does not reach the alveoli during respiration. As a general rule, the volume of air in the anatomical dead space in milliliters is approximately equal to the weight in pounds of the individual affected. Certain lung disorders, such as emphysema, increase the amount of anatomical dead space. Physiological dead space is an area in the respiratory system that includes the anatomical dead space together with the space in the alveoli occupied by air that does not contribute to the oxygen–carbon dioxide exchange.

dead space effect, any of several potential adverse effects, including hypoxemia and hypercapnia, produced by dead space in the lungs, particularly alveolar dead space.

deaf [AS], *adj.,* unable to hear; hard of hearing. –**deafness,** *n.*

deafferentation /dē·af'ərəntā″shən/ [L, *de,* from, *ad* + *ferre,* to bear], the elimination or interruption of afferent nerve impulses.

deafness, a condition characterized by a loss of hearing that makes it impossible for an individual to understand speech through hearing alone. In assessing deafness, the ears are examined for drainage, crusts, accumulation of cerumen, or structural abnormality. It is determined whether the hearing loss is conductive or sensory, temporary or permanent, and congenital or acquired in childhood, adolescence, or adulthood. The effect of aging is evaluated. A psychosocial assessment is conducted to ascertain whether the individual is well adjusted to hearing loss or reacts to the disability with fear, anxiety, frustration, depression, anger, or hostility. In all cases the degree of loss and the kind of impairment causing it are determined. See also **conductive hearing loss, sensorineural hearing loss.**

■ OBSERVATIONS: Many conditions and diseases may result in hearing loss. The person with a slight hearing loss may be initially unaware of the problem. Recognition, diagnosis, and early treatment may help prevent further impairment and prevent frustration, embarrassment, and danger for the person. An older person with a hearing impairment usually has a sensorineural loss. High-frequency sounds are hard to hear, and discernment of such softer speech sounds such as /s/ and /f/ becomes difficult. A severe or sudden hearing loss usually drives the person to seek help. If the loss is sudden, confusion, fear, and even panic are common. The person's speech becomes loud and slurred. There is new danger because the person cannot hear horns, whistles, or sirens and has not developed a way to cope with the impairment safely. The congenitally deaf person needs special speech and language intervention before reaching school age.

■ INTERVENTIONS: The treatment of hearing loss depends on the cause. Merely removing impacted cerumen from the external auditory canal may significantly improve hearing. Hearing aids, amplification of sound, or speech reading may be useful. Speech therapy is useful in teaching a person to speak or helping a person to retain the ability to speak.

■ PATIENT CARE CONSIDERATIONS: Caring for a deaf person who is hospitalized for treatment of another problem requires certain adjustments in communication between the health care provider and the patient. If the patient uses a hearing aid, its placement and operation are checked before the speaker begins to talk; the voice is modulated to a level that is comfortable for the patient, and the speaker stands or sits where the lips are visible to the deaf individual. If the patient uses sign language, an interpreter or another means of communication is sought; when a pad and pencil are used, a frequent practice with the newly deaf, the messages are written clearly in short, simple phrases, and adequate time is allowed for the patient to understand and answer.

deaminase /dē·am″inās/ [L, *de,* away, *amine,* ammonia; Fr, *diastase,* enzyme], one of the subclasses of enzymes that catalyze the hydrolysis of the NH_2 bond in amino compounds, usually with the concomitant removal of ammonia. The enzymes are usually named according to the substrate, such as adenosine deaminase, guanine deaminase, or guanosine deaminase. Also called **aminohydrolase.**

deamination /dē′aminā″shən/, the removal, usually by hydrolysis, of the NH_2 radical from an amino compound.

dean [L, *decanus,* chief of ten], chief executive and educational officer of a unit of a university, school, or college.

dearterialization /dē′ärtir′ē·əlīzā″shən/, **1.** conversion of oxygenated arterial blood into venous blood. **2.** interruption of the supply of arterial blood to an organ or body part.

death [AS], **1.** apparent death; the cessation of life as indicated by the absence of all vital functions. **2.** legal death; the total absence of activity in the brain and central nervous system, the cardiovascular system, and the respiratory system as observed and declared by a qualified professional. See also **cell death, emotional care of the dying patient, stages of dying, sudden infant death syndrome.**

death chill. See **algor mortis.**

death instinct, instinctive behavior that tends to be self-destructive.

death mask [AS, *death* + Fr, *masque*], an image or cast made of the face after death. The masks are generally made from clay, wax, plaster of paris, or other moldable material.

death rate, the number of deaths occurring within a specified population during a particular period, usually expressed in terms of deaths per 1000 persons per year.

death rattle, (*Informal*) a sound produced by air moving through mucus that has accumulated in the throat of a dying person who has lost the cough reflex. It is often accompanied by agonal respiration.

"death with dignity" [AS, *death* + L, *dignus,* worthy], the philosophical concept that a terminally ill client should be permitted to make choices about his or her death and to die naturally and comfortably.

DeBakey forceps, atraumatic tissue forceps used to grasp fine tissue.

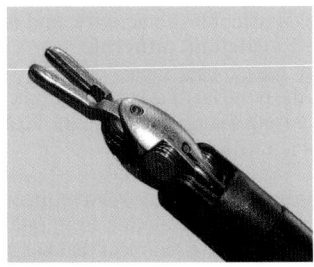

DeBakey forceps *(Courtesy Intuitive Surgical, Inc.)*

debility /dibil″itē/, frailness, weakness, or loss of strength. See also **asthenia.** *–debilitating, adj.*

debridement /debrēdmäN′/ [Fr, *debridle,* remove], **1.** the removal of dirt, foreign objects, damaged tissue, and cellular debris from a wound or a burn to prevent infection and to promote healing. In treating a wound, debridement is the first step in cleansing. It also allows thorough examination of the extent of the injury. In treating a burn, debridement of the eschar may be performed in a hydrotherapy bath. *–debride, v.* **2.** (in dentistry) the removal of supragingival and subgingival biofilms, calculus, plaque-retentive anomalies, and diseased root surfaces that harbor bacteria.

debris /dəbrē″/, the dead, diseased, or damaged tissue and any foreign material that is to be removed from a wound or other area being treated.

Debrox, a topical antiinfective agent. Brand name for **carbamide peroxide.**

debt /det/ [L, *debere,* to owe], something owed. Medical debt and the fear of medical debt have a significant impact on health care. See also **oxygen debt.**

debug /dibug″, dē″bug/ [L, *de* + Welsh, *bwg,* hobgoblin], to find and correct errors in computer software or hardware.

dec-, prefix meaning "tenth": *decigram, deciliter.*

Decaderm, a topical synthetic analog of cortisol in ointment form. Brand name for **dexamethasone.**

Decadron, a glucocorticoid. Brand name for **dexamethasone.**

Deca-Durabolin, an androgen. Brand name for *nandrolone decanoate.*

decalcification /dēkal′sifikā″shən/ [L, *de* + *calyx,* lime, *facere,* to make], loss of calcium salts from the teeth and bones caused by malnutrition, malabsorption, or other dietary or physiological factors, such as immobility. It may result, particularly in older people, from a diet that lacks adequate calcium. Malabsorption may be caused by a lack of vitamin D necessary for the absorption of calcium from the intestine; an excess of dietary fats that can combine with calcium to form an indigestible soaplike compound; the presence of oxalic acid, which can combine with calcium to form a relatively insoluble calcium oxalate salt; hormonal changes of menopause; or a relative lack of acid in the digestive tract, which can decrease the solubility of calcium. Other factors include the parathyroid hormone control of the calcium level in the bloodstream, the ratio of calcium to phosphorus in the blood, and the relative activity of osteoblast cells that form calcium deposits in the bones and teeth and osteoclast cells that absorb calcium from bones and teeth. Bone tissue tends to be maintained in quantities no greater than needed to meet current physical stress. Therefore inactive and, particularly, bedridden people lose calcium from their bones; osteoclastic activity exceeds osteoblastic activity, and decalcification occurs. See also **calcium, mineral.**

decannulation /dēkan′yəlā″shən/ [L, *de,* from, *cannula,* small reed], the removal of a cannula or tube that may have been inserted during a surgical procedure. Examples include the removal of a tracheostomy tube.

decanoic acid. See **capric acid.**

decant, to separate fluid from a solid sediment by gradually pouring the fluid sediment solution from one container into another without disturbing sediment that has settled onto the bottom of the container.

decapitation /dēkap′itā″shən/, literally, cutting off the head, as the head of a bone or the head of an organism, animal, or individual. Decapitation is a fatal injury.

decay /dikā″/, **1.** a gradual deterioration that accompanies the end of life. **2.** a gradual deterioration, usually caused by bacteria and other decomposers, of the body of an organism after death. **3.** the process of disintegration of a radioactive substance.

decay-accelerating factor (DAF), a protein inhibiting the complement system on the cell surface and the regulation of innate and adaptive immunity.

decay product [L, *de* + *cadere,* to fall, *producere,* to produce], a stable or radioactive nuclide formed by the disintegration of a radionuclide, either directly or as a result of successive transformation in a radioactive series. Also called **daughter product.**

decay time, the period required for a wavelength to go from peak amplitude to 0 volt (V).

deceleration /dēsel′ərā″shən/ [L, *de* + *accelerare,* to hasten], a decrease in the speed or velocity of an object or reaction. Compare **acceleration.**

deceleration injury, an injury resulting from a collision between a rapidly moving body part and a stationary object.

deceleration phase, (in obstetrics) the latter part of active labor, characterized by a decreased rate of dilation of the cervical os.

deceleration radiation. See **bremsstrahlung radiation.**

decerebrate /dēser″əbrāt/, **1.** lacking a cerebrum. **2.** lacking neural communication between the cerebrum and lower portions of the central nervous system.

decerebrate posture [L, *de* + *cerebrum,* brain, *ponere,* to place], the position of a patient, who is usually comatose, in which the arms are extended and internally rotated and the legs are extended with the feet in forced plantar flexion. It is usually observed in patients afflicted by compression of the brainstem at a low level. It may also be observed in children with brainstem damage. Also called **decerebrate rigidity.**

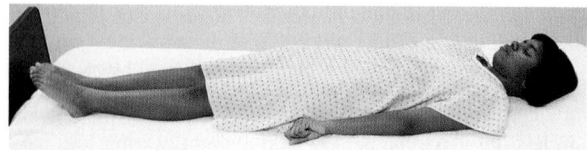

Patient with decerebrate posture (Ball et al, 2015)

decerebrate rigidity. See **decerebrate posture.**

decerebration /-brā″shən/ [L, *de,* from, *cerebrum*], the process of removing the brain or of cutting the brainstem of an animal above the level of the red nucleus, thus eliminating cerebral function.

deci-, prefix indicating one tenth.

decibel (dB) /des″əbəl/ [L, *decimus,* one tenth, *bel,* Alexander G. Bell, Canadian inventor, 1847–1922], a unit of measure of the intensity of sound. A decibel is one tenth of 1 bel (B); an increase of 1 B is perceived as a 10-fold increase in loudness, based on a sound-pressure reference level of 0.0002 dyne/cm², or 20 micropascals.

decidua /disij″o͞o·ə/ [L, *decidere,* to fall off], the epithelial tissue of the endometrium lining the uterus. It envelops the conceptus during gestation and is shed in the puerperium. It is also shed periodically with menstruation. Kinds include **decidua basalis, decidua capsularis, decidua vera.** See also **amniotic sac.**

decidua basalis, the decidua of the endometrium in the uterus that lies beneath the implanted ovum. Also called **decidua serotina.**

decidua capsularis, the decidua of the endometrium of the uterus covering the implanted ovum. Also called **decidua reflexa.**

decidual endometritis /disij″o͞o·əl/, an inflammation or infection of any portion of the decidua during pregnancy. See also **endometritis.**

decidua menstrualis, the endometrial mucosa shed during menstruation.

decidua parietalis. See **decidua vera.**

decidua reflexa. See **decidua capsularis.**

decidua serotina. See **decidua basalis.**

decidua vera, the decidua of the endometrium lining the uterus, except for those areas beneath and above the implanted and developing ovum called, respectively, the decidua basalis and the decidua capsularis. Also called **decidua parietalis.**

deciduoma /disij″o͞o·ō″mə/, a benign or malignant tumor of endometrial tissue. A deciduoma may develop after a pregnancy, regardless of the outcome. It may be detected by a Papanicolaou (Pap) test.

deciduous /də·sid′yo͞o·əs/ [L, *decidere,* to fall off], falling off or shedding at a certain stage of growth or maturity; lacking permanence.

deciduous dentition. Also called **primary dentition.**

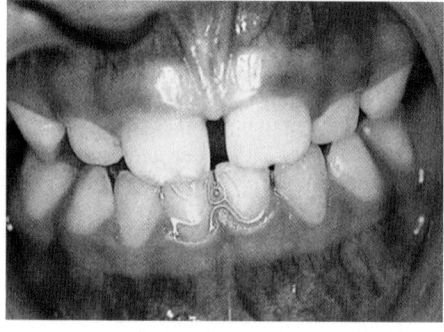

Deciduous dentition (Zitelli and Davis, 2007)

decigram (dg), a unit of mass in the metric system equal to 100 milligrams or one tenth of a gram.

deciliter (dL), a unit of volume in the metric system equal to 100 milliliters or one tenth of a liter.

decimeter (dm), a unit of length in the metric system equal to 10 centimeters or one tenth of a meter.

decision making, the process of evaluating available information and reaching a judgment or conclusion based on that information.

decision tree, a systematic method of managing a problem by graphically organizing the probabilities of outcomes of alternative treatments. At each decision node or branch, a possible alternative is matched with its relative worth, quality of life, freedom from disability, and other factors on which a prognosis may be based.

decitabine, an agent that prevents DNA methylation, halting growth of rapid proliferation blasts.
- INDICATIONS: This drug is used to treat naive and experienced myelodysplastic syndrome.
- CONTRAINDICATIONS: Pregnancy, lactation, severe neurotoxicity, severe blood dyscrasias, and known hypersensitivity to this drug prohibit its use. Its use is also contraindicated in children.
- ADVERSE EFFECTS: Adverse effects of this drug include confusion, abdominal pain, dyspepsia, hematoma, and cellulitis. Life-threatening side effects include neutropenia, thrombocytopenia, leukopenia, and anemia. Common side effects include headache; anxiety; dizziness; hypoesthesia; insomnia; edema; murmur; hypotension; nausea; anorexia; vomiting; diarrhea; constipation; stomatitis; alopecia; ecchymosis; erythema; pallor; petechiae; pruritus; rash; swelling of the face; urticaria; decreased potassium, sodium, magnesium, and albumin; increased or decreased glucose; myalgia; arthralgia; back pain; chest wall pain; pain in the limbs; cough; crackles; hypoxia; pharyngitis; pneumonia; and pulmonary edema.

declarative knowledge, knowing that something is the case; the ability to recite or describe information; an indication of recall of facts or steps in a task. Compare **procedural knowledge.**

declarative memory /dēkler″ətiv/, the mental registration, retention, and recall of past experiences, sensations, ideas, knowledge, and thoughts. The original information must be relayed through either the amygdala or hippocampal nuclear structures before long-term storage is possible.

Declomycin, an antibacterial agent. Brand name for **demeclocycline hydrochloride.**

decoction /dikok″shən/ [L, *de* + *coquere,* to cook], a liquid medicine made from an extract of water-soluble substances, usually with the aid of boiling water. Herbal remedies are usually decoctions. See also **concoction.**

decode /dikōd″/, to interpret coded information into a form usable by a receiver.

decoded message, (in communication theory) a message as translated by a receiver. If it is correctly interpreted within the context of the message as sent by the sender, the decoded message is the same as the encoded message. If it is not understood and interpreted as sent, it is not the same as the encoded message and is potentially misinterpreted.

decoic acid. See **capric acid.**

decoloration, the natural loss or removal of color, as by bleaching.

decompensation /dē′kəmpənsā″shən/ [L, *de* + *compensare,* to balance], **1.** the failure of a system, as cardiac decompensation in heart failure. **2.** (in psychology) the failure of a defense mechanism and/or the ability to cope or function.

decomposition /dē′kəmpəsish″ən/ [L, *de* + *componere,* to put together], **1.** the breakdown of a substance into simpler chemical forms. −*decompose, v.* **2.** the process of decay.

decompression /dē′kəmpresh″ən/ [L, *de* + *comprimere,* to press together], **1.** a technique used to readapt an individual to normal atmospheric pressure after exposure to higher pressures, as in diving. **2.** the removal of pressure caused by gas or fluid in a body cavity, such as the stomach or intestinal tract.

decompression sickness, a painful, sometimes fatal syndrome caused by the formation of nitrogen bubbles in the tissues of divers, caisson workers, and aviators who move too rapidly from environments of higher to those of lower atmospheric pressures. Nitrogen breathed in air under pressure dissolves in tissue fluids. When ambient pressure is reduced too rapidly, nitrogen goes out of solution faster than it can be circulated to the lungs for expiration. Gaseous nitrogen then accumulates in the joint spaces and peripheral circulation, impairing tissue oxygenation. Also called **bends, caisson disease, diver's palsy, diver's paralysis.** Compare **barotrauma.**
- OBSERVATIONS: The physiological effects include profound fatigue, disorientation, severe pain, and syncope. There are no specific laboratory tests for decompression sickness.
- INTERVENTIONS: When available, 100% oxygen is administered. Treatment entails rapid return of the patient to an environment of higher pressure (hyperbaric therapy) followed by gradual decompression. Rehydration with saline or Ringer's lactate solution is often required.
- PATIENT CARE CONSIDERATIONS: Relapses can occur without hyperbaric therapy even when patients respond well to oxygen and hydration. Admission to a facility with the capacity to administer hyperbaric therapy is a priority.

decongestant [L, *de* + *congerere,* to pile up], **1.** *adj.,* pertaining to a substance or procedure that eliminates or reduces congestion or swelling. **2.** *n.,* a decongestant drug. Adrenergic drugs (alpha$_1$ stimulants), such as ephedrine and pseudoephedrine, that cause vasoconstriction of nasal mucosa are used as decongestants.

decontamination /dā′kəntam′inā″shən/, the process of removing contaminants such as blood, body fluids, foreign materials, or radioactivity from an area, object, or person.

decorticate posture /dēkôr″tikāt/ [L, *de* + *cortex,* bark, *ponere,* to place], the position of a comatose patient in which the upper extremities are rigidly flexed at the elbows and at the wrists. The legs also may be flexed. The decorticate posture indicates a lesion in a mesencephalic region of the brain. In some instances the posture may be produced by applying a painful stimulus to a comatose patient. Also called *decorticate rigidity.*

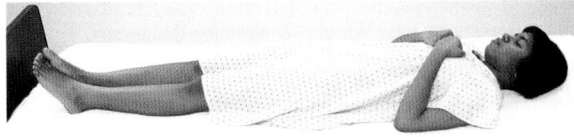

Patient with decorticate posture *(Ball et al, 2015)*

decortication /dēkôr′tikā″shən/ [L, *de* + *cortex,* bark], (in medicine) the removal of portions of the cortex or surface layer of an organ or structure, such as the kidney, the brain, or the lung. −*decorticate, adj., v.*

decrement /dek″rəmənt/ [L, *de* + *crescere,* to grow], a decrease or stage of decline, as of a uterine contraction.

decremental conduction /dek′rəmen″təl/, transmission of an electric impulse in which the amplitude of the impulse decreases with distance.

decrepitate percussion /dēkrep″itit/, a crackling noise produced by tapping the thoracic or abdominal wall of a patient with a respiratory disorder.

decrudescence /dē′krōōdes″əns/ [L, de, from, crudescere, to become bad], a decrease in the severity of symptoms.

decubital /dikyōō″bitəl/ [L, decumbere, to lie down], **1.** pertaining to a pressure ulcer caused by lying in a recumbent position. **2.** pertaining to a radiographic view obtained with the patient in a recumbent position.

decubitus /dikyōō″bitəs/ [L, decumbere, to lie down], a recumbent or horizontal position, as lateral decubitus, lying on one side.

decubitus angina, a condition characterized by periodic attacks of cardiac pain that occur when a person is lying down. Severe coronary artery disease, as well as fluid overload, causes strain on the heart, resulting in pain.

decubitus position, a position used in producing a radiograph of the chest or abdomen of a patient who is lying down, with the central ray horizontal. The patient may be prone (ventral decubitus), supine (dorsal decubitus), or on the left or right side (left or right lateral decubitus). See also **decubitus projection.**

decubitus posture, the position assumed by a bedridden patient to rest on his or her side to relieve the pressure of body weight on the sacrum, heels, or other areas vulnerable to pressure ulcers.

decubitus projection, (in radiology) the use of a horizontal beam with the patient in a decubitus position. See **decubitus position.**

decubitus ulcer, (Obsolete) now called **pressure ulcer,** pressure injury.

decussate /dəkus″āt/ [L, decussis, intersection], to cross in the form of an X as certain nerve fibers from the retina cross at the optic chiasm. –**decussation,** n.

decussation /di′kusā″shən/ [L, decussare, to make a cross], a crossing of central nervous system fibers in the brain, as some fibers on the left side cross to the right side and vice versa.

decussation of pyramids [L, decussare, to make a cross; Gk, pyramis], the crossing of nerve fibers of the corticospinal motor tract at the ventral side on the lower portion of the medulla oblongata.

dedifferentiation, regression of a cell from a specialized function to a simpler state, reminiscent of stem cells. See **anaplasia.**

deductible /dēduk″tibəl/, an amount paid each year by a health insurance plan enrollee before benefits begin. It is a mechanism for cost sharing. Should not be confused with **copayment.**

deduction [L, deducere, to lead], a system of reasoning that leads from a known principle to an unknown, or from the general to the specific. Deductive reasoning is used to test diagnostic hypotheses. See also **working diagnosis.**

deemed status /dēmd/ [AS, deman, to judge; L, status, a standing], a status conferred on a hospital or other organization by a professional standards review organization in formal recognition that the organization's review, continued-stay review, and medical care evaluation programs meet or exceed conditions of participation. Health care organizations with deemed status are exempt from the Medicare survey and certification process and can participate in and receive payment from the Medicare or Medicaid program.

deep artery of the thigh, (Nontechnical) the largest branch of the femoral artery and the major source of blood supply to the thigh. Also called **profunda femoris artery.**

deep auricular artery, a small branch of the maxillary artery that contributes to the blood supply of the external acoustic meatus.

deep bite. See **closed bite.**

deep brachial artery [As, dyppan, to dip; Gk, brachion, arm, arteria, airpipe], (Nontechnical) a branch of each of the brachial arteries, arising at the distal border of the teres major, passing deeply into the arm between the long and lateral heads of the triceps brachii, and supplying the humerus and muscles of the upper arm. It has five branches: ascending, radial collateral, middle collateral, muscular, and nutrient. Also called **superior profunda artery.**

deep brain stimulation (DBS), patient-controlled continuous high-frequency electrical stimulation of a specific area of the brain by means of an implanted electrode, which is controlled by a battery implanted just below the clavicle. The electrical signals block those signals from the brain causing tremors and some other related problems, such as occur in Parkinson disease, essential tremor, and dystonia.

deep breathing and coughing exercises, movements used to improve pulmonary gas exchange or to maintain respiratory function, especially after prolonged inactivity or general anesthesia. Incisional pain after surgery in the chest or abdomen often inhibits normal respiratory movements.
■ METHOD: The patient is assisted to a comfortable position, supine or sitting up. An analgesic may be given before the exercises if pain is present. Inhalation through the nose and exhalation through the mouth are encouraged. With the incision supported, the patient is asked to cough after a deep inhalation. If pain prevents the patient from producing a deep, effective cough, a series of short barklike coughs (also known as machine gun or huf-huf coughs) may be encouraged.
■ INTERVENTIONS: Simple techniques and encouragement significantly improve the effectiveness of the exercises. Positioning increases comfort, allows the abdominal contents to fall away from the diaphragm, and encourages full expansion of the chest wall on inspiration. If an incision is present, it may be supported with the hands or with a book or pillow held against the abdomen. The patient is often reluctant to breathe deeply or to cough. Adequate analgesia, encouragement, and explanation of the benefits of the exercises may overcome that resistance. Various devices are available for use in deep breathing and coughing, such as those used during atelectasis to strengthen the muscles used in expiration and to empty the alveoli of retained gas.
■ OUTCOME CRITERIA: When shallow breathing replaces deep breathing, mucus tends to dry in the airway, damaging the membranes that line the passages. Coughing and deep breathing improve ventilation and gas exchange by clearing the mucus and allowing moisturized air to enter the bronchi, bronchioles, and alveoli, preventing atelectasis and pneumonia.

deep circumflex iliac artery, a branch of the external iliac artery that, with the interior epigastric artery, supplies the inferior part of the abdominal wall.

deep dorsal vein, the vein that drains the erectile tissues of the clitoris and penis.

deep fascia, the most extensive of three kinds of fascia comprising an intricate series of connective sheets and bands that hold the muscles and other structures in place throughout the body, wrapping the muscles in gray, feltlike membranes. The deep fasciae comprise a continuous system, splitting and fusing in an elaborate network attached to the skeleton and divided into the outer investing layer, the internal investing layer, and the intermediate membranes. Compare **subcutaneous fascia, subserous fascia.**

deep heat, **1.** an over-the-counter preparation available as a cream, spray, and patch used in the treatment of muscular aches. **2.** (in occupational and physical therapy) the application of heat in the treatment of deep body tissues, particularly muscles and tendons. The thermal effects may be produced with shortwave therapy, phonophoresis, or ultrasound.

deepithelialization. See **epithelial debridement.**

deep lamellar endothelial keratoplasty (DLEK), a procedure in which a small incision is used to remove only the diseased tissue without transplanting the entire cornea. Only the inside layer of the cornea is replaced. This technique avoids the astigmatism that often occurs with penetrating keratoplasty and greatly reduces the risk of infection. Also called **lamellar transplant, split-thickness transplant.** See also **corneal grafting.**

deep massage, massage techniques whose purpose is to reach structures beneath the superficial tissue, using effleurage, direct pressure, or friction applied perpendicular to the fibers of the affected tissue.

deep palmar arch, the termination of the radial artery, joining the deep palmar branch of the ulnar artery in the palm of the hand.

deep perineal pouch, a thin space superior to the perineal membrane that contains a layer of skeletal muscle and various neurovascular elements.

deep pressure, 1. a tactile sensation of force applied to the skin, as in the feeling of the ischial tuberosities pressing into the seat of a chair. See also **deep sensation. 2.** (in occupational therapy) a tactile sensation of force, perceived, for example, when sensory end organs such as Pacinian corpuscles (located in the dermis of the skin) are activated. Occupational therapists who work with hyperactive children or children with autism sometimes employ deep pressure touch (DPT) as a therapeutic intervention designed to elicit calmer behavior.

deep petrosal nerve, a nerve formed in the internal carotid plexus that leaves the plexus in the middle cranial fossa and joins the greater petrosal branch of the facial nerve. It carries postganglionic sympathetic fibers destined mainly for blood vessels.

deep reflexes [ME, *dep,* hollow; L, *reflectere,* to bend back], any reflexes caused by stimulation of a deep body structure, such as a tendon reflex.

deep sedation, a state of a depressed level of consciousness with a partial loss of protective reflexes. The individual may not be able to maintain his or her airway and may not respond to verbal commands but responds purposefully following repeated or painful stimulation. This state is produced by pharmacological means. The patient maintains normal cardiovascular function.

deep sensation, the awareness or perception of pain, pressure, or tension in the deep layers of the skin, muscles, tendons, or joints. Such sensations are conveyed to the brain via the spinal column for interpretation. Compare **superficial sensation.** See also **deep pressure.**

deep temporal artery, one of the branches of the maxillary artery on each side of the head. It branches into the anterior portion and the posterior portion, both rising between the temporalis and the pericranium to supply the temporalis and to anastomose with the middle temporal artery. The anterior branch communicates with the lacrimal artery by small branches that pierce the zygomatic bone and the great wing of the sphenoid. Compare **middle temporal artery, superficial temporal artery.**

deep tendon reflex (DTR), a brisk contraction of a muscle in response to a sudden stretch induced by a sharp tap by a finger or rubber hammer on the tendon of insertion of the muscle. Absence of the reflex may be caused by damage to the muscle, peripheral nerve, nerve roots, or spinal cord at that level. A hyperactive reflex may indicate disease of the pyramidal tract above the level of the reflex arc being tested. Generalized hyperactivity of DTRs may be caused

by hyperthyroidism. Also called **myostatic reflex, tendon reflex.** Kinds include **Achilles tendon reflex, biceps reflex, brachioradialis reflex, patellar reflex, triceps reflex.**

deep transverse metatarsal ligaments, the ligaments that link together the distal heads of the metatarsals at the metatarsophalangeal joints.

deep transverse perineal muscle, a muscle on each side of the perineal membrane thought to stabilize the position of the perineal body, a midline structure along the posterior edge of the perineal membrane.

deep vein, one of the many systemic veins that accompany the arteries, usually enclosed in a sheath that wraps both the vein and the associated artery. Various structures, such as the skull, vertebral column, and liver, are served by less closely associated arteries and veins. Compare **superficial vein.**

deep vein thrombosis (DVT), a disorder involving a thrombus in one of the deep veins of the body, most commonly the iliac or femoral vein. Symptoms include tenderness, pain, swelling, warmth, and discoloration of the skin. A deep vein thrombus is potentially life threatening. Treatment includes the use of thrombolytic and anticoagulant drugs and interventional radiology. Treatment goals are directed to prevention of movement of the thrombus toward the lungs. See also **pulmonary embolism.**

■ OBSERVATIONS: It may be asymptomatic or may manifest as tenderness, pain, warmth, and swelling in the affected extremity with deep reddish or blue color. There is a positive Homans' sign in about 10% of cases, which affects a lower extremity. Serial compression ultrasonography is the initial test used for diagnosis. Magnetic resonance direct thrombus imaging may be used for thrombi undetectable on ultrasound. Contrast venography remains the gold standard for detection of lower extremity DVT. Chronic venous insufficiency and pulmonary embolus are the most common complications of thrombosis.

■ INTERVENTIONS: Initial treatment is heparin or enoxaparin followed by warfarin for maintenance treatment for 3 to 6 months. Continued monitoring of prothrombin time and partial thromboplastin time is done during anticoagulant therapy. Ligation, clipping, plication, and thrombectomy are surgical alternatives when thrombus fails to respond to anticoagulant therapy. An extravascular vena cava interruption with possible placement of intracaval filter is used for cases involving probable emboli. Analgesics are given for pain; however, aspirin is contraindicated because it interferes with platelet function. Enoxaparin may be used with patients at high risk for DVT to prevent thrombus formation.

■ PATIENT CARE CONSIDERATIONS: The immediate focus of the health care team is on prevention of pulmonary emboli, pain relief, prevention of skin breakdown, and prevention of complications related to anticoagulant therapy. Bed rest is no longer recommended. Early ambulation is encouraged, and compression stockings may be prescribed to reduce pain and swelling. Individuals are closely observed for signs of bleeding (e.g., gums, nasal mucosa, stool, and urine). Safety precautions are instituted to prevent bruising while on anticoagulants and to prevent skin ulceration of affected extremity. Individuals are monitored for manifestations of pulmonary emboli, including sudden dyspnea, tachypnea, and pleuritic chest pain. Education is important and includes effects and side effects of anticoagulant therapy; need for ongoing blood tests to monitor clotting and regulate anticoagulant dosage; avoidance of activities that may precipitate bleeding; avoidance of anticoagulant over-the-counter medications that may interfere with clotting (e.g., aspirin/aspirin products, NSAIDs, and herbal products). Education is needed about signs of pulmonary embolus and the need for immediate medical attention should they occur.

D

Instruction is provided to prevent pooled blood in the lower extremities, including regular use of compression garments and avoidance of prolonged standing, sitting, or walking. Teaching also includes prevention of future thrombosis episodes, such as avoidance or correction of modifiable risk factors (e.g., tobacco use or alcohol abuse, use of oral contraceptives or hormone replacement therapy, and prolonged periods of inactivity), regular exercise program, proper posture, and balanced diet with weight loss if indicated.

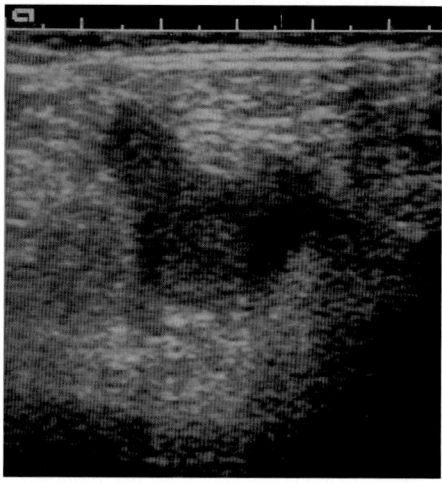

Deep vein thrombosis in pregnancy: ultrasound scan
(Greer et al, 2001)

deerfly fever. See **tularemia.**

DEET, an insect repellent. Abbreviation for *diethyltoluamide.*

defaecation. See **defecation.**

defamation /def′əmā″shən/ [L, *diffamare,* to discredit], any communication, written or spoken, that is untrue and that causes harm to the established good standing or reputability of another or that in any way brings that person into disrepute.

default judgment /difôlt′/ [L, *defallere,* to lack, *judicare,* to decide], (in law) a judgment rendered against a defendant as a result of the defendant's failure to appear in court or to answer the plaintiff's claim within the proper time.

defecation /def′ikā″shən/ [L, *defaecare,* to clean], the elimination of feces from the digestive tract through the rectum. Also spelled **defaecation.** See also **constipation, diarrhea, feces.** –*defecate, v.*

defecation reflex. See **rectal reflex.**

defecography /def′əkog″rəfē/, the radiographic examination of the rectum and anal canal of patients with defecative dysfunction. A barium sulfate paste is instilled directly into the rectum, and the patient is seated on a radiolucent commode in front of a fluoroscope. Lateral projections of the rectum and anal canal are recorded during defecation.

defective /difek″tiv/ [L, *defectus,* a failing], pertaining to something that is imperfect or inadequate.

defendant /difen″dənt/, (in law) the party named in a plaintiff's complaint and against whom the plaintiff's allegations are made. The defendant must respond to the allegations.

defense /də·fens′/ [L, *defendere,* to ward off], the practice of, or measures taken to ensure, protection.

defense mechanism [L, *defendere,* to repulse, *mechanicus,* machine; from the psychoanalytic theory of Sigmund Freud, Czech-Austrian neurologist and psychiatrist, 1856–1939], an unconscious intrapsychic reaction that offers protection to the self from stress or a threat. Defense mechanisms are of two types: those that diminish anxiety and are used by an individual to integrate more fully into society and those that do not reduce anxiety but simply postpone the effects of feeling it. Anxiety-reducing defenses include compensation, identification, introjection, some forms of repression, and sublimation. Defenses that postpone full expression of anxiety include denial, displacement, isolation, projection, reaction formation, rationalization, regression, some forms of repression, suppression, and undoing.

defense reflex, an autonomic defensive response by an animal when threatened. The response may consist of dilated pupils, baring of claws, or raising of feathers or hair.

defensin /difen″sin/, a peptide with natural antibiotic activity found within human neutrophils. Three types of defensins have been identified, each consisting of a chain of about 30 amino acids. Similar molecules occur in white blood cells of other animal species. They show activity toward viruses and fungi, in addition to bacteria.

defensive medicine, the ordering of unnecessary diagnostic tests and referrals to consultants by a physician or other primary health care provider to minimize the risk of malpractice.

defensive radical therapy /difen″siv/, (in psychology) a view of the therapeutic process in which the therapist begins at the patient's present state and encourages the patient to avoid self-defeating behavior as a survival tactic. The goal is to create social awareness that clients can use in coping with oppressive environments.

deferasirox, a rarely used heavy metal chelating agent.

■ INDICATIONS: This drug is used to treat chronic iron overload.

■ CONTRAINDICATIONS: Lactation, severe hepatic or renal disease, and known hypersensitivity to this drug prohibit its use. Its use is also contraindicated in children.

deferens /def″ərenz/ [L], carrying away. Also **deferent.**

deferent duct. See **vas deferens.**

deferoxamine mesylate /dĕ′fərok″səmēn/, a chelating agent with specific affinity for ferric iron and low affinity for calcium.

■ INDICATIONS: It is prescribed in the treatment of acute iron intoxication and chronic iron overload.

■ CONTRAINDICATIONS: Renal disease or anuria prohibits its use.

■ ADVERSE EFFECTS: Among the most serious adverse reactions are hypotension, tachycardia, dysuria, visual difficulties, and anaphylactoid reactions.

defervescence /di′fərves″əns/ [L, *defervescere,* to reduce heat], the diminishing or disappearance of a fever. –*defervescent, adj.*

defibrillate /difī″brilāt, difib″-/ [L, *de* + *fibrilla,* little thread], to stop fibrillation of the ventricles by delivering an electrical shock through the chest wall. See also **defibrillation.**

defibrillation /difī′brilā″shən/, the termination of ventricular fibrillation or pulseless ventricular tachycardia (inefficient, asynchronous contraction) by delivery of an electric shock to the patient's precordium. It is a common emergency measure generally performed by a physician, specially trained nurse, or paramedic. A device called an automated external defibrillator (AED) is designed for use by the lay public. In external defibrillation, one paddle is placed to the right of the upper sternum below the clavicle, and the other is applied to the midaxillary line of the left lower rib cage. In internal defibrillation, which may be performed during open-heart surgery, the paddles are placed directly on the heart. The defibrillator, usually a condenser-discharge system, is set to deliver between 200 and 360 J. If shocks fail to restore a perfusion rhythm, cardiopulmonary resuscitation is begun. Repeat shocks also are attempted periodically until ventricular fibrillation ceases or the efforts are deemed futile. See also **automated external defibrillator.** –**defibrillate,** *v.*

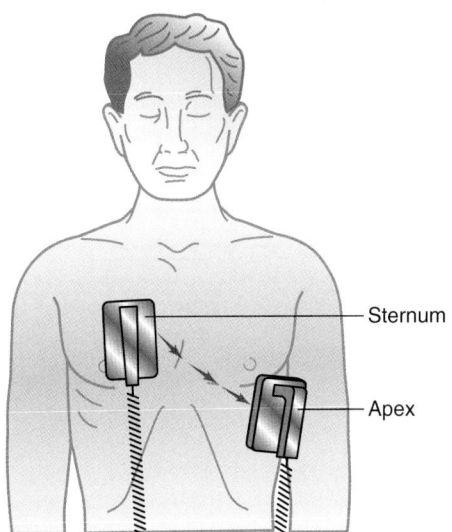

Paddle placement and current flow in defibrillation
(Sole et al, 2013)

defibrillator /difī″brilā′tər, difib″-/, a device that delivers an electrical shock at a preset voltage to the myocardium. It is used for restoring the normal cardiac rhythm and rate when the heart has stopped beating or is fibrillating. See also **implantable cardioverter-defibrillator, automated external defibrillator.**

defibrination, the in vitro removal of fibrin from blood to prevent clotting.

defibrination syndrome, *(Obsolete)* now called **disseminated intravascular coagulation.**

deficiency /difish″ənsē/, a lack or shortage of something.

deficiency disease [L, *de + facere,* to make, *dis,* opposite of; Fr, *aise,* ease], a condition resulting from the lack of one or more essential nutrients in the diet; from metabolic dysfunction; or from impaired digestion or absorption, excessive excretion, or increased biological requirements. Compare **malnutrition.** See also **avitaminosis.**

deficiency of sweating [AS, *swaetan*], *(Informal)* a failure of the sweat glands to secrete perspiration in normal amounts. Also called **anhidrosis, hypohidrosis.**

deficit /def′isit/, **1.** any deficiency or difference from what is normal, such as an oxygen deficit, a cause of hypoxia. **2.** a physical, emotional, or social limitation that interferes with activities of daily living.

defined formula diet, nutritional support provided by simple elemental nutritive components that require no further digestive breakdown and thus are readily absorbed. Examples include free amino acids from hydrolyzed protein and the simple sugar glucose, a carbohydrate. Also called **elemental formula,** *chemically defined formula diet.*

definitive /difin″ətiv/ [L, *definitivus,* a limiting], **1.** final; clearly established without doubt or question. **2.** (in embryology) fully formed in the final differentiation of a tissue, structure, or organ. Compare **primitive. 3.** (in parasitology) pertaining to the host in which the parasite undergoes the sexual phase of its reproductive cycle.

definitive host, any host organism in which a parasite reproduces sexually. The female Anopheles mosquito is the definitive host for malaria. Humans are definitive hosts for pinworms, schistosomes, and tapeworms. Also called **primary host.** Compare **dead-end host, intermediate host, reservoir host.** See also **host.**

definitive prosthesis, a permanent prosthetic device that replaces an immediate-fit appliance such as a pylon. In some cases a definitive prosthesis is used only when full weight-bearing on an artificial limb is feasible, which may follow amputation by 6 weeks or longer.

definitive treatment, any therapy generally accepted as a specific cure of a disease. Compare **expectant treatment, palliative treatment.**

defloration /def′lôrā″shən/ [L, *de + flos,* flower, *atio,* process], *(Obsolete)* disruption of the vaginal hymen by any means; most frequently associated with sexual intercourse.

deformity /difôr″mitē/ [L, *deformis,* misshapen], distortion, disfigurement, flaw, malformation, or misshape that affects the body in general or any part of it. It may be the result of disease, injury, or birth defect. Kinds include **clawfoot, syndactyly, cleft lip.**

deg, 1. abbreviation for **degeneration. 2.** abbreviation for **degree.**

degenerate /də·jen′er·āt/ [L, *degenerare*], **1.** *v.,* to change from a higher to a lower type or form. **2.** *(Slang) n.,* /də·jen′er·ət/, an individual who does not meet the expected moral standards in a society.

degeneration (deg) /dijen′ərā″shən/ [L, *degenerare,* to become unlike others], the gradual deterioration or loss of function of normal cells and body functions.

degenerative /dijen″ərətiv/ [L, *degenerare,* to become unlike others], pertaining to or involving degeneration or change to a lower or dysfunctional form.

degenerative chorea, *(Obsolete)* now called **Huntington disease.**

degenerative disease, any disease in which deterioration of structure or function of tissue occurs. Kinds include **arteriosclerosis, cancer, osteoarthritis.**

degenerative joint disease. See **osteoarthritis.**

degenerative neuralgia [L, *degenerare,* to become unlike others; Gk, *neuron,* nerve, *algos,* pain], a lack of sensation or abnormal sensations along a damaged nerve caused by degenerative changes, usually affecting older people.

degenerative neuritis [L, *degenerare,* to become unlike others; Gk, *neuron,* nerve, *itis,* inflammation], an inflammation caused by changes in nervous tissue.

degloving /dēglov″ing/ [L, *de + AS, glof*], **1.** an injury to an extremity—finger, hand, arm, leg, or foot—in which the soft tissue down to the bone, including neurovascular bundles and sometimes tendons, is traumatically peeled off. **2.** (in dentistry) the exposure of the bony mandibular anterior or posterior regions by oral surgery or trauma. **3.** removal of nitrile or vinyl hand coverings.

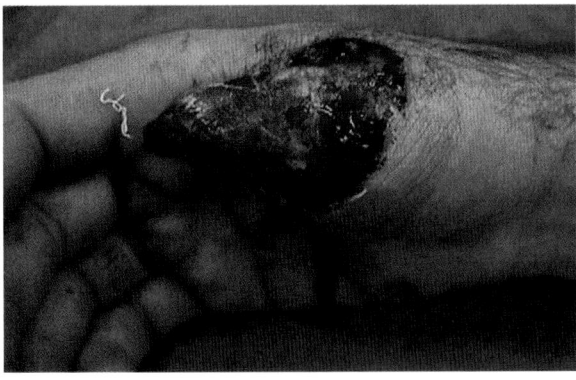

Degloving injury of the thumb *(Fatemi, 2007)*

deglutition /di'glo͞otish"ən/ [L, *deglutire*, to swallow], swallowing.

deglutition apnea, the normal absence of respiration during swallowing.

Degos disease. Also called **malignant atrophic papulosis.**

degradation /di'grədā"shən/ [L, *de + gradu*, step], **1.** the conversion of a chemical compound to a less complex compound, usually by splitting off one or more groups or subgroups of atoms, as in deamination. –*degrade, adj.* **2.** a decline to a lower condition, quality, or level. Decomposition of a compound, especially complex substances such as polymers and proteins, by stages, exhibiting well-defined intermediate products.

degranulation /dēgran'yəlā"shən/, the release of granules from cells, such as mast cells and basophils.

degree (deg) [Fr, *degre*], **1.** one of the divisions or intervals marked on a scale of units of measurement. See also **Celsius thermometer, Fahrenheit. 2.** a unit of measurement for an angle or arc of a circle.

degrees of freedom (df), a statistical measure of the number of independent observations or choices among members in a sample. It is used in determining the statistical significance of findings during data analysis.

degustation /dē'gəstā"shən/ [L, *degustare*, to taste], the act of tasting.

dehiscence /dihis"əns/ [L, *dehiscere*, to gape], the separation of a surgical incision or rupture of a wound closure.

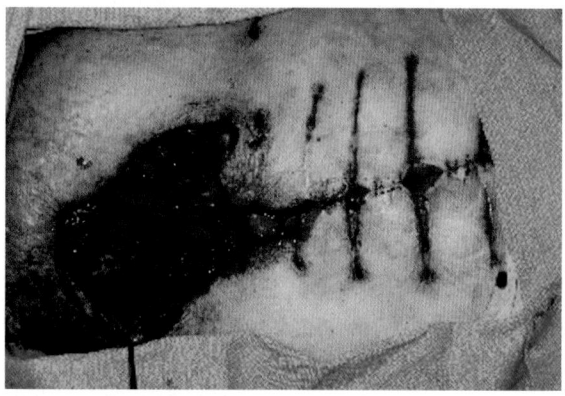

Partial wound dehiscence resulting in open wound healing by secondary intention *(Williams et al, 2007)*

dehumanization /dihyo͞o'mənīzā"shən/ [L, *de*, from, *humanitas,* human nature], the process of losing altruistic or individual qualities, as may occur in some psychotic states or in environments that produce emotional trauma (prisoner-of-war). It may be influenced by external forces.

dehumidifier /dē'hyo͞omid'ifī'ər/, an apparatus to remove moisture in the atmosphere.

dehydrate /dihī"drāt/ [L, *de* + Gk, *hydor,* water], **1.** to remove or lose water from a substance. **2.** to lose excessive water from the body, for example by excessive sweating, diarrhea, or vomiting.

dehydrated alcohol, a clear, colorless, highly hygroscopic liquid with a burning taste, containing at least 99.5% ethyl alcohol by volume. Also called **absolute alcohol.**

dehydration /di'hīdrā"shən/, **1.** excessive loss of water from body tissues. Dehydration is accompanied by a disturbance in the balance of essential electrolytes, particularly sodium, potassium, and chloride. It may follow prolonged fever, diarrhea, vomiting, acidosis, and any condition in which there is rapid depletion of body fluids. It is of particular concern among infants, young children, and the frail elderly because their electrolyte balance is normally precarious. Signs of dehydration include poor skin turgor (not a reliable sign in the elderly), flushed dry skin, coated tongue, dry mucous membranes, oliguria, irritability, and confusion. Normal fluid volume and balanced electrolyte values are the primary goals of therapy. **2.** rendering a substance free from water. Also called *anhydration.*

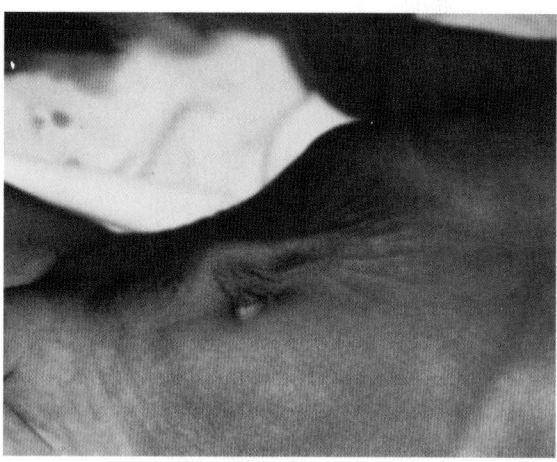

Dehydration resulting in poor skin turgor
(Zitelli and Davis, 2007)

dehydration fever, a fever associated with a significant loss of fluids, as from excessive sweating, vomiting, or diarrhea. Compare **inanition, starvation.**

dehydration of gingivae, the drying of gum tissue, often the result of mouth breathing. Dehydration lowers the resistance of the gingivae to infection.

dehydrogenate, to remove hydrogen atoms from compounds, as in the oxidation processes, typically to produce olefins from alkanes; a more specific example is to produce unsaturated fats from saturated fats.

deinstitutionalization /dē·in'stityo͞o'shənal'īzā"shən/ [L, *de + instituere,* to put in place], a movement beginning in the 1960s and carried through to the 1990s in the United States, Canada, and other countries worldwide, decommissioning large mental institutions with a goal of psychosocial rehabilitation and reintegration of their patients into community mental health settings and/or much smaller facilities. Community mental health clinics, group homes, and psychosocial day programs developed in response.

Deiters' nucleus /dī"tərz, dē"terz/ [Otto F.C. Deiters, German anatomist, 1834–1863], one of the vestibular nuclei located in the brainstem.

DEJ, abbreviation for **dentinoenamel junction.**

déjà vu /dāzhä vY", -vē", -vo͞o"/ [Fr, previously seen], the sensation or illusion that one is encountering a set of circumstances or a place that was previously experienced. The phenomenon is normal in everyone but occurs more frequently or continuously in certain emotional and organic disorders. Compare **jamais vu, paramnesia.**

Déjérine-Klumpke paralysis. See **Klumpke palsy.**

Déjérine-Roussy syndrome. See **thalamic syndrome.**

Déjérine-Sottas disease /dezh"ərin sot"əz, -sotäz"/ [Joseph J. Déjérine, French neurologist, 1849–1917; Jules Sottas, French neurologist, 1866–1943], a rare congenital spino-cerebellar

Clinical manifestations of dehydration

Manifestation	Isotonic (loss of water and salt)	Hypotonic (loss of salt in excess of water)	Hypertonic (loss of water in excess of salt)
Skin			
Color	Gray	Gray	Gray
Temperature	Cold	Cold	Cold or hot
Turgor	Poor	Very poor	Fair
Feel	Dry	Clammy	Thickened, doughy
Mucous membranes	Dry	Slightly moist	Parched
Tearing and salivation	Absent	Absent	Absent
Eyeball	Sunken	Sunken	Sunken
Fontanel	Sunken	Sunken	Sunken
Body temperature	Subnormal or elevated	Subnormal or elevated	Subnormal or elevated
Pulse	Rapid	Very rapid	Moderately rapid
Respirations	Rapid	Rapid	Rapid
Behavior	Irritable to lethargic	Lethargic or comatose; convulsions	Marked lethargy with extreme hyperirritability on stimulation

From Hockenberry MJ, Wilson D: *Wong's nursing care of infants and children,* ed 10, St Louis, 2015, Mosby

disorder characterized by the development of palpable thickenings along peripheral nerves, degeneration of the peripheral nervous system, pain, paresthesia, ataxia, and diminished sensation and deep tendon reflexes. Diagnosis is made by a histological examination of a peripheral nerve. Currently, there is no cure. Treatment is supportive. Also called **progressive interstitial hypertrophic neuropathy.**

deka-,   prefix indicating the multiple 10.

DEKA arm system,   a robotic prosthesis, developed with funding from DARPA (Defense Advanced Research Projects Agency), to restore functionality of a limb for individuals with an amputation. Muscular signals are translated by the prosthesis to allow for near-natural implementation of complex tasks, including grasp and fine-motor activities.

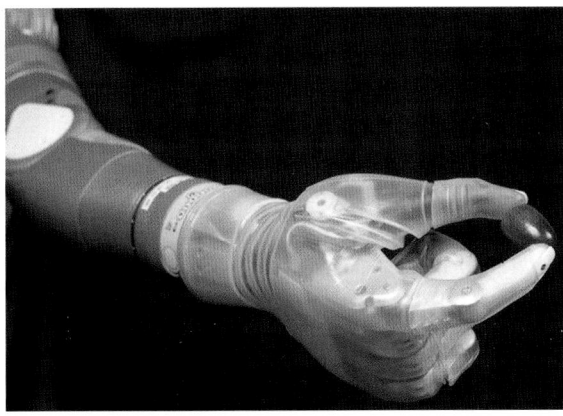

DEKA arm system *(© 2009 DEKA Research and Developmental Corporation. All rights reserved.)*

del,   abbreviation for **deletion.**

Delaney clause [James Delaney, New York Congressman, 1901–1987],   a 1960 amendment to the 1938 Federal Food, Drug, and Cosmetic Act regulating food additives. It prohibits the use of any food substance found to be carcinogenic in humans or animals. Food products used before 1958 not considered carcinogenic are classified as "Generally Regarded As Safe" (GRAS) and are exempt and not subject to testing. Additives after this time are subject to testing and evaluation.

Delano, Jane A.,   (1862–1919), an American nurse who organized the American Red Cross Nursing Service, an association formed to supply nurses to the military forces. She became director of the Nurses' Training School of the University of Pennsylvania in 1891 and was later appointed director of the Bellevue Hospital Training School for Nurses in New York, where she had been trained. On a trip to survey nursing conditions in Europe, she died after surgery for a mastoid infection at Base Hospital, Savenay, France, in March 1919.

delavirdine,   a nonnucleoside reverse transcriptase inhibitor.

■ INDICATIONS: It is used to treat HIV-1 in combination with zidovudine or didanosine.

■ CONTRAINDICATIONS: Known hypersensitivity to this drug or to atevirdine prohibits its use.

■ ADVERSE EFFECTS: Life-threatening effects are hepatotoxicity, neutropenia, leukopenia, thrombocytopenia, anemia, granulocytopenia, and nephrotoxicity. Other adverse effects include diarrhea, abdominal pain, nausea, fatigue, headache, rash, pain, myalgia, vomiting, and dyspepsia.

delayed dentition.   See **retarded dentition.**

delayed echolalia [Fr, *delai,* time extension; Gk, *echo,* sound, *lalein,* to babble],   a phenomenon, commonly seen in schizophrenia, involving the meaningless automatic repetition of overheard words and phrases. It occurs hours, days, or even weeks after the original stimulus.

delayed graft [ME, *delaein,* to leave; Gk, *graphein,* stylus],   **1.** a type of skin graft that is partially elevated and reinserted later in the same place. This procedure not only allows for an increase in the vascularization of the graft bed but also facilitates granulation tissue filling in anatomical defects. **2.** a technique employing a separate agent to create granulation tissue, followed by placement of a skin graft.

delayed graft function,   the need for the use of dialysis within 7 days of a renal transplant.

delayed hypersensitivity,   a type of hypersensitivity that (as opposed to immediate hypersensitivity) takes 24 to 72 hours to develop and is mediated by T lymphocytes rather than antibodies. Compare **immediate hypersensitivity.**

delayed hypersensitivity reaction,   the subset of type IV hypersensitivity reactions involving cytokine release and macrophage activation. The classic delayed hypersensitivity reaction is the tuberculin reaction observed in skin testing. See also **type IV hypersensitivity, hypersensitivity reaction.**

delayed-onset muscle soreness, muscle weakness, restricted range of motion, and tenderness on palpation, occurring 24 to 48 hours after intense or prolonged muscular activity.

delayed postpartum hemorrhage, hemorrhage occurring later than 24 hours after giving birth. It is most often caused by retained fragments of the placenta, a laceration of the cervix or vagina that was not discovered or was not completely sutured, or subinvolution of the placental site within the uterus. Characteristics of delayed postpartum hemorrhage are heavy bleeding and signs of impending shock and anemia. The cause is diagnosed and treated. A laceration is closed with suture, retained fragments of placenta are removed, infection is treated with antibiotics, or the relaxed uterus is caused to contract by the administration of ergonovine (Ergotrate) or oxytocin.

delayed sensation, a feeling or impression that is not experienced immediately after a stimulus. See also **sensation.**

delayed symptom [Fr, *delai* + Gk, *symptoma,* that which happens], a physiological or psychological sign that is not immediately apparent after an injury or incident. Examples include back pain the day after an automobile accident, headache two days after head trauma, or anxiety a week after after witnessing a traumatic event.

delayed treatment seeker, (in psychology) a person who delays seeking treatment for a problematic life event such as a sexual assault until months or years after the event, usually after a precipitating event such as an anniversary reaction.

delayed-type hypersensitivity (DTH), the subset of type IV hypersensitivity reactions involving cytokine release and macrophage activation. See also **type IV hypersensitivity.**

delayed vomiting, vomiting occurring much later than its stimulus, such as several hours after a meal or several days after a course of chemotherapy.

delegation, the transfer of responsibility for the performance of patient care while retaining accountability for the outcome.

deleterious /del'itir″ē·əs/ [Gk, *deleterios,* destroyer], harmful or dangerous.

deletion (del) /dilē″shən/ [L, *deletionum,* destruction], the loss of a piece of a chromosome.

deletion syndrome, any of a group of congenital autosomal anomalies that result from the loss of part of a chromosome as a result of breakage of a chromatid during meiosis. An example is cat-cry syndrome, which results from the absence of the short arm of chromosome 5.

Delhi boil. See **cutaneous leishmaniasis.**

deliberate hypotension, a technique in general anesthesia in which a short-acting hypotensive agent is administered to reduce blood pressure and thus bleeding during surgery. The procedure facilitates surgery by making vessels and tissues more visible and by reducing blood loss. Also called **controlled hypotension, hypotensive anesthesia, hypotensive technique.**

delinquency /diling″kwənsē/ [L, *delinquere,* to fail], **1.** negligence or failure to fulfill a duty or obligation. **2.** an offense, fault, misdemeanor, or misdeed; a tendency to commit such acts. See also **juvenile delinquency.**

delinquent /diling″kwənt/, **1.** *adj.,* characterized by neglect of duty or violation of law. **2.** *n.,* one whose behavior is characterized by persistent antisocial, illegal, violent, or criminal acts. See also **juvenile delinquent.**

délire de toucher /dālir″də tŏŏshā″/ [Fr], an abnormal desire or irresistible urge to touch objects.

delirious. See **delirium.**

delirious mania /dilir″ē·əs/, an extreme form of the manic state in which activity is so frenzied, confused, and incoherent that it is difficult to discern any link between affect and behavior.

delirium /dilir″ē·əm/ [L, *delirare,* to rave], **1.** a state of frenzied excitement or wild enthusiasm. **2.** an acute organic mental disorder characterized by confusion, disorientation, restlessness, clouding of the consciousness, incoherence, fear, anxiety, excitement, and, often, illusions; hallucinations, usually of visual origin; and, at times, delusions. The condition is caused by disturbances in cerebral functions that may result from a wide range of metabolic disorders, including nutritional deficiencies and endocrine imbalances; postpartum or postoperative stress; ingestion of toxic substances, such as various gases, metals, or drugs, including alcohol; and other causes of physical and mental shock or exhaustion. The symptoms are usually of short duration and reversible with treatment of the underlying cause; in extreme cases, however, in which the toxic condition is exceedingly severe or prolonged, permanent brain damage may occur. Compare **dementia.** Kinds include **acute delirium, chronic delirium, delirium tremens, exhaustion delirium,** *senile delirium,* **traumatic delirium. –delirious,** *adj.*

■ OBSERVATIONS: There is a rapid onset and acute change in mentation. Manifestations include fluctuating levels of consciousness; disorientation; impaired memory; inability to maintain or shift attention; irritability, agitation, restlessness, and hyperactivity; perceptual disturbance, hallucinations, and delusions; rambling and fragmented speech; and impaired sleep-wake cycle. There are typically lucid intervals with symptoms worsening at night. Duration of symptoms is limited. There are four diagnostic criteria for delirium: (1) disturbance of consciousness with reduced awareness and diminished abilities to focus and to maintain or shift attention; (2) a change in cognition, such as disorientation, memory loss, or language disturbance; (3) the development of the disturbance over a period of hours to days, with fluctuation during the day; and (4) evidence from clinical exam and/or lab findings that the disturbance is caused by physiological consequences of a medical condition. Delirium places medically ill individuals at greater risk for medical complications (pneumonia and decubitus) and is associated with functional decline and institutional placement. Delirium may lead to dementia.

■ INTERVENTIONS: Intervention centers around removal or withdrawal from toxic agents (alcohol and barbiturates) and IV sedation with antianxiety and antipsychotic agents for agitation, seizure activity, and tremors. Adequate fluid and electrolyte balance is also crucial.

■ PATIENT CARE CONSIDERATIONS: Care during an acute episode of delirium is aimed at support, reduction of confusion and agitated behavior, and prevention of injury. Interventions include seizure precautions, safety precautions (e.g., prevent wandering and climbing over bedrails), environmental control (adequate lighting, noise reduction, clear space, removal of hazards, avoidance of sensory extremes, and allowance for adequate sleep), reorientation procedures (e.g., clocks, calendars, familiar objects, use of glasses and hearing aids), consistency of caretakers, and family involvement. Restraints should be avoided. Tactics to prevent delirium are crucial in susceptible individuals (e.g., those with chronic or mental illness, altered sensory perception, or neurological disease; those with elevated ammonia, increased blood urea nitrogen, or hypoxia; those on CNS stimulants or depressants), and those in altered environments (e.g., ICU, isolation, incubators, and institutions). This is accomplished by assessing and removing noxious environmental stimuli while increasing meaningful stimuli. Reduction of risk factors (e.g., sleep deprivation, visual or hearing impediments, adverse medications, dehydration, and pain) and use of orienting features (e.g., clocks, calendars, windows, and familiar objects) are important, as is maintaining verbal and nonverbal contact, with judicious use of touch. Structuring and explaining routines and procedures and interpreting sights, sounds, and smells in the environment are also crucial in preventing delirium.

delirium tremens (DTs), an acute and sometimes fatal psychotic reaction caused by abrupt cessation of excessive intake of alcoholic beverages. Initial symptoms include loss of appetite, insomnia, and general restlessness, which are followed by agitation; excitement; disorientation; mental confusion; vivid and often frightening hallucinations; acute fear and anxiety; illusions and delusions; coarse tremors of the hands, feet, legs, and tongue; fever; increased heart rate; extreme perspiration; GI distress; and precordial pain. The episode, which usually constitutes a medical emergency, typically lasts from 3 to 6 days and is generally followed by a deep sleep. See also **alcohol withdrawal syndrome, Korsakoff psychosis.**

delivery /diliv″ərē/ [L, *de* + *liberare,* to free], (in obstetrics) the birth of a child. Also called **parturition.** See also **Bradley method, Lamaze method, Leboyer method of delivery, Read method.**

delivery room, a unit of a hospital used for childbirth and infant resuscitation.

DeLorme technique, a method of exercise with weights for the purpose of strengthening muscles in which sets of repetitions are repeated with rests between sets. The technique involves isotonic exercise and determination of the maximum level of resistance. See also **progressive resistance exercise.**

delousing /dēlou″sing/ [L, *de,* from; AS, *lus*], ridding a person or object of an infestation of lice.

delta /del″tə/, **1.** Δ, δ, fourth letter of the Greek alphabet. **2.** the fourth position in a series.

delta-1-testolactone. See **testolactone.**

delta-9-tetrahydrocannabinol (THC), a pharmacologically active ingredient of cannabis that has been used in treating some cases of nausea and vomiting associated with cancer chemotherapy. See also **cannabis, dronabinol.**

delta agent, a defective viral agent (hepatitis D) that occurs only in association with hepatitis B infection. It causes chronic hepatitis and progressive liver damage. The delta agent is able to induce infection only when it is a coinfection present along with hepatitis B. It occurs in 5% of people with hepatitis; it infects about 15 million people worldwide.

delta-aminolevulinic acid test, a urine test to diagnose porphyrias. It can also be used to diagnose lead or mercury poisoning in adults.

delta hepatitis. See **hepatitis D.**

delta optical density analysis [Gk, *delta,* fourth letter of Greek alphabet, *optikos,* of sight; L, *densus,* thick; Gk, a loosening], a technique used to diagnose hemolytic disease in a fetus by measuring the proportion of bilirubin decomposition products in the amniotic fluid. The method involves spectrographic examination of a fluid sample. It measures the bilirubin and bilirubin-products concentration according to the wavelengths of light absorbed by the hemolytic products, as the bilirubin products alter the normal color of the amniotic fluid. The data are sometimes expressed in terms of $\delta O_{D45} 0$, the number representing the wavelength in nanometers at which maximum absorption of light by bilirubin occurs. If the delta optical density analysis indicates the fetus is moderately to severely anemic, immediate delivery is usually recommended when the gestational age permits.

Otherwise, intrauterine fetal blood transfusions may be recommended.

Deltavirus /del″təvī″rəs/, a genus of satellite viruses that require a helper hepatitis B virus for their replication. An individual consists of spherical virion 35 to 37 nanometers in diameter with an envelope derived from the helper virus surrounding a spherical core 18 nm in diameter; the genome consists of a single molecule of single-stranded, negative-sense, circular RNA (size 1.7 kb). It contains a single species, hepatitis D virus. See also **hepatitis D.**

delta wave, 1. the slowest of several types of brain waves, characterized by a frequency of 4 Hz and a relatively high voltage. Delta waves are "deep-sleep waves" associated with a dreamless state from which an individual is not easily aroused. Also called *delta rhythm.* Compare **alpha wave, beta wave, theta wave. 2.** (in cardiology) a slurring of the QRS portion of an electrocardiogram tracing caused by pre-excitation in Wolff-Parkinson-White syndrome.

deltoid /del″toid/ [Gk, *delta,* triangular, *eidos,* form], **1.** triangular. **2.** pertaining to the deltoid muscle that covers the shoulder.

deltoid ligament [Gk, *delta* + L, *ligamentum*], the medial ligament of the ankle joint.

deltoid muscle, a large, thick triangular muscle that covers the shoulder joint. It is the prime mover of arm abduction. It is also a synergist of arm flexion, extension, and medial and lateral rotation. Also called *deltoideus.*

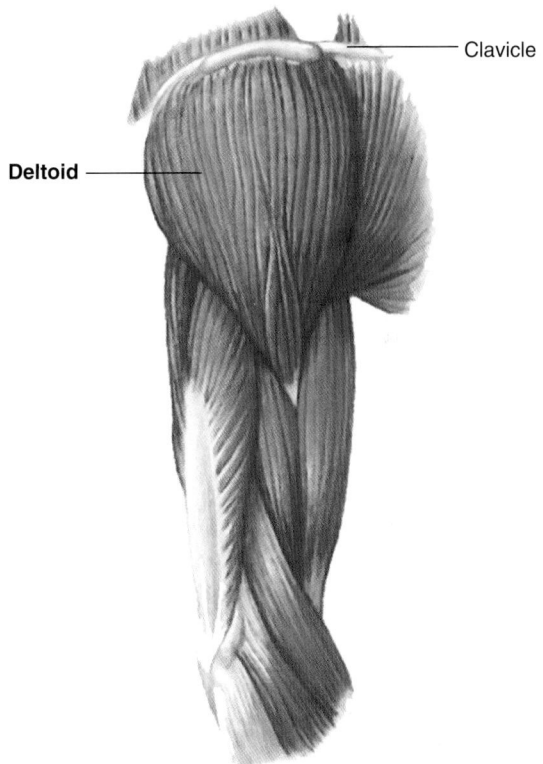

Clavicle

Deltoid

Deltoid muscle *(Patton and Thibodeau, 2010)*

deltopectoral triangle. See **clavipectoral triangle.**

deltoid tuberosity, the bony landmark on the proximal, lateral aspect of the humerus that serves as the location for the insertions for anterior, middle, and posterior deltoid muscles.

delusion /diloo″zhən/ [L, *deludere,* to deceive], a fixed false belief or perception unable to be changed despite evidence that refutes it. Delusions are found in persons with schizophrenia, bipolar disorder, and other mental disorders. While delusions may never completely be eliminated, some medications can minimize them such that they no longer predominate thought and disturb function. Compare **illusion.**

delusion of being controlled, the false belief that one's feelings, beliefs, thoughts, and acts are governed by some external force, as experienced in various forms of schizophrenia. See also **delusion.**

delusion of grandeur /grän″dyoor/, the gross exaggeration of one's importance, wealth, power, or talents, as manifested in such disorders as megalomania, dementia associated with late-stage syphilis, and paranoid schizophrenia. It may have a somatic or religious theme. See also **delusion.**

delusion of persecution, a morbid belief that one is being mistreated, harassed, or conspired against, as seen in paranoia and paranoid schizophrenia. The patient may single out a person or group as the source of persecution. See also **delusion.**

delusion of poverty, (in psychology) a false belief of a person that he or she is impoverished or will be deprived of material possessions.

delusion of reference. See **idea of reference.**

demand pacemaker [L, *demandere,* to give in charge, *passus,* step; ME, *maken*], a device used to stimulate the heart electrically when the heart's own impulses are not sufficient. The device measures the interval between the heart's native beats and delivers a stimulating pulse whenever that interval exceeds a set value.

demarcation /dē″märkā″shən/ [L, *de,* from, *marcare,* to mark], the process of setting limits or boundaries. See also **line of demarcation.**

demarcation current [L, *de + marcare,* to mark], an electrical current that flows from an uninjured to an injured end of a muscle. Also called **current of injury.**

deme /dēm/ [Gk, *demos,* common population], a small, local, closely related, interbreeding population of organisms, usually occupying a circumscribed area. Also called **genetic population.**

demecarium bromide /dē′məker″ē·əm/, an ophthalmic anticholinesterase agent.

■ INDICATIONS: It is prescribed in the treatment of open-angle glaucoma.

■ CONTRAINDICATIONS: Active uveal inflammation and/or glaucoma associated with iridocyclitis, bronchial asthma, peptic ulcer, epilepsy, recent myocardial infarction, pregnancy, or known hypersensitivity to this drug prohibits its use.

■ ADVERSE EFFECTS: Among the most serious adverse reactions are bradycardia, diarrhea, eye irritation, hypotension, headache, formation of cysts, and lens opacities.

demeclocycline hydrochloride /dēmek′lōsī″klēn/, a tetracycline antibiotic.

■ INDICATIONS: It is prescribed in the treatment of various gram-positive and gram-negative bacterial infections, including those in which use of penicillin is contraindicated.

■ CONTRAINDICATIONS: Renal or liver dysfunction, pregnancy, early childhood, or known hypersensitivity to this drug or to other tetracycline medication prohibits its use.

■ ADVERSE EFFECTS: Among the more serious adverse effects are GI disturbances, phototoxicity, potentially serious superinfections, and hypersensitivity reactions. Discoloration of teeth may occur in children exposed to the drug in utero or before 8 years of age.

demented /dimen″tid/ [L, *de,* away from, *mens,* mind], (*Informal*) pertaining to a form of mental disorder in which cognitive functions are affected. Central features are memory loss and inability to learn new material. Common causes are organic brain disorders.

dementia /dimen″shə/ [L, *de + mens,* mind], a progressive organic mental disorder characterized by chronic personality disintegration, confusion, disorientation, stupor, deterioration of intellectual capacity and function, and impairment of control of memory, judgment, and impulses. Kinds include **Pick disease, senile dementia–Alzheimer type, senile dementia, toxic dementia, dementia paralytica, secondary dementia.** Should not be confused with **delirium.**

■ OBSERVATIONS: There is more than one type of dementia, each slightly different from the others in presentation. In general, patients with dementia decline gradually, are confused, and do not have a change in their level of consciousness. The decline of cognitive function eventually becomes severe enough to impact social or occupational functioning.

■ INTERVENTIONS: Dementia caused by drug intoxication, hyperthyroidism, pernicious anemia, paresis, subdural hematoma, benign brain tumor, hydrocephalus, insulin shock, and tumor of islet cells of the pancreas can be reversed by treating the condition. Other organic forms of dementia such as Alzheimer disease are irreversible, progressive, and incurable. However, conditions that cause the decline may be treatable or partly reversible. Medications are available to slow the progression of some forms of dementia.

■ PATIENT CARE CONSIDERATIONS: As the ability to function effectively declines, care provision by others is increasingly necessary. The health care team should address the needs of dementia caregivers, as well as the patient. The increased burden of caregiving can contribute to numerous chronic health problems in the caregiver. For some patients with dementia, a long-term care facility can provide the most appropriate care. At the end stages, palliative care within a care facility is generally warranted.

dementia of the Alzheimer type, dementia occurring in Alzheimer disease, being of insidious onset and gradually progressive course, with histopathological changes characteristic of Alzheimer disease that are not due to other central nervous system, systemic, or substance-induced conditions known to cause dementia. It is characterized as early onset or late onset depending on whether or not it begins by the age of 65.

dementia paralytica, (*Obsolete*) now called **general paresis.**

dementia praecox, (*Obsolete*) now called **schizophrenia.**

dementia rating scale, a 0 to 3 scale used to quantify the severity of a patient's dementia. The rating is determined by a clinician based on assessment of a patient's cognitive and functional performance in six different areas.

dementia syndrome of depression, reversible dementia occurring in association with depression in the elderly, the cognitive deficits resolving with treatment of the depression.

Demerol, an opioid analgesic. Brand name for **meperidine hydrochloride.**

-demic, suffix meaning "relating to people or a district": *epidemic.*

demigauntlet bandage /dem′igônt″lit/ [L, *demidus,* half; Fr, *gant,* glove], a glovelike bandage over the hand that leaves the fingers free. See also **gauntlet bandage.**

demineralization /dēmin′əral′īzā″shən/ [L, *de + minera,* mine], a decrease in the amount of minerals or inorganic salts in tissues, as occurs in certain diseases.

demise /dimīz″/ [OFr, *demettre,* to put away], death, destruction, or end of existence.

democratic style /dem′okrat″ik/, people-centered leadership in which the group participates openly in decision making for group goals. In care facilities, shared governance is an example of the democratic style of leadership in which the residents exercise their rights to planning and decision making for care and for the facility as a whole. See also **shared governance.**

demography /dəmog″rəfē/ [Gk, *demos,* people, *graphein,* to record], the study of human populations, particularly the size, distribution, and characteristics of members of population groups. Demography is applied in studies of health problems involving ethnic groups, populations of a specific geographic region, religious groups with special dietary restrictions, and members of population groups that may represent a typical cross section of the entire nation. Compare **epidemiology.**

demonstrative /dimon″strətiv/, pertaining to a concept or an action that accompanies and illustrates speech, such as indication of the size of an object with the hands.

de Morsier syndrome. See **septooptic dysplasia.**

Demser, an antihypertensive drug. Brand name for **metyrosine.**

demulcent /dimul″sənt/ [L, *demulcere,* to stroke down], **1.** *n.,* any of several oily substances used for soothing and reducing irritation of surfaces that have been abraded or irritated, especially mucosal surfaces. **2.** *adj.,* soothing, as a counterirritant or balm.

Demulen, an oral contraceptive containing a progestin and an estrogen. Brand name for **ethynodiol diacetate and ethinyl estradiol.**

demyelinate /dēmī″əlināt′/, to remove or destroy the myelin surrounding the axons of nerve cells.

demyelination /dimī″əlinā″shən/ [L, *de* + Gk, *myelos,* marrow], the process of destruction or removal of the myelin sheath from a nerve or nerve fiber.

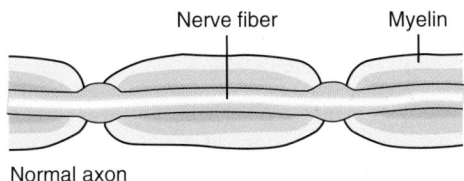

Nerve fiber   Myelin

Normal axon

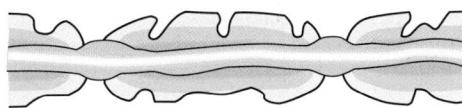

Disintegration of myelin

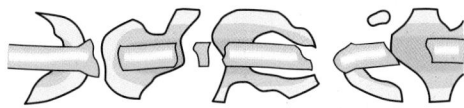

Disruption of axon function

Process of demyelination *(Monahan et al, 2007)*

denasality. See **hyponasality.**

denaturation /dēnā′chərā″shən/ [L, *de* + *natura,* natural], the alteration of the basic nature or structure of a substance.

denatured alcohol /dēnā″chərd/, ethyl alcohol made unfit for ingestion by the addition of acetone or methanol, used as a solvent and in chemical processes.

denatured protein [L, *de,* from, *natura, proteios,* first rank], a protein that has undergone change that causes its original properties to be lost. A protein can be denatured by radiation, heat, strong acids, or alcohol.

dendr-, prefix meaning "tree" or "branches": *dendrite.*

-dendria, suffix meaning the "twiglike branching of nerve fibers": *telodendria.*

dendrite /den″drīt/ [Gk, *dendron,* tree], a slender branching process that extends from the cell body of a neuron and that is capable of being stimulated by a neurotransmitter. Each neuron usually possesses several dendrites, which receive synapses where chemical transmission occurs from axons to dendrites (or an axon, in the case of unipolar neurons). The number of dendrites and thus the number of synapses varies with the functions of a neuron. Also called **cytodendrite.** Compare **axon.**

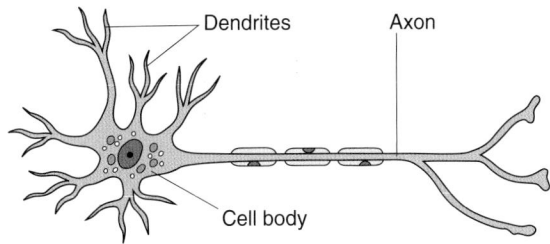

Dendrites   Axon

Cell body

Dendrite *(Coad and Dunstall, 2011)*

dendritic /dendrit″ik/, **1.** treelike, with branches that spread toward or into neighboring tissues, as dendritic keratitis. **2.** pertaining to a dendrite.

dendritic calculus [Gk, *dendron,* tree, *calculus,* pebble], a large calculus lodged in the pelvis of the kidney and shaped to fit the branches of the calyx. Also called **coral calculus.**

dendritic cell, a cell that captures antigens and migrates to the lymph nodes and spleen, where it presents the processed antigens to T cells.

dendritic keratitis, inflammation of the cornea and conjunctiva caused by herpesvirus type 1. Also called **herpetic keratitis.**

■ OBSERVATIONS: It is characterized by an ulceration of the surface of the cornea resembling a tree with knobs at the ends of the branches. Photophobia, the sensation of a foreign body in the eye, pain, and conjunctivitis are usual.

■ INTERVENTIONS: Treatment entails application of idoxuridine (IDU), chemical debridement with an iodine tincture, or surgical removal of the layer of corneal tissue cells affected.

■ PATIENT CARE CONSIDERATIONS: Untreated dendritic keratitis may cause permanent scarring of the cornea with impaired vision or blindness. Recurrent dendritic keratitis is often followed by disciform keratitis, which is characterized by clouding and deep swelling of the cornea and inflammation of the iris.

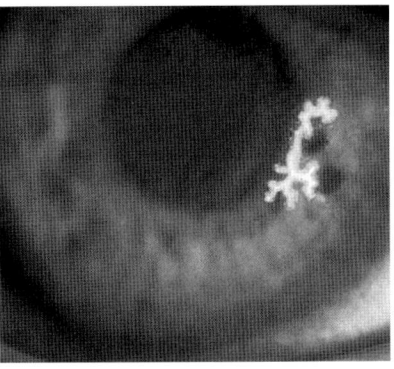

Dendritic keratitis *(Dehn and Asprey, 2014)*

dendrodendritic synapse /den′drōdendrit″ik/ [Gk, *dendron* + *dendron* + *synaptein*, to join], a type of synapse in which a dendrite of one neuron comes in contact with a dendrite of another neuron. Compare **axodendritic synapse.**

denervated /dēnur″vātid/ [L, *de* + *nervus*, nerve], having a nerve impulse route interrupted, as by excision or administration of a drug that blocks the pathway. The result is decreased or no transmission of impulses through this pathway.

dengue fever /deng″gē, den″gā/ [Sp, influenza; L, *febris*, fever], an acute Flavivirus infection caused by one of four antigenically distinct serotypes, which determines the severity of infection. It is transmitted to humans by the bite of an infected *Aedes aegypti* mosquito and occurs in tropical and subtropical regions. Also called **Aden fever, bouquet fever, breakbone fever, dandy fever,** *dengue,* **solar fever.** See also *Aedes*, **arbovirus, dengue hemorrhagic fever shock syndrome.**

- OBSERVATIONS: The disease usually produces a triad of symptoms: fever; rash; and severe head, back, and muscle pain. Manifestations of dengue usually occur in two phases separated by a day of remission. In the first phase the patient experiences fever, extreme weakness, headache, sore throat, muscle pains, and edema of the hands and feet. The second phase is marked by a return of fever and by a bright-red scarlatiniform rash. Occasionally shock and hemorrhage occur, leading to fatality.
- INTERVENTIONS: Treatment is symptomatic. Analgesics may be given to relieve headache and other pains.
- PATIENT CARE CONSIDERATIONS: Dengue is a self-limited illness, although recovery may require several weeks. A vaccine known as CYD-TDV (brand name Dengvaxia) is available.

dengue hemorrhagic fever shock syndrome (DHFSS), a grave form of dengue fever characterized by shock with collapse or prostration; cold, clammy extremities; a weak, thready pulse; respiratory distress; and all of the symptoms of dengue fever. Hemorrhages, bruises, and small reddish spots indicating bleeding from skin capillaries, as well as bloody vomit, urine, and feces, may be experienced and may precede circulatory collapse. This syndrome occurs when a person with immunity to one type of dengue virus becomes infected with another serotype. Treatment includes fluid and electrolyte replacement and blood, fresh frozen plasma, or platelet transfusions as needed. Oxygen and sedatives may be administered. See also **dengue fever.**

denial /dinī′əl/ [L, *denegare*, to negate], **1.** refusal or restriction of something requested, claimed, or needed, often causing physical or emotional deficiency. **2.** an unconscious defense mechanism in which emotional conflict and anxiety are avoided by refusal to acknowledge those thoughts, feelings, desires, impulses, or facts that are consciously intolerable.

denileukin diftitox, a miscellaneous antineoplastic agent.
- INDICATIONS: It is used to treat cutaneous T cell lymphoma that expresses the CD25 component of the IL-2 receptor.
- CONTRAINDICATIONS: Hypersensitivity to denileukin, diphtheria toxin, or interleukin-2 prohibits its use.
- ADVERSE EFFECTS: Life-threatening effects are thrombocytopenia and leukopenia. Other serious side effects include hematuria, albuminuria, pyuria, creatinine increase, anemia, hypoalbuminemia, edema, hypocalcemia, dehydration, hypokalemia, infection, chest pain, and flu-like symptoms. Common side effects include dizziness, paresthesia, nervousness, confusion, insomnia, hypotension, vasodilation, tachycardia, thrombosis, hypertension, dysrhythmias, nausea, anorexia, vomiting, diarrhea, constipation, dyspepsia, and dysphagia.

Denis Browne splint [Denis J.W. Browne, 20th-century Australian surgeon], a splint for the correction of clubfoot, composed of a bar attached to the soles of a pair of specialized shoes with screw receptacles on the soles. The splint is equipped with adapters for mounting the shoes to allow individual abduction of each foot. The splint is commonly applied nightly in late infancy after casting and manipulation have effectively reduced the deformity.

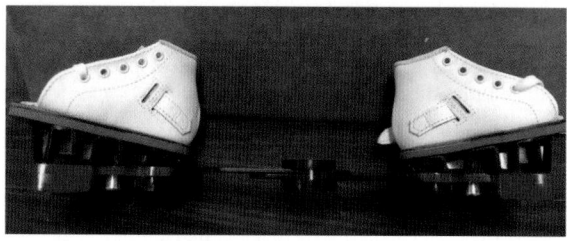

Denis Browne splint *(©2015 M.J. Markell Shoe Company)*

denitrogenation /dēnī′trōjənā″shən/, the elimination of nitrogen from the lungs and body tissues during a period of breathing pure oxygen. See also **nitrogen washout curve.**

dens /den″ēz/ [L, tooth], **1.** a tooth or toothlike structure or process. The term is sometimes modified to identify a particular tooth, such as dens caninus or dens molaris. **2.** the cone-shaped odontoid process of the axis, or second cervical vertebra. It receives the atlantal ring to act as a pivot for the atlas, or first cervical vertebra. See also **dentition, odontoid process, tooth.**

dense connective tissue, connective tissue characterized by closely compacted groups of fibers.

dense fibrous tissue [L, *densus*, thick], a fibrous connective tissue consisting of compact, strong, inelastic bundles of mostly parallel collagenous fibers that are glistening white. Dense regular fibrous tissue comprises the tendons, the aponeuroses, and the ligaments; dense irregular fibrous tissue comprises the fascial membranes, the dermis of the skin, the periosteum, and the capsules of organs. Compare **loose fibrous tissue.**

dens evaginatus, a developmental anomaly in which an extra enamel cusp (which may include pulp tissue) develops in the central groove or lingual ridge of molars or premolars. This cone-shaped elevation of enamel is subject to occlusal trauma and fracture. Removal of the cusp may often require pulp treatment. Should not be confused with **dens invaginatus.**

densimeter /densim′eter/. See **densitometer.**

dens in dente /den″tə/, an anomaly of the teeth, found chiefly in the maxillary lateral incisors and characterized by invagination of the enamel. The condition causes a radiographic image suggestive of a tooth within a tooth. Also called **dens invaginatus, gestant odontoma.**

dens invaginatus, a rare developmental anomaly of teeth resulting from infolding of the dental papilla before calcification. It may be confined to the crown or extend to the root of the teeth. Also called **dens in dente.** Should not be confused with **dens evaginatus.**

densitometer /den′sitom″ətər/ [L, *densus* + Gk, *metron*, measure], a device that uses a photoelectric cell to detect differences in the intensity of light transmitted through a substance, such as film, laminates, and substrates.

density (D) /den″sitē/ [L, *densus*, thick], **1.** the amount of mass of a substance in a given volume. The greater the mass in a given volume, the greater the density. See also **mass, volume. 2.** (in radiology) the degree of x-ray image blackening in film/screen radiography.

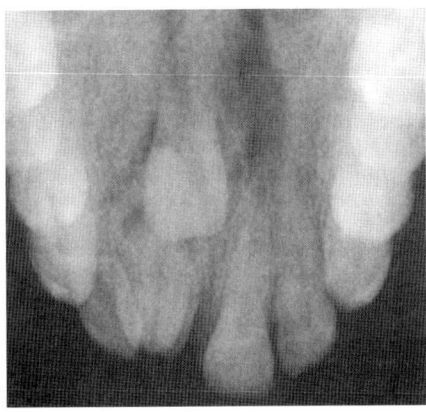

Dens in dente *(Regezi, Sciubba, and Pogrel, 2000)*

density gradient, a variation in the density of a solution caused by a change in concentration of a solute in a confined solution.

dens serotinus. See **wisdom tooth.**

dent-, denta-. See **dento-, dent-, denta-, denti-, dentia-.**

dental [L, *dens,* tooth], pertaining to a tooth or the teeth.

dental abscess. See **periapical abscess, periodontal abscess.**

dental alveolus /alvē″ələs/, a tooth socket in the mandible or maxilla.

dental amalgam, an alloy of silver, tin, and mercury with small amounts of cooper and sometimes zinc, used for restoring tooth surfaces affected by dental caries or trauma. See **amalgam,** def. 2.

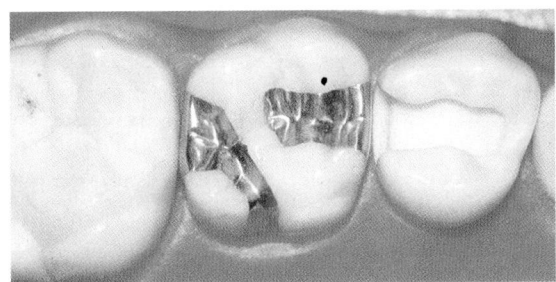

Dental amalgam *(Christensen, 2002)*

dental anesthesia, any of several methods to reduce or block the perception of pain and discomfort during a dental procedure. See also **awake anesthesia, inhalation anesthesia, local anesthesia, nitrous oxide, regional anesthesia, topical anesthesia, block anesthesia.**

dental anesthesiology /-ol″əjē/ [L, *dens,* tooth], one of the 10 specialties of dentistry; it deals with the advanced use of anesthesia, sedation, and pain management to facilitate dental procedures.

dental ankylosis, solid fixation of a tooth resulting from fusion of the cementum and alveolar bone, with obliteration of at least a portion of the periodontal ligament.

dental anomaly, an aberration in which one or more teeth deviate from the normal in form, function, or position.

dental appliance, any device placed in or on a patient by a dentist as part of a treatment protocol. Dental appliances include orthodontic, prosthetic, retaining, snoring/airway, and habit-modification devices.

dental arch, the curving shape formed by the arrangement of a normal set of teeth in each jaw. The inferior dental arch is formed by the mandibular teeth. The superior dental arch is formed by the maxillary teeth. See also **alveolar process.**

dental assistant, a person who performs highly technical skilled work under the supervision of dentists in a wide variety of tasks in the dental office, ranging from patient care to administrative duties to laboratory functions. See also **certified dental assistant, expanded function dental assistant.**

dental biomechanics, the study and use of mechanical devices and physical forces to effect desirable changes in oral structures.

dental bur, a rotary drill bit made of steel or diamond impregnated material attached to a steel shank, available in varying degrees of sharpness, lengths, shapes, and sizes, used in the preparation of teeth to receive a dental restoration.

dental calculus, a salivary deposit of calcium and magnesium phosphate, calcium carbonate, and other substances, with organic matter such as desquamated epithelium, mucin, and microorganisms, that adheres to the teeth or a dental prosthesis. See also **calculus.**

dental caries, a tooth disease caused by the complex interaction of food, especially starches and sugars, with saliva and the bacteria that form dental plaque. The term also refers to the tooth cavities that result from the disease. Plaque bacteria produce acids that cause demineralization of enamel and enzymes that attack the protein component of the tooth. This process, if untreated, ultimately leads to the formation of deep cavities and bacterial infection of the pulp chamber, which contains blood vessels and nerves. The development of dental caries in a debilitated patient is a concern because of the danger that infections of the teeth or gingival tissues may spread to the rest of the body. In addition, teeth that are decayed or painful inhibit mastication and can lead to dietary changes, which may in turn cause nutritional and digestive disorders. Dental caries may be prevented by a reduction in the frequency of sugar consumption, use of dental floss between the teeth, regular brushing of the teeth with a fluoridated toothpaste, drinking fluoridated water, topical application of fluorides to the teeth, and removal of plaque and calculus by a dental hygienist. Treatment of dental caries includes removal of the decayed material and restoration of the surface of the affected tooth with an amalgam or other restorative material. If the cavity has reached the pulp chamber, it may be necessary to remove the pulp tissues to alleviate pain, prevent the spread of infection to the rest of the body, and allow the continued use of the tooth. Alternatively, the entire tooth may be extracted. Kinds include **arrested dental caries, incipient dental caries, pit and fissure cavity, secondary dental caries, smooth surface cavity, primary dental caries.** See also **classification of caries.** −**carious,** *adj.*

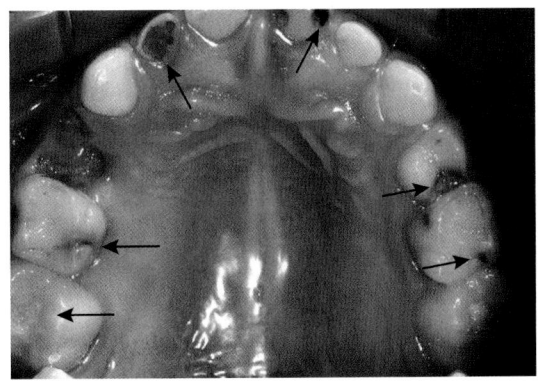

Dental caries *(Courtesy Dr. Frank Hodges)*

Black's system of classification of caries

Class I	Located in pits and fissures of the occlusal two thirds of posterior teeth or the lingual surface of anterior teeth
Class II	Located on the proximal surfaces of premolars and molars
Class III	Located on the proximal surfaces of central and lateral incisors and cuspids
Class IV	Located on the proximal surfaces of incisors and canines involving the incisal angle
Class V	Located in the gingival third on the labial, facial, or lingual surfaces of anterior or posterior teeth
Class VI	Located on cusp tips

dental chart, a simplified graphic representation of the teeth on which clinical, radiological, and forensic information may be recorded. See also **FDI numbering system, Palmer notation, universal tooth coding system.**

dental crypt, the space in the alveolar process occupied by a developing tooth.

dental emergency, an acute disorder of oral health that requires dental and/or medical attention, including broken, loose, or evulsed teeth caused by traumas; infections and inflammations of the soft tissues of the mouth; and complications of oral surgery, such as dry tooth socket.

dental engine, an apparatus consisting of a handpiece to which various burs (rotating drill bits) or other tools can be fitted. It is driven directly by an electric motor or by an electric motor via a continuous cordlike belt that runs over pulleys.

dental erosion, the chemical or mechanochemical destruction of tooth material that can involve enamel, dentin, and cementum and causes variously shaped concave depressions, generally at the cementoenamel junctions of teeth or the facial surface of the crown of the tooth. The erosion may be related to swimming in chlorinated pools or frequent sucking on citrus fruits held for a long period of time by the lips against the teeth. The surfaces of these depressions, unlike those of dental caries, are hard and smooth. See also **erosion.**

dental ethics [L, *dens,* tooth; Gk, *ethos,* ethics], a system of moral principles governing the professional conduct of dental professionals and dental practices ascribed by the American Dental Association Council on Ethics, state dental associations, and local dental societies. In Canada, these are governed by the Canadian Dental Association Code of Ethics and provincial dental regulatory bodies and called the CDA (Canadian Dental Association) principles of ethics.

dental examination, an inspection of the teeth and surrounding soft tissues of the oral cavity. The examiner generally uses an explorer, a slender steel instrument with a flexible, sharp point, to probe the minute indentations on tooth surfaces and around dental restorations for signs of demineralization and caries development. A radiographic record or imaging of the teeth and parts of the maxilla and mandible is usually made. The examiner may also insert a periodontal probe into the soft-tissue sulcus around each tooth to measure the depth of each sulcus and to explore for calculus and root defects. The examination should include inspection of the floor of the mouth, all surfaces of the tongue, the cheeks and soft tissue of the oral cavity, the salivary glands and ducts, and the lymph nodes of the neck in order to detect pathology. Also called **intraoral examination.**

dental extracting forceps, a hand instrument used for grasping teeth during their removal from the socket. Most forceps are designed for the extraction of a particular tooth in the maxilla or mandible.

dental film, an x-ray photograph of the teeth, exposed either intraorally or extraorally. Intraoral films are small double-emulsion films without screens but with a lead foil backing to reduce patient dose, enclosed in a moisture-resistant envelope. Extraoral films are large single-emulsion screen films.

dental fistula, an abnormal passage from a bacterially infected area of a tooth to the surface of the oral mucous membrane, permitting the discharge of inflammatory or suppurative material. Also called **alveolar fistula, alveolar sinus.**

dental floss, a thread used by hand to clean interproximal tooth surfaces and spaces between the teeth of plaque and biofilm. It may be waxed, unwaxed, or Teflon thread, and flavored or unflavored.

dentalgia. See **toothache.**

dental granuloma, an inflammatory formation of a microscopic grouping of macrophages, usually surrounded by lymphocytes and occasional plasma cells, that is attached to the apex of a tooth and surrounded by a fibrous capsule. On x-ray film or dental image it appears as a well-defined radiolucency.

dental handpiece, a dental instrument, either air driven or electrically driven, that holds various disks, cups, or burs, used to prepare a tooth to receive a restoration or to contour, clean, or polish a tooth or restoration.

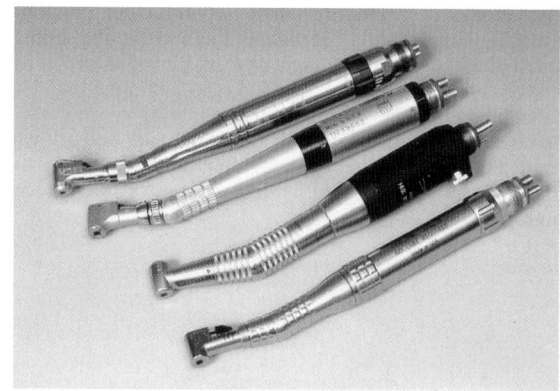

Dental handpieces *(Christensen, 2002)*

dental history, a record of a patient's oral health, general health, medical conditions, medical care, surgical treatments, current medication used, allergies, childhood diseases, radiographic history, and personal dental care, both past and present. An aid in treatment planning for a patient.

dental hygienist, a licensed oral health care professional authorized to provide clinical and therapeutic services under the supervision of a licensed dentist or, in some states, as a private practitioner in collaboration with a dentist. Duties include dental prophylaxis, radiography, administration of medications, and dental education at chairside and in the community. In some states, a dental hygienist with additional education may administer local anesthetics and nitrous oxide/oxygen analgesia, place and carve filling materials, conduct additional periodontal procedures, and function as a public health specialist. To practice as a registered dental hygienist, a person must complete at least 2 years of postsecondary education in an accredited community or dental college or university, successfully complete written and practical examinations, and be approved by a state or regional board of dental and dental hygiene examiners.

dental identification [L, *dens,* tooth, *idem,* the same, *facere,* to make], the process of establishing the unique characteristics of the teeth and dental work of an individual, thereby permitting the identification of the individual by comparison with his or her dental charts, records, plaster casts, radiographs or dental images, bite marks, and records. See also **forensic dentistry.**

dental impaction, the blocking of a tooth by a physical barrier, usually other teeth, so that it cannot erupt. See also **impacted tooth.**

dental implant, an artificial device surgically inserted into the jawbone to replace a missing tooth or to provide support for a prosthetic denture or fixed bridge. Components of the implant system include an implant body, composed of titanium or ceramic materials such as zirconia, which acts as the "root" of the implant restoration; the implant abutment or titanium post that attaches to the implant body and protrudes partially or completely through the gingival tissue into the mouth; and the crown or other prosthesis connected to the abutment either by a screw or by dental cement. The implant placement procedure includes drilling into the bone to place the implant body, which is allowed to heal for several weeks or months to allow osseointegration or bone generation to occur around the implant body. Osseointegration and implant stability are the major determinants for implant success. Disease can occur and disrupt the osseointegration around the implant body.

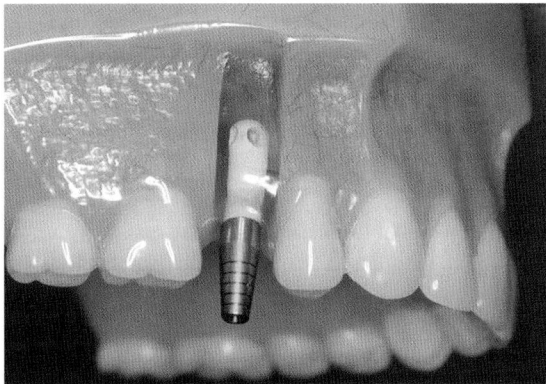

Dental implant *(Christensen, 2002)*

dental jurisprudence [L, *dens,* tooth, *jurisprudentia,* knowledge of the law], the study, knowledge, or science of law as it relates to the practice of dentistry and the actions of all dental professionals.

dental laboratory technician, a person who makes dental prostheses and orthodontic appliances as prescribed by a dentist. A dental laboratory technician may have a private laboratory or work in the premises of a dentist. Also called **dental technician.**

dental lamina, the histological primordial tissues found in the developing tooth within the jaw. Also called *tooth bud.*

dental laser, a device utilizing laser light of a certain frequency to remove pathological dental tissue and prepare the tooth to accept a dental restoration. Also a device used to remove or recontour oral soft tissue.

dental operculum [L, *dens,* tooth, *operculum,* a covering structure], a hood or flap of gingival tissue overlying the crown of an erupting tooth, commonly the mandibular third molars. This tissue will usually recede during tooth eruption. The tissue surrounding the operculum can become inflamed and painful. Also called **operculitis.**

dental papilla [L, *dens,* tooth, *papilla,* nipple], mesodermal tissue enclosed in the invaginated portion of the epithelial enamel organ and giving rise to three components of the tooth: dentin, formed by odontoblasts; cementum, formed by cementoblasts; and dental pulp.

dental pathology, the study of diseases, including causes and effects, of the oral cavity and the dentition.

dental plaque. See **bacterial plaque.**

dental plate [L, *dens,* tooth; OFr, *plate,* flat structure], *(Informal)* a dental prosthesis made to the shape of the maxilla or mandible jaw to support artificial teeth. See also **denture.**

dental porcelain, a type of high-temperature fusion glass used in dental restorations, either jacket crowns or inlays, artificial teeth, or metal-ceramic crowns. It is essentially a mixture of particles of feldspar, silica, and alumina (aluminum oxide), the feldspar melting first and providing a glass matrix for the silica and alumina. Porcelain, which comes in various shades, chemically and physically bonds to a metal coping and creates a tooth-colored restoration.

dental probe. See **periodontal probe.**

dental prophylaxis. See **oral prophylaxis.**

dental prosthesis [L, *dens,* tooth; Gk, *prosthesis,* an addition], a fixed or removable appliance used to replace one or more lost or missing natural teeth. Kinds include **complete denture, fixed bridgework, removable partial denture.**

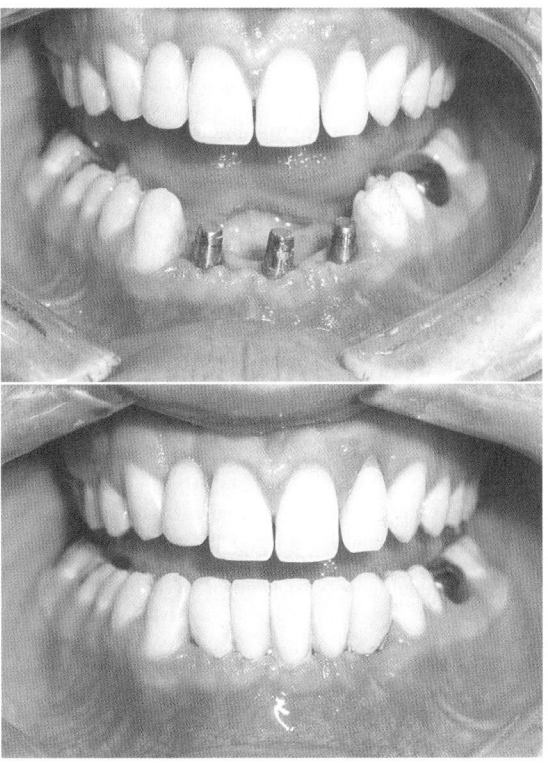

Fixed bridge prosthesis cemented over implants
(Christensen, 2002)

dental public health, a recognized specialty that is the science and art of preventing and controlling dental diseases and promoting dental health through organized community efforts. It is a form of dental practice that serves the community as a patient rather than the individual. It is concerned with the dental health education of the public, applied dental research, and the administration of group dental care programs, as well as the prevention and control of dental diseases on a community basis. Also called **public health dentistry.**

dental pulp, a small mass of loose connective tissue, blood vessels, and nerves located in a canal within the dentin layer of a tooth. The pulp chamber is found in the crown and the pulp canal within the root of a tooth. See also **pulp canal, pulp cavity, root canal.**

dental radiograph [L, *dens,* tooth, *radire,* to shine; Gk, *graphein,* to record],   an intraoral or extraoral x-ray film, picture, or image capture of teeth and the bone surrounding them. See also **bite wing radiograph, periapical radiograph.**

dental restoration.   See **restoration.**

dental sealant /sē″lənt/,   a plastic resin film coating that is applied to and adheres to the caries-free occlusal surfaces (chewing surfaces) of teeth to seal pits and fissures where plaque, food, and bacteria usually become trapped and cannot be physically reached to cleanse. The surface to be treated is isolated to ensure that it is not contaminated with saliva. It is then cleaned with a brush and pumice cleansing agent or micro-abraded, dried, and etched with a phosphoric acid solution. After the acid has been washed away and the tooth has been dried, the sealant is applied. Dental sealants are reported to reduce the incidence of caries in children's teeth by 50%. Also called **pit and fissure sealant.**

dental stone,   a calcined (strongly heated or processed) gypsum derivative similar to but stronger than plaster of paris; used for making dental casts and dies. Also called **artificial stone.**

dental surgeon [L, *dens,* tooth; Gk, *cheirourgos,* surgeon],   a dentist who is able to diagnose pathology and disease and who performs surgical procedures involving the teeth and surrounding oral tissues. Compare **dentist.** See also **dentistry.**

dental technician.   See **dental laboratory technician.**

dental therapist,   a licensed oral health care midlevel professional provider with distinct educational, examination, and practice requirements who may perform procedures as specified by state-specific laws. The position of dental therapist was created to help increase access to dental care in settings that serve low-income, uninsured, and underserved patients or in areas with a shortage of dental health professionals. There is also an advanced dental therapist (ADT) midlevel provider position; ADTs must earn a master's degree from an advanced dental therapy education program. Procedures performed may include oral health instruction and disease prevention education, including nutritional counseling and dietary analysis; preliminary charting of the oral cavity; the making of radiographs; mechanical polishing; application of topical preventive or prophylactic agents, including fluoride varnishes and pit and fissure sealants; pulp vitality testing; application of desensitizing medication or resin; fabrication of athletic mouthguards; placement of temporary restorations; fabrication of soft occlusal guards; tissue conditioning and soft reline; atraumatic restorative therapy; dressing changes; tooth reimplantation; administration of local anesthetic; and administration of nitrous oxide. Therapists' duties also may include emergency palliative treatment of dental pain, the placement and removal of space maintainers, cavity preparation, restoration of primary and permanent teeth, placement of temporary crowns, preparation and placement of preformed crowns, pulpotomies on primary teeth, indirect and direct pulp capping on primary and permanent teeth, stabilization of reimplanted teeth, extractions of primary teeth, suture removal, brush biopsies, repair of defective prosthetic devices, and recementing of permanent crowns, among others.

dental trephination,   surgical creation of a fistula by puncturing the soft tissue and bone overlying the root apex to provide drainage of infectious materials. Also called *apicostomy.*

dentinal tubules,   minute channels within dentin, extending from the pulp cavity to the cementum and enamel.

-dentate,   suffix meaning "possessing teeth": *edentate, multidentate, tridentate.*

dentate fracture /den″tāt/   [L, *dens*],   any fracture that causes serrated bone ends that fit together like the teeth of gears.

dentate nucleus,   a deep cerebellar nucleus that receives fibers from the lateral zone of the cerebellar cortex and

appears to act as a trigger for the motor cortex, governing intentional movements as well as properties of ongoing movements.

dentes.   See **dens.**

denti-, dentia-.   See **dento-, dent-, denta-, denti-, dentia-.**

dentibuccal /den″tibuk′əl/ [L, *dens,* tooth + *bucca,* cheek],   pertaining to the teeth and cheek.

denticle /den″tikəl/,   a calcified body found within the pulp chamber or pulp canal of a tooth. If it is composed of irregular dentin, it is known as a true denticle. Also called **endolith, pulp stone.**

denticulate /dentik″yəlit/ [L, *denticulus,* little tooth],   having very small teeth or toothlike projections.

dentifrice /den″tifris/ [L, *dens* + *fricare,* to rub],   a pharmaceutic compound used with a toothbrush for cleaning and polishing the teeth. It typically contains a mild abrasive, detergent, flavoring agent, fluoride, and binder. Other common ingredients are deodorants, humectants, desensitizers, mild bleaching agents, and various medications to prevent dental caries. Also called **toothpaste.**

dentigerous cyst /dentij″ərəs/ [L, *dens* + *gerere,* to bear],   one of three kinds of follicular cyst, consisting of an epithelium-lined sac filled with fluid or viscous material that surrounds the crown of an unerupted tooth or odontoma. It is the most common type of developmental odontogenic cyst that develops due to inflammation in contact with remnants of the enamel organ or follicular sac that surrounds an unerupted permanent tooth. Radiographically, it appears as a well-defined radiolucent lesion with a radiopaque border attached to the cervical area of an unerupted tooth. Treatment is excision. Compare **primordial cyst.**

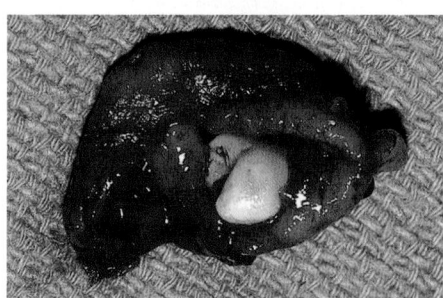

Dentigerous cyst *(Regezi, Sciubba, and Pogrel, 2000)*

dentin /den″tin/ [L, *dens*],   the chief material of teeth, consisting of calcium phosphate, surrounding the pulp, and situated inside the enamel and cementum. Harder and denser than bone, it consists of solid organic substratum infiltrated with lime salts. Nerves course throughout its structure. Also spelled **dentine.**

dentin eburnation /ē′burnā″shən/,   a change in carious teeth in which softened and decalcified dentin develops a hard, brown, polished appearance.

dentin globule,   a small spheric body in peripheral dentin, created by early calcification.

dentinoenamel /den′tinō·inam″əl/ [L, *dens* + OFr, *enesmail,* enamel],   pertaining to both the dentin and the enamel of the teeth.

dentinoenamel junction (DEJ),   the interface of the enamel and the dentin of a tooth crown, generally conforming to the shape of the crown. Also called **dentoenamel junction.**

dentinogenesis /den′tinōjen″əsis/ [L, *dens* + Gk, *genein,* to produce],   the formation of the dentin of the teeth. **–dentinogenic,** *adj.*

dentinogenesis imperfecta,   1. a genetic disturbance in the consistency of the dentin, characterized by early calcification of the pulp chambers, marked attrition, and an opalescent hue of the teeth. A form of dentin dysplasia. **2.** a localized form of mesodermal dysplasia affecting the dentin of the teeth. It may be hereditary and associated with osteogenesis imperfecta. **3.** a genetic condition that produces defective dentin but normal tooth enamel. Also called **hereditary opalescent dentin.**

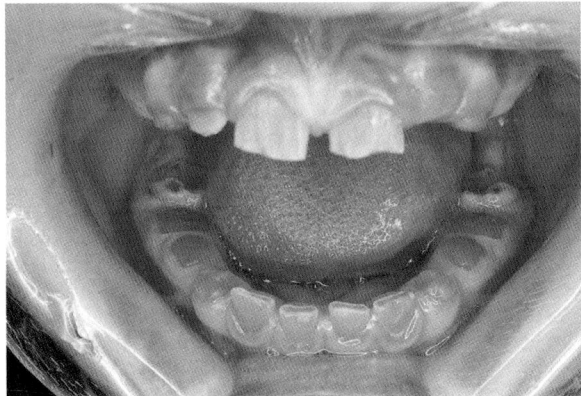

Dentinogenesis imperfecta *(Regezi, Sciubba, and Jordan, 2012)*

dentinogenic.   See **dentinogenesis.**

dentist [L, *dens*], a person who is qualified by training and licensed by a state or region to diagnose and treat abnormalities of the teeth, gingiva, face, head, neck, and underlying bone, including conditions caused by disease, trauma, and heredity. Required training in the United States consists of 3 to 4 years in an undergraduate college after fulfilling the undergraduate academic requirements for admission, a satisfactory score on a Dental Admission Test and 4 years at an American Dental Association–accredited dental college. After completing dental college, a dentist is awarded a degree of either Doctor of Dental Surgery (D.D.S.) or Doctor of Dental Medicine (D.M.D.); the two degrees are equivalent. A dentist must pass written and practical examinations to obtain a state license. Dental internships and residencies are not, as yet, required for general practice. See also **dentistry.**

dentistry /den″tistrē/ [L, *dens*], the art and science of practicing the diagnosis, prevention, and treatment of diseases and disorders of the teeth, face, head, neck, and all surrounding structures of the oral cavity. Responsibilities include the repair and restoration of teeth, the replacement of missing teeth, and the detection of diseases, such as blood dyscrasias and tumors, that require treatment by a dental specialist or physician. In addition to the general practice of dentistry, there are 10 recognized specialties, each requiring additional training after graduation from a dental college: dental public health, endodontics, oral and maxillofacial pathology, oral and maxillofacial radiology, oral and maxillofacial surgery, orthodontics, pediatric dentistry, periodontics, prosthodontics, and dental anesthesiology.

dentition /dentish″ən/ [L, *dentire*, to cut teeth], **1.** the development and eruption of the teeth. See also **teething. 2.** the arrangement, number, and kind of teeth as they appear in the dental arches of the mouth. **3.** the teeth of an individual or species as determined by their form and arrangement. See also **primary dentition, mixed dentition, natural dentition, permanent dentition, precocious dentition, retarded dentition, secondary dentition, predeciduous dentition.**

dento-, dent-, denta-, denti-, dentia-, prefix meaning "tooth" or "teeth": *dentalgia, denture.*

dentoalveolar abscess /den′tō-alvē″ələr/ [L, *dens + alveolus,* little hollow, *abscedere,* to go away], the formation and accumulation of pus in a tooth socket or the jawbone around the base of a tooth. The pus results from a bacterial infection that is usually secondary to an infection or injury to the tooth or alveolar tissues. It is polymicrobial, with an average of 4 to 6 different causative organisms. Also called **periapical abscess.**

dentoenamel junction.   See **dentinoenamel junction.**

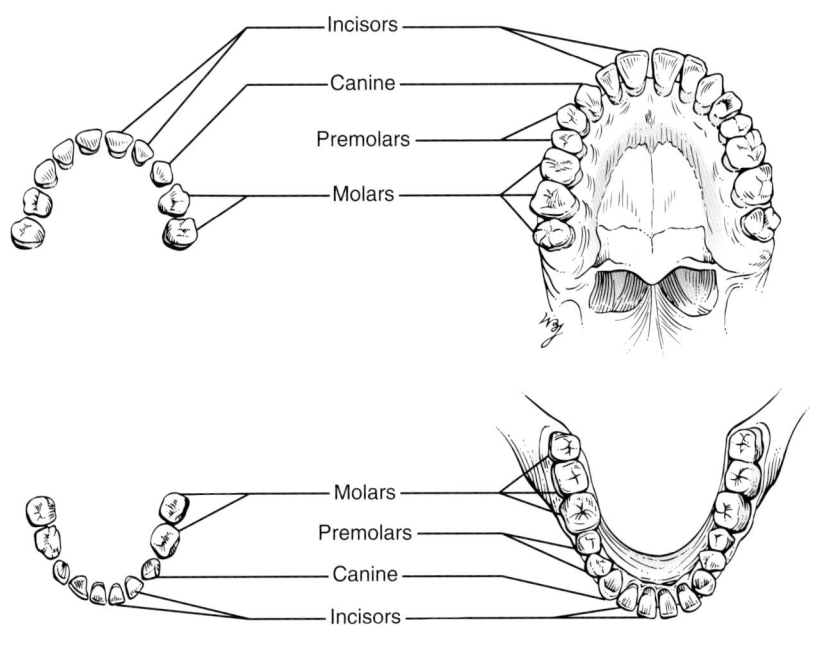

PRIMARY DENTITION   SECONDARY DENTITION

Primary dentition *(left)* and secondary dentition *(right)* *(Swartz, 2014)*

dentofacial /-fā″shəl/, pertaining to the mouth or the jaw.

dentofacial anomaly, a condition in which a mouth or jaw structure deviates from normal in form, function, or position.

dentofacial orthopedics. See **orthodontics and dentofacial orthopedics.**

dentogenesis imperfecta. See **dentinogenesis imperfecta.**

dentogingival fiber /-jinjī″vəl/ [L, *dens* + *gingiva,* gum], any of the many peridental connective tissue fibers (periodontal fibers) that emerge from the supraalveolar part of the cementum of a tooth, spread like a fan, and terminate in the free gingiva. See also **dentoperiosteal fiber.**

dentogingival junction, the interface between the junctional epithelium and the surface of the teeth.

dentoperiosteal fiber /den″tōper″ē·os″tē·əl/ [L, *dens* + Gk, *peri,* around, *osteon* bone], any of the many peridental connective tissue fibers that emerge from the supraalveolar part of the cementum of a tooth and extend apically beyond the alveolar crest into the mucoperiosteum of the attached gingiva.

dentulous /den″tyələs/ [L, *dens,* tooth, *-ulosus,* characterized by], possessing one or more natural teeth.

dentulous dental arch, a dental arch that contains one or more natural teeth.

denture /den″chər/ [L, *dens,* tooth], an artificial tooth or a set of artificial teeth not permanently fixed or implanted, used to replace a missing tooth or teeth. Compare **dental plate, fixed bridgework, implant denture.**

denture base, the part of a denture that covers the soft tissue of the mouth. It is commonly made of plastic, self-cured or heat-cured resin, or a combination of resin and metal to which artificial teeth are attached. Also called **saddle.**

denture-bearing area. See **stress-bearing area.**

denture flask, a sectional metal case in which plaster of paris or artificial stone is molded and in which dentures or other plastic resin restorations are heat-processed.

denture packing, the laboratory procedure of filling and compressing a denture-base material into a mold in a denture flask.

denturist /den″chərist/, a person other than a dentist who engages in the practice of dentistry, usually only to the extent of providing the fit, design, construction, insertion, and repair of complete or partial dentures without the ability to diagnose a patient's dental conditions. Most states in the United States have laws restricting such activity. In Canada, denturists are regulated under the health professions acts of provinces and territories. See also **dental laboratory technician.**

denucleated /dēnyoo″klē·ā′tid/ [L, *de,* from, *nucleus,* nut kernel], pertaining to a condition in which the nucleus has been removed.

denudation /den″oodā″shən/ [L, *denudare,* to make bare], **1.** the process of stripping bare. **2.** a condition of losing an outside layer, such as an epithelium.

Denver Articulation Screening Examination (DASE), a test for evaluating the clarity of pronunciation in children 2½ to 6 years of age. Each child's performance may be compared with a standardized norm for the age.

Denver classification, a system for identifying and classifying human chromosomes according to their size and the position of the centromere as determined during mitotic metaphase. The chromosomes are divided into seven major groups, designated A through G, which are arranged according to decreasing length. See also **chromosomal nomenclature, chromosome, karyotype.**

Denver Developmental Screening Test II (DDST), a test for evaluating development in children from 1 month to 6 years of age. The developmental level of motor, social, and language skills may be discovered by comparing the child's performance with the average performance of other children. The developmental age is expressed as a ratio in which the child's age is the denominator and the age at which the norm possesses skills equal to those of the child being tested is the numerator.

deodorant /dē·ō″dərənt/ [L, *de* + *odor,* smell], **1.** *adj.,* destroying or masking odors. **2.** *n.,* a substance that destroys or masks odors. Underarm deodorants are available as sprays, creams, solid gels, and liquids containing an antiperspirant, such as aluminum chloride, aluminum hydroxyl, aluminum sulfate, or aluminum zirconyl hydroxychloride. These aluminum salts may suppress sweat production and also form an obstructive hydroxide gel in sweat ducts. Vaginal deodorant sprays contain a fatty ester emollient, a masking fragrance, and an antimicrobial agent, such as benzethonium chloride, chlorhexidine hydrochloride, or triacetin; they are often associated with allergic reactions. Room and breath deodorants contain masking agents, such as mint, pine, eucalyptus, lemon, lavender, rosemary, sassafras, or thyme. Ozone masks odors by decreasing olfactory sensitivity. Chlorophyll has a deodorizing action that is enhanced by crotonic acid. Also called **antibromic.**

deodorized alcohol /dē·ō″dərīzd′/, a liquid, free of organic impurities, containing 92.5% absolute alcohol.

deodorizing douche, a stream of air or liquid that masks or absorbs foul odors, applied at moderate pressure into a body cavity or onto a body surface. See also **douche.**

deontologism /dē″ontol″əgiz′əm/ [Gk, *deon,* obligation, *logos,* science], a doctrine of ethics that states that moral duty or obligation is binding even though a moral action may be different or result in painful consequences, also, that what makes acts right are characteristics such as fidelity, veracity, justice, and honesty. Compare **natural law, utilitarianism.**

deorsumversion, turning downward, a downward gaze. See **infraversion.**

deossification /dē·os″ifikā″shən/, the loss of mineral matter from bones.

deoxidizer, an agent that removes oxygen. See also **reducing agent.**

deoxy-, desoxy-, prefix meaning "containing a decreased amount of oxygen": *deoxygenation, deoxyribose.*

deoxygenation /dē·ōk″sijənā″shən/ [L, *de,* from; Gk, *oxys,* sharp, *genein,* to produce], the removal of oxygen from a chemical compound.

deoxyribonucleic acid (DNA) /dē·ok″sirī′bōnooklē″ik/, a large, double-stranded, helical molecule that is the carrier of genetic information. In eukaryotic cells, it is found principally in the chromosomes of the nucleus. DNA is composed of four kinds of serially repeating nucleotide bases: adenine, cytosine, guanine, and thymine. Genetic information is coded in the sequence of the nucleotides. See also **nucleic acid, ribonucleic acid.**

deoxyribose /dē·ok″sē·rī′bōs/, ribose that has been transformed into a deoxy sugar, found in deoxyribonucleic acids (DNA). Also known as 2-deoxyribose, referring to the specific carbon atom that has been reduced. Compare **ribose.**

deoxy sugar /dē·ok″sē shoog′ər/, a sugar in which one or more carbon atoms have been reduced, thus losing its hydroxyl group.

Depakene, an anticonvulsant drug. Brand name for **divalproex sodium.**

Depakote, an anticonvulsant drug. Brand name for **divalproex sodium.**

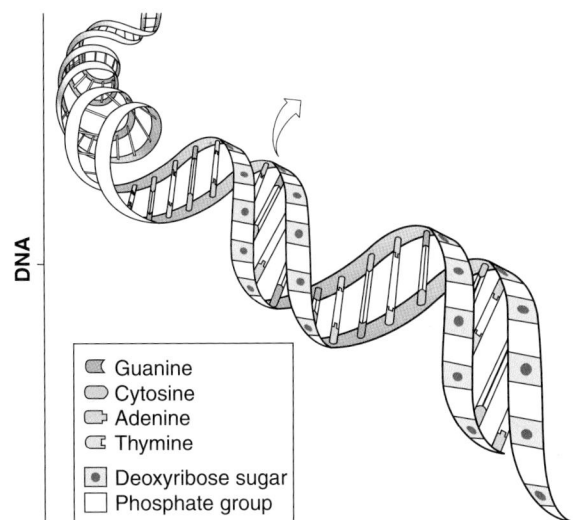

The structural relationship between DNA, chromatin, and chromosomes. *(Waugh and Grant, 2014)*

Department of Health and Human Services (DHHS), a cabinet-level department of the U.S. government with responsibility for the functions of various federal social welfare and health delivery agencies, such as the Food and Drug Administration. It also directs the U.S. Office of Consumer Affairs, Office of Civil Rights, Administration on Aging, Public Health Service, Indian Health Service, Social Security Administration, and National Institutes of Health.

Department of Transportation (DOT), a cabinet-level department of the U.S. government responsible for national transportation policies, including maritime, aviation, railroad, and highway safety and regulation of the transport of hazardous materials, such as medical gases.

dependence /dipen″dəns/ [L, *de* + *pendere,* to hang upon], **1.** the state of reliance on others to achieve self-care activities (such as feeding, dressing, hygiene, bathing, toileting). **2.** the total psychophysical state of one addicted to drugs or alcohol who must receive an increasing amount of the substance to prevent the onset of withdrawal symptoms.

dependency needs /dipen″dənsē/, the sum of the physical and emotional requirements of an infant for survival, including parenting, love, affection, shelter, protection, food, and warmth. Reliance on others to satisfy these needs decreases with age and maturity. Continuance in later years, in overt or latent form, is indicative of a pathological emotional disorder. These needs may increase under stress, as during physical illness, in which case they do not reflect a psychopathological condition. Compare **emotional need.**

dependent, pertaining to a condition of being reliant on someone or something else for help, support, favor, and other needs, as a child is dependent on a parent, an individual with a substance abuse disorder is dependent on a drug, or one variable is dependent on another. *−depend, v.*

dependent care, health care provided for persons, particularly children and disabled or elderly individuals, who are dependent on others for part or all of the activities of daily living.

dependent differentiation, the process of change of cells or structures mediated by an external factor. See also **correlative differentiation.**

dependent edema [L, *de,* from, *pendere,* to hand; Gk, *oidema,* swelling], a fluid accumulation in the tissues that is influenced by gravity. It is usually greater in the lower part of the body than in the part above the level of the heart.

dependent intervention, a therapeutic action based on the written or verbal prescription of another health professional. See also **intervention.**

dependent personality, behavior characterized by excessive or compulsive needs for attention, acceptance, and approval from other people to maintain security and self-esteem.

dependent personality disorder, **1.** a persistent mental state characterized by a lack of self-confidence and an inability to function independently. **2.** an overreliance on others to fulfill one's own physical, social, and emotional needs

dependent variable, (in research) a factor that is measured to learn the effect of one or more independent variables. For example, in a study of the effect of preoperative nursing intervention on postoperative vomiting, vomiting is the dependent variable measured to determine the effect of the nursing intervention. Compare **independent variable.**

depersonalization /dēpur′sənəlīzā″shən/ [L, *de* + *persona,* mask], a feeling of strangeness or unreality concerning oneself or the environment, often resulting from anxiety, stress, or fatigue. Some medications can also cause this sensation. Also called **self-alienation.** See also **alienation, depersonalization.**

depersonalization disorder, an emotional disturbance characterized by depersonalization feelings in which a dreamlike atmosphere pervades the consciousness. The body may not feel like one's own, and dramatic and important events may be watched with equanimity. The reaction is commonly seen in various forms of schizophrenia and in severe depression. Also called *depersonalization/derealization disorder.*

de Pezzer catheter. See **Pezzer catheter.**

depigmentation, lightening of the skin. See **dyspigmentation.**

depilation /dep′ilā″shən/ [L, *de* + *pilum,* hair], the removal or extraction of hair from the body, either temporarily by mechanical or chemical means or permanently by electrolysis, which destroys the hair follicle. Also called **epilation.** *−depilate, v.*

depilatory /dipil″ətôrē/, **1.** *adj.,* pertaining to a substance or procedure that removes hair. **2.** *n.,* a depilatory agent.

depilatory techniques [L, *depilare,* to deprive of hair; Gk, *technikos,* skillful], methods of removing unwanted body hair, such as plucking, external application of chemicals, electrolysis, application of melted wax, or laser treatments.

deplete /də·plēt′/ [L, *deplere,* to empty], to empty or unload; to cause nothing to be left.

depletion /də·plē′shən/ [L, *deplere,* to empty], **1.** the act or process of emptying or removing, such as of fluid from a body compartment. **2.** an exhausted state resulting from excessive loss of blood.

depolarization /dēpō′lərīzā″shən/, the reduction of a membrane potential to a less negative value. It is caused by the influx of cations, such as sodium and calcium, through ion channels in the membrane. In many neurons and muscle cells, depolarization may lead to an electric impulse called an action potential.

deposit /dəpoz′it/ [L, *de,* from + *ponere,* to place], **1.** sediment or dregs. **2.** extraneous inorganic matter collected in the tissues or in a viscus or cavity. **3.** hard or soft material laid down on a tooth surface, such as dental calculus or plaque.

deposition /dep′əzish″ən/ [L, *deponere,* to lay down], (in law) sworn pretrial testimony given by a witness in response to oral or written questions and cross-examination. The deposition is transcribed and may be used for further pretrial investigation. It may also be presented at the trial if the witness cannot be present. Compare **discovery, interrogatories.**

depot /dē″pō, dep′ō/ [Fr, depository], **1.** *n.,* any area of the body in which drugs or other substances such as fat are stored and from which they can be distributed. **2.** *adj.,* (of a drug) injected or implanted to be slowly absorbed into the circulation.

depot injection, an intramuscular injection of a drug in an oil suspension that results in a gradual release of the medication over several days.

depressant /dipres″ənt/ [L, *deprimere,* to press down], **1.** *adj.,* (of a drug) tending to decrease the function or activity of a system of the body. **2.** *n.,* such a drug. Kinds include **cardiac depressant, central nervous system depressant, respiratory depressant.**

depressed [L, *deprimere,* to press down], **1.** pertaining to a body structure that has been forced below the surface of surrounding parts, as in a skull fracture. **2.** pertaining to a condition in which general body activity is diminished, as in depressed urine output during dehydration. **3.** *(Informal)* pertaining to an emotional condition characterized by emotional dejection, loss of initiative, listlessness, loss of appetite, and difficulty with concentration. See also **depression.** **4.** *adj.,* (in psychiatry) the experience of a person diagnosed with depression, characterized by five or more specific symptoms of depression lasting for 2 or more weeks.

depressed fracture, any articular fracture in which fragments are pushed below the normal joint surface line, such as the tibial plateau, or a break in the skull in which bone fragments are pushed below the normal surface.

depression /dipresh″ən/ [L, *deprimere,* to press down], **1.** a depressed area, hollow, or fossa. **2.** downward or inward displacement. **3.** a decrease of vital functional activity. **4.** a mood disturbance characterized by feelings of sadness, despair, and discouragement resulting from and normally proportionate to some personal loss or tragedy. **5.** an abnormal emotional state characterized by exaggerated feelings of sadness, melancholy, dejection, worthlessness, emptiness, and hopelessness that are inappropriate and out of proportion to reality. Because the origin of depression can be genetic, pharmacological, endocrinal, infectious, nutritional, neoplastic, or neurological, the behavioral effects can appear as aggression or withdrawal, anorexia or overeating, anger or apathy, or any of myriad responses. Kinds include **depression with mixed features, depression with anxious distress.** Also called **major depressive disorder.** See also **bipolar disorder. –depressive,** *adj.*

■ OBSERVATIONS: Depression may be expressed in a wide spectrum of affective, physiological, cognitive, and behavioral manifestations. The varied behaviors represent the complex actions, reactions, and interactions of the person with depression to stimuli that may be either internal or external. Numerous symptoms representing a change from previous function are noted. The symptoms of depression are present during the same 2-week period, and at least one of the symptoms is depressed mood or loss of interest in pleasurable activities.
■ INTERVENTIONS: Depending on the root cause of the depression, a regime of antidepressant medication will be started to co-occur with individual and/or group psychotherapy. Depending on the severity of the depression, hospitalization may be warranted. In difficult-to-treat cases, a regimen of electroconvulsive therapy may be the treatment of choice, be followed by antidepressant medications and therapy.
■ PATIENT CARE CONSIDERATIONS: The condition is neurotic when the precipitating cause is an intrapsychic conflict or a traumatic situation or event that is identifiable, even though the person is unable to explain the overreaction to it. The condition is psychotic when there is severe physical and mental functional impairment caused by an unidentifiable intrapsychic conflict; it is often accompanied by hallucinations, delusions, and confusion concerning time, place, and identity.

depression with anxious distress, depression accompanied by anxiety, which may interfere with treatment or responses to treatment.

depression with mixed features, depression with manic symptoms in an individual who does not meet all of the criteria for a manic episode.

depression with psychotic features [L, *deprimere,* to press down; Gk, *psyche,* mind, *osis,* condition], a type of depressive disorder or mood disorder in which there are psychotic features, usually of a paranoid or somatic nature.

depressive. See **depression.**

depressive personality disorder, a condition characterized by a persistent and pervasive pattern of depressive cognitions and behaviors, such as chronic unhappiness, low self-esteem, pessimism, critical and derogatory attitudes toward oneself and others, feelings of guilt or remorse, and an inability to relax or feel enjoyment.

depressive pseudodementia, *(Obsolete)* a term whose use is discouraged as technically incorrect because the cognitive deficits are now believed to be real, if reversible. Now called **dementia syndrome of depression.**

depressive reaction, a condition of depressive emotional response to an external situation. The depressive state usually ends when the external situation is resolved.

depressor /dipres″ər/ [L, *deprimere,* to press down], any agent that reduces activity when applied to nerves and muscles. See also **depressant.**

depressor anguli oris, a muscle that is active during frowning, depressing the corner of the mouth.

depressor labii inferioris, a muscle that depresses the lower lip and moves it laterally.

depressor reflex [L, *deprimere,* to press down, *reflectere,* to bend back], a neural mechanism that produces an involuntary vasodilation and fall in arterial blood pressure in response to mechanical stimulation of the carotid sinus.

depressor septi /sep″tī/, one of the three muscles of the nose. Arising from the maxilla and inserting into the septum and the posterior aspect of the ala, it lies between the mucous membrane and the muscular structure of the lip and is a direct antagonist of the other muscles of the nose. It is innervated by buccal branches of the facial nerve and serves to draw down the ala, constricting the nostril. Compare **nasalis, procerus.**

deprivation /dep′rivā″shən/ [L, *deprivare,* to deprive], the lack of access to any of the essentials of life whether by circumstance or by the intentions of others to cause harm or gain control. In experimental psychology, animal or human subjects may be deprived of something desired or expected for a study of their reactions.

depth dose [AS, *diop* + Gk, *dosis,* giving], (in radiotherapy) the relationship between the dose of radiation at any depth within matter and the dose at a fixed reference point.

depth perception, the ability to judge depth or the relative distance of objects in space and to orient one's position in relation to them. Binocular vision is essential to this ability. Also called **stereopsis.**

depth psychology, any approach to psychology and psychological research that emphasizes the study of personality and behavior in relation to unconscious motivation. See also **psychoanalysis.**

depurative /depxu-ra″tiv/, a herb that has a detoxifying or purifying effect.

de Quervain fracture /dəkərvän″/ [Fritz de Quervain, Swiss surgeon, 1868–1940], a break in the navicular bone of the hand, with dislocation of the lunate bone.

de Quervain thyroiditis [Fritz de Quervain; Gk, *thyreos,* shield, *itis,* inflammation], an acute inflammatory condition of the thyroid characterized by swelling and tenderness of the gland. Also called **giant cell thyroiditis, granulomatous thyroiditis, subacute thyroiditis.** Should not be confused with **Graves disease.**

■ OBSERVATIONS: Symptoms associated with both hyperthyroid and hypothyroid disease may be present during the course of the inflammation. The condition is characterized by low-grade fever, difficulty swallowing, fatigue, and severe pain in the neck, ears, and jaw. The diagnosis may be made by a radiological scan showing depressed uptake of radioactive iodine in involved areas. Occasionally a fine-needle biopsy of the thyroid is performed.

■ INTERVENTIONS: Treatment may include antiinflammatory medication, such as aspirin or NSAIDs, if the condition continues for more than a few days. Corticosteroids are prescribed for prolonged or severe cases.

■ PATIENT CARE CONSIDERATIONS: The disorder often occurs after a viral infection of the upper respiratory tract. It tends to remit spontaneously and to recur several times.

der, abbreviation for **derivative chromosome.**

derailment /dirāl″mənt/, a pattern of speech in which incomprehensible, disconnected, and unrelated ideas replace logical and orderly thought.

derby hat fracture, a cranial concavity in infants sometimes, but not always, associated with a fracture. See **dishpan fracture.**

Dercum disease /dur″kəm/ [Francis X. Dercum, U.S. neurologist, 1856–1931], a potentially fatal disorder characterized by painful localized fatty swellings and nerve lesions. The disease mainly affects menopausal women. Also called **adiposis dolorosa.**

dereflection /dē′rəflek″shən/ [L, *de* + *reflectere,* to bend back], a technique of logotherapeutic psychology that is directed to taking a person's mind off a certain goal through a positive redirection to another goal, with emphasis on assets and abilities rather than the problems at hand. Dereflection often results in accomplishment of the original goal. See also **logotherapy.**

dereistic thought /dē′rē·is″tik/ [L, *de* + *res,* thing], a type of mental activity in which fantasy is not modified by logic, experience, or reality.

derivative /dəriv″ətiv/ [L, *derivare,* to turn away], anything that originates in another substance or object. For example, organs and tissues are derivatives of the primordial germ cells. Chemical derivatives may be produced to confirm identification of a compound or to aid in the analysis of a compound.

derivative chromosome (der), a chromosomal aberration caused by translocation.

derived protein /dirīvd″/, a small protein obtained by enzymatic or chemical hydrolysis of a larger protein source.

derived quantity, any secondary quantity, such as volume, derived from a combination of base quantities, such as mass, length, and time.

-derm, suffix meaning "skin": *bromoderma, mucoderm.*

derma-. See **dermato-, derma-, dermat-, dermo-.**

-derma, -dermia, -dermic, 1. suffix meaning "skin": *anetoderma.* **2.** suffix meaning a "(specified) skin ailment or skin condition": *pachyderma.* **3.** suffix meaning "related to the variety of skin": *hypodermic.*

dermabrasion /dur′məbrā″zhən/ [Gk, *derma,* skin; L, *abradere,* to scrape], a treatment for the removal of superficial scars on the skin by the use of revolving wire brushes or sandpaper. An aerosol spray is used to freeze the skin for this procedure. Dermabrasion is performed to reduce facial scars of severe acne. Compare **microdermabrasion.**

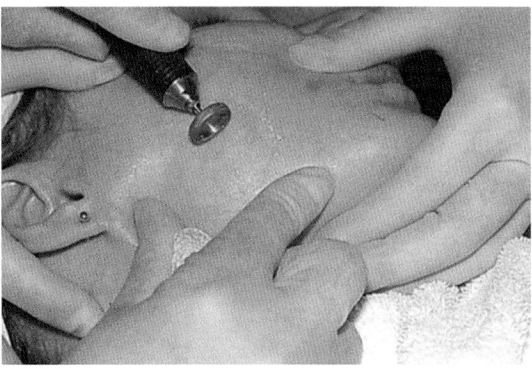

Dermabrasion *(Fewkes, Cheney, and Pollack, 1992)*

Dermacentor /dur′məsen″tər/, a widely distributed genus of ticks in the family Ixodidae, including a number that infest humans and other mammals. Several are vectors of diseases such as Colorado tick fever, anaplasmosis, Rocky Mountain spotted fever, tularemia, and brucellosis.

dermal. See **dermis.**

dermal graft [Gk, *derma,* skin, *graphion,* stylus], the transplantation of any living skin tissue that contains dermis and thus is capable of regenerating and secreting sweat and sebum and generating new hair growth.

dermal neurofibroma, a neurofibroma arising within the skin as a small, fleshy nodule that may become pedunculated, overlying a palpable subcutaneous lesion.

dermal papilla [Gk, *derma,* skin; L, *papilla,* nipple], any small elevation in the dermis, such as the elongated papilla seen in psoriasis.

dermat-. See **dermato-, derma-, dermat-, dermo-.**

dermatitis /dur′mətī″tis/ [Gk, *derma* + *itis,* inflammation], an inflammatory condition of the skin. Various cutaneous eruptions occur and may be unique to a particular allergen, disease, or infection. The condition may be chronic or acute; treatment is specific to the cause. Kinds include **actinic dermatitis, contact dermatitis, rhus dermatitis, seborrheic dermatitis.**

dermatitis exfoliativa neonatorum. Also called **staphylococcal scalded skin syndrome.** See **Ritter disease.**

dermatitis herpetiformis, a chronic, severely pruritic skin disease with symmetrically located groups of red papulovesicular, vesicular, bullous, or urticarial lesions. It is thought to be an immunological response to dietary gluten. Treatment may include a diet free of gluten and the administration of sulfone, dapsone, sulfapyridine, or antipruritic drugs.

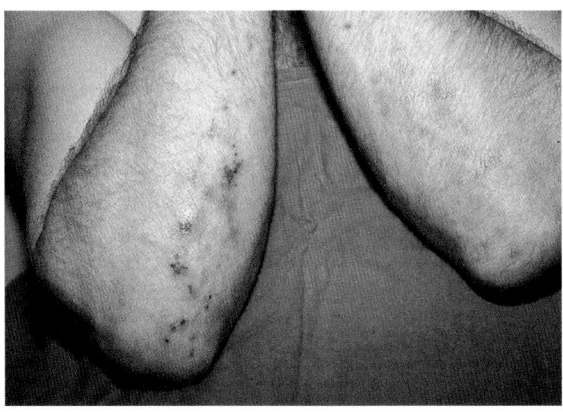

Dermatitis herpetiformis *(Cross, 2013)*

dermatitis medicamentosa, *(Obsolete)* now called **drug rash.**

dermatitis papillaris capillitii, *(Obsolete)* now called **keloid acne.**

dermatitis venenata, *(Obsolete)* now called **contact dermatitis.**

dermato-, derma-, dermat-, dermo-, prefix meaning "skin": *dermatome, dermatocellulitis, dermatocyst.*

dermatocellulitis /dur″mətōsel′yəlī″tis/, an inflammation of the skin and subcutaneous connective tissue.

dermatocyst /dur″mətōsist′/, a cystic tumor of cutaneous tissues.

dermatofibroma /dur′mətōfībrō″mə/ *pl. dermatofibromas, dermatofibromata* [Gk, *derma* + L, *fibra,* fiber, *oma,* tumor], a cutaneous nodule that is painless, round, firm, gray or red, elevated, and commonly found on the extremities. No treatment is required. Also called **fibrous histiocytoma.**

dermatofibrosarcoma /-fī′brōsärkō″mə/ [Gk, *derma,* skin; L, *fibra,* fiber; Gk, *sarx,* flesh, *oma,* tumor], a locally malignant dermal tumor of fibroblasts that begins as an indurated, slow-growing nodule. The back and front of the trunk are common sites. The tumor rarely metastasizes. Recurrences are the rule if the lesion is not widely excised.

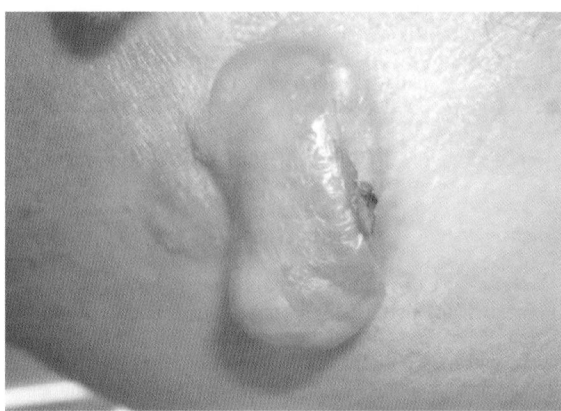

Dermatofibrosarcoma protuberans
(Lebwohl et al, 2014)

dermatoglyphics /dur′mətōglif″iks/ [Gk, *derma* + *glyphe,* a carving], the study of the skin ridge patterns on fingers, toes, palms of hands, and soles of feet. The patterns are used as a basis of identification and also have diagnostic value because of associations between certain patterns and chromosomal anomalies.

dermatographia /dur′mətōgraf″ē·ə/ [Gk, *derma* + *graphein,* to record], a benign dermatological condition characterized by raised wheals in a distinctive pattern consistent with the application of pressure from or scraping by the fingers in a word pattern or design. It is known informally as skin writing because the wheals can be caused by irritation from the fingers. See also **autographism, urticaria.**

dermatological agent /dur′mətoloj″ik/, a drug used to treat reactions or disorders of the skin.

dermatologist /dur′mətol″əjist/, a physician specializing in the skin, hair, and nails and their properties related to health and disease. Following an internship, a dermatologist receives at least 3 additional years of specialty medical training.

dermatology /-ol″əjē/ [Gk, *derma* + *logos,* science], the study of the skin, including its anatomical, physiological, and pathological characteristics and the diagnosis and treatment of skin disorders.

dermatoma /dur′mətō″mə/, **1.** a skin tumor. **2.** a patch of abnormally thick skin.

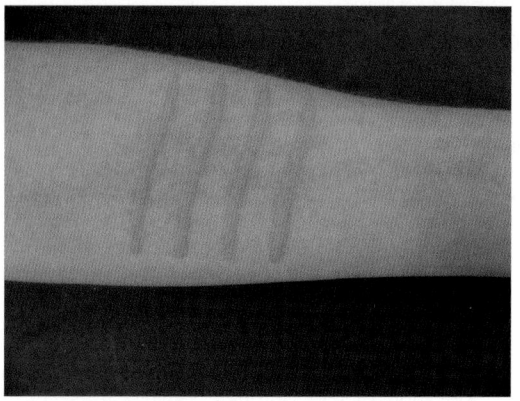

Dermatographia *(Abajian et al, 2014)*

dermatome /dur″mətōm/ [Gk, *derma* + *temnein,* to cut], **1.** (in embryology) the mesodermal layer in the early developing embryo that gives rise to the dermal layers of the skin. **2.** (in surgery) a small instrument used to cut thin slices of skin for grafting. **3.** an area on the surface of a body innervated by afferent fibers from one spinal root.

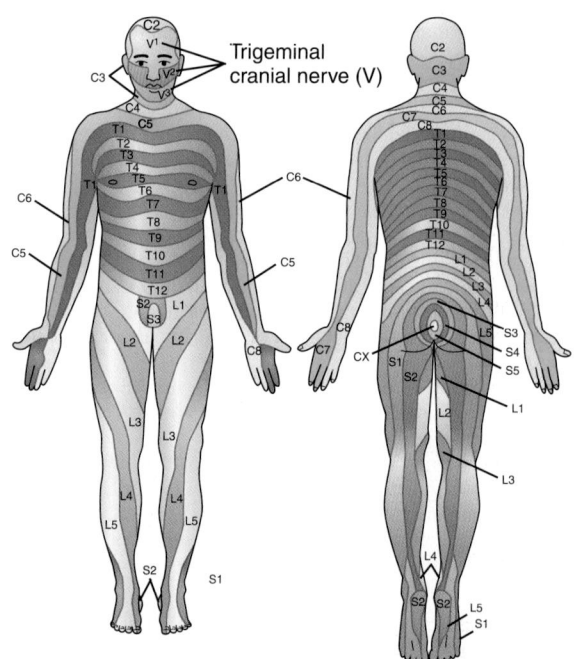

Dermatome distribution of spinal nerves
(Patton and Thibodeau, 2016)

dermatomycosis /dur′mətō′mīkō″sis/ [Gk, *derma* + *mykes,* fungus, *osis,* condition], a superficial fungal infection of the skin, characteristically found on parts that are moist and protected by clothing, such as the groin or feet. It is caused by a dermatophyte. See also **dermatophytosis.** –*dermatomycotic, adj.*

dermatomyositis /dur′mətōmī′ōsī″tis/ [Gk, *derma* + *mys,* muscle, *itis,* inflammation], a disease of the connective tissues, characterized by pruritic or eczematous inflammation of the skin and tenderness and weakness of the muscles.

■ OBSERVATIONS: Muscle tissue is destroyed, and loss is often so severe that the person may become unable to walk or to perform simple tasks. Swelling of the eyelids and face and loss of weight are common manifestations.

■ INTERVENTIONS: Treatment of this disease may include prescription of corticosteroids; immunosuppressants may be used in cases that are unresponsive. To prevent muscle wasting and preserve muscle function, physical therapy is required. Most cases respond to therapy, although the disease is usually more severe and treatment resistant in patients with pulmonary or cardiac issues.

■ PATIENT CARE CONSIDERATIONS: The cause is unknown, but in 15% of cases the condition develops with an internal malignancy. Viral infection and antibacterial medication are also associated with an increased incidence of dermatomyositis.

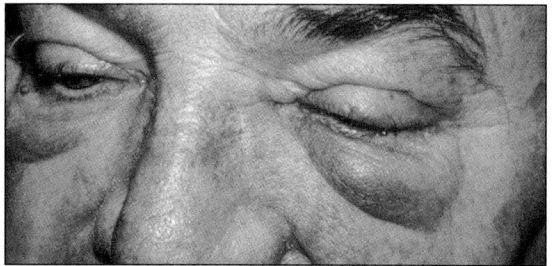

Swelling associated with dermatomyositis
(White and Cox, 2006)

dermatopathy /dur′mətop″əthē/, any disorder of the skin.

Dermatophagoides /-fagoi″dēz/ [Gk, *derma* + *phagein,* to eat, *eidos,* form], a genus of household dust mite responsible for allergic reactions in sensitive individuals. Protection against the microscopically small mite includes minimizing dust in the home, especially in the bedroom; encasing pillows and mattresses in allergen-proof coverings; controlling temperature; and keeping humidity below 70%. The mites thrive on skin scales, hair, pet foods, carpets, and bedding, in addition to ordinary house dust.

dermatophyte /dur″mətōfīt′, dərmat″əfīt/, any of several fungi that cause parasitic skin disease in humans. See also **dermatophytid,** *specific fungal infections.*

dermatophytid /dur′mətof″itid, dur′mətōfī″tid/ [Gk, *derma* + *phyton,* plant], an allergic skin reaction characterized by small vesicles and associated with dermatomycosis. The lesions result from sensitization to the infection elsewhere on the skin and do not contain fungi. See also **dermatomycosis, dermatophyte.**

dermatophytosis /dur′mətō′fītō″sis/ [Gk, *derma* + *phyton,* plant, *osis,* condition], a superficial fungus infection involving the stratum corneum of the skin, hair, and nails, caused by *Microsporum, Epidermophyton,* or *Trichophyton* species of dermatophyte. On the trunk and upper extremities it is commonly called "ringworm" infection and is characterized by round or oval scaly patches with slightly raised borders and clearing centers. On the feet, small vesicles, cracking, itching, scaling, and often secondary bacterial infections occur and are commonly called "athlete's foot." Treatment includes topical antifungal agents, such as tolnaftate, clotrimazole, and undecylenic acid, and oral griseofulvin. Fingernails and toenails respond poorly to topical treatment. Also called **epidermomycosis.** See also **tinea.**

dermatoplasty /dur″mətōplas′tē/, a surgical procedure in which skin tissue is transplanted to a body surface damaged by disease or injury.

dermatosclerosis /-sklərō″sis/ [Gk, *derma* + *sklerosis,* hardening], a skin disease characterized by fibrous thickening of the skin. See also **scleroderma.**

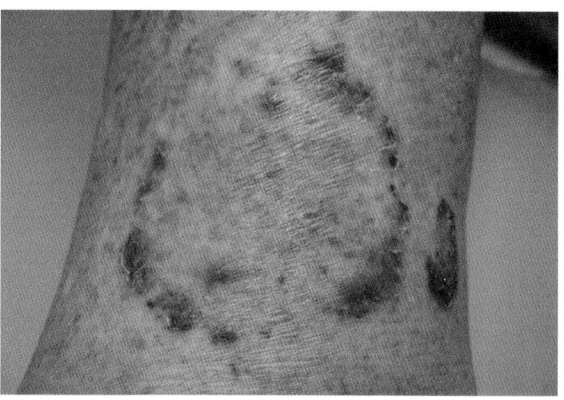

Dermatophytosis *(Brinster et al, 2011)*

dermatosis /dur′mətō″sis/ [Gk, *derma* + *osis,* condition], any disorder of the skin, especially those not associated with inflammation. Compare **dermatitis.**

dermatosis papulosa nigra, a common condition in individuals with darkly pigmented skin. It consists of multiple tiny, benign, skin-colored or hyperpigmented papules on the face, neck, and cheeks. The lesions increase in number with age.

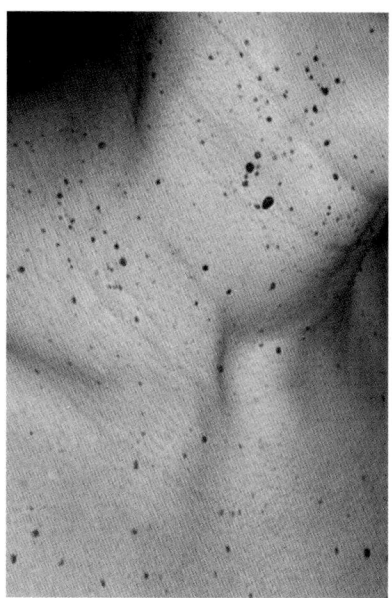

Dermatosis papulosa nigra *(Lawrence and Cox, 2002)*

dermis, the layer of the skin just below the epidermis, consisting of papillary and reticular layers and containing blood and lymphatic vessels, nerves and nerve endings, glands, and hair follicles. Formerly called **corium. −dermal,** *adj.*

-dermis, suffix meaning "tissue" or "skin": *epidermis.*

dermo-. See **dermato-, derma-, dermat-, dermo-.**

dermographism. See **dermatographia.**

dermoid /dur″moid/ [Gk, *derma* + *eidos,* form], **1.** *adj.,* pertaining to the skin. **2.** *(Informal) n.,* a dermoid cyst.

dermoid cyst, a tumor, derived from embryonal tissues, consisting of a fibrous wall lined with epithelium and a cavity containing fatty material, hair, teeth, bits of bone, and

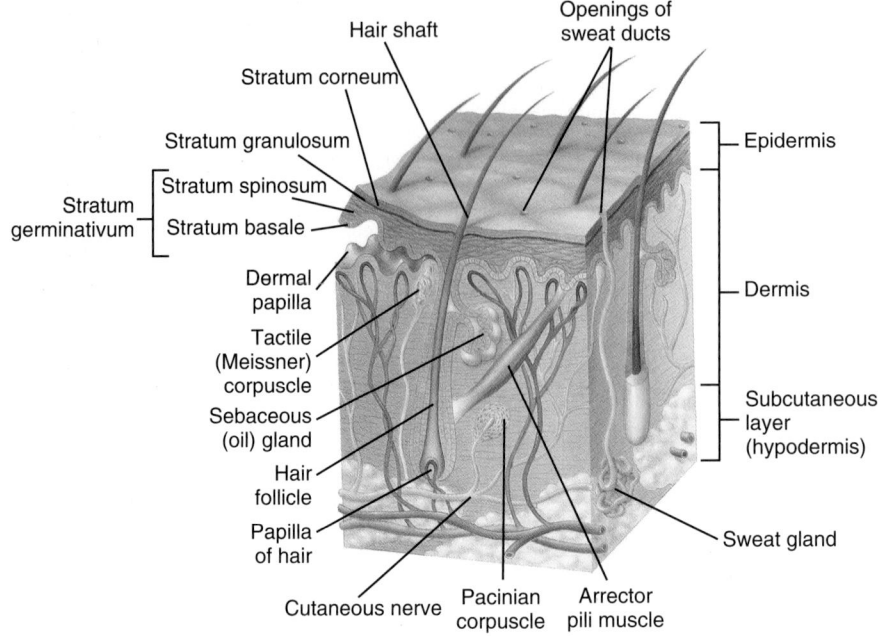

Hair shaft

Openings of sweat ducts

Stratum corneum

Stratum granulosum

Stratum spinosum

Stratum germinativum

Stratum basale

Epidermis

Dermal papilla

Dermis

Tactile (Meissner) corpuscle

Sebaceous (oil) gland

Subcutaneous layer (hypodermis)

Hair follicle

Papilla of hair

Sweat gland

Cutaneous nerve

Pacinian corpuscle

Arrector pili muscle

Dermis *(Thibodeau and Patton, 2003)*

cartilage. Also called **organoid tumor, teratoid tumor.** Kinds include **implantation dermoid cyst, inclusion dermoid cyst, thyroid dermoid cyst, tubal dermoid cyst.**

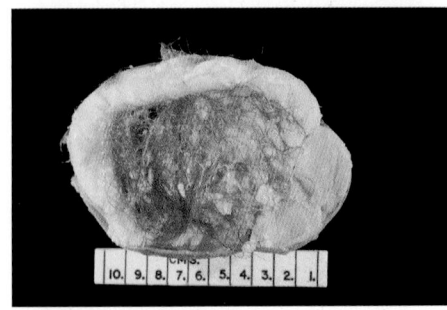

Dermoid cyst *(Greer et al, 2001)*

-**dermoma,** suffix meaning a "tumor of the skin layers": *bidermoma.*

derotation brace /dē′rōtā″shən/, a customized orthosis that provides stability at the knee joint. It consists of a single-joint hinged bar on one side and a rotating dial pad on the opposite side. The rotating pad can be placed on either the medial or the lateral side, depending on the location of the primary instability. Each brace is custom fitted.

DES, abbreviation for **diethylstilbestrol.**

desalination /dēsal′inā″shən/ [L, *de,* from, *sal,* salt], the process of removing salt from water or other substances.

desaturation /dēsach′ərā″shən/ [L, *de,* from, *saturare,* to fill], the formation of an unsaturated chemical compound from a saturated one.

Descemet membrane /desemā″/ [Jean Descemet, French physician, 1732–1810], a deep layer of the cornea, between the substantia propria externally and the endothelium internally.

descendens /disen″dənz/, **1.** the descending branch of the hypoglossal nerve. **2.** the cervicalis nerve formed by branches of the second and third cervical nerves.

descending aorta /disen″ding/ [L, *descendere,* to descend; Gk, *aerein,* to raise], the main portion of the aorta, consisting of the thoracic aorta and the abdominal aorta, which continues from the aortic arch into the trunk of the body. It supplies many structures, including the esophagus, lymph glands, ribs, stomach, liver, spleen, intestines, kidneys, reproductive organs, and, eventually, the lower limbs. See also **aorta.**

descending colon, the segment of the colon that extends from the end of the transverse colon at the splenic flexure on the left side of the abdomen down to the beginning of the sigmoid colon in the pelvis. See also **colon.**

descending current. See **centrifugal current.**

descending myelitis [L, *descendere,* to descend; Gk, *myelos,* marrow, *itis,* inflammation], a form of myelitis in which the pathological changes spread downward along the spinal cord.

descending neuritis [L, *descendere,* to descend; Gk, *neuron,* nerve, *itis,* inflammation], a form of neuritis that spreads downward from the upper part of the nervous system.

descending neuropathy [L, *descendere,* to descend; Gk, *neuron,* nerve, *pathos,* disease], a disease of the peripheral nervous system that spreads downward from the upper part of the body.

descending oblique muscle. See **external abdominal oblique muscle.**

descending tract [L, *descendere,* to descend, *tractus*], a nerve tract in the spinal cord that carries impulses away from the brain axis of the body or body part.

descensus /disen″səs/, the process of falling or descending. Also called **prolapse.**

descriptive anatomy /diskrip″tiv/ [L, *describere,* to write], the study of the morphological characteristics of the body by systems, such as the vascular system and the nervous system. Each system is composed of similar tissues that are essential to a particular function.

descriptive embryology, the study of the changes that occur in cells, tissues, and organs during the progressive stages of prenatal development.

descriptive epidemiology, the first stage of epidemiological investigation. It focuses on describing disease distribution by characteristics relating to time, place, and person.

descriptive psychiatry, the study of external, readily observable behavior. Compare **dynamic psychiatry.**

descriptive statistics, statistics that measure and describe characteristics of groups without drawing inferences about the population in general.

DES daughters, a group of women with increased susceptibility to cancer of the vagina and other reproductive organs because their mothers were given an estrogen medication, diethylstilbestrol (DES), from the 1940s through the 1960s to prevent miscarriage. Several other abnormalities have been reported among the DES daughters, including tissue that covers the cervix or a uterus that is too small to carry a pregnancy. Sons of women who took DES have an increased risk of undescended testes or other genital disorders.

desensitization. See **systemic desensitization.**

desensitize /dēsen″sitīz/ [L, _de_ + _sentire,_ to feel], **1.** (in immunology) to render an individual insensitive or less sensitive to any of the various antigens. **2.** (in psychiatry) to relieve an emotionally disturbed person of the stress of phobias and neuroses by encouraging discussion of the anxieties and the stressful experiences that cause the emotional problems involved. **3.** (in dentistry) to remove or reduce the painful response of vital exposed dentin to irritating substances and temperature changes.

desert fever, desert rheumatism. See **coccidioidomycosis.**

Desferal Mesylate, an iron-chelating agent. Brand name for **deferoxamine mesylate.**

desiccant /des″ikənt/ [L, _desiccare,_ to dry thoroughly], any agent or procedure that promotes the removal of water or the dehydration of substances whether gas, liquid, or solid. Also called **exsiccant, siccant.**

desiccate /des″ikāt/, **1.** to dry thoroughly by removing moisture. **2.** to preserve by drying, especially food. See also **exsiccate.**

designer drugs [L, _de_ + _signare,_ to mark], synthetic organic compounds that are designed as analogs of illicit drugs, with the same opioid or other dangerous effects. Because designer drugs are generally not listed as controlled substances by the U.S. Drug Enforcement Agency, prosecution of manufacturers, distributors, or users is frequently difficult.

desipramine hydrochloride /desip″rəmēn/, a tricyclic antidepressant.

■ INDICATIONS: It is prescribed in the treatment of mental depression and as adjunctive therapy for the treatment of chronic pain.

■ CONTRAINDICATIONS: Concomitant administration of monoamine oxidase inhibitors, heart block, recent myocardial infarction, or known hypersensitivity to this drug or to tricyclic medication prohibits its use. It is used with caution in patients who have seizure disorders or cardiovascular disease.

■ ADVERSE EFFECTS: Among the more serious adverse reactions are sedation as well as GI, cardiovascular, and neurological reactions. This drug interacts with many other drugs.

desired occupation, (in occupational therapy) those daily activities that are meaningful to a client and that give him or her a sense of identity.

desirudin, an anticoagulant.

■ INDICATIONS: This drug is used in prophylaxis for deep vein thrombosis in those undergoing hip replacement.

■ CONTRAINDICATIONS: Known hypersensitivity to natural or synthetic hirudins, active bleeding, and irreversible coagulation disorders prohibit this drug's use.

■ ADVERSE EFFECTS: Adverse effects of this drug include injection site mass, nausea, deep thrombophlebitis, anemia, and hypersensitivity. Life-threatening side effects include bleeding and hemorrhage.

desloratadine /des″lärat′ädēn/, a nonsedating antihistamine (H$_1$ receptor antagonist) used for treatment of allergic rhinitis and chronic idiopathic urticaria. It is administered orally.

-desma, suffix meaning "something bridging or connecting": _plasmodesma._

desmo-, prefix meaning "ligament": _desmoid tumor._

desmocyte. See **fibroblast.**

desmoid tumor /dez′moid/ [Gk, _desmos,_ band, _eidos,_ form], a fibrous neoplasm that may occur in the head, neck, upper arm, abdomen, or lower extremities. The tumor is usually a firm, rubbery mass.

desmopressin acetate /dez′mōpres″in/, a synthetic antidiuretic analog of arginine vasopressin, the naturally occurring human antidiuretic hormone.

■ INDICATIONS: It is prescribed as an antidiuretic in the treatment of diabetes insipidus and primary nocturnal enuresis and is used to control bleeding in hemophilia A and mild von Wildebrand's disease.

■ CONTRAINDICATIONS: Known hypersensitivity to this drug, hemophilia B, and severe von Wildebrand's disease (IIB) prohibit its use.

■ ADVERSE EFFECTS: Among the most serious adverse reactions are hyponatremia and water intoxication, which are seen more often when the drug is used for hemostatis. Mild effects, such as headache, cramps, and nasal congestion, also may occur.

desmosis /dezmō″sis/, any disease or disorder of the connective tissue.

desmosome /dez″məsōm/ [Gk, _desmos,_ band, _soma,_ body], a small, circular, dense area within the intercellular bridge that forms the site of adhesion between certain epithelial cells, especially the stratified epithelium of the epidermis. Also called **macula adherens.**

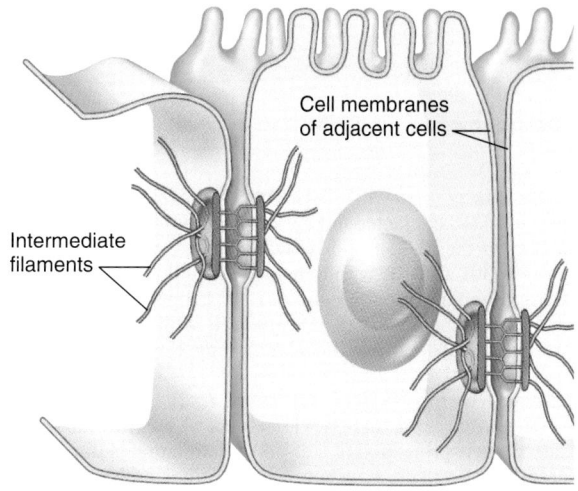

Desmosome

desogestrel /des″ojes′trel/, a progestational agent having little androgenic activity. It is used in combination with an estrogen component as an oral contraceptive.

Desonate, a topical steroid medication. Brand name for **desonide.**

desonide, an antiinflammatory topical cream, ointment, or liquid used to treat atopic dermatitis.

desoximetasone /desok′simet″əsōn/, a topical corticosteroid.

■ INDICATIONS: It is prescribed for the treatment of skin inflammation.

■ CONTRAINDICATIONS: Viral and fungal diseases of the skin, impaired circulation, or known hypersensitivity to this drug or to other steroid medication prohibits its use. Caution should be used in applying occlusive dressings over topical steroid medications.

■ ADVERSE EFFECTS: Among the more serious adverse reactions, usually occurring after prolonged or excessive application, are striae, hypopigmentation, or local irritation of the skin and various systemic effects.

desoxy-. See **deoxy-, desoxy-.**

Desoxyn, a central nervous system stimulant. Brand name for **methamphetamine hydrochloride.**

despair, a feeling of hopelessness.

desquamation /des′kwəmā″shən/ [L, *desquamare,* to take off scales], a normal process in which the cornified layer of the epidermis is sloughed in fine scales. Certain conditions, injuries, and medications accelerate desquamation and may cause peeling and the loss of deeper layers of the skin. Also called **exfoliation.** *−desquamative, adj., −desquamate, v.*

desquamative gingivitis /deskwam″ətiv/, a gingival inflammation characterized by peeling of the epithelium. In its chronic state it is most frequently associated with the hormonal changes of menopause. It may also be caused by biological stress, such as trauma to the epithelium, or by certain reactions to medications. Compare **eruptive gingivitis, pemphigus vulgaris.**

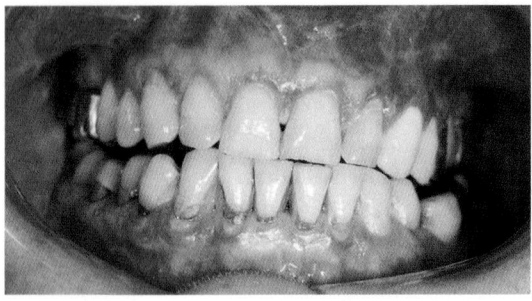

Desquamative gingivitis *(Ibsen and Phelan, 2014/Courtesy Dr. Edward V. Zegarelli)*

desquamative interstitial pneumonia (DIP), a respiratory disease characterized by an accumulation of cellular matter in the alveoli and bronchial tubes, affecting people in their 30s and 40s with a history of smoking. It leads to a fibrotic condition with symptoms of coughing, chest pain, weight loss, and dyspnea. Treatment is with corticosteroids, oxygen, and supportive medical therapy. Seventy percent of patients survive 10 years or longer.

destructive aggression /distruk″tiv/ [L, *destruere,* to destroy, *aggressio,* an attack], an act of hostility unnecessary for self-protection or self-preservation that is directed at an external object or person. See also **aggression, detachment, intermittent explosive disorder.**

destructive interference, a phenomenon affecting all types of waves (e.g., electromagnetic, acoustic, and radio waves) that results when propagated waves are out of phase, so that maximum compression for one wave occurs at the same point as maximum rarefaction for the second wave, causing the two waves to cancel each other out.

destructive lesion [L, *destruere,* to destroy, *laesio,* a hurting], a disorder that leads to the damage or necrosis of an organ or tissue.

desudation /des′ōodā″shən/, profuse sweating. It is sometimes followed by a skin rash.

desynchrony, a condition in which the environmental cues and patterns, such as sleeping and eating, conflict with an individual's existing pattern, as in jet lag.

Desyrel, an antidepressant. Brand name for **trazodone.**

detached retina. See **retinal detachment.**

detachment, separation. See also **destructive aggression.**

detection bias /ditek″shən/, a potential artifact in epidemiological data caused by the use of a particular diagnostic technique or type of equipment. As an example, cancer rates may vary in different regions or periods, not because of an actual difference in the incidence of the disease but because of different diagnostic technologies.

detector /detek″ter/, a device by which an object or condition can be discovered.

detergent /ditur″jənt/ [L, *detergere,* to cleanse], **1.** a cleansing agent. **2.** (in respiratory therapy) a wetting agent that is administered to mediate the removal of respiratory tract secretions from airway walls. See also **surfactant.**

deterioration /ditir′ē·ərā″shən/ [L, *deterior,* worse], a condition that is gradually worsening. Also called **retrogression.**

determinant evolution /ditur″minənt/ [L, *determinare,* to limit], the idea that evolution progresses according to a predetermined course. See also **orthogenesis.**

determinant of occlusion, one of the classifiable factors that influence proper closure of the teeth. The common fixed factors are intercondylar distance, anatomical characteristics, mandibular centricity, and the relationship of the jaws. Common changeable factors are tooth shape, tooth position, vertical dimensions of occlusion, cusp height, and fossa depth.

determinants of health. See **social determinants of health.**

determinate cleavage /ditur″minit/, mitotic division of the fertilized ovum into blastomeres that are each destined to form a specific part of the embryo. Damage to or destruction of any of these cells results in malformation of an organism. Also called **mosaic cleavage.** Compare **indeterminate cleavage.** See also **mosaic development.**

detoxification /dētok′sifikā″shən/ [L, *de* from + Gk, *toxikon,* poison; L, *facere,* to make], **1.** the removal of a poison or its effects from a patient. **2.** the purging or cleansing of the body of alcohol or drugs (illicit or prescribed).

detoxification service, a hospital service providing treatment to diminish or remove from a patient's body the toxic effects of chemical substances, such as alcohol or drugs, usually as an initial step in the treatment of a chemical-dependent person. The service may also be used to remove poisonous substances to which a person may have been exposed. See also **alcoholism, drug addiction.**

detoxification therapy, cleansing of the body through nutritional action, usually centering on GI function. It is claimed to assist in the transition to a healthier lifestyle by eliminating toxins. At the current time, there is no scientific evidence to support the efficacy of this treatment.

detoxify /dētok″sifī/ [L, *de,* from; Gk, *toxikon,* poison], **1.** to make a poisonous substance harmless or to overcome the effects of a poison. **2.** to cleanse the body of harmful substances such as drugs or alcohol.

detrition /dətrish′ən/ [L, *de,* from + *terere,* to wear], a wearing away, as of the teeth, by friction. See also **abrasion, attrition, erosion, abfraction.**

detrusor areflexia, failure of the detrusor muscle to respond to stimuli, usually owing to a lesion of a lower motoneuron, resulting in failure to empty the bladder completely on urination.

detrusor hyperactivity, detrusor hyperreflexia. See **detrusor overactivity.**

detrusor leak point pressure, as the bladder fills without an increase in abdominal pressure, the level of pressure at which leakage of urine through the urethra occurs. This is a measure of both strength of the urethral sphincters and compliance of the detrusor muscle.

detrusor muscle of bladder, the bundles of smooth muscle fibers forming the muscular coat of the urinary bladder, which are arranged in a longitudinal and a circular layer and, on contraction, serve to expel urine.

detrusor overactivity, involuntary contractions of the detrusor urinae muscle from any cause. Also called **detrusor hyperactivity, detrusor hyperreflexia.**

detrusor pressure, the pressure exerted inward by the detrusor urinae muscles of the bladder wall, one of the components of the total intravesical pressure.

detrusor-sphincter dyssynergia (DSD), contraction of the sphincter muscle of the urethra at the same time the detrusor muscle of the bladder is contracting, resulting in obstruction of normal urinary outflow.

detrusor urinae muscle /ditroo″zər/ [L, *detruder,* to thrust; Gk, *ouron,* urine; L, *musculus*], a complex of longitudinal fibers that form the external layer of the muscular coat of the bladder.

deuteranomaly /doo″terănom′älē/, a type of anomalous trichromatic vision in which the green-sensitive cones have decreased sensitivity. It is an X-linked trait, affecting about 5% of white males and 0.25% of females in the United States, and is the most common color vision deficiency.

deuteranopsia /doo″terănop′se·ä/, having only two types of functioning color receptors, resulting in retention of the sensory mechanism for two hues only (blue and yellow).

deuterium (²H or D) /dyōotir″ē·əm/ [Gk, *deuteros,* second], a stable isotope of the hydrogen atom, used as a kinetic tracer. Also called **heavy hydrogen.** See also **tritium.**

deutero-, deuto-, prefix meaning "second": *deutoplasm.*

deuteroplasm. See **deutoplasm.**

deuto-. See **deutero-, deuto-.**

deutoplasm /doo″təplaz′əm/ [Gk, *deuteros* + *plasma,* something formed], the inactive elements of the cytoplasm, primarily the stored nutritive material contained in yolk. Also called **deuteroplasm.**

DEV, abbreviation for **duck embryo vaccine.** See **rabies vaccine.**

devascularization /dēvas′kyələr′īzā″shən/ [L, *de,* from, *vasculum,* small vessel], the drawing away of blood from a body part or the stoppage of blood flow to it or the traumatic disruption of vascular supply to an organ.

developer fog, a defect in a film/screen radiographic image after processing, characterized by insufficient contrast. Causes include incorrect developer temperature, concentration, immersion time, or extraneous light.

development [Fr, *developper,* to unfold], **1.** the gradual process of change and differentiation from a simple to a more advanced level of complexity. In humans the physical, mental, and emotional capacities that allow complex adaptation to the environment and function within society are acquired through growth, maturation, and learning. Kinds include **arrested development, mosaic development, psychomotor development, psychosocial development, regulative development, psychosexual development. 2.** (in biology) the series of events that occur within an organism from the time of fertilization of the ovum to the adult stage. −*developmental, adj.*

developmental age (DA) /divel′əpmen″təl/, an expression of a child's maturational progress stated in age and determined by standardized measurements, such as body size and dimensions; by social and psychological functioning; by motor skills; and by mental and aptitude tests. Compare **achievement age, developmental quotient, mental age.**

developmental agraphia, a deficiency in a child's ability to learn to form letters and to write. Other learning is normal, and the child usually has no musculoskeletal or neurological problems.

developmental anatomy, the study of the differentiation and growth of an organism from one cell to birth. Also called **embryology.**

developmental anomaly, any congenital defect that results from interference with the normal growth and differentiation of the fetus. Such defects can arise at any stage of embryonic development, vary greatly in type and severity, and are caused by a wide variety of determining factors, including genetic mutations, chromosomal aberrations, teratogenic agents, and environmental factors. Developmental anomalies are classified either according to the organ system affected, such as congenital heart defects, or according to the way in which the defect occurred, such as developmental failure or arrest, failure to atrophy or subdivide, fusion, splitting, incorrect migration, and misplacement. Most developmental defects are apparent at birth, especially any structural malformation, but some, especially those involving the organ systems, do not become evident until days, weeks, or even years later.

developmental apraxia [L, *developper,* development; Gk, *a,* not, *prassein,* to do], a condition of ineffective motor planning and execution in children caused by immaturity of their central nervous system.

developmental arrest. See **arrested development.**

developmental coordination disorder, disorder characterized by motor coordination that is markedly below the chronological age and intellectual ability; significantly interferes with activities of daily living.

developmental crisis, severe, usually transient stress that occurs when a person is unable to complete the tasks of a psychosocial stage of development and is therefore unable to move on to the next stage. See also **psychosocial development.**

developmental disability (DD), an impairment caused by a neurological or physical deficit beginning before an individual reaches 22 years of age. It affects activities of daily living and significantly impairs the individual's general intellectual and/or adaptive functioning. Most developmental disabilities persist throughout the individual's life, although many can be effectively treated.

developmental disorder, a physical, cognitive, communication, social-emotional, and/or adaptive impairment that develops in an infant or toddler. It may affect one area of development or many. Early intervention programs to address the child's symptoms are essential to the well-being of the child and family. See also **pervasive developmental disorders.**

developmental dysplasia of the hip (DDH), instability of the hip joint leading to dislocation in the neonatal period. Although it may be associated with various neuromuscular disorders, such as myelodysplasia, or occur in utero, it most commonly occurs in neurologically normal infants and is multifactorial in origin. Usually there is laxity of the hip ligaments. Most affected infants are firstborn children, and 30% to 50% present in the breech position. About 90% of those affected are girls. DDH is the preferred term for babies and children with hip dysplasia because the condition can develop after birth. Formerly called **congenital dislocation of the hip.**

D

developmental dyspraxia, a disorder of sensory integration characterized by an impaired ability to plan skilled, non-habitual coordinated movements.

developmental frame of reference, (in occupational therapy) a framework guiding the practitioner in interventions at the current level of function and in the provision of subsequent slightly advanced challenges.

developmental groove, a fine, recessed line in the enamel of a tooth that marks the union of the lobes of the crown in its development.

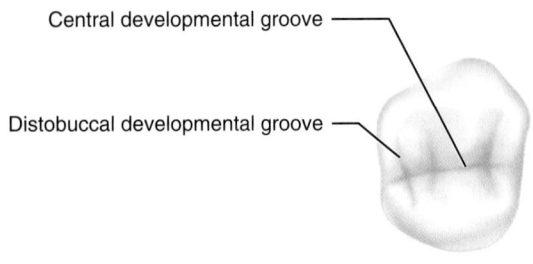

Central developmental groove

Distobuccal developmental groove

Developmental grooves *(Dean et al, 2011)*

developmental guidance, **1.** (in dentistry) comprehensive orthopedic control over the growth of the jaws and the eruption of the teeth. It may require precisely timed therapy with active appliances as well as supervisory examinations, including radiography and other diagnostic records. Guidance may be needed at various developmental stages throughout the entire growth and maturation of the face, beginning at the earliest detection of a developing malformation. **2.** educational interventions provided by the health care team and designed for the age and intellectual capacity of the individual that are related to coping with a disease or disability, planning for the future, or specific topics about making healthful decisions.

developmental horizon, any of 25 stages in the development of the human embryo from the one-cell stage at conception to the morphologically and physiologically complex organism at the end of the seventh week of gestation.

developmental model, **1.** a conceptual framework devised to be used as a guide in making a diagnosis, understanding a developmental process, and forming a prognosis for continued development. It has five components: The identifiable state describes the stage, level, phase, or period of the condition or process; the shift in state identifies qualities of change as progressive, sudden, abrupt, or recurrent; and the form of progression describes patterns of development as linear, spiral, or oscillating. The force that triggers the change or the step in development may be self-actualization or any form of stress. Development is ultimately constrained by the fifth component, potentiality, the genetic and environmental possibility of growth. **2.** (in nursing) a conceptual framework describing four stages, or processes, of development in the patient during therapy. In the first stage, called *orientation,* the patient begins a relationship with the nurse or other therapist and begins to clarify the problem with his or her help. In the second stage, called *identification,* the patient develops a sense of closeness and attachment to the therapist. During this period the patient and the therapist work comfortably together. In the third stage, called *exploitation,* the patient makes full use of the nursing services offered, begins to assume some control of the interactions, and becomes more independent. During the last stage, called *resolution,* the therapeutic relationship is terminated; the patient is independent and no longer needs the nurse or therapist. With this model the nurse therapist may plan nursing interventions appropriate to the patient's developmental level. The developmental model is one of the earliest nursing models to be developed. It views the person as a psychobiological being whose needs are expressed in behavior and who is unique and capable of learning and changing. Health is viewed as a forward movement of personality development and other ongoing processes, reflected by the person's creative, constructive, and productive community living. Thus the focus of nursing is to promote this forward movement by assisting the patient in self-repair and self-renewal.

developmental physiology, the study of the physiological processes as they relate to embryonic development.

developmental quotient (DQ), the numeric expression of a child's developmental level as measured by dividing the developmental age by the chronological age and multiplying by 100. Compare **intelligence quotient.** See also **developmental age.**

developmental sequence [Fr, *developper*; L, *sequi,* to follow], the order in which structure and function change during the process of growth and development of an organism. See also **ontogeny, phylogeny.**

developmental task, a physical or cognitive skill that a person must accomplish during a particular age period to continue development. An example is walking, which precedes the development of a sense of autonomy in the toddler period. The health care provider and therapist may also outline developmental tasks for families.

developmental theories of aging, concepts based on the identification of traits and characteristics that may be developed early in life or may change emphasis at different stages of development. Examples are theories of Jung, Erikson, and Havighurst.

deviance /dē″vē·əns/ [L, *deviare,* to turn aside], behavior that is contrary to the accepted standards and norms of a community or culture. See also **sexual deviance.**

deviant /dē″vē·ənt/ [L, *deviare,* to turn aside], pertaining to a person or object that departs from what is considered normal or standard.

deviant behavior, actions that exceed the usual limits of accepted behavior and involve failure to comply with the social norm of the group.

deviate /dē″vē·it/ [L, *deviare,* to turn aside], **1.** *n.,* a person or an act that varies from that which is considered standard, such as a social or sexual deviate, or that which is within a statistic norm. **2.** *v.,* to vary from that which is considered standard or within a statistic norm. **−deviant,** *adj.,* *−deviation, n.*

deviated septum, a shifted medial partition of the nasal cavity, a condition affecting many adults. The nasal septum more commonly shifts to the left during normal growth, but this deflection may be aggravated by a blow to the nose or by other trauma. A severe deflection of the septum may significantly obstruct the nasal passages and result in infection, sinusitis, shortness of breath, headache, or recurring nosebleeds. Severe septal deviation may be corrected by various surgical procedures, such as rhinoplasty or septoplasty. Postoperative care in such cases usually includes such measures as the maintenance of nasal packing, the administration of sedatives, and the placement of ice packs around the affected area to reduce swelling.

deviational nystagmus, a jerky movement of the eyes. See **end-positional nystagmus.**

deviation from normal, a quality, characteristic, symptom, or clinical finding that is different from what is commonly regarded as typical, such as an elevated temperature, multiple gestation, or an extra digit.

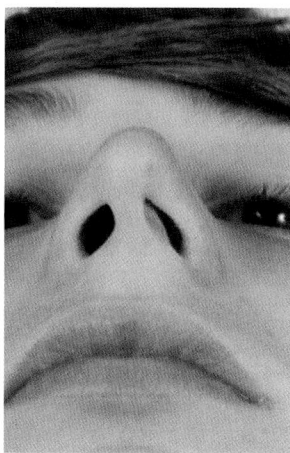

Deviated septum *(Haack and Papel, 2009)*

deviation of tongue [L, *deviare,* to turn aside; AS, *tunge*], a tendency of the tongue to turn away from the midline when extended or protruded. The condition is associated with a hypoglossal nerve defect, and the tongue deviates to the side of the injured nerve. Also called **tongue deviation.**

device /divīs´/ [OFr, *deviser,* to divide], an item other than a drug that has application in health care. The term is sometimes restricted by federal governments to items used directly by, on, or in the patient. Devices include orthopedic appliances, crutches, artificial heart valves, pacemakers, prostheses, wheelchairs, cervical collars, hearing aids, and eyeglasses. See also **medical device.**

Devic disease /dəvēk´/ [Eugène Devic, French physician, 1869–1930], combined, but not usually clinically simultaneous, demyelination of the optic nerve and the spinal cord, marked by diminution of vision and sometimes blindness, flaccid paralysis of the extremities, and sensory and genitourinary disturbances. Also called *neuromyelitis optica spectrum disorder.* Should not be confused with **multiple sclerosis.**

devil's claw, a perennial herb, *Harpagophytum procumbens,* native to southern Africa. Its dried tubular secondary roots and lateral tubers are used to improve digestion and generalized pain. It is also used in homeopathy for arthritic disorders and in folk medicine for a wide variety of disorders.

devil's grip. *(Informal)* See **epidemic pleurodynia.**

devitalized /dēvī´təlīzd/, pertaining to tissues with a reduced oxygen supply and blood flow.

devital tooth (devitalized tooth). See **pulpless tooth.**

dewar /dyoo¯´ər/, a double-walled chamber used to maintain the temperature of superconducting magnet coils near absolute zero. The outer chamber is filled with liquid nitrogen at a temperature of about −196° C (−321° F), and the inner chamber is filled with liquid helium at a temperature of −270° C (−454° F). A dewar is part of magnetic resonance imaging equipment.

dew point /dyoo¯/, the temperature at which air becomes saturated with water vapor and the water vapor condenses to liquid. In aerosol therapy, water may condense on containers, tubing, and other surfaces when the dew point is reached.

DEXA, abbreviation for **dual-energy x-ray absorptiometry.**

dexamethasone /dek´səmeth˝əsōn/, a long-acting synthetic adrenocorticoid with intense antiinflammatory activity and mineralocorticoid activity.

■ INDICATIONS: It is prescribed topically and systemically in the treatment of inflammatory conditions.

■ CONTRAINDICATIONS: Systemic fungal infections or known hypersensitivity to this drug prohibits its use.

■ ADVERSE EFFECTS: Among the more serious adverse reactions are GI, endocrine, neurological, fluid, and electrolyte disturbances.

dexamethasone (DST) suppression test, a test of the blood or urine after administration of dexamethasone, a synthetic steroid similar to cortisol, that is used to diagnose Cushing's syndrome.

dexchlorpheniramine maleate /deks´klôrfənir˝əmēn mal˝ē·it/, an antihistamine.

■ INDICATIONS: It is prescribed in the treatment of hypersensitivity reactions, including rhinitis, skin rash, and pruritus.

■ CONTRAINDICATIONS: Asthma or known hypersensitivity to this drug prohibits its use. It should not be given to newborns or lactating mothers.

■ ADVERSE EFFECTS: Drowsiness, skin rash, hypersensitivity reactions, dry mouth, and tachycardia may occur.

Dexedrine, a central nervous system stimulant with indications for narcolepsy and attention deficit hyperactivity disorder. Brand name for **dextroamphetamine sulfate.**

dexmedetomidine, an alpha$_2$ adrenoceptor agonist sedative.

■ INDICATIONS: It is used to sedate mechanically ventilated and intubated patients in the intensive care unit.

■ CONTRAINDICATIONS: Known hypersensitivity to this drug contraindicates its use.

■ ADVERSE EFFECTS: Life-threatening effects are atrial fibrillation and infarction. Other serious adverse effects include oliguria, hypertension, pulmonary edema, pleural effusion, hypoxia, leukocytosis, and anemia. Common side effects include nausea, bradycardia, and hypotension.

dexmethylphenidate, a central nervous system stimulant used to treat attention deficit hyperactivity disorder.

dexrazoxane, a cardioprotective agent.

■ INDICATIONS: It is prescribed in the protection of women from heart problems caused by doxorubicin treatment of breast cancer.

■ CONTRAINDICATIONS: It should not be given to patients with an allergy to dexrazoxane or any of its components or to those who are receiving chemotherapy that does not contain an anthracycline drug.

■ ADVERSE EFFECTS: The side effects most often reported include pain on or at the injection site, flushing, bruising, rash, numbness, or general body discomfort.

dexter (D) /deks´tər/ [L, *dexter,* right], right side; right.

dexterity /dekster´itē/ [L, *dexteritas*], skillfulness in the use of one's hands or body.

dextrad /deks´trad/ [L, *dexter,* right], toward the right side.

dextrad writing /deks˝trad/ [L, *dexter,* right; ME, *writen*], writing that moves from left to right.

dextrality. See **right-handedness.**

dextran fermentation /dek˝strən/ [L, *dexter,* right, *fermentare,* to cause to rise], the conversion of dextrose to dextran by the action of *Leuconostoc mesenteroides* dextran bacteria.

dextran preparation, any of a group of solutions containing polysaccharides, water, and, in some preparations, electrolytes. These solutions are used as plasma volume extenders in cases of hypovolemia from hemorrhage, dehydration, or another cause and are available for intravenous administration in several concentrations.

dextrin, a glucose polymer formed by the hydrolysis of starch. It is a tasteless, colorless, gummy substance, soluble in water. Dextrin is an intermediate substance formed during the conversion of starch into monosaccharides, such as glucose. It is used in a number of pharmaceutic products.

dextro-, dextr-, prefix meaning "right": *dextrocardia.*

D

dextroamphetamine sulfate /deks′trō·amfet″əmēn/, a central nervous system stimulant.

■ INDICATIONS: It is prescribed in the treatment of narcolepsy, hyperkinetic disorders, and attention deficit disorder in children and as an anorexiant in treating exogenous obesity.

■ CONTRAINDICATIONS: Cardiovascular disease, glaucoma, hypertension, hyperthyroidism, agitation, history of drug abuse, concomitant administration of a monoamine oxidase inhibitor within 14 days, or known hypersensitivity to this drug prohibits its use.

■ ADVERSE EFFECTS: Among the more serious adverse reactions are manifestations of central nervous system excitation, increased blood pressure, arrhythmias and other cardiovascular effects, nausea, anorexia, and drug dependence.

dextrocardia /-kär″dē·ə/, the location of the heart in the right hemithorax, either as a result of displacement by disease or as a congenital defect.

dextromethorphan hydrobromide /-methôr″fən/, an antitussive derived from morphine but lacking opioid effects.

■ INDICATIONS: It is prescribed for the suppression of nonproductive cough.

■ CONTRAINDICATIONS: Use of a monoamine oxidase inhibitor within the past 14 days or known hypersensitivity to this drug prohibits its use.

■ ADVERSE EFFECTS: The most serious adverse reaction is respiratory depression resulting from large doses.

dextrose /dek″strōs/ [L, *dexter,* right], glucose available in various solutions for IV administration.

■ INDICATIONS: It is prescribed for the treatment of calorie deficit, for hypoglycemia, and in solution for fluid deficit.

■ CONTRAINDICATIONS: Diabetic coma, intracranial or intraspinal hemorrhage, or delirium tremens prohibits its use.

■ ADVERSE EFFECTS: Among the more serious adverse reactions are hyperglycemia, glycosuria, and phlebitis.

dextrose and sodium chloride injection, a fluid, nutrient, and electrolyte replenisher. It is available for parenteral use in a variety of concentrations.

df, abbreviation for **degrees of freedom.**

DFA-TP test, abbreviation for **direct fluorescent antibody-*Treponema pallidum* test.**

dg, abbreviation for **decigram.**

D gene, one of a set of genes lying between the V and J genes, which code for the D region of heavy-chain or for the beta or delta chain of the T cell receptor.

D.H.E. 45, a vasconstrictor that works primarily by stimulating alpha-adrenergic receptors. Brand name for **dihydroergotamine mesylate.**

DHFSS, abbreviation for **dengue hemorrhagic fever shock syndrome.**

DHHS, abbreviation for **Department of Health and Human Services.**

dhobie itch /dō″bē/ [Hindi, *dhobie,* laundryman; AS, *giccan*], a fungal infection, such as jock itch or athlete's foot, that attacks moist parts of the body and causes an itching or burning sensation. Risk factors for infection include close-fitting or wet clothing or undergarments. Also called **tinea cruris.**

DHT, abbreviation for **dihydrotestosterone.**

di-, **1.** prefix meaning "two, twice": *dioxide.* **2.** prefix meaning "apart, thrugh": *diuresis.*

dia-, prefix meaning "apart, away from": *diastasis.*

DiaBeta, an oral antidiabetic drug. Brand name for **glyBURIDE.**

diabetes /dī′əbē″tēz/ [Gk, *diabainein,* to pass through], a clinical condition characterized by the excessive excretion of urine. The excess may be caused by a deficiency of antidiuretic hormone, as in diabetes insipidus, or it may be the polyuria resulting from the hyperglycemia that occurs in diabetes mellitus. See also **diabetes insipidus, diabetes mellitus.**

diabetes insipidus /insip″idəs/, a metabolic disorder caused by injury of the neurohypophyseal system. It is characterized by copious excretion of urine and excessive thirst, caused by deficient production or secretion of the antidiuretic hormone (ADH) or inability of the kidney tubules to respond to ADH. Rarely, the symptoms are self-induced by an excessive water intake. The condition may be acquired, familial, idiopathic, neurogenic, nephrogenic, or psychogenic.

■ OBSERVATIONS: The onset may be dramatic and sudden, and urinary output may exceed 10 L in 24 hours. Diagnosis is established by a water deprivation test in which urine volume increases and urine osmolality decreases. An MRI is performed to assess for abnormalities in or near the pituitary gland. A person with diabetes insipidus who is unconscious as a result of trauma or surgery continues to produce massive quantities of urine. If fluids are not administered in adequate amounts, the patient becomes severely dehydrated and hypernatremic.

■ INTERVENTIONS: In mild cases, no treatment is necessary. Vasopressin in an intramuscular injection or nasal spray is effective. Thiazide diuretics, by inducing a state of salt depletion, sometimes decrease the diuresis of water by as much as 50%.

■ PATIENT CARE CONSIDERATIONS: Infants, small children, and the elderly are particularly vulnerable to serious circulatory disturbances when dehydrated. Exceedingly careful monitoring is essential when the condition is suspected, especially after head surgery or trauma.

diabetes mellitus (DM) /məlī″təs/, a complex disorder of carbohydrate, fat, and protein metabolism that is primarily a result of a deficiency or complete lack of insulin secretion by the beta cells of the pancreas or resistance to insulin. The disease is often familial but may be acquired, as in Cushing's syndrome, as a result of the administration of excessive glucocorticoid. The various forms of diabetes have been organized into categories developed by the Expert Committee on the Diagnosis and Classification of Diabetes Mellitus of the American Diabetes Association. Type 1 diabetes mellitus in this classification scheme includes patients with diabetes caused by an autoimmune process, dependent on insulin to prevent ketosis. This group was previously called type I, insulin-dependent diabetes mellitus, juvenile-onset diabetes, brittle diabetes, or ketosis-prone diabetes. Patients with type 2 diabetes mellitus are those previously designated as having type II, non–insulin-dependent diabetes mellitus, maturity-onset diabetes, adult-onset diabetes, ketosis-resistant diabetes, or stable diabetes. Those with gestational diabetes mellitus are women in whom glucose intolerance develops during pregnancy. Other types of diabetes are associated with a pancreatic disease, hormonal changes, adverse effects of drugs, or genetic or other anomalies. A fourth subclass, the impaired glucose tolerance group, also called prediabetes, includes persons whose blood glucose levels are abnormal although not sufficiently above the normal range to be diagnosed as having diabetes. Contributing factors to the development of diabetes are heredity; obesity; sedentary lifestyle; high-fat, low-fiber diets; hypertension; and aging. See also **impaired glucose tolerance, potential abnormality of glucose tolerance.**

■ OBSERVATIONS: The onset of type 1 diabetes mellitus is sudden in children. Type 2 diabetes often begins insidiously. Characteristically, the course is progressive and includes increased urination, increased thirst, weight loss, polyphagia, hyperglycemia, and glycosuria. The eyes, kidneys, nervous system, skin, and circulatory system may be affected by the long-term complications of either type of diabetes. Infections are common. Atherosclerosis often develops. In type 1 diabetes mellitus, when no endogenous insulin is being secreted, ketoacidosis is a constant danger. The diagnosis is confirmed by fasting plasma glucose and history.

■ INTERVENTIONS: The goal of treatment is to maintain insulin glucose homeostasis. Type 1 diabetes is controlled by insulin, meal planning, and exercise. Studies have demonstrated that tight control of blood glucose levels (i.e., frequent monitoring and maintenance at as close to normal as possible to the level of nondiabetics) significantly reduces complications such as eye disease, kidney disease, and nerve damage. Type 2 diabetes is controlled by meal planning, weight loss, exercise, one or more oral agents, and insulin. Stress of any kind may require medication adjustment in both type 1 and type 2 diabetes.

diabetes mellitus autoantibody panel, a blood test to screen for diabetes in relatives of patients with type 1 diabetes mellitus. Antibodies often appear years before symptoms begin, allowing individuals to be closely monitored for the disease. The test is also helpful in determining the type of diabetes as patients with type 2 diabetes will not have the antibodies.

diabetic /dī′əbet″ik/, **1.** *adj.,* pertaining to diabetes. **2.** *adj.,* affected with diabetes. **3.** *n.,* a person who has diabetes mellitus.

diabetic acidosis [Gk, *diabainein,* to pass through; L, *acidus,* acid; Gk, *osis,* condition], a type of acidosis that may occur in diabetes mellitus as a result of excessive production of ketone bodies during oxidation of fatty acids. See also **diabetic ketoacidosis.**

diabetic amaurosis [Gk, *diabainein,* to pass through, *amauroein,* to darken], *(Obsolete)* blindness associated with diabetes mellitus, caused by a proliferative hemorrhagic form of retinopathy. Now called **diabetic retinopathy.**

diabetic coma, a life-threatening condition occurring in persons with diabetes mellitus. It is caused by undiagnosed diabetes; inadequate treatment; failure to take prescribed insulin; excessive food intake; or, most frequently, infection, surgery, trauma, or other stressors that increase the body's need for insulin. Without insulin to metabolize glucose, fats are used for energy, resulting in ketone waste accumulation and metabolic acidosis. The body's effort to counteract acidosis depletes the alkali reserve; causes a loss of sodium, chloride, potassium, and water; increases respiratory exhalation of carbon dioxide (Kussmaul breathing) and urinary excretion; and leads to dehydration and generalized hypoxia. Warning signs of diabetic coma include a dull headache, fatigue, inordinate thirst, epigastric pain, nausea, vomiting, parched lips, flushed face, and sunken eyes. The temperature usually rises and then falls, the systolic blood pressure drops, and circulatory collapse may occur. Immediate treatment consists of administering short-acting insulin and replacing

Target nutritional goals for patients with diabetes mellitus

Calories
Sufficient to achieve and maintain weight as close to desirable body weight as possible

Carbohydrate
Varies in relation to assessment and protein and fat intake; usually 40% to 60% of total calories
Liberalized, individualized emphasis on total carbohydrate intake versus eliminating simple sugars only
Carbohydrate consistency at meals
Modest amounts of sucrose and other refined sugars acceptable contingent on metabolic control and body weight

Protein
Usual dietary intake of protein double the amount needed
Exact ideal percentage of total calories debatable; usually 12% to 20% of total calories
Recommended dietary allowance (RDA): 0.8 g/kg body weight for adults; RDA modified for children, pregnant and lactating women, older adults, and those with special medical conditions
Avoidance of excess dietary protein intake in renal disease

Fat
Usually 30% or less of total calories, but may be as high as 40%
Polyunsaturated fats, 6% to 8%
Saturated fats, less than 10%
Monounsaturated fats, remaining percentage
Cholesterol, less than 300 mg/day
May need to be further modified, depending on lipid profile

Fiber
Up to 40 g/day
25 g/1000 kcal for low-calorie intakes

Alternative sweeteners
Use of various nutritive and nonnutritive sweeteners

Sodium
3000 mg/day or less
Modified for special medical conditions (e.g., hypertension, edema)

Alcohol
Two or less equivalents per day (1 equivalent = 1.5 ounces of distilled liquor, 4-ounce glass of wine, or 12-ounce glass of beer)

Vitamins and minerals
Despite a lack of scientific evidence that individuals with diabetes mellitus (DM) who eat a well-balanced diet require vitamin or mineral supplementation, the RDAs were developed based on a healthy population. Also, given that many vitamins and minerals are excreted in excess in the urine of individuals with DM, supplementation with a general multivitamin is prudent and rarely harmful.

From Monahan FD et al: *Phipps' medical-surgical nursing: health and illness perspectives,* ed 8, St Louis, 2007, Mosby.

Characteristics of types 1 and 2 diabetes mellitus

Characteristic	Type 1	Type 2
Age at onset	<20 yr	Increasingly occurring in younger children
Type of onset	Abrupt	Gradual
Sex ratio	Affects males slightly more than females	Females outnumber males
Percentage of diabetic population	5%–8%	85%–90%
Heredity:		
Family history	Sometimes	Frequently
Human leukocyte antigen	Associations	No association
Twin concordance	25%–50%	90%–100%
Ethnic distribution	Primarily Caucasians	Increased incidence in Native Americans, Hispanics, African-Americans
Presenting symptoms	3 Ps common: polyuria, polydipsia, polyphagia	May be related to long-term complications
Nutritional status	Underweight	Overweight
Insulin (natural):		
Pancreatic content	Usually none	>50% normal
Serum insulin	Low to absent	High or low
Primary resistance	Minimum	Marked
Islet cell antibodies	80%–85%	<5%
Therapy:		
Insulin	Always	20%–30% of patients
Oral agents	Ineffective	Often effective
Diet only	Ineffective	Often effective
Chronic complications	>80%	Variable
Ketoacidosis	Common	Infrequent

From Hockenberry MJ, Wilson D: *Wong's nursing care of infants and children,* ed 10, St Louis, 2015, Mosby.

electrolytes and fluids to correct the acidosis and dehydration. Nonketotic coma may occur in patients with poorly controlled type 2 diabetes mellitus and high levels of blood glucose but no fatty acid breakdown. The plasma hyperosmolarity causes water to leave cells, and the dehydration of cerebral cells results in coma. See also **diabetic ketoacidosis, insulin shock.**

diabetic diet,   a diet used to control blood glucose, weight, and cholesterol levels in individuals with diabetes mellitus. It usually contains limited amounts of simple sugars or readily digestible carbohydrates and amounts of proteins, complex carbohydrates, fiber, and unsaturated fats similar to those recommended for the general public. It is not a restrictive diet but rather a healthful eating plan that is coordinated with medication administration and exercise to control blood sugar levels. Dietary tools include carbohydrate counting, the use of exchange lists, and consideration of the glycemic index. See also **diabetes mellitus, Exchange Lists for Meal Planning, insulin, glycemic index.**

diabetic foot and leg care,   the special attention given to prevent the circulatory disorders and infections that frequently occur in the lower extremities of diabetic patients. ■ METHOD: The patient should be taught to examine the legs and feet daily for signs of dry, scaly, red, itching, or cracked skin; blisters; corns; calluses; abrasions; infection; blueness and swelling around varicosities; and thickened, discolored nails. The feet should be bathed daily in tepid water with mild or superfatted soap and dried gently but thoroughly with a soft towel. A lanolin-based lotion is then applied, although not between the toes; excess lotion is removed with a dry towel; vigorous rubbing and use of alcohol preparations are avoided because of drying and irritation of skin, which can lead to skin breakdown. Calluses and corns are removed, and thickened, deformed nails are cut by a podiatrist. Commercial remedies for removing calluses and corns should not be used. ■ INTERVENTIONS: The nurse provides foot and leg care while the diabetic patient is hospitalized. Before discharge the patient is instructed to examine and bathe the feet daily according to the recommended method, to report abnormalities, to keep the feet dry at all times, to wear cotton socks or stockings with cotton feet, and to place clean lamb's wool or cotton between the toes if they perspire. The patient is cautioned to avoid sustaining foot or leg trauma, walking barefoot, scratching insect bites, using a hot-water bottle or heating pad on the lower extremities, getting a sunburn, wearing constricting garments, remaining in the same position for long periods, sitting at more than a right-angle bend, and crossing the knees. The individual with diabetes is advised to alternate the wearing of two pairs of rubber-soled, well-fitted shoes wide enough to prevent pressure and rubbing; to air each pair of shoes between use; and to break in new shoes gradually. The patient often benefits from therapy to walk to tolerance daily, to plan exercise periods after meals, to bend and straighten the knees and rotate the ankles occasionally when sitting, and, when standing, to shift weight from time to time and walk in place. Patients may be referred to a certified diabetic educator for initial instruction about care. ■ OUTCOME CRITERIA: Meticulous care of the feet and legs can prevent serious complications, including local infection, skin ulcers, cellulitis, and gangrene.

diabetic gangrene [Gk, *diabainein,* to pass through, *gaggraina*],   gangrene, usually involving the lower extremities, that develops secondary to sensory peripheral neuropathy and peripheral vascular disease complications related to the diabetic disease process.

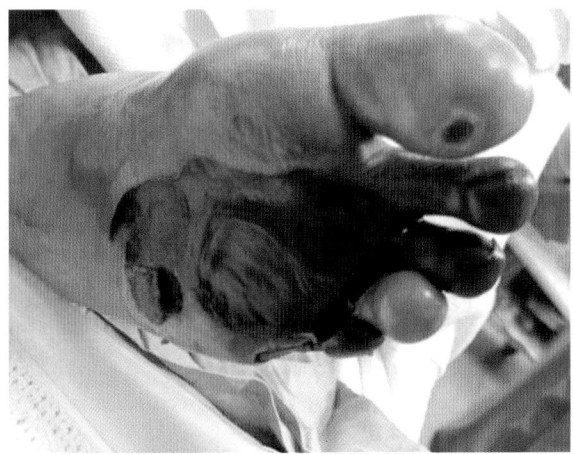

Diabetic gangrene *(Elsharawy, 2011)*

diabetic glycosuria [Gk, *diabainein,* to pass through, *glykys,* sweet, *ouron,* urine], excessive excretion of glucose into the urine as an effect of poorly controlled diabetes mellitus.

diabetic ketoacidosis (DKA), an acute, life-threatening complication of uncontrolled diabetes mellitus. In this condition extremely high blood glucose levels and urinary loss of water, potassium, ammonium, and sodium result in hypovolemia, electrolyte imbalance, and breakdown of free fatty acids, causing acidosis, often with coma. Compare **insulin shock.**

■ OBSERVATIONS: The person appears flushed; has hot, dry skin; is restless, uncomfortable, agitated, and diaphoretic; and has a fruity odor to the breath. Nausea, confusion, and coma are often noted. Persons with diabetes mellitus who produce no natural (endogenous) insulin are most often affected (type 1). Untreated, the condition invariably proceeds to coma and death.

■ INTERVENTIONS: IV insulin and hypotonic saline solution are administered immediately. Nasogastric intubation and bladder catheterization may be indicated. Blood glucose and ketone levels are determined hourly, and electrolyte and acid-base balance are monitored frequently. Bicarbonate may be given in dosages dependent on the degree of acidosis. Potassium is usually given because of intracellular potassium depletion. Plasma or a plasma expander may be necessary to prevent or correct shock resulting from hypovolemia.

■ PATIENT CARE CONSIDERATIONS: The cause of the episode of ketoacidosis is sought. The most common precipitating factors are undiagnosed type 1 diabetes mellitus, infection, GI upset, alcohol consumption, and failure to take insulin. Type 1 diabetes mellitus in childhood characteristically begins suddenly and progresses rapidly. Therefore, the diagnosis of type 1 diabetes is usually made when the child arrives at the hospital in diabetic ketoacidosis. Inpatient care after an episode of ketoacidosis is the same as for diabetes mellitus.

diabetic neuropathy, a noninflammatory disease process associated with diabetes mellitus and characterized by sensory and/or motor disturbances in the peripheral nervous system. Patients commonly experience degeneration of sensory nerves and pathways. Early symptoms, which include pain and loss of reflexes in the legs, may occur in patients with only mild hyperglycemia. Diabetes is associated with a wide range of neuropathies, including mononeuritis multiplex, compression and entrapment mononeuropathies, cranial neuropathies, and autonomic and small fiber neuropathies. Differential diagnosis is difficult because not all sensorimotor neuropathies are caused by diabetes.

diabetic polyneuritis, an inflammation involving many nerves. It usually occurs as a complication in long-term cases of diabetes mellitus.

diabetic polyneuropathy, a disorder involving a number of nerves, a long-term complication of diabetes mellitus. Central nervous system, autonomic, and peripheral nerves may be affected. Neuropathic ulcers commonly develop on the feet.

diabetic retinopathy, a disorder of retinal blood vessels. It is characterized by capillary microaneurysms, cotton-wool spots, hemorrhage, exudates, and the formation of highly permeable new vessels. The disorder occurs most frequently in patients with long-standing, poorly controlled diabetes mellitus. Repeated hemorrhage may cause permanent opacity of the vitreous humor, and blindness may eventually result. Photocoagulation of damaged retinal blood vessels by a laser beam may be performed to decrease retinal ischemia and to prevent hemorrhage from the vessels.

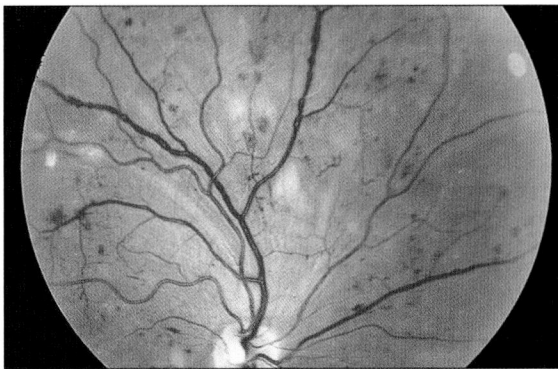

Diabetic retinopathy with cotton-wool exudates
(Goldman and Schafer, 2012)

diabetic tabes, a wasting condition associated with diabetic peripheral neuropathy. It may be accompanied by sharp pain, muscle weakness, atrophy of intrinsic foot muscles, and weakness of the toes' extensors and flexors. It may lead to foot drop because of ankle weakness. When these manifestations coexist with decreased proprioception in the feet, "pseudotabetic" gait may occur.

diabetic vulvovaginitis [Gk, *diabainein,* to pass through; L, *vulva,* wrapper, *vagina,* sheath; Gk, *itis,* inflammation], a mycotic infection of the vulva and vagina that is associated with diabetes.

diabetic xanthoma, an eruption of yellow papules or plaques on the skin in patients with uncontrolled diabetes mellitus. The lesion disappears as the metabolic functions are stabilized and the disease is controlled.

diabetogenic state /dī′əbet′ōjen″ik/, a health condition manifested by signs and symptoms of diabetes.

Diabinese, an oral antidiabetic drug. Brand name for **chlorproPAMIDE.**

diacetic acid. See **acetoacetic acid.**

diacetylmorphine. See **heroin.**

diacondylar fracture /dī′əkon″dilər/ [Gk, *dia,* through, *kondylos,* knuckle; L, *fractura,* break], any fracture that runs across the line of the rounded projection on a bone that articulates with another bone.

diadochokinesia /dī·ad′əkōkīnē″zhə/ [Gk, *diadochos,* successor, *kinesis,* motion], the normal ability of the muscles to move a limb alternately in opposite directions by flexion and extension. It is tested by asking the client to supinate and pronate the hands quickly and rhythmically.

D

diagnose /dī′agnōs/, to determine the type and cause of a health condition on the basis of signs and symptoms of the patient; data obtained from laboratory analysis of fluid, tissue specimens, and other tests; and family and occupational background information, such as recent injuries or exposure to toxic substances. See also **diagnosis.**

diagnosis /dī′agnō″sis/ [Gk, *dia* + *gnosis,* knowledge], **1.** identification of a disease or condition by a scientific evaluation of physical signs, symptoms, history, laboratory test results, and procedures. Kinds include **clinical diagnosis, differential diagnosis, laboratory diagnosis, nursing diagnosis, physical diagnosis. 2.** the art of naming a disease or condition. **–diagnostic,** *adj.,* **–diagnose,** *v.*

diagnosis by exclusion [Gk, *dia,* through, *gnosis,* knowledge; L, *excludere,* to shut out], diagnosis made by ruling out other possible causes of disease symptoms.

diagnosis-related group (DRG), a group of patients classified for measuring a medical facility's delivery of care. The classifications, used to determine Medicare payments for inpatient care, are based on primary and secondary diagnosis, primary and secondary procedures, age, and length of hospitalization. See also **prospective payment system.**

diagnostic /dī′agnos″tik/, pertaining to the identification of a disease or disorder.

Diagnostic and Statistical Manual of Mental Disorders, a manual published by the American Psychiatric Association listing the official diagnostic classifications of mental disorders. Each of the classifications of the mental disorders contains a code that provides a reference to the WHO International Classification of Diseases and offers such useful diagnostic criteria as essential and associated features of the disorder, age at onset, course, impairment, complications, predisposing factors, prevalence, sex ratio, familial patterns, and differential diagnoses. DSM-5, published in 2013, is the fifth edition of the manual.

diagnostic anesthesia, a procedure in which analgesia is induced to a depth adequate to permit comfortable performance of moderately painful diagnostic procedures of short duration. Awake anesthesia is often used for this purpose. See also **awake anesthesia.**

diagnostician /dī′agnostish″ən/, a person skilled and trained in identifying diseases, disorders, and conditions that interfere with health.

diagnostic medical sonographer, an allied health professional who provides patient services using diagnostic ultrasound under the supervision of a doctor of medicine or osteopathy responsible for the use and interpretation of ultrasound procedures.

diagnostic molecular scientist, an allied health professional who performs diagnostic tests on various specimen types after determining how the specimens will be handled. A baccalaureate degree is required, and a master's degree is usually completed.

diagnostic peritoneal lavage (DPL), a procedure used to detect intraabdominal bleeding or viscus perforation after abdominal trauma. The open or operative approach allows direct visual examination of the peritoneum when the catheter is inserted. Gastric and bladder decompression must precede performance of DPL.

diagnostic position of gaze. See **cardinal position of gaze.**

diagnostic process, the act of determining a patient's health status and evaluating the factors influencing that status.

diagnostic radiology, medical imaging using external sources of radiation.

diagnostic radiopharmaceutical, a radioactive drug administered to a patient as a diagnostic tracer to differentiate normal from abnormal anatomical structures or biochemical or physiological functions. Most, but not all, diagnostic radiopharmaceuticals emit gamma rays.

diagnostic sensitivity, the conditional probability that a person having a disease will be correctly identified by a clinical test (i.e., the number of true positive results divided by the total number with the disease, which is the sum of the numbers of true positive plus false negative results).

diagnostic services, activities related to treating or diagnosing a health care problem by monitoring existing conditions, evaluating new symptoms, and/or reviewing test results.

diagnostic specificity, the conditional probability that a person not having a disease will be correctly identified by a clinical test (i.e., the number of true negative results divided by the total number of those without the disease, which is the sum of the numbers of true negative plus false positive results).

diagonal artery, an inconstant artery, occasionally duplicated, arising from the trunk of the left anterior descending coronary artery and crossing the anterior aspect of the left ventricle diagonally, toward the left margin.

diagonal conjugate /dī·ag″ənəl/, a radiographic measurement of the distance from the inferior border of the symphysis pubis to the sacral promontory. The measurement, which averages around 12.5 to 13.0 cm in adult women, also may be determined by vaginal examination. See also **true conjugate.**

diakinesis /dī′əkinē″sis, dī′əkī-/ [Gk, *dia* + *kinesis,* motion], the final stage in the first meiotic prophase in gametogenesis in which the chromosomes achieve their maximum thickness. The chiasmata and nucleolus disappear, the nuclear membrane degenerates, and the spindle fibers form in preparation for the formation of dyads. See also **diplotene, leptotene, pachytene, zygotene.**

dial, a circular diagram with black lines radiating outward across a white background from the center, as is used in tests of astigmatism.

dialect /dī′əlekt/, a variation of spoken language different from other forms of the same language in pronunciation, syntax, and word meanings. A particular dialect is usually shared by members of an ethnic group, socioeconomic group, or people living together in a geographic area.

dialogue /dī′əlog/ [L, *dialogus,* philosophic conversation], a conversation between two people in which both listen intently to each other.

Dialose, a fixed-combination GI drug containing a stool softener and a laxative. Brand name for **docusate,** *sodium carboxymethylcellulose.*

dialy-, prefix meaning "dialysis or dissolution": *dialysate.*

dialysate, the material that passes through the membrane in dialysis.

dialysis /dī·al″isis/ [Gk *dia* + *lysis,* a loosening], **1.** the process of separating colloids and crystalline substances in solution by the difference in their rate of diffusion through a semipermeable membrane. **2.** a medical procedure for the removal of certain elements from the blood or lymph by virtue of the difference in their rates of diffusion through an external semipermeable membrane or, in the case of peritoneal dialysis, through the peritoneum. Dialysis may be used to remove poisons and excessive amounts of drugs, to correct serious electrolyte and acid-base imbalances, and to remove urea, uric acid, and creatinine in cases of chronic end-stage renal disease. Dialysis involves diffusion of particles from an area of high to lower concentration, osmosis of fluid across the membrane from an area of lesser to one of greater concentration of particles, and ultrafiltration or movement of fluid across the membrane as a result of an artificially created pressure differential. See also **hemodialysis, peritoneal dialysis.**

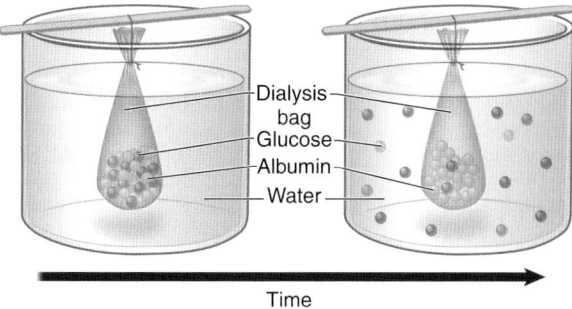

Dialysis *(Patton and Thibodeau, 2016)*

dialysis dementia, a neurological disorder that occurs in some patients undergoing dialysis. The precise cause is unknown, but the effect is believed to be related to chemicals in the dialyzing fluid, drugs administered to the dialysis patient, or both.

dialysis disequilibrium syndrome, a disorder caused by a rapid change in extracellular fluid composition during dialysis. It may be marked by cerebral or neurological disturbances, cardiac arrhythmias, and pulmonary edema.

dialysis fluid. See **dialysate.**

dialysis shunt [Gk, *dia,* through, *lysis,* loosening; ME, *shunten*], an external artificial link between a peripheral artery and a vein, in an arm or leg, for use in hemodialysis. Also called **arteriovenous fistula.**

dialysis technician [Gk, *dia,* through, *lysis,* loosening, *technikos,* skillful], an allied health professional who operates and maintains dialysis equipment for patients with kidney diseases. Dialysis technicians work under the supervision of a registered nurse or physician.

dialyzer /dī″əlī′zər/ [Gk, *dia + lysis,* loosening], **1.** a machine used in dialysis. **2.** a semipermeable membrane or porous diaphragm in a dialysis machine. See also **dialysis, hemodialysis, peritoneal dialysis.**

diameter (D) /dī·am′ə·tər/ [Gk, *diametros*], **1.** the length of a straight line passing through the center of a circle and connecting opposite points on its circumference. **2.** the distance between two specified opposite points on the periphery of a structure such as the cranium or pelvis.

Diameter-Index Safety System (DISS), a system of standardized connections between cylinders of medical gases and flowmeters or pressure regulators. Each gas has connections of a specific size to prevent accidental hookup of the wrong gas. Each type of gas and connector is assigned a DISS number, such as 1040 for nitrous oxide and 1240 for oxygen. See also **Pin-Index Safety System.**

diamine oxidase. See **histaminase.**

diaminovaleric acid. See **ornithine.**

Diamond-Blackfan syndrome, a rare congenital disorder evident in the first 3 months of life, characterized by severe anemia and a very low reticulocyte count but normal numbers of platelets and white cells. It is caused by a deficiency of erythrocyte precursors. Also called **congenital hypoplastic anemia.** See also **anemia.**

diamond bur /dī″(ə)mənd/, (in dentistry) a rotary device of differing shapes and sizes to shape and prepare teeth for restoration or extraction. It contains industrial diamond particles and is used as an abrasive.

Diamox, a carbonic anhydrase inhibitor. Brand name for **acetaZOLAMIDE.**

diapedesis /dī′əpidē″sis/ [Gk, *dia + pedesis,* an oozing], the passage of white blood cells through the walls of the blood vessels without damage to the vessels. See also **ameboid movement.**

diaper rash [ME, *diapre,* patterned fabric], an erythematous, papular, or scaly eruption in the diaper area of infants, caused by irritation from feces, moisture, heat, or ammonia produced by the bacterial decomposition of urine. Secondary infection by *Candida albicans* is common. Principles of treatment include frequent diaper changes, dryness, cleanliness, coolness, and ventilation of the affected area. Specific topical antimicrobial medication may be prescribed for secondary infection. Also called *diaper dermatitis.*

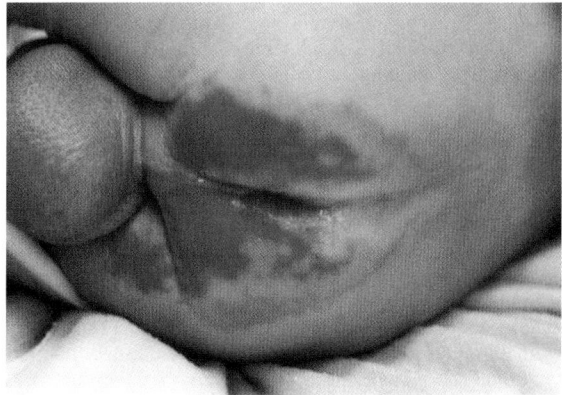

Infant with diaper rash *(Leifer, 2011)*

diaper restraint, a therapeutic device used for countertraction with lower extremity traction when other methods of countertraction are not effective. One device is used in treating children with orthopedic diseases and abnormalities. It is designed to fit over the pelvic area like diapers, with rings at each of four corners. A webbing strap is threaded through the rings and attached to the top side of the bedspring frame. Diaper restraints are used with Russell traction and with split Russell traction if additional countertraction is required but are not generally used with other kinds of traction. Compare **jacket restraint, sling restraint.**

diaphanography /dī·af·ənog″rəfē/ [Gk, *diaphanes,* shining through, *graphein,* to record], an imaging modality that uses selected wavelengths of light and special imaging equipment to examine the breast tissues. See also **diaphanoscopy.**

diaphanoscope /dī·af′ənoskōp′/, an instrument that transilluminates the interior of a cavity to determine the translucency of its walls.

diaphanoscopy /dī·af·ənos″kəpē/, examination of an internal structure with a diaphanoscope.

diaphoresis /dī′əfərē″sis/ [Gk, *dia + pherein,* to carry], the secretion of sweat, especially the profuse secretion associated with an elevated body temperature, physical exertion, exposure to heat, and mental or emotional stress. Sweating is centrally controlled by the sympathetic nervous system and is primarily a thermoregulatory mechanism. However, the sweat glands on the palms and soles respond to emotional stimuli and do not always participate in thermal sweating. The rate of sweating is generally not affected by water deficiency, but it may be reduced by severe dehydration; it also diminishes when salt intake exceeds salt loss. Also called **sweating.** See also **sudorific.**

diaphoretic. See **sudorific.**

diaphragm /dī″əfram/ [Gk, *diaphragma,* partition], **1.** (in anatomy) a dome-shaped musculofibrous partition that separates the thoracic and abdominal cavities. The convex cranial surface of the diaphragm forms the floor of the thoracic cavity; the concave surface forms the roof of the abdominal cavity. This partition is pierced by various openings through which pass the esophagus and inferior vena cava. The diaphragm aids respiration by moving up and down. During inspiration it moves down and increases the volume of the thoracic cavity. During expiration it moves up, decreasing the volume. During deep inspiration and expiration the range of diaphragmatic movement in the adult is about 30 mm on the right side and about 28 mm on the left side. The height of this structure also varies with the degree of distension of the stomach and the intestines and with the size of the liver. It is innervated by the phrenic nerve from the cervical plexus. **2.** See **contraceptive diaphragm. 3.** (in optics) an opening that controls the amount of light passing through an optical network. **4.** a thin, membranous partition, as that used in dialysis. **5.** (in radiography) a metal plate with a small opening that limits the diameter of the radiographic beam. **6.** See also **diaphragm stethoscope.** –*diaphragmatic, adj.*

diaphragma sellae. See **sellar diaphragm.**

diaphragmatic breathing /dī·əfragmat″ik/ [Gk, *diaphragma,* partition], a pattern of expiration and inspiration in which most of the ventilatory work is done with the diaphragm. Many males normally breathe diaphragmatically, whereas few females do. The technique is taught to patients with chronic obstructive pulmonary disease to facilitate respiration. The patient is trained to strengthen the contractile force of the abdominal wall muscles to elevate the diaphragm and empty the lungs. The patient places a hand on the epigastrium during training to focus attention on that portion of the body. Also called **diaphragmatic respiration.** Compare **abdominal breathing.**

diaphragmatic constriction, the narrowing in the esophagus where it crosses the diaphragm at the esophageal hiatus.

diaphragmatic flutter, rapid, rhythmic contractions of the diaphragm. The condition may simulate atrial flutter.

diaphragmatic hernia [Gk, *diaphragma,* partition; L, rupture], the protrusion of part of the stomach through an opening in the diaphragm, most commonly an abnormally enlarged esophageal hiatus. In some cases the intestines may also herniate into the chest. The enlargement of the normal opening for the esophagus may be caused by trauma, congenital weakness, increased abdominal pressure, or relaxation of ligaments of skeletal muscles, and it permits part of the stomach to slide into the thorax. A sliding hiatal hernia, one of the most common pathological conditions of the upper GI tract, may occur at any age but is most prevalent in elderly and middle-aged people. Kinds include **hiatal hernia.**

diaphragmatic node, a node in one of three groups of thoracic parietal lymph nodes, situated on the thoracic side of the diaphragm and consisting of the anterior set, the middle set, and the posterior set. The anterior set includes about three nodes dorsal to the base of the xiphoid process. The middle set of about three nodes on each side is close to the diaphragmatic entry of the phrenic nerves. The posterior set of diaphragmatic nodes consists of a few nodes on the crura of the diaphragm, connecting with the lumbar nodes and the posterior mediastinal nodes. Compare **intercostal node, sternal node.** See also **lymphatic system, lymph node.**

diaphragmatic peritonitis, an inflammation of the lower surface of the diaphragm.

diaphragmatic pleurisy, inflammation of the pleural covering of the diaphragm, which produces severe pain in the epigastric and hypochondrial regions and, occasionally, referred pain via the phrenic nerve to the shoulder.

diaphragmatic respiration. See **diaphragmatic breathing.**

diaphragm pessary. See **pessary.**

diaphragm stethoscope, an instrument for auscultation of bodily sounds. Originally designed by René Laënnec (1781–1826), it consists of a vibrating disk, or diaphragm, which transmits sound waves through tubing to two earpieces. Also called **binaural stethoscope.** See also **stethoscope.**

diaphyseal aclasis /dī″əfiz″ē·əl ak″ləsis/ [Gk, *dia + phyein,* to grow, *a, klasis,* not breaking], a relatively rare abnormal condition that affects the skeletal system. Characterized by multiple exostoses or bony protrusions, it is inherited as a dominant trait. Approximately half of the children of an individual with diaphyseal aclasis display varying degrees of its symptoms. The characteristic exostoses are radiographically and microscopically similar

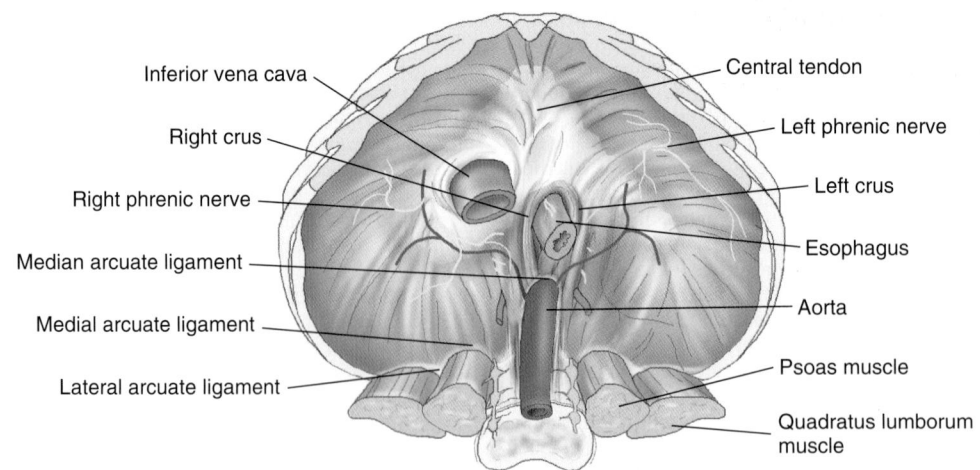

Inferior vena cava — Central tendon
Right crus — Left phrenic nerve
Right phrenic nerve — Left crus
Median arcuate ligament — Esophagus
Medial arcuate ligament — Aorta
Lateral arcuate ligament — Psoas muscle
— Quadratus lumborum muscle

Inferior view of the diaphragm *(Hagen-Ansert, 2012)*

to osteochondromas. Also called **hereditary deforming chondroplasia, multiple cartilaginous exostoses, multiple exostoses.**

■ OBSERVATIONS: Involvement is diffuse, with the long bones usually affected more severely and more frequently than the short bones. Depending on the specific area involved, various angular or rotational deformities may result. Diaphyseal aclasis is usually bilateral and occurs more frequently in boys than in girls. The major signs of the disease are the noticeable protrusions in the areas of the exostoses. Pain is not usually associated with the exostoses, but if present, it is usually minimal. Deformities of the extremities may be evident, depending on the severity and location of the exostoses. Radiographic examination reveals a broadened metaphyseal area, and the specific lesion is identified by abnormal continuity and decreased density. One form of the disorder, dyschondroplasia, results in dwarfism.

■ INTERVENTIONS: Asymptomatic lesions characteristic of diaphyseal aclasis usually require little or no treatment other than continued observation. The lesions located near the joints that interfere with joint motion or impair neurovascular function may be surgically excised. Angular and rotational deformities caused by the lesions may require physical therapy and surgical correction to facilitate function. Inequalities in the length of lower extremities resulting from unilateral involvement may require epiphysiodesis. A relatively small number of these lesions may become malignant.

■ PATIENT CARE CONSIDERATIONS: Although this disease is hereditary, its signs and symptoms are not usually evident until the affected individual is 2 years of age or older. Children of a parent who has the disease are often routinely examined for symptoms.

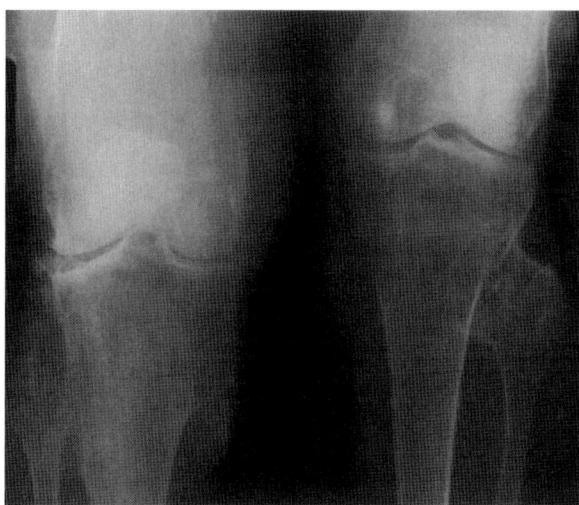

Diaphyseal aclasis: massive exostoses at muscle attachments of both knee joints (Moll, 1997)

diaphyseal-epiphyseal fusion, a surgical procedure to eliminate the epiphyseal line and unite the epiphyseal and diaphyseal bones.

diaphysis /dī·af″isis/ [Gk, *dia + phyein,* to grow], the shaft of a long bone, consisting of a tube of compact bone enclosing the medullary cavity.

diapositive. See **reversal film.**

diarrhea /dī′ərē″ə/ [Gk, *dia + rhein,* to flow], the frequent passage of loose, watery stools. The stool may also contain mucus, pus, blood, or excessive amounts of fat. Diarrhea is usually a symptom of some underlying disorder.

Conditions in which diarrhea is an important symptom are dysenteric disorders, malabsorption syndrome, lactose intolerance, irritable bowel syndrome, GI tumors, and inflammatory bowel disease. In addition to stool frequency, patients may complain of abdominal cramps and generalized weakness. Untreated, severe diarrhea may lead to rapid dehydration and electrolyte imbalance. It should be treated symptomatically until proper diagnosis can be made. Antidiarrheal preparations, such as diphenoxylate and paregoric, are helpful. If diarrhea is accompanied by vomiting, IV fluids may be necessary to prevent fluid depletion. Also spelled **diarrhoea.** See also **dehydration.** *–diarrheal, diarrheic, adj.*

diarrhoea. See **diarrhea.**

diarthroidial joints, a specialized form of articulation in which there is more or less free movement. The union of the bony elements is surrounded by an articular capsule enclosing a cavity lined by synovial membrane. Also called **synovial joint.**

diarthric. See **diarticular.**

diarthrosis. See **synovial joint.**

diarticular /dī′artik″yələr/ [Gk, *di,* twice; L, *articulare,* to divide into joints], having two joints. Also called **biarticular.**

Diasone Sodium Enterab, a leprostatic antibacterial drug. Brand name for *sulfoxone sodium.*

diastalsis /dī′əstal″sis/, a wave of alternating relaxation and contraction of the smooth muscles lining the walls of the small intestine in response to distension of the intestine, causing the movement of food through the intestine to facilitate digestion, absorption, and elimination.

diastasis /dī·as″təsis/ [Gk, separation], the forcible separation of two parts that are normally joined, such as parts of a bone at an epiphysis, two bones that lack a synovial joint, or two muscles, as in diastasis recti abdominis.

diastasis recti abdominis, the separation of the two rectus muscles along the median line of the abdominal wall. In a newborn the condition is the result of incomplete development. In an adult woman the abnormality is often caused by repeated pregnancies or multiple birth, such as the delivery of triplets.

diastatic fermentation /dī′əstat″ik/ [Gk, *diastasis,* separation; L, *fermentare,* to cause to rise], the conversion of starch to glucose by the enzyme ptyalin.

diastema /dī′əstē″mə/ [Gk, interval], a space between two teeth in the same dental arch not caused by the loss of a tooth between them. It occurs most commonly between the maxillary central incisors in adults.

diastole /dī·as″təlē/ [Gk, *dia + stellein,* to set], the period between contractions of the atria or the ventricles during which blood enters the relaxed chambers from the systemic circulation and the lungs. Ventricular diastole begins with the onset of the second heart sound and ends with the first heart sound. Compare **systole.** See also **adiastole.**

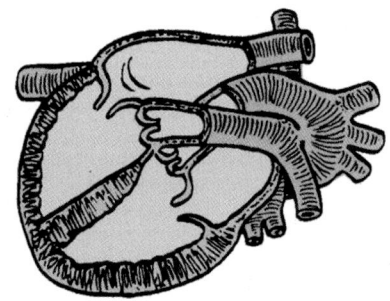

Filling of the heart chambers during diastole (Carlson and AACN, 2008)

-diastole, suffix meaning "the period of dilation of the heart shown as the lower blood pressure measurement": *adiastole, prediastole.*

diastolic /dī′əstol″ik/, pertaining to diastole, or the blood pressure at the instant of maximum cardiac relaxation.

diastolic augmentation, an increase in arterial diastolic blood pressure produced by a counterpulsation device such as an intraaortic balloon pump. A balloon-tipped catheter positioned in the aorta inflates during ventricular diastole, forcing blood back toward the heart, augmenting diastolic pressure, and assisting coronary artery filling. Balloon deflation at the onset of ventricular systole creates suction in the aorta, thereby assisting ventricular ejection and reducing systolic pressure.

diastolic blood pressure, the minimum level of blood pressure measured between contractions of the heart. It may vary with age, gender, body weight, emotional state, and other factors.

diastolic filling pressure, the blood pressure in a ventricle during diastole, resulting from venous return.

diastolic murmur [Gk, *dia,* between, *stellein,* to set; L, *murmur,* humming], a noise caused by turbulence of blood flow during ventricular relaxation. With few exceptions, diastolic murmurs are caused by organic heart disease.

diastolic pressure. See **diastolic blood pressure.**

diastolic thrill, a vibration felt over the heart during ventricular diastole. It may be caused by mitral valve stenosis, a patent ductus arteriosus, or severe aortic insufficiency.

diastrophic /dī′əstrof″ik/ [Gk, *diastrephein,* to distort], pertaining to a bent or curved condition of bones or distortion of other structures.

diastrophic dwarf, *(Obsolete)* now called **diastrophic dysplasia.**

diastrophic dysplasia, a condition in which a person has a short stature caused by osteochondrodysplasia. It is associated with various deformities of the bones and joints, including scoliosis, clubfoot, short limbs, hand defects, multiple joint contractures and subluxations, ear deformities, and cleft palate. The condition may be genetically related and transmitted as an autosomal-recessive trait.

diataxia /dī′ətak″sē·ə/, ataxia affecting both sides of the body.

diathermal /dī′əthur″məl/, **1.** the exchange of heat. **2.** pertaining to the use of elevated local temperature in the treatment of a disorder. The raised temperature may be produced by high-frequency electric current, ultrasound, or microwave radiation.

diathermy /dī′əthur″mē/ [Gk, *dia* + *therme,* heat], **1.** the production of heat in body tissues for therapeutic purposes by high-frequency currents that are insufficiently intense to destroy tissues or to impair their vitality. Diathermy is used in treating chronic arthritis, bursitis, fractures, and other musculoskeletal conditions. **2.** (in surgery) the use of extreme heat to destroy tissues (e.g., warts) or to cauterize a vessel to stop bleeding.

diathesis /dī·əthē″sis/ *pl. diatheses* [Gk, arrangement], a genetic predisposition to certain diseases or conditions.

diazepam /dī·az″əpam/, a benzodiazepine sedative and antianxiety agent.

■ INDICATIONS: It is prescribed in the treatment of anxiety, nervous tension, and muscle spasm and as an anticonvulsant. It may be used in withdrawal protocols for alcoholism.

■ CONTRAINDICATIONS: Acute narrow-angle glaucoma, psychosis, or known hypersensitivity to this drug or to any benzodiazepine medication prohibits its use. It is highly addictive and should be used with caution in persons challenged by addictions. Caution is required if used in patients going through alcohol withdrawal to prevent cross-addiction.

■ ADVERSE EFFECTS: Among the more serious adverse reactions are withdrawal symptoms resulting from discontinuation of treatment. Hypotonia, respiratory depression, drowsiness, and fatigue commonly occur.

diazo-, prefix indicating a chemical compound containing the group —N=N— *diazole, diazine.*

diazoxide /dī′əzok″sīd/, a vasodilator used as an antihypertensive. It also inhibits insulin release from the pancreas.

■ INDICATIONS: It is prescribed parenterally for emergency reduction of blood pressure in malignant hypertension and orally in some cases of hypoglycemia. This drug is for IV use in hospitalized patients only.

■ CONTRAINDICATIONS: Compensatory hypertension (e.g., coarctation of the aorta), cerebral bleeding, or known hypersensitivity to this drug or other thiazides prohibits its use. Caution is advised in heart disease, pregnancy, and impaired kidney function.

■ ADVERSE EFFECTS: Among the more serious adverse effects are tachycardia, sodium and water retention, hyperglycemia, and severe hypotension.

dibasic potassium phosphate, the dipotassium salt K_2HPO_4, used alone or in combination with other phosphate compounds as an electrolyte replenisher.

dibasic sodium phosphate, a salt of phosphoric acid. Used alone or in combination with other phosphate compounds, it is given intravenously as an electrolyte replenisher, orally or rectally as a laxative, and orally as a urinary acidifier and for prevention of kidney stones.

dibenzazepine /dī″benzaz″epēn/, any of a group of structurally related drugs, including the tricyclic antidepressants clomipramine, desipramine, imipramine, and trimipramine.

Dibenzyline, an alpha$_1$ receptor blocker. Brand name for **phenoxybenzamine hydrochloride.**

dibucaine /dī″bəkān/, a topical anesthetic ointment often used to treat pain and itch of hemorrhoids.

dic, abbreviation for **dicentric.**

DIC, abbreviation for **disseminated intravascular coagulation.**

dicalcium phosphate and calcium gluconate with vitamin D /dīkal″sē·əm/, a source of calcium and phosphorus.

■ INDICATIONS: It is prescribed for hypocalcemia, especially in pregnancy and lactation.

■ CONTRAINDICATIONS: Hypoparathyroidism or known hypersensitivity to the ingredients of this drug prohibits its use.

■ ADVERSE EFFECTS: There are no known adverse reactions.

dicarboxylic acid /dī′kär·bok·sil′ik as′id/, any of various organic acids that contain two carboxyl (COOH) groups, such as oxalic acid and tartaric acid.

dicentric (dic) /desen′trik/ [Gk, *di,* twice, *kentron,* center], (in genetics) pertaining to a structurally abnormal chromosome with two centromeres.

dicephalus, a fetus or twin with two heads.

dicephaly /dīsef″əlē/ [Gk, *di,* twice, *kephale,* head], a developmental anomaly in which a fetus has two heads. –*dicephalic, dicephalous, adj.*

dichlorodiphenyltrichloroethane. See **DDT.**

dichlorphenamide /dī″klôrfen″əmīd/, a carbonic anhydrase inhibitor.

■ INDICATIONS: It is prescribed in the treatment of chronic open-angle glaucoma and before surgery for angle-closure glaucoma.

■ CONTRAINDICATIONS: Liver and adrenocortical insufficiency, kidney failure, hyperchloremic acidosis, depressed sodium or potassium level, pulmonary obstruction, Addison's

disease, known or suspected pregnancy, or known hypersensitivity to this drug prohibits its use.
- ADVERSE EFFECTS: Among the more serious adverse reactions are anorexia, GI disturbances, acidosis, ureteral calculus formation, and aplastic anemia.

dichorial twins, dichorionic twins.   See **dizygotic twins.**

dichotomy /dīkot″əmē/ [Gk, *dicha,* in two, *temnein,* to cut], a division or separation into two equal parts.

dichromatic vision /dī′kromat″ik/ [Gk, *di,* twice, *chroma,* color; L, *visio*], a form of color vision in which only two of the three primary colors are perceived.

dichromic /di-kro′mik/, having, or pertaining to, two colors.

dichuchwa, endemic syphilis. See **bejel.**

Dick-Read method.   See **Read method.**

Dick test [George F. Dick, 1881–1967; Gladys R.H. Dick, 1881–1963; American physicians], a skin test formerly used for determining sensitivity to an erythrotoxin produced by the group A streptococci that cause scarlet fever.

diclofenac /diklo′fenak/, a nonsteroidal antiinflammatory drug used systemically as the potassium or sodium salt in the treatment of rheumatic and nonrheumatic inflammatory conditions and as the potassium salt to relieve pain and dysmenorrhea. It is also applied topically to the conjunctiva as a sodium salt to reduce ocular inflammation or photophobia after certain kinds of surgery and to the skin to treat actinic keratoses.

diclofenac potassium, the potassium salt of diclofenac, administered orally in the treatment of rheumatoid arthritis, osteoarthritis, ankylosing spondylitis, a variety of nonrheumatic inflammatory conditions, pain, and dysmenorrhea.

dicloxacillin sodium /dī′kloksəsil″in/, a penicillinase-resistant penicillin.
- INDICATIONS: It is prescribed in the treatment of bacterial infections, especially those caused by penicillinase-producing strains of staphylococci.
- CONTRAINDICATIONS: Known hypersensitivity to this drug or to any penicillin medication prohibits its use.
- ADVERSE EFFECTS: The most serious adverse effect is hypersensitivity reaction. Other side effects include nausea, vomiting, diarrhea, and epigastric distress.

DICOM, the standard used for the electronic transfer of digital image data, developed by a joint committee of the American College of Radiology and the National Electronics Manufacturers' Association. Abbreviation for *digital imaging and communications in medicine.*

Dicor, brand name for *castable ceramic dental material.*

dicrotic /dīkrot′ik/ [Gk, *dikrotos,* double beating], pertaining to a waveform that has two separate peaks. A dicrotic notch in a normal arterial waveform indicates aortic valve closure.

dicrotic notch /dīkrot″ik/, a small, downward deflection observed on the downstroke of an arterial pressure waveform. It represents closure of the aortic or pulmonic valve at the onset of ventricular diastole.

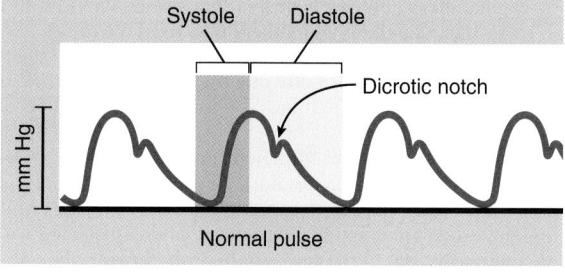

Dicrotic notch

dicrotic pulse, a pulse with two separate peaks, the second usually weaker than the first. Compare **bisferious pulse.**

dicrotic wave, in an arterial pulse recording, the portion of the descending limb following the aortic notch, including a second, smaller peak attributed to the reflected impulse of closure of the aortic valve.

dicumarol /dīkyoo″mərol/, an anticoagulant coumarin derivative.
- INDICATIONS: It is prescribed for the prophylaxis and treatment of thrombosis and embolism.
- CONTRAINDICATIONS: Risk of hemorrhage, peptic ulcer, ulcerative colitis, or known hypersensitivity to this drug prohibits its use.
- ADVERSE EFFECTS: Among the more serious adverse reactions are GI disturbances, nausea, bleeding, and diarrhea.

dicyclomine hydrochloride /dīsī″kləmin/, an anticholinergic/antispasmodic.
- INDICATIONS: It is prescribed as an adjunct to ulcer therapy and as a treatment for functional/irritable bowel syndrome.
- CONTRAINDICATIONS: Narrow-angle glaucoma, asthma, myasthenia gravis, obstruction of the genitourinary or GI tract, ulcerative colitis, or known hypersensitivity to this drug prohibits its use. It should not be used in infants.
- ADVERSE EFFECTS: Among the more serious adverse reactions are blurred vision, central nervous system effects, tachycardia, dry mouth, decreased sweating, and hypersensitivity reactions.

didactic /dīdak″tik/ [Gk, *didaskein,* to teach], pertaining to classroom teaching or instruction.

didanosine.   See **dideoxyinosine.**

dideoxycytidine /dī′dē·ok′sēsī″tidēn/.   See **zalcitabine.**

dideoxyinosine (ddI) /dī′dē·oksē·in″ōsēn/, an antiretroviral drug used in the treatment of human immunodeficiency virus infections. ddI inhibits the enzyme reverse transcriptase, thereby restricting viral replication activity. Inside the body, ddI is converted to dideoxyadenosine, which becomes incorporated into the deoxyribonucleic acid chain, interrupting its normal sequence and making viral replication impossible. Also called **didanosine.**

DIDMOAD syndrome, abbreviation for *diabetes insipidus, diabetes mellitus, optic atrophy, deafness syndrome.* See **Wolfram syndrome.**

Didrex, an anorexiant. Brand name for *benzphetamine hydrochloride.*

Didronel, a calcium regulator. Brand name for **etidronate disodium.**

didym-, 1. prefix meaning "testis": *didymitis, didymus.* 2. prefix meaning "paired" or "twin": *didymous.*

-didymis, suffix meaning "testicles": *epididymis.*

didymitis /did′əmī″tis/.   See **orchitis.**

didymous, growing or arranged in pairs.

didymus /did″iməs/, a testis.

-didymus, 1. suffix meaning "twins joined at a (specified) part of the body": *gastrodidymus.* 2. suffix meaning "a teratic fetus with supernumerary organ(s)": *pygodidymus.*

die, 1. to cease living. 2. a model of a prepared tooth made from a hard substance, usually dental stone.

diecious /dī·ē″shəs/ [Gk, *di + oikos,* house], pertaining to an organism that has either male or female reproductive organs. Also spelled **dioecious.**

dieldrin /dī·el″drin/, a highly toxic pesticide that is poisonous to humans and animals if ingested, inhaled, or absorbed through the skin. It causes dysfunction of the central nervous system and may be a carcinogen. Dieldrin is banned in Canada and the United States, but its usage before the 1980s has left residual toxins in a number of waterways.

dielectric /dī″elek′trik/, 1. *adj.,* transmitting electric effects by induction, but not by conduction. The term is applied to an insulating substance through or across which electric force is acting or may act by induction without conduction. **2.** *n.,* an insulating substance that transmits in this way (i.e., through or across which electric force is acting or may act by induction without conduction).

diencephalic syndrome /dis′ensəfal′ik/, failure to thrive in infants and young children associated with severe emaciation and central nervous system tumors. Intellectual development and linear growth are not affected.

diencephalon /dī′ənsef′əlon/ [Gk, *di* + *enkephalon,* brain], the portion of the brain between the cerebrum and the mesencephalon. It consists of the hypothalamus, thalamus, metathalamus, and the epithalamus and includes most of the third ventricle.

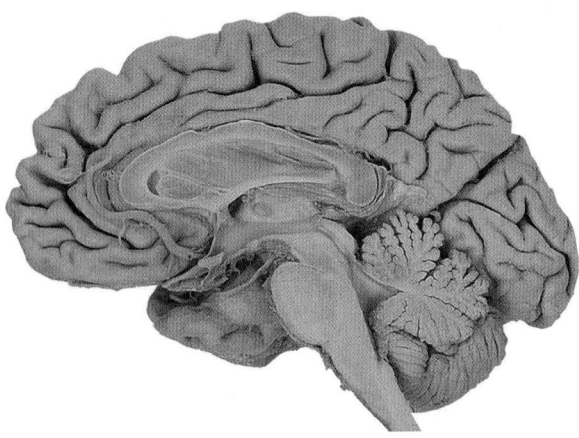

Diencephalon *(Nolte and Angevine, 2007)*

diener /dē″nər/ [Ger, man-servant], an individual who maintains the hospital laboratory or equipment and facilities. The morgue diener may also assist the pathologist in performing autopsies.

dieresis /dī·er″əsis/, separation of a structure's parts by surgery or other means.

diet /dī″it/ [Gk, *diaita,* way of living], **1.** food and drink considered with regard to their nutritional qualities, composition, and effects on health. **2.** nutrients prescribed, regulated, or restricted as to kind and amount for therapeutic or other purposes. **3.** the customary allowance of food and drink regularly provided or consumed. Compare **nutrition.** See also *specific diets.* —**dietetic,** *adj.*

dietary /dī″əter′ē/, pertaining to diet.

dietary allowances. See **recommended dietary allowances.**

dietary amenorrhea [Gk, *diaita,* way of living, *a,* absence, *men,* month, *rhoia,* to flow], an interruption of menstruation caused by malnutrition, starvation, or excessive voluntary dieting.

Dietary Approach to Stop Hypertension (DASH) diet, a diet high in fruits, vegetables, and low-fat dairy products; low in saturated and total fats; low in cholesterol; and high in fiber. Research studies support the hypothesis that this diet reduces blood pressure and may play a role in the prevention of high blood pressure.

dietary fiber, a generic term for nondigestible carbohydrate substances found in plant cell walls and surrounding cellular material, each with a different effect on the various GI functions, such as colon transit time, water absorption, and lipid metabolism. Dietary fiber may be water soluble or insoluble.

The soluble fibers include pectins, gums, mucilages, and algal products. They affect nutrient absorption and regulation. The insoluble fibers include cellulose, hemicellulose, and lignin and promote stool bulk and caloric motility. The main dietary fiber components are cellulose, lignin, hemicellulose, pectin, and plant gums. Foods high in dietary fiber are fruits; green, leafy vegetables, such as lettuce, spinach, celery, and cabbage; root vegetables, such as carrots, turnips, and potatoes; legumes; and whole-grain cereals and breads. The risk of development of constipation, hemorrhoids, diverticular disease, and colon cancer may be decreased by regular consumption of sufficient amounts of fiber. Most experts recommend intake of 20 to 30 g/day. Also called **bulk, roughage.**

dietetic, related to diet and nutrition. See **diet.**

dietetic food, 1. a specially prepared low-calorie food, often containing natural or artificial sweeteners. **2.** a food prepared for any specific dietary need or restriction, such as salt-free or vegetarian food. See also **dietetics.**

dietetic food diarrhea, an excessive intake of hexitols, sorbitol, and mannitol (used as sugar substitutes in candies, chewing gum, and dietetic foods), resulting in slow absorption and rapid small intestine motility and leading to osmotic diarrhea. See **osmotic diarrhea.**

dietetics /dī′itet″iks/, the science of applying nutritional principles to the planning and preparation of foods and regulation of the diet in relation to both health and disease.

dietetic technician, a person trained in food and nutrition who may work independently or on a team with a registered dietitian. Dietetic technicians often screen patients to identify nutrition problems, provide patient education and counseling, develop menus and recipes, supervise food service personnel, purchase food, and monitor inventory and food quality. A 2-year associate degree program is usually required. Those who complete the associate degree program and pass a registration exam become a Dietetic Technician, Registered (DTR).

diethyl ether. See **ether.**

diethylpropion hydrochloride /dī·eth′ilprō″pē·on/, an appetite suppressant; a central nervous system stimulant.

■ INDICATIONS: It is prescribed as a short-term adjunct in the treatment of exogenous obesity.

■ CONTRAINDICATIONS: Arteriosclerosis, hyperthyroidism, glaucoma, history of drug dependence or drug abuse, hypertension, concomitant administration of a monoamine oxidase inhibitor within 14 days, or known hypersensitivity to this drug prohibits its use.

■ ADVERSE EFFECTS: Among the more serious adverse reactions are restlessness and insomnia, increased blood pressure, arrhythmias, cardiovascular effects, nausea, dry mouth, and drug dependence.

diethylstilbestrol (DES) /-stilbes″trol/, a synthetic hormone with estrogenic properties. This agent was used extensively from 1948 to 1971 to decrease miscarriages, but it is now contraindicated because it is known to increase the risk of vaginal clear cell carcinoma in the women exposed to it in utero (i.e., daughters of mothers who used the drug). Also called **stilbestrol.**

dieting syndrome. See **chronic dieting syndrome.**

dietitian, registered dietitian. See **nutritionist, registered dietitian.**

Dietl crisis /dē″təl/ [Joseph Dietl, Polish physician, 1804–1878; Gk, *krisis,* turning point], episodic crampy upper abdominal pain, nausea, and vomiting caused by intermittent ureteropelvic junction obstruction, often associated with an aberrant vessel to the lower pole of the kidney. See also **hydronephrosis.**

diet therapy, the branch of dietetics concerned with the use of foods for therapeutic purposes. Compare **medical nutrition therapy.**

difenoxin /di″fĕnok′sin/, an agent used as the hydrochloride salt for its antiperistaltic action in treatment of diarrhea.

differential /dif′əren′shəl/, pertaining to or creating a condition that is not the same for all, as in the provision of a salary differential for individuals working on a weekend.

differential absorption [L, *differentia,* difference], the difference in absorption of x-rays by different body tissues. In a radiographic image of a body part, such as an arm, the image of the bone is produced because more x-rays are absorbed by bone than by the surrounding soft tissue. Also called **selective absorption.**

differential blood count. See **differential white blood cell count.**

differential diagnosis, the distinguishing between two or more diseases with similar symptoms by systematically comparing their signs and symptoms. See also **diagnosis.**

differential growth, a variance in the size or rate of growth of dissimilar organisms, tissues, or structures.

differential leukocyte count. See **differential white blood cell count.**

differential threshold, the lowest limit at which two stimuli can be differentiated or distinguished.

differential white blood cell count, enumeration and classification of the leukocytes in a Wright-stained blood film. The different categories of white blood cells are counted and reported as percentages of the total examined. Differential white blood cell count provides specific information related to infections and hematological diseases. Also called **differential leukocyte count.** Compare **complete blood count.** See also **leukocyte.**

differentiating agent, a substance, such as a retinoid, that induces a cell to stop dividing and to differentiate. Such agents may be capable of halting the proliferation of cancer cells.

differentiation /dif′əren′shē·ā″shən/ [L, *differentia,* difference], **1.** (in embryology) a process in development in which unspecialized cells or tissues are systemically modified and altered to achieve specific and characteristic physical forms, physiological functions, and chemical properties. Kinds include **correlative differentiation, functional differentiation, invisible differentiation, self-differentiation. 2.** progressive diversification leading to complexity. **3.** acquisition of functions and forms different from those of the original. **4.** distinguishing one thing or disease from another, as in differential diagnosis. **5.** (in psychology) mental autonomy or separation of intellect and emotions so that one is not dominated by reactive anxiety of a family or group emotional system. **6.** the first subphase of the separation-individuation phase in Mahler's system of preoedipal development. It generally occurs between 5 and 9 months of age, coinciding with the maturation of partial locomotor functioning and the beginning of the child's viewing the mother as a separate being. –*differentiate, v.*

differentiation therapy, a cancer therapy technique in which the malignant cell is regarded as having escaped the normal controls of cell growth and differentiation. The cancer cell is regarded as pathologically arrested at an early stage of differentiation, retaining the ability to proliferate. It is treated with agents that remove this block and allow the cells to differentiate along more normal lines until they eventually lose their ability to divide and replicate.

diffraction /difrak′shən/ [L, *dis,* opposite of, *frangere,* to break], the bending and scattering of wavelengths of light or other radiation as the radiation passes around obstacles or through narrow slits. X-ray diffraction is used in the study of the internal structure of cells. See also **refraction.**

diffuse /difyo͞oz″/ [L, *diffundere,* to spread out], becoming widely spread, such as through a membrane or fluid.

diffuse abscess, an abscess that spreads into neighboring tissues beyond fibrous walls.

diffuse angiokeratoma. See **angiokeratoma corporis diffusum.**

diffuse axonal injury (DAI), a type of brain injury caused by shearing forces that occur between different parts of the brain as a result of rotational acceleration. The corpus callosum and the brainstem are often affected. DAI most commonly occurs in motor vehicle crashes when the vehicle suddenly stops.

diffused light, light in which the precise source cannot be seen while the apparent area of the source is increased.

diffuse emphysema. See **panacinar emphysema.**

diffuse erythema, skin redness or inflammation that is spread over a large body surface.

diffuse esophageal spasm, abnormal contractions of the esophagus leading to difficult or painful swallowing and chest pain.

diffuse fibrosing alveolitis. See **interstitial pneumonia.**

diffuse goiter, an enlargement of all parts of the thyroid gland. Symptoms are those of hyperthyroidism.

diffuse hypersensitivity pneumonia, an immunologically mediated inflammatory reaction in the lungs induced by exposure to an allergen or a drug. Allergens that trigger the reaction may be derived from fungi, bird excreta, porcine or bovine proteins, wood dust, and fur. Drugs that induce hypersensity pneumonia include chlorproPAMIDE, hydrochlorothiazide, mecamylamine, mephenesin, methotrexate, nitrofurantoin, paraaminosalicylic acid, and penicillin. The disorder is characterized by cough, fever, dyspnea, malaise, pulmonary edema, and infiltration of the alveoli with eosinophils and large mononuclear cells. Also called **allergic alveolitis, allergic interstitial pneumonitis, extrinsic allergic pneumonia.** See also **bagassosis, pulmonary infiltrate with eosinophilia.**

diffuse idiopathic skeletal hyperostosis, a form of degenerative joint disease in which the ligaments along the spinal column become calcified and lose their flexibility.

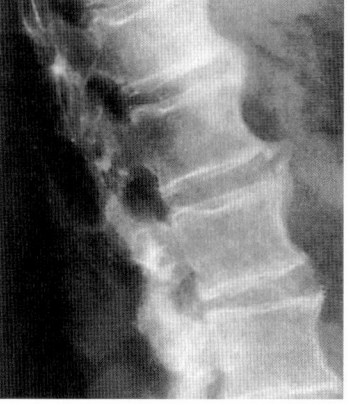

Diffuse idiopathic skeletal hyperostosis *(Moll, 1997)*

diffuse lipoma, diffuse lipomatosis. See **multiple lipomatosis.**

diffuse myelitis. See **disseminated myelitis.**

diffuse myocardial fibrosis,   a type of heart disease characterized by a generalized distribution of fibrous tissue that replaces normal heart muscle cells.

diffuse peritonitis [L, *diffundere,* to spread out; Gk, *peri,* near, *teinein,* to stretch, *itis,* inflammation], widespread peritonitis affecting most of the peritoneum, usually caused by a ruptured stomach or appendix. See also **generalized peritonitis, peritonitis.**

diffuse scleroderma.   See **scleroderma.**

diffuse sclerosis [L, *diffundere,* to spread out; Gk, *sklerosis,* hardening], a form of sclerosis that extends through much of the central nervous system. See also **sclerosis.**

diffusing capacity (D) /difyoo″sing/, the rate of gas transfer through a unit area of a permeable membrane per unit of gas pressure difference across it. It is affected by specific chemical reactions that may occur in the blood. Also called **diffusion factor, transfer factor of lungs.**

diffusing capacity of lungs (DL), the volume of a gas that diffuses from the lung across the alveolar-capillary membrane into the bloodstream per minute per mm Hg difference in pressure across the membrane. The normal DL for oxygen averages 20 mL/min/mm Hg. Also called **transfer factor of lungs.**

diffusion /difyoo″zhən/ [L, *diffundere,* to spread out], the process in which particles in a fluid move from an area of higher concentration to an area of lower concentration, resulting in an even distribution of the particles in the fluid. Little or no energy is required.

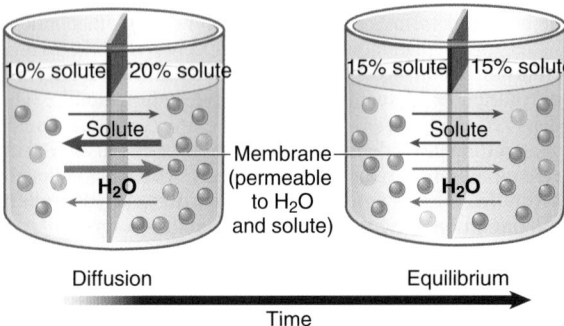

Diffusion *(Patton and Thibodeau, 2010)*

diffusion coefficient, the number of milliliters of a gas that will diffuse at a distance of 0.001 mm over a square centimeter surface per minute at 1 atm of pressure. The diffusion coefficient for any given gas is proportional to the solubility and molecular weight of the gas. See **coefficient.**

diffusion constant, a mathematical constant relating to the ability of a substance to disperse.

diffusion defect, any impairment in the diffusion of oxygen across the alveolar-capillary membrane caused by pathological changes in any of the structures of the membrane. Specific causes may include fibrosis, granuloma, interstitial edema, and proliferation of connective tissue.

diffusion deposition, the adsorption of an aerosol particle on the surface of an alveolar membrane or other airway structure.

diffusion factor.   See **diffusing capacity.**

diffusion of gases, a natural process, essential in respiration, in which molecules of a gas pass from an area of high concentration to one of lower concentration.

diflorasone diacetate /dīflôr″əsōn dī·as″ətāt/, a topical corticosteroid with high potency.

■ INDICATIONS: It is prescribed for the treatment of skin inflammation.

■ CONTRAINDICATIONS: Viral and fungal diseases of the skin, impaired circulation, or known hypersensitivity to this drug or to other steroidal medication prohibits its use.

■ ADVERSE EFFECTS: Among the more serious adverse reactions, usually occurring after prolonged or excessive application, are striae, hypopigmentation, local irritation of the skin, and various systemic effects.

Diflucan, a broad-spectrum antifungal agent. Brand name for **fluconazole.**

diflucortolone /diflookor″tählōn/, a synthetic corticosteroid used as the valerate salt and applied topically in treatment of inflammation and pruritus of dermatoses.

diflunisal /dīfloo″nisal/, a nonsteroidal antiinflammatory drug.

■ INDICATIONS: It is prescribed for the treatment of mild to moderate pain and inflammation in osteoarthritis and other musculoskeletal disorders.

■ CONTRAINDICATIONS: Hypersensitivity to aspirin and other nonsteroidal antiinflammatory drugs or known sensitivity to this drug prohibits its use.

■ ADVERSE EFFECTS: The most serious adverse reactions are GI pain, diarrhea, peptic ulcer, anorexia, anaphylactoid reactions with bronchospasm, and edema.

digastricus /dīgas″trikəs/ [Gk, *di,* twice, *gaster,* stomach], one of four suprahyoid muscles having two parts, an anterior belly and a posterior belly. The anterior belly acts to open the jaw and to draw the hyoid bone forward. The posterior belly acts to draw back and to raise the hyoid bone. Compare **geniohyoideus, mylohyoideus, stylohyoideus.**

DiGeorge syndrome /dijôrj″əz/ [Angelo M. DiGeorge, American physician, 1921–2009], a genetic disorder affecting chromosome 22. Now called **22q11.2 deletion syndrome.**

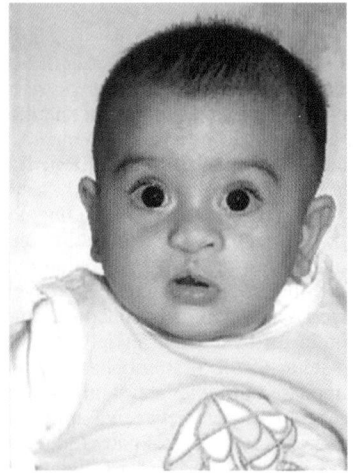

Typical appearance of child with DiGeorge syndrome
(Shearer et al, 2007)

digest /dijest′, dijest′, dī′jəst,/ [L, *digerere,* to break down], **1.** *v.,* to soften by heat and moisture. **2.** *v.,* to break into smaller parts and simpler compounds by mastication, hydrolysis, and action of intestinal secretions and enzymes, especially in the way the body digests food for the absorption of nutrients required in metabolism. The small intestine digests food by enzymatic actions that produce absorbable amino acids, emulsified fat particles, and monosaccharides. **3.** *n.,* any material that results from digestion or hydrolysis.

digestant /dijes″tənt/, a substance, such as pepsin, that is added to the diet as an aid to the digestion of food.

digestible /dijes″tibəl/, capable of being digested.

digestion /dijes″chən/ [L, *digerere,* to break down], the conversion of food into absorbable substances in the GI tract. Digestion is accomplished through the mechanical and chemical breakdown of food into increasingly smaller molecules with the help of glands located both inside and outside the gut. –*digestive, adj.*

digestive enzyme /dijes″tiv/ [L, *digerere,* to break down; Gk, *en* + *zyme,* ferment], any digestive system enzyme that hydrolyzes fats, proteins, or carbohydrates for absorption.

digestive fever, a slight rise in body temperature that normally accompanies the digestive process.

digestive gland, any one of the many structures that secrete agents involved in the breaking down of food into the constituent absorbable substances needed for metabolism. Some kinds of digestive glands are the salivary glands, gastric glands, intestinal glands, liver, and pancreas. Among important secretions produced by different digestive glands are hydrochloric acid, bile, mucus, and various enzymes.

digestive juice, thin, colorless secretion of the glands of the human stomach, composed mainly of hydrochloric acid, chymosin, pepsinogen, intrinsic factor, and mucus. Also called *digestive secretion.*

digestive system, the organs, structures, and accessory glands of the digestive tube of the body through which food passes from the mouth to the esophagus, stomach, and intestines. The accessory glands secrete the digestive enzymes, which break down food substances in preparation for absorption into the bloodstream. See also the *Color Atlas of Human Anatomy,* pp. A-32 to A-34.

digestive tract, a musculomembranous tube, about 9 meters long, extending from the mouth to the anus and lined with mucous membrane. Its various portions are the mouth, pharynx, esophagus, stomach, small intestine, and large intestine. The tube, which is part of the digestive system, includes numerous accessory organs. Also called **alimentary canal, alimentary tract, gastrointestinal tract, intestinal tract.** See also **digestive system.**

Digibind, the antibody used in the treatment of digoxin toxicity. Brand name for **digoxin immune FAB, ovine.**

digit /dij″it/ [L, *digitus*], a finger or a toe. Also called *dactylus.*

digit-, prefix meaning "finger" or "toe": *digitate.*

digital, **1.** the characterization or measurement of a signal in terms of a series of numbers rather than some continuously varying value. **2.** pertaining to a digit, that is, a finger or toe; resembling a finger or toe. See also **digitate. 3.** an electronic device that gives its reading/values in numbers (e.g., a digital clock). **4.** use of the binary system in computer technology or in computerized communications, such as digital telephone, pagers, and cellular telephones.

digital angiography, a technique of producing computer-enhanced radiographic images of the vascular system. Images are displayed on a video monitor after injection of contrast material. The displayed images can be recorded and stored.

digital compression [L, *digitus,* finger, *comprimere,* to press together], the act of pressing with the fingers, as when arresting the blood flow from a wound.

digital fluoroscopy, the projection of a radiographic image on an image-intensifying fluorescent screen coupled to a digital video image processor. The visible light from the energized phosphor is electronically amplified and directed into a

video camera. The video image is divided into pixels, which are in turn converted or digitized for storage or reproduction through an image processor.

digital image, a depiction recorded electronically, using pixels with attached data numerically coded to a color, to display photographic representations of objects and to allow viewing or transmission on a computer.

digitalis /dij′ital″is/ [L, *digitus,* finger or toe], a general term for cardiac glycoside. See also **digitoxin, digoxin.**
- INDICATIONS: It is prescribed in the treatment of congestive heart failure and certain cardiac arrhythmias.
- CONTRAINDICATIONS: Ventricular fibrillation, ventricular tachycardia, or known hypersensitivity to this drug prohibits its use.
- ADVERSE EFFECTS: The most serious reactions are cardiac arrhythmias that are more common with concomitant diuretics, disorientation, and visual disturbances.

digitalis glycoside, a potent cardiovascular drug with a low therapeutic index. See also **glycoside, digitalis.**

digitalis poisoning [L, *digitalis,* of the fingers, *potio,* drink], the toxic effects of digitalis medications prescribed for heart disorders such as heart failure and atrial fibrillation. Toxicity may result from the cumulative effect of the drug or from hypokalemia. Symptoms include vomiting, headache, serious dysrhythmias, disorientation, and visual color distortions.

digitalis therapy, the administration of a digitalis preparation to a person with a heart disorder to increase the force of myocardial contractions; produce a slower, more regular apical rate; and slow the transmission of impulses through the conduction system. It may be used in treating many cardiac disorders, including atrial fibrillation, atrial septal defect, coarctation of the aorta, congenital heart block, congestive heart failure, endocardial fibroelastosis, great vessel transposition, malformation of the tricuspid valve, myocarditis, paroxysmal atrial tachycardia, and patent ductus arteriosus.
- OUTCOME CRITERIA: In addition to promoting more forceful myocardial contractions and a slower, more regular apical beat, digitalis therapy can reduce venous pressure, improve pulmonary and systemic circulation, increase urinary output, reduce edema, and stop paroxysmal atrial tachycardia and atrial fibrillation.

digitalization /dij′ətal″īzā″shən/, the administration of digitalis in doses sufficient to achieve maximum pharmacological effects without producing toxic symptoms.

digitalized /dij″ətəlīzd′/, having a therapeutic total body level of digitalis, a cardiac glycoside.

digitalizing dose, the amount of digitalis needed to achieve a desired therapeutic effect.

digital radiography (DR) /dij″itəl/, any method of radiographic image formation that directly captures image data and uses a computer for image storage and manipulation. See also **digital angiography, digital fluoroscopy, digital tomosynthesis.**

digital reflex, **1.** a finger-jerk reaction produced by tapping the palmar aspect of the terminal phalanges of the fingers when they are slightly flexed. **2.** sudden flexion of the terminal phalanx of the thumb produced by tapping the terminal phalanx of the middle finger.

digital subtraction angiography (DSA), a method in which radiographic images of blood vessels filled with contrast material are digitized and then subtracted from images obtained before administration of the material. The method increases the contrast between the vessels and the background.

digital thermometer. See **thermometer.**

digital-to-analog converter, a device for translating digital information into a continuous form, as from an ohmmeter or thermometer. Also called **D/A converter,** *DAC, D/A, D2A.*

digital tomosynthesis, a system of tomography, using a computer and a digital fluoroscopy unit, that can synthesize any tomographic plane from a single tomographic pass. As only one tomographic pass is required, patient radiation exposure is reduced. Patient time in examination is also reduced as the recorded images can be synthesized and manipulated at a later time. See also **digital fluoroscopy.**

digitate /dij″ităt/ [L, *digitatus,* having fingers], having fingers or fingerlike projections. See also **digital,** def. 2.

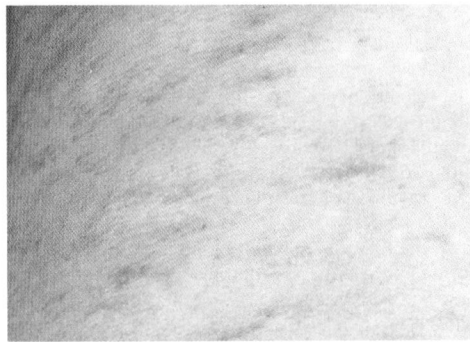

Digitate dermatosis *(du Vivier, 2002)*

digitate wart, a fingerlike horny projection that arises from a pea-shaped base. It is a benign viral infection of the skin and the adjacent mucous membrane. It may disappear spontaneously as an immune response develops in the host, or it may require treatment, such as by electrodesiccation and curettage. Also called **filiform warts.**

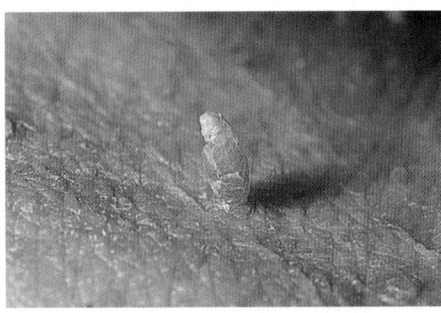

Digitate wart *(Habif, 2011)*

digitoxin /dij′itok″sin/, a cardiac glycoside obtained from leaves of *Digitalis purpurea.* Digitoxin differs in many ways from digoxin, including having a far greater half-life and a different route of elimination.

■ INDICATIONS: It is prescribed in the treatment of congestive heart failure and certain cardiac arrhythmias.

■ CONTRAINDICATIONS: Ventricular fibrillation, ventricular tachycardia, or known hypersensitivity to this drug prohibits its use.

■ ADVERSE EFFECTS: The most serious adverse reactions are cardiac arrhythmias and heart block, disorientation, and visual disturbances.

digit span test, an examination of the ability to recall a sequence of numbers just spoken.

diglyceride /dīglis″ərīd/, a chemical compound, a diester of glycerol in which the hydrogen in two of the hydroxyl groups is replaced by an acyl radical.

dignathus /dīnath″əs, dignā″thəs/, **1.** a fetus with a double lower jaw. **2.** a person with a cleft of the mandible.

digoxin /digok″sin/, a cardiac glycoside obtained from leaves of *Digitalis lanata.*

■ INDICATIONS: It is prescribed in the treatment of congestive heart failure and certain cardiac arrhythmias.

■ CONTRAINDICATIONS: Ventricular fibrillation, ventricular tachycardia, or known hypersensitivity to this drug prohibits its use.

■ ADVERSE EFFECTS: The most serious adverse reactions are cardiac arrhythmia and heart block, disorientation, and visual disturbances.

digoxin immune FAB, ovine, a preparation of antigen-binding fragments derived from specific antidigoxin antibodies produced in sheep that have been immunized with digoxin coupled as a hapten to human serum albumin. It is used as an antidote to life-threatening digoxin and digitoxin overdose and is administered intravenously.

■ INDICATIONS: It is prescribed for the treatment of life-threatening digoxin or digitoxin toxicity.

■ CONTRAINDICATIONS: Use of this product should be restricted to patients who are in shock or cardiac arrest or who show signs of severe ventricular arrhythmias, progressive bradycardia, or potassium concentrations exceeding 5 mEq/L.

■ ADVERSE EFFECTS: Among reported adverse reactions are low cardiac output, congestive heart failure exacerbated by withdrawal of the inotropic effect of digoxin, rapid ventricular response caused by withdrawal of the digitalis effect, and possible hypokalemia.

Di Guglielmo disease. See **erythroleukemia.**

Di Guglielmo syndrome. See **erythroleukemia.**

dihybrid /dī′hī″brid/ [Gk, *di,* twice; L, *hybrida,* mongrel offspring], pertaining to an individual, an organism, or a strain that is heterozygous for two specific traits, that is the offspring of parents differing in two specific gene pairs, or that is heterozygous for two particular traits or gene loci being followed.

dihybrid cross, the mating of two individuals, organisms, or strains that have different gene pairs that determine two specific traits or that have two particular characteristics or gene loci being followed.

dihydric alcohol /dīhī″drik/, an alcohol containing two hydroxyl groups. Also called **diol.**

dihydroergotamine mesylate /dīhī′drō·ərgot″əmēn me″si lāt/, an ergot alkaloid causing vasoconstriction through stimulation of several types of receptors, including alpha-adrenergic receptors and serotonin receptors.

■ INDICATIONS: It is prescribed for the treatment of migraine and vascular headache.

■ CONTRAINDICATIONS: Cardiovascular disease, hypertension, liver or kidney dysfunction, sepsis, pregnancy, or known hypersensitivity to this drug prohibits its use.

■ ADVERSE EFFECTS: Among the more serious adverse reactions are gangrene and the toxicity of the ergot alkaloids.

dihydrotachysterol /dīhī′drōtəkis″tərol/, a rapid-acting form of vitamin D.

■ INDICATIONS: It is prescribed in the treatment of hypocalcemia resulting from hypoparathyroidism and pseudohypoparathyroidism.

■ CONTRAINDICATIONS: Hypercalcemia, hypocalcemia with kidney insufficiency, hyperphosphatemia, or known hypersensitivity to this drug or to vitamin D prohibits its use. Caution is advised for lactating mothers.

■ ADVERSE EFFECTS: The most serious adverse reaction is hypercalcemia. With overdosage, calcification of soft tissues, including those of the heart, or cardiovascular or kidney failure may occur.

dihydrotestosterone (DHT) /di-hi″drōtestos′terōn/, an androgenic hormone formed in peripheral tissue from testosterone. It is thought to be the androgen responsible for development of the male primary sex characteristics during embryogenesis and of male secondary sex characteristics at puberty and for adult male sexual function.

diiodohydroxyquin. See **iodoquinol.**

dil-, -dil, combining form for the name of a vasodilator.

dilaceration /dī·las′ərā′shən/ [L. *di-,* apart or through + *lacerare,* to tear], **1.** a tearing apart, as of a cataract. **2.** (in dentistry) a condition resulting from injury to a tooth during its developmental period or as a result of insufficient space for a tooth to develop, with a crease or band at the junction of the crown and root, or with tortuous roots having abnormal curvatures. Should not be confused with *normal root curvature.*

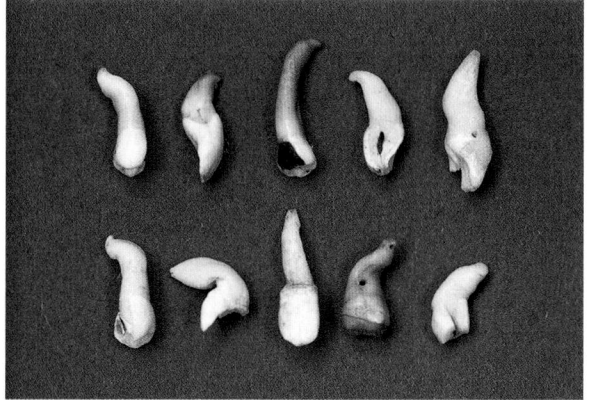

Dilaceration *(Regezi, Sciubba, and Jordan, 2012)*

Dilantin, an anticonvulsant used to control tonic-clonic and psychomotor seizures. Brand name for **phenytoin.**

dilatancy /dīlā′tənsē/ [L, *dilatare,* to widen], an unusual behavior observed in cytoplasm (and in some physical systems) during which its viscosity and applied force both increase.

dilatant, (in chemistry and physics) liquids or solutions whose viscosity increases as stress is applied.

dilatation. See **dilation.**

dilate /dī′lāt/, to cause a physiological increase in the diameter of a body opening, blood vessel, or tube, such as the widening of the pupil of the eye in response to decreased light or the widening of the uterine cervix during labor.

dilation /dīlā″shən/ [L, *dilatare,* to widen], **1.** the condition of being dilated or stretched. **2.** the process of causing a physiological increase in the diameter of a body opening, blood vessel, or tube. Examples include the widening of the pupil of the eye by the use of cycloplegic eyedrops for examination of the retina and opening of the uterine cervix to facilitate curettage by the use of a dilator. Also called **dilatation.**

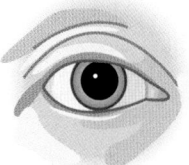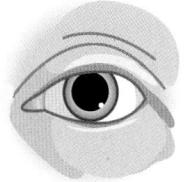

Bilateral dilated pupils *(AACN, 2008)*

dilation and curettage (D&C), widening of the uterine cervix and scraping of the endometrium of the uterus. It was once a common procedure used to diagnose disease of the uterus but has largely been supplanted by endometrial biopsy. See also **endometrial biopsy, fractional dilation and curettage, hysteroscopy.**

dilation and evacuation (D&E) [L, *dilatare,* to widen, *evacuare,* to empty], the removal of the products of conception, using suction and sharp curettage and forceps, usually associated specifically with pregnancies of 16 weeks or more in gestational age. The addition of forceps is to facilitate removal of fetal parts too large for the suction catheter.

dilation of the heart [L, *dilatare,* to widen; AS, *heorte*], an enlargement of the heart caused by stretching of a weakened myocardium. The condition is associated with acute pulmonary embolism and heart failure.

dilator /dī″lātər/ [L, *dilatare,* to widen], a device for expanding a body opening or cavity. Examples include a tent dilator, consisting of a sponge or bundle of seaweed that expands the cervical os, and a Barnes' bag (dilator), a rubber bag that can be inserted into a body cavity and filled with water to produce pressure on the cavity walls.

dilator naris, the alar portion of the nasalis muscle that dilates the nostril.

dilator pupillae, a muscle of the iris of the eye that dilates the pupil. It is composed of radial fibers, like spokes of a wheel, that converge from the circumference of the iris toward the center and blend with fibers of the sphincter pupillae near the margin of the pupil. The dilator pupillae is innervated primarily by nerve fibers from the sympathetic system (T_2 sympathetic chain ganglia) through axons along the ciliary arteries. Compare **sphincter pupillae.**

Dilaudid, an opioid analgesic. Brand name for **hydromorphone hydrochloride.**

Dilor, a bronchodilator. Brand name for **dyphylline.**

diltiazem /diltī″əzam/, a calcium channel blocker or calcium antagonist.

■ INDICATIONS: It is prescribed for the treatment of vasospastic and effort-associated angina, in addition to hypertension.

■ CONTRAINDICATIONS: Sick sinus syndrome, second- or third-degree atrioventricular block, or hypotension prohibits its use.

■ ADVERSE EFFECTS: Among the more serious adverse reactions are edema, arrhythmia, bradycardia, hypotension, syncope, rash, headache, and dizziness.

diluent /dil″oo·ənt, dil″yoo·ənt/ [L, *diluere,* to wash], a substance, generally a fluid, that makes a solution or mixture less concentrated, less viscous, or more liquid.

dilute /diloot′, dī″loot/ [L, *diluere,* to wash], **1.** *adj.,* pertaining to a solution that contains a relatively small amount of solute in proportion to solvent. **2.** *v.,* to make a solution less concentrated or to decrease a solution's concentration.

diluting agent /dilo͞o″ting/, a substance used to reduce the viscosity of respiratory tract secretions so that they can be removed easily. Examples include water and hypotonic saline solution, which can be aerosolized or nebulized.

dimenHYDRINATE /dim′ənhī″drināt/, an antiemetic.
■ INDICATIONS: It is prescribed in the treatment of nausea and motion sickness.
■ CONTRAINDICATIONS: Asthma or known hypersensitivity to this drug prohibits its use. It is not given to newborns or lactating mothers.
■ ADVERSE EFFECTS: Among the more serious adverse reactions are skin rash, hypersensitivity reactions, and tachycardia. Drowsiness and dry mouth are common.

dimension, a measure of the width, length, or height of a space, usually described in units of a linear scale.

dimer /dī″mər/ [Gk, *di,* twice, *meros,* parts], a compound formed by the union of two radicals or two molecules of a single simpler compound.

dimercaprol /dī′mərkap″rol/, a heavy-metal antagonist. Formerly called *British antilewisite (BAL).*
■ INDICATIONS: It is prescribed in the treatment of Wilson's disease and in the treatment of acute arsenic, mercury, or gold poisoning, as from an overdosage with mercurial diuretics, arsenics, or gold salts.
■ CONTRAINDICATIONS: Hepatic or renal insufficiency; poisoning with cadmium, iron, or selenium; or known hypersensitivity to the drug prohibits its use.
■ ADVERSE EFFECTS: Among the most serious adverse reactions are nephrotoxicity, acidosis, convulsions, and abnormal cardiovascular functions. Mild reactions include pain at the injection site, nausea, excessive salivation, and paresthesia.

Dimetane, an antihistamine. Brand name for **brompheniramine maleate.**

Dimetapp, a fixed-combination drug containing a decongestant and an antihistamine. Brand name for **brompheniramine maleate, phenylephrine hydrochloride.**

dimethoxymethylamphetamine (DOM) /dī″məthok′sēme th′iləmfet″əmēn/, a psychoactive or hallucinogenic agent.

dimethylamine $[(CH_3)_2NH]$, a secondary amine found in guano and decomposing fish.

dimethylaniline. See **auramine.**

dimethyl carbinol. See **isopropyl alcohol.**

dimethyl sulfoxide (DMSO) /dīmeth″il/, an organic solvent used as an antiinflammatory agent.
■ INDICATIONS: It is instilled into the bladder for the treatment of interstitial cystitis.
■ CONTRAINDICATIONS: Known hypersensitivity to this drug prohibits its use.
■ ADVERSE EFFECTS: Among the most serious adverse reactions are GI disturbances, photophobia, disturbance of color vision, and headache. A garliclike body odor and taste in the mouth may occur. When applied topically, it can cause local irritations and carry toxins into the systemic circulation.

Dimitri disease. See **Sturge-Weber syndrome.**

dimorphous /dīmôr″fəs/ [Gk, *di,* twice, *morphe,* form], pertaining to an organism or substance that exists in two distinct forms.

dimple, 1. a slight natural indentation or depression on a body surface, such as on the cheek. 2. a depression on a body surface resulting from contracting scar tissue or trauma.

dimpled sign, a physical diagnostic test to differentiate between a benign dermatofibroma lesion and a nodular melanoma. On pressure of the examiner's thumb and index finger benign tumors dimple, but malignant growths do not.

dimpling [ME, *dympull*], small, abnormal indentations or depressions on the surface of a body or organ.

dinitrochlorobenzene (DNCB) /dīnī′trōklôr′ōben″zēn/, a substance applied topically as a test for delayed hypersensitivity reactions. The compound has also been used as an immunotherapeutic agent to treat skin tumors.

2,4-dinitrophenol (DNP), 1. a dye used in biochemical research into oxidative processes. 2. a hapten commonly used to induce immune response.

dinucleotide, a compound containing two nucleotides.

dioctyl calcium sulfosuccinate, dioctyl potassium sulfosuccinate, dioctyl sodium sulfosuccinate. See **docusate.**

diode /dī″od/, 1. an electron tube or x-ray tube having a cathode and an anode. 2. an electrical device that has a higher conductance for current flowing in one direction than for current flowing in the opposite direction.

diode laser, a solid-state semiconductor used as a lasering medium.

dioecious. See **diecious.**

diol. See **dihydric alcohol.**

Dionysian /dē·onis″ē·ən/ [Gk, *Dionysos,* Greek god of wine], the personal attitude of one who is uninhibited, mystic, sensual, emotional, and irrational and who may seek to escape from the boundaries imposed by the limits of the senses.

diopter (D) /dī·op″tər/ [Gk, *dioptra,* optical measuring instrument], a metric measure of the refractive power of a lens. It is equal to the reciprocal of the focal length of the lens in meters. For example, a lens with a focal length of 0.5 m has a diopter measure of 2.0 (1/0.5) and, when prescribed as a corrective lens for the eye, should make printed matter most clearly focused when it is held 0.5 m (20 inches) from the eyes.

dioptric power /dī·op″trik/, the refractive power of an optic lens as measured in diopters.

diovular. See **binovular.**

diovulatory /dī·ov″yələtôr′ē/ [Gk, *di,* twice; L, *ovum,* egg], routinely releasing two ova during each ovarian cycle. Compare **monovulatory.**

dioxide /dī·ok″sīd/ [Gk, *di,* twice, *oxys,* sharp, *genein,* to produce], an oxide that contains two oxygen atoms.

dioxin /dī·ok″sin/, a contaminant of the herbicide 2,4,5-trichlorophenoxyacetic acid, widely used throughout the world in forestry, on grassland, against woody shrubs and trees on industrial sites, and for rice and sugarcane weed control. Because of its toxicity it is no longer manufactured in the United States. Exposure to dioxin is associated with chloracne and porphyria cutanea tarda. Dioxin was a contaminant of the jungle defoliant Agent Orange sprayed by the U.S. military aircraft over areas of Southeast Asia from 1965 to 1970. Also called **2,3,7,8-tetrachlorodibenzo-para-dioxin.**

DIP, abbreviation for **desquamative interstitial pneumonia.**

dipeptidases /dīpep″tidāzəs/, the final enzymes in the protein splitting system of digestion. They complete the task of breaking two-amino-acid dipeptides into single amino acids.

dipeptide, an organic compound formed by the union of two amino acids, with the link provided by the carboxyl group of one molecule and the amine group of the other.

diphallus, a rare congenital anomaly that occurs when two genital tubercles develop. The penis is partly or completely duplicated and may or may not be symmetrical. It is often associated with urogenital or other anomalies. Also called **double penis.**

diphasic /dīfā″zik/ [Gk, *di,* twice, *phasis,* appearance], pertaining to something that occurs in two stages or phases.

diphenhydrAMINE hydrochloride, an antihistamine.

■ INDICATIONS: It is prescribed in the treatment of hypersensitivity reactions, including rhinitis, skin rash, and pruritus, and in the treatment of motion sickness and insomnia.

■ CONTRAINDICATIONS: Asthma or known hypersensitivity to this drug prohibits its use. It is not given to newborns or lactating mothers.

■ ADVERSE EFFECTS: Among the more serious adverse reactions are skin rash, hypersensitivity reactions, and tachycardia. Drowsiness and dry mouth commonly occur.

diphenoxylate hydrochloride /dī′fənok″silāt/, an opioid antidiarrheal that contains subclinical amounts of atropine sulfate to limit abuse.

■ INDICATIONS: It is prescribed in the treatment of noninfectious diarrhea and intestinal cramping.

■ CONTRAINDICATIONS: Liver disease, antibiotic-associated diarrhea, or known hypersensitivity to this drug prohibits its use. It is not given to children less than 2 years of age.

■ ADVERSE EFFECTS: Among the more serious adverse reactions are abdominal discomfort, intestinal obstruction, skin rash, tachycardia, urinary retention, nausea, and addiction.

diphenylhydantoin. See **phenytoin.**

2,3-diphosphoglycerate test, a blood test used in the evaluation of nonspherocytic anemia.

2,3-diphosphoglyceric acid (DPG) /dīfos′fōgliser″ik/, a substance in the erythrocyte that affects the affinity of hemoglobin for oxygen. It is a chief end product of glucose metabolism and a link in the biochemical feedback control system that regulates the release of oxygen to the tissues.

diphosphonate /difos′fonāt/, any of a group of related phosphorus-containing compounds that are structurally similar to pyrophosphate but have enhanced stability to enzymatic and chemical hydrolysis and have affinity for sites of osteoid mineralization. They are used as sodium salts to inhibit bone resorption and are complexed with technetium-99m for bone imaging. The group includes alendronate, etidronate, and pamidronate. Also called **bisphosphonate.**

diphtheria /difthir′ē-ə, dipthir′ē-ə/ [Gk, *diphthera,* leather membrane], an acute contagious disease caused by the bacterium *Corynebacterium diphtheriae.* Untreated, the disease is often fatal from respiratory obstruction or heart and kidney failure.

■ OBSERVATIONS: Diphtheria is characterized by the production of a systemic toxin and an adherent false membrane lining of the mucous membrane of the throat. The toxin is particularly damaging to the tissues of the heart and central nervous system, and the dense pseudomembrane in the throat may interfere with eating, drinking, and breathing. The membrane may also be present in other body tissues. Lymph glands in the neck swell, and the neck becomes edematous.

■ INTERVENTIONS: Patients are usually hospitalized in isolation rooms. Treatment of the isolated patient may include administration of diphtheria antitoxin, antibiotics, rest, fluids, and an adequate diet. Tracheostomy is sometimes necessary.

■ PATIENT CARE CONSIDERATIONS: Recovery is slow, but it is usually complete. Immunization against diphtheria is available to all children in the United States and Canada and is usually given in conjunction with pertussis and tetanus immunization early in infancy.

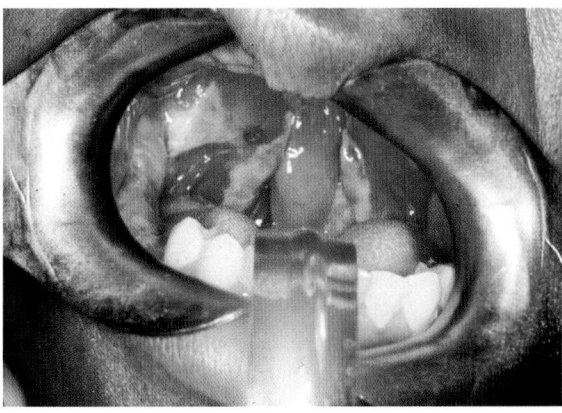

Diphtheria pseudomembrane *(Murray et al, 2010)*

diphtheria and tetanus toxoids (DT), an active immunizing agent.

■ INDICATIONS: It is prescribed for immunization against diphtheria and tetanus when pertussis vaccination is contraindicated.

■ CONTRAINDICATIONS: Immunosuppression, acute infection, or concomitant use of corticosteroids prohibits its use.

■ ADVERSE EFFECTS: The most serious adverse reaction is anaphylaxis.

diphtheria and tetanus toxoids and pertussis vaccine (DPT), an active immunizing agent.

■ INDICATIONS: It is prescribed for the routine immunization of children less than 6 years of age against diphtheria, tetanus, and pertussis.

■ CONTRAINDICATIONS: Immunosuppressive therapy, active infection, or neurological disorders prohibit its use.

■ ADVERSE EFFECTS: The most serious adverse reaction is anaphylaxis.

diphtheria and tetanus toxoids and pertussis vaccine adsorbed and *Haemophilus* **b conjugate vaccine,** a combination of diphtheria toxoid, tetanus toxoid, pertussis vaccine, and *Haemophilus* b conjugate vaccine, administered intramuscularly to children 18 months to 5 years of age for simultaneous immunization against diphtheria, tetanus, whooping cough, and infection by *Haemophilus influenzae* type b.

diphtheria antitoxin [Gk, *diphtheria,* leather membrane, *anti,* against, *toxikon,* poison], an antitoxin prepared by immunizing horses with diphtheria toxoid and extracting serum from the animal. The serum is standardized for strength and quality.

diphtherial cough /difthir′ē-əl/, a brassy, noisy, crouplike cough accompanied by stridor, observed mainly in children with laryngeal diphtheria.

diphtheritic croup /dif′thirit″ik/ [Gk, *diphtheria* + Scot, *croak,* to speak hoarsely], a diphtheritic inflammation of the larynx. Also called **laryngeal diphtheria.** See **diphtheritic laryngitis.**

diphtheritic laryngitis [Gk, *diphtheria, larynx, itis,* inflammation], inflammation of the larynx caused by the bacterium *Corynebacterium diphtheriae.* A serious complication is the formation of a false membrane. Also called **diphtheritic croup, laryngeal diphtheria.** See also **diphtheria.**

diphtheritic membrane, a membrane of coagulated fiber with bacteria and leukocytes. It is usually white or grayish yellow with well-defined margins. Airway obstruction or aspiration of the membrane is often the cause of death in diphtheria. See **diphtheria.**

diphtheritic pharyngitis [Gk, *diphtheria* + *pharynx,* throat, *itis,* inflammation], an inflammation of the pharynx caused by the bacterium *Corynebacterium diphtheriae* and associated with the formation of a false membrane. See also **diphtheria.**

diphtheritic sore throat, an inflammation of the pharynx or larynx caused by an infection of *Corynebacterium diphtheriae.* See **diphtheria.**

diphtheritic stomatitis, an inflammation of the mucous membrane of the mouth caused by *Corynebacterium diphtheriae.*

diphtheroid /dif″thəroid′/ [Gk, *diphthera,* leather membrane, *eidos,* form], **1.** pertaining to diphtheria. **2.** resembling the bacillus *Corynebacterium diphtheriae.*

diphyllobothriasis, a genus of tapeworm containing several species that is found in the intestine of fish, birds, and mammals, including man. Infection in humans is usually by eating uncooked fish. The larval stage is known as Sparganum. The species that most often infects humans is *Diphyllobothrium latum,* a giant freshwater fish tapeworm of North America and Europe. See **fish tapeworm infection.**

Diphyllobothrium /dəfil′ōboth″rē-əm/ [Gk, *di,* twice, *phyllon,* leaf, *bothrion,* pit], a genus of large parasitic intestinal flatworms having a scolex with two slitlike grooves. The species that most often infects humans is *Diphyllobothrium latum,* a giant freshwater fish tapeworm of North America and Europe. See also **fish tapeworm infection.**

-dipine, the generic stem suffix for the name of a phenylpyridine vasodilator (nifedipine type). See also **NIFEdipine.**

dipivefrin /dī′pivef″rin/, an ophthalmic sympathomimetic agent.

■ INDICATIONS: It is prescribed in the treatment of open-angle glaucoma.

■ CONTRAINDICATIONS: Narrow-angle glaucoma or known hypersensitivity to this drug prohibits its use.

■ ADVERSE EFFECTS: Among the most serious adverse effects are reactive hyperemia, conjunctivitis, allergic reactions, macular edema, tachycardia, arrhythmia, and hypertension.

diplegia /dīplē″jē-ə/ [Gk, *di,* twice, *plege,* stroke], paralysis of both sides of any body part or of like parts on the opposite sides of the body. Compare **hemiplegia.** Kinds include **cerebral palsy, facial diplegia.** –*diplegic, adj.*

diplo-, prefix meaning "double": *diplococcus, diplokaryon.*

diplococcus /dip′lōkok″əs/ *pl.* diplococci [Gk, *diploos,* double, *kokkos,* berry], **1.** *n.,* a member of the Coccaceae family that occurs in pairs because of incomplete cell division. Diplococci are often found as parasites or saprophytes. **2.** *adj.,* describing bacteria of the Coccaceae family, which occur as pairs of cocci. Kinds include *Streptococcus pneumoniae, Neisseria gonorrhoeae, Neisseria meningitidis.*

diploë /dip″lō-ē/, the loose tissue filled with red bone marrow between the two layers of the cranial bones.

diploid (2n) /dip′loid/ [Gk, *diploos* + *eidos,* form], having two complete sets of homologous chromosomes, such as are normally found in somatic cells and primordial germ cells before maturation. In humans the normal diploid number is 46. Compare **haploid, tetraploid, triploid.**

diploid nucleus, a nucleus having two sets of chromosomes, as normally found in the somatic cells of higher organisms.

diploidy /dip″loidē/, the state or condition of having two complete sets of homologous chromosomes.

diplokaryon /dip′lōker″ē-on/ [Gk, *diploos* + *karyon,* nut], a nucleus that contains twice the diploid number of chromosomes.

diploma program in nursing, a basic educational program that is designed to prepare nursing students for entry into practice, usually in 2 or 3 years. The recipient of a diploma is eligible to take the national certifying registration examination to become a registered nurse. In the United States, most diploma programs are conducted in hospitals, although some are located in community colleges. In Canada, diploma programs are conducted in community colleges or Collège d'Enseignement Général et Professionnel (in Quebec), as well as in a few hospital schools of nursing in the western provinces. These schools are negotiating collaboration with university schools of nursing. Once a significant venue for nursing education, diploma programs are increasingly rare.

diplomate /dip″ləmāt/, an individual who has earned a diploma or certificate, especially a physician who has been certified by a specialty board. See also **board certified.**

diplonema /dip′lənē″mə/ [Gk, *diploos,* + *nema,* thread], the looplike formation of the chromosomes in the diplotene stage of the first meiotic prophase in gametogenesis.

diplopagus /diplop″əgəs/ [Gk, *diploos* + *pagos,* something fixed], conjoined twins that are more or less equally developed, although one or several internal organs may be shared.

diplopia /diplō″pē-ə/ [Gk, *diploos* + *opsis,* vision], double vision caused by defective function of the extraocular muscles or a disorder of the nerves that innervate the muscles. It occurs when the object of fixation falls on the fovea in one eye and a nonfoveal point in the other eye or when the object of fixation falls on two noncorresponding points. Also called **ambiopia, double vision.** Compare **binocular vision.**

diplornavirus /dī′plôrnəvī″rəs/, a double-stranded ribonucleic acid virus that is the cause of Colorado tick fever. It is related to the reoviruses that are associated with various respiratory infections.

diplosomatia /dip′lōsōmā″shə/ [Gk, *diploos* + *soma,* body], *(Obsolete)* a congenital anomaly in which fully formed twins are joined at one or more areas of their bodies.

diplotene /dip″lətēn/ [Gk, *diploos* + *tainia,* ribbon], the fourth stage in the first meiotic prophase in gametogenesis in which chiasmata form between the chromatids of paired homologous chromosomes and crossing over occurs. The chromosomes then begin to repel each other and separate longitudinally, forming loops. See also **diakinesis, leptotene, pachytene, zygotene.**

dipodial symmelia /dīpō″dē-əl/ [Gk, *di,* twice, *pous,* foot, *syn,* together, *melosi,* limb], a developmental anomaly characterized by the fusion of the limbs and the presence of two feet. Compare **monopodial symmelia, sirenomelia, tripodial symmelia.** See also **sympus dipus.**

dipolar ion. See **zwitterion.**

dipole /dī″pōl/, **1.** a molecule whose ends carry opposite partial charges. **2.** a molecule with areas of opposing electrical charges, such as hydrogen chloride, which has a predominance of electrons and a partial negative charge about the chloride portion and a partial positive charge on the hydrogen side.

$$\delta^- \quad \delta^+ \qquad \delta^+ \quad \delta^-$$
$$\boxed{\text{Cl} - \text{H}} \; - - - - \; \boxed{\text{H} - \text{Cl}}$$

Dipole

diprosopus /dīpros″əpəs, dī′prəsō″pəs/ [Gk, *di,* twice, *prosopon,* face], a malformed fetus that has a double face showing varying degrees of development.

dipsesis /dipsē″sis/, extreme thirst.

-dipsia, -dipsy, suffix meaning "(condition of) thirst": *adipsia, hypodipsia.*

dipsomania /dip′sōmā″nē·ə/ [Gk, *dipsa,* thirst, *mania,* madness], an uncontrollable, often periodic craving for and indulgence in alcoholic beverages. Now called **alcoholism.**

dipstick, a chemically treated strip of paper used in the analysis of urine or other fluids.

-dipsy. See **-dipsia, -dipsy.**

dipus /dī″pəs/, conjoined twins who have only two feet.

dipygus /dīpī″gəs, dip″əgəs/ [Gk, *di,* twice, *pyge,* rump], a malformed fetus that has a double pelvis, one of which is usually not fully developed.

dipyridamole /dī′pirid″əmōl/, an antiplatelet agent.

■ INDICATIONS: When used in combination with coumarin anticoagulants, it is used to prevent postoperative thromboembolic complications of cardiac valve replacement.

■ CONTRAINDICATIONS: It should be used with caution in hypotension.

■ ADVERSE EFFECTS: The adverse reactions are mild and transient, such as headache, dizziness, rash, nausea, and flushing.

direct-access memory, access to computerized data independent of previously obtained data. The data transfer occurs directly between the computer memory and peripheral devices. See also **random-access memory.**

direct agglutination test, a test for the presence of antibodies to a specific antigen in which a dilute antiserum is mixed with the antigen in question.

direct amplification test, a method used to rapidly identify pathogenic organisms found in patient specimens. The RNA of an organism is copied (amplified) and then detected by using a nucleic acid probe. A small number of viruses and bacteria can be identified in a few hours in comparison to days or weeks needed for culturing.

direct antagonist [L, *diregere,* to direct; Gk, *antagonisma,* struggle], one of a pair or a group of muscles that pull in opposite directions, whose combined action prevents the part from moving.

direct bone conduction, the conduction of sound to the inner ear from a hearing aid implanted into the skull.

direct calorimetry, the measurement of the amount of heat directly generated by reaction. Compare **indirect calorimetry.**

direct causal association, a cause-and-effect relationship between a causative factor and a disease (or dependent factor) with no other factors intervening in the process.

direct contact, mutual touching of two individuals or organisms. Many communicable diseases may be spread by direct contact between an infected and a healthy person.

direct Coombs test, a blood test performed to identify hemolysis or to investigate hemolytic transfusion reactions. This test demonstrates whether the patient's red blood cells have been attacked by antibodies in the patient's own bloodstream. Compare **indirect Coombs test.**

direct costs, (in managed care) the costs of labor, supplies, and equipment to provide direct patient care services.

direct current (DC), an electric current that flows in one direction only and is substantially constant in value. Compare **alternating current.**

directed donation donor, Specific donor who makes a blood donation designated for transfusion to a specific recipient. The directed donor blood must meet the same criteria and undergo the same tests as any volunteer blood donor.

direct fluorescent antibody-*Treponema pallidum* **test (DFA-TP test),** a treponemal antibody test for syphilis using direct immunofluorescence to detect antibodies against *Treponema pallidum* in the serum.

direct fracture, any fracture occurring at a specific point of injury that is a direct result of that injury.

direct generation. See **asexual reproduction.**

direct gold, any form of 24-karat pure gold that may be compacted or condensed directly into a prepared tooth cavity to form a restoration. See also **gold foil.**

direct illumination, light from a distinct source focused directly on an object. Kinds include **slit lamp.** See also **illumination, transillumination.**

direct intervention, 1. (in occupational and physical therapy) hands-on therapy to increase the potential for new motor learning when there are deficits in movement and postural control that cannot be independently incorporated by the client. 2. a confrontation with a person with addictions at a surprise meeting planned by a family and/or concerned significant others and a therapist. It is designed to break the cycle of denial associated with the addiction and to encourage treatment. Also called **Johnson model of intervention.**

direct intraperitoneal insemination (DIPI), a method of assisted reproductive technology in which semen is injected into the pouch of Douglas.

directional atherectomy, the removal of plaque from a vessel using a specialized catheter for minimally invasive procedures. Blockages are identified and, if present, a catheter is advanced to cut the lesion. A low-pressure balloon is used to expose the lesion to the cutting surface. A stent may also be inserted to keep the vessel open.

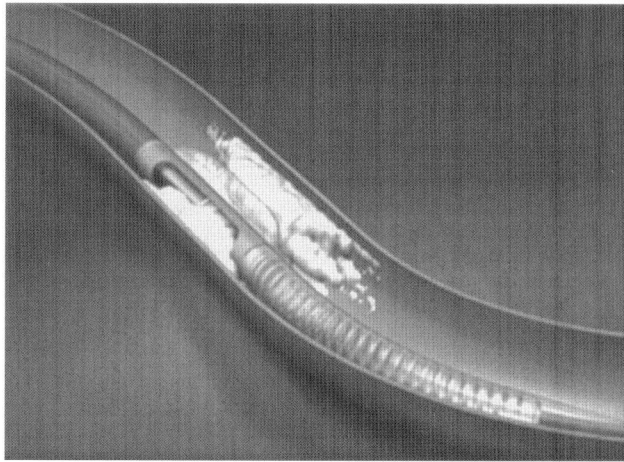

Directional atherectomy *(Norell et al, 2008)*

directional atherectomy catheter, a type of atherectomy catheter whose direction can be shifted to shave off additional plaque.

directive therapy [L, *diregere,* to direct, *therapeia,* treatment], a psychotherapeutic approach in which the psychotherapist directs the course of therapy by intervening to ask questions and offer interpretations. Compare **nondirective therapy.** See also **psychoanalysis.**

direct laryngoscopy [L, *diregere,* to direct, Gk, *larynx* + *skopein,* to watch], an examination of the larynx by means of a lighted instrument inserted through the mouth.

direct lead /lēd/, 1. an electrocardiographic conductor in which the exploring electrode is placed directly onto the surface of the exposed heart. 2. *(Informal)* a tracing produced by such a lead on an electrocardiograph.

direct light reflex, the constriction of a pupil receiving increased illumination, as by a light source during an ophthalmological examination. Also called **direct reaction to light.** Compare **consensual reaction to light.**

directly observed therapy (DOT), a strategy to ensure adherence to treatment is directly observed therapy. The patient meets with the health care provider, who observes the patient taking the medicine and explores any problems or side effects the patient may be experiencing.

direct measurement of blood pressure [L, *diregere,* to direct, *mensura,* to measure; ME, *blod* + L, *premere,* to press], measurement of blood pressure by means of a catheter inserted into an artery. The catheter is connected to a pressure transducer.

direct nursing care functions, liaison nursing activities that are focused on a particular patient, a patient's family, or a group for whom the nurse is directly responsible and accountable.

directory /direk″tərē/, **1.** (in computer processing) a listing of the files in a computer storage device, such as an area of a hard drive or other storage device. A device may contain many directories to facilitate organization of files. **2.** (for health or related reasons) a guide or listing to assist patients in locating health care professionals, services, and facilities.

direct patient care, care of a patient provided personally by a staff member and/or independent health care professional. Direct patient care may involve any aspects of the health care of a patient, including treatments, counseling, self-care, patient education, and administration of medication.

direct percussion. See **percussion.**

direct provider reimbursement, a method of direct payment for health care services, as fee-for-service.

direct pull-out services, the provision of professional services or interventions in a school in which specialists work closely with students outside the general education classroom. Instructional support or related services are provided in small groups or one-on-one in a separate setting.

direct-question interview, an inquiry that usually requires simple one- or two-word responses.

direct reaction to light. See **direct light reflex.**

direct reflex, a response that occurs on the same side of the body as the stimulus.

direct relationship, (in research). See **positive relationship.**

direct retainer, a clasp, attachment, or assembly fastened to an abutment tooth for the purpose of maintaining a removable restoration in its planned position in relation to oral structures. See also **precision rest.**

direct self-destructive behavior (DSDB), any form of suicidal activity such as suicide threats, attempts, or gestures and the act of suicide itself. The person is aware that death is the desired outcome of his or her act.

direct transfusion [L, *dirigere,* to direct, *transfundere,* to pour through], *(Obsolete)* the transfer of whole blood directly from a vein of the donor to a vein of the recipient in extraordinary circumstances. The practice has historical significance. The discovery of blood groups in the early 20th century, blood banking, and blood-borne pathogens made this method obsolete.

dirofilariasis /dī″rōfil′ərī″əsis/, a human infestation of the dog heartworm, *Dirofilaria immitis,* and the closely related *D. (Nochtiella) repens,* both of which may be transmitted through the bite of any of several species of mosquitoes. The filaria migrate through the bloodstream to the lung, producing pulmonary nodules and causing chest pain, coughing, and hemoptysis. The disease is rare among humans, but some species have been found to infect subcutaneous tissue and the eyes. Human disease is independent of dog ownership.

Humans are dead-end hosts for the parasites. Also called **zoonotic filariasis.**

dirty bomb, an explosive device that disperses radioactive material over a wide area, contaminating land, buildings, and people. Its purpose is to cause fear and to make an area unusable.

dis-, 1. prefix meaning "reversal," "apart," or "to separate": *dischronation, disinfect.* **2.** prefix meaning "opposite": *disease.*

disability /dis′əbil″itē/ [L, *dis,* opposite of, *habilis,* fit], impairment of function, either physically or mentally. It may be associated with a loss, absence, or impairment that limits full participation in major life activities. Formerly called *handicap.*

disablement model /disā″bəlmənt/, an evaluation and treatment model based on specific impairment, functional loss, and attainable quality of life rather than a medical diagnosis.

disaccharidase /disak′äridās″/, in humans, the enzyme that hydrolyzes disaccharides. The disaccharidases are located in the brush border membrane of the small intestine and hydrolyze the oligosaccharides and disaccharides produced after luminal digestion of starches and other carbohydrates. See also **disaccharide intolerance.**

disaccharidase deficiency. See **lactase deficiency.**

disaccharide /dīsak″ərīd/ [Gk, *di* + *sakcharon,* sugar], a general term for simple carbohydrates formed by the union of two monosaccharide molecules.

disaccharide intolerance, the inability to properly metabolize one or more disaccharides, usually resulting from deficiency of the corresponding disaccharidases, although it may have other causes such as impaired absorption. After ingestion of the disaccharide, there may be abdominal symptoms such as diarrhea, flatulence, borborygmus, distension, and pain. Kinds include **lactose intolerance.**

disadvantaged /dis′ədvan″tijd/ [L, *dis* + *abante,* superior position], (in health care) any group of people facing challenges that interfere with health and well-being, especially as they pertain to the social determinants of health. See also **social determinants of health.**

disarticulation /dis′ärtik′yəlā″shən/ [L, *dis* + *articulare,* to divide into joints], separation of a joint without cutting through a bone.

disaster [L, *dis,* apart, *astrum,* a star], any catastrophic event, mishap, or misfortune that is ruinous, distressing, or calamitous. The World Health Organization defines *disaster* as "an occurrence disrupting the normal conditions of existence and causing a level of suffering that exceeds the capacity of adjustment of the affected community."

disaster-preparedness plan [L, *dis* + *astrum,* favorable stars, *praeparare,* to prepare], (for health or related reasons) a formal plan of action, usually prepared in written form, for coordinating the response of a hospital staff or community agency in the event of a disaster within the hospital or the surrounding community.

disc. See **disk.**

discectomy. See **diskectomy.**

discernment, insight related to a patient problem or dilemma; the ability to analyze and understand a patient situation.

discharge (d/c) /dis″chärj/ [OFr, *deschargier,* to expel], **1.** *v.,* to release a substance or object. See also **evacuate, excrete, secrete. 2.** *v.,* to release a patient from a hospital. **3.** *v.,* to release an electric charge, which may be manifested by a spark or surge of electricity, from a storage battery, condenser, or other source. **4.** *v.,* to release a burst of energy from or through a neuron. **5.** *n.,* (in psychology) a release of emotions, often accompanied by a wide range of voluntary and involuntary reflexes, weeping, rage, or other emotional displays. Also called *affective discharge.* **6.** *n.,* a substance or object discharged. **7.** *n.,* the flow of a secretion or an excretion.

discharge abstract, items of information compiled from medical records of patients discharged from a hospital, organized and recorded in a uniform format to provide data for statistical studies, reports, or research.

discharge against medical advice (DAMA), the decision of a patient to leave a facility or agency despite the counsel of health care providers that additional care and treatment are necessary. See also **against medical advice.**

discharge coordinator, an individual who arranges with community agencies and institutions for the continuing care of patients after their discharge from a hospital or another health care facility.

discharge planning, the activities that facilitate a patient's movement from one health care setting to another, or to home. It is a multidisciplinary process involving physicians, nurses, social workers, and possibly other health professionals; its goal is to enhance continuity of care. It begins on admission.

discharge summary, a clinical report prepared by a physician or other health professional at the conclusion of a hospital stay or series of treatments. It outlines the patient's chief complaint, the diagnostic findings, the therapy administered and the patient's response to it, and recommendations on discharge.

discharging lesion [OFr, *deschargier* + L, *laesio,* hurting], an injury or infection of the central nervous system that causes sudden abnormal episodes of discharging nerve impulses.

dischronation /dis′krōnā″shən/, a disorder of time awareness. Also called **time agnosia.**

disciform keratitis /dis″ifôrm/ [Gk, *diskos,* flat plate; L, *forma,* form; Gk, *keras,* horn, *itis,* inflammation], an inflammatory condition of the eye that often follows an attack of dendritic keratitis, believed to be an immunological response to an ocular herpes simplex infection. The condition is characterized by disclike opacities in the cornea, usually with inflammation of the iris. See also **herpes simplex.**

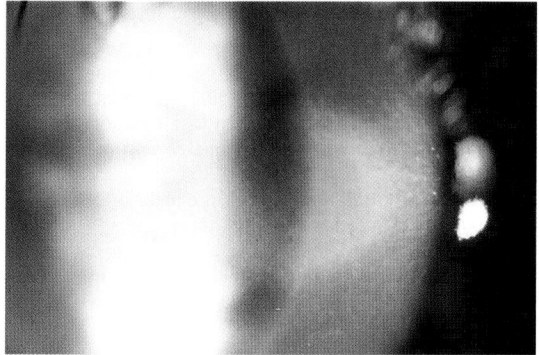

Disciform keratitis *(Kanski and Bowling, 2011)*

disclosing solution [L, *dis* + *claudere,* to close, *solutus,* dissolved], a vegetable-based dye solution, available in tablets or for topical application, used to stain and reveal plaque biofilm and other deposits on teeth.

disco-, prefix meaning "disk, disk-shaped": *discocyte.*

discoblastula /dis′kōblas″tyələ/ [Gk, *diskos,* flat plate, *blastos,* germ], a blastula formed from the partial cleavage

that occurs in a fertilized ovum containing a large amount of yolk. It develops from the blastodisc and consists of a cellular cap, or blastoderm, separated from the uncleaved yolk mass by a small cavity, the blastocele.

discocyte /dis″kəsīt/ [Gk, *diskos* + *kytos,* cell], a mature normal erythrocyte in the form of a biconcave disk without a nucleus.

discoid /dis″koid/ [Gk, *diskos,* flat plate, *eidos,* form], having a flat, round shape.

discoid lupus erythematosus (DLE) [Gk, *diskos* + *eidos,* form; L, *lupus,* wolf; Gk, *erythema,* redness, *osis,* condition], a chronic, recurrent disease, primarily of the skin, characterized by lesions that are covered with scales and extend into follicles. The lesions are typically distributed on the face but may also be present on other parts of the body. On healing the lesions often leave atrophic, hyperpigmented, or hypopigmented scars. If hairy areas are involved, alopecia may result. The cause of the disease is not established, but there is evidence that it may be an autoimmune disorder, and some cases seem to be induced by certain drugs. It is at least five times more common in women than in men and occurs most frequently in the third and fourth decades of life. Treatment includes use of a sunblock, hats, and protective clothing when exposure to sunlight cannot be avoided, application of steroids to the lesions, and use of systemic antimalarial drugs such as hydroxychloroquine; systemic corticosteroid agents may be used in severe cases. See also **systemic lupus erythematosus.**

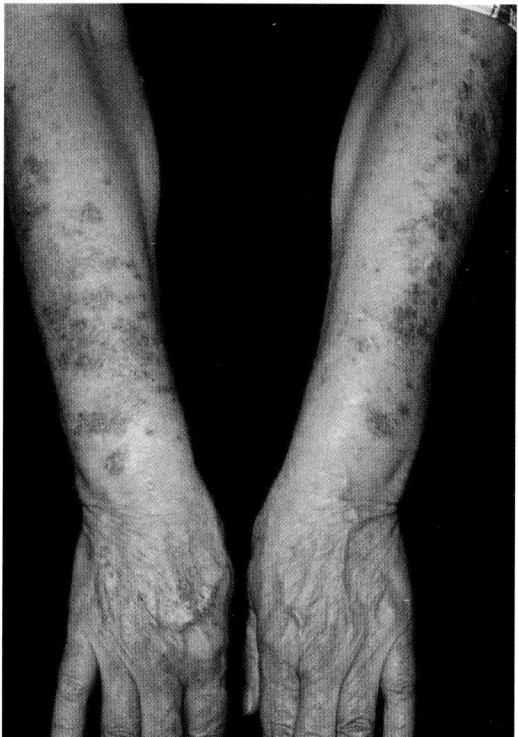

Discoid lupus erythematosus *(Courtesy Department of Dermatology, School of Medicine, University of Utah)*

discoid meniscus, an abnormal condition characterized by a discoid rather than a semilunar shape of the cartilaginous meniscus of the knee. The lateral meniscus is usually affected, although the medial meniscus may also become involved. The condition is a developmental anomaly that is asymptomatic in infants and young children; it appears most often between 6 and 8 years of age. Common complaints are that the knee joint clicks or gives way. These characteristics are often but not always associated with an injury to the knee. Examination demonstrates the clicking, usually during the last 15 to 20 degrees, when the knee is moved from flexion to extension. Surgical excision of the meniscus is seldom warranted in treating this benign condition.

discoid placenta [Gk, *diskos,* quoit, *eidos,* form; L, *placenta,* flat cake],   a round placenta.

disconfirmation /diskon'fərmā″shən/, a dysfunctional communication that negates, discounts, or ignores information received from another person.

discordance /diskôr″dəns/ [L, *discordare,* to disagree],   the expression of one or more specific traits in only one member of a pair of twins. Compare **concordance.** *–discordant, adj.*

discordant twins,   twins showing a marked difference in size (greater than 10% in weight) at birth. The condition is usually caused by overperfusion of one twin and underperfusion of the other. It is fairly common in identical twins but may also occur in dizygotic twins.

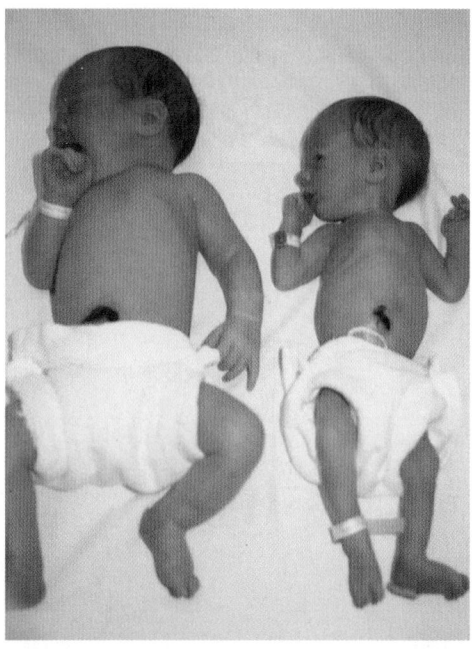

Discordant twins *(Clark, Thimpson, and Barkemeyer, 2000)*

discovery /diskov″ərē/ [L, *dis* + *coopiere,* to cover],   (in law) a pretrial procedure that allows one party to examine vital witnesses and documents held exclusively by the adverse party. Discovery is limited to materials, facts, and other resources that could not otherwise be reasonably expected to be discovered and that are necessary to the preparation of the case for trial. Also called **pretrial discovery.** Compare **deposition, interrogatories.**

discrete /diskrēt″/ [L, *discretus,* separated],   **1.** individually distinct. **2.** composed of distinct individual or unique parts.

discrete x-rays.   See **x-ray.**

discrimination /diskrim′inā″shən/ [L, *discrimen,* division],   (for health or related reasons) the act of distinguishing or differentiating. The ability to distinguish between touch or pressure at two nearby points on the body is known as two-point discrimination. See also **two-point discrimination test.**

discriminator /diskrim″inā′tər/,   an electronic device capable of accepting or rejecting a pulse of energy on the basis of the pulse's amplitude. It is used to separate low-energy from high-energy radionuclides.

disease [L, *dis* + Fr, *aise,* ease],   **1.** a condition of abnormal vital function involving any structure, part, or system of an organism. **2.** a specific illness or disorder characterized by a recognizable set of signs and symptoms attributable to heredity, infection, diet, or environment. Compare **condition, diathesis.**

disease-modifying antirheumatic drug (DMARD),   a classification of antirheumatic agents referring to their ability to modify the course of disease, as opposed to simply treating symptoms such as inflammation and pain. Agents in this group include auranofin, azathioprine, cyclosporine, gold salts, hydroxychloroquine, leflunomide, methotrexate, D-penicillamine, and sulfasalazine.

disease prevention,   activities designed to protect patients or other members of the public from actual or potential health threats and their harmful consequences.

disengagement /dis′engāj″mənt/   [Fr, *disengager,* to release from engagement],   **1.** an obstetric manipulation in which the presenting part of the baby is dislodged from the maternal pelvis as part of an operative delivery. See also **Kielland's rotation, version and extraction. 2.** the release or detachment of oneself from other persons or responsibilities. **3.** (in transactional family therapy) a role assumed by a trained psychologist or other qualified health professional in observing and restructuring intervention without becoming actively and directly involved in the problem.

disengagement theory,   the psychosocial concept that normally aging individuals and society mutually withdraw from normal interaction. The theory also assumes that older adults are a homogenous group whose members prefer the company of others of their own age. See also **activity theory.**

disequilibrium /disē′kwilib′rē·əm/ [L, *dis,* apart, *aequilibrium*],   the loss of balance or adjustment, particularly mental or psychological balance.

dishpan fracture [AS, *disc,* plate; L, *patina,* dish; *fractura,* break],   a fracture that depresses the skull. Also called **derby hat fracture.**

disinfect /dis′infekt″/ [L, *dis,* apart, *inficere,* to infect],   to eliminate many or all pathogenic microorganisms with the exception of bacterial spores.

disinfectant /dis′infek″tənt/,   a liquid chemical that can be applied to objects to eliminate many or all pathogenic microorganisms with the exception of bacterial spores. See also **antiseptic.**

disinfection /dis′infek″shən/,   the process of killing pathogenic organisms or rendering them inert.

disinfestation /dis′infestā″shən/ [L, *dis,* apart, *infestare,* to infest],   elimination of a threat of infestation by vermin, rodents, lice, or other noxious organisms.

disinhibition /dis′inhibish″ən/ [L, *dis,* apart, *inhibere,* to restrain],   the removal or loss of inhibition. See also **inhibition.**

disintegrative psychosis /disin″təgrā′tiv/,   a pervasive developmental disorder of childhood in which skills regress following normal development of speech, social behavior, and other traits. It usually occurs after the age of 3 years; the cause is unknown. Treatment includes early and intense educational interventions and therapy based on symptoms.

disjunction /disjungk″shən/ [L, *disjungere,* to disjoint],   the separation of paired homologous chromosomes during anaphase of the first meiotic division, or the separation of the chromatids of a chromosome during ana-phase of mitosis and the second meiotic division. Compare **nondisjunction.**

disk [Gk, *diskos,* flat plate], **1.** a flat, circular platelike structure, such as an articular disk or an optic disc. Also spelled **disc. 2.** *(Informal)* an intervertebral disk. **3.** media used to store data in a computerized format.

diskectomy /dis·kek′tə·me/ [Gk, *diskos,* flat plate + *ektome,* incision], excision of an intervertebral disk. Also spelled **discectomy.**

diskography /diskog″rəfē/, the radiographic examination of individual intervertebral disks after introduction of a radi-opaque contrast medium into the center of the disk. It is used in the investigation of ruptured disks but has largely been replaced by MRI and CT myelography.

dislocation /dis′lōkā″shən/ [L, *dis + locare,* to place], the displacement of any part of the body from its normal posi-tion, particularly a bone from its normal articulation with a joint. See also **incomplete dislocation.** *−dislocate, v.*

dislocation fracture, a fracture of the bony components of a joint associated with a displacement of a bone from its normal articulation with the joint.

dislocation of the clavicle [L, *dis,* apart, *locare,* to place, *clavicula,* little key], displacement of the collarbone. It may occur either at the sternal end or at the acromial or scap-ular extremity.

dislocation of the finger [L, *dis,* apart, *locare,* to place; AS, *finger*], displacement of a joint of the finger as a result of trauma. In the absence of an accompanying fracture the dis-located finger can usually be reduced by steadying the hand at the wrist and maneuvering the dislocated bone back into place.

dislocation of the hip [L, *dis,* apart, *locare,* to place; AS, *hype*], displacement of the femoral head out of the hip joint, usually accompanied by pain, edema, rigidity, shorten-ing of the leg, and loss of function. It may be congenital or acquired. Types of hip dislocation include obturator disloca-tion, in which the femoral head lies in the obturator foramen; perineal dislocation, in which the femoral head is displaced into the perineum; sciatic dislocation, in which the femoral head lies in the sciatic notch; and subpubic dislocation, in which the femoral head is displaced anteriorly.

dislocation of the jaw [L, *dis,* apart, *locare,* to place; ME, *jowe*], unilateral or bilateral displacement of the man-dibular condyle(s) from the mandibular fossa(e) over the articular tubercle(s) of the temporal bone, typically as a result of a blow, a fall, intubation, or yawning and accom-panied by severe muscle spasms. The mandible is fixed in an open position. If the mandible appears deviated to one side, the dislocation involves only one side. The disloca-tion is reduced manually with or without anesthetic seda-tion and with the possible use of a short-acting skeletal muscle relaxant. This is an extremely stressful and painful condition.

dislocation of the knee [L, *dis,* apart, *locare,* to place; AS, *cneow*], displacement of one of the bones of the knee joint. First aid treatment for the dislocation is the same as for a fracture: The joint is immobilized with splints; then it is urgent that the patient be moved to a health care facility to avoid potential vascular complications affecting both the limb and life.

dislocation of the shoulder [L, *dis + locare +* AS, *scul-der*], any of several kinds of displacement of the bones of the shoulder joint, including acromial joint disruption and separation and dislocation of the glenohumeral joint with the humeral head displaced anteriorly and inferiorly.

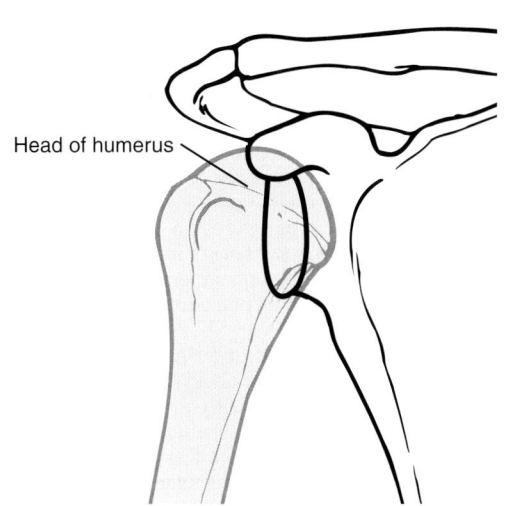

Head of humerus

Dislocation of the shoulder *(Miller-Keane and O'Toole, 1998)*

dislocation of the toe, displacement of a metatarsal bone at a joint.

dismembered pyeloplasty, **1.** a pyeloplasty procedure for redundancy of the renal pelvis, consisting of excision of the ureteropelvic junction and part of the pelvis and reat-tachment of the spatulated end of the ureter to the remaining pelvis. Also called **Anderson-Hynes pyeloplasty. 2.** a mini-mally invasive surgical procedure for correcting a kidney ureteropelvic junction obstruction.

dismiss [L, *dis + mittere,* to send], **1.** (in law) to discharge or dispose of an action, suit, or motion trial. *−dismissal, n.* **2.** to pay no attention to or give no merit to something because it is not seen as important or relevant.

disobliterative endarterectomy, surgical opening of a narrowed or blocked blood vessel by removing plaque from the arterial wall. See **endarterectomy.**

disodium edetate. See **edetate disodium.**

disopyramide phosphate /dī′sōpir″əmīd/, a cardiac antiarrhythmic.

■ INDICATIONS: It is prescribed in the treatment of atrial fi-brillation, atrial flutter, ventricular premature complexes, and coupled ventricular tachycardias.

■ CONTRAINDICATIONS: Cardiogenic shock, heart failure, preexisting second- or third-degree heart block in the ab-sence of a pacemaker, sick sinus syndrome, or known hyper-sensitivity to this drug prohibits its use.

■ ADVERSE EFFECTS: Among the more serious adverse reac-tions are severe hypotension, precipitation of heart failure, and aggravation of heart block. Urinary retention, dry mouth, and constipation commonly occur.

disorder [L, *dis,* apart, *ordo,* rank], a disruption of or inter-ference with normal functions or established systems, as a mental disorder or nutritional disorder. Compare **disease,** def. 2.

disordered metabolism, changes in metabolism that result from disease or medications administered to control dis-eases. Patients with acquired immunodeficiency syndrome, for example, may experience severe malnutrition, wasting, weight loss, hypermetabolism, or altered energy metabolism due to changes in the gut microbiome.

disorder of movement [L, *dis,* apart, *ordo,* rank, *movere,* to move], any perverse or abnormal function of muscular action that may result from infection, injury, or congenital disability, such as ataxia, involuntary grimacing, and chorea.

disorder of sleep [L, *dis* + *ordo* + AS, *slaep*], any condition that interferes with normal sleep patterns, such as sleep apnea, phase shift, use of alcohol and certain drugs, excessive sleepiness, sleepwalking, nightmares, sleep paralysis, restless legs syndrome, and narcolepsy. Treatment may include medications, relaxation, avoidance of stimulants, and referral to sleep disorder clinics.

disorder of written expression, a learning disorder in which the affected skill is written communication, characterized by errors in spelling, grammar, or punctuation; by poor paragraph organization; or by poor story composition or thematic development.

disorganized schizophrenia /disôr″gənīzd/ [L, *dis* + Gk, *organon,* organ], schizophrenia symptoms characterized by an earlier age of onset, usually at puberty, and a more severe disintegration of the personality than occurs in other forms of the disease. The essential features include incoherence, loose associations, gross disorganization of behavior, and flat or inappropriate affect. See also **schizophrenia.**

disorient /disôr″ē·ənt/, to cause to lose awareness or perception of space, time, or personal identity and relationships.

disorientation /-ā″shən/ [L, *dis* + *orienter,* to proceed from], a state of mental confusion characterized by inadequate or incorrect perceptions of place, time, or identity. Disorientation may occur in organic mental disorders, in drug and alcohol intoxication, and, less commonly, after severe stress.

disparate twins /dis″pərāt, disper″it/, twins who are distinctly different from each other in weight and other features.

disparities, (for health or related reasons) inequality in health status or in access to health services for a group of individuals based on racial, ethnic, or socioeconomic status.

dispense /dispens″/ [L, *dis,* apart, *pensare,* to weigh], to prepare and issue medications or medication mixtures from a pharmaceutical outlet or department.

disperse /dispərs″/ [L, *dis* + *spargere,* to scatter], to scatter the component parts, as of a tumor or of the fine particles in a colloid system; also the particles so scattered.

dispersing agent /dispur″sing/ [L, *dis* + *spargere,* to scatter, *agere,* to do], a chemical additive used in pharmaceutics to cause the even distribution of the ingredients throughout the product, such as in dermatological emulsions containing both oil and water. Dispersing agents commonly used in skin creams, lotions, and ointments include glyceryl monostearate, sodium lauryl sulfate, and polyethylene glycol derivatives. A dispersing agent may cause an allergic reaction or adverse effect in a hypersensitive person.

dispersion /dispur″shən/, the scattering or dissipation of finely divided material, as when particles of a substance are scattered throughout the volume of a fluid. Examples include colloids and gels, such as egg white, soap, and gelatin, which consist of large molecules or clumps of molecules that are able to attract and hold large numbers of water molecules.

dispersion forces. See **van der Waals forces.**

dispersion medium, a gas, liquid, or solid in which another substance is suspended. See **continuous phase, medium.**

displaced fracture /displāst/ [Fr, *deplacement,* to remove], a traumatic bone break in which two ends of a fractured bone are separated and out of their normal positions. The ends may pierce surrounding skin, as in a compound fracture, or may be contained within the skin, as in a closed fracture. These types of fractures usually require surgical intervention to restore the correct alignment of bony parts and for best postinjury outcome.

100% displaced fracture. See **complete fracture.**

displaced testis [Fr, *deplacement* + L, *testis,* testicle], a testis that is located in the pelvis, inguinal canal, or elsewhere after it normally would have descended into the scrotum.

displacement /displās″mənt/ [Fr, *deplacement,* to remove], **1.** the state of being displaced or the act of displacing. **2.** (in chemistry) a reaction in which an atom, molecule, or radical is removed from combination and replaced by another. **3.** (in physics) the displacing in space of one mass by another, as when the weight or volume of a fluid is displaced by a floating or submerged body. **4.** (in psychiatry) an unconscious defense mechanism for avoiding emotional conflict and anxiety by transferring emotions, ideas, or wishes from one object to a substitute that is less anxiety-producing. Compare **sublimation.** See also **percolation.** **5.** (in public health) the involuntary act of being removed from one's home or familiar surroundings as the result of a disaster, war, or other circumstance over which one has no control. This type of displacement leads to numerous health challenges.

displacement chromatography. See **chromatography.**

display /displā″/, something presented for viewing, such as on a computer screen.

disruptive behavior disorder, a condition characterized by socially inappropriate behavior, such as persistent disobedience, stubbornness, defiance, or irritability. This condition is typically more distressing to others than to the individual with the disorder. Kinds include **conduct disorder, oppositional defiant disorder.**

DISS, abbreviation for **Diameter-Index Safety System.**

dissect /disekt″/ [L, *dissecare,* to cut apart], **1.** to cut apart tissues for visual or microscopic study using a scalpel, a probe, or scissors. Compare **bisect. 2.** to tear away the intima of an artery, creating a false lumen that allows blood to flow into the wall of the artery. An aortic dissection that spreads to the coronary arteries can cause sudden death. **−dissection,** *n.*

dissecting aneurysm [L, *dissecare,* to cut apart; Gk, *aneurysma,* a widening], a localized dilation of an artery, most commonly the aorta, characterized by a longitudinal separation of the outer and middle layers of the vascular wall. Aortic dissecting aneurysms occur most frequently in men between 40 and 60 years of age and are preceded by hypertension in more than 90% of cases. Blood entering a tear in the intimal lining of the vessel causes a separation of weakened elastic and fibromuscular elements in the medial layer and leads to the formation of cystic spaces filled with matrix. Dissecting aneurysms in the thoracic aorta may extend into blood vessels of the neck. Rupture of a dissecting aneurysm may be fatal in less than 1 hour. Treatment consists of resection and replacement of the excised section of aorta with a synthetic prosthesis. See also **aortic aneurysm.**

dissection. See **dissect.**

disseminated /disem″inā″tid/, dispersed or spread throughout, as in an organ or the whole body.

disseminated intravascular coagulation (DIC) [L, *dis* + *seminare,* to sow, *intra,* within, *vasculum,* little vessel, *coagulare,* to curdle], a grave coagulopathy resulting from the activation of clotting and anticlotting processes in response to disease or injury, such as septicemia, acute shock, poisonous snakebites, neoplasms, obstetric emergencies, severe trauma, extensive surgery, and hemorrhage. The primary disorder initiates generalized intravascular clotting, which in turn activates fibrinolytic mechanisms. As a result, the initial hypercoagulability is succeeded by a deficiency in clotting factors with coagulopathy and hemorrhaging. Also called **consumption coagulopathy, defibrination syndrome.**

■ OBSERVATIONS: Purpura on the lower extremities and abdomen, reflecting fibrin deposits in capillaries, is a common first sign of DIC. Hemorrhagic bullae, cyanosis of the extremities, and focal gangrene in the skin and mucous membranes may follow. Hemorrhages from incisions or catheter or injection sites, GI bleeding, hematuria, pulmonary edema, pulmonary embolism, progressive hypotension, tachycardia, absence of peripheral pulses, restlessness, convulsions, or coma may occur. Laboratory studies generally show a marked deficiency of blood platelets, low levels of fibrinogen and other clotting factors, prolonged prothrombin and partial thromboplastin times, and abnormal erythrocyte morphological characteristics.

■ PATIENT CARE CONSIDERATIONS: The management of acute and chronic forms of DIC should primarily be directed at treatment of the underlying disorder. The care of a patient with life-threatening DIC requires careful monitoring, observation for evidence of bleeding, extremely gentle handling, maintenance of a safe environment, and emotional support.

disseminated myelitis, an inflammation of the spinal cord. Also called **diffuse myelitis.** See also **acute transverse myelitis.**

disseminated neuritis, inflammation of peripheral nerves with pain, tenderness, and loss of function. Lesions may affect the parenchyma of peripheral sensory and motor tracts. The condition may be caused by alcohol, infectious agents, or exposure to heavy metals. Compare **multifocal motor neuropathy.**

dissent /disent″/ [L, *dis* + *sentire,* to feel], **1.** *v.,* to differ in belief or opinion; to disagree. **2.** *n.,* (in law) a statement written by a judge who disagrees with the decision of the majority of the court. The dissent states explicit reasons for the contrary opinion. –*dissenting, adj.*

dissociation /disō′shē-ā″shən/ [L, + *sociare,* to unite], **1.** the act of separating into parts or sections. **2.** an unconscious defense mechanism by which an idea, thought, emotion, or other mental process is separated from the consciousness and thereby loses emotional significance. See also **dissociative disorder.** –*dissociative, adj.*

dissociation syndrome, a loss of the ability to sense painful and thermal stimuli while retaining the sense of touch, tactile discrimination, and position sense. The disorder occurs in syringomyelia and may also result from spinal tract lesions.

dissociative anesthesia /disō″shē·ətiv/, a unique anesthesia characterized by analgesia and amnesia with minimal effect on respiratory function. The patient does not appear to be anesthetized and can swallow and open eyes but does not process information. This form of anesthesia may be used to provide analgesia during brief, superficial operative procedures or diagnostic processes. Ketamine hydrochloride is a phencyclidine derivative that inhibits principally the NMDA (N-methyl-D-aspartate) receptor, used to induce dissociative anesthesia. Ketamine is used in combination with a benzodiazepine or alone for trauma patients with very unstable, low blood pressure or for elderly patients. Emergence may be accompanied by delirium, excitement, disorientation, and confusion.

dissociative disorder, a category of *DSM-5* disorder in which emotional conflicts are so repressed that a separation or split in the personality occurs, resulting in an altered state of consciousness or a confusion in identity. Symptoms may include amnesia, somnambulism, fugue, dream state, and dissociative identity disorder. It is caused by an inability to cope with severe stress or conflict and usually occurs suddenly, after a situation catastrophic to the person. Treatment may include hypnosis, especially when amnesia is the primary symptom; psychotherapy; and use of antianxiety medication. Also called **dissociative reaction.** Compare **conversion disorder.** See also **dissociation.**

dissociative identity disorder, a psychiatric disorder characterized by the existence of two or more distinct, clearly differentiated personality structures within the same individual, any of which may dominate at a particular time. Each personality is a complex unit with separate well-developed emotional and thought processes, behavior patterns, and social relationships. The various subpersonalities are usually dramatically different and may or may not be aware of the existence of the others. Formerly called **multiple personality disorder.**

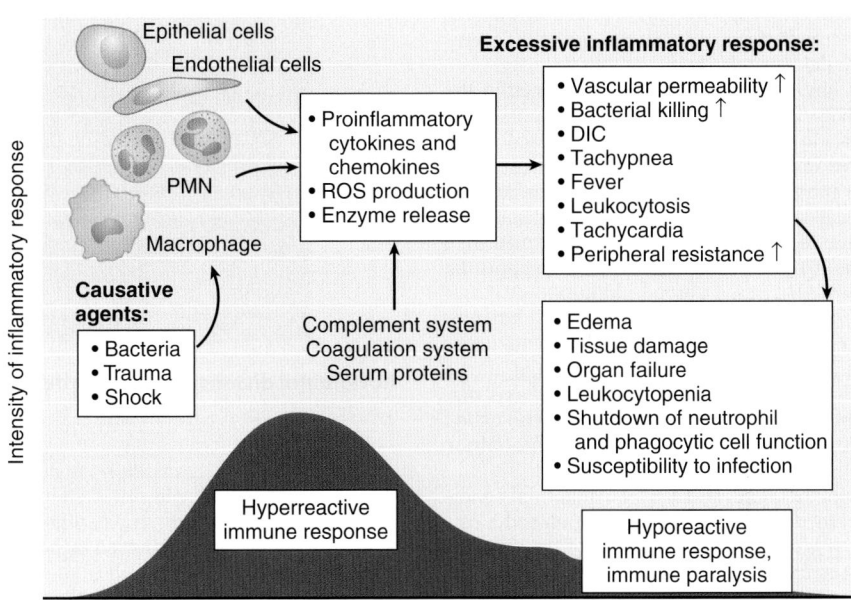

Dynamic time-course of the inflammatory response during sepsis

Disseminated intravascular coagulation (DIC) *(Walsh, 2009)*

dissociative reaction. See **dissociative disorder.**

dissolution /dis′əlōō″shən/ [L, *dis* + *solvere,* to loosen], **1.** the separation of a complex chemical compound into simpler molecules. **2.** the dissolving of chemical substances into a homogenous solution. **3.** the loss of mental powers.

dissolve, to disperse the molecules or ions of one substance throughout the bulk of another substance.

dissolved gas /disolvd″/ [L, *dis* + *solvere,* to loosen], gas in a simple physical solution, as distinguished from gas that has reacted chemically with a solvent or other solutes and is chemically combined.

dissonance, the interference between sound waves of different pitches.

distal /dis″təl/ [L, *distare,* to be distant], **1.** away from or the farthest from a point of origin or attachment. **2.** away from or the farthest from the midline or a central point, as a distal phalanx. Compare **proximal.**

distal acinar emphysema, one of the principal types of emphysema, limited to the distal ends of the alveoli along the interlobular septa and beneath the pleura, forming bullae. Also called **interlobular emphysema, paraseptal emphysema.** See also **bullous emphysema.**

distal convoluted tubule. See **distal tubule.**

distal latency, (in electroneuromyography) the interval between the stimulation of a compound muscle and the observed response. Normal nerve conduction velocity is above 40 m/sec in the lower extremities and above 50 m/sec in the upper extremities, but age, muscle disease, temperature, and other factors can influence the velocity.

distal muscular dystrophy, a rare form of muscular dystrophy that usually affects adults. It is characterized by moderate weakness and by wasting that begins in the arms and legs and then extends gradually to the proximal and facial muscles.

distal myopathy, an autosomal-dominant form of muscular dystrophy, appearing in two types. The first has onset in infancy, does not progress past adolescence, and is not incapacitating. The second has onset in adulthood and is called late distal hereditary myopathy. Also called **distal muscular dystrophy.**

distal part of prostatic urethra, the segment of the urethra that extends through the penis from the end of the membranous urethra to the navicular fossa.

distal phalanx, any one of the small distal bones in the third row of phalanges of the hand or the foot (second phalanx in the thumb and great toe). Each one at the end of the finger has a convex dorsal surface and a flat palmar surface, with a rough elevation at the end of the palmar surface that supports a fingernail and its sensitive pulp. The distal phalanx of each of the toes is smaller and more flattened than that of a finger; it also has a rough elevation to support the toenail and its pulp. Also called **ungual phalanx.**

distal radioulnar articulation, the pivotlike articulation of the head of the ulna and the ulnar notch on the lower end of the radius involving two ligaments. The joint allows rotation of the distal end of the radius around an axis that passes through the center of the head of the ulna. Also called **inferior radioulnar joint.** Compare **proximal radioulnar articulation.**

distal renal tubular acidosis (RTA), an abnormal condition characterized by excessive acid accumulation and bicarbonate excretion. It is caused by the inability of the kidney's distal tubules to secrete hydrogen ions, thus decreasing the excretion of titratable acids and ammonium and increasing the urinary loss of potassium and bicarbonate. The condition may cause hypercalciuria and the formation of kidney stones. Treatment is the same as for renal tubular acidosis.

Primary distal RTA occurs mostly in females, adolescents, older children, and young adults. It may occur sporadically or result from hereditary defects. Secondary distal RTA is associated with numerous disorders, such as cirrhosis of the liver, malnutrition, starvation, and various genetic abnormalities. Compare **primary proximal RTA, proximal renal tubular acidosis.**

distal sparing, a condition in which the spinal cord remains intact below a lesion. The reflex arc remains but is not modified by supraspinal influences. As a result, spastic movements distal to the level of the lesion may occur.

distal tubule, the portion of the nephron lying between the nephric (Henle's) loop and the collecting duct in the kidney. Also called **distal convoluted tubule.**

distance regulation [L, *distantia* + *regula,* rule], behavior that is related to the control of personal space. Most humans establish a quantum of space between themselves and others that offers security from either psychological or physical threat while not creating a feeling of isolation. The amount of social distance thus maintained varies with different individuals and in different cultures. For example, in Canadian and American culture, a distance of 3 feet from another person is the norm. In Asian countries it is much less. A wild animal generally maintains a flight distance, the minimum it will allow between itself and a potential enemy before fleeing. Animals of the same species also maintain a personal distance from each other.

distance vision, the ability to see objects clearly from a distance, usually from 20 feet (6 m) or more.

distemper /distem″pər/ [L, *dis,* apart, *temperare,* to regulate], **1.** any mental or physical disorder or indisposition. **2.** a potentially fatal viral disease of animals characterized by rhinitis, fever, and a loss of appetite.

distend /distend″/ [L, *distendere,* to stretch], to enlarge or dilate something.

distensibility /disten′sibil″itē/ [L, *distendere,* to stretch], the ability of something to become stretched, dilated, or enlarged.

distension /disten″shən/, the state of being distended or swollen.

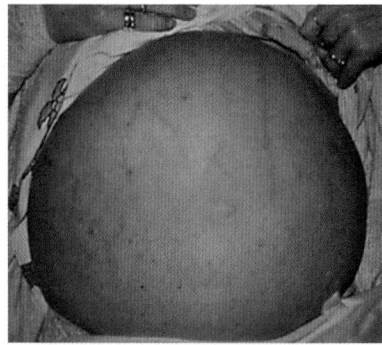

Abdominal distension from ascites *(Wilson and Giddens, 2013)*

distillate /distil″it/ [L, *distillare,* to drop down], the liquid vaporized, condensed, and collected in a distillation.

distillation /dis′tilā″shən/ [L, *distillare,* to drop down], the process of vaporization followed by condensation in another part of the system.

distilled water /distild″/ [L, *distillare,* to drop down; AS, *waeter*], water that has been purified by being heated to a vapor form and then condensed into another container as liquid water free of nonvolatile solutes.

distoclusion /dis'tə·klōō'zhən/ [L, *distare,* to be distant + *occludere,* to close up], malocclusion in which the mandibular arch is in a posterior position in relation to the maxillary arch, generally considered identical with Class II in Angle's classification of malocclusion. Also called **disto-occlusion, posterior occlusion.** See also **Angle's classification of malocclusion.**

distogingival /dis'tōjinjī''vəl/, pertaining to the surfaces of an anterior or a posterior tooth nearest the gum away from the midline and toward the back of the mouth.

distolabial /dis'tōlā''bē·əl/, pertaining to the surfaces of an anterior tooth away from the midline nearest the lips and toward the back of the mouth.

disto-occlusion. See **distoclusion.**

distortion /distôr''shən/ [L, *dis* + *torquere,* to twist], **1.** (in psychology) the process of shifting experience in one's perceptions. Distortions represent personal constructs of truth, validity, and right and wrong. The distortions of patients tend to influence their views of the world and themselves, as by altering a negative perception to one more favorable. **2.** (in radiology) radiographic image artifacts that may be caused by variations in the size and shape or position of the object. Thick or curved objects cause greater distortion than thin, flat objects because of unequal magnification. A shorter source-to-object distance results in greater image distortion, called magnification. Distortion also occurs when a three-dimensional structure is projected onto a two-dimensional structure.

distoversion /dis'tō-vər'zhən/ [L, *distare,* to be distant + *vertere,* to turn], the position of a tooth that is farther than normal from the median line of the face along the dental arch.

distractibility /distrak'tibil''itē/ [L, *dis* + *trahere,* to draw apart], a mental state in which attention does not remain fixed on any one subject but wavers or wanders.

distraction /distrak''shən/ [L, *dis* + *trahere,* to draw apart], **1.** a procedure that prevents or lessens the perception of pain by focusing attention on sensations unrelated to pain. **2.** a method of straightening a spinal column by the forces of axial tension pulling on the joint surfaces, such as applied by a Milwaukee brace.

distraught /distrôt'/ [OFr, *destrait,* inattentive], pertaining to a mental state of confusion, distraction, or absentmindedness.

distress /distres''/ [ME, *distressen,* to cause sorrow], an emotional or physical state of pain, sorrow, misery, suffering, or discomfort.

distributed processing /distrib''yətid/ [L, *distribuere,* to distribute], a combination of local and remote computer terminals in a network connected to a central computer to divide the workload.

distributing artery, an artery with a tunica media composed of circularly arranged smooth muscle. It receives blood from conducting arteries and distributes the blood to organs and tissues. Also called **muscular artery.**

distribution, the location of medications in various organs and tissues after administration. The concentration of highly water-soluble drugs may be greater in persons who are elderly, dehydrated, or febrile because they have less total body water for dilution of the substance. As the lean muscle mass decreases and body fat increases, drugs that are distributed primarily in body fat have a more prolonged effect.

distributive analysis and synthesis /distrib''yətiv/, the system of psychotherapy used by the psychobiological school of psychiatry. It involves an extensive and systematic investigation and analysis of a person's total past experiences to discover the emotional factors underlying personality problems and ways they can be synthesized into constructive behavioral patterns.

distributive care, a pattern of health care that is concerned with environment, heredity, living conditions, lifestyle, and early detection of pathological effects. The system is usually directed to continuous care of persons not confined to hospitals or other health care facilities.

district [L, *distringere,* to compel], **1.** (in hospital nursing) a group of patients in an area of the unit for whom a nurse manager or primary nurse is responsible. Patients are customarily assigned to a district on the basis of certain shared needs for nursing care. **2.** the area of a city or town assigned to a public health nurse.

district nurse. See **public health nursing.**

disulfiram /dīsul''firam/, an alcohol-use deterrent.

■ INDICATIONS: It is prescribed as a deterrent to drinking alcohol in the treatment of chronic alcoholism. It causes severe intestinal cramping, diaphoresis, and nausea and vomiting if alcohol is ingested. It requires that the patient explicitly know that, when combined with alcohol intake, death may occur.

■ CONTRAINDICATIONS: Alcoholic intoxication; recent or concomitant administration of metronidazole, paraldehyde, or alcohol; severe myocardial disease; coronary occlusion; psychosis; or known hypersensitivity to this drug prohibits its use.

■ ADVERSE EFFECTS: The most serious adverse reactions, which include optic neuritis, psychotic reaction, and polyneuritis, result from alcohol ingestion. Drowsiness, headache, and skin rash may occur. This drug interacts with several other drugs, such as metronidazole and warfarin.

disuse phenomena /disyōōs''/ [L, *dis* + *usus,* to make use of; Gk, *phainein,* to show], the physical and psychological changes, usually degenerative, that result from the lack of use of a body part or system. Disuse phenomena are associated with confinement and immobility, especially in orthopedics. Individuals deprived of sufficient interaction with the world around them may lose motivation and acquired abilities because of lack of practice. Pain and therapeutic narcotic drugs commonly associated with the treatment of many illnesses and abnormal conditions contribute to disuse phenomena. See also **hypostatic pneumonia.**

■ OBSERVATIONS: The physical changes often induced by continued bed rest constitute problems that affect many key areas and systems of the body, such as the skin, the musculoskeletal system, the GI tract, the cardiovascular system, and the respiratory system. Contractures are usually caused by flexion, because patients flex knees and hips whenever possible to relax muscles, especially when cold or in pain. The immobilized patient may experience bone demineralization caused by a restricted diet and decreased motility. The patient immobilized by a fracture, even if not confined to bed, may show signs of disuse phenomena. Muscle action is required to maintain blood flow to the bones, and the immobilized patient may not be capable of sufficient muscular activity to assure such blood flow, with its attendant delivery of critical nutrients and oxygen. The pooling of respiratory secretions is another disuse phenomenon caused by immobility and the horizontal position of the patient on bed rest.

■ INTERVENTIONS: Some common therapeutic measures for disuse phenomena are improvement of diet and nutrition, proper positioning and regular movement of the patient, meticulous hygiene, scrupulous skin care, and positive social interaction with the patient. Special alternating pressurized beds, a regular program of therapy, and range-of-motion machines for extremities may be used to improve circulation and muscle strength. The optimal care of patients with disuse phenomena, regardless of cause, requires a coordinated approach by a health care team.

■ PATIENT CARE CONSIDERATIONS: With appropriate rehabilitation this condition is usually curable and sometimes preventable.

Ditropan, an antispasmodic drug. Brand name for **oxybutynin chloride.**

Diucardin, a diuretic. Brand name for **hydroflumethiazide.**

Diupres, a fixed-combination drug containing a diuretic and an antihypertensive. Brand name for **chlorothiazide, reserpine.**

diurese /dī″yo͞orēs/, the act of increasing urine output. See also **diuresis.**

diuresis /dī″yo͞orē″sis/ [Gk, *dia,* through, *ouron,* urine], increased formation and secretion of urine. Diuresis occurs in conditions such as diabetes mellitus, diabetes insipidus, and acute renal failure. It is normal in the first 48 hours after giving birth. Coffee, tea, certain foods, diuretic drugs, anxiety, fear, and some steroids cause diuresis.

diuresis renography, the administration to a well-hydrated patient with an empty bladder of a radiopharmaceutical agent and 20 minutes later a diuretic, such as furosemide. The pattern of washout of the radiopharmaceutical is monitored to assess first the functioning of the collecting system and then the transport capacity of the upper urinary tract.

diuretic /dī″yo͞oret″ik/, **1.** *adj.,* (of a drug or other substance) tending to promote the formation and excretion of urine. **2.** *n.,* a drug that promotes the formation and excretion of urine. The more than 50 diuretic drugs available in the United States and Canada are classified by chemical structure and pharmacological activity into groups: carbonic anhydrase inhibitors, loop diuretics, mercurials, osmotics, potassium-sparing diuretics, and thiazides. A diuretic medication may contain drugs from one or more of these groups. Diuretics are prescribed to reduce the volume of extracellular fluid in the treatment of many disorders, including hypertension, congestive heart failure, and edema. The specific drug to be prescribed is selected according to the action desired and the patient's physical status. Hypersensitivity to sulfonamides prohibits use of many diuretic drugs, and diabetes mellitus may be aggravated by thiazide medications. Thus the presence of a particular condition may prohibit the use of a particular agent. Several adverse reactions, including hypovolemia and electrolyte imbalance, are common to all diuretics. Mercurial diuretics are rarely used because of their nephrotoxicity, and carbonic anhydrase inhibitors have only weak diuretic activity.

diuretic ceiling effect, the effect of possible increased drug toxicity without additional clinical benefit with the administration of more than a certain amount of diuretic drugs in a 24-hour period. Different diuretic drugs have different ceilings.

Diuril, a thiazide diuretic. Brand name for **chlorothiazide.**

diurnal /dīyo͞or″nəl/ [L, *diurnalis,* of a day], happening daily, as sleeping and eating.

diurnal enuresis [L, *diurnalis,* of a day; Gk, *enourein,* to urinate], a lack of control of urination during waking, daylight hours.

diurnal mood variation, a change in mood that is related to the time of day. Examples are commonly found in differences between "night people" and "morning people."

diurnal rhythm [L, *diurnalis,* of a day; Gk, *rhythmos*], patterns of activity or behavior that follow day-night cycles, such as breakfast-lunch-dinner schedules. See also **circadian rhythm.**

diurnal variation, **1.** the variability of output or excretion of a substance during the day versus the night or over a 12-hour interval. **2.** expected high and low levels of a substance during a 24-hour period. For example, blood cortisol is highest in the morning and lowest in the early evening.

divalent, (in chemistry) an atom with two additional or two missing electrons producing a dianion (e.g., O^{2-}) or a dication (e.g., Ca^{2+}), respectively.

divalproex sodium, an anticonvulsant drug used to treat epilepsy and seizures, controlling simple and complex absence seizures alone or in combination with other anticonvulsant drugs. It is also approved for the treatment of migraines.

■ INDICATIONS: It is prescribed to prevent or reduce the number of seizures by decreasing the activity of nerve impulses in the brain and central nervous system. It is converted to valproic acid in the body.

■ CONTRAINDICATIONS: It should not be given to patients with an allergy to valproic acid, sodium valproate, or divalproex or to those with liver disease.

■ ADVERSE EFFECTS: The side effects most often reported include changes in appetite, nausea, vomiting, stomach cramps, diarrhea, constipation, weakness, tiredness, clumsiness, drowsiness, or behavioral changes.

divergence /divur″jəns/ [L, *di* + *vergere,* to incline], a separation or movement of objects away from each other in the opposite direction, as in the simultaneous turning of the eyes outward as a result of an extraocular muscle defect.

divergent dislocation /divur″jənt/, the temporary displacement of two bones, such as the radius and ulna.

divergent squint. See **exotropia.**

divergent strabismus. See **exotropia.**

diverging lens. See **concave spherical lens.**

diver's palsy, diver's paralysis, (Nontechnical) now called **decompression sickness.**

diverticula, diverticular. See **diverticulum.**

Colonic diverticula *(Feldman, Friedman, and Brandt, 2016)*

diverticular disease, diverticulosis. See **diverticulitis, diverticulosis.**

diverticulectomy /dī′vurtik′yo͞olek″təmē/, surgical removal of a diverticulum.

diverticulitis /dī′vurtik′yo͞olī″tis/ [L, *diverticulare,* to turn aside; Gk, *itis,* inflammation], inflammation of one or more diverticula. The penetration of fecal matter through the thin-walled diverticula causes inflammation and abscess formation in the tissues surrounding the colon. With repeated inflammation the lumen of the colon narrows and may become obstructed. Compare **diverticulosis.**

■ OBSERVATIONS: During periods of inflammation the patient experiences crampy pain, particularly over the sigmoid colon; fever; and leukocytosis. Barium enemas and proctoscopy are used to rule out carcinoma of the colon, which exhibits some of the same symptoms.

■ INTERVENTIONS: Conservative treatment includes rest, IV fluids, antibiotics, and abstaining from eating and drinking. In acute cases bowel resection of the affected part greatly reduces mortality and morbidity rates.

■ PATIENT CARE CONSIDERATIONS: A high-fiber diet and the avoidance of red meats can decrease the development of diverticula and inflammation leading to diverticulits.

diverticulosis /dī′vurtik′yo͞olō″sis/ [L, *diverticulare,* to turn aside; Gk, *osis,* condition], the presence of pouchlike herniations through the muscular layer of the colon, particularly the sigmoid colon. Diverticulosis affects increasing numbers of people over 50 years of age and may be the result of the modern highly refined low-residue diet. Most patients with this condition have few symptoms except occasional bleeding from the rectum. Other reasons for bleeding, such as hemorrhoids, carcinoma, and inflammatory bowel disease, must be ruled out. Barium enemas and proctoscopic examination are used in establishing diagnosis. An increase in dietary fiber intake can aid in propelling the feces through the colon. Avoidance of foods with seeds and nuts decreases the risk of fecal material lodging in the diverticula. Hemorrhage from bleeding diverticula can become quite severe, and the patient may require surgery. Diverticulosis may lead to diverticulitis. See also **diverticulitis.**

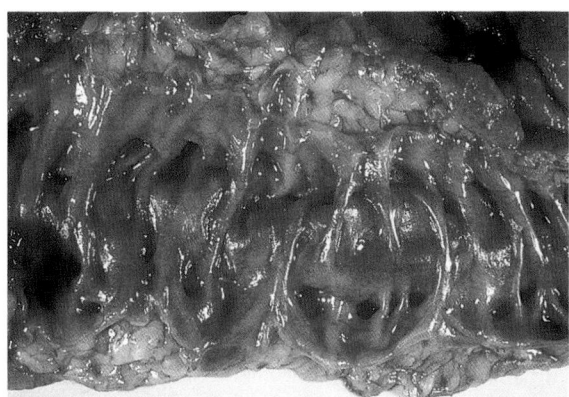

Diverticulosis of the sigmoid colon *(Cross, 2013)*

diverticulum /dī′vurtik″yo͞oləm/ *pl. diverticula* [L, *diverticulare,* to turn aside], a pouchlike herniation through the muscular wall of a tubular organ. A diverticulum may be present in the stomach, the small intestine, or, most commonly, the large intestine. It is typically detected by radiography after the ingestion of a radiopaque substance. See also **diverticulitis, diverticulosis, Meckel diverticulum.** −*diverticular, adj.*

divided dose, a measured fraction of a full dose of a medication, given at short intervals so that the full dose is eventually taken within a specified period.

diving, the act of work or recreation in an underwater environment. The main health effects are related to the increased pressure to which the person is subjected as the ambient pressure generally increases by 1 atm (14.7 pounds per square inch) for each 33 feet of descent below the water surface. Conditions that warrant caution about diving include obesity, diabetes, alcoholism, epilepsy, drug abuse, and respiratory disorders, including allergic rhinitis. See also **decompression sickness, diving reflex.**

diving goiter [AS, *dyypan,* to dip; L, *guttur,* throat], a large movable thyroid goiter located at times above the sternal notch and at other times below the notch. Also called **plunging goiter, wandering goiter.**

diving reflex, a neural mechanism that produces an automatic change in the cardiovascular system when the face and nose are immersed in cold water. The heart rate decreases and the blood pressure remains stable or increases slightly, while blood flow to all parts of the body except the brain is reduced, thereby helping the body to conserve oxygen. The reflex occurs in humans and other mammals. It is sometimes used in the treatment of paroxysmal tachycardias. The reflex extends the duration of the viability of brain cells during apnea beyond the usual period of 5 to 10 minutes. For this reason, cardiopulmonary resuscitation should always be attempted in drowning victims regardless of their time under water.

division [L, *dividere,* to divide], **1.** an administrative subunit in a hospital, such as a division of medical nursing or a division of surgical nursing. **2.** (in public health nursing) an area that encompasses several geographic districts. **3.** the separation of something into two or more parts or sections, such as cell division.

divorce therapy, a type of counseling that attempts to help divorced couples disengage from their former relationship and dysfunctional behavior toward each other or their children.

Dix, Dorothea Lynde [1802–1887], an American humanitarian who achieved fame as a social reformer primarily for her work in improving prison conditions and care of the mentally ill. During her lifetime she helped to establish mental institutions in 30 states and in Canada. During the U.S. Civil War she was appointed superintendent of army nurses for government hospitals.

Dix-Hallpike test /hôl′pīk/ [M.R. Dix, 20th-century otholaryngologist and C.S. Hallpike, English otologist, 1900–1979], a method for evaluating the function of the vestibule of the ear in patients with vertigo or hearing loss. The patient's position is quickly changed from sitting to lying down with the neck hyperextended and then returned to sitting or rotated 45 degrees to one side and then the other. Nystagmus can then be evaluated, and specific disorders of the vestibule may be diagnosed. See also **caloric test, electronystagmography, benign paroxysmal positional vertigo, nystagmus.**

dizygotic /dī′zīgot″ik/ [Gk, *di,* twice, *zygotos,* yolked together], pertaining to twins from two fertilized ova. Compare **monozygotic.** See also **twinning.**

dizygotic twins, two offspring born of the same pregnancy and developed from two ova that were released from the ovary simultaneously and fertilized at the same time. They may be of the same or opposite sex, differ both physically and genetically, and have two separate and distinct placentas and membranes, both amnion and chorion. The frequency of dizygotic twinning varies according to ethnic origin (the highest incidence occurs in African-Americans, the lowest in Asian-Americans, with Caucasians intermediate), maternal age (the highest rate occurs when the mother is 35 to 39 years of age), and heredity (showing an increase in the female genetic line rather than the male, although fathers may transmit the disposition to double ovulation to their daughters).

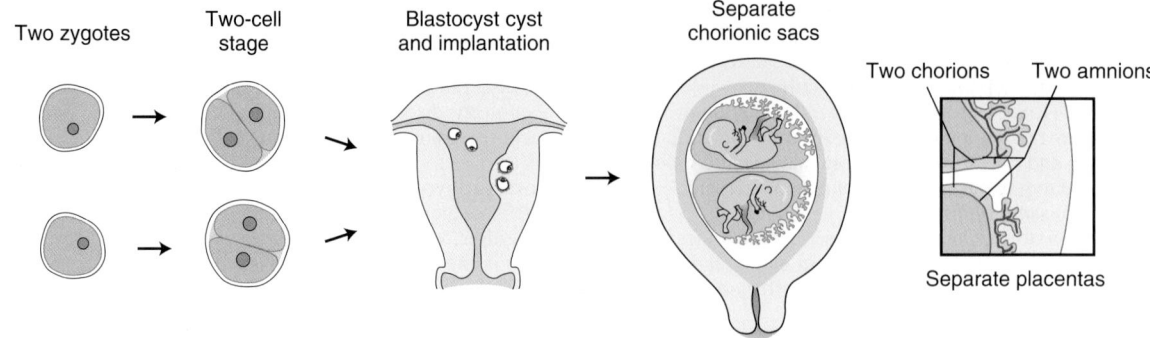

Development of dizygotic twins *(Hagen-Ansert, 2012)*

In general, the overall ratio is two thirds dizygotic twinning to one third monozygotic. Also called **binovular twins, false twins, fraternal twins, heterologous twins,** *dissimilar twins.*

dizziness [AS, *dysig,* stupid], a sensation of faintness and whirling or an inability to maintain normal balance in a standing or seated position, sometimes associated with giddiness, mental confusion, nausea, and weakness. Sometimes the room seems to spin, sometimes the individual (a sensation known as vertigo). A person who experiences dizziness should be carefully lowered to a safe position on a bed, chair, or floor because of the danger of injury from falling. Compare **syncope.** See also **vertigo.**

DKA, abbreviation for **diabetic ketoacidosis.**

dL, abbreviation for **deciliter.**

DLE, abbreviation for **discoid lupus erythematosus.**

DLEK, abbreviation for **deep lamellar endothelial keratoplasty.**

D log E curve. See *characteristic curve.*

DM, abbreviation for **diabetes mellitus.**

DMARD, abbreviation for **disease-modifying antirheumatic drug.**

D.M.D., a professional with a degree in the practice of oral medicine treatment, prevention, and maintenance. Abbreviation for *Doctor of Dental Medicine.* Compare **D.D.S.** See also **dentist.**

DMSO, abbreviation for **dimethyl sulfoxide.**

DNA, abbreviation for **deoxyribonucleic acid.**

DNA amplification, artificial increase in the number of copies of a particular DNA fragment into millions of copies through replication of the segment into which it has been cloned, a type of nucleic acid amplification.

DNA blotting, the transfer of separated DNA fragments from an electrophoretic gel to a membrane (e.g., nitrocellulose). Also called **Southern blot test.**

DNA chimera /kīmē″rə/, a recombinant molecule of DNA composed of segments from more than one source.

DNA-DNA hybridization, the formation of double-helical DNA from two complementary single strands. It is used to compare genome relationships between different species.

DNA fingerprint, the highly specific hybridization pattern generated by tandem repeats and other patterns of the DNA in an individual's genome.

DNA fingerprinting, a technique for comparing the nucleotide sequences of fragments of DNA from different sources. The fragments are obtained by treating the DNA with various endonucleases, enzymes that break DNA strands at specific sites. There is a chance of 1 in 30 billion that two persons who are not monozygotic twins would have identical DNA fingerprints. To resolve the complexities of the process, short, tandemly repeated, highly specific "minisatellite" genomic sequences are used. A wild-type M13 bacteriophage that identifies the differences is confined to two clusters of 15-base-pair repeats in the protein III gene of the bacteriophage. The specificity of the probe makes it applicable to questions of forensic science.

DNA gyrase, an enzyme that nicks and seals the DNA and relieves supercoiling.

DNA helicase, an enzyme that catalyzes the energy-dependent unwinding of the DNA double helix during DNA replication.

DNA library, a collection of DNA fragments of one organism, each carried by a plasmid or virus and cloned in an appropriate host. A DNA probe is used to locate a specific DNA sequence in the library. A collection representing the entire genome is called a genomic library. An assortment of DNA copies of messenger RNA produced by a cell is known as a complimentary DNA (cDNA) library. Also called **gene library.** See also **DNA probe.**

DNA ligase, an enzyme that can repair breaks in a strand of deoxyribonucleic acid (DNA) by synthesizing a bond between adjoining nucleotides. Under some circumstances the enzyme can join together loose ends of DNA strands, and in some cases it can repair breaks in ribonucleic acid (RNA). It serves as a catalyst.

DNA nucleotidyltransferase. Also called **DNA polymerase.**

DNA polymerase, (in molecular genetics) an enzyme that catalyzes the assembly of deoxyribonucleoside triphosphates into deoxyribonucleic acid, with single-stranded DNA serving as the template. The enzyme is often found in tumor cells. Also called **DNA nucleotidyltransferase.**

DNA probe, a labeled segment of DNA or RNA used to find a specific sequence of nucleotides in a DNA molecule. Probes may be synthesized in the laboratory with a sequence complementary to the target DNA sequence.

DNAR, abbreviation for **do not attempt resuscitation.**

DNCB, abbreviation for *2,4-dinitrochlorobenzene.*

DNP, 1. abbreviation for **2,4-dinitrophenol,** *2,4-dinitrophenyl.* **2.** initialism for **Doctor of Nursing Practice.**

DNR, abbreviation for **do not resuscitate.** See **no code.**

D.O., abbreviation for *Doctor of Osteopathy.* See also **physician.**

DOA, initialism for *dead on arrival.*

Dobie globule /dō″bē/ [William M. Dobie, English physician, 1828–1915], a very small stainable body in the transparent disk of a striated muscle fiber.

DOBUTamine hydrochloride /dōbyoo″təmēn/, a beta-adrenergic stimulating agent, acting primarily on beta$_1$ receptors.

■ INDICATIONS: It is prescribed to increase cardiac output in severe chronic congestive heart failure and to provide adjunct in cardiac surgery.

■ CONTRAINDICATIONS: Idiopathic hypertrophic subaortic stenosis or known hypersensitivity to this drug prohibits its use. It is not recommended for use in pregnancy.

■ ADVERSE EFFECTS: Among the most serious adverse reactions are cardiovascular effects, including tachycardia, hypertension, arrhythmias, and precipitation of angina. Nausea, vomiting, and headache may also occur.

Dobutrex, a synthetic catecholamine that stimulates beta-adrenergic receptors. It has many drug interactions. Brand name for **DOBUTamine hydrochloride.**

Dock, Lavinia Lloyd, an American public health nurse. A graduate of the Bellevue Hospital Training School for Nurses in New York in 1886, she started a visiting nurse service in Norwalk, Connecticut. She then joined the New York City Mission before becoming an assistant to Isabel Hampton Robb at Johns Hopkins Hospital in Baltimore. She returned to public health nursing when she joined the Henry Street Settlement in New York to work with Lillian Wald. She advocated an international public health movement and the improvement of education for nurses. With M. Adelaide Nutting, she wrote *History of Nursing,* a classic in nursing literature.

docosanol /doko′sänol/, an antiviral agent effective against activity viruses with a lipid envelope, including herpes simplex virus. It is used topically in the treatment of recurrent herpes labialis.

doctoral program in nursing, an educational program that offers preparation for a doctoral degree in the field of nursing designed to prepare nurses for advanced practice, academia, and research. On satisfactory completion of the course of study, the Ph.D. with a major in nursing, a degree of D.N.Sc. (Doctor of Nursing Science), D.S.N. (Doctor of Science in Nursing), or D.N.P. (Doctor of Nursing Practice) is awarded.

Doctor of Medicine, Doctor of Osteopathy. See **physician.**

Doctor of Nursing Practice (DNP), a terminal degree for advanced practice registered nurses (APRNs) and other registered nurses preparing for senior clinical positions.

Doctor of Occupational Therapy (DrOT, OTD), a postprofessional degree for occupational therapists preparing for leadership roles in the practice of occupational therapy.

Doctor of Physical Therapy (DPT), a terminal degree for physical therapists preparing for leadership roles in the practice of physical therapy.

Doctor of Public Health (DrPH), a terminal degree for public health professionals whose careers focus on research, education, and management within the public health sector.

documentation /dok′yəmentā″shən/ [L, *documentum,* proof], **1.** a written or electronic record of the health care provided to a patient. The specific requirements and format vary by profession, institution, and payer. See also **charting. 2.** written material associated with a computer or a program. Kinds of documentation include user documentation, an instruction manual that provides enough information to allow an individual to use the system; system documentation, a complete description of the hardware and software that make up a system; and program documentation, a description of what a program does and how it does it.

docusate /dok″yoosāt/, a stool softener. Also called **dioctyl calcium sulfosuccinate, dioctyl potassium sulfosuccinate, dioctyl sodium sulfosuccinate.**

■ INDICATIONS: It is prescribed in the treatment of constipation.

■ CONTRAINDICATIONS: Signs or symptoms of appendicitis, concomitant administration of mineral oil, or known hypersensitivity to the drug prohibits its use.

■ ADVERSE EFFECTS: No serious adverse reactions are known.

Dodd, Marylin J., a nursing theorist who, with Carolyn L. Wiener, developed the Theory of Illness Trajectory, which involves not only the patient but the family and caregivers. The theory helps elucidate how patients and families tolerate the states of uncertainty caused by the illness and manage the illness.

Döderlein's bacillus /dā″dərlīnz, dō″dərlēnz/ [Albert S. Döderlein, German physician, 1860–1941], a gram-positive bacterium present in normal vaginal secretions.

dofetilide, a class III antidysrhythmic.

■ INDICATIONS: It is used to treat atrial fibrillation and flutter.

■ CONTRAINDICATIONS: Known hypersensitivity to this drug, digitalis toxicity, aortic stenosis, pulmonary hypertension, QT syndromes, and severe renal disease prohibit its use. It is also contraindicated in children.

■ ADVERSE EFFECTS: Serious adverse effects include severe diarrhea, anorexia, angina, premature ventricular contractions, substernal pressure, transient hypertension, and precipitation of angina. Common side effects include syncope, dizziness, nausea, vomiting, hypotension, postural hypotension, and bradycardia.

doff /dôf/ [ME, contraction of *dooff,* take off], to take off (clothing).

Döhle-Heller disease. See **syphilitic aortitis.**

Döhle's inclusion bodies /dā″les, dōls/ [Karl G.P. Döhle, German pathologist, 1855–1928], blue inclusions in the cytoplasm of some leukocytes in May-Hegglin anomaly and in blood smears from patients with acute viral infections.

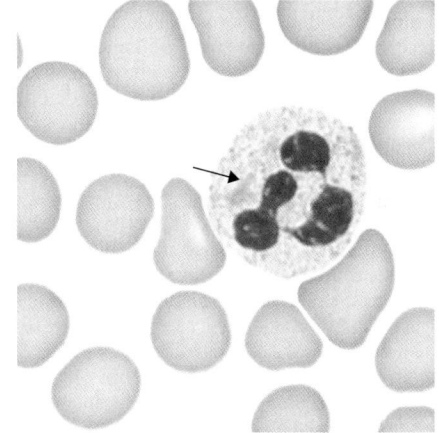

Döhle's inclusion bodies *(Carr and Rodak, 2013)*

dolasetron, an antiemetic.

■ INDICATIONS: It is used to prevent the nausea and vomiting associated with cancer chemotherapy and radiotherapy and to prevent postoperative nausea and vomiting.

■ CONTRAINDICATIONS: Known hypersensitivity prohibits its use.

■ ADVERSE EFFECTS: Bronchospasm and arrhythmias are life-threatening effects of this drug. Other adverse reactions include constipation, increased AST and ALT, abdominal pain, anorexia, dizziness, fatigue, drowsiness, rash, urinary retention, oliguria, electrocardiogram changes, hypotension, tachycardia, and hypertension. Common side effects include diarrhea and headache.

dolicho-, prefix meaning "long": *dolichocephaly.*

dolichocephaly, an elongated skull. See **scaphocephaly.**

doll's-eye reflex, a normal response in newborns to keep the eyes stationary as the head is moved to the right or left. The reflex disappears as ocular fixation develops. It is also evaluated in comatose children for assessment of cranial nerve (III, IV, VI) function. In adults, it is used to evaluate brainstem function in a comatose patient. After determining the absence of cervical injury, the examiner quickly moves the head to the side. The eyes should deviate in the direction opposite to the head's movement; loss of this reflex suggests dysfunction of brainstem or oculomotor nerves; inferolateral deviation of the eyes in combination with pupillary dilation implies dysfunction of the third cranial nerve, possibly due to tentorial herniation. See also **doll's head maneuver.**

doll's head maneuver, the rotation of the head from side to side to elicit the doll's-eye reflex. It is contraindicated if spinal cord injury is suspected. See also **doll's-eye reflex.**

Dolobid, a nonsteroidal antiinflammatory agent. Brand name for **diflunisal.**

Dolophine Hydrochloride, an opioid agonist analgesic. Brand name for **methadone hydrochloride.**

dolor /dō″lôr/ [L, pain], any condition of physical pain, mental anguish, or suffering. It is one of the four signs of inflammation. The others are calor (heat), rubor (redness), and tumor (swelling).

DOM, abbreviation for **dimethoxymethylamphetamine.**

domain, **1.** a region of a protein or polypeptide whose three-dimensional configuration enables it to interact specifically with particular receptors, enzymes, or other proteins. **2.** a sphere of knowledge, influence, or activity.

dome of pleura. See **cervical pleura.**

domestic abuse, abuse or violence commonly describing spouse or partner abuse, including physical and/or sexual violence (use of physical force) or threats of such violence or psychological and/or emotional abuse and/or coercive tactics. Also called **intimate partner violence.**

■ OBSERVATIONS: The individual may have no obvious signs of physical injury but may present with vague complaints, such as sleep and appetite disturbances, fatigue, dizziness, weight change, and symptoms associated with depression, anxiety, or posttraumatic stress. Illnesses, such as gastrointestinal and autoimmune disorders, have also been associated with abuse. Women also seek help for problems that are seemingly unrelated to abuse (e.g., a blood pressure check, a routine physical, treatment of allergies, or an upper respiratory infection). Physical abuse signs include bruising (face, neck, arms, legs, abdomen, or back), cuts, broken bones, black eyes, burns, marks of strangulation, wounds or bruises at different stages of healing, and swelling or puffiness in the face or around the eyes. Other signs include a history that does not match the presenting injuries and reports of being hit or injured. Signs of sexual abuse include bruising around the breasts or genitalia; genitalia, vaginal, or rectal swelling or lacerations; torn, stained, or bloody underclothing; and reports of being assaulted or raped. Manifestations of emotional abuse include reports of intimidation (such as looks, gestures, yelling, and throwing objects), threats to harm children, isolation from family and friends, and economic domination. The Abuse Assessment Screen is used for initial screening and is used for all high-risk individuals. Further definitive diagnosis is typically made by social service, health care, and legal experts after a more detailed history, investigation, and physical examination. Severe injury, disfigurement, and death are all complications of chronic and/or severe physical abuse.

■ INTERVENTIONS: Obvious signs of abuse should be reported immediately to appropriate local authorities for prompt investigation and victim protection. If the individual is perceived to be in immediate danger, protection should be sought through local Adult Protective Services or county Department of Social Services. Vague or inconsistent manifestations should be documented and referred for further evaluation and investigation.

■ PATIENT CARE CONSIDERATIONS: Health care providers serve as a frontline resource for the detection, intervention, and prevention of domestic abuse. This includes the identification of high-risk dependent domestic relationships, such as previous history of abuse or violence, feelings of worthlessness, inability to trust, high index of suspicion, substance abuse, depression, social isolation, financial dependence, poverty, homelessness, unemployment, intense family responsibilities, and inappropriate or fearful interaction patterns with spouse. Referrals for counseling to prevent or halt abuse and placement for safe haven are needed. Social agency referrals should be made for financial assistance, food, clothing, and shelter needs. Prevention activities center on raising individual and community awareness through education about the incidence and causes of domestic violence, provision of empowerment and assertiveness training, and screening of all women ages 14 and older as required of all health care settings by The Family Violence Prevention Fund and The Joint Commission on Healthcare.

dominance /dom″inəns/ [L, *dominari*, to rule], the property of an allele in which the allele is fully expressed in the phenotype, even when only one copy of the allele is present. See also **autosomal-dominant inheritance, recessive allele, segregation. –dominant,** *adj.*

dominant /dom″inənt/ [L, *dominari*, to rule], **1.** exerting a ruling or controlling influence. **2.** in genetics, capable of expression when carried by only one of a pair of homologous chromosomes. **3.** in coronary artery anatomy, supplying the posterior diaphragmatic part of the interventricular septum and the diaphragmatic surface of the left ventricle; said of the right and left coronary arteries.

dominant allele [L, *dominari*, to rule; Gk, *genein*, to produce], one of two or more alternative forms of a gene that is fully expressed in a heterozygote. Compare **recessive allele.**

dominant eye /dom″inənt/, the eye that is customarily used for monocular tasks. It may or may not be related to hand preference.

dominant group, a social group that controls the value system and rewards in a particular society.

dominant idiotype, a segment of an immunoglobulin molecule that is present on a large proportion of the immunoglobulins generated in response to a particular antigen. See also **idiotype.**

dominant trait, an inherited characteristic that is determined by a dominant allele. Polydactyly is an example of a dominant trait; individuals with either one or two copies of the polydactyly allele have extra fingers or toes.

don /don/ [ME, contraction of *doon,* put on], to put on (clothing).

Donath-Landsteiner syndrome /dō″notland″stīnər/ [Julius Donath, Austrian physician, 1870–1960; Karl Landsteiner, Austrian-American pathologist, 1868–1943], a rare blood disorder marked by hemolysis minutes or hours after exposure to cold. Systemic symptoms include the passage of dark urine, severe pain in the back and legs, headache, vomiting, diarrhea, and moderate reticulocytosis. Temporary hepatosplenomegaly and mild hyperbilirubinemia may follow the onset of an attack. The condition may occur with congenital or acquired syphilis, in which case antisyphilitic treatment is used. Also called **paroxysmal cold hemoglobinuria.**

donation /dōna′shun/, **1.** a gift. **2.** the act of giving.

Done nomogram, a graph on which a number of variables are plotted so that the value of a dependent variable can be read on the appropriate line when the values of the other variables are given.

donepezil, a reversible cholinesterase.
- INDICATIONS: It is used to treat mild to moderate dementia in Alzheimer disease.
- CONTRAINDICATIONS: Known hypersensitivity to this drug or to piperidine derivatives prohibits its use.
- ADVERSE EFFECTS: Life-threatening effects include seizures and atrial fibrillation. Other adverse effects are dizziness, somnolence, fatigue, abnormal dreams, syncope, hypotension or hypertension, anorexia, urinary frequency, urinary tract infection, incontinence, rash, flushing, rhinitis, upper respiratory infection, cough, pharyngitis, cramps, and arthritis. Common side effects include insomnia, headache, nausea, vomiting, and diarrhea.

dong quai, a perennial herb found in Japan, China, and Korea.
- INDICATIONS: It is used to promote women's health; for a variety of gynecological, menstrual, and menopausal symptoms; and to treat cirrhosis of the liver. Current research suggests it is ineffective for treating menopausal symptoms, and there are insufficient data to gauge its effectiveness for other indications.
- CONTRAINDICATIONS: It should not be used during pregnancy, in children, or in those with known hypersensitivity. It is contraindicated in people with bleeding disorders, excessive menstrual flow, or acute illness.

Donnatal, a fixed-combination drug containing a sedative and three anticholinergics, used to decrease the motility of the GI tract. Brand name for **phenobarbital, hyoscyamine, atropine, scopolamine.**

Donohue syndrome [William Donohue, Canadian pathologist], a rare autosomal-recessive genetic disorder marked by insulin resistance, causing slow physical and mental development with a characteristic elfin facies. Enlargement of the clitoris and breasts in females and the phallus in males also occurs. Formerly called **leprechaunism.**

donor /dō″nər/ [L, *donare,* to give], **1.** a human or other organism that gives living tissue to be used in another body, for example, blood for transfusion or a kidney for transplantation. See also **universal donor. 2.** a substance or compound that gives part of itself to another substance. Compare **acceptor.**

donor card [L, *donare,* to give, *charta*], wallet-size written documentation in which a person offers to make an anatomical gift of body parts at the time of death for transplantation to recipients needing replacement of vital organs or tissues. The information can also be found on a state driver's license. Consent for organ donation generally requires consent from family of the organ donor.

I wish to donate my organs and tissues. I wish to give:
❑ any needed organs and tissues
❑ only the following organs and tissues:
_____
Name: _____
Address: _____
Date Of Birth: _____
_____
Please share this card with family and friends
Signature: _____ Date: _____
Donate Life Missouri
573-522-2847 or 888-497-4564
www.missouriorgandonor.com

Donor card *(From the Missouri Department of Health and Senior Services)*

do not attempt resuscitation (DNAR), an advisory that resuscitation of a patient should not be attempted. Used more commonly in countries outside the United States. See **do not resuscitate.**

do not resuscitate (DNR), a part of an advanced directive that instructs health care providers that cardiopulmonary resuscitation and advanced cardiac life support should not be initiated. See **no code.**

Donovan bodies /don″əvan/ [Charles Donovan, Irish physician, 1863–1951], encapsulated gram-negative rods of the species *Calymmatobacterium granulomatis* present in the cytoplasm of mononuclear phagocytes obtained from the lesions of granuloma inguinale. They may be seen under the microscope in a Wright-stained smear of infected tissue. See also **granuloma inguinale.**

Donovanosis. See **granuloma inguinale.**

donut hole, *(Informal)* the gap between the initial phase of prescription medication coverage and catastrophic coverage related to Medicare Part D in the United States.

donut pad /dō″nut/, a pad designed to protect an injured joint. Cut to fit over the site of the injury, it causes the force on the body part to be transferred to surrounding areas. It is most effective for protecting small areas, such as heels or elbows.

doorknob comment, *(Informal)* a statement made by a patient or client alluding to something important in a vague way at the conclusion of an appointment.

DOOR syndrome, a rare syndrome of congenital deafness, onycho-osteodystrophy, and intellectual disability, existing in autosomal-dominant and autosomal-recessive forms.

dopa /dō″pə/, an amino acid, produced by oxidation of tyrosine that occurs naturally in plants and animals. It is a precursor of dopamine, epinephrine, norepinephrine, and melanin. See also **dopamine hydrochloride, levodopa.**

DOPamine /dō″pəmin/, a naturally occurring sympathetic nervous system neurotransmitter that is the precursor of norepinephrine. It is produced in the substantia nigra and transmitted to the putamen and caudate nucleus. It has an inhibitory effect on movement. A depletion of dopamine produces the symptoms of rigidity, tremors, and bradykinesia that are characteristic of Parkinson's disease. It is available as an intravenously injectable drug. Dopamine has potent dopaminergic, beta-adrenergic, and alpha-adrenergic receptor activity. See also **dopamine hydrochloride.**

dopamine hydrochloride, a sympathomimetic catecholamine. Lower doses preferentially stimulate peripheral dopamine receptors to cause primarily renal mesenteric vasodilation while higher doses also stimulate $beta_1$ and alpha adrenergic receptors and act to increase blood pressure.
- INDICATIONS: It is prescribed in the treatment of shock, hypotension, and low cardiac output to reduce the risk of renal failure.
- CONTRAINDICATIONS: Pheochromocytoma, tachyarrhythmias, ventricular fibrillation, or known hypersensitivity to this drug prohibits its use.
- ADVERSE EFFECTS: Among the more serious adverse reactions are arrhythmias, hypotension, hypertension, and tachycardia. These adverse reactions can be potentiated if dopamine is used concurrently with other drugs such as beta-blockers, MAO inhibitors, tricyclic antidepressants, or cocaine.

dopaminergic /dō′pəminur″jik/, having the effect of dopamine. See also **DOPamine.**

dopaminergic receptor, a protein on the surfaces of certain cells that binds specifically to the neurotransmitter dopamine. Such receptors on vascular epithelial cells, when stimulated by dopamine, cause the renal mesenteric, coronary, and cerebral arteries to dilate and the flow of blood to increase.

dopant /do′pant/, an impurity purposely added, as to a laser crystal or a semiconductor, during manufacturing to create a desired characteristic.

dope [AS, *dyppan*, to dip], *(Slang)* morphine, heroin, or another opioid; marijuana; or another substance illicitly bought or sold and often self-administered for sedative, hypnotic, euphoric, or other mood-altering purposes.

doped /dōpt/, **1.** having impurities (dopants) added purposely during manufacturing. **2.** *(Slang)* under the influence of drugs.

Doppler color flow /dop″lər/ [Christian J. Doppler, Austrian physicist and mathematician, 1803–1853], an ultrasonic technique for detecting anatomical details by color coding of velocity shifts. In cardiography blood flowing in one direction appears red, and blood flowing in the opposite direction appears blue. The technique can also indicate the velocity of red blood corpuscles moving through the circulatory system, which makes it possible to quantify the flow, measure the pressures within the heart chambers, and calculate the stroke volume. In laparoscopy, Doppler color flow allows for rapid identification and differentiation of ducts and valves in the viscera, particularly in detection and diagnosis of pancreatic and liver tumors and colorectal liver metastases. See also **Doppler ultrasonography.**

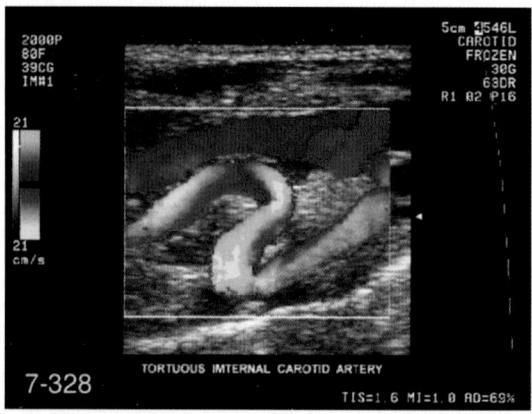

Image produced by Doppler color flow *(Hagen-Ansert, 2012)*

Doppler echocardiography [Christian J. Doppler], a technique in which Doppler ultrasonography is used to evaluate the direction and pattern of blood flow within the heart.

Doppler effect [Christian J. Doppler; L, *effectus*], the apparent change in frequency of sound or light waves emitted by a source as it moves away from or toward an observer. The frequency increases as the source moves toward the observer and decreases as it moves away, as the rising pitch of the whistle of an approaching train and the falling pitch of a departing train. The Doppler effect is also observed in electromagnetic radiation, such as light and radio waves. Also called **Doppler shift.** See also **electromagnetic radiation, ultrasonography, wavelength.**

Doppler-guided injection [Christian J. Doppler], the use of a handheld ultrasound detector to guide a needle or syringe for injecting fluid, such as in sclerotherapy to inject sclerosing fluid.

Doppler probe [Christian J. Doppler], a handheld diagnostic device that emits ultrasonic waves into the body. Reflection of the waves by a moving structure causes a change in their frequency. The Doppler probe has been used as a diagnostic tool since 1960 to study changes in blood flow in arteries and veins.

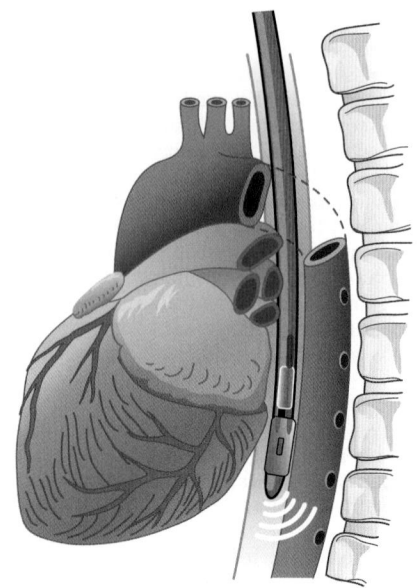

Esophageal Doppler probe *(Carlson and AACN, 2008)*

Doppler scanning. See **Doppler ultrasonography.**

Doppler shift. See **Doppler effect.**

Doppler ultrasonography [Christian J. Doppler], a technique used in ultrasound imaging to monitor moving substances or structures, such as flowing blood or a beating heart. The frequency of ultrasonic waves reflected by a moving surface is slightly different from that of the incident waves. The detected frequency shift yields information about the moving surface. The technique can be used to locate vessel obstructions, observe fetal heart sounds, localize the placenta, and image heart functions. Also called **Doppler scanning.**

Doribax, an antibiotic. Brand name for **doripenem.**

doripenem, a miscellaneous antibiotic.

■ INDICATIONS: This drug is used to treat serious infections caused by *Acinetobacter baumannii, Bacteroides caccae, B. fragilis, B. thetaiotaomicron, B. uniformis, B. vulgates, Escherichia coli, Klebsiella pneumoniae, Peptostreptococcus micros, Proteus mirabilis, Pseudomonas aeruginosa, Streptococcus contellatus, S. intermedius*; complicated urinary tract infections; pyelonephritis; and complicated intraabdominal infections.

■ CONTRAINDICATIONS: Viral infection and known hypersensitivity to this drug or to meropenem, imipenem, penicillin, or beta-lactam prohibit the use of this drug.

■ ADVERSE EFFECTS: Adverse effects of this drug include headache, diarrhea, nausea, vomiting, urticaria, phlebitis, erythema at the injection site, and pruritis. Life-threatening side effects include seizures, pseudomembranous colitis, hepatitis, Stevens-Johnson syndrome, toxic epidermal necrolysis, and anaphylaxis. A common side effect is rash.

Dormia basket, a tiny apparatus consisting of four wires that can be advanced through an endoscope into a body cavity or tube, manipulated to trap a calculus or other object, and withdrawn.

dornase alfa /dôr″nās/, a natural enzyme that depolymerizes DNA molecules. Because as much as 70% of the solid matter of purulent material consists of viscous DNA derived from the nuclei of neutrophils, dornase is used in respiratory therapy of disease such as cystic fibrosis to help break down purulent secretions in the airways. Dornase is produced with recombinant DNA technology in Chinese hamster ovary cells.

dorsal /dôr″səl/ [L, *dorsum*, the back], pertaining to the back or posterior. Compare **ventral.** See also **dorsiflect. –dorsum,** *n.*

-dorsal, suffix meaning "the back of something" or "the back": *thoracodorsal.*

dorsal column. See **posterior horn.**

dorsal decubitus position. See **supine.**

dorsal digital expansion, a triangular aponeurotic extension of the digital extensor tendon on the dorsum of the proximal phalanx of each digit to which the tendons of the lumbrical and interosseous muscles are also attached. It forms a movable hood around the metacarpophalangeal joint. Also called **extensor aponeurosis,** *hood.*

dorsal digital vein, one of the communicating veins along the sides of the fingers. The veins from the adjacent sides of the fingers unite to form three dorsal metacarpal veins, which end in a dorsal venous network on the back of the hand. Compare **basilic vein, cephalic vein, median antebrachial vein.**

dorsal flexure [L, *dorsalis,* back, *flectere,* to bend], the dorsal convexity of the thoracic region of the spine.

dorsalgia, back pain. See **dorsodynia.**

dorsal horn [L, *dorsalis,* back; AS, horn]. See **posterior horn.**

dorsal impaction syndrome, dorsal wrist pain after weight-bearing activities involving hyperextension, as may occur in weight lifting and gymnastics. Treatment includes rest, ice, antiinflammatory drugs, and technique modification.

dorsal inertia posture, a tendency of a debilitated or weak person to slip downward in bed when the head of the bed is raised. Because of loss of muscular strength or mental apathy, the person seems unable to adjust to a new position in bed.

dorsal interossei of the foot, the most superior muscles in the sole of the foot that abduct the second to fourth toes. These four muscles also act through the dorsal expansions to resist extension of the metatarsophalangeal joints and flexion of the interphalangeal joints.

dorsal interossei of the hand, four muscles between and attached to the shafts of the metacarpals.

dorsal interventricular artery, the arterial branch of the right coronary artery, branching to supply both ventricles. It runs down the dorsal sulcus two thirds of the way to the apex of the heart. Also called **right interventricular artery.**

dorsalis pedis artery, the continuation of the anterior tibial artery, starting at the ankle joint, dividing into five branches, and supplying various muscles of the foot and toes. Its branches are the lateral tarsal, medial tarsal, arcuate, first dorsal metatarsal, and deep plantar arteries.

dorsalis pedis pulse, the pulse of the dorsalis pedis artery, palpable at the prominent arch of the top of the foot between the first and second metatarsal bones. It is congenitally absent in approximately 10% of individuals.

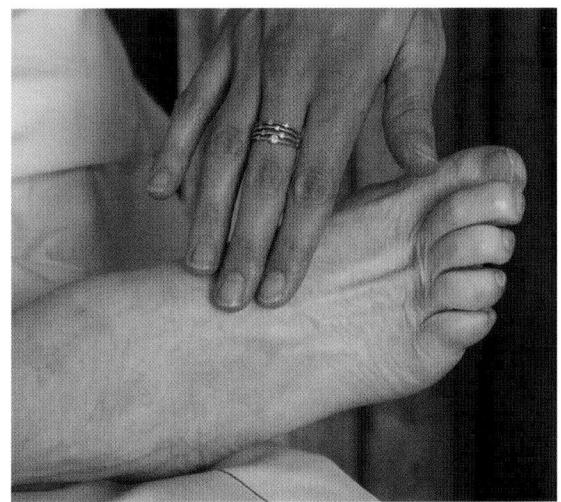

Palpating the dorsalis pedis pulse *(Ehrlich, 2013)*

dorsal lip, the marginal fold of the blastopore during gastrulation in the early stages of embryonic development of many animals. It marks the dorsal limit of the developing embryo, constitutes the primary organizer, gives rise to neural tissue, and corresponds to the primitive node in humans and higher animals.

dorsal nasal artery, a terminal branch of the ophthalmic artery that exits the orbit in the medial corner and supplies the dorsum of the nose.

dorsal position, lying on the back. See **supine position.**

dorsal recumbent [L, *dorsalis,* back; *recumbere,* to lie down], lying on the back, as in a supine position.

dorsal recumbent position [L, *dorsalis,* back, *positio*], the supine position with the person resting on the back, head, and shoulders.

dorsal reflex. See **erector spinae reflex.**

dorsal rigid posture, a position in which a patient lying in bed holds one or both legs drawn up to the chest. It often involves only the right leg and is intended to relieve the pain of appendicitis, peritonitis, kidney stones, or pelvic inflammation.

dorsal root [L, *dorsalis,* back; AS, *rot*], the sensory component or posterior root of a spinal nerve, attached centrally to the spinal cord.

dorsal root ganglion [L, *dorsalis* + AS, *rot* + Gk, *ganglion,* knot], a swelling consisting of sensory neuron cell bodies whose axons constitute the dorsal root of a spinal nerve.

dorsal scapular nerve, one of a pair of supraclavicular branches from the roots of the brachial plexus. It supplies the rhomboideus major and the rhomboideus minor and sends a branch to the levator scapulae.

dorsi-. See **dorso-, dorsi-.**

dorsiflect /dôr″siflekt/ [L, *dorsum* + *flectere,* to bend], to bend or flex backward, as in the upward bending of the fingers, wrist, foot, or toes.

dorsiflexion /dôr″siflek″shən/, to bend or flex backward, that is, to extend, as the wrist, from the anatomical position. See also **dorsiflexor.** −**dorsiflect,** *v.*

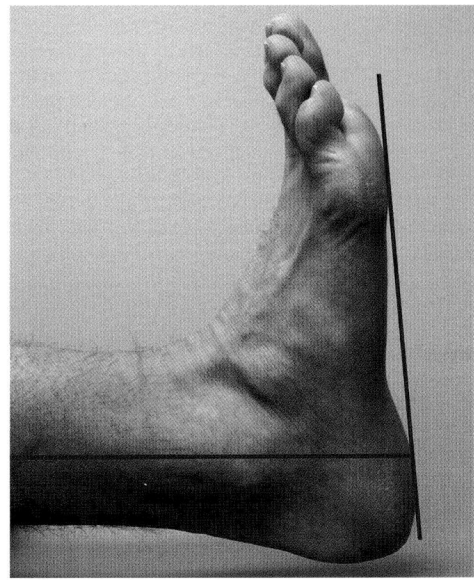

Dorsiflexion of the ankle *(Miller et al, 2009)*

dorsiflexor /dôr″siflek″sər/, a muscle causing backward flexion of a part of the body, as the hand or foot.

dorsiflexor gait, an abnormal gait caused by the weakness of the dorsiflexors of the ankle, characterized by footdrop during the entire gait cycle and excessive knee and hip flexion to allow clearance of the involved extremity during the swing phase. The sole of the affected foot also slaps forcibly against the ground at the moment of heel strike because of the inability of the dorsiflexor to decelerate the body weight as the heel strikes the ground. Compare **Trendelenburg gait.**

dorso-, dorsi-, prefix meaning "dorsum" or "back": *dorsolateral, dorsolumbar, dorsiflexion.*

dorsocuboidal reflex. See **Mendel's reflex.**

dorsodynia /dôr′sōdin″ē-ə/, back pain, particularly in the muscles of the upper back area. Also called **dorsalgia.**

dorsolateral /dôr′sōlat″ərəl/, pertaining to the back of the body and to the side.

dorsolumbar /dôr′sōlum″bər/, pertaining to the back of the body and the lumbar region.

dorsosacral /dôr′sōsā″krəl/, pertaining to the back of the body and the sacrum.

dorsosacral position. See **lithotomy position.**

dorsoventral /dôr′sōven″trəl/ [L, *dorsum,* back, *venter,* belly], pertaining to the axis that passes through the back of the body and the abdomen.

dorsum /dôr″səm/ [L, *dorsum,* back], the back of the body or the posterior or upper surface of a body part.

dorsum sellae /sel″ē/, the posterior boundary of the sella turcica of the sphenoid bone. It bears the posterior clinoid process and is an anatomical marker for the location of the pituitary gland at the base of the skull.

dorzolamide hydrochloride /dorzo′lämīd/, a carbonic acid anhydrase inhibitor used in treatment of open-angle glaucoma and ocular hypertension, administered topically to the conjunctiva as the hydrochloride salt.

■ INDICATIONS: It is prescribed in the treatment of glaucoma. It reduces intraocular pressure by decreasing the rate of fluid production.

■ CONTRAINDICATIONS: It should not be given to patients wearing soft contact lenses or those with allergy to dorzolamide, its components, or related substances.

■ ADVERSE EFFECTS: The side effects most often reported include ocular burning, stinging or discomfort following use; tearing; blurred vision; or light sensitivity.

dosage /dō′sij/ [Gk, *didonai,* to give], the regimen governing the size, amount, frequency, and number of doses of a therapeutic agent to be administered to a patient. Compare **dose.**

dosage compensation, a mechanism by which the expression of X-linked traits is equalized in males, who have one X chromosome, and females, who have two. In mammals it is accomplished by the inactivation of one of the X chromosomes in the somatic cells of females. See also **Lyon hypothesis.**

dose /dōs/ [GK, *didonai,* to give], the amount of a drug or other substance to be administered at one time. Compare **dosage.** See also **absorbed dose.**

dose area product (DAP), the product of the entrance skin dose and the cross-sectional area of the x-ray beam.

dose calculations, formulas for adjusting drug dosages for children, elderly adults, or other patients who may lack mechanisms for metabolizing and excreting average adult levels of medications. Infants, for example, have skin that is thin and permeable, a stomach that lacks gastric acid, body temperature that is poorly regulated, and immature liver and kidney function. See also **pediatric dosage.**

dose calibrator, an ionization chamber used in nuclear medicine to measure the amount of radioactivity of a radionuclide before injection into a patient.

dose equivalent (DE), a quantity used in radiation-safety work that expresses the amount of radiation dose and the physical damage that it may produce. It is the product of the dose (in gray or rad) and a quality factor specific to the type

and energy of the radiation delivering that dose. The unit of dose equivalent is the sievert (Sv) or the rem.

dose fractionation, division of a total dose into small increments delivered over several days rather than a large single dose delivered at one time. See **fractionation,** def. 5.

dose-limiting recommendations, the absorbed dose equivalent limit of radiation exposure, which may vary for different body or organ exposures. For example, the absorbed dose equivalent limit for the skin or forearms of a radiation worker is much higher than the whole-body exposure.

dose-limiting side effects, drug effects that prevent a drug from being administered in higher doses.

dose rate, the amount of delivered radiation absorbed per unit time.

dose ratemeter /rāt″mētər/, an instrument for measuring the dose rate of radiation.

dose response, a range of doses over which response occurs. Doses lower than the threshold produce no response while those in excess of the threshold exert no additional response. The shape of the curve is usually hyperbolic when plotted with linear axes and gives a sigmoidal curve when response is plotted versus the log of the dose. Beneficial drug responses are typically plotted on separate dose-response curves. Because the dose response and the chemotherapeutic index can overlap to some degree and may have different slopes, the margin of safety is often considered to be a better index.

dose-response relationship, a mathematic relationship between the dose of a drug or radiation and the body's reaction to it. In a linear dose-response relationship, the response is proportional to the dose. Thus, if the dose is doubled, the response is also doubled. In a linear nonthreshold relationship, any dose, regardless of size, can theoretically cause a response.

dose threshold, the minimum amount of a drug or absorbed radiation that produces a detectable effect.

dose to skin, the amount of absorbed radiation at the center of the irradiation field on the skin. It is the sum of the dose in the air and the scatter from body parts.

dosimeter /dōsim″ətər/ [L, *dosis* + Gk, *metron,* measure], an instrument used to detect and measure accumulated radiation exposure. One commonly used type consists of a pencil-sized ionization chamber with a self-reading electrometer; others include badges and rings.

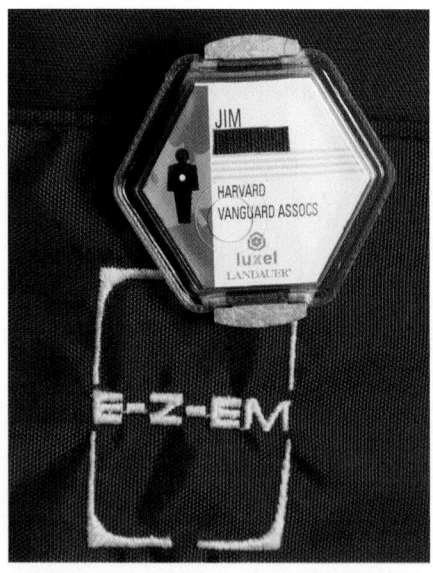

Optically stimulated luminescence (OSL) dosimeter
(Proctor and Adams, 2014)

dosimetry /dōsim″ətrē/ [Gk, *dosis,* giving, *metron,* measure], **1.** the determination of the amount, rate, and distribution of radiation or radioactivity from a source of ionizing radiation. **2.** the accurate determination of medicinal doses based on body size, sex, age, and other factors.

DOT, 1. initialism for **Department of Transportation. 2.** initialism for **directly observed therapy. 3.** abbreviation for *date of transfer.*

double [L, *duplus*], twice as much in strength, size, or amount.

double-approach conflict. See **approach-approach conflict.**

double-avoidance conflict. See **avoidance-avoidance conflict.**

double-barrel colostomy, a complete surgical division of the bowel. Two stomas are created; one stoma will discharge fecal material, and the second stoma will discharge mucoid material. Both stomas may be brought to the surface of the abdomen, or the mucous portion of the bowel may be ligated and remain in the abdomen to discharge mucus via the rectum. Compare **loop colostomy.**

double bind /bīnd/ [L, *duplus,* double; AS, *bindan,* to bind], a "no-win" situation resulting from two conflicting messages from a person who is crucial to one's survival, such as a verbal message that differs from a nonverbal message. An example is the insistence of a mother that she is not angry about a child's behavior although she is perceived as being obviously angry and hostile.

double-blind study, an experiment designed to test the effect of a treatment or substance by using groups of experimental and control subjects in which neither the subjects nor the investigators know which treatment or substance is being administered to which group. In a double-blind test of a new drug, the substance may be identified to the investigators by only a code. The purpose of a double-blind study is to eliminate the risk of prejudgment by the participants, which could distort the results. A double-blind study may be augmented by a cross-over experiment, in which experimental subjects unknowingly become control subjects, and vice versa, at some point in the study. See also **placebo.**

double-channel catheter [L, *duplus,* double; ME, *chanel* + Gk, *katheter,* a thing lowered into], a catheter with two lumens (channels) used to irrigate an internal cavity, with fluid entering one lumen and draining through the other. Also called **two-way catheter.**

double chin. *(Informal)* See **buccula.**

double collecting system, (of a body organ or system) a collecting system involving a double ureter. There may be either a duplex kidney or an ectopic kidney. Also called **duplicated collecting system.**

double-contrast arthrography, a method of making a radiographic image of a joint by injecting two contrast agents, usually a gaseous medium and a water-soluble iodinated agent, into the capsular space.

double-contrast barium enema [L, *duplus,* double, *contra,* against, *stare,* to stand; Gk, *barys,* heavy, *enienai,* to inject], an enema of radiopaque barium followed by evacuation and introduction of air. The purpose is to detail radiographically the mucosal lining of the large intestine. Also called *double-contrast enema, barium enema with air contrast.*

double-emulsion film, x-ray film that is coated with emulsion on both sides.

double-flap amputation [L, *duplus,* double; ME, *flappe,* flap; L, *amputare*], an amputation in which two flaps are made from the soft tissues to cover an area that has lost its integument from surgery or accident.

double fracture, a fracture consisting of breaks or cracks in two places in a bone, producing more than two bone segments.

double gel diffusion. See **immunodiffusion.**

double innervation, innervation of effector organs by fibers of the sympathetic and parasympathetic divisions of the autonomic nervous system. The pelvic viscera, bronchioles, heart, eyes, and digestive system are all doubly innervated. The fibers of the two divisions operate at cross-purposes to achieve a state of balance and maintain constancy in the body's internal environment. The mode of action of each division varies. In some structures one division is stimulating and the other inhibiting; in others, separate fibers from each division act to stimulate and inhibit complementary function.

double-lumen drain, a drain, such as a sump drain, consisting of two tubes, one inside the other.

double-needle entry, a technique for injecting a contrast medium or other agent with two needles, one with a larger bore. In diskography a 20-gauge needle is used to perform a spinal puncture and reach the anulus fibrosus of the disk, after which a longer 26-gauge needle is passed through the guide needle to the injection target area.

double penis. See **diphallus.**

double pneumonia, acute lobar pneumonia affecting both lungs.

double quartan fever, a form of malaria in which paroxysms of fever occur in a repeating pattern of 2 consecutive days followed by 1 day of remission. The pattern is usually the result of concurrent infections by two species of the genus *Plasmodium,* one causing paroxysms every 72 hours and the other every 48 hours. Compare **biduotertian fever.** See also **malaria.**

double setup, a practice in which an obstetric operating room is prepared for both vaginal delivery and cesarean section.

double system ureterocele, an outpouching of the distal ureter involving a double collecting system, seen most often in girls with an ectopic ureter.

double ureter, existence of a second ureter on one side that may be a complete connection from the kidney to the bladder or a partial tube forming a blind pouch. Most are asymptomatic, but some are accompanied by ectopic ureterocele. Also called **ureteral duplication.**

double vision. See **diplopia.**

double-void, a urinalysis procedure in which the first specimen is discarded and the second, obtained 30 to 45 minutes later, is tested. This method gives a more accurate measure of the amount of glucose in the urine at that particular time.

doubling dose, that dose of radiation expected to double the number of genetic mutations in a generation.

douche /doosh/ [Fr, shower-bath], **1.** *n.,* a procedure in which a liter or more of a solution of a medication or cleansing agent in warm water is introduced into the vagina under low pressure. Douches are also administered via prepackaged preparations of much smaller volume in flexible plastic bottles. Douching may be recommended in the treatment of various pelvic and vaginal infections. **2.** *v.,* to perform a douche.

doughnut pessary. See **pessary.**

Douglas's cul-de-sac [James Douglas, Scottish anatomist, 1675–1742; Fr, bottom of the bag], a rectouterine pouch or recess formed by a fold of peritoneum that extends between the rectum and the uterus. Also called *excavatio rectouterina.*

doula, a nonmedical person who specializes in the support of women during labor, birth, and the postpartum period. See also **labor coach.**

dowager's hump /dow″ijərz/, *(Nontechnical)* an abnormal backward curvature of the cervical spine as a result of compression fractures of osteoporosis. Though it may occur at any age, it is most common in elderly women. The term *dowager's hump* is in common usage in the clinical setting, but it is considered by some to be an impolite reference to a common problem associated with aging.

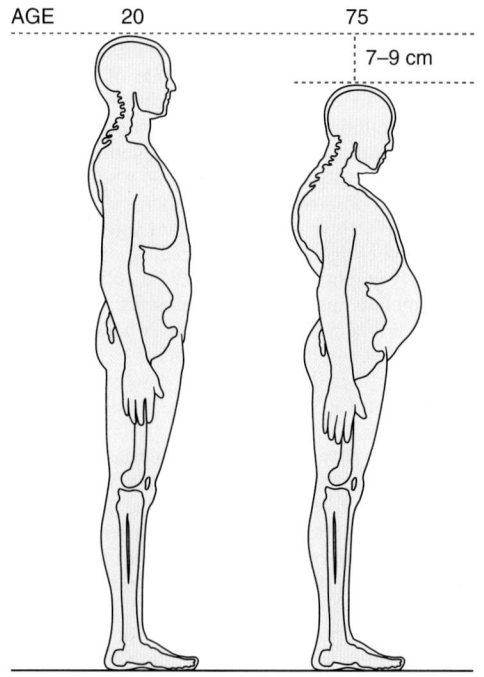

AGE   20   75

7–9 cm

Loss of height resulting from osteoporosis, leading to dowager's hump *(Magee, 2014)*

dowel /dow′əl/ [ME, *doule,* part of a wheel], **1.** (in dentistry) a small rod or pin, usually metal, fitted into a prepared hole within the root canal and cemented in place, serving to retain a dental restoration or a core, such as a crown. Also called *post and core.* **2.** a long, straight wooden stick used in many therapeutic exercises to strengthen muscles and improve coordination. **3.** (in orthopedic surgery) a rod, pin, or bone transplant material that is used to join structures or fill in a bone defect.

dowel graft, a cylindrical plug of bone used to immobilize adjacent vertebrae in anterior spinal fusion.

down [AS, *adune,* off hill], (of a computer) not operating as a result of malfunction or maintenance or for other reasons.

Downey cells [Hal Downey, American hematologist, 1877–1959], reactive (atypical) lymphocytes with enlarged nuclei exhibiting delicate chromatin and excessive, "stormy," and vacuolated cytoplasm. Downey cells are present in viral infections, infectious mononucleosis, and hepatitis.

download, to transfer data or programs from a central computer to a peripheral unit or drive.

down-regulation /doun reg-u-la′shun/, a decrease in the number of receptors for a chemical or drug on cell surfaces in a given area, usually caused by long-term exposure to the agent. See also **up-regulation.**

Down syndrome [John L. Down, English physician, 1828–1896], a congenital condition characterized by varying degrees of cognitive impairment and multiple defects. It is the most common chromosomal abnormality of a generalized syndrome and is caused by the presence of an extra chromosome 21 in the G group or, in a small percentage of cases, by the translocation of chromosome 14 or 15 in the D group and chromosome 21 or 22. Down syndrome occurs in approximately 1 in 600 to 650 live births and is associated with advanced maternal age, particularly over 35 years of age. The incidence is as high as 1 in 80 for offspring of women above 40 years of age. In cases caused by translocation, which is a genetic aberration that is hereditary rather than a chromosomal aberration caused by nondisjunction during cell division, the incidence is not associated with maternal age. The condition can be diagnosed prenatally by amniocentesis. A mosaic variant, in which there is a mixture of trisomy 21 and normal cells, causes fewer physical defects and less severe cognitive impairment depending on the degree of mosaicism. Also called **trisomy 21.** See also **nondisjunction.**

■ OBSERVATIONS: Infants with the syndrome are small and hypotonic, with characteristic microcephaly, brachycephaly, a flattened occiput, and typical facies with a characteristic slant to the eyes, depressed nasal bridge, low-set ears, and a large, protruding tongue that is furrowed and lacks a central fissure. The hands are short and broad with a transverse palmar or simian crease; the fingers are stubby and show clinodactyly, primarily of the fifth finger. The feet are broad and stubby with a wide space between the first and second toes and a prominent plantar crease. Other anomalies associated with the disorder are bowel defects, congenital heart disease (primarily septal defects), chronic respiratory infections, visual problems, abnormalities in tooth development, and susceptibility to acute leukemia.

■ INTERVENTIONS: The health care problems that affect physical health must be addressed. However, other issues can affect social and school success. A coordinated team approach will assist the individual with Down syndrome, and the caregivers, to achieve a maximal level of function and the best quality of life possible.

■ PATIENT CARE CONSIDERATIONS: The most significant feature of the syndrome is cognitive impairment, which varies considerably. The average IQ is in the range of 50 to 60, so the child is generally trainable and in most instances can be reared at home. The mortality rate is high within the first few years, especially in children with cardiac anomalies. Those who survive tend to be shorter than average and stocky in build; they show delayed or incomplete sexual development and can live to middle or old age, although adults with Down syndrome are prone to respiratory infections, pneumonia, and lung disease.

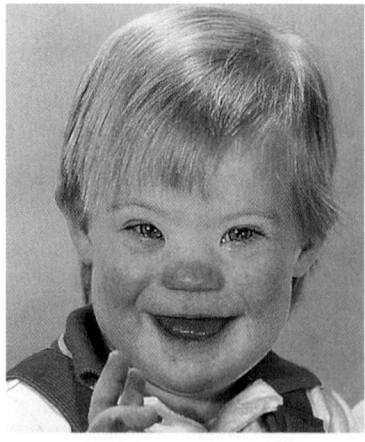

Typical facial appearance of a child with Down syndrome *(Patton and Thibodeau, 2014)*

down-time, a period during which a computer system is inoperable as a result of malfunction, for maintenance, or for other reasons.

doxacurium, a nondepolarizing neuromuscular blocker.

■ INDICATIONS: This drug is used to facilitate endotracheal intubation and skeletal muscle relaxation during mechanical ventilation, surgery, or general anesthesia.

■ CONTRAINDICATIONS: Known hypersensitivity to this drug prohibits its use. This drug must not be used in neonates.

doxapram hydrochloride /dok″səpram/, a respiratory stimulant.

■ INDICATIONS: It is prescribed to improve respiratory function after anesthesia, in drug-induced central nervous system depression, and for chronic pulmonary disease associated with acute hypercapnia.

■ CONTRAINDICATIONS: Seizure disorder, pulmonary disease, coronary artery disease, uncompensated heart failure, hypertension, or known hypersensitivity to this drug prohibits its use.

■ ADVERSE EFFECTS: Among the more serious adverse reactions are convulsions, bronchospasm, cardiovascular symptoms, and phlebitis.

doxepin hydrochloride /dok″səpin/, a tricyclic antidepressant.

■ INDICATIONS: It is prescribed in the treatment of depression. A topical preparation is also available for treating atopic dermatitis, and unlabeled uses include the treatment of neuropathic pain.

■ CONTRAINDICATIONS: Concomitant administration of monoamine oxidase inhibitors, recent myocardial infarction, seizure disorders, or known hypersensitivity to tricyclic medication prohibits its use.

■ ADVERSE EFFECTS: Among the more serious adverse reactions are GI, cardiovascular, and neurological disturbances. Sedation, dry mouth, and many drug interactions may occur.

doxercalciferol, a parathyroid agent (calcium regulator).

■ INDICATIONS: It is used to lower high parathyroid hormone levels in patients undergoing chronic kidney dialysis.

■ CONTRAINDICATIONS: Known hypersensitivity to this drug, hyperphosphatemia, hypercalcemia, and vitamin D toxicity prohibit its use.

■ ADVERSE EFFECTS: Adverse effects include drowsiness, headache, lethargy, nausea, diarrhea, vomiting, anorexia, dry mouth, constipation, cramps, metallic taste, myalgia, arthralgia, decreased bone development, polyuria, hypercalciuria, hyperphosphatemia, hematuria, and shortness of breath.

DOXOrubicin hydrochloride /dok″səroo″bisin/, an anthracycline antibiotic.

■ INDICATIONS: It is prescribed in the treatment of a wide variety of malignant neoplastic diseases, including leukemias, lymphomas, sarcomas, germ cell tumors, and carcinomas (e.g., lung, breast, prostate, ovary).

■ CONTRAINDICATIONS: Myelosuppression, heart disease, concurrent administration of daunorubicin, or known hypersensitivity to this drug prohibits its use.

■ ADVERSE EFFECTS: Among the more serious adverse reactions are myelosuppression and cardiomyopathy. Stomatitis, GI disturbances, and alopecia commonly occur.

doxycycline /dok″sisī″klēn/, a tetracycline antibiotic.

■ INDICATIONS: It is prescribed in the treatment of infections caused by susceptible bacterial strains, especially *Chlamydia*, *Rickettsia*, and *Mycoplasma*.

■ CONTRAINDICATIONS: Renal or liver dysfunction or known hypersensitivity to this drug or to other tetracycline medication prohibits its use. It is not given during pregnancy or to children less than 8 years of age.

■ ADVERSE EFFECTS: Among the more serious adverse reactions are GI disturbances, phototoxicity, potentially serious superinfections, and hypersensitivity reactions. Discoloration of teeth may occur in children exposed to the drug in utero or under 8 years of age.

doxylamine succinate /dok′silam″ēn/, an antihistamine.

■ INDICATIONS: It is prescribed for the treatment of acute allergic symptoms produced by the release of histamine.

■ CONTRAINDICATIONS: Known hypersensitivity to this drug prohibits its use. It is not recommended for use during pregnancy or lactation and is not given to children less than 6 years of age.

■ ADVERSE EFFECTS: Among the more serious reactions are sedation, ataxia, tachycardia, hemolytic anemia, and thrombocytopenia.

dP/dt, the rate of change of pressure with respect to time.

DPG, abbreviation for **2,3-diphosphoglyceric acid.**

DPL, abbreviation for **diagnostic peritoneal lavage.**

D.P.M., abbreviation for *Doctor of Podiatric Medicine.* See **podiatrist.**

DPT vaccine, abbreviation for **diphtheria and tetanus toxoids and pertussis vaccine.**

DQ, abbreviation for **developmental quotient.**

dr, abbreviation for **dram.**

Dr., abbreviation for *doctor.*

drachm. See **dram.**

dracunculiasis /drakun′kyoolī″əsis/ [Gk, *drakontion,* little dragon, *osis,* condition], a parasitic infection caused by infestation by the nematode *Dracunculus medinensis.* It is characterized by ulcerative skin lesions on the legs and feet that are produced by the emergence of one or more gravid female worms, which may be visible. People are infected by drinking contaminated water or eating contaminated shellfish. It is common in densely populated tropical and subtropical areas of the world. Treatment involves slow, progressive, mechanical removal of the worm over several days. Metronidazole may reduce inflammation and facilitate removal of the worm. Also called *dracontiasis,* **Guinea worm infection,** *dracunculosis.*

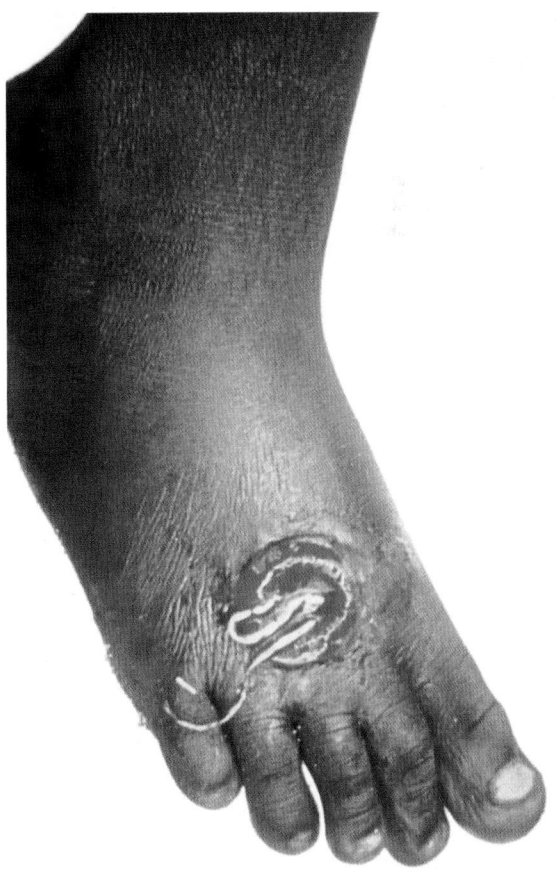

Dracunculiasis *(Bennett et al, 2015)*

Dracunculus medinensis /drakun″kyo͞oləs/, a parasitic nematode of the Mediterranean area that causes dracunculiasis. An American species is *Dracunculus insignis.* Also called **fiery serpent.**

dragon worm. See *Dracunculus medinensis.*

drag-to gait [ME, *dragen* + *gate,* path], a method of walking with crutches in which the feet are dragged rather than lifted with each step. See also **crutch gait.**

drain, a tube or other device used to remove air or a fluid from a body cavity or wound. The drain may be a closed system designed to provide complete protection against contamination, or an open system in which there is a continual exchange of material.

drainage /drā″nij/ [AS, *drachen,* teardrop], the removal of fluids from a body cavity, wound, or other source of discharge by one or more methods. Closed drainage is a system of tubing and other apparatus attached to the body to remove fluid in an airtight circuit that prevents environmental contaminants from entering the wound or cavity. Continuous bladder irrigation is drainage in which a body area is washed out by alternately flooding and then emptying it with the aid of gravity, a technique that may be used in treating a urinary bladder disorder. Open drainage is drainage in which discharge passes through an open-ended tube into a receptacle. Suction drainage uses a pump or other mechanical device to assist in extracting a fluid. See also **postural drainage, tidal drainage.**

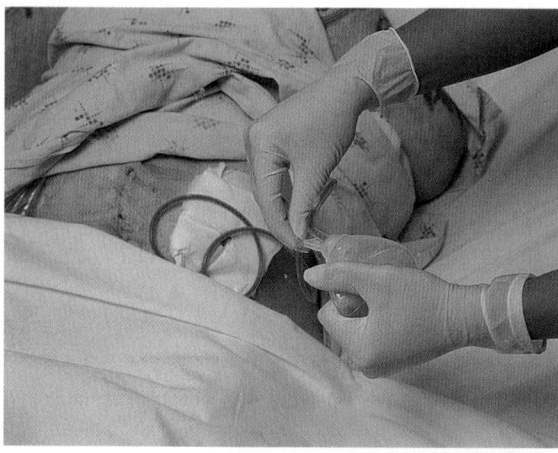

Drainage with a Jackson-Pratt drainage device
(deWit and O'Neill, 2014)

drainage tube, a heavy-gauge catheter used for the evacuation of air or a fluid from a cavity or wound in the body. The tube may be attached to a suction device or may allow flow by gravity into a receptacle.

draining sinus [AS, *drachen,* teardrop; L, *sinus,* hollow], an abnormal channel or fistula permitting the escape of exudate to the outside of the body.

Draize test /drāz/ [John Draize, American pharmacologist, 1900–1992)], a controversial method of testing the toxicity of pharmaceutic and other products to be used by humans by placing a small amount of the substance in the eyes of rabbits.

-dralazine, suffix for the name of an antihypertensive.

dram (dr.) /dram/ [Gk, *drachme,* weight of the same value], a unit of mass equivalent to an apothecary's

Types of wound drainage

Type	Appearance
A. Serous	Clear, watery plasma
	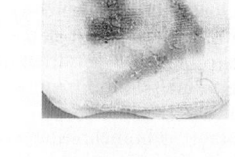
B. Purulent	Thick, yellow, green, tan, or brown
	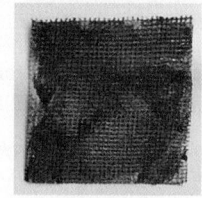
C. Serosanguineous	Pale, red, watery: mixture of serous and sanguineous
	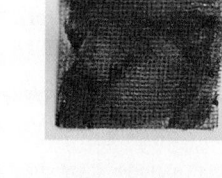
D. Sanguineous	Bright red: indicates active bleeding
	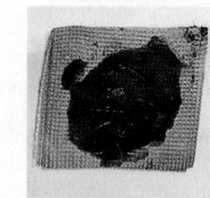

From Perry AG, Potter PA, Ostendorf WR: *Nursing interventions and clinical skills,* ed 6, St Louis, 2016, Elsevier.

measure of 60 grains or $\frac{1}{8}$ ounce and to $\frac{1}{16}$ ounce or 27.34 grains avoirdupois. Also spelled **drachm.**

Dramamine, an over-the-counter preparation used for motion sickness. Brand name for **dimenHYDRINATE.**

dramatic play /dramat″ik/ [Gk, *drama,* deed; AS, *plegan,* game], an imitative activity in which a child fantasizes and acts out various domestic and social roles and situations, such as rocking a doll, pretending to be a doctor or nurse, or teaching school. It is the predominant form of play among preschool children. One of its purposes is to allow for cognitive and behavioral rehearsals of adult roles.

drape [ME, *drap,* cloth], a sheet of fabric or paper, usually the size of a small bedsheet, for covering all or part of a person's body during a physical examination or treatment. It may also refer to the curtain pulled around a patient's bed or the examining area. −**drape,** *v.*

Drash syndrome /drash/ [Allan Lee Drash, American pediatrician, 1931–2009], a syndrome of male pseudohermaphroditism, nephropathy leading to renal failure, and, in most cases, Wilms tumor, caused by a genetic abnormality in chromosome 11. Also called *Denys-Drash syndrome.*

Draw-a-Person (DAP) Test [AS, *dragan* + L, *personalis* + *testum,* crucible], a psychoanalytic test based on the interpretation of drawings of human figures of both sexes. Interpretation depends on the subject's verbalizations, self-image, anxiety, sexual conflicts, and other factors. Also called **Machover Draw-a-Person Test.**

drawer sign [AS, *dragan,* to drag], a diagnostic sign of a ruptured or torn anterior cruciate or posterior cruciate ligament of the knee. Testing involves having the patient flex the knee at a right angle while the lower leg is grasped just below the knee and moved first toward, then away from the examiner. The test result is positive for the knee injury if the head of the tibia can be moved more than a half inch from the joint. See also **anterior drawer sign or test.**

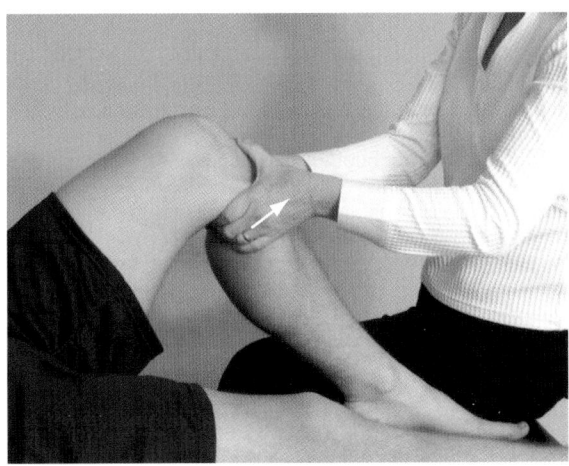

Assessing for drawer sign *(Magee, 2014)*

drawing, *(Informal)* a vague sensation of muscle tension, sometimes used to describe a pulling feeling with muscle movement in the arm.

drawsheet, a sheet that is smaller than a bottom or top sheet of a bed and that is usually placed over the middle of the bottom sheet to keep the mattress and bottom linens dry. The drawsheet can also be used to turn or move a patient in bed. Also called **turning sheet.** See also **log roll.**

dream [ME, *dreem,* joyful noise], **1.** a sequence of ideas, thoughts, emotions, or images that pass through the mind during the rapid eye movement stage of sleep. **2.** the sleeping state in which this process occurs. **3.** a visionary creation of the imagination experienced during wakefulness. **4.** (in psychoanalysis) the expression of thoughts, emotions, memories, or impulses repressed from the consciousness. **5.** (in analytic psychology) the wishes, emotions, and impulses that reflect the personal unconscious and the archetypes that originate in the collective unconscious. See also **dream analysis, dream state.**

dream analysis, a process of gaining access to the unconscious mind by means of examining the content of dreams, usually through the method of free association.

dream association, a relationship of thoughts or emotions discovered or experienced when a dream is remembered or analyzed. See also **dream analysis.**

dream state, a condition of altered consciousness in which a person does not recognize the environment and reacts in a manner opposed to his or her usual behavior, as by flight or an act of violence. The state is seen in epilepsy and certain disorders. See also **automatism, fugue.**

dress code [OFr, *dresser,* to arrange; L, *codex,* book], the standards set by an institution for the appropriate attire of its members.

dressing [OFr, *dresser,* to arrange], a clean or sterile covering applied directly to wounded or diseased tissue to absorb secretions, protect from trauma, administer medications, maintain wound cleanliness, or stop bleeding. Kinds include **absorbent dressing, antiseptic dressing, occlusive dressing, pressure dressing, wet dressing.**

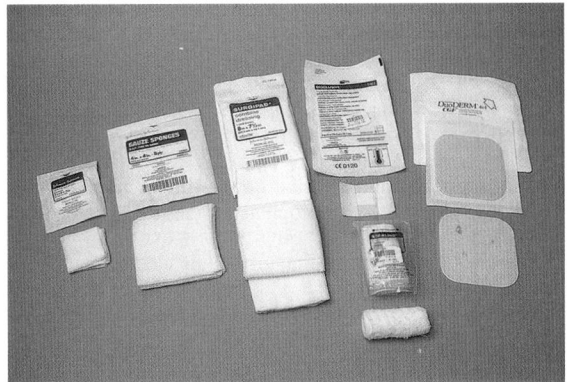

Various types of dressings *(deWit and O'Neill, 2014)*

dressing forceps, a kind of forceps that has narrow blades and blunt or notched teeth, designed for dressing wounds, removing drainage tubes, or extracting fragments of necrotic tissue.

Dressler syndrome /dres″lər/ [William Dressler, American physician, 1890–1969], an autoimmune disorder that may occur several days to several months after acute coronary infarction, characterized by fever, pericarditis, pleurisy, pleural effusions, and joint pain. It results from the body's immunological response to a damaged myocardium and pericardium. Treatment usually includes intensive aspirin therapy and, in severe cases, use of corticosteroids. A similar syndrome may occur after cardiac surgery. See also **postmyocardial infarction syndrome.**

DRG, abbreviation for **diagnosis-related group.**

DRI, initialism for *Dietary Reference Intake.*

drift [AS, *drifan,* to move forward], a gradual movement away from the original position. See also **antigenic drift, genetic drift.**

drifting tooth, a tooth that migrates from its normal position. Causes include a loss of proximal support or functional antagonists, occlusal traumatic tooth relationships, inflammatory and retrograde changes in the attachment apparatus, and oral habits, such as thumb-sucking and bruxism.

drill /dril/ [Dutch *drillen,* to bore], **1.** a rotating cutting instrument for making holes in hard substances, such as bones or teeth. See also **burr. 2.** (in dentistry) an instrument fitted into a handpiece used to remove dental caries, tooth and bone structure, and to prepare the teeth to properly accept dental restorations.

Drinker respirator [Philip Drinker, American engineer, 1894–1972], *(Obsolete)* an airtight respirator that consisted of a metal tank that enclosed the entire body except the head. Used for long-term therapy, it alternated positive and negative air pressure within the tank, providing artificial respiration by contracting and expanding the walls of the chest. It was widely used in the treatment of polio. Also called **artificial lung, iron lung.**

drip [AS, *dryppan,* to fall in drops], **1.** *n.,* the process in which a liquid or moisture forms and falls in drops. Kinds include **nasal drip, postnasal drip. 2.** *n.,* the slow but continuous infusion of a liquid into the body, as into the stomach peritoneum or a vein. **3.** *v.,* to infuse a liquid continuously into the body.

drip gavage, a method of enteral feeding of a liquid formula diet. The formula is contained in a bag suspended from a stand and slowly drips into the GI tract. It may also be administered with a feeding pump. See also **enteral tube feeding, tube feeding.**

drip system, (in IV therapy) an apparatus for delivering specific volumes of IV solutions within predetermined periods and at a specific flow rate. See also **macrodrip, microdrip.**

drive [AS, *drifan,* to move forward], **1.** a basic, compelling urge. A primary drive is one that is innate and in close contact with physiological processes. A secondary drive is one that evolves during the process of growth and that incites and directs behavior. **2.** an electromechanical device that holds a secondary storage medium and allows for the transfer of data to and from the computer, such as a disk drive or tape drive.

Drixoral, a fixed-combination drug containing an antihistamine and a vasoconstrictor, used for the relief of congestion of the upper respiratory tract. Brand name for *dexbrompheniramine maleate, pseudoephedrine sulfate.*

-drome, suffix meaning "that which runs or moves together" in a specified way: *syndrome.*

dromedary hump, a bulge on the lateral surface of a kidney (usually the left), resembling the hump of a dromedary camel, seen in persons whose spleen or liver presses down.

dromo-, prefix meaning "running" or "conduction": *dromotropic.*

dromostanolone propionate /drō'mostan″əlōn/, a synthetic androgen.

■ INDICATIONS: It is prescribed for the treatment of female breast cancer.

■ CONTRAINDICATIONS: It is not used for male breast cancer or in premenopausal women.

■ ADVERSE EFFECTS: Among the more serious adverse reactions are masculinization, edema, and hypercalcemia.

dromotropic, an agent that influences the conduction of electrical impulses. A positive dromotropic agent enhances the conduction of electrical impulses to the heart.

dronabinol /drōnab″inol/, an oral antiemetic that is a synthetic derivative of THC, the principal psychotropic constituent of marijuana.

■ INDICATIONS: It is prescribed for the treatment of refractory nausea and vomiting caused by cancer chemotherapy.

■ CONTRAINDICATIONS: It should not be given to persons with known hypersensitivity to the drug or to tetrahydrocannabinol, its active ingredient.

■ ADVERSE EFFECTS: Among adverse effects reported are drowsiness, dizziness, impaired coordination, and hallucinations. Dronabinol is a Schedule III controlled substance with a high potential for abuse. It can produce both physical and psychological dependence. It is not recommended for patients who are using a central nervous system depressant or other psychoactive drugs.

drooping eyelid, *(Nontechnical)* now called **ptosis.**

drooping lily sign, a deformity seen on IV urography of a duplex kidney, with the forcing of the lower collecting system and ureter outward and downward to resemble the shape of a drooping lily. It is caused by obstruction and dilation of the upper collecting system.

drop (gtt) [AS, *dropa*], a small spherical mass of liquid. A drop may vary in size with differences in temperature, viscosity, and other factors. For therapeutic purpose, a drop is regarded as having a volume of 0.06 to 0.1 mL, or 1 to 1.5 minims. 1.5 drops = 1 mL.

drop arm test, a diagnostic test for a tear in the supraspinatus tendon. The result is positive if the patient is unable to lower the affected arm slowly and smoothly from a position of 90 degrees of abduction.

drop attack, *(Informal)* a form of transient ischemic attack in which a brief interruption of cerebral blood flow causes a person to fall to the floor without losing consciousness. The fall may be caused by a disrupted sense of balance or decreased leg muscle tone. Weakness of the leg muscles or a hip or knee joint dysfunction may be a contributing factor.

droperidol /drəper″ədol/, an antipsychotic, sedative drug of the butyrophenone group, used most commonly with an opioid analgesic (fentanyl) in neuroleptanesthesia.

drop foot. See **footdrop.**

droplet infection [AS, *dropa* + L, *inficere,* to infect], an infection acquired by the inhalation of pathogenic microorganisms suspended in particles of liquid exhaled, sneezed, or coughed by another infected person or animal. Some diseases spread by droplets are chickenpox, common cold, influenza, measles, and mumps.

Droplet Precautions, guidelines recommended by the Centers for Disease Control and Prevention for reducing the risk of droplet transmission of infectious agents. Droplet transmission involves contact of the conjunctivae or the mucous membranes of the nose or mouth of a susceptible person with large-particle droplets (larger than 5 μm in size) containing microorganisms generated from a person who has a clinical disease or is a carrier of the disease. Droplets are generated from the source person primarily during coughing, sneezing, talking, and performance of certain procedures such as suctioning and bronchoscopy. Transmission of large-particle droplets requires close contact between source and recipient persons because droplets do not remain suspended in the air and generally travel only short distances (usually 3 feet or less). Special air handling and ventilation are not required to prevent droplet transmission because droplets do not remain suspended in the air. Droplet Precautions apply to any patient known or suspected to be infected with epidemiologically important pathogens that can be transmitted by infectious droplets. See also **Standard Precautions, Transmission-Based Precautions.**

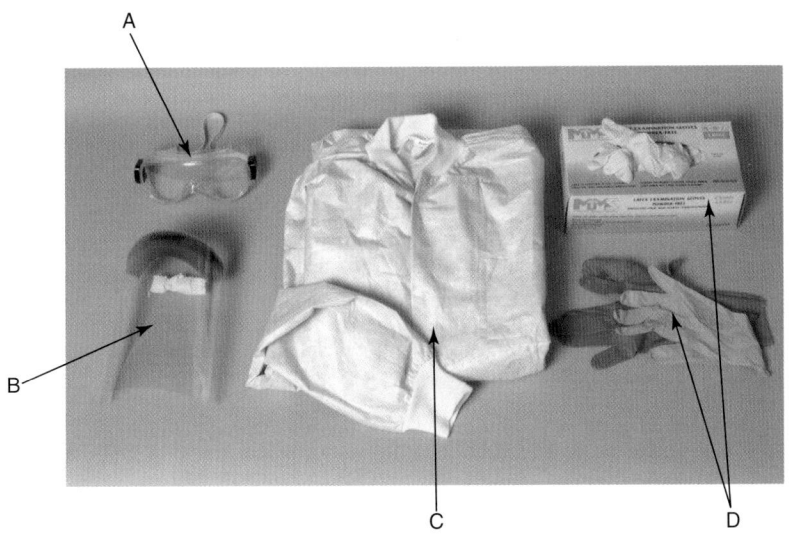

Personal protective equipment used for droplet infection. A, Goggles. B, Face shield. C, Fluid-impenetrable gown with elastic wristbands. D, Box of latex gloves and two pairs of colored nonlatex gloves *(Garrels and Oatis, 2011)*

dropped-beat pulse.   See **intermittent pulse.**

dropped wrist.   See **radial paralysis.**

dropper,   a glass or plastic tube narrowed at one end with a rubber bulb at the other end to dispense a liquid medication one drop at a time.

dropsy,   *(Obsolete)* now called **edema.**

Drosophila /drōsof″ilə/ [Gk, *drosos,* dew, *philein,* to love], a genus of fly that includes *Drosophila melanogaster,* the Mediterranean fruit fly. It is useful in genetic experiments because of the large chromosomes found in its salivary glands and its sensitivity to environmental effects, such as exposure to radiation.

drospirenone /drospi′rĕnōn/,   a spironolactone analog that acts as a progestational agent, used in combination with an estrogen component such as an oral contraceptive.

drotrecogin alfa,   a thrombolytic agent used to treat severe sepsis associated with organ dysfunction.

drowning [ME, *drounen*],   asphyxiation caused by submersion in a liquid. See also **near drowning.**

drowsiness,   a decreased level of consciousness characterized by sleepiness and difficulty in remaining alert but easy arousal by stimuli. It may be caused by a lack of sleep, medications, substance abuse, or a cerebral disorder.

drox,   abbreviation for *hydroxide anion.*

Dr. P.H.,   abbreviation for *Doctor of Public Health.*

DRS,   abbreviation for **dementia rating scale.** See also **Mattis Dementia Rating Scale.**

DRSP,   abbreviation for **drug-resistant** *Streptococcus pneumoniae.*

drug [Fr, *drogue*], **1.** any substance taken by mouth; injected into a muscle, the skin, a blood vessel, or a cavity of the body; or applied topically to treat or prevent a disease or condition. Also called **medicine. 2.** *(Informal)* any substance that can be abused for its stimulant, depressant, euphoric, or hallucinogenic effects.

drug absorption,   the process whereby a drug moves from the muscle, digestive tract, or other site of entry into the body toward the circulatory system.

drug abuse,   the use of a drug for a nontherapeutic effect. Some of the most commonly abused drugs are alcohol; nicotine; marijuana; amphetamines; barbiturates; cocaine; methaqualone; opium alkaloids; synthetic opioids; benzodiazepines, including flunitrazepam (Rohypnol); gamma-hydroxybutyrate; 3,4 methylenedioxymethamphetamine (MDMA, ecstasy); phencyclidine; ketamine; and anabolic steroids. Drug abuse may lead to organ damage, addiction, and disturbed patterns of behavior. Some illicit drugs, such as heroin, lysergic acid diethylamide, and phencyclidine hydrochloride, have no recognized therapeutic effect in humans. Use of these drugs often incurs criminal penalty in addition to the potential for physical, social, and psychological harm. See also **drug addiction.**

Drug Abuse Warning Network (DAWN),   a public health surveillance system designed to monitor information about admissions to emergency treatment facilities for drug abuse.

drug action,   the means by which a drug exerts a desired effect. Drugs are usually classified by their actions; for example, a vasodilator, prescribed to decrease blood pressure, acts by dilating blood vessels.

drug addiction,   a condition characterized by an overwhelming desire to continue taking a drug to which one has become habituated through repeated consumption because it produces a particular effect, usually an alteration of mental status. Addiction is usually accompanied by a compulsion to obtain the drug, a tendency to increase the dose, a psychological or physical dependence, and detrimental consequences for the individual and society. Common addictive drugs are barbiturates, alcohol, and morphine and other opioids, especially heroin, which has slightly greater euphorigenic properties than other opium derivatives. See also **alcoholism, drug abuse.**

drug agonist,   a drug that is capable of binding to a neurotransmitter or hormone receptor and causing a response similar to the endogenous hormone or neurotransmitter. Compare **antagonist.**

drug allergy,   hypersensitivity to a pharmacological agent. Manifestations range from a mild rash to anaphylactic shock, depending on the dose and the allergen sensitivity of the individual. The primary drug that produces allergy is penicillin. Others include aspirin, phenylbutazone, novobiocin, other antibiotics, and radiopaque contrast media containing iodine. See also **anaphylactic shock.** Should not be confused with **drug sensitivity.**

drug clearance, the elimination of a drug from the body. Drugs and their metabolites are excreted primarily by the kidneys into the urine, but other routes for elimination include bile, sweat, saliva, breast milk, and expired air. The rate of clearance helps determine the size and frequency of a dosage of a particular medication.

drug compliance, the reliability of the patient in using a prescribed medication exactly as ordered by the primary care provider. Noncompliance occurs when a patient forgets or neglects to take the prescribed dosages at the recommended times or decides to discontinue the drug without consulting the provider.

drug concentration, the amount of drug in a given volume of plasma (e.g., number of micrograms per milliliter). Toxic drug levels may be observed when the body's normal mechanisms for metabolizing and excreting drugs are impaired, as commonly occurs in patients with liver or kidney disorders and in infants with immature organs. Dosage adjustments should be made in such individuals to accommodate their impaired metabolism and excretion.

drug dependence, a psychological craving for, habituation to, abuse of, or physiological reliance on a chemical substance. See also **drug abuse, drug addiction.**

drug dispensing, the preparation, packaging, labeling, record keeping, and transfer of a prescription drug to a patient or an intermediary who is responsible for administration of the drug.

drug disposition, general term for the absorption, distribution, metabolism, and excretion of a drug that has been administered.

drug distribution, the pattern of distribution of drug molecules by various tissues after the chemical enters the circulatory system. Because of differences in pH, lipid content, cell membrane functions, and other individual tissue factors, most drugs are not distributed equally in all parts of the body. For example, the acidity of aspirin influences a distribution pattern that is different from that of an alkaline product such as amphetamine.

drug-drug interaction, a modification of the effect of a drug when administered with another drug. The effect may be an increase or a decrease in the action of either substance, or it may be an adverse effect that is not normally associated with either drug. The particular interaction may be the result of a chemical-physical incompatibility of the two drugs or a change in the rate of absorption or the quantity absorbed in the body, the binding ability of either drug, or an alteration in the ability of receptor sites and cell membranes to bind either drug. Most adverse drug-drug interactions are either pharmacodynamic or pharmacokinetic in nature.

Drug Enforcement Agency (DEA), an agency of the U.S. Drug Enforcement Administration of the federal government, empowered to enforce regulations that control the import or export of narcotic drugs and certain other substances or the traffic of these substances across state lines.

drug eruption. See **drug rash.**

drug fever, a fever caused by the pharmacological action of a medication, its thermoregulatory action, a local complication of parenteral administration, or, most commonly, an immunological reaction mediated by drug-induced antibodies. The onset of fever occurs usually between 7 and 10 days after the medication is begun. A return to normal is ordinarily seen within 2 or 3 days of discontinuance of the drug. The correct diagnosis of drug fever and the discontinuance of the medication are important to prevent further adverse reactions and possibly dangerous and expensive diagnostic and therapeutic interventions. See also **Jarisch-Herxheimer reaction.**

drug-food interaction, the effect produced when some drugs and certain foods or beverages are taken at the same time. For example, grapefruit juice blocks the metabolism of some drugs in the GI tract, an action that can cause normal dosages of a drug to reach toxic levels in the plasma.

drug holiday, a period of drug withdrawal to reverse ineffectiveness of a drug resulting from receptor desensitization or adverse effects that may result from chronic treatment. For example, after a 7- to 10-day drug holiday, levodopa responsiveness appears to be enhanced, and lower doses are required to produce a therapeutic effect.

drug-induced acne. See **acne medicamentosa.**

drug-induced cystitis, allergic inflammation of the bladder occurring in reaction to a medication.

drug-induced hepatopathy, toxic liver dysfunction in which the agent causing the liver damage is a drug. See also **toxic hepatopathy.**

drug-induced parkinsonism, a reversible syndrome with the clinical features of Parkinson's disease but caused by the acetylcholine-dopamine imbalance of antipsychotic drugs. See also **parkinsonism.**

drug-induced psychosis, a psychotic state induced by excessive dosage of certain therapeutic drugs as well as drugs of abuse. Therapeutic drugs often associated with drug-induced psychosis include atropine-like drugs, chloral hydrate, steroids, and isoniazid.

drug-induced teratogenesis, congenital anomalies that reflect toxic effects of drugs on the developing fetus. See also **fetal alcohol syndrome, thalidomide.**

drug interaction, alteration of the effects of a drug by reaction with another drug or drugs, with foods or beverages, or with a preexisting medical condition.

drug metabolism, the transformation of a drug by the body tissues, primarily those of the liver, into a more water-soluble metabolite that can be eliminated. This process inactivates many drugs, but some drugs have metabolites that are also biologically active and others are administered as pro-drugs that must undergo drug metabolism to become biologically active.

drug monograph, a statement that specifies the kinds and amounts of ingredients a drug or class of drugs may contain, the directions for the drug's use, the conditions in which it may be used, and the contraindications to its use.

drug overdose (OD) [Fr, *drogue,* drug; AS, *ofer*; Gk, *dosis,* giving], an accidental or purposeful dose of a drug large enough to cause severe adverse reactions.

drug potency, the amount of drug required to produce a given percentage of its maximal effect, irrespective of the size of maximal effect. A drug can have high potency but poor efficacy, meaning that response is seen at very low doses and remains small even at high doses. Drug potency is seldom an important clinical consideration.

drug profile, an outline or summary of the characteristics of a drug or drug family, listing dosage types, pregnancy category, prescription or over-the-counter forms, generics if available, contraindications, and classification if covered by controlled-substance laws.

drug rash, a skin eruption, usually an allergic reaction, that is caused by a particular drug. Nearly any drug can produce a skin reaction as a result of gradual accumulation of the drug or development of antibodies that reject a component of the medication. A drug rash that is a sensitivity reaction does not occur the first time the drug is taken; the effect is observed with subsequent uses. Also called **dermatitis medicamentosa.** See also **fixed drug eruption.**

drug reaction. See **adverse drug reaction.**

drug receptor, any part of a cell, usually a large protein molecule, on the cell surface or in the cytoplasm with which a drug molecule interacts to trigger a response or effect.

drug rehabilitation center, an agency that provides treatment for a person with a chemical or drug dependency.

drug resistance, the ability of disease organisms to resist effects of drugs that previously were toxic to them. Bacterial resistance to an antibiotic can result from mutation of a strain that has been exposed to an antibiotic or similar agent. Such acquired resistance may result from a chromosomal disruption or acquisition of a stray bit of deoxyribonucleic acid (DNA) on a resistant plasmid. It can also be caused by extrachromosomal pieces of DNA that carry codes for antibiotic-resistant genes from a transposon, a DNA segment capable of insertion into a bacterial chromosome-resistant plasmid, or both. Decreased permeability to an antimicrobial is a common form of intrinsic resistance. Alteration or inactivation of the antibiotic is perhaps the most common mechanism of drug resistance. Acquired resistance to beta-lactam antibiotics is determined by the production of enzymes that inactivate the antibiotic. Drug resistance may also result from a change in the target site on which it acts.

drug-resistant *Streptococcus pneumoniae,* a widespread strain of respiratory pathogen that is drug resistant. Until the 1960s *S. pneumoniae* was almost uniformly susceptible to penicillin alone. In 1967 resistance to penicillin and other microbial drugs was first reported in Australia. It has since spread worldwide. The introduction of pneumococcal conjugate vaccines has reduced the number of these infections substantially.

drug-seeking behavior (DSB), a pattern of seeking narcotic pain medication or tranquilizers with forged prescriptions, false identification, repeated requests for replacement of "lost" drugs or prescriptions, complaints of severe pain without an organic basis, and abusive or threatening behavior manifested when denied drugs.

drug sensitivity, an increase in the responsiveness of an individual to a medication because of variations in the way the drug is metabolized. Should not be confused with **drug allergy.**

drug sequestration, the process by which certain drugs are stored in the body tissues. Examples include tetracycline, which may be stored in bone tissue, and chloroquine, which is stored in the liver. Certain vitamins and other substances are stored in fat deposits.

drug tolerance, a condition of cellular adaptation to a pharmacologically active substance so that increasingly larger doses are required to produce the same physiological or psychological effect obtained earlier with smaller doses. Also called **metabolic tolerance.** See also **tachyphylaxis.**

drug trial, the process of determining an adequate and effective therapeutic dose or duration of treatment of a specific drug for a particular disease state. The trial culminates with (1) an acceptable clinical result, (2) intolerable adverse effects, (3) a poor response after an appropriate blood level is reached, or (4) administration of the drug for a specific time.

drum cartridge catheter technique, a method used in central vein cannulation. The vein is cannulated with an introducer cannula. The needle is removed and is replaced by the drum cartridge catheter, which is left in place.

drum electrode, an induction electrode that produces a strong magnetic field, used primarily with pulsed short-wave diathermy.

drusen /drooˈzən/ [Ger, *Drüse,* stony granule], small yellowish hyaline deposits that develop beneath the retinal pigment epithelium, sometimes appearing as nodules within the optic nerve head. They tend to occur most frequently in persons older than 60 years of age and are commonly associated with age-related macular degeneration. However, the presence of drusen does not indicate the person has age-related macular degeneration. There are several types of drusen, requiring different levels of caution and risk.

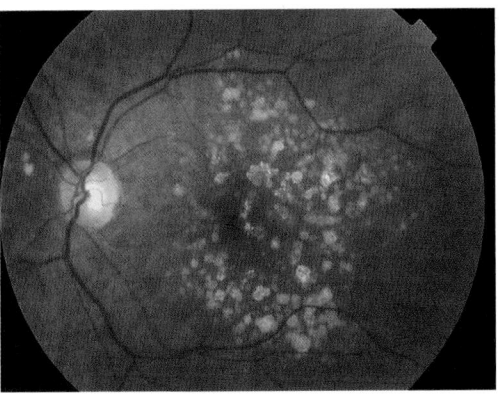

Retinal drusen *(Kanski and Bowling, 2011)*

DRVs, abbreviation for **Daily Reference Values.**

dry abscess, **1.** a collection of pus that disperses without reaching a point of bursting. **2.** the remains of an abscess after the pus is absorbed.

dry catarrh [AS, *dryge* + Gk, *kata,* down, *rhoia,* flow], a dry cough, accompanied by almost no expectoration, that occurs in severe coughing spells. It is associated with asthma and emphysema in older people.

dry cholera. See **cholera sicca.**

dry cough, a cough that does not produce sputum.

dry crackle, an abnormal chest sound produced by air passing through fibrotic alveolar sacs.

dry dressing, a plain dressing containing no medication, applied directly to an incision or a wound to prevent contamination or trauma or to absorb secretions.

dry eye syndrome, a dryness of the cornea and conjunctiva caused by a deficiency in tear production or altered tear film composition. It results in a sensation of a foreign body in the eye, burning eyes, keratitis, and erosion of the epithelial layers of the cornea and conjunctiva. See also **Sjögren syndrome.**

dry gangrene, a late complication of diabetes mellitus that is already complicated by arteriosclerosis, in which the affected extremity becomes cold, dry, and shriveled and eventually turns black. See also **gangrene.**

dry gas (D), a gas that contains no water vapor.

dry heat, a thermal effect produced by adding dry air or reducing the humidity of the environment.

dry heat sterilization [AS, *dryge* + *haetu* + L, *sterilis*], a method of sterilization that uses heated dry air at a temperature of 320° to 356° F (160° to 180° C) for 90 minutes to 3 hours.

dry heaves. *(Nontechnical)* See **retch.**

dry ice, solid carbon dioxide, with a temperature of about −140° F (−78° C). It is used in cryotherapy of various skin disorders, such as the removal of warts.

dry labor, *(Nontechnical)* a term used by the lay public to describe a labor in which amniotic fluid has already escaped. As amniotic fluid is continually produced, no labor is really dry.

dry mouth. *(Nontechnical)* See **xerostomia.**

dry pleurisy [AS, *dryge,* dry; Gk, *pleuritis*], inflammation of the pleura without effusion of serum. The cause may be a localized injury. Dry pleurisy may also be an early sign of tuberculosis.

dry rale, a fine sound associated with any of various interstitial lung diseases, such as idiopathic pulmonary fibrosis.

dry skin, epidermis that lacks moisture or sebum, often characterized by a pattern of fine lines, scaling, and itching.

Causes include too frequent bathing, low humidity, and decreased production of sebum in aging skin. Treatment includes decreased frequency of bathing, increased humidity, bath oils, emollients such as lanolin and glycerin, and hydrophilic ointments. Also called **xerosis.**

dry socket, an inflamed condition of a tooth socket (alveolus) after a tooth extraction. The socket is not actually dry but is filled with a degenerating, infective blood clot. Normally a blood clot forms over the alveolar bone at the base of the socket after an extraction. If the clot fails to form properly or becomes dislodged, bone tissue and nerve endings are exposed to the oral environment and can become infected, a usually painful condition. Analgesics, applied topical sedatives, and drainage are required, in addition to treatment with local or systemic antibiotic therapy to cure the infection. See also **alveolitis.**

dry vomiting [AS, *dryge* + L, *vomere,* to vomit], *(Nontechnical)* nausea with retching that does not produce vomitus. Also called **dry heaves.**

DSA, abbreviation for **digital subtraction angiography.**

DSB, abbreviation for **drug-seeking behavior.**

DSDB, abbreviation for **direct self-destructive behavior.**

DSM, abbreviation for *Diagnostic and Statistical Manual of Mental Disorders.*

DSM-5. See *Diagnostic and Statistical Manual of Mental Disorders.*

DSN, initialism for *Doctor of Science in Nursing.*

DSR, abbreviation for **dynamic spatial reconstructor.**

DT, abbreviation for **diphtheria and tetanus toxoids.**

DTaP, a vaccine in which the pertussis vaccine component is in the acellular rather than whole-cell form. Abbreviation for **diphtheria and tetanus toxoids and pertussis vaccine.**

DTH, abbreviation for **delayed-type hypersensitivity.**

DTIC-Dome, an antineoplastic. Brand name for **dacarbazine.**

DTP vaccine, a combination of diphtheria and tetanus toxoids and acellular pertussis, administered intramuscularly for active immunization against these diseases.

DTR, abbreviation for **deep tendon reflex.**

DTs, abbreviation for **delirium tremens.**

dual-energy x-ray absorptiometry (DEXA), 1. an imaging technique that uses two low-dose x-ray beams with different levels of energy to produce a detailed image of body components, used primarily to measure bone mineral density. **2.** an imaging technique for quantifying bone density, used in the diagnosis and management of osteoporosis.

dual-focus tube, an x-ray tube used for diagnostic imaging. It has one large and one small focal spot. The large focal spot is used when techniques that produce high heat are required; the small focal spot is used to produce fine, detailed images.

duality of central nervous system control /dyo͞o·al″itē/, a theory that the normal central nervous system is regulated by a check-and-balance feedback program. The theory is based on studies of posture-movement, mobility-stability, flexion-extension synergies, and similar action-reaction examples related to laws of basic physics. Duality theorists suggest that central nervous system disorders result from imbalances in the feedback system.

dual personality, a state of dissociation in which an individual presents personas to others at different times as two different persons, each with a different name and different personality traits. The two personalities are generally independent, contrasting, and unaware of the existence of the other. See also **dissociative disorder.**

Duane syndrome /dwān/ [Alexander Duane, American ophthalmologist, 1858–1926], an autosomal-dominant syndrome in which the affected eye shows limitation or absence of abduction, restriction of adduction, retraction of the globe on adduction, narrowing of the palpebral fissure on adduction and widening on abduction, and deficient convergence. It can be either unilateral or bilateral. It is caused by abnormal innervation of the third and sixth cranial nerves.

DUB, 1. abbreviation for **dysfunctional uterine bleeding. 2.** a genetically determined human blood factor that is associated with immunity to certain diseases.

Dubin-Johnson syndrome /do͞o″bin jon″sən/ [Isadore N. Dubin, American pathologist, 1913–1980; Frank B. Johnson, American pathologist, b. 1919], a rare chronic hereditary hyperbilirubinemia, characterized by nonhemolytic jaundice, abnormal liver pigmentation, and abnormal function of the gallbladder. It is caused by inability of the liver to excrete several organic anions. See also **hyperbilirubinemia of the newborn, Rotor's syndrome.**

dubnium (Db) [Joint Institute for Nuclear Research at Dubna, Russia], a transuranic element. Its atomic number is 105; the mass of its best-known isotope is 260. It is produced by an induced nuclear reaction.

DuBois formula /do͞oboiz″/ [Eugene DuBois, American physician 1882–1959], a logarithmic method of calculating the number of square meters of body surface area of an individual from the height in centimeters, the weight in kilograms, and a constant, 0.007184.

Dubowitz assessment [Victor Dubowitz, South African-English pediatrician, b. 1931], a method of clinical assessment of gestational age in the newborn that includes neurological criteria for the infant's maturity and other physical criteria to determine the gestational age of the infant; useful from birth to 5 days of life.

Duchenne-Aran disease /do͞oshen″äräN′/ [Guillaume B.A. Duchenne, French neurologist, 1806–1875; François A. Aran, French physician, 1817–1861], muscular atrophy caused by degeneration of the anterior horn cells of the spinal cord, primarily affecting the upper extremities. Chronic muscle wasting and weakness first appear in the hands and advance progressively to the arms and shoulders, eventually affecting the legs and other body areas. Several conditions may lead to this disease, such as the injection of toxins.

Duchenne-Erb paralysis. See **Erb's palsy.**

Duchenne disease /do͞oshen″/ [Guillaume B.A. Duchenne, French neurologist, 1806–1875], a series of three different neurological conditions. Kinds include **spinal muscular atrophy, bulbar paralysis, tabes dorsalis.** See also **muscular dystrophy.**

Duchenne muscular dystrophy [Guillaume B.A. Duchenne, French neurologist, 1806–1875], an abnormal congenital condition characterized by progressive symmetric wasting of the leg and pelvic muscles. This disease predominantly affects males and accounts for 50% of all muscular dystrophy diseases. Also called **pseudohypertrophic muscular dystrophy.**

■ OBSERVATIONS: It is an X-linked recessive disease that appears insidiously between 3 and 5 years of age and spreads from the leg and pelvic muscles to the involuntary muscles. Associated muscle weakness produces a waddling gait and pronounced lordosis. Muscles rapidly deteriorate, and calf muscles become firm and enlarged as a result of fatty deposits. Affected children experience contractures, have difficulty climbing stairs, often stumble and fall, and display winged scapulae when they raise their arms. Such persons are usually confined to wheelchairs by 12 years of age, and progressive weakening of cardiac muscle causes tachycardia and pulmonary problems. The patients affected may also have cardiac murmurs, faint heart sounds, and chest pain and may suffer arrhythmias or infections that produce overt heart failure.

■ INTERVENTIONS: There is no successful medical treatment of the disease. Orthopedic appliances, exercise, physical therapy, and surgery to correct contractures can help preserve mobility. Nursing care emphasizes psychological support of the patient and family and encouragement of the patient to prevent long periods of bed rest and inactivity. Occupational therapy to provide splints, braces, grab bars, and overhead slings helps the patient exercise and participate in activities of daily living. A wheelchair helps preserve mobility. Other devices that can increase comfort and help prevent footdrop include footboards, high-topped sneakers, and foot cradles. A team approach to the care of the patient that addresses the progress of the disease and both the short-term and long-term needs of the patient and family is necessary.

■ PATIENT CARE CONSIDERATIONS: Complications, especially in the later stages of this disease, can cause sudden death. Duchenne muscular dystrophy usually causes death within 10 to 15 years of symptom onset.

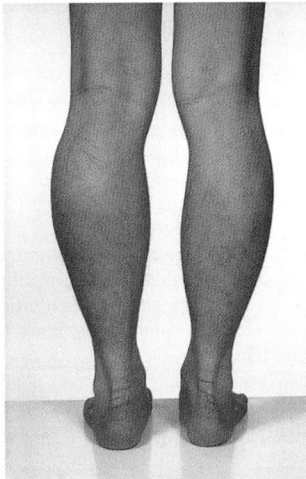

Duchenne muscular dystrophy: enlargement of calves *(Perkin, 2002)*

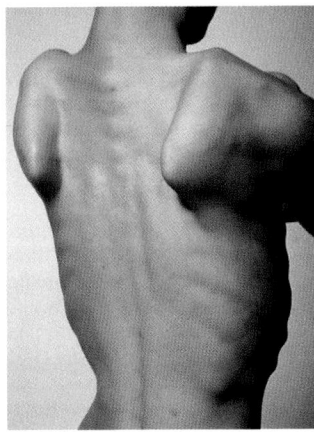

Duchenne muscular dystrophy: winged scapulae *(Mir, 2003)*

duck embryo vaccine, the first vaccine developed for pre-exposure and postexposure to the rabies virus. See **rabies vaccine.**

duck walk. *(Nontechnical)* See **metatarsus valgus.**

duct [L, *ducere*, to lead], a narrow tubular structure, especially one through which material is secreted or excreted.

ductal carcinoma, a neoplasm of the epithelium of ducts, especially in the breast or pancreas.

duct ectasia, an abnormal dilation of a duct by lipids and cellular debris. In a mammary duct the condition, which mainly tends to affect postmenopausal women, may be accompanied by inflammation and infiltration by plasma cells.

ductile, having the property of allowing metals to be drawn into the thinness of a wire.

ductility /duktil″itē/, the property of a material having a large elastic range and tending to deform before failing from stress.

duction /duk″shən/, the movement of an individual eyeball from the primary to secondary or tertiary position of gaze.

ductless gland /dukt″les/, a gland lacking an excretory duct, such as an endocrine gland, that secretes hormones directly into blood or lymph.

duct of Rivinus /rivē″nəs/ [L, *ducere*, to lead], one of the minor sublingual ducts. Compare **Bartholin duct.**

duct of Wirsung. See **pancreatic duct.**

ductoscopy, endoscopy with a microendoscope that facilitates assessment of changes in the breast ducts in women.

ductus /duk′tōōs/, the Latin term for *duct.*

ductus arteriosus, a vascular channel in the fetus that joins the pulmonary artery directly to the descending aorta. It normally closes after birth.

ductus deferens. See **vas deferens.**

ductus epididymidis, a tube into which the efferent ductules of the testes empty.

ductus venosus, the vascular channel in the fetus passing through the liver and joining the umbilical vein with the inferior vena cava. Before birth it carries highly oxygenated blood from the placenta to the fetal circulation. It closes shortly after birth as pulmonary circulation is established and as the vessels in the umbilical cord collapse and become occluded. See also **ductus arteriosus, foramen ovale.**

due diligence, efforts made by responsible persons to prevent causing harm to others or their property or organization.

due process, ability to take legal action when rights are violated; derived from the words due, owed, or owing as a natural or moral right, and process, to proceed against by law.

Duhring's disease. See **dermatitis herpetiformis.**

Duke longitudinal study, long-range, in-depth research into the normal aging process of middle-aged and older men and women conducted at Duke University Medical Center, Durham, NC. The Duke studies led to development of the "longevity quotient" used to evaluate an individual's rate of aging. It is calculated by the number of years a person survives beyond a given time divided by the expected number of years derived from actuarial tables.

Dukes classification, a staging system for colorectal tumors, from A to D, according to the degree of tissue invasion and metastasis. A Dukes A tumor is one that is confined to the mucosa and submucosa. A B tumor is one that has invaded the musculature but has not involved the lymphatic system. C tumors have invaded the musculature with metastatic involvement of the regional lymph nodes. D tumors are those that have metastasized to distant organ tissues. Compare **TNM staging system.**

Dulcolax, a stimulant laxative. Brand name for **bisacodyl.**

dull, **1.** blunt. **2.** sluggish. **3.** not sharp, vivid, or intense.

dull pain [ME, *dul*, not sharp; L, *poena*, penalty], a mildly throbbing acute or chronic pain, which may not deter the patient from expected or desired activity.

duloxetine, a miscellaneous antidepressant.

■ INDICATIONS: This drug is used to treat major depressive disorder and neuropathic pain associated with diabetic neuropathy.

■ CONTRAINDICATIONS: Narrow angle glaucoma and known hypersensitivity to this drug prohibit its use.

■ ADVERSE EFFECTS: Adverse effects of this drug include insomnia, anxiety, dizziness, tremor, fatigue, decreased appetite, decreased weight, thrombophlebitis, peripheral edema, constipation, diarrhea, dysphagia, nausea, vomiting, anorexia, dry mouth, colitis, gastritis, abnormal and delayed ejaculation, erectile dysfunction, urinary hesitation, photosensitivity, bruising, and swelling. A common side effect is abnormal vision.

dumb terminal [AS, *tumb,* mute; L, *terminalis,* end], a computer terminal that serves as an input or output device only and is incapable of performing any data-processing functions by itself. Compare **intelligent terminal.**

dumdum fever. See **kala-azar.**

dump [ME, *dumpen,* to throw down], **1.** to print out the contents of a computer memory or other computer-storage medium. **2.** the printout resulting from such an operation.

dumping syndrome [ME, *dumpen,* to throw down], the combination of profuse sweating, nausea, dizziness, and weakness experienced by patients who have had a subtotal gastrectomy. Symptoms are felt soon after eating, when the contents of the stomach empty too rapidly into the duodenum. The entrance of this hypertonic material into the small intestine causes fluid to shift into the intestine via osmosis. This increased volume causes peristalsis and diarrhea. The loss of fluid from capillaries causes hypotension with resulting weakness and dizziness. A high-protein, high-calorie diet, with small, dry meals taken frequently, should prevent discomfort and ensure adequate nutrition. See also **gastrectomy.**

Dunlop skeletal traction, an orthopedic mechanism that helps immobilize the upper arm in the treatment of contracture or supracondylar fracture of the elbow. The mechanism uses a system of traction weights, pulleys, and ropes and may be accompanied by skin traction. Dunlop skeletal traction is usually applied unilaterally but may also be applied bilaterally. Compare **Dunlop skin traction.**

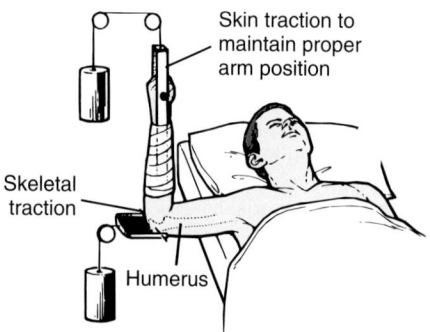

Dunlop skeletal traction *(Mir, 2003)*

Dunlop skin traction, an orthopedic mechanism consisting of adhesive or nonadhesive skin traction that helps immobilize the upper limb in the treatment of contracture or supracondylar fracture of the elbow. The mechanism uses a system of traction weights, pulleys, and ropes, usually applied unilaterally but sometimes bilaterally. Compare **Dunlop skeletal traction.**

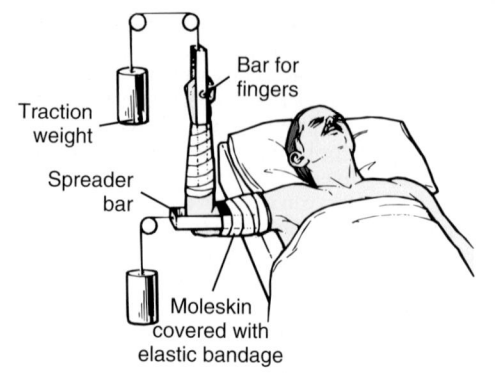

Dunlop skin traction *(Mir, 2003)*

Dunton, William R. [American psychiatrist, 1868–1966], one of the founders of the National Society for the Promotion of Occupational Therapy and a pioneer in the profession throughout his career. He advanced the idea that occupation must aim toward a useful end for it to effectively treat mental and physical disability. He authored two influential textbooks and numerous journal articles in occupational therapy (OT) and promoted quilting for his patients for its healing potential. He is often referred to as the father of occupational therapy. The National Society for the Promotion of Occupational Therapy became the American Occupational Therapy Association in 1921. See also **American Occupational Therapy Association.**

duodena. See **duodenum.**

duodenal /dōō′ədē″nəl/ [L, *duodeni,* 12 fingers], pertaining to the duodenum.

duodenal atresia, congenital absence or occlusion of a portion of the duodenum, characterized by vomiting a few hours after birth, cessation of bowel movements after 1 to 3 days, and usually distension of the epigastrium. It is often associated with Down syndrome.

duodenal bulb, the first part of the superior portion of the duodenum, which has a bulblike appearance on radiographic views of the small intestine.

duodenal digestion [L, *duodeni,* 12 fingers, *digere,* to separate], digestion that occurs in the first intestinal segment beyond the pylorus, where secretions of the liver and pancreas are received and mixed with the partially digested food from the stomach. Chyle is formed, fats are emulsified, starch is hydrolyzed, and proteolytic enzymes begin to break down proteins.

duodenal mesentery. See **mesoduodenum.**

duodenal switch (DS), a surgical treatment for morbid obesity consisting of resection of the greater curvature of the stomach, leaving in place the pylorus and a little of the duodenum, which are anastomosed to the ileum. The rest of the duodenum and jejunum simply empty their secretions into the distal ileum through a new anastomosis. Also called **biliopancreatic diversion, gastric reduction duodenal switch.**

duodenal ulcer, an ulcer in the duodenum, the most common type of peptic ulcer. See also **peptic ulcer.**

duodenectomy /dōō′ədenek″təmē/ [L, *duodeni,* 12 fingers; Gk, *ektomē,* excision], the total or partial excision of the duodenum.

duodenitis /dōō′ədēnī″tis/ [L, *duodeni,* 12 fingers; Gk, *itis,* inflammation], a condition of inflammation of the duodenum.

duodeno-, prefix meaning "duodenum": *duodenogastric, duodenography, duodenostomy.*

duodenogastric reflux /dōō′ədē′nōgas′trik/ [L, *duodeni,* 12 fingers + Gk, *gaster,* stomach; L, *refluere,* to flow back], reflux of the contents of the duodenum into the stomach, which may occur normally, especially during fasting.

duodenogastroesophageal reflux. See **gastroesophageal reflux.**

duodenography /dōō′ədənog″rəfē/ [L, *duodeni,* 12 fingers; Gk, *graphein,* to record], the radiographic examination of the duodenum and pancreas. It usually requires drug-induced paralysis of the duodenum to prevent peristaltic activity, use of a double-contrast medium, and maximum distension with the contrast medium so that the duodenum presses against and outlines the head of the pancreas. Also called **hypotonic duodenography.**

duodenojejunal flexure. See **angle of Treitz.**

duodenoscope /dōō′ədē″nəskōp′/, an endoscopic instrument, usually fiberoptic, inserted via the mouth for the visual examination of the duodenum.

duodenoscopy /dōō′ədənos″kəpē/, the visual examination of the duodenum by means of an endoscope.

duodenostomy /dōō′ədēnos″təmē/ [L, *duodeni,* 12 fingers; Gk, *stoma,* mouth], the surgical creation of a direct opening to the duodenum through the abdominal wall.

duodenum /dōō′ədē″nəm, dōō-od″inəm/ *pl.* **duodena, duodenums** [L, *duodeni,* 12 fingers], the shortest, widest, and most fixed portion of the small intestine, taking an almost circular course from the pyloric valve of the stomach so that its termination is close to its starting point. The majority of digestive enzymes secreted by the pancreas, as well as bile from the gallbladder, are ejected into the duodenum. It is about 25 cm long and is divided into superior, descending, horizontal, and ascending portions. The superior portion extends from the pylorus to the neck of the gallbladder. The descending portion extends from the neck of the gallbladder at the level of the first lumbar vertebra to the cranial border of the fourth lumbar vertebra. The horizontal portion passes from right to left, from the level of the fourth lumbar vertebra to the diaphragm. The ascending portion rises on the left side of the aorta to the level of the second lumbar vertebra, turning ventrally to become the jejunum at the duodenojejunal flexure. Compare **jejunum, ileum.**

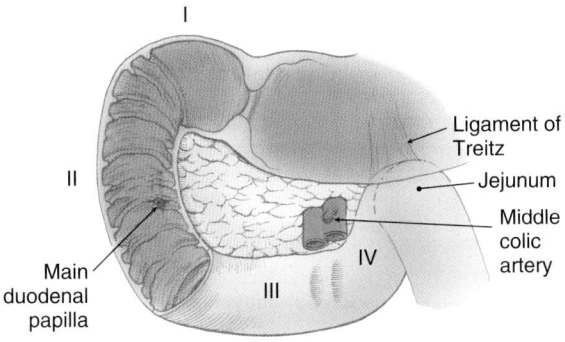

Duodenum *(Rothrock, 1992)*

dup, (in cytogenetics) abbreviation for *duplication.*

duplex inheritance. See **amphigenous inheritance.**

duplex kidney /dōō″pleks/, a kidney that has two separate collecting systems, with either a duplex ureter or a single ureter.

duplex scanner /dōō″pleks/, an ultrasound machine that generally combines a 7.5- or 10-MHz imaging probe with a 3-MHz pulsed Doppler to allow visualization of a portion of the venous system. The scanner can determine the direction of blood flow within the veins.

duplex transmission [L, *duplex,* twofold], the passage of a neural impulse in both directions along a nerve fiber.

duplex ultrasonography, a combination of real-time and Doppler ultrasonography. See also **duplex scanner.**

duplicated collecting system. See **double collecting system.**

duplicatus anterior, *(Obsolete)* conjoined twins. Now called **conjoined twins.**

dupp /dup/, a syllable used to represent the second heart sound in auscultation. It is shorter and higher-pitched than the first heart sound. See also **heart sound.**

Dupuytren contracture /dYpY·itraN″, dēpē·itran″/ [Guillaume Dupuytren, French surgeon, 1777–1835; L, *contractura* drawing together], a progressive, painless thickening and tightening of subcutaneous tissue of the palm, causing the fourth and fifth fingers to bend into the palm and resist extension. Tendons and nerves are not involved. Although the condition begins in one hand, both become symmetrically affected. Of unknown cause, it is most frequent in middle-aged males. Early surgical removal of the excess fibrous tissue under general anesthesia restores full use of the hand. An incision is made in the palm, and the thickened tissue is excised carefully to prevent injury to adjacent ligaments.

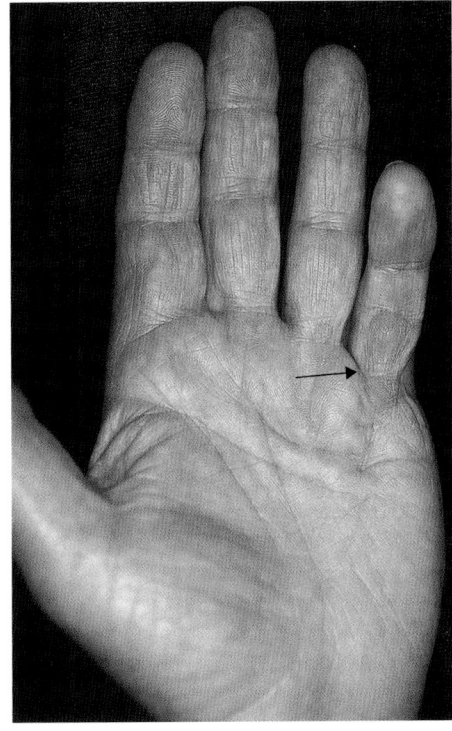

Dupuytren contracture *(Bolognia et al, 2014)*

Dupuytren fracture. See **Galeazzi fracture.**

dura. See **dura mater.**

durable medical equipment (DME), a medically necessary apparatus, device, or accessory that is prescribed by a physician, nurse practitioner, physician assistant, or clinical nurse specialist to improve the quality of life for an individual in his or her place of residence. Examples include wheelchairs and oxygen systems. See also **medical device.**

durable power of attorney for health care /dyo͞or′ə bəl/, a document that designates an agent or proxy to make health care decisions if the patient is no longer able to make them. The document directs the surrogate person to function as "attorney-in-fact" and make decisions regarding all treatment, including the final decision about cessation of treatment.

Durabolin, an anabolic steroid. Brand name for **nandrolone.**

dural sac /dyo͞or′əl/, the blind pouch formed by the lower end of the dura mater, at the level of the second sacral segment.

dural sheath, an extension of the dura mater covering the optic nerve and spinal nerve roots.

dural venous sinuses, endothelial-lined spaces between the outer periosteal and inner meningeal layers of the dura mater into which empty the cerebral veins, the cerebellar veins, and the veins draining the brainstem and that lead to the internal jugular veins.

dura mater /do͞o′rə mā″tər, dyo͞o′rə/ [L, *durus,* hard, *mater,* mother], the outermost and most fibrous of the three membranes surrounding the brain and spinal cord. The dura mater encephali covers the brain, and the dura mater spinalis covers the cord. See also **meninges.**

duration, the length of time a current is flowing. Also called **pulse width.**

duration tetany, a tetanic contraction occurring in response to the application of a galvanic current. See **tetany.**

duress /dyo͞ores′/ [L, *durus,* hard], (in law) an action compelling another person to do what he or she would not do voluntarily. A consent form signed under duress is not valid.

Durham-Humphrey Amendment, a 1952 modification of the 1938 U.S. Food, Drug, and Cosmetic Act. It differentiates between prescription and over-the-counter medications and specifies medications that can or cannot be refilled without a new prescription. It also identifies which original prescriptions and refills can be authorized over the telephone.

Duroziez' murmur /dY′rōzyäs, dir′-, do͞o′r-/ [Paul L. Duroziez, French physician, 1826–1897; L, *murmur*], a systolic murmur heard over the femoral or another large artery when the artery is compressed. The phenomenon is associated with high arterial pulse pressure or aortic insufficiency. A diastolic murmur may also be heard when pressure on the artery is increased distal to the stethoscope.

dust [AS], any fine, particulate, dry matter. Kinds include **inorganic dust, organic dust.**

dustborne infection, a disease in which the pathogenic organism is airborne in dust particles, as in coccidioidomycosis.

dutasteride, a sex hormone 5 alpha-reductase inhibitor used to treat benign prostatic hyperplasia in men with an enlarged prostate gland.

Dutch type periodic fever. See **hyperimmunoglobulinemia D syndrome.**

duty [ME, *duete,* conduct], (in law) an obligation owed by one party to another. Duty may be established by statute or other legal process, as by contract or oath supported by statute, or it may be voluntarily undertaken. Every person has a duty of care to all other people to prevent causing harm or injury by negligence.

duty cycle, the percentage of time that ultrasound is being generated (pulse duration) over one pulse period. Also called **mark:space ratio.**

Duverney fracture /do͞o′vərnā″/ [Joseph G. Duverney, French anatomist, 1648–1730], a break in the ilium just below the anterior superior spine.

Duvoid, a cholinergic receptor agonist. Brand name for **bethanechol chloride.**

DVD, an optical computer disk that is used to digitally store large graphic and video content. Abbreviation for *digital video disk.*

dV/dt, the rate of change of voltage with respect to time.

D.V.M., abbreviation for *Doctor of Veterinary Medicine.*

DVT, abbreviation for **deep vein thrombosis.**

dwarf /dwôrf/ [AS, *dweorge*], **1.** *n.,* a person of extremely short stature, especially one whose body parts are not proportional. Also called **nanus.** See also **achondroplastic dwarf, ateliotic dwarf, cretin dwarf, diastrophic dwarf, nanocephalic dwarf, phocomelic dwarf, pituitary dwarf, primordial dwarf, sexual dwarf, thanatophoric dwarf. 2.** *v.,* to prevent or retard, for example, normal growth.

dwarfism /dwôrf″izəm/, the underdevelopment of the body, characterized predominantly by extreme shortness of stature. At times the condition is associated with other defects and may involve varying degrees of intellectual disability. Dwarfism has multiple causes, including genetic defects and endocrine dysfunction involving either the pituitary or the thyroid gland.

dwarf tapeworm infection, a type of intestinal parasitic disease caused by an infestation of *Hymenolepis nana.* It occurs mainly in the southern United States and usually affects children who ingest eggs by placing contaminated materials into the mouth. It is the most common tapeworm infection diagnosed in the United States and throughout the world. The disease may be asymptomatic or may result in abdominal complaints and diarrhea. An infection may be treated with niclosamide or paromomycin. Prevention involves good hygiene practices. It is often seen in children subject to institutional living. See also *Hymenolepis.*

Dwayne-Hunt law /dwān″hunt″/, the principle that x-ray energy is inversely proportional to the photon wavelength. Thus, as the photon wavelength increases, photon energy decreases, and vice versa.

dwell time, 1. the time that something therapeutic or diagnostic remains inside a patient's body. **2.** in peritoneal dialysis, the time needed for the dialysis solution to remain in the body for equilibration to be reached on the two sides of the membrane.

dwindles, (*Informal*) a condition of physical deterioration involving several body systems, usually in an elderly person.

Dwyer instrumentation /dwī′ər/ [A.F. Dwyer, 1920–1975], a procedure for correcting the spinal curvature associated with scoliosis, involving a cable that is inserted to assist in maintaining the corrected curvature while the fusion heals. It is not usually removed unless there is postoperative indication of displacement or a pattern of associated symptoms. Dwyer cable instrumentation involves surgical intervention through the pulmonary cavity and the rib cage.

D-**xylose absorption test,** a serum, plasma, or urine test whose results reflect intestinal absorption of orally administered monosaccharide D-xylose, which is not a metabolic product found in the body. In malabsorption, blood levels and urine excretion are reduced. The test is used to separate patients with diarrhea caused by pancreatic or biliary dysfunction from those with diarrhea caused by malabsorption from conditions such as sprue, intrinsic factor deficiency, or Crohn disease.

D-xylose breath test, a breath test for bacterial overgrowth in the intestine in which the fasting patient is administered a dose of D-xylose labeled with carbon 14 and the amount of radiolabeled carbon dioxide in the breath is measured at regular time intervals. Excessive levels of carbon dioxide mean that there are high levels of anaerobic bacteria in the intestines breaking down the xylose.

Dy, symbol for the element **dysprosium.**

dyad /dī″ad/ [Gk, *dyas,* two], **1.** one of the paired homologous chromosomes, consisting of two chromatids, that result from the division of a tetrad in the first meiotic division of gametogenesis. –*dyadic, adj.* **2.** pertaining to two people engaged with each other.

dyadic interpersonal communication /dī·ad″ik/, a process in which two people interact face to face as senders and receivers, as in a conversation.

Dyazide, a fixed-combination drug formulated to maintain normal potassium levels by containing two diuretic agents. Brand name for **triamterene, hydrochlorothiazide.**

dyclonine hydrochloride /dī″klōnīn/, a local anesthetic, with bactericidal and fungicidal properties, for oral pain, pruritus, insect bites, and minor skin burns and injuries.

dye /dī/ [AS, *deag*], **1.** *v.,* to apply coloring to a substance. **2.** *n.,* a chemical compound capable of imparting color to a substance to which it is applied. Various dyes are used in medicine as stains for tissues, test reagents, therapeutic agents, and coloring agents in pharmaceutic preparations.

dye laser, a system of highly selective laser destruction of skin blemishes using various dyes at wavelengths at the longer oxygenated hemoglobin absorption peaks to overcome interference from overlying melanin.

-dynamia, -dynamy, suffix meaning "(condition of) strength": *adynamia.*

dynamic /dīnam″ik/ [Gk, *dynamis,* force], **1.** tending to change or to encourage change, such as a dynamic nurse-patient relationship. **2.** (in respiratory therapy) a condition of changing volume. Compare **static.**

dynamic cardiac work, the energy transfer that occurs during the ventricular ejection of blood.

dynamic compliance, the distensibility of the lungs, as measured by plethysmography during the breathing cycle. See also **lung compliance.**

dynamic electromyography, the study of patterns of muscle activity during activity.

dynamic equilibrium, the ability of a person to adjust to displacements of the body's center of gravity by changing its base of support.

dynamic ileus, an intestinal obstruction with associated recurrent and continuous muscle spasms. Also called **spastic ileus.**

dynamic imaging, the ultrasonographic imaging of an object in motion at a frame rate that does not cause significant blurring of images and at a repetition rate sufficient to represent the movement pattern adequately. Also called **real-time imaging.**

dynamic nurse-patient relationship, a conceptual framework in which the interpersonal aspects of the nurse-patient relationship are analyzed. Many factors affect the relationship. Elements in the process include the behavior of the patient, the reaction of the nurse, and the actions of the nurse that are intended to aid the patient. Also examined are the means for validating nurses' perceptions and interpretations and for evaluating the effects of the nursing actions taken.

dynamic orthosis, *pl. orthoses,* a medical device that allows movement in desired joint(s); a splint that assists an individual with movements. See **orthosis.**

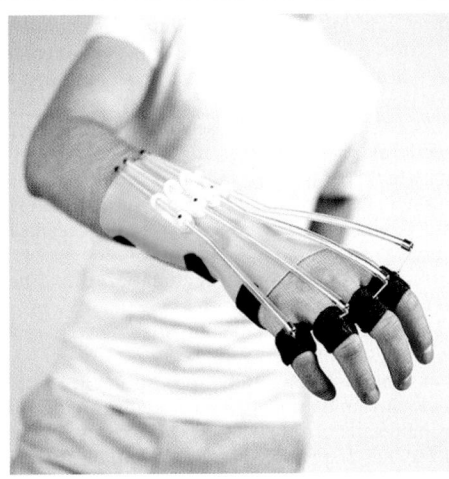

Dynamic metacarpophalangeal joint (MCP) orthosis
(Image courtesy Orfit.)

dynamic psychiatry, the study of motivational, emotional, and biological factors as determinants of human behavior.

dynamic range, 1. (in digital imaging) the range of gray shades that can be displayed by the system. **2.** the range of sound intensity from the faintest sound a person can hear to the level that causes pain.

dynamic retinoscopy, a type of retinoscopy in which the patient fixes the gaze on a target at a near distance. Accommodation is active.

dynamic spatial reconstructor (DSR), a computed tomography (CT)–based scanner that allows for high-resolution, three-dimensional imaging and visualization of cardiac cycles.

dynamic splint [Gk, *dynamis,* force; D, *splinte*], any brace or orthosis that incorporates springs, elastic bands, or other materials that produces a constant active force on a joint or joints and the surrounding tissue to increase joint range of motion or to compensate for loss of movement following muscle paresis or paralysis.

dynamic system theory, (in occupational therapy) a theory used as a framework to provide interventions for individuals with motor challenges proposing that multiple factors interact to make up movement.

dynamo-, prefix meaning "power" or "strength": *dynamometer.*

dynamometer /dī′nəmom″ətər/ [Gk, *dynamis,* force, *metron,* measure], a device for measuring the degree of force used in the contraction of a group of muscles, such as a squeeze dynamometer, which measures the gross grip strength of the hand muscles. Also called **ergometer.**

-dynamy. See **-dynamia, -dynamy.**

Dynapen, an antibiotic. Brand name for **dicloxacillin sodium.**

dyne /dīn/, a unit of force, specifically the force required to accelerate a free mass of 1 g at 1 cm/sec. One dyne equals 10^{-5} newton.

-dynia, suffix meaning "pain": *acrodynia, gastrodynia.*

dynode /dī″nōd/, one of a series of platelike elements that amplify electron pulses in a photomultiplier tube. Each electron that strikes a dynode causes several secondary electrons to be emitted. The dynode gain is the ratio of the number of secondary electrons to the number of incident electrons.

dynorphin /dīnôr″fən/, an endogenous opioid derived from the prohormone prodynorphin. It is a neuroactive peptide with potent analgesic effects.

dyphylline /dīfil″in/, a methylxanthine bronchodilator.

■ INDICATIONS: It can be prescribed in the treatment of bronchospasm in acute bronchial asthma, bronchitis, and emphysema but is no longer widely used.

■ CONTRAINDICATIONS: It is used with caution in patients with peptic ulcer or cardiovascular disease. Known hypersensitivity to this or to other xanthines prohibits its use.

■ ADVERSE EFFECTS: Among the more serious adverse reactions are GI distress, dizziness, tachycardia, headache, and palpitations.

Dyrenium, a potassium-sparing diuretic. Brand name for **triamterene.**

dys-, prefix meaning "bad, painful, disordered": *dyskinesia, dysarthria, dysarthrosis.*

dysacusis /dis′əkoo″sis/ [Gk, *dys,* difficult, *akouein,* to hear], **1.** any impairment of hearing involving difficulty processing details of sound as opposed to any loss of sensitivity to sound. **2.** pain or discomfort in the ear from exposure to sound.

dysaesthesia. See **dysesthesia.**

dysaphia, a disorder of touch sensation. See **paraphia.**

dysarthria /disär″thrē·ə/ [Gk, *dys + arthroun,* to articulate], difficult, poorly articulated speech, resulting from interference in the control and execution over the muscles of speech, usually caused by damage to a central or peripheral motor nerve.

■ OBSERVATIONS: There are many different types, depending on the location of the lesion. A universal finding is difficulty with the articulation of consonants. Intelligibility varies greatly, depending on the extent of neurological damage. Hypernasality is frequently present.

■ INTERVENTIONS: Treatment will vary depending on type; strengthening the oral musculature and improving breathing patterns are often required. A speech-language pathologist will conduct an evaluation and work with the individual patient to improve communication abilities and establish treatment goals.

■ PATIENT CARE CONSIDERATIONS: It is important for persons with dysarthria, their families and significant others, and the health care team to work together to establish good communication patterns.

dysarthrosis /dis′ärthrō″sis/ [Gk, *dys,* difficult, *arthron,* joint], any disorder of a joint, including disease, dislocation, or deformity, that makes movement of the joint difficult.

dysautonomia /disô′tənō″mē·ə/ [Gk, *dys + autonomia,* self-government], an autosomal-recessive disease of childhood characterized by defective lacrimation, skin blotching, emotional instability, motor incoordination, total absence of pain sensation, and hyporeflexia, seen almost exclusively in Ashkenazi Jews. Also called **familial autonomic dysfunction, familial dysautonomia, Riley-Day syndrome.**

dysbarism /dis″bäriz′əm/, a reaction to a sudden change in environmental pressure, such as rapid exposure to the lower atmospheric pressures of high altitudes. It is marked by symptoms similar to those of decompression sickness.

dysbasia /disbā″zhə/, difficulty in walking caused by a lesion in the nervous system or by mental illness.

dysbetalipoproteinemia /disbet′əlip′əprō′tinē″mē·ə/. See **broad beta disease.**

dyscholia /diskō″lē·ə/ [Gk, *dys + chole,* bile], any abnormal condition of the bile, related to either the quantity secreted or the condition of the constituents.

dyschondroplasia. See **enchondromatosis.**

dyschroic film fault /diskrō″ik/, a defect in a photograph or radiograph that appears as a pinkish coloration when the image is viewed by transmitted light and as a green coloration when the image is viewed by reflected light. It is usually caused by incomplete fixation of the film or by an overused fixing solution with a depleted acid concentration.

dyscrasia /diskrā″zhə/ [Gk, *dys + krasis,* mingling], pertaining to an abnormal condition of the blood or bone marrow, such as leukemia, aplastic anemia, or prenatal Rh incompatibility.

dyscrastic fracture /diskras″tik/, any fracture caused by the weakening of a specific bone as a result of a debilitating disease.

dysdiadochokinesia /dis′dī·ədō′kōkinē′zhə/ [Gk, *dys + diadochos,* working in turn, *kinesis,* movement], an inability to perform rapidly alternating movements, such as rhythmically tapping the fingers on the knee. The cause is a cerebellar lesion and is related to dysmetria, which also involves inappropriate timing of muscle activity.

dyseidetic /dis′idet′ik/, dyslexic regarding the sight or recognition of whole words.

dysenteric /dis′enter″ik/ [Gk, *dys + enteron,* intestine], pertaining to or resembling dysentery.

dysentery /dis″inter·ē/ [Gk, *dys + enteron,* intestine], an inflammation of the intestine, especially of the colon. The most common causes are bacterial (*Shigella* infection) and amebic (*Entamoeba histolytica* infection), although it can also be caused by chemical irritants. It is characterized by frequent and bloody stools, abdominal pain, and tenesmus. Dysentery is common in underdeveloped areas of the world and in times of disaster and social disorganization when sanitary living conditions, clean food, and safe water are not available. Treatment involves rehydration therapy. See also **amebic dysentery, shigellosis.**

dysentery toxin, an exotoxin produced by *Shigella dysenteriae.*

dysentry. See **dysentery.**

dysergia /disur″jē·ə/ [Gk, *dys + ergon,* work], a condition characterized by lack of muscle coordination caused by a defect of efferent nerve impulses.

dyserythropoiesis, defective development of erythrocytes.

dysesthesia /dis′esthē″zhə/, a common effect of spinal cord injury characterized by sensations of numbness, tingling, burning, or pain felt below the level of the lesion. It may also follow a dermatome distribution of a spinal nerve, as in the pain of shingles.

dysfibrogenemia /disfi″brojĕne′mīə/, the presence in the blood of abnormal fibrinogen; secondary to liver disease.

dysfluency /disfloo″ənsē/ [Gk, *dys-,* difficult + L, *fluere,* to flow], an interruption in the normal flow of speech. Kinds include **stuttering, hesitation dysfluencies.** −*dysfluent, adj.*

dysfunctional /disfungk″shənəl/ [Gk, *dys + L, functio,* performance], **1.** (of a body organ or system) unable to function normally. **2.** deviating from a prescribed behavior pattern in a way that is harmful. −*dysfunction, n.*

dysfunctional communication, a communication that results from inaccurate perceptions, faulty internal filters (personal interpretations of information), and social isolation. Communication behaviors of emotionally ill persons may have characteristics that prevent their establishing and maintaining relationships with others.

dysfunctional stereotype, a stereotype in which abnormal or impaired aspects of a culture are emphasized.

dysfunctional uterine bleeding (DUB), abnormal uterine bleeding that is not caused by a tumor, inflammation, or pregnancy. It may be characterized by painless, irregular heavy bleeding or intermenstrual spotting or periods of amenorrhea. The condition is associated with anovulation and unopposed estrogen stimulation. The plan of treatment depends on the patient's age and may include dilation and curettage and use of hormones and other medications.

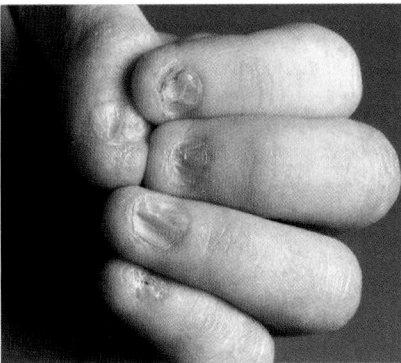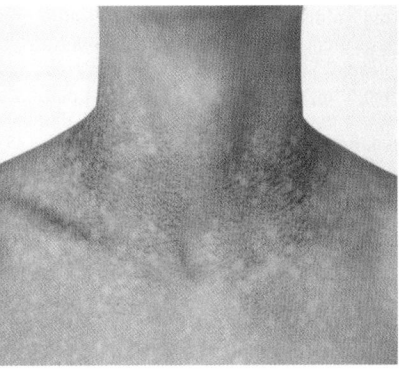

Nail dystrophy and cutaneous hyperpigmentation associated with dyskeratosis congenita
(Savage and Alter, 2009)

dysgammaglobulinemia /disgam′əglob′yəlinē″mē·ə/, an inherited immunodeficiency disease. Affected individuals do not produce adequate numbers of immunoglobulins, including antibodies, and therefore are susceptible to infection, cancer, and other diseases.

dysgenesis /disjen″əsis/ [Gk, *dys* + *genein,* to produce], defective or abnormal formation of an organ or part, primarily during embryonic development. Also called *dysgenesia.* −*dysgenic, adj.*

dysgenics /disjen″iks/, the study of factors or situations that are genetically detrimental to the future of a race or species. Compare **eugenics.**

dysgenitalism /disjen″itəliz′əm/ [Gk, *dys* + L, *genitalis,* belonging to birth], any condition involving the abnormal development of the genital organs.

dysgerminoma /dis′jərminō″mə/ *pl.* dysgerminomas, dysgerminomata [Gk, *dys* + L, *germen,* germ; Gk, *oma,* tumor], a rare malignant tumor of the ovary that occurs in young women and is believed to arise from the undifferentiated germ cells of the embryonic gonad. The tumor is histologically identical to seminoma. Dysgerminomas are extremely sensitive to irradiation and chemotherapy, and most patients retain their fertility. Also called **embryoma of the ovary, ovarian seminoma.**

dysgeusia /disgoō″zhə/ [Gk, *dys* + *geusis,* taste], an abnormal or impaired sense of taste.

dysglandular /disglan″dyələr/, caused by or related to excessive or inadequate secretion by a gland.

dysgnathia, malformation and/or abnormalities of the teeth that involve the jaws.

dysgnathic anomaly /disnath″ik/ [Gk, *dys* + *gnathos,* jaw], an abnormality that affects one or both jaws. Also called **dysgnathia.**

dysgraphia /disgraf″ē·ə/ [Gk, *dys* + *graphein,* to write], an impairment of the ability to write. Compare **agraphia.**

dyshidrosis /dishīdrō′sis/ [Gk, *dys,* difficult + *hidros,* sweat], any disorder of the eccrine sweat glands. Also spelled *dyshydrosis.*

dyskeratosis /dis′kerətō″sis/ [Gk, *dys* + *keras,* horn, *osis,* condition], an abnormal or premature keratinization of epithelial cells.

dyskeratosis congenita, an X-linked syndrome with onset in childhood, characterized by nail dystrophy, reticular cutaneous hyperpigmentation, mucosal leukokeratosis, and pancytopenia resembling that of Fanconi syndrome.

dyskinesia /dis′kinē″zhə/ [Gk, *dys* + *kinesis,* movement], an impairment of the ability to execute voluntary movements. See also **tardive dyskinesia.** −*dyskinetic, adj.*

dyskinesia intermittens, a condition of intermittent limping caused by circulatory impairment.

dyskinetic syndrome /dis′kinet″ik/, a form of cerebral palsy involving a basal ganglion disorder. Clinical features include athetoid movements of the extremities and sometimes the trunk. There may also be choreiform movements that tend to increase with emotional tension and diminish during sleep.

dyslexia /dislek″sē·ə/ [Gk, *dys* + *lexis,* word], an impairment of the ability to read, as a result of a variety of pathological conditions, some of which are associated with the central nervous system. Dyslexic persons often reverse letters and words, cannot adequately distinguish the letter sequences in written words, and have difficulty determining left from right. Compare **alexia.** −*dyslexic, adj.*

dyslipidemia /dislip′id·ē′mē·ə/ [Gk, *dys,* difficult + Fr, *lipide,* fat + Gk, *haemia,* blood], abnormality in, or abnormal amounts of, lipids and lipoproteins in the blood. See also **hyperlipemia, hypolipoproteinemia.**

dysmaturity /dis′machoor″itē/ [Gk, *dys* + L, *maturare,* to make ripe], **1.** the failure of an organism to develop, ripen, or otherwise achieve maturity in structure or function. **2.** the condition of a fetus or newborn who is abnormally small or large for its age of gestation. Compare **postmature infant, premature.** Kinds include **small for gestational age (SGA) infant, large for gestational age (LGA) infant.** −*dysmature, adj.*

dysmegalopsia /dis′megəlop″sē·ə/ [Gk, *dys,* difficult + *mega,* large], an inability to judge the size or measure of an object accurately. Compare **dysmetropsia.**

dysmelia /dismē″lyə/ [Gk, *dys* + *melos,* limb], an abnormal congenital condition characterized by missing or shortened extremities of the body associated with abnormalities of the spine in some individuals. It is caused by abnormal metabolism during the embryonic development of the limbs. See also **phocomelia.**

dysmenorrhea /dis′menərē″ə/ [Gk, *dys* + *men,* month, *rhein,* to flow], painful menstruation sufficiently severe that it prevents the performance of normal activities. Primary dysmenorrhea is associated with an excess of prostaglandins, primarily prostaglandin $F_{2\alpha}$ (PGF$_{2\alpha}$). Secondary dysmennorhea may be caused by a clinically identifiable cause or, if not, it is called idiopathic. These causes may be classified as extrauterine (endometriosis, benign and malignant tumors, inflammation, adhesions and, rarely, psychogenic), intramural (adenomyosis, leiomyomata), and intrauterine (leiomyomata, polyps intrauterine contraceptive devices, infection, and cervical stenosis). Treatment depends on identification of the specific cause. Also called **menorrhagia.** Also spelled *dysmenorrhoea.*

dysmetria /dismē″trē·ə/ [Gk, *dys* + *metron,* measure], a condition that prevents the affected individual from properly measuring distances associated with muscular acts and from controlling muscular action. It is associated with cerebellar lesions and typically characterized by overestimating or underestimating the range of motion needed to place the limbs correctly during voluntary movement. A person without neurological impairment and with eyes closed can move the arms from a position of 90 degrees of flexion to a position over the head and then return them to the 90-degree position; a person with dysmetria is unable to perform this test accurately. See also **hypermetria, hypometria.**

dysmetropsia, a visual illusion related to size. Also called **Alice in Wonderland syndrome.** Compare **dysmegalopsia.**

dysmnesic syndrome /disnē″sik/, a memory disorder characterized by an inability to learn simple new skills, although the person can still perform highly complex skills learned before the onset of the condition. The cause is a disease or injury that affects only certain brain tissues associated with memory. The victim often confabulates about events of the recent past for which there is no clear memory.

dysmorphogenesis /dis′môrfōjen″əsis/, the development of body structures that are not shaped according to expected standards.

dysmorphophobia /-fō″bē·ə/ [Gk, *dys + morphe,* form, *phobos,* fear], **1.** a fundamental delusion of body image. **2.** the morbid fear of deformity.

dysmyelination /dismī″ĕ-lina′shun/, breakdown or defective formation of a myelin sheath, usually involving biochemical abnormalities.

dysorexia /dis′ôrek″sē·ə/, **1.** an eating disorder associated with emotional or psychological impairment. **2.** a diminished, disordered, or unnatural appetite.

dysostosis /dis′ostō″sis/ [Gk, *dys + osteon,* bone, *osis*], an abnormal condition characterized by defective ossification, especially defects in the normal ossification of fetal cartilages. Kinds include **cleidocranial dysostosis, craniofacial dysostosis, mandibulofacial dysostosis, metaphyseal dysostosis, Nager's acrofacial dysostosis.**

dysostosis mandibularis. See **Nager acrofacial dysostosis.**

dyspareunia /dis′pəroo͞o″nē·ə/, an abnormal pain during sexual intercourse due to a spasm. It may result from abnormal conditions of the genitalia, dysfunctional psychophysiological reaction to sexual union, forcible coition, or incomplete sexual arousal. Dyspareunia is also associated with hormonal changes of menopause and lactation that result in drying of the vaginal tissues and with endometriosis, which may result in painful adhesions around the vagina and ligaments, decreasing their flexibility during intercourse. Dryness is commonly relieved by the local application of water-soluble lubricants. See also **vaginismus.**

dyspepsia /dispep″sē·ə/ [Gk, *dys + peptein,* to digest], a vague feeling of epigastric discomfort after eating. There is an uncomfortable feeling of fullness, heartburn, bloating, and nausea. Dyspepsia is not a distinct condition, but it may be a sign of an underlying intestinal disorder such as peptic ulcer, gallbladder disease, or chronic appendicitis. Symptoms usually increase in times of stress. −*dyspeptic, adj.*

dysphagia /disfā″jē·ə/ [Gk, *dys,* difficult + *phagia,* to swallow], a swallowing disorder, commonly associated with obstructive or motor disorders of the oropharynx, hypopharynx, or esophagus. Patients with obstructive disorders, such as esophageal tumor or lower esophageal ring, are unable to swallow solids but can tolerate liquids. Persons with motor disorders, such as achalasia, are unable to swallow solids or liquids. Diagnosis of the underlying condition is made through barium studies, the observed clinical signs, and evaluation of the patient's symptoms. See also **achalasia, aphagia, corkscrew esophagus.**

dysphagia lusoria [L, *lusus naturae,* freak of nature], an abnormal condition characterized by difficulty in swallowing, caused by the compression of the esophagus from an anomalous right subclavian artery that arises from the descending aorta and courses behind or in front of the esophagus. Compare **contractile ring dysphagia, vallecular dysphagia.**

dysphasia, difficulty swallowing. Compare **dysphagia.** Should not be confused with **aphasia.**

dysphonia /disfō″nē·ə/ [Gk, *dys + phone,* voice], any abnormality in the speaking voice, such as hoarseness. Dysphonia puberum refers to the voice changes that occur in adolescent boys.

dysphoria /disfôr″ē·ə/, a disorder of affect characterized by depression and anguish.

dysphylaxia /dis′filek″sē·ə/, a sudden awakening from deep sleep or a condition marked by too early awakening.

dyspigmentation /dispig′məntā″shən/, any abnormal increase or decrease in the production or distribution of skin pigment. See also **depigmentation.**

dysplasia /displā″zhə/ [Gk, *dys + plassein,* to form], any abnormal development of tissues or organs. An alteration in cell growth resulting in cells that differ in size, shape, and appearance, often as a result of chronic irritation. Common sites for dysplasia are the cervix and the respiratory tract in individuals with a history of smoking.

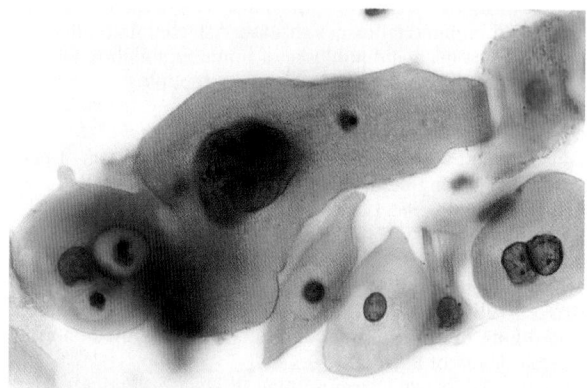

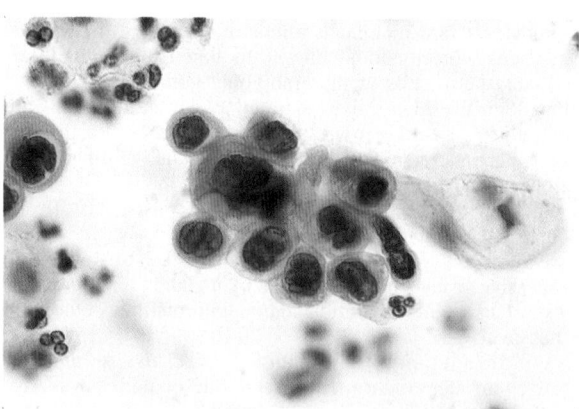

Top, **Mild dysplasia.** ***Bottom,*** **Severe dysplasia.**
(Damjanov and Linder, 2000)

-dysplasia, suffix meaning "(condition of) abnormal development": *chondrodysplasia, encephalodysplasia, osteomyelodysplasia.*

dysplasia epiphysealis hemimelica, a rare condition characterized by swellings in the extremities, usually on the inner and outer aspects of the ankles and knees, consisting of bone covered with epiphyseal cartilage, leading to limitation of motion of the joints. Also called **Trevor disease.**

dysplastic nevus, an acquired atypical nevus with an irregular border, indistinct margin, and mixed coloration, often occurring in large numbers and often a precursor of malignant melanoma.

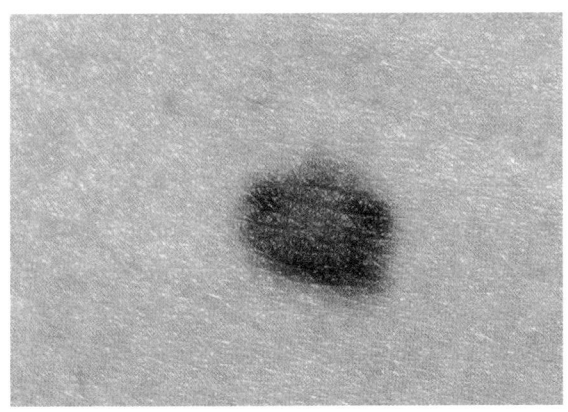

Dysplastic nevus *(Calonje et al, 2012)*

dysplastic nevus syndrome, an inherited genetic syndrome that causes the individual to have a large number of nevi (moles), often 100 or more. These nevi tend to become dysplastic and predispose the individual to the development of malignant melanoma. Also called **familial atypical mole-malignant melanoma syndrome (FAMMM), B-K mole syndrome.**

dyspnea /dispnē″ə/ [Gk, *dys* + *pnoia*, breathing], a distressful subjective sensation of uncomfortable breathing that may be caused by many disorders, including certain heart and respiratory conditions, strenuous exercise, or anxiety. Also called **breathlessness.** Also spelled *dyspnoea.* Compare **hyperpnea.** *−dyspneal, dyspneic, adj.*

dyspraxia /disprak″sē·ə/ [Gk, *dys* + *prassein*, to do], a partial loss of the ability to perform skilled, coordinated movements in the absence of any associated defect in motor or sensory functions. See also **apraxia.**

dysprosium (Dy) /disprō″sē·əm/ [Gk, *dys* + *prositos*, to approach], a rare-earth metallic element. Its atomic number is 66, and its atomic mass is 162.50. Dysprosium, in conjunction with other elements, is used in making laser materials, commercial lighting, neutron-absorbing control rods in nuclear reactors, and data-storage devices such as hard disks. It is employed as a source of infrared radiation. It is used in dosimeters for measuring ionizing radiation. Radioactive isotopes of dysprosium are used in radioisotope scanning, particularly in studies of the bones and joints.

dysproteinemia /disprō″tēnē″mē·ə/ [Gk, *dys* + *protos,* first, *haima,* blood], an abnormality of the protein content of the blood, usually involving the immunoglobulins.

dysraphia /disrā″fē·ə/ [Gk, *dys* + *raphe,* seam], failure of a raphe (an atomic seam) to fuse completely, as in incomplete closure of the neural tube. Also called **status dysraphicus.**

dysraphic syndrome /disraf″ik/, a developmental disorder, usually involving the spinal cord, such as encephalocele or myelomeningocele. See also **Arnold-Chiari malformation.**

dysregulation hypothesis /disreg″yəlā″shən/, the view that depression and affective disorders do not simply reflect decreased or increased catecholamine activity but that they are failures of the regulation of these systems.

dysrhythmia /disrith″mē·ə/, any disturbance or abnormality in a normal rhythmic pattern, specifically, irregularity in the brain waves, cardiac rhythm, or cadence of speech. Compare **arrhythmia.**

dyssebacea /disibā″shē·ə/ [Gk, *dys* + L, *sebum,* suet], a skin condition characterized by red, scaly, greasy patches on the nose, eyelids, scrotum, and labia. It results from a

deficiency of vitamin B$_2$ and is most commonly associated with chronic alcoholism, liver disease, chronic diarrhea, and protein malnutrition. Also called **shark skin.**

dyssymbolia, difficulty sharing thoughts and ideas using language.

dyssynergia /dis″inur″jē·ə/ [Gk, *dys* + *syn,* together, *ergein,* work], any disturbance in muscular coordination, as in cases of ataxia.

dystaxia /distak″sē·ə/ [Gk, *dys* + *taxis,* order], partial ataxia, such as dystaxia agitans, in which a spinal cord irritation causes a tremor but no paralysis.

dysthymia /disthim″ē·ə/ [Gk, *dys* + *thymos,* mind], a form of chronic unipolar depression that tends to occur in elderly persons with debilitating physical disorders, multiple interpersonal losses, and chronic marital difficulties. Several depressive episodes may merge into a low-grade chronic depressive state.

dysthymic disorder /disthim″ik/ [Gk, *dys* + *thymos,* mind], a disorder of mood in which the essential feature is a chronic disturbance of mood of at least 2 years' duration. It involves either depressed mood or loss of interest or pleasure in all or almost all usual activities and pastimes, and associated symptoms, but not of sufficient severity and duration to meet the criteria for a major depressive episode.

dysthyroid orbitopathy /disthī″roid or″bitop′əthē/ [Gk, *dys,* difficult, *thyreos,* shield, *eidos,* form; L, *orbita,* wheel track + Gk, *pathos,* disease], the inflammatory changes of the eye orbit associated with thyroid dysfunction, usually in Graves disease. Also called *dysthyroid ophthalmopathy,* **Graves orbitopathy.**

dystocia /distō″shə/ [Gk, *dys* + *tokos,* birth], abnormal labor, or a difficult labor or childbirth. It is characterized by abnormal progression of labor, either a protraction disorder (labor is slow to progress) or arrest disorder (labor ceases to progress). See also **cephalopelvic disproportion, fetal presentation, arrest disorders.**

dystonia /distō″nē·ə/ [Gk, *dys* + *tonos,* tone], any impairment of muscle tone. The condition commonly involves the head, neck, and tongue and often occurs as an adverse effect of a medication.

dystonia musculorum deformans (DMD), a rare abnormal condition characterized by intense, irregular torsion muscle spasms that contort the body. The muscles of the trunk, shoulder, and pelvis are commonly involved.

■ OBSERVATIONS: This disease appears in several forms, generally classified as autosomal recessive or autosomal dominant. The cause of this disorder is not known; a biochemical dysfunction is suspected. The autosomal-recessive form appears most often in Ashkenazic Jews and starts between 5 and 15 years of age, causing abnormalities of movement and speech. Muscle power and tone appear normal, but convulsive spasms make the involved muscles relatively useless. The autosomal-recessive form of the disease commonly begins with intermittent spasmodic inversion of the foot so that the affected individual has difficulty in placing the heel on the ground when walking and a distinctive, bowing gait develops. Lordosis and torsion of pelvis appear as the proximal muscles become more involved. Torticollis is often an early sign if the muscles of the neck and shoulder girdle are affected. The autosomal-dominant form of the disease appears in early adult life, generally affects the axial musculature, and progresses more slowly than the autosomal-recessive form.

■ INTERVENTIONS: Some muscle-relaxing drugs, such as the benzodiazepines, have been helpful in treating both forms of the condition. Mild cases have been successfully controlled for long periods with treatments that combine the use of muscle-relaxing drugs and physical therapy. Deep brain stimulation (DBS) may be employed, especially when medications do not sufficiently alleviate symptoms or the side effects are too severe. Speech therapy is helpful when the oral musculature is affected. Physical and occupational therapy, the use of splints, stress management, and biofeedback may benefit the patient.

■ PATIENT CARE CONSIDERATIONS: The care and support of the patient and family are complex. A coordinated team approach will assist in the management of the disorder. Genetic counseling should be considered for the family of a child with DMD.

dystonic /diston″ik/, referring to impairments of muscle tone, often excessive increase in tone, when the muscle is in action, and to hypotonia when it is at rest, often resulting in postural abnormalities.

dystrophia, a condition due to faulty or defective nutrition. See also **dystrophy.**

dystrophic /distrof″ik/ [Gk, *dys* + *trophe,* nourishment], pertaining to a usually congenital disorder of structure or function of an organ or tissue that is aggravated by defective nutrition, such as accumulation of calcium salts in the cornea.

dystrophic calcification [Gk, *dys* + *trophe,* nourishment; L, *calx,* lime, *facere,* to make], **1.** the pathological accumulation of calcium salts in necrotic or degenerated tissues. Compare **metastatic calcification. 2.** a response of the dental pulp to traumatic injury wherein the pulp produces reparative dentin, which can eventually obliterate the entire pulp chamber and root canal. Also called *pulpal dystrophic calcification.*

dystrophin /distrof″in/, a missing or defective protein in Duchenne's muscular dystrophy that is localized to the sarcolemma of the muscle cell membrane. Its absence results in abnormal cell permeability, which may lead to cell destruction.

dystrophin-glycoprotein complex (DGC), a large oligomeric complex of proteins and glycoproteins of the sarcolemma that is critical to the stability of muscle fiber membranes and to the linking of the actin cytoskeleton to the extracellular matrix. It includes dystrophin, sarcoglycans, dystroglycans, sarcospan, syntrophins, and dystrobrevin. Abnormalities of the plasma membranes of the muscle fibers that destroy this complex have been associated with several types of muscular dystrophy and with cardiomyopathy.

dystrophy /dis″trəfē/ [Gk, *dys* + *trophe,* nourishment], any abnormal condition caused by defective nutrition. It often entails a developmental change in muscles that does not involve the nervous system, such as fatty degeneration associated with increased size but decreased strength. Also called **dystrophia.** See also **muscular dystrophy.**

dysuria /disyoor″ē·ə/ [Gk, *dys* + *ouron,* urine], painful, burning urination, often caused by a bacterial infection, inflammation, or obstruction of the urinary tract. Laboratory examination of the urine may reveal the presence of blood, bacteria, or white blood cells. Dysuria is a symptom of cystitis, urethritis, prostatitis, urinary tract tumors, and some gynecological disorders and of the use of certain medications, such as opiates. Compare **hematuria, pyuria.**

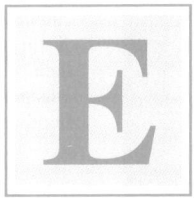

e-, prefix meaning "out from": *emollient.*

E, ε. See **epsilon.**

E, **1.** symbol for **elastance. 2.** symbol for **energy. 3.** symbol for *expectancy.* **4.** symbol for **electromotive force. 5.** symbol for **illumination.**

E₁, symbol for **monomolecular elimination reaction.**

E₂, symbol for **bimolecular reaction.**

Eakes, Georgene Gaskill, a nursing theorist who, with Mary Lermann Burke and Margaret A. Hainsworth, developed the Theory of Chronic Sorrow to describe the ongoing feelings of loss that arise from illness, debilitation, or death.

Eales' disease /ēlz/ [Henry Eales, British physician, 1852–1913], a condition marked by recurrent hemorrhages into the retina and vitreous, affecting mainly males in the second and third decades of life.

ear [AS, *eare*], one of two organs of hearing and balance, consisting of the external, middle, and internal ear. The external ear includes the skin-covered cartilaginous auricle visible on either side of the head and the part of the external auditory canal outside the skull. Together they form a funnel that directs sound waves toward the eardrum, or tympanic membrane, which marks the boundary between the external ear and the air-filled middle ear. The middle ear contains three very small bones, the malleus, incus, and stapes, which transmit vibrations caused by sound waves reaching the tympanic membrane to the oval window of the inner ear. The leverage

of the ossicles, or middle-ear bones, increases the intensity of sound vibrations by more than 25 dB. Because the inner ear is filled with fluid, the increased intensity helps compensate for the loss of signal normally caused by sound-wave reflection of the fluid. The inner ear contains two separate organs: the vestibular apparatus, which provides the sense of balance, and the cochlea, with the organ of Corti, which receives vibrations from the middle ear and translates them into nerve impulses, which are again interpreted by brain cells as specific sounds.

earache /ir″āk/ [AS, *eare* + *acan,* to hurt], a pain in the ear, sensed as sharp, dull, burning, intermittent, or constant. The cause is not necessarily a disease of the ear, because infections and other disorders of the nose, oral cavity, larynx, and temporomandibular joint can produce referred pain in the ear. Also called **otalgia, otodynia.** See also **referred pain.**

eardrop instillation, the instillation of a medicated solution into the external auditory canal of the ear. The patient is asked to turn the head to the side so that the ear being treated faces upward. The orifice is exposed, and the drops of medicine are directed toward the internal wall of the canal. The pinna is pulled upward and outward in a person more than 3 years of age and down and back in a younger child. The tragus is pushed against the ear canal to ensure that the drops stay in the canal.

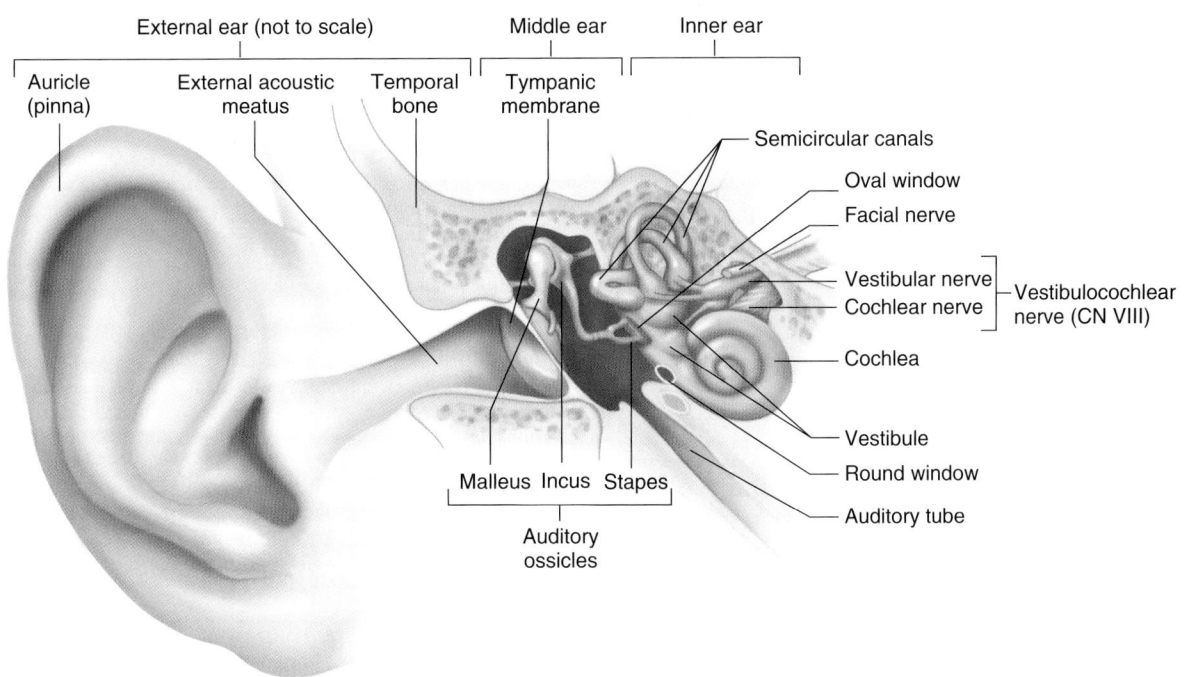

Structures of the ear *(Patton and Thibodeau, 2016)*

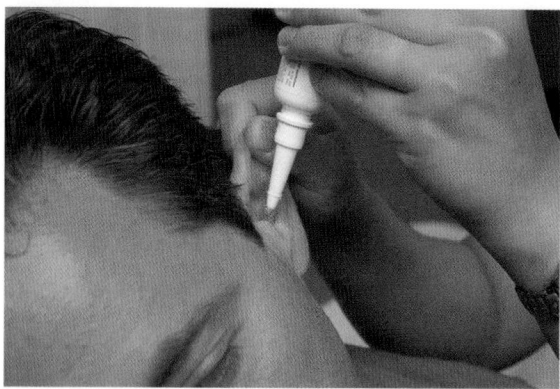

Eardrop instillation in an adult (deWit and O'Neill, 2014)

eardrops [AS, *eare* + *dropa*], a topical, liquid form of medication for the local treatment of various conditions of the ear, such as inflammation or infection of the lining of the external auditory canal or impacted cerumen (earwax).

eardrum. (*Nontechnical*) See **tympanic membrane.**

early adolescence, the period that encompasses the middle-school years (10 to 14 years of age). The majority of young people in this age group are experiencing puberty. See also **adolescence.**

Early and Periodic Screening Diagnosis and Treatment (EPSDT), a benefit of the U.S. Medicaid program for enrolled children under the age of 21 to ensure appropriate preventive, dental, and mental health care, as well as developmental and specialty services. All states are required to provide comprehensive services based on federal guidelines. See also **Medicaid.**

early childhood caries, a dental condition that occurs in children between 12 months and 3 years of age as a result of being given a bottle at bedtime, resulting in prolonged exposure of the teeth to milk or juice. Caries are formed because pools of milk or juice in the mouth break down to lactic acid and other decay-causing substances. Preventive measures include elimination of the bedtime feeding or substitution of water for milk or juice in the nighttime bottle. Formerly called **baby bottle tooth decay, nursing bottle caries, baby bottle caries.**

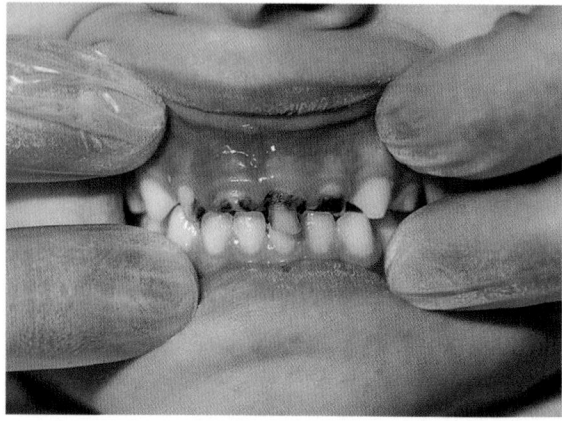

Early childhood caries (Sorrentino and Remmert, 2012)

early intervention program (EIP), **1.** educational and multidisciplinary support services for children with developmental delays and disabilities. The services involve families and caregivers to facilitate the achievement of a child's full potential. **2.** (in occupational therapy) programs that help children improve their abilities and learn new skills. They promote the function and engagement of infants and toddlers (birth to 3 years) and their families in everyday routines by addressing occupations.

early psychosis intervention, a specialized treatment program for individuals experiencing an initial psychotic episode. The treatment goals are to reduce the duration of untreated psychosis through early and appropriate detection and response and the minimization of social and societal impact.

ear oximeter [AS, *eare* + Gk, *oxys*, sharp, *genein*, to produce, *metron*, measure], a device placed over the earlobe that transmits a beam of light through the earlobe tissue to a receiver. It is a noninvasive method of measuring the level of saturated hemoglobin in the blood. As the amount of saturated hemoglobin alters the wavelengths of light transmitted through the earlobe, analysis of the light received is translated into percentage of oxygen saturation (SaO_2) of the blood. See also **pulse oximeter.**

ear speculum [AS, *eare* + L, *speculum*, mirror], a short, funnel-shaped tube attached to an otoscope for examining the ear canal.

ear thermometry, the measurement of the temperature of the tympanic membrane by detection of infrared radiation from the eardrum. See also **tympanic membrane thermometer.**

earwax. See **cerumen.**

East African sleeping sickness, now called **African trypanosomiasis.** See also **Rhodesian trypanosomiasis.**

eastern equine encephalitis (EEE), a form of encephalitis endemic to eastern regions of North America. The causative organism may be transmitted to humans via the bite of aedes mosquitoes. See **equine encephalitis.**

■ OBSERVATIONS: Symptoms of acute infection include the acute onset of fever, headache, disorientation, and seizures followed by coma in severe cases. Serologic testing remains the primary method for diagnosing infection.

■ INTERVENTIONS: Treatment is supportive.

■ PATIENT CARE CONSIDERATIONS: Mortality rates between 30% and 50% have been reported. Recovery may be marked by residual neurologic deficits and epilepsy.

eating, the ability to keep food and fluids in the mouth, move them around inside the mouth, and swallow them. Nurses, occupational therapists, and speech therapists play important and complementary roles in the assessment and management of eating for individuals who experience difficulty with this task.

eating disorders, a group of behaviors often fueled by unresolved emotional conflicts symptomized by altered food consumption. Compare **pica.** Kinds include **anorexia nervosa, bulimia, binge eating.**

Eating Disorders Inventory (EDI-3), a widely used self-report questionnaire measuring traits associated with eating disorders.

Eaton agent pneumonia. See **mycoplasma pneumonia.**

Eaton-Lambert syndrome [Lee M. Eaton, American neurologist; Edward H. Lambert, 20th-century American physiologist], a rare autoimmune disorder that is characterized by muscle weakness of the limbs. It is a form of myasthenia that tends to be associated with lung cancer. Also called **Lambert-Eaton myasthenic syndrome.**

EAV, abbreviation for **electroacupuncture after Voll.**

Ebbecke's reaction. See **autographism.**

EBCT, abbreviation for **electron beam computed tomography.**

Ebner's glands [Victor von Ebner, Austrian histologist, 1842–1925], serous glands of the tongue, opening at the bottom of the trough surrounding the circumvallate papillae.

Ebola virus disease /ēbō″lə/ [Ebola River District, Congo], an infection caused by a species of ribonucleic acid viruses of the *Filovirus* genus. There are four identified subtypes of Ebola virus: Côte d'Ivoire, Sudan, and Zaire, which have been associated with human disease, and Reston, which causes fatal hemorrhagic disease in nonhuman primates and originated in the Philippines. Also called **African hemorrhagic fever,** *Ebola hemorrhagic fever.* See also **Marburg virus disease.**

■ OBSERVATIONS: The incubation period ranges from 2 to 21 days. Initial symptoms include high fever, headache, chills, myalgia, sore throat, red itchy eyes, and malaise. Later symptoms include severe abdominal pain, chest pain, bleeding, shock, vomiting, and diarrhea. Maculopapular rash may occur in some patients.

■ INTERVENTIONS: Treatment is supportive; in nearly 90% of cases, death occurs within 1 week. It is not known why some patients are able to recover from the Ebola virus while others are not, but the latter have no detectable immune response to the infection.

■ PATIENT CARE CONSIDERATIONS: The natural reservoir and method of transmission of primary infections are unknown, but secondary infection is by direct contact with infectious blood or other body secretions, in research settings, or by airborne particles.

EBP, **1.** abbreviation for **epidural blood patch. 2.** abbreviation for **evidence-based practice.**

Ebstein's anomaly [Wilhelm Ebstein, German physician, 1836–1912; Gk, *anomalia,* irregularity], a congenital heart defect in which the tricuspid valve is displaced downward into the right ventricle. The abnormality is often associated with right-to-left atrial shunting and Wolff-Parkinson-White syndrome. See also **Wolff-Parkinson-White syndrome.**

EBV, abbreviation for **Epstein-Barr virus.**

EC, abbreviation for **Enzyme Commission.**

ec-, prefix meaning "out of": *eccentric, eccrine, ecchondroma.*

ECC, **1.** initialism for **emergency cardiac care. 2.** initialism for *external cardiac compression.*

eccentric /eksen″trik/ [Gk, *ek,* out, *centre,* center], **1.** pertaining to an object or activity that departs from the usual course or practice. **2.** pertaining to behavior that may appear to be odd or unconventional but does not necessarily reflect a disorder.

eccentric contraction, a type of muscle contraction that occurs as the muscle fibers lengthen, such as when a weight is lowered through a range of motion. The contractile force generated by the muscle is weaker than an opposing force, which causes the muscle to stretch. Compare **concentric contraction.**

eccentric exercise, a voluntary muscle activity in which there is an overall lengthening of the muscle in response to external resistance.

eccentric implantation [Gk, *ek,* out, *centre,* center], (in embryology) the embedding of the blastocyst within a fold or recess of the uterine wall, which then closes off from the main cavity.

eccentricity /ek′sentris″itē/, behavior that is regarded as odd or peculiar for a particular culture or community, although not unusual enough to be considered pathological.

eccentric jaw relation, any jaw relation other than centric relation at closure.

eccentric occlusion [Gk, *ek + centre* + L, *occludere,* to close up], a closed position of the teeth that does not coincide with centric relation, resulting in premature tooth contacts. Also called *acentric occlusion.*

ecchondroma /ek′əndrō″mə/ [Gk, *ek + chondros,* cartilage, *oma,* tumor], a benign tumor that develops on the surface of a cartilage or under the periosteum of bone. Also called *ecchondrosis.*

ecchymoma /ek′imō″mə/, a swelling caused by accumulation of blood on the site of a bruise.

ecchymosis /ek′imō″sis/ *pl. ecchymoses* [Gk, *ek + chymos,* juice], bluish discoloration of an area of skin or mucous membrane caused by the extravasation of blood into the subcutaneous tissues as a result of trauma to the underlying blood vessels or fragility of the vessel walls. Also called **bruise.** Compare **contusion, petechiae.**

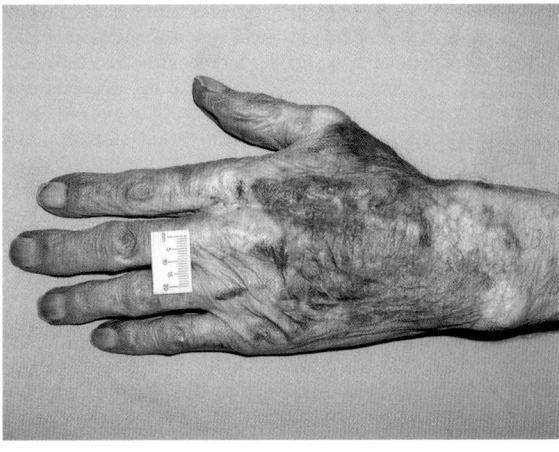

Ecchymosis of the hand *(Lynch, 2011)*

ecchymotic /ek′imot″ik/ [Gk, *ek,* out, *chymos,* juice], pertaining to a discolored area on the skin or membrane caused by blood seeping into the tissue as a result of a contusion. Compare **bruise.**

ecchymotic mask [Gk, *ek + chymos* + Fr, *masque*], a cyanotic or bluish discoloration of the face of a victim of traumatic asphyxia, as in strangulation or choking. The color is the result of petechial hemorrhages.

ecchymotic rash [Gk, *ek + chymos,* juice; OFr, *rasche,* scurf], a skin eruption characterized by black-blue spots caused by extravasation of blood into the tissues, usually as a result of a contusion.

eccrine /ek″rin/ [Gk, *ekkrinein,* to secrete], pertaining to a sweat gland that secretes outwardly through a duct to the surface of the skin. See also **exocrine.**

eccrine gland, one of the sudoriferous glands located in the dermis. Such glands are unbranched, coiled, and tubular. They promote cooling by evaporation of their secretion, which is clear, has a faint odor, and contains water, sodium chloride, and traces of albumin, urea, and other compounds. Compare **apocrine gland, sudoriferous gland.**

eccyesis, *(Obsolete)* now called **ectopic pregnancy.**

ECF, **1.** abbreviation for **extended care facility. 2.** abbreviation for **extracellular fluid.**

ECG, **1.** abbreviation for **electrocardiogram. 2.** abbreviation for **electrocardiograph. 3.** abbreviation for **electrocardiography. 4.** abbreviation for **echoencephalogram.**

-echia, suffix meaning a "condition of holding": *synechia.*

echinacea, a perennial herb used for medicinal purposes.

■ INDICATIONS: It is used for those with low immune status, for hard-to-heal superficial wounds, and as a sun protectant. It is most commonly used to treat the common cold and upper respiratory infections. It has no apparent protective effects but may decrease the duration and symptoms of the infection if started when symptoms are first noticed. There are insufficient reliable data for other indications.

■ CONTRAINDICATIONS: It is not recommended during pregnancy and lactation or in children. It is also contraindicated in people who have autoimmune diseases such as lupus erythematosus, multiple sclerosis, HIV/AIDS, or collagen disease and in people with tuberculosis or hypersensitivity to Bellis species or the Compositae family of herbs. Immunosuppression may occur after extended therapy with this herb. It should not be used for more than 8 weeks.

echino-, prefix meaning "spine" or "spiny": *echinostomiasis.*

echinococcosis /ekī′nōkokō″sis/ [Gk, *echinos,* prickly husk, *kokkos,* berry, *osis,* condition], an infestation, usually of the liver, caused by the larval stage of a tapeworm of the genus

Echinococcus. Dogs are the principal hosts of the adult worm; sheep, goats, horses, camels, cattle, rodents, and deer are the natural intermediate hosts for the larvae. Humans, especially children, can become infested with larvae by ingesting eggs shed in the stool of infected dogs and cats or by petting or handling household dogs or cats. The disease is most common in countries where livestock is raised with the help of dogs. Fluid-filled cysts form in affected organs such as the liver, lungs, brain, bones, or heart. Also called **hydatid disease, hydatidosis.** See also **cysticercosis, tapeworm infection.**

■ OBSERVATIONS: Clinical manifestations and prognosis vary, depending on the tissue invaded and the extent of infestation. Diagnosis is made by skin tests for sensitivity, serological tests, radiological evidence of cyst formation, and identification of larval cysts in infected tissue.

■ INTERVENTIONS: Treatment is an extended course of benzimidazole; puncture, aspiration, injection, and reaspiration of cysts; or careful removal of cysts, avoiding rupture of a cyst, which could cause severe allergic reactions or disseminate infection.

■ PATIENT CARE CONSIDERATIONS: The disease can be prevented by avoiding contact with infected dogs, deworming pet animals, and preventing dogs from eating carcasses of infected intermediate hosts.

Echinococcus /ekī'nōkok″əs/ [Gk, *echinos,* prickly husk, *kokkos,* berry], a genus of small tapeworms that primarily infect canines. See also **echinococcosis.**

echinocyte. See **burr cell.**

echinostomiasis, a food-borne infection caused by an intestinal trematode belonging to the family Echinostomatidae.

echo /ek″ō/, **1.** the reflection of an ultrasound wave back to the transducer from a structure in the plane of the sound beam. **2.** *(Informal)* echocardiography.

echo beat. See **reciprocal beat.**

echocardiogram /ek'ōkär″dē·əgram′/ [Gk, *echo,* sound, *kardia,* heart, *gramma,* record], a graphic outline of the movements of heart structures produced by ultrasonography; used to assess structure and function.

echocardiography /ek'ōkär″dē·og″rəfē/ [Gk, *echo* + *kardia,* heart, *graphein,* to record], a diagnostic, noninvasive procedure for studying the structure and motion of the heart. Ultrasonic waves directed through the heart are reflected backward, or echoed, when they pass from one type of tissue to another, such as from cardiac muscle to blood. The sound waves are transmitted from and received by a transducer and are recorded on a strip chart. Major diagnostic uses include the detection of atrial tumors and pericardial effusion, measurement of the ventricular septa and ventricular chambers, evaluation or monitoring of prosthetic valve function, and determination of mitral valve motion abnormalities and congenital lesions. Also called **ultrasonic cardiography.** See also **phonocardiograph, ultrasonography.**

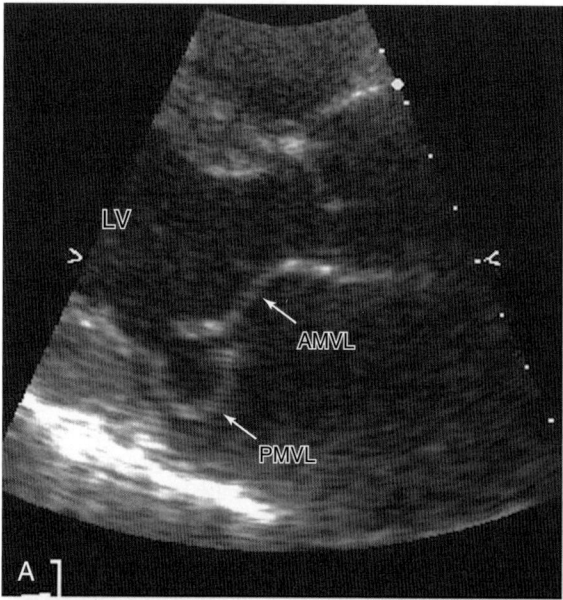

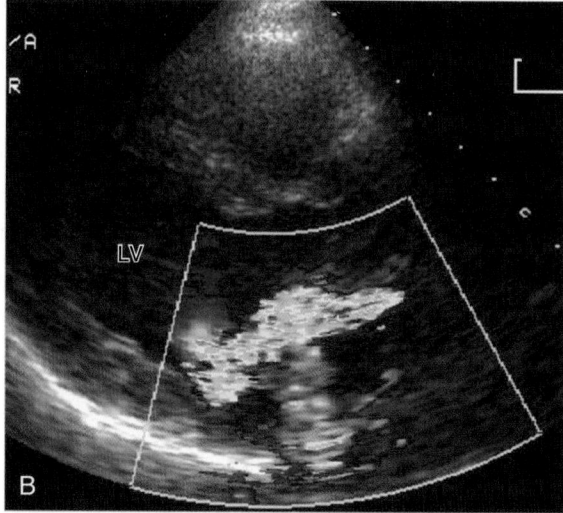

Mitral valve prolapse visualized with transthoracic echocardiography *(Andreoli, 2010)*

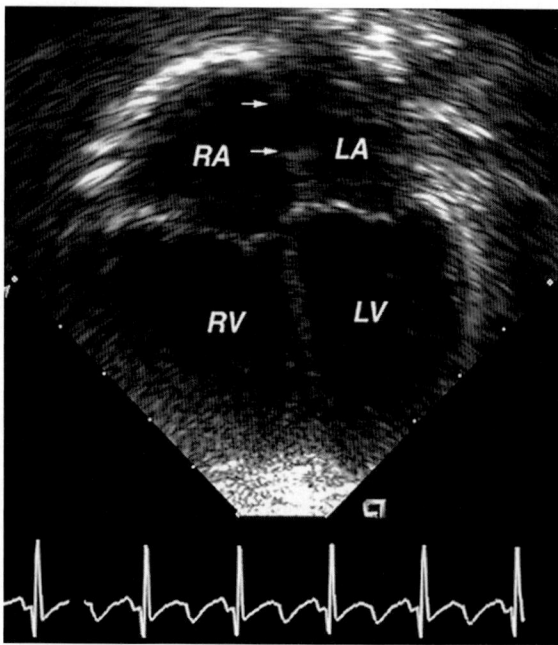

Four-chamber echocardiogram of an atrial septal defect *(Marcdante and Kliegman, 2015)*

echoencephalogram (EEG) /ek'ōensef″ələgram′/ [Gk, *echo* + *enkephalos,* brain, *gramma,* record], a recording produced by an echoencephalograph.

echoencephalography /ek′ō·ensef′əlog″rəfē/, the use of ultrasound to study the intracranial structures of the brain. The technique is useful for showing ventricular dilation and a major shift of midline structures caused by an expanding lesion. See also **ultrasonography.** −*echoencephalographic, adj.*

echogram /ek′ōgram/ [Gk, sound, record], a recording of ultrasound echo patterns of a body structure, such as a gravid uterus.

echographia. See **pseudoagraphia.**

echography. See **ultrasonography.**

echo home [Elder Cottage Housing Opportunity], (*Informal*) an independent housing facility for an older person in or near the family home.

echolalia /ek′ōlā″lyə/ [Gk, *echo* + *lalein,* to babble], **1.** (in psychiatry) the automatic and meaningless repetition of another's words or phrases, especially as seen in schizophrenia. Kinds include **delayed echolalia. 2.** (in pediatrics) a baby's imitation or repetition of sounds or words produced by others. It occurs normally in early childhood development. Also called *echophrasia,* **echo speech.** −*echolalic, adj.*

echo planar imaging (EPI), a fast magnetic resonance imaging mode.

echopraxia /ek′ōprak″sē·ə/ [Gk, *echo* + *prassein,* to practice], imitation or repetition of the body movements of another person, sometimes practiced by schizophrenic patients.

echo sign, **1.** a repeated sound heard on percussion of a hydatid cyst. **2.** an involuntary repetition of words heard. See also **echolalia.**

echo speech. See **echolalia.**

echothiophate iodide /-thī′ōfāt/, an anticholinesterase used for ophthalmic purposes.

■ INDICATIONS: It is prescribed for the treatment of chronic open-angle glaucoma and accommodative esotropia.

■ CONTRAINDICATIONS: Uveal inflammation, most types of angle-closure glaucoma, or known hypersensitivity to this drug prohibits its use.

■ ADVERSE EFFECTS: Among the more serious adverse effects are retinal detachment, nonreversible cataract, lens opacity, activation of iritis or uveitis, and iris cysts.

ECHO virus /ek″ō vī′rəs/ [enteric *c*ytopathogenic *h*uman *o*rphan + L, *virus,* poison], a picornavirus associated with many clinical syndromes but not identified as the causative organism of any specific disease. ECHO stands for *e*nteric, *c*ytopathic, *h*uman, *o*rphan. There are many ECHO viruses. More than 30 serotypes have been identified; many are harmless. Bacterial or viral disease may be complicated by ECHO virus infection, as aseptic meningitis accompanying some severe bacterial and viral infections.

e-cigarette or vaping associated lung injury (EVALI), acute lung injury occurring in individuals using electronic cigarettes (e-cigarettes), vape pens, or vape mods, most likely reflecting a spectrum of pulmonary disease rather than a single process. It is characterized by acute fibrinous pneumonitis, diffuse alveolar damage, or organizing pneumonia, usually bronchiolocentric and accompanied by bronchiolitis.

Eck's fistula [Nikoli V. Eck, Russian physiologist, 1849–1917], an artificial passage between the end of the hepatic portal vein and the side of the inferior vena cava. It is used to treat esophageal varices in portal hypertension.

eclampsia /iklamp″sē·ə/ [Gk, *ek,* out, *lampein,* to flash], a potentially life-threatening disorder characterized by hypertension, generalized edema, and proteinuria with seizures. It is the gravest form of pregnancy-induced hypertension. Bed rest in a quiet, dimly lighted room, the administration

of magnesium sulfate, and antihypertensive medications are prescribed. Vigilant monitoring of the condition, including deep tendon reflexes, is warranted as the danger is grave. The cause is unknown.

eclectic /iklek″tik/ [Gk, *eklektikos,* selecting], pertaining to a therapy that selects, combines, and incorporates diverse techniques from several systems or theories into an integrated approach.

eclipse scotoma /iklips″/ [Gk, *ekleipsis,* abandoning, *skotos,* darkness, *oma,* tumor], a small central area of depressed or lost vision caused by looking directly at the sun without adequate protection. Also called **solar maculopathy, solar retinopathy.**

ECM, initialism for *erythema chronicum migrans.*

ECMO, abbreviation for **extracorporeal membrane oxygenator.**

-ecoia, suffix meaning "(condition of the) sense of hearing": *bradyecoia.*

E. coli, abbreviation for *Escherichia coli.*

ecological chemistry /ikəloj″ik/, the study of chemical compounds synthesized by plants that influence ecological characteristics through chemical communication or toxic effects.

ecological fallacy, an inaccurate assignment of meaning to accurate statistical data that assigns characteristics of the group to each individual within that group. For example, if there is a very high incidence of breast cancer within a specific geographic region, it does not mean that every woman in that region will have breast cancer.

ecological model, a model that emphasizes the relationship between humans and their physical and social environments and assists in understanding the factors important to goal-directed motor actions.

ecology /ikol″əjē/ [Gk, *oekos,* house, *logos,* science], the study of the interaction between organisms and their environment.

econazole /ikon″əzōl/, a topical antifungal agent.

■ INDICATIONS: It is prescribed in the treatment of tinea pedis, tinea cruris, tinea corporis, tinea versicolor, and candidiasis.

■ CONTRAINDICATIONS: Known sensitivity to this drug prohibits its use.

■ ADVERSE EFFECTS: Among the most serious adverse effects are local irritation and hypersensitivity of the skin.

ecosystem /ek′ōsis″təm/, the total of all living things within a particular area and the nonliving things with which they interact.

ecstasy /ek″stəsē/ [Gk, *ekstasis,* derangement], **1.** an emotional state characterized by exultation, rapturous delight, or frenzy. It may be induced by a religious or deeply spiritual event, by medications, or by other substances. Compare **euphoria, mania.** −*ecstatic, adj.* **2.** (*Informal*) popular name for 3,4-methylenedioxymethamphetamine, a hallucinogenic drug of abuse. See also **drug abuse.**

ECT, **1.** abbreviation for **electroconvulsive therapy. 2.** abbreviation for **emission computed tomography.**

-ectasia, suffix meaning "dilatation, dilation, extension, or distension of an organ": *gastrectasia.*

ectatic emphysema. See **panacinar emphysema.**

ecthyma /ek″thimə/ [Gk, *ek,* out, *thyein,* to rush], an ulcerative pyoderma characterized by large pustules, crusts, and ulcerations surrounded by erythema. It is caused by a streptococcal infection after a minor trauma. The skin of the legs is most frequently affected. Treatment includes vigorous cleansing, application of compresses of cool Burow's solution to soften and remove crusts, and systemic administration of antibiotics. Compare **folliculitis, impetigo.**

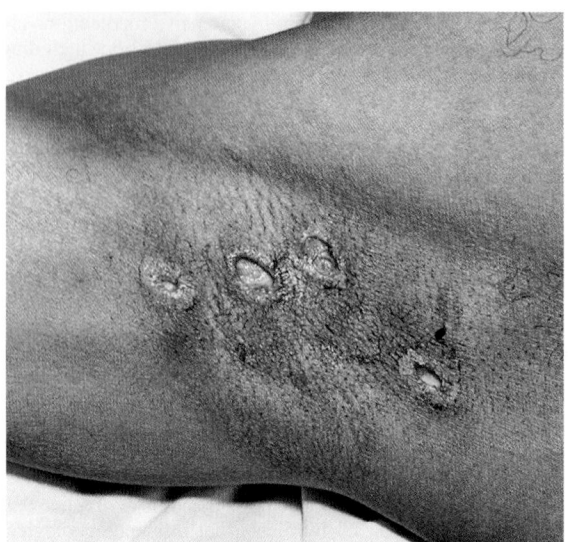

Ecthyma *(James, 2006)*

ecthyma contagiosum. See **contagious pustular dermatitis.**

ecto-, prefix meaning "outside": *ectoderm, ectoplasm.*

ectocytic /ek'təsit″ik/ [Gk, *ektos,* outside, *kytos,* cell], outside a cell and not part of its organization.

ectoderm /ek'tədurm/ [Gk, *ektos,* outside, *derma,* skin], the outermost of the three primary cell layers of an embryo. The ectoderm gives rise to the nervous system; the organs of special sense, such as the eyes and ears; the epidermis and epidermal tissue, such as fingernails, hair, and skin glands; and the mucous membranes of the mouth and anus. See also **embryo, endoderm, mesoderm.** *—ectodermal,* **ectodermic,** *adj.*

ectodermal cloaca /ek'tədur″məl/, a part of the cloaca in the developing embryo that lies external to the cloacal membrane and eventually gives rise to the anus and anal canal. Compare **endodermal cloaca.**

ectodermal dysplasia, any of a group of hereditary disorders involving tissues and structures derived from the embryonic ectoderm. Ectodermal dysplasia is a component of various syndromes, including anhidrotic ectodermal dysplasia and ectrodactyly-ectodermal dysplasia-clefting (EEC) syndrome.

ectodermic. See **ectoderm.**

ectodermoidal /ek'tədərmoi″dəl/ [Gk, *ektos,* outside, *derma,* skin, *eidos,* form], resembling or having the characteristics of ectoderm.

ectomorph /ek'təmôrf′/ [Gk, *ektos* + *morphe,* form], a type of body build characterized by slenderness, lean muscle mass, and long limbs. Compare **endomorph, mesomorph.** See also **asthenic habitus.**

-ectomy, suffix meaning the "surgical removal" of something specified: *lobectomy, thrombectomy, thyroidectomy.*

ectoparasite /ek'tōper″əsīt/ [Gk, *ektos* + *parasitos,* guest], (in medical parasitology) an organism that lives on the outside of the body of the host, such as a louse.

-ectopia, suffix meaning a "condition in which a (specified) organ or part is out of its normal place": *corectopia.*

ectopic /ektop″ik/ [Gk, *ek* + *topos,* place], **1.** (of an object or organ) situated in an unusual place, away from its normal location, for example, an ectopic pregnancy, which occurs outside the uterus. **2.** (of an event) occurring at the wrong time, as a premature heartbeat or premature ventricular contraction.

ectopic beat [Gk, *ek,* out, *topos,* place; AS, *beatan*], an impulse that originates in the heart at a site other than the sinus node. Also called **extrasystole.**

ectopic focus, an area in the heart that initiates abnormal beats. Ectopic foci may occur in both healthy and diseased hearts and are usually associated with irritation of a small area of myocardial tissue. They are produced in association with myocardial ischemia, drug (catecholamine) effects, emotional stress, and stimulation by foreign objects, including pacemaker catheters. Also called **ectopic pacemaker.**

ectopic kidney, a kidney not in the usual position. The most common types are abdominal, lumbar, pelvic, thoracic, and crossed fused ectopic kidneys.

ectopic myelopoiesis. See **extramedullary myelopoiesis.**

ectopic pacemaker. See **ectopic focus.**

ectopic pregnancy, an abnormal pregnancy in which the conceptus implants outside the uterine cavity or in the intramural portion of the uterus or cervix. Formerly called **eccyesis.** Kinds include **abdominal pregnancy, ovarian pregnancy, tubal pregnancy.**

ectopic rhythm [Gk, *ek* + *topos,* place, *rhythmos,* beat], an abnormal heart rhythm caused by the formation of impulses in a focus outside the sinus node. Such a rhythm may be protective in cases of failure of the sinus node or excessive slowing of its rhythm, or it may indicate an active abnormal focus.

ectopic tachycardia [Gk, *ek* + *topos,* place, *tachys,* swift, *kardia,* heart], an abnormally rapid heartbeat caused by excitation arising from a focus outside the sinus node.

ectopic teratism, a congenital anomaly in which one or more parts are misplaced, such as dextrocardia and transposition of the great vessels. See also **dextrocardia, transposition of the great vessels.**

ectopic testis, a testis that has descended from the abdominal cavity and settled in the suprapubic area, the thigh, or the perineum instead of the scrotum. Therapy requires surgery. See also **cryptorchidism.**

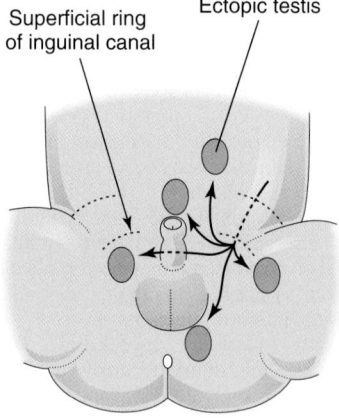

Usual locations of ectopic testes *(Moore and Persaud, 2008)*

ectopic ureter, a ureter that opens in a place other than the bladder wall. In women it may open into the vestibule, terminal urethra, vagina, cervix, or uterine cavity. In men it enters the genital or urinary tract above the level of the external sphincter.

ectoplasm, the compact, peripheral portion of the cytoplasm of a cell.

ectopy /ek″təpē/ [Gk, *ek,* out, *topos,* place], a condition in which an organ or substance is not in its natural or proper place, such as an ectopic pregnancy that develops outside the uterus or an ectopic heartbeat.

ectotoxin. See **exotoxin.**

ectro-, prefix meaning "loss or absence of, miscarriage, abortion"; used primarily to indicate a loss of limbs or body parts: *ectrodactyly, ectromelia.*

ectrodactyly /ek′trōdak″təlē/ [Gk, *ektrosis,* miscarriage, *daktylos,* finger], a congenital anomaly characterized by the absence of part or all of one or more of the fingers or toes. Also called *ectrodactylia, ectrodactylism.*

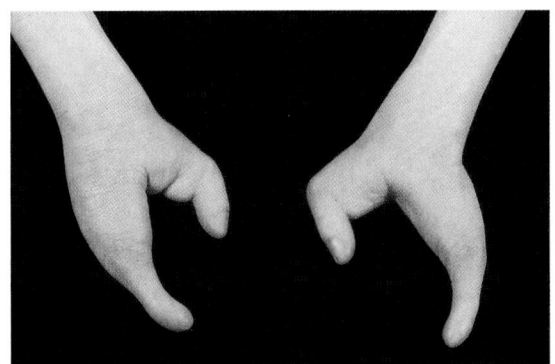

Ectrodactyly involving the hands *(Courtesy Dr. A.E. Chudley, Department of Pediatrics and Child Health, University of Manitoba, Children's Hospital)*

ectrodactyly-ectodermal dysplasia-clefting syndrome. See **EEC syndrome.**

ectrogenic. See **ectrogeny.**

ectrogenic teratism /-jen″ik/ [Gk, *ektrosis* + *genein,* to produce, *teras,* monster], a congenital anomaly caused by developmental failure in which one or more parts or organs are missing.

ectrogeny /ektroj″ənē/ [Gk, *ektrosis* + *genein,* to produce], the congenital absence or defect of any organ or part of the body. **−ectrogenic,** *adj.*

ectromelia /ek′trōmē″lyə/ [Gk, *ektrosis* + *melos,* limb], the congenital absence or incomplete development of the long bones of one or more of the limbs. Kinds include **amelia, hemimelia, phocomelia.** −*ectromelic,* *adj.,* −*ectromelus,* *n.*

ectropic /ektrop″ik/, inside out.

ectropion /ektrō″pē·on/ [Gk, *ek* + *trepein,* to turn], eversion, most commonly of the eyelid, exposing the conjunctival membrane lining the eyelid and part of the eyeball. The condition may involve only the lower eyelid or both eyelids. The cause may be paralysis of the facial nerve, scarring, neoplasia, or, in an older person, atrophy of the eyelid tissues. Compare **entropion.**

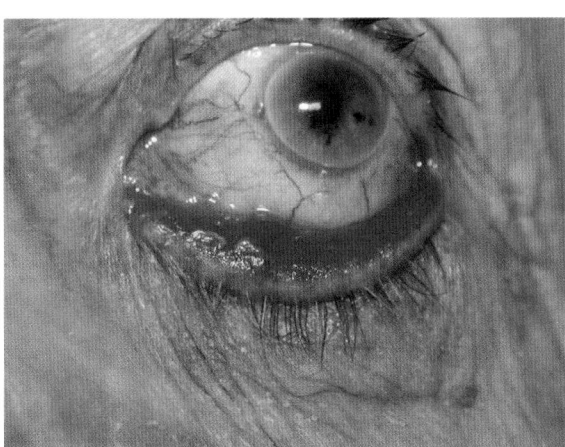

Ectropion *(Kanski, 2007/Courtesy A. Pearson)*

ectrosyndactyly /ek′trōsindak″təlē/ [Gk, *ektrosis* + *syn,* together, *daktylos,* finger], a congenital anomaly characterized by the absence of some but not all of the digits, with those that are formed webbed so as to appear fused. Also called *ectrosyndactylia.*

ECU, abbreviation for **environmental control unit.**

eculizumab, a monoclonal antibody.

■ INDICATIONS: This drug is used to treat paroxysmal nocturnal hemoglobinuria, a rare, genetic form of hemolytic anemia.

■ CONTRAINDICATIONS: Known hypersensitivity to this drug prohibits its use. Rapid discontinuation may result in serious hemolysis.

■ ADVERSE EFFECTS: Adverse effects of this drug include rash, dyspnea, calf or leg pain, chest pain, confusion, coughing up blood, sensitivity to light, fever, chills, persistent sore throat, mental changes, headache, nausea, vomiting, fever, stiff neck or back, mouth sores, fever blisters, and severe muscle aches. A life-threatening side effect is meningococcal infection. Common side effects are headache, nasopharyngitis, back pain, nausea, fatigue, and cough.

eczema /ek″simə/ [Gk, *ekzein,* to boil over], a general superficial dermatitis of unknown cause. In the early stage it may be pruritic, erythematous, papulovesicular, edematous, and weeping. Later it becomes crusted, scaly, thickened, or lichenified. Exacerbating factors include sudden temperature changes, humidity, psychological stress, illness, allergies, fibers, detergents, and perfumes. Eczema is not a distinct disease entity. See also **atopic dermatitis, nummular dermatitis. −eczematous,** *adj.*

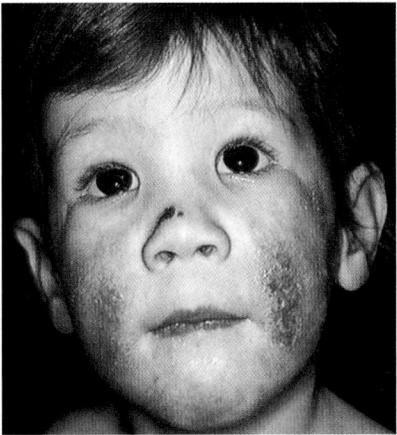

Child with infantile eczema *(Leifer, 2011)*

eczema herpeticum, a generalized vesiculopustular rash caused by herpes simplex virus or vaccinia virus infection of a preexisting rash such as atopic dermatitis. Also called **Kaposi varicelliform eruption.**

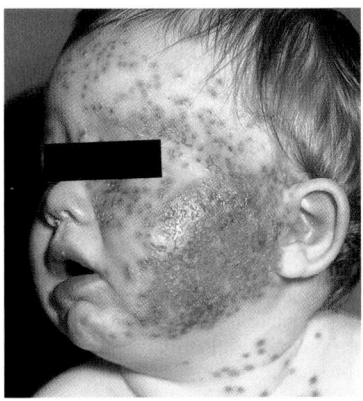

Child with eczema herpeticum *(Walker et al, 2014)*

eczema marginatum. See **tinea cruris.**

eczematous. See **eczema.**

eczematous conjunctivitis /eksem″ətəs/, conjunctival and corneal inflammation associated with multiple tiny ulcerated vesicles. The cause is believed to be a delayed hypersensitivity to bacterial protein. If untreated, the condition may lead to ingrowth of small blood vessels in the cornea, eventually obscuring vision. Treatment usually includes topical instillation of corticosteroids. Also called **staph marginal disease.**

eczopiclone, a sedative/hypnotic.

■ INDICATIONS: This drug is used to treat insomnia.

■ CONTRAINDICATIONS: Known hypersensitivity to this drug prohibits its use.

■ ADVERSE EFFECTS: Adverse effects of this drug include depression, hallucinations, headache, daytime drowsiness, peripheral edema, chest pain, dry mouth, bitter taste, and rash.

ED, **1.** abbreviation for **effective dose.** **2.** abbreviation for **emergency department.** **3.** abbreviation for **erectile dysfunction.**

ED₅₀, symbol for **median effective dose.**

ED₉₀, the dose of a therapeutic agent that eradicates 90% of the target pathogen.

edaphon /ed″əfon/, the composite of organisms that live in the soil. –*edaphic, adj.*

EDB, abbreviation for **ethylene dibromide.**

EDC, initialism for *expected date of confinement.* See **expected date of delivery.**

EDD, abbreviation for **expected date of delivery.**

eddy currents, small circular electric fields induced when a magnetic field is created. They result in intramolecular oscillation or vibration of tissue contents, causing generation of heat.

Edecrin Sodium, a loop diuretic. Brand name for **ethacrynate sodium.**

EDE limit, abbreviation for **effective dose equivalent limit.**

edema /idē″mə/ [Gk, *oidema,* swelling], the abnormal accumulation of fluid in interstitial spaces of tissues, such as in the pericardial sac, intrapleural space, peritoneal cavity, or joint capsules. Edema may be caused by increased capillary fluid pressure; venous obstruction such as occurs in varicosities; thrombophlebitis; pressure from casts, tight bandages, or garters; congestive heart failure; overloading with parenteral fluids; renal failure; hepatic cirrhosis; hyperaldosteronism such as in Cushing's syndrome; corticosteroid therapy; and inflammatory reactions. Edema may also result from loss of serum protein in burns, draining wounds, fistulas, hemorrhage, nephrotic syndrome, or chronic diarrhea; in malnutrition, especially kwashiorkor; in allergic reactions; and in blockage of lymphatic vessels caused by malignant diseases, filariasis, or other disorders. See also **anasarca, lymphedema.** –*edematose, edematous, adj.*

■ OBSERVATIONS: In the evaluation of tissue turgor, edema may be evaluated by position change, specific location, and response to pressure, as in pitting edema, when pressing the fingers into the edematous area causes a temporary indentation. An ultrasound evaluation of the affected extremity is indicated to rule out thrombosis.

■ INTERVENTIONS: Treatment of edema focuses on correcting the underlying cause. Potassium-sparing diuretics may be administered to promote excretion of sodium and water. Edematous parts of the body should be protected from prolonged pressure, injury, and temperature extremes. When a limb is edematous as a result of venous stasis, elevating the extremity and applying an elastic stocking or sleeve facilitate venous return.

■ PATIENT CARE CONSIDERATIONS: The patient may experience body image problems related to changes in size when edema is visible.

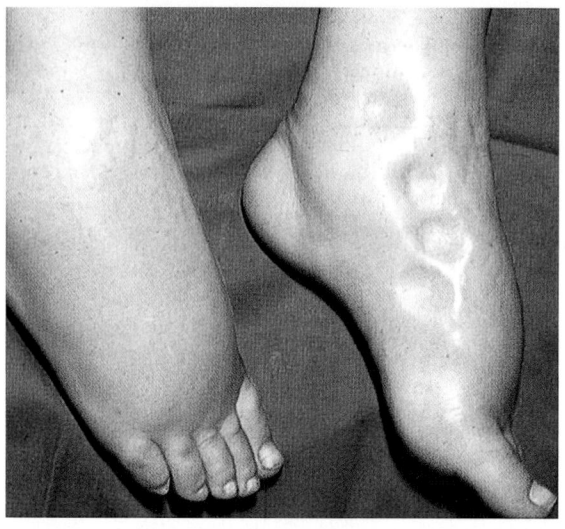

Pitting edema *(Bloom and Ireland, 1992)*

-edema, -edem, suffix meaning "swelling resulting from an excessive accumulation of serous fluid in the tissues of the body in (specified) locations": *cephaledema, dactyledema, papilledema.*

edema of glottis [Gk, *oidema,* swelling, *glossa,* tongue], a swelling caused by fluid accumulation in the soft tissues of the larynx. Symptoms include stridor, hoarseness, and dyspnea. The condition, usually inflammatory, may result from infection, injury, or inhalation of toxic gases. Also called **laryngeal edema.**

edematogenic /ēdem′ətōjen″ik/, causing edema.

edentulism /eden′tulizem/, the condition of being without natural teeth.

edentulous /ēden″chələs/, lacking natural teeth.

edetate calcium disodium (EDTA) /ed″ətāt/, a chelating agent used to treat lead poisoning. Should not be confused with **edetate disodium.**

edetate disodium, a parenteral chelating agent used to lower plasma calcium levels.

■ INDICATIONS: It should be prescribed only when clinical conditions such as hypercalcemic crisis or ventricular arrhythmia and heart block resulting from digitalis toxicity mandate aggressive therapy. It must be administered slowly and the recommended dosage should not be exceeded.

■ CONTRAINDICATIONS: Hypocalcemia, kidney disease, or known hypersensitivity to this drug prohibits its use.

■ ADVERSE EFFECTS: Among the more serious adverse effects are hypocalcemia, which can lead to tetany, arrhythmia, seizures, and death from respiratory arrest. Other adverse effects include nausea, vomiting, cramps, fever, thrombophlebitis, kidney damage, and hemorrhage associated with hypocoagulability.

edetic acid (EDTA) /idet″ik/, a chelating agent.

EDG, abbreviation for **electrodynograph.**

edge /ej/ [ME, *egge*], **1.** a thin side or border. **2.** the end of a surface (e.g., the edge of a surgical instrument).

edge enhancement, an image-processing filter used to enhance structure margins within an image. This feature is common in digital cameras, in the "sharpness" control of video monitors, and in computer printers to improve image quality.

edge response function (ERF), the ability of a computed tomography system to produce a sharp image of a high-contrast edge, such as the edge of the heart.

edgewise appliance, a fixed orthodontic appliance whose attachment brackets have a rectangular slot that engages a round or rectangular arch wire. The most widely prescribed orthodontic appliance, it is used to correct or improve malocclusion.

EDI, abbreviation for **Electronic Data Interchange.**

edible, pertaining to a substance that can be eaten.

EDRF, a term that is now used synonymously with nitric oxide. Abbreviation for **endothelial-derived relaxing factor.**

edrophonium chloride /ed′rōfō″nē·əm/, a cholinesterase inhibitor that acts as an antidote to curare and other nondepolarizing neuromuscular blockers and is an aid in the diagnosis of myasthenia gravis.

■ INDICATIONS: It is prescribed to reverse neuromuscular blockade, to treat curare toxicity, and to aid in the diagnosis of suspected myasthenia gravis.

■ CONTRAINDICATIONS: Obstruction of the GI or urinary tract, hypotension, bradycardia, or known hypersensitivity to this drug prohibits its use. Should be used with caution in patients with asthma and those taking cardiac glycosides.

■ ADVERSE EFFECTS: Among the most serious adverse effects are respiratory paralysis, hypotension, bradycardia, and bronchospasm.

edrophonium test, a test for myasthenia gravis in which an IV solution of edrophonium chloride is injected into a patient. A total of 10 mg of the cholinergic drug is prepared, and a 2-mg dose is injected. If there is no reaction in 30 seconds, the remaining 8 mg is administered. A brief improvement in muscle activity is regarded as a positive result. Edrophonium chloride is also used to distinguish between myasthenia gravis and a cholinergic crisis. Because edrophonium chloride can precipitate respiratory depression, the test should not be performed unless an anticholinergic antidote, such as atropine, and respiratory resuscitation equipment are available.

Edsall disease [David L. Edsall, American physician, 1869–1945], a cramping condition that is the result of excessive exposure to heat. Also called **heat cramp.**

EDTA, 1. abbreviation for *ethylene-diamineteraacetic acid (edetic acid).* 2. abbreviation for **edetate calcium disodium.** 3. acronym for **edetic acid.**

education, 1. (in occupational therapy) as an occupation, activities involved in learning and participating in the educational environment. See also **occupation. 2.** (for health or related reasons) activities that impart knowledge and information about health, illness, and well-being resulting in acquisition by the client of helpful behaviors, habits, and routines that may or may not require application.

educational psychology /ej′əkā″shənəl/ [L, *educatus,* to rear; Gk, *psyche,* mind, *logos,* science], the application of psychological principles, techniques, and tests to educational problems, such as the determination of more effective instructional methods, the assessment of student advancement, and the selection of students for specialized programs. See also **applied psychology.**

Edwards' syndrome. See **trisomy 18.**

EEC syndrome, an autosomal-dominant syndrome involving both ectodermal and mesodermal tissues, with ectodermal dysplasia associated with hypopigmentation of skin and hair, scanty hair and eyebrows, absence of lashes, nail dystrophy, small or missing teeth, missing digits, and cleft lip and palate. Also called **ectrodactyly-ectodermal dysplasia-clefting syndrome.**

EEE, abbreviation for **eastern equine encephalitis.** See **equine encephalitis.**

EEG, 1. abbreviation for **electroencephalogram.** 2. abbreviation for **electroencephalography.**

eelworm /ēl′werm/, a nematode, especially any of various small, free-living or plant parasitic roundworms.

EENT, initialism for *eyes, ears, nose, and throat.*

EEOC, abbreviation for **Equal Employment Opportunity Commission.**

ef-. See **ex-.**

EFA, abbreviation for **essential fatty acid.**

efavirenz, an antiviral.

■ INDICATIONS: It is used to treat HIV-1 in combination with other antiretroviral agents.

■ CONTRAINDICATIONS: Known hypersensitivity to this drug prohibits its use.

■ ADVERSE EFFECTS: Adverse effects include abdominal pain, headache, dizziness, fatigue, impaired concentration, insomnia, abnormal dreams, and depression. Common side effects include diarrhea, nausea, and rash.

effacement /ifās″mənt/ [Fr, *effacer,* to erase], thinning of the cervical shape and shortening of the cervical canal during labor from its normal 2 cm to a tissue-thin edge, which actually seems to disappear at full dilation (10 cm). Effacement is usually expressed as a percentage from the start of labor. See also **birth, cervix, dilation, station.**

effect, the result of an agent or cause.

effective atomic number, the average atomic number obtained from a weighted summation of the atomic constituents of a compound. See also **atomic number.**

effective compliance /ifek″tiv/ [L, *effectus,* performance], the ratio of tidal volume to peak airway pressure.

effective dose (ED), 1. on a graded dose-response curve in the laboratory, the dosage of a drug that may be expected to cause a response of the desired magnitude. See also **therapeutic dose. 2.** in a clinical setting, the dose needed to cause the desired response in a percentage of the people to whom it is given (e.g., an ED_{50} dosage of a drug is expected to produce a response in 50% of the patients receiving it).

effective dose equivalent limit (EDE limit), the largest amount of ionizing radiation a person may receive according to radiation protection guidelines. It combines both internal and external dose and has replaced the concept of maximum permissible dose for occupational exposures. The EDE limit

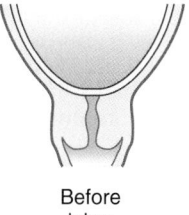

Before labor

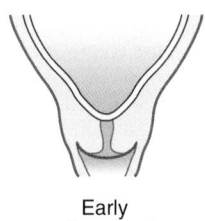

Early effacement

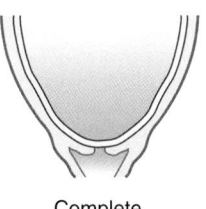

Complete effacement

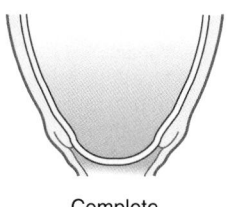

Complete dilation

Cervical effacement *(Bonewit-West, 2015)*

is prescribed for various organs as well as whole body and for various working conditions. Effective dose equivalent limits are regulated, and guidelines are published by the National Council of Radiation Protection (NCRP) and the FDA. See also **dose equivalent.**

effective half-life (ehl), the time required for a radioactive element in an animal body to be diminished by 50% as a result of radioactive decay and biological elimination. The effective half-life is equal to the product of the biological half-life *(bhl)* and the radioactive half-life *(rhl)* divided by the sum of the *bhl* and the *rhl*: $ehl = (bhl \times rhl)/(bhl + rhl)$.

effective osmotic pressure, the part of total osmotic pressure of a solution that determines the tendency of the solvent to pass through a boundary, such as a semipermeable membrane.

effective radiating area, the total area of the surface of the transducer that actually produces the sound wave.

effective refractory period. See **refractory period.**

effector /ifek″tər/ [L, *efficere,* to accomplish], **1.** an organ that produces an effect, such as glandular secretion, as a result of nerve stimulation. **2.** a molecule, such as an enzyme, that can start or stop a chemical reaction.

effector cell, **1.** a terminally differentiated leukocyte that performs more than one specific function. **2.** a muscle cell or gland cell.

effeminate /ifem″init/ [L, *effeminare,* to make womanish], a man with womanly or female characteristics not usually associated with men.

efferent /ef″ərənt/ [L, *effere,* to carry out], directed away from a center, such as certain arteries, veins, nerves, kidney, and lymphatic vessels. Compare **afferent.**

efferent duct, any duct through which a gland releases its secretions.

efferent nerve, a nerve that transmits impulses away or outward from a nerve center, such as the brain or spinal cord, usually causing a muscle contraction or release of a glandular secretion.

efferent pathway [L, *effere,* to carry out; ME, *paeth* + *weg*], **1.** the route of nerve fibers carrying impulses away from a nerve center. **2.** the system of blood vessels that conveys blood away from a body part. Compare **afferent.**

effervesce [Gk, *effervescere,* to foam up], to produce small bubbles or foam on the release of gas from a fluid.

effervescence /ef′ərves″əns/ [L, *effervescere,* to foam up], the production of small bubbles or foam associated with the escape of gas from a fluid.

effervescent /ef′ərves″ənt/, producing and releasing gas bubbles.

efficacy /ef″əkəsē/ [L, *effectus,* performance], **1.** (of a drug or treatment) the ability of a drug or treatment to produce a specific result, regardless of dosage. **2.** (in psychology) the personal ability to act upon and react to the world to achieve desired results. **3.** a person's beliefs about whether he or she can use his or her capacities to influence the course of events or circumstances in the external world; efficacy refers to how effective one feels about his or her abilities. See also **self-efficacy.**

efficiency /ifish″ənsē/, **1.** the production of desired results with the minimum waste of time and effort. **2.** the amount of achievement compared with the effort expended. **3.** (in radioassay) the counts perceived by a beta or gamma counter relative to the known disintegration rate of a comparable standard radioactive source.

effleurage /ef′ləräzh″/ [Fr, skimming the surface], a technique in massage in which long, light, or firm strokes are used, usually over the spine and back. Fingertip effleurage

is a light technique performed with the tips of the fingers in a circular pattern over one part of the body or in long strokes over the back or an extremity. Fingertip effleurage of the abdomen is a technique commonly used in the Lamaze method of natural childbirth. Compare **pétrissage, rolling effleurage.**

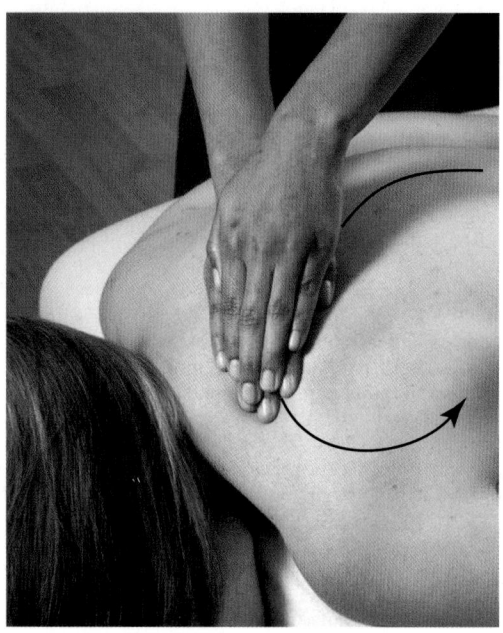

Effleurage *(Salvo, 2012)*

effluent /ef″lo̅o̅·ənt/, a liquid, solid, or gaseous emission that flows out, especially a discharge that carries waste products.

effluvium /iflo̅o̅″vē·əm/ [L, *effluvium,* a flowing out], an outflow of gas or vapor, usually malodorous or toxic.

effort syndrome [Fr, exertion; Gk, *syn,* together, *dromos,* course], an abnormal condition characterized by chest pain; dizziness; fatigue; palpitations; cold, moist hands; and sighing respiration. The condition is often associated with soldiers in combat but occurs also in other individuals. The pain often mimics angina pectoris but is more closely connected to anxiety states and occurs after rather than during exercise. Because angina may also be associated with anxiety, positive diagnosis of effort syndrome may require an exercise electrocardiogram. Other chest pains that mimic effort syndrome and angina may be caused by musculoskeletal problems, such as inflammation of the costochondral junctions, fractured ribs, or cervical spondylosis. Also called **neurocirculatory asthenia.**

effort thrombosis, an abnormal condition in which a clot develops within the subclavian or axillary vein following strenuous exercise. The condition is accompanied by pain, edema, and skin discoloration in the shoulder and upper arm. Also called **Paget-Schroetter syndrome, Paget-von Schroetter syndrome.**

effraction /ifrak″shən/, a breaking open or weakening.

effusion /ifyo̅o̅″zhən/ [L, *effundere,* to pour out], **1.** the escape of fluid, for example, from blood vessels as a result of rupture or seepage, usually into a body cavity. The condition is usually associated with a circulatory or renal disorder and is often an early sign of congestive heart disease. The term may be associated with an affected body area, as pleural or pericardial effusion. See also **edema, transudate. 2.** the outward spread of a bacterial growth.

eflornithine hydrochloride /eflôr″nithēn/,   an inhibitor of the enzyme ornithine decarboxylase, applied in creams by females over age 12 to limit unwanted facial hair growth and administered by injection to treat the meningoencephalitic stage (sleeping sickness) of a protozoal infection caused by *Trypanosoma brucei.*

EFM,   abbreviation for **electronic fetal monitor.**

Efudex,   an antineoplastic. Brand name for **fluorouracil.**

EGD,   abbreviation for **esophagogastroduodenoscopy.**

egest /ijest″/   [L, *egerere,* to expel],   *adj.,* to discharge or evacuate a substance from the body, especially to evacuate unabsorbed residue of foods from the intestines. −*egesta, n.*

EGF,   abbreviation for **epidermal growth factor.**

egg /eg/   [ONorse],   a female reproductive cell at any stage before fertilization. After fertilization and fusion of the pronuclei, it is called a zygote. Also called **ovum.**

eglandulous /ēglan″dyələs/,   describing an absence of glands.

ego /ē′gō, eg′ō/   [Gk, I or self],   **1.** the conscious sense of the self; those elements of a person, such as thinking, feeling, and willing, that distinguish him or her as an individual. **2.** (in psychoanalysis) the part of the psyche that experiences and maintains conscious contact with reality and tempers the primitive drives of the id and the demands of the superego with the social and physical needs of society. It represents the rational element of the personality, is the seat of such mental processes as perception and memory, and develops defense mechanisms against anxiety. See also **id, superego.**

ego-alien.   See **ego-dystonic.**

ego analysis,   (in psychoanalysis) the intensive study of the ego, especially the defense mechanisms.

ego boundary,   (in psychiatry) a sense or awareness that there is a distinction between the real and unreal. In some psychoses the person does not have an ego boundary and cannot differentiate his or her personal perceptions and feelings from those of other people.

egocentric /ē′gōsen″trik/   [Gk, *ego* + *kentron,* center],   **1.** *adj.,* regarding the self as the center, object, and norm of all experience and having little regard for the needs, interests, ideas, and attitudes of others. **2.** *n.,* a person possessing these characteristics.

ego-defense mechanism.   See **defense mechanism.**

ego-dystonic /ē′gōdiston″ik/,   describing elements of a person's behavior, thoughts, impulses, drives, and attitudes that are unacceptable to him or her and cause anxiety. Also called **ego-alien, self-alien.** Compare **ego-syntonic.**

ego-dystonic homosexuality,   a psychosexual disorder characterized by discomfort with one's sexuality and a persistent desire to change sexual orientation to heterosexuality. See also **homosexual.**

ego ideal,   the image of the self to which a person aspires both consciously and unconsciously and against which he or she measures himself or herself and judges personal performance. It is usually based on a positive identification with the significant and influential figures of the early childhood years. See also **identification.**

ego-integrity,   an acceptance of self, both successes and failure. It implies a healthy psychological state.

egoism /ē′gō·iz′əm, eg″-/,   **1.** selfishness, an overvaluation of the importance of the self, expressed as a willingness to gain an advantage at the expense of others. See also **egotism. 2.** the belief that individual self-interest is, or ought to be, the basic motive for all conscious behavior.

egoist /ē′gō·ist, eg″-/,   **1.** a selfish person, one who seeks to satisfy his or her own interests at the expense of others. See also **egotist. 2.** a person who believes in or acts in accordance with the concept that all conscious action is justifiably motivated by self-interest. −*egoistic, egoistical, adj.*

ego libido,   (in psychoanalysis) concentration of the libido on the self; self-love, narcissism.

egomania /ē′gōmā″nē·ə/   [Gk, *ego,* I + *mania,* madness],   a pathological preoccupation with the self and an exaggerated sense of one's own importance. Compare **narcissism.** −*egomaniac, n.*

egophony /ēgof″ənē/,   a change in the voice sound of a patient with pleural effusion or pneumonia as heard on auscultation. When the patient is asked to make /ē-ē-ē/sounds, they are heard over the peripheral chest wall as /ä-ä-ä/, particularly over an area of consolidated or compressed lung above the effusion. Also called **tragophony.**

ego strength,   (in psychotherapy) the ability to maintain the ego by a cluster of traits that together contribute to good mental health. The traits usually considered important include tolerance of the pain of loss, disappointment, shame, or guilt; forgiveness of those who have caused an injury, with feelings of compassion rather than anger and retaliation; acceptance of substitutes and ability to defer gratification; persistence and perseverance in the pursuit of goals; openness, flexibility, and creativity in learning to adapt; and vitality and power in the activities of life. The psychiatric prognosis for a client correlates positively with ego strength. A person with ego strength is better able to cope, adapt, and maintain mental health than one who does not have it.

ego-syntonic /ē′gō sinton″ik/,   describing those elements of a person's behavior, thoughts, impulses, drives, and attitudes that are acceptable to him or her and are consistent with the total personality. Compare **ego-dystonic.**

egotism /ē′gətiz′əm, eg″-/,   vanity, conceit, or overvaluation of the importance of the self and undervaluation or contempt of others. See also **egoism.** −*egotistic, egotistical, adj.*

egotist /ē′gətist, eg″-/,   one who is vain or conceited or who places too much importance on the self and is boastful, egocentric, and arrogant. See also **egoist.**

egotistic, egotistical.   See **egotism.**

egress /ē″gres/,   the act of emerging or moving forward.

Egyptian ophthalmia,   *(Obsolete)* eye inflammation. Now called **trachoma.**

EHD,   abbreviation for **electrohemodynamics.**

EHEC,   abbreviation for **enterohemorrhagic** *Escherichia coli.*

ehl,   abbreviation for **effective half-life.**

Ehlers-Danlos syndrome /ā″lərz dan″ləs/   [Edward Ehlers, Danish physician, 1863–1937; Henri A. Danlos, French physician, 1844–1912],   a hereditary disorder of connective tissue, marked by hyperplasticity of skin, tissue fragility, and hypermotility of joints. Minor trauma may cause a gaping wound with little bleeding. Sprains, joint dislocations, and synovial effusions are common. However, life expectancy is usually normal. Treatment includes symptomatic therapy, emotional support for the patient and family, and emphasis on avoiding trauma in childhood.

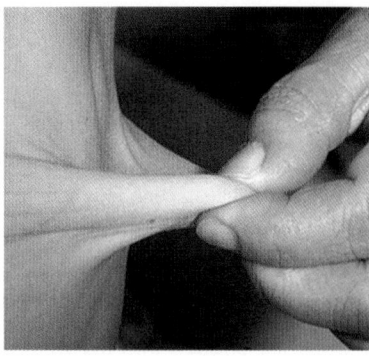

Skin laxity in Ehlers-Danlos syndrome *(Graham-Brown and Bourke, 2007)*

Ehrlichia, a genus of small spherical to ellipsoidal, nonmotile gram-negative bacteria. They occur singly or in compact inclusions in circulating mammalian leukocytes. Some species are the causative agents of ehrlichiosis and are transmitted by ticks. Two human tick-borne diseases have been associated with *Ehrlichia* species: human monocytic ehrlichiosis caused by *E. chaffeensis,* and human granulocytic ehrlichiosis caused by *E. equi.*

ehrlichiosis, a sometimes fatal tick-borne infection with symptoms similar to those of Lyme disease. The tick that carries the ehrlichiosis infection is the same species as the vector of Lyme disease, *Borrelia burgdorferi,* but the patient usually recovers within 8 weeks without the chronic arthritis symptoms associated with Lyme disease. Also called **human granulocytic ehrlichiosis, human monocytic ehrlichiosis.** See also *Ehrlichia.*

■ OBSERVATIONS: The great majority of infections are asymptomatic. Most cases present as mild to moderate acute febrile illness. The disease usually begins about 10 days after the bite of an infected tick, although some cases have begun abruptly, within hours, with influenza-like symptoms, including painful muscle aches, headaches, fever, chills, loss of appetite, and depressed blood cell counts.

■ INTERVENTIONS: Although similar to Lyme disease, the infection does not respond to the antibiotics used to treat Lyme disease. However, ehrlichiosis does respond to early treatment with tetracycline antibiotics.

■ PATIENT CARE CONSIDERATIONS: Diagnosis is difficult because of the similarities with Lyme disease, and cases of simultaneous infections of both types of bacteria have been reported.

eicosanoic acid /ī′kōsənō″ik/ [Gk, *eikosa,* twenty], a saturated fatty acid containing 20 carbon atoms in a straight chain, found in peanut oil, butter, and other fats. Also called *arachidic acid.*

eicosapentaenoic acid /ī·kō′sə·pen′tə·ē·nō′ik/, an omega-3, 20-carbon fatty acid found almost exclusively in fish and marine animal oils.

EID, abbreviation for **electronic infusion device.**

eidetic /īdet″ik/ [Gk, *eidos,* a form or shape seen], **1.** *adj.,* pertaining to or characterized by the ability to visualize and reproduce accurately the image of objects or events previously seen or imagined. **2.** *n.,* a person possessing such ability; said to have a photographic memory.

eidetic image, an unusually vivid, elaborate, and apparently exact mental image resulting from a visual experience and occurring as a fantasy, dream, or memory. See also **image.**

eighth cranial nerve. See **vestibulocochlear nerve.**

einsteinium (Es) /īnstī″nē·əm/ [Albert Einstein, German-born physicist and Nobel laureate, 1879–1955], a synthetic transuranic metallic element. Its atomic number is 99. The mass of its longest-lived, best-known isotope is 254. Einsteinium was first found in the debris from a hydrogen bomb explosion. It decays rapidly into berkelium.

Einthoven's formula /īnt″hōvənz/ [Willem Einthoven, Dutch physiologist, scientist, and Nobel laureate, 1860–1927; L, *forma,* pattern], a mathematical expression relating the voltages measured by electrocardiographic leads. The formula states that the sum of the voltages from lead I plus those from lead III minus those from lead II equals zero (I + III − II |m = 0). This formula is based on the principle that the sum of the voltages in any closed path equals zero. Because the positive and negative electrodes of lead II are reversed, the voltage from lead II is subtracted instead of added to the voltages from leads I and III. See also **Einthoven's triangle.**

Einthoven's triangle [Willem Einthoven], an equilateral triangle whose vertices lie at the left and right shoulders and the pubic region and whose center corresponds to the vector sum of all electrical activity occurring in the heart at any given moment, allowing for the determination of the electrical axis. Einthoven's triangle is approximated by the triangle formed by the axes of the bipolar electrocardiographic (ECG) limb leads I, II, and III. The center of the triangle offers a reference point for the unipolar ECG leads.

Eisenmenger complex /ī″sənmeng′ər/ [Victor Eisenmenger, German physician, 1864–1932; L, *complexus,* encirclement], a congenital heart disease characterized by a defect of the ventricular septum, a malpositioned aortic root that overrides the interventricular septum, and a dilated pulmonary artery.

Eisenmenger syndrome /i′sən·meng′ər/ [Victor Eisenmenger, German physician, 1864–1932], ventricular septal defect with pulmonary hypertension and cyanosis resulting from right-to-left (reversed) shunt of blood. It is sometimes defined as pulmonary hypertension and cyanosis, with the shunt being at the atrial, ventricular, or great vessel area.

ejaculate /ijak″yəlit/, *n.,* the semen discharged in a single emission. See also **ejaculation. –ejaculate,** *v.*

ejaculation /-ā″shən/ [L, *ejaculari,* to hurl out], the sudden emission of semen from the male urethra, usually during copulation, masturbation, or nocturnal emission. It is a reflex action in two phases. In the first phase, sperm, seminal fluid, and prostatic and bulbourethral gland secretions are moved into the urethra. In the second phase, strong spasmodic peristaltic contractions force ejaculation. The sensation of ejaculation is commonly also called orgasm. The fluid volume of the ejaculate is usually between 2 and 5 mL. Each milliliter usually contains 50 million to 150 million spermatozoa. **–ejaculatory,** *adj.*

ejaculator urinae. See **bulbospongiosus.**

ejaculatory duct /ijak″yəlatôr′ē/, the passage formed by the junction of the duct of the seminal vesicles and ductus deferens through which semen enters the urethra.

ejection /ijek″shən/ [L, *ejicere,* to cast out], forceful expulsion, as of blood from a ventricle of the heart.

ejection click, a sharp, clicking sound arising from near the heart. It may be caused by sudden swelling of a pulmonary artery, abrupt dilation of the aorta, or forceful opening of the aortic cusps. Ejection clicks are often heard during examination of individuals with septal defects or patent ductus arteriosus. Although they are associated with high pulmonary resistance and hypertension, they are common and of no clinical significance in pregnant women and in many other healthy people. Compare **systolic click.** See also **ejection sound.**

ejection fraction (EF), the fraction of the total ventricular filling volume that is ejected during each ventricular contraction. The normal EF of the left ventricle is 65%.

ejection murmur. See **systolic murmur.**

ejection period, the second phase of ventricular systole, when the semilunar valves are open and blood is being discharged into the aortic and pulmonary arteries. Also called **sphygmic interval.**

ejection sound, a sharp, clicking sound heard early in systole, coinciding with the onset of either right or left ventricular ejection. Aortic ejection sounds are commonly heard in aortic valvular stenosis, aortic insufficiency, coarctation of the aorta, and hypertension with aortic dilation. Pulmonary ejection sounds are heard in mild to moderate pulmonary stenosis, pulmonary hypertension, and dilation of the pulmonary artery. See also **ejection click.**

Ekbom syndrome. See **restless legs syndrome.**

EKC, abbreviation for **epidemic keratoconjunctivitis.**

EKG, abbreviation for **electrocardiogram.**

elaboration /ilab″ərāshən/ [L, *elaborare*, to work out], **1.** (in endocrinology) a process by which a gland synthesizes a complex substance from simpler substances and secretes it, usually under the stimulation of a tropic hormone from the pituitary gland. This process, regulated by a negative feedback system, which includes the hypothalamus, pituitary, and target gland, serves to maintain homeostasis in body function. **2.** the act of providing more context, details, or information. −*elaborate, adj.*

elaio-. See **eleo-.**

elapid /el′əpid/, **1.** *adj.,* pertaining to the members of a family of pit vipers that includes the genera *Micruroides* and *Micrurus.* **2.** *n.,* any of the members of this group.

Elaprase, enzyme replacement therapy. Brand name for **idursulfase.**

Elase, topical fixed-combination drug containing enzymes. Brand name for **fibrinolysin,** *desoxyribonuclease.*

Elase with Chloromycetin, a topical fixed-combination drug containing two lytic enzymes and an antibacterial agent. Brand name for **fibrinolysin,** *desoxyribonuclease,* **chloramphenicol.**

elastance /ilas′təns/ [Gk, *elaunein,* to drive], **1.** the quality of recoiling or returning to an original form after the removal of pressure. **2.** the degree to which an air- or fluid-filled organ, such as a lung, bladder, or blood vessel, can return to its original dimensions when a distending or compressing force is removed. **3.** the measurement of the unit volume of change in such an organ per unit of decreased pressure change. **4.** the reciprocal of compliance.

elastase, an enzyme that cleaves bonds adjacent to neutral amino acids in elastin.

elastic bandage /ilas″tik/ [Gk, *elaunein,* to drive; Fr, *bande,* strip], a bandage of stretchable fabric that provides support and allows movement. Among its uses is application to swollen extremities, such as knees or wrists, varicose veins, and broken ribs. Kinds include **Ace bandage™.**

elastic-band fixation, a method of treatment of fractures of the jaw using rubber bands to connect metal splints or wires that are attached to the maxilla and mandible. The rubber bands produce traction and draw the teeth into occlusion and proper alignment while the fracture is healing. Rubber bands are safer than rigid wires in the event of vomiting. See also **maxillomandibular fixation, nasomandibular fixation.**

elastic bougie, a flexible surgical instrument that can be passed through angular or winding channels. See also **bougie.**

elastic cartilage, the most pliant of the three kinds of cartilage, consisting of flexible and resilient fibers in an extracellular matrix. It is yellow and is located in various parts of the body, such as the external ear, the auditory tube, and the epiglottis. Also called **yellow cartilage.** Compare **hyaline cartilage, white fibrocartilage.**

elasticity /i′lastis″itē/, the ability of tissue to regain its original shape and size after being stretched, squeezed, or otherwise deformed. Muscle tissue is generally regarded as elastic because it is able to change size and shape and return to its original condition.

elastic membrane. See **cricothyroid membrane.**

elastic recoil /rē″koil/, the difference between intrapleural pressure and alveolar pressure at a given lung volume under static conditions.

elastic stocking, a type of hosiery that applies gradient pressure to the legs to prevent excessive blood accumulation in the lower extremities caused by faulty vein valves. The stockings are commonly prescribed for patients with varicose veins. Also called **gradient compression stockings.** Compare **antiembolism (AE) hose.**

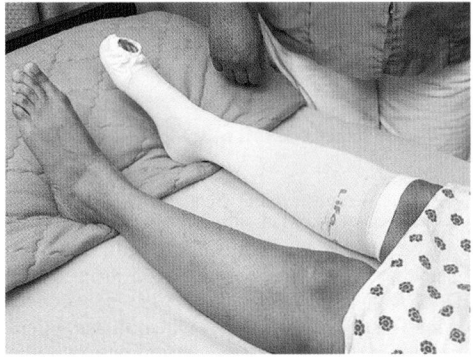

Elastic stocking *(Sorrentino, 2012)*

elastic tissue [Gk, *elaunein,* to drive; OFr, *tissu*], a type of connective tissue containing elastic fibers. It is found in ligaments of the spinal column, in the cartilage of the external ear, and in the walls of some large blood vessels.

elastic traction [Gk, *elaunein* + L, *trahere,* to draw], any therapeutic apparatus that uses an elastic device to pull on a limb.

elastin /ilas″tin/ [Gk, *elaunein,* to drive], a protein that forms the principal substance of yellow elastic tissue fibers.

elastofibroma /ilas′tōfībrō″mə/, a benign nonencapsulated mass of collagenous, fibrous, and elastic tissue that develops in subscapular fatty tissue in older persons.

elastomer /i·las′tōmər/ [Gk, *elaunein,* to drive + *meros,* part], a synthetic rubber; any of various soft, elastic, rubberlike polymers used in dentistry as an impression material and for maxillofacial extraoral prostheses. −*elastomeric, adj.*

elation /ilā″shən/ [L, *elatus,* a lifting up], an emotional reaction characterized by euphoria, excitement, extreme joyfulness, optimism, and self-satisfaction. It is considered to be of pathological origin when such a response does not realistically reflect a person's actual circumstances. Thus an elated mood may be characteristic of a manic state.

Elavil, a tricyclic antidepressant. Brand name for **amitriptyline.**

elbow [AS, *elboga*], the bend of the upper limb at the joint that connects the arm and the forearm. It is a common site of inflammation and injuries, such as those incurred during participation in various sports. See also **elbow joint.**

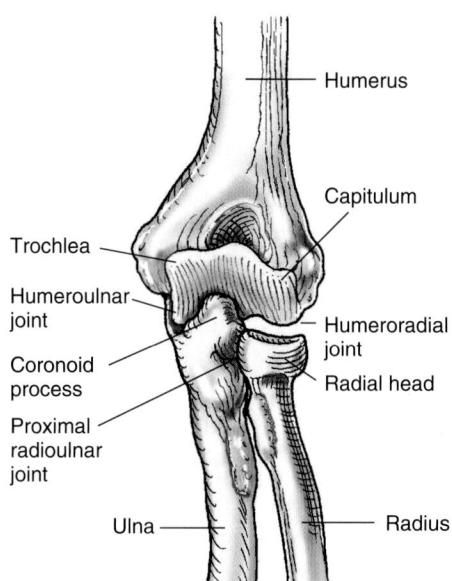

Humerus

Capitulum

Trochlea

Humeroulnar
joint

Humeroradial
joint

Coronoid
process

Radial head

Proximal
radioulnar
joint

Ulna

Radius

Anterior aspect of left elbow (Frank et al, 2012)

elbow bone. *(Nontechnical)* See **ulna.**

elbow jerk. See **triceps reflex.**

elbow joint, the hinged articulation of the humerus, the ulna, and the radius. It is covered by a protective capsule associated with three ligaments and an extensive synovial membrane. The elbow joint allows flexion and extension of the forearm and accommodates the radioulnar articulation. Also called *articulatio cubiti.*

elbow reflex. See **triceps reflex.**

elder, an herb found in the United States and Europe as a tall shrub.

■ INDICATIONS: This berry or flower may be useful for limiting the duration of symptoms from colds and flu; the flower is also used as a mouthwash and applied topically as an astringent for nasal and chest congestion, earache associated with chronic congestion, and hay fever.

■ CONTRAINDICATIONS: It is not recommended during pregnancy and lactation, in children, or in those with known hypersensitivity to this plant or similar plants. Raw or unripe fruit can cause nausea, vomiting, and severe diarrhea.

elder abuse, a reportable offense of physical, sexual, psychological, or material abuse, as well as violation of the rights of safety, security, and adequate health care of older adults. Contributing factors may include economic considerations, interpersonal conflicts, health, and dependency. Often the abused person denies that abusive acts occur and feels helpless and resigned to abuse. Health care workers are required to report suspected abuse, and perpetrators may be subject to criminal charges. Also called *abuse of the elderly.*

■ OBSERVATIONS: Manifestations are dependent on the form of abuse. Physical abuse signs include cuts; lacerations; bruises; welts; black eyes; broken bones and sprains; dislocations; injury incompatible with history; broken eyeglasses; torn clothing; physical signs of punishment or restraint; laboratory findings of medication overdose or underuse of prescription drugs; elder report of being hit, slapped, kicked, or maltreated; and caregiver's refusal to allow visitors to see elder alone. Sexual abuse signs include bruises around the breasts or genitalia; unexplained venereal disease or genital infections; unexplained vaginal or rectal bleeding; torn, stained, or bloody underclothing; and elder report of being assaulted or raped. Emotional abuse signs include emotional upset or agitation; hesitation to speak; extreme withdrawal; unusual behavior usually attributed to dementia; implausible stories; and reports of being verbally or emotionally abused. Neglect signs include dirty appearance; presence of feces and/or urine; environmental safety hazards; dehydration; malnutrition; untreated bed sores; poor personal hygiene; untreated health care problems; and elder report of mistreatment. Abandonment signs include desertion of an elder at a public institution or location such as a hospital, clinic, or shopping center, and elder self-report of abandonment. Signs of exploitation include unusual, sudden, or inappropriate activity in bank accounts; signatures on checks that do not resemble the older person's signature; unusual concern by caregiver that an excessive amount of money is being spent on care of the older person; numerous unpaid bills; overdue rent; abrupt changes in a will or other financial documents; unexplained disappearance of funds or valuable possessions; and unexplained or sudden transfer of assets to a family member or someone outside the family. Signs of self-neglect include dehydration; malnutrition; untreated or improperly attended medical conditions; poor personal hygiene; hazardous or unsafe living conditions; inappropriate or inadequate clothing; and overall lack of self-care. Diagnosis is typically made by social service, health care, and legal experts after history, investigation, and physical examination. Laboratory tests and drug screening may be done to determine the extent of malnutrition, dehydration, and medication drug levels. Severe injury, disfigurement, and death are all complications of chronic or severe physical abuse.

■ INTERVENTIONS: Obvious signs of abuse are reported to the local authorities for immediate investigation and elder protection. If the elder is perceived to be in immediate danger, elder protection should be sought through the local Adult Protective Services or the county Department of Social Services. If signs are vague or inconsistent, observations are documented and reported to appropriate local authorities for investigation.

■ PATIENT CARE CONSIDERATIONS: Health care professionals serve as a frontline resource for the detection, intervention, and prevention of elder abuse. This includes the identification of high-risk dependent elder relationships, such as those where an elder is dependent on caretakers; elders with functional impairments; previous history of abuse or neglect; evidence of substance abuse or polypharmacy; signs of depression; and lack of or limited financial and/or support resources. Members of the health care team need to do a thorough assessment for signs of coercive caretaker arrangements or lack of caretaker skills, identification of family crises that could trigger abuse or neglect, and identification of signs of abuse or neglect. All evidence should be carefully documented and reported to appropriate sources. The health care professional is also instrumental in assisting elder and family to seek respite care services, counseling, and support groups. Social agency referrals are needed for financial and functional assistance (e.g., housekeeping, cooking, and shopping). Skill-building workshops for family members, coordinated care of elderly needs, public education about the problem, and coordination among state agencies and service providers are all mechanisms for prevention. Education includes caregiver instruction about alternative forms of venting frustrations and information about available community resources.

elderly, *adj.,* pertaining to an older adult. See also **aging.**

elderly primigravida, a woman who becomes pregnant for the first time after the age of 34. Advances in obstetric care have greatly reduced the risks associated with conception after 34 years, which is of special importance as many more women are postponing pregnancy until their 30s for professional or personal reasons.

Eldopaque, a dermatological bleaching agent. Brand name for **hydroquinone.**

elective /ilek″tiv/ [L, *eligere,* to choose], pertaining to a procedure that is performed by choice and is not essential, such as elective surgery.

elective abortion, medically or surgically induced termination of a normally implanted and normal pregnancy prior to viability as a result of a personal decision of the woman. Compare **therapeutic abortion.** Kinds include **first-trimester abortion, second-trimester abortion.** See also **induced abortion.**

elective induction of labor, initiation of labor for maternal personal reasons when there is no medical indication and no complications are anticipated. See **induction of labor.**

Electra complex /ilek″trə/, (in psychiatry) the libidinous desire of a daughter for her father. Compare **Oedipus complex.** See also **phallic stage.**

electret /ilek″trət/, an insulator carrying a permanent charge similar to a permanent magnet.

electrical burn, the tissue damage resulting from heat of up to 5000° C generated by an electric current. The points of entrance and exit on the skin are burned, along with the muscle and subcutaneous tissues through which the current passes. Fatal cardiac arrhythmia may result from the current.

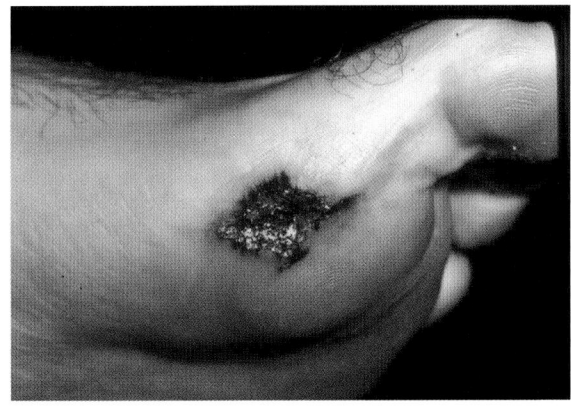

High-voltage electrical burn *(Lynch, 2011)*

electrically stimulated osteogenesis /ilek″triklē/ [Gk, *elektron,* amber; L, *stimulare,* to incite; Gk, *osteon,* bone, *genein,* to produce], a bone regeneration process induced by surgically implanted electrodes conveying electric current, especially at nonunion fracture sites. The process is effective because of the different electric potentials within bone tissue. Viable nonstressed bone is electronegative in the metaphyseal regions and over a fracture callus and electropositive in the diaphyses and other less active regions. Electrical stimulation of fractures can accelerate osteogenesis, forming bone more quickly in the area of a surgically inserted negative electrode. The precise mechanisms by which electricity induces osteogenesis are not understood, but research shows that when cathodes are implanted at a fracture site and an electric potential of less than 1 volt is applied, oxygen is consumed at the cathode, and hydroxyl ions are produced, decreasing the oxygen tension of the local tissue and increasing the alkalinity. Low tissue oxygen tension encourages bone formation, which follows a predominantly anaerobic metabolic pathway.

electrical silence, in electroencephalography and electromyography, absence of measurable electrical activity in tissue.

electric blood warmer, a device for heating blood before infusions, especially massive transfusions in which cold blood may cause a state of shock. The electric blood warmer includes a receptacle containing an electric heater and space for the insertion of a disposable blood-warming bag composed of parallel plastic tubes. The warmer is also equipped with a temperature indicator, which shows when the heating bag reaches the proper temperature of 99° F (37.6° C). An IV Y-set is commonly used in transfusions involving the electric blood warmer.

electrical cautery. See **electrocautery.**

electric circuit, the path of the electron flow from a generating source through various components and back to the generating source.

electric current, the net movement of electrons along a conducting medium.

electric field, the lines of force exerted on charged ions in the tissues by the electrodes that cause charged particles to move from one pole to another.

electric impedance, an opposition to electron flow in a conducting material.

electricity /i″lektris″itē/ [Gk, *elektron,* amber], a form of energy expressed by the activity of electrons and other subatomic particles in motion, as in dynamic electricity, or at rest, as in static electricity. Electricity can be produced by heat generated by a voltaic cell or produced by induction, rubbing of nonconductors with dry materials, or chemical activity. Electricity may be negative, when there is a surplus of electrons, or positive, when there is a surplus of protons or a deficiency of electrons.

electric muscle stimulator (EMS), a therapeutic electric current used to stimulate muscle directly, such as when the muscle is denervated and peripheral nerves are not functioning. See also **electrostimulation.**

electric potential, the potential difference between charged particles, usually expressed in the unit of volts. See also **potential.**

electric potential gradient. See **membrane potential.**

electric shock, a traumatic physical state caused by the passage of electric current through the body. It usually involves accidental contact with exposed parts of electric circuits in home appliances and domestic power supplies but may also result from lightning or contact with high-voltage wires. The resultant damage depends on the intensity of the electric current, the type of current, and the duration and the frequency of current flow. Alternating current (AC), direct current (DC), and mixed current cause different kinds and degrees of damage. High-frequency current produces more heat than low-frequency current and can cause burns, coagulation, and necrosis of affected body parts. Low-frequency current can burn tissues if the area of contact is small and concentrated. Severe electric shock commonly causes unconsciousness, respiratory paralysis, muscle contractions, bone fractures, and cardiac disorders. Even passage of small electric currents through the heart can cause fibrillation. Treatment may involve such measures as cardiopulmonary resuscitation, defibrillation, and IV administration of electrolytes to help stabilize vital functions. See also **cardiogenic shock, hypovolemic shock.**

electric shock therapy, *(Obsolete)* now called **electroconvulsive therapy.**

electric spinal orthosis (ESO), an electric device that helps control curvature of the spine by stimulating back muscles. The portable battery-powered machine does not correct scoliosis but prevents it from worsening.

electro-, prefix meaning "electricity": *electrocatalysis, electrocautery.*

electroacupuncture after Voll (EAV), a system of diagnosis and treatment based on the measurement of the electrical characteristics of acupoints, the results being used to determine a specific remedy.

electroanalgesia /ilek′trō·an′əljē″sē·ə/, the use of an electric current to relieve pain. See also **transcutaneous electrical nerve stimulation (TENS).**

electroanalytic chemistry /-an′əlit″ik/ [Gk, *elektron* + *analysis,* a loosening, *chemeia,* alchemy], the branch of chemistry concerned with the analysis of compounds by use of electrical properties to produce characteristic observable change in the substance being studied. See also **chemistry.**

electroanesthesia /-an′esthē″zhə/, the use of an electric current to produce local anesthesia.

electroaxonography. See **axonography.**

electrocardiogram (ECG, EKG) /-kär′dē·əgram′/ [Gk, *elektron* + *kardia,* heart, *gramma,* record], a recording of the heart's electrical activity. It may be displayed on a monitor or recorded on special tracing paper.

electrocardiograph (ECG) /-kär′dē·əgraf′/, a device used for recording the electrical activity of the myocardium to detect transmission of the cardiac impulse through the conductive tissues of the muscle. Electrocardiography allows diagnosis of specific cardiac abnormalities. Leads are affixed to certain anatomical points on the patient's chest, usually with an adhesive gel that promotes transmission of the electrical impulse to the recording device. –*electrocardiographic, adj.*

electrocardiographic technician /-kär′dē·ōgraf″ik/, an allied health worker with special training and experience in operating and maintaining electrocardiographic equipment and providing recorded data for diagnostic review by a physician.

electrocardiograph lead /lēd/, **1.** an electrode placed on part of the body and connected to an electrocardiograph. **2.** a record, made by the electrocardiograph, that varies with the site of the electrode. Electrocardiography is generally performed with the use of six limb leads and six leads placed on the precordium. The peripheral or extremity leads are designated I, II, III, AVR, AVL, and AVF. The chest leads are designated V1, V2, V3, V4, V5, and V6 to indicate the points on the precordium on which the electrodes are placed.

electrocardiography (ECG) /-kär′dē·og″rəfē/ [Gk, *elektron* + *kardia,* heart, *graphein,* to record], the study of records of electrical activity generated by the heart muscle. Also called **cardiography.**

electrocardiophonograph. See **phonocardiograph.**

electrocatalysis, the chemical decomposition of tissues caused by the application of electric current to the body.

electrocautery /ilek′trōkô″tərē/ [Gk, *elektron* + *kauterion,* branding iron], the application of a needle or snare heated by electric current for the destruction of tissue, such as for removing warts or polyps and cauterizing small blood vessels to limit blood loss during surgery. Also called **electric cautery, galvanic cautery, galvanocautery.** See also **diathermy.**

electrochemistry, the study of the electric effects that accompany chemical action and the chemical activity produced by electric influence.

electrocoagulation /-kō·ag′yəlā″shən/ [Gk, *elektron* + L, *coagulare,* to curdle], a therapeutic destructive form of electrosurgery in which tissue is hardened by the passage of high-frequency current from an electric cautery device. Also called **surgical diathermy.** Compare **electrodesiccation.**

electroconvulsive therapy (ECT) /-kənvul′siv/, the induction of a brief convulsion by passing an electric current through the brain for the treatment of affective disorders, especially in patients resistant to psychoactive-drug therapy. ECT is primarily used when rapid definitive response is required for either medical or psychiatric reasons, such as for a patient who is extremely suicidal and when the risks of other treatments outweigh the risk of ECT. A secondary use of ECT is treatment failure of other choices.

electrocution /-kyo͞o″shən/, death caused by the passage of electric current through the body. See also **electric shock.**

electrode /ilek″trōd/ [Gk, *elektron* + *hodos,* way], **1.** a contact for the induction or detection of electrical activity. **2.** a medium for conducting an electric current from the body to physiological monitoring equipment.

electrodermal /-dur″məl/, pertaining to electrical properties of the skin, particularly altered resistance.

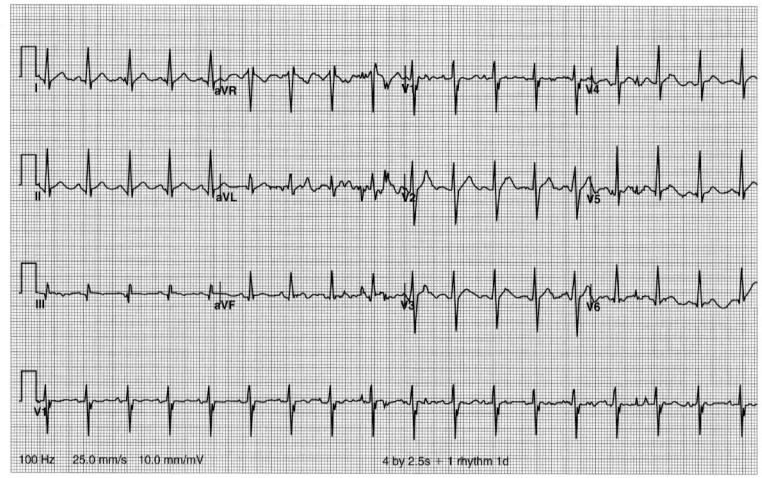

12-lead electrocardiogram *(Phalen and Aehlert, 2012)*

electrodermal activity therapy, a type of biofeedback therapy in which sensors attached to the palm or the palmar aspect of the fingers are used to monitor sweat output in response to stress. It is used in the treatment of stress, anxiety disorders, chronic pain, and hyperhidrosis.

electrodermal audiometry [Gk, *elektron* + *derma,* skin; L, *audire,* to hear; Gk, *metron,* measure], a method for determining hearing thresholds in which a harmless electric shock is used to condition the subject to a pure tone, which thereafter, coupled with the anticipation of a shock, elicits a brief electrodermal response. The lowest intensity of the sound that produces the skin response is considered the subject's hearing threshold. It is a very old procedure and rarely used today.

electrodesiccation /-des′ikā″shən/ [Gk, *elektron* + *desiccare,* to dry up], a technique in electrosurgery in which tissue is destroyed by burning with an electric spark. It is used primarily for eliminating small superficial growths but may be used with curettage to eradicate abnormal tissue deeper in the skin or to stop bleeding. In the latter case, layers of skin may be burned, then successively scraped away. The procedure is performed under local anesthesia.

electrodiagnosis /-dī′agnō″sis/ [Gk, *elektron* + *dia,* twice, *gnosis,* knowledge], the diagnosis of disease or injury by electrical stimulation of various nerves and muscles.

electrodynamics /-dīnam″iks/, the study of electrostatic charges in motion, such as the flow of electrons in an electric current. Compare **electrohemodynamics.**

electrodynograph (EDG) /-din″əgraf′/ [Gk, *elektron* + *dynamis,* force, *graphein,* to record], an electronic device used to measure pressures exerted in biological activity, such as those exerted by the human foot in walking, running, jogging, or climbing stairs.

electroencephalogram (EEG) /ilek′trō·ensef″ələgram′/ [Gk, *elektron* + *enkephalos,* brain, *gramma,* record], a graphic chart on which is traced the electric potential produced by the brain cells, as detected by electrodes placed on the scalp. The resulting brain waves are called alpha, beta, delta, and theta rhythms, according to the frequencies they produce, which range from 2 to 12 cycles per second with an amplitude of up to 100 μV. Variations in brain wave activity are correlated with neurological conditions, psychological states, and level of consciousness. See also **encephalography.**

electroencephalograph (EEG) /ilek′trō·ensef″ələgraf′/, an instrument for receiving and recording the electric potential produced by the brain cells. It consists of a vacuum tube amplifier that magnifies the electric currents received through electrodes placed on the scalp and electromagnetically records the patterns on a graphic chart. See also **electroencephalography.**

electroencephalographic technologist /ilek′trō·ensef′əl əgraf″ik/, a person trained in the management of an electroencephalographic laboratory with responsibility for the laboratory and equipment, including closed-circuit TV-EEG (CTV-EEG), the monitoring of patients with seizure disorders, and coordination of staffing. The technologist may supervise electroencephalographic technicians, who are generally responsible for the operation and maintenance of the equipment.

electroencephalography (EEG) /ilek′trō·ensef′əlog ″rəfē/, the process of recording brain wave activity. Electrodes are attached to various areas of the patient's head with collodion. During the procedure the patient remains quiet, with eyes closed, and refrains from talking or moving. In certain cases prescribed activities, especially hyperventilation, may be requested. The test is used to diagnose seizure disorders, brainstem disorders, focal lesions, and impaired consciousness. During neurosurgery the electrodes can be applied directly to the surface of the brain (intracranial electroencephalography) or placed within the brain tissue (depth electroencephalography) to detect lesions or tumors. See also **electroencephalogram.** −*electroencephalographic, adj.*

electrogram /ilek″trōgram′/ [Gk, *elektron* + *gramma,* record], a unipolar or bipolar record of the electrical activity of the heart as recorded by electrodes within the cardiac chambers or on the epicardium. Kinds include *atrial electrogram, ventricular electrogram,* **His bundle electrogram.**

electrohemodynamics (EHD) /ilek′trōhē″mōdīnam″iks/ [Gk, *elektron* + *haima,* blood, *dynamis,* force], a technique for noninvasively measuring the mechanical properties and hemodynamic characteristics of the vascular system, including arterial blood pressure, electric impedance, blood flow, and resistance to blood flow.

electroimmunodiffusion, an immunochemical method that combines electrophoretic separation with immunodiffusion by incorporating antibodies into the support medium. See also **immunodiffusion.**

electrolarynx /i·lek′troler′ingks/ [Gk, *elektron,* amber + *larynx*], an electromechanical device that enables a laryngectomized person to speak. When it is placed against the region of the laryngectomy a buzzing sound is produced, which is converted into simulated speech by movements of the organs of articulation (lips and tongue).

electrolysis /il′ektrol″isis/ [Gk, *elektron* + *lysis,* loosening], a process in which electrical energy causes a chemical change in a conducting medium, usually a solution or a molten substance, or the decomposition of a substance such as hair follicles. −**electrolytic,** *adj.*

electrolyte /ilek″trōlīt/ [Gk, *elektron* + *lytos,* soluble], an element or compound that, when melted or dissolved in water or another solvent, dissociates into ions and is able to conduct an electric current. Electrolytes differ in their concentrations in blood plasma, interstitial fluid, and cell fluid and affect the movement of substances between those compartments. Proper quantities of principal electrolytes and balance among them are critical to normal metabolism and function. For example, calcium (Ca) is necessary for relaxation of skeletal muscle and contraction of cardiac muscle; potassium (K) is required for contraction of skeletal muscle and relaxation of cardiac muscle. Sodium (Na) is essential in maintaining fluid balance. Certain diseases, conditions, and medications may lead to a deficiency of one or more electrolytes and to an imbalance among them; for example, certain diuretics and a low-sodium diet prescribed in hypertension may cause hypokalemic shock as a result of a loss of potassium. Diarrhea may cause a loss of many electrolytes, leading to hypovolemia and shock, especially in infants. Careful and regular monitoring of electrolytes and IV replacement of fluid and electrolytes are aspects of acute care in many illnesses. −**electrolytic,** *adj.*

electrolyte balance, the concentration of serum ions necessary to maintain equilibrium among electrolytes.

electrolyte imbalance, the serum concentrations of an electrolyte that are either higher or lower than normal.

electrolyte solution, any solution containing electrolytes prepared for oral, parenteral, or rectal administration for the replacement or supplementation of ions necessary for homeostasis. The loss of potassium ion (K⁺) by vomiting, by diarrhea, or by the action of certain medications, including diuretics and corticosteroids, may be corrected by

E

administering a solution high in potassium. Other electrolyte solutions containing combinations of sodium, potassium, calcium, magnesium, chloride, bicarbonate, phosphate, and/or lactate may be given to treat acid-base disturbance, as seen in chronic renal dysfunction or diabetic ketoacidosis. The solutions are available in a wide range of balanced formulas for replacement or maintenance, and most include various trace minerals.

electrolytic. See **electrolysis.**

electromagnetic /-magnet″ik/ [Gk, *elektron + Magnesia,* ancient source of lodestone], **1.** pertaining to magnetism that is induced by an electric current. **2.** pertaining to radiation such as light, microwaves, x-rays, gamma rays, or radio waves.

electromagnetic induction [Gk, *elektron + magnes,* lodestone; L, *inducere,* to bring in], the production of electric current in a circuit when it is passed through a changing magnetic field.

electromagnetic radiation, radiation that is produced with a combination of magnetic and electric forces. It exists as a continuous spectrum of radiation, from that with the highest energy level and shortest wavelength (gamma rays) to that with the lowest energy and longest wavelength (long radio waves). The visible part of the electromagnetic spectrum has a wavelength between 400 and 700 nm. Ultraviolet and infrared radiation have wavelengths just below the short end and above the long end of the visible spectrum, respectively. X-rays have wavelengths from about 0.005 to 10 nm. All forms of electromagnetic radiation travel at the speed of light.

electromagnetic spectrum, the range of frequencies and wavelengths associated with radiant energy.

electromallet condenser /-mal″ət/ [Gk, *elektron* + OFr, *mail,* maul; L, *condensare,* to make dense], an electromechanical device formerly used for compacting direct-filling gold, such as gold foil restorations in prepared tooth cavities.

electromechanical dissociation. See **pulseless electrical activity.**

electromotive force (EMF) /-mō″tiv/, the electric potential, or ability of electrical energy to perform work. EMF is usually measured in joules per coulomb, or volts. The higher the voltage, the greater the potential of electrical energy.

electromyogram (EMG) /ilek′trōmī″əgram′/, a record of the intrinsic electrical activity in a skeletal muscle. Such data aid the diagnosis of neuromuscular problems and are obtained by applying surface electrodes or by inserting a needle electrode into the muscle and observing electrical activity with an oscilloscope and a loudspeaker. Some electromyograms show abnormalities, such as spontaneous electric potentials within the muscle under study, and help pinpoint lesions of motor nerves. Electromyograms also measure electric potentials induced by voluntary muscular contraction. See also **electroneuromyography.**

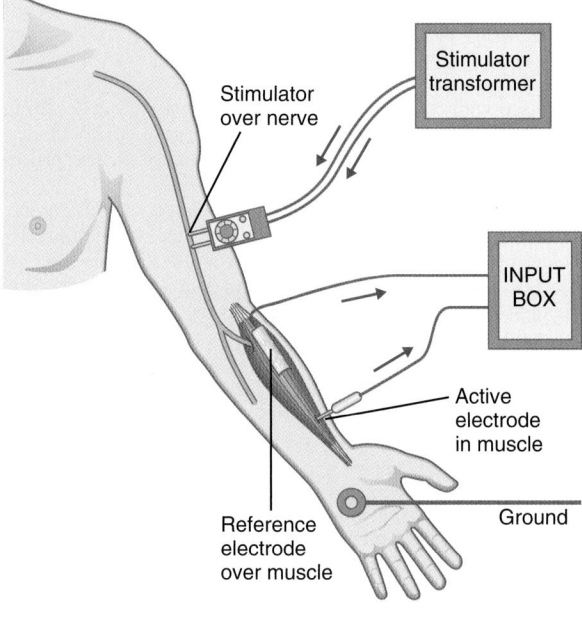

Electromyogram *(Mourad, 1991)*

Clinical manifestations of electrolyte imbalance

Imbalance	Clinical manifestations	Causes
Hyponatremia Na <135 mEq/L	Fatigue, abdominal cramps, diarrhea, weakness, hypotension, cool clammy skin	Excess sweating, excess intake of water, diuretics, adrenal insufficiency, renal failure
Hypernatremia Na >145 mEq/L	Thirst; dry, sticky mucous membranes; dry tongue and skin; flushed skin; increased temperature	Diarrhea, decreased water intake, saltwater ingestion, impaired renal function, febrile illness, inability to swallow, burns, diabetes insipidus
Hypokalemia K <3.5 mEq/L	Weakness, fatigue, anorexia, abdominal distention, cardiac arrhythmias	Diarrhea, vomiting, diuretics, burns, heat stress, ulcerative colitis, potassium-free IV fluids, metabolic acidosis, steroids
Hyperkalemia K >5.0 mEq/L	Cardiac arrhythmias, anxiety, increased bowel sounds, abdominal cramps	Acute/chronic renal failure, burns, crush injuries, metabolic acidosis, potassium-sparing diuretics
Hypocalcemia Ca <4.5 mg/dL	Abdominal cramps, tingling, muscle spasm, convulsions	Parathyroid dysfunction, vitamin D deficiency, pancreatitis
Hypercalcemia Ca >5.6 mg/dL	Bone pain, nausea, vomiting, constipation	Parathyroid tumor, bone cancer/metastasis, osteoporosis

Adapted from ENA: *Sheehy's emergency nursing: principles and practice,* ed 6, St. Louis, 2010, Mosby.

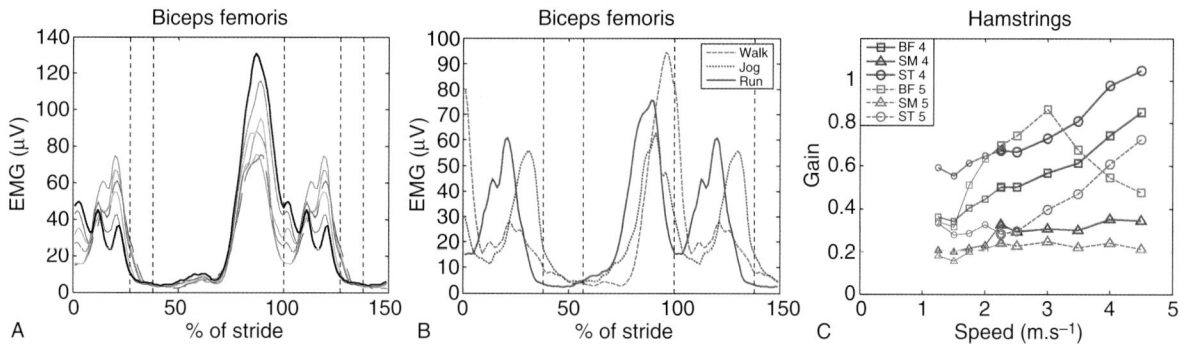

Electromyogram profile for walking (Gazendam et al, 2006)

electromyographic biofeedback /-mī′əgraf″ik/, a therapeutic procedure that uses electronic or electromechanical instruments to measure, process, and feed back reinforcing information with auditory and visual signals accurately. It is used to provide information about muscle activity during ambulation, for example, in clients with brain injury, stroke, or cerebral palsy.

electromyographic technician /-mī′əgraf″ik/, a health care provider with special training and experience to assist in evaluating, recording, and analyzing muscle action potentials with the use of various electronic devices.

electromyography (EMG) /-mī·og″rəfē/, the electrical recording of muscle action potentials.

electromyography of pelvic floor sphincter, an electrodiagnostic test performed to evaluate the neuromuscular function of the urinary or anal sphincter. It is done most often in patients with urinary or fecal incontinence.

electron /ilek″tron/ [Gk, *elektron,* amber], **1.** a negatively charged elementary particle that has a specific charge, mass, and spin. The number of electrons associated with an atom is equal to the atomic number of the element. **2.** a negative beta particle emitted from a radioactive substance. See also **atom, element, ion, neutron, proton.**

electronarcosis /ilek′trōnärkō″sis/ [Gk, *elektron* + *narkosis,* numbness], anesthesia produced by passing an electric current through the brain. The experimental procedure has been used in the former USSR. Compare **electrosleep therapy.**

electron beam computed tomography (EBCT), a specific type of computed tomography (CT) that was explicitly developed to better image heart structures, which never stop moving. The principal application advantage of EBCT is the increase in the speed of diagnostic recording due to a machine design that allows the x-ray source-point to be swept electronically, not mechanically.

electron capture, a radioactive decay process in which an atomic nucleus with an excess of protons draws an electron into itself, creating a neutron out of a proton and thus decreasing the atomic number by 1. Often the resulting nucleus is unstable and achieves stability by emitting a gamma ray.

electroneurodiagnostic technologist, an allied health professional who, in collaboration with an electroencephalographer, obtains interpretable recordings of a patient's nervous system function. The electrodiagnostic technologist takes a patient history; applies adequate recording electrodes and uses optimal EEG, EP, and PSG techniques; and documents the clinical condition of patients.

electroneurography, an electrodiagnostic test that assists in detecting and locating peripheral nerve injury or disease. This study is usually done in conjunction with electromyography.

electroneuromyography /ilek′trōno̅o̅r″ōmī·og″rəfē/ [Gk, *elektron* + *neuron,* nerve, *mys,* muscle, *graphein,* to record], a procedure for testing and recording neuromuscular activity by electrical stimulation of nerves. Needle electrodes are inserted into any skeletal muscle being studied, electric current is applied to the electrodes, and neuromuscular functions are observed and recorded by means of instruments, such as a cathode-ray oscilloscope and an appropriate recording device. The procedure is helpful in the study of neuromuscular conduction, the extent of nerve lesions, and reflex responses. Compare **nerve conduction test.** See also **electromyogram.**

electronic bulletin board /ilektron″ik/, a computerized communication system that allows users to compose and store information to be retrieved by other users of the system.

Electronic Data Interchange (EDI), a method by which two or more autonomous computer systems exchange computer-readable transaction data. It is possible even when the computers use different operating systems. It is the key factor in achieving automated medical records that can be shared electronically among providers. The Health Insurance Portability and Accountability Act includes security provisions that must be addressed in the exchange of protected health information.

electronic fetal monitor (EFM) [Gk, *elektron* + L, *fetus* + *monere,* to warn], a device that facilitates a more exact measurement of the fetal heart rate and pattern than auscultation of the fetal heart rate with a stethoscope. It also provides an evaluation of the strength of uterine contractions more efficiently than manual palpation. The fetal heart rate and pattern may be monitored externally by an ultrasound transducer or internally by the placement of an electrode directly on the fetal scalp if membranes are ruptured. The strength and pattern of uterine contractions may be monitored externally by the placement of a physical transducer measuring the "hardness" of the uterus or internally with the placement of a catheter that transmits intrauterine pressure to a pressure gauge on the device.

electronic health record (EHR), a comprehensive longitudinal collection of health information and encounter information about a patient. The EHR includes resources such as decision-support systems to analyze patient data and present evidence-based suggestions for treatment to the clinicians. Components include clinical decision support, electronic order entry, and order processing. The record is collected and stored in an electronic environment to aid providers in rendering high-quality, cost-efficient care. See also **charting, documentation, medical record.**

electronic infusion device (EID), an automated system of introducing a fluid other than blood into a vein. The device may have programmable settings that control the amount of fluid to be infused, rate, low-volume notification level, and a keep-vein-open rate. Some EIDs have titration modes that allow a change in the delivery rate without interrupting fluid flow. They also allow delivery in milliliters per hour.

electronic mail (email, e-mail, E-mail), messages sent by one user of a computerized communications system and retrieved almost instantaneously or at a later time by other users. Positive health outcomes are associated with this type of asynchronous communication between health care providers and patients. See also **electronic bulletin board.**

electronic stethoscope, an instrument designed and equipped to detect and amplify body sounds up to 18 times greater than a nonelectronic stethoscope. It also reduces ambient room noise through reduction technology.

electronic thermometer, a battery-powered thermometer that registers temperature by electronic means.

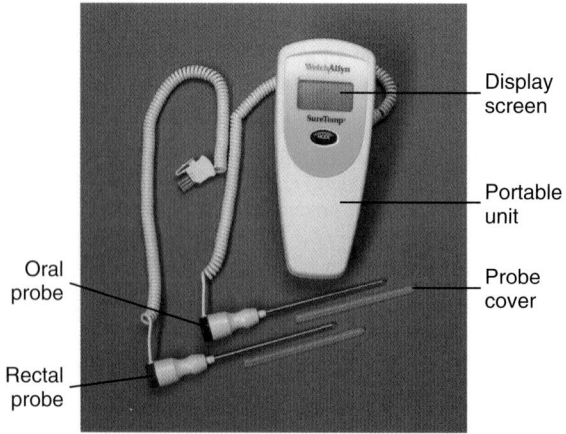

Display screen

Portable unit

Oral probe

Probe cover

Rectal probe

Electronic thermometer *(Bonewit-West, 2015)*

electron microscope, an electronic instrument that scans cell and tissue sections with a beam of electrons instead of visible light. The specimen is stained with electron-opaque dyes. With its high magnification power, it creates an image that can be photographed or viewed on a fluorescent screen. Compare **scanning electron microscope.** See also **electron microscopy.**

electron microscopy, a technique using an electron microscope in which a beam of electrons is focused by an electromagnetic lens and directed onto an extremely thin specimen. The electrons emerging are focused and directed by a second lens onto a fluorescent screen. The magnified image produced is 1000 times greater than that produced by an optic microscope and well resolved, but it is two-dimensional because of the thinness of the specimen. Compare **scanning electron microscopy, transmission scanning electron microscopy.**

electron scanning microscope. See **scanning electron microscope.**

electron transfer flavoprotein (ETF), a component of a side chain of redox reactions by which electrons are funneled to ubiquinone and thus the electron transport chain. Electrons from acyl coenzyme A (CoA) thioesters and choline are transferred via the flavin of acyl CoA dehydrogenases, dimethylglycine dehydrogenase, and sarcosine dehydrogenase to the flavin adenine dinucleotide prosthetic group of ETF, which is then oxidized by reduction of electron transfer flavoprotein ubiquinone oxidoreductase. Deficiency of ETF results in glutaric aciduria, type II.

electron volt (eV), a unit of energy equal to the energy acquired by an electron falling through a potential difference of 1 volt. One eV equals 1.6×10^{-12} erg or 1.6×10^{-19} J.

electronystagmography /ilek'trōnis'tagmog″rəfē/ [Gk, *elektron* + *nystagmos*, nodding, *graphein*, to record], a method of assessing and recording eye movements by measuring the electrical activity of the extraocular muscles. See also **electroencephalogram, nystagmus.**

electropalatography, a technique for recording the timing and location of tongue contact with the hard palate during speech, using an artificial palate that fits against the roof of the mouth and has electrodes embedded in the surface that faces the tongue. A computer records and displays the pattern of the pulses generated by contact of the tongue with the electrodes.

electrophoresis /ilek'trōfərē″sis/ [Gk, *elektron* + *pherein*, to bear], the movement of charged suspended particles through a liquid medium in response to changes in an electric field. Charged particles of a given substance migrate in a predictable direction and at a characteristic speed. The pattern of migration can be recorded in bands on an electrophoretogram. The technique is widely used to separate and identify serum proteins and other substances. *—electrophoretic, adj.*

electrophysiological study (EPS), an invasive electrodiagnostic or manometric procedure that uses electrode catheters to pace the heart and potentially induce arrhythmias. The test identifies defects in the heart conduction system and arrhythmias that are otherwise inapparent. It also is used to assess the effectiveness of antiarrhythmic drugs.

electrophysiology /-fis′ē-ol″əjē/ [Gk, *elektron* + *physis*, nature, *logos*, science], a branch of biology concerned with the relationship between electrical phenomena and biological function.

electropiezo activity. See **piezoelectric activity.**

electroplating /i·lek′trōplāt′ing/ [Gk, *electron* + Fr, *plat*, flat dish], plating or coating of an object with a layer of metal through the use of electrolytic processes.

electroporation /-pôrā″shən/, a type of osmotic transfection in which an electric current is used to produce temporary holes in cell membranes, allowing the entry of nucleic acids or macromolecules (a way of introducing new deoxyribonucleic acid into the cell). See also **transfection.**

electroresection /-risek″shən/ [Gk, *elektron* + L, *re*, again, *secare*, to cut], a technique for the removal of bladder tumors or prostate tissue by electrocautery. A wire is guided to the site through the urethra with the aid of an optic probe. Electricity is passed through the wire when the wire is properly located in the tissue to be destroyed. The procedure is performed after administration of an anesthetic.

electroshock [Gk, *elektron* + Fr, *choc*], a condition of shock caused by accidental contact with an electric current. The symptoms are similar to those of shock produced by thermal burns, trauma, or coronary thrombosis.

electroshock therapy, *(Obsolete)* now called **electroconvulsive therapy.**

electrosleep therapy [Gk, *elektron* + AS, *slaep* + Gk, *therapeia*, treatment], a technique designed to induce sleep, especially in psychiatric patients, by administering a low-amplitude pulsating current to the brain. The cathode is placed supraorbitally, and the anode is placed over the mastoid process. The current, which is discharged for 15 to 20 minutes, produces a tingling sensation but does not always induce sleep. The procedure is repeated from 5 to 30 times. Electrosleep therapy is said to be beneficial for patients with anxiety, depression, gastric distress, insomnia, personality disorders, and schizophrenia. Compare **electronarcosis.**

electrostatic imaging /-stat″ik/ [Gk, *elektron* + *stasis,* standing still; L, *imago,* image], a radiographic technique in which the ionic charge liberated during the irradiation process is converted into a visible image.

electrostimulation /-stim′yəlā″shən/, the application of electric current to stimulate muscle tissue for therapeutic purposes, such as facilitation of muscle activation and muscle strengthening. See also **electric muscle stimulator.**

electrosurgery /-sur″jərē/ [Gk, *elektron* + *cheiourgos,* surgeon], a surgical procedure performed with various electric instruments that operate on high-frequency electric current. Kinds include **electrocoagulation, electrodesiccation.**

electrotherapeutic current, any of three types of electric current, which, when introduced into biological tissue, is capable of producing specific physiological changes. The three types are direct monophasic, alternating biphasic, and pulsed polyphasic electric current.

electrotherapist /-ther″əpist/, a health care provider who has specific training and experience in the therapeutic use of electric current and frequency treatments. See also **transcutaneous electrical nerve stimulation (TENS), def. 1, electrotherapy.**

electrotherapy, the use of electrical energy as a medical treatment. Kinds include **TENS, deep brain stimulation.**

electrotonic current [Gk, *elektron* + *tonos,* tension], a current induced in a nerve sheath without the generation of new current by an action potential.

electrotonic synapse, a gap junction that transmits electrical impulses in electrically excitable tissue. See also **gap junction.**

electrovalence, the valence of an ion, equal to the absolute value of its charge. See also **valence, valence electron.**

eleidin /əlē″ədin/ [Gk, *elaia,* olive tree], a transparent, proteinaceous substance resembling keratin, found in the outer stratum lucidum of the epidermis.

element [L, *elementum,* first principle], one of more than 100 primary, simple substances that cannot be broken down by chemical means into any other substance. Each atom of any element contains a specific number of protons in the nucleus and an equal number of electrons outside the nucleus. In most elements, the nucleus may contain a variable number (high or low) of neutrons. An element with a disproportionate number of neutrons may be unstable, in which case the nucleus undergoes radioactive decay into a more stable element. See also **atom, compound, molecule, radioactivity.**

element 104. See **rutherfordium.**

element 105. See **dubnium.**

element 106. See **seaborgium.**

element 107, an element reportedly synthesized in 1976 by Russian scientists who bombarded isotopes of bismuth with heavy nuclei of chromium-54. The finding was not confirmed by scientists of other nations. It has been named bohrium (Bh).

elemental formula. See **defined formula diet.**

elementary particle, (in physics) a subatomic particle, such as an electron, neutron, or proton.

eleo-, prefix meaning "oil": *eleoma.*

eleoma /ē′lē-ō″mə/, a lipogranuloma, or swelling, usually caused by subcutaneous injection of oil.

elephantiasis /el′əfəntī″əsis/ [Gk, *elephas,* elephant, *osis,* condition], the end-stage lesion of filariasis, characterized by extensive swelling, usually of the external genitalia and the legs, resulting from obstruction of the lymphatics by filariae. The overlying skin becomes dark,

thick, and coarse. Elephantiasis results from filariasis of many years' duration. Nonfilarial elephantiasis occurring in the absence of filarial infection, seen mainly in the central African mountains, may be caused by persistent contact with volcanic ash. Nonfilarial elephantiasis is difficult to diagnose in the early stages, when it is most responsive to treatment. See also **filariasis.**

elephantine psoriasis /el′əfan″tīn/, a rare form of psoriasis that is characterized by thick, scaly plaques on the hips, thighs, and back.

elephantoid fever. See **elephantiasis, filariasis.**

eletriptan, an antimigraine agent used for the acute treatment of migraine with or without aura.

elevation /el′əva′shən/ [L, *elevare,* to lift], a raised area or a point of greater height.

elevator /el′əvā′tər/ [L, *elevare,* to lift], an instrument for lifting tissues, extracting teeth, removing bony fragments, or removing roots of teeth.

eleventh cranial nerve. See **accessory nerve.**

elfin facies syndrome, *(Obsolete)* now called **Williams syndrome.**

eligibility /el′əjəbil″itē/, entitlement of an individual to receive services based on that individual's enrollment in a health care plan.

Eligibility Guarantee Payment, a contract provision for guaranteeing payment from a health maintenance organization in the United States to the provider for services already delivered to enrollees whose coverage is terminated retroactively.

elimination /i·lim′i·nā′shən/ [L, *ex,* out + *limen,* threshold], **1.** the act of expulsion or of extrusion, especially of expulsion from the body. See also **clearance, defecation, excretion, urination. 2.** omission or exclusion, as in an elimination diet. See also **elimination diet.**

elimination diet /ilim′inā″shən/ [L, *eliminare,* to expel; Gk, *diata,* way of living], a procedure for identifying a food or foods to which a person is allergic by successively omitting from the diet certain foods in order to detect those responsible for the symptoms.

ELISA /əlī″zə/, a technology used to measure a variety of proteins and antigens. Abbreviation for **enzyme-linked immunosorbent assay.**

elixir /ilik″sər/ [Ar, *il-iksir,* seen as the philosopher's stone], a clear liquid containing water, alcohol, sweeteners, or flavors, used primarily as a vehicle for the oral administration of a drug.

Elixophyllin, a bronchodilator. Brand name for **theophylline.**

Elliot forceps. See **obstetric forceps.**

ellipsis /ilip″sis/, (in psychiatry) the omission by a patient of meaningful thoughts and ideas while undergoing therapy.

ellipsoidal, describing an object that has the shape of a spindle or an ellipse.

ellipsoid joint, a synovial joint in which a condyle is received into an elliptic cavity, as the wrist joint. A condyloid joint permits no axial rotation but allows flexion, extension, adduction, abduction, and circumduction. Also called **condyloid joint.** Compare **ball-and-socket joint, pivot joint, saddle joint.** See also **joint.**

elliptical trainer, exercise equipment designed to simulate motions such as stair-climbing and running by using pedals that move back and forth in an oval (elliptical) pattern to minimize the impact on the hips, back, and knees.

elliptocyte /ilip″təsīt/ [Gk, *elleipsis,* ellipse, *kytos,* cell], an oval red blood cell. Also called **ovalocytes.** See also **elliptocytosis.**

E

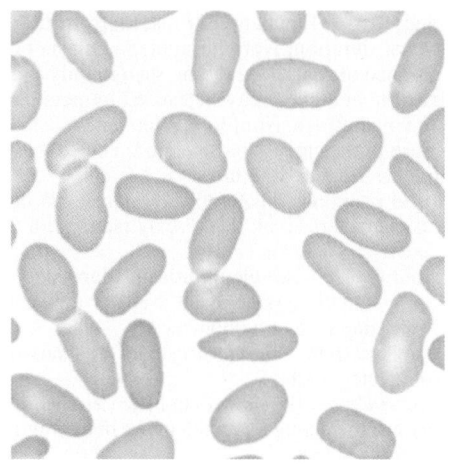

Elliptocyte *(Carr and Rodak, 2008)*

elliptocytic anemia, hereditary elliptocytosis. See also **elliptocytosis, ovalocytosis.**

elliptocytosis /ilip′tōsītō″sis/ [Gk, *elleipsis + kytos + osis*, condition], an abnormal condition of the blood characterized by increased numbers of elliptocytes. Less than 15% of the red blood cells appear in this form in normal blood; modest increases occur in a variety of anemias, including a rare congenital disorder, hereditary elliptocytosis. Also called **ovalocytosis.** Compare **spherocytosis.** See also **acanthocytosis, congenital nonspherocytic hemolytic anemia, sickle cell anemia, spherocytic anemia.**

Ellis–van Creveld syndrome. See **chondroectodermal dysplasia.**

elongation /i′longā″shən/ [L, *elongatio,* a prolonging], a state of being lengthened or extended.

elope /ilōp″/ [ME, *gantlopp,* to run away], *(Informal)* to leave a locked or secured psychiatric institution or inpatient health care facility without notice or permission.

Elspar, an antineoplastic. Brand name for **asparaginase.**

eluate /el″yoo·āt/ [L, *eluere,* to wash out], a solution or substance that results from an elution process. In column chromatography the eluate is collected as it drips from the column.

eluent /el″yoo·ənt/, a solvent or solution used in an elution process, such as column chromatography.

elution /eloo″shən/, the removal of an absorbed substance from a porous bed or chromatographic column by means of a stream of liquid or gas or the application of heat. The technique may consist of washing a material that dissolves out of just one component of a mixture. The term is also applied to the removal of antibodies or radioactive tracers from erythrocytes. In heat elution of antibodies, red cells in a saline solution are heated to 56° C and then centrifuged. Liquid elution of antibodies usually uses ether as the solvent.

em, abbreviation for **extrinsic muscle.**

EM, abbreviation for **erythema multiforme.**

em-, prefix meaning "in, on": *embolism, empathy.*

emaciation /imā′shi·ā″shən/ [L, *emaciare,* to make lean], **1.** excessive leanness caused by disease or lack of nutrition. **2.** an extreme loss of subcutaneous fat that results in an abnormally lean body, such as with starvation. *−emaciated, adj.*

e-mail. See **electronic mail.**

emancipated minor /iman″sipā′tid/ [L, *emancipare,* to set free], a person who is not legally an adult but who, because he or she is married, in the military, or otherwise no longer dependent on the parents, may not require parental permission for medical or surgical care. State and national laws vary in specific interpretations of the rule.

emasculation /imas′kyələ″shən/, surgical, chemical, or accidental loss of the organs of the male reproductive system. See also **castration.**

embalming /embä″ming/, the practice of applying antiseptics and preservatives and/or the injection of chemicals into a corpse to slow the natural decomposition of tissues.

Embden-Meyerhof defects /emb″den mī″ərhof/ [Gustav G. Embden, German biochemist, 1874–1933; Otto F. Meyerhof, German biochemist, 1884–1951], a group of hereditary hemolytic anemias caused by enzyme deficiencies. The most common form of the disorder is a pyruvate kinase deficiency. The condition is characterized by an absence of spherocytes and the presence of small numbers of crenated erythrocytes. The trait is transmitted as an autosomal-recessive gene, and the hemolytic anemia occurs only in homozygotes.

Embden-Meyerhof pathway. See **glycolysis.**

embedded tooth, an unerupted tooth. Also spelled **imbedded tooth.** Compare **impacted tooth.**

embol-, prefix meaning "to insert or plug": embolus, embolectomy.

embolectomy /em′bəlek″təmē/ [Gk, *embolos,* plug, *ektomē,* excision], a surgical incision into an artery for the removal of an embolus or clot, performed as emergency treatment for arterial embolism. The operation is done as soon as possible after a decrease in perfusion is detected. Thrombi tend to lodge at the juncture of major arteries. More than half lodge in the aorta, in arteries of the lower extremities, in the common carotid arteries, or in the pulmonary arteries. Before surgery, heparin may be administered, and an arteriogram may be used to identify the affected artery. A longitudinal incision is made in the artery, and the embolus is removed. After surgery the blood pressure is maintained close to the level of the preoperative baseline, as a decrease might predispose to new clot formation.

embolic. See **embolus.**

embolic gangrene [Gk, *embolos + gaggraina,* gangrene], the death and decay of body tissues caused by an embolus blocking the blood supply to that part.

embolic necrosis, death of a portion of tissue that results from an infarction caused by an embolus.

embolic thrombosis [Gk, *embolos,* plug, *thrombos,* lump, *osis,* condition], a clot that develops at the site of an impacted embolus (foreign body) in a blood vessel.

emboliform nucleus, a small cerebellar nucleus lying between the dentate nucleus and the globose nucleus and contributing to the superior cerebellar peduncles.

embolism /em″bəliz′əm/, an abnormal condition in which an embolus travels through the bloodstream and becomes lodged in a blood vessel. Symptoms vary with the character of the embolus, the degree of occlusion that results, and the size, nature, and location of the occluded vessel. Kinds include **air embolism, fat embolism, gas embolism. −embolic,** *adj.*

embolization agent, a substance used to occlude or drastically reduce blood flow within a vessel. Examples include microfibrillar collagen, absorbable gelatin sponge (Gelfoam), polyvinyl alcohol particles, tris-acryl gelatin microspheres, and silicone beads.

embolized atheroma, a fat particle lodged in a blood vessel. *−embolic,* *adj.*

emboloid. See **embolus.**

embolotherapy /em″bəlōther″əpē/, a technique of blocking a blood vessel with a balloon catheter. It is used for treating bleeding ulcers and blood vessel defects and for stopping blood flow to a tumor during surgery.

embolus /em″bələs/ *pl.* *emboli* [Gk, *embolos,* plug], a foreign object, quantity of air or gas, bit of tissue or tumor, or piece of a thrombus that circulates in the bloodstream until it becomes lodged in a vessel. –**embolic, emboloid,** *adj.*

embolysis /embol″isis/, the dissolution of an embolus, especially one caused by a blood clot. See also **thrombolysis.**

embrasure /embrā″zhər/, a normally occurring space between adjacent teeth on the same arch (maxillary or mandibular) resulting from variations in the positions and contours of teeth. Embrasures provide a spillway for the escape of food during mastication. See also **spillway.**

embryo /em″brē·ō/ [Gk, *en,* in, *bryein,* to grow], **1.** any organism in the earliest stages of development. **2.** in humans the stage of prenatal development from the time of fertilization of the ovum (conception) until the end of the eighth week. The period is characterized by rapid growth, differentiation of the major organ systems, and development of the main external features. Compare **fetus, zygote.** –**embryonoid, embryonal, embryonic,** *adj.*

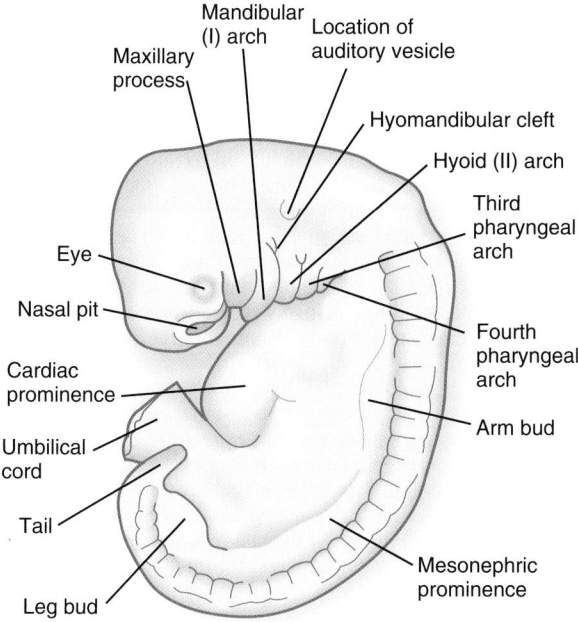

Maxillary process

Mandibular (I) arch

Location of auditory vesicle

Hyomandibular cleft

Hyoid (II) arch

Third pharyngeal arch

Eye

Nasal pit

Cardiac prominence

Umbilical cord

Tail

Leg bud

Fourth pharyngeal arch

Arm bud

Mesonephric prominence

Embryo: end of fourth week *(Carlson, 2009)*

embryo-, prefix meaning a "fetus": *embryology.*

embryocidal /em′brē·əsī″dəl/, pertaining to the killing of an embryo.

embryoctony /em′brē·ok″tənē/ [Gk, *en* + *bryein* + *kteinein,* to kill], the intentional destruction of a living embryo or fetus in utero. Also called **feticide.** See also **abortion.**

embryogenesis /em′brē·ōjen″əsis/ [Gk, *en* + *bryein* + *genein,* to produce], the process in sexual reproduction by which an embryo forms from the fertilization of an ovum. Also called *embryogeny.* See also **heterogenesis, homogenesis.** –**embryogenetic, embryogenic,** *adj.*

embryological development /-loj″ik/, the various intrauterine stages and processes involved in the growth and differentiation of the conceptus from the time of fertilization of the ovum until the eighth week of gestation. The stages are related to the biological status of the unborn child and

involve the differentiation of the various cells, tissues, and organ systems and the development of the main external features of the embryo. It occurs from approximately the end of the second week to the eighth week of intrauterine life. The fetal stage follows these stages, beginning at about the ninth week of gestation. The entire process of growth and development of the embryo and fetus is loosely called prenatal development. See also **prenatal development.**

embryologic, embryological. See **embryology.**

embryologist /em′brē·ol″əjist/, one who specializes in the study of organisms from conception to birth. See also **embryology.**

embryology /em′brē·ol″əjē/ [Gk, *en, bryein* + *logos,* science], the study of the origin, growth, development, and function of an organism from fertilization to birth. Kinds include **comparative embryology, experimental embryology, descriptive embryology.** –*embryologic, embryological, adj.*

embryoma /em′brē·ō″mə/ [Gk, *en* + *bryein* + *oma,* tumor], a tumor that arises from embryonic cells or tissues.

embryoma of the ovary. See **dysgerminoma.**

embryomorph /embrē″əmôrf′/ [Gk, *en* + *bryein* + *morphe,* form], any structure that resembles an embryo, especially a mass of tissue that may represent an aborted conceptus. –*embryomorphous, adj.*

embryonal. See **embryo.**

embryonal adenomyosarcoma, embryonal adenosarcoma. See **Wilms tumor.**

embryonal carcinoma /em″brē·ənal/, a malignant neoplasm derived from germinal cells that usually develops in gonads, especially the testes. The tumor, a firm nodular mass with hemorrhagic areas, is characterized histologically by large, undifferentiated cells with indistinct borders, eosinophilic cytoplasm, and prominent nucleoli in pleomorphic nuclei. Bodies resembling a 1- or 2-week-old embryo are occasionally seen in these tumors. The neoplasm is relatively resistant to radiation therapy. The tumor metastasizes by way of lymph channels. Surgery and chemotherapy are usually used in the treatment. See also **choriocarcinoma.**

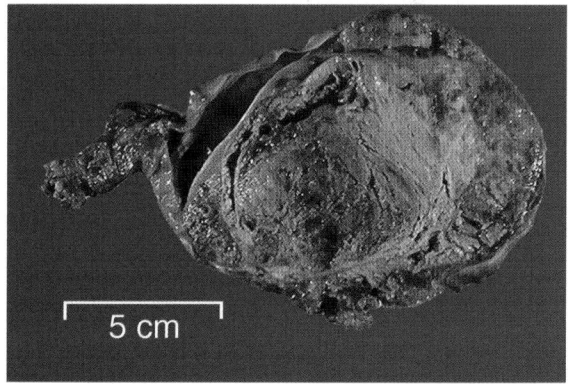

5 cm

Embryonal carcinoma *(Klatt, 2010)*

embryonal leukemia, *(Obsolete)* now called **stem cell leukemia.**

embryonate /em″brē·ənāt′/ [Gk, *en* + *bryein* + L, *atus,* shaped like], **1.** impregnate. **2.** pertaining to or resembling an embryo. **3.** containing an embryo.

embryonic. See **embryo.**

embryonic anideus [Gk, *en* + *bryein* + *an,* not, *eidos,* form], a blastoderm in which the axial elongation of the primitive streak and primitive groove fail to develop.

embryonic area.   See **embryonic disk.**

embryonic blastoderm,   the area of the blastoderm that gives rise to the primitive streak from which the embryonic body develops. Compare **extraembryonic blastoderm.**

embryonic competence,   the ability of an embryonic cell to react normally to the stimulation of an inductor, allowing continued normal growth or differentiation of the embryo.

embryonic disk,   the thickened plate from which the embryo develops in the second week of pregnancy. Scattered cells from the border of the disk migrate to the space between the trophoblast and yolk sac and become the embryonic mesoderm. The disk develops from the ectoderm and endoderm. Also called **embryonic area, gastrodisk, germ disk, germinal area.**

embryonic layer,   one of the three layers of cells in the embryo: the endoderm, the mesoderm, and the ectoderm. From these layers of cells arise all of the structures and organs and parts of the body. The endoderm and the ectoderm are the first to develop. During the third week of gestation the mesoderm arises between the ectoderm and the endoderm.

embryonic period,   the earliest period or phase of lung development in utero, lasting from the third week after conception to the sixth week. It is sometimes not named as a defined period of lung development, which is instead considered to begin with the following pseudoglandular period. During this period, a ventral respiratory diverticulum (lung bud) arises from the caudal end of the laryngotracheal groove and grows into bronchial buds and the primordial trachea. Also called *embryonic phase.*

embryonic pole,   the area of the blastocyst where the embryoblast and the trophoblast are in contact. The embryoblast attaches to the endometrial epithelium at this pole.

embryonic rest,   a portion of embryonic tissue that remains in the adult organism. Also called **epithelial rest,** *fetal rest.*

embryonic stage,   (in embryology) the interval of time from fertilization to the eighth week.

embryonic tissue   [Gk, *en* + *bryein,* to grow; OFr, *tissu*],   **1.** mucoid tissue; a loose, gelatinous mass of connective tissue cells. The gelatinous matrix is caused by the presence of mucopolysaccharides. Also called **mucous tissue, mucoid tissue. 2.** pertaining to tissue of an embryo.

embryoniform /em′brē·on′ifôrm′/   [Gk, *en* + *bryein* + L, *forma,* form],   resembling an embryo.

embryonoid.   See **embryo.**

embryoplastic /em′brē·ōplas″tik/   [Gk, *en* + *bryein* + *plassein,* to mold],   pertaining to the formation of an embryo, usually with reference to cells.

embryoscopy /em′brē·os′kəpē/,   the direct examination of an embryo by insertion of a lighted instrument through the mother's abdominal wall and uterus. The technique may be used to obtain tissue specimens for analysis or to perform needed surgery.

embryotome /em″brē·ətōm′/   [Gk, *en* + *bryein* + *temnein,* to cut],   a cutting instrument for the removal of a fetus when normal birth is not possible. See also **embryotomy.**

embryotomy /em′brē·ot″əmē/   [Gk, *en* + *bryein* + *temnein,* to cut],   **1.** the dismemberment or mutilation of a fetus for removal from the uterus when normal delivery is not possible. **2.** the dissection of an embryo for examination and analysis.

embryo transfer,   a technique in assisted reproduction in which fertilized ova are placed in the uterus adjacent to the endometrium, where it is hoped that implantation will occur. The biggest risk is multiple gestation, when two or more ova implant.

embryotroph /em″brē·ətrof′/   [Gk, *en* + *bryein* + *trophe,* nourishment],   the liquefied uterine nutritive material, composed of glandular secretions and degenerative tissue, that nourishes the mammalian embryo until placental circulation is established. Also called **histotroph, histotrophe, histotrophic nutrition.** Compare **hemotroph.**

embryotrophy /em′brē·ot″trəfē/,   the nourishment of the embryo. See also **embryotroph, hemotroph.** *−embryotrophic, adj.*

embryulcia /em′brē·ul″sē·ə/   [Gk, *en* + *bryein* + *elkein,* to draw],   the surgical extraction of the embryo or fetus from the uterus.

Emcyt,   an antineoplastic agent. Brand name for **estramustine phosphate sodium.**

eme-,   prefix meaning "to vomit": *emetic.*

emedastine /em″ědas′tēn/,   an antihistamine applied topically to the conjunctiva as emedastine difumarate in treatment of allergic conjunctivitis.

Emend,   an antiemetic. Brand name for **aprepitant.**

emergence /imur″jəns/   [L, *emergere,* to come forth],   the point in the process of recovery from general anesthesia at which a return of spontaneous respiration, protective airway reflexes, and consciousness occurs. It is also used to refer to the recovery from sedation. See also *postanesthesia care.*

emergency /imur″jənsē/   [L, *emergere,* to come forth],   a perilous situation that arises suddenly and threatens the life or welfare of a person or a group of people, as a natural disaster, medical crisis, or trauma situation.

emergency cardiac care (ECC) [L, *emergeere,* to come forth; Gk, *kardia* + ME, *caru,* sorrow],   the concentration of personnel and facilities organized to sustain the cardiovascular and pulmonary systems when a myocardial infarction or cardiac arrest occurs. The interventions assure prompt availability of basic life support, monitoring and treatment facilities, prevention of complications, and psychological reassurance. If cardiac arrest occurs outside a hospital, efforts are devoted to stabilizing the patient's cardiovascular and pulmonary systems while removing the individual to a hospital.

emergency childbirth,   a birth that occurs accidentally or precipitously in or out of the hospital, without standard obstetric preparations and procedures. Signs and symptoms of impending delivery include increased bloody show, frequent strong contractions, the mother's desire to bear down forcibly or her report that she feels as though she is going to defecate, visible bulging of the bag of waters, and crowning of the baby's head at the vaginal introitus.

■ METHOD: If time permits, equipment is readied, but the delivery is not delayed for such preparations. Useful equipment includes sterile gloves, towels, bulb syringe, receiving blankets, scissors, two Kelly clamps, cord clamp or tie, and a basin for the placenta. The mother's vital signs are taken, and the fetal heart sounds are listened to if time permits and if equipment is available. The mother is reassured that emergency deliveries are usually simple and that all procedures and events will be explained. Despite her compelling urge to push and to deliver quickly, the mother is encouraged to ease the baby out slowly by not pushing and by blowing air forcibly out through pursed lips as she feels the strength of the urge building. As the head emerges, it is supported but allowed to rotate naturally. A check is made immediately to determine whether or not the umbilical cord is wound around the neck. If it is, a gentle attempt is made to slip it over the baby's head; if it is too tight, it is immediately clamped with two Kelly clamps placed 2 or 3 inches apart, cut between the clamps, and unwound from the neck. If the baby does not deliver immediately, mucus and fluid in the nose and mouth are sucked out with a bulb syringe. The shoulders are delivered one at a time by guiding the head downward to deliver the anterior (upper) shoulder under the symphysis pubis, and then upward to deliver the posterior (lower) shoulder over the perineum. The rest of the baby is quickly born. If the membranes of the amniotic sac are intact, the sac is snipped or torn behind the baby's neck and peeled away from the face so that the baby can breathe. If necessary, the nares, nasopharynx, and mouth may be suctioned with the bulb syringe, taking care not to slow the heart rate by stimulating the vagus nerve with the tip of the syringe on the back of the throat. The baby is kept warm and held with the head lower than the chest; it may be laid skin-to-skin on the mother's abdomen. The baby may thus be positioned, observed, and warmed in one place as the nurse or other helper covers the mother and baby with a dry blanket or towel and continues to provide emergency care as necessary through the third stage of labor. There is no urgent need to cut the cord or to deliver the placenta. When it is desired, the cord may be cut by clamping it in two places several inches from the baby and cutting it between the clamps with sterile scissors. The cord clamp may be put on later. If possible, an Apgar score is taken first at 5 minutes of age, then at 10. The placenta is ready to be delivered when the cord is seen to advance a few inches, the uterus becomes firmer and rises in the abdomen, and a small gush of bright red blood emerges from the vagina. The mother may help expel it by bearing down. The placenta is lifted out of the vagina slowly, with care, so that all of the membranes are drawn out with it. The placenta and membranes are kept for further evaluation. The uterus is massaged to ensure that it is well contracted, and the baby is put to breast if the mother wishes. The uterus is palpated frequently, and it is massaged when necessary. The baby is kept with the mother and observed for warmth, color, activity, and respiration. After delivery of the placenta, the perianal area is rinsed with warm sterile water and dried with a clean towel or cloth, and an ice pack and a sanitary pad or small towel are applied in such a way that the mother can hold them in place by drawing her legs together.

■ OUTCOME CRITERIA: Almost all births are normal and do not constitute true medical emergencies. If a mother is healthy and is not bleeding, if her vital signs are normal, and if the fetal heart sounds are normal, there is no immediate cause for alarm, even if the birth is imminent. Emergency care is directed to ensuring that the newborn breathes well and is kept warm, that the mother is protected from hemorrhage, and that the mother's privacy is maintained. The nurse is likely to be the person who must initially evaluate the situation and decide whether to attempt to transfer or transport the mother or to prepare for emergency delivery. If a mother says the baby is coming, the attendant is advised to believe her and to act accordingly. Throughout the delivery and the third stage of labor, the nurse works to help the mother to feel calm, confident, and well cared for.

emergency contraceptive, medications given after unprotected intercourse to prevent pregnancy. Also called **postcoital contraceptive.** Kinds include **morning-after pill.**

emergency department (ED), (in a health care facility) a section of an institution that is staffed and equipped to provide rapid and varied emergency care, especially for those who are stricken with sudden and acute illness or who are the victims of severe trauma. The emergency department may use a triage system of screening and classifying clients to determine priority needs for the most efficient use of available personnel and equipment. The terms *Emergency Department (ED)* and *Emergency Room (ER)* are used interchangeably in Canada.

emergency doctrine, (in law) a doctrine that assumes a person's consent to medical treatment when he or she is in imminent danger and unable to give informed consent to treatment. Emergency doctrine assumes that the person would consent if able to do so. Also called **implied consent.**

emergency handling of radiation accidents. See **radiation exposure, emergency procedures.**

emergency medical identification. See **Medic Alert™®.**

emergency medical responder, an individual who administers immediate care to patients who access the emergency medical system. Responders are trained with the basic skills and knowledge needed to provide lifesaving interventions and to assist higher-level personnel at an emergency scene and during patient transport. Emergency medical responders function under medical oversight as part of a comprehensive emergency medical services response.

emergency medical services (EMS), a network of services coordinated to provide aid and medical assistance, from primary response to definitive care, involving personnel trained in the rescue, stabilization, transportation, and advanced treatment of traumatic or medical emergencies. Linked by a communication system that operates on both a local and a regional level, EMS is a tiered system of care, which is usually initiated by citizen action in the form of a telephone call to an emergency number. Subsequent stages include the emergency medical dispatch, first medical responder, ambulance personnel, medium and heavy rescue equipment, and paramedic units, if necessary. In the hospital, service is provided by emergency department nurses, emergency department physicians, specialists, and critical care nurses and physicians. See also **emergency medical technician–advanced life support, emergency medical technician–intermediate,** *emergency medical technician–intravenous, emergency medical technician–paramedic.*

emergency medical technician (EMT), a person trained in and responsible for the administration of specialized emergency care and the transportation of victims of acute illness or injury to a medical facility in compliance with national standards developed by the U.S. Department of Transportation. In addition to basic life-support skills, the EMT is trained in extrication, operation of emergency vehicles, basic anatomy, basic assessment of injury or illness, triage, care for specific injuries and illnesses, environmental emergencies, childbirth, and transport of the patient. Canadian EMT training and practice is similar but meets the regulatory standards for licensure in respective provinces or territories. See also **emergency medical services.**

emergency medical technician–advanced life support (EMT-ALS), an emergency medical technician with additional certification who may administer certain medications following the protocols or orders of the hospital physician, with whom radio contact is maintained. An EMT-ALS is also trained in the use of advanced life support systems, including electrical defibrillation equipment. See also **emergency medical services.**

emergency medical technician–intermediate (EMT-I), individuals with specialized training who provide emergency care, typically in an ambulance, until a patient can reach a hospital. There are two EMT-I levels, each with slightly different responsibilities. EMTs function as part of a comprehensive emergency medical services (EMS) response, with medical oversight. EMT licensure is provided by the National Registry of Emergency Medical Technicians (NREMT). Compare **emergency medical technician–advanced life support.** See also **emergency medical services.**

emergency medicine, a branch of medicine concerned with the diagnosis and treatment of conditions resulting from trauma or sudden illness. The patient's condition is stabilized, and care is transferred to the primary physician or to a specialist. Emergency medicine requires broad interdisciplinary training in the physiological and pathological characteristics of all body systems.

Emergency Nurses' Association (ENA), a national professional organization of emergency department nurses that defines and promotes emergency nursing practice. The association, which was founded in 1970, has written and implemented the Standards of Emergency Nursing Practice. The association offers a certification examination and awards the designation Certified Emergency Nurse (CEN) to nurses who successfully complete it. ENA publishes the *Journal of Emergency Nursing and Continuing Education Core Curriculum of Emergency Nursing Practice.* The association, which has headquarters in Chicago, works closely with its members and with related associations to define practice and to prepare professionals to deliver emergency care.

emergency nursing, nursing care provided to prevent imminent severe damage or death or to avert serious injury. Activities that exemplify emergency nursing are basic life support, advanced cardiac life support, cardiopulmonary resuscitation, and control of hemorrhage.

emergency readiness, a state of having made advance plans for coping with an unexpected natural disaster, civil disturbance, or military attack that may threaten death and injury to a local population. The planning includes educating the population about location of shutoff valves for utilities and about first aid, including cardiopulmonary resuscitation; ensuring that adequate sources of food, water, basic medical supplies, and bedding materials will be available; arranging for the disposal of human wastes when toilets are not functional; and establishing procedures for emergency care of the elderly, infants, small children, and women who may be pregnant. Plans for communication systems are also a part of emergency readiness. Also called *emergency preparedness.*

emergency room (ER, E.R.). *(Informal)* See **emergency department.**

emergent /imur″jənt/ [L, *emergens,* emerging], **1.** arising, often unexpectedly. **2.** changing or modifying an existing property, as when a mutation of a gene causes cell growth.

emergent evolution, the theory that evolution occurs in a series of major changes at certain critical stages and results from the total rearrangement of existing elements so that completely new and unpredictable characteristics appear within the species. See also **saltatory evolution.**

Emery-Dreifuss syndrome /em″ərē drī″fəs/ [Alan E.H. Emery, British geneticist, b. 1928; Fritz E. Dreifuss, 20th-century British physician, 1926–1997], an X-linked recessive form of muscular dystrophy that begins in early childhood and is characterized by joint contractures and cardiac conduction disorders. Cardiac pacemakers may be necessary to control arrhythmias. Muscle wasting and weakness in the shoulders, upper arms, and the calves usually appears by 10 years of age.

emesis. See **vomit,** def. 1.

-emesis, suffix meaning "to vomit": *hyperemesis.*

emesis basin /em″əsis, əmē″sis/ [Gk, *emesis,* vomiting; Fr, *bassin,* hollow vessel], a kidney-shaped bowl or pan that fits against the neck. It is used as a receptacle for vomitus.

emesis gravidarum, vomiting associated with pregnancy. See also **nausea and vomiting of pregnancy, hyperemesis gravidarum.**

Emete-con, an antiemetic. Brand name for **benzquinamide.**

emetic /imet″ik/, **1.** *adj.,* pertaining to a substance that causes vomiting. **2.** *n.,* an emetic agent.

-emetic, -emetical, suffix meaning "to cause vomiting": *antiemetic.*

Emetrol, a fixed-combination drug used to treat nausea and vomiting. Brand name for **fructose, glucose,** *orthophosphoric acid.*

EMF, abbreviation for **electromotive force.**

EMG, **1.** abbreviation for **electromyography. 2.** abbreviation for **electromyogram.**

EMG syndrome, a hereditary disorder transmitted as an autosomal-recessive trait, characterized by umbilical hernia (exomphalos), macroglossia, and gigantism, often accompanied by visceromegaly, dysplasia of the renal medulla, and enlargement of the cells of the adrenal cortex. Also called **Beckwith-Wiedemann syndrome, exophthalmos-macroglossia-gigantism syndrome.**

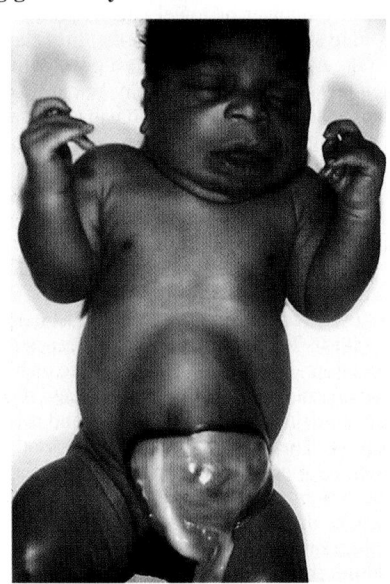

Infant with EMG syndrome *(Courtesy Dr. D. Becker)*

-emia, -aemia, -hemia, -haemia, a suffix meaning "blood condition": *anemia, polycythemia, hyperemia.*

emissary veins /em″əser′ē/ [L, *emittere,* to send forth], the small vessels in the skull that connect the sinuses of the dura mater with the veins on the exterior of the skull through a series of anastomoses.

emission /imish″ən/ [L, *emittere,* to send out], a discharge or release of something, such as a fluid from the body, electronic signals from a radio transmitter, or an alpha or beta particle from an atomic nucleus during radioactive decay.

emission computed tomography (ECT) [L, *emittere,* to send forth; *computare,* to count; Gk, *tome,* section, *graphein,* to record], a form of tomography in which the emitted decay products, such as positrons or gamma rays, of an ingested radioactive pharmaceutical are recorded in detectors outside the body. Computer reconstruction of the data yields a cross-sectional image of the body.

emit [L, *emittere,* to send out], to give or send out something, such as energy, sound, heat, or radiation.

emmetr-, prefix meaning "the correct measure": *emmetropia.*

emmetropia /em′ətrō″pē·ə/ [Gk, *emmetros,* proportioned, *opsis,* vision], a state of normal vision characterized by the proper relationship between the refractive system of the eyeball and its axial length. This correlation ensures that light rays entering the eye parallel to the optic axis are focused exactly on the retina. Compare **amblyopia, hyperopia, myopia.** *–emmetropic, adj.*

Emmet's operation, a surgical procedure for repair of a lacerated perineum or ruptured uterine cervix.

emollient /imol″yənt/ [L, *emolliere,* to soften], a substance that softens tissue, particularly the skin and mucous membranes.

emollient bath, a bath taken in water containing an emollient, such as bran, to relieve irritation and inflammation. See also **colloid bath.**

emotion /imō″shən/ [L, *emovere,* to disturb], **1.** the outward expression or display of mood or feeling states. **2.** the affective aspect of consciousness as compared with volition and cognition. Physiological alterations often occur with a marked change of emotion regardless of whether the feelings are conscious or unconscious, expressed or unexpressed. See also **emotional need, emotional response.**

emotional abuse /imō″shənəl/, the debasement of a person's feelings that causes the individual to perceive himself or herself as inept, not cared for, and worthless.

emotional age [L, *emovere,* to disturb; L, *aetas,* age], the age of an individual as determined by the stage of emotional maturity. It involves a comparison with chronological age (i.e., whether a person handles emotions as expected for his or her age).

emotional amalgam, an unconscious effort to deny or counteract anxiety.

emotional care of the dying patient, the compassionate, consistent support offered to help the terminally ill patient and his or her family cope with impending death. Family, friends, and health care professionals, including nurses, physicians, and hospice personnel, assist with the transition from life to death by offering a positive meaningful presence. See also **hospice, stages of dying.**

■ METHOD: The professional person providing emotional support for the terminally ill encourages the expression of personal feelings, anxieties, and experiences regarding death and empathizes with the patient and the family. To prevent conflicting statements, it is essential to know what the physician, other professionals, and family members tell the patient about the outcome. Effective support in terminal illness involves a nonjudgmental approach to the patient's relatives and significant others, an understanding of their problems, and efforts to assist them in the grieving process. The patient needs relief from pain, tender care, and continued attention through all the stages of dying.

■ INTERVENTIONS: Arrangements for hospice care or home care, when it is possible and desirable, can play a major role in assisting the patient and family to cope with impending death. Members of the health care team may teach methods of care required at home, may assist the family in realizing the patient's need to live as normally and as long as possible, and may refer the family to the social service department and to community resources for assistance.

■ OUTCOME CRITERIA: Sensitive emotional support appropriate to the stages of dying may help the person to move more rapidly to acceptance. The family usually goes through similar stages; therefore, support and counseling by an experienced person may greatly enhance the quality of life of the patient and family.

emotional deprivation [L, *emovere,* to disturb, *deprivare,* to deprive], a lack of adequate warmth, affection, and interest, especially of a parent or significant nurturer. It is a relatively common problem among institutionalized persons.

emotional diarrhea, *(Nontechnical)* the frequent passage of liquid stools caused by extreme emotional stress.

emotional hyperhidrosis, an autosomal-dominant disorder of the eccrine sweat glands, most often of the palms, soles, and axillae, in which emotional stimuli (e.g., anxiety) and sometimes mental or sensory stimuli elicit volar or axillary sweating (usually not both in the same individual). Eccrine sweat glands in other areas of the body are affected less often and are less sensitive to such stimuli.

emotional illness. See **mental illness.**

emotional intelligence (EI), the ability to monitor one's own reactions and the reactions of others and to appropriately manage those reactions. Skills involved in emotional intelligence include awareness, problem solving, and interpersonal relationship management.

emotional lability, a condition of excessive emotional reactions and frequent mood changes. Also called *emotionally labile, adj.*

emotional need, a psychological or mental requirement of intrapsychic origin that usually centers on such basic feelings as love, fear, anger, sorrow, anxiety, frustration, and depression and involves the understanding, empathy, and support of one person for another. Such needs normally occur in everyone but usually increase during periods of excessive stress or physical and mental illness and during various stages of life, such as infancy, early childhood, and old age. If these needs are not routinely met by appropriate, socially accepted means, they can precipitate psychopathological conditions. Appropriate measures common in health care for anticipating and satisfying the emotional needs of patients in stress include physical closeness, especially remaining with the person during periods when the feeling is acute; empathetic listening as the patient discusses the feeling; encouragement to verbalize feelings; and planning activities that provide a constructive outlet for the feeling or the situation causing it. Compare **dependency needs.** See also **emotion.**

emotional response, a reaction to a particular intrapsychic feeling or feelings, accompanied by physiological changes that may or may not be outwardly manifested but that motivate or precipitate some action or behavioral response. See also **emotion.**

emotional support, the sensitive, understanding approach that helps patients accept and deal with their illnesses; communicate their anxieties and fears; derive comfort from a gentle, sympathetic, caring person; and increase their ability to care for themselves.

■ METHOD: Essential in providing emotional support are recognizing and respecting the individuality, personal preferences, and human needs of each patient. Understanding the sick and appreciating the psychological effects on the patient of the transition from health to illness are also important. The patient is encouraged to verbalize feelings and concerns, and the attentive listener avoids interjecting clichés, such as "Don't worry," "Take it easy," or "Everything will be all right." The nurse and other health team members realize that the patient may express some fears but may act out others through anger, hostility, silence, or assumed joviality. Efforts to change the patient, negative criticism, a judgmental attitude, and facial expressions that may indicate rejection are carefully avoided. Opportunities to listen to the troubled patient and provide compassionate and realistic counseling and care are sought.

■ INTERVENTIONS: The nurse establishes means of communication, provides an atmosphere that invites the patient to discuss worrisome feelings, and presents a caring attitude. This is especially important when the illness damages the person's body image or self-concept.

■ OUTCOME CRITERIA: Emotional support frequently improves the patient's psychological and physical state, often enabling him or her to accept the illness and to adjust with less anxiety to the changes required.

emotional support animal (ESA), a pet that provides emotional support and comfort, assisting individuals with serious mental health issues in coping with challenges that might otherwise compromise quality of life. When an individual secures a prescription for an ESA from a mental health professional, the ESA is allowed to travel with fewer restrictions and to stay in pet-free housing.

empathic /empath″ik/ [Gk, *en,* into, *pathos,* feeling], pertaining to or involving the entering of one person into the emotional state of another while remaining objective and distinctly separate.

empathy /em″pəthē/ [Gk, *en,* in, *pathos,* feeling], the ability to recognize and to some extent share the emotions and states of mind of another and to understand the meaning and significance of that person's behavior. It is an essential quality for effective psychotherapy. Compare **sympathy.** −**empathic,** *adj.,* −*empathize, v.*

emphysema /em″fəsē″mə/ [Gk, *en* + *physema,* a blowing], *adj.,* an abnormal condition of the pulmonary system, characterized by overinflation and destructive changes in alveolar walls. It results in a loss of lung elasticity and decreased gas exchange. When emphysema occurs early in life, it is usually related to a rare genetic deficiency of serum alpha-1-antitrypsin, which inactivates the enzymes leukocyte collagenase and elastase. More common causes are air pollution and cigarette smoking. Acute emphysema may be caused by the rupture of alveoli during severe respiratory efforts, as may occur in acute bronchopneumonia, suffocation, whooping cough, and, occasionally, labor. Patients with chronic emphysema may also have a component of chronic bronchitis. Emphysema also occurs after asthma or tuberculosis, conditions in which the lungs are overstretched until the elastic fibers of the alveolar walls are destroyed. In old age the alveolar membranes atrophy and may collapse, producing large, air-filled spaces and a decreased total surface area of the pulmonary membranes. Kinds include **centriacinar emphysema, distal acinar emphysema, panacinar emphysema.** −**emphysematous,** *adj.*

■ OBSERVATIONS: The patient may have dyspnea on exertion or at rest, cough, orthopnea, unequal chest expansion, tachypnea, tachycardia, diminished breath sounds caused by air trapping, or, atypically, an elevated temperature and breath sounds if there is an infection. Anxiety, increased $PaCO_2$, restlessness, confusion, weakness, anorexia, hypoxemia, and respiratory failure are common in advanced cases. Chronic emphysema is characterized by increased anterior-posterior chest diameter secondary to hyperinflation and air trapping and use of accessory muscles.

■ INTERVENTIONS: The primary treatment consists of breathing exercises, oxygen administration, and avoiding infection. The airway is kept open, and oxygen is administered to maintain an arterial oxygen saturation of 92%. Bronchodilators, antibiotics, expectorants when bronchitis is also present, methylxanthines, and corticosteroids may be prescribed. Sedation is to be avoided because sedatives depress respiratory function.

■ PATIENT CARE CONSIDERATIONS: The patient is taught breathing exercises and encouraged to drink between 2 and 3 L of fluids daily, if not contraindicated by cardiac function. Activity is encouraged to the limit of the patient's tolerance. Fatigue, constipation, and upper respiratory tract infection and irritation are to be avoided. Mechanical ventilation and oxygen therapy may be prescribed for use at home. The patient is taught the adverse role that smoking plays in the disease and is encouraged to stop smoking.

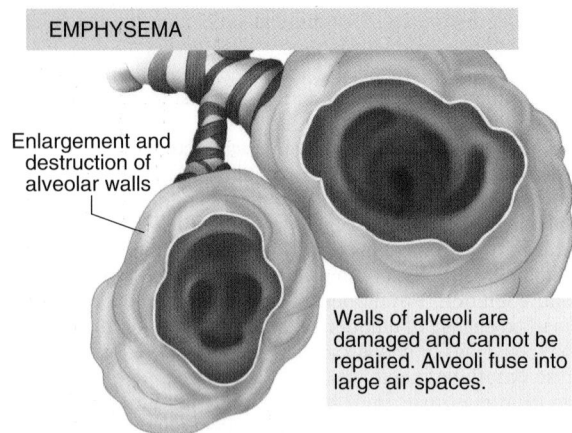

EMPHYSEMA

Enlargement and destruction of alveolar walls

Walls of alveoli are damaged and cannot be repaired. Alveoli fuse into large air spaces.

Panacinar emphysema: ruptured alveoli *(Kumar et al, 2010)*

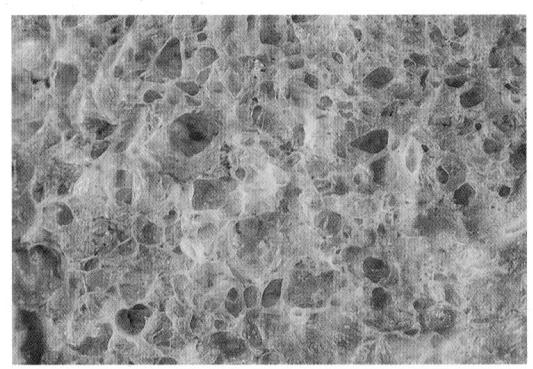

Emphysema *(Patton and Thibodeau, 2016)*

emphysematous /em″fisem″ətəs/ [Gk, *en,* in, *physema,* a blowing], pertaining to or affected with emphysema.

emphysematous abscess, an abscess in which air or gas is present.

emphysematous chest. See **barrel chest.**

emphysematous gastritis, infectious gastritis in which the infectious agents are gas-producing bacteria. Radiologically it resembles gastric emphysema but is much more serious, even life threatening.

emphysematous pyelitis, pyelitis with air or gas only in the collecting system.

empiric /empir″ik/ [Gk, *empeirikos,* experimental], pertaining to a method of treating disease based on observations and experience without an understanding of the cause or mechanism of the disorder or the way the therapeutic agent or procedure affects improvement or cure. The empiric treatment of a new disease may be based on observations and experience gained in the management of analogous disorders. −*empirical, adj.*

empirical, a fact or set of facts verified by observation or data.

empirical formula, a chemical formula that shows the smallest whole number ratio of atoms of different elements in a molecule. It does not indicate structural linkage. An example is CH_2O, a carbohydrate.

empiricism /empir″isiz′əm/, a form of therapy based on the therapist's personal experience and that of other practitioners. −*empiricist, n.*

empiric treatment. See **treatment.**

Employment Retirement Income Security Act (ERISA), a federal law, enacted in 1974, regulating employee welfare benefit plans, including group health plans.

empowerment, the act of promoting self-actualization and understanding one's influence over a situation.

emprosthotonos /em′prosthot″ənəs/ [Gk, *emprosthen,* forward, *tenein,* to cut], a position of the body characterized by forward, rigid flexure at the waist. The position is the result of a prolonged involuntary muscle spasm that is most commonly associated with tetanus infection or strychnine poisoning.

empty follicle syndrome, a condition in which oocytes are absent from stimulated follicles.

empty sella syndrome [AS, *oemettig,* unoccupied; L, *sella,* saddle], an abnormal enlargement of the sella turcica filled with cerebrospinal fluid. The pituitary gland may be smaller than normal and flattened, or it may be absent. Signs and symptoms of hormonal imbalance (for example, hypopituitarism) may be present, as may headache, but some patients are asymptomatic. The diagnosis may be made by computed axial tomography scan, skull radiographic study, or pneumoencephalography.

empyema /em′pī·ē″mə, em′pē·ē″mə/ [Gk, *en* + *ipyon,* pus], an accumulation of pus in the pleural space, as a result of bacterial infection, such as pleurisy or tuberculosis. It is usually removed by surgical incision, aspiration, and drainage. Antibiotics, usually penicillin or vancomycin, are administered to combat the underlying infection. Oxygen therapy may also be administered.

EMS, 1. abbreviation for **electric muscle stimulator. 2.** abbreviation for **emergency medical services. 3.** abbreviation for **eosinophilia-myalgia syndrome, tryptophan-induced.**

EMS standing orders, routine medical procedures approved in advance for emergency medical services (EMS) crews to perform before consulting a physician.

EMT, abbreviation for **emergency medical technician.**

EMT-ALS, abbreviation for **emergency medical technician–advanced life support.**

EMT-P, abbreviation for *emergency medical technician–paramedic.*

emtricitabine, an antiretroviral drug.
■ INDICATIONS: This drug is used with other antiretroviral drugs to treat HIV infection.
■ CONTRAINDICATIONS: Known hypersensitivity to this drug prohibits its use.
■ ADVERSE EFFECTS: Adverse effects of this drug include headache, abnormal dreams, depression, dizziness, insomnia, neuropathy, paresthesia, arthralgia, myalgia, cough, change in body fat distribution, rash, and skin discoloration. Common side effects include nausea, vomiting, diarrhea, anorexia, abdominal pain, and dyspepsia.

Emtriva, an antiviral drug. Brand name for **emtricitabine.**

emulsification /imul′sifikā″shən/, the breakdown of large fat globules into smaller, uniformly distributed particles. It is accomplished mainly by bile acids in the small intestine. Emulsification is the first preparation of fat for chemical digestion by specific enzymes. See also **emulsify.**

emulsifier /imul″sifī′ər/ [L, *emulgere,* to milk out, *facere,* to make], a substance such as egg yolk or gum arabic that can cause oil to be suspended in water.

emulsify [L, *emulgere,* to milk out, *facere,* to make], to disperse a liquid into another liquid with which it is immiscible, making a colloidal suspension. Soaps and detergents emulsify by surrounding small globules of fat, preventing them from settling out. Bile acts as an emulsifying agent in the digestive tract by dispersing ingested fats into small globules. **–emulsification,** *n.*

emulsion /imul″shən/ [L, *emulgere,* to milk out], **1.** a system consisting of two immiscible liquids, one of which is dispersed in the other in the form of small droplets or micelles. **2.** a composition sensitive to actinic rays of light, consisting of one or more silver halides suspended in gelatin applied in a thin layer to film.

en-, prefix meaning "in, on": *enanthema, enostosis.*

ENA, abbreviation for **Emergency Nurses' Association.**

E

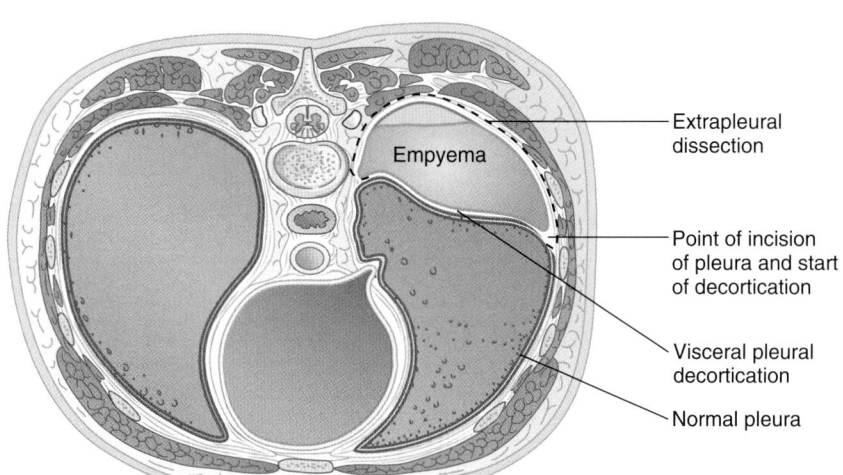

Cross section of thorax with empyema *(AACN, 2008)*

- Extrapleural dissection
- Empyema
- Point of incision of pleura and start of decortication
- Visceral pleural decortication
- Normal pleura

Common distinguishing features of emphysema and chronic bronchitis*

Patient data	Emphysema (Type A: pink puffer)	Bronchitis (Type B: blue bloater)
History		
Lifestyle	Smoker	Smoker
Weight	Weight loss	Overweight
Onset of symptoms	Usually after age 50	Usually after age 40
Sputum	Mild, mucoid	Excessive, purulent
Cough	Minimal or absent	Chronic; more severe in mornings
Dyspnea	Progressive exertional dyspnea	Mild to moderate, but may gradually progress to severe exertional dyspnea
Patient complaints	Dyspnea on exertion, fatigue, insomnia	Chronic cough with mucopurulent sputum, chills, malaise, muscle aches, fatigue, insomnia, loss of libido
Physical signs		
Edema	Absent	Present
Central cyanosis	Absent	Present in advanced disease
Use of accessory muscles to breathe	Present	Absent until end stage
Body build	Thin, wasted	Stocky, overweight
Anteroposterior chest diameter	'Barrel chest,' 1:1 ratio anteroposterior chest diameter	Normal
Auscultation of chest	Decreased breath sounds, decreased heart sounds, prolonged expiration	Wheezes, crackles, rhonchi, depending on the severity of disease
Percussion	Hyperresonance	Normal
Jugular vein distention	Absent	Present
Other	Pursed-lip breathing	Evidence of right-sided heart failure (cor pulmonale)
General diagnostic tests		
Chest radiography	Narrowed mediastinum; normal or small vertical heart; hyperinflation; low, flat diaphragm; presence of blebs or bullae	Congested lung fields, increased bronchial vascular markings, enlarged horizontal heart
Arterial blood gas analysis	Decreased PaO_2 (60–80 mm Hg); normal or increased $PaCO_2$ (increases with advancing disease)	Decreased PaO_2 (65 mm Hg); increased $PaCO_2$
Electrocardiography	Normal or tall symmetrical P waves; tachycardia, if hypoxic	Right axis deviation, right ventricular hypertrophy, atrial arrhythmias
Hematocrit	Normal	Polycythemia
Pulmonary function tests		
Functional residual capacity	Increased	Normal or slight increase
Residual volume	Increased	Increased
Total lung capacity	Increased	Normal
Forced expiratory volume	Decreased	Decreased
Vital capacity	Decreased	Normal or slight decrease
Static lung compliance	Increased	Normal

From Copstead-Kirkhorn LE, Banasik JL: *Pathophysiology,* ed 5, Philadelphia, 2014, Saunders.
*Clinically, features of bronchitis and emphysema are not always clear-cut because many patients have a combined disease process.

enabler /enā″blər/, a significant other of a substance abuser who provides either implicit or explicit support of substance-abusing or dysfunctional behavior.

enalapril maleate /enal″əpril/, an angiotensin-converting enzyme (ACE) inhibitor used as an oral antihypertensive drug.
■ INDICATIONS: It is prescribed in the treatment of hypertension or heart failure or as a preventive for myocardial infarction, stroke, or cardiovascular death.
■ CONTRAINDICATIONS: It should be used with caution in patients suffering severe salt or fluid depletion or in combination with a potassium-sparing diuretic. ACE inhibitors should not be used during pregnancy, especially during the second and third trimesters.
■ ADVERSE EFFECTS: Among the more serious adverse effects are hyperkalemia, cough, hypotension, dizziness, and headache.

enamel /inam″əl/ [OFr, *esmail*], the hard, white crystalline substance of the minerals hydroxyapatite and/or fluorapatite that forms the outermost covering of the clinical and anatomical crown of a tooth. It contains no nerves or blood vessels and is the hardest bony substance in the body. It is produced by epithelial cells called ameloblasts.

enamel cell. See **ameloblast.**

enamel hypocalcification, a defect in which the enamel of the teeth is soft and undercalcified and opaque in appearance but normal in quantity. It is caused by defective maturation of ameloblasts. The teeth are chalky in consistency, their surfaces wear down rapidly and are more susceptible to caries, and a yellowish brown stain appears on the teeth as the underlying dentin is exposed. The condition affects both primary and secondary teeth. Compare **enamel hypoplasia.** See also **amelogenesis imperfecta.**

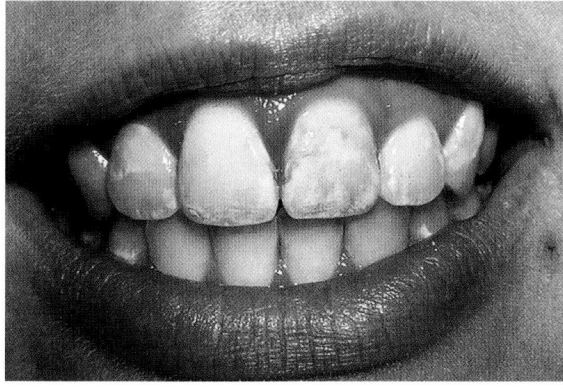

Enamel hypocalcification *(Heymann and Swift, 2006)*

enamel hypoplasia, the incomplete or defective formation of enamel, resulting in the alteration of tooth form or color. Compare **enamel hypocalcification.** See also **amelogenesis imperfecta.**

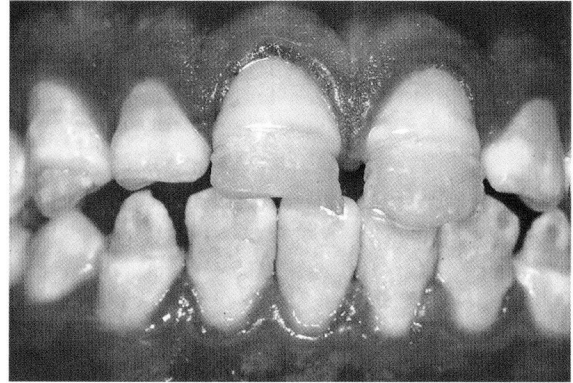

Severe enamel hypoplasia *(Sapp, 2004)*

enamel niche, either of two depressions on a tooth, located between the lateral dental lamina and the developing dental germ.

enamel organ, a complex epithelial structure on the dental papilla. It produces enamel for the developing tooth.

enanthema /en'anthē″mə/ [Gk, *en* + *anthema*, blossoming], a sudden eruptive lesion of the surface of a mucous membrane. Also called *enanthem.*

enantiomer, (in physical science) one of the two nonsuperimposable mirror-image forms of a chiral compound.

enarthrosis. See **ball-and-socket joint.**

en bloc /enblok″, äNblôk″/ [Fr, in a block], all together, or as a whole.

encapsulated /enkaps″yəlā'tid/ [Gk, *en* + L, *capsula,* little box], (of arteries, muscles, nerves, and other body parts) enclosed in fibrous or membranous sheaths. It refers to organisms that form a protective capsule. See also **Tenon's capsule, synovial sheath.**

-ence. See **-ency, -ance, -ancy, -ence.**

encephal-, prefix meaning "the brain": *encephalalgia, encephalitis.*

encephalalgia /ənsef'əlal″jə/, *(Obsolete)* now called **headache.**

-encephalia, -encephaly, suffix meaning "(condition of the) brain": *anencephaly, holoprosencephaly, micrencephalia.*

encephalitis /ensef'əlī″tis/ *pl. encephalitides* [Gk, *enkephalos,* brain, *itis,* inflammation], an inflammatory condition of the brain. The cause is usually an arbovirus infection transmitted by the bite of an infected mosquito, but it may be the result of lead or other poisoning or of hemorrhage. Certain protozoal infections such as toxoplasmosis can cause encephalitis in immunocompromised patients. Postinfectious encephalitis occurs as a complication of another infection, such as chickenpox, influenza, or measles, or after smallpox vaccination. Compare **meningitis.** See also **equine encephalitis.**

■ OBSERVATIONS: The condition is characterized by headache, neck pain, fever, nausea, and vomiting. Neurological disturbances, including seizures, personality change, irritability, lethargy, paralysis, weakness, and coma, may occur.

■ INTERVENTIONS: Medical management will depend on the cause. Nursing care during the acute period will focus on lowering fever, providing hydration, and monitoring the patient for increased intracranial pressure and seizures. Complications associated with encephalitis can be significant. The health care team must be vigilant and coordinated to minimize these complications.

■ PATIENT CARE CONSIDERATIONS: The outcome depends on the cause, the age and condition of the person, and the extent of inflammation. Severe inflammation with destruction of nerve tissue may result in a seizure disorder, loss of a special sense or other permanent neurological problem, or death. Usually the inflammation involves the spinal cord and brain; hence, in most cases a more accurate term is encephalomyelitis.

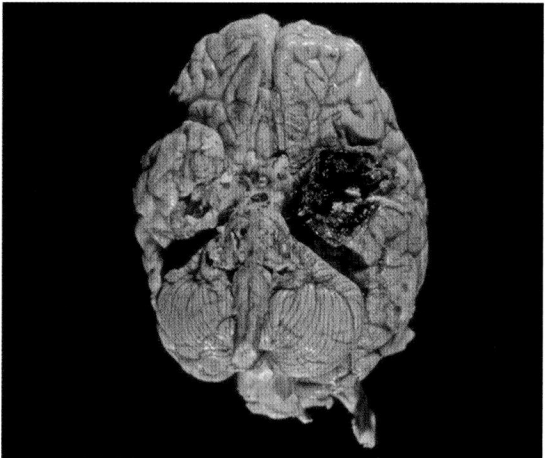

Viral encephalitis infection at base of brain *(Fugate et al, 2014)*

encephalitis lethargica. See **epidemic encephalitis.**

encephalitis neonatorum. See **neonatorum encephalitis.**

encephalitis periaxialis diffusa. See **Schilder disease.**

encephalocele /ensef'ələsēl'/ [Gk, *enkephalos* + *koilia,* cavity], **1.** protrusion of the brain through a congenital defect in the skull. **2.** hernia of the brain. See also **neural tube defect.**

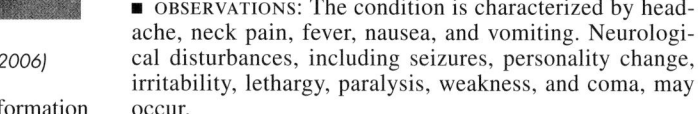

E

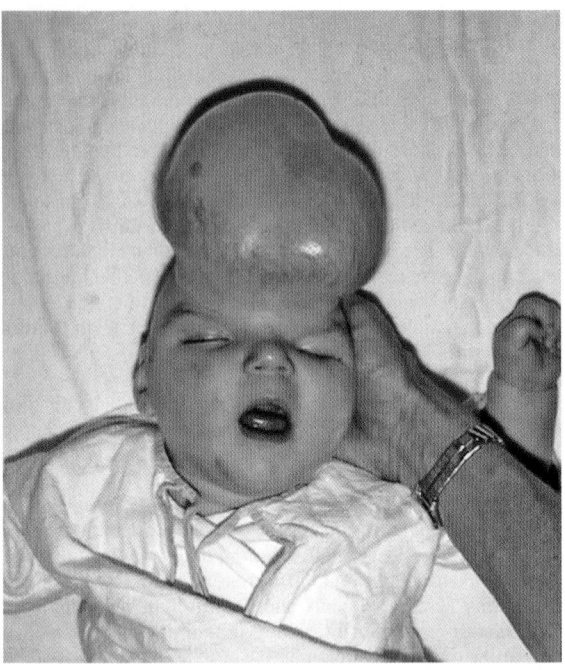

Infant with encephalocele *(Cohen and Lemire, 1982)*

encephalodysplasia, any congenital anomaly of the brain.

encephalogram /ensef″ələgram′/ [Gk, *enkephalos* + *gramma,* record], a radiograph of the brain made during encephalography.

encephalography /ensef′əlog″rəfē/, *(Obsolete)* a procedure no longer performed that resulted in radiographic delineation of the structures of the brain containing fluid after the cerebrospinal fluid was withdrawn and replaced by a gas, such as air, helium, or oxygen. The procedure was used mainly for indicating the site of cerebrospinal fluid obstruction in hydrocephalus or structural abnormalities of the posterior fossa. Compare **echoencephalography, electroencephalography.** −*encephalographic, adj.*

encephaloid carcinoma. See **medullary carcinoma.**

encephalomeningitis /-men′inji″tis/ [Gk, *enkephalos,* brain, *meninx,* membrane, *itis,* inflammation], an inflammation of the brain and meninges.

encephalomeningocele. See **meningoencephalocele.**

encephalomyelitis /ensef′əlōmī′əli″tis/ [Gk, *enkephalos* + *myelos,* marrow, *itis*], an inflammatory condition of the brain and spinal cord that damages myelin, characterized by fever, headache, stiff neck, back pain, and vomiting. Depending on the cause, the age and condition of the person, and the extent of the inflammation and irritation to the central nervous system, seizures, paralysis, personality changes, a decreased level of consciousness, coma, or death may occur. Sequelae, such as seizure disorders or decreased mental ability, may occur after severe inflammation that causes extensive damage to the cells and tissues of the nervous system. See also **acute disseminated encephalomyelitis, encephalitis, equine encephalitis.**

encephalomyocarditis /ensef′əlōmī′ōkärdī″tis/ [Gk, *enkephalos* + *mys,* muscle, *kardia,* heart, *itis,* inflammation], an infectious disease of the central nervous system and heart tissue caused by a group of small ribonucleic acid picornaviruses. Rodents are a major reservoir of the infection. Human illness ranges from asymptomatic infection to severe encephalomyeli-

tis. Symptoms are generally similar to those of poliomyelitis. Myocarditis is not a feature of infection in humans, and most victims recover promptly without sequelae. Treatment is supportive. See also **picornavirus.**

encephalon [Gk, *enkephalos,* brain], **1.** the cerebrum and its related structures of cerebellum, pons, and medulla oblongata. **2.** the contents of the cranium.

encephalopathy /ensef′əlop″əthē/ [Gk, *enkephalos* + *pathos,* disease], any abnormal condition of the structure or function of brain tissues, especially chronic, destructive, or degenerative conditions. Kinds include **Wernicke's encephalopathy, Schilder's disease.**

encephalotrigeminal angiomatosis. See **Sturge-Weber syndrome.**

-encephaly. See **-encephalia, -encephaly.**

enchondroma /en′kəndrō″mə/ *pl. enchondromas, enchondromata* [Gk, *en* + *chondros,* cartilage, *oma,* tumor], a benign, slowly growing tumor of cartilage cells that arises in the extremity of the shaft of tubular bones in the hands or feet. The growth of the neoplasm may distend the bone. Also called **enchondrosis, true chondroma.**

enchondromatosis /en′kəndrō′mətō″sis/ [Gk, *en* + *chondros,* cartilage, *oma,* tumor, *osis,* condition], a congenital disorder characterized by the proliferation of cartilage within the extremity of the shafts of bones, causing thinning of the cortex and distortion in length. Also called **dyschondroplasia, Ollier disease.** Compare **Maffucci syndrome.**

enchondromatous myxoma /en′kondrō″mətəs/, a tumor of the connective tissue, characterized by the presence of cartilage between the cells of connective tissue. See also **myxoma.**

enchondrosarcoma. See **central chondrosarcoma.**

enchondrosis. See **enchondroma.**

enchylema. See **hyaloplasm.**

-enchyma, suffix meaning the "liquid that nourishes tissue, or tissue itself": *karyenchyma, mesenchyma, parenchyma.*

enclave /en″klāv, enklāv″/, a detached mass of tissue enclosed in an organ or in a different kind of tissue.

encode /enkōd″/ [Gk, *en* + L, *caudex,* book], **1.** to translate a message, signal, or stimulus into a code. **2.** to rewrite information into a form that can be interpreted by a computer manually or automatically, as by a computer program.

encoded message, (in communication theory) the product of using a word, phrase, gesture, or symbol to communicate to another person. The receiver will decode it. For example, if the sender simply uses plain language, the receiver of the same language will easily decode it and interpret the message.

encopresis /en′kōprē″sis/, fecal holding with constipation and fecal soiling. −*encopretic, adj.*

encounter [Gk, *en* + L, *contra,* against], (in psychotherapy) the interaction between a patient and a psychotherapist, such as occurs in existential therapy, or among several members of a small group, such as encounter or sensitivity training groups. In an encounter emotional change and personal growth are affected by participants' expression of strong feelings. See also **existential therapy.**

encounter data, information showing use of provider services by health plan enrollees that is used to develop cost profiles of a particular group of enrollees and then to guide decisions about or provide justification for the maintenance or adjustment of premiums.

encounter group, (in psychology) a small group of people who meet to increase self-awareness, promote personal growth, and improve interpersonal communication. Members focus on becoming aware of their feelings and on developing the ability to express those feelings openly, honestly, and clearly. See also **group therapy, psychotherapy, sensitivity training group.**

en coup de sabre [Fr, cut from a sword], a type of linear scleroderma characterized by a thickened white line of collagen on the face or scalp. See also **localized scleroderma.**

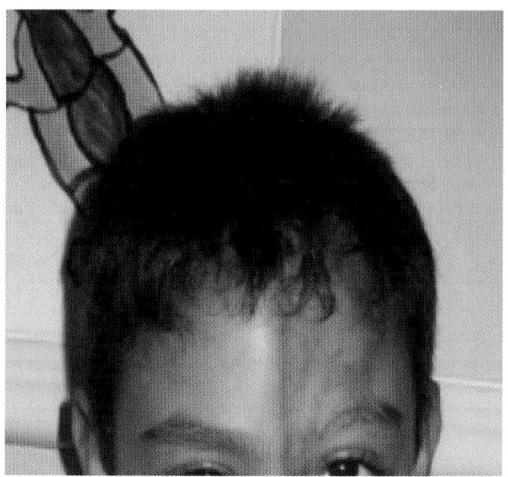

Child with en coup de sabre *(Gómez et al, 2012)*

encourager role, a group member whose task is to agree with, praise, and support the suggestions, opinions, beliefs, and overall contributions of other group members.

enculturation /enkul′chərā″shən/ [Gk, *en* + L, *cultura,* cultivation], the process of learning the concepts, values, and behavioral standards of a particular culture.

-ency, -ance, -ancy, -ence, **1.** suffixes meaning a "quality or state": *deficiency, urgency.* **2.** suffixes meaning a "person or thing in a state": *latency.* **3.** suffixes meaning an "instance of a quality or state": *emergency.*

encyst /ensist′/, to form a cyst or capsule. See also **cyst.** −*encysted,* adj.

encysted pleurisy, a form of pleurisy with adhesions that surround the effused material. Also called **blocked pleurisy, circumscribed pleurisy.**

end, abbreviation for **endoreduplication.**

end-. See **endo-, end-, ent-, ento-.**

Endameba, any ameba of the genus *Endamoeba.*

endamebiasis. See **amebiasis.**

Endamoeba, a genus of amebic parasites in invertebrates, originally described from cockroaches.

endamoebiasis. See **amebiasis.**

endarterectomy /en′därtərek″təmē/ [Gk, *endon,* within, *arteria,* airpipe, *ektomē,* excision], the surgical removal of the intimal lining of an artery. The procedure is done to clear a major artery that may be blocked by plaque accumulation. Kinds include **disobliterative endarterectomy, gas endarterectomy.**

endarteritis /en′därtərī″tis/ [Gk, *endon* + *arteria* + *itis,* inflammation], inflammation of the inner layer of one or more arteries, which may become partially or completely occluded. Also called **acute endarteritis.**

endarteritis deformans. See **chronic endoarteritis.**

endarteritis obliterans, an inflammatory condition of the lining of the arterial walls in which the intima proliferates, narrowing the lumen of the vessels and occluding the smaller vessels. Also called **arteritis obliterans.**

end artery, a blood vessel that does not join with any other vessel. Also called **terminal artery.**

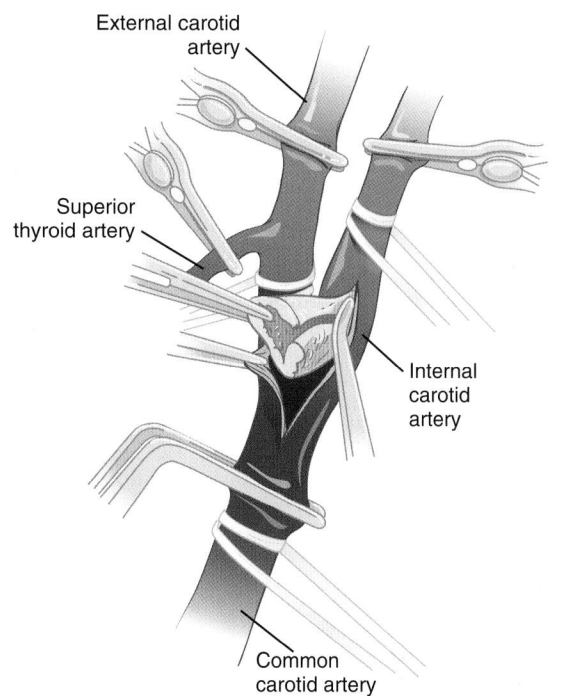

Endarterectomy *(AACN, 2008)*

end bud [AS, *ende* + Gk, *bolbos,* onion], a mass of undifferentiated cells produced from the remnants of the primitive node and the primitive streak at the caudal end of the developing embryo after formation of the somites is completed. In lower animals it gives rise to the tail or any other caudal appendage and part of the trunk. In humans it forms the caudal portion of the trunk. Also called **tail bud.**

end bulbs of Krause. See **Krause's corpuscles.**

end-diastolic pressure /-dī·əstol″ik/ [AS, *ende* + Gk, *dia* + *stellein,* to set; L, *premere,* to press], the pressure of the blood in the ventricles at the end of diastole.

endemic /endem″ik/ [Gk, *endemos,* native], (of a disease or microorganism) the expected or "normal" incidence indigenous to a geographic area or population. See also **epidemic, pandemic.**

endemic disease, a physical or mental disorder caused by health conditions usually present within a community. It usually describes an infection that is transmitted directly or indirectly between humans and is occurring at the usual expected rate.

endemic goiter, an enlargement of the thyroid gland caused by the intake of inadequate amounts of dietary iodine. Iodine deprivation leads to diminished production and secretion of thyroid hormone by the gland. The pituitary gland, operating on a negative feedback system, senses the deficiency and secretes increased amounts of thyroid-stimulating hormone, causing hyperplasia and hypertrophy of the thyroid gland.

■ OBSERVATIONS: The goiter may grow during the winter months and shrink during the summer months when the person eats more iodine-containing fresh vegetables. Initially the goiter is diffuse; later it becomes multinodular.

■ INTERVENTIONS: The use of iodized salt is a prophylactic treatment. Desiccated thyroid given orally may prevent further growth of adult goiters and may reduce the size of diffuse goiters.

■ PATIENT CARE CONSIDERATIONS: Endemic goiter occurs occasionally in adolescents at puberty and widely in population groups in geographic areas in which limited amounts of iodine are present in soil, water, and food. A large goiter may cause dysphagia, dyspnea, tracheal deviation, and cosmetic problems.

endemic syphilis, a chronic infectious skin disease that is closely related to *Treponema pallidum* and is frequently contracted in childhood without venereal contact. It is known as bejel in heavily populated communities of developing countries. Also called **nonvenereal syphilis.** See also **bejel.**

endemic typhus. See **murine typhus.**

end-feel, the sensation imparted to the examiner's hands at the end point of the available range of motion. It varies according to the limiting structure or tissue. Types of end-feel include capsular, bone-on-bone, spasm, and springy block. Empty end-feel is the absence of an end-feel during a range of motion examination when the patient stops further movement of a joint before the examiner senses any organic resistance to the movement.

endo-, end-, ent-, ento-, prefix meaning "inward, within": *endocarditis, endoparasite, endodermal.*

endobronchitis /en'dōbrongkī″tis/, inflammation of the smaller bronchi, often caused by a bronchial mucosal infection.

endocardia. See **endocardium.**

endocardial. See **endocardium.**

endocardial candidiasis. See *Candida* **endocarditis.**

endocardial cushion defect /en'dōkär″dē·əl/, any cardiac defect resulting from the failure of the endocardial cushions in the embryonic heart to fuse and form the atrial septum. It is common in Down syndrome. See also **atrial septal defect, congenital cardiac anomaly.**

endocardial cushions, a pair of thickened tissue sections in the embryonic atrial canal. During embryonic development they meet and fuse to form a septum dividing the canal into two channels, which eventually become the atrioventricular orifices.

endocardial fibroelastosis /fī'brō·ē′lastō″sis/ [Gk, *endon* + *kardia,* heart; L, *fibra,* fiber; Gk, *elaunein,* to drive, *osis,* condition], an abnormal condition characterized by the development of a thick, fibroelastic endocardium that can cause failure of the heart to pump blood.

endocardial murmur, a continuous, soft sound made by an abnormality within the heart.

endocardial pacing. See **pacing.**

endocardial tubes, paired, longitudinal, endothelial-lined channels formed from the cardiogenic mesoderm in embryonic development that fuse to form the primordial heart tube.

endocarditis /en'dōkärdī″tis/ [Gk, *endon* + *kardia,* heart, *itis,* inflammation], an inflammation of the endocardium and heart valves. The condition is characterized by lesions caused by a variety of diseases. Kinds of endocarditis are bacterial endocarditis, nonbacterial thrombotic endocarditis, and Libman-Sacks endocarditis. All types of endocarditis are rapidly lethal if untreated, but most patients with endocarditis are successfully treated by various antibacterial and surgical measures. See also **bacterial endocarditis, subacute bacterial endocarditis.**

endocardium /en'dōkär″dē·əm/ *pl.* **endocardia,** the innermost lining of the heart chambers containing small blood vessels and a few bundles of smooth muscle. It is continuous with the endothelium of the great blood vessels. Compare **epicardium, myocardium.**

endocervical /-sur″fikəl/ [Gk, *endon* + L, *cervix,* neck], pertaining to that portion of the cervical canal dominated by endometrial columnar cells rather than flat squamous cells. Its special importance is the junction of the two, the squamocolumnar junction, which is the most common site of cervical dysplasia. Also called **intracervical.** See also **squamocolumnar junction.**

endocervicitis /en'dōsur′visī″tis/, an abnormal condition characterized by inflammation of the epithelium and glands of the canal of the uterine cervix. See also **cervicitis.**

endocervix /en'dōsur″viks/, **1.** the membrane lining the canal of the uterine cervix. **2.** the opening of the cervix into the uterine cavity.

endochondral /-kon″drəl/ [Gk, *endon,* within, *chondros,* cartilage], pertaining to something within the cartilage.

endochondral bone. See **cartilaginous bone.**

endocrinasthenia /-krin'asthē″nē·ə/, a neural deficit caused by an alteration of the endocrine system.

endocrine /en'dəkren, -krīn/ [Gk, *endon* + *krinein,* to secrete], pertaining to a process in which a group of cells secretes into the blood or lymph circulation a substance (for example, hormone) that has a specific effect on tissues in another part of the body.

endocrine diabetes mellitus [Gk, *endon,* within, *krinein,* to secrete, *diabainein,* to pass through, *mellitus,* honeyed], a form of diabetes associated with diseases of other glands, such as the adrenals, pituitary, or thyroid, classified under other specific types in the American Diabetes Association Classification. Compare **diabetes mellitus.**

endocrine fracture /-krēn/, *(Informal)* any fracture that results from weakness of a specific bone caused by an endocrine disorder such as hyperparathyroidism, in which calcium loss from bone is accelerated.

endocrine gland, a ductless gland that produces and secretes hormones into the blood or lymph nodes, affecting metabolism and other body processes. The endocrine glands include the pituitary, pineal, hypothalamus, thymus, thyroid, parathyroid, adrenal cortex, medulla, pancreatic islands of Langerhans, and gonads. Cells in other structures, such as the GI mucosa, the kidneys, the heart, and the placenta, also have endocrine functions. Compare **exocrine gland.**

endocrine system [Gk, *endon* + *krinein,* to secrete; *systema*], the network of ductless glands and other structures that elaborate and secrete hormones directly into the bloodstream, affecting various processes throughout the body, such as metabolism, growth, and secretions from other organs. Glands of the endocrine system include the thyroid, the parathyroid, the anterior pituitary, the posterior pituitary, the pancreas, the suprarenal glands, and the gonads. The pineal gland is also considered an endocrine gland because it is ductless, although its precise endocrine function is not established beyond its involvement in daily, monthly, and annual rhythms. Various other organs have some endocrinological function. See also the *Color Atlas of Human Anatomy,* pp. A-18 to A-19. Compare **exocrine.**

endocrino- [Gk, *endon,* within, *krinein,* to secrete], prefix meaning "endocrine system, endocrine structures or function": *endocrinology, endocrinopathy.*

endocrinologist /en'dōkrinol″əjist/, a physician who specializes in the endocrine system and its disorders.

endocrinology /-krinol″əjē/ [Gk, *endon* + *krinein,* to secrete, *logos,* science], the study of the anatomical, physiological, and pathological characteristics of the endocrine system and of the treatment of endocrine problems.

endocrinopathy /-krinop″əthē/ [Gk, *endon,* within, *krinein,* to secrete, *pathos,* disease], a disease involving an endocrine gland or a dysfunction that decreases the quality or quantity of the gland's secretion or response to a hormone.

endocytosis /en'dōsītō″sis/ [Gk, *endon,* within, + *kytos,* cell], uptake by a cell of material from the environment by invagination of its plasma membrane, which may be either phagocytosis or pinocytosis. Compare **exocytosis.**

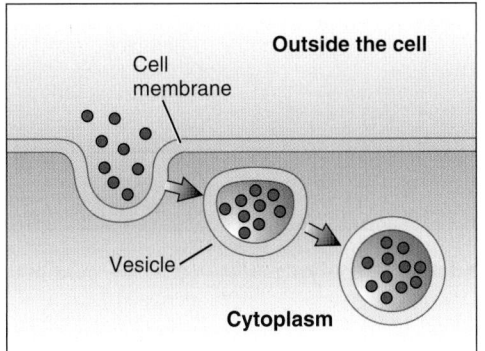

Endocytosis *(Herlihy, 2014)*

endoderm /en″dədurm/ [Gk, *endon* + *derma,* skin], (in embryology) the innermost of the cell layers that develop from the embryonic disk of the inner cell mass of the blastocyst. From the endoderm arises the epithelium of the trachea, bronchi, lungs, GI tract, liver, pancreas, urinary bladder, anal canal, pharynx, thyroid, tympanic cavity, tonsils, and parathyroid glands. The endoderm thus comprises the lining of the cavities and passages of the body and the covering of most of the internal organs. Compare **ectoderm, hypoblast, mesoderm.**

endodermal /-dur″məl/ [Gk, *endon,* within, *derma,* skin], pertaining to the inner of the three layers of the embryo and the epithelial lining of the respiratory system, the digestive tract, and other tissues.

endodermal cloaca, a part of the cloaca in the developing embryo that lies internal to the cloacal membrane and gives rise to the bladder and urogenital ducts. Compare **ectodermal cloaca.** See also **urogenital sinus.**

endodermal sinus tumor, yolk sac tumor.

endodontics [Gk, *endon,* within, *odous,* tooth], the branch of dentistry that specializes in the diagnosis and treatment of diseases of the dental pulp, tooth root, and surrounding tissues and in the associated practice of root canal therapy. Also called *endodontia,* **endodontology, pulpodontia.**

endodontist /-don″tist/ [Gk, *endon,* within, *odous,* tooth], a dentist who specializes in endodontics.

endodontology. See **endodontics.**

endogenous /endoj″ənəs/ [Gk, *endon* + *genein,* to produce], **1.** growing within the body. **2.** originating from within the body or produced from internal causes, such as a disease caused by the structural or functional failure of an organ or system. Compare **exogenous.** *–endogenic, adj.*

endogenous carbon dioxide, carbon dioxide produced within the body by metabolic processes.

endogenous hypertriglyceridemia. See **hyperlipidemia type IV.**

endogenous infection, an infection caused by the reactivation of previously dormant organisms, as in coccidioidomycosis, histoplasmosis, and tuberculosis. Compare **mixed infection, retrograde infection, secondary infection.**

endogenous iritis. See **primary iritis.**

endogenous obesity, obesity resulting from dysfunction of the endocrine or metabolic system. Compare **exogenous obesity.** See also **obesity.**

endogenous opioid, an opiate-like substance, such as an endorphin, produced by the body.

endogenous uric acid [Gk, *endon,* within + *genein,* to produce + *ouron,* urine; L, *acidus*], uric acid produced by the metabolism of purines in the body's own nucleoproteins, as distinguished from metabolism of purine products in foods.

endointoxication /en′dō·intok″sikā″shən/, poisoning caused by a toxin produced within the body, such as from dead and infected tissue in gangrene.

endolymph /en″dəlimf/ [Gk, *endon* + *lympha,* water], the pale fluid in the membranous labyrinth (cochlear duct) of the internal ear. Compare **perilymph.**

endolymphatic appendage, an outgrowth of the otic vesicle that forms the endolymphatic duct and sac during embryonic development.

endolymphatic duct /-limfat″ik/, a labyrinthine passage in the inner ear joining an endolymphatic sac with the utricle and saccule.

endolymphatic sac, the blind end of an endolymphatic duct.

endomastoiditis /-mas′toidī″tis/, an inflammation within the mastoid cavity and cells.

endometrial /en′dōmē″trē·əl/ [Gk, *endon* + *metra,* womb], pertaining to endometrium.

endometrial biopsy, a biopsy specimen of the endometrium, performed with a very thin suction cannula introduced through the cervical os. Common indications for the procedure include infertility, multiple spontaneous abortions, abnormal or irregular vaginal bleeding, menopausal vaginal bleeding, and ovulation induction and infertility therapy.

endometrial cancer, a carcinoma of the endometrium of the uterus. It is the most prevalent gynecological malignancy, most often occurring in the fifth or sixth decade of life. Although the cause of endometrial cancer is not clear, some of the risk factors associated with an increased incidence of the disease are a medical history of infertility, anovulation, late menopause (52 years), administration of unopposed exogenous estrogen, uterine polyps, and a combination of diabetes, hypertension, and obesity. Adenocarcinomas constitute roughly 90% of all endometrial tumors; the remaining 10% comprise mixed carcinomas, sarcomas, and benign adenoacanthomas.

■ OBSERVATIONS: Abnormal vaginal bleeding, especially in a postmenopausal woman, is the cardinal symptom. Lower abdominal and low back pain may also be present; a large, boggy uterus is often a sign of advanced disease. Fewer than half the patients with endometrial cancer have a positive finding on Papanicolaou's (Pap) test of the cervix and vagina because the tumor cells rarely exfoliate in early stages of the lesion. A Pap test of cells removed from the endometrium obtained from jet washings of the uterine cavity provides more accurate data. Vacuum curettage is also used to extract endometrial cells for study, but the diagnostic technique most frequently recommended is dilation and curettage, in which each section of the uterus is examined and curetted for biopsy specimens.

■ INTERVENTIONS: Endometrial lesions may spread to the cervix but rarely invade the vagina. They metastasize to the broad ligaments, fallopian tubes, and ovaries so frequently that bilateral salpingo-oophorectomy with abdominal hysterectomy is the usual treatment. Radiotherapy is usually administered before and after surgery. High doses of a progestogen may be prescribed for palliation in advanced or inoperable cases. Chemotherapy may also be used.

■ PATIENT CARE CONSIDERATIONS: Survival rates are high if the disease is identified at an early stage.

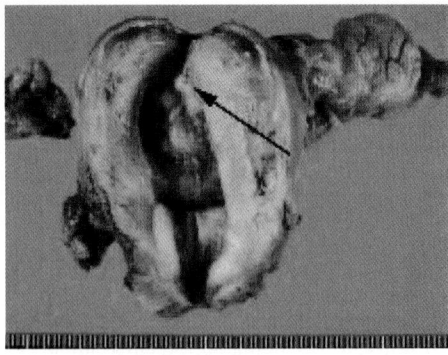

Endometrial cancer *(Koo et al, 2014)*

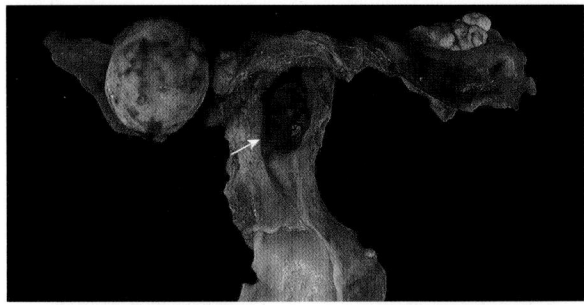

Endometrial polyp *(Finkbeiner, Ursell, and Davis, 2009)*

endometrial cyst [Gk, *endon*, within, *metra*, womb, *kystis*, bag], an ovarian cyst that develops as a distension of an endometrial gland.

endometrial hyperplasia, an abnormal condition characterized by overgrowth of the endometrium resulting from sustained stimulation by estrogen (of endogenous or exogenous origin) that is not opposed by progesterone. Estrogen acts as a growth hormone for the endometrium. Through a complex intercellular mechanism, endometrial cells bind estrogen preferentially and undergo changes characteristic of the proliferative phase of the menstrual cycle. If estrogen stimulation continues for 3 to 6 months without periodic cessation or counteractive progesterone stimulation, as occurs in anovulatory or perimenopausal women and in those receiving replacement estrogen without added progestogen, the endometrium becomes abnormally thickened and glandularized. The causative relationship between estrogen and endometrial hyperplasia is well established; there is some indication but no proof that estrogen also provokes the change from hyperplasia to neoplasia and malignancy. Endometrial hyperplasia often results in abnormal uterine bleeding.

■ OBSERVATIONS: Unremitting estrogen stimulation eventually causes cystic or adenomatous endometrial hyperplasia. The latter is a premalignant lesion that undergoes malignant degeneration in approximately 25% of cases.

■ INTERVENTIONS: Progestogen therapy is effective in reversing the abnormal histopathological changes of endometrial hyperplasia. If hyperplasia is adenomatous, hysterectomy is commonly performed.

■ PATIENT CARE CONSIDERATIONS: Bleed, particularly in older women, constitutes an indication for biopsy or curettage of the endometrium to establish histopathological diagnosis and to rule out malignancy. A functioning estrogen-secreting tumor is suspected if the woman is not taking estrogen medication.

endometrial polyp, a pedunculated overgrowth of endometrium, usually benign. Polyps are a common cause of vaginal bleeding in perimenopausal women and are often associated with other uterine abnormalities, such as endometrial hyperplasia or fibroids. They may occur singly or in clusters and are usually 1 cm or less in diameter, but they may become much larger and prolapse through the cervix. Treatment for the condition includes surgical dilation and curettage.

endometriosis /en′dōmē′trē·ō″sis/ [Gk, *endon* + *metra*, womb, *osis,* condition], endometrial tissue located outside the uterine cavity, most commonly in the posterior cul-de-sac and adnexae but rarely found in areas far removed from the pelvis. Multiple etiologies have been suggested, including direct spread, hematogenous spread, and spontaneous formation from multipotential tissue. The condition may cause chronic pelvic pain. Multiple hormonal and surgical therapies are available, depending on the severity of symptoms and whether infertility is involved.

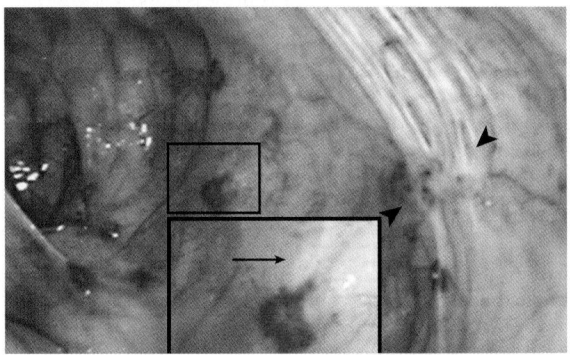

A hemorrhagic area of the right cul-de-sac (small box) is seen on magnification to lie adjacent to a clear macule of endometriosis (large box) and may contain a gland/stroma complex of endometriosis obscured beneath the hemorrhage. The base of the right uterosacral ligament demonstrates thickening of whitish fibrosis and entrapment of old dark blood between the arrowheads. *(Rothrock, 2015)*

endometriosis interna. See **primary endometriosis.**

endometritis /en′dōmitrī″tis/ [Gk, *endon*, within + *metra*, womb, *itis,* inflammation], an inflammatory condition of the endometrium or decidua, with extension into the myometrium and parametrial tissues. It is usually caused by bacterial infection, commonly by gonococci or hemolytic streptococci. The condition is characterized by fever, abdominal pain, tachycardia, malodorous discharge, tenderness, and enlargement of the uterus. It occurs most frequently after childbirth or abortion and is associated with the use of an intrauterine contraceptive device. It can also be the result of caesarean delivery. Compare **pelvic inflammatory disease.** Kinds include **decidual endometritis.**

■ OBSERVATIONS: Diagnosis may be made by physical examination, history, laboratory analysis revealing an elevated white blood cell count, ultrasound, and bacteriological identification of the pathogen.

■ INTERVENTIONS: Treatment includes antibiotics, rest, analgesia, adequate fluid intake, and, if necessary, surgical drainage of a suppurating abscess, hysterectomy, or salpingo-oophorectomy.

■ PATIENT CARE CONSIDERATIONS: Endometritis may be mild and self-limited, chronic or acute, and unilateral or bilateral. It may cause sterility if scar formation occludes the passage of the fallopian tubes. Septic abortion and puerperal fever are forms of endometritis that caused many deaths before asepsis and antibiotics became commonly available.

endometrium /en′dōmē″trē·əm/ [Gk, *endon* + *metra,* womb], the mucous membrane lining of the uterus, consisting of the stratum compactum, the stratum spongiosum, and the stratum basale. The endometrium changes in thickness and structure with the menstrual cycle. The stratum compactum and the stratum spongiosum constitute the pars functionalis and are shed with each menstrual flow. The pars functionalis is known as the decidua during pregnancy, when it underlies the placenta. Compare **myometrium, parametrium.**

endomorph /en″dəmôrf′/ [Gk, *endon* + *morphe,* form], a type of body build characterized by a soft, rounded physique with a large trunk and thighs. Compare **ectomorph, mesomorph.** See also **pyknic.**

endomyocardial fibrosis [Gk, *endon,* within + *mys,* muscle + *kardia,* heart; L, *fibra,* fiber + *osis,* condition], idiopathic myocardiopathy occurring endemically in various parts of Africa and rarely in other areas, characterized by cardiomegaly; marked thickening of the endocardium with dense, white fibrous tissue that frequently extends to involve the inner third or half of the myocardium; and congestive heart failure.

endomyocarditis /-mī′ōkärdī″tis/ [Gk, *endon,* within, *mys,* muscle, *kardia,* heart, *itis,* inflammation], an inflammation of the lining of the heart.

endoneurial nerve sheath. See **nerve sheath.**

endonuclease, an enzyme that cleaves or hydrolyzes phosphodiester bonds within a polynucleotide chain.

endoparasite /en′dōper″əsīt/ [Gk, *endon* + *parasitos,* guest], (in medical parasitology) an organism that lives within the internal organs or tissues of the host, such as a tapeworm.

endopathy /endop″əthē/, any disease originating within the person.

endopeptidase /en′dōpep″ti·dās/ [Gk, *endon,* within + Gk, *peptein,* to digest + *ase,* enzyme suffix], any peptidase that catalyzes the cleavage of internal peptide bonds in a polypeptide or protein. Endopeptidases are divided into subclasses on the basis of catalytic mechanism and comprise the serine endopeptidases, cysteine endopeptidases, aspartic endopeptidases, metalloendopeptidases, and other endopeptidases.

endophthalmitis /endof′thalmī″tis/ [Gk, *endon* + *ophthalmos,* eye, *itis*], an infectious condition of the internal eye in which the primary signs are decreased vision, vitritis, and development of a hypopyon. Patients usually complain of pain. Other symptoms include erythema and edema. It may result from bacterial or fungal infection or from trauma. Depending on the cause, therapy requires surgical intervention or administration of an intraocular antibiotic. Also called *endophthalmia.*

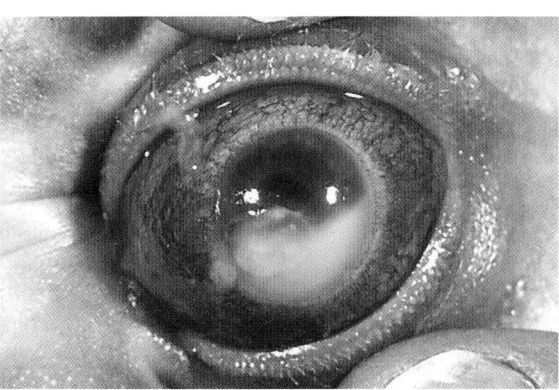

Endophthalmitis with hypopyon *(Hoyt and Taylor, 2013)*

endophthalmitis phacoanaphylactica /fak′ō·an′əfilak″-təkə/. See **phacolytic glaucoma.**

endophytic /en′dōfit″ik/ [Gk, *endon* + *phyton,* plant], pertaining to the tendency to grow inward, such as a tumor that grows into the wall of a hollow organ.

endoplasm /en″dōplaz′əm/ [Gk, *endon,* within, *plasma,* plasm], the inner portion of cytoplasm.

endoplasmic reticulum (ER) /-plaz″mik/ [Gk, *endon* + *plassein,* to mold], an extensive network of membrane-enclosed tubules in the cytoplasm of cells. The structure functions in the synthesis of proteins and lipids and in the transport of these metabolites within the cell. It is the site where some proteins get glycosylated.

endoprosthesis /-prosthē″sis, -pros″thəsis/ [Gk, *endon* + *prosthesis,* addition], a prosthetic device installed within the body, such as an internal cardiac pacemaker.

endopyelotomy /en″dopi′ĕlot″äme/, a minimally invasive surgical procedure to correct a stenosed ureteropelvic junction by cutting from within with an instrument inserted through an endoscope.

endoreduplication (end) /en′dōridoo͞″plikā′shən/ [Gk, *endon* + L, *re,* again, *duplicare,* to duplicate], replication of the chromosomes without subsequent cell division.

end-organ [AS, *ende* + Gk, *organon,* instrument], a nerve ending in which the terminal nerve filaments are encapsulated.

endorphin /endôr″fin/ [Gk, *endon* + *morphe,* shape], one of the three groups of endogenous opioid peptides composed of many amino acids, elaborated by the pituitary gland and other brain areas, and acting on the central and the peripheral nervous systems to reduce pain. There are three known, designated *alpha, beta,* and *gamma.* Beta-endorphin has been isolated in the brain and in the GI tract and seems to be the most potent of the endorphins. Beta-endorphin is composed of 30 amino acids that are identical to part of the sequence of 91 amino acids of the hormone beta-lipotropin, also produced by the pituitary gland. Behavioral tests indicate that beta-endorphin is a powerful analgesic in humans and animals. Brain-stimulated analgesia in humans releases beta-endorphin into the cerebrospinal fluid. Compare **enkephalin.**

endorsement /endôrs″mənt/ [Gk, *en* + L, *dorsum,* the back], a statement of recognition of the license of a health practitioner in one state by another state. An endorsement relieves the health practitioner of the necessity of completing the full licensing procedure of the state in which practice is to be undertaken.

endoscope /en″dəskōp′/ [Gk, *endon* + *skopein*, to look], an illuminated optic instrument for the visualization of the interior of a body cavity or organ. Instruments are available in varying lengths and may have attachments for diagnostic and therapeutic procedures. The fiberoptic endoscope has great flexibility, reaching previously inaccessible areas. Although the endoscope is generally introduced through a natural opening in the body, it may also be inserted through an incision. Instruments are designed for viewing specific areas of the body. Kinds include **bronchoscope, cystoscope, gastroscope, laparoscope, otoscope.** See also **fiberoptics.** −*endoscopic, adj.*

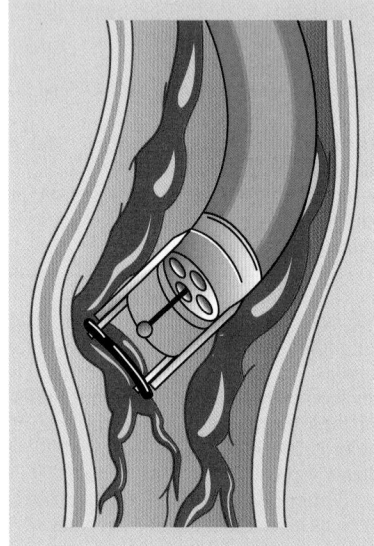

The endoscope with an attached ligating device *(AACN, 2008)*

endoscopic laser cholecystectomy. See **cholecystectomy.**

endoscopic retrograde cholangiopancreatography (ERCP), a diagnostic and therapeutic combination-use of endoscopy and fluoroscopy used to evaluate the biliary and pancreatic ducts. Through the endoscope the physician can see the interior of the stomach and duodenum, attain access to the biliary tree and pancreas, and inject radiographic contrast medium to facilitate visibility via fluoroscopy and on radiographic images. Stones in the biliary tree can be retrieved via the endoscope. See also **cholangiography.**

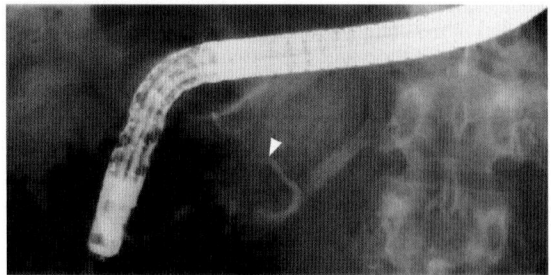

Endoscopic retrograde cholangiopancreatogram
(Courtesy Riverside Methodist Hospitals)

endoscopy /endos″kəpē/, the visualization of the interior of organs and cavities of the body with an endoscope. The GI structures that can be examined through this procedure include the esophagus, stomach, duodenum, colon, and pancreas and the biliary tract with the aid of x-ray film and fluoroscopy. Endoscopy can also be used to obtain samples for cytological and histological examination and to follow the course of a disease, such as the assessment of the healing of gastric and duodenal ulcers. See also **abdominoscopy, bronchoscopy, cystoscopy, gastroscopy, laparoscopy.**

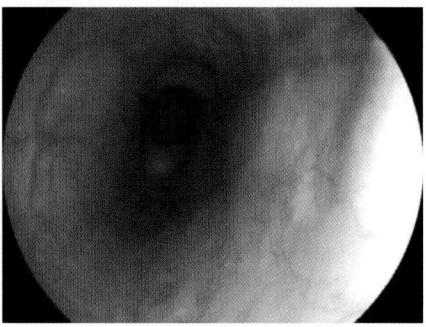

Upper endoscopy images *(Canard et al, 2011)*

endoskeletal prosthesis /-skel″ətəl/ [Gk, *endon* + *skeletos*, dried up, *prosthesis*, addition], a lower-limb support consisting of an internal pylon usually covered with a lightweight material, such as plastic foam. See also **pylon.**

endoskeleton, the internal network of bones, to which muscles are attached. Compare **exoskeleton.**

endosseous implant. See **dental implant.**

endosteal hyperostosis /endos″tē·əl/, an inherited bone disorder characterized by an overgrowth of the mandible and brow areas. The excessive bone growth can lead to entrapment of cranial nerves, causing facial palsy and loss of hearing. Also called **Van Buchem's syndrome.**

endosteal implant [Gk, *endon*, within + *osteon*, bone], a dental implant made of metal, ceramic, or polymeric material, consisting of a blade, screw, pin, or vent, inserted into the jawbone through the alveolar or basal bone, with a post protruding through the mucoperiosteum into the oral cavity to serve as an abutment for dentures, single tooth replacement, or orthodontic appliances.

endostomy therapist. See **enterostomal therapist.**

endothelial /en′dōthē″lē·əl/ [Gk, *endon*, within, *thele*, nipple], pertaining to endothelium.

endothelial cell [Gk, *endon*, within, *thele*, nipple; L, *cella*, storeroom], a lining cell of a body cavity or of the cardiovascular system. It is usually seen as a flat, nucleated cell.

endothelial-derived relaxing factor (EDRF), nitric oxide or related substances produced by the endothelial cells lining blood vessels. Its vasodilatory effect on neighboring vascular smooth muscle cells is an important regulator of local blood flow.

endothelial myeloma. See **Ewing sarcoma.**

endothelin (ET) /-thē″lin/, any of a group of vasoconstrictive peptides produced by endothelial cells. Three known endothelins, designated ET-1, ET-2, and ET-3, are chemically related to asp venom. ET-1 is the most potent vasoconstrictor yet discovered, being 10 times stronger than the second-most potent vasoconstrictor known, angiotensin II.

-endothelioma, suffix meaning "a tumor of endothelial tissue": *hemangioendothelioma, chondroendothelioma.*

endothelium /en′dōthē″lē·əm/ [Gk, *endon* + *thele*, nipple], the layer of simple squamous epithelial cells that lines the heart, the blood and lymph vessels, and the serous cavities of the body. It is highly vascular, heals quickly, and is derived from the mesoderm.

endothoracic fascia /-thôras″ik/,   a sheet of connective tissue within the thorax; the outer boundary of the thoracic cavity. It separates the parietal pleura from the chest wall and the diaphragm. A thickened portion also attaches to the medial border of the first rib.

endotoxin /en′dōtok″sin/   [Gk, *endon* + *toxikon,* poison],   a toxin contained in the cell walls of some microorganisms, especially gram-negative bacteria, that is released when the bacterium dies and is broken down in the body. Fever, chills, shock, leukopenia, and a variety of other symptoms result, depending on the particular organism and the condition of the infected person. Compare **exotoxin.**

endotoxin shock [Gk, *endon,* within, *toxikon,* poison; Fr, *choc*],   a septic shock in response to the release of endotoxins produced by gram-negative bacteria. The toxin is released on the death of the bacterial cell, especially *Escherichia coli.*

endotracheal /en′dōtrā″kē·əl/   [Gk, *endon* + *tracheia* + *arteria,* airpipe],   within or through the trachea.

endotracheal anesthesia,   general anesthesia that includes an endotracheal tube as a method for controlling ventilation. Anesthesia may be maintained using inhalational anesthetic agents or with a combination that includes intravenous agents. See also **laryngeal mask airway, King airway.**

endotracheal intubation,   the management of the patient with an airway catheter inserted through the mouth or nose into the trachea. An endotracheal tube may be used to maintain a patent airway, to prevent aspiration of material from the digestive tract in the unconscious or paralyzed patient, to permit suctioning of tracheobronchial secretions, or to administer positive-pressure ventilation that cannot be given effectively by a mask. Endotracheal tubes may be made of rubber or plastic and usually have an inflatable cuff to maintain a closed system with the ventilator.

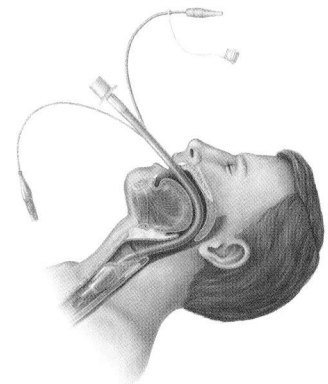

Endotracheal intubation *(Courtesy Mallinckrodt, Inc.)*

endotracheal tube,   a large-bore catheter inserted through the mouth or nose and into the trachea to a point above the bifurcation of the trachea. It is used for delivering oxygen under pressure when ventilation must be totally controlled and in general anesthetic procedures. See also **endotracheal intubation.**

endovasculitis /-vas′kyəli″tis/,   inflammation of the tunica intima of a blood vessel.

endoxin /endok″sin/,   an endogenous analog of digoxin that occurs naturally in humans. It is a hormone that may regulate the excretion of salt.

end plate [AS, *ende* + ME, *plat*],   the motor end plate in the nervous system, located at the terminal membrane of an axon and the postjunctional membrane of the adjoining muscle tissue. Also called **myoneural junction.**

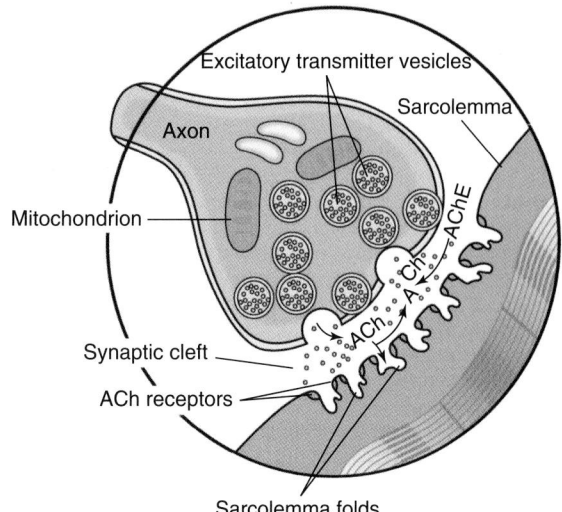

End plate *(Phipps et al, 2003)*

end point,   **1.** (in chemistry) the point at which the condition of equivalence is reached during a titration. This may be indicated by reaching a maximum value in the slope of a titration curve, for example. **2.** the point or time at which an activity is finished. **3.** the point at which a chemical indicator changes color, for example, in an acid-base titration.

end-positional nystagmus,   a horizontal rhythmic oscillation of the eyes on extreme lateral gaze. It occurs in normal eyes when the fixation point is outside the binocular field. Also called **deviational nystagmus, pseudonystagmus.**

end product /endprod′əkt/,   the chemical compound resulting from completion of a sequence of metabolic reactions.

end-stage disease [AS, *ende* + OFr, *estage* + L, *dis* + Fr, *aise,* ease],   a disease condition that is essentially terminal because of irreversible damage to vital tissues or organs. Kidney or renal end-stage disease is defined as a point at which the kidney is so badly damaged or scarred that dialysis or transplantation is required for patient survival.

end-tidal capnography /end″tīdəl/,   the process of continuously recording the level of carbon dioxide in expired air. The percentage of carbon dioxide at the end of expiration can be estimated and gives a close approximation of the alveolar carbon dioxide concentration. The process, which requires the use of infrared spectroscopy, is used to monitor critically ill patients and in pulmonary function testing. The data are typically recorded automatically on a strip of graph paper on a bedside patient monitor.

end-tidal CO_2,   the partial pressure or maximal concentration of carbon dioxide (CO_2) at the end of an exhaled breath, which is expressed as a percentage of CO_2 or mm Hg. The normal values are 5% to 6% CO_2, which is equivalent to 35 to 45 mm Hg. See **capnometry.**

end-tidal CO_2 determination,   the concentration of carbon dioxide in a patient's end-tidal breath, assumed to reflect arterial carbon dioxide tension. A significant difference may indicate a change in ventilation/perfusion matching.

end-to-end anastomosis.   See **anastomosis.**

end-to-side anastomosis,   an anastomosis connecting the end of one vessel or piece of bowel with the side of another one.

endurance /endyŏŏr″əns/,   the ability to continue an activity despite increasing physical or psychological stress, as in

E

the effort to perform additional numbers of muscle contractions before the onset of fatigue. Although endurance and strength are different qualities, weaker muscles tend to have less endurance than do strong muscles.

Enduron, a thiazide diuretic used to treat hypertension. Brand name for **methyclothiazide.**

Enduronyl, a fixed-combination cardiovascular drug containing a diuretic and an antihypertensive agent. Brand name for **methyclothiazide,** *deserpidine.*

-ene, suffix used for naming hydrocarbons: *xanthene.*

enema /en″əmə/ [Gk, *enienai,* to send in], the introduction of a solution into the rectum for cleansing or therapeutic purposes. Enemas may be commercially packed disposable units or reusable equipment prepared just before use.

energy /en′ərjē/ [Gk, *energia*], the capacity to do work or to perform vigorous activity. Energy may occur in the form of heat, light, movement, sound, or radiation. Human energy is usually expressed as muscle contractions and heat production, made possible by the metabolism of food that originally acquired the energy from sunlight. Chemical energy is that released as a result of a chemical reaction, as in the metabolism of food. −*energetic, adj.*

energy conservation, a principle that energy cannot be created or destroyed although it can be changed from one form into another, as when heat energy is converted to light energy. It is now superseded by the special relativity equation $E = mc^2$, but it is still applicable to chemical changes.

energy conservation techniques, strategies to save energy and make tasks easier to complete. An example is sitting to complete self-care.

energy cost of activities, the metabolic cost in calories or kilojoules of various forms of physical activity. For example, the average metabolic equivalent (MET) of walking at a rate of 3 km/hr is 2 METs per minute, and the energy cost of walking at a speed of 6 km/hr is 5 METs per minute. See also **metabolic equivalent of task.**

energy field, the flow of energy surrounding a person.

energy output, the amount of energy expended by work or activity by the body per specified period.

energy-protein malnutrition. See **protein-energy malnutrition.**

energy subtraction, a radiographic technique in which two different x-ray beams are used alternately to provide a subtraction image resulting from differences in photoelectric interaction.

enervation /en′ərvā″shən/ [L, *enervare,* to weaken], **1.** reduction or lack of nervous energy; weakness; lassitude; languor. **2.** removal of a complete nerve or a section of nerve.

en face /äNfäs″, enfäs″/, "face-to-face"; a position in which the mother's face and the infant's face are approximately 8 inches apart and on the same plane, as when the mother holds the infant up in front of her face or when she nurses the child. Studies of maternal and infant bonding have shown that mothers seek eye-to-eye contact and that they will instinctively move the baby to an en face position. In addition, infants have been shown to prefer a human face to other visual stimuli and to be best able to focus at a distance of 8 to 10 inches (20 to 25 cm).

enflurane /en″flo͞orān/, a halogenated volatile liquid; a nonflammable anesthetic gas of the ether family. Its use has been supplanted by newer, shorter acting agents.

enfuvirtide, an antiretroviral drug.

■ INDICATIONS: This drug is used in combination with other antiretrovirals to treat HIV-1 infection.

■ CONTRAINDICATIONS: Known hypersensitivity to this drug prohibits its use.

■ ADVERSE EFFECTS: Adverse effects of this drug include anxiety, peripheral neuropathy, taste disturbance, insomnia, depression, abdominal pain, anorexia, constipation, pancreatitis, injection site reactions, influenza, cough, conjunctivitis, lymphadenopathy, myalgia, hyperglycemia, and pneumonia. Life-threatening side effects include glomerulonephritis, renal failure, Guillain-Barré syndrome, thrombocytopenia, and neutropenia.

engagement /engāj″mənt/ [Fr, a bonding], **1.** (in labor) fixation of the fetal head in the maternal midpelvis with the biparietal diameter of the fetal head level with the plane of the ischial spines (i.e., the greatest transverse diameter of the fetal head has negotiated the pelvic inlet). **2.** (in occupational therapy) active participation in activities, occupations, and daily living. The goal of occupational therapy services is to enable persons to engage in desired occupations.

English position. See **lateral recumbent position.**

engorged /in·gôrjd′/ [Fr, *engorger,* to fill up], distended or swollen with fluids.

engorgement /engôrj″mənt/ [Fr, *engorger,* to fill up], distension or vascular congestion of body tissues, such as the swelling of breast tissue caused by an increased flow of blood and lymph before true lactation.

engram /en″gram/, **1.** a hypothetical neurophysiological storage unit in the cerebrum that is the source of a particular memory. **2.** an interneuronal circuit involving specific neurons and muscle fibers that can be coordinated to perform specific motor activity patterns. Thousands of repetitions may be needed to establish an engram. **3.** the permanent trace left by a stimulus in nerve tissue.

engrossment. See **bonding.**

enhancement /enhans″mənt/ [ME, *enhauncen,* to raise], the act of improving, heightening, or augmenting.

enkephalin /enkef″əlin/ [Gk, *enkepalos,* brain, *in,* within], one of two pain-relieving pentapeptides produced in the body, located in the pituitary gland, brain, and GI tract. Axon terminals that release enkephalins are concentrated in the posterior horn of the gray matter of the spinal cord, in the central part of the thalamus, and in the amygdala of the limbic system of the cerebrum. Enkephalins function as neurotransmitters or neuromodulators and inhibit neurotransmitters in the pathway for pain perception, thereby reducing the emotional as well as the physical impact of pain. Methionine-enkephalin and isoleucine-enkephalin are each composed of five amino acids, four of which are identical in both compounds. These two neuropeptides can depress neurons throughout the central nervous system. Although it is not known exactly how these neuropeptides function, the enkephalins are natural pain killers and may be involved, with other neuropeptides, in the development of psychopathological behavior in some cases. Compare **endorphin.**

enkephalinergic neuron /enkef′əlinur″jik/, a nerve cell that releases the peptide neurotransmitter enkephalin. Such neurons are widespread in the central nervous system.

enol /ē″nol/, an organic compound with an alcohol or hydroxyl group directly attached (bonded) to a double bond. By transfer of the hydrogen atom from oxygen to carbon, the enol form becomes the (usually more stable) keto form. Such compounds usually exist as enol-keto tautomers.

enophthalmos /en′əfthal″məs/ [Gk, *en,* in, *ophthalmos,* eye], backward displacement of the eye in the bony socket, caused by traumatic injury or developmental defect. Ptosis may cause an incorrect diagnosis of enophthalmos. Compare **ptosis.** −*enophthalmic, adj.*

enoxacin /ĕ-nok′säsin/, an antibacterial effective against many gram-positive and gram-negative bacteria, administered orally in the treatment of gonorrhea and urinary tract infections.

enoxaparin /e-nok″säpar′in/, a low-molecular-weight heparin used as the sodium salt to prevent pulmonary embolism and deep venous thrombosis after hip or knee replacement or high-risk abdominal surgery, administered subcutaneously as the sodium salt. It is also used together with warfarin in the treatment of deep venous thrombosis and together with aspirin in the prevention of coronary thrombosis associated with unstable angina or certain kinds of myocardial infarction.

enoximone /enok′sīmōn/, a vasodilator similar to inamrinone, used as a cardiotonic in the short-term management of congestive heart failure. It is administered intravenously.

enriched, **1.** (in nutrition) pertaining to foods to which vitamins or minerals have been added within limits specified by the U.S. Food and Drug Administration, usually to replace nutrients lost during processing. For example, enriched grain products have four B vitamins (B_1, B_2, B_3, and folic acid) and iron added. **2.** (in chemistry) pertaining to a substance containing a proportion of isotope greater than that found in the naturally occurring form of the same element. **3.** (in chemistry) pertaining to a compound containing a greater proportion of one of two possible forms.

enrollee, an individual who has signed up to receive health care under a particular type of plan. Not applicable in Canada. Also called **beneficiary member, participant.**

ensiform cartilage, ensiform process. See **xiphoid process.**

ensulizole /ensul′īzōl/, a water-soluble absorber of ultraviolet B radiation, used topically as a sunscreen.

Ensure, a lactose-free nutritional supplement containing protein, carbohydrates, fat, vitamins, and minerals.

ENT, initialism for *ear, nose, and throat.* See **ENT specialist.**

entacapone, an antiparkinson agent.
■ INDICATIONS: It is used to treat parkinsonism in patients who are experiencing end-of-dose decreased effect.
■ CONTRAINDICATIONS: Known hypersensitivity to this drug prohibits its use.
■ ADVERSE EFFECTS: Serious adverse effects include psychosis, hallucination, hypomania, severe depression, dizziness, gastritis, GI disorders, alopecia, dark urine, back pain, dyspnea, purpura, fatigue, asthenia, and bacterial infection. Common side effects include involuntary choreiform movements, hand tremors, fatigue, headache, anxiety, twitching, numbness, dyskinesia, hypokinesia, hyperkinesia, weakness, confusion, agitation, nightmares, nausea, vomiting, anorexia, abdominal distress, dry mouth, flatulence, bitter taste, diarrhea, constipation, dyspepsia, and orthostatic hypotension.

ental /en″tal/ [Gk, *entos,* within], central or inner; interior or inside.

Entameba, any ameba of the genus *Entamoeba.*

entamebiasis. See **amebiasis.**

Entamoeba /en′təmē″bə/ [Gk, *entos,* within, *amoibe,* change], a genus of intestinal amebic parasites of which several species are pathogenic to humans. See also *Entamoeba histolytica.*

Entamoeba coli, a common nonpathogenic amebic parasite found in the intestines of humans and other mammals. It is similar to and sometimes confused with *E. histolytica,* the causal agent of amebic dysentery. However, *E. coli* organisms tend to be slightly larger, have more pseudopods, and be sluggish in movement.

Entamoeba gingivalis, a temperature-resistant species of ameba found in the mouth of humans and other mammals. As a causal agent of gingivitis, it is associated with poor dental hygiene.

Entamoeba histolytica /his′təlit″ikə/, a pathogenic species of ameba that causes amebic dysentery and hepatic amebiasis in humans. See also **amebiasis, amebic dysentery, hepatic amebiasis.**

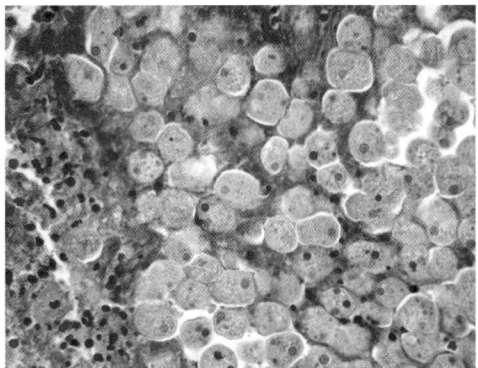

***Entamoeba histolytica* in the colon** *(Kumar et al, 2007)*

entamoebiasis. See **amebiasis.**

entecavir, an antiviral drug.
■ INDICATIONS: This drug is used to treat chronic hepatitis B.
■ CONTRAINDICATIONS: Known hypersensitivity to this drug prohibits its use.
■ ADVERSE EFFECTS: Adverse effects of this drug include fatigue, dizziness, insomnia, nausea, vomiting, and diarrhea. Life-threatening side effects include lactic acidosis and severe hepatomegaly with stenosis. Common side effects include headache and dyspepsia.

enter-. See **entero-, enter-.**

enteral /en′tərəl, enter″əl/ [Gk, *enteron,* bowel], within the small intestine or via the small intestine.

enteral feeding, a mode of feeding that uses the GI tract, such as oral or tube feeding.

enteral nutrition, the provision of nutrients through the GI tract when the client cannot ingest, chew, or swallow food but can digest and absorb nutrients.

enteral tube feeding [Gk, *enteron,* bowel; L, *tubus* + AS, *faedan*], the introduction of nutrients directly into the GI tract by feeding tube. Routes include both nonsurgical and surgically placed. Kinds include **nasogastric feeding, gastrostomy feeding, jejunostomy feeding.** See also **drip gavage, tube feeding.**

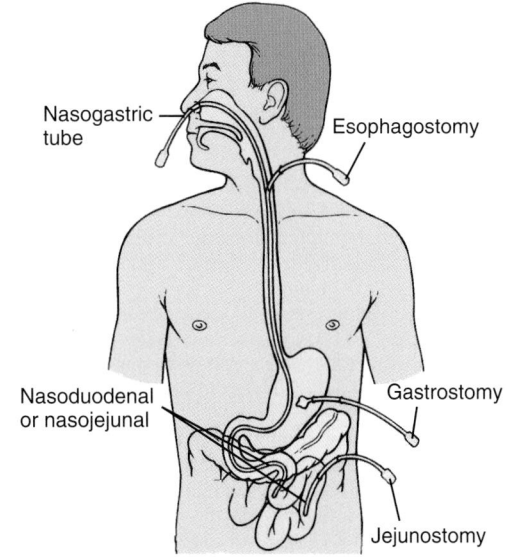

Common placement locations for enteral feeding tubes *(Lewis et al, 2007)*

Common problems of patients receiving tube feedings

Problems and possible causes	Corrective measures
Vomiting and/or aspiration	
Improper placement of tube	Replace tube in proper position. Check tube position before beginning feeding and every 8 hr if continuous feedings.
Delayed gastric emptying, increased residual volume	If gastric residual volume is ≥250 mL after second gastric residual check, a promotility agent should be considered. If gastric residual volume is >500 mL, hold enteral nutrition and reassess patient tolerance.
Potential for aspiration	Keep head of bed elevated to 30- to 45-degree angle. Have patient sit up on side of bed or in chair. Encourage ambulation unless contraindicated.
Diarrhea	
Feeding too fast	Decrease rate of feeding. Change to continuous drip feedings.
Medications	Check for drugs that may cause diarrhea (e.g., antibiotics).
Low-fiber formula	Change to formula with more fiber.
Tube moving distally	Properly secure tube before beginning feeding. Check before each feeding or at least every 24 hr if continuous feedings.
Contamination of formula	Refrigerate unused formula and record date opened. Discard outdated formula every 24 hr. Discard formula left standing for longer than manufacturer's guidelines: 8 hr for ready-to-feed formulas (cans), 4 hr for reconstituted formula, or 24–48 hr for closed-system enteral formulas. Use closed system to prevent contamination. Use sterile water for flushes.
Constipation	
Formula components	Consult health care provider for change in formula to one with more fiber content. Obtain laxative order.
Poor fluid intake	Increase fluid intake if not contraindicated. Give free water, as well as formula. Give total fluid intake of 30 mL/kg body weight.
Drugs	Check for drugs that may be constipating.
Impaction	Perform rectal examinations to check and manually remove feces if present.
Dehydration	
Excessive diarrhea, vomiting	Decrease rate or change formula. Check drugs that patient is receiving, especially antibiotics. Take care to prevent bacterial contamination of formula and equipment.
Poor fluid intake	Increase intake and check amount and number of feedings. Increase amount of intake if appropriate.
High-protein formula	Change formula.
Hyperosmotic diuresis	Check blood glucose levels frequently. Change formula.

From Lewis SL et al: *Medical-surgical nursing: assessment and management of clinical problems,* ed 9, St Louis, 2014, Mosby.

enterectomy /en'tərek″təmē/ [Gk, *enteron,* intestine, *ektomē,* excision], the surgical removal of a portion of intestine.

enteric /enter″ik/ [Gk, *enteron,* bowel], pertaining to the intestinal tract.

enteric coating, a layer added to oral medications that allows the medication to pass through the stomach and be absorbed in the intestinal tract. The coating protects against the effects of stomach juices, which can interact with, destroy, or degrade these drugs.

enteric cytopathogenic human orphan virus. See **ECHO virus.**

enteric fever. See **typhoid fever.**

enteric infection, a disease of the intestine caused by any infection. Symptoms similar to those caused by pathogens may be produced by chemical toxins in ingested foods and by allergic reactions to certain food substances. Among bacteria commonly involved in enteric infections are *Escherichia coli, Vibrio cholerae,* and several species of *Salmonella, Shigella,* and anaerobic streptococci. Enteric infections are characterized by diarrhea, abdominal discomfort, nausea and vomiting, and anorexia. A significant loss of fluid and electrolytes may result from severe vomiting and diarrhea. Oral rehydration therapy with clean water and electrolyte solution may be given. Medication for sedation and relief of abdominal cramps may be prescribed. Antibiotics may be recommended, depending on the specific microorganism causing the infection.

enteric intussusception, intussusception involving two segments of the small intestine.

entericoid fever /enter″ikoid/ [Gk, *enteron* + *eidos,* form], a typhoidlike febrile disease characterized by intestinal inflammation and dysfunction. See also **enteric infection, typhoid fever.**

enteric orphan virus [Gk, *enteron,* bowel, *orphanos,* bereft; L, *virus,* poison], an enterovirus isolated from humans and other animals that was not originally associated with the disease. See also **ECHO virus.**

enteritis /en'tərī″tis/, inflammation of the mucosal lining of the small intestine, resulting from a variety of causes—bacterial, viral, functional, and inflammatory. Involvement of both small and large intestines is called enterocolitis. Compare **gastroenteritis.** See also **enterocolitis.**

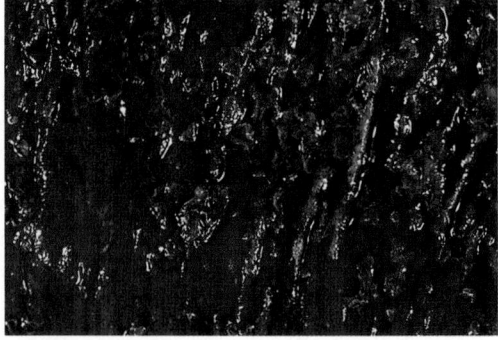

Fungal enteritis *(Damjanov and Linder, 2000)*

entero-, enter-, combining form meaning "intestines": *enteric, enterobacterial, enterobiasis.*

Enterobacter cloacae /en′tirōbak″tər klō·ā″kē, klō·ā″sē/ [Gk, *enteron* + *bakterion,* small staff; L, *cloaca,* sewer], a common species of gram-negative rod-shaped bacteria of the family Enterobacteriaceae found in human and animal feces, dairy products, sewage, soil, and water. *E. cloacae* are important nosocomial pathogens responsible for a number of infections such as bacteremia, lower respiratory tract infections, urinary tract infections, and septic arthritis.

Enterobacteriaceae /en′tirōbaktir′ē·ā″si·ē/ [Gk, *enteron* + *bakterion,* small staff], a family of aerobic and anaerobic gram-negative bacteria that includes both normal and pathogenic enteric microorganisms. Among the significant genera of the family are *Escherichia, Klebsiella, Proteus,* and *Salmonella.*

enterobacterial /-baktir″ē·əl/ [Gk, *enteron* + *bakterion,* small staff], pertaining to a species of bacteria found in the digestive tract.

enterobiasis /en′tirōbī″əsis/ [Gk, *enteron* + *bios,* life, *osis,* condition], a parasitic infestation with *Enterobius vermicularis,* the common pinworm, causing a crawling sensation and pruritus. The nematodes infect the large intestine, and the females deposit eggs in the perianal area, causing pruritus and disturbed sleep. Reinfection commonly results from transfer of eggs to the mouth by contaminated fingers. Airborne transmission is possible because eggs remain viable for 2 weeks in contaminated clothing, bedding, or objects. Five hundred million cases are reported annually worldwide, and 50% of children will be infected at some point in their lives. Also called **oxyuriasis.**

■ OBSERVATIONS: To diagnose enterobiasis, the sticky side of an adhesive cellophane tape swab is pressed against the perianal skin and then examined for eggs under a microscope.

■ INTERVENTIONS: Therapy for the whole family may be necessary. Effective anthelmintics include pyrantel pamoate, mebendazole, albendazole, and thiabendazole.

■ PATIENT CARE CONSIDERATIONS: Personal hygiene, including handwashing, is the best preventive measure. The CDC recommends daily morning bathing and daily changing of underwear. Careful handling and frequent changing of underclothing, nightclothes, towels, and bedding can help reduce infection, reinfection, and environmental contamination with pinworm eggs. Items should be laundered in hot water, especially after each treatment of the infected person and after each usage of washcloths until infection is cleared.

Enterobius vermicularis /en′tərō″bē·əs/ [Gk, *enteron* + *bios,* life; L, *vermiculus,* small worm], a common parasitic nematode that resembles a white thread between 0.5 and 1 cm long. Also called *Oxyuris vermicularis,* **pinworm, seatworm, threadworm.** See also **enterobiasis.**

enterocele /en′tirōsēl′/, **1.** a hernia of the intestine. **2.** posterior vaginal hernia. Compare **enterocoele.**

enterochromaffin cell. See **argentaffin cell.**

enteroclysis /en′tərok″lisis/, a radiographic procedure in which a contrast medium is injected into the duodenum to permit examination of the small intestine. To improve visualization of the bowel wall, air is sometimes injected into the small intestine after the contrast medium has reached the cecum.

enterococcemia /en″terokokse′meä/, blood infection by enterococci.

Enterococcus /en″terokok′us/ *pl.* enterococci [Gk, *enteron* + *kokkos,* berry], a genus of gram-positive, facultatively anaerobic bacteria of the family Streptococcaceae, formerly classified in the genus *Streptococcus. E. faecalis* and *E. faecium* are normal inhabitants of the human intestinal tract that occasionally cause urinary tract infections, infective endocarditis, bacteremia, and life-threatening nosocomial infections (vancomycin-resistant *Enterococci* infection). *E. avium* is found primarily in the feces of chickens and may

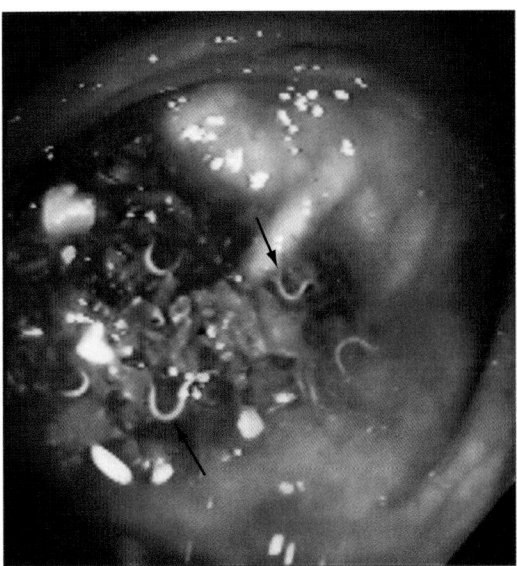

Pinworms *(Enterobius vermicularis) (arrows)* found on screening colonoscopy *(Feldman et al, 2010)*

be associated with appendicitis, otitis, and brain abscesses in humans.

enterocoele, the abdominal cavity.

enterocolitis /-kōlī″tis/ [Gk, *enteron* + *kolon,* bowel, *itis*], an inflammation involving both the large and small intestines. Also called **coloenteritis.**

enterocutaneous fistula, a cutaneous fistula connecting the body surface and some parts of the intestine.

enterocystoplasty /en″terosis′toplas″te/, the most common type of augmentation cystoplasty, using a portion of intestine for the graft. Kinds include **ileocystoplasty, ileocecocystoplasty, sigmoid cystoplasty.**

enterodynia /-din″ē·ə/, intestinal pain.

enteroenterostomy /en′tərō·en′təros″təmē/, the surgical creation of an artificial connection between two segments of the intestine.

enterogastritis. See **gastroenteritis.**

enteroglucagon /-gloo″kəgon/, any of a group of glucagon-like hyperglycemic peptides, released by cells in the mucosa in the upper intestine in response to the ingestion of carbohydrates and fat and stimulating intestinal epithelial cell preparation and renewal. Enteroglucagons are similar to pancreatic glucagons but immunologically different. Glicentin and oxyntomodulin are the principal enteroglucagons.

enterohemorrhagic *Escherichia coli* /-hem′ôraj″ik/, a strain of *E. coli* that causes hemorrhage in the intestines. The organism produces shiga toxin, which damages bowel tissue, causing intestinal ischemia and colonic necrosis. Symptoms are stomach cramping and bloody diarrhea. An infectious dose may be as low as 10 organisms. Spread by contaminated beef, unpasteurized milk and juice, sprouts, lettuce, and salami, as well as contaminated water, the infection can be serious although there may be no fever. Treatment consists of antibiotics and maintenance of fluid and electrolyte balance. In advanced cases, surgical removal of portions of the bowel may be required.

enterohepatic circulation /en′tərōhəpat″ik/, a route by which part of the bile produced by the liver enters the intestine, is resorbed by the liver, and then is recycled into the intestine. The remainder of the bile is excreted in feces.

enterokinase /en′tirōkī″nās/ [Gk, *enteron* + *kinesis,* movement, *ase,* enzyme], an intestinal juice enzyme that activates the proteolytic enzymes in pancreatic juice as they enter the duodenum.

enterolith /en′tərōlith′/ [Gk, *enteron* + *lithos,* stone], a stone consisting of ingested material found within the intestine. See also **calculus.**

enterolithiasis /en′tərōlithī′əsis/, the presence of enteroliths in the intestine.

enteron, small intestine. See **digestive tract, small intestine.**

enteropathic *Escherichia coli* /-path′ik/, a strain of *E. coli* that is the cause of epidemic infantile diarrhea. See also **epidemic diarrhea in newborns.**

enteropathy /en′tərop″əthē/, a disease or other disorder of the intestines.

enterostomal therapist /-stō″məl/, a registered nurse who is qualified by education in an accredited program in enterostomal therapy to provide care for persons with stomas, draining wounds, fistulae, incontinence, and actual or potential alterations in tissue integrity. Also called **endostomy therapist.** See also **Wound, Ostomy and Continence Nurses (WOCN) Society.**

enterostomy /en′təros″təmē/ [Gk, *enteron* + *stoma,* mouth], a surgical procedure that produces an artificial anus or fistula in the intestine through an incision in the abdominal wall. See also **colostomy.**

enterotoxigenic /-tok′sijen″ik/, producing an enterotoxin.

enterotoxigenic *Escherichia coli,* a strain of *E. coli* that is a frequent cause of diarrhea in travelers. See also **traveler's diarrhea.**

enterotoxin /-tok″sin/, a toxic substance that causes an adverse reaction by cells of the intestinal mucosa. Most enterotoxins are produced by certain species of bacteria, such as *Staphylococcus.*

enterovesical fistula, a fistula connecting some part of the intestine with the urinary bladder. Also called **vesicoenteric fistula.**

Enterovirus /-vī″rəs/ [Gk, *enteron* + L, *virus,* poison], a genus of Picornaviridae that preferentially replicates in the mammalian intestinal tract. Kinds include **coxsackie virus, ECHO virus, poliovirus.** –*enteroviral, adj.*

enthesitis /en′thəsī″tis/, an inflammation of the insertion of a muscle with a strong tendency toward fibrosis and calcification. It is usually only painful when the involved muscle is activated.

enthesopathy /en′thəsop″əthē/, an arthritic condition affecting tendons and ligaments rather than joint membranes.

ento-. See **endo-, end-, ent-, ento-.**

entodermal. See **endodermal.**

entomophthoromycosis basidiobolae, a chronic infection caused by *Basidiobolus ranarum,* a filamentous fungus, in which gradually enlarging granulomas form in the subcutaneous tissues of the arms, chest, and trunk. Multiple purulent ulcers may develop. The infection is seen in children and adolescents in tropical areas of Indonesia, India, and Africa. Also called **subcutaneous chronic zygomycosis.**

entopic /entop″ik/, occurring in the proper place. Compare **ectopic.**

entopic phenomena, sensations perceived for mechanical reasons within the eye, such as floaters or flashes caused by retinal changes.

entrainment /entrān″mənt/ [Fr, *entrainer,* to drag along], **1.** the synchronization of rhythmic cycles. For example, infants have been observed to move in time to the rhythms of adult speech but not to random noises or disconnected words or vowels. Entrainment is thought to be an essential factor in maternal-infant bonding. **2.** a technique for identifying the slowest pacing necessary to terminate an arrhythmia, particularly atrial flutter.

entrance block [Fr, *entrer,* to enter; AS, *blok*], a theoretic zone that surrounds a pacemaker focus and protects it from discharge by an extraneous impulse that might trigger ectopic ventricular contractions.

entrance exposure, the skin dose of radiation as the beam enters the patient. It may be expressed in milligrays, milliroentgens, or C/kg.

entrapment neuropathy /entrap″mənt/ [OFr, *entraper,* to catch in a trap; Gk, *neuron,* nerve, *pathos,* disease], injury or inflammation of single nerves caused by pressure from surrounding tissues, such as ligaments and fascia.

entropion /entrō″pē·on/ [Gk, *en* + *tropos,* a turning], turning inward or turning toward, usually a condition in which the eyelid turns inward toward the eye. In either the upper or lower eyelid, cicatricial entropion can result from scar tissue formation. Spastic entropion results from an inflammation or other factor that affects tissue tone. An inflammation of the eyelid may be the result of an infectious disease or irritation from an inverted eyelash. Compare **ectropion.** See also **blepharitis.**

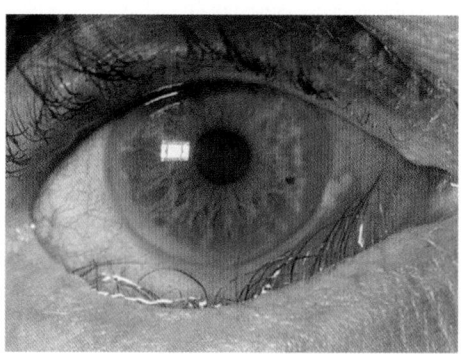

Entropion *(Kanski and Nischal, 1999)*

entropy /en′trəpē/ [Gk, *en* + *tropos,* a turning], the tendency of a system to change from a state of order to a state of disorder, expressed in physics as a measure of the part of the energy in a thermodynamic system that is not available to perform work. According to the principles of evolution, living organisms tend to go from a state of disorder to a state of order in their development and thus appear to reverse entropy. However, maintaining a living system requires the expenditure of energy, leaving less energy available for work, with the result that the entropy of the system and its surroundings increases.

ENT specialist. See **otolaryngologist.**

enucleation /inoo′klē·ā″shən/ [L, *e,* without, *nucleus,* nut], **1.** removal of an organ or tumor in one piece. **2.** removal of the entire eyeball, performed for malignancy, severe infection, extensive trauma, or control of pain in glaucoma. Local or general anesthesia is used. The optic nerve and muscle attachments are cut; if possible, the surrounding layer of fascia is left with the muscles. A round implant of hydroxyapatite (coralline or syntetic) is inserted, and the muscles are sutured around it, providing a permanent stump to give support and motion to an artificial eye, or an implant of porous polyethylene is inserted, allowing the rectus muscle to be sutured directly to the implant. After surgery, pressure dressings are kept in place for 1 or 2 days to prevent hemorrhage. Other possible complications include thrombosis of nearby blood vessels, which may lead to infection, including meningitis.

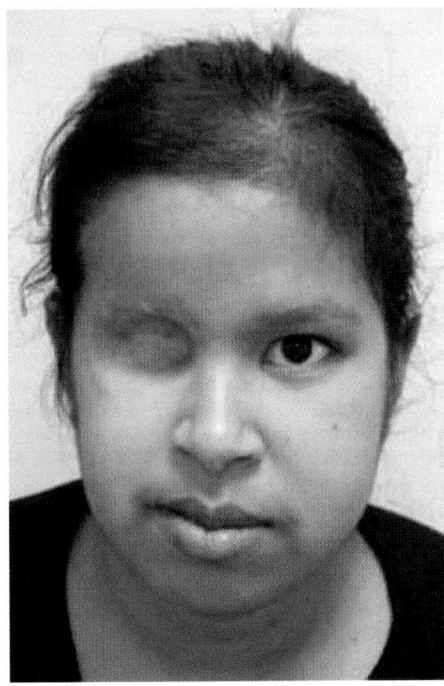

Young woman with enucleation of eye *(Tummawanit et al, 2013)*

enucleator /inoo″klē·ā′tər/ [L, *e*, without, *nucleus,* nut], a procedure or device for removing a nucleus from a cell.

enuresis /en′yoorē″sis/ [Gk, *enourein,* to urinate], incontinence of urine, especially nocturnal bed-wetting.

envenomation /enven′əmā″shən/, the injection of snake, arachnid, or insect venom into the body.

environment [Gk, *en,* in; L, *viron,* circle], **1.** all of the many factors, both physical and psychological, that influence or affect the life and survival of a person. See also **biome, climate.** –*environmental, adj.* **2.** (in occupational therapy) the physical and social features of the specific context in which a client engages in occupations.

environmental carcinogen /envī′rənmen″təl/, any of the natural or synthetic substances that can cause cancer. Such agents may be divided into chemical agents, physical agents, hormones, and viruses. Some environmental carcinogens are arsenic, asbestos, uranium, vinyl chloride, ionizing radiation, ultraviolet rays, x-rays, and coal tar derivatives. Carcinogenic effects of chemicals may be delayed for as long as 30 years. Other carcinogens produce more immediate effects. Some studies indicate that the carcinogens in cigarette smoke are involved in 80% of all lung cancer. Most carcinogens are unreactive or secondary carcinogens but are converted to primary carcinogens in the body. Numerous factors, such as heredity, affect the susceptibilities of different individuals to cancer-causing agents.

environmental control unit (ECU), an apparatus designed for individuals with functional limitations that controls devices such as lamps, televisions, radios, telephones, and alarm systems. Similar to television remote control devices, they are typically switches manipulated by the lips, chin, or other body movements. A voice-activated smart speaker equipped with a far-field microphone that supports voice recognition can also be used for environmental control when wirelessly connected to appliances and devices.

environmental health, the total of various aspects of substances, forces, and conditions in and about a community that affect the health and well-being of the population.

environmental health technician, a health care professional who performs technical assistance under professional supervision in monitoring environmental health hazards such as radioactive contamination, air and water pollution, and disposal of chemical wastes of industry.

environmentally induced disorder, an atypical condition that results from an environmental toxin (such as lead).

environmental medicine, a practice of medicine in which the major focus is on cause-and-effect relationships in health. Evaluations are made of such factors as eating and living habits and types of air breathed. Testing in the patient's own environment is performed to determine what precipitators are present that may be related to disease or other health problems. A treatment protocol is developed from this information.

Environmental Protection Agency (EPA), an agency of the United States federal government charged with the protection of human health and the environment.

environmental services, a functional unit of a health care facility. It has the responsibility for laundry, liquid and solid waste control, safe disposal of materials contaminated by radiation or pathogenic organisms, and general maintenance of safety and housekeeping.

enzacamene /en″zah-kam′ēn/, an absorber of ultraviolet radiation, used topically as a sunscreen.

enzygotic twins. See **monozygotic twins.**

enzymatic debridement /en′zīmat″ik/, the use of nonirritating, nontoxic vegetable enzymes to remove dead tissue from a wound without destroying normal tissue.

enzymatic detergent asthma, an allergic reaction experienced by persons who have become sensitized to alcalase, an enzyme contained in some laundry detergents. Alcalase is produced by the bacterium *Bacillus subtilis,* and persons sensitive to the enzyme are also usually allergic to the bacterium. Asthmatic symptoms may progress in severe cases to an allergic alveolitis. The most serious cases were originally among workers in plants that manufacture laundry detergents.

enzyme /en″zīm/ [Gk, *en,* in, *zyme,* ferment], a protein produced by living cells that catalyzes chemical reactions in organic matter. Most enzymes are produced in tiny quantities and catalyze reactions that take place within the cells. Digestive enzymes, however, are produced in relatively large quantities and act outside the cells in the lumen of the digestive tract. The substance that is acted upon by an enzyme is called a substrate. See also **substrate.**

Enzyme Commission (EC), the International Commission on Enzymes, a committee established in 1956 by the International Union of Biochemistry to standardize enzyme classification and nomenclature.

enzyme deficiency anemia, a deficiency of enzymes in the pathways that metabolize glucose and adenosine triphosphate (Embden-Meyerhof and pentose phosphate shunt pathways), which frequently leads to premature red blood cell destruction.

enzyme induction [Gk, *en* + *zyme,* ferment; L, *inducere,* to lead in], the increase in the rate of a specific enzyme synthesis from basal to maximum level caused by the presence of a substrate or substrate analog that acts as an inducer. The inducer may be a substance that inactivates a repressor chemical in the cell.

enzyme-linked immunosorbent assay (ELISA), a laboratory technique for detecting specific antigens or antibodies by using enzyme-labeled immunoreactants and a solid-phase binding support, such as a test tube. A number of different enzymes can be used, including carbonic anhydrase, glucose oxidase, and alkaline phosphatase. Labeling is done by covalently binding the enzyme to the test substance through an enzyme-protein coupling agent such as glutaraldehyde. Products of the reaction may be detected by fluorometry or photometry. ELISA is nearly as sensitive as radioimmunoassay and more sensitive than complement fixation, agglutination, and other techniques.

enzyme therapy, in complementary medicine, the oral administration of proteolytic enzymes for the purpose of improving immune system function. It is used for a wide variety of disorders, including trauma, inflammation, autoimmune diseases, and viral infection, and as adjunctive therapy in cancer treatment.

enzymology /en′zīmol″əjē/, the study of enzymes and their actions.

enzymolysis /en′zīmol″isis/ [Gk, *en,* in, *zyme,* ferment, *lysis,* loosening], destruction or change of a substance caused by means of enzymatic action.

enzymopenia /en′zīmōpē″nē-ə/, the deficiency of an enzyme.

enzymuria /en′zīmŏŏr′ē-ə/, the presence of enzymes in urine.

EOA, abbreviation for **esophageal obturator airway.**

EOM, 1. abbreviation for **extraocular muscles. 2.** abbreviation for **extraocular movement.**

eosin /ē″əsin/, a group of red acidic xanthine dyes often used in combination with a blue-purple basic dye such as hematoxylin to stain tissue slides in the laboratory.

eosin-, prefix meaning "a rose, red, or dawn color": *eosinopenia, eosinophil, eosinophilic.*

eosinoblast. See **myeloblast.**

eosinopenia /ē″əsinəpē″nē-ə/, an abnormally low number of eosinophil leukocytes in the blood.

eosinophil /ē′əsin″əfil/ [Gk, *eos,* dawn, *philein,* to love], a granulocytic bilobed leukocyte characterized by large numbers of regular refractile cytoplasmic granules that stain bright orange with the acid dye eosin. Eosinophils constitute 1% to 3% of the white blood cells in peripheral blood films. They increase in number with allergy and some parasitic conditions and decrease with steroid administration. Compare **basophil, neutrophil. –eosinophilic,** *adj.*

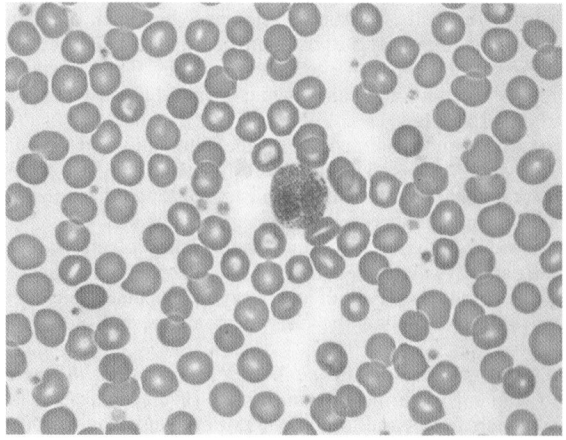

Eosinophil *(Courtesy Zane Amenhotep, MS, University of California—San Francisco)*

eosinophilia /ē′əsin′ōfil″yə/, abnormal increase in blood film eosinophils, accompanying an allergic response or parasitic infestation.

eosinophilia-myalgia syndrome, tryptophan-induced, a potentially fatal disorder resulting from ingestion of tryptophan. It is characterized by a symptom complex of severe muscle pain, tenosynovitis, muscle edema, and skin rash lasting several weeks.

eosinophilic /ē′əsin′əfil″ik/, **1.** the tendency of a cell, tissue, or organism to be readily stained by the dye eosin. **2.** pertaining to an eosinophilic leukocyte.

eosinophilic adenoma. See **acidophilic adenoma.**

eosinophilic cellulitis. See **Wells syndrome.**

eosinophilic cholangitis, a rare type of cholangitis resulting from eosinophilic infiltration and characterized by multiple strictures in the bile ducts. The cause is unknown.

eosinophilic enteropathy, a rare form of food allergy that is characterized by nausea, crampy abdominal pain, diarrhea, urticaria, an elevated eosinophil count in the blood, and eosinophilic infiltrates in the intestine. Diagnosis is made by an elimination diet. Symptoms usually disappear when the offending food is removed from the diet.

eosinophilic fasciitis, inflammation of fasciae of the limbs, associated with eosinophilia, edema, and swelling. The cause is unknown, but the condition often occurs after strenuous exercise. Also called **Shulman syndrome.**

eosinophilic gastroenteritis, a disorder marked by infiltration of the mucosa of the small intestine by eosinophils, with edema but without vasculitis, and by eosinophilia of the peripheral blood. Symptoms, including abdominal pain, diarrhea, nausea, fever, and malabsorption, depend on the site and extent of the disorder. The stomach is also frequently involved. The disorder is commonly associated with intolerance to specific foods.

eosinophilic granuloma, 1. a simple or multiple growth in the bone or lung characterized by numerous eosinophils and histiocytes. Eosinophilic granulomas occur most frequently in children and adolescents. **2.** See **anisakiasis.**

eosinophilic leukemia, a malignant neoplasm of the blood-forming tissues in which eosinophils are the predominant cells. The disease resembles chronic myelocytic leukemia but may have an acute course, even when no blast forms are present in the peripheral blood.

eosinophilic leukocyte. See **eosinophil.**

eosinophilic meningitis, meningitis with an increase in lymphocytes and a high percentage of eosinophils in the cerebrospinal fluid. It usually results from infection with *Angiostrongylus cantonensis.*

eosinophilic myeloencephalitis, a complex of neurological symptoms produced by invasion of the central nervous system by *Gnathostoma spinigerum,* including severe nerve root pain, followed by paralysis of extremities and sudden sensorial impairment, accompanied by increased number of eosinophils in the cerebrospinal fluid, which is often bloody or yellowish.

eosinophilic pneumonia, inflammation of the lungs, characterized by infiltration of the alveoli with eosinophils and large mononuclear cells, pulmonary edema, fever, night sweats, cough, dyspnea, and weight loss. The disease may be caused by a hypersensitivity reaction to fungi spores; plant fibers; wood dust; bird droppings' porcine, bovine, or piscine proteins; *Bacillus subtilis* enzyme in detergents; or certain drugs. Treatment consists of removal of the offending allergen and symptomatic and supportive therapy. Compare **bronchopneumonia.** See also **asthmatic eosinophilia.**

-eous, suffix meaning "like" or "composed of" or "relating to" something specified: *cutaneous, osseous.*

EP, abbreviation for **evoked potential.**

ep-. See **epi-, ep-.**

EPA, abbreviation for **Environmental Protection Agency.**

epaxial muscles, the intrinsic muscles of the back.

elementary body, an infectious, nonreplicative, morphologically distinct form of certain bacteria.

EPEC, abbreviation for **enteropathic** *Escherichia coli.*

ependyma /ipen″dimə/ [Gk, an upper garment], a layer of ciliated epithelial membrane that lines the central canal of the spinal cord and the ventricles of the brain. −*ependymal, adj.*

ependymal glioma, a large vascular fairly solid tumor in the fourth ventricle, composed of malignant glial cells.

ependymitis /ipen′dimī″tis/, an inflammation of the ependymal tissue, the epithelial lining of the ventricles of the brain, and of the canal of the spinal cord.

ependymoblastoma /ipen′dimōblastō″mə/, a malignant neoplasm composed of primitive cells of the ependyma. Also called **malignant ependymoma.**

ependymoma /ipen′dimō″mə/ [Gk, *ependyma,* an upper garment, *oma,* tumor], a neoplasm composed of differentiated cells of the ependyma. The tumor, which is usually a benign pale, firm, encapsulated, somewhat nodular mass, commonly arises from the roof of the fourth ventricle and may extend to the spinal cord. Primary lesions may also develop in the spinal cord. Also called *ependymocytoma.*

ephapse /ef″aps/ [Gk, *ephasis,* a touching], a point of lateral contact between nerve fibers across which impulses may be transmitted directly through the cell membranes rather than across a synapse. Compare **synapse.** −*ephaptic, adj.*

ephaptic transmission /ifap″tik/, the passage of a neural impulse from one nerve fiber, axon, or dendrite to another through the membranes. The mechanism may be a factor in epileptic seizures. Compare **synaptic transmission.**

ephebiatrics /ēfeb′ē·at″riks/ [Gk, *ephebos,* puberty, *iatros,* physician], a branch of medicine that specializes in the health of adolescents.

ephedra, an evergreen herb found throughout the world. Also called *ma huang.*

■ INDICATIONS: The sale of ephedra was banned in the United States by the U.S. Food and Drug Administration in December 2003 because of safety concerns (e.g., highlighted by the death of baseball pitcher Steve Bechler), making it the first over-the-counter nutritional supplement to be banned. This herb was used for seasonal and chronic asthma, nasal congestion, and cough. It is not banned in Canada but is highly restricted in its use.

■ CONTRAINDICATIONS: People cultivating their own ephedra should be aware that it is contraindicated in those with known hypersensitivity to sympathomimetics, women who are pregnant or lactating, children less than 12 years of age, and people with narrow-angle glaucoma, seizure disorders, hyperthyroidism, diabetes mellitus, prostatic hypertrophy, arrhythmias, heart block, hypertension, psychosis, tachycardia, and angina pectoris.

ephedrine /ef″ədrēn/, an alpha- and beta-adrenergic agonist that also promotes the release of norepinephrine from sympathetic nerve terminals.

■ INDICATIONS: It is prescribed in the treatment of asthma and bronchitis and is used topically as a nasal decongestant. The drug is historically important, but its use is now limited because of the availability of more selective beta$_2$ agonists for treating asthma.

■ CONTRAINDICATIONS: Concomitant administration of monoamine oxidase inhibitors, hypertension, cardiac artery disease, cardiac arrhythmia, or known hypersensitivity to this drug prohibits its use.

■ ADVERSE EFFECTS: Among the more serious adverse effects are nervousness, insomnia, anorexia, and increased blood pressure.

ephemeral /ifem″ərəl/ [Gk, *epi,* above, *hemera,* day], pertaining to a short-lived condition, such as a fever.

EPI, 1. abbreviation for **echo planar imaging. 2.** abbreviation for **early psychosis intervention.**

epi-, ep-, prefix meaning "on, upon": *epicanthus, epidural.*

epiblast /ep″iblast′/ [Gk, *epi,* upon, *blastos,* germ], the primordial outer layer of the blastocyst or blastula, before differentiation of the germ layers, that gives rise to the ectoderm and contains cells capable of forming the endoderm and mesoderm. See also **ectoderm.** −*epiblastic, adj.*

epicanthus /ep′ikan″thəs/ [Gk, *epi*+ *kanthos,* lip of a vessel], a vertical fold of skin over the angle of the inner canthus of the eye. It may be slight or marked, covering the canthus and the caruncle. It is a hereditary trait in people of Asian descent and is of no clinical significance. Some infants with Down syndrome have marked epicanthal folds. Also called *epicanthal fold, epicanthic fold.* −*epicanthal, epicanthic, adj.*

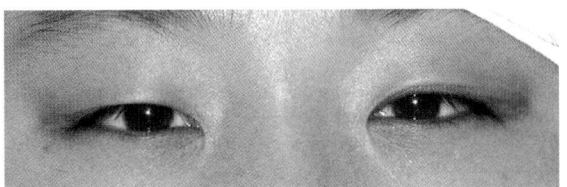

Individual with moderate epicanthus *(Chen et al, 2009)*

epicardia /-kär″dē·ə/ [Gk, *epi,* above, *kardia,* heart], the part of the esophagus that lies between the cardiac orifice of the stomach and the esophageal opening of the diaphragm.

epicardial. See **epicardium.**

epicardial pacing. See **pacing.**

epicardium /ep′ikär″dē·əm/ [Gk, *epi* + *kardia,* heart], the outermost of the three layers of tissue that form the heart wall. It is composed of a single sheet of squamous epithelial cells overlying delicate connective tissue. The epicardium is the visceral portion of the serous pericardium and folds back on itself to form the parietal portion of the serous pericardium. Compare **myocardium.** See also **pericardium.** −**epicardial,** *adj.*

epicondylar. See **epicondyle.**

epicondylar fracture /-kon″dilər/, any fracture that involves the medial or lateral epicondyle of a specific bone, such as the humerus.

epicondyle /ep′ikon″dəl/ [Gk, *epi* + *kondylos,* knuckle], a projection on the surface of a bone above its condyle; site for muscular or ligamentous attachment. −**epicondylar,** *adj.*

epicondylitis /ep′ikon′dilī″tis/, a painful and sometimes disabling inflammation of the muscle and surrounding tissues of the elbow, caused by repeated strain on the forearm near the medial or lateral epicondyle of the humerus. The strain may result from violent extension or supination of the wrist against a resisting force, such as may occur in playing tennis or golf, twisting a screwdriver, or carrying a heavy load with the arm extended. Treatment usually includes rest, injection of procaine with or without hydrocortisone, stretching and strengthening of the muscle, and, in some cases, surgery to release part of the muscle from the epicondyle. See also **golfer's elbow, lateral humeral epicondylitis.**

epicranial. See **epicranium.**

E

epicranial aponeurosis /-krā″nē·əl/ [Gk, *epi* + *kranion,* skull, *apo,* away, *neuron,* tendon], a fibrous membrane that covers the cranium between the occipital and frontal muscles of the scalp. Also called **galea aponeurotica.**

epicranium /-krā″nē·əm/ [Gk, *epi* + *kranion,* skull], the complete scalp, including the integument, the muscular sheets, and the aponeuroses. Compare **epicranius. –epicranial,** *adj.*

epicranius [Gk, *epi* + *kranion,* skull], the broad muscular and tendinous layer of tissue covering the top and sides of the skull from the occipital bone to the eyebrows. It consists of broad, thin muscular bellies, connected by an extensive aponeurosis. Innervation of the epicranius by branches of the facial nerves can draw back the scalp, raise the eyebrows, and move the ears. Compare **epicranium.** See also **epicranial aponeurosis, occipitofrontalis, temporoparietalis.**

epicritic /-krit″ik/, pertaining to the somatic sensations of fine discriminative touch, vibration, two-point discrimination, stereognosis, and conscious and unconscious proprioception.

epidemic /-dem″ik/ [Gk, *epi* + *demos,* people], **1.** *adj.,* affecting a significantly large number of people at the same time. **2.** *n.,* a disease that spreads rapidly through a demographic segment of the human population, such as everyone in a given geographic area, a military base, or similar population unit, or everyone of a certain age or sex, such as the children or women of a region. **3.** *n.,* a disease or event whose incidence is beyond what is expected. Compare **endemic, epizootic, pandemic.**

epidemic cerebrospinal meningitis. See **meningococcal meningitis.**

epidemic diarrhea in newborns [Gk, *epi,* above, *demos,* the people, *dia,* through, *rhein,* flow; ME, *newe* + *beren*], any severe gastroenteritis epidemic among a community of newborns, as may occur in a hospital nursery.

epidemic encephalitis, any diffuse inflammation of the brain occurring in epidemic form. Also called **von Economo encephalitis.** Kinds include **Japanese encephalitis, St. Louis encephalitis.** See also **encephalitis.**

epidemic hemoglobinuria. See **hemoglobinuria.**

epidemic hemorrhagic conjunctivitis [Gk, *epi,* above, *demos,* the people, *haima,* blood, *rhegnynei,* to gush; L, *conjunctivus,* connecting; Gk, *itis,* inflammation], a highly contagious infection, commonly involving an enterovirus, that begins with eye pain accompanied by swollen eyelids and hyperemia of the conjunctiva. It is a self-limiting disorder that has no specific remedy.

epidemic hemorrhagic fever, a severe viral infection marked by fever and bleeding. The disorder develops rapidly and is characterized initially by fever and muscle ache, possibly followed by hemorrhage, peripheral vascular collapse, hypovolemic shock, and acute kidney failure. The arbovirus or other pathogen is believed to be transmitted by mosquitoes, ticks, mites, or rodents. The pathophysiological characteristics of the hemorrhagic effect are uncertain, although it is assumed the disease organism causes damage to the lining of the capillaries. Kinds include **Argentine hemorrhagic fever, Bolivian hemorrhagic fever, dengue fever, Lassa fever, yellow fever.** See also *specific viral infections.*

epidemic hysteria. See **mass hysteria.**

epidemic keratoconjunctivitis (EKC) [Gk, *epi,* above, *demos,* the people, *keras,* horn; L, *conjunctivus;* Gk, *itis,* inflammation], an adenovirus infection consisting of an acute, severely painful conjunctivitis followed by keratitis. In the western world, EKC strikes predominantly in selected environments: industry eye clinics, emergency rooms, nursing homes, schools, camps, and child-care centers. The virus is often found on the hands of people with active EKC. Hand-to-eye transmission is felt to be a common method of spread, especially in the medical setting. Swimming pools and schools have been implicated in transmission, and it can spread through inanimate objects. In the eye clinic and emergency room, instruments and contaminated eyedrops can transmit the virus. EKC is quite contagious and prone to epidemics that may be quite large. It is treated by lubrication with artificial tears.

epidemic myalgia, a disease caused by coxsackie B virus. It is characterized by sudden acute chest or epigastric pain and fever lasting 3 to 14 days, followed by complete spontaneous recovery. Also called **devil's grip, epidemic myositis.** Formerly called **epidemic pleurodynia.**

epidemic myositis. See **epidemic myalgia, epidemic pleurodynia.**

epidemic parotitis. See **mumps.**

epidemic pleurodynia, an acute infectious disease caused by strains of enterovirus *Coxsackie,* type B, mainly affecting children. It is characterized by severe intermittent pain in the abdomen or lower chest, fever, headache, sore throat, malaise, and extreme myalgia. The symptoms may continue for weeks or subside after a few days and recur for a period of weeks. Transmission is through the fecal-oral route. Treatment is symptomatic; complete recovery is usual. Also called **Bornholm disease, devil's grip, epidemic myositis.** Now called **epidemic myalgia.**

epidemic typhus, an acute severe rickettsial infection characterized by prolonged high fever, headache, and a dark maculopapular rash that covers most of the body. The causative organism, *Rickettsia prowazekii,* is transmitted indirectly as a result of the bite of the human body louse or squirrel flea or louse; the pathogen is contained in feces of the louse and enters the body tissues as the bite is scratched. Disease is manifested by the abrupt onset of an intense headache and a fever reaching 40° C (104° F) beginning after an incubation period of 1 week. The rash follows on the fifth day of onset. Complications may include vascular collapse, renal failure, pneumonia, or gangrene. Mortality rate is as high as 40% depending on preexisting clinical conditions. Treatment may include antipyretics and supportive symptomatic care. Health care workers are at risk of acquiring this infection from louse bites or louse feces. Also called **classic typhus, European typhus, jail fever, louse-borne typhus.** Compare **murine typhus.** See also **Brill-Zinsser disease,** *Rickettsia,* **typhus.**

epidemic vomiting, an episode of sudden vomiting by members of a group of people in close contact. The vomiting, caused by infection with the Norwalk virus (containing a ribonucleic acid genome), usually begins without previous signs or symptoms of illness and may continue for several hours, ending abruptly. The vomiting may be accompanied by headache, abdominal pain, and diarrhea. The patients are frequently children who are attending the same school.

epidemiological. See **epidemiology.**

epidemiologist /-dē′mē·ol″əjist/, a specialist in the study, treatment, and prevention of diseases. The epidemiologist may lead or oversee specialty programs, such as the prevention of disease in a target population or the treatment of illnesses unique to certain populations.

epidemiology /-dē′mē·ol″əjē/ [Gk, *epi* + *demos,* people, *logos,* science], the study of the determinants of disease events in populations. **–epidemiological,** *adj.*

epiderm-, epidermo-, prefix *(epi-)* plus a combining form *(-derm, -dermo)* meaning "epidermis": *epidermoid, epidermolysis, epidermolytic.*

epidermal growth factor (EGF) /ep′idur″məl/, a mitogenic polypeptide produced by many cell types and made in large amounts by some tumors. It promotes growth and differentiation, is essential in embryogenesis, and is also important in wound healing. It has been found to be part of a family of compounds that includes also transforming growth factor.

epidermal inclusion cyst.   See **epidermoid cyst.**

epidermal nevus /-dur″məl/ [Gk, *epi* + *derma,* skin; L, *naevus,* birthmark], a discrete discolored congenital lesion caused by an overgrowth of epidermis. It may be seen in newborns. Also called **epithelial nevus, hard nevus.**

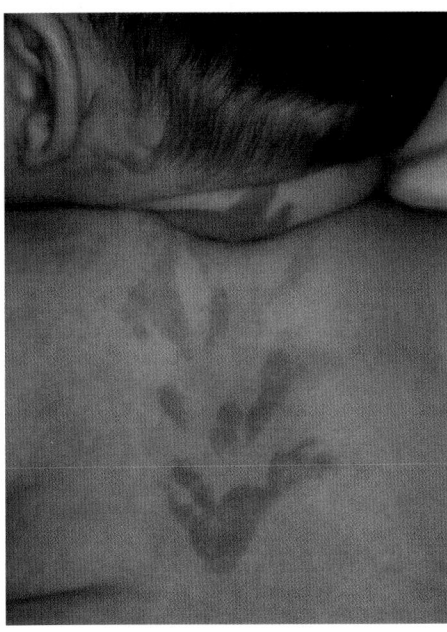

Infant with epidermal nevi *(Bolognia et al, 2014)*

epidermis /ep′idur″mis/ [Gk, *epi* + *derma,* skin], the superficial avascular layers of the skin, made up of an outer dead, cornified part and a deeper living, cellular part. Each layer is named for its unique function, texture, or position. The deepest layer is the stratum basale. It anchors the more superficial layers to the underlying tissues, and it provides new cells to replace those lost by abrasion from the outermost layer. The cells of each layer migrate upward as they mature. Above the stratum basale lies the stratum spinosum. As the cells migrate to the next layer, the stratum granulosum, they become flat, lying parallel with the surface of the skin. Over this layer, such as in the thick skin of the palms of the hands and soles of the feet, lies a clear, thin band of homogenous tissue called the stratum lucidum. The outermost layer, the stratum corneum, is composed of scaly, squamous plaques of dead cells that contain keratin, a waterproofing protein that hardens over several days. This horny layer is thick over areas of the body subject to abrasion, such as the palms of the hands, and thin over other more protected areas. Altogether these layers are between 0.5 and 1.1 mm in thickness. Also called **cuticle.** See also **skin.** *−epidermal, epidermoid, adj.*

epidermoid carcinoma /-dur″moid/ [Gk, *epi* + *derma* + *eidos,* form], a malignant neoplasm in which the tumor cells tend to differentiate in the manner of epidermal cells, then form horny cells called prickle cells. Also called *squamous cell skin cancer.*

epidermoid cyst, a common benign cavity lined by keratinizing epithelium and filled with a cheesy material composed of sebum and epithelial debris. The cyst is in the skin, connected to the surface by a pore. Treatment is surgical excision. Also called **sebaceous cyst, epidermal inclusion cyst.** Compare **pilar cyst.**

epidermolysis bullosa /ep′idərmol″isis/ [Gk, *epi* + *derma* + *lysis,* loosening], a group of rare hereditary skin diseases in which vesicles and bullae develop, usually at sites of trauma. Severe forms may also involve mucous membranes and may leave scars and contractures on healing. Basal cell and squamous cell carcinomas sometimes develop in the scar tissue.

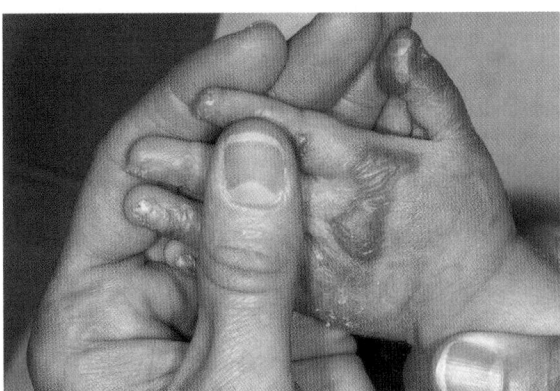

Junctional epidermolysis bullosa *(Weston, 2007)*

epidermolytic hyperkeratosis [Gk, *epi* + *derma,* skin + *lysis,* loosening; Gk, *hyper,* excess + *keras,* horn + *osis,* condition], a rare autosomal-dominant form of ichthyosis with a high frequency of spontaneous mutations. Present at birth, it is characterized by generalized erythroderma and severe hyperkeratosis with small wartlike scales over the entire body, especially in body folds, and sometimes on the palms and soles. There are also recurrent bullae on the lower limbs. If sepsis and electrolyte imbalances are not treated correctly in neonates, morbidity can occur. Also called **bullous congenital ichthyosiform erythroderma.** See also **ichthyosis.**

epidermomycosis.   See **dermatophytosis.**

epidermophytosis /ep′idur′mōfītō″sis/, a superficial fungus infection of the skin.

epididym-, prefix meaning "epididymis": *epididymoorchitis, epididymitis.*

epididymal appendix, a cystic structure sometimes found on the head of the epididymis. It represents a remnant of the mesonephros. Also called **appendix epididymidis.**

epididymis /ep′idid″imis/ *pl. epididymides* [Gk, *epi* + *didymos,* pair], one of a pair of long, tightly coiled ducts that carry sperm from the seminiferous tubules of the testes to the vas deferens.

epididymitis /ep′idid′imī″tis/ [Gk, *epi* + *didymos* + *itis,* inflammation], acute or chronic inflammation of the epididymis. It may result from venereal disease, urinary tract infection, prostatitis, prostatectomy, or prolonged use of indwelling catheters. Symptoms include fever and chills; pain in the groin; and tender, swollen epididymides. Treatment includes bed rest, scrotal support, antiinflammatory medications, and antibiotics, as appropriate.

epididymoorchitis /ep′idid′imō′ôrkī″tis/ [Gk, *epi* +, *didymos* + *orchis,* testis, *itis*], inflammation of the epididymis and of the testis. See also **epididymitis, orchitis.**

epididymovesiculography /ep′idid′imōves′ikyəlog″rəfē/, the radiographic examination of the seminal ducts. It is usually performed in cases of sterility, cysts, tumors, abscesses, or inflammation. The contrast medium may be injected through a catheter in the urethra or placed directly in the ducts through a surgical incision in the upper part of the scrotum.

epidural /ep′idoo̅r″əl/ [Gk, *epi* + *dura,* hard], outside or above the dura mater, which surrounds the central nervous system.

epidural abscess, a disorder characterized by inflammation and a collection of pus between the dura mater of the brain and skull, or between the dura mater of the spinal cord and the vertebral canal. It is called an intracranial epidural abscess if the infection is inside the skull. The infection is usually caused by a bacterium such as *Staphylococcus,* but it can also be secondary to a fungal or viral infection, which can occur secondary to a chronic ear or sinus infection, a penetrating head injury, or mastoiditis. Fever, headache, and neurological symptoms are common. Surgery to remove the purulent material and treatment with antibiotics are the usual treatments.

epidural anesthesia/analgesia, a type of anesthesia block in which a local anesthetic is injected into the epidural space surrounding the dural sac, which contains CSF and the spinal cord. Epidurals are most commonly performed in the lumbar area by an injection of medication through a catheter placed in the epidural space. Analgesia is maintained by either intermittent dosing or a continuous infusion into the catheter. Close monitoring of vital signs, respirations, pain, and sensation is important. Epidurals have a wide application in anesthesia and pain management because of their safety and versatility. Epidural anesthesia or analgesia can be tailored to affect an area of the body from the lower extremities to the upper abdomen (thoracic epidural). Epidurals are often used for labor and birth and in postoperative pain management. The most common adverse effects include unintentional dural membrane puncture, postdural puncture headache, and hypotension from sympathetic nerve block and vascular dilation. Severe complications may include intravascular injection of local anesthetic, seizures, or hematoma of the epidural space. See also **caudal anesthesia, epidural hematoma, regional anesthesia.**

epidural blood patch (EBP), a treatment for postdural puncture headache caused by an inadvertent puncture of the dura mater during an epidural anesthetic in which 15 to 20 mL of a patient's autologous blood is injected into the epidural space at or near the location of a dural puncture. The volume injected displaces cerebrospinal fluid (CSF) from the lumbar CSF space into the area surrounding the brain, often yielding immediate relief. When the blood clots, it seals the dural puncture, prohibiting further leakage of CSF from the subarachnoid space.

epidural hematoma, accumulation of blood in the epidural space, caused by damage to and leakage of blood from the middle meningeal artery, producing compression of the dura mater and thus of the brain. Unless evacuated, it may result in herniation through the tentorium and death.

epidural hemorrhage, a hemorrhage that produces a collection of blood outside the dura mater of the brain or spinal cord. It usually results from tearing of the middle meningeal artery and may be rapidly life threatening. Also called **extradural hemorrhage.**

epidural space, the space immediately above and surrounding the dura mater of the brain or spinal cord, beneath the endosteum of the cranium and the spinal column.

epifascial /ep′ifash′ē·əl/ [Gk, *epi* + L, *fascia,* band], on a fascia.

epifolliculitis /ep′ifolik′yəlī″tis/, an inflammation of the hair follicles of the head. See also **folliculitis.**

epigastric /-gas″trik/ [Gk, *epi,* above, *gaster,* stomach], pertaining to the epigastrium, the area above the stomach.

epigastric arteries, the arteries (superficial, superior, and inferior) that supply the medial abdominal wall.

epigastric hernia, the protrusion of an internal organ through the linea alba.

epigastric node [Gk, *epi* + *gaster,* stomach; L, *nodus,* knot], a node in one of the seven groups of parietal lymph nodes serving the abdomen and the pelvis, comprising about four nodes along the caudal portion of the inferior epigastric vessels. See also **lymph, lymphatic system, lymph node.**

epigastric pain [Gk, *epi,* above, *gaster,* stomach; L, *poena,* penalty], pain in the upper middle part of the abdomen.

epigastric reflex [Gk, *epi,* above, *gaster,* stomach; L, *reflectere,* to bend back], a contraction of the rectus abdominis muscle that occurs when the skin surface in the upper and middle abdominal region is stimulated. The reflex also may be induced by stimulation of the axillary region of the fifth and sixth dorsal nerves.

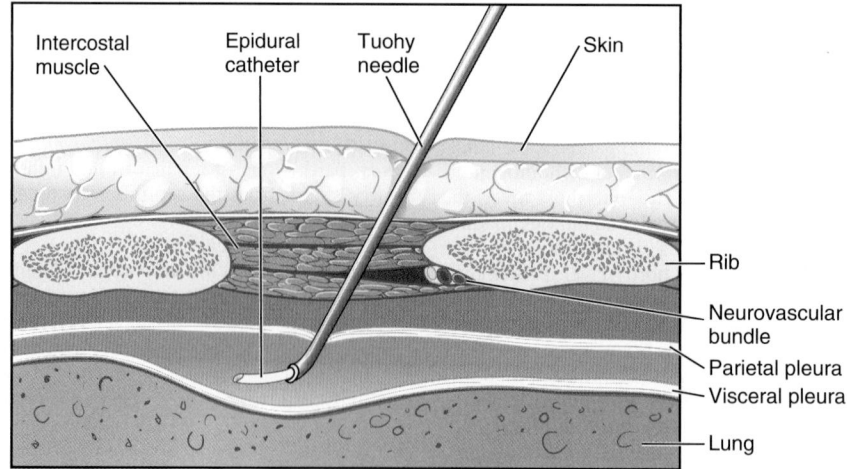

Epidural catheter *(AACN, 2008)*

epigastric region, the part of the abdomen in the upper zone between the right and left hypochondriac regions. Also called **antecardium, epigastrium.** See also **abdominal regions.**

epigastric sensation, a weak, sinking feeling of undefined nature that is usually localized in the pit of the stomach but may occur throughout the abdominal region. See also **sensation,** def. 1.

esophageal dilators, devices consisting of a series of radiopaque flexible tubes of graded diameter for stretching strictures in the esophagus or the cardioesophageal sphincter. Also called *esophageal bougies.*

epigastrium. See **epigastric region.**

epigenesis /ep′ijen″əsis/ [Gk, *epi + genein,* to produce], (in embryology) a theory of development in which the organism grows from a simple to more complex form through the progressive differentiation of an undifferentiated cellular unit. Compare **preformation.** –*epigenetic, adj.,* –*epigenesist, n.*

epigenetics, biological mechanisms that affect gene expression without a change in the DNA sequence. See also **methylation.**

epiglott-, prefix meaning "epiglottis": *epiglottitis.*

epiglottic vallecula, a depression between the lateral and median glossoepiglottic folds on each side.

epiglottiditis. See **epiglottitis.**

epiglottis /ep′iglot″is/ [Gk, *epi + glossa,* tongue], the thin, leaf-shaped cartilaginous structure that overhangs the larynx like a lid and prevents food from entering the larynx and the trachea while swallowing.

epiglottitis /ep′iglotī″tis/ [Gk, *epi + glossa,* tongue, *itis,* inflammation], an inflammation of the epiglottis. Acute epiglottitis is a severe form of the condition, which primarily affected children 2 to 7 years of age before a significant decrease in the occurrence of the disease resulting from the introduction of the *Haemophilus influenzae* B vaccine in 1985. It is characterized by fever; sore throat; drooling; stridor; croupy cough; and an erythematous, swollen epiglottis. The patient may become cyanotic and require an emergency tracheostomy to maintain respiration. The causative organism is usually *Haemophilus influenzae,* type B, but it can also be caused by *Streptococcus,* groups A, B, and C; *S. pneumoniae*; *Klebsiella pneumoniae*; *Candida albicans*; *Staphylococcus aureus*; *Neisseria meningitides*; *Varicella zoster*; and other viruses. Antibiotics, rest, oxygen, and supportive care are usually included in treatment. Also called **epiglottiditis.** See also **acute epiglottitis.**

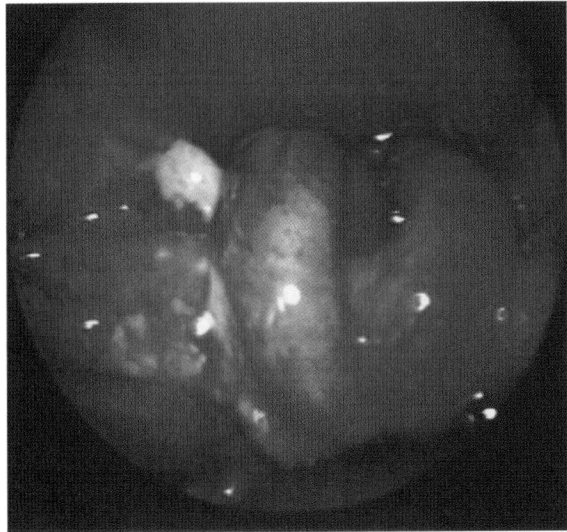

Acute epiglottitis *(Marx et al, 2014)*

epilating forceps /ep′ilā′ting/ [L, *e + pilus,* without hair], a kind of small spring forceps, used for removing unwanted hair.

epilation. See **depilation.**

epilepsy /ep′ilep′sē/ [Gk, *epilepsia,* seizure], a group of neurological disorders characterized by recurrent episodes of convulsive seizures, sensory disturbances, abnormal behavior, loss of consciousness, or all of these. Common to all types of epilepsy is an uncontrolled electrical discharge from the nerve cells of the cerebral cortex. Although most epilepsy is of unknown cause, it is sometimes associated with cerebral trauma, intracranial infection, brain tumor, vascular disturbances, intoxication, or chemical imbalance. See also **absence seizure, focal seizure, psychomotor seizure, tonic-clonic seizure.**

■ OBSERVATIONS: The frequency of attacks may range from many times a day to intervals of several years. In predisposed individuals, seizures may occur during sleep or after physical stimulation, such as by a flickering light or sudden loud sound. Emotional disturbances also may be significant triggers. Some seizures are preceded by an aura, but others have no warning symptoms. Most epileptic attacks are brief. They may be localized or general, with or without clonic movements, and are often followed by drowsiness or confusion. Diagnosis is made by observation of the pattern of seizures and abnormalities on an electroencephalogram. Diagnosis is also aided by a system of classification of the criteria that characterize the different types of epileptic seizures. One major category in the classification scheme encompasses the partial seizures, which often begin focally, then spread to other brain areas. A second major category includes the generalized seizures, which usually begin deep in the brain and impair consciousness.

■ INTERVENTIONS: The kind of epilepsy determines the selection of preventive medication. Correctable lesions and metabolic causes are eliminated when possible. During a seizure the patient should be protected from injury without being severely restrained.

■ PATIENT CARE CONSIDERATIONS: In addition to protecting the patient from injury, a health care provider observing an epileptic seizure should carefully note and accurately describe the sequence of seizure activity. The patient and family must be fully informed and counseled about the disorder; about the importance of regularly taking prescribed medication, never discontinuing treatment without professional advice, and using a medical identification tag; on the toxic effects of medication; and on the importance of maintaining the most normal lifestyle possible. Health care providers also have a responsibility to correct any misunderstanding of this condition that could limit educational or occupational opportunities for individuals who are affected by it.

epileptic dementia [Gk, *epilepsia,* seizure; L, *de + mens,* mind], epileptic events in dementia. They are often unrecognized because they are usually nonconvulsive.

epileptic march. See **cortical march.**

epileptic stupor, *(Obsolete)* the state of unawareness and unresponsiveness that follows an epileptic seizure or postepileptic state. Now called **postictal.**

epileptic vertigo [Gk, *epilepsia,* seizure; L, *vertigo,* dizziness], an aura of dizziness that may precede, accompany, or follow an epileptic seizure.

epileptogenic /ep′ilep′tōjen″ik/, causing epileptic seizures.

epiloia, *(Obsolete)* now called **tuberous sclerosis.**

epimysium /ep′imiz″ē·əm/ [Gk, *epi + mys,* muscle], the outermost fibrous sheath that covers a muscle, continuous

E

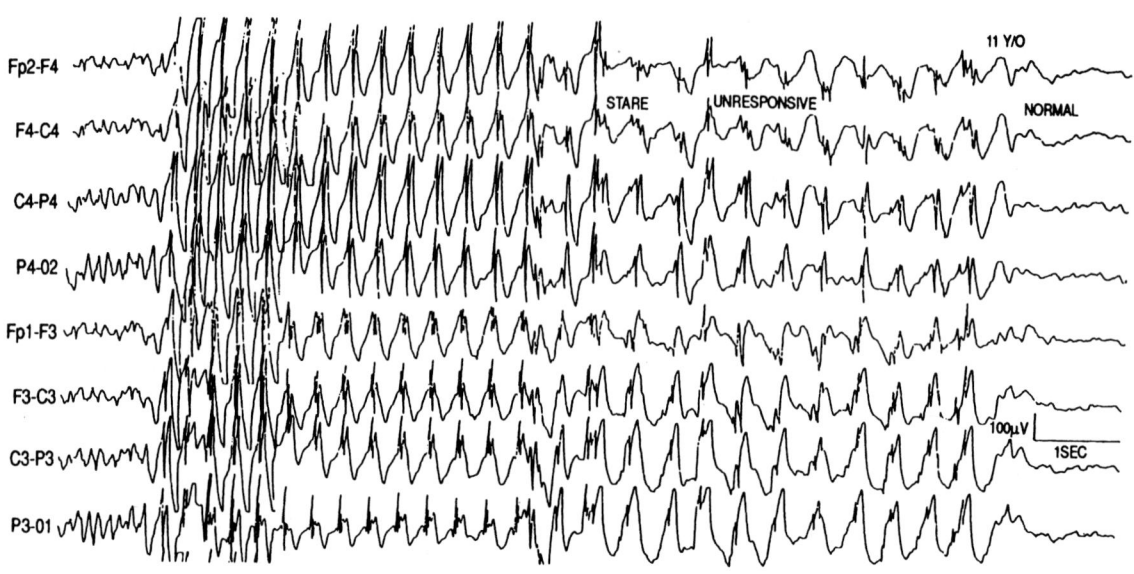

Childhood absence epilepsy: typical EEG pattern *(Goldman et al, 2004)*

Classification of seizures

Type of seizure	Effect on consciousness	Signs and symptoms	Postictal state
Partial seizures			
Simple partial (focal)	Not impaired	Focal twitching of extremity Speech arrest Special visual sensations (e.g., seeing lights) Feeling of fear or doom	No
Complex partial (formerly psychomotor or temporal lobe seizures)	Impaired	May begin as simple partial and progress to complex Automatic behavior (e.g., lip smacking, chewing, or picking at clothes)	Yes
Complex partial progressing to generalized tonic-clonic	Impaired	Begins as complex partial as above, then progresses to tonic-clonic as described below	Yes
Generalized seizures			
Absence (formerly petit mal)	Impaired	Brief loss of consciousness, staring, unresponsiveness	No
Tonic-clonic (formerly grand mal)	Impaired	Tonic phase involving rigidity of all muscles, followed by clonic phase involving rhythmic jerking of muscles, and possibly tongue biting and urinary and fecal incontinence May be any combination of tonic and clonic movements	Yes
Atonic	Impaired for only a few seconds	Brief loss of muscle tone, which may cause patient to fall or drop something; referred to as drop attacks	No
Myoclonic	Impaired for only a few seconds or not at all	Brief jerking of a muscle group, which may cause patient to fall	No

From Monahan FD et al: *Phipps' medical-surgical nursing: health and illness perspectives,* ed 8, St Louis, 2007, Mosby.

with the perimysium. It is sturdy in some areas but more delicate in others, such as those areas where the muscle moves freely under a strong sheet of fascia. The epimysium may also fuse with fascia that attaches a muscle to a bone.

epinephrine /ep′ənef″rin/ [Gk, *epi* + *nephros,* kidney], an endogenous adrenal hormone and synthetic adrenergic agent. It acts as an agonist at alpha₁, alpha₂, beta₁, and beta₂ receptors. Also called **adrenaline.**
■ INDICATIONS: It is prescribed to treat anaphylaxis, acute bronchial spasm, and nasal congestion and to increase the effectiveness of a local anesthetic.

■ CONTRAINDICATIONS: Known hypersensitivity to this drug prohibits its use. It must be used with extreme caution with patients who have cardiac disease or conditions.
■ ADVERSE EFFECTS: Among the most serious adverse effects are arrhythmias, increases in blood pressure, rebound congestion (when it is used as a decongestant), tachycardia, and nervousness.

epiotic /ep′ē·ot″ik/, **1.** pertaining to the portion of the temporal bone that is the ossification center for the mastoid. **2.** above the ear.

epipastic /ep′ipas″tik/ [Gk, *epipassein,* to sprinkle about], dusting powder.

epiphora. See **tearing.**

epiphyseal /epʹifiz″ē·əl, ipifʹəsē″əl/ [Gk, *epi,* above, *phyein,* to grow], pertaining to or resembling the epiphysis of a bone. It is the rounded end of a long bone located at its joint with adjacent bone. The epiphysis of the bone is covered in hyaline cartilage. Also spelled **epiphysial.** See also **bone.**

epiphyseal fracture [Gk, *epi + phyein,* to grow, *fractura,* break], a fracture involving the epiphyseal plate (or growth plate) of a long bone, which causes separation or fragmentation of the plate. Also called **Salter-Harris fracture.**

epiphyseal plate [Gk, *epi,* above, *phyein,* to grow, *platys,* flat], a thin layer of cartilage between the epiphysis and the diaphysis of a bone. It is the bone-forming center responsible for growth in bone length. Epiphyseal plates remain open until late adolescence. Also called **growth plate.**

epiphysial. See **epiphyseal.**

epiphysis /epifʹisis/ *pl. epiphyses* [Gk, *epi + phyein,* to grow], the enlarged proximal and distal ends of a long bone. See also **epiphyseal plate.** –**epiphysial,** *adj.*

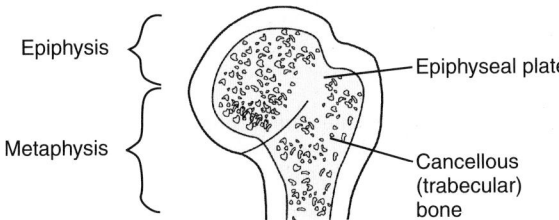

Epiphysis *(Rakel and Rakel, 2011)*

epiphysis cerebri. See **pineal body.**

epiphysitis /ipifʹisīʹtis/, an inflammation of the epiphysis, usually of a long bone, such as the femur or humerus. The disorder mainly affects children.

epipial /epʹi·piʹəl/ [Gk, *epi + L, pia,* soft or tender], situated on the pia mater.

epiploic /epʹiplōʹik/, pertaining to the omentum.

epiploic appendix, one of the fat pads, 2 to 10 cm long, scattered through the peritoneum along the colon and the upper part of the rectum, especially along the transverse and sigmoid colon.

epiploic foramen [Gk, *epiploon,* caul; L, *foramen,* a hole]. See **omental foramen.**

epipygus. See **pygomelus.**

epiretinal /epʹiretʹinal/, overlying the retina.

epiretinal membrane, a pathological membrane partially covering the surface of the retina, probably originating from the retinal pigment epithelial and glial cells. Membranes peripheral to the macula are generally asymptomatic, but those involving the macula or adjacent to it may cause reduction in vision, visual distortion, and diplopia.

epirubicin, an antibiotic antineoplastic drug.

■ INDICATIONS: It is used as an adjuvant therapy to treat breast cancer with axillary node involvement following resection.

■ CONTRAINDICATIONS: Factors that prohibit its use include severe hepatic disease, baseline neutrophil count less than 1500 cells/mm³, severe myocardial insufficiency, recent myocardial infarction, pregnancy, lactation, systemic infections, and known hypersensitivity to this drug, anthracyclines, or anthracenediones.

■ ADVERSE EFFECTS: Life-threatening effects are thrombocytopenia, leukopenia, anemia, neutropenia, secondary acute myelocytic leukemia, sinus tachycardia, premature ventricular contractions, bradycardia, and extrasystoles. Other serious adverse effects include increased blood pressure and chest pain. Common side effects include nausea, vomiting, anorexia, mucositis, diarrhea, amenorrhea, hot flashes, hyperuricemia, rash, necrosis at the injection site, reversible alopecia, infection, febrile neutropenia, lethargy, fever, and conjunctivitis.

episcleritis /epʹisklərīʺtis/, inflammation of the outermost layers of the sclera and the tissues overlying its posterior parts.

episcope, a skin surface microscope that uses the technology of epiluminescence microscopy (the application of oil to produce translucence of the epidermis on a skin lesion). The episcope is placed gently over the lesion to observe its general appearance, surface, pigment pattern, border, and depigmentation.

episi-, prefix meaning "vulva": *episiotomy.*

episiotomy /epēʹzē·otʺəmē/ [Gk, *episeion,* pubic region, *temnein,* to cut], a surgical procedure in which an incision is made in a woman's perineum to enlarge her vaginal opening for delivery. It is performed most often electively to prevent tearing of the perineum, to hasten or facilitate birth of the baby, or to prevent stretching of perineal muscles and connective tissue thought to predispose to subsequent abnormalities of pelvic outlet relaxation, as cystocele, rectocele, and uterine prolapse. Its prophylactic efficacy is debated. It is usually required for a forceps delivery. The incision into the vaginal and perineal tissue is closed with absorbable sutures that need not be removed. Deep incisions require closure in two or more layers. Immediate complications include hemorrhage and extension of the incision along the vaginal sulcus or into the anal sphincter or rectum. Delayed complications include hematoma and abscess. Application of cold packs to the perineum for several hours immediately after delivery minimizes swelling. Later alternating applications of heat and cold and warm sitz baths reduce discomfort, but sitz baths longer than 10 minutes soften tissue and prolong healing time. See also **mediolateral episiotomy, median episiotomy.**

episode /epʺisōd/ [Gk, *episodion,* coming in besides], an incident or event that stands out from the continuity of everyday life, such as an episode of illness or a traumatic event in the course of a child's development. –**episodic,** *adj.*

episode of hospital care, the services provided by a hospital in the continuous course of care of a patient with a health condition. It may cover a sequence from emergency through inpatient to outpatient services.

episodic, occurring at intervals. See **episode.**

episodic care /-sodʹik/, a pattern of health care in which services are provided to a person for a particular problem without an ongoing relationship being established between the person and health care professionals. Emergency departments provide episodic care.

episodic memory, a type of long-term, declarative memory in which are stored memories of personal experiences that are tied to particular times and places. See also **declarative memory.**

episome /epʹisōm/ [Gk, *epi + soma,* body], an extrachromosomal replicating unit that exists autonomously or functions with a chromosome. See also **colicinogen, conjugon, F factor, plasmid, R factor.**

epispadias /epʹispāʺdē·əs/ [Gk, *epi + spadon,* a rent], a congenital defect in which the urethra opens on the dorsum of the penis at any point below the internal sphincter. Other pelvic abnormalities may be present. Treatment focuses on correcting or managing urinary incontinence, which occurs because the urinary sphincters are defective, and on permitting sexual function. The corresponding defect in women, in which the urethra opens by the separation of the labia minora and a fissure of the clitoris, is quite rare.

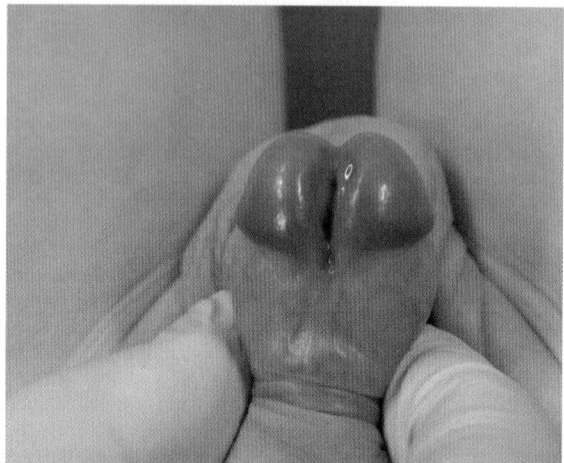

Infant with epispadias (Bos et al, 2013)

epistasis /epis″təsis/ [Gk, a standing], **1.** suppression of a secretion or excretion, as of blood, menses, or lochia. **2.** an interaction between genes at different loci in which one gene masks or suppresses the expression of the other. Epistasis, which is nonallelic and therefore different from dominance, may be caused by the presence of homozygous recessive alleles at one gene pair, as occurs in the Bombay phenotype, or by the presence of a dominant allele at one locus that counteracts the expression of a dominant allele at the other locus. Compare **dominance.** *−epistatic, adj.*

epistaxis /ep′istak″sis/ [Gk, a dropping], bleeding from the nose caused by local irritation of mucous membranes, violent sneezing, fragility or manipulation of the mucous membrane, chronic infection, trauma, hypertension, coagulopathy, vitamin K deficiency, or thrombocytopenia. Also called **nosebleed.**

■ OBSERVATIONS: Epistaxis may result from the rupture of tiny vessels in the anterior nasal septum. This occurs most frequently in early childhood and adolescence. In adults it occurs more commonly in men than in women; may be severe in elderly persons; may be accompanied by respiratory distress, apprehension, restlessness, vertigo, and nausea; and may lead to syncope.

■ INTERVENTIONS: The patient suffering epistaxis is instructed to breathe through the mouth, to sit quietly with the head tilted slightly backward. The bleeding may be controlled by inserting a cotton ball soaked in a topical vasoconstrictor and applying pressure to the skin on both sides of the nose, occluding the blood supply to the nostrils; or by placing an ice compress over the nose. The nasal mucosa may be anesthetized with topical lidocaine, cauterized with a silver nitrate stick or an electrical cautery, and then sprayed with epinephrine. Severe bleeding, especially from the posterior nasal septum, may be treated by packing, which is left in place for 1 to 3 days. Persistent or recurrent profuse epistaxis

may be treated by ligating an artery supplying the nose, such as the external carotid, ethmoid, or internal maxillary artery.

episternal /ep′istur″nəl/, situated on or over the sternum.

epistropheus. See **axis.**

epithalamus /ep′ithal″əməs/ [Gk, *epi* + *thalamos,* chamber], the uppermost portion of the diencephalon. It includes the trigonum habenulae, the pineal body, the posterior commissure, and the medullary layers of thalamus. Compare **hypothalamus, metathalamus, subthalamus, thalamus.** *−epithalamic, adj.*

epithecium, a layer of tissue that covers the hymenium in many fungi.

epithelial /-thē″lē·əl/ [Gk, *epi,* above, *thele,* nipple], pertaining to or involving the outer layer of the skin.

epithelial cancer [Gk, *epi,* above, *thele,* nipple; L, *cancer,* crab], a carcinoma that develops from epithelium or related tissues in the skin, hollow viscera, and other organs. Also called **epithelioma.**

epithelial cell, any one of several cells arranged in one or more layers that form part of a covering or lining of a body surface. The cells usually adhere to one other along their edges and surfaces. One surface is free, and the other rests on a noncellular basement membrane. See also **epithelial tissue.**

epithelial cuff. See **junctional epithelium.**

epithelial cyst, 1. any cyst lined by keratinizing stratified squamous epithelium, found most often in the skin. **2.** epidermal cyst.

epithelial debridement [Gk, *epi,* above, *thele,* nipple; Fr, *débridement,* incision], the removal of the entire inner lining and the attachment from the gingival or periodontal pocket with a gingival curettage. Also called *soft tissue curettage,* **deepithelialization.**

epithelialization /-thē′lē·al′izā″shən/ [Gk, *epi,* above, *thele,* nipple; L, *ization,* process], the regrowth of skin over a wound.

epithelial nevus. See **epidermal nevus.**

epithelial peg [Gk, *epi* + *thele,* nipple], any of the papillary projections of the epithelium that penetrate the underlying stroma of connecting tissue and normally develop in mucous membranes and dermal tissues. Also called **rete peg.**

epithelial rest. See **embryonic rest.**

epithelial tissue [Gk, *epi,* above, *thele,* nipple; OFr, *tissu*], a closely packed single or stratified layer of cells covering the body and lining its cavities, with the exception of the blood and lymph vessels.

epithelioblastoma /ep′ithē′lē·ō′blastō″mə/, a tumor composed of epithelial cells.

epitheliofibril. See **tonofibril.**

epithelioid leiomyoma /ep′ithē″lē·oid/ [Gk, *epi* + *thele* + *eidos,* form], an uncommon neoplasm of smooth muscle in which the cells are polygonal. It usually develops in the stomach. Also called **bizarre leiomyoma, leiomyoblastoma.**

epithelioma /-thē′lē·ō″mə/ [Gk, *epi* + *thele* + *oma,* tumor], a neoplasm derived from the epithelium of the skin.

-epithelioma, suffix meaning a "tumor of epithelial tissue": *adenoepithelioma, fibroepithelioma, trichoepithelioma.*

epithelioma adamantinum. See **ameloblastoma.**

epithelioma adenoides cysticum. See **trichoepithelioma.**

epithelium /-thē′lē·əm/ [Gk, *epi* + *thele,* nipple], the covering of the internal and external organs of the body and the lining of vessels, body cavities, glands, and organs. It consists of cells bound together by connective material and varies in the number of layers and the kinds of cells. The stratified squamous epithelium of the

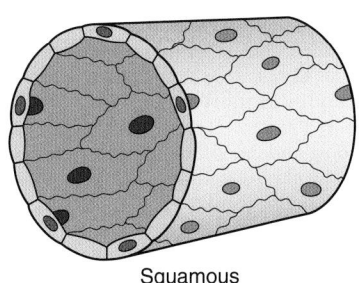 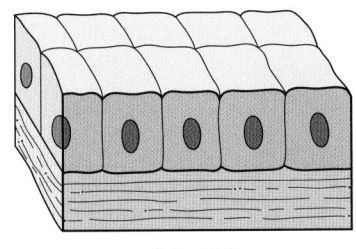 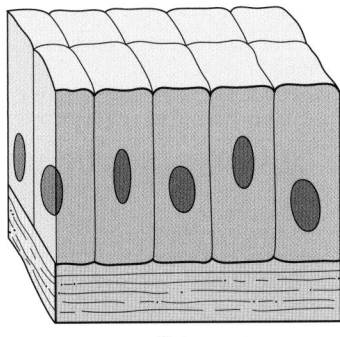

Squamous   Cuboidal   Columnar

Types of epithelial cells (*Coad and Dunstall, 2011*)

E

epidermis comprises five different cellular layers. **—epithelial,** *adj.*

epitope /ep″itōp/ [Gk, *epi + topos,* place]. See **antigenic determinant.**

epitympanic recess /-timpan″ik/ [Gk, *epi + tympanon,* drum], the area of the tympanic cavity cranial to the tympanic membrane. It contains the upper half of the malleus and greater part of the incus. Also called **attic.**

epizootic /ep′izō-ot″ik/, a disease or condition that occurs at about the same time in many animals of the same species in a geographic area.

eplerenone, an antihypertensive agent.

Epley maneuver, a four-step exercise that helps to treat the symptoms of benign paroxysmal positional vertigo (BPPV). Step 1: The individual sits up on a bed, with legs flat on the bed and out front; the head is then turned 45 degrees to the left. Step 2: The individual lies down, keeping the head turned to the left and waits 30 seconds. Step 3: The individual turns the head to the right 90 degrees, until it's facing 45 degrees to the right side and waits 30 seconds. Step 4: The individual rolls over onto the right side before sitting up.

EPO, **1.** abbreviation for **erythropoietin. 2.** abbreviation for **Exclusive Provider Organization.**

eponychium. See **cuticle,** def. 3.

eponym /ep″ənim/ [Gk, *epi,* above, *onyma,* name], a name for a disease, organ, procedure, or body function that is derived from the name of a person, usually a physician or scientist who first identified the condition or devised the object bearing the name. Kinds include **fallopian tube, Parkinson's disease, Billings method.**

epoophoron /ep′ō-of″əron/ [Gk, *epi + oophoron,* ovary], a rudimentary structure that is situated in the mesosalpinx between the ovary and the uterine tube. The epoophoron is a persistent portion of the embryonic mesonephric duct. Also called **parovarium.**

epoprostenol /e″popros′těnol/, name for prostacyclin when used pharmaceutically. It is used in the form of the sodium salt as an inhibitor of platelet aggregation for blood contacting nonbiological systems, as in renal dialysis; as a pulmonary antihypertensive; and as a vasodilator.

epoxy, an organic chemical substructure consisting of a three-membered ring derived from the union of an oxygen atom and two carbon atoms. Epoxy resins are used as bonding agents.

eprosartan /ep″rosar′tan/, an angiotensin II antagonist that causes vasodilation and decreases the effects of aldosterone. It is used as an antihypertensive and is administered orally.

EPS, abbreviation for **electrophysiological study.**

EPSDT, abbreviation for **Early and Periodic Screening Diagnosis and Treatment.**

epsilon /ep″silon/, E, ε, the fifth letter of the Greek alphabet.

Epsom salt. See **magnesium sulfate.**

EPSP, abbreviation for *excitatory postsynaptic potential.*

Epstein-Barr virus (EBV) /ep″stīnbär″/ [Michael A. Epstein, b. 1921, English pathologist; Yvonne M. Barr, 20th-century English virologist; L, *virus,* poison], the herpesvirus that causes infectious mononucleosis and is associated with nasopharyngeal sarcoma, Hodgkin disease, B cell lymphoma, leukoplakia, central nervous system lymphoma in AIDS, and Burkitt lymphoma, especially in immunodeficient patients such as posttransplantation patients on immunosuppressive therapy. It is also thought to cause oral hairy leukoplakia. One of the most common human viruses, it resides in the salivary glands, is transmitted with saliva, and continues to be shed. EBV is ubiquitous. By 40 years of age 99% of the U.S. population has serological evidence of EBV infection. Infection is often asymptomatic. There is no specific treatment. No antiviral drugs are available. The scientific name is human herpesvirus 4 (HHV 4).

Epstein-Barr virus (EBV) titer, a blood test to indicate chronic EBV and associated illnesses.

Epstein pearls [Alois Epstein, Czechoslovakian physician, 1849–1918; L, *perla,* a mussel], small, white pearl-like epithelial cysts that occur on both sides of the midline of the hard palate of the newborn. They are normal and usually disappear within a few weeks. Compare **Bednar aphthae, thrush.**

e.p.t., a brand name for a human pregnancy test kit that uses monoclonal antibody technology to detect the presence of human chorionic gonadotropin in urine.

EP test, abbreviation for *erythrocyte protoporphyrin test.* See **zinc protoporphyrin.**

eptifibatide, an antiplatelet agent.

■ INDICATIONS: It is used to treat acute coronary syndrome, including patients with percutaneous coronary intervention.

■ CONTRAINDICATIONS: The following factors prohibit its use: known hypersensitivity to this drug, active internal bleeding, history of bleeding, stroke within 1 month, major surgery with severe trauma, severe hypotension, history of intracranial bleeding, intracranial neoplasm, arteriovenous malformation/aneurysm, aortic dissection, and dependence on renal dialysis.

■ ADVERSE EFFECTS: Life-threatening effects of this drug are stroke and bleeding. Hypotension is another serious adverse reaction.

epulis /epyōō′lis/ *pl. epulides* [Gk, *epi* + *oulon*, gum], any tumor or growth on the gingiva.

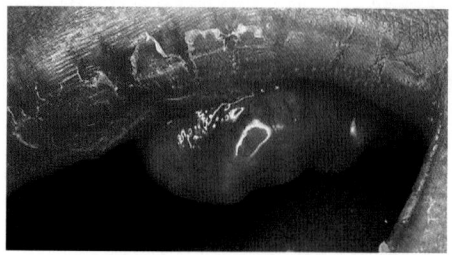

Epulis *(Zitelli and Davis, 2012)*

epulosis /ep′yəlō″sis/, a healing process by scar formation, resulting in the production of a cicatrix.

Equagesic, a fixed-combination central nervous system drug that contains an analgesic and a sedative. Brand name for **aspirin, meprobamate.**

equal cleavage /ē′kwəl/ [L, *aequare*, to make alike; AS, *cleofan*], mitotic division of the fertilized ovum into blastomeres of identical size, as occurs in humans and most other mammals. Compare **unequal cleavage.**

equal distribution, a capitation method used by some health care systems in the United States in which income is distributed equally among health care providers. It is used when the patient population is geographically and clinically homogeneous. See also **capitation.**

Equal Employment Opportunity Commission (EEOC), a body appointed by the president of the United States to administer the Civil Rights Act of 1964, particularly to investigate complaints of discrimination in employment in businesses engaged in interstate commerce. Discrimination based on race, color, creed, or national origin is forbidden, but certain kinds of employers and certain conditions of employment allow exceptions to the act.

Equanil, a sedative. Brand name for **meprobamate.**

equation [L, *aequare*, to make equal], an expression in symbols of equality or equivalence.

equator /ē·kwā′tər/ [L, *aequator*, equalizer], an imaginary line encircling a globe, equidistant from the poles, used in anatomical nomenclature to designate such a line on a spherical organ, dividing the surface into two approximately equal parts.

equatorial plane /ēk′wətôr″ē·əl/ [L, *aequare*, to make alike; Fr, *flat* + *vessel*], the plane at the center of the spindle in which the chromosomes are arranged during metaphase of mitosis and meiosis.

equi-, prefix meaning "equal" or "equality": *equilibrate, equilibrium.*

equianalgesic dose /ē′kwē·an′əljē″sik/, a dose of one analgesic that is equivalent in pain-relieving effects to that of another analgesic. This equivalence permits substitution of medications to prevent possible adverse effects of one of the drugs. The term is also applied to equivalent alternative dose sizes and routes of administration.

equifinality, 1. the capacity of an individual to reach a goal from different starting points and in different ways. 2. the inability to predict how a given situation or event in the present will develop in the future. Systems can change in an infinite number of ways.

equilbrium responses, complex postural reactions that enable the body to recover balance. Equilibrium reactions begin to develop around 6 months of age. They include righting reactions and are essential for volitional movement and mobility. These reactions consist of subtle movements or changes in muscle tone in response to changes in center of gravity. Also called **equilibrium reaction.**

equilibration /ē′kwilibrā″shən/ [L, *aequus,* equal, *libra,* balance], the balancing and integrating of new experiences with those of the past in the psychological development of an individual.

equilibrium /ē′kwilib″rē·əm/ [L, *aequilibrium*], 1. a state of balance or rest resulting from the equal action of opposing forces such as calcium and phosphorus in the body. 2. (in psychiatry) a state of mental or emotional balance. 3. (in radiotherapy) a point at which the rate of production of a daughter element is equal to the rate of decay of the parent element and the activities of parent and daughter are identical.

equilibrium reaction, automatic, reflexive, compensatory movements of body parts that restore and maintain the center of gravity over the base of support when the center of gravity of the supporting surface is displaced. Equilibrium reactions begin to develop around 6 months of age.

equilin /ek′wəlin/, an estrogen isolated from the urine of pregnant horses. It is used in hormone replacement therapy. See also **conjugated estrogen.**

equin-, equino-, prefix meaning "characteristic of a horse": *equinovarus.*

equine antitoxin, an antitoxin derived from the blood of healthy horses immunized against a specific bacterial toxin.

equine encephalitis /ē′kwin, ek′win/ [L, *equus,* horse; Gk, *enkephalon,* brain, *itis,* inflammation], an arbovirus infection with a member of the Togaviridae family, Alphavirus, characterized by inflammation of the nerve tissues of the brain and spinal cord. Other characteristics include high fever, headache, nausea, vomiting, myalgia, and neurological symptoms, such as visual disturbances, tremor, lethargy, and disorientation. The virus is transmitted by the bite of an infected mosquito. Horses are the primary host of the viruses that cause the infection; humans are secondary hosts. Because horses are deadend hosts, they are not a significant risk factor for human infection. Eastern equine encephalitis (EEE) is a severe form of the infection, with a mortality rate of 33%. The main EEE transmission cycle is between mosquitoes and birds, specifically the mosquito *Culiseta melanura.* EEE occurs primarily along the eastern seaboard of the United States and lasts longer and causes more deaths and residual morbidity than western equine encephalitis (WEE), which occurs throughout the United States and produces a mild, brief illness, as does Venezuelan equine encephalitis (VEE), which is common in Central and South America, Florida, and Texas. See also **encephalitis, encephalomyelitis, eastern equine encephalitis, western equine encephalitis, Venezuelan equine encephalitis.**

equine gait [L, *equus,* horse; ONorse, *gate,* a way], a manner of walking characterized by footdrop. The condition is the result of damage to the peroneal nerve, which causes the foot to hang in a toes-downward position.

equinovarus. See **clubfoot.**

equinus /ēkwī′nəs/ [L, horse], a condition characterized by tiptoe walking on one or both feet. It is usually associated with clubfoot.

equipotential, 1. (in physics) indicating bodies that have the same electrical potential. 2. pertaining to lines of force that have the same electrical potential.

equity model /ek″witē/, an organizational model for medical providers in the United States that offers the provider equity in a company instead of cash payments.

equitherapy, the use of horses in animal-assisted therapy for physical, mental, or emotional difficulties.

equivalence /ikwiv″ələns/, a state of being equal in value.

equivalent weight [L, *a* + *aequus* + *valere,* equal value; AS, *gewiht*], **1.** the weight of an element in any given unit (such as grams) that will displace a unit weight of hydrogen from a compound or combine with or replace a unit weight of hydrogen. **2.** the weight of an acid or base that will produce or react with 1.008 grams of hydrogen ion. **3.** the weight of an oxidizing or reducing agent that will produce or accept one electron in a chemical reaction.

equivocal symptom [L, *aequus,* equal, *vocare,* to call; Gk, *symptoma,* that which happens], a symptom that may be attributed to more than one cause or that may occur in several diseases.

Er, symbol for the element **erbium.**

eradication /irad′ikā″shən/, the process of completely removing or destroying something.

Eraxis, an antifungal drug. Brand name for **anidulafungin.**

Erb-Duchenne paralysis. See **Erb palsy.**

Erbitux, an epidermal growth factor receptor used in the treatment of malignancies. Brand name for **cetuximab.**

erbium (Er) /ur″bē·əm/ [Ytterby, Sweden], a metallic rare earth element. Its atomic number is 68; its atomic mass is 167.26.

Erb muscular dystrophy [Wilhelm H. Erb], a form of muscular dystrophy that first affects the shoulder girdle and later often involves the pelvic girdle. It is a progressively disabling disease with onset in childhood or adolescence and is usually inherited as an autosomal-recessive trait. It affects both sexes. In males, differential diagnosis of Erb muscular dystrophy and Duchenne muscular dystrophy may be difficult. Also called **scapulohumeral muscular dystrophy.**

Erb palsy [Wilhelm H. Erb, German neurologist, 1840–1921], a kind of paralysis caused by traumatic injury to the upper brachial plexus. It occurs most commonly as a result of forcible traction during childbirth, with injury to one or more cervical nerve roots. The signs of Erb palsy include loss of sensation in the arm and paralysis and atrophy of the deltoid, the biceps, and the brachialis muscles. The arm on the affected side hangs loosely with the elbow extended and the forearm pronated. Treatment initially requires that the arm and shoulder be immobilized to allow the swelling and inflammation of the associated neuritis to resolve. Physical therapy, occupational therapy, and splinting may be necessary to improve muscle function and to prevent flexion contracture of the elbow. Also called **Erb-Duchenne paralysis.**

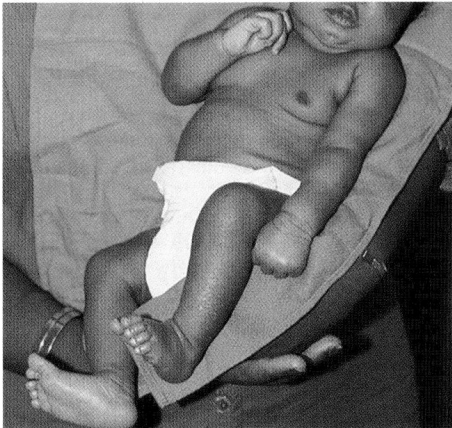

Infant with Erb palsy *(Hockenberry and Wilson, 2015)*

Erb's point [Wilhelm H. Erb], a landmark of the brachial plexus on the upper trunk, located about 1 inch (2.5 cm) above the clavicle at about the level of the sixth cervical vertebra. The point is the location of an angle between the posterolateral border of the sternocleidomastoid muscle and the clavicle. Electrical stimulation at Erb's point causes contractions of the biceps, deltoid, and other arm muscles.

ERCP, abbreviation for **endoscopic retrograde cholangiopancreatography.**

erectile /irek″til, -tīl/ [L, *erigere,* to erect], capable of being erected or raised to an erect position. The term is usually used to describe spongy tissue of the penis or clitoris that becomes turgid and erectile when filled with blood. It also may be used when referring to the epidermal tissue involved in the appearance of "goose bumps" (piloerection) in response to fear, anger, cold, or other stimuli.

erectile dysfunction, failure by a male to attain or maintain erection until completion of sexual relations on an ongoing basis. The cause may be physical or psychological in nature. See **impotence.**

erectile myxoma, an angioma that contains areas of myxomatous tissue.

erection /irek″shən/ [L, *erigere,* to erect], the condition of hardness, swelling, and elevation observed in the penis and to a lesser degree in the clitoris, usually caused by sexual arousal but also occurring during sleep or after physical stimulation. It results when additional blood enters the organ and blood pressure within the organ increases, and it is influenced by psychic and nerve stimulation. Erection enables the penis to enter the vagina and to emit semen. See also **ejaculation, nocturnal emission, priapism.**

erector spinae. See **sacrospinalis.**

erector spinae reflex [L, *erigere,* to erect, *spina,* spine, *reflectere,* to bend back], a reflex characterized by contraction of the sacrospinalis and other back muscles when the overlying skin is stimulated. Also called **dorsal reflex, lumbar reflex.**

ERF, abbreviation for **edge response function.**

erg /urg, erg/, a unit of energy in the centimeter-gram-second system equal to the work done by a force of 1 dyne through a distance of 1 cm. 1 erg |m = 10^{-7} J. See also **joule.**

-erg-, combining form denoting an ergot alkaloid derivative.

ergastoplasm /ərgas″təplaz′əm/ [Gk, *ergaster,* worker, *plassein,* to mold], a network of cytoplasmic structures that show basophilic staining properties. See also **endoplasmic reticulum.**

-ergic, -ergetic, suffix meaning an "effect of activity": *allergic, adrenergic, cholinergic.*

ergo-, combining form meaning "work": *ergometer, ergotherapy.*

ergocalciferol. See **calciferol.**

ergogenic /ur′gōjen″ik/, a tendency to increase work output.

ergogenic aid, a technique or substance used by athletes with the expectation that it will provide a competitive edge. Classifications of ergogenic aids include nutritional, pharmacologic, physiologic, or psychologic. The aids range from the use of accepted techniques, such as carbohydrate loading, to illegal approaches, such as anabolic-androgenic steroid use.

ergoloid mesylate /ur″gōloid/, an ergot alkaloid preparation with psychotropic actions but lacking significant vasoconstrictor or vasodilator effects.

■ INDICATIONS: It is occasionally prescribed in the treatment of symptomatic age-related decline in mental capacity with an unknown cause, as in senile dementia, but its efficacy is not well established.

■ CONTRAINDICATIONS: Psychosis or known sensitivity to this drug prohibits its use.

■ ADVERSE EFFECTS: Among the most serious adverse effects are sublingual irritation, transient nausea, and gastric disturbance.

Ergomar, an ergot alkaloid. Brand name for **ergotamine tartrate.**

ergometer. See **dynamometer.**

ergometrine maleate. See **ergonovine maleate.**

ergometry /ərgom″ətrē/, the study of physical work activity of the body in motion, including activity performed by specific muscles or muscle groups. Studies may involve testing with equipment such as stationary bicycles, treadmills, or rowing machines.

ergonomics /ur′gōnom″iks/ [Gk, *ergon,* work, *nomos,* law], a scientific discipline devoted to the study and analysis of human work, especially as it is affected by individual anatomical, psychological, and other human characteristics. —*ergonomic, adj.*

ergonovine maleate /ur′gōnō″vēn/, an oxytocic ergot alkaloid. Also called **ergometrine maleate.**

■ INDICATIONS: It is prescribed to contract the uterus in the treatment or prevention of postpartum or postabortion hemorrhage caused by uterine atony.

■ CONTRAINDICATIONS: Pregnancy, peripheral vascular disease, elevated blood pressure, or known hypersensitivity to this drug prohibits its use.

■ ADVERSE EFFECTS: Among the more serious adverse effects are hypertension, nausea, headache, blurred vision, and hypersensitivity reactions. Fetal death may result from use of the drug in pregnancy.

ergosome. See **polysome.**

ergosterol /ərgos″tərôl/, an unsaturated hydrocarbon of the vitamin D group isolated from yeast, mushrooms, ergot, and other fungi. When treated with ultraviolet irradiation it is converted into vitamin D_2. See also **calciferol, viosterol, vitamin D.**

ergot /ur″gət/ [L, *ergota,* a grain fungus], a fungus structure that replaces the seed of rye and other cereal grasses infested with the parasitic fungus *Claviceps purpurea.* Ergot contains ergot alkaloids, the agents responsible for what was known as St. Anthony's fire in people who consumed the contaminated grain in the Middle Ages. Effects included hallucinations and such intense vasoconstriction in the extremities that portions of the limbs often developed gangrene and fell off before the person died.

ergot alkaloid, one of a large group of alkaloids derived from a common fungus, *Claviceps purpurea.* The alkaloids comprise three groups: the amino acid alkaloids typified by ergotamine, the dihydrogenated amino acid alkaloids such as dihydroergotamine, and the amine alkaloids such as ergonovine.

■ INDICATIONS: Ergotamine and dihydroergotamine are less effective oxytocics than ergonovine. Therefore ergonovine, given orally or intravenously, is currently used in obstetrics to treat or prevent postpartum uterine atony and to complete an incomplete or missed abortion. Ergotamine is prescribed to relieve migraine headache. It acts by reducing the amplitude of arterial pulsations in the external carotid branches of the cranial arteries resulting from stimulation of vasoconstrictive alpha receptors, and it may also act as a serotonin antagonist.

■ CONTRAINDICATIONS: Peripheral vascular disease, coronary artery disease, hypertension, renal or hepatic dysfunction, and sepsis are contraindications for ergot alkaloids. Pregnancy prohibits their use because they may cause contractions of the uterus, decreased blood flow to the fetus, and fetal death.

■ ADVERSE EFFECTS: Ergot poisoning may result from prolonged or excessive use of the drug or accidental ingestion of contaminated grain. Signs of toxicity are thirst, diarrhea, dizziness, chest pain, abnormal and variable rate of cardiac contraction, nausea and vomiting, digital paresthesia, severe cramping, and seizures. Tissue anoxia and gangrene of the extremities may occur as a result of prolonged vasoconstriction if poisoning is severe.

ergotamine tartrate /ərgot″əmēn/, a vasoconstrictor that binds to several receptor populations (e.g., alpha-adrenergic, dopamine, serotonin) and, depending upon the receptor, can be an agonist or antagonist.

■ INDICATIONS: It is prescribed to abort or prevent vascular headaches such as migraines.

■ CONTRAINDICATIONS: Pregnancy, peripheral vascular disease, infectious disease, or known hypersensitivity to this drug prohibits its use.

■ ADVERSE EFFECTS: Among the more serious adverse effects are vomiting, diarrhea, thirst, tingling of fingers and toes, and increased blood pressure. Fetal death may occur if it is used during pregnancy.

ergotherapy /ur′gōther″əpē/ [Gk, *ergon,* work, *therapeia,* treatment], the use of physical activity and exercise in the treatment of disease. By extension the therapy includes any procedure that increases the blood supply to a diseased or injured part, such as massage or various types of hot baths. —*ergotherapeutic, adj.*

ergotism /ur′gətiz″əm/ [L, *argota,* a grain fungus], **1.** an acute or chronic disease caused by excessive dosages of medications containing ergot. Symptoms may include cerebrospinal manifestations such as spasms, cramps, and dry gangrene. **2.** a chronic disease caused by ingestion of cereal products made with rye flour contaminated by ergot fungus.

ergot poisoning [L, *argota,* a grain fungus; L, *potio,* drink], the toxic effects of ingesting food or medications containing ergot alkaloids, particularly ergotamine. See also **ergotism.**

ergotropic /ur′gōtrop″ik/, **1.** pertaining to an activity or work state involving somatic muscle, sympathetic nervous system, and cortical alpha rhythm activity. **2.** pertaining to the administration of medications or other therapies to energize the power of the body's blood and other tissues to resist infections.

-ergy, **1.** suffix meaning an "action": *energy, synergy.* **2.** suffix meaning an "effect" or "result": *allergy, photoallergy.*

-eridine, suffix denoting an analgesic of the meperidine group.

Erikson, Erik [1902–1994], a psychologist who described the development of identity of the self and the ego through successive stages that naturally unfold throughout the lifespan. The eight stages are trust vs. mistrust (infancy); autonomy vs. shame and doubt (toddlerhood); initiative vs. guilt (preschool); industry vs. inferiority (middle childhood); identity vs. role confusion (adolescence); intimacy vs. isolation (young adulthood); generativity vs. stagnation (middle adulthood); and ego integrity vs. despair (older adulthood).

Eriksson, Katie, a nursing theorist who developed the Theory of Caritative Care, which distinguishes between caring ethics, the practical relation between the patient and the nurse, and nursing ethics, the ethical principles and rules that guide decision-making. Caritative caring consists of love and charity, or caritas, and respect and reverence for human holiness and dignity. Suffering related to lack of caritative care violates human dignity.

ERISA, abbreviation for **Employment Retirement Income Security Act.**

erlotinib, a miscellaneous antineoplastic drug.

■ INDICATIONS: This drug is used in the treatment of non–small cell lung cancer.

■ CONTRAINDICATIONS: Pregnancy and known hypersensitivity to this drug prohibit its use.

■ ADVERSE EFFECTS: A life-threatening side effect of this drug is interstitial lung disease. Common side effects include nausea, diarrhea, vomiting, anorexia, mouth ulceration, rash, conjunctivitis, eye pain, fatigue, infection, cough, and dyspnea.

erogenous /iroj′ənəs/ [Gk, *eros,* love, *genein,* to produce], pertaining to the production of erotic sensations or sexual excitement. Also called **erotogenic.**

erogenous zones, areas of the body in which sexual tension tends to become concentrated and can be relieved by manipulation of the region. The areas include the mouth, anus, nipples, and genitals.

Eros /ir′os, er′os/ [Gk, mythic love-inciting son of Aphrodite], a Freudian term for the drive or instinct for love, creativity, and survival, including self-preservation and continuation of the species through reproduction. Compare **Thanatos.**

erosion /irō′zhən/ [L, *erodere,* to consume], **1.** the wearing away or gradual destruction of a surface. For example, a mucosal or epidermal surface may erode as a result of inflammation, injury, or other causes, usually marked by the appearance of an ulcer. See also **necrosis. 2.** the action of acid (low pH) substances dissolving tooth structure. Can be due to habitual sucking on citrus fruits such as lemons, from acidic swimming pool water, or gastroesophageal reflux.

erosive gastritis /irō′siv/, an inflammatory condition characterized by multiple erosions of the mucous membrane lining the stomach. Nausea, anorexia, pain, and gastric hemorrhage may occur. Acute erosive gastritis involves erosions of the full thickness of the stomach mucosa, usually with some degree of hemorrhaging; it may be either localized or diffuse. Chronic erosive gastritis is a type of chronic gastritis with mild symptoms, characterized by multiple punctate or aphthous ulcers, found by endoscopy. Some patients have nausea and vomiting, but others are symptom free. Complications include perforation, penetration into a surrounding organ, and hemorrhage. The cause may be a reaction to nonsteroidal antiinflammatory drugs, a complication of Crohn's disease or a viral infection, or an unknown factor. Also called **varioliform gastritis.** See also **chemical gastritis, corrosive gastritis.**

erosive osteoarthritis, a form of osteoarthritis affecting the proximal and distal interphalangeal joints, the first metatarsophalangeal and carpometacarpal joints, the knees, and the spine. The absence of rheumatoid factor and rheumatoid nodules and the lack of systemic involvement differentiate this syndrome from rheumatoid arthritis. Also called **Kellgren syndrome.**

-erotic, suffix meaning "sexual love or desire": *autoerotic, eroticism.*

eroticism /irot′isiz′əm/ [Gk, *erotikos,* sexual love], **1.** sexual impulse or desire. **2.** the arousal or attempt to arouse the sexual instinct through suggestive or symbolic means. **3.** the expression of sexual instinct or desire. **4.** an abnormally persistent sexual drive. Also called *erotism.* See also **anal eroticism, oral eroticism.**

eroto- /irot′ə-/, prefix meaning "sexual love or desire": *erotogenic.*

erotogenic. See **erogenous.**

erratic /irat′ik/ [L, *erraticus,* wandering], deviating from the normal but with no apparent fixed course or purpose.

error [L, *errare,* to wander], **1.** (in research) a defect in the design of a study, in the development of measurements or instruments, or in the interpretation of findings. **2.** a mistake.

error message, a brief statement rendered by a computer and recorded for review, sometimes displayed to the user by way of a peripheral device, such as a monitor or printer, often indicating that a procedure or command has failed to complete. Messages that are not displayed in real time can be reviewed by developers by way of an error log.

error theory of aging, a theory of aging that ascribes aging to the accumulation of errors in the process of information flow from genes to proteins. The errors create faulty proteins that do not function normally, resulting in impaired cell function and death. See also **theories of aging.**

ERT, abbreviation for **external radiation therapy.**

ertapenem, an antiinfective agent to treat adults with moderate to severe infections, complicated skin and skin structure infections, and complicated urinary tract infections.

erucic acid /erōō′sik/, a fatty acid that has been associated with heart disease. It is present in rapeseed oil that is used in some countries as a vegetable oil for salad dressings, margarines, and mayonnaise. Canola oil is a rapeseed oil from which virtually all erucic acid has been removed through breeding.

eructation /ē′ruktā′shən/ [L, *eructare,* to belch], the act of drawing up air from the stomach with a characteristic sound through the mouth. Also called **belching.**

eruption /irup′shən/ [L, *eruptio,* bursting forth], the appearance of rapidly forming skin lesions, especially of a viral exanthem, or of a rash that commonly accompanies a drug reaction.

eruptive fever /irup′tiv/ [L, *eruptio,* bursting forth; *febris*], a febrile disease of Mediterranean regions, Africa, the Crimea, and India, caused by infection with *Rickettsia conorii.*

eruptive gingivitis, inflammation of the gums that may occur when the secondary teeth (adult dentition) break through into the oral cavity.

eruptive xanthoma, a skin disorder associated with elevated triglyceride levels in the blood. Numerous erythematous or pale, raised papules suddenly appear on the trunk, legs, arms, and buttocks.

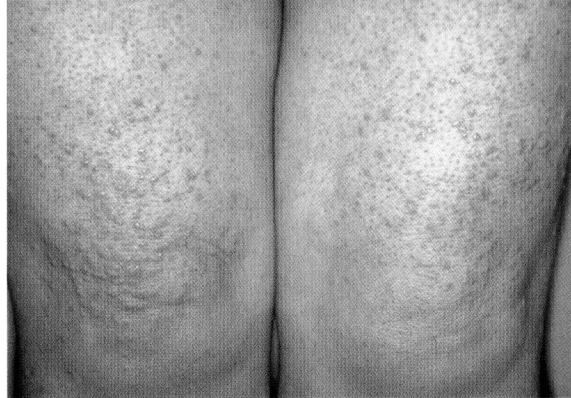

Eruptive xanthoma *(James and Elston, 2018)*

ERV, abbreviation for **expiratory reserve volume.**

erysipelas /er′isip′ələs/ [Gk, *erythros,* red, *pella,* skin], an infectious skin disease characterized by redness, swelling, vesicles, bullae, fever, pain, and lymphadenopathy. It is caused by a species of group A beta-hemolytic streptococci. Predisposing conditions include diabetes, HIV, and nephrotic syndrome, as well as immunocompromised conditions. It is also seen in those with vagrant lifestyles. Treatment includes antibiotics, analgesics, and packs or dressings applied locally to the lesions.

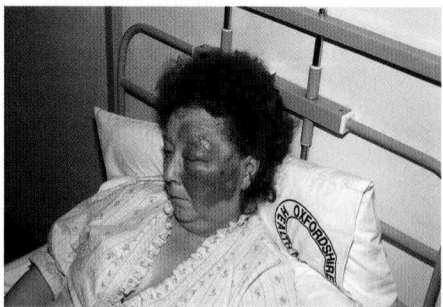

Woman with erysipelas *(Conlon and Snydman, 2000)*

erysipeloid /er′isip″əloid/ [Gk, *erhthros + pella + eidos,* form], an infection of the hands characterized by blue-red patches and occasionally by erythema. It is acquired by handling meat or fish infected with *Erysipelothrix rhusiopathiae.* The disease is self-limited, lasting about 3 weeks, but responds to penicillin. Also called **fish-handler's disease.** Should not be confused with **erysipelas.**

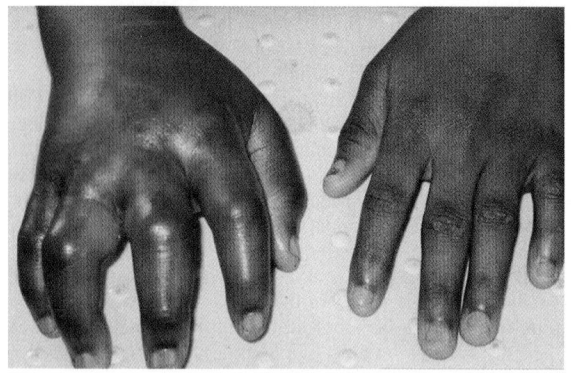

Patient with erysipeloid infection *(Habif, 2016)*

erythema /er′ithē″mə/ [Gk, *erythros,* red], redness or inflammation of the skin or mucous membranes that is the result of dilation and congestion of superficial capillaries. Examples of erythema are nervous blushes and mild sunburn. See also **erythroderma, rubor. –erythematous,** *adj.*

erythema infectiosum, an acute benign infectious disease, mainly of childhood, characterized by fever and an erythematous rash that begins on the cheeks and later appears on the arms, thighs, buttocks, and trunk. As the rash progresses, earlier lesions fade. Sunlight aggravates the eruption, which usually lasts about 10 days but may recur in 1 to 3 weeks or longer after exposure to sunlight or heat. For a period the rash may reappear whenever the skin is irritated. It is caused by parvovirus B$_{19}$. Morbidity is more significant in adults, immunocompromised patients, pregnant women, and those with uremia. Isolation of patients is not required. Also called **fifth disease.**

erythema marginatum, a skin disorder seen in acute rheumatic fever, sepsis, hereditary angioedema, and other conditions; it is characterized by temporary disk-shaped nonpruritic reddened macules that fade in the center, leaving raised margins.

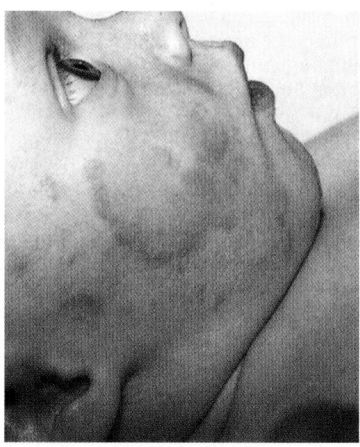

Infant with erythema marginatum *(Weston, Lane, and Morrelli, 2007)*

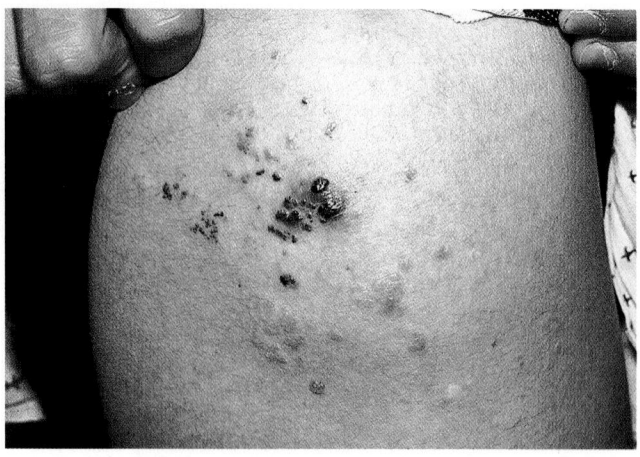

Erythema infectiosum *(Cohen, 2013)*

erythema migrans (EM), a disease that begins as small papules that spread peripherally, characterized by a raised, red margin and clearing in the center. It may mark the site of a tick bite and is a diagnostic sign of Lyme disease. Also called **bullseye rash.** See also **Lyme disease.**

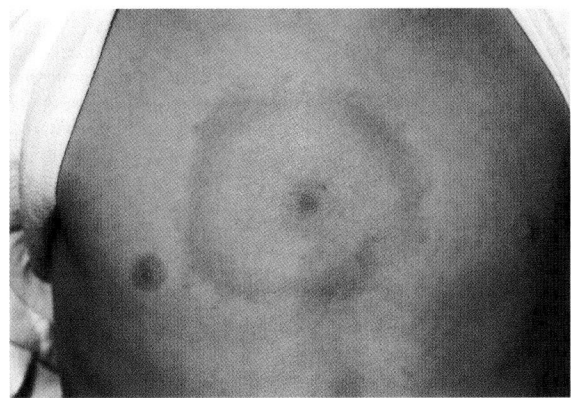

Erythema migrans associated with Lyme disease *(Paller and Mancini, 2011)*

erythema multiforme (EM) /mul′tifôr″mē, mōōl′tēfôr″mā/, any of three major clinical syndromes characterized by lymphocytic infiltrates in the skin that cause keratinocyte necrosis. The patient may experience polymorphous eruption of skin and mucous membranes. Macules, papules, nodules, vesicles or bullae, and target (bullseye-shaped) lesions are seen. The three major classifications of erythema multiforme are EM minor, EM major, and pure plaque toxic epidermal necrosis. EM minor is an acute form of the disease, characterized by three-ring target lesions on the extremities. Symptoms often follow an infection of herpes simplex. The patient may have raised lesions but no fever and no blistering. EM major is characterized by the presence of target lesions, blistering, and detachment of the skin and mucous membranes. EM major also tends to follow herpes simplex virus infections. Plaque toxic epidermal necrolysis may not be associated with target lesions. However, the condition is associated with detachment of large sheets of skin. It is generally drug induced. Definitive and preventive treatment depends on finding the specific cause. Supportive treatment includes the normalization of electrolytes, hydration, and topical steroids and emollients.

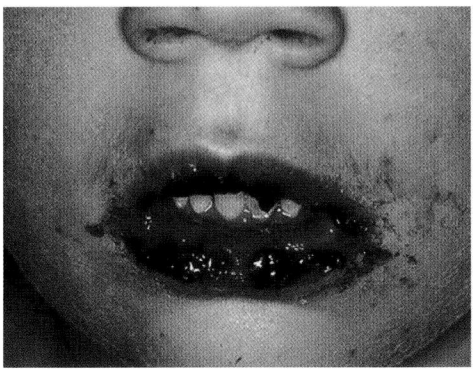

Child with erythema multiforme *(Bolognia et al, 2014)*

erythema neonatorum, a common skin condition of neonates characterized by a pink papular rash frequently superimposed with vesicles or pustules. The rash appears within 24 to 48 hours after birth and disappears spontaneously after several days. A smear of the papules that reveals the presence of eosinophils rather than neutrophils differentiates the condition from neonatal pustular melanosis. Also called **toxic erythema of the newborn.**

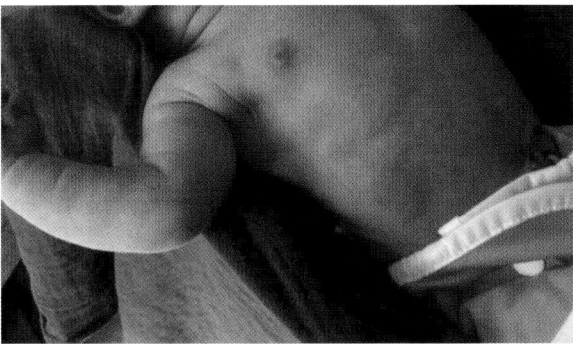

Erythema neonatorum *(Gleason and Juul, 2018).*

erythema nodosum, a hypersensitivity reaction characterized by reddened, tender, subcutaneous nodules on the extensor aspects of the extremities, such as the shins. The nodules last for several days or weeks, never ulcerate, and are often associated with mild fever, malaise, and pain in muscles and joints. This condition may accompany streptococcal infections, tuberculosis, sarcoidosis, drug sensitivity, ulcerative colitis, and pregnancy. A course of corticosteroids is usually effective in diminishing the symptoms.

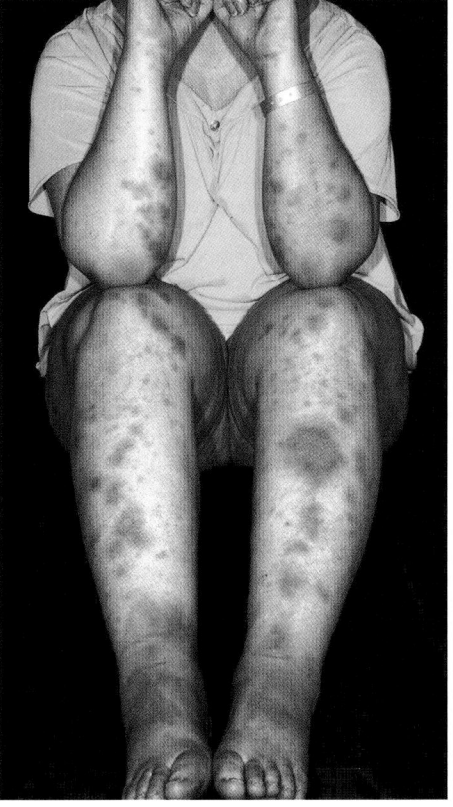

Patient with erythema nodosum *(Habif, 2010)*

erythema perstans, a persistent local redness of the skin, characteristically annular.

erythematous. See **erythema.**

erythematous pemphigus [Gk, *erythros,* red, *pemphix,* bubble], a skin disorder characterized by bullous eruptions on the trunk and a facial eruption that resembles that of lupus erythematosus. The condition may be accompanied by seborrheic dermatitis. Also called **pemphigus erythematosus,** *Senear-Usher syndrome.*

erythemo-, combining form meaning "red": *erythematous, erythemogenic.*

erythemogenic /er″ithe″mojen′ik/, producing or causing erythema.

erythralgia /er′ithral′jə/ [Gk, *erythros,* red, *algos,* pain], a skin disorder characterized by a painful burning sensation, raised skin temperature, and redness, generally of the lower limbs.

erythrasma /er′ithraz″mə/ [Gk, *erythros,* red], a bacterial skin infection caused by *Corynebacterium minutissimum,* common in the axillary or inguinal region and characterized by irregular reddish-brown areas. An asymptomatic disease, it is more common in diabetics and responds quickly to oral erythromycin. Compare **intertrigo, tinea cruris.**

erythremia /er′ithrē′mē·ə/ [Gk, *erythros* + *haima,* blood], an abnormal increase in the number of red blood cells. See **polycythemia.**

erythro-, combining form meaning "red": *erythroblast, erythrocyte.*

erythroblast /erith″rəblast′/, a nucleated immature form of a red blood cell found only in bone marrow.

erythroblastoma /-blastō″mə/ [Gk, *erythros,* red, *blastos,* germ, *oma,* tumor], a myeloma tumor (osteolytic neoplasm) in which the cells resemble erythroblasts.

erythroblastosis /-blastō′sis/, the presence of abnormally large numbers of erythroblasts in the peripheral blood.

erythroblastosis fetalis /-blastō″sis/ [Gk, *erythros* + *blastos,* germ, *osis,* condition; L, *fetus,* bringing forth], a type of hemolytic anemia in newborns that results from maternal-fetal blood group incompatibility, specifically involving the Rh factor and the ABO blood groups. The condition is caused by an antigen-antibody reaction in the bloodstream of the infant resulting from placental transmission of maternally formed antibodies against the incompatible antigens of the fetal blood. In Rh factor incompatibility, the hemolytic reaction occurs only when the mother is Rh negative and the infant is Rh positive. The isoimmunization process rarely occurs in the first pregnancy, but there is increased risk with each succeeding pregnancy. See also **hydrops fetalis, hyperbilirubinemia of the newborn, Rh factor, hemolytic disease of the fetus and newborn.**

erythrochromia /-krō″mē·ə/, **1.** a red coloration or stain. **2.** red pigmentation in spinal fluid caused by the presence of blood.

Erythrocin, an antibiotic. Brand name for **erythromycin.**

erythrocyanosis /-sī′ənō′sis/, a condition characterized by bluish-red discoloration of skin accompanied by swelling, burning, and itching. It is caused by exposure to cold.

erythrocyte /erith″rəsīt′/ [Gk, *erythros* + *kytos,* cell], mature red blood cell; a biconcave disk about 7 μm in diameter that contains hemoglobin confined within a lipoid membrane. It is the major cellular element of the circulating blood and transports oxygen as its principal function. The number of red blood cells per microliter of blood is 4.5 to 5.5 million in men and 4.2 to 4.8 million in women. The red blood cell count varies with age, activity, and environmental conditions. An erythrocyte normally survives for 110 to 120 days, when it is removed from the bloodstream and broken down by the reticuloendothelial system. New erythrocytes are produced at a rate of slightly more than 1% a day; thus a constant level is usually maintained. Acute blood loss, hemolytic anemia, or chronic oxygen deprivation may cause erythrocyte production to increase greatly. Erythrocytes originate in the marrow of the flat bones or at the end of long bones. Also called **red cell, red corpuscle.** Compare **normoblast, reticulocyte.** See also **erythropoiesis, hemoglobin, red cell indexes.**

erythrocyte reinfusion, the process of injecting into an individual's bloodstream red blood cells previously taken from that individual and preserved temporarily by freezing. The process is managed in the same manner as when an individual donates his or her own blood for later retransfusion. Also called **autologous transfusion.**

erythrocyte sedimentation rate (ESR), the rate at which red blood cells settle out in a vertical column of anticoagulated whole blood, expressed in millimeters per hour. Blood is collected in an anticoagulant and allowed to form a sediment in a calibrated glass column. At the end of 1 hour the laboratory technician measures the distance the erythrocytes have fallen in the tube. Elevated sedimentation rates are not specific for any disorder but most commonly indicate the presence of inflammation. Inflammation causes an alteration of the blood proteins, which makes the red blood cells aggregate, becoming heavier than normal. The speed with which they fall to the bottom of the tube corresponds to the degree of inflammation. Serial evaluations of erythrocyte sedimentation rate are useful in monitoring the course of inflammatory activity in rheumatic diseases and, when performed with a white blood cell count, can indicate infection. Certain noninflammatory conditions, such as pregnancy, are also characterized by high sedimentation rates. The Westergren ESR is determined with a 200-mm Westergren tube. Values are higher for women in both methods and vary according to the method used. Normal findings by the Westergren method are up to 20 mm/hr for females and up to 15 mm/hr for males. Other diseases that alter blood proteins can also cause abnormal ESRs. Also called **sedimentation rate.** See also **inflammation.**

erythrocythemia /erith″rōsīthē″mē·ə/ [Gk, *erythros* + *kytos* + *haima,* blood], an increase in the number of erythrocytes circulating in the blood.

erythrocytosis /erith″rōsītō″sis/ [Gk, *erythros* + *kytos* + *osis,* condition], an abnormal increase in the number of circulating red cells. See also **polycythemia.**

erythroderma /erith″rōdur″mə/ [Gk, *erythros* + *derma,* skin], an abnormal redness of the skin. Compare **erythema, rubor.**

erythroderma desquamativum. See **Leiner disease.**

erythroderma polyneuropathy. See **acrodynia.**

erythrogenesis, the creation of red blood cells. See also **erythropoiesis.**

erythroid /erith″roid/, **1.** reddish in color. **2.** pertaining to erythrocytes.

erythroleukemia /-lookē″mē·ə/ [Gk, *erythros* + *leukos,* white, *haima,* blood], a malignant blood disorder characterized by a proliferation of erythropoietic elements in bone marrow, erythroblasts with bizarre lobulated nuclei, and abnormal myeloblasts in peripheral blood. The disease may have an acute or chronic course. Also called **Di Guglielmo disease, Di Guglielmo syndrome, erythromyeloblastic leukemia.**

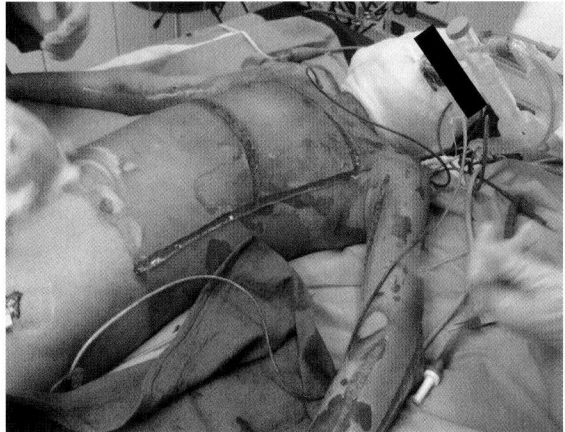

Erythroleukemia *(Carr and Rodak, 2008)*

erythroleukosis, an abnormal increase in numbers of granulocytes and red blood cells.

erythromelalgia /erith′rōmilal″jə/ [Gk, *erythros + melos,* limb, *algos,* pain], a rare disorder characterized by a paroxysmal dilation of the peripheral blood vessels. It occurs bilaterally, usually in the extremities, and is associated with burning, redness of the skin, and pain. −*erythromelalgic, adj.*

erythromycin /erith′rōmī″sin/, an antibiotic (of the macrolide type).

■ INDICATIONS: It is prescribed in the treatment of many bacterial and mycoplasmic infections, particularly those that cannot be treated by penicillin.

■ CONTRAINDICATIONS: Liver disease or known hypersensitivity to this drug prohibits its use.

■ ADVERSE EFFECTS: The more serious adverse effects result from its effects on the metabolism of other drugs, which have led to fatalities. Cholestatic hepatitis, hypersensitivity reactions, and GI discomfort are other adverse effects associated with its use.

erythromyeloblastic leukemia. See **erythroleukemia.**

erythron /erith′ron/, the total mass of circulating red blood cells (RBCs) and the RBC-forming tissues from which they are derived.

erythropathy /er′ithrop″əthē/, any disease involving the red blood cells (erythrocytes).

erythropenia. See **hypocythemia.**

erythrophage /erith″rəfāj/, a phagocyte that ingests red blood cells or blood pigment.

erythrophobia /-fō″bē-ə/ [Gk, *erythros + phobos,* fear], **1.** an anxiety disorder characterized by an irrational fear of blushing or of displaying embarrassment. **2.** a symptom manifested by blushing at the slightest provocation. **3.** a morbid fear of or aversion to the color red. −*erythrophobic, adj.*

erythroplasia of Queyrat /erith′rōplā″zhə/ [Gk, *erythros + plasis,* forming; Louis A. Queyrat, French dermatologist, 1856–1933], an in situ squamous cell carcinoma on the glans or corona of the penis. It is a shiny, velvety, well-circumscribed reddish patch on the skin. It is usually excised surgically. See also **Bowen's disease.**

erythropoiesis /erith′rōpō-ē″sis/ [Gk, *erythros + poiein,* to make], the process of erythrocyte production in the bone marrow involving the maturation of a nucleated precursor into a hemoglobin-filled, nucleus-free erythrocyte that is regulated by erythropoietin, a hormone produced by the kidney. Compare **erythrogenesis.** See also **erythrocyte, erythropoietin, hemoglobin, leukopoiesis.** −*erythropoietic, adj.*

erythropoietic porphyria. See **porphyria.**

erythropoietic protoporphyria (EPP), an autosomal-dominant disorder that is a form of erythropoietic porphyria. It is characterized by increased levels of protoporphyrin in the erythrocytes, plasma, liver, and feces and a wide variety of photosensitive skin changes, ranging from a burning or pruritic sensation to erythema, plaquelike edema, and wheals.

erythropoietin (EPO) /erith′rōpō-ē″tin/ [Gk, *erythros + poiein,* to make], a glycoprotein hormone synthesized mainly in the kidneys and released into the bloodstream in response to anoxia. The hormone acts to stimulate and to regulate the production of erythrocytes and thus increases the oxygen-carrying capacity of the blood. See also **erythropoiesis.**

erythropoietin (EPO) test, a blood test measuring the hormone erythropoietin, used in the diagnosis of anemia and polycythemia.

Erythrovirus /e-rith′rōvi″rus/, a genus of parvoviruses containing viruses that infect erythrocyte progenitor cells. It includes the species B19 virus.

Es, symbol for the element **einsteinium.**

ESADDI, abbreviation for **Estimated Safe and Adequate Daily Dietary Intake.**

escape beat [ME, *escapen,* to flee; *beten,* to beat], an automatic beat of the heart that occurs after an interval equal to or longer than the duration of its normal cycle. Escape beats function as safety mechanisms, and anything that produces a long pause in the prevailing heart cycle may allow an escape to occur. Pauses in which escape beats occur may be caused by sinoatrial block, atrioventricular (AV) block, or sinus bradycardia. Escape beats may arise from the atria, the AV junction, or the ventricles.

escape rhythm [OFr, *escaper + Gk, rhythmos,* beat], a sustained heartbeat that occurs when the sinus or atrioventricular (AV) node is depressed. Under such conditions, the heart rate is controlled by the AV junction or the His-Purkinje system.

escarronodulaire. See **Marseilles fever.**

-escent, suffix meaning "beginning to be": *adolescent, convalescent, incandescent.*

eschar /es″kär/ [Gk, *eschara,* scab], a dry crust that results from trauma, such as a thermal or chemical burn, infection, or excoriating skin disease. −**escharotic,** *adj.*

escharonodulaire. See **Marseilles fever.**

escharotic. See **eschar.**

escharotomy /es′kärot″əmē/, a surgical incision into necrotic tissue resulting from a severe burn. The procedure is sometimes necessary to prevent edema from generating sufficient interstitial pressure to impair capillary filling, causing ischemia.

Patient with burns requiring escharotomy *(Vincent et al, 2011)*

Escherichia coli /eshĭrĭ″kē·ə kō″lī/ [Theodor Escherich, German physician, 1857–1911; Gk, *kolon*, colon], a species of coliform bacteria of the family Enterobacteriaceae, normally present in the intestines and common in water, milk, and soil. *E. coli* is the most frequent cause of urinary tract infection and is a serious gram-negative pathogen in wounds. *E. coli* septicemia may rapidly result in shock and death through the action of an endotoxin released from the bacteria. See also **enterohemorrhagic *Escherichia coli*.**

escitalopram, an antidepressant, selective serotonin reuptake inhibitor used to treat major depressive disorders.

Escobar syndrome. See **multiple pterygium syndrome.**

escutcheon /eskuch″ən/ [L, *scutum*, shield], the pattern of distribution of coarse, adult pubic hair, rhomboid in the male and triangular in the female.

-esis, suffix meaning "an action," "a process," or "result of": *enuresis, genesis, synthesis.*

Eskalith, a medication used to treat bipolar affective disorders. Brand name for **lithium carbonate.**

Esmarch bandage /es″märk/ [Johann F.A. von Esmarch, German surgeon, 1823–1908], a broad, flat elastic bandage wrapped around an elevated limb to force blood out of the limb. It is used before certain surgical procedures to create a blood-free field.

ESO, abbreviation for **electric spinal orthosis.**

eso-, prefix meaning "within": *esophagitis, esotropia, esophagus.*

esomeprazole /es″omep′räzōl/, a proton pump inhibitor administered orally as the magnesium salt in treatment of gastroesophageal reflux disease and in the treatment of duodenal ulcer associated with *Helicobacter pylori* infection.

esophageal. See **esophagus.**

esophageal atresia /əsof′əjē″əl, es′ofā″jē·əl/ [Gk, *oisophagos*, gullet], an abnormal esophagus that ends in a blind pouch or narrows to a thin cord and thus does not provide a continuous passage to the stomach. It usually occurs as a congenital anomaly. Treatment varies by severity. Surgical intervention of some type is required to maintain nutrition.

esophageal cancer, a rare malignant neoplastic disease of the esophagus that peaks at about 60 years of age, occurs three times more frequently in men than in women, and is found more often in Asia and Africa than in North America. Risk factors associated with the disease are heavy consumption of alcohol, tobacco smoking, betel-nut chewing, Plummer-Vinson syndrome, Barrett esophagus, and achalasia. Aflatoxin in moldy grain and peanuts or a dietary deficiency, especially of molybdenum, may be involved. See also **esophagectomy.**

■ OBSERVATIONS: Esophageal cancer does not often cause any symptoms in the early stages, but in later stages produces painful dysphagia, chest pain, anorexia, weight loss, regurgitation, cervical adenopathy, and, in some cases, persistent cough. Left vocal cord paralysis and hemoptysis indicate an advanced stage of the disease. Diagnostic measures include barium swallow, fiberoptic esophagoscopy, and biopsy and cytological examination of the primary lesion and regional nodes. Most esophageal tumors are poorly differentiated squamous cell carcinomas; adenocarcinomas occur less frequently and are usually found in the lower third of the esophagus.

■ INTERVENTIONS: Surgical treatment may require total or partial esophagectomy. Radiotherapy may eradicate early local tumors and may effectively palliate the symptoms of an advanced lesion. Chemotherapy may be used in palliation of advanced disease or as an adjuvant to surgery or radiation therapy.

■ PATIENT CARE CONSIDERATIONS: Esophageal cancer metastasizes rapidly and thus has a poor prognosis. The tumor may spread locally to invade the trachea, bronchi, pericardium, great blood vessels, and thoracic vertebrae or may metastasize to lymph nodes, the lungs, and the liver.

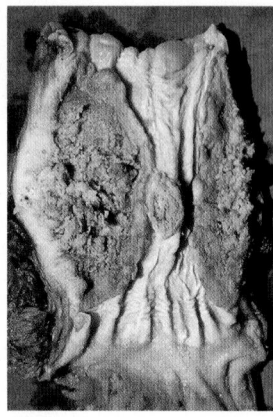

Esophageal cancer *(Fletcher, 2007)*

esophageal dilator, a bougie or similar instrument for dilation of an esophageal stricture or the lower esophageal sphincter.

esophageal dysfunction, any disturbance, impairment, or abnormality that interferes with the normal functioning of the esophagus, such as dysphagia, esophagitis, or sphincter incompetence. The condition is one of the primary symptoms of scleroderma.

esophageal function studies, manometric tests used to assess esophageal function. These include tests for acid reflux, acid clearing, and acid perfusion.

esophageal lead /lēd/, **1.** an electrocardiographic conductor in which the exploring electrode is placed within the lumen of the esophagus. It is used to detect sizable atrial deflections as an aid in identifying cardiac arrhythmias. **2.** *(Informal)* a tracing produced by such a lead on an electrocardiograph.

esophageal obturator airway (EOA), an emergency device that consists of a large tube that is inserted into the mouth through an airtight face mask. Holes in the tube open into the oropharynx when properly placed. The esophagus is blocked by inflating a balloon at the end of the tube. Because of the design, air passes only into the trachea.

esophageal peristalsis, strong, uncoordinated nonpropulsive contractions of the esophagus evoked by swallowing. On barium radiography, the lumen of the esophagus appears as a series of concentric narrowings or as a spiral coil.

esophageal speech. See **alaryngeal speech.**

esophageal varices, a complex of longitudinal tortuous veins at the lower end of the esophagus, enlarged and swollen as the result of portal hypertension. These vessels are especially susceptible to hemorrhage. Conditions that can cause portal hypertension include cirrhosis and chronic hepatitis.

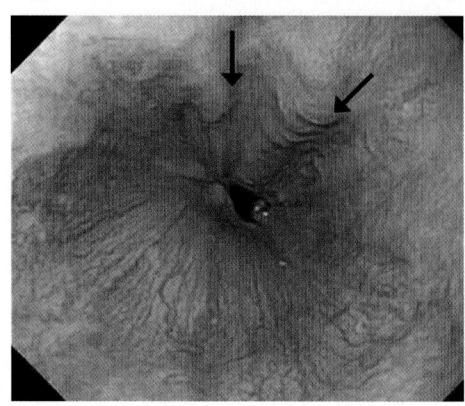

Esophageal varices *(Simonetto et al, 2014)*

esophageal web, a thin membrane that may develop across the lumen of the esophagus, usually near the level of the cricoid cartilage. The abnormal condition is generally associated with iron deficiency anemia and usually disappears when the underlying problem is resolved. See also **Plummer-Vinson syndrome.**

esophagectomy /esof′əjek″təmē/ [Gk, *oisophagos* + *ektomē,* excision], a surgical procedure in which all or part of the esophagus is removed, as may be required to treat severe recurrent bleeding, esophageal varices, or esophageal cancer.

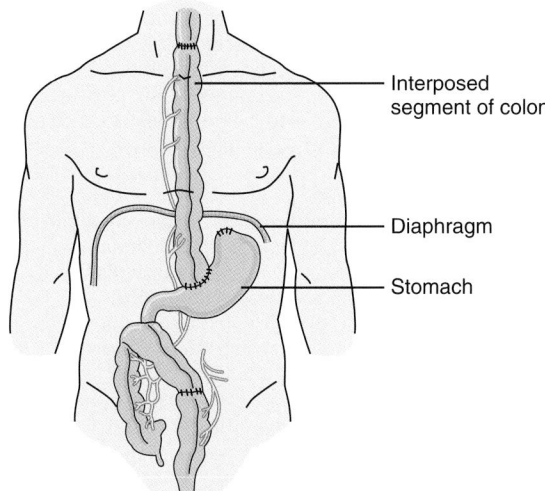

Esophagectomy with colon interposition *(Monahan et al, 2007)*

esophagitis /esof′əjī″tis/ [Gk, *oisophagos*+*itis*], inflammation of the mucosal lining of the esophagus caused by infection, irritation from a nasogastric tube, or, most commonly, backflow of gastric juice from the stomach.

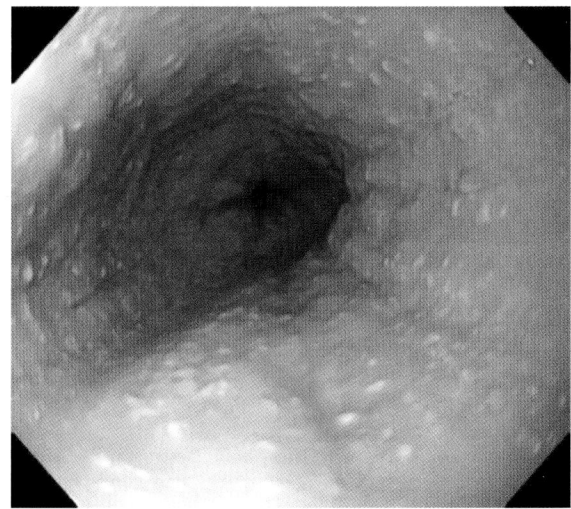

Eosinophilic esophagitis *(Marcdante and Kliegman, 2015)*

esophagocele /esof″əgōsēl′/, a hernia of the mucous membrane through a weakened area in the wall of the esophagus.

esophagogastroduodenoscopy (EGD) /ə·sof′əgōgas′trōdoo′odənos′kəpe/, an endoscopic test that permits direct visualization of the upper GI tract. Insertion of a long, flexible, fiberoptic-lighted scope allows examination of tumors, varices, mucosal inflammations, hiatal hernias, polyps, ulcers, and obstructions. This test evaluates patients with dysphagia, weight loss, early satiety, upper abdominal pain, ulcer symptoms, or dyspepsia and is also used therapeutically for electrocoagulation, laser coagulation, or injection of sclerosing agents.

esophagogastronomy /esof′əgō′gastron″əmē/ [Gk, *oisophagos,* gullet, *gaster,* stomach, *stoma,* mouth], the surgical creation of a passage between the esophagus and the stomach.

esophagography, a radiographic study of the esophagus using contrast (barium) to outline the esophagus for the identification of structural and functional abnormalities.

esophagogastroscopy /-gastros″kəpē/ [Gk, *oisophagos,* gullet, *gaster,* stomach, *skopein,* to watch], the examination with an endoscope of the esophagus and stomach.

esophagogastrostomy /-gastros″təmē/, an artificial connection of the esophagus to the stomach.

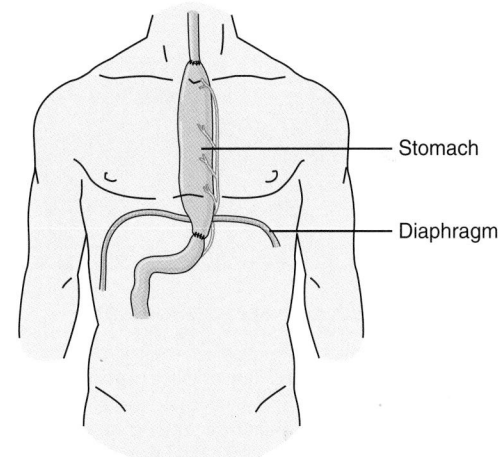

Esophagogastrostomy for esophageal cancer *(Monahan et al, 2007)*

esophagojejunostomy /-jij′oonos″təmē/ [Gk, *oisophagos,* gullet; L, *jejunum,* empty, *stoma,* mouth], the surgical creation of a direct passage from the esophagus to the jejunum, bypassing the stomach. The procedure is used after total gastrectomy.

esophagomyotomy /-mī′ot″əmē/, a longitudinal incision in the lower part of the esophageal muscle made to treat esophageal achalasia, an obstruction to the passage of food.

esophagoscopy /esof′əgos″kəpē/ [Gk, *oisophagos* + *skopein,* to look], examination of the esophagus with an endoscope.

esophagospasm /esof′əgōspaz′əm/ [Gk, *oisophagos,* gullet, *spasmos*], spasmodic contractions of the walls of the esophagus. The symptoms are substernal chest pain similar to angina pectoris and dysphagia for both liquids and solid food.

esophagostomy /esof′əgos″təmē/, a surgical opening into the esophagus for enteral tube feeding.

esophagus /esof′əgəs/ [Gk, *oisophagos*], the musculomembranous canal, about 24 cm long, extending from the pharynx to the stomach. It begins in the neck at the inferior border of the cricoid cartilage, opposite the sixth cervical vertebra, and descends to the cardiac sphincter of the stomach in a vertical path with two slight curves. The esophagus is composed of a fibrous coat, a muscular coat, and a submucous coat and is lined with mucous membrane. Also called **gullet.** –**esophageal,** *adj.*

esophoria /es′əfôr″ē·ə/ [Gk, *eso,* inward, *pherein,* to bear], the latent medial deviation of the visual axis of one eye in the absence of visual stimuli for fusion. Also called **cross-eye.** Compare **esotropia, exophoria.** –*esophoric, adj.*

esotropia /es′ətrō″pē·ə/ [Gk, *eso* + *tropos,* turning], a medial deviation of one eye relative to the other fixating eye such that fusion is not maintained. Also called **convergent squint, convergent strabismus, internal strabismus.** Compare **esophoria, exotropia.** See also **strabismus.** –*esotropic, adj.*

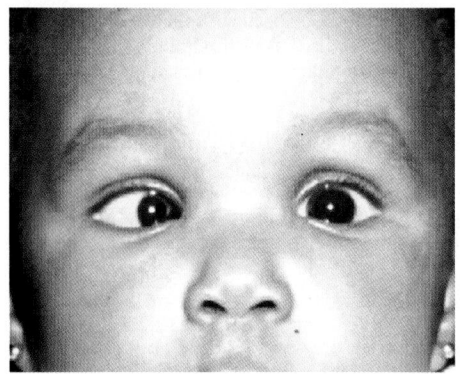

Child with esotropia *(Kliegman, 2011)*

ESP, abbreviation for **extrasensory perception.**

espundia /espun″dē·ə/ [Sp, cancerous ulcer], a cutaneous form of American leishmaniasis most common in Brazil, caused by *Leishmania brasiliensis.* The primary lesion often disappears spontaneously, followed by mucocutaneous lesions that destroy the mucosal surface of the nose, pharynx, and larynx. If the condition is untreated, potentially fatal secondary bacterial infections and disfigurement may occur. Also called **Breda disease.**

ESR, abbreviation for **erythrocyte sedimentation rate.**

essential /esen″shəl/, a necessary part of a thing without which it could not exist.

essential amino acid [L, *essentia,* quality], an organic compound not synthesized in the body that is essential for protein synthesis in adults and optimal growth in infants and children. Adults require isoleucine, leucine, lysine, methionine, phenylalanine, threonine, tryptophan, and valine. Infants need these amino acids plus arginine and histidine. Cysteine and tyrosine are derived from methionine and phenylalanine, respectively, and are considered semiessential. See also **amino acid, nonessential amino acid.**

essential fatty acid (EFA), a polyunsaturated acid, such as linoleic, alpha-linolenic, and arachidonic acids, essential in the diet for proper growth, maintenance, and functioning of the body. EFAs are prostaglandin precursors that play important roles in metabolism. They are also necessary for the normal functioning of the reproductive and endocrine systems and the breaking up of cholesterol deposits on arterial walls. The best dietary sources are natural vegetable oils, such as soy and corn oils; margarines blended with vegetable oils; wheat germ; edible seeds, such as pumpkin, sesame, and

sunflower; and fish oils, especially cod liver and other fish body oil. Although rare, a deficiency of EFAs causes changes in cell structure and enzyme function, resulting in decreased growth and other disorders. Symptoms include brittle and lusterless hair, nail problems, dandruff, allergic conditions, and dermatoses, especially eczema in infants. Also excessive amounts may reduce the level of vitamin E in tissues and cause other metabolic disturbances.

essential fever, a fever occurring in the absence of a known infectious disease.

essential hypertension, an elevated systemic arterial pressure for which no cause can be found. It is often the only significant clinical finding. Individuals with elevated blood pressure are at risk for cardiovascular disease. In examining patients with essential hypertension, clinicians consider the complex mechanisms that control blood pressure, such as the arterial baroreflex, body fluid regulators, the renin-angiotensin system, and vascular autoregulation. Also called **primary hypertension.** See also **benign hypertension, malignant hypertension.**

essential mixed cryoglobulinemia, a rare condition characterized by deposition of type II cryoglobulins without a detectable cause, inducing cutaneous vasculitis, synovitis, and glomerulonephritis. See also **cryoglobulin.**

essential nutrients, the carbohydrates, proteins, fats, minerals, vitamins, and water necessary for growth, normal function, and body maintenance. These substances must be supplied by food because most are not synthesized by the body in the quantities required for normal health.

essential oils, **1.** a class of generally aromatic volatile oils. **2.** the essences extracted from plants for use in flavoring foods, perfumes, and medicines. Some essential oils have been used therapeutically for thousands of years.

essential pruritus [L, *essentia,* quality, *prurire,* to itch], localized or generalized pruritus that begins without a preexisting skin disorder. Underlying causes may include renal disease, liver disease, thyroid disease, anemia, or lymphoma/leukemia.

essential thrombocythemia, a myeloproliferative neoplasm characterized by extreme thrombocytosis. Approximately 50% of essential thrombocythemia cases are characterized by presence of the JAK2 mutation. See **thrombocytosis.**

essential tremor, an involuntary fine shaking of the hand, the head, and the face, especially during routine body movements. It is a familial disorder inherited as an autosomal-dominant trait and appears during adolescence or in middle age, slowly progressing as a more pronounced disorder. The precise cause of this condition is not known. Essential tremor is aggravated by activity and emotion and can be reduced in some patients by the administration of mild sedatives, such as propranolol and diazepam, or with alcohol consumption. Also called **benign essential tremor, familial tremor.** Compare **parkinsonism.**

essential vertigo [L, *essentia,* quality, *vertigo,* dizziness], a form of vertigo for which no organic cause has been found.

established name, the name assigned to a drug by the U.S. Adopted Names Council. The established name, generally shorter than the chemical name, is the name by which the drug is known to health practitioners. Also called **generic name.** See also **chemical name, trademark.**

Estar, a topical agent used to treat eczema and psoriasis. Brand name for **coal tar.**

estazolam /estaz′olam/, a benzodiazepine used as a sedative and hypnotic in the treatment of insomnia. It is administered orally.

ester /es″tər/ [Ger, *Essigäther,* acetic ether], a class of chemical compounds formed by the bonding of an alcohol and one or more organic acids, with the loss of a water molecule for each ester group formed. Fats are esters produced by the bonding of fatty acids with the alcohol glycerol.

esterase /es″tərās/, any enzyme that splits esters.

esterification, the process of combining an organic acid (RCOOH) with an alcohol (ROH) to form an ester (RCOOR) and water.

esterified estrogen /ester″ifĭd/, an ester of natural estrogen.

■ INDICATIONS: It is prescribed for menstrual irregularities, contraception, and menopausal symptoms.

■ CONTRAINDICATIONS: It should not be used in anticipation of cardiovascular benefits because results from a clinical trial (HERS) found that its use was associated with an increased risk of unstable angina and myocardial infarction. Pregnancy, known or suspected breast cancer, thrombophlebitis, vaginal bleeding of unknown origin, or known hypersensitivity to this drug prohibits its use.

■ ADVERSE EFFECTS: Among the more serious adverse effects are gallbladder disease, thromboembolic disease, and a possible increase in risk of cancer.

esterify, to convert into an ester.

ester local anesthetic, a class of local anesthetics with an ester chemical group that differentiates it from the amide group of local anesthetics. They are metabolized primarily by pseudocholinesterase. Because of rapid metabolism, most ester local anesthetics have a relatively short duration of action with the exception of tetracaine. Kinds include **benzocaine, chloroprocaine, cocaine hydrochloride, procaine hydrochloride, Nesacaine™, tetracaine hydrochloride.**

esthesia /esthē″zhə/, **1.** capacity for perception. **2.** sensitivity or feeling. **3.** any disorder of the nervous system that affects perception or sensitivity.

esthesio-, prefix meaning "feeling or perceptive faculties": *esthesiophysiology.*

esthesiophysiology /esthē″zē·ōfiz′ē·ol′əjē/, the study of sense organ function.

-esthetic, -esthetical, -esthes, -aesthetic, -aesthetical, suffix meaning "a person's consciousness of something (e.g., a sensation)": *anesthetic, kinesthetic.*

esthetics /esthet″iks/ [Gk, *aisthetikos,* sensitivity], the branch of philosophy dealing with the forms and psychological effects of beauty. In medicine, esthetics may be applied to dental reconstruction and plastic surgery.

estimated date of delivery (EDD), an approximate date for the birth of a child. It is calculated by adding 280 days (40 weeks) to the date of the first day of the last menstrual period. It can also be calculated by an ultrasound scan, which provides an estimate of gestational age.

estimated hepatic blood flow (EHBF), an estimate of the rate of blood flow through the liver in a liver function test, such as by calculating indocyanine green clearance.

Estimated Safe and Adequate Daily Dietary Intake (ESADDI), nutrient intake recommendations, made by the National Academy of Sciences' Food and Nutrition Board, that give what is considered a safe range of intake for some nutrients because not enough information is available to set recommended dietary allowance values for them.

Estinyl, an estrogen. Brand name for **ethinyl estradiol.**

estr-, prefix for the name of an estrogen, a female hormone.

Estrace, an estrogen. Brand name for **estradiol.**

estradiol /es′trədī″ôl/, the most potent naturally occurring human estrogen.

estramustine /es″trämus″tēn/, an antineoplastic agent containing estradiol joined to mechlorethamine and administered orally for palliative treatment of metastatic or progressive

carcinoma of the prostate. It is used as estramustine phosphate sodium.

estramustine phosphate sodium /es′trəmus″tēn/, an antineoplastic agent.

■ INDICATIONS: It is prescribed for palliative treatment of metastatic or progressive carcinoma of the prostate.

■ CONTRAINDICATIONS: Thromboembolytic disorders or known hypersensitivity to this drug prohibits its use.

■ ADVERSE EFFECTS: The most serious adverse effects are cerebrovascular accident, myocardial infarction, thrombophlebitis, pulmonary emboli, and congestive heart failure.

estrangement /estrānj″mənt/ [L, *extraneus,* not belonging], **1.** a psychological effect of the separation of a mother from her newborn required when the infant is ill or premature or has a congenital defect, thereby diverting the mother from establishing a normal relationship with her child. **2.** the feeling that external objects have a strange, unfamiliar, or unreal quality, caused by a failure of cathexis of the external ego boundary, one of whose functions is to identify external objects as real and familiar.

Estratab, brand name for **esterified estrogen.**

estrin. See **estrogen.**

estriol /es″trē·ôl/, a relatively weak, naturally occurring human estrogen found in high concentrations in urine.

estrogen /es″trojən/ [Gk, *oistros,* gadfly, *genein,* to produce], one of a group of hormonal steroid compounds that promote the development of female secondary sex characteristics. Human estrogen level is elaborated in the ovaries, adrenal cortices, testes, and fetoplacental unit. During the menstrual cycle, estrogen renders the female genital tract suitable for fertilization, implantation, and nutrition of the early embryo. Pharmaceutic preparations of estrogen are used in oral contraceptives to prevent pregnancy, palliate certain types of postmenopausal breast cancer and prostatic cancer, inhibit lactation, and treat threatened abortion and ovarian disease. Estrogen replacement therapy may be prescribed to relieve the vasomotor symptoms of menopause. Its long-term continued use increases the risk of endometrial carcinoma. Also spelled **oestrogen.** Formerly called **estrin.** Kinds include **conjugated estrogen, esterified estrogen, estradiol, estriol, estrone.**

estrogen fractions test, a 24-hour urine or blood test that measures levels of the three major estrogens. Test results aid in the evaluation of menopausal status, sexual maturity, gynecomastia or feminization syndromes, certain ovarian tumors, and placental function and fetal normality in high-risk pregnancies.

estrogen receptor assay, a microscopic examination of breast tumor tissue used to determine the probable response of a tumor to endocrine therapy.

estrogen replacement therapy, administration of an estrogen to treat estrogen deficiency, such as that occurring after menopause. There are a number of indications, including treatment of vasomotor symptoms, such as hot flashes, and of thinning of the skin and vaginal epithelium, atrophic vaginitis, and vulvar atrophy. In women with a uterus, a progestational agent is usually included to prevent endometrial hyperplasia. Also called **hormone replacement therapy.**

estrone /es″trōn/, a relatively potent endogenous estrogen.

estropia, strabismus in which one or both eyes turn inward.

estropipate /es′trəpip″āt/, an estrogen.

■ INDICATIONS: It is prescribed in the treatment of vasomotor symptoms of menopause, atrophic vaginitis, kraurosis vulvae, female hypogonadism, female castration, and primary ovarian failure. Estrogens should be used topically whenever possible for treating symptoms of menopause (e.g., vaginal atrophy).

E

■ CONTRAINDICATIONS: Should not be used to prevent coronary vascular disease. Known or suspected cancer of the breast or estrogen-dependent neoplasia, pregnancy, thrombophlebitis or thromboembolic disorders, undiagnosed abnormal genital bleeding, or complications of previous administration of estrogen prohibit its use.

■ ADVERSE EFFECTS: Among the most serious adverse effects are a possible increased risk of cancer, gallbladder disease, and thromboembolic disorders.

estrus /es″trəs/, the cyclic period of sexual receptivity in mammals other than primates, marked by intense sexual urge and coinciding with the time that fertilization can take place.

estrus cycle [Gk, *oistros*, gadfly, *kyklos*, circle], the periodic changes in the female body that occur under the influence of sex hormones.

ESWL, abbreviation for **extracorporeal shock-wave lithotripsy.**

ET, 1. abbreviation for **endothelin. 2.** abbreviation for **endotracheal tube.**

eta /ē″tə, ā″tə/, H, η, the seventh letter of the Greek alphabet.

etanercept, a biological agent.

■ INDICATIONS: It is used to treat acute or chronic rheumatoid arthritis that has not responded to other treatments.

■ CONTRAINDICATIONS: Known hypersensitivity and sepsis prohibit its use.

■ ADVERSE EFFECTS: Adverse effects include abdominal pain, dyspepsia, headache, asthenia, dizziness, injection site reaction, cough, upper respiratory infection, non-upper respiratory infection, and sinusitis. Common side effects include rash, pharyngitis, and rhinitis.

-etanide. See **-eridine.**

état criblé /ātä″ krēblā″/ [Fr, sievelike state], a condition or state of multiple sievelike perforations in swollen lymphatic nodules in the intestine. It is a frequently fatal complication of untreated typhoid fever.

etching /ech″ing/, the cutting of a hard surface, such as metal or glass, by a corrosive chemical, usually an acid, to create a design.

ETEC, abbreviation for **enterotoxigenic *Escherichia coli.***

ETF, abbreviation for **electron transfer flavoprotein.**

ethacrynate sodium. See **ethacrynic acid.**

ethacrynic acid /eth′əkrin″ik/, a loop diuretic.

■ INDICATIONS: It is prescribed as a treatment for severe edema, such as nephrotic syndrome, hepatic cirrhoses, and ascites of malignancy. Unlike many other diuretics, ethacrynic acid is not a sulfonamide derivative and can therefore be tolerated by some people who develop hypersensitivity reactions to other diuretics.

■ CONTRAINDICATIONS: Pregnancy, anuria, or known hypersensitivity to this drug prohibits its use. It is not given to infants.

■ ADVERSE EFFECTS: Among the more serious adverse effects are tetany, muscle weakness, cramps, and excessive diuresis. Hearing loss may occur.

ethambutol /etham′butol/, an antibacterial agent specifically effective against *Mycobacterium tuberculosis.* It is administered orally as the hydrochloride salt, in conjunction with one or more other antituberculous drugs, in the treatment of pulmonary tuberculosis.

ethambutol hydrochloride /eth′əmbyoo̅″təl/, a tuberculostatic antibiotic.

■ INDICATIONS: It is prescribed in the treatment of pulmonary tuberculosis in combination with other drugs.

■ CONTRAINDICATIONS: Optic neuritis or known hypersensitivity to this drug prohibits its use. It is not recommended for small children.

■ ADVERSE EFFECTS: Among the most serious adverse effects are diminished visual acuity and allergic reactions, such as rashes.

ethanedioic acid. See **oxalic acid.**

ethanoic acid. See **acetic acid.**

ethanol /eth″ənol/, ethyl alcohol. See also **alcohol.**

ethanolamine, an amino alcohol formed by the decarboxylation of serine. It is a component of certain cephalins and phospholipids and is used as a surfactant in pharmaceutic products.

ethanol test, a blood, urine, saliva, or breath test usually performed to evaluate alcohol-impaired drivers or those with alcohol overdose.

ethaverine hydrochloride /eth′əver″ēn/, a smooth muscle relaxant.

■ INDICATIONS: It is prescribed to relieve spasm of the GI or genitourinary tract, arterial vasospasm, cerebral insufficiency, and peripheral and cerebrovascular insufficiency.

■ CONTRAINDICATIONS: Liver disease, atrioventricular dissociation, or known hypersensitivity to this drug prohibits its use. It is prescribed with caution to patients who have glaucoma.

■ ADVERSE EFFECTS: Among the more serious adverse effects are hypotension, abdominal distress, cardiac arrhythmia, and headache.

ethene. See **ethylene.**

ether /ē″thər/ [Gk, *aither*, air], **1.** any of a class of organic compounds in which two hydrocarbon groups are linked by an oxygen atom. **2.** a nonhalogenated volatile liquid no longer used in clinical practice as a general anesthetic. Also called **diethyl ether, ethyl oxide.**

ethereal /ithir″ē-əl/ [Gk, *aither*, air], **1.** pertaining to or resembling ether. **2.** (in chemistry) referring to a solvent that contains diethyl ether.

ether screen. See **anesthesia screen.**

ethical dilemma, (for health or related reasons) a challenge that health care providers face when there is a struggle to decide what course of action to take in a difficult situation.

ethical distress, (for health or related reasons) the discomfort a health care provider experiences when he or she is prevented from doing what is believed to be right.

ethics /eth″iks/ [Gk, *ethikos*, moral duty], the science or study of moral values or principles, including ideals of autonomy, beneficence, and justice. –*ethical, adj.*

Ethics in Patient Referrals Act, a U.S. federal law, the Stark Law, enacted in 1989, that prohibits referrals for Medicare and Medicaid patients by a physician to a clinical laboratory in which the physician has a financial interest. A 1994 amendment includes other services and equipment such as physical and occupational therapy; radiology and other diagnostic services; radiation therapy; parenteral and enteral nutrients, equipment, and supplies; and home health services.

ethinyl estradiol /eth″inil/, an estrogen.

■ INDICATIONS: It is prescribed in the treatment of postmenopausal breast cancer, menstrual cycle irregularities, prostatic cancer, and hypogonadism and for contraception and relief of menopausal vasomotor symptoms.

■ CONTRAINDICATIONS: Thrombophlebitis, abnormal genital bleeding, known or suspected pregnancy, or known hypersensitivity to this drug prohibits its use.

■ ADVERSE EFFECTS: Among the more serious adverse effects are thrombophlebitis, embolism, and hypercalcemia.

ethionamide /eth′ē·ənam″īd/, a tuberculostatic antibacterial.

■ INDICATIONS: It is prescribed for the treatment of tuberculosis in conjunction with other drugs when frontline therapy has failed.

■ CONTRAINDICATIONS: Existing liver damage or known hypersensitivity to this drug prohibits its use.

■ ADVERSE EFFECTS: Among the more serious adverse effects are skin rash, jaundice, mental depression, and GI side effects.

ethmocarditis /eth′mōkärdī″tis/, a chronic inflammation of the cardiac connective tissue.

ethmoid /eth″moid/ [Gk, *ethmos,* sieve, *eidos,* form], **1.** pertaining to the ethmoid bone. **2.** having a large number of sievelike openings.

ethmoidal air cell /ethmoi′dəl/ [Gk, *ethmos,* sieve, *eidos,* form], one of the numerous small thin-walled cavities in the ethmoid bone of the skull. The cavities are lined with mucous membrane continuous with that of the nasal cavity and lie between the upper part of the nasal cavities and the orbits. Compare **frontal sinus, maxillary sinus, sphenoidal sinus.**

ethmoidal process, an outgrowth on the superior border of the inferior concha that articulates with the uncinate process of the ethmoid.

ethmoid bone, the very light, sievelike, and spongy bone at the base of the cranium, also forming the roof and most of the walls of the superior part of the nasal cavity. It consists of four parts: a horizontal plate, a perpendicular plate, and two lateral labyrinths.

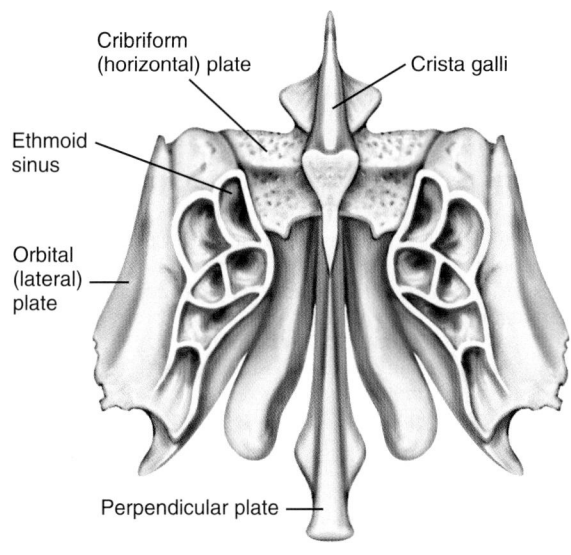

Cribriform (horizontal) plate

Crista galli

Ethmoid sinus

Orbital (lateral) plate

Perpendicular plate

Ethmoid bone

ethmoid cells, paranasal sinuses occurring in groups within the ethmoid bone and communicating with the ethmoidal infundibulum and bulla and the superior and highest meatus. They are often subdivided into anterior, middle, and posterior ethmoid cells, groups of air cells named according to where they open into the nasal meatus. Compare **frontal sinus, maxillary sinus, sphenoidal sinus.**

ethmoidectomy. See **sinus surgery.**

ethmoidofrontal suture /ethmoi′dōfron″təl/, a line in the skull between the cribriform plate of the ethmoid and the orbital plate and posterior margin of the nasal process. Also called **frontoethmoidal suture.**

ethmoidolacrimal suture /-lak″rimәl/, a line in the skull between the orbital plate of the ethmoid and the posterior margin of the lacrimal bone.

ethmosphenoid suture /eth′mōsfē″noid/, a line in the skull between the crest of the sphenoid bone and the perpendicular and cribriform plates of the ethmoid. Also called **sphenoethmoidal suture.**

ethnic group /eth″nik/, a population of individuals organized on the basis of an assumed common cultural origin.

ethnocentrism /eth′nōsen″trizm/ [Gk, *ethnos,* nation, *kentron,* center], **1.** a belief in the inherent superiority of the group to which one belongs. **2.** a proclivity to consider other ethnic groups in terms of one's own origins. See also **cultural relativism.**

ethnography /ethnog″rəfē/ [Gk, *ethnos,* nation, *graphein,* to record], a qualitative study describing the cultural practices of individuals and cultural groups.

ethnomedicine, the scientific study of the health care practices and beliefs of different cultures.

ethoheptazine /eth″o-hep′tah-zēn/, an analgesic used as the citrate salt to control mild to moderate pain, administered orally.

ethology /ethol″əjē/ [Gk, *ethos,* character, *logos,* science], **1.** (in zoology) the scientific study of the behavioral patterns of animals, specifically in their native habitat. **2.** (in psychology) the empiric study of human behavior, primarily social customs, manners, and mores. −*ethologic, ethological, adj.,* −*ethologist, n.*

ethosuximide /eth′ōsuk″simīd/, an anticonvulsant drug.

■ INDICATIONS: It is prescribed in the treatment of absence seizures.

■ CONTRAINDICATIONS: Known hypersensitivity to this drug or to any succinimide medication prohibits its use.

■ ADVERSE EFFECTS: Among the more serious adverse effects are blood dyscrasias, GI disturbance, and hematopoietic complications.

ethotoin /eth′ōtō″in/, an anticonvulsant drug.

■ INDICATIONS: It is prescribed in the treatment of generalized tonic-clonic and complex-partial seizures.

■ CONTRAINDICATIONS: Liver disease, hematologic disorders, or known hypersensitivity to this drug or to any hydantoin prohibits its use. It is not recommended for use during pregnancy or lactation.

■ ADVERSE EFFECTS: Among the more serious adverse effects are blood disorders, nausea, fatigue, skin rash, alopecia, erythema multiforme, exfoliative dermatitis, and chest pain.

ethyl alcohol. See **alcohol.**

ethyl aminobenzoate. See **benzocaine.**

ethyl chloride /eth″il/, a topical anesthetic used in short operations.

■ INDICATIONS: It is prescribed in the treatment of skin irritations and in minor skin surgery; the skin is sprayed until the surface turns white with frost. It is highly flammable.

■ CONTRAINDICATIONS: Known hypersensitivity to this drug prohibits its use. It is not used on broken skin or on mucous membrane.

■ ADVERSE EFFECTS: Among the more serious adverse effects are pain, muscle spasm, and, as a result of excessive use, frostbite.

ethylene /eth″əlēn/ [Gk, *aither,* air, *hyle,* stuff], a colorless flammable gas that is just lighter than air and has a slightly sweet odor and taste. It was previously used as an inhaled general anesthetic and is slightly more potent than nitrous oxide. It is now used in the food industry for control of fruit ripening, flower opening, and the shedding of leaves. Also called **ethene, olefiant gas.**

E

ethylenediamine /eth′əlēndi·am″ēn/, a clear, thick liquid having the odor of ammonia. It is used as a solvent, an emulsifier, and a stabilizer with aminophylline injections.

ethylene dibromide (EDB), a volatile liquid used as an insecticide and gasoline additive. Because it has been found to be a cause of cancer in animals, the Environmental Protection Agency no longer allows the use of EDB to control insect pests in grains and fruits intended for human use.

ethylene dichloride poisoning, the toxic effects of exposure to ethylene dichloride, a hydrocarbon solvent, diluent, and fumigant, which is one of the most abundant of all chlorinated organic chemicals. It is an eye, ear, nose, throat, and skin irritant and has produced cancers in laboratory animals. Inhalation or ingestion can lead to serious illness or death. The compound is metabolized into 2-chloroethanol and monochloroacetic acid, both more toxic than the original chemical.

ethylene glycol poisoning, the toxic reaction to ingestion of ethylene glycol or diethylene glycol, chemicals used in automobile antifreeze preparations. Symptoms in mild cases may resemble those of alcohol intoxication but without the breath odor produced by alcoholic beverages. Vomiting, carpopedal spasm, lumbar pain, renal failure, respiratory distress, convulsions, and coma may also occur.

ethylene oxide (CH_2CH_2O), a highly flammable gas used to sterilize surgical instruments and other supplies; the simplest epoxide.

ethylestrenol, an anabolic steroid.

ethyl oxide. See **ether.**

ethyne. See **acetylene.**

ethynodiol diacetate and ethinyl estradiol, an oral estrogen-progestin combination contraceptive.

■ INDICATIONS: It is prescribed for prevention of pregnancy.

■ CONTRAINDICATIONS: Thrombophlebitis, cardiovascular disease, breast or reproductive organ cancer, or known hypersensitivity to either ingredient prohibits its use.

■ ADVERSE EFFECTS: Among the more serious adverse effects are thrombophlebitis, uterine fibroma, gallbladder disease, embolism, and hepatic lesions.

-etic, suffix used as the equivalent of -ic in forming adjectives: *genetic, kinetic.*

etidronate disodium /etid″rənāt/, a regulator of calcium metabolism. Also called **sodium etidronate.**

■ INDICATIONS: It is prescribed in the treatment of Paget's disease and heterotopic ossification caused by injury to the spinal cord and after total hip replacement.

■ CONTRAINDICATIONS: There are no known contraindications.

■ ADVERSE EFFECTS: Among the more serious adverse effects are bone pain both at pagetic sites and at previously asymptomatic sites, GI disturbances, and elevated serum phosphate concentrations.

etio-, prefix meaning "causation": *etiology.*

etiology /ē′tē·ol″əjē/ [Gk, *aitia,* cause, *logos,* science], **1.** the study of all factors that may be involved in the development of a disease, including the susceptibility of the patient, the nature of the disease agent, and the way in which the patient's body is invaded by the agent. **2.** the cause of a disease. Compare **pathogenesis.** –*etiological, adj.*

etodolac /etodo′lak/, a nonsteroidal antiinflammatory drug used as an analgesic and antiinflammatory agent, especially to treat arthritis. It is administered orally.

etomidate /etom″idāt/, a short-acting, hypnotic nonbarbiturate intravenous agent used for induction of general anesthesia. It has minimal adverse cardiovascular and respiratory effects, thus providing a greater margin of safety in patients with or at risk for heart disease. Adverse effects include

transient reduction in adrenal gland cortisol release, pain on injection, and involuntary muscle movements.

etoposide, an antineoplastic or chemotherapeutic agent and mitotic inhibitor.

■ INDICATIONS: It is prescribed in the treatment of several forms of cancer, including lymphomas, testicular cancer, prostate cancer, and small-cell lung cancer, to prevent tumor cells from dividing and spreading.

■ CONTRAINDICATIONS: It should not be used if there is an allergy to etoposide or podophyllum. There is a potential adverse effect to the fetus if used by a pregnant patient, and the drug should not be used if breastfeeding.

■ ADVERSE EFFECTS: The side effects most often reported include chills, rapid heartbeat, painful or difficult breathing, decreased blood pressure, hair loss, rash, itching, skin discoloration, and digestive disorders.

etoposide phosphate, the phosphate salt of etoposide, having the same actions and uses as the base, administered intravenously.

Etrafon, a central nervous system fixed-combination drug containing an antipsychotic and an antidepressant. Brand name for **perphenazine,** *amitriptyline hydrochloride.*

etretinate /etret″ināt/, a synthetic derivative of vitamin A used as an oral drug to treat psoriasis.

■ INDICATIONS: It is prescribed for severe recalcitrant psoriasis, including generalized pustular and erythrodermic psoriasis.

■ CONTRAINDICATIONS: It is contraindicated for women who are of childbearing age unless a pregnancy test within 2 weeks of the start of therapy has negative results. Because of the risk of hyperostosis, the drug should not be given to children unless all alternative therapies have been exhausted. Intolerance to vitamin A derivative is another contraindication.

■ ADVERSE EFFECTS: Adverse effects may include benign intracranial hypertension, hepatitis, visual abnormalities including corneal damage, skeletal hyperostosis, peeling skin, alopecia, muscle cramps, and headache.

etymology [Gk, *etymos,* base; L, *logos,* words], **1.** the study of the origin and development of words. **2.** analysis of how parts of speech developed and are used.

etymon, pl. *etyma,* an earlier form of a word. See also **etymology.**

Eu, symbol for the element **europium.**

eu-, prefix meaning "well," "easily," "good," "true": *eubiotics, eugamy, euthyroid.*

Eubacterium /yoo′baktir″ē·əm/, a large genus of nonsporulating gram-positive anaerobic rod-shaped bacteria normally found in soil and water. The organisms are also found in the skin and cavities of humans and other mammals, where they may cause soft-tissue infections. One species has been found in dental tartar; another synthesizes vitamin B_{12}. *Eubacterium* is susceptible to penicillin, cliridamycin, and metronidazole.

eubiotics /yoo′bī·ot″iks/ [Gk, *eu,* well, *bios,* life], the science of healthy living.

eucalyptol /yoo′kəlip″tol/, a substance with an aromatic odor obtained from the volatile oil of *Eucalyptus* and used in nasal emollients. Also called **cajeputol.**

eucaryocyte. See **eukaryocyte.**

eucaryon. See **eukaryon.**

eucaryosis. See **eukaryosis.**

eucaryote, eucaryotic. See **eukaryote.**

eucholia /yookō″lyə/ [Gk, *eu,* well, *chole,* bile], the normal state of the bile as to the quantity secreted and the condition of the constituents.

euchromatin /yookrō″mətin/ [Gk, *eu* + *chroma,* color], the part of a chromosome that is active in gene expression. It stains most deeply during mitosis, when it is in a coiled, condensed state during each repetition of the cell cycle. It alternates between condensation and dispersion. Compare **heterochromatin.** See also **chromatin.** —*euchromatic, adj.*

euchromosome. See **autosome.**

eugamy /yoo′gəmē/ [Gk, *eu* + *gamos,* marriage], the union of gametes that contain the same haploid number of chromosomes. —*eugamic, adj.*

eugenics /yoojen″iks/ [Gk, *eu* + *genein,* to produce], the study of methods for controlling the characteristics of populations through selective breeding.

euglobulin /yooglob″yəlin/ [Gk, *eu* + L, *globulus,* small sphere], that fraction of serum globulin that is insoluble in distilled water but soluble in saline solutions. This is one of a number of different properties used to classify proteins. Compare **albumin, cryoglobulin.** See also **electrophoresis, plasma protein.**

euglobulin lysis time test, a test, performed on blood plasma, that is a highly complex global nonspecific assay of the fibrinolytic system; it is designed to detect hyperfibrinolysis associated with inflammation, trauma, liver disease, malignancy, or thrombolytic therapy. This test has been largely replaced by specific fibrinolytic pathway component assays, including fibrinogen, factor XIII, plasminogen, tissue plasminogen activator, plasminogen activator inhibitor 1 and D-dimer.

eugnathia /yoona′thē·ə/ [Gk, *eu,* well + *gnathos,* jaw], an abnormality of the oral cavity that is limited to the teeth and their immediate alveolar supports and does not include the jaws. Compare **dysgnathic anomaly.**

eugnathic anomaly /yoonath″ik/ [Gk, *eu* + *gnathos,* jaw; *anomalia,* irregularity], an abnormality of the teeth and their alveolar supports. Compare **dysgnathic anomaly.**

eukaryocyte /yooker″ē·ōsīt′/ [Gk, *eu* + *karyon,* nut, *kytos,* cell], a cell that has a true nucleus, found in all organisms except bacteria.

eukaryon /yooker″ē·on/ [Gk, *eu,* good, *karyon,* nut], a cell nucleus that is highly complex and organized and is surrounded by a double membrane.

eukaryosis /yooker′i·ō″sis/ [Gk, *eu* + *karyon,* nut, *osis,* condition], the state of having a eukaryon. Compare **prokaryosis.**

eukaryote /yooker″ē·ot/ [Gk, *eu* + *karyon,* nut], *adj.,* an organism whose cells contain a true nucleus. All organisms except bacteria are eukaryotes. Also spelled **eucaryote.**

eukaryotic cell, a cell with a true nucleus. See also **cell.**

Eulexin, an antiandrogen antineoplastic agent. Brand name for **flutamide.**

eunuch /yoo″nək/ [Gk, *eune,* couch, *echein,* to guard], a male whose testicles have been destroyed or removed. If this occurs before puberty, secondary sex characteristics fail to develop, and symptoms such as a feminine voice and absence of facial hair can result from the reduced level of male hormones in the blood. See also **secondary sex characteristic.**

eunuchism /yoo″nəkiz′əm/, the condition of being a eunuch, with the lack of male hormones caused by castration.

eunuchoidism /yoo″nəkoidiz′əm/, a condition resulting from a deficiency in the production or effectiveness of male hormones. The deficiency leads to sterility, abnormal tallness, small testes, and impaired development of secondary sexual characteristics, libido, and sexual potency.

euphoretic /yoo′fəret″ik/ [Gk, *eu* + *pherein,* to bear], **1.** *adj.,* (of a substance or event) tending to produce a condition of well-being or elation. **2.** *n.,* a substance tending to produce a feeling of well-being or elation, such as ecstasy and cocaine.

euphoria /yoofôr″ē·ə/ [Gk, *eu* + *pherein,* to bear], **1.** a feeling or state of well-being or elation. **2.** an exaggerated or abnormal sense of physical and emotional well-being not based on reality or truth, disproportionate to its cause, and inappropriate to the situation, as commonly seen in the manic stage of bipolar disorder, some forms of schizophrenia, organic mental disorders, and toxic and drug-induced states. Compare **ecstasy.**

euploid /yoo″ploid/ [Gk, *eu* + *ploos,* multiple], **1.** *n.,* an individual, organism, strain, or cell whose chromosome number is an integral multiple of the normal haploid number characteristic of the species. Euploids may be as diploid, triploid, tetraploid, or polyploid. **2.** *adj,* pertaining to such an individual, organism, strain, or cell. Compare **aneuploid.** —*euploidy, n.*

euploidy /yoo″ploidē/, the state or condition of having a variation in chromosome number that is an exact multiple of the characteristic haploid number. Compare **aneuploidy.**

eupnea /yoop·nē″ə/ [Gk, *eu,* well, *pnein,* to breathe], normal, quiet breathing at a rate of 12 to 20 breaths per minute in adults.

Eurax, a scabicide. Brand name for **crotamiton.**

European blastomycosis. See **cryptococcosis.**

European typhus. See **epidemic typhus.**

europium (Eu) /yoorō″pē·əm/ [Europe], a metallic rare earth element. Its atomic number is 63; its atomic mass is 151.96.

eury-, prefix meaning "wide, broad": *eurycephalic.*

eurycephalic, having a wide cranial diameter.

Eurytrema, the genus name for low pathogenic parasites known as trematodes.

Eustachian cushion. See **torus tubarius.**

eustachian salpingitis, an inflammation of the eustachian tube.

eustachian tube /yoostā″shən/ [Bartolomeo Eustachio, Italian anatomist, 1524–1574; L, *tubus*], a tube lined with mucous membrane that joins the nasopharynx and the middle ear cavity. It is normally closed but opens during yawning, chewing, and swallowing to allow equalization of the air pressure in the middle ear with atmospheric pressure.

eustress /yoo″stres/, **1.** a positive form of stress. **2.** a balance between selfishness and altruism through which an individual develops the drive and energy to care for others.

euthanasia /yoo′thənā″zhə/ [Gk, *eu,* good; *thanatos,* death], **1.** the deliberate causing of the death of a person who is suffering from an incurable disease or condition. It may be active, such as by administration of a lethal drug, or passive, such as by withholding of treatment. Legal authorities, church leaders, philosophers, and commentators on ethics and morality usually distinguish passive euthanasia from active euthanasia. Passive euthanasia is now legal in Belgium, Switzerland, France, Mexico, Germany, and the states of Oregon, Vermont, and Washington. Active euthanasia is now legal in Ireland, Australia, and the state of Montana. Passive and active euthanasia are now legal in the Netherlands (Holland) and Canada. Also called **mercy killing.** Compare **assisted suicide. 2.** an easy, quiet, painless death.

euthenics /yoothen″iks/ [Gk, *eu* + *tithenai,* to place], the science that deals with improvement of the human species through the control of environmental factors, such as pollution, malnutrition, disease, and drug abuse. Compare **eugenics.**

euthymia, 1. a pleasant, relaxed state of tranquility. **2.** stable mood.

euthymic, pertaining to a normal mood in which the range of emotions is neither depressed nor highly elevated.

E

euthymism /yōōthī″mizəm/ [Gk, *eu* + *thymos*, thyme flowers], the characteristic of normal mood responses.

euthyroid /yōōthī″roid/ [Gk, *eu*, well, *thyreos*, oblong shield], pertaining to a normal thyroid gland and normal thyroid gland function.

eV, abbreviation for **electron volt.**

evacuant /ivak″yōō·ənt/ [L, *evacuare*, to empty], any medicine or other agent, such as an emetic or laxative, that causes an organ to discharge its contents.

evacuate /ivak″yōō·āt/ [L, *evacuare*, to empty], **1.** *v.*, to discharge or to remove a substance from a cavity, space, organ, or tract of the body. **2.** *n.*, a substance discharged or removed from the body, such as evacuation of stool. −*evacuation, n.*

evacuator /ivak″yōō·ā′tər/, an instrument for emptying a cavity, such as removing a calculus from the urinary bladder.

evagination /ēvaj′inā″shən/, the turning inside out or protrusion of a body part or organ.

EVALI, acronym for e-cigarette or vaping associated lung injury,

evaluating /ival′yōō·ā″ting/ [L, *ex*, away, *valare*, to be strong], **1.** (in five-step nursing process) a category of nursing behavior in which the extent to which the established goals of care have been met is determined and recorded. To make this judgment, the nurse estimates the degree of success in meeting the goals, evaluates the implementation of nursing interventions, investigates the patient's adherence to therapy, and records the patient's response to therapy. The nurse evaluates effects of the interventions used, the need for change in goals of care, the accuracy of the implementation of nursing interventions, and the need for change in the patient's environment or in the equipment or procedures used. The impact of the care or treatment on the patient, the patient's family, and the staff is evaluated; the accuracy of tests and measurements is checked; and the patient's and family's understanding of the information given them is evaluated. The patient's expressed and observed response to care is recorded. Although evaluation is considered the final step of the five-step nursing process, in practice it is integral to effective nursing practice at all steps of the process. See also **analyzing, assessing, implementing, nursing process, planning. 2.** (for health or related reasons) the assessment of clients to establish goals and intervention plans. All health care providers and practitioners evaluate the effectiveness of interventions to determine how best to help clients achieve their goals.

evaluation, 1. assessment of performance against an established set of goals or objectives. **2.** a critical appraisal or assessment; a judgment of the value, worth, character, or effectiveness of something; measurement of progress. A broad view of evaluation in health care includes three approaches, directed toward structure, process, and outcome, depending on the focus of evaluation and the criteria or standards being used.

evaporate. See **evaporation.**

evaporated milk /ivap″ərā′tid/, homogenized whole milk from which 50% to 60% of the water content has been evaporated. It is fortified with vitamin D, canned, and sterilized. When it is diluted with an equal amount of water, its nutritional value is comparable to that of fresh whole milk.

evaporation /ivap′ərā″shən/ [L, *ex* + *vapor*, steam], the change of a substance from a liquid state to a gaseous state. The process of evaporation is hastened by an increase in temperature and a decrease in atmospheric pressure. See also **boiling point.** −**evaporate,** *v.*

evening primrose oil, an oil produced by cold extraction from the ripe seeds of *Oenothera biennis*, the evening primrose, used internally in the treatment of mastalgia, premenstrual syndrome, and atopic eczema. There is insufficient evidence to support its efficacy.

eventration /ē′vəntrā″shən/, the protrusion of the intestines from the abdomen.

event-related potential (ERP) [L, *evenire*, to happen, *relatus*, carry back, *potentia*, power], a type of brain wave that is associated with a response to a specific stimulus, such as a particular wave pattern observed when a patient hears a clicking sound. See also **evoked potential.**

evergreen contract, a health care contract that is automatically renewed for the term of the contract unless it is renegotiated. Not applicable in Canada.

eversion /ivur″zhən/, a turning outward or inside out, such as a turning of the foot outward at the ankle.

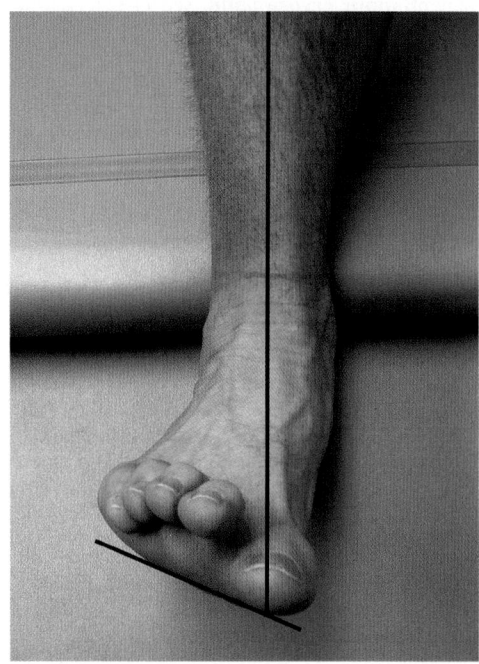

Eversion range of motion *(Miller et al, 2009)*

evidence-based dentistry, a systematic practice of dentistry in which the dentist finds, assesses, and implements methods of diagnosis and treatment on the basis of the best available current research, the dentist's clinical expertise, and the needs and preferences of the patient.

evidence-based medicine, the practice of medicine in which the physician finds, assesses, and implements methods of diagnosis and treatment on the basis of the best available current research, the physician's clinical expertise, and the needs and preferences of the patient.

evidence-based nursing, the practice of nursing in which the nurse makes clinical decisions on the basis of the best available current research evidence, the nurse's clinical expertise, and the needs and preferences of the patient.

evidence-based pharmacy, the practice of pharmacy in which the pharmacist makes decisions on the basis of the best available current research evidence, the pharmacist's expertise, and the needs and preferences of the patient.

evidence-based practice (EBP), the practice of health care in which the practitioner systematically finds, appraises, and uses diagnostic and treatment guidelines based on the most valid outcomes-based research. EBP incorporates the best evidence available with clinician expertise to treat patients.

evisceration /ivis′ərā″shən/ [L, *ex* + *viscera*, entrails], **1.** the removal of the viscera from the abdominal cavity; disembowelment. **2.** the removal of the contents from an organ or the removal of an organ from its cavity. **3.** the protrusion of an internal organ through a wound or surgical incision, especially in the abdominal wall. –*eviscerate, v.*

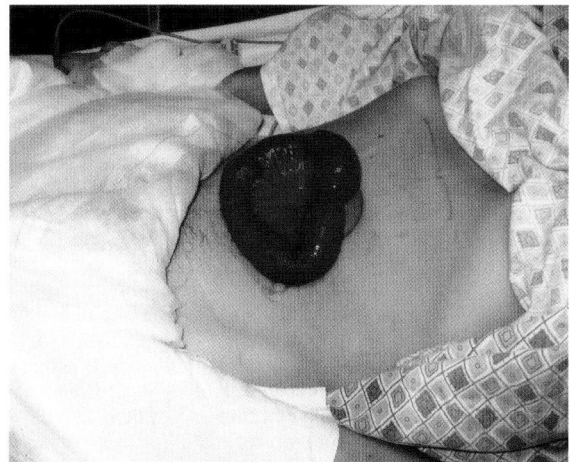

Patient with bowel evisceration *(Choo and McElroy, 2008)*

evocation /ev′ōkā″shən/ [L, *evocare*, to call forth], a specific morphogenetic change within a developing embryo that results from the action of a single hormone or other chemical. See also **induction.**

evocator /ev″ōkā′tər/ [L, *evocare*, to call forth], a specific chemical substance or hormone that is emitted from the organizer part of the embryonic tissue and acts as a morphogenetic stimulus in the developing embryo.

evoked potential (EP) /ivōkt″/ [L, *evocare*, to call forth, *potentia*, power], an electrical response in the brainstem or cerebral cortex that is elicited by a specific stimulus. The stimulus may affect the visual, auditory, or somatosensory pathway, producing a characteristic brain wave pattern. The activity and function of the system may be monitored during surgery while the patient is unconscious. The surgeon is thus able to prevent damage to the nerves during operative procedures. Evoked potentials are also used to diagnose multiple sclerosis and various disorders of hearing and sight. Kinds include **brainstem auditory evoked response, somatosensory evoked potential, visual-evoked potential.** See also **brain electric activity map.**

evoked potential (EP) studies, an electrodiagnostic test indicated for patients with suspected sensory deficit who are unable to indicate or unreliable in indicating stimulus recognition. Evoked potential studies are used to evaluate areas of the cortex that receive incoming stimulus from the eyes, ears, and lower/upper extremity sensory nerves; to monitor natural progression or treatment of deteriorating neurological diseases; and to identify histrionic or malingering patients with sensory deficit complaints. These studies include visual evoked responses, auditory brainstem evoked potentials, and somatosensory evoked responses.

evoked response audiometry, a method of testing hearing ability at the level of the brainstem and auditory cortex. Evoked response audiometry is useful in diagnosing possible defects in the vestibulocochlear nerve and brainstem auditory pathways.

evolution /ev′əlōō″shən/ [L, *evolvere*, to roll forth], **1.** a gradual, orderly, and continuous process of change and development from one condition or state to another. It encompasses all aspects of life, including physical, psychological, sociological, cultural, and intellectual development, and involves a progressive advancement from a simple to a more complex form or state through the processes of modification, differentiation, and growth. **2.** a change in the genetic composition of a population of organisms over time. **3.** the appearance over long periods of time of new taxonomic groups of organisms from preexisting groups. Kinds include **convergent evolution, determinant evolution, emergent evolution, organic evolution, orthogenic evolution, saltatory evolution.** –*evolutionist, n.*

evolution of infarction, the normal healing process after a myocardial infarction, as demonstrated on successive electrocardiograms.

evulsed tooth. See **avulsed tooth.**

Ewing sarcoma /yōō″ing/ [James Ewing, American pathologist, 1866–1943], a malignant tumor that develops from bone marrow, usually in long bones or the pelvis. It occurs most frequently in adolescent boys and is characterized by pain, swelling, fever, and leukocytosis. The tumor, a soft, crumbly grayish mass that may invade surrounding soft tissues, may be difficult to distinguish histologically from a neuroblastoma or a lymphoma. Surgery, chemotherapy, and radiotherapy are often used in treatment. Also called **endothelial myeloma,** *Ewing tumor.* See also **neuroblastoma, histiocytic malignant lymphoma.**

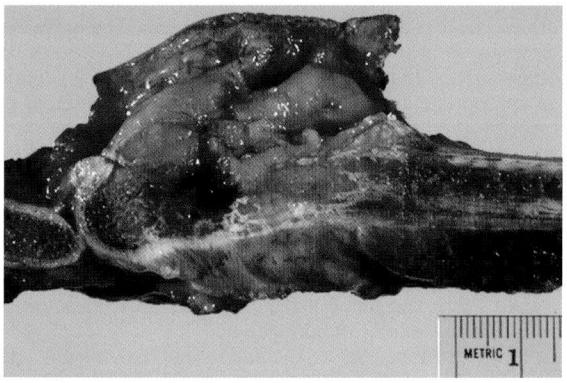

Ewing sarcoma of clavicle *(Folpe and Inwards, 2010)*

ex-, prefix meaning "away from," "outside," "without": *excoriation, exfoliation, exocrine.*

exa-, prefix of a Standard International unit that indicates 10^{18}.

exacerbation /igzas′ərbā″shən/ [L, *exacerbare*, to provoke], an increase in the seriousness of a disease or disorder as marked by greater intensity in the signs or symptoms of the patient being treated.

examination, a critical inspection and investigation, usually following a particular method, performed for diagnostic or investigational purposes.

exanthem /ig″zan″thəm/ [Gk, eruption], a rapidly erupting rash that may have specific diagnostic features of an infectious disease. Chickenpox, measles, roseola infantum, and rubella are usually characterized by a particular type of exanthem. Also called *exanthema.* Compare **enanthema.** –**exanthematous,** *adj.*

exanthema subitum. See **roseola infantum.**

exanthematous /ig′zɘnthem″ɘtɘs/ [Gk, *ex,* out, *anthema,* blossoming], pertaining to an eruptive disease (such as measles) or the skin rash that accompanies it.

exanthem subitum, exanthema subitum. See **roseola infantum.**

excavator /eks′kɘvāt′ɘr/ [L, *ex,* out + *cavus,* hollow], **1.** an instrument for hollowing out something by removing the center or inner part, or for making a hole or cavity such as the removal of dental caries or granulation tissue. **2.** a scoop, spoon, or gouge for surgical use.

exceptional education need, the determination that a disability or condition exists and interferes with the child's or adolescent's ability to participate in an educational program.

excess /ek′ses/, an amount more than is normal or necessary.

excessive sweat /ikses″iv/ [L, *excedere,* to go out; AS, *swaeaten*], perspiration greater than normal for the ambient environment. It is usually a sign of septic fever, pulmonary tuberculosis, hyperthyroidism, chronic renal disease, or malaria. Abnormal sweating of the hands and feet is often a sign of anxiety or other emotional stress.

excess mortality /ikses″/ [L, *excedere,* to go out, *mortalis,* mortal], a premature death, or one that occurs before the average life expectancy for a person of a particular demographic category.

Exchange Lists for Meal Planning, a grouping of foods in which the carbohydrates, fats, proteins, and calories are similar for the serving sizes listed. The lists, published by the American Dietetic Association and the American Diabetes Association, are used in meal planning for various diseases as well as for weight reduction. Foods are divided into three different groups or lists: carbohydrates, meat and meat substitutes, and fats. The carbohydrate group is subdivided into lists of starch, fruit, milk, other carbohydrates, and vegetables. A dietitian can create an appropriate dietary program prescribing the number of calories and units of each exchange category to be consumed daily, as well as a plan for when they should be eaten. The patient selects preferred foods from the lists. Other countries such as Canada use similar lists, for example, Food Choices.

exchanges. See **health insurance marketplace.**

exchange transfusion, the removal of all or most of a patient's diseased blood and its simultaneous replacement with an equal volume of normal blood.

exchange transfusion in the newborn /iks·chāng″/ [L, *ex* + *cambire,* to change], the introduction of whole blood in exchange for a large amount of an infant's circulating blood, which is repeatedly withdrawn in small amounts and replaced with equal amounts of donor blood. The procedure is performed to improve the oxygen-carrying capacity of the blood in the treatment of erythroblastosis fetalis by removing Rh and ABO antibodies, sensitized erythrocytes that produce hemolysis, and accumulated bilirubin.

excimer laser /ek″simɘr/, one of a class of lasers with output in the ultraviolet range of the electromagnetic spectrum. The name is derived from the symbol formed by the combination of xenon atoms (Xe) and halogen atoms (X) to yield xenon-halide compounds as XEX.

excision /iksish″ɘn/ [L, *ex* + *caedere,* to cut], **1.** the process of cutting out or off. **2.** (in molecular genetics) the process by which a genetic element is removed from a strand of deoxyribonucleic acid. Compare **resection.** −*excise, v.*

excitability /iksī′tɘbil″itē/ [L, *excitare,* to arouse], the property of a cell that enables it to react to irritation or stimulation, such as the ability of a nerve or muscle cell to react to an electrical stimulus.

excitant /eksī′tɘnt/, a drug or other agent that arouses the central nervous system or other body system in a particular manner. Excitants may be drugs or other substances, such as caffeine, or visual or auditory stimuli.

excitation /ek′sitā″shɘn/ [L, *excitare,* to arouse], nerve or muscle action as a result of impulse propagation; a state of mental or physical excitement.

excitatory amino acids /eksī″tɘtôr′ē/, one of a group of amino acids that affect the central nervous system by acting as neurotransmitters and in some cases as neurotoxins. Examples include glutamate and aspartate, which cause depolarization but may also trigger the death of neurons. Some excitatory amino acids are produced by plants and fungi and may be responsible for hypoxic or hypoglycemic brain damage.

excitatory impulse, a sudden force that stimulates activity.

excited state /eksī″tid/ [L, *excitare,* to rouse, *status*], **1.** (in chemistry and physics) an energy level of a system that is higher than the ground state. The system decays to the ground state and emits the energy difference, usually in the form of photons. **2.** (in psychology) a higher state of consciousness; hyperalertness; a state in which thinking and behavior may be frenzied or agitated.

excitement /eksīt″mɘnt/, **1.** a mental and physiological state of arousal that temporarily interrupts homeostasis or a sense of calm. It is a strong emotion that cannot be ignored and that may lead to spontaneous action (positive or negative). **2.** a pathological state. Excitement in mania can lead to greater unpredictability, lack of impulse control, and potential aggression. Excitement for dementia patients can lead to an increase in confusion and potentially a catastrophic reaction.

exciting eye, (in sympathetic ophthalmia) the eye that sustains a penetrating injury and causes an inflammatory reaction in the fellow eye. Also called **inciting eye.**

exclusion from base price, a health care contract provision in the United States in which high-cost variable items beyond the control of the provider, such as organ procurement costs, are excluded from the base price.

Exclusive Provider Organization (EPO), a type of managed health care organization in which no coverage is typically provided for services received outside the EPO. However, some EPOs incorporate the primary care physician gatekeeper concept along with prospective approval of referrals to specialists of providers outside the EPO.

excoriation /ekskôr′ē·ā″shɘn/ [L, *excoriare,* to flay], an injury to a surface of the body caused by trauma, such as scratching, abrasion, or a chemical or thermal burn.

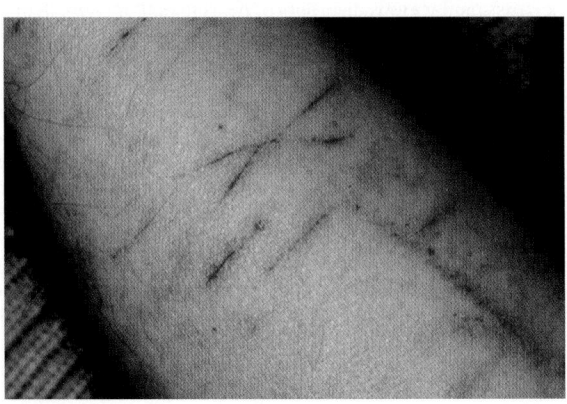

Excoriations from tree branch scratches *(Lemmi and Lemmi, 2000)*

excrement /eks″krəment/, any waste matter, particularly feces, discharged from the body.

excreta /ekskrē′tə/ [L, *excernere,* to separate], any waste matter discharged from the body.

excrete /ekskrēt′/ [L, *excernere,* to separate], to evacuate a waste substance from the body, often via a normal secretion; for example, a drug that may be excreted in breast milk.

excretion /ekskrē′shən/, the process of eliminating, shedding, or getting rid of substances by body organs or tissues, as part of a natural metabolic activity. Excretion usually begins at the cellular level, where water, carbon dioxide, and other waste products of cellular life are emptied into the capillaries. The epidermis excretes dead skin cells by shedding them daily.

excretory /eks″krətôr′ē/ [L, *excernere,* to separate], relating to the process of excretion. Often used in combination with another term to identify an object or procedure associated with excretion, such as excretory urography.

excretory duct, a duct that is conductive but not secretory.

excretory organ, an organ that is concerned primarily with the production and discharge of body wastes.

excretory urography [L, *excernere,* to separate; Gk, *ouron,* urine, *graphein,* to record], the radiographic imaging of the urinary tract. Conventional radiography, computed tomography (CT) urography, and magnetic resonance (MR) urography are used to capture images of the urinary tract after use of an intravenous contrast material. Also called **intravenous urography.**

excursion /ikskur″zhən/ [L, *ex,* out, *currere,* to run], a departure or deviation from a direct or normal course.

execute /ek″səkyo͞ot/, (of a computer) to follow a set of instructions to complete a program or specified function.

executive functioning, higher order reasoning and planning functions, such as forming goals, planning, implementing plans, and performing effectively.

executive physical /iksek″yətiv/, a physical examination that includes extensive laboratory, radiographic, and other tests that may be provided periodically to management-level personnel at employer expense. Such examinations may be detailed and expensive.

exemestane, an antineoplastic drug.
■ INDICATIONS: It is used to treat advanced breast cancer in postmenopausal patients whose cancer is unresponsive to other therapies.
■ CONTRAINDICATIONS: Its use is prohibited in premenopausal women, pregnant women, and clients with known hypersensitivity to this drug.
■ ADVERSE EFFECTS: Adverse effects include fatigue, diarrhea, constipation, abdominal pain, increased appetite, hypertension, depression, insomnia, anxiety, cough, and dyspnea. Common side effects include nausea, vomiting, hot flashes, and headache.

exenatide, an antidiabetic drug.
■ INDICATIONS: This drug is given in combination with metformin or a sulfonylurea to treat type 2 diabetes mellitus.
■ CONTRAINDICATIONS: Known hypersensitivity to this drug prohibits its use.
■ ADVERSE EFFECTS: Adverse effects of this drug include feeling jittery, restlessness, weakness, nausea, vomiting, diarrhea, dyspepsia, anorexia, gastroesophageal reflux, and weight loss. A life-threatening side effect is hypoglycemia. Common side effects include headache and dizziness.

exencephaly /ek′sənsef′əlē/ [L, *ex,* out + Gk, *enkephalos,* brain], a developmental anomaly characterized by a lack of all or part of the skull so that the brain is exposed. See also **anencephaly.**

exenteration /eksen″terā′shun/, **1.** surgical removal of the inner organs; evisceration. **2.** (in ophthalmology) removal of the entire contents of the orbit.

exercise /ek″sərsiz/ [L, *exercere,* to exercise], **1.** *n.,* the performance of any physical activity for the purpose of conditioning the body, improving health, or maintaining fitness or as a means of therapy for correcting a deformity or restoring the organs and body functions to a state of health. **2.** *n.,* any action, skill, or maneuver that causes muscle exertion and is performed repeatedly to develop or strengthen the body or any of its parts. **3.** *v.,* to use a muscle or part of the body in a repetitive way to maintain or develop its strength. Exercise has a beneficial effect on each of the body systems, although in excess it can lead to the breakdown of tissue and cause injury. Kinds include **active assisted exercise, active exercise, active resistance exercise, aerobic exercise, anaerobic exercise, isometric exercise, isotonic exercise, muscle-setting exercise, passive exercise, progressive resistance exercise, range-of-motion exercise, therapeutic exercise, underwater exercise.**

exercise amenorrhea, absence of menses associated with high-intensity athletics leading to a lack of estrogen from body fat and anovulation. See also **stress amenorrhea, hypothalmic-pituitary amenorrhea.**

exercise electrocardiogram (ECG), a record of the electrical activity of the heart taken during graded increases in the rate of exercise. It is important in the diagnosis of coronary artery disease. Abnormal changes in cardiac function that are absent during rest may occur with exercise. See also **stress test.**

exercise-induced anaphylaxis, a rare severe allergic reaction brought on by strenuous exercise. Cessation of physical activity usually results in immediate improvement. See also **anaphylaxis.**

exercise-induced asthma /-indyo͞ost′/, a form of asthma that produces symptoms after strenuous exercise. The condition usually occurs in persons who already have asthma, hay fever, or related hypersensitivity reactions. The effect may be acute but is reversible.

exercise prescription [L, *exercere + prae + scribere,* to write], an individualized schedule for physical fitness exercises.

exercise tolerance, the level of physical exertion an individual may be able to achieve before reaching a state of exhaustion. Exercise tolerance tests are commonly performed on a treadmill under the supervision of a health professional who can stop the test if signs of distress are observed.

exeresis /ekser″əsis/ [Gk, *ex + eresis,* removal], *(Obsolete)* the surgical excision of a part, organ, or body structure.

exertional headache /igzur″shənəl/ [L, *exserere,* to stretch out; AS, *heafod + acan,* headache], an acute headache that occurs during strenuous exercise. It usually recedes when the level of effort is reduced, when an analgesic medication is taken, or both.

exfoliation /eksfō′lē·ā″shən/ [L, *ex + folium,* leaf], peeling and sloughing off of tissue cells. This is a normal process that may be exaggerated in certain skin diseases or after a severe sunburn or may be done deliberately, such as with microdermabrasion. See also **desquamation, exfoliative dermatitis.** −*exfoliative, adj.*

exfoliative cytology /eksfō″lē·ətiv/, the microscopic examination of desquamated cells for diagnostic purposes. The cells are obtained from lesions, sputum, secretions, urine,

E

and other material by aspiration, scraping, a smear, or washings of the tissue. Compare **aspiration biopsy cytology.**

exfoliative dermatitis, any inflammatory skin disorder characterized by excessive peeling or shedding of skin. The cause is unknown in about half of cases. Known causes include drug reactions, scarlet fever, leukemia, lymphoma, and generalized dermatitis. Treatment is individualized, but care is essential to prevent secondary infection, avoid further irritation, maintain fluid balance, and stabilize body temperature.

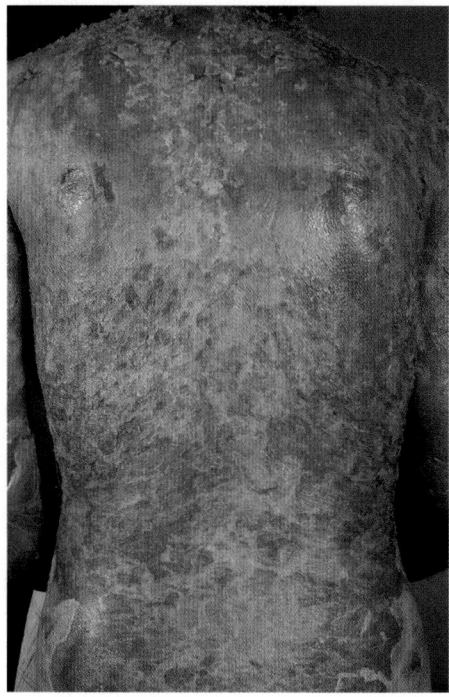

Exfoliative dermatitis *(Bolognia et al, 2014)*

exhalation. See **expiration.**

exhale, to move air out of the lungs. Also called **expire.**

exhaustion /igzôs″chən/ [L, *exhaurire,* to drain away], a state of extreme loss of physical or mental abilities caused by fatigue or illness. Multiple causes are possible, including extreme cases of mania. Exhaustion can be life-threatening.

exhaustion delirium, a delirium that may result from prolonged physical or emotional stress, fatigue, or shock associated with severe metabolic or nutritional problems. See also **delirium.**

exhaustion psychosis [L, *exhaurire,* to drain out; Gk, *psyche,* mind, *osis,* condition], an abnormal mental condition attributable to physical exhaustion. The main symptom, a delirious state, may develop in some explorers, mountain climbers, persons lost in the wilderness, and terminally ill and/or manic patients. See also **exhaustion delirium.**

exhibitionism /ek′sibish″əniz′əm/ [L, *exhibere,* to exhibit], **1.** the flaunting of oneself or one's abilities to attract attention. **2.** (in psychiatry) a psychosexual disorder that occurs primarily in men in which the repetitive act of exposing the genitals in socially unacceptable situations is the preferred means of achieving sexual excitement and gratification. See also **paraphilia, scopophilia.** *–exhibitionist, n.*

existential humanistic psychotherapy. See **humanistic existential therapy.**

existential psychiatry /eg′zisten″shəl/ [L, *existere,* to spring forth; Gk, *psyche,* mind, *iatreia,* medical care], a school of psychiatry based on the philosophy of existentialism that emphasizes an analytic, holistic approach in which mental disorders are viewed as deviations within the total structure of an individual's existence rather than as results of any biologically or culturally related factors.

existential therapy, a kind of psychotherapy that emphasizes the development of a sense of self-direction through choice, awareness, and acceptance of individual responsibility.

exit block [L, *exire,* to depart; Fr, *bloc*], the failure of an expected impulse to emerge from its focus of origin and cause depolarization of cardiac muscle.

exit dose, the amount of radiation at the surface of the body opposite that to which the radiation is directed.

Exjade, an iron chelator. Brand name for **deferasirox.**

exo-, prefix meaning "outside, outward": *exocrine, exogenous.*

exocoelom. See **extraembryonic coelom.**

exocrine /ek″səkrin/ [Gk, *exo,* outside, *krinein,* to secrete], pertaining to the process of secreting outwardly through a duct to the surface of an organ or tissue or into a vessel. Compare **endocrine system.** See also **exocrine gland, eccrine.**

exocrine gland, a gland that discharges its secretions through ducts opening on internal or external surfaces of the body. Kinds include **lacrimal gland.** See also **gland.**

exocytosis /ek′sōsītō′sis/ [Gk, *exos,* outside + *kytos,* a hollow vessel], discharge from a cell of particles that are too large to diffuse through the wall. Compare **endocytosis.**

exodondist. See **dental surgeon.**

exoenzyme /ek′sō·en″zīm/, an enzyme that does not function within the cells from which it is secreted.

exogenous /igzoj″ənəs/ [Gk, *exo* + *genein,* to produce], **1.** outside the body. **2.** originating outside the body or an organ of the body or produced from external causes, such as a disease caused by a bacterial or viral agent foreign to the body. Compare **endogenous.** *–exogenic, adj.*

exogenous hypertriglyceridemia. See **hyperlipidemia type I.**

exogenous infection [Gk, *exo,* outside, *genein,* to produce; L, *inficere,* to infect], an infection that develops from bacteria normally outside the host that have gained access to the body.

exogenous obesity, obesity caused by a caloric intake greater than needed to meet the metabolic needs of the body. Compare **endogenous obesity.** See also **obesity.**

exogenous uric acid [Gk, *exo,* outside, *genein,* to produce, *ouron,* urine; L, *acidus*], the accumulation of uric acid in the body produced by the metabolism of purine-rich foods.

exon /ek″son/ [Gk, *exo* + *genein,* to produce], the part of a DNA molecule that contains the code for the final messenger RNA.

exonuclease /ek′sōno͞o″klē·ās/ [Gk, *exo* + L, *nucleus,* nut; *ase,* enzyme], an enzyme that digests DNA or RNA from the ends of the strands.

Exophiala /ek′sofī′ə·lə/, a widespread genus of saprobic Fungi Imperfecti. *E. jeanselmei* is commonly found in soil and sewage and causes mycetoma and opportunistic infections in humans. *Hortae werneckii* (formerly classified as *E. werneckii*) is the cause of tinea nigra. Because it is so variable, some authorities have proposed dividing it into more than one species. Infection usually results from traumatic implantation and is associated with local or systemic immunosuppression.

exophoria /ek′səfôr″ē·ə/ [Gk, *exo* + *pherein,* to bear], the latent lateral deviation of the visual axis of one eye outward. Also called **divergent strabismus.** Compare **exotropia.** −*exophoric, adj.*

■ OBSERVATIONS: Occurs in the absence of visual stimuli for fusion and when fatigued. When concentrating on an image, the eyes function normally, but eyestrain may cause a headache or other unpleasant symptoms, such as blurred vision and mild nausea.

■ INTERVENTIONS: Eye exercises usually help, but if the condition is severe, surgery is indicated.

■ PATIENT CARE CONSIDERATIONS: For the most part, vision is unaffected although blurred vision or double vision is not uncommon.

exophthalmia /ek′softhal″mē·ə/ [Gk, *exo* + *ophthalmos,* eye], an abnormal condition characterized by a marked protrusion of the eyeballs (exophthalmos), usually resulting from the increased volume of the orbital contents caused by a tumor; swelling associated with cerebral, intraocular, or intraorbital edema or hemorrhage; paralysis of or trauma to the extraocular muscles; or cavernous sinus thrombosis. It may also be caused by endocrine disorders such as hyperthyroidism and Graves disease, varicose veins within the orbit, or injury to orbital bones. Visual acuity may be impaired in exophthalmia; keratitis, ulceration, infection, and blindness may also occur. Treatment depends on the underlying cause. Acute advanced exophthalmia is often irreversible. Also called **protrusio bulbi.** See also **proptosis.** −*exophthalmic, adj.*

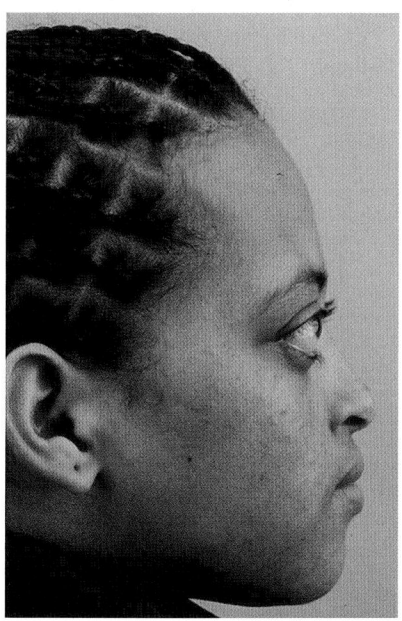

Young woman with exophthalmia associated with Graves disease *(Schaaf et al, 2009)*

exophthalmic goiter /ek′softhal″mik/, exophthalmos that occurs in association with goiter, as in Graves disease.

exophthalmometer /ek′səfthalmom″ətər/ [Gk, *exo* + *ophthalmos,* eye, *metron,* measure], an instrument used for measuring the degree of forward displacement of the eye in exophthalmos. The device allows measurement of the forward distance of the lateral orbital rim to the front of the cornea.

exophthalmos. See **exophthalmia.**

exophthalmos-macroglossia-gigantism syndrome. See **EMG syndrome.**

exophytic /ek′səfit″ik/ [Gk, *exo* + *phyton,* plant], pertaining to the tendency to grow outward, such as a tumor that grows into the lumen of a hollow organ rather than into the wall.

exophytic carcinoma, a malignant epithelial neoplasm that resembles a papilloma or wart.

exoskeletal prosthesis /ek′səskel″ətəl/ [Gk, *exo* + *skeletos,* dried up, *prosthesis,* addition], a prosthetic device in which support is provided by an outside structure (not an implant), such as an artificial limb. See also **prosthesis.**

exoskeleton /ek′səskel″ətən/ [Gk, *exo,* outside, *skeletos,* dried up], the hard outer covering of many invertebrates, such as crustaceans, which lack the bony internal skeleton of vertebrates. Compare **endoskeleton.**

exostosis /ek′sostō″sis/ [Gk, *exo* + *osteon,* bone], **1.** an abnormal benign growth on the surface of a bone. Also called **hyperostosis.** −*exostosed,* **exostotic,** *adj.* **2.** (in dentistry) asymptomatic bony hard nodules on the buccal aspect of the maxillary or mandibular alveolar ridges. No treatment is indicated unless they interfere with the fabrication of a prosthetic appliance. Palatal or mandibular tori are examples of exostoses that occur in specific locations.

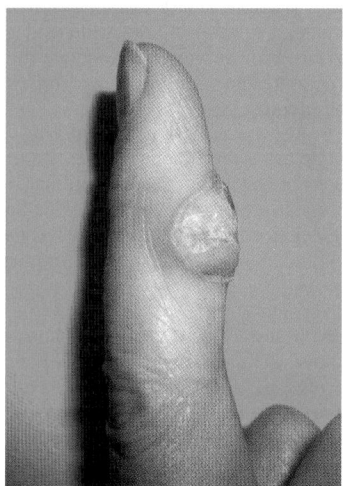

Exostosis *(Cañueto et al, 2010)*

exostosis cartilaginea [Gk, *ex,* out, *osteon,* bone; L, *cartilago,* cartilage], an outgrowth of cartilage at the ends of long bones. Also called **cartilage capped exostosis.**

exostotic. See **exostosis.**

exoteric /ek′səter″ik/ [Gk, *exoterikos,* external], lying outside an organism.

exothermic, indicating a chemical process accompanied by the release of heat, such as the loss of body surface heat.

exotosis, a nonmalignant bony overgrowth on the surface of a bone. Also called *bone spur.*

exotoxin /ek'sətok″sin/ [Gk, *exo* + *toxikon,* poison], a toxin that is secreted or excreted by a living microorganism. Compare **endotoxin.**

exotropia /ekstrō″fēə/, a deviation of the lines of sight between the two eyes in which the nonfixating eye is pointed outward. The eye has defective vision. Also called **divergent squint, divergent strabismus.** Compare **exophoria.**

expanded function dental assistant, a dental assistant with training beyond basic dental assisting, who has passed a competency examination and who has state-granted permission to perform certain dental procedures other than the removal, altering, or shaping of human tissue. Examples of some expanded functions are placement of post-extraction and sedative dressings; placing periodontal dressings; sizing stainless steel crowns; placing and condensing amalgam for Class I, V, and VI restorations; carving amalgam; placing composite for Class I, V, and VI restorations; polishing the coronal surfaces of teeth; minor palliative care of dental emergencies (placing sedative filling); preliminary bending of archwire; removal of orthodontic bands and bonds; final cementation of any permanent appliance or prosthesis; minor palliative care of orthodontic emergencies (bend/clip wire, remove broken appliance); making impressions for the fabrication of removable prosthesis; placement of temporary soft liners in a removable prosthesis; placing retraction cord in preparation for fixed prosthodontic impressions; making impressions for the fabrication of fixed prosthesis; extraoral adjustment of fixed prosthesis; extraoral adjustment of removable prosthesis during and after insertion; placement and cementation of orthodontic brackets or bands; monitoring sedation and general anesthesia; assisting with airway maintenance and emergency care of the patient; and monitoring and possibly initiating nitrous oxide therapy.

expanded role [L, *expandere,* to spread out; OFr, *rolle,* an assumed character], the functions of a health care professional that are not specified in the traditional limits of practice legislation. An example is the role of nurse practitioner, necessitating legal coverage through the establishment of standardized procedures or amendments or changes in nursing practice acts.

expansion /ekspan'shən/ [L, *expandere,* to spread out], **1.** the process or state of being increased in extent, surface, or bulk. **2.** a region or area of increased bulk or surface.

expectant treatment /ekspek″tənt/ [L, *exspectare,* to wait for; Fr, *traitment*], application of therapeutic measures to relieve symptoms as they arise in the course of a disease, rather than treatment of the cause of illness. Some kinds of expectant treatment are amputations for gangrene in a patient with diabetes, coronary bypass procedures in a patient with generalized atherosclerosis, and transplantation of tendons in a patient with severe rheumatoid arthritis. Compare **definitive treatment, palliative treatment, treatment.**

expectation /eks'pektā″shən/ [L, *exspectare,* to wait for], **1.** anticipation by the staff of a patient's behavior that is based on a knowledge and understanding of the person's abilities and problems. **2.** anticipation of the performance of health care professionals in defined roles, such as role expectation.

expectation of life. See **life expectancy.**

expected date of delivery (EDD), the predicted date of a pregnant woman's delivery. Pregnancy lasts approximately 266 days, or 38 weeks from the day of fertilization, but is considered clinically to last 280 days, or 40 weeks, or 10 lunar months, or $9\frac{1}{3}$ calendar months from the first day of the last menstrual period (LMP). The EDD is usually calculated on the basis of $9\frac{1}{3}$ calendar months, but if a woman is certain that coitus occurred only once during the month and if she knows the date on which it occurred, the EDD may be calculated as 38 weeks from that date. In the absence of a special calendar or device for calculating the EDD, it is arrived at by counting back 3 months from the first day of the LMP and then adding 7 days and 1 year; thus, if the first day of a woman's LMP was July 18, 2014, one counts back 3 months to April 18, 2014, then adds 7 days and 1 year to arrive at an EDD of April 25, 2015 (Nägele's rule). Because calendar months differ in length, this calculation may give a date that is a few days more or less than 280 days from the first day of the LMP, but it provides a very close approximation, and a trivial error will not be of clinical significance because of the variability of the actual durations of normal pregnancies. The expectant mother is advised that the EDD is only an estimate and that the chances are that she will give birth within 2 weeks before or, more commonly, after the calculated date. Also called *expected date of birth, expected date of confinement.*

expectorant /ikspek″tərənt/ [Gk, *ex,* out, *pectus,* breast], **1.** pertaining to a substance that promotes the ejection of mucus or other exudates from the lung, bronchi, and trachea. **2.** an agent that promotes expectoration by reducing the viscosity of pulmonary secretions or by decreasing the tenacity with which exudates adhere to the lower respiratory tract. Also called **mucolytic.** Kinds include **acetylcysteine, guaifenesin,** *terpin hydrate.* −*expectorate, v.*

expectoration /ekspek″tərā″shən/, the ejection of mucus, sputum, or fluids from the trachea and lungs by coughing or spitting.

experience rating /ikspir″ē·əns/ [L, *experientia,* testing, *rata,* proportion], a system used by insurance companies in the United States to set the premium to be paid by the insured on the basis of the risk to the company of providing the insurance. Experience rating may lead to very high malpractice premiums in some medical specialties, for the insurance company calculates the premium on the basis of settlements made in related malpractice cases during a specified period. Experience rating is also used to set annual membership health maintenance fees in organizations in which the cost of providing the services in a previous accounting period is used to determine the premiums for the next fiscal year. Compare **community rating.**

experiment, an investigation in which one or more variables may be altered under controlled circumstances to study the effects of altering variables.

experimental design /eksper'imen″təl/ [L, *experimentum* + *designare,* to mark out], (in research) a study design used to test cause-and-effect relationships between variables. The classic experimental design specifies an experimental group and a control group. The independent variable is administered to the experimental group and not to the control group, and both groups are measured on the same dependent variable. Subsequent experimental designs have used more groups and more measurements over longer periods. True experiments must have control, randomization, and manipulation.

experimental embryology, the study and analysis through experimental techniques of the factors, mechanisms, and relationships that determine and influence prenatal development.

experimental epidemiology, a type of epidemiological investigation that uses an experimental model for studies to confirm a causal relationship suggested by observational studies.

experimental group, a set of items or people under study to determine the effect of an event, a substance, or a technique. Compare **control group.**

experimental medicine, a branch of the practice of medicine in which new drugs or treatments are evaluated for safety and efficacy in a clinical laboratory setting by using animals or, in certain cases, human subjects.

experimental pathology, the study of diseases deliberately induced in laboratory animals.

experimental physiology, a branch of the study of physiology in which the functions of various body systems are evaluated in a clinical laboratory setting by using animals or, in some cases, human subjects.

experimental psychology, the study of mental processes and phenomena by observation in a controlled environment using various tests, manipulations, and experiments. Compare **analytic psychology.**

experimental variable. See **independent variable.**

expertise /eks′pərtēz″/ [L, *experiri,* to try], special skills or knowledge acquired by a person through education, interactions with evidence, or experience.

expert panel, a group convened for the purpose of providing specialized expertise related to a specific topic or area of interest.

expert witness /ikspurt″, ek″spərt/ [L, *experiri,* to try; AS, *witnes,* knowledge], a person who has special knowledge of a subject about which a court requests testimony. Special knowledge may be acquired by experience, education, observation, or study but is not possessed by the average person. An expert witness provides testimony or informed opinions on evidence. This evidence often serves to educate the court and the jury in the subject under consideration.

expiration /ik′spirā″shən/ [L, *expirare,* to breathe out], **1.** breathing out, normally a passive process, depending on the elastic qualities of lung tissue and the thorax. Also called **exhalation.** Compare **inspiration.** −*expiratory, adj.* **2.** the end of a predefined period. **3.** termination or death.

expiration date, the date beyond which a food, drug, blood or blood product, or other substance used in health care is considered unsafe or ineffective.

expiratory center [L, *expirare,* to breath out; Gk, *kentron,* center], one of several regions of the medulla, responsible for control of respiration. It is a subregion specifically involved in carrying out the activity of expiration.

expiratory phase, the portion of the respiratory cycle that involves exhalation, or moving air out of the lungs. In normal circumstances, it is passive. In a ventilated patient the expiratory phase may be passive, depending on the recoil of elastic tissues in the lung to move air out, or active, applying positive pressure to the abdominal area or negative pressure to the upper airway.

expiratory reserve volume (ERV), the maximum volume of gas that can be exhaled after a resting volume exhalation. See also **vital capacity.**

expiratory retard, (in respiratory care) a mode of mechanical ventilation that mimics the prolonged expiratory phase and pursed-lip breathing of emphysema. The method adds

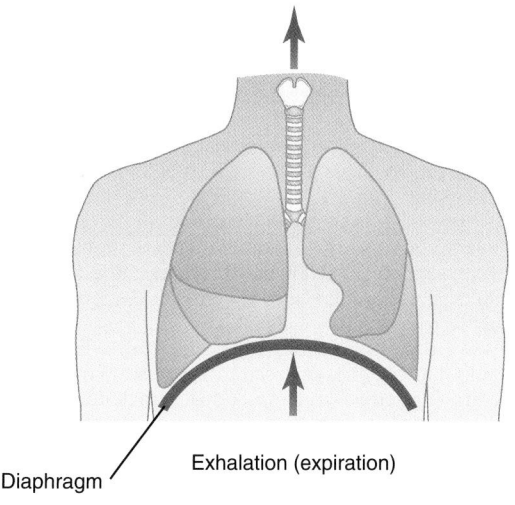

Diaphragm   Exhalation (expiration)

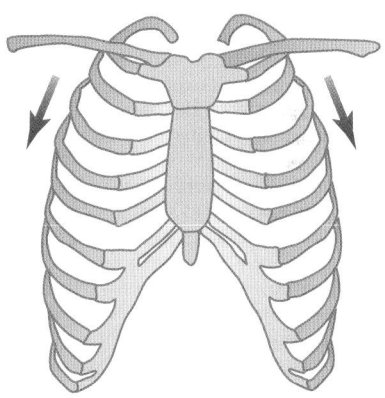

Chest cavity becomes smaller

Expiration *(Bonewit-West, 2015)*

some resistance to expiration. Low levels of positive end-expiratory pressure may produce a similar effect. Also called *expiratory resistance.*

expire /ikspī″ər/ [L, *expirare,* to breathe out], **1.** to breathe out. Also called **exhale. 2.** to die.

expired gas (E), any gas exhaled from the lungs.

explantation /ex-plan-ta′shun/, the removal of an implant.

exploration stage, the period of infancy or early childhood (0 to 2 years) in which a child seeks out stimuli. The child in this stage is just beginning to move and perform skills.

exploratory /iksplôr″ətôr′ē/ [L, *explorare,* to search out], pertaining to investigation, as in exploratory surgery.

exploratory operation [L, *explorare,* to search out, *operari,* to work], surgical intervention to find the cause of a disorder by opening a body cavity or organ and examining the interior.

explosion, **1.** a sudden and violent decomposition of a chemical compound. **2.** a sudden radical breakout.

explosive personality /iksplō″siv/ [L, *ex,* out, *plaudere,* to clap], behavior characterized by episodes of uncontrolled rage and physical abusiveness in reaction to relatively minor stressors. See **intermittent explosive disorder.**

E

explosive speech, *(Nontechnical)* abnormal speech characterized by slow, jerky articulation interspersed with sudden loud enunciation of words, often seen in brain disorders. The term is rarely used by speech-language pathologists. See also **logospasm.**

exponent /ikspō″nənt/, a superscript on a number that indicates how many times a number is to be multiplied by itself (for example, $3^4 = 3 \times 3 \times 3 \times 3 = 81$). In medical or scientific reports, powers of 10 are commonly used to indicate very large or very small numbers, such as in the examples 10^6 representing 1,000,000 or 10^{-6} representing 1/1,000,000. Exponents also are indicated by prefixes, such as *mega-* for 10^6 and *micro-* for 10^{-6}.

exposed pulp [L, *exponere,* to lay out, *pulpa,* flesh], dental pulp that becomes exposed to the oral environment and potential bacterial infection. Causes include fracture of the crown through trauma and loss of a tooth crown, the advance of dental caries to the pulp chamber, or penetration through the dentin during restorative preparation or caries excavation.

exposure /ikspō″zhər/ [L, *exponere,* to lay out], **1.** a measure of the ionization of air produced by a beam of radiation. It is expressed as coulombs per kilogram of air. **2.** a state of being in the presence of or subjected to a force or influence (e.g., viral exposure, heat exposure).

exposure angle, the angle of the arc described by the movement of a radiographic tube and image receptor during a tomographic exposure. It is usually less than the tomographic angle. The exposure angle influences the thickness of the tomographic section: smaller angles produce thicker sections.

exposure switch, (in radiology) a control device designed to interrupt the power automatically when pressure by the operator's hand or foot is released. The purpose is to prevent accidental continuing exposure of the patient to radiation. A common exposure switch is a foot pedal.

exposure unit, any of the conventional or SI units used to measure radiation exposure. Kinds include **roentgen, rad, rem, curie, gray, sievert, becquerel.**

expression /ikspresh″ən/ [L, *exprimere,* to express], **1.** the indication of a physical or emotional state through facial appearance or vocal intonation. **2.** the act of pressing or squeezing to expel something, such as milk from the breast when lactating or the fetus from the uterus by exertion of pressure on the abdominal wall. **3.** (in genetics) the detectable effect or appearance in the phenotype of a particular trait or condition. See also **expressivity.** *−express, v.*

expressive aphasia, a knowledge of what is to be communicated, but an inability to communicate it. See **motor aphasia.**

expressive language disorder, a communication disorder in children and adults, characterized by problems with expression of language, either oral or signed. It includes difficulties such as limited speech or vocabulary, vocabulary errors, difficulty or hesitation in word selection, oversimplification of grammatical or sentence structure, omission of parts of sentences, unusual word order, and slowed acquisition of language skills. Two types are recognized, *acquired* and *developmental.*

expressivity /eks′presiv″itē/ [L, *exprimere,* to make clear], the variability with which basic patterns of inheritance are modified, both in degree and in variety, by the effect of a given gene in people of the same genotype. For example, polydactyly may be expressed as extra toes in one generation and extra fingers in another.

expulsive stage of labor /ikspul″siv/ [L, *expellere,* to drive out, *stare,* stand, *labor,* work], the second stage of labor, during which the mother's uterine contractions are accompanied by a bearing-down reflex. It begins after full dilation of the cervix and continues to the complete birth of the infant.

exsanguinate /eksang″gwināt/ [L, *ex + sanguis,* blood], to drain away or deprive an organ of blood.

exsanguination /eksang′gwinā″shən/, a massive loss of blood.

exsiccant. See **desiccant.**

exsiccate. See **desiccate.**

exstrophy /ek″strōfē/ [Gk, *ekstrephein,* to turn inside out], a congenital malformation in which a hollow organ has its wall turned inside out, establishing a communication with the exterior. An example is exstrophy of the bladder with eversion of the posterior bladder wall, which causes urine to drain to the exterior.

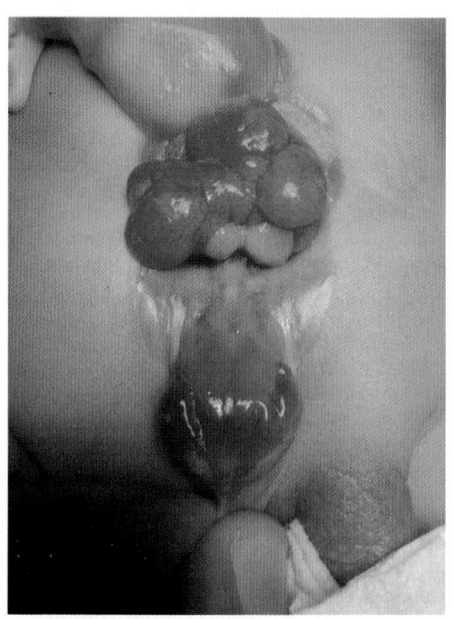

Boy with exstrophy *(Nelson, 2013)*

exstrophy-epispadias complex, a group of congenital defects of the anterior abdominal wall, including exstrophy of the bladder, exstrophy of cloaca, and epispadias, under the theory that they are all expressions of the same developmental anomaly.

exstrophy of the bladder, a developmental anomaly marked by absence of part of the lower abdominal wall and the anterior wall of the urinary bladder, with eversion of the posterior wall of the bladder through the defect, as well as an open pubic arch and widely separated ischia connected by a fibrous band.

extended arm. See **reacher.**

extended care facility (ECF) [L, *extendere,* to stretch], an institution devoted to providing medical, nursing, or custodial care for an individual over a prolonged period, such as during the course of a chronic disease or the rehabilitation phase after an acute illness. Also called **convalescent home, nursing home.** Kinds include **intermediate care facility, skilled nursing facility.**

extended family, a family group consisting of the biological or adoptive parents, their children, the grandparents, and other family members. The extended family is the basic family group in many societies. Among its characteristics are exchange of information from experienced older members to less experienced younger ones, care of the older family members in the home by the younger ones, and care of younger members' children by older members. Compare **nuclear family.**

extended insulin-zinc suspension, a long-acting insulin that is slowly absorbed and slow to act.

extended-wear contact lens, a refractive index device that fits over the cornea, designed to permit air permeation. Oxygen may pass between the lens and the cornea, thereby reducing the risk of corneal irritation.

extender, **1.** something that causes an increase in time or size, such as a substance added to a medication to stretch the time required for the drug to be absorbed. **2.** (in occupational therapy) a device or tool that lengthens reach. Also called **reacher.**

Extendryl, a fixed-combination nasal decongestant drug containing an adrenergic, an antihistaminic, and an anticholinergic. Brand name for **phenylephrine hydrochloride, chlorpheniramine maleate,** *methscopolamine nitrate.*

extension /iksten″shən/ [L, *extendere,* to stretch], a "straightening" movement allowed by certain joints of the skeleton that increases the angle between two adjoining bones, such as extending the leg, which increases the posterior angle between the femur and the tibia. Compare **flexion.**

extension partial denture. See **partial denture.**

extensor /iksten″sər/ [L, *extendere,* to stretch out], any muscle that extends a body part, such as the extensor indicis, which extends the index finger.

extensor aponeurosis, a flattened tendon serving as a connective attachment for a muscle tendon in the hand or foot.

extensor carpi radialis brevis [L, *extendere* + Gk, *karpos,* wrist; L, *radius,* ray, *brevis,* short], one of the muscles of the posterior forearm. It inserts into the dorsal surface of the third metacarpal bone and functions to extend the hand and forearm.

extensor carpi radialis longus, one of the seven superficial muscles of the posterior forearm. It inserts into the dorsal surface of the second metacarpal bone and serves to extend the hand and flex the forearm.

extensor carpi ulnaris, one of the muscles of the lateral forearm. It inserts by a tendon into the ulnar side of the fifth metacarpal bone and functions to extend and adduct the hand.

extensor digiti minimi, an extensor muscle of the posterior forearm. It is a slender muscle that arises from the common extensor tendon and joins the expansion of the extensor digitorum tendon on the back of the first phalanx of the little finger. It functions to extend the little finger and hand.

extensor digitorum, a muscle of the posterior forearm. It divides distally into four tendons that pass under the extensor retinaculum and diverge on the back of the hand, inserting into the second and third phalanges of the medial four fingers. It functions to extend the phalanges and, by continued action, the wrist. Also called *extensor digitorum communis.*

extensor digitorum brevis, a muscle that flexes the three middle toes and the proximal metatarsophalangeal joint of the great toe.

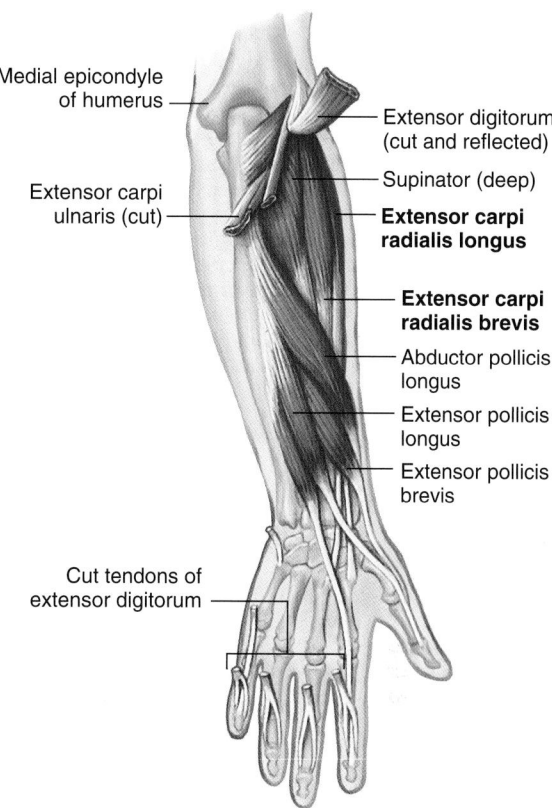

Medial epicondyle of humerus

Extensor carpi ulnaris (cut)

Extensor digitorum (cut and reflected)

Supinator (deep)

Extensor carpi radialis longus

Extensor carpi radialis brevis

Abductor pollicis longus

Extensor pollicis longus

Extensor pollicis brevis

Cut tendons of extensor digitorum

Extensor carpi radialis *(Patton and Thibodeau, 2016)*

extensor digitorum longus, a penniform muscle located at the lateral part of the anterior leg. It is one of four anterior crural muscles. It extends the proximal phalanges of the four small toes and dorsiflexes the foot.

extensor hallucis longus, a muscle that extends the great toe and dorsiflexes the foot at the ankle joint.

extensor indicis. See **extensor.**

extensor lag, the loss of active extension range of motion evident at a joint that can extend fully only with passive motion.

extensor pollicis brevis, a muscle that extends the metacarpophalangeal and carpometacarpal joints of the thumb.

extensor pollicis longus, a muscle that extends all the joints of the thumb.

extensor retinaculum of the ankle, either of two thick layers of fascia holding dorsiflexor tendons in place in the ankle.

extensor retinaculum of the hand, the thick band of antebrachial fascia that wraps tendons of the extensor muscles of the forearm at the distal ends of the radius and the ulna. Also called **retinaculum extensorum manus, superficial dorsal carpal ligament.**

extensor thrust, a spinal-level reflex present in a human in the first 2 months of life. It is an exaggeration of the positive support reflex and consists of an uncontrolled extension of a flexed leg when the sole of the foot is stimulated.

extern /eks″turn/ [L, *externus,* outward], students in the health professions who spend additional time in the clinical area providing care under the supervision of qualified professionals to refine clinical skills. Compare **intern,** def. 2.

E

external /ikstur″nəl/ [L, *externus,* outward], **1.** being on the outside or exterior of the body or an organ. **2.** acting from the outside, such as an external influence or exogenous factor. **3.** pertaining to the outward or visible appearance. Compare **internal.**

external abdominal oblique muscle, one of a pair of muscles that are the largest and the most superficial of the five anterolateral muscles of the abdomen. It is a broad, thin four-sided muscle that acts to compress the contents of the abdomen and assists in micturition, defecation, emesis, parturition, and forced expiration. Both sides acting together serve to flex the vertebral column, drawing the pubis toward the xiphoid process. One side alone functions to bend the vertebral column laterally and to rotate it, drawing the shoulder of the same side forward. Also called **obliquus externus abdominis.** Compare **internal abdominal oblique muscle.**

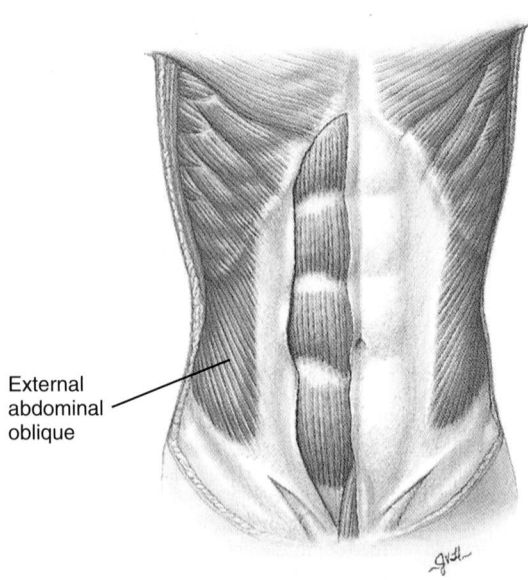

External abdominal oblique muscle *(Thibodeau and Patton, 2003)*

external abdominal region. See **lateral region.**

external absorption, the taking up of substances through the mucous membranes or the skin.

external acoustic meatus, the canal of the external ear, composed of bone and cartilage, extending from the auricle to the tympanic membrane. Also called **external auditory canal, external auditory meatus.**

external aperture of aqueduct of vestibule, an external opening for the small canal extending from the vestibule of the inner ear, located on the internal surface of the petrous part of the temporal bone lateral to the opening for the internal acoustic passage.

external aperture of canaliculus of cochlea, an external opening of the cochlear channel on the margin of the jugular opening in the temporal bone.

external aperture of tympanic canaliculus, the lower opening of the tympanic channel on the inferior surface of the petrous part of the temporal bone.

external auditory canal, external auditory meatus. See **external acoustic meatus.**

external beam radiotherapy, treatment by radiation emitted from a source located outside the body. Also called **beam therapy,** *external beam therapy.*

external carotid artery, one of a pair of arteries with eight major temporal or maxillary branches, rising from the common carotid arteries. It supplies various parts and tissues of the head and neck.

external carotid plexus, a network of nerves around the external carotid artery, formed by the external carotid nerves from the superior cervical ganglion. It supplies sympathetic fibers associated with branches of the external carotid artery. Compare **common carotid plexus, internal carotid plexus.**

external cervical os, an external opening of the uterus that leads into the cavity of the cervix. Compare **internal cervical os.**

external conjugate, the distance measured with obstetric calipers from the depression below the lowest lumbar vertebra posteriorly to the upper border of the symphysis anteriorly (usually about 21 cm).

external counterpulsation, a noninvasive technique for providing counterpulsation (assisted heart pumping). In one technique the limbs are placed in inflatable trousers. Inflation and deflation are synchronized with the cardiac cycle, generating augmented blood flow during diastole and assisted ejection during systole.

external cuneiform bone. See **lateral cuneiform bone.**

external ear, the outer structure of the ear, consisting of the auricle and the external acoustic meatus. Sound waves are funneled through the external ear to the middle ear. Compare **inner ear, middle ear.**

external fertilization, the union of male and female gametes outside the bodies from which they originated, such as occurs in frogs and most fish.

external fistula, an abnormal passage between an internal organ or structure and the cutaneous surface of the body. It can be surgically created or caused by delayed wound healing or necrotizing tumors.

external fixation, a method of holding together the fragments of a fractured bone by using transfixing metal pins through the fragments and a compression device attached to the pins outside the skin surface. Care includes regular cleansing of the skin around the pins and, in certain cases, application of antibiotic solutions or ointments. The pins are removed in a later procedure when the fracture is healed. Compare **internal fixation.**

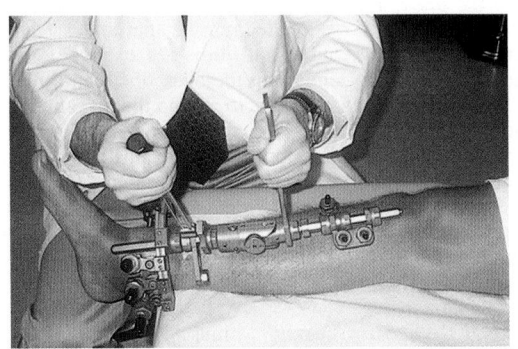

External fixation *(Courtesy Zimmer, Inc.)*

external iliac artery, the larger, more superficial division of the common iliac artery, which descends into the thigh and becomes the femoral artery. The external iliac artery supplies the lower limb. Compare **internal iliac artery.**

external iliac node, a node in one of the seven groups of parietal nodes serving the lymphatic system in the abdomen and the pelvis. Compare **common iliac node, iliac circumflex node, internal iliac node.** See also **lymph, lymphatic system, lymph node.**

external iliac vein, one of a pair of veins in the lower body that join the internal iliac veins to form the two common iliac veins. Compare **internal iliac vein.**

external jugular vein, the more superficial and lateral of a pair of large vessels on each side of the neck that receive most of the blood from the exterior of the cranium and the deep tissues of the face. Compare **internal jugular vein.**

external locus of control. See **locus of control.**

external malleolus /male″ōlas/ [L, *externus,* outward, *malleolus,* little hammer], a rounded bony prominence on either side of the ankle joint. Also called **malleolus fibulae.**

external occipital crest, a ridge extending downward from the external occipital protuberance.

external occipital protuberance, a midline projection of the occipital bone with curved lines extending laterally from it.

external pacemaker [L, *externus,* outward, *passus,* step; ME, *maken,* to make], **1.** a device used to stimulate the heartbeat electrically by means of impulses conducted through the chest wall, as used in emergency care of significant bradyarrhythmias. **2.** a device in which the impulse generator is outside the chest but is connected with the heart by wires that pass under the skin. The wires are placed during a surgical procedure and are removed after surgery, when the risk of bradycardia has diminished.

external perimysium, connective tissue surrounding muslce fibers. See **epimysium.**

external phase, the fluid phase of a colloid within which a solid or fluid particles are distributed or suspended. See **continuous phase.**

external pin fixation, a method of holding together the fragments of a fractured bone by means of pins that are attached to the bone and that protrude from the skin. See also **skeletal fixation.**

external pterygoid muscle, one of the four short, thick, somewhat conical muscles of mastication that function to open the jaws, protrude the mandible, and move the mandible from side to side. Also called **pterygoideus lateralis.**

external radiation therapy (ERT), the therapeutic application of ionizing radiation from a source of radiation outside the body, such as a kilovoltage radiographic machine, a megavoltage cobalt 60 machine, or a supervoltage linear accelerator, cyclotron, or betatron. ERT is used most frequently in the treatment of cancer but is also used in the therapy of keloids and some dermatological conditions and in counteracting the body's physiological rejection of transplanted organs.

external resorption, dissolving of the tooth structures progressing from the outside of the tooth to the inside of the tooth, not related to caries and often idiopathic in nature. Compare **internal resorption.**

external respiration, the part of the respiratory process that involves the exchange of gases in the alveoli of the lungs.

external rotation, turning outwardly or away from the midline of the body, such as when a leg is externally rotated with the toes turned outward or away from the body's midline.

external secretion. See **exocrine gland.**

external shunt, a device for the passage of body fluid from one compartment to another. It consists of a tube or catheter (or a series of such containers) that passes from one compartment or cavity to another over the body surface rather than inside the body. See also **hemodialysis, hydrocephalus.**

external sphincter of female urethra, a sphincter muscle that compresses the central part of the urethra in females. It originates in the ramus of the pubis and is innervated by the perineal nerves.

external sphincter of male urethra, a sphincter muscle that compresses the membranous part of the urethra in males. It originates in the ramus of the pubis and is innervated by the perineal nerves.

external urethral orifice. See **urinary meatus.**

external ventricular drain, a ventricular catheter connected to a drainage system and a closed collection bag. It allows the clinician to control fluid flow and, to some extent, pressure in the cranial vault.

external version, an obstetric procedure in which a fetus is turned, usually from a breech or transverse presentation to a vertex presentation, by external manipulation through the abdominal wall. Usually performed between 36 and 38 completed weeks of gestation. Compare **version and extraction.**

exteroceptive /ek′stərōsep″tiv/ [L, *externus,* outside, *recipere,* to receive], pertaining to stimuli that originate from outside the body or to the sensory receptors that they activate. Compare **interoceptive, proprioception.**

exteroceptor /ek′stərōsep″tər/ [L, *externus,* outside, *recipere,* to receive], any sensory nerve ending, such as those located in the skin, mucous membranes, or sense organs, that responds to stimuli originating outside the body, such as touch, pressure, or sound. Compare **interoceptor, proprioceptor.** See also **chemoreceptor.**

extinction /iksting″shən/, a state of being lost or destroyed.

extirpation /ek′stərpā″shən/ [L, *extirpare,* to root out], the total removal of a diseased organ or body part.

extra-, extro-, prefix meaning "outside," "beyond," "in addition to": *extracorporeal, extradural, extraocular.*

extraarticular /ek′strə·ärtik″yələr/ [L, *extra,* outside, *articulare,* to divide into joints], pertaining to the area outside a joint. For example, an extraarticular distal radius fracture is a fracture of the distal radius bone that does not include the articular surface.

extra beat [L, *extra,* outside; AS, *beatan*], an extra heart contraction. It is indicated by a premature atrial, junctional, or ventricular complex on an electrocardiogram.

extracapsular /-kaps″yələr/ [L, *extra,* outside, *capsula,* little box], pertaining to something outside a capsule, such as the articular capsule of the knee joint.

extracapsular ankylosis. See **false ankylosis.**

extracapsular dendrite [L, *extra + capsula +* Gk, *dendron,* tree], pertaining to dendrites of some autonomic nerves that penetrate the capsule boundary and extend some distance from the cell body.

extracapsular fracture [L, *extra + capsula,* little box], any fracture that occurs near a joint but does not directly involve the joint capsule. This type of fracture is extremely common in the hip.

extracellular /-sel″yələr/ [L, *extra + cella,* storeroom], occurring outside a cell or cell tissue or in cavities or spaces between cell layers or groups of cells. See also **cell, edema, interstitial.**

extracellular fluid (ECF), the portion of the body fluid comprising the interstitial fluid and blood plasma. The adult body contains about 11.2 L of interstitial fluid, constituting about 16% of body weight, and about 2.8 L of plasma, constituting about 4% of body weight. Plasma and interstitial fluid are very similar chemically and, in conjunction with intracellular fluid, help control the movement of water and electrolytes throughout the body. Some of the important ionized components of extracellular fluid are protein, magnesium, potassium, chlorine, calcium, and certain sulfates.

extracellular matrix, a substance containing collagen, elastin, proteoglycans, glycosaminoglycans, and fluid, produced by cells and in which the cells are embedded. The matrix secreted by chondroblasts, for example, is responsible for the properties of cartilage.

extracellular space. See **extracellular.**

extrachromosomal /-krō'məsō″məl/, occurring without direct involvement of the chromosomes. See **epigenesis.**

extracoronal /eks'trəkor'ənəl/ [L, *extra* + *corona,* crown], outside the crown of a tooth.

extracoronal retainer /-kôr″ənəl/ [L, *extra* + *corona,* crown, *retinere,* to hold], **1.** a dental anchor that incorporates a cast restoration lying largely external to the coronal portion of a tooth and complements the contour of the tooth crown. Resistance to displacement is developed between the inner surfaces of the casting and the external walls of the prepared tooth. The restoration incorporating an extracoronal retainer may be a complete or partial crown. **2.** a direct clasp-type retainer that engages an abutment tooth on its external surface, used to retain and stabilize a removable partial denture. **3.** a manufactured direct retainer, the protruding portion of which is attached to the external surface of a cast crown on an abutment tooth.

extracorporeal /ek'strakôr'pôr″ē·əl/ [L, *extra* + *corpus,* body], something that is outside the body, such as extracorporeal circulation in which venous blood is diverted outside the body to a heart-lung machine and returned to the body through a femoral or other artery.

extracorporeal membrane oxygenator (ECMO), a device that oxygenates a patient's blood outside the body and returns the blood to the patient's circulatory system. The technique may be used to support an impaired respiratory system.

extracorporeal oxygenation, the use of an artificial membrane outside the body to provide for oxygenation of the blood in a patient with severe lung disease.

extracorporeal photochemotherapy, a procedure for treating T-cell lymphoma, graft-versus-host disease, and systemic sclerosis by the removal of whole blood in patients who have previously ingested the photosensitizing agent 8-methoxypsoralen (8-MOP), followed by leukapheresis and exposure of the 8-MOP–containing leukocytes outside the body to ultraviolet A light before their return to the patient. See also **photochemotherapy.**

extracorporeal shock-wave lithotripsy (ESWL) [L, *extra,* outside, *corpus,* body; Fr, *choc* + AS, *wafian* + Gk, *lithos,* stone, *tribein,* to wear away], use of vibrations of powerful sound waves to break up calculi in the urinary tract or gallbladder. Also called **shock-wave lithotripsy.**

extracorporeal technician. See **perfusion technologist.**

extracranial /-krā″nē·əl/ [L, *extra,* outside; Gk, *kranion,* skull], pertaining to something outside or unconnected with the skull.

extract [L, *ex,* out, *trahere,* to draw], **1.** *n.,* a substance, usually a biologically active ingredient, prepared by the use of solvents or evaporation to separate the substance from the original material. **2.** a concentrated form of an herb that is derived when the crude herb is mixed with water, alcohol, or another solvent and distilled or evaporated. Extracts may be either fluid or solid. **3.** *v.,* to remove a tooth from the oral cavity by means of elevators or forceps or both. – *extraction, n.*

extractor /ikstrak″tər/, a medical instrument, such as a forceps, used to remove a foreign body, tissue sample, or medical device placed in a body cavity.

extradural /ek'trədo͞or″əl/ [L, *extra* + *dura,* hard], outside the dura mater.

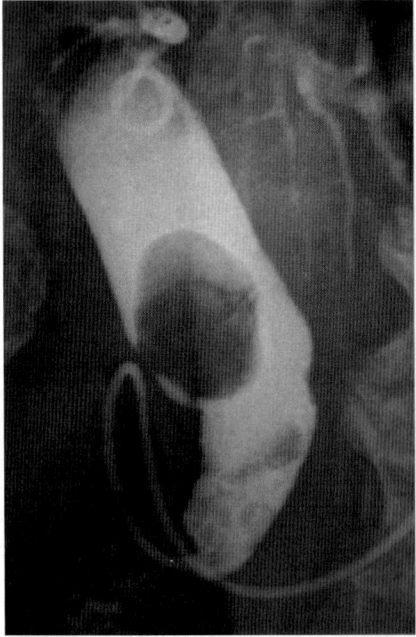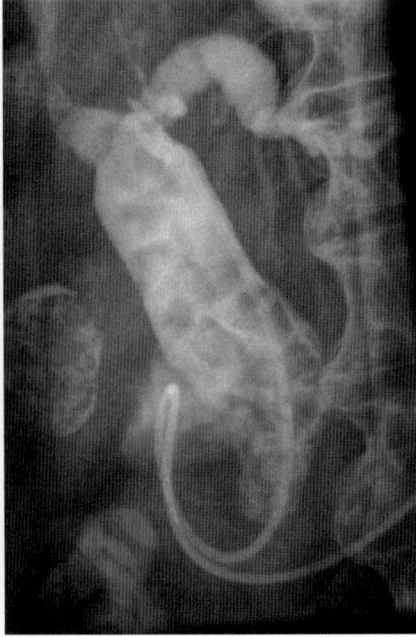

Large bile duct stone before and after fragmentation with extracorporeal shock-wave lithotripsy (ESWL)
(Amplatz et al, 2006)

extradural anesthesia, anesthetic nerve block achieved by the injection of a local anesthetic solution into the space in the spinal canal outside the dura mater of the spinal cord. Kinds include **caudal anesthesia, epidural anesthesia/analgesia, paravertebral block.**

extradural hemorrhage. See **epidural hemorrhage.**

extradural space, the space between the cranial cavity and the outer layer of dura mater.

extraembryonic blastoderm /-em′brē·on″ik/ [L, *extra* + Gk, *en,* in, *bryein,* to grow], the area of the blastoderm outside the embryo that gives rise to the membranes that surround the embryo during gestation. Compare **embryonic blastoderm.** See also **allantois, amnion, chorion, yolk sac.**

extraembryonic coelom, a cavity external to the developing embryo that forms between the mesoderm of the chorion and that covers the amniotic cavity and yolk sac. Also called **exocoelom.**

extraembryonic mesoderm [L, *extra,* outside; Gk, *en* + *bryein,* to grow, *mesos,* middle, *derma,* skin], any mesoderm in the uterus that is not involved with the embryo itself. Included are mesoderms in the amnion, chorion, yolk sac, and connecting stalk.

extrahepatic cholestasis, cholestasis occurring outside the liver, caused by blockage of a bile duct or ducts. It may be caused by a tumor or stricture, a gallstone or other damage in the duct, pancreatitis, or other causes.

extramammary Paget disease /-mam″ərē/ [L, *extra,* outside, *mamma,* breast; James Paget, English surgeon, 1814–1899; L, *dis* + Fr, *aise,* ease], a gradually spreading red, scaly, and crusted lesion resembling that of Paget disease but not occurring on the breast. A common area is the vulva. The lesions give rise to carcinoma in approximately 50% of the cases.

extramarital /-mer″itəl/, happening outside a marriage, such as an extramarital affair. Not within the boundary of the legal union of partners in marriage.

extramedullary /-med″yəler′ē/ [L, *extra* + *medulla,* marrow], pertaining to something outside or unrelated to any medulla.

extramedullary myeloma [L, *extra* + *medulla,* marrow], a plasma cell tumor most often associated with multiple myeloma that occurs outside the bone marrow, usually affecting the visceral organs or the nasopharyngeal and oral mucosa. Also called **extramedullary plasmacytoma, peripheral plasma cell myeloma, plasma cell tumor.**

extramedullary myelopoiesis, the formation and development of myeloid tissue outside the bone marrow. Also called **ectopic myelopoiesis.**

extramedullary plasmacytoma. See **extramedullary myeloma.**

extraneous /exstrā′nē·əs/ [L, strange], **1.** originating or entering from outside the organism. **2.** (in a health history) information that is given but not necessarily pertinent to the situation at hand.

extraocular /-ok″yo͞olər/ [L, *extra* + *oculus,* eye], outside the eye.

extraocular movement. See **cardinal position of gaze.**

extraocular muscle palsy, an abnormal condition characterized by paralysis of the extrinsic muscles of the eye, such as the superior, inferior, medial, and lateral rectus muscles, and the superior and the inferior oblique muscles. See also **strabismus.**

extraocular muscles (EOMs), the six sets of muscles that control movements of the eyeball. They are the superior rectus and inferior rectus, which move the eye up and down; the medial rectus and the lateral rectus, which move the eye to either side; and the superior oblique and inferior oblique,

which move the eye downward and inward, and upward and inward, respectively.

extraoral anchorage /-ôr″əl/ [L, *extra* + *oralis,* mouth, *ancora,* hook], an orthodontic holding device outside the mouth, typically linking dental attachments to a wire bow or to hooks extending between the lips and attached by elastic to a cap, neck strap, or other device outside the mouth. Also called *extraoral orthodontic appliance.*

extraperitoneal /-per′itonē″əl/ [L, *extra* + Gk, *peri,* near, around, *teinein,* to stretch], occurring or located outside the peritoneal cavity.

extraperitoneal cesarean section, *(Obsolete)* a method for surgically delivering a baby through an incision in the lower uterine segment without entering the peritoneal cavity. This operation dates from the era before antibiotics. The procedure was performed to prevent the spread of infection from the uterus into the peritoneal cavity. Compare **classic cesarean section, low cervical cesarean section.** See also **cesarean section.**

extrapleural /-plo͞or″əl/, outside the pleural cavity.

extrapleural pneumothorax, a condition in which a pocket of air or gas forms between the endothoracic fascia-pleura layer and the adjacent chest wall. See also **pneumothorax.**

extrapsychic conflict /-sī″kik/ [L, *extra* + Gk, *psyche,* mind; L, *confligere,* to strike together], an emotional conflict that usually occurs when one's inner needs and desires do not coincide with the restrictions of the environment or society. Compare **intrapsychic conflict.** See also **conflict.**

extrapulmonary /-pul″məner′ē/, outside of or unrelated to the lungs.

extrapulmonary small cell carcinoma, a primary small cell cancer with a histological diagnosis of small cell carcinoma but located in body areas outside the lungs. It occurs most frequently around the head and neck; in the pancreas, colon, and rectum; and in the genitourinary tract.

extrapyramidal /ek′strəpiram″ədəl/ [L, *extra* + Gk, *pyramis,* pyramid], **1.** pertaining to the tissues and structures outside the cerebrospinal pyramidal tracts of the brain that are associated with movement of the body, excluding motor neurons, the motor cortex, and the corticospinal and corticobulbar tracts. **2.** pertaining to the function of these tissues and structures.

extrapyramidal disease, any of a large group of conditions affecting the extrapyramidal tracts and characterized by involuntary movement, changes in muscle tone, and abnormal posture. Kinds include **tardive dyskinesia, chorea, athetosis, Parkinson's disease.**

extrapyramidal side effects, side effects that mimic extrapyramidal disease and are caused by drugs (usually first-generation antipsychotics) that block dopamine receptor sites in the extrapyramidal system tract. See also **parkinsonism.**

extrapyramidal system, the part of the nervous system that includes the basal nuclei (e.g., substantia nigra, subthalamic nucleus), part of the midbrain, and the motor neurons of the spine. See also **extrapyramidal tracts.**

extrapyramidal tracts, the uncrossed tracts of motor nerves from the brain to the anterior horns of the spinal cord, except the crossed fibers of the pyramidal tracts. Within the brain, extrapyramidal pathways comprise various relays of motoneurons between motor areas of the cerebral cortex, the basal nuclei, the thalamus, the cerebellum, and the brainstem. The extrapyramidal pathways are functional rather than anatomical units, comprising the nuclei and the fibers and excluding the pyramidal tracts. They especially control and coordinate the postural, static, supporting, and locomotor mechanisms and cause contractions of muscle groups sequentially or simultaneously. The extrapyramidal pathways include the corpus striatum, the subthalamic nucleus, the substantia nigra, and the red nucleus, together with their interconnections with the reticular formation, the cerebellum, and the cerebrum. Compare **pyramidal tract.**

extrarenal uremia. See **prerenal uremia.**

extrasensory /-sen″sərē/ [L, *extra* + *sentire*, to feel], pertaining to alleged awareness of events that cannot be observed by any of the five basic senses. Kinds include **telepathy, psychokinesis, clairvoyance.**

extrasensory perception (ESP) [L, *extra* + *sentire*, to feel, *percipere*, to perceive], alleged awareness or knowledge acquired without using the physical senses. See also **clairvoyance, parapsychology, telepathy.**

extrasystole. See **ectopic beat.**

extrauterine /-yoo″tərīn/ [L, *extra* + *uterus*, womb], occurring or located outside the uterus.

extravasation /ikstrav′əsā″shən/ [L, *extra* + *vas*, vessel], **1.** a passage or escape into the tissues, usually of blood, serum, lymph, or infusion. Compare **bleeding. 2.** passage or escape into tissue of antineoplastic chemotherapeutic drugs. Signs and symptoms may be sudden onset of localized pain at an injection site, sudden redness or extreme pallor at an injection site, or loss of blood return in an IV needle. Tissue sloughing and necrosis may occur if the condition is severe. Treatment depends on the causative agent. Nursing responsibilities include maintaining the patient IV line, elevating the affected area, applying ice packs, and notifying the physician of the need for antidote injections, if applicable. See also **exudate, transudate.** −*extravasate, v.*

extravascular fluid /-vas″kyələr/ [L, *extra*, outside, *vasculum*, small vessel, *fluere*, to flow], fluid in the body that is outside the blood vessels. Kinds include **lymph, cerebrospinal fluid.**

extraventricular hydrocephalus. See **hydrocephalus.**

extraversion. See **extroversion.**

extravert. See **extrovert.**

extraverted personality. See **extroverted personality.**

extremity /ikstrem″itē/ [L, *extremitas*], a limb or appendage. The arm may be identified by the layperson as an upper extremity and the leg as a lower extremity.

extrinsic /ikstrin″sik/ [L, *extrinsecus*, on the outside], pertaining to anything external or originating outside a structure or organism, including parts of an organ that are not wholly contained within it, as an extrinsic muscle.

extrinsic allergic alveolitis. See **hypersensitivity pneumonitis.**

extrinsic allergic pneumonia. See **diffuse hypersensitivity pneumonia.**

extrinsic asthma. See **allergic asthma.**

extrinsic factor. See **cyanocobalamin.**

extrinsic muscle (em) [L, *extrinsecus*, on the outside], **1.** a muscle that is outside the organ it controls, as the extraocular muscles that control eye movements. Extrinsic muscles of the hand include 20 muscles outside the hand and include long flexors and extensors of the wrist and fingers, the pronators, and the supinator. **2.** a muscle that links a limb to the trunk of the body.

extrinsic pathway of coagulation, the mechanism that produces fibrin after tissue injury, beginning with formation of an activated complex between tissue factor and activated factor VII and leading to activation of factor X, which induces the reactions of the common pathway of coagulation. Compare **intrinsic pathway of coagulation.** See also **coagulation cascade, common pathway of coagulation.**

extro-. See **extra-, extro-.**

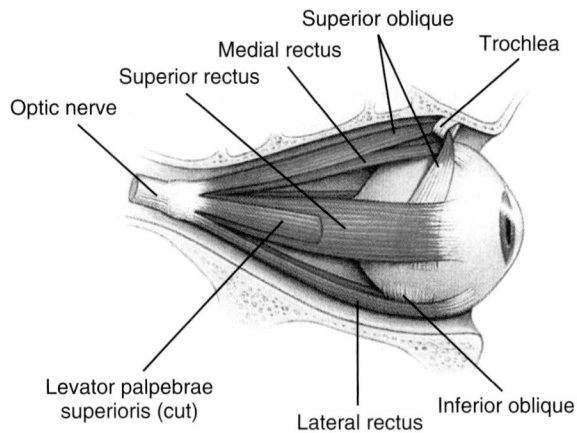

Superior view

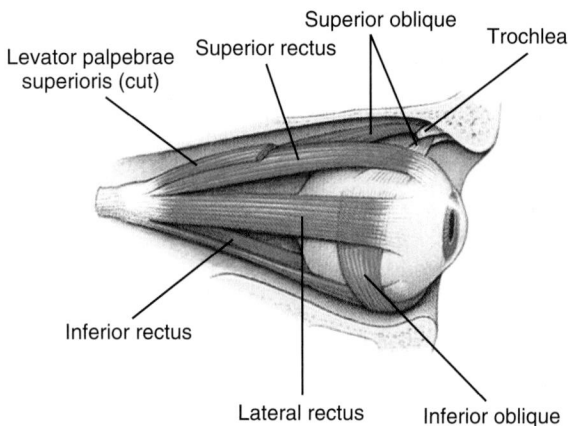

Inferior view

Extrinsic muscles of the eye *(Patton and Thibodeau, 2016)*

extroversion /-vur″zhən/ [L, *extra* + *vertere*, to turn], **1.** the tendency to direct one's interests and energies toward external values or things outside the self. **2.** the state of being totally or primarily concerned with what is outside the self.

extrovert /ik″strəvurt′/, a person whose interests are directed away from the self and concerned primarily with external reality and the physical environment rather than with inner feelings and thoughts. This person is usually highly sociable, outgoing, and emotionally expressive.

extroverted personality /-vur″tid/ [L, *extra*, outside, *vertere*, to turn, *personalis*, of a person], a persona that is directed to a greater degree toward the outer world of people and events rather than the subjective inner world experience. Also called **extraverted personality.**

extrude /ekstrōōd″/ [L, *extrudere*, to push out], to thrust out from a surface or from alignment.

extrusion /ek·strōō′zhən/ [L, *extrudere*, to push out], **1.** thrusting or pushing out; expulsion by force. **2.** the overeruption or movement of a tooth beyond its normal occlusal plane in the absence of opposing occlusal force. **3.** an orthodontic technique for the elongation or elevation of a tooth. Compare **intrusion.**

extrusion reflex /ekstroo″zhən/ [L, *extrudere,* to push out, *reflectere,* to bend back], a normal response in infants to force the tongue outward when it is touched or depressed. The reflex begins to disappear by about 3 or 4 months of age. Constant protrusion of a large tongue may be a sign of Down syndrome.

extubation /iks′t(y)ōōbā″shən/ [L, *ex,* out, *tuba,* tube], the process of withdrawing a tube from an orifice or cavity of the body. *–extubate, v.*

exuberant callus. See **heterotopic ossification.**

exudate /eks″yōōdāt/ [L, *exsudare,* to sweat out], fluid, cells, or other substances that have been slowly exuded, or discharged, from cells or blood vessels through small pores or breaks in cell membranes. Perspiration, pus, and serum are sometimes identified as exudates.

exudation /eks′yədā″shən/ [L, *exudare*], the oozing of fluid, pus, or serum. The exudate may or may not contain fibrous or coagulated material.

exudative /igzōo″dətiv/, relating to the oozing of fluid and other materials from cells and tissues, usually as a result of inflammation or injury.

exudative enteropathy, diarrhea that occurs in diseases characterized by inflammation or destruction of intestinal mucosa. Crohn's disease, ulcerative colitis, tuberculosis, and some lymphomas cause an increased amount of plasma, blood, mucus, and protein to accumulate in the intestine, adding to fecal bulk and frequency. See also **diarrhea.**

exudative inflammation [L, *exudare,* to sweat out, *inflammare,* to set afire], an inflammation of a serous or raw cavity in which fluid is released from the inflamed surface.

exudative retinopathy, a condition marked by masses of white or yellowish exudate in the posterior part of the fundus oculi, with deposits of cholesterol and blood debris from retinal hemorrhage, that leads to destruction of the macula and blindness. Also called **Coats disease, Coats retinitis,** *exudative retinitis.*

eye [AS, *eage*], one of a pair of organs of sight, contained in a bony orbit at the front of the skull, with retrobulbar fat, and innervated by four cranial nerves: optic, oculomotor, trochlear, and abducens. Associated with the eye are certain accessory structures, such as the muscles, the fasciae, the eyebrow, the eyelids, the conjunctiva, and the lacrimal gland. The bulb of the eye is composed of segments of two spheres with nearly parallel axes that constitute the outside tunic and one of three fibrous layers enclosing two internal cavities separated by the crystalline lens. The smaller cavity anterior to the lens is divided by the iris into two chambers, both filled with aqueous humor. The posterior cavity is larger than the anterior cavity and contains the jellylike vitreous body that is divided by the hyaloid canal. The outside tunic of the bulb consists of the transparent cornea anteriorly, constituting one fifth of the tunic, and the opaque sclera posteriorly, constituting five sixths of the tunic. The intermediate vascular, pigmented tunic consists of the choroid, the ciliary body, and the iris. The internal tunic of nervous tissue is the retina. Light waves passing through the lens strike a layer of rods and cones in the retina, creating impulses that are transmitted by the optic nerve to the brain. The transverse and the anteroposterior diameters of the eye bulb are slightly greater than the vertical diameter; the bulb in women is usually smaller than the bulb in men. Eye movement is controlled by six muscles: the superior and inferior oblique muscles and the superior, inferior, medial, and lateral rectus muscles. Also called **bulbus oculi,** *eyeball.*

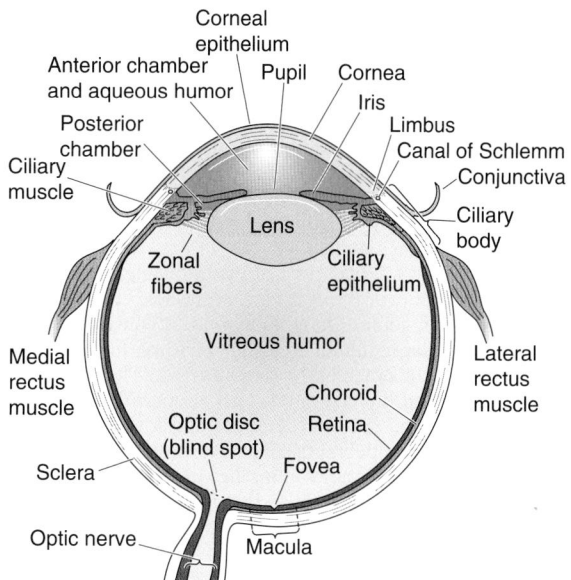

Cross section of right eye *(Boron and Boulpaep, 2012)*

eye bank [AS, *eage* + It, *banca,* bench], a facility for collecting and storing corneas and other ocular tissues for transplantation to recipients.

eyebrow [AS, *eage* + *bru*], **1.** the supraorbital arch of the frontal bone that separates the orbit of the eye from the forehead. **2.** the arch of hairs growing along the ridge formed by the supraorbital arch of the frontal bone.

eye-closure reflex. See **wink reflex.**

eyecup, a small vessel or cup that is shaped to fit over the eyeball and used to bathe the exposed surface of the eye.

eye deviation [AS, *eage* + L, *deviare,* to turn aside], **1.** a movement of one or both eyes, singly or jointly, from the median line or from the original direction of fixation. Manifest deviation is the number of degrees by which the visual axis of one eye deviates from that of the other in cases of squint, when both eyes are open. **2.** (in strabismus) the departure of the foveal line of sight of one eye from the point of fixation.

eye dominance, an unconscious preference to use one eye rather than the other for certain purposes, such as looking through a microscope or telescope.

eyedrops, a liquid medicine that is administered by allowing it to fall in drops onto the conjunctival surface.

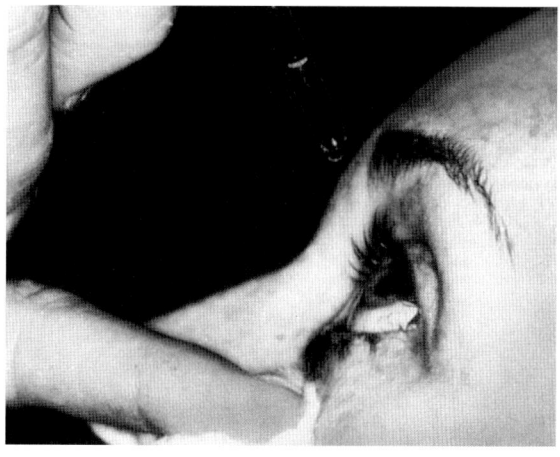

Instillation of eyedrops *(Stein et al, 2013)*

eye glasses, transparent lenses held in metal or plastic frames in front of the eyes to correct refractive errors or to protect the eyes from harmful electromagnetic waves or flying objects.

eyeground, the fundus of the eye as revealed by ophthalmoscopic examination.

eyelash [AS, *eage* + ME, *lasche*], one of many stiff hairs growing in double or triple rows along the border of the eyelids in front of a row of ciliary glands that are in front of a row of meibomian glands.

eyelid [AS, *eage* + *hlid*], one of two movable folds of protective thin skin over the eye, with eyelashes, ciliary glands, and meibomian glands along its margin. It consists of loose connective tissue containing a thin plate of fibrous tissue lined with mucous membrane (conjunctiva). The orbicularis oculi muscle and the oculomotor nerve control the opening and closing of the eyelid. The upper and lower eyelids are separated by the palpebral fissure. Also called **palpebra.**

eyelid myoclonia, rapid blinking of the eyelids with upward deviation of the eyes and extension of the head.

eye memory. See **visual memory.**

eye patching, **1.** placement of a soft patch over a closed eye to restrict lid movement during corneal reepithelialization or a similar healing procedure in progress. **2.** occlusion of the better eye by patch placement in young patients with amblyopia to force greater use of the amblyopic eye. **3.** patching used in cases of diplopia (double vision).

eye reanimation, microsurgical restoration of function of a paralyzed iris sphincter.

eye shielding, protection of an injured eye by securing a metal or plastic eye shield or a disposable cup over the eye to prevent further injury.

eye wash, an apparatus for irrigating the eyes after exposure to dust or other debris or chemical contamination. The shower directs one or two streams of water so that they flush over the eyes and lids. The person being treated should blink the eyes and move the head in different directions with the eyes open, continuing the irrigation as needed.

eye worm. See ***Loa loa.***

ezetimibe, an antilipemic agent used to treat hypercholesterolemia, homozygous low-density lipoprotein receptor disorder, and homozygous sitosterolemia.

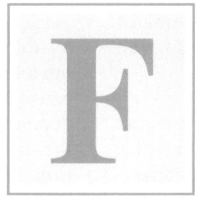

f, **1.** symbol for *breaths per unit time.* **2.** symbol for *respiratory frequency.*

F, **1.** abbreviation for **Fahrenheit. 2.** abbreviation for **farad. 3.** symbol for **fluorine. 4.** abbreviation for **frequency.**

F$_1$, symbol for **first filial generation.**

F$_2$, symbol for **second filial generation.**

F$_c$, a part of a molecule of an antibody that has been split by a proteolytic enzyme. It represents the relatively constant region, as distinguished from the Fab portion, that contains the binding sites. The F$_c$ portion is sometimes identified as the crystallizable fragment.

FA, **1.** abbreviation for **fatty acid. 2.** abbreviation for **femoral artery. 3.** abbreviation for **folic acid.**

FAAN, abbreviation for **Fellow of the American Academy of Nursing.**

Fab fragment, the region of an antibody molecule that contains the antigen-binding site, consisting of a light chain and part of a heavy chain. Such fragments are produced when antibodies are digested by enzymes, such as the protease papain. Fab fragments are used as an antidote for treating toxicity caused by digoxin, digitoxin, and oleander tea. See also **F$_c$, Digibind.**

FAB classification, a classification of acute leukemia produced by a three-nation joint collaboration (French-American-British). Acute lymphoblastic leukemia is subdivided into three types, and acute myelogenous leukemia is subdivided into eight types.

fabere, a measurement based on several types of extremity movements. Abbreviation for *flexion, abduction, external rotation, then extension.* See also **Patrick test.**

fabere sign. See **Patrick test.**

Fabrazyme, an enzyme replacement. Brand name for **agalsidase beta.**

fabrication /fab′rikā″shən/, a psychological reaction in which false statements are contrived to mask memory defects. It is a clinical feature of Korsakoff's syndrome and other disorders. See also **confabulation.**

Fabry disease. See **angiokeratoma corporis diffusum.**

Fabry syndrome. See **angiokeratoma corporis diffusum.**

FAC, an anticancer drug combination of fluorouracil, doxorubicin, and cyclophosphamide.

F.A.C.D., abbreviation for *Fellow of the American College of Dentists.*

face [L, *facies*], **1.** *n.,* the front of the head from the chin to the brow, including the skin and muscles and structures of the forehead, eyes, nose, mouth, cheeks, and jaw. **2.** *n.,* the visage or countenance. **3.** *v.,* to direct the face toward something. See also **en face. –facial,** *adj.*

face-bow [L, *facies* + AS, *boga*], a device resembling a caliper for measuring the relationship of the maxilla to the temporomandibular joints. The measurement is used in the fabrication of denture casts and major restorative procedures involving natural teeth. See also **articulator.**

face lift, a plastic surgery procedure in which wrinkles and other signs of aging skin are eliminated. Also called **rhytidectomy, rhytidoplasty.**

face presentation [L, *facies,* face, *praesentare,* to show], an obstetric presentation in which the chin of the fetus is the first feature to appear in labor.

facet /fas″it/ [Fr, *facette,* little face], **1.** (in dentistry) a flattened, highly polished wear pattern on a tooth. **2.** a small, smooth-surfaced process for articulation.

facetectomy /fas″itek″təmē/, surgical removal of a facet, particularly the articular facet of a vertebra.

facet joint, synovial joint between articular processes (zygapophytes) of the vertebrae. Also called **zygapophyseal joint.**

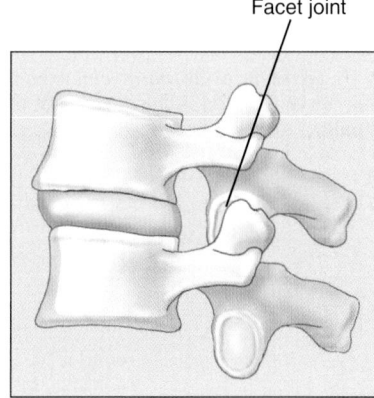

Facet joint *(Muscolino, 2011)*

facial. See **face.**

facial angle /fāshəl/ [L, *facies* + *angulus,* a corner], the degree of protrusion of the lower face, assessed by measuring the inclination of the facial plane relative to the horizontal reference plane.

facial artery, one of a pair of tortuous arteries that arise from the external carotid arteries, divide into four cervical and five facial branches, and supply various organs and tissues in the head. The cervical branches of the facial artery are the ascending palatine, tonsillar, glandular, and submental. The facial branches are the inferior labial, superior labial, lateral nasal, angular, and muscular.

facial bones, the 14 bones that form the face of the skull. They include two each of the nasal, palatine, inferior nasal concha, maxilla, lacrimal, and zygomatic bones, plus the mandible and vomer.

facial diplegia, a rare neuromuscular condition characterized by bilateral paralysis of various muscles of the face. See also **Möbius' syndrome.**

facial hemiplegia,   paralysis of the muscles of one side of the face, usually causing a facial droop and associated with a stroke.

facial hemispasm.   See **Bell's spasm.**

facial muscle,   one of numerous muscles of the face that seldom remains distinct over its entire length because of a tendency to merge with a neighboring muscle at its termination or its attachment. The five groups of facial muscles are the muscles of the scalp, the extrinsic muscles of the ear, the muscles of the nose, the muscles of the eyelid, and the muscles of the mouth. The platysma is one of the facial group but is classified among the muscles of the neck. Also called **muscle of expression.**

facial nerve,   either of a pair of mixed sensory and motor cranial nerves that arise from the brainstem at the base of the pons and divide immediately in front of the ear into six branches, innervating the scalp, forehead, eyelids, muscles of facial expression, cheeks, and jaw. Also called **seventh cranial nerve.**

facial nerve paralysis,   a loss of voluntary control of the muscles of the face, usually on one side. The condition may be caused by a lesion involving the facial muscles or a nerve peripheral to the nucleus or by damage elsewhere in the brainstem or cerebrum. Weakness may be limited to the lower portion of the face, depending on the site of the lesion and the tracts involved.

facial neuralgia,   the occurrence of pain in the middle ear and auditory canal caused by inflammation of the otic ganglion.

facial palsy [L, *facies,* face; Gk, *paralyein,* to be palsied],   a loss of motor nerve function in the muscles of the face. See also **Bell's palsy.**

facial paralysis,   an abnormal condition characterized by the partial or total loss of the functions of the facial muscles or the loss of sensation in the face. It may be caused by disease or by trauma. The degree of paralysis depends on the nerves affected. Brain injury above the facial nerve nucleus usually does not block the innervation of the brow and the forehead muscles. Injury to the nucleus of the facial nerve or injury to its peripheral neurons paralyzes all the ipsilateral facial muscles. See also **Bell's palsy.**

facial perception,   the ability to judge the distance and direction of objects through the sensation felt in the skin of the face. The phenomenon is commonly experienced by those who are blind and is rarely experienced in the dark by those with sight. Also called **facial vision.**

facial reanimation,   the use of surgical procedures to improve facial appearance and motion in facial paralysis.

facial tic [L, *facies,* face; Fr, *tic,* twitching],   any repetitive, spasmodic, and involuntary contraction of groups of facial muscles. See also **tic douloureux, trigeminal neuralgia.**

facial vein,   one of a pair of superficial veins that drain deoxygenated blood from the superficial structures of the face. The facial vein anastomoses with the cavernous sinus through various veins, such as the angular, the supraorbital, and the superior ophthalmic. Because the vein has no valves that prevent the backflow of blood, infections of the skin near the nose and mouth may progress into deeper tissues and lead to meningitis. Blood-borne organisms can reach the cavernous sinus through the anastomoses.

facial vision.   See **facial perception.**

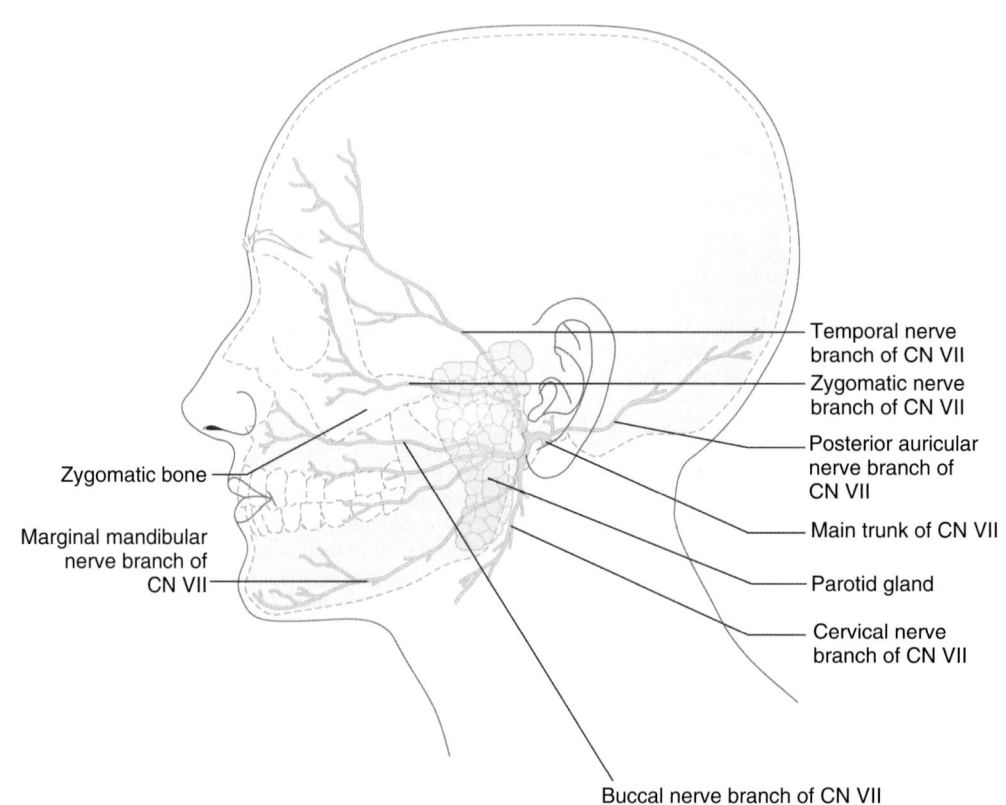

Main branches of the facial nerve (CN VII) *(Kouba and Moy, 2008)*

facies /fā″shē·ēs/ *pl. facies* [L, face], **1.** the face. **2.** the surface of any body structure, part, or organ. **3.** facial expression or appearance.

facilitation /fəsil′itā″shən/ [L, *facilitas,* easiness], **1.** the enhancement or reinforcement of any action or function so that it can be performed more easily. Compare **inhibition. 2.** (in neurology) the phenomenon whereby two or more afferent impulses that individually are not strong enough to elicit a response in a neuron can collectively produce a reflex discharge greater than the sum of the separate responses. See also **summation.**

facilitation/excitation, planned, graded physical guidance techniques used to improve movement coordination by increasing inadequate muscle tone, altering sensory responsiveness, and/or altering behavioral states (e.g., hands-on facilitation techniques that are targeted key postural points such as the shoulders, trunk, and hips).

facilitory casting /fəsil′itôr′ē/, a method of making prosthetic casts with materials that increase muscle tone in a specific group while increasing or decreasing range of motion.

facio-, prefix meaning "face": *faciolingual.*

faciodigitogenital syndrome, faciogenital dysplasia. See **Aarskog's syndrome.**

faciolingual /fā′shōling″gwəl/, pertaining to the face and tongue.

F.A.C.O.G., abbreviation for *Fellow of the American College of Obstetricians and Gynecologists.*

F.A.C.P., abbreviation for *Fellow of the American College of Physicians.*

F.A.C.S., abbreviation for *Fellow of the American College of Surgeons.*

facsimile (fax), a method of transmitting images or printed matter by electronic means. Images are scanned, converted into electronic signals, and sent over telephone lines to a fax receiver, which reconverts the electronic data into a duplicate of the original image.

F.A.C.S.M., abbreviation for *Fellow of the American College of Sports Medicine.*

-faction, suffix meaning "a process of making": *liquefaction, putrefaction.*

factitial /fakti″shəl/ [L, *facticius,* artificial], artificial or self-induced, such as a factitial dermatitis.

factitial dermatitis, self-induced skin lesions resulting from habitual rubbing, scratching, hair pulling, malingering, or mental disturbance.

factitious diarrhea, diarrhea caused by something the patient is doing to his or her own body, usually surreptitious laxative abuse.

factitious disorder /faktish″əs/, a *DSM-5* diagnosis marked by disease symptoms caused by deliberate efforts of a person to gain attention. Such actions may be repeated, even when the individual is aware of the hazards involved. See also **Münchausen's syndrome.**

Factive, a synthetic broad-spectrum antibacterial agent. Brand name for **gemifloxacin.**

-factive, -fying, suffix meaning "making": *intensifying, putrefactive.*

factor, **1.** one of a number of elements contributing to a whole. **2.** a number by which another number is exactly divisible. **3.** one of a number of elements that affect a specific result.

factor I. See **fibrinogen.**

factor II. See **prothrombin.**

factor IIa. See **thrombin.**

factor III, *(Obsolete)* designation for a membrane protein normally found in subendothelial tissue. When exposed to blood, it forms a complex with factor VIIa to activate extrinsic coagulation. Now called **tissue factor.**

factor IV, a designation for calcium that is involved in the process of blood coagulation.

factor V, coagulation cofactor to factor Xa; forms a complex that converts prothrombin rapidly to thrombin. Also called **proaccelerin.**

factor VII, a serine protease procoagulant present in the plasma and synthesized in the liver in the presence of vitamin K. Also called **proconvertin.**

factor VIII, a coagulation factor present in normal plasma but deficient from the blood of persons with hemophilia A. Acts as a cofactor to factor IX in intrinsic coagulation. Also called **antihemophilic factor.**

factor IX, a serine protease coagulation factor present in normal plasma but deficient from the blood of persons with hemophilia B. Factor IX forms a complex with its cofactor, factor VIII, to activate factor X. Also called **Christmas factor.**

factor IX complex, a hemostatic containing factors II, VII, IX, and X.

■ INDICATIONS: It is prescribed in the treatment of hemophilia B. It is a vitamin K–dependent protein synthesized in the liver.

■ CONTRAINDICATIONS: Liver disease with associated intravascular coagulation and fibrinolysis is the only contraindication.

■ ADVERSE EFFECTS: Among the more serious adverse effects are hepatitis, intravascular coagulation, circulatory collapse, and hypersensitivity reaction.

factor X, a serine protease coagulation factor in normal plasma that forms a complex with its cofactor, factor V, to convert prothrombin to thrombin. Also called **Stuart-Prower factor.**

factor XI, a serine protease coagulation factor present in normal plasma that activates factor IX. Deficiency results in Rosenthal disease.

factor XII, a serine protease coagulation factor present in normal plasma that activates factor XI in the presence of prekallikrein and high molecular weight kininogen. Factor XII is activated in vitro by contact with negatively charged surfaces, such as glass, kaolin, or ellagic acid. Deficiencies of factor XII do not cause clinical bleeding disorders but may prolong laboratory coagulation tests. Also called **Hageman factor.**

factor XIII, a transamidase coagulation factor present in normal plasma that crosslinks fibrin polymer to produce a stable fibrin clot. Also called *fibrin stabilizing factor.*

factor-searching study, (in nursing research) a study design that produces a qualitative narrative description that includes categories or classifications of phenomena. It may be used to describe various aspects of nursing practice, characteristics of a population, or both. Factor searching is often a preliminary step in a study at a higher level of inquiry.

factor V Leiden (FVL) test, a molecular diagnostic test on DNA derived from whole blood that tests for the factor V Leiden mutation, an amino acid substitution in the coagulation factor V molecule that renders it resistant to activated protein C digestion, resulting in an increased thrombotic risk.

factor Xa, a serine endopeptidase that catalyzes the conversion of prothrombin to active thrombin.

facultative /fak′əltā″tiv/ [L, *facultas,* capability], **1.** not obligatory. **2.** having the ability to adapt to more than one condition, such as a facultative anaerobe. Compare **obligate.**

facultative aerobe, an organism that is able to grow under anaerobic conditions but that develops most rapidly in an aerobic environment. Compare **obligate aerobe.** See also **aerobe.**

facultative anaerobe, an organism that is able to grow under aerobic conditions but that develops most rapidly in an anaerobic environment. Compare **obligate anaerobe.** See also **anaerobic infection, anaerobe.**

facultative parasite. See **parasite.**

faculty /fak′əltē/ [L, *facultas,* capability], **1.** any normal physiological function or natural ability of a living organism, such as the digestive faculty or the ability to perceive and distinguish sensory stimuli. **2.** an ability to do something specific, such as learn languages or remember names. **3.** any mental ability or power, such as memory or thought. **4.** a department in an institution of learning or the people who teach in a department of such an institution.

FAD, abbreviation for *fetal activity determination.* See **non-stress test.**

fading assistance, a method of grading an activity by gradually reducing the level of support given until the individual performs the activity independently.

fading time, the time required for a constant stimulus applied to a fixed area of the peripheral visual field to stop.

faecal. See **fecal.**

faeces, faex. See **feces.**

Faget sign /fazhā′/ [Jean C. Faget, French physician, 1818–1884], a falling pulse rate associated with a constant temperature, or a constant pulse associated with a rising temperature. It is an unusual sign found in yellow fever. Also called *Faget law.*

fagicladosporic acid /faj′iklad′ōspôr″ik/, a toxin produced by *Cladosporium epiphyllum,* a member of a genus of fungi that cause "black spot" in stored meat, tinea nigra, and black degeneration of the brain.

Fahrenheit (F) /fer″ənhīt/ [Daniel G. Fahrenheit, German physicist, 1686–1736], a scale for the measurement of temperature in which the boiling point of water is 212° F and the freezing point of water is 32° F at sea level. To convert to Celsius, subtract 32, then divide by 1.8. Compare **Celsius.**

failed forceps, a situation in which the use of obstetric forceps to assist the birth powers fails in obtaining a vaginal birth. Compare **trial forceps.** See also **double setup, forceps delivery.**

failure to thrive (FTT) /fāl″yər/ [L, *fallere,* to deceive; ME, *thriven,* to grasp], the abnormal delay of growth and development of an infant resulting from conditions that interfere with normal metabolism, appetite, and activity. Causative factors include chromosomal abnormalities, as in Turner's syndrome and the various trisomies; major organ system defects that lead to deficiency or malfunction; systemic disease or acute illness; physical deprivation, primarily malnutrition; and various psychosocial factors, as in severe cases of maternal deprivation syndrome. Metabolic disturbances of short duration, as occur during acute illness, usually have no long-term effects on development and are usually followed by a period of rapid growth. Prolonged nutritional deficiency may cause permanent and irreversible delay of physical, mental, or social development.

faint [OFr, *faindre,* to feign], **1.** *(Nontechnical) v.,* to lose consciousness, often causing a fall, as in a syncopal attack. See also **syncope. 2.** *adj.,* a subjective feeling of light-headedness and weakness, as if one will fall. **3.** *adj.,* barely perceptible, as a *faint* symptom.

fainting. See **syncope.**

faith healing [L, *fidere,* to trust; AS, *hoelen,* to make whole], alleged healing through the power to cause a cure or recovery from an illness or injury without the aid of conventional medical treatment. The healer is believed to have been given that power by a supernatural force.

falciform body. See **sporozoite.**

falciform ligament /fal″sifôrm/, a triangular or sickle-shaped ligament of the body, such as the broad ligament of the liver.

falciform ligament of liver. See **broad ligament of the liver.**

falcine herniation, a herniation of the brain beneath the falx cerebri, caused by focal cerebral edema.

falciparum malaria /falsip″ərəm/ [L, *falx,* sickle, *forma,* form; It, *mal,* bad, *aria,* air], the most severe form of malaria, caused by the protozoon *Plasmodium falciparum.* The condition is characterized by extremely grave systemic symptoms, mild jaundice, mental confusion, enlarged spleen and liver, increased respiratory rate, edema, GI symptoms, and anemia. The parasite replicates so rapidly in erythrocytes that cerebral vessels may be obstructed. Falciparum malaria episodes do not last as long as other forms of malaria; if treatment is begun promptly, the disease may be mild and the recovery uneventful. Relapses are uncommon, but death may result from dehydration and anemia. The usual treatment is chloroquine, but patients known to have contracted malaria in an area that harbors drug-resistant *P. falciparum* are often treated with a combination of quinine, pyrimethamine, and mefloquine. Compare **quartan malaria, tertian malaria.** See also **algid malaria, blackwater fever, malaria.**

fall /fawl/, a coming down freely, usually under the influence of gravity.

fallectomy /fəlek″təmē/. See **salpingectomy.**

fallen arch, a flattened foot arch, which often results in a flat deformity or splayfoot. The condition may involve the longitudinal arch, the transverse arch, or both. When the longitudinal arch is involved, the condition is called flatfoot. See also **flatfoot.**

fallopian canal [Gabriello Fallopio, Italian anatomist, 1523–1562; L, *canalis*], a passageway for the facial nerve through the petrous bone.

fallopian tube /fəlō″pē·ən/ [Gabriello Fallopio], one of a pair of ducts opening at one end into the uterus and at the other end into the peritoneal cavity, over the ovary. Each tube serves as the passage through which an ovum is carried to the uterus and through which spermatozoa move out toward the ovary. The tube lies in the upper border of the broad ligament (the mesosalpinx). Each tube has four parts: the fimbriae, the infundibulum, the ampulla, and the isthmus. The fimbriae drape in fingerlike projections from the infundibulum over the ovary. Immediately proximal to the infundibulum is the ampulla, the widest portion of the tube. The ampulla is connected to the fundus of the uterus by the isthmus. Also called **oviduct, uterine tube.** See also **tubal ligation.**

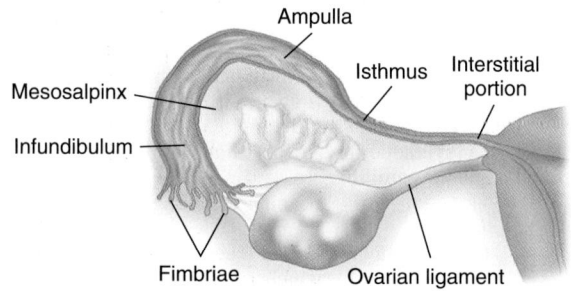

Parts of the fallopian tube *(Hagen-Ansert, 2012)*

Fallot's syndrome. See **tetralogy of Fallot.**

fallout [AS, *feallan,* to fall, *ut*], the deposition of radioactive debris after a nuclear explosion. The waste products of an atmospheric explosion of an atomic bomb may travel thousands of miles in the atmosphere and be deposited over a large geographic area.

false ankylosis [L, *fallere,* to deceive; Gk, *agkylosis,* joint stiffness], a type of joint immobility that results from abnormal inflexibility of body parts outside the joint. Also called **extracapsular ankylosis.**

false anorexia. See **pseudoanorexia.**

false cyst. See **pseudocyst.**

false diverticulum [L, *fallere,* to deceive, *diverticulare,* to turn aside], a protrusion of mucous membrane through a muscular coat defect of a hollow organ.

false glottis, the triangular opening between the two adjacent vestibular folds at the entrance to the middle chamber of the laryngeal cavity. Also called **glottis spuria, rima respitoria, rima vestibule.**

false imprisonment [L, *falsus,* deceptive; ME, *imprisonen*], (in law) an intentional tort; the intentional unjustified, nonconsensual detention or confinement of a person within fixed boundaries for any length of time. Restraint may be physical, chemical, or emotional (e.g., intimidation or threat).

false joint [L, *fallere,* to deceive, *jungere,* to join], a joint that develops at the site of a former fracture. Also called **nonunion, pseudoarthrosis.**

false labor, discoordinate albeit painful uterine contractions, usually experienced in the late third trimester, that do not result in progressive dilation and effacement of the cervix and descent of the fetus (true labor). See **Braxton Hicks contractions.**

false negative, a result of a diagnostic test or procedure that incorrectly indicates the absence of a finding, condition, or disease. All tests and procedures generate false positive (false alarm) and false negative (miss) results. Test and procedure designers establish levels of clinical specificity and sensitivity that minimize false results. Screening tests and procedures are designed to be sensitive, producing high false positive rates. Confirmatory tests and procedures follow to substantiate the findings. Screening and confirmatory tests and procedures are used in sequence to generate the best clinical validity. Compare **false positive.**

false-negative rate [L, *fallere,* to deceive, *negare,* to deny, *ratum,* calculate], the rate of occurrence of negative test results in subjects known to have the disease or behavior for which an individual is being tested.

false neuroma, 1. a neoplasm that does not contain nerve elements. **2.** See **cystic neuroma.**

false nucleolus. See **karyosome.**

false pelvis, the part of the pelvis superior to a plane passing through the linea terminalis.

false personification, (in psychiatry) the labeling and prejudgment of others without validating evidence.

false positive, a test result that wrongly indicates the presence of a disease or other condition the test is designed to reveal. Compare **false negative.**

false-positive rate [L, *fallere,* to deceive, *positivus* + *ratum,* calculate], the rate of occurrence of positive test results in subjects known to be free of a disease or disorder for which an individual is being tested.

false pregnancy. See **pseudocyesis.**

false rib, vertebrocostal rib. See **rib, vertebrocostal rib.**

false suture, an immovable fibrous joint in which rough articulating surfaces form the connection between certain bones of the skull. Compare **true suture.** Kinds include **sutura plana, sutura squamosa.**

false transactions, (in transactional analysis), transactions in which communication is stopped or distorted when one individual relates from a different ego state than what is expected.

false twins. See **dizygotic twins.**

false vertebra, one of the vertebral segments that form the sacrum and the coccyx. Also called **fixed vertebra.**

false vocal cord, either of two thick folds of mucous membrane in the larynx separating the ventricle from the vestibule. Each fold encloses a narrow band of fibrous tissue (the ventricular ligament). Also called **vestibular fold.** Compare **vocal cord.**

falx /falks, fôlks/ *pl. falces* [L, sickle], **1.** *n.,* a sickle-shaped structure. **2.** *adj.,* sickle-shaped.

falx cerebelli. See **cerebellar falx.**

falx cerebri. See **cerebral falx.**

falx inguinalis. See **inguinal falx.**

falx ligamentosa, the broad ligament of the liver.

FAM, an anticancer drug combination of fluorouracil, doxorubicin, and mitomycin.

famciclovir, an antiviral drug.

■ INDICATIONS: It is prescribed in the treatment of acute herpes zoster and recurrent genital herpes.

■ CONTRAINDICATIONS: It should not be given to patients with kidney disease or an allergy to famciclovir. The safety of the drug in children or in women who are pregnant or breastfeeding has not been established.

■ ADVERSE EFFECTS: The side effects most often reported include fatigue, fever, pain, chills, headache, dizziness, nausea, diarrhea, vomiting, and constipation.

familial /fəmil′yəl/ [L, *familia,* household], pertaining to a characteristic, condition, or disease that is present in some families and not others or that occurs in more family members than would be expected by chance. It is usually but not always hereditary. Compare **acquired, congenital, hereditary.**

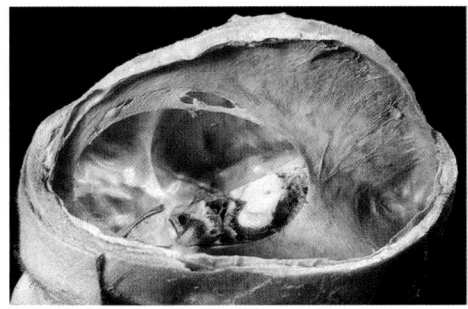
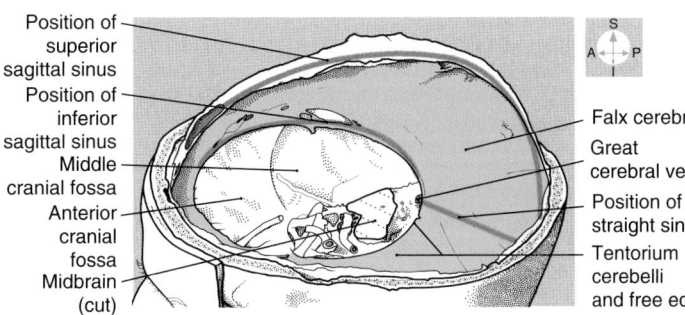

Falx cerebri and tentorium cerebelli revealed by removal of the vault of the cranium *(Gosling et al, 2008)*

familial adenomatous polyposis (FAP), an inherited disorder characterized by the development of myriad polyps in the colon beginning in late adolescence or early adulthood. Untreated, the condition nearly always leads to colon cancer. See also **adenomatous polyposis coli.**

familial atypical mole-malignant melanoma syndrome (FAMMM). See **dysplastic nevus syndrome.**

familial autonomic dysfunction. See **dysautonomia.**

familial centrolobar sclerosis. See **Pelizaeus-Merzbacher disease.**

familial cretinism, a rare genetic disorder caused by an inborn error of metabolism resulting from an enzyme deficiency that interferes with thyroid hormone biosynthesis. Clinical manifestations include lethargy, stunted growth, and cognitive impairment. The condition is transmitted as an autosomal-recessive trait and is treated by early administration of thyroid hormone, if possible in utero, to reduce the abnormalities of mental development. See also **cretinism.**

familial dysautonomia. See **dysautonomia.**

familial hemophagocytic lymphohistiocytosis [L, *familia,* household; Gk, *histion,* web, *kytos,* cell; L, *reticulum,* little net; Gk, *osis,* condition], an autosomal-recessive disease, characterized by anemia, granulocytopenia, and thrombocytopenia. Phagocytosis of blood cells and infiltration of bone marrow by macrophages commonly cause death in childhood. Also called *familial hemophagocytic reticulosis.*

familial Hibernian fever, a periodic syndrome associated with a mutation in a receptor for tumor necrosis factor. This defect causes recurrent high fevers, rash, and abdominal pain. Mean age of first episode is 3 years but varies from patient to patient.

familial hypercholesterolemia. See **low-density lipoprotein (LDL) receptor disorder.**

familial hyperglyceridemia. See **hyperlipidemia type I.**

familial iminoglycinuria. See **iminoglycinuria.**

familial juvenile nephronophthisis. See **medullary cystic disease.**

familial lipoprotein lipase deficiency. See **hyperchylomicronemia.**

familial Mediterranean fever, an autosomal-recessive intestinal disorder usually occurring in people of Mediterranean descent, characterized by short recurrent attacks of fever with pain in the abdomen, chest, or joints and erythema resembling that seen in erysipelas. It is sometimes complicated by secondary amyloidosis. The age of onset is usually between 5 and 15 years. Also called **benign paroxysmal peritonitis, familial recurrent polyserositis, periodic peritonitis, periodic polyserositis, recurrent polyserositis.**

familial multiple endocrine. See **multiple endocrine adenomatosis.**

familial nonhemolytic jaundice. See **Gilbert's syndrome.**

familial osteochondrodystrophy. See **Morquio's disease.**

familial periodic fever, a rare autosomal-dominant syndrome that includes an abnormality on the cell receptor for tumor necrosis factor. It is characterized by periodic fever and a variety of skin disorders. The fever lasts for 4 days to 3 weeks with mild systemic manifestations such as abdominal pain, headache, and chest pain. Also called **tumor necrosis factor receptor–associated periodic syndrome.**

familial periodic paralysis [L, *familia,* household; Gk, *peri,* near, *hodos,* way, *paralysein,* to be palsied], a rare inherited disorder in which clients suffer attacks of general flaccid paralysis after attacks of hypokalemia (potassium depletion). The episodes may follow administration of glucose and are relieved by administration of potassium chloride.

familial polyposis, an abnormal condition characterized by multiple polyps in the colon and rectum. The disease has high malignancy potential and is inherited as a heterozygous, autosomal-dominant trait. Total proctocolectomy eliminates the risk of cancer, which, if untreated, occurs before 40 years of age. Genetic counseling is advised. Kinds include **Gardner's syndrome.** See also **polyposis.**

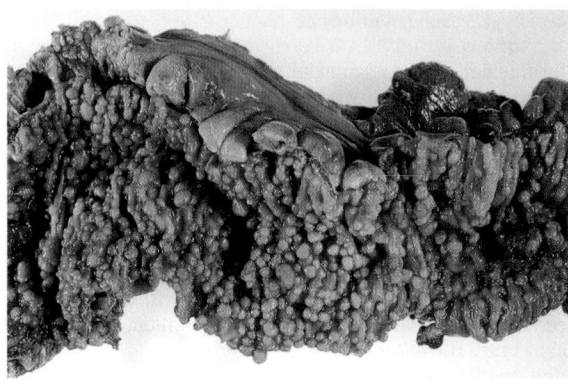

Familial polyposis *(Walker et al, 2014)*

familial recurrent polyserositis. See **familial Mediterranean fever.**

familial spinal muscular atrophy. See **Werdnig-Hoffmann disease.**

familial tremor. See **essential tremor.**

familial visceral amyloidosis, a rare autosomal-dominant type of amyloidosis characterized by nephropathy, arterial hypertension, hepatosplenomegaly, albuminuria, hematuria, and pitting edema. Affected patients usually die within 10 years of onset of clinical manifestations. Also called *Ostertag, Ostertag type a.*

family [L, *familia,* household], a group of people related by heredity, such as parents, children, and siblings. The term sometimes is broadened to include persons related by marriage or those living in the same household, who are emotionally attached, interact regularly, and share concerns for the growth and development of the group and its individual members.

family Apgar, a family therapy rating system in which the name Apgar contains the first letters of five words *a*daptability, *p*artnership, *g*rowth, *a*ffection, and *r*esolve—that represent the questionnaire categories. Each family member indicates a degree of satisfaction in each of the five categories on a scale of 0 to 2. The system is used most frequently in studies of families with a geriatric member. See also **Apgar score.**

family care leave, absence from a job that is permitted for an employee to care for a family member who is ill, disabled, or pregnant. The U.S. Family and Medical Leave Act of 1993 provides 12 weeks of unpaid leave per year from a job for the birth or adoption of a child; for the care of a seriously ill child, spouse, or parent; or for a serious illness affecting the employee. The law applies only to companies with 50 or more employees. Employers must guarantee that a worker can return to the same or a comparable job.

family-centered care, primary health care that includes an assessment of the health of an entire family, identification of actual or potential factors that might influence the health of its members, and implementation of interventions needed to maintain or improve the health of the unit and its members.

family-centered maternity care, a system for the delivery of safe, high-quality health care adapted to the physical and psychosocial needs of the patient, the patient's entire family, and the newly born offspring.

family-centered nursing care, nursing care directed to improving the potential health of a family or any of its members by assessing individual and family health needs and strengths, by identifying problems influencing the health care of the family as a whole and those influencing the individual members, by using family resources, by teaching and counseling, and by evaluating progress toward stated goals.

family counseling, a program of providing information and professional guidance to members of a family concerning specific health matters, such as the care of a child with severe developmental disabilities or the risk of transmitting a known genetic defect.

family disorganization, a breakdown of a family system. It may be associated with parental overburdening or loss of significant others who served as role models for children or support systems for family members. Family disorganization can contribute to the loss of social controls that families usually impose on their members.

family dynamics, the forces at work within the family that produce particular behaviors or symptoms.

family functions, processes by which the family operates as a whole, including communication and manipulation of the environment for problem solving.

family health. See **family history.**

family history, an essential part of a patient's medical history in which he or she is asked about the health of members of the immediate family in a series of specific questions to discover any disorders to which the patient may be particularly vulnerable, such as "Has anyone in your family had tuberculosis? Diabetes mellitus? Breast cancer?" Hereditary and familial diseases are especially noted. The age and health of each person, age at death, and causes of death are charted. Often a genogram is developed for pictoral documentation. The family health history is obtained from the patient or family in the initial interview and becomes a part of the permanent record. Other questions, such as those concerning the age, sex, relationships of others in the household, and marital history of the patient, may also be asked if the information has not already been secured.

family medicine, the branch of medicine that is concerned with the diagnosis and treatment of health problems in people of either sex and any age. Practitioners of family medicine are often called family practice physicians, family physicians, or, formerly, general practitioners. They often act as the primary health care providers, referring complex disorders to a specialist.

family myths, myths that are constructed to deny the reality or idealize an aspect of family situations.

family nurse practitioner (FNP), a nurse practitioner possessing skills necessary for the detection and management of acute self-limiting conditions and management of chronic stable conditions. An FNP provides primary ambulatory care for families in collaboration with primary care physicians. The FNP gives direct health care and guides or counsels families as required. Consultation, copractice, and referral to associated physicians are aspects of the FNP's practice.

family of origin, the family into which a person is born.

family of procreation, the family a person forms through marriage and/or childbearing.

family physician, a medical practitioner with a specialty in family medicine. Also called **family practice physician.**

Formerly called **general practitioner.** See also **family medicine.**

family planning. See **contraception.**

family planning, natural, methods of preventing conception without the use of artificial contraceptive means. Also called **fertility awareness methods.** See also **contraception.**

family practice [L, *familia,* household; Gk, *praktikos,* ready for action], a medical specialty that encompasses several branches of medicine, including internal medicine, preventive medicine, pediatrics, surgery, psychiatry, and obstetrics and gynecology. It includes client management, counseling, problem solving, and coordination of total health care delivery to all members of a family, regardless of sex or age.

family practice physician, a practitioner of family medicine, usually one who has completed a residency program in the specialty. See also **family medicine.**

family processes, the psychosocial, physiological, and spiritual functions and relationships within the family unit.

family structure, the composition and membership of the family and the organization and patterning of relationships among individual family members. In planning health care for a family member or the entire family, an awareness of that family's structure may be important.

family therapy, (in psychiatry) a therapy modality that focuses treatment on the process between family members that supports and perpetuates symptoms; a way of conceptualizing human relationship problems that focuses on the context in which an emotional problem is generated.

famine fever. See **relapsing fever.**

famotidine /famot″idēn/, an oral and parenteral antiulcer drug; an H_2-receptor antagonist.

■ INDICATIONS: It is prescribed in treatment of duodenal ulcer and pathological hypersecretory conditions and for stress-ulcer prophylaxis.

■ CONTRAINDICATIONS: Famotidine should be used with caution in patients with impaired kidney function.

■ ADVERSE EFFECTS: Among adverse effects reported are headache, dizziness, constipation, diarrhea, and temporary irritation of the injection site.

Famvir, an antiviral drug. Brand name for **famciclovir.**

fan beam, a geometric pattern produced by collimating a spatially extended x-ray beam with a long, narrow slit. Also called *fan x-ray beam.*

FANCAP, (United States) a mnemonic device for helping student nurses learn to assess, provide, and evaluate direct patient care. It stands for *f*luids, *a*eration, *n*utrition, *c*ommunication, *a*ctivity, and *p*ain. Occasionally a variant, FANCAS, is substituted, in which the *S* represents *s*timulation.

Fanconi anemia /fankō″nē/ [Guido Fanconi, Swiss pediatrician, 1892–1979], a rare, usually congenital disorder transmitted as an autosomal-recessive trait, characterized by aplastic anemia in childhood or early adult life, bone abnormalities, chromatin breaks, and developmental anomalies. Children begin to show symptoms between 4 and 12 years of age. Also called **congenital pancytopenia, pancytopenia-dysmelia.** Also spelled *Fanconi anaemia.*

Fanconi syndrome [Guido Fanconi], a group of disorders that includes pancytopenia, renal tubular dysfunction, glycosuria, phosphaturia, and bicarbonate wasting. The condition is often marked by osteomalacia, acidosis, rickets, and hypokalemia. Two main types of the syndrome have been differentiated. Idiopathic Fanconi syndrome is an inherited autosomal-recessive disorder and usually accompanies other genetic disorders such as Wilson disease, galactosemia, or glycogen storage disease. Acquired Fanconi syndrome is usually the result of toxicity from various sources, including ingestion of outdated tetracycline, heavy metal poisoning, or vitamin D deficiency. Because of numerous variations of the syndrome, different alleles are believed responsible for the different recessively inherited factors expressed as signs and symptoms of the group of disorders.

fango /fän″gō/ [It, mud], mud taken from thermal springs at Battaglia, Italy, and used to treat gout and other rheumatic diseases.

fan lateral projection, a technique for making a radiographic image of the hand without superimposition of the phalanges. The patient places the fingers around a sponge wedge shaped so that each finger appears separately, in a fan-like pattern, on the x-ray image.

Fansidar, a fixed-combination antimalarial agent. Brand name for **pyrimethamine, sulfadoxine.**

fantasy /fan″təsē/ [Gk, *phantasia,* imagination], **1.** the unrestrained free play of the imagination; fancy. **2.** a mental image, which may be distorted or grotesque, that is often the result of the action of drugs or a disease of the central nervous system. **3.** the mental process of transforming undesirable experiences into imagined events or into a sequence of ideas in order to fulfill an unconscious wish, need, or desire or to give expression to unconscious conflicts, such as a daydream.

F.A.O.T.A., abbreviation for *Fellow of the American Occupational Therapy Association.*

FAP, abbreviation for **familial adenomatous polyposis.** See **adenomatous polyposis coli.**

F.A.P.T.A., abbreviation for *Catherine Worthingham Fellow of the American Physical Therapy Association.*

farad (F) /fer″əd/ [Michael Faraday, English scientist, 1791–1871], a unit of capacitance that increases the potential difference between the plates of a capacitor by 1 volt with a charge of 1 coulomb.

Faraday cage /fer″ədā/, a wire-mesh cage that surrounds a magnetic resonance (MR) scanner and shields it from stray radiofrequency waves. Such waves would otherwise distort the results of MR imaging.

Farber disease, Farber lipogranulomatosis /fär″bər/ [Sidney Farber, American pediatrician, 1903–1973], a lysosomal storage disease of ceramide metabolism resulting from defective ceramidase. The disease is marked by hoarseness; aphonia; a brownish desquamating dermatitis that begins at about 3 months of age; foam cell infiltration of bones and joints that causes deformations; granulomatous reaction in lymph nodes, heart, lungs, and kidneys; and psychomotor delay. Also called **ceramidase deficiency.**

Farber test, a microscopic examination of newborn meconium for lanugo and squamous cells. The fetus normally swallows amniotic fluid containing these large proteins, which then pass through the digestive system to be excreted, usually after birth, in the first stools. The absence of hair or skin cells is suggestive of intestinal obstruction or atresia and requires further evaluation.

Far Eastern hemorrhagic fever, a form of epidemic hemorrhagic fever, indigenous to Asia, that is transmitted by a virus carried by Asian rodents and causes hemorrhagic fever with renal syndrome. The infection is characterized by four phases: febrile phase, hypotensive phase, oliguric phase, and polyuric phase. Hypotensive shock may occur as the fever subsides. Thirst continues into the second week, oliguria develops, and the blood pressure returns to normal. Blood urea nitrogen levels increase hyperphosphatemia and hypercalcemia, and other complications occur. Diuresis follows the oliguric phase, generating a urine output of as much as 8 L/day and causing electrolyte imbalance. The mortality rate may be as high as 33%. There is no specific treatment.

far field. See **Fraunhofer zone.**

farmer's lung [L, *firmare,* to make firm], an allergy-related respiratory disorder caused by the inhalation of actinomycetes or other microbes in dusts from moldy crops. It is a form of hypersensitivity pneumonitis that affects individuals in whom antibodies to the mold spores have developed. It exists in acute, subacute, and chronic forms. It is characterized by coughing, dyspnea, cyanosis, tachycardia, nausea, chills, and fever. Lengthy exposure to dust from moldy crops can lead to permanent lung damage, physical disability and, in some cases, death. There is no cure; once a hypersensitivity develops, it persists for years and possibly the entire life-span of the individual. Treatment may include cromolyn sodium and a corticosteroid.

far point [ME, *farr* + L, *punctus,* pricked], **1.** the farthest distance from the eye at which an object can be seen clearly when the eye is at rest and accommodation is fully relaxed. **2.** the point at which the visual axes of the two eyes meet when at rest.

farsightedness. See **hyperopia.**

FAS, abbreviation for **fetal alcohol syndrome.**

fasci-, prefix meaning "band or bundle of fibrous tissue": *fascicular, fasciitis.*

fascia /fash″ē·ə/ *pl. fasciae* [L, band], the fibrous connective membrane of the body that may be separated from other specifically organized structures, such as the tendons, the aponeuroses, and the ligaments, and that covers, supports, and separates muscles. It varies in thickness and density and in the amounts of fat, collagenous fiber, elastic fiber, and tissue fluid it contains. Kinds include **deep fascia, subcutaneous fascia, subserous fascia.** –*fascial, adj.*

fascia bulbi. See **Tenon capsule.**

fasciae, fascial. See **fascia.**

fascia lata, deep fascia in the thigh and gluteal region.

fascial cleft /fash″ē·əl/ [L, *fascia* + ME, *clift*], a place of cleavage between two contiguous fascial surfaces, such as the deep fasciae and the subcutaneous fasciae. A fascial cleft is rich in fluid but poor in traversing fibers. Thus two fascial surfaces may move or be separated easily. Compare **fascial compartment, fascial membrane lamination.**

fascial compartment, a part of the body that is walled off by fascial membranes, usually containing a muscle or group of muscles or an organ, just as the heart is contained by the mediastinum. Compare **fascial cleft, fascial membrane lamination.**

fascial membrane lamination, a pad of connective tissue that contains fat and an occasional blood vessel or lymph node. It is found where a fascial membrane splits into two sheets, such as at the division of the outer cervical fascia above the sternum. Compare **fascial cleft, fascial compartment.**

fascia of piriform muscle, an extension of the parietal pelvic fascia that surrounds the piriform muscle. Also called **piriform fascia.**

fascicle. See **fasciculus.**

fascicular /fəsik″yələr/ [L, *fasciculus,* little bundle], pertaining to something arranged as a bundle of rods, such as groups of nerve or muscle fibers.

fascicular neuroma, a neoplasm composed of myelinated nerve fibers. Also called **medullated neuroma.**

fascicular twitching. See **twitching.**

fasciculation /fasik′yo͞olā″shən/ [L, *fasciculus,* little bundle, *atio,* process], a localized uncoordinated, uncontrollable twitching of a single muscle group innervated by a single motor nerve fiber or filament that may be palpated and seen under the skin. In anesthesia it refers to muscle twitches that occur with administration of the depolarizing muscle relaxant succinylcholine. It also may be symptomatic of a number of disorders, including dietary deficiency, cerebral palsy, fever, neuralgia, polio, rheumatic heart disease, sodium deficiency, tic, or uremia. Fasciculation of the heart muscle is known as fibrillation. –**fascicular,** *adj.,* –*fasciculate, v.*

fasciculus /fəsik″yələs/ [L, little bundle], a small bundle of muscle, tendon, or nerve fibers wrapped by a layer of connective tissue called the perimysium (muscle) or perineurium (nerve fiber). The arrangement of fasciculi in a muscle is correlated with the power of the muscle and its range of motion. The patterns of muscular fasciculi are penniform, bipenniform, multipenniform, and radiated. Also called **fascicle. –fascicular,** *adj.*

fasciitis /fas′ē·ī″tis/, **1.** an inflammation of the connective tissue that may be caused by streptococcal or other types of infection, an injury, or an autoimmune reaction. **2.** an abnormal benign growth (pseudosarcomatous fasciitis) resembling a tumor that develops in the subcutaneous oral tissues, usually in the cheek. Commonly growing rapidly and then regressing, it consists of young fibroblasts and many capillaries and may be mistaken for fibrosarcoma.

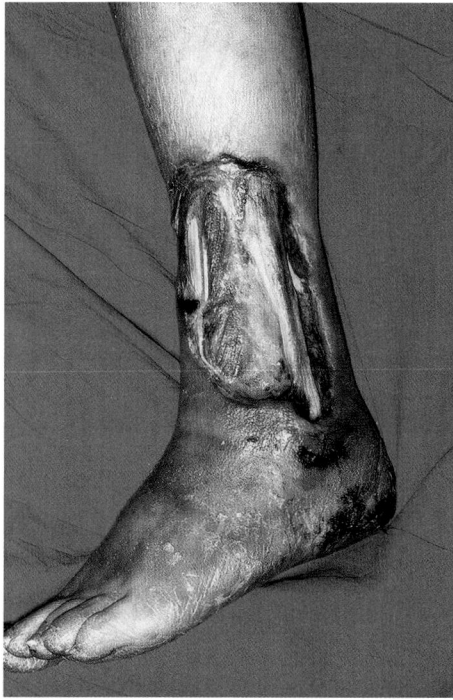

Necrotizing fasciitis *(Courtesy Dr. R.A. Marsden)*

fasciodesis /fā′sē·ōdē″sis/, a surgical procedure in which a fascia is attached to another fascia or to a tendon.

fascioliasis /fas′ē·ōlī″əsis/ [L, *fasciola,* little band; Gk, *osis,* condition], infection by a liver fluke of the species *Fasciola hepatica* or *F. gigantica.* It is characterized by epigastric pain, fever, hepatomegaly, jaundice, eosinophilia, urticaria, and diarrhea. Fibrosis of the liver is a consequence of prolonged infection. It is acquired by ingestion of encysted forms of the fluke found on aquatic plants, such as raw watercress grown in water contaminated by sheep or cattle dung. The disease is prevalent in many parts of the world, including the southern and western United States. Incidence of infection has increased over the last 20 years. Bithionol or triclabendazole, given orally, is the usual treatment.

fasciolopsiasis /fas′ē·ōlopsī″əsis/ [L, *fasciola,* little band; Gk, *opsis,* appearance, *osis,* condition], an intestinal infection of humans and pigs, prevalent in Asia. It is characterized by abdominal pain, diarrhea, constipation, eosinophilia, ascites, and sometimes edema. It is caused by the fluke *Fasciolopsis buski,* the largest intestinal fluke affecting humans. The disease is usually acquired by eating contaminated water plants such as raw water chestnuts but is also possibly acquired by drinking untreated water. Most infections are light and asymptomatic. Symptomatic infection is easily treated with anthelmintics, such as praziquantel.

Fasciolopsis buski /fas′ē·əlop″sis bus″kē/, a species of large fluke that is an important intestinal parasite endemic in Asia and the tropics. In the United States and other countries, it is occasionally found in imported food products such as water chestnuts and other vegetation contaminated with infective metacercariae. See also **fasciolopsiasis.**

fascioscapulohumeral muscular dystrophy /fas′ē·ō-skap′yəlōhyoo″mərəl/ [L, *fasciculus,* little bundle, *scapula,* shoulderblade, *humerus,* shoulder], an abnormal congenital condition that is one of the main types of muscular dystrophy. It is characterized by progressive symmetric wasting of the skeletal muscles, especially the muscles of the face, the shoulders, and the upper arms, without any associated neural or sensory disorders. This disease is not usually fatal but spreads to all the voluntary muscles and commonly produces a pendulous lower lip and the absence of the nasolabial fold. It is an autosomal-dominant disease that may be transmitted to males and females. Also called **Landouzy-Dejerine muscular dystrophy.** Compare **Duchenne's muscular dystrophy.**

fasciotomy /fas′ē·ot″əmē/, a surgical incision into an area of fascia.

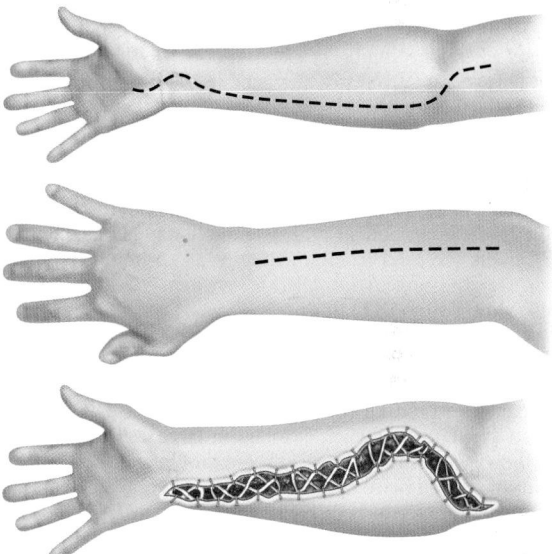

Delayed closure of a fasciotomy of the arm using vascular loops and staples *(Cioffi et al, 2014)*

fascitis. See **fasciitis.**

F.A.S.R.T., abbreviation for *Fellow of the American Society of Radiologic Technologists.*

fast, 1. *adj.,* resistant to change, especially to the action of a specific medication or chemical, as a staining agent. **2.** *n.,* abstinence from all or certain foods. See also **fasting. 3.** *adj.,* occurring quickly and in a short span of time.

fast-acting insulin. See **short-acting insulin.**

fast brushing, the use of a battery-powered brush to stimulate C fibers (group IV afferent neurons), which send many collaterals to the reticular activating system.

fast channel, a protein channel, such as a sodium channel, that becomes activated relatively quickly. A fast voltage-gated channel has a much lower activation potential than does the slow type. See also **slow channel.**

fastigial nucleus /fastij″ē·əl/, one of a group of deep cerebellar nuclei that receive input from the medial zone of the cerebellum. It is involved in the control of posture and equilibrium.

fastigium /fastij″ē·əm/ [L, ridge], **1.** the highest point in the course of a fever, or the most symptomatic point in the course of an illness. **2.** the angle at the top of the roof of the fourth ventricle in the brain. **3.** the highest point.

fasting [AS, *foestan,* to observe], **1.** the act of abstaining from food for a specific period, usually for therapeutic or religious purposes. **2.** the elimination of foods with the addition of fluids such as mineral water, herbal and fruit teas, broth, and fruit juices for a limited period of time. This therapy requires the supervision of a health professional experienced in this form of therapy.

fasting blood sugar, a determination of blood glucose levels after an 8-hour period of fasting.

fasting plasma glucose (FPG), a measurement of the concentration of glucose in the plasma after the patient has not eaten for at least 8 hours. See also **blood glucose test.**

fasting serum gastrin, measurement of the levels of gastrin in blood serum after the patient has fasted for 12 hours so that presence of food is not a factor. It is markedly increased in certain conditions such as Zollinger-Ellison syndrome and G cell hyperplasia.

fast neutron therapy, a radiotherapeutic technique used in the treatment of certain soft tissue sarcomas.

fast pain, a localized sensation of discomfort felt immediately after a noxious stimulus is delivered. It usually disappears when the stimulus ceases.

fast spin-echo (FSE), a magnetic resonance imaging technique that uses multiple spin-echoes to reduce imaging times in comparison to spin-echo imaging. See also **spin-echo.**

fast-twitch (FT) fiber, a muscle fiber that can develop high tension rapidly. It is usually innervated by a single alpha neuron and has low fatigue resistance, low capillary density, low levels of aerobic enzymes, and low oxygen availability. FT fibers are used in such activities as sprinting, jumping, and weightlifting. Also called *fast-twitch muscle fiber.* See also **slow-twitch (ST) fiber.**

fat [AS, *faett*], **1.** a substance composed of lipids or fatty acids and occurring in various forms or consistencies ranging from oil to tallow. **2.** a type of body tissue composed of cells containing stored fat (depot fat). Stored fat is usually identified as white fat, which is found in large cellular vesicles, or brown fat, which consists of lipid droplets. Stored fat contains more than twice as many calories per gram as sugars and serves as a source of body energy. In addition, stored fat helps cushion and insulate vital organs. See also **adipose, obesity.**

fatal /fā′təl/ [L, *fatum,* what has been spoken], causing death.

fatality /fātal″itē/ [L, *fatalis,* preordained], **1.** an individual case of death. **2.** a condition, disease, accident, or disaster resulting in death.

fatality rate, the death rate observed in a specified group of people involved in a simultaneous event such as a disease or disaster.

fat cell lipoma. See **hibernoma.**

fat embolism, a circulatory condition characterized by the blocking of an artery by a plug of fat. The plug enters the circulatory system after the fracture of a long bone or, less commonly, after traumatic injury to adipose tissue or to a fatty liver. Fat embolism usually occurs suddenly 12 to 36 hours after an injury and is characterized by symptoms related to the site occluded, such as severe chest pain, pallor, dyspnea, tachycardia, delirium, prostration and, in some cases, coma. Anemia and thrombocytopenia are common. Systemic fat embolism may occur after extensive trauma, since lipid metabolism is altered by the injury and free fatty acids are released, resulting in vasculitis with obstruction of many small pulmonary and cerebral arteries. Classic signs of systemic fat embolism are petechial hemorrhages on the neck, shoulders, axillae, and conjunctivae that appear 2 or 3 days after the injury. Radiographic findings include patchy diffuse opacities throughout the lungs. There is no specific therapy for systemic fat embolism. The patient is placed in a high Fowler's position and given oxygen, corticosteroids, blood transfusion, respiratory assistance, or other supportive care as needed. Compare **air embolism, gas embolism.**

FA test, abbreviation for **fluorescent antibody test.**

father complex [L, *pater* + *complecti,* to embrace], *(Nontechnical)* a repressed desire for an incestuous relationship with one's father.

father fixation, an arrest in psychosexual development characterized by an abnormally persistent, close, and often paralyzing emotional attachment to one's father. Compare **mother fixation.** See also **freudian fixation.**

fatigability /fat′igəbil″itē/, a tendency to become tired or exhausted quickly or easily. It may occur in certain types of cells that undergo periods of excessive activity.

fatigue /fətēg″/ [L, *fatigare,* to tire], **1.** a state of exhaustion or a loss of strength or endurance, such as may follow strenuous physical activity. **2.** loss of ability of tissues to respond to stimuli that normally evoke muscular contraction or other activity. Muscle cells generally require a refractory or recovery period after activity, when cells restore their energy supplies and excrete metabolic waste products. **3.** an emotional state associated with extreme or extended exposure to psychic pressure, as in battle or combat fatigue.

fatigue fever, a benign episode of fever and muscle pain after overexertion. The symptoms are caused by an accumulation of the metabolic waste products of muscle contractions and may persist for several days.

fatigue fracture, any fracture that results from excessive physical activity and not from any specific injury, as commonly occurs in the metatarsal bones of runners. See also **stress fracture.**

fatigue state [L, *fatigare,* to tire, *status,* condition], the state of lowest energy of a system. See also **ground state.**

fat-induced hyperlipidemia. See **hyperlipidemia type I.**

fat injection, transplantation of a patient's own fat to other areas on the body, as to the face to minimize wrinkles or to the lips or penis to augment size. The procedure is discouraged in breast augmentation, because it can hamper the detection of early breast cancer, causing false-positive test results.

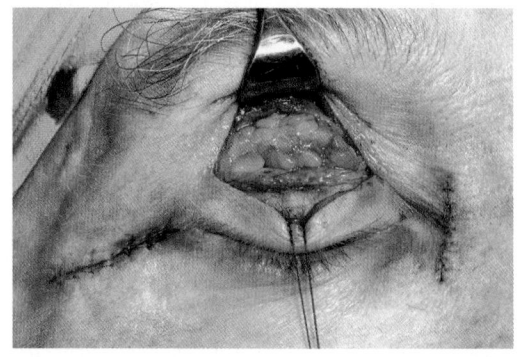

Fat graft to the upper eyelid *(Tyers and Collin, 2008)*

fat metabolism, the biochemical process by which fats are broken down, incorporated, and used by the cells of the body. Fats provide more food energy (9 kcal/g) than carbohydrates (4.1 kcal/g). Fat catabolism begins with the hydrolysis of fats (triglycerides) into glycerol and fatty acids. Glycerol is converted into a compound that can enter the citric acid cycle. Catabolism of fatty acids continues by beta-oxidation to produce acetylcoenzyme A, which also enters the citric acid cycle. The body synthesizes fats from fatty acids and glycerol or from compounds derived from excess glucose or from amino acids. The body can synthesize only saturated fatty acids; essential unsaturated fatty acids can be supplied only by diet. Fat metabolism is controlled by hormones such as insulin, growth hormone, adrenocorticotropic hormone, and glucocorticoids. The rate of fat catabolism is inversely related to the rate of carbohydrate catabolism, and in some conditions, such as diabetes mellitus, the secretion of these hormones increases to counter a decrease in carbohydrate catabolism.

fat necrosis [AS, *faett* + Gk, *nekros,* dead, *osis,* condition], a condition caused by trauma or infection in which neutral tissue fats are broken down into fatty acids and glycerol. Fat necrosis occurs most commonly in the breasts and subcutaneous areas. It also may develop in the abdominal cavity after an episode of pancreatitis causes a release of enzymes from the pancreas.

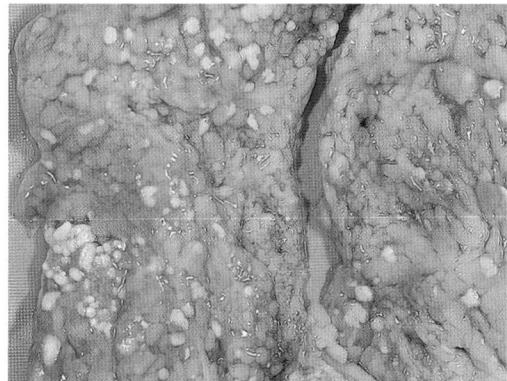

Fat necrosis *(Kumar et al, 2007)*

fat overload syndrome, a condition of hepatosplenomegaly, anemia, GI disturbances, and very high triglyceride levels resulting from IV administration of fat emulsion.

fat pad, a mass of closely packed fat cells surrounded by fibrous tissue septa. Fat pads may be generously supplied with capillaries and nerve endings. Intraarticular fat pads are also covered by a layer of synovial cells. An example is the buccal pad of fat seen in nursing babies.

fat solvent. See **nonpolar solvent.**

fatty acid (FA) [AS, *faett* + L, *acidus,* sour], any of several organic acids produced by the hydrolysis of neutral fats and consisting of a long hydrocarbon chain ending in a carboxyl group. The hydrocarbon chains may be fully saturated or contain varying degrees of unsaturation (exhibited by C=C bonds). In cells, fatty acids usually occur in combination with another molecule rather than in a free state. Essential fatty acids, including linoleic acid and linolenic acid, are unsaturated molecules that cannot be produced by the body and must therefore be included in the diet. See also **saturated fatty acid, unsaturated fatty acid.**

fatty alcohol, a hydroxy derivative of a hydrocarbon from the paraffin series.

fatty ascites. See **chylous ascites.**

fatty cirrhosis [AS, *faett* + Gk, *kirrhos,* yellow-orange, *osis,* condition], a form of cirrhosis that develops over a long period of poor nutrition, resulting in fatty infiltration of the liver. See also **cirrhosis.**

fatty degeneration [AS, *faett* + L, *degenerare,* to deviate], the abnormal deposition of fat within cells or the invasion of organs by fatty tissue. Also called **adipose degeneration.**

fatty diarrhea, the excretion of fatty, foul-smelling stools that float on water. The condition is associated with chronic pancreatic disease and other malabsorption disorders. Also called **pimelorrhea.**

fatty infiltration, a normal phase of breast development, characterized by accumulation of increased amounts of fat around the parenchymal breast tissue. It is normally followed later in life by involution.

fatty infiltration of heart [AS, *faett* + L, *in* + *filtrare* + AS, *heorte*], an accumulation of large amounts of fat within the cells of the heart. The heart muscle may be marked by irregular, pale streaks representing areas of fatty infiltration. The condition is sometimes associated with severe and prolonged anemia.

fatty liver, an accumulation of triglycerides in the liver. The causes include obesity, diabetes, excessive consumption of alcohol, IV administration of drugs such as tetracycline and corticosteroids, and exposure to toxic substances such as carbon tetrachloride and yellow phosphorus. Fatty liver is also seen in kwashiorkor and is a rare complication of unknown origin in late pregnancy. The symptoms are anorexia, hepatomegaly, and abdominal discomfort. Fat cells can be seen under the microscope after liver biopsy. The condition is usually reversible after the underlying condition is corrected or the offending drug is withdrawn. See also **cirrhosis.**

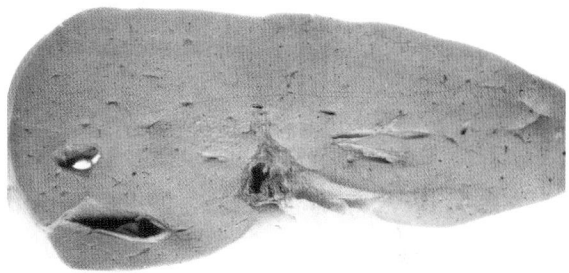

Alcoholic fatty liver *(Saxena, 2011)*

fatty stool [AS, *faett* + *stol,* seat], feces containing an abnormally large amount of fat, as indicated by their floating on water. See also **celiac disease, steatorrhea.**

fatty tissue [AS, *faett* + OFr, *tissu*], loose connective tissue with many cells that contain fat vacuoles. Also called **adipose tissue.**

faucial isthmus /fô″shəl/, the aperture of the mouth into the pharynx. The anterior pillars of the fauces form the glossopalatine arch; the posterior pillars form the pharyngopalatine arch. Also called **oropharyngeal isthmus.**

faulty restoration /fôl″tē/ [L, *fallere,* to deceive, *restaurare,* to renew], any dental filling or fabrication that contains flaws, such as overhanging or incomplete fillings, voids, or incorrect anatomical characteristics of occlusal and marginal ridge areas. Such flaws may mar individual tooth fillings and fixed bridges or clasps of removable prosthetics and may cause inflammatory and dystrophic diseases of the teeth and periodontium. See also **restoration.**

favism /fā″vizəm/ [It, *fava,* bean], an acute hemolytic anemia caused by ingestion of the beans or inhalation of the pollen from the *Vicia faba* (fava) plant. Sensitive individuals have a genetic deficiency of glucose-6-phosphate dehydrogenase, usually the result of a hereditary biochemical abnormality of the erythrocytes. Symptoms include dizziness, headache, vomiting, fever, jaundice, eosinophilia, and often diarrhea. The condition occurs primarily in persons of southern Italian extraction and is treated by blood transfusion and avoidance of fava beans and pollen. See also **glucose-6-phosphate dehydrogenase (G6PD) deficiency.**

favus /fā″vəs/ [L, honeycomb], a fungal infection of the scalp, skin, or nails, more common in children than adults. It is caused by *Trichophyton* fungi. Favus is characterized by thick yellow crusts with suppuration, a honeycomb appearance, a distinct "mousy" odor, permanent scars, and alopecia. It is rarely seen in North America but is common in the Middle East and Africa.

fax, abbreviation for **facsimile.**

FBS, abbreviation for **fasting blood sugar.** See **blood glucose test.**

F.C.A.P., abbreviation for *Fellow of the College of American Pathologists.*

FCC, abbreviation for **Federal Communications Commission.**

F.C.C.P., abbreviation for *Fellow of the American College of Chest Physicians.*

FDA, abbreviation for **Food and Drug Administration.**

FDI numbering system [Fr, *Féderation Dentaire Internationale*], an internationally used two-digit system for identifying and referring to teeth, established through the FDI and headquartered in Paris, France. See also **Palmer notation, universal tooth coding system.**

Fe, symbol for the element **iron.**

fear-tension-pain syndrome, a concept formulated by Grantly Dick-Read, MD, (1890–1959) to explain the pain commonly expected and reported in childbirth. The concept proposes that attitudes induce anxiety before labor and cause fear in labor. This fear causes muscular and psychological tension that interferes with the natural processes of dilation and delivery, resulting in pain. He advocated education, exercise, and warm emotional and physical support in labor to counteract the syndrome and coined the term *natural childbirth* for a labor or delivery in which the well-trained woman joyfully, comfortably, and with a calm, cooperative attitude participates in a natural experience. Elements of his method of psychophysical preparation for childbirth are incorporated into most other methods of natural childbirth. See also **Bradley method, Lamaze method, Read method, natural childbirth.**

febri-, prefix meaning "fever": *febrile, febrifacient.*

febrifacient /feb′rifā″shənt/, an agent that induces a fever.

febrifuge. See **antipyretic.**

febrile /fē″bril, feb″ril/ [L, *febris,* fever], pertaining to or characterized by an elevated body temperature, such as a febrile reaction to an infectious agent. A body temperature above 100° F (37.8° C), or 99.6° F (37.6° C) rectally, is commonly regarded as febrile. Compare **afebrile.** –**febrility,** *n.*

-febrile, suffix meaning "fever": *afebrile.*

febrile/cold agglutinins test, blood tests used to diagnose infectious diseases and some neoplastic diseases. The febrile agglutinins serological studies are used to diagnose salmonellosis, rickettsial diseases, brucellosis, tularemia, and some leukemias and lymphomas, whereas cold agglutinins are found in patients infected by *Mycoplasma pneumoniae,* influenza, mononucleosis, rheumatoid arthritis, and lymphomas.

febrile delirium [L, *febris,* fever, *delirare,* to rave], a symptom of disordered central nervous system function, with excitement, restlessness, and disorientation accompanying some acute fevers.

febrile response. See **fever.**

febrile seizure, a seizure associated with a febrile illness. Treatment depends on the age of the patient and the number of seizures. Generalized recurrent febrile seizures in children may be treated as grand mal epilepsy.

febrile state [L, *febris,* fever, *status,* condition], a significant increase in body temperature accompanied by increased pulse and respiration rates, anorexia, constipation, insomnia, headache, pains, and irritability.

febrile urine, a deep orange-colored, strong smelling urine of a patient with a fever, usually caused by concentration of the urine as a result of dehydration.

febrility. See **febrile.**

fecal. See **feces.**

fecal fat test, a stool test performed to confirm the diagnosis of steatorrhea.

fecal fistula [L, *faex,* waste matter, *fistula,* pipe], an abnormal passage from the colon to the external surface of the body, for discharging feces. Fistulas of this kind are usually created surgically in operations involving the removal of malignant or severely ulcerated bowel segments. See also **colostomy.**

fecal impaction, an accumulation of hardened or inspissated feces in the rectum or sigmoid colon that the individual is unable to move. Diarrhea may be a sign of fecal impaction, since only liquid material is able to pass the obstruction. Occasionally fecal impaction may cause urinary incontinence through pressure on the bladder. Treatment includes oil and cleansing enemas and manual breaking up and removal of the stool by a gloved finger. Persons who are dehydrated; nutritionally depleted; on long periods of bed rest; receiving constipating medications such as iron or opiates; or undergoing barium radiographic studies are at risk of developing fecal impaction. Prevention includes adequate ingestion of bulk food, fluids, exercise, regular bowel habits, privacy for defecation, and occasionally stool softeners or laxatives. See also **constipation, obstipation.**

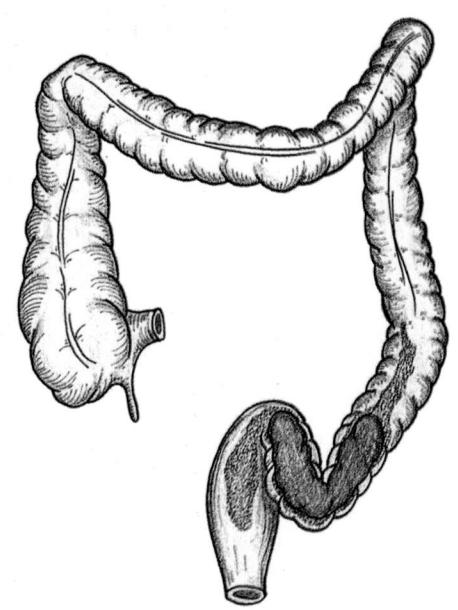

Fecal impaction (Potter and Perry, 2003)

fecalith /fē″kəlith/ [L, *faex* + Gk, *lithos,* stone], a hard, impacted mass of feces in the colon. To allow evacuation, an oil retention enema is usually administered. If it is ineffective, manual removal can be performed. See also **atonic constipation, constipation.**

fecal softener, a drug that lowers the surface tension of the fecal mass, allowing the intestinal fluids to penetrate and soften the stool. Also called **stool softener.**

feces /fē″sēz/ *sing. faex* [L, *faex,* waste matter], waste or excrement from the digestive tract that is formed in the intestine and expelled through the rectum. Feces consist of water, food residue, bacteria, and secretions of the intestines and liver. Gross examination of feces for color, odor, quantity, and consistency and microscopic examination for the presence of blood, fat, mucus, or parasites are common diagnostic procedures. Also called **stool.** Also spelled *faeces.* See also **defecation. –fecal,** *adj.*

fecund. See **fecundity.**

fecundation /fē′kəndā″shən, fek′-/ [L, *fecundare,* to make fruitful], impregnation or fertilization; the act of fertilizing. See also **artificial insemination.** *–fecundate, v.*

fecundity /fikun″ditē/, the ability to produce offspring, especially in large numbers and rapidly; fertility. **–fecund,** *adj.*

Federal Communications Commission (FCC), a U.S. federal agency that regulates interstate and international communications by radio, television, wire, satellite, cable, and 911.

federally qualified heath center (FQHC), an organization receiving grants under Section 330 of the Public Health Service Act. The designation is provided by the Department of Health and Human Services and the Centers for Medicare and Medicaid Services and indicates approval to receive reimbursement. The main purpose of the FQHC program is to enhance the provision of primary care services in underserved areas. FQHCs must offer a sliding fee scale, provide comprehensive services, have an ongoing quality assurance program, and have a governing board of directors.

federally qualified health center look-alike (FQHC-Look-Alike), a health center certified by the Centers for Medicare and Medicaid Services as meeting all requirements for a health center program but not receiving grant funding. It may receive special Medicare and Medicaid reimbursement. See also **federally qualified heath center.**

Federal Register, a document published by the U.S. government each working day to inform the public of executive regulations, presidential orders, hearings and meeting schedules of various federal agencies, and related matters. The Federal Register contains announcements of the U.S. Food and Drug Administration, the Environmental Protection Agency, and other governmental bureaus that regulate matters of health and safety.

Federal Tort Claims Act, a statute passed in 1946 that allows the U.S. federal government to be sued for the wrongful action or negligence of its employees. The act, for most purposes, eliminates the doctrine of governmental immunity, which formerly prohibited the bringing of a suit against the federal government.

Federal Trade Commission (FTC), an agency in the executive branch of the U.S. federal government created to promote trade and to prevent practices that restrain free enterprise and competition. In the area of health care, the commission successfully challenged the American Medical Association's ban on physician advertising. The FTC held that competition among physicians and the free choice of the consumer were impaired by the antiadvertising policy.

Fede disease. See **Riga-Fede disease.**

feedback [AS, *faedan + baec*], **1.** information produced by a receiver and perceived by a sender that informs the sender of the receiver's reaction to the message. Feedback is a cyclic part of the process of communication that regulates and modifies the content of messages. **2.** the return of some of the output so as to exert some control in the process.

feedback loop, the circular path seen in a system that has feedback, such that the output of the system participates in the control of the system. It can be positive or negative.

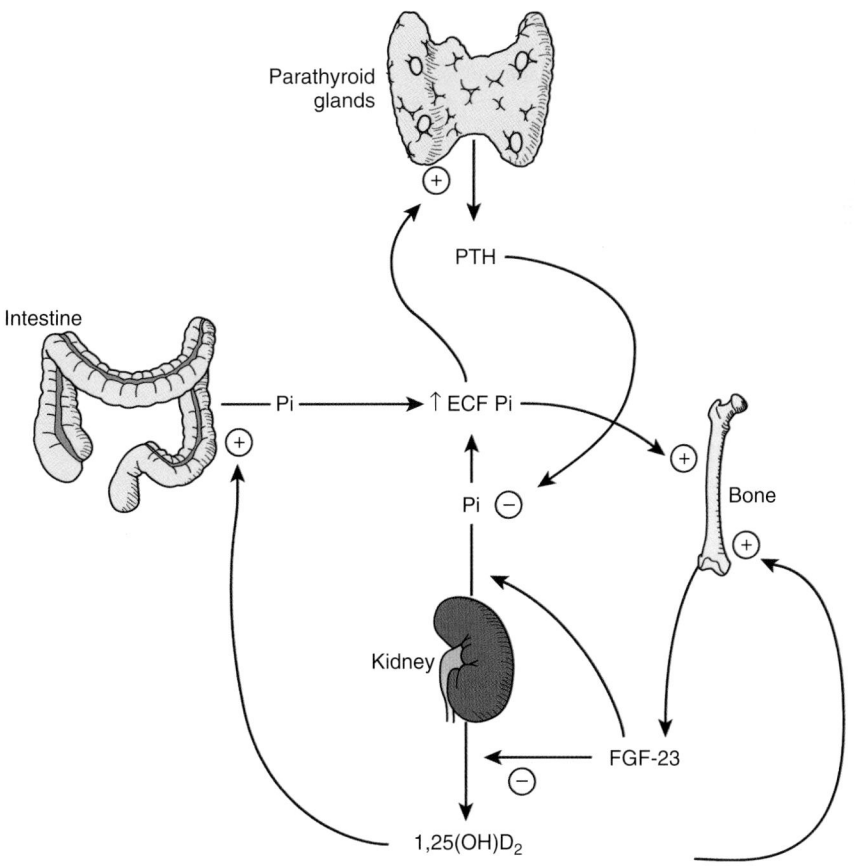

Endocrine feedback loops for regulation of electrolytes *(Bindels et al, 2012)*

feed backward, a concept in motor control theory that incorporates concepts from systems theory. It refers to the neurological pathway that enables the motor system to react to sensory input that indicates deviations from the planned movement. For example, when lifting something that looks heavy but is not, sensory feedback to the muscles is necessary to quickly adjust the force output to improve control and accuracy with task performance.

feedforward control, anticipatory movement to prepare for motor response (e.g., deciding where to run to catch a ball).

feeding [AS, *faedan*], the act or process of taking or giving food or nourishment. Kinds include **breastfeeding, tube feeding.** See also **alimentation, parenteral nutrition.**

feeding tube, a tube for introducing fluids of high caloric value into the stomach. See also **tube feeding.**

fee-for-service [AS, *feoh,* property; L, *servitum,* slavery], **1.** a charge made for a professional activity, such as a physical examination, the fitting of a contraceptive diaphragm, or the monitoring of a person's blood pressure. **2.** a system for the payment of professional services in which the practitioner is paid for the particular service rendered rather than receiving a salary for providing professional services as needed during scheduled hours of work or time on call.

fee-for-service equivalent, (in U.S. managed care) a specialty capitation method in which a fee schedule is developed for service and providers are paid a percentage of the fee schedule. Periodically the overall value of services provided is compared with payments received, and the balance is distributed proportionately to participating providers.

feeling, **1.** a quality of mood. **2.** a subjective experience caused by stimulation of a sensory nerve.

Feer disease. See **acrodynia.**

FEES, abbreviation for **fiberoptic endoscopic evaluation of swallowing.**

fee schedule, (in U.S. managed care) the specific dollar amount to be charged for each service offered.

fee screen system, a method of establishing payment for physician services that is based on the usual, customary, or reasonable charge according to a regional evaluation. It allows physicians to establish their own reimbursement level for units of service.

feet. See **foot.**

FEF, abbreviation for **forced expiratory flow.**

Fehling's solution /fā″lingz/ [Hermann C. von Fehling, German chemist, 1812–1885], a solution containing cupric sulfate, sodium hydroxide, and potassium sodium tartrate, used for testing for the presence of glucose and other reducing substances in the urine. Also called *Fehling's reagent.*

Feingold diet /fīn″gōld/ [Benjamin Feingold, American pediatrician, 1900–1982], a diet developed to treat hyperactive children that excludes foods manufactured with synthetic colorings, flavorings, and preservatives and limits the intake of fruits and vegetables that contain salicylates, such as oranges, apricots, peaches, cucumbers, and tomatoes. Research studies have not supported the efficacy of this diet.

felbamate /fel′bämāt″/, an anticonvulsant used in treatment of epilepsy; administered orally.

Feldene, a nonsteroidal antiinflammatory drug. Brand name for *piroxicam.*

FeldenKrais method /fel″dənkrīs/, **1.** (in psychiatry) a proprietary system that uses an exploratory technique to enable patients to relearn dysfunctional movement patterns. Therapy takes two forms: awareness through movement, in which the patient is guided verbally through increasingly complex structured movements, and functional integration, in which the practitioner introduces new motion patterns to the patient by gentle manipulation. **2.** a bodywork technique that integrates principles of physics, judo, and yoga. The practitioner directs sequences of movement using verbal or hands-on techniques or teaches a system of self-directed exercises to treat physical impairments through the learning of new movement patterns.

feldspar /feld″spär/ [Ger, *feld,* field, *spath,* spar], a crystalline mineral of aluminum silicate with potassium, sodium, barium, and calcium. It melts over a range of 593.5° C to 1093° C (1100° F to 2000° F) and is an important component of dental porcelain.

F element. See **F factor.**

fellatio /fəlā″shē·ō/, oral stimulation of the male genitalia.

fellow [AS, *feolaga,* friendly association], **1.** a member of a learned society. **2.** a graduate student who holds a position in a university or college. **3.** a peer, associate, or person of the same class or rank.

Fellow of the American Academy of Nursing (FAAN), a member of the American Academy of Nursing. The Academy was established in 1966 by the House of Delegates of the American Nurses Association to recognize significant contributions of individuals to the nursing profession. See also **American Academy of Nursing.**

fellowship /fel″ōship/ [As, *feolaga,* friendly association], a grant given to a person to pay for study or training or to allow payment for work on a special project. It provides a stipend and, in some cases, the miscellaneous expenses involved in the study, training, or project.

felon /fel″ən/ [L, *fel,* venom], a suppurative abscess on the distal phalanx of a finger.

felonious assault. See **felony.**

felony /fel″ənē/, (in criminal law) a crime declared by statute to be more serious than a misdemeanor and deserving of a more severe penalty. Conviction usually requires imprisonment in a penitentiary for longer than 1 year. Crimes of murder, rape, burglary, and arson are tried as felonies in most cases. In many states there is current, pending, or new legislation that essentially bars applicants from taking the nursing licensure exam NCLEX-RN® or NCELX-PN® if certain felonies exist in their history. Criminal background checks, state and federal, are required of all graduate nurses and, in some states, of nursing students before clinical rotations.

Felty syndrome /fel″tē/ [Augustus R. Felty, American physician, 1895–1963], a group of pathological changes that occur in adults with rheumatoid arthritis, characterized by splenomegaly, leukopenia, frequent infections, and sometimes thrombocytopenia and anemia. The cause of the syndrome is unknown. Surgical resection of the spleen offers temporary improvement in about one half of the cases. See also **hypersplenism.**

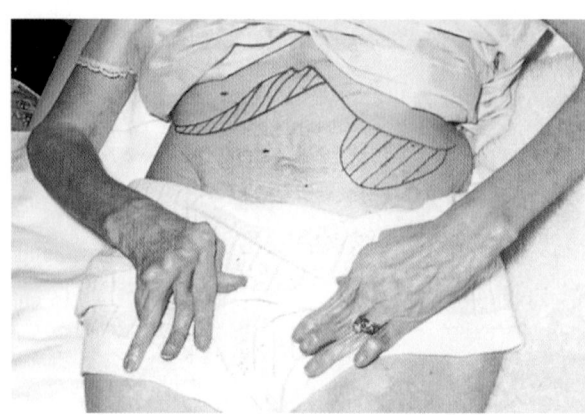

Splenomegaly associated with Felty syndrome *(Moll, 1997)*

female [L, *femella,* young woman], **1.** *adj.,* pertaining to the sex that has the ability to become pregnant and bear children; feminine. **2.** *n.,* a female person.

female catheterization, a procedure for removing urine by means of a urinary catheter introduced through the urinary meatus and urethra into the bladder. The procedure is performed for relief of distension if voluntary micturition is not possible (such as after trauma or surgery), as a preparation for and during anesthesia, or if a specimen of urine from the bladder is required or medication is to be instilled into the bladder. A straight catheter or a retention catheter with a balloon may be used. A 12 to 16 Fr catheter is usually selected for straight drainage. See also **catheterization, male catheterization.**

■ METHOD: The necessary sterile equipment is usually available in a sterile catheterization kit and includes cotton swabs, a bowl for collecting urine, a disposable catheter, a sponge stick for holding the swabs, a disinfectant for washing the urinary meatus and the perineal area adjacent to it, gloves, a lubricant for the catheter tip, and a drape. Often a preassembled kit of disposable sterile equipment is available, leaving only the separately packaged catheter to be selected. A clean, rather than sterile, technique can be used for self-catheterization.

■ OUTCOME CRITERIA: Catheterization predisposes the urinary tract to infection, and traumatic catheterization further increases the risk. Care, gentleness, and asepsis are essential. If the bladder is distended with urine, it may cause damage to the bladder, chills, and shock. Certain conditions, including radical vulvectomy, postoperative swelling, or structural anomalies, may obscure the urinary meatus. The indication for catheterization, the age of the patient, and the condition and size of the urethra affect the choice of catheter style and size.

female circumcision. See **clitoridectomy.**

female condom, a sheath worn inside the vagina, extending outward to cover the vulva. It is used to prevent pregnancy and/or transmission of sexually transmitted diseases.

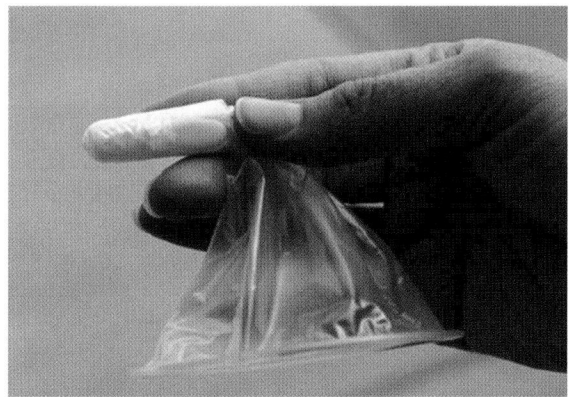

Female condom *(Berksinska et al, 2011)*

female factor infertility, infertility because of an anatomical or physiological problem with the female reproductive or immune system. See also **tubal factor infertility.**

female genital mutilation, the ritual practice of altering the genital structures, at times excising the entire clitoris without anesthetic. The practice is recognized internationally as a violation of the human rights of girls and women. Female genital mutilation is classified into four major types:

(1) clitoridectomy, the partial or total removal of the clitoris or in very rare cases only the prepuce; (2) excision, the partial or total removal of the clitoris and the labia minora, with or without excision of the labia majora; (3) infibulation, the narrowing of the vaginal opening through the creation of a covering seal formed by cutting and repositioning the inner or outer labia, with or without removal of the clitoris; and (4) all other harmful procedures to the female genitalia for nonmedical purposes (e.g., pricking, piercing, incising, scraping, and cauterizing the genital area). Also called **clitoridectomy.**

female pseudohermaphroditism, a form of congenital gonadal disorder in which ovaries are present irrespective of the condition of the external genitals. See also **pseudohermaphroditism.**

female reproductive system assessment, an evaluation of a patient's genital tract and breasts with an investigation of past and present disorders that may be factors in the individual's current gynecological condition. A careful assessment of the patient's reproductive system is essential for establishing an early diagnosis and providing prompt treatment of any abnormalities. See also **pelvic examination.**

female sexual dysfunction, impaired or inadequate ability of a woman to engage in or enjoy satisfactory sexual intercourse and orgasm. Symptoms include dyspareunia, vaginismus, persistent inability to reach orgasm, and inhibition in sexual arousal, so that congestion and vaginal lubrication are minimal or absent. Causes may include anxiety, fear, negative emotions associated with sexual arousal and intercourse, and interpersonal problems. Neurological dysfunction may also be present. Treatment is focused on eliminating physical problems and sexual anxieties and on enhancing erotic sensitivities. Compare **male sexual dysfunction.** See also **sexual dysfunction.**

female sterility [L, *femella,* young woman, *sterilis,* barren], the condition of being incapable of attaining pregnancy for any reason involving the female reproductive system or physiology or as a result of a surgical sterilization procedure such as tubal ligation or hysterectomy.

female urethra, a narrow duct about 3.7 cm long, extending from the neck of the bladder above the anterior vaginal wall to the urinary meatus.

feminist therapy, an alternative therapy that is both a philosophical approach to the conduct of therapy and a specific type of therapy. The focus of both types is a consciousness raising that focuses on the presence of sexism and sex role stereotyping in society.

feminization /fem′inīzā″shən/ [L, *femina,* woman], **1.** the normal development or induction of female secondary sex characteristics. **2.** the induction of female sex characteristics in a genotypic male. Compare **virilization.** See also **pseudohermaphroditism. 3.** testicular feminization in males with an X and a Y chromosome and a female phenotype caused by fetal hypogonadism. It is often familial. Individuals with this condition usually have undescended or labial testes, a short blind vaginal pouch, no uterus, well-developed breasts, sparse or absent axillary and pubic hair, normal plasma levels of testosterone and follicle-stimulating hormone, and increased concentrations of estradiol and luteinizing hormone. **4.** secondary female sex characteristics caused by an adrenocortical estrogen-secreting tumor, failure of the liver to inactivate endogenous estrogens such as in advanced alcoholism, or the administration of estrogen therapy for androgen-dependent neoplasms.

feminizing adrenal tumor /fem″inī′zing/, a rare neoplasm of the adrenal cortex, characterized in males by gynecomastia, hypertension, diffuse pigmentation, a high level of estrogen in urine, and loss of potency. Testicular atrophy frequently occurs, but the prostate and penis are usually normal in size. The tumor may be large enough to be palpated or to be diagnosed by IV urography or arteriography. In most cases it is a carcinoma. Treatment includes surgical resection and chemotherapy with mitotane. In women these tumors, which are extremely rare, are associated with precocious puberty.

femora. See **femur.**

femoral /fem″ərəl/ [L, *femur,* thigh], pertaining to the femur or the thigh.

femoral angle. See **neck shaft angle.**

femoral anteversion, inward twisting of the femur so that the knees and feet turn inward, usually seen in children or in persons with osteoarthritis of the hip.

femoral artery (FA), an extension of the external iliac artery into the lower limb, starting immediately distal to the inguinal ligament and ending at the junction of the middle and lower thirds of the thigh. It divides into seven branches, continuing as the popliteal artery, and supplies various parts of the lower limb and trunk, such as the groin and its organs.

femoral catheter, a central venous catheter inserted through the femoral vein.

femoral condyle, one of a pair of large flared prominences on the distal end of the femur. Identified as lateral and medial femoral condyles, they are covered with a thick layer of hyaline cartilage and articulate with the patella and the tibia at the knee joint.

femoral epiphysis, a secondary bone-forming center of the femur, separated from the main part of the bone by cartilage during the period of bone immaturity. In overweight adolescents, there may be bone slippage along the femoral capital epiphysis, marked by pain and loss of range of motion.

femoral hernia, a hernia in which a loop of intestine descends through the femoral canal into the groin. Surgical repair, herniorrhaphy, is the usual treatment. See also **hernia.**

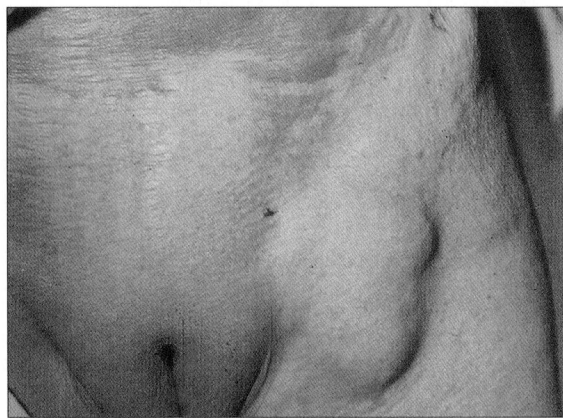

Femoral hernia causing a bulging enlargement of the femoral canal (Hagen-Ansert, 2012)

femoral nerve, the largest of the seven nerves stemming from the lumbar plexus and the main nerve of the anterior part of the thigh. Also called **anterior crural nerve.**

femoral pulse, the pulse of the femoral artery, palpated in the groin.

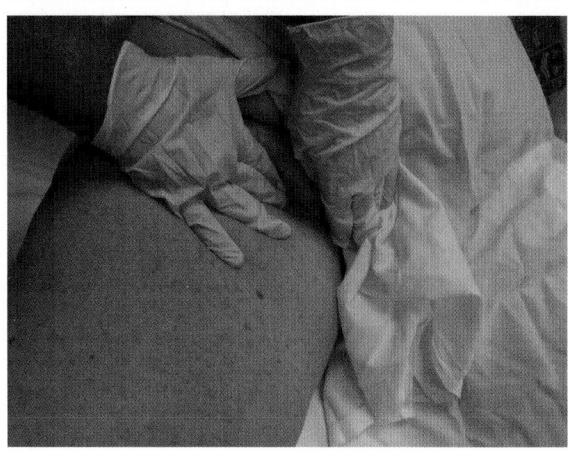

Femoral pulse

femoral reflex [L, *femur,* thigh, *reflectere,* to bend back], an extension of the knee and a plantar flexion of the toes of the foot that occurs when the skin on the upper anterior third of the thigh is stimulated.

femoral stem, in arthroplasty of the hip or knee, the part of the prosthesis that inserts into the end of the trimmed and prepared femur.

femoral-to-popliteal artery bypass, grafting with a saphenous vein or straight synthetic graft to bypass an occluded section of the femoral artery and restore blood flow to the leg. Surgery is performed with the patient in a supine position, with the hip externally rotated and abducted and the knee flexed. An in situ femoral-to-popliteal bypass uses the patient's saphenous vein, which stays in place. Contraindications for this procedure are varicose veins or previous saphenous vein ligation and stripping.

femoral torsion, an extreme lateral or medial twisting rotation of the femur on its longitudinal axis, which may be caused by the action of the gluteal or other muscles. Compare **tibial torsion.**

femoral triangle, a wedge-shaped depression formed by the muscles in the upper thigh at the junction between the anterior abdominal wall and the lower limb through which the femoral nerve, artery, and vein and lymphatic vessels pass.

femoral vein, a large vein in the thigh that is a continuation of the popliteal vein and that accompanies the femoral artery in the proximal two thirds of the thigh. Its distal portion lies lateral to the artery, and its proximal portion lies deeper to the artery. Near its termination, it is joined by the great saphenous vein. At the inguinal ligament it becomes the external iliac vein.

femoro-, a prefix meaning relationship to the femur.

Femstat, an antifungal drug. Brand name for **butoconazole nitrate.**

femur /fē″mər/ *pl. femora, femurs* [L, thigh], the thigh bone, which extends from the pelvis to the knee. It is largely cylindric and is the longest and strongest bone in the body. It has a large round head that fits the acetabulum of the hip, and it displays a large neck and several prominences and ridges for muscle attachments. In an erect posture it inclines medially, drawing the knee joint near the line of gravity of the body.

FE$_{Na}$, abbreviation for **fractional excretion of sodium.**

FeNO, abbreviation for **fractional exhaled nitric oxide.**

fenestra /fines″trə/ *pl. fenestrae* [L, window], **1.** an aperture, as in a bandage or cast, that is cut out to relieve pressure or to administer regular skin care. **2.** a microscopic opening in certain capillaries specialized in filtration, as in the glomerular capillaries of the kidney often covered by membrane.

fenestra cochlea. See **round window.**

fenestrae. See **fenestra.**

fenestra rotunda. See **round window.**

fenestrate. See **fenestration.**

fenestrated drape, a drape with a round or slitlike opening in the center.

fenestration /fen′əstrā″shən/ [L, *fenestra,* window], **1.** a surgical procedure in which an opening is created to gain access to the cavity within an organ or a bone. **2.** an opening created surgically in a bone or organ of the body. **3.** (in dentistry) a procedure to expose a root tip of a tooth to permit drainage of exudate or to allow access to place a retrograde filling at the apex of a tooth root. **4.** (in dentistry) bone loss that resembles a "window" because it is bordered by alveolar bone along its coronal aspect and is located on the facial or lingual aspect of a tooth. The exposed root surface is in direct contact with gingiva or alveolar mucosa. Also called **window. –fenestrate,** *v.*

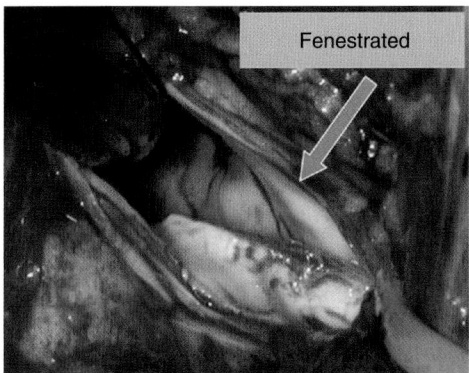

Open fenestration of aorta (Roselli et al, 2011)

fenofibrate /fen′ofi′brāt/, an agent chemically related to clofibrate used to treat hyperlipidemia, administered orally.

fenoldopam, an antihypertensive drug.

■ INDICATIONS: It is used to treat hypertensive crisis when an urgent decrease of pressure is required, including malignant hypertension.

■ CONTRAINDICATIONS: Known hypersensitivity to this drug and sulfite sensitivity prohibit its use.

■ ADVERSE EFFECTS: Life-threatening effects are hypotension, myocardial infarction, ischemic heart disease, and leukocytosis. Other adverse effects include anxiety, dizziness, ST-T wave changes, angina pectoris, palpitations, nausea, vomiting, constipation, diarrhea, bleeding, and increased levels of blood urea nitrogen, glucose, lactic dehydrogenase, creatinine, and hypokalemia. Headache is a common side effect.

fenoprofen calcium /fē′nəprō″fen/, a nonsteroidal antiinflammatory agent and analgesic.

■ INDICATIONS: It is prescribed in the treatment of arthritis and other painful inflammatory conditions.

■ CONTRAINDICATIONS: Renal dysfunction, upper GI disease, or known hypersensitivity to this drug, to aspirin, or to nonsteroidal antiinflammatory medication prohibits its use.

■ ADVERSE EFFECTS: Among the more serious adverse effects are GI disturbances, gastric or duodenal ulceration, dizziness, skin rash, and tinnitus.

fenoterol /fen′ōter″ol/, a beta$_2$-adrenergic receptor agonist used as a bronchodilator for the treatment and prophylaxis of reversible bronchospasm, administered by inhalation as the hydrobromide salt.

fentanyl citrate, a general anesthetic. See also **buccal fentanyl.**

■ INDICATIONS: It is prescribed as an adjunct to general anesthesia, as a preoperative and postoperative analgesic, and as a component in neuroleptanesthesia and analgesia.

■ CONTRAINDICATIONS: Myasthenia gravis, use of a monoamine oxidase inhibitor within 14 days, or known hypersensitivity to this drug prohibits its use.

■ ADVERSE EFFECTS: Among the more serious adverse effects are drug dependence, hypotension, pruritus, respiratory depression, and laryngospasm.

fenugreek, an annual herb found in Europe and Asia.

■ INDICATIONS: It is used for loss of appetite, skin inflammation, water retention, cancer, constipation, diarrhea, high cholesterol, high blood glucose, and calcium oxalate stones. It may be effective at lowering blood glucose (slow intestinal absorption) and as a poultice for local inflammation, but there are insufficient reliable data on its efficacy for other uses.

■ CONTRAINDICATIONS: It should not be used during pregnancy because it can cause premature labor. It is also contraindicated during lactation, in children, and in those with known hypersensitivity to this herb.

Feosol, an iron supplement prescribed to help increase hemoglobin production. Brand name for **ferrous sulfate.**

-fer, suffix meaning "producing or carrying something specified": *buffer, transfer.*

Fergon, an iron supplement prescribed to help increase red blood cell production. Brand name for *ferrous gluconate.*

Ferguson's reflex, a contraction of the uterus after the cervix is stimulated, usually associated with the release of prostaglandins.

fermentation /fur′məntā″shən/ [L, *fermentare,* to cause to rise], a chemical change that is brought about in a substance by the action of an enzyme or microorganism, especially the anaerobic conversion of foodstuffs to certain products. Kinds include **acetic fermentation, alcoholic fermentation, ammoniacal fermentation, amylic fermentation, butyric fermentation, caseous fermentation, dextran fermentation, diastatic fermentation, lactic acid fermentation, propionic fermentation,** *storing fermentation,* **viscous fermentation.**

fermentative dyspepsia /fərmen″tətiv/, an abnormal condition characterized by impaired digestion associated with the fermentation of digested food. See also **dyspepsia.**

fermium (Fm) /fur″mē·əm/ [Enrico Fermi, Italian physicist, 1901–1954], a synthetic transuranic metallic element. Its atomic number is 100; the mass of its longest-lived, best-known isotope is 257. Fermium was first detected in the debris from a hydrogen bomb explosion and later produced in a reactor.

ferning test /fur″ning/ [AS, *faern,* fern; L, *testum,* crucible], a technique used to determine the presence of estrogen in the uterine cervical mucus. It is often used to test for ovulation. High levels of estrogen cause the cervical mucus to dry in a fernlike pattern on a slide. Also called **arborization test.**

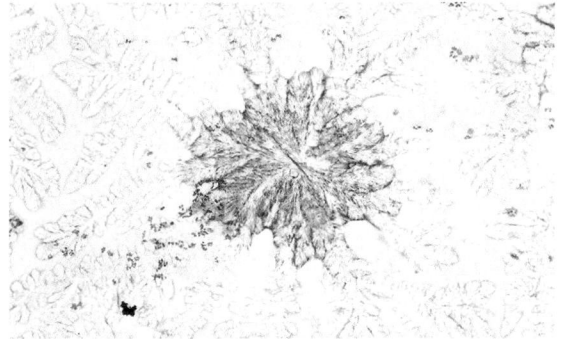

Ferning (McKee, 1997)

-ferous, suffix meaning "producing or carrying" something specified: *lactiferous, luminiferous.*

ferr-, ferri-. See **ferro-, ferr-, ferri-.**

ferredoxin, a nonheme protein containing equal amounts of iron and sulfur. Ferredoxins are involved in electron transport in photosynthesis and nitrogen fixation.

ferric /fer″ik/, pertaining to a cation of iron in which the metal is trivalent, as in ferric chloride and ferric hydroxide. Also called *iron (III).*

ferritin /fer″itin/ [L, *ferrum,* iron], an iron compound formed in the intestine and stored in the liver, spleen, and bone marrow for eventual incorporation into hemoglobin. Serum ferritin levels are used as an indicator of the body's iron stores. Normal adult blood levels are 12 to 300 ng/mL for males and 10 to 150 ng/mL for females.

ferritin test, a blood test used to determine available iron stores in the body. It is used to diagnose iron-deficiency anemia and, when combined with the serum iron level and total iron-binding capacity tests, can differentiate and classify various kinds of anemias.

ferro-, ferr-, ferri-, prefix meaning "iron": *ferromagnetic, ferritin, ferric.*

ferrokinetics /fer″ōkinet″iks/, the study of iron metabolism.

ferromagnetic /fer″ōmagnet″ik/, pertaining to substances, such as iron, nickel, and cobalt, that are strongly affected by magnetism and may become magnetized by exposure to a magnetic field.

ferrotherapy /fer″ōther″əpē/, the use of iron and iron compounds in the treatment of illness.

ferrous /fer″əs/, pertaining to a compound of iron in which the metal is divalent, such as ferrous ammonium sulfate. See also **iron.**

ferrous sulfate, an antianemia (hematinic) agent. See also **iron.**

■ INDICATIONS: It is prescribed in the treatment of iron-deficiency anemia.

■ CONTRAINDICATIONS: Hemochromatosis, hemosiderosis, hemolytic anemias, and hypersensitivity to any of the ingredients prohibit its use.

■ ADVERSE EFFECTS: Among the most serious adverse effects are GI irritation, diarrhea, and constipation.

fertile /fur″təl/ [L, *fertilis,* fruitful], **1.** capable of reproducing or bearing offspring. **2.** (of a gamete) capable of inducing fertilization or being fertilized. **3.** prolific; fruitful; not sterile. –**fertility,** *n.,* –**fertilize,** *v.*

fertile eunuch syndrome, a hypogonadotropic hormonal disorder of males in which the levels of testosterone and follicle-stimulating hormone are inadequate to induce spermatogenesis and the development of secondary sexual characteristics. If supplemental hormones are not prescribed, the affected person acquires the appearance of a eunuch. Also called **Pasqualini syndrome.**

fertile period, the time in the menstrual cycle during which fertilization may occur. Spermatozoa can survive for approximately 5 days; the ovum lives for approximately 24 hours. Thus the fertile period begins up to approximately 6 days before ovulation and lasts for approximately 1 day afterward. It may be identified by observation of the changes in the quantity and character of the cervical mucus or changes in the basal body temperature, or it may be determined from a calendar record of six or more menstrual cycles, applying the knowledge that ovulation usually occurs 14 days before menstruation.

fertility /fərtil″itē/, the ability to reproduce.

fertility awareness methods. See **natural family planning method.**

fertility factor. See **F factor.**

fertility rate, the number of live births divided by the number of females aged 15 through 44 years of age. It is usually expressed as the number per 1000 women.

fertilization /fur″tilīzā″shən/ [L, *fertilis,* fruitful], the union of male and female gametes to form a zygote from which the embryo develops. See also **in vitro fertilization, oogenesis, spermatogenesis.**

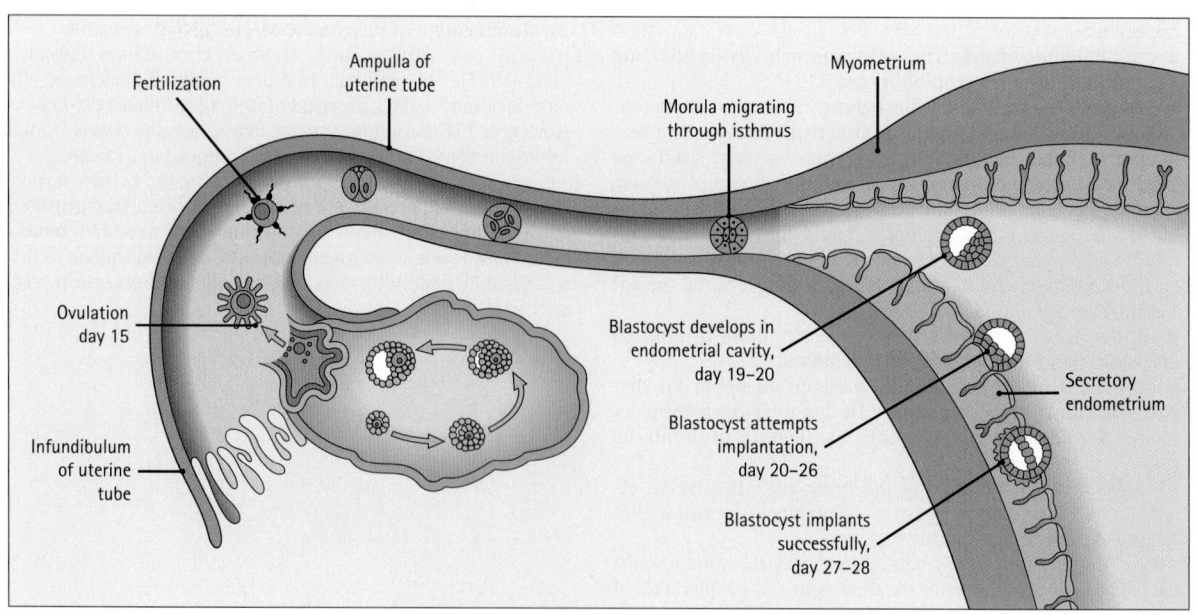

Fertilization cycle *(Lowe and Anderson, 2015)*

fertilization age. See **fetal age.**

fertilization membrane, a viscous membrane surrounding a fertilized ovum that prevents penetration of additional spermatozoa. It is formed by granules that are released by the fertilized ovum and adhere to the vitelline membrane.

fertilize. See **fertile.**

fertilizin /fərtil″izin/, a glycoprotein found on the plasma membrane of the ovum in various species. See also **acrosomal reaction.**

Festal, a fixed-combination GI drug that contains a group of digestive enzymes and bile constituents. Brand name for **pancreatin,** *bile components, hemicellulase.*

fester, 1. to become superficially inflamed and pus-producing. **2.** to become increasingly virulent.

festinant /fes″tinənt/, pertaining to a gait pattern that accelerates involuntarily as a result of a nervous system disorder. The increased rate of walking represents an automatic attempt by the body to overtake a displaced center of gravity. See also **extrapyramidal disease, festinating gait.**

festinating gait /fes″tinā′ting/ [L, *festinare,* to hasten], a manner of walking in which a person's speed increases in an unconscious effort to "catch up" with a displaced center of gravity. It is a common characteristic of Parkinson's disease.

festoon [Fr, *feston,* scallop], a carving in the base material of a denture that simulates the contours of the external root curvatures as seen in natural gingival tissues. See also **gingival festoon, McCall's festoon.**

FET, abbreviation for **forced expiratory time.**

fetal /fē″təl/ [L, *fetus,* fruitful], pertaining to the final stage of development of a prenatal mammal. In humans the fetal period extends from the first day of the ninth week of intrauterine life until birth.

fetal age, the age of the conceptus computed from the time elapsed since fertilization. Also called **fertilization age.** Compare **gestational age.**

fetal alcohol syndrome (FAS) [L, *fetus* + Ar, *alkohl,* essence; Gk, *syn,* together, *dromos,* course], a set of congenital psychological, behavioral, and physical abnormalities that tend to appear in infants whose mothers consumed alcohol during pregnancy. It is characterized by typical craniofacial and limb defects, cardiovascular defects, intrauterine growth impairment, and delayed development. The most serious cases have involved infants born to mothers who were chronic alcoholics and drank heavily during pregnancy. Women who drank less reportedly gave birth to infants with less serious malformations, or fetal alcohol effects (FAEs), but it is not known whether there is a lower limit to alcohol consumption during pregnancy or a particular period in embryonic life when the offspring is most vulnerable to effects of alcohol.

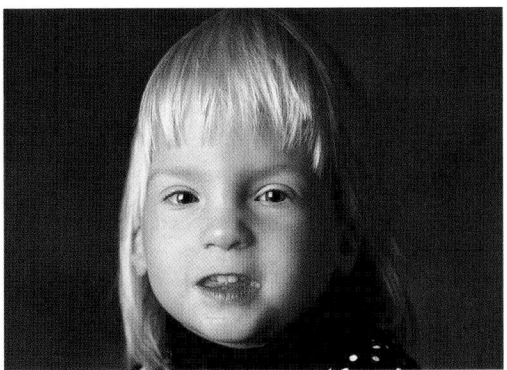

Child with fetal alcohol syndrome *(Fortinash and Holoday Worret, 2008)*

fetal alveoli, the terminal pulmonary sacs of a fetus, which are filled with fluid before birth. The fluid is a transudate of fetal plasma.

fetal asphyxia, a situation of damaging fetal acidemia, hypoxia, and metabolic acidosis.

fetal attitude, a nonspecific term describing the intrapartum relationship of the fetal parts to each other. Compare **fetal position, fetal presentation.**

fetal biophysical profile, an ultrasound method of evaluating fetal status during the antepartal period based on five variables originating within the fetus: fetal heart rate, breathing movement, gross movements, muscle tone, and amniotic fluid volume. It is indicated in cases of postdate pregnancy, maternal hypertension, diabetes mellitus, vaginal bleeding, maternal Rh sensitization, maternal history of stillbirth, and premature membrane rupture.

fetal bradycardia, a fetal heart rate in utero of less than 110 beats per minute.

fetal circulation, the pathway of blood circulation in the fetus. Oxygenated blood from the placenta travels through the umbilical vein to the heart. The blood enters the right atrium at a pressure sufficient to direct most of the flow across the atrium and through the foramen ovale into the left atrium; thus oxygenated blood is available for circulation through the left ventricle to the head and upper extremities. The blood returning from the head and arms enters the right atrium via the superior vena cava. It flows through the atrium at a relatively low pressure. Passing the tricuspid valve, it falls into the right ventricle, from which most of it is pumped through the pulmonary artery and the ductus arteriosus into the descending aorta for circulation to the lower parts of the body. A small amount of blood in the pulmonary artery is not shunted through the ductus and is carried to the lungs. The blood is returned to the placenta through the umbilical arteries.

fetal death, the intrauterine death of a fetus, or the death of a fetus weighing at least 500 g or after 20 or more weeks of gestation.

fetal distress, *(Informal)* a compromised condition of the fetus. Now called **nonreassuring fetal status.**

fetal dose, the estimated amount of radiation received by a fetus during a radiographic examination of a pregnant woman. It is expressed in milligrays (mGy).

fetal face syndrome. See **Robinow syndrome.**

fetal fibronectin test, an analysis of vaginal secretions of a pregnant woman to determine the risk of preterm delivery.

fetal heart rate (FHR), the number of heartbeats in the fetus that occur in a given unit of time. The FHR varies in cycles of fetal rest and activity and is affected by many factors, including maternal fever, uterine contractions, maternal-fetal hypotension, and many drugs. The normal FHR is between 110 beats/min and 160 beats/min. In labor the FHR is monitored with a fetoscope, an electronic fetal monitor for detecting abnormal alterations in the heart rate, especially recurrent decelerations that continue past the end of uterine contractions.

fetal heart sounds [L, *fetus,* fruitful; AS, *heorte* + L, *sonus,* sound], sounds produced by the heart of a fetus, as detected by auscultation or by electronic fetal monitoring. The heart forms at about 21 to 22 days of gestation. Complete innervation of the heart resulting in contraction occurs at approximately 5 weeks, allowing for auscultation.

fetal hemoglobin (HgbF), the predominate hemoglobin found in later pregnancy, composed of two alpha chains and two beta chains physiologically different from adult hemoglobin A (HgbA) in that, at any given oxygen tension, HgbF has a higher oxygen affinity and oxygen saturation than HgbA.

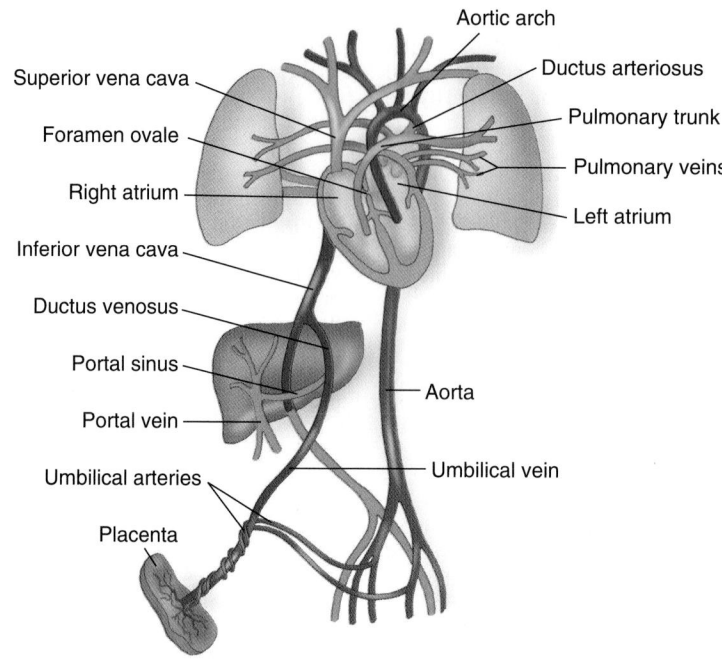

Aortic arch
Ductus arteriosus
Pulmonary trunk
Pulmonary veins
Left atrium
Superior vena cava
Foramen ovale
Right atrium
Inferior vena cava
Ductus venosus
Portal sinus
Portal vein
Aorta
Umbilical arteries
Umbilical vein
Placenta

Fetal circulation *(Hagen-Ansert, 2012)*

Thus, although the partial pressure of oxygen in the fetal arterial blood supply is only 20 to 25 mm Hg, the fetus remains adequately oxygenated in utero and the early neonatal period.

fetal hemoglobin test, a test of maternal blood to detect leakage of fetal cells into the maternal circulation, an indication of fetal-maternal hemorrhage.

fetal hydantoin syndrome (FHS), a complex of birth defects associated with prenatal maternal ingestion of hydantoin derivatives. Symptoms of FHS include microcephaly, hypoplasia or absence of nails on the fingers or toes, abnormal facies, mental and physical impairment, and cardiac defects. The syndrome occurs to some degree in 10% to 40% of infants born of mothers who use this anticonvulsant. Hydantoin is sometimes associated with hemorrhage and, more rarely, with neural crest tumors in the newborn.

fetal hydrops. See **hydrops fetalis.**

fetal lie, the relationship of the long axis of the fetus to the long axis of the mother. See also **fetal presentation.**

fetal lipoma. See **hibernoma.**

fetal membranes, the structures that protect, support, and nourish the embryo and fetus, including the yolk sac, allantois, amnion, and chorion.

fetal microchimerism, persistence in the mother's circulation after pregnancy of a low number of fetal cells. It may play a role in some autoimmune disorders.

fetal monitor. See **electronic fetal monitor.**

fetal mortality rate, the number of fetal deaths per 1000 births, or per live births.

fetal movements [L, *fetus* + *movere,* to move], muscular motions produced by the fetus in utero. See also **quickening.**

fetal nonstress test, an electrodiagnostic test to evaluate the viability of a fetus. It documents the function of the placenta in its ability to supply adequate blood to the fetus.

fetal oxygen saturation monitoring. See **fetal scalp blood pH test.**

fetal placenta [L, *fetus* + *placenta,* flat cake], the portion of the placenta that is formed from the shaggy chorion frondosum, the villi of which invade the decidua basalis. Also called **pars fetalis.**

fetal position, **1.** the relationship of the orientation of the presenting part of the fetus to the four quadrants of the maternal pelvis, identified by initial L (left), R (right), A (anterior), and P (posterior). The presenting part is also identified by initial O (occiput), M (mentum), and S (sacrum). If a fetus presents with the occiput directed to the posterior aspect of the mother's right side, the fetal position is right occiput posterior (ROP). Compare **fetal attitude, fetal presentation.** **2.** the assumption of a posture by a child or adult resembling that of the fetus in the womb. The limbs are drawn in closely to the body, the head is bent forward, and the back is curled.

fetal presentation, the part of the fetus that lies closest to or has entered the true pelvis. Types of presentation include cephalic (vertex, brow, face, and chin), breech (frank breech, complete breech, incomplete breech, and single or double footling breech), shoulder, and compound, involving more than one part in the true pelvis. See also **fetal attitude, fetal lie, fetal position.**

fetal respiration, the exchange of gases and metabolic products between the blood of the mother and the fetus by means of the placental interface in utero.

fetal rickets. See **achondroplasia.**

fetal rotation [L, *fetus* + *rotare,* to rotate], the turning of the head as it begins the descent through the birth canal. See **cardinal movements of labor.**

fetal scalp blood pH test, a measurement of fetal scalp blood pH used to diagnose fetal distress. Also called **fetal oxygen saturation monitoring.**

fetal stage, (in embryology) the interval from the end of the embryonic stage, at the end of the seventh or eighth week of gestation, to birth, 38 to 42 weeks after the first day of the last menstrual period.

fetal tachycardia, a fetal heart rate that continues at 160 beats/min or more for more than 10 minutes.

fetal viability, that point in fetal development, and indirectly in age, when a fetus is able to survive, with or without artificial life support, after birth. See **viable infant.**

feti-, feto-, foeti-, foeto-, prefix meaning "fetus" or "fetal": *feticide, fetochorionic, fetoscope.*

feticide. See **embryoctony.**

fetid /fet″id, fē″tid/ [L, *fetere,* to stink], pertaining to something that has a foul or putrid odor.

fetish [Fr, *fetiche,* artificial], **1.** any object or idea given unreasonable or excessive attention or reverence. **2.** (in psychology) any inanimate object or any body part not of a sexual nature that arouses erotic feelings or fixation. The erotic symbolism is unique to the fetishist and results from unconscious associations. See also **paraphilia.** –*fetishism, n.*

fetishist /fet″ishist/, a person who believes in or receives erotic gratification from fetishes.

fetochorionic /fē″tōkôr′ē·on″ik/ [L, *fetus,* fruitful; Gk, *chorion,* skin], pertaining to the fetus and the chorion.

fetofetal transfusion. See **twin-to-twin transfusion.**

fetoglobulins /fē″tōglob″yəlinz/, proteins found in fetal blood and normally in small amounts in adult blood. The group includes alpha-fetoprotein. In certain diseases, fetoglobulins may be present in adult blood in larger concentrations.

fetography /fētog″rəfē/ [L, *fetus* + Gk, *graphein,* to record], roentgenography of the fetus in utero. See also **fetometry.**

fetology /fētol″əjē/ [L, *fetus* + Gk, *logos,* science], the branch of medicine that is concerned with the fetus in utero, including the diagnosis of congenital anomalies, the prevention of teratogenic influences, and the treatment of certain disorders. Also called *embryatrics.*

fetometry /fētom″ətrē/ [L, *fetus* + Gk, *metron,* measure], the measurement of the size of the fetus, especially the diameter of the head and circumference of the trunk. Kinds include **roentgen fetometry.**

fetoplacental /-pləsen″təl/ [L, *fetus* + *placenta,* flat cake], pertaining to the fetus and the placenta.

fetoprotein /-prō″tēn/ [L, *fetus* + Gk, *proteios,* first rank], an antigen that occurs naturally in fetuses and occasionally in adults as the result of certain diseases. An increased amount of alpha-fetoprotein in the fetus is diagnostic for neural tube defects. The presence of beta-fetoprotein in the blood of adults is associated with leukemia, hepatoma, sarcoma, and other neoplasms. See also **alpha-fetoprotein, beta-fetoprotein.**

fetor ex ore. See **halitosis.**

fetor hepaticus [L, stench, *hēpar,* liver], foul-smelling breath associated with severe liver disease. Also called **liver breath.**

fetor oris. See **halitosis.**

fetoscope /fē″təskōp′/ [L, *fetus* + Gk, *skopein,* to look], **1.** a thin catheter inserted through a small incision to allow for direct visualization of the fetus, the placenta, and the umbilical cord. **2.** a specialized stethoscope for monitoring the fetal heartbeat.

fetoscopy /fētos″kəpē/, an endoscopic procedure in which an instrument is inserted through the abdominal wall and uterine wall for observation of the fetus, the amniotic cavity, the amniotic fluid, the umbilical cord, and the fetal side of the placenta and for access for the sampling of tissues or fluids, including fetal blood.

fetotoxic /-tok″sik/ [L, *fetus* + Gk, *toxikon,* poison], pertaining to anything that is poisonous to a fetus.

fetus /fē″təs/ [L, fruitful], the unborn offspring of any viviparous animal after it has attained the particular form of the species; more specifically the human being in utero after the embryonic period and the beginning of the development of the major structural features, from the ninth week after fertilization until birth. Kinds of fetal anomalies include anideus, lithopedion, mummified fetus, parasitic fetus, and sirenomelia. Also spelled **foetus.** Compare **embryo.** See also **prenatal development.** –*fetal, foetal, adj.*

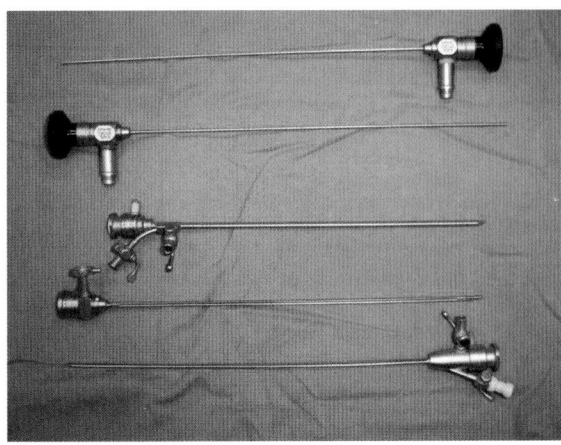

Fetoscopes *(Chang, 2012)*

fetus acardiacus, fetus acardius. See **acardia.**

fetus amorphus, a shapeless conceptus that has no formed or recognizable parts.

fetus anideus. See **anideus.**

fetus in fetu /infē″too/, a fetal anomaly in which a small, imperfectly formed twin, incapable of independent existence, is contained within the body of the normal twin, the autosite.

fetus papyraceus, a twin fetus that has died in utero early in development and has been pressed flat against the uterine wall by the living fetus. Also called **paper-doll fetus, papyraceous fetus.**

fetus sanguinolentis /sang′gwinəlen″tis/, a darkly colored, partly macerated fetus that has died in utero.

FEV, abbreviation for **forced expiratory volume.**

FEVC, abbreviation for **forced expiratory vital capacity.**

fever [L, *febris*], an elevation of body temperature above the normal circadian range as a result of an increase in the body's core temperature. Fever is a temperature above 37.2° C (98.9° F) in the morning or above 37.7° C (99.9° F) in the evening. Fever results from an imbalance between the elimination and the production of heat. Exercise, anxiety, and dehydration may increase the temperature of healthy people. Infection, neurological disease, malignancy, pernicious anemia, thromboembolic disease, paroxysmal tachycardia, congestive heart failure, crushing injury, severe trauma, and many drugs may cause fever. No single theory explains the mechanism whereby the temperature is increased. Fever has no recognized function in conditions other than infection. It increases metabolic activity by 7% per degree Celsius, requiring a greater intake of food. Convulsions may occur in children whose fevers tend to rise abruptly, and delirium is seen with high fevers in adults and in children. Very high temperatures, as in heatstroke, may be fatal. The course of a fever varies with the cause, the condition of the patient, and the treatment given. The onset may be abrupt or gradual, and the period of maximum elevation, called the stadium or fastigium, may last for a few days or up to 3 weeks. The fever may resolve suddenly, by crisis, or gradually, by lysis. Certain diseases and conditions are associated with fevers that begin, rise, and fall in such characteristic curves that diagnosis may be made by studying a graphic record of the course of the fever. Also called **febrile response.** Kinds include **habitual fever, intermittent fever, relapsing fever.** See also **fever treatment, hyperpyrexia, quartan malaria, remittent fever, septic fever, tertian malaria.**

fever blister, a cold sore caused by herpesvirus 1. It generally appears around the mouth or nasal mucous membranes following a febrile episode or cold. See also **herpes simplex.**

F

feverfew, a perennial herb found throughout the world.

■ INDICATIONS: It is used for migraines, cluster headaches, fever, psoriasis, and inflammation. It is probably safe and effective when used over short terms at recommended levels of migraine prophylaxis and possibly safe for long-term use; it does not abort migraine attacks. There are insufficient reliable data for other uses.

■ CONTRAINDICATIONS: Chewing the leaves, one of the traditional methods for ingesting the herb, can lead to mouth ulcerations. It should not be used during pregnancy and lactation, in children, or in those with known hypersensitivity to this herb.

fever of unknown origin (FUO), a febrile illness of at least 3 weeks' duration with a temperature of at least 38.3° C (100.9° F) on at least three occasions and failure to establish a diagnosis in spite of intensive inpatient or outpatient evaluation (three outpatient visits or 3 days' hospitalization). The duration of febrile illness required to establish a diagnosis of FUO varies among authorities and is sometimes given as shorter than 3 weeks.

fever treatment, the care and management of a person who has an elevated temperature.

■ METHOD: The patient is observed for symptoms of fever, such as tachycardia; a full, bounding pulse or a weak, thready pulse; rapid breathing; hot, dry, hyperemic skin; chills; headache; diaphoresis; restlessness; delirium; dehydration; tremors; convulsions; and coma. Diagnostic studies such as blood, urine, and sputum cultures and visualization procedures may be ordered to determine fever causation. Treatment may include the administration of antibiotic, antipyretic, and sedative drugs. If the temperature is extremely high, a hypothermia blanket may be prescribed. The patient's temperature is checked every 2 to 4 hours or as condition and protocol indicate. Antipyretic and sedative therapy is continued as ordered. Increased amounts of fluids are given orally or parenterally, physical activity is reduced, and the skin is exposed to air, with care taken to prevent chilling.

■ INTERVENTIONS: The nurse observes and records the symptoms accompanying fever, administers the ordered medication and cooling measures, reassures the patient, and explains the importance of therapy and adequate fluid intake.

■ OUTCOME CRITERIA: Antipyretic drugs and cooling measures usually reduce the temperature, but the patient may require additional fluids and treatment for the underlying cause of the fever.

Fèvre-Languepin syndrome. See **popliteal pterygium syndrome,** def. 2.

fexofenadine, an antihistamine.

■ INDICATIONS: It is used to treat rhinitis and allergy symptoms.

■ CONTRAINDICATIONS: Known hypersensitivity to this drug and severe hepatic disease prohibit its use. Its use is also contraindicated in lactating women and in newborn or premature infants.

■ ADVERSE EFFECTS: Life-threatening effects are hemolytic anemia, thrombocytopenia, leukopenia, agranulocytosis, pancytopenia, and arrhythmias (rare). Other adverse effects are urinary frequency, dysuria, urinary retention, impotence, thickening of bronchial secretions, dry nose and throat, nausea, diarrhea, abdominal pain, vomiting, constipation, headache, stimulation, drowsiness, sedation, fatigue, confusion, blurred vision, tinnitus, restlessness, tremors, paradoxical excitation in children or the elderly, rash, eczema, photosensitivity, urticaria, hypotension, palpitations, bradycardia, and tachycardia.

FFA, abbreviation for **free fatty acid.**

F factor, an extrachromosomal segment of DNA that is present in conjugating male bacteria but absent in females. Also called **F element, fertility factor, sex factor.**

¹⁸F-FDG, symbol for [¹⁸F],-2-fluoro-2-deoxy-D-glucose, a sugar analog used in positron emission tomography to determine the local cerebral metabolic rate of glucose as a measure of neural activity in the brain.

FG syndrome [FG, initials of family names of patients in whom it was first observed], an X-linked recessive syndrome of cognitive impairment, an abnormally large brain structure, imperforate anus and other GI defects, delayed motor development, congenital hypotonia, characteristic facies and personality, short stature, skeletal anomalies, and congenital cardiac defects.

FHR, abbreviation for **fetal heart rate.**

FHS, abbreviation for **fetal hydantoin syndrome.**

FI, abbreviation for *fixed interval.*

fiber /fī″bər/, **1.** a long, filmlike, threadlike, acellular structure found in plant and animal tissues. Plant fibers usually consist of structural carbohydrates such as cellulose in cell walls. Composed of repeating glucose units in long, single strands, cellulose cannot be digested by enzymes in the human intestine. Other plant fiber components include hemicellulose and pectin. Animal fibers are composed mainly of the protein collagen, which forms elastic threads of loose connective tissue in skin and other organs. See also **dietary fiber. 2.** a skeletal muscle cell. **3.** the axon of a nerve cell.

fiberglass dermatitis, a pruritic papular skin disease produced by mechanical irritation from glass fibers. Body folds and areas covered by tight-fitting clothing are among common sites of the pruritic dermatitis. Hardening of the sites usually occurs after several weeks.

fiber-modified diet, a diet that contains more or less fiber than a normal diet.

fiberoptic bronchoscopy /-op″tik/ [L, *fibra* + Gk, *optikos,* sight], the visual examination of the tracheobronchial tree through a fiberoptic bronchoscope. Also called **bronchofibroscopy.** See also **bronchoscopy, fiberoptics.**

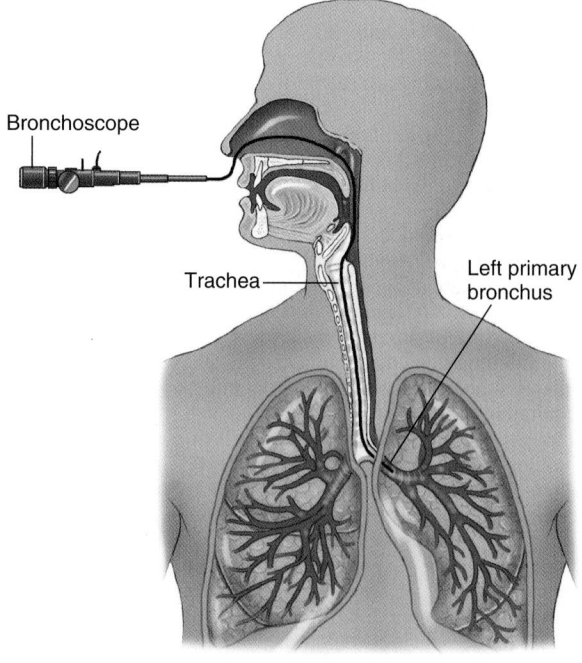

Bronchoscope

Trachea

Left primary bronchus

Fiberoptic bronchoscopy *(LaFleur, 2011)*

fiberoptic colonoscope, a colonoscope that uses fiberoptic technology.

fiberoptic duodenoscope, an instrument for visualizing the interior of the duodenum, consisting of an eyepiece, a flexible tube incorporating bundles of coated glass or plastic fibers with special optic properties, and a terminal light. When the duodenoscope is introduced into the patient's mouth and threaded through the upper digestive tract to the duodenum, the light illuminates the internal structures and any lesions present, and the fiberoptic bundles transmit the image to the observer's eyepiece.

fiberoptic endoscopic evaluation of swallowing (FEES), diagnosis and treatment of swallowing disorders by means of a flexible fiberoptic endoscope introduced transnasally into the hypopharynx. It allows direct observation of the pharyngeal and laryngeal structures during swallowing and enables the examiner to suggest swallowing maneuvers and posture changes to improve function.

fiberoptics /-op″tiks/, the technical process by which an internal organ or cavity can be viewed, using glass or plastic fibers to transmit light through a specially designed tube and reflect a magnified image. Also spelled **fibreoptics.** –*fiberoptic, adj.*

fiberscope /fī″bərskōp/ [L, *fibra* + Gk, *skopein,* to look], a flexible fiberoptic instrument having an inner shaft coated with light-conveying glass or plastic fibers for visualization of internal structures. Fiberscopes are specially designed for the examination of particular organs and cavities of the body and are used in bronchoscopy, endoscopy, and gastroscopy.

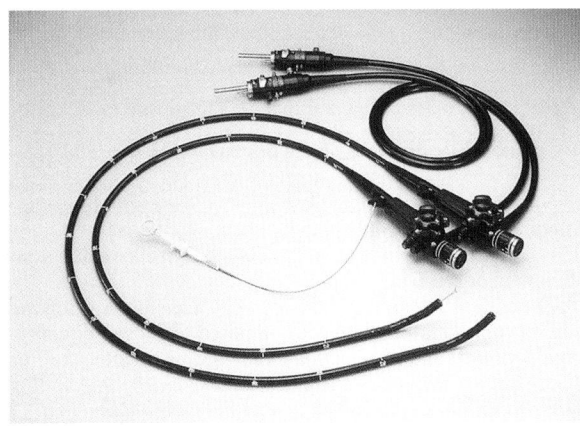

Flexible colon fiberscopes *(Monahan et al, 2007)*

-fibrate, suffix for clofibrate-type compounds.

fibrates /fī″brāts/, a general term for fibric acid derivatives, such as gemfibrozil.

fibreoptics. See **fiberoptics.**

fibril /fī″bril/ [L, *fibrilla,* small fiber], a small filamentous fiber that often is a component of a cell, as in a mitotic spindle or a myofibril. –*fibrillary, adj.*

fibrillation /fī″brilā″shən/ [L, *fibrilla,* small fiber, *atio,* process], involuntary recurrent contraction of a single muscle fiber or of an isolated bundle of nerve fibers. Fibrillation of a chamber of the heart results in inefficient random contraction of that chamber and disruption of the normal sinus rhythm of the heart. Fibrillation is usually described by the part that is contracting abnormally, such as atrial fibrillation or ventricular fibrillation.

fibrillin /fibri″lin/ [L, *fibrilla,* small fiber], a major component of elastin-associated microfibrils. Mutations in the fibrillin-1 protein gene are associated with Marfan's syndrome. See also **Marfan's syndrome.**

fibrin /fī″brin/ [L, *fibra,* fiber], a stringy insoluble protein produced by the action of thrombin on fibrinogen in the clotting process. Fibrin is responsible for the semisolid character of a blood clot. Compare **fibrinogen.** See also **blood clotting, coagulation, fibrinolysis, thrombin.**

fibrinocellular /fī″brinōsel″yələr/, composed of fibrin and cells, as occurs in some exudates that result from inflammation.

fibrinogen /fībrin″əjən/ [L, *fibra,* fiber; Gk, *genein,* to produce], a plasma protein that is converted into fibrin by thrombin in the presence of calcium ions. Also called **factor I.** Compare **fibrin.** See also **afibrinogenemia, blood clotting, fibrinolysis, thrombin.**

fibrinogenic. See **fibrinogenous.**

fibrinogenopenia /fī″brinōjen″ōpē″nē·ə/ [L, *fibra* + Gk, *genein,* to produce, *penia,* poverty], a deficiency of fibrinogen in the blood.

fibrinogenous /fī″brinoj″ənəs/ [L, *fibra,* fiber; Gk, *genein,* to produce], pertaining to the characteristics or properties of fibrinogen or the production of fibrin.

fibrinogen test, a blood test that evaluates the blood clotting mechanism. Increased concentrations of fibrinogen may indicate tissue inflammation or necrosis and may predict increased risk of coronary artery or cerebrovascular disease. Low levels are seen with liver disease, malnutrition, and consumptive coagulopathy.

fibrinokinase /fī″brinōkī″nās/ [L, *fibra* + Gk, *kinesis,* motion], a non–water-soluble enzyme in animal tissue that activates plasminogen. Also called **tissue kinase, tissue plasminogen activator.**

fibrinolysin /fī″brinol″isin/ [L, *fibra* + Gk, *lysein,* to loosen], a proteolytic enzyme that dissolves fibrin. It is formed from plasminogen in the blood plasma. Also called **plasmin.** See also **fibrinolysis.**

fibrinolysis /fī″brinol″isis/, the process of fibrin digestion by plasmin that is the normal mechanism for the removal of fibrin clots. It is stimulated by adhesion of plasmin and tissue plasminogen activator to fibrin. –*fibrinolytic, adj.*

fibrinopeptide /fī″brinōpep″tīd/ [L, *fibra* + Gk, *peptein,* to digest], either of two peptides (A and B) split off from fibrinogen by the action of thrombin. See also **fibrinogen, thrombin.**

fibrinoscopy /fī″brinos″kəpe/. See **inoscopy.**

fibrinous pericarditis [L, *fibra,* fiber; Gk, *peri,* near, *kardia,* heart, *itis,* inflammation], a condition in which a lymphoid exudate accumulates on the pericardium and coagulates. The coagulated exudate may acquire a thick, buttery appearance.

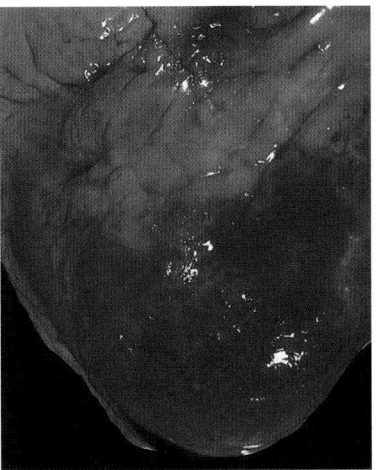

Fibrinous pericarditis *(Kumar et al, 2010)*

fibrin-stabilizing factor.   See **factor XIII.**

fibro-, prefix meaning "fiber": *fibroadenoma, fibroblast, fibroelastosis.*

fibroadenoma /fī′brō·ad′inō″mə/ *pl. fibroadenomas, fibroadenomata* [L, *fibra* + Gk, *aden,* gland, *oma,* tumor], a benign tumor composed of dense epithelial and fibroblastic tissue. A fibroadenoma of the breast is nontender, encapsulated, round, movable, and firm. It is usually located in the upper outer quadrant of the breast and occurs most frequently in women younger than 30 years of age. Surgical excision is usually performed to ensure that it is not cancerous.

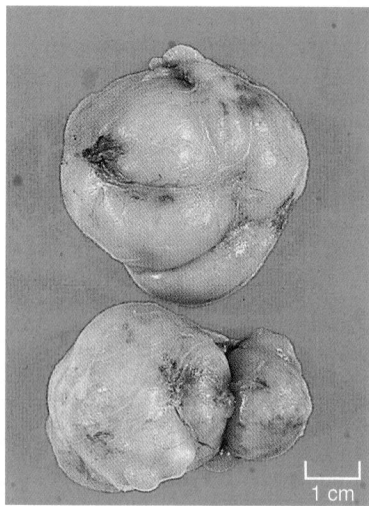

Fibroadenoma *(Cross, 2013)*

fibroangioma.   See **angiofibroma.**

fibroareolar tissue.   See **areolar tissue.**

fibroblast /fī′brəblast/ [L, *fibra* + Gk, *blastos,* germ], a flat, elongated undifferentiated cell in the connective tissue that gives rise to various precursor cells, such as the chondroblast, collagenoblast, and osteoblast, which form the fibrous, binding, and supporting tissue of the body. Also called **desmocyte, fibrocyte.** *–fibroblastic, adj.*

fibroblastoma /-blastōma/ [L, *fibra* + Gk, *blastos,* germ, oma, *tumor*], a tumor derived from a fibroblast, now differentiated as a fibroma or a fibrosarcoma.

fibrocarcinoma.   See **scirrhous carcinoma.**

fibrocartilage /-kär″tilij/ [L, *fibra* + *cartilago*], cartilage that consists of a dense matrix of white collagenous fibers. Of the three kinds of cartilage in the body, fibrocartilage has the greatest tensile strength. Fibrocartilaginous disks between the vertebrae help cushion the jolts to which the vertebral column is continually subjected. See also **hyaline cartilage.** *–fibrocartilaginous, adj.*

fibrocartilaginous joint.   See **symphysis,** def. 1.

fibrochondritis /-kondrī″tis/, an inflammation of fibrocartilage.

fibrochondroma /-kondrō″mə/, a tumor composed of mixed fibrous and cartilaginous tissues.

fibrocyst /fī″brəsist/, **1.** any cystic lesion within a fibrous connective tissue. **2.** a cystic fibroma.

fibrocystic /-sis″tik/, pertaining to a fibrocyst or cystic fibroma.

fibrocystic disease of the breast /-sis″tik/ [L, *fibra* + Gk, *kystis,* bag], the presence of single or multiple cysts that are palpable in the breasts. The cysts are benign and fairly common, yet must be considered potentially malignant and observed carefully for growth or change. The client may report unilateral or bilateral breast pain and tenderness that frequently begin 7 to 10 days before menses and resolve as the menses progresses. The cysts can be aspirated and a biopsy performed. In most cases no treatment is required. Decreasing caffeine in the diet and taking supplemental vitamin E have been effective in helping to alleviate breast tenderness. Women should be taught how to perform frequent breast examinations. A woman is shown any cysts present and is taught palpation, and the importance of any change is emphasized. Reassurance should also be given that the condition is very common and generally not associated with cancer. Only about 5% of fibrocystic conditions could be considered a risk factor for later development of cancer. Also called **chronic cystic mastitis.** See also **cystic fibrosis.**

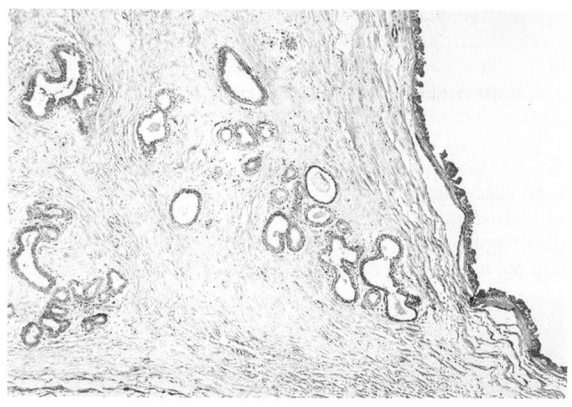

Fibrocystic disease of the breast *(Kumar et al, 2007)*

fibrocystic disease of the pancreas.   See **cystic fibrosis.**

fibrocyte.   See **fibroblast.**

fibrodysplasia ossificans progressiva.   See **myositis ossificans progressiva.**

fibroelastic membrane of larynx, a membrane linking the laryngeal cartilages that is composed of a lower cricothyroid ligament and an upper quadrangular ligament.

fibroelastic tissue.   See **fibrous tissue.**

fibroepithelial papilloma /-ep′ithē″lē·əl/ [L, *fibra* + Gk, *epi,* above, *thele,* nipple; L, *papilla,* nipple; Gk, *oma,* tumor], a benign epithelial tumor containing extensive fibrous tissue. Also called **fibropapilloma.**

fibroepithelial polyp.   See **acrochordon.**

fibroepithelioma /fī′brō·ep′ithē′lē·ō″mə/ *pl. fibroepitheliomas, fibroepitheliomata* [L, *fibra* + Gk, *epi,* above, *thele,* nipple, *oma,* tumor], a neoplasm consisting of fibrous and epithelial components.

fibrofolliculoma /-folik′yəlō″mə/, a benign tumor derived from the dermal part of a hair follicle. It may appear as a dome-shaped yellowish papule on the skin, accompanied by strands of follicular epithelium.

fibrogenous.   See **fibrinogenous.**

fibrogliosis /-glī·ō″sis/, the formation of scar tissue in the brain in reaction to a penetrating injury. The scar is produced by fibroblasts and astrocytes, a type of glial cell.

fibroid /fī″broid/ [L, *fibra* + Gk, *eidos,* form], **1.** having fibers. **2.** *(Informal)* a fibroma or myoma, particularly of the uterus.

fibroidectomy /fī′broidek″təmē/ [L, *fibra,* fiber; Gk, *eidos,* form, *ektomē,* excision], the surgical removal of a fibrous tumor, such as a uterine fibromyoma.

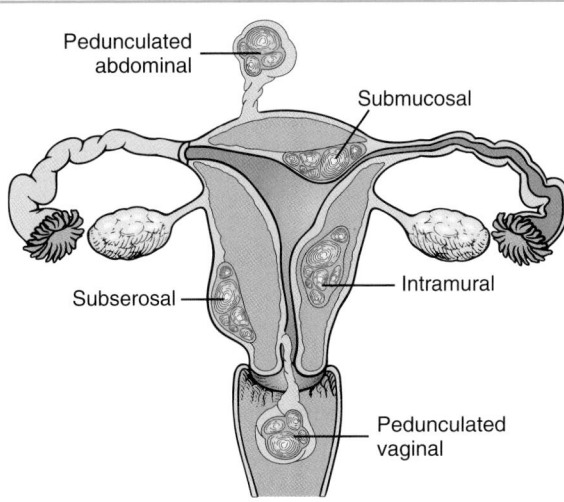

Common locations of fibroids *(Damjanov, 2012)*

fibroid tumor.   See **fibroma.**

fibrolipoma /fī′brōlipō″mə/,   a fibrous tumor that also contains fatty material. Also called **lipofibroma.**

fibroma /fībrō″mə/ *pl. fibromas, fibromata*   [L, *fibra* + Gk, *oma,* tumor],   a benign neoplasm consisting largely of fibrous or fully developed connective tissue.

fibroma cavernosum,   a tumor that contains large vascular spaces, an excessive amount of fibrous tissue, and blood or lymph vessels.

fibroma cutis,   a fibrous tumor of the skin.

fibroma durum.   See **hard fibroma.**

fibroma molle.   See **soft fibroma.**

fibroma mucinosum,   a fibrous tumor in which degenerating mucoid material is present.

fibroma myxomatodes.   See **myxofibroma.**

fibroma of the breast [L, *fibra,* fiber; Gk, *oma,* tumor; AS, *braest*],   a tumor of the breast, usually benign and composed of connective tissue. See also **fibroma.**

fibroma pendulum,   a pendulous fibrous tumor of the skin.

fibroma sarcomatosum.   See **fibrosarcoma.**

fibromata.   See **fibroma.**

fibroma thecocellulare xanthomatodes.   See **theca cell tumor.**

fibromatosis /-mətō″sis/   [L, *fibra* + Gk, *oma,* tumor, *osis,* condition],   **1.** a gingival enlargement believed to be hereditary or idiopathic, manifested in the secondary dentition. It is characterized by a firm hyperplastic tissue that covers the surfaces of the teeth. Differentiation between this condition and phenytoin hyperplasia is based on a history of phenytoin ingestion. The gums consist of fibrous lesions that demonstrate an infiltrative growth pattern and aggressive clinical behavior. Histologically, it presents as dense hypocellular and hypovascular collagenous tissue, which forms interlacing bundles running in all directions. See also **gingival hyperplasia. 2.** a benign tumor of soft tissue. Should not be confused with **neurofibromatosis.**

fibromuscular dysplasia (FMD) /-mus″kyələr/,   an arterial disorder sometimes associated with strokes or transient ischemic attacks (TIAs). The condition, which may appear as either fibromuscular hyperplasia or perimuscular fibrosis, is characterized by intraluminal folds of fibrous endothelial tissue. They appear as vertical bars on angiography and become the originating site of platelet adherence aggregation and thrombus formation. The condition commonly involves the renal arteries and is associated with hypertension.

fibromyalgia,   a form of nonarticular rheumatism characterized by musculoskeletal pain, spasms, stiffness, fatigue, and severe sleep disturbance. Common sites of pain or stiffness include the lower back, neck, shoulder region, arms, hands, knees, hips, thighs, legs, and feet. These sites are known as trigger points. Physical therapy, nonsteroidal antiinflammatory drugs, and muscle relaxants provide temporary relief. Also called **fibrositis, soft tissue rheumatism.**

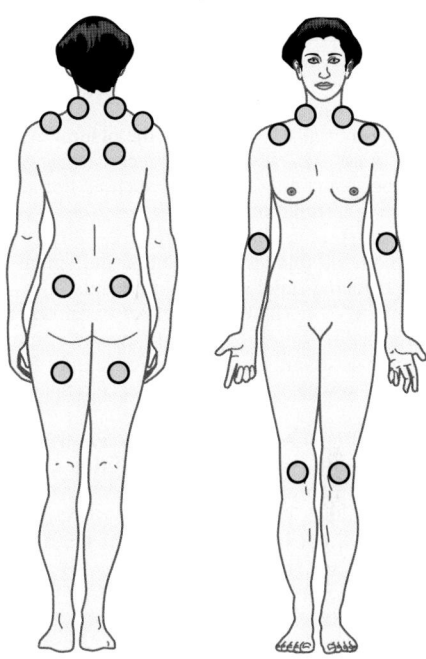

Fibromyalgia tender points *(Young-Adams and Proctor, 2011)*

fibromyoma uteri.   See **leiomyoma uteri.**

fibromyomectomy /fī′brōmī′ōmek″təmē/,   a surgical procedure for removing a uterine fibroma or other type of fibromyoma.

fibromyositis /fī′brōmī′əsī″tis/   [L, *fibra* + Gk, *mys,* muscle, *itis,* inflammation],   any one of a large number of disorders characterized by stiffness and joint or muscle pain, accompanied by localized inflammation of muscle and fibrous connective tissues. The condition may develop after climatic change, infection, or physical or emotional trauma. It may recur and become chronic. Treatment includes rest, heat, massage, salicylates, and, in severe cases, intraarticular injections of a corticosteroid and procaine. Kinds include **lumbago, pleurodynia, torticollis.** See also **rheumatism.**

fibropapilloma.   See **fibroepithelial papilloma.**

fibroplasia /-plā″zhə/,   the formation of a scar during the fibroblastic repair phase of healing.

fibrosarcoma /-särkō″mə/ *pl. fibrosarcomas, fibrosarcomata*   [L, *fibra* + Gk, *sarx,* flesh, *oma,* tumor],   a sarcoma that contains fibrous connective tissue.

fibrosing alveolitis /fī′brōsing/   [L, *fibra* + *alviolus,* small hollow; Gk, *itis,* inflammation],   a severe form of alveolitis characterized by dyspnea and hypoxia. It occurs in advanced rheumatoid arthritis and other autoimmune diseases. X-ray films show thickening of the alveolar septa and diffuse pulmonary infiltrates. See also **alveolitis.**

fibrosis /fībrō″sis/   [L, *fibra* + Gk, *osis,* condition],   **1.** a proliferation of fibrous connective tissue that occurs normally in the formation of scar tissue to replace tissue lost through injury or infection. **2.** an abnormal condition in which fibrous connective tissue spreads over or replaces normal smooth muscle or other normal organ tissue. Fibrosis is most common in the heart, lung, peritoneum, and kidney. See also **cystic fibrosis, fibromyalgia.**

fibrosis of the lungs [L, *fibra* + Gk, *osis,* condition; AS, *lungen*], the formation of scar tissue in the connective tissue of the lungs as a sequel to any inflammation or irritation caused by tuberculosis, bronchopneumonia, or a pneumoconiosis. Localized fibrosis may be complicated by infarction, abscess, or bronchiectasis. Also called **pulmonary fibrosis.**

fibrositis. See **fibromyalgia.**

fibrothorax /-thôr″aks/, fibrosis of the pleural membranes.

fibrous /fī″brəs/ [L, *fibra,* fiber], consisting mainly of fibers or fiber-containing materials, such as fibrous connective tissue. See also **fibrosis.**

fibrous astrocyte, a glial cell with long, fibrous processes found in the white matter of the brain and spinal cord. Its cytoplasm contains bundles of glial filaments.

fibrous capsule, 1. the external layer of an articular capsule. It surrounds the articulation of two adjoining bones. **2.** the external, tough membranous envelope surrounding some visceral organs, such as the liver. Compare **synovial membrane.**

fibrous connective tissue. See **connective tissue.**

fibrous dysplasia, an abnormal condition characterized by the fibrous displacement of the osseous tissue within the bones affected. The specific cause of fibrous dysplasia is unknown, but indications are that the disease is of developmental or congenital origin. The distinct kinds of fibrous dysplasia are monostotic fibrous dysplasia, polyostotic fibrous dysplasia, and polyostotic fibrous dysplasia with associated endocrine disorders. Any bone may be affected with monostotic fibrous dysplasia. The polyostotic type usually displays a segmental distribution of the involved bones, all of which show varying degrees of the characteristic fibrous replacement of the osseous tissue. The onset of fibrous dysplasia is usually during childhood, and the disorder progresses beyond puberty and through adulthood. The onset of symptoms is usually during childhood, although diagnosis may be delayed until adolescence or even early adulthood if symptoms are minimal. The initial signs may be a limp, a pain, or a fracture on the affected side. Girls affected may have an early onset of menses and breast development and early epiphyseal closure. Albright's syndrome is usually diagnosed on the basis of a triad of symptoms, including the polyostotic type of fibrous dysplasia, café-au-lait patches on the skin, and precocious puberty. Pathological fractures are frequently associated with this process, and angulation deformities may follow. The involved extremity may be shortened, and the classic "shepherd's crook" deformity is common. Radiographic examination usually reveals a well-circumscribed lesion occupying all or a portion of the shaft of the long bone involved. Pathological fractures in patients with fibrous dysplasia usually heal with conservative treatment, but residual deformities often remain. When symptoms are mild and limited, this disease usually progresses slowly. Radiation therapy is not used because it may provoke malignant degeneration. Biopsies are commonly performed if pain increases or if alterations are seen on radiographic examination.

fibrous goiter, an enlargement of the thyroid gland, characterized by hyperplasia of the capsule and connective tissue.

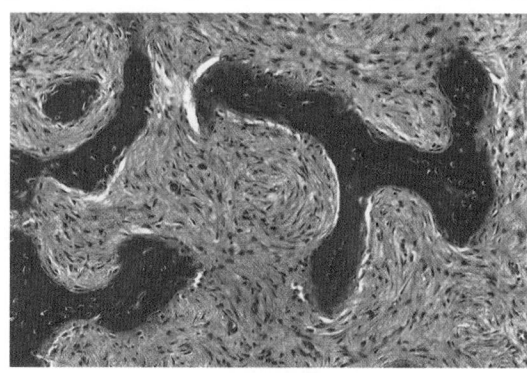

Fibrous dysplasia *(Fletcher, 2007)*

fibrous hamartoma of infancy, a benign, nonencapsulated tumor, sometimes present at birth but usually appearing during the first year of life, most frequently in the shoulder, axilla, or upper arm. It is a firm, painless, skin-colored nodule composed of well-defined fibrous trabeculae, immature mesenchymal tissue, and mature adipose cells; invasion of the surrounding subcutaneous tissue frequently occurs.

fibrous histiocytoma. See **dermatofibroma.**

fibrous joint, any one of many slightly movable joints, such as those of the skull segments, in which a fibrous tissue or sometimes a form of cartilage connects the bones. The three kinds of articulation associated with fibrous joints are syndesmosis, sutura, and gomphosis. Also called **junctura fibrosa, synarthrosis.** Compare **cartilaginous joint, synovial joint.**

fibrous thyroiditis, a rare disorder characterized by slowly progressive fibrosis of an enlarged thyroid, with replacement of normal thyroid tissue by dense fibrous tissue. The gland eventually becomes fixed to the adjacent muscles, nerves, blood vessels, and trachea by means of this fibrous tissue. The disease occurs more frequently in women than in men and usually arises after 40 years of age. Obstructive symptoms are uncommon but can include a choking sensation, dyspnea, and dysphagia. Hypothyroidism may occur, but in most patients the gland functions normally. Treatment includes surgical excision and thyroid hormone administered postoperatively, as required. Also called **ligneous thyroiditis, Riedel's struma, Riedel's thyroiditis.**

fibrous tissue, the connective tissue of the body, consisting of closely woven elastic fibers and fluid-filled areolae. Also called **fibroelastic tissue.** Compare **areolar tissue.** See also **connective tissue.**

fibrous trigone, a thickened area of tissue between the aortic ring and the atrioventricular ring. The right fibrous trigone is between the aortic ring and the right atrioventricular ring. The left fibrous trigone is between the aortic ring and the left atrioventricular ring.

fibrovascular proliferation /-vas″kyələr/, the growth of new blood vessels and fibrous tissues on the surface of the retina and optic nerve in diabetic retinopathy. The growths can vary from barely visible vessels to dense sheets of avascular fibrous tissue.

fibula /fib″yələ/ [L, buckle], one of the two bones of the lower leg, lateral to and smaller in diameter than the tibia. In proportion to its length, it is the most slender of the long bones and presents three borders and three surfaces for attaching various muscles, including the peronei longus and brevis and the soleus longus. Also called **calf bone.**

fibular /fib″yələr/ [L, *fibula,* clasp], pertaining to the fibula.

fibular collum, neck of fibula; the portion of the fibula between the head and shaft.

fibularis brevis, a muscle that assists in eversion of the foot. It is innervated by the superficial fibular nerve.

fibularis longus, a muscle that everts and plantarflexes the foot and helps to support the arches of the foot, mainly the lateral and transverse arches. It is innervated by the superficial fibular nerve.

fibularis tertius, a part of the extensor digitorum longus that assists in dorsiflexion and possibly eversion of the foot. It is innervated by the deep fibular nerve.

fibular notch, a depression on the lateral surface of the lower end of the tibia, which articulates with the lower end of the fibula.

Fick's law [Adolf E. Fick, German physiologist, 1829–1901], **1.** (in chemistry and physics) an observed law stating that the rate at which one substance diffuses through another is directly proportional to the concentration gradient of the diffusing substance. **2.** (in medicine) an observed law stating that the rate of diffusion across a membrane is directly proportional to the concentration gradient of the substance on the two sides of the membrane and inversely related to the thickness of the membrane.

Fick principle, a method for making indirect measurements, based on the law of conservation of mass. It is used specifically to determine cardiac output, in which the amount of oxygen uptake of each unit of blood as it passes through the lungs is equal to the oxygen concentration difference between arterial and mixed venous blood. Cardiac output is calculated by measuring the uptake of oxygen for a given period, noted as milliliters per minute, then dividing that ratio by the difference in oxygen saturation of arterial and mixed venous blood samples in milliliters per 100 mL of blood and multiplying the total by 100.

F.I.C.S., abbreviation for *Fellow of the International College of Surgeons.*

fictive kin /fik″tiv/, people who are regarded as being part of a family even though they are not related by either blood or marriage bonds. Fictive kinship may bind people together in ties of affection, concern, obligation, and responsibility.

FID, abbreviation for **free-induction decay.**

fidelity, (for health or related reasons) the quality or state of being faithful; for health professionals, this may involve the commitment to follow through on proposals and to keep promises to coworkers, clients, and organizations.

field [AS, *feld*], **1.** a defined space, area, or distance. The field of vision represents the total area that can be seen with one fixed eye. The binocular field is the area that can be seen with both eyes. **2.** an area within a computer record where a specified type of data is stored.

field fever, a form of leptospirosis caused by *Leptospira grippotyphosa,* which primarily affects agricultural workers. It is characterized by fever, abdominal pain, diarrhea, vomiting, stupor, and conjunctivitis. Also called *canefield fever,* **harvest fever, mild fever, 7-day fever.** See also **leptospirosis.**

field of vision [AS, *feld* + L, *visio,* seeing], the area of space in which objects are visible at the same time when the eye is fixed and the face is turned so as to exclude the limiting effects of the orbital margins and nose.

fiery serpent. See *Dracunculus medinensis,* **dracunculiasis.**

fièvre boutonneuse. See **African tick typhus.**

fifth cranial nerve. See **trigeminal nerve.**

fifth disease. See **erythema infectiosum.**

fight-or-flight. See **flight-or-fight reaction.**

FIGLU, abbreviation for **formiminoglutamic acid.**

FIGO staging system, a classification system for cancers of the uterine cervix established by the French Fédération Internationale de Gynécologie et d'Obstétrique. Tumors are classified by Roman numerals from I to IV, representing a range from precancerous or in situ to highly malignant. Classification subdivisions are represented by letters and numbers.

figure-eight bandage, a bandage with successive laps crossing over and around each other to resemble the numeric figure eight. See also **bandage.**

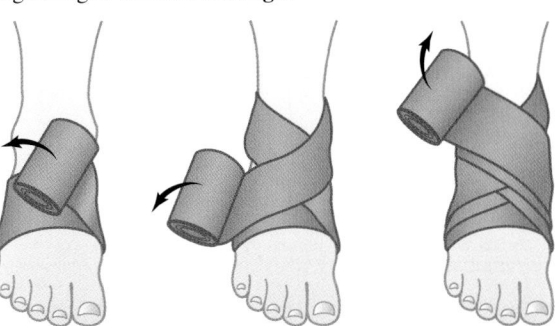

Figure-eight bandage *(Bonewit-West, 2015)*

figure-eight suture [L, *sutura*], a suture that begins at the deepest layer on each side of a wound, then crosses over to pass through the superficial layers on the opposite side before being tied.

figure-four test. See **Patrick test.**

figure-ground relationship /fig″(y)ər/ [L, *figura,* form; AS, *grund* + L, *relatus,* carry back], a perceptual field that is divided into a figure, which is the object of focus, and a diffuse background. See also **ground.**

fila-, prefix meaning "thread" or "threadlike": *filamentous, Filaria.*

filament /fil′əmənt/ [L, *filare,* to spin], a fine threadlike fiber. Filaments are found in most tissues and cells of the body and serve various morphological or physiological functions.

filamentous /fil′əmen″təs/ [L, *filare,* to spin], pertaining to something that is threadlike or capable of being drawn out into a threadlike structure.

Filaria /filarē·ə/ *pl. filariae* [L, *filum,* thread], a genus of slender nematodes of the superfamily Filarioidea. There are many species, some of which are parasitic in animals.

filariasis /fil′ərī″əsis/ [L, *filum,* thread; Gk, *osis,* condition], a disease caused by the presence of filariae or microfilariae in body tissues. Filarial worms are round, long, and threadlike and are common in most tropic and subtropic regions. They tend to infest the lymph nodes, lymphatics, subcutaneous tissues, and skin after entering the body as microscopic larvae through the bite of a mosquito, blackfly, or midge. The infection is characterized by occlusion of the lymphatic vessels, with swelling and pain of the limb distal to the blockage. After many years the limb may become greatly swollen and the skin coarse and tough. Treatment is by oral administration of diethylcarbamazine, ivermectin, albendazole, or mebendazole. Apheresis, antihistamines, and corticosteroid therapy may be performed before the administration of antihelmenthic agents to reduce the risk of reaction associated with heavy worm burden. The most effective means of preventing infestation is flying insect control. See also **elephantiasis,** *Loa loa, Mansonella,* **onchocerciasis,** *Wuchereria.*

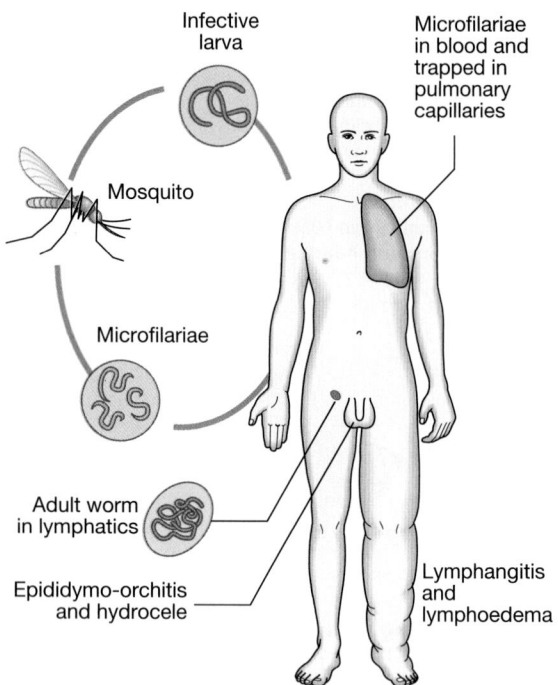

Life cycle of lymphatic filariasis *(Walker et al, 2014)*

filariform /filer″ifôrm/,   pertaining to a structure or organism that is threadlike.

Filarioidea /filar′ē·oi′dē·ə/   [L, *filum*, thread + Gk, *eidos*, form],   the filariae, a superfamily or order of nematode parasites, the adults being threadlike worms that invade the tissues and body cavities where the female deposits embryonated eggs (prelarvae) known as microfilariae. These microfilariae are ingested by blood-sucking insects in whom they pass their developmental stage and are returned to humans when the insects bite. Genera infecting humans include *Brugia, Loa, Mansonella, Onchocerca,* and *Wuchereria.*

file,   **1.** (in dentistry) a tool for scaling or removing plaque and calcified deposits from the teeth, or in the preparation of the root canal during endodontic therapy. **2.** a collection of related data or information, assembled for a specified purpose and stored as a unit.

filial generation /fil″ē·əl/   [L, *filius*, son, *generare*, to beget],   the offspring produced from a given mating or cross. See also **first filial generation, second filial generation.**

filiform bougie /fil″ifôrm/   [L, *filum*, thread, *forma*, form; Fr, *bougie*, candle],   an extremely thin device for passage through a narrow pathway, such as a sinus tract. See also **bougie.**

filiform catheter,   a catheter with a slender, threadlike tip that allows the wider portion of the instrument to be passed through canals that are constricted or irregular because of an obstruction or an angulation in the canal. It may bypass obstructions or dilate strictures.

filiform papilla.   See **papilla.**

filiform warts.   See **digitate wart.**

filling,   a dental restoration consisting of a silver amalgam, composite, glass ionomer, porcelain, gold, or other material that is inserted into a prepared tooth cavity to repair a carious lesion.

filling factor [AS, *fyllan*, filling; L, *factor*, a maker],   a measure of the geometric relationship between a magnetic resonance (MR) imaging coil and the body. This relationship affects the MR signal-to-noise ratio and, ultimately, image quality. Achieving a high filling factor requires fitting the coil closely to the body, thus potentially decreasing patient comfort.

filling pressure.   See **end-diastolic pressure.**

film [AS, *filmen*, membrane],   **1.** a thin sheet or layer of any material, such as a coating of oil on a metal part. **2.** (in photography and radiography) a thin, flexible transparent sheet of cellulose acetate or polyester plastic material coated with a light-sensitive emulsion, used to record images, such as organs, structures, and tissues, that may be involved in disease and diagnosis.

film badge dosimeter,   a photographic film packet, sensitive to ionizing radiation, used for estimating the exposure of personnel working with x-rays and other radioactive sources; film badge dosimeters have been largely replaced by thermoluminescent dosimeters. See **thermoluminescent dosimetry.**

film development,   the processing of photographic or x-ray films to manifest the latent image resulting from exposure of the chemically treated emulsion to electromagnetic radiation. Development involves wetting the film to loosen the emulsion, followed by a series of chemical baths that reduce the exposed silver ions to black metallic silver. The reducing agents for radiographic films generally contain hydroquinone to produce black tones slowly and phenidone to produce shades of gray rapidly.

film fault,   a defect in a photograph or radiograph, usually caused by a chemical, physical, or electrical error in its production. See also **artifact.**

film screen mammography,   a breast radiographic technique in which a special single-emulsion film and high-detail intensifying screens are used. The technique provides a fine detail image at radiation exposure levels of less than 1 rad, compared with older methods that generated radiation levels of as much as 16 rad. Film screen mammography has largely been replaced by digital mammography.

filopressure,   the temporary compression of a blood vessel by a ligature. The ligature is removed when the blood flow has stopped.

Filovirus,   a genus of single-stranded negative-sense ribonucleic acid viruses in the Filoviridae family that targets primates and causes hemorrhagic fevers. It is one of the most destructive viruses known to man. The genus includes the Ebola and Marburg viruses.

filter [Fr, *filtrer*, to strain],   **1.** a device or material through which a gas or liquid is passed to separate out unwanted matter. **2.** (in radiology) a device added to radiographic equipment that selectively removes low-energy x-rays that have no chance of reaching the image receptor. Examples include bow-tie, compensating, and conic filters.

filtered back projection,   a mathematical technique used in magnetic resonance imaging and computed tomography to create images from a set of multiple projection profiles.

filtration /filtrā″shən/   [Fr, *filtrer*, to strain],   the addition of sheets of metal to a beam of x-rays for the purpose of altering the energy spectrum and thus the imaging characteristics and penetrating ability of the radiation. Filtration is generally accomplished with aluminum or copper at low to medium energy and with tin, copper, or aluminum at higher energy.

filtration angle.   See **angle of iris.**

filum /fī″ləm/,   a threadlike structure, as the filum terminale, which extends from the lower end of the spinal cord.

fimbria /fim″brē·ə/   [L, *fringe*],   any structure that forms a border or edge or that resembles a fringe. Kinds include **fimbria hippocampi, fimbria ovarica,** *fimbriae tubae terminale (spinal cord).* See also **pilus,** def. 2.

fimbriae of uterine tube, the branched fingerlike projections at the distal end of each of the fallopian tubes. The projections are connected to the ovary and have epithelial cells with cilia that serve to move the ovum toward the uterus. Also called *fimbriae tubae.*

fimbria hippocampi, a band of efferent fibers in the brain formed by the alveus hippocampi that is continuous with the posterior pillar of the fornix.

fimbrial tubal pregnancy /fim″brē-əl/, an ectopic tubal pregnancy in which implantation occurs in the fimbriated distal end of a fallopian tube. See also **tubal pregnancy, ectopic pregnancy.**

fimbria ovarica, the longest of the fimbriae tubae. It extends from the infundibulum to the ovary. Also called **fimbriated extremity.**

fimbriated /fim″brē-ā′tid/ [L, *fimbria,* a fringe], having fimbria, or the fringelike projection of the ovaries or the nerve fibers along the border of the hippocampus.

fimbriated extremity. See **fimbria ovarica.**

fimbriated fold, a rough fold lateral to the lingual vein on either side of the frenulum of the tongue.

finasteride /fin″əstərīd, finas″tərīd/, a drug used to treat benign prostatic hyperplasia by blocking the production of dihydrotestosterone, a major hormone stimulating prostate growth. It is also used as a hair growth stimulant in the treatment of androgenetic alopecia. It is administered orally.

finding, **1.** an observation made about a particular disease state, usually in relation to physical examination and laboratory tests. **2.** a conclusion drawn from an examination, study, or experiment.

fine motor skills [Fr, *fin,* thin; L, *movere* + ONor, *skilja,* to cut apart], the use of precise coordinated movements in such activities as writing, buttoning, cutting, tracing, or visual tracking.

fine-needle aspiration, a diagnostic technique that uses a very thin needle and gentle suction to obtain tissue samples, most commonly used for breast and thyroid biopsies. The needle is thinner than that used for venipuncture, and the procedure is less painful than drawing of blood. Usually the procedure is done on an outpatient basis, and no anesthetic is used. The aspirated tissue is examined by a pathologist.

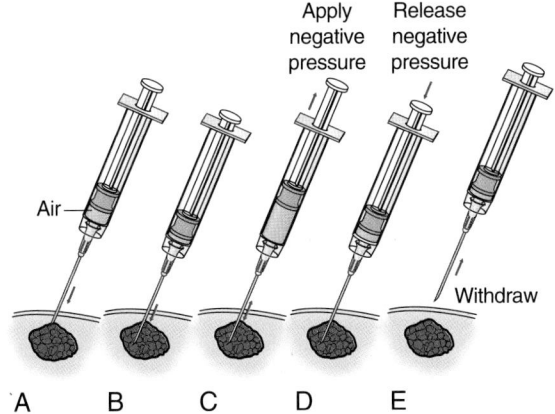

Fine-needle aspiration *(Pfenninger, 2011)*

fineness /fīn″nes/ [Fr, *fin,* thin], a means of grading alloys in relation to their gold content. The fineness of an alloy is designated in parts per thousand of pure gold, which is 1000 fine. Gold alloys and pure gold may be used in dental restorations, such as tooth crowns and prepared tooth-cavity fillings.

fine tremor [Fr, *fin,* thin; L, *tremor,* to tremble], a vibration that occurs after a voluntary movement or one that results from fatigue in the corresponding muscle group.

finger [AS, *fingar*], any of the digits of the hand. The fingers are composed of three bony phalanges. Some anatomists regard the thumb as a finger, since its metacarpal bone ossifies in the same way as a phalanx. Other anatomists regard the thumb as being composed of a metacarpal bone and two phalanges. The digits of the hand are anatomically numbered 1 to 5, starting with the thumb. See also **nail,** def. 1.

finger agnosia, a neurological disorder in which a patient is unable to distinguish between stimuli applied to two different fingers without visual clues; to recognize his or her own digits, for example, finger versus thumb; or to recognize or identify another person's fingers. It is seen most often in Gerstmann syndrome. See also **Gerstmann syndrome.**

finger goniometer [AS, *finger* + Gk, *gonia,* angle, *metron,* meter], an instrument for measuring the angle of a finger joint.

finger-nose test [AS, *finger* + *nosu* + L, *testum,* crucible], a test of the coordination of the arms. The patient is asked to draw the tip of the index finger quickly to the nose, then to touch the examiner's finger, and then to go back and forth quickly. An inability to perform the test accurately may be an indication of cerebellar disease.

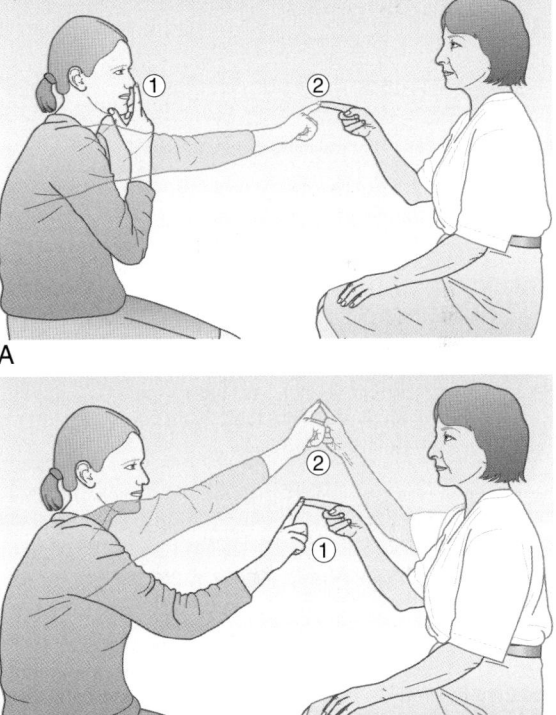

Finger-nose test *(Douglas et al, 2013)*

finger percussion. See **percussion.**

finger phenomenon, a diagnostic test for organic hemiplegia. With the patient's elbow on the table, the examiner grasps the patient's wrist and uses the thumb to put pressure on the radial side of the patient's pisiform bone. If the hemiplegia is organic, the patient's fingers spread fanwise.

fingerprint, an image left on a smooth surface by the pattern of the pad of a distal phalanx. The distinctive pattern of loops and whorls represents the fine ridges marking the skin. Because each individual's fingerprints are unique, a classification system of the patterns is useful in identifying individuals.

finger pulse therapy, a form of biofeedback therapy in which a sensor attached to the finger monitors cardiac activity. It is used in the treatment of anxiety, hypertension, and some cardiac arrhythmias.

finger stick, the act of puncturing the tip of the finger to obtain a small sample of capillary blood. In some procedures the hand may be first immersed in warm water for 10 minutes to "arterialize" the capillary blood or give it characteristics similar to those of arterial blood.

finger sweep, a technique for clearing a mechanical obstruction from the upper airway of an unconscious patient. The rescuer opens the victim's mouth by grasping the lower jaw and tongue between the thumb and fingers. The rescuer then attempts to sweep the foreign object out of the victim's mouth with a finger. Care must be taken to visualize the object before performing a finger sweep as the object can be pushed deeper into the airway.

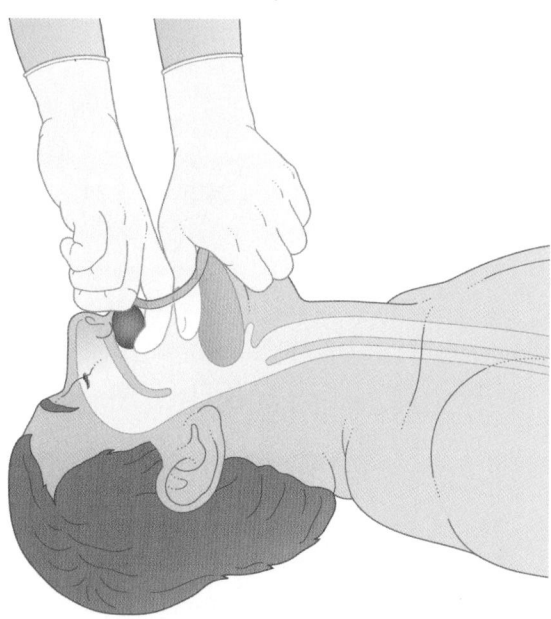

Finger sweep *(Stein et al, 2013)*

Finnish bath. See **sauna bath.**

FiO₂, abbreviation for **fraction of inspired oxygen.**

Fiorinal, a group of fixed-combination drugs containing a sedative-hypnotic; an analgesic, antipyretic, and antiinflammatory; and a central nervous system stimulant. Brand name for *butalbital,* **aspirin, caffeine.**

fire ant sting, a potentially lethal venomous injection of piperidine alkaloids by a fire ant. The ant attaches itself to the skin with its mandibles and injects venom through a stinger in the posterior part of its abdomen. The ant injects repeatedly as it rotates its body around the attachment site. All victims experience a local wheal and flare reaction that lasts up to an hour, followed by formation of a sterile pustule. The pustule sloughs off after about 48 hours but is followed by itching that may last for days. Fire ant stings are a common cause of anaphylaxis in the southern United States.

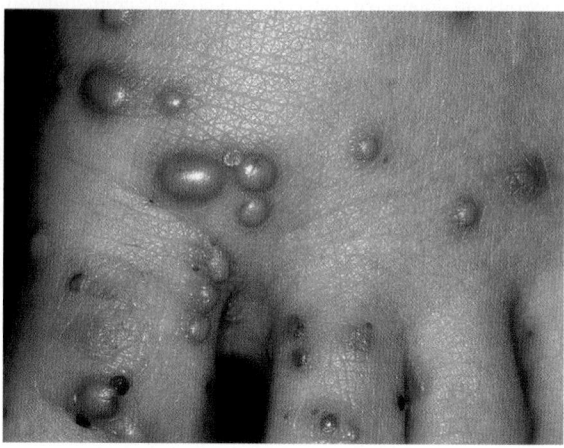

Pustules at the site of fire ant stings *(James et al, 2016)*

fire damp. See **damp.**

fireman's cramp. See **heat cramp.**

first aid [AS, *fyrst* + Fr, *aider,* to help], the immediate care that is given to an injured or ill person before treatment by medically trained personnel. Attention is directed first to the most critical problems: evaluation of the patency of the airway, the presence of bleeding, and the adequacy of cardiac function. The patient is kept warm and as comfortable as possible. The conscious patient is reassured and queried for significant details of his or her medical history, such as diabetes, a known heart condition, or allergic reactions to drugs. If the patient is unconscious, a medical identification card, bracelet, or necklace is sought. The patient is moved as little as possible, particularly if there is a possibility of fracture. If vomiting occurs, the patient's head is moved to a position for the vomitus to exit easily to prevent aspiration. See also **cardiopulmonary resuscitation, control of hemorrhage, emergency medicine, emergency nursing.**

first cranial nerve. See **olfactory nerve.**

first cuneiform. See **medial cuneiform bone.**

first-degree burn, a burn that affects the epidermis only, causing erythema and, in some cases, mild edema, without vesiculation.

first dentition. See **primary dentition.**

first-dollar coverage, an insurance plan under which the third-party payer assumes liability for covered services as soon as the first dollar of expense for such services is incurred, without requiring the insured to pay a deductible.

first filial generation (F₁), the heterozygous offspring produced by the crossing of a homozygous dominant strain with a homozygous recessive strain.

first-generation scanner, an early type of computed tomography device that used a finely collimated (pencil) x-ray beam and a single detector moving in a translate-rotate mode. It required 180 translations, each separated by a 1-degree rotation, and up to 5 minutes for one image.

first intention. See **intention.**

first-line therapy. See **induction therapy.**

first metacarpal bone, the metacarpal bone of the thumb.

first-order change, a change within a system that itself remains unchanged.

first-order kinetics, a chemical reaction in which the rate of decrease in the number of molecules of a substrate is proportional to the concentration of substrate molecules remaining. In first-order reactions involving two substances, only one of the concentrations affects the rate. The rate of metabolism of most drugs follows the rule of first-order kinetics and is independent of the dose. Also called *first-order reaction.* See also **kinetics.**

first responder, the first emergency person to arrive at the scene of a traumatic or medical situation. This person is trained according to a national standard curriculum set up by the U.S. Department of Transportation.

first rib, the highest rib of the thoracic cage. It moves about the axis of its neck, raising and lowering the sternum. First rib movement during quiet breathing is negligible, but under conditions of stress it can increase the anteroposterior diameter of the chest.

first stage of labor [ME, *fyrst* + OFr, *estage* + L, *labor,* work], the interval from the start of labor until full cervical dilation (10 cm). It is divided into two phases. The first phase is the latent phase, encompassing early effacement and dilation. Second is the active phase, when more rapid dilation occurs, usually beginning at approximately 4 cm dilation.

first-trimester abortion, the termination of a pregnancy prior to 12 completed weeks of gestation. See also **elective abortion, therapeutic abortion.**

FISH, abbreviation for **fluorescent in situ hybridization.**

Fishberg concentration test /fish′berg/, a test for renal function. The patient is given supper with not more than 200 mL of fluid and nothing thereafter. Urine voided during the night is discarded. The morning urine is saved, the patient is kept in bed, and the urine of 1 hour later and of 2 hours later is saved. If the specific gravity of any of these three specimens is less than 1.024, there is impairment of renal concentration.

fish-handler's disease. See **erysipeloid.**

fish poisoning, poisoning caused by ingestion of poisonous fish, some of which have the poison in their muscles, skin, or other organs, while others secrete poisons. It is marked by various gastrointestinal and neurological disturbances that sometimes can be fatal. Kinds include **ciguatera poisoning, tetraodon poisoning.**

fish skin disease. See **ichthyosis.**

fish tapeworm infection [AS, *fisc,* fish], an infection caused by the tapeworm *Diphyllobothrium latum* that is transmitted to humans when they eat contaminated raw or undercooked freshwater fish. Fish tapeworm infection is common in temperate zones throughout the world and is found in the Great Lakes region of the United States and Alaska. Endemic foci have been found among Eskimos in Alaska and Canada. Most infections are asymptomatic. However, persons may exhibit abdominal discomfort, vomiting, diarrhea, weight loss, and vitamin B_{12} deficiency. Treatment is praziquantel and vitamin B_{12}, if indicated, for deficiency. In severe cases intestinal obstruction may result. Also called **diphyllobothriasis.** See also *Diphyllobothrium,* **tapeworm infection.**

fiss-, prefix meaning "split" or "cleft": *fission, fissiparous, fissure.*

fission /fish″ən/ [L, *fissio,* splitting], **1.** the act or process of splitting or breaking up into two or more parts. **2.** a type of asexual reproduction common in bacteria, protozoa, and other simpler forms of life in which the cell divides into two or more equal components, each of which eventually develops into a complete organism. Kinds include **binary fission, multiple fission. 3.** (in physics) the splitting of the nucleus of an atom and subsequent release of energy. Also called **nuclear fission.**

fissiparous /fisip″ərəs/, reproduced by fission.

fissura. See **fissure.**

fissural angioma /fish′ərəl/ [L, *fissura,* cleft], a tumor composed of a cluster of dilated blood vessels found on the lip, face, or neck in an embryonal fissure.

fissure /fish″ər/ [L, *fissura,* cleft], **1.** a cleft or groove on the surface of an organ, often marking its division into parts, such as the lobes of the lung. **2.** a cracklike lesion of the skin, such as an anal fissure. **3.** a lineal fault on a bony surface that occurs during the development of a part, such as a fissure in the enamel of a tooth. A fissure is usually deeper than a sulcus, but in the terminology of anatomy *fissure* and *sulcus* are often used interchangeably. Also called **fissura.** –*fissured, adj.*

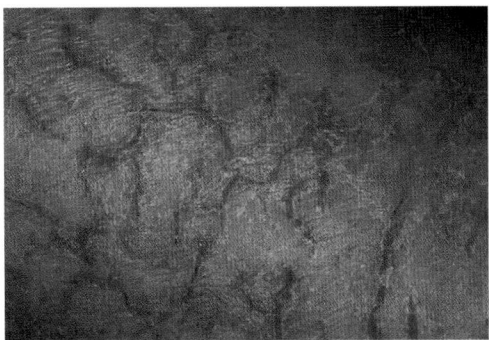

Fissures *(Lemmi and Lemmi, 2000)*

fissured tongue /fish″ərd/ [L, *fissura,* cleft; AS, *tunge*], a tongue with deep surface furrows that may radiate outward. The condition may be inherited as an autosomal-dominant trait.

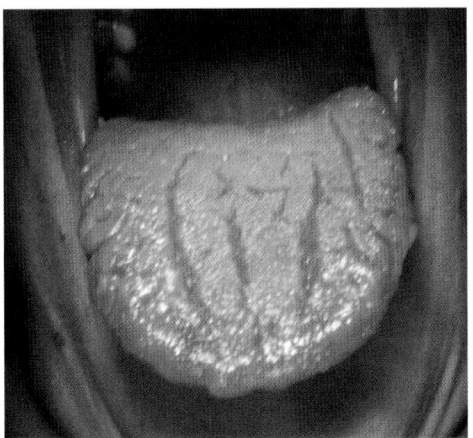

Fissured tongue *(Ibsen and Phelan, 2009)*

fissure fracture, any fracture in which a crack extends into the cortex of the bone but not through the entire bone. See also **greenstick fracture.**

fissure-in-ano. See **anal fissure.**

fissure of Bichat. See **transverse fissure.**

fissure of Rolando. See **central sulcus.**

fissure of Sylvius. See **lateral cerebral sulcus.**

fistula /fis″choolə, -chələ/ *pl. fistulae, fistulas* [L, pipe], an abnormal passage from an internal organ to the body surface or between two internal organs, such as a hepatopleural or pulmonoperitoneal fistula. Fistulas may occur in many sites from the gingiva to the anus. They may be caused by a congenital defect, injury, infection, spreading of a malignant lesion, surgery, radiotherapy of a cancerous growth, or trauma during childbirth. They also may be created to achieve therapeutic purposes or obtain body secretions for physiological studies. An arteriovenous fistula is commonly created to gain access to the patient's bloodstream for hemodialysis. Anal fistulas that result from rupture or drainage of abscesses may be treated by fistulectomy or fistulotomy; fistulas between the vagina and bladder, urethra, ureter, or rectum may be repaired surgically, but the results are not always successful. –**fistulous,** *fistular, fistulate, adj.*

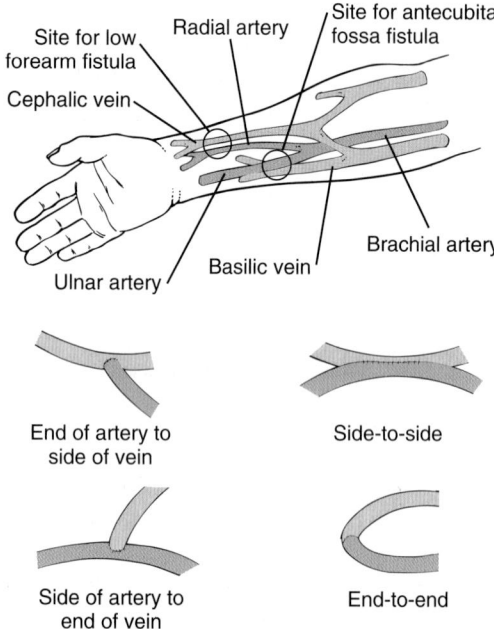

Arteriovenous fistula *(Miller-Keane and O'Toole, 1998)*

fistula-in-ano. See **anal fistula.**

fistular, fistulas, fistulate. See **fistula.**

fistulectomy /fis′chəlek″təmē/ [L, *fistula,* pipe; Gk, *ektomē,* excision], the surgical removal of a fistula.

fistulous. See **fistula.**

fit, **1.** *(Nontechnical)* a paroxysm or seizure. **2.** the sudden onset of an episode of symptoms, such as a fit of coughing. **3.** the manner in which one surface is aligned to another, such as the alignment of a denture with the gingiva and jaw.

Fitbit, an activity tracker designed to help an individual achieve better health by gaining an awareness of his or her exact level of daily activities.

fitness, a measure of the ability of a person to perform certain tasks. See also **physical fitness.**

fit testing, a protocol conducted by a clinical facility to ensure that a respirator fits an employee correctly and comfortably.

Fitzgerald factor. See **high-molecular-weight kininogen.**

Fitzgerald treatment. See **zone therapy.**

Fitz-Hugh–Curtis syndrome /fitz′-hyoō–kər′tis/ [Thomas Fitz-Hugh, Jr., American physician, 1894–1963; Arthur H. Curtis, American gynecologist, 1881–1955], perihepatitis occurring as a complication of gonorrhea or chlamydial infection in women, marked by fever, upper quadrant pain, tenderness and spasm of the abdominal wall, and

occasionally by friction rub over the liver. This syndrome is characterized by adhesions between the liver and other sites in the peritoneum. The treatment used is that appropriate to gonorrhea or chlamydia infection.

Fitzpatrick, Joyce J., a nursing theorist who derived her Life Perspective Rhythm Model from Martha Rogers' conceptualization of unitary man. She began publishing in 1970. Fitzpatrick proposes that the process of human development is characterized by rhythms that occur within the context of continuous person-environment interaction. Nursing activity focuses on enhancing the developmental process toward health. Fitzpatrick believes a central concern of nursing science and the nursing profession is the meaning attributed to life as the basic understanding of human existence. The four major concepts in this model are expressed as nursing, person, health, and environment. The person is viewed as a unified open rhythmic system with temporal patterns, consciousness patterns, and motion and perceptual patterns. Health is a human dimension under continuous development, interacting with the environment. It is seen as a heightened awareness of the meaningfulness of life. See also **Rogers, Martha E.**

5-day fever. See **trench fever.**

five elements, in Ayurvedic tradition, the basic entities (earth, air, fire, water, and space) whose interaction gives rise to material existence.

five-in-one repair, medial meniscectomy, medial collateral ligament repair, vastus medialis advancement, semitendinosus advancement, and pes anserinus transfer. See **Nicholas procedure.**

five phases, in traditional Chinese medicine, a set of dynamic relations (designated earth, metal, water, wood, and fire) that can be used to categorize relationships among phenomena. They are sometimes called the five elements because of their superficial resemblance to the elements of alchemy.

five-step nursing process, a nursing process comprising five broad categories of nursing behaviors: assessing, analyzing, planning, implementing, and evaluating. The nurse gathers information about the patient, identifies his or her specific needs, develops a plan of care with the patient to answer these needs, implements the plan of care, and evaluates the effects of the implementation. The nurse involves the patient, the patient's family, and significant others in each step of the process to the greatest extent possible and compensates for and acknowledges the factors that may influence the provision of care by the nurse and staff. Implicit in the nursing process is the therapeutic and personal relationship of the nurse, the patient, the patient's family, and significant others. See also **nursing process.**

fixate, fixated. See **fixation.**

fixating eye /fik″sāting/ [L, *figere,* to fasten; AS, *eage*], in strabismus, the eye that is directed to a given object to position that object on the fovea. Compare **squinting eye.**

fixation /fiksā″shən/ [L, *figere,* to fasten, *atio,* process], (in psychoanalysis) an arrest at a particular stage of psychosexual development, such as anal fixation. –*fixated, adj.,* –*fixate, v.*

fixational ocular movements /fiksā″shənəl/, rotation of the eyes during voluntary fixation on an object.

fixation muscle, a muscle that acts to hold a part of the body in appropriate position. Compare **antagonist, prime mover, synergist.**

fixative /fik″sətiv/ [L, *figere,* to fasten], **1.** any substance used to bind, glue, or stabilize. **2.** any substance used to preserve gross or histological specimens of tissue for later examination.

fixator, a device composed of rods and pins designed to provide stabilization of a body part. The external skeletal apparatus may be attached directly to the bone.

fixed anions /fikst/, anions that are not part of the body's buffer anions.

fixed bridgework, a dental prosthetic constructed to replace missing teeth that incorporates artificial teeth permanently attached to natural teeth or implants in the jaw.

fixed cantilever. See **partial denture.**

fixed cations, cations that are not part of the body's metabolic buffering system.

fixed-combination drug [L, *figere,* to fasten, *combinare,* to combine; Fr, *drogue*], any of a group of multiple-ingredient preparations that provide concomitant administration of specific amounts of two or more medications.

fixed coupling, the occurrence of a normal and an ectopic heartbeat with a constant interval between the two each time the ectopic beat occurs.

fixed delusion [L, *figere,* to fasten, *deludere,* to deceive], a delusion that is consistent, unaltered, and difficult to interrupt.

fixed-dose combination. See **fixed-combination drug.**

fixed dressing, a dressing usually made of gauze impregnated with a hardening agent, such as plaster of paris, sodium silicate, starch, or dextrin, applied to support or immobilize a part of the body. The dressing is soaked in water, applied to the part to be immobilized, and allowed to harden. See also **cast, splint.**

fixed drug eruption, well-defined red to purple lesions that appear at the same sites on the skin and mucous membranes each time a particular drug is used. The reaction occurs most commonly in patients who are using tetracycline or phenolphthalein.

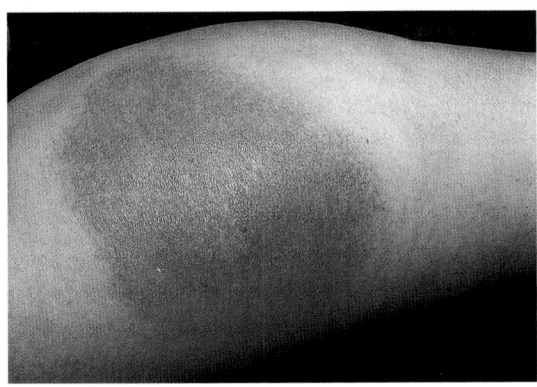

Fixed drug eruption *(Callen et al, 2009)*

fixed fulcrum, a tomographic fulcrum that remains at a fixed height.

fixed idea, **1.** a persistent, obsessional thought or notion. **2.** in certain mental disorders, especially obsessive-compulsive disorder, an idea that dominates mental activity and persists despite contrary evidence or rational refutation. Also called **idée fixe.**

fixed interval (FI) reinforcement, (in psychiatry) reinforcement given after a specific amount of time has elapsed.

fixed macrophage [L, *figere,* to fasten; Gk, *makros,* large, *pagein,* to eat], a nonmotile mononuclear phagocyte found in connective tissue, liver sinuses, spleen, lymph glands, and bone marrow.

fixed noncirculating phagocyte. See **phagocyte.**

fixed orthodontic appliance, a mechanical device cemented to the teeth or attached by adhesive material, used for changing or stabilizing the relative positions of the teeth.

fixed partial denture, a dental prosthesis permanently held in position by attachments to adjacent prepared natural teeth, roots, or implants. Compare **removable partial denture.**

fixed-performance oxygen delivery system. See **high-flow oxygen delivery system.**

fixed phagocyte. See **phagocyte.**

fixed pupil [L, *figere,* to fasten, *pupilla,* little girl], an abnormal condition in which the pupils fail to dilate or contract when stimulated. The cause is commonly adhesions binding the iris to the lens capsule or acute glaucoma causing interference with the nerve supply of the iris.

fixed-rate pacemaker [L, *figere,* to fasten, *ratum,* calculate, *passus,* step; ME, *maken*], an electronic cardiac stimulator that delivers impulses to the cardiac muscle at a preset rate regardless of the heart's independent activity.

fixed ratio (FR) reinforcement, (in psychiatry) reinforcement given after a specific number of responses have occurred.

fixed torticollis [L, *figere,* to fasten, *tortus,* twisted, *collum,* neck], a condition in which neck muscles on one side are so short that the head is held continuously in the same position. See also **torticollis.**

fixed vertebra. See **false vertebra.**

flaccid /flak″sid/ [L, *flaccus,* flabby], weak, soft, and flabby; lacking normal muscle tone, such as flaccid muscles associated with peripheral neuritis, poliomyelitis, and early stroke. –*flaccidity, flaccidness, n.*

flaccid bladder, a bladder that is unable to contract sufficiently to empty. It may be secondary to neural deficiencies or chronic obstruction. The bladder can be emptied by pressure applied to the area or via catheterization. Also called **atonic bladder, autonomous bladder, nonreflex bladder.** Compare **spastic bladder.**

flaccid dysarthria. See **lower motor neuron dysarthria.**

flaccidity, flaccidness /flaksid″itē/. See **flaccid.**

flaccid paralysis, an abnormal condition characterized by the weakening or the loss of muscle tone. It may be caused by disease or by trauma affecting the nerves associated with the involved muscles. Compare **spastic paralysis.**

flagell-, prefix meaning "whiplike process, tapping": *flagellation, flagellum, flagellant.*

flagella. See **flagellum.**

flagellant /flaj″ələnt/, a person who receives sexual gratification from the practice of flagellation.

flagellate /flaj″əlāt′, -lit/ [L, *flagellum,* whip], a protozoon or alga that propels itself with flagella. Kinds include *Giardia, Leishmania, Trichomonas, Trypanosoma.* See also **protozoon.**

flagellation /flaj′əlā″shən/, **1.** the act of whipping, beating, or flogging. **2.** a type of massage administered by tapping the body with the fingers. See also **massage. 3.** a type of sexual deviation in which a person is erotically gratified by being whipped or by whipping another. See also **masochism, sadism. 4.** the arrangement of flagella on an organism; exflagellation.

flagellum /flajel″əm/ *pl. flagella* [L, whip], a long, hairlike projection that extends from some unicellular organisms and from the sperm of animals, algae, and some plants. Flagellar motion is a complex, whiplike undulation that propels cells through a fluid environment.

Flagyl, an antibiotic and antiprotozoal drug. Brand name for **metronidazole.**

flail chest /flāl/ [ME, *fleyl,* whip; AS, *cest,* box], a thorax in which there are two fractures on at least two adjacent ribs causing instability in part of the chest wall and paradoxic breathing, with the lung underlying the injured area contracting on inspiration and bulging on expiration. If it is uncorrected, hypoxia will result.

■ OBSERVATIONS: Flail chest is characterized by sharp pain; uneven chest expansion; shallow, rapid respirations; and decreased breath sounds. Tachycardia and cyanosis may be present. Potential complications include atelectasis, pneumothorax, hemothorax, cardiac tamponade, shock, and respiratory arrest. Often other traumatic injuries are present in a patient with a flail chest.

■ INTERVENTIONS: The treatment of choice is internal stabilization of the chest wall through the use of positive pressure. Bilevel positive pressure or mechanical ventilation may be used. If the patient breathes against the automatic ventilator, a sedative and muscle relaxant may be ordered to achieve ventilatory control. Chest tubes may be required to remove air or fluid that is preventing expansion of the affected lung, and a nasogastric tube may be ordered to provide food and fluids. The patient's vital signs and breath sounds are frequently evaluated, and arterial blood gases are monitored.

■ PATIENT CARE CONSIDERATIONS: The patient with flail chest usually requires a long period of care involving frequent repositioning, scrupulous attention to the patency and cleanliness of the tracheostomy or endotracheal tube, skin care, oral hygiene, pain management, and emotional support. Members of the health care team perform passive range-of-motion exercises involving the extremities, explain the various procedures, and provide a pad and pencil or a magic slate with which the patient can communicate.

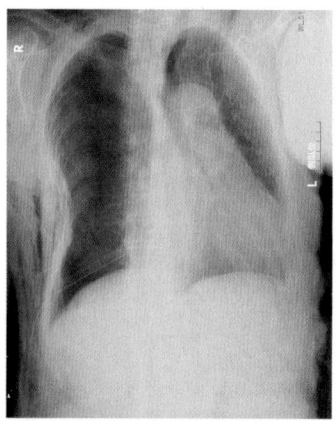

Computed tomography scan of flail chest showing multiple rib fractures *(Mori et al, 2020)*

flame photometry [L, *flagrare*, to burn; Gk, *phos*, light, *metron*, measure], measurement of the wavelength of light rays emitted by excited metallic electrons exposed to the heat energy of a flame, used to identify characteristics in clinical specimens of body fluids. The intensity of the emitted light is proportional to the concentration of atoms in the fluid, and a quantitative analysis can be made on that basis. In the clinical laboratory, flame photometry was once used to measure sodium, potassium, and lithium levels but is no longer used routinely.

flammable, the property of igniting and burning easily and rapidly. See also **inflammable.**

flange /flanj/, **1.** the part of a denture base that extends from the cervical ends of the teeth to the border of the denture. It can be used for retention of the denture upon the residual alveolar ridge by utilizing the contours of the labial and buccal musculature and mucosa. **2.** a prosthesis with a lateral vertical extension designed to direct a resected mandible into centric occlusion. **3.** the barrier around a stoma that protects the skin and provides support for the adherence of the appliance.

flank, the posterior portion of the body between the ribs and the ilium. Flank pain is sometimes associated with the kidney.

flap, a layer of skin or other tissue surgically separated from deeper structures for transplantation, coverage of an area that has been injured, or examination of deeper tissues.

flapping tremor. See **asterixis.**

flap reconstruction, an alternative to skin expansion as a method of breast reconstruction after mastectomy. It involves creation of a skin flap using tissue from another part of the body, such as the back or abdomen. The flap is attached to the chest to create a pocket for implantation or to build a breast mound.

flap surgery, a type of breast reconstruction that is performed in a single stage, in some cases at the same time as a mastectomy.

flare /fler/, **1.** a red blush on the skin at the periphery of an urticarial lesion seen in immediate hypersensitivity reactions. **2.** an expanding skin flush spreading from an infective lesion or extending from the principal site of a reaction to an irritant. **3.** the sudden intensification of a disease.

flaring of nostrils, nasal widening during inspiration, a sign of air hunger or respiratory distress.

flash, a sudden or intermittent brief burst of intense heat or light. See also **hot flash, rush.**

flashback, a phenomenon experienced by persons who have taken a hallucinogenic drug or had psychological trauma and unexpectedly reexperience its effects. This is also suffered by patients with posttraumatic stress disorder.

flash burn, a lesion caused by exposure to an extremely intense source of radiant energy or heat. Flash burn commonly occurs on the corneas of arc welders.

flashover phenomenon, an effect of a lightning strike or other intense electric discharge in which the electric current passes over the body instead of through it. The result is a red, featherlike branching pattern on the skin.

flask, **1.** a narrow-neck glass vessel used for heating liquids, distilling chemicals, or culturing fluid media. **2.** a small glass receptacle for holding liquids or powders.

flask closure [L, *vasculum*, small vessel, *claudere*, to close], the joining of two halves of a flask that encloses and forms a mold for a denture base.

flasking /flask'ing/ [L, *vasculum*, small vessel], **1.** the act of investing in a flask. **2.** the process of investing the cast and a wax denture in a flask preparatory to molding the denture base material into the form of the denture.

flat affect, the absence or near absence of emotional response to a situation that normally elicits emotion. It is observed in schizophrenia and some depressive disorders. Also called **flattened affect.**

Flatau-Schilder disease. See **Schilder disease.**

flat bone [AS, *flet*, floor], any of the bones that provide structural contours of the skeleton. Examples include ribs and bones of the cranium.

flat electroencephalogram, a graphic chart on which no tracings are recorded during electroencephalography, indicating a lack of brain wave activity. Flat readings are indicative of brain death except in cases of profound hypothermia and central nervous system depression. Also called **isoelectric electroencephalogram.** See also **brain death.**

flatfoot, an abnormal but relatively common condition characterized by the flattening out of the arch of the foot. Also called **pes planus.** See also **fallen arch.**

flat spring contraceptive diaphragm, a kind of contraceptive diaphragm in which the flexible metal spring that forms the rim is a thin, light, flat band made of stainless steel. The rubber dome is approximately 3.8 cm deep, and the diameter of the rubber-covered rim is between 55 and 100 mm. Seven sizes, in increments of 5 mm, allow the clinician to fit the diaphragm to a particular woman. This kind of

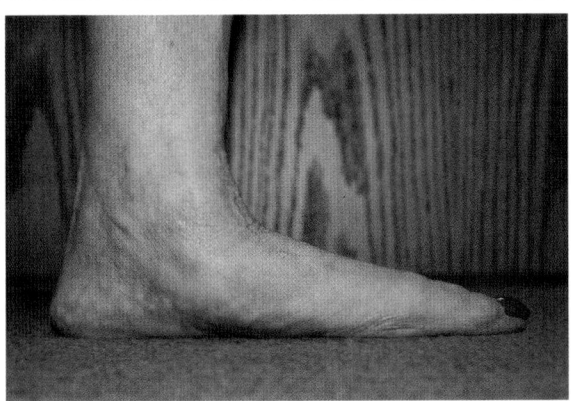

Flatfoot demonstrating collapse of the arch
(Coughlin et al, 2014)

diaphragm is prescribed for a woman whose vaginal musculature provides good support, whose uterus is in the normal
position and not acutely retroflexed or anteflexed, and whose
vagina, neither very long nor very short, has a shallow arch
behind the symphysis pubis.

flattened affect. See **flat affect.**

flatulence /flach′ələns/ [L, *flatus,* a blowing], the presence of an excessive amount of air or gas in the stomach and
intestinal tract, causing distension of the organs and in some
cases mild to moderate pain.

flatulent /flach′ələnt/ [L, *flatus,* a blowing], pertaining to
gas or air in the digestive tract.

flatus /flā″təs/ [L, a blowing], air or gas in the intestine
that is passed through the rectum. See also **aerophagy.**

flat wart. See **verruca plana.**

flav-, prefix meaning "yellow": *flavone, Flavivirus,
flavoprotein.*

flaval ligaments [L, *ligare + flavus,* yellow], the bands of
yellow elastic tissue connecting the laminae of adjacent vertebrae from the axis to the first segment of the sacrum. They
are thin, broad, and long in the cervical region, thicker in the
thoracic region, and thickest in the lumbar region. They help
hold the body erect.

Flavivirus, a genus of a family of Flaviviridae single-
stranded positive-sense ribonucleic acid viruses, including species that cause yellow fever, dengue, and St. Louis
encephalitis. Most are arboviruses transmitted by mosquitoes
or ticks. Also called **group B arbovirus.**

flavocoxid, an oral nutritional supplement.
■ INDICATIONS: This drug is used for dietary management of
osteoarthritis.
■ CONTRAINDICATIONS: Known hypersensitivity to this drug
prohibits its use.
■ ADVERSE EFFECTS: Adverse effects of this drug include
hypertension, increase in varicose veins, psoriasis, and fluid
accumulation in the knees.

flavone /flā″vōn/ [L, *flavus,* yellow], a colorless crystalline flavonoid derivative and component of bioflavonoid.

flavoprotein, a group of conjugated proteins that make yellow enzymes essential for cellular respiration. They also are
involved in liberation of hydrogen from oxidation of fatty acids
and function as electron acceptors in oxidative phosphorylation.

flavoxate hydrochloride /flavok″sāt/, a smooth muscle
relaxant.
■ INDICATIONS: It is prescribed for spastic conditions of the
urinary tract.
■ CONTRAINDICATIONS: GI hemorrhage or obstruction, urinary tract obstruction, or known hypersensitivity to this drug
prohibits its use.

Superior

Flaval ligamenta

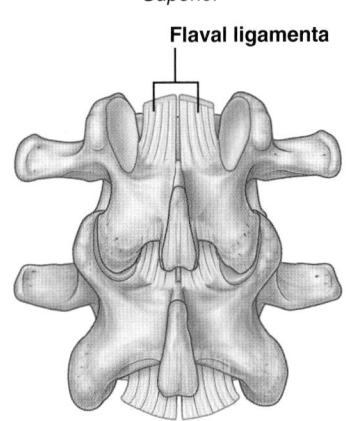

Inferior

Flaval ligamenta *(Drake, Vogl, and Mitchell, 2005)*

■ ADVERSE EFFECTS: Among the more serious adverse effects are nervousness, nausea, abdominal pain, fever, and
tachycardia.

flax, a flowering annual herb found in the United States,
Canada, and Europe.
■ INDICATIONS: The seeds are used for constipation and as a
source of omega-3 fatty acids.
■ CONTRAINDICATIONS: It is contraindicated in people with
bowel obstruction and dehydration. It is also not recommended during pregnancy and lactation, in children, or in
those with known hypersensitivity to this product. It should
not be used as a poultice on open wounds.

fl. dr., abbreviation for **fluid dram.**

flea [AS], a wingless, bloodsucking insect of the order
Siphonaptera, some species of which transmit arboviruses to
humans by acting as host or vector to the organism.

flea bite, a small puncture wound produced by a blood-
sucking flea. Certain species of fleas transmit plague, murine
typhus, and probably tularemia.

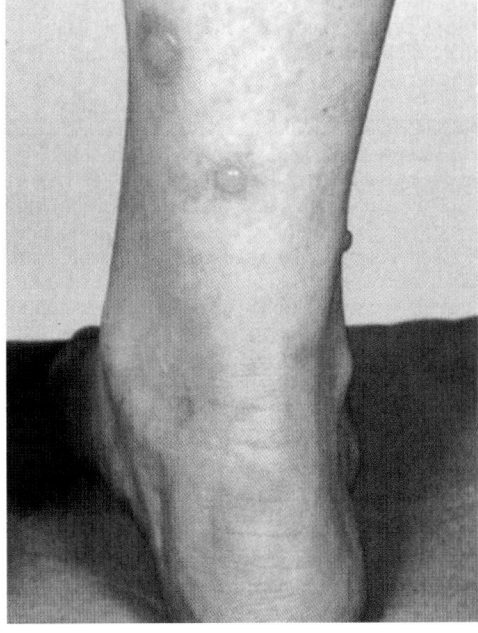

Flea bite *(du Vivier, 2002)*

F

flea-borne typhus. See **murine typhus.**

flecainide /flĕka′nīd/. See **flecainide acetate.**

flecainide acetate /flekā″nīd/, an oral antiarrhythmic drug. Also called **flecainide.**

- INDICATIONS: It is prescribed for the treatment of ventricular arrhythmias (e.g., sustained ventricular tachycardia) and for treating supraventricular tachycardia in the absence of conduction defects when other drugs have failed.

- CONTRAINDICATIONS: Preexisting second- or third-degree atrioventricular block, right bundle-branch block associated with a left hemiblock in the absence of a pacemaker, cardiogenic shock, and coronary artery disease prohibit its use. Concurrent therapy with disopyramide and verapamil is not recommended, and there is insufficient experience with concurrent use with nifedipine or diltiazem to recommend concurrent use. Should not be administered with other drugs that are highly dependent on CYP3A or CYP2D6 for metabolism such as ritonavir and amprenavir.

- ADVERSE EFFECTS: Among adverse effects reported are new or increased arrhythmias or congestive heart failure, dizziness, visual disturbances, dyspnea, headache, nausea, fatigue, tremor, constipation, and edema.

fleck dystrophy of the cornea. See **speckled dystrophy of the cornea.**

-flect, -flex, suffix meaning "to bend": *dorsiflect, reflex.*

Fleet Enema, a manufactured enema formula containing 16 g sodium biphosphate and 6 g sodium phosphate per 100 mL solution. It is available in disposable plastic pouches fitted with prelubricated rectal tubes.

Fleischner method /flīsh″nər/ [Felix Fleischner, American radiologist, 1893–1969], a technique for producing lordotic x-ray projections of the lungs. The patient leans backward from the waist to a nearly 45-degree posterior inclination with his or her back against the x-ray image receptor.

flesh, the soft, muscular tissues of the body. See also **muscle.**

Fletcher factor, a prekallikrein blood coagulation substance that interacts with both factor XII and Fitzgerald factor, activating both and accelerating thrombin formation.

Flexeril, a muscle relaxant. Brand name for **cyclobenzaprine hydrochloride.**

Flex-Foot, a stored-energy foot prosthesis containing a J-shaped plastic beam that acts like a spring when the wearer walks or runs. See also **stored-energy foot.**

flexibilitas cerea. See **cerea flexibilitas.**

flexibility /flek″sibil′i·tē/ [L, *flectere,* to bend], the quality of being readily bent without breaking.

flexible, **1.** the ability to bend without breaking, a characteristic describing an individual who is able to easily adapt to new situations. **2.** movement of a joint with ease.

flexion /flek″shən/ [L, *flectere,* to bend], **1.** a movement allowed by certain joints of the skeleton that decreases the angle between two adjoining bones, such as bending the elbow, which decreases the angle between the humerus and the ulna. Compare **extension. 2.** a resistance to the descent of the fetus through the birth canal that causes the neck to flex so the chin approaches the chest. Thus the smallest diameter (suboccipitobregmatic) of the vertex presents.

flexion jacket, a corset designed to provide spinal immobility. It is typically fashioned of a rigid material and, like a Griswald brace, provides three-point fixation in opposite directions.

flexitime. See **flextime.**

flexor /flek″sər/ [L, bender], a muscle that flexes a joint.

flexor carpi radialis [L, *flexor,* bender], a slender, superficial muscle of the forearm that lies on the ulnar side of the pronator teres. It functions to flex and to help abduct the hand. Compare **flexor carpi ulnaris, palmaris longus.**

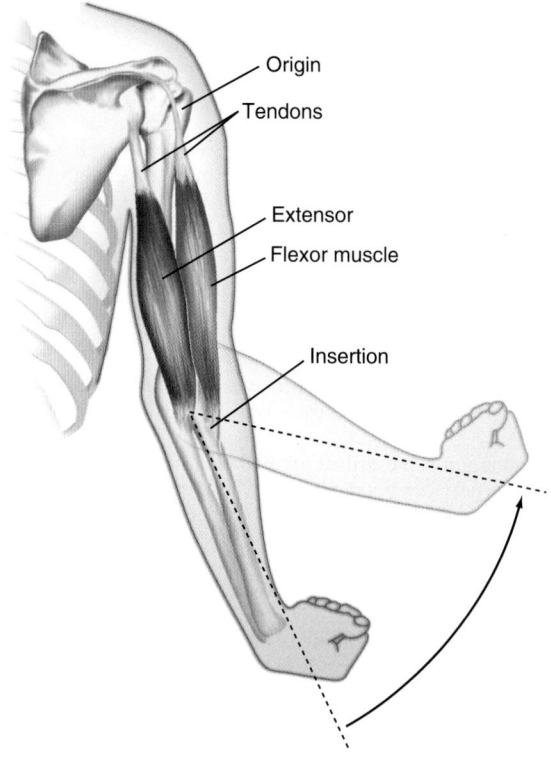

Flexion of the elbow *(Koeppen and Stanton, 2010)*

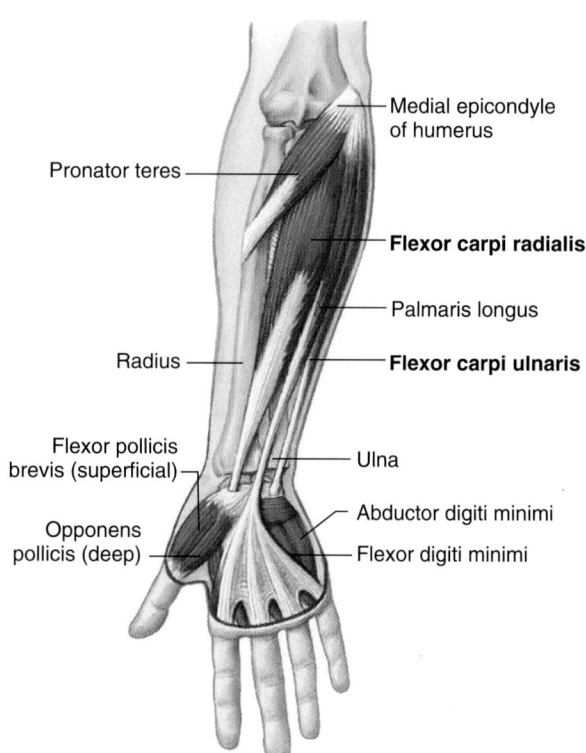

Flexor carpi radialis and flexor carpi ulnaris *(Patton and Thibodeau, 2016)*

flexor carpi ulnaris, a superficial muscle lying along the ulnar side of the forearm. It functions to flex and adduct the hand. Compare **flexor carpi radialis, palmaris longus.**

flexor digiti minimi brevis, 1. short flexor muscle of little finger; a muscle that inserts on the medial side of the proximal phalanx of the finger to flex it and is innervated by the ulnar nerve. **2.** short flexor muscle of little toe; a muscle that inserts on the lateral surface of the base of the proximal phalanx of the toe to flex it and is innervated by the lateral plantar nerve.

flexor digitorum brevis, short flexor muscle of toes; a muscle that inserts on the middle phalanges of the four lateral toes and flexes them. It is innervated by the medial plantar nerve.

flexor digitorum longus, the muscle that flexes the lateral four toes. It is involved with gripping the ground during walking and propelling the body forward off the toes at the end of the stance phase of gait. It is innervated by the tibial nerve.

flexor digitorum profundus, one of two deep flexor muscles of the fingers; a muscle that inserts on the distal phalanges of the fingers and flexes them. It is innervated by the ulnar and anterior interosseous nerves.

flexor digitorum superficialis, the largest superficial muscle of the forearm, lying in the second of four layers. The muscle flexes the second phalanx of each finger and, by continued action, the hand. Also called *flexor digitorum sublimis.* Compare **flexor carpi radialis, flexor carpi ulnaris, palmaris longus, pronator teres.**

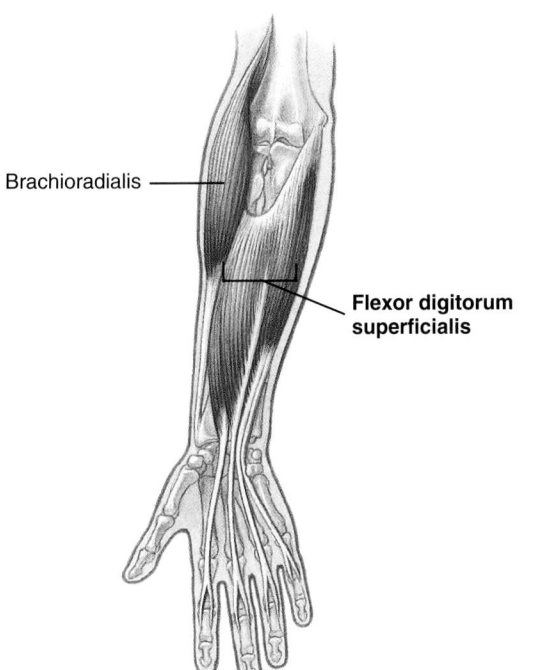

Flexor digitorum superficialis *(Patton and Thibodeau, 2016)*

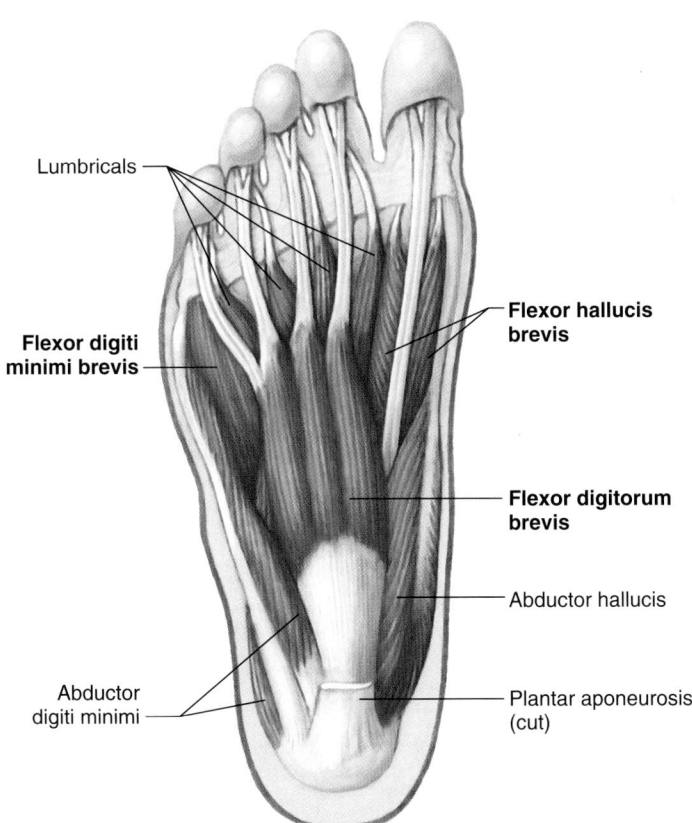

Flexor digiti minimi brevis, flexor digitorum brevis, and flexor hallucis brevis muscles of the foot *(Patton and Thibodeau, 2016)*

flexor hallucis brevis, short flexor muscle of great toe; a muscle that inserts in the base of the proximal phalanx of the great toe and flexes it. It is innervated by the medial plantar nerve.

flexor hallucis longus, the muscle that flexes the great toe. It is particularly active during the toe-off phase of walking when the body is propelled forward of the stance leg and the great toe is the last part of the foot to leave the ground. It can also contribute to plantarflexion of the foot at the ankle joint. It is innervated by the tibial nerve.

flexor pollicis brevis, a thenar muscle that flexes the thumb. It is innervated by the anterior interosseous nerve, a branch of the median nerve.

flexor pollicis longus, the muscle that flexes the metacarpophalangeal joint of the thumb.

flexor retinaculum of ankle [L, *flexor,* bender, *retinaculum,* halter; AS, *ancleow*], **1.** a strong band of fascia from the medial malleolus to the calcaneum, passing over the three long flexor tendons and blood vessels and nerves of the posterior leg. **2.** the roof of the tarsal tunnel.

flexor retinaculum of wrist [L, *flexor,* bender, *retinaculum,* halter; AS, *wrist*], a strong ligament across the front of the hollow of the carpus and over the flexor tendons of the fingers and median nerve.

flexor withdrawal reflex, a common cutaneous reflex consisting of a widespread contraction of physiological flexor muscles and relaxation of physiological extensor muscles. It is characterized by abrupt withdrawal of a body part in response to painful or injurious stimuli. A relatively innocuous stimulation of the skin may result in a weak contraction of one or more flexor muscles and a minimal withdrawal reflex.

FlexPen, a device to administer insulin that is prefilled and color-coded. It allows for accurate measurement by dialing the number of units to be administered.

flextime /fleks″tīm/ [L, *flectere,* to bend; AS, *tima*], a system of staffing that allows the individualization of work schedules. A person working days may choose to work from 7:00 to 3:00, 9:00 to 5:00, or other hours. Full staffing must be maintained, but within the group flextime can be arranged. Use of the system tends to improve morale and decrease turnover. Also called **flexitime.**

flexure /flek″shər/, a normal bend or curve in a body part, such as the colic flexure of the colon or the dorsal flexure of the spine.

flight into health [AS, *fleogan,* to fly], **1.** an abnormal but common reaction to an unpleasant physical sensation or symptom in which the person denies the feeling or observation, insisting that there is nothing wrong. See also **illness experience. 2.** voluntary and temporary suppression of mental or physical symptoms to prevent further analysis of the patient's emotional state.

flight of ideas, (in psychiatry) a continuous stream of talk in which the patient switches rapidly from one topic to another and each subject is incoherent and unrelated to the preceding one or is stimulated by some environmental circumstance. The condition is frequently a symptom of acute manic states and schizophrenia. Compare **circumstantiality.**

flight-or-fight reaction [AS, *fleogan,* to fly, *feohtan,* to fight; L, *reagere,* to act again], **1.** (in physiology) the reaction of the body to stress, in which the sympathetic nervous system and the adrenal medulla act to increase the cardiac output, dilate the pupils of the eyes, increase the rate of the heartbeat, constrict the blood vessels of the skin, increase the levels of glucose and fatty acids in the circulation, and induce an alert, aroused mental state. **2.** (in psychiatry) a person's reaction to stress by either fleeing from a situation or remaining and attempting to deal with it.

flight to illness, the effort of the patient to convince the therapist that he or she is too ill to terminate therapy and that continued support is needed.

flip angle, in magnetic resonance imaging, the degree of rotation of the macroscopic magnetization vector produced by a radiofrequency pulse with respect to the direction of the static magnetic field.

floater [AS, *flotian,* to float], a spot that appears to drift in front of the eye, caused by a shadow cast on the retina by vitreous debris. Most floaters are benign and represent remnants of a network of blood vessels that existed prenatally in the vitreous cavity. The sudden onset of several floaters may indicate serious disease. Hemorrhage into the vitreous humor may cause a large number of big and little shadows and a red discoloration of vision. The cause is often traumatic injury, but spontaneous intraocular hemorrhage is observed in proliferative diabetic retinopathy, hypertension, or increased intracranial pressure. Cancer, detachment of the retina, occlusion of a retinal vein, and other purely ocular diseases may also cause hemorrhage into the vitreous cavity. Inflammation of the retina resulting from chorioretinitis may cause entry of inflammatory cells into the vitreous humor. Inflammatory debris may adhere to the vitreous framework in netlike masses that are very disruptive of normal vision. Retinal detachment also causes a sudden appearance of flashes of light and/or floaters and a diminished field of vision as a shower of red cells and pigment is released into the vitreous humor. Careful ophthalmological examination through a well-dilated pupil is recommended for all people who experience a sudden occurrence of floaters because each of the pathological causes can be treated in the early stages and loss of vision can usually be prevented. Also called **musca volitans,** *musca volitantes.*

floating head [AS, *flotian,* to float, *heafod*], a condition that exists when the biparietal diameter of the fetal head is above the plane of the pelvic inlet. The term comes from the ease with which the fetal head is pushed upward on pelvic examination (i.e., it "floats away") as compared to the engaged fetal head, when such movement is difficult if not impossible. See also **ballottement, engagement.**

floating kidney, a kidney that is not securely fixed in the normal anatomical location because of congenital malplacement or traumatic injury. Compare **ptotic kidney.**

floating patella [AS, *flotian,* to float + L, *patella,* small pan], a patella that has been forced away from the femoral condyle by an effusion into the knee joint.

floating ribs, vertebral rib. See **rib, vertebral rib.**

floating spleen, a spleen that is displaced and abnormally movable. Also called **wandering spleen.**

float nurse, a nurse who is available for assignment to duty on an ad hoc basis, usually to assist in times of unusually heavy workloads or to assume the duties of absent nursing personnel. A float nurse is recruited from a group of nurses called a float pool. Also called **contingent nurse.** See also **nurses' registry.**

flocculant /flok″yo̅o̅lənt/, an agent or substance that causes flocculation.

flocculate, flocculation. See **flocculent.**

flocculation test /flok′yo̅o̅lā″shən/ [L, *floccus,* flock of wool], a serological test in which a positive result depends on the degree of flocculent precipitation produced in the material being tested. Some tests for syphilis, including the Venereal Disease Research Laboratories slide test, are flocculation tests.

flocculent /flok″yo̅o̅lənt/ [L, *floccus,* flock of wool], clumped or tufted, such as a cloud, or covered with a woolly, fuzzy surface. –*floccule, flocculation,* n., –*flocculate,* v.

flood fever. See **typhus.**

flooding [AS, *flod*], **1.** (*Informal*) profuse bleeding from the uterus, especially after childbirth, or prolonged menses. **2.** a technique used in behavioral therapy for the reduction of anxiety associated with various phobias. Exposure to a stimulus that usually provokes anxiety desensitizes a person to that stimulus, thereby reducing fear and anxiety. It is similar to implosive therapy except that the stimulus is real, whereas in implosive therapy, it is suggested. Compare **implosive therapy, systemic desensitization.**

floor, the lower inner surface of any cavity or organ.

floppy epiglottis, a condition in which the epiglottis is sucked into the glottis during inspiration. It is a common cause of laryngeal stridor in infants. Adult onset is rare. When present in adults, it is most often associated with head injury or cerebrovascular accident.

floppy-valve syndrome. See **Barlow's syndrome.**

flora /flôr′ə/, microorganisms that live on or within a body to compete with disease-producing microorganisms and provide a natural immunity against certain infections. Also called **normal flora.**

florid /flôr″id/ [L, *floridus,* flowery], in human skin complexion or wound appearance, a bright red color.

Florone, a topical corticosteroid. Brand name for **diflorasone diacetate.**

Floropryl, an inhibitor of cholinesterase, used ophthalmically. Brand name for *isoflurophate.*

flossing, the mechanical cleansing of proximal tooth surfaces, subgingivally and supragingivally, by dental tape, Teflon thread, or waxed or unwaxed dental floss.

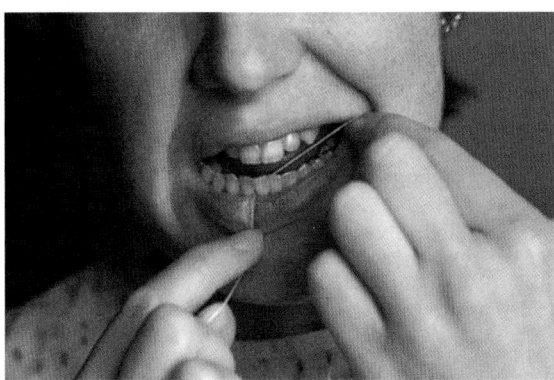

Flossing *(Potter and Perry, 2005)*

flotation device /flōtā″shən/ [Fr, *flotter,* to float], a foam mattress with a gellike pad located in its center, designed to protect bony prominences and distribute pressure evenly against the skin's surface.

flotation therapy, a state of semi-weightlessness produced by various types of hospital equipment and used in the treatment and prevention of pressure ulcers.

flow, **1.** the movement of a liquid or gas. **2.** (*Slang*) copious menstruation but less profuse than flooding.

flow chart [AS, *flowan* + L, *charta,* paper], **1.** a graphic representation of a computer program sequence. It is developed before the writing of a computer program. **2.** a diagram representing a workflow process.

flow cycling, the delivery of gas under positive pressure during inspiration until flow drops to a specified terminal level.

flow cytometry, a technique in which cells suspended in a fluid flow one at a time through a focus of exciting light, which is scattered in patterns characteristic to the cells and their components. They are often labeled with fluorescent markers so that light is first absorbed and then emitted at altered frequencies. A sensor detecting the scattered or emitted light measures the size and molecular characteristics of individual cells. Tens of thousands of cells can be examined per minute, and the data gathered are processed by computer.

flower essences, aqueous extracts of the fresh flowers of various plants chosen for their effects on specific mental or emotional symptoms, combined with brandy as a preservative. They are used to address spiritual, mental, and emotional as well as physical problems.

flowmeter, a device that regulates and measures the flow of a fluid or gas. In an anesthetic gas machine it is the flowmeter that measures gases by speed of flow, according to their viscosity and density. Also called **rotameter,** *Thorpe tube.*

flow sheet, (in a patient record) a graphic summary of several changing factors, especially the patient's vital signs or weight and the treatments and medications given. For example, in labor the flow sheet displays the progress of labor, including centimeters of cervical dilation, cervical effacement, position of the baby's head, baby's heart rate, frequency of contractions, mother's temperature and blood pressure, and medications given or procedures performed.

flow study. See **uroflowmetry.**

flow transducer, a measuring device that calculates volume by dividing flow by time.

flow trigger, a trigger for initiating assisted ventilation, consisting of a mechanism for measuring the patient's inspiratory effort and starting assisted ventilation when flow reaches a given level.

flow-volume curve, a graphic of the instantaneous rate of airflow during a forced expiration. It is plotted as a function of the volume. It may be a maximum expiratory flow-volume curve or a partial expiratory flow-volume curve.

flow-volume dysequilibrium, the lower than normal solute content of blood that has just gone through dialysis. Dialysis tends to draw solutes out of other fluid-containing body compartments, such as cells. Urea rebound is one result.

flow-volume loop, a graph of the rate of airflow as a function of lung volume during a complete respiratory cycle consisting of a forced inspiration followed by a forced expiration. The plotted curve appears as a loop and is used in assessing pulmonary function.

floxuridine /floksyoor″ədēn/, an antineoplastic agent.

■ INDICATIONS: It is prescribed in the treatment of metastases to the liver from colon, stomach, and other GI cancers.

■ CONTRAINDICATIONS: Bone marrow depression, infection, poor nutritional state, or known hypersensitivity to this drug prohibits its use.

■ ADVERSE EFFECTS: Among the more serious adverse effects leading to drug discontinuation are severe depression of the bone marrow; acute GI disturbances, including nausea, vomiting, diarrhea, and stomatitis; and myocardial ischemia. Alopecia and dermatitis commonly occur.

fl. oz., abbreviation for **fluid ounce.**

flu /floo/, **1.** (*Informal*) influenza. **2.** any viral infection, especially of the respiratory or intestinal system.

fluconazole /floo koe′ na zole/, an antifungal medication that can be administered by the oral and intravenous routes.

■ INDICATIONS: It is prescribed in the treatment of *Candida* infections and fungal infections of the central nervous system.

■ CONTRAINDICATIONS: Sensitivity to azole compounds; concomitant administration of quinidine, cisapride, and/or SSRIs prohibit its use.

■ ADVERSE EFFECTS: Most commonly, abdominal pain, diarrhea, dizziness, headache, nausea, rash, vomiting, and/or elevated liver enzymes. High doses are associated with birth defects.

fluctuant /fluk″chōō·ənt/, pertaining to a wavelike motion that is detected when a structure containing a liquid is palpated.

fluctuation /fluk·chōō·ā″shən/ [L, *fluctuare,* to wave], **1.** a wavelike motion of fluid in a body cavity that follows a shaking motion. **2.** a variation in a fixed value or mass.

flucytosine /flōōsī″təsēn/, an antifungal drug.

■ INDICATIONS: It is prescribed as an adjunct in the treatment of certain serious fungal infections, usually Candida or Cryptococcus.

■ CONTRAINDICATIONS: Known hypersensitivity to this drug prohibits its use. Close monitoring is required when administering it to patients with renal disorders, bone marrow depression, or AIDS.

■ ADVERSE EFFECTS: Among the more serious adverse effects are GI disturbances, including enterocolitis, abnormal liver function, hepatomegaly, and bone marrow depression. Also causes hallucinations, confusion and other CNS effects, respiratory depression, peripheral neuropathy, and hearing loss.

Fludara, an antineoplastic drug. Brand name for **fludarabine.**

fludarabine, an antimetabolite used to treat neoplasia.

■ INDICATIONS: It is prescribed in the treatment of patients with B cell chronic lymphocytic leukemia and as salvage therapy for non-Hodgkin's lymphoma and acute leukemias.

■ CONTRAINDICATIONS: It should not be given to patients who are pregnant or hypersensitive to this drug or its components. Patients should be closely observed for signs of hematological and nonhematological toxicity (e.g., edema, fatigue, myalgias).

■ ADVERSE EFFECTS: It is a potent antineoplastic agent with potentially significant side effects. The side effects most often reported include myelosuppression, fever and chills, nausea, and vomiting.

fludeoxyglucose F 18 /flōō″de·ok″seglōō′kōs/, radiolabeled 2-deoxy-D-glucose. It is used in positron emission tomography in the diagnosis of brain disorders, cardiac disease, and tumors of various organs.

fluency disorder. See **stuttering.**

fluent /flōō′ənt/ [L, *fluens* flowing], flowing effortlessly. It is said of speech.

-fluent, suffix meaning "flowing": *effluent, confluent.*

fluent aphasia /flōō″ənt/ [L, *fluere,* to flow; Gk, *a,* not, *phasis,* speech], a form of aphasia in which the patient articulates words easily, although the message may be unintelligible or may not be related to a particular stimulus. Kinds include **Wernicke's aphasia, conduction aphasia.**

fluid /flōō′id/ [L, *fluere,* to flow], **1.** a substance, such as a liquid or gas, that is able to flow and to adjust its shape to that of a container because it is composed of molecules that are able to change positions with respect to each other without separating from the total mass. **2.** a body fluid, either intracellular or extracellular, involved in the transport of electrolytes and other vital chemicals to, through, and from tissue cells. See also **blood, cerebrospinal fluid, lymph.**

fluid balance, a state of equilibrium in which the amount of fluid consumed equals the amount lost in urine, feces, perspiration, and exhaled water vapor.

fluid dram (fl. dr.), a unit of liquid measure equal to 3.696 mL, 60 minims, or ⅛ fluid ounce.

fluidic ventilator /flōō·id″ik/, a device used in respiratory therapy that applies the Coanda effect to the movement of the flow of air or gases. As the airstream passes a wall, a pocket of turbulence forms a low-pressure bubble next to the wall,

causing the airstream to adhere to the wall. As a gas travels faster over the pocket of turbulence, the surrounding gas molecules not in the stream acquire a higher pressure, holding the stream against the wall. The gas flow tends to remain in that pattern until it is diverted by a different input pressure. See also **Coanda effect.**

fluid intelligence, the speed and accuracy with which one can reason abstractly and problem solve.

fluidized air bed, a bed that minimizes pressure and distributes weight evenly over the support surface. A gentle flow of temperature-controlled air is projected upward through numerous tiny openings called ceramic microspheres. Also called **Clinitron bed™.**

fluidotherapy /flōō′idōther″əpē/, a modality of dry heat that uses a suspended airstream flowing through finely divided solid particles to emulate the properties of a liquid. It simultaneously performs the functions of applied heat, massage, sensory stimulation, and pressure oscillations. The goal is to relieve pain and discomfort associated with musculoskeletal disorders of the extremities.

fluid ounce (fl. oz.), a measure of liquid volume in the apothecaries' system that is equal to 8 fluid drams or 29 mL, 480 minims, ½₀ imperial pint, or the volume occupied by 437.5 grains of distilled water at a temperature of 16.7° C. See also **apothecaries' measure, metric system.**

fluid overload, an excessive accumulation of fluid in the body caused by excessive parenteral infusion or deficiencies in cardiovascular or renal fluid volume regulation. Compare **circulatory overload, hypervolemia.**

fluid retention, a failure to excrete excess fluid from the body. Causes may include renal, cardiovascular, or metabolic disorders. In uncomplicated cases the condition can sometimes be corrected with diuretics and a low-salt diet.

fluid therapy, the regulation of water balance in patients with impaired renal, cardiovascular, or metabolic function by careful measurement of fluid intake against daily losses.

fluid volume, the volume of the body fluids, including both intracellular fluid and extracellular fluid.

fluid volume imbalance, abnormally decreased or increased fluid volume or rapid shift from one compartment of body fluid to another.

fluke /flōōk/, a parasitic flatworm of the class Trematoda, including the genus *Schistosoma.*

flunisolide, an intranasal and oral inhalation adrenal corticosteroid.

■ INDICATIONS: It is prescribed in the treatment of seasonal or continuing allergic rhinitis that involves inflammation of the mucous membranes of the nasal passages and for the treatment of asthma.

■ CONTRAINDICATIONS: It should not be given to patients with allergy to this drug or any of its components or to patients with status asthmaticus or untreated bacterial, viral, or fungal infections of the respiratory tract or nasal mucosa.

■ ADVERSE EFFECTS: The side effects most often reported include nasal or throat irritation, stinging, burning, or dryness; nosebleed; sneezing; bloody mucus; congestion; asthma; increased coughing; sore throat; or lesions in the nose or throat.

fluocinolone acetonide /flōō′ōsin″əlōn/, a topical glucocorticoid.

■ INDICATIONS: It is prescribed for severe dermatoses.

■ CONTRAINDICATIONS: Impaired circulation, viral and fungal diseases of the skin, or known hypersensitivity to this drug or to other steroid medication prohibits its use.

■ ADVERSE EFFECTS: Among the more serious adverse effects are systemic side effects that result from prolonged use or excessive application. Various hypersensitivity reactions may occur.

fluocinonide /floo͞o′ōsin″ənīd/, a topical corticosteroid.

■ INDICATIONS: It is prescribed to reduce skin inflammation and the associated pruritus.

■ CONTRAINDICATIONS: Viral and fungal diseases of the skin, tuberculosis of the skin, or known hypersensitivity to this drug prohibits its use.

fluorescein dilaurate, an ester of fluorescein with two molecules of laurate, used in the pancreolauryl test of pancreatic function.

fluorescence /floo͞ores″əns/ [L, *flux,* a discharge], the emission of light of one wavelength by a substance when it is exposed to electromagnetic radiation of a shorter wavelength. Fluorescent substances that emit visible light appear luminous. –*fluoresce, v.*

fluorescent /floo͞ores′ent/, pertaining to or characterized by fluorescence.

fluorescent antibody test (FA test) /floo͞ores″ənt/, a test in which a fluorescent dye is used to stain an antibody for identification of clinical specimens. Fluorescent dyes conjugate with immunoglobulins without altering the antibody-antigen reaction, making the dyed organisms glow visibly when examined under a fluorescent microscope. The fluorescent antibody technique can be used in identification of *Mycobacterium tuberculosis* and in the most common serological screening test for syphilis. Also called **immunofluorescence test.** Kinds include **fluorescent treponemal antibody absorption test.**

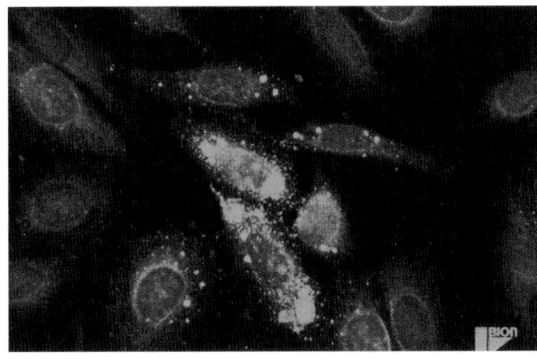

Fluorescent antibody test showing mumps virus *(Forbes, Sahm, and Weissfeld, 2007/Courtesy Bion Enterprises, Ltd.)*

fluorescent in situ hybridization (FISH), a genetic mapping technique using fluorescent tags for analysis of chromosomal aberrations and genetic abnormalities. Also called **chromosome painting.**

fluorescent microscopy, examination with a fluorescent microscope equipped with a source of ultraviolet light rays, used to study specimens, such as tissues or microorganisms, that have been stained with fluorescent dye. Also called **ultraviolet microscopy.** See also **fluorescent antibody test.**

fluorescent treponemal antibody absorption test (FTA-ABS test), the standard treponemal antigen test for syphilis. Nonspecific antibodies are removed from patient serum, which is then reacted with *Treponema pallidum* fixed to a glass slide. Specific antibodies adhering to the treponemes are demonstrated with fluorescein-labeled antihuman globulin. Positive tests are seen in about 85% of cases of primary syphilis, 100% in secondary syphilis, and 98% in late syphilis. The test remains positive for life even after syphilis has been successfully treated. See also **fluorescent antibody test.**

fluoridation /floor′idā″shən/ [L, *fluere,* to flow], the process of adding fluoride, especially to a public water supply, to reduce tooth decay. See also **fluoride.**

fluoride /floor″īd/, an anion of fluorine. Fluoride compounds are introduced into drinking water or applied directly to the teeth to prevent tooth decay.

fluoride application, fluoride dental treatment [L, *fluere,* to flow, *dens,* tooth; Fr, *traitment*], the direct oral application of fluoride compounds to reduce the incidence of dental caries.

fluoride poisoning [L, *fluere,* to flow, *potio,* drink], **1.** See **fluorosis. 2.** the toxic effects of contact with compounds of fluorine, an intensely poisonous pale yellow gas. Sodium fluoroacetate is a powerful rodent poison; methyl fluoroacetate is regarded as too toxic to use as a pesticide. The fluoroacetate compounds inhibit enzymes of the citric acid cycle. Inhalation of hydrogen fluoride can lead to bronchospasm, laryngospasm, and pulmonary edema.

fluorination /floor′inā″shən/, the addition of fluorine to a compound, such as those commonly found in topical corticosteroids.

fluorine (F) /floor″ēn, floo͞o′ərēn/ [L, *fluere,* to flow], an element of the halogen family and the most reactive of the nonmetals. Its atomic number is 9, and its atomic mass is 19.00. It occurs in nature only as a component of substances such as fluorspar, cryolite, and phosphate rocks. It can be prepared by the electrolytic decomposition of hydrogen fluoride and in its pure form is a pale yellow toxic gas 1.6 times heavier than air. It is also a component of very stable fluorocarbons used in the manufacture of resins and plastics. As a component of fluorides, it is widely distributed throughout the soils of the earth, enters plants, is ingested by humans, and is absorbed from the GI tract. Fluorides in the atmosphere and industrial dust are absorbed by the lungs and the skin. Relatively soluble compounds, such as sodium fluoride, are almost completely absorbed by humans. The relatively insoluble compounds, such as cryolite, are poorly absorbed. Small amounts of sodium fluoride are added to the water supply of many communities to harden tooth enamel and decrease dental caries. Excessive amounts of fluoride can mottle tooth enamel and cause osteosclerosis. Acute fluoride poisoning and death can result from the accidental ingestion of insecticides and rodenticides containing fluoride salts.

fluoroacetic acid (FCH$_2$COOH) /floor′ō·asē″tik, -aset″ik/, a colorless water-soluble, highly toxic compound that blocks the citric acid cycle, causing convulsions and ventricular fibrillation. It is derived from a South African tree and is used in some potent pesticides.

fluorocarbons /floor′ōkär″bəns/ [L, *fluere,* to flow, *carbo,* coal], hydrocarbons where some or all of the hydrogens are replaced by fluorine. Fluorocarbons are generally colorless, nonflammable gases, but some are liquids at room temperature. The compounds can produce mild upper respiratory tract irritation, and excessive exposure has been cited as a cause of central nervous system depression.

fluorochrome stain, a fluorescent dye used to stain the cell walls of fungi and bacteria. The organisms then fluoresce when exposed to UV light rays. It is commonly used to visualize acid-fast bacilli (mycobacteria) in specimens. Kinds include **auramine O, acridine.**

fluorodopa F 18 /floor′odo′pə/, a radiolabeled compound of fluorine and levodopa, used for positron emission tomography of the cerebrum.

fluorometry /floo͞orom″ətrē/ [L, *fluere* + Gk, *metron,* measure], measurement of fluorescence emitted by compounds when exposed to ultraviolet or other intense radiant energy. The atoms of certain substances produce fluorescence of a characteristic color and wavelength, allowing identification and quantification of several clinically significant compounds in biological specimens. Although fluorometry is a highly sensitive method of analysis, test interference by other compounds, especially drugs, may limit its usefulness in some situations. –*fluorometric, adj.*

Fluoroplex, a topical preparation of an antineoplastic drug. Brand name for **fluorouracil.**

fluoroquinolone /floo″okwin′olōn/, any of a subgroup of quinolones that contain one or more fluorine atoms attached to the central ring system that have a broader spectrum of antibiotic activity than quinolones. Kinds include **nalidixic acid,** *ciprofloxacin (Cipro).*

fluoroscope /floor″əskōp′/ [L, *fluere* + Gk, *skopein,* to look], a device used to project a radiographic image on a fluorescent screen for visual examination. –*fluoroscopic, adj.*

fluoroscopic compression device /floor′əskop″ik/, any of several objects that can be placed on a specific area of a patient's abdomen to compress the abdomen and separate loops of bowel during fluoroscopy of the digestive tract.

fluoroscopy /flooros″kəpē/, the visual examination of a part of the body or the function of an organ with a fluoroscope. The technique offers continuous imaging of the motion of internal structures and immediate serial images. It is invaluable in many clinical procedures, such as cardiac catheterization.

fluorosis /floorō″sis/ [L, *fluere* + Gk, *osis,* condition], the condition that results from excessive prolonged ingestion of fluorine. Unusually high concentration of fluorine in the drinking water typically causes mottled discoloration and pitting of the enamel of the secondary and primary dentition in children whose teeth developed while maternal intake of fluorinated water was high. Severe chronic fluorine poisoning leads to osteosclerosis and other pathological bone and joint changes in adults. See also **fluoridation, fluoride.**

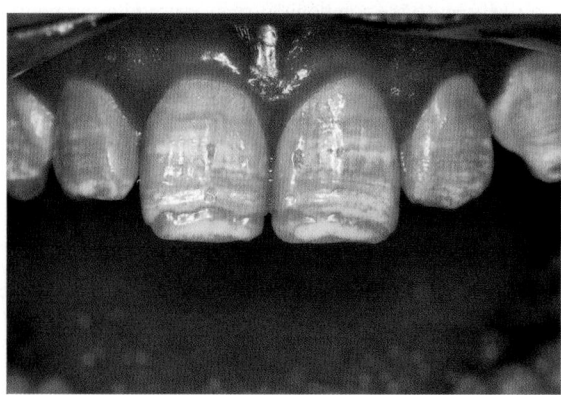

Moderate fluorosis (Sapp, 2004)

fluorouracil /floor′ōyoor″əsil/, an antimetabolite antineoplastic drug.

■ INDICATIONS: It is prescribed in the treatment of malignant neoplastic disease of the skin, breast, and internal organs.

■ CONTRAINDICATIONS: Bone marrow depression, infection, poor nutritional status, or known hypersensitivity to this drug prohibits its use.

■ ADVERSE EFFECTS: Among the more serious adverse effects are severe depression of the bone marrow and acute GI disturbances, including nausea, vomiting, diarrhea, and stomatitis. Alopecia and dermatitis commonly occur. Effects of topical application include photosensitivity, rash, and scarring.

Fluothane, an inhalational general anesthetic. Brand name for **halothane.**

fluoxetine hydrochloride /floo·ok″sətēn/, an oral antidepressant that acts by selectively preventing serotonin reuptake.

■ INDICATIONS: It is prescribed for major depressive disorder, obsessive-compulsive disorder, and bulimia nervosa.

■ CONTRAINDICATIONS: Known hypersensitivity to this drug prohibits its use.

■ ADVERSE EFFECTS: Serious adverse effects include seizures, hemorrhage, tachycardia, bradycardia, myocardial infarction, and thrombophlebitis.

fluoxymesterone /floo·ok′simes″tərōn/, an androgenic and anabolic steroid.

■ INDICATIONS: It is prescribed in the treatment of testosterone deficiency, breast cancer in females, and delayed puberty in males.

■ CONTRAINDICATIONS: Male breast or prostate cancer, liver disease, known or suspected pregnancy, or known hypersensitivity to this drug prohibits its use.

■ ADVERSE EFFECTS: It commonly causes priapism in males, menstrual irregularities in females, edema, and acne. Among the more serious adverse effects are anaphylaxis, hypercalcemia, and jaundice.

flupenthixol decanoate, a long-acting ester of flupenthixol, administered intramuscularly as a depot injection.

flupenthixol hydrochloride, the hydrochloride salt of flupenthixol, administered orally.

fluphenazine hydrochloride /floofen″əzēn/, a phenothiazine antipsychotic drug.

■ INDICATIONS: It is prescribed in the treatment of schizophrenia and other psychotic disorders.

■ CONTRAINDICATIONS: Parkinson disease, concurrent administration of central nervous system depressants, liver or renal dysfunction, severe hypotension, or known hypersensitivity to this drug or to other phenothiazine medication prohibits its use.

■ ADVERSE EFFECTS: The most common adverse reactions are movement disorders and hypotension. Among the more serious adverse effects are liver toxicity, blood dyscrasias, and hypersensitivity reactions.

flurandrenolide /floo′rəndren″əlīd/, a topical glucocorticoid.

■ INDICATIONS: It is prescribed for the treatment of eczema and dermatitis.

■ CONTRAINDICATIONS: Impaired circulation, viral and fungal diseases of the skin, or known hypersensitivity to this drug or to steroid medication prohibits its use.

■ ADVERSE EFFECTS: Among the more serious adverse effects are systemic side effects that result from prolonged use or excessive application and hypersensitivity.

flurazepam hydrochloride /flooraz″əpam/, a benzodiazepine sedative-hypnotic agent.

■ INDICATIONS: It is prescribed in the short-term treatment of insomnia.

■ CONTRAINDICATIONS: Liver or kidney insufficiency, sleep apnea, or known hypersensitivity to this drug prohibits its use.

■ ADVERSE EFFECTS: Among the most serious adverse effects are possible physical and psychological dependence. Dizziness and drug hangover may also occur, and there have been instances of anterograde amnesia with aggressive behavior.

flurbiprofen /floorbi′profen/, a nonsteroidal antiinflammatory drug, administered orally in the treatment of arthritis, ankylosing spondylitis, bursitis, tendinitis, soft tissue injuries, and dysmenorrhea. The sodium salt is applied topically to the conjunctiva to inhibit miosis during, and inflammation after, ophthalmic surgery.

flurbiprofen sodium, the sodium salt of flurbiprofen, applied topically to the conjunctiva to inhibit miosis during, and as an antiinflammatory after, ophthalmic surgery.

flush [ME, *fluschen*], **1.** a blush or sudden reddening of the face and neck. **2.** a sudden subjective feeling of heat. **3.** a prolonged reddening of the face such as may be seen with fever, use of certain drugs, or hyperthyroidism. **4.** a sudden rapid flow of water or other liquid.

flush device, an apparatus in a hemodynamic monitoring system used to infuse normal saline to remove air bubbles, clear blood, and assure line patency. This ensures transmission of a clear pressure wave from a catheter to a transducer to provide accurate arterial or venous pressure measures.

flutamide, a hormonal (antiandrogen) antineoplastic agent.

■ INDICATIONS: It is prescribed along with leuprolide in the treatment of metastatic prostate cancer and other cancers stimulated by male hormones and is sometimes used to treat female hirsutism.

■ CONTRAINDICATIONS: It should not be given to patients who are allergic to the product. Hormonal medications should be avoided or used with extreme caution by women who are breastfeeding or who may be pregnant. Anticoagulants may interact with flutamide.

■ ADVERSE EFFECTS: The side effects most often reported include hot flashes, loss of sex drive, impotence, nausea, vomiting, breast enlargement, and stomach upset.

fluticasone /flōotik´äsōn″/, a steroid antiinflammatory agent, used topically as the propionate salt in treatment of itching or inflammation, intranasally in the treatment of allergic rhinitis and other inflammatory nasal conditions and of nasal polyps, and by inhalation in treatment of asthma.

flutter, a rapid vibration or pulsation that may interfere with normal function.

flutter-fibrillation [AS, *fleotan*, to move quickly; L, *fibrilla*, small fiber], a type of atrial fibrillation (involuntary recurrent contraction) in which the irregular fibrillatory line resembles atrial flutter mixed with atrial fibrillatory waves.

fluvastatin, an HMG-CoA reductase inhibitor used to treat dyslipidemia.

■ INDICATIONS: It is used as an adjunct treatment in primary hypercholesterolemia (types Ia and Ib) and in coronary atherosclerosis associated with coronary artery disease.

■ CONTRAINDICATIONS: Factors that prohibit its use include known hypersensitivity to this drug, pregnancy, lactation, and active liver disease.

■ ADVERSE EFFECTS: Adverse effects include myalgias, myopathy, and rhabdomyolysis; liver dysfunction; gastrointestinal effects; and headache.

fluvoxamine /flōovok´sämēn/, a selective serotonin reuptake inhibitor used as the maleate salt to relieve the symptoms of obsessive-compulsive disorder, administered orally.

fluvoxamine maleate, a selective serotonin reuptake inhibitor antidepressant.

■ INDICATIONS: It is prescribed in the treatment of obsessive-compulsive disorder in adult patients and has unlabeled uses for treating depression and panic attacks in adults and anxiety in children.

■ CONTRAINDICATIONS: It should not be given to patients with allergy to fluvoxamine maleate, patients who use monoamine oxidase inhibitors, or patients with a history of seizures, suicide attempts, or mania.

■ ADVERSE EFFECTS: The side effects most often reported include headache, sleepiness or insomnia, nausea, vomiting, and sexual dysfunction.

flux /fluks/ [L, *fluere,* to flow], **1.** an excessive flow or discharge. **2.** a substance that maintains the cleanliness of metals to be united and facilitates the easy flow and attachment of solder.

flux gain /fluks/, the ratio of the number of light photons at the output phosphor of a radiographic image intensifier tube to the number at the input phosphor.

fly [AS, *flyge*], a two-winged insect of the order Diptera, some species of which transmit arboviruses to humans.

fly bites, bites that may be caused by species of deerflies, horseflies, blackflies, or sand flies. Such bites produce a small painful wound with swelling caused by substances in the insect's saliva that are injected beneath the surface of the skin. Emergency treatment for fly bites includes cleaning the site and placing ice on it. The bite should be monitored for possible infections, as biting flies often transmit diseases.

Fm, symbol for the element **fermium.**

FMD, abbreviation for **fibromuscular dysplasia.**

FMET, abbreviation for **formylmethionine.**

FMG, abbreviation for **foreign medical graduate.**

FMIA, abbreviation for **Frankfurt-mandibular incisor angle.**

FML®, an ophthalmic glucocorticoid agent. Brand name for *fluorometholone.*

FMR-1, the symbol for a gene associated with the cognitive impairment of fragile X syndrome. The normal function of the gene has not been determined.

fMRI, abbreviation for **functional magnetic resonance imaging.**

FNP, abbreviation for **family nurse practitioner.**

foam /fōm/, **1.** *n.,* a dispersion of gas in a liquid or solid, such as pumice or whipped cream. **2.** *n.,* frothy saliva, produced particularly on exertion or pathologically. **3.** *v.,* to produce or cause production of such a substance.

foam bath [AS, *fam + baeth*], a bath taken in water containing a saponin substance that covers the surface of the liquid and through which air or oxygen is blown to form the foam.

foam test. See **shake test.**

focal /fō″kəl/ [L, *focus,* hearth], pertaining to a focus.

focal dermal hypoplasia, an autosomal-dominant X-linked disorder found exclusively in females, characterized by linear areas of dermal hypoplasia with herniation of underlying tissue through the defects. There are also telangiectasias, areas of discoloration, localized fatty deposits, papillomas of mucous membranes around orifices, and limb anomalies such as syndactyly, adactyly, and oligodactyly. Also called **Goltz syndrome.**

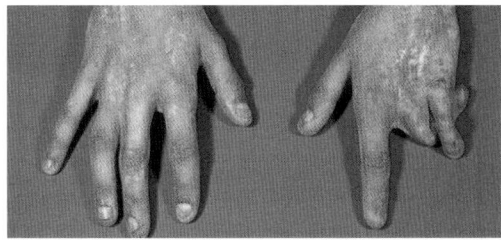

Focal dermal hypoplasia *(Hordinsky, Sawaya, and Scher, 2000)*

focal emphysema, centriacinar emphysema associated with inhalation of environmental dusts, producing dilation of the terminal and respiratory bronchioles. Also called *focal dust emphysema.*

focal glomerular sclerosis, focal sclerosing lesions of renal glomeruli with proteinuria, hematuria, hypertension, and the nephrotic syndrome. It may be idiopathic or secondary to other conditions, including heroin-abuse nephropathy, chronic interstitial nephritis, and malignancies. Exacerbations and remissions may occur, most often in children; progression to renal failure occurs at a variable and unpredictable rate. Also called *focal glomerulosclerosis.*

focal illumination. See **illumination.**

focal lesion [L, *focus* hearth + *laesio,* hurting], an infection, tumor, or injury that develops at a restricted or circumscribed area of tissue.

focal plane, the plane of tissue that is in focus on a tomogram.

focal point [L, *focus, punctus,* pricked], a point at which rays of light meet when deflected, either by reflection or refraction.

focal seizure [L, *focus,* hearth; OFr, *seisir*], a transitory disturbance in motor, sensory, or autonomic function that results from abnormal neuronal discharges in a localized part of the brain, most frequently motor or sensory areas adjacent to the central sulcus. Focal motor seizures commonly begin as spasmodic movements in the hand, face, or foot. Abnormal neuronal discharges that arise in the motor area that controls mastication and salivation may be manifested by chewing, lip smacking, swallowing movements, and profuse salivation. Abnormal electrical activity in the sensory strip of the cortex may be evident initially as a numb, prickling, tingling, or crawling feeling, and the neuronal discharge may spread to motor areas. See also **epilepsy, motor seizure.**

focal spot, the area on the anode of an x-ray tube or the target of an accelerator that is struck by electrons and from which the resulting x-rays are emitted. The shape and size of a focal spot influence the resolution of a radiographic image. An increase in focal spot size, which may accompany deterioration of the x-ray tube, reduces the ability to image small structures. Also called *actual focal spot.*

focal symptom [L, *focus,* hearth; Gk, *symptoma,* that which happens], a body function disturbance centered on a specific body system or part.

focal zone, (in ultrasonography) the distance along the beam axis of a focused transducer assembly, from the point where the beam area first becomes equal to four times the focal area to the point beyond the focal surface where the beam area again becomes equal to four times the focal area.

focus /fō″kəs/ [L, hearth], **1.** a specific location, as the site of an infection or the point at which an electrochemical impulse originates. **2.** the point at which light rays converge after passing through a lens.

focused activity /fō″kəst/, a therapeutic technique of actively leading the patient to adaptive coping skills and away from maladaptive ones.

focused grid, an x-ray grid that has lead foils placed at an angle so that they all point to a focus at a specific distance.

foetal. See **fetal.**

foeti-, foeto-. See **feti-, feto-, foeti-, foeto-.**

foetus. See **fetus.**

Fogarty catheter, a type of balloon-tip catheter used to remove thrombi and emboli from blood vessels.

fogged film fault /fogd/ [Dan, *spray* + AS, *filmen,* membrane; L, *fallere,* to deceive], a defect in a photograph or radiograph that appears as a foggy area. It is usually caused by stray light or radiation, use of expired film, or an unsafe darkroom light. See also **artifact.**

fogging [ME, *fogge*], an optical method of determining refractive error by placing excessively convex lenses in front

of the eyes. The patient is made artificially hyperopic by means of the spheres in order to relax all accommodation.

fog nebulizer /neb″yəlī′zer/, (in respiratory care) a device that humidifies by producing large volumes of particles.

foil pellet, a loosely rolled piece of gold foil, used for making various dental restorations, such as permanent tooth cavity fillings and tooth crowns. See also **gold foil.**

folacin. See **folic acid.**

folate /fō″lāt/, **1.** a salt of folic acid. **2.** any of a group of substances found in some foods and in mammalian cells that act as coenzymes and promote the chemical transfer of single carbon units from one molecule to another. See also **folic acid.**

folate deficiency, a deficiency of folic acid. See also **folic acid.**

fold. See **plica.**

folded cravat sling, a bandage suspended from the neck, usually for supporting a forearm. It is prepared by placing a broad fold of cloth on the chest vertically with one end over the shoulder of the affected arm. The other end hangs in front of the chest, and the lower end is moved up and over the shoulder and tied.

Foley catheter /fō″lē/ [Frederick E.B. Foley, American physician, 1891–1966], a rubber catheter with a balloon tip that is filled with a sterile liquid after it has been placed in the bladder. This kind of catheter is used when continuous drainage of the bladder is desired, such as in surgery, or when repeated urinary catheterization would be necessary if an indwelling catheter were not used. Sterile technique is used in placing the catheter. See also **catheterization.**

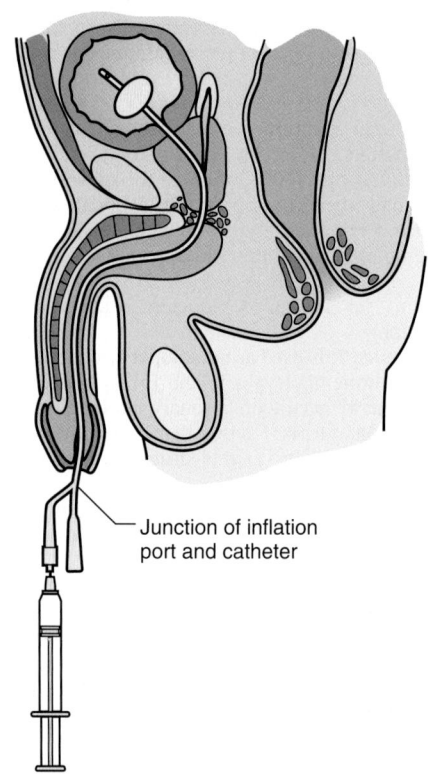

Junction of inflation port and catheter

Foley catheter *(Pfenninger, 2011)*

Foley Y-V pyeloplasty, pyeloplasty for repair of an obstructed and high ureteropelvic junction. A V-shaped flap is made from part of the renal pelvis and inserted into a Y-shaped incision whose angle is at the junction.

foliate papillae /fō″lē·āt/, a series of nipplelike processes that occur in folds along the lateral margins and in the front of the palatoglossus muscle of the tongue.

folic acid (FA) /fō″lik, fol″ik/, a yellow crystalline water-soluble vitamin essential for cell growth and reproduction. It functions as a coenzyme with vitamins B_{12} and C in the metabolism and use of proteins and in the formation of nucleic acids and heme for hemoglobin. Deficiency results in poor growth, graying of hair, glossitis, stomatitis, GI lesions, and diarrhea, and it may lead to megaloblastic anemia. Deficiency is caused by inadequate dietary intake of the vitamin, malabsorption, metabolic abnormalities, or drug-nutrient interactions. Need for folic acid increases in pregnancy, infancy, and periods of stress. A daily intake of 400 mg before conception and during early pregnancy has been found to lower the risk of fetal neural tube defects. Rich dietary sources include spinach and other green leafy vegetables, liver, kidney, asparagus, lima beans, nuts, orange juice, and whole-grain cereals. It is both heat- and light-labile, and considerable loss of the vitamin occurs during cooking and when it has been stored for a long period. Also called **folacin, pteroylglutamic acid, vitamin B_9.**

folic acid deficiency anemia, a form of megaloblastic (macrocytic) anemia caused by a lack of folic acid in the diet.

folic acid test (folate), a blood test performed to evaluate hemolytic disorders and to detect anemia caused by folic acid deficiency.

folie /fōlē″/ [Fr, madness], a psychiatric condition in a person who has previously been in good mental health. Kinds include **folie à deux, folie circulaire, folie du doute, folie du pourquoi, folie gemellaire, folie musculaire, folie raisonnante.**

folie à deux. See **shared paranoid disorder.**

folie circulaire. See **bipolar disorder.**

folie du doute /dYdo͞ot″/ [Fr, madness of doubts], an extreme obsessive-compulsive reaction characterized by persistent doubting, vacillation, repetition of a particular act or behavior, and pathological indecisiveness to the point of being unable to make even the most trifling decision.

folie du pourquoi /dYpo͞orkwô·ä″/ [Fr, madness of why], a psychopathological condition characterized by the persistent tendency to ask questions, usually concerning unrelated topics.

folie gemellaire /zhemeler″/ [Fr, madness in twins], a psychotic condition that occurs simultaneously in twins, sometimes in those not living together or closely associated at the time.

folie musculaire /mYskYler″/, severe chorea.

folie raisonnante /rezônäNt″/ [Fr, deliberating reason], a delusional form of any psychosis marked by a thought process that seems logical but lacks common sense.

folinic acid /fōlin″ik/, an active form of folic acid. It is used to treat megaloblastic anemias that are not caused by vitamin B_{12} deficiency and to counteract the toxic effects of antineoplastic folic acid antagonists, such as methotrexate. Also called **citrovorum factor, leucovorin.**

folk illnesses /fōk/, health disorders that are attributed to nonscientific causes. The major categories are naturalistic illnesses caused by impersonal factors such as yin-yang forces, and personalistic illnesses caused by evil eye or other "magic."

follicle /fol″ikəl/ [L, *folliculus,* small bag], **1.** a small, secretory sac, such as the dental follicles that enclose the teeth before eruption or the hair follicles within the epidermis. **2.** a

fluid- or colloid-filled ball of cells in some glands such as the thyroid and the ovaries. –**follicular,** *adj.*

follicle recruitment, the process by which certain primordial ovarian follicles begin growing in a given menstrual cycle.

follicles of Lieberkühn. See **Lieberkühn's glands.**

follicle-stimulating hormone (FSH), a gonadotropin that stimulates the growth and maturation of graafian follicles in the ovary and promotes spermatogenesis in the male. It is secreted by the anterior pituitary gland. FSH-releasing hormone produced in the median eminence of the hypothalamus controls the release of FSH by the pituitary. Increasing amounts of FSH are secreted in the postmenstrual or resting phase of the menstrual cycle, causing a primordial follicle to develop into a mature graafian follicle containing a mature ovum. The graafian follicle produces estrogen, which reaches a high level before ovulation and suppresses release of FSH. In males FSH maintains the integrity of the seminiferous tubules and influences all the stages of spermatogenesis. It may be used to treat some conditions. One form with luteinizing hormone (menotropins) is derived from the urine of postmenopausal women.

follicle-stimulating hormone–releasing factor (FSH-RF) [L, *folliculus,* small bag, *stimulare,* to incite; Gk, *horaein,* to set in motion], a hormone from the hypothalamus that stimulates the synthesis and release of FSH and luteinizing hormone from the anterior pituitary. See also **gonadorelin acetate.**

follicle-stimulating hormone surge, a sharp increase in serum levels of follicle-stimulating hormone seen around the middle of the menstrual cycle about 1 to 2 days before ovulation.

follicular /fōlik′yo͞olər/ [L, *folliculus,* small bag], of or pertaining to a follicle or follicles.

follicular adenocarcinoma /fōlik′yo͞olər/, a neoplasm characterized by a follicular arrangement of cells often seen in the thyroid gland, occurring most often in older individuals. The follicular thyroid carcinoma has a tendency to metastasize distantly to the lungs and bones. Surgery is the preferred treatment. If complete excision of the primary tumor is not feasible, radioiodine therapy is indicated. See also **medullary carcinoma, papillary adenocarcinoma.**

follicular antrum, a cavity filled with follicular fluid on one side of a vesicular ovarian follicle in its later stages of growth just before ovulation.

follicular cyst, a tooth-forming sac that arises from the epithelium of a tooth bud and dental lamina. Kinds include **dentigerous cyst, multilocular cyst, primordial cyst.**

follicular goiter, an enlargement of the thyroid gland characterized by proliferation of the follicles and epithelial tissue.

follicular phase, the first of the three phases of the reproductive cycle, consisting of menstruation and the follicular phase. During menstruation, dominant ovarian follicles develop in response to rising follicle-stimulating hormone (FSH) and luteinizing hormone (LH) levels. Nondominant follicles undergo atresia. Compare **ovulation, luteal phase.**

follicular stigma, a spot on the surface of an ovary where the vesicular ovarian follicle will rupture and permit passage of the ovum during ovulation. Also called **macula folliculi.**

follicular tonsillitis [L, *folliculus,* a small bag, *tonsilla* + Gk, *itis,* inflammation], inflammation of the tonsils accompanied by a purulent infection of the tonsillar crypts.

follicular vulvitis [L, *folliculus,* a small bag, *vulva,* a wrapper; Gk, *itis,* inflammation], an inflammation of the skin follicles of the vulva.

folliculitis /fōlik′yo͞olī″tis/, inflammation of hair follicles, caused by an infection, such as in sycosis barbae.

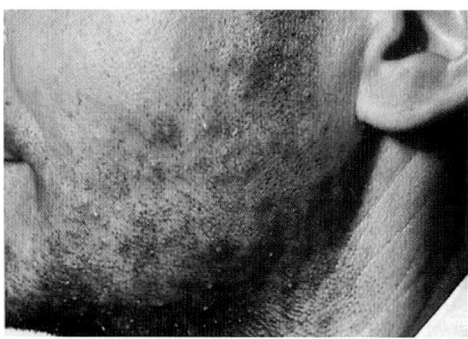

Folliculitis *(Courtesy American Academy of Dermatology and Institute for Dermatologic Communication and Education)*

folliculitis keloidalis. See **keloid acne.**

folliculogenesis /fōlik′yōōlōjen″əsis/, **1.** the stimulation of follicle development in the ovary by hormones or drugs. **2.** the development of follicles in the ovary, normally under the influence of the follicle-stimulating hormone secreted by the anterior pituitary gland.

folliculoma. See **granulosa cell tumor.**

folliculosis /fōlik′yōōlōsis/, a condition characterized by the development of a large number of lymph follicles, which may or may not be associated with an infection. In conjunctival folliculosis the large number of lymph follicles may give the conjunctival sac a granular appearance.

follitropin /folitro″pin/, a follicle-stimulating hormone. Follitropin alfa and follitropin beta are forms produced by genetically modified hamster cells and used in the treatment of infertility.

follitropin alfa/follitropin beta, an ovulation stimulant.

■ INDICATIONS: It is used to induce ovulation during assisted reproductive technologies such as in vitro fertilization.

■ CONTRAINDICATIONS: Factors that prohibit its use include known hypersensitivity, pregnancy, undiagnosed vaginal bleeding, intracranial lesion, and ovarian cyst not caused by polycystic ovarian disease.

■ ADVERSE EFFECTS: The most common side effects are ovarian hyperstimulation, nausea, abdominal pain, and multiple birth pregnancies.

follow-up, **1.** an act of renewing contact with sources of information and reviewing data needed to reinforce or evaluate a previous action or report, such as reexamination of an earlier diagnosis or prognosis. **2.** some further action taken after a procedure is finished, such as contact by a health care agency days or weeks after a patient has undergone treatment.

fomentation /fō′mentā″shən/ [L, *fomentare,* to apply a poultice], **1.** a topical treatment for pain or inflammation that uses a warm, moist application. **2.** a substance or poultice that is used as a warm, moist application.

fomite /fō″mīt/ [L, *fomes,* tinder], nonliving material such as bed linen that may transmit microorganisms.

fomivirsen /fomiv′ersin/, an antiviral agent administered by intravitreal injection in the treatment of cytomegalovirus retinitis associated with acquired immunodeficiency syndrome (AIDS); used as the sodium salt.

fondaparinux, a low-molecular-weight heparin used as an anticoagulant for the prevention of deep vein thrombosis and pulmonary emboli in hip and knee replacement and in hip fracture surgery.

Fones method /fōnz/ [Alfred C. Fones, American dentist, 1869–1938], a toothbrushing technique that uses large, sweeping, scrubbing circles over occluded teeth, with the toothbrush held at right angles to the tooth surfaces. With the jaws parted, the palatal and lingual surfaces of the teeth are scrubbed in smaller circles. Occlusal surfaces of the teeth are scrubbed in an anteroposterior direction.

Fonsecaea /fon″sese′ə/, a genus of imperfect fungi. *F. compactum* and *F. pedrosoi* are causal agents of chromoblastomycosis.

font, a set of type of one size and face.

fontanel /fon′tənel″/ [Fr, *fontaine,* fountain], a space covered by tough membranes between the bones of an infant's cranium. The anterior fontanel, roughly diamond-shaped, usually closes between the ages of 12 and 18 months. The posterior fontanel, triangular in shape, closes about 2 to 3 months after birth. Increase in intracranial pressure may cause a fontanel to become tense or bulge, as evidenced in infection such as meningitis. A fontanel may be soft and depressed as a result of dehydration. Also called *fonticulus.* Also spelled *fontanelle.*

food [AS, *foda*], **1.** any substance, usually of plant or animal origin, consisting of carbohydrates, proteins, fats, and such supplementary elements as minerals and vitamins, that

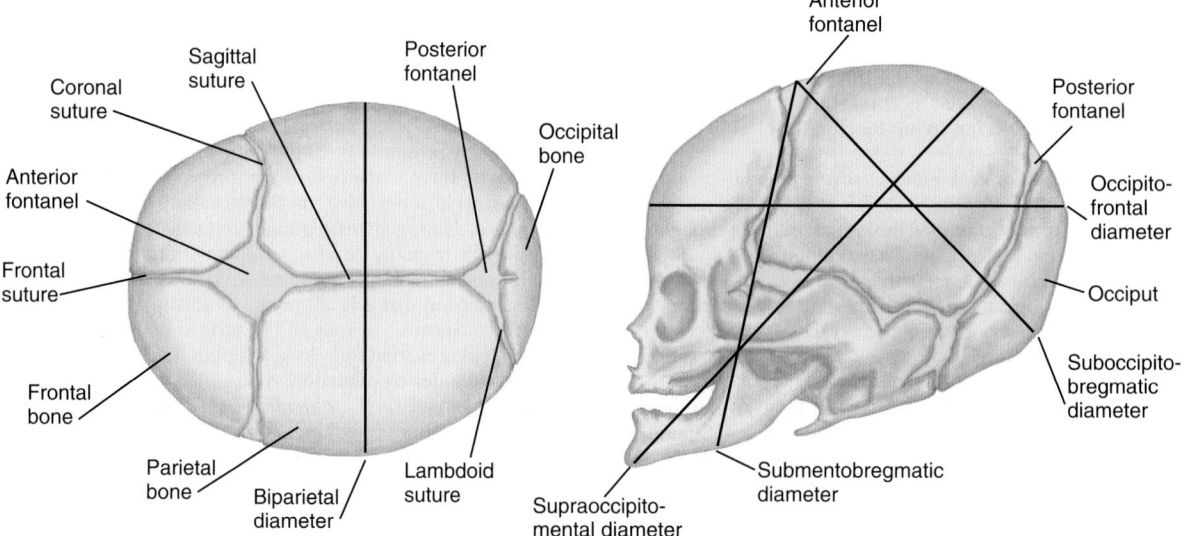

A   B

Fontanels and sutures *(McKinney et al, 2013)*

is ingested or otherwise taken into the body and assimilated to provide energy and to promote the growth, repair, and maintenance essential for sustaining life. **2.** nourishment in solid form, as contrasted with liquid form. **3.** a particular kind of solid nourishment, such as breakfast food or snack food.

food additive, any of a large variety of substances added to foods to prevent spoilage, improve appearance, enhance flavor or texture, or increase nutritional value. Most food additives must be approved by the U.S. Food and Drug Administration to determine whether they can cause cancer, birth defects, or other health problems. Examples include butylated hydroxyanisole and butylated hydroxytoluene in vitro, antioxidants that are added to fats to slow rancidity.

food allergy, a hypersensitive state that results from the ingestion, inhalation, or other contact with a specific food antigen. Symptoms of sensitivity to specific foods can include allergic rhinitis, bronchial asthma, urticaria, angioneurotic edema, dermatitis, pruritus, headache, labyrinthitis and conjunctivitis, nausea, vomiting, diarrhea, pylorospasm, colic, spastic constipation, mucous colitis, and perianal eczema. Food allergens are protein in nature and elicit an immunoglobulin response. The most common foods that cause allergic reactions are wheat, milk, eggs, fish and other seafoods, chocolate, corn, nuts (particularly peanuts), strawberries, chicken, pork, legumes, tomatoes, cucumbers, garlic, and citrus fruits. Foods that are rarely allergenic are rice, lamb, gelatin, peaches, pears, lettuce, artichokes, sesame oil, and apples. Diagnosis of a specific food allergy is obtained by a detailed food history, food diary, elimination diet, cutaneous tests, and blood examination for an immunoglobulin response. Compare **gastrointestinal allergy.**

Food and Drug Administration (FDA), a U.S. federal agency responsible for the enforcement of federal regulations on the manufacture and distribution of food, drugs, medical devices, and cosmetics. The regulations are intended to prevent the sale of impure or dangerous substances.

food and drug interactions, adverse health effects of certain combinations of foods and medications. Examples include reduced activity of drug-metabolizing enzymes (e.g., grapefruit juice is an inhibitor) or interference with the absorption of a drug (e.g., calcium inhibits tetracycline absorption from the GI tract).

food-borne botulism. See **botulism.**

food chain [AS, *foda* + *chaine*], an ecological sequence in which the various organisms within a community subsist on organisms lower in the sequence, as the human eats the fish that eats the worm, and so on. Each level within the chain has a fundamental role, and destruction of any one member affects the rest of the chain negatively.

food challenge, a challenge test for determining food allergens. A small amount of the suspected allergen is administered orally, and the patient is monitored for reactions such as rash, rhinorrhea, or diarrhea. Also called *food challenge test.*

food contaminants /kəntam″inənts/, substances that make food unfit for human consumption. Examples include bacteria, toxic chemicals, carcinogens, teratogens, and radioactive materials. Basically harmless substances, such as water, that may be added to food to increase its weight are also regarded as contaminants.

food exchange list. See **Exchange Lists for Meal Planning.**

food insecurity, a concern that a lack of money or access will interfere with the ability to secure adequate food for an individual or a family.

food poisoning, any of a large group of toxic processes that result from the ingestion of a food contaminated by toxic substances or by bacteria that contain toxins. Kinds include **ciguatera poisoning, shellfish poisoning, Minamata disease, mushroom poisoning,** *Salmonella* **gastroenteritis.** See also **botulism, ergot alkaloid, phalloidine, toadstool poisoning.**

food pyramid, a diagrammatic proportional representation of human nutritional needs updated in 2005 by the U.S. Department of Agriculture to replace the previous food pyramid created in 1992. Replaced in 2011 with the "My Plate" icon.

food sensitivity/hypersensitivity reaction, sensitivity to food items that is not a food allergy and does not involve the immune system. Kinds include **lactose intolerance.** See also **food allergy.**

food service administrator, a member of a hospital staff who is responsible for the planning and management of the food service system of the facility.

food service department, the section of a hospital or similar health facility that is responsible for food preparation and services to patients and personnel. It also provides nutritional care to patients.

foot [AS, *fot*], the distal extremity of the leg, consisting of the tarsus, the metatarsus, and the phalanges.

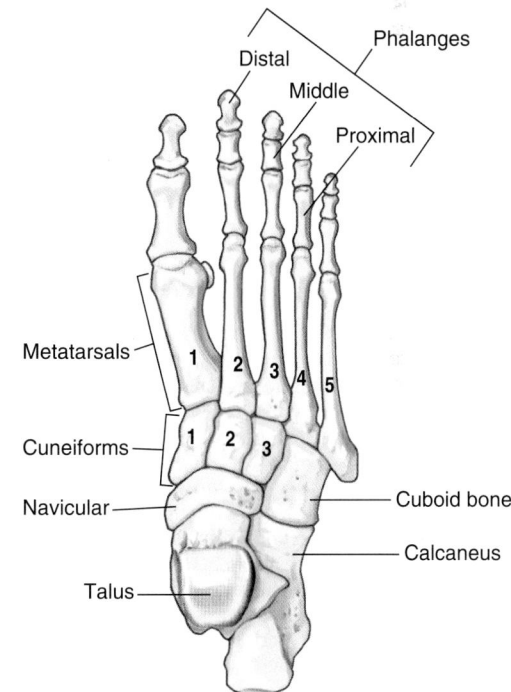

Bones of the foot *(Patton and Thibodeau, 2016)*

foot-and-mouth disease, an acute extremely contagious rhabdovirus, specifically vesicular stomatitis virus, infection, primarily of cloven-hooved animals. It is characterized by the development of ulcers on the skin around the mouth, on the mucous membrane in the mouth, and on the udders. Horses are immune. The virus is transmitted to humans by direct contact with infected animals or their secretions or with contaminated milk, although this is rare. It should not be confused with hand-foot-and-mouth disease, which is caused by a different virus (coxsackie A). Symptoms and signs in humans include headache, fever, malaise, and vesicles on the tongue, oral mucous membranes, hands, and feet. Generalized pruritus and painful ulcerations may occur; however, the temperature soon falls, the lesions subside in about a week, and total healing without scars is complete by 2 or 3 weeks. Treatment is symptomatic. Also called **aphthous fever.** See also **picornavirus.**

footboard, a board, device or open box placed at the end of a patient's bed and at a level above the top of the mattress to prevent the weight of the top sheet and blankets from resting on the feet. It is situated so that the soles of the feet are positioned firmly against the board with the legs at right angles to it. Its purposes are to help the bedridden patient retain normal posture and prevent footdrop.

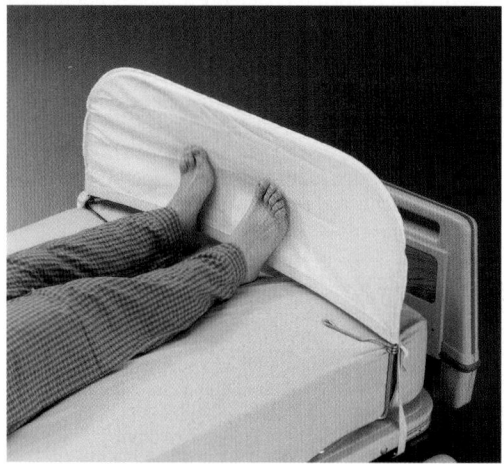

Footboard *(Courtesy Posey Company)*

foot-candle /fŏŏt′kandəl/ [AS, *fot*; L, *candela,* light], a unit of illumination being 1 lumen per square foot or equivalent to 1.0764 milliphots. Compare **lux.** See also **phot.**

footdrop /fŏŏt″drop/ [AS, *fot* + *dropa*], an abnormal neuromuscular condition of the lower leg and foot characterized by an inability to dorsiflex, or evert, the foot, caused by damage to the common peroneal nerve.

-footed, suffix meaning "having feet" of a specified sort or number: *clubfooted, flatfooted.*

footling breech [AS, *fot* + ME, *brech*], an intrauterine position of the fetus in which one or both feet are positioned below the buttocks at the inlet of the maternal pelvis. One foot presents in a single footling breech, both in a double footling breech. Compare **frank breech.** See also **breech birth.**

foot-pound, a unit for the measurement of work or energy. One foot-pound is the amount of work required to move 1 pound a distance of 1 foot in the same direction as that of the applied force.

footprinting, a method for determining the location of binding between a protein and a DNA molecule. The technique involves nuclease digestion of the unbound and therefore unprotected sequences of DNA. The protected DNA fragment that remains can be identified electrophoretically.

for-, prefix meaning "an opening": *foramen.*

foramen /fôrā″mən/ *pl. foramina* [L, hole], an opening or aperture in a membranous structure or bone, such as the apical dental foramen and the carotid foramen.

foramen caecum, a foramen immediately posterior to the frontal crest that may transmit emissary veins connecting the nasal cavity with the superior sagittal sinus.

foramen diaphragmatis. See **pacchionian foramen.**

foramen lacerum, an irregular opening in the temporal bone that is filled with cartilage.

foramen of Monro /monrō″/, a passage between the lateral and third ventricles of the brain.

foramen of Vesalius. See **venous foramen.**

foramenotomy, surgical removal of small pieces of bone around an intervertebral foramen, allowing more room for the spinal nerve. The procedure usually accompanies a laminectomy.

foramen ovale. See **oval foramen.**

foramen spinosum, a small opening near the posterior angle of the greater wing of the sphenoid bone. It is the smallest of three pairs of sphenoidal foramina that transmit nerves and blood vessels.

foramina. See **foramen.**

foramina transversarium, openings in the transverse processes of the vertebrae that together form a longitudinal passage on each side of the cervical spine for the vertebral artery and veins.

Forbes-Albright syndrome /fôrbs-ôl″brīt/ [Anne P. Forbes, American physician, 1911–1992; Fuller Albright, American physician, 1900–1969], an endocrine disease characterized by amenorrhea, prolactinemia, and galactorrhea, caused by an adenoma of the anterior pituitary. Diagnosis is made by radiographic examination of the anterior pituitary and a blood test for prolactin. Surgical resection of the adenoma is usually indicated. See also **galactorrhea, pituitary gland.**

Forbes disease. See **Cori disease.**

forbidden clone hypothesis [AS, *forbeodan* + Gk, *klon,* a cutting, *theoria,* speculation], a proposed explanation for autoimmunity that postulates that clones of cells that can react against the body persist after birth and can be activated by a viral infection or by some metabolic change. It holds that most cells of the immune system attack only foreign antigens, but these clones of cells attack the tissues of the body. Compare **sequestered antigens hypothesis.**

force [L, *fortis,* strong], **1.** energy applied so that it initiates motion, changes the speed or direction of motion, or alters the size or shape of an object. **2.** a push or pull defined as mass times acceleration. If the force on an object produces movement, it is called dynamic. If the force does not produce movement, it is called static.

forced expiratory flow (FEF), the average volumetric flow rate during any stated volume interval while a forced expired vital capacity test is performed. It is usually expressed as a percentage of vital capacity.

forced expiratory time (FET), the time required to exhale a given volume of air.

forced expiratory vital capacity (FEVC), the maximum volume of gas that can be forcibly and rapidly exhaled after a full inspiration. Also called **forced vital capacity, timed vital capacity.**

forced expiratory volume (FEV), the volume of air that can be forcibly expelled in a fixed period after full inspiration. Compare **vital capacity.** See also **expiratory reserve volume.**

forced-inhalation abdominal breathing, a respiratory therapy technique in which the patient inhales through the nose with an effort forceful enough to lift small sandbag weights placed on the abdomen. The technique is said to resemble closely the abdominal effort involved in normal breathing.

forced vital capacity. See **forced expiratory vital capacity.**

forceps *pl. forceps* [L, pair of tongs], a pair of any of a large variety and number of surgical instruments, all of which have two handles or sides, each attached to a dull blade. The handles may be joined at one end, such as a pair of tweezers, or the two sides may be separate to be drawn together in use, such as obstetric forceps. Forceps are used to grasp, handle, compress, pull, or join tissue, equipment, or supplies. Kinds include **thumb forceps, Adson-Brown forceps, Magill forceps, Kocher's forceps, suture forceps, tying forceps.**

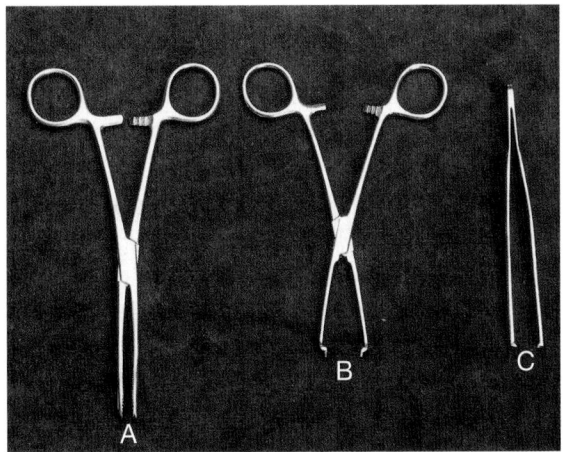

A and B, Ring-handle forceps. C, Spring-handle thumb forceps (Proctor and Adams, 2014)

forceps delivery, an obstetric operation in which instruments are used to assist the normal expulsive forces to deliver a baby. Prerequisites to forceps delivery include full dilation of the cervix, engagement of the fetal head, certain knowledge of the position of the head, and ruptured membranes. The blades of the forceps are introduced into the vagina one at a time and applied symmetrically to opposite sides of the baby's head; the handles of the forceps are pulled together so that the head is held firmly between the blades; and traction force is applied to facilitate vaginal delivery. When the head has been delivered, the forceps are removed and the delivery is completed manually. Because cesarean section is performed more often now than formerly, forceps deliveries are increasingly uncommon. Low forceps pertain to assisted birth in which the head is at the perineum in either the anterior or posterior presentation. Mid forceps are less common and involve application of the forceps above the station for low forceps but where the head is engaged, sometimes with rotation of the head. High forceps are of historical interest only, involving application of forceps to a floating head, and are proscribed in modern obstetric practice. Compare **forceps rotation, trial forceps.** See also **obstetric forceps.**

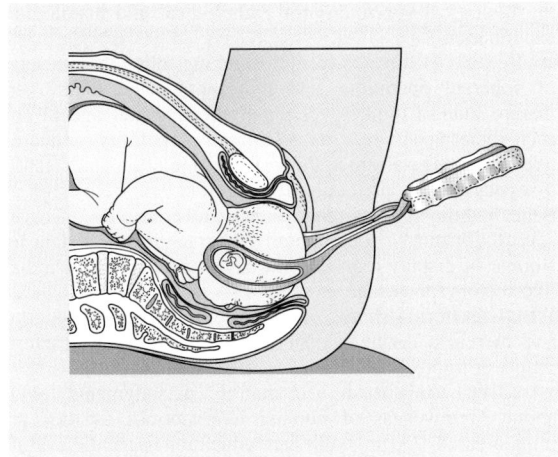

Forceps delivery (Greer et al, 2001)

forceps rotation, an obstetric operation in which forceps are used to turn a baby's head that is arrested in transverse or posterior position in the birth canal, facilitating the natural birth forces to allow vaginal delivery. Compare **forceps delivery, manual rotation.** Kinds include **Kielland's rotation,** *Scanzoni's rotation.* See also **obstetric forceps.**

forceps tenaculum. See **tenaculum.**

forcible inspiration [L, *fortis,* strong, *inspirare*], breathing that is assisted by a mechanical ventilator that forces air into the lungs during inhalation but allows the patient to exhale passively.

Fordyce-Fox disease /fôr″dis-foks′/ [G.H. Fox, American dermatologist, 1846–1937; John A. Fordyce, American dermatologist, 1858–1925], an apocrine gland disorder. Also called **apocrine miliaria, Fox-Fordyce disease.**

Fordyce spots [John A. Fordyce, American dermatologist, 1858-1925], the presence of enlarged oil glands in the mucosal membranes of the lips, cheeks, gums, and genitalia that appear as tiny, whitish-yellow raised lesions. It is a common condition and may be symptomless.

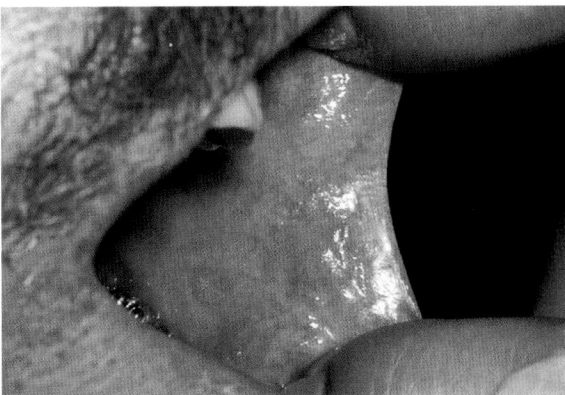

Fordyce spots on the buccal mucosa (Sapp, 2004)

fore-, prefix meaning "front" or "before": *forearm, foregut, forewaters.*

forearm, the portion of the upper extremity between the elbow and the wrist. It contains two long bones, the radius and ulna. Also called **antebrachium.**

forearm crutch, also called **lofstrand crutch.**

forebrain. See **prosencephalon.**

forefinger, the first, or index, finger.

forefoot, the portion of the foot that includes the metatarsus and toes.

foregut /fôr″gut/ [AS, *fore,* in front, *guttas*], the cephalic portion of the embryonic alimentary canal. It consists of endodermal tissue and gives rise to the pharynx, esophagus, stomach, liver, pancreas, most of the small intestine, and respiratory ducts. Compare **hindgut, midgut.**

forehead /fôr′hed/ [AS, *fore,* in front + *heafod,* head], the region of the face superior to the eyes.

foreign body /fôr″in/ [Fr, *forain,* alien; AS, *bodig*], any object or substance found in an organ or tissue in which it does not belong under normal circumstances, such as a bolus of food in the trachea or a particle of dust in the eye.

foreign body granuloma [OFr, *forain* + AS, *bodig* + L, *granulum,* little grain; Gk, *oma,* tumor], a chronic inflammatory mass of tissue that accumulates around foreign bodies such as gravel, splinters, or bits of sutures.

foreign body in airway, anything found in the airway that is not normally present. Examples include food, coins, small pieces of toys, and bones. It is crucial to determine the extent of airway obstruction. The patient may be asymptomatic or may exhibit dyspnea or changes in breathing pattern or color (cyanosis). Removal of the foreign body is generally performed with a fiberoptic laryngoscope and forceps or by bronchoscopy.

foreign body in ear [OFr, *forain* + AS, *bodig* + *eare*], any object found in the ear canal that is not normally part of it, such as a bean, insect, or pebble.

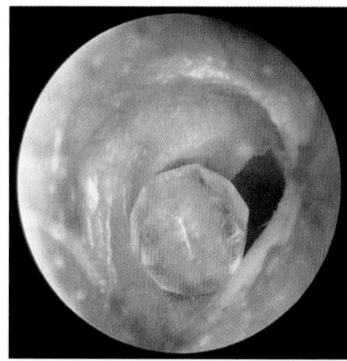

Foreign body in the ear *(Swartz, 2009)*

foreign body in esophagus [OFr, *forain* + AS, *bodig* + Gk, *oisophagos,* gullet], anything found in the esophagus that is not normally a part of the tissue.

foreign body in eye [OFr, *forain* + AS, *bodig* + *eage*], anything found in the eye that is not a normal part of the tissue. Foreign bodies may be superficially embedded in the tissue surfaces or may penetrate the globe.

foreign body in throat [OFr, *forain* + AS, *bodig* + *throte*], anything found in the throat that is not normally present. A common foreign body in the throat is a posteriorly displaced tongue.

foreign body obstruction, a disturbance in normal function or a pathological condition caused by an object lodged in a body orifice, passage, or organ. Most cases occur in children who suddenly inhale or swallow a foreign object or insert it into a body opening. Large boluses of hastily eaten food frequently lodge in the esophagus, causing coughing, choking, and, if the airway is obstructed, asphyxia. Forceful blows to the victim's back between the shoulder blades or the Heimlich maneuver may dislodge the bolus. Esophageal foreign bodies usually produce an immediate reaction but occasionally result in a long asymptomatic period before signs of obstruction or infection are evident. Laryngeal foreign bodies usually cause hoarseness, wheezing, and dyspnea; a sharp object, such as a chicken bone, may perforate the larynx and cause swelling and infection. A foreign body in the trachea may cause wheezing, an audible slap, coughing, and dyspnea. A small object may become lodged in a bronchus, producing coughing, which is often followed by an asymptomatic period before signs of obstruction and inflammation appear.

foreign medical graduate (FMG), a physician trained in and graduated from a medical school outside the United States and Canada. U.S. citizens who graduated from medical schools outside the United States and Canada are also classified as FMGs.

forensic /fôren″sik/ [L, *forum,* public place], **1.** pertaining to courts of law. **2.** relating to or dealing with the application of scientific knowledge to legal problems.

forensic dentistry, the branch of dentistry that deals with the legal aspects of professional dental practices and treatment, with particular emphasis on the use of dental records to identify victims of crimes or accidents.

forensic medicine [L, *forum,* public place, *medicinus,* physician], a branch of medicine that deals with the legal aspects of health care (e.g., autopsies, investigation, and determination of time and cause of death).

forensic nursing, a nursing specialty involving provision of care to victims of crime, such as sexual and other types of assaults, as well as collecting evidence, performing certain types of death investigations, and working with prison inmates.

forensic psychiatry [L, *forum,* public place; Gk, *psyche,* mind, *iatreia,* treament], a branch of psychiatry concerned with the application of psychiatry to law, including criminal responsibility, guardianship, and competence to stand trial.

foreplay /fôr″plā/, sexual activities, such as kissing and fondling, that precede coitus.

foreshortened image. See **image foreshortening.**

foreskin /for″skin/ [AS, *fore* + *skinn*], a loose fold of skin that covers the end of the penis or clitoris. Its removal constitutes circumcision. Also called **prepuce.**

Forestier disease /fō′restē·ā′/ [Jacques Forestier, French neurologist,1890–1978], hyperostosis of the anterolateral part of the vertebral column, especially in the thoracic region.

forestomach, a constricted passage from the esophagus to the stomach lying just inside the opening formed by the cardiac sphincter.

forest yaws /for″ist/ [L, *foris,* outside; Afr, *yaw,* strawberry], a cutaneous form of American leishmaniasis, common in South and Central America, caused by *Leishmania guyanensis.* The disease is chronic, with multiple deep skin ulcers that occasionally spread to the nasal mucosa. Also called **pian bois.**

forewaters /fôr″wôtərs/ [AS, *fore* + *waeter*], the part of the amniotic sac that pouches into the cervix in front of the presenting part of the fetus.

fork /fôrk/ [L, *furca*], **1.** an instrument with prongs. **2.** something resembling such an instrument.

forked tongue /fôrkt/ [L, *furca* + AS, *tunge*], a tongue divided by a longitudinal fissure. Also called **bifid tongue, slit tongue.**

-form, -forme, suffix meaning "having a (specified) shape or form": *acneiform, coliform.*

formaldehyde (HCHO) /fərmal″dəhīd/, a toxic, colorless foul-smelling gas that is soluble in water and used in that form as a disinfectant, fixative, or preservative. Also called **methanol.**

formalin /fôr″məlin/, a clear solution of formaldehyde in water. A 37% solution is used for fixing and preserving biological specimens for pathological and histological examination.

formal operations, a form of thinking following the stage of concrete operations and representing the final, most mature state of thinking. It usually occurs after age 11 and is characterized by true logical thought, capability for deductive reasoning, abstract thinking, formulation and testing of hypotheses, appreciation for multiple perspectives on an issue, and the manipulation of ideas and concepts.

format /fôr″mət/, a computerized arrangement of data for storage or display requiring the division of space on a disk into sectors for storage.

formation /fôrmā″shən/, **1.** a cluster of people who occupy and therefore define a quantum of space. **2.** a structure, shape, or figure.

formative evaluation /fôr″mətiv/, **1.** judgments made about effectiveness of nursing interventions as they are implemented. **2.** (in health care education) periodic evaluation of a student during a course, usually a clinical practicum.

formboard, equipment used in tactile performance testing. It consists of a board with cutouts of various shapes and sizes and blocks of corresponding geometric characteristics. Subjects are tested on their ability to fit the blocks into the proper cutout spaces.

form constancy, the ability to visually manipulate forms, to recognize that a shape remains the same despite changes in size and orientation, and to anticipate outcomes of visual manipulation.

forme fruste /fôrm″ frYst″, fôrm″ fr○̄○st′/ *pl.* **formes frustes** [Fr, rough form], **1.** an incomplete or atypical form of a disease or a disease that is spontaneously arrested before it has run its usual course. **2.** (in genetics) an inherited disorder in which there is minimal expression of an abnormal trait.

formic acid (HCOOH) /fôr″mik/, a colorless, pungent liquid found in nature in nettles, ants, and other insects. It is prepared commercially from oxalic acid and glycerin and from the oxidation of formaldehyde. Formerly used as a vesicant, it currently has no therapeutic applications. Also called *methanoic acid.*

formiminoglutamic acid (FIGLU) /fôrmim′inōgl○̄○tam″ik/, a compound formed in the metabolism of histidine, present in urine in elevated levels in folic acid deficiency. Increased excretion of FIGLU may indicate folic acid deficiency.

-formin, suffix for phenformin-type oral hypoglycemics.

forming, the first stage of group development. This stage encompasses the transition from a group of individuals to a functioning team; members build confidence and trust in one another as well as in their leader.

formol. See **formaldehyde.**

formoterol fumarate, a long-acting beta$_2$-adrenergic agonist bronchodilator; used to maintain and treat asthma and to prevent exercise-induced bronchospasm.

formula /fôr″m(y)ələ/ [L, *forma,* pattern], **1.** a simplified statement, generally using numerals and other symbols, expressing the constituents of a chemical compound, a method for preparing a substance, or a procedure for achieving a desired value or result. *–formulaic, adj.* **2.** *(Informal)* a specially formulated milk mixture or substitute for feeding an infant.

formulary /fôr″myələ′rē/ [L, *forma,* pattern], a listing of drugs intended to include a large enough range of medications and sufficient information about them to enable health practitioners to prescribe treatment that is medically appropriate. Hospitals maintain formularies that list all drugs commonly stocked in their pharmacies. Third-party organizations such as insurance companies usually maintain formularies that list drugs that the company will cover under plan benefits. See also **compendium,** *United States Pharmacopeia.*

formulation /fôr′myələ″shən/ [L, *forma,* pattern], **1.** a pharmacological substance prepared according to a formula. **2.** a systematic and precise statement of a problem, a theory, or a method of analysis in research.

formylmethionine (FMET) /fôr′milməthī″ənēn/, (in molecular genetics) the first amino acid in a protein sequence.

fornication /fôr′nikā″shən/ [L, *fornix,* arch], (in law) sexual intercourse between two people who are not married to each other. The specific legal definition varies from jurisdiction to jurisdiction. In some, both persons are unmarried; in some, one is unmarried; in some, the charge is adultery rather than fornication if the woman is married, regardless of the man's marital status.

fornix /fôr″niks/ *pl.* **fornices** [L, arch], an archlike structure or space, such as the fornix cerebri, the superior or inferior conjunctival fornices, or the vaginal fornices.

fornix cerebri /ser″əbrī/, an archlike body of nerve fibers that lies beneath the corpus callosum of the cranium and serves as the efferent pathway from the hippocampus.

forskolin (FSK), an activator of adenylate cyclase. FSK interacts directly with ion channels, increasing glutamate responses and amplitude and decay time of spontaneous excitatory postsynaptic currents.

Fortaz, a cephalosporin antibiotic. Brand name for **ceftazidime.**

Fort Bragg fever. See **pretibial fever.**

fortified milk [L, *fortis,* strong; AS, *milc*], pasteurized milk enriched with one or more nutrients, usually vitamins A and D, that has been standardized at 400 International Units per quart (fortified vitamin D milk).

fortify, addition of a substance to a food product to increase its nutritional benefit.

forward chaining, a method of measuring rehabilitation performance. The patient performs the first step independently, and the therapist helps the patient perform the rest of the steps. The routine is then repeated with the patient performing the first two steps independently, then the first three steps, and so on.

forward-leaning posture, a respiratory therapy technique intended to reduce or eliminate the involvement of the accessory muscles of respiration in ambulatory patients with breathing difficulty. It involves walking while bent forward in a slightly stooped posture. For patients unable to tolerate functional walking, a special high walker with wheels may be used.

fosamprenavir, a protease inhibitor antiretroviral.
■ INDICATIONS: This drug is used in combination with other antiretrovirals to treat HIV-1 infection.
■ CONTRAINDICATIONS: Known hypersensitivity to protease inhibitors prohibits the use of this drug.
■ ADVERSE EFFECTS: Adverse effects of this drug include rash, pruritus, headache, fatigue, depression, oral paresthesia, and redistribution or accumulation of body fat. Common side effects include nausea, diarrhea, vomiting, and abdominal pain.

Foscavir, an antiviral drug used in the treatment of cytomegalovirus retinitis in conjunction with ganciclovir and for the treatment of herpes simplex infections when acyclovir fails. Brand name for *foscarnet.*

fosfomycin, a urinary antiinfective drug.
■ INDICATIONS: It is used to treat infections of the urinary tract caused by *Enterococcus faecalis* and *Escherichia coli.*
■ CONTRAINDICATIONS: Known hypersensitivity to this drug prohibits its use.
■ ADVERSE EFFECTS: Adverse effects include vaginitis, dysuria, hematuria, menstrual disorder, fever, insomnia, somnolence, migraine, asthenia, nervousness, constipation, dry mouth, flatulence, increased SGPT, dyspepsia, and pruritus. Common side effects are headache, dizziness, nausea, vomiting, anorexia, diarrhea, and rash.

fosinopril, an angiotensin-converting enzyme inhibitor. It inhibits the formation of the hormone angiotensin II, which is a powerful vasoconstrictor that also stimulates the release of the sodium-retaining hormone aldosterone.
■ INDICATIONS: It is prescribed alone or in combination for the treatment of high blood pressure, congestive heart failure, and left ventricular dysfunction following myocardial infarction.
■ CONTRAINDICATIONS: It should not be given to patients with allergy to angiotensin-converting enzyme inhibitors. It should be used with caution in patients with kidney diseases or diabetes or with potassium-containing products.
■ ADVERSE EFFECTS: The side effects most often reported include "first-dose effect," including dizziness and fainting caused by lowered blood pressure, persistent dry nonproductive cough, depression, headache, palpitations, breathing difficulty, and fluid retention.

fosphenytoin, an anticonvulsant drug.

■ INDICATIONS: It is used to treat generalized tonic-clonic seizures and status epilepticus.

■ CONTRAINDICATIONS: Factors that prohibit its use include known hypersensitivity to this drug, psychiatric conditions, pregnancy, bradycardia, sinoatrial and atrioventricular block, and Stokes-Adams syndrome.

■ ADVERSE EFFECTS: Life-threatening effects are ventricular fibrillation, nephritis, agranulocytosis, leukopenia, aplastic anemia, thrombocytopenia, megaloblastic anemia, and Stevens-Johnson syndrome. Other adverse effects include drowsiness, dizziness, insomnia, paresthesias, depression, suicidal tendencies, aggression, headache, confusion, hypotension, nystagmus, diplopia, blurred vision, nausea, vomiting, constipation, anorexia, weight loss, hepatitis, jaundice, gingival hyperplasia, urine discoloration, rash, lupus erythematosus, hirsutism, and hypocalcemia.

Fosrenol, a drug used to reduce serum phosphate in patients with end-stage renal disease. Brand name for **lanthanum (La).**

fossa /fos″ə/ *pl. fossae* [L, ditch], a hollow or depression, especially on the surface of the end of a bone, such as the olecranon fossa or the coronoid fossa.

fossa of vestibule of vagina. See **vestibular fossa.**

Foster bed, a special bed used in the care and treatment of severely injured patients, especially those with spinal injuries. It consists of two Bradford frames mounted on a castered base. The assembly is attached to a rotary bearing mechanism, permitting horizontal turning of the patient without moving the spine. The patient can be rotated to supine and prone positions while maintaining proper immobilization and alignment of injured body structures. A horizontal turning frame permits hyperextension and traction at each end of the frame, and either end of the bed can be elevated to provide countertraction. It can be used in posttraumatic management of patients with spinal instability, with or without cord damage, and in the management of the postoperative patient with multilevel spinal fusion when weight-bearing or ambulation is contraindicated. The Foster bed is also used for halo-femoral traction and maintenance of continuous cervical traction in flexion for patients with unstable cervical neck problems. Compare **CircOlectric (COL) bed™, hyperextension bed, Stryker wedge frame.** See also *Bradford frame.*

Foster Kennedy syndrome /fos′tər ken′ə·dē/ [Robert Foster Kennedy, American neurologist, 1884–1952], a syndrome characterized by retrobulbar neuritis, central scotoma, optic disc atrophy on the side of the lesion, and papilledema on the opposite side, occurring in tumors of the frontal lobe of the brain that press downward.

fo-ti, a climbing perennial herb found in China.

■ INDICATIONS: It is used for tiredness, constipation, cancer, and elevated cholesterol. It appears to be safe and effective as a laxative, but proof of efficacy for other indications is lacking.

■ CONTRAINDICATIONS: It is contraindicated during pregnancy and lactation, in children, and in those with known hypersensitivity to this product or with diarrhea.

foulage. See **pétrissage.**

foundation [L, *fundamentum*], (in dentistry) any device or material added to a remaining tooth structure to enhance the stability and retention of an overlying cast restoration, such as a pin retainer, amalgam, or casting.

foundation model, a health maintenance organization or other health system that is legally established as a tax-exempt, not-for-profit corporation organized to operate as a charitable institution.

fourchette /fŏŏrshet″/ [Fr, fork], a tense band of mucous membranes at the posterior angle of the vagina that connects the posterior ends of the labia minora.

four-handed dentistry, a technique in which a dental assistant or dental hygienist works directly with the dentist on the procedures being done in the mouth of a patient. The technique reduces fatigue and improves the effectiveness of dental procedures.

Fourier transform (FT) /fŏŏryā′/ [Jean B.J. Fourier, French mathematician, 1768–1830; L, *transformare,* to change form], a mathematical procedure that separates out the frequency components of a signal from its amplitudes as a function of time, or vice versa.

Fourier transform imaging [Jean B.J. Fourier], (in medical physics) nuclear magnetic resonance (NMR) imaging techniques in which at least one dimension is phase encoded by applying variable gradient pulses along that dimension before "reading out" the NMR signal with a gradient magnetic field perpendicular to the variable gradient. The Fourier transform is then used to reconstruct an image from the set of encoded NMR signals.

Fournier gangrene /fŏŏrnyā′/ [Jean A. Fournier, French syphilographer, 1832–1914], a rare fulminant infective gangrene of the scrotum or vulva associated with diabetes or alcohol abuse. It occurs after local trauma, operative procedures, underlying urinary tract disease, or a distant acute inflammatory process. It has also been associated with the administration of sodium-glucose cotransporter-2 (SGLT2) inhibitors for the management of type 2 diabetes. Also called *necrotizing fasciitis of the perineum.*

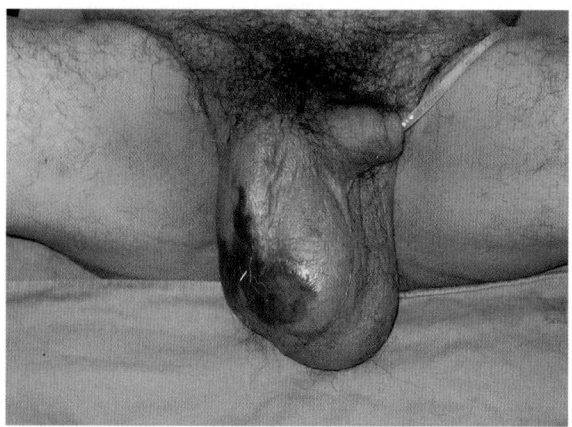

Fournier gangrene of scrotum *(Kobayashi, 2008)*

four-poster orthosis, an orthosis to immobilize the cervical vertebrae. It contains four vertical posts or poles on the anterior and posterior lateral sides of the head and is placed over the shoulders. The head is supported under the chin and occiput, and the posts prevent movement.

four-tailed bandage, a narrow piece of cloth with two ties on each end for wrapping a joint, such as an elbow or knee, or a prominence, such as the nose or chin.

fourth cranial nerve. See **trochlear nerve.**

fourth-degree burn, a burn that extends deeply into the subcutaneous tissue, completely destroying the skin, subcutaneous fat, and underlying tendons and sometimes involving muscle, fascia, or bone.

fourth-generation cephalosporin, a broad-spectrum cephalosporin having the greatest activity against gram-negative organisms of any of the cephalosporins. Cefepime is often so classified, although it is sometimes included with the third-generation cephalosporins.

fourth-generation scanner, a computed tomography machine in which the x-ray source rotates but the detector assembly does not. Radiation detection is accomplished through a fixed, circular array of up to 1000 detectors. Fourth-generation scanners may have scanning times as short as 1 second.

fourth stage of labor [ME, *feower,* four; OFr, *estage* + L, *labor,* work], a postpartum period of about 4 hours after the third stage, or delivery of the placenta. Some complications, especially hemorrhage, occur at this time, necessitating careful observation of the mother.

fourth ventricle [ME, *feower,* four; L, *ventriculus,* little belly], a cavity with a diamond-shaped floor in the hindbrain, communicating below with the central canal of the spinal cord and above with the cerebral aqueduct of the midbrain. At the bottom of the ventricle are surfaces of the pons and medulla.

fovea capitis /fō′vē·ə/ [L, *fovea,* pit], 1. a depression on the proximal surface of the head of the radius where it meets the capitulum of the humerus. 2. a fovea on the head of the femur, where the round ligament is attached.

fovea centralis, an area at the center of the retina where cone cells are concentrated and there are no rod cells. See also **macula lutea.**

Fowler position /fou′lərz/ [George R. Fowler, American surgeon, 1848–1906], the posture assumed by the patient when the head of the bed is raised 90 degrees and his or her knees are elevated slightly. See also **high-Fowler position.**

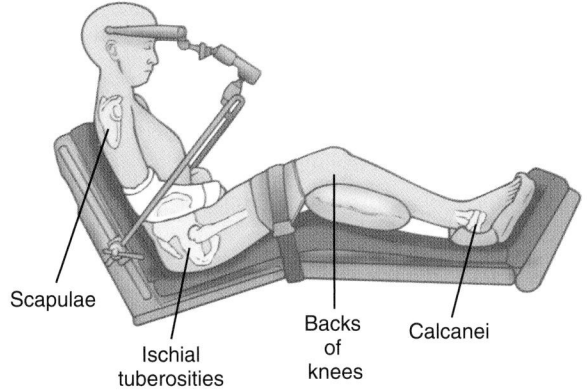

Scapulae

Ischial tuberosities

Backs of knees

Calcanei

Potential pressure areas in the Fowler position
(Rothrock, 2011)

Fox-Fordyce disease /foksfôr′dīs/ [G.H. Fox, American dermatologist, 1846–1937; John Addison Fordyce, American dermatologist, 1858–1925], a chronic skin disease, usually seen in women, characterized by small papular eruptions and other skin changes of apocrine gland-bearing areas, especially the axillae and genitalia, caused by obstruction and rupture of the intraepidermal part of the ducts of the glands. Also called **apocrine miliaria, Fordyce-Fox disease.**

foxglove /foks′glov/, the common name for *Digitalis purpura,* the plant that is a source of digitalis, a powerful cardiac stimulant.

Fox's knife, a flat metallic device used to visualize the relationships of denture baseplate/wax rims to facial landmarks, aiding in the placement of artificial teeth in wax during denture construction.

FPG, abbreviation for **fasting plasma glucose.**

Fr, 1. symbol for the element **francium.** 2. abbreviation for **French scale.**

FR, abbreviation for *fixed ratio.*

fract-, prefix meaning "a breaking": *fractionation, fracture.*

fractional dilation and curettage /frak′shənəl/, a diagnostic procedure in which each section of the uterus is examined and curetted to obtain specimens of the endometrium from all parts of the organ.

fractional excretion of sodium (FE$_{Na}$), an assessment of acute renal failure comparing the sodium clearance with the creatinine clearance.

fractional exhaled nitric oxide (FeNO), a measurement of exhaled nitric oxide, a gas associated with inflammation of the airways.

fractionation /frak′shənā″shən/ [L, *frangere,* to break], 1. (in neurology) a mechanism within the neural arch of the vertebrae whereby only a portion of the efferent nerves innervating a muscle reacts to a stimulus, even when the reflex requirement is maximal, so that a reserve of neurons remains to respond to additional stimuli. Through this phenomenon muscle tension is maintained. 2. (in chemistry) the separation of a substance into its basic constituents by using such procedures as fractional distillation or crystallization. 3. (in bacteriology) the process of isolating a pure culture by successive culturing of a small portion of a colony of bacteria. 4. (in histology) the process of isolating the different components of living cells by centrifugation. 5. (in radiology) the process of administering a dose of radiation in smaller units over time (rather than in a single large dose) to minimize surrounding tissue damage. Also called **dose fractionation.**

fraction of inspired oxygen (FiO$_2$) [L, *frangere,* to break, *inspirare,* to breathe in; Gk, *oxys,* sharp, *genein,* to produce], the proportion of oxygen in the air that is inspired.

fracture /frak″chər/ [L, *frangere,* to break], 1. the breaking of a part, especially of a bone or tooth. 2. a traumatic injury to a bone in which the continuity of the bone tissue is broken. A fracture is classified by the bone involved, the part of that bone, and the nature of the break, such as a comminuted fracture of the head of the tibia. See also *specific types of fractures.*

fracture-dislocation, a break in the bony structures of any joint, with associated dislocation of the same joint.

fracture of clavicle [L, *frangere + clavicula,* little key], a break in the long bone of the shoulder girdle. It is typically accompanied by pain, swelling, and a protuberance and depression over the site of the injury. The patient usually supports the arm on the injured side at the elbow. Treatment generally involves application of a clavicle strap or a figure-eight bandage.

fracture of olecranon [L, *frangere + Gk, olekranon,* point of the elbow], a break in the bony prominence of the ulna at the elbow joint. Different types of olecranon fractures may occur, depending on the articular surfaces involved. The triceps, which normally extends the elbow, may become spastic as a result of the injury.

fracture of patella [L, *frangere + patella,* small pan], a break in the sesamoid knee cap. The fracture often occurs in automobile accidents in which the knee strikes the dashboard. The damage is complicated by reflex bracing of the quadriceps femoris muscle, which pulls the fragments apart. Treatment includes suturing the bone fragments and confining the patient in a long-leg cast.

fracture of radius [L, *frangere + ray*], a break in the radius, usually with backward and radial displacement of the wrist and hand. The fracture commonly occurs when a

Types and causes of fractures

Type	Description	Cause
Avulsion	Fracture that pulls bone and other tissues from usual attachments	Direct energy or force, with resisted extension of bone and joint
Bucket-handle	Double vertical fractures of pelvis on same side, resulting in pelvic dislocation	Direct blow or anterior compression force, with or without sacral torsion
Butterfly	Butterfly-shaped piece of fractured bone, usually accompanying comminuted fracture	Direct, indirect, or rotational force to bone
Comminuted	Fracture with more than two pieces; may have significant associated soft tissue trauma	Direct crushing injury or force to tissues and bone
Compound (open)	Skin broken over fracture; possible soft tissue trauma	Moderate to severe energy that is continuous and exceeds tissue tolerances
Compression	Fracture is squeezed or wedged together at one side	Compressive, axial energy or force applied directly from above fracture site
Displaced	Fracture with one, both, or all fragments out of normal alignment	Direct energy or force to site
Greenstick	Break in only one cortex of bone	Minor direct or indirect energy
Impacted	Fracture with one end wedged into opposite end or inside fractured fragment	Compressive axial energy or force directly to distal fragment
Intraarticular	Fracture involving bones inside a joint	Direct or indirect energy or force to joint
Lead pipe (torus)	Fracture of one cortex of shafts of radius and ulna (one cortex of each bone), shown as wrinkle or buckle	Direct blow to forearm or indirect compressive force, as from a fall
Linear	As a line, so can be transverse or oblique	Minor or moderate energy of force directly to bone
Neoplastic (pathological)	Transverse, oblique, or spiral fracture of bone weakened by tumor pressure or presence	Minor energy or force, which may be direct or indirect
Oblique	Fracture at oblique angle across both cortices	Direct or indirect energy, with angulation and some compression
Occult	Fracture that is hidden or not readily discernible	Minor force or energy
Segmental	Fracture with two or more pieces or segments	Direct or indirect moderate to severe force

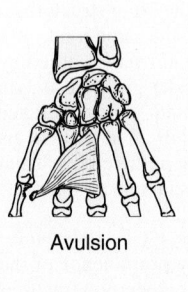
Avulsion
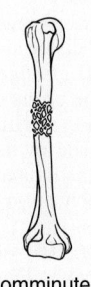
Comminuted
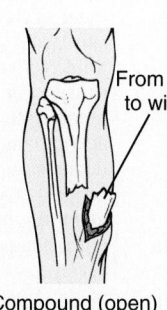
From within to without
Compound (open)
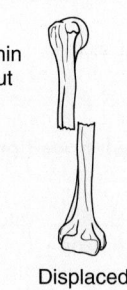
Displaced
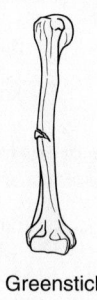
Greenstick
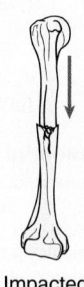
Impacted
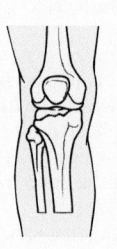
Intraarticular
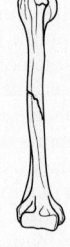
Oblique
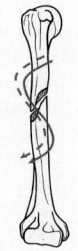
Spiral
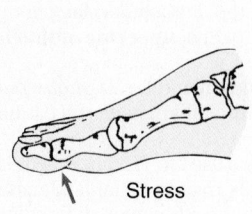
Stress
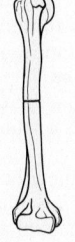
Transverse

Types and causes of fractures—cont'd

Type	Description	Cause
Spiral	Fracture that curves around cortices and may become displaced by twisting	Direct or indirect twisting energy or force with distal part held or unable to move
Stellate	Central fracture point from which fissures radiate	Direct blow or force of moderate energy
Stress	Crack in one cortex of bone	Repetitive direct energy or force, as from jogging, running, or striking a lever, or from osteoporosis
Transverse	Horizontal break through bone	Direct or indirect energy toward bone

Illustrations from Lewis SL et al: *Medical surgical nursing: assessment and management of clinical problems,* ed 8, St Louis, 2011, Mosby; and Lewis SL et al: *Medical surgical nursing: assessment and management of clinical problems,* ed 7, St. Louis, 2007 Mosby.

falling person extends the arm and hand in an effort to cushion the impact. See also **Colles' fracture.**

fracture of skull [L, *frangere* + AS, *skulle,* bowl], a break in one or more of the cranial bones. A fracture in the vault of the skull is usually a compound fracture and is complicated by possible damage to brain tissue, particularly if shards of bone are driven into the brain by the force of the trauma.

fracture pan, a bedpan in which the upper edge is flattened to facilitate correct placement for patients who have difficulty raising their hips. It allows the bedpan to be slid under the patient.

fracture threshold, a measure of bone density used in predicting osteoporosis risk factors. Various investigators have established different methods of interpreting bone density data. One method predicts that 95% of women will have vertebral fractures if their trabecular bone volume is less than 14% of the mean.

fragile X syndrome /fraj′əl/, a reproductive disorder characterized by a nearly broken X chromosome, which has a tip hanging by a flimsy thread. It is the most common inherited cause of cognitive impairment. Only about 75% of the results of tests for the broken chromosome are accurate. Some healthy individuals may possess fragile X chromosomes without exhibiting symptoms and may transmit the condition to children or grandchildren.

fragilitas ossium. See **osteogenesis imperfecta.**

fragment /frag′mənt/ [L, *frangere,* to break], one of the small pieces into which a larger entity has been broken.

fragmented fracture. See **comminuted fracture.**

Fragmin, a low-molecular-weight heparin. Brand name for **dalteparin sodium.**

frail elder, an older person (usually above 85 years of age) who has multiple physical or mental disabilities that may interfere with the ability to perform activities of daily living independently.

fraise /frāz/ [Fr, strawberry], a smooth hemispheric or conic burr with cutting edges. It is used for enlarging trephine openings or cutting osteopathic flaps.

Fraley syndrome, nephralgia with dilation of the upper pole renal calices around the kidney caused by compression of the adjacent infundibulum, usually caused by pressure from vessels serving that part of the kidney.

frambesia, framboesia. See **yaws.**

frame /frām/, a structure, usually rigid, designed for giving support to or for immobilizing a part.

frame of reference [AS, *framian,* to help; L, *referre,* to carry back], **1.** the personal guidelines of an individual, taken as a whole. An individual frame of reference reflects the person's social status, cultural norms, and concepts. **2.** (in occupational therapy) the framework that assists the occupational therapy practitioner in identifying problems, completing evaluations, developing interventions, and measuring outcomes.

Franceschetti syndrome /fran′chesket″ēz/ [Adolphe Franceschetti, Swiss ophthalmologist, 1896–1968], a complete form of mandibulofacial dysostosis. See also **Treacher Collins syndrome.**

franchise dentistry /fran″chīz/ [Fr, exemption; L, *dens,* tooth], the practice of dentistry under a trade name purchased from another dentist or dental practice. Under a franchise license agreement, the franchiser may use the trade name, associated marketing products, and treatment techniques for a sum of money, in accordance with the franchise rules and regulations.

Francisella, a genus of nonmotile, nonspore-forming gram-negative aerobic bacteria that is a facultative intracellular pathogen of macrophages. Frequently found in natural waters, it can be parasitic in humans, other mammals, birds, and arthropods. The organism causes tularemia in humans.

francium (Fr) /fran″sē·əm/ [France], a metallic element of the alkali metal group. Its atomic number is 87, and the mass of its longest-lived isotope is 223. Formed from the decay of actinium, all of its 20 isotopes are radioactive and short-lived.

frank [L, *francus,* forthright], obvious or clinically evident, such as the unequivocal presence of a condition or a disease. Kinds include *frank bleeding.*

Frank biopsy guide, a trademark for a device consisting of a long needle containing a hooked wire used to obtain biopsy samples of breast tissue. The needle is inserted into the breast until its tip nearly touches the lesion observed by mammography. The needle is withdrawn, but the hooked wire remains to locate the tissue site. The surgeon cuts along the wire or otherwise approaches the hooked end of the wire and removes the tissue. See also **Kopan's needle.**

frank breech [L, *francus* + ME, *brec*], an intrauterine position of the fetus in which the buttocks present at the maternal pelvic inlet, the legs are straight up in front of the body, and the feet are at the shoulders. Compare **complete breech, footling breech.** See also **breech birth.**

Frankfurt horizontal plane [Frankfurt-am-Main (anthropological) Agreement, 1882], (in dentistry) a craniometric surface determined by the inferior borders of the bony orbits and the upper margin of the auditory meatus. It passes through the two orbitales and the two tragions and is commonly used as a reference surface in orthodontic diagnosis and treatment planning.

Frankfurt line. See **Reid's base line.**

Frankfurt-mandibular incisor angle (FMIA), (in dentistry) the precumbency of the mandibular incisor to the Frankfurt horizontal plane. The angle is formed by the intersection of the long axis of the lower central incisor with the Frankfurt-mandibular plane.

Frank-Starling relationship [Otto Frank, German physiologist, 1865–1944; Ernest H. Starling, English physiologist, 1866–1927], a mathematical expression stating that stroke volume increases with diastolic volume. The relationship is based on the principle that the force exerted by the myocardial fibers during contraction is directly proportional to their length or degree of stretch at the start of contraction. Because there are no adequate in vivo methods of measuring fiber length or diastolic volume, pulmonary artery obstructive pressure or pulmonary artery end-diastolic pressure is used as an index of diastolic volume. The relationship holds over a range of diastolic volumes. Beyond that range, the myocardial fibers are stretched past the point of maximal overlap between thick and thin filaments, and contractile force and stroke volume decrease. Also called **Starling's law of the heart,** *Frank-Starling mechanism.*

Fraser syndrome /frā′zer/ [George Robert Fraser, Czechoslovakian-born American geneticist, b. 1932], an autosomal-recessive abnormality characterized by absence of an opening in the eyelids, disorganization of one or both ocular globes, malformed ears, cleft palate, laryngeal stenosis, syndactyly, meningoencephalocele, imperforate anus, cardiac defects, and maldeveloped kidneys. Also called **cryptophthalmos syndrome.**

fraternal twins. See **dizygotic twins.**

F-ratio [Sir Ronald Aylmer *Fisher,* British statistician, 1890–1962], **1.** the variance between the means of several groups relative to the variance within the groups, used in the *F*-test in the analysis of variance. **2.** the variance between or within treatments.

fraud /frôd/ [L, *fraudare,* to cheat], (in law) the act of intentionally misleading or deceiving another person by any means so as to cause him or her legal injury, usually the loss of something valuable or the surrender of a legal right resulting from the action of that person on the misrepresentation.

Fraunhofer lines, absorption bands or lines seen in a spectrum, caused by the absorption of groups of light rays in their passage through solids, liquids, or gases.

Fraunhofer zone /froun′hōfer/ [Joseph von Fraunhofer, German optician, 1787–1826], the zone farthest from the face of an ultrasound transducer. It is characterized by a divergence of the ultrasound beam and a more uniform ultrasound intensity. Also called **far field.** See also **Fresnel zone.**

FRC, abbreviation for **functional residual capacity.**

F.R.C.P., abbreviation for *Fellow of the Royal College of Physicians of London.*

F.R.C.S., abbreviation for *Fellow of the Royal College of Surgeons.*

freckle [ME, *freken*], a brown or tan macule on the skin that results from exposure to sunlight. There is an inherited tendency to freckling, and it is most frequently seen in persons with red hair. Freckles are harmless, but people who freckle easily should avoid excessive sun exposure or use protective sunscreens because they have a tendency toward development of more serious actinic skin changes. Compare **lentigo.**

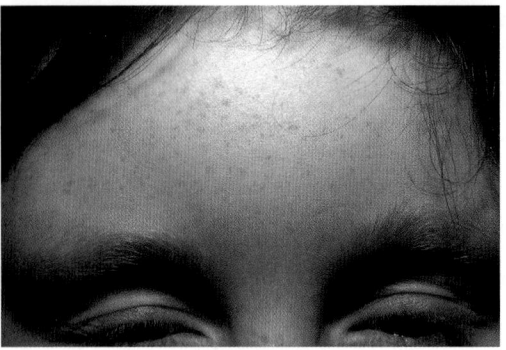

Child with freckles *(Pride et al, 2008)*

Fredet-Ramstedt operation. See **pyloromyotomy.**

free-air chamber [AS, *freo,* free; Gk, *aer,* air; L, *camera,* vault], an ionization device used as a primary standard for calibrating x-ray exposure.

free, appropriate public education (FAPE), free public education that is mandated for all children, adolescents, and young adults who have disabilities and are between 3 and 21 years of age.

free association, **1.** spontaneous, consciously unrestricted association of ideas, feelings, or mental images. **2.** spontaneous verbalization of thoughts and emotions that enter the consciousness during psychoanalysis. It is the basis of classical freudian analysis and also of jungian-type analysis.

freebase. See **crack.**

freebasing, a chemical process (e.g., ether extraction, addition of ammonia) used to increase the stimulating effect of illicit drugs, such as cocaine, by converting the salt of the drug into its noncharged base form that can more readily enter the brain. The resulting product is smoked.

free circulating phagocyte. See **phagocyte.**

free clinic, a clinic or health program, usually located in a neighborhood setting, that provides health care for ambulatory patients at nominal or no cost.

Freedom of Information Act, a law requiring federal agencies to provide access to information, with some exceptions, upon request. Amendments to the original law have made it easier for individuals to review agency records. The Department of Health and Human Services makes many records available on the Web sites of its offices.

freedom to suspend reality, (in occupational therapy) the ability to participate in "make-believe," or activities in which the participants pretend; the ability to create new play situations and to interact with materials, space, and people in ways that are fluid, flexible, and not bound to the constraints of real life.

free fatty acid (FFA) [AS, *freo* + *faett* + L, *acidus,* sour], a nonesterified fatty acid, released by the hydrolysis of triglycerides within adipose tissue. Free fatty acids can be used as an immediate source of energy by many organs and can be converted by the liver into ketone bodies.

free-floating anxiety, a generalized, persistent, pervasive fear that is not attributable to any specific object, event, or source. See also **anxiety.**

free-form foot orthosis, an orthosis that is molded directly to a patient's foot. It requires less material and time to produce than other orthoses but does not provide a positive model for a more exact fabrication of a balanced orthosis.

free gingiva, the unattached portion of the gum coronal to the junctional epithelium. It encircles each tooth and forms a gingival sulcus or crevice.

free gingival groove,   a shallow line or depression on the gingival surface at the junction of the free and attached gingivae. Also called **mucogingival line.**

free graft [AS, *freo* + Gk, *graphein,* stylus], a graft completely removed from its original site and replaced at a new site in a single one-stage operation.

free-induction decay (FID), a signal emitted by the atomic nuclei in a tissue after a radiofrequency pulse has excited the nuclear spins at resonance. The decaying oscillation of the nuclei back to their normal state causes them to emit photons, which provide the signal from which a magnetic resonance image is made.

free macrophage [AS, *freo* + Gk, *makros,* large, *phagein,* to eat], a motile macrophage derived from a monocyte. It responds to chemotactic stimuli and migrates from blood vessels to tissue spaces.

Freeman-Sheldon syndrome /frē′mən shel′dən/ [Ernest Arthur Freeman, British orthopedic surgeon, 1900–1975; Joseph Harold Sheldon, British physician, 1920–1964], a congenital anomaly, transmitted as an autosomal-dominant trait, consisting of characteristic flattened, masklike facies; small mouth, the lips protruding as in whistling; deep-set eyes with hypertelorism; camptodactyly with ulnar drift of the fingers; and clubfoot. Also called **craniocarpotarsal dystrophy, whistling face syndrome, whistling face-windmill vane hand syndrome.**

free nerve ending, a receptor nerve ending that is not enclosed in a capsule. A typical free nerve ending consists of a bare axon that may be myelinated or unmyelinated. It is often found in fibrous capsules, ligaments, or synovial spaces and may be sensitive to mechanical or biochemical stimuli.

free phagocyte. See **phagocyte.**

free radical, an atom or molecule with at least one unpaired electron. Oxygen is a stable diradical, but most other free radicals are unstable and react readily with other molecules.

free-radical theory of aging, a concept of aging based on the premise that the main causative factor is an imbalance between the production and elimination in the body tissues of free chemical radicals from oxygen metabolism.

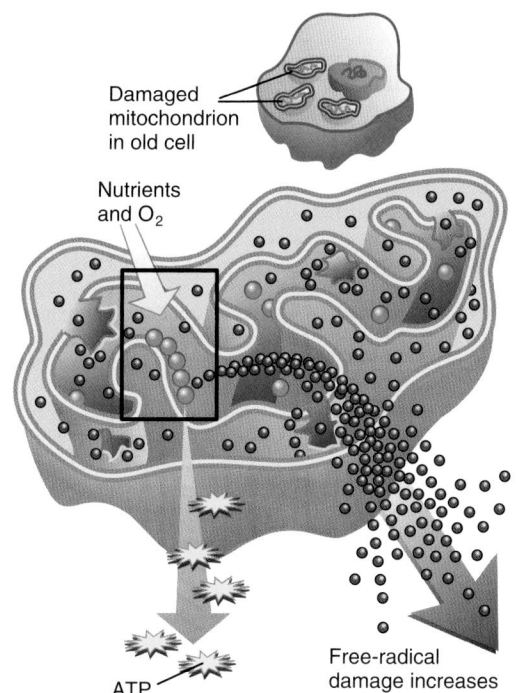

Damaged mitochondrion in old cell

Nutrients and O_2

ATP

Free-radical damage increases

Free-radical theory of aging *(McCance and Huether, 2010)*

free-standing tax-exempt clinic, (in U.S. managed care) an organization that may employ physicians or make arrangements with physicians as independent contractors. It is usually organized as a not-for-profit, tax-exempt corporation. It is the direct provider of health care and holds preferred provider organization and health maintenance organization contracts, bills and collects in its own name, and owns the accounts receivable department.

free thyroxine, the amount of the unbound, active thyroid hormone thyroxine circulating in the blood, measured by specific laboratory procedures. See also **free thyroxine index.**

free thyroxine index, the amount of unbound, physiologically active thyroxine (T_4) in serum. This amount is determined by direct assay or, more frequently, calculated on the basis of an in vitro uptake test. In this test the uptake (by resin or charcoal) of labeled triiodothyronine (T_3) is measured; because T_3 is less strongly bound by serum, it is used instead of T_4. The free T_4 index is then obtained by multiplying the T_3 uptake by the total concentration of T_4 in serum.

free thyroxine (FT_4) test, a blood test used to determine thyroid function, especially when the patient has concurrent clinical situations that may alter protein blood levels. Abnormal levels indicate either hyper- or hypothyroid states.

free water, that portion of the water in body tissue that is not bound by macromolecules or organelles.

free-water clearance, the calculated volume of water that must be added to a given volume of urine to make it isotonic to the plasma.

freeway space [AS, *freo* + *wegan* + L, *spatium*], the separation between the occlusal surfaces of the maxillary and mandibular teeth when the mandible is in its rest position. Also called **interocclusal distance, interocclusal gap.**

freezing, a sudden inability of patients with Parkinson's disease to initiate or continue repetitive motor activity. The patient may be unable to take the first step in walking or, if walking, may find a real or imagined obstacle that causes the feet to remain in one spot.

freezing point [ME, *fresen,* to be cold; L, *punctus,* pricked], the temperature at which a substance changes from a liquid to a solid state. The freezing point for water is 32° on the Fahrenheit scale and 0° on the Celsius scale.

Freiberg infraction [Albert H. Freiberg, American surgeon, 1868–1940; L, *infarcire,* to stuff], an abnormal orthopedic condition characterized by osteochondritis or aseptic necrosis of bone tissue, most commonly affecting the head of the second metatarsal.

Frei test /frī/ [William S. Frei, German dermatologist, 1885–1943], *(Obsolete)* a test that was performed to confirm a diagnosis of lymphogranuloma venereum. Killed antigen, originally derived from infected patients, was injected intradermally in one forearm, and a control material was injected into the other arm. If a red, thickened papule developed at the site of injection of antigen, the test result was positive. The test is now of historical significance only.

Frejka splint /frā″kə/, a corrective device used to maintain abduction and articulation of the head of the femur with the acetabulum in a baby born with dislocated hips. It consists of a pillow that is belted between the legs. See also **congenital dislocation of the hip.**

fremitus /frem″itəs/ [L, a growling], a tremulous vibration of the chest wall caused by vocalization that is primarily palpated during physical examination. Kinds include **tactile fremitus, vocal fremitus.**

frena. See **frenum.**

French scale (Fr), a method of sizing catheters, tubules, and sounds in which each Fr unit is equivalent to 1.3 mm.

frenectomy /frənek″təmē/ [L, *frenum,* bridle; Gk, *ektomē,* excision], a surgical procedure for excising a frenum or frenulum, such as the excision of the lingual frenum from its attachment into the mucoperiosteal covering of the alveolar process to correct ankyloglossia. Compare **frenotomy.**

frenga. See **bejel.**

Frenkel exercises [Heinrich S. Frenkel, Swiss neurologist, 1860–1931], a system of slow, repetitious exercises of increasing difficulty, developed to treat ataxia in multiple sclerosis and similar disorders.

frenotomy /frənot″əmē/ [L, *frenum* + Gk, *temnein,* to cut], a surgical procedure for repairing a defective frenum, such as the cutting or lengthening of the lingual frenum to correct ankyloglossia. Compare **frenectomy.**

frenulum. See **frenum.**

frenulum linguae. See **frenulum of the tongue.**

frenulum of labia minora, the small transverse fold formed by the union of the labia minora posterior to the vestibule.

frenulum of the clitoris. See **labia minora.**

frenulum of the ileal orifice, a fold formed by the joined extremities of the ileal orifice, extending partly around the lumen of the colon. It was called frenulum of ileocecal valve before it was discovered that the valve was found only in cadavers.

frenulum of the lips /fren′yələm/, a fold of movement-limiting mucous membrane running from the gums to the lips or tongue. The frenulum of the lower lip is called the frenulum labii inferioris. That of the upper lip is the frenulum labii superioris.

frenulum of the tongue [L, *frenum,* bridle; AS, *tunge*], a longitudinal fold of mucous membrane connecting the floor of the mouth to the underside of the tongue in midline. A congenital defect causes an abnormal shortness of the frenulum, causing tongue-tie, which can be surgically corrected. Also called **frenulum linguae, lingual frenum.**

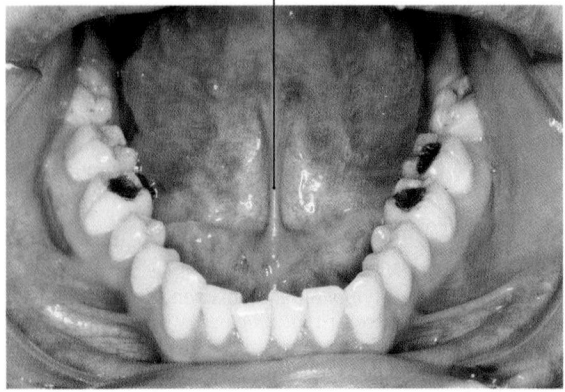

Frenulum of tongue

Frenulum *(Paulson, 2013)*

frenum /frē″nəm/ *pl. frenums, frena* [L, *frenum,* bridle], a restraining portion or structure; a fold of mucous membrane that connects two parts, one more or less movable. Also called **frenulum.**

frequency (F) /frē″kwənsē/ [L, *frequens,* frequent], **1.** the number of repetitions of any phenomenon within a fixed period, such as the number of heartbeats per minute. **2.** (in biometry) the proportion of the number of persons having a discrete characteristic to the total number of persons being studied. **3.** (in electronics) the number of

cycles of a periodic quantity, such as alternating current, that occur in a period of 1 second. Electromagnetic frequencies, formerly expressed in cycles per second (cps), are now expressed in hertz (Hz).

freshening, a step in the process of wound repair in which fibrin, granulation, and early scar tissue are removed in preparation for secondary closure.

fresh frozen plasma (FFP) [ME, *fresen,* to be cold; Gk, *plassein,* to mold], plasma separated from whole blood and frozen within 8 hours of collection. FFP has a shelf life of 12 months when stored at minus 18° C or below. It contains normal levels of all the coagulation proteins, including the labile factors V and VIII. See also **plasma.**

Fresnel zone /freznel′/ [Augustine J. Fresnel, French physicist, 1788–1827], the region nearest the face of an ultrasound transducer. It is characterized by a highly collimated beam with great variation in ultrasound intensity and is generally the area of best image resolution. Also called **near field.**

freudian /froi″dē·ən/ [Sigmund Freud], **1.** *adj.,* pertaining to Sigmund Freud; his theories and doctrines, which stress the formative years of childhood as the basis for later psychoneurotic disorders, primarily through the unconscious repression of instinctual drives and sexual desires; and his system of psychoanalysis, based on free association and dream analysis, for treating such disturbances. **2.** *adj.,* pertaining to anything that is easily interpreted according to the theories of Freud or in psychoanalytic terms. **3.** *adj.,* pertaining to the school of psychiatry based on Freud's teachings. **4.** *n.,* one who adheres to Freud's school of psychiatry. See also **psychoanalysis.**

freudian fixation [Sigmund Freud], an arrest in psychosexual development characterized by a firm emotional attachment to another person or object. Kinds include **father fixation, mother fixation.**

freudianism /froi″dē·əniz′əm/, the school of psychiatry based on the psychoanalytic theories and psychotherapeutic methods of treating disorders developed by Sigmund Freud and his followers. Also called **freudism.** See also **psychoanalysis.**

freudian slip, (in freudian psychology) a behavioral error in speech or action that is believed to reveal a hidden motive in the unconscious thoughts or feelings of the perpetrator.

freudism. See **freudianism.**

Freud, Sigmund /froid/ [Austrian neurologist, 1856–1939], founder of a complex integrated theory of psychological causes of mental disorders, some, such as hysteria, with physical symptoms. Among tenets of freudian theory are that human beings are motivated by a pleasure principle; receive internal stimulation from a sex instinct and a death instinct; have personality structures that can be divided into ego, superego, and id; and have unconscious, preconscious, and conscious levels of mental activity. See also **freudian, freudian fixation, freudianism.**

friable /frī′əbəl/ [L, *friare,* to crumble], easily shattered, crumbled, or pulverized, such as tissues of the liver.

fricative /frik″ətiv/, a consonant speech sound such as an /f/ or /s/, made by forcing an airstream through a constricted opening.

Fricke dosimeter, a meter that quantifies radiation dose by measuring the change in the concentration of ferric ions in a solution subject to irradiation.

friction /frik″shən/ [L, *fricare,* to rub], **1.** the act of rubbing one object against another. See also **attrition. 2.** a type of massage in which deeper tissues are stroked or rubbed, usually through strong circular movements of the hand. See also **massage.**

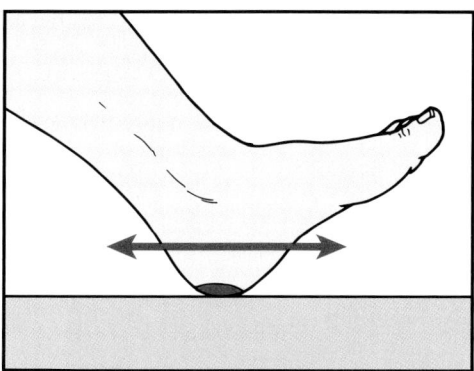

Friction as a cause of pressure ulcers
(Cameron and Monroe, 2011)

frictional force /frik″shənəl/, the force component parallel to the surfaces at the point of contact between two objects. The frictional component, in contact between curved objects, may be tangential to the surfaces. Frictional force may be increased or decreased by such factors as moisture on a surface.

friction burn, tissue injury caused by abrasion of the skin. See also **abrasion.**

friction rub, a dry, grating sound heard with a stethoscope during auscultation. It is a normal finding when heard over the liver and splenic areas. A friction rub auscultated over the pericardial area is suggestive of pericarditis; a rub over the pleural area may be a sign of lung disease.

Friedländer's bacillus /frēd″lendərz/ [Carl Friedländer, German pathologist, 1847–1887]. See *Klebsiella pneumoniae.*

Friedländer pneumonia [Carl Friedländer; Gk, *pneumon,* lung], a form of bronchopneumonia with a high mortality rate, particularly among older patients, caused by the bacterium *Klebsiella pneumoniae.* The pneumonic patches tend to become confluent, and those who survive may experience pulmonary abscesses and necrosis.

Friedman curve /frēd″mən/ [Emanuel A. Friedman, American obstetrician, b. 1926], a graph depicting the progress of labor, often used in reference to the normal progress of labor and a vaginal delivery. The labor curve is divided into latent and active phases, with the latter subdivided into latent, acceleration, maximum slope, and deceleration. A deviation from this graph may be indicative of an abnormality of labor, which may require intervention.

Friedman's test [Maurice H. Friedman, American physiologist, 1903-1991], **1.** *(Obsolete)* an early method of testing for pregnancy in which a sample of urine from a woman was injected into a mature unmated female rabbit, also called the *rabbit test.* If the woman was pregnant, the rabbit's ovaries would change in response to the presence of human chorionic gonadotropin. Modern pregnancy tests are still based on the presence of human chorionic gonadotropin, but a live animal is no longer required. **2.** (in statistics) a nonparametric alternative to the one-way analysis of variance (ANOVA), with repeated measures used to test for differences between groups when the dependent variable is ordinal.

Friedreich ataxia /frēd″rīsh/ [Nikolaus Friedreich, German physician, 1825–1882], a condition characterized by muscular weakness, loss of muscular control, weakness of the lower extremities, and an abnormal gait. It may be hereditary and exhibits both dominant and recessive inheritance patterns. The primary pathological feature is pronounced sclerosis of the posterior columns of the spinal cord with possible involvement of the spinocerebellar tracts and the corticospinal tracts. Friedreich's ataxia usually affects individuals between 5 and 20 years of age. The highest incidence of onset is at puberty. The characteristically ataxic gait may progress to severe disability. Over a period of years a child who is affected may also have ataxia of the upper extremities and difficulty in performing simple maneuvers such as writing or handling eating utensils. The characteristic gait of this disease is caused by a cavus deformity, or clawfoot. The gait and the stance of the affected individual are unsteady. A positive Romberg sign may be evident, and Babinski sign is present with absent or decreased deep reflexes. The condition may also cause slurred speech, head tremors, tachycardia, and cardiac failure. Thoracic scoliosis is present in approximately 80% to 90% of the patients afflicted. All the signs and symptoms are progressive. There is no cure. Treatment is supportive. Orthoses may be useful to varying degrees in prevention of associated deformities and maintenance of an ambulatory status. Correction of the foot deformity allows the patient to remain ambulatory as long as possible and is performed when the disease process does not appear to be progressing, thereby reducing the potential for recurrence. Spinal fusion may correct the associated scoliosis. In progression of this disease, death usually results from myocardial failure.

Friedreich's sign [Nikolaus Friedreich; L, *signum,* sign], the diastolic collapse of the jugular veins in adherent pericardium.

Fried's rule, a method of estimating the dose of medicine for a child by multiplying the adult dose by the child's age in months and dividing the product by 150. See also **Clark's rule.**

frigid /frij″id/ [L, *frigidus,* cold], **1.** lacking warmth of feeling; unemotional; unimaginative; without passion or ardor and stiff or formal in manner. **2.** (of a woman) unresponsive to sexual advances or stimuli, abnormally indifferent or averse to sexual intercourse, or unable to have an orgasm during sexual intercourse. Compare **impotence.** See also **orgasm.** –*frigidity, n.*

fringe field /frinj/, in magnetic resonance imaging, the part of the magnetic field that extends away from the confines of the magnet and cannot be used for imaging. It may affect nearby equipment and personnel.

frit /frit, frē/ [Fr, fried], a partially or wholly fused porcelain that is cracked by plunging into water while hot. It is used to make dental porcelain powders.

frog leg position. See **Lauenstein method.**

frog sign, *(Nontechnical)* prominent neck vein palpitations associated with cardiac rhythm abnormalities. See also **cannon A wave.**

Fröhlich syndrome. See **adiposogenital dystrophy.**

frôlement /frôlmäN″/ [Fr, brushing], **1.** the rustling type of sound often heard on auscultating the chest in diseases of the pericardium. **2.** a kind of massage that uses a light brushing stroke with the hand. See also **massage.**

Froment sign, the flexing of the terminal phalanx of the thumb against the flexed index finger. See **thumb sign.**

front-, prefix combining form meaning "forehead" or "front": *frontal bone.*

frontal bone /fron″təl/ [L, *frons,* forehead], a single cranial bone that forms the front of the skull from above the orbits posteriorly to a junction with the parietal bones at the coronal suture and sagittal suture (bregma).

frontal crest, a midline ridge of bone extending from the surface of the frontal bone. It is a point of attachment for the falx cerebri.

frontal lobe, the largest of five lobes constituting each of the two cerebral hemispheres. It lies beneath the frontal bone; occupies part of the lateral, medial, and inferior surfaces of each hemisphere; and extends posteriorly to the central sulcus and inferiorly to the lateral fissure. It is responsible for voluntary control over most skeletal muscles. The frontal lobe significantly influences personality and is

F

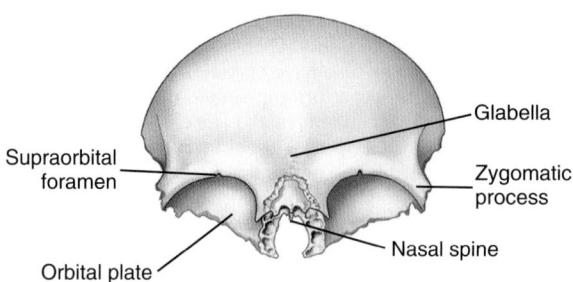

Frontal bone

associated with the higher mental activities, such as planning, judgment, emotion, and conceptualization. Compare **central lobe, occipital lobe, parietal lobe, temporal lobe.**

frontal lobe dementia, any of various dementias caused by frontal lobe lesions, such as that seen in Pick's disease.

frontal lobe syndrome, behavioral and personality changes usually observed after a neoplastic or traumatic frontal lobe lesion. The patient may become sociopathic, boastful, hypomanic, uninhibited, exhibitionistic, and subject to outbursts of irritability or violence. In other cases the person may become depressed, apathetic, lacking in initiative, negligent about personal appearance, and inclined to perseverate. Partial frontal lobectomy was formerly performed by some psychosurgeons to reduce drive in extremely disturbed psychotic patients, but the results were highly questionable.

frontal nerve, the largest branch of the ophthalmic nerve. Its two terminal branches are the supratrochlear nerve and the supraorbital nerve.

frontal plane, **1.** any of the vertical planes passing through the body from the head to the feet, perpendicular to the sagittal planes. **2.** the plane parallel to the long axis of the body and at right angles to the median sagittal plane, dividing the body into front and back portions. Also called **coronal plane.** Compare **median plane, sagittal plane, transverse plane.** See also **frontal section.**

frontal pole [L, *frons,* forehead, *polus*], the anterior extremity of the frontal lobe of the cerebrum.

frontal section [L, *frons,* forehead, *sectio,* a cutting], a section of the head or other body part cut into anterior and posterior portions. Also called **coronal section.** See also **frontal plane.**

frontal sinus, one of a pair of small cavities in the frontal bone of the skull that communicate with the nasal cavity and lie above the orbits. The frontal sinuses are situated behind the superciliary arches and are lined with a mucous membrane that is continuous with that of the nasal cavity. Each sinus opens into the anterior part of the middle meatus through the frontonasal duct. The frontal sinuses are absent at birth, become well developed between the seventh and eighth years, and reach their full size after puberty. Compare **ethmoidal air cell, maxillary sinus, sphenoidal sinus.**

frontal-temporal dementia, any of several degenerative conditions of the frontal and anterior temporal lobes that cause personality and behavioral changes sometimes mistaken for those of Alzheimer disease and may eventually progress to immobility and loss of speech. There is not the memory loss seen in Alzheimer disease, but there is often hyperorality.

frontal vein, one of a pair of superficial veins of the face, arising in the plexus of the forehead. Each frontal vein communicates with the frontal tributaries of the superficial temporal vein and lies near the vein of the opposite side as it courses toward the root of the nose. Compare **angular vein, facial vein.**

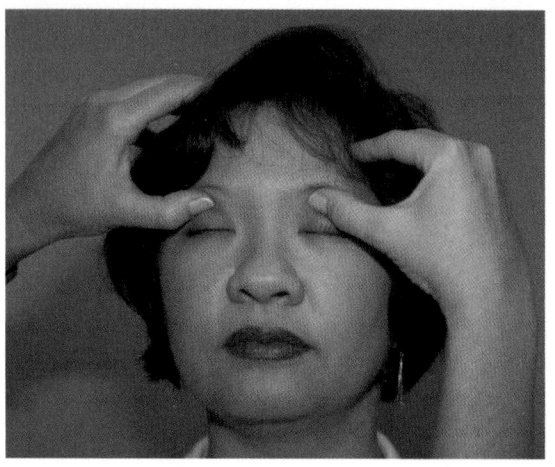

Assessment of the frontal sinuses *(Lemmi and Lemmi, 2000)*

frontocortical aphasia. See **motor aphasia.**

frontoethmoidal suture. See **ethmoidofrontal suture.**

frontonasal dysplasia, a hereditary form of defective midline development of the head and face, including ocular hypertelorism, occult cleft nose and maxilla, and sometimes cognitive impairment or other defects. Also called **median cleft facial syndrome.**

frontotemporal dementia (FTD), a rare brain disorder that affects the frontal and temporal lobes of the brain, affecting personality, behavior, and language.

front-tap reflex, in spinal irritability, contraction of the gastrocnemius muscle caused by a tap on the skin muscles of the extended leg.

frostbite [AS, *frost + bitan*], a traumatic effect of extreme cold on skin and subcutaneous tissues that is first recognized by distinct pallor of exposed skin surfaces, particularly the nose, ears, fingers, and toes. Vasoconstriction and damage to blood vessels impair local circulation and cause anoxia, edema, vesiculation, and necrosis. Gentle warming is appropriate first-aid treatment; rubbing of the affected part is avoided. Later therapy is similar to treatment of thermal burns. Iatrogenic frostbite is the result of excessive use of ethyl chloride sprays for local anesthesia for the relief of muscle and tendon strains. Compare **chilblain, immersion foot.**

■ OBSERVATIONS: Manifestations for superficial frostbite present as a white, waxy, soft, and numb appearance of the injured area while it is still cold. As thawing occurs, the area becomes flushed, edematous, and painful, and may become mottled and purple. Within 24 hours, large blisters form and remain for about 2 weeks before turning into a hardened eschar, which separates in about a month. As the eschar separates, it leaves painful, sensitive new skin that often sweats excessively. In deep frostbite, the injured part remains hard, cold, mottled, and blue-gray after thawing; edema forms in entire limb and may remain for months. Blisters may or may not form weeks after the injury. After several weeks, dead tissue blackens and sloughs off and a line demarcates dead from live tissue. Diagnosis is made by clinical evaluation plus a history of exposure to cold. Loss of digits, ears, nose, and extremities is possible, as is secondary infection and long-term residual symptoms, such as neuropathic pain, sensory deficits, hyperhidrosis, hair and nail deformities, and arthritis.

■ INTERVENTIONS: Acute treatment centers around rapid rewarming by immersion in water (40° C to 42° C) for 15 to 30 minutes. Intravenous analgesics are used for pain. Immunological agents (tetanus) and antiinfective drugs are given for prophylaxis. Fluid and electrolytes are replaced. After the affected area has thawed, plasma expanders are used to reduce sludge and thrombus formation. Whirlpool hydrotherapy is used 20 to 30 minutes three to four times a day. Physical therapy is used to increase function after edema resolves. In deep and severe cases, escharotomy may be performed with debridement after retraction of viable tissue. Amputation is done for nonviable extremities. Sympathectomy may be performed for severe vasospasm. ■ PATIENT CARE CONSIDERATIONS: Immediately after injury, constrictive and wet clothing should be removed and the affected area should be insulated and immobilized. The area should never be massaged or rubbed or subjected to dry heat. Associated hypothermia must be stabilized with heated saline; warming blankets; and warmed, humidified oxygen. Long-term precautions should be taken with injured area to prevent dislodgement of eschar and further damage. An exercise program may be needed to prevent joint restriction. Counseling may be needed for altered body image from loss of digits or limbs. Education is needed about adequate protection when exposed to cold temperatures and use of preventive measures, such as carrying extra clothing, coats, blankets, fluids, high carbohydrate foods, cell phone, and hazard markers in the car when traveling in cold weather.

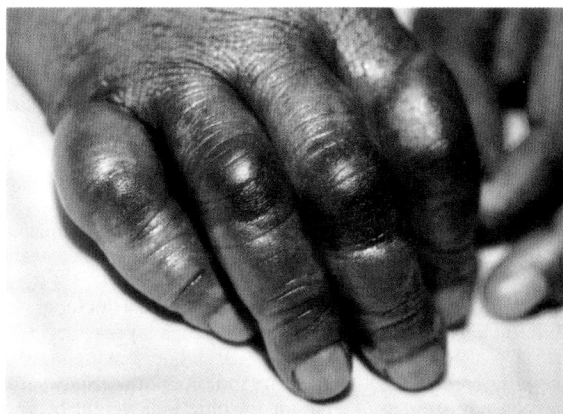

Frostbite of the fingers *(Cameron, 2014)*

frottage /frôtäzh″/ [Fr, rubbing], **1.** sexual gratification obtained by rubbing (especially the genital area) against the clothing of another person, as can occur in a crowd. **2.** a massage technique using rubbing.

frotteur /frôtœr″/ [Fr], a person who obtains sexual gratification by the practice of frottage.

frovatriptan, an antimigraine agent used for the acute treatment of migraine with or without aura.

frozen red blood cells, red cells cryopreserved with glycerol and stored frozen at minus 65° C for up to 10 years. Also called **glycerolized red cells**.

frozen section [ME, *fresen* + L, *sectio*], a histological section of tissue that has been frozen by exposure to dry ice.

frozen section method [AS, *freosan,* to freeze; L, *sectio,* a cutting; Gk, *meta,* order, *hodos,* path], (in surgical pathology) a method used in preparing a selected portion of tissue for pathological examination. The tissue is moistened and, fixed or unfixed, is rapidly frozen and cut by a microtome in a cryostat. This method is very rapid, allowing the pathologist to examine the specimen during a surgical procedure.

F.R.S.C., abbreviation for *Fellow of the Royal Society of Canada.*

fructokinase /fruk′tōkī″nās/, an enzyme that catalyzes the transfer of a high-energy phosphate group from adenosine triphosphate to D-fructose.

fructosamine test /frŏōktōs′əmēn/, determination of the glycated albumin level by measuring the reduction of nitroblue tetrazolium to purple under alkaline conditions, used as an index of the average glycemic state over the preceding 2 to 3 weeks. It is not widely used; however, it is useful when glycosylated hemoglobin (hemoglobin A1C) cannot be reliably measured.

fructose /fruk′tōs, frŏōk″-/, a yellowish-to-white, crystalline, water-soluble levorotatory ketose monosaccharide that is sweeter than sucrose. It is found in honey and several fruits and combines with glucose to form the disaccharide sucrose. Also called **fruit sugar, levulose.** See also **high-fructose corn syrup.**

fructose intolerance [L, *fructus,* fruit, *in* + *tolerare,* to bear], an inherited disorder marked by an absence of enzymes needed to metabolize fructose. Symptoms include sweating, tremors, confusion, digestive distress with vomiting, and failure of infants to grow. The condition is transmitted as an autosomal-recessive trait. Also called **hereditary fructose intolerance.**

fructosemia /frŏōk′tōsē″mē-ə/ [L, *fructus,* fruit; Gk, *haima,* blood], the presence of fructose in the blood.

fructose test, a laboratory fertility examination of the semen of azoospermic men. Fructose comes primarily from the seminal vesicles. The purpose of the test is to rule out possible ejaculatory duct obstruction or agenesis of seminal vesicles.

fructosuria /frŏōk′tōsŏor″ē-ə/, presence of the sugar fructose in the urine. This usually harmless and asymptomatic condition is caused by the hereditary absence of the enzyme fructokinase, which normally assists fructose metabolism. Essential fructosuria is associated with symptoms of diabetes mellitus. Also called **levulosuria.**

fruit sugar. See **fructose.**

frustration /frustrā″shən/, a feeling that results from interference with one's ability to attain a desired goal or satisfaction.

FSE, abbreviation for **fast spin-echo.**

FSF, abbreviation for **fibrin-stabilizing factor.** See **factor XIII.**

FSH, abbreviation for **follicle-stimulating hormone.**

FSH-RF, abbreviation for **follicle-stimulating hormone– releasing factor.**

FSK, abbreviation for **forskolin.**

FT, initialism for *fast-twitch.* See **fast-twitch (FT) fiber.**

FT₄, abbreviation for **free thyroxine.**

FTA-ABS test, abbreviation for **fluorescent treponemal antibody absorption test.**

FTC, abbreviation for **Federal Trade Commission.**

F-test [Sir Ronald Aylmer *Fisher,* British statistician, 1890– 1962], a statistical test comparing the means of more than two groups simultaneously by comparing two different measures of variance of the observations. One statistic measures the variations between the means of the groups (the between-groups variation), the other the variations within the groups (the within-group variation). If the two measures of variance yield similar results and their ratio, the F-ratio, approximates 1.0, the null hypothesis that all observations came from the same population cannot be rejected, whereas under the alternative hypothesis, the F-ratio is expected to be larger than 1.0. The test is the first step in the analysis of variance.

FTT, initialism for **failure to thrive.**

fuchsin bodies. See **Russell bodies.**

Fuchs method, a technique for a radiographic examination of the odontoid process projected through the foramen magnum. It is used when it is difficult to visualize the tip of the process on an image obtained by using the conventional open mouth method. See also **Judd method.**

fucosidosis /fyōō′kōsidō″sis/, a hereditary lysosomal storage disorder that results from the absence of the enzyme required to metabolize fucoside moieties. It causes cognitive impairment, neurological deterioration, coarse facial features, thickened skin, and hepatosplenomegaly.

FUDR, an antiviral and antineoplastic drug. Brand name for **floxuridine.**

fugue /fyōōg/ [L, *fuga,* running away], a state of dissociative reaction characterized by amnesia and physical flight from an intolerable situation. During the episode the person appears normal and seems consciously aware of what may be very complex activities and behavior, but afterward he or she has no recollection of the actions or behavior. The condition may last for only a few days or weeks, or it may continue for several years, during which the person wanders away from the customary environment, enters a new occupation, and undertakes an entirely different way of life. The syndrome appears to be caused by an inability to cope with a severe conflict or with a chronically stressful life situation. A form of fugue also occurs briefly after an epileptic seizure. See also **ambulatory automatism, automatism, dissociative reaction.**

Fukuhara syndrome. See **MERRF syndrome.**

Fukuyama type congenital muscular dystrophy /fōō′kōōya′ma/ [Yukio Fukuyama, 20th-century Japanese physician], an autosomal-recessive type of muscular dystrophy evident in infancy. Muscle abnormalities resemble those of Duchenne's muscular dystrophy, and patients are cognitively impaired with microgyria and other cerebral abnormalities. Also called *Fukuyama's syndrome.* See also **Duchenne's muscular dystrophy.**

fulcrum /fōōl″krəm, ful″-/ [L, *fulcire,* to support], **1.** the stable point or the position on which a lever, such as the ulna or the femur, turns. Numerous common body movements, such as raising the arm and walking, are combinations of lever actions involving fulcrums. The muscles provide the forces that move the numerous bones acting as levers. **2.** (in radiology) an imaginary pivot point about which the x-ray tube and image receptor move. During computed tomography the fulcrum lies in the focal, or object, plane, and only anatomical areas lying in this plane are focused and imaged.

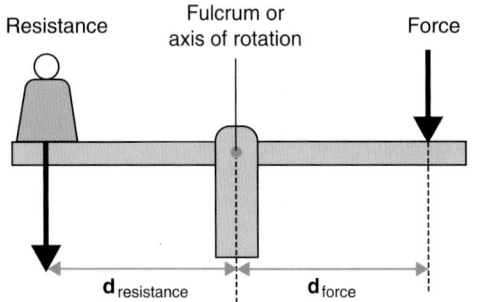

Fulcrum *(Everett and Kell, 2010)*

fulfillment [AS, *fullfyllan,* to make full], a perception of harmony in life that results when an individual has found meaning and acts purposefully.

fulgurate /ful″gyərāt/ [L, *fulgur,* lightning], **1.** *adj.,* pertaining to sudden, intense, sharp pain. **2.** *v.,* to use a movable electrode to destroy superficial tissue.

fulguration. See **electrodesiccation.**

full-arch wire, a wire that is attached to the teeth and extends from the molar region of one side, across the front of the mouth, to the molar region on the other side. It is used to cause or guide orthodontic tooth movement. A sectional arch wire or shorter version of the full-arch wire may also be used.

A section arch usually spans three to four posterior teeth in the same dental arch.

full denture [AS, *fol* + L, *dens,* tooth], a removable dental prosthesis that replaces all of the natural teeth in the maxillary or mandibular dental arch. The denture is usually made of methyl methacrylate along with synthetic artificial teeth, and is completely supported by the mouth tissues. Also called **complete denture.**

full-liquid diet, a diet consisting of only liquids and foods that liquefy at body temperature. It includes milk, milk drinks, carbonated beverages, coffee, tea, strained fruit juices, broth, strained cream soup, eggs cooked to liquid consistency or pasteurized, egg substitutes, cream, melted butter or margarine, strained precooked infant cereals in milk, thin custards, gelatin desserts, ice cream, sherbet, strained vegetables in soup, honey, syrups, sugar, and dry skim milk dissolved in liquids. The diet is prescribed after surgery, in some acute infections of short duration, in the treatment of acute GI disorders, and for patients too ill to chew. See also **liquid diet.**

full-lung tomography, a technique for producing general tomographic surveys of both lungs for the purpose of detecting possible occult nodules of metastases. Such lesions usually cannot be visualized with conventional radiological methods.

full pulse [AS, *fol* +, *pulsare,* to beat], a large-volume pulse with a low pulse pressure. Also called **pulsus magnus.**

full-risk HMO, (in U.S. managed care) a health maintenance organization in which the hospital receives capitation (money paid) for all facility and hospital-based physician services. The physician group receives capitation and shares the deficit or surplus of the hospital risk pool. The HMO retains premium dollars and assumes risk for out-of-area emergencies, pharmacy benefits, and vision benefits.

full term [AS, *fol* + Gk, *terma,* limit], pertaining to the normal period of human gestation between 39 weeks, 0 days and 40 weeks, 6 days.

full-thickness graft, a tissue transplant that includes the full thickness of the skin and subcutaneous layers.

full weight-bearing (FWB) [AS, *fol* + *gewiht* + ME, *beren*], relating to a view in radiology that shows the response to stresses of a natural posture. Full weight-bearing views of the foot are useful in studying flatfoot and clawfoot.

full-width half maximum (FWHM), a measure of resolution equal to the width of an image line source at points where the intensity is reduced to half the maximum.

fulminant hepatitis, a rare and frequently fatal form of acute hepatitis B in which the patient's condition rapidly deteriorates, with hepatic encephalopathy, necrosis of the hepatic parenchyma, coagulopathy, renal failure, and coma.

fulminating /ful″minā′ting/ [L, *fulminare,* lightning flash], (of a disease or condition) rapid, sudden, and severe, such as an infection, fever, or hemorrhage. Also called *fulminant. –fulminate , v.*

fulvestrant, an antineoplastic agent used to treat advanced breast carcinoma in estrogen-receptor–positive patients.

Fulvicin, an antifungal drug. Brand name for **griseofulvin.**

fumigate /fyōō″migāt/, to disinfect by exposing an area or object to pesticidal smoke or fumes.

fuming, producing a visible vapor.

function /fungk″shən/ [L, *functio,* performance], **1.** *n.,* an act, process, or series of processes that serve a purpose. **2.** *v.,* to perform an activity or to work properly and normally.

functional /fungk″shənəl/ [L, *functio,* performance], **1.** pertaining to a function. **2.** affecting the functions but not the structure of an organism or organ system.

functional age, a combination of the chronological, physiological, mental, and emotional ages.

functional analysis, (in psychiatry) a type of therapy that traces the sequence of events involved in producing and maintaining undesirable behavior.

functional antagonism, (in pharmacology) a situation in which two agonists interact with different receptors and produce opposing effects.

functional assessment, a focused evaluation of the activities performed and involved in daily living to determine an individual's well-being in regard to mental and physical condition, independence, and lifestyle. See **health history.**

functional bowel syndrome, *(Obsolete)* now called **irritable bowel syndrome.**

functional capacities, (in occupational therapy) the abilities and skills that people possess that allow them to perform an activity or task.

functional contracture. See **hypertonic contracture.**

functional differentiation, (in embryology) the specialization or diversification that results from the particular function of a cell or tissue.

functional disease, 1. a disease that affects function or performance. **2.** a condition marked by signs or symptoms of an organic disease or disorder although careful examination fails to reveal any evidence of structural or physiological abnormalities. The symptoms of a functional disorder are as real as those of an organic disease. Headache, impotence, certain heart murmurs, and constipation may be symptoms either of organic disease or of functional disease.

functional dyspepsia, a condition characterized by impaired digestion caused by an atonic or a neurological problem. See also **dyspepsia.**

functional foods, foods and food supplements marketed for presumed health benefits, such as vitamin supplements and certain herbs.

functional group, (in occupational therapy) groups that result in end products or that help members achieve desired skills and abilities.

functional health history. See **complete health history.**

functional hearing loss, hearing loss that lacks any organic lesion. Also called **nonorganic hearing loss.**

functional illness, a physical disorder with no known structural explanation for the symptoms. See also **disorder, functional disease.**

Functional Independence Measure (FIM), the most widely used standardized evaluation tool for physical disabilities. The tool is used to assess 18 areas of functioning, including self-care, sphincter control, transfers, locomotion, communication, and social cognition, scoring each on a scale ranging from 1 (total assistance) to 7 (complete independence). Also available in a pediatric form (WeeFIM).

functional imaging, a diagnostic procedure in which a sequence of radiographic or scintillation camera images of the distribution of an administered radioactive tracer delineates one or more physiological processes in the body.

functional impotence. See **impotence.**

functional magnetic resonance imaging (fMRI), a radiographic technique for imaging brain activity. In fMRI the technologist takes a rapid succession of scans designed to detect increases in oxygen consumption in various regions of the brain, which reflects small changes in blood flow and increased activity in certain cells.

functional method, a type of nursing care delivery system.

functional mobility, the ability to move within one's environment in order to participate in activities of daily living and instrumental activities of daily living, such as moving from one place to another in a home, moving around in bed, and performing transfers.

functional murmur [L, *functio,* performance], a heart murmur caused by an alteration of function without structural heart disease or damage, as in a murmur related to anemia. Also called **physiological murmur.**

functional nursing, an organizational mode for assigning nursing personnel that is task- and activity-oriented, using auxiliary health workers trained in a variety of skills. Each person is assigned specific functions performed for all patients in a given unit, and all report to the nurse responsible for care.

functional overlay, an emotional aspect of an organic disease. It may occur as an overreaction to an illness and is characterized by symptoms that continue long after clinical signs of the disease have ended.

functional pathology [L, *functio,* performance; Gk, *pathos,* disease, *logos,* science], a study of the functional changes that result from structural alterations in tissues.

functional position of the hand, a position for splinting the hand, including the wrist and fingers. It consists of dorsiflexing both the wrist between 20 and 35 degrees and the proximal interphalangeal joints between 45 and 60 degrees. The thumb is abducted and in opposition and alignment with the pads of the fingers.

functional progression, a rehabilitative sequence for a musculoskeletal or similar injury. With variations for individual cases, the program usually progresses from immobilization for primary healing through protection of range of motion to endurance and strengthening activities related to the patient's work and play requirements.

functional psychosis, a severe emotional disorder characterized by personality derangement and loss of ability to function in reality but without evidence that the disorder is related to the physical processes of the brain.

functional residual capacity (FRC), the volume of gas in the lungs at the end of a normal tidal volume exhalation. The functional residual capacity is equal to the residual volume plus the expiratory reserve volume. In anesthesia FRC serves as an oxygen reservoir in an apneic patient. FRC is reduced in obesity due to the cephalad position of the diaphragm.

functional splint [L, *functio,* performance; ME, *splent*], an orthopedic device that allows or assists a patient's movements. Also called **ambulatory splint, dynamic splint.** See also **splint.**

functional visual skills, various normal eye activities, such as depth perception, eye aiming and alignment, oculomotility, convergence and divergence, and accommodative ability.

functional vomiting, vomiting whose physiological cause is unknown.

fundal height /fun″dəl/ [L, *fundus,* bottom; AS, *heightho*], the height of the fundus of the uterus, measured in centimeters from the top of the symphysis pubis to the highest point in the midline at the top of the uterus. Fundal height is measured at each prenatal visit with large blunt calipers or with a tape measure. From the twentieth to the thirty-second week of pregnancy the height in centimeters is roughly equal to the gestational age in weeks in a woman with normal body habitus and a vertex presentation. Thereafter the one-to-one ratio often varies, depending on engagement of the fetal head.

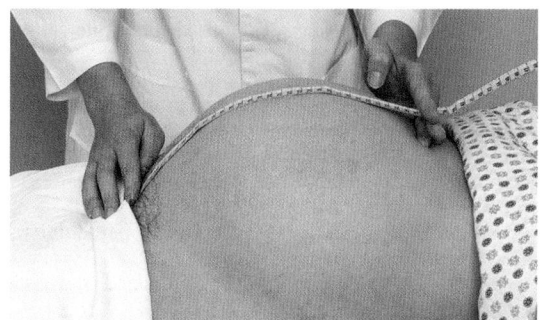

Measurement of fundal height *(Seidel et al, 2011)*

fundal placenta [L, *fundus,* bottom, *placenta,* flat cake],   a placenta that is attached to the fundus of the uterus.

fundamentals of nursing /fun′dəmen″təls/,   the basic principles and practices of nursing as taught in educational programs for nurses. In a course on the fundamentals of nursing, traditionally required in the first semester of the program, the student attends classes and gives care to selected patients. A fundamentals of nursing course emphasizes the importance of the fundamental needs of humans as well as competence in basic skills as prerequisites to providing comprehensive nursing care.

fundi.   See **fundus.**

fundic gastritis,   gastritis whose focus is in the gastric fundus.

fundiform ligament of the penis /fun″difôrm/,   a band of fibrous and elastic fibers blending with the fascia surrounding the penis. It extends from the linea alba above the pubic symphysis and attaches to the penile fascia.

fundoplication /fun′dəplikā″shən/   [L, *fundus,* bottom, *plicare,* to fold],   a surgical procedure involving making tucks (plication) in the fundus of the stomach around the lower end of the esophagus. The operation is used in the treatment of gastroesophageal and paraesophageal hernias. See also **plication.**

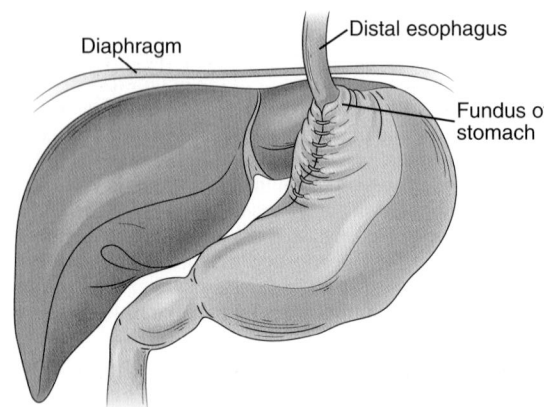

Labels: Diaphragm · Distal esophagus · Fundus of stomach

Nissen fundoplication for hiatal hernia
(Cooper and Gosnell, 2015)

fundoscopy.   See **ophthalmoscopy.**

fundus /fun″dəs/ *pl. fundi*   [L, bottom],   **1.** the base or the deepest part of an organ. **2.** the portion farthest from the mouth of an organ, such as the fundus of the uterus or the fundus of an eye.

funduscope.   See **ophthalmoscope.**

funduscopy.   See **ophthalmoscopy.**

fundus microscopy,   examination of the interior of the eye using an instrument that combines an ophthalmoscope and a lens with high magnifying power for observing minute structures on the retina.

fundus of the gallbladder,   the closed end of the gallbladder, adjacent to the inferior border of the liver.

fundus of the stomach,   a cul-de-sac of the stomach that lies above the level of the cardiac orifice, where the esophagus joins the stomach. It contains a gas bubble, the magenblassen.

fundus of the urinary bladder,   the bottom of the bladder, formed by the convex posterior wall.

fungal /fung″gəl/   [L, *fungus,* mushroom],   pertaining to or resembling a fungus or fungi.

fungal abscess,   a collection of pus produced by a fungal infection.

fungal antibody tests,   a relatively unreliable blood test to detect fungal infections.

fungal infection [L, *fungus,* mushroom, *inficere,* to stain],   any inflammatory condition caused by a fungus. Most fungal infections are superficial and mild, though persistent and difficult to eradicate. Some, particularly in older, debilitated, or immunosuppressed or immunodeficient people, may become systemic and life threatening. Kinds include **aspergillosis, blastomycosis, candidiasis, coccidioidomycosis, histoplasmosis.**

fungal infection of nail,   an infection of the horny cutaneous plates on the dorsal tips of the fingers and toes. The infection is commonly caused by *Tricophyton* organisms and treated with oral terbinafine or itraconazole. The infection is defined by the part of the nail that is infected.

fungal pneumonia,   pneumonia caused by inhaled fungi, usually *Blastomyces dermatitidis, Coccidioides immitis,* or *Histoplasma capsulatum.* Numerous other fungi, such as *Aspergillus* and *Candida,* infect immunocompromised patients. See also **blastomycosis, histoplasmosis.**

fungal septicemia [L, *fungus* + Gk, *septikos,* putrid, *haima,* blood],   a form of systemic infection in which the causative agent is a fungus in the circulatory bloodstream.

fungemia /funjē″mē·ə/ [L, *fungus* + Gk, *haima,* blood],   the presence of fungi in the blood, mostly seen in immunocompromised patients. Diagnosis is difficult because routine blood cultures have poor sensitivity. Compare **bacteremia, parasitemia, viremia.**

fungi /fun′ji/,   in the classification of living organisms, one of the kingdoms of eukaryotic organisms. See also **fungus.**

fungicide /fun″jisīd/,   a drug that kills fungi. See also **antifungal,** def. 2. –*fungicidal, adj.*

fungiform /fun″jifôrm/   [L, *funis + forma*],   shaped like a mushroom.

fungiform papilla.   See **papilla.**

-fungin,   suffix for antifungal antibiotics.

fungistatic /fun′jēstat″ik/,   having an inhibiting effect on the growth of fungi.

Fungizone,   an antifungal drug. Brand name for **amphotericin B.**

fungus /fun′gəs/ *pl. fungi* [L, *fungus,* mushroom],   a eukaryotic, thallus-forming organism that feeds by absorbing organic molecules from its surroundings. Fungi lack chlorophyll and therefore are not capable of photosynthesis. They may be saprophytes or parasites. Unicellular fungi (yeasts) reproduce by budding; multicellular fungi, such as molds, reproduce by spore formation. Fungi may invade living organisms, including humans, as well as nonliving organic substances. See also **fungal infection. –fungal,** *fungous, adj.*

funic presentation /fyo͞o″nik/   [L, *funis,* cord, *praesentare,* to show],   (in obstetrics) the appearance of the umbilical cord before the main presenting part of the fetus. Also called **cord presentation,** *funis presentation,* **presentation.**

funic souffle /fyo͞o″nik so͞o″fəl/   [L, *funis,* cord; Fr, *souffle,* breath],   a soft, muffled, blowing sound produced by blood rushing through the umbilical vessels and synchronous with the fetal heart sound.

funicular hernia,   a type of indirect inguinal hernia.

funicular part of ductus deferens,   a middle part of the ductus deferens, where it is within the spermatic cord.

funiculitis /fənik′yəlī″tis/,   any abnormal inflammatory condition of a cordlike structure of the body, such as the spinal cord or spermatic cord. Inflammation of the umbilical cord is usually associated with chorioamnionitis.

funiculopexy /fənik″yəlōpek′sē/, a surgical procedure for correcting an undescended testicle in which the spermatic cord is sutured to surrounding tissue.

funiculus /fənik″yələs/ [L, little cord], a division of the white matter of the spinal cord, consisting of fasciculi or fiber tracts.

funiculus umbilicalis. See **umbilical cord.**

funis /fyoo″nis, foo″nis/, a cordlike structure, such as the umbilical cord.

funnel chest [L, *fundere,* to pour], a skeletal abnormality of the chest characterized by a depressed sternum. The deformity may not interfere with breathing, but surgical correction is often recommended for cosmetic reasons. Also called **pectus excavatum.**

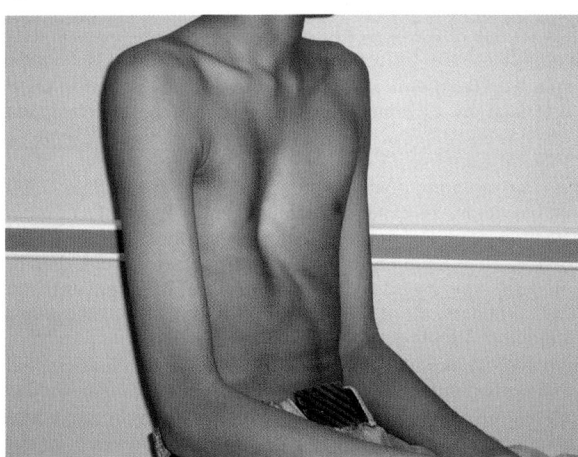

Funnel chest *(Kelly, 2008)*

funny bone, a popular name for a point at the lower end of the humerus where the ulnar nerve crosses the elbow joint near the surface and, if subjected to external pressure, produces a tingling sensation.

FUO, abbreviation for **fever of unknown origin.**

Furadantin, an antibacterial drug. Brand name for **nitrofurantoin.**

furazolidone /foo′rəzol″idōn/, an antibiotic with antibacterial and antiprotozoal activity.

■ INDICATIONS: It is prescribed for the treatment of diarrhea caused by susceptible bacterial or protozoal infections (e.g., *Giardiasis, Vibrio)* of the GI tract.

■ CONTRAINDICATIONS: Known hypersensitivity to this drug prohibits its use. It is not given to children less than 1 month of age, and it is not used with drugs that are contraindicated with monoamine oxidase inhibitors. Foods high in tyramine and concurrent use of alcohol should be avoided.

■ ADVERSE EFFECTS: Among the more serious adverse effects are hemolytic anemia and fever, skin rash, and abdominal pain.

furcation /fərkā″shən/ [L, *furca,* fork], the region of division of tooth root. It is a bifurcation if there are two roots or a trifurcation if there are three roots.

furcation probe. See **periodontal probe.**

furfuraceous desquamation /fur′fərā″sē·əs/ [L, *furfur,* bran, *desquamare,* to scale off], the shedding of epidermis in large scales.

furosemide /foorō″səmīd/, a loop diuretic.

■ INDICATIONS: It is prescribed in the treatment of edema caused by congestive heart failure, renal failure, or liver failure and alone or in combination for the treatment of hypertension.

■ CONTRAINDICATIONS: Anuria, pregnancy, lactation, electrolyte depletion, or known hypersensitivity to this drug or other sulfonylureas prohibits its use.

■ ADVERSE EFFECTS: Among the more serious adverse effects are fluid and electrolyte imbalances.

Furoxone, an antibacterial antiprotozoal drug. Brand name for **furazolidone.**

furred tongue. See **coated tongue.**

furrow /fur″ō/ [AS, *furh*], a groove, such as the atrioventricular furrow that separates the atria from the ventricles of the heart.

furuncle /fyoor″ungkəl/ [L, *furunculus,* petty thief], a localized suppurative staphylococcal skin infection originating in a gland or hair follicle and characterized by pain, redness, and swelling. Necrosis deep in the center of the inflamed area forms a core of dead tissue that is spontaneously extruded, eventually resorbed, or surgically removed. It is important to avoid irritating or squeezing the lesion to prevent spread of the infection. Treatment may include antibiotics, local moist heat, and, when there is definite fluctuation and the hard white core is evident, incision and drainage. Also called **boil.** Compare **carbuncle.** –**furunculous,** *adj.*

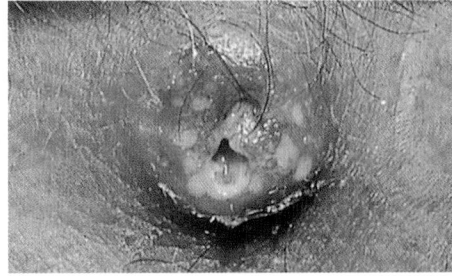

Furuncle *(Courtesy Dr. Jaime A. Tschen, Baylor College of Medicine, Department of Dermatology)*

furunculosis /fyoorung′kyoolō″sis/, an acute skin disease characterized by boils or successive crops of boils that are caused by staphylococci or streptococci.

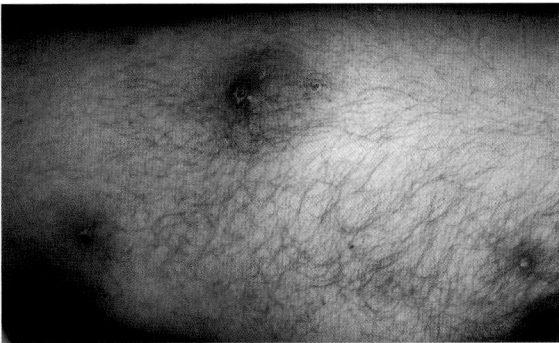

Furunculosis *(Lebwohl et al, 2014)*

furunculous. See **furuncle.**

-fuse, suffix meaning "to pour or flow": *diffuse, profuse.*

fused teeth /fyoozd/ [L, *fundere,* to melt], partial or complete fusion of two or more individual teeth caused by union of two adjacent tooth buds by either enamel or cementum. Not to be confused with germination or "twinning" of a single tooth bud.

fusiform /fyoo″sifôrm/ [L, *fusus,* spindle, *forma,* form], a structure that is tapered at both ends.

fusiform aneurysm, a localized dilation of an artery in which the entire circumference of the vessel is distended. The result is an elongated, tubular, or spindlelike swelling. Also called **Richet's aneurysm.** Compare **saccular aneurysm.**

fusiform gyrus [L, *fusus,* spindle, *forma,* form; Gk, *gyros,* turn], a convolution of the cerebral hemispheres that lies below the collateral fissures and joins the occipital and temporal lobes.

fusiform megalourethra, a huge diverticulum of the anterior urethra resulting from absence of an entire section of the corpus spongiosum.

fusimotor /fyoo″zimō′tər/ [L, *fusus* + *motare,* to move about], pertaining to the motor nerve fibers, or gamma efferent fibers, that innervate the intrafusal fibers of the muscle spindle.

fusion /fyoo″zhən/ [L, *fusio,* outpouring], **1.** the joining into a single entity, as in optic fusion. **2.** See **ankylosis. 3.** the surgical joining of two or more vertebrae, performed to stabilize a segment of the spinal column after severe trauma, herniation of a disk, or degenerative disease. Under general anesthesia the cartilage pads are removed from between the posterior parts of the involved vertebrae. Bone chips are cut from one of the patient's iliac crests and inserted in place of the cartilage, fusing the articulating surfaces into one segment of bone. **4.** (in psychiatry) the tendency of two people who are experiencing an intense emotion to unite.

fusional amplitude. See **amplitude of convergence.**

fusional movement /fyoo″zhənəl/, a reflex that moves the visual axes to the point of fixation, producing stereoscopic vision.

fusion beat, in an electrocardiogram, a P wave or QRS complex resulting from the concurrent activation of the atria or the ventricles by two stimuli in the same chamber. An atrial fusion beat results when the sinus beat coincides with an atrial ectopic beat, when two atrial ectopic beats coincide, or when an atrial or sinus beat coincides with retrograde conduction from a junctional focus. A ventricular fusion beat results when a ventricular beat coincides with a sinus beat, a ventricular ectopic beat, or a junctional beat.

fusion imaging, a combination of two images from different modalities into a single image, such as computed tomography and positron emission tomography.

Fusobacterium, a large cigar-shaped anaerobic bacillus genus, only some of which are pathogenic to humans. *F. fusiforme* is found in cavities of humans and other animals. It is sometimes associated with Vincent's angina. *F. nucleatum* is associated with pleuropulmonary infection and disease and also is one of the causes of gingivitis.

fusospirochetal disease /fyoo′zōspī′rōkē″təl/ [L, *fusus,* spindle; Gk, *speira,* coil, *chaite,* hair], any infection characterized by ulcerative lesions in which both a fusiform bacillus and a spirochete are found, such as trench mouth or Vincent's angina.

FVIII, a large glycoprotein containing more than 2300 amino acids, 24 cysteine residues, and 25 potential glycosylation sites. The factor is used to treat blood-clotting disorders, such as hemophilia A, in which the factor is deficient or missing. Also called **recombinant factor VIII concentrate.**

FVL, abbreviation for *factor V–Leiden.* See **factor V–Leiden (FVL) test.**

F wave, a waveform recorded in electroneuromyographic and nerve conduction tests. It appears on supramaximal stimulation of a motor nerve and is caused by antidromic transmission of a stimulus. The F wave is used in studies of motor nerve function in the arms and legs.

f waves, in an electrocardiogram, wavy deflections at a rate of 400 or more per minute that represent atrial fibrillation.

FWB, abbreviation for **full weight-bearing.**

FWHM, abbreviation for **full-width half maximum.**

-fy, suffix meaning "to make into" something specified: *acidify, clarify.*

-fying. See **-factive, -fying.**

-fylline, suffix for theophylline derivatives.

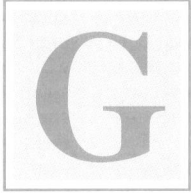

g, **1.** abbreviation for **gram. 2.** abbreviation for **standard gravity.**

G1, a phase in the cell cycle during which the cell's future can be influenced by various positive and negative signals, such as growth factors. The signals determine whether the cell will advance beyond a certain checkpoint. Once beyond the checkpoint, the cell is committed to entering a phase during which it replicates its DNA in preparation for mitosis.

G2, a phase in the cell cycle that follows DNA replication. During G2, the cell checks the accuracy of DNA replication and prepares for mitosis.

G6PD deficiency, abbreviation for **glucose-6-phosphate dehydrogenase (G6PD) deficiency.**

Ga, symbol for the element **gallium.**

GA, abbreviation for **general anesthesia.**

GABA, abbreviation for **gamma-aminobutyric acid.**

gabapentin /gab″əpen′tin/, an anticonvulsant chemically related to alpha-aminobutyric acid. It is administered orally and used in the treatment of partial seizures and chronic neuropathic pain. In veterinary medicine, gabapentin is being used to treat anxiety and phobic disorders in dogs and cats.

GABHS, abbreviation for *group A beta-hemolytic streptococcal skin disease.*

GAD, abbreviation for **generalized anxiety disorder.**

gadolinium (Gd) /gad′əlin″ē·əm/ [Johan Gadolin, Finnish chemist, 1760–1852], **1.** a rare earth metallic element. Its atomic number is 64, and its atomic mass is 157.25. It is now widely used as an MRI contrast agent. **2.** (in radiology) a phosphor used for its fluorescent properties in the manufacture of extraoral radiography intensifying screens. **3.** an element used for shielding in neutron radiography.

GAF, abbreviation for **Global Assessment of Functioning (GAF) scale.**

gag [ME, *gaggen,* to strangle], **1.** *n.,* a dental device for holding the jaws open during oral surgery or dental restoration. Also called **mouth prop, bite block. 2.** *v.,* to retch or attempt to vomit.

gag reflex [ME, *gaggen,* to strangle; L, *reflectere,* to bend back], a normal neural reflex elicited by touching the soft palate or posterior pharynx in which the responses are symmetric elevation of the palate, retraction of the tongue, and contraction of the pharyngeal muscles. The reflex is used as a test of the integrity of the vagus and glossopharyngeal nerves. Also called **pharyngeal reflex.**

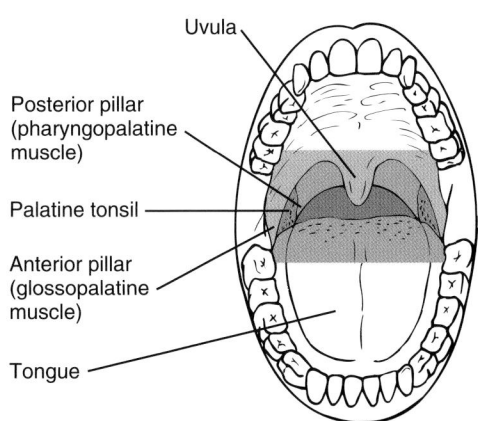

Areas that react in a gag reflex when touched *(Miller-Keane and O'Toole, 1998)*

Labels: Uvula; Posterior pillar (pharyngopalatine muscle); Palatine tonsil; Anterior pillar (glossopalatine muscle); Tongue

Gail model, a collection of epidemiological and risk factor data used to calculate the risk of breast cancer.

gain of function mutation, a genetic mutation causing the altered gene to possess a new molecular function or a new pattern of gene expression.

gait [ONorse, *geta,* a way], the manner or style of walking, including rhythm, pattern, cadence, and speed.

gait analysis, evaluation of the manner or style of walking, normally done by observing an individual walking in a straight line. Objective measurement systems that include video recordings, infrared cameras, specialized floor systems, and electromyography may be employed when deviations from normal are present.

Gait Assessment Rating Scale (GARS), a standardized test or inventory of 16 abnormal aspects of gait that may be observed by an examiner as a patient walks at a self-selected pace. The abnormalities are commonly seen in elderly people who fall. Each aspect is graded on a scale of 0-1-2-3, with lower numbers indicating less abnormality. Often used as a screening tool to identify patients who are at risk for falls.

gait belt, a specialized canvas, nylon, or leather belt from 1 to 4 inches wide, placed around a client's waist in order to support the client when he or she is ambulating or transferring.

gait determinant, one of a number of the kinetic anatomical factors that govern an individual's locomotion in the process of walking. Pelvic rotation, pelvic tilt, knee and hip flexion, knee and ankle interaction, and lateral pelvic displacement are the main determinants of gait. Such descriptions are often important in analyzing and correcting pathological gaits of patients afflicted by orthopedic diseases, deformities, or abnormal bone conditions.

gait disorder, an abnormality in the manner or style of walking that results in an inconsistent flow of ambulation. Gait disorders usually result from neuromuscular, arthritic, or other body changes. The body's center of gravity may change over the years, causing a change in the degree of knee flexion needed to maintain one's balance when walking. Some individuals with neuromuscular disorders walk with a shuffling gait or move with lurching actions. At times a gait disorder may be the result of a medication that causes confusion or loss of coordination or an eye or ear disturbance that affects the sense of balance.

galact-, galacta-. See **galacto-, galact-, galacta-.**

-galactia, suffix meaning "a condition involving secretion of milk": *oligogalactia.*

galacto-, galact-, galacta-, prefix meaning "milk": *galactocele, galactorrhea.*

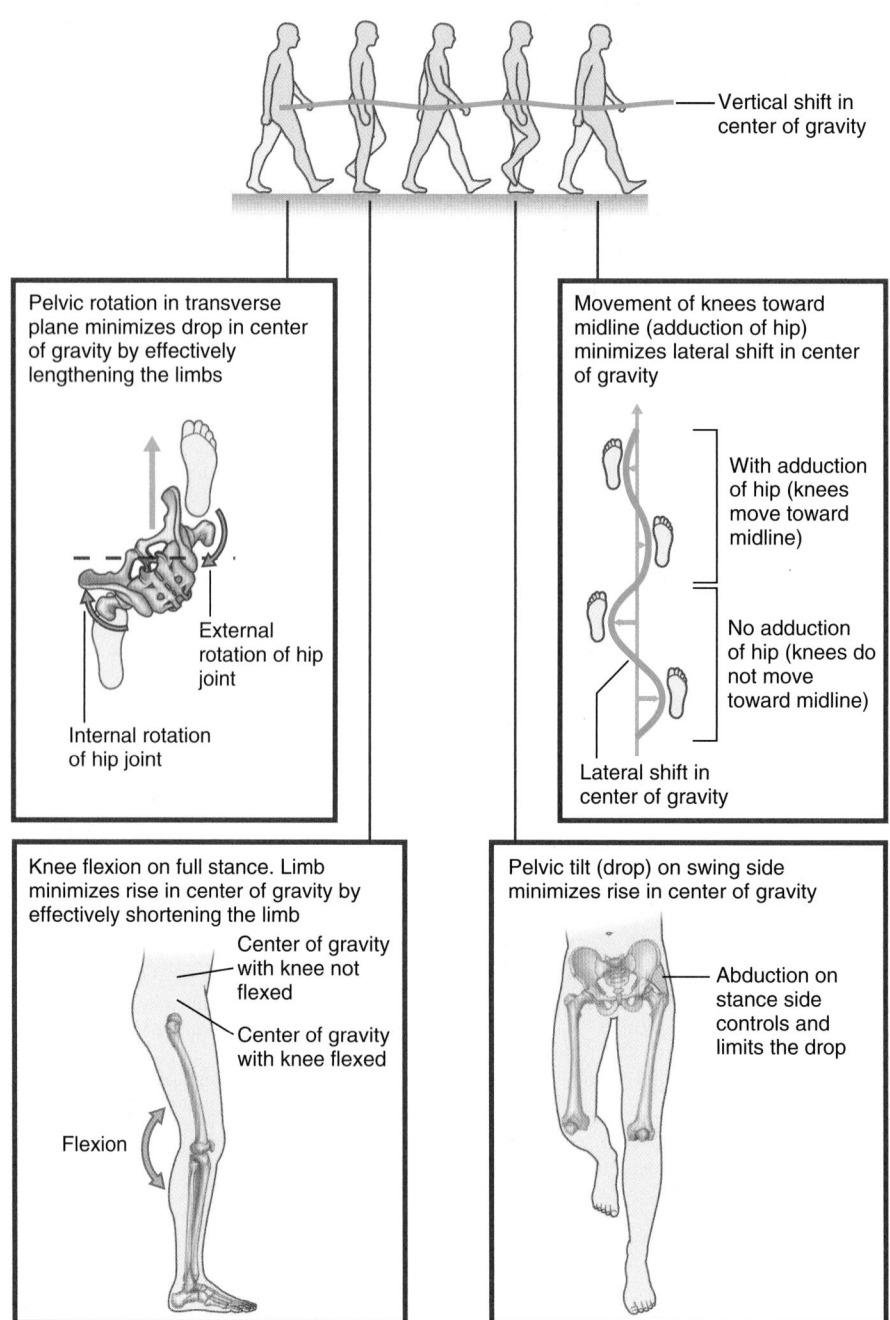

Gait determinants *(Drake, Vogl, and Mitchell, 2015)*

galactocele /gəlak″təsēl′/, a postpartum breast cyst caused by blockage of a mammary gland milk duct. A woman with a galactocele experiences unilateral, localized pain.

galactokinase /gəlak″tōkī″nās/ [Gk, *gala,* milk, *kinesis,* movement; Fr, *diastase,* enzyme], an enzyme that functions in the metabolism of glycogen. Galactokinase catalyzes a metabolic step involving the transfer of a high-energy phosphate group from a donor molecule to a molecule of galactose, producing a molecule of D-galactose 1-phosphate.

galactokinase deficiency, an autosomal-recessive inherited disorder of carbohydrate metabolism in which the enzyme galactokinase is deficient or absent. As a result, dietary galactose is not metabolized, galactose accumulates in the blood, and cataracts may develop rapidly. Food containing galactose, such as milk and certain milk products, must be eliminated from the diet. Compare **lactase deficiency.**

galactophorous duct /-fôr″əs/ [Gk, *gala* + *pherein,* to bear; L, *ducere,* to lead], a passage for milk in the lobes of the breast.

galactopoiesis, the maintenance of milk production. Also called **lactogenesis.**

galactorrhea /gəlak″tərē″ə/ [Gk, *gala* + *rhoia,* flowing], **1.** a spontaneous flow of milk from the nipple. **2.** lactation not associated with childbirth or nursing. The condition is sometimes a symptom of a pituitary gland tumor. See also **Forbes-Albright syndrome.**

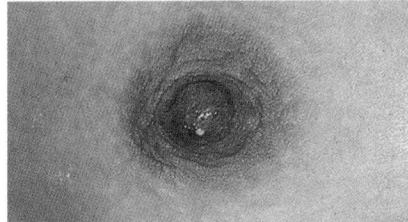

Galactorrhea *(Belchetz and Hammond, 2003)*

galactosamine, galactose that contains an amine group on the second group.

galactose /gəlak″tōs/ [Gk, *gala* + *glykys,* sweet], a simple sugar found in the dextrorotatory form in lactose (milk sugar), nerve cell membranes, sugar beets, gums, and seaweed and in the levorotatory form in flaxseed mucilage. Prepared galactose, a white crystalline substance, is less sweet and less soluble in water than glucose but is similar in other properties.

galactose breath test, a breath test of liver function, in which the fasting subject is administered a dose of galactose labeled with carbon 13 and levels of labeled carbon dioxide in the breath are measured at specific time intervals. Low levels of carbon dioxide indicate that the galactose is not being metabolized properly, indicating either an enzyme deficiency or liver dysfunction, such as the fibrosis accompanying hepatitis.

galactosemia /gəlak″tōsē″mē·ə/ [Gk, *gala* + *glykys,* sweet, *haima,* blood], a group of inherited autosomal-recessive disorders of galactose metabolism. It is characterized by a deficiency of an enzyme involved in galactose metabolism, galactose-1-phosphate uridyl transferase. Shortly after birth an intolerance to milk occurs; it is evidenced by anorexia, nausea, vomiting, and diarrhea and causes failure to thrive. Hepatosplenomegaly, cataracts, and cognitive impairment develop. Greater than normal amounts of galactose are present in the blood, the galactose tolerance test result indicates an abnormality, and the red cells show deficient galactose enzyme activity. Because the elimination of galactose from the diet results in the rapid decrease of all symptoms except cognitive impairment, early diagnosis and prompt therapy are essential.

Pregnant women known to be carriers should exclude lactose and galactose from their diet. Compare **glycogen storage disease.** See also **galactose, inborn error of metabolism.**

galactose tolerance test, a test of the ability of the liver to remove galactose from the blood and convert it to glycogen. The test, which is used to estimate impaired liver function, measures the rate of galactose excretion after ingestion or injection of a measured amount of galactose.

galactosidase, an enzyme that catalyzes the metabolism of galactosides.

galactoside /gəlak″tō″sīd′/, a glycoside containing galactose.

galactoside permease, an enzyme that catalyzes the transport of lactose into the cell.

galactosis /gal′əktōsis/, lactation; the formation of breast milk by the lacteal glands.

galactosuria /-sōōr″ē·ə/, the presence of galactose, a simple sugar, in the urine.

galactosyl ceramide lipidosis /gəlak″təsil/ [Gk, *gala* + *glykys,* sweet; L, *cera,* wax, *lipos,* fat, *osis,* condition], a rare, fatal inherited disorder of lipid metabolism, present at birth. Infants become paralyzed, blind, and deaf, and experience increasing levels of cognitive impairment; eventually they die of bulbar paralysis. There is no known treatment for the disorder, but it can be detected in pregnancy by amniocentesis. Also called **globoid leukodystrophy, Krabbe disease.** Compare **Tay-Sachs disease.**

galactosyl transferase, an enzyme in the head of sperm that is required for sperm to bind to eggs.

galactozymase /-zī″māz/, an enzyme in milk that is able to hydrolyze starch.

galacturia /gal′əktōōr″ē·ə/ [Gk, *gala,* milk, *ouron,* urine], a condition in which the urine has a milky color caused by the abnormal presence of galactose, a monosaccharide, in the urine.

galanin /galan″in, gal″ənin/, a neuropeptide in the small intestine and central and peripheral nervous systems that has a role in bowel motility, pancreas activity, and prolactin and growth hormone release.

galantamine /gälan′tämēn/, a reversible competitive inhibitor of acetylcholinesterase used as the hydrobromide salt in the treatment of mild to moderate Alzheimer disease. It is administered orally.

Galant reflex /gəlant″/, a normal response in the neonate when held in ventral suspension (face down) to move the hips toward the stimulated side when the back is stroked along the spinal cord. The reflex disappears by about 4 weeks of age. Absence of the reflex may indicate spinal cord lesion. Also called **trunk incurvation reflex.**

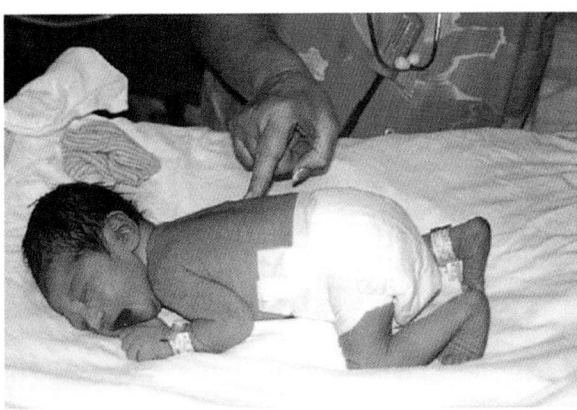

Elicitation of the Galant reflex *(Courtesy Marjorie Pyle, RNC, Lifecircle)*

galea aponeurotica. See **epicranial aponeurosis.**

Galeazzi fracture /gal'ē·at″sē/ [Riccardo Galeazzi, Italian surgeon, 1866–1952], a break in the distal radius accompanied by dislocation of the radioulnar joint. Also called **Dupuytren fracture.**

Galen's vein /gā″lənz/ [Claudius Galen, Greek physician, circa AD 130–200], the large vein formed by the union of the two terminal cerebral veins. It curves around the splenium of the corpus callosum and continues as the straight sinus of the brain. Also called **great cerebral vein of Galen.**

gall, 1. See **bile. 2.** a lump or ball that forms most often on the stems, leaves, or roots of plants at the site of injuries caused by insects, fungi, bacteria, or other organisms. An example is the oak gall, which contains tannin.

gallamine triethiodide /gal'ämēn tri″ēthi′odīd/, a quaternary ammonium compound, the triethiodide salt used as a skeletal muscle relaxant during surgery and other procedures, such as endoscopy or intubation. It is administered intravenously.

gallbladder (GB) /gôl″blad′ər/ [ME, gal + AS, blaedre], a pear-shaped excretory sac lodged in a fossa on the visceral surface of the right lobe of the liver. It stores and concentrates bile, which it receives from the liver via the hepatic duct. In an adult it holds about 32 mL of bile. During digestion of fats the gallbladder contracts, ejecting bile through the common bile duct into the duodenum. The gallbladder is divided into a fundus, body, and neck and is covered by the peritoneum. Obstruction of the biliary system by gallstones may lead to jaundice and pain and may require surgical or other intervention. See also **lithotripsy.**

gallbladder carcinoma, a malignant neoplasm of the bile reservoir, characterized by anorexia, nausea, vomiting, weight loss, progressively worsening right upper quadrant pain, and eventually jaundice. Tumors of the gallbladder are predominantly adenocarcinomas. Often associated with biliary calculi and chronic cholecystitis, they are three to four times more common in women than in men and rarely occur before 40 years of age. Physical examination reveals an enlarged gallbladder in about half of the cases. Ultrasound or radiographic tests may aid in making a diagnosis. Complete removal of the gallbladder may sometimes be curative, but partial hepatectomy may be required because the tumor typically infiltrates the liver and ducts. Palliative surgery is often needed. Radiotherapy may be palliative. Chemotherapy is usually ineffective.

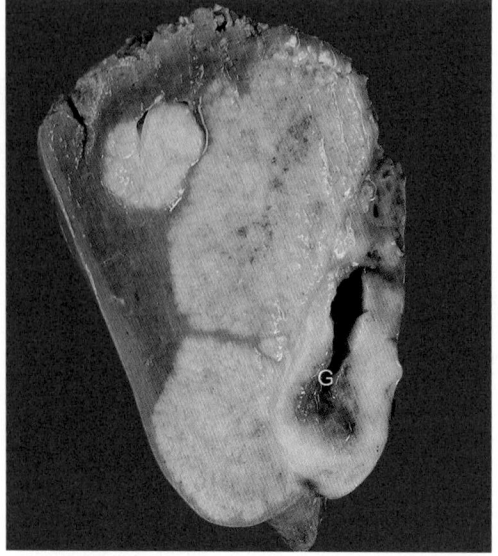

Gallbladder and liver carcinoma (Ahn et al, 2006)

gallbladder lithiasis. See **cholecystolithiasis.**

gallbladder nuclear scanning, a nuclear scan used to evaluate the biliary tract. This test may also be used to evaluate the gallbladder for obstruction of the cystic duct, cholecystitis, and common bile duct obstruction.

gallium (Ga) /gal″ē·əm/ [L, Gallia, Gaul], a metallic element. Its atomic number is 31, and its atomic mass is 69.72. The melting point of gallium is 29.8° C (88.6° F); it will melt if held in the hand. Because of its high boiling point (2403° C or 4357.4° F), it is used in high-temperature thermometers. Radioisotopes of gallium are used in total body scanning procedures. Many of its compounds are poisonous.

gallium scan, a nuclear scan of the total body performed after an IV injection of radioactive gallium, a radionuclide that concentrates in areas of inflammation and infection, abscess, and benign and malignant tumor. It is useful in detecting metastatic tumor, especially lymphoma.

gallop /gal″əp/ [Fr, galop], a third or fourth heart sound, which at certain heart rates sometimes sounds like the gait of a horse. Also called gallop rhythm. See also S_3, S_4, **summation gallop.**

gallstone. See **biliary calculus, cholelithiasis.**

gallstone pancreatitis, acute pancreatitis accompanied by presence of gallstones, one of the most common types.

galoche chin /gəlosh/ [Fr, galosh + AS, cin], a narrow protruding or thrusting chin. It is a congenital condition.

galvanic /galvan″ik/ [Luigi Galvani, Italian physician, 1737–1798], pertaining to electrical currents produced by chemical activity.

galvanic cautery. See **electrocautery.**

galvanic electric stimulation [Luigi Galvani], the use of a high-voltage electric stimulator to treat muscle spasms, edema of acute injury, myofascial pain, and certain other disorders. See also **transcutaneous electrical nerve stimulation (TENS).**

galvanic skin response (GSR) [Luigi Galvani; AS, scinn + L, respondere, to reply], a reaction to certain stimuli as indicated by a change in the electrical resistance of the skin. The effect is related to subconscious activity of the sweat glands and may result from pleasant as well as unpleasant stimuli. The GSR is used in some polygraph examinations.

galvanocautery. See **electrocautery.**

galvanoionization. See **iontophoresis.**

galvanometer /gal″vənom″ətər/ [Luigi Galvani], an instrument used to measure the strength and direction of flow of an electric current. Its action depends on the deflection of a magnetic needle in the field produced by current passing through a coil. A simple galvanometer is used mainly to detect the presence of an electric current. Galvanometers are used in certain diagnostic instruments, such as electrocardiographs.

Galveston Orientation and Amnesia Test (GOAT), a series of 10 questions asked of a patient to help evaluate post-traumatic amnesia. The test is repeated on a weekly basis and is scored on a scale of 0 to 100. A patient is determined to be out of the amnesic state when the score exceeds 75.

gam-. See **gamo-, gam-.**

Gambian trypanosomiasis /gam″bē·ən/, a usually chronic form of African trypanosomiasis, caused by the parasite Trypanosoma brucei gambiense. An infected individual may have relatively mild symptoms for months or years before developing the neurological symptoms of the terminal stage. Also called *Trypanosoma brucei gambiense,* **West African sleeping sickness.** Compare **Rhodesian trypanosomiasis.** See also **African trypanosomiasis.**

game knee [ME, gamen + AS, cneow], an informal term for any injury or condition that interferes with normal function of the knee joint.

gamet-. See **gameto-, gamet-.**

gamete /gam″ēt/ [Gk, marriage partner], **1.** a mature male or female germ cell that is capable of functioning in fertilization or conjugation and contains the haploid number of chromosomes of the organism. **2.** an ovum or a spermatozoon. See also **meiosis.** –**gametic,** *adj.*

gamete intrafallopian transfer (GIFT), a human fertilization technique in which male and female gametes are injected through a laparoscope into the fimbriated ends of the fallopian tubes.

gametic /gəmat″ik/, pertaining to a reproductive cell such as a spermatozoon or ovum forming the gamete.

gametic chromosome, any of the chromosomes contained in a haploid cell, specifically a spermatozoon or an ovum, as contrasted with those in a diploid, or somatic, cell.

gameto-, gamet-, prefix meaning "reproductive cell": *gametocyte, gametogenesis.*

gametocide /gəmē″tōsīd/ [Gk, *gamete* + L, *caedere,* to kill], any agent that is destructive to gametes or gametocytes. The term is most often used to refer to agents specific for gametocytes of the protozoon *Plasmodium,* which causes malaria. –**gametocidal,** *adj.*

gametocyte /gəmē″tōsīt/ [Gk, *gamete* + *kytos,* cell], any cell capable of dividing into or in the process of developing into a gamete.

gametogenesis /gam″itōjen″əsis/ [Gk, *gamete* + *genein,* to produce], the origin and maturation of gametes, which occurs through meiosis. See also **oogenesis, spermatogenesis.** –**gametogenous, gametogenic,** *adj.*

gametophyte /gəmē″tōfīt/ [Gk, *gamete* + *phyton,* plant], a cell in the reproductive stage when the nuclei are in a haploid condition.

gamma /gam″ə/, Γ, γ, the third letter of the Greek alphabet. It is a symbol for photon, heavy-chain immunoglobulins, or the third component in a series of certain chemical groups, such as the gamma-chain of hemoglobin.

gamma-aminobutyric acid (GABA), an amino acid that functions as an inhibitory neurotransmitter in the brain and spinal cord. It is also found in the heart, lungs, and kidneys and in certain plants.

gamma-benzene hexachloride. See **lindane.**

gamma camera [Gk, *gamma,* third letter of Greek alphabet; L, *camera,* vault], a device that uses the emission of light from a crystal struck by gamma rays to produce an image of the distribution of radioactive material in a body organ. The light is detected by an array of light-sensitive electronic components and is converted into electric signals, which are processed to produce the image. The gamma camera is a workhorse of nuclear medicine departments, where it is used to produce scans of patients who have been injected with small amounts of radioactive materials.

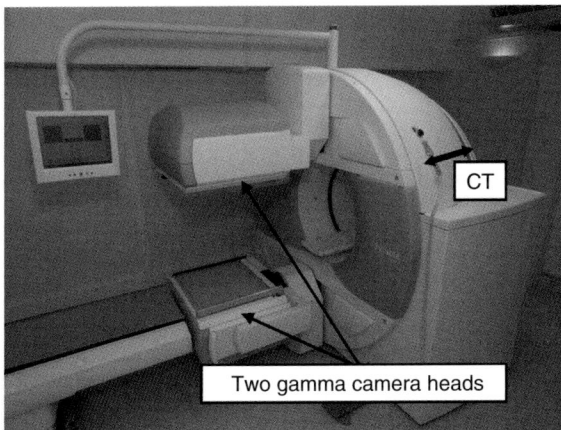

CT

Two gamma camera heads

Combined gamma camera, with two detector heads and CT scan *(Papathanassiou and Liehn, 2008)*

gamma efferent fiber [Gk, *gamma* + L, *efferre,* to carry out, *fibra,* fiber], any of the motor nerve fibers that transmit impulses from the central nervous system to the intrafusal fibers of the muscle spindle. The gamma efferent fibers are responsible for deep tendon reflexes, spasticity, and rigidity, but not for the degree of contractile response. They function in regulating the sensitivity of the spindle and the total tension of the muscle.

gamma globulin. See **immune gamma globulin.**

gamma-glutamyltransferase (GGT), an enzyme that appears in the serum of patients with several types of liver or gallbladder disorders, including drug hepatotoxicity, biliary tract obstruction, alcohol-induced liver disease, and liver carcinoma. Normal adult (after 45 years of age) GGT blood levels are 8 to 38 U/L.

gamma-glutamyltransferase (GGT) test, a blood test that measures GGT and is used to detect liver cell dysfunction. It accurately indicates cholestasis, biliary obstruction, cholangitis, or cholecystitis. It can also detect chronic alcohol ingestion and therefore is useful in the screening or evaluation of patients with alcoholism. Levels of GGT are also elevated after acute myocardial infarction.

gamma interferon. See **interferon gamma.**

gamma knife, an apparatus for precisely aimed intersecting beams of gamma rays that delivers radiation therapies as treatment for intracranial lesions, either tumors or vascular anomalies. It is used in stereotactic radiosurgery.

gamma knife stereotaxic radiosurgery, a method for destroying deep-seated brain tumors with a focused beam of gamma radiation. By using three-dimensional stereoscopic techniques to aim the radiation from several angles, it is possible to concentrate the energy on the tumor while minimizing damage to surrounding tissues.

gamma radiation [Gk, *gamma* + L, *radiare,* to emit rays], a very-high-frequency form of electromagnetic radiation consisting of photons emitted by radioactive elements in the course of nuclear transition. The wavelength of gamma radiation is characteristic of the radioactive elements involved and ranges from about 4×10^{-10} to 5×10^{-13} m. Gamma radiation can penetrate thousands of meters of air and several centimeters of soft tissue and bone. It is more penetrating than alpha radiation and beta radiation but has less ionizing power and is not deflected in electric or magnetic fields. Like x radiation, gamma radiation can injure and destroy body cells and tissue, especially cell nuclei. However, controlled application of gamma radiation is important in the diagnosis and treatment of various conditions, including skin cancer and malignancies deep within the body. Also called *gamma rays.* See also **x-ray.**

gammopathy /gamop″əthē/, an abnormal condition characterized by the presence of markedly increased levels of gamma globulin in the blood. Two different types of hypergammaglobulinemia can be distinguished. Monoclonal gammopathy is commonly associated with an electrophoretic pattern showing one sharp, homogenous electrophoretic band in the gamma globulin region. This reflects the presence of excessive amounts of one type of immunoglobulin secreted by a single clone of B lymphocytes. Polyclonal gammopathy reflects the presence of a diffuse hypergammaglobulinemia in which all immunoglobulin classes are proportionally increased. See also **Bence Jones protein, multiple myeloma.**

gamo-, gam-, prefix meaning "marriage" or "sexual union": *gamogenesis, gamont, gamone.*

gamogenesis /gam″ōjen″əsis/ [Gk, *gamos,* marriage, *genein,* to produce], sexual reproduction through the fusion of gametes. –**gamogenetic,** *adj.*

gamone /gam″ōn/ [Gk, *gamos,* marriage], a chemical substance secreted by ova and spermatozoa that is believed to attract the gametes of the opposite sex and facilitate union. Kinds include **androgamone, gynogamone.**

gampsodactyly. See **clawfoot.**

-gamy, 1. suffix meaning a "(specified) type of marriage": *monogamy.* **2.** suffix meaning "possession of organs for reproduction": *autogamy.* **3.** suffix meaning a "union for propagation": *allogamy.*

ganciclovir /gansik′lōvir/, an antiviral drug structurally related to acyclovir, used to prevent cytomegalovirus disease after transplantation and to treat or prevent cytomegalovirus retinitis in persons with acquired immunodeficiency syndrome.

gangli-. See **ganglio-, gangli-.**

ganglia. See **ganglion.**

gangliated. See **ganglionated.**

ganglio-, gangli-, prefix meaning "ganglion": *gangliocytoma, ganglionated.*

gangliocytoma /gang′glē·ō′sītō″mə/, a benign tumor involving ganglion cells. These tumors are frequently found in the pituitary gland, where they are associated with hypersecretion of growth hormone–releasing hormone (ganglioneuroma).

ganglion /gang′glē·on/ *pl. ganglia* [Gk, knot], **1.** a knot or knotlike mass of nervous tissue. **2.** one of the nerve cell bodies, chiefly collected in groups outside the central nervous system. Very small groups abound in association with alimentary organs. The two types of ganglia in the body are the sensory ganglia on the dorsal roots of spinal nerves and on the sensory roots of the trigeminal, facial, glossopharyngeal, and vagus nerves and the autonomic ganglia of the sympathetic and parasympathetic systems.

ganglionar neuroma /gang·glē″ənər/ [Gk, *ganglion* + *neuron,* nerve, *oma,* tumor], a tumor composed of a solid mass of ganglia and nerve fibers, usually found in abdominal tissues and occurring most commonly in children. Chemotherapy or surgery is often recommended. Also called **ganglionated neuroma, ganglionic neuroma.**

ganglionated, having ganglia. Also called **gangliated.**

ganglionated nerve, a nerve of the sympathetic nervous system.

ganglionated neuroma. See **ganglionar neuroma.**

ganglionic blockade /gang′glē·on″ik/, the blocking of nerve impulses at synapses of autonomic ganglia, usually by the administration of ganglionic blocking agents.

ganglionic blocking agent, any one of a group of drugs prescribed to produce controlled hypotension, as required in certain surgical procedures or in emergency management of hypertensive crisis. The drugs act by occupying receptor sites (nicotinic neuronal receptors) on sympathetic and parasympathetic autonomic ganglia, preventing a response of these nerves to the action of acetylcholine liberated by the presynaptic nerve endings. Mecamylamine is the most commonly prescribed ganglionic blocking agent. These drugs are used with great caution in treating patients who are affected with coronary, cerebrovascular, or renal insufficiency or who have a history of severe allergy. Adverse reactions to the drugs include sudden marked hypotension, paralytic ileus, urinary retention, constipation, visual disturbances, heartburn, and nausea.

ganglionic crest. See **neural crest.**

ganglionic cyst, a swollen area of the synovial sheath of a tendon that is common at the back of the wrist.

ganglionic glioma [Gk, *ganglion* + *glia,* glue, *oma,* tumor], a nervous system tumor composed of glial cells and ganglion cells that are nearly mature. See also **neuroblastoma.**

ganglionic neuroma. See **ganglionar neuroma.**

ganglionic ridge. See **neural crest.**

ganglion impar, the union of the two sympathetic trunks anterior to the coccyx.

ganglionitis /gang′glē·ənī″tis/, an inflammation of a nerve or lymph ganglion.

ganglioside /gang″glē·əsīd′/, a glycosphingolipid found in the brain and other nervous system tissues. Gangliosides are members of a group of galactose-containing cerebrosides with a basic composition of ceramide-glucose-galactose-*N*-acetyl neuraminic acid. Accumulation of gangliosides caused by an inborn error of metabolism results in gangliosidosis or Tay-Sachs disease.

gangliosidosis type I. See **Tay-Sachs disease.**

gangliosidosis type II. See **Sandhoff's disease.**

gang rape, sexual intercourse against the will of the victim by a group of assailants. Gang sex attacks usually, but not always, are committed by several males who take turns assaulting a female, but the victim may be another male, as in a prison. See also **rape, statutory rape.**

gangrene /gang″grēn/ [Gk, *gangraina,* a gnawing sore], necrosis or death of tissue, usually the result of ischemia (loss of blood supply), bacterial invasion, and subsequent putrefaction. The extremities are most often affected, but it can occur in the intestines and gallbladder. Internally gangrene may be a complication of strangulated hernia, appendicitis, cholecystitis, or thrombosis of the mesenteric arteries to the gut. In all types of gangrene, surgical debridement is necessary to remove the necrotic tissue before healing can progress. Cleanliness and maintenance of good circulation are considerations essential in preventing this condition. See also **gas gangrene, open amputation, dry gangrene, moist gangrene.** *–gangrenous, adj.*

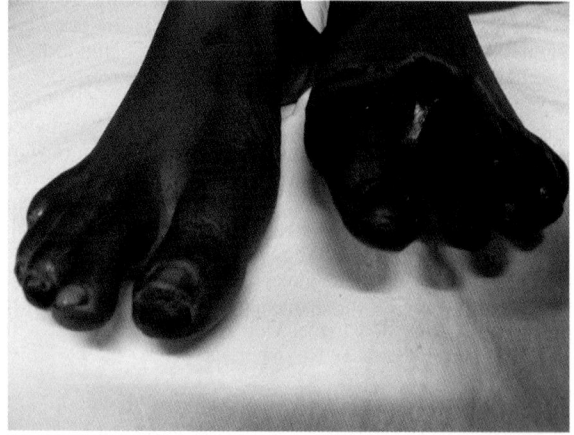

Gangrene of the feet *(Misra et al, 2013)*

gangrenous appendicitis /gang″grənəs/ [Gk, *gangraina,* a gnawing sore; L, *appendere,* to hang upon; Gk, *itis,* inflammation], a condition in which the appendix becomes gangrenous because obstruction of its lumen blocks the flow of blood to that body part.

gangrenous necrosis. See **necrosis.**

gangrenous stomatitis. See **noma.**

gangrenous vulvitis [Gk, *gangraina* + L, *vulva,* wrapper; Gk, *itis,* inflammation], tissue necrosis of the vulva, usually associated with inadequate blood supply and often with bacterial infection as well.

ganirelix, a gonadotropin-releasing hormone antagonist.

- INDICATIONS: It is used to inhibit premature luteinizing hormone surges in women undergoing controlled ovarian hyperstimulation.
- CONTRAINDICATIONS: Pregnancy, lactation, latex allergy, and known hypersensitivity to this drug prohibit its use.
- ADVERSE EFFECTS: Fetal death is a life-threatening consequence of this drug's use. Other adverse effects include headache, ovarian hyperstimulation syndrome, gynecological abdominal pain, nausea, and pain on injection. Common side effects include spotting and breakthrough bleeding.

ganja. See **cannabis.**

Gantanol, a sulfa antibiotic. Brand name for **sulfamethox-azole.**

Gantrisin, a sulfa antibiotic. Brand name for **sulfiSOXA-ZOLE.**

gantry assembly /gan″trē/, a subsystem of the computed tomography apparatus consisting of the x-ray tube, the detector array, the high-voltage generator, the patient support and positioning couch, and the mechanical support for each.

gap [OE, *gapa,* a hole], **1.** a short, missing segment in one strand of a DNA molecule. **2.** a break in development caused by physical, social, or emotional deficits. **3.** an opening in a solid structure or surface.

gap junction, a type of junction between cells, consisting of a narrowed portion of the intercellular space that contains channels or pores composed of hexagonal arrays of membrane-spanning proteins around a central lumen (connexon), through which pass ions and small molecules. In electrically excitable tissues such as myocardial tissue and the central nervous system, gap junctions serve to transmit electrical impulses by movement of ions and are known as electrotonic synapses. Also called **nexus.** See also **connexon.**

gap phenomenon, a situation in which a premature cardiac stimulus encounters a block where an earlier or later stimulus could be conducted.

Garamycin, an aminoglycoside antibacterial drug. Brand name for **gentamicin sulfate.**

Gardner-Diamond syndrome [Frank H. Gardner, American physician, b. 1919; Louis K. Diamond, American physician, b. 1902], a condition resulting from autoerythrocyte sensitization, marked by large, painful transient skin discolorations that appear without apparent cause but often accompany emotional upsets, various collagen disorders, and abnormalities of protein metabolism. Treatment includes topical and systemic corticosteroids. Also called **autoerythrocyte sensitization syndrome.**

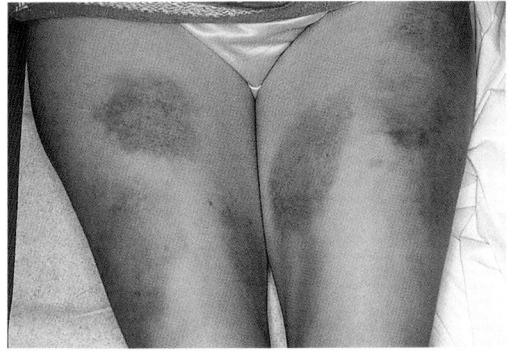

Skin discolorations associated with Gardner-Diamond syndrome *(Callen et al, 2000)*

Gardnerella vaginalis /gärd′nərel″ə/ [Herman L. Gardner, 20th-century American bacteriologist; L, *vagina,* sheath], a genus of rod-shaped gram-negative bacteria normally found in the female genital tract. Overgrowth is associated with polymicrobial infection. See also **bacterial vaginosis.**

Gardnerella vaginalis vaginitis [Herman L. Gardner; L, *vagina,* sheath; Gk, *itis,* inflammation], a chronic inflammation of the vagina caused by the bacterium *Gardnerella vaginalis.*

Gardner, Mary Sewell [1871–1961], an American public health nurse who wrote the classic text *Public Health Nursing.* She directed the Providence, Rhode Island, District Nursing Association and was instrumental in the development of the National Organization for Public Health Nursing and of public health nursing in the American Red Cross.

Gardner syndrome [Eldon J. Gardner, American geneticist, 1909–1989], a form of familial polyposis of the large bowel, with fibrous dysplasia of the skull, extra teeth, osteomas, fibromas, and epidermal cysts. The condition is inherited as an autosomal-dominant trait, and malignancies occur more often than usual in families having this syndrome.

Gardner-Wells tongs, pins that are attached to the skull of patients immobilized with cervical injuries. The pins are used to apply traction to reduce a fracture or dislocation while the patient is in a bed with a traction setup.

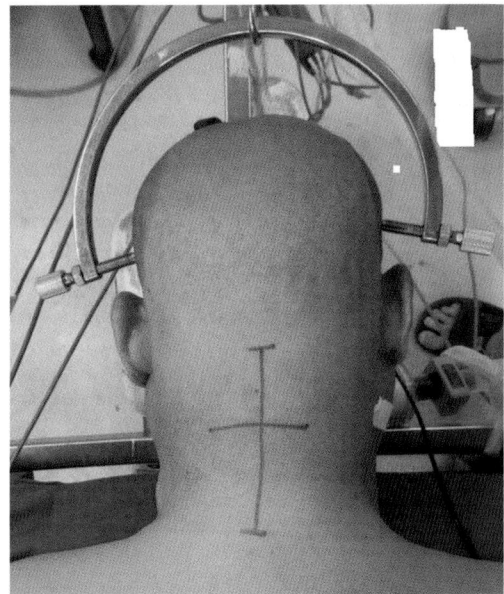

Patient with Gardner-Wells tongs *(Kumar et al, 2014)*

gargle /gär″gəl/ [Fr, *gargouille,* drainpipe], **1.** *v.,* to hold and agitate a liquid at the back of the throat by tilting the head backward and forcing air through the solution. The procedure is used for cleansing or medicating the mouth and oropharynx. **2.** *n.,* a solution used to rinse the mouth and oropharynx.

gargoylism. See **Hurler syndrome.**

garlic, an herbal product taken from a perennial bulb grown throughout the world.
- INDICATIONS: It is used for vascular disease, elevated LDL, elevated triglycerides, low HDL, high blood pressure, poor circulation, risk of cancer, inflammatory disorders,

G

childhood ear infection, and yeast infection. The allicin of fresh garlic may cause a small decrease in LDL cholesterol and slight decrease in blood pressure and may have some antibacterial properties, but garlic is not nearly as effective as prescribed drugs for these purposes. Its influence on cancer risk and efficacy for other uses has not been adequately documented. Allicin is very labile, and there is concern that many commercial products contain less than the advertised amount of allicin.

■ CONTRAINDICATIONS: In normal amounts, garlic is likely safe during pregnancy and for children. Garlic should not be used in large amounts during pregnancy, because it may be fatal to the fetus or stimulate labor. Large amounts also should not be given to children directly or via breast milk because it may cause colic in infants or be fatal to children through uncharacterized mechanisms. It is contraindicated in those with known hypersensitivity, stomach inflammation, or gastritis. People who have had or are about to have surgery should also avoid it, since clotting time may be increased.

GARS, abbreviation for **Gait Assessment Rating Scale.**

Garth method [William P. Garth, American orthopedic surgeon], a positioning method for producing x-ray images of the scapulohumeral joint and identifying shoulder dislocations, scapular fractures, and bony defects involving the humeral head. The patient faces the x-ray tube with the affected shoulder joint centered to the midline of the image receptor (IR). The affected elbow is flexed and the forearm is placed across the patient's chest. The opposite shoulder is angled 45 degrees away from the IR. The central ray is directed at a 45-degree angle toward the patient's feet and passes through the affected shoulder joint.

Gartner's cyst [Hermann T. Gartner, Danish anatomist, 1785–1827], a remnant of the mesonephric (Wolffian) ducts that develop, from predetermined structures, and later regress. The remnant may develop a secretory mechanism, causing dilation of surrounding cells, and transform into a duct cyst, usually during late adolescence.

Gartner's duct, one of two vestigial closed ducts, each parallel to a uterine tube.

gas [Gk, *chaos*], an aeriform fluid that possesses complete molecular mobility and the property of indefinite expansion. A gas has no definite shape, and its volume is determined by its container and by temperature and pressure. Compare **liquid, solid. –gaseous,** *adj.*

GAS, abbreviation for **general adaptation syndrome.**

gas bacillus [Gk, *chaos* + L, *bacillum,* small rod], any of several bacillus-shaped species that produce a gas as a byproduct of their metabolism. Examples include *Escherichia coli,* which ferments lactose and glucose, and the clostridial species that produces gas gangrene.

gas chromatography, the separation and analysis of different substances according to their different affinities for a standard absorbent. In the process a gaseous mixture of the substances is passed through a glass cylinder containing the absorbent, which may be dampened with a nonvolatile liquid solvent for one or more of the gaseous components. As the mixture passes through the absorbent, each substance is absorbed to a different extent and leaves a characteristic pigment. The bands of different colors left when all the gaseous mixture has moved through the absorbent constitute a chromatograph for analysis. Compare **column chromatography, ion exchange chromatography.**

gas distension, a visual and measurable expansion of abdominal girth due to an accumulation of air within the gastrointestinal tract.

gas embolism, an occlusion of one or more small blood vessels, especially in the muscles, tendons, and joints, caused by expanding gas bubbles. Gas emboli can rupture tissue and blood vessels, causing decompression sickness and death. This phenomenon commonly affects deep-sea divers who rise too quickly to the surface without adequate decompression. Gas emboli are most dangerous in the central nervous system because of associated neurological changes, such as syncope, paralysis, and aphasia. Such emboli are extremely painful. The prevention and treatment of gas emboli involve gradual decompression of atmospheric gases, especially nitrogen, that are dissolved in the blood. Compare **air embolism, fat embolism.** See also **decompression sickness.**

gas endarterectomy. See **endarterectomy.**

gaseous. See **gas.**

gas gangrene, necrosis accompanied by gas bubbles in soft tissue after surgery or trauma. It is caused by anaerobic organisms, such as various species of *Clostridium,* particularly *C. perfringens.* Symptoms include pain, swelling, and tenderness of the wound area; moderate fever; tachycardia; and hypotension. The skin around the wound becomes necrotic and ruptures, revealing necrotic muscle. A characteristic finding is toxic delirium. Spontaneous gas gangrene is most often caused by the spread of *C. septicum* from the GI tract of colon cancer patients. Because of its aerotolerant nature, *C. septicum* can infect normal tissues. If untreated, gas gangrene is rapidly fatal. Prompt treatment, including excision of gangrenous tissue and IV administration of penicillin G, saves 80% of patients. The disease is prevented by proper wound care. Also called **anaerobic myositis.**

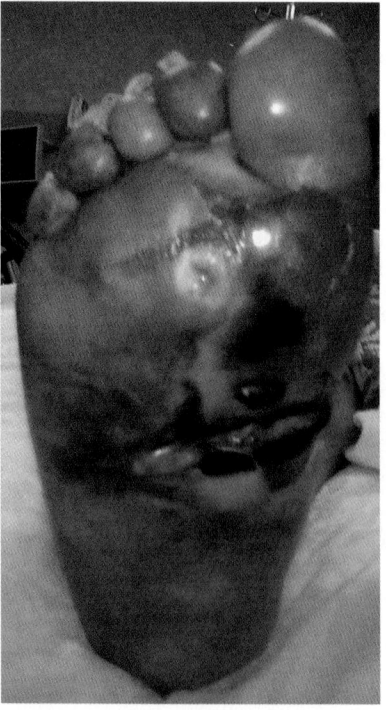

Foot of patient with gas gangrene *(Brucato et al, 2014)*

gasoline poisoning. See **petroleum distillate poisoning.**

gas pains. See **flatulence.**

gas permeable contact lens. See **rigid gas permeable (RGP) contact lens.**

gas-scavenging system, the equipment used to prevent waste anesthetic gases from escaping into the atmosphere of the operating room. Also called **scavenging system.** See also **trace gas.**

Gasser syndrome. See **hemolytic uremic syndrome.**

gas sterilization [Gk, *chaos,* gas; L, *sterilis,* barren], the use of a gas such as ethylene oxide, C_2H_4O, to sterilize medical equipment.

Gastaut disease. See **Lennox-Gastaut syndrome.**

gaster-. See **gastro-, gaster-, gastr-.**

gas therapy, the use of medical gases in respiratory therapy. Kinds include **carbon dioxide therapy, controlled oxygen therapy, helium therapy, hyperbaric oxygenation.**

gastr-. See **gastro-, gaster-, gastr-.**

gastralgia. See **stomachache.**

gastrectasia /gas′trektā″zhə/ [Gk, *gaster,* stomach, *ektasis,* stretching], an abnormal dilation of the stomach that may be accompanied by pain, vomiting, rapid pulse, and falling body temperature. Causes include overeating, obstruction of the pyloric valve, or a hernia.

gastrectomy /gastrek″təmē/, surgical excision of all or, more commonly, part of the stomach, performed to remove a chronic peptic ulcer, to stop hemorrhage in a perforating ulcer, or to remove a malignancy. Before surgery a GI series is done and a nasogastric tube is inserted. With the patient under general anesthesia, one half to two thirds of the stomach is removed, including the ulcer and a large area of acid-secreting mucosa. A gastroenterostomy is then done, joining the remainder of the stomach to the jejunum or duodenum. After surgery the nurse observes the drainage from the nasogastric suction tube for bright red blood, indicative of hemorrhage. Blockage of the tube is reported at once, because gastric distension strains the suture lines. Irrigation is done only according to surgeon's orders, gently and with small amounts of fluid, if at all. Adequate medication for pain allows deeper breathing and coughing because the incision is close to the diaphragm. The nurse encourages the patient to breathe deeply and, if necessary, to cough. With the return of peristalsis, water is given orally, and, if tolerated without pain or nausea, the nasogastric tube is removed. The diet gradually progresses to six small bland meals a day with 120 mL of fluid hourly between meals. A temperature elevation or dyspnea may indicate leakage of oral fluids or gastric leaks from the incision around the anastomosis. The most common complication of gastrectomy is dumping syndrome, with fullness and discomfort after meals. Other possible complications include marginal peptic ulcer, in which gastric acids come into contact with a suture line; afferent loop syndrome, in which the duodenal loop is blocked and pancreatic juices and bile flow back into the stomach; vitamin B_{12} and folic acid deficiency; reduced absorption of calcium and vitamin D; and functional hyperinsulinism, in which carbohydrates now passing directly into the small bowel cause an outpouring of insulin into the bloodstream and a resultant hypoglycemia within 2 hours. See also **dumping syndrome, gastric resection, gastroenterostomy, nasogastric tube, peptic ulcer.**

-gastria, suffix meaning "(condition of) possessing a stomach or stomachs": *agastria, microgastria.*

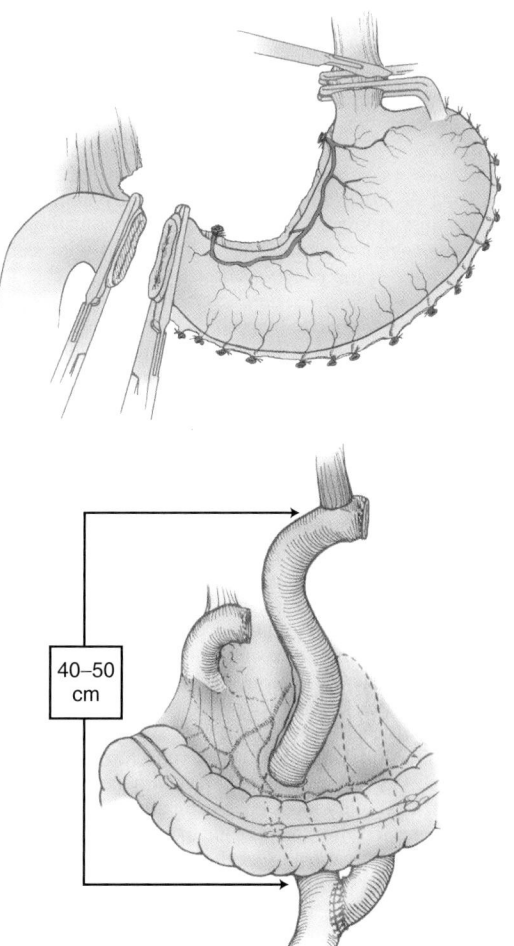

Total gastrectomy *(Rothrock, 2015)*

gastric /gas″trik/ [Gk, *gaster,* stomach], pertaining to the stomach.

-gastric, suffix meaning a "pertaining to the stomach": *hypogastric, mesogastric.*

gastric acid pump inhibitor. See **proton pump inhibitor.**

gastric analysis, examination of the contents of the stomach, primarily to determine the quantity of acid present and incidentally to ascertain the presence of blood, bile, bacteria, and abnormal cells. It may also be done to detect acid-fast bacillus in a client with undiagnosed tuberculosis. A sample of gastric secretion is obtained via a nasogastric tube. The technique used varies according to the information desired. The total absence of hydrochloric acid is diagnostic of pernicious anemia. Patients with gastric ulcer and gastric cancer may secrete less acid than normal whereas patients with duodenal ulcers secrete more. The composition and volume of the secretions may also provide diagnostic information. This procedure is rarely performed.

gastric antacid. See **antacid.**

gastric antral vascular ectasia, a rare vascular anomaly of the gastric antrum consisting of dilated and thrombosed capillaries and veins that form lines in the antrum that radiate toward the pylorus, resembling the stripes on a watermelon, seen most often in elderly women or patients with chronic liver disease. It may result in chronic blood loss and anemia. Also called *watermelon stomach.*

gastric areas, small patches of gastric mucosa, 1 to 5 mm in diameter, separated by the plicae villosae and containing the gastric pits.

gastric atrophy. See **atrophic gastritis.**

gastric banding, a surgical treatment for weight reduction consisting of creation of a gastric pouch by application to the proximal stomach of a silicone band, sometimes with an accompanying reservoir that can be filled with saline to adjust the size of the pouch's stoma.

gastric bypass, bariatric surgery performed to reduce stomach capacity and allow food to bypass part of the small intestine.

gastric cancer, a malignancy of the stomach. Approximately 97% of stomach tumors are adenocarcinomas, which may be ulcerating, polypoid, diffuse, and fibrous, or superficial spreading lesions. Lymphomas and leiomyosarcomas account for less than 3%. Symptoms of gastric cancer are vague epigastric discomfort, dysphagia, anorexia, weight loss, back pain, and unexplained iron-deficiency anemia. However, many cases are asymptomatic in the early stages, and metastases may cause the first symptoms. Diagnostic measures include a test for occult blood in the stool, an upper GI series, a computed tomographic examination of the gastric mucosa with a flexible endoscope, and biopsy and cytological studies of exfoliated tumor cells. Surgery is usually recommended for suitable lesions. Radiotherapy and chemotherapy are usually not effective in adenocarcinoma but are often used in gastric lymphoma. Chemotherapy is used in treating advanced metastatic gastric adenocarcinoma. Gastric cancer is declining in incidence in North America and Western Europe but is common in Japan. Dietary factors, such as nitrates, smoked and salted fish and meats, and moldy foods containing aflatoxin, and infection with *Helicobacter pylori* are thought to cause gastric cancer, but the cause remains unknown. Genetic factors also play a role. The incidence is higher in men than in women and peaks in individuals 50 to 59 years of age. The risk increases in workers exposed to asbestos and in patients with pernicious anemia.

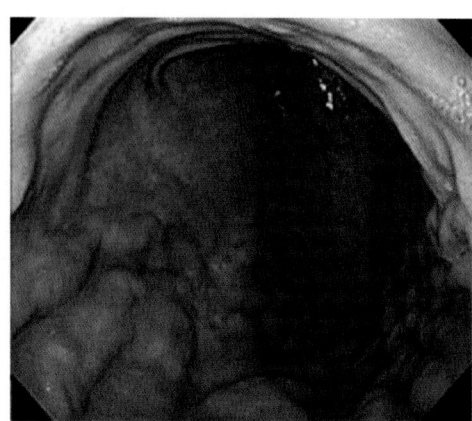

Gastric cancer *(Sugano, 2008)*

gastric digestion [Gk, *gaster,* stomach; L, *digere,* to separate], digestion by gastric juice in the stomach.

gastric dumping, excessively rapid movement of partially digested food from the stomach into the jejunum, occurring most often in patients who have had partial gastrectomy with gastrojejunostomy.

gastric dyspepsia, pain or discomfort localized in the stomach. See also **dyspepsia.**

gastric emesis [Gk, *gaster,* stomach, *emesis,* vomiting], vomiting associated with a stomach disorder, such as stomach cancer, stomach ulcer, or severe gastritis.

gastric fistula, an abnormal passage into the stomach, communicating most frequently with an opening on the external surface of the abdomen. A gastric fistula may be created surgically to provide tube feeding for patients with severe esophageal disorders. See also **gastrostomy, gastrostomy feeding.**

gastric fundus, that part of the stomach to the left and above the level of the entrance of the esophagus.

gastric glands, the secreting glands of the stomach, including the fundic, cardiac, and pyloric glands; sometimes used specifically to denote the fundic glands.

gastric inhibitory polypeptide (GIP), a GI hormone found in the mucosa of the small intestine. Release of the hormone, mediated by the presence of glucose or fatty acids in the duodenum, results in the release of insulin by the pancreas and inhibition of gastric mobility acid secretion.

gastric intubation, a procedure in which a Levin tube or other small-caliber catheter is passed through the nose into the esophagus and stomach. It may be used for the introduction into the stomach of liquid formulas to provide nutrition for unconscious patients or for premature or sick newborns. Medication or a contrast medium may be instilled for treatment or for radiological examination. See also **gastric lavage, Levin tube.**

gastric juice, digestive secretions of the gastric glands in the stomach, consisting chiefly of pepsin, hydrochloric acid, rennin, and mucin. The pH is strongly acid (0.9 to 1.5). Achlorhydria (a deficiency of hydrochloric acid in gastric juice) is present in pernicious anemia and stomach cancer. Excessive secretion of gastric juice may lead to mucosal irritation and peptic ulcer. See also **achlorhydria, gastric analysis, peptic ulcer.**

gastric lavage, the washing out of the stomach with sterile water or a saline solution. The procedure is performed to remove irritants or toxic substances and possibly before such examinations as endoscopy or gastroscopy. See also **irrigation.**

gastric motility, the spontaneous peristaltic movements of the stomach that aid in digestion, moving food through the stomach and out through the pyloric sphincter into the duodenum. Excess gastric motility causes pain that is usually treated with antispasmodic medication. Below normal motility is common in labor, after general anesthesia, and as a side effect of some sedative hypnotics.

gastric mucin [Gk, *gaster,* stomach; L, *mucus*], a viscous secretion of glycoproteins produced from the mucous membrane lining of swine stomachs and formerly used in the treatment of peptic ulcers.

gastric node, a node in one of three groups of lymph glands associated with the abdominal and pelvic viscera supplied by branches of the celiac artery. The gastric nodes accompany the left gastric artery and are divided into the superior and inferior gastric nodes. Compare **hepatic node, pancreaticolienal node.**

gastric pacing, surgical implantation of pacing wires attached to the stomach; an emerging therapy for gastroparesis.

gastric reduction duodenal switch (GRDS), a surgical procedure for weight reduction. See **duodenal switch.**

gastric resection [Gk, *gaster,* stomach; L, *re + secare,* to cut], the surgical removal of part or all of the stomach, usually performed in the treatment of stomach cancer or intractable peptic ulcer. See also **gastrectomy, gastroenterostomy.**

gastric restriction, any of various surgical treatments for morbid obesity in which part of the stomach is closed off from the flow of nutrients through the alimentary canal, such as gastric banding, gastric bypass, and gastric partitioning.

gastric sleeve, a surgical procedure to reduce the size of the stomach. It reduces the amount of food that can be consumed and reduces hunger. It may be the first stage prior to a duodenal switch; some patients lose enough weight that a second surgical procedure is not required. See also **bariatric surgery, duodenal switch.**

gastric ulcer. See **peptic ulcer.**

gastrin /gas″trin/ [Gk, *gaster,* stomach], a polypeptide hormone, secreted by the pylorus, that stimulates the flow

G

of gastric juice and contributes to the stimulus for bile and pancreatic enzyme secretion. Normal findings of blood levels of gastrin are less than 200 pg/mL.

gastrinoma /gas′trinō″mə/, a tumor found in the pancreas and in the duodenum associated with the presence of peptic ulcers.

gastrin-releasing peptide, a 27-amino acid linear neuropeptide, structurally and functionally related to bombesin, that mediates neural release of antral gastrin, causes bronchoconstriction and respiratory tract vasodilation, stimulates growth and mitogenesis of cells in culture, and may act as an excitatory neurotransmitter of enteric interneurons.

gastrin stimulation test following calcium infusion, a serum test for gastrin, a gastric or pancreatic secretion. Blood is collected before and sequentially after calcium infusion and measured for gastrin. The presence of a gastrinoma (Zollinger-Ellison syndrome) is reflected in a sharp rise in gastrin production.

gastritis /gastrī″tis/, an inflammation of the lining of the stomach that occurs in two forms. Acute gastritis may be caused by severe burns; major surgery; aspirin or other antiinflammatory agents (nonsteroidal antiinflammatory drugs); corticosteroids; drugs; food allergens; or viral, bacterial, or chemical toxins. Symptoms include anorexia, nausea, vomiting, and discomfort after eating. They usually abate after the causative agent has been removed. Chronic gastritis is usually a sign of underlying disease, such as peptic ulcer, stomach cancer, Zollinger-Ellison syndrome, or pernicious anemia. Differential diagnosis is by endoscopy with biopsy. Compare **peptic ulcer.** Kinds include **atrophic gastritis, hemorrhagic gastritis, hypertrophic gastritis.** See also **acute erosive gastritis, alkaline reflux gastritis.**

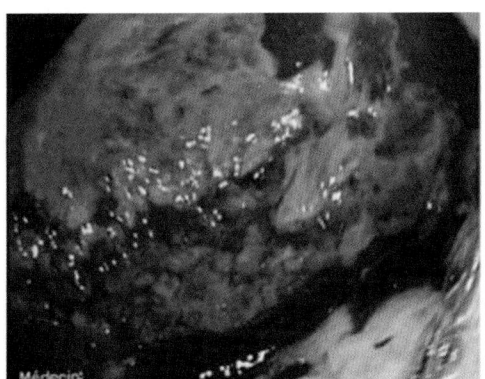

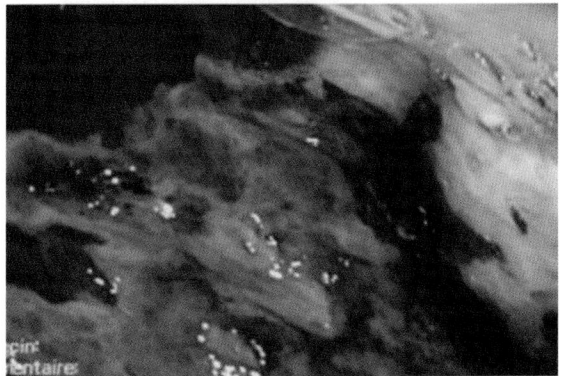

Severe gastritis *(Amielh et al, 2009)*

gastro-, gaster-, gastr-, prefix meaning "stomach" or "abdomen": *gastrocoele, gastroenteritis.*

gastrocamera /gas′trōkam″ərə/, a small camera that can be lowered into the stomach through the esophagus and retrieved after recording images of the stomach lining.

gastrocnemius /gas′trōnē″me·us/ [Gk, *gastroknemia,* calf of the leg], the most superficial calf muscle in the posterior part of the leg. It joins the tendon of the soleus as part of the tendo calcaneus. It flexes the leg and plantarflexes the foot. Compare **plantaris, soleus.**

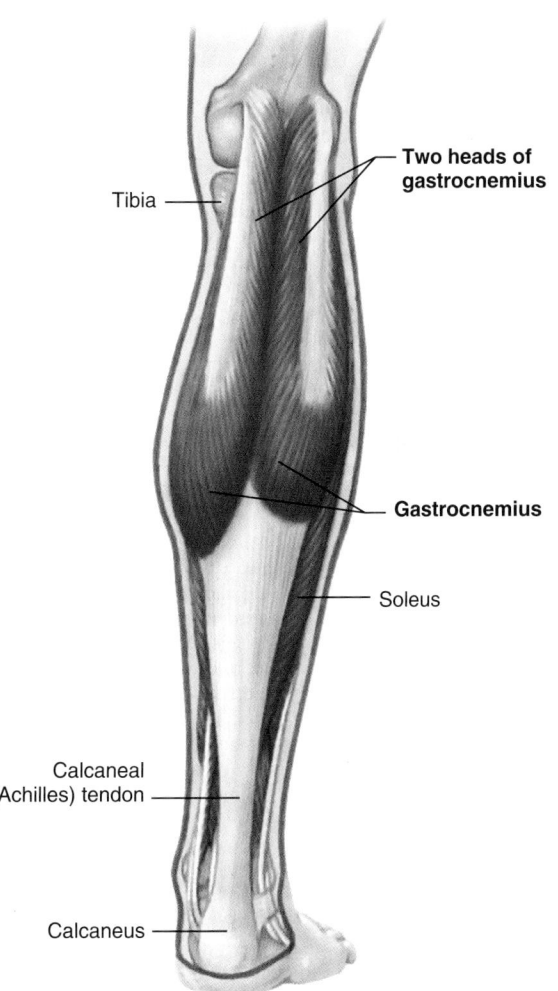

Gastrocnemius *(Patton and Thibodeau, 2016)*

gastrocnemius gait, an abnormal gait associated with a weakness of the gastrocnemius, characterized by the dropping of the pelvis on the affected side at the last moment of the stance phase in the walking cycle, accompanied by lagging or slowness in forward pelvic movement.

gastrocnemius test, a test of the function of the gastrocnemius muscle by ankle plantar flexion while the patient is in a prone position. The examiner places fingers for palpation on the posterior side of the calf while the patient pulls the heel upward, thus plantar flexing the ankle. Flexion of the toes and forefoot before movement of the heel is evidence of muscle substitution.

gastrocoele. See **archenteron.**

gastrocolic omentum. See **greater omentum.**

gastrocolic reflex /-kol″ik/ [Gk, *gaster* + *kolon,* colon; L, *reflectere,* to bend backward], a mass peristaltic movement of the colon that often occurs 15 to 20 minutes after food enters the stomach. When an infant is fed, this reflex may cause bowel movement.

gastrocystoplasty /gas″trosis′toplas″te/, augmentation cystoplasty using a portion of the stomach for the graft.

gastrodidymus /-did″iməs/ [Gk, *gaster* + *didymos,* twin], conjoined, equally developed twins united at the abdominal region. Also called **omphalodidymus.**

gastrodisciasis /gas′trōdiskī″əsis/ [Gk, *gaster* + *diskos,* disk, *eidos,* form, *osis,* condition], an infection of trematodes of the genus *Gastrodiscoides,* which are digestive tract parasites. The species *G. hominis,* a reddish-orange fluke averaging 1 cm in length, is endemic in the hog populations of Southeast Asia and is transmitted to humans.

gastrodisk. See **embryonic disk.**

gastroduodenal /-do͞o′ədē″nəl/ [Gk, *gaster* + L, *duodeni,* 12 fingers], pertaining to the stomach and duodenum.

gastroduodenitis /-do͞o′ədenī″tis/ [Gk, *gaster,* stomach; L, *duodeni,* 12 fingers; Gk, *itis,* inflammation], inflammation of the stomach and duodenum.

gastroduodenoscopy /-do͞o′ədenos″kəpē/, inspection of the stomach and duodenum by means of a gastroscope passed through the oral cavity and esophagus.

gastroduodenostomy /-do͞o′ədenos″təmē/, surgical establishment of a passageway between the stomach and the duodenum. It may be done, for example, to bypass a pyloric obstruction.

gastrodynia. See **stomachache.**

gastroenteritis /gas′trō·en′tərī″tis/ [Gk, *gaster* + *enteron,* intestine, *itis,* inflammation], an inflammation of the stomach and intestines accompanying numerous GI disorders. Symptoms are anorexia, nausea, vomiting, fever (depending on causative factor), abdominal discomfort, and diarrhea. The condition may be caused by bacterial enterotoxins, bacterial or viral invasion, chemical toxins, or miscellaneous conditions, such as lactose intolerance. The onset may be slow, but more often it is abrupt and violent, with rapid loss of fluids and electrolytes caused by persistent vomiting and diarrhea. Hypokalemia and hyponatremia, acidosis, or alkalosis may develop. Treatment is supportive and includes bed rest, sedation, IV replacement of electrolytes, and antispasmodic medication to control vomiting and diarrhea. With a precise diagnosis, medication and treatment can be specific and curative, such as an antitoxin prescribed for gastroenteritis resulting from a bacterial endotoxin. After the acute phase, water may be given by mouth. If it produces no vomiting or diarrhea, clear fluids may be added, followed, if tolerated, by a diet of foods that appeal to the patient and do not cause symptoms. Also called **enterogastritis.**

■ OBSERVATIONS: Onset is often sudden, with abdominal pain and cramping, nausea and vomiting, diarrhea with or without blood and mucus, anorexia, general malaise, and muscle aches. Dehydration, hypokalemia, and hyponatremia occur with persistent vomiting and diarrhea. Diagnosis relies on identification of the causative agent through stool and blood cultures, Gram's stain, and direct swab rectal cultures. Complications of gastroenteritis include dehydration, shock, vascular collapse, and renal failure. In rare instances, complications may lead to death. Infants, small children, the elderly, and debilitated individuals are at greatest risk.

■ INTERVENTIONS: Most gastroenteritis is self-limiting and does not require therapy. Adequate rehydration is the primary treatment. Fluids are limited until vomiting ceases, then oral rehydration is instituted. IV fluid and electrolyte replacement may be necessary if dehydration is severe. Antidiarrheal agents may be used to slow diarrhea. Antibiotic agents may be used for gastroenteritis with systemic involvement. Antimicrobials are not generally recommended for simple gas-

troenteritis because these drugs may prolong the carrier state and contribute to the emergence of drug-resistant organisms. Antiemetics may be used for moderate to severe vomiting unless the causative agent is viral or bacterial, in which case antiemetics are not given to avoid impairment of GI motility.

■ PATIENT CARE CONSIDERATIONS: Nursing focus is on the replacement and monitoring of fluid and electrolytes. Accurate monitoring of intake and output is essential. Strict medical asepsis should be instituted when indicated by the causative agent. The importance of rest and increased fluid intake should be stressed along with the self-limiting nature of the disease. Education about proper food handling and storage is necessary after acute symptoms have ceased.

gastroenterologist /gas′trō·en′tərol″əjist/, a physician who specializes in diseases affecting the GI tract.

gastroenterology /gas′trō·en′tərol″əjē/ [Gk, *gaster* + *enteron,* intestine, *logos,* science], the study of diseases affecting the GI tract, including the stomach, intestines, gallbladder, and bile duct.

gastroenterostomy /gas′trō·en′təros″təmē/ [Gk, *gaster* + *enteron,* intestine, *stoma,* mouth], surgical formation of an artificial opening between the stomach and the small intestine, usually at the jejunum. The operation is performed with a gastrectomy to route food from the remainder of the stomach into the small intestine or alone to treat a perforating ulcer of the duodenum. A GI series is done before surgery, and a nasogastric tube is inserted. The jejunum is pulled up and anastomosed with the stomach. A new opening is then made for food to pass from the stomach directly into the jejunum. Pancreatic juices and bile are still secreted into the duodenum and pass through its distal end to the jejunum. Postsurgical complications and care are the same as for gastrectomy. Compare **gastrectomy.**

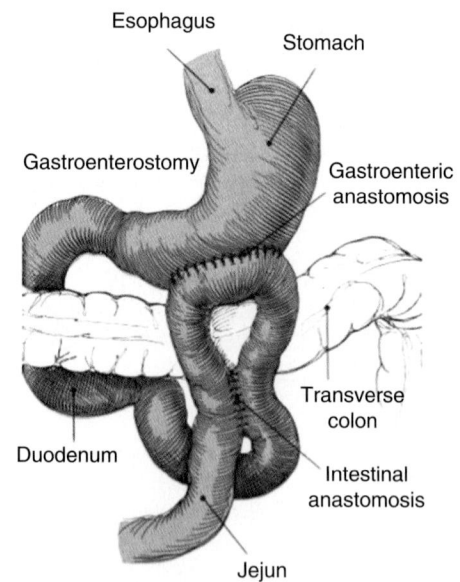

Gastroenterostomy *(Chopita et al, 2007)*

gastroesophageal /gas′trō·isof′əjē″əl/ [Gk, *gaster* + *oisophagos,* gullet], pertaining to the stomach and esophagus.

gastroesophageal hemorrhage. See **Mallory-Weiss syndrome.**

gastroesophageal reflux, a backflow of contents of the stomach into the esophagus that is often the result of incompetence of the lower esophageal sphincter. Gastric juices are acidic and therefore produce burning pain in the esophagus. Repeated episodes of reflux may cause esophagitis, peptic esophageal stricture, or esophageal ulcer. In uncomplicated cases treatment consists of elevation of the head of the bed, avoidance of acid-stimulating foods, and regular administration of antacids. In complicated cases surgical repair may provide relief. Also called **GERD.** See also **chalasia, esophagitis, heartburn, hiatal hernia, reflux esophagitis.**

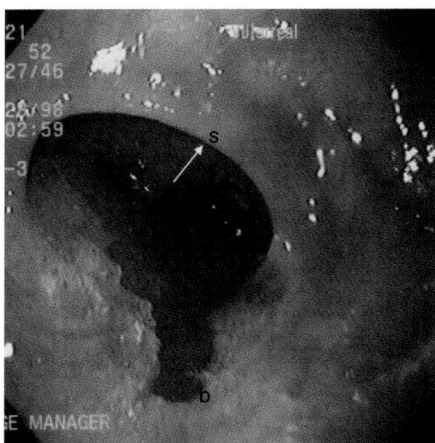

Gastroesophageal reflux: endoscopic view *(Goldman et al, 2008)*

gastroesophageal reflux scan, a nuclear scan that is used to evaluate patients with symptoms of heartburn, regurgitation, vomiting, and dysphagia and to evaluate the medical or surgical treatment of patients with gastroesophageal reflux.

gastroesophagitis /gas′trō·isof′əjī″tis/, inflammation of the stomach and esophagus.

gastrofiberscope /-fī″bərskōp′/, a flexible fiber endoscope for examination of the stomach.

gastrohepatic omentum. See **lesser omentum.**

gastrointestinal (GI) /gas′trō·intes″tinəl/ [Gk, *gaster* + L, *intestinum,* intestine], pertaining to the organs of the GI tract, from mouth to anus.

gastrointestinal allergy, an immediate hypersensitivity reaction of the digestive system after the ingestion of certain foods or drugs. GI allergy differs from food allergy, which can affect other organ systems. Compare **food allergy.** See also **lactose intolerance.**

■ OBSERVATIONS: Characteristic symptoms include itching and swelling of the mouth and oral passages, nausea, vomiting, diarrhea (sometimes containing blood), severe abdominal pain, and, in severe cases, anaphylactic shock.

■ INTERVENTIONS: Treatment includes identification and removal of the allergen. In an acute attack epinephrine may be administered as a stimulant, and muscle relaxants may be given to reduce intestinal spasms that cause abdominal pain.

■ PATIENT CARE CONSIDERATIONS: In childhood, GI allergy is most often caused by hypersensitivity to cow's milk and is characterized by diarrhea and colicky pain, sometimes with vomiting, eczema, respiratory distress, and thrombocytopenia.

gastrointestinal anthrax. See **anthrax.**

gastrointestinal bleeding, any bleeding from the GI tract. The most common underlying conditions are peptic ulcer, Mallory-Weiss syndrome, esophageal varices, diverticulosis, ulcerative colitis, and carcinoma of the stomach and colon. Vomiting of bright red blood or passage of coffee-ground vomitus indicates upper GI bleeding, usually from the esophagus, stomach, or upper duodenum. Aspiration of the gastric contents, lavage, and endoscopy are performed to determine the site and rate of bleeding. Tarry black stools indicate a bleeding source in the upper GI tract; bright red blood from the rectum usually indicates bleeding in the distal colon. GI bleeding is treated as a potential emergency. Patients may require transfusions, fluid replacement, endoscopic treatment, or gastric lavage and are watched carefully so as to prevent shock and hypovolemia. In all patients blood loss is evaluated and ability to coagulate is tested. See also **coffee-ground vomitus, hematochezia, melena.**

gastrointestinal bleeding scan, a nuclear scan that is used to localize the site of bleeding in patients who are having active gastrointestinal hemorrhage. It may also be used in patients with suspected intraabdominal (nongastrointestinal) hemorrhage of unknown origin.

gastrointestinal gas. See **flatulence.**

gastrointestinal infection, any infection of the digestive tract caused by bacteria, viruses, or parasites. All may have common clinical features of nausea, vomiting, diarrhea, and anorexia. Treatment in most cases includes rest, ready access to a bathroom, and food and beverages to replenish loss of fluid and electrolytes.

gastrointestinal obstruction, any obstruction of the passage of intestinal contents, caused by mechanical blockage or failure of motility. Mechanical blockage may be caused by adhesions resulting from surgery or inflammatory bowel disease, an incarcerated hernia, fecal impaction, tumor, intussusception, volvulus, or foreign body ingestion. Failure of motility may follow anesthesia, abdominal surgery, or occlusion of any of the mesenteric arteries to the gut. Symptoms vary with the cause of obstruction but generally include vomiting, abdominal pain, and increasing abdominal distension. Dehydration and prostration may follow. Characteristically bowel sounds are diminished or absent, especially distal to the obstruction, and abdominal guarding is prominent. A barium enema may be performed, but barium is never given by mouth because it increases the volume of the obstruction. The objective of therapy is to remove the obstruction as quickly and safely as possible. A tube is inserted into the stomach or small intestine to aspirate contents and relieve distension. During these procedures the patient is monitored for proper fluid and electrolyte balance. Surgical intervention may be necessary. Medication for pain can aggravate the condition by further decreasing motility of the GI tract, and it may not be prescribed in the acute period, before the location and extent of the obstruction are discovered.

gastrointestinal series, an examination of the upper GI tract using barium as the contrast medium for a series of x-ray films. Also called **barium meal.**

gastrointestinal system assessment, an evaluation of the patient's digestive system and symptoms.

■ METHOD: Discussion of symptoms is encouraged. The patient is asked whether there is or has been pain or tenderness in the oral cavity, gums, tongue, lips, abdomen, or rectum, and whether there have been instances of dysphagia, belching, heartburn, anorexia, nausea, vomiting, constipation, diarrhea, or painful defecation. Information is elicited about changes in eating; bowel habits; the color, character, and frequency of stools and urine; the use of laxatives or enemas; and the occurrence of fatigue, hemorrhoids, and edema of the extremities. The patient's general appearance, weight, and temperature are noted; the blood pressure, pulse, and respirations are checked in the supine, sitting, and standing positions; and the urinary output and color are determined. The presence of allergies, stomatitis, and halitosis and the condition of the tongue, gums, oral mucosa, and teeth are recorded. The abdomen is examined for distension, rigidity, ascites, symmetry, organomegaly, keloid tissue, visible peristalsis, bowel sounds, masses, and the presence of an ostomy. The perianal area is inspected for its general condition, color, odor, and hemorrhoids; the sclera for signs of jaundice; and the skin for pruritus, spider angioma, purpura, palmar erythema, peripheral edema, jaundice, and distended, tortuous blood vessels. Relevant to the assessment are concurrent endocrine, cardiovascular, and neurological disorders; severe burns; psychological problems; carcinoma; alcohol or drug abuse; and previous GI surgery and illnesses such as hepatitis, liver cirrhosis, or pancreatitis. The patient's personality type; attitude toward work; and use of tobacco, antacids, laxatives, anticholinergics, steroids, antidiarrheals, antiemetics, sedatives, tranquilizers, barbiturates, antihypertensives, antibiotics, and aspirin are investigated. The family history, especially of GI disease, carcinoma, and diabetes mellitus, is an important aspect of the evaluation. Diagnostic aids include a complete blood count, stool examination, prothrombin time, and determinations of levels of alkaline phosphatase, serum and urine bilirubin, aspartate aminotransferase, alanine aminotransferase, lactic acid dehydrogenase, blood urea nitrogen, serum lipase, cholinesterase, calcium, albumin, and glucose. Additional laboratory studies for evaluation are total protein level; serum electrolyte profile; serum carotene, delta-xylose tolerance, galactose tolerance, hippuric acid, and bromsulphalein tests; the albumin-globulin ratio, serum flocculation, and thymol turbidity tests; urobilinogen level; the polyvinylpyrrolidone test for protein loss; Sulkowitch's test for calcium in urine; and Schilling test for GI absorption of vitamin B_{12}. Procedures that may be required for the diagnosis include upper GI, small bowel, and gallbladder series; esophageal and gastric endoscopy and biopsy; scans of the liver and pancreas; biopsy of the liver, colon, or rectum; gastric analysis, sigmoidoscopy, abdominal x-ray images, ultrasound, fluoroscopy, percutaneous transhepatic cholangiography, endoscopic retrograde cholangiopancreatography, magnetic resonance cholangiopancreatography, hepatobiliary iminodiacetic acid scan, splenoportography, and digital rectal examinations.

■ INTERVENTIONS: Health care providers conduct the interview, record observations of the patient, and assemble the results of the diagnostic laboratory studies and procedures.

gastrointestinal tract. See **digestive tract.**

gastrojejunostomy. See **Billroth's operation II.**

gastrokinetic drugs /-kinet″ik/, chemicals that stimulate salivation, increase lower esophageal sphincter pressure, and improve esophageal clearance in the supine, but not in the upright, position. Cisapride, once the widely used drug in this category, has been taken off the market because of fatal arrhythmias. Metoclopramide, another agent in this category, has side effects that make it undesirable, and its efficacy is questionable in comparison to the now widely used proton pump inhibitors. Also called **prokinetic.**

gastromalacia /-məlā″shə/ [Gk, *gaster,* stomach, *malakia,* softness], autolytic rupture of the stomach, usually occurring postmortem.

gastromegaly /-meg″əlē/ [Gk, *gaster* + *megas,* large], an abnormal enlargement of the stomach or abdomen.

gastroparesis /-pərē″sis/, **1.** paralysis of the stomach. **2.** failure of the stomach to empty caused by decreased gastric motility. The major causes are various kinds of abdominal inflammation, scleroderma, diabetic autonomic neuropathy, vagotomy, and the use of anticholinergic medications.

gastropericardial fistula, a fistula connecting the stomach with the pericardium, usually a complication after gastroesophageal surgery.

gastroplasty /gas″troplas′tē/ [Gk, *gaster* + *plassein,* to mold], any surgery performed to reshape or repair any stomach defect or deformity.

gastropore. See **blastopore.**

gastroschisis /gastros″kəsis/ [Gk, *gaster* + *schisis,* division], a congenital defect characterized by incomplete closure of the abdominal wall with protrusion of the viscera. Compare **omphalocele.**

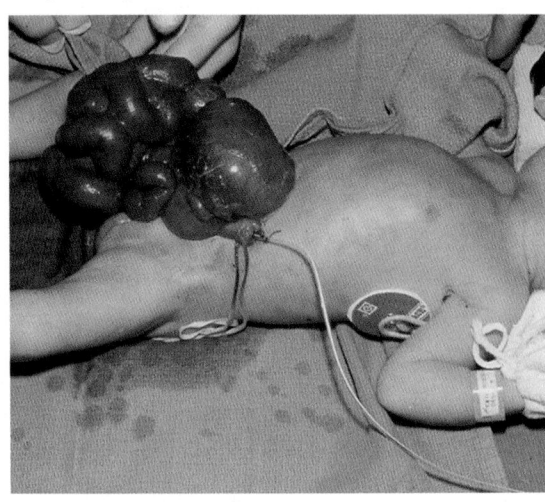

Neonate with gastroschisis *(Courtesy Dr. A.E. Chudley, Department of Pediatrics and Child Health, University of Manitoba, Children's Hospital)*

gastroscope /gas″trōskōp′/ [Gk, *gaster* + *skopein,* to look], *n.,* a fiberoptic instrument for examining the interior of the stomach.

gastroscopy /gastros″kəpē/, the visual inspection of the interior of the stomach by means of a gastroscope inserted through the esophagus to visualize the esophagus, stomach, and duodenum. See also **endoscopy, fiberoptics.** –*gastroscopic, adj.*

gastrostomy /gastros″təmē/ [Gk, *gaster* + *stoma,* mouth], surgical creation of an artificial opening into the stomach through the abdominal wall. It is performed to prevent malnutrition and starvation in patients who have esophageal cancer or tracheoesophageal fistula, who may be unconscious for a prolonged period, or who are unable to swallow as a result of a cerebrovascular accident, Alzheimer disease, or another disorder. It also permits retrograde dilation of an esophageal stricture. The anterior wall of the stomach is drawn forward and sutured to the abdominal wall. A Foley catheter or other tube or a special prosthesis is then inserted into an incision in the stomach, and the opening is tightly sutured to prevent leakage of the stomach contents. The device is clamped and is opened when liquid food supplement is instilled. After surgery glucose water may be given, followed by a slow continuous feeding of a warm blended formula to increase absorption. The skin is kept clean and dry around the site. Skin irritation indicates leakage of gastric secretions and digestive enzymes.

gastrostomy feeding, the introduction of a nutrient solution through a tube that has been surgically inserted into the stomach through the abdominal wall. See also **enteral tube feeding.**

gastrostomy tube, a tube used to introduce nutrients into the stomach, to remove fluids and ingested poisons, or to decompress the stomach. Also called **stomach tube.**

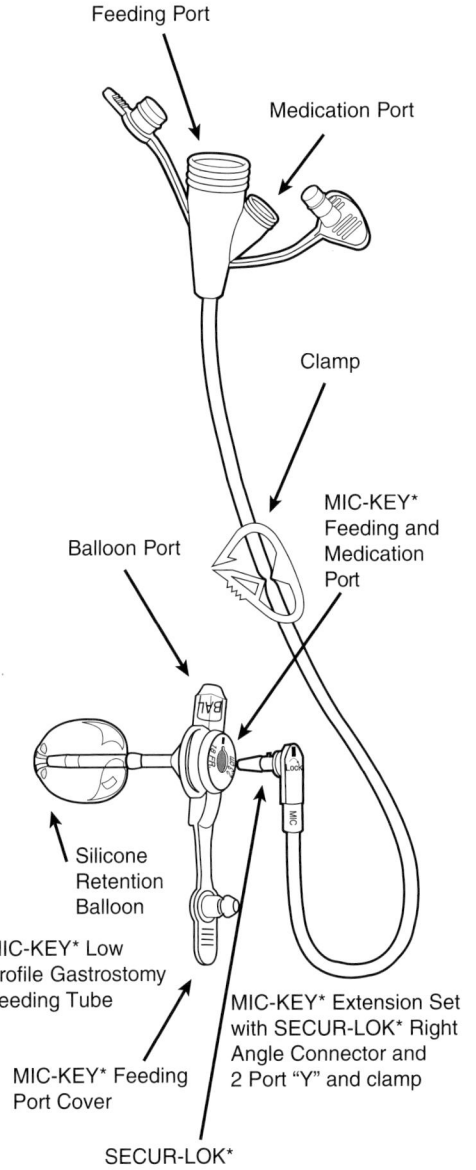

Feeding Port

Medication Port

Clamp

MIC-KEY* Feeding and Medication Port

Balloon Port

Silicone Retention Balloon

MIC-KEY* Low Profile Gastrostomy Feeding Tube

MIC-KEY* Feeding Port Cover

MIC-KEY* Extension Set with SECUR-LOK* Right Angle Connector and 2 Port "Y" and clamp

SECUR-LOK* Connector

Gastrostomy tube: Ballard Mic-Key *(Courtesy Kimberly-Clark Worldwide, Inc.)*

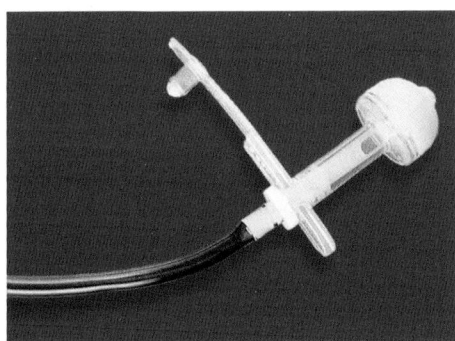

Gastrostomy tube: Bard button *(Courtesy C.R. Bard, Inc.)*

gastrothoracopagus /gas′trōthôr′əkop″əgəs/ [Gk, *gaster* + *thorax,* chest, *pagos,* fixture], conjoined twins who are united at the thorax and abdomen.

gastrula /gas″troõlə/ [Gk, *gaster,* stomach], the early embryonic stage formed by the invagination of the blastula. The cup-shaped gastrula consists of an outer layer of ectoderm and an inner layer of mesentoderm that subsequently differentiate into the mesoderm and endoderm. See also **blastula, embryonic layer.**

gastrulation /gas′trəlā″shən/ [Gk, *gaster,* stomach], the development of the gastrula in lower animals and the formation of the three germ layers in the embryo of humans and higher animals. It is characterized by an extensive series of coordinated morphogenetic movements within the blastula or blastocyst by which the primitive body plan of the organism is established and by which the areas that later differentiate into various structures and organs are in their proper position for development.

Gatch bed /gach/ [William D. Gatch, American surgeon, 1878–1961; AS, *bedd*], a bed that has an adjustable joint, allowing the knees to be flexed and the legs supported.

gate /gāt/, **1.** *n.,* an electronic circuit that passes a pulse only when a signal (the gate pulse) is present at a second input. **2.** *n.,* a mechanism for opening or closing a protein channel in a cell membrane, regulated by a signal such as increased concentration of a neurotransmitter, change in electrical potential, or physical binding of a ligand molecule to the protein to cause a conformational change in the protein molecule. **3.** *v.,* to open and close selectively and function as a gate.

Gate Control Theory of Pain, a theory first published by Canadian psychologist Robert Melzak (b. 1929) and British neuroscientist David Patrick Walls (1925–2001) in 1962 that posits that nonpainful input closes the gates to painful input, thereby ending transmission of the sensation of pain.

gatekeeper, a health care professional who is the patient's first contact with the health care system and triages the patient's further access to the system.

gatekeeper effect, a contraction of the endothelium mediated by immunoglobulin G. It permits components of the blood to gain access to the extravascular space as a result of the increased vascular permeability.

gateway drugs, minor substances of abuse, such as inhalants, used in general by children or young people before they experiment with marijuana or hard drugs; entry drugs.

gatifloxacin, a broad-spectrum fluoroquinolone antiinfective.
■ INDICATIONS: It was previously used to treat acute bacterial exacerbation of chronic bronchitis, acute sinusitis, community-acquired pneumonia, gonorrhea, and infections, but systemic formulations were withdrawn from the market due to serious dysglycemia. Topical ophthalmic agents remain.
■ CONTRAINDICATIONS: Known hypersensitivity to quinolones prohibits its use.
■ ADVERSE EFFECTS: Common side effects of topical use include local tearing and burning.

gating, the organizing of image data so that information used to construct an image originates in the same point in the cycle of a repeating movement, such as a heartbeat. The moving object is thus frozen at that phase of its movement, and image blurring is minimized.

gating mechanism, **1.** the increasing duration of an action potential from the atrioventricular node to a point in the distal Purkinje system, beyond which it decreases. **2.** a process that controls the opening and closing of cell-membrane ion channels.

Gaucher disease /gôshā″/ [Phillipe C.E. Gaucher, French physician, 1854–1918], a rare autosomal-recessive familial

G

disorder of lipid metabolism caused by an enzyme deficiency, characterized by widespread reticulum cell hyperplasia in the liver, spleen, lymph nodes, and bone marrow. Beginning in infancy or early childhood, splenomegaly, hepatomegaly, and abnormal bone growth develop. Diagnosis is made through biopsy of the liver, spleen, or bone marrow. Mortality rate is high, but children who survive adolescence may live for many years. Also called **glucosyl cerebroside lipidosis.**

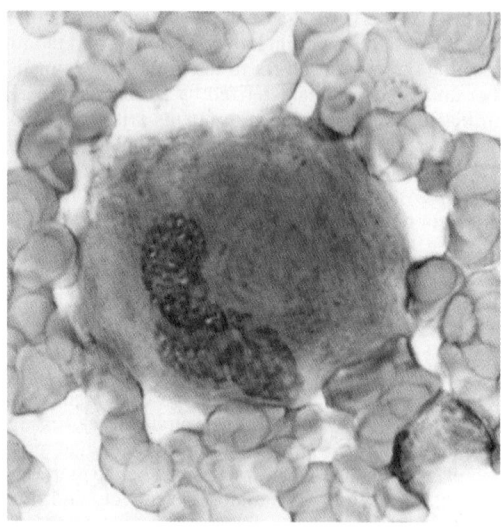

Bone marrow smear in Gaucher disease *(Carr and Rodak, 2008)*

gauge /gāj/ [ME], an instrument for determining physical properties of anything, including caliber, dimensions, or pressure.

gauntlet bandage /gônt″lit/ [Fr, *gantlet*, small glove, *bande*, strip], a glovelike bandage covering the hand and the fingers. See also **demigauntlet bandage.**

gauss /gôs, gous/ [J.K.F. Gauss, German physicist, 1777–1855], a unit of magnetic field strength. It is equal to 10^{-4} tesla.

gauze /gôz/ [Fr, *gaze*], a transparent fabric of open weave and differing degrees of fineness, most often cotton muslin, used in surgical procedures and for bandages and dressings. It may be sterilized and permeated by an antiseptic or lotion. Kinds include **absorbable gauze, absorbent gauze, petrolatum gauze.** See also **bandage.**

gauze sponge [Fr, *gaze* + Gk, *spoggia*], a piece of folded gauze used during surgery to wipe up bleeding surfaces and thereby help locate any sources of blood loss. Gauze sponges used in surgery have a radiographic strip that can be detected on an x-ray image.

gavage /gäväzh″/ [Fr, *gaver*, to gorge], the process of feeding a patient through a nasogastric tube. Also called *gavage feeding*, **nasogastric feeding.** See also **drip gavage, enteral tube feeding.**

gavage feeding of the newborn, a procedure in which a tube passed through the nose or mouth into the stomach is used to feed a newborn with weak sucking, uncoordinated sucking and swallowing, respiratory distress, tachypnea, or repeated apneic spells.

gay [Fr, *gai*, merry], **1.** *n.*, a person with a preference for same-sex relationships. **2.** *adj.*, pertaining to homosexuality.

Gay-Lussac's law /gā″ ləsaks″/ [Joseph L. Gay-Lussac, French scientist, 1778–1850; L, *legu*, a rule], (in physics) a law stating that the volume of a specific mass of a gas increases as the temperature increases if the pressure remains constant in a rigid container. See also **Charles' law.**

gaze /gāz/ [ME, *gazen*, to stare], a state of looking in one direction. A person with normal vision has six basic positions of gaze, each determined by control of different combinations of contractions of extraocular muscles. See also **cardinal position of gaze.**

gaze palsy. See **supranuclear gaze disturbance.**

gaze paresis, a disturbance of eye conjugate movement in which gaze tends to be tonically deviated in the direction of normal gaze. For example, in left frontal lobe damage the patient cannot voluntarily look to the right and the eyes spontaneously deviate to the left. The patient may be able to return the gaze voluntarily to the midline but cannot move the eyes past the midline into the paretic field of gaze.

gaze test, a test of ocular and vestibular functioning. Movements of the eye are recorded with the patient gazing straight at an object and at positions off to different sides of it; then with eyes closed for 20 seconds, the patient must perform a small mental exercise. The eyes normally should assume a center gaze while they are closed.

GB, abbreviation for **gallbladder.**

GBIA, abbreviation for **Guthrie bacterial inhibition assay.**

g.c., *(Informal)* abbreviation for **gonococcus.**

G cell hyperplasia, increased numbers of G cells in the gastric mucosa, causing marked hypergastrinemia resembling that seen in Zollinger-Ellison syndrome.

G-CSF, abbreviation for **granulocyte colony-stimulating factor.**

Gd, symbol for the element **gadolinium.**

GDM, abbreviation for **gestational diabetes mellitus.**

GDNF, abbreviation for **glial cell line–derived neurotrophic factor.**

GDS, abbreviation for **Geriatric Depression Scale.**

Ge, symbol for the element **germanium.**

gefitinib, a tyrosine kinase inhibitor; an antineoplastic drug.
■ INDICATIONS: This drug is used for targeted therapy of non–small cell lung cancer.
■ CONTRAINDICATIONS: Pregnancy and known hypersensitivity to this drug prohibit its use.
■ ADVERSE EFFECTS: Adverse effects of this drug include nausea, diarrhea, vomiting, anorexia, mouth ulceration, rash, pruritus, acne, dry skin, cough, dyspnea, peripheral edema, amblyopia, conjunctivitis, eye pain, corneal erosion, and ulcer. Life-threatening side effects include pancreatitis, toxic epidermal neurolysis, angioedema, and interstitial lung disease.

gegenhalten /gā″gənhäl′tən/ [Ger, counterpressure], the involuntary resistance to passive movement of the extremities. It may occur as a symptom of catatonia, in which there is passive resistance to stretching movements, even when the patient attempts to cooperate. The effect may be psychogenic in origin or may be a sign of dementia or cerebral deterioration. Also called **paratonia.**

Geiger-Müller (GM) counter /gī″gər mil′ər/ [Hans Geiger, German physicist, 1882–1945; Walther Müller, 20th-century German physicist; Fr, *conter*, to tell], an electronic device that indicates the level of radioactivity of a substance by counting the number of ionizing subatomic particles emitted by the substance. As the particles pass through a gas-filled tube inside the counter, they ionize the gas and cause an electric discharge. The tube cannot identify the type or energy of a particle. Also called *Geiger counter.*

gel /jel/ [L, *gelare,* to congeal], a colloid that is firm although it contains a large amount of liquid, used in many medicines as a demulcent, a vehicle for other drugs, an antacid, or an astringent, depending on the drug from which it is derived. Also called **jelly.**

-gel, suffix meaning "jellylike substances" formed by cooling a colloid into a semisolid state.

gelat-, prefix meaning "to freeze, congeal": *gelatinous.*

gelatin buildup /jel″ətən/, an x-ray film artifact that may appear as a sharp area of either increased or reduced density.

gelatin film, absorbable, a hemostatic.
- INDICATIONS: It is used to attain hemostasis during surgery, particularly neurological, thoracic, and ophthalmic procedures.
- CONTRAINDICATIONS: Infection or gross contamination of the surgical wound prohibits its use.
- ADVERSE EFFECTS: There are no known adverse effects.

gelatiniform carcinoma. See **mucinous carcinoma.**

gelatinous /jəlat″ənəs/ [L, *gelare,* to congeal], pertaining to or resembling a viscous, jellylike substance.

gelatinous carcinoma. See **mucinous carcinoma.**

gelatin sponge, an absorbable local hemostatic.
- INDICATIONS: It is prescribed to control surgical bleeding and treat pressure ulcers.
- CONTRAINDICATIONS: Frank infection, extensive and abnormal bleeding, postpartum bleeding, or menorrhagia prohibits its use.
- ADVERSE EFFECTS: There are no known adverse effects.

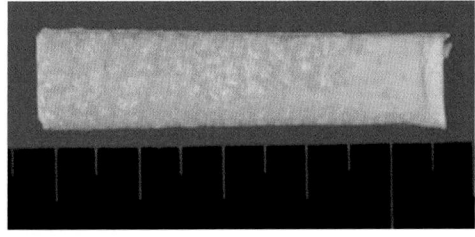

Macroscopic image of gelatin sponge (Igai et al, 2007)

gel diffusion. See **immunodiffusion.**

gel filtration, a method of separating molecules by size. A solution containing molecules of various sizes is passed through a filter consisting of a porous material, generally a polyacrylamide or polysaccharide. The larger molecules are excluded from the interior of the filter and thus emerge from it earlier than the smaller molecules.

Gelfoam, brand name for an absorbable hemostatic gelatin sponge.

Gell and Coombs classification /jel; ko͞omz/, a classification of immune mechanisms of tissue injury, comprising four types of hypersensitivity reactions: *type I* (anaphylactic reactions), immediate hypersensitivity reactions mediated by interaction of immunoglobulin E antibody and antigen and release of histamine and other mediators; *type II* (cytotoxic reactions), antibody-mediated hypersensitivity reactions caused by antibody-antigen interactions on cell surfaces; *type*

III (immune complex reactions), mediated hypersensitivity reactions, local or general inflammatory responses caused by formation of circulating immune complexes and their deposition in tissues; and *type IV* (cell-mediated hypersensitivity reactions), delayed hypersensitivity reactions initiated by sensitized T lymphocytes either by release of lymphokines or by T-cell–mediated cytotoxicity.

Gellhorn pessary. See **pessary.**

gemcitabine, an antimetabolite antineoplastic drug.
- INDICATIONS: It is used to treat adenocarcinoma of the pancreas (nonresectable Stages II and III or metastatic Stage IV) and non–small-cell lung cancer (Stages IIIA or B and IV). It is also used in combination with cisplatin to treat inoperable, advanced, or metastatic non–small-cell lung cancer.
- CONTRAINDICATIONS: Known hypersensitivity and pregnancy prohibit its use.
- ADVERSE EFFECTS: Life-threatening effects are leukopenia, anemia, neutropenia, thrombocytopenia, and hemorrhage. Other adverse effects include diarrhea, nausea, vomiting, anorexia, constipation, stomatitis, irritation at the site of administration, rash, alopecia, dyspnea, fever, and infection.

gemellary /jem″əler′ē/ [L, *gemellus,* twin], pertaining to twins.

gemellipara /jem″əlip″ərə/ [L, *gemellus* + *parare,* to give birth], a woman who has given birth to twins.

gemellology /jem″əlol″əjē/ [L, *gemellus* + Gk, *logos,* science], the study of twins and the phenomenon of twinning.

gemellus /jəmel″əs/, either of a pair of small muscles arising from the ischium. They rotate the thigh laterally and blend with the obturator internus tendon.

gemellus test, a test of the function of the gemellus superior and gemellus inferior in hip external rotation while the patient is seated with the knees flexed. The examiner places one hand on the lateral aspect of the knee to prevent flexion or abduction of the hip while the patient rotates the thigh outward by moving the foot medially.

gemfibrozil /jemfī″brəzil/, a fibric acid derivative that acts as a dyslipidemic agent.
- INDICATIONS: It is used to treat dyslipidemia, specifically elevated triglycerides.
- CONTRAINDICATIONS: Hepatic dysfunction, gallbladder disease, or known hypersensitivity to this drug prohibits its use.
- ADVERSE EFFECTS: Among the adverse effects are abdominal or epigastric pain, urticaria, dizziness, anemia, and elevated liver function tests.

gemifloxacin, a fluoroquinolone antiinfective.
- INDICATIONS: This drug is used to treat acute bacterial exacerbation of chronic bronchitis caused by *Streptococcus pneumoniae, Haemophilus influenzae, H. parainfluenzae,* and *Moraxella catarrhalis* and community-acquired pneumonia caused by *S. pneumoniae* (including multidrug-resistant strains), *H. influenzae, M. catarrhalis, Mycoplasma pneumoniae, Chlamydia pneumoniae,* and *Klebsiella pneumoniae.* The drug should be reserved for the treatment of complicated infections.
- CONTRAINDICATIONS: Known hypersensitivity to quinolones prohibits the use of this drug.
- ADVERSE EFFECTS: Adverse effects include dizziness, headache, and nausea. QT interval prolongation has also been observed. This group of agents now bears an additional black box warning of long-term central nervous system toxicity that is possible even after short-course treatment

and may present as tendinitis, tendinopathy, or peripheral neuropathy. Life-threatening side effects include pseudo-membranous colitis, anaphylaxis, and Stevens-Johnson syndrome.

gemin-, prefix meaning "a twin or double": *gemination.*

gemination, (in dentistry) the "twinning" of a single tooth bud. Geminated teeth usually have a single common root, a common pulp canal, and visible partial cleavage of the enamel crown. The normal quantity of teeth is present in the dental arch. Not to be confused with **fusion.**

gemistocyte /gemis″təsīt/, an astrocyte with an eccentric nucleus and swollen cytoplasm, as seen in areas of nervous tissue affected by edema, demyelination, or infarction.

gemma /jem″ə/ *pl. gemmae* [L, bud], **1.** a budlike projection produced by some organisms during budding, a type of asexual reproduction. Also called **gemmule. 2.** any budlike or bulblike structure, such as a taste bud or end bulb. −*gemmaceous, adj.*

gemmate /jem″āt/ [L, *gemma + atus,* function], **1.** *adj.,* having buds or gemmae. **2.** *v.,* to reproduce by budding.

Age of onset of selected genetic disorders

Age of onset	Disorder
Lethal during prenatal life	Some chromosome abnormalities Some extensive malformations Osteogenesis imperfecta
At birth (congenital)	Congenital malformations Chromosome abnormalities (e.g., Down syndrome) Some forms of hereditary deafness Osteogenesis imperfecta
Soon after birth or after feeding is initiated	Phenylketonuria Galactosemia Maple syrup urine disease Lactase insufficiency
Infancy	Sickle cell disease Tay-Sachs disease Werdnig-Hoffmann disease Hereditary clotting disorders Osteogenesis imperfecta Mucopolysaccharidoses
Early childhood	Cystic fibrosis Various muscular dystrophies Fragile X syndrome
Near puberty	Limb-girdle muscular dystrophy Adrenogenital syndrome Turner syndrome Klinefelter syndrome
Young adulthood	Acute intermittent porphyria Hereditary juvenile glaucoma
Variable age of onset	Diabetes mellitus Huntington disease Myotonic dystrophy Macular degeneration Hereditary amyotrophic lateral sclerosis

From Hockenberry MJ, Wilson D: *Wong's nursing care of infants and children,* ed 8, St Louis, 2007, Mosby.

gemmation /jemā″shən/ [L, *gemmare,* to produce buds], the process of reproduction by budding. Also called **gemmulation.**

gemmiferous /jemif″ərəs/ [L, *gemma + fer,* bearing], having buds or gemmae; gemmiparous.

gemmiform /jem″ifôrm′/, resembling a bud or gemma.

gemmipara /jemip″ərə/ [L, *gemma + parare,* to give birth], an animal that produces gemmae or reproduces by budding, such as a hydra. −*gemmiparous, adj.*

gemmulation. See **gemmation.**

gemmule. See **gemma.**

gemtuzumab ozogamicin /gemtoo͞′zoo͞mab″ o″zo-gah-mi′sin/, a recombinant DNA-derived monoclonal antibody conjugated with a cytotoxic antitumor antibiotic used as an antineoplastic in the treatment of relapsed acute myelogenous leukemia; administered intravenously.

gen-, geno-, prefix meaning "to become or produce": *generic, genogram.*

-gen, -gene, **1.** suffix meaning "that which generates": *carcinogen.* **2.** suffix meaning "that which is generated": *immunogen.*

gender /jen″dər/ [L, *genus,* kind], **1.** a classification of the sex of a person, denoted as male, female, or nonbinary. **2.** the specific sex of a person. See also **sex.**

gender identity, the inner sense of maleness or femaleness. Differentiation of gender identity begins in infancy, continues throughout childhood, and is reinforced during adolescence. Also called **core gender identity.**

gender dysphoria, a condition characterized by a persistent feeling of discomfort or anxiety related to the assigned sex of an individual and the individual's gender identity.

gender panic, fear or anxiety associated with challenges to the "naturalness" of a male-female gender binary, as when a transgender individual enters a restroom inconsistent with the individual's anatomy.

gender role, the expression of a person's gender identity; the image that a person presents to both himself or herself and others.

gender testing [L, *genus,* kind, *testum,* crucible], a procedure for validating the sex of an individual by examining a tissue sample, usually obtained from oral mucous membrane cells, for the presence of a Y chromosome.

gene /jēn/ [Gk, *genein,* to produce], the biological unit of inheritance, consisting of a particular nucleotide sequence within a DNA sequence that occupies a precise locus on a chromosome and codes for a specific polypeptide chain. In diploid organisms, which include humans and other mammals, genes occur as paired alleles. Kinds include **complementary gene, mutant gene, operator gene, pleiotropic gene, regulator gene, structural gene, supplementary gene.** See also **chromosome, cistron, deoxyribonucleic acid, operon.**

-gene. See **-gen, -gene.**

gene amplification [Gk, *genein,* to produce; L, *amplus,* large], a process in which a specific gene or set of genes is duplicated many times in certain cells in response to defined signals or environmental stresses.

gene amplification technique, a term sometimes used to denote a nucleic acid amplification technique, although the segment of DNA or RNA undergoing amplification does not necessarily correspond to a single entire gene. See also **polymerase chain reaction.**

gene expression,   **1.** the flow of genetic information from gene to protein. **2.** the process, or the regulation of the process, by which the effects of a gene are manifested. **3.** the manifestation of a heritable trait in an individual carrying the gene or genes that determine it.

gene library.   See **DNA library.**

gene marker.   See **genetic marker.**

gene pool [Gk, *genein,* to produce; AS, *pol*],   the total number of genes in a population. If the population reproduces by random sexual selection, there will be a normal (bell-shaped) distribution of genes in the gene pool.

gene probe,   a device used in molecular biology for locating a particular gene on a chromosome. It involves pairing a short known segment of deoxyribonucleic acid or ribonucleic acid with a matching sequence of bases on a chromosome.

genera.   See **genus.**

general adaptation syndrome (GAS) [L, *genus,* kind; L, *adaptare,* to fit; Gk, *syn,* together, *dromos,* course],   the defense response of the body or the psyche to injury or prolonged stress, as described by Hans Selye (1907–1982). It consists of an initial stage of shock or alarm reaction, followed by a phase of increasing resistance or adaptation in which the various defense mechanisms of the body or mind are used, and culminates in a state of adjustment and healing or of exhaustion and disintegration. Also called **adaptation syndrome.** See also **alarm reaction, crisis, posttraumatic stress disorder, stress.**

general anesthesia (GA),   the absence of sensation and consciousness as induced by various anesthetic medications, given by inhalation or IV injection. The components of general anesthesia are analgesia, amnesia, muscle relaxation, control of vital signs, and unconsciousness. The depth of anesthesia is planned to allow the surgical procedure to be performed without the patient experiencing pain, moving, or having any recall of the procedure. Endotracheal intubation or insertion of another artificial airway device and respiratory support are often necessary. General anesthesia may be administered only by an anesthesiologist with or without an assistant or a certified registered nurse anesthetist and by a dentist with postgraduate training and licensing. Compare **local anesthesia, regional anesthesia, topical anesthesia.** See also **anesthesia.**

generalization /jen′(ə)rəlīzā″shən/ [L, *genus,* kind; Gk, *izein,* to cause],   **1.** the reasoning by which a basic conclusion is reached, with application to different items that have a common factor. **2.** the process of reducing or subsuming under a general rule or statement, such as classifying items in general categories. **3.** a principle with general application. **4.** (in occupational therapy) the ability of a patient to apply knowledge and skills learned in therapy to a variety of similar but new situations.

generalized anaphylaxis /jen″(ə)rəlīzd′/,   a severe reaction to an allergen characterized by itching, edema, wheezing respirations, apprehension, cyanosis, dyspnea, pupillary dilation, falling blood pressure, and rapid, weak pulse that may quickly produce shock and death. The reaction is mediated by immunoglobulin E antibodies that form in response to an initial sensitizing dose of an allergen and render the individual hypersensitive to the allergen by binding it to mast cells and basophils. A subsequent challenging dose of the allergen causes the cells to release histamine, bradykinin, and other vasoactive amines, producing anaphylaxis. See also **anaphylactic shock, anaphylaxis,** *reagin-mediated disorder.*

generalized anxiety disorder (GAD),   an anxiety reaction characterized by persistent apprehension. The symptoms range from mild, chronic tenseness, with feelings of timidity, fatigue, apprehension, and indecisiveness, to more intense states of restlessness and irritability that may lead to aggressive acts. In extreme cases the overwhelming emotional discomfort is accompanied by physical reactions, including tremor, sustained muscle tension, tachycardia, dyspnea, hypertension, increased respiration, and profuse perspiration. Other physical signs include changes in skin color, nausea, vomiting, diarrhea, restlessness, immobilization, insomnia, and changes in appetite, all occurring without underlying organic cause. The symptoms of anxiety may be controlled with medication, such as tranquilizers, but psychotherapy is the preferred treatment. Also called **anxiety reaction, anxiety state.** See also **anxiety, anxiety attack.**

generalized emphysema.   See **panacinar emphysema.**

generalized morphea,   large skin patches associated with the deposition of collagen. Generalized morphea covers large areas of the body. Skin thickening over joints may affect function. Compare **morphea.** See also **localized scleroderma.**

generalized peritonitis [L, *genus,* kind; Gk, *peri,* near, *teinein,* to stretch, *itis,* inflammation],   a bacterial infection of the peritoneum secondary to an infection in another organ, as when an appendix ruptures or an ulcer perforates the gastric wall. The symptoms are usually acute and severe. See also **peritonitis.**

generalized scleroderma.   See also **scleroderma.**

generally recognized as effective (GRAE),   one of the statutory criteria that must be met by a drug before it can be approved as a new drug. Meeting these criteria relieves the manufacturer of the necessity of obtaining premarket approval as required by the Federal Food, Drug, and Cosmetic Act. To be recognized as effective, the drug must be, according to the act, considered safe and effective by "experts qualified by scientific training and experience."

generally recognized as safe (GRAS),   a 1958 rule established by the U.S. Food and Drug Administration (FDA) to identify foods regarded as safe to use because of lack of evidence that they may be harmful. Originally the rule was applied to all foods that were in use in 1958 and were not then known to be hazardous. Later, because of improved scientific techniques for detecting mutagens and carcinogens, items that had been classified as safe, such as caffeine, were further tested by the FDA to determine whether they should remain on the GRAS list.

general paresis [L, *genus,* kind; Gk, paralysis],   a neurological disorder that results from chronic syphilitic infection. It is characterized by degeneration of the cortical neurons; progressive dementia, tremor, and speech disturbances; muscular weakness; and ultimately generalized paralysis. It is often accompanied by periods of exultation and delusions of grandeur. Treatment usually consists of large doses of penicillin, without which the outcomes are almost invariably progressive deterioration and death. Also called **paretic dementia, syphilitic meningoencephalitis.**

general practice,   in some countries, the term for comprehensive medical care regardless of age of the patient or presence of a condition that may require the services of a specialist. This term has now largely been replaced by the term *family practice.*

general practitioner (GP) [L, *genus,* kind; Gk, *praktikos,* practical],   a family practice physician. See also **family medicine, family practice, family practice physician.**

G

general relaxation [L, *genus,* kind, *relaxare,* to ease], a slackening of strain or tension of the entire body, particularly of the muscles.

general sensory disorganization, disorders in which sensory systems are providing inaccurate information; may be associated with impairments in the tactile, vestibular, and/or auditory systems; also associated with infants who are characterized as "fussy babies."

general symptom [L, *genus* + Gk, *symptoma,* that which happens], a symptom that affects the entire body rather than a specific organ or location. Also called **constitutional symptom.**

generation /jen'ərā″shən/ [L, *generare,* to beget], **1.** the act or process of reproduction; procreation. **2.** a group of contemporary individuals who have descended through the same number of life cycles from a common ancestor. **3.** the period between the birth of one individual and the birth of its offspring. Kinds include **alternate generation, filial generation, parental generation.**

generative /jen″ərā′tiv/ [L, *generare,* to beget], pertaining to activity that generates new physical or mental growth, such as creative problem solving.

generic /jəner″ik/ [L, *genus,* kind], **1.** pertaining to a genus. **2.** pertaining to a substance, product, or drug that is not protected by trademark. **3.** pertaining to the nontrademarked name assigned to a drug by the U.S. Adopted Names (USAN) Council.

generic equivalent, a drug product sold under its generic name with the same active ingredients, route of administration, dosage form, strength, and indications as one or more others sold under trademark. Inactive ingredients may not be the same. The performance of the drug (its safety and efficacy) must be similar to the brand product as well.

generic name, the official established nonproprietary name assigned to a drug. A drug is licensed under its generic name, and all manufacturers of the drug list it by its generic name. However, a drug is usually marketed under trademark chosen by the manufacturer. See also **chemical name, established name, trademark.**

generic nursing program, a program that prepares people with no professional nursing experience for entry into the field of nursing. It can lead to a licensed practical nurse degree, an associate degree of nursing, or a bachelor of science in nursing degree.

-genesia, suffix meaning a "(specified) condition concerning information": *agenesia.*

genesis /jen″əsis/ [Gk, origin], **1.** the origin, generation, or developmental evolution of anything. **2.** the act of producing or procreating.

-genesis. See **-genesia.**

gene splicing /jēn/, a process by which a segment of DNA is attached to or inserted into a strand of DNA from another source. In recombinant DNA technology, DNA from humans or other organisms is spliced into bacterial plasmids.

gene therapy, a procedure that involves injection of "healthy genes" into the bloodstream of a patient to cure or treat a hereditary disease or similar illness. Blood is withdrawn from the patient; the white cells are separated and cultured in a laboratory. Normal genes from a volunteer are inserted into modified viruses, which, in turn, transfer the normal gene into the chromosomes of the patient's white cells. The white cells containing the normal genes are finally injected into the patient's bloodstream. A clinical application of gene therapy may be found in the treatment of thalassemia, a genetically determined disease, in which efforts have been made to increase hemoglobin F production and improve the level of anemia. Research goals include changing the actual hemoglobin genes in red blood cell precursors or transplantation of normal hemoglobin genes into the bone marrow of thalassemia patients. Also called **somatic-cell gene therapy.**

genetic /jənet″ik/ [Gk, *genesis,* origin], **1.** pertaining to reproduction, birth, or origin. **2.** pertaining to genetics or heredity. **3.** pertaining to or produced by a gene; inherited.

-genetic, 1. suffix meaning "generation by (specified) agents": *mitogenetic.* **2.** suffix meaning "generating": *osteogenetic.* **3.** suffix meaning "something generated by a (specified) agent": *amphigenetic.*

genetic affinity, relationship by direct descent.

genetically significant dose (GSD) /jənet″iklē/, **1.** an arbitrary measure of the estimated annual gonadal radiation received by the population gene pool. In the United States the estimated GSD is 20 mrad. The figure is not intended to suggest possible genetic effects of exposure to that level of radiation. **2.** an estimate of the genetic significance of gonad radiation doses, which takes into account the number of offspring expected for each individual on the basis of age and sex.

genetic association, a condition in which specific genotypes are associated with other factors, such as specific diseases.

genetic carrier, a person who carries an allele without exhibiting its effects. Such an allele is usually recessive, but it may also be dominant and latent, with symptoms that do not appear until adulthood.

genetic code, the information carried by DNA that determines the specific amino acids and their sequence in each protein synthesized by an organism. The code consists of the sequence of nucleotides in the DNA molecule of each chromosome in the nucleus of every cell. During transcription, a specific part of the code is transcribed into a sequence of nucleotides in the messenger RNA (mRNA). The mRNA travels from the nucleus to the cytoplasm, where it is translated into protein by the ribosomes. A codon consisting of three consecutive nucleotides in the mRNA codes for each amino acid in the protein. A change in the code may result in an incorrect sequence of the amino acids in the protein, causing a mutation. See also **anticodon, transcription, translation.**

genetic colonization, the process by which a parasite introduces into its host genetic information that induces the host to synthesize products solely for the use of the parasite.

genetic counseling, the process of determining the occurrence or risk of occurrence of a genetic disorder in a family and of providing information and advice about topics such as care of an affected child, prenatal diagnosis, termination of a pregnancy, sterilization, and artificial insemination. Effective genetic counseling begins with an accurate diagnosis of the condition because many of the more than 3000 known inherited disorders have similar clinical manifestations. Special biochemical cytogenetic or molecular genetic tests may be required. A genetic counselor also must prepare a careful, detailed family history, recorded in the form of a pedigree chart, and must have an understanding of genetic principles, especially a knowledge of the risks related to multifactorial inheritance. The most efficient counseling services consist of a group of specialists, including physicians, geneticists, psychologists, biochemists, cytologists, nurses, and social workers. Nurses must be especially alert to situations in which persons may need genetic counseling, must become familiar with facilities in the area that provide genetic counseling, and must help couples arrive at tentative decisions regarding family planning or the care of a child with a genetic disorder. See also **genetic screening, prenatal diagnosis.**

genetic counselor, a health professional academically and clinically prepared to communicate genetic, medical, and technical information about the occurrence, or risk of occurrence, of a genetic condition or birth defect. As part of a genetic delivery services team, the genetic counselor consults with individuals, and/or their families, about their birth defects or genetic disorders, their risk for inherited conditions, and their options. A master's degree in genetic counseling is usually required; the American Board of Genetic Counseling provides certification.

genetic death, 1. the failure of an organism to survive as a result of its genetic makeup. 2. the removal of an allele or genotype from the gene pool of a population or from a given familial descent because of the sterility, failure to reproduce, or death before sexual maturity of all individuals bearing that allele or genotype.

genetic disorder. See **inherited disorder.**

genetic drift, a gradual change in the allelic frequencies within a population as a result of chance. The smaller a population is, the greater is the tendency for variation within each generation so that eventually small, isolated, inbreeding groups become genetically quite different from their ancestors. Also called **random genetic drift.**

genetic engineering, the process of producing recombinant DNA for the purposes of altering and controlling the genotype and phenotype of organisms. Restriction enzymes are used to break a DNA molecule into fragments so that genes from another organism can be inserted into the DNA. Genetic engineering has been used to produce a variety of human proteins, including growth hormone, insulin, and interferon, in bacteria. At present, it represents a powerful tool for medical research but is possible only in microorganisms. In the future, genetic engineering may be applicable to more complex organisms, offering the possibility of controlling and eliminating genetic disorders and malformations in humans.

genetic equilibrium, the state within a population at which the frequency of alleles and genotypes does not change from generation to generation. It routinely occurs in large, interbreeding populations in which mating is random and there are no or relatively few mutations. See also **Hardy-Weinberg equilibrium principle.**

genetic homeostasis, the maintenance of genetic variability within a population through adaptation to varied or changing environments and conditions of life as a result of shifts or resistance to shifts in allelic frequencies.

genetic immunity. See **natural immunity.**

genetic isolate, a group of individuals that are genetically separated by geographic, racial, social, cultural, or other barriers that prevent them from interbreeding with those outside the group. Depending on the size of the group and the amount of inbreeding that occurs, genetic isolates may show an increased incidence of otherwise rare inherited defects. See also **deme.**

geneticist /jənet″isist/, a scientist who specializes in the study or application of genetics.

genetic load, the average number of accumulated detrimental genes per individual within a population, including those caused by mutation and selection within a recent generation and those inherited from ancestors. Genetic load is expressed in lethal equivalents.

genetic map, the graphic representation of the linear arrangement of genes on a chromosome and the relative distances between them in map units or morgans. Also called **linkage map.**

genetic marker, any specific gene that produces a readily recognizable genetic trait that can be used in family and population studies or in linkage analysis. Also called **gene marker, marker gene.**

genetic polymorphism, the recurrence within a population of two or more discontinuous genetic variants of a specific trait in such proportions that they cannot be maintained simply by mutation. Examples include the sickle cell trait, the Rh factor, and the blood groups. Compare **balanced polymorphism.**

genetic population. See **deme.**

genetics /jənet″iks/, 1. the science that studies the principles and mechanics of heredity, specifically the means by which traits are passed from parents to offspring and the causes of the similarities and differences between related organisms. 2. the total genetic makeup of a particular individual, family, group, or condition. Kinds include **clinical genetics, molecular genetics, population genetics.** See also **cytogenetics, Mendel's laws.**

genetic screening, the process of investigating a specific population of persons for the purpose of detecting the presence of disease, either incipient or overt, such as the generalized screening of all newborns for phenylketonuria. Genetic screening may be used to identify those who possess defective genes, gain information concerning the incidence of a disorder in the population, and provide reproductive information, specifically to those at risk, such as the close relatives of persons affected with inborn errors of metabolism or those in certain ethnic groups who have a high incidence of a particular disease, specifically sickle cell anemia in African-Americans and Tay-Sachs disease in Ashkenazic Jews. When accompanied by education and counseling, mass screening programs can be effective in the management of genetic disorders. See also **genetic counseling.**

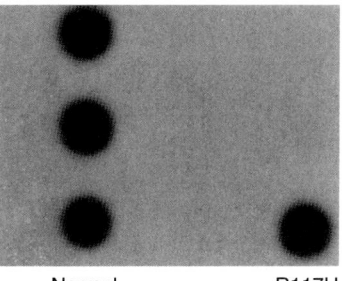

Normal   R117H

Genetic screening (Courtesy Lesa Nelson and Dr. Kenneth Ward, University of Utah Health Sciences Center)

gene transfer [Gk, *genein,* to produce; L, *transferre,* to bring across], a type of gene therapy in which a gene is transplanted from a donor organism into a recipient organism.

-genic, 1. suffix meaning "causing, forming, producing": *acnegenic.* 2. suffix meaning "produced by or formed from": *biogenic.* 3. suffix meaning "related to a gene": *allogenic.*

geniculate neuralgia /jənik″yəlāt/ [L, *geniculum,* little knee; Gk, *neuron,* nerve, *algos,* pain], a severe debilitating inflammatory condition of the geniculate ganglion of the facial nerve. It is characterized by pain in the ear, loss of the sense of taste, facial paralysis, and a decrease in salivation and lacrimation. It sometimes follows herpes zoster infection. It may be treated with Tegretol or Sansert. If surgery is required, microvascular decompression to relieve abnormal compression of the nerve may be needed.

geniculate zoster. See **herpes zoster.**

genio-, prefix meaning "chin": *geniohyoideus.*

genioglossus,   one of the thick, fan-shaped extrinsic muscles that depress the central part of the tongue and protrude the anterior part of the tongue out of the oral fissure. The genioglossus muscles are innervated by the hypoglossal nerves.

geniohyoideus /jē′nē·ōhī·oi″dē·əs/   [Gk, *genion,* chin, *hyoides,* Y-shaped],   one of the four suprahyoid muscles that draw the hyoid bone and the tongue forward. Also called *geniohyoid muscle.* Compare **digastricus, mylohyoideus, stylohyoideus.** See also **suprahyoid muscles.**

genit-,   **1.** prefix meaning "birth" or "reproduction": *genitalia.* **2.** prefix meaning "generative organs" or "sexual reproduction": *genitourinary.*

genital.   See **genitals.**

genital herpes.   See **herpes genitalis, herpes simplex.**

genitalia.   See **genitals.**

genital reflex.   See **sexual reflex.**

genitals /jen″itəlz/   [L, *genitalis*],   the sex, or reproductive, organs visible on the outside of the body. In the female they include the vulva, mons pubis, labia majora, labia minora, clitoris, and vaginal vestibule. The male genitals include the penis, scrotum, and testicles. Also called **genitalia.** –**genital,** *adj.*

genital stage /jen″itəl/   [L, *genitalis* + Fr, *stage,* trial period],   (in psychoanalysis) the final period in freudian psychosexual development, beginning with adolescence and continuing through the adult years, when the genitals are the predominant source of pleasurable stimulation. The most significant feature of this stage is direction of sexual interest not just toward self-satisfaction but toward establishment of a stable and meaningful relationship. See also **psychosexual development.**

genital tract.   See **reproductive system.**

genital wart [L, *genitalis* + AS, *wearte*],   a small, soft, moist pink or red swelling of the genitals that becomes pedunculated and may be painless, caused by a sexually transmitted disease, human papillomavirus (HPV), which accounts for over 50% of all cases of sexually transmitted disease. The growth may be solitary, or a cauliflower-like group may be present in the same area of the genitalia. Atypical genital warts should be biopsied and examined as possible carcinomas because they are associated with cervical cancer. No therapy has been shown to eradicate HPV. One third of lesions disappear without treatment. Treatment may include topical applications of podofilox, podophyllin resin, or trichloracetic acid; cryotherapy with liquid nitrogen; laser treatment; or surgical removal. A vaccine (Gardasil) to help prevent HPV infections protects against four types of HPV. Also called **condyloma, condyloma acuminatum, venereal wart, verruca acuminata.**

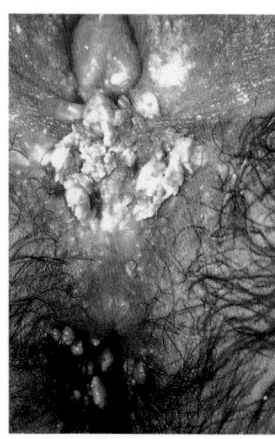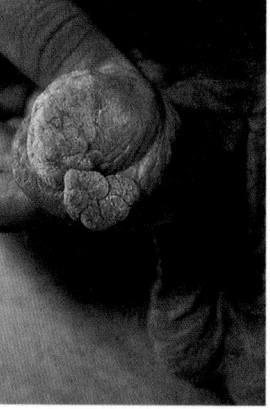

Genital warts *(Graham-Brown and Bourke, 2007)*

genitourinary (GU) /jen′itō·yŏŏr″iner′ē/   [L, *genitalis* + Gk, *ouron,* urine],   referring to the genital and urinary systems of the body: the organ structures, functions, or both. Also called **urogenital.**

genitourinary fistula,   an abnormal communication between organs of the urogenital system or between organs of the urogenital system and some other system.

genitourinary system,   all of the urinary and genital organs and their associated structures, including the kidneys, ureters, bladder, and urethra; the ovaries, fallopian tubes, uterus, clitoris, and vagina (in women); and the testes, seminal vesicles, seminal ducts, prostate, and penis (in men). Also called **urogenital system.** See also *Color Atlas of Human Anatomy,* pp. A-39 to A-41.

genocide /jen″əsīd/,   the systematic extermination of a national, ethnic, political, religious, or other population.

genogram /jē″nōgram/,   a diagram that depicts family relationships over at least three generations. It is useful as a tool for studying the process of a family system or hereditary disease over time.

genome /jē″nōm/   [Gk, *genein,* to produce],   the complete set of genes in the chromosomes of each cell of a specific organism. –**genomic,** *adj.*

genome map,   a graphic representation of the locations of genes in a genome. The human genome map, completed in 1996, locates 5264 markers for genes and has led to the discovery of 223 genes linked to more than 200 diseases. The mouse genome map locates 7377 markers on 20 chromosomes.

genomic /jēnō″mik/,   pertaining to the genome.

genomic imprinting,   differential expression of a gene or genes as a function of whether they were inherited from the male or the female parent (e.g., a deletion on chromosome 15 that causes Prader-Willi syndrome if inherited from the father causes instead Angelman's syndrome if inherited from the mother).

genotoxic /jē′nōtok″sik/,   capable of altering DNA, thereby causing cancer or mutation.

genotoxic carcinogens,   cancer-causing agents that can alter deoxyribonucleic acid (DNA) molecules. Genotoxic carcinogens include organic compounds that induce mutations directly, organic compounds that alter DNA after activating metabolism, and metals or metal salts that can alter DNA.

genotype /jē″nōtīp′/   [Gk, *genos,* birth, *typos,* mark],   **1.** the complete genetic constitution of an organism or group, as determined by the specific combination and location of the genes on the chromosomes. **2.** the alleles situated at one or more sites on homologous chromosomes. A pair of alleles is usually designated by letters or symbols, such as *AA* when the alleles are identical and *Aa* when they are different. **3.** a group or class of organisms having the same genetic makeup; the type species of a genus. Compare **phenotype.** –*genotypic, adj.*

-genous,   suffix meaning "to originate from" or "to contain": *homogenous.*

gentamicin sulfate /jen′təmī″sin/,   an aminoglycoside antibiotic.

■ INDICATIONS: It is prescribed for the treatment of severe infections caused by organisms sensitive to gentamicin, especially gram-negative organisms.

■ CONTRAINDICATIONS: Concomitant administration of other potentially ototoxic or nephrotoxic drugs or known hypersensitivity to this drug or to other aminoglycoside medications prohibits its use. It is used with caution in patients with impaired renal function. It cannot be coadministered with a variety of other drugs. It can be given in combination with penicillins but not physically through the same parenteral tubing.

■ ADVERSE EFFECTS: Among the more serious adverse effects are nephrotoxicity, auditory or vestibular ototoxicity, impairment of neuromuscular transmission, and hypersensitivity reactions.

gentian violet /jen″shən/, a topical antibacterial and antifungal agent.

■ INDICATIONS: It is used to treat superficial *Candida* infections of the skin and vagina. It is also effective against some superficial bacterial infections such as those caused by *Staphylococcus*.

■ CONTRAINDICATIONS: Known hypersensitivity to this drug prohibits its use. It is not applied to ulcerative lesions of the face.

■ ADVERSE EFFECTS: Permanent discoloration of the skin may occur after topical exposure.

gentiotannic acid /jen′shē·ətan″ik/, a form of tannic acid once used as an astringent and in the treatment of burns but no longer recommended because of its hepatotoxicity.

Gentran 40, a plasma volume extender. Brand name for *dextran 40.*

Gentran 70, a plasma volume extender. Brand name for *dextran 70.*

genu /jē″nōō/ [L, knee], the knee or any angular structure resembling the flexed knee.

genupectoral position /je′nōōpek″tərəl/ [L, *genu,* knee, *pectus,* breast, *positio*], knee-chest position. To assume the genupectoral position the person kneels so that the weight of the body is supported by the knees and chest, with the buttocks raised. The head is turned to one side and the arms are flexed so that the upper part of the body can be supported in part by the elbows. The position is sometimes used for rectal or gynecological examinations.

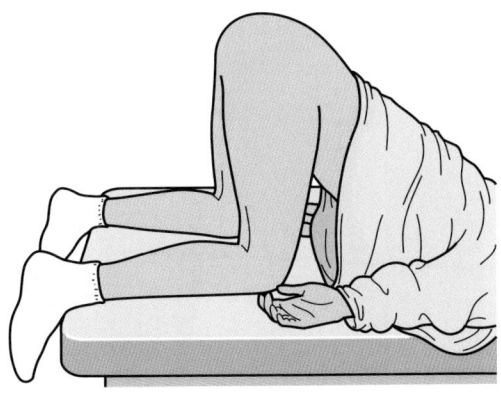

Genupectoral position *(Roberts, 2014)*

genu recurvatum [L, *genu,* knee, *recurvare,* to bend back], a deformity in which the lower leg is hyperextended at the knee joint. Also called *back knee.*

genus /jē″nəs/ *pl. genera* [L, kind], a subdivision of a family of organisms. A genus usually is composed of several closely related species. The genus *Homo* has only one species, *Homo sapiens* (humans). See also **family.**

genu valgum [L, *genu,* knee, *valgus,* bent inward], a deformity in which the legs are curved inward at the knee so that the knees are close together and strike each other as the person walks and the ankles are widely separated. Also called **knock-knee,** *valgus deformity.*

genu varum [L, knee, *varus,* bent outward], a deformity in which one or both legs are bent outward at the knee. Also called **bowleg.** Compare **genu valgum.**

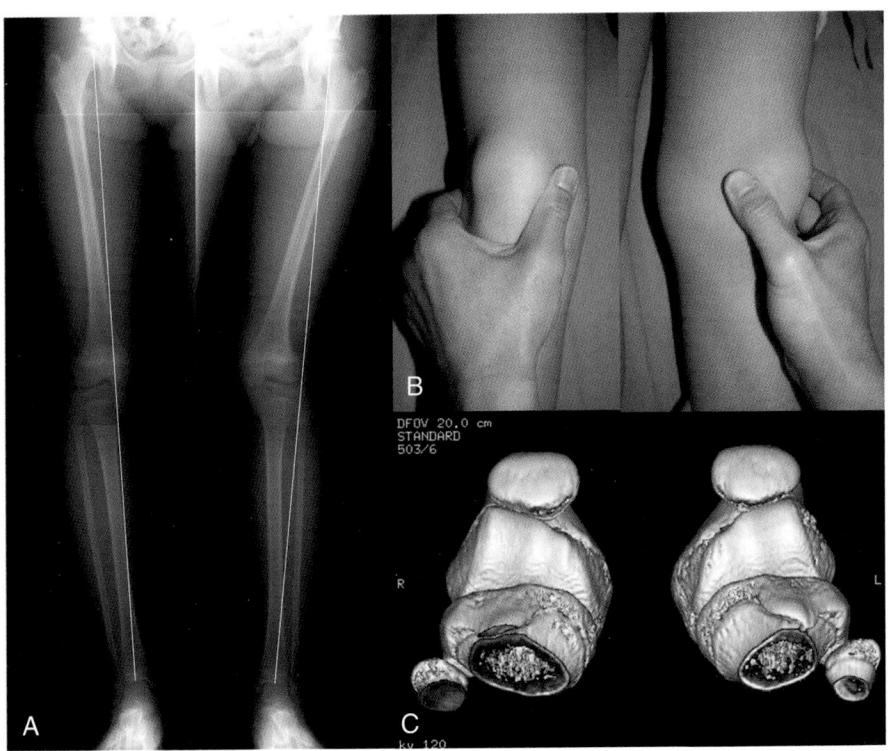

Recurrent patellar dislocation with spontaneous genu valgum deformity treated by distal femoral osteotomy alone *(Suzuki et al, 2020)*

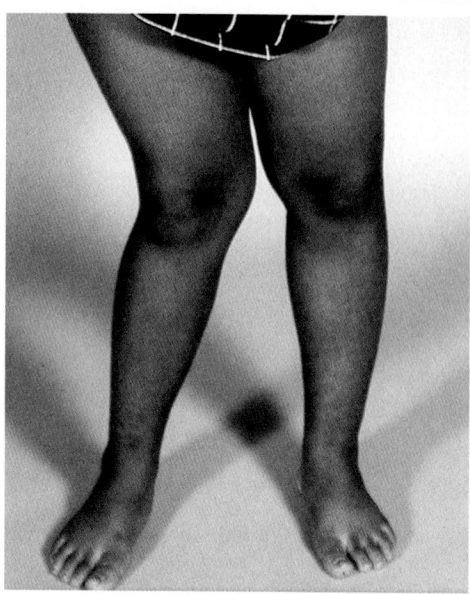

Genu varum *(Herring, 2008)*

-geny, suffix meaning "production, generation, origin": *homogeny, phylogeny, morphogeny.*

geo-, prefix meaning "earth" or "soil": *geobiology, geophagia, geotropism.*

geobiology, an interdisciplinary field of study examining the interaction of living organisms and the Earth.

Geocillin, extended-spectrum penicillin antibacterial drug. Brand name for *carbenicillin indanyl sodium.*

geographic retinal atrophy, a pattern of well-demarcated epithelial atrophy of retinal pigment leading to vision loss, most often associated with age-related macular degeneration.

geographic tongue /jē′əgraf′ik/ [Gk, *ge,* earth, *graphein,* to record; AS, *tunge*], a common benign condition of the tongue seen in 1%-3% of the population, more frequently seen in females, in which the dorsum of the tongue possesses multiple zones of erythema surrounded by slightly elevated yellow-white borders. The pattern of lesions can change in appearance every few days or weeks. Patients may experience no sensation, or tenderness with a burning sensation. Also called **benign migratory glossitis, erythema migrans,** *wandering rash of the tongue, erythema areata migrans, stomatitis areata migrans.*

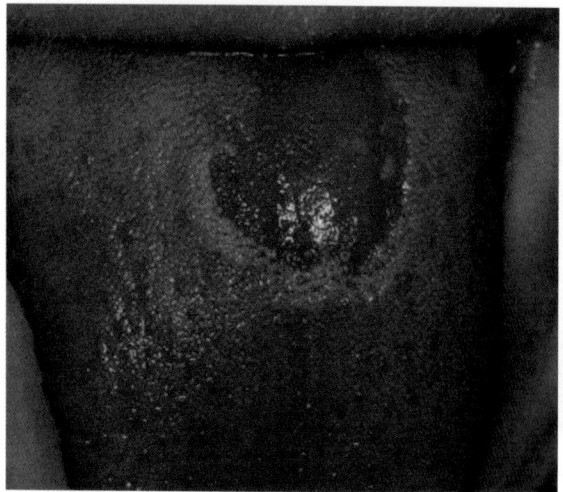

Geographic tongue of a child *(Stoopler et al, 2015)*

geometric mean. See **mean.**

geometric unsharpness, image blur resulting from the finite size of the x-ray tube focal spot (as opposed to a point source).

geophagia, the practice of eating clay or dirt. A form of pica, the compulsion is thought by some to be associated with disorders of mineral balance. Some patients with pica have been found to suffer from an iron deficiency and to respond to iron therapy.

geotrichosis /jē′ōtrikō″sis/ [Gk, *ge,* earth, *thrix,* hair, *osis,* condition], a condition associated with a rare fungus *Geotrichum candidum,* which can cause oral, bronchial, pharyngeal, and intestinal disorders. *G. candidum* is normally found in healthy individuals, soil, and dairy products and is not necessarily pathogenic. Geotrichosis most commonly occurs in immunosuppressed individuals with diabetes. Bronchopulmonary complications associated with this disorder may produce a cough with thick, bloody sputum. Geotrichosis has been associated with allergic asthmatic reactions similar to allergic aspergillosis and a type of intestinal disorder characterized by abdominal pain, diarrhea, and rectal bleeding. Oral lesions that may occur with this disorder are commonly treated with a solution of gentian violet; associated abdominal lesions are treated with the oral administration of gentian violet capsules. Associated pulmonary lesions are treated with the oral administration of potassium iodide.

geotropism /je-ot′ro-pizm/ [L, *pro,* earth], growth influenced by gravity.

gEq, abbreviation for **gram-equivalent weight.**

Gerbich blood group /gər′bich/, a blood group consisting of three high-prevalence erythrocytic antigens, Ge 2, Ge 3, and Ge 4, and five antigens of very low prevalence.

GERD /gərd/, acronym for *gastroesophageal reflux disease.* See **gastroesophageal reflux.**

geriatric day care /jer′ē-at″rik/ [Gk, *geras,* old age; AS, *daeg* + L, *garrire,* chatter], an ambulatory health care facility for older adults who require continual supervision or assistance. It usually offers a broad range of professional and community services to maximize functional independence of the patients and may provide respite from care for family members during the day.

geriatric dentistry. See **gerodontics.**

Geriatric Depression Scale (GDS), a brief depression screening inventory composed of 30 items that require yes or no answers. A score of 11 or above indicates depressed individuals. There is a 15-item short version. Scores of 5 or more may indicate depression.

geriatric education for emergency medical services (GEMS), a continuing education program, developed by the American Geriatrics Society and the National Council of State Emergency Medical Services Training Coordinators, to train first responders, EMTs, paramedics, and other emergency care providers to deliver state-of-the-art prehospital care to older adults.

geriatrician /jer′ē-ətrish″ən/, a physician who has specialized postgraduate education and experience in the medical care of older persons.

geriatric nurse practitioner (GNP), a registered nurse with additional education obtained through a master's degree program in nursing that prepares the nurse to deliver primary health care to elderly adults.

geriatrics /jer′ē-at″riks/, the branch of medicine dealing with the physiological characteristics of aging and the diagnosis and treatment of diseases affecting the aged.

germ /jurm/ [L, *germen,* sprout], **1.** *(Nontechnical)* any microorganism, especially one that is pathogenic. **2.** a unit of living matter able to develop into a self-sufficient organism, such as a seed, spore, or egg. **3.** (in embryology) the first stage in development, such as a spermatozoon or other germ cell.

German cockroach, *Blattella germanica,* a small light-brown species found as a household pest in North America and Europe.

germanium (Ge) /jərmā″nē·əm/ [Germany], a metallic element with some nonmetallic semiconductor properties. Its atomic number is 32; its atomic mass is 72.61.

German measles. See **rubella.**

germ cell, 1. a sexual reproductive cell in any stage of development from the primordial embryonic form to the mature gamete. **2.** an ovum or spermatozoon or any of their preceding forms. **3.** any cell undergoing gametogenesis. Also called **gonoblast, gonocyte.** Compare **somatic cell.**

germ disk. See **embryonic disk.**

germ-free animal, a laboratory animal raised under sterile conditions, free of exposure to microorganisms. The diet is controlled, preventing exposure to microorganisms that may be in food. Germ-free animals have lymphoid tissue that is not fully developed and may have a deficiency of serum immunoglobulin.

germicide /jur″misīd/ [L, *germen,* sprout, *caedere,* to kill], a drug that kills pathogenic microorganisms. See also **antibacterial, antifungal, antiviral.** –*germicidal, adj.*

germinal /jur″minəl/ [L, sprout], pertaining to or characteristic of a germ cell or to the early stages of development.

germinal area. See **embryonic disk.**

germinal center [L, *germen,* sprout; Gk, *kentron,* center], an antigen-localizing follicle of lymphoid tissue, occupying the center of the lymphatic nodules of the spleen, tonsils, and lymph nodes. It reacts to antigens, enlarging and becoming filled with lymphoblasts and macrophages at the center of a ring of small lymphocytes.

germinal cords, the precursors to the embryonic ovary or testis, derived from the gonadal cords.

germinal disk. See **embryonic disk.**

germinal epithelium, 1. the epithelial layer covering the genital ridge from which the gonads are derived in early embryonic development. **2.** the epithelial covering of the ovary, formerly thought to be the site of the formation of the oogonia. See also **oogenesis.**

germinal membrane. See **blastoderm.**

germinal nucleus. See **pronucleus.**

germinal pole. See **animal pole.**

germinal stage, (in embryology) the interval of time from fertilization to implantation during which the ovum undergoes cell division several times, travels to the uterus, and, in the form of a blastocyst, begins to implant itself in the endometrium. The germinal stage is over at about 10 days of gestation.

germination /jur″minā″shən/ [L, *germen,* sprout], **1.** the initial growth and development of an organism from the time of fertilization to the formation of the embryo. **2.** the sprouting of a spore or the seed of a plant. –*germinate, v.*

germinoma /jur″minō″mə/, a neoplasm of the germinal tissue of the gonads, the mediastinum, or the pineal region. It is commonly associated with pituitary disorders.

germ layer, one of the three primordial cell layers formed during gastrulation in the early stages of embryonic development from which the entire range of body tissue is derived. Each germ layer has the potential for forming different cell types that differentiate into the various structures of the body. See also **ectoderm, endoderm, mesoderm.**

germ line, genetic material in a cell lineage that is passed down through the gametes before it is modified by somatic recombination or maturation.

germ nucleus. See **pronucleus.**

germ plasm, 1. the part of a germ cell that contains the reproductive and hereditary material; the total of the DNA in a specific cell or organism. **2.** (*Nontechnical*) germ cells

in any stage of development together with the tissues from which they originated.

germ theory [L, *germen,* sprout; Gk, *theoria,* speculation], the concept that all infectious and contagious diseases are caused by living microorganisms. The science of bacteriology developed after establishment of this theory. Also called **pathogenic theory of medicine.**

gero-, geronto-, prefix meaning "old age" or "the aged": *gerodontics.*

geroderma /jer′ədur″mə/ [Gk, *geron,* old man, *derma,* skin], **1.** the atrophic skin of aging. **2.** skin that is thin and wrinkled as a result of a defective state of nutrition. **3.** any condition characterized by skin that is thin and wrinkled, resembling the skin of old age.

gerodontics /jer′ōdon′tiks/ [Gk, *geron,* old man + *odous,* tooth], **1.** the delivery of dental care to aging persons. **2.** the diagnosis, prevention, and treatment of dental problems peculiar to advanced age. Also called **geriatric dentistry,** *gerodontia, gerodontology.*

geri-, gero-, prefix meaning "old age": *geriatrician.*

gerontic nursing, nursing care pertaining to an older person that combines geriatric nursing (nursing care primarily for older persons who are ill) and gerontological nursing (a more holistic view of the nursing care of older persons).

geront(o) [word element, Gk.], old age; the aged.

geronto-. See **gero-, geronto-.**

gerontogen /jeron″təjən/, an environmental agent that contributes to the aging process by accelerating the onset and/or rate of progression of aging. Examples include age-dependent cellular and biochemical responses to oxidant damage to aging of cells. Kinds include **cigarette smoking, ultraviolet (UV) rays.**

gerontological rehabilitation nursing, a nursing specialty whose focus is helping elderly individuals affected by chronic illness or physical disability to adapt to their disabilities and to achieve their optimal level of physical, mental, and psychosocial well-being. It takes into consideration both normal age-related changes and functional limitations brought about by illness or injury.

Gerontological Society of America (GSA), an organization of scientific and academic professionals interested in studies of the nature of the aging process and the clinical manifestations of disease in the aging organism. GSA members participate with the International Association of Gerontology in periodic seminars at which worldwide research on longevity is presented.

gerontology /jer′əntol″əjē/ [Gk, *geras,* old age, *logos,* science], the study of all aspects of the aging process, including the clinical, psychological, economic, and sociological issues encountered by older persons and their consequences for both the individual and society.

gerontotoxon, an abnormal white or gray opaque ring at the outer edge of the cornea. Sometimes it is present at birth or appears in childhood and is called *arcus juvenilis.* It is particularly common in people over 50 years old and is then given the name *arcus senilis.* It results from deposits of cholesterol in the cornea or from degeneration of the cornea's supporting framework. See also **arcus senilis.**

geropsychiatry /jer′ōsīkī″ətrē/ [Gk, *geras,* old age, *psyche,* mind], the study and treatment of psychiatric aspects of aging and mental disorders of elderly people or the functional/mental disorders of people in their 50s and 60s if they qualify.

-gerous, suffix meaning "bearing, producing, or containing" something specified: *dentigerous cyst.*

Gerson diet, a detoxification diet, claimed to be useful in the treatment of cancer, allergies, and a wide variety of degenerative diseases, consisting of large quantities of organically grown fruits and vegetables, consumed mainly in the form of juice. It is often combined with other complementary therapies. The Gerson therapy has not been approved by the FDA for use as a treatment for cancer or any other disease.

Gerstmann syndrome /gerst'män/ [Josef Gerstmann, Austrian neurologist, 1887–1969], a combination of finger agnosia, right-left disorientation, agraphia, acalculia, and often constructional apraxia. It is often associated with dominant parietal lobe lesions. See also **acalculia, agraphia, constructional apraxia, finger agnosia.**

Gerstmann-Sträussler-Scheinker syndrome /gerst'män shtrois'lershĭn'ker/, an extremely rare group of prion diseases, inherited as an autosomal-dominant trait but linked to different mutations of the prion protein gene. All forms of the syndrome have the common characteristics of cognitive and motor disturbances and the presence of numerous amyloid plaques in the brain. Three forms have been recognized: the ataxic form, which is accompanied by progressive cerebellar ataxia and dementia; the telencephalic form, which is accompanied by dysarthria, dementia, rigidity, tremor, and hyperreflexia; and Gerstmann-Sträussler-Scheinker syndrome with neurofibrillary tangles, in which there is progressive short-term memory loss and clumsiness. Death usually occurs in 1 to 5 years.

Gerstmann-Sträussler syndrome. See **transmissible spongiform encephalopathy.**

Gesell Developmental Assessment [Arnold L. Gesell, American pediatrician and psychologist, 1880–1961], an evaluation program that provides information by direct observation on gross motor, fine motor, language, personal-social, and cognitive development. There are no right or wrong answers.

Gestalt /gəshtält'/ *pl. Gestalts, Gestalten* [Ger, form], a single physical, psychological, or symbolic configuration, pattern, or experience that consists of a number of elements and that has an effect as a whole different from that of the sum of its parts.

Gestalt psychology, a school of psychology, originating in Germany, that maintains that a psychological phenomenon is perceived as a total configuration or pattern, rising from the relationships among its constituent elements, rather than as discrete elements possessing attributes of their own, and that the pattern, or Gestalt, cannot be derived from the summation of its constituents. Thus learning is regarded as resulting from insight, defined as a process or reorganization, rather than from association or trial and error, and behavior is seen as an integrated response to a unitary situation rather than as a series of reflexes and sensations. Also called **configurationism,** *Gestaltism.* See also **Gestalt.**

Gestalt therapy, a form of psychotherapy that stresses the unity of self-awareness, behavior, and experience. It incorporates elements of psychoanalytic, behavioristic, and humanistic existential therapy. See also **Gestalt psychology.**

gestant anomaly. See **odontoma.**

gestant odontoma. See **dens in dente.**

gestate /jes'tāt/ [L, *gestare,* to bear], **1.** to carry a developing fetus in the womb. **2.** to grow and develop slowly toward maturity, such as a fetus in the womb.

gestation /jestā'shən/ [L, *gestare,* to bear], in a viviparous animal, the period from the fertilization of the ovum until birth. Gestation varies with the species. In humans the average duration is 266 days, or approximately 280 days from the onset of the last menstrual period. A gestation time of less than 37 weeks is regarded as premature; one that continues beyond 42 weeks is considered postmature, regardless of the size of the fetus or other factors. See also **pregnancy.**

gestational age /jestā'shənəl/ [L, *gestare* + *aetas,* time of life], the age of a fetus or a newborn, usually expressed in weeks dating from the first day of the mother's last menstrual period.

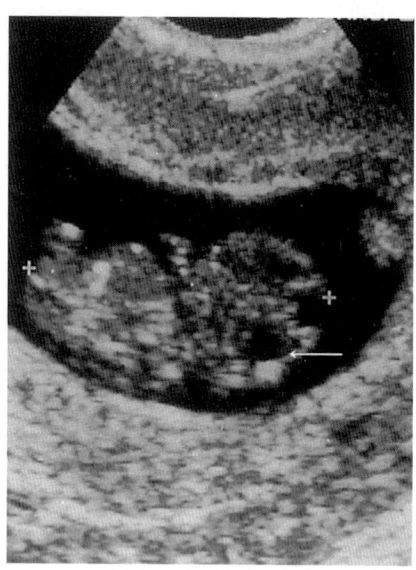

Ultrasound assessment of gestational age *(Murray and McKinney, 2006)*

gestational assessment [L, *gestare,* to bear, *assidere,* to sit beside], calculation of the fetal age of the offspring on the basis of such factors as the menstrual history of the mother, the date when fetal heart sounds are first detected, and the evaluation of ultrasound data. The information is important in planning emergency care in the event of premature birth signs.

gestational diabetes mellitus (GDM), a disorder characterized by an impaired ability to metabolize carbohydrates, usually caused by a deficiency of insulin or insulin resistance, occurring in pregnancy. It disappears after delivery of the infant but in a significant number of cases returns years later as type 2 diabetes mellitus. There are two classes of gestational diabetes. Class A1 can be managed with diet and exercise; class A2 requires management with insulin or other medications. Self-monitoring of blood glucose and a meal plan that controls the amount of carbohydrates eaten are also important. See also **diabetes mellitus.**

gestational hypertension, hypertension that develops after 20 weeks of gestation in the absence of proteinuria; generally over 139/89 mm Hg. Gestational hypertension may be transient but often precedes preeclampsia, which is hypertension with proteinuria after 20 weeks' gestational age. Also called **pregnancy-induced hypertension.**

gestational sac, the structure enclosing an early pregnancy.

gestation period [L, *gestare,* to bear; Gk, *peri,* near, *hodos,* way], the time span between conception and labor. In humans the period is approximately 38 weeks.

gestures in physical examination /jes'chərs/, physical appearance clues in diagnosis, such as a patient's pressing a clenched fist against the sternum as a "body language" message of the pain experienced during a myocardial infarction.

Getman visuomotor theory [Gerald Getman], a concept that visual perception is based on developmental sequences of physiological actions in children. The sequence of eight stages begins with innate response systems and advances to cognitive integration of perceptions, abstractions, and higher symbolic activity.

-geusia, -geustia, suffix meaning "(condition of the) sense of taste": *dysgeusia, hemigeusia, parageusia.*

gFOBT, abbreviation for *guaiac fecal occult blood test.*

GFP, abbreviation for **green fluorescent protein.**

GFR, abbreviation for **glomerular filtration rate.**

GGT, abbreviation for **gamma-glutamyltransferase.**

GH, abbreviation for **growth hormone.**

Ghon focus, the primary parenchymal lesion of primary pulmonary tuberculosis in children. When it is associated with a corresponding lymph node focus, it is known as Ghon's complex. See also **Ghon's complex.**

Ghon's complex [Anton Ghon, Czechoslovakian pathologist, 1866–1936], a combination of pleural surface-healed granulomas, calcifications, or scars on the middle lobe of the lung together with hilar lymph node granulomas. The complex is evidence that a primary tuberculosis case, usually from a childhood infection, has healed.

ghost cells [AS, *gast* + L, *cella,* storeroom], enlarged epithelial cells that have no nucleus so that only the plasma membranes are observed in microscopic examinations. Also called **shadow cells.**

ghost teeth. See **odontodysplasia.**

GHRF, abbreviation for *growth hormone–releasing factor.*

GH-RH, abbreviation for **growth hormone–releasing hormone.**

GHRIH, abbreviation for **growth hormone release–inhibiting hormone.** See **somatostatin.**

GI, abbreviation for **gastrointestinal.**

Gianotti-Crosti syndrome /jänot′ē kros′tē/ [Fernando Gianotti, Italian dermatologist, 1920–1984; Agostino Crosti, 20th-century Italian dermatologist], a generally benign and self-limited disease of young children that had previously been associated with hepatitis B virus but is now known to occur in other viral illnesses. It is characterized by the appearance of crops of usually nonpruritic, dusky or coppery red, flat-topped, firm papules forming a symmetric eruption on the face, buttocks, and limbs, including the palms and soles, and associated with malaise, low-grade fever, and a few other symptoms. Also called **acrodermatitis papulosa infantum, infantile acrodermatitis, papular acrodermatitis of childhood.**

giant axonal neuropathy, an autosomal-recessive neuropathy of childhood characterized by enlarged axons made up of masses of tightly woven neurofilaments.

giant cell /jī″ənt/ [L, *gigas,* huge, *cella,* storeroom], an abnormally large tissue cell that often contains more than one nucleus and may appear as a merger of several normal cells.

giant cell arteritis. See **temporal arteritis.**

giant cell carcinoma, a malignant epithelial neoplasm characteristically containing many large anaplastic cells. A small percentage of adenocarcinomas of the lung and liver also contain such cells. Also called **carcinoma gigantocellulare.**

giant cell hepatitis. See **neonatal hepatitis.**

giant cell interstitial pneumonia. See **interstitial pneumonia.**

giant cell myeloma, a bone tumor of multinucleated giant cells that resembles osteoclasts scattered in a matrix of spindle cells. Myelomas of this kind may be benign or malignant and may cause pain, functional disability, and pathological fractures. Also called **giant cell tumor of bone.**

giant cell sarcoma, osteoblastic sarcoma. See **giant cell myeloma, osteoblastic sarcoma.**

giant cell thyroiditis. See **de Quervain's thyroiditis.**

giant cell tumor of bone. See **giant cell myeloma.**

giant chromosome, any of the excessively large chromosomes found in insects and certain other animals, including the lampbrush and polytene chromosomes.

giant condyloma, a destructive tumor resembling squamous cell carcinoma but actually a form of condyloma acuminatum, usually on the penis, but sometimes present elsewhere in the anogenital area in either men or women. It presents as a large verrucous to fungating, cauliflowerlike mass that erodes the involved skin and progresses to penetrate and destroy deeper tissues. Also called **Buschke-Löwenstein tumor.**

giant follicular lymphoma, a nodular, well-differentiated lymphocytic malignant lymphoma in which nodules distort the normal structure of a lymph node. Also called **Brill-Symmers disease,** *giant follicular lymphadenopathy,* **Symmers disease.**

giant hypertrophic gastritis, a rare disease characterized by large folds of nodular gastric rugae that may cover the wall of the stomach, causing anorexia, nausea, vomiting, and abdominal distress. Endoscopic examination may be necessary for diagnosis. The disease is associated with an increased incidence of stomach cancer. Also called **Ménétrier disease.**

giant peristaltic contraction, a propulsive contraction of the bowel that normally occurs periodically in the distal small intestine and colon. The contractions are 1.5 to 2 times larger than normal in amplitude and 4 to 6 times longer in duration than usual. In certain disease states, giant peristaltic contractions may start in the proximal small intestine and proceed uninterrupted. They may also be induced by a variety of stimuli including certain antibiotics, radiation therapy, and parasitic infections.

Gianturco coil, a mechanism for occluding a patent ductus arteriosus and for permanent vascular occlusion of other major arteries.

Giardia /jē·är″dē·ə/ [Alfred Giard, French biologist, 1846–1908], a common genus of flagellate protozoans and a major cause of nonbacterial diarrhea in North America and of intestinal disease globally. Many species of *Giardia* normally inhabit the digestive tract and cause inflammation in association with other factors that produce rapid proliferation of the organism. See also **giardiasis.**

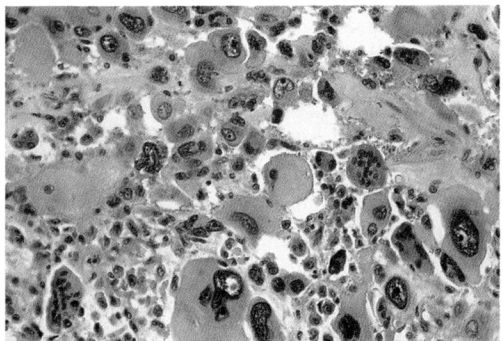

Giant cell carcinoma of the bladder *(Fletcher, 2007)*

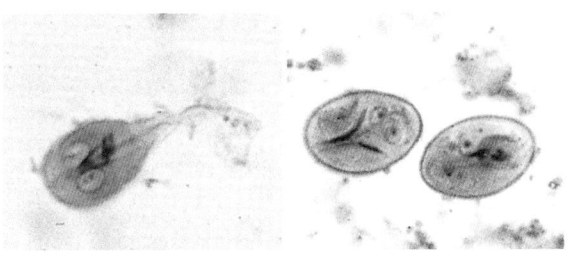

***Giardia lamblia* trophozoite and cyst** *(Murray et al, 2004)*

giardiasis /jē·ärdī″əsis/ [Alfred Giard; Gk, *osis,* condition], a diarrheal illness caused by infection with the protozoan *Giardia lamblia.*
- OBSERVATIONS: Infection may be asymptomatic or may cause nausea; abdominal cramps; foul-smelling, greasy diarrhea; fatigue; and weight loss.
- INTERVENTIONS: Often, the infection resolves without treatment. When treatment is required, metronidazole, tinidazole, furazolidone, or paromomycin may be used.
- PATIENT CARE CONSIDERATIONS: The source of infection is usually fecally contaminated water. Cases have occurred in day care facilities with poor hygienic practices. Infants and children are at greatest risk for complications.

gibbus /gib″əs, jib″əs/ [L, hump], a hump, swelling, or enlargement on a body surface, usually confined to one side.

gibbus deformity, a form of structural kyphosis, usually secondary to tuberculosis infection of the thoracic vertebral body, in which the vertebral column becomes sharply angulated at the site of the lesion.

Gibraltar fever. See **brucellosis.**

Gibson murmur [George A. Gibson, Scottish physician, 1854–1913], a heart murmur that is heard continuously throughout the cardiac cycle in patients with patent ductus arteriosus. It waxes at the end of systole and wanes near the end of diastole and is often described as a "machinery-like" murmur. It is often accompanied by a thrill. It is usually localized in the second left interspace near the sternum and usually is indicative of patent ductus arteriosus. Also called **machinery murmur.**

Gibson walking splint, a kind of Thomas splint that enables a patient to be ambulatory.

Giemsa stain /gē·em″sə/ [Gustav Giemsa, German chemist, 1867–1948; Fr, *teindre,* to dye], an azure dye used as a stain in the microscopic examination of the blood for certain protozoan parasites, viral inclusion bodies, and rickettsia and, more routinely, in the preparation of a smear for a differential white cell count. It is modified and combined with Wright stain to better detect organisms.

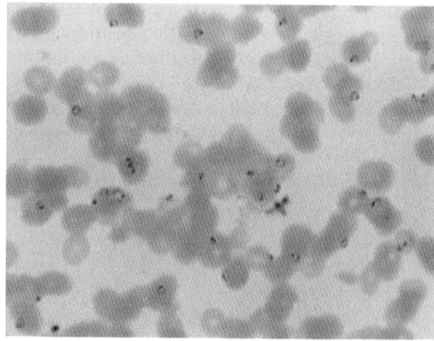

Giemsa stain showing *Plasmodium falciparum* trophozoites *(Conlon and Snydman, 2000)*

GIFT, abbreviation for **gamete intrafallopian transfer.**

giga-, prefix meaning "one billion (¹09)": *gigabit, gigabyte, gigahertz.*

gigantism /jigan″tizəm/ [L, *gigas,* giant], an abnormal condition characterized by excessive size and stature. It is caused most frequently by hypersecretion of growth hormone (GH) that occurs before the closure of the bone epiphyses; it occurs to a lesser degree in hypogonadism and in certain genetic disorders. Gigantism with normal body proportions and normal sexual development usually results from hypersecretion of GH in early childhood. Hypogonadism, by delaying puberty and closure of the epiphyses, may lead to gigantism. Excessive linear growth often occurs in males with more than one Y chromosome, and it may accompany Klinefelter syndrome, Marfan syndrome, and some cases of generalized lipodystrophy. Children with cerebral gigantism are cognitively impaired and have a large head and extremities and an awkward gait. Growth is rapid during their first few years and then reverts to a normal rate. Appropriate gonadal hormones may be administered to control abnormal growth of children with hypogonadism. The treatment of acromegalic gigantism is usually irradiation or surgical removal of the GH-secreting adenoma. Compare **acromegaly.** See also **eunuchoidism.**

giganto-, prefix meaning "huge": *gigantocellulare.*

Gilbert syndrome [Nicolas A. Gilbert, French physician, 1858–1927], a benign hereditary condition characterized by hyperbilirubinemia and jaundice. See also **hyperbilirubinemia of the newborn.**

Gilchrist disease. See **blastomycosis.**

Gilles de la Tourette syndrome /zhēl″də lä toorets″/ [George Gilles de la Tourette, French neurologist, 1857–1927], an abnormal condition characterized by facial grimaces, vocalizations, tics, and involuntary arm and shoulder movements. In adolescence the condition worsens. The patient may grunt, snort, and shout involuntarily. Coprolalia can develop. In adulthood the condition usually lessens and tends to wax and wane. Treatment with dopamine antagonists has been found to be very effective. Also called **Tourette syndrome.** See also **aboiement.**

Gillies' operation /gil″ēz/ [Harold D. Gillies, English surgeon, 1882–1960], a surgical procedure for reducing fractures of the zygoma and zygomatic arch by making an incision in the temporal hairline.

Gil-Vernet technique, a surgical procedure in which both ureters are excised from their normal attachments to the bladder and reattached medially near each other within the trigone.

ginger, an herb native to the tropics of Asia and now cultivated in the tropics of South America, China, India, Africa, the Caribbean, and parts of the United States.
- INDICATIONS: It is considered safe when consumed in food. Medicinal amounts of the herb are used for nausea, motion sickness, indigestion, and inflammation. It may be effective against motion sickness but does not help treat nausea from other causes (e.g., opioid analgesia, chemotherapy). Its efficacy as an antiinflammatory drug has not been established.
- CONTRAINDICATIONS: It is not recommended during pregnancy (it may be an abortifacient when taken in large amounts) or lactation, in children, or in those with known hypersensitivity to this product. It should not be used in cholelithiasis unless directed by a physician. Safety when large amounts of ginger are ingested for medicinal purposes has not been established.

ginger paralysis /jin″jər/, a polyneuropathy that primarily affected upper motor nerves to the distal parts of the extremities, caused by a neurotoxin found in an extract of Jamaican ginger (Jake) in the early part of the 20th century. Also called **Jake paralysis.**

gingiva /jinjī″və/ *pl. gingivae* [L, gum], the gum tissues of the mouth, consisting of a mucous membrane with supporting fibrous tissue that overlies the crowns of unerupted teeth and encircles the necks of teeth that have erupted. **–gingival,** *adj.*

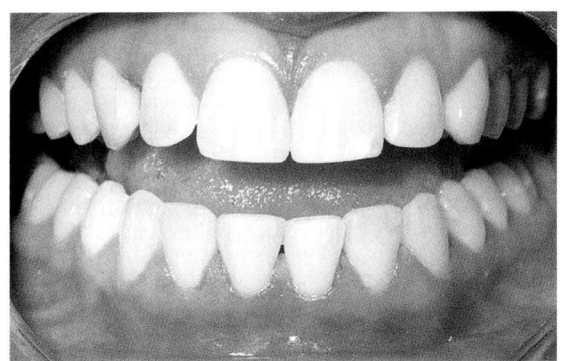

Healthy gingiva *(Christensen, 2002)*

gingival /jin′jival/, pertaining to the gingivae.

gingival blanching [L, *gingiva* + Fr, *blanchir*, to whiten], the lightening of gum color, usually temporary, caused by stretching or pressure upon gum tissue and decreased blood supply.

gingival blood supply, the vascular supply to the gums. It rises from blood vessels that pass along the outer periosteum of bone and anastomose with vessels of the periodontal membrane as well as intraalveolar blood vessels.

gingival cavity, a tooth cavity that occurs in the third of the clinical crown nearest the gum. A gingival cavity is in Class V of Black's Classification of Caries.

gingival color, the color of gum tissue. It is affected by the thickness and degree of keratinization of the epithelium, blood supply, pigmentation, medications, and periodontal, gingival, and systemic diseases.

gingival consistency, the combination of tactile and visual characteristics of healthy gum tissue. The tissue should be firm and resilient and should resemble smooth velvet or a finely or coarsely grained orange peel. Compare **gingival color.**

gingival corium, the most stable connective tissue of the gingiva, which lies between the periosteum and the lamina propria mucosae.

gingival crater, a depression in the gum tissue, especially in the area of the former apex of interdental papilla. It is commonly a result of acute inflammation of the gingival tissue, such as in cases of necrotizing ulcerative gingivitis. It can also result due to food impaction against the tissue subjacent to the contact areas of adjacent teeth.

gingival crevice, a normal space located around a tooth between the wall of the unattached gum tissue and the enamel and/or cementum of the tooth. Also called **gingival sulcus.**

gingival cuff, the protective mucosa around enamel at the neck of a tooth. See **junctional epithelium.**

gingival cyst, a developmental nonkeratinizing odontogenic cyst found in the oral soft tissue of adults. A variation of the lateral periodontal cyst.

gingival discoloration, a change in the normal color of the gum tissue, associated with inflammation, reduced blood supply, abnormal pigmentation, and other problems.

gingival disease, any disease of the gingivae, such as gingivitis. The American Academy of Periodontology classifies gingival disease as a major group of periodontal diseases and distinguishes two main subgroups: those gingival diseases induced by dental plaque and those attributed to other causes. The plaque-induced diseases may be associated with endocrine changes, medications, systemic disease, or malnutrition. Other causes of gingival lesions include viral infections, fungal infections, genetic predispositions, systemic conditions, allergic reactions, and traumatic lesions, among others.

gingival festoon, the distinct rounding and enlargement of the margins of the gum tissue found in early gingival involvement. Compare **festoon, McCall's festoon.**

gingival hormonal enlargement, swelling of the gums associated with poor oral hygiene and hormonal imbalance during pregnancy, puberty, or postmenopausal therapy. Also called **pregnancy epulis.**

gingival hyperplasia, an increase in the number of cells of the gum tissues, resulting in an overgrowth that may partially or totally cover the teeth; may be generalized or localized. Causes include hereditary and metabolic disorders, or drugs such as: the anticonvulsants phenytoin and carbamazepine; cyclosporine, a potent immunosuppressant used for organ transplant recipients; calcium channel blockers, such as nifedipine and amlodipine, used for the treatment of hypertension; the antibiotic erythromycin; and oral contraceptives. While the cause is considered to be multifactorial, the presence of gingival inflammation due to poor oral hygiene can contribute to the development. The presence of malpositioned teeth or orthodontic bands can exaggerate the condition. Treatment includes surgical excision of the enlarged tissue, followed by meticulous oral hygiene.

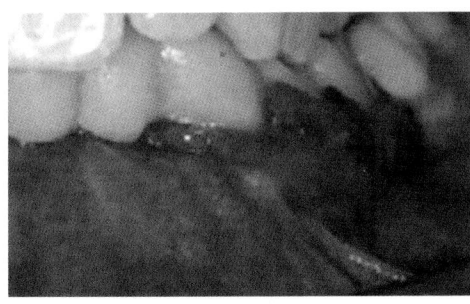

Gingival hyperplasia *(Ciocca et al, 2007)*

gingival hypertrophy, an increase in the size of gum tissue encircling the teeth. It may be caused by gum inflammation and periodontal disease.

gingival line [L, *gingiva,* gum, *linea*], the scalloped line formed by the edge of the unattached gum tissue at the margin of the soft tissues beside the teeth. The line is called marginal gingiva when viewed labially, buccally, or lingually. Between the teeth in the interproximal area, the line is called interdental gingiva or interdental papilla. Also called **gum line.**

gingival massage, the mechanical rubbing of the gum tissues for cleansing purposes, for improvement of tissue tone and blood circulation, and for keratinization of the surface epithelium.

gingival mat, the connective tissue of the gum, composed of coarse, broad collagen fibers that attach the gingivae to the teeth and hold the unattached gum close to the teeth.

gingival papilla. See **interdental gingiva.**

gingival physiology, the function of the gum tissue as supportive and protective investments of the teeth and subjacent tissues. The gingival fiber apparatus serves as a barrier to apical migration of the junctional epithelium and binds the gingival tissues to the teeth. Normal gingival topography permits the free flow of food away from the occlusal surfaces and from the cervical and interproximal areas of the teeth.

gingival pocket. See **periodontal pocket.**

gingival position, the level of the gum margin in relation to the teeth.

gingival shrinkage, the reduction in the mass and height of the gum tissue, especially as a result of the therapeutic elimination of subgingival deposits, curettage of the soft tissue wall of the gingival pocket, and resolution of inflammation as a result of periodontal therapy.

gingival stippling, numerous small dimples or depressions in the surface of healthy gum tissue, producing an appearance that varies from that of smooth velvet to that of an orange peel. See also **epithelial peg, gingival consistency.**

gingival sulcus. See **gingival crevice.**

gingivectomy /jin′jīvek″təmē/ [L, *gingiva* + Gk, *ektomē,* excision], surgical removal of infected and diseased gum tissue, performed to arrest the progress of periodontal disease, or the removal of healthy tissue for aesthetic purposes. With the patient under local anesthesia, possibly along with sedation or nitrous oxide, the affected tissue is removed, and the accessible root surfaces are debrided of calculus and necrotic cementum. This procedure eliminates periodontal pockets. The healthy gingival tissues are sutured into place, and a periodontal pack may be placed on the surgical site to prevent trauma during eating and to allow new tissue growth to fill in the area. Bleeding, discomfort, and pain are generally associated with the procedure. After surgery the patient is closely monitored for signs of hemorrhage, frequency in swallowing, or a rise in pulse rate. The periodontal pack is removed after 1 week. Compare **gingivoplasty.**

gingivitis /jin′jivī″tis/ [L, *gingiva* + Gk, *itis,* inflammation], inflammation of the gingiva, with symptoms that may include redness, swelling, and bleeding. Gingivitis is generally the result of poor oral hygiene and of the accumulation of bacterial plaque on the teeth, but it may be a sign of other conditions, such as diabetes mellitus, leukemia, hormonal changes, or vitamin deficiency. It is common in pregnancy, is usually painless, and may be acute or chronic. Research is finding associations between the occurrence of periodontal disease and heart disease, stroke, asthma, and low birth weight neonates. Frequent removal of plaque and regular visits to the dentist or dental hygienist along with proper oral hygiene may help in prevention. Compare **necrotizing ulcerative gingivitis.**

■ OBSERVATIONS: This gum inflammation is usually painless in its early stages and manifests as redness, swelling, and bleeding of the gums. Halitosis and bluish gum discoloration may also be present. Complications include development of pus pockets and abscess formation and pain. Diagnosis is made on oral examination.

■ INTERVENTIONS: Treatment is targeted at plaque removal and antibiotics for signs of infection. Soft tissue debridement may be indicated for chronic or severe cases.

■ PATIENT CARE CONSIDERATIONS: Interventions should focus on education about appropriate oral hygiene (brushing, flossing, and gum massage) and regular dental care with professional teeth cleaning.

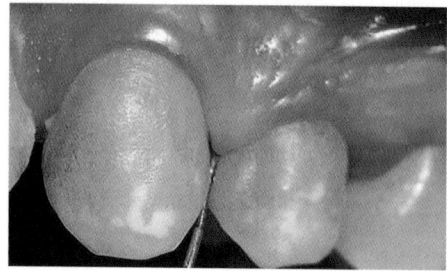

Mild edematous gingivitis *(Newman et al, 2015)*

gingivo-, prefix meaning "gingiva": *gingivoplasty, gingivostomatitis.*

gingivoplasty /jin″jivōplas′tē/ [L, *gingiva* + Gk, *plassein,* to shape], the surgical contouring of the gum tissues and interdental papillae to restore gingival tissue to more normal form and function. Compare **gingivectomy.**

gingivostomatitis /jin′jivōstŏ′mətī″tis/ [L, *gingiva* + Gk, *stoma,* mouth, *itis,* inflammation], multiple painful ulcers on the gums and mucous membranes of the mouth, the result of a herpesvirus infection. The condition most frequently affects infants and young children. It usually subsides after 1 week to 10 days, but in rare cases it may progress to a systemic viral infection. It may disguise other more serious mouth ulcers. See also **herpes simplex.**

ginglymus joint. See **hinge joint.**

ginkgo, an herbal product harvested from a tree that is native to China and Japan.

■ INDICATIONS: It is used for poor circulation, diabetes, vascular disease, cancer, inflammatory disorders, impotence, and degenerative nerve conditions. It is also used for age-related declines in cognition and memory. Ginkgo is generally considered to have some efficacy against dementia.

■ CONTRAINDICATIONS: It is contraindicated in people with coagulation or platelet disorders or hemophilia, in children, and in those with known hypersensitivity to this product. Caution must be taken if administered to patients taking antiplatelet agents such as aspirin or anticoagulants such as heparin and warfarin.

ginseng, an herb with red or yellow fruits that is native to the Far East and is now found throughout the world. One species is native to North America.

■ INDICATIONS: It is used for physical and mental exhaustion, stress, viral infections, diabetes, sluggishness, fatigue, weak immunity, and convalescence and may have some efficacy (e.g., better stress tolerance, reaction times, abstract thinking).

■ CONTRAINDICATIONS: It should not be used during pregnancy and lactation or in children. It is also contraindicated in those with known hypersensitivity, hypertension, and cardiac disorders.

Giordano-Giovannetti diet /jôrdä″nō jō′vənet″ē/, a low-protein, low-fat, high-carbohydrate diet with controlled potassium and sodium intake, used in chronic renal insufficiency and liver failure. Protein is given only in the form of essential amino acids so that the body will use excess blood urea nitrogen to synthesize the nonessential amino acids for the production of tissue protein. The foods included are eggs, small amounts of milk, low-protein bread, and some fruits and vegetables low in potassium, such as green beans, summer squash, cabbage, pears, grapefruit, and fresh or frozen blackberries, blueberries, and boysenberries. There are many modified forms of this diet, depending on patient requirements and tolerance and usually varying in the amount and origin of the protein. Also called *Giovannetti diet.* See also **renal diet.**

GIP, abbreviation for **gastric inhibitory polypeptide.**

gipoma /gipō″mə/ gastric inhibitory polypeptide-secreting tumor, GIP-oma, a pancreatic tumor that causes changes in secretion of gastric inhibitory polypeptide.

girdle /gur″dəl/, any curved or circular structure, such as the hipline formed by the bones and related tissues of the pelvis.

girdle pad, a covering that fits over the iliac crests and sacrum to protect the hip area in contact sports. Also called *sports girdle.*

GI tract, abbreviation for **gastrointestinal tract.** See **digestive tract.**

glabella /gləbəl″ə/ [L, *glabrum,* bald], a flat triangular area of bone between the two superciliary ridges of the forehead. It is sometimes used as a baseline for cephalometric measurements.

glabella tap, a rapid tap between the eyebrows with the finger. Normally, the patient stops blinking after the second or third tap, but in Parkinson disease and certain kinds of cerebral degeneration the blinking continues even after many taps. It can also occur with normal aging. Also called *glabella tap sign, orbicularis oculi sign, blinking reflex.*

glabrous skin /glā″brəs/ [L, *glaber,* smooth; AS, *scinn*], smooth, hairless skin.

glacial acetic acid /glā″shəl/, a clear, colorless liquid or crystalline substance (CH_3COOH) with a pungent odor. It is obtained by the destructive distillation of wood, by oxidation of acetylene and water by air, or by the oxidation of ethyl alcohol by aerobic bacteria, as in the production of vinegar. Glacial acetic acid is strongly corrosive and potentially flammable, having a low flash point. It is miscible in alcohol, ether, glycerol, and water and is used as a solvent for organic compounds. Also called **vinegar acid.**

gladiate, shaped like a sword. See **xiphoid.**

gland [L, *glans,* acorn], any one of many organs in the body comprising specialized cells that secrete or excrete materials not related to their ordinary metabolism. Some glands lubricate; others, such as the pituitary gland, produce hormones; hematopoietic glands, such as the spleen and certain lymph nodes, take part in the production of blood components. Exocrine glands discharge their secretions into ducts. They may be classified by the shape and complexity of their duct systems. Endocrine glands are ductless and discharge their secretions directly into the blood or interstitial fluid. See also **exocrine gland, endocrine gland. –glandular,** *adj.*

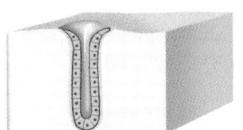

Simple tubular

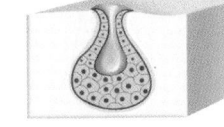

Simple coiled tubular

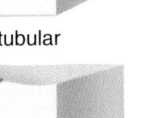

Simple branched tubular

Simple alveolar

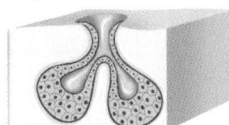

Simple branched alveolar

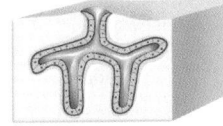

Compound tubular

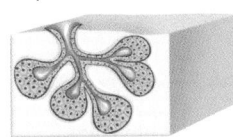

Compound alveolar

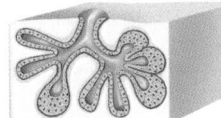

Compound tubuloalveolar

Exocrine glands: structural classification

glanders [OFr, neck gland swelling], an infection caused by the bacillus *Burkholderia mallei* (formerly called *Pseudomonas mallei),* transmitted to humans from horses and other domestic animals. It is characterized by purulent inflammation of the mucous membranes and development of skin nodules that ulcerate. If untreated with antibiotics, the infection may spread to the bones, liver, central nervous system, and other tissues and cause death. It is endemic in Africa, Asia, and South America but has been eradicated in Europe and North America. Infection has been seen in laboratory workers because of the low infectious dose. It is considered a potential agent for bioterrorism.

glandes, **1.** a small rounded body or mass. **2.** See **glans.**

gland of Montgomery. See **areolar gland.**

glands of bile duct, tubuloacinar glands in the mucosa of the bile ducts and the neck of the gallbladder. Also called **biliary glands.**

glands of Moll Zeis. See **ciliary gland.**

glandular. See **gland.**

glandular carcinoma. See **adenocarcinoma.**

glandular epithelium [L, *glandula,* small gland; Gk, *epi,* above, *thele,* nipple], epithelium that contains glandular cells.

glandular fever. See **infectious mononucleosis.**

glandular hypospadias [L, *glandula,* small gland, *hypo,* under, *spadōn,* a rent], the most common type of hypospadias in which the urethral orifice opens at the site of the frenum, which may be rudimentary or absent. The normal site of the urinary meatus is represented on the glans penis as a blind pit. Also called **balanic hypospadias.**

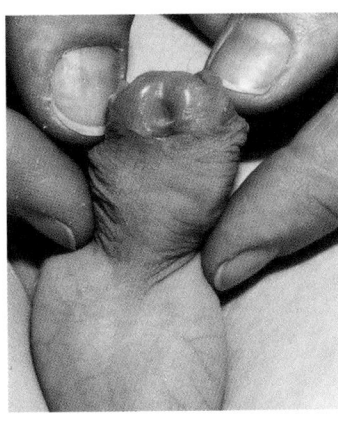

Glandular hypospadias *(Courtesy Dr. A.E. Chudley, Department of Pediatrics and Child Health, University of Manitoba, Children's Hospital)*

glandular tissue [L, *glandula,* small gland; OFr, *tissu*], a group of epithelial secreting cells composing a definitive glandular organ, such as the thyroid.

glandula vestibularis major. See **Bartholin gland.**

glans /glanz/ *pl. glandes* [L, acorn], **1.** a general term for a small rounded mass or a glandlike body. **2.** erectile tissue, as on the ends of the clitoris and the penis.

glans of clitoris [L, *glans* + Gk, *kleitoris*], the erectile tissue at the end of the clitoris. It comprises two corpora cavernosa enclosed in a dense, fibrous membrane and connected to the pubis and ischium. Also called *glans clitoridis.*

glans penis, the conical tip of the penis that covers the end of the corpora cavernosa penis and the corpus spongiosum like a cap. The urethral orifice is normally located at the distal tip of the glans penis. The corona glandis, the widest part of the glans penis, is around the base of the proximal portion. A fold of thin, hairless skin forms the foreskin covering the glans penis.

Glanzmann thrombasthenia, severe mucocutaneous bleeding disorder caused by one of a series of mutations in platelet glycoprotein IIb or IIIa with a defect of fibrinogen-dependent platelet aggregation. See **thrombasthenia.**

glare, a strong, dazzling light that may cause discomfort to the eye. Visual problems that result from glare often involve inadequate lighting conditions; they particularly affect individuals with cataracts or other disease conditions. The condition is relieved somewhat by using incandescent rather than fluorescent lighting, wearing a visor, wearing special anti-glare lenses, and using a matte-black cardboard typoscope for reading words on a glaring white paper.

Glasgow Coma Scale, a quick, practical standardized system for assessing the degree of consciousness in the critically ill and for predicting the duration and ultimate outcome of coma, primarily in patients with head injuries. The system involves eye opening, verbal response, and motor response, all of which are evaluated independently according to a rank order that indicates the level of consciousness and degree of dysfunction. The degree of consciousness is assessed numerically by the best response. The results may be plotted on a

G

graph to provide a visual representation of the improvement, stability, or deterioration of a patient's level of consciousness, which is crucial to predicting the eventual outcome of coma. The sum of the numeric values for each parameter can also be used as an overall objective measurement, with 15 indicative of no impairment, 3 compatible with brain death, and 7 usually accepted as a state of coma. The test score can also function as an indicator for certain diagnostic tests or treatments, such as the need for a computed tomography scan, intracranial pressure monitoring, and intubation. The scale has a high degree of consistency even when used by staff with varied experience.

Glasgow Coma Scale scoring

Eyes Open

4	Spontaneously
3	On request
2	To pain stimuli (supraorbital or digital)
1	No opening

Best Verbal Response

5	Oriented to time, place, person
4	Engages in conversation, confused in content
3	Words spoken but conversation not sustained
2	Groans evoked by pain
1	No response

Best Motor Response

6	Obeys a command ("Hold out three fingers.")
5	Localizes a painful stimulus
4	Withdraws in response to pain
3	Flexes either arm
2	Extends arm to painful stimulus
1	No response

Glasgow Outcome Scale, a functional assessment inventory used after brain injury. It predicts five global categories: death, persistent vegetative state, severe disability, moderate disability, and good recovery. Should not be confused with **Glasgow Coma Scale.**

glass ionomer cement, a dental cement used for small restorations on the proximal surfaces of anterior teeth, for restoration of eroded areas at the gingival margin, as base material under dental restorations, and as a luting agent for restorations and orthodontic bands. It releases fluoride ions, which can provide some anticaries activity.

glatiramer, an immunomodulator drug used for multiple sclerosis.

■ INDICATIONS: It is used to reduce the frequency of relapses in patients with relapsing-remitting multiple sclerosis.

■ CONTRAINDICATIONS: Known hypersensitivity to this drug or to mannitol prohibits its use.

■ ADVERSE EFFECTS: Common adverse effects include injection site reactions, nausea, vomiting, diarrhea, anorexia, gastroenteritis, ecchymosis, chills, and arthralgia.

glauco-, prefix meaning "gray or silver": *glaucoma, glaucomatous halo.*

glaucoma /glôkō′mə, glou-/ [Gk, cataract], an abnormal condition of elevated pressure within an eye that occurs when aqueous production exceeds aqueous outflow, resulting in damage to the optic nerve. Acute (angle-closure, closed-angle, or narrow-angle) glaucoma occurs if the pupil in an eye with a narrow angle between the iris and cornea dilates markedly, causing obstruction of aqueous humor drainage from the anterior chamber. Primary open-angle glaucoma (POAG) is much more common in the United States and develops slowly and insidiously without a narrow angle. Peripheral visual field losses are most common, developing often without the patient's awareness

until there is very serious disease. The obstruction is believed to occur within the trabecular meshworks. **–glaucomatous,** *adj.*

■ OBSERVATIONS: Acute angle-closure glaucoma is accompanied by extreme ocular pain, blurred vision, redness of the eye, and dilation of the pupil. Nausea and vomiting may occur. If untreated, acute glaucoma causes complete and permanent blindness within 2 to 5 days. Chronic open-angle glaucoma may produce no symptoms except gradual loss of peripheral vision over a period of years. Sometimes present are headaches, blurred vision, and dull pain in the eye. Cupping of the optic discs may be noted on ophthalmoscopic examination. Halos around lights and central blindness are late manifestations. Both types are characterized by elevated intraocular pressure indicated by tonometry.

■ INTERVENTIONS: Acute glaucoma is treated with eyedrops to constrict the pupil and draw the iris away from the cornea; osmotic agents such as mannitol or glycerol given systemically to lower intraocular pressure; acetazolamide to reduce fluid formation; and surgical iridectomy to produce a filtration pathway for aqueous humor. Chronic glaucoma can usually be controlled with eyedrops such as beta-blockers, alpha-agonists, topical carbonic anhydrase inhibitors, and prostaglandin analogs.

Rapidly rising intraocular pressure

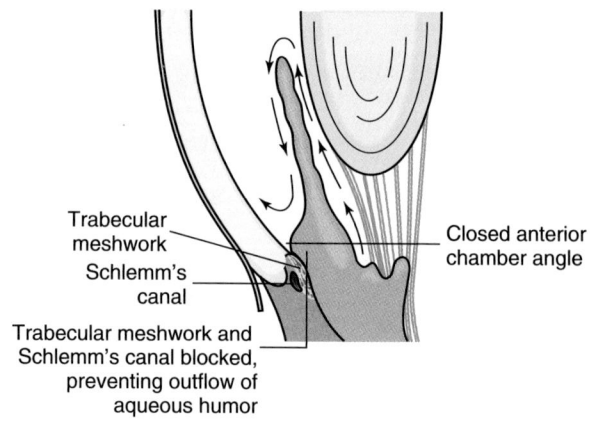

Acute angle-closure glaucoma *(Monahan et al, 2007)*

Slowly rising intraocular pressure

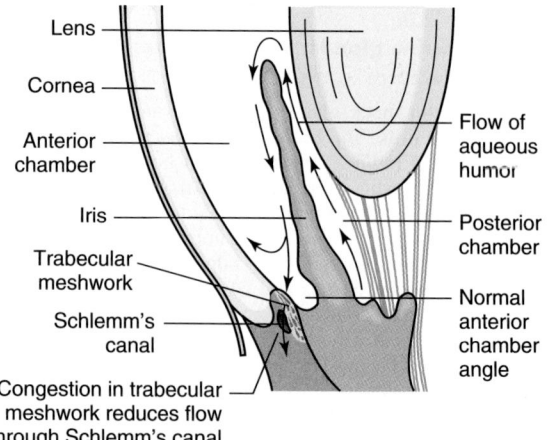

Chronic open-angle glaucoma *(Monahan et al, 2007)*

glaucoma consummatum, *(Obsolete)* now called **absolute glaucoma.**

glaucomatocyclitic crisis /glôkom′ətōsiklit″ik/, an episodic rise in intraocular pressure in one eye resembling acute angle-closure glaucoma, associated with minimal signs of uveitis. Also called **Posner-Schlossman syndrome.**

glaucomatous. See **glaucoma.**

glaucomatous halo /glôkom″ətəs/, **1.** an illusion of a circle of brightness surrounding a light, observed by patients with acute glaucoma, which is caused by edema of the corneal epithelium. **2.** a yellowish white ring surrounding the optic disc, a sign of atrophy of the choroid in glaucoma.

glaze /glāz/ [ME, *glasen*], **1.** *v.,* to cover with a glossy, smooth surface or coating. **2.** *n.,* a ceramic veneer added to a dental porcelain restoration after it has been fired, to give a completely nonporous, glossy, or semiglossy surface. **3.** *n.,* the final firing (in air) of dental porcelain, when formation of a thin, vitreous, glossy surface takes place.

-glea, -glia, suffix meaning "a binding gelatinous medium": *zooglea.*

glenohumeral /glē′nōhyoō″mərəl/ [Gk, *glene,* joint socket; L, *humerus,* shoulder], pertaining to the glenoid cavity and the humerus at the shoulder joint.

glenohumeral joint, the shoulder joint, formed by the glenoid cavity of the scapula and the head of the humerus.

glenohumeral ligaments [Gk, *glene,* joint socket, *humerus,* shoulder], three thickened bands of connective tissue attached proximally to the anterior margin of the glenoid cavity and distally to the neck of the humerus.

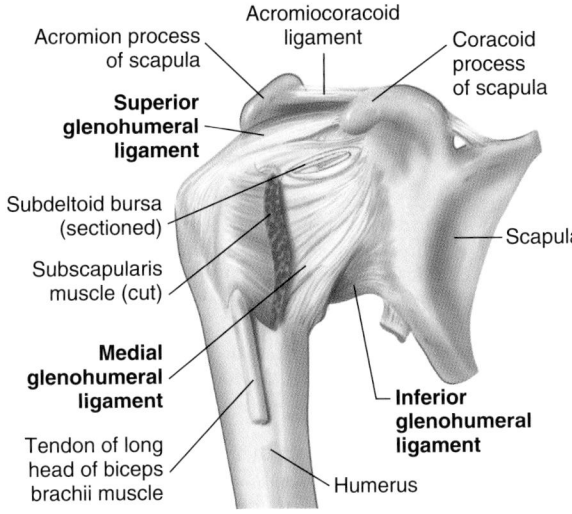

Glenohumeral ligaments *(Patton and Thibodeau, 2016)*

glenoid cavity /glē″noid/ [Gk, *glene,* joint socket, *eidos,* form; L, *cavum*], a shallow socket with which the head of the humerus articulates below the acromion at the junction of the superior and axillary borders. Also called **glenoid fossa.**

glenoid fossa, mandibular fossa. See **glenoid cavity, mandibular fossa.**

glenoid labrum, a fibrocartilaginous collar that deepens and expands the glenoid cavity.

glia. See **neuroglia.**

glia cells /glī″ə, glē″ə/ [Gk, *glia,* glue; L, *cella,* storeroom], neural cells that have a connective-tissue-supporting function in the central nervous system. Examples include astrocytes and oligodendroglial cells of ectodermal origin and microglial cells of mesodermal origin.

gliadin /glī″ədin/ [Gk, *glia,* glue], a fraction of the gluten protein that is found in wheat and rye and to a lesser extent in barley and oats. Its solubility in diluted alcohol distinguishes it from another grain protein, glutenin. Those with celiac disease are sensitive to this substance, and it is excluded from their diet. See also **celiac disease.**

gliadin and endomysial antibodies testing, a blood test to assist in the identification of celiac disease and to monitor disease status and dietary compliance.

glial cell line–derived neurotrophic factor (GDNF) /glī″əl/, a nerve growth drug that has been used in laboratory animals to reverse the progression of symptoms of Parkinson's disease and other brain diseases. GDNF is believed to act as a biological shield, protecting nerve cells from damage that normally would destroy them.

gliding [AS, *glidan,* to glide], **1.** one of the four basic movements allowed by the various joints of the skeleton. It is common to all movable joints and permits one surface to move smoothly over an adjacent surface, regardless of shape. Gliding is the only motion allowed by most of the wrist and the ankle joints. **2.** a smooth, continuous movement. Compare **angular movement, circumduction, rotation.**

gliding contusion, a brain injury caused by displacement of the gray matter of the cerebral cortex during angular acceleration of the head. Most of the damage occurs at the junction between the gray matter and the white matter. Such contusions are associated with diffuse axonal injuries and acute subdural hematomas.

gliding joint, a synovial joint in which articulation of contiguous bones allows only gliding movements, as in the wrist and the ankle. The ligaments or the osseous processes around each gliding joint limit movements of apposed plane surfaces or concavoconvex articulations. Also called *arthrodia, articulatio plana.* Compare **hinge joint, pivot joint.**

gliding testis, an undescended testis that can reach the top of the scrotum but then glides back up.

gliding zone, an articular cartilage surface area immediately adjacent to a joint space. It consists of a thin layer of densely packed collagen fibers lying parallel to the surface and covered by a fine acellular, afibrillar membrane. At the periphery the fibrous components merge with the fibrous periosteum of the adjacent bone.

glimepiride /glimep′irīd/, a sulfonylurea compound used as a hypoglycemic in treatment of type 2 diabetes mellitus, administered orally.

glio-, prefix meaning "neuroglia" or "a gluey substance": *glioma, gliosarcoma, gliosis.*

glioblastoma. See **spongioblastoma.**

glioblastoma multiforme /glī″ōblastō″mə mul′tifôr′mē/ [Gk, *glia,* glue, *blastos,* germ, *oma,* tumor; L, *multus,* many, *forma,* form], a malignant, invasive, rapidly growing pulpy or cystic tumor of the cerebrum or the spinal cord. The lesion spreads with pseudopod-like projections. It is composed of a mixture of monocytes, pyriform cells, immature and mature astrocytes, and neural ectodermal cells with fibrous or protoplasmic processes. Also called **anaplastic astrocytoma, glioma multiforme.**

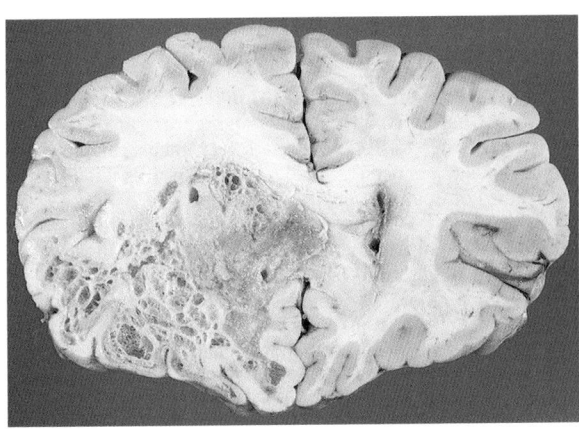

Glioblastoma multiforme *(Finkbeiner, Ursell, and Davis, 2009)*

G

glioma /glī·ō″mə/ *pl.* **gliomas, gliomata** [Gk, *glia* + *oma,* tumor], any of the largest group of primary tumors of the brain, composed of malignant glial cells. Kinds include **astrocytoma, ependymoma, glioblastoma multiforme, medulloblastoma, oligodendroglioma.**

-glioma, suffix meaning a "tumor arising from the neuroglia": *angioglioma, oligodendroglioma, paraganglioma.*

glioma multiforme. See **glioblastoma multiforme.**

glioma retinae. See **retinoblastoma.**

glioma sarcomatosum. See **gliosarcoma.**

gliomata. See **glioma.**

glioneuroma /glī′ōnō̄ōrō″mə/ *pl.* **glioneuromas, glioneuromata** [Gk, *glia* + *neuron,* nerve, *oma,* tumor], a neoplasm composed of nerve cells and elements of their supporting connective tissue.

gliosarcoma /glī′ōsärkō″mə/ *pl.* **gliosarcomas, gliosarcomata** [Gk, *glia* + *sarx,* flesh, *oma,* tumor], a tumor composed of spindle-shaped cells in the delicate supporting connective tissue of nerve cells. Also called **glioblastoma, glioma, spongioblastoma, spongiocytoma.**

gliosarcoma retinae. See **retinoblastoma.**

gliosis /glī·ō″sis/, a proliferation of astrocytes that may appear as a sign of healing after a central nervous system injury. See also **fibrogliosis.**

glipiZIDE /glip″izīd/, an oral antidiabetic drug.

■ INDICATIONS: It is prescribed as an adjunct to diet and exercise to lower blood glucose levels of patients with type 2 diabetes mellitus.

■ PROCEDURE: The dosage is adjusted in patients with renal dysfunction.

■ ADVERSE EFFECTS: Common adverse effects include nausea, heartburn, hypoglycemia, and weight gain.

Glisson's capsule /glis″ənz/ [Francis Glisson, English physician, 1597–1677; L, *capsula,* little box], the fibrous outer tissue sheath around lobules of the liver that carry branches of the hepatic artery, portal vein, and bile duct. Also called **hepatobiliary capsule.**

glitter cells [ME, *gliteren,* to shine], white blood cells in which movement of granules is observed in their cytoplasm. They are seen in microscopic examination of urine samples in cases of pyelonephritis or disorders marked by low osmolality.

GLMA, a nonprofit, professional membership organization of health care providers advancing the health and well-being of lesbian, gay, bisexual, and transgender (LGBT) individuals and families.

Gln, abbreviation for **glutamine.**

global aphasia /glō″bəl/ [L, *globus,* ball; Gk, *a* + *phasis,* without speech], a loss of ability to use or comprehend any form of written or spoken language. The condition involves both sensory and motor nerve tracts and is a relatively more severe form of aphasia. Communication is attempted through gestures or the use of automatic words and phrases. Also called **mixed aphasia.**

Global Assessment of Functioning (GAF) scale, a scale used to assess psychiatric status, ranging from 1 (lowest level of functioning) to 100 (highest level), measuring psychologic, social, and occupational functioning. It is widely used in studies of treatment effectiveness.

global mental functions, part of the classification of bodily functions from the International Classification of Functioning, Disability and Health (ICF); also included in the *Occupational Therapy Practice Framework* (3rd ed.). Global mental functions include consciousness, orientation, sleep, temperament and personality, and energy and drive.

global warming, an ecological model of world climate changes based on the greenhouse effect, exacerbated by burning of fossil fuels, massive deforestation, and conversion of cropland to industrial and other urban uses, all contributing to an increase in the earth's temperature. Major shifts in climate are not unusual in the history of the earth, which has undergone global warming in previous periods of geological history.

globin /glō″bin/ [L, *globus,* ball], a group of four protein molecules that become bound by the iron in heme molecules to form hemoglobin or myoglobin.

-globin, suffix meaning "containing protein": *hemoglobin, myoglobin.*

-globinuria, suffix meaning "(condition involving) the presence of complex proteins in the urine": *hemoglobinuria, methemoglobinuria, myoglobinuria.*

globoid leukodystrophy. See **galactosyl ceramide lipidosis.**

globose nucleus, one of four deeply placed cerebellar nuclei, located medially to the emboliform nucleus. It receives input from the intermediate zone of the cerebellar cortex, and its axons exit through the superior cerebellar peduncle. The globose nucleus is involved in posture control and voluntary movement.

globule /glob″yōol/ [L, *globulus,* small ball], a small spheric mass. Kinds include **dentin globule, Dobie globule, Marchi globule, milk globule, Morgagni globule, myelin globule.**

globulin /glob″yōolin/, one of a broad category of simple proteins classified by solubility, electrophoretic mobility, and molecular weights. Compare **albumin.** See also **euglobulin, plasma protein.**

globulinuria /-ōōr″ē·ə/ [L, *globulus,* small ball; Gk, *ouron,* urine], the presence of globulin-class proteins in the urine.

globus hystericus /glō″bus/ [L, small ball; Gk, *hystera,* womb], a transitory sensation of a lump in the throat that cannot be swallowed or coughed up, often accompanying emotional conflict or acute anxiety. The condition is thought to be caused by a functional disturbance of the ninth cranial nerve and spasm of the inferior constrictor muscle that encircles the lower part of the throat. The physical examination result tends to be normal, as does the result of barium esophagography.

globus pallidus /pal″idəs/ [L, small ball, pale], the smaller and more medial part of the lentiform nucleus of the brain, separated from the putamen by the lateral medullary lamina and divided into external and internal portions closely connected to the striatum, thalamus, and mesencephalon.

-gloea. See **-glea, -glia.**

glomangioma /glōman′jē·ō″mə/ *pl.* **glomangiomas, glomangiomata** [L, *glomus,* ball of thread; Gk, *angeion,* vessel, *oma*], a benign tumor that develops from a cluster of blood cells in the skin. Also called **angiomyoneuroma, angioneuroma.**

glomera. See **glomus.**

glomerular. See **glomerulus.**

glomerular capsule. See **Bowman's capsule.**

glomerular disease, any of a group of diseases in which the glomerulus of the kidney is affected. Depending on the particular disease, there may be hyperplasia, atrophy, necrosis, scarring, or deposits in the glomeruli. The symptoms may be abrupt in onset or slowly progressive. Compare **acute tubular necrosis.** See also **glomerulonephritis.**

glomerular endothelium, the visceral layer of the kidney, composed of modified squamous epithelium.

glomerular filtration, the renal process whereby fluid in the blood is filtered across the capillaries of the glomerulus and into the urinary space of Bowman's capsule.

glomerular filtration rate (GFR) [L, *glomerulus,* small ball; Fr, *filtre* + L, *ratus*], a kidney function test in which results are determined from the amount of ultrafiltrate formed by plasma flowing through the glomeruli of the kidney. The amount is calculated from inulin and creatinine clearance, serum creatinine, and blood urea nitrogen. The GFR can also be estimated from equations that include creatinine, age, gender, and ethnicity.

glomerular proteinuria, the most common kind of proteinuria, caused by glomerular disease and abnormal permeability of the glomerular capillaries to protein.

glomeruli. See **glomerulus.**

glomerulo-, prefix meaning "glomerulus," the functional unit of the kidney: *glomerulonephritis, glomerulosclerosis.*

glomerulonephritis /glōmer″yo͞olōnəfrī″tis/ [L, *glomerulus,* small ball; Gk, *nephros,* kidney, *itis*], an inflammation of the glomerulus of the kidney, characterized by proteinuria, hematuria, decreased urine production, and edema. Kinds include **acute glomerulonephritis, chronic glomerulonephritis, subacute glomerulonephritis.**

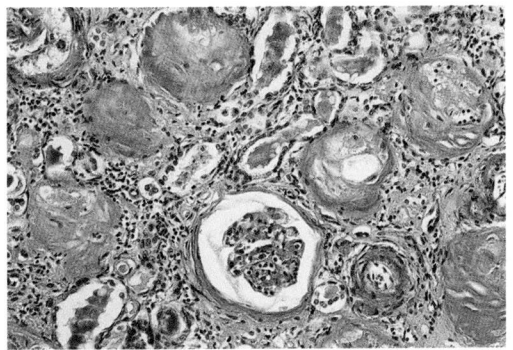

Chronic glomerulonephritis *(Courtesy Dr. M.A. Venkatachalam, Department of Pathology, University of Texas Health Sciences Center)*

glomerulosclerosis /-sklərō″sis/ [L, *glomerulus,* small ball; Gk, *sklerosis,* a hardening, *osis,* condition], a severe kidney disease in which glomerular function of blood filtration is lost as fibrous scar tissue replaces the glomeruli. The disease commonly follows an infection or arteriosclerosis.

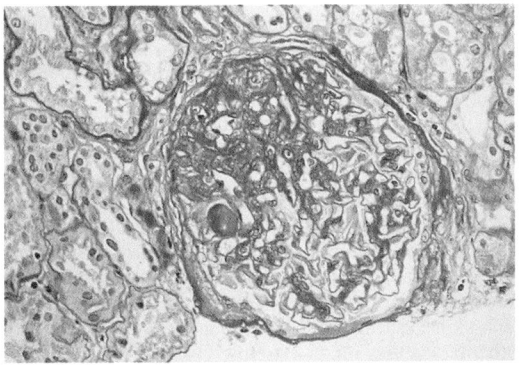

Glomerulosclerosis *(Courtesy Dr. H. Rennke, Department of Pathology, Brigham and Women's Hospital)*

glomerulotubular balance, the balance between reabsorption of solutes in the proximal renal tubules and glomerular filtration, which must be as constant as possible. If the glomerular filtration rate rises or falls, the rate of tubular reabsorption must rise or fall proportionally. Balance is maintained by neural, hormonal, and other mechanisms.

glomerulus /glōmer″yo͞oləs/ *pl. glomeruli* [L, small ball], **1.** a tuft or cluster. **2.** a structure composed of blood vessels or nerve fibers, such as a renal glomerulus. **–glomerular,** *adj.*

glomus /glō″məs/ [L, ball of thread], a small group of arterioles connecting directly to veins and having a rich nerve supply.

glomus cell, 1. an epithelioid cell surrounding a coiled arteriovenous anastomosis of a glomus body. **2.** a modified smooth muscle cell.

glomus tumor, a benign, frequently painful neoplasm involving the arteriovenous anastomoses of the skin, frequently found under the nailbed. It contains many small vascular channels surrounded by glomus cells.

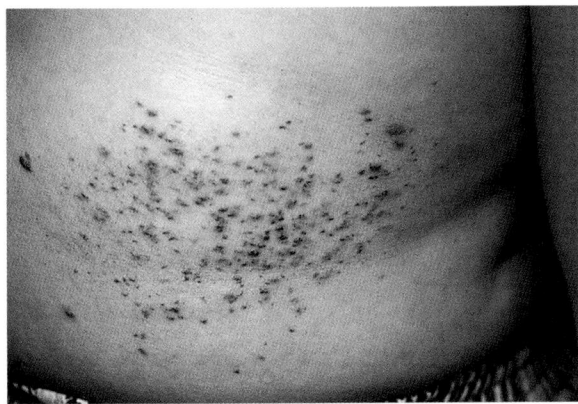

Glomus tumors *(Callen et al, 2000)*

gloss-. See **glosso-, gloss-.**

glossa. See **tongue.**

glossalgia. See **glossodynia.**

glossectomy /glosek″təmē/ [Gk, *glossa,* tongue, *ektomē,* excision], the surgical removal of all or a part of the tongue.

-glossia, 1. suffix meaning "related to the tongue": *macroglossia.* **2.** suffix meaning the "possession of a specified number of tongues": *aglossia.*

glossitis /glosī″tis/ [Gk, *glossa,* tongue, *itis*], inflammation of the tongue. Acute glossitis, characterized by swelling, intense pain that may be referred to the ears, salivation, fever, and enlarged regional lymph nodes, may develop during an infectious disease or after a burn, bite, or other injury. Glossitis in which there is smooth atrophy of the surface and edges of the tongue is seen in pernicious anemia. Glossitis in which irregular, bright red patches appear on the tip or sides of the tongue (Moeller's glossitis) occurs in menopausal women. The condition causes pain or a burning sensation and sensitivity to hot or spicy foods; it often resists treatment. In congenital glossitis there is a flat or slightly elevated patch or plaque anterior to the circumvallate papillae in the midline of the dorsal surface of the tongue.

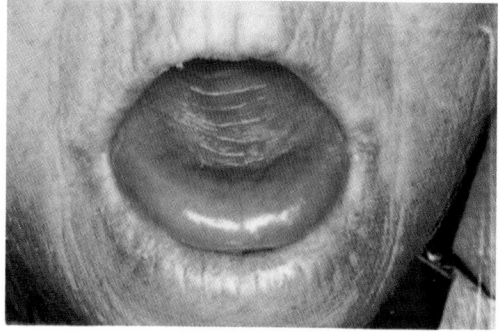

Severe atrophic glossitis *(Feldman, Friedman, and Brandt, 2010)*

glossitis parasitica.   See **parasitic glossitis.**

glossitis rhomboidea mediana.   See **median rhomboid glossitis.**

glosso-, gloss-,   prefix meaning "tongue": *glossodynia, glossectomy.*

glossodynia   /glos'ōdin″ē·ə/ [Gk, *glossa + odyne,* pain],   pain in the tongue caused by acute or chronic inflammation, abscess, ulcer, or trauma. Also called **glossalgia.**

glossodynia exfoliativa.   See **Moeller glossitis.**

glossoepiglottic   /glos'ō·ep'iglot″ik/,   pertaining to the epiglottis and the tongue.

glossohyal.   See **hyoglossal.**

glossolalia   /glos'ōlā″lyə/ [Gk, *glossa + lalein,* to babble],   speech in an unknown "language," as in "speaking in tongues" during a state of religious ecstasy when the message being transmitted through the speaker is believed to be a message from a celestial spirit or from God.

glossoncus   /glosong″kəs/ [Gk, *glossa + onkos,* swelling],   a local swelling or general enlargement of the tongue.

glossopalatine arch,   one of the folds of mucous membrane on either side of the mouth enclosing the palatoglossus muscle. See **palatoglossus.**

glossopathy   /glosop″əthē/ [Gk, *glossa + pathos,* disease],   a pathological condition or disease of the tongue, such as acute inflammation caused by a burn, bite, injury, or infectious disease; enlargement resulting from congenital lymphangioma; or a disorder produced by mycotic infection, malignant lesion, or congenital anomaly.

glossopexy   /glos″əpek'sē/ [Gk, *glossa + pexis,* fixation],   a procedure in which the tongue is anchored to the lower lip and mandible to relieve upper airway obstruction in infants.

glossopharyngeal   /glos'ōfərin″jē·əl/ [Gk, *glossa + pharynx,* throat],   pertaining to the tongue and pharynx. See also **glossopharyngeal nerve.**

glossopharyngeal breathing (GPB),   a technique of forcing air into the lungs with the pharynx and tongue muscles. The technique can be taught to patients whose respiratory muscles are weak.

glossopharyngeal nerve,   either of a pair of cranial nerves essential to the sense of taste, sensation in some viscera, and secretion from certain glands. The nerve has both sensory and motor fibers that pass from the tongue, parotid gland, and pharynx; communicate with the vagus nerve; and connect with two areas in the brain. Also called **Hering's nerve, nervus glossopharyngeus, ninth cranial nerve.**

glossopharyngeal neuralgia,   a disorder of unknown origin characterized by recurrent attacks of severe pain in the

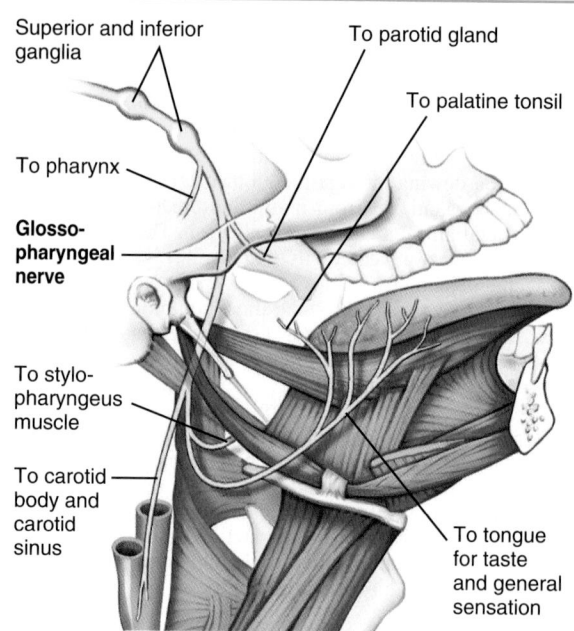

Glossopharyngeal nerve

back of the pharynx, the tonsils, the base of the tongue, and the middle ear. It tends to affect more men than women, with an onset after 40 years of age. Attacks lasting from a few seconds to minutes may be triggered by swallowing. The symptoms may be similar to those of trigeminal neuralgia. Treatment is usually pharmaceutic, but surgery may be recommended to sever involved nerve tracts.

glossophytia   /glos'əfit″ē·ə/ [Gk, *glossa + phyton,* plant],   a condition of the tongue characterized by a blackish patch on the dorsum on which filiform papillae are greatly elongated and thickened like bristly hairs. The usually painless condition may be caused by heavy smoking or the extensive use of broad-spectrum antibiotics. See also **parasitic glossitis.**

glossoplasty   /glos'ōplas'tē/ [Gk, *glossa + plassein,* to mold],   a surgical procedure or plastic surgery on the tongue performed to correct a congenital anomaly, repair an injury, or restore a measure of function after excision of a malignant lesion.

glossoptosis   /glos'optō″sis/ [Gk, *glossa + ptosis,* falling],   the retraction or downward displacement of the tongue.

glossopyrosis   /glos'ōpīrō″sis/ [Gk, *glossa + pyr,* fire, *osis,* condition],   a burning sensation in the tongue caused by chronic inflammation, exposure to extremely hot or spicy food, or psychogenic glossitis.

glossorrhaphy   /glosôr″əfē/ [Gk, *glossa + rhaphe,* seam],   the surgical suturing of a wound in the tongue.

glossotrichia   /glos'ətrik″ē·ə/ [Gk, *glossa + thrix,* hair],   a condition of the tongue characterized by a hairlike appearance of the papillae. Also called **hairy tongue.**

glossy skin [ONorse, *glosa,* smooth and shiny; AS, *scinn*],   a shiny skin that is usually secondary to neuritis and may be associated with other integumentary disorders, including alopecia, skin fissuring, and ulceration. It usually begins as an erythematous area on an extremity, usually the hands.

glott-,   prefix meaning "pertaining to the glottis": *glottal fry, glottal stop.*

glottal fry,   the raspy or croaking ("froglike") quality of the voice in its lowest register. It results from loose closure of the glottis that allows air to bubble through, giving rise to a series of low-pitched pops and rattles.

glottal stop /glot′əl stop/, **1.** a speech sound made by closure of the glottis or vocal folds and then an explosive release. **2.** an abnormal sound substitution with a guttural quality.

glottis, *pl.* **glottises, glottides** [Gk, opening to larynx], **1.** true glottis; a slitlike opening between the true vocal cords (plica vocalis). Also called **rima glottidis, true glottis. 2.** the phonation apparatus of the larynx, composed of the true vocal cords and the opening between them (rima glottidis). −*glottic, glottal, adj.*

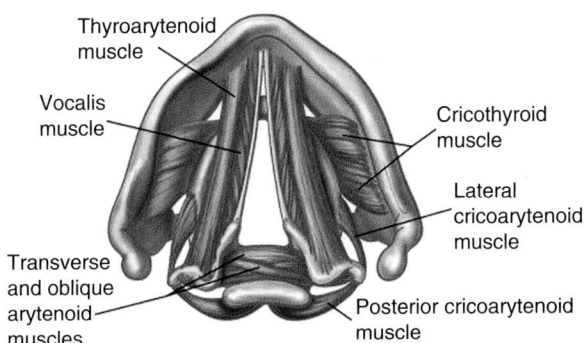

Thyroarytenoid muscle

Vocalis muscle

Cricothyroid muscle

Lateral cricoarytenoid muscle

Transverse and oblique arytenoid muscles

Posterior cricoarytenoid muscle

Glottis *(Thurnher et al, 2007)*

glottis spuria. See **false glottis.**

gloves, sterile or clean fitted coverings for the hands, usually with a separate sheath for each finger and thumb. Clean gloves are worn to protect health care personnel from urine, stool, blood, saliva, and drainage from wounds and lesions of patients and to protect patients from health care personnel who may have cuts. Sterile gloves are worn when there is contact with sterile instruments or sterile body sites.

glow curve, (in thermoluminescence dosimetry) the graphic representation of the emitted light intensity that increases with the increasing phosphor temperature.

GLP-1, abbreviation for **glucagon-like peptide 1.**

Glu, abbreviation for **glutamic acid.**

glucagon /gloo′kəgon/ [Gk, *glykys,* sweet, *agaein,* to lead], a polypeptide hormone, produced by pancreatic alpha cells in the islets of Langerhans, that stimulates the conversion of glycogen to glucose in the liver. Secretion of glucagon is stimulated by hypoglycemia and by growth hormone from the anterior pituitary. A preparation of purified crystallized glucagon is used in the treatment of certain hypoglycemic states. Also called **hyperglycemic-glycogenolytic factor.**

glucagon-like peptide 1 (GLP-1), an appetite-suppressing substance found in the brain and intestine. In the brain, GLP-1 acts as a satiety signal. In the intestine it slows emptying of the stomach and stimulates the release of insulin from the pancreas.

glucagonoma syndrome /gloo′kəgonō″mə/ [Gk, *glykys* + *agaein* + *oma,* tumor], a disease associated with a glucagon-secreting tumor of the islet cells of the pancreas. It is characterized by hyperglycemia, stomatitis, glossitis, anemia, weight loss, and a characteristic rash. Treatment is surgical removal of the tumor.

glucagon (recombinant), a form of pancreatic hormone produced by recombinant DNA technology, having the same functions and uses as that of animal origin. Glucagon stimulates the conversion of glycogen into glucose.

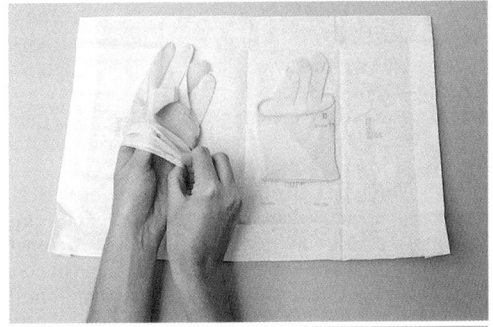
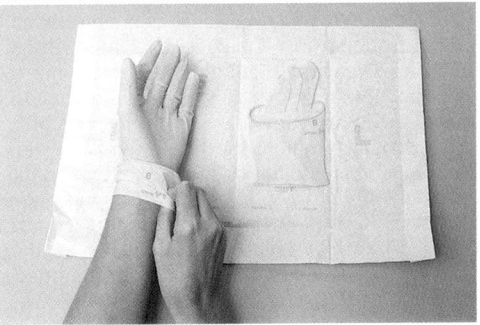
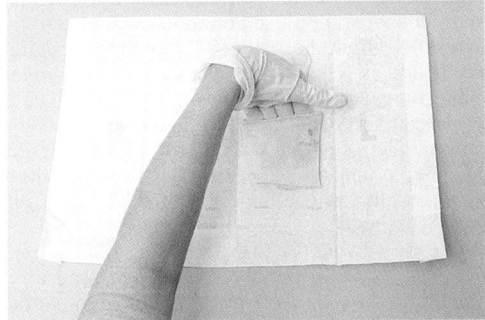
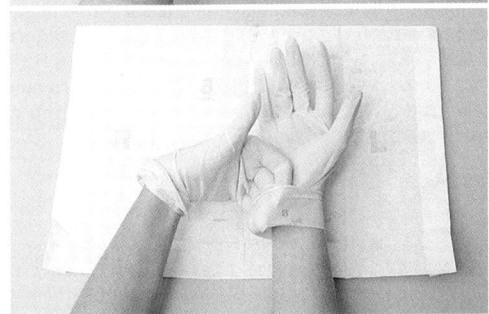
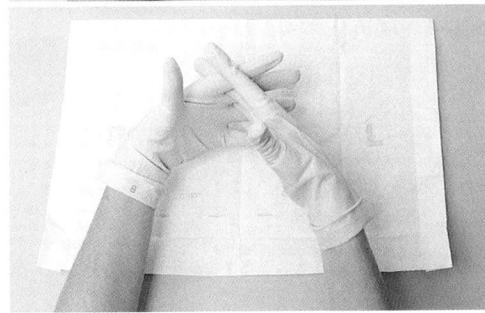

Technique for putting on sterile gloves *(Potter et al, 2011)*

G

glucagon test, a blood test measuring the hormone glucagon that is used to help diagnose glucagonoma, glucagon deficiency, diabetes mellitus, pancreatic insufficiency, renal failure, and other conditions.

gluco-, glyco-, prefix meaning "sweetness" or "glucose": *glucocorticoid, glucogenesis, glucosuria, glycogenesis.*

glucocorticoid /gloo̅′kōkôr″təkoid/ [Gk, *glykys* + L, *cortex,* bark; Gk, *eidos,* form], an adrenocortical steroid hormone that increases gluconeogenesis, exerts an anti-inflammatory effect, and influences many body functions. The most important of the three glucocorticoids is cortisol (hydrocortisone). Corticosterone is less active, and cortisone is inactive until converted to cortisol. Glucocorticoids promote the release of amino acids from muscle, mobilize fatty acids from fat stores, and increase the ability of skeletal muscles to maintain contractions and avoid fatigue. These hormones are known to stabilize mitochondrial and lysosomal membranes, increase the production of adenosine triphosphate, promote the formation of certain liver enzymes, and decrease antibody production and the number of circulating eosinophils. A deficiency of glucocorticoids is characterized by hyperpigmentation (bronzing) of the skin, fasting hypoglycemia, weight loss, and apathy. An excess is associated with elevated serum glucose levels, thinning of the skin, ecchymosis, osteoporosis, poor wound healing, increased susceptibility to infection, and obesity. Glucocorticoid secretion is stimulated by the adrenocorticotropic hormone of the anterior pituitary, which in turn is regulated by the corticotropin-releasing hormone of the hypothalamus and circulating cortisol levels (negative feedback). Synthetic or semisynthetic glucocorticoids, derived chiefly from cortisol, include prednisone, prednisolone, dexamethasone, methylprednisolone, triamcinolone, and betamethasone. Compare **mineralocorticoid.**

glucogenesis, giving rise to or producing glucose.

glucometer, a small portable instrument used to calculate blood glucose levels. Newer glucometers work with apps on smartphones to manage and track blood sugar levels and monitor them over time. Also called *blood glucose monitor.*

gluconeogenesis /gloo̅′kōnē′ōjen″əsis/, the formation of glucose from glycerol and proteins rather than from carbohydrates. Also called **glyconeogenesis.**

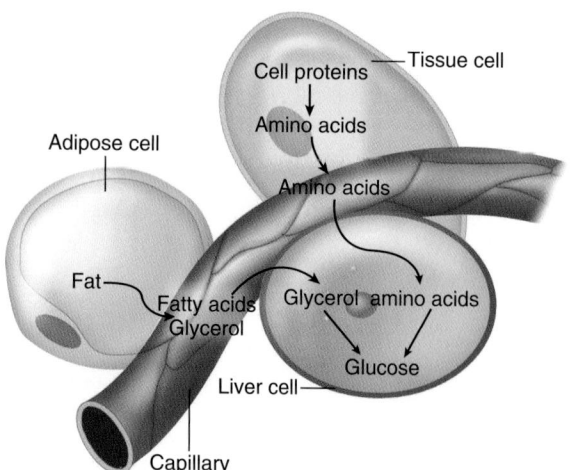

Gluconeogenesis *(Patton and Thibodeau, 2016)*

Glucophage, a biguanide antidiabetic agent, taken orally. Brand name for **metformin hydrochloride.**

glucosamine sulfate, **1.** the sulfate salt of glucosamine, prepared artificially as a nutritional supplement that is a popular home remedy for osteoarthritis. **2.** a chemical found in the body that produces a variety of other chemicals involved in building tendons, ligaments, cartilage, and synovial fluid.

glucosan /gloo̅′kəsan/ [Gk, *glykys,* sweet], any of a large group of anhydrous polysaccharides that on hydrolysis yields a hexose, primarily anhydrides of glucose. Kinds include **cellulose, glycogen, starch, dextrin.**

glucose /gloo̅′kōs/ [Gk, *glykys,* sweet], a simple sugar found in certain foods, especially fruits, and a major source of energy present in the blood and animal body fluids. Glucose, when ingested or produced by the digestive hydrolysis of double sugars and starches, is absorbed into the blood from the intestines by a facilitated transport mechanism using carrier proteins. Excess glucose in circulation is normally polymerized within the liver and muscles as glycogen, which is hydrolyzed to glucose and liberated as needed. The determination of blood glucose levels is an important diagnostic test in diabetes and other disorders. Prepared glucose is a syrupy sweetening agent. Pharmaceutic preparations of glucose are widely used in the treatment of many disorders. Normal adult blood glucose levels range from 70 to 115 mg/dL (4 to 6 mmol/L), with generally higher levels after 50 years of age. See also **dextrose, glycogen.**

glucose electrode, a specialized electric terminal that contains incorporated enzyme for glucose determination.

glucose-galactose malabsorption, a disorder of transport clinically characterized by the neonatal onset of profuse, acidic, watery diarrhea leading to severe dehydration and death if untreated, resulting from a selective defect in the intestinal transport of glucose and galactose. It can be treated by a glucose- and galactose-free diet.

glucose intolerance, inability to properly metabolize glucose, a type of carbohydrate intolerance. Compare **diabetes mellitus.** See also **glucose tolerance test, impaired glucose tolerance.**

glucose 1-phosphate, an intermediate compound in carbohydrate metabolism; specifically it is the product formed in glycogenolysis when glycogen phosphorylase cleaves a molecule of glucose from the glycogen storage molecule.

glucose 6-phosphate, an intermediate compound in carbohydrate metabolism. G6P is produced in the first step of glycolysis when a hexokinase enzyme regiospecifically phosphorylates glucose at carbon-6 hydroxyl group.

glucose-6-phosphate dehydrogenase (G6PD) deficiency, an inherited disorder characterized by red cells partially or completely deficient in G6PD, an enzyme critical in aerobic glycolysis. A sex-linked disorder, the defect is fully expressed in affected males despite a heterozygous pattern of inheritance. The disorder is associated with episodes of acute hemolysis under conditions of stress or in response to certain chemicals or drugs, particularly quinine. The anemia that results is a nonspherocytic hemolytic anemia. See also **congenital nonspherocytic hemolytic anemia, favism.**

glucose-6-phosphate dehydrogenase (G6PD) test, a blood test to diagnose G6PD deficiency in suspected individuals. Deficiency of this enzyme causes precipitation of hemoglobin and cellular membrane changes, possibly resulting in hemolysis of variable severity, a sex-linked trait carried on the X chromosome.

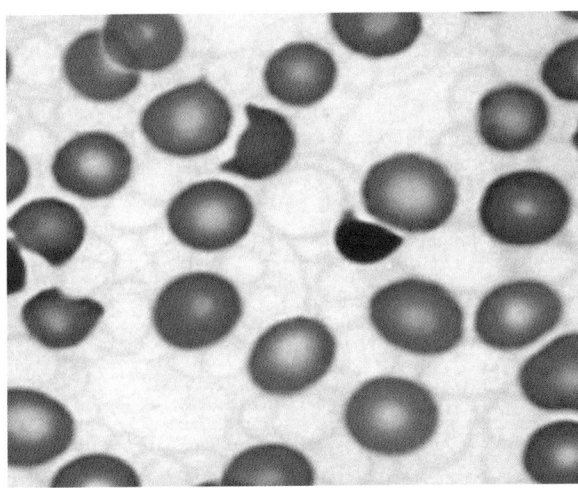

Glucose-6-phosphate dehydrogenase (G6PD) disease
(Gilbert-Barness, 2007)

glucose tolerance test (GTT), a test of the body's ability to metabolize carbohydrates by administering a standard dose of glucose and measuring the blood and urine for glucose level at regular intervals thereafter. The patient usually eats normally in the days before testing and fasts for 8 hours before the test. A fasting blood glucose level is obtained; then the patient drinks a dose of glucose based on his or her weight. Blood and urine are collected periodically for up to 6 hours. The glucose tolerance test is most often used to assist in the diagnosis of diabetes, hypoglycemia, or other disorders that affect carbohydrate metabolism.

glucosuria /glōō′kōsōōr″ē·ə/ [Gk, *glykys* + *ouron,* urine], abnormal presence of glucose in the urine resulting from the ingestion of large amounts of carbohydrate or from a metabolic disease, such as diabetes mellitus. See also **glycosuria.** –*glucosuric, adj.*

glucosyl, **1.** pertaining to glucose. **2.** a glucose radical.

glucosyl cerebroside lipidosis. See **Gaucher disease.**

Glucotrol, an oral antidiabetic drug in the sulfonylurea drug class. Brand name for **glipiZIDE.**

glue sniffing [Gk, *gloios* + ME, *sniffen*], the practice of inhaling the vapors of toluene, a volatile organic compound used as a solvent in certain glues. The glue is squeezed into a plastic bag, which is then placed over the nose and mouth. Intoxication and dizziness result. Prolonged accidental or occupational exposure or repeated recreational use may damage a variety of organ systems. Death has resulted from asphyxiation and heart failure. See also **huffing, inhalant abuse.**

glutamate /glōō″təmāt/, a salt of glutamic acid. In addition to being one of the 20 major amino acids incorporated into the peptide chains of proteins, it is a major excitatory amino acid of the central nervous system.

glutamic acid (Glu) /glōōtam″ik/ [L, *gluten,* glue, *amine,* ammonia; *acidus,* sour], a nonessential amino acid that occurs widely in a number of proteins. Preparations of glutamic acid are used as aids for digestion. See also **amino acid, protein.**

glutamic acid decarboxylase autoantibody, an antibody found in patients with insulin-dependent diabetes mellitus. The antibody recognizes glutamic acid decarboxylase, an intracellular enzyme.

glutamic acidemia /glōōtam′ik as′idē″mē·ə/, an inherited disorder of amino acid metabolism in which the body is

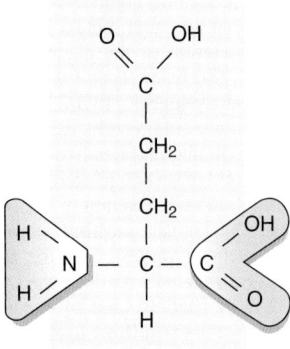

Chemical structure of glutamic acid

unable to process certain proteins. Mutations in the GCDH gene prevent production of the enzyme or result in the production of a defective enzyme that cannot function to break down amino acids. The deficiency of this enzyme allows lysine, hydroxylysine, and tryptophan and their intermediate breakdown products to build up to abnormal levels. The condition is characterized by cognitive and growth impairments, seizures, and fragile hair growth. Strict dietary control may help limit progression of the neurological damage.

glutamic acid hydrochloride, a gastric acidifier.
■ INDICATIONS: It is prescribed for the treatment of hypoacidity. It is also used as a food additive and flavor enhancer.
■ CONTRAINDICATIONS: Hyperacidity, peptic ulcer, or known hypersensitivity to this drug prohibits its use.
■ ADVERSE EFFECTS: The most serious adverse effect is systemic acidosis that results from overdose.

glutamic oxaloacetic transaminase. See **aspartate aminotransferase.**

glutamic pyruvic transaminase. See **alanine aminotransferase.**

glutamine (Gln) /glōō″təmēn/ [L, *gluten* + *amine,* ammonia], a nonessential amino acid found in the juices of many plants and in many proteins in the body. It functions as an amino donor for many reactions. It is also a nontoxic transport for ammonia because it is readily hydrolyzed to glutamic acid and free ammonia, the latter excreted in the urine. See also **amino acid, protein.**

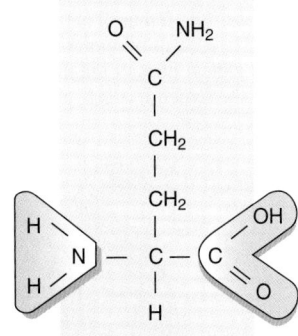

Chemical structure of glutamine

glutaraldehyde /glōō′täral″dəhīd/, a histological fixative and sterilant for medical instruments.

glutargin /glōōtär″gin/, arginine glutamate. See also **arginine.**

glutaricaciduria /glōōtar′ikas′idyōō′rē·ə/, **1.** an autosomal-recessive disorder of amino acid metabolism characterized by accumulation and excretion of the dicarboxylic acid glutaric acid and occurring in two types. Type I is characterized by progressive dystonia and dyskinesia, hypoglycemia, mild ketosis and acidosis, opisthotonus, choreoathetosis, motor delay, cognitive impairment, hypotonia, and death within the first decade. Type II is caused by any of several related defects and is characterized by accumulation and excretion of various organic acids, hypoglycemia without ketosis, metabolic acidosis, and many phenotypic manifestations varying with the specific defect. A later age of onset is correlated with decreased severity, whereas neonatal onset may be accompanied by congenital anomalies and is rapidly fatal. See also **multiple acyl CoA dehydrogenation deficiency. 2.** excretion of glutaric acid in the urine.

glutathione /glōō′təthī′ōn/ [L, *gluten* + Gk, *theione,* sulfur], a tripeptide of glutamic acid, cysteine, and glycine whose deficiency is commonly associated with hemolytic anemia. It functions by taking up and giving off hydrogen. It transports amino acids across cell membranes and conjugates to drugs enabling excretion.

gluteal /glōō′tē·əl/ [Gk, *gloutos,* buttocks], pertaining to the buttocks or to the muscles that form the buttocks.

gluteal fold, 1. a fold of the buttock. **2.** the horizontal lower margin of the buttock at its junction with the thigh.

gluteal gait. See **Trendelenburg gait.**

gluteal reflex, contraction of the gluteus muscles elicited by stroking the back.

gluteal region, the region overlying the gluteal muscles.

gluteal tuberosity, a ridge on the lateral posterior surface of the femur to which is attached a fourth of the gluteus maximus.

gluten /glōō′tən/ [L, glue], the insoluble protein constituent of wheat and other grains (rye, oats, and barley). It is obtained from flour by washing out the starch and is used as an adhesive agent, giving to dough its tough, elastic character. For some people, ingestion of gluten results in potentially life-threatening malabsorption. See also **gliadin, food sensitivity/hypersensitivity reaction, celiac disease.**

gluten-induced enteropathy. See **celiac disease.**

gluteus /glōō′tē′əs/, any of the three muscles that form the buttocks: the gluteus maximus, gluteus medius, and gluteus minimus. The gluteus maximus is a large muscle with an origin in the ilium, the sacrum, and the sacrotuberous ligament and an insertion in the gluteal tuberosity of the femur and the fascia lata. It acts to extend the thigh. The gluteus medius originates between the anterior and posterior gluteal lines of the ilium and inserts in the greater trochanter of the femur. It acts to abduct and medially rotate the thigh. The gluteus minimus originates between the inferior and anterior gluteal lines of the ilium and inserts in the greater trochanter of the femur. It acts to abduct the thigh.

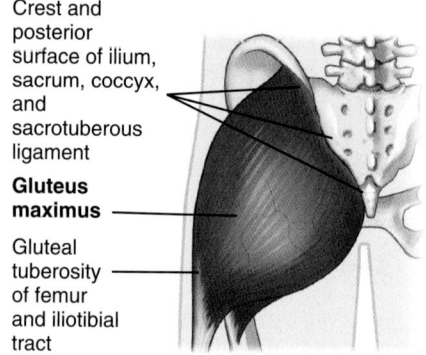

Crest and posterior surface of ilium, sacrum, coccyx, and sacrotuberous ligament

Gluteus maximus

Gluteal tuberosity of femur and iliotibial tract

Gluteus maximus muscle

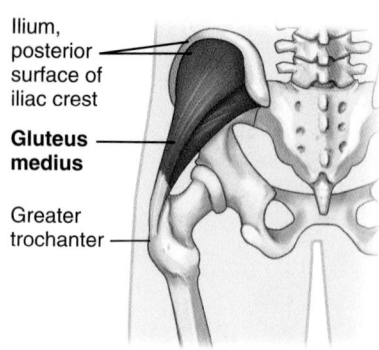

Ilium, posterior surface of iliac crest

Gluteus medius

Greater trochanter

Gluteus medius muscle

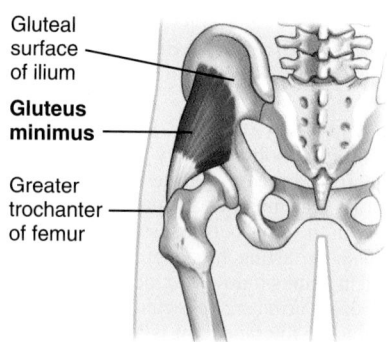

Gluteal surface of ilium

Gluteus minimus

Greater trochanter of femur

Gluteus minimus muscle

Gly, abbreviation for **glycine.**

glyBURIDE /glī″bərīd/, an oral antidiabetic drug in the sulfonylurea drug class.

■ INDICATIONS: It is prescribed as an adjunct to diet and exercise to lower blood glucose levels of patients with type 2 diabetes mellitus.

■ CONTRAINDICATIONS: Because of its long duration of action, it may produce prolonged hypoglycemia; there is also a risk of severe hypoglycemia in elderly, debilitated, or malnourished patients. The dosage may require adjustment for patients taking other drugs that increase blood glucose levels.

■ ADVERSE EFFECTS: Among the more serious adverse effects are nausea, hypoglycemia, weight gain, and skin allergies.

glycate, the product of a nonenzymatic reaction between a sugar and a free amino group of a protein.

glycated hemoglobin. See **glycosylated hemoglobin.**

-glycemia, suffix meaning a "condition of sugar in the blood": *hyperglycemia.*

glycemic index, a ranking of foods based on the response of postprandial blood glucose levels as compared with a reference food, usually either white bread or glucose.

glycemic load (GL), a formula that combines both the quantity and quality of carbohydrates: GL = Glycemic index (GI) of food × Amount (g) of available carbohydrate per serving/100.

glycerin /glis″ərin/ [Gk, *glykys,* sweet], a sweet, colorless oily fluid that is a pharmaceutic grade of glycerol. Glycerin is used as a moistening agent for chapped skin, an ingredient of suppositories for constipation, and a sweetening agent and vehicle for drug preparations.

glycerol $(C_3H_8O_3)$ /glis″ərôl/ [Gk, *glykys,* sweet], an alcohol that is a component of fats. Glycerol is soluble in ethyl alcohol and water. Also called *1, 2, 3-propanetriol.* See also **glycerin.**

glycerol kinase, an enzyme in the liver and kidneys that catalyzes the transfer of a phosphate group from adenosine triphosphate to form adenosine diphosphate and L-glycerol-3-phosphate.

glyceryl alcohol. See **glycerin.**

glyceryl guaiacolate. See **guaifenesin.**

glyceryl triacetate. See **triacetin.**

glyceryl trinitrate. See **nitroglycerin.**

glycine (Gly) /glī″sin/ [Gk, *glykys* + L, *amine,* ammonia], a nonessential amino acid occurring widely as a component of animal and plant proteins. Synthetically produced glycine is used in solutions for irrigation, in the treatment of various muscle diseases, and as an antacid and dietary supplement. It is the only amino acid lacking an R group side chain and therefore also lacking stereochemistry. See also **amino acid, protein.**

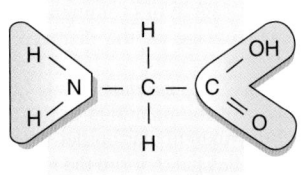

Chemical structure of glycine

glyc(o) [Gk, *glukys,* sweet], combining form for sweetness or sugar.

glyco-. See **gluco-, glyco-.**

glycocholic acid /glīkōkol″ik/ [Gk, *glykys,* sweet; L, *acidus,* sour], a substance in bile, formed by glycine and cholic acid, that aids in digestion and absorption of fats. Glycocholic acid is used as a food additive and an emulsifying agent. Also called **cholylglycine.**

glycogen /glī″kəjən/ [Gk, *glykys,* sweet, *genein,* to produce], a polysaccharide that is the major carbohydrate stored in animal cells. It is formed from repeating units of glucose and stored chiefly in the liver and, to a lesser extent, in muscle cells. Glycogen is depolymerized to glucose, which is released into the circulation as needed by the body. Also called *animal starch,* **hepatin, tissue dextrin.** See also **glucose.**

glycogenesis /glī″kōjen″əsis/, the synthesis of glycogen from glucose.

glycogenolysis /glī″kōjenol″isis/ [Gk, *glykys* + *genein* + *lysis,* loosening], the breakdown of glycogen to glucose.

glycogen storage disease [Gk, *glykys* + *genein* + L, *instaurare,* to renew, *dis,* opposite of; Fr, *aise,* ease], any of a group of inherited disorders of glycogen metabolism. An enzyme deficiency or defect in glycogen transport causes glycogen to accumulate in abnormally large amounts in various parts of the body. Biopsy and chemical analysis reveal the missing enzyme. Also called *glycogenosis.*

glycogen storage disease, type Ia. See **von Gierke disease.**

glycogen storage disease, type Ib, a form of glycogen storage disease in which excessive amounts of glycogen are deposited in the liver and leukocytes. Some symptoms are similar to, but less severe than, those of glycogen storage disease, type Ia (von Gierke's disease). Additional symptoms include neutropenia and recurrent GI inflammatory disease.

Biopsy of the affected organs reveals the absence of glucose-6-phosphatase translocase, an enzyme necessary for glycogen metabolism.

glycogen storage disease, type II. See **Pompe disease.**

glycogen storage disease, type III. See **Cori disease.**

glycogen storage disease, type IV. See **Andersen disease.**

glycogen storage disease, type V. See **McArdle disease.**

glycogen storage disease, type VI. See **Hers disease.**

glycogen storage disease, type VII. See **Tarui disease.**

glycohemoglobin. See **glycosylated hemoglobin.**

glycolipid /glī″kōlip″id/ [Gk, *glykys,* sweet, *lipos,* fat], a compound that consists of a lipid and a carbohydrate, usually galactose, found primarily in the tissue of the nervous system, especially the myelin sheath and the ganglion cells.

glycolysis /glīkol″isis/ [Gk, *glykys* + *lysis,* loosening], a series of enzymatically catalyzed reactions by which glucose and other sugars are broken down to yield lactic acid (anaerobic glycolysis) or pyruvic acid (aerobic glycolysis). The breakdown releases energy in the form of adenosine triphosphate (ATP). Also called **Embden-Meyerhof pathway.** See also **citric acid cycle, lactic acid.**

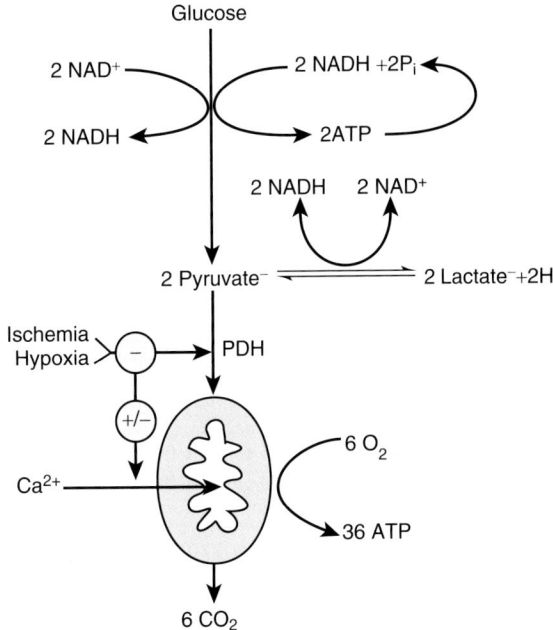

Glycolysis *(Fuhrman and Zimmerman, 2011)*

glycolytic myopathy, any metabolic myopathy resulting from a defect of glycolytic enzyme activity, marked by exercise intolerance and cramping, the accumulation of glycogen in muscle, and recurrent myoglobinuria.

glycometabolism /glī″kōmətab″əliz′əm/, the metabolism of sugar and other carbohydrates.

glyconeogenesis. See **gluconeogenesis.**

glycopenia /-pē″nē·ə/, **1.** See **hypoglycemia. 2.** a deficiency of sugar in the blood or tissues.

glycopeptides /-pep″tīdz/, a class of peptides that contain sugars linked with amino acids, as in bacterial cell walls.

glycophorin /-fôr″in/, one of a group of proteins (A-E) that projects through the membrane of red blood cells (RBCs). The outside end of glycophorins A and B carries antigens of the MNS blood group. The sialic acid component of glycophorins contributes to the negative charge of the outer erythrocyte plasma membrane. Influenza virus can attach to sialic acid present on glycophorin A, B, C, D, and E and produce agglutination (does not enter RBCs). Malaria virus can attach to glycophorin A and C and infect RBCs. See also **blood group.**

glycoprotein /glī′kōprō″tēn/ [Gk, *glykys*, sweet, *proteios*, first rank], any of the large group of conjugated proteins in which the nonprotein substance is a carbohydrate. Kinds include **mucin, mucoid.**

glycoprotein IIb/IIIa, 1. a transmembrane protein of platelets. **2.** an integrin that binds fibrinogen, von Willebrand's factor, and other adhesive ligands playing a role in platelet aggregation and thrombus formation.

glycopyrrolate /glī′kōpir″əlāt/, an anticholinergic.

■ INDICATIONS: It is prescribed as an adjunct to ulcer therapy and parenterally to reduce secretions before surgery.

■ CONTRAINDICATIONS: Narrow-angle glaucoma, asthma, obstruction of the genitourinary or GI tract, ulcerative colitis, or known hypersensitivity to this drug prohibits its use.

■ ADVERSE EFFECTS: Among the more serious adverse effects are blurred vision, central nervous system effects, tachycardia, dry mouth, decreased sweating, and hypersensitivity reactions.

glycoside /glī′kəsīd/ [Gk, *glykys*, sweet], any of several carbohydrates that yield a sugar and a nonsugar on hydrolysis. The plant *Digitalis purpurea* yields a glycoside used in the treatment of heart disease.

glycosphingolipids /glī′kōsfing′gōlip″ids/, compounds formed from carbohydrates and ceramide, a fatty substance, found in tissues of the central nervous system and also in erythrocytes. Deficiency of an enzyme needed to metabolize glycosphingolipids leads to a potentially fatal nervous system disorder.

glycosuria /glī′kōsŏŏr″ē·ə/ [Gk, *glykys* + *ouron*, urine], abnormal presence of a sugar, especially glucose, in the urine. Glycosuria can result from the ingestion of large amounts of carbohydrate, or it may be caused by endocrine or renal disorders. It is a finding most routinely associated with diabetes mellitus. –*glycosuric, adj.*

glycosyl /glī′kōsil/, the radical formed from a saccharide, such as glucose, by removal of a specific hydroxyl group.

glycosylated hemoglobin (GHb/Hb A$_{1c}$) /glīkō″silā′tid/, a hemoglobin A molecule with a glucose group on the N-terminal valine amino acid unit of the beta chain. The glycosylated hemoglobin concentration represents the average blood glucose level over the previous several weeks. In controlled diabetes mellitus the concentration of glycosylated hemoglobin is within the normal range, but in uncontrolled cases the level may be three to four times the normal concentration. Assays of Hb A$_{1c}$, which normally has a 4-month life span, reveal whether glucose levels have been properly controlled during a period of several weeks before the test. The normal range is 1.8% to 4.0% for children; 2.2% to 4.8% for adults. Also spelled *glycosylated haemoglobin.*

glycosylated hemoglobin (GHb, GHB) test, a blood test used to monitor diabetes treatment. It measures the amount of hemoglobin A$_{1c}$ in the blood and provides an accurate long-term index of the patient's average blood glucose level.

glycosylation /glīkə′səlā′shən/, the formation of linkages with glycosyl groups, covalently attaching a carbohydrate to another molecule.

glycyl alcohol. See **glycerin.**

glycyrrhiza /glis′iri′zə/, licorice.

glycyrrhizic acid /glis′iriz″ik/, a sweet compound containing potassium and calcium salts derived from licorice root. It is used as an expectorant and as a flavoring for pharmaceutics. See also **licorice.**

GM, abbreviation for *Geiger-Müller.*

gm, abbreviation for **gram.**

GM-2, a carbohydrate found in much larger quantities in cancer cells than in normal cells, used in some experimental cancer therapy. When it is mixed with bacille Calmette-Guérin and injected into melanoma patients, some patients make antibodies against the cancer cells.

GM-CSF, abbreviation for **granulocyte-macrophage colony-stimulating factor.**

GMP, abbreviation for **guanosine monophosphate.**

GN, abbreviation for **graduate nurse.**

gnath-. See **gnatho-, gnath-.**

gnathalgia. See **gnathodynia.**

-gnathia, suffix meaning a "condition of the jaw": *micrognathia, retrognathia.*

gnathic /nath″ik/ [L, *gnathos*, jaw], pertaining to the jaw or cheek.

gnathic index, the degree of prominence of the upper jaw, expressed as a percentage of the distance from basion to nasion.

gnathion /nā″thē·on/ [L, *gnathos*, jaw], the lowest point in the lower border of the mandible in the median plane. It is found on the bony mandibular border when palpated from below and naturally lies posterior to the tegumental border of the chin. It is a common reference point in the diagnosis and orthodontic treatment of various kinds of malocclusion and is an anthropometric landmark.

gnatho-, gnath-, prefix meaning "jaw": *gnathodynamometer, gnathodynia.*

gnathodynamometer /nā′thōdī′nəmom″ətər/ [Gk, *gnathos* + *dynamis*, force, *metron*, measure], an instrument used for measuring the biting pressure of the jaws of an individual. Also called **occlusometer.**

gnathodynia /nā′thōdin″ē·ə/ [Gk, *gnathos* + *odyne*, pain], pain in the jaw, such as that commonly associated with an impacted wisdom tooth. Also called **gnathalgia.**

gnathology /nāthol″əjē/ [Gk, *gnathos* + *logos*, science], a field of dental or medical study that deals with the entire chewing apparatus, including its anatomical, histological, morphological, physiological, and pathological characteristics. Diagnostic, therapeutic, and rehabilitative procedures result from these studies.

gnathoschisis. See **cleft palate.**

gnathostatic cast /nā′thōstat″ik/ [Gk, *gnathos* + *statike*, weighing; ME, *casten*], a cast or mold of the teeth trimmed so that its occlusal plane is in its normal oral attitude when the cast is set on a horizontal surface. It is used in orthodontic diagnosis based on gnathostatics.

gnathostatics /nā′thōstat″iks/ [Gk, *gnathos* + *statike*, weighing], a technique of orthodontic diagnosis based on an analysis of the relationships between the teeth and certain reference points on the skull. See also **gnathostatic cast.**

Gnathostoma /nathos′tomə/ [Gk, *gnathos* + *stoma*, mouth], a genus of parasitic nematodes of the family Gnathostomatidae characterized by distinct jaws. *G. spinigerum* is parasitic in cats, dogs, and humans after they eat raw fish containing the larvae, causing gnathostomiasis. See also **gnathostomiasis.**

gnathostomiasis /nath′ōstōmī′əsis/ [Gk, *gnathos* + *stoma*, mouth + *osis*, condition], infection with the nematode *Gnathostoma spinigerum*, occurring when undercooked fish harboring the larvae is eaten. Because of its consumption of raw fish, the population of Southeast Asia, especially residents of Thailand and Japan, is particularly at risk. The larvae migrate, often in the subcutaneous tissue, causing a creeping eruption associated with intense eosinophilia. Occasionally they migrate to deeper tissues and cause abscesses or to the central nervous system, where they cause eosinophilic myeloencephalitis. The infection is treated by surgical removal or treatment with albendazole or ivermectin. See also **cutaneous larva migrans.**

gno-, prefix meaning "to know or discern": *gnotobiotic.*

-gnomonic, -gnomonical, suffix meaning "signs or experience in knowing or judging (a condition)": *pathognomonic.*

-gnomy, suffix meaning the "science or means of judging" something specified: *physiognomy.*

-gnosia, suffix meaning a "(condition of) perceiving or recognizing": *acognosia, simultanagnosia, autotopagnosia.*

-gnosis, suffix meaning "knowledge": *abarognosis, diagnosis, topognosis.*

gnotobiotic /nō′tōbī·ot″ik/, pertaining to a germ-free animal or an animal or an environment in which all the microorganisms are known. See also **germ-free animal.**

GNP, abbreviation for **geriatric nurse practitioner.**

GnRH, abbreviation for **gonadotropin-releasing hormone.**

goal /gōl/ [ME, *gol,* limit], the purpose toward which an endeavor is directed, such as the outcome of diagnostic, therapeutic, and educational management of a patient's health problem.

goal attainment scale (GAS), an individualized outcome measure involving goal selection and goal grading; it is standardized in order to calculate the extent to which a patient's goals are met by defining levels of achievement and assigning numbers to them (−2, −1, 0, +1, +2).

goal-oriented movements, voluntary movements that are organized around behavioral goals, environmental context, and task specificity.

GOAT, abbreviation for **Galveston Orientation and Amnesia Test.**

goblet cell [ME, *gobelet,* small bowl], one of the many specialized epithelial cells that secrete mucus and form glands of the epithelium of the stomach, the intestine, and parts of the respiratory tract. Also called **beaker cell, chalice cell.** See also **gland.**

goiter /goi′ter/ [L, *guttur,* throat], an enlarged thyroid gland, usually evident as a pronounced swelling in the neck. It may be cystic or fibrous, containing nodules or an increased number of follicles. The goiter may surround a large blood vessel, or a part of the enlarged gland may be situated beneath the sternum or in the thoracic cavity. Also spelled *goitre.* See also **diffuse goiter, Basedow goiter, cystic goiter, fibrous goiter, toxic goiter, wandering goiter.** −*goitrous, adj.*

■ OBSERVATIONS: The enlargement may be associated with hyperthyroidism, hypothyroidism, or normal levels of thyroid function.

■ INTERVENTIONS: Treatment may include total or subtotal surgical removal, the administration of antithyroid drugs or radioiodine, or use of thyroid hormone to block the pituitary mechanism that releases thyroid-stimulating hormone.

■ PATIENT CARE CONSIDERATIONS: After thyroidectomy, maintenance therapy with thyroid hormone may be required.

goitrogenic glycoside /goi′trəjen″ik/, a compound found in mustard, horseradish, and cruciferous vegetables such

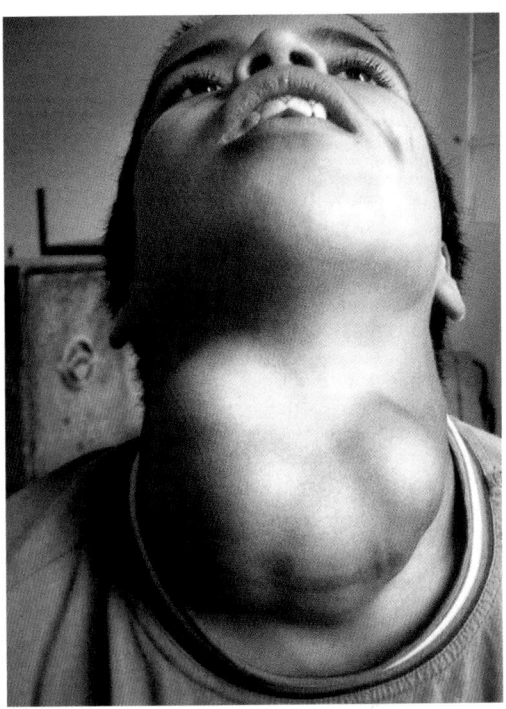

Child with large nodular goiter *(Kliegman et al, 2016)*

as cabbage that interferes with iodine uptake in the thyroid gland, leading to the development of goiter.

goitrous thyroiditis. See **Hashimoto disease.**

gold (Au) [AS, *geolu,* yellow], a yellowish soft metallic element that occurs naturally as a free metal and as the telluride $AuAgTe_4$. Its atomic number is 79; its atomic mass is 196.97. Gold has been highly valued since antiquity and has been and is used for currency, for ornamentation, and as a dental restorative material. It is usually hardened by alloying it with small amounts of nickel or copper. It is highly resistive to oxidation but can be dissolved in aqua regia and aqueous potassium cyanide. Gold salts, in which gold is attached to sulfur, are often used in the treatment, or chrysotherapy, of patients with rheumatoid arthritis, as well as other rheumatic and autoimmune diseases. Chrysotherapy is often associated with serious side effects. See also **chrysotherapy.**

gold-198, a radioactive gold antineoplastic drug.

■ INDICATIONS: It is prescribed for treatment of cancer of the prostate, cervix, and bladder and for reduction of fluid accumulation secondary to a cancer.

■ CONTRAINDICATIONS: Ulcerative tumors, pregnancy, lactation, or unhealed surgical wounds prohibit its use. It is not prescribed for patients less than 18 years of age.

■ ADVERSE EFFECTS: The most serious adverse effect is radiation sickness.

Goldblatt kidney, an abnormal kidney in which constriction of a renal artery leads to ischemia and release of renin, a pressor substance associated with hypertension.

gold compound, a drug containing gold salts, usually administered with other drugs in the treatment of rheumatoid arthritis. Gold is potentially toxic and is administered only under the supervision of a specialist in chrysotherapy. Toxic reactions range from mild dermatoses to lethal poisoning. Various radioisotopes of gold have been used in diagnostic radiology and in radiological treatment of certain malignant neoplastic diseases.

Goldenhar syndrome /gōl′dən·härz/ [Maurice Goldenhar, 20th-century Swiss physician], a congenital condition characterized by colobomas of the upper eyelid, dermoids on the eyeball, bilateral accessory auricular appendages anterior to the ears, and vertebral anomalies, frequently associated with characteristic facies, consisting of asymmetry of the skull, prominent frontal bossing, low hairline, mandibular hypoplasia, low-set ears, and sometimes smallness of the mouth on one side. Also called **OAV syndrome, oculoauriculovertebral dysplasia.**

goldenseal, a perennial herb found in the Ohio River Valley.
- INDICATIONS: It is used for high blood pressure, poor appetite, infections, menstrual problems, minor sciatic pain, and muscle spasms. It is also used as an eye wash and by some hoping to hide the presence of marijuana, cocaine, or other illicit drugs in the urine. Goldenseal is ineffective at masking illicit drugs in urine tests. There is insufficient reliable information to gauge its efficacy for other uses.
- CONTRAINDICATIONS: It is probably not safe when used at high doses or long term. The active constituent berberine can cause significant toxicity. Goldenseal is contraindicated in women who are pregnant (it is a uterine stimulant) or breastfeeding, and it should not be used in infants. It also should not be used in people with known hypersensitivity to this herb or with cardiovascular conditions such as heart block, arrhythmias, or hypertension. It should not be used locally for purulent ear discharge or in a ruptured eardrum.

gold foil, pure gold that has been rolled and beaten into a very thin sheet, used for making foil pellets, which are a direct dental restorative material. The main types of gold foil are cohesive, semicohesive, and noncohesive.

gold inlay, an intracoronal cast restoration of gold alloy that restores one or more tooth surfaces within the cusp prominences of a posterior tooth. It is held in place by the internal walls of the tooth and dental cements.

Goldman applanation tonometer (GAT) [Hans Goldman, Austrian opthamologist 1899–1991], a device mounted on a slit lamp used to measure intraocular presssure (IOP) in which the force required to flatten, or applanate, a constant area of the cornea is measured and related to the IOP using the Imbert–Fick principle. The patient sits upright for the examination.

Goldman-Fox knife, a dental surgical instrument with a sharp cutting edge, designed for the incision and contouring of gingival tissue.

gold sodium thiomalate, an antirheumatic drug.
- INDICATIONS: It is prescribed for the treatment of rheumatoid arthritis.
- CONTRAINDICATIONS: Severe debilitation, systemic lupus erythematosus, renal or liver disease, blood dyscrasias, Sjögren's syndrome (in rheumatoid arthritis), or known hypersensitivity to this drug or to other gold or heavy metal salts prohibits its use.
- ADVERSE EFFECTS: Among the most serious adverse effects are various blood dyscrasias, renal damage, and allergic reactions. Dermatitis, stomatitis, and lesions of the mucous membranes also may occur.

gold standard, **1.** an accepted test that is assumed to be able to determine the true disease state of a patient regardless of positive or negative test findings or sensitivities or specificities of other diagnostic tests used. **2.** an acknowledged measure of comparison of the superior effectiveness or value of a particular medication or other therapy as compared with that of other drugs or treatments.

gold therapy. See **chrysotherapy.**

golfer's elbow, an informal term for inflammation of the medial epicondyle of the humerus, associated with repeated use of the wrist flexors.

Golgi apparatus /gôl′jē/ [Camillo Golgi, Italian histologist and Nobel laureate, 1843–1926; L, *ad,* toward, *praeparare,* to prepare], one of many small membranous structures found in most cells, composed of various elements associated with the formation of carbohydrate side chains of glycoproteins, mucopolysaccharides, and other substances. Saccules within each structure migrate through the plasma membrane and release substances associated with external and internal secretion. Also called *Golgi body, Golgi complex.*

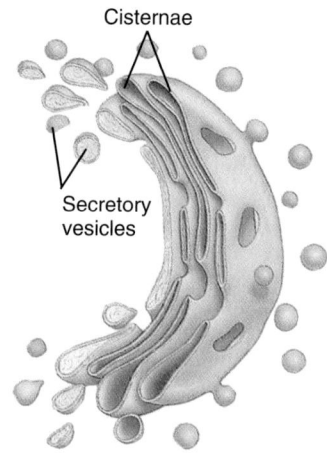

Cisternae

Secretory vesicles

Golgi apparatus *(Thibodeau and Patton, 2007)*

Golgi-Mazzoni corpuscles /gôl′jē matsō′nē/ [Camillo Golgi; Vittori Mazzoni, Italian physiologist, 1880–1940], a number of thin capsules enveloping terminal nerve fibrils in the subcutaneous tissue of the fingers. They have thicker cores than Pacini corpuscles but are similar special sensory end organs. Compare **Krause corpuscles, Pacini corpuscles, Ruffini corpuscles.**

Golgi cells [Camillo Golgi; L, *cella,* storeroom], either of two types of cells. Golgi type I neurons are nerve cells that have long axons that leave the local neurophil area of the parent cell body, traverse the white matter, and project to the rest of the nervous system. Golgi type II neurons are nerve cells with short trajectory axons, like stellate cells of the cerebral and cerebellar cortex. They generally do not enter white matter but remain within the local neurophil in the cerebral and cerebellar cortices and the retina.

Golgi tendon organ [Camillo Golgi], a sensory nerve ending that is sensitive to both tension and excessive passive stretch of a skeletal muscle.

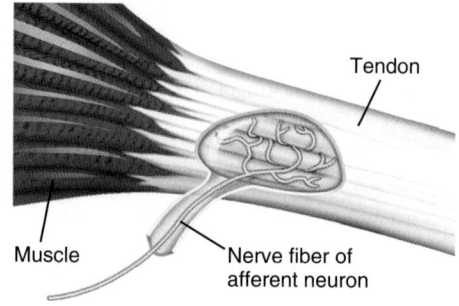

Tendon

Muscle

Nerve fiber of afferent neuron

Golgi tendon organ

Golgi type I neurons, Golgi type II neurons.   See **Golgi cells.**

Goltz syndrome.   See **focal dermal hypoplasia.**

gomphosis /gomfō″sis/ *pl. gomphoses* [Gk, *gomphos,* bolt],   an articulation by the insertion of a conical process into a socket, such as the insertion of a root of a tooth into an alveolus of the mandible or the maxilla. Gomphosis is not a connection between true bones but is considered a type of fibrous joint. Compare **sutura, syndesmosis.**

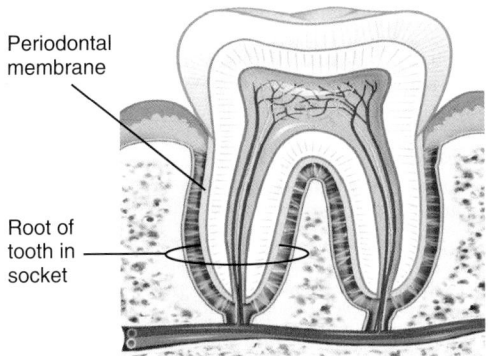

Periodontal membrane

Root of tooth in socket

Gomphosis

gon-, gono-,   prefix meaning "semen" or "seed": *gonococcus, gonorrhea, gonocyte.*

gonad /gō″nad/ [Gk, *gone,* seed],   a gamete-producing gland, such as an ovary or a testis. −*gonadal, adj.*

gonadal aplasia /gō″nədəl/,   a congenital state in which there is defective development of the germinal tissues of the gonads.

gonadal cords,   epithelial cells derived from the coelomic epithelium that penetrate the underlying mesenchyme, where they form cords. Also called **primordial sex cords.**

gonadal dose,   the amount of radiation received by the gonads as a result of a radiographic examination. It may vary from less than 0.01 mGy for a dental or chest radiograph to 2.25 mGy for a lumbar spine radiograph. During pelvimetry a fetus receives 8 mGy.

gonadal dysgenesis,   a general designation for a variety of conditions involving anomalies in the development of the gonads. Kinds include **Turner syndrome, hermaphroditism, gonadal aplasia.**

gonadal shield,   a specially designed contact or shadow shield used to protect the gonadal area of a patient from the primary radiation beam during radiographic procedures. It is generally used for patients who are potentially reproductive, including women under 50 years of age and all males.

gonado-,   prefix meaning relationship to the gonads: *gonadotropic.*

gonadoblastoma /gō″nədōblastō′mə/ [Gk, *gone,* seed + *blastos,* germ + *oma,* tumor],   a rare benign type of germ cell tumor, usually occurring in patients with gonadal dysgenesis, and often bilateral. It contains all gonadal elements and is frequently associated with an abnormal chromosomal karyotype. It may give rise to a dysgerminoma or other more malignant germ cell tumor. See also **dysgerminoma, gonadal dysgenesis.**

gonadorelin acetate,   the acetate ester of gonadorelin, having the same actions and uses as the hydrochloride salt. It is also used in the treatment of delayed puberty, female infertility, and amenorrhea; it is administered subcutaneously or intravenously.

gonadotrophic /gō′nədōtrof″ik/,   **1.** pertaining to genitalia. **2.** capable of influencing the gonads. **3.** relating to the state in which the gonads exert influence on the body.

gonadotropic /gō′nədōtrop″ik/,   acting on or stimulating the gonads. Also called **gonadotrophic.** See also **gonadotropin.**

gonadotropin /gō′nədōtrop″in/ [Gk, *gone* + *trophe,* nourishment],   a hormonal substance that stimulates the function of the testes and the ovaries. The gonadotropic follicle-stimulating hormone and luteinizing hormone are produced and secreted by the anterior pituitary gland. In early pregnancy, human chorionic gonadotropin is produced by the placenta (basis for early pregnancy detection). It acts to sustain the function of the corpus luteum of the ovary, forestalling menstruation and thus maintaining pregnancy. Gonadotropins are prescribed to induce ovulation in infertility that is caused by inadequate stimulation of the ovary by endogenous gonadotropic hormones. Excessive stimulation of the ovary may result in vast enlargement of the gland, maturation of many follicles, multiple pregnancy, bleeding into the abdomen, and pain. While named for their effects on the ovaries, follicle-stimulating hormone and luteinizing hormone are also major gonadotropins in the testes, causing the Leydig cells to secrete testosterone and facilitating spermatogenesis. Also called *gonadotrophin.* −**gonadotrophic, gonadotropic,** *adj.*

gonadotropin-releasing hormone (GnRH) [Gk, *gone,* seed, *trope,* a turn; ME, *relesen*; Gk, *hormaein,* to set in motion],   a decapeptide hypophysiotropic hormone secreted by the hypothalamus. It stimulates the release of luteinizing hormone and follicle-stimulating hormone by the anterior pituitary.

gonial angle.   See **angle of mandible.**

-gonic,   suffix meaning "work required to facilitate a specified reaction": *schizogonic.*

gonio-,   prefix meaning "angle": *goniometer, gonioscope, gonion.*

goniometer /gon′ē·om″ətər/,   an instrument used to measure angles, particularly range-of-motion angles of a joint.

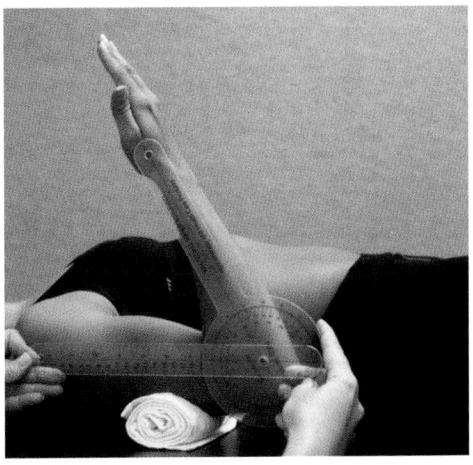

Goniometer *(Andrews et al, 2012)*

goniometry /gon′ē·om″ətrē/ [Gk, *gonia,* angle, *metron,* measure],   **1.** a system for measuring angles of a joint. **2.** a system for measuring angles during testing for various labyrinthine diseases that affect the sense of balance. One test uses a plank, one end of which may be raised to any desired height. The patient stands on the plank as one end

G

is gradually raised, and the point at which he or she can no longer maintain balance is noted. *–goniometric, adj.*

gonion /gō'nē·on/ [Gk, *gonia,* angle], an anthropometric landmark located at the most inferior, posterior, and lateral point on the external angle of the mandible, being the apex of the maximum curvature of the mandible, where the ascending ramus becomes the body of the mandible. See also **mandible.**

gonioscope /gō'nē·əskōp'/ [Gk, *gonia* + *skopein,* to look], a mirrored optical instrument used to examine the filtration angle of the anterior chamber of the eye. The mirrors permit visualization of the angle by means of a reflected image.

goniotomy /gōn'ē·ot'əmē/, an operation performed to remove any obstruction to the flow of aqueous humor in the front chamber of the eye. The procedure is commonly done in patients with congenital glaucoma.

gon(o) [Gk, *gōnía,* angle], combining form meaning *angle.*

gonoblast. See **germ cell.**

gonococcal /gon'əkok″əl/ [Gk, *gone,* seed, *kokkos,* berry], pertaining to or resembling gonococcus.

gonococcal pyomyositis [Gk, *gone,* seed, *kokkos,* berry, *pyon,* pus, *mys,* muscle, *itis,* inflammation], an acute inflammatory condition of a muscle caused by infection with *Neisseria gonorrhoeae,* characterized by abscess formation and pain. It is an unusual form of gonorrhea and must be differentiated from sarcoma. Diagnosis is made by the discovery of the gonococcal diplococci within the abscess when a bacterial culture of a specimen is prepared after exploratory surgery. The patient is then usually found to be asymptomatically infected in the urogenital organs. Antibiotic treatment, most often with ceftriaxone, is rapidly effective in curing the infection.

gonococcal salpingitis [Gk, *gone,* seed, *kokkos,* berry, *salpigx,* tube, *itis,* inflammation], infection of the fallopian tubes and immediately adjacent area by *Neisseria gonorrhoeae.* Also called **gonorrheal salpingitis.**

gonococcal urethritis [Gk, *gone,* seed, *kokkos,* berry, *ourethra,* urethra, *itis,* inflammation], inflammation of the urethra caused by an infection of *Neisseria gonorrhoeae.*

gonococcus /gon'əkok″əs/ *pl.* **gonococci** [Gk, *gone* + *kokkos,* berry], a gram-negative intracellular diplococcus of the species *Neisseria gonorrhoeae,* the cause of gonorrhea.

gonocyte. See **germ cell.**

gonorrhea /gon'ərē″ə/ [Gk, *gone* + *rhoia,* flow], a common sexually transmitted disease that most often affects the genitourinary tract and occasionally the pharynx or rectum. Infection results from contact with an infected person or with secretions containing the causative organism *Neisseria gonorrhoeae.* Infants born to infected women may acquire conjunctival infection from passage through the birth canal. Gonorrheal infections must be reported to local health departments in the United States. The Centers for Disease Control and Prevention estimate that more than 700,000 new infections occur annually. Also spelled *gonorrhoea.*

■ OBSERVATIONS: Urethritis; dysuria; purulent, greenish-yellow urethral or vaginal discharge; red or edematous urethral meatus; and itching, burning, or pain around the vaginal or urethral orifice are characteristic. The vagina may be massively swollen and red, and the lower abdomen may be tense and very tender. As the infection spreads, as occurs more commonly in women than in men, nausea, vomiting, fever, and tachycardia may occur as salpingitis, oophoritis, or peritonitis develops. Inflammation of the tissues surrounding the liver also may occur, causing pain in the upper right quadrant of the abdomen. Severe disseminated infection is also more common in women than in men and is characterized by signs of septicemia with polyarthritis, tender papillary lesions on the skin of the hands and feet, and inflammation of the tendons of the wrists, knees, and ankles. Gonococcal ophthalmia involves infection of the conjunctiva and

may lead to scarring and blindness. Gonorrhea is diagnosed by bacteriological culture of the organism from a smear obtained from a specimen of exudate. In men a microscopic study of a Gram-stained specimen of exudate that reveals gram-negative intracellular diplococci is diagnostic of gonorrheal infection, but this finding is not diagnostic in women.

■ INTERVENTIONS: Guidelines currently recommend dual therapy with ceftriaxone and azithromycin. Alternatives would include cefixime, gentamicin, or gemifloxacin. Emerging resistance patterns and the need for appropriate therapy may modify the therapeutic approach. Generally patients with gonorrheal infections should be treated simultaneously for presumptive chlamydial infections. The routine instillation of 1% solution of silver nitrate or topical ophthalmic antibiotic into the eyes of the newborn provides effective prophylaxis against conjunctival infection in the newborn period that might otherwise result from contact with the infected secretions of an asymptomatic infected mother during vaginal delivery.

■ PATIENT CARE CONSIDERATIONS: It is important that the patient's sexual contacts be treated. Before administration of any antibiotic it is ascertained that the patient does not have any known sensitivity to the drug being given and that equipment and drugs are available to treat any hypersensitivity reaction that may occur. Precaution against spread of the disease is recommended through condom use or monogamous sexual relations.

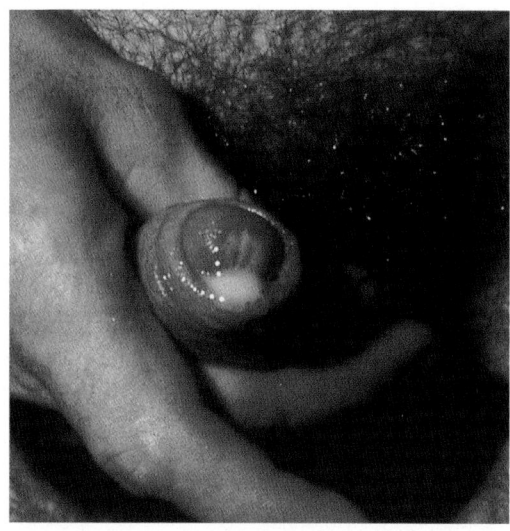

Gonorrhea in the male patient *(Morse et al, 2010)*

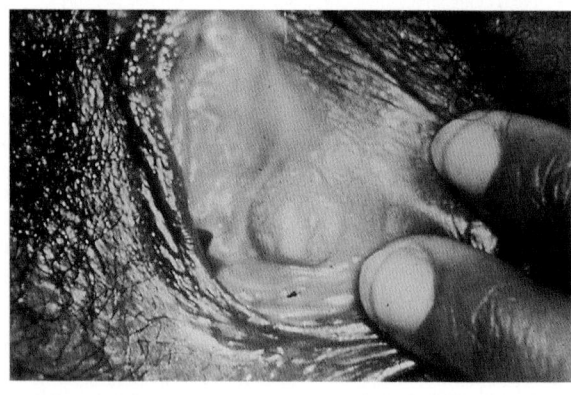

Gonorrhea in the female patient *(Morse et al, 2010)*

gonorrheal /gonˈərēˈəl/ [Gk, *gone,* seed, *kokkos*], pertaining to or resembling gonorrhea.

gonorrheal arthritis [Gk, *gone,* seed, *kokkos,* berry, *arthron,* joint, *itis,* inflammation], a blood-borne gonococcal infection of the joints. It may affect one or several joints, may occur as a chronic or acute form, and often leads to joint fusion. Infection may result in pus formation in an affected joint.

gonorrheal conjunctivitis, a severe, destructive form of purulent conjunctivitis caused by the gonococcus *Neisseria gonorrhoeae.* Prompt treatment by the IV administration of antibiotics is required to prevent scarring of the cornea and blindness. Newborns receive routine prophylaxis of a topical ophthalmic instillation of 1% solution of silver nitrate or an antibiotic ophthalmic ointment. The treatment has largely eradicated the infection in infants. See also **ophthalmia neonatorum.**

gonorrheal proctitis [Gk, *gone,* seed, *rhoia,* flow, *proktos,* anus, *itis,* inflammation], an inflammation of the rectum caused by an infection of gonorrhea.

gonorrheal salpingitis. See **gonococcal salpingitis.**

gonorrheal urethritis. See **gonococcal urethritis.**

-gony, suffix meaning "birth," "origin," or "procreation": *amphigony, schizogony, sporogony.*

Gonyaulax catenella /gonˈē·ô″laks/, a species of toxin-producing planktonic protozoa ingested by shellfish along the coasts of North America that causes shellfish poisoning. It colors the sea red in an infected area. The phenomenon is called red tide. See also **shellfish poisoning.**

Goodell's sign /gŏŏdelzˈ/ [William Goodell, American gynecologist, 1829–1894], softening of the uterine cervix, a probable sign of pregnancy.

Goodman syndrome /gŏŏdˈmənz/ [Richard M. Goodman, Israeli physician, 20th century], an autosomal-recessive form of acrocephalopolysyndactyly characterized also by congenital heart defects, sideward deviation and abnormal flexion of digits, and ulnar drift, but with unimpaired intelligence. Also called **Carpenter syndrome, Noack syndrome, Sakati-Nyhan syndrome.**

Goodpasture syndrome /gŏŏd″pas·chər/ [Ernest W. Goodpasture, American pathologist, 1886–1960], a chronic relapsing pulmonary hemosiderosis, an autoimmune disease usually associated with glomerulonephritis and characterized by a cough with hemoptysis, dyspnea, anemia, and progressive renal failure. Mild forms may respond to corticosteroids or immunosuppressive drugs. Severe recurrent cases have a poor prognosis; hemodialysis and kidney transplantation are the only treatments.

Goodrich, Annie Warburton [1866–1954], an American nursing educator who was instrumental in advancing nursing from an apprenticeship to a profession. She was superintendent of nurses at several New York hospitals before going to Teachers College, Columbia University, in 1914. In addition to teaching, she was associated with the Henry Street Settlement and the Nursing Department of the U.S. Army. In 1923 she became dean of the newly formed School of Nursing at Yale University, which awarded a degree similar to that awarded in other professions.

Good Samaritan legislation /səmarˈitən/ [good Samaritan, from New Testament parable; L, *lex,* law, *lator,* proposer], laws enacted in most states to protect physicians, dentists, nurses, and some other health professionals from liability while rendering emergency medical or dental aid, unless there is proven willful wrong or gross negligence.

gooseflesh. See **pilomotor reflex.**

Gopalan syndrome. See **burning feet syndrome.**

Gordon reflex [Alfred Gordon, American neurologist, 1874–1953], **1.** an abnormal variation of the Babinski reflex, elicited by compressing the calf muscles, characterized by dorsiflexion of the great toe and fanning of the other toes. It is evidence of disease of the pyramidal tract. **2.** an abnormal reflex, elicited by compressing the forearm muscles, characterized by flexion of the fingers or of the thumb and index finger. It is seen in diseases of the pyramidal tract. Compare **Chaddock reflex, Oppenheim reflex.** See also **Babinski reflex.**

Gordon syndrome /gôrˈdən/ [Richard D. Gordon, 20th-century Australian physician], a type of pseudohypoaldosteronism with hypertension and hyperkalemia but without salt wasting, thought to be caused by abnormally increased absorption of chloride by the renal tubules. See also **pseudohypoaldosteronism.**

Gorham disease /gorˈəm/ [Lemuel Whittington Gorham, American physician, 1885–1968], a gradual, but often complete, resorption of a bone or group of bones, which may be associated with multiple hemangiomas. It usually occurs in children or young adults, sometimes following trauma, but its cause is unknown.

Gosselin fracture /gôslaN″/ [Leon A. Gosselin, French surgeon, 1815–1847], a V-shaped break in the distal tibia, extending to the ankle.

GOT, abbreviation for **glutamic oxaloacetic transaminase.** See **aspartate aminotransferase.**

gotu kola, a creeping herb found in swamps of Africa, Sri Lanka, and Madagascar.

■ INDICATIONS: It is taken systemically to treat venous insufficiency and for a variety of other reasons, including improving memory and intelligence, and it is used topically to treat chronic wounds and psoriasis. It may be effective for its topical indications and for treating venous insufficiency. There are insufficient reliable data for any of its other uses.

■ CONTRAINDICATIONS: It should not be used during pregnancy and lactation or in children until more research is available. Those with known hypersensitivity to this herb or to members of the celery family should not use this product.

goundou /gŏŏn″dŏŏ/ [West African], a condition characterized by bony exostoses of the nasal and maxillary bones, usually occurring as a late sequela of yaws in people in Africa and Latin America. Also called **anakhré.** See also **yaws.**

gout [L, *gutta,* drop], a disease associated with an inborn error of uric acid metabolism that increases production or interferes with excretion of uric acid. Excess uric acid is converted to sodium urate crystals that precipitate from the blood and become deposited in joints and other tissues. Men are more often affected than premenopausal women. The great toe is a common site for the accumulation of urate crystals. The condition can cause exceedingly painful swelling of a joint, accompanied by chills and fever. The symptoms are recurrent. Episodes become longer each year. See also **chondrocalcinosis, Lesch-Nyhan syndrome, tophus.**

■ PATIENT CARE CONSIDERATIONS: The disorder is disabling and, if untreated, can progress to the development of destructive joint changes, such as tophi. Acute treatment usually includes administration of colchicine, phenylbutazone, indomethacin, or glucocorticoid drugs and a diet that excludes purine-rich foods such as organ meats. It may include surgical removal of ulcerated tophi. Chronically, probenecid, allopurinol, colchicine, or febuxostat may be used to decrease uric acid levels. Acquired gout is a condition having the signs and symptoms of gout but resulting from another disorder or treatment for a different condition. Diuretic drugs can alter the concentration of uric acid so that uric acid salts precipitate from the blood and are carried to the joints.

G

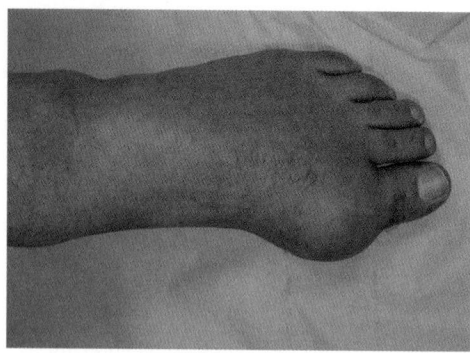

Gout in the first metatarsal joint *(Tanner et al, 2014)*

gouty /gou′tē/ [L, *gutta,* drop], pertaining to or resembling the condition of gout.

gouty arthritis. See **gout.**

GP, abbreviation for **general practitioner.**

gp160, a glycoprotein found on the outer surface, or envelope, of the human immunodeficiency virus. It is composed of gp120, which protrudes from the envelope, and gp41, which is embedded in the envelope.

GPB, abbreviation for **glossopharyngeal breathing.**

GPT, abbreviation for **glutamic pyruvic transaminase.** See **alanine aminotransferase.**

GPWW, abbreviation for **group practice without walls.**

gr, abbreviation for **grain.**

graafian follicle /grä″fē·ən, -grā″-/ [Reijnier de Graaf, Dutch physician, 1641–1673; L, *folliculus,* small bag], a mature ovarian vesicle, measuring about 10 to 12 mm in diameter, that ruptures during ovulation to release the ovum. Many primary ovarian follicles, each containing an immature ovum about 35 µm in diameter, are embedded near the surface of the ovary, just below the tunica albuginea. Under the influence of the follicle-stimulating hormone from the adenohypophysis, one ovarian follicle ripens into a graafian follicle during the proliferative phase of each menstrual cycle. The cells that form the graafian follicle are arranged in a layer three to four cells thick around a relatively large volume of follicular fluid. Within the follicle the ovum grows to about 100 µm in diameter, ruptures, and is swept into the fimbriated opening of the uterine tube. The cavity of the follicle collapses when the ovum is released, and the remaining follicular cells greatly enlarge to become the corpus luteum. If the ovum is fertilized, the corpus luteum grows and becomes the corpus luteum of pregnancy, which degenerates by the end of 9 months and has a diameter of about 30 mm. As the ovarian follicle ripens into the graafian follicle, it produces estrogen, which stimulates the proliferation of the endometrium and the enlargement of the uterine glands. The growing corpus luteum produces progesterone, which triggers endometrial gland secretion and prepares the uterus to receive the fertilized ovum. If the ovum is not fertilized, the graafian follicle forms the corpus luteum of menstruation, which degenerates before the next menstrual cycle, leaving the small scarred corpus albicans.

grab bar, a short length of metal or heavy plastic secured firmly to a wall to enhance safety, mobility, and balance for individuals needing additional support. Grab bars are usually placed in bathrooms.

gracile /gras″il/, long, slender, and graceful.

gracilis /gras″ilis/, the most superficial of the five medial femoral muscles. It is a thin, flattened muscle that is broad proximally and narrow distally. It functions to adduct the thigh and flex the leg and to assist in the medial rotation of

the leg after it is flexed. Compare **adductor brevis, adductor longus, adductor magnus, obturator externus.**

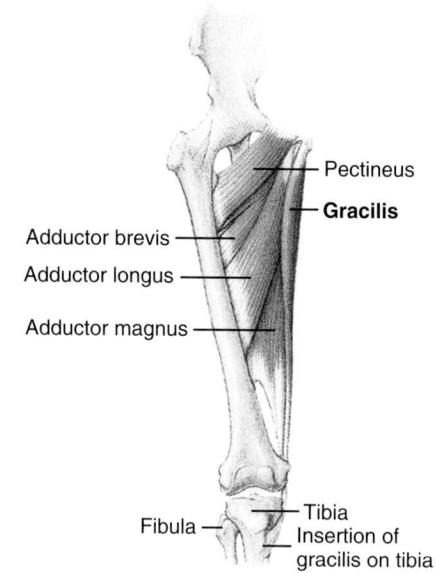

Gracilis muscle *(Patton and Thibodeau, 2016)*

gradation, (in occupational therapy) a systematic progression of activities.

gradation of activity /gradā′shən/, therapeutic activities that are appropriately paced and modified to demand maximal capacities at any point in progression or regression of the patient's condition.

graded exercise test (GXT), a test given to a cardiac patient during rehabilitation to assess prognosis and quantify maximal functional capacity. The test is given before discharge to determine guidelines for activity programs at home and work during convalescence. See also **exercise electrocardiogram.**

gradient /grā′dē·ənt/ [L, *gradus,* step], **1.** the rate of increase or decrease of a measurable phenomenon, such as temperature or pressure. **2.** a visual representation of the rate of change of a measurable phenomenon; a curve.

gradient compression stockings, a garment designed to prevent the accumulation of fluids in an extremity. The amount of pressure is greatest at the distal end of the garment and gradually decreases toward the proximal end. Kinds include **Jobst garment™.**

gradient former, a device for the preparation of linear-density gradient medium in a column for gradient electrophoresis.

gradient gel electrophoresis, gel electrophoresis performed in a concentration gradient gel with progressively decreasing pore size.

gradient magnetic field, a magnetic field that changes in strength in a given direction. Such fields are used in magnetic resonance imaging (MRI) to select a region for imaging and to encode the location of MRI signals received from the object being imaged.

gradient plate technique, a method for isolating antibiotic-resistant bacteria mutants by exposing an agar plate containing concentration gradient of antibiotic to an inoculation of bacteria to be tested.

grading activities, (in occupational therapy) changing the process, environment, tools, or materials of activities to increase or decrease the performance demands on the client.

graduated bath /graj″oo·a′tid/ [L, *gradus,* step; AS, *baeth*], a hydrotherapy treatment in which the temperature of the water is slowly reduced.

graduated muscular contractions, controlled shortening of muscle units in properly timed and adequate response to a stimulus. The contractions may be induced by the central nervous system or by electric stimulation. Contractile force can be controlled by varying the number of units that contract or by increasing the frequency of contractions.

graduated resistance exercise. See **progressive resistance exercise.**

graduate medical education (GME) /graj″oo·it/, formal medical education pursued after receipt of the doctor of medicine (M.D.) or other professional degree in the medical sciences, usually as an intern, resident, or fellow.

graduate nurse (GN) [L, *gradus,* step, *nutrix,* nurse], a nurse who is a graduate of an accredited school of nursing, but not yet licensed.

Graduate Record Examination (GRE), an examination administered to graduates of institutions of higher learning. The scores are used as criteria for admission to master's and doctoral programs in many institutions and areas of specialization, including the health sciences. The examination tests verbal and mathematical aptitudes and abilities.

GRAE, abbreviation for **generally recognized as effective.**

graft [Gk, *graphion,* stylus], a tissue or an organ taken from a site or a person and inserted into a new site or person, performed to repair a defect in structure. The graft may be temporary, such as an emergency skin transplant for extensive burns, or permanent with the grafted tissue growing to become a part of the body. Skin, bone, cartilage, blood vessel, nerve, muscle, cornea, and whole organs, such as the kidney or the heart, may be grafted. Preoperative care focuses on a high-protein diet and vitamins to ensure optimal physical condition and on freedom from infection. With the patient under general or local anesthesia, the tissue is transferred and sutured into place. Rejection of a nonautograft is the major complication: fever, pain in the graft area, and evidence of loss of function 4 to 15 days after the procedure are indicative of rejection. Immunosuppressive drugs are given in large doses to suppress antibody production and rejection. Even if an early reaction is prevented, late rejection may occur 1 year or more after the graft is done. Also called **transplant.** See also **allograft, autograft, isograft, skin graft, xenograft.**

graft facilitation, a method for extending the survival of a graft by conditioning the recipient with an immunoglobulin-blocking factor, which suppresses graft rejection.

graft rejection, the immunological destruction of transplanted organs or tissues. The rejection may be based on both cell-mediated and antibody-mediated immunity against cells of the graft by a histoincompatible recipient. First-set rejection usually occurs within 10 days. Second-set rejection occurs within 1 week after a second graft with the same antigenic specificity as the first is placed in the same host.

graft-versus-host disease (GVHD), a rejection response of certain grafts, especially of bone marrow. It is commonly associated with inadequate immunosuppressive therapy of the donor, which allows immunocompetent cells in the donated tissue to recognize the recipient's tissues as foreign and to attack them. Because the recipient is totally immunosuppressed, the recipient's immune system cannot defend against the attack. Characteristic signs may include skin lesions with edema, erythema, ulceration, scaling, loss of hair, lesions of the joints and the heart, and hemolytic anemia with a positive Coombs' test reaction. Also called *graft-versus-host reaction,* **homologous disease.**

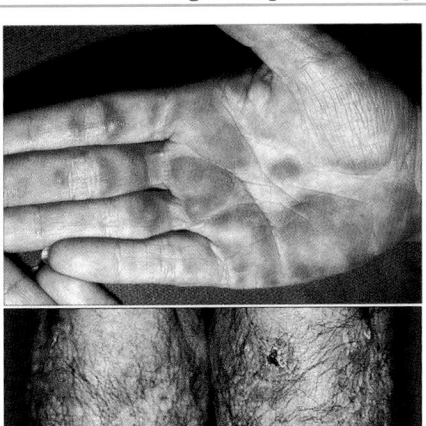
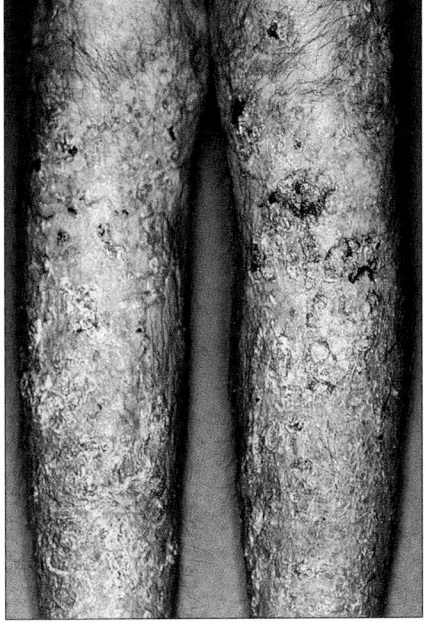

Acute graft-versus-host disease *(top)* and chronic graft-versus-host disease *(bottom)* *(Cohen, 2005)*

Graham's law /grā′əmz/ [Thomas Graham, English chemist, 1805–1869], the law stating that the rate of diffusion of a gas through a liquid (or the alveolar-capillary membrane) is directly proportional to its solubility coefficient and inversely proportional to the square root of its density.

Graham Steell murmur [Graham Steell, British physician, 1851–1942], an early diastolic murmur heard in the second intercostal space to the left of the sternum. It is associated with pulmonary valve regurgitation in pulmonary hypertension.

grain (gr) [L, *granum,* seed], the smallest unit of mass in avoirdupois, troy, and apothecaries' weights formerly based on the weight of a plump grain of wheat. The grain is the same and is equal to 65 mg. The troy and apothecaries' ounces contain 480 grains; the avoirdupois ounce contains 437.5 grains.

gram (g, gm) [L, *gramma,* small weight], a unit of mass in the metric system equal to 1/1000 kilogram, 15.432 grains, and 0.0353 ounce avoirdupois. 453.6 g = 1 lb. The preferred abbreviation is *g.*

-gram, -gramme, **1.** suffix meaning "a drawing" or "a written record": *electroencephalogram, mammogram.* **2.** suffix identifying a basic unit of mass: *centigram, kilogram.*

gram calorie. See **calorie.**

gram-equivalent weight (gEq), an equivalent weight of a substance calculated as the gram mass that contains, replaces, or reacts (directly or indirectly) with the Avogadro number of hydrogen atoms. Because 1 atom of sulfur (atomic mass 32) combines with 2 atoms of hydrogen (atomic mass 1), the gram-equivalent weight of sulfur is 32/2 = 16.

gram-molecular mass, a mass in grams numerically equal to the molecular weight of a substance or the sum of all the atomic masses in its molecular formula. For example, the gram-molecular weight of carbon dioxide (CO_2) is 12 (atomic mass of carbon) + (2 × 16) (atomic mass of oxygen), or 44 g. See also **mole, molecular weight.**

gram-negative [Hans C.J. Gram, Danish physician, 1853–1938; L, *negare,* to say no], having the pink color of the counterstain used in Gram's method of staining microorganisms. This property is a primary method of characterizing organisms in microbiology. Some of the most common gram-negative pathogenic bacteria are *Bacteroides fragilis, Salmonella typhi, Shigella dysenteriae,* and *Yersinia pestis.*

gram-positive [Hans C.J. Gram; L, *positivus*], retaining the violet color of the stain used in Gram's method of staining microorganisms. This property is a primary method of characterizing organisms in microbiology. Some of the most common kinds of gram-positive pathogenic bacteria are *Bacillus anthracis, Clostridium* species, *Mycobacterium leprae, Mycobacterium tuberculosis, Staphylococcus aureus, Streptococcus pneumoniae,* and *Streptococcus pyogenes.*

Gram stain [Hans C.J. Gram, Danish bacteriologist, 1853-1938], the method of staining microorganisms by using a violet stain, followed by an iodine solution; decolorizing with an alcohol or acetone solution; and counterstaining with safranin. The retention of either the violet color of the stain or the pink color of the counterstain serves as a primary means of identifying and classifying bacteria. Also called *Gram's method.* See also **gram-negative, gram-positive.**

gram-variable, gram-positive bacteria that can become gram-negative after culturing.

grandiose /gran″dē·ōs′/ [L, *grandis,* great], **1.** pertaining to something or somebody imposing, impressive, magnificent; pompous and showy. **2.** pertaining to behavior or beliefs seen in a mania.

grandiosity. See **megalomania.**

grand mal seizure. *(Informal)* See **generalized tonic-clonic seizure.**

grand multipara /grand/ [L, *grandis,* great, *multus,* many, *parere,* to give birth], a woman who has carried six or more pregnancies to a viable stage.

grand rounds [L, *grandis* + *rotundus,* wheel], a formal conference in which an expert presents a lecture concerning a clinical issue intended to be educational for the listeners. In some settings, grand rounds may be formal teaching rounds conducted by an expert at the bedsides of selected patients.

granisetron /granis′etron/, an antiemetic used in conjunction with cancer chemotherapy or radiotherapy, administered orally or intravenously as the hydrochloride salt.

grant [ME, *granten,* to believe a request], a monetary award given to an institution, a project, or an individual by the federal government, a foundation, a private business, or an institution to provide financial support for research, service, or training. The applicant usually writes a formal application (proposal) for the grant, which is reviewed by the granting agency and compared with other proposals. The grantee is usually accountable to the grantor for reporting the outcomes as a result of the awarded resources.

granul-, prefix meaning "grains or granules": *granular cast, granulocyte, granuloma.*

granular /gran″yələr/ [L, *granulum,* little grain], **1.** macroscopically resembling or feeling like sand. **2.** microscopically appearing to have a few or many particles within or on its surface, such as a stained granular leukocyte. –**granularity,** *n.*

granular cast [L, *granulum,* little grain; ONorse, *kasta*], a mass of pathological debris composed of cells filled with protein and fatty granules.

granular conjunctivitis. See **trachoma.**

granular degeneration, swelling of cells caused by accumulation of intracellular water in response to cell injury. Also called **ballooning degeneration hydropic degeneration, cloudy swelling.**

granular endoplasmic reticulum, the presence of ribosomes over the surface of endoplasmic reticulum. See **endoplasmic reticulum.**

granular induration, fibrosis of an organ, characterized by the formation of localized granular areas, as seen in cirrhosis of the liver.

granularity. See **granular.**

granulation tissue /gran″yəlā″shən/ [L, *granulum,* little grain], any soft pink fleshy projections that form during the healing process in a wound that does not heal by primary intention. The tissue consists of many capillaries surrounded by fibrous collagen. Overgrowth of granulation tissue causes proud flesh growing above the skin. See also **pyogenic granuloma.**

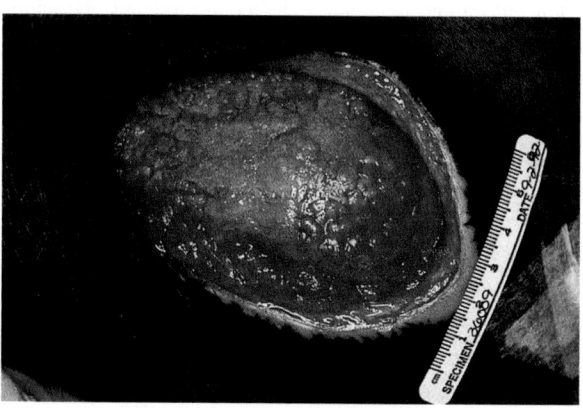

Granulation tissue *(Elkin, Perry, and Potter, 2007)*

granule /gran′yool/ [L, *granulum,* little grain], a particle, grain, or other small dry mass capable of free movement. Unlike powders, granules are usually free-flowing because of small surface forces involved.

granulocyte /gran″yoolosīt′/ [L, *granulum* + Gk, *kytos,* cell], a type of leukocyte characterized by the presence of cytoplasmic granules. Compare **agranulocyte.** Kinds include **basophil, eosinophil, neutrophil, monocyte.** –*granulocytic, adj.*

granulocyte colony-stimulating factor (G-CSF), a glycoprotein secreted by a variety of cells that stimulates the growth of hematopoietic stem cells and their differentiation into granulocytes. It is often used to treat patients who have become severely neutropenic as a result of chemotherapy or irradiation. See also **growth factor.**

granulocyte-macrophage colony-stimulating factor (GM-CSF), a glycoprotein secreted by several different immune cell types that stimulates the growth of myeloid progenitor cells and their differentiation into granulocytes and monocytes. See also **growth factor.**

granulocyte transfusion, the use of specially prepared leukocytes for the treatment of severe granulocytopenia and for prophylaxis in the prevention of serious infection in patients with leukemia or those receiving cancer chemotherapy. The procedure has the same risks as a blood transfusion.

granulocytic leukemia. See **chronic myelogenous leukemia.**

granulocytic sarcoma. See **chloroma.**

granulocytopenia /gran′yŏōlōsī′tōpē″nē·ə/ [L, *granulum* + Gk, *kytos,* cell, *penia,* poverty], an abnormal decrease in the total number of granulocytes in the blood. Also called **granulopenia, neutropenia.** Compare **granulocytosis.** See also **leukopenia.** −*granulocytopenic, adj.*

granulocytosis /gran′yŏōlōsītō″sis/ [L, *granulum* + Gk, *kytos,* cell, *osis,* condition], an abnormal increase in the total number of granulocytes in the blood, as occurs in response to infection. Compare **granulocytopenia.**

granuloma /gran′yŏōlō″mə/ *pl.* *granulomas, granulomata* [L, *granulum* + Gk, *oma,* tumor], a chronic tumorlike mass of inflammatory lesion consisting of a central collection of macrophages, often with multinucleated giant cells, surrounded by lymphocytes. Granulomas most often occur in the lungs, but they can also occur in other parts of the body. Granulomas form as a defense mechanism of walling off foreign invaders such as bacteria or fungi. They may resolve spontaneously, remain static, become gangrenous, spread, or act as a focus of infection. Treatment depends on the cause and probable course of the particular granuloma.

-granuloma, suffix meaning a "tumorlike mass or nodule of granulation tissue": *lipogranuloma, xanthogranuloma.*

granuloma annulare, a self-limited chronic skin disease of unknown cause that consists of reddish papules or nodules arranged in a ring with a normal or sunken center. It most commonly occurs on the distal portions of the extremities. It is not contagious.

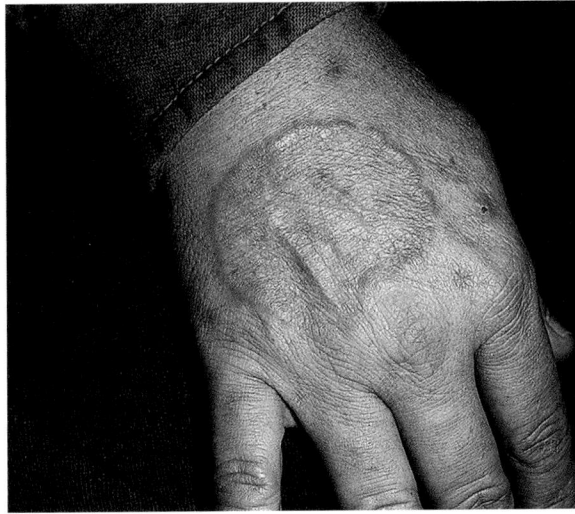

Granuloma annulare (Callen et al, 2000)

granuloma fissuratum. See **acanthoma fissuratum.**

granuloma gluteale infantum, a skin condition of the neonate characterized by large elevated bluish or brownish red nodules on the buttocks. It often occurs as a secondary reaction to the application of strong topical ointments over time. The lesions routinely disappear within a couple of months after the use of the preparations is discontinued.

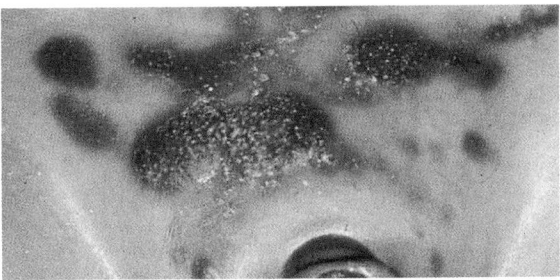

Granuloma gluteale infantum (Courtesy Dr. David Atherton)

granuloma inguinale, a sexually transmitted disease characterized by ulcers of the skin and subcutaneous tissues of the groin and genitalia. It is caused by infection with *Calymmatobacterium granulomatis,* a small gram-negative rod-shaped bacillus. It occurs more frequently in men than in women and is associated with anal intercourse. Diagnosis is made by microscopic examination and identification of characteristic "safety-pin"-shaped bodies known as Donovan bodies in the cytoplasm of phagocytes taken from a lesion and dyed with Wright's or Giemsa stain or by histological examination of a biopsy specimen. Untreated, the lesions spread, deepen, multiply, and become secondarily infected, resulting in mutilation and destruction of genital tissue. Streptomycin is usually effective in treating the infection. All patients who have or are suspected of having granuloma inguinale are also tested for syphilis because concurrent infection is common. Also called **Donovanosis.**

granulomatosis /gran′yŏōlōmətō″sis/ [L, *granulum* + Gk, *oma,* tumor, *osis,* condition], a condition or disease characterized by the development of granulomas. Kinds include **berylliosis, pulmonary Wegener granulomatosis.**

granulomatosis with polyangiitis (GPA), an uncommon disease occurring mainly in the fifth decade and characterized by granulomatosis vasculitis of the upper and lower respiratory tract, necrotizing glomerulonephritis, and varying degrees of small-vessel vasculitis. Symptoms may include sinus pain; bloody, purulent nasal discharge; saddle-nose deformity; chest discomfort and cough; weakness; anorexia; weight loss; and skin lesions. Renal involvement is seen in 80% of cases. Use of cytotoxic drugs, especially cyclophosphamide, has produced long-term remissions in many patients. The cause of the disease is unknown. Formerly called **Wegener granulomatosis.**

granulomatous /gran′yəlom″ətəs/ [L, *granulum,* little grain], pertaining to or resembling granulomas.

granulomatous amebic encephalitis, chronic encephalitis, usually seen in debilitated or immunocompromised patients, caused by infection with species of *Acanthamoeba.* It is marked by the formation of granulomas. Headache, seizures, nausea, and vomiting frequently occur.

granulomatous gastritis, chronic gastritis with granulomas of the stomach mucosa. It is seen with Crohn's disease, sarcoidosis, or certain other conditions.

granulomatous prostatitis, prostatitis with granuloma formation, such as from infection with *Mycobacterium tuberculosis,* parasites, or fungi.

granulomatous thyroiditis. See **de Quervain thyroiditis.**

granulopenia. See **granulocytopenia.**

granulopoiesis /gran′yŏōlōpōī·ē′sis/, the production or formation of granulocytes.

granulopoietin /gran′yoo̅lō′pō·ē″tin/, cytokines or growth factors acting on granulocytes. See also **granulocyte colony-stimulating factor.**

granulosa cell tumor /gran′yoo̅lō′sə/ [L, *granulum,* little grain], a fleshy ovarian tumor with yellow streaks that originates in cells of the primordial membrana granulosa and may grow to a large size. Excessive production of estrogen, resulting in endometrial hyperplasia and menorrhagia, may be associated with the tumor. Also called *granulosa cell carcinoma.*

granulosa-lutein cells, lutein cells of the corpus luteum derived from granulosa cells.

granulosa-theca cell tumor, an ovarian tumor composed of granulosa (follicular) cells or theca cells or both. The tumor is associated with excessive production of estrogen and hyperplasia of the breast and endometrium. See also **luteoma.**

granulosis /gran′yoo̅lō″sis/, any disorder characterized by an accumulation of granules in an area of body tissue, such as a skin eruption marked by tiny granules beneath the surface.

grapeseed, an herb found throughout the world.

■ INDICATIONS: It is used as a chronic disease preventative and an antiinflammatory, and it is a source of essential fatty acids and antioxidant tocopherols. It is used orally for the prevention of atherosclerosis and cancer and in folk medicine for the treatment of circulatory disorders. It may improve venous tone; there are insufficient reliable data for any other indications.

■ CONTRAINDICATIONS: Its use should be avoided during pregnancy and lactation and in children until more research is available.

-graph, **1.** suffix meaning the "product of drawing or writing": *radiograph.* **2.** suffix meaning a "machine for making something drawn": *actigraph, pneumograph.*

graphanesthesia /graf′anəsthē″zhə/, inability to feel writing on the skin, usually caused by a central nervous system lesion, typically tested by writing numbers in the palm and asking the patient to tell the number. Also called **agraphesthesia.**

-grapher, suffix meaning "one who writes about" something specified: *sonographer, syphilographer.*

graphesthesia /graf′esthē″zhə/, ability to feel writing on the skin.

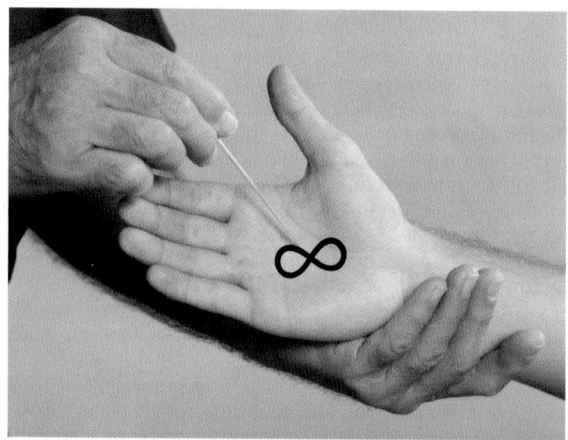

Testing for graphesthesia *(Evans, 2009)*

-graphia, suffix meaning "an abnormality revealed through handwriting": *dysgraphia, pseudoagraphia.*

graphing /graf″ing/, the organization of data consisting of two or more variables along horizontal and vertical axes of a graph to show relationships between specific quantities or other specific factors.

graphite /graf′īt/ [L, *graphites,* from Gk, *graphis,* a writing instrument], a form of native mineralized carbon whose dust causes a form of pneumoconiosis when it is inhaled. See also **pneumoconiosis.**

graphite pneumoconiosis /noo′mōkō′nē·ō′sis/, silicosis resulting from inhalation of graphite dust, which often contains up to 10% silica. Also called *graphite fibrosis, graphitosis.*

grapho-, prefix meaning "writing": *graphospasm.*

graphospasm. See **writer's cramp.**

-graphy, suffix meaning a "kind of printing" or "process of recording": *arteriography, cardiography, dermography.*

GRAS, abbreviation for **generally recognized as safe.**

Grashey method, a positioning method for producing true anteroposterior x-ray images of the scapulohumeral joint. The patient faces the x-ray tube with the affected shoulder centered to the midline of the image receptor (IR). The affected elbow is flexed, and the forearm is placed across the patient's chest. The opposite shoulder is rotated 45 degrees away from the IR, and the central ray is directed perpendicularly through the affected shoulder joint.

grasping forceps, any forceps for grasping tissue and exerting traction, having finger rings and a locking mechanism.

grasp reflex [ME, *graspen,* grab; L, *reflectere,* to bend back], a reflex induced by stroking the palm or sole with the result that the fingers or toes flex in a grasping motion. The reflex is a pathological manifestation of diseases of the premotor cortex. In young infants the tonic grasp reflex is normal; the child can grasp the examiner's fingers so firmly that he or she can be lifted into the air. Also called **darwinian reflex.**

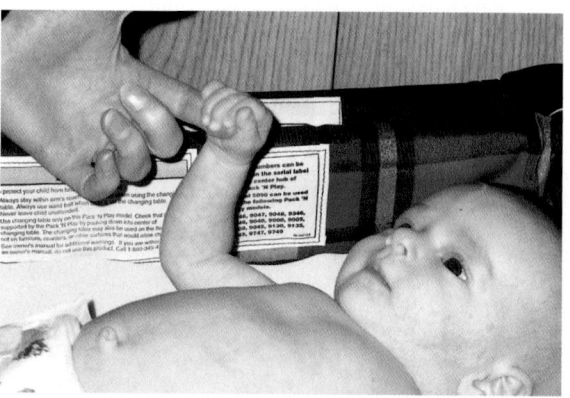

Grasp reflex in an infant *(Leifer, 2003)*

grass. See **cannabis.**

grass-line ligature [AS, *graes* + L, *linea,* thread, *ligare,* to bind], a fine cord made from the fibers of a grass-cloth plant, used in orthodontics for minor adjustments or movement of the teeth. The ligature exerts traction by shrinking when wetted by saliva.

Graves disease /grāvz/ [Robert J. Graves, Irish physician, 1796–1853], a multisystem autoimmune disorder characterized by pronounced hyperthyroidism, usually associated with an enlarged thyroid gland and exophthalmos (abnormal protrusion of the eyeball). The origin is unknown, but the disease is familial and is usually associated with thyroid-stimulating autoantibodies that bind to TSH receptors and stimulate thyroid secretion. The disease, which is five times more common in women than in men, occurs most frequently when the individual is between 30 and 60 years of age and can arise after an infection or physical or emotional stress. Typical signs, which are related to hyperthyroidism, are nervousness, a fine tremor of the hands, weight loss, fatigue, breathlessness, palpitations, increased heat intolerance, increased metabolic rate, and GI motility. An enlarged thymus, generalized hyperplasia of the lymph nodes, blurred or double vision, localized myxedema, atrial arrhythmias, and osteoporosis may occur. The diagnosis may be established by tests that measure TSH, thyroxine, and triiodothyronine levels in serum. If necessary, radioactive iodine uptake in the gland is tested. Treatment may include prescription of antithyroid drugs, such as methimazole, propylthiouracil, and iodine preparations. Radioactive iodine may be administered, but hospitalization for a few days is recommended for patients treated with a large dose. Occasionally subtotal thyroidectomy may be indicated. In patients with inadequately controlled disease, infection or stress may precipitate a life-threatening thyroid storm. The exophthalmia may or may not resolve with the treatment of the disease. Also called **exophthalmic goiter, thyrotoxicosis, toxic goiter.**

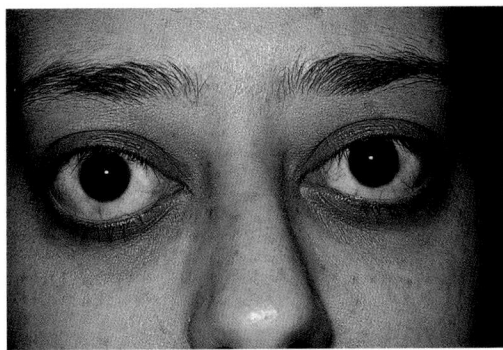

Bilateral proptosis in individual with Graves disease
(Tyers and Collin, 2008)

Graves orbitopathy /grāvz/ [Robert J. Graves, Irish physician, 1796–1853; L, *orbita,* wheel track + Gk, *pathos,* disease], An ocular disease usually occurring in patients with hyperthyroidism or a history of hyperthyroidism due to Graves disease. The most common clinical features are upper eyelid retraction, redness and swelling of the periorbital tissues and conjunctivae, and bulging eyes. Also called *Graves ophthalmopathy.*

gravid /grav′id/ [L, *gravidus,* pregnant], pregnant or capable of becoming pregnant. −*gravidness, gravidity, n.*

gravid-, prefix meaning "pregnancy" or "pregnant": *gravida, gravid, gravidarum chloasma.*

gravida /grav′idə/ [L, *gravidus,* pregnant], a woman who is pregnant or who has been pregnant, regardless of the pregnancy outcome. The patient may be identified more specifically as gravida I if pregnant for the first time, for example, or gravida II if pregnant a second time.

-gravida, suffix meaning "pregnant woman with (specified) quantity of pregnancies": *nulligravida, primigravida.*

gravida I or 1. See **primigravida.**

gravida II or 2, a woman who has been pregnant twice, regardless of outcome. See also **secundigravida.**

gravidarum chloasma /grav′ider″əm, gräv′idär″-/ [L, *gravidus,* pregnant; Gk, *chloazein,* to be green], hyperpigmentation in circumscribed areas of the skin associated with pregnancy. See also **chloasma.**

gravidum gingivitis /grav′idəm/ [L, *gravidus,* pregnant, *gingiva,* gums, *itis,* inflammation], a nonspecific, noninfectious inflammation of the gums during pregnancy. Also called **pregnancy gingivitis.**

gravimetric analysis. See **quantitative analysis.**

gravitational insecurity, refers to an excessive fear of ordinary movement, being out of an upright position, or having one's feet off the ground.

gravity /grav′itē/ [L, *gravis,* heavy], the universal effect of the attraction between any body of matter and any planetary body. The force of the attraction depends on the relative masses of the bodies and on the inverse of the square of the distance between them.

gravity-eliminated plane, a supported position or plane in which the effect of gravity is absorbed or neutralized. In evaluation of muscle strength, certain tests are conducted in the gravity-eliminated plane. Other tests may involve movements against the force of gravity.

gravity goniometer, an instrument used for measuring joint angles, consisting of a device that rests on or is strapped to the part to be measured and a dial that rotates behind a weighted pointer that remains vertical by force of gravity.

gray (Gy), the SI unit of absorbed radiation dose. One gray equals the energy equivalent of 1 J/kg of matter; 1 Gy equals 100 rad. See also **radiation absorbed dose.**

gray baby syndrome. See **gray syndrome.**

gray column, any of the three longitudinally oriented thickenings in the spinal cord, composed of gray nervous tissue and containing the nerve cell bodies. They are commonly referred to as *horns* because in transverse sections of the spinal cord they have the appearance of horns. See also **anterior horn, lateral horn, posterior horn.**

gray hepatization. See **hepatization.**

gray matter, the gray nervous tissue found in the cortex of the cerebrum and cerebellum and the core of the spinal cord. It is predominantly composed of neuron cell bodies and unmyelinated axons. The gray color is produced by cytoplasmic elements seen in all cell bodies and processes not covered by whitish myelin. Nuclei in the gray substance of the spinal cord function as centers for all spinal reflexes. Also called **gray substance.** Compare **white matter.** See also **cerebellum, cerebral cortex, cerebrum, spinal cord, spinal nerves.**

gray ramus communicans, the communicating branch of nerves that connects the sympathetic trunk or a ganglion to the anterior ramus and contains the postganglionic sympathetic fibers.

gray scale, 1. the property in which intensity information in ultrasonography is recorded as changes in the brightness of the gray scale display. 2. (in radiology) the number of shades of gray displayed in an image.

gray scale display, in ultrasonography, a signal-processing method for selectively amplifying and displaying the level echoes from soft tissues at the expense of the larger echoes. Also called **compression amplification.**

gray substance. See **gray matter.**

gray syndrome, a toxic condition in neonates, especially premature infants, caused by a reaction to chloramphenicol. Because the body's mechanisms for detoxification and excretion of drugs are immature, the infant has limited ability to conjugate and thus eliminate the chloramphenicol. The condition is named for the characteristic ashen-gray cyanosis, which is accompanied by abdominal distension, hypothermia, vomiting, respiratory distress, and vascular collapse. The syndrome, which is fatal if the drug is continued, can be prevented by conservative dosages of the drug and by restriction of its use in women during late pregnancy or labor (because chloramphenicol readily crosses the placental barrier) and in lactating mothers. Also called **gray baby syndrome.**

GRE, abbreviation for **Graduate Record Examination.**

great auricular nerve [AS, large; L, *auricula,* little ear, *nervus,* nerve], one of a pair of cutaneous branches of the cervical plexus, arising from the second and the third cervical nerves. It is distributed to the skin of the face and the skin of the mastoid process. It also communicates with the lesser occipital nerve, the auricular branch of the vagus nerve, and the posterior auricular branch of the facial nerve.

great calorie.   See **Calorie.**

great cardiac vein,   one of the five tributaries of the coronary sinus, beginning at the apex of the heart and ascending along the anterior interventricular sulcus to the base of the ventricles. It then curves left in the coronary sulcus, reaches the back of the heart, and opens into the left part of the coronary sinus. It receives various tributaries from the left atrium. The great cardiac vein drains the blood through its tributaries from the capillaries of the myocardium. Also called **vena cordis magna.** Compare **middle cardiac vein, small cardiac vein.**

great cerebral vein of Galen.   See **Galen's vein.**

greater circulation.   See **systemic circulation.**

greater multangular.   See **trapezium.**

greater omentum [AS, *great,* large; L, *omentum,* entrails], a filmy, transparent double fold of the peritoneum, draping the transverse colon and coils of the small intestine. It is attached along the greater curvature of the stomach and the first part of the duodenum. It is a readily movable structure that spreads easily into areas of trauma, often sealing hernias and walling off infections that would otherwise cause general peritonitis, as can occur from a ruptured vermiform appendix. It also contains fat and maintains the temperature of the intestines. Also called **gastrocolic omentum.** Compare **lesser omentum.**

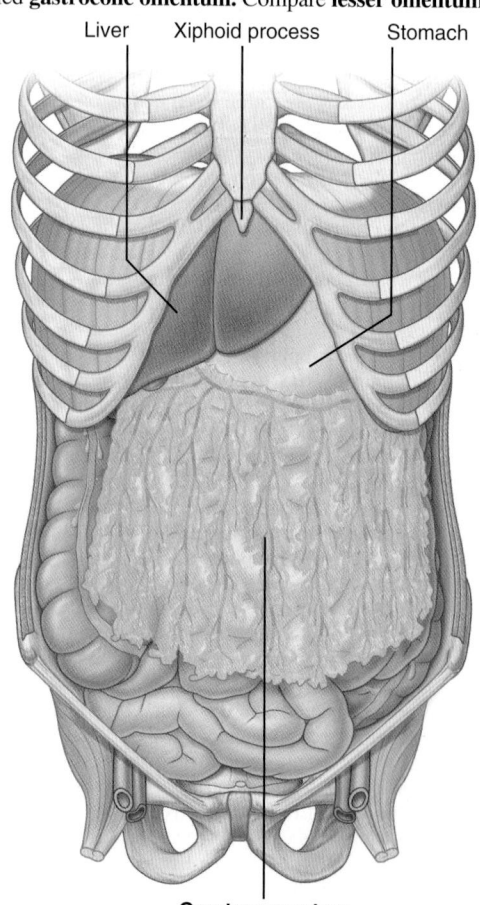

Liver   Xiphoid process   Stomach

Greater omentum

Greater omentum *(Drake, Vogl, and Mitchell, 2015)*

greater palatine artery,   a branch of the maxillary artery that supplies anterior regions of the medial wall and adjacent floor of the nasal cavity. It anastomoses with the septal branch of the sphenopalatine artery.

greater petrosal nerve,   a branch of the facial nerve that innervates all the salivary glands above the level of the oral fissure, as well as all mucus glands in the nose and the lacrimal gland in the orbit.

greater saphenous vein,   one of a pair of the longest veins in the body, which contains 10 to 20 valves along its course through the leg and the thigh before ending in the femoral vein. It begins in the medial marginal vein of the dorsum of the foot and ascends anteriorly to the tibial malleolus and up the medial side of the leg in relation to the saphenous nerve. It runs posteriorly to the medial condyles of the tibia and the femur and passes through the saphenous hiatus immediately before joining the femoral vein. It contains more valves in the leg than in the thigh and receives many cutaneous veins and numerous tributaries, such as those from the sole of the foot. Near the saphenous hiatus it is joined by the superficial epigastric vein, the superficial epigastric circumflex, and the superficial external pudendal veins. Also called **saphenous vein.** Compare **common iliac vein, femoral vein.**

greater sciatic foramen [AS, *great* + Gk, *ischiadikos,* hip joint; L, *foramen,* hole], a major route of communication between the pelvic cavity and the lower limb, formed by the greater sciatic notch in the pelvic bone, the sacrotuberous and sacrospinous ligaments, and the spine of the ischium.

greater sciatic notch [AS, *great,* large; Gk, *ischiadikos,* hip joint; OFr, *enochier,* notch], a notch on the posterior border of the hip bone between the posterior inferior iliac spine and the spine of the ischium.

greater trochanter,   a large projection of the femur to which are attached various muscles, including the gluteus medius, gluteus maximus, and obturator internus. The greater trochanter projects from the angle formed by the neck and body of the femur.

greater vestibular gland.   See **Bartholin gland.**

great foramen,   a passage in the occipital bone through which the spinal cord enters the spinal column.

great membrane,   the external components of a membrane, such as the layer of carbohydrate molecules on the outer surface.

great vessel,   one of the large arteries and veins entering and leaving the heart. They include the aorta, the pulmonary arteries and veins, and the superior and inferior vena cava.

Greenfield filter [L. Greenfield, 20th-century American surgeon], a filter placed in the inferior vena cava under fluoroscopic guidance. It is used in patients who are particularly vulnerable to pulmonary embolism, such as those diagnosed with deep venous thrombosis with contraindications to anticoagulation, to prevent venous emboli from entering the pulmonary circulation.

Greenfield disease [Joseph G. Greenfield, British pathologist, 1884–1958], a disorder of the white matter of the brain tissue, characterized by an accumulation of sphingolipid in both parenchymal and supportive tissues and a diffuse loss of myelination. An infantile form usually begins by the third year of life, with symptoms that include loss of vision, rigidity, motor disorders, and mental deterioration. A juvenile form usually begins before 10 years of age and an adult form after 16 years of age; the adult form is marked by psychiatric symptoms that progress to dementia. See also **leukodystrophy.**

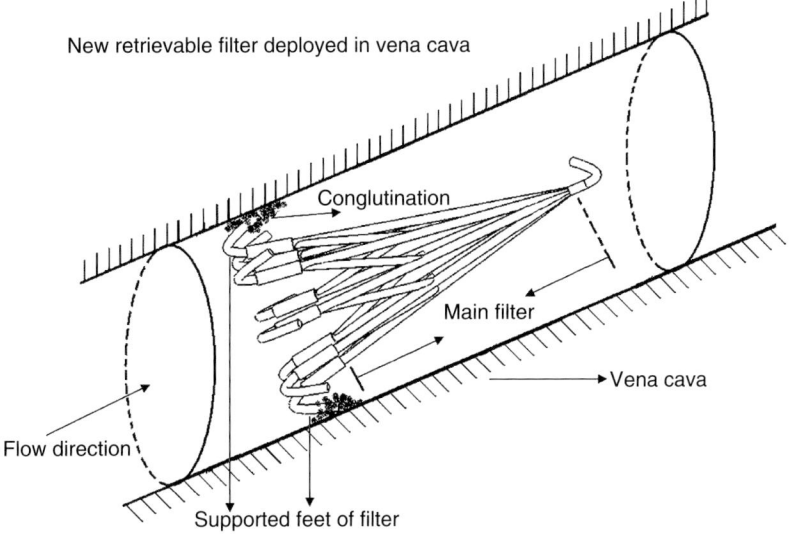

New retrievable filter deployed in vena cava

Conglutination

Main filter

Vena cava

Flow direction

Supported feet of filter

Greenfield filter *(Chen et al, 2012)*

green fluorescent protein (GFP), a protein obtained from the jellyfish *Aequorea victoria* that emits a bright green fluorescence when illuminated. GFP is used to monitor gene expression, gene transfer across plasma membranes, and cell surface activity.

greenhouse effect, a theorized change in the earth's climate caused by accumulation of solar heat in the earth's surface and atmosphere. Human activity contributes increasing amounts of the so-called greenhouse gases, such as carbon dioxide, methane, and chlorofluorocarbon, to the atmosphere. Some of the particles and gases in the atmosphere also allow more sunlight to filter through to the earth's surface but reflect much of the radiant infrared energy that otherwise would escape through the atmosphere back into space. See also **global warming.**

Greenough microscope. See **stereoscopic microscope.**

green soap [AS, *grene* + L, *sapo*], a soft soap made from vegetable oils with sodium or potassium hydroxide in concentrations adjusted to retain glycerol. The soap actually may be any color, depending on the oils added.

green soap tincture [AS, *grene* + L, *sapo*, soap, *tinctura*, dyeing], an alcoholic solution of green soap with lavender oil added.

greenstick fracture [AS, *grene* + *stician*], an incomplete fracture in which the bone is bent but broken only on the outer arc of the bend. Children, especially those with rickets, are particularly likely to have greenstick fractures. Immobilization is usually effective, and healing is rapid. Also called **bent fracture, hickory stick fracture.** See also **fracture.**

green tea, an herb that grows as a native shrub in Asia.
■ INDICATIONS: It is used to prevent cancer and heart disease, for hypercholesterolemia, and as an antidiarrheal. It is effective as an antidiarrheal, and there is some epidemiological evidence of efficacy related to its other uses.
■ CONTRAINDICATIONS: It is contraindicated in those with known hypersensitivity to this product and in those with kidney inflammation, GI ulcers, insomnia, cardiovascular disease, and increased intraocular pressure.

green tobacco sickness, a nicotine-induced illness of tobacco harvest workers characterized by headache, dizziness, vomiting, and prostration. It is caused by skin contact with wet tobacco leaves.

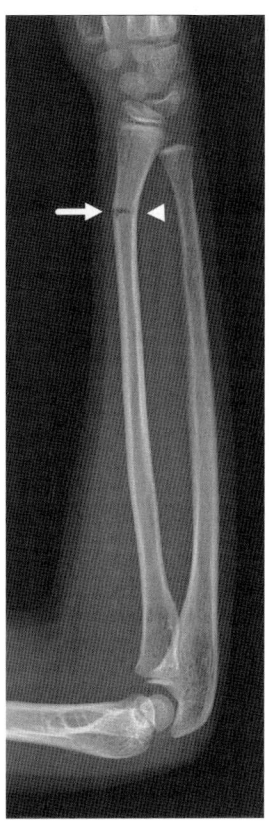

Greenstick fracture *(Ho-Fung et al, 2017)*

-grel, suffix for a platelet antiaggregate.

grenz rays [Ger, *Grenze*, boundary; L, *radius*, ray], low-energy x-rays with very little penetrating ability that are frequently applied by dermatologists, rather than by radiotherapists, for the treatment of skin conditions.

Greulich-Pyle method /groi″lish pīl″, grōō″lik-/, a technique for evaluating the bone age of children by using a single frontal radiograph of the left hand and wrist.

Grey Turner sign [George Grey Turner, English surgeon, 1877–1951], bruising of the skin of the loin in acute hemorrhagic pancreatitis. Also called **Turner sign.**

grid [ME, *gredire,* grate], a device used during a radiographic examination to absorb radiation that is not heading along a straight line from the x-ray source to the image receptor. Such scattered radiation does not contribute useful information and thus constitutes a source of unwanted density. A linear grid consists of alternating parallel strips of radiopaque and radiolucent material. Linear grids may cause variations in image density because of primary-photon attenuation. Density is at a maximum in the center of the image receptor and decreases toward the edges.

grid cutoff, an undesirable absorption of primary-beam x-rays by a grid, which prevents useful x-rays from reaching the image receptor. It is an effect of improper grid positioning and occurs most commonly with linear grids.

grid ratio, (in radiology) the ratio of the height of the lead strips to the width of the interspacing of a grid.

grief [L, *gravis,* heavy], a nearly universal pattern of physical and emotional responses to bereavement, separation, or loss. It is time linked and must be differentiated from depression. The physical components are similar to those of fear, rage, and pain: Stimulation of the sympathetic portion of the autonomic nervous system can cause increased heart and respiratory rates, dilated pupils, sweating, bristling of the hair, increased blood flow to the muscles, and increased energy reserves. Digestion slows. The emotional components proceed in stages from alarm to disbelief and denial, to anger and guilt, to a search for a source of comfort, and, finally, to adjustment to the loss. The way in which a grieving person behaves is greatly affected by the culture in which he or she has been reared. See also **bereavement, parental grief.**

grief reaction, a complex of somatic and psychological symptoms associated with extreme sorrow or loss, specifically the death of a loved one. Somatic symptoms include feelings of tightness in the throat and chest with choking and shortness of breath, abdominal distress, lack of muscular power, and extreme tiredness and lethargy. Psychological reactions involve a generalized awareness of mental anguish and discomfort accompanied by feelings of guilt, anger, hostility, extreme restlessness, inability to concentrate, and lack of capacity to initiate and maintain organized patterns of activities. Such symptoms may appear immediately after a crisis, or they may be delayed, exaggerated, or apparently absent, depending on the degree of involvement of the relationship and the physical and mental status of the person. Although both the somatic and psychological reactions have the potential for developing into pathological conditions, appropriate adaptive behavior and normal responses, such as sobbing or talking about the dead person or tragedy, are methods of working through the acute grief and lead to successful resolution of the crisis. Most acute grief reactions are resolved within 4 to 6 weeks, although the period varies and may be much longer, especially in cases of unexpected and sudden death. Intervention by health care professionals, especially nurses, is necessary when individuals exhibit maladaptive behavioral patterns that prevent the resolution of grief and can lead to morbid reactions, including such accepted psychosomatic illnesses as asthma and ulcers.

griffe des orteils. See **clawfoot.**

Grifulvin, an antifungal drug. Brand name for **griseofulvin.**

grinder's asthma /grīn′dərz/ [ME, *grinden,* to crush; Gk, panting], a condition characterized by asthmatic symptoms caused by inhalation of fine particles produced by industrial grinding processes. See also **pneumoconiosis.**

grinder's disease. See **silicosis.**

grinding-in, a clinical corrective adjustment of one or more natural or artificial teeth to improve centric and eccentric occlusions. Compare **occlusal adjustment, selective grinding.**

grip and pinch strength, the measurable ability to exert pressure with the hand, fingers, or both. It is measured by having a patient forcefully squeeze, grip, or pinch dynamometers; results are expressed in either pounds or kilograms of pressure.

gripes /grīps/ [AS, *gripan,* to grasp], severe and usually spasmodic pain in the abdominal region caused by an intestinal disorder. Also called *griping.*

grippe. *(Obsolete)* See **influenza.**

Grisactin, an antifungal drug. Brand name for **griseofulvin.**

griseofulvin /gris′ē·ōful″vin/, an antifungal drug.

■ INDICATIONS: It is prescribed in the treatment of certain fungal infections of the skin, hair, and nails.

■ CONTRAINDICATIONS: Liver dysfunction, porphyria, or known hypersensitivity to this drug prohibits its use.

■ ADVERSE EFFECTS: The most serious adverse effects are blood dyscrasias. Headache, GI symptoms, and rashes also may occur.

generalized tonic-clonic seizure, an epileptic seizure characterized by a generalized involuntary muscular contraction and cessation of respiration followed by tonic and clonic spasms of the muscles. Breathing resumes with noisy respirations. The teeth may be clenched, the tongue bitten, and control of the bladder or bowel lost. As this phase of the seizure passes, the person may fall asleep or experience confusion. Usually the person has no recall of the seizure on awakening. A sensory warning, or aura, can precede each tonic-clonic seizure. These seizures may occur singly, at intervals, or in close succession. Anticonvulsant medications are usually prescribed as prophylaxis against tonic-clonic seizures. Also called **grand mal seizure.** Compare **absence seizure, focal seizure, psychomotor seizure.**

Griswald brace, an orthosis for the control of vertebral body compression fractures, designed with two anterior forces that are each equal to one half the posterior force to extend the spine. Also called **Jewett brace.**

Grocco sign, Grocco triangle. See **Korányi sign.**

grocer's itch [AS, *gican,* itch], a dermatitis caused by contact with mites found in grain, cheese, or dried foods. Also called *Glycyphagus domesticus.*

groin [ME, *grynde*], each of two areas where the abdomen joins the thighs; the inguinal area.

grommet /grom′et/, a tube inserted through the tympanic membrane for drainage of the middle ear.

Grönblad-Strandberg syndrome /grōn″blad strand″bərg/ [Ester E. Grönblad, Swedish ophthalmologist, 1898–1942; James V. Strandberg, Swedish dermatologist, 1883–1942], an autosomal-recessive disorder of connective tissue characterized by premature aging and breakdown of the skin (first affecting the neck), gray or brown streaks on the retina, and hemorrhagic arterial degeneration, including retinal bleeding that causes vision loss. Angina pectoris and hypertension are common. Weak pulse, episodic cramplike pains in the calves, and fatigue with exertion may affect the extremities. The prognosis depends on vessel involvement, but life expectancy is shortened. Treatment is symptomatic. Also called **pseudoxanthoma elasticum.**

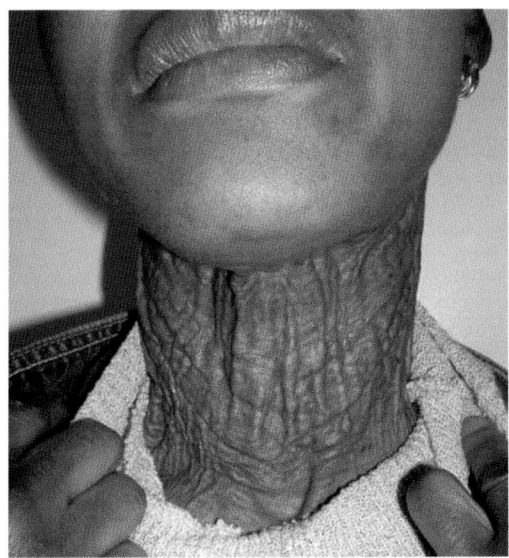

Neck skin of woman with Grönblad-Strandberg syndrome *(Akram et al, 2007)*

groove [AS, *grafan,* to dig], a shallow, linear depression in various structures throughout the body, such as those that form channels for nerves along the bones, those in bones for the insertion of muscles, and those between certain areas of the brain.

grooved pegboard test, a method for evaluating psychomotor function by measuring how quickly a subject can insert pegs into grooved holes. The test is reported to be sensitive to the effects of various neurotoxins that can affect perception and dexterity.

Groshong catheter, a modification of the Hickman catheter with a valve that is closed when the catheter is not in use. It is used for long-term administration of substances such as antibiotics, total parenteral nutrition, or chemotherapeutic agents.

gross [OFr, *gros,* large], macroscopic, as in gross pathology; the study of tissue changes without magnification by a microscope. Compare **microscopic.**

gross anatomy, the study of the organs or parts of the body large enough to be seen with the naked eye. Also called **macroscopic anatomy.**

Grossman principle, (in tomography) the principle that when the fulcrum or axis of rotation remains at a fixed point, the focal plane is changed by raising or lowering the table top through this point to the desired height.

gross motor skills [Fr, *gros,* big; L, *movere,* ONorse, *skilja,* to cut apart], the ability to use large muscle groups that coordinate body movements involved in activities such as walking, running, jumping, throwing, and maintaining balance.

gross sensory testing, an evaluation procedure that includes assessment of passive motion sense in the shoulder, elbow, wrist, and fingers and the ability to localize touch stimuli to specific fingers. It usually precedes motor evaluation of a patient.

gross visual skills, the general ability of a person to track a large, bright object side to side or up to down without jerkiness, nystagmus, or convergence and to discriminate among various basic shapes and colors.

ground [AS, *grund*], **1.** (in electricity) a connection between the electric circuit and the ground, which becomes a part of the circuit. **2.** (in psychology) the background of a visual field that can enhance or inhibit the ability of a patient to focus on an object.

grounding pad, an inactive electrode, part of a monopolar electrocautery, that is attached to the patient and returns the current distributed from the active electrode to the generator through an attached cable to complete the electrical circuit.

ground itch, pruritic papules and/or urticarial vesiculopustular lesions secondary to penetration of the skin by hookworm or threadworm larvae. The condition is prevalent in tropical and subtropical climates and may be prevented by wearing shoes and by establishing sanitary disposal of feces. See also **hookworm.**

ground state, **1.** the lowest energy level of a physical system. See also **fatigue state. 2.** the most energetically stable form of an atom or molecule.

ground substance. See **matrix.**

group [Fr, *groupe,* cluster], (in research) any set of items or people under study. See also **control group, experimental group.**

group B arbovirus. *(Obsolete)* See *Flavivirus.*

group dynamics [Fr, *groupe* + Gk, *dynamis,* force], the interactions and relationships that take place among group members as well as between the group and the rest of society. It includes interdependence of group members, collective problem solving and decision making, and group conformity.

grouper /grōōp′er/, any of various, usually large marine fish of the genera *Epinephelus* and *Mycteroperca,* found in tropical waters. They are often eaten by humans but sometimes contain ciguatoxin and can cause ciguatera.

group function, (in dentistry) the simultaneous contacting of opposing teeth in a segment or a unit, used to stabilize a full maxillary and mandibular denture during eccentric motion of the mandible in relation to the maxilla.

group-model HMO, a health maintenance organization (HMO) in which a contract is established with multispecialty medical groups for medical services. The HMO is responsible for marketing and developing contracts with enrollees and hospitals. Care is provided at hospitals where the physicians have admitting privileges or at ancillary facilities with which the HMO subcontracts.

group practice, two or more physicians, advanced practice nurses, and/or physician assistants who work together and share facilities. The physicians may practice different specialties. Physicians who are part of a group often are prohibited from becoming independent contractors and earning money by providing medical care outside the group.

group practice without walls (GPWW), a medical practice formed to share economic risk, expenses, and marketing efforts. Physicians retain separate offices and finances. Often a central site is established to house administrative services and some or all ancillary services.

group specificity, **1.** an enzyme property that is specific to both the type of bond and structure. See **specificity. 2.** (in epidemiology) a proportion of persons without disease who are correctly identified by a screening test or case definition as not having disease.

group therapy, the application of psychotherapeutic techniques within a group of people (usually 10 or fewer) who are experiencing similar difficulties. Generally a group leader directs the discussion of problems in an attempt to promote individual psychological growth and favorable personality change. The procedure provides opportunities for treating a greater number of people in a shorter time than would be possible with individual therapy, and it is used in clinics, in institutions, and in private practice. Group therapy has been found to be particularly effective in the treatment of various

G

substance abuse disorders. Kinds include **psychodrama.** See also **Gestalt therapy, psychotherapy, self-help group, transactional analysis.**

growing fracture [AS, *growan* + L, *fractura,* to break], a fracture, usually linear, in which consecutive radiographic images show a gradual separation of the fracture edges over time. The separation is often caused by the pressure of soft tissues, as when arachnoid tissues expand through the edges of a skull fracture.

growing pains, **1.** aches and a throbbing sensation that occur in the muscles of children or adolescents usually at night. There is no evidence that growth is painful, and the cause of growing pains is unknown. Growing pains may be a result of fatigue, emotional problems, postural defects, or other causes that are unrelated to growth. Most often, there is no identifiable cause and no treatment is required. **2.** *(Informal)* emotional and psychological problems experienced during adolescence.

growth [AS, *growan,* to grow], **1.** an increase in the size of an organism or any of its parts, as measured in increments of weight, volume, or linear dimensions, that occurs as a result of hyperplasia or hypertrophy. **2.** the normal progressive anatomical, physiological development from infancy to adulthood that is the result of gradual and normal processes of accretion and assimilation. The total of the numerous changes that occur during the lifetime of an individual constitutes a dynamic and complex process that involves many interrelated components, notably heredity, environment, nutrition, hygiene, and disease, all of which are subject to a variety of influences. In childhood growth is categorized according to the approximate age at which distinctive physical changes usually appear and at which specific developmental tasks are achieved. Such stages include the prenatal period, infancy, early childhood (including the toddler and the preschool periods), middle childhood, and adolescence. There are two periods of accelerated growth: (1) the first 12 months, in which the infant triples in weight, increases the height at birth by approximately 50%, and undergoes rapid motor, cognitive, and social development; and (2) the second, and the months around puberty, when the child approaches adult height and secondary sexual characteristics emerge. Physical growth may be abnormally accelerated or slowed by a defect in the hypophyseal or pituitary gland. **3.** any abnormal localized increase of the size or number of cells, as in a tumor or neoplasm. **4.** a proliferation of cells, specifically a bacterial culture or mold. Compare **development, differentiation, maturation.**

growth charts, graphic displays of normal progressive changes in height, weight, and head circumference. They consider the range of growth as expressed in percentiles or as standard deviation from the mean for average height, weight, and BMI for age. Head circumference measurements are common from birth to 2 years of age.

growth curve, a graphic display of data showing proliferation of cell numbers in a culture as a function of time.

growth factor, any protein that stimulates the division and differentiation of specific types of cells. Growth factors specifically involved in the division and differentiation of bone marrow stem cells are classified as colony-stimulating factors. Platelets are a rich source of growth factors, some of which may be involved in the cellular proliferation that occurs in diseases such as rheumatoid arthritis and glomerulonephritis. Kinds include *platelet-derived growth factor,* **epidermal growth factor, nerve growth factor.** See also **cytokine.**

growth factor receptor, a plasma membrane–spanning protein that binds with a specific growth factor on the external surface of a cell and transduces a signal that triggers cell division.

growth failure, a lack of normal physical and psychological development that results from genetic, nutritional, pathological, or psychosocial factors. See also **failure to thrive, maternal deprivation syndrome.**

growth hormone (GH), a single-chain peptide secreted by the anterior pituitary gland in response to GH-releasing hormone. Its secretion is controlled in part by the hypothalamus. GH promotes protein synthesis in all cells, increases fat mobilization and use of fatty acids for energy, and decreases use of carbohydrate. Growth effects depend on the presence of thyroid hormone, insulin, and carbohydrate. Somatomedins, proteins produced chiefly in the liver, play a vital role in GH-induced skeletal growth. GH cannot cause elongation of long bones after the epiphyses close, however, so stature does not increase after puberty. GH accelerates the transport of specific amino acids into cells, stimulates the synthesis of messenger ribonucleic acid (RNA) and ribosomal RNA, influences the activity of several enzymes, increases the storage of phosphorus and potassium, and promotes a moderate retention of sodium. GH secretion, controlled almost exclusively by the central nervous system, occurs in bursts, with more than half of the total daily amount released during early sleep. Somatostatin, an anterior pituitary regulating hormone produced in the hypothalamus, inhibits GH secretion as well as secretion of insulin and gastrin. A deficiency of GH causes dwarfism; an excess results in gigantism in children or acromegaly in adults. Also called **somatotropic hormone, somatotropin.** See also **acromegaly, dwarfism, gigantism, somatostatin.**

growth hormone release–inhibiting hormone. See **somatostatin.**

growth hormone–releasing hormone (GH-RH), a neuropeptide released by the hypothalamus that travels to the anterior pituitary to stimulate growth hormone release. Also called *somatocrinin,* **somatoliberin, somatotropin-releasing hormone.**

growth hormone (GH) test, a blood test, usually after an arginine infusion followed by insulin-induced hypoglycemia, used to identify growth hormone deficiency in adolescents who have short stature, delayed sexual maturity, or other growth deficiencies. It is also used to document the diagnosis of GH excess in gigantic or acromegalic patients and to screen for pituitary hypofunction.

growth phase, one of the stages in the growth of a neoplasm.

growth plate. See **epiphyseal plate.**

growth retardation, failure of an individual to develop at a normal rate of height and weight for his or her age. See also **intrauterine growth retardation.**

grunting [ME, *grunten*], abnormal, short, deep, hoarse sounds in exhalation that often accompany severe chest pain. The grunt occurs because the glottis briefly stops the flow of air, halting the movement of the lungs and their surrounding or supporting structures. Grunting is most often heard in a person who has pneumonia, pulmonary edema, or fractured or bruised ribs. Atelectasis in the newborn also causes grunting, which results from the effort required to fill the lungs.

GSA, abbreviation for **Gerontological Society of America.**

GSD, abbreviation for **genetically significant dose.**

GSR, abbreviation for **galvanic skin response.**

GSW, abbreviation for **gunshot wound.**

G syndrome. See **Smith-Lemli-Opitz syndrome.**

gt, abbreviation for **gutta.**

GTP, abbreviation for **guanosine triphosphate.**

GTPase, enzyme activity that catalyzes the hydrolysis of guanosine triphosphate to guanosine diphosphate and orthophosphate.

GTT, abbreviation for **glucose tolerance test.**

gtt, gtts, GTTS, abbreviation for **guttae.**

G tube, Also called **stomach tube.** See **gastrostomy tube.**

GU, abbreviation for **genitourinary.**

guaiac /gwī′ak/, a wood resin, formerly used as a reagent in laboratory tests for the presence of occult blood.

guaiacol poisoning. See **phenol poisoning.**

guaiac test, a test, using guaiac as a reagent, formerly performed on feces and urine for detecting occult blood in the intestinal and urinary tracts.

guaifenesin /gwī′əfen″əsin/, glyceryl guaiacolate, a white to slightly gray powder with a bitter taste and faint odor, widely used as an expectorant. Guaifenesin increases the flow of fluid in the respiratory tract, reducing the viscosity of bronchial and tracheal secretions and facilitating their removal by the cough reflex and ciliary action. It may increase the risk of hemorrhage in patients taking heparin.

guanabenz acetate /gwan′abenz/, a centrally acting alpha$_2$ adrenergic agonist that decreases sympathetic nervous system tone.
- INDICATIONS: It is prescribed in the treatment of hypertension.
- CONTRAINDICATIONS: Known hypersensitivity to this drug prohibits its use.
- ADVERSE EFFECTS: Among adverse effects are dizziness, sedation, and dry mouth.

guanadrel /gwä′nädrel/, an adrenergic neuron blocking agent used in the treatment of hypertension and used as the sulfate salt.

guanadrel sulfate /gwan′ədril/, an antihypertensive agent.
- INDICATIONS: It is prescribed in the treatment of hypertension in patients who do not respond to first-line agents, usually in combination with a diuretic.
- CONTRAINDICATIONS: Pheochromocytoma, administration of monoamine oxidase inhibitors, frank congestive heart failure, or known sensitivity to this drug prohibits its use.
- ADVERSE EFFECTS: Among the most serious adverse effects are orthostatic hypotension and syncope.

guanase. See **guanine deaminase.**

guanethidine sulfate /gwaneth′idēn/, a peripherally acting antiadrenergic antihypertensive.
- INDICATIONS: It is prescribed in the treatment of moderate and severe hypertension.
- CONTRAINDICATIONS: Heart failure, concomitant administration of monoamine oxidase inhibitors, pheochromocytoma, or known hypersensitivity to this drug prohibits its use. It should be avoided in elderly patients.
- ADVERSE EFFECTS: Among the more serious adverse effects are orthostatic hypotension, salt and water retention, bradycardia, diarrhea, and inability to ejaculate.

guanine /gwan′ēn/, a purine base that is a component of DNA and RNA. In free or uncombined form it occurs in trace amounts in most cells, usually as a product of the enzymatic hydrolysis of nucleic acids and nucleotides. On hydrolysis it is first converted into xanthine and finally into uric acid. See also **adenine.**

guanine deaminase, an enzyme that catalyzes the hydrolysis of guanine to xanthine and ammonia. It is present in the liver, kidney, spleen, and other tissues. Also called **guanase.**

guanosine /gwan″ōsēn/, a nucleoside composed of guanine and a sugar, D-ribose. It is a major component of the nucleotides guanosine monophosphate and guanosine triphosphate and of RNA. A related nucleoside, deoxyguanosine, is a major component of DNA.

guanosine deaminase. See **deaminase.**

guanosine monophosphate (GMP), a nucleotide that plays an important role in various metabolic reactions and in the formation of RNA from DNA templates.

guanosine triphosphate (GTP), a high-energy nucleotide, similar to adenosine triphosphate, that functions in various metabolic reactions, such as the activation of fatty acids and the formation of peptide bonds in protein synthesis.

guaranine /gwərä′nin/, caffeine.

guardian ad litem /ad lī′təm/ [L, *ad litem,* to litigate], (in law) a person who is appointed by a court to prosecute or defend a suit for an infant or an incapacitated person. A guardian ad litem is sometimes appointed when a person's life is in imminent danger and that person refuses treatment.

guardianship, a legal status that places the care and property of an individual in the hands of another person. Implementation of the law varies in different cases and jurisdictions.

guarding. See **abdominal splinting.**

Guarnieri bodies /gŏŏ′ärnyer″ēz/ [Giuseppi Guarnieri, Italian physician, 1856–1918], acidophilic inclusion bodies that are formed in the cytoplasm of cells infected with cowpox or vaccinia virus. Now called *B-type inclusions.*

Gubbay test of motor proficiency, a screening test for the identification of developmental dyspraxia, consisting of eight activities, such as whistling, throwing a tennis ball, and fitting shapes into appropriate slots. The results of the test discriminate between impaired motor function and normal development in children.

gubernaculum, a fetal ligament that passes through the anterior abdominal wall and connects the inferior pole of each gonad with primordia of the scrotum in men and the labia majora in women.

Guedel's signs /gŏŏ′dəlz/ [Arthur E. Guedel, American anesthesiologist, 1883–1956]. See **stages of anesthesia.**

Guérin's fracture /gāraNz″/ [Alphonse F.M. Guérin, French surgeon, 1816–1895], a break in the maxilla. Also called **LeFort I fracture.**

guggul, an herb that is native to India.
- INDICATIONS: It is used for high LDL cholesterol, elevated triglycerides, and weight loss.
- CONTRAINDICATIONS: Its use is contraindicated during pregnancy, because it can cause uterine contractions. It also should not be used during lactation, in children, and in those with known hypersensitivity to this product.

guided imagery /gī′did/, a therapeutic technique in which the patient enters a relaxed state and focuses on an image related to the issue being confronted. The therapist uses the image as the basis of an interactive dialogue to help the person resolve the issue. It is used for a wide variety of indications, including relaxation and stress management, behavior modification, pain management, and the treatment of life-threatening and terminal illness.

guide dog [ME, *guiden,* to guard; OE, *docga*], a dog trained to aid in the mobility of a blind or visually impaired individual. Guide dogs are usually recruited from certain compatible breeds and tested at 13 weeks of age. If qualified, the dog is then specially trained in private hands for 1 year and retested. Most dogs selected for training pass the final test. Guide dogs also may be trained to serve as "ears" for people who are deaf or hearing impaired. Also called **companion animal, Seeing Eye dog.**

guided reminiscence, in reminiscence therapy, the eliciting of recollections of past experiences by the use of open-ended questions.

guide plane [ME, *guiden,* to guard; L, *planum,* level ground], **1.** a part of an orthodontic appliance that has an established inclined plane for changing the occlusal relation of the maxillary and mandibular teeth and for permitting their movement to normal positions. **2.** a plane that is developed on the occlusal surfaces of occlusion rims for positioning the mandible in centric relation. **3.** two or more parallel vertical surfaces of abutment teeth shaped to direct the path of placement and removal of a partial denture.

guide-shoe marks, a radiographic image artifact caused by pressure of the guide shoes, the curved metal lips that guide x-ray film in automatic developing systems. The guide shoes leave scratches called ridge lines in the image.

guidewire /gīd'wī·ər/ [ME, *guiden,* to guard; AS, *wir*], a device used to position an IV catheter, endotracheal tube, central venous line, or gastric feeding tube or to localize a tumor during open breast biopsy.

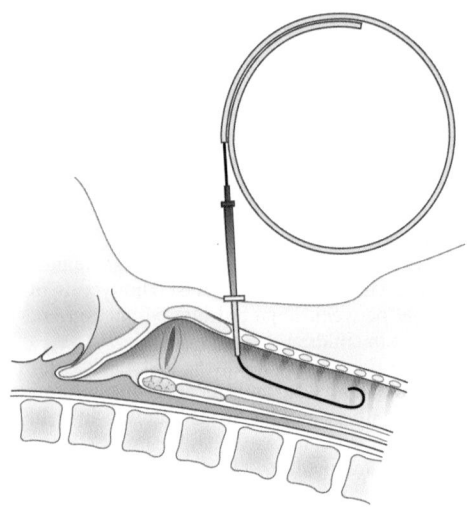

Guidewire insertion *(Hagberg, 2013)*

guiding, (in occupational therapy) a method in which therapists assist their patients in perceiving the environment by directing movement of their hands and bodies in functional activities. An example is hand-over-hand guiding in which the therapist's hand is over the patient's hand and assists in performance of a task.

Guillain-Barré syndrome /gēyan″bärā″/ [Georges Guillain, French neurologist, 1876–1951; Jean A. Barré, French neurologist, 1880–1967], an idiopathic, peripheral polyneuritis that may occur 1 to 3 weeks after a mild episode of fever associated with a viral infection or with immunization but that can also occur with no preceding illness. Symmetric pain and weakness affect the extremities, and paralysis may develop. The neuritis may spread to the trunk and face. Symptoms vary in intensity from mild to severe enough to require critical nursing care, including ventilator assistance. Immediate treatment consists of supportive care and high IV doses of immunoglobulins. Recovery depends on the extent of neuritis and may take weeks to many months. A coordinated interprofessional approach that considers long-term rehabilitation during the acute phases of the disease is necessary for optimal outcomes. Also called **acute febrile polyneuritis, acute idiopathic polyneuritis, infectious polyneuritis.**

■ OBSERVATIONS: Manifestations may range from mild to severe and generally develop 1 to 3 weeks after an upper respiratory or gastrointestinal infection. The first sign is symmetric muscle weakness in the distal extremities accompanied by paresthesia. This weakness spreads upward to the arms and trunk and then to the face. This ascension usually peaks about 2 weeks after onset. Deep tendon reflexes are com-

monly absent. Difficulty chewing, swallowing, and speaking may occur, and respiratory paralysis may develop. Signs of autonomic nervous system dysfunction, such as facial flushing, profuse diaphoresis, bowel and bladder atony, postural hypotension, hypertension, tachycardia, and heart block, may develop. Deep, aching muscle pain is also common. The diagnosis is based on history and clinical presentation. Lumbar puncture results typically reveal an increase in cerebrospinal fluid protein without an increase in lymphocyte count. Electromyography is markedly abnormal with reduced nerve conduction velocity. A small percentage of those affected die of respiratory failure. Some have permanent residual neurological deficits. Most patients make a full recovery, but the recovery time may be as long as 3 years.

■ INTERVENTIONS: Treatment is supportive, with the use of IV immunoglobulins or plasmapheresis to counteract neurological defect and speed recovery of neurological deficit. Subcutaneous heparin is given to prevent thromboembolism. Tracheostomy and mechanical ventilation are necessary to treat respiratory paralysis, and breathing function tests should be performed and followed closely. Continuous cardiac monitoring is done to detect possible sinus tachycardia and/or bradyarrhythmias. Physical and occupational therapy interventions can ameliorate the impact of neurologic deficits and prevent many of the problems associated with immobility.

■ PATIENT CARE CONSIDERATIONS: Care for patients with Guillain-Barré disease is complex and multifaceted. In acute disease, careful assessment of ascending paralysis and monitoring of respiratory function to ensure airway patency and adequate gas exchange are imperative. Continuing assessments are needed of corneal, gag, and swallow reflexes. Blood pressure is monitored for fluctuations; cardiac rate and rhythm are monitored for tachycardia, bradycardia, heart block, and asystole. Pain assessment and management are required for paresthesias, hyperesthesias, muscle cramps, and deep muscle aches. Complications related to autonomic dysfunction, paralysis, and immobility (e.g., pressure sores, thromboemboli, aspiration, urinary retention, fecal impaction, and nerve palsies) must be prevented. This includes a rigorous turning and positioning schedule, regular passive range-of-motion exercises, careful pulmonary toilet and feeding routines, application of thromboembolic stockings, and institution of bowel and bladder programs. Communication systems may be needed if the individual is on a ventilator or has facial paralysis. Emotional and social support are needed to reduce fear and anxiety. Rehabilitation may be indicated for recovery of functional abilities and long-term adaptation to permanent neurological deficit.

guilt [AS, *gylt,* delinquency], **1.** a feeling caused by tension between the ego and superego when one falls below the standards set for oneself. **2.** a remorseful awareness of having done something wrong.

guilty, (in criminal law) a verdict by the court that to a moral certainty it is beyond reasonable doubt that the defendant committed the crime and is responsible for the offense as charged.

guinea worm. See **_Dracunculus medinensis._**

Guinea worm infection. See **dracunculiasis.**

Gulf War syndrome, a group of medical and psychological complaints, including fatigue, skin rash, memory loss, and headaches, experienced by men and women who served in the 1991 Persian Gulf War. Researchers observed similar physical effects in laboratory animals exposed to a mixture of cholinesterase inhibitor insecticides and pyridostigmine; soldiers were exposed to both agents during the war.

gullet. See **esophagus.**

gum, 1. a sticky excretion from certain plants. **2.** a firm layer of flesh covering the alveolar processes of the jaws and the base of the teeth. See also **gingiva.**

gum arabic.   See **acacia gum.**

gumboil [AS, *goma,* gum + *byl*],   an abscess of the gingiva and periosteum resulting from injury, infection, or dental decay. The gum is characteristically red, swollen, and tender. The abscess may rupture spontaneously, or it may require incision. Treatment may include antibiotics and hot mouthwashes. Also called **parulis.**

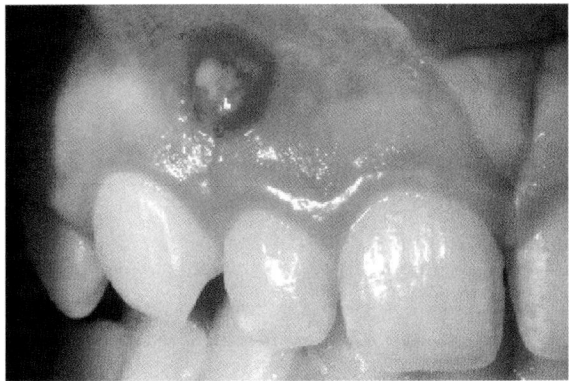

Gumboil *(Neville et al, 2015)*

gum camphor.   See **camphor.**

gum line.   See **gingival line.**

gumma /gum″ə/ *pl.* **gummas, gummata** [AS, *goma,* gum],   **1.** a granuloma, characteristic of tertiary syphilis, varying from 1 mm to 1 cm in diameter. It is usually encapsulated and contains a central necrotic mass surrounded by inflammatory and fibrotic zones of tissue. Infectious organisms of the genus *Treponema* may be found in a gumma. The lesion may be localized or diffuse, occurring on the trunk, legs, and face and on various internal organs, especially the liver. It can also form in the brain, leading to neurological problems. Rupture of a gumma produces a shallow ulcer that heals slowly. **2.** a soft granulomatous lesion that sometimes accompanies tuberculosis.

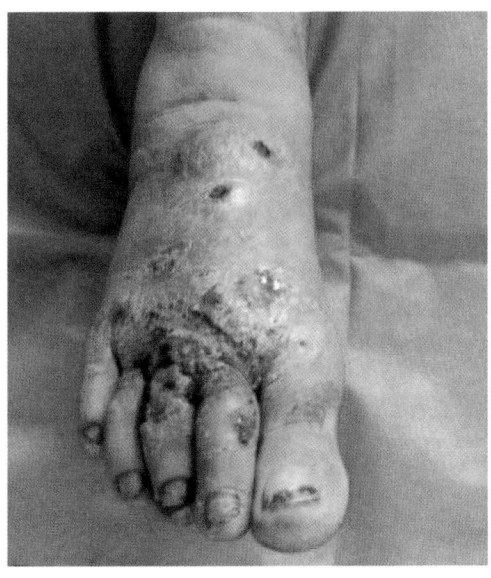

Tuberculous gummas *(Hadj et al, 2013)*

gun-barrel vision.   See **tunnel vision.**

Gunning splint [Thomas B. Gunning, American dentist, 1813–1889; D, *splinte,* split],   a splint used to support the maxilla and the mandible during jaw surgery.

Gunn syndrome.   See **jaw-winking.**

gunshot fracture [ME, *gunne* + AS, *sceotan,* to shoot; L, *fractura,* break],   a fracture caused by a bullet or similar projectile.

gunshot wound (GSW),   penetration of the body by a bullet, commonly marked by a small entrance wound and a larger exit wound. The wound is usually accompanied by damage to blood vessels, bones, and other tissues. There is high risk of infection caused by exposure of the wound to the external environment and debris carried inside the body by the bullet. Additional complications depend on the part of the body wounded.

Gunson method,   a method of radiographic examination of the pharynx and upper esophagus during swallowing. A dark-colored shoestring is tied around the patient's throat just above the thyroid cartilage. The movement of the larynx is then shown by the elevation of the shoestring as the thyroid cartilage moves anteriorly, followed immediately by displacement of the shoestring as the cartilage passes superiorly.

Günther disease /gun″thər/   [Hans Günther, German physician, 1884–1956],   a rare congenital disorder of porphyrin metabolism that is associated with sunlight-induced skin lesions. See also **porphyria.**

gurgle [Fr, *gargouiller,* to gurgle],   an abnormal coarse sound heard during auscultation, especially over large cavities or a trachea nearly filled with secretions.

gurney /gur″nē/,   a cot with wheeled legs, used in hospitals to transport patients.

Gurvich radiation.   See **mitogenetic radiation.**

gustation /gustā″shən/   [L, *gustare,* to taste],   the sense and act of tasting foods, beverages, or other substances.

gustatory /gus″tətôr′ē/   [L, *gustare,* to taste],   pertaining to the act or sense of taste or the organs of taste.

gustatory anosmia,   the inability to smell foods.

gustatory hallucination [L, *gustare,* to taste, *alucinari,* wandering mind],   a false taste sensation of either food or beverage on the mucous membrane lining the empty mouth.

gustatory organ.   See **taste bud.**

gustatory papilla [L, *gustare,* to taste, *papilla,* nipple],   any of the small tissue elevations in the mouth that contain sense organs of taste, such as the circumvallate papilla of the tongue.

gut [AS, *guttas*],   **1.** intestine. **2.** *(Informal)* digestive tract. **3.** suture material manufactured from the intestines of sheep.

gut-associated lymphoid tissue,   lymphoid tissue associated with the gut, including the tonsils, Peyer's patches, lamina propria of the GI tract, and appendix.

Guthrie bacterial inhibition assay (GBIA) /guth″rē/,   a screening for phenylketonuria (PKU) used to detect the abnormal presence of phenylalanine metabolites in the blood. A small amount of blood is obtained and placed in a medium with a strain of *Bacillus subtilis,* a bacterium that cannot grow without phenylalanine. If phenylalanine metabolites are present, the bacteria reproduce, and the test result is positive, indicating that the patient has phenylketonuria. Routine screening of newborns for PKU is now mandatory in the United States and Canada. The Guthrie blood test has normally been done before discharging the newborn from the hospital. However, it is important to note that this test is not valid until the newborn has ingested an ample amount (for 2 or 3 days) of the amino acid phenylalanine, which is a constituent of both human and cow's milk. Although the GBIA is still widely used, tandem mass spectrometry, which can screen for a wider variety of congenital diseases, is more common. Both methods still use Guthrie cards to store the dried blood of infants for testing. Also called **Guthrie test.** See also **phenylketonuria.**

G

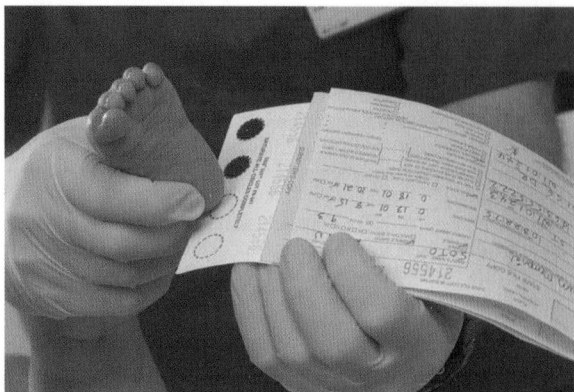

Guthrie bacterial inhibition assay *(Zakus, 2001)*

Guthrie test /guth′re/, a screening tool used with infants to determine the level of phenylalanine in the blood. Blood is placed on filter paper, which is then placed on agar plates with a strain of *Bacillus subtilis* that requires phenylalanine for growth. If there is excessive phenylalanine in the blood sample, a halo will form around the filter paper, and additional tests are required to determine the seriousness of the hyperphenylalaninemia.

gutta (gt) /gut″ə, gōōt″ä/ [L, drop], one drop, or about 1 minim, of a medication.

guttae (gtt, gtts, GTTS) [L, drops], the plural of *gutta*; more than one drop, as in *guttae pro auribus,* or ear drops, or *guttae ophthalmicae,* or eyedrops. See also **gutta.**

gutta-percha /gut′ə pur″chə/ [Malay, *getah-percha,* latex sap], the coagulated rubbery sap of various tropical trees, used along with a sealer to fill the prepared root canal in endodontic treatment and for temporarily sealing the dressings of prepared tooth cavities. When combined with fillers and coloring materials, it may be rolled into sheets and used to make temporary bases for dentures.

gutta-percha point, a small cone of gutta-percha, which, along with endodontic sealer, may be used to fill a root canal. The radiopacity of gutta-percha points permits them to be used also as probes for determining the depth and topographic characteristics of periodontal pockets and fistulas by means of radiography or dental imaging.

guttate psoriasis /gut′āt/ [L, *gutta,* drop; Gk, itch], an acute form of psoriasis that consists of teardrop-shaped red scaly papules and patches measuring 3 to 10 mm all over the body. A beta-hemolytic streptococcal pharyngitis or other upper respiratory infection may precipitate this reaction in susceptible individuals. Treatment is essential to prevent a more severe form of psoriasis. Compare **pustular psoriasis.** See also **psoriasis.**

guttural /gut′ərəl/ [L, *guttur,* throat], pertaining to or belonging to the throat, including low-pitched, raspy voice quality.

Guyon tunnel [Felix J. Guyon, French surgeon, 1831–1920], a fibroosseous tunnel formed in part by the pisohamate ligament of the hand. It contains the ulnar artery and nerve and may be the site of a compression injury.

GVHD, abbreviation for **graft-versus-host disease.**

G-Well. See **lindane.**

GXT, abbreviation for **graded exercise test.**

Gy, an SI unit. Abbreviation for **gray.**

gymnema, an herb found in India and Africa.

■ INDICATIONS: It is used to reduce high blood glucose levels; it may have some efficacy.

■ CONTRAINDICATIONS: There is insufficient reliable information on the safety of gymnema. It should not be used

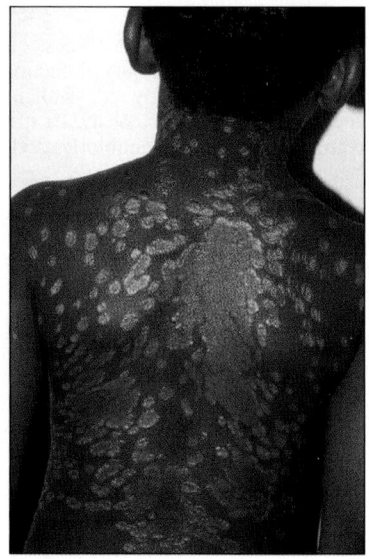

Guttate psoriasis *(White and Cox, 2006)*

during pregnancy and lactation, in children, or in those with known hypersensitivity to this product.

gymno-, prefix meaning "nakedness."

gyn, 1. *(Slang)* abbreviation for **gynecologist. 2.** initialism for **gynecology.**

gyn-. See **gyneco-, gyn-, gyne-, gyno-.**

-gyn. See **-gyne, -gyn.**

gynaecology, British spelling for gynecology. See **gynecology.**

gynaecomastia, British spelling for gynecomastia. See **gynecomastia.**

gynandrous /gīnan″drəs, jī-/ [Gk, *gyne,* woman, *aner,* man], describing a man or a woman who has some of the physical characteristics usually attributed to the other sex, as a female pseudohermaphrodite. Compare **androgynous.** *−gynandry, n.*

gyne-. See **gyneco-, gyn-, gyne-, gyno-.**

-gyne, -gyn, word element meaning "(specified) female characteristics": *OB-Gyn.*

gynec(o) [word element, Gk], *woman.*

gyneco-, gyn-, gyne-, gyno-, prefix meaning "woman" or "female gender": *gynecoid, gynecomastia, gynandrous.*

gynecography /gī′nə-, jin′əkog″rəfē/, the radiographic examination of the female pelvic organs.

gynecoid obesity, obesity in which fat is localized in the lower half of the body, most frequently seen in women and having a better prognosis for morbidity and mortality than the android type. Compare **android obesity.**

gynecoid pelvis /gī′nəkoid, jin′ək-/ [Gk, *gyne + eidos,* form; L, *pelvis,* basin], a type of pelvis characteristic of the normal female and associated with the smallest incidence of fetopelvic disproportion. The inlet is nearly round, the sacrum is parallel to the posterior aspect of the symphysis pubis, the sidewalls are straight, and the ischial spines are blunt and do not encroach on the space in the true pelvis. It is the ideal pelvic type for childbirth. It is one of the four classic Caldwell-Moloy pelvic types. Also spelled *gynaecoid pelvis.*

gynecological /gī′nə-, jin′əkəloj″ik/ [Gk, *gynaikos,* of a woman], pertaining to gynecology, or the study of diseases of the female reproductive organs and the breasts.

gynecological examination, examination of the breasts, external genitalia, and internal pelvic organs. See also **pelvic examination.**

gynecological operative procedures [Gk, *gynaikos,* of a woman; L, *operari,* to work, *procedere,* to proceed], surgery of the female reproductive system.

gynecologist /gī′nəkol″əjist, jī′-, jin′-/, a physician who specializes in the health care of women, including pregnancy and diseases of the reproductive organs and breasts.

gynecology (gyn) /gī′nəkol″əjē, jī′-, jin′-/ [Gk, *gyne* + *logos,* science], the evaluation and treatment of diseases of the female reproductive organs, including the breasts. Unlike most specialties in medicine, gynecology encompasses surgical and nonsurgical expertise. It is usually practiced in conjunction with obstetrics.

gynecomastia /gī′nəkōmas″tē·ə, jī′-, jin′-/ [Gk, *gyne* + *mastos,* breast], an abnormal enlargement of one or both breasts in males. Milk production may or may not be present. The condition is usually temporary and benign. It may be caused by hormonal imbalance; a tumor of an adrenal gland, testis, or pituitary; use of medication that contains estrogens or steroidal compounds; or failure of the liver to inactivate circulating estrogen, as in alcoholic cirrhosis. Less commonly the gynecomastia may be caused by a hormone-secreting tumor of the breast, lung, or other organ. It tends to subside spontaneously but, if marked, may be corrected surgically for cosmetic or psychological reasons. Biopsy may be performed to rule out cancer.

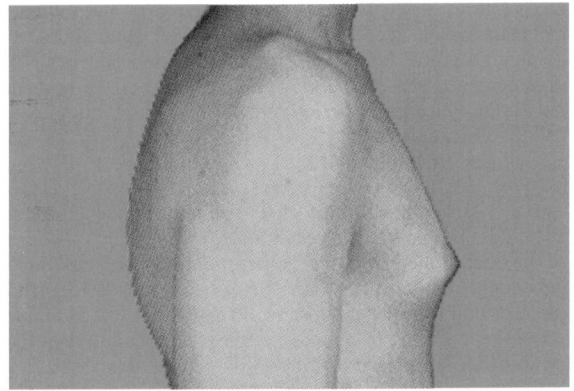

Young man with adolescent gynecomastia *(Hammond, 2009)*

Gyne-Lotrimin, an antifungal drug. Brand name for **clotrimazole.**

gynephobia /gī′nəfō″bē·ə, jī′-, jin′-/ [Gk, *gyne* + *phobos,* fear], an anxiety disorder characterized by a morbid fear of women or by a morbid aversion to the society of women. It is an obsessive, phobic phenomenon that occurs almost entirely in men and may usually be traced to some frightening experience involving women that occurred in childhood. Treatment consists of psychotherapy to uncover the causative emotional conflict, followed by behavior therapy, specifically systemic desensitization and flooding to reduce anxiety.

-gynic, -gynous, suffix meaning "human female" or "female characteristics": *androgynous, hologynic.*

gyno-. See **gyneco-, gyn-, gyne-, gyno-.**

gynogamone /gī′nōgam″ōn/ [Gk, *gyne* + *gamos,* marriage], a chemical secreted by female gametes that is believed to attract male gametes.

gypsum /jip′səm/, a mineral composed mainly of crushed calcium sulfate hemihydrate. It is the main ingredient in making plaster of paris surgical casts, dental casts, and impressions for dentures. Gypsum dust has an irritant action on the mucous membranes of the respiratory tract and the conjunctiva.

gyrase /jī″rās/, an enzyme that promotes the unwinding of the closed circular deoxyribonucleic acid helix of bacteria.

gyri. See **gyrus.**

-gyria, suffix meaning "spiral" or "convolution": *agyria, microgyria, ulegyria.*

gyromagnetic ratio (γ), a value characteristic of any magnetic nucleus that determines the Larmor frequency, f_L, in a given magnetic field B ($f_L = \gamma B$).

gyrus /jīrəs/ *pl. gyri* [Gk, *gyro,* circle], one of the winding convolutions of the cerebral hemisphere of the brain. They are caused by infolding of the cortex and are separated by the shallow grooves (sulci) or deeper grooves (fissures). See also **cerebral cortex.**

G

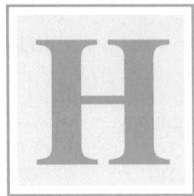

[H+], symbol for **hydrogen ion.**

h, **1.** abbreviation for **haustus. 2.** abbreviation for **hecto-. 3.** abbreviation for **height. 4.** abbreviation for *hora,* the Latin word for *hour.* **5.** abbreviation for *horizontal.* **6.** abbreviation for **hyperopia. 7.** symbol for **Planck constant.**

H, **1.** symbol for the element **hydrogen. 2.** abbreviation for **henry.**

¹H, an isotope of hydrogen. Symbol for **protium.**

²H, an isotope of hydrogen containing one proton and one neutron. Symbol for **deuterium.**

³H, an isotope of hydrogen containing one proton and two neutrons. Symbol for **tritium.**

H₀, symbol for **null hypothesis.**

HA, abbreviation for **hepatitis A.**

HA-1A, a genetically engineered antibody used in the treatment of gram-negative bacteremia and septic shock. The antibody binds to bacterial lipopolysaccharide. It is relatively free of side effects.

HAAg, abbreviation for *hepatitis A antigen.* See **hepatitis A.**

HAART, abbreviation for **highly active antiretroviral therapy.**

Haas method, a technique for producing radiographic images of the interior of the skull. The patient rests the forehead and nose on the table so that the x-ray beam enters the skull near the base of the occipital bone and emerges on the frontal bone above the nasal bone.

habeas corpus /hā′bē·əs kôr′pəs/ [L, you have the body], (for health or related reasons) a principle of law in the United States designed to prevent arrest or confinement without just cause. Individuals have the right to question the cause and legality of detention.

Habermann disease. See **Mucha-Habermann disease.**

habilitation /həbil′itā″shən/, health care services designed to assist patients or clients with the skills, function, or performance needed for participation in occupational and daily life activities. Habilitation may involve, for example, acquiring or maintaining skills, minimizing the deterioration of skills, or compensating for an impairment. Compare **rehabilitation.**

habit [L, *habitus,* condition], **1.** a customary or particular practice, manner, or mode of behavior. **2.** an acquired tendency to respond and perform in a consistent way in a familiar environment or situation. **3.** *(Informal)* the habitual use of drugs or narcotics. See also **habit spasm, habit training.**

habitat /hab′itat/ [L, *habitare,* to dwell], a natural environment where an organism, including a human being, may live and grow normally.

habit spasm, an involuntary twitching or tic. It usually involves a small muscle group of the face, neck, or shoulders and causes movements such as spasmodic blinking or rapid jerking of the head to the side. The movements are often generated by emotional conflicts rather than by organic disorder. They may serve as a release for tension or anxiety.

habit tic [L, *habitus,* condition; Fr, *tic*], a brief recurrent movement of a muscle group, such as a blink, grimace, or sudden head turning, that is of psychogenic rather than organic origin.

habit training, the process of teaching a child how to adjust to the demands of the external world by forming certain habits, primarily those related to eating, sleeping, elimination, and dress.

habitual abortion /həbich′ōō·əl/ [L, *habituare,* to become used to], *(Obsolete)* spontaneous abortion of three successive pregnancies before the twentieth week of gestation. Now called **recurrent pregnancy loss.** See also **cerclage, incompetent cervix.**

habitual dislocation [L, *habitus,* condition, *dis* + *locare,* to place], a dislocation that recurs repeatedly after reduction.

habitual fever, habitual hyperthermia. See **fever, habitual hyperthermia.**

habitual hyperthermia, a rare condition of unknown cause that occurs in young females, characterized by body temperatures of 99° F to 100.5° F regularly or intermittently for years, associated with fatigue, malaise, vague aches and pains, insomnia, bowel disturbances, and headaches. No organic cause can be found. The diagnosis is usually made only after a prolonged period of study and observation. Also called **habitual fever.**

habituation /həbich′ōō·ā″shən/ [L, *habituare,* to become used to], **1.** an acquired tolerance gained by repeated exposure to a particular stimulus such as alcohol. **2.** a decline and eventual elimination of a conditioned response by repetition of the conditioned stimulus. **3.** psychological and emotional dependence on a drug, tobacco, or alcohol that results from the repeated use of the substance but without the addictive, physiological need to increase dosage. Also called **negative adaptation.** Compare **addiction. 4.** (in occupational therapy) internal readiness to demonstrate a consistent pattern of behavior guided by habits and roles; this readiness is associated with specific temporal, physical, or social environments.

habitus /hab″itəs/, a person's appearance or physique, as an athletic habitus.

HACEK, acronym for *Haemophilus, Actinobacillus, Cardiobacterium, Eikenella,* and *Kingella,* microorganisms associated with infective endocarditis.

hacking cough [AS, *haeccan* + *cohettan*], a short, weak repeating cough, often caused by irritation of the larynx by a postnasal drip. It can also result from side effects of angiotensin-converting enzyme inhibitor therapy and smoking.

Haeckel law. See **recapitulation concept.**

haemangioma. See **hemangioma.**

haemarthros. See **hemarthros.**

haematemesis. See **hematemesis.**

haematocele, British spelling for hematocele. See **hematocele.**

haematocrit. See **hematocrit.**

haematocytoblast. See **hematocytoblast.**

haematology. See **hematology.**

haematoma. See **hematoma.**

haematomyelia. See **hematomyelia.**

haematuria. See **hematuria.**

haeme. See **heme.**

-haemia. See **-emia, -aemia, -hemia, -haemia.**

haemochromatosis. See **hemochromatosis.**

haemoconcentration. See **hemoconcentration.**
haemodialysis. See **hemodialysis.**
haemodilution. See **hemodilution.**
haemofiltration. See **hemofiltration.**
haemoglobin. See **hemoglobin.**
haemoglobinometer. See **hemoglobinometer.**
haemoglobinopathy. See **hemoglobinopathy.**
haemoglobinuria. See **hemoglobinuria.**
haemolysin. See **hemolysin.**
haemolysis. See **hemolysis.**
haemolytic anemia. See **hemolytic anemia.**
haemoperfusion. See **hemoperfusion.**
haemopericardium. See **hemopericardium.**
haemoperitoneum. See **hemoperitoneum.**
haemophilia. See **hemophilia.**

Haemophilus /hēmof″iləs/ [Gk, *haima,* blood, *philein,* to love], a genus of gram-negative rod-shaped pathogenic bacteria frequently found in the respiratory tract of humans and other animals. Examples are *H. influenzae,* which causes respiratory tract infections and one form of meningitis; *H. haemolyticus,* a hemolytic species pathogenic in the upper respiratory tract of humans; and *H. ducreyi,* which causes chancroid. *Haemophilus* species are generally sensitive to cephalosporins, tetracyclines, and sulfonamides.

Haemophilus influenzae, a small gram-negative nonmotile parasitic bacterium that occurs in two forms, encapsulated and nonencapsulated, and in six types, a, b, c, d, e, and f. Almost all infections are caused by encapsulated type b organisms. *H. influenzae* is found in the nasopharynx of approximately 75% of healthy children and adults. In children and in debilitated older people, severe destructive inflammation of the larynx, trachea, and bronchi may result from infection. Subacute bacterial endocarditis, purulent meningitis, and pneumonia also may be caused by it. Secondary infection by *H. influenzae* occurs in influenza and in many other respiratory diseases. Several *H. influenzae* B conjugate vaccines are available.

Haemophilus influenzae pneumonia, bacterial pneumonia caused by infection with *H. influenzae,* seen mainly in young children and debilitated or immunocompromised adults. It sometimes progresses to life-threatening conditions such as meningitis, pericarditis, endocarditis, and epiglottitis that can cause obstruction of the airway.

haemoptysis. See **hemoptysis.**
haemorrhage. See **hemorrhage.**
haemorrhagic disease of newborn. See **hemorrhagic disease of newborn.**
haemorrhoid. See **hemorrhoid.**
haemorrhoidectomy. See **hemorrhoidectomy.**
haemosiderin. See **hemosiderin.**
haemostasis. See **hemostasis.**
haemostatic. See **hemostatic.**
haemothorax. See **hemothorax.**

hafnium (Hf) /haf″nē-əm/ [Hafnia, Medieval Latin name of Copenhagen, Denmark], a hard, brittle, silver-gray metallic element of the third transition series. Its atomic number is 72; its atomic mass is 178.49. Elements in this group show some nonmetallic chemical characteristics.

Hagedorn needle /hä″gedôrn/ [Werner Hagedorn, German physician, 1831–1894], a flat surgical needle with a cutting edge near its point and a very large eye at the other end.

Hageman factor. See **factor XII.**

Haglund deformity [Sims E.P. Haglund, Swedish orthopedist, 1870–1937], a foot disorder characterized by an enlarged posterosuperior lateral aspect of the calcaneus, often associated with an inverted subtalar joint. It is a common cause of posterior Achilles bursitis.

Hailey-Hailey disease. See **benign familial chronic pemphigus.**

Hainsworth, Margaret A., a nursing theorist who, with Mary Lermann Burke and Georgene Gaskill Eakes, developed the Theory of Chronic Sorrow to describe the ongoing feelings of loss that arise from illness, debilitation, or death.

hair [AS, *haer*], a filament of keratin consisting of a root and a shaft formed in a specialized follicle in the epidermis. There are three stages of hair development: (1) anagen, the active growing stage; (2) catagen, a short interlude between the growth and resting phases; and (3) telogen, the resting (club) stage before shedding. Scalp hair grows at an average rate of 1 mm every 3 days, with body and eyebrow hair growing at a much slower rate. Hair plucking does not stop hair growth. See also **hirsutism, lanugo.**

hair analysis [AS, *haer* + Gk, a loosening], chemical analysis of a hair sample to find possible evidence of exposure to a toxic substance. Molecules of lead compounds and other chemicals are absorbed and stored in hair shafts. Hair analysis is also used to determine possible causes of malnutrition. Samples for analysis are taken from areas close to the scalp to eliminate chances that toxic chemicals found in the hair may have been absorbed from air pollutants.

hair cycle, the successive phases of the production and then loss of hair, consisting of growth (anagen), regression (catagen), and quiescence (telogen).

hair follicle [AS, *haer* + L, *folliculus,* a small bag], a tube-like opening in the epidermis where the hair shaft develops and into which the sebaceous glands open.

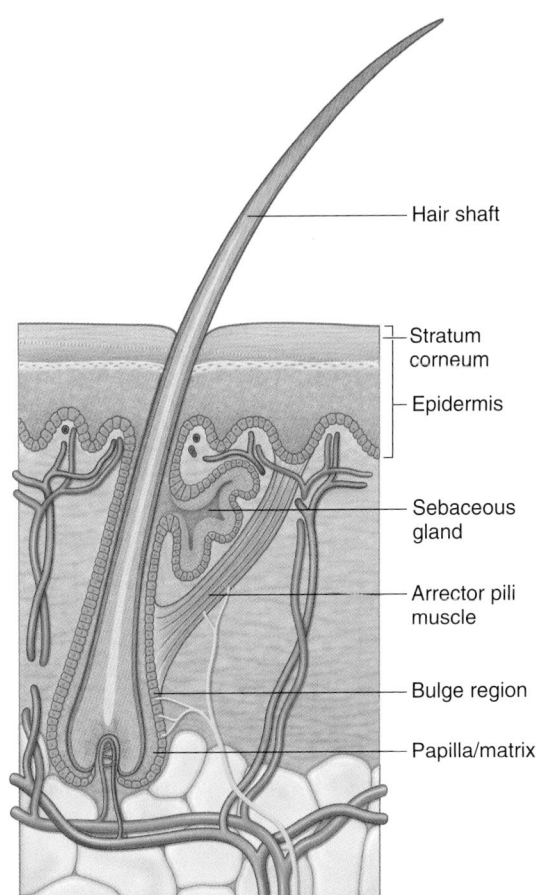

Hair shaft

Stratum corneum

Epidermis

Sebaceous gland

Arrector pili muscle

Bulge region

Papilla/matrix

Hair follicle *(Robinson et al, 2010)*

hairline fracture [AS, *haer* + L, *linea* + *fractura*], a minor fracture that appears on an x-ray image as a thin line between two segments of a bone. The segments remain in alignment and the fracture may not extend completely through the bone. A fatigue hairline fracture may develop without apparent injury and in the absence of trauma.

hair matrix carcinoma. See **basal cell carcinoma.**

hair pulling. See **trichotillomania.**

hair transplantation, a form of dermatological surgery and plastic surgery, performed to correct scalp hair deficiencies caused by hormonal changes, burns, or injuries. The procedure uses existing hair to fill in bald areas. Several sessions are usually required to achieve the level of hair fullness desired by the patient. The sessions consist of grafting the hair-bearing tissue over the bald area directly or using micrografts of follicles to restore the hairline. It is important that the patient have healthy hair growth on other parts of the head to serve as donor areas and that color, texture, and other aspects of a matching transplant be compatible.

hairy-cell leukemia [AS, *haer* + L, *cella,* storeroom; Gk, *leukos,* white, *haima,* blood], an uncommon neoplasm of blood-forming tissues, characterized by pancytopenia, enlargement of the spleen, and many fine projections on the surface of reticulum cells in the blood and bone marrow. The disease occurs six times more frequently in men than in women and usually appears in the fifth decade with an insidious onset and a variable course marked by anemia, thrombocytopenia, and spontaneous bruising. Some cases may achieve long-term remission through alpha-interferon administration or chemotherapy using vincristine and prednisone. Also called **leukemic reticuloendotheliosis.**

hairy leukoplakia, a form of leukoplakia associated with the opportunistic presence of the Epstein-Barr virus and characterized by a white plaque. It presents as a well-demarcated white lesion that can vary in appearance from flat and plaquelike to a papillary/filiform corrugated lesion. It can often be seen on one or both lateral margins of the tongue. It is associated with patients who are infected with the human immunodeficiency virus (HIV) or patients with other forms of immunosuppression. Lesions usually improve or resolve with improvement of the patient's immune system.

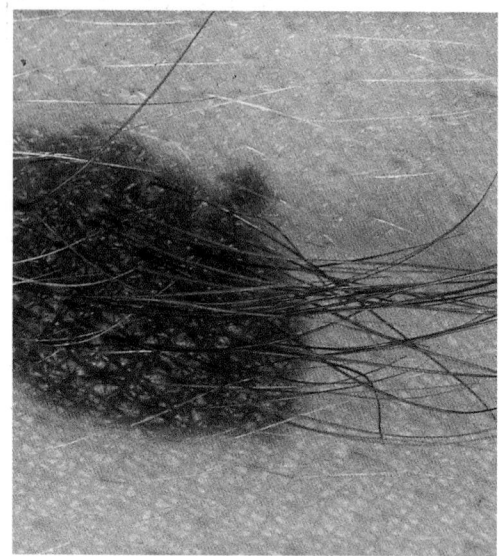

Hairy nevus *(du Vivier, 2002)*

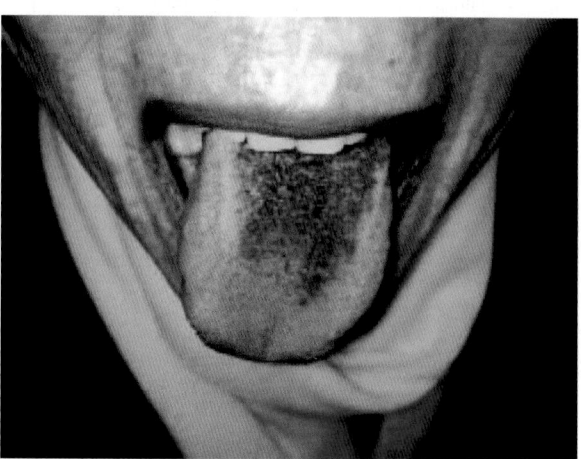

Hairy tongue *(Arab et al, 2015)*

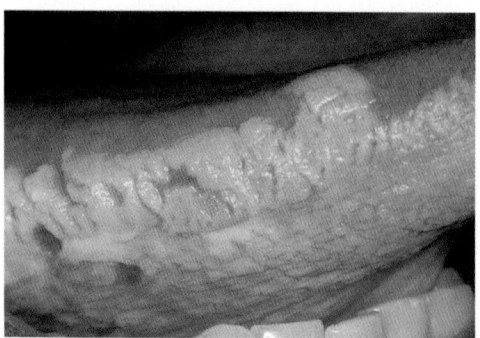

Hairy leukoplakia *(Regezi, Sciubba, and Jordan, 2008)*

hairy nevus [AS, *haer* + L, *naevus,* birthmark], a mole, usually pigmented, that has hairs growing from it.

hairy tongue, a dark, pigmented overgrowth of the filiform papillae of the tongue that has a thickened, furry appearance. It is a benign and frequent side effect of use of some antibiotics. The condition gradually subsides, and no treatment is indicated. See also **glossotrichia.**

halcinonide /həlsin′ənīd/, a topical glucocorticoid.

■ INDICATIONS: It is prescribed topically for the treatment of inflammation.

■ CONTRAINDICATIONS: Viral and fungal diseases of the skin, impaired circulation, or known hypersensitivity to this drug or to steroid medication prohibits its use.

■ ADVERSE EFFECTS: Among the more serious adverse effects are skin reactions and systemic side effects that result from prolonged or excessive application.

Halcion, a hypnotic agent. Brand name for **triazolam.**

Haldol, a tranquilizer. Brand name for **haloperidol.**

half-kneel, a resting position whereby an individual has the foot of one leg and the knee of the other leg supported on the ground, with one thigh and the trunk upright.

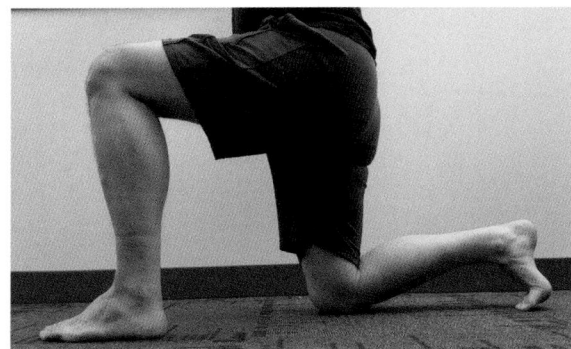

Half-kneel

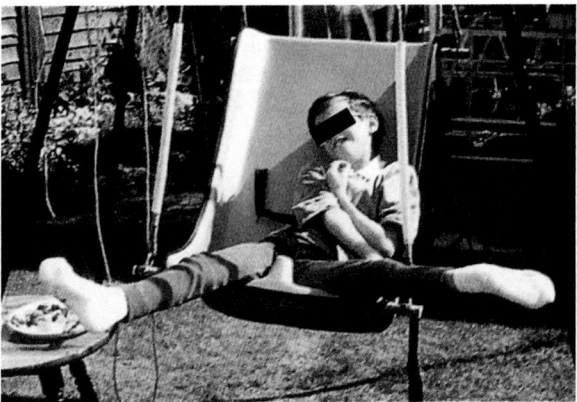

Child with Hallervorden-Spatz syndrome: abnormal posturing *(Newton, 1995)*

half-life (t₁/₂) [AS, *haelf* + *lif*], **1.** the time required for a radioactive substance to lose 50% of its activity through decay. Each radionuclide has a unique half-life. Also called **radioactive half-life. 2.** the amount of time required to reduce a drug level to half of its initial value. Usually the term refers to time necessary to reduce the plasma value to half of its initial value. After five half-lives, 97% of a single drug dose will be eliminated. See also **biological half-life, effective half-life.**

half-normal saline, a solution of 0.45% NaCl used for mucosal hydration. As the water in the solution evaporates, the saline concentration increases, achieving nearly normal saline concentration in the respiratory tract.

half-sibling, one of two or more children who have one parent in common (a half-brother or half-sister).

half-value layer (HVL), the amount of absorbing material required to attenuate a beam of radiation to half its original level. Quantities are indicated by length, as millimeters of aluminum or centimeters of soft tissue.

halfway house, a specialized treatment facility, usually for psychiatric patients who no longer require complete hospitalization but who need some care and time to adjust to living independently. Halfway houses are also used for substance abuse recovery.

halisteresis /həlis″tərē′sis/ [Gk, *hals*, salt, *steresis*, absence of], a theoretic process of bone resorption in which bone salts are removed by humoral mechanisms and returned to body tissue fluids, leaving behind a decalcified bone matrix. See also **osteolysis.**

halitosis /hal′itō″sis/ [L, *halitus*, breath; Gk, *osis*, condition], offensive breath resulting from poor oral hygiene; dental or oral infections; ingestion of certain foods, such as garlic or alcohol; use of tobacco; or some systemic diseases, such as the odor of acetone in diabetes and ammonia in liver disease.

Hallervorden-Spatz syndrome /hol″ərfôr′dən shpots/ [Julius Hallervorden, German neurologist, 1882–1965; H. Spatz, German neurologist, 1888–1969], a progressive degenerative neurological disease of children, with symptoms of parkinsonism. It is characterized by rigidity, athetosis, and dementia. The cause is an accumulation of iron pigments in the globus pallidus and substantia nigra. Treatment is similar to that of Parkinson disease and Huntington's chorea.

hallex. See **hallux.**

Hall, Lydia E., (1906–1969), a nursing theorist who presented her Care, Core, and Cure Model in "Nursing: What Is It?" in *The Canadian Nurse* (1964). Hall believed that nursing functions differently in three overlapping circles that constitute aspects of patients. She labeled the circles *the body* (the care), *the disease* (the cure), and *the person* (the core). Hall viewed nursing in relation to the core aspect as concerned with the therapeutic use of self in communicating with the patient. Care is the nurturing, comforting component, the "hands-on" care of the patient. Cure is the aspect of nursing involved with treatments and administration of medications. Hall's concept includes adult patients who have passed the acute stage of illness and have rehabilitation and feelings of self-actualization as their goal.

Hallpike test. See **Dix-Hallpike test.**

halluces. See **hallux.**

hallucination /həloo′sinā″shən/ [L, *alucinari,* to wander in mind], a sensory perception that does not result from an external stimulus and that occurs in the waking state. It can occur in any of the senses and is classified accordingly as auditory, gustatory, olfactory, tactile, or visual. It is a symptom of psychotic behavior, often noted during schizophrenia, as well as of other mental or organic disorders and conditions. –*hallucinations, adj.,* –*hallucinate, v.*

hallucinogen /həloo″sənəjen′, hal′əsin″əjən, hal′yəsin″əjən/ [L, *alucinari,* to wander in mind + Gk, *genein,* to produce], a substance that causes excitation of the central nervous system, characterized by hallucination, mood change, anxiety, sensory distortion, delusion, and depersonalization; increased pulse, temperature, and blood pressure; and dilation of the pupils. The ingestion of hallucinogenic substances may cause psychic dependence and depressive or suicidal psychotic states. Kinds include **lysergide, mescaline, phencyclidine hydrochloride, psilocybin.**

hallucinogenesis /-jen′əsis/ [L, *alucinari,* to wander in mind; Gk, *genein,* to produce], a cause or source of hallucinations.

hallucinosis /həloo′sinō″sis/ [L, *alucinari* + Gk, *osis,* condition], a pathological mental state in which awareness consists primarily or exclusively of hallucinations. Kinds include **alcoholic hallucinosis.**

hallux /hal″əks/ *pl. halluces* [L, *hallex,* large toe], the great toe.

hallux rigidus, a painful deformity of the great toe, limiting motion at the metatarsophalangeal joint.

hallux valgus, a deformity in which the great toe is angled away from the midline of the body toward the other toes. In some cases the great toe rides over or under the other toes. Compare **hallux varus.**

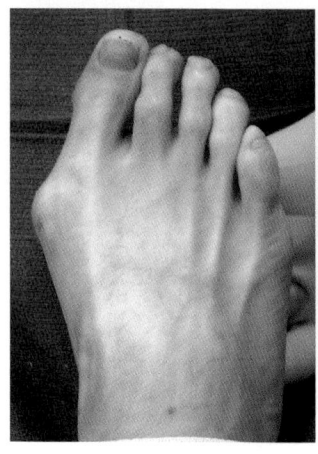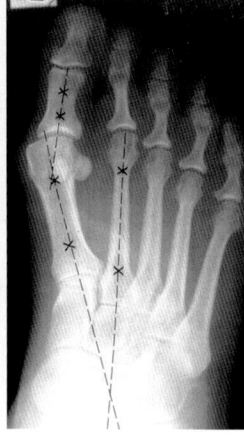

Hallux valgus deformity (Coughlin et al, 2014)

hallux varus, a deformity in which the great toe is angled away from the other toes. Compare **hallux valgus.**

halo- /hal′ō-/, prefix meaning "salt": *halogen.*

halobetasol /hal″oba′täsol/, a very high-potency synthetic corticosteroid used topically in the form of the propionate as an antiinflammatory and antipruritic agent.

halo cast. See **halo vest.**

halo effect, the beneficial effect of an interview or other encounter, as may occur in the course of a research project or a health care visit. The halo effect cannot be attributed to the content of the interview or to any specific act or treatment; it is the result of indefinable interpersonal factors present in the interaction.

halofantrine, an antimalarial drug.
- INDICATIONS: It is used to treat mild to moderate malaria.
- CONTRAINDICATIONS: Known hypersensitivity to halofantrine prohibits its use.
- ADVERSE EFFECTS: Common side effects include nausea, vomiting, anorexia, diarrhea, and arrhythmias.

Halog, a topical glucocorticoid. Brand name for **halcinonide.**

halogen /hal′ōjən/ [Gk, *hals,* salt, *genein,* to produce], any member of group 17 (or Group VIIA) in the periodic table: fluorine, chlorine, bromine, iodine, and astatine. With the exception of astatine, they are found in seawater as the corresponding halide ion.

halogenated hydrocarbon /həloj″ənā′tid/ [Gk, *hals,* salt, *genein,* to produce, *hydor,* water; L, *carbo,* coal], a volatile liquid used as an inhalation anesthetic, administered in combination with oxygen and/or nitrous oxide. The only halogenated hydrocarbon used for anesthesia is halothane. See also **halothane.**

halogenoderma /hal′ōdur″mə/, skin changes caused by ingestion or injection of halogen, usually a bromide or an iodide.

halo nevus, a benign melanocytic nevus that appears as a central brown mole surrounded by a circle of depigmented skin. There are sometimes multiple nevi. Over a period of months the central nevus becomes flat and loses its pigment, leaving a round white macule. Eventually the halo repigments.

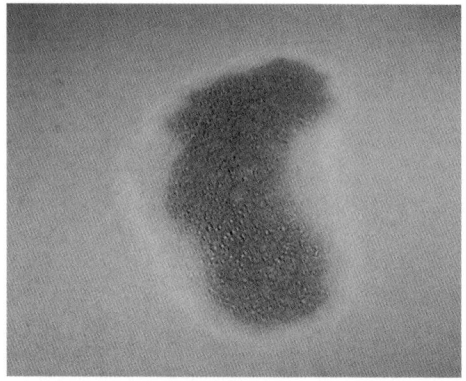

Halo nevus (Aouthmany et al, 2011)

haloperidol /hal′ōper″ədôl/, a butyrophenone antipsychotic drug.
- INDICATIONS: It is prescribed in the treatment of schizophrenia, in the control of tics and verbal utterance of Tourette syndrome, in the treatment of severe behavioral problems in children, and as a sleep aid.
- CONTRAINDICATIONS: Parkinson disease, concurrent administration of central nervous system depressants, liver or renal dysfunction, severe hypotension, or known hypersensitivity to this drug prohibits its use.
- ADVERSE EFFECTS: There is a wide range of adverse effects. Among the more serious adverse effects are hypotension and hypersensitivity reactions. It also has comparatively high risk for a variety of extrapyramidal effects, including pseudoparkinson signs and symptoms, tardive dyskinesia, dystonia, and akathisia.

halo sign [Gk, *halos,* circular floor; L, *signum,* mark], **1.** (in radiography) a halo effect produced in the radiograph of the fetal head between the subcutaneous fat and the cranium. It is said to be indicative of intrauterine death of the fetus. **2.** (in computed tomography) ground glass opacity surrounding a pulmonary nodule or mass, representing hemorrhage. **3.** (in mammography) a radiolucent rim around a lesion that is generally but not always indicative of a benign breast lesion. **4.** (in ultrasound) the appearance of a peripheral rim clearly different from the central portions of a lesion; useful in interpreting images of the hepatobiliary system. Also called *hypoechogenic rim.*

Halotestin, an androgen. Brand name for **fluoxymesterone.**

halothane /hal′əthān/, an inhalation anesthetic.
- INDICATIONS: It is prescribed for induction and maintenance of general anesthesia.
- CONTRAINDICATIONS: It is not recommended for obstetric anesthesia unless uterine relaxation is required.
- ADVERSE EFFECTS: Among the more serious but rare adverse reactions are hepatic necrosis, cardiac arrest or arrhythmia, hypotension, malignant hyperthermia, nausea, and emesis.

halothane-related hepatitis, an adverse reaction of some patients to inhalation of halothane, a general anesthetic, characterized by hepatitis and a severe fever that develops several days after exposure to the anesthetic. The risk is higher for obese patients, possibly because body fat tends to store the chemical.

halo vest [Gk, *halos,* circular floor; AS, *kasta*], an orthopedic device used to help immobilize the neck and head, providing traction to the cervical spine. It incorporates a vest, usually with shoulder straps, and metal bars within the cast that connect the vest to secure pins to a band around the skull. The halo is attached to the skull by pins or screws. The halo vest is used to aid the healing of injuries and cervical dislocations and to position and immobilize a patient after cervical surgery.

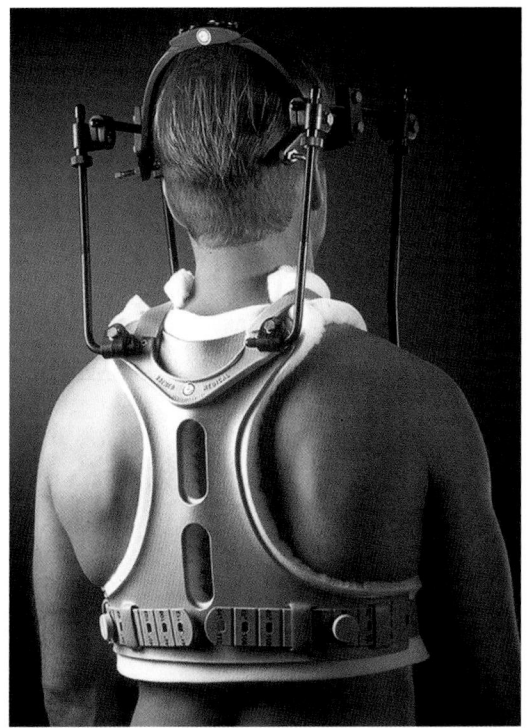

Halo vest (Courtesy DePuy Spine, a Johnson & Johnson Co)

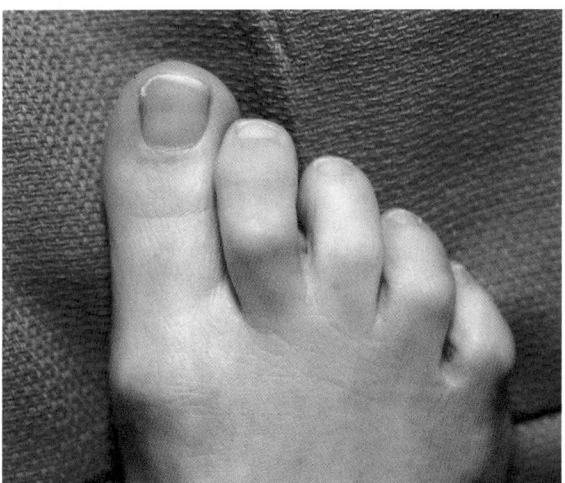

Hammer toe (Canale and Beaty, 2008)

radiograph of the lung that is a manifestation of a pulmonary infarction.

Ham test, a rarely performed blood test used in the diagnosis of paroxysmal nocturnal hemoglobinuria.

hamstring muscle [AS, *hamm + streng*], any one of three muscles at the back of the thigh: medially the semimembranosus and the semitendinosus and laterally the biceps femoris.

Halsted forceps /hal″stedz/ [William S. Halsted, American surgeon, 1852–1922], **1.** a small pointed hemostatic forceps. See also **mosquito forceps. 2.** a forceps with slender jaws for grasping arteries and other blood vessels.

Halsted suture [William S. Halsted, American surgeon, 1852–1922], the union of two adjoining skin surfaces by a suture placed through the subcuticular fascia.

hamamelis water. See **witch hazel.**

hamartoma, a new tissue growth resembling a tumor. It results from a defective overgrowth in tissue formation.

hamartoma syndrome. See **Cowden disease.**

hamate bone /ham″āt/ [L, *hamatus,* hooked], a carpal (wrist) bone that rests on the fourth and fifth metacarpal bones and projects a hooklike process, the hamulus, from its palmar surface. Its dorsal surface is rough for ligamentous attachment. The hamate bone articulates with the lunate proximally, the fourth and fifth metacarpal distally, the triangular medially, and the capitate laterally. Also called **os hamatum, unciform bone.**

Hamman-Rich syndrome. See **interstitial pneumonia.**

Hamman disease. See **pneumomediastinum.**

hammer finger [AS, *hamer + finger*], a permanently flexed terminal phalanx caused by an injury to the extensor tendon. Also called **mallet finger.**

hammer toe [AS, *hamer + ta*], a foot digit permanently flexed at the proximal phalangeal joint and hyperextended at the distal interphalangeal joint, producing a clawlike appearance. The anomaly may be present in more than one digit but is most common in the second toe. It may accompany clawfoot.

Hampton's hump [Aubrey O. Hampton, American radiologist, 1900–1955], a soft-tissue image in a

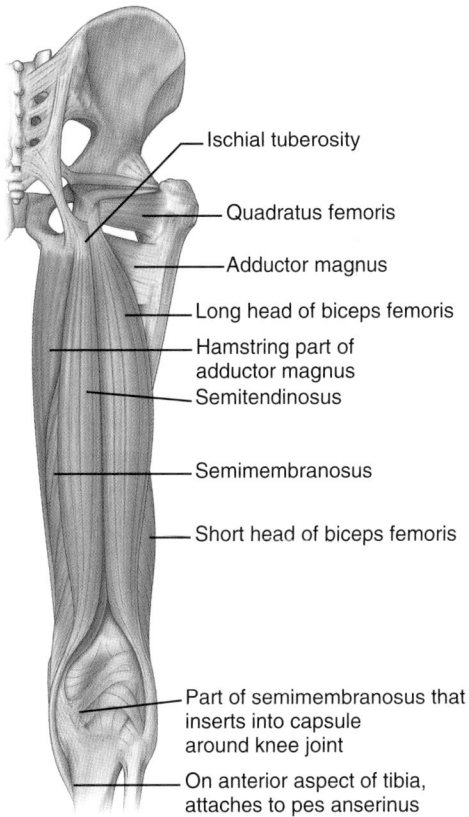

Hamstring muscles (Drake, Vogl, and Mitchell, 2010)

Ischial tuberosity

Quadratus femoris

Adductor magnus

Long head of biceps femoris

Hamstring part of adductor magnus

Semitendinosus

Semimembranosus

Short head of biceps femoris

Part of semimembranosus that inserts into capsule around knee joint

On anterior aspect of tibia, attaches to pes anserinus

H

hamstring reflex, a normal deep tendon reflex elicited by tapping one of the hamstring tendons behind the knee, causing contraction of the tendon and flexion of the knee. The patient should be lying in the supine position with the knee and hip partially flexed and the leg supported by the examiner's hand. An accentuated hamstring reflex may result from a lesion of the pyramidal system above the level of the fourth lumbar nerve root. See also **deep tendon reflex.**

hamstring tendon, one of the three tendons from the three hamstring muscles in the back of the thigh. The one lateral and the two medial hamstring tendons connect the hamstring muscles to the knee.

hamular notch. See **pterygomaxillary notch.**

hamulus /ham′yoo·ləs/ *pl. hamuli* [L, little hook], **1.** a general term denoting a hook-shaped process. **2.** hook of the hamate carpal bone of the hand.

hand [AS, *hand*], the part of the upper limb distal to the forearm. It is the most flexible part of the skeleton and has a total of 29 bones, 8 forming the carpus, 5 forming the metacarpus, 14 forming the phalangeal section, and 2 sesamoid bones. Also called **manus.**

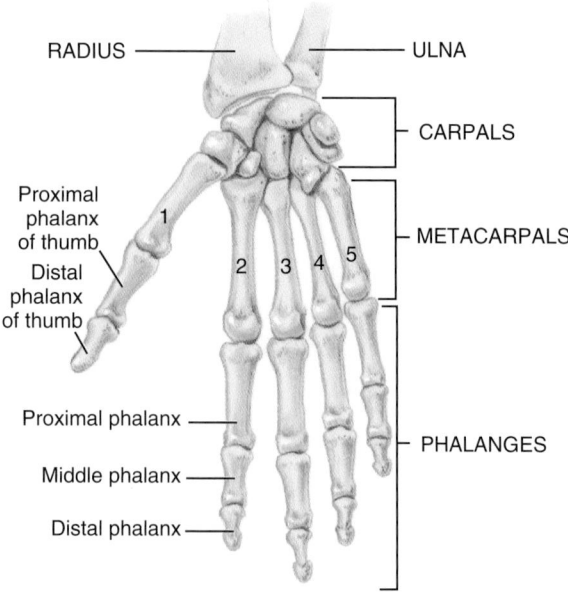

Hand (right, palmar aspect)

Bones of the hand and wrist *(Cummings, 2008)*

handblock [AS, *hand* + Fr, *bloc*], a device made of a wood block that is several inches high with a firm handle. The device can assist an individual with impaired mobility in sitting push-ups, an exercise that can enhance transfers or mobility in bed. Also called **push-up block.**

Hand-Schuller-Christian disease (HSC), a disease primarily seen in infants and children in which there is a classic triad of symptoms in one third of individuals: exophthalmos, diabetes insipidus, and lesions in the skull. It is one of three diseases characterized by an increase in the number of histocytes. See also **eosinophilic granuloma, Letterer-Siwe syndrome.**

hand condenser, (in dentistry) an instrument for compacting amalgams or composite resin, or to place gold foil, using force applied by the operator, with or without supplementary force from a mallet wielded by an assistant.

handedness /han′didnes/ [AS, *hand* + *ness,* condition], a preference for use of either the left or right hand. The preference is related to cerebral dominance: left-handedness corresponds to dominance of the right side of the brain, and vice versa. Also called **chirality, laterality.**

hand-foot-and-mouth disease, a viral infection usually caused by coxsackie A virus but also by enterovirus 71. It is characterized by the appearance of painful ulcers and vesicles on the mucous membranes of the mouth and on the hands and feet. The disease is very contagious and mainly affects children, including infants. There is no specific treatment. It is spread through contact with oral secretions (respiratory droplets) or stool. Lesions usually resolve in 1 week. Antiseptic mouthwashes and simple analgesics can be used to relieve discomfort of eating. It should not be confused with foot-and-mouth disease, which is primarily an animal disease.

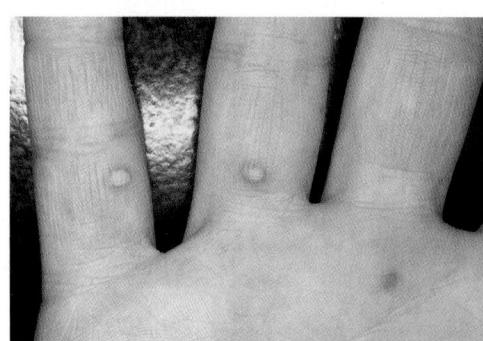

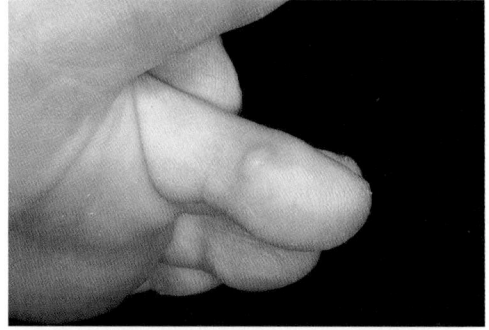

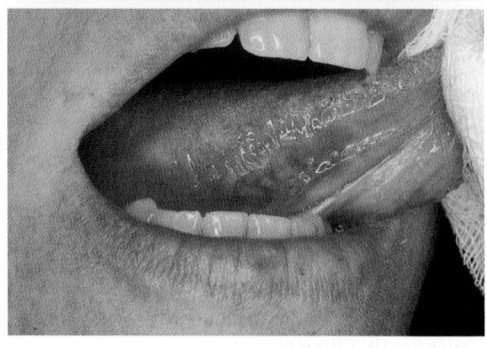

Hand-foot-and-mouth disease *(Regezi et al, 2008/Courtesy Steven K. Young, MD)*

hand-foot syndrome. See **palmoplantar erythrodysesthesia**.

handicapped /han′dikapt/ [hand in cap, a 17th-century game with forfeits], **1.** *(Nontechnical)* historic term used to refer to a person with a disability. Compare **disability. 2.** pertaining to spaces or equipment designed for individuals with disabilities.

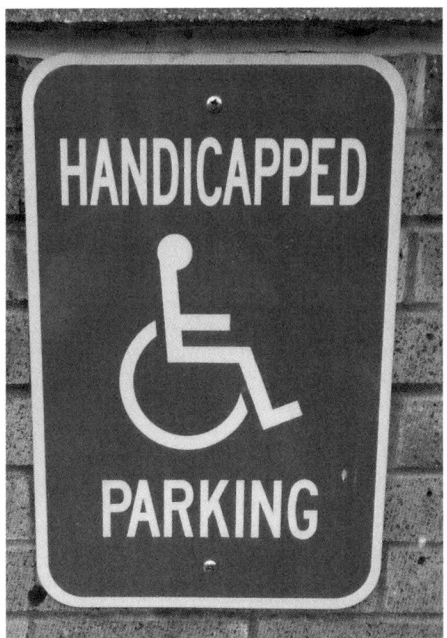

Handicapped parking placard

handpiece /hand′pēs/, a handheld extraoral or intraoral device for holding rotary instruments in a dental engine or condensing points in mechanical condensing units. It can be driven by an arm, cable, belt, or tube to a power source, such as a motor, directly to a motor, or to an air-pressure driven motor.

hand scaling, the manual removal of plaque and calculus from the surface of a tooth by an instrument.

hands-only CPR, a lifesaving technique involving no mouth-to-mouth contact in the revival of an individual with a witnessed cardiac arrest outside a health care facility. Chest compressions that are at least 2 inches deep and delivered at a rate of at least 100 compressions per minute are administered until appropriate lifesaving measures are available.

handwriting group, (in occupational therapy) a group designed to help its members build a solid foundation of skills required for efficient and legible handwriting.

hanging drop preparation [ME, *hangen,* to hang; AS, *dropa,* to fall; L, *praeparer,* to make ready], a technique used for the examination and identification of certain microorganisms, such as spirochetes or trichomonads. The technique requires a coverslip, a microscope, and a special slide that has a central concavity. A specimen suspected of containing the microorganism is diluted with a sterile isotonic solution. A drop of this fluid mixture is placed on a glass coverslip, which is then inverted carefully and placed over the slide so that the drop is hanging from the slip into the concavity in the slide. The delicate structures and the method of movement characteristic of the species may then be viewed through the microscope.

hangman's fracture, a break in the posterior elements of the cervical vertebrae with dislocation of C2.

hangnail [AS, *angnaegl,* troublesome nail], a piece of partially disconnected epidermis of the cuticle or nail fold. Tearing the skin fragment causes a red, painful, easily infected sore. Early treatment is to trim the hangnail close with nail clippers. For inflamed cases an antibiotic ointment and protective bandage are used.

hangover, a popular term for a group of disagreeable physical effects, including nausea, thirst, fatigue, headache, and irritability, resulting from the heavy consumption of alcohol and/or certain drugs.

Hanhart syndrome /hän′härt/ [Ernst Hanhart, Swiss physician, 1891–1973], any of several syndromes of variable inheritance, characterized chiefly by severe micrognathia, high nose root, small eyelid fissures, low-set ears, and variable absence of digits or limbs, usually below the elbow or knee.

Hanot disease /hanō′/ [Victor C. Hanot, French physician, 1844–1896]. See **primary biliary cholangitis**.

Hansel stain, a stain used to detect eosinophils in urine or other body fluids, the eosinophils staining red against a background of blue.

Hansen bacillus [Gerard H.A. Hansen, Norwegian physician, 1841–1912; L, *bacillum,* a small rod], the acid-fast *Mycobacterium leprae,* which is the cause of leprosy.

Hansen disease. See **leprosy.**

Hantaan virus, a virus of the genus *Hantavirus* that causes severe epidemic hemorrhagic fever (Korean hemorrhagic fever) in Asia.

Hantavirus, a genus of RNA viruses in the Bunyaviridae family. *Hantavirus* is the cause of several different forms of hemorrhagic fever with renal syndrome. Some people appear to be more susceptible than others who are presumed to have had similar exposure to the virus. About half of all reported cases have been fatal. A *Hantavirus* infection begins with flulike symptoms and may be mistaken for other diseases. Some patients were diagnosed originally as having hepatitis or inflammation of the pancreas, or both. The disease can be spread by several common rodent species via rodent excreta. Most U.S. cases have been reported in the western United States, but confirmed hantavirus cases have also been found in the New York City suburbs. *Hantavirus* includes the Hantaan, Seoul, Puumala, Prospect Hill, Sin Nombre, and Porogia strains. See also **hemorrhagic fever.**

hantavirus pulmonary syndrome, a sometimes fatal febrile illness caused by a virus of the genus *Hantavirus,* characterized by variable respiratory symptoms followed by acute respiratory distress, sometimes progressing to respiratory failure.

hepadnavirus /hapad′nəvī″rəs/, any virus belonging to the family Hepadnaviridae, which is made up of viruses that can cause liver infections.

-haphia. See **-aphia, -haphia.**

haplo-, prefix meaning "single," "simple": *haploid.*

haploid /hap″loid/ [Gk, *haploos,* single, *eidos,* form], having only one complete set of nonhomologous chromosomes. Also called **monoploid, monoploidic. –haploidy,** *n.*

haploid nucleus [Gk, *haploos,* single, *eidos,* form; L, nut], a nucleus possessing only half the normal somatic number of chromosomes. It may occur in a germ cell after meiosis and before fertilization. Also called **hemikaryon.**

haploidy. See **haploid.**

Habsburg jaw, a lower jaw (mandible) that projects forward in advance of the upper jaw (maxilla), resulting in a skeletal Class III malocclusion according to Angle's classification of malocclusion. The term relates to the Habsburg royal family in which that facial pattern was dominant. See also **Angle's classification of malocclusion.**

H

Habsburg lip, an overdeveloped, thick lower lip, which often accompanies the Habsburg jaw (a jaw that projects forward). This kind of lip was characteristic of many members of the royal German-Austrian family that produced several European rulers between 1278 and 1918.

hapten /hap″tən/ [Gk, *haptein,* to grasp], a small molecule that acts as an antigen by combining with particular bonding sites on an antibody. By itself it cannot induce an immune response, but when bonded to a carrier protein it may cause an immune response.

haptics /hap′tiks/ [Gk, *haptein,* to grasp], the science concerned with studying the sense of touch. –haptic, *adj.*

haptoglobin /hap′tōglō″bin/ [Gk, *haptein,* to grasp; L, *globus,* ball], a plasma protein that irreversibly binds free hemoglobin and is removed by macrophages conserving iron. The quantity of haptoglobin is increased in certain chronic diseases and inflammatory disorders and is decreased or absent in hemolytic anemia. Normal adult findings range from 100 to 150 mg/dL. Compare **transferrin.** See also **hemoglobinemia, hemoglobinuria.**

haptoglobin test, a blood test primarily used to detect hemolysis, the intravascular destruction of red blood cells. Abnormally low levels of haptoglobin may indicate hemolytic anemias, whereas high levels are found in primary liver disease, many inflammatory diseases, acute myocardial infarction, and some cancers.

harborage transmission /här′bərij/, a mode of infection transmission in which the organism does not undergo morphological and physiological changes in the vector.

hard chancre [AS, *heard* + Fr, *canker*], a syphilitic chancre or primary lesion that develops at the site of a syphilis infection. The lesion begins as a small red papule that gradually hardens and erodes into an extremely contagious, although painless, ulcer. A secretion exuded by the sore contains *Treponema pallidum,* the organism that is the causative agent of syphilis in humans.

hard contact lens [AS, *heard* + L, *contingere,* to touch, *lentil*], a polymethylmethacrylate, or rigid gas-permeable, contact lens that retains its form without support, in contrast with a soft contact lens, which readily yields to pressure.

hard data, information about a patient that is obtained by observation and measurement, including laboratory data, as opposed to information collected by interview of the patient or others.

hard disk, a computer data storage medium that consists of a rigid disk with an electromagnetic coating allowing information to be transcribed onto and from it. Permanently mounted in a dust-proof container, a hard disk has a storage capacity many times that of other storage devices. Also called *hard drive.*

hardening /här′dəning/ [AS, *heard,* hard], **1.** sclerosis. See **induration, sclerosis. 2.** the procedure of rendering tissue firm so that it may be more readily cut for purposes of microscopic examination.

hardening of the arteries. *(Informal)* See **arteriosclerosis.**

hard fibroma, a neoplasm composed of fibrous tissue in which few cells are present. Also called **fibroma durum.**

hard metal disease, pneumoconiosis caused by inhalation of fine particles of cobalt, usually in conjunction with tungsten carbide. In early stages reversible hyperplasia and metaplasia of the bronchial epithelium are seen. Later, subacute alveolitis and then chronic interstitial fibrosis develop. Also called **cobalt lung.**

hardness /härd′nəs/ [AS, *heard,* hard], **1.** a quality of water produced by soluble salts of calcium and magnesium or other substances that form a precipitate with soap and thus interfere with its cleansing power. **2.** the quality of firmness produced by cohesion of the particles composing a substance, as evidenced by its inflexibility or resistance to indentation, distortion, or scratching. **3.** (in radiography) the quality of the primary beam.

hardness of x-rays, the relative energy or penetrating power of x-rays. In general, the hardness increases as the wavelength of the x-rays decreases. Also called **hard radiation.** Compare **soft radiation.**

hard nevus. See **epidermal nevus.**

hard palate [AS, *heard,* hard; L, *palatum*], the bony portion of the roof of the mouth, continuous posteriorly with the soft palate and bounded anteriorly and laterally by the alveolar arches and the gums. The hard palate is covered with stratified squamous epithelium and furnished with numerous palatal glands lying between the mucous membrane and the surface of the bone. Compare **soft palate.**

hard radiation. See **hardness of x-rays.**

hard soap, a cleansing agent made with natural oils/fats and sodium hydroxide or sodium carbonate.

HARDE syndrome. See **Walker-Warburg syndrome.**

hardware, the tangible parts of a computer, such as chips, boards, wires, transformers, and peripheral devices. See also **software.**

hard water [AS, *heard* + *waeter*], water that contains certain cations, particularly calcium and magnesium, that precipitate with soap solutions. The term is generally applied to tap water, and the degree of hardness varies with the source and previous treatment.

Hardy-Weinberg equilibrium principle /här″dē wīn″bərg/ [G.H. Hardy, English mathematician, 1877–1947; Wilhelm Weinberg, German physician, 1862–1937; L, *aequilibris,* equal weight, *principium,* a beginning], a principle stating that the frequency of alleles and genotypes remains relatively unchanged from generation to generation in a large, interbreeding population characterized by random mating, Mendelian inheritance, and the absence of migration, mutation, and selection. Under such conditions, the ratio of individuals homozygous for a dominant allele to those heterozygous to those homozygous for a recessive allele is 1:2:1. See also **genetic equilibrium.**

harelip. *(Obsolete)* See **cleft lip.**

hare eye. See **lagophthalmos.**

harlequin color /här″lək(w)in/ [It, *arlecchino,* goblin; L, *color,* hue], a temporary flushing of the skin on one side lower side of the body with pallor on the other side. Commonly seen in normal young infants, it disappears as the child matures.

harlequin fetus, an infant whose skin at birth is completely covered with thick, horny scales that resemble armor and are divided by deep red fissures. The condition is the most severe form of lamellar exfoliation of the newborn. In the neonatal period, the newborn is at risk for secondary sepsis and dehydration. There is no cure at the present time.

harlequin ichthyosis, the ichthyosis affecting a harlequin fetus. See also **ichthyosis.**

harlequin snake. See **coral snake.**

Harrington rod /har′ingtən/ [Paul R. Harrington, American orthopedic surgeon, 1911–1980], one of the rigid, contoured metal rods inserted surgically, along with metal hooks, in the posterior elements of the spine to provide distraction and compression in the treatment of scoliosis and other deformities.

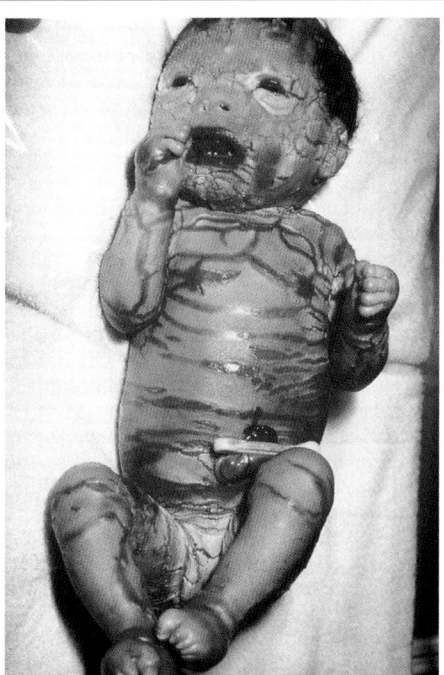

Infant with harlequin ichthyosis *(Rennie, 2012)*

Harrison's groove [Edward Harrison, English physician, 1776–1838], a deformity of the thorax that develops as a result of the pull of the diaphragm on ribs weakened by rickets or some other calcium deficiency disorder.

Harris tube [Franklin Harris, American surgeon, b. 1895], a mercury-weighted single-lumen tube formerly used for gastric and intestinal decompression. It is not in current use because of the danger of mercury poisoning.

Hartmann's curet [Arthur Hartmann, German physician, 1849–1931], a curet used for the removal of adenoids. See also **curet.**

Hartmann pouch, a bulbous region of the neck of the gallbladder. When a gallstone lodges in this area, the gallbladder cannot empty normally and contractions of the gallbladder wall produce severe pain.

Hartmann's solution. See **Ringer's lactate solution.**

Hartnup disease [Hartnup, family name of first patients diagnosed in England, 1956], a rare autosomal-recessive genetic metabolic disorder characterized by pellagra-like skin lesions, transient cerebellar ataxia, and hyperaminoaciduria. It is caused by defects in intestinal absorption and renal reabsorption of neutral amino acids. Bacterial degradation of unabsorbed amino acids in the gut leads to the absorption of breakdown products and their appearance in urine; the unavailability of tryptophan leads to a deficiency of niacin, the antipellagra vitamin. Common symptoms of the disease are dry, scaly, well-circumscribed skin lesions; glossitis; stomatitis; diarrhea; psychiatric problems; and pronounced photosensitivity. Brief exposure to the sun may cause erythema, edema, and vesiculation. Treatment consists of oral nicotinamide, a high-protein diet containing proteins composed of more easily absorbed small peptides, and avoidance of sun exposure.

Harvard apparatus, a small pump that can be adjusted to deliver small amounts of medication in solution through an IV infusion set. It is commonly used to administer oxytocin in the induction or augmentation of labor.

harvest fever. See **leptospirosis.**

harvest mite. See **chigger.**

Hashimoto disease /hä′shimō″tō/ [Hakaru Hashimoto, Japanese surgeon, 1881–1934], a progressive autoimmune thyroid disorder, characterized by the production of antibodies in response to thyroid antigens and the replacement of normal thyroid structures with lymphocytes and lymphoid germinal centers. The disease shows a marked hereditary pattern, but it is 20 times more common in women than in men. It occurs most frequently between 30 and 50 years of age but may arise in young children. The thyroid, typically enlarged, pale yellow, and lumpy on the surface, shows dense lymphocytic infiltration and follicular hyperplasia. The goiter is usually asymptomatic, but occasionally patients have difficulty swallowing and a feeling of local pressure. The thymus is usually enlarged, and regional lymph nodes often show hyperplasia. A definitive diagnosis can be made if a fluorescent scan shows a decrease or absence of thyroid-stable iodine and if the result of a hemagglutination test for thyroid antigens is positive. Replacement therapy with thyroid hormone is indicated for patients with thyroid deficiency and can prevent further enlargement of the goiter. Also called *Hashimoto struma, Hashimoto thyroiditis,* **lymphocytic thyroiditis, struma lymphomatosa.**

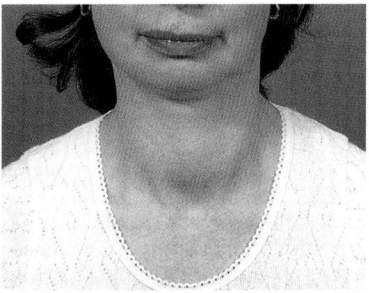

Enlargement of the thyroid gland associated with Hashimoto disease *(Belchetz and Hammond, 2003)*

hashish. See **cannabis.**

hashitoxicosis /hash″itok″siko′sis/, excessive functional activity of the thyroid gland in patients with Hashimoto disease, in whom decreased thyroid function would ordinarily be expected.

Hasner fold. See **lacrimal fold.**

hatchet /hach′ət/, (in dentistry) a bibeveled or single beveled cutting dental hand instrument having its cutting edge in line with the axis of its blade. It is used for breaking down tooth structure undermined by caries, smoothing cavity walls, removing unsupported enamel, and sharpening line and point angles.

hatha yoga, the area of raja yoga best known in the West, based on physical purification and strengthening as a means of self-transformation. It encompasses a system of over 1000 asanas (postures), designed to promote mental and physical well-being and to allow the mind to focus and become free from distraction for long periods of meditation, along with pranayama (breath control). A number of styles of yoga founded on hatha yoga have been developed.

haustrum /hôs′trəm/ *pl. haustra* [L, *haustor,* drawer], a general term denoting a recess or sacculation, as of the colon.

haustus (h) /hôs′təs/, *(Obsolete)* a draft of medicine; a quantity ordered as a single dose.

HAV, initialism for *hepatitis A virus.* See **hepatitis A.**

Haverhill fever /hā″vəril/ [Haverhill, Massachusetts, disorder first diagnosed, 1925], a febrile disease caused by infection with *Streptobacillus moniliformis,* usually transmitted by the bite of a rat but sometimes transmitted by secretion from the mouth, nose, or urine of an infected rodent. The spirochete-like bacterium is normally present in rat saliva. Characteristically the wound from the bite heals, but within 10 days fever, chills, vomiting, headache, and muscle and joint pain occur, followed within 3 days by a rash. Treatment with antibiotics is effective. *S. moniliformis* is identified by laboratory analysis using fluorescent antibody screening. Also called **streptobacillary rat-bite fever.**

Havers glands. See **haversian glands.**

haversian canal /havur″shən/ [Clopton Havers, English physician, 1650–1702], one of the many tiny longitudinal canals in bone tissue, averaging about 0.05 mm in diameter. Each contains blood vessels, connective tissue, nerve filaments, and occasionally lymphatic vessels. The canals are interconnected and part of an intricate network. See also **haversian canaliculus, haversian system, Volkmann's canal.**

haversian canaliculus /kan′əlik″yələs/ [Clopton Havers], any of the many tiny passages radiating from the lacunae of bone tissue to larger haversian canals. See also **haversian canal, haversian system.**

haversian glands [Clopton Havers; L, *glans,* acorn], extrasynovial fat pads that may project into the joint space. Also called **Havers glands.**

haversian lamella [Clopton Havers; L, *lamella,* a small plate], one of a series of lamellae (circular layers) arranged around the central haversian canal of an osteon, or cylindrical unit of bone structure. Also called **Havers lamella.**

haversian system [Clopton Havers], a circular unit of bone tissue, consisting of concentric rings of osteocytes and lamellae in the bone around a central blood vessel canal. See also **haversian canal, haversian canaliculus, Volkmann's canal.**

Havers lamella. See **haversian lamella.**

Hawley retainer /hô′lē/ [C.A. Hawley, American dentist, early 20th century], an orthodontic appliance consisting of a removable labial wire and an acrylic biteplate resting against the palate, used to stabilize teeth after their movement or as a basis for tooth movement by providing anchorage for other attachments. Also called *Hawley appliance.*

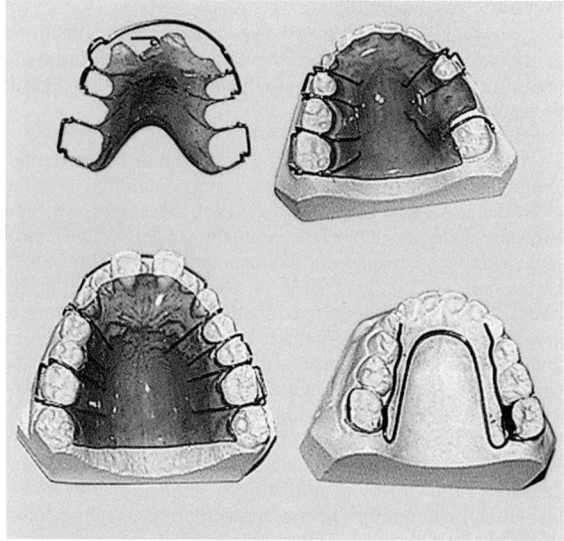

Examples of Hawley retainers *(Bird and Robinson, 2015)*

hawthorn, an herbal product taken from a bush or tree found throughout the United States, Canada, Europe, and Asia.
■ INDICATIONS: It is used for poor circulation, chest pain, irregular heartbeat, high blood lipids, and high blood pressure.

Several studies have shown beneficial effects of hawthorn in heart failure; there are insufficient reliable data for its other uses.
■ CONTRAINDICATIONS: It should not be used during pregnancy and lactation or in children. It is also contraindicated in those with known hypersensitivity to this herb or other members of the Rosaceae family.

Hawthorne effect /hô′thôrn/, an unintentional, usually beneficial, effect on a person, a group of people, or the function of the system being studied. It is the effect of an encounter, as with an investigator or health care provider, or of a change in a program or facility, as by painting of an office or change in the lighting system. The Hawthorne effect is likely to confound the results of a study or investigation because it is usually present and difficult to identify. It was named for a study in industrial management at the Hawthorne (Illinois) facility of the Western Electric Company.

hay fever [AS, *heawan,* to hew; L, *febris,* fever], *(Informal)* an acute seasonal allergic rhinitis stimulated by tree, grass, or weed pollen. Also called **pollen coryza, pollinosis.** See also **allergic rhinitis, organic dust.**

Hayflick limits [Leonard Hayflick, American microbiologist, b. 1928; L, *limes,* border], the concept that the life span of living organisms is limited by the number of times that somatic cells will subdivide. On the basis of human cells in cultures, where divisions occur about 50 times, it is estimated that the average human life span is limited to around 115 years. See also *deliberate biological programming.*

Hay-Wells syndrome /hā welz/ [R.J. Hay, British dermatologist, 20th century; Robert Stuart Wells, British dermatologist, 20th century], an autosomal-dominant syndrome of ectodermal dysplasia, cleft lip and palate, and ankyloblepharon. It is also characterized by hypodontia, palmar and plantar keratoderma, partial anhidrosis, sparse wiry hair, and sometimes otological defects. Also called **AEC syndrome, ankyloblepharon–ectodermal dysplasia–clefting syndrome.**

hazard /haz′ərd/ [Fr, *hasard,* chance], a condition or phenomenon that increases the probability of a loss. A hazard can increase the chances of a loss that does not necessarily result in illness or injury. –*hazardous, adj.*

hazardous materials, substances or materials that have been determined by the government to pose an unreasonable risk to health, safety, or property when transported in commerce, such as toxins, marine pollutants, and substances at high temperatures.

Hb, abbreviation for **hemoglobin.**

HB, abbreviation for **hepatitis B.**

Hb A, abbreviation for **hemoglobin A.**

Hb A₂, abbreviation for **hemoglobin A₂.**

Hb C, abbreviation for **hemoglobin C.**

HBE, abbreviation for **His bundle electrogram.**

Hb F, abbreviation for **hemoglobin F.**

HBIG, abbreviation for **hepatitis B immune globulin.**

HBP, abbreviation for **high blood pressure.** See **hypertension.**

Hb S, abbreviation for **hemoglobin S.**

HBsAG, abbreviation for **hepatitis B surface antigen.** See **Australia antigen.**

Hb SC, abbreviation for *hemoglobin SC.*

HBV, initialism for *hepatitis B virus.* See **hepatitis B.**

HC, abbreviation for **hepatitis C.**

HCFA, abbreviation for **Health Care Financing Administration.**

hCG, abbreviation for **human chorionic gonadotropin.** See **chorionic gonadotropin.**

H chain, heavy chain, any of the large polypeptide chains of five classes that, paired with the L or light chains, make up the antibody molecule of an immunoglobulin. Heavy chains bear the antigenic determinants that differentiate the classes of immunoglobulins. See also **heavy chain disease.**

HCl, 1. chemical formula for **hydrochloric acid. 2.** chemical formula for *hydrogen chloride.*

HCP, abbreviation for **hereditary coproporphyria.** See **coproporphyria.**

HCV, initialism for *hepatitis C virus.* See **hepatitis C.**

HD, 1. abbreviation for **hepatitis D. 2.** abbreviation for **hemodialysis.**

HDCV, abbreviation for **human diploid cell rabies vaccine.**

H deflection, a deviation observed on the His bundle electrogram that represents activation of the bundle of His.

HDI, abbreviation for **high-definition imaging.**

HDL, abbreviation for **high-density lipoprotein.**

HDL-C, abbreviation for *high-density lipoprotein cholesterol.* See **cholesterol.**

HDV, initialism for *hepatitis D virus.* See **hepatitis D.**

He, symbol for the element **helium.**

HE, abbreviation for **hepatitis E.**

head [AS, *heafod*], **1.** the uppermost extremity, containing the brain, special sense organs, mouth, nose, ears, and related structures. Most of the tissues are enclosed within the skull, composed of 22 bones. At birth the head is about half the size of an adult head; the greatest changes after infancy involve growth of the facial area. **2.** a rounded, usually proximal portion of some long bones.

headache /hed′āk/ [AS, *heafod* + *acan,* to hurt], a pain in the head from any cause. Also called **cephalalgia, cephalgia.** Kinds include **cluster headache,** *functional headache,* **histamine headache, migraine, organic headache,** *sinus headache,* **tension headache.**

head and neck cancer, any malignant neoplasms of the upper aerodigestive tract, facial features, and structures in the neck, which appear as masses, ulcerations, or flat lesions that usually produce early symptoms. See also *specific cancers.*

head banging, a form of physical exertion observed during some temper tantrums. It usually occurs near the peak of excitement and may be associated with other physical or muscular movements.

head bobbing, a sign of respiratory distress in an infant. It occurs when the infant uses the scaleni and sternocleidomastoid muscles to assist ventilation. The contraction of these muscles causes the head to bob because the neck extensor muscles are not strong enough to stabilize the head.

head box, a clear plastic chamber that fits over a patient's head with an adjustable seal around the neck for mechanical ventilation. Humidified gas enters the chamber, and excess gas is released through an outlet valve. The device may help prevent the need for intubation.

headcap. See **headgear.**

head, eye, ear, nose, and throat (HEENT), a specialty in medicine concerned with the anatomical, physiological, and pathological characteristics of the head, eyes, ears, nose, and throat and with the diagnosis and treatment of disorders of those structures.

headgear /hed′gēr/, a harnesslike device fitting over the top of the head, back of the head, or both, serving as a source of resistance for extraoral anchorage for an orthodontic appliance. Also called **headcap.**

head injury, any traumatic damage to the head resulting from blunt or penetrating trauma of the skull. Blood vessels, nerves, and meninges can be torn. Bleeding, edema, and ischemia may result. See also **concussion.**

head kidney. See **pronephros.**

head louse. See **lice,** *Pediculus humanus capitis.*

head nurse. See **nurse manager.**

head of rib, the head of a rib that articulates with a vertebral body.

head process, a strand of cells that extends forward from the primitive node in the early stages of embryonic development in vertebrates. It is the precursor of the notochord and forms the primitive axis around which the embryo develops. Also called **notochordal plate.**

heads-up tilt table test (HUTT), a method of evaluating patients with neurocardiac syncope. After baseline signs are recorded with the patient in the supine position, the patient is tilted to an 80-degree angle for 30 minutes or until neurocardiac syncope signs appear.

head-tilt, chin-lift airway technique, a method of providing maximum airway opening in an unconscious person. With the victim lying on his or her back, the rescuer pushes down on the victim's forehead with the palm of the hand, tilting the victim's head back. With the other hand, the rescuer lifts the victim's lower jaw near the chin. The technique opens the airway by moving the tongue away from the back of the throat and the epiglottis away from the opening of the trachea. This technique is not recommended if a cervical spine injury is suspected. See also **cardiopulmonary resuscitation.**

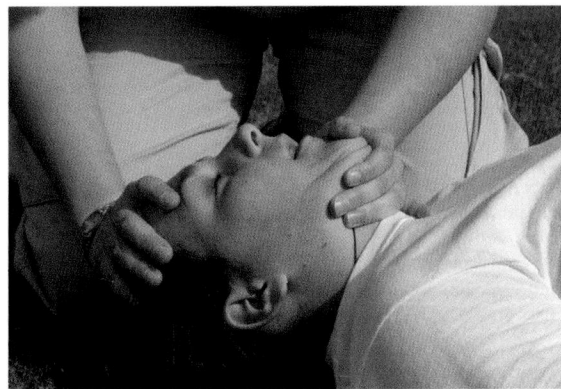

Head-tilt, chin-lift airway technique *(Cummings, 2008)*

head traction. *(Informal)* See **cervical traction.**

Heaf test /hēf/ [Frederick R.G. Heaf, English physician, 1894–1973], *(Obsolete)* a tuberculin skin test that used a multiple puncture technique; it is no longer available. See also **tuberculin test.**

healing [AS, *haelan,* to cure], **1.** the act or process in which the normal structural and functional characteristics of health are restored to diseased, dysfunctional, or damaged tissues, organs, or systems of the body. See also **intention, wound repair. 2.** the process of helping individuals to achieve a state in which they are able to function physically, mentally, socially, and spiritually in ways that facilitate the expression of their full potential and realize individual goals for health.

healing by third intention, a method of closing a grossly contaminated wound in which the wound is left open until contamination has been markedly reduced and inflammation has subsided and then is closed by first intention. Also called *delayed closure.* See also **intention.**

health [AS, *haelth*], a condition of physical, mental, and social well-being and the absence of disease or other abnormal condition; not a static condition. See also **high-level wellness, homeostasis.**

health assessment, an evaluation of the health status of an individual by performing a physical examination after obtaining a health history. Various laboratory tests may also be ordered to confirm a clinical impression or to screen for dysfunction. The depth of investigation and the frequency of the assessment vary with the condition and age of the client and the facility in which the assessment is performed. The person's response to any dysfunction present is observed and noted. The techniques of the health assessment include inspection, palpation, percussion, and auscultation.

health behavior, an action taken by a person to maintain, attain, or regain good health and to prevent illness. Health behavior reflects a person's health beliefs. Some common health behaviors are exercising regularly, eating a balanced diet, and obtaining necessary inoculations.

health belief model, a conceptual framework that describes a person's health behavior as an expression of health beliefs. The model was designed to predict a person's health behavior, including the use of health services, and to justify intervention to alter maladaptive health behavior. Components of the model include the person's own perception of susceptibility to a disease or condition, the perceived likelihood of contracting that disease or condition, the perceived severity of the consequences of contracting the condition or the disease, the perceived benefits of care and barriers to preventive behavior, and the internal or external stimuli that result in appropriate health behavior by the person.

health care consumer, any actual or potential recipient of health care, such as a patient in a hospital, a client in a community mental health center, or a member of a prepaid health maintenance organization.

Health Care Financing Administration (HCFA), a U.S. agency that was renamed in July 2001 as the Centers for Medicare and Medicaid Services. See **Centers for Medicare and Medicaid Services.**

health care industry, the complex of preventive, remedial, and therapeutic services provided by hospitals and other institutions, nurses, doctors, dentists, medical administrators, government agencies, voluntary agencies, noninstitutional care facilities, pharmaceutic and medical equipment manufacturers, and health insurance companies.

health care provider, any individual, institution, or agency that provides health services to health care consumers.

health care proxy [AS, *haelth* + ME, *caru,* sorrow; L, *procuratio,* a deputy], a person designated to make health care decisions for a patient who has become incapacitated.

health center, **1.** a site for the provision of preventive and primary health care. **2.** a community-based public or private nonprofit health care organization that complies with Federal requirements. Kinds include **federally qualified heath center, Federally qualified health center look-alike.**

health care system, the complete network of agencies, facilities, and all providers of health care in a specified geographic area. Nursing services are integral to all levels and patterns of care, and nurses form the largest number of providers in a health care system.

health certificate, a statement signed by a health care provider that attests to the state of health of a person.

health consumer. See **health care consumer.**

health councils, (in Canada) organizations that plan and allocate health care facilities to optimize limited funding resources.

health culture, a system that attempts to explain and treat sickness and to maintain health. Health cultures are a component of the larger culture or tradition of a people and may be a popular or folk system or a technical or scientific one.

health disparities, preventable differences in the achievement of optimal physiological and psychological health experienced by underserved and/or marginalized populations.

health economics, a social system that studies the supply and demand of health care resources and the effect of health services on a population.

health education, educational programs directed to the public that attempt to improve, maintain, and safeguard the health of the community.

health hazard [AS, *haelth* + OFr, *hasard*], a danger to health resulting from exposure to environmental pollutants, such as asbestos or ionizing radiation, or to a lifestyle choice, such as cigarette smoking or chemical abuse.

health history, a collection of information obtained from the patient and from other sources concerning the patient's physical status as well as his or her psychological, social, and sexual function. The history provides a database on which a diagnosis, a plan for management of the diagnosis, treatment, care, and follow-up observation of the patient may be made. The first part of the history describes the chief complaint; the history of the present illness, including its signs and symptoms, onset and character; and any factors or behaviors that aggravate or ameliorate the symptoms. The patient's own words often serve as the best description and may be quoted. The second part of the history comprises an account of previous illnesses and health-promotion behaviors, allergies, transfusions, immunizations, screening tests, and hospitalizations. An occupational history, describing the patient's work and exposure to stress, toxins, radiation, or other occupational hazards, should be included. The effect of the current illness on the patient's work is also noted. A social history is taken in which the patient's social, cultural, environmental, and familial milieu are outlined, focusing on aspects that might have an effect on the current illness. In some instances a sexual history may be relevant. A review of systems, including mental health, may follow or be incorporated into the health history. Also called **functional assessment, personal and social history.** Kinds include **complete health history, interval health history.** See also **family history, occupational history, past health, present health, review of systems, sexual history.**

health information administrator, a graduate of a baccalaureate degree program in health information management who contributes to the development or management of computer-based clinical and administrative record systems.

health information exchange (HIE), a secure system for sharing clinical information and electronic health records among hospital systems and health care providers to enable rapid confidential access to clinical information.

health information technician, a graduate of an associate degree program who performs tasks related to computer-based management of health care data.

health insurance marketplace, A Web site (http://healthcare.gov) for individuals, families, and small businesses in the United States to explore coverage options, compare health insurance plans, choose a plan, enroll in coverage, or change and update a plan. Individuals and families may apply for coverage online, by phone, or with a paper application.

Health Insurance Portability and Accountability Act (HIPAA), an act of Congress, passed in 1996, that affords certain protections to persons covered by health care plans, including continuity of coverage when changing jobs, standards for electronic health care transactions, and privacy safeguards for individually identifiable patient information.

health maintenance, a systematic program or procedure planned to prevent illness, maintain maximum function, and promote health. It is central to health care, especially to nursing care at all levels (primary, secondary, and tertiary) and in all patterns (preventive, episodic, acute, chronic, and catastrophic).

health maintenance organization (HMO), a type of group health care practice that provides basic and supplemental health maintenance and treatment services to voluntary enrollees who prepay a fixed periodic fee that is set without regard to the amount or kind of services received. In addition to diagnostic and treatment services, including hospitalization and surgery, an HMO often offers supplemental services, such as dental, mental, and eye care, and prescription drugs. Federal financial support for the establishment of HMOs was provided under Title XIII of the 1973 U.S. Public Health Service Act.

health nurse, a community or visiting nurse assigned primarily to promote health maintenance and preventive health measures within the community.

health outcomes, indicators that measure the health status of an individual or a community, especially in response to a targeted intervention. Kinds include **glycosylated hemoglobin, fetal mortality rate.**

health physicist, a health scientist who directs research, training, and management of programs in which patients and health professionals are exposed to potential hazards associated with the use of diagnostic and therapeutic equipment, such as radioactive materials.

health physics, the study of the effects of ionizing radiation on the body and the methods for protecting people from the undesirable effects of the radiation. Health physics is concerned with the development and evaluation of methods, techniques, materials, and procedures to be used to protect people from these untoward effects. Also called **medical physics.**

health policy, 1. a statement of a decision regarding a goal in health care and a plan for achieving that goal. For example, to prevent an epidemic, a program for inoculating a population is developed and implemented. **2.** a field of study and practice in which the priorities and values underlying health resource allocation are determined.

health professional, any person who has completed a course of study in a field of health, such as a registered nurse, physical therapist, or physician. The person is usually licensed by a government agency or certified by a professional organization.

health professional shortage area, a designation made by the federal government to identify geographic areas, populations, and/or facilities that have a shortage of health care providers.

health-related services, actions of a health facility other than providing medical care that may contribute directly or indirectly to the physical or mental health and well-being of patients. These actions may include personal or social services, for example.

health resources, all materials, personnel, facilities, funds, and any other resources that can be used for providing health care and services.

Health Resources and Services Administration (HRSA), a U.S. federal agency with responsibility for improving health care access for people who are uninsured, isolated, or medically vulnerable. HRSA also oversees organ, tissue, and bone marrow donation. It supports programs that prepare against bioterrorism, compensates individuals harmed by vaccination, and maintains databases that protect against health care malpractice and health care waste, fraud, and abuse.

health risk, a disease precursor associated with a higher-than-average morbidity or mortality rate. Health risks include demographic variables, certain individual behaviors, familial and individual histories, and certain physiological changes.

health risk appraisal, a process of gathering, analyzing, and comparing an individual's or community's characteristics prognostic of health with those of a standard age group or community group, thereby predicting the likelihood that a person or a member of the community may prematurely experience a health problem associated with higher-than-average morbidity and mortality rates.

health savings account (HSA), a mechanism to set aside money for medical expenses and reduce taxable income for U.S. citizens with qualifying high-deductible health plans.

health screening, a program designed to evaluate the health status and potential of an individual. In the process it may be found that a person has a particular disease or condition or is at greater-than-normal risk of its development. Health screening may include taking a personal and family health history and performing a physical examination, tests, laboratory tests, or radiological examination and may be followed by counseling, education, referral, or further testing.

health service area, a geographic region designated under the U.S. National Health Planning and Resources Development Act of 1974, by means of such factors as geographic features, political boundaries, population, and health resources, for the effective planning and development of health services.

health supervision, health teaching, counseling, or monitoring of the status of a patient's health other than for physical care. Such supervision occurs in health care agencies, clinics, physicians' offices, or a patient's home.

health systems agency (HSA), a body established under the terms of the U.S. National Health Planning and Resources Development Act of 1974. Health planning agencies are intended to provide networks of health planning and resource development services in each of several health service areas established by the Act. Health systems agencies are nonprofit. They may include private organizations, public regional planning bodies, local government agencies, and consumers. See also **health systems plan.**

health systems plan, a plan specifying long-range goals of a health services area. Health systems plans are prepared by health systems agencies. See also **health policy.**

health unit coordinator, a person who ensures the efficient operation of hospital and medical offices by performing administrative and clerical tasks, such as maintaining medical records, scheduling appointments and medical tests, transcribing doctor's orders, keeping supplies stocked, and communicating with other health care professionals.

healthy, a condition of physical, mental, and social well-being and of absence of disease or another abnormal condition.

Healthy People 2020, a government-sponsored statement of national health objectives in 28 focus areas designed to identify and reduce the most significant preventable health threats within the United States. The overall goals of the program are to increase the quality and length of life and to eliminate health disparities. Goals are developed for each decade.

hearing [AS, *hieran*], the sense that enables sound to be perceived. It is a major function of the ear. Any reduction in the ability to perceive sounds results in hearing loss, which can range from mild impairment to complete deafness. See also **deafness.**

hearing aid, an electronic device that amplifies sound used by people with impaired hearing. The device consists of a microphone, a battery power supply, an amplifier, and a receiver. The microphone receives sound waves directed toward the person with hearing loss, then converts the sound waves to electrical impulses that are amplified with the aid of the power supply, and the receiver converts the electrical impulses back into sound vibrations. Newer programmable hearing aids can be customized on the basis of the characteristics of an individual's hearing loss. Types of hearing aids include in-the-canal (ITC) hearing aids, completely-in-the-canal (CIC) hearing aids, in-the-ear (ITE) hearing aids, behind-the-ear (BTE) hearing aids, receiver-in-canal hearing aids, extended-wear hearing aids, and middle ear implants. Most of the hearing aids sold are in-the-canal, completely-in-the-canal, and in-the-ear models. Behind-the-ear hearing aids are most common for babies and young children.

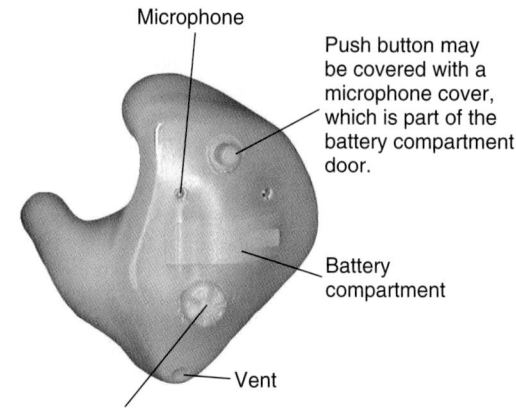

Microphone

Push button may be covered with a microphone cover, which is part of the battery compartment door.

Battery compartment

Vent

On/Off switch/Volume control

Hearing aid *(Courtesy Siemens Hearing Instruments, Inc.)*

hearing impairment, a loss of hearing. The terms *deaf* or *hard of hearing* are preferred by the deaf community as the term *hearing impairment* focuses on what an individual cannot do and establishes hearing as the standard and anything different as "impaired."

hearing loss, an inability to perceive the normal range of sounds that are usually audible. Hearing loss may be greater at some frequencies than others, or all frequencies may be equally affected. Conductive hearing loss is a result of damage to the outer or middle ear, whereas sensorineural hearing loss results from damage to the cochlea or auditory nerve. The loss is measured in decibels and may be described as mild, moderate, severe, or profound. See also **conductive hearing loss, sensorineural hearing loss.**

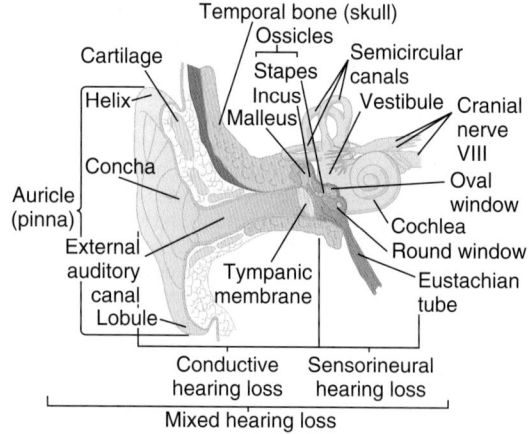

Temporal bone (skull)
Ossicles
Cartilage
Stapes
Semicircular canals
Helix
Incus
Vestibule
Malleus
Cranial nerve VIII
Concha
Auricle (pinna)
Oval window
External auditory canal
Cochlea
Round window
Tympanic membrane
Eustachian tube
Lobule

Conductive hearing loss | Sensorineural hearing loss
Mixed hearing loss

Types of hearing loss *(Black and Hawks, 2009)*

heart [AS, *heorte*], the muscular cone-shaped hollow organ, about the size of a clenched fist, that pumps blood throughout the body and beats normally about 70 times per minute by coordinated nerve impulses and muscular contractions. Enclosed in pericardium, it rests on the diaphragm between the lower borders of the lungs, occupying the middle of the mediastinum. It is covered ventrally by the sternum and the adjoining parts of the third to the sixth costal cartilages. The organ is about 12 cm long, 8 cm wide at its broadest part, and

6 cm thick. The weight of the heart in men averages between 280 and 340 g and in women, between 230 and 280 g. The layers of the heart, starting from the outside, are the epicardium, the myocardium, and the endocardium. The chambers include two ventricles with thick muscular walls, making up the bulk of the organ, and two atria with thin muscular walls. A septum separates the ventricles and extends between the atria (interatrial septum), dividing the heart into the right and the left sides. The left side of the heart pumps oxygenated blood into the aorta and on to all parts of the body. The right side receives deoxygenated blood from the vena cava and pumps it into the pulmonary arteries. The valves of the heart include the tricuspid valve, the bicuspid (mitral) valve, the semilunar aortic valve, and the semilunar pulmonary valve. The sinoatrial node in the right atrium of the heart (under the control of the medulla oblongata in the brainstem) initiates the cardiac impulse, causing the atria to contract. The atrioventricular (AV) node near the septal wall of the right atrium spreads the impulse over the AV bundle (bundle of His) and its branches, causing the ventricles to contract. Both atria contract simultaneously, followed quickly by the simultaneous contraction of the ventricles. The sinoatrial node of the heartbeat sets the rate. Other factors affecting the heartbeat are emotion, exercise, hormones, temperature, pain, and stress. See also **endocardium, epicardium, heart valve, myocardium.**

heart attack. See **myocardial infarction.**

heartbeat, a complete cycle of cardiac muscle contraction and relaxation.

heart block, an interference with the normal conduction of electrical impulses that control activity of the heart muscle. Heart block is usually specified by the location of the block and the type, such as a first-degree atrioventricular (AV) block, in which atrial impulses are delayed by a fraction of a second before being conducted to the ventricles. Heart block can occur in the sinus node, atria, AV node, AV bundle, fascicles, or a combination of these structures. See also **atrioventricular block, bundle branch block, cardiac conduction defect, infranodal block, intraatrial block, intraventricular block, sinoatrial (SA) block.**

heartburn, a painful burning sensation in the esophagus just below the sternum. Heartburn is usually caused by the reflux of gastric contents into the esophagus but may result from gastric hyperacidity or peptic ulcer. Antacids relieve the symptoms but do not cure the condition. Also called **pyrosis.** See also **gastroesophageal reflux, hiatal hernia.**

heart disease risk factor [AS, *heorte,* heart; L, *dis* + Fr, *aise,* ease, *risquer,* chance of injury; L, *facere,* to make], one of several hereditary, lifestyle, and environmental influences that increase one's chance of developing heart disease. Examples include cigarette smoking, high blood pressure, diabetes, obesity, high cholesterol level, lack of routine exercise, and hereditary factors as signified by family history.

heart failure, a condition in which the heart cannot pump enough blood to meet the metabolic requirements of body tissues. Many of the symptoms associated with heart failure are caused by the dysfunction of organs other than the heart, especially the lungs, kidneys, and liver. Ventricular dysfunction is usually the basic disorder in congestive heart failure. It often triggers compensatory mechanisms that preserve cardiac output but produce symptoms and signs such as dyspnea, orthopnea, rales, and edema. Heart failure is closely associated with many forms of heart disease, most of which initially affect the left side of the heart. Hence, clinicians commonly divide associated heart failure into left-sided heart failure and right-sided heart failure. Peripheral edema is associated with right-sided heart failure, and dyspnea and other respiratory disorders with left-sided heart failure. Heart failure in infants and children is usually the result of congenital heart disease but also may be caused by

Anterior view of the heart *(Patton and Thibodeau, 2016)*

myocarditis and ectopic tachycardia. Rheumatic mitral disease and aortic valve disease frequently cause congestive heart failure in young adults. Mitral valve disease, especially mitral stenosis, is the most common cause of heart failure in young adults and affects more young women than men. The common causes of heart failure after 40 years of age are coronary atherosclerosis with myocardial infarction, anemia, diastolic hypertension, hypervolemia, valvular heart disease, pulmonary disease, renal disease, and diffuse myocardial disease. Some individuals may suffer heart failure caused by a combination of congenital heart disease and acquired disease. After 50 years of age, a common cause of heart failure, especially in men, is calcific aortic stenosis. Some of the extracardiac signs of heart failure are ascites, bronchial wheezing, hydrothorax, edema, liver enlargement, moist rales, and splenomegaly. Cardiac signs associated with heart failure are abnormalities in the jugular venous pulsation, the carotid pulse, and the apex wave on cardiographic tracings. Treatment for heart failure commonly involves reduction of the heart's workload, administration of drugs such as beta-blockers, digitalis to increase myocardial contractility and cardiac output, salt-restricted diet, diuretics, angiotensin-converting enzymes to decrease afterload, and surgical intervention. Also called **cardiac failure.** See also **compensated heart failure, congestive heart failure.**

heart-hand syndrome. See **Holt-Oram syndrome.**

heart-lung machine, an apparatus consisting of a pump and an oxygenator that takes over the functions of the heart and lungs, especially during open heart surgery. The blood is shunted from the venous system through an oxygenator and returned to the arterial circulation.

heart massage. See **cardiac massage.**

heart murmur. See **cardiac murmur.**

heart rate, the frequency with which the heart beats, calculated by counting the number of QRS complexes or ventricular beats per minute. See also **pulse.**

heart scan, a radiographic scan of the heart, performed after the injection of a radioactive material into a vein. It is used for determining the size, shape, and location of the heart; for diagnosing pericarditis; and for viewing the chambers of the heart. See also **electrocardiography, echocardiography.**

heart sound, a noise produced within the heart during the cardiac cycle that can be heard over the precordium. It may reveal abnormalities in cardiac structure or function. Cardiac auscultation is performed systematically from the apex to the base of the heart or from base to apex, using a stethoscope to listen, initially with the diaphragm and then with the bell of the instrument. Standard heart sounds include S_1, produced by the closure of the atrioventricular valves; S_2, produced by the closure of the semilunar valves; S_3; and S_4. Additional heart sounds include clicks, gallops, murmurs, rubs, and snaps.

heart surgery, any surgical procedure involving the heart, performed to correct acquired or congenital defects, replace diseased valves, open or bypass blocked vessels, or graft a prosthesis or a transplant. Two major types of heart surgery are performed: closed and open. The closed technique is done through a small incision, without use of the heart-lung machine. In the open technique the heart chambers are open and fully visible, and blood is detoured around the surgical field by the heart-lung machine. Preoperative care focuses on correcting metabolic imbalances and cardiac and pulmonary ailments and on performing diagnostic and laboratory tests. General anesthesia is used, the chest cavity is opened, and the heart-lung machine is connected. Hypothermia also is used to decrease the metabolic rate and the need of the tissues for oxygen. After surgery, constant observation is required in an intensive care unit for signs of hemorrhage and shock, cardiac arrhythmias, sudden chest pain, organ failure, and pulmonary edema. The blood pressure and all pulses, respirations, and venous and pulmonary artery pressures and cardiac rhythm (ECG) are monitored. If the blood pressure is high enough to ensure cerebral profusion, the head of the patient's bed is elevated to a semi-Fowler position to encourage chest drainage and lung expansion. The patient is quickly extubated. Oxygen is provided. Chest tube drainage, urinary output, and temperature are noted hourly; IV infusions and sometimes blood transfusions are given. Narcotics help control pain so the patient can effectively cough, deep breathe, and become quickly mobile. Antibiotics are given to prevent infection. Mortality rate is highest during the first 48 hours after surgery. Kinds include **coronary bypass, endarterectomy.** See also **arrhythmia, fibrillation, heart-lung machine, hypothermia, pulmonary edema.**

heart transplantation [AS, *hoerte* + L, *transplantare*], the surgical removal of a donor heart and transfer of the organ to a recipient. The donor heart is usually obtained from an accident victim who was healthy before dying, and it is used to replace the severely diseased heart of another person. Total ischemic time for the transplanted heart is dependent on donor age, with greater tolerance for prolonged ischemic times among grafts from younger donors. The heart is transplanted with anastomoses of the aorta, pulmonary artery, and atria; venous return is provided by an anastomosis between the recipient's right atrium and that of the transplanted organ. Most recipients survive for more than 1 year, and nearly three fourths are able to return to work. The three-year survival rate approaches 75%.

heart valve, one of the four structures within the heart that prevent backflow of blood by opening and closing with each heartbeat. The valves include two semilunar valves, the aortic and pulmonary; the mitral or bicuspid valve; and the tricuspid valve. The valves permit blood flow in only one direction; any of the valves may become defective, permitting the backflow associated with heart murmurs. Also called **cardiac valve.** See also **heart, mitral valve, semilunar valve, tricuspid valve.**

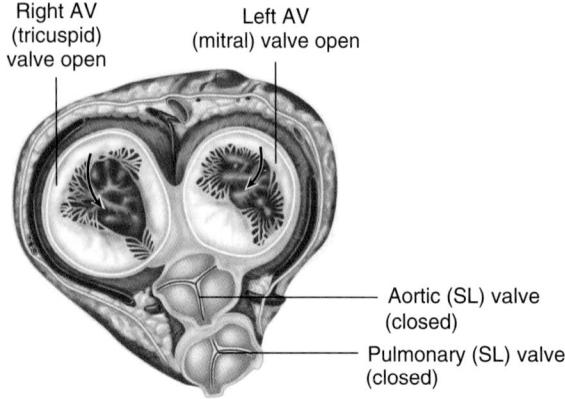

Heart valves *(Patton and Thibodeau, 2016)*

heat and moisture exchanger, a device placed within the patient's breathing circuit and the endotracheal tube, used to preserve moisture and heat. Fresh gas flow can evaporate moisture from mucous membranes in the respiratory tract.

heat cramp [AS, *haetu* + *crammian,* to fill], any painful spasm of the voluntary muscles in the arm, leg, or abdomen caused by depletion in the body of both water and salt. It usually occurs after vigorous physical exertion in an extremely hot environment or under other conditions that cause profuse sweating and depletion of body fluids and electrolytes. The individual should be moved to a cooler place and given salt-containing fluids. Also called *cane-cutter's cramp,* **fireman's cramp, miner's cramp, stoker's cramp.** See also **heat exhaustion.**

heated nebulization, a method of inhalation therapy that uses a heating device with a nebulizer that produces a spray with a higher water content than that of a cold atomizer. The mist may be administered through a mask or in a tent.

heat exhaustion, an abnormal condition characterized by weakness, vertigo, nausea, muscle cramps, and loss of consciousness, caused by depletion of body fluid and electrolytes that results from exposure to intense heat or inability to acclimatize to heat. Body temperature is near normal; blood pressure may drop but usually returns to normal as the person is placed in a recumbent position. The skin is cool, damp, and pale. The person usually recovers with rest and replacement of water and electrolytes. Also called **heat prostration.** Compare **heat hyperpyrexia.** See also **heat cramp.**

heat hyperpyrexia, a severe and sometimes fatal condition resulting from failure of the temperature-regulating capacity of the body, caused by prolonged exposure to sun or to high temperature. Reduction or cessation of sweating is sometimes an early symptom. Body temperature of 105° F or higher, tachycardia, hot and dry skin, headache, altered mental status, and seizures may occur. Treatment includes cooling, sedation, and fluid replacement. Also called **heatstroke, siriasis, sunstroke, thermic fever.** Compare **heat exhaustion.** See also **hyperpyrexia.**

heat labile [L, *labilis,* liable to slip], readily destroyed by heat. See also **thermolabile.**

heat-labile antibody, an immunoglobulin that loses its ability to interact with antigens when heated above 56° C.

heat prostration. See **heat exhaustion.**

heat rash, a finely papular or vesicular inflammation of the skin that results from prolonged exposure to heat and high humidity. Tingling and prickling sensations are common. Prevention and treatment include cool, dry temperatures; ventilation; and absorbent powders. See also **miliaria.**

heat shock protein (HsP), an intracellular protein that increases in concentration during metabolic stress, such as exposure to heat. HsPs affect protein assembly, folding, sorting, and uptake into organelles. There are various kinds of HsPs, each performing different functions.

heatstroke. See **heat hyperpyrexia.**

heaves /hēvz/ [AS, *hebban,* to lift], **1.** a chronic pulmonary disease, similar to human pulmonary emphysema, characterized by wheezing, coughing, and dyspnea on exertion. The cause of the condition is unknown. **2.** *(Informal)* vomiting and retching.

heavy chain, a high-molecular-weight polypeptide that is part of an immunoglobulin molecule. Different types of heavy chains characterize the various categories of immunoglobulins (Igs), such as IgG and IgA. See **immunoglobulin.**

heavy chain disease [AS, *heafig* + L, *catena,* chain; *dis,* opposite of; Fr, *aise,* ease], a plasma cell disorder characterized by a proliferation of immunoglobulin heavy chains. Excessive levels of alpha, gamma, delta, and mu chains are produced, and effects tend to vary according to the predominant type of heavy chain. Alpha heavy chain disease mainly affects children living in the Middle East, causing diffuse abdominal lymphoma and malabsorption disorders. Most gamma heavy chain disease patients are elderly men who have symptoms resembling those of malignant lymphoma: enlarged liver and spleen, fever, anemia, and increased susceptibility to infections. Delta heavy chain disease is rare and marked by symptoms similar to those of multiple myeloma. Mu heavy chain disease presents symptoms of chronic lymphocytic leukemia, and treatment is symptomatic.

heavy function, (in dentistry) increased functional activity of the teeth, which enhances occlusal force.

heavy hydrogen. See **deuterium.**

Comparison of heat-related illness

	Heat cramps	Heat exhaustion	Heat hyperexia (heat stroke)
Cramps	✓	✓	
Fever		✓(<104° F)	✓(>104° F)
Nausea		✓	✓
Headache			✓
Skin	Normal to warm	Cool and clammy	Hot and dry

heavy metal, a metallic element with a specific gravity five or more times that of water. The heavy metals include antimony, arsenic, bismuth, cadmium, cerium, chromium, cobalt, copper, gallium, gold, iron, lead, manganese, mercury, nickel, platinum, silver, tellurium, thallium, tin, uranium, vanadium, and zinc. Small amounts of many of these elements are common and necessary in the diet. Large amounts of any of them may cause poisoning.

heavy metal nephropathy, the kidney damage resulting from any of various forms of heavy metal poisoning, usually in the form of tubulointerstitial nephritis. The most common metals involved are cadmium, lead, and mercury.

heavy metal poisoning, poisoning caused by the ingestion, inhalation, or absorption of various toxic heavy metals. Kinds include **antimony poisoning, arsenic poisoning, cadmium poisoning, lead poisoning, mercury poisoning.** See also **heavy metal.**

heavy vaginal bleeding. (Informal) See **menorrhagia, menometrorrhagia.**

heavy water, water in which the hydrogen component is deuterium (^{2}H), or heavy hydrogen. It has properties different from those of ordinary water. Because of its ability to absorb neutrons, heavy water is used as a moderator in nuclear reactions. Also written as D_2O.

hebephrenia, hebephrenic schizophrenia. See **disorganized schizophrenia.**

Heberden node /hē″bərdən/ [William Heberden, English physician, 1710–1801; L, *nodus,* knot], an abnormal cartilaginous or bony enlargement of a distal interphalangeal joint of a finger, usually occurring in degenerative diseases of the joints. Compare **Bouchard node.**

hebetude /heb″itoōd′/ [L, *hebeo,* to be blunt], a state of dullness or lethargy, characteristic of some forms of schizophrenia.

heboid paranoia. See **paranoid schizophrenia.**

hectic fever, a fever that recurs each day, with profound sweating, chills, and facial flushing.

hecto- (h) [Gk, *hekaton,* one hundred], prefix in the metric system indicating 100 units. For example, 1 hectometer equals 100 meters.

-hedonia, suffix meaning "(condition of) pleasure, cheerfulness": *anhedonia.*

-hedron, suffix meaning a "geometric figure with (specified) sides": *decahedron, octahedron, polyhedron.*

heel [AS, *hela*], the posterior part of the foot, formed by the largest tarsal bone, the calcaneus.

heel cup, a plastic device designed to help relieve the pain of a heel spur or contusion by pushing the fat pad of the heel under the calcaneus to increase the cushioning effect.

heel effect, (in radiology) x-ray intensity that is greater at the cathode end of the x-ray field and lower at the anode end because of absorption in the target material. The heel effect is more pronounced with a shorter distance between the source and image receptor.

heel-knee test [AS, *hela* + *cneow,* knee; L, *testum,* crucible], a method of assessing coordination of movements of the extremities. In the test the patient, lying supine, is asked to touch the knee of one leg with the heel of the other.

heel lift, a foot orthosis, usually made of sheets of cork, to correct a dysfunction that results from anatomical limb length differences or decreased flexibility.

heel puncture [AS, *hela* + L, *punctura*], a method of obtaining a blood sample from a newborn or premature infant by a puncture in the lateral or medial areas of the plantar surface of the heel. Care must be exercised to prevent puncture of the posterior curvature of the heel and to make the puncture as shallow as feasible.

heel-shin test [AS, *hela* + *scinu,* shin; L, *testum,* crucible], a cerebellar test for assessing coordination of movements of the extremities. In the test, the patient, lying supine, is asked to pass the heel of one leg slowly down the shin of the other leg from the knee to the ankle.

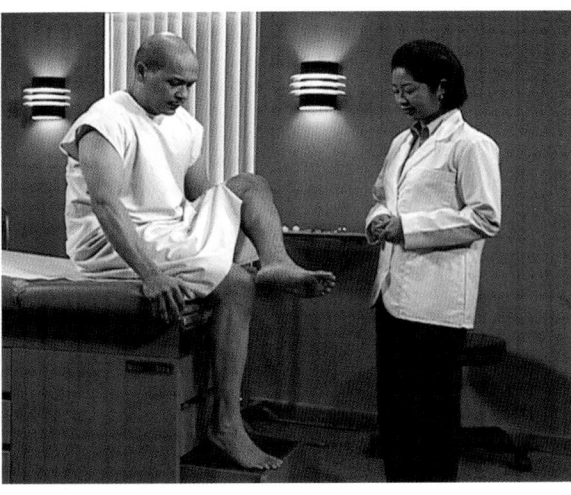

Heel-shin test *(From Elsevier, Clinical Skills: Essentials Collection)*

heel spur. See **calcaneal spur.**

HEENT, abbreviation for **head, eye, ear, nose, and throat.**

Hegar's dilators /hā″gərz/ [Alfred Hegar, German gynecologist, 1830–1914], instruments used to forcibly dilate the cervix. The instruments have blunt ends and come in sets with a range of diameters. See also **bougie.**

Hegar sign [Alfred Hegar; German gynecologist, 1830-1914; L, *signum,* sign], a softening of the isthmus of the uterine cervix that often is discernible on bimanual examination in early gestation. It is historically a probable sign of pregnancy.

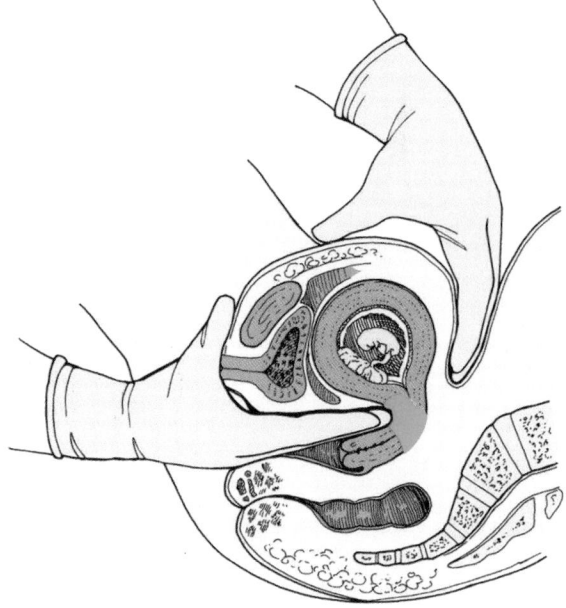

Hegar sign *(Lowdermilk et al, 2016)*

height (h, ht) /hīt/ [AS, *hiehtho*], the vertical measurement of a structure, organ, or other object from bottom to top, when it is placed or projected in an upright position.

height of contour, the greatest convexity of a tooth surface, viewed from a predetermined position.

Heimlich maneuver /hīm′lik, -lish/ [H.J. Heimlich, American physician, 1920–2016; Fr, *manjuvre,* work done by hand], an emergency procedure for dislodging a bolus of food or another obstruction from the trachea to prevent asphyxiation. The choking person is grasped from behind by the rescuer, whose fist, thumb side in, is placed just below the victim's xiphoid with the other hand placed firmly over the fist. The rescuer then pulls the fist firmly and abruptly upward into the epigastrium, forcing the obstruction up the trachea. If repeated attempts do not clear the airway, an emergency cricothyrotomy may be necessary. Also called **abdominal thrust.**

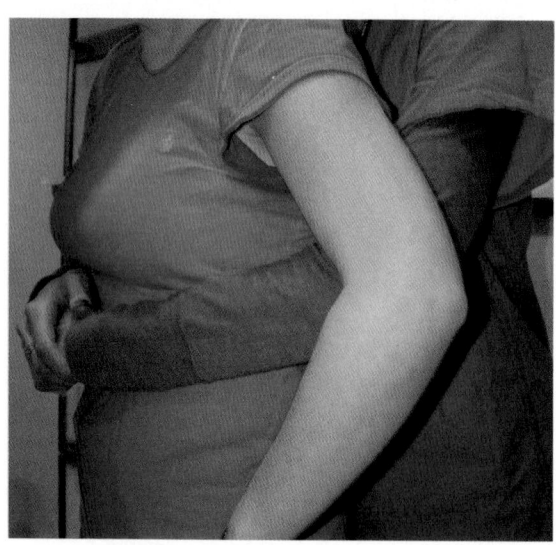

Heimlich maneuver *(Ehrlich, 2013)*

Heimlich sign [H.J. Heimlich; L, *signum*], a universal distress signal that a person is choking and unable to speak, made by grasping the throat with a thumb and index finger, thereby attracting the attention of others nearby. Also called **universal choking signal.**

Heimlich valve, a small one-way valve used for chest drainage that empties into a flexible collection device and prevents return of gases or fluids into the pleural space. The Heimlich valve is less than 13 cm (5 inches) long and facilitates patient ambulation. It can be used in many patients instead of a traditional water seal drainage system.

Heinz bodies /hīnts/ [Robert Heinz, German pathologist, 1865–1924], irregularly shaped bits of altered hemoglobin found in the red blood cells of people who are hypersensitive to certain chemicals, such as aniline, phenylhydrazine, and primaquine.

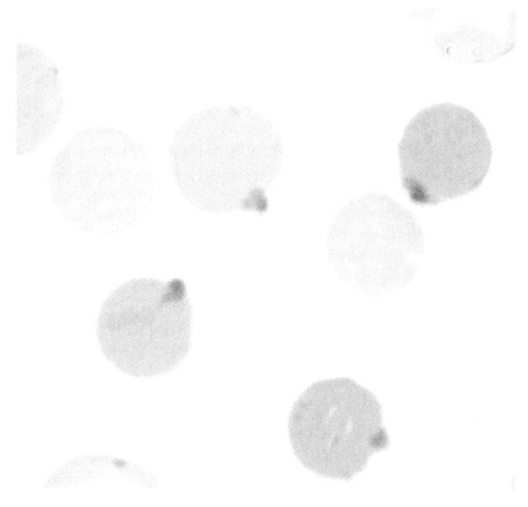

Heinz bodies *(Carr and Rodak, 2008)*

Helen, Sister (Helen Bowden), a nurse who received her education in England and became the first director of the newly formed Bellevue Hospital Training School for Nurses in New York in 1873. Although she had not trained under Florence Nightingale, she set up the Bellevue school according to Nightingale's principles. She was a member of the All Saints Sisterhood. After several years at Bellevue, having established one of the leading nursing schools in the United States, she went to South Africa.

helical computed tomography, computed tomography that combines continuous gantry rotation with continuous table movement to form a helical or spiral path of scan data. Also called **spiral computed tomography.**

helical virus /hel′ikəl/, a virus in which the protein capsid appears in a coiled pattern.

Helicobacter /hel′ikōbak′tər/ [Gk, *helix,* coil + *bakterion,* small staff], a genus of gram-negative, rod-shaped, microaerophilic bacteria of the family Spirillaceae, consisting of motile, spiral organisms with multiple sheathed flagella; formerly classified in the genus *Campylobacter.* The bacteria are found in the gastric mucosal layer; many people are infected without showing any symptoms. *H. pylori* is the causative agent of stomach ulcers, gastritis, and duodenitis. It causes 90% of duodenal ulcers and 80% of gastric ulcers. Infection significantly increases the risk of developing gastric cancer or mucosa-associated lymphoid tissue (MALT) lymphoma. Antibiotics can eliminate the infection and ulcer.

Helicobacter pylori, a species of spiral or straight gram-negative bacteria with multiple sheathed flagella found in the gastric mucosa of humans and other animals and associated with gastric and peptic ulcers as well as gastric cancers. Formerly called ***Campylobacter pylori.***

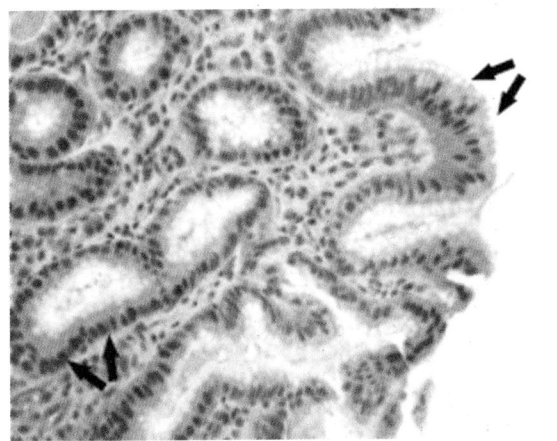

Gastric mucosa infected with *H. pylori* *(Wei et al, 2008)*

***Helicobacter pylori* antibodies test,** a test to detect the presence of *H. pylori.* The most accurate method of testing is microscopic examination of a gastric mucosal biopsy specimen. Other kinds of tests include breath test, rapid urease testing, and serological testing.

***Helicobacter pylori* gastritis,** gastritis caused by the presence of *H. pylori* in the stomach mucosa. *H. pylori* may be present for many years as chronic gastritis before finally causing an attack of acute gastritis.

helicopod gait /hel″ikōpod′/ [Gk, *helix,* coil, *pous,* foot], a manner of walking in which the feet trace half circles. It is associated with some mental disorders. Also called *helicopodia.*

helicotrema, a narrow slit at the apex of the cochlea where the two canals of the cochlear duct, the scala vestibuli and the scala tympani, communicate.

heliotherapy. See **solar therapy.**

heliox therapy, inhalation of a gaseous mixture of oxygen and helium to provide relief from the shortness of breath associated with upper airway obstructive disease. It reduces turbulence in the airway.

helium (He) /hē′lē·əm/ [Gk, *helios,* sun], a colorless, odorless gaseous element; the second-lightest element. Its atomic number is 2; its atomic mass is 4.00. Helium is classified as a noble gas in group 18 (group VIIIA) on the periodic table. It is one of the rare or inert gases and does not combine with other elements. It occurs in the atmosphere at concentrations of five parts per million. Because of its lightness and lack of flammability, it is also used to lift airships and balloons. In the liquid state it is used for low-temperature activities. The main physiological and medical uses of helium are in respiratory therapy and testing and the prevention of nitrogen narcosis and decompression sickness in hyperbaric environments. Helium is one third as soluble in lipids as is nitrogen. That characteristic accounts for its preferred use in hyperbaric atmospheres, such as those associated with deep-sea diving. A mixture of 80% helium and 20% oxygen is commonly breathed by deep-sea divers to prevent gas emboli and by patients undergoing treatment to clear obstruction of the respiratory tract. Problems associated with such uses involve the high velocity of acoustic transmission in helium and the high thermal conductivity of the gas. These characteristics produce voice distortions and hypothermia in persons who inhale it. The low density of helium reduces the effort of

breathing any gas mixture of which it is a component. Helium is used in pulmonary function testing to calculate the diffusion and residual capacities of the lungs.

helium therapy, the use of helium-oxygen gas mixtures to treat patients with airway obstruction. Because of its low density, helium can negotiate an obstruction more easily than nitrogen can, so less driving pressure is required to move the gas mixture in and out of the lungs.

helix /hē′liks/ [Gk, coil], **1.** a coiled, spiral-like formation characteristic of many organic molecules, such as DNA and certain proteins. **2.** the large outside rim of the auricle.

Hellerwork structural integration, a bodywork technique that consists of deep pressure on soft tissues to improve alignment, movement reeducation to avoid unnecessary stress on the body structure, and dialogue with a practitioner to enhance the individual's awareness of how attitude affects structure and movement pattern.

Hellin's law, a generalized formula for calculating the ratio of multiple births in any population, stating that if twin births occur at the rate of 1:*N*, then the rate of triplet births is approximately 1:N^2, the rate of quadruplet births is approximately 1:N^3, and so on. The value of *N* varies greatly but is generally close to 80. Also called *Hellin-Zeleny law.*

HELLP syndrome /help/, abbreviation for a form of severe preeclampsia, a hypertensive complication of late pregnancy. The letters stand for *h*emolysis, *e*levated *l*iver enzymes, and *l*ow *p*latelet level.

helmet cells, fragmented red blood cells that appear "scooped out" so that they resemble helmets. They are found in patients with microangiopathic hemolytic anemia and thrombotic thrombocytopenic purpura. Helmet cells can also be seen in the blood samples of people with prosthetic heart valves and in individuals with unstable hemoglobin conditions that produce Heinz bodies.

helminth /hel′minth/ [Gk, *helmins,* worm], a worm, especially one of the pathogenic parasites of the division Metazoa, including flukes, tapeworms, and roundworms.

-helminth, suffix meaning "worm": *platyhelminth.*

helminthemesis /hel′minthem″əsis/ [Gk, *helmins,* worm, *emesis,* vomiting], the vomiting of intestinal worms.

helminthiasis /hel′minthī″əsis/ [Gk, *helmins,* worm, *osis,* condition], a parasitic infestation of the body by helminths that may be cutaneous, visceral, or intestinal. Ascariasis, bilharziasis, filariasis, hookworm, and trichinosis are common forms of the disease.

helminthic /helmin″thik/ [Gk, *helmins,* worm], pertaining to worms.

helminthology /hel′minthol″əjē/, a branch of medicine concerned with parasitic worms.

helper T cell, a T lymphocyte that promotes the immune response of other lymphocytes to foreign antigens by releasing soluble proteins called helper factors. It is essential in determining B cell antibody class switching and maximizing bacteriocidal activity of phagocytes, as well as in growth and activation of cytotoxic T cells. Helper T cells have no cytotoxic or phagocytic activity. See also **T cell.**

helper virus, a virus that allows the replication of a coinfecting defective virus by supplying or restoring viral gene activity or allowing the defective virus to form a protein coat. Hepatitis B acts as a helper virus to delta agent, a defective RNA virus.

helplessness /help″ləsnəs/, a feeling of a loss of control or ability, usually after repeated failures, or of being immobilized or frozen by circumstances beyond one's control with the result that one is unable to make autonomous choices.

H

Helsinki Accords /helsing′kē/, a declaration signed by the representatives of 35 member nations of the Conference on Security and Cooperation in Europe in Helsinki, Finland, on August 1, 1975. The declared goals of the nonbinding document comprised four principal aspects of European security: economic cooperation, humanitarian issues, contact between the East and West, and provision for a later follow-up conference (held in Belgrade in 1978). Follow-up conferences were planned in part to allow the member nations to monitor each other's performance on humanitarian issues, such as the right to self-determination of all people and respect for fundamental freedoms, including thought, conscience, and religion or belief, without regard to race, language, sex, or religion. The Helsinki Accords grew from the precedent set by the judgments at the Nuremberg tribunals—that crimes against humanity are offenses subject to criminal prosecution. The principle and the practice of informed consent in health care grew from this precedent. Also called *Helsinki Declaration.* See also **Nuremberg tribunal.**

hema-, hemat-, prefix meaning "blood": *hematoma, hematemesis.*

Hemabate, a prostaglandin abortifacient; also used to treat refractory postpartum bleeding. Brand name for *carboprost tromethamine.*

hemacytometer /he′məsītom′ətər/ [Gk, *haima,* blood, *kytos,* cell, *metron,* measure], a device for visually counting the number of cells in a known volume of blood or other fluid.

hemadsorption /hē′madsôrp″shən, hem′-/ [Gk, *haima,* blood; L, *ad,* to, *sorbere,* to swallow], the adherence of red blood cells to other cells or surfaces; a process in which a substance or an agent, such as certain viruses and bacilli, adheres to the surface of an erythrocyte. The process occurs naturally, or it may be induced for laboratory identification of bacteriological specimens.

hemagglutination /hē′məgloo̅′tinā″shən, hem′-/ [Gk, *haima* + L, *agglutinare,* to glue], the agglutination of erythrocytes by an antigen-antibody reaction.

hemagglutination inhibition (HI), **1.** the inhibition of virus-induced hemagglutination as a procedure for identifying hemagglutinating viruses. HI is used in the diagnosis of infections by certain viruses, such as rubella, herpes zoster, and herpes simplex. **2.** a method for measuring the concentration of soluble antigens in biological specimens in which the specimen is incubated first with homologous antibodies and then with antigen-coated erythrocytes.

hemagglutinin [Gk, *haima* + L, *agglutinare*], a type of antibody that agglutinates red blood cells. It is classified according to the source of cells agglutinated as autologous (from the same organism), homologous (from an organism of the same species), and xenogeneic (from an organism of a different species).

hemangi-, combining form meaning "blood vessel" or "a collection of blood vessels": *hemangioma, hemangiectasis.*

hemangiectasis, dilation of a blood vessel.

hemangioblast /hēman″jē·ōblast′/, an embryonic mesodermal cell that gives rise to vascular endothelium and blood-forming cells.

hemangioblastoma /hēman′jē·ōblastō″mə/ *pl. hemangioblastomas, hemangioblastomata* [Gk, *haima* + *angeion,* vessel, *blastos,* germ, *oma,* tumor], a brain tumor composed of a proliferation of capillaries and of disorganized clusters of capillary cells or angioblasts, usually occurring in the cerebellum.

hemangioendothelioma /hēman′jē·ō·en′dōthē′lē·ō″mə/ *pl. hemangioendotheliomas, hemangioendotheliomata* [Gk, *haima* + *endon,* inside, *thele,* nipple, *oma,* tumor], **1.** a tumor, consisting of endothelial cells, that grows around an artery or a vein. The benign form occurs in children and is usually cured by local excision. The tumor rarely becomes malignant. Also called **angioendothelioma. 2.** malignant hemangioendothelioma. See also **angiosarcoma.**

hemangiofibroma /-fībrō′mə/ [Gk, *haima,* blood; L, *fibra,* fiber; Gk, *oma,* tumor], a tumor that has the characteristics of both a hemangioma and a fibroma.

hemangioma /hēman′jē·ō′mə/ *pl. hemangiomas, hemangiomata* [Gk, *haima* + *angeion,* small vessel, *oma*], a benign tumor consisting of a mass of blood vessels.

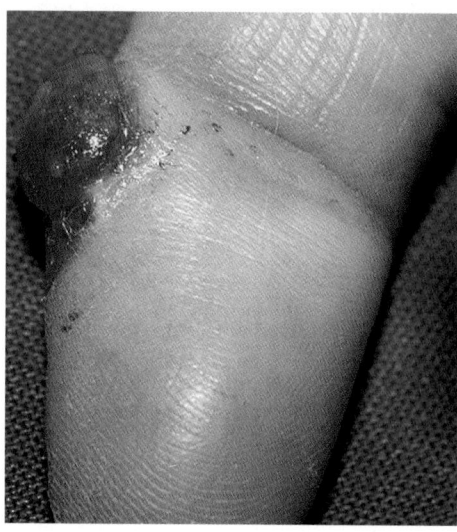

Hemangioma *(James, Berger, and Elston, 2011)*

hemangioma simplex. See **capillary hemangioma.**

hemangioma-thrombocytopenia syndrome, a blood disorder usually occurring in the first few months of life in which severe thrombocytopenia and other evidence of intravascular coagulation are accompanied by rapidly expanding hemangiomas of the trunk, extremities, and abdominal viscera, sometimes associated with bleeding and anemia. Bleeding is thought to result from the trapping and destruction of platelets within the tumor and depletion of circulating clotting factors. Also called **Kasabach-Merritt syndrome.**

hemangiosarcoma. See **angiosarcoma.**

hemapoiesis /hem′əpō·ē′sis/ [Gk, *haima,* blood, *poiein,* to make], the formation of blood cells.

hemarthros /hem′är″thrəs/ [Gk, *haima,* blood, *arthron,* joint], the extravasation of blood into a joint.

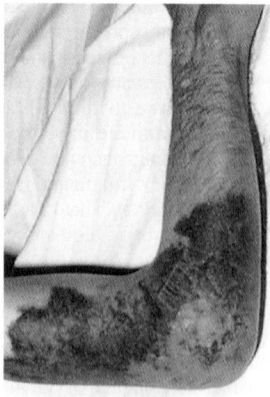

Hemarthros *(Moll, 1997)*

hemarthrosis, blood in a joint cavity. Also called **hemarthros.**

hematemesis /hē′mətem″əsis, hem′-/ [Gk, *haima + emesis*, vomiting], vomiting of bright red blood, indicating rapid upper GI bleeding, commonly associated with esophageal varices or peptic ulcer. The rate and the source of bleeding are determined by endoscopic examination. Any blood found in the stomach is removed by nasogastric suction. Treatment requires replacement of blood by transfusion, administration of IV fluids for maintenance of fluid and electrolyte balance, and possible gastric lavage. Surgery may be necessary. The patient is usually anxious and needs quiet, warmth, and reassurance. Also spelled **haematemesis.** See also **gastrointestinal bleeding.**

hematic. See **hemic.**

hematinic /hem′ətin″ik/, a therapeutic agent that produces an increase in the number of erythrocytes and/or hemoglobin concentration in erythrocytes, such as iron or B complex vitamins.

hematinuria /hem′ətino͞or″ē·ə/ [Gk, *haima*, blood, *ouron*, urine], a dark-colored urine resulting from the presence of hematin or hemoglobin. See also **hemoglobinuria.**

hemat(o) [word element, Gk, blood], combining form for terms relating to blood or blood vessels.

hematocele /hem″ətōsēl′/, a cystlike accumulation of blood within the tunica vaginalis of the scrotum. It is usually caused by injury and may require surgery if the blood is not readily resorbed.

hematochezia /hem′ətōkē″zhə/ [Gk, *haima + chezo*, feces], the passage of blood in the feces. The cause is usually bleeding in the colon or rectum, but it may result from the loss of blood higher in the digestive tract, although blood passed from the stomach or small intestine generally loses its red coloration. Cancer, colitis, and ulcers are among causes of hematochezia. Compare **melena.**

hematocrit /hemat″ōkrit/ [Gk, *haima + krinein*, to separate], a measure of the packed cell volume of red cells, expressed as a percentage of the total blood volume. The normal range is between 43% and 49% in men and between 37% and 43% in women.

hematocrit reading. See **packed cell volume.**

hematocyte /hem″ətōsīt/ [Gk, *haima*, blood, *kytos*, cell], a blood cell, particularly a red blood cell. Also called **hemocyte.**

hematocytoblast /hem′ətōsī″təblast′/ [Gk, *haima*, blood, *kytos*, cell, *blastos*, germ], a large nucleated reticuloendothelial cell found in bone marrow. It is believed to be a common precursor of various blood elements. Also called **hemocytoblast.**

hematogenesis /-jen′əsis/ [Gk, *haima*, blood, *genein*, to produce], the formation of blood cells or an increase in the production of blood elements. Also called **hemapoiesis.**

hematogenic shock. See **hemorrhagic shock.**

hematogenous /hēmətoj″ənəs/ [Gk, *haima + genein*, to produce], originating or transported in the blood.

hematogenous pigment [Gk, *haima*, blood, *genein*, to produce; L, *pingere*, to paint], the red color of erythrocytes caused by the presence of hemoglobin.

hematogenous tuberculosis [Gk, *haima*, blood, *genein*, to produce; L, *tuberculum*, a small swelling; Gk, *osis*, condition], a form of tuberculosis that is blood-borne.

hematoid /hem″ətoid/, bloodlike or resembling blood.

hematologic, hematological. See **hematology.**

hematologic death syndrome /hem′ətoloj″ik/, a group of clinical signs and symptoms of radiation damage to the blood cells. The condition is characterized by nausea, vomiting, fever, diarrhea, infections, anemia, leukopenia, and hemorrhage. It can result from exposure to a dose of 200 to 1000 rad. The mean survival time for a person with hematologic death syndrome is estimated at between 10 and 60 days.

hematologic effect, the response of blood cells to radiation exposure. All types of blood cells are destroyed by radiation, and the degree of cell depletion increases with increasing dose. Lymphocytes are affected first and are reduced in number within minutes or hours after exposure. Erythrocytes are less sensitive than other types of blood cells and may not show radiation effects for several weeks.

hematologist /hē′mətol″əjist, hem′-/, a medical specialist in the field of blood cells and blood-forming organs.

hematology /hē′mətol″əjē, hem′-/ [Gk, *haima + logos*, science], *adj.,* the scientific study of blood and blood-forming tissues. Also spelled **haematology. –hematologic, hematological,** *adj.*

hematolysis. See **hemolysis.**

hematoma /hē′mətō″mə, hem′-/ *pl. hematomas, hematomata* [Gk, *haima + oma*, tumor], a collection of extravasated blood trapped in the tissues of the skin or in an organ, resulting from trauma or incomplete hemostasis after surgery. Initially there is frank bleeding into the space; if the space is limited, pressure slows and eventually stops the flow of blood. The blood clots, serum collects, the clot hardens, and the mass becomes palpable to the examiner and is often painful to the patient. A hematoma may be drained early in the process and bleeding arrested with pressure or, if necessary, with surgical ligation of the bleeding vessel. Considerable blood may be lost, and infection is a serious complication.

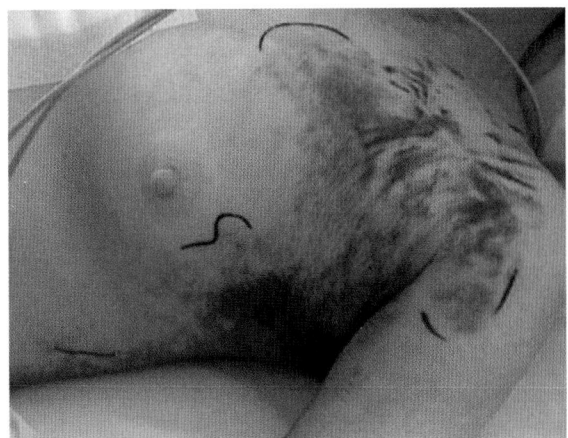

Large hematoma on left upper chest *(Vetrugno, Muzzi, and Giordano, 2007)*

-hematoma, suffix meaning "a swelling containing blood": *cephalhematoma.*

hematometra /hē′mətōmē″trə/, an accumulation of fluid or menstrual blood in the uterine cavity.

hematometry /hem′ətom″ətrē/, an examination of a blood sample to determine the number, type, and properties of blood cells and platelets and the amount of hemoglobin.

hematomyelia /hē′mətōmē″lē·ə/ [Gk, *haima + meylos*, marrow], the appearance of frank blood in the fluid of the spinal cord.

hematopathology /-pəthol″əjē/, the division of pathology that specializes in blood cell diseases and diseases of the blood-forming organs.

hematopericardium. See **hemopericardium.**

hematoperitoneum /-per'itənē″əm/ [Gk, *haima*, blood, *peri*, near, *tenein*, to stretch], the effusion of blood into the peritoneal cavity.

hematophagous /hem'ətof″əgəs/, **1.** pertaining to the feeding on blood by insects or other parasites. **2.** pertaining to the destruction of erythrocytes by phagocytes.

hematopoiesis /hē'mətōpō·ē″sis, hem'-/ [Gk, *haima* + *poiein*, to make], the normal formation and development of blood cells in the bone marrow. In severe anemia and other hematological disorders, cells may be produced in organs outside the marrow (extramedullary hematopoiesis). See also **erythropoiesis.** –**hematopoietic,** *adj.*

hematopoietic, related to the formation of blood.

hematopoietic growth factor /-pō·et″ik/, any protein, including erythropoietin, interleukins, and colony-stimulating factors, that promotes the proliferation, maturation, and differentiation of hematopoietic stem cells.

hematopoietic malignancies, diseases such as leukemia that arise as a result of unregulated clonal proliferation of hematological cells.

hematopoietic stem cell, an actively dividing cell that is capable of self-renewal and of differentiation into any blood cell lineage.

hematopoietic syndrome, a group of clinical features associated with effects of radiation on the blood and lymph tissues. It is characterized by nausea and vomiting, anorexia, lethargy, hemolysis and destruction of the bone marrow, and atrophy of the spleen and lymph nodes.

hematopoietic system [Gk, *haima*, blood, *poiein*, to make; L, *systema*], body organs and tissues involved in the formation and functioning of blood elements; includes the bone marrow and spleen.

hematospermia /-spur″mē·ə/, the presence of blood in the semen. Causes include many conditions affecting the genitourinary tract, most commonly prostatic biopsy. The condition is rarely serious. Treatment is dependent on the underlying cause.

hematothorax. See **hemothorax.**

hematoxylin-eosin /hē'mətok″silin/ [*Haematoxylon campechianum*, logwood; Gk, *eos*, dawn], a stain commonly used to treat tissue sections on microscope slides.

hematuria /hē'mətoō̄r″ē·ə, hem'-/ [Gk, *haima* + *ouron*, urine], *adj.,* abnormal presence of blood in the urine. It is symptomatic of many renal diseases and disorders of the genitourinary system and is detected by microscopic examination of urine sediment and chemical analysis using a reagent chemical.

heme /hēm/ [Gk, *haima*, blood], the pigmented iron-containing nonprotein part of the hemoglobin molecule. There are four heme groups in a hemoglobin molecule, each consisting of a cyclic structure of four pyrrole residues, called protoporphyrin, and an iron ion in the center. Heme binds and carries oxygen in the red blood cells, releasing it to tissues.

heme iron, iron occurring in a heme complex, as in hemoglobin and myoglobin. Dietary sources of iron are meat, fish, and poultry.

hemeralopia /hem'ərəlō″pē·ə/ [Gk, *hemera*, day, *alaos*, blind, *ops*, eye], an abnormal visual condition in which bright light causes blurring of vision. Also called **day blindness, night sight.** –*hemeralopic, adj.*

■ OBSERVATIONS: Hemeralopia is an unpleasant side effect of certain anticonvulsant medications, including trimethadione, prescribed in the treatment of petit mal seizures.

■ INTERVENTIONS: Identification of the underlying cause is important. In addition to being a side effect of medication, it may be associated with cataracts, genetic disorders, or brain injury.

■ PATIENT CARE CONSIDERATIONS: Sunglasses and adjustment of lighting will help patients be more comfortable.

hemi-, prefix meaning "half": *hemiataxia, hemiopia, hemiplegia.*

-hemia. See **-emia, -aemia, -hemia, -haemia.**

hemiacephalus /hem'ē·āsef″ələs/ [Gk, *hemi*, half, *a*, without, + *kephale*, head], a fetus in which the brain and most of the cranium are lacking. See also **anencephaly.**

hemiachromatosia /hem'ē-ak'rōmətō″zhə/, a state of being color blind in only one half of the visual field.

hemialgia /hem'ē-al″jē·ə/, pain that affects one side of the body.

hemiamblyopia /hem'ē-am'blē-ō″pē·ə/ [Gk, *hemi*, half, *amblys*, dull, *ops*, eye], blindness in half of the normal visual field. Also called **hemianopia, hemianopsia.**

hemianalgesia /hem'ē-an'əljē″sē·ə/ [Gk, *hemi*, half, *a*, without, *algos*, pain], a loss of feeling or sensitivity to pain affecting half of the body or one side of the body.

hemianesthesia /hem'ē-an'esthē″zhə/ [Gk, *hemi* + *anaisthesia*, absence of feeling], a loss of feeling on one side of the body.

hemianopia, hemianopsia. See **hemiamblyopia.**

hemiarthroplasty /hem'ē-är″thrəplas'tē/, a surgical procedure for repair of an injured or diseased hip joint involving replacing the head of the femur with a prosthesis without reconstruction of the acetabulum.

hemiataxia /hem'ē-ətak″sē·ə/, a loss of muscle control affecting one side of the body, usually as a result of a stroke or cerebellar injury. The condition may be ipsilateral or contralateral.

hemiazygous vein /hem'ē-əzī″gəs/ [Gk, *hemi* + *a*, without, + *zygon*, yoke], one of the tributaries of the azygous vein of the thorax. It starts in the left ascending lumbar vein, enters the thorax through the left crus of the diaphragm, ascends on the left side of the vertebral column as high as the ninth thoracic vertebra, and passes dorsal to the aorta to enter the azygous. The hemiazygous vein receives about four of the caudal intercostal veins, the left subcostal vein, and some of the esophageal and mediastinal veins.

hemiballismus. See **ballismus.**

hemiblock, a failure to conduct a cardiac impulse down one division of the left bundle branch, such as an anterior superior or a posterior inferior hemiblock.

hemic /hem″ik, hē″mik/, pertaining to blood. Also called **hematic.**

hemicellulose /hem'ēsel″yoōlōs/ [Gk, *hemi* + L, *cellula*, little cell], any of a group of polysaccharides that constitute the chief part of the skeletal substances of the cell walls of plants. They resemble cellulose but are soluble and more easily extracted and decomposed. See also **dietary fiber.**

hemicephalia /-sefā″lyə/ [Gk, *hemi* + *kephale*, head], a congenital anomaly characterized by the absence of half of the cerebrum, caused by severe arrest of brain development in the fetus. The cerebellum and basal ganglia may be present in rudimentary form.

hemicephalus [Gk, *hemi*, half, *kephale*, head], a fetus with congenital absence of half of the cerebrum.

hemicolectomy /hem'ikōlek'təme/ [Gk, *hemi*, half + *kolon*, colon + *ektome*, excision], excision of approximately half of the colon.

hemicrania /-krā″nē·ə/ [Gk, *hemi* + *kranion*, skull], **1.** a headache, usually migraine, that affects only one side of the head. **2.** a congenital anomaly characterized by the absence of half of the skull in the fetus; incomplete anencephaly.

hemicraniectomy /-kran′ē·ek″təmē/ [Gk, *hemi,* half, *kranion,* skull, *ektomē,* excision], a surgical procedure in which part or all of one half of the skull is excised and reflected as a preliminary step to certain types of brain operations.

hemidiaphragm /-dī″əfram/, either the left or right functional half of the diaphragm. Although the diaphragm is a single anatomical unit, it is divided by the union of its central tendon and the pericardium into separate leaves, each with its own nerve supply, and each hemidiaphragm can function independently.

hemidystrophy /-dis″trəfē/, a condition in which the two sides of the body do not develop equally.

hemiectromelia /hem′ē·ek′trōmē″lyə/ [Gk, *hemi* + *ektosis,* miscarriage, *melos,* limb], a congenital anomaly characterized by the incomplete development of the limbs on one side of the body. −*hemiectromelus, n.*

hemiepilepsy /hem′ē·ep″əlepsē/, a rare condition in which clonic seizures affect only one side of the body.

hemifacial spasm. See **convulsive tic.**

hemigastrectomy /-gastrek″təmē/, surgical removal of one half of the stomach.

hemigeusia, absence of the sense of taste on one side of the tongue.

hemiglossal /-glos″əl/, pertaining to one side of the tongue. Also called **hemilingual.**

hemignathia /hem′ēnā″thē·ə/ [Gk, *hemi* + *gnathos,* jaw], **1.** a congenital anomaly characterized by incomplete development of the lower jaw on one side of the face. **2.** a condition of having only one jaw. −*hemignathus, n.*

hemihyperplasia /-hī′pərplā″zhə/ [Gk, *hemi* + *hyper,* excessive, *plassein,* to form], overdevelopment or excessive growth of half of a specific organ or part or all of the organs and parts on one side of the body.

hemihypertonia /-hī′pərtō″nē·ə/ [Gk, *hemi* + *hyper* + *tonikos,* stretching], exaggerated tension in the muscles on one side of the body. In one form of the disorder, spasms may occur occasionally in different muscle groups on one side of the body.

hemihypertrophy /-hīpur″trəfē/ [Gk, *hemi* + *hyper* + *trophe,* nourishment], an unusual enlargement or overgrowth of half of the body or half of a body part.

hemihypoplasia /-hī′pōplā″zhə/ [Gk, *hemi* + *hypo,* under, *plassein,* to form], partial or incomplete development of half of a specific organ or part or all of the organs and parts on one side of the body.

hemikaryon. See **haploid nucleus.**

hemilaminectomy /hem′ilam′inek′təme/ [Gk, *hemi,* half; L, *lamina,* plate; Gk, *ektome,* excision], surgical removal of one side of the vertebral lamina.

hemilateral /-lat″ərəl/, pertaining to one side.

hemilingual. See **hemiglossal.**

hemimelia /-mē′lyə/ [Gk, *hemi* + *melos*], a developmental anomaly characterized by the absence or gross shortening of the lower portion of one or more of the limbs. The condition may involve either or both of the bones of the distal arm or leg and is designated according to which is absent or defective, as fibular, radial, tibial, or ulnar hemimelia. See also **ectromelia, phocomelia.**

hemiopia /hem′ē·ō″pē·ə/ [Gk, *hemi,* half, *ops,* eye], a condition involving only one eye or half the visual field.

hemipagus /hemip″əgəs/ [Gk, *hemi* + *pagos,* fixture], symmetric twins who are conjoined at the thorax.

hemiparesis /-pərē′sis/ [Gk, *hemi* + *paralyein,* to be palsied], muscular weakness of one half of the body. Compare **hemiplegia.**

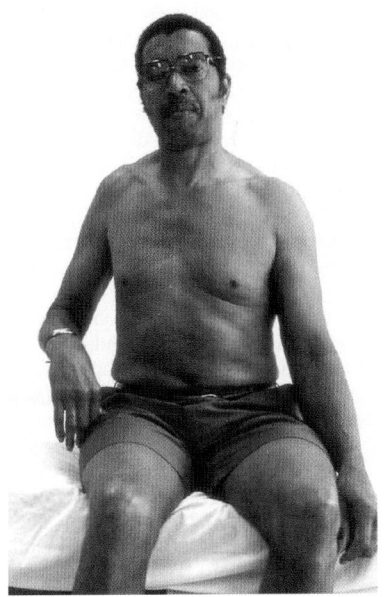

Posture typical in hemiparesis *(Frownfelter and Dean, 2006)*

hemiparesthesia /-per′esthē″zhə/ [Gk, *hemi,* half, *para,* beside, *aisthesis,* sensation], a numbness or other abnormal or impaired sensation that is experienced on only one side of the body.

hemiplegia /hem′iplē″jə/ [Gk, *hemi* + *plege,* stroke], paralysis of one side of the body. Also called **unilateral paralysis.** Compare **diplegia, paraplegia, tetraplegia.** Kinds include **cerebral hemiplegia, facial hemiplegia, spastic hemiplegia.** −*hemiplegic, adj.*

hemiplegic gait /-plē″jik/ [Gk, *hemi,* half, *plege,* stroke; ONorse, *gata,* a way], a manner of walking in which an affected limb moves in a semicircle with each step.

hemisection /-sek″shən/ [Gk, *hemi,* half; L, *sectare,* to cut], half of a body or other object divided along a longitudinal plane, producing two lateral halves.

hemisectomy /hem′ēsek′tämē/, amputation of one root of a two-rooted mandibular tooth. See also **apicoectomy, hemisection.**

hemisomus /hem′isō″məs/ [Gk, *hemi* + *soma,* body], a fetus or individual in whom one side of the body is malformed, defective, or absent.

hemisphere /hem″isfir/ [Gk, *hemi* + *sphaira,* sphere], **1.** one half of a sphere or globe. **2.** the lateral half of the cerebrum or of the cerebellum. −*hemispheric, adj.*

hemispherectomy /hem″i·sfēr·ek′tə·mē/, resection of one hemisphere of the brain, an extremely rare surgery performed to treat intractable seizure disorders in children. Although this surgery results in some physical debilitation, such as loss of use of the hand opposite the resected hemisphere and some visual dysfunction, it does not affect cognitive abilities.

hemiteras /hem′ēter″əs/ *pl.* **hemiterata** [Gk, *hemi* + *teras,* monster], any individual with a congenital malformation that is not severe or disabling. −*hemiteratic, adj.*

hemithorax /-thôr″aks/, one side of the chest.

hemithyroidectomy /-thī′roidek″təmē/, surgical removal of one lobe of the thyroid gland.

hemivertebra /-vur″təbrə/, an abnormal condition characterized by the congenital failure of a vertebra to develop completely. It is possibly caused by the complete failure of the

H

growth center of one vertebral body. Usually half of the vertebra involved is completely or partially developed, and the other half is absent. One or more vertebrae may be involved. The different conditions produce varying degrees of balanced or unbalanced scoliosis. As a result of the developmental abnormality of the spine, a wedge-shaped vertebra develops, and adjacent vertebral bodies expand to fit the deformity or tilt to accommodate wedge-shaped articulation. Hemivertebra may be classified according to the degree of developmental failure of involved vertebral growth centers. When two vertebral bodies are involved and growth centers on the same side fail to develop, moderate to severe unbalanced congenital scoliosis results. When growth centers fail to develop on opposite sides, balanced congenital scoliosis results. Singular hemivertebra may cause few if any signs and symptoms. Depending on the degree of congenital scoliosis involved, any associated deformity may become more apparent with growth. Other types of hemivertebra, especially those involving unbalanced congenital scoliosis, usually progress markedly with growth and have a relatively poor prognosis unless early spinal fusion prevents further spinal curvature. No treatment may be required for the form of the condition associated with balanced congenital scoliosis.

hemizona assay, an in vitro test of sperm function in which a human zona pellucida is divided in half and one half is incubated with sperm from a donor known to be normal and the other half with sperm from the patient being tested. The number of sperm bound to each half is calculated. The number from the patient's sperm is divided by that from the donor's sperm. A figure of less than 0.60 indicates abnormal patient sperm.

hemizygote /-zī″gōt/ [Gk, *hemi* + *zygon,* yoke], an individual, organism, or cell that has only one allele for a specific characteristic. The trait specified by the allele is expressed regardless of whether the allele is dominant or recessive. Such alleles include those on the single X chromosome in males, which have no corresponding alleles on the Y chromosome. –*hemizygotic, hemizygous, adj.,* –*hemizygosity, n.*

hemlock (poison hemlock), the common name for *Conium maculatum,* a plant indigenous to most of Europe and the source of a poisonous alkaloid, coniine. It is considered unsafe for any use, but an extract of the leaves and flowers of conium has been used as a respiratory sedative and its hydrochloride salts have been used as an antispasmodic. Also called **conium.** Compare **water hemlock.**

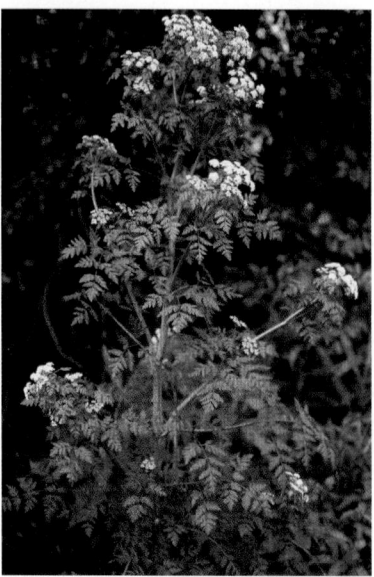

Hemlock *(From the U.S. Department of Agriculture)*

hemo-, prefix relating to blood or blood vessels: *hemostasis.*

hemoagglutination. See **hemagglutination.**

hemoagglutinin. See **hemagglutinin.**

hemobilinuria /hē′mōbil′inoor″ē·ə/, the presence of the brown pigment urobilin in the blood and urine.

hemoblastic leukemia. See **stem cell leukemia.**

hemochromatosis /hē′mōkrō′mətō″sis, hem′-/ [Gk, *haima,* blood, *chroma,* color, *osis,* condition], an inherited disease of iron metabolism, characterized by excess iron deposits throughout the body. Hepatomegaly, skin pigmentation, diabetes mellitus, and cardiac failure may occur. Multiple phlebotomies are required to deplete excess iron. Also spelled **haemochromatosis.** Compare **hemosiderosis.** See also **iron metabolism, siderosis, thalassemia.**

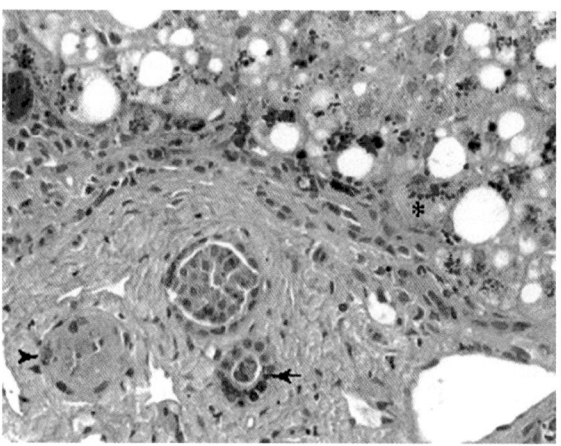

Hemochromatosis in liver biopsy tissue *(Saxena, 2011)*

hemoclip, a malleable metal clip used to ligate small blood vessels during surgery and to mark the location of body structures in radiographic procedures.

hemoconcentration /-kon′səntrā″shən/ [Gk, *haima* + L, *cum,* together with, *centrum,* center], an increase in the number of red blood cells resulting from either a decrease in plasma volume or increased production of erythrocytes.

hemocyanin /hē′mōsī″ənin/, an oxygen-carrying protein molecule present in certain lower animals, particularly arthropods and mollusks. The molecule is similar to the hemoglobin molecule of human blood but uses copper atoms, rather than iron, and is less efficient than hemoglobin in requiring many more atoms to bind a single molecule of oxygen.

hemocyte, hematocytoblast. See **hematocyte, hematocytoblast.**

hemocytoblast. See **hematocytoblast.**

hemocytoblastic leukemia. See **stem cell leukemia.**

hemocytology /-sītol″əjē/ [Gk, *haima,* blood, *kytos,* cell, *logos,* science], the study of the components of blood.

hemodiafiltration /-dī′əfiltrā″shən/, a technique similar to hemofiltration, used to treat uremia by convective transport of the solute rather than diffusion.

hemodialysis /hē′mōdī·al″isis, hem′-/ [Gk, *haima* + *dia,* apart, *lysis,* loosening], a procedure in which impurities or wastes are removed from the blood, used in treating patients with renal failure and various toxic conditions. The patient's blood is shunted from the body through a machine for diffusion and ultrafiltration and then returned to the patient's circulation. Hemodialysis requires access to the patient's bloodstream, a mechanism for the transport of the blood to and from the dialyzer, and a dialyzer. Also spelled **haemodialysis.** See **arteriovenous fistula,** def. 2, **external shunt.**

■ METHOD: Access may be achieved by an external shunt or an arteriovenous fistula. When hemodialysis is being performed, cannulas are separated, allowing the arterial blood to flow to the dialyzer and the dialyzed blood to return from the dialyzer to the circulation through the cannula in the vein. An arteriovenous fistula is created by the anastomosis of a large vein to an artery. Large-bore needles are threaded into superficial vessels enlarged by the increased flow caused by the fistula. Various dialyzers may be used. Hemodialysis takes from 3 to 8 hours depending on the patient's condition, weight, and laboratory values and may be necessary daily in acute conditions or two to three times a week in chronic renal failure.

■ INTERVENTIONS: A decrease in blood flow through the shunt may cause clotting. Therefore, any factor that may result in a slowing of the flow should be avoided. Some of these factors are systemic hypotension, infection of the shunt or fistula, compression of the shunt or fistula, thrombophlebitis, and prolonged inflation of a blood pressure cuff. Infection is prevented in the area around an external shunt by placing a sterile dressing over the shunt and changing the dressing daily. Before the procedure is begun, the patient is told how long it will take, what pain or discomfort may be expected, what will be felt afterward, what food or activity will be allowed during the procedure, and whether family or friends may be present during treatment. Headache, nausea, and muscle cramps are common, especially during the procedure and for a few hours afterward. The patient usually feels best on the day after hemodialysis. Rest, an antiemetic,

and a mild analgesic may make the procedure more comfortable. Most patients need emotional support and some physical assistance during hemodialysis. The physical status of the patient is monitored frequently throughout. Blood pressure, pulse, and blood tests for electrolyte and acid-base balance are performed. Normal saline solution may be administered to counteract hypotension that results from rapid removal of fluid from the intravascular compartment. The patient is weighed before and after the treatment to determine the amount of fluid lost during the procedure. An anticoagulant is usually given to prevent coagulation of the blood in the dialyzer, cannulas, or catheters. To prevent hemorrhage, protamine sulfate may be administered after the procedure to reverse the effect of the anticoagulant. Any treatment that causes tissue trauma, such as dental extraction, venipuncture, or intramuscular injection, is not recommended during or immediately after dialysis.

■ OUTCOME CRITERIA: The discomfort before, during, and just after dialysis; the prolonged time of relative immobility during the procedure; and the dietary restrictions necessary in renal insufficiency all cause considerable stress in the patient. Adjustments in the patterns of daily life are necessary and require the assistance of professionals with experience and training.

hemodialysis technician, a health professional who has received special training in the operation of hemodialysis equipment and the treatment of patients with kidney failure.

hemodialyzer. See **dialyzer.**

hemodilution /-dilōō″shən/ [Gk, *haima,* blood; L, *diluare,* to wash away], a condition in which the concentration of

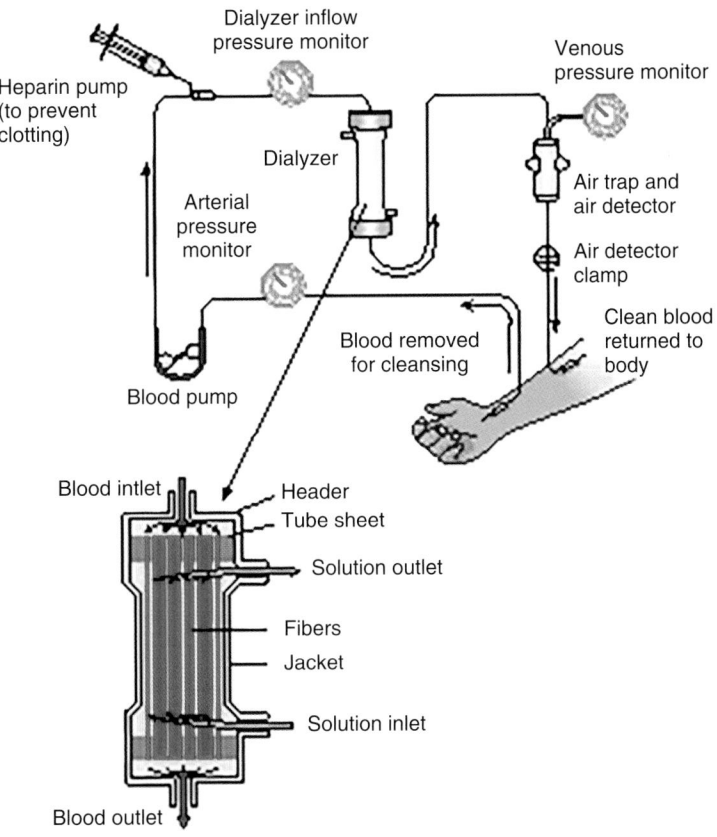

Dialyzer for hemodialysis *(Nix, 2013)*

erythrocytes or other blood elements is lowered, usually resulting from an increase in plasma volume, often secondary to the use of plasma.

hemodynamics /-dīnam″iks/ [Gk, *haima* + *dynamis,* force], the study of the physical aspects of blood circulation, including cardiac function and peripheral vascular physiological characteristics.

Hemofil M, brand name for *human antihemophilic factor.*

hemofiltration /-filtrā″shən/, a type of hemodialysis in which there is convective transport of the solute through ultrafiltration across the membrane. It is reported to be more effective than diffusion in removing higher molecular-weight solutes from the blood, particularly in the treatment of uremia.

hemoglobin (Hb, Hgb) /hē″məglō″bən/ [Gk, *haima* + L, *globus,* ball], a complex protein-iron compound in the blood that carries oxygen to the cells from the lungs and carbon dioxide away from the cells to the lungs. Each erythrocyte contains 200 to 300 molecules of hemoglobin, each molecule of hemoglobin contains four heme groups, and each heme carries one molecule of oxygen. A hemoglobin molecule contains four globin polypeptide chains. Each polypeptide chain is composed of 141 to 146 amino acids. The absence, replacement, or addition of only one amino acid modifies the properties of the hemoglobin. Different kinds of hemoglobin are identified by their specific combination of polypeptide chains. Normal adult hemoglobin is composed of alpha and beta chains. About 2% of adult hemoglobin is composed of alpha and delta chains, called hemoglobin A_2 (Hb A_2). Fetal hemoglobin is composed of alpha and gamma globin. The normal concentrations of hemoglobin in the blood are 12 to 16 g/dL in women and 13.5 to 18 g/dL in men. In an atmosphere of high oxygen concentration, such as in the lungs, hemoglobin binds with oxygen to form oxyhemoglobin. In an atmosphere of low oxygen concentration, such as in the peripheral tissues of the body, oxygen is replaced by carbon dioxide to form carboxyhemoglobin. Hemoglobin releases carbon dioxide in the lungs and picks up oxygen for transport to the cells.

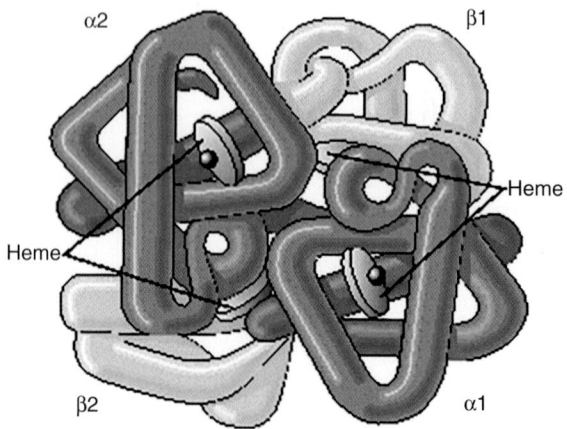

Molecular structure of hemoglobin *(Copstead-Kirkhorn and Banasik, 2014)*

hemoglobin A (Hb A), normal adult hemoglobin composed of alpha and beta globin chains. Also called

adult hemoglobin. Compare **hemoglobin F.** See also **hemoglobinopathy.**

hemoglobin A₁c. See **glycosylated hemoglobin.**

hemoglobin A₂, a normal hemoglobin present in small amounts in adults, characterized by the substitution of delta chains for beta chains. Its concentration in the blood increases in various hematological diseases. It normally constitutes 1.5% to 3.5% of the total hemoglobin.

hemoglobin Bart's, an abnormal hemoglobin that is detectable only during the newborn period. It is composed of four gamma chains having high oxygen affinity. Its presence indicates that one or more of the four genes that produce alpha globin chains are dysfunctional, resulting in alpha-thalassemia. The more alpha genes affected, the more significant the thalassemia and clinical symptoms.

hemoglobin C (Hb C), an autosomal-recessive qualitative hemoglobinopathy in which lysine is substituted for glutamic acid at position 6 of the beta globin chain. Deoxygenated red cells crystallize to form a hexagonal "bar of gold" crystal that slows their passage. Target cells are prominent. Hemoglobin C migrates slowly in hemoglobin electrophoresis, a trait used to identify its presence.

hemoglobin C disease, an inherited hemoglobinopathy caused by hemoglobin C. The heterozygous form is asymptomatic; homozygous hemoglobin C disease causes a mild to moderate hemolytic anemia. In the homozygous form, target cells and hemoglobin C crystals are seen in microscopic examination of a blood film. See also **hemoglobin C, hemoglobin SC (Hb SC) disease.**

hemoglobin E, a qualitative hemoglobinopathy in which lysine becomes substituted for glutamic acid at position 26 of the beta chain. Prevalent in Africa and Southeast Asia, especially Thailand. The homozygous state causes a mild to moderate anemia. The heterozygous state is clinically silent.

hemoglobin E disease [Gk, *haima,* blood; L, *globus,* ball; E; Gk, *dis,* not; Fr, *aise,* ease], a mild form of anemia caused by a genetic abnormality of the hemoglobin molecule. Worldwide it is the third most common form of hemoglobin disorder, primarily affecting people of Southeast Asian and African descent.

hemoglobin electrophoresis, a test to identify various abnormal hemoglobins in the blood, including certain genetic disorders, such as sickle cell anemia.

hemoglobinemia /hē″mōglō″binē″mē·ə, hem′-/, presence of free hemoglobin in the blood plasma, usually associated with intravascular hemolysis.

hemoglobin F (Hb F), normal fetal hemoglobin. Hb F is replaced by hemoglobin A in the first weeks after birth. Hb F has an increased capacity to carry oxygen and is present in increased amounts in sickle cell disease, thalassemia, and hereditary persistence of hemoglobin F.

hemoglobin G, any of various abnormal hemoglobins with an amino acid substitution on the alpha chain. The most common one is hemoglobin G Philadelphia.

hemoglobin Gower, a normal hemoglobin present in early embryonic life and disappearing before birth. It occasionally consists entirely of epsilon chains (ε_4), but the usual forms are hemoglobin Gower-1, consisting of two zeta and two epsilon chains ($\zeta_2\varepsilon_2$), and hemoglobin Gower-2, consisting of two alpha and two epsilon chains ($\alpha_2\varepsilon_2$).

hemoglobin H, hemoglobin composed of four beta chains, found in alpha thalassemia. Infants may be born with a mixture of hemoglobin H and hemoglobin Bart's.

hemoglobin H disease, alpha-thalassemia in individuals heterozygous for hemoglobin H, characterized by chronic hemolytic anemia associated with splenomegaly. Red blood cell microcytosis and hypochromia are accompanied by inclusion bodies resembling Heinz bodies, detectable by supravital staining.

hemoglobin Kansas, an abnormal hemoglobin with threonine substituted for asparagine at position 102 of the beta chain, resulting in decreased oxygen affinity and cyanosis.

hemoglobin Köln, an unstable hemoglobin that has methionine substituted for valine at position 95 of the beta chain, usually resulting in hemolytic anemia with Heinz bodies in the erythrocytes.

hemoglobin M, hemoglobin in which the iron, normally in the bivalent ferrous state, is oxidized to the trivalent ferric state, usually as a result of smoking or other inflammatory conditions; rarely an inherited hemoglobinopathy.

hemoglobin M disease [Gk, *haima*, blood; L, *globus,* ball; M; Gk, *dis*, not; Fr, *aise,* ease], a mild to moderate anemia in which a percentage of the hemoglobin contains iron in the Fe^{+++} state and is unable to combine with oxygen. The patient may experience cyanosis. See also **methemoglobin.**

hemoglobinometer /-om″ətər/ [Gk, *haima*, blood; L, *globus,* ball; Gk, *metron*, measure], any of several types of instruments designed to measure the concentration of hemoglobin in a blood sample. Some convert hemoglobin to stable measurable cyanmethemoglobin; others employ a detergent such as sodium dodecyl sulfate to lyse red blood cells and release hemoglobin for measurement.

hemoglobinometry /he″moglob'inom'ĕtre/, measurement of blood hemoglobin concentration, usually with a hemoglobinometer, after the hemoglobin has been converted to cyanmethemoglobin or freed from red blood cells by sodium dodecyl sulfate.

hemoglobinopathy /hē′mōglō′binop″əthē, hem′-/ [Gk, *haima* + L, *globus,* ball; Gk, *pathos,* disease], a group of inherited disorders characterized by structural variations of the hemoglobin molecule. An abnormality may occur in the heterozygous or the homozygous form. The alteration appears as the substitution of one or more amino acids in the globin portion of the molecule at selected positions in the two alpha or two beta polypeptide chains. Although more than 100 variants have been described, only hemoglobins S and C are commonly seen. In the heterozygous form the normal adult pigment, hemoglobin A, and the variant both appear in the red cell. Little or no clinical manifestation of disease may be present. In the homozygous form only the variant hemoglobin is present, and the characteristic symptoms of that hemoglobinopathy appear. Mixed heterozygous forms are also known to occur. The normal hemoglobin A may be absent, and two or three hemoglobin variants may be present. Also spelled **haemoglobinopathy.** Compare **thalassemia.** Kinds include **hemoglobin C disease, hemoglobin SC (Hb SC) disease, sickle cell anemia.** See also **hemoglobin, hemoglobin A, sickle cell thalassemia, sickle cell trait.**

hemoglobin Portland, a normal hemoglobin present in the fetus late in the first trimester of pregnancy, consisting of zeta and gamma chains ($\zeta_2\gamma_2$). It disappears in utero.

hemoglobin S (Hb S), hemoglobinopathy characterized by the substitution of the amino acid valine for glutamic acid at position 6 in the beta chain of the hemoglobin molecule. Hemoglobin S migrates to between hemoglobin C and hemoglobin A in hemoglobin electrophoresis. As the hemoglobin S becomes deoxygenated, red cells become sickle-shaped, occluding capillaries. If the proportion of Hb S to Hb A is large, as in sickle cell anemia, local infarction occurs. See also **sickle cell anemia, sickle cell crisis, sickle cell trait.**

hemoglobin SC (Hb SC) disease, a genetic anemia in which abnormal alleles, one for hemoglobin S and one for hemoglobin C, are inherited. The disorder is characterized by a clinical course considerably less severe than that of sickle cell anemia despite the absence of normal hemoglobin. Also called **sickle cell–hemoglobin C disease.** See also **hemoglobin C disease, sickle cell anemia.**

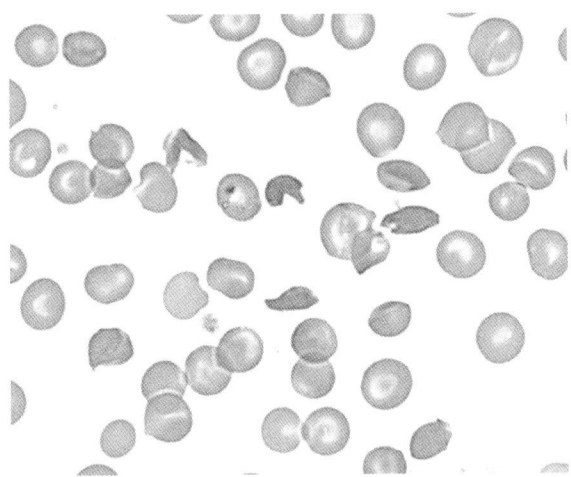

Hemoglobin SC in peripheral blood sample *(Hisi, 2012)*

hemoglobin SD disease, a genetically determined anemia in which the erythrocytes contain both hemoglobin S and hemoglobin D, with symptoms like those of mild sickle cell anemia. Also called **sickle cell–hemoglobin D disease.** See also **sickle cell anemia.**

hemoglobin Seattle, an abnormal hemoglobin in which glutamic acid replaces alanine at position 76 of the beta chain, decreasing the hemoglobin molecule's affinity for oxygen.

hemoglobin (Hb, Hgb) test, a blood test that measures the total amount of hemoglobin in the peripheral blood, which reflects the number of red blood cells in the blood. The test is normally performed as part of a complete blood count. Abnormal levels indicate anemia, erythrocytosis, and sickle cell disease, among others.

hemoglobinuria /-o͞or″ē·ə/ [Gk, *haima* + L, *globus,* ball; Gk, *ouron,* urine], *adj.,* abnormal presence in the urine of hemoglobin that is not attached to red blood cells. Hemoglobinuria can result from various autoimmune diseases or episodic hemolytic disorders. It can be diagnosed by using a dipstick reagent that is sensitive to free hemoglobin.

hemoglobinuric /-o͞or″ik/ [Gk, *haima,* blood; L, *globus,* ball; Gk, *ouron,* urine], pertaining to the presence of hemoglobin in the urine.

hemogram /hē″məgram/ [Gk, *haima* + *gramma,* record], a written or graphic record of a differential blood count that emphasizes the size, shape, special characteristics, and numbers of the solid components of the blood. See also **complete blood count.**

hemolith /-lith/, a calculus in the wall of a blood vessel.

hemolysin /himol″əsin/ [Gk, *haima* + *lysis,* loosening], any one of the numerous substances that lyse or dissolve red blood cells. Hemolysins are produced by bacterial strains, including staphylococci and streptococci, and are contained in venoms and vegetables. Bacterial hemolysins are divided into those that are filterable and those that cluster around the bacterial colony on a culture medium containing red blood cells. Hemolysins appear to aid the invasive power of bacteria. Also spelled **haemolysin.** See also **hemoglobin, hemolysis.**

hemolysis /himol″isis/ [Gk, *haima* + *lysis,* loosening], *adj.,* the breakdown of red blood cells and the release of hemoglobin that occur normally at the end of the life span of a red cell. Hemolysis may occur in antigen-antibody reactions, metabolic abnormalities of the red cell that significantly shorten red cell life span, and mechanical trauma, such as cardiac prosthesis. Dilution of the blood by IV administration of excessive amounts of hypotonic solutions, which causes progressive swelling and eventual rupture of the erythrocyte, also results in hemolysis. Also spelled **haemolysis.** −*hemolytic, adj.*

hemolytic anemia /-lit″ik/ [Gk, *haima* + *lysis* + *a,* without, + *haima,* blood], a disorder characterized by acute or chronic premature destruction of red blood cells. Anemia may be partially compensated by bone marrow production. The condition may be associated with some infectious diseases, certain inherited red cell disorders, or neoplastic diseases. It may be a response to drugs or other toxic agents. Also spelled **haemolytic anemia.** Compare **aplastic anemia, congenital nonspherocytic hemolytic anemia, iron-deficiency anemia,** *myelophthisic anemia.* See also **anemia, hemolysis, spherocytosis.**

hemolytic disease of the fetus and newborn, alloimmune hemolytic anemia caused by placental transfer of IgG blood group antibodies from an immunized mother to the fetus, whose red cells carry an antigen inherited from the father. Hemolysis of fetal red cells can cause severe anemia, jaundice, and enlargement of the liver and spleen, which, without intervention, can lead to hypoxia, cardiac failure, generalized edema, respiratory distress, and death.

hemolytic jaundice, a yellowish discoloration of the skin and conjunctiva caused by a breakdown of red blood cells, which causes excessive amounts of bilirubin. See also **hyperbilirubinemia.**

hemolytic jaundice of the newborn. See **icterus gravis neonatorum.**

hemolytic uremic syndrome, a kidney disorder marked by renal failure, microangiopathic hemolytic anemia, and platelet deficiency. The syndrome, the cause of which is unknown, usually occurs in infancy. With conservative management, including dialysis, most infants and children recover. The prognosis in adults is uncertain.

hemoperfusion /-pərfyoo″zhən/, the perfusion of blood through a sorbent device, such as activated charcoal or resin beads, rather than through dialysis equipment. Hemoperfusion may be used in treating uremia, liver failure, and certain forms of drug toxicity.

hemopericardium /-per′ikär″dē·əm/ [Gk, *haima* + *peri,* near, *kardia,* heart], an accumulation of blood within the pericardial sac surrounding the heart that may result in cardiac tamponade.

hemoperitoneum /-per′itōnē″əm/ [Gk, *haima* + *peri,* around, *tenein,* to stretch], the presence of extravasated blood in the peritoneal cavity caused by surgical procedures, necrotizing tumors, fistulas, or laparoscopy procedures.

hemophil /hē″mōfil/ [Gk, *haima,* blood, *philein,* to love], **1.** bacteria of the genus *Haemophilus,* which thrive in culture media containing blood. **2.** an organism thriving on blood.

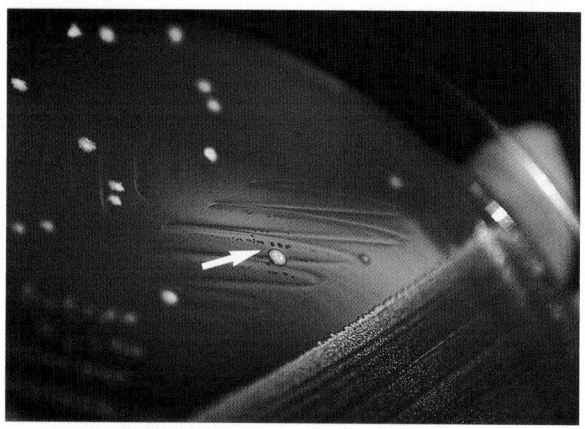

Hemophil *(Forbes, Sahm, and Weissfeld, 2007)*

hemophilia /hē″mōfē″lyə, hem′-/ [Gk, *haima* + *philein,* to love], a group of hereditary bleeding disorders characterized by a deficiency of one of the factors necessary for coagulation of the blood. The two most common forms of the disorder are hemophilia A and hemophilia B. Hemophilia A (classic hemophilia) is the result of a deficiency or absence of coagulation factor VIII. Hemophilia B (Christmas disease) results from a deficiency of factor IX. Hemophilia C (Rosenthal disease) is a factor XI deficiency. The clinical severity of the disorder varies with the extent of the deficiency. Anatomical bleeding—bleeding into joints, muscles, and soft tissue—is typical of hemophilia. Greater-than-usual loss of blood during dental procedures, epistaxis, hematoma, and hemarthrosis are common problems in patients with hemophilia. Also spelled **haemophilia.** See also **von Willebrand disease,** *specific blood factors.* −*hemophilic, adj.,* −*hemophiliac, n.*

■ OBSERVATIONS: The primary presenting sign in hemophilia is excessive, poorly controlled bleeding. The rate of bleeding depends on the amount of factor activity and the severity of the injury that caused the bleeding. A factor activity level below 1% can cause spontaneous bleeding or severe bleeding from even minor trauma. When the factor activity level is more than 5%, bleeding is usually caused by trauma and is more easily controlled. The bleeding is anatomical, involving subcutaneous and muscle tissue, or deep bleeding into joints and organ systems. Laboratory tests reveal a normal prothrombin time, a prolonged partial thromboplastin time, and a normal platelet function. Assays are used to determine the factor affected and the level of factor activity. A common cause of death is intracranial bleeds, which occur in about 10% of hemophiliacs and are fatal 30% of the time. Other complications of repeat bleeds include joint and musculoskeletal deformities, pericardial tamponade, airway compression, and uncontrolled hemorrhage.

■ INTERVENTIONS: Replacement of deficient factors with recombinant factor products or plasma-derived factor concentrates is the primary treatment. This may be used as prophylaxis or to stop bleeding episodes. Desmopressin acetate is used to stimulate factor VIII in mild hemophilia A. Aminocaproic acid is given in cases of persistent bleeding unresponsive to treatment. Pain is controlled with acetaminophen or codeine. Aspirin and NSAID use and intramuscular injections should be avoided because they may precipitate bleeding. Extreme care must be exercised when individuals with hemophilia need surgery or dental work.

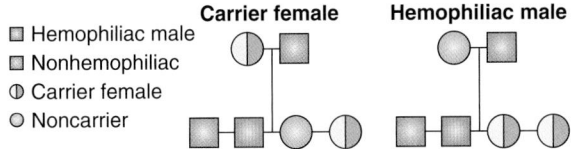

□ Hemophiliac male
□ Nonhemophiliac
⊕ Carrier female
○ Noncarrier

Carrier female   **Hemophiliac male**

Inheritance patterns in hemophilia *(Beare and Myers, 1998)*

hemophilia A, a hereditary blood disorder usually expressed in males that is transmitted as an X-linked recessive mutation causing a deficiency of coagulation factor VIII. Hemophilia A is sometimes named classic hemophilia. See also **coagulation factor, hemophilia.**

hemophilia B, a hereditary blood disorder, transmitted as an X-linked recessive trait and caused by a deficiency of factor IX. The condition is clinically similar to but less severe than hemophilia A. Also called **Christmas disease.** See **coagulation factor, hemophilia.**

hemophilia C, a hereditary blood disorder, transmitted as an X-linked recessive trait and caused by a deficiency of factor XI, the plasma thromboplastin antecedent. The condition is clinically similar to but may be less severe than hemophilia A. Also called *Rosenthal syndrome.* See also **coagulation factor, hemophilia.**

hemopneumopericardium /hē′mōnoo̅′mōper′ikär″dē·əm/ [Gk, *haima,* blood, *pneuma,* air, *kardia,* heart], an accumulation of blood and air in the pericardium. Also called **pneumohemopericardium.**

hemopneumothorax /hē′mōnoo̅′mōthôr″aks/ [Gk, *haima,* blood, *pneuma,* air, *thorax,* chest], an accumulation of blood and air in the pleural cavity.

hemoptysis /himop″tisis/ [Gk, *haima* + *ptyein,* to spit], the coughing up of blood from the respiratory tract. Blood-streaked sputum often is present in minor upper respiratory infections or bronchitis. More profuse bleeding may indicate *Aspergillus* infection, lung abscess, tuberculosis, or bronchogenic carcinoma, in which the blood loss is caused by erosion of the pulmonary vessels. Hemoptysis is normal after some endoscopic procedures. Radiographic examination, endoscopy, and bronchoscopy are often used to diagnose hemoptysis.

hemorheology /-rē·ol″əjē/ [Gk, *haima,* blood, *rhoia,* flow, *logos,* science], the study of the effects of blood flow pressure on the cellular components of blood and on the walls of blood vessels.

hemorrhage /hem′ərij/ [Gk, *haima* + *rhegnynei,* to gush], a loss of a large amount of blood in a short period, either externally or internally. Hemorrhage may be arterial, venous, or capillary. Also spelled **haemorrhage.** –*hemorrhagic, adj.*

■ OBSERVATIONS: Symptoms of massive hemorrhage are related to hypovolemic shock: rapid, thready pulse; thirst; cold, clammy skin; sighing respirations; dizziness; syncope; pallor; apprehension; restlessness; and hypotension. If bleeding is contained within a cavity or joint, pain will develop as the capsule or cavity is stretched by the rapidly expanding volume of blood.

■ INTERVENTIONS: Effort is directed to stopping the hemorrhage. If hemorrhage is external, pressure is applied directly to the wound or to the appropriate pressure points. The part of the body that is wounded may be elevated. Ice, applied directly to the wound, may slow bleeding by causing vasoconstriction. Body temperature may be maintained by keeping the person covered and flat. If an extremity is wounded, and if the bleeding is severe, a tourniquet may be applied proximal to the wound.

hemorrhagic cholecystitis, cholecystitis with hemorrhage into the gallbladder. It is usually acalculous, but sometimes there are gallstones.

hemorrhagic cystitis, bladder inflammation with a large amount of blood in the urine secondary to chemotherapy, radiation, mechanical trauma, or passage of a kidney stone.

hemorrhagic diathesis /-raj″ik/, an inherited predisposition to any of a number of abnormalities characterized by excessive bleeding. See also **Fanconi syndrome, hemophilia, von Willebrand disease.**

hemorrhagic disease of newborn, a bleeding disorder of neonates that is usually caused by a deficiency of vitamin K. Also spelled **haemorrhagic disease of newborn.**

hemorrhagic familial angiomatosis. See **hereditary hemorrhagic telangiectasia.**

hemorrhagic fever, a group of viral infections characterized by fever, chills, headache, malaise, and respiratory or GI symptoms, followed by capillary hemorrhages and, in severe infection, by oliguria, kidney failure, hypotension, and possibly death. Many forms of the disease occur in specific geographic areas. See also **dengue fever, dengue hemorrhagic fever shock syndrome, Ebola virus disease, Lassa fever, Marburg virus disease.**

hemorrhagic gastritis, a form of acute gastritis usually caused by a toxic agent, such as alcohol, aspirin or other drugs, or bacterial toxins that irritate the lining of the stomach. Nausea, vomiting, and epigastric distress may persist after the irritant is removed. Treatment is symptomatic.

hemorrhagic infarct [Gk, *haima,* blood, *rhegnynei,* to gush; L, *infarcire,* to stuff], an area of necrosis that has accumulated so much blood that it resembles a red, swollen bruise.

hemorrhagic jaundice [Gk, *haima,* blood, *rhegnynei,* to gush; Fr, *jaune,* yellow], a form of jaundice that occurs in Weil disease or other forms of leptospirosis in which capillary injury and anemia are present.

hemorrhagic lung. See **adult respiratory distress syndrome.**

hemorrhagic measles [Gk, *haima,* blood, *rhegnynei,* to gush; ME, *masalas*], a severe form of measles characterized by bleeding into the skin and mucous membranes. Also called **black measles.**

hemorrhagic pericarditis [Gk, *haima,* blood, *rhegnynei,* to gush, *peri,* near, *kardia,* heart, *itis,* inflammation], inflammation of the pericardium accompanied by a bloody effusion. The condition is frequently caused by tuberculosis or a tumor.

hemorrhagic plague [Gk, *haima,* blood, *rhegnynei,* to gush; L, *plaga,* stroke], a severe form of bubonic plague in which bleeding occurs under the skin. Also called **bubonic plague.**

hemorrhagic pleurisy [Gk, *haima,* blood, *rhegnynei,* to gush, *pleuritis*], an inflammation of the pleura in which effusion of blood into the tissues occurs.

hemorrhagic purpura [Gk, *haima,* blood, *rhegnynei,* to gush; L, *purpura,* purple], bruises or purple skin discolorations of 1 cm in diameter or greater, suggesting systemic bleeding; usually associated with diminished strength of vascular walls, thrombocytopenia, von Willebrand disease, and platelet disorders. See **immune thrombocytopenic purpura, thrombopenic purpura.**

hemorrhagic shock, shock associated with the sudden and rapid loss of significant amounts of blood. Severe traumatic injuries often cause such blood losses. This results in inadequate perfusion to meet the metabolic demands of cellular function. Death occurs within a relatively short time unless transfusion quickly restores normal blood volume.

Hemorrhagic shock often accompanies secondary shock. Compare **primary shock.**

hemorrhagic urticaria [Gk, *haima,* blood, *rhegnynei,* to gush; L, *urtica,* nettle], a skin eruption characterized by bleeding in the wheals, usually as a complication of another disease such as nephritis. In some cases the bleeding occurs first and the wheals become superimposed. Also called **urticaria hemorrhagica.**

hemorrheology. See **hemorheology.**

hemorrhoid /hem′əroid/ [Gk, *haima + rhoia,* flow], a varicosity in the lower rectum or anus caused by congestion in the veins of the hemorrhoidal plexus.

■ OBSERVATIONS: Internal hemorrhoids originate above the internal sphincter of the anus. If they become large enough to protrude from the anus, they become constricted and painful. Small internal hemorrhoids may bleed with defecation. External hemorrhoids appear outside the anal sphincter. They are usually not painful, and bleeding does not occur unless a hemorrhoidal vein ruptures or thromboses.

■ INTERVENTIONS: Treatment includes local application of a topical medication to lubricate, anesthetize, and shrink the hemorrhoid. Sitz baths and cold or hot compresses are also soothing. The hemorrhoids may require sclerosing by injection, ligation, or surgical excision. Ligation is increasingly the preferred treatment because it is simple and effective and does not require anesthesia. The hemorrhoid is grasped with a forceps, and a rubber band is slipped over the varicosity, causing tissue necrosis and sloughing of the hemorrhoid, usually within 1 week.

■ PATIENT CARE CONSIDERATIONS: Constipation, straining to defecate, and prolonged sitting contribute to the development of hemorrhoids. The client is counseled about ways to prevent these predisposing factors. Because pregnancy is associated with an increased incidence of hemorrhoids, women who are pregnant are counseled on how to avoid constipation.

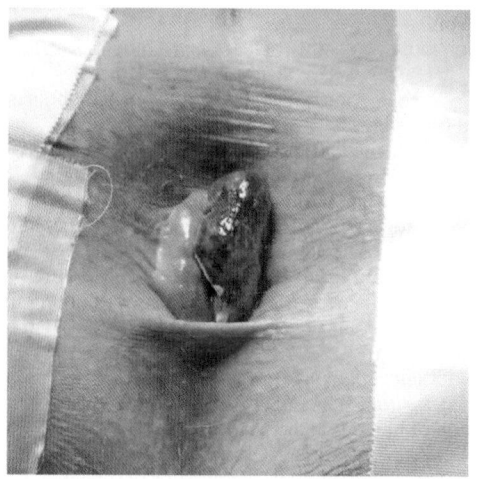

Internal hemorrhoid *(Mounsey et al, 2011)*

hemorrhoidal tag, an anal skin tag that was originally part of hemorrhoidal tissue.

hemorrhoidectomy /hem′əroidek″təmē/ [Gk, *haimorrhois,* a vein that discharges blood, *ektomē,* excision], the removal of dilated veins in the anal region to mitigate pain and bleeding. Most hemorrhoidectomies are outpatient procedures. Rubber band ligation, which can be done through an anoscope without sedation, is the most popular outpatient therapy. Surgery may be indicated for larger symptomatic external and internal hemorrhoids. The patient is usually placed in the lithotomy or jackknife position and receives spinal, caudal, epidural, or local anesthesia. Possible postoperative complications include constipation, pain, fecal impaction, hemorrhage, infection, and urinary retention.

hemosalpinx /hē′mōsal″pinks/ [Gk, *haima,* blood, *salpinx,* tube], a collection of blood in a fallopian tube. The most common cause is a tubal pregnancy. Endometriosis can also cause this condition.

hemosiderin /hē′mōsid″ərin/ [Gk, *haima + sideros,* iron], an iron-rich pigment that is a product of red cell hemolysis. Iron is often stored in this form.

hemosiderosis /hē′mōsid′ərō″sis, hem′-/ [Gk, *haima + sideros,* iron, *osis,* condition], an increased deposition of iron in a variety of tissues, usually in the form of hemosiderin and usually without tissue damage. It is often associated with diseases involving chronic, extensive destruction of red blood cells, such as thalassemia major. Compare **hemochromatosis, sideroblastic anemia.** See also **ferritin, iron transport, siderosis, thalassemia, transferrin.**

hemostasis /himos″təsis, hē′məstā″sis/ [Gk, *haima + stasis,* halting], **1.** the process of maintaining the blood in a fluid state within the confines of the circulatory system. A complex interaction of processes consisting of vasoconstriction, platelet aggregation, thrombin and fibrin generation, coagulation regulation, and fibrinolysis. **2.** the arrest of the escape of blood by compression or ligation.

hemostat, an instrument used as a clamp that stops hemorrhage by compressing a bleeding vessel. See **Halsted forceps.**

hemostatic /-stat″ik/ [Gk, *haima + stasis,* halting], pertaining to a procedure, device, or substance that arrests the flow of blood. Direct pressure, tourniquets, and surgical clamps are mechanical hemostatic measures. Cold applications, including the use of an ice bag on the abdomen to halt uterine bleeding and irrigation of the stomach with an iced solution to check gastric bleeding, are hemostatic. Gelatin sponges, solutions of thrombin, and microfibrillar collagen, which cause the aggregation of platelets and the formation of clots, are used to arrest bleeding in surgical procedures. Aminocaproic acid is administered orally or intravenously in the treatment of excessive bleeding caused by systemic hyperfibrinolysis. Phytonadione (vitamin K_1) is used in the prevention and treatment of hemorrhagic disease in newborns and the treatment of prothrombin deficiency induced by anticoagulants or other drugs.

hemostatic forceps. See **artery forceps.**

hemotherapeutics /-ther′əpyoō″tiks/, a form of treatment that involves the use of fresh blood plasma or serum. Also called *hemotherapy.*

hemothorax /hē′mōthôr″aks, hem′-/ [Gk, *haima + thorax,* chest], an accumulation of blood and fluid in the pleural cavity, between the parietal and visceral pleura, usually the result of trauma. Blood can also accumulate in the thoracic cavity as a result of erosion of pulmonary vessels, the rupture of blebs, or granulomas. Hemothorax also may be caused by the rupture of small blood vessels in inflammation caused by pneumonia, tuberculosis, or tumors. Shock from hemorrhage, pain, and respiratory failure follow if emergency care is not available.

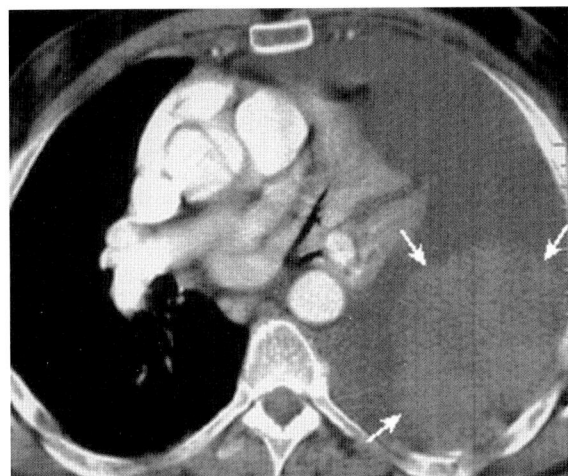

CT scan of a patient with a large left hemothorax
(Leonard, 2009)

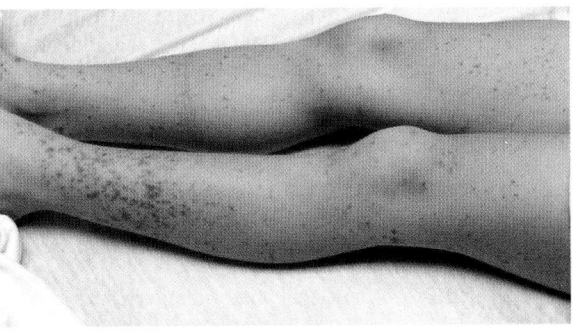

Henoch-Schönlein purpura *(Marcdante and Kliegman, 2015)*

hemotroph /hē′mətrof/, the total nutritive substances supplied to the embryo from the maternal circulation after the development of the placenta. Also called *hemotrophic nutrition*. Also spelled *hemotrophe*. Compare **embryotroph.** −*hemotrophic, adj.*

Henderson-Hasselbalch equation [Lawrence J. Henderson, American chemist, 1878–1942; Karl A. Hasselbalch, Danish biochemist, 1874–1962], the relationship among pH, the pK_a of a buffer system, and the ratio of the concentrations of the weak acid and its conjugate base.

Henderson, Virginia [1897–1996], a nursing theorist who introduced a holistic approach to the profession in 1966. The theory is based on the concepts that the body and mind are inseparable, no two individuals are alike, and the role of nursing is independent of the functions of the physician. The Henderson theory proposes that 14 components of basic nursing care contribute to the health of a patient. They relate to (1) breathing, (2) eating and drinking, (3) elimination, (4) movement and posture, (5) sleep and rest, (6) clothing, (7) maintenance of body temperature, (8) cleaning and grooming of the body, (9) avoidance of environmental dangers and injury, (10) communication, (11) worship, (12) work, (13) play and recreation, and (14) learning and discovery.

Henle fissure /hen″lē/ [Friedrich Gustav Henle, German anatomist, 1809–1885], one of many patches of connective tissue between the muscle fibers of the heart.

Henle's loop. See **loop of Henle.**

Henoch-Schönlein purpura /hen″ôkh shœn″līn/ [Eduard H. Henoch, German physician, 1820–1910; Johannes L. Schönlein, German physician, 1793–1864], a self-limited hypersensitivity vasculitis, chiefly of children, characterized by purpuric skin lesions that appear predominantly on the lower abdomen, buttocks, and legs and are usually associated with pain in the knees and ankles. Other joint involvement, GI bleeding, and hematuria are also common findings. The disease lasts up to 6 weeks and has no sequelae if renal involvement is not severe. Immunosuppressive drugs, such as corticosteroids, may help relieve the nephropathy. Also called **anaphylactoid purpura, Henoch-Schönlein syndrome, Schönlein-Henoch purpura.**

Henoch-Schönlein purpura nephritis, a type of glomerulonephritis sometimes seen with Henoch-Schönlein purpura. Clinical characteristics usually resemble those of IgA nephropathy, and a rapidly progressive form can lead to renal failure.

Henoch-Schönlein syndrome. See **Henoch-Schönlein purpura.**

henry (H) [Joseph Henry, American physicist, 1797–1878], an International System unit of electrical inductance equal to 1 volt-second per ampere.

Henry's law [William Henry, English chemist, 1774–1836], (in physics) a law stating that the solubility of a gas in a liquid is proportional to the pressure of the gas if the temperature is constant and the gas does not chemically react with the liquid.

Henschen method, a technique for positioning a patient's head in a true lateral position to produce a radiographic image of the mastoid and petrous portions of the skull.

Hensen's knot, Hensen's node. See **primitive node.**

hen worker's lung. See **pigeon breeder's lung.**

HEP, abbreviation for **hepatoerythropoietic porphyria.**

HEPA, abbreviation for *high-efficiency particulate air* filters.

heparin /hep″ərin/ [Gk, *hēpar*, liver], a naturally occurring mucopolysaccharide that acts in the body as an antithrombin factor to prevent intravascular clotting. The substance is produced by basophils and mast cells, which are found in large numbers in the connective tissue surrounding capillaries, particularly in the lungs and liver. In the form of sodium salt, heparin is used therapeutically as an anticoagulant. See also **heparin sodium.**

heparin-induced thrombocytopenia with thrombosis (HIT), arterial and venous clots that may develop after five days of unfractionated heparin therapy; caused by the production of anti-heparin-platelet factor 4 antibodies.

heparin lock flush solution (USP) [Gk, *hēpar*, liver; OE, *loc* + ME, *fluschen* + L, *solutus*, dissolved], a sterile solution of heparin sodium, saline solution, and benzyl alcohol that is intended for use in maintaining patency in IV equipment. It is not used in anticoagulant therapy.

heparin rebound, the reactivation of heparin effect that occurs from 5 minutes to 5 hours after neutralization with protamine sulfate.

heparin sodium, an anticoagulant.

■ INDICATIONS: It is prescribed in the treatment and prophylaxis of a variety of thromboembolic disorders. It inhibits blood clotting and prevents recurring coronary artery occlusion.

■ CONTRAINDICATIONS: Known hypersensitivity to this drug prohibits its use. It is given only when frequent monitoring of the coagulation status of the patient's blood is possible.

■ ADVERSE EFFECTS: The most serious adverse reaction is hemorrhage. Vasospastic disorders may occur.

hepat-. See **hepato-, hepat-, hepatico-.**

hepatectomy /hep′ətek″təmē/ [Gk, *hēpar,* liver, *ektomē,* excision], a surgical procedure performed to remove a portion of the liver.

hepatic /hepat″ik/ [Gk, *hēpar,* liver], pertaining to the liver.

hepatic acinus, a functional unit of the liver, smaller than a portal lobule; a diamond-shaped mass of liver parenchyma surrounding a portal tract.

hepatic adenoma, a rapidly growing tumor of the liver that may become very large and rupture, causing a lethal internal hemorrhage. The incidence is frequently associated with the use of oral contraceptives.

hepatic amebiasis, a disorder characterized by enlargement and tenderness of the liver that is often associated with amebic dysentery. The inflammation results from direct infection with *Entamoeba histolytica,* ingested in water or food contaminated with human feces. See also **amebiasis, amebic dysentery.**

hepatic amyloidosis, a type of primary amyloidosis in which amyloid fibrils invade the liver, causing hepatomegaly. The prognosis is grave, with many patients dying within a year.

hepatic bile, bile obtained from a duodenal drainage tube after the gallbladder has been emptied.

hepatic cells. See **hepatic cord.**

hepatic coma, a neuropsychiatric manifestation of extensive liver damage caused by chronic or acute liver disease. Either endogenous or exogenous waste toxic to the brain is not neutralized in the liver before being shunted back into the peripheral circulation of the blood, or substances required for cerebral function are not synthesized in the liver and therefore are not available to the brain. Commonly, ammonia, a by-product of protein metabolism that is toxic to the brain, is not converted to urea by the liver. The condition is characterized by variable consciousness, including lethargy, stupor, and coma; a tremor of the hands; personality change; memory loss; hyperreflexia; and hyperventilation. Respiratory alkalosis, mania convulsions, and death may occur. The outcome varies according to the pathogenesis of the condition and the treatment. Also called **portal-systemic encephalopathy.** See also **cirrhosis, hepatitis.**

■ INTERVENTIONS: Treatment in most cases includes cleansing enemas, low-protein diet, parenteral hydration with a balanced electrolyte solution, and specific treatment for the underlying cause. It may also include the use of neomycin orally to kill off bacteria and thus prevent elevated blood urea nitrogen levels.

hepatic cord, a mass of cells, arranged in irregular radiating columns and plates, spreading outward from the central vein of the hepatic lobule. The cells are many-sided and contain one or sometimes two distinct nuclei. Many such cords join to form the parenchyma of the liver lobule. Each cell usually contains granules, some protoplasmic and others consisting of glycogen, fat, or an iron compound. Also called **hepatic cells.**

hepatic dyspepsia, a digestive difficulty caused by a liver disorder.

hepatic encephalopathy. See **hepatic coma.**

hepatic fistula, an abnormal passage from the liver to another organ or body structure.

hepatic insufficiency, a failure or partial failure of normal liver function.

hepatic ischemia, injury to liver cells resulting from a deficiency of blood or oxygen, caused by hypotension from decreased cardiac output, shock, or some other cause. Also called *hypoxic hepatitis, ischemic hepatitis,* **shock liver.**

herpetic keratitis. See **dendritic keratitis.**

hepatic lobes [Gk, *hēpar,* liver, *lobos,* lobes], the large divisions of the liver: caudate, quadrate, left, and right.

hepatic node, a node in one of three groups of lymph glands associated with the abdominal and pelvic viscera supplied by branches of the celiac artery. The hepatic nodes are divided into the hepatic and subpyloric groups. The hepatic group, on the stem of the hepatic artery, extends along the common bile duct, between the two layers of the lesser omentum, as far as the porta hepatis. The subpyloric group comprises about five nodes closely relating to the division of the gastroduodenal artery. Both groups receive materials from the stomach, the duodenum, the liver, the gallbladder, and the pancreas. Their efferent vessels join the celiac set of preaortic nodes. Compare **gastric node, pancreaticolienal node.**

hepatico-. See **hepato-, hepat-, hepatico-.**

hepaticoduodenostomy /hepat′ikōdoo′ōdənos″təmē/, surgical establishment of a passageway between the hepatic duct and the duodenum.

hepaticoenterostomy /hepat′ikō·en′teros″təmē/, surgical establishment of a passageway between the hepatic duct and the intestine.

hepaticolithotomy /-lithot″əmē/, an incision made in the hepatic bile duct for the removal of gallstones.

hepaticolithotripsy /-lith″ətrip′sē/, a surgical procedure in which gallstones in the bile duct are crushed for removal.

hepatic porphyria. See **porphyria.**

hepatic portal circulation. See **portal circulation.**

hepatic portal vein, a large vein through which all venous blood from the gastrointestinal system enters the inferior surface of the liver. The vein then ramifies like an artery to distribute blood to small endothelial-lined hepatic sinusoids, which form the vascular exchange network of the liver.

hepatic pulse, pulsation of the liver, such as may occur in tricuspid incompetence.

hepatic steatosis. See **nonalcoholic fatty liver disease.**

hepatic vein catheterization, the introduction of a long, fine catheter into a hepatic venule for the purpose of recording intrahepatic venous pressure. The catheter is inserted through a vein in the arm and is passed through the right atrium, inferior vena cava, and hepatic vein into the small hepatic vessel.

hepatic veins [Gk, *hēpar,* liver; L, *vena*], the three main veins, the right, middle, and left, that drain the blood returned from the liver into the inferior vena cava.

hepatin. See **glycogen.**

hepatitis /hep′ətī″tis/ [Gk, *hēpar* + *itis,* inflammation], an inflammatory condition of the liver, characterized by jaundice, hepatomegaly, anorexia, abdominal and gastric discomfort, abnormal liver function, clay-colored stools, and tea-colored urine. The condition may be caused by bacterial or viral infection, parasitic infestation, alcohol, drugs, toxins, or transfusion of incompatible blood. It may be mild and brief or severe, fulminant, and life-threatening. The liver usually is able to regenerate its tissue, but severe hepatitis may lead to cirrhosis and chronic liver dysfunction. Compare **anicteric hepatitis.** See also **viral hepatitis.**

Characteristics of hepatitis viruses

	Incubation period	Mode of transmission	Sources of infection and spread of disease	Infectivity
Hepatitis A virus (HAV)	15–50 days (average 28)	Fecal-oral (fecal contamination and oral ingestion)	Crowded conditions (e.g., day care); poor personal hygiene; poor sanitation; contaminated food, milk, water, and shellfish; persons with subclinical infections; infected food handlers; sexual contact; IV drug users	Most infectious during 2 wk before onset of symptoms; infectious until 1–2 wk after the start of symptoms
Hepatitis B virus (HBV)	45–180 days (average 56–96)	Percutaneous (parenteral)/permucosal exposure to blood or blood products Sexual contact Perinatal transmission	Contaminated needles, syringes, and blood products; sexual activity with infected partners; asymptomatic carriers Tattoo/body piercing with contaminated needles; bites	Before and after symptoms appear; infectious for 4–6 mo; in carriers continues for patient's lifetime
Hepatitis C virus (HCV)	14–180 days (average 56)	Percutaneous (parenteral)/mucosal exposure to blood or blood products High-risk sexual contact Perinatal contact	Blood and blood products, needles and syringes, sexual activity with infected partners	1–2 wk before symptoms appear; continues during clinical course; 75%–85% go on to develop chronic hepatitis C
Hepatitis D virus (HDV)	2–26 wk; HBV must precede HDV; chronic carriers of HBV are always at risk	Can cause infection only when HBV is present; routes of transmission same as for HBV	Same as HBV	Blood is infectious at all stages of HDV infection
Hepatitis E virus (HEV)	15–64 days (average 26–42 days)	Fecal-oral Outbreaks associated with contaminated water supply in developing countries	Contaminated water; poor sanitation; found in Asia, Africa, and Mexico; not common in United States and Canada	Not known; may be similar to HAV

From Lewis SL et al: *Medical-surgical nursing: assessment and management of clinical problems,* ed 9, St Louis, 2014, Mosby.

hepatitis A (HA), a viral hepatitis caused by the hepatitis A virus (HAV), a picornovirus; it is characterized by slow onset of signs and symptoms. The virus may be spread through fecally contaminated food or water. The infection most often occurs in young adults; it is usually followed by complete recovery and does not result in chronic infection. Disease duration is from 15–45 days. Relapses 6–12 months after the initial diagnosis are seen in 15% of patients. Prophylaxis with immune globulin is effective in household and sexual contacts. A vaccine for immunization is available. Standard precautions should be used for diapered or incontinent patients. Also called **acute infective hepatitis.** See also **viral hepatitis.**

hepatitis A vaccine inactivated, an inactivated whole virus vaccine derived from an attenuated strain of hepatitis A virus grown in cell culture; administered intramuscularly.

hepatitis B (HB), a viral hepatitis caused by the hepatitis B virus (HBV), a hepadnavirus. The virus is transmitted by transfusion of contaminated blood or blood products, by sexual contact with an infected person, by the use of contaminated needles and instruments, or in utero. It can cause acute and chronic hepatitis. Ninety-five percent of patients clear the infection and develop antibodies to HBV. The remaining 5% who are unable to clear the virus develop chronic infections that put them at risk for long-term complications.

Severe infection may cause prolonged illness, destruction of liver cells, cirrhosis, increased risk of liver cancer, or death. A vaccine is available and recommended for infants, teenagers, and adults at risk for exposure. Treatment may involve transplantation. Also called **serum hepatitis.** See also **viral hepatitis.**

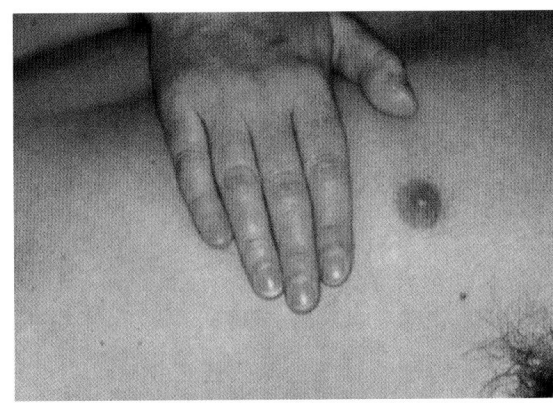

Jaundice in a patient with hepatitis
(Emond, Welsby, and Rowland, 2003)

hepatitis B immune globulin (HBIG), a passive immunizing agent.

- INDICATIONS: It is prescribed for postexposure prophylaxis against infection by the hepatitis B virus.
- CONTRAINDICATIONS: Known hypersensitivity to the drug or to gamma globulin prohibits its use.
- ADVERSE EFFECTS: Among the most serious adverse reactions are severe hypersensitivity reactions. Pain and inflammation at the site of injection may also occur.

hepatitis B surface antigen. See **Australia antigen.**

hepatitis B vaccine, a vaccine prepared from the blood plasma of asymptomatic human carriers of hepatitis B virus. A series of three doses is recommended to achieve immunity. The vaccine is advised particularly for people who are likely to have contact with blood or fluids of affected people, such as nurses, physicians, dentists, dental hygienists, and laboratory personnel.

hepatitis B vaccine (recombinant), a genetically engineered vaccine produced in yeast cells by recombinant deoxyribonucleic acid technology.

hepatitis B vaccine inactivated, a preparation of formalin-treated hepatitis B surface antigen isolated from plasma of human carriers of hepatitis B. It has been superseded by the recombinant form of the vaccine in the United States.

hepatitis C (HC), a type of hepatitis transmitted most commonly by blood transfusion or percutaneous inoculation, as when IV drug users share needles or when drug users share straws for nasal inhalation of cocaine. It is transmitted less commonly by sexual intercourse. The disease progresses to chronic hepatitis in up to 80% of the patients acutely infected, culminating in cirrhosis. Diagnosis is made through identification of antibodies of HCV or PCR. Treatment is alpha-interferon and ribavarin. Those infected with hepatitis C can remain asymptomatic for 10 to 20 years. Because hepatitis C carriers are vulnerable to severe hepatitis if they contract hepatitis A or B, vaccination against hepatitis A and B is recommended. Also called *parenterally transmitted non-A non-B hepatitis.*

hepatitis D (HD), a form of acute or chronic hepatitis, caused by the hepatitis delta virus, that occurs only in patients co-infected with hepatitis B. Hepatitis D virus (HDV) relies on hepatitis B virus (HBV) replication and cannot replicate independently. The disease usually develops into a chronic state. Diagnosis is made by detecting serum antibodies to HDV. It is transmitted sexually and through needle sharing. The only treatment is prevention of HBV. Also called **delta hepatitis.**

hepatitis E (HE), a self-limited type of hepatitis occurring primarily in Asia and Africa, acquired by ingestion of fecally contaminated water or food. Symptoms are similar to those of hepatitis A. Also called *enterically transmitted non-A non-B hepatitis.*

hepatitis F (HF), a hypothetical virus linked to hepatitis, possibly a mutation of the hepatitis B virus. The most recent finding was in 1994, when novel viral particles were discovered in the feces of posttransfusion patients without hepatitis A, B, C, or E. When injected into the bloodstream of rhesus monkeys, these particles caused hepatitis. When further investigations failed to confirm the existence of the virus, it was delisted as a cause of infectious hepatitis. Also called **Toga virus.**

hepatitis G (HG), a form of hepatitis, caused by the hepatitis G virus (HGV), that is transmitted by infected blood or blood products. It can also be transmitted by sharing personal items contaminated with the virus, by vertical transmission (mother to newborn), and by various sexual activities. Infection is of widespread occurrence and causes generally asymptomatic to mild disease. It is seen in patients after drug transfusions, in patients undergoing hemodialysis, and in IV drug abusers. It is also seen in infants born to infected mothers. The virus is not primarily replicated in the liver and may only be associated with hepatitis rather than the cause of infection.

hepatitis virus studies, a series of tests used to detect antigens and antibodies to hepatitis B surface antigen (HBsAg), hepatitis B surface antibody (HBsAb), hepatitis B core antibody (HBcAb), hepatitis B e-antigen (HBeAg), hepatitis B e-antibody (HBeAb), and hepatitis C antibodies (HCV IgG).

hepatization /hep′ətīzā″shən/ [Gk, *hepatizein,* like the liver], transformation of lung tissue into a solid mass resembling the liver, as in early pneumococcal pneumonia, in which consolidation and effusion of red blood cells in the alveoli produce red hepatization. In later stages of pneumococcal pneumonia, when white blood cells fill the alveoli, the consolidation becomes gray hepatization, or yellow hepatization, when infiltrated by fat deposits.

hepato-, hepat-, hepatico-, prefix meaning "liver": *hepatobiliary, hepatectomy, hepatocellular.*

hepatobiliary capsule. See **Glisson's capsule.**

hepatoblastoma /hep′ətō′blastō″mə/, a cancer of the liver that tends to occur in children. It is usually detected during examination for causes of failing health and for the presence of a mass in the upper abdomen. Hepatoblastoma may be associated with precocious puberty.

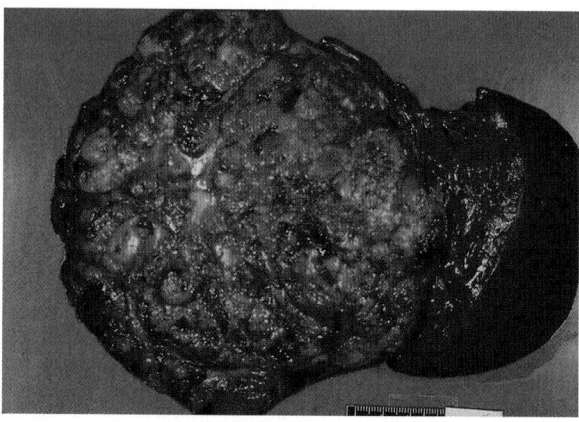

Hepatoblastoma *(Skarin, 2010)*

hepatocarcinogen /-kärsin″əjən/, an agent that causes carcinoma of the liver.

hepatocarcinoma. See **malignant hepatoma.**

hepatocele [Gk, *hēpar,* liver, *kele,* hernia], a hernia of a portion of the liver through the diaphragm or the abdominal wall.

hepatocellular carcinoma. See **malignant hepatoma.**

hepatocellular jaundice /-sel″yələr/, jaundice resulting from disease or injury to liver cells.

hepatocholangitis /hep′ətōkō′lanjī″tis/, an inflammation of both the liver and the bile ducts.

hepatocyte /hep″ətōsīt/ [Gk, *hēpar* + *kytos,* cell], a parenchymal liver cell that performs all the functions ascribed to the liver.

hepatocyte growth factor (HGF), a potent mitogen and inducer of hepatocyte proliferation, produced in the liver by cells other than hepatic cells and in many other organs by cells of the mesenchyme. It is also multifunctional and regulates cell growth and motility.

hepatoduodenal ligament /hep′ətōdoo̅o̅′ədē″nəl, -doo̅·od″inəl/ [Gk, *hēpar* + L, *duodeni,* twelve fingers], the portion of the lesser omentum between the liver and the duodenum, containing the hepatic artery, the common bile duct, the portal vein, the lymphatics, and the hepatic plexus of nerves. These structures are enclosed within a fibrous capsule between the two layers of the ligament. Compare **hepatogastric ligament.**

hepatoerythropoietic porphyria (HEP) /hep′ə·tō·ərith′rōpoi·et′ik/ [Gk, *hēpar,* liver + *erythros,* red + *poiein,* to make], a severe homozygous form of porphyria cutanea tarda (PCT) believed to result from an autosomal-recessive defect in the same enzyme activity as PCT. It is clinically identical to PCT, but onset is in early childhood, and activity of the affected enzyme in liver, erythrocytes, and fibroblasts is virtually absent.

hepatogastric ligament /hep′ətōgas″trik/ [Gk, *hēpar* + *gaster,* stomach], the portion of the lesser omentum between the liver and the stomach. Compare **hepatoduodenal ligament.**

hepatogenous jaundice /hep′ətoj″ənəs/ [Gk, *hēpar,* liver, *genein,* to produce; Fr, *jaune,* yellow], a type of jaundice caused by a condition of the liver.

hepatogram /hep″ətōgram′/, **1.** a sphygmographic tracing of the liver pulse. **2.** a radiographic image of the liver.

hepatography /hep′ətog″rəfē/, **1.** the recording of the liver pulse. **2.** the radiographic or isotope scintigraphic visualization of the liver.

hepatojugular /hep′ətōjug″yoo̅lər/ [Gk, *hēpar,* liver; L, *jugulum,* neck], pertaining to the liver and the jugular vein.

hepatojugular reflux [Gk, *hēpar* + L, *jugulum,* neck], an increase in jugular venous pressure when pressure is applied for 30 to 60 seconds over the abdomen, suggestive of right-sided heart failure.

hepatolenticular degeneration /həpat′ōlentik″yoo̅lər/ [Gk, *hēpar* + L, *lens,* lentil], an abnormal autosomal-recessive condition associated with defective copper metabolism in the body, characterized by decreased serum ceruloplasmin and copper levels and increased secretion of urinary copper. In individuals with this condition, tissue deposits of copper associated with hepatic cirrhosis, deep marginal pigmentation of the cornea (known as Kayser-Fleischer rings), and extensive degeneration of the central nervous system, especially the basal ganglions, develop. Also called **Wilson disease.** See also **Kayser-Fleischer ring.**

hepatolienal fibrosis. See **congestive splenomegalia.**

hepatolithiasis /-lithī″əsis/, the presence of stones in the liver.

hepatologist /hep′ətol″əjist/, a physician who specializes in diseases of the liver.

hepatology /hep′ətol″əjē/, the branch of medicine that is concerned primarily with diseases of the liver.

hepatoma /hep′ətō″mə/ *pl. hepatomas, hepatomata* [Gk, *hēpar* + *oma,* tumor], a primary malignant tumor of the liver, which is relatively rare in the United States, characterized by hepatomegaly, pain, hypoglycemia, weight loss, anorexia, and ascites, as well as elevated serum alpha-fetoprotein levels, portal hypertension, and jaundice in the plasma. It occurs most commonly in the sixth decade, and its incidence is higher in African-Americans than in Caucasians. It occurs most frequently in association with hepatitis or cirrhosis of the liver and in those parts of the world where the mycotoxin aflatoxin is found. It is treated with surgical resection when isolated to one lobe of the liver. The prognosis is poor. Chemotherapy and liver transplantation are used in some centers.

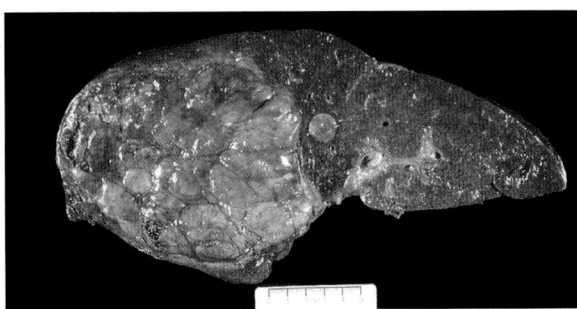

Subdural hepatoma *(Kumar, Abbas, and Fausto, 2005)*

hepatomegaly /hep′ətōmeg″əlē/ [Gk, *hēpar* + *megas,* large], abnormal enlargement of the liver that is usually a sign of disease, often discovered by percussion and palpation as part of a physical examination. In hepatomegaly the liver is easily palpable below the ribs in the right upper quadrant of the abdomen and may be tender to the touch. Hepatomegaly may be caused by hepatitis or other infection; fatty infiltration, as in alcoholism; biliary obstruction; or malignancy.

hepatonecrosis /-nekrō″sis/, **1.** the death of liver cells. **2.** gangrene of the liver.

hepatopancreatic ampulla /-pan′krē·at″ik/ [Gk, *hēpar* + *pan,* all, *kreas,* flesh], the dilation formed by the junction of the pancreatic and bile ducts as they open into the lumen of the duodenum. Also called **ampulla of the bile duct, ampulla of Vater, Vater's ampulla.**

hepatopulmonary syndrome, arterial hypoxemia caused by pulmonary vasodilation in conjunction with chronic liver disease, usually occurring as a result of portal hypertension in cirrhosis.

hepatorenal /hep′ətōrē″nəl/ [Gk, *hēpar,* liver; L, *ren,* kidney], pertaining to the liver and the kidneys.

hepatorenal syndrome, a type of kidney failure characterized by a gradual loss of function without signs of tissue damage. It is associated with hepatitis or cirrhosis of the liver; its exact cause is unknown.

hepatosplenomegaly /-splē′nōmeg″əlē/ [Gk, *hēpar,* liver, *splen* + *megas,* large], enlargement of the spleen and liver.

hepatotoxic /-tok″sik/, destructive to the liver.

hepatotoxicity /hep′ətōtoksis″itē/ [Gk, *hēpar* + *toxikon,* poison], the tendency of an agent, usually a drug or alcohol, to have a destructive effect on the liver.

hepatotropic /hep′ə-totrop′ik/, having a special affinity for or exerting a specific effect on the liver.

hepatotropic virus, a virus that primarily affects the liver, such as the hepatitis viruses.

Hepatovirus /hep′ə-tovi′rus/, a genus of picornaviruses. This genus includes viruses that cause hepatitis A, among other diseases.

hepatoxin /-tok″sin/, a poison that damages parenchymal cells of the liver.

hepta-, hept-, prefix meaning "seven": *heptaploid, heptavalent.*

heptachlor poisoning /hep′təklôr′/ [Gk, *hepar,* seven, *chloros,* green; L, *potio,* drink], a form of chlorinated organic insecticide poisoning.

heptaploid. See **polyploid.**

heptavalent /hep′tivā′lənt/, pertaining to a chemical that has a valence of 7. Also called **septivalent.**

herald patch. See **pityriasis rosea.**

herb /(h)urb/ [L, *herba,* grass], **1.** any plant that is used for culinary or medicinal purposes. **2.** a leafy plant without a wooden stem whose parts growing above the ground die back after the growing season.

herbalist /hur′bəlist/, **1.** a person who specializes in the study of herbs and their health benefits. **2.** a practitioner or individual who uses plants or parts of plants for therapeutic benefit. **3.** an individual who grows and harvests herbal plants for medicinal purposes.

herbal medicine, the use of medicinal products containing as active ingredients exclusively plant material and/or vegetable drug preparations used to treat various health conditions. Also called **phytotherapy.**

herb bath [L, *herba,* grass; AS, *baeth*], a medicinal bath taken in water that contains a mixture of aromatic herbs.

herbicide /er′-, her′bisīd/, an agent that is destructive to weeds or causes an alteration in their normal growth.

herbicide poisoning /her″bisīd/ [L, *herba,* grass, *caedere,* to kill], a poisoning caused by the ingestion, inhalation, or absorption of a substance intended for use as a weed killer or defoliant. Many of the commonly used agricultural herbicides can produce symptoms ranging from skin irritation to hypotension, liver and kidney damage, and coma or convulsions. Estimated fatal doses may be as small as 1 to 10 g. Some herbicides contain extremely toxic substances; poisoning is characterized by dysphagia, burning stomach pain, throat constriction, diarrhea, or other severe symptoms.

herbivore /hərbivōr/ [L, *herba,* grass, *vorare,* to devour], an animal that subsists mostly or entirely on plants. –*herbivorous, adj.*

herb tea, a medicinal beverage prepared by the infusion of a water-soluble extract of leaves, roots, bark, or other parts of an herb. The vegetable matter is commonly macerated and steeped in boiling water, which is strained and served hot. Cold water may be used for herbs containing readily soluble active principles.

herd immunity [ME, *heord,* group; L, *immunis,* free from], a form of immunity that occurs when prior illness or vaccination of a significant portion of a population provides a measure of protection for individuals who have not developed this immunity.

herd instinct [ME, *heord* + L, *instinctus,* impulse], the basic need of social animals, including humans, for the companionship of peers and a tendency to find compatibility with the behavioral standards of others in the group.

hereditability /hәred′itəbil″itē/ [L, *hereditas,* inheritance], the degree to which a specific trait is controlled by inheritance.

hereditary /hәred″iter′ē/ [L, *hereditas,* inheritance], transmitted from parent to offspring; inborn; inherited. Compare **acquired, congenital, familial.**

hereditary angioedema, an inherited autosomal-dominant disorder characterized by the episodic appearance of nonpitting edema involving any part of the body, including mucosal surfaces. The attacks last 48 to 72 hours and can be life-threatening if edema obstructs the airway.

hereditary ataxia, one of a group of inherited degenerative diseases of the spinal cord, cerebellum, and often other parts of the nervous system, characterized by tremor, spasm, muscle wasting, skeletal change, and sensory disturbances resulting in impaired motor activity. Kinds include **ataxia-telangiectasia syndrome, Friedreich's ataxia.**

hereditary brown enamel. See **amelogenesis imperfecta.**

hereditary coproporphyria. See **coproporphyria.**

hereditary deforming chondroplasia. See **diaphyseal aclasis.**

hereditary disorder. See **inherited disorder.**

hereditary elliptocytosis. See **elliptocytosis.**

hereditary enamel hypoplasia. See **amelogenesis imperfecta.**

hereditary essential tremor. See **essential tremor.**

hereditary fructose intolerance. See **fructose intolerance.**

hereditary hemochromatosis, an autosomal-recessive disorder of metabolism that involves the deposition of iron-containing pigments in the tissues. Iron accumulation is lifelong, with symptoms that include joint or abdominal pain, weakness, and fatigue appearing usually in the fifth or sixth decades of life. If untreated, the disorder may lead to bronzing of the skin, arthritis, diabetes, cirrhosis, or heart disease. It typically affects men more often than women. See also **hemochromatosis.**

hereditary hemorrhagic telangiectasia, a vascular anomaly, inherited as an autosomal-dominant trait, characterized by hemorrhagic telangiectasia of the skin and mucosa. Small red-to-violet lesions are found on the lips, oral and nasal mucosa, tongue, and tips of fingers and toes. The thin, dilated vessels may bleed spontaneously or as a result of only minor trauma, and this condition becomes progressively more severe. Bleeding from superficial lesions is often profuse and may result in severe anemia. No specific treatment is known, but accessible bleeding lesions may be treated with pressure, styptics, and topical hemostatics. Transfusions may be indicated for acute hemorrhage, and iron-deficiency anemia may require continuous treatment. Also called **hemorrhagic familial angiomatosis, Osler-Weber-Rendu syndrome, Rendu-Osler-Weber syndrome.**

hereditary hyperuricemia. See **Lesch-Nyhan syndrome.**

hereditary multiple exostoses, a rare familial dyschondroplastic disease in which bony protuberances form on the shafts of the long bones and eventually develop into caps of cartilage covering the ends of the bones. The affected joints lose their mobility, and the bones stop growing. The disease begins in childhood and has no cure. Very rarely a chondrosarcoma may develop from the cap of an exostosis. See also **Ollier dyschondroplasia.**

hereditary opalescent dentin. See **dentinogenesis imperfecta.**

hereditary oral disease, any abnormal condition characterized by genetic defects of structures in or around the mouth, such as deformed dentition, ankyloglossia, hereditary gingival fibromatosis, or cleft palate. Many hereditary oral diseases, including Crouzon's disease, sickle cell anemia, gargoylism, familial amyloidosis, and achondroplasia, are associated with generalized defects as well as oral and facial characteristics.

hereditary osteoonychodysplasia. See **nail-patella syndrome.**

hereditary protoporphyria. See **porphyria.**

hereditary renal adysplasia, an autosomal-dominant condition in which a kidney is severely dysplastic, nonfunctional, and often ectopic. If bilateral, as in the oligohydramnios sequence, the infant usually dies soon after birth.

hereditary spherocytosis. See **spherocytic anemia.**

hereditary tyrosinemia. See **tyrosinemia.**

heredity /hәred″itē/ [L, *hereditas,* inheritance], **1.** the process by which particular traits or conditions are genetically transmitted from parents to offspring, causing resemblance of individuals related by descent. It involves the separation and recombination of genes during meiosis and fertilization and the further interaction of developmental influences and genetic material during embryogenesis. **2.** the total genetic constitution of an individual; the sum of the qualities inherited from ancestors and the potentialities of transmitting these qualities to offspring.

Hering-Breuer reflex /her″ing broi″ər/ [Heinrich E. Hering, German physiologist, 1866–1948; Joseph Breuer, Austrian physician, 1842–1925], a neural mechanism that terminates inspiration and initiates expiration. The reflex is triggered by impulses that originate in stretch receptors of the bronchi and bronchioles in response to distension of the airway, increased intratracheal pressure, or pulmonary inflation. The impulses travel via afferent fibers of the vagus nerves to the medullary respiratory center. The Hering-Breuer reflex is well developed at birth and is hyperactive in conditions of restrictive ventilatory insufficiency.

Hering's nerve. See **glossopharyngeal nerve.**

Hermansky-Pudlak syndrome /hərmän′skē pood′läk/ [F. Hermansky, Czechoslovakian internist, 20th century; P. Pudlak, Czechoslovakian internist, 20th century], an autosomal-recessive form of albinism, with a predisposition to hemorrhage secondary to a platelet defect and accumulation of a ceroid-like substance in the reticuloendothelial system, oral mucosa, and urine.

hermaphroditism /hərmaf″rəditiz′əm/ [Gk, *Hermaphroditos,* son of Hermes and Aphrodite], a rare condition resulting from a chromosomal abnormality in which both testicular and ovarian tissue exist in the same person. The testicular tissue contains seminiferous tubules or spermatozoa, and the ovarian tissue contains follicles or corpora albicantia. Also called *hermaphrodism.* Compare **pseudohermaphroditism.** −*hermaphroditic, adj.*

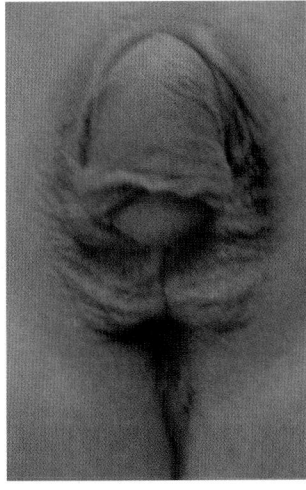

Hermaphroditism *(Podesta and Urcullo, 2008)*

hermetic /hərmet″ik/ [Gk], from use in alchemy, pertaining to sealing a container to make it airtight.

hernia /hur″nē-ə/ [L, rupture], protrusion or projection of an organ through an abnormal opening in the muscle wall of the cavity that surrounds it. A hernia may be congenital, may result from the failure of certain structures to close after birth, or may be acquired later in life as a result of obesity, muscular weakness, surgery, or illness. Kinds include **abdominal hernia, diaphragmatic hernia, femoral hernia, hiatal hernia, inguinal hernia, umbilical hernia.** See also **herniorrhaphy.**

hernial /hur″nē-əl/, pertaining to or resembling a hernia.

hernial ring, a ring through which a hernia protrudes, such as a dilated internal inguinal ring.

hernial sac [L, *hernia,* rupture; Gk, *sakkos,* sack], a pouch of peritoneum into which organs or other tissues pass to form a hernia.

herniated /hur″nē-ā′tid/, pertaining to a tear or abnormal bulge of an organ or organ part through a retaining tissue.

herniated disk, a rupture of the fibrocartilage surrounding an intervertebral disk, releasing the nucleus pulposus that cushions the vertebrae above and below. The resultant pressure on spinal nerve roots may cause considerable pain and damage the nerves, resulting in restriction of movement. The condition most frequently occurs in the lumbar region. Also called *herniated intervertebral disk, herniated nucleus pulposus,* **ruptured intervertebral disk, slipped disk.**

herniation /hur″nē-ā″shən/, a protrusion of a body organ or portion of an organ through an abnormal opening in a membrane, muscle, or other tissue. See also **hernia, hiatal hernia.**

herniography /hur′nē-og″rəfē/, the radiographic examination of a hernia after it has been injected with a contrast medium.

herniorrhaphy /hur′nē-ôr′əfē/, the surgical repair of a hernia.

herniotomy /hur′nē-ot″əmē/ [L, *hernia* + Gk, *temnein,* to cut], a surgical procedure to reduce a hernia.

heroin /her″ō·in/ [Ger, *heroine,* originally trademark for diacetylmorphine], a morphine-like drug with no currently acceptable medical use in the United States. Heroin is included in Schedule I of the Controlled Substances Act of 1970. Like other opium alkaloids, it can produce analgesia, respiratory depression, GI spasm, and physical dependence. It produces its major effects on the central nervous system and bowel and alters the endocrine and autonomic nervous systems. Heroin, which loses much of its analgesic power when taken orally, is more powerful than morphine and acts more rapidly. Repeated use of this drug produces tolerance

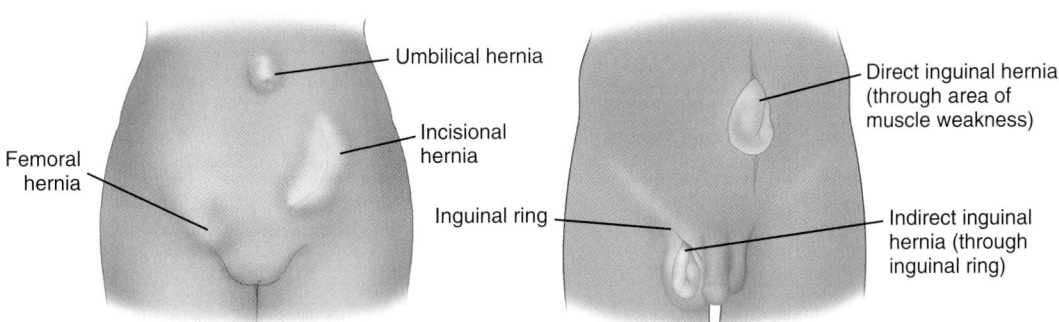

Common locations of hernias *(Leonard, 2012)*

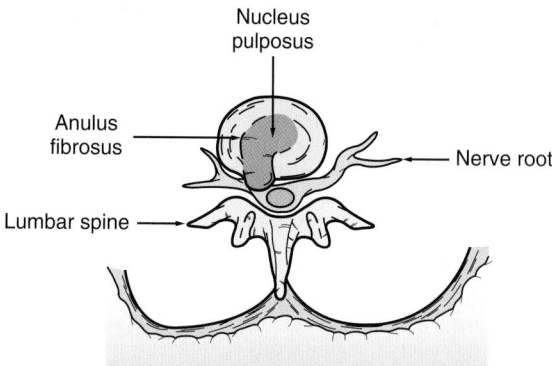

Herniated disk

to most of the acute opioid effects; physical dependence develops concurrently with tolerance. Withdrawal from heroin after relatively few exposures commonly produces acute abstinence syndrome. Withdrawal signs are usually observed shortly before the next planned dose and commonly include anxiety, restlessness, irritability, and craving for another dose. Other withdrawal signs that may appear 8 to 15 hours after the last dose include lacrimation, perspiration, yawning, and restless sleep. On awakening from such sleep the severely addicted heroin user may experience withdrawal signs, such as vomiting, pain in the bones, diarrhea, convulsions, and cardiovascular collapse. Withdrawal signs usually peak at between 36 and 48 hours and gradually subside during the following 10 days. Methadone is commonly used as a substitute drug in the treatment of heroin addiction (methadone maintenance therapy). Also called **diacetylmorphine.**

herpangina /hur′panjī″nə/ [Gk, *herpein,* to creep; L, *angina,* quinsy], a viral infection, usually of young children, characterized by sore throat, headache, anorexia, and pain in the abdomen, neck, and extremities. Febrile convulsions and vomiting may occur in infants. Papules or vesicles may form in the pharynx and on the tongue, the palate, or the tonsils. The lesions evolve into shallow ulcers that heal spontaneously. The disease usually runs its course in less than 1 week. Treatment is symptomatic. The cause is often infection by a strain of coxsackie virus, typically coxsackie virus A. If similar shallow, blister-like lesions appear on the soles of the feet or the palms of the hands, it is called hand-foot-and-mouth disease.

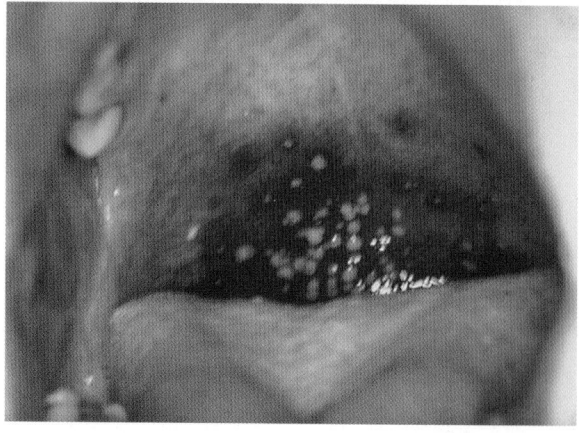

Herpangina *(Cohen, Opal, and Powderly, 2010)*

herpes genitalis /hur″pēz jen′ital″is/ [Gk, *herpein,* to creep; L, *genitalis,* genitalia], a chronic infection caused by type 2 herpes simplex virus (HSV2), usually transmitted by sexual contact. It causes painful vesicular eruptions on the skin and mucous membranes of the genitalia of males and females. When acquired during pregnancy, HSV2 may be transmitted through the placenta to the fetus and to the newborn by direct contact with infected tissue during birth. It can be a precursor of cervical cancer.

■ OBSERVATIONS: In the male, herpes genitalis infections may resemble penile ulcers. A small group of vesicular lesions surrounded by erythematous tissue may occur on the glans or prepuce. The lesions erupt into superficial ulcers that often heal in 5 to 7 days, although they also may become the sites of secondary infections. The lesions are painful and are often associated with a burning sensation, urinary dysfunction, fever, malaise, and swelling of the lymph nodes in the inguinal area. The female patient may exhibit the same or similar systemic effects, and members of both sexes may complain of painful sexual intercourse. In the female, herpes genitalis lesions are likely to appear as multiple superficial eruptions on the surfaces of the cervix, vagina, or perineum. There may be a discharge from the cervix. Vaginal lesions may appear as mucous patches with grayish ulcerations. Laboratory tests from smears of fluid taken from the base of lesions show a positive Tzanck reaction with multiple nucleated giant cells, which distinguishes HSV2 infections from other venereal diseases. Infection tends to recur.

■ INTERVENTIONS: Acyclovir taken orally results in partial control of the symptoms and signs of herpes episodes. The drug accelerates healing but does not eradicate the infection. The antiviral agents valacyclovir, penciclovir, and famciclovir may suppress reaction and also may lessen the severity and duration of the outbreak.

■ PATIENT CARE CONSIDERATIONS: The provider teaches patients with genital herpes about the potential for recurrent episodes of lesions and advises them to abstain from sexual activity while the lesions are present. Sexual transmission has been documented during phases when no lesions were present. Women of childbearing age with genital herpes should inform their health care provider if they become pregnant.

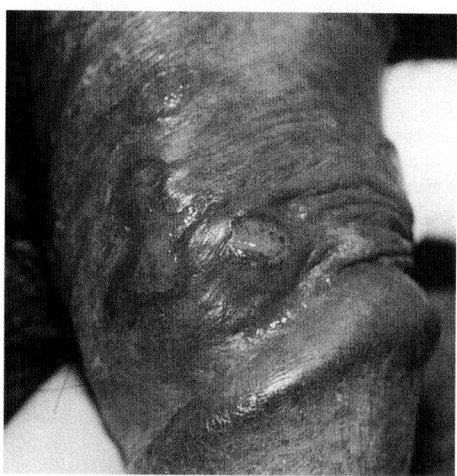

Herpes genitalis *(Morse et al, 2010)*

herpes gestationis [Gk, *herpein* + L, *gestare,* to bear], a generalized pruritic vesicular or bullous rash that appears in the second or third trimester of pregnancy and disappears several weeks after delivery. The lesions often recur with succeeding pregnancies and are associated with premature birth and increased fetal mortality rate. Herpes gestationis has no relation to herpesvirus infection.

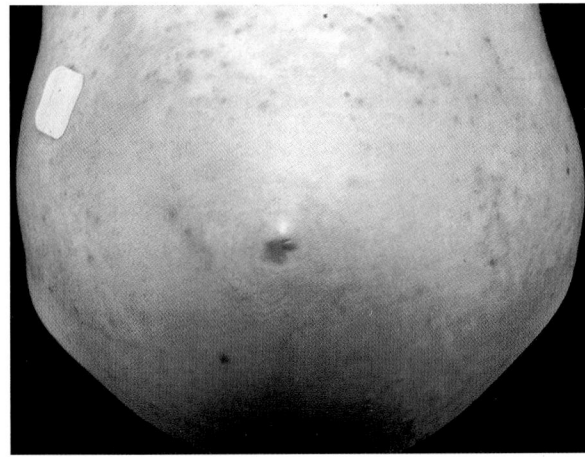

Herpes gestationis *(Black et al, 2008)*

herpes labialis.   See **herpes simplex.**

herpes menstrualis [Gk, *herpein,* to creep; L, *menstruare*],   a form of herpes simplex that tends to erupt during menstrual periods.

herpes simplex [Gk, *herpein* + L, *simplex,* uncomplicated],   an infection caused by a herpes simplex virus (HSV), which has an affinity for the skin and nervous system and usually produces small, transient, irritating, and sometimes painful fluid-filled blisters on the skin and mucous membranes. HSV1 (oral herpes, herpes labialis, cold sore) infections tend to occur in the facial area, particularly around the mouth and nose; HSV2 (herpes genitalis) infections are usually limited to the genital region.

■ OBSERVATIONS: The initial symptoms of an HSV1 infection usually include burning, tingling, or itching sensations about the edges of the lips or nose within 1 or 2 weeks after contact with an infected person. Several hours later, small red papules develop in the irritated area. Later, small vesicles, or fever blisters, filled with fluid erupt. Several small vesicles may merge to form a larger blister. The vesicles generally are associated with itching, pain, or similar discomfort. Other effects often include a mild fever and enlargement of the lymph nodes in the neck. Laboratory analysis of the vesicular fluid usually shows the presence of herpesvirus particles and the absence of pyogenic bacteria. Within 1 week after the onset of symptoms, thin yellow crusts form on the vesicles as healing begins. In skin areas that are moist or protected and in severe cases, healing may be delayed. HSV2 infections in adolescence are associated with an increased incidence of cervical cancer in adulthood.

■ INTERVENTIONS: Treatment of herpes simplex is symptomatic. The lesions may be washed gently with soap and water to reduce the risk of secondary infection. Topical penciclovir cream may speed healing. When secondary infections have begun, antibiotics are prescribed. Although there is no cure, treatment includes oral acyclovir or valacyclovir.

■ PATIENT CARE CONSIDERATIONS: Because herpesviruses are extremely contagious, the nurse follows all appropriate procedures in contacts with patients to avoid acquiring and transmitting the infection. Washing the hands and wearing disposable gloves when in contact with oral secretions or genitalia help prevent transmission of the virus. Once acquired, the virus tends to remain latent in the tissues of the nervous system and may be reactivated by a variety of stimuli, including a febrile illness, physical or emotional stress, exposure to sunlight, or ingestion of certain foods or drugs. Topical sunscreen preparations offer some protection against exposure to the sun, and patients are advised to avoid repeated exposure to stimuli to which they are sensitive. The complications of herpetic infections may include encephalitis, herpes simplex keratitis, and gingivostomatitis. In cases involving systemic complications, IV acyclovir, blood transfusions, IV solutions, and other therapy may be required. In uncomplicated cases the herpes attack is usually self-limiting and runs its course in 3 weeks or less.

herpes simplex encephalitis,   a necrotizing inflammation of the brain that follows an infection with herpes simplex virus. It is a common acute form of encephalitis and is similar to other viral encephalitis infections. Repeated seizures occur early in the course, and there is severe hemorrhagic necrosis. Affected areas of the brain are usually the orbital portions of the frontal lobes and the inferomedial portions of the temporal lobe. Persons of any age may be infected, but cerebral sequelae (caused by HSV2) are more likely to occur in infants. The mortality rate varies, but even desperately ill patients may recover completely.

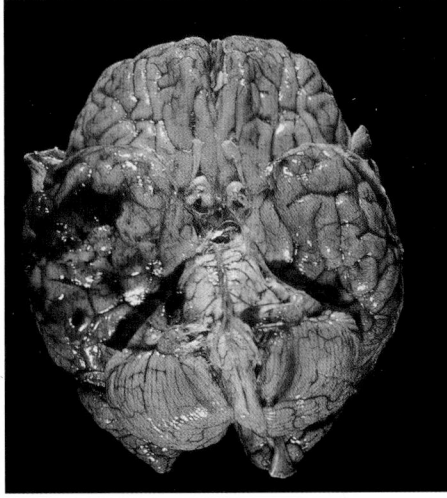

Herpes simplex encephalitis *(Goljan, 2013)*

herpes simplex keratitis.   See **ocular herpes.**

herpes simplex (HSV) test,   a blood test or microscopic culture done to detect types 1 and 2 of the herpes simplex virus. HSV1 is primarily responsible for the oral lesions known as "cold sores" whereas HSV2 is a sexually transmitted viral infection of the urogenital tract, although crossover of the two types can occur. Culture is the more accurate of the two types of tests.

herpesvirus /hur′pēzvī″rəs/   [Gk, *herpein* + L, *virus,* poison],   any of the viruses from the family Herpesviridae. At least eight species of herpesvirus are known to be infectious to humans: herpes simplex viruses 1 and 2, varicella zoster virus, Epstein-Barr virus, cytomegalovirus, human herpesvirus 6, and human herpesvirus 7. Human herpesvirus 8 causes Kaposi sarcoma.

herpesvirus hominis.   See **herpes simplex.**

herpesvirus simiae encephalomyelitis,   an infection of the central nervous system by a B form of herpes simplex virus that usually affects simians. Persons most likely to be infected by the monkey virus are veterinarians and animal laboratory workers. Some cases of simian B virus may be life threatening.

H

herpes zoster /zos'tər/ [Gk, *herpein* + *zoster,* girdle], an acute infection caused by reactivation of the latent varicella zoster virus, which mainly affects adults. The cause of reactivation is unknown, but it is linked to stress, aging, and immune impairment. It is characterized by the development of painful vesicular skin eruptions that follow the underlying route of cranial or spinal nerves inflamed by the virus. Prompt treatment with antivirals can speed healing and reduce the risk of postherpetic neuralgia. Also called **shingles.** See also **herpes simplex, varicella zoster virus.**

herpes zoster ophthalmicus, a form of herpes zoster in which the virus invades the gasserian ganglion, causing pain and skin eruptions along the ophthalmic branch of the fifth cranial nerve. There also may be involvement of the third cranial nerve. The infection frequently leads to corneal ulceration or other ocular complications. Also called **ophthalmic herpes zoster.**

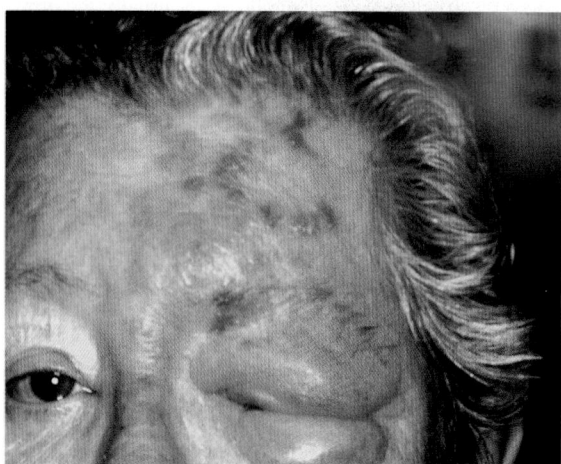

Herpes zoster ophthalmicus involving the fifth cranial nerve *(Yanoff and Duker, 2014)*

herpes zoster oticus, a herpes zoster infection of the eighth cervical (vestibulocochlear) nerve ganglia and geniculate ganglion, causing severe pain in the external ear structures and pain or paralysis along the facial nerve. The disease also may cause hearing loss and vertigo. The vertigo is usually transient, but the hearing loss and facial paralysis may be permanent. Vesicular eruptions may occur along the external ear canal and ear pinna. Treatment is generally symptomatic, with diazepam administered for vertigo, analgesics for pain, and corticosteroids for other symptoms. Acyclovir may be prescribed.

herpes zoster virus. See **chickenpox.**

herpetic encephalitis /hərpet'ik/ [Gk, *herpein,* to creep + *enkephalos,* brain + *itis,* inflammation], the most common form of acute encephalitis, caused by a herpesvirus and characterized by hemorrhagic necrosis of parts of the temporal and frontal lobes. Onset is over several days and involves fever, headache, seizures, stupor, and often coma, frequently with a fatal outcome.

herpetic gingivostomatitis, primary herpetic gingivostomatitis is the most common viral infection of the gum tissue due to herpes simplex type I virus (HSV-1), presenting with fragile vesicles that rapidly progress to painful ulcerations of the gingival tissue. Primary infection also presents with fever, lymphadenopathy, and fatigue. Herpes infections are transmitted by physical contact and typically arise in early childhood. Recurrent herpetic gingivostomatitis occurs in 15% to 45% of the infected population. Treatment includes antiviral medications initiated within the first 3 symptomatic days of lesion onset.

herpetic keratitis. See **dendritic keratitis.**

herpetic neuralgia /hərpet'ik/ [Gk, *herpein,* to creep, *neuron,* nerve, *algos,* pain], a form of neuralgia with intractable pain that develops at the site of a previous eruption of herpes zoster. It more frequently occurs in the elderly.

herpetic sore throat, a herpes inflammation that develops in the region of the pharynx.

herpetic stomatitis [Gk, *herpein,* to creep, *stoma,* mouth, *itis,* inflammation], a form of inflammation of the mouth caused by a herpesvirus infection, also characterized by ulcers.

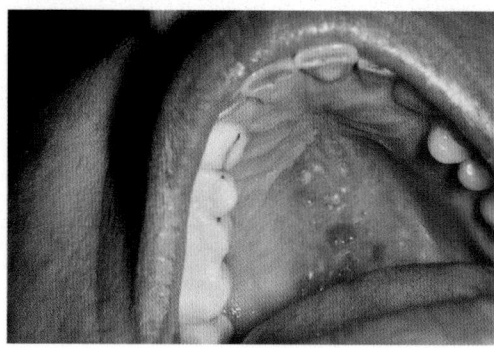

Herpetic stomatitis *(Swartz, 2009)*

herpetic whitlow, cutaneous herpes simplex on the terminal segment of a finger, resulting in formation of deep coalescing vesicles with tissue destruction.

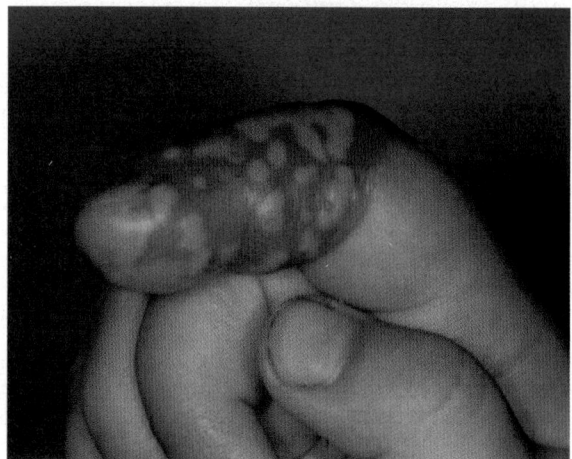

Infant's finger with herpetic whitlow *(Hoff and Gerber, 2012)*

herpetiform /hərpet'ifôrm'/ [Gk, *herpein* + L, *forma,* form], having clusters of vesicles that resemble the skin lesions of some herpesvirus infections.

Herplex, a topical antiviral drug. Brand name for **idoxuridine.**

Hers disease /herz, hurz/ [H.G. Hers, 20th-century Belgian physiologist; L, *dis,* opposite of; Fr, *aise,* ease], an uncommon metabolic disorder of glycogen storage involving a deficiency of glycogen phosphorylase. It is characterized by hepatomegaly and an accumulation of abnormally large amounts of glycogen in the liver as a result of its inability to break down glycogen. The condition is inherited as an autosomal-recessive trait. Genetic counseling may be of benefit. Other treatment is symptomatic and supportive. Also called

glycogen storage disease, type VI. See also **glycogen storage disease.**

hertz (Hz) /hurts, herts/ [Heinrich R. Hertz, German physicist, 1857–1894], a unit of measurement of wave frequency equal to 1 cycle per second.

HERV, abbreviation for **human endogenous retroviruses.**

Herxheimer reaction /herks″hī″mər/ [Karl Herxheimer, German dermatologist, 1861–1944], a reaction to endotoxin-like products released by the death of harmful microorganisms within the body during antimicrobial treatment. The reaction was originally discovered in penicillin treatment of syphilis, but it has been found to occur with other diseases as well.

Herzog taping protocol, a procedure for immobilizing and balancing a foot with tape after a musculoskeletal injury. The protocol consists of step-by-step instructions for applying tape, beginning with the lateral aspect of the head of the fifth metatarsal and continuing through the lateral plantar aspect of the foot.

Heschl's gyrus /hesh″əl/ [Richard L. Heschl, Austrian pathologist, 1824–1881; Gk, *gyros,* turn], any of several small gyri that run transversely on the upper surface of the temporal operculum of the insula of the cortex.

hesitation dysfluencies, the excessive use of *ahs, ums, uhs, OK,* or other fillers used by a speaker of the English language. See also **dysfluency.**

hesperidin /hesper″idin/, a crystalline flavone glycoside present in most citrus fruits, especially in the spongy casing of oranges and lemons.

Hesselbach hernia /hes″əlbaks, -bäkhs/ [Franz K. Hesselbach, German surgeon, 1759–1816], a protrusion of diverticula through the femoral sheath, usually associated with direct inguinal hernia.

Hesselbach's triangle. See **inguinal triangle.**

hetastarch /het″əstärch/, a plasma volume expander.

■ INDICATIONS: It is prescribed to treat hypovolemia in shock and is used in leukapheresis to help increase the yield of granulocytes.

■ CONTRAINDICATIONS: Severe bleeding, severe heart or kidney dysfunction with oliguria or anuria, or known hypersensitivity to this drug prohibits its use.

■ ADVERSE EFFECTS: Among the more serious adverse reactions are influenza-like symptoms, muscle pain, edema, and anaphylaxis.

heter-. See **hetero-, heter-.**

heterauxesis. See **allometric growth.**

hetero-, heter-, prefix meaning "another" or "different": *heteroblastic, heteroeroticism.*

heteroallele /het″ərō·əlēl″/ [Gk, *heteros,* different, *alleolon,* of one another], one of a pair of alleles at a specific locus on homologous chromosomes that differs from the other of the pair. *−heteroallelic, adj.*

heteroantibody /het″ərō·an″tibod′ē/, an antibody that recognizes an antigen from a species other than that of the antibody producer.

heteroantigen /he″tərō·an″təjən/, an antigen that originates in a different species and is foreign to the antibody producer.

heteroblastic /het″ərōblas″tik/ [Gk, *heteros + blastos,* germ], developing from different germ layers or kinds of tissue rather than from a single type. Compare **homoblastic.**

heterocellular /-sel″yələr/, pertaining to a structure formed by more than one kind of cell.

heterocephalus /-sef″ələs/ [Gk, *heteros + kephale,* head], a malformed fetus that has two heads of unequal size. *−heterocephalous, heterocephalic, adj.*

heterochromatin /-krō″mətin/ [Gk, *heteros,* different, *chroma,* color], the part of a chromosome that is inactive in gene expression but may function in controlling metabolic activities, transcription, and cell division. It stains most intensely during interphase and usually remains in a condensed state throughout the cell cycle. It consists of two types: constitutive heterochromatin, which is present in all cells and is characteristic of the Y chromosome, and facultative heterochromatin, which is present in the inactivated X chromosome of the mammalian female. Compare **euchromatin.** See also **chromatin.** *−heterochromatic, adj.*

heterochromatinization /-krō″mətīnəzā″shən/, the transformation of genetically active euchromatin into genetically inactive heterochromatin. It occurs during the inactivation of one of the X chromosomes in the mammalian female during the early stages of embryogenesis. See also **Lyon hypothesis.**

heterochromia iridis /het″ər·ōkrō″mē·ə ī′ridis/ [Gk, *heteros,* different, *chroma,* color, *iris,* rainbow], difference of color in the two irides or in different areas of the same iris.

heterochromosome /-krō″məsōm/, a sex chromosome. See also **heterotypic chromosomes.** *−heterochromosomal, adj.*

heterodidymus /het″ərōdid″iməs/ [Gk, *heteros + didymos,* twin], a conjoined twin fetus in which the parasitic elements consist of a head, neck, and thorax attached to the thoracic wall of the autosite. Also called **heterodymus.**

heteroduplex /-doo″pleks/ [Gk, *heteros* + L, *duoplicare,* to double], a DNA molecule in which the two strands are derived from different individuals, with the result that some base pairs may not be complementary.

heteroduplex mapping, a method for determining the location of insertions, deletions, and other heterogeneities in the two strands of a DNA molecule.

heterodymus. See **heterodidymus.**

heteroenzyme /het″ərō·en″zīm/, a functionally identical enzyme from a different species.

heteroeroticism /het″ərō·irot″isiz′əm/ [Gk, *heteros,* different, *eros,* love], sexual feeling or activity directed toward another individual. Also called **alloeroticism, alloerotism,** *heteroerotism.* Compare **autoeroticism.**

heterofermentation /-fur″məntā″shun/, fermentation that produces major products that are different.

heterogamete. See **anisogamete.**

heterogametic /-gamet′ik/, pertaining to the sex that produces gametes of different kinds in terms of their sex chromosomes. In human beings the male, who possesses X-bearing and Y-bearing sperm, is the heterogametic sex.

heterogamy /het″ərog″əmē/ [Gk, *heteros + gamos,* marriage], **1.** See **anisogamy. 2.** See **heterogenesis,** def. 1. *−heterogamous, adj.*

heterogeneic antigen, xenogeneic antigen.

heterogeneity /-jənē″itē/, **1.** a quality of being dissimilar in kind. **2.** a state of having different characteristics and qualities.

heterogeneous /het″əroj″ənəs/ [Gk, *heteros,* different, *genos,* kind], **1.** consisting of dissimilar elements or parts; unlike; incongruous. **2.** not having a uniform quality throughout. Compare **homogeneous.** *−heterogeneity, adj.*

heterogenesis /-jen″əsis/ [Gk, *heteros + genein,* to produce], *reproduction* that differs in successive generations, such as the alternation of sexual and asexual reproduction, so that offspring have characteristics different from those of the parents. In the asexual stage, it often involves one or more parthenogenetic or hermaphroditic generations, often with various hosts, as in the case of many trematode parasites. Also called **heterogamy,** *heterogeny, heterogony.* Compare **homogenesis.** See also **asexual reproduction, abiogenesis, metagenesis.** *−heterogenic, heterogenetic, adj.*

heterogenous /het′əroj″ənəs/ [Gk, *heteros* + *genos,* kind], **1.** having a nonuniform composition throughout. **2.** derived or developed from another source or from two different sources.

heterogenous vaccine [Gk, *heteros,* different, *genein,* to produce; L, *vaccinus,* cow], a vaccine made against the same species of pathogen from a source other than the patient's own tissues.

heterograft. See **xenograft.**

heteroinfection /-infek″shən/ [Gk, *heteros,* different; L, *inficere,* to stain], infection by a microorganism originating outside the body.

heterolactic acid fermentation /-lak″tik/, bacterial fermentation that produces a mixture of lactic acid and other products.

heterologous. See **xenogeneic.**

heterologous insemination. See **artificial insemination.**

heterologous tumor [Gk, *heteros* + *logos,* relation], a neoplasm consisting of tissue different from that of its site. Compare **homologous tumor, organoid neoplasm.**

heterologous twins. See **dizygotic twins.**

heterologous vaccine, a vaccine that confers protective immunity against a pathogen that shares cross-reacting antigens with the microorganisms in the vaccine.

heterometropia /-mətrō″pē-ə/ [Gk, *heteros,* different, *metron,* measure, *ops,* eye], a generally mild visual disorder in which one eye refracts differently from the other, causing slightly different images to be perceived by the right and left eyes.

heteronymous /het′əron″iməs/ [Gk, *heteros,* different, *onyma,* name], **1.** having different names; the opposite of synonymous. **2.** pertaining to an optical phenomenon in which two images are produced by one object.

heterophil /het″ərofil′/ [Gk, *heteros* + *philein,* to love], a granulocyte; in humans, called a neutrophil.

heterophil antibody, an antibody induced by an external antigen that can cross-react with self-antigens.

heterophil antibody test [Gk, *heteros* + *philein,* to love], a test for the presence of heterophil antibodies in the serum of patients suspected of having infectious mononucleosis, based on an agglutination reaction between heterophil antibodies in a person's serum and heterophil antigen, a normal component of sheep erythrocytes. This antibody eventually appears in the serum of more than 80% of the patients with mononucleosis caused by the Epstein-Barr virus; hence it is highly diagnostic of the disease. See also **Epstein-Barr virus.**

heterophilic leukocyte /-fil″ik/ [Gk, *heteros,* different, *philein,* to love, *leukos,* white, *kytos,* cell], a neutrophil of certain animal species that takes an acid stain.

Heterophyes /het″erofi′ēz/, a genus of minute trematodes found in the middle third of the small intestine of humans and certain other mammals. Various species are found in Egypt and Turkey, throughout Asia, and in Japan and the Philippines.

heteroplastic transplantation /-plas″tik/ [Gk, *heteros,* different, *plassein,* to mold; L, *transplantare*], the transfer of tissue from one animal to another of a different species. Compare **homoplastic transplantation.**

heteroploid /het″ərəploid′/ [Gk, *heteros* + *ploos,* times, *eidos,* form], **1.** *n.,* an individual, organism, strain, or cell that has a variation in the number of chromosomes characteristic of somatic cells of the species. The change may involve entire sets of chromosomes or single chromosomes. **2.** *adj.,* pertaining to such an individual, organism, strain, or cell. See also **aneuploid, euploid. –heteroploidy,** *n.*

heteroploidy /het″ərəploi′dē/, the state or condition of having an abnormal number of chromosomes, either more or less than that characteristic of the somatic cell of the species.

heteropolymer /-pol″imir/ [Gk, *heteros* + *polys,* many, *meros,* part], a compound formed from subunits that are not all the same, such as a protein composed of various amino acid subunits.

heterosexual /-sek″shəl/ [Gk, *heteros,* different; L, *sexus,* male or female], **1.** *n.,* a person whose sexual desire or preference is for people of the opposite sex. **2.** *adj.,* pertaining to sexual desire or preference for people of the opposite sex. See also **sexual orientation. –heterosexuality,** *n.*

heterosis /het′ərō″sis/ [Gk, *heteros* + *osis,* condition], the superiority of first-generation hybrid plants and animals with respect to one or more traits when compared with either of the parent strains or with corresponding inbred strains. Also called **hybrid vigor.**

heterotaxy syndrome, a variable set of complex congenital anomalies of the GI and cardiovascular systems that results from the transposition of the abdominal and thoracic viscera.

heterotopic ossification /-top″ik/ [Gk, *heteros* + *topos,* place], a nonmalignant overgrowth of bone, frequently occurring after a fracture, that is sometimes confused with certain bone tumors when visualized on x-ray images. Also called **exuberant callus, myositis ossificans.**

heterotopic pain, pain that is perceived in a part of the body that is not the source of the pain, such as pain originating in the gallbladder that may be felt in the right shoulder. The phenomenon seems to be caused by projection of sensory neurons from different parts of the body into the same regions of the central nervous system. Also called **referred pain.**

heterotopic pregnancy, a pregnancy that is both intrauterine and extrauterine.

heterotopic transplantation [Gk, *heteros,* different, *topos,* place; L, *transplantare*], the transfer of tissue from one part of a body of a donor to another area of the body of a recipient.

heterotransplant /-trans″plant/ [Gk, *heteros,* different; L, *transplantare*], the transfer of tissue from one animal to another of a different species.

heterotypic /het′ərōtip″ik/ [Gk, *heteros* + *typos,* pattern], pertaining to or characteristic of a type differing from the usual or the normal, specifically regarding the first meiotic division of germ cells in gametogenesis as distinguished from the second meiotic division or a mitotic division. Also called *heterotypical.* Compare **homeotypic.**

heterotypic chromosomes, any unmatched pair of chromosomes, specifically the sex chromosomes.

heterotypic mitosis, the division of bivalent chromosomes, as occurs in the first meiotic division of germ cells in gametogenesis; a reduction division. Compare **homeotypic mitosis.**

heterozygosis /het′ərōzīgō″sis/ [Gk, *heteros* + *zygotos,* yoked, joined], **1.** the formation of a zygote by the union of two gametes that have dissimilar pairs of alleles. **2.** the production of hybrids through crossbreeding. **–heterozygotic,** *adj.*

heterozygote /-zī″gōt/ [Gk, *heteros,* different, *zygotos,* yoked], an organism whose somatic cells have two different allelomorphic genes on the same locus of each pair of chromosomes. It can produce two different types of gametes.

heterozygote detection, the use of amniocentesis and other techniques to identify potential inherited X-linked recessive disorders, such as Hunter syndrome or Duchenne muscular dystrophy.

heterozygotic. See **heterozygosis.**

heterozygous /het′ərəzī″gəs/ [Gk, *heteros* + *zygotos,* yoked], having two different alleles at corresponding loci on homologous chromosomes. An individual who is heterozygous for a trait has inherited an allele for that trait from one parent and an alternative allele from the other parent. An individual who is heterozygous for a genetic disease caused by a dominant allele, such as Huntington disease, manifests the disorder. A person who is heterozygous for a hereditary disorder produced by a recessive allele, such as sickle cell anemia, is asymptomatic or exhibits reduced symptoms of the disease. The offspring of a heterozygous carrier of a genetic disorder have a 50% chance of inheriting the allele associated with the disorder if the other parent does not carry the allele. Compare **homozygous.**

heuristic /hyo͞oris″tik/ [Gk, *heuriskein,* to discover], **1.** serving to stimulate interest for further investigation. **2.** pertaining to a teaching method in which an individual is encouraged to learn through independent research and investigation.

HEV, initialism for *hepatitis E virus.*

hex-, hexa-, prefix meaning "six": *hexadactyly, hexose.*

hexachlorophene /hek′səklôr″əfēn/, a topical bacteriostatic cleansing agent. The skin should be rinsed thoroughly to prevent systemic absorption.

■ INDICATIONS: It is used as an antiseptic scrub and as a disinfectant to clean inanimate objects of gram-positive bacteria. It is not effective against gram-negative bacteria such as *Pseudomonas aeruginosa* or *Escherichia coli.*

■ CONTRAINDICATIONS: Known hypersensitivity to this drug prohibits its use. Systemic absorption can occur when it is used on burns, broken skin, mucous membranes, and infant skin, with hemotoxic effects. Hexachlorophene washing of disposable gloves prior to reusing them is not recommended; if reusing gloves is absolutely necessary, chlorhexidine 4% liquid soap or povidone-iodine 7.5% liquid soap are far superior choices.

■ ADVERSE EFFECTS: Among the more serious adverse effects are skin rash and neurological abnormalities.

hexacosanol. See **ceryl alcohol.**

hexadactyly /hek′sədak′təle/ [Gk, *hex,* six + *daktylos,* finger], the occurrence of six digits on the hand or foot.

hexadecanoic acid. See **palmitic acid (CH₃[CH₂]₁₄COOH).**

hexadecanol. See **cetyl alcohol.**

Hexadrol, brand name for **dexamethasone.**

hexamethylenamine. See **methenamine.**

hexamethylmelamine /-meth′ilmel″əmēn/. See **altretamine.**

hexanoic acid. See **caproic acid.**

hexaploid. See **polyploid.**

hexavalent /hek′sivā″lənt/, pertaining to a chemical with a valence of 6. Also called **sexivalent.**

hexenmilch. See **witch's milk.**

hexokinase /hek′səkī″nās/ [Gk, *hex,* six, *glykys,* sweet, *kinein,* to move, *ase,* enzyme], a transferase enzyme present in all tissue that catalyzes the transfer of a phosphate group from adenosine triphosphate to glucose 6-phosphate. It is also found in yeast.

hexosaminidase test, a blood test used to detect the presence of the enzyme hexosaminidase, which is present in Tay-Sachs disease and in Sandhoff disease, a variant of Tay-Sachs.

hexose /hek″sōs/ [Gk, *hex,* six, *glykys,* sweet], a monosaccharide that contains six carbon atoms in the molecule. Glucose, mannose, and fructose are the principal hexoses found in nature, as well as being the principal absorbable end products of carbohydrate digestion.

hexylcaine hydrochloride /hek″silkān/, a local anesthetic for use on intact mucous membranes of the respiratory, upper GI, and urinary tracts.

hexylresorcinol /hek′silrəsôr″sənol/, an antiseptic and anthelmintic.

Hf, symbol for the element **hafnium.**

HF, abbreviation for **hepatitis F.**

HFJV, abbreviation for **high-frequency jet ventilation.** See **high-frequency ventilation.**

HFO, abbreviation for **high-frequency oscillation.**

HFV, abbreviation for **high-frequency ventilation.**

Hg, symbol for the element **mercury.**

HG, abbreviation for **hepatitis G.**

Hgb, abbreviation for **hemoglobin.**

HgbF. See **fetal hemoglobin.**

HGE, abbreviation for **human granulocytic ehrlichiosis.** See **ehrlichiosis.**

HGF, **1.** initialism for *human growth factor.* **2.** abbreviation for **hyperglycemic-glycogenolytic factor.** See **glucagon.**

Home Health Care Classification system (HHCC), a computerized classification system for home health care that assessed and classified home health Medicare patients to predict their need for nursing and other home health care services and evaluate their outcomes of care. Now called **Clinical Care Classification.**

HI, abbreviation for **hemagglutination inhibition.**

hiatal hernia, protrusion of a portion of the stomach upward through the diaphragm. The condition occurs in about 40% of the population, and most people display few, if any, symptoms. The major difficulty in symptomatic patients is gastroesophageal reflux, the backflow of the acid contents of the stomach into the esophagus. Diagnosis is made easily on x-ray films and may be an incidental finding of a chest radiogram. Surgical treatment is usually unnecessary, and efforts should be directed to alleviating the discomfort associated with reflux. See also **diaphragmatic hernia, gastroesophageal reflux, heartburn.**

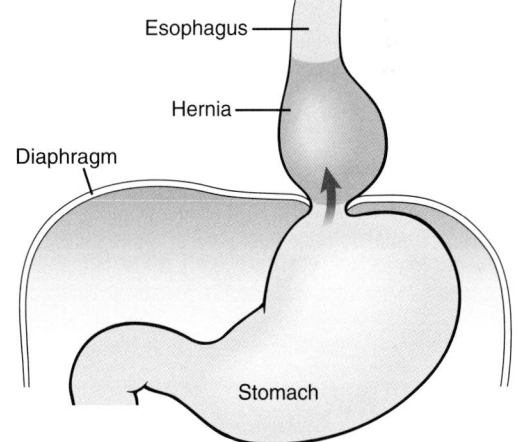

Hiatal (diaphragmatic) hernia *(Salvo, 2014)*

hiatus /hī·ā″təs/ [L, *hiare,* to stand open], a usually normal opening in a membrane or other body structure. –*hiatal, adj.*

hiatus esophagus [L, *hiare,* to stand open; Gk, *oisophagos,* gullet], the opening in the diaphragm for the esophagus.

hibakusha /hē′bäkoo″shä/ [Japanese], people who were exposed to the atomic bomb explosions in Hiroshima and Nagasaki, Japan.

Hib disease, an infection caused by *Haemophilus influenzae* type B (Hib), which mainly affects children in the first 5 years of life. It is a leading cause of bacterial meningitis, as well as childhood bacterial pneumonia, joint or bone infections, and throat inflammations. More than two thirds of the U.S. cases of Hib disease have been attributed to exposure in day-care centers. It is fatal in about 5% of infections. The infection can generally be prevented with a vaccine, given in infancy, usually at 2, 4, and 6 months of age and at 12 to 15 months of age.

hibernation /hī″bərnā″shun/ [L, *hibernare,* to winter], a natural physiological state or process wherein a generalized slowdown in metabolic and body functions produces a somnolescent condition and in which body temperature is maintained at a lower level than normal. It is a survival mechanism used by some species of birds and mammals to cope with periods of low temperature and reduced food supply.

hibernoma /hī″bərnō″mə/ *pl.* hibernomas, hibernomata [L, *hibernus,* winter; Gk, *oma,* tumor], a benign tumor, usually on the hips or the back, composed of fat cells that are partly or entirely of fetal origin. Also called **fat cell lipoma, fetal lipoma.**

Hibiclens®, a topical antibiotic and cleanser for the skin and mucous membranes.

hiccup /hik″əp/, a characteristic sound that is produced by the involuntary contraction of the diaphragm, followed by rapid closure of the glottis. Hiccups have various causes, including indigestion, rapid eating, certain types of surgery, and epidemic encephalitis. They can also be caused by or associated with abdominal distension. Most episodes of hiccups do not persist longer than a few minutes, but recurrent and prolonged attacks sometimes occur. The condition is most often seen in men. Sedatives are used in extreme cases.

Hickman catheter /hik′mən/ [R.O. Hickman, 20th-century American surgeon], a type of central venous catheter used for the long-term administration of substances via the venous system, such as antibiotics, total parenteral nutrition, or chemotherapeutic agents. It can be used for continuous or intermittent administration and may have either a single or a double lumen.

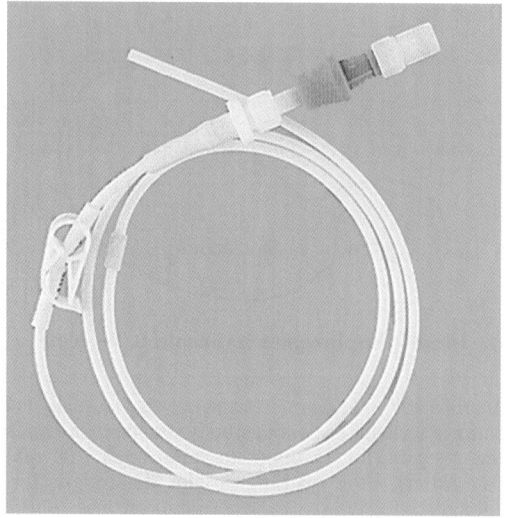

Hickman catheter *(Tighe, 2012)*

hickory stick fracture. See **greenstick fracture.**

HICPAC, abbreviation for **Hospital Infection Control Practices Advisory Committee.**

hidradenitis. See **hydradenitis.**

hidradenitis suppurativa /hī′dradənī′tis sup′yoorətē′və/ [Gk, *hydos,* water + *aden,* gland + *itis,* inflammation; L, *suppurare,* to form pus], a chronic disease of the apocrine gland–bearing areas, chiefly the axillae (especially in young women) and anogenital region (especially in men), caused by occlusion of the pores with secondary bacterial infection of apocrine sweat glands. It is characterized by the development of one or more tender red abscesses that enlarge and eventually break through the skin, yielding purulent or seropurulent drainage. Healing occurs with fibrosis, and recurrences lead to sinus tract formation and progressive scarring.

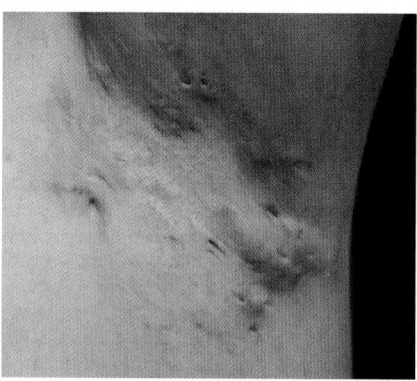

Hidradenitis suppurativa in the axilla
(Roberson et al, 2015)

hidro-, prefix meaning "sweat" or "sweat gland": *hidrosis.*

hidrosis /hidrō″sis, hī-/ [Gk, *hidros,* sweat], sweat production and secretion. Also spelled **hydrosis.** Compare **anhidrosis, hyperhidrosis.** *−hidrotic, adj.*

hieralgia /hī′əral″jə/ [Gk, *hieron,* sacrum, *algos,* pain], a painful sacrum.

hiero-, hier-, prefix meaning "sacrum" or "something sacred": *hieralgia, hierarchy.*

high. See **rush.**

high-altitude pulmonary edema [ME, *heigh,* high + L, *altitudo* + Gk, *oidema,* swelling], a form of pulmonary edema that occurs in people who move rapidly to higher altitudes. Fluid accumulates in the lungs as atmospheric pressure decreases.

high blood pressure (HBP). See **hypertension.**

high-calorie diet, a diet that provides 1000 or more calories a day beyond what is ordinarily recommended. It may be prescribed for nursing mothers, patients with severe weight loss caused by illness, or people with abnormally high metabolic rates or energy requirements, such as certain athletes or outdoor workers.

high-copy number, a large number of repetitive copies of a gene, such as may be produced by cloning.

high-definition imaging (HDI), an ultrasound technique used in breast cancer diagnosis to determine without biopsy whether a lump is a solid tumor or a relatively harmless fluid-filled cyst. HDI also provides a clear picture of lumps, revealing such details as irregular colors and edges.

high-density lipoprotein (HDL) [ME, *heigh,* high; L, *densus,* thick; Gk, *lipos,* fat, *proteios,* first rank], a plasma protein made mainly in the liver and containing about 50% lipoprotein (apoprotein) along with cholesterol, triglycerides, and phospholipid. It is involved in transporting cholesterol and other lipids to the liver to be disposed. Higher levels of high-density lipoprotein are associated with decreased cardiac risk profiles. See also **low-density lipoprotein, very low–density lipoprotein.**

high-dose tolerance, the absence of an expected immunological response after repeated injections of large amounts of an antigen.

high enema [ME, *heigh* + Gk, *einienai,* to send in], an enema that is inserted into the colon through a long catheter with the goal of cleansing the entire bowel.

high-energy phosphate compound, a chemical compound containing an easily hydrolyzed phosphoric anhydride group. The hydrolysis of this group liberates considerable energy, and coupling of this reaction to an endothermic reaction provides the energy necessary for the endothermic reaction to proceed. Adenosine triphosphate is the most powerful and ubiquitous of the high-energy phosphate compounds found in the body. All of these compounds liberate energy to fuel muscle contraction, active transport across cell membranes, and synthesis of many substances in the body.

highest intercostal vein [ME, *heigh* + L, *inter,* between, *costa,* rib, *vena,* vein], one of a pair of veins that drain the blood from the upper two or three intercostal spaces. The right vein descends and opens into the azygous vein. The left vein crosses the arch of the aorta and opens into the left brachiocephalic vein, usually receiving the left bronchial vein.

high-flow oxygen delivery system, a respiratory care apparatus that supplies inspired gases at a consistent preset oxygen concentration. It is generally not affected by changes in the ventilatory pattern. Also called **fixed-performance oxygen delivery system.**

high forceps, an obstetric procedure in which forceps are used to deliver a baby whose head is not engaged in the birth canal. It is no longer considered acceptable or meeting the standard of care. Compare **low forceps, mid forceps.** See also **forceps delivery, obstetric forceps.**

high-Fowler position [ME, *heigh,* high; George R. Fowler, American surgeon, 1848–1906], placement of the patient in a semisitting position by raising the head and trunk 90 degrees. The knees may or may not be flexed.

high-frequency hearing loss [ME, *heigh* + L, *frequens*; AS, *deaf*], a loss of ability to hear high-frequency sounds. It is most commonly associated with aging or noise exposure. Examples of high-frequency sounds are a whistle, the chirping of a bird, and the "s" sound in *sun.* Hearing loss may begin in early adulthood with a loss of hearing to frequencies in the range of 18 to 20 kHz. At about 60 years of age, loss of hearing may begin to affect lower frequencies, in the range of 4 to 8 kHz, thus interfering with the ability to understand speech. Hearing loss caused by noise exposure is often greatest at or near 4 kHz.

high-frequency jet ventilation, a type of high-frequency ventilation characterized by delivery of gas through a small catheter in the endotracheal tube.

high-frequency oscillation, **1.** a type of high-frequency ventilation characterized by the use of active expiration. **2.** the use of an inflatable vest connected to an air-pulse generator that causes rapid inflation and deflation, creating pressure on the chest similar to clapping. The resultant vibrations loosen secretions from the chest wall. Compare **clapping and vibrating.**

high-frequency percussive ventilation, a type of high-frequency ventilation characterized by delivery of pressure-limited breaths in short bursts of gas from a Venturi mask.

high-frequency positive pressure ventilation, a type of high-frequency ventilation characterized by low compressible volume circuit and tidal volume delivery of 3 to 4 mL/kg.

high-frequency ventilation (HFV), a technique for providing ventilatory support to patients at a rate of at least 60 breaths per minute with small tidal volumes. It may be used during intraoperative procedures such as laryngoscopy or bronchoscopy, as well as for ventilation in patients with a bronchopleural fistula or advanced respiratory distress syndrome, or in respiratory distress of the neonate. Kinds of HFV include high-frequency jet ventilation (HFJV) and high-frequency oscillation (HFO). HFJV uses a high-pressure gas source that can produce short, rapid jets of gas through a small-bore cannula into the airway above the carina at a rate of 100 to 400 per minute. HFO forces small impulses of gas into and out of the airway at a rate of 400 to 4000 per minute. See also **high-frequency jet ventilation, high-frequency oscillation.**

high-fructose corn syrup, a sweetener made by processing corn syrup to increase the level of fructose, usually to between 42% and 55% of the total sugar, with the balance being glucose. It is used extensively as a sweetener in processed foods and soft drinks, particularly soda and baked goods, but it is included also in many foods not normally thought of as sweet foods. See also **fructose.**

high labial arch, (in dentistry) a labial arch wire adapted to lie gingivally to the anterior tooth crowns with auxiliary springs that extend downward in contact with the teeth to be moved.

highland moccasin. See **copperhead.**

high-level wellness, a concept of optimal health that emphasizes the integration of body, mind, and environment to maximize the function of an individual.

high lithotomy, a suprapubic approach for surgical removal of urinary bladder stones that are not easily removed by ultrasonic crushing. Also called **suprapubic lithotomy.**

highly active antiretroviral therapy (HAART), the aggressive use of extremely potent antiretroviral agents in the treatment of human immunodeficiency virus infection.

high-molecular-weight kininogen, a high-molecular-weight plasma protein that plays a role in the coagulation process.

high-potassium diet, a diet that contains foods rich in potassium, including all leafy green vegetables, brussels sprouts, citrus fruits, bananas, dates, raisins, legumes, meats, and whole grains. It is indicated for any condition that causes loss of extracellular fluid such as acute diarrhea, congenital renal alkalosis, aldosteronism, hypokalemia, hypertension, and diabetic coma. It is also indicated for individuals who are receiving some diuretics, such as thiazide and furosemide, or corticosteroid therapy.

high-pressure liquid chromatography, a method of chromatography for separating and quantitating mixtures of substances in a solution. The procedure uses a high-resolution column, pressure, and gradient elution systems for separation of solutes by absorption, partition, ion exchange, and size exclusion. Also called *high-performance liquid chromatography.*

high-protein diet, a diet that contains large amounts of protein, consisting largely of meats, fish, milk, legumes, and nuts. It may be indicated in protein depletion that results from any cause, as a preoperative preparation, or for patients with severe burns and sepsis. It is sometimes used for short-term weight loss. High-protein diets may be contraindicated in liver failure or when kidney function is so impaired that added protein could result in azotemia and acidosis.

high-residue diet /-rez″idyo͞o/ [ME, *heigh* + L, *residuum,* remaining; Gk, *diaita,* way of living], a diet that contains a greater than usual proportion of substances that the digestive tract will not metabolize and absorb, such as soluble and insoluble dietary fiber.

high-resolution, the quality and accuracy of detail presented by a graphics system display, such as on a computer monitor screen or a computer printout. Generally, resolution quality increases as the number of pixels, or image-forming units in the display, increases.

high-risk infant, any neonate, regardless of birth weight, size, or gestational age, who has a greater than average chance of morbidity or mortality, especially within the first 28 days of life. Risk factors include preconceptual, prenatal, natal, or postnatal conditions or circumstances that interfere with the normal birth process or impede adjustment to extrauterine growth and development. See also **neonatal period, premature infant.**

high-speed handpiece, a handheld dental cutting instrument that rotates at up to 450,000 rpm. Modern high-speed handpieces are powered by miniature turbines driven by compressed air or an electric motor.

high-vitamin diet, a dietary regimen that includes a variety of foods containing therapeutic amounts of all of the vitamins necessary for the metabolic processes of the body. It is often ordered in combination with other therapeutic diets that contain larger than usual amounts of protein or calories, especially in the treatment of severe or chronic infection, malnutrition, or vitamin deficiency.

hila. See **hilum.**

hilar /hī'lär/ [L, *hilum,* a trifle], pertaining to a hilum.

Hilgenreiner line, a line connecting the superior aspect of the triradiate cartilages of the acetabula, used in radiographic assessment of the hip joint.

Hill-Burton Act, a 1946 amendment to the U.S. Public Health Service Act authorizing grants to states for surveying their hospital and public health center needs and for planning and constructing additional facilities. Subsequent amendments authorized federal funding for as much as two thirds of the cost of construction projects and broadened the scope of the legislation to include diagnostic and treatment centers, long-term treatment centers, and nursing homes and to aid in modernization of existing hospitals. Also called **Hospital Survey and Construction Act.**

Hill-Burton programs, a cluster of programs created by U.S. legislation included in the National Health Planning and Resources Development Act of 1974. The programs allow federal monetary assistance for modernization of health facilities, construction of outpatient health centers, construction of inpatient facilities in underserved areas, and conversion of existing health care facilities for the provision of new health services.

hilum /hī'ləm/ *pl.* **hila** [L, *hilum,* a trifle], a depression or recess at that part of an organ where vessels and nerves enter and leave.

hilum of the lung, an area of the lung where the mediastinal pleura is continuous with the visceral pleura.

hindbrain /hīnd'brān/ [ME, *hind* + AS, *bragen*], the division in the brain of an embryo that eventually becomes the pons, the medulla oblongata, and the cerebellum.

hindgut /hīnd'gut/ [ME, *hind* + AS, *guttas*], the caudal portion of the embryonic alimentary canal. It is formed by the development of the tail fold and eventually gives rise to part of the small and large intestines, rectum, bladder, and urogenital ducts. Compare **foregut, midgut.** See also **cloaca.**

hind kidney. See **metanephros.**

hinge axis, a line that passes through the left and right mandibular condyles and coincides with the center of rotation of the mandible. Determining the hinge axis is essential in constructing dental prostheses and correcting occlusal interferences.

hinge axis-orbital plane, a reference plane for the diagnosis of various types of malocclusions and for the development of associated prostheses. It is usually determined by marking three points on a patient's face. Two of the points, one on each side of the face, are located on the hinge axis. The third point is located on the face at the level of the orbital rim just beneath the eye.

hinge bow. See **kinematic face-bow.**

hinged knee, an appliance designed to protect and support the knee during activity. It consists of an elastic sleeve with medial and lateral steel or aluminum bars hinged at the axis of the knee joint. The hinged bars are stabilized with leather or self-adhesive (Velcro) straps.

hinged knee brace, an orthotic device. See **hinged knee.**

hinge joint [ME, *henge,* hinge; ME, *jointe,* a connection], a synovial joint providing a connection in which articular surfaces are closely molded together in a manner that permits extensive motion in one plane. The distal bone of a hinge joint seldom moves in the same plane as that of the axis of the proximal bone. The interphalangeal joints are hinge joints. Also called **ginglymus joint.** Compare **gliding joint, pivot joint.**

hip. See **coxa.**

HIPAA, abbreviation for **Health Insurance Portability and Accountability Act.**

hip bath. See **sitz bath.**

hipbone. See **innominate bone.**

hip joint. See **coxal articulation.**

hip-joint disease [AS, *hype* + L, *jungere,* to join; Gk, *dis,* not; Fr, *aise,* ease], any abnormal condition of the hip joint, such as Legg-Calvé-Perthes disease or congenital dislocation of the hip.

Hip Knee Ankle Foot Orthosis (HKAFO), a device to provide stability to the hips and lower extremity. It is used in the treatment of muscular imbalance and/or weakness, paralysis, cerebral palsy, muscular dystrophy, and multiple sclerosis. It reduces unwanted motion and energy expenditure.

hippocampal /hip'ōkam''pəl/ [Gk, *hippokampos,* seahorse], pertaining to the hippocampus.

hippocampal commissure [Gk, *hippokampos,* seahorse; L, *commissura,* a joint], a thin triangular sheet of transverse fibers that connects the medial edges of the posterior pillars of the fornix in the brain.

hippocampal fissure, a fissure reaching from the posterior aspect of the corpus callosum to the tip of the temporal lobe.

hippocampal formation [Gk, *hippokampos,* seahorse; L, *formatio*], a part of the rhinencephalon, including the dentate gyrus, longitudinal striae, and hippocampus.

hippocampal gyrus [Gk, *hippokampos,* seahorse, *gyros,* turn], a convolution on the medial side of the temporal lobe of the cerebral cortex.

hippocampus /hip'ōkam''pəs/ *pl.* **hippocampi** [Gk, *hippokampos,* seahorse], a curved convoluted elevation of the floor of the inferior horn of the lateral ventricle of the brain. It is composed of gray substance covered by a layer of white fibers, the alveus, and functions as an important component of the limbic system and of memory processing. Its efferent projections form the fornix of the cerebrum. Also called **Ammon's horn,** *hippocampus major.*

hippocampus minor. See **calcar avis.**

Hippocrates /hipok''rətēz/, a Greek physician born about 460 BC on the island of Cos, a center for the worship of Aesculapius. Called the "Father of Medicine," Hippocrates introduced a scientific approach to healing by seeking physical causes of disease rather than magic or mythic relationships used by members of the Aesculapian cults of the time. He also compiled case records of illnesses, including results of treatments administered, and developed the art of ethical bedside care. See also **Hippocratic oath.**

Hippocrates bandage. See **capeline bandage.**

hippocratic facies, a drawn, pinched, and pale appearance of the face, indicative of approaching death.

Hippocratic oath /hip′əkrat″ik/, an oath, attributed to Hippocrates, that serves as an ethical guide for the medical profession. It may be incorporated into the graduation ceremonies of medical colleges and reads as follows: I swear by Apollo the physician, by Æsculapius, Hygeia, and Panacea, and I take to witness all the gods, and all the goddesses, to keep according to my ability and my judgment the following Oath: To consider dear to me as my parents him who taught me this art; to live in common with him and if necessary to share my goods with him; to look upon his children as my own brothers, to teach them this art if they so desire without fee or written promise; to impart to my sons and the sons of the master who taught me and the disciples who have enrolled themselves and have agreed to the rules of the profession, but to these alone, the precepts and the instruction. I will prescribe regimen for the good of my patients according to my ability and my judgment and never do harm to anyone. To please no one will I prescribe a deadly drug, nor give advice which may cause his death. Nor will I give a woman a pessary to procure abortion. But I will preserve the purity of my life and my art. I will not cut for stone, even for patients in whom the disease is manifest; I will leave this operation to be performed by practitioners (specialists in this art). In every house where I come I will enter only for the good of my patients, keeping myself far from all intentional ill-doing and all seduction, and especially from the pleasures of love with women or with men, be they free or slaves. All that may come to my knowledge in the exercise of my profession or outside of my profession or in daily commerce with men, which ought not to be spread abroad, I will keep secret and will never reveal. If I keep this oath faithfully, may I enjoy my life and practice my art, respected by all men and in all times; but if I swerve from it or violate it, may the reverse be my lot. See also **Hippocrates.**

hippuric acid [Gk, *hippos,* horse, *ouron,* urine; L, *acidus,* sour], a detoxication product in the urine of some animals; used as a medication in the treatment of arthritic diseases.

hip replacement [AS, *hype*], substitution of an artificial ball and socket joint for the hip joint. Hip replacement is performed to relieve a chronically painful and stiff hip in advanced osteoarthritis, an improperly healed fracture, degenerative joint disease, or rheumatoid arthritis. Antibiotic therapy is begun before surgery, and the patient is taught to walk with crutches or a walker. During surgery the femoral head, neck, and part of the shaft are removed, and the contours of the socket are smoothed. A prosthesis of a durable, hard metal alloy or stainless steel is attached to the femur. A metal or a plastic acetabulum is implanted. The affected leg is kept abducted and in straight alignment with pillows; external rotation of the leg must be prevented. The nurse observes nerve function and circulation in the leg frequently during the first postoperative day. The most frequent complications are infection requiring removal of the new joint and dislocation. Ambulation begins gradually, with frequent short walks. Sitting for more than 1 hour is to be prevented, and hip flexion beyond 60 degrees may cause dislocation of the prosthesis. The patient continues an exercise program after discharge to maintain functional motion of the hip joint and to strengthen the abductor muscles. Weight-bearing may be modified according to the type of prosthesis implanted.

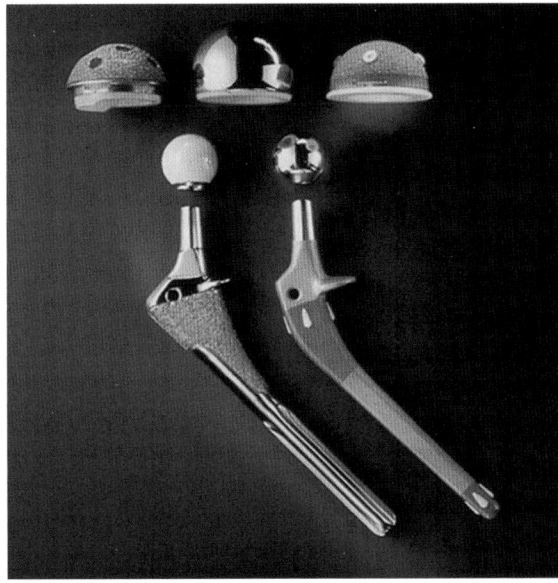

Hip replacements *(Courtesy Zimmer, Inc.)*

Hiprex, a urinary antibacterial drug. Brand name for **methenamine.**

Hirschberg test /hursh″bərgz/, a screening test for strabismus.

Hirschfeld method [Isador Hirschfeld, American dentist, 1881–1965], a tooth-brushing technique in which the bristles are vigorously rotated in very small circles against the gingivae and the axial surfaces of the teeth at a slight incisal or occlusal angle.

Hirschsprung disease /hirsh″sprŏŏng/ [Harald Hirschsprung, Danish physician, 1830–1916], the congenital absence of autonomic ganglia in the smooth muscle wall of the distal part of the colon, which causes poor or absent peristalsis in the involved segment of colon, accumulation of feces, and dilation of the bowel (megacolon). Symptoms include intermittent vomiting, diarrhea, and constipation. The abdomen may become distended to several times its normal size. The condition is usually diagnosed in infancy, but it may not be recognized until much later in childhood, when anorexia, lack of urge to defecate, distension of the abdomen, and poor health occur. Diagnosis is confirmed by barium enema; biopsy of the affected tissue shows the absence of ganglia. Surgical repair in early childhood is usually successful. A temporary colostomy is performed, and the aganglionic portion of the bowel is resected. The colostomy is almost always reversed a few months later. Also called **aganglionic megacolon, congenital megacolon.**

■ OBSERVATIONS: Manifestation patterns vary according to the length of the affected bowel. Neonates may be asymptomatic during the first few months of life. In a complete obstruction, signs include delayed passage of meconium, obstipation, massive abdominal distension, refusal to feed, and bilious vomiting. In a partial obstruction there are cycles of constipation and diarrhea with thin ribbon-like stools, intermittent vomiting, abdominal distension, and possible failure to thrive. If the condition goes undiagnosed until childhood, there are signs of anorexia, abdominal distension, lack of urge to defecate, and general poor health. Diagnosis is made through observation of clinical signs of obstruction and barium enema results that reveal narrowing of the colon distal to obstruction and enlargement of the colon proximal

H

to the obstruction. Diagnosis is confirmed by a rectal suction biopsy that reveals no evidence of ganglion cells. Enterocolitis or toxic megacolon is the most serious complication and is marked by sudden onset of fever, abdominal distension, and explosive bloody diarrhea. Enterocolitis causes death in about 20% of the cases.

■ INTERVENTIONS: The treatment is relief of the obstruction by one of several procedures, including a Soave endorectal pull through, a Duhamel procedure to create a neorectum, a Swenson procedure to resect the aganglionic segment, a laparoscopic pull-through procedure, or a transanal endorectal coloanal anastomosis. A myectomy may be performed if only the anal segment is involved. A myectomy/myotomy may be indicated if the entire intestine is involved. A temporary ostomy is created to relieve obstruction and to promote healing after surgery. Antiinfectives are used to treat or prevent infection. Analgesics are used to control pain, and antiemetics are used for nausea and vomiting.

■ PATIENT CARE CONSIDERATIONS: Acute care focuses on routine preoperative and postoperative care, including saline enemas to prep the bowel for surgery, comfort measures, IV hydration, I and O, abdominal measurements, support and reassurance to child and family, colostomy care, and wound care. Instruction is needed for care and cleaning of the colostomy, and a home health care referral will help establish continuity of such care. Caregivers should be educated to expect continuing soiling incidents after surgery. Genetic counseling is needed for the parents.

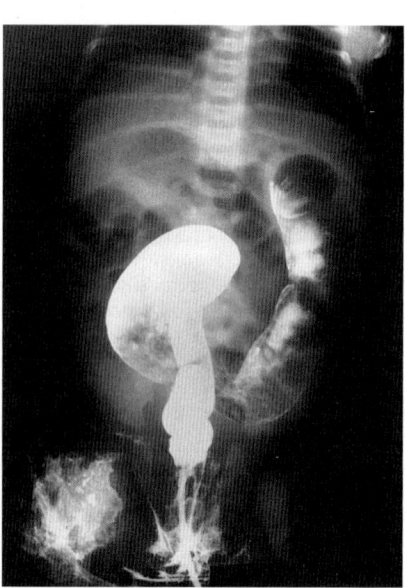

Hirschsprung disease: barium enema
(Courtesy American College of Radiology)

hirsutism /hur″sōōtiz′əm/ [L, *hirsutus,* hairy], excessive body hair in a masculine distribution pattern as a result of heredity, hormonal dysfunction, porphyria, or medication. Treatment of the specific cause usually stops growth of more hair. Excess hair may be removed by laser, electrolysis, chemical depilation, shaving, or waxing. Fine facial hair may be most effectively minimized by bleaching. Topical eflornithine (Vaniqa) can slow hair growth, as can oral medications. Compare **hypertrichosis.** *–hirsute, adj.,* *–hirsuteness, n.*

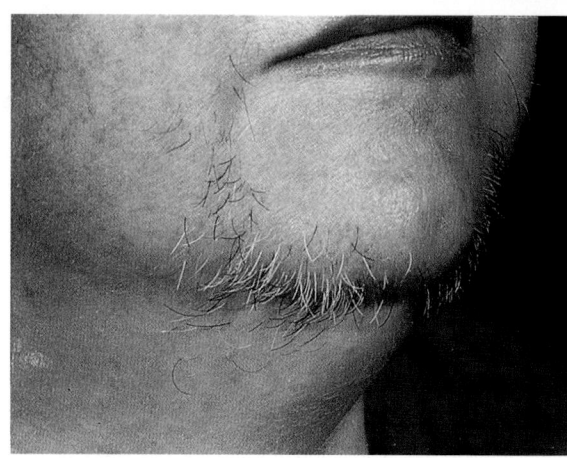

Hirsutism in a woman as a result of hormonal dysfunction *(Ferri, 2009)*

hirsutoid papilloma of the penis /hur″sōōtoid/ [L, *hirsutus,* shaggy; Gk, *eidos,* form], a condition characterized by clusters of small white papules on the coronal edge of the glans penis. Also called **papillomatosis coronae penis, pearly penile papules.**

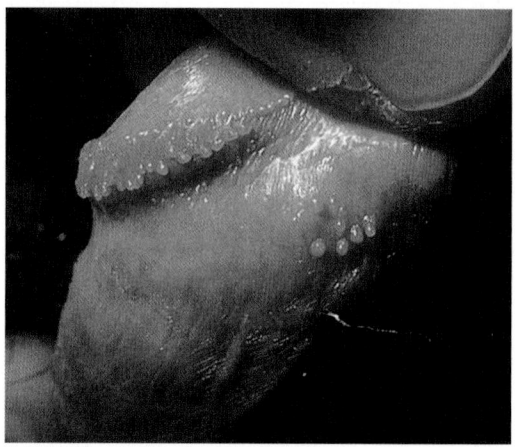

Hirsutoid papilloma of the penis *(Morse, Holmes, and Ballard, 2003)*

His, abbreviation for **histidine.**

His bundle. See **bundle of His.**

His bundle electrogram (HBE) [Wilhelm His, Jr., German physician, 1863–1934], a direct recording of the electrical activity in the atrioventricular bundle (bundle of His). It is no longer routinely performed.

His-Purkinje system /his′pərkin″jē/ [Wilhelm His, Jr.; Johannes E. Purkinje, Czechoslovakian physiologist, 1787–1869], the conduction system in the heart from the atrioventricular bundle (bundle of His) to the distal Purkinje fibers.

hist-. See **histo-, hist-.**

histaminase /histam″inās/, a soft tissue enzyme found in various body tissues. It catalyzes the decarboxylation of histamine and converts histamine into inactive imidazolacetic acid. Also called **diamine oxidase.**

histamine /his″təmēn, -min/ [Gk, *histos,* tissue; L, *amine,* ammonia], a compound, found in all cells, that is produced by the breakdown of histidine. It is released in allergic inflammatory reactions. Cellular receptors of hista-mine include the H$_1$ receptors, which are responsible for the dilation of blood vessels and the contraction of smooth mus-cle; the H$_2$ receptors, which are responsible for the stimulation of heart rate and gastric secretion; and H$_3$ receptors, which are believed to play a role in regulation of the release of histamine and other neurotransmitters from neurons. H$_1$ and H$_2$ receptors also mediate the contraction of vascular smooth muscle.

histamine-blocking agent, a substance that interferes with the stimulation of cells by histamine, which is a substance produced by nearby cells to cause, among other things, inflammation and acid release in the stomach.

histamine headache, a headache associated with the release of histamine from the body tissues and marked by symptoms of dilated carotid arteries, fluid accumulation under the eyes, tearing or lacrimation, and rhinorrhea (runny nose). Symptoms include sudden sharp pain on one side of the head, involving the facial area from the neck to the temple. Treatment includes the use of preparations of antihistamines and ergot that help constrict the arteries. Also called **cluster headache, Horton histamine cephalalgia.** See also **cephalalgia.**

histenzyme /histen″zīm/, a renal tissue enzyme that splits hippuric acid into glycine and benzoic acid.

histidine (His or H) /his″tidēn/ [Gk, *histos,* tissue], a basic amino acid found in many proteins and a precursor of histamine. It is an essential amino acid in infants. See also **amino acid, protein.**

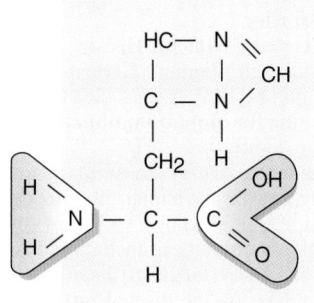

Chemical structure of histidine

histidinemia /his″tidinē″mē·ə/, an inherited metabolic disor-der caused by an enzyme defect involving L-histidine ammo-nia lyase and affecting the amino acid histidine. The condition leads to cognitive impairment and nervous system disorders. It is controlled by diet that limits the intake of histidine.

histio- [word element, Gk, web], a combining form mean-ing *tissue.*

histioblast /his″tē-/, a tissue-forming cell.

histiocyte, a tissue macrophage or dendritic cell that plays a role in the body's immune system. See **macrophage.**

histiocytic leukemia. See **monocytic leukemia.**

histiocytic malignant lymphoma /his″tē-ōsit″ik/ [Gk, *his-tos* + *kytos,* cell], a lymphoid neoplasm containing undif-ferentiated primitive cells or differentiated reticulum cells. Also called **reticulum cell sarcoma.**

histiocytic necrotizing lymphadenitis. See **Kikuchi lymphadenitis.**

histiocytosis X /his″tē-ōsītō″sis/, a cluster of conditions encompassing benign eosinophilic granuloma and several malignant lymphomatous diseases. Also called **eosino-philic granuloma,** *pulmonary histiocytosis X, pulmonary Langerhans cell histiocytosis.*

histiotypic growth /his″tē-ōtip″ik/ [Gk, *histos* + *typos,* mark], the uncontrolled proliferation of cells, as occurs in tissue cultures, bacterial cultures, and molds. Compare **organotypic growth.**

histo-, hist-, prefix meaning "tissue": *histocompatability, histolysis, histoplasmosis.*

histocompatibility /his″tōkəmpat′ibil″itē/ [Gk, *histos,* tis-sue; L, *compatibilis,* agreeing], the biological elements that determine acceptance or rejection of a transplanted tis-sue from one individual to another; in particular, the alleles that code for major histocompatibility complex (MHC) proteins.

histocompatibility antigen [Gk, *histos* + L, *compatibi-lis,* agreeable], cell surface antigens encoded by a large gene family that are usually referred to as minor and major histocompatibility complex. They are the cause of most graft rejections that occur in organ transplantation between two genetically different individuals. See also **isoantigen.**

histocompatibility gene [Gk, *histos,* tissue; L, *compati-bilis* + *genein,* to produce], the HLA complex gene that determines an antigen that governs histocompatibility of the donor and recipient of transplanted tissue. See also **human leukocyte antigen.**

histogram /his″təgram′/ [Gk, *histos* + *gramma,* record], (in research) a graph showing the values of one or more variables plotted against time or against frequency of occurrence. A graph of a patient's temperature, pulse, and respiration is an example of a histogram.

histography /histog″rəfē/ [Gk, *histos* + *graphein,* to record], the process of describing or creating visualizations of tissues and cells. –*histographic, adj.,* –*histographically, adv.,* –*histographer, n.*

histoincompatible /his″tō·in′kəmpat″əbəl/, pertaining to host and donor tissues that have different genotypes and are therefore likely to induce an immune response, leading to rejection of a tissue graft or organ transplant.

histological [Gk, *histos,* tissue, *logos,* science], pertaining to the study of the microscopic anatomical and physiological characteristics of tissues and the cells found therein. See also **histology.**

histological technician, an allied health professional who prepares tissue specimens of human and animal origin for a pathologist to examine for diagnostic, research, or teach-ing purposes. Histological technicians process sections of body tissue by fixation, dehydration, embedding, sectioning, decalcification, microincineration, mounting, and routine and special staining. The minimum educational requirement is an associate's degree. Also called **histotechnician.** See also **histotechnologist.**

histologist /histol″əjist/, a medical scientist who specializes in the study of the structure of organ tissues, including the composition of cells and their organization into various body tissues. See also **histology.**

histology /histol″əjē/ [Gk, *histos* + *logos,* science], **1.** the science dealing with the microscopic identification of cells and tissue. **2.** the structure of organ tissues, including the composition of cells and their organization into various body tissues. –**histological,** *histologic, adj.*

histolysis [Gk, *histos,* tissue, *lysis,* loosening], breakdown or dissolution of living organic tissue. –**histolytic,** *adj.*

histolytic /his″tōlit″ik/, pertaining to or causing the break-down or dissolution of living organic tissue. See also **histolysis.**

histone /his″tōn/ [Gk, *histos,* tissue], any of a group of strongly basic, low-molecular-weight proteins that are sol-uble in water and insoluble in dilute ammonia and combine with DNA to form nucleoproteins. They are found in the nucleus of eukaryotic cells, where they form a complex with

DNA in the chromatin and function in regulating gene activity. See also **nucleosome**.

histopathology /his'tōpəthol'əjē/ [Gk, *histos,* tissue, *pathos,* disease, *logos,* science], the study of diseases involving the tissue cells.

Histoplasma capsulatum [Gk, *histos* + *plasma* + L, *capsula,* little box], a dimorphic fungal organism that is a single budding yeast at body temperature and a mold at room temperature. It is the causative organism in histoplasmosis, common in the Mississippi River Valley. The fungus, spread by airborne spores from soil contaminated with excreta from birds or infected bats, acts as a parasite on the cells of the reticuloendothelial system. See also **histoplasmosis.**

histoplasmin test /-plaz″min/, a skin test for diagnosis of an infection caused by *Histoplasma capsulatum* fungus.

histoplasmosis /his'tōplazmō″sis/ [Gk, *histos* + *plasma* + *osis,* condition], an infection caused by inhalation of spores of the fungus *Histoplasma capsulatum.* Most cases are asymptomatic. Individuals who experience symptoms are usually either immunocompromised or have been exposed to a high inoculum. Primary histoplasmosis is characterized by fever, malaise, cough, and lymphadenopathy. Spontaneous recovery is usual; small calcifications remain in the lungs and affected lymph glands. Progressive histoplasmosis, the sometimes fatal disseminated form of the infection, is characterized by ulcerating sores in the mouth and nose; enlargement of the spleen, liver, and lymph nodes; and severe and extensive infiltration of the lungs. The severe form is treated with amphotericin B, and less severe cases may be treated with ketoconazole. Infection confers immunity. A histoplasmin skin test may be performed to identify people who may safely work with contaminated soil. The disease is most common in the Mississippi and Ohio River Valleys. Also called **Darling disease.**

history /his″tərē/ [L, *historia,* inquiry], **1.** a record of past events. **2.** a systematic account of the medical, emotional, and psychosocial occurrences in a patient's life and of factors in the family, ancestors, and environment that may have a bearing on the patient's condition.

history of present illness, an account obtained during the interview with the patient of the onset, duration, and character of the present illness, as well as of any acts or factors that aggravate or ameliorate the symptoms. The patient is asked what he or she considers to be the cause of the symptoms and whether a similar condition has occurred in the past. See also **health history.**

histotechnician. See **histological technician.**

histotechnologist, an allied health professional who prepares tissue specimens of human and animal origin for a pathologist to examine for diagnostic, research, or teaching purposes. Histotechnologists perform all functions of the histological technician as well as identifying tissue structures, cell components, and their staining characteristics and relating them to physiological functions; implementing and testing new techniques and procedures; making judgments concerning the results of quality control measures; instituting proper procedures to maintain accuracy; and sometimes supervising and teaching. A 4-year baccalaureate degree program is usually required. See also **histological technician.**

histotoxin /-tok″sin/ [Gk, *histos* + *toxikon,* poison], any substance that is poisonous to body tissues. Histotoxins are usually generated within the body rather than being introduced externally. An example is the tissue-destroying enzymes formed by bacteria such as *Clostridium perfringens.*

histotroph, histotrophe, histotrophic nutrition. See **embryotroph.**

histrionic /his'trē·on″ik/ [L, *histrio,* actor], pertaining to exaggerated facial expressions, speech, or body movements, such as used on the stage.

histrionic paralysis [L, *histrio,* actor; Gk, *paralyein*], *(Obsolete)* now called **conversion disorder.**

histrionic personality [L, *histrio,* actor, *persona,* role played], a personality characterized by behavioral patterns and attitudes that are overreactive, emotionally unstable, overly dramatic, and self-centered, exhibited as a means of attracting attention, either consciously or unconsciously. Also called **hysteric personality.** See also **histrionic personality disorder.**

histrionic personality disorder, a disorder characterized by dramatic, reactive, and intensely exaggerated behavior, which is typically self-centered. It results in severe disturbance in interpersonal relationships that can lead to psychosomatic disorders, depression, alcoholism, and drug dependency. Symptoms include emotional excitability, such as irrational angry outbursts or tantrums; abnormal craving for activity and excitement; overreaction to minor events; manipulative threats and gestures; egocentricity; inconsiderateness; inconsistency; and continuous demand for reassurance generated by feelings of helplessness and dependency. A person with this disorder is perceived by others as vain, demanding, superficial, self-centered, and self-indulgent. The disorder is more prevalent in women than in men and is treated by various psychotherapies, depending on the individual and the severity of the condition. See also **narcissistic personality disorder.**

His-Werner disease [Wilhelm His, Jr., German physician, 1863–1934; Heinrich Werner, German physician, 1874–1947; Gk, *dis,* not; Fr, *aise,* ease]. See **trench fever.**

HIV, abbreviation for **human immunodeficiency virus.**

HIV-associated dementia (HAD), a usually rapidly progressive dementia that is the primary manifestation of encephalopathy caused by human immunodeficiency virus type I infection. It is marked by a variety of cognitive, motor, and behavioral abnormalities, including loss of retentive memory, inattentiveness, language disorders, apathy, incoordination, and ataxia. As the disease progresses, paraplegia, urinary and bowel incontinence, abulia, and mutism may occur. Survival after the onset of dementia is usually 3 to 6 months but is occasionally longer.

HIV-associated fever of unknown origin, a fever of at least 38.3° C occurring on several occasions over a period of 4 weeks of outpatient care or 3 days of hospitalization in a patient with human immunodeficiency virus infection, for which a cause cannot be determined after 3 days of investigation, including 2 days of incubation of cultures.

HIV-associated nephropathy, renal pathology in patients infected with the human immunodeficiency virus, similar to focal glomerular sclerosis, with proteinuria, enlarged kidneys, and dilated tubules containing proteinaceous casts. It may progress to end-stage renal disease within weeks. Formerly called **AIDS nephropathy.**

HIV-associated retinopathy, a usually asymptomatic microangiopathy affecting the retina, seen in human immunodeficiency virus infection. It is manifested by transient cotton-wool exudate and occasionally by hemorrhages, microaneurysms, and other lesions of the microvasculature. Also called **AIDS-associated retinopathy.**

hives, skin eruptions. See **urticaria.**

Hivid, an antiretroviral nucleoside analog. Brand name for **zalcitabine.**

HIV protease inhibitor /prō'tē·ās inhib'itər/ [*protein* + *-ase,* enzyme suffix; L, *inhibere,* to restrain], any of a group of antiretroviral drugs active against the human immunodeficiency virus that prevent protease-mediated cleavage of viral polyproteins, causing production of immature viral particles that are noninfective. Kinds include *indinavir sulfate, nelfinavir mesylate,* **ritonavir, saquinavir.** See also **protease inhibitor.**

H⁺,K⁺-ATPase /ā·tē·pē′ās/, a membrane-bound enzyme occurring on the secretory surfaces of parietal cells that uses the energy derived from the hydrolysis of ATP to drive the exchange of ions across the cell membrane, secreting acid into the gastric lumen. Protons and chloride ions are pumped against gradients across the apical membranes of activated parietal cells into the gastric lumen in exchange for potassium ions. See also **adenosine triphosphatase.**

HLA, abbreviation for **human leukocyte antigen.**

HLA-A, abbreviation for *human leukocyte antigen A.* See **human leukocyte antigen.**

HLA-B, abbreviation for *human leukocyte antigen B.* See **human leukocyte antigen.**

HLA complex, antigens formed from genes on chromosome 6. HLA genes code for proteins that enable the immune system to differentiate tissues or proteins between "self" and "nonself." These loci are identified by numbers and letters, such as HLA-B27. Antigens are divided into three classes. Class I antigens (HLA-A, -B, and -C) occur on the surface of all nucleated cells and platelets and are important in tissue transplantation. If donor and recipient HLA antigens do not match, the nonself antigens are recognized and destroyed by killer T cells. Class II antigens occur only on immunocompetent cells and normally recognize foreign proteins. Class III antigens are nonhistocompatibility antigens, such as some complement components, that map in the HLA complex. Also called **major histocompatibility complex,** *histocompatibility complex.*

HLA-D, abbreviation for *human leukocyte antigen D.* See **human leukocyte antigen.**

HLH, initialism for *human luteinizing hormone.*

HLHS, abbreviation for **hypoplastic left heart syndrome.**

HMD, abbreviation for **hyaline membrane disease.** See **respiratory distress syndrome of the newborn.**

HME, abbreviation for **human monocytic ehrlichiosis.** See **ehrlichiosis.**

HMG-CoA reductase, a rate-controlling enzyme of cholesterol synthesis. Activity of the enzyme may be as much as 60 times higher than normal in patients with low-density lipoprotein receptor disorder.

HMG-CoA reductase inhibitor, any of a group of drugs that competitively inhibit the enzyme catalyzing the rate-limiting step in cholesterol biosynthesis and that are used to lower plasma lipoprotein levels in the treatment of hyperlipoproteinemia. Also called **statin.**

HMO, abbreviation for **health maintenance organization.**

HMS Liquifilm, an ophthalmic preparation containing a glucocorticoid. Brand name for **medrysone.**

Ho, symbol for the element **holmium.**

H₂O, chemical formula for **water.**

hoarseness /hôrs′nəs/, an unnatural condition marked by a deep or rough, harsh, grating voice, indicating an inflammation of the throat and larynx.

hod-, combining form meaning "pathway": *method.*

Hodgkin disease, Hodgkin lymphoma /hoj′kinz/ [Thomas Hodgkin, English physician, 1798–1866], a malignant disorder characterized by painless, progressive enlargement of lymphoid tissue, usually first evident in cervical lymph nodes; other early signs may include splenomegaly and the presence of Reed-Sternberg cells, large binucleate CD20 (B cell marker)-positive lymphoid/histiocytic cells. Symptoms include anorexia, weight loss, generalized pruritus, low-grade fever, night sweats, anemia, and leukocytosis. The disease is diagnosed in about 7100 Americans annually and causes approximately 1700 deaths a year. It affects twice as many males as females, and it most often occurs in individuals who are 25 to 30 years of age or older than 50 years of age. The diagnosis is established by biopsy. The patient undergoes staging to determine the extent of the disease, including computed tomography of the chest and abdomen, complete blood count, biopsy of distant lymph nodes, liver function studies, and bilateral bone marrow biopsies. Radiotherapy, using a covering mantle to protect other organs, is the treatment of choice for early stages of the disease; combination chemotherapy is the treatment for advanced disease. Long-term remissions are achieved in more than half of the patients treated, and 60% to 90% of those with localized disease may be cured. There is a threefold increased risk of development of Hodgkin disease in first-degree relatives, suggesting an unknown genetic mechanism.

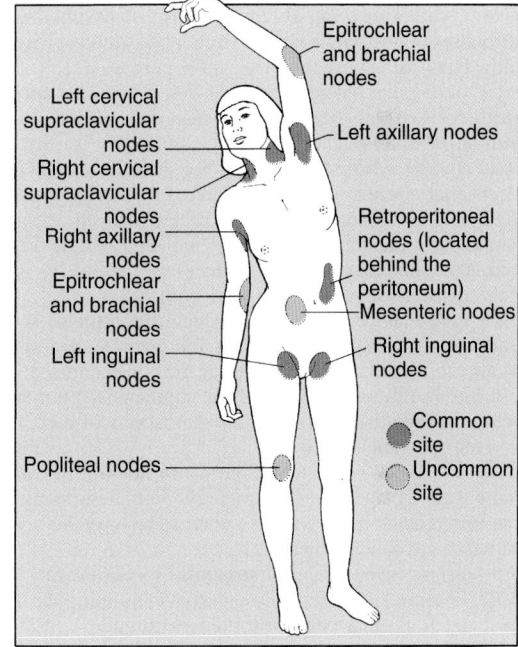

Lymph node sites for Hodgkin disease
(Huether and McCance, 2012)

Hodgson's disease /hoj′sənz/ [Joseph Hodgson, English physician, 1788–1869; Gk, *dis,* not; Fr, *aise,* ease], an aneurysmal dilation of the aorta.

Hoffmann disease. See **Werdnig-Hoffmann disease.**

Hoffmann reflex [Johann Hoffmann, German neurologist, 1857–1919], an abnormal reflex elicited by sudden forceful flicking of the nail of the index, middle, or ring finger, which causes flexion of the thumb and of the middle and distal phalanges of one of the other fingers. It is indicative of pyramidal tract disease above the level of the seventh or eighth cervical and first thoracic vertebrae. Also called *Hoffmann sign.*

hol-. See **holo-, hol-.**

holandric /holan″drik/ [Gk, *holos*, whole, *aner*, man], **1.** referring to genes located on the nonhomologous portion of the Y chromosome. **2.** pertaining to traits or conditions transmitted only through the paternal line. Compare **hologynic.**

holandric inheritance, the acquisition or expression of traits or conditions only through the paternal line, transmitted by genes located on the nonhomologous portion of the Y chromosome. Compare **hologynic inheritance.**

hold-relax, a technique of facilitating neuromuscular sensation and awareness, used in treating hypertonicity or motor dysfunction. It is often applied when there is muscle tightness on one side of a joint and when immobility is the result of pain.

holism /hō″lizəm/ [Gk, *holos*, whole], a philosophical concept in which an entity is seen as more than the sum of its parts. Holism is prominent in current approaches to psychology; biology; medicine; nursing; allied health professions; and other scientific, sociological, and educational fields of study and practice. Also spelled **wholism.**

holistic /hōlis″tik/ [Gk, *holos*], pertaining to the whole; considering all factors, as holistic medicine.

holistic counseling, an alternative form of psychotherapy that focuses on the whole person (mind, body, and spirit) and health. The goal is growth of the whole person.

holistic dentistry, dental practice that takes into account the effect of dental treatment and materials on the overall health of the individual.

holistic health /hōlis″tik/ [AS, *hal*, whole, *haelth*], a concept that concern for health requires a perception of the individual as an integrated system rather than one or more separate parts, including physical, mental, spiritual, and emotional. Also spelled *wholistic health.*

holistic health care, a system of comprehensive or total patient care that considers the physical, emotional, social, economic, and spiritual needs of the person; his or her response to illness; and the effect of the illness on the ability to meet self-care needs. Holistic nursing is the modern nursing practice that expresses this philosophy of care. Also called **comprehensive care.**

holistic nurse, a nurse who focuses on healing the whole person as the goal of care. In practicing holistic nursing, the nurse implements interventions aimed at bio-psycho-social-spiritual-environmental healing.

Hollenback condenser. See **pneumatic condenser.**

Holliday-Segar formula, a method of estimating the daily caloric needs of the average hospital patient under conditions of bed rest, based on the body weight in kilograms of the patient. Beginning at 100 kcal/kg for an infant, the formula plots a curve to 1500 kcal plus 20 kcal/kg for each kilogram over 20 kg.

hollow /hol′ō/ [OE, *holh*], a depressed area or concavity.

hollow cathode lamp [ME, *holwe* + Gk, *kata*, down, *hodos*, way, *lampas*], a lamp consisting of a metal cathode and an inert gas. When an electric current is passed through the cathode, electrons in the metal are excited so as to emit a line spectrum of specific wavelengths related to the metal of the cathode.

holmium (Ho) /hōl″mē·əm/ [L, *Holmia*, Stockholm, Sweden], a rare earth metallic element. Its atomic number is 67; its atomic mass is 164.93.

holo-, hol-, prefix meaning "entire" or "the whole": *holodiastolic, holistic, holoacardius.*

holoacardius /hol′ō·ākär″dē·əs/ [Gk, *holos* + *kardia*, heart], a separate, seriously defective monozygotic twin fetus. It is usually a shapeless, nonformed mass in which the heart is absent and the circulation in utero is accomplished

totally by the heart of the viable twin through a vascular shunt.

holoacardius acephalus, a seriously defective separate twin fetus that lacks a heart, a head, and most of the upper portion of the body.

holoacardius acormus, a separate twin fetus in which the trunk is malformed and little more than the head is recognizable.

holoacardius amorphus, a malformed separate twin fetus in which there are no recognizable or formed parts.

holoarthritis /-ärthrī″tis/, a form of arthritis that involves all or most of the joints.

holoblastic /hol′əblas″tik/ [Gk, *holos* + *blastos*, germ], pertaining to an ovum that contains little or no yolk and undergoes total cleavage. Compare **meroblastic.**

holocephalic /hō′lōsifal″ik/ [Gk, *holos* + *kephale*, head], pertaining to a malformed fetus in which several parts are deficient, although the head is complete.

holocrine /hol′əkrēn/ [Gk, *holos*, whole, *krienein*, to secrete], pertaining to the secretion of a gland or the gland itself as well as the accumulated gland secretions.

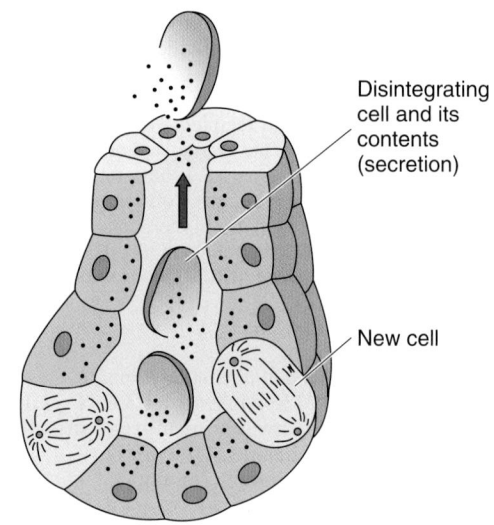

Disintegrating cell and its contents (secretion)

New cell

Holocrine gland *(Gartner and Hiatt, 2007)*

holocrine gland [Gk, *holos*, whole, *krienein*, to secrete], a gland whose discharge contains disintegrated or altered cells of the gland. Compare **apocrine gland, merocrine gland.**

holodiastolic. See **pandiastolic.**

holoendemic /hol′ō·endem″ik/, pertaining to an intensely endemic disease area.

holoenzyme /hol′ō·en″zīm/ [Gk, *holos* + *en*, in, *zymos*, ferment], a complete enzyme-cofactor complex that gives rise to full catalytic activity.

holographic reconstruction /-graf″ik/, a method of producing three-dimensional images with diagnostic ultrasound equipment.

hologynic /hol′ōjin″ik/ [Gk, *holos* + *gyne*, female], **1.** referring to genes located on attached X chromosomes. **2.** pertaining to traits or conditions transmitted only through the maternal line. Compare **holandric.**

hologynic inheritance, the acquisition or expression of traits or conditions only through the maternal line, transmitted by genes located on attached X chromosomes. The phenomenon is not known to occur in humans. Compare **holandric inheritance.**

holoprosencephaly /hol′ōpros′ensef″əlē/ [Gk, *holos* + *pro,* before, *enkephalos,* brain], a congenital defect caused by the failure of the prosencephalon to divide into hemispheres during embryonic development. It is characterized by multiple midline facial defects, including cyclopia in severe cases. It can also be caused by an extra chromosome in the 13–15 or D group, manifested as one of many developmental defects. See also **trisomy 13.** –*holoprosencephalous, holoprosencephalic, adj.*

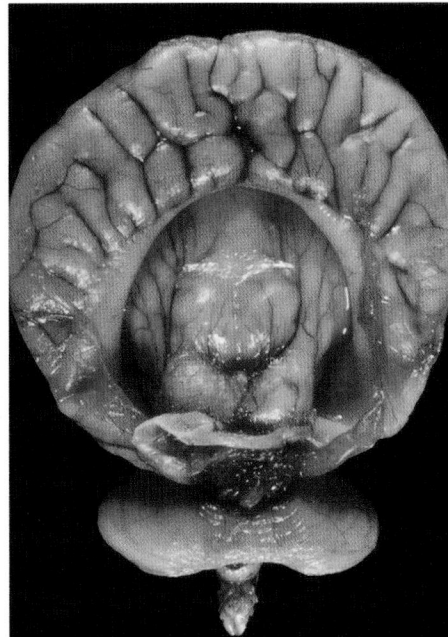

Holoprosencephaly: view of dorsal surface
(Kumar, Abbas, and Fausto, 2005)

holorachischisis. See **complete rachischisis.**
holosystolic. See **pansystolic.**
Holter monitor [Norman J. Holter, American biophysicist, 1914–1983; L, *monere,* to remind], a device for making prolonged electrocardiograph recordings (usually 24 hours) on a portable recorder while the patient conducts normal daily activities. The patient also may keep an activity diary for the purpose of comparing daily events with electrocardiographic tracings. Also called **ambulatory electrocardiograph.**
Holthouse hernia. See **inguinocrural hernia.**
Holt-Oram syndrome /hōlt or′əm/ [Mary Clayton Holt, British cardiologist, 20th century; Samuel Oram, English cardiologist, b. 1913], autosomal-dominant heart disease of varying severity, usually an atrial or ventricular septal defect associated with skeletal malformation (hypoplastic thumb and short forearm). Also called **heart-hand syndrome.**
Holtzman inkblot technique, a modification of the Rorschach test in which many more pictures of inkblots are used, the subject is permitted only one response to each design, and the scoring is predominantly objective rather than subjective.
Homans sign [John Homans, American surgeon, 1877–1954; L, *signum,* mark], pain in the calf with dorsiflexion of the foot, indicating the presence of a blood clot. Although often utilized in a clinical evaluation, it is no longer considered a reliable indicator and should always be supplemented by more conclusive studies if a clot is suspected. See also **Doppler ultrasonography, venography.**

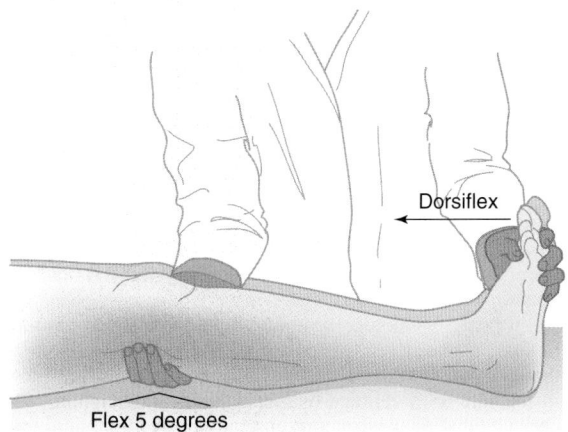

Testing for Homans sign *(Leifer, 2011)*

home assessment [AS, *ham,* village; L, *assidere,* to sit beside], an examination of the living area of a physically challenged person to make recommendations for the elimination of safety hazards and suggestions for architectural or other modifications that would allow for independent functioning.
home care [AS, *ham,* village; L, *garrire,* to chatter], a health service provided in the patient's place of residence for the purpose of promoting, maintaining, or restoring health or minimizing the effects of illness and disability. Service may include such elements as medical, dental, and nursing care; speech and physical therapy; homemaking services of a home health aide; and provision of transportation. The nature and extent of care needed and the ability of the patient's family and friends to assume responsibility for that care are assessed. Nursing may be provided by a registered nurse, licensed practical nurse, or home health aide. Some hospitals have home care services that include regular visits by a nurse and a physician to patients in the home.
home health agency, an organization that provides health care in the home. Medicare certification for a home health agency in the United States requires provision of skilled nursing services and at least one additional therapeutic service.
home health aide, an individual, often certified, who provides personal care and services to the elderly, persons with disabilities, and individuals experiencing chronic or terminal illness in the home to augment self-care and/or care provided by family members.
home health nurse, a registered nurse who visits patients in the home. The nurse works primarily in the area of secondary or tertiary care, providing hands-on care and educating the patient and family on care and prevention of future episodes.
homeless person, an individual who has no permanent home, haven, or domicile. Such individuals usually are indigent and depend on charity or public assistance for temporary lodging and medical care. An estimated 30% of homeless persons suffer from some type of mental disorder. See also **indigence.**
home establishment and management activities, the tasks that are necessary to obtain personal and household possessions and to maintain a household and its environment (e.g., home, yard, garden, appliances, and vehicles); such tasks would include the maintenance and repair of personal possessions, such as clothing and household items, and knowing how to seek help when needed.
homeo-, homoeo-, homoio-, prefix meaning "sameness, similarity": *homeopathy, homeomorphous, homeotypic.*

homeodynamics /hō′mē·ədīnam″iks/ [Gk, *homoios,* similar, *dynamis,* force], the constantly changing interrelatedness of body components while an overall equilibrium is maintained.

homeomorphous /-môr″fəs/, similar in appearance but different in composition.

Homeopathic Pharmacopoeia of the United States, one of the three official drug compendia specified in the Federal Food, Drug, and Cosmetic Act. See also **compendium, *National Formulary.***

homeopathist /hō′mē-op″əthist/, a physician who practices homeopathy.

homeopathy /hō′mē-op″əthē/ [Gk, *homoios,* similar, *pathos,* disease], a system of therapeutics based on the theory that "like cures like." The theory was advanced in the late 18th century by Dr. Samuel Hahnemann, who believed that a large amount of a particular drug may cause symptoms of a disease whereas moderate dosage may reduce those symptoms; thus some disease symptoms may be treated by very small doses of medicine. Compare **allopathy.** *−homeopathic, adj.*

homeostasis /hō′mē·əstā″sis/ [Gk, *homoios + stasis,* standing still], a relative constancy in the internal environment of the body, naturally maintained by adaptive responses that promote healthy survival. Various sensing, feedback, and control mechanisms function to effect this steady state. Some of the key control mechanisms are the reticular formation in the brainstem and the endocrine glands. Some of the functions controlled by homeostatic mechanisms are heartbeat, hematopoiesis, blood pressure, body temperature, electrolytic balance, respiration, and glandular secretion. *−homeostatic, adj.*

homeotherapy /-ther″əpē/, the treatment or prevention of disease by homeopathic methods.

homeotic mutation /hō′mē-ot″ik/, a mutation that causes tissues to alter their normal differentiation pattern, producing integrated structures but in unusual locations. For example, a homeotic mutation in the fruit fly, *Drosophila,* causes legs to develop where antennae normally form.

homeotypic /hō′mē·ōtip″ik/ [Gk, *homoios + typos,* mark], pertaining to or characteristic of the regular or usual type, specifically regarding the second meiotic division of germ cells in gametogenesis as distinguished from the first meiotic division. Also called *homeotypical.* Compare **heterotypic.**

homeotypic mitosis, the separation of sister chromatids, as occurs in the second meiotic division of germ cells in gametogenesis. Compare **heterotypic mitosis.**

homicide /hom″isīd/ [L, *homo,* man, *caedere,* to kill], the death of one human being caused by another.

hominal physiology /hom″inəl/ [L, *hominis,* human; Gk, *physis,* nature, *logos,* science], the study of the specific physical and chemical processes involved in the normal functioning of humans; human physiology.

hominid /hom″inid/ [L, *homo,* man; Gk, *eidos,* form], pertaining to the primate family Hominidae, which includes humans.

homo-, **1.** prefix meaning "the same": *homogenesis, homogenized, homozygous.* **2.** prefix meaning "the addition of one CH$_2$ group to the main compound": *homocarnosine, homocystine.*

homoblastic /hō′mōblas″tik/ [Gk, *homos + blastos,* germ], developing from the same germ layer or from a single type of tissue. Compare **heteroblastic.**

homocarnosine /hō′mōkär′nōsēn/, a dipeptide consisting of gamma-aminobutyric acid and histidine. In humans it is found in the brain but not in other tissues.

homochronous inheritance /hōmok″rənəs/ [Gk, *homos + chronos,* time], the appearance of traits or conditions in offspring at the same age when they appeared in the parents.

homocysteine /-sis″tēn/, an amino acid containing sulfur and a homolog of cysteine, produced in the demethylation of methionine. It is also an intermediate product in the biosynthesis of cysteine from L-methionine via L-cystathionine in the breakdown of proteins. High levels of homocysteine are associated with an increased risk of collagen cardiovascular disorders, particularly thromboembolic stroke. It is believed the amino acid may have a toxic effect on cells lining the blood vessels. Studies also indicate that low levels of homocysteine are found in people with high intake of B vitamins. See also **homocystine.**

homocysteine (HCY) test, a blood test used to detect levels of homocysteine, which, if increased, may act as an independent risk factor for ischemic heart disease, cerebrovascular disease, peripheral arterial disease, and venous thrombosis. This test should be considered for screening in individuals with progressive and unexplained atherosclerosis despite normal lipoproteins and in the absence of other risk factors and in those with an unusual family history of atherosclerosis.

homocystine /-sis″tin/, a disulfide analog of homocysteine produced by the oxidation of homocysteine. See also **homocysteine.**

homocystinemia /-sis′tinē″mē·ə/, an amino acid disorder that causes an excess of homocystine in the blood. See also **homocystinuria.**

homocystinuria /hō′mōsis′tinoor″ē·ə/ [Gk, *homos +* (cystine); Gk, *ouron,* urine], a rare biochemical abnormality characterized by the abnormal presence of homocystine, an amino acid, in the blood and urine, which is caused by any of several enzyme deficiencies in the metabolic pathway of methionine to cystine. The disease is inherited as an autosomal-recessive trait. Its clinical signs are similar to those of Marfan syndrome, including cognitive impairment, osteoporosis leading to skeletal abnormalities, dislocated lenses, and thromboembolism. Treatment may include a diet low in methionine and supplementation with large doses of vitamin B. Long-term results of treatment are not available. *−homocystinuric, adj.*

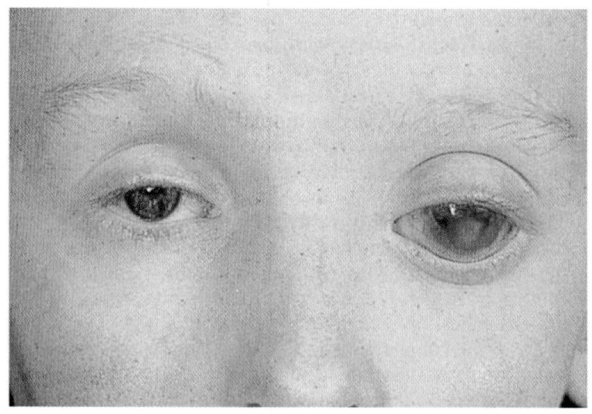

Homocystinuria: lens dislocation *(Newton, 1995)*

homoeo-. See **homeo-, homoeo-, homoio-.**

homogametic /hō″mōgamet″ik/ [Gk, *homos* + *gamete,* spouse], pertaining to the sex that produces gametes of only one kind in terms of their sex chromosomes. In human beings, the female is the homogametic sex.

homogenate /hōmoj″ənit/, a tissue that is or has been made homogenous, as by grinding cells into a creamy consistency for laboratory studies. A homogenate usually lacks cell structure. Also called **broken cell preparation.**

homogeneous /hō″mōjē″nē·əs/ [Gk, *homos* + *genos,* kind], **1.** consisting of similar elements or parts. **2.** having a uniform quality throughout. Also spelled **homogenous.** Compare **heterogeneous.** −*homogeneity, adj.*

homogenesis /hō″mōjen″əsis/ [Gk, *homos* + *genesis,* origin], reproduction by the same process in succeeding generations so that offspring are similar to the parents. Also called **homogeny.** Compare **heterogenesis.**

homogenetic /-jenet″ik/, pertaining to homogenesis.

homogenized /hōmoj″ənīzd/ [Gk, *homos,* same, *genein,* to produce], the state of having undergone homogenization; having a uniform texture or consistency throughout.

homogenized milk [Gk, *homos* + *genos,* kind], milk that has been mechanically treated to reduce and emulsify the fat globules so that the cream cannot separate.

homogenous /hōmoj″ənəs/ [Gk, *homos* + *genos,* kind], **1.** See **homogeneous. 2.** having a likeness in form or structure as a result of a common ancestral origin. Also called **homogenetic.** Compare **heterogenous.**

homogenous graft. See **allograft.**

homogentisic acid, a compound that is an intermediate product of the metabolism of tyrosine. It forms a melanin-like staining substance in the urine of people who have alkaptonuria.

homogeny /hōmoj″ənē/ [Gk, *homos* + *genos,* kind], **1.** See **homogenesis. 2.** a likeness in structure or form that results from a common ancestral origin. Compare **homoplasty.**

homograft. See **allograft.**

homoio-. See **homeo-, homoeo-, homoio-.**

homoiothermal. See **warm-blooded.**

homoiothermic /hom″ē·əthur″mik/ [Gk, *homos,* same, *therme,* heat], pertaining to the ability of warm-blooded animals to maintain a relatively stable internal temperature regardless of the temperature of the environment. This ability is not fully developed in newborn humans.

homolateral /hō″mōlat″ərəl/, pertaining to the same side of the body.

homolateral limb synkinesis, a condition of hemiplegia in which there appears to be a mutual dependency between the affected upper and lower limbs. Efforts at flexion of an upper extremity cause flexion of the lower extremity.

homolog /hom″əlog/ [Gk, *homos,* same], **1.** any organ corresponding in function, origin, and structure to another organ, as the flippers of a seal correspond to human hands. **2.** (in chemistry) one of a series of compounds, each formed by an added common atom or atom combination. For example, CH_4, methane, is followed by C_2H_6, ethane, with the addition of a CH_2 group. Also spelled **homologue.** Compare **analog.** −*homologous, adj.*

homologous /hōmol″əgəs/ [Gk, *homos,* same, *logos,* relation], pertaining to corresponding attributes; similar in structure. Compare *analogous.* See also **homolog.**

homologous anaphylaxis [Gk, *homos,* same, *logos,* relation, *ana,* back, *phylaxis,* protection], a form of passive anaphylaxis resulting from the transfer of serum between animals of the same species.

homologous chromosomes [Gk, *homos,* same, *chroma* color, *soma* body], any two chromosomes in a diploid somatic cell that are identical in size, shape, and gene loci. In humans there are 22 pairs of homologous chromosomes and 1 pair of sex chromosomes, with 1 member of each pair derived from the mother and the other from the father.

homologous disease. *(Obsolete)* See **graft-versus-host disease.**

homologous graft [Gk, *homos,* same, *logos,* relation, *graphein,* stylus], a tissue removed from a donor for transplantation to a recipient of the same species. Also called **homogenous graft.** Compare **autograft, isograft, xenograft.**

homologous insemination. See **artificial insemination— husband.**

homologous organs [Gk, *homos,* same, *logos,* relation, *organon,* instrument], body parts of different species (or sexes) that are structural equivalents, such as the arms of humans and the forelegs of dogs and cats.

homologous transplantation. See **homoplastic transplantation.**

homologous tumor, a neoplasm made up of cells resembling those of the tissue in which it is growing. Compare **heterologous tumor, organoid neoplasm.**

homologue. See **homolog.**

homonymous /hōmon″iməs/ [Gk, *homos,* same, *onyma,* name], having the same name or sound.

homonymous diplopia [Gk, *homos,* same, *onyma,* name, *diploos,* double, *opsis,* vision], a type of diplopia in which the image observed by the right eye is located to the right of the image observed by the left eye.

homonymous hemianopia [Gk, *homos* + *onyma,* name], blindness or defective vision in the right or left halves of the visual fields of both eyes.

homophobia /hō″mōfō″bē·ə/ [Gk, *homos,* same, *phobos,* fear], fear of or prejudice against homosexuals.

homoplastic. See **homoplasty.**

homoplastic transplantation [Gk, *homos,* same, *plassein,* to mold; L, *transplantare,* to transplant], the homologous transplantation of tissue from one human to another or from one animal to another of the same species. Also called **homologous transplantation.**

homoplasty /hō″məplas″tē/ [Gk, *homos* + *plassein,* to mold], having a likeness in form or structure acquired through similar environmental conditions or parallel evolution rather than resulting from common ancestral origin. Compare **homogeny.** −*homoplastic, adj.*

homopolymer /hō″mōpol″imir/ [Gk, *homos* + *poly,* many, *meros,* part], a compound formed from subunits that are the same, such as a carbohydrate composed of a series of glucose units.

homosalate /hō″mōsal″āt/, a sunscreen effective against ultraviolet B rays, applied topically to the skin.

Homo sapiens /hō″mō sā″pē·əns, sä″pē·ens/ [L, *homo,* human, *sapere,* to know or taste], the scientific name of the human species.

homosexual /-sek″shəl/ [Gk, *homos* + L, *sexus,* sex, gender], **1.** *adj.,* pertaining to or denoting the same sex. **2.** *n.,* a person who is sexually attracted to members of the same sex. Compare **heterosexual.** See also **lesbian.**

homosexuality. See **sexual orientation.**

homosexual intercourse [Gk, *homos,* same; L, *sexus,* male or female, *intercursus,* interposition], sexual activity of members of the same sex, ranging from feelings and fantasies to kissing and genital, oral, or anal contact.

homothermal. See **warm-blooded.**

H

homotopic pain /hō′mōtop″ik/, pain experienced at the point of injury.

homotype /hō′mōtīp/, any structure or body part, such as a hand or foot, that appears in reversed symmetry with a similar part.

homovanillic acid (HVA) /hō′mōvənil″ik/, an acid that is produced by the normal metabolism of dopamine and that may occur at an elevated level in urine in association with tumors of the adrenal gland. Its normal accumulation in a 24-hour collection urine sample is 15 mg.

homozygosis /hō′mōzīgō″sis/ [Gk, *homos* + *zygon,* yoke], **1.** the formation of a zygote by the union of two gametes that have one or more pairs of identical alleles. **2.** the production of purebred organisms or strains through inbreeding.

homozygote /hō′məzī″gōt/ [Gk, *homos,* same, *zygon,* yoke], an organism whose somatic cells have identical genes on the same locus on one of the chromosome pairs.

homozygous /hō′məzī″gəs/ [Gk, *homos* + *zygon,* yoke], having two identical alleles at corresponding loci on homologous chromosomes. An individual who is homozygous for a trait has inherited from each parent one allele for that trait. A person who is homozygous for a genetic disease caused by a pair of recessive alleles, such as sickle cell anemia, manifests the disorder. All of his or her offspring will inherit the allele for the disease. Compare **heterozygous.**

homunculus /hōmung″kyələs/ *pl. homunculi* [L, little man], **1.** (in early embryological theories of development, primarily preformation) a minute and complete human being contained in each of the germ cells that after fertilization grows from the microscopic to normal size. **2.** a small anatomical model of the human form; a manikin, specifically, one described in fictional literature as having been produced by an alchemist. **3.** (in psychiatry) a little man created by the imagination who possesses magical powers.

hook grasp, a type of prehension in which an object is grasped with the fingers alone, without use of the thumb and palm.

hookworm [AS, *hok* + *wyrm*], *(Nontechnical)* a nematode of the genera *Ancylostoma, Necator,* or *Uncinaria.* Most hookworm infections in the western hemisphere are caused by the species *Necator americanus.* Infection occurs when the larvae invade exposed skin, mostly the feet. Individuals may be asymptomatic carriers.

hookworm disease [AS, *hok* + *wyrm* + Gk, *dis,* not; Fr, *aise,* ease], a roundworm infestation that may involve either of two important intestinal parasites of humans, *Ancylostoma duodenale* or *Necator americanus.* Both forms of the disease, ancylostomiasis and necatoriasis, are characterized by abdominal pain, in heavy infection, and iron-deficiency anemia. The worm enters the human body as a larva by penetrating the skin, traveling to the lungs via the circulatory system, and ascending the respiratory tract to the pharynx, where it is swallowed. In the intestinal tract the hookworm attaches its mouth to the mucosa and subsists on the blood of the host. Hookworm is believed to infect 800 million people globally. It is treated with cryotherapy when still in the skin. Albendazole is effective against both the intestinal stages and skin infestation.

hops, a perennial herb cultivated throughout the world.
■ INDICATIONS: It is used as a flavoring (e.g., beer), mild sedative, diuretic, and weak antibiotic. It is also used to improve appetite and to treat insomnia, hyperactivity, pain, fever, and jaundice. It may be effective against restlessness; there are insufficient reliable data on its efficacy for other indications.

■ CONTRAINDICATIONS: It should not be used in people who are hypersensitive to this product; who have breast, uterine, or cervical cancers; or who suffer from a depressive condition.

hordeolum /hôrdē″ələm/ [L, *hordeum,* barley], a furuncle of the margin of the eyelid originating in the sebaceous gland of an eyelash. Treatment includes hot compresses and antibiotic ophthalmic preparations; incision and drainage are occasionally required. Also called **sty.** Compare **chalazion.**

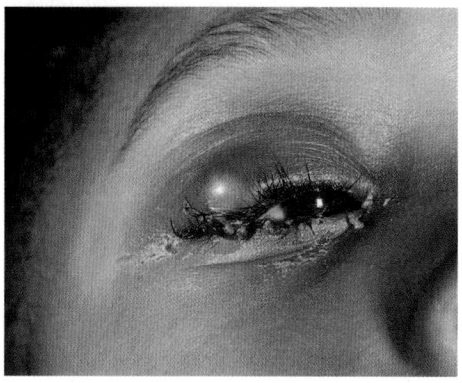

Hordeolum *(Roberts and Hedges, 2010)*

horizon /hôrī″zən/ [Gk, *horizein,* to encircle], a specific stage of human embryonic development determined by the appearance and ultimate formation of certain anatomical characteristics. The classification comprises 23 stages, each lasting 2 to 3 days, beginning with the fertilization of the ovum and ending 7 to 9 weeks later with the initiation of the fetal period of intrauterine life.

horizontal abdominal position /hôr′izon″təl/, prone position.

horizontal angulation [Gk, *horizein,* to encircle; L, *angularis,* angle], the angle within the occlusal plane, relative to a reference in the vertical or sagittal plane, at which the central x-ray beam is directed during radiography or dental imaging of oral structures. Compare **vertical angulation.**

horizontal fissure of the right lung, a cleft that marks the separation of the upper and middle lobes of the right lung.

horizontal overlap. See **overjet.**

horizontal plane [Gk, *horizein,* to encircle; L, *planum,* level ground], **1.** any plane of the erect body parallel to the horizon, dividing the body into upper and lower parts. **2.** a plane passing through a tooth at right angles to its long axis.

horizontal position, a position in which the patient lies on the back with the legs extended.

horizontal pursuit, a visual screening test in which the patient is asked to follow with both eyes a target moving in a horizontal plane while the examiner observes accuracy of alignment and supportive head movements.

horizontal resorption, a pattern of bone reduction in marginal periodontitis wherein the marginal crest of the alveolar bone between adjacent teeth remains level and the bases of the periodontal pockets are above the crest. Compare **vertical resorption.** See also **resorption.**

horizontal transmission, the spread of an infectious agent from one person or group to another, usually through contact with contaminated material, such as sputum or feces.

horizontal vertigo, a feeling of instability or a spinning sensation experienced while lying down, frequently caused by a labyrinthine disorder.

horizontal violence, violence directed toward one's peers.

horm-, prefix meaning "an impulse, to urge or stimulate": *hormic, hormonal.*

hormic psychology /hôr″mic/ [Gk, *hormaien,* to begin action], (in psychology) the school that stresses the purposive, goal-oriented nature of human behavior.

hormonal /hôr″mōnəl/ [Gk, *hormaein,* to set in motion], pertaining to or resembling hormones.

hormonal therapy. See **hormone therapy.**

hormone /hôr″mōn/ [Gk, *hormaein,* to set in motion], a complex chemical substance produced in one part or organ of the body that initiates or regulates the activity of an organ or a group of cells in another part. Hormones secreted by the endocrine glands are carried through the bloodstream to the target organ. Secretion of these hormones is regulated by other hormones, by neurotransmitters, and by a negative feedback system in which an excess of target organ activity or hormone signals a decreased need for the stimulating hormone. Other hormones are released by organs for local effect, most commonly in the digestive tract.

-hormone, 1. suffix meaning "a chemical substance possessing a regulatory effect," classified by source: *parahormone.* **2.** suffix meaning "a chemical substance possessing a regulatory effect," classified by activity affected: *neurohormone.*

hormone replacement therapy, the administration of sex hormones following menopause or hysterectomy or in amenorrhea. There are a number of indications, including the induction of menses in amenorrhea. If used for postmenopausal symptoms, it should be given in the smallest effective dose for the shortest period of time. Following the completion of the Women's Health Initiative study, hormone replacement therapy is no longer used for the prevention of osteoporosis or coronary artery disease.

hormone-sensitive lipase, an enzyme that catalyzes the release of fatty acids from adipose tissues.

hormone therapy, the treatment of diseases with hormones obtained from endocrine glands or substances that simulate hormonal effects. Also called *endocrine therapy,* **hormonal therapy.**

horn, a projection or protuberance on a body structure. Examples include the horn of the hyoid bone and the iliac horn.

Horner syndrome [Johann F. Horner, Swiss ophthalmologist, 1831–1886], a neurological condition characterized by a constricted (miotic) pupil, ptosis, and facial anhidrosis, associated with a lesion in the spinal cord, with damage to a cervical nerve or any ascending part of the sympathetic outflow to the face/head. Signs are ipsilateral (same side) to the injury.

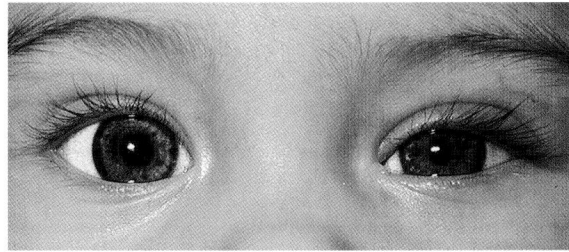

Child with Horner syndrome: ptosis of the right eyelid
(Taylor and Hoyt, 2005)

horny /hôr′nē/, having the nature or appearance of a projection. Also called **corneous, keratic.**

horny layer. See **stratum corneum.**

horripilation. See **pilomotor reflex.**

horse chestnut, a herbal product taken from a tree or shrub found worldwide. Its bark, flowers, leaves, and seeds may be harvested.

■ INDICATIONS: It is used for fever, fluid retention, frostbite, hemorrhoids, inflammation, lower extremity swelling, phlebitis, varicose veins, and wounds. Horse chestnut seeds may have efficacy in the treatment of varicose veins and other forms of venous insufficiency. There is insufficient reliable information regarding efficacy of the bark, flower, or leaf products for other indications.

■ CONTRAINDICATIONS: It is contraindicated during pregnancy and lactation and in children until more research has been completed.

horse serum [AS, *hors* + L, *serum,* whey], immune serum prepared from the blood of a horse that has developed immunity to toxins. Because many people are sensitive to horse serum, a skin test for sensitivity is recommended before passive immunization with horse antibodies. Tetanus immune globulin prepared from human immune serum is preferred.

horseshoe fistula /hôrs″shoo/ [AS, *hors* + *scoh,* shoe], an abnormal semicircular passage in the perianal area with both openings on the surface of the skin.

horseshoe kidney, a relatively common congenital anomaly characterized by an isthmus of parenchymal tissue connecting the two kidneys at the lower poles. The condition may cause obstruction of the ureters, hydronephrosis, and abdominal pain. It is corrected by surgery to separate and reposition the kidneys.

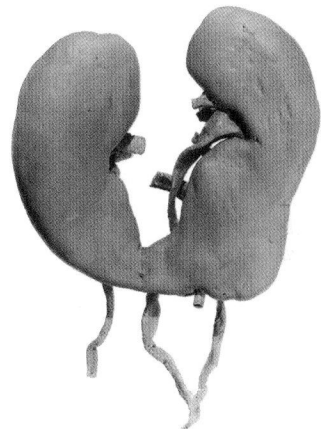

Horseshoe kidneys: posterior view
(Moore, Persaud, and Shiota, 2000)

horsetail, a perennial herb known as a pteridophyte, found throughout the world.

■ INDICATIONS: It is probably unsafe and should not be used for any purpose. It is used as a diuretic, a genitourinary astringent, and an antihemorrhagic. It is also used for Bell's palsy and for healing broken bones. There are no studies confirming its efficacy.

■ CONTRAINDICATIONS: People ignoring personal safety concerns should be aware that it should not be used during pregnancy and lactation or in children. It is also contraindicated in those with known hypersensitivity, edema, cardiac or renal disease, or nicotine sensitivity. It should not be used for prolonged periods of time.

Hortega cells. See **microglia.**

Horton arteritis. See **temporal arteritis.**

Horton headache. See **migrainous cranial neuralgia.**

Horton histamine cephalalgia. See **histamine headache.**

hospice /hos″pis/ [L, *hospes,* host], a system of family-centered care designed to assist the terminally ill person to be comfortable and to maintain quality of life through the phases of dying. Hospice care is multidisciplinary and includes home visits, professional health care available on call, teaching and emotional support of the family, and physical care of the client. Some hospice programs provide care in a center, as well as in the home or in a nursing home. Services are typically used within the last 6 months of life expectancy. Hospice also offers bereavement counseling for the family. See also **emotional care of the dying patient, stages of dying.**

hospital /hos″pitəl/ [L, *hospitium,* guesthouse], a health care facility that provides inpatient beds, continuous nursing services, and an organized medical staff.

hospital-acquired infection. See **nosocomial infection.**

hospital clinic, an ambulatory care site owned by a hospital where persons who do not require hospitalization receive health care. It may be primary care or subspecialty care.

Hospital Infection Control Practices Advisory Committee (HICPAC), a committee established in 1991 by the U.S. government with members appointed by the Secretary of Health and Human Services. It provides advice and guidance related to isolation practices and serves as an advisory committee to the U.S. Centers for Disease Control and Prevention for updating guidelines and policy statements related to control of nosocomial infection.

hospitalism /hos″pitəliz′əm/, the physical or mental effects of hospitalization or institutionalization on patients, especially infants and children in whom the condition is characterized by social regression, personality disorders, and stunted growth. See also **anaclitic depression.**

hospitalist /hos′pi·təl·ist/, a physician specializing in hospital inpatient care.

Hospital Survey and Construction Act. See **Hill-Burton Act.**

host /hōst/ [L, *hospes*], **1.** an organism in which another, usually parasitic, organism is nourished and harbored. A definitive host is one in which the adult parasite lives and reproduces. An intermediate host is one in which the parasite exists in its nonsexual, larval stage. A reservoir host is a primary animal host for organisms that are sometimes parasitic in humans and through which humans may become infected. **2.** the recipient of a transplanted organ or tissue. Compare **donor.**

host defense mechanisms, a group of body protective systems, including physical barriers and the immune response, that normally guard against infection.

hostility /hostil″itē/ [L, *hostilis,* hostile], an emotional state characterized by enmity toward others and a desire to harm those at whom the antagonism is directed. The hostility may be expressed passively or actively.

host-modulating therapy, efforts to control periodontal disease by directly targeting the host response. An example is the use of drugs that do this, such as subgingival antimicrobial doses of doxycycline, NSAIDs, or bisphosphonates.

hot bath [AS, *hat* + *baeth*], a bath in which the temperature of the water is gradually raised to about 106° F (41.11° C).

hot compress [AS, *hat* + L, *comprimere,* to press together], a heated pad of damp, thickly folded cloth applied to an area to reduce pain or inflammation. See also **fomentation.**

hot flash, a transient sensation of warmth experienced by some women during or after menopause. Hot flashes result from autonomic vasomotor disturbances that accompany changes in the neurohormonal activity of the ovaries, hypothalamus, and pituitary. The exact causative mechanism is not known. All menopausal women do not experience hot flashes; among those who do, the frequency, duration, and intensity vary widely. Although physically harmless, the symptom may be extremely disturbing or, rarely, disabling. Hot flashes may be alleviated by cyclic or continuous administration of exogenous estrogen. Also called *hot flush.* See also **menopause.**

hot line, a means of contacting a trained counselor or specific agency for help with a particular problem, such as a rape hot line or a battered child hot line. The person needing help calls a telephone number and speaks to a counselor, who remains anonymous and who offers emotional support, specific recommendations for action, and referral to other medical, social, or community services. Such services are usually maintained by volunteers and are accessible 24 hours a day, 7 days a week.

hot spot, 1. a site in a gene sequence at which mutations occur with an unusually high frequency. **2.** an area on a nuclear medicine image that represents an abnormally high absorption of radiation.

Hounsfield unit /hounz″fēld/ [Godfrey N. Hounsfield, 20th-century English scientist], the numeric information contained in each pixel of a CT image. It is related to the composition and nature of the tissue imaged and is used to represent the density of tissue. Also called **CT number,** *Hounsfield number.*

hourglass uterus [Gk, *hora* + AS, *glaes*], a uterus in which a segment of circular muscle fibers contracts during labor, causing constriction ring dystocia. The condition is marked by lack of progress despite adequate labor contractions and by recession rather than descent of the presenting part during a contraction.

housekeeping department, a unit of a hospital staff responsible for cleaning the hospital premises and furnishings and for disinfecting surfaces to reduce the presence of pathogenic organisms. See also **environmental services.**

housemaid's knee [AS, *hus* + *maeden* + *cneow,* knee], *(Informal)* a chronic inflammation of the bursa in front of the kneecap, characterized by redness and swelling. It is caused by prolonged and repetitive pressure of the knee on a hard surface.

house organ, a publication designed for distribution to the employees or members of an institution or business. It may be prepared by a staff within the institution or business or by an outside agency.

house physician [AS, *hus* + Gk, *physikos,* natural], a physician on call and immediately available in a hospital or other health care facility.

house staff, the interns and residents who are employed at a hospital while receiving additional training after graduation from medical college.

house surgeon, a surgeon on call and immediately available on the premises of a hospital.

Houston's valves. See **transverse rectal folds.**

Hovius plexus. See **Leber plexus.**

Howell-Jolly bodies /hou″əl jol″ē/ [William H. Howell, American physiologist, 1860–1945; Justin M.J. Jolly, French histologist, 1870–1953], deep purple spherical erythrocyte nucleic acid inclusions observed on microscopic examination of stained blood films. They are most commonly seen in people who have hemolytic or megoblastic anemia, leukemia, thalassemia, or congenital absence of the spleen and in those who have had a splenectomy.

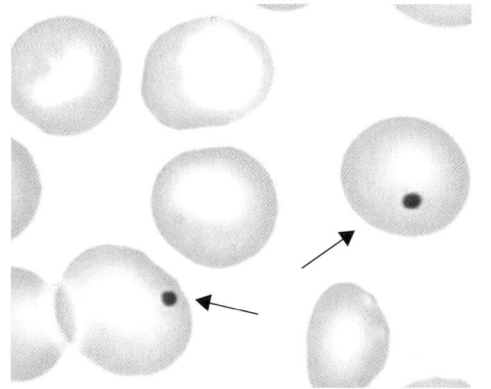

Howell-Jolly bodies *(Carr and Rodak, 2009)*

HPG, initialism for *human pituitary gonadotropin.*

HPL, abbreviation for **human placental lactogen.**

HPV, 1. abbreviation for **human papillomavirus. 2.** abbreviation for **human parvovirus.**

hr, abbreviation for *hour.*

H₁ receptor, a type of histamine receptor present in smooth muscles, on vascular endothelial cells, in the heart, and in the central nervous system. Triggering of H_1 receptors by histamine mediates vasodilation, smooth muscle contraction, and gastric acid secretion. See also **antihistamine, histamine blocking agent.**

H₂ receptor, a type of histamine receptor on various kinds of cells through which histamine mediates bronchial constriction in asthma and GI constriction in diarrhea. See also **antihistamine, histamine blocking agent.**

H₁ receptor antagonist, any of a large number of agents that block the action of histamine by competitive binding to the H_1 receptor. Such agents also have sedative, anticholinergic, and antiemetic effects, the exact effect varying from drug to drug, and are used for the relief of allergic symptoms and as antiemetics, antivertigo agents, sedatives, and antidyskinetics in parkinsonism. This group is traditionally called the antihistamines. See also **antihistamine.**

H₂ receptor antagonist, an agent that blocks the action of histamine by competitive binding to the H_2 receptor. It is used to inhibit gastric secretion in the treatment of peptic ulcer.

HRF, 1. abbreviation for *histamine-releasing factor.* **2.** abbreviation for *homologous restriction factor.*

HRIG, abbreviation for *human rabies immune globulin.*

HRSA, abbreviation for **Health Resources and Services Administration.**

hs, h.s., short form for the Latin phrase *hora somni,* meaning *at bedtime.* Because hs (h.s.) is considered an error-prone abbreviation (it could be confused to mean half-strength), it should no longer be used as an abbreviation for *at bedtime.*

HSA, abbreviation for **health systems agency.**

HSP, abbreviation for **heat shock protein.**

HSV, initialism for *herpes simplex virus.* See **herpes genitalis, herpes simplex.**

HSV1, initialism for *herpes simplex virus type 1.* See **herpes simplex.**

ht, abbreviation for **height.**

HTLV, abbreviation for *human T-cell lymphotropic virus.* See **human T-cell lymphotropic virus (HTLV) type I/II antibody test.**

HTLV-I, abbreviation for **human T-cell lymphotropic virus type I.**

HTLV-II, abbreviation for **human T-cell lymphotropic virus type II.**

HTLV-III, abbreviation for **human T-cell lymphotropic virus type III.** See **human immunodeficiency virus.**

Hu antigen, a family of four RNA-binding proteins (HuD, HuC/ple21, Hel-N1, and Hel-N2) that are expressed in neurons and are believed to play an important role in the development and maintenance of the nervous system. They are also expressed in the cells of small cell lung carcinoma, sarcoma, and neuroblastoma, and antibodies to them are associated with neurological paraneoplastic syndromes.

Hubbard tank [Carl P. Hubbard, American engineer, 1857–1938), a water tank in which patients can perform underwater exercise. The patient's trunk and extremities are submerged on a stretcher. The water provides buoyancy and heat for the benefit of weakened or painful muscles or joints with limited active range of motion. The tank also may be used for wound debridement. See also **whirlpool bath.**

huffing, forced expiration with an open glottis used to clear secretions from the airway when pain limits normal coughing.

HUGO /hyo͞o′gō/, abbreviation for **Human Genome Organization.**

Huhner test /ho͞o′nər/ [Max Huhner, American urologist, 1873–1947], a test for male fertility in which a semen sample aspirated from the vagina within an hour after coitus is examined for spermatozoal activity.

human /h(y)o͞o′mən/ [L, *humanus*], a member of the genus *Homo* and particularly of the species *H. sapiens.*

human bite [L, *humanus* + AS, *bitan*], a wound caused by the piercing of skin by human teeth. Bacteria are usually present, and serious infection often follows. The area is thoroughly washed with an antiseptic and rinsed well. The wound is examined frequently, and appropriate antibiotic therapy instituted, if necessary.

human chorionic gonadotropin. See **chorionic gonadotropin.**

human chorionic somatomammotropin (HCS), a hormone produced by the syncytiotrophoblast during pregnancy. It regulates carbohydrate and protein metabolism of the mother to ensure delivery to the fetus of glucose for energy and protein for fetal growth. HCS, an insulin antagonist, also may have a diabetogenic effect in the mother, who therefore may have an increased blood glucose level. Also called *chorionic growth hormone-prolactin,* **human placental lactogen.**

human diploid cell rabies vaccine (HDCV), an inactivated rabies virus vaccine prepared from rabies virus grown in human diploid cell cultures. Active immunization with HDCV begins on the day of exposure, followed by four or five additional injections. Passive immunization with human rabies immune globulin may be given concurrently with HDCV.

human ecology, the study of the interrelationships between people and their environments, as well as among individuals within an environment.

human endogenous retroviruses (HERV), retrovirus-like sequences found in the human genome, thought to constitute the remains of true retroviruses that were absorbed through evolution. At least one is thought to be linked to expression of tumor cells. They are also thought to be involved in autoimmune disorders such as multiple sclerosis.

Human Genome Organization (HUGO), an international group established in 1989 to coordinate activities concerned with the human genome project, including the distribution of funding and dissemination of information.

human granulocytic ehrlichiosis (HGE). See **ehrlichiosis.**

human growth hormone (synthetic). See **synthetic human growth hormone.**

human herpesvirus 6, a T-cell lymphotrophic virus belonging to the subfamily Betaherpesvirinae that has a high affinity for CD4 lymphocytes. It exists as two variants, A and B. Variant A is isolated mainly in immunocompromised individuals. Variant B causes roseola infantum. Most healthy adults carry the virus and are asymptomatic; infection results in lifelong persistence. See also **herpesvirus, roseola infantum.**

human herpesvirus 7, a virus belonging to the subfamily Betaherpesvirinae, closely related to human herpesvirus 6 but not known to be associated with any disease. See also **human herpesvirus 6.**

human herpesvirus 8, a virus in the family Herpesviridae that has been implicated as the causative agent of Kaposi sarcoma, a rare form of cancer occasionally seen in patients with AIDS, and primary effusion lymphoma. The predominant route of transmission is sexual activity. The virus may also be transmitted through blood contact in IV drug use. Treatment is currently experimental. Also called **Kaposi sarcoma–associated herpesvirus.** See also **Kaposi sarcoma, primary effusion lymphoma.**

human immunodeficiency virus (HIV) /im′yo͞onō′difish″ə nsē/ [L, *humanus* + *immunis,* free from, *de,* from, *facere,* to make, *virus,* poison], a retrovirus that causes acquired immunodeficiency syndrome (AIDS). Retroviruses produce the enzyme reverse transcriptase, which allows the viral RNA genome to be transcribed into DNA inside the host cell. HIV is transmitted through contact with an infected individual's blood, semen, breast milk, cervical secretions, cerebrospinal fluid, or synovial fluid. It infects CD4-positive helper T cells of the immune system and causes infection with an incubation period that averages 10 years. With the immune system destroyed, AIDS develops as opportunistic infections such as candidiasis, Kaposi sarcoma, *Pneumocystis pneumonia,* and tuberculosis that attack organ systems throughout the body.

Aside from the initial antibody tests (enzyme-linked immunosorbent assay and Western blot) that establish the diagnosis for HIV infection, the most important laboratory test for monitoring the level of infection is the CD4 lymphocyte test, which determines the percentage of T lymphocytes that are CD4 positive. Patients with CD4 cell counts greater than $500/mm^3$ are considered most likely to respond to treatment with alpha-interferon and/or zidovudine. A significant drop in the CD4 cell count is a signal for therapeutic intervention with antiretroviral therapy. Vaccines based on the HIV envelope glycoproteins gp120 and gp160, intended to boost the immune system of people already infected with HIV, are being investigated. Formerly called **human T-cell leukemia virus type III, human T-cell lymphotropic virus type III.** See also **acquired immunodeficiency syndrome.**

human insulin, a biosynthetic product manufactured from *Escherichia coli* by recombinant deoxyribonucleic

---

Signs and symptoms of HIV infection

- Chills and fever
- Night sweats
- Dry, productive cough
- Dyspnea
- Lethargy
- Confusion
- Stiff neck
- Seizures
- Headache
- Malaise
- Fatigue
- Oral lesions
- Skin rash
- Abdominal discomfort
- Diarrhea
- Weight loss
- Lymphadenopathy
- Progressive generalized edema

From Monahan FD et al: *Phipps' medical-surgical nursing: health and illness perspectives,* ed 8, St Louis, 2007, Mosby.

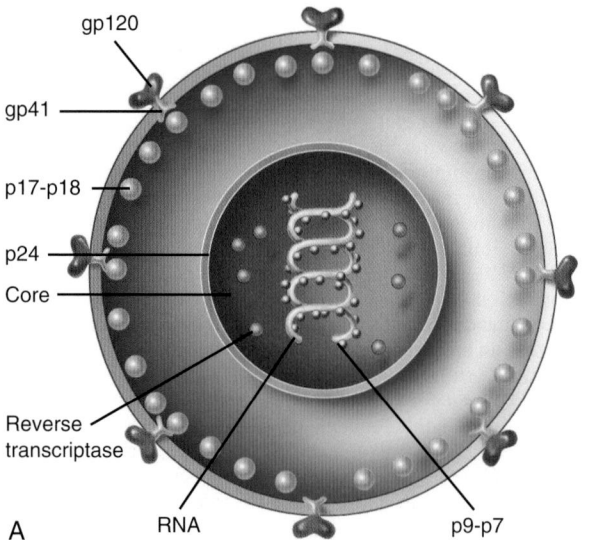

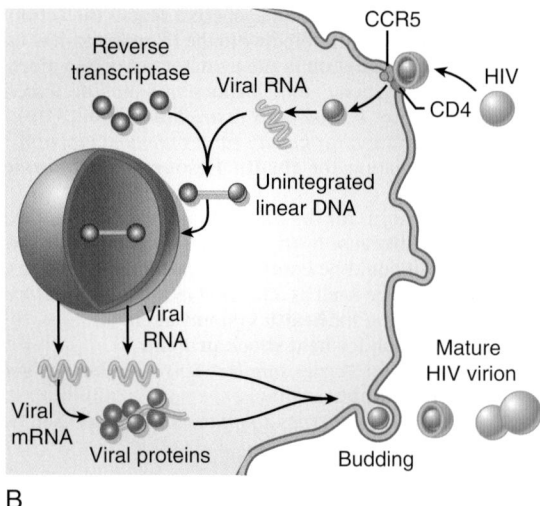

A, Diagram of a retrovirus with essential envelope glycoproteins, core enzymatic proteins, and RNA chromatin. B, Process of replication of human immunodeficiency virus (HIV) *(Sapp, 2004)*

acid technology. The advantage of human insulin is that it eliminates allergic reactions that occur with the use of animal insulins. See also **insulin,** def. 2.

human investigations committee, a group established in a hospital, school, or university to review research proposals involving human subjects to protect the rights of the people to be studied and to ensure that ethical principles are appropriately followed. Also called **human subjects review committee, institutional review board.**

humanism /h(y)ōō′məniz′əm/, a system of thought pertaining to the interests, needs, and welfare of human beings. The concept that human needs and values are of utmost importance.

humanistic existential therapy /hyōō′mənis″tik/, a kind of psychotherapy that promotes self-awareness and personal growth by stressing current reality and by analyzing and altering specific patterns of response to help a person realize his or her potential. This process may be facilitated in a group setting, where additional aspects of problems are revealed through interaction with others. Also called **existential humanistic psychotherapy.** Kinds include **client-centered therapy, existential therapy, Gestalt therapy.**

humanistic nursing model, a conceptual framework in which the nurse-patient relationship is analyzed as a human-to-human event rather than a nurse-to-patient interaction. The nurse makes therapeutic use of herself or himself, understanding the effects of nursing actions. Four phases are recognized in the development of the therapeutic relationship. The encounter phase is followed by the phase in which the identities of the nurse and patient emerge. The nurse empathizes and then sympathizes with the patient. The meaning of the patient's experience is important; hope and suffering are seen as central to that experience. Self-knowledge and self-awareness of the nurse are essential. Nursing intervention proceeds in five steps: observation of the need for intervention; validation of this observation; determination of the ability of the nurse to facilitate any necessary referral; formulation of a plan for meeting the need; and evaluation of the degree to which the need is met.

humanistic psychology, a branch of psychology that emphasizes a person's struggle to develop and maintain an integrated, harmonious personality as the primary motivational force in human behavior. See also **self-actualization.**

human leukocyte antigen (HLA), antigens formed from genes on chromosome 6. The loci are identified by numbers and letters, such as HLA-B27. Antigens are divided into three classes. Class I antigens (HLA-A, -B, and -C) occur on the surface of all nucleated cells and platelets and present endogenous antigen peptides to CD8 T cells (in other mammals: major histocompatibility complex [MHC] class I molecules). If donor and recipient HLA complexes do not match, the nonself antigens are recognized as foreign and destroyed by CD8 T cells. Class II antigens occur only on antigen-presenting cells and present exogenous antigens (in nonhumans MHC class II molecules). Class III antigens are nonhistocompatibility antigens, such as some complement components, that map in the HLA complex. Also called **major histocompatibility complex.** See also **HLA complex.**

human liver fluke. See **liver fluke.**

human lymphocyte antigen B27 (HLA-B27) test, a blood test done as part of paternity investigations to indicate tissue compatibility with tissue transplantation and to assist in the diagnosis of Reiter syndrome and other conditions.

human metapneumovirus, a species that causes respiratory infection in humans that is clinically similar to but less severe than that caused by respiratory syncytial virus.

human monocytic ehrlichiosis. See **ehrlichiosis.**

human natural killer cell, a lymphocyte that is able to lyse tumor and virally infected cells as part of the body's natural defense against malignancy and invasion by pathogens.

human papillomavirus (HPV), a virus that is the cause of common warts of the hands and feet, as well as lesions of the mucous membranes of the oral, anal, and genital cavities. More than 50 types of HPV have been identified, some of which are associated with cancerous and precancerous conditions. The virus can be transmitted through sexual contact, and specific types of the virus are a precursor to cancer of the cervix. Transmission has taken place without the presence of warts, indicating that it may occur through body fluids, such as semen or cervical secretions. There is no specific cure for an HPV infection, but the virus often can be controlled by podophyllin or interferon and the warts can be removed by cryosurgery, laser treatment, or conventional surgery. A vaccine is available for young girls, boys, and women (9–26 years) that protects against four types of HPV. The optimal time for administration is at age 11 or 12.

human papillomavirus (HPV) test, a fluid analysis of a cervical mucous specimen, performed to identify genital HPV in women who have abnormal Pap smears.

human parvovirus (HPV), a small single-stranded deoxyribonucleic acid virion that has been associated with several diseases, including erythema infectiosum and aplastic crises of chronic hemolytic anemias. Parvoviruses of various types also infect wild and domestic animals and may replicate in susceptible cells without a helper virus. See also **helper virus, virion.**

human placental lactogen (HPL), a placental hormone that may be deficient in certain abnormalities of pregnancy. The normal concentrations of this hormone in serum after the fifth week of pregnancy are 0.5 mcg/mL and increase to approximately 8 mcg/mL at the time of delivery. Also called **human chorionic somatomammotropin.**

human placental lactogen (HPL) test, a blood test to measure HPL, useful in monitoring placental function.

human prion diseases. See **transmissible spongiform encephalopathy.**

human rhinovirus 14, the common cold virus. It has a complex protein coat containing "sticky sites" that help attach the virus to cell receptors in the upper respiratory system. Because of the more than 100 strains of the virus that are known, devising a vaccine that would protect against all variations is difficult.

human subjects review committee. See **human investigations committee.**

human T-cell leukemia virus, human T-cell lymphotropic virus, *(Obsolete)* now called **human T-cell lymphotropic virus type I.**

human T-cell leukemia virus type I. See **human T-cell lymphotropic virus type I.**

human T-cell leukemia virus type II. See **human T-cell lymphotropic virus type II.**

human T-cell leukemia virus type III. See **human immunodeficiency virus.**

human T-cell lymphotropic virus type I (HTLV-I), a type C oncovirus of worldwide distribution, but most common in Japan, Africa, and the Caribbean basin, having an affinity for CD4 T lymphocytes; it causes chronic infection and is associated with adult T-cell leukemia and lymphoma and tropical spastic paraparesis. Also called **human T-cell leukemia virus type I.**

human T-cell lymphotropic virus type II (HTLV-II), a type C oncovirus having extensive serological cross-reactivity with HTLV-I, isolated from an atypical T-cell variant of hairy cell leukemia and also from patients with other hematological disorders. Also called **human T-cell leukemia virus type II.**

human T-cell lymphotropic virus type III (HTLV-III). See **human immunodeficiency virus.**

human T-cell lymphotropic virus (HTLV) type I/II antibody test, a blood test used to detect the antibodies produced when an individual has an HTLV infection. HTLV viruses may also be directly identified using molecular tests (polymerase chain reaction, or PCR) that detect the genetic material of the viruses.

Humatin, an amebicide. Brand name for **paromomycin sulfate.**

Humatrope, a brand of human synthetic growth hormone produced with recombinant deoxyribonucleic acid techniques. It is a polypeptide hormone with 191 amino acids in the same sequence as somatotropin. Brand name for **growth hormone.**

humectant /hyōōmek″tənt/, a substance that promotes retention of moisture.

humer-, prefix meaning "the humerus": *humeral stem.*

humeral. See **humerus.**

humeral articulation. See **shoulder joint.**

humeral stem, in arthroplasty of the shoulder or elbow, the part of the prosthesis that inserts into the end of the trimmed and prepared humerus.

humerus /hyōō″mərəs/ *pl. humeri* [L, shoulder], the bone of the upper arm, from the elbow to the shoulder joint where it articulates with the scapula. It comprises a body, a head, and two condyles. The body is almost cylindric proximally and prismatic and flattened distally and has two borders and three surfaces. The nearly hemispheric head articulates with the glenoid cavity of the scapula and has a constriction called the surgical neck, frequently the seat of a fracture. The condyles at the distal end have several features that articulate with the radius and ulna. Also called **arm bone. –humeral,** *adj.*

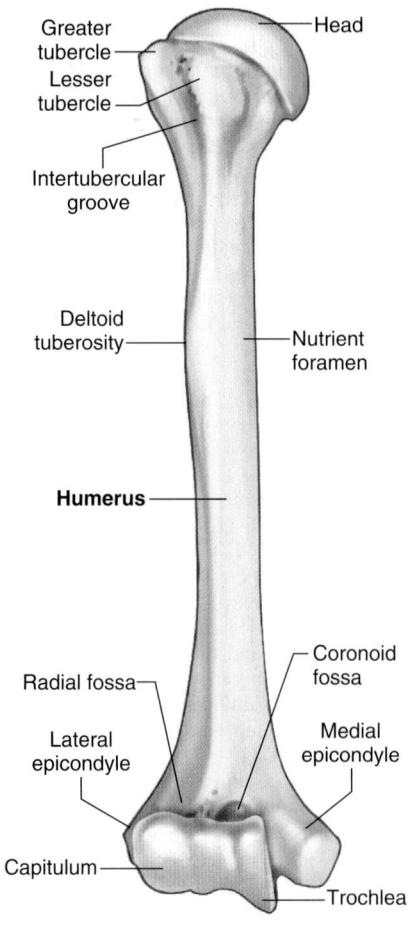

Greater tubercle
Lesser tubercle
Head
Intertubercular groove
Deltoid tuberosity
Nutrient foramen
Humerus
Radial fossa
Coronoid fossa
Lateral epicondyle
Medial epicondyle
Capitulum
Trochlea

Humerus *(Patton and Thibodeau, 2016)*

humidification /hyōōmid′ifikā″shən/ [L, *humidus,* moist, *facere,* to make], the process of increasing the relative humidity of the atmosphere around a patient through the use of aerosol generators or steam inhalers that exert an antitussive effect. Humidification acts by decreasing the viscosity of bronchial secretions, whereas added medications or sodium chloride may stimulate coughing by an irritant effect.

humidifier /hyōōmid′ifī′ər/ [L, *humidus,* moist, *facere,* to make], a medical device designed to adjust the amount of moisture in the atmosphere of a room or respiratory device.

humidifier lung, hypersensitivity pneumonitis caused by inhalation of air that has been passed through humidifiers, dehumidifiers, or air conditioners contaminated by any variety of fungi, amebas, or thermophilic bacteria.

humidity /hyōōmid″itē/ [L, *humidus,* moist], the level of moisture in the atmosphere, which varies with the temperature. The percentage is usually represented in terms of relative humidity, with 100% the point of air saturation, or the level at which the air can absorb no additional water.

humor /hyōō″mər/ [L, *humidus,* moist], any body fluid or semifluid substance such as blood or lymph. The term is often used in reference to the aqueous humor or the vitreous humor of the eye.

humoral hypercalcemia of malignancy, hypercalcemia of malignancy caused by bone resorption mediated by circulating osteoclast-activating factors released from distant tumor cells.

humoral immunity /hyōō″mərəl/ [L, *humor,* liquid, *immunis,* freedom], an immune response that is mediated by antibodies (immunoglobulins IgA, IgD, IgE, IgG, and IgM) produced by plasma cells that can recognize bacteria or parasite antigens and subsequently coat these microorganisms. The microorganisms are either (1) neutralized, (2) recognized by the complement system and destroyed, or (3) recognized and phagocytosed by phagocytes and subsequently destroyed. Compare **cell-mediated immunity.**

Humorsol, an ophthalmic anticholinesterase agent. Brand name for **demecarium bromide.**

humpback /hump″bak/ [Du, *homp,* thick slice; AS, *baec*], *(Obsolete)* now called **kyphosis.**

Humulin, brand name for *human insulin of recombinant deoxyribonucleic acid origin.*

Hungarian Medical Association of America, a voluntary organization of physicians and scientists of Hungarian heritage; founded in 1968.

hunger, a physical sensation usually associated with a craving or desire for food.

hunger contractions, strong contractions of the stomach usually associated with a desire for food.

hunger pain, epigastric cramps often associated with a desire for food.

hung-up reflex, a deep tendon reflex in which, after a stimulus is given and the reflex action takes place, the limb slowly returns to its neutral position. This prolonged relaxation phase is characteristic of reflexes in persons with hypothyroidism. See also **deep tendon reflex.**

Hunner's ulcer [Guy LeRoy Hunner, American surgeon, 1868–1957], a deep hemorrhagic lesion in the bladder associated with interstitial cystitis.

Hunter's canal. See **adductor canal.**

Hunter syndrome [Charles Hunter, Canadian physician, 1873–1955; Gk, *syn,* together, *dromos,* course], a hereditary defect in mucopolysaccharide metabolism affecting only males, characterized by dwarfism, kyphosis, gargoylism, and cognitive impairment. It is transmitted as an X-linked recessive trait. Females who carry the gene can be identified by biochemical tests. Also called **MPS II, X-linked mucopolysaccharidosis.** See also **mucopolysaccharidosis.**

Huntington disease [George S. Huntington, American physician, 1851–1916],　a rare abnormal hereditary condition characterized by chronic progressive chorea and mental deterioration that results in dementia. An individual afflicted with the condition usually shows the first signs in the fourth decade of life and dies within 15 years. It is transmitted as an autosomal trait and becomes progressively worse in severity as the trinucleotide repeats grow in successive generations. There is no known effective treatment, but symptoms can be relieved with medication.

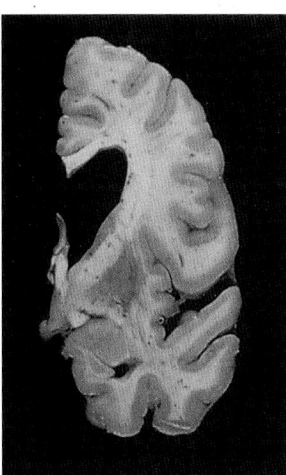

Huntington disease: dilated lateral ventricle with caudate and lentiform atrophy *(Perkin, 2002)*

Hurler syndrome [Gertrude Hurler, German physician, 1889–1965],　a type of mucopolysaccharidosis, transmitted as an autosomal-recessive trait, that produces severe cognitive impairment. Symptoms appear within the first few months of life. Characteristic signs of the disease are enlargement of the liver and spleen, often with cardiovascular involvement. Facial characteristics include a low forehead and enlargement of the head, sometimes resulting from hydrocephalus. Corneal clouding is common, and the neck is short. Marked kyphosis is apparent at the dorsolumbar level, and the hands and the fingers are short and broad. Flexion contractures are common. The disease process usually results in death during childhood from cardiac complications or pulmonary disorders. Also called **gargoylism, lipochondrodystrophy, MPS I.** See also **mucopolysaccharidosis.**

Hürthle cell adenoma /hirt′lə, hōorth′lē/ [Karl W. Hürthle, German histologist, 1860–1945],　a benign tumor of the thyroid gland composed of large cells with granular eosinophilic cytoplasm (Hürthle cells). Compare **Hürthle cell carcinoma.**

Hürthle cell carcinoma [Karl W. Hürthle],　a malignant neoplasm of the thyroid gland composed of Hürthle cells. These tumors, which occur more often in women than in men, are encapsulated, resemble adenomas, and are locally invasive. Compare **Hürthle cell adenoma.**

Hürthle cell tumor [Karl W. Hürthle],　a neoplasm of the thyroid gland composed of large cells with granular eosinophilic cytoplasm (Hürthle cells) that may be benign (Hürthle cell adenoma) or malignant (Hürthle cell carcinoma).

husband-coached childbirth.　See **Bradley method.**

Husted, Gladys L. and James H.,　nursing theorists who developed the Symphonological Bioethical Theory and the Symphonological Model for Ethical Decision Making. Symphonology is the system of ethics inherent in the mutual commitments and obligations agreed upon by the health care professional and patient. Central to this implicit agreement are the needs of the patient. Bioethical standards include autonomy, beneficence, fidelity, freedom, objectivity, and self-assertion. The model is designed to provide nurses and other health care professionals with theoretical guidelines for ethical delivery of care.

Hutch diverticulum,　herniation of bladder mucosa through a weak point in the wall near the ureterovesical junction, often caused by chronically high intravesical pressure.

Hutchinson-Gilford syndrome.　See **progeria.**

Hutchinson disease.　See **angioma serpiginosum.**

Hutchinson freckle [Jonathan Hutchinson, English surgeon, 1828–1913],　a tan patch on the skin that grows slowly and becomes mottled, dark, thick, and nodular. The lesion is usually seen on one side of the face of an elderly person. Local excision is recommended because it often becomes malignant. Also called **lentigo maligna.** See also **melanoma.**

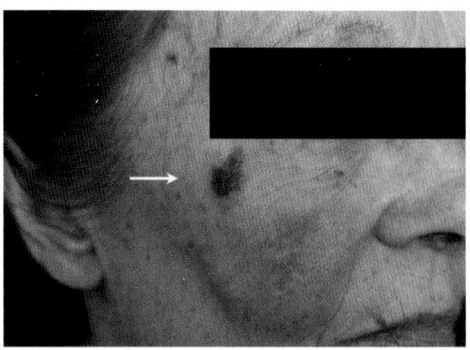

Hutchinson freckle *(Tiodorovic-Zivkovic et al, 2015)*

Hutchinson teeth [Jonathan Hutchinson],　a characteristic of congenital syphilis in which the adult secondary central and lateral incisors are peg-shaped or screwdriver-shaped, widely spaced, and notched at the end, with a central crescent-shaped deformity. Also called *Hutchinson incisors.* See also **syphilis.**

Hutchinson triad [Jonathan Hutchinson],　the interstitial keratitis, notched teeth, and deafness characteristic of congenital syphilis. See also **syphilis.**

Hutchison-type neuroblastoma [Robert G. Hutchison, English pediatrician, 1871–1960; Gk, *typos,* mark],　a neuroblastoma that has metastasized to the cranium.

HUTT,　acronym for **heads-up tilt table test.**

HVA,　abbreviation for **homovanillic acid.**

HV interval /in′tərvəl/,　the conduction time of an impulse traveling through the His-Purkinje system. It is measured from the onset of the atrioventricular bundle potential to the onset of ventricular activation as recorded on an electrogram.

HVL,　abbreviation for **half-value layer.**

hyal-.　See **hyalo-, hyal-.**

hyaline /hī″əlin/ [Gk, *hyalos,* glass],　pertaining to substances that are clear or glasslike.

hyaline bodies [Gk, *hyalos* + AS, *bodig*],　**1.** the residue of colloidal degeneration found in some cells. **2.** globules of neurosecretory material found in the posterior lobe of the pituitary. **3.** deposits of homogenous eosinophilic material found in renal tubular epithelium and representing excess protein molecules that cannot be metabolized or transported.

hyaline cartilage [Gk, *hyalos,* glass; L, *cartilago*],　a type of connective tissue composed of specialized cells in a translucent, pearly blue matrix. Hyaline cartilage thinly covers the articulating ends of bones, connects the ribs to the sternum, and supports the nose, the trachea, and part of the larynx. It is covered by a membranous perichondrium, except where it coats the ends of bones, and tends to calcify in advanced age. Compare **elastic cartilage, white fibrocartilage.**

hyaline cast, a transparent cast composed of mucoprotein.

hyaline membrane [Gk, *hyalos,* glass; L, *membrana*], a fibrous covering of the alveolar membranes in infants, caused by a lack of pulmonary surfactant associated with prematurity and low-birth-weight delivery. See also **respiratory distress syndrome of the newborn.**

hyaline membrane disease. See **respiratory distress syndrome of the newborn.**

hyaline thrombus, a transparent mass of hemolyzed erythrocytes.

hyalinization /hī′əlin′īzā″shən/ [Gk, *hyalos,* glass], the development of glassy homogenous material within a cell.

hyalinuria /-ōōr″ē·ə/ [Gk, *hyalos,* glass, *ouron,* urine], the presence of hyaline casts of protein in the urine, indicative of renal disease.

hyalo-, hyal-, prefix meaning "resembling glass": *hyalinization, hyaloplasm, hyaloid.*

hyalohyphomycosis /hī′əlohi″fomiko′sis/, a hyphomycosis caused by mycelial fungi with colorless walls, most of which are opportunistic. It usually occurs as a result of steroid therapy, indwelling catheters, immunosuppressive drugs, or cytotoxins.

hyaloid /hī″əloid/ [Gk, *hyalos,* glass, *eidos,* form], pertaining to or resembling hyaline.

hyaloid artery [Gk, *hyalos + eidos,* form], an embryonic blood vessel that branches to supply the vitreous body of the eye and develops part of the blood supply to the capsula vasculosa lentis. The hyaloid artery disappears from the fetus in the ninth month of pregnancy, leaving a vestigial remnant, the hyaloid canal, which persists in the adult as a narrow passage through the vitreous body from the optic disc to the posterior surface of the crystalline lens.

hyaloid membrane [Gk, *hyalos,* glass; L, *membrana*], a surface layer of the vitreous body of the eye, at the interface between the primary and secondary vitreous, and at the boundaries of the hyaloid canal.

hyaloplasm /hī″əlōplaz′əm/ [Gk, *hyalos + plasma,* formation], the portion of the cytoplasm that is clear and more fluid than the granular and reticular part. Also called **cytohyaloplasm, cytolymph, enchylema, interfibrillar mass of Flemming, interfilar mass, paramitome.**

hyaluronate /hī′əlōōronāt′/, a salt, anion, or ester of hyaluronic acid. The sodium salt and a derivative of it are used as analgesics in the treatment of osteoarthritis of the knee, administered by intraarticular injection.

hyaluronate sodium, the sodium salt of hyaluronic acid; a preparation obtained from chicken combs used as an analgesic in the treatment of osteoarthritis of the knee, administered by intraarticular injection.

hyaluronate sodium derivative, a polymeric derivative of hyaluronate sodium, having the same actions and uses.

hyaluronic acid /hī′əlyōōron′ik/, a mucopolysaccharide formed by the polymerization of acetylglucosamine and glucuronic acid, which occurs in vitreous humor, synovial fluids, and various tissues. Known as the cement substance of tissues, it forms a gel in intercellular spaces.

hyaluronidase /hī′əlyōōron′ədās/, an enzyme that hydrolyzes hyaluronic acid, a component of the extracellular matrix.

■ INDICATIONS: It is prescribed to increase the absorption and dispersion of parenteral drugs that have extravasated (e.g., vesicant chemotherapeutics), for hypodermoclysis, and for improvement of resorption of radiopaque agents.

■ CONTRAINDICATIONS: Acute inflammation, infection, or known hypersensitivity to this drug prohibits its use.

■ ADVERSE EFFECTS: The most serious adverse effect is hypersensitivity.

hybrid /hī″brid/ [L, *hybrida,* offspring], **1.** *n.,* an offspring produced by mating organisms from different species, varieties, or genotypes. **2.** *adj.,* pertaining to such an offspring.

hybridization /hī′bridīzā″shən/, **1.** the process of producing hybrids by crossbreeding. **2.** the process of combining single-stranded nucleic acids from different sources to form stable, double-stranded molecules. The technique involves fragmentation and separation of the source nucleic acids by heating, followed by recombination through cooling. The resulting hybrids can be DNA-DNA, DNA-RNA, or RNA-RNA duplexes.

hybridoma /hī′bridō″mə/, a hybrid cell formed by the fusion of a myeloma cell and an antibody-producing cell. Hybridomas are used to produce monoclonal antibodies.

hybrid subtraction, a method for producing digitized radiographic images that requires at least four images. It uses both energy and temporal subtraction steps to mitigate patient motion artifacts.

hybrid vigor. See **heterosis.**

Hycodan, a fixed-combination antitussive/anticholinergic medication. Brand name for **hydrocodone bitartrate,** *homatropine.*

Hycomine, a fixed-combination drug containing an decongestant and an antitussive. Brand name for *phenylpropanolamine hydrochloride,* **hydrocodone bitartrate.**

hydantoin /hīdan″tō·in/, any one of a group of anticonvulsant medications, chemically and pharmacologically similar to the barbiturates, that acts to limit seizure activity and reduce the spreading of abnormal electrical excitation from the focus of the seizure. A primary hydantoin in the management of almost all forms of epilepsy is phenytoin, formerly known as diphenylhydantoin. Frequent determination of the blood concentration of hydantoin is necessary.

hydatid /hī″dətid/ [Gk, *hydatis,* water drop], a cyst or cystlike structure that usually is filled with fluid, especially the cyst formed around the developing scolex of the dog tapeworm. Humans and sheep can become hosts to the larval stage by ingesting the eggs. Hydatid cysts may be identified by palpation. They occur most commonly in the liver. An acute anaphylactoid allergic reaction may occur if the cyst ruptures. See also **hydatid cyst, hydatid mole, hydatidosis.** *–hydatic, adj.*

hydatid cyst, a cyst in the liver that contains larvae of the tapeworm *Echinococcus granulosus,* whose eggs are carried from the intestinal tract to the liver via the portal circulation. Patients are generally asymptomatic, except for hepatomegaly and a dull ache over the right upper quadrant of the abdomen. Radiological tests are used in diagnosis, and, because no medical treatment is available, surgical removal of the cyst or percutaneous aspiration-injection-reaspiration drainage is indicated. Should not be confused with **hydatid mole.**

hydatid disease. See **echinococcosis.**

hydatidiform /hī′dətid′ifôrm/ [Gk, *hydatis,* water drop; L, *forma*], having the appearance or form of a hydatid.

hydatid mole, an intrauterine neoplastic mass of grapelike enlarged chorionic villi that occurs in approximately 1 in 1500 pregnancies in the United States and eight times more frequently in some Asian countries. Molar pregnancies are more common in older and younger women than in those between 20 and 40 years of age. The cause of the degenerative disorder is not known. It may be the result of a primary ovular defect, an intrauterine abnormality, or a nutritional deficiency. Also called *hydatidiform mole,* **vesicular mole.** See also **trophoblastic cancer.**

■ OBSERVATIONS: Characteristic signs are extreme nausea, uterine bleeding, anemia, hyperthyroidism, an unusually large uterus for the duration of pregnancy, absence of fetal heart sounds, edema, and high blood pressure. Diagnostic measures include ultrasonography, amniography, and measurement of chorionic gonadotropin level in the blood. In most cases the mole is discovered when abortion is threatened or in progress.

■ INTERVENTIONS: Oxytocin may be used to stimulate evacuation of a mole that is not spontaneously aborted, and curettage is usually performed several days later to be certain that no molar tissue remains in the uterus.

■ PATIENT CARE CONSIDERATIONS: It is important that pregnancy be avoided for at least 1 year and that assays for chorionic gonadotropin be performed to monitor for the risk of development of gestational trophoblastic disease.

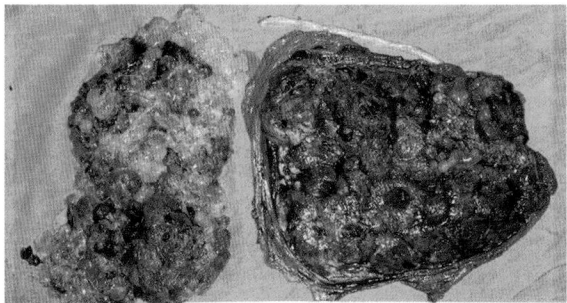

Gross appearance of the hydatid mole *(Peng et al, 2014)*

hydatidosis /hī′dətidō″sis/ [Gk, *hydatis* + *osis,* condition], infestation with the tapeworm *Echinococcus granulosus.*

hydatiform. See **hydatidiform.**

Hydeltrasol, a glucocorticoid. Brand name for *prednisolone sodium phosphate.*

Hydeltra TBA, a glucocorticoid. Brand name for *prednisolone tebutate.*

Hydergine, brand name for a fixed-combination drug containing various ergoloids used to treat dementia. Brand name for **ergoloid mesylate.**

hydr-. See **hydro-, hydr-.**

hydradenitis /hī′dradəni″tis/ [Gk, *hydor,* water, *aden,* gland, *itis,* inflammation], an infection or inflammation of the sweat glands.

hydrALAZINE hydrochloride /hīdral″əzēn/, a vasodilator used in hypertension.

■ INDICATIONS: It is prescribed in the treatment of moderate to severe hypertension, primary pulmonary hypertension, and hypertension of preeclampsia, and during the treatment of congestive heart failure.

■ CONTRAINDICATIONS: Coronary artery disease, mitral valvular rheumatic heart disease, or known sensitivity to this drug prohibits its use.

■ ADVERSE EFFECTS: Among the most serious adverse effects are angina pectoris, palpitations, tachycardia, hypotension, anorexia, tremors, blood dyscrasias, depression, nausea, peripheral neuritis, and a drug-induced lupuslike syndrome.

hydramnios /hīdram″nē·əs/ [Gk, *hydor* + *amnos,* lamb's caul], an abnormal condition of pregnancy characterized

by an excess of amniotic fluid. It occurs in less than 1% of pregnancies and is diagnosed by palpation, ultrasound, or radiographic examination. It is associated with maternal disorders, including toxemia of pregnancy and diabetes mellitus, and some fetal disorders, including anomalies of the GI tract, respiratory tract, and cardiovascular system, which may interfere with normal exchange of amniotic fluid. Fetal hydrops and multiple gestation are also associated with the condition. The incidence of premature rupture of the membranes, premature labor, and perinatal mortality is increased. Periodic amniocentesis may be necessary. Also called *hydramnion,* **polyhydramnios.** Compare **oligohydramnios.**

hydranencephaly /hīdran′ənsef″əlē/, a neurological disorder in which the cerebral hemispheres are lacking although the cerebellum, brainstem, and other central nervous system tissues may be intact. The newborn with hydranencephaly may have normal neurological functions but does not develop, and computed tomographic scans indicate an absence of cerebral tissue. Treatment is supportive. See also **anencephaly.**

hydrargyrism. See **mercury poisoning.**

hydrate /hī″drāt/ [Gk, *hydor,* water], **1.** a combination of a substance with one or more water molecules. **2.** a molecular association of a substance with water.

hydration /hīdrā″shən/ [Gk, *hydor,* water], a chemical process in which water is added to a substance. Hydration may or may not involve breaking bonds in the substance.

Hydrea, an antineoplastic drug. Brand name for **hydroxyurea.**

hydremic ascites /hīdrem″ik/ [Gk, *hydor* + *haima,* blood, *askos,* bag], an abnormal accumulation of fluid within the peritoneal cavity accompanied by hemodilution, as in protein calorie malnutrition. See also **ascites.**

-hydria, suffix meaning "level of fluid in the body": *chlorhydria, hyperchlorhydria.*

hydro-, hydr-, prefix meaning "water" or "hydrogen": *hydrocele, hydramnios.*

hydroa /hīdrō″ə/ [Gk, *hydor* + *oon,* egg], an unusual vesicular and bullous skin condition of childhood that recurs each summer after exposure to sunlight, sometimes accompanied by itching, lichenification, and scars. It usually disappears soon after puberty. Treatment includes use of sunscreen and avoidance of exposure to sunlight.

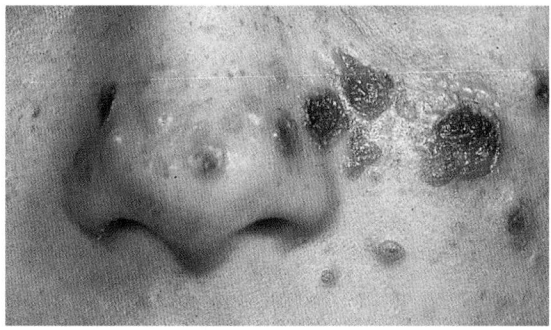

Hydroa vacciniforme *(du Vivier, 2002)*

hydroalcoholic /hi″dro·al″kähol′ik/, pertaining to or containing both water and alcohol.

hydrobilirubin /hī′drōbil′iroo″bin/ [Gk, *hydor,* water; L, *bilis,* bile, *ruber,* red], a reddish-brown bile pigment produced by the reduction of bilirubin.

hydrocarbon /-kär″bən/ [Gk, *hydor* + L, *carbo,* charcoal], any of a large group of organic compounds whose molecules are composed of hydrogen and carbon, many of which are derived from petroleum. Brief incidental exposures to low concentrations of solvent vapors that contain carbon, such as gasoline, lighter fluids, aerosol sprays, and spot removers, may be relatively harmless, but exposures to concentrations of hydrocarbon vapors often found in the home and in manufacturing environments may be dangerous.

hydrocele /hī″drōsēl′/ [Gk, *hydor* + *kele*, hernia], an accumulation of fluid in any saclike cavity or duct, specifically in the tunica vaginalis testis or along the spermatic cord. The condition is caused by inflammation of the epididymis or testis or by lymphatic or venous obstruction in the cord. Congenital hydrocele is caused by failure of the canal between the peritoneal cavity and the scrotum to close completely during prenatal development. In some newborns the defect may resolve spontaneously after neonatal obliteration of the communication. Treatment for persistent hydrocele is surgery. Aspiration is only a temporary measure and may induce secondary infection. See also **hydrocephalus, inguinal hernia.**

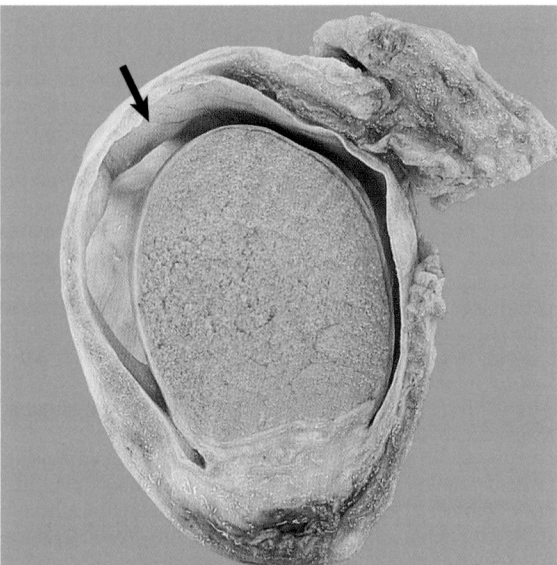

Hydrocele: The tunica vaginalis is dilated *(arrow)*
(Cross, 2013)

hydrocephalic cry /-səfal″ik/, an involuntary loud nighttime cry of a child who has acquired hydrocephalus.

hydrocephalocele, a hernia consisting of a watery sac of brain tissue protruding through a fissure into the skull.

hydrocephalus /-sef″ələs/ [Gk, *hydor* + *kephale,* head], a pathological condition characterized by an abnormal accumulation of cerebrospinal fluid, usually under increased pressure, within the cranial vault and subsequent dilation of the ventricles. Interference with the normal flow of cerebrospinal fluid may result from increased secretion of the fluid, obstruction within the ventricular system (noncommunicating or intraventricular hydrocephalus), or defective resorption from the cerebral subarachnoid space (communicating or extraventricular hydrocephalus). Hydrocephalus may be caused by developmental anomalies, infection, trauma, or brain tumors. Also called *hydrocephaly.* See also **macrocephaly.** —*hydrocephalic, adj., n.*

■ OBSERVATIONS: The condition may be congenital, with rapid onset of symptoms, or it may progress slowly so that neurological manifestations do not appear until early to late childhood or even early adulthood. In infants the head grows at an ab-

normal rate with separation of the sutures, bulging fontanels, and dilated scalp veins. The face becomes disproportionately small, and the eyes appear depressed within the sockets. Typical behavior includes irritability with lethargy and vomiting, opisthotonos, lower extremity spasticity, and failure to perform normal reflex actions. If the condition progresses, lower brainstem function is disrupted; the skull becomes enormous; the cortex is destroyed; and the infant displays somnolence, seizures, and cardiopulmonary obstruction and usually does not survive the neonatal period. At later onset, after the cranial sutures have fused and the skull has formed, symptoms are primarily neurological and include headache, edema of the optic disc, strabismus, and loss of muscular coordination. Hydrocephalus in infants is suspected when head growth is observed to be in excess of the normal rate. In all age groups, diagnosis is confirmed by such procedures as cerebrospinal fluid examination, computed tomography, air encephalography, arteriography, and echoencephalography.

■ INTERVENTIONS: Treatment consists almost exclusively of surgical intervention to correct the ventricular obstruction, reduce the production of cerebrospinal fluid, or shunt the excess fluid by ventricular bypass to the right atrium of the heart or to the peritoneal cavity. Surgically treated hydrocephalus with continued neurosurgical and medical management has a survival rate of approximately 80%, although prognosis depends largely on the cause of the condition. Hydrocephalus is frequently associated with myelomeningocele, in which case there is a less favorable prognosis.

■ PATIENT CARE CONSIDERATIONS: Primary care of the child with hydrocephalus consists of maintaining adequate nutrition, proper positioning and support to prevent extra strain on the neck, and assistance with diagnostic evaluation and procedures. After surgery, in addition to routine care and observation to prevent complications, especially infection, the nurse gives support to the parents and teaches them how to care for a child with a functioning shunt, specifically how to recognize signs that indicate shunt malfunction or infection and how to pump the shunt.

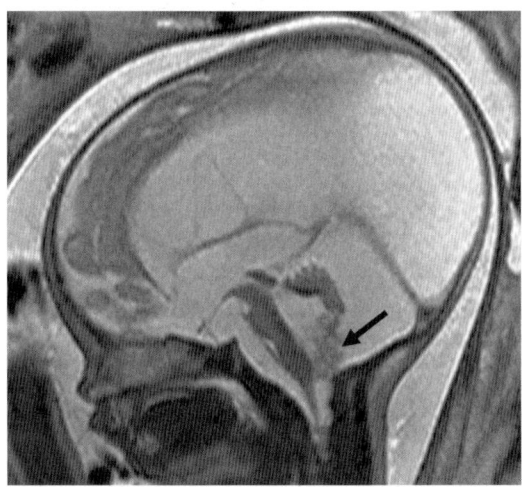

Hydrocephalus *(Lyons et al, 2015)*

hydrochloric acid (HCl) /-klôr″ik/ [Gk, *hydor* + *chloros,* green], an aqueous solution of hydrogen chloride or hydrogen ions and chloride ions. Hydrochloric acid is secreted in the stomach and is a major component of gastric juice.

hydrochlorothiazide /-klôr′ōthī″əzīd/, a thiazide diuretic.

■ INDICATIONS: It is prescribed in the treatment of mild to moderate hypertension and edema caused by congestive heart failure or protein loss by the kidney (nephritic syndrome).

■ CONTRAINDICATIONS: Anuria or known hypersensitivity to this drug, to other thiazide medication, or to sulfonamide derivatives prohibits its use.

■ ADVERSE EFFECTS: Among the more serious adverse effects are hypoglycemia, hyperglycemia, hyperuricemia, and hypersensitivity reactions.

hydrocholeretics /-kō′lərет″iks/ [Gk, *hydor* + *chloe,* bile, *eresis,* removal], drugs that stimulate the production of bile with a low specific gravity or with a minimal proportion of solid constituents.

Hydrocil Instant, a laxative. Brand name for *psyllium hydrophilic mucilloid.*

hydrocodone bitartrate /-kō″dōn/, an opioid antitussive and analgesic.

■ INDICATIONS: It is prescribed in the treatment of cough and moderate to severe pain.

■ CONTRAINDICATIONS: Drug dependence or known hypersensitivity to this drug prohibits its use.

■ ADVERSE EFFECTS: Among the more serious adverse effects are drug dependence and respiratory and circulatory depression.

hydrocolloid, a gelatinous suspension in which water is the dispersion material. It is used in dentistry as an impression material.

hydrocortisone /-kôr″tisōn/, a topical corticosteroid.

■ INDICATIONS: It is prescribed for the topical treatment of skin inflammation.

■ CONTRAINDICATIONS: Viral and fungal diseases of the skin that occur where circulation is impaired or known hypersensitivity to steroids prohibits its use.

■ ADVERSE EFFECTS: Among the more serious adverse effects are various systemic side effects that may result from prolonged or excessive use. Local irritation of the skin may occur.

hydrocortisone enema, an aqueous solution of hydrocortisone administered rectally as an antiinflammatory in the treatment of ulcerative colitis.

hydrocortisone, hydrocortisone acetate, hydrocortisone cyclopentylpropionate. See **cortisol.**

hydrocortisone probutate, an ester of hydrocortisone used topically for the relief of inflammation and pruritus in corticosteroid-responsive dermatoses.

hydrocortisone sodium succinate. See **cortisol.**

Hydrocortone, a glucocorticoid. Brand name for *hydrocortisone acetate.*

hydrocytosis /hi″drōsito′sis/. See **stomatocytosis.**

HydroDIURIL, a diuretic. Brand name for **hydrochlorothiazide.**

hydroencephalocele /hi″drō-ensef′älosēl″/. See **hydrocephalocele.**

hydroflumethiazide /-floo″methī″əzīd/, a diuretic.

■ INDICATIONS: It is prescribed in the treatment of mild to moderate hypertension and edema caused by congestive heart failure or protein loss in the urine (nephrotic syndrome).

■ CONTRAINDICATIONS: Anuria or known hypersensitivity to this drug, to other thiazide medication, or to sulfonamide derivatives prohibits its use.

■ ADVERSE EFFECTS: Among the more serious adverse effects are blood disorders, hypotension, hypokalemia, hyperglycemia, hyperuricemia, and hypersensitivity reactions.

hydrofluoric acid /hi″drōfloor″ik/, a term applied to aqueous solutions of hydrogen fluoride, an organic acid used in dilute solutions for cleaning and etching. It is extremely poisonous, as well as corrosive to the skin.

hydrogel, a gel in which water is the dispersion medium.

hydrogen (H) /hi″drəjən/ [Gk, *hydor* + *genein,* to produce], a gaseous monovalent element. Its atomic number is 1; its atomic mass is 1.008. It is the simplest and the lightest of the elements and is a colorless, odorless, highly flammable diatomic gas. It occurs in pure form only sparsely in the earth and the atmosphere but is plentiful in the sun and in many other stars. Hydrogen is a component of numerous compounds, many of them produced by the body. As a component of water, hydrogen is crucial in the metabolic interaction of acids, bases, and salts within the body and in the fluid balance necessary for the body to survive.

hydrogenase /hi″drōjənās′/ [Gk, *hydor,* water, *genein,* to produce, *ase,* suffix indicating an enzyme], an enzyme that catalyzes reduction of molecules by combining them with two atoms of hydrogen.

hydrogenation. See **reduction,** def. 1.

hydrogen bonding, a type of dipole-dipole intermolecular force in which a hydrogen atom covalently linked to an electronegative element such as oxygen, nitrogen, or fluorine has a large degree of positive character relative to the electronegative atom, thereby causing the compound to possess a large dipole and to associate strongly with other like molecules.

hydrogen carbonate. See **bicarbonate.**

hydrogen cyanide (HCN), an extremely poisonous, colorless, toxic, volatile liquid or gas with the aroma of bitter almonds. It occurs naturally in almonds and in the stone pits of peaches, plums, and other fruits. Inhalation of the gas can cause death within a minute. When dissolved in water, it is called hydrocyanic acid or prussic acid.

hydrogen donor, a compound that gives up hydrogen (usually H^+, a proton) to another compound.

hydrogen ion, a positively charged hydrogen atom or proton $[H^+]$.

hydrogen ion concentration of blood, a measure of blood pH and its effect on the ability of the hemoglobin molecule to hold oxygen. See also **Bohr effect.**

hydrogen peroxide, a disinfectant and sterilizing agent without antiseptic properties because it is rapidly inactivated by enzymes in the skin. However, the frothing that occurs is beneficial since it loosens debris in wounds.

hydrogen sulfide poisoning, poisoning by excessive exposure to hydrogen sulfide gas, seen primarily in those who work with petroleum or petrochemicals. The gas is a potent inhibitor of cytochrome-*c* oxidase, and poisoning is characterized by metabolic acidosis and anoxia. Severe cases may result in coma with death from respiratory paralysis. Treatments include immediate inhalation of amyl nitrate, injections of sodium nitrate, inhalation of oxygen, administration of bronchodilators, and, in severe cases, hyperbaric oxygen therapy.

hydroglossa. See **ranula.**

hydrokinetics /-kinet″iks/ [Gk, *hydor,* water, *kinesis,* motion], the study of movement of fluids.

hydrolase /hi″drōlās/, an enzyme that cleaves ester bonds by the addition of water.

hydrolysis /hidrol″isis/ [Gk, *hydor* + *lysis,* loosening], the chemical alteration or decomposition of a compound with water.

hydrolytic /-lit″ik/ [Gk, *hydor,* water, *lysis,* loosening], pertaining to or having the ability to produce hydrolysis.

hydrolyze /hi″drōlīz/ [Gk, *hydor,* water, *lysis,* loosening], **1.** to cause or bring about hydrolysis. **2.** to cause a substance to split into component parts by the addition of water.

hydrometer /hidrom″ətər/ [Gk, *hydor* + *metron,* measure], a device that determines the specific gravity or density of a liquid by a comparison of its weight with that of an equal volume of water. A calibrated hollow glass device is placed in the liquid being examined, and the depth to which the device settles in the liquid is noted.

hydromorphone hydrochloride /-môr′fōn/, an opioid analgesic.

■ INDICATIONS: It is used to treat moderate to severe pain.

■ CONTRAINDICATIONS: It is used with caution in many conditions, including head injuries, asthma, impaired renal or hepatic function, or unstable cardiovascular status. Known hypersensitivity to this drug prohibits its use.

■ ADVERSE EFFECTS: Among the most serious adverse effects are drowsiness, dizziness, nausea, constipation, respiratory and circulatory depression, and drug addiction.

hydromyelia /hī′drōmī·ē′lē·ə/ [Gk, *hydor*, water + *myelos*, marrow], a pathological condition characterized by dilation of the central canal of the spinal cord with increased fluid accumulation. Compare **syringomyelia.**

hydronephrosis /hī′drōnefrō″sis/ [Gk, *hydor* + *nephros*, kidney, *osis*, condition], distension of the pelvis and calyces of the kidney by urine that cannot flow past an obstruction in a ureter. Ureteral obstruction may be caused by a tumor, a calculus lodged in the ureter, inflammation of the prostate gland, or edema caused by a urinary tract infection. Symptoms include pain in the flank and, in some cases, hematuria, pyuria, and hyperpyrexia. IV pyelography, cytoscopy, or retrograde pyelography may be used in diagnosis. Surgical repair or removal of the obstruction may be necessary. Prolonged hydronephrosis causes atrophy and eventual loss of kidney function. Also called **ureterohydronephrosis.** See also **urinary calculus.** –*hydronephrotic, adj.*

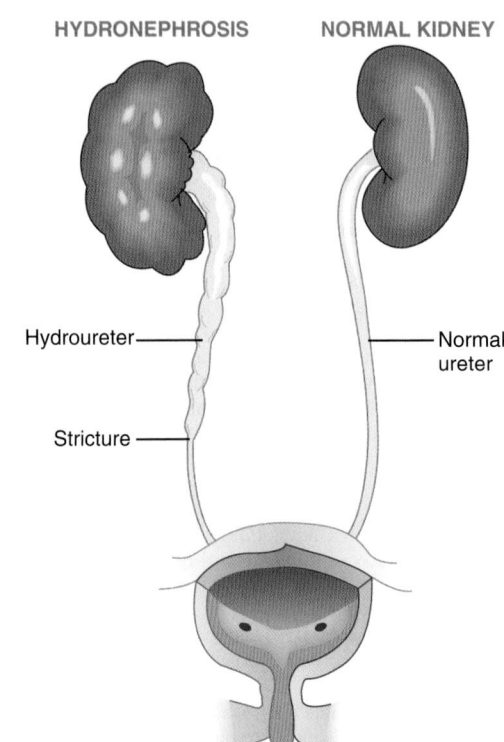

HYDRONEPHROSIS   **NORMAL KIDNEY**

Hydroureter   Normal ureter

Stricture

Hydronephrosis *(Proctor and Adams, 2014)*

hydropenia /-pē′nē·ə/, **1.** the process of removing water from a living thing. **2.** a condition resulting from lack of water in the body tissues.

hydropericarditis, inflammation of the pericardium accompanied by excessive accumulation of serous fluid.

hydropericardium. See **pericardial effusion.**

hydroperitoneum /-per′itōnē″əm/, an accumulation of fluid in the peritoneum.

hydrophilic /-fil″ik/ [Gk, *hydor* + *philein*, to love], pertaining to the property of attracting or associating preferentially with water molecules, a quality possessed by polar radicals or ions. Compare **hydrophobic.**

hydrophobia /-fō′bē·ə/ [Gk, *hydor* + *phobos*, fear], **1.** one of the later symptoms of a rabies infection, when muscle spasms in the throat make drinking anything extremely painful. **2.** a morbid, extreme fear of water.

hydrophobic [Gk, *hydor* + *phobos*, fear], pertaining to the property of repelling or preferentially excluding water molecules, a quality possessed by nonpolar radicals or molecules that are more soluble in organic solvents than in water. Compare **hydrophilic.**

hydrophone /hī′drəfōn/, a small-diameter probe with a piezoelectric element, usually about 0.5 mm in diameter, at one end. When placed in an ultrasound beam, the hydrophone produces an electric signal.

hydrophthalmos, **1.** a type of glaucoma characterized by enlargement and distension of the fibrous coats of the eyeball. **2.** See **congenital glaucoma.**

hydropic /hīdrop″ik/ [Gk, *hydrops*], containing an excess of water or watery fluid.

Hydropres, a fixed-combination drug containing a diuretic and an antihypertensive drug. Brand name for **hydrochlorothiazide, reserpine.**

hydrops /hī″drops/ [Gk, dropsy], an abnormal accumulation of clear watery or serous fluid in a body tissue or cavity, such as a joint, a graafian follicle, a fallopian tube, the abdomen, the middle ear, or the gallbladder. Hydrops in the entire body may occur in infants born with thalassemia or severe Rh sensitization. Formerly called **dropsy.**

hydrops fetalis, massive edema in the fetus or newborn, usually in association with severe erythroblastosis fetalis. Severe anemia and effusions of the pericardial, pleural, and peritoneal spaces also occur. The condition usually leads to death, even with immediate exchange transfusions after delivery. Also called **fetal hydrops.**

hydrops gravidarum [Gk, *hydor*, water; L, *gravidus*, pregnant], edema caused by pregnancy.

hydrops tubae profluens, blocking of the fallopian tube. See **intermittent hydrosalpinx.**

hydroquinone /hī′drōkwin″ōn/, a dermatological bleaching agent.

■ INDICATIONS: It is prescribed to reduce pigmentation of the skin in certain conditions in which an excess of melanin causes hyperpigmentation.

■ CONTRAINDICATIONS: Sunburn, prickly heat, other irritation of the skin, or known hypersensitivity to this drug prohibits its use.

■ ADVERSE EFFECTS: Among the more serious adverse effects are tingling, erythema, burning, and severe inflammation of the skin.

hydrosalpinx /hī′drōsal″pingks/ [Gk, *hydor* + *salpinx*, tube], an abnormal condition of the fallopian tube in which it is cystically enlarged and filled with clear fluid. It is the result of an infection that has previously occluded the tube at both ends. The purulent material produced by the infection undergoes liquefaction during resolution of the acute phase of the inflammatory process.

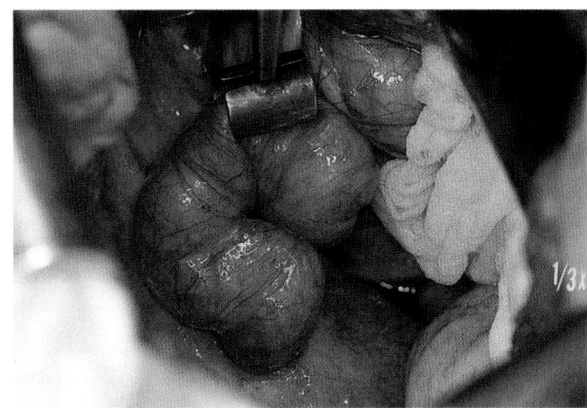

Hydrosalpinx *(Baggish and Karram, 2011)*

hydrosis [Gk, *hydor,* water, *osis,* condition], pertaining to the production of sweat.

Hydro-Sphere Nebulizer, a trademark for a type of nebulizer in which a source gas enters a hollow sphere coated with a film of water. The gas exits through slits at the top of the sphere as an aerosol jet, carrying particles of fluid from the sphere's surface.

hydrostatic /-stat″ik/ [Gk, *hydor,* water, *statos,* standing], pertaining to fluids at rest or in equilibrium and the pressure they exert.

hydrostatic densitometry, the weighing of a person under water to determine the ratio of lean tissue to body fat.

hydrostatic pressure, the pressure exerted by a liquid.

hydrostatics, the study of pressures in liquids at rest or in equilibrium.

hydrotherapy /-ther″əpē/ [Gk, *hydor + therapeia,* treatment], the use of water in the treatment of various disorders. Hydrotherapy may include continuous tub baths or shower sprays.

hydrothorax /-thôr″aks/ [Gk, *hydor + thorax,* chest], a noninflammatory accumulation of serous fluid in one or both pleural cavities.

hydrotropism /-trō″pizəm/ [Gk, *hydor + trope,* turning], the tendency of a cell or organism to turn or move in a certain direction under the influence of a water stimulus.

hydrous /hī′drəs/ [Gk, *hydor,* water], pertaining to a substance or object that contains water or is moist.

hydrous wool fat. See **lanolin.**

hydroxide (OH⁻) /hīdrok″sīd/, an ion.

hydroxyamphetamine hydrobromide /hīdrok′sē·əmfet″ə mēn/, an adrenergic agonist.
- INDICATIONS: It is prescribed for short-term dilation of the pupil for ophthalmoscopy and as a diagnostic aid in Horner syndrome.
- CONTRAINDICATIONS: Narrow-angle glaucoma or known hypersensitivity to this drug prohibits its use.
- ADVERSE EFFECTS: Among the more serious adverse effects are increased intraocular pressure and photophobia.

hydroxyandrosterone /hīdrok′sē·andros″tərōn/ [Gk, *hydor + andros,* male, *stereos,* solid], a sex hormone secreted by the testes and adrenal glands. Its normal accumulation in the urine of men after 24-hour collection is 0.1 to 8 mg; in women, 0 to 0.5 mg.

hydroxyapatite /hīdrok′sē·ap″ətīt/, an inorganic compound composed of calcium, phosphate, and hydroxide, found in the bones and teeth in a crystallized latticelike form that gives these structures rigidity.

hydroxybenzene. See **carbolic acid.**

hydroxychloroquine sulfate /-klôr″əkwīn/, a drug initially developed to treat malaria that also has efficacy against autoimmune diseases.
- INDICATIONS: It is prescribed in the treatment of malaria and the suppression of acute paroxysmal attacks of the disease; in the treatment of extraintestinal, usually hepatic, amebiasis; and in conjunction with salicylate to reduce the symptoms of lupus erythematosus and rheumatoid arthritis.
- CONTRAINDICATIONS: Concurrent use of other 4-aminoquinolones or of gold salts or a known hypersensitivity to this drug or to other 4-aminoquinolones prohibits its use. It is used with caution in cases of alcoholism, blood dyscrasia, severe neurological disorder, retinal or visual field damage, psoriasis, or porphyria. The drug is not usually recommended in pregnancy because it has been associated with damage to the central nervous system of the fetus.
- ADVERSE EFFECTS: Among the many severe adverse effects are retinopathy, corneal opacity, polyneuritis, seizure, agranulocytosis, and hepatitis. The incidence and severity of these and many other adverse effects increase with the dosage and prolonged duration of treatment.

17-hydroxycorticosteroid /-kôr′tikos″təroid/, any steroid hydroxylated at carbon-17 secreted by adrenal glands and occasionally measured in the urine in a test for determining adrenal function and diagnosing hypoadrenalism or hyperadrenalism. The normal accumulation in the urine of men after 24-hour collection is 5.5 to 14.5 mcg; in women, 4.9 to 12.9 mcg; and in children, slightly less. The levels are normally two to four times higher in all cases after injection of 25 USP units of adrenocorticotropic hormone.

17-hydroxycorticosteroids test (17-OCHS), an obsolete 24-hour urine test formerly used to detect abnormal levels of 17-OCHS. Elevated levels are seen in hyperfunction of the adrenal gland (Cushing syndrome), whereas low levels are seen in hypofunction (Addison disease).

11-hydroxyetiocholanolone /hīdrok′sē·ē′tē·ōkolan″ə lōn/, a sex hormone secreted by the testes and adrenal glands. The normal accumulation in the urine after 24-hour collection is 0.2 to 0.6 mg in men and 0.1 to 1 mg in women.

5-hydroxyindoleacetic acid (5-HIAA) /hīdrok′sē·in′dōlē· əset″ik/, an acid produced by serotonin metabolism, measured in the blood and urine to aid in the diagnosis of certain kinds of tumors. It commonly rises above normal levels in whole blood in association with asthma, diarrhea, rapid heartbeat, and other symptoms and is elevated in the urine of patients with carcinoid syndrome. Its normal concentration in whole blood is 0.05 to 0.20 g/mL; its normal accumulation in urine after 24-hour collection is 1 to 5 mg.

5-hydroxyindoleacetic acid test, a 24-hour urine test used to detect and follow the clinical course of patients with carcinoid tumors, which may grow in the appendix, intestine, lung, or any tissue derived from the neuroectoderm.

hydroxyl (OH) /hīdrok″sil/, a monovalent radical consisting of an oxygen atom and a hydrogen atom. The hydroxyl radical is an extremely reactive species capable of damaging DNA.

hydroxyproline /-prō′lēn/, an amino acid whose level in the urine is elevated in diseases of the bone and in certain genetic disorders, such as Marfan syndrome. Its normal accumulation in urine after a 24-hour collection is 10 to 75 mg.

hydroxypropyl cellulose /hīdrok″sēpro′pil sel′u-lōs/, a water-soluble derivative of cellulose, used as a pharmaceutic

H

aid and applied topically to the conjunctiva to protect and lubricate the cornea in the treatment of dry eye.

5-hydroxytryptamine (5-HT). See **serotonin.**

hydroxyurea /hīdrok′siyo͞ore̅″ə/, an antineoplastic.

■ INDICATIONS: It is prescribed in the treatment of a variety of neoplasms and other conditions involving the blood and by itself or as a radiosensitizer for the treatment of other cancers, including those involving the brain, head and neck, lungs, kidneys, ovaries, and prostate.

■ CONTRAINDICATIONS: Bone marrow depression or known hypersensitivity to this drug prohibits its use. It is not to be given to women who are or may become pregnant.

■ ADVERSE EFFECTS: The most serious adverse effect is bone marrow depression. GI disturbances and dermatitis also may occur.

hydrOXYzine hydrochloride /hīdrok″səzēn/, an antihistamine.

■ INDICATIONS: It is prescribed for the relief of anxiety, nervous tension, hyperkinesis, itching, and motion sickness.

■ CONTRAINDICATIONS: Known hypersensitivity to this drug is the only contraindication.

■ ADVERSE EFFECTS: No serious adverse effects have been observed. Decreased mental alertness sometimes occurs.

hygiene /hī″jēn/ [Gk, *Hygieia,* the goddess of health], **1.** the principles and science of the preservation of health and prevention of disease. **2.** sanitation.

hygienist /hī″jənist, hījē″nist/ [Gk, *Hygieia*], one who practices the principles and laws of hygiene. See also **hygiene.**

hygro-, prefix for terms relating to moistness or moisture.

hygroma /hī·grō′mə/ *pl. hygromas, hygromata* [Gk, *hygros,* moist + *-oma,* tumor], a sac, cyst, or bursa distended with a fluid.

hygrometer /hīgrom″ətər/ [Gk, *hygros,* moist, *metron,* measure], an instrument that directly measures relative humidity of the atmosphere or the proportion of water in a specified gas or gas mixture, without extracting the moisture.

hygroscopic humidifier /-skop″ik/, a humidifying device attached to the tubing circuit of a mechanical ventilator or anesthesia gas machine to maintain a constant rate of humidity in the trachea.

Hygroton, a diuretic. Brand name for **chlorthalidone.**

Hylorel, an antihypertensive drug. Brand name for **guanadrel sulfate.**

hymen /hī″mən/ [Gk, membrane], a fold of mucous membrane, skin, and fibrous tissue that covers the introitus of the vagina. It may be absent; small; thin and pliant; or, rarely, tough and dense, completely occluding the introitus. When the hymen is disrupted, small rounded "tags" of tissue remain. See also **carunculae hymenales.**

hymenal /hī″mənəl/ [Gk, *hymen,* membrane], pertaining to the hymen.

hymenal tag, normal redundant hymenal tissue protruding from the floor of the infant's vagina during the first weeks after birth. It eventually disappears without treatment.

hymenectomy /hī″mənek″təmē/ [Gk, *hymen,* membrane, *ektomē,* excision], the surgical excision of a membrane, particularly the hymen.

hymenolepiasis, heavy infestation by *Hymenolepis nana,* a rat tapeworm that may cause abdominal pain, bloody stools, and disorders of the nervous system, especially in children. Contaminated food spreads the disease, which is endemic in the United States. Quinacrine hydrochloride or hexylresorcinol is used to treat the infestation. Praziquantel is the drug of choice for treatment of this infection. Also called **rat tapeworm infection.**

Hymenolepis /hī″mənol′əpis/ [Gk, *hymen,* membrane + *lepis,* rind], a genus of tapeworms of the family

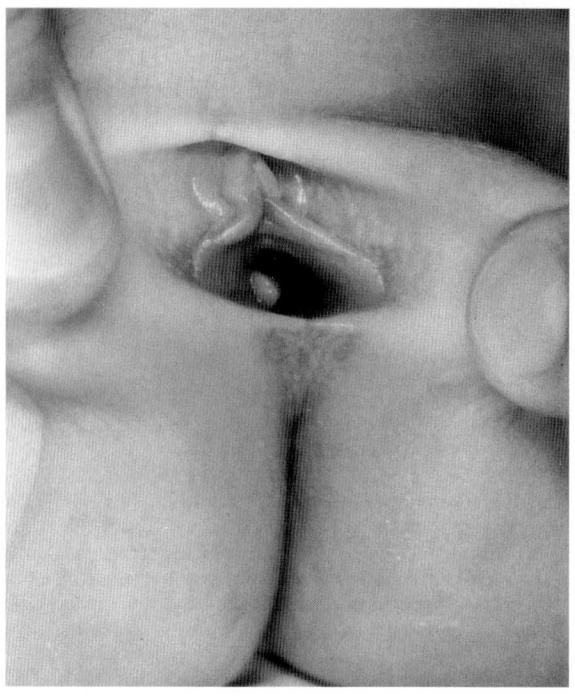

Infant with hymenal tag *(Wein et al, 2012)*

Hymenolepididae, which parasitize birds and mammals, including humans. See also **hymenolepiasis.**

hymenotomy /hī″mənot″əmē/ [Gk, *hymen* + *temnein,* to cut], the surgical incision of the hymen.

hyo-, prefix meaning "shaped like the letter *u* or pertaining to the hyoid bone": *hyoepiglottic, hyoglossus.*

hyoepiglottic ligament, a ligament that extends from the midline of the epiglottis anterosuperiorly to the body of the hyoid bone.

hyoglossal /hī′ō-glos″əl/ [Gk, *hyoeides,* upsilon, U-shaped; *glossa,* tongue], pertaining to the tongue and the horseshoe-shaped hyoid bone at the base of the tongue immediately above the thyroid cartilage.

hyoglossal membrane, a widening of the lingual septum connecting the root of the tongue to the hyoid bone.

hyoglossus /-glos″əs/ [Gk, *hyoeides* + *glossa,* tongue], a depressor muscle of the tongue that arises from the hyoid bone.

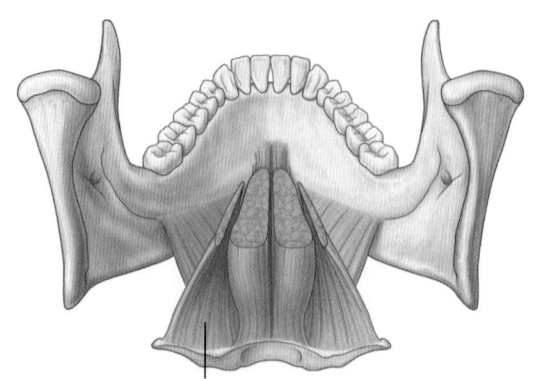

Hyoglossus muscle

Hyoglossus muscle *(Drake, Vogl, and Mitchell, 2015)*

hyoid /hī′oid/ [Gk, *hyoeides,* upsilon, U-shaped], **1.** *n.,* the hyoid bone. **2.** *adj.,* pertaining to the hyoid bone.

hyoid arch [Gk, *hyoeides* + L, *arcus,* bow], the second pharyngeal or branchial arch. It is present in typical form in the embryo, but the skeletal elements develop into the stapes and styloid process of the temporal bone of the adult.

hyoid bone /hī′oid/ [Gk, *hyoeides,* upsilon, U-shaped; AS, *ban,* bone], a single U-shaped bone suspended from the styloid processes of the temporal bones. The body of the hyoid is square and flat; its ventral surface is convex and angled cranially. Two greater wings of the bone attach to the lateral thyroid ligaments, and the body of the bone attaches to various muscles, such as the hypoglossus and the sternohyoideus. The hyoid is palpable in the neck. Also called **lingual bone, os hyoideum.**

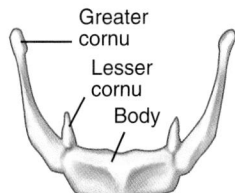

Greater cornu
Lesser cornu
Body

Hyoid bone

hyoscine. See **scopolamine.**

hyoscine hydrobromide. See **scopolamine.**

hyoscyamine /hī′əsī″əmēn/, an anticholinergic/antispasmodic drug.

■ INDICATIONS: It is prescribed in the treatment of hypermotility of the GI and lower urinary tracts and is used preoperatively to reduce secretions and block vagal inhibitory effects on the heart.

■ CONTRAINDICATIONS: Narrow-angle glaucoma, asthma, obstruction of the genitourinary or GI tract, severe ulcerative colitis, or known hypersensitivity to this drug prohibits its use.

■ ADVERSE EFFECTS: Among the more serious adverse effects are blurred vision, central nervous system effects, tachycardia, dry mouth, decreased sweating, and hypersensitivity reactions.

hyp-. See **hypo-, hyp-.**

hypalgesia /hī′paljē″zē·ə/ [Gk, *hypo,* below, *algesis,* pain], diminished sensibility to pain. −*hypalgesic, adj.*

hypaxial muscles, muscles of the limbs and trunk.

hyper-, prefix meaning "excessive," "above," or "beyond": *hyperacuity, hyperalkalinity, hyperemesis.*

Hyperab, a passive immunizing agent. Brand name for **rabies immune globulin.**

hyperacidity /hī′pərəsid′itē/ [Gk, *hyper,* excess; L, *acidus,* sour], an excessive amount of acidity, as in the stomach. See also **hyperchlorhydria.**

hyperactive child syndrome, *(Obsolete)* now called **attention deficit–hyperactivity disorder.**

hyperactivity /-aktiv″itē/ [Gk, *hyper* + L, *activus,* active], any abnormally increased motor activity or function involving either the entire organism or a particular organ, as the heart or thyroid. Compare **hypoactivity.** See also **attention deficit disorder.**

hyperacuity /-akyōō′itē/ [Gk, *hyper* + *akouien,* to hear], excessive sensitivity to sounds.

hyperadenosis /-ad′ənō″sis/ [Gk, *hyper* + *aden,* gland, *osis,* condition], a condition characterized by enlarged glands.

hyperadrenalism. See **Cushing disease.**

hyperadrenocorticism. See **Cushing syndrome.**

hyperalbuminemia /-albyōō′minē″mē·ə/, an excessive amount of albumin in the blood.

hyperaldosteronism. See **aldosteronism.**

hyperalgia /-al″jə/, extreme sensitivity to pain.

hyperalimentation /-al′iməntā″shən/ [Gk, *hyper* + L, *alimentum,* nourishment], **1.** overfeeding or the ingestion or administration of an amount of nutrients that exceeds the demands of the appetite. **2.** See **total parenteral nutrition.**

hyperalkalinity /-al′kəlin″itē/, a condition of excessive alkalinity.

hyperammonemia /hī′pəram′ōnē″mē·ə/ [Gk, *hyper* + L, *sal ammoniacus* + Gk, *haima,* blood], abnormally high levels of ammonia in the blood. Ammonia is produced in the intestine, absorbed into the blood, and detoxified in the liver. It is also generated as a by-product of protein metabolism. An increased production of ammonia or a decreased ability to detoxify it increases the blood levels of ammonia. The disorder is controlled by low-protein diets, including essential amino acid mixtures. Untreated, the condition leads to hepatic encephalopathy, characterized by asterixis, vomiting, lethargy, coma, and death.

hyperammonuria /hī′peram′ōnu′re·ə/, increased excretion of ammonia in the urine, as with hyperammonemia.

hyperbaric chamber /-ber″ik/ [Gk, *hyper,* excess, *baros,* weight, *kamara,* arched roof], an airtight chamber containing an oxygen atmosphere under high pressure. A patient may be placed in the chamber for the treatment of certain infections, tumors, and cardiovascular diseases in which atmospheric oxygen pressures up to three times normal may have therapeutic value.

hyperbaric oxygen, oxygen under greater than atmospheric pressure.

hyperbaric oxygenation [Gk, *hyper* + *baros,* weight, *oxys,* sharp, *genein,* to produce], the administration of oxygen at greater-than-normal atmospheric pressure. The procedure is performed in specially designed chambers that permit the delivery of 100% oxygen at atmospheric pressure that is three times normal. The technique is used to overcome the natural limit of oxygen solubility in blood, which is about 0.3 mL of oxygen per 100 mL of blood. In hyperbaric oxygenation, dissolved oxygen can be increased to almost 6 mL per 100 mL and the PO_2 in blood may be nearly 2000 mm Hg at 3 atmospheres absolute. Hyperbaric oxygenation has been used to treat carbon monoxide poisoning, air embolism, smoke inhalation, acute cyanide poisoning, decompression sickness, wounds, clostridial myonecrosis, and certain cases of blood loss or anemia in which increased oxygen transport may compensate in part for hemoglobin deficiency. Factors limiting the usefulness of hyperbaric oxygenation include the hazards of fire and explosive decompression, pulmonary damage and neurological toxicity at high atmospheric pressures, cardiovascular debility of the patient, and the need to interrupt treatments repeatedly because exposures at maximum atmospheric pressures must be limited to 90 minutes. Also called *hyperbaric oxygen therapy.*

hyperbaric solution [Gk, *hyper,* excess, *baros,* weight], a type of spinal anesthetic that has a specific gravity greater than that of cerebrospinal fluid so that it will settle into the lowest parts of the spinal canal.

hyperbarism /-ber″izəm/, any disorder resulting from exposure to increased ambient pressure, usually caused by sudden exposure to or a significant increase in pressure. See also **barotrauma, decompression sickness.**

hyperbetalipoproteinemia /hī′pərbā′təlip′ōprō′tēnē″mē·ə/ [Gk, *hyper* + *beta,* second letter of Greek alphabet, *lipos,* fat, *proteios,* first rank, *haima,* blood], type II hyperlipoproteinemia, a genetic disorder of lipid metabolism characterized by abnormally high levels of serum cholesterol and the appearance of xanthomas on the tendons of the heels, knees, and fingers. There is a marked tendency to development of atherosclerosis and early myocardial infarction, especially among males. Treatment attempts to reduce blood cholesterol levels in the hope of lowering the risk of early death from heart disease. The patient is usually counseled to avoid most meats, eggs, milk products, and all saturated fats and is encouraged to eat fish, grains, fruits, vegetables, lean poultry, and unsaturated fats. Exercise may be recommended, and drugs may be prescribed in some cases. See also **cholesteremia.**

hyperbilirubinemia /hī′pərbil′iroo′binē″mē·ə/ [Gk, *hyper* + L, *bilis,* bile, *ruber,* red; Gk, *haima,* blood], greater-thannormal amounts of the bile pigment bilirubin in the blood, often characterized by jaundice, anorexia, and malaise. Hyperbilirubinemia is most often associated with liver disease or biliary obstruction, but it also occurs when there is excessive destruction of red blood cells, as in hemolytic anemia. Treatment is specific to the underlying condition. When bilirubin levels are high, treatment includes phototherapy and hydration.

hyperbilirubinemia of the newborn, an excess of bilirubin in the blood of the neonate. It is usually caused by a deficiency of an enzyme that results from physiological immaturity or by increased hemolysis, especially that produced by blood group incompatibility, which, in severe cases, can lead to kernicterus. Also called **neonatal hyperbilirubinemia.** See also **breast milk jaundice, cholestasis, Crigler-Najjar syndrome, Dubin-Johnson syndrome, erythroblastosis fetalis, Gilbert syndrome, kernicterus, phototherapy in the newborn, Rotor syndrome.**

■ OBSERVATIONS: The elevation of serum bilirubin levels in the normal newborn is caused by the greater concentration of circulating erythrocytes and the infant's diminished ability to conjugate and excrete bilirubin because of a lack of the enzyme glucuronyl transferase, a reduced albumin concentration, and a lack of intestinal bacteria. Jaundice appears when blood levels of bilirubin exceed 5 mg/dL, usually not before 24 hours in full-term neonates. Clinically observable jaundice or serum bilirubin level exceeding 5 mg/dL within the first 24 hours of life is abnormal and indicates a pathological cause of hyperbilirubinemia. In erythroblastosis fetalis, jaundice is evident shortly after birth, and bilirubin levels rise rapidly. Severely affected infants also show hepatosplenomegaly and signs of anemia, which quickly worsen, causing a decrease in oxygen-carrying capacity that may lead to cardiac failure and shock. Early symptoms of kernicterus are lethargy, poor feeding, and vomiting, followed by severe neurological excitation or depression, including tremors, twitching, convulsion, opisthotonos, a high-pitched cry, hypotonia, diminished deep tendon reflexes, and absence of Moro and sucking reflexes. Brain damage generally does not occur at serum bilirubin levels below 20 mg/dL in an otherwise healthy term infant. Factors such as metabolic acidosis, lowered albumin levels, hypoxia, hypothermia, free fatty acids, and certain drugs, especially salicylates and sulfonamides, increase the risk at much lower levels. The mortality rate may reach 50%. Sequelae of kernicterus include cognitive impairment, minimal brain dysfunction, cerebral palsy, delayed or abnormal

motor development, hearing loss, ataxia, athetosis, perceptual problems, and behavioral disorders.
■ INTERVENTIONS: Such preventive measures as frequent feedings during the first 6 to 12 hours of life to increase GI motility have little justification. Infants with mild jaundice require no treatment, only observation. Phototherapy is the usual treatment for severe or increasing hyperbilirubinemia. If hyperbilirubinemia is the result of increased hemolysis caused by blood group incompatibility, exchange transfusion may be done. It is usually indicated if laboratory analysis reveals a positive antiglobulin test result, a hemoglobin concentration of the cord blood below 12 g/dL, or a bilirubin level of 20 mg/dL or more in a full-term infant or 15 mg/dL or more in a premature infant. Phototherapy may be used in conjunction with exchange transfusion, except in cases of Rh incompatibility. If used immediately after the initial exchange transfusion, phototherapy may remove enough bilirubin from the tissues to make subsequent transfusions unnecessary. Clinical practice nomograms using major and minor risk factors are useful for predicting worsening hyperbilirubinemia and need for phototherapy or exchange transfusion.
■ PATIENT CARE CONSIDERATIONS: An initial concern is to identify high-risk infants in whom hyperbilirubinemia and kernicterus may develop. The nurse may monitor the serum bilirubin levels and observe for evidence of jaundice, anemia, central nervous system irritability, and such conditions as acidosis, hypoxia, and hypothermia. In erythroblastosis fetalis, exchange transfusion may be necessary. The amounts of blood infused and withdrawn, the vital signs, and any signs of exchange reactions are noted. Resuscitative equipment is kept available. Optimal body temperature is maintained: Hypothermia increases oxygen and glucose consumption, causing metabolic acidosis, and hyperthermia damages the donor's erythrocytes, causing an elevation in the amount of free potassium, which may lead to infant cardiac arrest. After the procedure a sterile dressing is applied to the catheter site.

hypercalcemia /hī′pərkalsē″mē·ə/ [Gk, *hyper* + L, *calx,* lime; Gk, *haima,* blood], *adj.,* greater-than-normal amounts of calcium in the blood, most often resulting from excessive bone resorption and release of calcium, as occurs in hyperparathyroidism, metastatic tumors of bone, Paget disease, and osteoporosis. Clinically patients with hypercalcemia experience confusion, anorexia, abdominal pain, muscle pain, and weakness. Extremely high levels of blood calcium may result in coma, shock, kidney failure, and death. Hypercalciuria is also found in most patients with elevated blood calcium level. Prednisone, diuretics, isotonic saline solution, and other drugs may be used in treatment.

hypercalcemia of malignancy, an abnormal elevation of serum calcium associated with malignant tumors, resulting from osteolysis caused by bone metastases or by the action of circulating osteoclast-activating factors released from distant tumor cells (known as humoral hypercalcemia of malignancy).

hypercalcemic nephropathy /-kalsē″mik/ [Gk, *hyper,* L, *calx,* lime, *haima,* blood; Gk, *nephros,* kidney, *pathos,* disease], a progressive disorder of kidney function caused by an excessive level of calcium in the blood. The calcium causes cumulative functional and histological abnormalities that lead to a decreased glomerular filtration rate and kidney failure.

hypercalciuria /hī′pərkal′sēyoor″ē·ə/ [Gk, *hyper* + L, *calx,* lime; Gk, *ouron,* urine], the presence of abnormally great amounts of calcium in the urine, resulting from conditions such as sarcoid, hyperparathyroidism, or certain types of arthritis that are characterized by augmented bone resorption. Immobilized patients are often hypercalciuric. Some people absorb more calcium than is normal and therefore excrete greater than normal amounts into their urine. Concentrated amounts of calcium in the urinary tract may form kidney stones. Treatment is directed to correcting any underlying disease condition and limiting dietary intake of calcium. Also called *hypercalcinuria.* Compare **hypercalcemia.** *−hypercalciuric, adj.*

hypercapnia /hī'pərkap″nē·ə/ [Gk, *hyper* + *kapnos,* vapor], greater-than-normal amounts of carbon dioxide in the blood. Also called **hypercarbia.**

hypercapnic acidosis /-kap″nik/ [Gk, *hyper* + *kapnos,* vapor; L, *acidus,* sour, *osis,* condition], an excessive acidity in body fluids caused by an increase in carbon dioxide tension in the blood. The condition may be secondary to pulmonary insufficiency. As carbon dioxide accumulates in the blood, its acidity increases.

hypercarbia. See **hypercapnia.**

hypercarotenemia, an excessive amount of carotene in the blood usually associated with a yellow discoloration of the skin.

hypercementosis, a nonneoplastic deposition of excessive cementum that is continuous with normal radicular cementum.

hyperchloremia /-klôrē″mē·ə/ [Gk, *hyper* + *chloros,* green, *haima,* blood], an excessive level of chloride in the blood that results in acidosis. Also spelled *hyperchloraemia.* See also **acidosis.**

hyperchlorhydria /-klôrhid″rē·ə/ [Gk, *hyper* + *chloros* + *hydor,* water], the excessive secretion of hydrochloric acid by cells lining the stomach, resulting in gastric acid levels higher than the reference range. Also called **chlorhydria.** See also **hyperacidity.**

hypercholesterolemia /-kōles′tərōlē″mē·ə/ [Gk, *hyper* + *chole,* bile, *stereos,* solid, *haima,* blood], a condition in which greater-than-normal amounts of cholesterol are present in the blood. High levels of cholesterol and other lipids may lead to the development of atherosclerosis. Hypercholesterolemia may be reduced or prevented by avoiding saturated fats, which are found in red meats, eggs, and dairy products, or by certain medications. Inherited hypercholesterolemia is caused by a defect in the low-density lipoprotein receptor or apolipoprotein B; in such cases diet is a less effective factor.

hypercholesterolemic xanthomatosis. See **low-density lipoprotein (LDL) receptor disorder.**

hyperchromatic. See **hyperchromia.**

hyperchromia /-krō″mē·ə/ [Gk, *hyper* + *chroma,* color], an increase of hemoglobin in the erythrocytes.

hyperchylomicronemia /-kī′lōmī′krōnē″mē·ə/ [Gk, *hyper* + *chylos,* juice, *mikros,* small, *haima,* blood], type I hyperlipoproteinemia, a rare congenital deficiency of an enzyme essential to fat metabolism. Fat accumulates in the blood as chylomicron. The condition affects children and young adults, in whom xanthomas (fatty deposits) in the skin, hepatomegaly, and abdominal pain develop. Pancreatitis is the most significant complication. Strict limitation of dietary fat may allow the person to prevent discomfort and complications. Also called **familial lipoprotein lipase deficiency.** See also **chylomicron.**

hypercoagulability /-kō·ag′yələbil″itē/ [Gk, *hyper* + L, *coagulare,* to curdle, *habilis,* able], a tendency of the blood to clot more rapidly than is normal.

hyperdactyly. See **polydactyly.**

hyperdiploid. See **hyperploid.**

hyperdipsia, intense thirst of relatively brief duration.

hyperdontia, an excess number of teeth. See **supernumerary teeth.**

hyperdynamic circulation, abnormally increased circulatory volume with low vascular resistance and often tachycardia, a condition sometimes accompanying septic shock, preeclampsia, and other conditions.

hyperdynamic syndrome /-dīnam″ik/ [Gk, *hyper* + *dynamis,* force], a cluster of symptoms that signals the onset of septic shock, often including a shaking chill, rapid rise in temperature, flushing of the skin, galloping pulse, and alternating rise and fall of the blood pressure. This is a medical emergency treated by keeping the patient warm, elevating the legs to assist venous return, administering IV fluids and antibiotics, and managing blood pressure. Nothing is given by mouth. The patient's head is turned to the side to prevent aspiration if there is vomiting. See also **septic shock.**

hyperemesis /hī′per·em′ə·sis/ [Gk, *hyper,* excess + *emesis,* vomit], excessive vomiting.

hyperemesis gravidarum /hī′pərem″isis/ [Gk, *hyper* + *emesis,* vomiting; L, *gravida,* pregnant], an abnormal condition of pregnancy characterized by protracted vomiting, weight loss, and fluid and electrolyte imbalance. If the condition is severe and intractable, brain damage, liver and kidney failure, and death may result. The cause of the condition is not known; an increase in levels of chorionic gonadotropins or other hormones, an immunological sensitivity to products of conception, or aggravation of preexisting emotional conflicts has been suggested, but a causal relationship has not been proved. It occurs in approximately 3 of every 1000 pregnancies. Its incidence has diminished in recent years.

■ OBSERVATIONS: Dry mucous membranes are a sign of dehydration. Other signs include decreased skin elasticity, a rapid pulse, and falling blood pressure. The specific gravity of the urine rises, and the volume of urine excreted falls. The hematocrit is elevated because of hemoconcentration. Loss of electrolytes in vomitus leads to metabolic acidosis with hypokalemia, hypochloremia, and hyponatremia. Severe potassium deficit alters myocardial function; the electrocardiogram may show prolonged P-R and Q-T intervals and inverted T waves. In addition to weight loss, undernourishment causes fever, ketosis, and acetonuria. Severe vitamin B deficiency may result in encephalopathy manifested by confusion and eventually coma. Laboratory analyses of blood indicate increased concentrations of metabolic products normally cleared by the liver and kidneys. Forceful vomiting may cause retinal hemorrhages that impair vision and gastroesophageal tears that bleed, causing hematemesis or melena.

■ INTERVENTIONS: Effective therapy arrests vomiting and achieves rehydration, adequate nutrition, and emotional stabilization. Bed rest is instituted. Antiemetics safe for the fetus are sometimes administered. Fluids, electrolytes, nutrients, and vitamins are given parenterally if the woman is unable to retain fluids by mouth. The fetal heart rate is measured frequently. Psychiatric consultation and therapy are sometimes beneficial. Termination of pregnancy is curative but almost never required.

■ PATIENT CARE CONSIDERATIONS: Women are often frightened of and uncomfortable about their illness at a time when they worry about the health of their unborn child as well as their own health. Visitors are encouraged; isolation, formerly recommended, is not desirable. Sympathetic listening and supportive, nonjudgmental care are provided. The woman and her family are told often that the prognosis is excellent

H

for both mother and baby. The woman is weighed regularly, and her weight is accurately recorded, for the best evidence of recovery is steady weight gain.

hyperemia /hī′pərē″mē·ə/   [Gk, *hyper* + *haima,* blood],   an excess of blood in part of the body, caused by increased blood flow, as in the inflammatory response, local relaxation of arterioles, or obstruction of the outflow of blood from an area. Skin overlying a hyperemic area usually becomes reddened and warm. −*hyperemic, adj.*

hyperesthesia /-esthē″zhə/,   an extreme sensitivity of one of the body's sense organs, such as pain or touch receptors in the skin.

hyperextension /-exten″shən/   [Gk, *hyper* + L, *extendere,* to stretch out],   movement at a joint to a position beyond the joint's normal alignment in anatomical position, increasing the resting angle between two articulating bones.

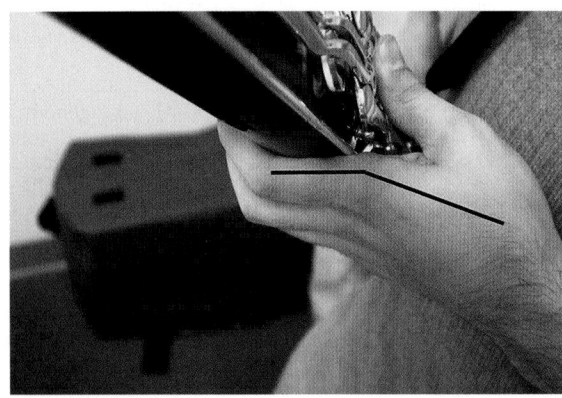

Hyperextension *(© 2008 – Jan Dommerholt)*

hyperflexia /-flek″shə/   [Gk, *hyper* + L, *flectere,* to bend],   the forcible overflexion or bending of a limb.

hyperfunction /-fungk″shən/   [Gk, *hyper* + L, *functio,* performance],   increased function of any organ or system.

hypergenesis /-jen″əsis/   [Gk, *hyper* + *genesis,* origin],   excessive growth or overdevelopment. The condition may involve the entire body, as in gigantism, or any part, or it may result in the formation of extra parts, such as additional fingers or toes. −*hypergenetic, adj.*

hypergenetic teratism /-jənet″ik/   [Gk, *hyper* + *genesis* + *tera,* monster],   a congenital anomaly in which there is excessive growth of a part, an organ, or the entire body.

hypergenitalism /-jen″itəliz′əm/,   the presence of abnormally large external genitalia. The condition is usually associated with precocious puberty.

hyperglobulinemia /-glob′yəlinē″mē·ə/   [Gk, *hyper,* L, *globulus,* small globe, *haima,* blood],   an excess of globulin in the plasma.

hyperglycemia /hī′pərglīsē″mē·ə/   [Gk, *hyper* + *glykys,* sweet, *haima,* blood],   a greater-than-normal amount of glucose in the blood. Most frequently associated with diabetes mellitus, the condition may also occur in newborns, after the administration of glucocorticoid hormones, or with an excess infusion of IV solutions containing glucose, especially in poorly monitored long-term hyperalimentation.

hyperglycemic-glycogenolytic factor.   See **glucagon.**

hyperglycemic-hyperosmolar nonketotic syndrome /-glīsē″mik/   [Gk, *hyper* + *glykys* + *hyper* + *osmos,* impulse; L, *non,* not, (ketone)],   a diabetic syndrome caused by

hyperosmolarity of extracellular fluid and resulting in severe osmotic diuresis causing dehydration. HHS is often a consequence of dehydration, stress, or diabetogenic medication given to an elderly person with undiagnosed or diagnosed type 2 diabetes. Also called *hyperglycemic-hyperosmolar syndrome (HHS).*

hyperglyceridemia /-gli′səridē″mē·ə/   [Gk, *hyper* + *glykys* + *haima,* blood],   an excess of glycerides, particularly triglycerides, in the blood. It is caused by a congenital defect in the ability to metabolize the amino acid glycine.

hyperglycinemia,   an increased concentration of glycine in the blood.

hyperglycogenolysis /-gli′kōjənol″isis/,   excessive breaking down of glycogen to glucose in animal tissue.

hyperglycosuria /-gli′kōso͞or″ē·ə/,   an excess of sugar in the urine.

hyperglysemia /-gli′kəsē″mē·ə/,   an excess of sugar in the blood. See also **hyperglycemia.**

hypergonadism /-gō″nədiz′əm/   [Gk, *hyper* + *gone,* seed],   excessive secretion of hormones from the ovaries or testes.

hyperhidrosis /hī′pərhīdrō″sis, -hidrō″sis/   [Gk, *hyper* + *hidros,* perspiration],   excessive perspiration often caused by heat, hyperthyroidism, strong emotion, menopause, or infection. Symptomatic therapy usually includes topical antiperspirants and anticholinergics or Botox. Severe cases may be treated with surgery. Also called **hyperidrosis, polyhidrosis, polyidrosis.**

hyperhydration.   See **overhydration.**

hyperidrosis.   See **hyperhidrosis.**

hyperimmune /-imyo͞on″/   [Gk, *hyper* + L, *immunis,* freedom],   having a greater-than-normal immunity because of an unusual abundance of antibodies.

hyperimmune globulin,   any of various immune globulin preparations especially high in antibodies against certain specific diseases.

hyperimmune plasma,   plasma containing high levels of antibodies after donors are vaccinated to stimulate an immune response. The plasma is then administered to recipients unable to make antibodies. It confers passive immunity.

hyperimmunoglobulinemia D,   an abnormal elevation of immunoglobulin D in the serum.

hyperimmunoglobulinemia D syndrome (HIDS),   a periodic fever inherited as an autosomal-recessive trait, caused by mutations in the gene for mevalonate kinase and having onset usually before 1 year of age. It is characterized by attacks of high fever preceded by chills, occurring at intervals of approximately 4 to 8 weeks and lasting 4 to 6 days, often accompanied by headache, arthritis and arthralgia, erythematous lesions, and hepatosplenomegaly. Serum IgD levels are continuously high. Also called **Dutch type periodic fever.**

hyperinsulinism /-in″səliniz′əm/   [Gk, *hyper* + L, *insula,* island],   an excessive amount of insulin in the body. It may be caused by administration of an insulin dose greater than required or the presence of an insulin-secreting tumor in the islets of Langerhans or insulin reference. If there is hypoglycemia, symptoms include hunger, shakiness, and diaphoresis. See also **insulin shock.**

hyperirritability /-irit′əbil″itē/   [Gk, *hyper;* L, *irritare,* to tease],   excessive excitability or sensitivity; exaggerated response to a stimulus.

hyperkalemia /hī′pərkəlē″mē·ə/   [Gk, *hyper* + L, *kalium,* potassium; Gk, *haima,* blood],   greater-than-normal amounts of potassium in the blood. This condition is seen frequently in acute renal failure, massive trauma, major burns, and Addison disease. Early signs are nausea, diarrhea, and muscle weakness. As potassium levels increase, marked cardiac changes are observed in the electrocardiogram due to changes in membrane potential. Treatment of severe hyperkalemia includes oral administration of Kayexalate (sodium polystyrene sulfonate) and IV administration of sodium bicarbonate, calcium salts, and dextrose. Hemodialysis is used if these measures fail.

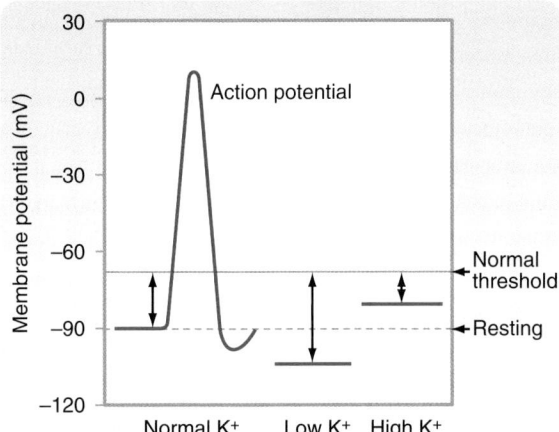

Hyperkalemia causes the membrane potential to become less negative, which decreases excitability by inactivating the fast Na⁺ channels responsible for the depolarizing phase of the action potential
(Koeppen and Stanton, 2010)

hyperkalemic periodic paralysis. See **adynamia episodica hereditaria.**

hyperkeratinization /-ker′ətinīzā″shən/ [Gk, *hyper,* excessive, *keras,* horn], an abnormal horny thickening of the epithelium of the palms and soles.

hyperkeratosis /-ker′ətō″sis/ [Gk, *hyper* + *keras,* horn, *osis,* condition], overgrowth of the cornified epithelial layer of the skin. See also **callus, corn.** –*hyperkeratotic, adj.*

hyperketonemia /-kē′tōnē″mē-ə/, an abnormally high level of ketone bodies in the blood.

hyperketonuria /-kē′tōnoo̅o̅r″ē-ə/, an abnormally high level of ketone bodies in the urine.

hyperkinesis. See **attention deficit disorder.**

hyperlactation /-laktā″shən/, a condition in which lactation continues beyond the usual period of breastfeeding. Also called **superlactation.**

hyperlipemia /-lipē″mē-ə/, cloudy or opaque plasma caused by fat particles called chylomicrons seen subsequent to a fat-laden meal caused by a lipoprotein lipase deficiency or a defect in the conversion of low-density lipoprotein to high-density lipoprotein.

hyperlipidemia /-lip′idē″mē-ə/ [Gk, *hyper* + *lipos,* fat, *haima,* blood], an excess of lipids, including glycolipids, lipoproteins, and phospholipids, in the plasma.

hyperlipidemia type I, a condition of elevated blood lipid levels characterized by an increase in both cholesterol and triglycerides and caused by the presence of chylomicrons. It is inherited as an autosomal-recessive trait and has a low risk of atherosclerosis. It results in recurrent bouts of acute pancreatitis. The symptoms begin in childhood. The accumulation of triglycerides is generally proportional to the amount of dietary fat. Treatment is primarily dietary. Both saturated and unsaturated fats are restricted to amounts that produce less than 500 mg/dL of blood, evaluated after an overnight fast. Also called **exogenous hypertriglyceridemia, familial hyperglyceridemia, fat-induced hyperlipidemia.**

hyperlipidemia type IIA, hyperlipidemia type IIB. See **low-density lipoprotein (LDL) receptor disorder.**

hyperlipidemia type III. See **broad beta disease.**

hyperlipidemia type IV, a relatively common form of hyperlipoproteinemia characterized by a slight elevation in cholesterol levels, a moderate elevation of triglyceride levels, and an elevation of the triglyceride carrier protein (very-low-density lipoprotein) level. It is sometimes familial and is associated with an increased risk for coronary atherosclerosis. The condition is controlled with weight reduction, a low-carbohydrate diet, medications, niacin, and avoidance of alcohol. Also called **endogenous hypertriglyceridemia.**

hyperlipidemia type V, a condition of elevated blood lipid levels, characterized by slightly increased cholesterol level, greatly increased triglyceride level, elevation of the triglyceride carrier protein (very-low-density lipoprotein) level, and above-normal levels of chylomicrons. It is a genetically heterogenous disorder that apparently does not increase the risk of atherosclerosis. Treatment includes weight control, a low-fat diet, drugs, niacin, and abstinence from alcohol. Also called **mixed hyperlipemia, mixed hypertriglyceridemia.**

hyperlipoproteinemia /hī′pərlip′ōprō′tēnē″mē-ə/ [Gk, *hyper* + *lipos,* fat, *proteios,* first rank, *haima,* blood], any of a large group of inherited and acquired disorders of lipoprotein metabolism characterized by greater than normal amounts of certain protein-bound lipids and other fatty substances in the blood and usually low levels of high-density lipoprotein cholesterol. Hyperlipoproteinemia causes atherosclerosis and pancreatitis. The treatment includes dietary control of fats and/or saturated fats and cholesterol. Diet may reduce specific lipoprotein levels in the blood. Medication and other treatment vary according to the specific metabolic defect, its cause, and its prognosis. Also called **dyslipidemia.** Formerly called **hyperlipidemia.**

hyperlysinemia, a genetic mutation affecting enzymes that break down lysine, resulting in elevated levels of lysine in the blood and urine. This disorder is not commonly associated with health problems.

hypermagnesemia /hī′pərmag′nisē″mē-ə/ [Gk, *hyper* + *magnesia,* magnesium, *haima,* blood], a greater-than-normal amount of magnesium in the plasma, found in people with kidney failure and in those who use large doses of drugs containing magnesium, such as antacids. Toxic levels of magnesium cause cardiac arrhythmias and depression of deep tendon reflexes and respiration. Treatment often includes IV fluids, a diuretic, and hemodialysis.

hypermature cataract /-məchoo̅o̅r″/ [Gk, *hyper,* L, *maturare,* to make ripe; Gk, *katarrhaktes,* portcullis], an opaque lens that has become soft and reduced in size.

hypermenorrhea. See **menorrhagia.**

hypermetabolic state /-met′əbol″ik/, an abnormally increased rate of metabolism, as in a high fever or hyperthyroidism.

hypermetabolism /-mətab″əliz′əm/, increased metabolism, usually accompanied by excessive body heat.

hypermetaplasia /-met′əplā″zhə/,   an abnormal increase in the rate of transformation of one kind of tissue into another, as in the development of tumors.

hypermetria /hī′pərmē″trē·ə/   [Gk, *hyper* + *metron,* measure],   an abnormal form of coordination characterized by a dysfunction of the power to control the range of muscular action and causing movements that overreach the intended goal. Compare **hypometria.**

hypermetropia, hypermetropy. See **hyperopia.**

hypermimia, a highly animated use of gestures in communication.

hypermnesia /hī′pərm·nē″zhə/,   an extraordinarily good state of memory.

hypermobility /-mōbil″itē/   [Gk, *hyper;* L, *mobilis,* movable],   an abnormally wide range of movement of the joints. The condition is seen in children and may be associated with Marfan syndrome.

hypermorph /hī″pərmôrf′/   [Gk, *hyper* + *morphe,* form], **1.** a person whose arms and legs are disproportionately long in relation to the trunk and whose sitting height is disproportionately short compared to the standing height. **2.** a mutant allele that has an increased effect on the expression of a trait. Compare **amorph, antimorph, hypomorph.**

hypermotility /-motil″itē/,   an excessive movement of the involuntary muscles, particularly in the GI tract.

hypernasality /hī′pərnāzal′itē/   [Gk, *hyper,* excess + *nasus,* nose],   excessively nasal speech resonance, which may result in unintelligible speech. It occurs when there is too much vibration from sound energy in the nasal cavity during the production of voiced oral sounds. Also called **open rhinolalia.** See also **velopharyngeal insufficiency.**

hypernatremia /hī′pərnatrē″mē·ə/   [Gk, *hyper* + L, *natrium,* sodium],   a greater-than-normal concentration of sodium in the blood, caused by excessive loss of water and electrolytes that results from polyuria, diarrhea, excessive sweating, or inadequate water intake. It may also be a result of a large intake of salt, either orally or intravenously. When water loss is caused by kidney dysfunction, urine is profuse and dilute. If water loss is not through the kidneys, such as in diarrhea and excessive sweating, the urine is scanty and highly concentrated. People with hypernatremia may become mentally confused, have seizures, and lapse into coma. The treatment is restoration of fluid and electrolyte balance by mouth or by IV infusion. Care must be taken to restore water balance slowly because further electrolyte imbalances may occur and complications from correcting sodium concentration may arise.

hyperopia (h) /-ō″pē·ə/   [Gk, *hyper* + *ops,* eye],   farsightedness, or an inability of the eye to focus on nearby objects. It results from an error of refraction in which rays of light entering the eye are brought into focus behind the retina. Also called **farsightedness, hypermetropia, hypermetropy.** Compare **myopia.**

hyperorchidism /-ôr″kidiz′əm/   [Gk, *hyper,* excessive, *orchis,* testis],   excessive endocrine activity of the testes.

hyperornithinemia /-ôr′nithinē″mē·ə/,   a metabolic disorder involving the amino acid ornithine, which tends to accumulate in the tissues, causing seizures and cognitive impairment. Treatment is a low-protein diet.

hyperosmia /-oz″mē·ə/,   an abnormally increased sensitivity to odors. Compare **anosmia.**

hyperosmolarity /-oz′məler″itē/   [Gk, *hyper* + *osmos,* impulse],   a state or condition of abnormally increased osmolarity. −*hyperosmolar, adj.*

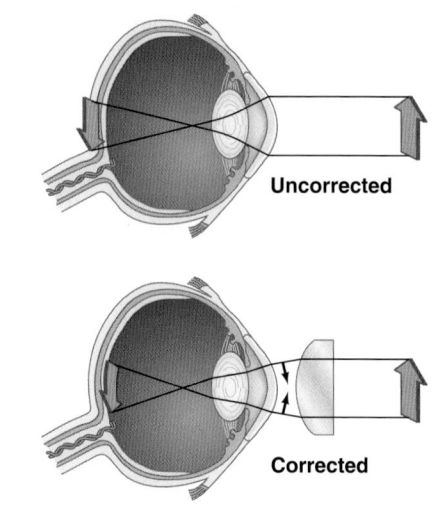

Hyperopia *(Patton and Thibodeau, 2016)*

hyperosmotic /-osmot″ik/,   pertaining to a solution that has a higher solute concentration than another solution. Compare **hypoosmotic, isosmotic.**

hyperostosis. See **exostosis.**

hyperostosis frontalis interna, thickening of the inner table of the frontal bone, which may be associated with hirsutism and obesity. It most commonly affects women near menopause. It is thought to be a generalized disorder of bone metabolism and may cause neuropsychological sequelae. Also called **Morel's syndrome.**

hyperoxaluria /-ok′səloor″ē·ə/,   an excessive level of oxalic acid or oxalates, primarily calcium oxalate, in the urine. The cause is usually an inherited deficiency of an enzyme needed to metabolize oxalic acid, which is present in many fruits and vegetables, or a disorder of fat absorption in the small intestine. An excess of oxalates may lead to the formation of renal calculi and renal failure. Treatments include high fluid intake and long-term coadministration of pyridoxine and inhibitors of calcium oxalate crystallization.

hyperoxemia /-oksē″mē·ə/   [Gk, *hyper,* excess, *oxys,* sharp, *haima,* blood],   increased oxygen content of the blood.

hyperoxia /-ok″sē·ə/,   abnormally high oxygen tension in the blood.

hyperoxygenation /-ok′sijənā″shən/   [Gk, *hyper* + *oxys,* sharp, *genein,* to produce],   the use of high concentrations of inspired oxygen before and after endotracheal aspiration.

hyperparathyroidism /-per′əthī″roidiz′əm/   [Gk, *hyper* + *para,* beside, *thyreos,* shield, *eidos,* form],   an abnormal endocrine condition characterized by hyperactivity of any of the four parathyroid glands with excessive secretion of parathyroid hormone (PTH), which causes increased resorption of calcium from the skeletal system and increased absorption of calcium by the kidneys and GI system. The condition may be primary, originating in one or more of the parathyroid glands and usually caused by an adenoma, or secondary, resulting from an abnormal hypocalcemia-producing condition in another part of the body, which causes a compensatory hyperactivity of the parathyroid glands.

■ OBSERVATIONS: Hypercalcemia in primary hyperparathyroidism results in dysfunction of many body systems. In the kidneys, tissue calcifies, calculi form, and renal failure may ensue. In addition, excess phosphorus is excreted, and excess 1,25 (OH)2 D (vitamin D) is synthesized. In the bones and joints, osteoporosis develops, causing pain and fragility;

fractures, synovitis, and pseudogout often occur. In the GI tract, chronic, piercing epigastric pain may develop as a result of pancreatitis and increased gastrin production; anorexia and nausea may occur; and vomiting of blood may result if peptic ulceration occurs. In the neuromuscular system, generalized weakness and atrophy develop if the condition is not corrected, and changes in the central nervous system produce alteration of consciousness, coma, psychosis, abnormal behavior, and disturbances of personality. Secondary hyperparathyroidism may result in many of these signs of calcium imbalance and in various abnormalities of the long bones, such as rickets. The diagnosis of primary hyperparathyroidism is made by laboratory findings of increased levels of PTH and calcium in the blood and by the characteristic appearance of the bones on radiographic films. Calcium in the blood and urine and chloride and alkaline phosphatase in the blood are present in excessive amounts; phosphorus is present in the serum in less than normal amounts.

■ INTERVENTIONS: Primary parathyroidism that is the result of an adenoma of one of the glands is treated by excision of the tumor; other causes of primary disease may require excision of up to one half of the glandular tissue. In asymptomatic patients over 50, noninterventional observation may be indicated. Dietary intake of calcium may be limited, and adequate hydration must be maintained. Estrogens may be used in postmenopausal females. Bisphosphates may be administered in severe hypercalcemia to lower the serum calcium level. After surgery, calcium levels in the blood may drop rapidly to dangerously low levels if frequent laboratory evaluations are not made and supplemental calcium is not given as required. Secondary hyperparathyroidism is managed by treating the underlying cause of hypertrophy of the gland. Vitamin D is frequently given, and peritoneal dialysis may be necessary to remove excess calcium from the circulation.

■ PATIENT CARE CONSIDERATIONS: Frequent laboratory evaluations of blood levels of calcium, phosphorus, potassium, and magnesium are necessary throughout the course of treatment. Because fractures occur easily and are common, great care is taken to prevent trauma to the patient. IV hydration is usually performed to dilute the concentration of calcium, and the lungs are assessed regularly to detect pulmonary edema in its earliest stages. Tetany is a warning sign of severe hypoglycemia; calcium gluconate is kept available for immediate use after surgery. Walking and moving about cause pain but accelerate healing of the affected bones and are therefore encouraged.

hyperperistalsis /-per′istal″sis/ [Gk, *hyper,* excess, *peristellein,* to clasp], a state of excessive motility of the waves of alternate contractions and relaxations that propel contents forward through the digestive tract. See also **peristalsis.**

hyperphagia. See **polyphagia.**

hyperphenylalaninemia /hī′pərfen′ilal′əninē″mē·ə/ [Gk, *hyper* + (phenylalanine), *haima,* blood], an abnormally high concentration of phenylalanine in the blood. This symptom may be the result of one of several defects in the metabolic process of breaking down phenylalanine. See also **phenylketonuria.**

hyperphoria /hī′pərfôr″ē·ə/ [Gk, *hyper* + *pherein,* to bear], the tendency of an eye to deviate upward.

hyperphosphoremia /-fos′fərē″mē·ə/, an abnormally high level of phosphorus compounds in the blood.

hyperpigmentation /-pig′məntā″shən/ [Gk, *hyper* + L, *pigmentum,* paint], a darkening of the skin. Causes include heredity, medications, exposure to the sun, trauma, and adrenal insufficiency. Compare **hypopigmentation.** See also **chloasma, melanocyte-stimulating hormone.**

hyperpituitarism /-pityoo″itəriz′əm/ [Gk, *hyper,* excess; L, *pituita,* phlegm], overactivity of the anterior lobe of the pituitary gland, resulting in increased secretion of its hormones and leading to such conditions as acromegaly

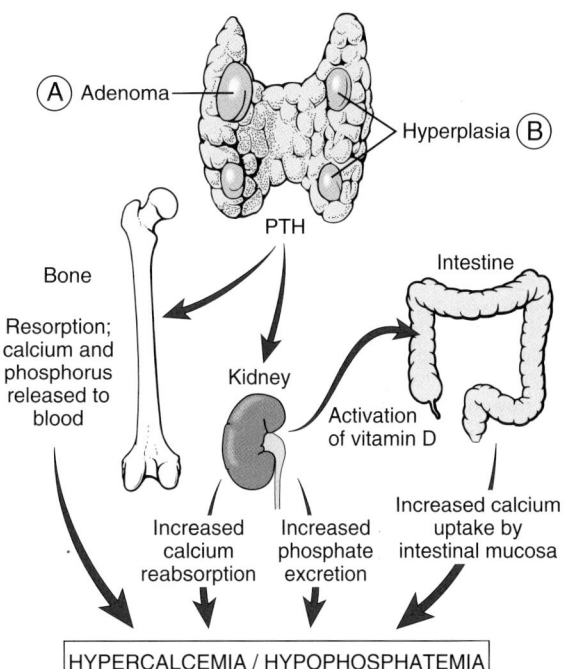

Metabolic consequences of hyperparathyroidism
(Damjanov, 2011)

and Cushing disease. See also **gigantism,**   **acromegaly, Cushing disease.**

hyperplasia /hī′pərplā″zhə/ [Gk, *hyper* + *plassein,* to mold], an increase in the number of cells of a body part that results from an increased rate of cellular division. Types of hyperplasia include compensatory, hormonal, and pathological. Compare **aplasia, hypertrophy, hypoplasia.**

hyperplastic gingivitis [Gk, *hyper,* excess, *plassein,* to mold; L, *gingiva,* gum; Gk, *itis,* inflammation], inflammation and enlargement of the gums caused by an increase in the number of cells, usually because of bacterial plaque accumulation. Compare **hypertrophic gingivitis.**

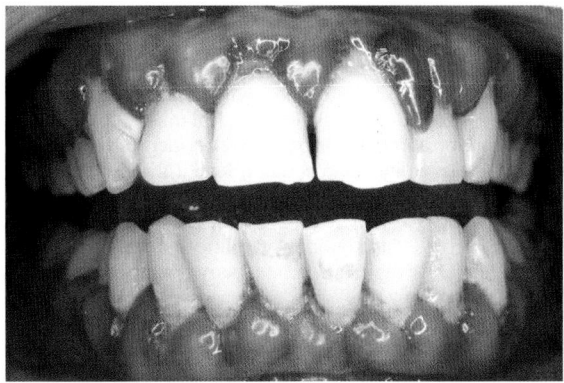

Patient with chronic hyperplastic gingivitis
(Neville et al, 2016)

hyperplastic obesity. See **obesity.**

hyperploid /hī″pərploid/ [Gk, *hyper* + *eidos,* form], **1.** *n.,* an individual, organism, strain, or cell that has one or more chromosomes in excess of the haploid number or of an exact multiple of the haploid number characteristic of the species. The result is one or more unbalanced sets of chromosomes, which are referred to as hyperdiploid, hypertetraploid, hypertriploid, and so on, depending on the number of multiples of the haploid number they contain. **2.** *adj.,* pertaining to such an individual, organism, strain, or cell. Compare **hypoploid.** See also **trisomy. –hyperploidy,** *adj.*

hyperploidy /hī″pərploi′dē/, any increase in chromosome number that involves individual chromosomes rather than entire sets, resulting in more than the normal haploid number characteristic of the species, as in Down syndrome. Compare **hypoploidy.**

hyperpnea /hī′pərpnē″ə/ [Gk, *hyper* + *pnoe,* blowing], an exaggerated deep, rapid, or labored respiration. It occurs normally with exercise and abnormally with aspirin overdose, pain, fever, hysteria, or any condition in which the supply of oxygen is inadequate, such as cardiac disease and respiratory disease. Also spelled *hyperpnoea.* Compare **dyspnea, hypopnea, orthopnea, tachypnea.** See also **respiratory rate. –***hyperpnoic, hyperpneic, adj.*

hyperpolarized helium /-pō″lərīzd/, a gas used in magnetic resonance imaging studies of respiratory disorders to produce images of the air spaces in the lungs.

hyperprolactinemia /-prōlak′tinē″mē-ə/ [Gk, *hyper* + L, *pro,* before, *lac,* milk; Gk, *haima,* blood], an excessive amount of prolactin in the blood, usually caused by a pituitary adenoma but sometimes caused by endocrine side effects related to certain antipsychotic medications. In women it is usually associated with galactorrhea and secondary amenorrhea; in men it may be a factor in gynecomastia, decreased libido, and impotence.

hyperprolinemia /hī′pərprō′linē′mē-ə/, an autosomal-recessive aminoacidopathy characterized by an excess of proline in the body fluids and occurring as two types, I and II, each of which is caused by deficiency in a different enzyme involved in proline metabolism. Type 1 is associated with renal disease and type 2 with cognitive impairment and convulsions.

hyperproteinemia /-prō′tēnē″mē-ə/ [Gk, *hyper,* excessive, *proteios,* first rank, *haima,* blood], an abnormally high concentration of protein in the blood.

hyperptyalism. See **ptyalism.**

hyperpyrexia /hī′pərpīrek″sē-ə/ [Gk, *hyper* + *pyressein,* to be feverish], an extremely elevated temperature that sometimes occurs in acute infectious diseases, especially in young children. Malignant hyperpyrexia, characterized by a rapid rise in temperature, tachycardia, tachypnea, sweating, rigidity, and blotchy cyanosis, occasionally occurs in patients undergoing general anesthesia. A high temperature may be reduced by sponging the body with tepid water, giving a tepid tub bath, using a hypothermia blanket, administering hydration, or administering antipyretic medication, such as aspirin or acetaminophen, or dantrolene if the cause is malignant hyperthermia. See also **fever.** *–hyperpyretic, adj.*

hyperreactivity /-rē′aktiv″itē/ [Gk, *hyper* + L, *re,* again, *activus,* active], an abnormal condition in which responses to stimuli are exaggerated. For example, asthma involves hyperreactive airways.

hyperreflection /-riflek″shən/, a compulsion to devote excessive attention to oneself.

hyperreflexia /-riflek″sē-ə/ [Gk, *hyper* + L, *reflectere,* to bend back], increased reflex reactions. See also **autonomic hyperreflexia.**

hypersalivation. See **sialorrhea.**

hypersensibility /-sen′səbil″itē/, excessive ability to perceive or feel, as excessive sensibility to pain.

hypersensitivity /-sen′sətiv″itē/ [Gk, *hyper* + L, *sentire,* to feel], **1.** an abnormal condition characterized by an exaggerated response of the immune system to an antigen. See also **allergy. 2.** increased sensitivity (reactions to tactile,

auditory, vestibular, or proprioceptive sensations) or awareness. *–hypersensitive, adj.*

hypersensitivity pneumonitis, an inflammatory form of interstitial pneumonia that results from an immunological reaction in a hypersensitive person. The reaction may be provoked by a variety of inhaled organic dusts, often those containing fungal spores. The disease can be prevented by avoiding contact with the causative agents. Classification of the disease is based solely on the character of the immune response rather than on its clinical manifestations. A wide variety of symptoms may occur, including asthma, fever, chills, malaise, and muscle aches, which usually develop 4 to 6 hours after exposure. Laboratory examination of the blood commonly reveals leukocytosis. Recovery is usually spontaneous. In an acute attack, corticosteroids may be given to diminish the inflammatory response. Also called **extrinsic allergic alveolitis.** Kinds include **bagassosis, cork worker's lung, farmer's lung, humidifier lung, mushroom worker's lung.** See also **Arthus reaction.**

hypersensitivity reaction, an inappropriate and excessive response of the immune system to a sensitizing antigen, called an allergen. Several factors determine the degree of the response: the person's genetic predisposition for an exaggerated response, the amount of allergen, the kind of allergen, its route of entrance into the body, the timing of the exposures to the allergen, and the site of the allergen–immune mediator reaction. Hypersensitivity reactions are classified into four types according to the components of the immune system involved in their mediation. Kinds include **type I hypersensitivity, type II hypersensitivity, type III hypersensitivity, type IV hypersensitivity.**

hypersensitization /-sen′sitīzā″shən/ [Gk, *hyper,* excess; L, *sentire,* to feel], a state of increased reactivity or sensitivity to a stimulus.

hypersomnia /hī′pərsom″nē-ə/ [Gk, *hyper* + L, *somnus,* sleep], **1.** sleep of excessive depth or abnormal duration, usually caused by psychological rather than physical factors and characterized by a state of confusion on awakening. **2.** extreme drowsiness, often associated with lethargy. **3.** a condition characterized by periods of deep, long sleep. Compare **narcolepsy.**

hyperspadias. See **epispadias.**

hypersplenism /hī′pərsplē″nizəm/ [Gk, *hyper* + *splen,* spleen], a syndrome consisting of splenomegaly and a deficiency of one or more types of blood cells. Causes may include portal hypertension, the lymphomas, the hemolytic anemias, malaria, tuberculosis, and various connective tissue and inflammatory diseases. Patients complain of abdominal pain of the left upper and middle quadrant. Patients often experience a sensation of fullness after small meals secondary to an enlarged spleen pressing against the stomach. On physical examination the enlarged spleen is felt and abnormal bruits (vascular sounds) may be auscultated over the epigastric area. Treatment of the underlying disorder may relieve the syndrome and its secondary effects. Splenectomy is considered when hemolytic anemias or splenic enlargement is severe, in treatment failures, or if the danger of vascular accident is significant. See also **splenectomy.**

Hyperstat, an emergency vasodilator. Brand name for **diazoxide.**

hypersthenic /hī′pərsthen″ik/, **1.** pertaining to a condition of excessive strength or tonicity of the body or a body part. **2.** pertaining to a body type characterized by massive proportions.

hypersystole /-sis″təlē/, abnormal force or duration of ventricular contraction.

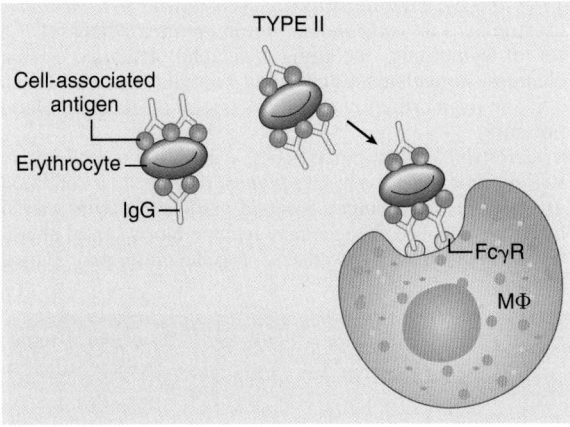

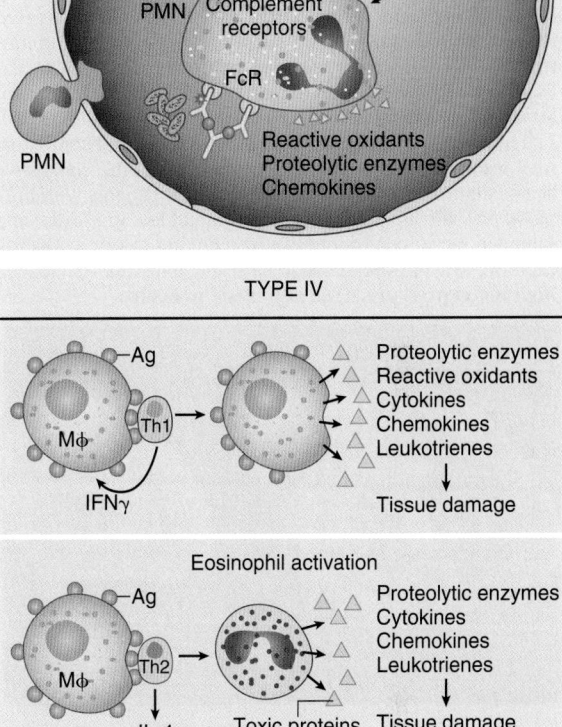

Hypersensitivity reactions *(Goldman et al, 2008)*

hypertaurodontism /hī′pərtô′rōdon′tizəm/ [Gk, *hyper,* excess; L, *taurus,* bull; Gk, *odous,* tooth], taurodontism (grossly enlarged pulp chamber) in which the tooth roots do not branch. See also **mesotaurodontism, taurodontism.**

hypertelorism /hī′pərtel″əriz′əm/ [Gk, *hyper* + *tele,* far, *horizo,* separate], a developmental defect characterized by an abnormally wide space between two organs or parts. Compare **hypotelorism.** Kinds include **ocular hypertelorism.**

hypertelorism-hypospadias syndrome. See **Smith-Lemli-Opitz syndrome.**

hypertension /-ten″shən/ [Gk, *hyper* + L, *tendere,* to stretch], a common disorder that is a known cardiovascular disease risk factor, characterized by elevated blood pressure over the normal values of 120/80 mm Hg in an adult over 18 years of age. This elevation in blood pressure can be divided into three classes of hypertension. Prehypertension describes blood pressure measurements of greater than 120 mm Hg systolic or 80 mm Hg diastolic and less than 130 mm Hg systolic or 90 mm Hg diastolic. Persons exhibiting prehypertension are encouraged to explore lifestyle modifications to lower blood pressure, but blood-pressure lowering agents are not generally prescribed without compelling indications. The second classification of hypertension is Stage 1 hypertension and is defined by a blood pressure of over 130 mm Hg systolic or 90 mm Hg diastolic but less than 160 mm Hg systolic or 100 mm Hg diastolic. Patients with Stage 1 hypertension are also encouraged to make lifestyle modifications, and initial drug therapy may include thiazide-type diuretics, ACE inhibitors, calcium channel blockers, beta-blockers, and angiotensin-receptor blockers, or a combination of these. Stage 2 hypertension is defined by a blood pressure greater than 160 mm Hg systolic or 100 mm Hg diastolic. Persons with Stage 2 hypertension are encouraged to make lifestyle modifications. Two-drug combination therapies (of thiazide-type diuretics, ACE inhibitors, calcium channel blockers, beta-blockers, and angiotensin-receptor blockers) are indicated for these patients. Essential hypertension, the most common kind, has no single identifiable cause, but risk for the disorder is increased by obesity, a high serum sodium level, hypercholesterolemia, and a family history of high blood pressure. Known causes of secondary hypertension include sleep apnea, chronic kidney disease, primary aldosteronism, renovascular disease, chronic steroid therapy, Cushing syndrome, pheochromocytoma, coarctation of the aorta, and thyroid or parathyroid disease. The incidence of hypertension is higher in men than in women and is twice as great in African-Americans as in Caucasians. People with mild or moderate hypertension may be asymptomatic or may experience suboccipital headaches, especially on rising; tinnitus; light-headedness; ready fatigability; and palpitations. With sustained hypertension, arterial walls become thickened, inelastic, and resistant to blood flow, and the left ventricle becomes distended and hypertrophied as a result of its efforts to maintain normal circulation against the increased resistance. Inadequate blood supply to the coronary arteries may cause angina or myocardial infarction. Left ventricular hypertrophy may lead to congestive heart failure. Malignant hypertension, characterized by a diastolic pressure higher than 120 mm Hg, severe headaches, blurred vision, and confusion, may result in fatal uremia, myocardial infarction, congestive heart failure, or a cerebrovascular accident. Patients with high blood pressure are advised to follow a diet low in sodium and saturated fat; to control obesity by reducing caloric intake; to exercise; to avoid stress; and to have adequate rest. Also called **high blood pressure.** See also **blood pressure.**

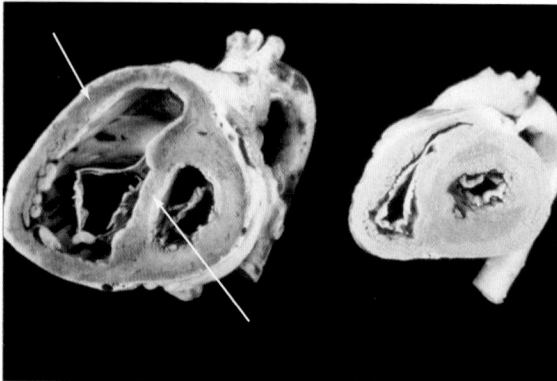

Ventricular hypertrophy in heart on left associated with hypertension; normal size heart on right *(Taussig and Landau, 2008)*

hypertensive /-ten″siv/ [Gk, *hyper,* excessive; L, *tendere,* to stretch], pertaining to high blood pressure, its cause, or its effects.

hypertensive arteriosclerosis, a form of arteriosclerosis complicated by a buildup of the muscular and elastic tissues of the arterial walls caused by hypertension.

hypertensive crisis [Gk, *hyper* + L, *tendere,* to stretch; Gk, *krisi,* turning point], a sudden, severe increase in blood pressure to a level exceeding 200/120 mm Hg, occurring most frequently in individuals who have untreated hypertension or who have stopped taking prescribed antihypertensive medication. See also **malignant hypertension.**

■ OBSERVATIONS: Characteristic signs include severe headache, vertigo, diplopia, tinnitus, photophobia, nosebleed, twitching of muscles, tachycardia or other cardiac arrhythmia, distended neck veins, narrowed pulse pressure, nausea, and vomiting. The patient may be confused, irritable, or stuporous, and the condition may lead to convulsions, coma, myocardial infarction, renal failure, cardiac arrest, or stroke.

■ INTERVENTIONS: Treatment consists of antihypertensive drugs and diuretics; anticonvulsants, sedatives, and antiemet-

ics may be used if indicated. The patient is usually placed on a cardiac monitor in a bed with the head elevated and is maintained in a quiet environment. The diet is low in calories, and sodium and fluids may be restricted. As the patient's condition improves, progressive ambulation is permitted, but the patient is carefully observed for symptoms of orthostatic hypotension, such as pallor, diaphoresis, or faintness, which may be side effects of the antihypertensive drugs.

■ PATIENT CARE CONSIDERATIONS: The major concerns of the health care providers in the acute-care setting are to observe and report any sign of hypertension. In preparation for discharge the nurses and physicians advise the patient to recognize symptoms of any dramatic increase or decrease in blood pressure, to adhere to the prescribed diet and medication, and to avoid fatigue, heavy lifting, use of tobacco products, and stressful situations. The pharmacist, dietitian, and therapists also provide instructions to assist the patient in controlling his or her blood pressure.

hypertensive encephalopathy [Gk, *hyper* + L, *tendere,* to stretch; Gk, *enkephalos,* brain, *pathos,* disease], a set of symptoms, including headache, lethargy, vision changes, convulsions, and coma secondary to end-organ damage from critically elevated systolic or diastolic blood pressure.

hypertensive retinopathy [Gk, *hyper* + L, *tendere,* to stretch, *rete* + *net,* web; Gk, *pathos,* disease], a condition in which retinal changes occur in association with arterial hypertension. The changes may include blood vessel alterations, hemorrhages, exudates, papilledema, and retinal edema.

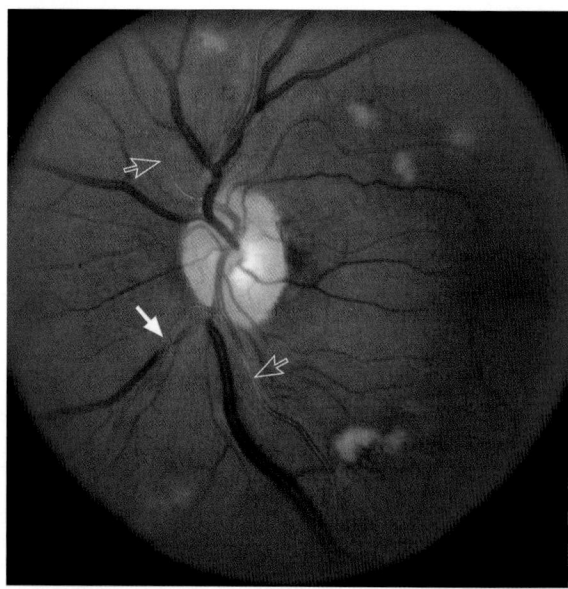

Hypertensive retinopathy with cotton wool spots, arteriovenous nicking (solid arrow), and "silver wiring of vessels" (open arrows) *(Liu, Volpe, and Galetta, 2010)*

hypertetraploid. See **hyperploid.**

hyperthermia /hī′pərthur″mē·ə/ [Gk, *hyper* + *therme,* heat], **1.** a much higher than normal body temperature induced therapeutically or iatrogenically. **2.** *(Nontechnical)* malignant hyperthermia. **3.** the use of various heating methods, such as electromagnetic therapy, to produce temperature elevations of a few degrees in cells and tissues. It is believed to lead to an antitumor effect. Hyperthermia may be used in conjunction with radiotherapy or chemotherapy for cancer treatment.

hyperthyroidism /-thī″roidiz′əm/ [Gk, *hyper* + *thyreos,* shield, *eidos,* form], a condition characterized by hyperactivity of the thyroid gland. The gland is usually enlarged, secreting greater-than-normal amounts of thyroid hormones, and the metabolic processes of the body are accelerated. Nervousness, exophthalmos, tremor, constant hunger, weight loss, fatigue, heat intolerance, palpitations, and diarrhea may develop. Antithyroid drugs, such as propylthiouracil or methimazole, are usually prescribed. Radioactive iodine may be prescribed in certain cases. Surgical ablation of the gland is sometimes necessary. Untreated hyperthyroidism may lead to death from cardiac failure. See also **Graves disease, thyroid storm.**

hypertonia /-tō″nē·ə/, **1.** abnormally increased muscle tone or strength. The condition is sometimes associated with genetic disorders, such as trisomy 18, and may be expressed in arm or leg deformities. **2.** a condition of excessive pressure, such as the intraocular pressure of glaucoma.

hypertonic /hī′pərton″ik/ [Gk, *hyper* + *tonos,* stretching], **1.** *adj.,* pertaining to a solution that causes cells to shrink. **2.** *n.,* a solution that increases the degree of osmotic pressure on a semipermeable membrane. Compare **hypotonic, isotonic. 3.** *adj.,* exhibiting increased muscle tone, characterized by stiffness or a lack of flexibility.

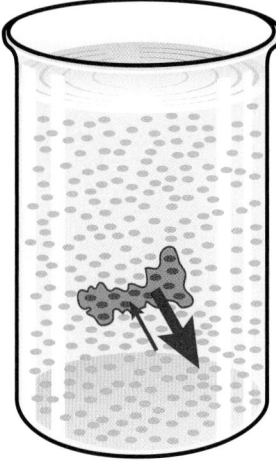

Red blood cell in hypertonic solution
(Waugh and Grant, 2014)

hypertonic bladder [Gk, *hyper,* excess, *tonos,* tone; AS, *blaedre*], a condition of excessive tension in the detrusor muscle of the bladder, often caused by an irritant such as a calculus or occurring after surgery.

hypertonic contracture, prolonged muscle contraction that results from continuous nerve stimulation in spastic paralysis. Anesthesia or sleep eliminates this condition. Also called **functional contracture.**

hypertonicity /-tənis″itē/ [Gk, *hyper,* excess, *tonos,* tone], **1.** excessive tone, tension, or activity. **2.** (in ophthalmology) increased intraocular pressure. **3.** excessive tension of the arteries or muscles. **4.** increase in osmotic pressure.

hypertonic saline, a saline solution that contains 1% to 23.4% sodium chloride (compared with normal saline solution at 0.9%).

hypertonus /-tō″nəs/, an excessive level of skeletal muscle tension or activity. See also **clonus.**

hypertrichosis, excessive hair growth anywhere on a person's body. Compare **hirsutism.**

hypertriglyceridemia. See **hyperchylomicronemia.**

hypertriploid. See **hyperploid.**

hypertrophic /-trof″ik/ [Gk, *hyper,* excess, *trophe,* nourishment], pertaining to an increase in size, structure, or function.

hypertrophic angioma. See **hemangioendothelioma.**

hypertrophic cardiomyopathy, an abnormal condition characterized by gross hypertrophy of the interventricular septum and left ventricular free wall of the heart. Ventricular hypertrophy results in impaired diastolic filling and reduced cardiac output. Signs and symptoms, such as fatigue and syncope, are often associated with exercise when the demand for increased cardiac output cannot be met. This is commonly a genetic disease, with numerous genes implicated. It is also frequently seen in individuals with chronic uncontrolled hypertension. Also called **hypertrophic obstructive cardiomyopathy.**

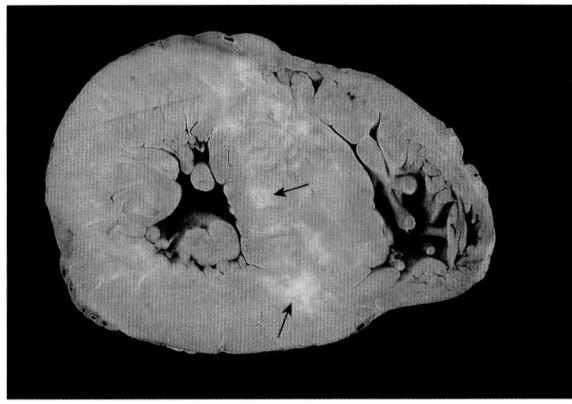

Hypertrophic cardiomyopathy
(Finkbeiner, Ursell, and Davis, 2009)

hypertrophic catarrh [Gk, *hyper* + *trophe,* nourishment, *kata,* down, *rhoia,* flow], a chronic condition characterized by inflammation and discharge from a mucous membrane, accompanied by the thickening of the mucosal and submucosal tissue. Compare **atrophic catarrh.** See also **catarrh.**

hypertrophic cicatrization. See **hypertrophic scarring.**

hypertrophic cirrhosis, a stage of cirrhosis characterized by an overgrowth of liver tissue.

hypertrophic gastritis, a premalignant condition characterized by inflammation of the gastric mucosa associated with gastric albumin wasting. Symptoms include epigastric pain, nausea, vomiting, weight loss, and abdominal distension. It is differentiated from other forms of gastritis by the presence of prominent rugae (folds), enlarged glands, excess mucus production, and nodules on the wall of the stomach. This condition often accompanies peptic ulcer, Zollinger-Ellison syndrome, or gastric hypersecretion.

hypertrophic gingivitis [Gk, *hyper,* excess, *trophe,* nourishment], inflammation and enlargement of the gums resulting from an increase in the size of cells, usually because of an underlying systemic disorder. Compare **gingivitis, hyperplastic gingivitis.**

hypertrophic obesity. See **obesity.**

hypertrophic obstructive cardiomyopathy. See **hypertrophic cardiomyopathy.**

hypertrophic pulmonary osteopathy. See **Marie's hypertrophy.**

hypertrophic scarring, excessive overgrowth of dense collagen tissue, often red, pink, or purple in appearance, at the site of a healed skin defect. It resembles a keloid but is usually temporary, most often regresses without treatment, and remains confined to the site of injury. Also called **hypertrophic cicatrization.**

hypertrophic subaortic stenosis, a form of hypertrophic cardiomyopathy, in which the left ventricle is hypertrophied (commonly with disproportionate involvement of the interventricular septum) and the cavity is small. It is marked by obstruction to left ventricular outflow. Also called *idiopathic hypertrophic subaortic stenosis, muscular subaortic stenosis.*

hypertrophy /hīpur″trəfē/ [Gk, *hyper + trophe,* nourishment], an increase in the size of an organ caused by an increase in the size of the cells rather than the number of cells. The cells of the heart and kidney are particularly prone to hypertrophy. Also called **overgrowth.** Compare **atrophy, auxesis, hyperplasia.** Kinds include **adaptive hypertrophy, compensatory hypertrophy, Marie's hypertrophy, physiological hypertrophy, unilateral hypertrophy.** −**hypertrophic,** *adj.*

hypertrophy of heart [Gk, *hyper,* excess, *trophe,* nourishment; AS, *heorte*], an increase in the size of the heart resulting from enlargement of the heart muscle, but without an increase in the capacity of the heart chambers. It is a compensatory mechanism in heart failure associated with increased afterload, such as that caused by hypertension or aortic stenosis.

hypertropia. See **anoopsia.**

hyperuricaemia, hyperuricemia. See **gout.**

hyperuricosuria /hi′peru′rĭkosu′re·ä or re·ə/, an excess of uric acid or urates in the urine. Also called **hyperuricuria, uricosuria.**

hyperuricuria. See **hyperuricosuria.**

hypervalinemia /hī′pərval′inē′mē·ə/, **1.** an autosomal-recessive aminoacidopathy, probably caused by a defect in an enzyme necessary for valine catabolism, characterized by elevated levels of valine in the plasma and urine and by failure to thrive. **2.** elevated levels of valine in the plasma. Hypervalinemia is often associated with maple sugar urine disease. Also called **valinemia.**

hyperventilation /-ven′tilā″shən/ [Gk, *hyper + ventilare,* to fan], pulmonary ventilation rate greater than that metabolically necessary for gas exchange, resulting from an increased respiration rate, an increased tidal volume, or both. Hyperventilation causes an excessive intake of oxygen and elimination of carbon dioxide and may cause hyperoxygenation. Hypocapnia and respiratory alkalosis then occur, leading to dizziness, faintness, numbness of the fingers and toes, possibly syncope, and psychomotor impairment. Causes of hyperventilation include asthma or early emphysema; increased metabolic rate caused by exercise, fever, hyperthyroidism, or infection; lesions of the central nervous system, as in cerebral thrombosis, encephalitis, head injuries, or meningitis; hypoxia or metabolic acidosis; use of hormones and drugs, such as epinephrine, progesterone, and salicylates; difficulties with mechanical respirators; and psychogenic factors, such as acute anxiety or pain. Compare **hypoventilation.** See also **respiratory center.**

hyperventilation tetany, a disorder characterized by muscle twitches, cramps, or spasms caused by abnormally low blood levels of CO_2 from forced overbreathing. See also **tetany.**

hyperviscosity /-viskos″itē/ [Gk, *hyper,* excess; L, *viscosus,* sticky], extreme viscosity or thickness of fluid.

hyperviscosity syndrome, several syndromes associated with increased thickness and slowed flow rate of blood. One type, which results from serum hyperviscosity, is caused by increased proteins and is characterized by neurological and ocular disorders. Another type is polycythemia, causing organ congestion, reduced capillary perfusion, and increased cardiac effort. A third group includes conditions in which the deformability of erythrocytes is impaired, such as sickle cell anemia.

hypervitaminosis /-vī′təminō″sis/, an abnormal condition resulting from excessive intake of toxic amounts (self-prescribed, usually from supplements) of one or more vitamins, especially over a long period. Serious effects may result from overdoses of fat-soluble vitamins A, D, E, or K, but adverse reactions are less likely with the water-soluble B and C vitamins, except when taken in megadoses. Compare **avitaminosis.** See also **megadose,** *specific vitamins.*

hypervolemia /-vōlē″mē·ə/ [Gk, *hyper* + L, *volumen,* paper roll; Gk, *haima,* blood], an increase in the amount of intravascular fluid, particularly in the volume of circulating blood or its components. See also **congestive heart failure.**

hypesthesia /hī′pisthē″zhə/ [Gk, *hypo,* under, *aisthesis,* feeling], a decrease in sensitivity to stimuli, especially touch. Also called **hypoesthesia.** −*hypesthetic, adj.*

hypha /hī″fə/ [Gk, *hyphe,* web], a threadlike structure in the mycelium in a fungus.

hyphema /hīfē″mə/ [Gk, *hypo,* under, *haima,* blood], a hemorrhage into the anterior chamber of the eye, usually caused by a blunt trauma. The patient is treated by an ophthalmologist, who evaluates the need for evacuation of the blood and the use of mydriatic or miotic medications or a carbonic anhydrase inhibitor. Glaucoma may result from recurrent bleeding.

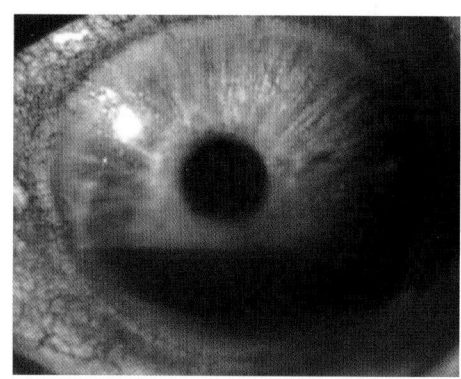

Hyphema *(Palay and Krachmer, 2005)*

hyphomycosis /hi″fomiko′sis/, any infection caused by an imperfect fungus of the form-class Hyphomycetes. The group has been divided into hyalohyphomycosis and phaeohyphomycosis on the basis of the color of the mycelium and wall of the fungus. It is a disease of horses and mules, rarely of humans.

hypnagogic. See **hypnagogue.**

hypothalmic-pituitary amenorrhea, the cessation of menses associated with functional causes (weight loss, excessive exercise, obesity); drug-induced causes (marijuana or psychoactive drugs, including antidepressants); neoplastic causes (prolactin-secreting pituitary adenomas, craniopharyngioma); psychogenic causes (chronic anxiety, pseudocyesis, or anorexia nervosa); or other causes, such as head injury or chronic medical illness.

hypnagogic hallucination /hip′nəgoj″ik/ [Gk, *hypnos,* sleep, *agogos,* leading], a vivid image that occurs while falling asleep.

hypnagogue /hip″nəgog/ [Gk, *hypnos + agogos,* leading], an agent or substance that tends to induce sleep or the feeling of dreamy sleepiness, as occurs before falling asleep. See also **hypnotic. –hypnagogic,** *adj.*

hypno-, prefix meaning "sleep": *hypnagogic, hypnosis.*

hypnoanalysis /hip′nə·anal″isis/ [Gk, *hypnos* + *analyein,* to loosen], the use of hypnosis as an adjunct to other techniques in psychoanalysis.

hypnogenic zone /hip′nəjen″ik/, a specific area on the body that, when stimulated, can cause a person to enter a sleeplike state.

hypnopomic hallucination, an image perceived while awakening from sleep.

hypnosis /hipnō″sis/ [Gk, *hypnos,* sleep], a passive, trancelike state that resembles normal sleep during which perception and memory are altered, resulting in increased responsiveness to suggestion. The condition is usually induced by the monotonous repetition of words and gestures while the subject is completely relaxed.

hypnotherapy /hip′nəther″əpē/ [Gk, *hypnos* + *therapeia,* treatment], the induction of a specific altered state (trance) for memory retrieval, relaxation, or suggestion. Hypnotherapy is often used to alter habits (e.g., smoking, obesity), treat biological mechanisms such as hypertension or cardiac arrhythmias, deal with the symptoms of a disease, alter an individual's reaction to disease, and affect an illness and its course through the body.

hypnotic /hipnot″ik/ [Gk, *hypnos,* sleep], one of a class of drugs often used as sedatives. See also **hypnagogue.**

-hypnotic, suffix meaning "sleep" or "hypnosis": *posthypnotic.*

hypnotic sleep /hipnot″ik/ [Gk, *hypnos,* sleep; ME, *slep*], sleep induced through the administration of hypnotic medicines.

hypnotic suggestion [Gk, *hypnos,* sleep; L, *suggerere,* to suggest], a suggestion implanted in the mind of a person under hypnosis.

hypnotic trance, an artificially induced sleeplike state, as in hypnosis.

hypnotism /hip″nətiz′əm/ [Gk, *hypnos,* sleep], the study or practice of inducing hypnosis.

hypnotist /hip″nətist/, one who practices hypnotism.

hypnotize /hip″nətīz/, **1.** to put into a state of hypnosis. **2.** to fascinate, entrance, or control through personal characteristics.

hypo-, hyp-, prefix meaning "under, below, beneath, deficient" or, in chemistry, "lacking oxygen": *hypochlorite, hypodermic, hypodontia.*

hypoacidity /hī′pō·əsid″itē/, a deficiency of acid.

hypoactivity /-aktiv″itē/ [Gk, *hypo,* under; L, *activus,* active], any abnormally diminished activity of the body or its organs, such as decreased cardiac output, thyroid secretion, or peristalsis. Compare **hyperactivity.**

hypoacusis /-əkoō″sis/ [Gk, *hypo,* under, *akouein,* to hear], a reduced sensitivity to sounds.

hypoadrenalism. See **Addison disease.**

hypoalbuminemia /-alboō′minē″mē·ə/, a condition of abnormally low levels of albumin in the blood. It may occur in celiac disease, tropical sprue, malnutrition, and some forms of liver or kidney impairment.

hypoalimentation /-al′iməntā″shən/ [Gk, *hypo* + L, *alimentum,* nourishment], a condition of insufficient or inadequate nourishment.

hypoallergenic /-al′ərjen″ik/ [Gk, *hypo,* under, *allos,* other, *ergein,* to work], having a lowered potential for producing an allergic reaction.

hypobarism /-ber″izəm/, air pressure that is significantly less than the sea-level normal of 760 mm Hg. See also **barotrauma, decompression sickness.**

hypobetalipoproteinemia /-hī′pōbā′təlip′ōprō′tēnē″mē·ə/ [Gk, *hypo* + *beta,* second letter of Greek alphabet, *lipos,* fat, *proteios,* first rank, *haima,* blood], an inherited disorder in which there are less than normal amounts of beta-lipoprotein in the serum. Blood lipids and cholesterol are present at less than the expected levels regardless of dietary intake of fats. There are no clinical signs, and treatment is unnecessary. Compare **hyperbetalipoproteinemia.**

hypoblast /hī″pōblăst/ [Gk, *hypo* + *blastos,* germ], the lower layer of the bilaminar embryonic disk in a human embryo, present during the second week of gestation, that gives rise to the endoderm.

hypocalcemia /hī′pōkalsē″mē·ə/ [Gk, *hypo* + L, *calx,* lime; Gk, *haima,* blood], a deficiency of calcium in the serum that may be caused by hypoparathyroidism, vitamin D deficiency, kidney failure, acute pancreatitis, or inadequate amounts of plasma magnesium and protein. Normal serum calcium levels range from 8.5 to 10.5 mg/dL. Mild hypocalcemia is asymptomatic. Severe hypocalcemia is characterized by cardiac arrhythmias and tetany with hyperparesthesia of the hands, feet, lips, and tongue. The underlying disorder is diagnosed and treated, and calcium is given by mouth or IV infusion. Hypocalcemia is also seen in dysmature newborns, in infants born of mothers with diabetes, or in normal babies of normal mothers delivered after a long or stressful labor and delivery. The condition is signaled by vomiting, twitching of extremities, poor muscle tone, high-pitched crying, and difficulty in breathing. Also spelled *hypocalcaemia.* See also **Chvostek sign, Chvostek-Weiss sign, tetany.** –*hypocalcemic, adj.*

hypocalcemic tetany /-kalsē″mik/ [Gk, *hypo,* under; L, *calx,* calcium, *haima,* blood, *tetanos,* convulsive tension], a disease caused by an abnormally low level of calcium in the blood. It is characterized by hyperexcitability of the neuromuscular system and results in carpopedal spasms. A common cause is a deficiency of parathyroid hormone secretion.

hypocalciuria /-kal′siuoōr″ē·ə/ [Gk, *hypo,* under; L, *calx,* lime; Gk, *ouron,* urine], a diminished level of calcium in the urine.

hypocapnia /-kap″nē·ə/, an abnormally low arterial carbon dioxide level. Also called *hypocarbia.*

hypochloremia /-klôrē″mē·ə/ [Gk, *hypo* + *chloros,* green, *haima,* blood], a decrease in the chloride level in the blood serum below 95 mEq/L. The condition may result from prolonged gastric suctioning. Also spelled *hypochloraemia.*

hypochloremic alkalosis /-klôrē″mik/, a metabolic disorder resulting from an increase in blood bicarbonate level secondary to loss of chloride from the body.

hypochlorhydria /-klôrhid″rē·ə/ [Gk, *hypo* + *chloros,* green, *hydor,* water], a deficiency of hydrochloric acid in gastric secretions.

hypochlorite poisoning /-klôr″īt/, toxic effects of ingestion of or skin contact with household or commercial bleaches or similar chlorinated products. Symptoms include pain and inflammation of the mouth and digestive tract, vomiting, and breathing difficulty. Skin contact may produce blisters.

hypochlorous acid /-klôr″əs/ [Gk, *hypo* + *chloros,* green; L, *acidus,* sour], a compound, HOCl, that is stable only in the form of a dilute aqueous solution formed by dissolving chlorine gas in water to yield a greenish-yellow solution. An unstable compound that decomposes to hydrochloric acid and oxygen, it is used as a bleaching agent and disinfectant.

hypocholesteremia /-kəles′tərē″mē·ə/, an abnormally low level of cholesterol in the blood. Also called *hypocholesterolemia.*

hypochondria. See **hypochondriasis.**

hypochondriac /-kon″drē·ak/ [Gk, *hypo,* under, *chondros,* cartilage], **1.** *adj.,* pertaining to the regions of the upper abdomen beneath the lower ribs and lateral to the epigastric region. See also **hypochondriac region. 2.** *n.,* a person who is so preoccupied with matters of ill health that the state of mind itself becomes a disability. –*hypochondriacal, adj.*

hypochondriac region [Gk, *hypo* + *chondros,* cartilage; L, *regio,* direction], the part of the abdomen in the upper zone on both sides of the epigastric region and beneath the cartilages of the lower ribs. Also called **hypochondrium.** See also **abdominal regions.**

hypochondriasis /hī′pōkəndrī″əsis/ [Gk, *hypo* + *chondros,* cartilage, *osis,* condition], a chronic abnormal concern about the health of the body. It is characterized by extreme anxiety, depression, and an unrealistic interpretation of real or imagined physical symptoms as indications of a serious illness or disease despite rational medical evidence that no disorder is present. The condition is caused by some unresolved intrapsychic conflict and may involve a specific organ, such as the heart, lungs, or eyes, or several body systems at various times or simultaneously. In severe cases the distorted body-mind relationship is so strong that actual symptoms may develop. Treatment usually consists of psychotherapy to uncover the underlying emotional conflict. Also called **hypochondria.**

hypochondrium. See **hypochondriac region.**

hypochondroplasia /-kon′drōplā″zhə/, an inherited form of dwarfism that resembles a mild form of achondroplasia. It is relatively uncommon and is transmitted as an autosomal-dominant trait.

hypochromic /hī′pōkrō″mik/ [Gk, *hypo* + *chroma,* color], pale-staining red blood cells with a broadened central zone of pallor; most often associated with hypochromic, microcytic anemia; thalassemia; and anemia of chronic inflammation. Compare **normochromic.** See also **hypochromic anemia, red cell indexes.**

hypochromic anemia, 1. a group of anemias characterized by a decreased concentration of hemoglobin in the red blood cells. **2.** a decrease in hemoglobin characterized by hypochromic, microcytic red blood cells, such as iron-deficiency anemia, thalassemia, and anemia of chronic inflammation. See also **anemia, red cell indexes.**

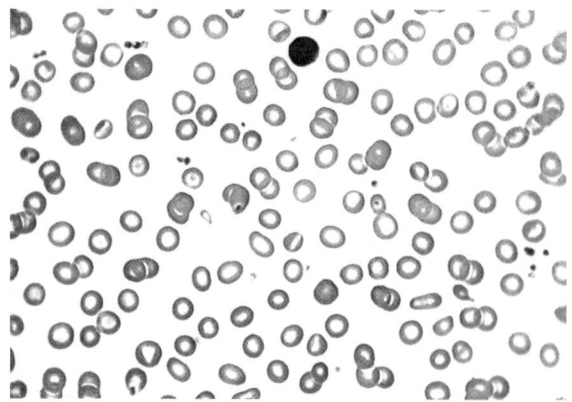

Peripheral blood smear with hypochromic microcytic anemia *(Aster, Pozdnyakova, and Kutok, 2013)*

hypocitraturia /hī″pōsĭtratu′re·ə/, excretion of urine containing an abnormally small amount of citrate, a significant risk factor for kidney stone formation and recurrence.

hypocycloidal motion /-sī″kloidəl/, a complex circular movement of the x-ray tube and image receptor during the acquisition of tomographic images. It is used to blur structures outside the focal plane and eliminate ghost images.

hypocythemia, deficiency in the number of red blood cells. Also called **erythropenia.**

hypocytic leukemia. See **aleukemic leukemia.**

hypodermatoclysis. See **hypodermoclysis.**

hypodermic /-durmik/ [Gk, *hypo* + *derma,* skin], pertaining to the area below the skin, such as in a hypodermic injection.

hypodermic implantation [Gk, *hypo,* under, *derma,* skin; L, *implantare,* to set into], the introduction of a solid medicine under the skin, usually on the chest or abdominal wall, to ensure local action or slow absorption.

hypodermic needle, a short, thin hollow needle of varying sizes and lengths that attaches to a syringe for injecting a drug or medication under the skin or into vessels and for withdrawing a fluid, such as blood, for examination.

hypodermic syringe [Gk, *hypo,* under, *derma,* skin, *syrigx,* tube], an instrument designed to direct fluid under the skin through a fine hollow needle.

hypodermic tablet, a compressed or molded dosage form of a medication that can be dissolved for IV administration.

hypodermoclysis /hī′pōdərmok″lisis/ [Gk, *hypo* + *derma,* skin, *klysis,* flushing out], the injection of an isotonic or hypotonic solution into subcutaneous tissue to supply a continuous and large amount of fluid, electrolytes, and nutrients. The procedure is used to replace the loss or inadequate intake of water and salt during illness or surgery or after shock or hemorrhage. It is performed only when a patient is unable to take fluids intravenously, orally, or rectally. The rate of absorption into the circulatory system is increased with the addition to the solution of the enzyme hyaluronidase. The most common sites of administration are the anterior thighs, the abdominal wall along the crest of the ilium, below the breasts in women, and directly over the scapula in children; sites should be changed when multiple infusions are given. The patient is placed in a comfortable position because the procedure takes a long time. The patient is observed for signs of circulatory collapse, respiratory difficulty, and edema at the site of injection. Also called **hypodermatoclysis, interstitial infusion, subcutaneous infusion.**

hypodiploid. See **hypoploid.**

hypodipsia /-dip″sē·ə/, a condition in which homeostasis is threatened by an abnormally low fluid intake. It is often related to dysfunction of the thirst osmoreceptor in the anterior hypothalamus.

hypodontia /hī′pōdon′shə/. See **partial anodontia.**

hypoechogenic rim. Also called **halo sign,** def. 4.

hypoesthesia. See **hypesthesia.**

hypofertility. See **subfertility.**

hypofibrinogenemia /-fī′brinōjənē″mē·ə/ [Gk, *hypo* + L, *fibra,* fiber; Gk, *genein,* to produce, *haima,* blood], plasma fibrinogen deficiency. It may be inherited or acquired, as in disseminated intravascular coagulation or liver disease.

hypofunction /-fungk″shən/ [Gk, *hypo,* under; L, *functio,* performance], a diminished or inadequate level of activity of an organ system or its parts.

hypogammaglobulinemia /-gam′əglō′byəlinē″mē·ə/ [Gk, *hypo* + *gamma,* third letter in Greek alphabet; L, *globus,* small sphere; Gk, *haima,* blood], lower than normal concentration of plasma gamma globulin, usually the result of increased protein catabolism or loss of protein via the urine. It is associated with a decreased resistance to infection.

hypogastric /-gas″trik/ [Gk, *hypo,* under, *gaster,* stomach], pertaining to the hypogastrium, the lower abdominal region below the umbilical region and between the right and left iliac regions.

hypogastric artery.   See **internal iliac artery.**

hypogastric pain,   pain in the lower abdomen.

hypogastric plexus,   a complex of nerve fibers in the pelvic area near the termination of the aorta and the beginning of the common iliac artery.

hypogastric region, hypogastrium.   See **pubic region.**

hypogenitalism /-jen″itəliz′əm/ [Gk, *hypo* + L, *genitalis,* fruitful],   a condition of delayed sexual development caused by a defect in male or female hormonal production in the testis or ovary.

hypogeusia /-gōō″zē·ə/,   reduced taste, often a consequence of Parkinson or Alzheimer disease, as well as a side effect of multiple medications.

hypoglossal /-glos″əl/ [Gk, *hypo,* under, *glossa,* tongue],   pertaining to nerves or other structures under the tongue.

hypoglossal nerve [Gk, *hypo* + *glossa,* tongue],   either of a pair of cranial nerves essential for swallowing and for moving the tongue. Each nerve has four major branches, communicates with the vagus nerve, and arises from nucleus XII in the brain. Damage to the nerve will affect the tongue. Also called **nervus hypoglossus, twelfth cranial nerve.**

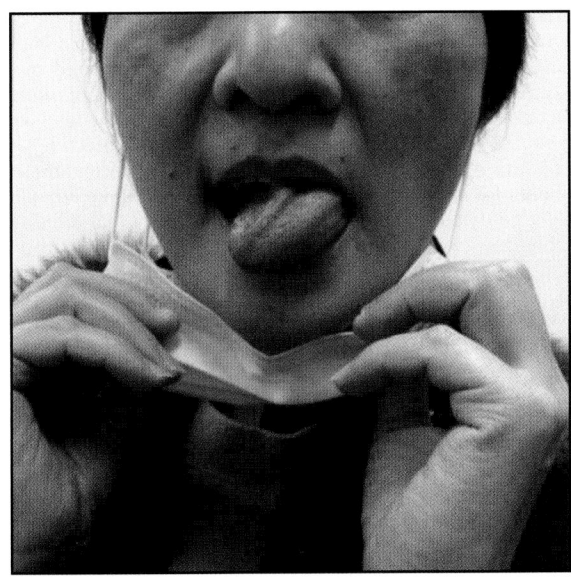

Assessment of the hypoglossal nerve with deviation suggesting nerve damage *(Chen et al, 2014)*

hypoglossus /-glos″əs/,   **1.** a muscle that retracts and pulls down the side of the tongue. **2.** the hypoglossal nerve.

hypoglycemia /hī′pōglīsē″mē·ə/ [Gk, *hypo* + *glykys,* sweet, *haima,* blood],   a low level of glucose in the blood. It may be caused by administration of too much insulin, excessive secretion of insulin by the islet cells of the pancreas, or dietary deficiency. The condition may cause weakness, headache, hunger, visual disturbances, ataxia, anxiety, personality changes, and, if untreated, delirium, coma, and death. The treatment is the administration of glucose by mouth if the patient is conscious or IV glucose supplementation if the person is unconscious or uncooperative. Glycogen or complex carbohydrates may also be given. Also called **glycopenia.** Also spelled *hypoglycaemia.* Compare **diabetic coma.**

Signs and symptoms of hypoglycemia

Adrenergic symptoms
- Pallor
- Diaphoresis
- Tachycardia
- Piloerection
- Palpitations
- Nervousness
- Irritability
- Sensation of coldness
- Weakness
- Trembling

Hunger neuroglycopenic symptoms
- Headache
- Mental confusion
- Circumoral paresthesia
- Fatigue
- Incoherent speech
- Coma
- Diplopia
- Emotional lability
- Convulsions

From Monahan FD et al: *Phipps' medical-surgical nursing: health and illness perspectives,* ed 8, St Louis, 2007, Mosby.

hypoglycemic /-glīsē″mik/ [Gk, *hypo,* under, *glykys,* sweet, *haima,* blood],   pertaining to or resembling a state of low blood glucose level.

hypoglycemic agent,   any of various synthetic drugs that lower the blood glucose level and are used to treat type 2 diabetes mellitus. They may stimulate synthesis of insulin by pancreatic beta cells, inhibit glucose production, facilitate transport of glucose to muscle cells, and sometimes increase the number of receptor sites where insulin can be bound and can initiate the process of breaking down glucose. Most are sulfonylureas, including acetohexamide, chlorpropamide, glipizide, tolazamide, and tolbutamide. Patients should be advised that these drugs are not a cure for diabetes but only a means of controlling it and that it is important to continue to comply with dietary and exercise prescriptions.

hypoglycemic coma [Gk, *hypo,* under, *glykys,* sweet, *koma,* deep sleep],   a loss of consciousness that results from abnormally low blood glucose levels.

hypoglycogenolysis /-glī′kōjənol″isis/,   a metabolic disorder in which deficient or defective splitting of glycogen molecules results in decreased formation of glucose.

hypogonadism /-gō″nədiz′əm/,   a deficiency in the secretory activity of the ovary or testis. The condition may be primary or caused by a gonadal dysfunction involving the Leydig cells in the male, or it may be secondary to a hypothalamus or pituitary disorder. Secondary hypogonadism is sometimes further differentiated into pituitary hypogonadism and hypothalamic hypogonadism.

hypohidrosis,   diminished sweat production as a result of a congenital condition, or a blockage of the sweat ducts as a sequela to prickly heat, excessive heat, autonomic neuropathy, or conditions such as hemorrhage or diarrhea that cause body fluid loss. See also **anhidrosis.**

hypohidrotic ectodermal dysplasia.   See **anhidrotic ectodermal dysplasia.**

hypoinsulinism /-in″səliniz′əm/ [Gk, *hypo,* under; L, *insula,* island (of Langerhans)],   a deficiency of insulin secretion by cells of the pancreas, with associated signs and symptoms of diabetes.

hypokalemia /hī′pōkəlē″mē·ə/ [Gk, *hypo* + L, *kalium,* potassium; Gk, *haima,* blood], a condition in which an inadequate amount of potassium, the major intracellular cation, is found in the circulating bloodstream. Hypokalemia is characterized by abnormal electrocardiographic findings, weakness, confusion, mental depression, and flaccid paralysis. The cause may be starvation, treatment of diabetic acidosis, adrenal tumor, or diuretic therapy. Mild hypokalemia may resolve itself when the underlying disorder is corrected. Severe hypokalemia may be treated by the administration of potassium chloride, orally or parenterally, and by a diet high in potassium. Also called **kaliopenia.** Also spelled *hypokalaemia.* Compare **hyperkalemia.** See also **electrolyte balance.** –*hypokalemic, adj.*

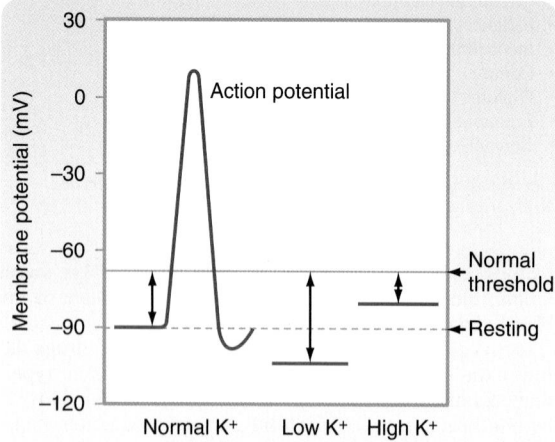

Hypokalemia hyperpolarizes the membrane potential and thereby reduces excitability
(Koeppen and Stanton, 2010)

hypokalemic alkalosis /-kalē″mik/, a pathological condition resulting from the accumulation of base or the loss of acid from the body, associated with a low level of serum potassium. The retention of alkali or the loss of acid occurs primarily in extracellular fluid, but the pH of intracellular fluid may also be subnormal. See also **hypokalemia.**

hypokalemic nephropathy, nephropathy with hypokalemia, interstitial nephritis, swelling and vacuolization of proximal renal tubules, and progressive renal failure, resulting from long-term conditions, such as oncotic overloading of the kidney filtration mechanisms by sugars.

hypokalemic periodic paralysis [Gk, *hypo,* under; L, *kalium,* potassium; Gk, *peri,* near, *hodos,* way, *paralyein,* to be palsied], a state of recurring attacks of muscular weakness associated with low blood levels of potassium.

hypokinesia. See **hypomotility.**

hypokinetic /-kinet″ik/ [Gk, *hypo,* under, *kinesis,* movement], pertaining to diminished power of movement or motor function, which may or may not be accompanied by a mild form of paralysis.

hypolipoproteinemia /hī′pōlip′ōprō′tēnē″mē·ə/ [Gk, *hypo* + *lipos,* fat, *proteios,* first rank, *haima,* blood], a group of defects of lipoprotein metabolism that cause varying complexes of signs. Primary, or hereditary, hypolipoproteinemia factors include abnormal transport of triglycerides in the blood, low levels of high-density lipoproteins, and abnormal fat deposits in the body, especially in the kidneys and the liver. In some of the syndromes ocular, cardiovascular intestinal, and neurological effects are also present. The condition also may be secondary to anemia, malabsorption syndromes, or malnutrition.

hypomagnesemia /hī′pōmag′nise″mē·ə/, an abnormally low concentration of magnesium in the blood plasma, which causes nausea, vomiting, muscle weakness, tremors, tetany, and lethargy. Tachycardia and arrhythmia may also occur. Mild hypomagnesemia is usually the result of inadequate absorption of magnesium in the kidney or intestine, although it is also seen after prolonged parenteral feeding and during lactation. A more severe form is associated with malabsorption syndrome, protein malnutrition, and parathyroid disease. Magnesium salts to correct the deficiency may be given orally or intravenously.

hypomania /-mā″nē·ə/ [Gk, *hypo* + *mania,* madness], a mild degree of mania characterized by optimism; excitability; energetic, productive behavior; marked hyperactivity and talkativeness; heightened sexual interest; quick anger and irritability; and a decreased need for sleep. It may be observed before a full-blown manic episode. –*hypomanic, adj.,* –*hypomaniac, n.*

hypomelanosis of Ito. See **incontinentia pigmenti achromians.**

hypometria /hī′pōmē″trē·ə/ [Gk, *hypo* + *metron,* measure], an abnormal form of dysmetria characterized by a dysfunction of the power to control the range of muscular action, resulting in movements that fall short of the intended goals of the affected individual. Compare **hypermetria.**

hypomobility /-mōbil″itē/, a decrease in the normal movement of a joint or body part, as may result from an articular surface dysfunction or from disease or injury that affects a bone, muscle, or joint.

hypomorph /hī″pōmôrf/ [Gk, *hypo* + *morphe,* form], **1.** a person whose arms and legs are disproportionately short in relation to the trunk and whose sitting height is disproportionately tall compared to the standing height. **2.** a mutant allele that has a reduced effect on the expression of a trait but does not cause abnormal development. Also called **leaky gene.** Compare **amorph, antimorph, hypermorph.**

hypomotility /-mōtil″itē/ [Gk, *hypo,* under; L, *motare,* to move frequently], a state of diminished motility or loss of power to move about. Also called **hypokinesia.**

hyponasality /hī′pōnāzal′itē/ [Gk, *hypo,* under + *nasus,* nose], a speech characteristic caused by insufficient resonance of air in the nasal cavity so that speakers sound as if they have a cold. Consonant sounds /m/, /n/, and /ng/ are affected. Also called **denasality.**

hyponatremia /hī′pōnatrē″mē·ə/ [Gk, *hypo* + L, *natrium,* sodium; Gk, *haima,* blood], a lower-than-normal concentration of sodium in the blood, caused by inadequate excretion of water or by excessive water in the circulating bloodstream. In a severe case the person may experience water intoxication, with confusion and lethargy, leading to muscle excitability, convulsions, and coma. Fluid and electrolyte balance may be restored by IV infusion of a balanced solution or a fluid-restricted diet.

hyponychial /hī′ponik′e·al/. See **subungual.**

hypoosmolality [Gk, *hypo* + *osmos,* impulse], a state or condition of abnormally reduced osmolality. The normal serum concentration (millimoles per liter) is 0.43–0.50 times the serum osmolality (milliosmoles per kilogram). A decrease in this ratio is caused by an increase in other osmolutes, such as glucose or ketone bodies in diabetes mellitus, urea in uremia, or salicylate in salicylic poisoning. See also **osmolality.**

hypoosmotic /hī′pō-ozmot″ik/, pertaining to a solution that has a lower solute concentration than another solution. Compare **hyperosmotic, isosmotic.**

hypoosmotic swelling, swelling of sperm in a hypoosmotic solution because of shifts in free water.

hypoparathyroidism /-per′əthī′roidiz′əm/ [Gk, *hypo* + *para*, beside, *thyreos*, shield, *eidos*, form], a condition of insufficient secretion of the parathyroid glands. It can be caused by primary parathyroid dysfunction or by elevated serum calcium level.

hypoperistalsis /-per′istal″sis/ [Gk, *hypo*, under, *peristellein*, to clasp], a state of abnormally slow motility of waves of alternate contraction and relaxation that propel contents forward through the digestive tract. See also **peristalsis.**

hypopharyngeal /-fərin″jē-əl/ [Gk, *hypo* + *pharynx*, throat], **1.** pertaining to the hypopharynx. **2.** situated below the pharynx.

hypopharyngeal eminence. See **copula.**

hypopharynx /-fer″ingks/, the inferior portion of the pharynx between the epiglottis and the larynx. It corresponds to the height of the epiglottis and is a critical dividing point in separating solids and fluids from air entering the region.

hypophonia /-fō″nē-ə/ [Gk, *hypo*, under, *phone*, voice], a weak or whispered voice.

hypophoria /-fôr″ē-ə/, a type of strabismus in which the patient may not show signs of ocular muscle imbalance until the affected eye is covered, resulting in a downward deviation. Otherwise the central nervous system may attempt to compensate for the defect through a fusion of the images received from both of the eyes.

hypophosphatasia /hī′pōfos′fətā″zhə/ [Gk, *hypo* + *phosphoros*, lightbearing], congenital absence of alkaline phosphatase, an enzyme essential to the calcification of bone tissue. Complications include vomiting, growth delay, and often death in infancy. Children who survive have numerous skeletal abnormalities and suffer from dwarfism. There is no known treatment.

hypophosphatemic rickets /hī′pōfos′fətē″mik/, a rare familial disorder characterized by impaired resorption of phosphate in the kidneys and poor absorption of calcium in the small intestine, which result in osteomalacia, delayed growth, skeletal deformities, and pain. Treatment includes replacement of phosphate and vitamin D to be taken by mouth.

hypophyseal /-fizē″əl, -fiz″ē-əl/ [Gk, *hypo*, under, *phyein*, to grow], pertaining to the hypophysis (pituitary body).

hypophyseal cachexia. See **panhypopituitarism.**

hypophyseal dwarf. See **pituitary dwarf.**

hypophyseal hormones, pituitary hormones that are associated with body growth and exercise effects, such as luteinizing hormone, which stimulates testosterone production and muscular hypertrophy; growth hormone; and antidiuretic hormone.

hypophyseal portal system, a set of vessels (arteries and capillaries) that carry blood and regulatory hormones from the hypothalamus to the adenohypophysis, where the target cells of the releasing hormones are located.

hypophysectomy /hīpof′əsek″təmē/ [Gk, *hypo* + *phyein*, to grow, *ektomē*, excision], surgical removal of the pituitary gland. It may be performed to slow the growth and spread of endocrine-dependent malignant tumors or to excise a pituitary tumor. The gland is removed only if other treatment, such as x-ray therapy, radioactive implants, or cryosurgery, fails to destroy all pituitary tissue. With general anesthesia, the gland is completely removed. Postoperative nursing care is as for a craniotomy. Levels of hormones, including thyroid-stimulating hormone, adrenocorticotropic hormone, and antidiuretic hormone, are monitored, and replacement therapy is begun as needed. Urinary output is measured every 2 hours for several days to monitor for diabetes insipidus, and an amount in excess of 300 mL in any 2-hour period is reported. The patient is closely monitored for early signs of thyroid crisis, Addisonian crisis, electrolyte imbalance, hemorrhage, hypothermia, and meningitis. −*hypophysectomize, v.*

hypophyseoprivic /-fiz′ē-ōpriv″ik/ [L, *privus*, deprived], pertaining to a deficiency of hormone secretions by the pituitary gland (hypophysis). The condition may be caused by functional inactivity or surgical removal of the gland.

hypophysial fossa, the deep central area of the sella turcica that contains the pituitary gland.

hypophysis /hīpof″isis/ [Gk, *hypo*, under, *phyein*, to grow], the pituitary body (gland). The anterior lobe is sometimes identified as the adenohypophysis and the posterior lobe as the neurohypophysis.

hypophysis cerebri. See **pituitary gland.**

hypopigmentation /-pig′məntā″shən/ [Gk, *hypo* + L, *pigmentum*, paint], unusual lack of skin color, but not complete lack of pigment as seen in albinism. Compare **hyperpigmentation.**

hypopituitarism /-pityōō″iteriz′əm/ [Gk, *hypo* + L, *pituita*, phlegm], an abnormal condition caused by diminished activity of the pituitary gland resulting in decreased secretion of its hormones. Symptoms vary depending on which hormones are affected. The manifestations depend on the hormone(s) and target tissues involved. Serum levels of pituitary hormones are lower than normal.

hypoplasia /hī′pōplā″zhə/ [Gk, *hypo* + *plassein*, to mold], underdevelopment of an organ or a tissue, usually resulting from the presence of a smaller-than-normal number of cells. Also called **hypoplasty.** Compare **aplasia, hyperplasia.** Kinds include **cartilage-hair hypoplasia, enamel hypoplasia.** See also **oligomeganephronia, osteogenesis imperfecta.** −**hypoplastic,** *adj.*

hypoplasia of the mesenchyme. See **osteogenesis imperfecta.**

hypoplastic. See **hypoplasia.**

hypoplastic anemia /-plas″tik/, anemias characterized by inadequately functioning bone marrow. Compare **aplastic anemia, polycythemia.**

hypoplastic dwarf. See **primordial dwarf.**

hypoplastic left heart syndrome (HLHS), any of a group of congenital anomalies consisting of hypoplasia or atresia of the left ventricle and of the aortic or mitral valve or both and hypoplasia of the ascending aorta. It is characterized by respiratory distress and extreme cyanosis, with cardiac failure and death in early infancy.

hypoplasty. See **hypoplasia.**

hypoploid /hī″pəploid/ [Gk, *hypo* + *eidos*, form], **1.** *n.*, an individual, organism, strain, or cell that has fewer than the haploid number or than an exact multiple of the haploid number of chromosomes characteristic of the species. The result is one or more unbalanced sets of chromosomes, which are referred to as hypodiploid, hypotriploid, hypotetraploid, and so on, depending on the number of multiples of the haploid chromosomes they contain. **2.** *adj.*, pertaining to such an individual, organism, strain, or cell. Also called *hypoploidic.* Compare **hyperploid.** See also **monosomy.** −**hypoploidy.** *n.*

hypoploidy /hī″pəploi′dē/, any decrease in chromosome number that involves individual chromosomes rather than entire sets so that fewer than the normal haploid number of chromosomes characteristic of the species are present, as in Turner syndrome. Compare **hyperploidy.**

hypopnea /hīpop″nē·ə, hī′pōnē″ə/ [Gk, *hypo* + *pnoe,* breath], abnormally shallow and slow respiration. In well-conditioned athletes it may be appropriate and is often accompanied by a slow pulse. Otherwise, it is apparent when pleuritic pain limits excursion and is characteristic of damage to the brainstem. Accompanied by a rapid, weak pulse, it is a grave sign. See also **respiration rate.**

hypopotassemia /-pot′əsē″mē·ə/ [Gk, *hypo* + Ð, *potasch,* potash; Gk, *haima,* blood], a deficiency of potassium in the blood. See also **hypokalemia.**

hypoproliferative anemias /-prolif″ərətiv′/, a group of anemias caused by inadequate production of erythrocytes. The condition is associated with protein deficiencies, renal disease, and myxedema.

hypoproteinemia /hī′pōprō′tēnē″mē·ə/ [Gk, *hypo* + *proteios,* first rank, *haima,* blood], abnormally decreased plasma protein, accompanied by edema, nausea, vomiting, diarrhea, and abdominal pain. It may be caused by renal failure and *burns.*

hypoprothrombinemia /hī′pōprōthrom′binē″mē·ə/ [Gk, *hypo* + L, *pro,* before; Gk, *thrombos,* lump, *haima,* blood], abnormally reduced plasma prothrombin, characterized by bleeding, poor clot formation, and prolonged prothrombin and partial thromboplastin times. It is usually caused by inadequate synthesis of prothrombin in the liver, vitamin K deficiency, or most often by anticoagulant therapy. Also spelled *hypoprothrombinaemia.* See also **blood clotting.**

hypoptyalism. See **hyposalivation.**

hypopyon /hīpō″pē·on/ [Gk, *hypo* + *pyon,* pus], the presence of leukocytes and an accumulation of pus in the anterior chamber of an eye, which appears as a whitish or gray fluid between the cornea and the iris. It may occur as a complication of a penetrating wound to the eye, conjunctivitis, herpetic keratitis, or corneal ulcer.

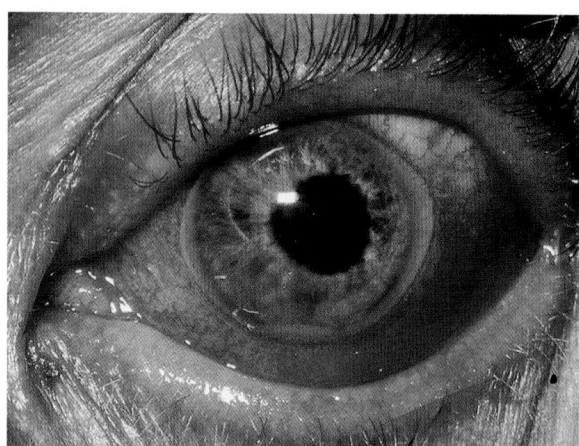

Hypopyon *(Spalton et al, 2005)*

hyporeflexia /-riflek″sē·ə/ [Gk, *hypo* + L, *reflectere,* to bend back], decreased reflex reactions.

hyposalivation /-sal′ivā″shən/ [Gk, *hypo* + L, *saliva,* spittle], a decreased flow of saliva associated with dehydration; radiation therapy of the salivary gland regions; anxiety; menopause; the use of drugs such as atropine, glycopyrrolate,

and antihistamines; vitamin deficiency; inflammation or infection of the salivary glands; or various syndromes, such as Plummer-Vinson syndrome. Also called **asialorrhea.** See also **xerostomia.**

hyposensitization, a form of immunotherapy that can either reduce or eliminate hypersensitivity. See also **immunotherapy.**

hypospadias /hī′pōspā′dē·əs/ [Gk, *hypo,* under, *spadōn,* a rent], a developmental anomaly in the male in which the urethra opens on the ventral aspect of the penis or on the perineum.

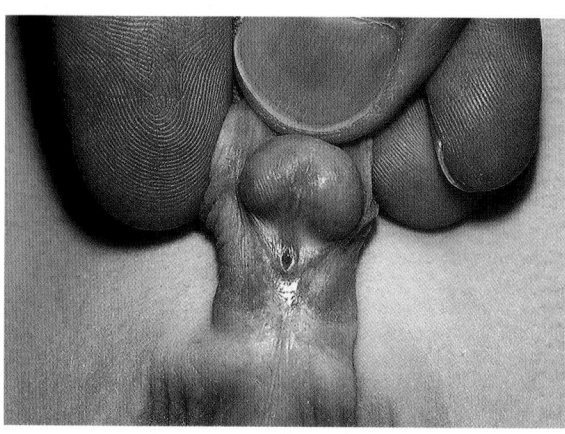

Infant with hypospadias *(Rothrock, 2015)*

hypospermatogenesis /hi″pōsper″mätojen′ĕsis/, a reduction in the number of germ cells (spermatogonia, spermatocytes, and spermatids), resulting in a low sperm count. Compare **aspermatogenesis.**

hypostatic /-stat″ik/ [Gk, *hypo* + *stasis,* standing still], pertaining to an accumulation of deposits of substances or congestion in a body area that results from a lack of activity.

hypostatic lung collapse [Gk, *hypo,* under, *stasis,* standing still; AS, *lungen* + L, *collabi,* to fall together], a disorder in which fluids or suspended solids pool or settle in a part of the lung, resulting in congestion.

hypostatic pneumonia, a type of pneumonia associated with elderly or debilitated people who remain in the same position for long periods. Fluids tend to settle in one area of the lungs, increasing the susceptibility to infection.

hyposthenic /hī′pōsthen″ik/, **1.** pertaining to a lack of strength or muscle tone. **2.** describing a body type characterized by a slender build.

hypotelorism /hī′pōtel″əriz′əm/ [Gk, *hypo* + *tele,* far, *horizo,* separate], a developmental defect characterized by an abnormally decreased distance between two organs or parts. Compare **hypertelorism.** Kinds include **ocular hypotelorism.**

hypotension /-ten″shən/ [Gk, *hypo* + L, *tendere,* to stretch], an abnormal condition in which the blood pressure is not adequate for normal perfusion and oxygenation of the tissues. An expanded intravascular space, hypovolemia, or diminished cardiac output may be the cause.

hypotensive /-ten″siv/ [Gk, *hypo,* under; L, *tendere,* to stretch], pertaining to abnormally low blood pressure.

hypotensive anesthesia, hypotensive technique. See **deliberate hypotension, controlled hypotension.**

hypotetraploid. See **hypoploid.**

hypothalamic. See **hypothalamus.**

hypothalamic amenorrhea /-thalam″ik/ [Gk, *hypo + thalamos,* chamber], cessation of menses caused by disorders that inhibit the hypothalamus from initiating the cycle of neurohormonal interactions of the brain, pituitary, and ovary necessary for ovulation and subsequent menstruation. Examples of causes are stress, anxiety, and acute weight loss. See also **amenorrhea.**

hypothalamic hormones, a group of hormones secreted by the hypothalamus, including vasopressin, oxytocin, and releasing and inhibitory hormones that act on the anterior pituitary.

hypothalamic obesity [Gk, *hypo,* under, *thalamos,* chamber; L, *obesitas,* fatness], obesity caused by damage or a functional disturbance involving the hypothalamus.

hypothalamic-pituitary-adrenal axis, the combined system of neuroendocrine units that in a negative feedback network regulate the adrenal gland's hormonal activities.

hypothalamus /hī′pōthal″əməs/ [Gk, *hypo + thalamos,* chamber], a portion of the diencephalon of the brain, forming the floor and part of the lateral wall of the third ventricle. It activates, controls, and integrates the peripheral autonomic nervous system, endocrine processes, and many somatic functions, such as body temperature, sleep, and appetite. Compare **epithalamus, metathalamus, subthalamus, thalamus. –hypothalamic,** *adj.*

hypothenar eminence /hīpoth″ənär, hī′pōthē″när/ [Gk, *hypo + thenar,* palm], a fleshy pad on the ulnar side of the palm of the hand.

hypothermal /-thur″məl/ [Gk, *hypo,* under, *therme,* heat], **1.** pertaining to a condition in which the body temperature is significantly below normal as a result of external exposure to cold or has been reduced markedly for surgical or therapeutic purposes. **2.** pertaining to temperatures that are tepid to slightly warm.

hypothermia /hī′pōthur″mē·ə/ [Gk *hypo+ therme,* heat], **1.** an abnormal and dangerous condition in which the oral temperature is below 95° F (35° C) or the rectal temperature is below 96° F (35.5° C), usually caused by prolonged exposure to cold or damp conditions. Symptoms include drowsiness, lack of coordination, confusion, and uncontrolled shivering. Respiration is shallow and slow, and the heart rate is faint and slow. The person may appear to be dead. People who are very old or very young; people who have cardiovascular problems; and people who are hungry, tired, or under the influence of alcohol are most susceptible to hypothermia. Hospitalization is necessary for evaluating and treating any metabolic abnormalities that may result from hypothermia. Hypothermic patients in cardiac arrest should be rewarmed to 32° C (92° F) before resuscitation efforts are abandoned. **2.** the deliberate and controlled reduction of body temperature with cooling mattresses or ice as preparation for some surgical procedures or in other situations in which a reduction in the metabolic rate is necessary. Also called *therapeutic hypothermia.*

hypothermia blanket, a covering or pad used to lower the body temperature to decrease metabolism and oxygen consumption during a surgical procedure or to induce therapeutic hypothermia.

hypothermia therapy, the reduction of a patient's body temperature to counteract prolonged high fever caused by an infectious or neurological disease or, less frequently, as an adjunct to anesthesia in heart or brain surgery.
■ METHOD: Hypothermia may be produced by autotransfusing blood after it is circulated through coils submerged in a refrigerant or, most commonly, by applying cooling blankets or vinyl pads containing coils through which cold water and alcohol are circulated by a pump. The cooling unit is placed in an open area. Any kinks or twists in the tubing are removed, and the blanket is checked for leaks. The patient is wrapped in bath blankets and then covered with the cooling blanket. The patient's temperature, registered by means of a probe inserted into the rectum, is read and recorded before hypothermia is initiated, every 5 minutes until the desired reduction is achieved, and then every 15 minutes. The blood pressure, pulse, respirations, and neurological status are checked every 5 to 10 minutes until the temperature is stabilized, then every 30 minutes for 2 hours, every 4 hours for the next 24 hours, and subsequently as required. Every 1 to 2 hours the patient is assisted in turning, coughing, and deep breathing. At similar intervals the chest is auscultated for breath sounds, and oral, nose, and skin care are administered; the skin is lubricated with oil or lotion before and during the procedure. An indwelling catheter is connected to a closed gravity drainage system, as ordered, and fluid intake and output are measured; if less than 30 mL of urine per hour is excreted, the physician is notified. If the patient's oral temperature is less than 90° F (32.2° C), the gag reflex is tested before any oral fluids or foods are administered. Nasooral suction is performed as indicated, body alignment is maintained, and passive or active range-of-motion exercises are performed every 4 hours. Because shivering increases body heat, medication for its prevention, such as chlorpromazine hydrochloride, may be ordered. The patient is observed for medication reactions, decrease in blood pressure, bradycardia, arrhythmias, bradypnea, respiratory failure, unequal pupils, increase in intracranial pressure, changes in consciousness, intestinal ileus, and frostbite. Any changes in skin color or signs of edema and induration are reported to the physician immediately. At the termination of therapy, the cooling blanket is replaced by regular blankets, and the patient usually warms at his or her own rate. As the patient's temperature approaches normal, the blankets are removed, but the temperature probe remains in place until the body temperature is stable.
■ INTERVENTIONS: The technician administers hypothermia, carefully monitoring the patient's vital signs and any evidence of complications.
■ OUTCOME CRITERIA: Hypothermia therapy used in the treatment of high fever associated with generalized severe infections reduces body heat by decreasing metabolism and inhibits the multiplication of the causative pathogenic organisms. Patients with a high temperature caused by a neurological disease may be maintained in a state of mild hypothermia (87° F to 95° F or 30.6° C to 35° C) for as long as 5 days. The procedure is successful if the fever is broken and complications do not occur.

hypothesis /hīpoth″isis/ [Gk, groundwork], (in research) a statement derived from a theory that predicts the relationship among variables representing concepts, constructs, or events. Kinds include **causal hypothesis, null hypothesis, predictive hypothesis.**

hypothyroid /-thī″roid/ [Gk, *hypo,* under, *thyreos,* shield, *eidos,* form], pertaining to or resembling thyroid deficiency.

hypothyroid dwarf. See **cretin dwarf.**

hypothyroidism /-thī″roidiz′əm/ [Gk, *hypo + thyreos,* shield, *eidos,* form], a condition characterized by decreased activity of the thyroid gland. It may be caused by surgical removal of all or part of the gland, overdosage with antithyroid medication, decreased effect of thyroid-releasing hormone secreted by the hypothalamus, decreased secretion of thyroid-stimulating hormone by the pituitary gland, atrophy of the thyroid gland itself, or peripheral resistance to thyroid hormone. See also **Hashimoto disease, myxedema.**
■ OBSERVATIONS: Manifestations include weight gain; cold, pale, dry, rough hands and feet; reduced attention span with

memory impairment, slowed speech, and loss of initiative; swelling in extremities and around the eyes, eyelids, and face; menstrual irregularities; muscle aches and weakness; joint aches and stiffness; clumsiness; hyperstiff reflexes; decreased pulse; decreased blood pressure; agitation; depression; and paranoia. Hypothyroidism is diagnosed through lab testing. Serum and serum-free triiodothyronine and thyroxine (T_3, T_4) are decreased. Serum thyroid-stimulating hormone (TSH) is increased in primary hypothyroidism and decreased or normal in secondary hypothyroidism. Serum lipids and cholesterol levels are increased. Myxedema coma is a life-threatening complication of hypothyroidism that necessitates immediate treatment. It is preceded by gradual or sudden onset of mental sluggishness, drowsiness, and lethargy. Other complications include ischemic heart disease, congestive heart failure, pleural and pericardial effusion, deafness, psychosis, and anemia.
■ INTERVENTIONS: The primary treatment for hypothyroidism is oral replacement of the thyroid hormone, with lifelong monitoring of TSH level at least annually. Triiodothyronine may be added to the replacement therapy regimen in patients who continue to have mood or memory problems.
■ PATIENT CARE CONSIDERATIONS: Nursing care centers around education and includes instruction about signs and symptoms of hypothyroidism and hyperthyroidism, drug effects and side effects, and the need for thyroid hormone replacement therapy and monitoring for life. Nurses also play a role in early detection by advising patients to undergo thyroid screening every 2 to 3 years.

hypotonia /-tō″nē·ə/ [Gk, *hypo,* under, *tonos,* stretching], a condition of diminished tone or tension that may involve any body structure.

hypotonic /hī′pŏton″ik/ [Gk, *hypo,* under, *tonos,* stretching], **1.** *adj.,* pertaining to a lower or lessened tone or tension in any body structure, as in paralysis. **2.** *n.,* a solution having a lower concentration of solute than another solution, hence exerting less osmotic pressure than that solution. **3.** *adj.,* pertaining to a solution that causes cells to swell. Compare **hypertonic, isotonic.**

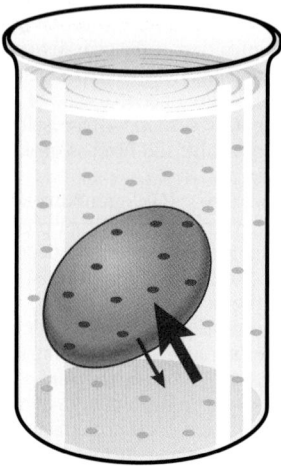

Red blood cell in hypotonic solution
(Waugh and Grant, 2014)

hypotonic duodenography. See **duodenography.**
hypotonic saline [Gk, *hypo,* under, *tonos,* tone; L, *sal,* salt], a saline solution that is less than isotonic in strength.
hypotriploid. See **hypoploid.**

hypoventilation /-ven′tilā″shən/ [Gk, *hypo* + L, *ventilare,* to fan], an abnormal condition of the respiratory system that occurs when the volume of air that enters the alveoli and takes part in gas exchange is not adequate for the body's metabolic needs. It is characterized by cyanosis, polycythemia, increased $PaCO_2$, and generalized decreased respiratory function. Hypoventilation may be caused by an uneven distribution of inspired air (as in bronchitis), obesity, neuromuscular or skeletal disease affecting the thorax, decreased response of the respiratory center to carbon dioxide, or a reduced amount of functional lung tissue, as in atelectasis, emphysema, and pleural effusion. The results of hypoventilation are hypoxia, hypercapnia, pulmonary hypertension with cor pulmonale, and respiratory acidosis. Treatment includes weight reduction in cases of obesity, artificial respiration, and possibly tracheostomy. Compare **hyperventilation.** See also **respiratory center.**
hypovitaminosis. See **avitaminosis.**
hypovolemia /-vōlē″mē·ə/ [Gk, *hypo* + L, *volumen,* whirl; Gk, *haima,* blood], an abnormally low circulating blood volume. Also spelled *hypovolaemia.* −*hypovolemic, adj.*
hypovolemic shock /-vōlē·mik/, a state of physical collapse and prostration caused by massive blood loss, about one fifth or more of total blood volume. The common signs include low blood pressure, thready pulse, clammy skin, tachycardia, rapid breathing, and reduced urinary output. The associated blood losses may stem from GI bleeding, internal or external hemorrhage, or excessive reduction of intravascular plasma volume and body fluids. Disorders that may cause hypovolemic shock are dehydration from excessive perspiration, severe diarrhea, protracted vomiting, intestinal obstruction, peritonitis, acute pancreatitis, and severe burns, which deplete body fluids. Associated effects may include metabolic acidosis with the accumulation of lactic acid, irreversible cerebral and renal damage, and disseminated intravascular coagulation. Treatment of hypovolemic shock focuses on prompt replacement of blood and fluid volumes, identification of bleeding sites, and control of bleeding. Without fast, aggressive treatment, further collapse that can cause death ensues. Compare **cardiogenic shock.** See also **electric shock, shock.**
hypoxemia /hī′poksē″mē·ə/ [Gk, *hypo* + *oxys,* sharp, *genein,* to produce, *haima,* blood], an abnormal deficiency in the concentration of oxygen in arterial blood. Symptoms of acute hypoxemia are cyanosis, restlessness, stupor, coma, Cheyne-Stokes respiration, apnea, increased blood pressure, tachycardia, and an initial increase in cardiac output that later falls, producing hypotension and ventricular fibrillation or asystole. Chronic hypoxemia stimulates red blood cell production by the bone marrow, leading to secondary polycythemia. Hypoxemia caused by decreased alveolar oxygen tension or underventilation improves with oxygen therapy. Hypoxemia resulting from shunting of blood from the right side of the heart to the left side without exchange of gases in the lungs is treated with bronchial hygiene and positive end-expiratory pressure. Also spelled *hypoxaemia.* Compare **hypoxia.** See also **anoxia, asphyxia.**
hypoxia /hīpok″sē·ə/ [Gk, *hypo* + *oxys,* sharp, *genein,* to produce], inadequate oxygen tension at the cellular level, characterized by tachycardia, hypertension, peripheral vasoconstriction, dizziness, and mental confusion. Mild hypoxia stimulates peripheral chemoreceptors to increase heart and respiration rates. The central mechanisms that regulate breathing fail in severe hypoxia, leading to irregular respiration, Cheyne-Stokes respiration, apnea, and respiratory and cardiac failure. Increased sensitivity to the depressant effect of opiates on the respiratory system is common in chronic hypoxia, causing severe depression of respiration or apnea from relatively small doses. If the availability of oxygen is inadequate

for aerobic cellular metabolism, energy is provided by less efficient anaerobic pathways that produce metabolites other than carbon dioxide and water. The tissues most sensitive to hypoxia are the brain, heart, pulmonary vessels, and liver. Treatment may include cardiotonic and respiratory stimulant drugs, oxygen therapy, mechanical ventilation, and frequent analysis of blood gases. Compare **hypoxemia.** See also **acute hypoxia, anoxia, chemoreceptor, chronic hypoxia, hyperventilation, respiratory center.** –*hypoxic, adj.*

hypoxic drive /-hīpok″sik/, stimulation of respiration by low PaO₂, mediated through the carotid and aortic bodies.

hypsi-, prefix meaning "high": *hypsibrachycephaly, hypsicephaly.*

hypsibrachycephaly /hips′ibrakisef″əlē/ [Gk, *hypsi,* high, *brachys,* short, *kephale,* head], the condition of having a skull that is high with a broad forehead. See also **brachycephaly, oxycephaly.** –*hypsibrachycephalic, adj., n.*

hypsicephaly. See **oxycephaly.**

hypso-, prefix meaning "height": *hypsophobia.*

hypsophobia, fear of heights.

hyster-. See **hystero-, hyster-.**

hysteralgia. See **metralgia.**

hysterectomy /his′tərek″təmē/ [Gk, *hystera,* womb, *ektomē,* excision], surgical removal of the uterus, performed to remove fibroid tumors of the uterus or to treat chronic pelvic inflammatory disease, severe recurrent endometrial hyperplasia, uterine hemorrhage, and precancerous and cancerous conditions of the uterus. Types of hysterectomy include total hysterectomy, in which the uterus and cervix are removed, and radical hysterectomy, in which ovaries, oviducts, lymph nodes, and lymph channels are removed with the uterus and cervix. Menstruation ceases after either type is performed. A vaginal irrigation may be given preoperatively. During surgery the uterus is excised and removed, either through the abdominal wall or through the vagina. In some cases it may be removed laparoscopically. One or both ovaries and oviducts may be removed at the same time. After surgery the nurse frequently observes the abdominal dressing and vaginal pad for bleeding. The lower half of the bed is kept flat, and the patient is advised to avoid sharply flexing the thighs or knees, because thrombophlebitis of the blood vessels of the pelvis and upper thigh is a frequent complication. Leg exercises, as well as use of sequential compression devices to prevent deep vein thrombosis, are encouraged. Low back pain or scanty urine may indicate a ligated ureter. Compare **hysterosalpingo-oophorectomy.** Kinds include **cesarean hysterectomy.** –*hysterectomize, v.*

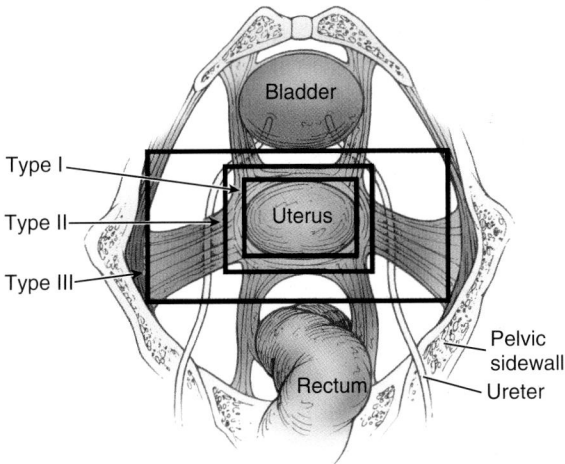

Types of hysterectomy: Type I—simple hysterectomy; Type II—modified radical hysterectomy; Type III—radical hysterectomy *(Rothrock, 2015)*

hysteresis /his′tərē″sis/ [Gk, *hysterein,* to be late], **1.** a lagging or slowing of one of two associated phenomena or a failure to act in unison. **2.** the influence of the previous condition or treatment of the body on its subsequent response to a given force, as in the elastic property of a lung. At any given lung volume the elastic recoil pressure within the airways during expiration is less than that which exists at the same lung volume during inspiration.

hysteria /histir″ē·ə/ [Gk, *hystera,* womb], a general state of tension or excitement in a person or a group, characterized by unmanageable fear and temporary loss of control over the emotions.

hysteric /hister″ik/ [Gk, *hystera,* womb], pertaining to or resembling hysteria.

hysteric amaurosis [Gk, *hystera* + *amauroein,* to darken], monocular or, more rarely, binocular blindness that follows an emotional shock. It may last for hours, days, or months.

hysteric aphonia. *(Obsolete)* See **conversion dysphonia.**

hysteric ataxia [Gk, *hystera,* womb, *ataxia,* without order], a loss of control over voluntary movements in walking or standing, although the involved muscles function normally when the person is lying or sitting. See also **astasia-abasia.**

hysteric blindness. See **psychic blindness.**

hysteric chorea [Gk, *hystera,* womb, *choreia,* dance], a condition in which an individual has choreiform movements, although the actions are psychogenic rather than the result of true chorea.

hysteric convulsion, a violent involuntary contraction and relaxation of the skeletal muscles marked by spasmodic muscular contractions with no organic cause.

hysteric dyspepsia, difficulty in digestion caused by emotional disturbances.

hysteric lethargy [Gk, *hystera* + *lethargia,* drowsiness], a sleep induced by hypnosis. See also **hypnosis, lethargy.**

hysteric paralysis [Gk, *hystera,* womb, *paralyein,* to be palsied], a loss of movement or muscular weakness that is psychogenic rather than the result of an identifiable organic defect.

hysteric personality. See **histrionic personality.**

hysteric syncope, a temporary loss of consciousness or a fainting spell caused by emotional agitation.

hysteric tremor [Gk, *hystera,* womb; L, *tremere,* to tremble], **1.** a fine rhythmic shaking in one extremity or of a generalized nature that may be an expression of fear, anxiety, or hysteria. **2.** a coarse, irregular shaking that increases with voluntary movements. **3.** a shaking that is transient and is caused by exposure to drugs or toxic substances rather than an organic disorder.

hysteric vertigo, a giddiness or loss of stability, often with a sensation of rotation, with no organic cause.

hystero-, hyster-, prefix meaning "uterus": *hysterectomy, hysterogram, hysterotome.*

hysterodynia. See **metralgia.**

hysterogram /his″tərōgram′/ [Gk, *hystera* + *gramma,* record], a radiographic image of a uterus made after the injection of a contrast medium into the uterine cavity. See also **hysterosalpingogram.**

hysterography /his′tərog″rəfē/ [Gk, *hystera,* womb, *graphein,* to record], the use of x-ray images and other instruments to make a medical assessment of the condition of the uterus.

hysterolaparotomy /his′tərōlap′ərot″əmē/ [Gk, *hystera* + *lapara,* loin, *temnein,* to cut], *(Obsolete)* now called **abdominal hysterectomy.**

hystero-oophorectomy /-ō′əfərek″təmē/ [Gk, *hystera,* womb, *oophoron,* ovary, *ektomē,* excision], the surgical removal of the uterus and both ovaries.

hysterosalpingogram /his′tərō′salping″gōgram′/ [Gk, *hystera* + *salpinx,* tube, *gramma,* record], an x-ray image of the uterus and the fallopian tubes using gas or a radiopaque substance introduced through the cervix to allow visualization of the cavity of the uterus and the passageway of the tubes. A blockage of a structure is demonstrated on the film because the radiopaque substance cannot pass to the more distal structures and escape from the ends of the tubes into the peritoneal cavity. Serial hysterosalpingography is useful in the diagnosis of the cause of infertility.

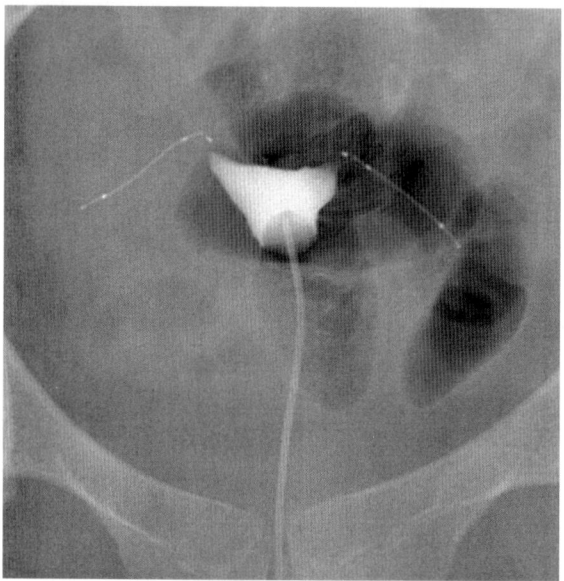

Hysterosalpingography used to evaluate the patency of the fallopian tubes *(Fielding et al, 2011)*

hysterosalpingography /his′tərōsal′ping·gog″rəfē/, a method of producing radiographic images of the uterus and fallopian tubes as part of the diagnosis of abnormalities in the reproductive tract of a nonpregnant woman. The technique outlines the size, shape, and position of the organs, including any tumors, fistulas, or polyps. It also reveals any obstructions in the fallopian tubes.

hysterosalpingo-oophorectomy /-salping′gō·ō′əfərek″təmē/ [Gk, *hystera* + *salpinx,* tube, *oophoron,* ovary, *ektomē,* excision], surgical removal of one or both ovaries and oviducts along with the uterus, performed commonly to treat malignant neoplastic disease of the reproductive tract and chronic endometriosis. Removal of the ovaries and oviducts is routinely done with a hysterectomy on menopausal or postmenopausal women. To prevent the severe symptoms of sudden menopause in premenopausal women, a portion of one ovary is left, unless a malignancy is present. If both ovaries are removed and no malignancy is present, estrogen replacement therapy is often begun immediately. Elastic stockings or bandages may be applied to the legs to prevent circulatory stasis because thrombophlebitis of the blood vessels of the pelvis or thigh is a frequent complication. The lower half of the bed is kept flat, and the patient is instructed not to flex the thighs or knees. Low back pain or scanty urine may indicate a ligated ureter. Compare **hysterectomy.**

hysteroscope /his′tərōskōp′/ [Gk, *hystera,* womb + *skopein,* to look to view], an endoscope used in direct visual examination of the canal of the uterine cervix and the cavity of the uterus.

hysteroscopy /his′təros″kepē/ [Gk, *hystera* + *skopein,* to look], direct visual inspection of the cervical canal and uterine cavity through a hysteroscope. Hysteroscopy is performed to examine the endometrium, to secure a specimen for biopsy, to remove an intrauterine device, or to excise cervical polyps. The endoscope is passed through the vagina and into the uterus, and the surrounding tissues are examined. The procedure is contraindicated in pregnancy, acute pelvic inflammatory disease, chronic upper genital tract infection, recent uterine perforation, and known or suspected cervical malignancy. *−hysteroscopic, adj.,* **−hysteroscope,** *n.*

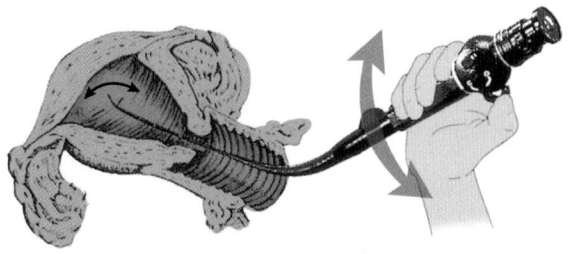

Hysteroscopic examination of the uterine cavity
(Pfenninger, 2011)

hysterotome /his″tərotōm′/ [Gk, *hystera,* womb, *temnein,* to cut], a surgical knife used for certain procedures involving the uterus.

hysterotomy /his′tərot″əmē/ [Gk, *hystera* + *temnein,* to cut], surgical incision of the uterus, performed as a method of abortion in a pregnancy beyond the first trimester of gestation when a saline injection abortion was incomplete or a tubal sterilization is to be done with the abortion. During surgery the lower segment of the uterus is incised, and the products of conception are withdrawn.

hysterovaginoenterocele /-vaj′inō·en″tərōsēl′/ [Gk, *hystera,* womb; L, *vagina,* sheath; Gk, *enteron,* bowel, *kele,* hernia], a hernia involving the uterus, vagina, and intestines. Prolapse of the pelvic organs may be caused by pregnancy or an inherent weakness of the supporting structures. It is also common after menopause. Treatment may include surgical repair or the use of a pessary.

Hytone, a glucocorticoid. Brand name for **hydrocortisone.**

Hz, abbreviation for **hertz.**

HZV, abbreviation for **herpes zoster virus.** See **chickenpox.**

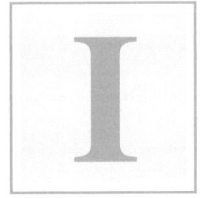

I, symbol for the element **iodine.**

-i, 1. plural-forming suffix used in native and later scientific Latin words: *bacilli, bronchi.* **2.** plural-forming suffix used in scientific terms derived through Latin from Greek: *pylori.*

[131]**I, symbol** for *radioactive iodine, isotopic (atomic) mass 131.*

[132]**I, symbol** for *radioactive iodine, isotopic (atomic) mass 132.*

-ia, suffix meaning "a specified condition of a disease or process": *aboulia, acarbia, syringobulbia.*

IABC, abbreviation for *intraaortic balloon counterpulsation.* See **intraaortic balloon pump.**

IABP, abbreviation for **intraaortic balloon pump.**

IADL, abbreviation for **instrumental activities of daily living.**

IADR, abbreviation for **International Association for Dental Research.**

IAH, abbreviation for **idiopathic diffuse alveolar hemorrhage.**

I and O, abbreviation for **intake and output.**

-iasis, suffix meaning "the formation or presence of an abnormal condition or disease": *amebiasis, elephantiasis.*

-iatria. See **-iatry, -iatria.**

-iatric, -iatrical, suffix meaning "relating to medicine, physicians, or medical treatment": *bariatric, psychiatric, pediatric.*

-iatrist, -iatrician, suffix meaning "one who treats" or "a physician": *physiatrist, pediatrician, podiatrist.*

iatro-, prefix meaning "physician" or "treatment": *iatrogenic, iatropic.*

iatrogenic /ī′atrōjen″ik, yat-/ [Gk, *iatros,* physician, *genein,* to produce], *adj.,* caused by treatment or diagnostic procedures. An iatrogenic disorder is a condition that is caused by medical personnel or procedures or that develops through exposure to the environment of a health care facility. Examples include bleeding or infection from a diagnostic aspiration, or an allergic reaction to a dye used as a contrast agent. See also **nosocomial. –iatrogeny,** *iatrogenesis, n.*

iatrogenic diabetes mellitus, a form of diabetes that develops as an adverse effect of treatment for a different medical problem. As an example, individuals who are administered high doses of corticosteroids often develop iatrogenic diabetes mellitus. Also called **secondary diabetes.**

iatrogenic pneumothorax, a condition in which air or gas is present in the pleural cavity as a result of mechanical ventilation, tracheostomy tube placement, or other therapeutic intervention.

iatrogeny. See **iatrogenic.**

iatrology, *(Obsolete)* the science of medicine.

iatropic /ī′atrop″ik/ [Gk, *iatros,* physician, *trepein,* to turn], causing an individual to seek medical attention, especially when precipitated by a medical intervention.

iatropic stimulus, the symptoms that induce a patient to seek professional health care. See also **chief complaint.**

-iatry, -iatria, suffix meaning "a (specified) type of medical treatment, medical profession, or physicians": *neuropsychiatry, geropsychiatry, podiatry.*

I band [ME, *band,* flat strip], an isotropic band within a striated muscle fiber that appears dark in polarized light but light when stained. The I band lengthens with muscle contraction. Compare **A band.** See also **sarcomere.**

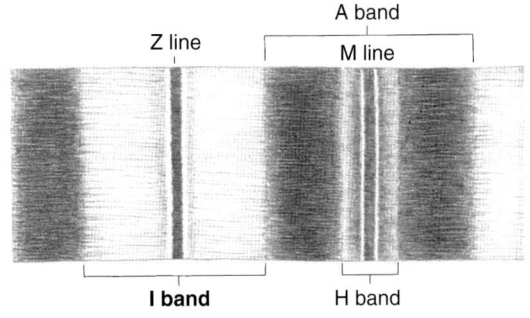

I band *(Thompson, Porter, and Fernandez, 2002)*

ibandronate, a bone-resorption inhibitor and electrolyte modifier.

■ INDICATIONS: This drug is used to prevent and treat osteoporosis.

■ CONTRAINDICATIONS: Achalasia, esophageal stricture, hypocalcemia, intraarterial administration, renal failure, vitamin D deficiency, and known hypersensitivity to bisphosphonates prohibit the use of this drug.

■ ADVERSE EFFECTS: Adverse effects of this drug include fever, insomnia, dizziness, headache, hypertension, ocular pain or inflammation, uveitis, constipation, nausea, vomiting, diarrhea, dyspepsia, rash, injection site reaction, bone pain, and myalgia. Common side effects include hypomagnesemia, hypophosphatemia, and hypocalcemia.

IBC, abbreviation for **iron-binding capacity.**

IBD, abbreviation for **inflammatory bowel disease.** See **ulcerative colitis.**

-ible. See **-able, -ible.**

ibritumomab tiuxetan, a monoclonal antibody radioimmunotherapy used as part of a regimen for non-Hodgkin lymphoma.

IBS, abbreviation for **irritable bowel syndrome.**

ibuprofen /ī″byo͞o″prōfin/, a COX-1 over-the-counter nonsteroidal antiinflammatory agent.

■ INDICATIONS: It is used for the treatment of fever, headaches, and pain from rheumatoid arthritis and osteoarthritis, muscle aches, and menstrual cramps.

■ CONTRAINDICATIONS: Renal dysfunction, disorders of the GI tract, or known hypersensitivity to this drug, to other nonsteroidal antiinflammatory drugs, or to aspirin prohibits its use.

■ ADVERSE EFFECTS: Among the more serious adverse effects are GI disturbances, gastric or duodenal ulceration, dizziness, skin rash, and tinnitus.

ibutilide /ibu'tilīd/, a cardiac depressant used in the treatment of atrial arrhythmias; it is administered by IV infusion.

ibutilide fumarate, a drug used to treat heart arrhythmias.

■ INDICATIONS: It is prescribed in an effort to convert atrial fibrillation and atrial flutter of recent onset to normal sinus rhythm.

■ CONTRAINDICATIONS: If it does not result in conversion after an initial 10-minute infusion, a second 10-minute infusion may be given, but not sooner than 10 minutes after the first dose has been completed.

■ ADVERSE EFFECTS: The side effects most often reported include life-threatening arrhythmias, including ventricular tachycardia.

IBW, abbreviation for **ideal body weight.**

IC, 1. abbreviation for **inspiratory capacity. 2.** abbreviation for **interstitial cystitis.**

-ic, -ac, suffix meaning "pertaining to, similar to": *iththyotic, cadaveric, hypochondriac.*

ICA, abbreviation for **islet cell antibody.**

-icam, suffix for antiinflammatory agents of the isoxicam group.

ICD, abbreviation for **implantable cardioverter-defibrillator.**

ICD, abbreviation for *International Classification of Diseases.*

ice burn, partial-thickness thermal necrosis of the skin caused by prolonged therapy entailing applications of ice.

Iceland disease /īs"land/, a group of symptoms associated with effects of a viral infection of the nervous system, including muscular pain and weakness, depression, and sensory changes. It mainly affects young adults, women more than men. Its exact cause is unknown. Also called **benign myalgic encephalomyelitis, chronic fatigue syndrome, Royal free disease.**

Iceland moss, *Cetraria islandica,* a lichen native to Iceland.

I cell disease, a form of lysosomal disease characterized by progressive mental deterioration, heart disease, and respiratory failure in the first 10 years of life. A number of lysosomal enzymes are lacking, and fibroblasts display numerous coarse inclusions. Also called **inclusion cell disease, mucolipidosis II.**

ice pack [ME, *is + pakke*], a container of crushed ice placed on the body to reduce tissue temperature, relieve pain, soothe inflamed tissue, or control bleeding.

ICF, 1. abbreviation for **intermediate care facility. 2.** abbreviation for **intracellular fluid.**

ICF/IID, abbreviation for *intermediate care facilities for individuals with intellectual disabilities.* Formerly called *ICF/MR.* See **intermediate care facility.**

ICH, abbreviation for **intracerebral hemorrhage.**

ichor /ī"kôr/, a thin, watery fluid discharged from a sore.

ichthyo-, prefix meaning "fish": *ichthyosis, ichthyoid, ichthyotic.*

ichthyoid /ik"thē·oid/ [Gk, *ichthys,* fish, *eidos,* form], pertaining to objects or structures that are fish-shaped or fishlike.

ichthyosis /ik"thē·ō"sis/ [Gk, *ichthys,* fish, *osis,* condition], any of several inherited dermatological conditions in which the skin is dry and hyperkeratotic, resembling fish scales. It usually appears at or shortly after birth and may be part of one of several rare syndromes. Some types respond temporarily to urea or lactic acid emollients. A rare, acquired variety accompanying a lymphoma or multiple myeloma occurs in adults. Also called **fish skin disease, xeroderma.** –**ichthyotic,** *adj.*

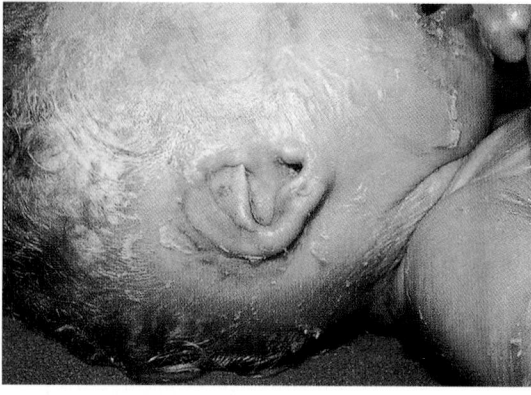

Lamellar ichthyosis *(Weston, Lane, and Morrelli, 2007)*

ichthyosis congenita, ichthyosis fetalis, See **lamellar exfoliation.**

ichthyosis fetus. See **harlequin fetus.**

ichthyosis hystrix [Gk, *ichthys,* fish + *osis,* condition + *hystrix,* porcupine], a localized form of epidermolytic hyperkeratosis having the appearance of linear epidermal nevi. See also **epidermolytic hyperkeratosis.**

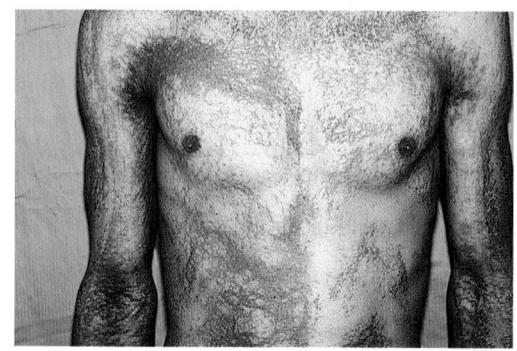

Ichthyosis hystrix *(Callen et al, 2000)*

ichthyosis vulgaris [Gk, *ichthys + osis + L, vulgaris,* common], a hereditary skin disorder characterized by large, dry, dark scales that cover the face, neck, scalp, ears, back, and extensor surfaces but not the flexor surfaces of the body. The condition is transmitted as an autosomal-dominant trait; it appears several months to 1 year after birth. Management consists of topical application of emollients and use of keratolytic agents to facilitate removal of the scales. Also called *ichthyosis simplex.* See also **sex-linked ichthyosis.**

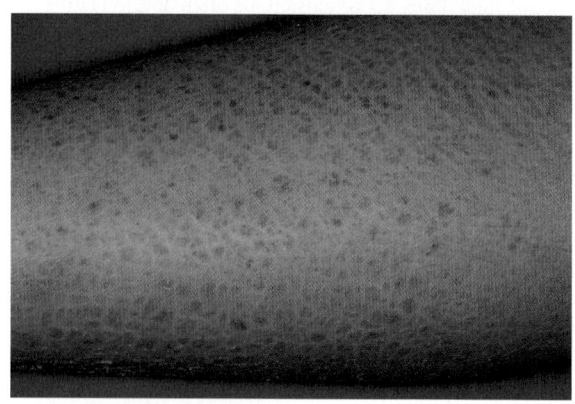

Ichthyosis vulgaris *(Paller and Mancini, 2011)*

ichthyotic. See **ichthyosis.**

-ician, suffix meaning "a specialist in a field": *clinician, pediatrician, technician.*

ICN, abbreviation for **International Council of Nurses.**

icon /ī″kən/, an image on the screen of a computer terminal representing a specific command or point for data entry.

ICP, abbreviation for **intracranial pressure.**

-ics, suffix meaning the "systematic formulation of a body of knowledge": *cytogenetics, bionics, eugenics.*

ICSH, abbreviation for **interstitial cell-stimulating hormone.** See **luteinizing hormone.**

ICSI, abbreviation for **intracytoplasmic sperm injection.**

ictal /ik″təl/ [Gk, *ikteros,* jaundice], pertaining to a sudden acute onset, as convulsions of an epileptic seizure.

-ictal, suffix meaning "a sudden attack or stroke": *postictal.*

icter-, prefix meaning "jaundice": *icterogenic.*

icteric /ikter″ik/ [Gk, *ikteros,* jaundice], pertaining to or resembling jaundice.

icterogenic /ik″tərōjen″ik/, causing jaundice.

icterus. See **jaundice.**

icterus gravis neonatorum /ik″tərəs/ [Gk, *ikteros,* jaundice; L, *gravis,* weight, *neonatus,* newborn], a hemolytic jaundice of the newborn caused by incompatibility between the mother's serum and the infant's red corpuscles.

icterus neonatorum, a jaundiced condition in a newborn.

ictus /ik″təs/ *pl. ictuses, ictus* [L, stroke], **1.** a seizure. **2.** a cerebrovascular accident. −**ictic, ictal,** *adj.*

ICU, abbreviation for **intensive care unit.**

id [L, it], **1.** (in freudian psychoanalysis) the part of the psyche, functioning in the unconscious, that is the source of instinctive energy, impulses, and drives. It is based on the pleasure principle and has strong tendencies toward self-preservation. Compare **ego, superego. 2.** the true unconscious.

ID, abbreviation for **infectious disease.**

-id, **1.** suffix meaning "structure" or "body": *plasmid.* **2.** suffix meaning "a member of a group": *tuberculid.*

idarubicin, an antibiotic and antineoplastic drug.

■ INDICATIONS: This drug is used in combination with other antineoplastics for acute myelocytic leukemia in adults.

■ CONTRAINDICATIONS: Pregnancy, hypersensitivity, lactation, and myelosuppression prohibit the use of this drug.

■ ADVERSE EFFECTS: Adverse effects of this drug include hypertension, extrasystoles, ventricular tachycardia, bundle branch block, atrioventricular block, palpitations, supraventricular extrasystoles, syncope, and nausea. Common side effects include headache, hypotension, and bradycardia. Life-threatening side effects include sinus arrest, congestive heart failure, and arrhythmias.

IDDM, abbreviation for **insulin-dependent diabetes mellitus.** See **type 1 diabetes mellitus.**

-ide, suffix meaning "a compound of": *chloride, monoxide, sulfide.*

idea [Gk, form], any thought, concept, intention, or impression that exists in the mind as a result of awareness, understanding, or other mental activity.

ideal body weight (IBW), the weight statistically determined to be associated with the lowest mortality for an average individual, adjusting for some combination of height, age, frame size, and gender. Which factors should be included and how it should be determined remain controversial.

ideal gas law /īdē″əl/ [Gk, *idea,* form, *chaos,* gas; AS, *lagu,* law], the rule that $PV = nRT$, with the product of pressure *(P)* and volume *(V)* equal to the product of the number of moles of gas *(n),* absolute temperature *(T),* and a gas constant *(R).*

idealized image /īdē″əlīzd/, a concept of a person characterized by a sense of perfection and admiration that results in unrealistically high and unattainable goals.

idea of influence, an idea held less firmly than a delusion, often seen in paranoid disorders, that external forces or persons are controlling one's thoughts, actions, and feelings.

idea of persecution, an idea held less firmly than a delusion, often seen in paranoid disorders, that one is being threatened, discriminated against, or mistreated by other persons or external forces.

idea of reference, a delusion that the statements, events, or actions of others, usually interpreted as deprecatory, refer to oneself. It is often seen in paranoid disorders. Also called **delusion of reference, referential idea.**

ideational apraxia /ī″dē·ā″shənəl/ [Gk, *idea,* form, *a* + *prassein,* not to do], a condition in which the conceptual process is lost, often because of a lesion in the parietal lobe. The individual is unable to formulate a plan of movement and does not know the proper use of an object because of a lack of perception of its purpose. There is no loss of motor movement or strength, but the reason for the movement is confused. Also called **sensory apraxia.** See also **apraxia.**

idée fixe. See **fixed idea.**

identical twins. See **monozygotic twins.**

identification /īden′tifikā″shən/ [L, *idem,* the same, *facere,* to make], an unconscious defense mechanism by which a person patterns his or her personality on that of another person, assuming the person's qualities, characteristics, and actions. The process is a normal function of personality development and learning, specifically of the superego, and it contributes to the acquisition of interests and ideals. Identification first occurs in early childhood when 3- to 5-year-olds identify with parental same-sex figures. It resurges in adolescence as a major task of identifying with peers.

identity /īden″titē/, a component of self-concept characterized by one's persisting consciousness of being oneself, separate and distinct from others. Identity diffusion, or identity confusion, is a lack of clarity and consistency in one's perception of the self, which produces a high degree of anxiety.

identity crisis [L, *idem,* the same; Gk, *krisis,* turning point], a period of confusion concerning an individual's sense of self and role in society, which occurs most frequently in the transition from one stage of life to the next. It is often expressed by isolation, negativism, extremism, and rebelliousness.

identity diffusion. See **identity.**

identity disorder of childhood, a mental disturbance of childhood in which the person is abnormally uncertain and concerned about long-term goals such as career choice or sexual preference to the point that the concerns interfere with educational and social functions. See also **identity crisis.**

ideo-, prefix meaning "idea": *ideology.*

ideokinetic apraxia. See **ideomotor apraxia.**

ideology /ī″de·ol″əjē/ [Gk, *idea*], a scheme of ideas or a systematic organization of ideas associated with doctrine and philosophy.

ideomotor apraxia /īdē″əmō″tor/ [Gk, *idea* + L, *motare,* to move about; Gk *a* + *prassein,* not to do], the inability to translate an idea into motion, resulting from some interference with the transmission of the appropriate impulses from the brain to the motor centers. There is no loss of the ability to perform an action automatically, such as tying the shoelaces, but the action cannot be performed on request. The condition is often caused by diffuse cortical disease. Also called **ideokinetic apraxia, limb kinetic apraxia, transcortical apraxia.** See also **apraxia.**

ideophobia /-fō″bē·ə/ [Gk, *idea* + *phobos,* fear], an anxiety disorder characterized by the irrational fear or distrust of ideas or reason. See also **phobia.**

idio-, prefix meaning "private," "distinctive," "peculiar": *idiopathic.*

idiocrasy. See **idiosyncrasy.**

idiogram /id″ē·əgram′/, a diagram or graphic representation of a karyotype, showing the number, relative sizes, and morphological characteristics of the chromosomes of a species, individual, or cell.

idiojunctional rhythm /-jungk″shənəl/ [Gk, *idios,* own; L, *jungere,* to join; Gk, *rhythmos*], a heart rhythm emanating from the junction of the atrioventricular (AV) node and the AV bundle but without retrograde conduction to the atria.

idiomere. See **chromomere.**

idiopathic /-path″ik/ [Gk, *idios* + *pathos,* disease], without a known cause.

idiopathic diffuse alveolar hemorrhage (IAH), bleeding into the alveoli of the lungs caused by any of a number of disorders, including Goodpasture's syndrome, Wegener's granulomatosis, and collagen vascular disease.

idiopathic disease, a disease that develops without an apparent or known cause, although it may have a recognizable pattern of signs and symptoms and may be curable.

idiopathic edema, edema of unknown cause, usually affecting women, occurring intermittently over a period of years, and usually worse during the premenstrual phase. It is associated with increased aldosterone secretion.

idiopathic gangrene [Gk, *idios,* own, *pathos,* disease, *gag-graina*], a gangrenous condition of unknown cause.

idiopathic guttate hypomelanosis /hī′pōmel″ənō″sis/, one of many drop-shaped hypopigmented macules of unknown origin. It is a common benign condition occurring in adults. In most instances, no treatment is required.

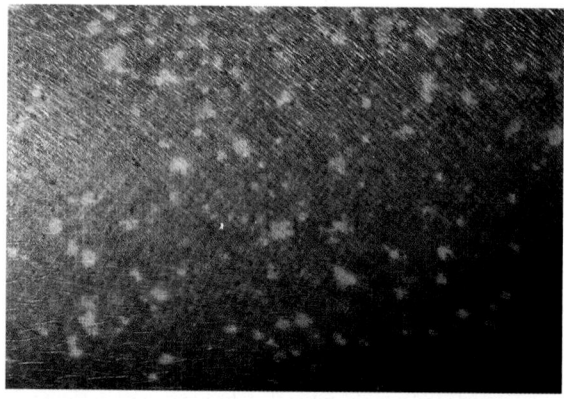

Idiopathic guttate hypomelanosis *(James et al, 2016)*

idiopathic hemosiderosis, the accumulation of iron-containing deposits in cells of the lungs as a result of bleeding in the lungs.

idiopathic hypercalciuria, elevated urine calcium of unknown cause, often with formation of renal calculi. It is characterized by a normal concentration of calcium in the blood, the absence of diseases that cause increased urine calcium, and calcium excretion that is above 250 mg/day in women and 300 mg/day in men. Patients experience increased gut calcium absorption, decreased renal calcium reabsorption, and have a tendency to lose calcium from bone.

idiopathic hypoventilation, a disorder of unknown cause associated with deficient ventilation of the alveoli of the lungs.

idiopathic intracranial hypertension, increased intracranial pressure in the absence of disease.

idiopathic midline destructive disease (IMDD), a disorder of unknown cause characterized by ulceration and necrosis of the midline facial tissues and obstruction of the upper airways. IMDD develops without systemic involvement.

idiopathic multiple pigmented hemorrhagic sarcoma. See **Kaposi sarcoma.**

idiopathic nephrotic syndrome [Gk, *idios,* own, *pathos,* disease, *nephros,* kidney], a kidney disease of unknown origin characterized by hematuria, albuminuria, edema, and hypertension resulting from damaged glomerular capillaries.

idiopathic neuralgia [Gk, *idios,* own, *pathos,* disease, *neuron,* nerve, *algos,* pain], a form of neuralgia that occurs without any identifiable structural nerve lesion.

idiopathic pericarditis [Gk, *idios,* own, *pathos,* disease, *peri,* near, *kardia,* heart, *itis,* inflammation], an inflammation of unknown cause associated with the membrane enclosing the heart.

idiopathic postpartum renal failure, kidney failure that begins 1 day to several weeks after a delivery that follows an uneventful gestation. Symptoms include oliguria or anuria, which progresses to azotemia, with complications of hemolytic anemia or coagulopathy. Treatment is supportive but aimed primarily at reducing blood pressure.

idiopathic pulmonary fibrosis [Gk, *idios,* own, *pathos,* disease; L, *pulmoneus,* the lungs, *fibra,* fiber], a disorder of unknown cause characterized by fibrosis of the lungs. It may follow an earlier inflammation or disease, such as tuberculosis or pneumoconiosis.

idiopathic pulmonary hemorrhage, bleeding in the lungs without a known cause. It may be a cause of secondary spontaneous pneumothorax.

idiopathic reactive hypoglycemia, a condition of diminished blood glucose level that occurs after the ingestion of carbohydrates that has no known cause. It may be related to increased insulin sensitivity or decreased counterregulatory hormone secretion or action. Treatment is dietary and includes eating frequent meals of moderate size that are reasonably high in protein with a low glycemic load.

idiopathic respiratory distress syndrome. See **respiratory distress syndrome of the newborn.**

idiopathic scoliosis, an abnormal condition characterized by a lateral curvature of the spine. It is the most common type of scoliosis, evident in 70% of all patients with scoliosis and up to 80% of those with structural scoliosis. It may occur at any age, but three types are commonly associated with certain age groups. The infantile type affects 1- to 3-year-olds. The juvenile type affects 3- to 10-year-olds. The adolescent type affects preadolescents and adolescents. The main factors in diagnosing idiopathic scoliosis are the degree, balance, and rotational component of the curvature. The rotational component may contribute to rib cage deformities and impingement on the pulmonary and cardiac systems.

■ OBSERVATIONS: The most common type is the adolescent type. Early diagnosis is difficult because the associated curvature is often hidden by clothing. Preadolescent screening is encouraged in schools. The signs commonly associated with scoliosis include unlevel shoulders, a prominent scapula, a prominent breast, a prominent flank area, an unlevel or prominent hip, poor posture, and an obvious curvature. During diagnosis it is necessary to view the patient from the front and from the back and while the patient is bending.

Other signs that may be associated with idiopathic scoliosis are occasional transient pain and fatigue and decreased pulmonary function. Radiographic films of the spine in the bending position are important in ascertaining the flexibility of the curvature and the potential for spontaneous correction. Neurological deficits are commonly associated with severe curvature and vary according to the extent to which the curvature has impinged on the spinal cord. Some signs of such impingement are reflex, sensation, and motor alterations of the lower extremities.

■ INTERVENTIONS: Nonsurgical intervention commonly uses observation, an exercise program, and a Milwaukee brace. Observation consists of frequent physical examinations and radiographic monitoring of the progress of the curvature. Exercise programs are designed to promote the maximum correction possible, as indicated by the degree of flexibility shown in the initial radiographic examination. Observation and the exercise program are used with patients who have a curvature less than 15 to 20 degrees. Greater degrees of curvature usually require the use of a Milwaukee brace in addition to observation and an exercise program. The brace, which is usually worn 23 hours a day, is used to control the progress of the curvature. The exercise program is implemented when the adolescent is out of the brace, and additional exercises are performed while in the brace. Surgical intervention may be required if the curvature has progressed to 40 degrees or more at the time of diagnosis or if a slightly lesser degree of curvature exists with a high degree of rotational component or imbalance. Approximately 5% to 10% of patients with idiopathic scoliosis require surgical intervention, which involves fusing of the involved vertebrae to prevent progress of the deformity.

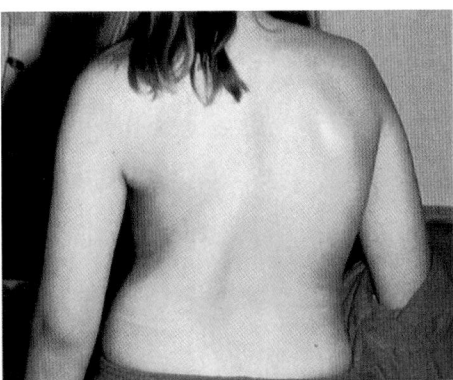

Idiopathic scoliosis: scapular asymmetry *(Nymberg and Crawford, 1996)*

idiopathic steatorrhea [Gk, *idios,* own, *pathos,* disease, *stear,* fat, *rhoia,* flow], excess fat in the stool, particularly as in celiac disease in adults.

idiopathic tetanus [Gk, *idios,* own, *pathos,* disease, *tetanos,* convulsive tension], **1.** a tetanus infection of unknown cause. **2.** a tetanus infection occurring without a wound.

idiopathic ventricular tachycardia, an accelerated heart rhythm (greater than 100 beats/min) that originates in a focus within a ventricle but is of unknown cause.

idiopathy /id′ē·op″əthē/, any primary disease that arises without an apparent cause. **–idiopathic,** *adj.*

idiosyncrasy /-sin″krəsē/ [Gk, *idios* + *synkrasis,* mixing together], **1.** a physical or behavioral characteristic or manner that is unique to an individual or to a group. **2.** an

individual's unique hypersensitivity to a particular drug, food, or other substance. Also called **idiocrasy.** See also **allergy.**

idiosyncratic /-sinkrat″ik/ [Gk, *idios,* own, *synkrasis,* mixing together], pertaining to personal peculiarities or mannerisms.

idiosyncratic drug effect [Gk, *idios,* own, *synkrasis,* mixing together; Fr, *drogue*], an uncommon response to a drug because of a genetic predisposition. It usually manifests as an abnormally short or abnormally large or long response to the drug, but it is possible for the response to be qualitatively different.

idiotope /id′ē·ətōp′/, an antigenic determinant on a variable region of an immunoglobulin molecule.

idiotrophic /-trof″ik/, describing an organism capable of obtaining its own nourishment.

idiot savant /idē·ō″ savänt″/, an individual with cognitive impairment who is nonetheless capable of performing certain unusual mental feats, primarily those involving music, puzzle solving, or manipulation of numbers.

idiotype /id′ē·ətīp′/ [Gk, *idios* + *typos,* mark], unique differences between immunoglobulins of different antigen-binding specificities. Idiotypes are determined by the structure of the variable regions of the immunoglobulins. This also applies to T-cell receptors.

idioventricular /-ventrik″yələr/ [Gk, *idios* + L, *ventriculus,* little belly], originating in a ventricle.

idioventricular rhythm [Gk, *idios,* own; L, *ventriculus,* little belly; Gk, *rhythmos*], an independent cardiac rhythm caused by a repeated discharge of impulses at a rate of less than 100 beats/min from a focus within a ventricle.

-idium, noun-forming suffix: *Clostridium, miracidium.*

IDL, abbreviation for **intermediate-density lipoprotein.**

IDM, abbreviation for *infant of a diabetic mother.*

idoxuridine /ī′doksyoor″ədēn/, an ophthalmic antiviral drug.

■ INDICATIONS: It is prescribed for the treatment of herpes simplex keratitis.

■ CONTRAINDICATIONS: Deep ulceration of the cornea or known hypersensitivity to this drug prohibits its use.

■ ADVERSE EFFECTS: Among the more serious adverse effects are visual disturbances and eye discomfort.

id reaction, the autosensitization resulting from any inflammatory condition that causes pruritus and vesicular lesions. These secondary lesions are caused by circulating antigens and are usually distant from the primary infection.

IDSA, abbreviation for *Infectious Disease Society of America.*

idursulfase, a rarely used enzyme replacement.

■ INDICATIONS: This drug is used to treat mucopolysaccharidosis II.

■ CONTRAINDICATIONS: Known hypersensitivity to this drug or other systemic antifungal or azoles, fungal meningitis, and onchomycosis or dermatomycosis in cardiac function prohibit its use.

■ ADVERSE EFFECTS: Adverse effects of this drug include insomnia, fever, rigors, weakness, anxiety, hypertension, hypotension, tachycardia, anemia, cramps, abdominal pain, flatulence, gynecomastia, impotence, decreased libido, malaise, hypokalemia, and tinnitus. Life-threatening side effects include GI bleeding, hepatotoxicity, toxic epidermal necrolysis, and rhabdomyolysis. Common side effects include headache, dizziness, nausea, vomiting, anorexia, diarrhea, pruritus, rash, edema, and fatigue.

I:E ratio, the ratio of the duration of inspiration to the duration of expiration. A range of 1:1.5 to 1:2 for an adult is considered acceptable for mechanical ventilation. Ratios of 1:1

or higher may cause hemodynamic complications, whereas ratios lower than 1:2 indicate lower mean airway pressure and fewer associated hazards.

-ifene, suffix for antiestrogen products of the clomiphene and tamoxifen groups.

-iform, suffix meaning "in the form of": *bulbiform.*

ifosfamide, an antineoplastic alkylating agent.

■ INDICATIONS: This drug is used to treat testicular cancer, soft tissue sarcoma, Ewing sarcoma, non-Hodgkin lymphoma, lung sarcoma, and pancreatic sarcoma.

■ CONTRAINDICATIONS: Pregnancy, bone marrow suppression, and known hypersensitivity to this drug prohibit its use.

■ ADVERSE EFFECTS: Adverse effects of this drug include facial paresthesia, fever, malaise, somnolence, confusion, depression, hallucinations, dizziness, disorientation, cranial nerve dysfunction, nausea, vomiting, anorexia, stomatitis, constipation, diarrhea, dysuria, urinary frequency, dermatitis, alopecia, and pain at the injection site. Life-threatening side effects include seizures, coma, hepatoxicity, hematuria, nephrotoxicity, hemorrhagic cystitis, thrombocytopenia, leukopenia, and anemia.

Ig, abbreviation for **immunoglobulin.**

IgA, abbreviation for **immunoglobulin A.**

IgA deficiency, now called **selective IgA deficiency.**

IgD, abbreviation for **immunoglobulin D.**

IgE, abbreviation for **immunoglobulin E.**

IGF, abbreviation for **insulin-like growth factor.**

IgG, abbreviation for **immunoglobulin G.**

IgM, abbreviation for **immunoglobulin M.**

ignipeditis /ig′nĕpedī′tis/ [L, *ignis,* fire, *pes,* foot], a burning pain in the soles of the feet caused by peripheral neuropathy.

IGT, abbreviation for **impaired glucose tolerance.**

I.H., abbreviation for **infectious hepatitis.**

IL-1, abbreviation for **interleukin-1.**

IL-2, abbreviation for **interleukin-2.**

IL-3, abbreviation for **interleukin-3.**

IL-4, abbreviation for **interleukin-4.**

IL-5, abbreviation for **interleukin-5.**

IL-6, abbreviation for **interleukin-6.**

IL-7, abbreviation for **interleukin-7.**

IL-8, abbreviation for **interleukin-8.**

IL-9, abbreviation for **interleukin-9.**

IL-10, abbreviation for **interleukin-10.**

IL-11, abbreviation for **interleukin-11.**

IL-12, abbreviation for **interleukin-12.**

IL-13, abbreviation for **interleukin-13.**

IL-14, abbreviation for **interleukin-14.**

IL-15, abbreviation for **interleukin-15.**

ILD, abbreviation for **interstitial lung disease.**

Ile, abbreviation for **isoleucine.**

ilea, ileac, ileal. See **ileum.**

ileal atresia, atresia of the ileum, the most common type of intestinal atresia.

ileal bypass /il″ē·əl/ [L, *ileum,* intestine; AS, *bi,* near; Fr, *passer*], a surgical procedure for treating obesity by anastomosis of the upper portion of the small intestine to a more distal segment of the small intestine, thereby bypassing much of the length of the ileum that normally absorbs nutrients. See also **intestinal bypass.**

ileal conduit [Fr, *conduire,* to guide], a method of urinary diversion using intestinal tissue. The ureters are implanted in a section of dissected ileum. This section is sutured closed on one end; the other end is drawn through the abdominal wall (right lower quadrant) to create a stoma. The patient wears a pouch to collect the urine.

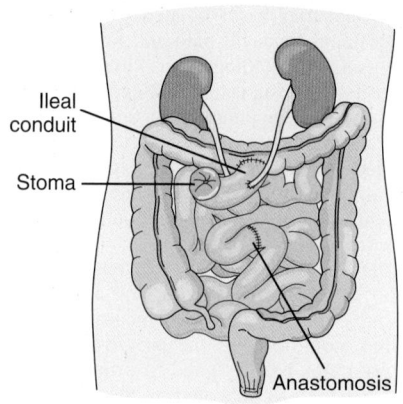

Ileal conduit *(Monahan and Neighbors, 2007)*

ileal diverticulum. See **Meckel diverticulum.**

ileal intussusception, intussusception involving two segments of the ileum.

ileal neobladder, a neobladder made from a section of ileum. Also called **continent ileal reservoir.**

ileal valve. See **ileocecal valve.**

ileectomy /il′ē·ek″təmē/, surgical removal of the ileum.

ileitis /il′ē·ī″tis/ [L, *ileum,* intestine; Gk, *itis*], inflammation of the ileum. See also **Crohn's disease.**

ileo-, prefix meaning "the ileum": *ileocecal, ileoanal.*

ileoanal /il′ē·ō·ā′nal/, pertaining to or connecting the ileum and the anus.

ileoanal anastomosis /il′ē·ō·ā′nəl/, a surgical procedure in which the colon and rectum are removed but the anus and anal sphincter are left intact. An anastomosis is formed between the lower end of the small intestine and the anus. The operation is an alternative to proctocolectomy for the treatment of ulcerative colitis.

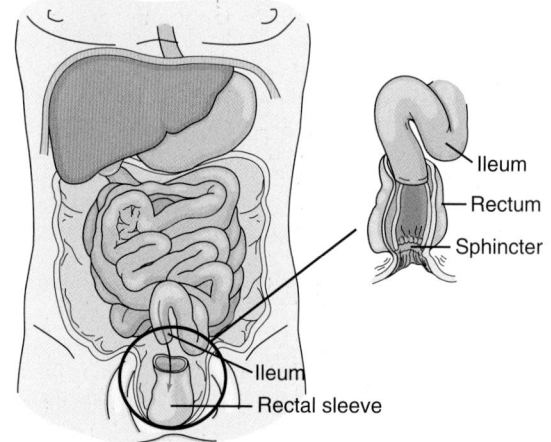

Ileoanal anastomosis *(Monahan and Neighbors, 2007)*

ileoanal reservoir, a pouch for the collection of feces, created surgically in a two-stage operation. The first stage involves removal of the rectal mucosa, an abdominal colectomy, and construction of a fecal reservoir from loops of ileum. A temporary ileostomy is created at this time to allow the ileoanal reservoir to heal. Several months later the patient returns for closure of the ileostomy so that discharge of feces through the anus is possible.

ileocecal /il′ē·ōsē″kəl/ [L, *ileum,* intestine, *caecus,* blind], pertaining to both the ileum and the cecum and the region where they are joined.

ileocecal fold, two flaps surrounding the opening of the ileum into the large intestine where the cecum and ascending colon join together. The flaps project into the lumen of the large intestine and come together at their end, forming ridges. Musculature from the ileum continues into each flap, forming a sphincter. Possible functions of the ileocecal fold include preventing reflux from the cecum to the ileum and regulating the passage of contents from the ileum to the cecum.

ileocecal incompetence. See **incompetence.**

ileocecal intussusception, a telescoping of one section of the bowel into another at the ileocecal junction, with the cecum being drawn back into the ileum.

ileocecal lip of ileal orifice, the inferior of the two lips forming the ileal orifice.

ileocecal orifice, ostium ileale.

ileocecal syndrome. See **appendicitis.**

ileocecal valve [L, *ileum,* intestine, *caecus,* blind, *valvarum,* folding door], the sphincter muscle between the ileum of the small intestine and the cecum of the large intestine. It consists of two flaps that project into the lumen of the large intestine, immediately above the vermiform appendix, preventing food from reentering the small intestine.

ileocecocystoplasty /il″e·ose″kosis′toplas″te/, augmentation cystoplasty using an isolated segment of the ileum and cecum for the graft.

ileocecostomy. See **cecoileostomy.**

ileocolic intussusception, intussusception at the ileocecal junction, with the distal ileum being drawn forward into the colon.

ileocolic lip of ileal orifice, the superior of the two lips forming the ileal orifice.

ileocolic node /il′ē·ōkol″ik/ [L, *ileum* + Gk, *kolon,* colon; L, *nodus,* knot], a node in one of three groups of superior mesenteric lymph glands, forming a chain of approximately 15 nodes around the ileocolic (mesenteric) artery. They tend to form in two main groups, one near the duodenum and the other on the lower part of the ileocolic artery. The chain breaks into several groups where the artery divides into its terminal branches. The ileocolic nodes receive materials from the jejunum, ileum, cecum, vermiform appendix, ascending colon, and transverse colon. Their efferent vessels pass to the preaortic nodes. Compare **mesenteric node, mesocolic node.**

ileocolitis /-kōlī″tis/, an inflammation of the ileum and colon.

ileocystoplasty /-sis″təplas′tē/ [L, *ileum* + Gk, *kystis,* bag, *plassein,* to mold], a surgical procedure in which the bladder is reconstructed by using a segment of the ileum for the bladder wall.

ileocystostomy /-sistos″təmē/ [L, *ileum,* intestine; Gk, *kystis,* bag, *stoma,* mouth], a surgical procedure to form a passage to direct urine through the abdominal wall by using a segment of small intestine as a conduit from the bladder.

ileopectineal eminence. See **iliopubic eminence.**

ileorectal /-rek″təl/, pertaining to the ileum and rectum.

ileosigmoid knotting, a severe type of volvulus consisting of twisting together of the ileum and the sigmoid colon.

ileosigmoidostomy /-sig′moidos″təmē/, surgical formation of a passageway between the ileum and the sigmoid colon.

ileostomate /il′ē·os″təmāt/, a person who has undergone an ileostomy.

ileostomy /il′ē·os″təmē/ [L, *ileum* + Gk, *stoma,* mouth, *temnein,* to cut], surgical formation of an opening of the ileum onto the surface of the abdomen through which fecal matter is emptied. The operation is performed in advanced or recurrent ulcerative colitis, Crohn disease, or cancer of the large bowel. A low-residue diet is given before surgery and is reduced to fluids 24 hours before surgery to decrease intestinal residue. Intestinal antibiotics are given to decrease the bacterial count. A nasogastric or intestinal tube is passed. The diseased portion of the large bowel is removed in a permanent ileostomy. Occasionally, the distal and proximal segments of bowel may be reconnected after ulcerated areas have healed. A loop of the proximal ileum is then drawn out onto the abdomen and sutured in place, and a stoma is formed. A pouch may be made with part of the terminal ileum, in which the open end is woven through the rectus muscles to form a valve and then opens onto the abdomen. After surgery the patient wears a disposable bag to collect the semiliquid fecal matter, which begins to drain once peristalsis is restored and the nasogastric tube is removed. Because the secretions contain digestive enzymes that can ulcerate the skin around the stoma, it is important to ensure that nothing leaks from the bag. The patient is instructed on application and care of the stoma and the ileostomy bag. If a pouch is present, it is drained three or four times a day through a small irrigating catheter through the valve. Compare **colostomy.** See also **enterostomy, ostomy irrigation, stoma.**

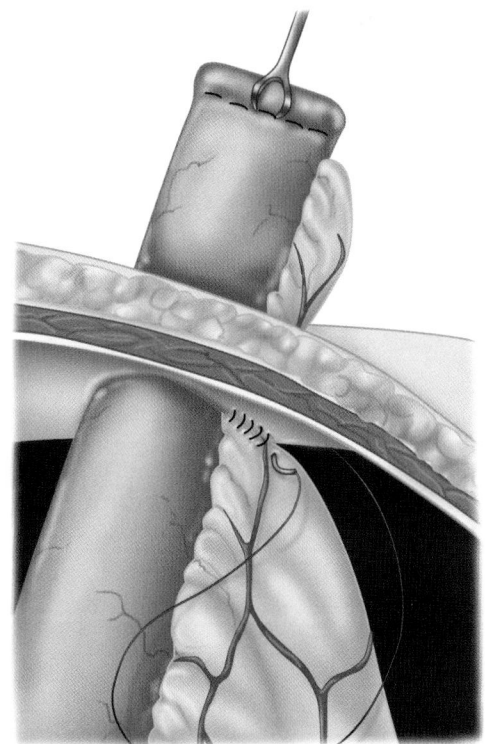

Ileostomy *(Fleshman et al, 2013)*

ileum /il′ē·əm/ *pl. ilea* [L, intestine], the lower-third distal portion of the small intestine, extending from the jejunum to the cecum. Internally it has a few small circular folds and numerous clusters of lymphatic tissues. It ends in the right iliac fossa, opening into the medial side of the large intestine. See also **ileocecal valve.** *—ileal, ileac, adj.*

ileus /il′ē·əs/ [L; Gk, *eilein,* to pack close together], an obstruction of the intestines, such as an adynamic ileus caused by immobility of the bowel or a mechanical ileus in which the intestine is blocked by mechanical means. See also **paralytic ileus.**

ilia.   See **ilium.**

-iliac,   suffix meaning "the ilium": *sacroiliac.*

iliac circumflex node /il′ē·ak/ [L, *ilium,* flank, *circum,* around, *flectere,* to bend, *nodus,* knot],   a node in one of the seven clusters of parietal lymph nodes of the abdomen. This node is one of a group found along the course of the deep iliac circumflex vessels. Compare **common iliac node, external iliac node, internal iliac node.** See also **lymph, lymphatic system, lymph node.**

iliac crest [L, *ilia,* intestines; ME, *creste*],   the upper elevated margins of the ilium.

iliac fascia,   the portion of the endoabdominal fascia that is attached with the iliacus to the crest of the ilium and passes under the inguinal ligament into the thigh.

iliac horns,   accessory bony spurs on the posterior of the ilium, one of the symptoms of nail-patella syndrome.

iliac part of iliopsoas fascia,   the part of the fascia that invests the iliac muscle.

iliac region.   See **inguinal region.**

iliac tuberosity,   a rough elevation of the posterior iliac crest to which the posterior sacroiliac ligaments are attached. It is also a point of origin of the erector spinae and multifidus muscles.

iliacus /ilī′əkəs/ [L, *ilium,* flank],   a flat triangular muscle that covers the inner curved surface of the iliac fossa. It arises from the inner aspect of the superior iliac crest, from the anterior and the iliolumbar ligaments, and from the sacrum. It joins the psoas major to form the iliopsoas at the inguinal ligament. The iliacus is innervated by branches of the femoral nerve that contain fibers from the second and third lumbar nerves. It acts to flex and laterally rotate the thigh. Compare **psoas major, psoas minor.**

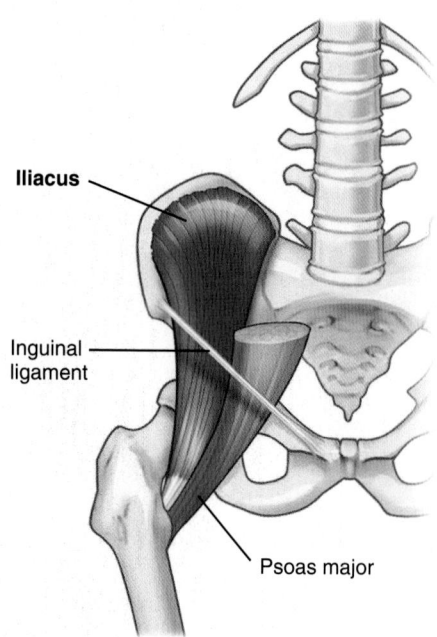

Iliacus muscle

ilio-,   prefix meaning "ilium" or "flank": *iliocostalis, iliolumbar, ilioinguinal.*

iliocostalis,   the most laterally placed column of erector spinae muscles, including the iliocostalis lumborum, iliocostalis thoracis, and iliocostalis cervicis.

iliofemoral /il′ē·ōfem″ərəl/,   pertaining to the ilium and femur.

iliofemoral ligament [L, *ilium* + *femur,* thigh, *ligamentum*],   a triangular band of connective tissue attached by its apex to the anterior inferior spine of the ilium and acetabular margin and by its base to the intertrochanteric line of the femur.

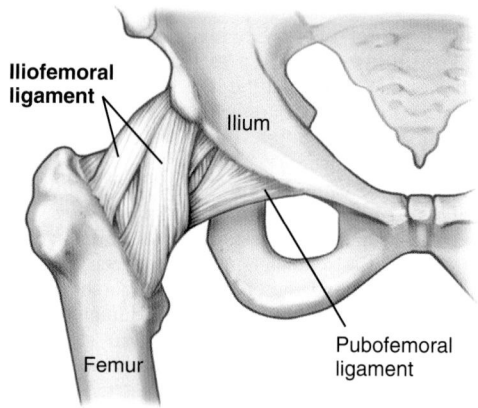

Iliofemoral ligament

iliofemoral thrombosis,   an abnormal vascular condition in which a clot develops in the iliofemoral circulation.

iliohypogastric nerve,   a nerve with branches that innervate the posterolateral gluteal skin and the skin in the pubic region, as well as the abdominal musculature.

ilioinguinal /il′ē·ō·ing″gwinəl/ [L, *ilium* + *inguen,* groin],   pertaining to the hip and inguinal regions.

ilioinguinal nerve,   a nerve that provides cutaneous innervation to the upper medial thigh, the root of the penis and the anterior surface of the scrotum in men, or the mons pubis and labia majora in women. Through its course, it also supplies branches to the abdominal musculature.

iliolumbar artery,   a branch of the posterior trunk of the internal iliac artery that supplies muscle and bone.

iliolumbar ligament /-lum″bər/ [L, *ilium* + *lumbus,* loin, *ligare,* to bind],   one of a pair of ligaments forming part of the connection between the vertebral column and the pelvis. Each iliolumbar ligament attaches to a transverse process of the fifth lumbar vertebra and laterally to the ilium and inferiorly passes to the base of the sacrum, where it blends with the sacroiliac ligament.

iliopectineal eminence.   See **iliopubic eminence.**

iliopectineal line /-pek″tənəl/ [L, *ilium* + *pectus,* breast, *linea*],   a bony ridge on the inner surface of the ilium and pubic bones that divides the true and false pelves. Also called **brim of true pelvic cavity, inlet.**

iliopectineal tubercle.   See **iliopubic eminence.**

iliopsoas /il′ē·ōsō″əs/ [L, *ilium* + Gk, *psoa,* loin muscle],   one of the pair of muscle complexes that flex, adduct, and laterally rotate the thigh and the lumbar vertebral column, consisting of the psoas major and the iliacus. The psoas minor is often absent.

iliopsoas abscess [L, *ilium*],   a collection of pus in the iliopsoas muscle, possibly tuberculous in origin, that spreads from the thoracic or lumbar spine to the upper leg muscles, usually caused by staphylococcus infection.

iliopubic eminence, a diffuse enlargement just anterior to the acetabulum, marking the junction of the ilium with the superior ramus of the pubis. Also called **iliopectineal eminence, iliopectineal tubercle.**

iliorenal bypass, a technique of renal revascularization involving insertion of a saphenous vein graft between an iliac artery and a renal artery to serve as a passage around an occluded segment of renal artery.

iliotibial tract /-tib″ē·əl/ [L, *ilium,* flank, *tibia,* shinbone], a band of connective tissue that extends from the iliac crest to the knee and links the gluteus maximus to the tibia.

ilium /il″ē·əm/ *pl. ilia* [L, flank], the uppermost of the three bones that make up the innominate bone (hip bone). The ilium forms the superior part of the acetabulum and provides attachment for several muscles, including the obturator internus, the gluteals, the iliacus, and the sartorius. Compare **ischium, pubis.** *–iliac, adj.*

illegal abortion, an abortion performed contrary to the laws regulating abortion. Illegal abortions are often associated with life-threatening complications. See also **septic abortion.**

illegitimate /il′ejit″imit/ [L, *in,* not, *lex,* law], **1.** not authorized by law. **2.** not in accordance with accepted standards or customs. **3.** *(Informal)* an individual not recognized as a lawful offspring. Most states and governments no longer use this term to describe someone whose parents were not married at the time of their birth.

illicit /ilis″it/ [L, *in,* not, *lex,* law], pertaining to an act that is unlawful or otherwise not permitted.

illiterate /ilit″ərit/, unable to read and write.

illness [ME, unhealthy condition], an abnormal process in which aspects of the social, physical, emotional, or intellectual condition and function of a person are diminished or impaired compared with that person's previous condition.

illness behavior, the manner in which individuals monitor the structure and functions of their own bodies, interpret symptoms, take remedial action, and make use of health care facilities.

illness experience, the process of being ill. A commonly used model is Suchman's stages of illness, comprising five stages: stage I, experiencing a symptom; stage II, assuming a sick role; stage III, making contact for health care; stage IV, being dependent (a patient); and stage V, recovering or being rehabilitated. Each stage is characterized by certain decisions, behaviors, and end points. During stage I, in which a symptom is experienced, the person decides that something is wrong and seeks a remedy. Stage I ends with the person's accepting the reality of the symptom, no longer delaying any action toward help or denying the symptom (flight into health). During stage II the person decides that the illness is real and that care is necessary. Advice, guidance, and validation are sought. This stage gives the person permission to act sick and to be excused temporarily from usual obligations. The outcome of this stage is acceptance of the role—or denial of its necessity. In stage III, professional advice is sought. Authoritative declarations identify and validate the illness and legitimize the sick role. The person usually asks for help and negotiates for treatment. Denial may still occur, and the patient may "shop" further for medical care or may accept the illness, the medical authority, and the plan for treatment. In stage IV, professional treatment is performed and accepted by the person, who is now perceived as a patient. At any time during this stage the dependent patient may experience ambivalent feelings and may decide to reject the treatment, the caregiver, and the illness. More often care is accepted with ambivalence. The patient has a particular need to be informed and to be given emotional support during this stage. During stage V the patient relinquishes the sick role. The usual tasks and roles are reassumed to the greatest degree possible. Some people do not willingly give up the sick role, becoming in their own eyes chronically ill, or they may, for secondary gain, malinger, acting sick. Most people accept recovery and work toward rehabilitation.

illness prevention, **1.** a system of health education programs and activities directed at protecting patients from real or potential health threats, minimizing risk factors, and promoting healthy behavior. **2.** actions taken by individuals to prevent illness in themselves and/or their families.

illumination /iloo″minā″shən/ [L, *illuminare,* to make light], the lighting of a part of the body or of an object under a microscope for the purpose of examination. *–illuminate, v.*

illumination assessment, evaluation of the quality of lighting in the workplace.

illusion /iloo″zhən/ [L, *illudere,* to mock], a false interpretation of an external sensory stimulus, usually visual or auditory, such as a mirage in the desert or voices on the wind.

Ilosone, an antibacterial drug. Brand name for *erythromycin estolate.*

IM, abbreviation for **intramuscular.**

image /im″ij/ [L, *imago,* likeness], **1.** a representation or visual reproduction of the likeness of someone or something, such as a painting, photograph, or sculpture. **2.** an optic representation of an object, such as that produced by refraction or reflection. **3.** a person or thing that closely resembles another; semblance. **4.** a mental picture, representation, idea, or concept of an objective reality. **5.** (in psychology) a mental representation of something previously perceived and subsequently modified by other experiences, resulting from intrapsychic or extrapsychic stimuli, or both.

image acquisition time, the time required to acquire the data used in producing a magnetic resonance image. It does not include the time involved in constructing the image from the data. In comparing sequential plane imaging and volume imaging techniques, the equivalent image acquisition time per slice must be considered, as well as the actual image acquisition time.

image compression, reduction of the space required to store or the time required to transfer a digital image.

image detector, any recording medium used in radiology.

image foreshortening, a type of shape distortion in which a radiographic image appears shorter and wider than the actual structure it represents. It results from misalignment of the x-ray tube relative to the patient, of the patient relative to the image receptor, or of the tube relative to the image receptor.

image format, the manner in which a digital image is stored, such as on a computer disk, magnetic tape, or film.

image intensifier, an electronic device used to produce a fluoroscopic image with a low-radiation exposure. A beam of x-rays passing through the patient is converted into a pattern of electrons in a vacuum tube. The electrons are accelerated and concentrated onto a small fluorescent screen, where they present a bright image, which is generally displayed on a video monitor.

image matrix, an arrangement of columns and rows of cells, or pixels, forming a digital image.

image receptor (IR), a device that captures the remnant x-ray beam so that it can be processed and transformed into a visible image. An image receptor may be a radiographic film and cassette, a phosphorescent screen (used in fluoroscopy or computed radiography), or a special detector placed in a table or upright bucky diaphragm (used in digital radiography).

imagery /im″ijrē/ [L, *imago*], (in psychiatry) the formation of mental concepts, figures, or ideas; any product of the imagination. An imagery technique is applied therapeutically to decrease anxiety. See also **guided imagery.**

imagination /imaj′inā″shən/ [L, *imaginare,* picture to oneself], **1.** the ability to form, or the act or process of forming, mental images or conscious concepts of things that are not immediately available to the senses. **2.** (in psychology) the ability to reproduce images or ideas stored in the memory by the stimulation or suggestion of associated ideas or to regroup former ideas and concepts to form new images and ideas concerned with a particular goal or problem. See also **fantasy.**

imaging /im″ijing/ [L, *imago*], the formation of a mental picture or representation of someone or something using the imagination. See also **fantasy.**

imaging platean, an image receptor similar to a film/screen cassette that houses a photostimulable phosphor screen used in computed radiography.

imago /imā″gō/ [L, likeness], (in analytic psychology) an unconscious, usually idealized mental image of a significant individual, such as one's mother, in a person's early formative years. See also **identification.**

imatinib /imā″tĭnib″/, an inhibitor acting specifically on an abnormal enzyme form that is created by the Philadelphia chromosome abnormality and present in chronic myeloid leukemia. It is administered orally as the mesylate salt in the treatment of chronic myeloid leukemia during blast crisis, accelerated phase, or chronic phase after failure of interferon-alpha therapy.

imbalance /imbal″əns/ [L, *im,* not, *bilanx,* having two scales], **1.** a lack of balance between opposing muscle groups, such as in the imbalance of extraocular muscles leading to strabismus. **2.** an abnormal balance of fluid and electrolytes in the body tissues. **3.** the unequal distribution of subjects in a population group, such as the only girl in a large family of boys. **4.** a lack of balance in a person with mental abilities that are remarkable in one area but deficient in others, as in an idiot savant.

imbedded tooth. See **embedded tooth.**

imbricate /im″brikāt/ [L, *imbrex,* roofing tile], to build a surface with overlapping layers of material. Surgeons may imbricate with layers of tissue when closing a wound or other opening in a body part. –**imbrication,** *n.*

IMDD, abbreviation for **idiopathic midline destructive disease.**

Imferon, an injectable hematinic. Brand name for **iron dextran.**

imide-, imido-, prefix indicating the presence in a chemical compound of the bivalent group NH: *imidogen.*

imiglucerase, an analog of a human enzyme produced by recombinant deoxyribonucleic acid technology.
- INDICATIONS: It is prescribed as enzyme replacement therapy for patients with type I Gaucher disease.
- CONTRAINDICATIONS: There are no known contraindications to the use of imiglucerase by injection.
- ADVERSE EFFECTS: The side effects most often reported include headache, nausea, abdominal discomfort, dizziness, and rash.

imino-, prefix indicating the presence of the bivalent group NH attached to a nonacid radical: *iminoglycinuria.*

iminoglycinuria /im′inōglī′sinoͦor″ē-ə/, a benign familial condition characterized by the abnormal urinary excretion of the imino acids glycine, proline, and hydroxyproline.

imipenem-cilastatin sodium /im′ipē″nəm sil′əstat″in/, a broad-spectrum parenteral antibiotic.
- INDICATIONS: It is prescribed for the treatment of infections caused by susceptible organisms in the lower respira-

tory or urinary tracts, skin, abdomen, reproductive organs, bones, or joints. It is also used in the treatment of endocarditis and septicemia.
- CONTRAINDICATIONS: It is not recommended for children. Caution should be used in administering it to patients with pseudomembranous colitis, hypersensitivity reactions, or a history of seizures.
- ADVERSE EFFECTS: The most common adverse effects are phlebitis, thrombophlebitis, nausea, vomiting, diarrhea, rash, fever, and central nervous system symptoms.

imipramine hydrochloride /imip″rəmēn/, a tricyclic antidepressant.
- INDICATIONS: It is prescribed in the treatment of mental depression.
- CONTRAINDICATIONS: Concomitant administration of monoamine oxidase inhibitors, recent myocardial infarction, cardiovascular disease or seizure disorder, or known hypersensitivity to this drug or to other tricyclic medication prohibits its use.
- ADVERSE EFFECTS: Among the more serious adverse effects are sedation, GI disturbances, and cardiovascular and neurological reactions. It should not be withdrawn abruptly. This drug interacts with many other drugs.

imiquimod /im″ĭkwim′od/, a biological response modifier used topically in the treatment of venereal warts of the external genitalia and perianal region.

imitation, (in therapies) the physical or motor modeling or demonstration of the desired action.

imitative behavior, (in occupational therapy) mimicking the actions of peers, in particular the actions of a group leader and other group members who are modeling appropriate, socially acceptable interactions.

immature baby /iməchoͦor″/ [L, *im,* not, *maturus,* ripe], a term sometimes applied to an infant who weighs less than 1134 g (2.5 lb) and who is significantly underdeveloped at birth.

immature cataract [L, *im + maturus,* ripe; Gk, *katarrhaktes*], a cataract at an early stage of development when the lens, partially opaque, absorbs fluid and increases by swelling. Only part of the lens is opaque.

immature erythrocyte [L, *im + maturus,* ripe; Gk, *erythros,* red, *kytos,* cell], a nucleated precursor red blood cell in the erythrocyte series: pronormoblast, basophilic normoblast, polychromatophilic normoblast, or orthochromic normoblast. The orthochromic normoblast appears on peripheral blood films of newborns, in uncompensated hemolytic anemia, and in hematological neoplasms.

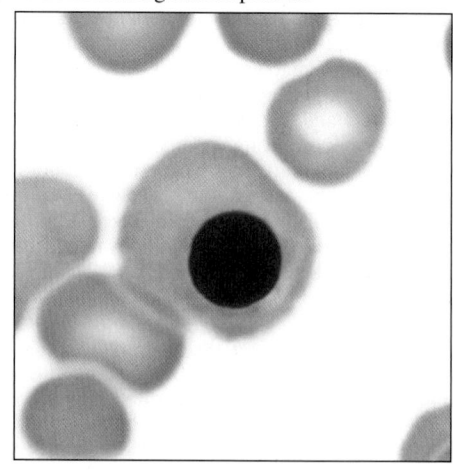

Immature erythrocyte: the orthochromatic normoblast
(McPherson and Pincus, 2011)

immediate auscultation /imē″dē·it/ [L, *im* + *medius,* middle, *auscultare,* to listen], a method of examining a patient by placing an ear or stethoscope on the skin directly over the body part being studied.

immediate automatism, a state in which a person acts spontaneously and automatically and later has no recollection of the behavior.

immediate denture [L, *im* + *medius* + *dens,* tooth], a removable artificial denture that is placed in the mouth immediately after the surgical removal of all remaining teeth at the same appointment as the tooth extractions to maintain normal appearance, act as a compression and protective dressing, and allow the ability to chew food. It may be a complete or a partial denture.

immediate hypersensitivity, an allergic reaction that occurs within minutes after exposure to an allergen and is mediated by antibodies. Compare **delayed hypersensitivity.**

immediate hypersensitivity reaction. See **hypersensitivity reaction.**

immediate postoperative fit (IPOF) prosthesis, a temporary or preparatory prosthesis, such as a pylon.

immediate posttraumatic automatism, a state following a highly stressful event in which a person acts spontaneously and automatically and later has no recollection of the behavior.

immersion /imur″zhən/ [L, *im* + *mergere,* to dip], the placing of a body or an object into water or other liquid so that it is completely covered by the liquid. –**immerse,** *v.*

immersion foot, an abnormal condition of the feet characterized by damage to the muscles, nerves, skin, and blood vessels. It is caused by prolonged exposure to dampness or by prolonged immersion in cold water. See also **frostbite, trench foot.**

Immerslund-Gräsbeck syndrome, a familial form of megaloblastic anemia and cobalamin deficiency. It is characterized by selective intestinal malabsorption of vitamin B_{12}, uninfluenced by intrinsic factor. About 90% of the cases are associated with a mild, nonspecific form of proteinuria.

imminent abortion. See **inevitable abortion.**

immiscible /imis″əbəl/ [L, *im* + *miscere,* to mix], not capable of being mixed, such as oil and water. Compare **miscible.**

immobilization /imō′bəlīzā″shən/, **1.** fixation of a body part so that it cannot move during surgery or after setting of a fracture. **2.** prolonged inactivity of an individual, as with bed rest for neurological injury such as coma or quadriplegia. –**immobile,** *adj.*

immobilization test, a procedure for identifying antibodies to motile microorganisms by measuring the ability of the antibodies to restrict the motility of the microorganisms.

immotile cilia syndrome /imō″til/ [L, *im* + *motilis,* movable, *cilia,* eyelashes; Gk, *syn,* together, *dromos,* course], a condition in which cilia, the hairlike processes of epithelial cells, fail to function normally. As a result, the patient has difficulty in filtering dust and other airborne debris from the respiratory system. See also **Kartagener syndrome.**

immune /imyoon″/ [L, *immunis,* free from], having resistance to infection by a particular pathogen because of the presence of specific antibodies and white blood cells capable of recognizing the same pathogen.

immune complex, a multimolecular complex formed when an antibody binds to a specific antigen. The complex is capable of activating complements and is a factor in diseases such as arthritis, vasculitis, serum sickness, and glomerulonephritis.

immune complex hemolytic anemia, the destruction of red blood cells caused by the formation of specific antigen-antibody complexes in the presence of complement.

immune cytolysis, cell destruction mediated by a specific antibody that activates the complement system, resulting in rupture of the cell membrane.

immune deviation, modification of an immune response to an antigen.

immune exclusion, the prevention of an antigen from entering the body by a specific immune response—for example, the binding of secretory IgA to antigens to neutralize them. The neutralized antigens are unable to interact with the epithelium.

immune gamma globulin, passive immunizing agent obtained from pooled human plasma. Also called immune globulin. See also **immunoglobulin G.**

■ INDICATIONS: It is prescribed for immediate short-lived protection against measles, poliomyelitis, chickenpox, serum hepatitis after transfusion, hepatitis A, and other disease-causing organisms to which the person has been recently exposed or may be exposed and as replacement therapy for patients with agammaglobulinemia or hypogammaglobulinemia.

■ CONTRAINDICATIONS: Known hypersensitivity to gamma globulins prohibits its use.

■ ADVERSE EFFECTS: Among the more serious adverse effects are pain and inflammation at the site of injection, allergic reactions, and headache.

immune hemolysis, *(Obsolete)* now called **immune complex hemolytic anemia, immunohemolytic anemia.**

immune human globulin, a sterile solution of globulins derived from adult human blood that is used as a passive immunizing agent.

immune human serum globulin. See **immunoglobulin.**

immune reaction. See **immune response.**

immune recognition, recognition of nonself antigens by the immune system. Cells of the innate (or nonspecific) immune system contain receptors that can recognize conserved products of microorganisms. T and B cells of the adaptive (or specific) immune system recognize nonself antigens via B or T cell receptors.

immune response, a response of the body to protect itself against invading pathogens, foreign tissues, and malignancies. It consists of the innate (or nonspecific) immune response and the adaptive (or specific/acquired) immune response. Cells of the innate immune system recognize and respond to pathogens in a generic way, and the response is short-lasting. B and T cells of the adaptive immune system are highly specific for a specific antigen of a pathogen. They can provide long-lasting protection (memory). Also called **immune reaction.** See also **humoral immunity, immune system.**

immune serum. See **antiserum.**

immune serum globulin (ISG). See **immunoglobulin.**

immune surveillance. See **immunological surveillance.**

immune system, a system of tissues, organs, and cells that protects the body against pathogenic organisms and other foreign bodies. The principal components of the immune system include the primary lymphoid tissues (bone marrow, thymus) and the secondary lymphoid tissues (lymph nodes, spleen, tonsils, mucosa-associated lymphoid tissue [MALT]). The immune system protects the body initially by creating local barriers and inflammation. The local barriers provide chemical and mechanical defenses through the skin, the mucous membranes, and the conjunctiva. Inflammation draws polymorphonuclear leukocytes and neutrophils to the site of injury, where these phagocytes engulf the invading pathogens (innate immunity). If these first-line defenses fail or are inadequate to protect the body, the humoral immune response and the cell-mediated immune response are

Comparison of humoral immunity and cell-mediated immunity

Characteristics	Humoral immunity	Cell-mediated immunity
Cells involved	B lymphocytes	T lymphocytes, macrophages
Products	Antibodies	Sensitized T cells, cytokines
Memory cells	Present	Present
Protection	Bacteria Viruses (extracellular) Respiratory and gastrointestinal pathogens	Fungus Viruses (intracellular) Chronic infectious agents Tumor cells
Examples	Anaphylactic shock Atopic diseases Transfusion reaction Bacterial infections	Tuberculosis Fungal infections Contact dermatitis Graft rejection Destruction of cancer cells

From Lewis SL et al: *Medical-surgical nursing: assessment and management of clinical problems,* ed 9, St. Louis, 2014, Mosby.

activated (adaptive immunity). See also **immune response, humoral immunity, cell-mediated immunity.**

immune thrombocytopenic purpura /-sī′təpē″nik/ [Gk, *thrombos + kytos,* cell, *penia,* poverty; L, *purpura,* purple], mucocutaneous bleeding of thrombocytopenia, caused by a platelet membrane-specific autoantibody that shortens the platelet life span. It is diagnosed by exclusion of drug effects, inflammatory disorder, thrombotic thrombocytopenic purpura, DIC, or hematological disorder. It affects middle-aged adults and is more prevalent in women than in men. Acute immune thrombocytopenic purpura is a side effect of viral infection in children 2 to 6 years of age, and although the thrombocytopenia is profound, the disorder resolves spontaneously within a few weeks. Also called *autoimmune thrombocytopenic purpura.* Compare **disseminated intravascular coagulation.** Formerly called *idiopathic thrombocytopenic purpura.* See also **hemophilia, hemorrhagic diathesis, thrombasthenia.**

■ OBSERVATIONS: Common manifestations include petechiae and ecchymoses on the skin, particularly the lower extremities; easy bruising; bleeding from the nose and gums; melena in stools; hematemesis; heavy menses and breakthrough bleeding; and hematuria. Jaundice, fever, and decreased levels of consciousness may be seen in thrombotic thrombocytopenic purpura. Diagnosis focuses on obtaining a history of bleeding symptoms and on ruling out other causes of thrombocytopenia, such as medications, ethanol abuse, HIV, or hematological disorder. Lab findings include decreased platelet count. Bleeding time is prolonged, but coagulation time is normal. Capillary fragility is increased. Bone marrow aspiration shows an abundance of megakaryocytes. In thrombotic thrombocytopenic purpura there is severe anemia, elevated BUN, elevated creatinine, elevated reticulocytes, elevated LDH, decreased haptoglobin, and fragmented RBCs on peripheral smear. Platelet size and morphological appearance may be abnormal in thrombotic thrombocytopenic purpura. Complications include hemorrhage into organs, such as the brain, gastrointestinal tract, or heart, which can be fatal without treatment.

■ INTERVENTIONS: Medications that may be causing or contributing to the thrombocytopenia are discontinued. Treatment is determined by platelet count and bleeding status. Corticosteroids are used to enhance platelet production and promote capillary integrity. Immunosuppressants are used if the disease does not respond to steroids. Platelet transfusions are used in cases of severe bleeding in idiopathic thrombocytopenic purpura. Plasma exchange or plasmapheresis is the treatment of choice in thrombotic thrombocytopenic purpura. Vincristine may be used in thrombotic thrombocy-

topenic purpura cases that are refractory to plasmapheresis. Splenectomy may be considered for severe unresponsive thrombocytopenia. Immune globulin is given to prepare severely thrombocytic individuals for surgery. Platelet counts and bleeding episodes are monitored closely. Stool softeners are administered to prevent constipation.

■ PATIENT CARE CONSIDERATIONS: Goals are aimed at eliminating gross or occult bleeding, maintaining vascular integrity, decreasing risk for injury, and reducing complications. Safety precautions are instituted to prevent bruising (e.g., mouth swabs and soft-bristle toothbrush for oral care; electric razor for shaving; insertion of IV access device for blood draws; padding of bed rails and hard surfaces). Emesis, sputum, stool, urine, and other secretions for occult blood and pad counts during menstruation are frequently assessed and tested. Active bleeding is controlled with ice packs, gentle pressure, or packing. Rest and activity should be carefully balanced to conserve energy. Education is needed on trauma prevention and safety precautions, including the avoidance of contact sports; the avoidance of the Valsalva maneuver; the necessity for gentle coughing, sneezing, and nose blowing; and the necessity for increased fluid intake and balanced periods of rest and exercise. Instruction in infection precautions is given for those taking immunosuppressants. Education includes instruction to avoid anticoagulant over-the-counter medications, such as aspirin or aspirin products and other NSAIDs.

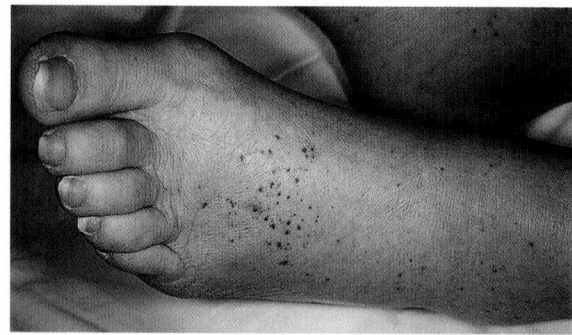

Immune thrombocytopenic purpura *(Callen et al, 2000)*

immunity /imyŏŏ″nitē/ [L, *immunis,* free from], **1.** (in civil law) exemption from a duty or an obligation generally required by law, as an exemption from taxation or from penalty for wrongdoing or protection against liability. **2.** the quality of being insusceptible to or unaffected by a particular disease or condition. Kinds include **acquired immunity, active immunity, passive immunity. –immune,** *adj.*

immunization /im′yənīzā″shən/ [L, free], a technique used to induce an immune response to a specific disease by exposing an individual to an antigen to raise antibodies to that antigen. See also **vaccination.**

immunoablative /im″mu·no·ab′lätiv/, immunosuppressant with removal and destruction of a cell population, such as in the ablative step preceding bone marrow transplantation.

immunoabsorbent /im′yənō′absôr″bənt/, a gel or other inert substance used to absorb antibodies from a solution or to purify them.

immunoabsorption /im′yənō′absôrp″shən/, **1.** removal of a specific group of antibodies by antigens. **2.** removal of antigen by interaction with specific antibodies.

immunoadsorbent /im′yənō′adsôr″bənt/, an insoluble preparation of antigens or antibodies used to bind homologous antibodies or antigens and remove them from a mixture of substances.

immunoassay /im′yənō·as″ā/ [L, *immunis* + Fr, *essayer,* to try], a commonly employed assay in which a solid-phase target antigen is designed to bind with an antibody in vitro to reveal its presence. When a conjugated antihuman immunoglobulin is added, it binds the antibody of interest. The conjugate, usually an enzyme, then reacts with its substrate to generate color or fluorescence that is proportional to antibody concentrations. See also **enzyme-linked immunosorbent assay, radioimmunoassay, sandwich technique.**

immunoaugmentative therapy. an unproven cancer treatment that proposes that cancer cells can be arrested by the use of four different blood proteins. Should not be confused with **cancer immunotherapy.**

immunobead /im′yənōbēd″/, a tiny, inert, plastic sphere coated with antigens or antibody, used for immunoassays, such as the isolation of B cells from T cells.

immunobead assay, an assay for any of various types of antibodies or antigens, using immunobeads coated with a corresponding antigen or antibody that aggregates or agglutinates in the presence of the one in question.

immunoblastic lymphoma /-blas″tik/, a proliferation of immunoblasts involving the lymph nodes.

immunoblastic lymphadenopathy, Also called **angioimmunoblastic T-cell lymphoma.**

immunoblotting /-blot″ing/, a method for identifying antigens. The antigens are allowed to adhere to cellulose sheets and are identified by staining with labeled antibodies. The method is also used to detect monoclonal proteins. See also **Western blot test.**

immunochemistry, the study of the chemical properties of antigens and antibodies, complement, and T cell receptors.

immunochemotherapy /-kem′ōther″əpē/, a combination of biotherapy and chemotherapy. See also **chemotherapy, immunotherapy.**

immunocompetence /-kom′pətəns/, the ability of an immune system to mobilize and deploy its antibodies and other responses to stimulation by an antigen. Immunocompetence may be weakened in older individuals as a result of age-related attenuation in T cell function. It may also be diminished by viruses, radiation, and chemotherapeutic drugs. –*immunocompetent, adj.*

immunocomplex assay, a laboratory assessment of the amounts of components in multimolecular antigen-antibody complexes. The assay is used in various diagnostic tests for collagen-vascular disorders, glomerulonephritis, vasculitis, hepatitis, and neoplastic diseases.

immunocomplex hypersensitivity [L, *immunis,* free from, *complexus,* embrace; Gk, *hyper,* excess; L, *sentire,* to feel], *(Obsolete)* now called **type III hypersensitivity.**

immunocomplex-mediated hypersensitivity reaction, *(Obsolete)* now called **hypersensitivity reaction.**

immunocompromised /-kom″prəmīzd′/ [L, *immunis,* free from, *compromittere,* to promise mutually], pertaining to an immune response that has been weakened by a disease or an immunosuppressive agent.

immunocompromised host, an individual whose immune response is weakened as a result of an immunodeficiency disorder or exposure to immunosuppressive drugs or irradiation.

immunodeficiency. See **immunocompromised.**

immunodeficiency disease /-difish″ənsē/, any of a group of diseases caused by a defect in the immune system and generally characterized by susceptibility to infections and chronic diseases. Such diseases are sometimes classified as B cell (antibody) deficiencies, T cell (cellular) deficiencies, combined T and B cell deficiencies, defects of cell movement, and defects of microbicidal activity. See also **severe combined immunodeficiency disease.**

immunodeficient /-difish″ənt/ [L, *immunis* + *de,* from, *facere,* to make], pertaining to an abnormal condition of the immune system in which cellular or humoral immunity is inadequate and resistance to infection is decreased. Kinds include **hypogammaglobulinemia, lymphoid aplasia.** See also **immunocompromised.**

immunodiagnosis. See **serological diagnosis.**

immunodiagnostic /-dī′əgnos″tik/ [L, *immunis* + Gk, *dia,* through, *gnosis* knowledge], pertaining to or characterizing a diagnosis based on an antigen-antibody reaction. In many cases a tumor releases a discrete antigenic substance into the blood. Detection of a particular antigen can provide an immunodiagnostic sign of the presence of the tumor associated with that antigen.

immunodiffusion /-dify̅o̅o̅″zhən/ [L, *immunis* + *diffundere,* to spread], a technique for the identification and quantification of any of the immunoglobulins. It is based on the presence of a visible precipitate that results from an antigen-antibody combination under certain circumstances. Gel diffusion is a technique that involves evaluation of the precipitin reaction in a clear gel, seen when an antigen placed in a hole in the agarose diffuses evenly into the medium. An obvious ring forms where the antigen meets the antibody. Electroimmunodiffusion is a gel diffusion to which an electrical field is applied, accelerating the reaction. Double gel diffusion is a technique that permits identification of antibodies in mixed specimens. In an agar plate, antigen is placed in one well, antibody in another. Antigen and antibody diffuse out of their wells. In mixed antigen specimens each antigen-antibody combination forms a separate line; observation of the location, shape, and thickness of a line permits identification and quantification of the antibody.

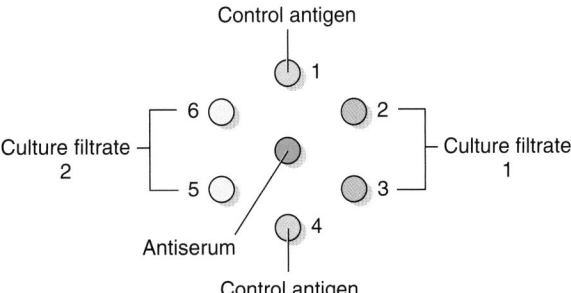

Immunodiffusion *(Mahon, Lehman, and Manuselis, 2011)*

immunoelectroadsorption /im′yənō′ilek′trō·adsôrp″shən/, an antibody assay technique in which antigens are adsorbed onto a metal-coated glass slide with an electric current. Serum containing antibodies is then applied to the slide.

immunoelectrodiffusion. See **immunodiffusion.**

immunoelectron microscopy /im′yənō′ilek″tron/, electron microscopy of specimens labeled with antibodies that have been conjugated with gold. The gold makes the antibody labels electron-dense.

immunoelectrophoresis /-ilek′trōfôrē″sis/ [L, *immunis* + Gk, *elektron,* amber, *pherein,* to bear], a technique that combines electrophoresis and immunodiffusion to separate and allow identification of complex proteins. The proteins in the test serum are spread out in agar and separated by electrophoresis. Wells or troughs are then cut into the agar, and parts of antibody are placed in the troughs and allowed to diffuse toward the separated proteins. A visible precipitin will form in a series of arcs in the agar when an antigen-antibody reaction occurs. The shape and location of each arc are specific for known proteins. Unusual arcs are representative of abnormal or unknown protein. Although the density of the precipitation corresponds to the concentration of protein in each electrophoretic band, immunoelectrophoresis does not accurately quantify the amount of protein in the test serum. *—immunoelectrophoretic, adj.*

immunoenhancement /im′yənō′enhans″mənt/, the augmentation of immune responsiveness by immunization or other means.

immunoferritin /-fer″itin/, an antibody labeled with ferritin used to identify specific antigens in electron microscopy.

immunoferritin technique, a method of labeling antibody molecules with ferritin, an electron-dense material. The ferritin renders the sites of antibody attachment visible in electron microscopy.

immunofixation /-fiksā″shən/, a process by which antigens in a protein mixture are separated on an electrophoretic gel and identified by the application of labeled antibodies.

immunofixation electrophoresis, a blood or urine test used to detect monoclonal gammopathies.

immunofluorescence /-floores″əns/ [L, *immunis* + *fluere,* to flow], a technique used for the rapid identification of an antigen by exposing it to known antibodies tagged with the fluorescent dye fluorescein and observing the characteristic antigen-antibody reaction of precipitation. As the fluorescent antibody reacts with its specific antigen, the precipitate appears luminous in the ultraviolet light projected by a fluorescent microscope. Many of the most common infectious organisms can be identified by this technique. Among them are *Candida albicans, Haemophilus influenzae, Neisseria gonorrhoeae, Shigella, Staphylococcus aureus,* and several viruses, including rabies virus and many enteroviruses. See also **fluorescent antibody test, fluorescent microscopy.** *—immunofluorescent, adj.*

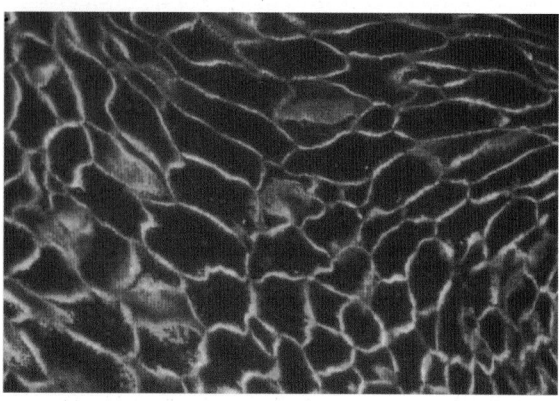

Immunofluorescence *(Courtesy Dr. Troy E. Daniels)*

immunofluorescence test. See **fluorescent antibody test.**

immunofluorescent. See **immunofluorescence.**

immunofluorescent microscopy. See **fluorescent microscopy, immunofluorescence.**

immunogen /imyōō″nəjən/ [L, *immunis* + Gk, *genein,* to produce], any agent or substance capable of provoking an immune response or producing immunity. *—immunogenic, adj.*

immunogenetics /-jənet″iks/, a branch of medicine concerned with the role of genetics in tissue transplantation and immunological response.

immunogenicity. See **antigenicity.**

immunoglobulin (Ig) /-glob″yəlin/ [L, *immunis* + *globus,* small sphere], any of five structurally distinct classes of proteins (IgA, IgD, IgE, IgG, IgM) produced by B cells. Immunoglobulins are present in two physical forms: membrane-bound (B cell receptors) and secreted. The B cell receptor can recognize foreign antigens and subsequently activate the B cell to become plasma or memory B cell with the help of CD4 T cells. Antibodies are produced by plasma cells and can identify and neutralize foreign antigens such as bacteria and viruses. They are the main mediators of the humoral immune response. Also called **immune serum globulin.** See also **antibody, antigen, immunity.**

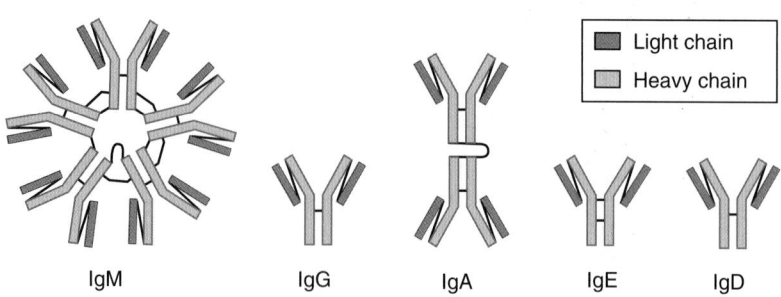

Immunoglobulins *(Patton and Thibodeau, 2016)*

Properties of immunoglobulin classes

Property	Immunoglobulin class				
	IgG	IgM	IgA	IgE	IgD
Principal site	Internal body fluids	Serum	Serum and exocrine secretions	Tissue bound	Bound to lymphocyte surface
Fixed complement	Yes	Yes	No	No	No
Crosses placenta	Yes	No	No	No	No
Principal functions	Agglutination, detoxification, virus neutralization; enhancement of phagocytosis	Agglutination, cytolysis; enhancement of phagocytosis	Protection of mucosal surfaces	Mediation of immediate type of hypersensitivity	Control of lymphocytic activation and suppression

immunoglobulin A (IgA), one of the most prevalent of the five classes of antibodies produced by the body. It is found in all secretions of the body and is the major antibody in the tears, saliva, and mucous membranes lining the intestines and bronchi. IgA combines with a protein in the mucosa and defends body surfaces by seeking out foreign microorganisms and triggering an antigen-antibody reaction. The normal concentration of IgA in serum is 50 to 250 mg/dL. Compare **immunoglobulin D, immunoglobulin E, immunoglobulin G, immunoglobulin M.** See also **IgA deficiency.**

immunoglobulin D (IgD), one of the five classes of antibodies produced by the body. It is found in small amounts in serum tissue. Although its precise function is not known, IgD increases in quantity during allergic reactions to milk, insulin, penicillin, and various toxins. The normal concentration of IgD in serum is 0.5 to 3 mg/dL. Compare **immunoglobulin A, immunoglobulin E, immunoglobulin G, immunoglobulin M.**

immunoglobulin E (IgE), one of the five classes of antibodies produced by the body. It is concentrated in the lungs, skin, and mucous membranes. It provides the primary defense against parasites, such as parasitic worms, but can also recognize allergens (such as pollen, dust mites). After binding with receptors on mast cells and basophils, it can release histamines and leukotrienes from these cells and cause anaphylactic hypersensitivity reactions characterized by wheal and flare. The normal concentration of IgE in serum is 0.01 to 0.04 mg/dL. Compare **immunoglobulin A, immunoglobulin D, immunoglobulin G, immunoglobulin M.**

immunoglobulin electrophoresis, a blood test done to detect and identify the various immunoglobulins (antibodies), such as IgG, IgA, IgM, IgE, and IgD. Serum immunoelectrophoresis is used to detect and monitor the course of diseases.

immunoglobulin G (IgG), one of the five classes of antibodies produced by the body and the most abundant antibody isotype found in the circulation. It is synthesized in response to invasions by bacteria, fungi, and viruses. IgG crosses the placenta and can protect the fetus from invading microorganisms. The normal concentration of IgG in serum is 800 to 1600 mg/dL. Compare **immunoglobulin A, immunoglobulin D, immunoglobulin E, immunoglobulin M.**

immunoglobulin M (IgM), one of the five classes of antibodies produced by the body and the largest in molecular structure. It is found in circulating fluids and is the first immunoglobulin to appear on the cell surface of B cells and the first to be produced when the body is challenged by antigens. It does not cross the placenta. IgM triggers the increased production of immunoglobulin G and the complement fixation required for effective immune responses. It is the dominant antibody in ABO blood group incompatibilities. The normal concentration of IgM in serum is 40 to 120 mg/dL. Compare **immunoglobulin A, immunoglobulin D, immunoglobulin E, immunoglobulin G.**

immunohematology /-hem′ətol″əjē/ [L, *immunis* + Gk, *haima,* blood, *logos,* science], the study of antigen-antibody reactions and their effects on blood.

immunohemolytic anemia. See **immune complex hemolytic anemia.**

immunoincompetence /im′yənō′inkom″pətəns/, the inability to develop an immune reaction. See also **immunocompromised host. –immunoincompetent,** *adj.*

immunoincompetent /im′yənō′inkom″pətənt/, pertaining to the inability to develop an immune response to the challenge of antigens.

immunological barrier /-loj″ik/, an apparent protection against an immune response afforded by certain areas of the body, as, for example, the placenta between mother and child.

immunological disease [L, *immunis,* free from; Gk, *logos,* science; L, *dis* + Fr, *aise,* ease], any condition caused by an abnormal immune system.

immunological granuloma, a small, organized, compact collection of mononuclear phagocytes that develops within 2 or 3 weeks after the introduction of a foreign material, provoking an inflammatory response. Such materials include sea urchin toxin, chemicals used in making tattoos, and antigens associated with leprosy, tuberculosis, and cat-scratch fever.

immunological infertility, any of several types of female factor infertility believed to be caused by the presence of antibodies that interfere with functioning of the sperm, such as antisperm antibody.

immunologically competent cell, a cell of the lymphoid series that can react with antigen to produce antibody or to become active in cell-mediated immunity or delayed hypersensitivity reactions.

immunological model of aging, the hypothesis that a decline in the function of T cells and B cells causes normal cells to be unrecognized as such, thereby triggering immune reactions against an individual's own tissues.

immunological pregnancy test, a method of detecting pregnancy through an increase in the concentration of human chorionic gonadotropin (HCG) in the plasma or urine, as determined by the reaction of HCG with a specific antiserum.

immunological surveillance [L, *immunis,* free from; Gk, *logos,* science; Fr, *surveiller,* to watch over], the constant monitoring by the immune system of microorganisms, foreign tissue, and diseases caused by altered cells, especially cancer cells. Also called **immune surveillance, immunosurveillance.**

immunological test [L, *immunis* + *testum,* crucible], a test based on immunological principles. Kinds include **direct agglutination test, complement assay, Western blot test.**

immunologist /im′yənol″əjist/, a specialist in immunology.

immunological memory, the ability of the immune system to respond rapidly to a pathogen that has been encountered previously. Also called *immunologic memory.*

immunology /im′yənol″əjē/ [L, *immunis* + Gk, *logos,* science], the study of the reaction of tissues of the immune system of the body to antigenic stimulation.

immunomodulator /-mod″yəlā′tər/ [L, *immunis* + *modulus,* little measure], a substance that alters the immune response by augmenting or reducing the ability of the immune system to respond to antigens. Immunomodulators include corticosteroids, cytotoxic agents, thymosin, and immunoglobulins. Some immunomodulators are naturally present in the body, and some of these are available in pharmacological preparations. –*immunomodulation, n.*

immunopathology /-pəthol″əjē/, **1.** the study of disease processes that have an immunological cause. **2.** injury induced by antibodies or other products of an immune response.

immunophenotypic analysis /-fē′nōtip″ik/, a method for dividing lymphomas and leukemias into clonal subgroups on the basis of differences in cell surfaces and cytoplasmic antigens. The antigenic differences are detected with monoclonal antibodies and flow cytometry.

immunopotency /-pō′tənsē/ [L, *immunis* + *potentia,* power], the ability of an antigen to elicit an immune response.

immunoprecipitation /-prisip′itā″shən/, a procedure used to isolate target molecules with which antibodies react. Precipitation results when insoluble antigen-antibody complexes are formed by the reaction between soluble antigens and antibodies.

immunoproliferative disorder, a condition characterized by the continuous proliferation of a subset of immune cells, such as lymphocytes or plasma cells, that is associated with autoimmune and immunoglobulin disorders.

immunoproliferative small intestine disease (IPSID), a disorder characterized by small, diffuse lesions composed of cells that have features of plasma cells, histiocytes, and atypical lymphocytes. The disease mainly affects the duodenum and proximal jejunum. Patients experience diarrhea, weight loss, abdominal pain, and clubbing of the fingers and toes. Also called **alpha chain disease, Mediterranean lymphoma.**

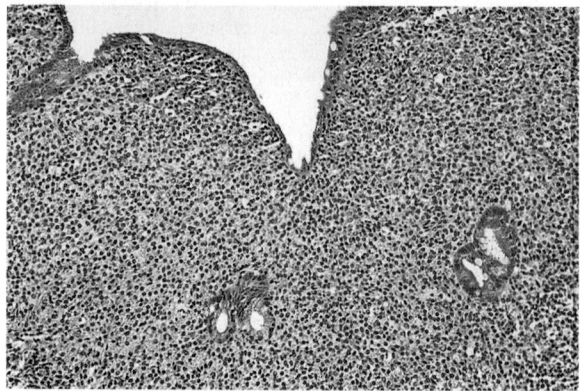

Immunoproliferative small intestine disease *(Fletcher, 2007)*

immunoprophylaxis /-prō′filak″sis/, the introduction of active immunization through vaccines or passive immunization through antisera.

immunoradiometric assay /-rā′dē·ōmet″rik/, a method for measuring certain plasma proteins by using radiolabeled antibodies.

immunoreactant, a substance that participates in an immune response; an antigen or antibody. –*immunoreactive, adj.*

immunoregulation /-reg′yəlā″shən/, control of the immune response to prevent tissue damage, autoimmune diseases, or allergic reactions, as by manipulation of pathways involving regulatory immune cells.

immunoregulatory hormones /-reg″yələtôr′ē/, chemical substances secreted by endocrine glands and lymphocytes that influence activities of the immune system.

immunosecretory disorders, a group of disorders characterized by monoclonal proliferation of immunoglobulin-producing cells that resemble lymphocytes or plasma cells. Kinds include **primary amyloidosis, cryoglobulinemia, heavy chain disease, multiple myeloma,** *benign monoclonal gammopathy, plasma cell dyscrasia.*

immunoselection /-silek″shən/ [L, *immunis* + *seligere,* to select], the survival of certain cells as a result of their lack of surface antigens that would otherwise make them vulnerable to attack and destruction by antibodies. See also **erythroblastosis fetalis, Rh factor.**

immunosorbent /-sôr″bənt/, a substance containing attached antigens used to remove homologous antibodies from a solution. See also **enzyme-linked immunosorbent assay.**

immunostimulant /-stim′yələnt/, an agent, such as bacille Calmette-Guérin vaccine, that induces an immune response at the site of injection, a response that sometimes can be beneficial in the treatment of cancer and other disease.

immunosuppression /-səpresh″ən/ [L, *immunis* + *supprimere,* to press down], **1.** the administration of agents that significantly interfere with the ability of the immune system to respond to antigenic stimulation by inhibiting cellular and humoral immunity. Corticosteroids; cytotoxic drugs, including antimetabolites and alkylating agents; antilymphocytic antibodies; and irradiation may produce immunosuppression. Immunosuppression may be deliberate, such as in preparation for bone marrow or other transplantation to prevent rejection by the host of the donor tissue, or incidental, such as often results from chemotherapy for the treatment of cancer. **2.** an abnormal condition of the immune system characterized by markedly inhibited ability to respond to antigenic stimuli. –*immunosuppressed, adj.*

immunosuppressive /-səpres″iv/, **1.** *adj.,* pertaining to a substance or procedure that lessens or prevents an immune response. **2.** *n.,* an immunosuppressive agent. The immunosuppressive drugs used most frequently to prevent allograft rejection are the interleukin 2 production inhibitors cyclosporine and tacrolimus, the cytotoxic purine antimetabolite azathioprine, the alkylating agent cyclophosphamide, and the adrenocorticosteroid prednisone. Methotrexate, cytarabine, dactinomycin, and thioguanine are also potent immunosuppressive drugs. Monoclonal antibodies against the T cell receptor (muromonab-CD3) and interleukin 2 receptors (basiliximab and daclizumab) are also administered for immunosuppression. The use of some of these agents is being explored for the treatment of autoimmune diseases such as rheumatoid arthritis and systemic lupus erythematosus.

immunosurveillance. See **immunological surveillance.**

immunotherapy /-ther″əpē/ [L, *immunis* + Gk, *therapeia,* treatment], the application of immunological knowledge and techniques to prevent and treat disease. Examples include the administration of increasing doses of allergens in the treatment of allergies, the use of immunostimulants and immunosuppressants, the transfer of immunocompetent cells and tissues from one person to another, some treatments for cancer, and the use of interferon for its antiviral and antitumor properties. –*immunotherapeutic, adj.*

immunotoxin (IT) /-tok″sin/, a toxin that is chemically attached to a monoclonal antibody and used to destroy a specific type of target cell. An example is the plant toxin ricin, which inhibits protein synthesis in tumor cells that are recognized by the antibodies to which ricin is attached.

Imodium, an antidiarrheal drug. Brand name for **loperamide hydrochloride.**

Imovax, a rabies virus vaccine. Brand name for *rabies human diploid cell vaccine.*

impacted /impak″tid/ [L, *impingere,* to drive against], tightly or firmly wedged in a limited amount of space. **–impaction,** *n.,* **–impact,** *v.*

impacted cerumen, accumulated cerumen forming a solid mass that adheres to the wall of the external auditory canal.

impacted fracture, a bone break in which the adjacent fragmented ends of the fractured bone are wedged together and the bone is shortened.

impacted tooth, a tooth so positioned against another tooth, bone, or soft tissue that its complete and normal eruption is impossible or unlikely. An impacted third molar tooth may be further described according to its position, such as buccoangular, distoangular, or vertical. Compare **embedded tooth.**

impaction /impak″shən/ [L, *impingere,* to drive against], **1.** an obstacle or malposition that prevents a tooth from erupting. **2.** the presence of a large or hard fecal mass in the rectum or colon.

impaired glucose tolerance (IGT) /imperd″/ [L, *impejorare,* to make worse; Gk, *glykys,* sweet; L, *tolerare,* to endure], a condition in which fasting plasma glucose levels are higher than normal but lower than those diagnostic of diabetes mellitus. In some people this represents a stage in the natural history of diabetes. Individuals with IGT are encouraged to lose weight and make lifestyle changes to delay the development of diabetes. Not all people will progress to diabetes mellitus, and glucose levels can return to normal. Also called *pre-diabetes.* See also **diabetes mellitus.**

impairment [L, *impejorare,* to make worse], any disorder in structure or function resulting from anatomical, physiological, or psychological abnormalities that interfere with normal activity.

impedance /impē″dəns/ [L, *impedire,* to entangle], a form of electric resistance observed in an alternating current that is analogous to the classic electric resistance that occurs in a direct current circuit. It is expressed as a ratio of voltage applied to a circuit to the current it produces, as an alternating current oscillates ahead of or behind the voltage.

impedance audiometry. See **audiometry.**

impedance plethysmography, a technique for detecting blood vessel occlusion that determines volumetric changes in the limb by measuring changes in its girth as indicated by changes in the electric impedance of mercury-containing polymeric silicone (Silastic) tubes in a pressure cuff. The method is based on the principle that any circumferential rate of change in a limb segment is directly proportional to the volumetric rate of change, which in turn reflects occlusion of venous and arterial blood flow. However, the technique does not accurately indicate the presence or absence of partially obstructing thrombi in major vessels.

imperative conception /imper″ətiv/ [L, *imperare,* to command], a thought or impression that appears spontaneously in the mind and cannot be eliminated, such as an obsession.

imperative idea. See **compulsive idea.**

imperforate /impur″fərit/ [L, *im,* not, *perforare,* to pierce], lacking a normal opening in a body organ or passageway. An infant may be born with an imperforate anus. Compare **perforate.**

imperforate anus, any of several congenital developmental malformations of the anorectal portion of the GI tract.

■ OBSERVATIONS: The most common form is anal agenesis, in which the rectal pouch ends blindly above the surface of the perineum. An anal fistula is present in 80% to 90% of cases. Other forms include anal stenosis, in which the anal aperture is small, and anal membrane atresia, in which the anal membrane covers the aperture, creating an obstruction.

■ INTERVENTIONS: The defect is usually discovered at birth; inspection reveals absence of the anus or the presence of a thin translucent membrane covering it. Digital and endoscopic examination allows identification of the anatomical character of the malformation. Radiographic examination is performed to outline the rectal pouch. A radiopaque marker is placed at the usual site of the anus, and the infant is held upside down. Air moving through the intestines into the distal portion of the bowel or the rectum is visible on the x-ray film. Anal stenosis is treated with daily digital dilation begun in the hospital and continued at home by the parents. An imperforate anal membrane is excised, and digital dilation is performed daily as the skin heals. Surgical reconstruction is performed to treat anal agenesis in infants in whom the pouch is below the puborectalis of the levator ani; an anus is created surgically by an anoplasty. Anal atresia in which the pouch at the end of the bowel is high above the perineum may require a colostomy.

■ PATIENT CARE CONSIDERATIONS: Often it is the nurse who identifies the anal malformation during the routine newborn assessment. A newborn who does not pass any stool in the first 24 hours requires further evaluation for the possibility of the defect. The passage of meconium from the vagina or urinary meatus clearly indicates the presence of anal fistula and usually occurs in association with an imperforate anus. Postoperative care in the newborn treated surgically for any of these conditions requires scrupulous attention to the perineal area.

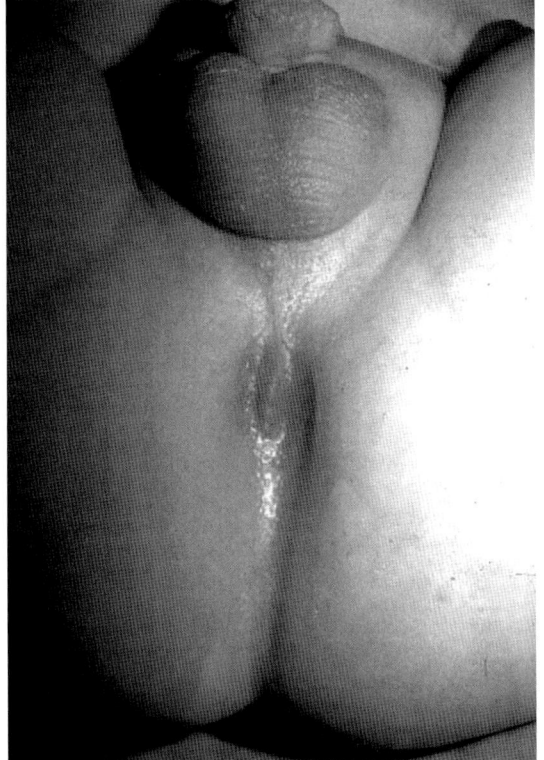

Imperforate anus *(Wyllie, Hyams, and Kay, 2016)*

imperforate hymen [L, *im + perforare,* to pierce; Gk, *hymen,* membrane], a hymen that completely encloses the external orifice of the vagina.

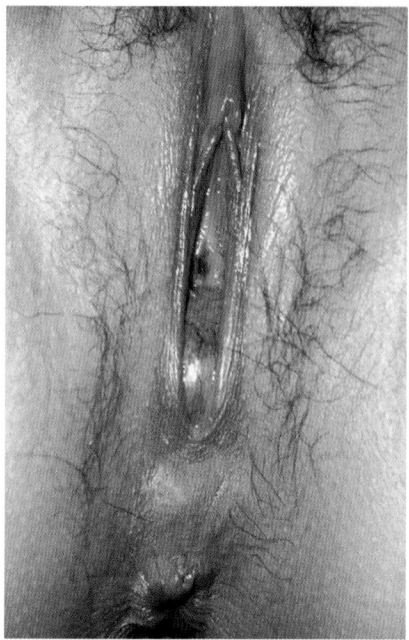

Imperforate hymen *(Falcone and Hurd, 2007)*

impermeable /impur″mē·əbəl/ [L, *im,* not, *permeare,* to pass through], (of a tissue, membrane, or film) preventing the passage of a substance through it; impervious.

impetigo /im′pətī″gō/ [L, *impetus,* attack], a streptococcal, staphylococcal, or combined infection of the skin beginning as focal erythema and progressing to pruritic vesicles, erosions, and honey-colored crusts. Lesions usually form on the face and spread locally. The disorder is highly contagious through contact with the discharge from the lesions. Acute glomerulonephritis is an occasional complication. Treatment includes thorough cleansing with antibacterial soap and water, compresses of Burow's solution, and topical or oral antibiotics. Treatment of the sores, use of individual washcloths and linens, and scrupulous handwashing help prevent spread of the infection. *—impetiginous, adj.*

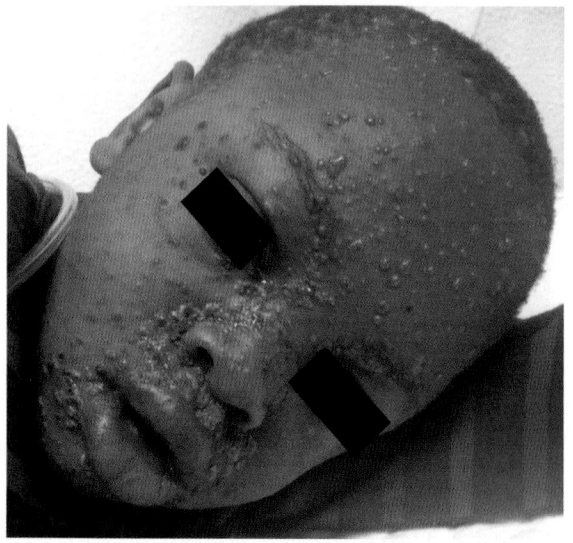

Child with perioral impetigo *(Dias et al, 2015)*

impetigo contagiosa [L, *impetus,* attack, *contingere,* to touch], an acute contagious superficial infection of the skin. It is characterized by vesicles that rupture, leaving a purulent exudate that dries into golden crusts.

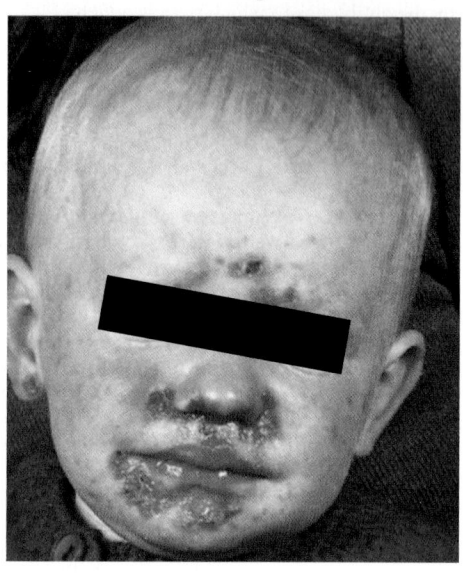

Toddler with impetigo contagiosa *(du Vivier, 2002)*

impetigo herpetiformis [L, *impetus,* attack; Gk, *herpein,* to creep; L, *forma*], a rare skin disorder that mainly affects pregnant women, beginning as an eruption in the genitofemoral area and spreading to other areas. The eruptions are usually irregular or circular groups of pustules that tend to coalesce.

impingement injection test /impinj″mənt/, an appraisal of shoulder injury in which the injection of 10 mL of lidocaine into the subacromial space reduces the painful arc of abduction by more than 50%.

impingement sign, a painful arc produced by forceful abduction of the internally rotated arm against the acromion in evaluation of a shoulder injury.

impingement syndrome, a progressive condition of shoulder pain and dysfunction, usually caused by repetitive placement of the arm in overhead positions. The disorder is a common sports injury, particularly among persons who participate in baseball, tennis, swimming, and volleyball.

implant /im″plant, implant′/ [L, *implantare,* to set into], **1.** (in radiotherapy) an encapsulated radioactive substance embedded in tissue for therapy. Seeds containing iodine-125 may be implanted permanently in prostate and chest tumors, and seeds of iridium-192 in ribbons or wire may be embedded temporarily in head and neck cancers. Sealed sources of cesium-137 or radium-226 may be implanted in the body cavity temporarily in the treatment of gynecological malignancies; strontium-90 in sealed sources may be embedded for a brief period (usually less than 2 minutes) in the treatment of eye tumors; needles containing radium-226 may be used as temporary interstitial implants. Patients with radioactive implants are isolated from other patients whenever possible. **2.** (in surgery) material inserted or grafted into an organ or structure of the body. The implant may be of tissue, such as in a blood vessel graft, or of an artificial substance, such as in a hip prosthesis, a cardiac pacemaker, or a container of radioactive material.

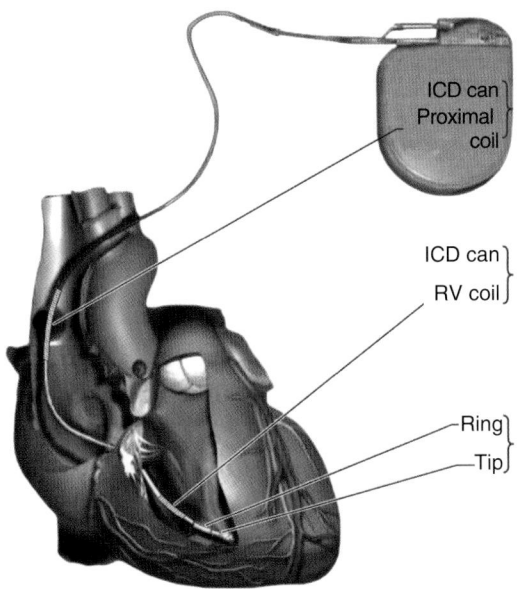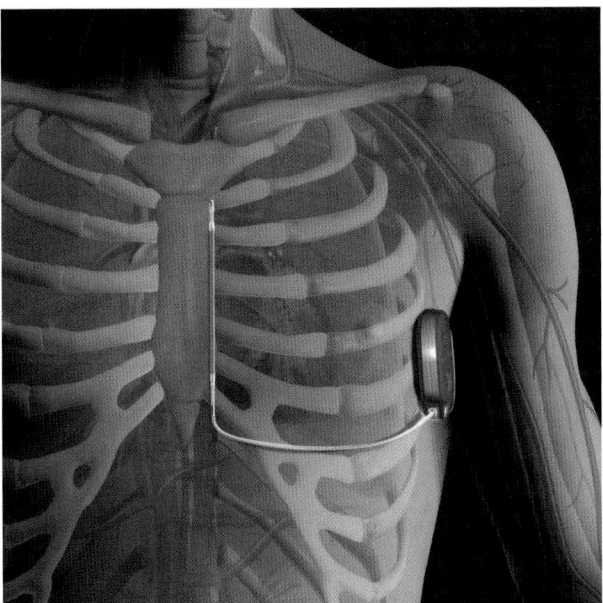

Transvenous ICD device *(Mann et al, 2015)*

implantable cardioverter-defibrillator (ICD), a surgically implanted electric device that automatically terminates lethal ventricular arrhythmias by delivering low-energy shocks to the heart, restoring proper rhythm when the heart begins beating rapidly or erratically. About the size of an audiotape cassette, the device can be implanted without thoracotomy in many cases. It is attached to the abdomen or chest wall with a wire link to the heart.

implantable loop recorder (ILR), a subcutaneous electrocardiographic (ECG) monitoring device used for diagnosis in patients with cardiac disease.

implantation, (in embryology) the process involving the attachment, penetration, and embedding of the blastocyst in the lining of the uterine wall during the early stages of prenatal development. It may be artificial or natural. Also called **nidation.** Kinds include **eccentric implantation, interstitial implantation, superficial implantation.**

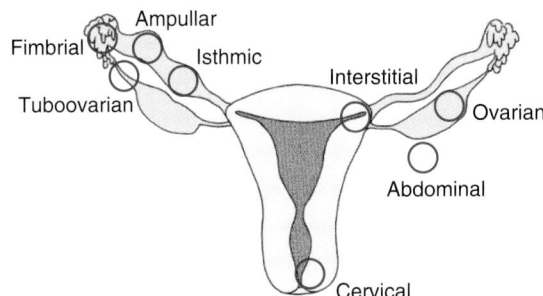

Sites of ectopic pregnancy implantation *(Lowdermilk et al, 2012)*

implantation dermoid cyst, a tumor derived from embryonal tissues, caused by an injury that forces part of the ectoderm into the body.

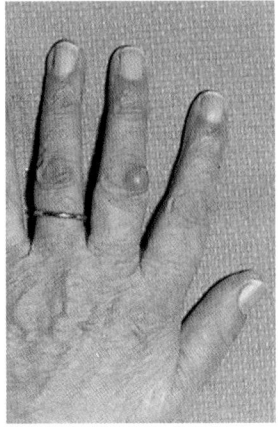

Implantation dermoid cyst *(Moll, 1997)*

implantation endometriosis [L, *implantare,* to set into; Gk, *endon,* within, *metra,* womb, *osis,* condition], ectopic endometrial tissue prevalent throughout the peritoneal cavity. Also called **peritoneal endometriosis.**

implant denture, a complete or partial denture that includes a subperiosteally or intraperiosteally implanted framework in contact with alveolar bone. The denture attaches to one or more posts that project from the framework through the connective tissues and mucous membranes. A variety of designs are available. This type of solution to the loss of natural teeth requires a strong commitment by the patient to practice effective oral hygiene measures.

implanted infusion port, a self-sealing silicone septum encased in a metal or plastic case with an attached silicone catheter that is threaded intravenously. It is implanted subcutaneously and used for long-term venous access for infusion of medications, parenteral nutrition, or IV solutions.

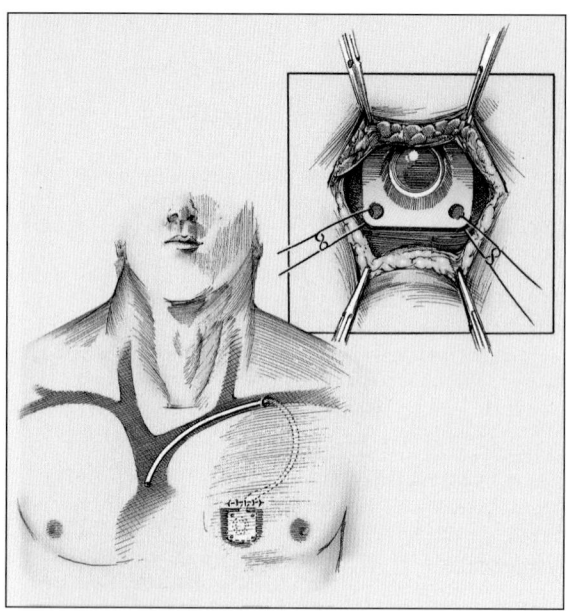

Placement of implanted infusion port into a subcutaneous pocket *(Mansour and Niederhuber, 2014)*

implanted suture [L, *implantare*, to set into, *sutura*], a suture formed by inserting pins on opposite sides of a wound and drawing the edges of the wound together by winding thread tightly around the pins.

implant restoration, a single- or multiple-tooth implant crown or bridge that replaces a missing tooth or teeth.

implementation /im'pləməntā″shən/ [L, *implere*, to fill], **1.** a deliberate action performed to achieve a goal, such as carrying out a plan in caring for a patient. **2.** the fourth step, or phase, of the nursing process.

implementation mechanism, the means by which innovations are transferred from a concept to a product that can be used to improve health.

implementing /im″pləmen′ting/ [L, *implere*, to fill], (in five-step nursing process) a category of nursing behavior in which the actions necessary for accomplishing the health care plan are initiated and completed. Implementing includes performing or assisting in the performance of the patient's activities of daily living, if necessary; counseling and teaching the patient or the patient's family; giving care to achieve patient comfort and therapeutic goals and to optimize the patient's achievement of health goals; supervising and evaluating the work of staff members; and recording and exchanging information relevant to the patient's continued health care. The nurse helps the patient and the patient's family recognize and manage the emotional and psychological stress attendant on the patient's condition and facilitates the relationships of the patient, patient's family, staff, and other significant people. Correct principles, procedures, and techniques of health care are taught, and the patient is informed about the current status of his or her health. If necessary, the patient or the patient's family is referred to a health or social resource in the community. Care is given to achieve therapeutic goals, including acting to compensate for adverse reactions; using preventive and precautionary measures and correct technique in administering care; preparing the patient for surgery, delivery, or other procedure; and initiating lifesaving measures in emergencies. Care is given to the patient in a manner and to a degree that best promotes the patient's attainment of the goals by providing an environment that is conducive to attaining them, by adjusting the care given according to the patient's needs, by stimulating and motivating the patient to achieve independence, by encouraging the patient to comply with and accept the regimen of care, and by compensating for the staff reactions to factors that influence the relationship with the patient and the therapy planned. Implementing follows planning and precedes evaluating in the five-step nursing process. See also **analyzing, assessing, evaluating, nursing process, planning.**

implied consent /implīd″/ [L, *implicare*, to involve, *consentire*, to feel], the granting of permission for health care without a formal agreement between the patient and health care provider. An example is emergency care rendered to an adult patient who is unconscious and requires immediate lifesaving care. It is implied that consent would be granted if the patient were able. Compare **informed consent.**

implosion /implō″zhən/ [L, *im* + *plaudere*, to strike], **1.** a bursting inward. **2.** a psychiatric treatment for people disabled by phobias and anxiety in which the person is desensitized to anxiety-producing stimuli by repeated intense exposure in imagination or reality, until the stimuli are no longer stressful. Also called **flooding.** *–implode, v.*

implosive therapy, a form of therapy in which exposure to a stimulus that usually provokes anxiety desensitizes a person to that stimulus, thereby reducing fear and anxiety. It is similar to flooding, except that the stimuli is suggested, not real. Compare **flooding,** def. 2.

impotence /im″pətəns/ [L, *im,* not, *potentia,* power], **1.** weakness. **2.** inability of the adult male to achieve or sustain a penile erection or, less commonly, to ejaculate after achieving an erection. Several forms are recognized. Functional impotence has a psychological basis. Organic impotence includes vasculogenic, neurogenic, endocrinic, and anatomical factors. Anatomical impotence results from physically defective genitalia. Atonic impotence involves disturbed neuromuscular function. Poor health, old or advancing age, drugs, smoking, trauma, and fatigue can induce impotence. Also called **erectile dysfunction,** *impotency.* *–impotent, adj.*

impregnate /impreg″nāt/ [L, *impregnare*, to make pregnant], **1.** to inseminate and make pregnant; to fertilize. **2.** to saturate or mix with another substance. *–impregnable, adj., –impregnation, n.*

impression /impresh″ən/ [L, *imprimere*, to press into], **1.** (in dentistry and prosthetic medicine) a mold of a part of the mouth or other part of the body from which a dental restoration or prosthesis may be constructed. **2.** (in the medical record) the examiner's diagnosis or assessment of a problem, disease, or condition. **3.** a strong sensation or effect on the mind, intellect, or feelings. **4.** a slight indentation or depression, as one produced on the surface of one organ by pressure exerted by another. **5.** use of an elastomeric material to physically record a prepared tooth impression. Artificial dental stone (gypsum) is poured into the impression, making an exact replica of the tooth/mouth for the construction of a prosthesis. See also **indirect restorative method.**

impression material [L, *imprimere*, to press into, *materia*, stuff], any substance used for making a directly constructed mold of teeth and oral structures to produce dental restorations.

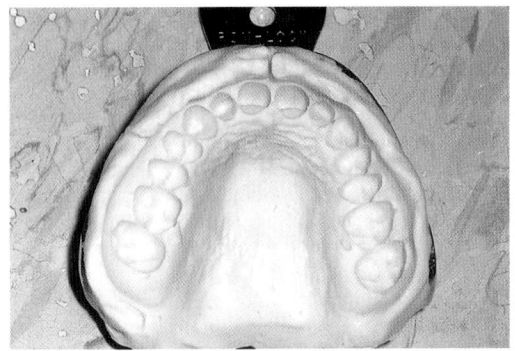

Dental impression *(Bird and Robinson, 2012)*

impression tray, a rounded, contoured tray that holds the substance used in creating a mold of the teeth. It is used in dentistry.

imprinted gene, a gene whose expression has been affected by genomic imprinting so that only a single allele functions, the other being turned off by epigenetic mechanisms during embryonic development.

imprinting [Fr, *empreindre,* to impress], (in ethology) a special type of learning that occurs at critical points during the early stages of development in animals. It involves behavioral patterning and social attachment, is characterized by rapid acquisition and irreversibility, and is usually species-specific, although animals exposed to members of a different species during this short period may become attached to and identify with that particular species instead of their own. See also **bonding.**

imprisonment /impriz″ənment/ [Fr, *emprisonner,* to confine], (in law) the act of confining, detaining, or arresting a person or in any way restraining personal liberty and preventing free exercise of movement. See also **false imprisonment.**

impulse /im″puls/ [L, *impellere,* to drive], **1.** (in psychology) a sudden, irresistible, often irrational inclination, urge, desire, or action resulting from a particular feeling or mental state. **2.** (in physiology) the electrochemical process involved in neural transmission. Also called **nerve impulse, neural impulse. –impulsive,** *adj.*

impulse-conducting system [L, *impellere,* to drive, *conducere,* to conduct; Gk, *systema*], the Purkinje fibers within the heart muscle that conduct impulses controlling the contractions of the atria and ventricles.

impulse control disorder, a behavior in which the individual fails to resist performing a potentially harmful act. The individual usually has a sense of tension or arousal before committing the act and a sense of relief or pleasure when it is committed.

impulsion /impul″shən/ [L, *impellere,* to drive], an urge to act without consideration of consequences.

impulsive. See **impulse.**

Imuran, an immunosuppressive drug. Brand name for **azathioprine.**

IMV, abbreviation for **intermittent mandatory ventilation.**

In, symbol for the element **indium.**

in-, 1. prefix meaning "in, on, within, into or toward": *inborn, inbreeding.* **2.** prefix meaning "not, lack of, opposite of": *insoluble.*

-in, 1. suffix meaning "neutral substance": *albumin, zinc gelatin.* **2.** suffix meaning "an antibiotic": *bacitracin, penicillin, streptomycin.* **3.** suffix meaning "a pharmaceutic product": *aspirin, niacin.* **4.** suffix meaning "a chemical compound": palmitin. **5.** suffix meaning "an enzyme": pepsin.

inactivated measles virus vaccine /inak″tivā′tid/ [L, *in,* not, *activus* + OE, *masala,* blister; L, *virus,* poison, *vaccinus,* of a cow], a measles vaccine virus that was treated so that it was no longer capable of replication. It was available in the 1960s and 1970s as an alternative to live attenuated measles vaccine. Some individuals who received inactivated vaccine are at risk of developing severe atypical measles syndrome when exposed to the natural virus. Revaccination with live vaccine is important.

inactivation, the halting of biological activity.

inactive colon /inak″tiv/ [L, *in,* not, *activus,* active; Gk, *kolon,* colon], hypotonicity of the bowel that results in decreased contractions and propulsive movements and a delay in the normal 12-hour transit time of luminal contents from the cecum to the anus. Colonic inactivity may be caused by acquired or congenital megacolon, anticholinergic drugs, depression, faulty habits of elimination, inadequate fluid intake, lack of exercise, a low-residue or starvation diet, neuroendocrine response to surgical stress, prolonged bed rest, or a neurological disease such as diabetic visceral neuropathy, multiple sclerosis, parkinsonism, or spinal cord lesions. Normal motility of the colon is frequently compromised by the continued use of laxatives. Acquired megacolon, characterized by an abnormally large, inactive bowel and chronic constipation, is common in cognitively impaired children and adults with chronic mental illness. In congenital megacolon (Hirschsprung disease), congenital absence of myenteric innervation in a distal segment of the colon causes loss of motility and massive dilation of the proximal segment of the large bowel and extreme constipation. The disorder is more common in males than females and in severe cases slows growth. Treatment of colonic inactivity includes a stimulus-response training program to establish regular bowel habits, the use of stool softeners and hydrophilic colloids to increase fecal bulk, and a diet containing adequate roughage.

inactive electrode, in electrocautery, the electrode through which current distributed through the active electrode is returned to the generator.

inadequate personality /inad″əkwit/ [L, *in,* not, *adaequare,* to equal, *personalis,* of a person], a personality characterized by a lack of physical stamina; emotional immaturity; social instability; poor judgment; reduced motivation; ineptness, especially in interpersonal relationships; and an inability to adapt or react effectively to new or stressful situations.

inamrinone lactate /am″rinōn/, an IV cardiac inotropic drug. Formerly called **amrinone lactate.**

■ INDICATIONS: It is prescribed in the short-term management of congestive heart failure in patients who do not respond to therapy with digitalis, diuretics, and vasodilators.

■ CONTRAINDICATIONS: Concomitant use with disopyramide and any combination therapy should be closely monitored for potential interactions.

■ ADVERSE EFFECTS: Among the more serious adverse effects are thrombocytopenia, arrhythmias, hypotension, nausea, vomiting, liver impairment, and hypersensitivity effects.

inanimate /inan″imit/ [L, *in,* not, *animus,* life spirit], not alive; lacking signs of life.

inanition /in′ənish″ən/ [L, *inanis,* empty], **1.** an exhausted condition resulting from lack of food and water or a defect in assimilation; starvation. **2.** a state of lethargy characterized by a loss of vitality or vigor in all aspects of social, moral, and intellectual life.

inborn /in″bôrn/ [L, *in,* within; AS, *beran,* to bear], innate; acquired or occurring during intrauterine life, with reference to both normally inherited traits and developmental or genetically transmitted anomalies. See also **congenital, hereditary, inborn error of metabolism.**

inborn error of metabolism, one of many abnormal metabolic conditions caused by an inherited defect of a single enzyme or other protein. Although people with such diseases are defective in only one protein, they generally display a large number of physical signs that are characteristic of the genetic trait and are related to excesses or deficiencies of the substrate on which the enzyme acts. The diseases are rare. Kinds include **galactosemia, glucose-6-phosphate dehydrogenase (G6PD) deficiency, Lesch-Nyhan syndrome, phenylketonuria, Tay-Sachs disease.**
■ OBSERVATIONS: Inborn errors of metabolism may be detected in the fetus in utero by the examination of squamous and blood cells obtained by amniocentesis and fetoscopy. Laboratory tests after birth often show higher than normal levels of particular metabolites in the blood and urine, such as phenylpyruvic acid and phenylalanine in phenylketonuria (PKU) and galactose in galactosemia. The values are higher in homozygous than in heterozygous carriers. Signs of the various defects are usually seen only in homozygous carriers.
■ INTERVENTIONS: Treatment for some pathological inborn errors may be removal of food in the diet containing the nondegradable metabolite to prevent its accumulation. Removal of dietary phenylalanine in PKU and galactose in galactosemia is effective in preventing the development of symptoms if treatment is begun early. In those cases of inborn errors of metabolism in which the nondegradable metabolite is endogenous, such as in the mucopolysaccharidoses, treatment is focused on the management of complications and is not specific for the underlying abnormality.

inborn lysosomal disease, one of many inherited disorders of metabolism involving degradative enzymes normally located in lysosomes. The condition leads to storage of abnormal amounts of lysosomal agents. Also called **lysosomal storage disease.**

inborn reflex. See **unconditioned response.**

inbreeding /in″brēding/ [L, *in,* within; AS, *bredan,* to reproduce], the production of offspring by the mating of closely related organisms, the most extreme form being self-fertilization, which occurs in certain plants and animals. Inbreeding increases the chance that recessive alleles for both desirable and undesirable traits will become homozygous and be expressed phenotypically. In humans the amount of inbreeding in a specific population is largely controlled by tradition and cultural practices. Inbreeding is a standard agricultural method for developing desirable genotypes and pure lines in plants and animals. Compare **outbreeding.**

incandescent [L, *incandescere,* to begin to glow], hot to the point of glowing or emitting intense light rays, as an incandescent light bulb.

incapacitating agents, drugs that interfere with the ability to think clearly or cause unconsciousness or some other altered state of consciousness. Their primary use is not to kill, although they can be lethal in high doses. They include aerosolized opioids and the anticholinergic BZ. Treatment of exposure to incapacitating agents is supportive.

incarcerate /inkar″sərāt/ [L, *in,* within, *carcerare,* to imprison], to trap, imprison, or confine, such as a loop of intestine in an inguinal hernia. See also **hernia.**

incarcerated hernia [L, *in* + *carcerare,* to imprison, *hernia,* rupture], a loop of bowel with ends occluded so that solids cannot pass. The herniated bowel will not return to its normal position without manipulation or surgery. It is essential to correct the condition before the bowel becomes strangulated. Also called **irreducible hernia.**

incentive spirometry /insen″tiv/, a method of encouraging voluntary deep breathing by providing visual feedback about inspiratory volume. Using a specially designed spirometer, the patient inhales until a preset volume is reached, then sustains the inspiratory volume by holding his or her breath for 3 to 5 seconds. Incentive spirometry reduces the risk of atelectasis and pulmonary consolidation.

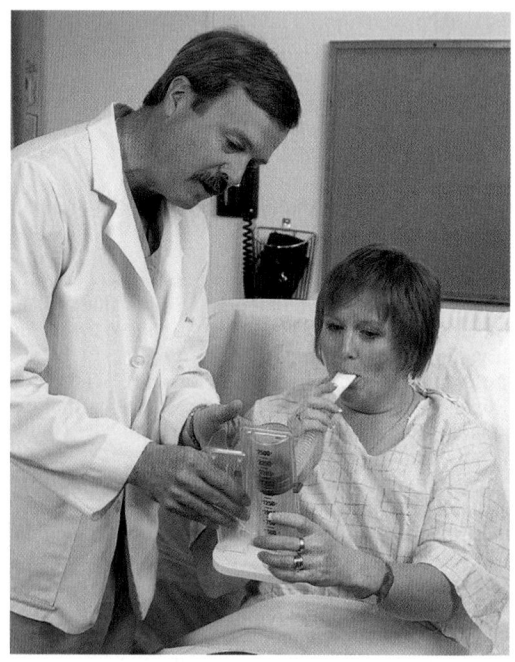

Teaching use of the incentive spirometer *(deWit and O'Neill, 2014)*

inception /insep″shən/ [L, *incipere,* to begin], the origin or beginning of anything.

incest /in″sest/ [L, *incestum,* defiled], sexual intercourse between persons closely related. −*incestuous, adj.*

incidence /in″sidəns/ [L, *incidere,* to happen], **1.** the number of times an event occurs. **2.** (in epidemiology) the number of new cases in a particular period. Incidence is often expressed as a ratio, in which the number of cases is the numerator and the population at risk is the denominator. See also **rate.**

incidence rate, the rate of new cases of a disease in a specified population over a defined period.

incidental additives /in′siden″təl/ [L, *incidere,* to happen, *additio,* something added], material added to food by the use of pesticides, herbicides, or chemicals used in food processing.

incident report, a document, usually confidential (protected from discovery by a plaintiff in a lawsuit), that describes any accident or deviation from policies or orders involving a patient, employee, visitor, or student on the premises of a health care facility. Also called *unusual occurrence report.*

incineration /insin′ərā″shən/ [L, *incinerare,* to burn to ashes], the removal or reduction of materials by burning.

incipient /insip″ē·ənt/ [L, *incipire,* to commence], coming into existence; at an initial stage; beginning to appear, such as a symptom or disease.

incipient carious lesion. See **primary dental caries.**

incipient dental caries, the earliest detectable signs of tooth decay. At this stage, the lesion has not penetrated the dentin.

incisal /insī′zəl/ [L, *incidere,* to cut into], pertaining to the cutting edge of an anterior tooth.

incisal angle /insī′səl/ [L, *incidere,* to cut into, *angulus,* corner], the angle between the hinge axis-orbital plane and the discluding surface of the maxillary incisors.

incisal guide. See **anterior guide.**

incisal guide pin, a metal rod, attached to the upper member of a dental articulator, that touches the incisal guide table to maintain the established vertical separation of the upper and lower members of the articulator. See also **articulator.**

incision /insizh′ən/ [L, *incidere,* to cut into], a cut produced surgically by a sharp instrument that creates an opening into an organ or space in the body.

incisional hernia /insish′ənəl/ [L, *incidere,* to cut into, *hernia,* rupture], a herniation through a surgical scar.

incisive canal cyst. See **nasopalatine duct cyst.**

incisive papilla. See **palatine raphe.**

incisor /insī′zər/, one of the four anterior teeth in each dental arch. Primary incisors appear during infancy and are replaced during childhood by secondary incisors. The crown of each incisor is chisel shaped and has a sharp cutting edge. Its labial surface is convex, smooth, and highly polished; its lingual surface is concave and, in many individuals, is marked by an inverted V-shaped basal ridge near the gingiva of the maxillary arch. The neck of an incisor is constricted, and the root is single, long, and conic. The upper incisors are larger and stronger than the lower and are directed downward and forward. Compare **canine tooth, molar, premolar.**

incisura /in′sisyoo̅′rə/ [L, *incidere,* to cut into], a notch or incision on an organ or body part.

inciting eye. See **exciting eye.**

inclusion /inkloo̅′zhən/ [L, *in,* within, *claudere,* to shut], **1.** the act of enclosing or the condition of being enclosed. **2.** a structure within another, such as an inclusion in the cytoplasm of the cells. **3.** models based on the premise that children with special needs should be educated in a regular classroom (instead of a self-contained classroom) with support personnel or services provided in that classroom.

inclusion bodies, normal or abnormal objects of various shapes and sizes observed in the nucleus or cytoplasm of blood cells or other tissue cells.

inclusion body myositis, a progressive inflammatory myopathy primarily involving muscles of the pelvic region and legs, usually seen in older people. The muscles are infiltrated by mononuclear inflammatory cells, sarcoplasmic vacuoles, masses of filaments and filamentous microtubules, and sometimes eosinophilic bodies.

inclusion cell disease. See **I cell disease.**

inclusion conjunctivitis, an acute purulent conjunctival infection caused by *Chlamydia* organisms. It occurs in two forms. The infection in infants is characterized by bilateral swelling of the conjunctiva, redness, and purulent discharge. The adult variety is unilateral, less severe, and less purulent and is associated with preauricular lymphadenopathy. Local instillation of antibiotics is effective treatment.

inclusion dermoid cyst, a tumor derived from embryonal tissues, caused by the inclusion of foreign tissue when a developmental cleft closes.

inclusive, (in therapies) a therapeutic model that requires the practitioner to provide direct services for all students in a classroom, incorporating their unique needs.

inclusiveness principle /inkloo̅′sivnəs/ [L, *in,* within, *claudere,* to shut, *principium,* a beginning], a rule that there is active, intentional, and ongoing engagement with diverse populations in the community.

inclusive rate /inkloo̅′siv/, a method of calculating inpatient hospital charges in which a fixed amount covers all services, regardless of the number or intensity of services provided.

incoercible /in′kō-ur′sibəl/, pertaining to something that cannot be restrained or willfully terminated, as a siege of hiccups.

incoercible vomiting, forcible emptying of the stomach that is intractable or uncontrollable. See also **pernicious vomiting.**

incoherent /in′kōhir′ənt/ [L, *in,* not, *cohaere,* to hold together], **1.** disordered; without logical connection; disjointed; lacking orderly continuity or relevance. **2.** unable to express one's thoughts or ideas in an orderly, intelligible manner, usually as a result of emotional stress.

incompatibility /in′kəmpat′ibil′itē/ [L, *in,* not, + *compatibilus,* agreeing], not capable of coexistance, as in a transfusion of blood group A donor cells to a blood group O recipient, resulting in a transfusion reaction.

incompatible /in′kəmpat′əbəl/ [L, *in,* not, *compatibilus,* agreeing], unable to coexist. A tissue transplantation may be rejected because recipient and donor antibody factors are incompatible.

incompetence /inkom′pətəns/ [L, *in,* not, *competentia,* capable], **1.** lack of ability to function. Kinds include **ileocecal incompetence, aortic incompetence, valvular incompetence.** —**incompetent,** *adj.* **2.** (in law) inability to function at a safe level or to provide care that is consistent with standards of practice. **3.** legal status of a person declared to be unable to provide for his or her own needs and protection. The status must be proved in a court hearing.

incompetent. See **incompetence.**

incompetent cervix [L, *in,* not, *competentia,* capable, *cervix,* neck], (in obstetrics) a condition characterized by painless dilation of the cervical os of the uterus before term without labor or contractions of the uterus. Miscarriage or premature delivery may result. Incompetent cervix is treated prophylactically by cerclage or another procedure in which the cervix is held closed by a surgically implanted suture.

incomplete abortion /in′kəmplēt′/ [L, *in,* not, *complere,* to fill, *ab,* away from, *oriri,* to be born], termination of pregnancy in which the products of conception are not entirely expelled or removed. It often causes hemorrhage that may require surgical evacuation by curettage, oxytocics, and blood replacement. Infection is also a frequent complication of incomplete abortion. Compare **complete abortion.**

incomplete dislocation [L, *in* + *complere,* to fill, *dis* + *locare,* to place], a partial abnormal separation of the articular surfaces of a joint. Also called **subluxation.**

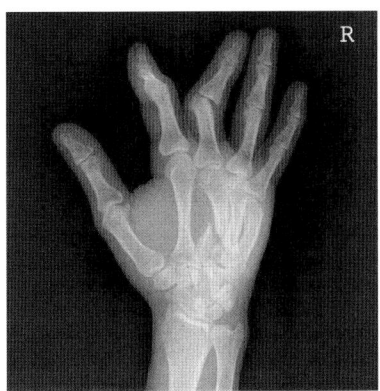

Fracture and incomplete dislocation of the third digit
(Kowalczyk and Mace, 2009)

incomplete fistula.   See **blind fistula.**

incomplete fracture,   a bone break in which the crack in the osseous tissue does not completely traverse the width of the affected bone but may angle off in one or more directions.

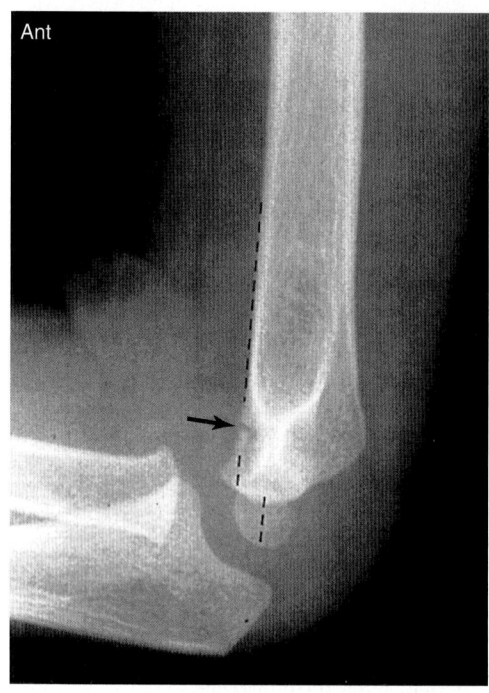

Incomplete cortical fracture *(arrow)* **and displacement of the humerus** *(Mettler, 2014)*

incomplete hemianopia,   a form of hemianopia, a disorder that results in blindness in half of the visual field of one or both eyes. In incomplete hemianopia, less than half of the visual field is affected by blindness. See also **hemiamblyopia.**

incomplete hernia [L, *in + complere,* to fill up, *hernia,* rupture],   a hernia that has not yet protruded through a weak spot or opening.

incomplete protein,   a food that is inadequate in one or more of the nine amino acids essential for normal growth and maintenance of tissue when used as the sole source of protein.

incongruent communication /inkong″grōo·ənt/,   a communication pattern in which the sender gives conflicting messages on verbal and nonverbal levels and the listener does not know which message to accept. See also **double bind.**

inconspicuous penis,   a categorical term denoting a penis that appears to be abnormally small, although the shaft can be abnormal or normal in size. The category includes a variety of anomalies, including webbed penis, concealed penis, and micropenis.

incontinence /inkon″tinəns/ [L, *incontinentia,* inability to retain],   the inability to control urination or defecation. Urinary incontinence may be caused by physiological, psychological, or pathological factors. Treatment depends on the diagnosed cause. Fecal incontinence may result from relaxation of the anal sphincter or disorders of the central nervous system or spinal cord and may be treated by a program of bowel training. See also **bowel training, urinary incontinence. −incontinent,** *adj.*

incontinent.   See **incontinence.**

incontinentia pigmenti /inkon′tinen′shə pigmen′tī/,   an X-linked dominant syndrome with onset at birth or shortly thereafter that is usually lethal in males. It is characterized by the presence of brown or slate-brown bands, whorls, swirls, or splatter-like hyperpigmented cutaneous lesions that are preceded by vesiculobullous and verrucous inflammatory changes and are often associated with developmental anomalies involving other structures, such as the hair, eyes, and skeletal and central nervous systems. Also called **Bloch-Sulzberger incontinentia pigmenti, Bloch-Sulzberger syndrome.**

incontinentia pigmenti achromians,   a congenital neurocutaneous syndrome, not present at birth but appearing in early life, characterized by the presence of peculiar whorled, linear, and splatter-like patterns of hypopigmentation and often associated with other abnormalities, including hair loss and ocular, musculoskeletal, and mental disturbances. Also called **hypomelanosis of Ito.** Should not be confused with **incontinentia pigmenti.**

Increlex,   brand name for **mecasermin.**

increment /ing′krəmənt/ [L, *incresere,* to grow],   **1.** an increase or gain. **2.** the act of growing or increasing. **3.** the amount of an increase or gain in intrauterine pressure as uterine contractions begin in labor. −*incremental, adj.*

incremental line /ing′krəmen″təl/,   **1.** one of a series of lines showing successive layers deposited in a tissue. **2.** a very fine line of cementum that follows the contours of a tooth.

incremental lines of Ebner [Victor von Ebner, Austrian histologist, 1842–1925],   delicate lines seen on ground sections of a tooth, demarcating increments of dentin.

incretin,   metabolic hormones whose functions include the regulation of glucose metabolism by stimulating the release of insulin by the β cells and, at the same time, inhibiting the release of glucagon by pancreatic α cells, resulting in a decrease in blood glucose levels.

incrustation,   hardened exudate, scale, or scab.

incubation period /in″kyəbā′shən/   [L, *incubare,* to lie on; Gk, *peri,* around, *hodos,* way],   **1.** the time between exposure to a pathogenic organism and the onset of symptoms of a disease. **2.** the time required to induce the development of an embryo in an egg or to induce the development and replication of tissue cells or microorganisms being grown in culture media or other special laboratory environment. **3.** the time allowed for a chemical reaction or process to proceed.

incubator /in″kyəbā′tər/,   an apparatus used to provide a controlled environment, especially temperature. Other environmental components, such as darkness, light, oxygen, moisture, and dryness, may also be controlled, as in an incubator for the cultivation of eggs or microorganisms in a laboratory or an incubator for premature infants.

incud-,   prefix meaning "an anvil (the incus)": *incudectomy.*

incudectomy /in″kyōodek″təmē/   [L, *incus,* anvil, *ektomē,* excision],   surgical removal of the incus, performed to treat conductive hearing loss that results from necrosis of the tip of the incus. The defective incus is excised and replaced with a bone chip graft so that sound vibrations are again transmitted. After surgery the patient is instructed to change position slowly to avoid dizziness, to avoid blowing the nose and sneezing, and to report any fever, headache, dizziness, or ear pain.

incurable /inkyōo″rəbəl/,   not responding to medical or surgical treatment.

incus /ing″kəs/ *pl. incudes*   [L, anvil],   one of the three ossicles in the middle ear, resembling an anvil. It transmits sound vibrations from the malleus to the stapes. Compare **malleus, stapes.** See also **middle ear.**

IND, abbreviation for **investigational new drug.**

indanedione derivative /indāne″dē·ōn/, one of a small group of oral anticoagulants (e.g., anisindione) designed for long-term therapeutic use in patients who cannot tolerate other oral anticoagulants. Anticoagulation using indanediones is difficult to control, and these agents may cause grave adverse effects, including severe renal and hepatic toxicity, agranulocytosis, and leukopenia. For this reason coumarin derivatives are preferred. Regular evaluations of prothrombin time are necessary. Extreme fatigue, sore throat, chills, and fever are signs of impending toxicity and require discontinuation of the drug. Compare **coumarin.**

Indego®, a powered exoskeleton that serves as a lower limb orthosis. It is used in gait training for individuals with impaired mobility.

indemnify /indem″nifī/, to protect against liability for loss or injury by guaranteeing compensation for the loss or injury.

indentation /in′dəntā″shən/ [L, *in,* within, *dens,* tooth], a notch, pit, or depression in the surface of an object, such as toothmarks on the tongue or skin. −*indent, v.*

independence /in′dəpen″dəns/ [L, *in,* not, *de,* from, *pendere,* to hang], **1.** the state or quality of being independent; autonomy; freedom from the influence, guidance, or control of a person or a group. **2.** a lack of requirement or reliance on another for physical existence or emotional needs. −*independent, adj.*

independent assortment. See **Mendel's laws.**

independent intervention. See **intervention.**

independent living center, rehabilitation facility in which people with disabilities can receive individualized education and training in the performance of all or most activities of daily living. A typical independent living center may contain a completely furnished multiroom apartment, including a kitchen with cabinets and cooking facilities that can be reached easily by a person in a wheelchair, designed for training patients in homemaking skills.

independent practice, (in nursing) the practice of certain aspects of professional nursing that are encompassed by applicable licensure and law and require no supervision or direction from others. Nurses in independent practice may have an office in which they see patients and charge fees for service. In all nursing settings, state practice acts define certain aspects of nursing practice that are independent and may define those that must be done only under supervision or direction of another individual, usually a physician.

Independent Practice Association (IPA), a U.S. type of physician alliance in which the physicians own the practice, as opposed to physicians employed by an entity such as a health maintenance organization. Physicians in the IPA are legally organized as a corporation, partnership, professional corporation, or foundation to contract as a group to provide services. Economic risk is shared, but overhead is not. The IPA may contract with a health maintenance organization (HMO) to service enrollees but will usually still see non-HMO clients. See also **health maintenance organization.**

independent variable, (in research) a variable that is manipulated (controlled) by the researcher and evaluated by its measurable effect on the dependent variable or variables. For example, in a study of the effect of nursing intervention on postoperative vomiting, nursing intervention is the independent variable evaluated by its effect on the dependent variable, the incidence of postoperative vomiting. Also called **experimental variable, predictor variable.** Compare **dependent variable.**

Inderal, a nonselective beta-adrenergic blocking agent. Brand name for **propranolol hydrochloride.**

indeterminate cleavage /in′ditur″minit/ [L, *in,* not, *determinare,* to fix limits; AS, *cleofan,* to split], mitotic division of the fertilized ovum into blastomeres that have similar developmental potential and, if isolated, can each give rise to a complete individual embryo. Also called **regulative cleavage.** Compare **determinate cleavage.** See also **regulative development.**

index /in′deks/ *pl. indexes, indices* [L, that which points out], **1.** index finger, the second digit of the hand, the finger adjacent to the thumb. Also called **forefinger,** *index finger.* **2.** a unitless quantity, usually a ratio of two measurable quantities having the same dimensions, or such a ratio multiplied by 100. **3.** a core or mold used in dentistry to record or maintain the relative position of a tooth or teeth to one another and/or to a cast, to ensure reproduction in the dental prosthesis of their original position. **4.** a directory, in particular an alphabetized list of terms, each term accompanied by page numbers or other notations telling where it appears in a given work or set of works.

index astigmatism [L, *indicare,* to make known, *a + stigma,* point], an astigmatism caused by unequal refractive indices in different parts of the lens.

index case [L, *indicare,* to make known], (in epidemiology) the first case of a disease, as contrasted with subsequent cases. See also **propositus.**

index myopia, a kind of nearsightedness caused by a variation in the index of refraction of the eye media.

India ink test, a test used to detect *Cryptococcus* in wet preparations of patient specimens. The capsule of the yeast resists colorization by the India ink, resulting in clear organisms against dark background. The appearance of encapsulated yeast cells in cerebrospinal fluid is diagnostic for cryptococcal meningitis.

Indiana pouch, a type of continent urinary diversion in which part of the ileum and cecum is modified to form a pouch with modification of the ileocecal orifice to maintain continence. Also called **continent urostomy.**

Indian Health Service, a bureau of the Department of Health and Human Services for providing public health and medical services to Native Americans and Alaska natives in the United States. In Canada the services are provided by the Ministry of Indian Affairs.

Indian tick fever. See **Marseilles fever.**

indican /in″dikən/ [Gk, *indikon,* indigo], a substance (potassium indoxyl sulfate) produced in the intestine by the decomposition of tryptophan, absorbed by the intestinal wall, and excreted in the urine. Its level may be elevated in the urine of patients on high-protein diets or those suffering from GI disease. The normal accumulation of indican in urine is 10 to 20 mg/24 hr.

indication /in′dikā″shən/ [L, *indicare,* to make known], a reason to prescribe a medication or perform a treatment. A bacterial infection may be an indication for the prescription of a specific antibiotic; appendicitis is an indication for appendectomy. −*indicate, v.*

indicator /in″dikā′tər/, a tape, paper, tablet, or other substance that is used to test for a specific reaction because it changes in a predictable visible way. Also called **reagent.** Kinds include *autoclave indicator,* **dipstick, litmus paper.**

indicator-dilution method, a method for measuring blood volume. A known amount of a substance that dissolves freely in blood but does not leave the capillaries is injected intravenously. After a few minutes a sample of blood is withdrawn, and the volume of blood in the body is calculated from the concentration of the substance in the sample, the sample's volume, and the hematocrit.

indices. See **index.**

indigenous /indij″ənəs/ [L, *indigena,* a native], **1.** native to or occurring naturally in a specified area or environment, as certain species of bacteria in the human digestive tract. **2.** referring to the first people of a land; aboriginals or natives.

indigestible /in′dijes″təbəl/ [L, *in,* not, *digerere,* to separate], pertaining to a food substance that cannot be broken down within the digestive tract and converted into an absorbable nutrient.

indigestion. See **dyspepsia.**

indinavir, an antiretroviral protease inhibitor.

■ INDICATIONS: It is prescribed in the treatment of human immunodeficiency virus infection.

■ CONTRAINDICATIONS: It should not be given to patients with a risk of kidney stones. It should be administered with other medications to reduce the risk of resistance development.

■ ADVERSE EFFECTS: Protease inhibitors increase plasma glucose, cholesterol, and triglyceride levels and cause a redistribution of body fat toward the center. Indinavir also can cause nephrolithiasis and hyperbilirubinemia.

indirect calorimetry, the measurement of the amount of heat generated in an oxidation reaction by determining the intake or consumption of oxygen or by measuring the amount of carbon dioxide or nitrogen released and translating these quantities into a heat equivalent. Compare **direct calorimetry.**

indirect Coombs test [Robert Coombs, British immunologist 1921—2006], a blood test used during blood compatibility crossmatching to detect the presence of circulating antibodies against red blood cells. The major purpose of this test is to determine whether the patient has serum antibodies (besides the major ABO/Rh system) to red blood cells that he or she might receive by blood transfusion. Compare **direct Coombs test.**

indirect division. See **mitosis.**

indirect laryngoscopy [L, *in,* not, *directus,* straight; Gk, *larynx + skopein,* to view], a method of examining the larynx with a mirror. Compare **direct laryngoscopy.**

indirect nursing care functions, activities that are not associated with face-to-face contact with a patient or his or her family but are an important component of care. Kinds include **documentation.**

indirect ophthalmoscope, an ophthalmoscope with a biconvex lens that produces a reversed inverted and magnified stereoscopic image.

indirect percussion, a technique in physical examination in which the examiner taps on an intermediate surface, such as the examiner's finger, rather than directly on the body surface being examined. See also **percussion.**

indirect provider reimbursement, a method of payment to an agency for health services delivered by providers, such as nurses.

indirect restorative method, a technique for fabricating a restoration on a cast of the original tooth, such as the indirect construction of an inlay. After a die is made from an impression of the prepared tooth, a wax pattern is formed and the inlay is cast. The cast inlay is then fitted and finished on the die and then cemented into the tooth.

indirect retainer, that part of a removable partial denture that resists movement of a free-end denture base away from its tissue support by means of lever action on the opposite side of the fulcrum line.

indirect services, therapy services that are related to modification of the environment to help the client succeed and achieve goals.

indirect vision [L, *in + directus,* straight, *visio,* seeing], a visual sensation caused by stimulation of the extramacular portion of the retina. Also called **peripheral vision.**

indium (In) [L, *indicum,* indigo], a silvery metallic element with some nonmetallic chemical properties. Its atomic number is 49; its atomic mass is 114.82. It is used in electronic semiconductors.

indium 111 in ibritumomab tiuxetan, a chelate of indium 111 and the immunoconjugate ibritumomab tiuxetan, used in the treatment of non-Hodgkin lymphoma. It is administered intravenously.

individual education program (IEP), a written plan developed by a team of parents, teachers, special educators, occupational and physical therapy practitioners, nurses, primary health care providers, and others that specifies the educational services that are needed by a student, particularly a student with special needs, and how these services will be provided.

individual immunity /in′divij″o͞o·əl/ [L, *individuus,* indivisible, *immunis,* free from], a form of natural immunity not shared by most other members of the race and species. It is rare and probably occurs as the result of an infection that was not recognized when it occurred. Compare **species immunity.**

individualized family service plan (IFSP), a written intervention plan for children from birth to 3 years of age;

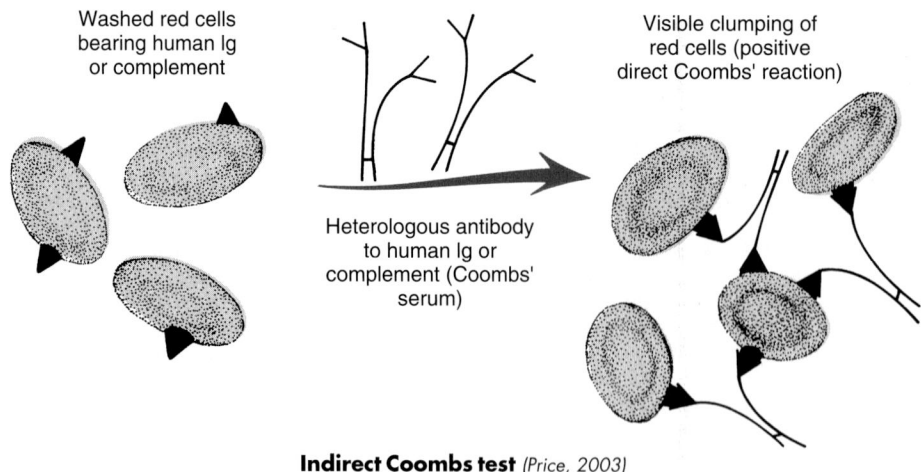

Washed red cells bearing human Ig or complement

Visible clumping of red cells (positive direct Coombs' reaction)

Heterologous antibody to human Ig or complement (Coombs' serum)

Indirect Coombs test *(Price, 2003)*

the plan is developed by a specialized team to focus on family priorities and resources.

individual practice associations (IPA), a health maintenance organization (HMO) in which individual physicians contract directly and independently with the HMO.

individual psychology, a modified system of psychoanalysis, developed by Alfred Adler, that views maladaptive behavior and personality disorders as resulting from a conflict between the desire to dominate and feelings of inferiority. See also **adlerian psychology, inferiority complex.**

Indocin, a nonsteroidal antiinflammatory agent. Brand name for **indomethacin.**

indocyanine green /in′dōsī′ənēn/, a dye occurring as an olive-brown, dark green, dark blue, or black powder, used intravenously as a diagnostic aid in the determination of blood volume, cardiac output, and hepatic function.

indocyanine green clearance, the hepatic clearance of indocyanine green, calculated in liver function tests.

indole /in″dōl/, a volatile chemical produced during serotonin metabolism. It is partly responsible for the odor of feces.

indoleacetic acid (IAA) /in′dōləsē″tik, -əset″ik/, a major terminal metabolite of tryptophan that is present in very small amounts in normal urine and excreted in elevated quantities by patients with carcinoid tumors. It is measured as 5-hydroxyindoleacetic acid (5-HIAA).

indolent /in″dələnt/ [L, *in + dolere,* to suffer pain], **1.** pertaining to an organic disorder that is accompanied by little or no pain. **2.** slow to heal or grow, as in wounds that heal very slowly.

indomethacin /in′dōmeth″əsin/, a nonsteroidal antiinflammatory agent.

■ INDICATIONS: It is prescribed in the treatment of arthritis, gout attacks, and certain other inflammatory conditions.

■ CONTRAINDICATIONS: Upper GI disease or known hypersensitivity to this drug or to aspirin prohibits its use. It is not given to children less than 15 years of age or to pregnant or lactating women.

■ ADVERSE EFFECTS: The most serious adverse effect is peptic ulcers. GI upset, dizziness, tinnitus, and rashes also may occur.

induce /ind(y)o͞os″/ [L, *inducere,* to lead in], to cause or stimulate the start of an activity, as an enzyme induces a metabolic activity. See also **induced fever. –induction, inducer,** *n.*

induced abortion, an intentional termination of pregnancy before the fetus has developed enough to live if born. Pregnancies may be terminated deliberately at the request of the mother or for medical indications during the first trimester by vacuum aspiration and/or curettage or during the second trimester by dilation and evacuation, induction of labor, or hysterotomy. Compare **spontaneous abortion.** See also **septic abortion, therapeutic abortion.**

■ METHOD: The type of procedure depends on stage of pregnancy and may be either medical or surgical in nature.

■ OUTCOME CRITERIA: Ultrasound or tissue evidence and a physical exam are used to confirm complete removal of all uterine contents. Intercourse and use of tampons are discouraged. Normal activity can be resumed within a day or two if no complications occur. Potential complications include heavy bleeding, infection, abdominal pain, incomplete removal of all uterine contents, perforation of uterus, scar tissue in uterus, trouble becoming pregnant in the future, and psychological sequelae. Follow-up is routinely scheduled about 2 weeks after the procedure.

induced lethargy, a trancelike state produced during hypnosis. See also **hypnosis, lethargy.**

induced mutation [L, *inducere,* to lead in, *mutare,* to change], a mutation that is produced by treatment with a physical or chemical agent that affects the deoxyribonucleic acid molecules of a living organism.

induced phagocytosis [L, *inducere,* to lead in; Gk, *phagein,* to eat, *kytos,* cell], the ingestion of microorganisms and other foreign particles by cells (mostly macrophages) of the reticuloendothelial system because of a stimulus from the microorganisms or particles.

induced psychotic disorder, a severe mental disturbance in which there is a withdrawal from reality, resulting from exposure to a toxic agent such as a drug or hallucinogen.

induced trance, a somnambulistic state resulting from hypnotism.

induced vomiting [L, *inducere,* to lead in; *vomere,* to vomit], vomiting produced by administration of an emetic or by insertion of a finger or blunt instrument into the throat. Vomiting is no longer medically indicated and can lead to esophageal or stomach damage, but it may be self-induced by patients afflicted with bulimia. See also **bulimia.**

inducer /indo͞o″sər/, a substance, usually a substrate of a specific enzyme, that combines with and inactivates the repressor produced by a regulator gene in bacteria. This combination prevents the repressor from blocking activation of the operator gene, allowing one or more structural genes to be transcribed.

induction /induk″shən/ [L, *inducere,* to lead in], the process of stimulating and determining morphogenetic differentiation in a developing embryo through the action of chemical substances transmitted from one embryonic part to another. See also **evocation.**

induction chemotherapy, chemotherapy as the initial treatment for cancer, typically before radiation or surgical intervention.

induction of anesthesia, **1.** the administration of a drug or combination of drugs at the beginning of an anesthetic that results in a state of general anesthesia. **2.** the process of causing general anesthesia by the administration of pharmaceutics.

induction of labor, an obstetric procedure in which labor is initiated artificially by means of amniotomy or administration of oxytocics. It is performed electively or for fetal or maternal indications. Elective induction is carried out for the convenience of the mother or the obstetrician, often to avert the possibility of delivery outside the hospital when labor is judged to be imminent and the mother is expected to have an unusually rapid birth. Elective inductions are performed less often now than in the past. Prerequisites for elective induction are a term gestation, a fetal weight of at least 2500 g, a cervix judged ready to dilate, a vertex presentation, and engagement of the presenting part of the fetus in the pelvis. Errors in the estimation of gestational age and fetal weight may result in the delivery of an unexpectedly immature or low-birth-weight infant. Indicated induction is performed when its risk is judged to be less than that of continuing the pregnancy in such conditions as premature rupture of the membranes, severe maternal diabetes, and intractable preeclampsia. Surgical induction is effected by amniotomy, often with stripping of the membranes and digital stretching of the cervix; it is very often carried out in conjunction with medical induction. Medical induction is achieved through the administration of oxytocin, almost always by IV infusion, in a carefully controlled manner using microdrip equipment or an infusion pump. Beginning with very small amounts of oxytocin in an IV solution, the dosage is increased by gradual increments of the rate or concentration of infusion until effective labor is established. With IV oxytocin inductions a secondary, piggyback infusion without medication is always attached to the tubing so that an unmedicated infusion can be maintained if oxytocin is stopped. Prostaglandins are more commonly used to induce labor in the second trimester, particularly for therapeutic abortions. Electronic fetal and uterine monitoring is usually instituted during induction of labor to prevent hyperstimulation of the uterus and fetal distress. Ideally induced labor mimics natural labor, but in practice it usually does not. Longer and harder contractions commonly occur. In addition to unexpected fetal immaturity, complications of induction of labor include umbilical cord prolapse after amniotomy, tumultuous labor, tetanic uterine contractions, rupture of the uterus, placental abruption, fetal maternal hypotension, water intoxication, postpartum uterine atony and hemorrhage, and fetal asphyxia, hypoxia, or death. If the induction fails to produce effective labor, cesarean section is often required to prevent the adverse sequelae of the procedures used in the induction. For this reason it is usually recommended that induction of labor not be attempted unless delivery must be accomplished to prevent severe fetal or maternal morbidity.

induction phase, the period during which a normal cell becomes transformed into a cancerous cell.

induction therapy, the first therapeutic measure used to treat a disease, especially when combined modality therapy is planned. Also called **first-line therapy.**

inductive approach /induk″tiv/, the analysis of data and examination of practice problems within their own context rather than from a predetermined theoretical basis. The approach moves from the specific to the general.

inductor /induk″tər/ [L, *inducere,* to lead in], (in embryology) a tissue or cell that emits a chemical substance that stimulates some morphogenetic effect in the developing embryo. See also **evocator, organizer.**

induration /in′dyərā″shən/ [L, *indurare,* to make hard], hardening of a tissue, particularly the skin, caused by edema, inflammation, or infiltration by a neoplasm. −*indurated, adj.*

industrial health [L, *industria,* diligence; ME, *helthe*], the health concerns associated with the workplace, such as exposure to asbestos, mining and milling dusts, and metal and acid vapors; lighting; and ergonomic factors.

industrial psychology [L, *industria,* diligence], the application of psychological principles and techniques to the problems of business and industry, including the selection of personnel, the motivation of workers, and the development of training programs. See also **applied psychology.**

indwelling catheter /in″dweling/ [L, *in,* within; AS, *dwellan,* to remain], a urinary catheter designed to be left in place for continuous drainage of urine. It is held in place by an inflatable balloon that prevents expulsion. Compare **straight catheter.** Kinds include **Foley catheter, three-way irrigation catheter, suprapubic catheter.** See also **self-retaining catheter.**

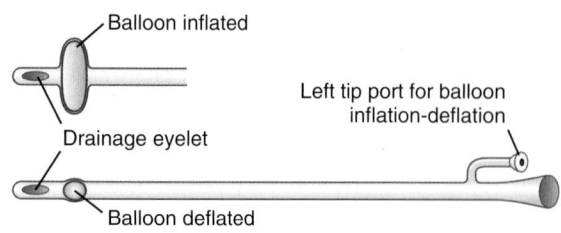

Foley

Indwelling catheter *(Dehn and Asprey, 2013)*

-ine, suffix meaning a "chemical substance": *chlorine, strychnine.*

inebriant /inē″brē·ənt/ [L, *inebriare,* to make drunk], a substance that induces inebriation or intoxication, as does ethanol.

inebriate /inē″brē·āt/, to make intoxicated.

inert /inurt′/ [L, *iners,* idle], 1. not moving or acting, such as inert matter. 2. (of a chemical substance) not taking part in a chemical reaction. 3. (of a medical ingredient) not active pharmacologically; serving only as a bulking, binding, or sweetening agent or other excipient in a medication.

inert gas, neutral monotomic elements with completely filled outer electron shells. These elements are all gaseous and extremely nonreactive. The inert gases are argon, helium, neon, and radon. Compounds are known for krypton and xenon, so they are no longer considered inert.

inertia /inur″shə/ [L, idleness], 1. the tendency of a body at rest to remain at rest unless acted on by an outside force, and the tendency of a body in motion to remain at motion in the direction in which it is moving unless acted on by an outside force. 2. an abnormal condition characterized by a general inactivity or sluggishness, such as colonic inertia or uterine inertia.

inertial impaction /inur″shəl/, the deposition of large aerosol particles on the walls of an airway conduit. The impaction tends to occur where the airway direction changes. Small particles have less inertia and are more likely to be carried around corners and continue in the path of the airflow.

inevitable abortion /inev″itəbəl/ [L, *inevitabilis,* unavoidable], a condition of pregnancy in which spontaneous termination is imminent and cannot be prevented. It is characterized by bleeding, uterine cramping, dilation of the cervix, and presentation of the conceptus in the cervical os. If heavy bleeding supervenes, immediate evacuation of the uterus may be required. Transvaginal ultrasound makes it possible to determine presence or absence of fetal heart movement at 5 weeks' gestation. Compare **incomplete abortion, threatened abortion.**

inevitable personal event, (in occupational therapy) naturally occurring communication, reaction processes, tasks, or general circumstances that occur during therapy and that have the potential to detract from or strengthen the therapeutic relationship.

in extremis [L, *extremus,* outermost], 1. a difficult situation. 2. at the point of death.

infant /in″fənt/ [L, *infans,* unable to speak], 1. *n.,* a child who is in the earliest stage of extrauterine life, a time extending from the first month after birth to approximately 12 months of age, when the baby is able to assume an erect posture. 2. *n.,* (in law) a person not of full legal age; a minor. 3. *adj.,* pertaining to infancy; in an early stage of development. −**infantile,** *adj.*

infant botulism, an intoxication by neurotoxins produced by *Clostridium botulinum* that occurs in children under 6 months of age. The condition is characterized by severe hypotonicity of all muscles, constipation, lethargy, and feeding difficulties, and it may lead to respiratory insufficiency. The botulism neurotoxin is usually found in the GI tract rather than in the blood, indicating that it is probably produced in the gut rather than ingested. The epidemiological and pathophysiological characteristics of the syndrome are not clearly understood.

■ INTERVENTIONS: Treatment is supportive, including optimal management of fluids, electrolytes, and nutrition. Ventilatory support may also be necessary. An antitoxin, botulism immune globulin intravenous (BIGIV), should be given as soon as possible.

infant death, (*Informal*) (in epidemiology) the death of a live-born child before the first birthday. See also **infant mortality.**

infant feeding. See **bottle feeding, breastfeeding.**

infanticide /infan″tisīd/ [L, *infans,* unable to speak, *caedere,* to kill], the killing of an infant or young child. The act is usually a psychotic reaction and is often associated with severe depression, such as that occurring in bipolar disorder and occasionally in extreme postpartum disturbances. −*infanticidal, adj.*

infantile /in″fəntīl/ [L, unable to speak], **1.** characteristic of infants or infancy. **2.** lacking maturity, sophistication, or reasonableness. **3.** affected with infantilism. **4.** being in a very early stage of development.

infantile acrodermatitis. See **Gianotti-Crosti syndrome.**

infantile amnesia, (in psychology) the inability of adults to remember events from early childhood. It is explained by a theory that a memory for skills develops earlier than a fact-memory system, which may not develop until the third year. Thus a person may learn skills without remembering how the skills were acquired. Also called *childhood amnesia.*

infantile autism, a pervasive developmental disorder characterized by disturbances in emotional, social, and linguistic development in a child before the age of 30 months. Symptoms include deviations in customary ways of relating to people, objects, and situations. It may result from organic brain dysfunction. See also **autistic disorder.**

infantile celiac disease. See **celiac disease.**

infantile cerebral ataxic paralysis [L, *infans,* unable to speak, *cerebrum,* the brain; Gk, *ataxia,* without order, *paralyein,* to be palsied], a form of congenital symmetrical paralysis characterized by cerebral maldevelopment, ataxia, spasticity of the legs, and possibly cognitive impairments.

infantile cerebral sphingolipidosis. See **Tay-Sachs disease.**

infantile cirrhosis, a progressive fibrous liver disorder caused by protein malnutrition.

infantile colic [L, *infans,* unable to speak; Gk, *kolikos,* pain in the colon], a descriptive term for a suggested intestinal cause of discomfort in a newborn. Specific causes and mechanisms have not been defined. The typical infantile colic patient eats and gains weight but may also appear excessively hungry. Aerophagia caused by crying may lead to flatulence and abdominal distension.

infantile cortical hyperostosis, a familial disorder characterized in an infant by subperiosteal bone formation over many bones, causing swellings and tenderness in the affected areas. The child also tends to be feverish and irritable. The mandible is most commonly involved. Radiographs indicate areas of new bone growth beneath the periosteum. The disorder appears before 6 months of age and disappears during childhood. Also called **Caffey disease.**

infantile dwarf, a person whose mental and physical development is greatly delayed as a result of various causes, such as genetic or developmental defects.

infantile eczema. See **atopic dermatitis.**

infantile encephalitis [L, *infans,* unable to speak; Gk, *enkephalos,* brain, *itis,* inflammation], any of a group of brain inflammation conditions affecting infants. The cause may be a direct viral infection or a secondary encephalitis that is a complication of measles, chickenpox, rubella, or other diseases.

infantile fibromatosis. See **congenital generalized fibromatosis.**

infantile hemiplegia, paralysis of one side of the body that may occur at birth as a result of a cerebral hemorrhage, in utero as a result of lack of oxygen, or during a febrile illness in infancy.

infantile hydrocele [L, *infans* + Gk, *hydor,* water, *kele,* hernia], an accumulation of fluid in the tunica vaginalis. It may be present at birth or acquired.

infantile myofibromatosis, a condition present at birth or occurring soon after, characterized by one or more firm, rubbery, spherical or ovoid nodules in the skin and subcutaneous tissue. The nodules are composed of myofibroblasts and may undergo ulceration and calcification. In about half of patients, skeletal fibromas also occur. When lesions are limited to the skin and bones (a condition sometimes known as congenital multiple fibromatosis), prognosis is good and lesions resolve spontaneously. Visceral involvement may also occur (congenital generalized fibromatosis) and is highly lethal.

infantile neuroaxonal dystrophy, progressive hereditary degenerative encephalopathy transmitted as an autosomal-recessive trait, beginning in infancy with muscular hypotonia and arrest of development in late infancy, followed by dementia, blindness, spasticity, and ataxia. Pathologically it is characterized by widespread focal swellings and degeneration of the axons with scattered globular bodies in the brain. Also called **Seitelberger disease.**

infantile paralysis. See **poliomyelitis.**

infantile pellagra. See **kwashiorkor.**

infantile poliomyelitis. See **acute atrophic paralysis.**

infantile spasms, a syndrome of severe myoclonus appearing in the first 18 months of life and associated with general cerebral deterioration. It is marked by severe flexion spasms of the head, neck, and trunk and extension of the arms and legs. Also called *infantile massive spasms, jackknife seizures, jackknife spasms.*

infantile spinal muscular atrophy. See **Werdnig-Hoffmann disease.**

infantile spinal paralysis [L, *infans,* unable to speak, *spina* + Gk, *paralyein,* to be palsied], acute anterior poliomyelitis, a viral infection characterized by nonspecific illnesses, aseptic meningitis, and flaccid weakness of muscle groups.

infantile uterus, a uterus that has failed to attain adult characteristics.

infantilism /infan″tiliz′əm/ [L, *infans,* unable to speak], **1.** a condition in which various anatomical, physiological, and psychological characteristics of childhood persist in the adult. It is characterized by cognitive impairment, underdeveloped sexual organs, and usually small stature. Compare **progeria. 2.** a condition, usually of psychological rather than organic origin, characterized by speech and voice patterns in an older child or adult that are typical of very young children.

infant mortality, the statistical rate of infant death during the first year after live birth, expressed as the number of such deaths per 1000 live births in a specific geographic area or institution in a given period.

infant of chemically dependent mother, a newborn who shows withdrawal symptoms, usually within the first 24 hours of life, most commonly caused by maternal antepartum dependence on heroin, methadone, diazepam, phenobarbital, or alcohol. Also called **neonatal abstinence syndrome.** See also **fetal alcohol syndrome.**

■ OBSERVATIONS: Characteristic symptoms include tremors, irritability, hyperactive reflexes, increased muscle tone, twitching, increased mucus production, nasal congestion, respiratory distress, excessive sweating, elevated temperature, vomiting, diarrhea, and dehydration. The infants cry shrilly, often sneeze, frantically suck their fists but feed poorly, and frequently yawn but have difficulty falling asleep. They are usually pale, are often born with or develop nose and knee abrasions from fussiness and irritability, and are subject to convulsions.

■ INTERVENTIONS: The infant is kept warm, snugly swaddled in a padded crib, and exposed to minimal visual, auditory, and tactile stimulation. The baby is handled only when necessary and is then held firmly, close to the body.

■ PATIENT CARE CONSIDERATIONS: These high-risk infants require special attention, and the mother should be encouraged to participate in her baby's care as soon as possible. The health care team can play a major role in the promotion of parent-child bonding. A multidisciplinary early-intervention program can assess and intervene if the infant experiences developmental delays.

infarct /infärkt′/ [L, *infarcire,* to stuff], a localized area of necrosis in a tissue resulting from anoxia. It is caused by an interruption in the blood supply to the area or, less frequently, by circulatory stasis produced by the occlusion of a vein that ordinarily carries blood away from the area. Some infarcts are pale and white because of the lack of circulation. Others may resemble a red, swollen bruise because of hemorrhage and an accumulation of blood in the area. Also called **infarction.**

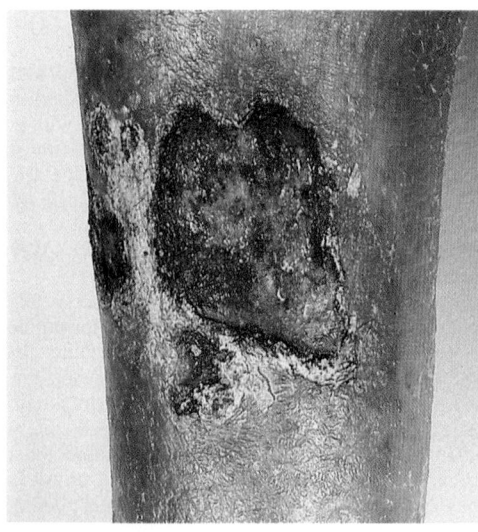

Infarct *(du Vivier, 2002)*

infarct extension, a myocardial infarction that has spread beyond the original area, usually as a result of the death of cells in the ischemic margin of the infarct zone.

infarction /infärk′shən/ [L, *infarcire,* to stuff], **1.** See **infarct. 2.** the development and formation of an infarct. Kinds include **myocardial infarction, pulmonary infarction.**

infect [L, *inficere,* to stain], to transmit a pathogen that may induce development of an infectious disease in another person.

infected abortion, a spontaneous or induced termination of an immature pregnancy in which the products of conception have become infected, causing fever and requiring antibiotic therapy and evacuation of the uterus. Compare **septic abortion.**

infected hydronephrosis, a dilation of the renal pelvis and calyces that has become complicated by bacterial infection.

infection /infek′shən/ [L, *inficere,* to stain], **1.** the invasion of the body by pathogenic microorganisms that reproduce and multiply, causing disease by local cellular injury,

secretion of a toxin, or antigen-antibody reaction in the host. **2.** a disease caused by the invasion of the body by pathogenic microorganisms. Compare **infestation. –infectious,** *adj.*

infection control, programs of disease surveillance, generally within health care facilities, designed to investigate, prevent, and control the spread of infections and their causative microorganisms. Infection control can include the policies and procedures of a hospital or other health facility to minimize the risk of spreading nosocomial or community-acquired infections to patients or members of the staff.

infection control committee, a group of hospital health professionals composed of infection control personnel, with medical, nursing, administrative, and occasionally dietary and housekeeping department representatives, who plan and supervise infection control activities.

infection control nurse, a registered nurse who is assigned responsibility for surveillance and infection prevention, education, and control activities.

infectious /infek′chəs/, **1.** capable of causing an infection. **2.** caused by an infection.

infectious arthritis [L, *inficere,* to stain; Gk, *arthron,* joint + *itis,* inflammation], arthritis caused by bacteria, rickettsiae, mycoplasmas, viruses, fungi, or parasites. See also **septic arthritis.**

infectious bulbar paralysis [L, *inficere,* to stain, *bulbus,* swollen root; Gk, *paralyein,* to be palsied], a viral disease of animals (swine, cattle, dogs, cats, and rats) that may cause a mild pruritus when transmitted to humans. Also called **pseudorabies.**

infectious disease (ID) [L, *inficere,* to stain, *dis* + Fr, *aise,* ease], any clinically evident communicable disease, or one that can be transmitted from one human being to another or from animal to human by direct or indirect contact. Compare **communicable disease.**

infectious endocarditis, endocarditis caused by infection with microorganisms, especially bacteria and fungi. It was formerly classified according to course as acute and subacute. Because underlying causes and available therapies have changed, this division has little current clinical validity and has been largely replaced by classification on the basis of cause or underlying anatomy. Infectious endocarditis is common in IV drug abusers.

infectious gastritis, any type of inflammation of the gastric mucosa, usually chronic, caused by a bacterial infection in the stomach, the most common type being *Helicobacter pylori* gastritis. Many cases are asymptomatic, but symptoms can include dyspepsia and gastrointestinal bleeding. In immunocompromised patients, gastritis may occur as a complication of tuberculosis, syphilis, or other conditions.

infectious granuloma [L, *inficere,* to stain, *granulum,* little grain; Gk, *oma,* tumor], a lumpy lesion of granuloma tissue that may develop in diseases such as tuberculosis, syphilis, and actinomycosis.

infectious hepatitis (I.H.). See **hepatitis A.**

infectious isolation [L, *inficere,* to stain; It, *isolare,* to detach], a practice of confining a patient with a particularly virulent disease to an isolated room or other area to reduce the risk of contact and spread of the disease among hospital personnel.

infectious mononucleosis [L, *inficere,* to stain; Gk, *monos,* single; L, *nucleus,* nut; Gk, *osis,* condition], an acute herpesvirus infection caused by the Epstein-Barr virus (EBV). The disease is usually transmitted by droplet infection but is not highly or predictably contagious. Young people are most often affected. In childhood the disease is mild and usually unnoticed; the older the person, the more severe the symptoms are likely to be. Infection confers permanent immunity, although the virus continues to replicate and can be transmitted. When infection lasts more than 6 months it is called chronic EBV. See also **Epstein-Barr virus, viral infection.**

■ OBSERVATIONS: The hallmark signs of mononucleosis are profound fatigue; a fever that peaks in the late afternoon at 101° F to 105° F (38.3° C to 40.6° C); severely painful and exudative pharyngitis; and symmetric lymphadenopathy. Splenomegaly is usually present in the second or third week. Mild hepatomegaly may also be present. A maculopapular rash, palatal petechiae, and periorbital edema are less common signs. Fatigue and general malaise may persist for months after infection clears. Diagnosis is made by the presence of clinical manifestations plus a differential WBC count showing lymphocytes and monocytes more than 50%; a heterophil agglutination antibody test with an antibody titer greater than 1:40; and an EBV-immunoglobulin M test with antibodies more than 1:80. Liver function tests (aspartate aminotransferase [AST], alanine aminotransferase [ALT], and bilirubin) will be elevated if the liver is involved. Complications are rare but include splenic rupture, anemia, Guillain-Barré syndrome, meningitis, and encephalitis.

■ INTERVENTIONS: Treatment is supportive in nature, with bed rest during the acute phase; saline throat gargles; adequate hydration; nonaspirin analgesics and antipyretics; and steroids for treating impending airway obstruction, severe thrombocytopenia or hemolytic anemia. Transfusions may be indicated for severe anemia or thrombocytopenia. Splenectomy is indicated for splenic rupture.

■ PATIENT CARE CONSIDERATIONS: The focus is on stressing rest to prevent injury to the liver and the spleen and supportive care, such as gargles to ease sore throat and antipyretics, cool cloths, and sponge baths to relieve fever. Education should stress the avoidance of heavy lifting and contact sports for at least 2 months after acute recovery to prevent injury to the spleen.

infectious myringitis, an inflammatory contagious condition of the eardrum caused by viral or bacterial infection. *Mycoplasma* is a common cause of this infection. It is characterized by the development of painful vesicles on the eardrum, very often linked to otitis media. The pain begins suddenly, with a duration of 24 to 48 hours. Also called **bullous myringitis.**

infectious nucleic acid, deoxyribonucleic acid or, more commonly, viral ribonucleic acid that is able to infect the nucleic acid of a cell and induce the host to produce viruses.

infectious parotitis. See **mumps.**

infectious polyneuritis. See **Guillain-Barré syndrome.**

infective endocarditis. See **bacterial endocarditis.**

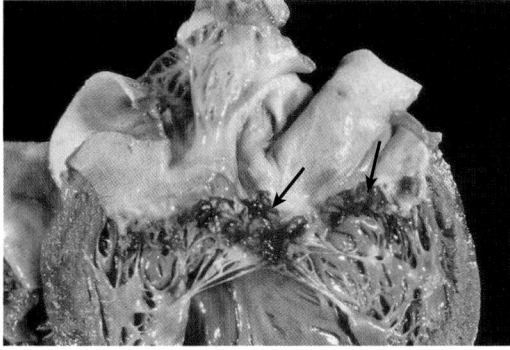

Bacterial infective endocarditis *(Kumar et al, 2010)*

infective tubulointerstitial nephritis [L, *inficere,* to stain, *tubulus,* tubule, *interstitium,* space between], an acute inflammation of the kidneys usually caused by an infection by *Escherichia coli* or another pyogenic pathogen. The condition is characterized by chills, fever, nausea and vomiting, flank pain, dysuria, proteinuria, and hematuria. The kidney may become enlarged, and portions of the renal cortex may be destroyed. Infection is usually the result of bacterial contamination of a urinary catheter, but it may occur in any condition characterized by urinary stasis.

infectivity /infektiv″itē/ [L, *inficere,* to stain], the ability of a pathogen to spread rapidly from one host to another.

inferior /infir″ē·ər/ [L, *inferus,* lower], **1.** situated below a given point of reference, as the feet are inferior to the legs. **2.** of poorer quality or value. Compare **superior.**

inferior alveolar artery, an artery that descends with the inferior alveolar nerve from the first or mandibular portion of the maxillary artery to the mandibular foramen on the medial surface of the ramus of the mandible. It enters the mandibular canal and continues to the first premolar tooth, where it divides into the mental and incisor branches. Also called *arteria alveolaris inferior.*

inferior aperture of minor pelvis, an irregular opening bounded by the coccyx, the sacrotuberous ligaments, part of the ischium, the sides of the pubic arch, and the pubic symphysis.

inferior aperture of thorax, an irregular opening bounded by the twelfth thoracic vertebra, the eleventh and twelfth ribs, and the edge of the costal cartilages as they meet the sternum.

inferior carotid triangle [L, *inferior,* lower; Gk, *karos,* heavy sleep; L, *triangulus,* three-cornered], a triangular area bounded by the midline of the neck, the superior belly of the omohyoid muscle above, and the sternocleidomastoid muscle behind. Also called **muscular triangle.**

inferior cervical ganglion, a ganglion at the lower end of the cervical part of the sympathetic trunk that combines with the first thoracic ganglion to form the stellate ganglion.

inferior conjunctival fornix, the space in the fold of conjunctiva created by the reflection of the conjunctiva covering the eyeball and the lining of the lower eyelid. Compare **superior conjunctival fornix.**

inferior gastric node, a node in one of two groups of gastric lymph glands lying between the two layers of the lesser omentum along the pyloric half of the greater curvature of the stomach. Compare **hepatic node, superior gastric node.**

inferior gluteal artery, a large terminal trunk of the internal iliac artery that contributes to the blood supply of the gluteal region and anastomoses with a network of vessels around the hip joint.

inferior gluteal nerve, a nerve that supplies the gluteus maximus.

inferiority complex /infir″ē·ôr″itē/, **1.** a personal feeling or sense of being inadequate. It is largely unconscious and influences attitudes and behaviors. **2.** (in psychoanalysis) a complex characterized by striving for unrealistic goals to compensate for low self-esteem, usually related to childhood trauma.

inferior kidney, inferior segment of kidney; the renal segment located most inferiorly.

inferior maxillary bone. See **mandible.**

inferior mesenteric artery, a visceral branch of the abdominal aorta, arising just above the division into the common iliacs and supplying the left half of the transverse colon, all of the descending and iliac colons, and most of the rectum. It has left colic, sigmoid, and superior rectal branches.

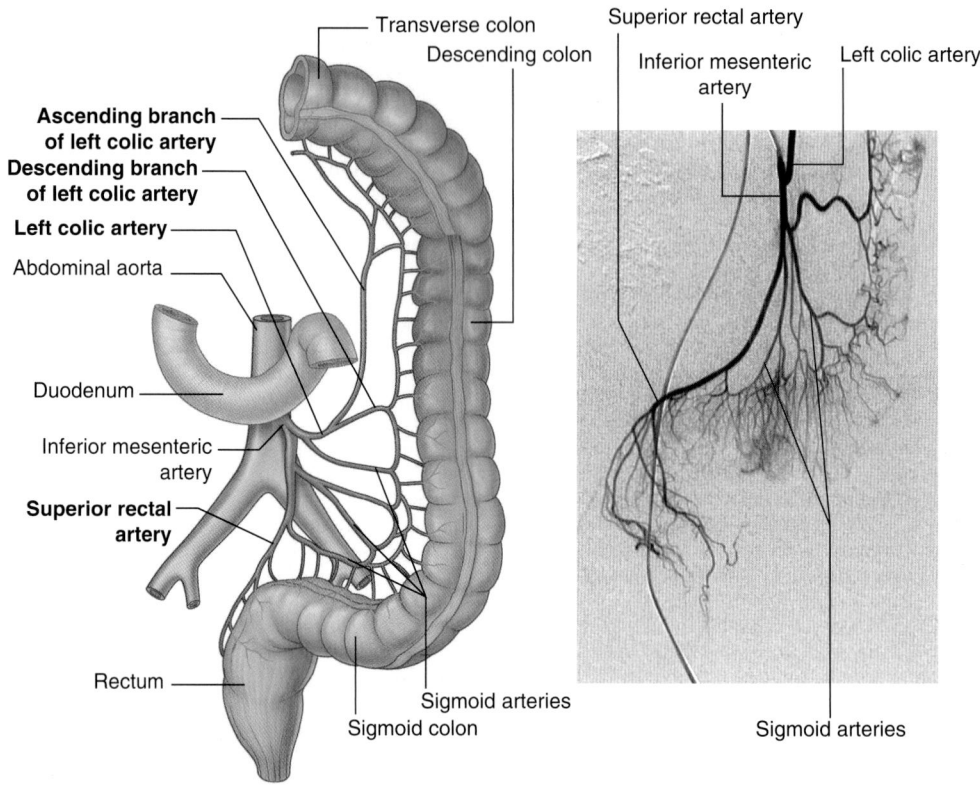

Inferior mesenteric artery *(Drake, Vogl, and Mitchell, 2010)*

inferior mesenteric node, a node in one of the three groups of visceral lymph glands serving the viscera of the abdomen and the pelvis. The inferior mesenteric nodes are associated with the branches of the inferior mesenteric artery. The inferior mesenteric nodes drain the descending colon, the iliac and sigmoid parts of the colon, and the upper part of the rectum. Their efferent vessels pass to the preaortic nodes. Compare **gastric node, superior mesenteric node.**

inferior mesenteric vein, the vein in the lower body that returns the blood from the rectum, the sigmoid and descending colons, and part of the transverse colon. It receives the sigmoid veins from the sigmoid colon and the iliac colon and the left colic vein from the descending colon and the left colic flexure. Compare **superior mesenteric vein.**

inferior olivary nucleus [L, *inferior,* lower, *oliva,* olive, *nucleus,* nut kernel], a small purse-shaped collection of nerve cells lying posterolateral to the pyramid, just below the level of the pons. It is a source of cerebellar climbing fibers.

inferior orbital fissure, a groove in the inferolateral wall of the orbit that contains the infraorbital and zygomatic nerves and the infraorbital vessels.

inferior phrenic artery, a small visceral branch of the abdominal aorta that arises from the aorta itself, the renal artery, or the celiac artery. It divides into the medial and lateral branches and supplies the diaphragm. A few vessels of the inferior vena cava stem from the lateral branch of the right phrenic artery. Some branches of the left phrenic artery supply the esophagus.

inferior pole of kidney. See **poles of kidney.**

inferior radioulnar joint. See **distal radioulnar articulation.**

inferior rectal plexus, the subcutaneous portion of the rectal venous plexus, below the pectinate line.

inferior right lateral flexure of rectum, the fourth bend of the rectum, where it deviates laterally to the right.

inferior sagittal sinus, one of the six venous channels of the posterior dura mater, draining blood from the brain into the internal jugular vein. It receives deoxygenated blood from several veins from the falx cerebri and, in some individuals, from a few veins from the cerebral hemispheres. Compare **straight sinus, superior sagittal sinus, transverse sinus.**

inferior subscapular nerve /subskap″yŏŏlər/, one of three small nerves that arise from the posterior cord of the brachial plexus. It supplies part of the subscapularis and ends in the teres major. Compare **superior subscapular nerve.**

inferior thyroid vein, one of the few veins that arise in the venous plexus on the thyroid gland and form a plexus ventral to the trachea, under the sternothyroideus muscle. A left vein descends from this plexus to join the left brachiocephalic trunk; a right vein descends obliquely to open into the right brachiocephalic vein at its junction with the superior vena cava.

inferior ulnar collateral artery, one of a pair of branches of the deep brachial arteries, arising about 5 cm from the elbow, passing inward to form an arch with the deep brachial artery, and carrying blood to the muscles of the forearm. Compare **superior ulnar collateral artery.**

inferior vena cava, the large vein that returns deoxygenated blood to the heart from parts of the body below the diaphragm. It is formed by the junction of the two common iliac veins to the right of the fifth lumbar vertebra and ascends along the vertebral column, pierces the diaphragm, and opens into the right atrium of the heart. As it passes through the diaphragm, it receives a covering of serous pericardium. The inferior vena cava contains a semilunar valve that is rudimentary in the adult but very large and important in the fetus. The vessel receives blood from the two common iliacs, the lumbar veins, and the testicular veins. Compare **superior vena cava.**

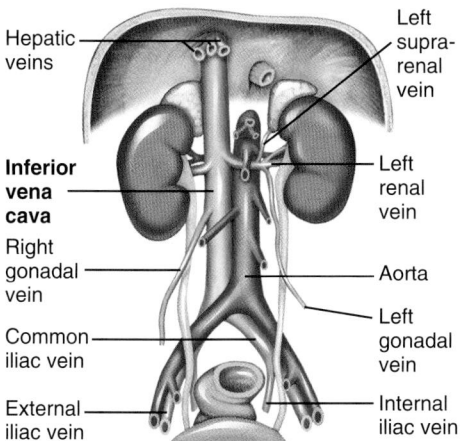

Labels: Hepatic veins; Left suprarenal vein; **Inferior vena cava**; Left renal vein; Right gonadal vein; Aorta; Common iliac vein; Left gonadal vein; External iliac vein; Internal iliac vein

Inferior vena cava and its tributaries

inferior vesical artery, an artery in men that supplies branches to the bladder, ureter, seminal vesicle, and prostate.

infero-, prefix meaning "low": *inferolateral, inferomedial.*

inferolateral /in′fərōlat″ərəl/ [L, *inferus,* lower, *latus,* side], pertaining to a location situated below and to the side.

inferomedial /in′fərōmē″dē·əl/ [L, *inferus,* lower, *medius,* middle], pertaining to a location situated below and toward the center.

infertile /infur″təl/ [L, *in,* not, *fertilis,* fruitful], denoting the inability to produce offspring. This condition may be present in one or both sex partners and may be temporary and reversible. The cause may be physical, including immature sexual organs, abnormalities of the reproductive system, hormonal imbalance, and dysfunction or anomalies in other organ systems, or it may result from psychological or emotional problems. The condition is classified as primary, in which pregnancy has never occurred, and secondary, when one or more pregnancies have occurred. Compare **sterile.**

infertility /in′furtil″itē/, the condition of being unable to produce offspring. Compare **sterility.**

infest /infest″/, to attack, invade, and subsist on the skin or in the internal organs of a host. Compare **infect.**

infestation /in′festā″shən/ [L, *infestare,* to attack], the presence of animal parasites in the environment, on the skin, or in the hair of a host.

infiltrate /infil″trāt/, **1.** *v.,* to penetrate the interstices of a tissue or substance. **2.** *n.,* the material or solution so deposited.

infiltration /in′filtrās″hən/ [L, *in,* within, *filtare,* to strain through], the process whereby a fluid passes into the tissues, such as when a local anesthetic is administered or an IV solution infuses into the tissues surrounding the venipuncture site.

infiltrative disorder /infil″trətiv/, a condition caused by the diffusion or accumulation in cells or tissues of substances not normally found in those cells or tissues, as in granulomatous diseases.

infirmary /infur″mərē/ [L, *infirmus,* weak], a place that provides care for sick or convalescing individuals, sometimes within a larger residential facility (e.g., a college dormitory or prison) and sometimes as a specialized clinic within a larger hospital system.

inflammable, capable of spontaneously bursting into flame. See also **flammable.**

inflammation [L, *inflammare,* to set afire], the protective or destructive response of body tissues to irritation or injury. Inflammation may be acute or chronic. Its cardinal signs are redness (rubor), heat (calor), swelling (tumor), and pain (dolor), often accompanied by loss of function. The process begins with a transitory vasoconstriction, then is followed by a brief increase in vascular permeability. The second stage is prolonged and consists of sustained increase in vascular permeability, exudation of fluids from the vessels, clustering of leukocytes along the vessel walls, phagocytosis of microorganisms, deposition of fibrin in the vessel, disposal of the accumulated debris by macrophages, and finally migration of fibroblasts to the area and development of new, normal cells. The severity, timing, and local character of any particular inflammatory response depend on the cause, the area affected, and the condition of the host. Histamine, kinins, and various other substances mediate the inflammatory process. −*inflammatory, adj.*

inflammatory autobullectomy, spontaneous regression of a bulla caused by inflammation in patients with bullous emphysema.

inflammatory bowel disease. See **ulcerative colitis.**

inflammatory cell, a neutrophil, macrophage, monocyte, eosinophil, or basophil that participates in the inflammatory response to a foreign substance.

inflammatory dysmenorrhea [L, *inflammare* + Gk, *dys* + *men,* month, *rhein,* to flow], menstrual pain that accompanies pelvic infection, fibroids, or endometritis. Also called **secondary dysmenorrhea.**

inflammatory fracture [L, *inflammare,* to set afire, *fractura,* break], a break in bone tissue weakened by inflammation.

inflammatory response, a tissue reaction to injury or an antigen that may include pain, swelling, itching, redness, heat, and loss of function. The response may involve dilation of blood vessels and consequent leakage of fluid, causing edema; leukocytic exudation; and release of plasma proteases and vasoactive amines such as histamine.

inflammatory scoliosis [L, *inflammare* + Gk, *skoliosis,* curvature], a form of scoliosis caused by muscle spasms associated with acute inflammation.

inflatable pessary. See **pessary.**

inflatable splint /inflā″təbəl/ [L, *in,* within, *flare,* to blow; ME, *splente*], a tubular device that is placed around a patient's extremity and inflated with air to maintain rigidity. Also called **pneumatic splint.**

inflection, **1.** the act of bending inward or the state of being bent inward. **2.** the intonation or pitch of the voice.

infliximab, a monoclonal antibody.

■ INDICATIONS: It is used to treat moderate to severe fistulizing Crohn's disease.

■ CONTRAINDICATIONS: Known hypersensitivity to murines prohibits its use.

■ ADVERSE EFFECTS: Life-threatening effects include anaphylaxis, anemia, and tachycardia. Other adverse effects include dry skin, sweating, flushing, hematoma, pruritus, upper respiratory infection, pharyngitis, bronchitis, cough, dyspnea, sinusitis, myalgia, back pain, arthralgia, dysuria, urinary frequency, chest pain, hypertension, and hypotension. Common side effects include nausea, vomiting, abdominal pain, stomatitis, constipation, dyspepsia, flatulence, headache, dizziness, depression, vertigo, fatigue, anxiety, fever, rash, dermatitis, and urticaria.

influenza /inˈflo͞o·enˈzə/ [It, influence], a highly contagious infection of the respiratory tract caused by orthomyxovirus and transmitted by airborne droplet infection. It occurs in isolated cases, epidemics, and pandemics. Symptoms include sore throat, cough, fever, muscular pains, and weakness. The incubation period is brief (from 1 to 3 days), and the onset is usually sudden, with chills, fever, respiratory symptoms, headache, myalgia, and extreme fatigue. Treatment is symptomatic and usually involves bed rest, acetaminophen, and drinking of fluids. Fever and constitutional symptoms distinguish influenza from the common cold. Complete recovery in 3 to 10 days is the rule, but bacterial pneumonia may occur among high-risk patients, such as the elderly, the very young, and people who have chronic pulmonary disease, and lead to death. On average, 5% to 20% of the population suffer influenza infection annually, and approximately 56,000 die. Three main strains of influenza virus have been recognized: type A, type B, and type C. New strains of the virus emerge at regular intervals. Yearly vaccination with the currently prevalent strain of influenza virus is recommended. Treatment or prophylaxis in high-risk patients may be achieved with rimantadine. Oseltamivir (oral) and Zanamivir (aerosol), when administered within 48 hours of onset, may lessen the severity and duration of symptoms. Also called **flu, grippe, la grippe.**

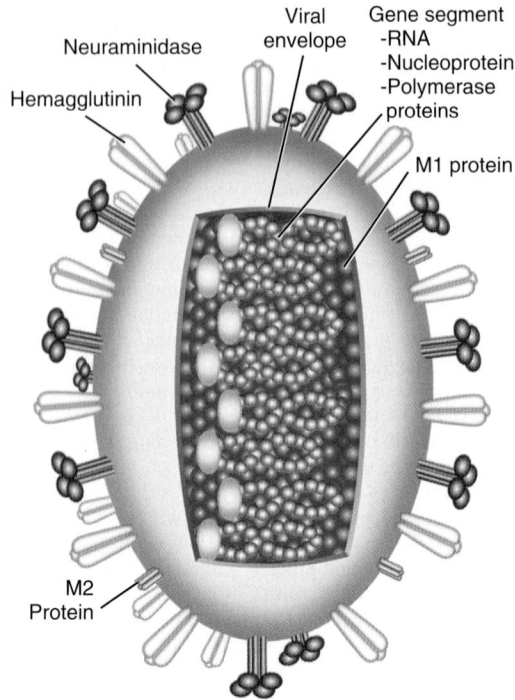

Schematic model of influenza A virus *(Rakel and Rakel, 2011)*

influenza A virus, influenza B virus, influenza C virus, species in the genera *Influenzavirus A, Influenzavirus B,* and *Influenzavirus C.*

influenza-like illness, nonspecific respiratory illness whose symptoms resemble those of influenza but that are usually caused not by influenza virus infection but by other viruses or by bacteria.

Influenzavirus /inˈflo͞o·enˈzäviˈrəs/, former genus name for the viruses that cause influenza, now found to be two different genera, which are named *Influenzavirus A* and *Influenzavirus B.*

Influenzavirus A, a genus of viruses of the family Orthomyxoviridae containing the agent of influenza A. It is usually the cause of epidemics and pandemics. It is divided into subgroups based on two surface proteins: neuraminidase and haemoglutinin. Vaccination against influenza A is available. See also **influenza.**

Influenzavirus B, a genus of viruses of the family Orthomyxoviridae containing the agent of influenza B. It affects only humans. It can cause epidemics, albeit not as severe as those caused by influenza A. Vaccination against influenza B is available. See also **influenza.**

Influenzavirus C, a genus of viruses of the family Orthomyxoviridae containing the agent of influenza C, a very mild infection. See also **influenza.**

influenza-virus vaccine, an active immunizing agent.
- INDICATIONS: It is prescribed for immunization against influenza.
- CONTRAINDICATIONS: Acute infection or allergy to eggs prohibits its use.
- ADVERSE EFFECTS: Among the more serious adverse effects are anaphylaxis and Guillain-Barré syndrome.

informal admission, a type of admission to a psychiatric hospital in which there is no formal or written application and the patient is free to leave at any time. Also called *voluntary admission.* Compare **involuntary patient.**

informal instructional environment, (in occupational therapy) a learning milieu characterized by freedom in choosing activities with a minimal emphasis on assessment or the use of external motivators, fostering thoughtful and creative learners who learn to develop solutions through problem solving.

informatics, computerized automated delivery and manipulation of information to and by users of computer systems.

information systems director [L, *informatio,* idea], a person who directs and administers a data processing facility. Also called *chief information officer (CIO).*

informed consent [L, *informare,* to give form, *consentire,* to sense], permission obtained from a patient to perform a specific test or procedure. Informed consent is required before most invasive procedures are performed and before a patient is admitted to a research study. The document used must be written in a language understood by the patient and be dated and signed by the patient and have at least one witness. Signed consent should be obtained by the person performing the procedure. Included in the document are clear, rational statements that describe the procedure or test. Also required is a statement that care will not be withheld if the patient does not consent. Informed consent is voluntary. By law, informed consent must be obtained more than a given number of days or hours before certain procedures, including therapeutic abortion and sterilization, and must always be obtained when the patient is fully competent. An individual must be of a certain legal age to give consent; laws vary from state to state and from country to country. Compare **implied consent.**

infra-, prefix meaning "situated," "formed," or "occurring beneath": *infraclavicular.*

infrabony pocket. See **periodontal pocket.**

infraclavicular fossa /inˈfrəkləvikˈyələr/, a small pocket or indentation just below the clavicle on both sides of the body.

infraclusion /inˈfrəkloōˈzhən/ [L, *infra*, below + *occludere*, to close up], malocclusion in which a tooth has failed to erupt fully and reach the line of occlusion and is out of contact with the opposing tooth. Also called **infraversion.**

infraction fracture /infrakˈshən/ [L, *infractio*, a breaking, *fractura*, break], a neoplastic fracture characterized by a small radiolucent line in radiographs and most commonly associated with a disorder of metabolism. See also **greenstick fracture.**

infradentale /inˈfrədentāˈlē/, a bone measurement landmark, being the highest anterior point on the gingiva between the mandibular central incisors.

infradian rhythm /inˈfrāˈdē·ən/ [L, *infra*, below, *dies*, day; Gk, *rhythmos*], a biorhythm that has a period shorter than 24 hours.

infraglenoid tubercle, a large triangular roughening inferior to the glenoid cavity in the scapula that is the site of attachment for the long head of the triceps brachii muscle.

infraglottic. See **subglottic.**

infrahyoid /inˈfrəhīˈoid/, pertaining to the area below the hyoid bone, particularly the group of muscles attached to it.

inframammary fold (IMF), the angle of deflection where the breast tissue meets the chest wall below the breast.

inframammary region, the part of the pectoral region inferior to the breast, bordered inferiorly by the hypochondriac region of the abdomen.

inframandibular. See **submandibular.**

inframaxillary, **1.** pertaining to the mandible, or lower jaw. **2.** lying below the maxilla, or upper jaw.

infranodal block /inˈfrənōˈdəl/ [L, *infra*, below, *nodus*, knot; Fr, *bloc*], a type of atrioventricular (AV) block caused by an abnormality below the AV node, either in the bundle of His or in both bundle branches. An infranodal block has more serious clinical implications than a block at the level of the AV node. The condition is often the result of arteriosclerosis, degenerative diseases, a defect in the conduction system, or a tumor. It most often occurs in older persons. Symptoms include frequent episodes of fainting and a pulse rate of 20 to 40 beats/min. Diagnosis is made by an electrocardiogram, which shows intraventricular conduction disturbances during sinus rhythm and distinguishes nodal from infranodal block. The usual therapy is implantation of a demand pacemaker. Compare **bundle branch block, intraventricular block.** See also **Adams-Stokes syndrome, atrioventricular block, cardiac conduction defect, heart block, intraatrial block, sinoatrial (SA) block.**

infranodal disease, a cardiac disorder involving the electrical conduction system of the heart below the atrioventricular node. Kinds include **bundle branch block.**

infraorbital /inˈfrə·ôrˈbitəl/ [L, *infra*, below, *orbita*, wheeltrack], pertaining to the area beneath the floor of the bony cavity in which the eyeball is located.

infraorbital foramen [L, *infra*, below, *orbita*, wheeltrack, *foramen*, hole], an opening on the anterior aspect of the maxilla. Through it pass the inferior orbital nerves and blood vessels.

infrapatellar fat pad /inˈfrəpətelˈər/, an area of palpable soft tissue in front of the joint space on either side of the patellar tendon.

infrapatellar synovial joint. See **alar fold.**

infrared radiation /inˈfrəredˈ/ [L, *infra* + AS, *read*, red; L, *radiare*, to emit rays], electromagnetic radiation with wavelengths between about 700 nm and 1 mm, longer than those of visible light but shorter than those of microwaves and radio waves. Infrared radiation that strikes the body surface is perceived as heat.

infrared therapy, treatment by exposure to various wavelengths of infrared radiation. Hot water bottles and heating pads of all kinds emit longwave infrared radiation; incandescent lights emit shortwave infrared radiation. Infrared treatment is performed to relieve pain and to stimulate circulation of blood.

infrared thermography, measurement of temperature through the detection of infrared radiation emitted by heated tissue. Temperature measurement from multiple body areas can be used to generate an image of the body in real time.

infrasonics /inˈfrəsonˈiks/, sound frequencies that are below the range of human hearing.

infraspinatus. See **infraspinous muscle.**

infraspinous fossa, a large triangular region of the posterior scapula below the spine.

infraspinous muscle /inˈfrə·spīˈnos/ [L, *infra*, below + *spina*, spine], the muscle arising from the infraspinous fossa and inserting in the greater tubercle of the humerus. It functions to rotate the humerus laterally. Also called **infraspinatus.**

infraversion /inˈfrəverˈzhən/ [L, *infra*, below + *vertere*, to turn], **1.** See **infraclusion. 2.** the downward deviation of one eye. **3.** conjugate downward rotation of both eyes. Also called **deorsumversion.**

infundibula. See **infundibulum.**

infundibular stalk /inˈfundibˈyələr/ [L, *infundibulum*, funnel; ME, *stalke*], an elongated funnel-shaped structure that connects the hypothalamus with the pituitary gland.

infundibulopelvic ligament, the suspensory ligament of the ovary.

infundibulum /inˈfundibˈyələm/ *pl. infundibula* [L, funnel], a funnel-shaped structure or passage, such as the cavity formed by the fimbriae tubae at the distal end of the fallopian tubes, the stalk that extends from the hypothalamus to the posterior lobe of the pituitary gland, or the passage connecting the middle meatus of the nose with the frontal sinus.

infundibulum of gallbladder, the tapering part of the gallbladder, ending at the neck.

infusate /infyoōˈsāt/, a parenteral fluid slowly introduced into a patient over a specific period.

infusate contamination, the introduction of pathogens into a sterile container, the contents of which are to be infused through a sterile setup with tubing into a patient's intravascular system during surgery or other procedures.

infused oil, a mixture comprised of the herb's volatile oils and another oil. The so-called carrier oil is used to extract an herb's volatile oils by soaking plant parts in it for a specified time period.

infusion /infyoōˈzhən/ [L, *in*, within, *fundere*, to pour], **1.** the introduction of a substance, such as a fluid, electrolyte, nutrient, or drug, directly into a vein or interstitially by means of gravity flow. Sterile techniques are maintained, the equipment is periodically checked for mechanical difficulties, and the patient is observed for swelling at the site of injection and for cardiac or respiratory difficulties. Compare **injection, instillation, insufflate. 2.** the substance introduced into the body by infusion. **3.** the steeping of a substance, such as an herb, to extract its medicinal properties. **4.** a liquid preparation made by pouring water over plant parts (such as dried or fresh leaves, flowers, fruits) and allowing the mixture to steep. Boiling water is usually used, but cold water may also be used. Making a cup of herbal tea is an example. *–infuse, v.*

infusion pump, an apparatus designed to deliver measured amounts of a drug or IV solution through IV injection over time. Some kinds of infusion pumps can be implanted surgically.

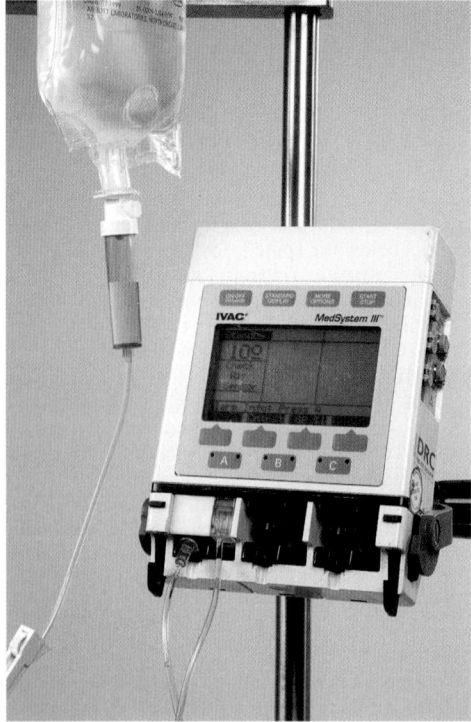

Local anesthetic infusion pump *(Courtesy Breg, Inc.)*

ingestion /injes″chən/ [L, *in,* within, *gerere,* to carry], the oral taking of substances into the body. The term is generally applied to both nutrients and medications.

ingrown hair [L, *in,* within; AS, *growen,* to grow, *haer*], a hair that fails to follow the normal follicle channel to the surface, with the free end becoming embedded in the skin. The hair then acts like a foreign body, and inflammation and suppuration follow.

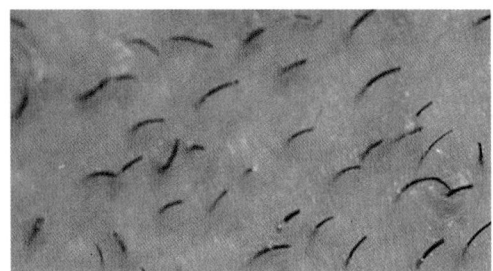

Ingrown hair *(du Vivier, 2002)*

ingrown toenail, a toenail whose distal lateral margin grows or is pressed into the skin of the toe, causing an inflammatory reaction. Granulation tissue may develop, and secondary infection is common. Treatment includes use of wider shoes, proper trimming of the nail, and various surgical procedures to narrow the nail or to reduce the size of the lateral nail fold.

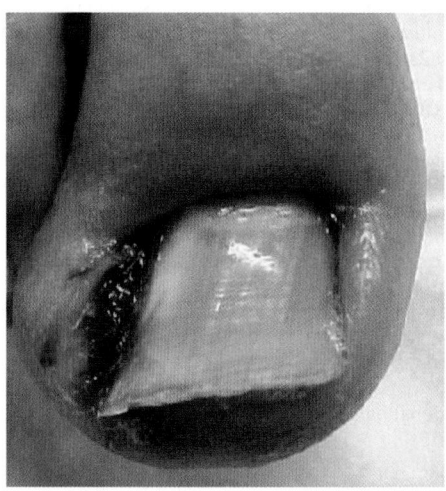

Ingrown toenail *(Marks and Miller, 2006)*

inguinal /ing″gwinəl/ [L, *inguen,* groin], pertaining to the groin.

inguinal canal, the tubular passage through the lower muscular layers of the abdominal wall that contains the spermatic cord in the male and the round ligament in the female. It is a common site for hernias.

inguinal falx, the inferior terminal portion of the common aponeurosis of the internal abdominal oblique and the transverse abdominis. It is inserted into the crest of the pubis, just below the superficial inguinal ring, and strengthens that part of the anterior abdominal wall. The width and the strength of the inguinal falx vary. Also called **conjoined tendon, falx inguinalis.**

inguinal hernia, a hernia in which a loop of intestine enters the inguinal canal. In a male it sometimes fills the scrotal sac. An inguinal hernia is usually repaired surgically to prevent the herniated segment from becoming strangulated, gangrenous, or obstructive, thereby blocking passage of waste through the bowel. Of all hernias, 75% to 80% are inguinal hernias. See also **hernia.**

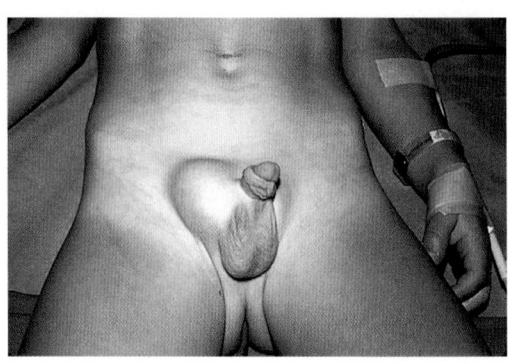

Inguinal hernia *(Brandt, 2008)*

inguinal ligament, a band of fibrous tissue that spans the gap between the anterior superior iliac spine and the pubic tubercle. Also called **crural ligament.**

inguinal node, any of the approximately 18 nodes in the group of lymph glands in the upper femoral triangle of the thigh. These nodes are divided into the superficial inguinal nodes and the subinguinal nodes. Compare **anterior tibial node, popliteal node.**

inguinal part of ductus deferens, a middle part of the ductus deferens, located within the inguinal canal.

inguinal region, the part of the abdomen surrounding the inguinal canal in the lower zone on both sides of the pubic region. Also called **iliac region.** See also **abdominal regions.**

inguinal ring, either of the two apertures of the inguinal canal, the internal end opening into the abdominal wall and the external end opening into the aponeurosis of the obliquus externus abdominis above the pubis.

inguinal ring, external, superficial inguinal ring.

inguinal ring, internal, deep inguinal ring.

inguinal triangle, a triangular area in the lower abdominal wall bounded laterally by the inferior epigastric artery, medially by the rectus abdominis muscle, and inferiorly by the inguinal ligament.

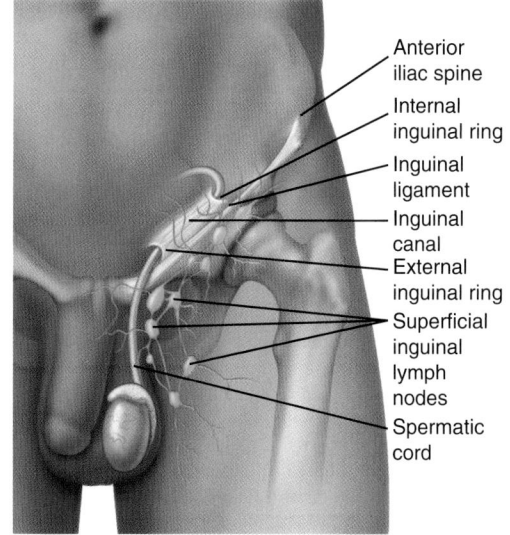

Structures of the inguinal region *(Harkreader, Hogan, and Thobaben, 2007)*

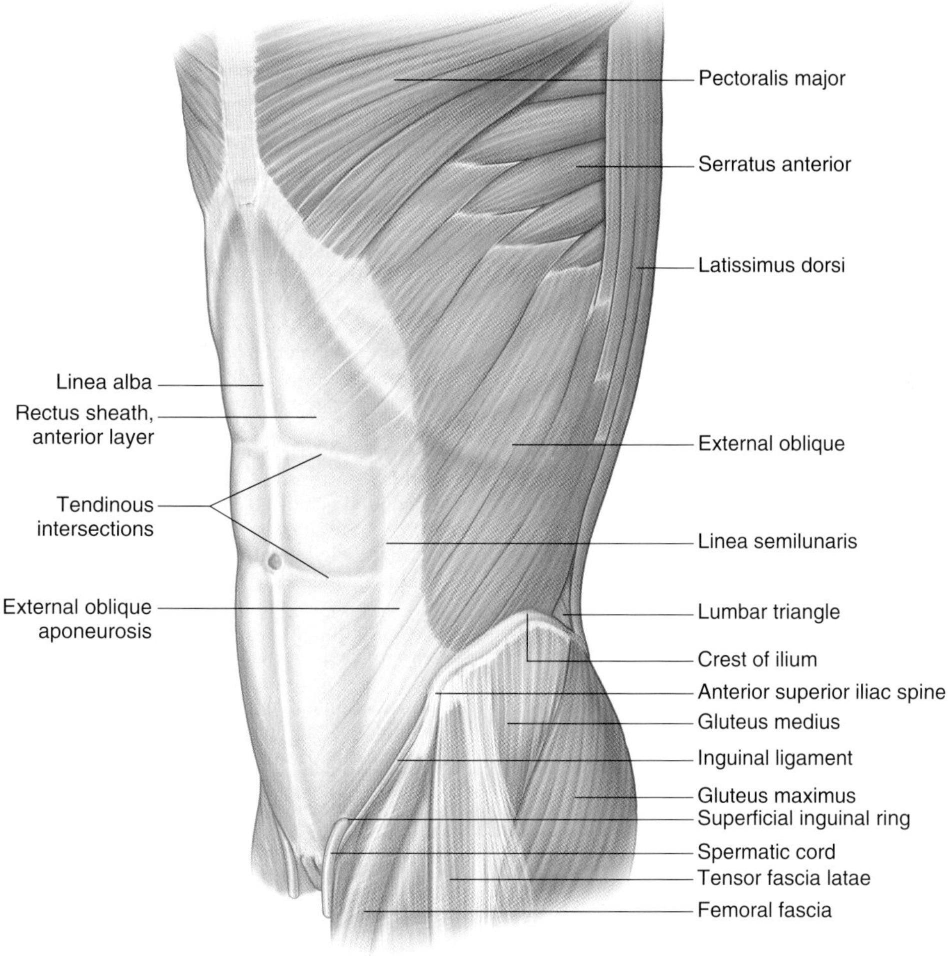

Superficial (external) inguinal ring and spermatic cord *(Standring, 2008)*

inguino-, combining form meaning "groin": *inguinocrural.*

inguinocrural hernia /ing′gwinōlkrōō″rəl/ [L, *inguen,* groin, *crus,* thigh, *hernia,* rupture], an intestinal outpouching that has turned outward from the inguinal canal into the folds of the groin. Also called **Holthouse hernia.**

INH, abbreviation for *isonicotinic acid hydrazide.* See **isoniazid.**

inhalant /inhā′lənt/, a substance introduced into the body by inhalation. It may be a medication, such as an aerosol administered in respiratory therapy, or a volatile chemical that is abused, such as toluene, used in glue sniffing.

inhalant abuse, the deliberate inhalation or sniffing of household products such as glue, gasoline, or aerosols for their psychoactive properties. Serious side effects are associated with the practice, and death is possible. See also **glue sniffing, huffing.**

inhalation, **1.** the drawing of air or other substances into the airways and lungs. See also **inspiration. 2.** any drug or solution of drugs administered (as by means of nebulizers or aerosols) by the nasal or oral respirator route.

inhalation administration of medication /in′həlā″shən/ [L, *in,* within, *halare,* to breathe], the administration of a drug by inspiration of the vapor released from a fragile ampule packed in a fine mesh that is crushed for immediate administration. Ammonia inhalants in first aid kits are often packaged in this fashion to be used in fainting episodes. The medication is absorbed into the circulation through the mucous membrane of the nasal passages. An increasing number of medications are being formulated as vaporized drugs, or V-drugs, that can be administered as fine nasal mist for a quicker onset of action. Medications may also be administered into the respiratory tract using inhalation therapy techniques. See also **inhalation therapy, respiratory therapy, V-drugs.**

inhalational challenge test, a type of challenge test done to determine reactivity to drugs or causative allergens in allergic asthma, in which a dilute concentrate of the suspected substance is inhaled and the patient is assessed for bronchial reactivity, which may be either early or late. Also called *inhalational challenge,* **bronchoprovocation inhalation test.**

inhalation anesthesia, anesthesia achieved by the inhalation of an anesthetic gas or a vapor. Although general anesthesia by inhalation has been used to permit surgical operations for over a century, the mechanism by which these anesthetics act is not completely understood. In adults, administration of an inhalation anesthetic is usually initiated during the induction phase of anesthesia after IV administration of a short-acting hypnotic drug, such as sodium pentothal, etomidate, or propofol. In pediatrics, inhalation anesthesia is often used to initiate anesthesia by using a mask induction with a nonpungent inhalational agent such as sevoflurane and nitrous oxide. The procedure may require endotracheal intubation or other methods of maintenance of airway patency and control. Among the principal inhalation anesthetics are nitrous oxide, desflurane, sevoflurane, and isoflurane.

inhalation anthrax. See **anthrax.**

inhalation injury, damage to the pulmonary parenchyma caused by inhalation of substances such as very hot air, toxic gas, asbestos, and chemical products of plastic manufacture.

inhalation therapy, a treatment in which a substance is introduced into the respiratory tract with inspired air. Oxygen, water, and various drugs may be administered by techniques of inhalation therapy. The goals of treatment are varied, such as improved strength of respiratory function in a bedridden patient, bronchodilation in an asthmatic patient, or liquefaction of mucus in a person with chronic obstructive lung disease.

inhalation toxicity, **1.** a severe neuromuscular disorder with symptoms like those of Parkinson disease, caused by prolonged inhalation of manganese dust. **2.** adverse effects from breathing in airborne particles of an irritating or poisonous substance.

inhale /inhāl′/ [L, *in,* within, *halare,* to breathe], to breathe in or to draw in with the breath. Also called **inspire.**

inhaler [L, *in* + *halare,* to breathe], a device for administering medications to be inhaled, such as vapors, fine powders, or volatile substances. An inhaler also may be designed to administer anesthetic gases.

in-hand manipulation, moving objects within the hand.

inherent /inhir″ənt/ [L, *inhaerere,* to cling to], inborn, innate; natural to an environment. Compare **indigenous.**

inherent rate, the frequency of impulse formation attributed to a given pacemaker location within the heart. The following rates are representative of the adult heart: sinus node, 60 to 100 beats/min; atrioventricular junction, 40 to 60 beats/min; ventricle, 15 to 40 beats/min. In adults a rate above 100 beats/min is normal during exercise, exertion, strong emotion, or pain. Most clinicians are alert to possible problems when the sinus rate is greater than 90 beats/min and are not concerned unless it drops to less than 50 beats/min. In children the normal sinus rate is higher, decreasing as the age of the child increases.

inheritance /inher′itəns/ [L, *in,* within, *hereditare,* to inherit], **1.** the acquisition or expression of traits or conditions by transmission of genetic material from parents to offspring. **2.** the sum of the genetic qualities or traits transmitted from parents to offspring; the total genetic makeup of a fertilized ovum. Kinds include **alternative inheritance, amphigenous inheritance, autosomal inheritance, blending inheritance, codominant inheritance, complemental inheritance, crisscross inheritance, cytoplasmic inheritance, holandric inheritance, hologynic inheritance, homochronous inheritance, maternal inheritance, monofactorial inheritance, multifactorial inheritance, supplemental inheritance, X-linked inheritance.** —*inherited, adj.,* —*inherit, v.*

inherited disorder /inher″itid/, any disease or condition that is genetically determined and involves a single gene mutation, a multifactorial inheritance, or a chromosomal aberration. Also called **genetic disorder, hereditary disorder.**

inherited trait [L, *in,* within, *hereditare,* to inherit; Fr, *trait,* a draft], a distinguishing quality or characteristic that is transmitted genetically from one generation to the next.

inhibin /inhib″in/, a gonadal hormone that inhibits activity of the follicle-stimulating hormone secreted by the anterior pituitary gland.

inhibiting gene /inhib″iting/ [L, *inhibere,* to restrain; Gk, *genein,* to produce], a gene that prevents the expression of another gene. See also **epistasis.**

inhibiting hormone. See **hormone.**

inhibition /in′hibish″ən/ [L, *inhibere,* to restrain], **1.** (in psychology) the unconscious restraint of a behavioral process, usually resulting from the social or cultural forces of the environment; the condition inducing such restraint. **2.** (in psychoanalysis) the process in which the superego prevents the conscious expression of an unconscious instinctual drive, thought, or urge. **3.** (in physiology) the restraint, checking, or arrest of the action of an organ or cell or the reduction of a physiological activity by antagonistic stimulation. **4.** (in chemistry) the stopping or slowing of the rate of a chemical reaction. Formerly called **negative catalysis.**

inhibition assay, an immunoassay in which an excess of antigens prevents or inhibits the completion of either the initial or the indicator phase of the reaction.

inhibition of reflexes [L, *inhibere,* to restrain, *reflectere,* to bend back], **1.** the prevention of a reflex action, requiring a series of biochemical mechanisms to restrict the flow of excitatory impulses at presynaptic and postsynaptic points in the system. **2.** a negative reflex effect that may become established during differential conditioning. The negative conditioned reflex represents an inhibition of a conditioned reflex.

inhibitor /inhib″itər/, a drug or other agent that prevents or restricts a certain action.

inhibitor of apoptosis protein (IAP), any of a class of proteins that play a regulatory role in cell death in many species by inhibiting caspase activity, which in turn blocks apoptosis. Such proteins are also expressed abnormally in many tumors.

inhibitory /inhib″itôr′ē/ [L, *inhibere,* to restrain], tending to stop or slow a process, such as a neuron that suppresses the intensity of a nerve impulse. Compare **induce.**

inhibitory enzyme [L, *inhibere,* to restrain; Gk, *en,* within; *zyme,* ferment], an enzyme that blocks rather than catalyzes a chemical reaction.

inio-, prefix meaning "the occiput": *inion.*

inion /in″ē·on/ [Gk]. See **external occipital protuberance.**

initial contact stance stage /inish″əl/ [L, *initium,* beginning, *contigere,* to touch], one of the five stages in the stance phase of walking or gait, specifically associated with the moment when the foot touches the ground or floor and the leg prepares to accept the weight of the body. The initial contact stance stage figures in the diagnoses of many abnormal orthopedic conditions and is often correlated with electromyographic studies of the muscles used in walking, such as the pretibial muscle and the gluteus maximus. Compare **loading response stance stage, midstance, preswing stance stage, terminal stance.** See also **swing phase of gait.**

initial lesion. See **primary lesion.**

initiation codon /inish″ē·ā″shən kō″don/ [L, *initium,* beginning, *caudex,* book], the triplet of nucleotides, usually adenine-uracil-guanine (AUG) or, in some cases, guanine-uracil-guanine (GUG), that in eukaryotes and archea code for methionine and in bacteria code for formylmethionine, the first amino acids in all protein sequences. Also called *initiator codon,* **start codon.**

initiator /inish″ē·ā″tər/, a cocarcinogenic factor that causes a usually irreversible genetic mutation in a normal cell and primes it for uncontrolled growth. Kinds include **radiation, aflatoxins, nitrosamines,** *urethane.*

initiator-contributor role, (in occupational therapy) a role assumed by a therapist in which the therapist suggests goals or shares ideas on how to solve problems or accomplish specific tasks.

inject. See **injection.**

injectable contraceptive /injek″təbəl/, medroxyprogesterone acetate, a progestin used as a contraceptive, administered intramuscularly at a dose sufficient to prevent ovulation. The muscle into which the hormone is injected serves as a depot from which the hormone is slowly released so that injections need to be given only every 3 months. This is a very convenient and highly effective method of contraception.

injection /injek″shən/ [L, *in,* within, *jacere,* to throw], **1.** the act of forcing a liquid into the body by means of a needle and syringe. Injections are designated according to the anatomical site involved; the most common are intraarterial, intradermal, intramuscular, intravenous, and subcutaneous. Parenteral injections are usually given for therapeutic reasons, although they may be used diagnostically. Sterile technique is maintained. Compare **infusion, instillation, insufflate. 2.** the substance injected. **3.** redness and swelling observed in the physical examination of a part of the body, caused by dilation of the blood vessels secondary to an inflammatory or infectious process. **–inject,** *v.*

injection cap, a rubber diaphragm under a plastic cap. It permits needle insertion into a catheter or vial.

injection technique. See **intradermal injection, intramuscular injection, intrathecal injection, intravenous injection, subcutaneous injection.**

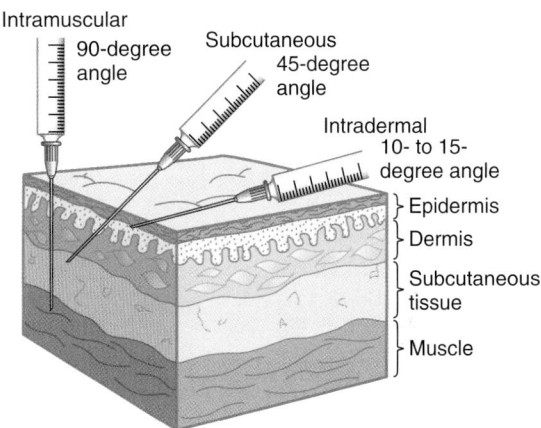

Different angles of insertion for injection *(Bonewit-West, 2012)*

injunction /injungk″shən/ [L, *injungere,* to enjoin], a court order that prevents a party from performing a specified act.

injury severity score (ISS), an evaluation system developed to predict the outcomes of traumas, including mortality and length of hospital stay. See also **Glasgow Coma Scale.**

inlay /in′lā/ [L, *in,* within; AS, *lecan,* lay], **1.** material, such as bone or skin, inserted into a tissue defect. **2.** (in dentistry) a restoration made outside of a tooth to correspond with the form of a prepared cavity and then cemented into the tooth. An inlay is placed within the cusps of posterior teeth. Compare **onlay.**

inlay splint [L, *in,* within; AS, *lecan,* lay], a casting for fixing or supporting one or more approximating teeth. It is composed of either a single casting or two or more inlays soldered together.

inlet [L, *in,* within; ME, *leten*], a passage leading into a cavity, such as the pelvic inlet that marks the brim of the pelvic cavity.

inlet contraction. See **contraction.**

in loco parentis /in lō″kō pəren″tis/ [L, in the parents' place], the assumption by a person or institution of the parental obligations of caring for a child without adoption.

innate /in″āt, ināt′/ [L, *innatus,* inborn], **1.** existing in or belonging to a person from birth; inborn; hereditary; congenital. **2.** a natural and essential characteristic of something or someone; inherent. **3.** originating in or produced by the intellect or the mind.

innate immunity, also called **natural immunity.** See **immune response.**

inner cell mass [AS, *innera,* within; L, *cella,* storeroom, *massa,* lump], a cluster of cells localized at the animal pole of the blastocyst of placental mammals from which the embryo develops. Also called **cell mass.** See also **trophoblast.**

inner ear, the complex inner structure of the ear, containing receptors for hearing and balance. The maculae and crystae cells help maintain equilibrium; the organ of Corti cells translate sound vibrations into impulses for the sense of hearing. The auditory receptor cells are innervated by the cochlear nerve. Also called **internal ear, labyrinth.** Compare **external ear, middle ear.**

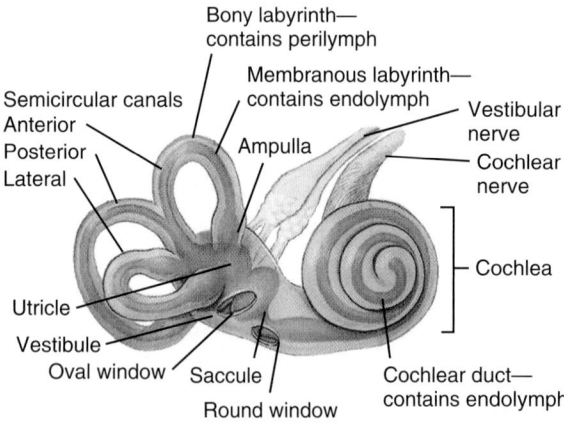

Bony labyrinth—
contains perilymph
Membranous labyrinth—
contains endolymph
Semicircular canals
Anterior
Posterior
Lateral
Ampulla
Vestibular nerve
Cochlear nerve
Cochlea
Utricle
Vestibule
Oval window
Saccule
Round window
Cochlear duct—
contains endolymph

Inner ear *(Applegate, 2011)*

inner layer of glomerular capsule, the visceral layer of glomerular capsule.

innervate /in″ərvāt/ [L, *in + nervus*], to supply a body part or organ with nerves or nervous stimuli.

innervation /in′ərvā″shən/ [L, *in,* within, *nervus,* nerve], the distribution or supply of nerve fibers or nerve impulses to a body part. –**innervate,** *v.*

innervation apraxia. See **motor apraxia.**

inner zone of renal medulla, the part of the renal medulla farthest in from the cortex, containing the innermost part of the loop of Henle and medullary collecting tubule.

innidation. See **nidation.**

innocent /in″əsənt/ [L, *innocens,* harmless], benign, innocuous, or functional, such as an innocent heart murmur.

innocuous /inok″yo͞o·əs/ [L, *innocuus,* harmless], pertaining to use of a substance or procedure that causes no ill effects.

innominate /inom″ināt/ [L, *innominatum,* nameless], without a name or unnamed. The term is traditionally applied to certain anatomical structures, often identified by their descriptive name, such as the hip bone and brachiocephalic artery.

innominate artery, one of the three arteries branching from the arch of the aorta, running about 5 cm from the level of the cranial border of the second right costal cartilage; ascending cranially, dorsally, and obliquely to the right; and dividing into the right common carotid and the right subclavian arteries. Also called **brachiocephalic artery, brachiocephalic trunk.**

innominate bone, the hip bone. It consists of the ilium, ischium, and pubis and unites with the sacrum and coccyx to form the pelvis. Also called **os coxae.**

innominate substance, a region of the forebrain that lies ventral to the anterior half of the lentiform nucleus. It contains the basal forebrain, which receives afferent input from the reticular formation, hypothalamus, and limbic cortex. Also called **substantia innominata.**

innominate vein, a large vein on either side of the neck that is formed by the union of the internal jugular and subclavian veins. The two veins drain blood from the head, neck, and upper extremities and unite to form the superior vena cava. Also called **brachiocephalic vein.**

Inocor, a cardiac inotropic drug. Brand name for **inamrinone lactate.**

inocula, innoculant. See **inoculum.**

inoculation /inok″yəlāshən/ [L, *inoculare,* to graft], the introduction of a substance (inoculum) into the body to produce or to increase immunity to the disease or condition associated with the substance. It is performed by making multiple scratches in the skin after placement of a drop of the substance on the skin, by puncture of the skin with an implement bearing multiple short tines, or by intradermal, subcutaneous, or intramuscular injection. Inoculation can also be intranasal or oral. –*inoculate, v.*

inoculum /inok″yo͞oləm/ *pl. inocula* [L, *inoculare,* to graft], a substance introduced into the body to cause or to increase immunity to a specific disease or condition. It may be a toxin; a live, attenuated, or killed virus or bacterium; or an immune serum. Also called *inoculant.* See also **immune system.**

inoperable /inop″ərəbəl/ [L, *in + operari,* to work], pertaining to a medical condition that would not benefit from surgical intervention or for which the risk outweighs the benefits.

inorganic /in′ôrgan″ik/ [L, *in,* not; Gk, *organikos,* natural], (in chemistry) pertaining to a chemical compound that is not primarily based on or derived from hydrocarbons.

inorganic acid, a compound containing no carbon that is composed of hydrogen and one or more electronegative elements, such as chlorine. Kinds include **hydrochloric acid.**

inorganic chemistry, the study of the properties and reactions of all chemical elements and compounds other than hydrocarbons or their derivatives.

inorganic dust, dry, finely powdered particles of an inorganic substance, especially dust, which, when inhaled, can cause abnormal conditions of the lungs. See also **anthracosis, asbestosis, berylliosis, pneumoconiosis, silicosis.**

inorganic phosphorus, phosphorus that may be measured in the blood as phosphate ions. Its increased concentration may indicate bone, kidney, or glandular disease; decreased concentration may be associated with alcoholism, vitamin deficiency, and other problems. Normal concentrations in the serum of adults are 1.8 to 2.6 mEq/L. See also **phosphorus.**

inoscopy, microscopic examination of the fibers or fibrinous matter of the sputum, blood, effusions, or other biological material. Also called **fibrinoscopy.**

inosine /in″əsēn, -sīn/, a nucleoside derived from animal tissue, especially intestines, originally used in food processing and flavoring. It has been used in the treatment of cardiac disorders and is now under investigation in studies of cancer and virus chemotherapy. See also **inosiplex.**

inosiplex /inō″sipleks/, a form of inosine that acts as a stimulator of the immune system. It is currently under investigation for use in cancer therapy, in the treatment of herpesvirus and rhinovirus infections, and in immune restoration in preAIDS patients. Also called **methisoprinol.**

inositol /inō″sətōl, inos″-/, an isomer of glucose that occurs widely in plant and animal cells. Although inositol has no current therapeutic use, it is an essential cell constituent.

inotropic /in″ōtrop″ik/ [Gk, *inos,* fiber, *trope,* turning], pertaining to the force or energy of muscular contractions, particularly those of the heart. An inotropic agent increases myocardial contractility.

inotropic agent, 1. a substance that influences the force of muscular contractions. 2. an agent that increases the force of muscular contractions of the heart.

inpatient /in″pāshənt/ [L, *in,* within, *patior,* to suffer], 1. *n.,* a patient who has been admitted to a hospital or other health care facility for at least an overnight stay. 2. *adj.,* pertaining to the treatment or care of such a patient or to a health care facility to which a patient may be admitted for 24-hour care. Compare **outpatient.**

inpatient care unit, a hospital unit organized for the provision of medical and nursing services to a group of inpatients. Units are usually grouped according to diagnosis or other common characteristics, such as maternity or surgical patients.

input, the information or material that enters or is manually entered, for example, with a keyboard.

input device [L, *in,* within; ME, *putten,* to place], an implement that allows for the entry of commands or information for processing in a form acceptable to a computer, often from a peripheral, such as a mouse, keyboard, tape drive, disk drive, microphone, or light pen.

inquest /in″kwest/ [L, *in,* within, *quaerere,* to seek], a legal inquiry or examination.

INR, abbreviation for **International Normalized Ratio.**

insane /insān″/ [L, *in,* not, *sanus,* sound], a legal term describing unsound, diseased, or deranged mental functioning, particularly as it pertains to a person who is unable to provide adequate self-care if there is a need to protect the patient and the public from each other. In the United States the precise definition of this legal term varies from state to state.

insanity /insan″itē/ [L, *in,* not, *sanus,* sound], *(Informal)* a term used more in legal and social situations than in health care. It refers to those mental illnesses that are of such a serious or debilitating nature as to interfere with one's capability of functioning within the legal limits of society and performing the normal activities of daily living.

insatiable /insā″shē·əbəl/ [L, *insatiatus,* not satisfied], pertaining to an appetite for food or other needs that cannot be satisfied.

insect bite [L, *in,* within, *secare,* to cut], the bite of any parasitic or venomous arthropod such as a louse, flea, mite, tick, or arachnid. Many arthropods inject venom that produces poisoning or severe local reaction, saliva that may contain viruses, or substances that produce mild irritation. The degree of irritation produced by an insect's bite is affected by the design and shape of its mouth parts: A horsefly, for example, makes a short lateral and coarse wound whereas a tick takes hold with its backward curved teeth, making its removal difficult. Spiders inflict a sharp pinprick bite that may remain unnoticed until the injected venom has begun to produce a painful reaction. Treatment of a bite depends on the species of insect, the reaction to the bite, and the risk of sequelae from it. First aid treatment is generally symptomatic and includes ice or cold packs, careful cleaning of the wound, and antihistamines or specific antivenin as necessary.

insecticide /insek″tisīd/, a chemical agent that kills insects.

insecticide poisoning. See **chlorinated organic insecticide poisoning.**

insemination /insem′inā″shən/, the injection of semen into the vagina. It may involve an artificial process unrelated to sexual intercourse.

insenescence /in′sines″əns/ [L, *insenescere,* to begin to grow old], 1. the process of aging. 2. the state of being chronologically old but retaining the vitality of a young person.

insensible /insen″sibəl/ [L, *in* + *sentire,* to feel], 1. pertaining to a person who is unconscious for any reason. 2. pertaining to a person who is apathetic or deprived of normal sense perceptions.

insensible perspiration [L, *in,* not, *sentire,* to feel, *per,* through, *spirare,* to breathe], the loss of body fluid by evaporation, such as normally occurs during respiration. A small amount of perspiration is continually excreted by the sweat glands in the skin. The portion that evaporates before it may be observed also contributes to insensible perspiration. Also called **insensible water loss.**

insensible water loss, the amount of fluid lost on a daily basis from the lungs, skin, respiratory tract, and water excreted in the feces. The exact amount cannot be measured, but it is estimated to be between 40 and 600 mL in an adult under normal circumstances.

insertion /insur″shən/ [L, *inserere,* to introduce], (in anatomy) the place of attachment, such as that of a muscle to the bone it moves.

insertion forceps. See **point forceps.**

insertion site, the point in a vein where a needle or catheter is inserted.

inservice education [L, *in,* within, *servus,* a slave, *educare,* to rear], a program of instruction or training provided by an agency or institution for its employees. The program is held in the institution or agency and is intended to increase the skills and competence of the employees in a specific area. Inservice education may be a part of any program of staff development. See also **staff development, def. 1.**

insheathed /inshēthd″/ [L, *in,* within; AS, *scaeth,* sheath], enclosed within a sheath.

insidious /insid″ē·əs/ [L, *insidiosus,* cunning], describing a development that is gradual, subtle, or imperceptible. Certain chronic diseases, such as glaucoma, can develop insidiously with symptoms that are not detected by the patient until the disorder is established. Compare **acute.**

insight /in″sīt/ [L, *in,* within; AS, *gesihth,* sight], 1. the capacity for comprehending the true nature of a situation or for penetrating an underlying truth. 2. an instance of penetrating or comprehending an underlying truth, primarily through intuitive understanding. 3. (in psychology) a type of self-understanding encompassing both intellectual and emotional awareness of the unconscious nature, origin, and mechanisms of one's attitudes, feelings, and behavior. It is one of the most important goals of psychotherapy and, with integration, leads to modification of maladaptive behavioral patterns. See also **integration.**

insipid /insip″id/ [L, *in* + *sapidus,* savory], dull, tasteless, or lifeless.

in situ /in sī″too, sit″oo/ [L, *in,* within, *situs,* position], 1. in the natural or usual place. 2. describing a cancer that has not metastasized or invaded neighboring tissues, such as carcinoma in situ.

insoluble /insol″yəbəl/ [L, *in,* not, *solubilis,* soluble], unable to be dissolved, usually in a specific solvent, such as a substance that is insoluble in water.

insoluble fiber, fiber that is not soluble in water, composed mainly of lignin, cellulose, and hemicelluloses and primarily found in the bran layers of cereal grains. Its actions include increasing fecal bulk and decreasing free radicals in the GI tract.

insomnia /insom″nē·ə/ [L, *in,* not, *somnus,* sleep], chronic inability to sleep or to remain asleep throughout the night;

wakefulness; sleeplessness. Insomnia may be the symptom of a psychiatric disorder.

insomniac /insom″nē·ak/, **1.** *n.,* a person with insomnia. **2.** *adj.,* pertaining to, causing, or associated with insomnia. **3.** *adj.,* characteristic of or occurring during a period of sleeplessness.

inspiration /in′spirā″shən/ [L, *inspirare,* to breathe in], the act of drawing air into the lungs. The major muscle of inspiration is the diaphragm, the contraction of which creates a reduced pressure in the chest, causing the lungs to expand and air to flow inward. Accessory inspiratory muscles include the external intercostals, scaleni, scapular elevators, and sternocleidomastoids. Since expiration is usually a passive process, these muscles of inspiration alone produce normal respiration. Lungs at maximal inspiration have an average total capacity of 5.5 to 6 L of air. Also called **inhalation.** Compare **expiration.** See also **inspiratory reserve volume. –inspiratory,** *adj.*

inspiratory /inspī″rətôr′ē/ [L, to breathe in], pertaining to inspiration.

inspiratory capacity (IC), the maximum volume of gas that can be inhaled from the end of a resting exhalation. Equal to the sum of the tidal volume and the inspiratory reserve volume, it is measured with a spirometer.

inspiratory dyspnea [L, *inspirare,* to breathe in; Gk, *dys,* without, *pnoia,* breath], a form of breathing difficulty caused by an obstruction in the larynx, trachea, or bronchi.

The patient attempts to compensate for this deficiency with prolonged, deep inspirations.

inspiratory gas flow rate, the amount of gas delivered per minute to a patient's lungs by mechanical ventilation.

inspiratory hold, either of two kinds of modification in an inhalation produced by intermittent positive-pressure breathing: (1) a pressure hold, in which a preset pressure is reached and held for a designated period, or (2) a volume hold, in which a predetermined volume is delivered and then held for a designated period.

inspiratory muscle fatigue, weakness or exhaustion of the muscles that produce inspiration, resulting in a condition of threatened acute respiratory failure.

inspiratory reserve volume (IRV), the maximum volume of gas that can be inhaled beyond a normal resting inspiration.

inspiratory resistance muscle training, exercises that require inhalation against some type of resisting force. An example of such training is abdominal breathing practice with the Pflex or threshold inspiratory muscle trainer. The amount of resistance is gradually increased over several weeks of abdominal muscle training. Resistance may also be used against expansion of the rib cage by the intercostal musculature during inspiration. The resistance may be provided by a therapist pushing against the ribs or by applying a belt or swathe tightly about the costal margin.

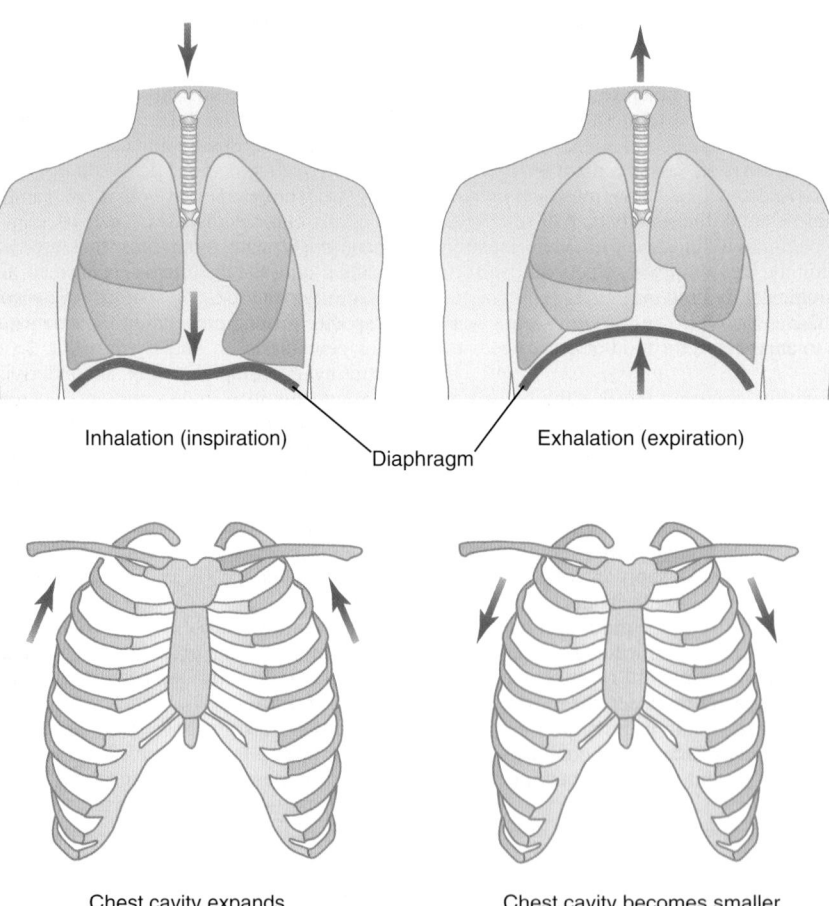

Inhalation (inspiration)　　Exhalation (expiration)

Diaphragm

Chest cavity expands　　Chest cavity becomes smaller

Inspiration *(Bonewit-West, 2015)*

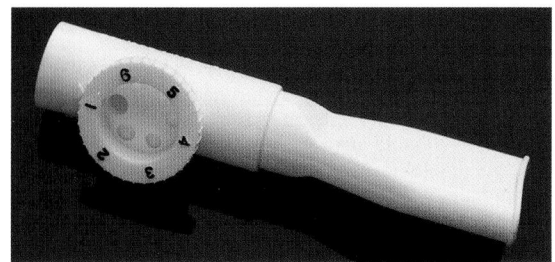

Inspiratory muscle trainer *(Courtesy Philips Respironics, Inc.)*

inspiratory waveform, one of several flow patterns during inspiration associated with mechanical ventilation. These patterns include a square wave, in which the inspiratory flow rises rapidly to a preset level and stays at that level until expiration begins; a sinusoidal wave, in which the flow gradually increases and decreases throughout inspiration; and a descending ramp wave, in which the flow increases very rapidly and then decreases gradually until the end of inspiration. The last pattern is most similar to normal breathing.

inspire. See **inhale.**

inspirometer /in′spirom″ətər/ [L, *inspirare,* to breathe in; Gk, *metron,* measure], an apparatus used to measure the volume, force, and frequency of a patient's inspirations.

inspissate /inspis″āt/ [L, *inspissare,* to thicken], (of a fluid) to thicken or harden through the absorption or evaporation of liquid, such as milk in an inspissated milk duct. −*inspissation, n.*

instillation /in′stilā″shən/ [L, *instillare,* to drip], **1.** a procedure in which a fluid is slowly introduced into a cavity or passage of the body and allowed to remain for a specific length of time before being drained or withdrawn. It is performed to expose the tissues of the area to the solution, to warmth or cold, or to a drug or substance in the solution. **2.** a solution so introduced. Compare **infusion, injection, insufflate.** −*instill, v.*

instinct /in″stingkt/ [L, *impulse*], a genetic predisposition to act without thought and in an automatic fashion in certain situations, particularly those that preserve or protect life.

instinctive reflex. See **unconditioned response.**

institutionalism syndrome /in′stityoo″shənəliz′əm/, a condition characterized by apathy, withdrawal, submissiveness, and lack of initiative. A patient with this syndrome may resist leaving a hospital, even when the surroundings are barely adequate, because it is familiar and predictable and demands are minimal.

institutionalize /in′stityoo″shənəliz′/ [L, *instituere,* to put in place], to place a person in an institution for psychological or physical treatment or for the protection of the person or society. −*institutionalized, adj.,* −*institutionalization, n.*

institutional review board (IRB), an organizational committee that reviews and approves biomedical research that uses humans as subjects.

instrument /in″strəmənt/ [L, *instrumentum,* tool], a surgical tool or device designed to perform a specific function, such as cutting, dissecting, grasping, holding, retracting, or suturing. Surgical instruments are usually made of steel and are specially treated to be durable, heat-resistant, rust-resistant, and stainproof. Kinds include **clamp, needle holder, retractor, speculum.**

instrumental activities of daily living (IADL) /in′strəmen″təl/, activities that support life within the home and community and that often require more complex interactions than those used in a category called activities for daily living, or

ADL. IADL include care of others, care of pets, child rearing, communication management, driving and community mobility, financial management, health management and maintenance, home establishment and management, meal preparation and cleanup, religious and spiritual activities, implementation of safety and emergency precautions, and shopping. Compare **activities of daily living.**

instrumental conditioning. See **operant conditioning.**

instrumental labor [L, *instrumentum,* tool, *labor,* work], child delivery in which the use of instruments, such as forceps or perforators, is required.

instrumentation /in′strəmentā″shən/, the use of sensors and medical devices for treatment and diagnosis.

insufficiency /in′səfish″ənsē/ [L, *in,* not, *sufficere,* to be adequate], inability to perform a necessary function adequately. Kinds include **adrenal insufficiency, aortic insufficiency, pulmonary insufficiency,** *valvular insufficiency.*

insufficient sleep syndrome /in′səfish″ənt/, a neurological disorder in which individuals persistently fail to obtain enough sleep to support normal wakefulness.

insufflate /in″səflāt, insuf′lāt/ [L, *insufflare,* to blow into], to blow a gas or powder into a tube, cavity, or organ to allow visual examination, to remove an obstruction, or to apply medication. See also **Rubin's test.** −*insufflation, n.*

insufflator /in″səflā′tər/ [L, *insufflare,* to blow into], an apparatus used to blow air or gas into a body cavity.

insul-, prefix meaning "island" or "island-shaped": *insulation, insulin, insulinoma.*

insulation /in′səlā″shən/, a nonconducting substance that offers a barrier to the passage of heat or electricity.

insulin /in″səlin/ [L, *insula,* island], **1.** a naturally occurring polypeptide hormone secreted by the beta cells of the islets of Langerhans in the pancreas in response to increased levels of glucose in the blood as well as to the parasympathetic nervous system and other stimuli. The hormone acts to regulate the metabolism of glucose and the processes necessary for the intermediary metabolism of fats, carbohydrates, and proteins. Insulin lowers the blood glucose level and promotes transport of glucose into the muscle cells and other tissues. Inadequate secretion of insulin causes elevated blood glucose and triglyceride levels and ketonemia, as well as the characteristic signs of diabetes mellitus, including increased desire to eat, excessive thirst, increased urination, and eventually lethargy and weight loss. Uncorrected severe deficiency of insulin is incompatible with life. Normal findings of insulin assay in adults are levels of 5 to 24 mmU/mL. **2.** a pharmacological preparation of the hormone administered in treating diabetes mellitus. The various preparations of insulin available for prescription vary in onset, intensity, and duration of action. Animal source insulins, pork and beef, have been discontinued in the U.S. market. Human insulin is derived by recombinant DNA technology and is termed quick acting, intermediate acting, or long acting. Most replacement insulin is given by subcutaneous injection in individualized dosage schedules and insulin pumps, but insulin also can be replaced intravenously. Adverse reactions include hypoglycemia and insulin shock that result from excess dosage and hyperglycemia and diabetic ketoacidosis from inadequate dosage. Fever, stress, infection, pregnancy, surgery, and hyperthyroidism may significantly increase insulin requirements; liver disease, hypothyroidism, vomiting, and renal disease may decrease them. Blood tests for glucose and ketones are performed to determine the need for adjustment of the dosage or of the schedule of administration. See also **human insulin.**

insulin allergy, a hypersensitivity reaction to insulin, usually a reaction to its protein components. More purified

Insulins

Type	Description	Effect on blood glucose (hours after administration)		
		Onset	Peak	Duration
Ultra-short acting	Clear	15 min	1 hr	4 to 5 hr
Short acting				
Regulate (crystalline zinc)	Clear	30 to 60 min	2 to 4 hr	6 to 8 hr
Semilente (SL)	Cloudy: amorphous insulin zinc suspension, no protamine	1 hr	4 to 6 hr	12 to 16 hr
Intermediate acting				
NPH	Cloudy: crystalline zinc insulin suspension, 50% saturated with protamine	2 to 3 hr	8 to 12 hr	18 to 24 hr
Lente	Cloudy: mixture 30% SL + 70% UL, no protamine	2 to 3 hr	8 to 12 hr	18 to 24 hr
Long acting				
PZI	Cloudy: excess protamine	6 hr	14 to 20 hr	24 to 36 hr
Ultralente (UL)	Cloudy: crystalline insulin suspension, high zinc content, no protamine	6 hr	16 to 18 hr	30 to 36 hr

insulins have now been developed that are less likely to cause an allergic reaction and other complications. Human insulin, prepared by recombinant genetic engineering, eliminates many problems associated with repeated insulin injections because of reduced antibody concentrations.

insulin antibody test, a blood test used to detect the presence of insulin antibodies, which develop in nearly all patients treated with exogenous insulin. These antibodies may reduce the amount of insulin available for glucose metabolism and may contribute to insulin resistance. See also **blood glucose test, fasting plasma glucose.**

insulinase, an enzyme that inactivates insulin.

insulin aspart, a rapid-acting analog of human insulin created by recombinant DNA technology, in which an aspartate residue has been substituted for the usual proline at position 28 on the insulin B chain. It is administered subcutaneously for the treatment of diabetes mellitus.

insulin assay, a blood test used to diagnose insulinoma (tumor of the islets of Langerhans) and to evaluate patients with fasting hypoglycemia. It is often combined with a fasting plasma glucose test to increase its diagnostic value.

insulin-dependent diabetes mellitus. See **type 1 diabetes mellitus.**

insulinemia /in′səlinēmē·ə/ [L, *insula,* island; Gk, *haima,* blood], an abnormally high level of insulin in the blood.

insulin glargine, an analog of human insulin produced by recombinant DNA technology, differing from human insulin in that the asparagine at position A21 is replaced by glycine and two arginines are added to the C-terminus of the B-chain. It is administered subcutaneously for once-daily insulin replacement therapy.

insulin human zinc suspension, an intermediate-acting insulin consisting of a sterile suspension of human insulin in buffered water with the addition of a suitable zinc salt such that the solid phase of the suspension contains a 7:3 ratio of crystalline to amorphous insulin. It is administered subcutaneously.

insulin injection sites, body tissue areas that allow optimal use of subcutaneous injections of insulin. The choice of sites can affect the rate of absorption and peak action times, but repeated use of the same injection site can lead to localized tissue damage, resulting in malabsorption of insulin. These problems are minimized by systematic rotation of injection sites within the selected anatomical area.

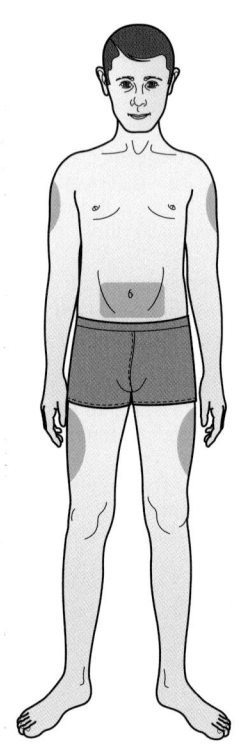

■ **Injection sites** – check for lipohypertrophy or lipoatrophy

Insulin injection sites for children (Lissauer, Clayden, and Craft, 2012)

insulin-like growth factor (IGF), hormones that stimulate protein synthesis and sulfation. IGF I and II play a role in uterine and placental growth and early fetal growth during pregnancy. Also called **somatomedin C.**

insulin lipodystrophy [L, *insula,* island; Gk, *lipos,* fat; *dys,* bad, *trophe,* nourishment], the loss of local fat deposits in patients with diabetes as a complication of repeated insulin injections into the same subcutaneous tissue.

insulin lispro, a pancreatic hormone.

■ INDICATIONS: It is used to treat ketoacidosis types I and II and types 1 and 2 diabetes mellitus.

■ CONTRAINDICATIONS: Known hypersensitivity to this drug or to protamine prohibits its use.

■ ADVERSE EFFECTS: Anaphylaxis is a life-threatening effect of this drug. Other adverse effects include blurred vision, dry mouth, flushing, rash, urticaria, warmth, lipohypertrophy, swelling, redness, and rebound hyperglycemia (the Somogyi effect). Lipodystrophy and hypoglycemia are common side effects.

insulinogenic /in′səlin′ōjen″ik/ [L, *insula* + Gk, *genein,* to produce], promoting the production and release of insulin by the islets of Langerhans in the pancreas.

insulinoma /in′səlinō″mə/ *pl. insulinomas, insulinomata* [L, *insula* + Gk, *oma,* tumor], a tumor, often benign, arising from the insulin-secreting cells of the islets of Langerhans or the ductular/acinar system of the pancreas. The most common symptom is hypoglycemia due to overproduction of insulin. Surgical resection of the tumor may be possible, thus limiting the development of hypoglycemic episodes. Also called **insuloma, islet cell adenoma.** Compare **islet cell tumor.**

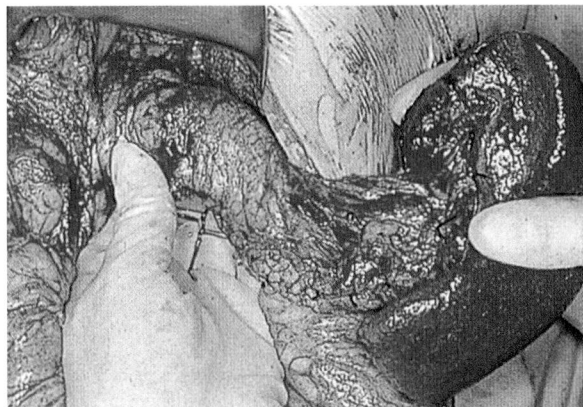

Insulinoma *(Greig and Garden, 1996)*

insulin pump [L, *insula,* island; ME, *pumpe*], a portable battery-powered instrument that delivers a measured amount of insulin to the layer of fat under the skin, typically located on the abdominal wall. It can be programmed to deliver varied doses of insulin according to the body's needs at the time.

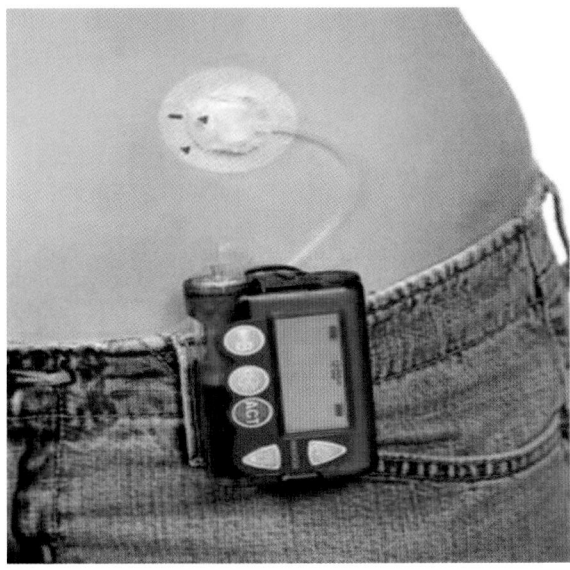

Insulin pump *(Kerr and Partridge, 2011)*

insulin reaction, the adverse effects caused by excessive levels of circulating insulin, causing hypoglycemia. See also **hyperinsulinism.**

insulin rebound, extreme fluctuations in blood glucose levels as a result of overreaction of the body's homeostatic feedback mechanisms for control of glucose metabolism. When exogenous insulin is given, the hypoglycemia triggers an outpouring of glucagon and epinephrine, both of which raise the blood glucose concentration markedly, so that, although the patient may actually have periods of hypoglycemia, urine and blood glucose tests will show hyperglycemia.

■ INTERVENTIONS: Treatment is aimed at modifying the extremes by gradually lowering the insulin dosage so as to reduce stimulation of the feedback system of glucose regulation.

■ PATIENT CARE CONSIDERATIONS: The patient may need to take smaller doses of insulin or take it at more frequent intervals and at different times during the day.

insulin resistance, a cause of type 2 diabetes mellitus characterized by a need for an increased amount of insulin per day to control hyperglycemia and ketosis. It is associated with decreased or ineffective glucose transporter proteins with insulin-sensitive cells or insulin-binding by high levels of antibody. Insulin-resistant states also may occur with acanthosis nigrans, Werner syndrome, ataxia telangiectasia, Alström syndrome, pineal hyperplasia syndrome, and various lipodystrophic disorders.

insulin shock, a condition of severe hypoglycemia caused by an overdose of insulin, decreased intake of food, or excessive exercise. Compare **diabetic coma, ketoacidosis.**

■ OBSERVATIONS: It is characterized by sweating, trembling, chilliness, nervousness, irritability, hunger, hallucination, numbness, and pallor. Uncorrected, it progresses to convulsions, coma, and death.

■ INTERVENTIONS: Treatment requires an immediate dose of glucose orally or parenterally or glucagon IM or IV.

■ PATIENT CARE CONSIDERATIONS: Individuals taking medications that lower their blood sugar, including insulin and oral hypoglycemic agents, should wear a device such as a medical ID bracelet or necklace stating that they have diabetes and are using these agents.

insulin tolerance test, a test of the body's ability to use insulin, in which insulin is given and blood glucose is measured at regular intervals. Thirty minutes after the insulin is administered, blood glucose level is usually lower but not less than half of the fasting glucose level. Glucose levels usually return to normal after about 90 minutes. In people who have hypoglycemia, the glucose levels may drop lower and be slower to return to normal.

insulintropin /in′səlintrop″in/ [L, *insula,* island], a naturally occurring hormone produced in the intestines when food is ingested. It causes the release of insulin from the pancreas, which in turn regulates blood glucose levels. Also called **incretin.**

insulitis /in′səlī″tis/, a lymphocytic infiltration of the pancreatic beta cells in the islets of Langerhans. The condition is associated with the development of type 1 diabetes mellitus. Also called **isletitis.**

insuloma. See **insulinoma.**

intake [L, *in,* within; AS, *tacan,* to take], **1.** the process in which a person is admitted to a clinic or hospital or is signed in for an office visit. The reason for the visit and various identifying data about the patient are noted. Certain routine preliminary procedures may be performed, such as obtaining a blood pressure reading or a urine specimen. In some clinical settings the intake may also include obtaining such additional information as the patient's basic health history and previous source of care. **2.** the amount of food or fluid ingested or infused in a given period. Intake is measured and noted in milliliters or grams per 8-, 12-, or 24-hour period.

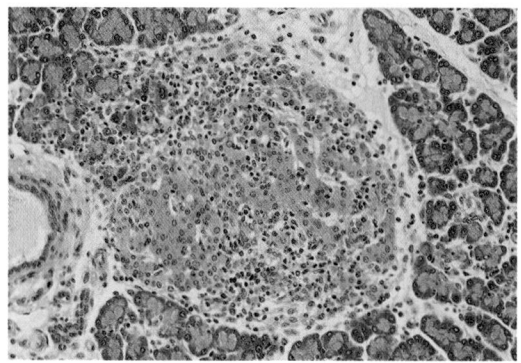

Insulitis *(Kumar et al, 2010)*

intake and output (I & O), the recording of all fluids that enter the body, both by mouth and intravenously, and all measurable fluids expelled (urine, liquid stool, and vomitus).

Intal, an antiasthmatic mast cell inhibitor agent. Brand name for **cromolyn sodium.**

integral dose /in″təgrəl/ [L, *integrare,* to make whole; Gk, *dosis,* giving], the total amount of energy absorbed by a patient or object during exposure to radiation. Also called **volume dose.**

integrate. See **integration.**

integrated circuit, a circuit, such as a computer chip, whose components are fabricated on a single semiconductor substrate.

Integrated Group Without Walls /in″təgrā′tid/, a network of physicians who have merged legally but continue to practice individually. Selected functions, such as information management, are centralized.

Integrated Health Care Delivery System, a managed care system in the United States that includes a hospital organization that provides acute patient care, a multispecialty medical care delivery system, the capability of contracting for any other needed services, and a payer. Services are provided to enrollees of the health plan.

Integrated Multispecialty Group, a managed care system similar to a single-specialty medical group, except that various specialties and usually primary care are also provided. Also called **Multispecialty Medical Group.**

integrated system, **1.** (in managed care) a legal partnership between groups of physicians and hospitals that contract and share risk while working together. It may include foundations, management service organizations, and physician-hospital organizations. **2.** a group of interconnected units that form a functioning computer system.

integrating dose meter /in″təgrā′ting/, a device that measures the total amount of radiation administered to a patient during a radiotherapy exposure. It is usually placed on the patient's skin and may terminate the exposure when the desired amount is reached.

integration /in′təgrā″shən/ [L, *integrare,* to make whole], **1.** the act or process of unifying or bringing together. **2.** (in psychology) the organization of all elements of the personality into a coordinated functional whole that is in harmony with the environment, one of the primary goals in psychotherapy. It involves the assimilation of insight and the coordination of new and old data, experiences, and emotional reactions so that an effective change can occur in behavior, thinking, or feeling. See also **insight. –integrate,** *v.*

integration of self, one of the components of high-level wellness. It is a prerequisite for the achievement of maturity and is characterized by the integration of mind, body, and spirit into one harmoniously functioning unit.

integrative babbling, the last stage of babbling development for speech. It begins when the child is between 10 and 15 months old. Words that are comprehensible typically occur around the first birthday, and complex babbling combines with a few real words. Intonation is present, and it is possible to discern questions and commands. Also called **jargon,** *conversational babble, modulated babble.*

integrin /integ″rin/, **1.** a protein that links the outside of a cell with its interior. **2.** a heterodimeric molecule involved in cell-substate and cell-cell adhesion.

integument /integ″yoomənt/ [L, *integumentum,* a covering], a covering or skin. *–integumentary, adj.*

integumentary system /integ′yəmen″tərē/, the skin and its appendages, hair, nails, and sweat and sebaceous glands.

integumentary system assessment, an evaluation of the general condition of a patient's integument and of factors or abnormalities that may contribute to the presence of a dermatological disorder.

■ METHOD: The patient is asked to supply subjective information about itching, pain, rashes, blisters, or boils; whether the skin usually is dry, oily, thin, rough, bumpy, or puffy; or whether it feels hot or cold, peels, changes in color, or is marked with dark liver (aging) spots. Objective information is gleaned from inspecting the skin. Observations are made of the intactness, turgor, elasticity, temperature, cleanliness, odor, wetness or dryness, and color of the skin. Cyanosis of the lips, circumoral area, mucous membranes, earlobes, or nailbeds; jaundice of the sclera; paleness of conjunctivae; and distribution of pigment are noted. Evidence of rashes, edema, needle marks, insect bites, scabies, acne, sclerema, decubiti, uremic frost on the beard or eyebrows, or pressure areas over bony prominences is recorded. The nails are examined for brittleness, lines, a convex ram's horn or concave spoon shape, and the condition of surrounding tissue, including clubbing of the fingers and toes. The existence and characteristics of lesions such as maculae, papules, vesicles, pustules, bullae, hives, warts, moles, ulcers, scars, keloids, petechiae, lipomas, crusts of dried exudate, flakes of dead epidermis, excoriations, blackheads, and chancres are noted. The patient's exposure to parasites, to internal allergens in food and drugs, and to external allergens in cosmetics, soaps, topical medication, and plants, as well as a family history of allergies, is investigated, as well as currently used medication, creams, lotions, ointments, hygienic measures, and sexual practices. Diagnostic aids contributing to the evaluation are skin and lesion cultures, punch biopsies, skin tests for allergies, a lupus erythematosus preparation, and a blood culture.

■ PATIENT CARE CONSIDERATIONS: The health care practitioner conducts the interview to obtain subjective data on the patient's condition, makes the necessary observations, and assembles the background information and results of the diagnostic tests.

■ OUTCOME CRITERIA: A well-conducted assessment of the patient's integument is a valuable aid in diagnosing a dermatological disorder or a disease with dermatological manifestations, such as palmar rash in syphilis.

intellect /in′təlekt/ [L, *intellectus,* perception], **1.** the power and ability of the mind for knowing and understanding, as contrasted with feeling or with willing. **2.** a person possessing a great capacity for thought and knowledge. *–intellectual, adj., n.*

intellectual disability, below-average cognitive functioning that causes developmental delays and impairments in multiple areas of occupation, including social participation, education, activities of daily living and instrumental activities of daily living, and play/leisure.

intellectualization /in′təlek′choo·əlīzā″shən/ [L, *intellectus* + Gk, *izein,* to cause], **1.** (in psychiatry) a defense mechanism in which reasoning is used as a means of blocking a confrontation with an unconscious conflict and the emotional stress associated with it. **2.** the overuse of abstract thinking or generalizations to control or minimize painful feelings.

intelligence /intel′ijəns/ [L, *intelligentia,* perception], **1.** the potential ability to acquire, retain, and apply experience, understanding, knowledge, reasoning, and judgment in coping with new experiences and in solving problems. **2.** the manifestation of such ability. See also **intelligence quotient. –intelligent,** *adj.*

intelligence quotient (IQ), a numeric expression of a person's intellectual level as measured against the statistical average of his or her age group. On several of the traditional scales, it is determined by dividing the mental age, derived through psychological testing, by the chronological age and multiplying the result by 100. Average IQ is considered to be 100. Compare **achievement quotient.** See also *accomplishment quotient.*

intelligence test, any of a variety of standardized tests designed to determine the mental age of an individual by measuring the relative capacity to absorb information and to solve problems. Compare **achievement test, aptitude test, personality test, psychological test.**

intelligent. See **intelligence.**

intelligent terminal, a computer terminal that can function as a processing device in addition to providing input/output facilities, whether operated independently or connected to a main computer. Compare **dumb terminal.**

intemperance /intem″pərəns/ [L, *in,* not, *temperare,* to moderate], excessive indulgence in eating, drinking, or other lifestyle functions.

intensifying screen /inten″sifĭ′ing/ [L, *intensus,* tighten, *facere,* to make; ME, *screne*], a device consisting of fluorescent material, which is placed in contact with the film in a radiographic cassette. Radiation interacts with the fluorescent phosphor, releasing light photons. These photons expose the film with greater efficiency than would the radiation alone. Thus patient exposure to radiation can be reduced.

intensity-modulated radiation therapy (IMRT), a specialized method of delivering radiation so that the beam enters the body from many different angles to get to the tumor with pinpoint accuracy while sparing much of the surrounding healthy tissue.

intensive care /inten″siv/ [L, *intensus,* tighten, *garrire,* to chatter], constant complex health care as provided in various acute life-threatening conditions such as multiple trauma, severe burns, or myocardial infarction or after certain kinds of surgery. Care is most frequently given by specially trained personnel in a unit equipped with various technologically sophisticated machines and devices for treating and monitoring the condition of the patient. Also called **critical care.**

intensive care unit (ICU), a hospital unit for patients requiring close monitoring and intensive care. An ICU contains highly technical and sophisticated monitoring devices and equipment and is staffed by personnel trained to deliver critical care. A large tertiary care facility usually has separate units specifically designed for the intensive care of adults, infants, children, or newborns or for other groups of patients requiring a certain kind of treatment. See also **coronary care unit.**

intention /inten″shən/ [L, *intendere,* to aim], a kind of healing process. Healing by primary intention is the initial union of the edges of a wound, progressing to complete healing without granulation. Healing by secondary intention is wound closure in which the edges are separated, granulation tissue develops to fill the gap, and epithelium grows in over the granulations, producing a scar. Healing by tertiary intention, also called delayed closure, is wound closure that is postponed due to poor circulation, a contaminated or infected wound. The wound is left open until contamination has been reduced and inflammation has subsided and then is closed. See also **healing.**

intentional additives, substances that are deliberately added in the manufacture of food or pharmaceutic products to improve or maintain flavor, color, texture, or consistency or to enhance or conserve nutritional value. Compare **incidental additives.**

Intentional Relationship Model (IRM), (in occupational therapy) a model to explain therapeutic relationships developed by Renee Taylor, Ph.D., that involves six modes of interpersonal style (advocating, empathizing, collaborating, problem-solving, encouraging, and instructing). IRM provides descriptions of inevitable interpersonal events, along with strategies to enhance the therapeutic use of self.

intention tremor, fine, rhythmic, purposeless movements that tend to increase during voluntary movements. Compare **resting tremor.** See also **tremor.**

inter-, prefix meaning "situated," "formed," or "occurring between": *interarticular, intercalary, intercapillary.*

interactional model /-ak″shənəl/ [L, *inter,* between, *agere,* to do], a therapy model that views the family as a communication system comprising interlocking subsystems of family members. Family dysfunction occurs when the rules governing family interaction become vague and ambiguous. The therapeutic goal is to help the family clarify the rules governing their relationships.

interactionist theory /-ak″shənist/, an aging theory that views age-related changes as resulting from the interactions among the individual characteristics of the person, the circumstances in society, and the history of social interaction patterns of the person.

interaction processes, a component of the theory of effective practice. The processes consist of a series of interactions between a nurse and a patient. The series occurs in a sequence of actions and reactions until the patient and the nurse both understand what is wanted and the desired behavior or act is achieved.

interactive guided imagery, the focusing of a patient's attention on a target visual stimulus to produce a specific physiological change that can promote healing. Imagery is effective in almost all of the major physiological systems of the body, including respiration, heart rate, blood pressure, metabolic rates in cells, gastrointestinal mobility and secretion, sexual function, cortisol levels, and immune responsiveness.

interactive perceptual mode, (in therapies) a means of learning through group discussion.

interalveolar /-alvē″ələr/ [L, *inter,* between, *alveolus,* little hollow], pertaining to the area between alveoli.

interalveolar septum, **1.** the tissue between adjacent pulmonary alveoli, consisting of a dense capillary network covered on both sides by thin alveolar epithelial cells. Also called **alveolar septum. 2.** a bony partition between adjacent tooth sockets.

interarticular /-ärtik″yələr/ [L, *inter,* between, *articulus,* joint], pertaining to the areas between two joints or between facing surfaces of a joint.

interarticular fibrocartilage [L, *inter* + *articulus,* joint], one of four kinds of fibrocartilage, consisting of flattened fibrocartilaginous plates between the articular cartilage of the most active joints, such as the sternoclavicular, wrist, and knee joints. The synovial surfaces extend over the fibrocartilaginous plates and attach to surrounding ligaments. The fibrocartilaginous plates absorb shocks and increase mobility. Compare **circumferential fibrocartilage, connecting fibrocartilage, stratiform fibrocartilage.**

interarytenoid fold, a fold of mucosa forming the base of the rima glottidis at the bottom of the interarytenoid notch.

interatrial /in′tər·ā′trē·əl/ [L, *inter,* between + *atrium,* hall], situated between the atria of the heart.

intercalary /intur″kəler′ē, in′tərkal′ərē/ [L, *intercalare,* to insert], occurring between two others, such as the absence of the middle part of a bone with the proximal and the distal parts present.

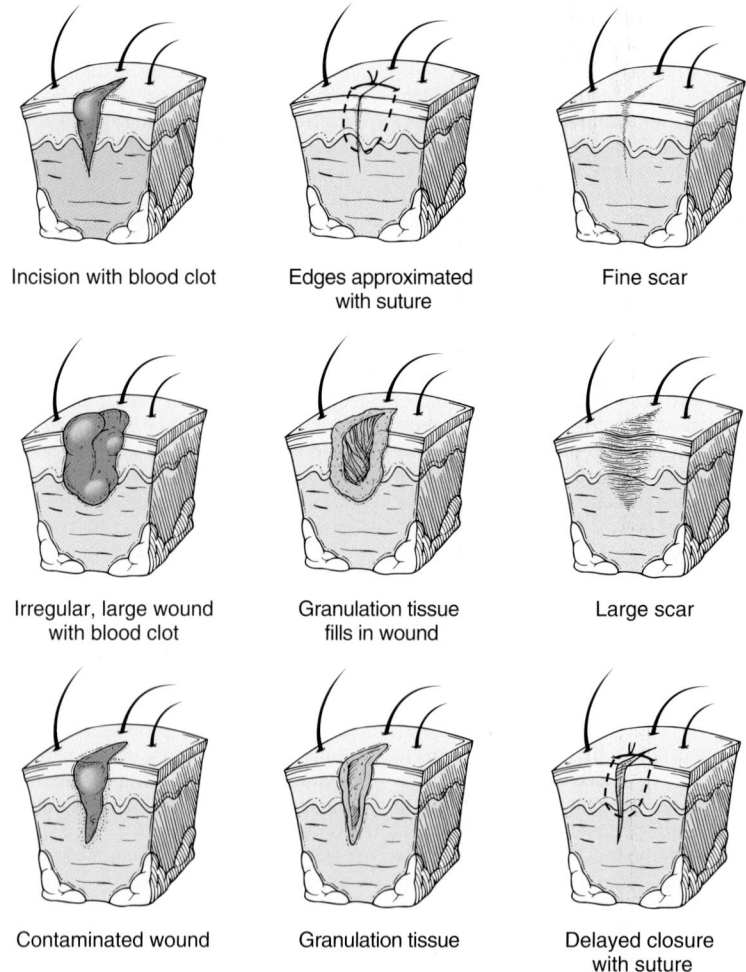

Incision with blood clot | Edges approximated with suture | Fine scar

Irregular, large wound with blood clot | Granulation tissue fills in wound | Large scar

Contaminated wound | Granulation tissue | Delayed closure with suture

Types of wound healing. A, Primary intention. B, Secondary intention. C, Tertiary intention *(Christensen, 2010)*

intercalate /intur″kəlāt/ [L, *intercalare*], to insert between adjacent surfaces or structures. —*intercalation, n.*

intercalated disks /in·tur′kə·lā·təd/, dense bands running between myocardial cells both transversely and longitudinally, forming a stepped configuration. They contain intercellular junctions that link adjacent cells both electrically and mechanically.

intercapillary /in′tər·kap′i·lar·ē/ [L, *inter,* between + *capillaris,* hairlike], among or between capillaries.

intercapillary glomerulosclerosis /-kap″iler′ē/ [L, *inter* + *capillaris,* hairlike, *glomerulus,* small ball; Gk, *sklerosis,* a hardening], an abnormal condition characterized by degeneration of the renal glomeruli. It is associated with diabetes and often produces albuminuria, nephrotic edema, hypertension, and renal insufficiency. Also called **Kimmelstiel-Wilson syndrome.**

intercavernous sinuses /-kav″ərnəs/ [L, *inter,* between, *caverna,* cavity, *sinus,* curve], the cavities through which the cavernous sinuses of the dura mater communicate.

intercellular /-sel′yələr/ [L, *inter* + *cella,* storeroom], pertaining to the area between or among cells.

intercellular bridge, a structure that connects adjacent cells, occurring primarily in the epithelium and other stratified squamous epithelia. It consists of slender strands of cytoplasm that project from the surfaces of adjacent cells and merge at the desmosome. Also called **cytoplasmic bridge.**

interceptive orthodontics /in′tər·sep′tiv/, that phase of orthodontics concerned with elimination of a condition such

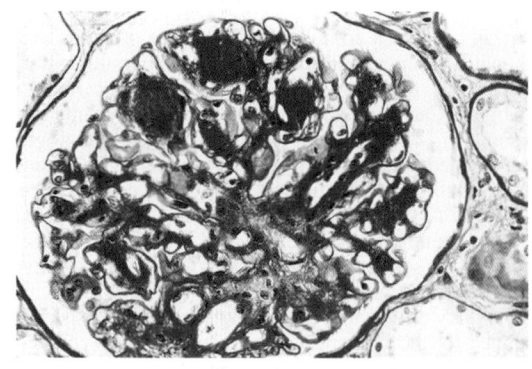

Intercapillary glomerulosclerosis *(Kumar et al, 2010)*

as crossbite or spacing that might lead to the development of malocclusion.

intercerebral /-ser″əbrəl/ [L, *inter,* between, *cerebrum,* brain], pertaining to the area between the left and right cerebral hemispheres.

interchange. See **reciprocal translocation.**

interchondral articulation, the articulation of the cartilage of adjacent ribs, mainly between the costal cartilages of ribs VII to X but sometimes involving the costal cartilages of ribs V and VI. Interchondral joints provide indirect anchorage to the sternum and contribute to the formation of a smooth inferior costal margin. They are usually synovial, and the thin fibrous capsules are reinforced by interchondral ligaments.

interclavicular /-kləvik″yələr/ [L, *inter,* between, *clavicula,* little key], pertaining to the area between the clavicles.

interconceptional gynecological care /-kənsep″shənəl/ [L, *inter* + *concipere,* to take in], health care of a woman during her reproductive years, between pregnancies, and 6 weeks after delivery. Screening tests for cervical cancer, breast and pelvic examinations, evaluation of general health, and laboratory determination of glucosuria and proteinuria and of the hematocrit or hemoglobin are common and routine aspects of interconceptional care. Testing and treatment for pelvic, vaginal, or genital infections may be required. A contraceptive method may also be discussed, taught, prescribed, or provided. Ordinarily the basic examination is performed annually. The method of contraception may be adjusted or changed at interim visits. Infections or other complaints are investigated, diagnosed, and treated as symptoms appear. Interconceptional care is increasingly given by nurse practitioners or nurse midwives who follow protocols for treatment and referral formulated in consultation with a supervising gynecologist.

intercondylar fracture /-kon″dilər/ [L, *inter* + Gk, *kondylos,* knuckle], a longitudinal fracture of the humerus between its two condyles.

intercostal /-kos″təl/ [L, *inter* + *costa,* rib], pertaining to the space between two ribs.

intercostal bulging, the visible expansion of the soft tissues between the ribs that occurs when increased expiratory effort is needed to exhale, as in asthma, cystic fibrosis, or obstruction of an airway by a foreign body. Compare **retraction of the chest.**

intercostal muscles, the muscles between adjacent ribs. They are designated as external and internal and function as secondary ventilatory muscles.

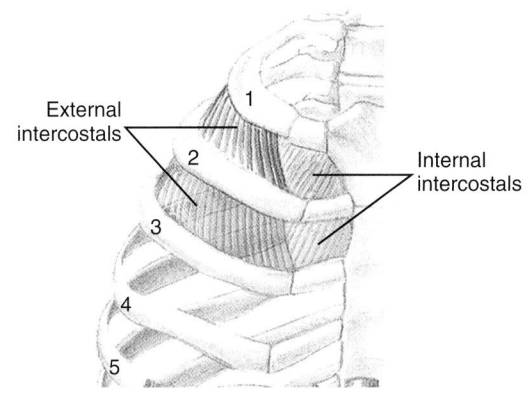

External
intercostals

Internal
intercostals

Intercostal muscles *(Thibodeau and Patton, 2003)*

intercostal neuralgia, pain in the intercostal spaces of the chest wall, involving intercostal nerves.

intercostal node, a node in one of three groups of thoracic parietal lymph nodes situated near the dorsal parts of the intercostal spaces. The nodes are associated with lymphatic vessels that drain the posterolateral area of the chest. The efferent vessels from the nodes in the caudal four or five spaces form a descending trunk that opens into the dilated origin of the thoracic duct. The efferent vessels from the nodes in the upper intercostal spaces on the left side connect with the thoracic duct. Those on the right side end in the right lymphatic duct. Compare **diaphragmatic node, sternal node.** See also **lymphatic system, lymph node.**

intercostal space [L, *inter,* between, *costa,* rib, *spatium*], the region between the ribs.

intercostobrachial nerve, a branch of the second intercostal nerve that contributes to cutaneous innervation of the medial surface of the upper arm.

intercourse. See **coitus.**

intercristal /-kris″təl/ [L, *inter* + *crista,* ridge], pertaining to the space between two crests.

intercurrent disease /-kur″ənt/ [L, *intercurrere,* to run between], a disease that develops in and may alter the course of another disease.

interdental canal /-den″təl/ [L, *inter* + *dens,* tooth], a channel in the alveolar process of the mandible, between the roots of the medial and lateral incisors, for the passage of anastomosing blood vessels between the sublingual and inferior dental arteries. Also called **nutrient canal.**

interdental gingiva, the supporting gingival tissues, containing prominent horizontal collagen fibers, that normally fill the space between two approximating teeth. Also called **gingival papilla.**

interdental groove, a linear vertical depression on the surface of the interdental papillae, which functions as a channel for the egress of food from the interproximal areas.

interdental spillway, a channel formed by the interproximal contours of adjoining teeth and their investing tissues.

interdependence, **1.** (for health or related reasons) mutual dependence and/or reliance upon members of a group in reciprocal relationships. **2.** (in biology) relationships within and between biological and physical environments to sustain life.

interdependent intervention. See **intervention.**

interdigestive migrating motor complex /-dijes″tiv/, a pattern of small bowel cyclic motor activity that follows completion of food digestion and absorption. It consists of periods of inactivity alternating with segmental or propulsive contractions.

interdigestive period, a period of relative inactivity in the alimentary tract between two periods of digestive activity.

interdisciplinary, working with a variety of disciplines or professions to serve a client, patient, or community.

interests, (in occupational therapy) the tasks that one finds enjoyable and satisfying.

interest tests, psychological tests designed to clarify an individual's vocational potential or to compare an individual's performance with the average scores of a specific population.

interface /in″tərfās/ [L, *inter* + *facies,* face], **1.** the connection between different elements of a computer system or between different computers. **2.** the method by which a computer user interacts with a computer system as displayed on a monitor screen, such as a graphic user interface.

interfemoral /in′tərfem′ərəl/ [L, *inter,* between + *femur,* thigh], between the thighs.

interference /-fir″əns/ [L, *inter* + *ferire,* to strike], **1.** (in physics) the combination of electromagnetic, light, or sound waves of the same frequency that prevent expected transmission. **2.** the erratic transmission of signals from a medical device caused by the simultaneous reception of signals from a source other than that being monitored; for example, the reception of electrical impulses from a nearby IV pump when monitoring the electrical activity of the heart.

interferent /-fir″ənt/ [L, *inter* + *ferire,* to strike], any chemical or physical phenomenon that can interfere with or disrupt a reaction or process.

interferential current therapy /-fərən″shəl/, a form of electrical stimulation therapy using two or three distinctly different currents that are passed through a tissue from surface electrodes. Portions of each current are canceled by the other, resulting in the application of a different net current to the target tissue. It is used in pain management and to relieve muscle spasms.

interferon /-fir"on/ [L, *inter* + *ferire,* to strike], a natural glycoprotein formed by cells exposed to a virus or another foreign particle of nucleic acid. It induces the production of translation inhibitory protein (TIP) in noninfected cells. TIP blocks translation of viral RNA, thus giving other cells protection against both the original and other viruses. Interferon is species specific.

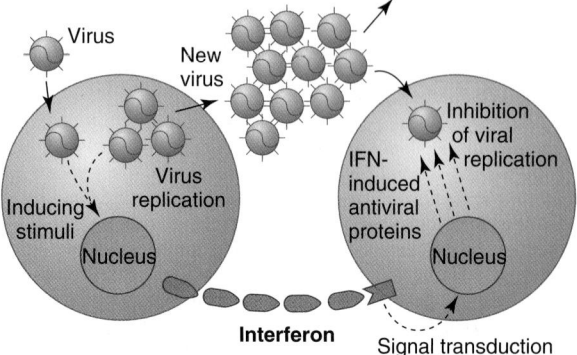

Mechanisms of action of interferon *(Lewis et al, 2014)*

interferon alfa-2a, a synthetic form of interferon-α produced by recombinant technology that acts as a biological response modifier. It is used as an antineoplastic in the treatment of hairy cell leukemia and AIDS-related Kaposi sarcoma. It is administered intramuscularly or subcutaneously.

interferon alfa-2a, recombinant, a parenteral antineoplastic drug.
- INDICATIONS: It is administered in the treatment of AIDS-related Kaposi sarcoma, hairy cell and chronic myelogenous leukemia, and chronic hepatitis C. It also has a variety of unlabeled or investigational uses.
- CONTRAINDICATIONS: Caution is recommended in prescribing this product for patients with severe cardiovascular disease.
- ADVERSE EFFECTS: Among reported adverse effects are influenza-like symptoms, particularly at the beginning of therapy with the drug; confusion; dizziness; nervousness; depression; anorexia; nausea; vomiting; diarrhea; throat inflammation; dry and itching skin; alopecia; diaphoresis; blood pressure changes; and tachycardia.

interferon alfa-2b, a synthetic form of interferon-α produced by recombinant technology that acts as a biological response modifier, used in the treatment of venereal warts, hepatitis B, chronic hepatitis C, and as an antineoplastic in the treatment of hairy cell leukemia, malignant melanoma, non-Hodgkin lymphomas, multiple myeloma, mycosis fungoides, and AIDS-related Kaposi sarcoma. It is administered intramuscularly, subcutaneously, or intralesionally.

interferon alfa-2b, recombinant, a parenteral antineoplastic drug with indications, contraindications, and adverse effects similar to those of interferon alfa-2a, recombinant.

interferon alfacon-1, a recombinant type 1 interferon.
- INDICATIONS: It is used to treat chronic hepatitis C infections. It is being used investigationally to treat hairy cell leukemia in combination with granulocyte colony–stimulating factor.
- CONTRAINDICATIONS: Hypersensitivity to alpha interferons or to products derived from *Escherichia coli* prohibit its use.
- ADVERSE EFFECTS: Life-threatening effects include granulocytopenia, thrombocytopenia, and leukopenia. Other adverse effects include headache, rigors, insomnia, dizziness, nausea, diarrhea, anorexia, vomiting, constipation, hemorrhoids, decreased salivation, musculoskeletal pain, dysmenorrhea, vaginitis, menstrual disorders, alopecia, pruritus, rash, erythema, tinnitus, earache, conjunctivitis, eye pain,

granulocytopenia, ecchymosis, hypertension, palpitations, nervousness, depression, anxiety, emotional lability, abnormal thinking, upper respiratory infection, respiratory tract congestion, and bronchitis.

interferon alfa-n1 lymphoblastoid, a recombinant type 1 interferon.
- INDICATIONS: It is used to treat chronic hepatitis C infections.
- CONTRAINDICATIONS: Factors that prohibit its use include known hypersensitivity to alpha interferons and a history of anaphylactic reactions to bovine or ovine immunoglobulins, egg protein, polymyxin B, or neomycin sulfate.
- ADVERSE EFFECTS: Life-threatening effects include granulocytopenia, thrombocytopenia, and leukopenia. Other adverse effects include ecchymosis and epistaxis. Common side effects include headache, fever, insomnia, dizziness, anxiety, hostility, lability, nervousness, depression, confusion, abnormal thinking, amnesia, abdominal pain, nausea, diarrhea, anorexia, vomiting, back pain, alopecia, pruritus, rash, erythema, dry skin, pharyngitis, upper respiratory infection, cough, dyspnea, and bronchitis.

interferon alfa-n3, a highly purified mixture of natural human interferon proteins that acts as a biological response modifier, used in the treatment of venereal warts. It is administered intralesionally.

interferon-alpha, 1. a signaling protein that activates host cells; involved in the innate immune response against viral infections. Also spelled *interferon-alfa.* 2. a biological therapy drug obtained from the leukocyte fraction of human blood. It may be used to treat renal carcinoma, melanoma, carcinoid tumors, and some types of lymphoma and leukemia. The trade name is Multiferon®.

interferon-beta, the major interferon produced by double-stranded RNA-induced fibroblast cultures. Interferon-beta is produced mainly by fibroblasts, epithelial cells, and macrophages.

interferon beta-1a, an antiviral and immune system regulator.
- INDICATIONS: It is prescribed in the treatment of relapsing forms of multiple sclerosis. It can help reduce the number of neurological attacks and slow the progress toward physical disability.
- CONTRAINDICATIONS: It should not be given to patients with allergy or sensitivity to interferon beta-1a or components of its formulation.
- ADVERSE EFFECTS: The side effects most often reported include headache, muscle aches, chills, fever, weakness, and influenza-like symptoms.

interferon beta-1b, a synthetic modified form of interferon-beta produced by recombinant DNA techniques, used as a biological response modifier in the treatment of relapsing forms of multiple sclerosis. It is administered subcutaneously.

interferon beta-2. See **interleukin-6.**

interferon gamma (IFN gamma), a cytokine critical for innate and adaptive immunity against viral, bacterial, and protozoal infections. IFN gamma is produced predominantly by natural killer cells and activated CD8 T cells.

interferon gamma-1b, a synthetic form of interferon-beta produced by recombinant technology that acts as a biological response modifier and antineoplastic. It is used to reduce the frequency and severity of serious infections associated with chronic granulomatous disease; it is administered subcutaneously.

interferon nomenclature, a system recommended by the International Interferon Nomenclature Committee for identifying interferon compounds. For a specific interferon, the name consists of "interferon" followed by a Greek letter (spelled out), a hyphen, an Arabic number, and a lowercase letter, as in interferon alfa-2a.

interfibrillar mass of Flemming, interfilar mass. See **hyaloplasm.**

interim rate /in″tərim/ [L, meanwhile, *ratum,* calculate], a method of third-party payment for costs of hospital services in which an amount is paid periodically pending an accounting of actual costs at the end of a designated period.

interior /in·tēr′ē·ər/ [L, inner], **1.** situated inside; inward. **2.** an inner part or cavity.

interiorization /intir′ē·ərīzā″shən/ [L, *interior,* inner; Gk, *izein,* to cause], the merging of reflex and cognitive processes as a response to the environment.

interior mesenteric artery [L, inner; Gk, *mesos,* middle, *enteron,* intestine, *arteria,* airpipe], a visceral branch of the abdominal aorta, arising just above the division into the common iliacs and supplying the left half of the transverse colon, all of the descending and iliac colons, and most of the rectum. It has left colic, sigmoid, and superior rectal branches.

interkinesis /in″tərkinē″sis, -kīnē″sis/ [L, *inter* + Gk, *kinein,* to move], the interval between the first and second nuclear divisions in meiosis. See also **interphase.**

interleukin /-loo͞″kin/, cytokines mainly produced by leukocytes. Interleukins participate in communication among leukocytes and are important in the inflammatory response. Most interleukins direct other cells to divide and differentiate. Each acts on a particular group of cells that have receptors specific to that interleukin.

interleukin-1 (IL-1), IL-1 alpha is produced by activated macrophages, neutrophils, epithelial cells, and endothelial cells. It is responsible for the production of inflammation and the promotion of fever and sepsis. IL-1 beta is produced by activated macrophages as a proprotein, which is proteolytically processed to its active form by caspase 1. It is an important mediator of the immune response and involved in cell proliferation, differentiation, and apoptosis.

interleukin-2 (IL-2), a cytokine with various immunological functions, including the ability to initiate proliferation of activated T cells. IL-2 is used in the laboratory to grow T cell clones with specific helper, cytotoxic, and regulatory functions.

interleukin-3 (IL-3), a cytokine that supports the growth of pluripotent bone marrow stem cells. It is produced by activated T cells and basophils.

interleukin-4 (IL-4), a cytokine that induces differentiation of naive CD_4 T cells (TH_0) to Th_2 cells (important for activation and differentiation of B cells). IL-4 stimulates the activation of B cells and the differentiation of B cells into plasma cells. Also called **B cell stimulating factor-1.**

interleukin-5 (IL-5), a cytokine produced by helper T cells (Th2) and mast cells. It stimulates B cells and eosinophils and facilitates the differentiation of B cells that secrete immunoglobulin A.

interleukin-6 (IL-6), a cytokine produced by T cells, macrophages, dendritic cells, and fibroblasts. It has both proinflammatory and antiinflammatory functions. It is an important mediator of fever and of the acute phase response. Also called **beta$_2$-interferon.**

interleukin-7 (IL-7), a cytokine produced by bone marrow and thymic stromal cells that causes lymphoid stem cells to differentiate into progenitor B and T cells and stimulates the killing of foreign cells by T cells and monocytes.

interleukin-8 (IL-8), a chemokine produced mainly by macrophages and epithelial and endothelial cells. IL-8 attracts and activates neutrophils.

interleukin-9 (IL-9), a cytokine produced by CD4 T cells that acts as a regulator of several hematopoietic cells.

interleukin-10 (IL-10), a cytokine expressed by CD4 and CD8 T cells, monocytes, macrophages, and activated B cells. It inhibits cytokine synthesis and suppresses the function of inflammatory immune cells.

interleukin-11 (IL-11), a cytokine produced by bone marrow stromal cells. IL-11 stimulates megakaryocytopoiesis, activates osteoclasts, inhibits epithelial cell proliferation and apoptosis, and inhibits macrophage function.

interleukin-12 (IL-12), a cytokine produced by activated dendritic cells. IL-12 induces differentiation of naive CD4 T cells to Th1 cells (important for activation and differentiation of CD8 T cells). Also stimulates cell-mediated killing by natural killer cells and lymphocytes.

interleukin-13 (IL-13), a cytokine produced mainly by CD4 T helper (Th2) cells (important for activation and differentiation of B cells). It is closely related to IL-4.

interleukin-14 (IL-14), a cytokine produced by T cells and some malignant B cells. It enhances the proliferation of B cells and induces memory B cell production and maintenance.

interleukin-15 (IL-15), a cytokine that enhances peripheral blood T cell production.

interlobular arteries of kidney. See **cortical radiate arteries.**

interlobular duct /-lob′yələr/ [L, *inter* + *lobulus,* small lobe], any duct connecting or draining the lobules of a gland.

interlobular ductules, interlobular bile ducts; small channels between the hepatic lobules, draining into the biliary ductules.

interlobular emphysema. See **distal acinar emphysema.**

interlobular pleurisy, encysted inflammation of the pleura between the lobes of the lung.

interlocked twins [L, *inter* + AS, *loc,* a fastening], monozygotic twins so positioned in the uterus that the neck of one becomes entwined with that of the other during presentation, making vaginal delivery impossible. Such interlocking occurs when one fetus is a breech presentation and the other a vertex presentation. Also called *interlocking twins.*

intermaxillary segment, median palatine process.

intermediary /-mē″dē·er′ē/ [L, *inter* + *mediare,* to divide], a private insurance company or public or private agency selected by health care providers to pay claims under the Medicare program.

intermediary metabolism [L, *inter,* between, *mediare,* to divide; Gk, *metabole,* change], the metabolic processes involved in the synthesis of cellular components between digestion of food and excretion of waste products.

intermediate-acting insulin [L, *inter* + *mediare,* to divide, *activus,* active], a preparation of synthetic human insulin to which zinc has been added under specific chemical conditions that has an intermediate duration of action. Intermediate-acting insulin has an onset of action in 1 to 3 hours, a duration of action up to 24 hours, and peak action from 6 to 8 hours. Kinds include **NPH insulin.** See also **insulin.**

intermediate care /-mē″dē·it/, **1.** a level of medical care for certain chronically ill or disabled individuals in which room and board are provided but skilled nursing care is not. Title XI of U.S. Medicaid legislation mandates standards and federal subsidies for intermediate care of the recipients of public assistance. **2.** a unit for patients who do not require intensive care but who are not yet ready to receive care and monitoring on a regular medical-surgical unit.

intermediate care facility (ICF), a health facility that provides medically related services to persons with a variety of physical or emotional conditions requiring institutional facilities but without the degree of care provided by a hospital or skilled nursing facility. An example is an intermediate care facility for cognitively impaired or other developmentally disabled persons.

intermediate care unit, a transitional unit for patients from critical care units that provides close monitoring and provision of noncritical care before discharge.

intermediate cell mass. See **nephrotome.**

intermediate column. See **lateral horn.**

intermediate cuneiform bone, the smallest of the three cuneiform bones of the foot, located between the medial and the lateral cuneiform bones. Also called **middle cuneiform bone, second cuneiform bone.**

intermediate-density lipoprotein (IDL), a lipid-protein complex with a density between those of very-low-density lipoprotein and low-density lipoprotein. The product has a relatively short half-life and is normally in the blood in very low concentrations. In a type III hyperlipoproteinemic state the IDL concentration in the blood is elevated.

intermediate disk. See **Z line.**

intermediate host, any animal in which the larval or intermediate stage of a parasite develops but does not sexually reproduce. Certain snails are intermediate hosts for liver flukes and schistosomes. Humans are intermediate hosts for malaria parasites. Also called **secondary host.** Compare **dead-end host, definitive host, reservoir host.** See also **host.**

intermediate left lateral flexure of rectum, the third bend of the rectum, where it deviates laterally to the left.

intermediate mass, the connecting mass of nervous tissue between two lobes of the diencephalon.

intermediate mesoderm. See **nephrotome.**

intermediate nerve, the smaller root of the facial nerve, lying between the main root and the vestibulocochlear nerve. It consists of parasympathetic and sensory fibers, and its branches supply the lacrimal, nasal, palatine, submandibular, and sublingual glands, as well as the anterior two thirds of the tongue.

intermenstrual /-men″stroo·əl/ [L, *inter* + *menstruum,* menstrual fluid], pertaining to the time between menstrual periods.

intermenstrual fever, the normal slight elevation of temperature that marks ovulation, usually occurring about 14 days before the onset of menses.

intermenstrual pain. See **mittelschmerz.**

intermittent /-mit″ənt/ [L, *inter* + *mittere,* to send], **1.** occurring at intervals. **2.** alternating between periods of signs and symptoms followed by periods of remission.

intermittent acute porphyria. See **acute intermittent porphyria.**

intermittent assisted ventilation (IAV), a system of respiratory therapy in which assisted ventilation is combined with spontaneous breathing. Also called **intermittent demand ventilation.**

intermittent claudication. See **claudication.**

intermittent compression, external compression used to control and reduce accumulation of lymph in body tissues. Devices to provide intermittent compression in an on-off timing sequence include inflated pressure sleeves and linear compression pumps. Some devices provide cold temperatures with compression to assist in controlling edema. Intermittent compression is also used to decrease acute bleeding.

intermittent demand ventilation. See **intermittent assisted ventilation.**

intermittent explosive disorder, a psychological disturbance beginning in childhood and characterized by discrete episodes of violence and aggressive behavior or destruction of property in otherwise normal individuals. The acts may occur as an overreaction to an ordinarily minor event.

intermittent fever, a fever that recurs in cycles of paroxysms and remissions, such as in malaria. Kinds include **biduotertian fever, double quartan fever, quartan malaria.**

intermittent hydrosalpinx [L, *inter,* between, *mittere,* to send; Gk, *hydor,* water, *salpinx,* tube], a fluid accumulation in a fallopian tube. The fluid is released periodically through the uterine cavity. Also called **hydrops tubae profluens.**

intermittent incontinence [L, *inter,* between, *mittere,* to send, *incontinentia,* inability to retain], urinary incontinence that occurs only when there is pressure on the bladder or muscular exertion. See also **incontinence.**

intermittent mandatory ventilation (IMV), a mode of mechanical ventilation in which the patient is allowed to breathe independently except during certain prescribed intervals, when a ventilator delivers a breath either under positive pressure or in a measured volume. Compare **intermittent positive-pressure breathing.** See also **respiratory therapy.**

intermittent positive-pressure breathing (IPPB), a form of assisted or controlled respiration produced by a ventilatory apparatus in which compressed gas is delivered under positive pressure into a person's airways until a preset pressure is reached. Passive exhalation is allowed through a valve, and the cycle begins again as the flow of gas is triggered by inhalation. Also called **intermittent positive-pressure ventilation.**

■ METHOD: The use of the IPPB unit involves the combined efforts of the physician, the respiratory therapist or technician, and the nurse. The specific pressure and volume and the use of nebulizing or other attachments are ordered individually. The equipment is tested and introduced to the patient by the respiratory therapist. The nurse observes that the patient closes the lips around the mouthpiece and does not allow air to escape from the nose or mouth during inspiration and determines whether the therapy is effective. Exhaled tidal volume is measured, with a goal of achieving 10-15 mL/kg of body weight.

■ INTERVENTIONS: The patient may require reassurance that the machine will automatically shut off airflow at the end of inspiration and encouragement to relax and allow the lungs to be completely filled by the machine. The patient is cautioned not to manipulate any of the controls.

■ OUTCOME CRITERIA: Ventilation may be greatly improved by the use of the IPPB unit. Secretions may be thinned and cleared, and the passages may be humidified, allowing greater comfort and a better exchange of gases.

intermittent positive-pressure breathing unit. See **IPPB unit.**

intermittent positive-pressure ventilation. See **intermittent positive-pressure breathing.**

intermittent pulse [L, *inter,* between, *mittere,* to send, *pulsare,* to beat], a pulse in which an occasional beat is absent. It tends to occur with second-degree heart block or extrasystole. Also called **dropped-beat pulse.**

intermittent torticollis [L, *inter,* between, *mittere,* to send, *tortus,* twisted, *collum,* neck], intermittent, powerful spasms of the neck muscles, drawing the head to one side. The spasms usually occur in the sternocleidomastoid muscle.

intermittent tremor [L, *inter,* between, *mittere,* to send, *tremere,* to tremble], a rhythmic involuntary shaking that is not continuous or constant.

intern /in″turn/ [L, *internus,* inward], **1.** *n.,* a physician in the first postgraduate year who is learning medical practice under supervision before beginning a residency program. **2.** *n.,* any immediate postgraduate trainee in a clinical program. **3.** *v.,* to work as an intern.

internal /intur″nəl/ [L, *internus,* inward], within or inside. −**internally,** *adv.*

internal abdominal oblique muscle, one of a pair of anterolateral muscles of the abdomen, lying under the external oblique muscle in the lateral and ventral part of the abdominal wall. It is smaller and thinner than the external oblique muscle. It functions to compress the abdominal contents and assists in micturition, defecation, emesis, parturition, and forced expiration. Both muscles acting together serve to flex the vertebral column, drawing the costal cartilages toward the pubis. One side acting alone bends the vertebral column laterally and rotates it, drawing the shoulder of the opposite side downward. Also called **obliquus internus abdominis.** Compare **external abdominal oblique muscle.**

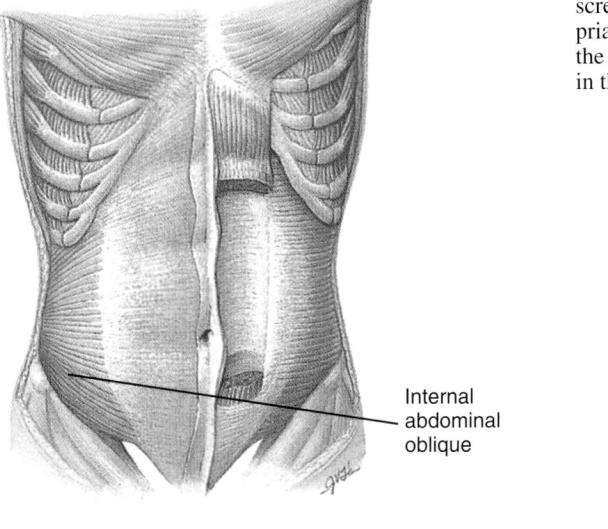

Internal oblique muscle *(Thibodeau and Patton, 2003)*

internal acoustic meatus, an opening in the petrous portion of the temporal bone through which the facial, intermediate, and vestibulocochlear nerves and the labyrinthine artery pass. Also called **meatus acusticus internus.**

internal aperture of tympanic canaliculus, the upper opening of the tympanic channel in the temporal bone, leading to the tympanum.

internal bleeding [L, *internus,* inward; AS, *blod*], hemorrhage into an internal organ, tissue, or body cavity (e.g., intraperitoneal bleeding or intestinal bleeding).

internal carotid artery, each of two arteries starting at the bifurcation of the common carotid arteries, opposite the cranial border of the thyroid cartilage, through which blood circulates to many structures and organs in the head.

internal carotid plexus, a network of nerves on the internal carotid artery, formed by the internal carotid nerve. The internal carotid plexus supplies sympathetic fibers to the branches of the internal carotid artery, the tympanic plexus, the nerves of the cavernous sinus, and the cranial parasympathetic ganglia through which the fibers pass. Compare **common carotid plexus, external carotid plexus.**

internal cervical os, an internal opening of the uterus that corresponds to the slight constriction or isthmus of that organ about midway in its length. The internal cervical os separates the body of the uterus from the cervix. Compare **external cervical os.**

internal control, (in occupational therapy) the extent to which individuals are in charge of their own actions and the outcome of an activity.

internal cuneiform bone. See **medial cuneiform bone.**

internal ear. See **inner ear.**

internal fertilization, the union of gametes within the body of the female after insemination. See also **artificial insemination.**

internal fistula, an abnormal passage between two internal organs or structures.

internal fixation, any method of holding together the fragments of a fractured bone without the use of appliances external to the skin. After open reduction of the fracture, smooth or threaded pins, Kirschner wires, screws, plates attached by screws, or medullary nails may be inserted through an appropriate incision to stabilize the fragments. In some instances the device is removed at a later operation, but it may remain in the body permanently. Compare **external pin fixation.**

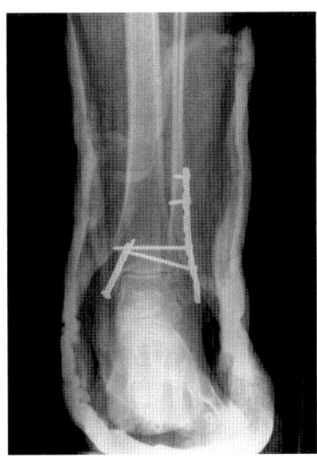

Internal fixation *(Courtesy Ohio State University Medical Center)*

internal hemorrhage, bleeding into a serous cavity, a hollow viscus, or tissues.

internal hemorrhoid, a fold of mucous membrane at the anorectal junction, caused by edema or dilation of the interior rectal vein.

internal hernia, a protrusion of an intraperitoneal viscus into a recess or compartment within the peritoneal cavity.

internal iliac artery, a division of the common iliac artery, supplying the walls of the pelvis, the pelvic viscera, the genital organs, and part of the medial thigh. In the fetus the internal iliac artery is twice as large as the external iliac artery and is the direct continuation of the common iliac artery. After birth the internal iliac artery becomes smaller than the external iliac artery. Also called **hypogastric artery.** Compare **external iliac artery.**

internal iliac node, a node in one of seven groups of parietal lymph nodes serving the abdomen and the pelvis. The internal iliac nodes surround the internal iliac vessels and receive lymphatic vessels corresponding to the branches of the internal iliac artery. Their afferent vessels drain lymph from the pelvic viscera, the buttocks, and the dorsal portions of the thighs. Their efferent vessels end in the common iliac nodes. Compare **external iliac node, iliac circumflex node.** See also **lymph, lymphatic system, lymph node.**

internal iliac vein, one of the pair of veins in the lower body that join the external iliac vein to form the two common iliac veins. Each vein begins at the greater sciatic foramen and, at the pelvic brim, joins the external iliac vein. Compare **external iliac vein.**

internal injury [L, *internus,* inward, *injuria*], a wound, trauma, or damage to the viscera.

internalization /intur′nəlīzā″shən/ [L, *internus* + Gk, *izein,* to cause], the process of adopting within the self, either unconsciously or consciously through learning and socialization, the attitudes, beliefs, values, and standards of another person or more generally of the society or group to which one belongs. See also **socialization.**

internal jugular catheter, a central venous catheter inserted through the internal jugular vein.

internal jugular vein, one of a pair of veins in the neck. Each vein collects blood from one side of the brain, the face, and the neck, and both unite with the subclavian vein to form the brachiocephalic vein. Each internal jugular vein is continuous with the sigmoid in the posterior part of the jugular foramen at the base of the skull. Compare **external jugular vein.**

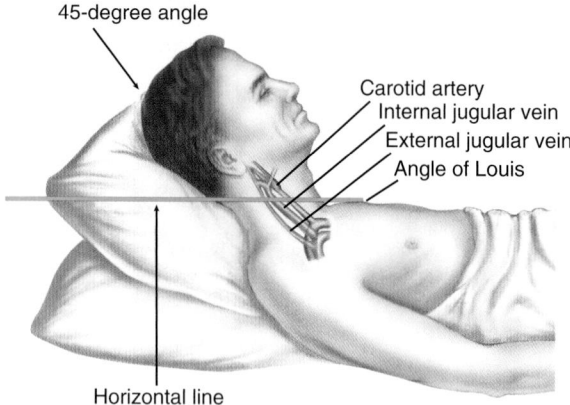

Internal jugular vein *(Thompson, Porter, and Fernandez, 2002)*

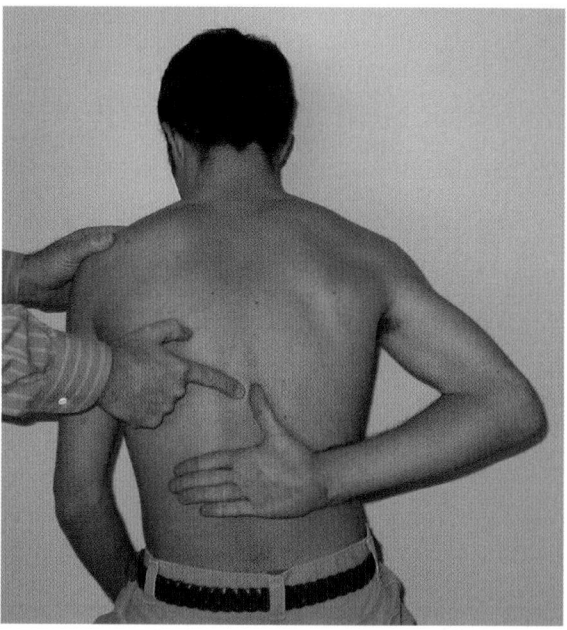

Assessment of internal rotation of the shoulder
(Waldman, 2010)

internal locus of control. See **locus of control.**

internally. See **internal.**

internal malleolus. See **medial malleolus.**

internal mammary artery. See **internal thoracic artery.**

internal mammary artery bypass, a surgical procedure to correct a coronary artery obstruction. The internal mammary artery in situ and still attached to the subclavian artery is anastomosed to the coronary artery beyond the obstruction.

internal mammary node. See **sternal node.**

internal medicine, the branch of medicine concerned with the study of the physiological and pathological characteristics of the internal organs and with the medical diagnosis and treatment of individuals with disorders of these organs.

internal os, the internal opening of the cervical canal.

internal podalic version and total breech extraction. See **version and extraction.**

internal pterygoid muscle, one of the four muscles of mastication. It acts to close the jaws. Also called **pterygoideus medialis.** See also **external pterygoid muscle.**

internal pudendal artery, a branch of the anterior trunk of the internal iliac artery in the pelvis with branches that supply the rectum and perineum and the erectile tissues of the penis and clitoris.

internal respiratory nerve of Bell. See **phrenic nerve.**

internal resorption, a rare dental condition occurring when dentin and pulpal walls begin to resorb the tooth structure within the root canal.

internal rotation, 1. the turning of a limb about its axis of rotation toward the midline of the body. **2.** medial rotation.

internal secretion [L, *internus,* inward, *secernere,* to separate], a type of secretion in which substances pass directly from a gland into the bloodstream.

internal sphincter muscle of urethra, a circular layer of smooth muscle fibers, innervated by the vesical nerve, that surrounds the internal urethral orifice in males and acts to close it. No such structure exists in females.

internal standard, an element or compound added in a known amount to yield a signal against which an instrument or an analyte to be measured can be calibrated.

internal strabismus. See **esotropia.**

internal strangulation [L, *internus,* inward, *strangulare,* to choke], a state of extreme constriction of an organ, such as a loop of intestine trapped in an opening, resulting in an interruption in the blood supply and ischemia. See also **inguinal hernia, intestinal strangulation.**

internal thoracic artery, one of a pair of arteries that arise from the first portions of the subclavian arteries, descend to the margin of the sternum, and divide into the musculophrenic and superior gastric arteries at the level of the sixth intercostal space. The artery supplies the pectoral muscles, the breasts, the pericardium, and the abdominal muscles. In females, it is also called the internal mammary artery.

internal thoracic vein, one of a pair of veins that accompanies the internal thoracic artery, receiving tributaries that correspond to those of the artery. It forms a single trunk that runs up on the medial side of the artery and ends in the corresponding brachiocephalic vein. The superior phrenic vein usually opens into the internal thoracic vein.

International Agency for Research on Cancer (IARC), an agency established in 1965 by the World Health Assembly as an autonomous agency of the World Health Organization with the aim of promoting international collaboration in cancer research. Its mission is to coordinate international studies on the causes of human cancer, the mechanisms of carcinogenesis, and strategies for cancer prevention, with a particular focus on promoting research in regions of the world where it is lacking.

International Association for Dental Research (IADR), an international organization concerned with research in dentistry and the exchange of information regarding such research.

International Classification of Diseases, an official list of categories of diseases, physical and mental, issued by the World Health Organization (WHO). It is used primarily for statistical purposes in the classification of morbidity and mortality data. Any nation belonging to WHO may adjust the classification to meet specific needs. See also *Diagnostic and Statistical Manual of Mental Disorders.*

International Commission on Radiation Protection (ICRP), a nongovernmental organization founded in England in 1928 to provide general guidance on the safe use of radiation sources, including appropriate protective measures and codes of practice for medical radiology. The ICRP was originally established as a source of information about the hazards of x-rays and radium in medicine but was reorganized in 1950 to include effects of nuclear energy.

International Council of Nurses (ICN), the oldest international health organization. It is a federation of nurses' associations from 112 countries and was one of the first health organizations to develop strict policies of nondiscrimination on the basis of nationality, race, creed, color, politics, sex, or social status. The objectives of the ICN include promotion of national associations of nurses, improvement of standards of nursing and competence of nurses, improvement of the status of nurses within their countries, and provision of an authoritative international voice for nurses. The following ICN definition of the nurse is accepted internationally and serves as a pattern in developing nursing practice and nursing education throughout the world: "A nurse is a person who has completed a program of basic education and is qualified and authorized in her/his country to practice nursing. Basic nursing education is a formally recognized program of study that provides a broad and sound foundation for the practice of nursing, and for postbasic education, which develops specific competency. At the first level, the educational program prepares the nurse, through study of behavior, life, and nursing sciences and clinical experience, for effective practice and direction of nursing care and for the leadership role. The first level nurse is responsible for planning, providing, and evaluating nursing care in all settings for the promotion of health, prevention of illness, care of the sick, and rehabilitation; and functions as a member of the health team. In countries with more than one level of nursing personnel, the second level program prepares the nurse, through study of nursing theory and clinical practice, to give nursing care in cooperation with and under the supervision of a first level nurse." The ICN is active in the World Health Organization, the United Nations Educational, Scientific, and Cultural Organization, and other international organizations.

International Normalized Ratio (INR), a comparative rating of a patient's prothrombin time (PT) ratio, used as a standard for monitoring the effects of warfarin.

International Federation of Red Cross and Red Crescent Societies (IFRC), an international organization based in Geneva, Switzerland, that coordinates activities among the National Red Cross and Red Crescent Societies. The federation leads and organizes international activities in cooperation with the national societies to provide relief assistance in response to large-scale emergencies. See **American Red Cross, Canadian Red Cross.**

International Sign Language, a sign language composed of a blending of vocabulary signs from numerous different countries, sometimes used at international meetings and events of deaf persons.

International Society of Surgery (ISS), an international professional organization of surgeons. Also called *Société Internationale de Chirurgie.*

International System of Units (SI), an internationally accepted scientific system of expressing length, mass, and time in base units (IU) of meters, kilograms, and seconds, replacing the old centimeter-gram-second system. The SI system includes as standard measurements the ampere, candle, Kelvin scale, and mole.

International Union Against Cancer (UICC) [Fr. *Union Internationale Contre le Cancer*], an international, nongovernmental organization founded in 1933 addressing all aspects of cancer control. See also **cancer.**

International Unit (IU, I.U.), a unit of measure in the International System of Units. See also **SI units.**

interneuron /-nōor″on/, a nerve cell whose axon and dendrite lie entirely within the central nervous system and whose function is to relay impulses within the central nervous system.

internist /intur″nist, in″turnist/ [L, *internus,* inward], a physician who specializes in internal medicine.

internship /in″turnship′/, a period of apprenticeship for a medical school graduate. Interns serve in a hospital for a specified period before beginning a professional practice. Some hospitals also offer internships for new graduates in nursing or for senior nursing students.

internuncial neuron /-nun″sē-əl/ [L, *inter* + *nuntius,* messenger], a connecting neuron in a neural pathway, usually serving as a link between two other neurons.

interocclusal distance, interocclusal gap. See **freeway space.**

interocclusal record /-əklōo″səl/, an imprint of the positional relation of opposing teeth or jaws to each other, made of the surfaces of occlusal rims or teeth with a material such as plaster of paris, wax, zinc oxide-eugenol paste, an elastomeric material, or acrylic resin.

interoceptive /in′tərōsep″tiv/ [L, *internus,* inward, *capere,* to take], pertaining to stimuli originating from within the body that are related to the functioning of the internal organs or the receptors they activate. Compare **exteroceptive, proprioception.**

interoceptor /-sep″tər/ [L, *internus* + *capere,* to take], any sensory nerve ending located in cells in the viscera that responds to stimuli originating from within the body in relation to the function of the internal organs, such as digestion, excretion, and blood pressure. Compare **exteroceptor, proprioceptor.**

intraoperative lymphatic mapping (ILM), the use of injected dyes or nuclear-imaging agents to identify diseased nodes during operative procedures for cancers of the oral cavity and breast, as well as melanoma. See also **sentinel node biopsy.**

interosseous /-os″ē-əs/ [L, *inter,* between, *os,* bone], pertaining to an area between bones or a structure, such as a ligament, connecting two bones.

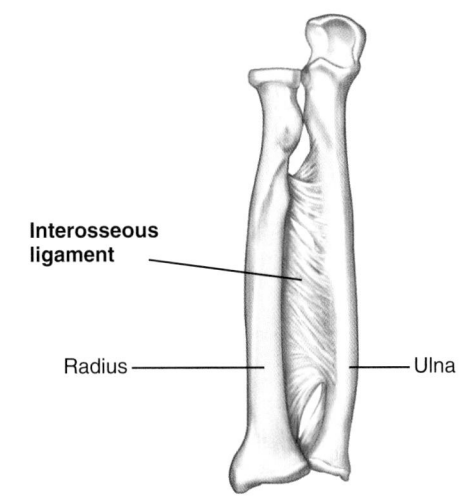

Interosseous ligament

Radius — — Ulna

Interosseous ligament

interparietal fissure. See **intraparietal sulcus.**

interparoxysmal /-per′əksis′məl/ [L, *inter,* between, *paroxysmos,* irritation], pertaining to something that happens between sudden recurrences of diseases or symptoms.

interperiosteal fracture /in′tərper′ē·os″tē·əl/ [L, *inter* + Gk, *peri,* around, *osteon,* bone], an incomplete fracture in which the periosteum is not disrupted.

interpersonal /-pur′sənəl/ [L, *inter,* between, *personalis*], pertaining to the interactions of individuals.

interpersonal characteristics, (for health or related reasons) relevant aspects of the personality that the health care provider and client/patient bring into a therapeutic relationship.

interpersonal event, (in occupational therapy) a naturally occurring communication, reaction, process, task, or general circumstance that occurs during therapy that has the potential to detract from or strengthen the therapeutic relationship.

interpersonal event cascade, (in occupational therapy) an occasion in which more than one interpersonal event follows a therapist's initial response to a single interpersonal event.

interpersonal focusing, (in occupational therapy) a therapeutic strategy that emphasizes "feeling" and "relating" issues over "doing" issues.

interpersonal learning, (in therapies) the process of becoming more aware of one's behavior and interaction skills and how one's behavior affects others.

interpersonal psychiatry [L, *inter* + *persona,* mask], a theory of psychiatry introduced by Harry Stack Sullivan (1892–1949) that stresses the nature and quality of relationships with significant others as the most critical factor in personality development.

interpersonal reasoning, (in therapies) the process by which a therapist consciously and reflectively monitors both the therapeutic relationship and the interpersonal events of therapy in order to decide on and enact appropriate interpersonal strategies.

interpersonal self-discipline, the ability to anticipate, measure, and respond to the effects of ongoing communications with a client/patient.

interpersonal skill base, the interpersonal skills that are judiciously applied by the therapist to build a functional working relationship with a client.

interpersonal therapy, a kind of psychotherapy that views faulty communications, interactions, and interrelationships as basic factors in maladaptive behavior. Kinds include **transactional analysis.**

interphase /in″tərfās′/ [L, *inter* + Gk, *phasis,* phase], the stage in the cell cycle during which the cell is not dividing, the chromosomes are not individually distinguishable, and such biochemical and physiological activities as DNA synthesis occur. Interphase follows telophase of one cell division and extends to the beginning of prophase of the next division. See also **anaphase, interkinesis, metaphase, mitosis, prophase, telophase, karyostasis.**

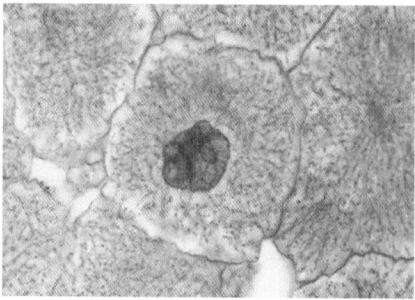

Interphase (© Ed Reschke; Used with permission)

interpleural space /-ploor″əl/ [L, *inter,* between; Gk, *pleura,* rib; L, *spatium*], the potential space of the mediastinum between the two pleural linings, which contains serous fluid. Also called **pleural cavity.**

interpolated premature ventricular contraction /intur″pəlā′tid/ [L, *interpolare,* to refurbish], a ventricular extrasystole that occurs between two consecutive sinus-conducted beats. It is not followed by a compensatory pause.

interpolation /intur′pəlā″shən/, **1.** the transfer of tissues, as in plastic surgery or transplantation. **2.** (in statistics) the introduction of an estimated intermediate value of a variable between known values.

interpreter /intur″prətər/ [Fr, *interpreter,* to translate], **1.** an individual who facilitates communication between a patient and a health care professional who do not speak or sign the same language. **2.** a computer program that remains in the source and translates or executes higher level language.

interprofessional, *adj.,* describing collaborative initiatives in which health care professionals work together to overcome fragmentation and traditional disciplinary boundaries to improve educational and service outcomes.

interproximal film image. See **bite wing film image.**

interpubic disk /-pyoo″bik/ [L, *inter* + *os pubis,* pubic bone; Gk, *diskos,* flat plate], the fibrocartilaginous plate connecting the opposed surfaces of the bodies of the pubic bones. Varying in thickness, it is strengthened by interlacing fibers and often contains a cavity that usually appears after the tenth year of life. Also called **discus interpubicus.**

interpulse interval /-puls″/, the time elapsed between successive nerve impulses; the reciprocal of impulse frequency.

interradicular septum. See **interalveolar septum.**

interradicular space /-radik′yələr/ [L, *inter* + *radix,* root, *spatium*], the area between the roots of a multirooted tooth, normally occupied by a bony septum and the periodontal membrane.

interrogatories /in′tərog″ətôr′ēz/ [L, *inter* + *rogare,* to ask], (in law) a series of written questions submitted to a witness or other person having information of interest to the court. The answers are transcribed and are sworn to under oath. Interrogatories are used during the pretrial period as a means of discovery. They differ from depositions in that there is no opportunity for cross-examination. Compare **deposition, discovery.**

interrupted suture /in′tərup″tid/ [L, *interrumpere,* to sever, *sutura*], a single suture tied separately, as distinguished from a continuous suture.

intersection syndrome, a condition of pain, crepitus, and a squeaky sensation in the dorsal radial forearm. It occurs most commonly among weight lifters and rowers and is treated with splinting, analgesics, and steroid injection as needed.

intersex /in″tərseks′/ [L, *inter* + *sexus,* sex, gender], any individual who has anatomical characteristics of both sexes or whose external genitalia are ambiguous or inappropriate for either the normal male or female. See also **intersexuality, pseudohermaphroditism.**

intersexuality /-sek′shoo·al″itē/ [L, *inter* + *sexus,* male or female], the condition in which an individual has both male and female anatomical characteristics to varying degrees or in which the appearance of the external genitalia is ambiguous or differs from that characteristic of the gonadal or genetic sex. See also **hermaphroditism, pseudohermaphroditism.** −*intersexual, adj.*

intersphincteric groove, an indistinct groove in the anal canal, forming the lower border of the pecten analis and marking the change between the subcutaneous part of the external anal sphincter and the border of the internal anal sphincter.

interspinales, the true segmental muscles of the back.

interspinal ligament /-spī″nəl/ [L, *inter* + *spina,* spine, *ligare,* to bind], one of many thin, narrow membranous ligaments that connect adjoining spinous processes of the vertebrae and extend from the root of each process to the apex. The interspinal ligaments are only slightly developed in the neck.

interspinous /-spī″nəs/ [L, *inter* + *spina,* spine], pertaining to the space between any spinous processes.

interstitial /in′tərstish″əl/ [L, *inter* + *sistere,* to stand], pertaining to the space between cells, as interstitial fluid, or between organs. Also called **intercellular.**

interstitial cell-stimulating hormone (ICSH), a hormone secreted by the anterior pituitary gland that stimulates the production of testosterone by the Leydig, or interstitial, cells of the testis. Also called **luteinizing hormone.**

interstitial cystitis (IC), an inflammation of the bladder, believed to be associated with an autoimmune or allergic response. The bladder wall becomes inflamed, ulcerated, and scarred, causing frequent painful urination. Hematuria may occur. Treatment may include distension of the bladder and cauterization of the ulcers (if present), dietary modification, oral or intravesical medication, pain management, and alternative therapies such as acupuncture. Cystectomy with urinary diversion is rarely indicated. The condition occurs most often in women and may resemble the early stages of bladder cancer. Diagnosis is often by exclusion and may require cystoscopy and biopsy. Also called **painful bladder syndrome.** See also **Hunner's ulcer.**

interstitial emphysema, a form of emphysema in which air or gas escapes into the interstitial tissues of the lung after a penetrating injury or a rupture in an alveolar wall. Because the alveoli must be decompressed, there is danger that the pleura will be torn, causing a pneumothorax. The condition is diagnosed by chest x-ray films. See also **pneumothorax.**

interstitial fibroid [L, *interstitium,* space between, *fibra,* fiber; Gk, *eidos,* form], a fibrous tumor that develops in the muscular wall of the uterus and tends to grow inward.

interstitial fluid, an extracellular fluid that fills the spaces between most of the cells of the body and provides a substantial portion of the liquid environment of the body. Formed by filtration through the blood capillaries, it is drained away as lymph. It closely resembles blood plasma in composition but contains less protein. Compare **intracellular fluid, lymph, plasma.**

interstitial growth, an increase in size by hyperplasia or hypertrophy within the interior of a part or structure that is already formed. Compare **appositional growth.**

interstitial hypertrophic neuropathy. See **Déjérine-Sottas disease.**

interstitial implantation, (in embryology) the complete embedding of the blastocyst within the endometrium of the uterine wall.

interstitial inflammation [L, *interstitium,* space between, *inflammare,* to set afire], an inflammation in an area of connective tissues.

interstitial infusion. See **hypodermoclysis.**

interstitial keratitis, an uncommon inflammation within the layers of the cornea. The first symptom is a diffuse haziness. Blood vessels may grow into the area and cause permanent opacities. The causes are syphilis, tuberculosis, leprosy, and vascular hypersensitivity. Treatment is specific to the infection or condition.

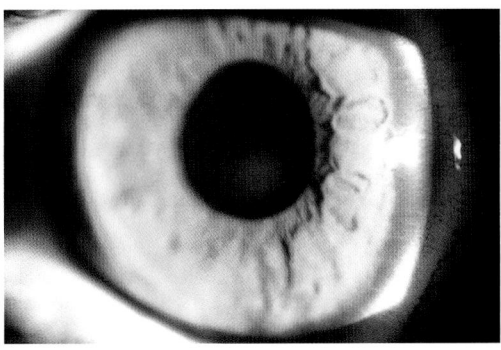

Interstitial keratitis *(Spalton, Hitchings, and Hunter, 2005)*

interstitial lung disease (ILD), a respiratory disorder characterized by a dry, unproductive cough and dyspnea on exertion. The patient may have swallowing disorders or joint and muscle pain and a history of industrial exposure to inorganic dusts, such as asbestos or silica. X-ray films usually show fibrotic infiltrates in the lung tissue, usually in the lower lobes. The fibrosing or scarring of lung tissue is often the result of an immune reaction to an inhaled substance. However, interstitial lung disease may result from viral, bacterial, or other infections; uremic pneumonitis; cancer; a congenital or inherited disorder; or circulatory impairment. The condition may be self-limiting, progress to respiratory or cardiac failure, or undergo spontaneous recovery.

interstitial mastitis [L, *interstitium,* space between; Gk, *mastos,* breast], an inflammation of the connective tissue between ducts of the breast.

interstitial myositis. See **myositis fibrosa.**

interstitial nephritis, inflammation of the interstitial tissue of the kidney, including the tubules. The condition may be acute or chronic. Acute interstitial nephritis is an immunological adverse reaction to certain drugs, often sulfonamide or methicillin (allergic interstitial nephritis). Acute renal failure, fever, rash, and proteinuria are characteristic of this condition. Most people regain normal kidney function when the offending drug is discontinued. Chronic interstitial nephritis is a syndrome of interstitial inflammation and structural changes, sometimes associated with such conditions as ureteral obstruction, pyelonephritis, exposure of the kidney to a toxin, rejection of a transplant, and certain systemic diseases. Gradually renal failure, nausea, vomiting, weight loss, fatigue, and anemia develop. Acidosis and hyperkalemia may follow. The nurse watches carefully for signs of electrolyte imbalance, dehydration, and hypovolemia, especially if there is frequent vomiting. Fluids and electrolytes may be replaced intravenously. Treatment includes correction of the underlying cause. If the cause is an obstruction of the urinary tract, rapid recovery may follow removal of the obstruction. In other cases, hemodialysis and kidney transplantation may be necessary.

interstitial plasma cell pneumonia. See **pneumocystosis.**

interstitial pneumonia, a condition of diffuse, chronic inflammation of the lungs beyond the terminal bronchioles, characterized by fibrosis and collagen formation in the alveolar walls and by the presence of large mononuclear cells in the alveolar spaces. The symptoms are progressive dyspnea, clubbing of the fingers, cyanosis, and fever. The disease may result from a hypersensitive reaction to busulfan, chlorambucil, hexamethonium, or methotrexate. It may also be an autoimmune reaction, because it often accompanies celiac disease, rheumatoid arthritis,

Sjögren's syndrome, and systemic sclerosis. X-ray films of the lungs show patchy shadows and mottling, as in bronchopneumonia. Later stages of the disease reveal bronchiectasis, dilation of the bronchi, and shrinkage of the lungs. Treatment includes bed rest, oxygen therapy, and corticosteroids. Most patients die within 6 months to a few years, usually as a result of cardiac or respiratory failure. Also called **diffuse fibrosing alveolitis, giant cell interstitial pneumonia, Hamman-Rich syndrome.** Compare **bronchopneumonia.**

interstitial pregnancy, See **ectopic pregnancy.**

interstitial therapy, radiotherapy in which needles or wires that contain radioactive material are implanted directly into tumor areas. See also **brachytherapy.**

interstitial tissue [L, *interstitium,* space between; OFr, *tissu*], the connective and supporting tissue within and surrounding major functional elements of an organ.

interstitial tubal pregnancy, a kind of tubal pregnancy in which implantation occurs in the proximal interstitial portion of one of the fallopian tubes. See also **tubal pregnancy.**

interstitium /-stish″ē·əm/, the space between cells in a tissue.

intertransverse ligament /-transvurz″/ [L, *inter + transversus,* cross-direction], one of many fibrous bands connecting the transverse processes of vertebrae. In the cervical region, intertransverse ligaments consist of a few scattered fibers; in the thoracic region they are rounded cords intimately connected with the deep muscles of the back. In the lumbar region they are thin and membranous.

intertrigo /in′tərtrī″gō/ [L, *inter + terere,* to scour], an erythematous irritation of opposing skin surfaces caused by friction, moisture, warmth, or sweat retention. Common sites are the axillae, the folds beneath large or pendulous breasts, and the inner aspects of the thighs. Maceration and candidal infection may be complications if the area is also warm and moist. Prevention is by weight reduction, powdering, cleansing, and use of antifungal topical medication when necessary. —*intertriginous, adj.*

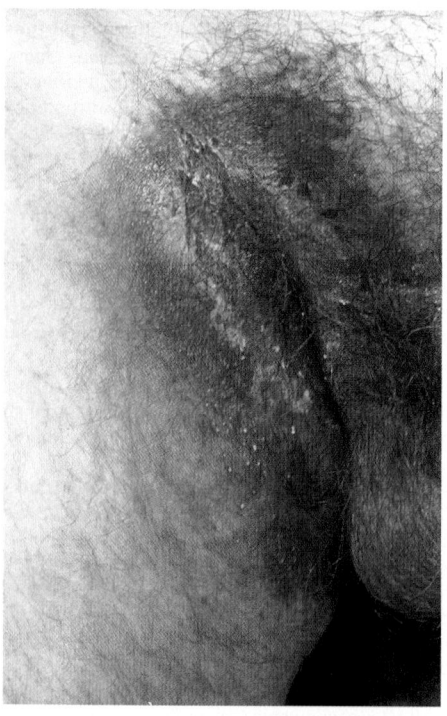

Candidal intertrigo *(Lim, 2007)*

intertrochanteric crest /in′tərtrō′kanter″ik/ [L, *inter + trochanter,* runner, *crista,* ridge], one of a pair of ridges along the thigh bones, curving obliquely from the greater to the lesser trochanter.

intertrochanteric fracture, a crack in the proximal femur between the greater and the lesser trochanters that usually requires surgical intervention.

intertrochanteric line, a line that runs across the anterior surface of the thigh bone from the greater to the lesser trochanter, winding around the medial surface and ending in the linea aspera. The proximal half of the intertrochanteric line is the attachment for the iliofemoral ligament; the distal half holds the vastus medialis muscle.

intertuberous diameter /-tŏŏ″bərəs/ [L, *inter + tuber,* swelling; Gk, *dia,* across, *metron,* measure], the distance between the ischial tuberosities, a factor used in determining the dimensions, including the narrowest diameter, of the pelvic outlet.

interureteral /in″terure′teral/, situated between the ureters.

interval /in′tərval/ [L, *intervallum,* space between], a space between things or events, or a break or interruption in an otherwise continuous flow.

interval health history [L, *intervallum,* space between], a kind of health history that notes the general condition of a client during the period between visits and is not limited to facts relevant to a particular condition. The interval health history provides an ongoing account of a person's health, serving to bring the database up to date.

intervention /in′tərven″shən/ [L, *inter + venire,* to come], **1.** an act performed to prevent harm to a patient or to improve the mental, emotional, or physical function of a patient. A physiological process may be monitored or enhanced, or a pathological process may be arrested or controlled. Independent intervention is any health care activity pertaining to aspects of professional practice that are encompassed by licensure and law and require no supervision or direction from others. Interdependent intervention refers to any health care activity carried out by one health care professional in collaboration with another. See also **nursing intervention. 2.** (in occupational therapy) the process and skilled actions taken by occupational therapy practitioners in collaboration with clients to facilitate engagement in occupation related to health participation. The intervention process includes the plan, implementation, and review.

intervention approaches, (in occupational therapy) strategies and guidelines based on theory and research evidence that are selected to direct the process of intervention.

interventional cardiology, the subspecialty of cardiology that uses intravascular catheter-based techniques with fluoroscopy to treat coronary artery, valvular, and congenital cardiac disease.

interventricular /-ventrik″yələr/ [L, *inter,* between, *ventriculus,* little belly], pertaining to the location between the ventricles, as the septum of the heart.

interventricular septum [L, *inter,* between, *ventriculus,* little belly, *saeptum,* fence], the wall between the ventricles of the heart. Also called **ventricular septum.**

intervertebral /in′tərvur″təbrəl/ [L, *inter + vertebra,* back joint], pertaining to the space between any two vertebrae, such as the fibrocartilaginous disks.

intervertebral disk, one of the fibrous, broad, and flattened disks found between adjacent spinal vertebrae, except the axis and the atlas. The disks vary in size, shape, thickness, and number, depending on the location in the back and the particular vertebrae they separate.

intervertebral fibrocartilage, See **intervertebral disk.**

intervertebral foramen, any of the passages between adjacent vertebrae through which the spinal nerves and vessels pass.

intervertebral ganglion [L, *inter,* between, *vertebra,* back joint; Gk, *ganglion,* knot], the ganglionic enlargement of a spinal nerve root between adjacent vertebrae.

interview /inˈtərvyo͞o/, a verbal interaction with a patient initiated for a specific purpose and focused on a specific content area. A problem-seeking interview is an inquiry that focuses on gathering data to identify problems the patient needs to resolve. A problem-solving interview focuses on problems that have been identified by the patient or health care professional.

intervillous space /inˈtərvilˈəs/ [L, *inter* + *villus,* hair, *spatium*], one of many spaces between the chorionic villi of the endometrium of the gravid uterus, beneath the placenta. The intervillous spaces act as small reservoirs for oxygenated maternal blood from which the fetal circulation may take up the nutrients and gases by osmosis, hydrostatic pressure, and diffusion.

intestinal. See **intestine.**

intestinal absorption [L, *intestinum,* intestine, *absorbare,* to swallow], the passage of the products of digestion from the lumen of the small intestine into the blood and lymphatic vessels in the wall of the gut. The surface area of the intestine is greatly increased by the presence of fingerlike projections called villi, each of which contains capillaries and a lymphatic vessel, or lacteal. Most dissolved nutrients pass quickly into the capillary bed for transport through the portal circulation to the liver. Lipids enter the lymphatic channels, which eventually rejoin the venous circulation at the thoracic duct in the neck.

intestinal amebiasis. See **amebic dysentery.**

intestinal angina, chronic vascular insufficiency of the mesentery caused by atherosclerosis and resulting ischemia of the smooth muscle of the small bowel. Also called **chronic intestinal ischemia.**

intestinal apoplexy, the sudden occlusion of one of the three principal arteries to the intestine by an embolism or a thrombus. This condition leads rapidly to necrosis of intestinal tissue and is often fatal. Treatment is usually surgical. The occlusion is removed, and often the affected portion of the bowel is resected. See also **atherosclerosis.**

intestinal atresia [L, *intestinum* + Gk, *a* + *tresis,* boring], a pathological obstruction of the continuous lumen of the intestinal tract caused by a defect of development in utero.

intestinal bypass [L, *intestinum* + AS, *bi* + Fr, *passer* + Gk, *cheirourgos*], a surgical procedure to shorten the digestive tract. It is performed so that less intestinal surface will be available to absorb nutrients from the digested food passing through, as in morbid obesity, or to bypass a blocked or diseased portion of the intestine. The technique usually involves anastomosing the jejunum to the ileum. See also **ileal bypass.**

intestinal colic [L, *intestinum* + Gk, *kolikos,* colonic pain], spasmodic pain in intestinal disorders.

intestinal dyspepsia, an abnormal condition characterized by impaired digestion associated with a disorder that originates in the intestines. See also **dyspepsia.**

intestinal fistula, an abnormal passage from the intestine to other internal organs or to an external abdominal opening or stoma, usually created surgically for the exit of feces after removal of a malignant, severely ulcerated, or diseased segment of the bowel. See also **colostomy.**

intestinal flora [L, *intestinum* + *flos,* flowers], the natural bacterial content of the inside of the digestive tract.

intestinal flu, a viral gastroenteritis, an inflammation of the stomach and intestines, usually caused by infection by an enterovirus. It is characterized by abdominal cramps, diarrhea, nausea, and vomiting. Outbreaks may be sporadic or epidemic, and the disease usually is mild and self-limited. Treatment is symptomatic. Control of diarrhea may be achieved with antidiarrheal medication and a diet limited to clear fluids. See also **enteric infection, gastroenteritis.**

intestinal fluke [L, *intestinum* + AS, *floc*], any internal parasite of the genera *Fasciolopsis, Heterophyes,* and *Metagonimus* in North America and of other genera in Asia and in tropical countries. They enter the body through the mouth as encysted larvae in aquatic vegetation or freshwater fish. Symptoms of intestinal fluke infestation usually include abdominal pain and obstruction and diarrhea.

intestinal gas [L, *intestinum*], vapors in the digestive tract arising from three sources—swallowed air, gas produced by digestive processes, and blood gases diffused into the intestinal lumen. Gases produced in the intestine and diffused from blood are mainly hydrogen (H_2), most of which is a bacterial fermentation product of ingested carbohydrates, carbon dioxide (CO_2), and methane (CH_4).

intestinal glands. See **Lieberkühn's glands.**

intestinal infarction. See **intestinal strangulation.**

intestinal juices, the secretions of glands lining the intestine.

intestinal lipodystrophy. See **lipodystrophy.**

intestinal lipophagic granulomatosis. See **Whipple disease.**

intestinal lymphangiectasia. See **hypoproteinemia.**

intestinal obstruction, any obstruction that results in failure of the contents of the intestine to progress through the lumen of the bowel. The most common cause is a mechanical blockage resulting from adhesions, impacted feces, tumor of the bowel, hernia, intussusception, volvulus, or the strictures of inflammatory bowel disease. Obstruction may also be the result of paralytic ileus. Obstruction of the small bowel may cause severe pain, vomiting of fecal matter, dehydration, and eventually a drop in blood pressure. Obstruction of the colon causes less severe pain, marked abdominal distension, and constipation. Radiographic examination may reveal the level of obstruction and its cause. Treatment includes the evacuation of intestinal contents by means of an intestinal tube. Surgical repair is sometimes necessary. Fluid balance and electrolyte balance are restored by carefully monitored IV infusion. Nonnarcotic analgesics are usually prescribed to prevent the decrease in intestinal motility that often accompanies the administration of narcotic analgesics. Also called **ileus.** See also **hernia, intussusception, volvulus.**

intestinal perforation [L, *intestinum* + *perforare,* to pierce], the escape of digestive tract contents into the peritoneal cavity as the result of trauma or a disease condition such as a ruptured appendix or perforated ulcer. The condition inevitably leads to peritonitis.

intestinal pseudoobstruction [L, *intestinum,* intestine; Gk, *pseudes,* false; L, *obstruere,* to build against], a condition characterized by constipation, colicky pain, and vomiting, but without evidence of organic obstruction.

intestinal strangulation, the arrest of blood flow to the bowel, causing edema, cyanosis, and gangrene of the affected loop of bowel. This condition is usually caused by a hernia, intussusception, or volvulus. Early signs of intestinal strangulation resemble those of intestinal obstruction, but peritonitis, shock, and the presence of a tender mass in the abdomen are important findings in making a differential diagnosis. In addition to surgery, treatment includes

I

the immediate correction of fluid and electrolyte imbalance. Also called **intestinal infarction.**

intestinal tonsil, one of a group of lymphatic nodules forming a single layer in the mucous membrane of the ileum opposite the mesenteric attachment. The nodules are oval patches about 1 cm wide and extend for about 4 cm along the intestine. In most individuals they appear in the distal ileum, but they also appear in the jejunum of a few individuals. Also called **Peyer's patches.** Compare **lingual tonsil, palatine tonsil, pharyngeal tonsil.**

intestinal tract [L, *intestinum* + *tractus*], the segments of the small and large intestines between the pyloric valve and the rectum. The intestinal tract forms part of the digestive tract.

intestinal tube [L, *intestinum* + *tubus*], a specialized flexible, hollow cylindrical device inserted into the gastrointestinal tract for therapeutic measures, such as decompression or nutritional support.

intestinal villi, the multitudinous threadlike projections that cover the surface of the mucosa of the small intestine and serve as the sites of absorption (by active transport and diffusion) of fluids and nutrients.

intestine /intes″tin/ [L, *intestinum*], the portion of the alimentary canal extending from the pyloric opening of the stomach to the anus. It includes the small and large intestines. Also called **bowel.** –**intestinal,** *adj.*

intima /in″timə/ [L, *intimus,* innermost], the innermost layer of a structure, such as the lining membrane of an artery, vein, lymphatic vessel, or organ. –**intimal,** *adj.*

intimal fibroplasia, a type of fibromuscular dysplasia that affects mainly children and young adult men, characterized by short localized areas of smooth stenosis of the tunica intima, either symmetric or asymmetric. Sometimes it is a result of trauma, surgery, or infection.

intimal sclerosis [L, *intimus,* innermost; Gk, *sklerosis,* hardening], a hardening of the innermost layer of a blood vessel wall. See also **atherosclerosis.**

intimate partner violence. See **domestic abuse.**

intoe. See **metatarsus varus.**

intolerance /intol″ərəns/ [L, *in,* not, *tolerare,* to bear], a condition characterized by inability to absorb or metabolize a nutrient or medication. Exposure to the substance may cause an adverse reaction, as in lactose intolerance. Compare **allergy, atopic.**

intoxicant /intok″sikənt/ [L, *in* + Gk, *toxikon,* poison], any agent that can cause intoxication or poisoning.

intoxication /intok″sikā″shən/ [L, *in,* within; Gk, *toxikon,* poison], **1.** the state of being poisoned by a drug or other toxic substance. **2.** the state of being inebriated as a result of an excessive consumption of alcohol. **3.** a state of mental or emotional hyperexcitability, usually euphoric.

intra-, prefix meaning "situated, formed, or occurring within": *intrabronchial, intracutaneous, intramatrical.*

intraabdominal infection /in″trə·abdom″inəl/, a disease caused by organisms, usually bacterial or fungal, situated within the cavity of the abdomen. The infection may be in the retroperitoneal space or the peritoneal cavity and can arise as a result of surgery. Intraperitoneal infections may be diffuse or localized in one or more abscesses in recesses such as the pelvic space or perihepatic spaces. Abscesses also form about diseased viscera. Treatment depends on the type of infectious organism and the site of the infection.

intraabdominal pressure [L, *intra,* within, *abdomen,* belly], the degree of pressure within the abdominal cavity.

intraalveolar pocket. See **periodontal pocket.**

intraaortic balloon pump (IABP) /in″trə·ā·ôr″tik/ [L, *intra* + *aeirein,* to rise], a counterpulsation device that provides temporary cardiac assist in the management of refractory left ventricular failure that may follow myocardial

infarction or occur in preinfarction angina. The balloon is attached to a catheter inserted into the aorta and is automatically inflated during diastole and deflated during systole. Also called **aortic balloon pump,** *intraaortic balloon counterpulsation.* See also **counterpulsation.**

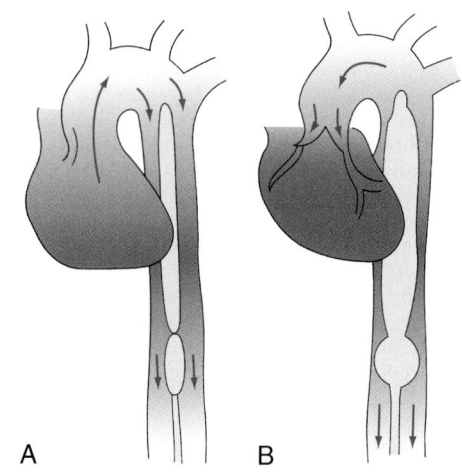

Intraaortic balloon pump. The balloon is (A) deflated during systole and (B) inflated during diastole. *(Sole, Klein, and Moseley, 2013)*

intraarterial /in″trə·ärtir″ē·əl/, pertaining to a structure or action inside an artery.

intraarticular /in″trə·ärtik″yələr/ [L, *intra* + *articulus,* joint], within a joint.

intraarticular fracture, a fracture involving the articular surfaces of a joint.

intraarticular injection, the injection of a medication into a joint space, usually to reduce inflammation, such as in bursitis or fibromyositis. With the same technique abnormally excessive fluid may be withdrawn from the joint space. The fluid may be a result of trauma or inflammation.

intraarticular ligament, a ligament that forms part of the joints between 16 of the 24 ribs, dividing the joints into two cavities, each containing a synovial membrane. Each intraarticular ligament consists of a short, flattened band of fibers inside the joint, attached by one extremity to the rib and by the other to the intervertebral disk. Intraarticular ligaments are not present in the joints of the first, tenth, eleventh, and twelfth ribs, each of which has only one synovial cavity. Compare **radiate ligament.**

intraatrial /in″trə·ā″trē·əl/ [L, *intra* + *atrium,* hall], pertaining to the space or substance within an atrium of the heart.

intraatrial block, delayed or abnormal conduction of the cardiac impulse within the atria. It is identified on an electrocardiogram by a prolonged and often a notched P wave. Also called **sinoatrial (SA) block.** See also **atrioventricular block, heart block, intraventricular block.**

intrabony pocket. See **periodontal pocket.**

intracanalicular fibroma /-kan′əlik″yələr/ [L, *intra* + *canaliculus,* small channel], a tumor containing glandular epithelium and fibrous tissue, occurring in the breast.

intracanicular papilloma /-kənik″yələr/, a benign warty growth in certain glands, especially the breast.

intracapsular fracture /-kap″syələr/ [L, *intra* + *capsula,* little box], a fracture within the capsule of a joint.

intracardiac /-kar″dē·ak/ [L, *intra,* within; Gk, *kardia,* heart], pertaining to the interior of the heart chambers.

intracardiac catheter. See **cardiac catheter.**

intracardiac electrogram, a record of changes in the electric potentials of specific cardiac loci as measured by electrodes placed within the heart via cardiac catheters. It is used for loci that cannot be assessed by body surface electrodes, such as the bundle of His or other regions within the cardiac conducting system.

intracardiac lead /lēd/ [L, *intra* + Gk, *kardia,* heart; AS, *laedan,* lead], **1.** an electrocardiographic conductor in which the exploring electrode is placed within one of the cardiac chambers, usually by means of cardiac catheterization. **2.** *(Informal)* a tracing produced by such a lead on an electrocardiograph.

intracartilaginous endochondral ossification. See **ossification.**

intracatheter /-kath″ətər/ [L, *intra* + Gk, *katheter,* something lowered], a thin, flexible, plastic catheter introduced through a stainless steel needle and threaded into a blood vessel to infuse blood, fluid, or medication. Also called *intracath.*

intracavernosal injection, introduction of a hypodermic needle into the corpus cavernosum of the penis in order to administer a medication. It is used for treatment of erectile dysfunction.

intracavitary /in′trəkav″itər′ē/ [L, *intra* + *cavum,* cave], pertaining to the space within a body cavity.

intracavitary therapy, a kind of radiotherapy in which one or more radioactive sources are placed, usually with the help of an applicator or holding device, within a body cavity to irradiate the walls of the cavity or adjacent tissues.

intracellular /-sel″yələr/ [L, *intra,* within, *cella,* storeroom], **1.** pertaining to the interior of a cell. **2.** within a cell.

intracellular fluid (ICF) [L, *intra* + *cella,* storeroom, *fluere,* to flow], a fluid within cell membranes throughout most of the body, containing dissolved solutes that are essential to electrolytic balance and to healthy metabolism. Also called *intracellular water.* Compare **extracellular fluid, interstitial fluid, lymph, plasma.**

intracerebral /-ser″əbrəl/ [L, *intra* + *cerebrum,* brain], pertaining to the area or substance within the cerebrum.

intracerebral hematoma, a localized collection of extravasated blood within the cerebrum, associated with a cerebral laceration resulting from a contusion. See also **intracerebral hemorrhage.**

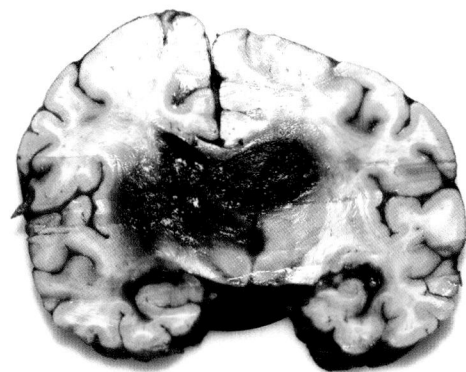

Intracerebral hemorrhage *(Purrucker et al, 2014)*

intracerebral hemorrhage (ICH), a type of hemorrhagic stroke in which bleeding directly into the brain occurs. It is most often caused by hypertension and is associated with increased intracranial pressure. ICH usually occurs in the basal ganglia, thalamus, pons, and cerebral and cerebellar white matter.

intracervical. See **endocervical.**

intracistronic /in′trəsistron″ik/ [L, *intra* + *cis,* this side, *trans,* across], within a cistron.

intracoronal retainer /-kôr″ənəl/ [L, *intra* + *corona,* crown], **1.** a cast restoration, such as an inlay, that lies largely within the contour of the tooth crown. The retention to displacement is developed between the restoration and the walls of the prepared tooth cavity. **2.** a direct retainer used in the construction of removable partial dentures. It consists of a female portion within the coronal segment of the crown of an abutment and a male portion attached to the denture proper. See also **inlay.**

intracostal /-kos″təl/, pertaining to the inner surface of a rib.

intracranial /-krā″nē·əl/ [L, *intra,* within; Gk, *kranion,* skull], pertaining to the area within the cranium (the bony skull).

intracranial abscess. See **brain abscess.**

intracranial aneurysm, localized dilation of any of the cerebral arteries. Characteristics of the condition include sudden severe headache, stiff neck, photophobia, nausea, vomiting, and sometimes loss of consciousness. Rupture of an intracranial aneurysm produces a mortality rate approaching 50%, and survivors face a high risk of recurrence. Some forms of intracranial aneurysm may be treated surgically. Kinds include **berry aneurysm, fusiform aneurysm, mycotic aneurysm.**

intracranial hemorrhage [L, *intra,* within; Gk, *kranion,* skull, *haima,* blood], a hemorrhage within the cranium.

intracranial pneumatocele. See **pneumocephalus.**

intracranial pressure (ICP), pressure that occurs within the brain and cerebral spinal fluid.

intractable /intrak″təbəl/ [L, *intractabilis,* hard to manage], having no relief, such as a symptom or a disease that is not relieved by the therapeutic measures used.

intractable pain [L, *intractabilis,* hard to manage, *poena,* penalty], pain that is not relieved by ordinary medical, surgical, and nursing measures. The pain is often chronic and persistent and can be psychogenic in nature.

intracutaneous /-kyo͞otā″nē·əs/ [L, *intra* + *cutis,* skin], within the skin, particularly the dermis.

intracystic papilloma /-sis″tik/ [L, *intra* + Gk, *kystis,* bag], a benign epithelial tumor formed within a cystic adenoma.

intracytoplasmic sperm injection (ICSI), a micromanipulation technique used in male factor infertility, in which a single spermatocyte is inserted into an oocyte by micropuncture.

intradermal /-dur″məl/ [L, *intra,* within; Gk, *derma,* skin], in the skin.

intradermal injection, the introduction of a hypodermic needle into the dermis for the purpose of instilling a substance, such as a serum or vaccine.

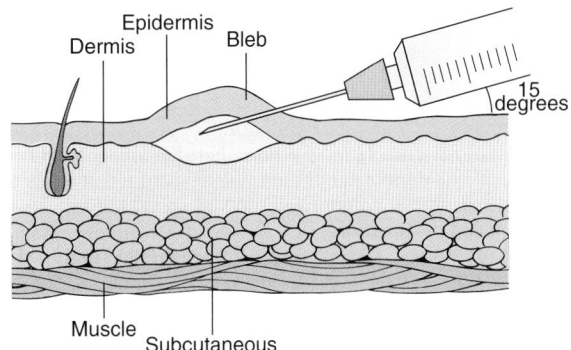

Intradermal injection technique *(Clayton and Willihnganz, 2013)*

intradermal test [L, *intra* + Gk, *derma,* skin], a procedure used to identify suspected allergens by subcutaneously injecting the patient with small amounts of extracts of the suspected allergens. The injections are made at spaced intervals, usually in the forearm or the scapular region. The patient is concurrently injected with the diluent alone as a control procedure. The test result is positive if within 15 to 30 minutes the injection of extract produces a wheal surrounded by erythema and the control injection produces no symptoms. The intradermal test is started with highly diluted solutions; if the initial test result is negative, the procedure is repeated with stronger solutions. This gradual method is used to prevent a systemic reaction, which is more of a risk with intradermal testing than with other kinds of allergy testing, such as the scratch test. The intradermal test tends to be more accurate than the scratch test and is often performed if scratch test results are negative or unclear. Intradermal testing also limits to between 20 and 30 the number of suspected allergens that can be examined simultaneously in the skin of one patient. Also called **subcutaneous test.** Compare **patch test, scratch test.** See also **conjunctival test, use test.**

intradialytic hypotension, hypotension sometimes seen as a complication of hemodialysis.

intradiscal electrothermal therapy, a minimally invasive procedure for the treatment of discogenic low back pain.

intraductal /-duk″təl/, within a duct.

intraductal carcinoma [L, *intra* + *ductus,* duct], a neoplasm that occurs most often in the breast but can occur elsewhere, as in the salivary glands. The lesion on cross section usually shows well-differentiated tumor cells in calcified and dilated ducts.

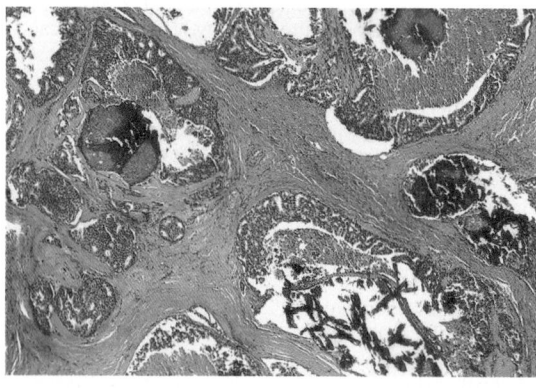

Intraductal carcinoma of the salivary gland (Fletcher, 2007)

intraductal papilloma, a small benign epithelial tumor in a milk duct of the breast, occasionally marked by bleeding from the nipple. See also **papilloma.**

intradural lipoma [L, *intra* + *dura,* hard], a fatty tumor in or beneath the dura mater of the spine or sacrum that tends to infiltrate the dorsal column and roots of spinal nerves, causing pain and dysfunction.

intraepidermal carcinoma /in′trə·ep′idur″məl/ [L, *intra* + Gk, *epi,* above, *derma,* skin], a neoplasm of squamous epidermal cells that does not proliferate into the basal area and often occurs in many sites simultaneously. The lesions, which enlarge slowly, are resistant to chemotherapy and to radiation. Also called **precancerous dermatitis.**

intraepidermal vesicle, a fluid-filled, blisterlike cavity within the epidermis, usually less than 1 cm in diameter.

intraepithelial carcinoma. See **carcinoma in situ.**

intrafollicular insemination (IFI), a method of assisted reproductive technology in which semen is injected into the fluid-filled sac that contains an oocyte.

intrafusal muscle fiber /-fyoo″zəl/, the striated muscle fiber within a muscle spindle.

intrahepatic cholestasis, a result of some condition inside the liver, such as an infection, sepsis, cirrhosis, an abscess, a tumor, or a complication from medication.

intrahepatic cholestasis of pregnancy, a type of intrahepatic cholestasis sometimes seen during the third trimester of pregnancy, characterized by severe itching, hepatomegaly, and sometimes jaundice. It clears up after delivery. The cause is unknown, but because it occurs far more in certain ethnic groups than in others, there may be a genetic link.

intraluminal /-loo″minəl/, **1.** within the lumen of any tubular structure or organ. **2.** between or among tubes.

intraluminal coronary artery stent, a device permanently inserted into a coronary artery to maintain patency of the lumen of the vessel.

intramammary abscess /-mam″ərē/, a collection of pus within a mammary gland.

intramembranous ossification. See **ossification.**

intramenstrual pain /-men″stroo·əl/ [L, *intra,* within, *menstrualis,* monthly, *poena,* penalty]. See **mittelschmerz.**

intramural /-myoo″rəl/ [L, *intra,* within, *murus,* wall], pertaining to events or structures within the walls of an organ, body part, or cavity.

intramural part of male urethra, the short, most proximal part of the urethra, running almost vertically down from the bladder to where it enters the prostate.

intramural part of ureter, the short distal portion of the ureter after it bends to run obliquely through the wall of the bladder.

intramuscular (IM) /-mus″kyələr/ [L, *intra,* within, *musculus,* muscle], pertaining to the interior of muscle tissue.

intramuscular injection [L, *intra* + *musculus*], the introduction of a hypodermic needle into a muscle to administer a medication.

■ METHOD: The equipment is selected and the medication drawn up into the syringe. The selected site is prepared by cleansing with alcohol. Care must be taken to identify landmarks and select sites to prevent damage to nerves and adjacent structures.

■ PATIENT CARE CONSIDERATIONS: Infection may result from nonaseptic technique; care is taken not to contaminate the needle before injection or to suffer a needlestick. Certain medications can cause tissue necrosis if injected into the subcutaneous tissues. Many medications may be given intravenously or intramuscularly, but the intravenous dose may be much smaller. Inadvertent injection into a blood vessel can cause severe systemic reactions of an overdose. Often biologicals, such as antigens, serums, or vaccines, may leave a knot in the muscle that is not painful and that subsides slowly over several weeks or months, though it may cause concern in the patient or in the parents of younger patients. The lump should not grow larger or become more painful. If it does, one may assume that an abscess has formed.

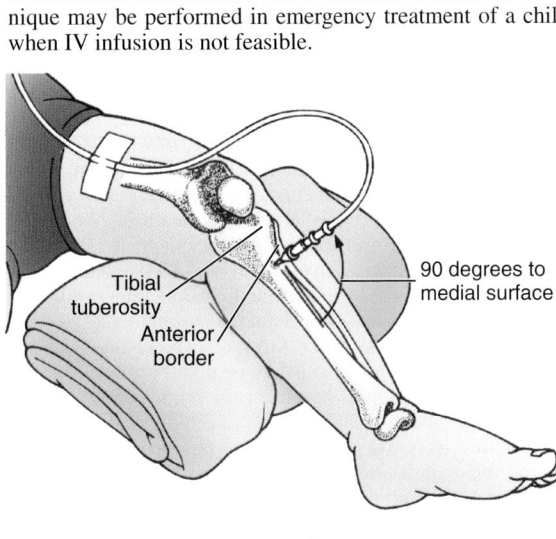

Intramuscular injection technique *(Clayton and Willihnganz, 2013)*

intraocular /-ok″yələr/ [L, *intra* + *oculus*, eye], pertaining to structures or substances within the eye.

intraocular lens (IOL), a plastic artificial lens generally inserted into the capsule of the lens after cataract removal.

intraocular pressure, the internal pressure of the eye, regulated by resistance to the flow of aqueous humor through the fine sieve of the trabecular meshwork. Contraction or relaxation of the longitudinal muscles of the ciliary body affects the size of the opening in the meshwork. In older persons the trabecular meshwork may become sclerotic and obstructed, preventing the normal flow of aqueous humor from passing out at the proper rate and causing an increase in the intraocular pressure. See also **glaucoma.**

intraoperative /-op″ərətiv′/ [L, *intra* + *operari*, to work], pertaining to the period during a surgical procedure. Compare **perioperative.**

intraoperative hyperthermia [L, *intra* + *operari*, to work], a rapid rise in temperature during a surgical procedure. Causes may include dehydration, premedication with anticholinergic drugs, excessive surgical draping, malignant hyperthermia, thyroid storm, neuroleptic syndrome, septicemia, blood transfusion reaction, or excessive heat delivery from radiant warmers.

intraoperative lymphatic mapping. See **sentinel node biopsy.**

intraoperative radiotherapy (IORT), the use of a single high dose of radiation at the time of surgery as adjuvant therapy in tumor resection.

intraoperative ultrasound, a diagnostic technique that uses a portable ultrasound device to scan the spinal cord during spinal surgery. The method enables surgeons to locate and identify tumors of the central nervous system that may not be detected by computed tomography or other techniques. Intraoperative ultrasound can distinguish between syrinxes, or fluid-filled cysts, and neoplastic growths in nervous system tissue.

intraoral examination. See **dental examination.**

intraoral orthodontic appliance /in′trə-ôr″əl/ [L, *intra* + *oralis*, mouth], a device placed inside the mouth to correct or alleviate malocclusion.

intraosseous /in′trə-os″ē-əs/ [L, *intra*, within, *os*, bone], pertaining to the interior of bone.

intraosseous infusion, the injection of blood, medications, or fluids into bone marrow rather than into a vein. The technique may be performed in emergency treatment of a child when IV infusion is not feasible.

Intraosseous infusion technique *(Rothrock, 2015)*

intraparietal sulcus /-perī″ətəl/ [L, *intra* + *paries*, wall, *sulcus*, groove], an irregular groove on the convex surface of the parietal lobe that marks the division of the inferior and superior parietal lobules of the cerebrum. Also called **interparietal fissure.**

intrapartal care /-pär″təl/ [L, *intra* + *partus*, birth], care of a pregnant woman from the onset of labor to the completion of the fourth stage of labor with the expulsion of the placenta. See also **antepartal care, emergency childbirth, newborn intrapartal care, postpartal care.**

■ METHOD: The signs and symptoms of true labor are observed. Uterine contractions increase in frequency, duration, and strength. Pressure of the presenting part of the fetus causes dilation and effacement of the cervix and contractions of the amniotic sac, producing a bloody discharge called "bloody show." A physical examination of the mother is performed. Urine is measured regularly through labor and may be tested for levels of ketones, protein, and glucose to determine specific gravity. A microhematocrit is often done. The position, attitude, and presentation of the fetus are ascertained by abdominal palpation. The cervical effacement and dilation and the station of the presenting part of the fetus are determined periodically by vaginal examination, using careful aseptic technique. If the amniotic sac has broken, the color, character, and quantity of the amniotic fluid are noted. The fetal heart rate is counted, and variations are noted in relation to the timing and intensity of contractions.

intrapartal period, the period spanning labor and birth.

intrapartum /-pär″təm/, pertaining to the period of labor and birth.

intrapartum hemorrhage, copious bleeding, usually caused by abruptio placentae or placenta previa during labor. See also **hemorrhage.**

intraperiosteal fracture /in′trəper′ē-os″tē-əl/ [L, *intra* + Gk, *peri*, around, *osteon*, bone], a fracture that does not rupture the periosteum.

intrapleural space /-ploor″əl/ [L, *intra*, within; Gk, *pleura*, rib; L, *spatium*], the cavity of the pleura.

intrapsychic conflict /-sī″kik/ [L, *intra* + Gk, *psyche*, mind], an emotional clash of opposing impulses within oneself, for example, the id versus the ego or the ego versus the superego. See also **conflict.**

intrapulmonary /-pul″məner′ē/ [L, *intra*, within, *pulma*, lung], pertaining to the interior of the lungs.

intrapulmonary shunt [L, *intra* + *pulmoneus*, relating to the lung], (in respiratory therapy) a condition in which a region of the lungs is perfused with little or no ventilation. It is indicated by a low ratio of QS/QT, in which QS represents the difference between end capillary oxygen content and mixed venous oxygen content and QT represents cardiac output. The condition may occur in atelectasis, pneumonia, pulmonary edema, and adult respiratory distress syndrome.

intrarenal azotemia, an elevated blood urea concentration caused by a reduced glomerular filtration rate resulting in acute or chronic diseases of the renal parenchyma.

intrarenal hemodynamics /-rē″nəl/ [L, *intra* + *ren*, kidney], the pattern of blood flow or distribution in the various parts of the kidney. Normally the renal cortex and outer medulla receive the major portion of renal blood flow.

intraspinal hypodermic /-spī″nəl/ [L, *intra*, within, *spina*, spine, *hypo*, under, *derma*, skin], pertaining to the injection of a substance into the spinal canal.

intrathecal /in′trəthē″kəl/ [L, *intra* + *theca*, sheath], pertaining to a structure, process, or substance within a sheath, such as within the spinal canal.

intrathecal injection, the introduction of a hypodermic needle into the subarachnoid space for the purpose of instilling a material for diffusion throughout the spinal fluid.

intrathoracic goiter /-thôras″ik/ [L, *intra* + Gk, *thorax*, chest; L, *guttur*, throat], an enlargement of the thyroid gland that protrudes into the thoracic cavity.

intrathoracic kidney, an ectopic kidney that partially or completely protrudes above the diaphragm into the posterior mediastinum. Also called *thoracic kidney.*

intratubal insemination (ITI), method of assisted reproductive technology in which washed semen is injected into the fallopian tube.

intrauterine /in′trəyoo″tərin/ [L, *intra*, within, *uterus*, womb], pertaining to the inside of the uterus.

intrauterine catheter. See **catheter.**

intrauterine device (IUD) [L, *intra* + *uterus*, womb; Fr, *devise*], (*Informal*) a contraceptive device, consisting of a bent strip of radiopaque plastic with a fine monofilament tail. The addition of copper wire and/or bands increases the effectiveness. Progesterone-filled IUDs are also available. The mechanism of action is not known. Insertion into the cervix is performed during or just after menstruation when the cervix is slightly open and menstruation assures that a pregnancy does not exist. The tail string of the IUD is left projecting a few centimeters from the cervix. By feeling the string with her finger at least once each menstrual cycle the wearer can be sure the device is in place. The string also provides a hold for removing the IUD. The rate of failure for the IUD method of contraception is approximately one to five unplanned pregnancies in 100 women using the device for 1 year. IUDs can cause complications; the most serious is pelvic inflammatory disease. When such infections occur in pregnancy, they may be overwhelming and lethal; therefore the IUD is removed if pregnancy is suspected. Some other complications are cervicitis, perforation of the uterus, salpingitis that causes sterility, ectopic pregnancy, abortion, embedding of the device in the wall of the uterus, endometritis, bleeding, pain, cramping, undetected expulsion, and irritation of the penis. Also called **coil, loop,** *intrauterine contraceptive device.*

intrauterine fracture, a fracture that occurs during fetal life.

intrauterine growth curve, a line on a standardized graph representing the mean weight for gestational age through pregnancy to term. It provides a method for classifying infants according to their state of maturity and fetal development.

intrauterine growth retardation, an abnormal process in which the development and maturation of the fetus are impeded or delayed more than two deviations below the mean for gestational age, sex, and ethnicity. It may be caused by genetic factors, maternal disease, or fetal malnutrition that results from placental insufficiency. See also **growth retardation, small for gestational age (SGA) infant.**

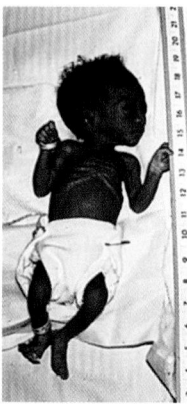

Infant with intrauterine growth retardation (*Courtesy TALC, Institute of Child Health*)

intrauterine insemination (IUI), artificial insemination in which specially washed sperm is injected through the cervix directly into the uterus.

intrauterine transfusion, direct transfer of Rh-negative blood cells into a fetus in utero in cases of isoimmunization. See also **transfusion.**

intravascular /-vas″kyələr/ [L, *intra* + *vasculum*, little vessel], pertaining to the inside of a blood vessel.

intravascular coagulation test, a test for detecting coagulation of blood within the blood vessels.

intravascular fluid, a term sometimes used to refer to that part of the extracellular fluid that is within the blood vessels (i.e., the plasma).

intravenous (IV) /-vē″nəs/ [L, *intra* + *vena*, vein], pertaining to the inside of a vein, as of a thrombus or an injection, infusion, or catheter.

intravenous alimentation. See **total parenteral nutrition.**

intravenous bolus, a relatively large dose of medication administered into a vein in a short period, usually within 1 to 30 minutes. The IV bolus is commonly used when rapid administration of a medication is needed, such as in an emergency; when the drugs being given cannot be diluted, such as many cancer chemotherapeutic drugs, are administered; and when the therapeutic purpose is to achieve a peak drug level in the bloodstream of the patient. The IV bolus is not used when the medication must be diluted in a large-volume parenteral fluid before entering the bloodstream or when the rapid administration of a medication, such as potassium chloride, may be life-threatening. The IV bolus is normally not used for patients who have decreased cardiac output, decreased urinary output, pulmonary congestion, or systemic edema. Such patients have decreased tolerance to medications, which therefore must be diluted more than usual and administered at slower rates. A wristwatch with a second hand is recommended for the timing of all IV bolus injections. The amount of medication to be delivered per minute is determined by dividing the total amount to be injected by the prescribed time for delivery. The IV bolus site is prepared with an appropriate antiseptic, and sterile technique is used to enter the site with a venipuncture needle. A winged-tip needle is used for administering an IV bolus because it is small enough to lessen the risk of collapsing the vein and causing trauma and is more stable than a syringe needle. If a primary IV line is already established, the IV bolus is administered by mixing the prescribed drug with the appropriate amount of diluent and then administering the drug into the primary line, after first determining whether it is compatible with the primary IV solution. Also called **intravenous push.**

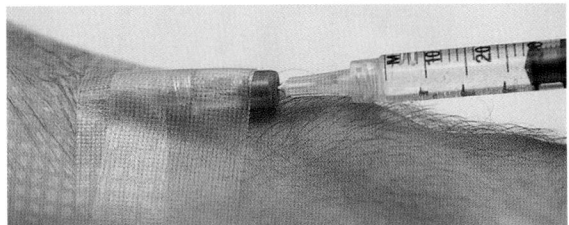

Administration of medication by intravenous bolus
(Potter and Perry, 2005)

intravenous catheter [L, *intra,* within, *vena,* vein; Gk, *katheter,* a thing inserted], a catheter that is inserted into a vein for supplying medications or nutrients directly into the bloodstream or for diagnostic purposes such as studying blood pressure.

intravenous cholangiography (IVC), (in diagnostic radiology) a procedure for outlining the major bile ducts. A radiopaque contrast material is injected intravenously, and serial radiographic images are taken. See also **cholangiography.**

intravenous controller, any of several devices that automatically deliver IV fluid at selectable flow rates. The controller is commonly equipped with a rate selector, drop sensor, and alarm. When the infusion does not flow at the prescribed rate, the drop alarm emits a visual and an audible signal. The IV controller works by gravity, so the IV container must be placed at least 30 inches (76.20 cm) above the venipuncture site. The controller cannot exert the positive pressure of a true pump and is not recommended for the delivery of highly viscous fluid or for maintenance of an open arterial line. Compare **intravenous peristaltic pump, intravenous piston pump, intravenous syringe pump.**

intravenous digital subtraction angiography (IV-DSA), a procedure for the radiographic visualization of arteries after injection of a radiopaque contrast medium into a vessel.

intravenous fat emulsion, a preparation of 10% fat administered into a vein to help maintain the weight of an adult patient or the weight and growth of a younger patient. Such fat emulsions are prepared from refined soybean oil and egg-yolk phospholipids and may contain such major fatty acids as linoleic, oleic, palmitic, and linolenic acids. The IV fat emulsion is isotonic and may be administered into a peripheral vein, but it is not mixed with other solutions used in parenteral alimentation. IV fat emulsions are often administered when hyperalimentation is not sufficient to maintain adequate treatment of a patient

or when the patient needs calories but cannot tolerate the high percentage of dextrose contained in hyperalimentation solutions. Such emulsions may also be administered to patients who need more essential fatty acids than are contained in hyperalimentation solutions or who need general nutritional improvement, especially postoperative patients. IV emulsions are not administered to patients suffering from disturbances of normal fat metabolism (such as hyperlipemia), severe hepatic diseases, blood coagulation defects caused by decreased blood-platelet counts, pulmonary diseases, lipoid nephrosis, hepatocellular damage, or bone marrow dyscrasia or to those being treated with anabolic inhibitory drugs. If possible, the IV fat emulsion is usually administered during the day so that the patient may follow a normal eating pattern with rest during the night and lower nocturnal urinary flow. Once the primary IV line has been established, IV fat emulsions are usually administered with the aid of an electronic control device to maintain an even flow rate and prevent fatty-acid overload. The patient's fluid intake and output are regularly measured during the delivery of such an emulsion, and daily blood studies are conducted to determine the level of free-floating triglycerides. Hepatic function tests are performed if the patient receives consecutive IV fat emulsion infusions over a long period. Immediate adverse reactions or those that may occur up to 2½ hours after the onset of the infusion may include temperature rise, flushing, sweating, pressure sensations over the eyes, nausea, vomiting, headache, chest and back pain, dyspnea, and cyanosis. Delayed adverse reactions or those that occur within 10 days of the onset of such infusions may include hepatomegaly, splenomegaly, thrombocytopenia, focal seizures, hyperlipemia, hepatic damage, jaundice, hemorrhagic diathesis, and gastroduodenal ulcer.

intravenous feeding, the administration of nutrients through a vein or veins.

intravenous infusion, **1.** a solution administered into a vein through an infusion set that includes a plastic or glass vacuum

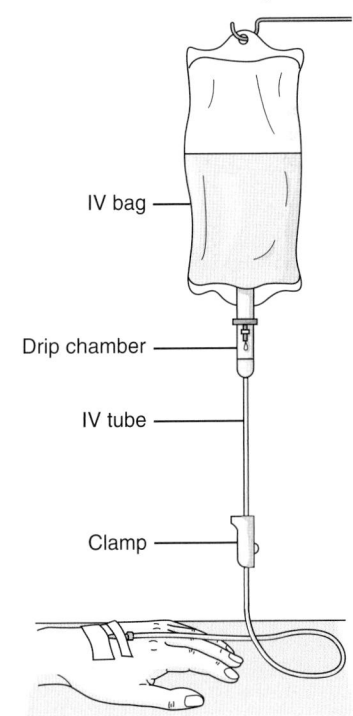

Intravenous infusion *(Sorrentino, 2008)*

bottle or bag containing the solution and tubing connecting the bottle to a catheter or a needle in the patient's vein. **2.** the process of administering a solution intravenously. Swelling of the limb around and distal to the site of injection may indicate that the tip of the catheter or needle is in the subcutaneous tissue and not in the vein. The fluid may be infiltrating the tissue spaces. It should be withdrawn and the limb elevated. Redness, swelling, heat, and pain around the vein at the site of injection or proximal to it may indicate thrombophlebitis. The infusion should be discontinued and the inflammatory condition treated. The infusion is usually begun again at another site. See also **venipuncture.**

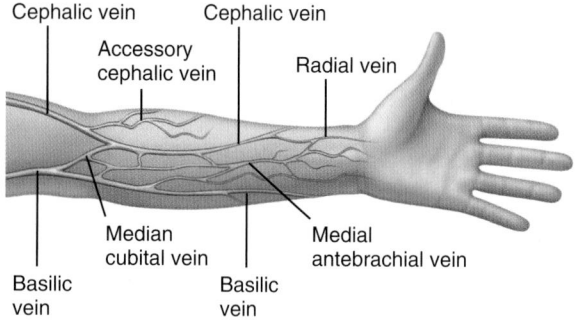

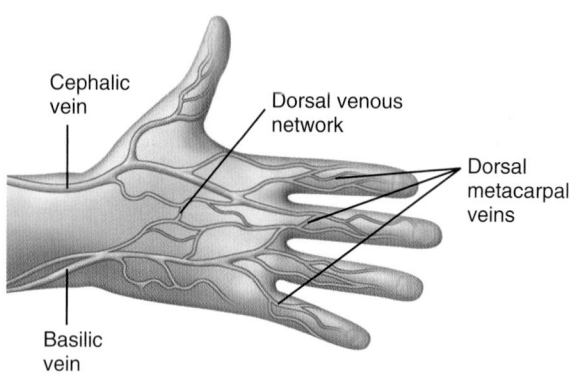

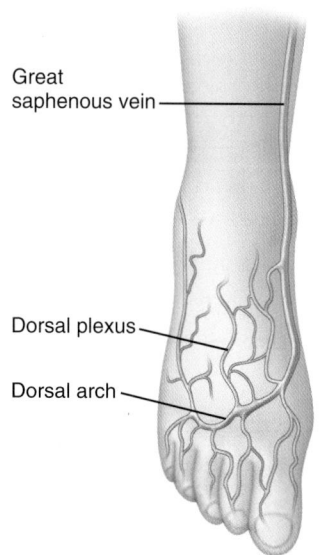

Common intravenous infusion sites *(Harkreader, Hogan, and Thobaben, 2007)*

intravenous infusion filter,   any of the numerous devices used to help ensure the purity of an IV solution. IV filters strain the solution to remove such contaminants as dissolved impurities (detergents, proteins, and polysaccharides), extraneous salts, microorganisms, particles, precipitates, and undissolved drug powders. Any such contaminants may complicate the IV therapy and patient recovery. Some filters are built into the primary IV tubing; others must be attached. One of the main criteria for selecting a filter is the assurance that the filter is not too fine for the IV solution to be strained; filters that are too fine clog. The size of filter membranes varies from 5 to 0.22 μm. Filters of 1 to 5 μm will remove most particulate debris but not most fungi or bacteria. Filters that are 0.45 μm or less remove fungi and most bacteria; filters that are 0.22 μm remove all fungi and bacteria but also reduce the flow rate of the IV solution, which is crucial when rapid delivery is required. See also **needle filter.**

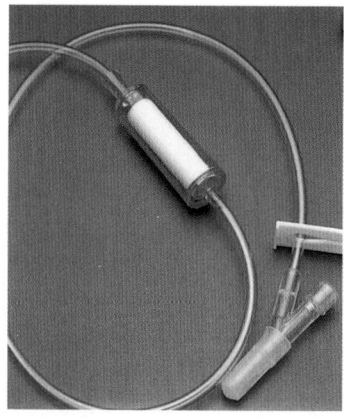

Intravenous infusion filter *(Courtesy Millipore Corporation)*

intravenous infusion technique,   the calculations for determining the delivery rate of IV fluid for the individual patient and the necessary spiking of the container and priming of the tubing before venipuncture and fluid administration.
- METHOD: The rate at which solution is to be administered by IV infusion can be determined from the procedure formula. The hands are washed thoroughly before assembling the container of IV solution, the IV pole, and the proper tubing with the flow clamp placed in a position directly beneath the drip chamber and clamped. If a bottle with a rubber stopper is used, the protective metal cap is removed, and, with the bottle held securely on a stable surface, the spike of the tubing is pushed firmly into the stopper. To spike an IV bottle with an indwelling vent and latex diaphragm, the metal cap and diaphragm are removed and the spike is inserted into the nonvented hole. If a hiss, indicating a vacuum, does not follow, the bottle is contaminated and should be discarded. Nonvented tubing is used with this kind of bottle. A plastic bag of IV fluid is hung on a hook for spiking, the cap is removed by pulling it smoothly to the right, and a nonvented spike is inserted into the port by using one quick, even motion to prevent the escape of fluid. An IV bag with a firm, easily grasped port with a lip to prevent touch contamination may be spiked before hanging by grasping the port firmly; squeezing the bag may expel air and is carefully prevented. After the hanging bag or bottle is spiked, the drip chamber is gently squeezed until it is half full before the tubing is primed. The end of the tubing is held over a sink or clean receptacle as the protective cap is removed, and the cap is kept uncontaminated for reuse. The flow clamp is released, and the tubing is allowed to fill with fluid until all air bubbles

Complications of intravenous fluid therapy

Observations	Nursing actions
Circulatory overload Bounding pulse, venous distension, hoarseness, dyspnea, cough, pulmonary rales, restlessness	Notify physician. Reduce flow to "keep open" rate. Raise head of bed to facilitate breathing.
Local infiltration Decreased rate or cessation of fluid flow Tissue around needle or catheter site cold, pale, swollen, hard Complaint of local pain	Stop infusion. Arrange to restart infusion at another site. Apply moist heat. Elevate lower arm.
Thrombophlebitis Pain, redness, warmth, edema along vein	Same as for local infiltration. Cold compress may be applied initially.
Pyrogenic reaction Fever, chills, general malaise, nausea, and vomiting 30 min after infusion started Hypotension (if severe)	Switch to another infusion solution and run at "keep open" rate. Notify physician. Monitor vital signs. Save infusion fluid for culture.
Anaphylactic reaction (with proteins) Apprehension, dyspnea, wheezing, tightness of chest, itching, hypotension	Switch infusion to nonprotein solution and run at "keep open" rate. Notify physician. Monitor vital signs.

From Monahan FD et al: *Phipps' medical-surgical nursing: health and illness perspectives,* ed 8, St Louis, 2007, Mosby.

are expelled; if a back check valve is on the tubing, the valve is inverted during priming. The flow clamp is then closed, the protective cap is replaced, and the tubing is looped over the IV pole so that it does not interfere with venipuncture. Once the needle or intracatheter is inserted and connected to the tubing, the fluid container is hung securely from the IV pole or hook above the insertion site. The flow clamp is opened, and the proper fluid delivery rate is adjusted by counting the number of drops entering the drip chamber in a minute. Throughout the administration of IV fluid, rate of flow is checked periodically and any necessary readjustments of the clamp are made. IV fluids also may be delivered via IV pump. IV pump tubing is then used, and the flow rate is calculated in mL/hr.

■ INTERVENTIONS: The nurse assembles the apparatus for the IV infusion, spikes the fluid container, primes the tubing, calculates the proper rate for the patient, and ensures that the rate of delivery and asepsis are maintained. The nurse carefully observes the patient for signs of circulatory overload, such as a bounding pulse, engorged peripheral veins, dyspnea, cough, and pulmonary edema, indicating that the infusion rate is too rapid and requires adjustment.

■ OUTCOME CRITERIA: IV solutions administered to maintain normal body fluid levels and electrolyte balance do not overload the circulation when delivered at the flow rate required by the individual patient.

intravenous injection, a hypodermic injection into a vein for the purpose of instilling a single dose of medication, injecting a contrast medium, or beginning an IV infusion of blood, medication, or a fluid solution, such as saline or dextrose in water. See also **venipuncture.**

intravenous (IV) therapy, the administration of fluids into a vein through a needle or small-caliber catheter. Ongoing assessment and attention to patient comfort are important.

intravenously, through a vein.

intravenous medication [L, *intra,* within, *vena,* vein, *medicare,* medicine], a pharmaceutical delivered directly into the bloodstream via a vein.

intravenous peristaltic pump, any one of several devices for administering IV fluids by exerting pressure on the IV tubing rather than on the fluid itself. Most peristaltic pumps operate with normal IV tubing and deliver fluid at a selectable cubic centimeter per hour rate. This device is equipped with a drop sensor, rate selector, power switch indicator lamp, and drop indicator and alarm. The alarm sounds when the infusion does not flow at the prescribed rate. Compare **intravenous controller, intravenous syringe pump, intravenous piston pump.**

intravenous piston pump, any of several devices that accurately control the infusion of IV fluids by piston action. Most IV piston pumps can be operated by battery, as well as by electric current, and require special tubing. Some models are portable. IV piston pumps are commonly equipped with controls that allow selectable flow rates and indicators that display flow rates, dose limits, and cumulative fluid volumes. Such pumps commonly monitor the patient's skin for infiltration by IV fluid and are equipped with infiltration and flow alarms. The IV piston pump monitors the actual volume of IV fluid administered instead of counting drops of fluid; hence, its accuracy is not affected by drop size, temperature, or fluid viscosity. The pump is designed to reduce the delivery rate to a keep-vein-open rate if the proper flow rate or the dose limit is exceeded. The pump also stops delivery of the IV fluid if the line is clogged or if infiltration is detected. Compare **intravenous controller, intravenous peristaltic pump, intravenous syringe pump.**

intravenous pump, a pump designed to regulate the rate of flow of a fluid administered through an IV catheter. See also **Harvard apparatus.**

intravenous push. *(Informal)* See **intravenous bolus.**

intravenous urography, a radiographic technique for examining the structure and function of the urinary system. A contrast medium is injected intravenously, and serial x-ray images are taken as the medium is cleared from the blood by the kidneys. The renal calyces, renal pelvis, ureters, and urinary bladder are all visible on the radiographs. Tumors, cysts, stones, and many structural and functional abnormalities may be diagnosed with this technique. Fasting and bowel cleansing with a cathartic or an enema before the procedure improve visualization of the urinary tract. The patient may also be asked to void immediately before injection of the contrast medium to prevent dilution of the medium in the bladder and immediately afterward to check residual urine in the bladder. Also called *descending urography,* **excretory urography, intravenous urography, pyelography.**

intravenous syringe pump, any one of several devices that automatically compress a syringe plunger at a controlled rate. Such devices are used with disposable syringes that can deliver blood, medications, or nutrients by IV, arterial, or subcutaneous routes. IV syringe pumps can deliver small volumes of fluid at rates as low as 0.01 mL/hr. They are often used in the treatment of infants and are especially useful in the care of ambulatory patients. They are ideal for keeping arterial lines open and are usually battery operated and portable. Compare **intravenous controller, intravenous peristaltic pump, intravenous piston pump.**

intravenous team, a group of registered nurses and licensed practical nurses with special training who administer IV therapy. State laws may restrict practice of IV therapy to specific categories of health professionals.

intravenous urography. See **intravenous pyelography.**

intraventricular /-ventrik″yələr/ [L, *intra* + *ventriculus,* little belly], pertaining to the space within a ventricle or to the conduction system within the walls of a ventricle.

intraventricular block, altered conduction of the cardiac impulse within the ventricles. The block can occur as a right bundle branch block, left bundle branch block, hemiblock, left anterior or posterior fascicular block, or bifascicular block. Intraventricular blocks are identified on an electrocardiogram when the QRS duration is greater than normal. They can be caused by coronary artery disease, valvular heart disease, ventricular hypertrophy and fibrosis, cardiomyopathy, or degeneration of the conduction system. Prognosis is based on the underlying cardiac condition. Also called **sinoatrial (SA) block.** See also **bundle branch block, heart block, hemiblock, intraatrial block.**

intraventricular conduction defect, a delay in conduction of a ventricular impulse within the ventricles that does not correspond to either a right bundle branch block or a left bundle branch block.

intraventricular hydrocephalus. See **hydrocephalus.**

intraventricular pressure [L, *intra,* within, *ventriculus,* little belly], the pressure of the blood within the heart's ventricles. It varies with the phase of the cardiac cycle.

intraventricular sulcus, one of the two sulci (anterior and posterior) that separate the two ventricles of the heart. The anterior intraventricular sulcus contains the anterior interventricular artery and the great cardiac vein. The posterior interventricular sulcus contains the posterior interventricular artery and the middle cardiac vein.

intravesical pressure, the pressure exerted on the contents of the urinary bladder, being the sum of the intraabdominal pressure from outside the bladder and the detrusor pressure exerted by the bladder wall musculature itself. Also called *bladder pressure, vesical pressure.*

intravesical ureterocele, a prolapse of the terminal part of the ureter into the bladder. Also called **orthotopic ureterocele.**

intrinsic /intrin″sik/ [L, *intrinsecus,* inside], **1.** denoting a natural or inherent part or quality. **2.** originating from or situated within an organ or tissue.

intrinsic asthma, a nonseasonal, nonallergic form of asthma, which usually first occurs later in life than allergic asthma and tends to be chronic and persistent rather than episodic. Precipitating factors include inhalation of irritating pollutants, such as dust particles, smoke, aerosols, strong cooking odors, and paint fumes and other volatile substances. Intrinsic asthma may also be triggered by exposure to cold, damp weather; sudden inhalation of cold, dry air; physical exercise; violent coughing or laughing; respiratory infections, such as the common cold; or psychological factors, such as anxiety. Compare **allergic asthma.** See also **asthma.**

intrinsic factor, a substance secreted by the gastric mucosa that is essential for the intestinal absorption of cyanocobalamin. Intrinsic factor forms a bond with molecules of cyanocobalamin, and this complex is transported across the ileal membrane. A deficiency of intrinsic factor, caused by gastrectomy, myxedema, or atrophy of the gastric mucosa, causes pernicious anemia. See also **pernicious anemia.**

intrinsic minus hand deformity, an abnormality that results from interruption of the ulnar and median nerves at the wrist. It causes metacarpophalangeal joint hyperextension and interphalangeal joint flexion.

intrinsic motivation, a prompt to action that comes from within the individual; a drive to action that is rewarded by doing the activity itself, rather than deriving some external reward from it.

intrinsic muscles, muscles that are entirely within the body part or segment moved by them, as the tongue muscles.

intrinsic muscles of the tongue, the superior longitudinal, inferior longitudinal, transverse, and vertical muscles that alter the shape of the tongue by lengthening and shortening it, curling and uncurling its apex and edges, and flattening and rounding its surface.

intrinsic pathway of coagulation, an in vitro sequence of reactions leading to fibrin formation, beginning with the contact activation of factor XII, followed by the sequential activation of factors XI, IX, and VIII, and resulting in the activation of factor X, which in activated form initiates the common pathway of coagulation. Compare **extrinsic pathway of coagulation.** See also **coagulation cascade, common pathway of coagulation.**

intrinsic PEEP, abbreviation for **intrinsic positive end-expiratory pressure.**

intrinsic positive end-expiratory pressure (intrinsic PEEP), elevated positive end-expiratory pressure and dynamic pulmonary hyperinflation caused by insufficient expiratory time or a limitation on expiratory flow. It cannot be routinely measured by a ventilator's pressure monitoring system but only by an expiratory hold maneuver done by the clinician. Its presence increases the work required to trigger the ventilator, causes errors in the calculation of pulmonary compliance, may cause hemodynamic compromise, and complicates interpretation of hemodynamic measurements. Also called **auto-PEEP.**

intro-, prefix meaning "into" or "within": *introitus, introjection, introspection.*

introitus /intrō″itəs/ [L, *intro,* inside, *ire,* to go], an entrance or orifice in a cavity or a hollow tubular structure of the body, such as the vaginal introitus.

introjection /-jek″shən/ [L, *intro* + *jacere,* to throw], an ego defense mechanism whereby an individual unconsciously incorporates into his own ego structure the qualities of another person, usually a significant other. It happens early in life and continues less intensely throughout.

intromission /-mish″ən/, the insertion of one object into another, such as the introduction of the penis into the vagina.

intron /in″tron/ [L, *intra*, within, *regin*, region], a sequence of nucleotides in eukaryotic DNA that does not code for amino acids and interrupts the coding sequence of a gene. Some genes contain numerous long introns.

Intron A, a parenteral antineoplastic drug. Brand name for **interferon alfa-2b, recombinant.**

Intropin, an adrenergic drug. Brand name for **dopamine hydrochloride.**

introspection /-spek″shən/ [L, *introspicere*, to look into], **1.** the act of examining one's own thoughts and emotions. **2.** a tendency to look inward and view the inner self. −*introspective, adj.*

introsusception /-susep″shən/ [L, *intro*, inside, *suscipere*, to receive], the telescoping or invagination of one segment of the digestive tract into another segment, usually a lower segment. The process can cause obstruction and strangulation of the bowel.

introversion /-vur″zhən/ [L, *intro* + *vertere*, to turn], **1.** the tendency to direct one's interests, thoughts, and energies inward or toward things concerned with the self. **2.** the state of being totally or primarily concerned with one's own intrapsychic experience.

introvert /in′trəvurt/ [L, *intro* + *vertere*, to turn], **1.** *n.,* a person whose interests are directed inward and who is emotionally reserved and quiet in social situations. **2.** *v.,* to turn inward or to direct one's interests and thoughts toward oneself. Compare **ambivert, extrovert.** See also **egocentric.**

introverted personality /-vur″tid/ [L, *intro*, inside, *vertere*, to turn, *personalis*], a personality that is focused on inner thoughts and that derives more energy from being alone than from the company of others.

intrusion /in·trŏŏ′zhən/ [L, *intrudere*, to push or force in], an orthodontic technique of depressing a tooth back into the occlusal plane or attempting to prevent its eruption or elongation during correction of an excessive overbite. Compare **extrusion,** def. 3.

intubate /in″tyŏŏbāt/ [L, *in*, within, *tubus*, tube], to catheterize or insert a tube into an organ or body part.

intubation [L, *in*, within, *tubus*, tube, *atio*, process], passage of a tube into a body aperture, specifically the insertion of a breathing tube through the mouth or nose into the trachea to ensure a patent airway for the delivery of anesthetic gases and oxygen or both. Blind intubation is the insertion of a breathing tube without the use of a laryngoscope. Kinds include **endotracheal intubation,** *nasotracheal intubation.*

intussusception /in′təsəsep″shən/ [L, *intus*, within, *suscipere*, to receive], prolapse of one segment of bowel into the lumen of another segment. This kind of intestinal obstruction may involve segments of the small intestine, the colon, or the terminal ileum and cecum. Intussusception occurs most often in infants and small children and is characterized by abdominal pain, vomiting, and presence of bloody mucus in the stool (currant jelly stool). Barium enema is used to confirm the diagnosis, and surgery is usually necessary to correct the obstruction. See also **intestinal obstruction.**

intussusceptum, the portion of the intestine that has been invaginated within another part in intussusception.

inulin /in″yŏŏlin/, a fructose-based starch derived from rhizomes of plants from the Compositae family. It is used as a diagnostic aid in tests of kidney function, specifically glomerular filtration. It is not metabolized or absorbed by the

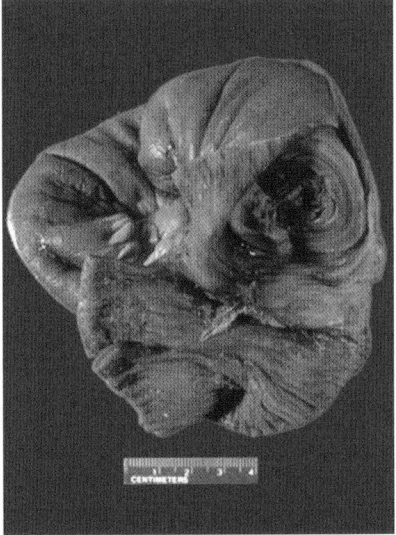
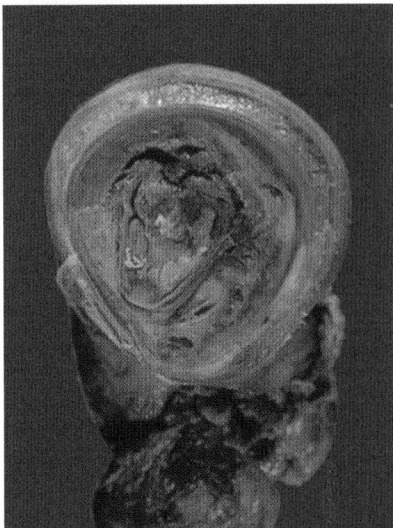

Intussusception *(Klatt, 2010)*

body. It is freely filtered by the glomeruli of the kidney but is neither secreted nor reabsorbed by the tubules, making its clearance equivalent to the glomerular filteration rate.

inulin clearance, a test of the rate of filtration of a starch, inulin, in the glomerulus of the kidney. Inulin is given by mouth, and the glomerular filtration rate can be estimated from the amount of inulin that appears in the urine. The clearance rate of inulin in urine for adults with normal renal function is 100 to 150 mL/min.

inunction /inungk′shən/ [L, *in*, within, *ungere*, to smear], **1.** the rubbing of a drug mixed with an oil or fatty substance into the skin, with absorption of the active ingredient. **2.** any compound so applied.

inundation fever. See **scrub typhus.**

in utero /inyŏŏ′tərō/, inside the uterus.

invagination /invaj′ənā″shən/ [L, *in*, within, *vagina*, sheath], **1.** a condition in which one part of a structure telescopes into another, as the intestine during peristalsis. If the invagination is extensive or involves a tumor or polyp, it may cause an intestinal obstruction, necessitating surgery.

2. surgery for repair of a hernia by replacement of the contents of the hernial sac in the abdominal cavity. General or spinal anesthesia may be used. See also **hernia, intestinal obstruction, intussusception, peristalsis.** −*invaginate, v.*

invariable behavior /inver′ē·əbəl/ [L, *in,* not, *variare,* to vary], behavior that results from physiological response to a stimulus and that is not modified by individual experience, such as a reflex. Compare **variable behavior.**

invasion /invā′zhən/ [L, *in,* within, *vadere,* to go], the process by which malignant cells move through the basement membrane and gain access to blood vessels and lymphatic channels.

invasion of privacy, (in law) the violation of another person's right to be left alone and free of unwarranted publicity and intrusion. See also **HIPAA.**

invasive /invā′siv/ [L, *in,* within, *vadere,* to go], characterized by a tendency to spread, infiltrate, and intrude.

invasive carcinoma, a malignant neoplasm composed of epithelial cells that infiltrate and destroy surrounding tissues and may metastasize.

invasive mole. See **chorioadenoma destruens.**

invasive procedure [L, *in + vadere,* to go, *procedere,* to proceed], a diagnostic or therapeutic technique that requires entry of a body cavity or interruption of normal body functions. Kinds include **colonoscopy, endoscopy.**

invasive thermometry, measurement of tissue temperature using probes placed directly into the tissue.

Invega, brand name for **paliperidone.**

inverse I:E ratio, an inspiratory/expiratory ratio in mechanical ventilation in which the duration of inspiration is prolonged relative to that of expiration. This condition is sometimes instituted to improve oxygenation, as in the care of infants with idiopathic respiratory distress syndrome and of adults in whom conventional ventilator techniques fail. I:E ratios in such cases may be approximately 2:1 or 3:1. Also called **reversed I:E ratio.** See also **I:E ratio.**

inverse Marcus Gunn syndrome. See **Marin Amat syndrome.**

inverse relationship. See **negative relationship.**

inverse square law, a law stating that the amount of radiation reaching a surface is inversely proportional to the square of the distance between the source and the surface. For example, a person standing 1 m from a patient being treated with radium is exposed to four times more radiation than a person standing 2 m from the patient.

Inversine, a ganglionic blocking agent. Brand name for **mecamylamine hydrochloride.**

inversion /invur′zhən/ [L, *invertere,* to turn over], **1.** an abnormal condition in which an organ is turned inside out, such as a uterine inversion. **2.** a chromosomal defect in which a segment of a chromosome breaks off and then reattaches to the chromosome in the reverse orientation, causing the genes carried on that part of the chromosome to be in an abnormal position and sequence.

inversion recovery (IR), a magnetic resonance pulse sequence designed to emphasize T_1 differences.

inversion traction, a positional form of traction for the prevention and treatment of back disorders. Special equipment is used to lengthen the spinal column while the patient is in an inverted position. A similar effect is achieved by hanging upside down from a chinning bar.

invert /in′vurt/ [L, *invertere,* to turn over], to turn something upside down or inside out.

invertebrate /invur″təbrit/, an animal that lacks a vertebral column. Invertebrates comprise more than 95% of all species of animals.

invert sugar [L, *invertere,* to turn over; Gk, *sakcharon*], a mixture of equal amounts of dextrose and fructose, obtained by hydrolyzing sucrose. It is used in solution as a parenteral nutrient.

investigational device exemption (IDE) /inves′tigā″shənəl/ [L, *investigare,* to search for], an agreement through which the federal government permits the testing of new medical devices.

investigational new drug (IND), a drug not yet approved for marketing by the U.S. Food and Drug Administration (FDA) and available only for use in experiments to determine its safety and effectiveness. The use of an investigational new drug in human subjects requires approval by the FDA of an application that includes reports of animal toxicity tests, descriptions of proposed clinical trials, and a list of the investigators and their qualifications.

investing fascia, a layer of fascia that closely invests a muscle or ligament.

Invirase, an antiretroviral protease inhibitor. Brand name for **saquinavir.**

invisible differentiation /inviz′ibəl/ [L, *in,* not, *visibilis,* visible, *differentia,* difference], (in embryology) a fixed determination for specialization and diversification that exists in embryonic cells but is not yet visibly apparent. See also **chemodifferentiation.**

in vitro /invē″trō/ [L, *in,* within, *vitreus,* glassware], occurring in a laboratory apparatus. Compare **in vivo.**

in vitro fertilization (IVF), a method of fertilizing human ova outside the body by collecting the mature ova and placing them in a dish with a sample of spermatozoa. After an incubation period of 48 to 72 hours, the fertilized ova are injected into the uterus through the cervix. The procedure takes from 2 to 3 days. See also **gamete intrafallopian transfer.**

in vitro susceptibility testing, a laboratory trial of the sensitivity of microorganisms, particularly fungi, to potential therapeutic chemicals.

in vivo /invē″vō/ [L, *in,* within, *vivo,* alive], occurring in an organism. Compare **in vitro.**

in vivo fertilization, a method of fertilization of an ovum within a fallopian tube of a fertile female donor for transplantation into an infertile recipient.

in vivo tracer study, a diagnostic procedure in which a series of images of an administered radioactive tracer demonstrates normal or abnormal structures or processes as the tracer passes through a patient's body. A strip-chart recording of the procedure, such as a radionuclide angiocardiogram, shows the passage of the tracer through body.

involucrum /in′vəloo″krəm/ *pl.* involucra [L, *involvere,* to wrap up], a sheath or coating, such as that encasing a sequestrum of necrotic bone.

involuntary /invol″əntər′ē/ [L, *in,* not, *voluntas,* will], occurring without conscious control or direction. See also **autonomy.**

involuntary muscle. See **smooth muscle.**

involuntary nervous system. See **visceral nervous system.**

involuntary patient, a person admitted to a psychiatric facility against his or her will. Compare **informal admission.**

involution /in′vəloo″shən/ [L, *involvere,* to wrap up], **1.** a normal process of turning or rolling inward characterized by a decrease in the size of an organ caused by a decrease in the size of its cells, as in postpartum involution of the uterus. **2.** (in embryology) a developmental process in which a group of cells grows over the rim at the border of the organ or part and, rolling inward, rejoins the organ or part to form a tube, such as in the heart or bladder.

In vitro fertilization *(Carlson, Eisenstat, and Ziporyn, 2004)*

1. Hormonal stimulation of egg maturation
2. Removal of eggs by laparoscopy
3. Collection of sperm sample and concentration of most active sperm
4. In vitro fertilization
5. Early cleavage in vitro
6. Extra embryos frozen
7. Reimplantation of up to three embryos

involutional melancholia, *(Obsolete)* a term for a state of depression that occurs during the climacteric (menopause of women). It is now treated as a major depressive episode. See also **depression.**

inward aggression /in'wərd/ [AS, *inweard*], destructive behavior that is directed against oneself. See also **aggression, masochism.**

iodide /ī'ədīd/ [Gk, *ioeides,* violet], an anion of iodine. Sodium and potassium iodide are the salts most commonly used in medicine.

iodinated serum albumin /ī'ədinā'tid/, a sterile, buffered, isotonic solution containing radioiodinated normal human serum used in diagnostic tests of blood volume and cardiac output. It is adjusted to provide not more than 1 mCi of radioactivity per milliliter.

iodine (I) /ī'ədīn/ [Gk, *ioeides,* violet], a nonmetallic element of the halogen group. Its atomic number is 53; its atomic mass is 126.90. Iodine is a bluish black solid that becomes a violet vapor on heating without going through a liquid phase. Iodine is an essential micronutrient or trace element. Almost 80% of the iodine present in the body is in the thyroid gland, mostly in the form of thyroglobulin. Iodine deficiency can result in goiter or cretinism. Iodine is found in seafood, iodized salt, and some dairy products. It is used as a contrast agent for blood vessels in computed tomography scans. Radioisotopes of iodine are used in radioisotope scanning procedures and in palliative treatment of cancer of the thyroid.

iodine poisoning [Gk, *ioeides,* violet; L, *potio,* drink], toxic effects of ingesting iodine, a potent antiseptic with low tissue toxicity. Symptoms include burning pain in the mouth and esophagus, abdominal pain, vomiting, diarrhea, delirium, shock, nephritis, laryngeal edema, and circulatory collapse. The mucous membranes are stained brown by the iodine.

iodism /ī'ədiz'əm/ [Gk, *ioeides* + *ismos,* process], a condition produced by excessive amounts of iodine in the body. It is characterized by increased lacrimation and salivation, rhinitis, weakness, and skin eruption.

iodize /ī'ədīz/ [Gk, *ioeides* + *izein,* to cause], to treat or impregnate with iodine or an iodide. Table salt is iodized to prevent the occurrence of goiter in areas with insufficient iodine in the drinking water or food. Iodized oil, a viscous liquid with the odor of garlic, has been used as a contrast medium in radiology.

iodized oil, a preparation of oil that contains covalently bound iodine. It is commonly used as a radiocontrast agent. It is also used as a suspension medium for chemotherapy.

iodized salt [Gk, *ioeides,* violet; AS, *sealt*], table salt to which potassium or sodium iodide has been added to protect against goiter, particularly in regions where soil and drinking water have low iodine content. The iodides are added to achieve approximately 100 ppm.

iodo-, prefix meaning "iodine": *iododerma, iodophor, iodotherapy.*

iododerma /ī·ō·dōdur'mə/ [Gk, *ioeides* + *derma,* skin], a skin rash of follicular papules and pustules caused by a hypersensitivity to ingested iodides. The lesions may be acneiform, bullous, or fungating. Treatment requires removal of iodides.

iodophor /ī·ōdəfôr/ [Gk, *ioeides* + *phoros,* bearer], an antiseptic or disinfectant that combines iodine with another agent, such as a detergent.

iodopsin /ī'ōdop'sin/ [Gk, *ioeides* + *optikos,* vision], a photosensitive chemical in the cones of the retina that reacts in association with other chemicals and plays a part in color vision. Iodopsin is more stable when exposed to bright light than rhodopsin, which is found in the rods of the retina. Color vision, a synthesis of red, green, and blue light, is induced by changes within the pigments of different types of cones during a photochemical process in which coded nerve impulses are sent to the brain. Research on the exact role of iodopsin in color vision, which is still unknown, is ongoing.

iodoquinol /ī'ōdō'kwinol/, an amebicide.

■ INDICATIONS: It is prescribed in the treatment of intestinal amebiasis. It is also used as a preventative in high-risk people.

■ CONTRAINDICATIONS: Hepatic disease and known hypersensitivity to iodine or 8-hydroxyquinoline prohibit its use.

■ ADVERSE EFFECTS: Among the most serious adverse effects are dizziness, thyroid enlargement, optic neuropathy, optic atrophy, and peripheral neuropathy.

iodotherapy /ī·ō'dōther'əpē/, a treatment that uses iodine or an iodide.

ion /ī″ən, ī′on/ [Gk, *ienai,* to go], an atom or group of atoms that has acquired an electrical charge through the gain or loss of an electron or electrons.

-ion, **1.** suffix meaning "an electrically charged particle": *anion, cation.* **2.** a noun-forming suffix: *basion, osteopedion, opinion.*

ion exchange chromatography, the process of separating and analyzing different substances according to their affinities for chemically stable but very reactive synthetic exchangers, which are composed largely of polystyrene and cellulose. The process uses an absorbent containing ionizing groups and accommodates the exchange of ions between a solution of substances to be analyzed and the absorbent. Ion exchange chromatography is often used to separate components of nucleic acids and proteins elaborated by various structures throughout the body. Different ions deposited in the absorbent during the exchange produce bands of different colors, which constitute a chromatograph. Compare **column chromatography, gas chromatography.**

ionic bonding /ī·on′ik/ [Gk, *ienai* + ME, *band,* to bind], an electrostatic force between ions. Ionic compounds do not form true molecules; in aqueous solution they separate into their hydrated constituent ions.

ionic dissociation, a phenomenon whereby ions in ionic compounds in an aqueous solution are freed from their mutual attractions and distribute themselves uniformly throughout the solvent.

ionic strength, the sum of the concentrations of all ions in a solution multiplied by the square of their charge.

ionization /ī′ənīzā″shən/ [Gk, *ienai* + *izein,* to cause], the process in which a neutral atom or molecule gains or loses electrons and thus acquires a negative or positive electrical charge. Ionizing radiation produces ionization in its passage through body tissue or other matter. Ionization can also cause cell death or mutation.

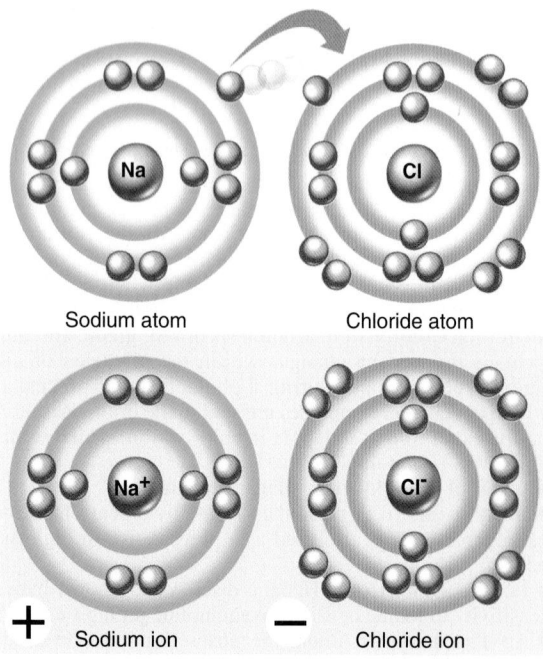

Sodium atom · Chloride atom

Sodium ion · Chloride ion

Ionization

ionization chamber, a small cavity filled with air that collects the ionic charge liberated during irradiation. The exposure and dose of radiation can be calculated from the amount of change liberated and the mass of air in the chamber.

ionization constant (K), after establishment of ionic equilibrium, the product of the molar concentration of the ions divided by the molar concentration of the nonionized molecules.

ionize /ī″ənīz/ [Gk, *ienai* + *izein,* to cause], to separate or change into ions. See also **ion.**

ionized calcium, the ionized, unbound, noncomplexed fraction of serum calcium that is biologically active.

ionizing energy /ī″ənī′zing/, the average energy lost by ionizing radiation in producing an ion pair in a gas. In air the value is approximately 33.73 electron volts.

ionizing radiation, high-energy electromagnetic waves (such as x-rays and gamma rays) and particles (such as alpha and beta particles, neutrons, protons, and heavy nuclei) that cause substances in their paths to dissociate into ions. The spatial distribution of the ionization depends on the kind of radiation, its penetrating power, the location of the source, and the nature of the irradiated material. High-energy x-rays penetrate deeply, most beta particles penetrate only a few millimeters, and alpha particles penetrate only a fraction of a millimeter. However, all three produce intense ionization along their tracks. Ionizing radiation directly affects living organisms by killing cells or slowing their development and by producing gene mutations and chromosome breaks. Tissues containing elements with relatively high atomic masses, such as calcium in bones and teeth, absorb much higher doses of ionizing radiation than do soft tissues.

ionizing radiation injury [Gk, *ion,* going; L, *radiare,* to shine, *injuria*], damage or ill effects suffered by exposure to ionizing radiation. The risk of cell death or injury from radiation depends on the type of tissue cells, the stage of cell division at the time of exposure, the intensity and time span of exposure, and the type of radiation administered. See also **radiation burn.**

ion-selective electrode, a potentiometric electrode that develops a potential in the presence of one ion (or class of ions) but not in the presence of a similar concentration of other ions.

iontophoresis /ī·on′tōfôrē′·sis/ [Gk, *ion,* going, *pherein,* to carry], the introduction of ions of soluble salts into the tissues by direct current. Also called **galvanoionization, ionophoresis, medical ionization.**

iontophoretic pilocarpine test [Gk, *ienai* + *pherein,* to carry], a sweat test used in the diagnosis of cystic fibrosis. Pilocarpine iontophoresis is used to stimulate production of sweat, which is absorbed from the forearm in a previously weighed gauze pad. The sweat sample is then analyzed for concentrations of sodium and chloride electrolytes. Now largely replaced by genetic analysis.

ion transfer, a method of transporting chemicals across a membrane by using an electric current as a driving force.

iopromide /ī″opro′mīd/, a nonionic, low-osmolality, radiopaque medium used for cardiovascular imaging, excretory urology, and contrast enhancement in computed tomography.

iota /ī·ō″tə/, **1.** I, ι, the ninth letter of the Greek alphabet. **2.** something tiny, such as one iota.

ioversol /ī″over′sol/, a nonionic contrast medium used in angiography and urography and for contrast enhancement in computed tomography.

Iowa trumpet /ī′əwə/, a kind of needle guide used in performing a pudendal block. It consists of a long, thin cylinder through which a needle may be passed. A ring is attached to the proximal end of the guide, allowing the operator to hold it securely.

ioxilan /iok'slan/, a low-viscosity, low-osmolality, nonionic contrast agent used in arteriography, excretory urography, and computed tomography.

IPA, abbreviation for **Independent Practice Association.**

IPAA, abbreviation for *International Psychoanalytical Association.*

IPA-Model HMO, a health maintenance organization (HMO) that contracts with an independent practice association (IPA) for physician services. The IPA processes and adjudicates claims. The HMO provides enrollees and hospital contracts.

ipecac /ip'əkak/, an emetic once widely used. It has not been manufactured since 2010 because of a lack of evidence of effectiveness when administered to induce vomiting for poisoning. It delayed or interfered with more effective treatments.

IPOF, abbreviation for *immediate postoperative fit.* See **immediate postoperative fit (IPOF) prosthesis.**

ipomea /ipəmē″ə/, a resin prepared from the dried root of *Ipomoea orizabensis,* formerly used as a cathartic.

IPPB, abbreviation for **intermittent positive-pressure breathing.**

IPPB unit, a pressure-cycled ventilator providing a flow of air into the lungs at a predetermined pressure. As the pressure is attained, the flow is stopped, pressure is released, and the patient exhales. The IPPB device is used to prevent postoperative atelectasis, to promote full expansion of the lungs, to improve oxygenation, and to administer nebulized medications into the respiratory passages.

IPPV, abbreviation for **intermittent positive-pressure ventilation.** See **intermittent positive-pressure breathing.**

Iprivask, brand name for **desirudin.**

ipsi-, prefix meaning "the same, or self": *ipsilateral.*

IPSID, abbreviation for **immunoproliferative small intestine disease.**

ipsilateral [L, *ipse,* same, *latus,* side], affecting the same side of the body. Compare **contralateral.**

IPSP, abbreviation for *inhibitory postsynaptic potential.*

IPV, abbreviation for **poliovirus vaccine, inactivated.** See **poliovirus vaccine.**

IQ, abbreviation for **intelligence quotient.**

Ir, symbol for the element **iridium.**

IR, **1.** abbreviation for **image receptor. 2.** abbreviation for *interventional radiology.* **3.** abbreviation for **inversion recovery.**

IRB, abbreviation for **institutional review board.**

irbesartan, an antihypertensive drug.

■ INDICATIONS: It is used to treat hypertension, either alone or in combination with other drugs. It is also used investigationally to treat heart failure and hypertension in patients with diabetic nephropathy caused by type 2 diabetes mellitus.

■ CONTRAINDICATIONS: Known hypersensitivity and second- and third-trimester pregnancy prohibit its use.

■ ADVERSE EFFECTS: Anxiety, headache, fatigue, diarrhea, and dyspepsia are among the adverse effects. Common side effects include dizziness, cough, and upper respiratory infection.

Iressa, brand name for **gefitinib.**

Ir g, abbreviation for *immune response function gene.* See **immune response.**

irid-, prefix for terms pertaining to the iris: *iridectomy.*

iridectomy /ī'ridek″təmē/ [Gk, *iris,* rainbow, *ektomē,* excision], surgical removal of part of the iris of the eye. It is performed most often to restore drainage of the aqueous humor in glaucoma or to remove a foreign body or a malignant tumor. An incision is made through the cornea, and the iris is grasped with forceps or a hook and drawn out through the incision. The affected area is cut away, and the elastic iris is allowed to slip back into place. Subjunctival antibiotics may be instilled, and an eye pad is applied. After surgery, the patient is observed for signs of local hemorrhage or excessive pain.

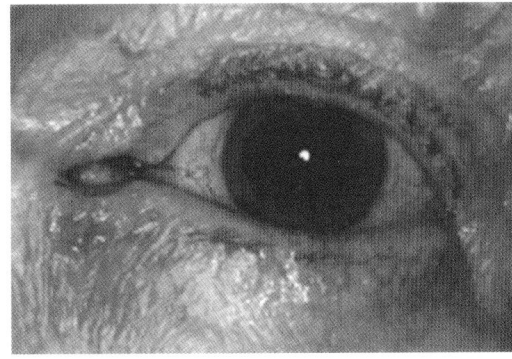

Irregular pupil caused by iridectomy *(Lemmi and Lemmi, 2000)*

iridemia /ī'ridē″mēə/, hemorrhage from the iris.

iridescence /ir'ides″əns/ [L, *iridescere,* to shine like a rainbow], the property of light interference or ability to break up light waves into colors of the spectrum.

iridic. See **iris.**

iridium (Ir) /irid'ē·əm/ [Gk, *iris,* rainbow], a silvery-bluish metallic element. Its atomic number is 77; its atomic mass is 192.22.

irido-, iro-, prefix meaning "the iris" or "a colored circle": *iridopathy, iridotomy, iridoplegia.*

iridology /ī'ridol″əjē/ [Gk, *iris,* rainbow, *logos,* science], the science that specializes in relations between disease and the shape, color, and other individual characteristics of the iris. There is considerable controversy over its validity.

iridopathy /ī'ridop″əthē/, any disease of the iris.

iridoplegia /ī'ridōplē″jə/ [Gk, *iris,* rainbow, *plege,* stroke], a condition of paralysis of the sphincter muscle of the iris or the dilator muscle or both.

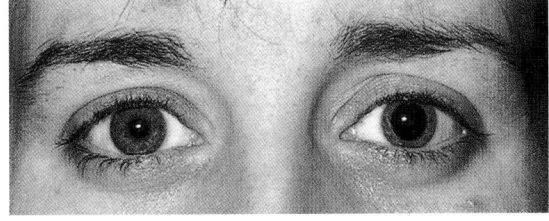

Iridoplegia *(Perkin, 2002)*

iridotomy /ī'ridot″əmē/ [Gk, *iris* + *temnein,* to cut], a surgical incision into the iris of the eye. It is performed to relieve occlusion of the pupil, to enlarge the pupil in cataract extraction, or to treat postoperative glaucoma. Topical anesthetic drops are used. An incision is made through the cornea, and a cut is made transversely across the sphincter fibers of the iris. Atropine and an antibiotic may be instilled, and a dressing and shield are applied. After surgery the dressing is observed for signs of drainage. See also **iridectomy, iris.**

irinotecan, an antineoplastic hormone.

■ INDICATIONS: It is used to treat metastatic carcinoma of the colon or rectum.

■ CONTRAINDICATIONS: Pregnancy and known hypersensitivity to this drug prohibit its use.

■ ADVERSE EFFECTS: Life-threatening effects include leukopenia, anemia, and neutropenia. Other adverse effects include fever, headache, chills, dizziness, diarrhea, nausea, vomiting, anorexia, constipation, cramps, flatus, stomatitis, dyspepsia, site irritation, rash, sweating, dyspnea, increased cough, rhinitis, vasodilation, edema, asthenia, and weight loss.

iris /ī′ris/ [Gk, rainbow], an annular, colored membrane shaped like a disc, suspended in aqueous humor between the cornea and the crystalline lens of the eye and enclosing a circular pupil. Smooth muscle fibers of the iris contract and relax to allow more or less light to enter the eye through the pupil. The periphery of the iris is continuous with the ciliary body and is connected to the cornea by the pectinate ligament. The iris divides the space between the lens and the cornea into an anterior and a posterior chamber. The involuntary muscle of the iris is composed of circular fibers and radiating fibers. Dark pigment cells under the translucent tissue of the iris are variously arranged in different people to produce different colored irises. The pigment is absent in albinos. In blue eyes the pigment cells are confined to the posterior surface of the iris, but in gray eyes, brown eyes, and black eyes the pigment cells appear in the anterior layer of epithelium and in the stroma. See also **dilator pupillae, sphincter pupillae. −iridic,** *adj.*

iritis /īrī′tis/ [Gk, *iris* +*itis*], an inflammatory condition of the iris of the eye characterized by pain, lacrimation, photophobia, and, if severe, diminished visual acuity. On ophthalmic examination the eye looks cloudy, the iris bulges, and the pupil is contracted. The underlying cause is treated if identified, but the condition is most often idiopathic. The pupil is dilated, usually with atropine, and a corticosteroid may be prescribed to reduce inflammation. If the inflammation is allowed to continue and the pupil is left constricted, permanent scarring may occur, causing an opacity over the lens and diminished vision.

iro-. See **irido-, iro-.**

iron (Fe) /ī′ərn/ [AS, *iren*], a common metallic element essential for the synthesis of hemoglobin. Its atomic number is 26; its atomic mass is 55.85. Iron salts and complexes, including ferrocholinate, ferrous fumarate, ferrous gluconate, ferrous sulfate, and iron dextran are used to treat iron-deficiency anemias.

iron-binding capacity (IBC), the extent to which transferrin in the serum of a given patient can bind serum iron.

iron-deficiency anemia, a microcytic hypochromic anemia caused by inadequate supplies of iron needed to synthesize hemoglobin. Symptoms are pallor, fatigue, anorexia, malaise, and weakness. Laboratory diagnosis includes hemoglobin, hematocrit, transferrin saturation, ferritin, and serum iron concentration. Iron deficiency may be the result of an inadequate dietary supply of iron, poor absorption of iron by the digestive system, chronic bleeding, or compensated hemolytic anemia. Replacement iron can be supplied by oral ferrous sulfate. The anemia corrects in 2 months, but therapy is continued for another 4 months to replace tissue stores. Compare **hemolytic anemia, hypoplastic anemia.** See also **iron metabolism, nutritional anemia, red cell indexes.**

iron dextran, an injectable hematinic.

■ INDICATIONS: It is prescribed in the treatment of iron-deficiency anemia that is not responsive to oral iron therapy.

■ CONTRAINDICATIONS: Early pregnancy, anemias other than iron-deficiency anemia, or known hypersensitivity to this drug prohibits its use.

■ ADVERSE EFFECTS: Among the more serious adverse effects are severe hypersensitivity reactions, including fatal anaphylaxis. Inflammation or phlebitis at the site of injection, arthralgia, headache, GI distress, fever, and lesser hypersensitivity reactions may occur.

iron level and total iron-binding capacity test, a blood test used to diagnose iron-deficiency anemia and hemochromatosis (iron overload or poisoning), among other conditions.

iron lung. See **Drinker respirator.**

iron metabolism, a series of processes involved in the entry of iron into the body and its absorption, transport, storage, use in the formation of hemoglobin and other iron compounds, and eventual excretion. Iron normally enters through the intestinal mucosa and is oxidized from ferrous to ferric iron in the process. The rate at which iron enters is modulated by this absorption mechanism. When iron stores are high, iron no longer passes through but is trapped by the mucosal cells of the intestine to be eliminated. Once in the blood, iron cycles between the plasma and the reticuloendothelial or erythropoietic system. For hemoglobin synthesis, plasma iron is delivered to the normoblast, where it remains up to 4 months, functioning in the hemoglobin molecules of a mature red cell. Senescent red cells then deteriorate. The iron is released from the hemoglobin by the reticuloendothelial

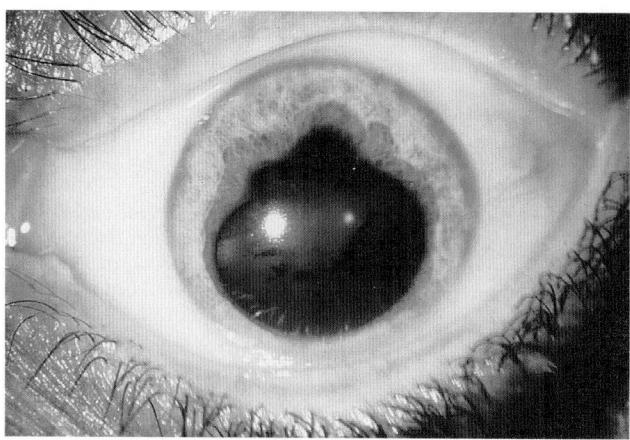

Iritis *(McIntosh et al, 2008)*

system to reenter the transport pool for recycling. The normal iron distribution in a 70-kg adult (male) totals approximately 3.7 g, more than 65% in circulating hemoglobin. Another 27% is found in the storage pool as hemosiderin or ferritin. The body normally conserves iron so well that loss, usually only through the feces, is normally limited to about 1 mg/day. This amount is easily provided by a dietary intake of only 10 mg/day. Iron deficiency may follow extended intervals of inadequate iron intake (especially in women), in pregnancy when higher levels of iron are needed, or with excessive blood loss. Iron overload sometimes occurs in disorders in which normal regulation of iron absorption is impaired, called hemochromatosis. Hemochromatosis may be inherited or acquired in long-term transfusion therapy for chronic anemias.

iron overload, an excess of iron in the body. See also **hemochromatosis, hemosiderosis, siderosis.**

iron poisoning [AS, *iren* + L, *potio,* drink], toxic effects of ingesting iron salts, particularly ferrous sulfate and ferrous chloride. Ferrous sulfate tablets, sometimes mistaken for candy, can cause vomiting, collapse, and liver necrosis. Ferrous chloride, a corrosive substance, causes vomiting, diarrhea, and hemorrhage when taken internally. Iron encephalopathy has resulted from excessive use of iron preparations.

iron-polysaccharide. See **polysaccharide-iron complex.**

iron-rich food, any food item containing a relatively large amount of iron. One of the best sources of dietary iron is liver. Oysters, clams, heart, kidney, lean meat, seafood, and iron-fortified foods are other good sources. Leafy green vegetables, whole grains, and legumes are among the best plant sources. See also **iron, iron-deficiency anemia.**

iron salt poisoning, poisoning caused by overdose of ferric or ferrous salt, characterized by vomiting, bloody diarrhea, cyanosis, and gastric and intestinal pain.

iron-storage disease, an abnormal accumulation of iron in the parenchyma of many organs, as in hemosiderosis.

iron sucrose, a complex of ferric hydroxide, $Fe(OH)_3$, in sucrose, used intravenously to treat iron-deficiency anemia in hemodialysis patients receiving supplemental erythropoietin therapy.

iron transport, the process whereby iron is carried from the intestinal mucosa to sites of use and storage. Iron binds with transferrin and shuttles to storage and utilization sites. Transferrin becomes attached to exogenous iron that enters through the intestinal villi or that reenters the plasma from the sinusoids of the spleen. The iron is then released to the normoblasts, and the transferrin is freed for additional transport functions that may involve iron stored as ferritin or hemosiderin. See also **hemosiderosis, iron metabolism, transferrin.**

irradiation /irā′dē·ā″shən/ [L, *irradiare,* to beam upon], exposure to any form of electromagnetic energy, such as heat, light, or x-rays. Radioactive sources of electromagnetic energy, such as x-rays or isotopes of iodine or cobalt, are used diagnostically to examine internal body structures. The same or similar sources of radioactivity in larger amounts are used to destroy microorganisms or tissue cells that have become cancerous. Infrared or ultraviolet light may be used to produce heat in body tissues for pain relief or to treat acne, psoriasis, or other skin ailments. Ultraviolet light is also used to identify certain bacteria and toxic molds. See also **radiation sickness, radioactivity, ultraviolet.** –**irradiate,** *v.*

irrational /irash′ənəl/ [L, *irrationalis,* contrary to reason], pertaining to events, conditions, or behavior that may be considered unreasonable.

irreducible /ir′əd(y)oo̅″sibəl/ [L, *in,* not, *reducere,* to bring back], unable to be returned to the normal position or condition, as an irreducible hernia. See also **incarcerate.**

irreducible hernia. See **incarcerated hernia.**

irregular pulse /ireg′yələr/ [L, *in,* not, *regula,* rule, *pulsare,* to beat], a variation in the force or rhythm of impulses in an artery, caused by cardiac arrhythmia.

irreversible /ir′əvur″sibəl/ [L, *irrevertere,* to not turn back], pertaining to a situation or condition that cannot be reversed or undone.

irreversible coma. See **brain death.**

irreversible shock, a condition in which shock does not respond to available forms of treatment and in which recovery is impossible as a result of massive cellular damage.

irrigate /ir′igāt/ [L, *irrigare,* to supply water], to flush with a fluid, usually with a slow, steady pressure on a syringe plunger. It may be done to cleanse a wound or to clear tubing.

irrigation /ir′igā″shən/, the process of washing out a body cavity or wounded area with a stream of water or other fluid. It is also used to cleanse a tube or drain inserted into the body, such as an indwelling catheter. The procedure is most commonly performed with water, saline, aminoacetic acid, or antiseptic solution on the eye, ear, throat, vagina, or urinary tract. Gentle pressure is applied in the introduction of the fluid, except in the debridement of wounds, and the solution is removed from internal cavities through suction or drainage. See also **lavage.** –**irrigate,** *v.*

irrigator /ir′igā″tər/, an apparatus with a flexible tube for flushing or washing out a body cavity.

irritability /ir′itəbil″itē/ [L, *irritare,* to tease], a condition of abnormal excitability or sensitivity.

irritable bladder /ir′itəbəl/ [L, *irritare,* to tease; AS, *blaedre*]. See **overactive bladder.**

irritable bowel syndrome (IBS) [L, *irritare,* to tease; OFr, *boel* + Gk, *syn,* together, *dromos,* course], abnormally increased motility of the small and large intestines, of unknown origins. Most of those affected are young adults who complain of diarrhea and, occasionally, pain in the lower abdomen. The pain is usually relieved by passing flatus or stool. In diagnosing irritable bowel syndrome, other conditions, such as dysentery, lactose intolerance, and the inflammatory bowel diseases, must be ruled out. Many persons benefit from the use of bulk-producing agents in the diet because bulk tends to stabilize the water content of the stool. Antidiarrheal drugs are helpful in decreasing the frequency of stool. Mild tranquilizers or antidepressants are sometimes given to relieve anxiety or depression. Also called **functional bowel syndrome, mucous colitis, spastic colon.**

irritant /ir′itənt/ [L, *irritare,* to tease], an agent that produces inflammation or irritation.

irritant poison [L, *irritare,* to tease, *potio,* drink], any of a large number of toxic substances in the environment that can cause pain in the digestive tract, diarrhea, vomiting, abdominal cramps, and urinary tract disorders. Some irritant chemicals are industrial gases, such as ammonia, chlorine, phosgene, sulfur dioxide, hydrogen sulfide, and nitrogen dioxide, which may leak into the atmosphere.

irritation fibroma /ir′itā″shən/, a localized broad-based persistent exophytic lesion composed of dense scarlike connective tissue containing few blood vessels. Caused by episodes of prolonged irritation or by trauma. It can commonly develop on the buccal mucosa, gingiva, tongue, lips, or palate.

IRV, abbreviation for **inspiratory reserve volume.** See **pulmonary function test.**

Irving technique, a method of tubal ligation in which the uterine tubes are ligated and severed and the proximal ends are sewn into the myometrium. Also called *Irving operation, Irving procedure.*

Isaacs syndrome /ī′zəks/ [H. Isaacs, 20th-century American neurologist], progressive muscle stiffness and spasms, with continuous muscle fiber activity similar to that seen with neuromyotonia. Compare **stiff-man syndrome.**

ischaemic contracture. See **Volkmann contracture.**

ischemia /iskē″mē·ə/ [Gk, *ischein,* to hold back, *haima,* blood], a decreased supply of oxygenated blood to a body part. The condition is often marked by pain and organ dysfunction, as in ischemic heart disease. Some causes of ischemia are arterial embolism, atherosclerosis, thrombosis, and vasoconstriction. Also spelled *ischaemia.* Compare **infarction.** −*ischemic, adj.*

ischemic contracture. See **Volkmann contracture.**

ischemic heart disease /iskē′mik/, a pathological condition caused by lack of oxygen in cells of the myocardium.

ischemic lumbago, a pain in the lower back and buttocks caused by vascular insufficiency, as in occlusion of the abdominal aorta.

ischemic necrosis. See **coagulation necrosis.**

ischemic pain, unpleasant, often excruciating pain associated with decreased blood flow caused by mechanical obstruction, constricting orthopedic casts, or insufficient blood flow that results from injury or surgical trauma. Ischemic pain caused by occlusive arterial disease is often severe and may not be relieved, even with narcotics. The individual with peripheral vascular disease may experience ischemic pain only while exercising because the metabolic demands for oxygen cannot be met as a result of occluded blood flow. The ischemic pain of partial arterial occlusion is not as severe as the abrupt, excruciating pain associated with complete occlusion, such as by an embolus or thrombus. See also **pain intervention.**

ischemic paralysis, loss of motor control in a body area caused by an interruption in the blood supply to the area's muscles or nerves.

ischemic penumbra, an area of moderately ischemic brain tissue surrounding an area of more severe ischemia. Theoretically, blood flow to this area may be enhanced in order to prevent the spread of a cerebral infarction.

ischemic pericarditis [Gk, *ischein,* to hold back, *haima,* blood, *peri,* near, *kardia,* heart, *itis,* inflammation], inflammation of the pericardium caused by interruption of its blood supply during myocardial infarction.

ischemic stroke, a cerebrovascular disorder caused by deprivation of blood flow to an area of the brain, generally as a result of thrombosis, embolism, or reduced blood pressure.

ischia. See **ischium.**

ischial spines /is″kē·əl/ [Gk, *ischion,* hip joint; L, *spina,* thorn], two relatively sharp posterior bony projections into the pelvic outlet from the ischial bones that form the lower border of the pelvis.

ischial tuberosity [Gk, *ischion,* hip joint; L, *tuber,* swelling], a rounded protuberance of the lower part of the ischium. It forms a bony area on which the human body rests when in a sitting position.

ischio-, prefix meaning "the ischium" or "the hip": *ischioanal, ischiocele, ischiocavernosus.*

ischioanal fossae, gutters in the anal triangle, one on each side of the anal aperture, formed by the levator ani muscles and adjacent pelvic walls as the two structures diverge inferiorly.

ischiocavernosus, one of two muscles that cover the crura of the penis and clitoris and force blood from the crura into the body of the erect penis and clitoris.

ischiocele. See **sciatic hernia.**

ischiococcygeal muscle, a muscle originating in the ischial spine. It inserts into the lateral border of the lower part of the sacrum and the upper coccyx that supports and raises the coccyx. It is innervated by the third and fourth sacral nerves.

ischiofemoral ligament, a ligament that reinforces the posterior aspect of the fibrous membrane that encloses the hip. It is attached medially to the ischium, just posteroinferior to the acetabulum, and laterally to the ischial tuberosity deep to the iliofemoral ligament. It helps to stabilize the hip joint and reduce the amount of muscle energy required to maintain a standing position. See also **iliofemoral ligament, pubofemoral ligament.**

ischium /is″kē·əm/ *pl.* **ischia** [L; Gk, *ischion,* hip joint], one of the three parts of the hip bone, which joins the ilium and the pubis to form the acetabulum. The ischium comprises the dorsal part of the hip bone and is divided into the body of the ischium, which forms the posteroinferior two fifths of the acetabulum, and the ramus, which joins the inferior ramus of the pubis. The spine of the ischium provides attachment for various muscles, such as the gemellus superior, the coccygeus, and the levator ani. The greater sciatic notch above the spine transmits the superior and inferior gluteal vessels and various nerves, such as gluteal nerves and the sciatic nerve. A notch below the spine of the ischium transmits various ligaments, vessels, and nerves for other parts. The large dorsal tuberosity of the ischium provides attachment for various muscles, such as the adductor longus, the semimembranosus, the biceps femoris, and the semitendinosus. Compare **ilium, pubis.**

isch-, prefix meaning "restraint" or "suppression": *ischemia.*

ISCLT, abbreviation for *International Society of Clinical Laboratory Technologists.*

Isentress, brand name for **raltegravir.**

ISG, abbreviation for **immune serum globulin.** See **immunoglobulin.**

ISH, abbreviation for **isolated systolic hypertension.**

Ishihara chart, the pseudoisochromatic chart used in the Ishihara test for color vision deficiencies.

Ishihara color test /ish′ēhä″rə/ [Shinobu Ishihara, Japanese ophthalmologist, 1879–1963], a test of color vision that uses a series of plates on which are printed pseudoisochromatic round dots in a variety of colors and patterns. People with normal color vision are able to discern specific numbers or patterns on the plates; the inability to pick out a given number or shape is symptomatic of a specific deficiency in color perception.

ISID, abbreviation for *International Society of Infectious Diseases.*

island /ī′lənd/ [OE, *īegland,* island]. See **islet.**

island fever. *(Informal)* See **scrub typhus.**

island of Reil. See **central lobe.**

islands of Langerhans /lang″gərhanz/ [L, *insula,* island; Paul Langerhans, German pathologist, 1847–1888], clusters of cells within the pancreas that produce insulin, glucagon, and pancreatic polypeptide. They form the endocrine portion of the gland, and their hormonal secretions released into the bloodstream are balanced, important regulators of carbohydrate metabolism. The islands of Langerhans are scattered throughout the pancreas; the beta cells, which secrete insulin, usually appear in the center of each of the lobules. Alpha cells secrete glucagon, and pancreatic peptide cells secrete pancreatic peptide. The cells the islands comprise are arranged in plates interspersed by capillaries. Also called **islets of Langerhans.**

islet /ī′lət/ [MFr, *islette,* little island], a cluster of cells or an isolated piece of tissue. Also called **island.**

islet cell adenoma. See **insulinoma.**

islet cell antibody (ICA) /ī'lit/ [MFr, *islette*, little island], an immunoglobulin that reacts with cytoplasmic components of pancreatic islet cells. These antibodies occur in about 60% to 70% of newly diagnosed patients with insulin-dependent diabetes mellitus, providing strong evidence for an autoimmune origin and pathogenesis of the disease. The presence of ICA can be demonstrated years before the occurrence of symptoms. The antibody tends to disappear with time.

islet cell tumor, any tumor of the islets of Langerhans. Kinds include **insuloma, gastrinoma,** *glucagonoma, somatostatinoma.*

isletitis. See **insulitis.**

islets of Langerhans. See **islands of Langerhans.**

-ism, -ismus, suffix meaning "condition of," "practice of," "theory of": *hyperthyroidism, hypopituitarism, strabismus.*

iso- /ī'sō-/, prefix meaning "equal": *isobar, isoantibody, isohydric.*

isoagglutination /ī'sō·əgloo̅'tinā″shən/ [Gk, *isos,* equal; L, *agglutinate,* to glue], the clumping of erythrocytes by agglutinins from the blood of another individual of the same species.

isoagglutinin /ī'sō·əgloo̅'tinin/ [Gk, *isos,* equal; L, *agglutinate,* to glue], an antibody that causes agglutination of erythrocytes in other members of the same species that carry the corresponding antigen on their erythrocytes.

isoamyl alcohol. See **amyl alcohol.**

isoantibody /ī'sō·an″tibod'ē/ [Gk, *isos + anti,* against; AS, *boding,* body], an antibody to isoantigens found in other members of the same species. See also **autoimmune disease, tissue typing.**

isoantigen /ī'sō·an″tijən/ [Gk, *isos + anti,* against; AS, *boding,* body; Gk, *Geenen,* to produce], a substance present in some members of a species that stimulates production of antibodies in other members of the species. Also called **alloantigen.** Compare **autoantigen, autoimmune disease.** Kinds include *blood group antigen.* See also **antigen.**

isobar /ī'səbär/ [Gk, *isos + barrios,* weight], **1.** a line connecting points of equal pressure on a graph, such as lines connecting points of equal carbon dioxide tension on a pH-bicarbonate diagram. **2.** (in nuclear medicine) one of a group of nuclides having the same total number of neutrons and protons in the nucleus but so proportioned that their atomic numbers have different values.

isobaric /-bär'ik/ [Gk, *isos,* equal, *barrios,* weight], **1.** pertaining to two substances or solutions of the same specific gravity. **2.** pertaining to two isotopes that have the same mass number but different atomic numbers. **3.** having the same barometric pressure.

isobutyl alcohol ($C_4H_{10}O$) /ī'soby̅oo̅'til/ [Gk, *isos + butyrin,* butter, *hyl,* matter; AR, *alcohol,* essence], a clear colorless liquid that is miscible with ethyl alcohol or ether. Also called *2-methyl-1-propanol.*

isocapnic /-kap'nik/, pertaining to a level of carbon dioxide in the tissues that remains steady despite changing levels of ventilation.

isocarboxazid /-kärbok″səzid/, a monoamine oxidase inhibitor.

■ INDICATIONS: It is prescribed in the treatment of mental depression.

■ CONTRAINDICATIONS: Liver or kidney dysfunction; congestive heart failure; pheochromocytoma; concomitant use of a sympathomimetic drug or foods high in tryptophan, tyramine, or caffeine; or known hypersensitivity to the drug prohibits its use. Must be used with caution in patients with suicidal ideation.

■ ADVERSE EFFECTS: Among the more serious adverse effects are hyperactivity, cardiac arrhythmia, hypotension, vertigo, dryness of mouth, constipation, and blurred vision. Monoamine oxidase inhibitors produce many adverse drug interactions.

isochromosome /-krō″məsōm/, a chromosome whose arms are of equal length.

isochronic tones, regular beats of a single tone that are quickly turned on and off.

isocrotic, describing the separation of a mixture by chromatography using a single solvent or solvent mixture.

isodiametric, measuring the same in all diameters.

isodose chart /ī'sədōs/ [Gk, *isos + doss,* giving, *charta,* paper], a graphic representation of the distribution of radiation in a medium in which lines are drawn through points receiving equal doses. Isodose charts are determined for x-rays traversing the body, for radium applicators used in intracavitary or interstitial treatment, and for working areas where x-rays or radionuclides are used.

isodynamic law /ī'sōdīnam'ik/, the rule that, for energy purposes, different foods may replace one another in accordance with their caloric values, as determined when burned in a calorimeter.

isoeffect lines /ī'sō·ifekt″/, lines on a graph representing doses of radiation that have tumoricidal effects in normal tissues.

isoelectric /ī'sō·ilek″trik/ [Gk, *isos + electron,* amber], pertaining to the electric baseline of an electrocardiogram, which is the period between the end of the T wave and the beginning of the P wave.

isoelectric electroencephalogram. See **flat electroencephalogram.**

isoelectric focusing, the ordering and concentration of substances according to their isoelectric points.

isoelectric period, a period in physiological activity, such as nerve conduction or muscle contraction, when there is no variation in electric potential.

isoelectric point, the pH at which a molecule containing two or more ionizable groups is electrically neutral. The average number of positive charges equals the average number of negative charges.

isoenzyme /ī'sō·en″zīm/ [Gk, *isos + en,* in, *syme,* ferment], a chemically distinct form of an enzyme. The various forms are distinguishable in analysis of blood samples, which aids in the diagnosis of disease. Different enzymes that catalyze the same physiological reaction may also exist as isoenzymes in different animal species. Also called **isozyme.**

isoetharine, isoetharine hydrochloride. See **isoetharine mesylate.**

isoetharine mesylate /ī'sō·eth″ərēn/, a beta-adrenergic bronchodilator.

■ INDICATIONS: It is prescribed in the treatment of bronchial asthma, bronchitis, and emphysema.

■ CONTRAINDICATIONS: A history of cardiac arrhythmia or known hypersensitivity to this drug or to sympathomimetic medications prohibits its use.

■ ADVERSE EFFECTS: Among the more serious adverse effects are palpitations, tachycardia, arrhythmias, vertigo, nervousness, and headache.

isoexposure line /ī'sō·ikspō″zhər/, an imaginary line representing positions of equal exposure to radiation around a fluoroscopic instrument.

isoflows /ī'sōflōz/, a measure of early small airway dysfunction in a patient made by comparing forced expiratory flow rates of air and helium at fixed points in time.

isogamete /ī'sōgam″ēt/ [Gk, *isos* + *gamete,* wife], a reproductive cell of the same size and structure as the one with which it unites. Compare **anisogamete.** –*isogametic, adj.*

isogamy /īsog″əmē/ [Gk, *isos* + *gamos,* marriage], sexual reproduction in which there is fusion of gametes of the same size and structure, such as in certain algae, fungi, and protists. Compare **anisogamy.** –*isogamous, adj.*

isogeneic. See **syngeneic.**

isogenesis /-jen″əsis/ [Gk, *isos* + *genein,* to produce], development from a common origin and according to similar processes. Also called *isogeny.* –*isogenic, isogenetic, adj.*

isograft /ī″səgraft′/ [Gk, *isos* + *graphion,* stylus], surgical transplantation of histocompatible tissue between genetically identical individuals, such as monozygotic twins. Compare **allograft, autograft, xenograft.** See also **graft.**

isohemagglutinin. See **isoagglutinin.**

isohydric shift [Gk, *isos* + *hydor,* water; AS, *sciftan,* to divide], the series of reactions in red blood cells in which CO_2 is taken up and oxygen is released without the production of excess hydrogen ions.

isoimmunization /ī′sō·im′yənīzā″shən/, the development of antibodies against antigens from the same species, such as anti-Rh antibodies in an Rh-negative person. See also **erythroblastosis fetalis.**

isokinetic /-kinet″ik/, pertaining to a concentric or eccentric contraction that occurs at a set speed against a force of maximal resistance produced at all points in the range of motion.

isokinetic exercise [Gk, *isos,* equal, *kinesis,* motion; L, *exercere,* to keep at work], a form of exercise in which maximum force is exerted by a muscle at each point throughout the active range of motion as the muscle contracts. The effort of the patient to resist the movement is measured.

isolate /ī″səlāt/ [It, *isolare,* to detach], **1.** to separate a pure chemical substance from a mixture. **2.** to derive from any source a pure culture of a microorganism. **3.** to prevent an individual from having contact with the rest of a population.

isolated systolic hypertension (ISH), a type of hypertension in which only the systolic blood pressure is elevated. The condition, which usually affects the elderly, increases the risk of stroke or heart attack.

isolation /-lā″shən/ [L, *insula,* island], the separation of a seriously ill patient from others to prevent the spread of an infection or to protect the patient from irritating or infectious environmental factors. A patient undergoing radiation therapy may also be isolated to reduce the exposure of hospital personnel to effects of radioactive materials. Types of isolation include airborne, droplet, contact, and infectious.

isolation incubator, a crib with a controlled environment maintained for premature or other infants who require separation from other infants in the nursery.

isolation precautions, special precautionary measures, practices, and procedures used in the care of patients with contagious or communicable diseases. The U.S. Centers for Disease Control and Prevention provides explicit and comprehensive guidelines for control of the spread of infectious disease in the care of hospitalized patients. The type of infectious disease a patient has dictates the kind of isolation precautions necessary to prevent spread of the disease to others.

isolation ward [It, *isolare,* to detach; ME, *warden*], a room or section of a hospital in which certain categories of patients, particularly those infected with acute contagious diseases, can be treated with a minimum of contact with the rest of the patients and hospital personnel.

Isolette, a trademark for a self-contained incubator unit that provides a controlled heat, humidity, and oxygen microenvironment for the isolation and care of premature and low-birth-weight neonates. The apparatus is made of a clear plastic material and has a large door and portholes for easy access to the infant with a minimum of heat and oxygen loss. A sensor mechanism constantly monitors the infant's temperature and controls the heat within the unit.

isoleucine (Ile) /ī'sōlōō″sēn/ [Gk, *isos* + *leukos,* white], an amino acid that occurs in most dietary proteins and is essential for proper growth in infants and for nitrogen balance in adults.

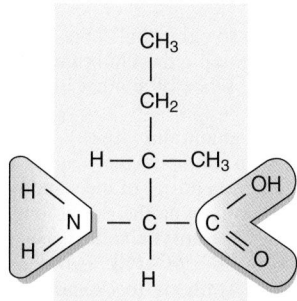

Chemical structure of isoleucine

isologous graft /īsol′əgəs/ [Gk, *isos,* equal, *logos,* relation, *graphion,* stylus], a tissue transplant between two individuals who are genetically identical, as identical twins.

isomeric /-mer″ik/ [Gk, *isos,* equal, *meros,* part], pertaining to a chemical phenomenon in which two compounds of the same chemical formula may differ in chemical and physical properties. The difference is the result of the arrangement of atoms in the respective molecules, either the connections between the atoms or their arrangements in three-dimensional space.

isomers /ī″səmərz/, compounds that have the same formula but different structures, resulting in different properties.

isometheptene hydrochloride /-məthep″tēn/, an antispasmodic and vasoconstrictor drug that is a component in some fixed-combination drugs used to treat migraine.

isometric /ī″səmet″rik/ [Gk, *isos* + *metron,* measure], maintaining the same length or dimension.

isometric contraction [Gk, *isos,* equal, *metron,* measure; L, *contractio,* a drawing together], muscular contraction not accompanied by movement of the joint. Resistance applied to the contraction increases muscle tension without producing movement of the joint. Also called **muscle-setting exercise.**

isometric exercise, a form of active exercise in which muscle tension is increased while pressure is applied against stable resistance. This exercise may be accomplished by pushing or pulling against an immovable object or by simultaneously contracting opposing muscles, such as by pressing the hands together. There is no joint movement, and muscle length remains unchanged, but muscle strength and tone are maintained or improved. Compare **isotonic exercise.** See also **exercise.**

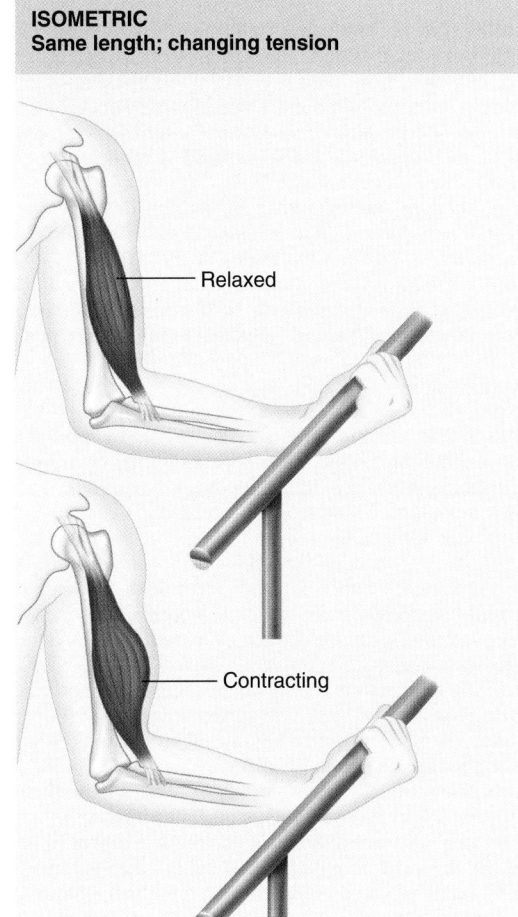

ISOMETRIC
Same length; changing tension

Relaxed

Contracting

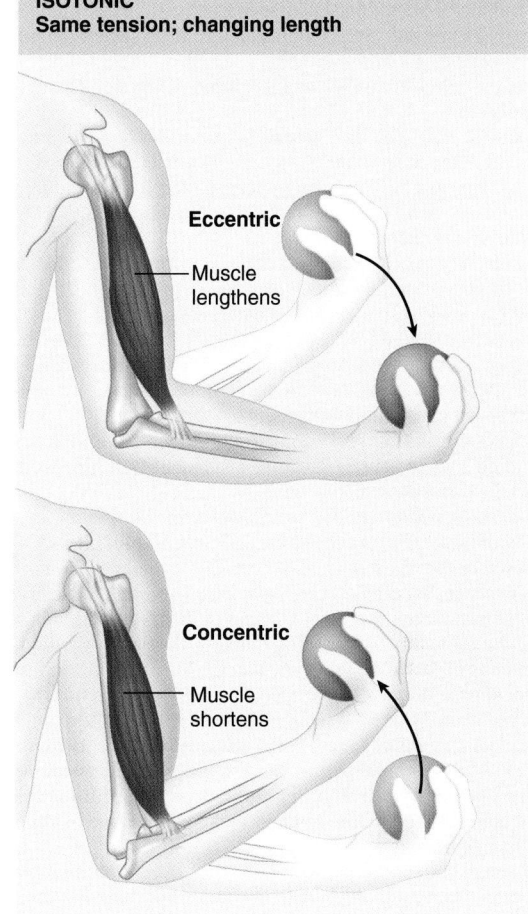

ISOTONIC
Same tension; changing length

Eccentric

Muscle
lengthens

Concentric

Muscle
shortens

Isometric exercise *(Patton and Thibodeau, 2016)*

isometric growth, an increase in the size of different organs or parts of an organism at the same rate. Compare **allometric growth.**

isoniazid /ī'sənī″əzid/, a tuberculostatic antibacterial. Also called **INH.**

■ INDICATIONS: It is prescribed for prophylaxis for those who have been exposed to tuberculosis and is used in combination with other agents in the treatment of tuberculosis caused by mycobacteria sensitive to the drug.

■ CONTRAINDICATIONS: Liver disease, a previous history of a hepatotoxic reaction to isoniazid, or known hypersensitivity to this drug prohibits its use.

■ ADVERSE EFFECTS: Among the more serious adverse effects in long-term treatment are hepatotoxicity and peripheral neuropathy. Rashes, fever, and central nervous system effects commonly occur.

isoosmotic. See **isosmotic.**

isopentoic acid. See **isovaleric acid.**

isophane insulin suspension /ī'səfān/ [Gk, *isos* + *phanein*, to show; L, *insula*, island; *suspendere*, to hang up], a modified form of protamine zinc insulin suspension. It is an intermediate-acting insulin that is a stable, commonly prescribed preparation. Also called **NPH insulin™.**

isoprenaline. See **isoproterenol hydrochloride.**

isopropanol. See **isopropyl alcohol.**

isopropylacetic acid. See **isovaleric acid.**

isopropyl alcohol (C_3H_8O) /ī'sōprō″pil/, a clear, colorless bitter aromatic liquid that is miscible with water, ether, chloroform, and ethyl alcohol. A solution of approximately 70% isopropyl alcohol in water is used as a rubbing compound. Also called *avantin,* **dimethyl carbinol, isopropanol, 2-propanol, rubbing alcohol.** See also **alcohol.**

isopropylaminoacetic acid. See **valine.**

isoproterenol hydrochloride /ī'sōprəter″ənol/, a beta-adrenergic stimulant.

■ INDICATIONS: It is used as a bronchodilator and as a cardiac stimulant.

■ CONTRAINDICATIONS: Cardiac arrhythmia or known hypersensitivity to this drug prohibits its use.

■ ADVERSE EFFECTS: Among the more serious adverse effects are arrhythmias, tachycardia, hypotension, and intensification of angina.

Isoptin, a calcium channel blocker or calcium ion antagonist. Brand name for **verapamil.**

Isopto Atropine, an anticholinergic agent. Brand name for **atropine sulfate.**

Isopto Carbachol, a cholinergic drug. Brand name for *carbachol.*

Isopto Carpine, a cholinergic drug. Brand name for **pilocarpine hydrochloride.**

Isopto Cetamide, an antibacterial drug. Brand name for *sulfacetamide sodium.*

Isopto Homatropine, an anticholinergic drug. Brand name for *homatropine hydrobromide.*

Isopto Hyoscine, an anticholinergic drug. Brand name for *scopolamine hydrobromide.*

Isordil, an antianginal agent. Brand name for **isosorbide dinitrate.**

isosmotic /ī′sozmot″ik/, pertaining to a solution that has the same solute concentration (osmolality) as another solution. Also called **isoosmotic.** Compare **hyperosmotic, hypoosmotic.**

isosorbide dinitrate /-sôr″bīd/, an antianginal agent. Its prototype is nitrogycerin.

■ INDICATIONS: It is prescribed as a coronary vasodilator in the treatment of angina pectoris and congestive heart failure and esophageal spasm caused by GI reflux.

■ CONTRAINDICATIONS: Closed-angle glaucoma, known hypersensitivity to this drug, concurrent use of drugs for erectile dysfunction, narrow-angle glaucoma, head trauma, or severe anemia prohibits its use.

■ ADVERSE EFFECTS: The most serious effect is occasional marked hypotension. Flushing, headache, light-headedness, and dizziness may also occur.

isosorbide mononitrate, an active metabolite of isosorbide dinitrate, having the same actions and uses. It is administered orally.

Isospora /ī·sos′pə·rə/ [Gk, *isos,* equal + *sporos,* seed], a genus of coccidian protozoa found in birds, amphibians, reptiles, and mammals, including humans, that infects the epithelial cells of the small intestine. It is the least common cause of coccidiosis. It includes the species *I. belli* and *I. hominis.*

isosporiasis /ī·sos′pə·rī′ə·sis/, infection with *Isospora.* Two species, *I. hominis* and *I. belli,* affect humans, causing diarrhea with abdominal pain and cramping. See also **coccidiosis.**

isosthenuria /i″sos-thĕ-nu′re-ah/, excretion of urine that is not concentrated by the kidneys and has the same osmolality as that of plasma.

isotachophoresis /-tak′ōfôrē″sis/ [Gk, *isos* + *tachos,* speed, *pherein,* to bear], the ordering and concentration of substances of intermediate effective mobilities between an ion of high effective mobility and one of much lower effective mobility, followed by their migration at a uniform speed.

isothermal /-thur″məl/ [Gk, *isos,* equal, *therme,* heat], having the same temperature. See also **synthermal.**

isotones /ī″sətōnz′/, atoms that have the same number of neutrons but different numbers of protons.

isotonic /ī″səton″ik/ [Gk, *isos* + *tonikos,* stretching], pertaining to a solution that causes no change in cell volume. Compare **hypotonic, hypertonic.**

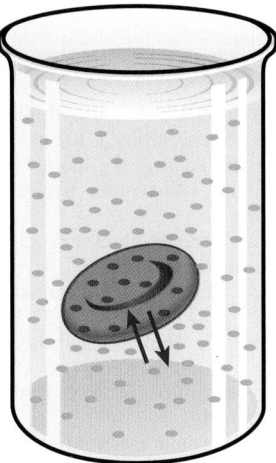

Red blood cell in isotonic solution *(Waugh and Grant, 2014)*

isotonic exercise, a form of active exercise in which muscles contract and cause movement. There is no significant change in resistance throughout the movement, so the force of contraction remains constant. Such exercise greatly enhances joint mobility and helps improve muscle strength and tone. Two examples of isotonic exercise are rising on tiptoes and stretching arms overhead. Compare **isometric exercise.** See also **exercise.**

isotonicity law /ī′sətonis″itē/, a law that describes a state of equal osmotic pressure in extracellular body fluids that results from equal concentrations of electrolytes and other solute particles in the fluid. If a hypertonic solution is ingested, additional water will be drawn from surrounding blood plasma to dilute the intestinal contents and maintain tonicity.

isotope /ī″sətōp/ [Gk, *isos* + *topos,* place], one of two or more forms of an atom having the same number of protons in the atomic nucleus but different numbers of neutrons and thus a different atomic mass. For example, two common isotopes of carbon are ^{12}C, which has six neutrons, and ^{14}C, which has eight. Many isotopes are used in diagnostic and therapeutic procedures.

isotopic tracer /ī′sətop″ik/ [Gk, *isos* + *topos,* place; Fr, *tracer,* to track], an isotope or mixture of isotopes of an element incorporated into a sample to permit observation of the course of the element through a chemical, physical, or biological process. The observations may be made by measuring the radioactivity or the abundance of the isotope.

isotretinoin /-trətin″ō·in/, an antiacne agent.

■ INDICATIONS: Subject to significant restrictions, it is prescribed for the treatment of severe cystic acne.

■ CONTRAINDICATIONS: Pregnancy or sensitivity to the medication or any of its components prohibits its use.

■ ADVERSE EFFECTS: Because this drug is a powerful teratogen, young females must be thoroughly educated about the risk of pregnancy and are often placed on birth control pills. The most serious adverse effects to users are epistaxis, cheilitis, conjunctivitis, paresthesia, dizziness, and serum lipid and hematological disturbances. It may also lower bone mineral density, a consideration for those participating in sports. Some patients become severely depressed or psychotic, which can make them aggressive or suicidal.

isotype /ī′sətīp/, the class of an immunoglobulin. The five major immunoglobulin classes are IgA, IgD, IgE, IgG, and IgM. They differ in their heavy chains (mu, delta, gamma, epsilon, or alpha).

isovaleric acid /-vəler″ik/ [Gk, *isos* + L, *valeriana,* herb, *acidus,* sour], a fatty acid with a pungent taste and disagreeable odor that is found in valerian and other plant products, as well as in cheese. It also occurs as a metabolite of the amino acid leucine and is found in the sweat of feet and in the urine of patients with smallpox, hepatitis, and typhus. It has been used commercially in a variety of drugs, perfumes, and flavorings. Isovaleric acidemia occurs in patients who have abnormally high levels of isovaleric acid in the blood and urine as a result of an inherited deficiency of the enzyme isovaleryl coenzyme A dehydrogenase. The condition is treated with diets that contain low-leucine foods. Also called **isopentoic acid, isopropylacetic acid.**

isovolume pressure-flow curve /-vol″yəm/, a curve on a graph describing the relationship of driving pressure to the resulting volumetric flow rate in the airways at any given lung inflation.

isovolumic contraction /-vəloo̅″mik/ [Gk, *isos* + L, *volumen,* paper roll, *contractio,* drawing together], the early phase of systole, in which the myocardial muscle fibers have begun to shorten but have not developed enough pressure in the ventricles to overcome the aortic and pulmonary end-diastolic pressures and open the aortic and pulmonary valves. During this period of muscle fiber contraction, the ventricular volumes do not change. See also **afterload.**

isoxsuprine hydrochloride /ī´sok″səprēn/, a peripheral vasodilator.

■ INDICATIONS: It is prescribed for the symptomatic relief of cerebrovascular insufficiency and improvement of circulation in arteriosclerosis, Raynaud disease, and Buerger disease.

■ CONTRAINDICATIONS: Known hypersensitivity to this drug or arterial bleeding prohibits its use.

■ ADVERSE EFFECTS: Among the more serious adverse effects are tachycardia, hypotension, chest pain, and dermatitis.

isozyme. See **isoenzyme.**

isradipine /israd´ipēn/, a calcium channel blocking agent used alone or with a thiazide diuretic for the treatment of hypertension.

ISS, **1.** abbreviation for **International Society of Surgery. 2.** abbreviation for **injury severity score.**

-ist, suffix meaning "a practitioner of a science": *audiologist, pharmacist, radiologist.*

isthmus /is´məs/ *pl. isthmuses, isthmi* [Gk, *isthmos,* a narrow connection, passage, or constriction], a constriction between two larger parts of an organ or anatomical structure, such as the isthmus of the thyroid.

isthmus of gastric gland, the part of a gastric gland immediately adjacent to the opening into the gastric pit.

isthmus of thyroid [Gk, *isthmos + thyreos + eidos,* form], the part of the thyroid gland, anterior to the trachea, that joins the two lateral lobes of the gland.

Isuprel, a beta-adrenergic stimulant. Brand name for **isoproterenol hydrochloride.**

IT, abbreviation for **immunotoxin.**

itch [AS, *giccan*], **1.** *v.,* to feel a sensation, usually on the skin, that makes one want to scratch. **2.** *n.,* a tingling, annoying sensation on an area of the skin that makes one want to scratch it, caused in some people, for example, by rhus dermatitis, a mosquito bite, or an allergic reaction. **3.** *n.,* the pruritic condition of the skin caused by infestation with the parasitic mite *Sarcoptes scabiei.*

itch mite [AS, *giccan + mite*], a tiny arachnid with piercing and sucking mouthparts. At least three genera of itch mites are recognized: *Chorioptes, Notoedres,* and *Sarcoptes.*

itchy. See **itch.**

-ite, **1.** suffix meaning "compounds": *nitrite, apatite, anabolite.* **2.** suffix meaning "a body part": *chondriomite, somite, autosite.*

-itic, suffix meaning "related to something specified": *nephritic, syphilitic.*

-itis, suffix meaning an "inflammation of a (specified) organ": *carditis, bursitis, pyelitis.*

ITP, abbreviation for **immune thrombocytopenic purpura.**

IU, I.U., **1.** abbreviations on the "Do Not Use" abbreviation list because of their potential for misinterpretation. **2.** abbreviation for **International Unit.**

IUD, abbreviation for **intrauterine device.**

-ium, **1.** suffix used to name metallic elements: *radium, sodium.* **2.** suffix for quaternary ammonium derivatives.

IUPAC, abbreviation for *International Union of Pure and Applied Chemistry.*

IUPC, abbreviation for *intrauterine pressure catheter.*

IV, **1.** abbreviation for **intravenous, intravenously. 2.** *(Informal)* equipment consisting of a bottle or bag of fluid, infusion set with tubing, and intravenous catheter, used in intravenous therapy. **3.** intravenous administration of fluids or medication by injection into a vein.

IVAC pump, a trademark for a portable IV pump that electronically regulates and monitors the flow of IV fluid. It is usually attached to the IV stand. See also **intravenous pump.**

IVC, abbreviation for **intravenous cholangiography.**

Ivemark syndrome /ē´vəmärk, ī´v″märk/, a rare congenital defect in which the internal organs of the chest and abdomen are not in anatomically correct positions.

IVF, abbreviation for **in vitro fertilization.**

ivory bones. See **osteopetrosis.**

IVP, abbreviation for **intravenous pyelography.**

IV push. *(Informal)* See **intravenous bolus.**

IVT, initialism for *intravenous transfusion.*

IV-type traction frame, a metal structure for holding traction equipment. It consists of two metal uprights, one at each end of the bed, which support an overhead metal bar. The base of each upright is clamped to a horizontal bar that fits into holders inserted at the corners of the bed. Compare **claw-type traction frame.** See also **traction frame.**

ivy poisoning. See **rhus dermatitis.**

ixabepilone, a miscellaneous antineoplastic drug.

■ INDICATIONS: This drug is used to treat breast cancer.

■ CONTRAINDICATIONS: Known hypersensitivity to drugs with polyoxyethylated castor oil, pregnancy, and breastfeeding prohibit the use of this drug.

■ ADVERSE EFFECTS: adverse effects of this drug include bradycardia, abnormal ECG, angina, atrial flutter, cardiomyopathy, chest pain, edema, MI, vasculitis, abdominal pain, anorexia, colitis, constipation, coagulopathy, gastritis, jaundice, gastroesophageal reflux disease, hepatic failure, infections, rash, hypokalemia, metabolic acidosis, impaired cognition, chills, fatigue, fever, flushing, headache, insomnia, bronchospasm, cough, dyspnea, and dehydration. Life-threatening side effects include neutropenia, thrombocytopenia, anemia, and anaphylaxis. Common side effects include hypotension, nausea, vomiting, diarrhea, alopecia, arthralgia, myalgia, peripheral neuropathy, and hypersensitivity reactions.

Ixempra, brand name for **ixabepilone.**

Ixodes /iksō´dēz/ [Gk, sticky], a genus of parasitic hard-shelled ticks associated with the transmission of a variety of infections, such as Rocky Mountain spotted fever, Lyme disease, erlichiosis, and babesiosis.

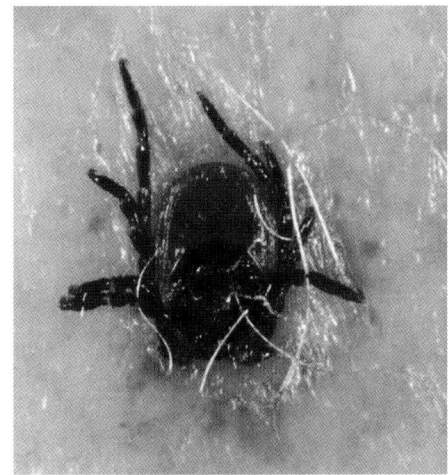

Ixodes scapularis *(Marks and Miller, 2006)*

ixodi-,   prefix meaning "ticks": *ixodiasis.*

ixodiasis /ik′sōdī″əsis/,   **1.** skin lesions created by the bites of ixodid ticks. **2.** any tick-transmitted disease.

ixodid /iksod″id, iksō″did/,   pertaining to hard ticks of the family Ixodidae.

Iyengar yoga,   a style of yoga that emphasizes correct body alignment in the asanas (postures) and holding the asanas for extended periods of time. It also uses props, such as wooden blocks and belts, to help achieve and support the asanas.

-ize,   suffix to form verbs from adjectives and nouns. Verbs mean "to make, become, engage in, or use" or "to treat or combine with": *oxidize, anesthetize.*

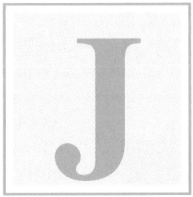

J

J, abbreviation for **joule.**

Jaccoud dissociated fever /zhäk$\overline{oo}$″/ [Sigismond Jaccoud, French physician, 1830–1913], a form of febrile meningitic fever accompanied by a paradoxical slow pulse rate; it is seen in patients with tuberculous meningitis.

jacket [Fr, *jaquette*], a supportive or confining therapeutic casing or garment for the torso. It is also used to prevent edema in the extremities. See also **Minerva cast.**

jacket restraint, an orthopedic device used to help immobilize the trunk of a patient in traction and to discourage the patient from sitting up in bed. The jacket restraint is attached to both sides of the bedspring frame by means of buckled webbing straps that are sewn into the side seams of the restraint. The jacket restraint may be used with most kinds of traction but is not usually used with Dunlop skin traction, Dunlop skeletal traction, Bryant traction, halo-femoral traction, or halo-pelvic traction. A restraint of any kind should be used only when the risk of activity outweighs the benefits, and even then with extreme caution. Compare **diaper restraint, sling restraint.**

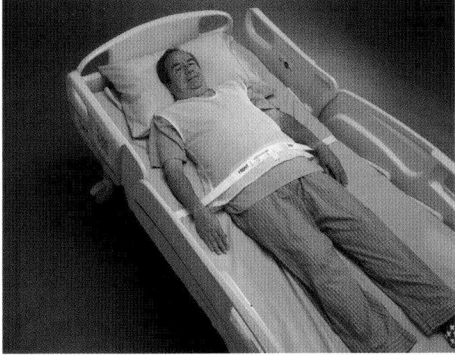

Jacket restraint *(Courtesy of Posey Company)*

jackknife position /jak″nīf/, an anatomical position in which the patient is placed on the stomach with the hips flexed and the knees bent at a 90-degree angle and the arms outstretched in front of the patient. Examination and instrumentation of the rectum are facilitated by this position.

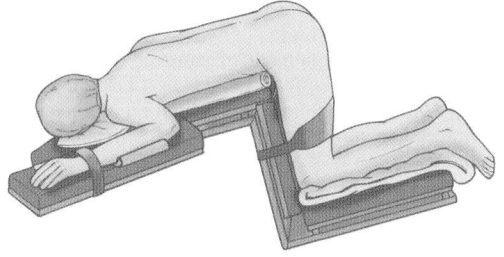

Jackknife position *(Rothrock, 2011)*

jackscrew /jak′skr$\overline{oo}$/, a threaded device used in orthodontic appliances for the separation or approximation of teeth or jaw segments.

Jackson crib, a removable orthodontic appliance retained in position by crib-shaped wires.

jacksonian epilepsy /jaksō′nē·ən/ [John H. Jackson, English neurologist, 1835–1911], epilepsy characterized by focal motor seizures with unilateral clonic movements that start in one group of muscles and spread systematically to adjacent groups, reflecting the march of the epileptic activity through the motor cortex (jacksonian march). The seizures are due to a discharging focus in the contralateral motor cortex.

jacksonian march. See **cortical march.**

jacksonian seizure, a series of focal seizures with unilateral clonic movements that start in one group of muscles and spread systematically to adjacent groups, reflecting the march of the epileptic activity through the motor cortex. See also **focal seizure.**

Jackson sign [John H. Jackson, English neurologist, 1835–1911], (in hemiparesis) an observation that during quiet respiration the movement of the paralyzed side of the chest may be greater than that of the opposite side. However, the paralyzed side moves less under forced respiration.

jackstone calculus, a urinary calculus with spikes like those of the toy in the game of jacks.

Jacob x membrane. See **retina.**

Jacquemier's sign /zhäkmē·āz″/ [Jean M. Jacquemier, French obstetrician, 1806–1879], a deepening of the color of the vaginal mucosa just below the urethral orifice. It may sometimes be noted after the fourth week of pregnancy, but it is not a reliable sign of pregnancy.

jactitation /jak″titā″shən/ [L, *jactare,* show off, display], twitchings or spasms of muscles or muscle groups, as observed in the restless body movements of a patient with a high fever.

JAK2, a gene that provides instructions for making a protein that promotes the growth and division of cells.

JADA, abbreviation for *The Journal of the American Dental Association.*

jail fever. See **epidemic typhus.**

Jake paralysis, (of historic significance) upper motor neuron damage resulting in a characteristic walk. It was first observed in the 1930s during Prohibition in the United States and was caused by drinking an alcoholic extract of Jamaican ginger adulterated by the neurotoxin tri-ortho-cresyl phosphate (Jake). See **ginger paralysis.**

Jakob-Creutzfeldt disease. See **Creutzfeldt-Jakob disease.**

JAMA /jä″mä, jam″ə, jā″ā′em′ā″/, acronym for *Journal of the American Medical Association.*

jamais vu /zhämāvY″, -vē″, -v$\overline{oo}$″/ [Fr, never seen], the sensation of being a stranger when with a person one knows or when in a familiar place. The phenomenon occurs occasionally in healthy people but more frequently in those who have temporal lobe epilepsy. Compare **déjà vu.**

Janeway lesion /jān″wā/ [Edward G. Janeway, American physician, 1841–1911; L, *laedere,* to injure], a small, painless erythematous or hemorrhagic macule on the palms or soles. It is diagnostic of subacute bacterial endocarditis.

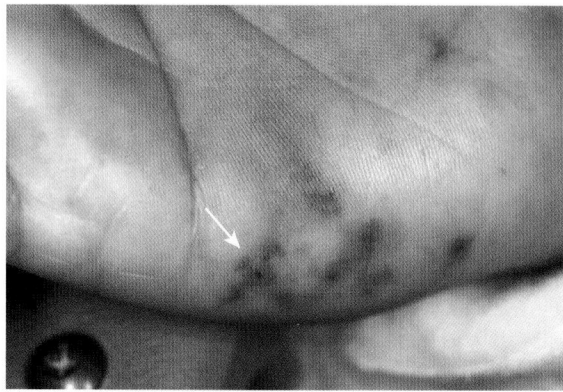

Janeway lesions *(Ferri, 2016)*

janiceps /jan″əseps/ [L, *Janus,* two-faced Roman god, *caput,* head], a conjoined twin fetus in which the heads are fused, with the faces looking in opposite directions. The faces and bodies of both twins may be fully formed, or one member may be only partially formed and act as a parasite on the more fully developed fetus.

Jansen disease. See **metaphyseal dysostosis.**

Jansky-Bielschowsky disease /yahn′skē byelschov′ske/ [Jan Janský, Czech physician, 1873–1921, and Max Bielschowsky, German neuropathologist, 1869–1940], the late infantile form of neuronal ceroid lipofuscinosis, occurring between 2 and 4 years of age and characterized by abnormal accumulation of lipofuscin. It begins as myoclonic seizures and progresses to neurological and retinal degeneration and death, usually by the age of 8 to 12 years.

janus particle /ˈjā-nəs/ [Janus, two-faced Roman deity], a nanoparticle consisting of two distinct properties.

Januvia, an incretin-based oral hypoglycemic. Brand name for **sitagliptin.**

Japanese encephalitis (JE), a severe epidemic infection of brain tissue seen in East and Southeast Asia and the South Pacific, including Australia and New Zealand. The virus is carried by domestic pigs and wild birds. The disease is characterized by shaking chills, paralysis, and weight loss and is caused by *Flavivirus* transmitted by the mosquito *Culex tritaeniorhynchus.* Symptoms include headache, fever, neck stiffness, tremors, seizures, spastic paralysis, and coma. Mortality rate ranges widely from 0.3% to 60%. Various neurological and psychiatric sequelae are common. An inactivated JE vaccine is available and recommended for travel to endemic areas. Treatment is supportive. Also called *Japanese B encephalitis.*

Japanese flood fever, Japanese river fever. See **scrub typhus.**

Japanese spotted fever, an acute infection occurring in Japan caused by *Rickettsia japonica* and transmitted by Ixodidae. It is characterized by fever and headache and the appearance of an eschar and rash.

JAPHA /jaf″ə, jā″ā′pē″āch′ā′/, abbreviation for *Journal of the American Public Health Association.*

jar, **1.** *v.,* to shake or jolt. **2.** *n.,* a cylindrical container.

Jarcho-Levin syndrome /jär′kō lev′in/ [Saul Wallenstein Jarcho, American physician, 1906-2000; Paul M. Levin, 20th-century American physician], an autosomal-recessive disorder consisting of multiple vertebral defects, short thorax, rib abnormalities, camptodactyly, fused fingers, and, occasionally, urogenital abnormalities. Death from respiratory insufficiency usually occurs in infancy. Also called **spondylothoracic dysplasia.**

jargon (jar.) /jär″gən/ [Fr, *jargonner,* to speak indistinctly], **1.** incoherent speech or gibberish. **2.** a terminology used by scientists, artists, or others of a professional subculture that is not understood by the general population. **3.** a state in child language acquisition characterized by strings of babbled sounds paired with gestures. As children master language, the use of jargon will diminish; continued use may be indicative of difficulty with language acquisition, requiring evaluation by a speech-language pathologist. See also **integrative babbling.**

jargon aphasia [Fr, *jargonner* + Gk, *a* + *phasis,* speech], a form of speech in which several words are combined in a single word but in a jumbled manner with incorrect accents or words mixed with neologisms.

Jarisch-Herxheimer reaction /jä″ris herks″hīmər/ [Adolph Jarisch, Austrian dermatologist, 1850–1902; Karl Herxheimer, German dermatologist, 1861–1944], a transient, short-term, immunological reaction commonly seen after antibiotic treatment of early and later stages of syphilis and less often in other diseases, such as borreliosis, brucellosis, typhoid fever, and trichinosis. It is seen in 50% of patients with primary syphilis and 90% of those with secondary syphilis. Manifestations include fever, chills, headache, myalgias, and exacerbation of cutaneous lesions. The reaction has been attributed to liberation of endotoxin-like substances or antigens from the killed or dying microorganisms, but its exact pathogenesis is unclear.

Jarvik-7 [Robert K. Jarvik, American cardiologist, b. 1946], *(Obsolete)* an artificial heart designed by R.K. Jarvik for use in humans. The Jarvik-7 was an early model that depended on air pressure to drive the ventricles. It is no longer in use in clinical practice.

jaundice /jôn″dis, jän″dis/ [Fr, *jaune,* yellow], a yellow discoloration of the skin, mucous membranes, and sclerae of the eyes caused by greater-than-normal amounts of bilirubin in the blood. Jaundice is a symptom of many disorders, including liver diseases, biliary obstruction, and the hemolytic anemias. Also called **icterus.** See also **anicteric hepatitis, hyperbilirubinemia.** *–jaundiced, adj.*

■ OBSERVATIONS: Because persons with dark skin sometimes have yellow-tinged sclerae, the hard palate of the mouth is often the best place to assess for jaundice. Persons with jaundice may experience nausea, vomiting, and abdominal pain and may pass dark urine and clay-colored stools. Useful diagnostic procedures include a clinical evaluation of the signs and symptoms, tests of liver function, and techniques for direct or indirect visualization, such as x-ray imaging, computed tomographic scan, ultrasound, endoscopy or exploratory surgery, and biopsy.

■ INTERVENTIONS: Treatment of jaundice as a symptom of disease depends on the underlying cause. Discomfort due to itching, if present, may be treated with oral antihistamines if not contraindicated and topical lotions, medicated baths, or phototherapy.

■ PATIENT CARE CONSIDERATIONS: Physiological jaundice commonly develops in newborns and disappears after a few days. Rarer disorders causing jaundice are Crigler-Najjar syndrome and Gilbert syndrome.

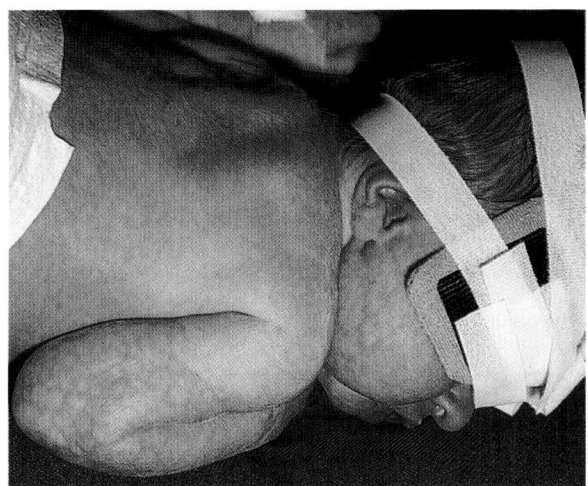

Infant undergoing phototherapy for physiological jaundice *(Eichenfield et al, 2015)*

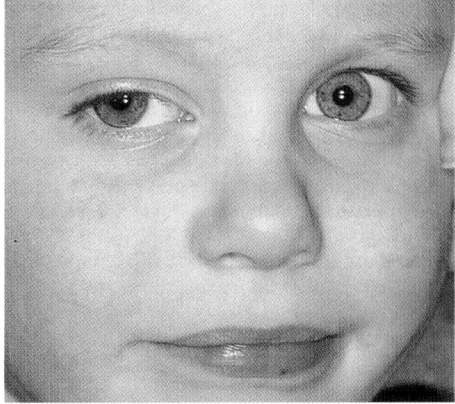

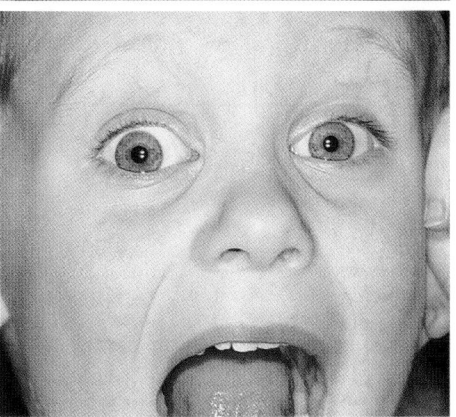

Child demonstrating the phenomenon of jaw-winking
(Yanoff and Sassani, 2008)

jaw [AS, *ceowan,* to chew],   a common term used to describe the maxillae and the mandible and the soft tissue that covers these structures, which contain the teeth and form the framework for the mouth. See also **jaw relation.**

jaw jerk,   an abnormal reflex elicited by tapping the chin with a rubber hammer while the mouth is half open and the jaw muscles are relaxed. A quick snapping shut of the jaw implies damage to the area of cerebral cortex governing motor activity of the fifth cranial nerve. Also called **chin reflex, chin-jerk reflex, mandibular reflex.**

jaw relation,   any alignment related to the position of the mandible to the maxilla.

jaw-winking,   an involuntary facial movement phenomenon in which the eyelid droops, usually on one side of the face, when the jaw is closed but rises when the jaw is opened or when the jaw is moved from side to side. The raising of the eyelid often appears exaggerated. Also called **Gunn syndrome, Marcus Gunn syndrome.** See also **Marin Amat syndrome.**

J chain,   a polypeptide chain that holds immunoglobulin A (IgA) dimers and IgM pentamers together.

JC virus (JCV),   a virus common in the general population. In patients with immunodeficiencies it is associated with progressive multifocal leukoencephalopathy. It is also known as the John Cunningham virus, so named for the patient from whom the virus was first isolated.

J/deg,   abbreviation for *joules per degree.*

JE,   abbreviation for **Japanese encephalitis.**

Jebsen hand function test,   a short standardized test providing objective measurements of fine and gross motor hand function using simulated activities of daily living (writing, card turning, picking up small objects, simulated feeding, stacking, picking up large lightweight objects, and picking up large heavy objects), with norms for patient comparison.

Jefferson fracture,   a fracture characterized by bursting of the ring of the first cervical vertebra.

jejuna.   See **jejunum.**

jejunal /jijo͞o′nəl/ [L, *jejunus,* empty],   pertaining to the jejunum, the length of intestine between the duodenum and the ileum. See also **jejunum.**

jejunal atresia,   a narrowing of the part of the small intestine between the duodenum and ileum.

jejunal feeding tube,   a hollow tube inserted into the jejunum through the abdominal wall for administration of liquefied foods to patients who have a high risk of aspiration. See also **enteral tube feeding, tube feeding.**

jejunectomy /jij′o͞onek″təmē/,   the surgical removal of all or part of the small intestine between the duodenum and ileum.

jejuno-,   prefix meaning "the jejunum": *jejunogastric, jejunocolostomy, jejunotomy.*

jejunocolostomy /jijo͞o′nōkəlos″təmē/,   the surgical creation of an anastomosis between the jejunum and colon.

jejunogastric intussusception,   the prolapse of an anastomosed jejunum into the stomach; a complication sometimes seen after gastrojejunostomy.

jejunoileitis.   See **Crohn's disease.**

jejunostomy /jij′o͞onos″təmē/,   a surgical procedure to create an artificial opening to the jejunum through the abdominal wall. It may be a permanent or a temporary opening.

jejunostomy feeding.   See **tube feeding.**

jejunotomy /jij′o͞onot″əmē/,   a surgical incision in the jejunum.

jejunum /jijo͞o′nəm/ [L, *jejunus,* empty],   the intermediate or middle of the three portions of the small intestine, connecting proximally with the duodenum and distally with the ileum. The jejunum has a slightly larger diameter, a deeper color, and a thicker wall than the ileum and contains heavy, circular folds that are absent in the lower part of the ileum. The jejunum also has larger villi than the ileum. Compare **ileum. –jejunal,** *adj.*

jelly,   a semisolid nonliquid colloidal mass. See also **gel, contraceptive jelly, Wharton jelly, petroleum jelly.**

jellyfish sting [L, *gelare,* to congeal; AS, *fisc + stingan*],   a wound caused by skin contact with a jellyfish, a sea animal with a bell-shaped gelatinous body and numerous suspended long tentacles containing stinging structures.

■ OBSERVATIONS: In most cases a tender red welt develops on the affected skin. In some cases, depending on the sensitivity

J

of the person and the species of jellyfish, severe localized pain and nausea, weakness, excessive lacrimation, nasal discharge, muscle spasm, perspiration, difficulty in swallowing, and dyspnea may occur.

■ INTERVENTIONS: First-aid guidelines published by the American Red Cross and the American Heart Association recommend rinsing the area of the sting with vinegar. Vinegar neutralizes the venom and prevents its spread. This should be followed by soaking the affected area in warm water for 20 minutes.

■ PATIENT CARE CONSIDERATIONS: Emergency personnel should be contacted if the person shows signs of a severe allergic reaction.

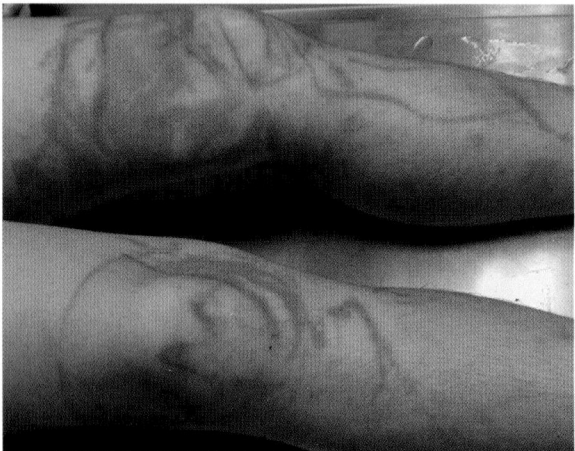

Jellyfish sting *(Lebwohl et al, 2018)*

Jendrassik maneuver /yendrä″shiks/ [Ernst Jendrassik, Hungarian physician, 1858–1921; Fr, *manoeuvre*, action], (in neurology) a distracting maneuver in which the patient hooks the flexed fingers of the two hands together and forcibly tries to pull them apart; it is used to overcome the voluntary suppression of reflexes. While this tension is being exerted, the lower extremity reflexes are tested.

Jenner, Edward [1749–1823], an English physician who discovered the principle of smallpox vaccination in 1796. He is known as the father of immunology for his pioneering work and his discovery of the first successful vaccine.

jerk, **1.** a sudden abrupt motion such as a thrust, yank, push, or pull. **2.** a quick muscular contraction induced when a tendon over a bone is tapped. See also **spasm.**

jerk finger. See **trigger finger.**

jerk nystagmus, a slow drift of the eyes in one direction, followed by a rapid recovery movement in the other direction.

jerks, a form of choreomania, or a morbid desire to make rhythmic movements, sometimes associated with emotional fervor.

jet humidifier, a humidifier that increases the surface area for exposure of water to gas by breaking the water into small aerosol droplets. Air or a gas passes through a restriction after entering the humidifier, producing a foaming mixture of liquid and gas. Gas issuing from the unit has a maximum amount of water vapor and a minimum of liquid water particles.

jet lag [L, *jacere*, to throw; Scand, *lagga*, to fall behind], a condition of desynchrony with disruption of the normal circadian rhythm, caused by rapid travel across several time zones. It is characterized by fatigue, insomnia, and disturbances in body function.

jet nebulizer [L, *nebula*, mist], a humidifier that uses Bernoulli's principle to convert a pool of liquid into a fine mist of aerosol particles. A jet stream of gas is projected at high velocity across the end of a capillary tube. The gas jet reduces the pressure at the top of the tube, causing the liquid to move to the top, where it is continuously drawn off as aerosol particles that enter the outflow passage of the humidifier.

Jeune syndrome /zhœn, zhōōn/ [Mathis Jeune, French pediatrician, 1910–1983], a rare genetic disorder that affects the way a child's cartilage and bones develop. Constriction of the upper thorax may affect breathing. The child's limbs are short, and overall height is affected. Kidney and liver dysfunction is not uncommon in this disorder. It is inherited as an autosomal-recessive trait. Also called **asphyxiating thoracic dysplasia.**

jeweler's forceps, a thumb forceps with very fine, pointed tips, used for microvascular and ophthalmic procedures.

Jewett brace. See **Griswald brace.**

jigger. See **chigoe.**

jimson weed /jim″sən/, a common name for *Datura stramonium,* a poisonous plant with large trumpet-shaped flowers. It is a member of solanaceous plants and a natural source of cholinergic blockers. Its chief components are the anticholinergics hyoscyamine and scopolamine.

jitters, **1.** irregularities in ultrasound echo locations caused by mechanical or electronic disturbances. **2.** *(Informal)* an uneasy, nervous feeling.

J/kg, abbreviation for *joules per kilogram.*

Joanna Briggs Institute (JBI), an international research and development organization located at the University of Adelaide, South Australia, that supports the synthesis, transfer, and utilization of evidence.

Jobst garment, a type of pressure wrap applied to control hypertrophic scar formation or lymphedema. Brand name for **gradient compression stockings.**

jock itch. *(Informal)* See **tinea cruris.**

JOD, abbreviation for **juvenile-onset diabetes, juvenile onset-type diabetes.** See **type 1 diabetes mellitus.**

Jod-Basedow phenomenon /jod′ bä″zədō′/ [Ger, *Jod,* iodine; Karl A. von Basedow, German physician, 1799–1854], thyrotoxicosis that may occur when dietary iodine is given to a patient with endemic goiter in an area of environmental iodine deficiency. It is presumed that iodine deficiency protects some patients with endemic goiter from development of thyrotoxicosis. The phenomenon may also occur when large doses of iodine are given to patients with nontoxic multinodular goiter in areas with sufficient environmental iodine. Also called *iodine-induced hyperthyroidism.*

Joffroy reflex /zhôfrô·ä″, jof″roi/ [Alexis Joffroy, French physician, 1844–1908], a reflex contraction of the gluteus muscles produced when firm pressure is applied to the buttocks of patients with spastic paralysis of the lower limbs.

Joffroy sign [Alexis Joffroy, French neurologist, 1844–1908], **1.** an absence of forehead creases when a patient with Graves disease looks upward with the head bent forward. **2.** an inability to perform simple mathematical exercises, such as addition or multiplication, caused by an organic brain disease.

jogger's heel [ME, *joggen,* to shake; AS, *hela,* heel], a painful condition characterized by bruising, bursitis, fasciitis, or calcaneal spurs that results from repetitive and forceful striking of the heel on the ground. It is common among joggers and distance runners. Judicious selection of well-fitting running shoes and avoidance of running on hard surfaces are recommended to prevent occurrence or recurrence of the condition.

Johnson, Dorothy E. [Dorothy E. Johnson, American nurse, 1919–1999], a nursing theorist who developed a behavioral systems model presented in *Conceptual Models for Nursing Practice* (Riehl and Roy, eds., 1973). Johnson's theory addresses two major components: the patient and nursing. The patient is a behavioral system with seven interrelated subsystems. Each subsystem has structural and functional requirements. Johnson considered that problems in nursing are caused by disturbances in the structure or functions of the subsystems or the system. Her behavioral systems theory provides a conceptual framework for nursing education, practice, and research.

Johnson method, (in dentistry) a technique for filling root canals, in which gutta-percha cones are dissolved in a chloroform-rosin solution in the root canal to form a plastic mass. The plastic material is forced toward the apex of the root canal, and more is added until the canal is sealed. Compare **lateral condensation method.**

Johnson model of intervention [Vernon Johnson, Episcopal priest and addiction researcher, 1920–1999], a system that makes the consequences of addiction clear through a meeting with family members and significant others. See also **direct intervention,** def. 2.

joint [L, *jungere,* to join], any one of the articulations between bones. Each is classified according to structure and movability as fibrous, cartilaginous, or synovial. Fibrous joints are immovable, cartilaginous joints are slightly movable, and synovial joints are freely movable. Typical immovable joints are those connecting most of the bones of the skull with a sutural ligament. Typical slightly movable joints are those connecting the vertebrae and the pubic bones. Most of the joints in the body are freely movable and allow gliding, circumduction, rotation, and angular movement. Also called **articulation.** See also **cartilaginous joint, fibrous joint, synovial joint.**

Classification of joints

Type of joint	Example	Description
Fibroid (synarthrosis)		No movement is permitted
Suture	Cranial sutures	United by thin layer of fibrous tissue
Synchondrosis	Joint between the epiphysis and diaphysis of long bones	Temporary joint in which the cartilage is replaced by bone later in life
Cartilaginous (amphiarthrosis)		Slightly movable joint
Symphysis	Symphysis pubis	Bones are connected by a fibrocartilage disk
Syndesmosis	Radius-ulna articulation	Bones are connected by ligaments
Synovial (diarthrosis)		Freely movable; enclosed by joint capsule and synovial membrane
Ball and socket	Shoulder	Widest range of motion; movement in all planes
Hinge	Elbow	Motion limited to flexion and extension in a single plane
Pivot	Atlantoaxis	Motion limited to rotation
Condyloid	Wrist between radius and carpals	Motion in two planes at right angles to each other, but no radial rotation
Saddle	Thumb at carpal-metacarpal joint	Motion in two planes at right angles to each other, but no axial rotation
Gliding	Intervertebral: between the articular surfaces of successive vertebrae	Motion limited to gliding

Adapted from Seidel et al: *Mosby's guide to physical examination,* ed 6, St. Louis, 2006, Mosby. Illustrations from Thibodeau GA, Patton KT: *Anatomy & physiology,* ed 7, St. Louis, 2010, Mosby.

joint and several liability, (in law) a condition in which several persons share the liability for a plaintiff's injury and may be found liable individually or as a group.

joint appointment, **1.** a faculty appointment to two institutions within a university or system, as to the schools of health sciences and medicine of the same university. **2.** (in academic nursing) the appointment of a member of the faculty of a university to a clinical service of an associated service institution. A psychiatric nurse might hold appointment in a university as an assistant professor and might also be a clinical nurse specialist in a service institution. The practice of joint appointments began at Case Western Reserve University, University Hospital, Cleveland. See also **unification model.**

joint audit. See **nursing audit.**

joint capsule [L, *jungere,* to join, *capsula,* little box], a fibrous saclike structure of dense, irregular connective tissue that envelops the end of bones in a diarthrodial joint and contains synovial fluid. It contains an outer fibrous membrane and an inner synovial membrane.

joint chondroma, a cartilaginous mass that develops in the synovial membrane of a joint.

joint conference committee, a hospital organization composed of the governing board, administration, and medical staff representatives whose purpose is to facilitate communication between the groups.

joint fracture. See **intraarticular fracture.**

joint instability, an abnormal increase in joint mobility. See also **hypermobility.**

joint mouse, a small, movable stone, such as a loose fragment of cartilage, formed in or near a joint, usually a knee. See also **loose body.**

joint planning, the development by two or more health care providers of a strategic plan to serve the health care needs of an area while sharing clinical or administrative services or data but not assets.

joint practice, **1.** the practice of one or more physicians, nurses, and other health professionals, usually private, who work as a team, sharing responsibility for a group of patients. **2.** (in inpatient nursing) the practice of making joint decisions about patient care by committees of the physicians and nurses working on a division.

joint protection, the use of orthotics with therapeutic exercise to prevent damage or deformity of a joint during rehabilitation to restore power and range of motion. An example is an ankle-foot orthosis that allows weight-bearing on an extended knee.

joint replacement. See **arthroplasty.**

Jones criteria /jōnz/ [T. Duckett Jones, American physician,1899–1954], a standardized set of guidelines for the diagnosis of rheumatic fever, as recommended by the American Heart Association (and most recently revised in 2015). See also **rheumatic fever.**

Joseph disease. See **Machado-Joseph disease.**

Joubert syndrome /zhoo·bār′/ [Marie Joubert, 20th-century Canadian neurologist], a disorder of brain development consisting of partial or complete agenesis of the cerebellar vermis and a malformed brainstem. Characteristics include weak muscle tone, abnormal breathing patterns, developmental delay, and abnormal eye movements. Inheritance is usually autosomal-recessive, but on rare occasions it may also be X-linked recessive. Treatment is supportive. Also called *cerebelloparenchymal disorder.*

joule (J) /jool/ [James P. Joule, English physicist, 1818–1889], a unit of energy or work in the meter-kilogram-second system and the SI system. It is equivalent to 10^7 ergs.

journaling, **1.** a therapeutic technique using the written word as a method of introspection. **2.** the recording of all foods consumed in a written diary or in a digital format to assist in weight loss or to maintain a healthy weight with adequate nutritional intake.

joystick, **1.** a vertical stick or lever that can be manipulated in various directions to control a cursor or other movements on a computer screen. It is used mainly in playing computer games. **2.** a vertical stick or lever that can be manipulated in various directions to drive an electric wheelchair.

J-pouch, a fecal reservoir formed surgically by folding over the distal end of the ileum in an ileoanal anastomosis.

JRA, abbreviation for **juvenile rheumatoid arthritis.**

Judd method, a technique for positioning a patient for radiographic examination of the atlas and odontoid process.

judgment /juj″mənt/ [L, *judicare,* to judge], **1.** (in law) the final decision of the court regarding the case before it. **2.** the reason given by the court for its decision; an opinion. **3.** an award, penalty, or other sentence of law given by the court. **4.** the ability to recognize the relationships of ideas and to form correct conclusions from those data as well as from those acquired from experience.

judgment call, (Slang) a decision based on experience, especially a judgment that resolves a serious problem in which the data are inconclusive or equivocal.

jug-, **1.** prefix meaning "a yoke type of connection": *jugal, jugum.* **2.** prefix meaning "collarbone, throat, neck": *jugular.*

jugal /joo″gəl/ [L, *jugum,* yoke], pertaining to structures attached or yoked, as the zygomatic bone or malar bone.

jugu-, prefix meaning "to kill": *jugulate.*

jugular /jug″yələr/ [L, *jugulum,* neck], **1.** *adj.,* pertaining to or involving the throat. **2.** (Informal) n., the jugular vein.

jugular foramen [L, *jugulum,* neck, *foramen,* hole], one of a pair of openings between the lateral part of the occipital bone and the petrous part of the temporal bones in the skull. The foramen contains the inferior petrosal sinus; the transverse sinus; some meningeal branches of the occipital and ascending pharyngeal arteries; and the glossopharyngeal, vagus, and accessory nerves.

jugular foramen syndrome. See **Vernet syndrome.**

jugular fossa, a deep depression adjacent to the interior surface of the petrosa of the temporal bone of the skull.

jugular notch of the sternum, the large notch in the manubrium of sternum. Also called **suprasternal notch.**

jugular process, a portion of the occipital bone that projects laterally from the squamous part to the temporal bone. On its anterior border a deep notch forms the posterior and medial boundary of the jugular foramen.

jugular pulse, a pulsation in the jugular vein caused by conditions that inhibit diastolic filling of the right side of the heart.

jugular trunk, one of the two lymphatic vessels, right and left, that drain the head and neck.

jugular tubercle, a large rounded mound of the occipital bone medial to the jugular foramen.

jugular venous pressure (JVP), blood pressure in the jugular vein, which reflects the volume and pressure of venous blood. If the neck veins are filled only to a point a few millimeters above the clavicle at the end of exhalation, JVP is usually normal. With an elevated JVP the neck veins may be distended as high as the angle of the jaw. An elevated JVP is typically a sign of congestive heart failure.

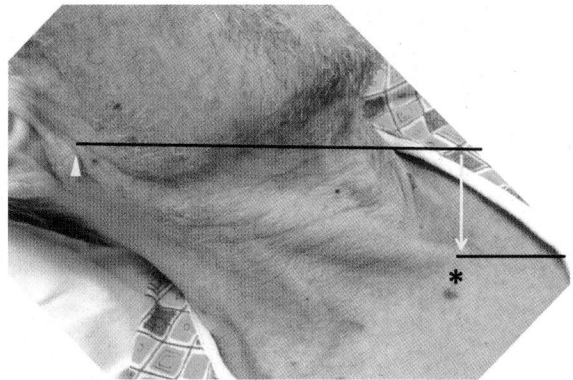

Evaluation of JVP. With the patient lying at about 45 degrees, the highest point of pulsation of the jugular vein is identified (*arrowhead*)**. This is then related to the angle of Louis, found at the junction of the manubrium with the body of the sternum** (*asterisk*)**. The vertical distance to the top of the jugular venous wave** (*arrow*) **can be determined and reported in centimeters as the JVP** (*Beigel et al, 2013*)

jugulate, to kill by slitting the throat.

jugum /jōo″gəm/ [L, yoke], a ridge or furrow joining two points.

juice /jōos/ [L, *jus*, broth], **1.** *n.,* any fluid secreted by the tissues of animals or plants. In humans it usually refers to the secretions of the digestive glands. Kinds include **gastric juice, intestinal juices, pancreatic juice. 2.** *v.,* to extract fluids from fruits and vegetables.

juice therapy, the use of concentrated nutritional elixirs of fruit extracts and vegetables for nutritional maintenance.

jumentous /jōomen″təs/ [L, *jumentum*, beast of burden], (*Obsolete*) a term used to describe urine with a strong odor, like that of a horse.

jumping disease, any of several disorders characterized by exaggerated responses to small stimuli, muscle tics (including jumping), automatic obedience even to dangerous suggestions, and sometimes coprolalia or echolalia. It is unclear whether the responses are neurogenic or psychogenic in origin. Kinds include **Gilles de la Tourette syndrome, jumping Frenchmen of Maine syndrome.**

jumping Frenchmen of Maine syndrome, a form of jumping disease observed in a group of lumbermen of French-Canadian descent working in a remote area of Maine. Affected individuals had exaggerated startle responses, automatic obedience, and often echolalia. It is believed to have represented a form of operant conditioning rather than a true disease. See also **jumping disease.**

jumping gene. See **transposon.**

junction /jungk″shən/ [L, *jungere,* to join], an interface or meeting place for tissues or structures.

junctional bigeminy /jungk″shənəl/ [L, *jungere,* to join, *bis,* twice, *geminus,* twin], cardiac arrhythmia in which each sinus beat is followed by a junctional beat after a constant delay.

junctional epithelium [L, *jungere,* to join; Gk, *epi + thele,* nipple], an area of epithelial soft tissue surrounding the abutment post of a tooth. Also called **attached epithelial cuff, epithelial cuff, gingival cuff.**

junctional extrasystole [L, *jungere,* to join, *extra,* beyond; Gk, *systole,* contraction], a premature heartbeat that usually arises from the junction of the atrioventricular (AV) node

and the AV bundle, the primary junctional pacing site, but may also arise from within the AV bundle.

junctional parenchymal defect, on ultrasound of the kidney, an echogenic mass sometimes seen in the parenchyma, resembling a cortical scar but indicating only a benign collection of fat at the junction where two of the fetal lobes of the kidney fuse.

junctional rhythm, a cardiac rhythm usually originating at the junction of the atrioventricular (AV) node and the AV bundle. It may be a normal escape rhythm (rate between 40 and 60 beats/min) or an active focus (rate 60 beats/min or greater).

junctional tachycardia, a junctional rhythm with a rate greater than 100 beats/min. The mechanism may be enhanced normal automaticity, abnormal automaticity, or triggered activity caused by digitalis toxicity.

junction lines, vertical lines that appear in the mediastinum on a posterior-anterior projection radiographic image of the chest.

junction nevus [L, *jungere,* to join, *naevus,* birthmark], a hairless flat or slightly raised brown skin blemish arising from pigment cells at the epidermal-dermal junction. A junctional nevus may be found anywhere on the surface of the body. Malignant change may be signaled by increase in size, hardness or darkening, bleeding, or appearance of satellite discoloration around the nevus. Junctional nevi undergoing these changes and lesions found in areas subject to trauma should be evaluated by a dermatologist.

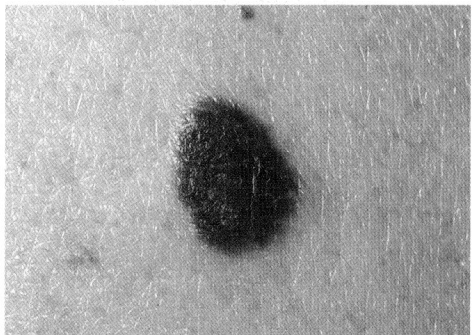

Junction nevus (*Habif, 2010*)

junctura cartilaginea. See **cartilaginous joint.**

junctura fibrosa. See **fibrous joint.**

junctura synovialis. See **synovial joint.**

juncture, a joint or union of two parts.

Jung, Carl G., the Swiss-born psychologist and psychiatrist who is known as the founder of analytic psychology. Jung attached importance to the analysis and interpretation of aspects of an individual's dreams and fantasies. Jung's view of the dynamics of personality represented an attempt to interpret human behavior from a philosophic, religious, and mystical, as well as scientific, perspective. In Jung's work titled *Psychological Types,* published in 1921, he proposed the personality types of introversion and extroversion and the four mental processes or functions of thinking, feeling, sensation, and intuition. See also **analytic psychology.**

Jungian psychology. See **analytic psychology.**

Junin fever. See **Argentine hemorrhagic fever.**

juniper tar /jōo″nipər/ [L, *juniperus* + AS, *teoru*], a dark, oily liquid obtained by the destructive distillation of the wood of *Juniperus oxycedrus* trees, used as an antiseptic stimulant in ointments for skin disorders such as psoriasis and eczema. Also called **cade oil.**

junk. *(Slang)* See **heroin.**

jurisprudence /joo͞′risproo͞″dəns/ [L, *jus,* law, *prudentia,* knowledge], the science and philosophy of law. Medical jurisprudence relates to the interfacing of medicine with criminal and civil law.

justice [L, *justus,* sufficient], **1.** a principle of bioethics that addresses fair and equal treatment for all, with due reward and honor. Equitability and appropriateness of treatment are used in the interpretation of this principle. **2.** (in research) equitable distribution of benefits and burdens of research. **3.** the treatment of people in a nonprejudicial manner.

juvenile /joo͞″vənəl, -vənīl/ [L, *juvenus,* youthful], **1.** *n.,* a young person; a youth; a child; a youngster. **2.** *adj.,* pertaining to, characteristic of, or suitable for a young person; youthful. **3.** *adj.,* physiologically underdeveloped or immature. **4.** *adj.,* denoting psychological or intellectual immaturity; childish.

juvenile alveolar rhabdomyosarcoma, a rapidly growing tumor of striated muscle occurring in children and adolescents, chiefly in the extremities. The prognosis is grave.

juvenile angiofibroma. See **nasopharyngeal angiofibroma.**

juvenile aponeurotic fibroma. See **aponeurotic fibroma.**

juvenile delinquency, persistent antisocial, illegal, or criminal behavior by children or adolescents to the degree that it cannot be controlled or corrected by the parents. It endangers others in the community, and it becomes the concern of a law enforcement agency.

juvenile delinquent, a person who performs illegal acts and who has not reached an age at which treatment as an adult can be accorded under the laws of the community having jurisdiction. Also called **juvenile offender, young offender.**

juvenile diabetes. *(Obsolete)* See **type 1 diabetes mellitus.**

juvenile glaucoma [L, *juvenus,* young; Gk, *glaukcos,* bluish-gray], increased intraocular tension in a young adult caused by developing structural defects that restrict the outflow of fluid. There is a strong genetic influence.

juvenile kyphosis. See **Scheuermann disease.**

juvenile laryngeal respiratory papillomatosis, multiple squamous cell tumors that develop in the larynx, usually in young children. The growths are transmitted by a papilloma virus and may be acquired from the mother. The laryngeal papillomas tend to undergo periods of remission and recurrence over a period of several years.

juvenile lentigo. See **lentigo.**

juvenile myoclonic syndrome, a condition in which myoclonic seizures begin to appear around the time of puberty. The myoclonic jerks are more likely to occur immediately after awakening and are often associated with sleep deprivation and photosensitivity.

juvenile myxedema. See **childhood myxedema.**

juvenile offender. See **juvenile delinquent.**

juvenile-onset diabetes, juvenile onset-type diabetes. *(Obsolete)* See **type 1 diabetes mellitus.**

juvenile rheumatoid arthritis (JRA), a form of rheumatoid arthritis, usually affecting the larger joints of children younger than 16 years of age and often accompanied by systemic manifestations. As bone growth in children is dependent on the epiphyseal plates of the distal epiphyses, skeletal development may be impaired if these structures are damaged. Treatment is supportive and includes analgesia, antiinflammatory medication, and rest. *Also called juvenile idiopathic arthritis,* **Still disease.**

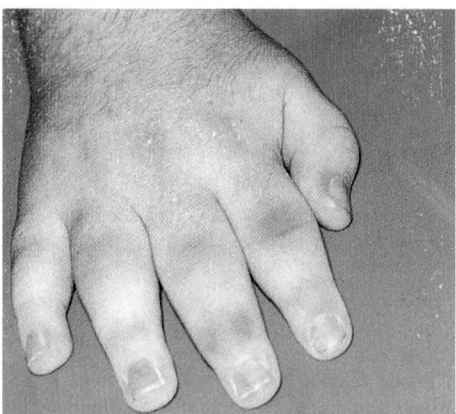

Juvenile rheumatoid arthritis: deformity of the fingers
(Zitelli and Davis, 2002)

juvenile spinal muscular atrophy, a disorder beginning in childhood in which progressive degeneration of anterior horn and medullary nerve cells leads to skeletal muscle wasting. The condition usually begins in the legs and pelvis. Also called **Wohlfart-Kugelberg-Welander disease.**

juvenile xanthogranuloma, a skin disorder characterized by groups of yellow, red, or brown papules or nodules on the extensor surfaces of the arms and legs and, in some cases, on the eyeball, meninges, and testes. The lesions typically appear in infancy or early childhood and usually disappear in a few years.

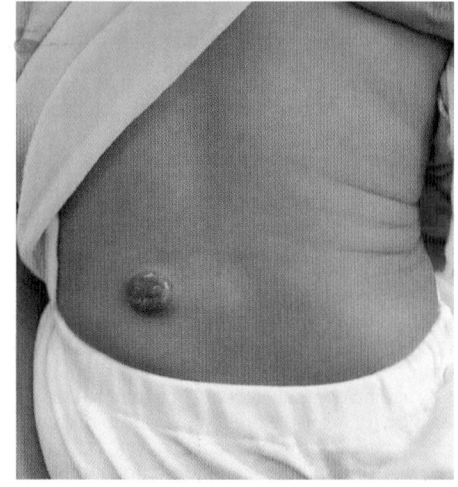

Juvenile xanthogranuloma *(Numajiri et al, 2006)*

juxta-, prefix meaning "near": *juxtaglomerular, juxtaposition.*

juxtaarticular /juk′stə-ärtik″yələr/ [L, *juxta,* near, *articulus,* joint], pertaining to a location near a joint.

juxtacrine /juks″təkrin/, describing a hormonal relationship in which the secretory cell is adjacent to an effector cell.

juxtaglomerular /-glōmer″ələr/ [L, *juxta,* near, *glomerulus,* small ball], pertaining to an area near or adjacent to the afferent and efferent arterioles of the kidney glomerulus.

juxtaglomerular apparatus, a collection of cells located beside each renal glomerulus, consisting of a portion of the distal convoluted tubule arising from that glomerular capsule, segments of the afferent and efferent arterioles closest to the glomerulus, and cells lying between these structures. It is involved in the secretion of renin and EPO in response to blood pressure changes and is important in autoregulation of certain kidney functions. Also called **juxtaglomerular complex.**

juxtaglomerular cells [L, *juxta,* near, *glomerulus,* small ball, *cella,* storeroom], smooth myoepithelioid cells lining the glomerular end of the afferent arterioles in the kidney that are in opposition to the macula densa region of the early distal tubule. These cells synthesize and store renin and release it in response to decreased renal perfusion pressure, increased sympathetic nerve stimulation of the kidneys, or decreased sodium concentration in fluid in the distal tubule.

juxtaglomerular complex. See **juxtaglomerular apparatus.**

juxtamedullary /-med″əler′ē/, near the border of a medulla.

juxtamedullary cortex, the part of the renal cortex nearest to the medulla.

juxtamedullary glomerulus, a renal glomerulus located particularly close to the corticomedullary border.

juxtamedullary nephron, one whose proximal convoluted tubule is close to the corticomedullary border and whose loop of Henle extends deep into the renal medulla.

juxtaposition /-pəzish″ən/, the placement of objects side by side or end to end.

JVP, abbreviation for **jugular venous pressure.**

J wave. See **Osborn wave.**

J

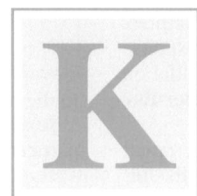

k, a symbol for the metric measurement prefix *kilo-*, which is equal to 1000 or 10^3.

K, 1. symbol for **ionization constant. 2.** symbol for **Kelvin scale. 3.** symbol for the element **potassium. 4.** abbreviation for **kilobyte. 5.** symbol in electronics for 1024 (2^{10}). **6.** abbreviation for **katal.**

Km. See **Michaelis-Menten kinetics.** Symbol for *Michaelis-Menten constant.*

kA, abbreviation for *kiloampere.*

-kacin, suffix for antibiotics derived from *Streptomyces kanamyceticus.*

Kaffir pox. See **alastrim.**

kainite /kī″nāt/, a mineral found in marine deposits and volcanic vapors; it is used as a fertilizer and as a source of potassium and magnesium compounds.

kak-, prefix meaning "bad": *kakosmia.*

kakosmia. See **cacosmia.**

kala-azar /kä″lə äzär″/ [Hindi, *kala,* black; Assamese, *azar,* fever], a chronic and potentially fatal disease caused by a protozoal infection transmitted to humans, particularly to children, by the bite of the sand fly. Kala-azar occurs primarily in Asia, parts of Africa, several South and Central American countries, and the Mediterranean region. Global travel has increased the incidence of this disease in nonendemic countries. Symptoms vary depending on the infecting species. Treatment is based on presentation as well as the extent and progression of the disease. Pentavalent antimonials have been the mainstay of treatment for decades. Newer therapeutic options include liposomal amphotericin B, miltefosine, fluconazole, and ketoconazole. Also called *Assam fever,* **black fever, dumdum fever, ponos, visceral leishmaniasis.** See also **leishmaniasis.**

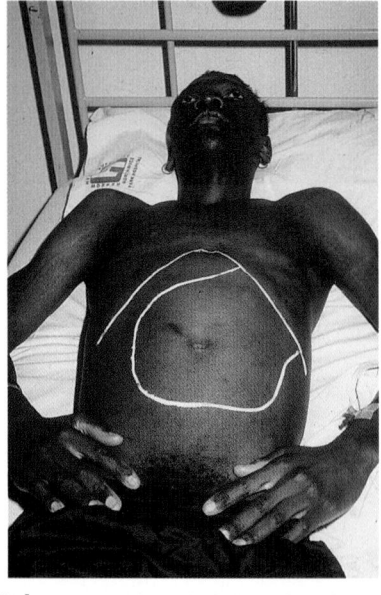

Kala-azar *(Cohen, Powderly, and Opal, 2010)*

kalemia /kəlē″mē·ə/, the presence of potassium in the blood.

kali-, prefix meaning "potassium": *kaliopenia, kalium.*

kaliopenia. See **hypokalemia.**

kalium (K) /kā″lē·əm/ [Ar, *quali,* potash], potassium.

kaliuresis /kal′iyo͞orē″sis/, the excretion of potassium in the urine.

kallak /kal″ak/, a pustular skin disease observed among the Inuit people of the northern and Arctic regions of North America.

kallikrein-kinin system /kalik″rē·in-/, a proposed hormonal system that functions within the kidney, with the enzyme kallikrein in the renal cortex mediating production of bradykinin, which acts as a vasodilator peptide. Kallikrein is present in blood plasma, urine, and tissues in an inactive state. Also spelled *kallikren-kinin system.*

Kallmann syndrome [Franz J. Kallmann, American psychiatrist, 1897–1965], a condition characterized by the absence of the sense of smell and longer-than-average limbs. It is caused by agenesis of the olfactory bulbs and secondary hypogonadism related to a decrease of luteinizing hormone–releasing hormone (interstitial cell-stimulating hormone).

kanamycin /kan′əmī″sin/, an aminoglycoside antibiotic derived from *Streptomyces kanamyceticus.*

kanamycin sulfate, an aminoglycoside antibiotic.

■ INDICATIONS: It is prescribed in the treatment of certain severe infections (especially those caused by gram-negative aerobes) and as second-line therapy for tuberculosis.

■ CONTRAINDICATIONS: Concomitant administration of ototoxic drugs or known hypersensitivity to this drug or to other aminoglycoside antibiotics prohibits its use. It is used with caution in patients having impaired renal function and in the elderly.

■ ADVERSE EFFECTS: Among the more serious adverse effects are nephrotoxicity, vestibular and auditory ototoxicity, neuromuscular blockade, and hypersensitivity reactions.

kangaroo care, the practice in which a caregiver holds a diapered infant, particularly a preterm infant, with skin-to-skin contact.

Kanner syndrome [Leo Kanner, Austrian-born American child psychiatrist, 1896–1981], now called **autism spectrum disorders.**

Kantian theory, the ethical theory of the 18th-century German philosopher Immanuel Kant (1724–1804). It focuses on the rightness or wrongness of actions in and of themselves, rather than on the consequences of those actions. According to Kant, the principles by which actions are judged right or wrong can be determined by reason, and the individual has a duty to act in accordance with these principles.

Kantrex, an aminoglycoside antibacterial drug. Brand name for **kanamycin sulfate.**

Kaochlor, an oral electrolyte replacement solution. Brand name for **potassium chloride.**

kaodzera. See **Rhodesian trypanosomiasis.**

kaolin /kā″əlin/ [Chin, *kao-ling,* high ridge], an absorbent and protective emollient used topically in an ointment.

kaolinosis /kā′əlinō″sis/, a form of pneumoconiosis acquired by inhaling clay dust (kaolin). Kaolin is used in the manufacture of paper, ceramics, heat-resistant wood, soaps, toothpaste, and some medicines.

Kaon Cl, an oral electrolyte replacement solution. Brand name for **potassium chloride.**

Kaopectate, an antidiarrheal drug. Its formulations have varied over the years; current formulations include bismuth subsalicylate. Additionally, ingredients differ from country to country.

Kaposi disease /kap″əsē/ [Moritz K. Kaposi, Austrian dermatologist, 1837–1902; L, *dis* + Fr, *aise,* ease], a rare inherited skin disorder that begins in childhood and mainly involves exposed skin areas. Exposure to sunlight results in erythema and vesiculation, followed by increased pigmentation and telangiectasia, skin ulcers, warts, and malignant epitheliomas. Also called **xeroderma pigmentosum.**

Kaposi sarcoma (KS, ks) [Moritz K. Kaposi], a malignant, multifocal neoplasm of reticuloendothelial cells that begins as soft brownish or purple papules on the feet or hard palate and slowly spreads in the skin, metastasizing to the lymph nodes and viscera. It occurs most often in men and is associated with diabetes, malignant lymphoma, human immunodeficiency virus (HIV)/acquired immunodeficiency syndrome (AIDS), or other disorders. Radiotherapy and chemotherapy are usually recommended. Also called **idiopathic multiple pigmented hemorrhagic sarcoma, multiple idiopathic hemorrhagic sarcoma.**

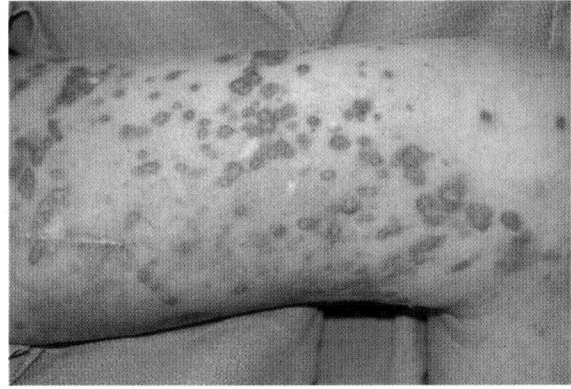

Papules associated with Kaposi sarcoma
(Nooshin et al, 2011)

Kaposi sarcoma–associated herpesvirus. See **human herpesvirus 8.**

Kaposi varicelliform eruption. See **eczema herpeticum.**

kappa /kap″ə/, **1.** K, κ, the tenth letter of the Greek alphabet, used to denote (in chemistry) the tenth carbon atom in a chain. **2.** one of two light chains in an immunoglobulin molecule. **3.** a type of killer particle present in certain strains of *Paramecium.* **4.** the angle between the visual axis and the pupillary axis.

kappa chain, a type of light polypeptide chain of immunoglobulin molecules.

kappa light chain, one of two kinds of smaller peptide chains present in an immunoglobulin molecule. See also **lambda light chain.**

kaps-. See **caps-, kaps-, capsul-, capsulo-.**

karat, the proportion of gold in 24 parts of a gold alloy; 24-karat gold is pure gold.

karaya powder /kär″äyä/ [Hindi, *karayal,* resin; L, *pulvis,* dust], a dried form of *Sterculia urens* or other species of *Sterculia,* used as a bulk cathartic. The use of such a bulk-forming cathartic may also increase the loss of sodium, potassium, and water. With some individuals the use of karaya powder may cause allergic reactions such as urticaria, rhinitis, dermatitis, and asthma. Methylcellulose has largely replaced this drug in modern use. Externally it is used as a drying agent for stage I and stage II pressure ulcers.

kardex, a generic term for a card-filing system that allows quick reference to the particular needs of each patient for certain aspects of nursing care; the system is often used for change-of-shift reports. Increasingly, electronic documentation systems are incorporating information recorded on the kardex.

Kartagener syndrome /kärtag″ənərz/ [Manes Kartagene, Swiss physician, 1897–1975], an inherited disorder characterized by bronchiectasis, chronic paranasal sinusitis, and transposed viscera, usually dextrocardia. *Also called immotile cilia syndrome, Kartagener type.*

karyenchyma. See **karyolymph.**

karyo-, prefix meaning "nucleus": *karyocyte, karyokinesis, karyolymph.*

karyoclasis, karyoclastic. See **karyoklasis.**

karyocyte /ker″ē·əsīt′/ [Gk, *karyon,* nut + *kytos,* cell], a normoblast, or developing red blood cell, with a nucleus condensed into a homogenous staining body. It is normally found in the red bone marrow. The term is not in common usage.

karyogamy /ker′ē·og″əmē/ [Gk, *karyon,* nut + *gamos,* marriage], the fusion of cell nuclei, as in conjugation and zygosis. *–karyogamic, adj.*

karyogenesis /ker′ē·ōjen″əsis/ [Gk, *karyon* + *genein,* to produce], the formation and development of the nucleus of a cell. *–karyogenetic, adj.*

karyokinesis /ker′ē·ōkinē″sis, -kinē″sis/ [Gk, *karyon* + *kinesis,* motion], the division of the nucleus and equal distribution of nuclear material during mitosis and meiosis. The process involves the four stages of prophase, metaphase, anaphase, and telophase. It precedes the division of the cytoplasm. Also called **karyomitosis.** See also **cytokinesis.** *–karyokinetic, adj.*

karyoklasis /ker′ē·ok″ləsis/ [Gk, *karyon* + *klasis,* breaking], **1.** the disintegration of a cell nucleus or nuclear membrane. **2.** the interruption of mitosis. Also spelled *karyoclasis. –karyoklastic, karyoclastic, adj.*

karyology /ker′ē·ol″əjē/ [Gk, *karyon* + *logos,* science], the branch of cytology that concentrates on the study of the cell nucleus, especially the structure and function of the chromosomes. *–karyological, karyologic, adj., –karyologist, n.*

karyolymph /ker″ē·əlimf′/ [Gk, *karyon* + *lympha,* water], the clear, usually nonstaining, fluid substance of a cell nucleus. It consists primarily of proteinaceous, colloidal material in which the nucleolus, chromatin, linin, and various submicroscopic particles are dispersed. Also called **karyenchyma, nuclear hyaloplasm, nuclear sap, nucleochyme, linin.** *–karyolymphatic, adj.*

karyolysis /ker′ē·ol″isis/ [Gk, *karyon* + *lysis,* loosening], the dissolution of a cell nucleus. It occurs normally, both as a form of necrobiosis and during the generation of new cells through mitosis and meiosis.

K

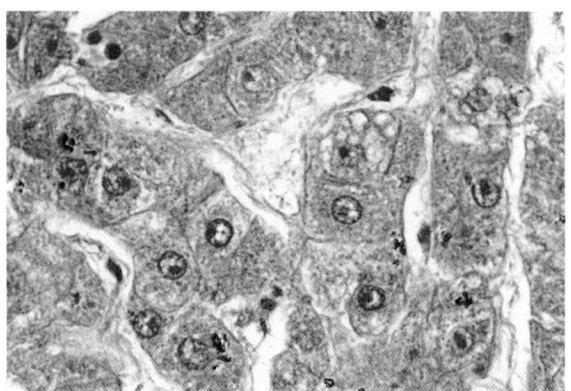

Normal cell with visible nucleolus and karyolysis leaving the cell as a mass with complete dissolution of the nucleus (Stevens, Lowe, and Scott, 2009)

karyolytic /ker′ē·əlit″ik/, **1.** *adj.*, pertaining to karyolysis. **2.** *n.*, something that causes the destruction of a cell nucleus.

karyomegaly /ker′ē·ōmeg″əlē/ [Gk, *karyon,* nut + *megas,* large], an increase in the nuclear size of tissue cells.

karyomere /ker″ē·əmir′/ [Gk, *karyon + meros,* part], **1.** a saclike structure containing an unequal portion of the nuclear material after atypical mitosis. **2.** a segment of a chromosome. See also **chromomere.**

karyometry /ker′ē·om″ətrē/, the measurement of the nucleus of a cell. −*karyometric, adj.*

karyomit /ker″ē·əmit′/ [Gk, *karyon + mitos,* thread], **1.** a single chromatin fibril of the network within the nucleus of a cell. **2.** a chromosome.

karyomitome /ker′ē·om″itōm/ [Gk, *karyon + mitos,* thread], the fibrillar chromatin network within the nucleus of a cell. Also called **karyoreticulum.**

karyomitosis. See **karyokinesis.**

karyomorphism /-môr″fizəm/ [Gk, *karyon + morphe,* form], the shape or form of a cell nucleus, especially that of a leukocyte. −*karyomorphic, adj.*

karyon /ker″ē·on/ [Gk, nut], the nucleus of a cell. −*karyontic, adj.*

karyophage /ker″ē·ōfāj′/ [Gk, *karyon + phagein,* to eat], an intracellular protozoan parasite that destroys the nucleus of the cell it infects. −*karyophagous, karyophagic, adj.*

karyoplasm. See **nucleoplasm.**

karyoplasmic ratio. See **nucleocytoplasmic ratio.**

karyopyknosis /-piknō″sis/ [Gk, *karyon + pyknos,* thick], the state of a cell in which the nucleus has shrunk and the chromatin has condensed into solid masses, as in cornified cells of stratified squamous epithelium. −*karyopyknotic, adj.*

karyoreticulum. See **karyomitome.**

karyorrhexis /-rek″sis/ [Gk, *karyon + rhexis,* rupture], the disintegration of the nucleus in a cell. −*karyorrhectic, adj.*

karyosome /ker′ē·əsōm′/ [Gk, *karyon + soma,* body], a dense, irregular mass of chromatin filaments in a cell nucleus. It is often seen during interphase and may be confused with the nucleolus because of similar staining properties. Also called **chromatin nucleolus, chromocenter, false nucleolus, prochromosome.**

karyospheric /-sfer″ik/ [Gk, *karyon + sphaira,* ball], **1.** *n.,* a spheric nucleus. **2.** *adj.,* pertaining to such a nucleus.

karyostasis /ker′ē·os″təsis/ [Gk, *karyon + stasis,* standing], the resting stage of the nucleus between cell division. See also **interphase.** −*karyostatic, adj.*

karyotheca. See **nuclear envelope.**

karyotin. See **chromatin.**

karyotype /ker″ē·ətīp′/ [Gk, *karyon + typos,* mark], **1.** the number, form, size, and arrangement within the nucleus of the somatic chromosomes of an individual or species, as determined by a microphotograph taken during metaphase of mitosis. **2.** a diagrammatic representation of the chromosome complement of an individual or species, in which the chromosomes are arranged in pairs in descending order of size and according to the position of the centromere. See also **chromosome, Denver classification, idiogram.** −*karyotypic, adj.*

Kasabach-Merritt syndrome. See **hemangioma-thrombocytopenia syndrome.**

Kasabach method /kas″əbak/ [H.H. Kasabach, American radiologist, 1899–1943], (in radiology) a technique for positioning a patient for radiographic examination of the odontoid process.

Kasai operation. See **portoenterostomy.**

Kashin-Bek disease [Nikolai I. Kashin, Russian orthopedist, 1825–1872; E.V. Bek; L, *dis* + Fr, *aise,* ease], a chronic disease of joints affecting bone growth in children living in China, Tibet, Korea, and eastern Siberia. Range of motion is usually restricted. Also spelled *Kaschin-Beck disease.*

kat, abbreviation for **katal.**

kat-, kata-, cat-, cata-, prefix meaning "to go down," "to go against," or "to reverse": *katadidymus.*

katadidymus /kat′ədid″əməs/ [Gk, *kata,* down + *didymos,* twin], conjoined twins united in the lower portion of the body and separated at the top.

katal (K, kat) /kat″al/ [Gk, *kata,* down], an enzyme unit in moles per second defined by the SI system: 1 K lm = 6.6 × 10⁹ U.

Katz index /kats/ [Sidney Katz, American physician, 1924–2012], a tool for assessing a patient's ability to perform activities of daily living in the areas of bathing, dressing, toileting, transferring, continence, and feeding. In each category, a score of one indicates complete independence in performing the activity and zero indicates that assistance is required, so that the total score ranges from 0 to 6.

kava, an herb that is harvested from the root of a shrub that grows in the South Sea islands.

■ INDICATIONS: It may be useful for nervous anxiety, restlessness, sleep disturbances, and stress.

■ CONTRAINDICATIONS: Kava should not be used during pregnancy and lactation, in children under 12 years of age, or in persons with known hypersensitivity, major depressive disorder, or Parkinson disease.

Kawasaki disease. See **mucocutaneous lymph node syndrome.**

Kay Ciel, an oral electrolyte replacement solution. Brand name for **potassium chloride.**

Kayser-Fleischer ring /kī″zər flī″shər/ [Bernhard Kayser, German ophthalmologist, 1869–1954; Bruno Fleischer, German ophthalmologist, 1874–1904], a gray-green to red-gold pigmented ring at the outer margin of the cornea (limbal border), pathognomonic of hepatolenticular degeneration, a rare progressive disease caused by a defect in copper metabolism and transmitted as an autosomal-recessive trait. The disease is characterized by cerebral degenerative changes, liver cirrhosis, splenomegaly, involuntary

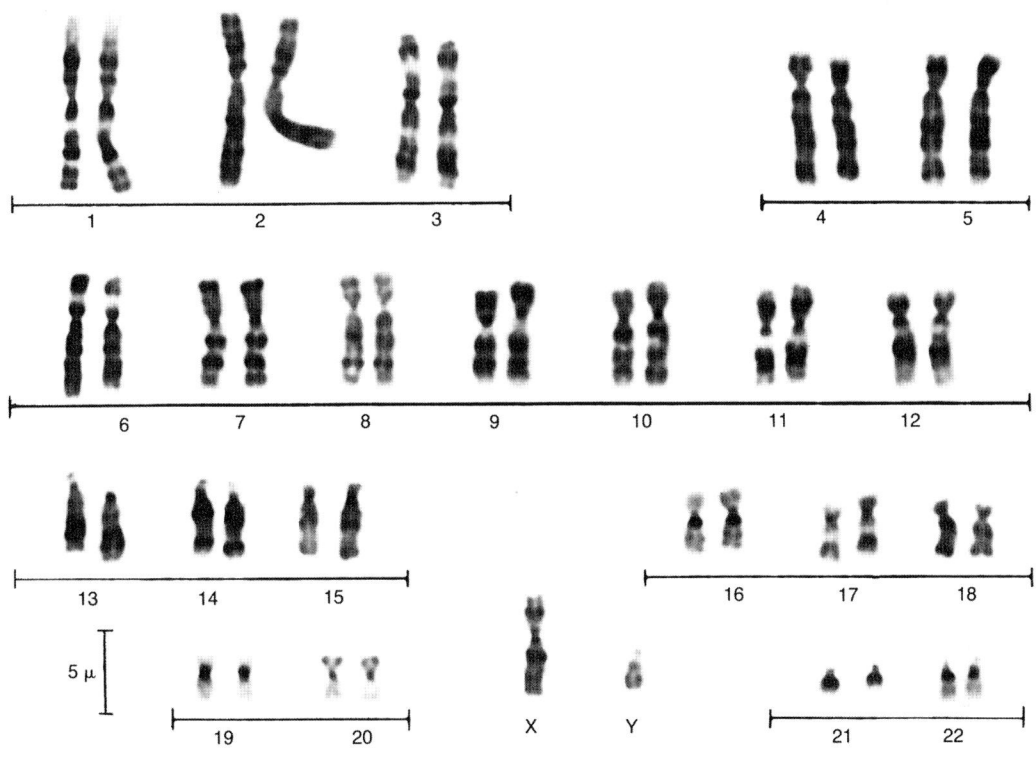

Human karyotype *(Gartner and Hiatt, 2007)*

K

movements, muscle rigidity, psychic disturbances, and dysphagia. See also **Wilson disease.**

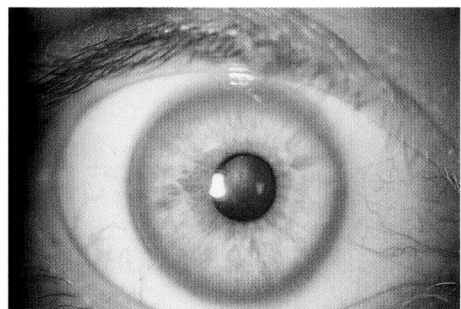

Kayser-Fleischer ring *(Swartz, 2006)*

Kazanjian operation /kasanʺjē·ən/ [Varaztad J. Kazanjian, Armenian-born maxillofacial surgeon in U.S., 1879–1974], a surgical procedure for extending the vestibular sulcus to improve the prosthetic foundation of toothless dental ridges.

kb, **1.** abbreviation for **kilobase. 2.** abbreviation for **kilobyte.**

kbp, abbreviation for **kilobase pair.**

kcal, abbreviation for **kilocalorie.**

kcalorie. See **calorie.**

kCi, abbreviation for *kilocurie.*

KCl, symbol for **potassium chloride.**

KE, abbreviation for **kinetic energy.**

Kearns-Sayre syndrome /kernz sār/ [Thomas P. Kearns, American ophthalmologist, 1922–2011; George P. Sayre, American pathologist, 1911–1991], progressive ophthalmoplegia, pigmentary degeneration of the retina, myopathy, ataxia, and cardiac conduction defect, with onset before the age of 20 years. Almost all patients have large mitochondrial DNA deletions, and ragged red fibers are seen on muscle biopsy. Also called **ophthalmoplegia plus.**

Kedani fever. See **scrub typhus.**

K-edge, a discontinuity in the absorption coefficient at an energy level corresponding to the binding energy of K-shell electrons.

keel, (in prosthetics) a device in a stored-energy foot prosthesis that bends the foot upward when weight is applied to the toe. See also **carina, Seattle Foot, stored-energy foot.**

kefir /kefʺər/ [Russ, fermented milk], a slightly effervescent, acidulous beverage prepared from the milk of cows, sheep, or goats through fermentation by kefir grains, which contain yeasts and lactobacilli. The probiotic properties of kefir provide a source of bacteria necessary in the GI tract. Also spelled **kephir.**

Keflex, a cephalosporin antibacterial drug. Brand name for **cephalexin.**

Kefzol, an antibacterial drug. Brand name for **cefazolin sodium.**

Kegel exercises. See **pubococcygeus exercises.**

Keith bundle, Keith-Flack node. Also called **sinoatrial node.** See **sinus node.**

Keith-Wagener-Barker classification system [Norman M. Keith, Canadian physician, b. 1885; Henry P. Wagener, American physician, b. 1890; N.W. Barker, 20th-century American physician], a method of classifying the degree of hypertension in a patient on the basis of retinal changes. The stages are group 1, identified by constriction of the retinal arterioles; group 2, constriction and sclerosis of the retinal arterioles; group 3, characterized by hemorrhages and exudates in addition to group 2 conditions; and group 4, papilledema of the retinal arterioles.

kel-, prefix meaning "tumor" or "fibrous growth": *keloid, keloidosis.*

Kellgren syndrome /kel″grin/ [Henry Kellgren, Swedish physician, b. 1827]. See **erosive osteoarthritis.**

Kelly clamp [Howard A. Kelly, American gynecologist, 1858–1943; AS, *clam,* to fasten], a curved hemostat without teeth, used primarily for grasping vascular tissue in gynecological procedures.

Kelly plication, an operation for correction of stress incontinence in women. The connective tissue between the vagina and the urethra and the floor of the bladder are sutured to form a wide shelf of firm tissue supporting the urethra and bladder.

Kelly pad, a horseshoe-shaped inflatable rubber drainage pad used in a bed or on the operating table.

keloid /kē″loid/ [Gk, *kelis,* spot + *eidos,* form], an overgrowth of collagenous scar tissue at the site of a skin injury, particularly a wound or a surgical incision. The new tissue is elevated, rounded, and firm. People with darker skin are particularly susceptible to keloid formation, but it can occur in all skin types. A tendency to develop keloids runs in families. Types of therapy include solid carbon dioxide, liquid nitrogen, intralesional corticosteroid injections, radiation, silicon gel, and surgery. Treatment may worsen the condition. Also spelled *cheloid.* Compare **hypertrophic scarring.** —*cheloidal,* **keloidal,** *adj.*

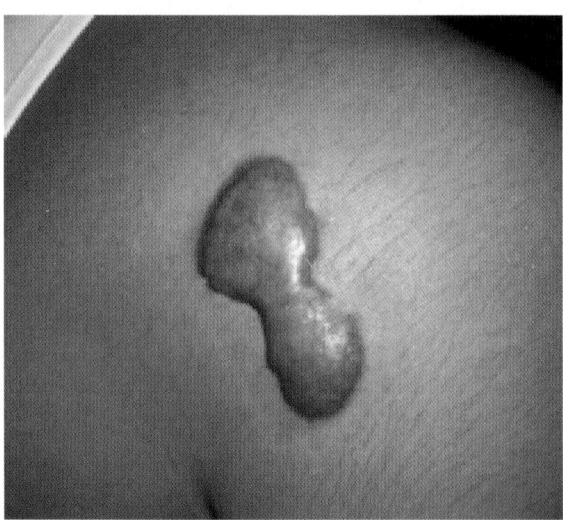

Keloid *(Ogawa, 2008)*

keloid acne [Gk, *kelis,* spot + *eidos,* form + *akme,* point], pyoderma in and around the pilosebaceous structures, resulting in keloid scarring. People with darker skin are most susceptible. Also called **dermatitis papillaris capillitii, folliculitis keloidalis.**

keloidal. See **keloid.**

keloidal scar. See **keloid scar.**

keloidosis /kē″loidō″sis/ [Gk, *kelis* + *eidos,* form + *osis,* condition], habitual or multiple formation of keloids.

keloid scar [Gk, *kelis,* spot + *eidos,* form + *eschara,* scab], an overgrowth of tissue in a scar at the site of skin injury, particularly a wound or a surgical incision. The amount of tissue growth is in excess of that necessary to repair the wound and is partially caused by an accumulation of collagen at the site. Also called **keloidal scar.**

kelp /kɛlp/ [ME, *culp*], **1.** any of the brown seaweed species of *Laminaria* found on the Atlantic coast of Europe. **2.** the ashes of *Laminaria* seaweed burned in a process of extracting iodine and potassium salts.

Kelvin scale (K) [Lord Kelvin (William Thomson), British physicist, 1824–1907], an absolute temperature scale calculated in Celsius units from the point at which molecular activity apparently ceases, −273.15° C. To convert Celsius degrees to Kelvin, add 273.15.

Kemadrin, an antiparkinsonial muscle relaxant from the anticholinergic drug class. Brand name for **procyclidine hydrochloride.**

Kempner rice-fruit diet. See **rice diet.**

Kenalog, a glucocorticoid. Brand name for *triamcinolone acetonide.*

Kennedy classification [Edward Kennedy, American dentist, b. 1883], a method of classifying partial edentulous conditions and partial dentures, based on the position of the spaces once occupied by the missing teeth in relation to the remaining teeth. It is useful in the construction of and planning for removable partial dentures.

Kenny treatment. See **Sister Kenny's treatment.**

keno-, prefix meaning "empty": *kenophobia, kenogenesis.*

kenogenesis. See **cenogenesis.**

kenophobia /kē″nōfō″bē·ə/ [Gk, *kenos,* empty + *phobos,* fear]. See **agoraphobia.**

Kent bundle [Albert F.S. Kent, English physiologist, 1863–1958; AS, *byndel,* to bind], an accessory pathway between an atrium and a ventricle outside the conduction system. This congenital anomaly causes Wolff-Parkinson-White syndrome. The term "accessory pathway" is preferred because the one Kent described had a precise location (anterior and near the fibrous ring of the tricuspid valve). See also **Wolff-Parkinson-White syndrome.**

Kenya fever. See **Marseilles fever.**

kephal-. See **cephalo-, cephal-.**

kephir. See **kefir.**

kera-, prefix meaning "horn": *keratitis, keratoma, keratosis, keratin.*

kerasin /ker″əsin/ [L, *cera,* wax], a cerebroside, found in brain tissue, that consists of a fatty acid, galactose, and sphingosine.

kerat-, kerato-, 1. prefix meaning "horny, cornified": *keratolysis, keratoma, keratonosis.* **2.** prefix meaning "cornea, corneal": *keratoiritis, keratome.*

keratectomy /ker′ətek″təmē/ [Gk, *keras,* horn + *ektomē,* excision], an opthalmological surgical procedure to remove part of the cornea, performed to excise a small, superficial lesion that does not warrant a corneal graft. Local anesthesia is used. The scar is excised, and an antibiotic is injected under the conjunctiva. A topical steroid is given and a light pressure dressing applied. After surgery, the dressings are changed daily. Corneal epithelium grows rapidly, filling a small surgical area in about 60 hours.

keratic /kərat″ik/ [Gk, *keras,* horn + L, *icus,* like], **1.** pertaining to keratin. **2.** pertaining to the cornea.

keratic precipitate, a group of inflammatory cells deposited on the endothelial surface of the cornea after trauma or inflammation, sometimes obscuring vision.

keratin /ker″ətin/ [Gk, *keras,* horn], a fibrous sulfur-containing protein that is the primary component of the epidermis, hair, nails, enamel of the teeth, and horny tissue of animals. The protein is insoluble in most solvents, including gastric juice. For this reason, it is often used as a coating for pills that must pass through the stomach unchanged to be dissolved in the intestines.

keratin cyst, an epithelial cyst containing keratin. Also called **keratinous cyst.**

keratinization /-īzā″shən/ [Gk, *keras* + L, *izein,* to cause], a process by which epithelial cells lose their moisture and are replaced by horny tissue.

keratinize /ker′ətinīz/, to make or become horny tissue.

keratinocyte /kerat″inōsīt′/ [Gk, *keras* + *kytos,* cell], an epidermal cell that synthesizes keratin and other proteins and sterols. These cells constitute 95% of the epidermis, being formed from undifferentiated, or basal, cells at the dermal-epidermal junction. Its characteristic intermediate filament protein is cytokeratin. In its various successive stages, keratin forms the prickle cell layer and the granular cell layer, in which the cells become flattened and slowly die to form the final layer, the stratum corneum, which gradually exfoliates.

keratinophilic /kerat′inōfil″ik/, describing a type of fungi that uses keratin as a substrate.

keratinous cyst. See **keratin cyst.**

keratitis /ker′ətī″tis/, any inflammation of the cornea. Compare **keratopathy.** Kinds include **dendritic keratitis, interstitial keratitis, keratoconjunctivitis sicca, trachoma. –keratic,** *adj.*

keratoacanthoma /ker′ətō·ak′anthō″mə/ [Gk, *keras* + *akantha,* thorn + *oma,* tumor], a benign, rapidly growing, flesh-colored papule or nodule of the skin with a central plug of keratin. The lesion is most common on the face or the back of the hands and arms. It disappears spontaneously in 4 to 6 months, leaving a slightly depressed scar. Biopsy is often necessary to differentiate it from a squamous cell carcinoma.

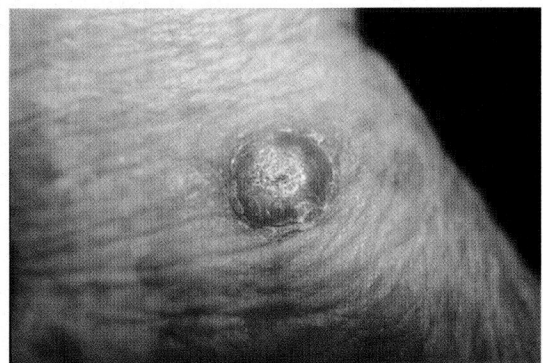

Keratoacanthoma *(Courtesy Department of Dermatology, School of Medicine, University of Utah)*

keratocele /ker′ətōsēl′/, a hernia of Descemet's membrane through an ulcer in the outer layers of the cornea.

keratoconjunctivitis /ker′ətōkənjungk′tivī″tis/ [Gk, *keras* + L, *conjunctivus,* connecting + Gk, *itis,* inflammation], inflammation of the cornea and the conjunctiva. Kinds include **eczematous conjunctivitis, epidemic keratoconjunctivitis, keratoconjunctivitis sicca.**

keratoconjunctivitis sicca, dryness of the cornea caused by a deficiency of tear secretion in which the corneal surface appears dull and rough and the eye feels gritty and irritated. The condition may be associated with erythema multiforme, Sjögren's syndrome, trachoma, and vitamin A deficiency. Methylcellulose artificial tears may give some relief, as can insertion of plugs into the punctae and use of cyclosporine drops.

keratoconus /ker′ətōkō″nəs/ [Gk, *keras* + *konos,* cone], a noninflammatory protrusion of the central or paracentral region of the cornea. It is worse in allergy sufferers and may result in marked irregular astigmatism. It is also associated with Down syndrome. Gas permeable contact lenses often significantly improve visual acuity as compared with spectacles, although a corneal transplant is indicated in about 15% of patients with this condition. The cause of the condition is unknown, but it likely has a genetic basis.

keratocyst /ker″ətōsist′/, a thin-walled, tooth-forming cyst lined by keratinizing epithelium. It may be solitary or part of a multiple lesion, most frequently in the posterior body or ramus of the mandible, and may or may not be associated with teeth. See also **odontogenic keratocyst.**

keratocyte. See **corneal corpuscle.**

keratoderma /ker′ətōdur″mə/ [Gk, *keras,* horn + *derma,* skin], **1.** a horny skin or covering. **2.** hypertrophy of the horny layer of the skin. See also **callus, hyperkeratosis.**

keratoderma blennorrhagica /-durmə/, the development of hyperkeratotic skin lesions (pustules and crusts) of the palms, soles, and nails. The condition tends to occur in some patients with Reiter syndrome.

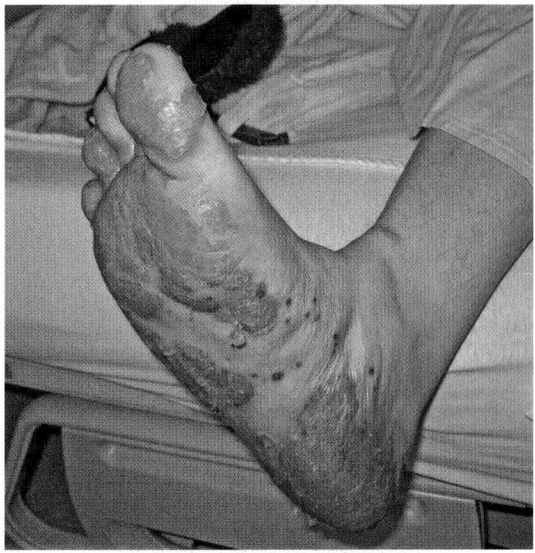

Keratoderma blennorrhagica *(Fitzpatrick and High, 2018)*

keratodermatitis /-dur′mətī″tis/, an inflammation and proliferation of the cells of the horny layer of the skin.

keratoectasia /ker′ətō·ektā″zha/, a forward bulging or protrusion of the cornea. Also called **kerectasis.**

keratoepithelioplasty /-ep′ithē″lē·əplas′tē/, a surgical procedure for the repair of corneal epithelial defects. The defective cornea is removed and replaced with small pieces of donor cornea, which proliferate and replace the original tissue.

keratogenesis /-jen″əsis/, the formation of horny tissue caused by the growth of keratin-producing cells.

keratogenic /-jen″ik/, pertaining to an agent that induces a growth of horny tissue.

keratogenous /ker′ətoj″ənəs/, pertaining to development of the horny layer of the skin or the growth of cells that produce keratin, which results in the formation of horny tissue, such as fingernails and scales.

keratoglobus /-glō″bəs/, a congenital anomaly characterized by distension of the cornea and the anterior segment of the eye. Also called **megalocornea.**

keratohyalin /-hī″əlin/ [Gk, *keras + hyalos,* glass], a substance in the granules found in keratinocytes of the epidermis. The keratohyalin granule develops within and around the fibrillar protein, contributing in an unknown manner to the functional maturity of keratin.

keratoid /ker″ətoid/ [Gk, *keras,* horn, *eidos,* form], resembling horny or corneal tissue.

keratoiritis /ker′ətōīrī″tis/, an inflammation of the cornea in association with inflammation of the iris.

keratolysis /ker′ətol″ə-sis/ [Gk, *keras + lysis,* loosening], the loosening and shedding of the outer layer of the skin, which may occur normally by exfoliation or as a congenital condition in which the skin is shed at periodic intervals. *−keratolytic, adj.*

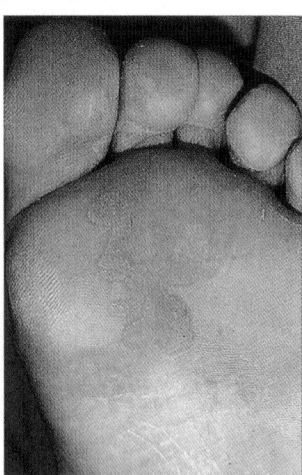

Keratolysis *(Lawrence and Cox, 2002)*

keratoma /ker′ətō″mə/, a hard, thick epidermal growth caused by hypertrophy of the horny layer of the skin. See also **callus,** def. 2.

keratomalacia /-məlā″shə/ [Gk, *keras + malakia,* softness], a condition characterized by xerosis and ulceration of the cornea, resulting from severe vitamin A deficiency. It commonly occurs as a secondary result of diseases that affect vitamin A absorption or storage, such as ulcerative colitis, celiac syndrome, cystic fibrosis, and sprue. Also at risk are infants and children who are given dilute formula, who are malnourished, or who are allergic to whole milk and fed skimmed milk, which is a poor source of vitamin A. See also **vitamin A.**
■ OBSERVATIONS: Early symptoms include night blindness; photophobia; swelling and redness of the eyelids; and drying, roughness, pain, and wrinkling of the conjunctiva.
■ INTERVENTIONS: Treatment consists of vitamin A supplements. The dosage is determined by the severity of the condition, although prolonged daily administration of large doses, especially to infants, may result in hypervitaminosis. An adequate diet containing whole milk and foods high in vitamin A or carotenes prevents the condition.
■ PATIENT CARE CONSIDERATIONS: In advanced deficiency, Bitot's spots appear; the cornea becomes dull, lusterless, and hazy, and without adequate therapy it eventually softens and perforates, resulting in blindness.

keratome, a surgical instrument used in ophthalmic surgery to make an incision in the cornea.

keratomycosis /-mīkō″sis/, a fungal disease of the cornea.

keratopathy /ker′ətop″əthē/ [Gk, *keras + pathos,* disease], any noninflammatory disease of the cornea. Compare **keratitis.**

keratophakia /-fā″kē·ə/, the surgical implantation of donor cornea to the anterior cornea to modify a refractive error.

keratoplasty. See **corneal grafting.**

keratorrhexis /ker″atorek′sis/, rupture of the cornea. Also spelled *keratorhexis.*

keratosis /ker′ətō″sis/ [Gk, *keras + osis,* condition], any skin lesion in which there is overgrowth and thickening of the cornified epithelium. Approximately 20% of these skin lesions develop into squamous cell carcinoma. Prevention includes limits on time in the sun, avoidance of tanning beds, and consistent use of sunscreen. Kinds include **actinic keratosis, seborrheic keratosis.** *−keratotic, adj.*

keratosis follicularis, a group of several skin disorders characterized by keratotic papules that coalesce to form brown or black crusted, wartlike patches. These vegetations may spread widely, ulcerate, and become covered with a purulent exudate. Treatment includes large doses of topical or oral retinoids and oral or topical corticosteroids. Also called **Darier disease.**

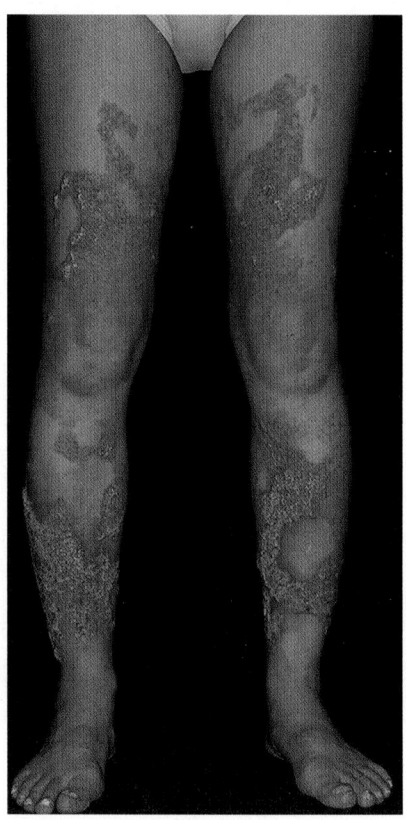

Patient with keratosis follicularis *(Moriuchi et al, 2008)*

keratosis seborrheica. See **seborrheic keratosis.**
keratosis senilis, keratotic. See **keratosis.**
kerectasis. See **keratoectasia.**
kerion /kir″ē·on/ [Gk, honeycomb], an inflamed boggy granuloma or secondary infected lesion that develops as an immune reaction to a superficial fungus infection, generally in association with tinea capitis of the scalp. Treatment can be challenging; in addition to the use of topical treatments,

oral administration of griseofulvin, terbinafine, itraconazole, or fluconazole is often required.

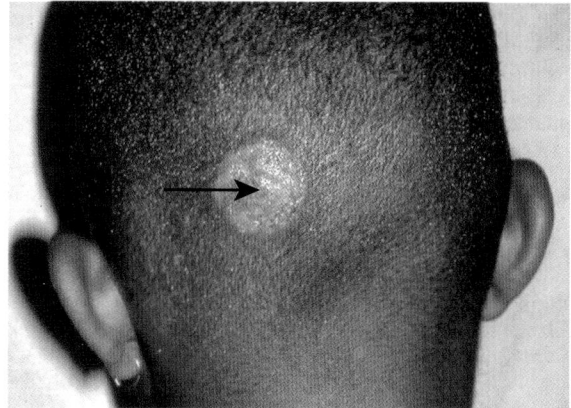

Kerion *(Cordoro and Ganz, 2005)*

Kerley lines /kur″lē/ [Peter J. Kerley, English radiologist, 1900-1979], a fine threading of opaque lines that appears on chest x-ray images. This radiographic finding is consistent with fluid in the interstitial tissue of the lungs associated with certain disease conditions, such as congestive heart failure and pleural lymphatic engorgement. Also called **septal lines.**

KERMA, a unit of quantity referring to the kinetic energy transferred from photons to charged particles, such as electrons in Compton interactions, per unit mass. The SI unit for the KERMA is the gray, and the special unit is the rad. Abbreviation for *kinetic energy released in the medium, kinetic energy released in matter.*

kernicterus /kərnik″tərəs/ [Ger, *kern,* kernel; Gk, *ikteros,* jaundice], an abnormal toxic accumulation of bilirubin in central nervous system tissues caused by hyperbilirubinemia. See also **hyperbilirubinemia of the newborn.**

Kernig sign /ker″nik/ [Vladimir M. Kernig, Russian physician, 1840–1917], a diagnostic sign for meningitis marked by a loss of the ability of a supine patient to completely straighten the leg when it is fully flexed at the knee and hip. Pain in the lower back and resistance to straightening the leg constitute a positive Kernig sign. Usually the patient can extend the leg completely when the thigh is not flexed on the abdomen. Compare **Brudzinski sign.**

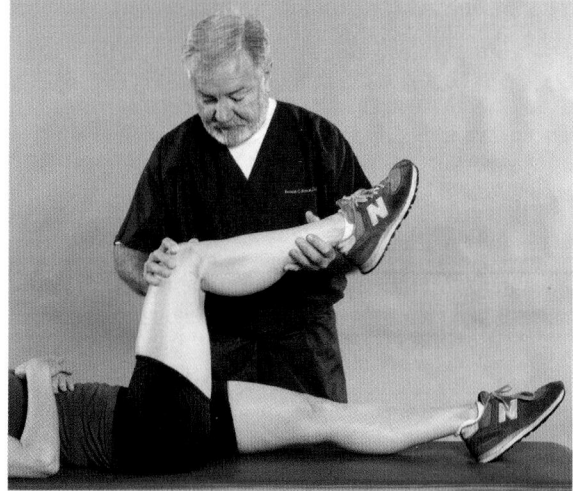

Assessment of Kernig sign *(Evans, 2009)*

kerosene poisoning /ker″əsēn/ [Gk, *keros,* wax; L, *potio,* drink], a toxic condition caused by the ingestion of kerosene or the inhalation of its fumes. See also **petroleum distillate poisoning.**
- OBSERVATIONS: Symptoms after ingestion include drowsiness, fever, a rapid heartbeat, tremors, and severe pneumonitis if the fluid is aspirated.
- INTERVENTIONS: Vomiting is not induced. If the person breathed in kerosene fumes, he or she should be moved to fresh air. Local emergency services and a poison control center should be contacted if kerosene poisoning is suspected. Emergency care will largely depend on the route and amount of the poisoning. It may include intubation, gastric lavage, and debridement of tissue if burned.
- PATIENT CARE CONSIDERATIONS: Damage can continue to occur after the immediate episode. Kerosene, and all fuel oils, should be kept in a safe place to prevent accidental exposure.

Ketalar, a general anesthetic. Brand name for **ketamine hydrochloride.**

ketamine hydrochloride /kē′təmēn/, a rapid-acting nonbarbiturate general anesthetic induction agent, administered parenterally to achieve dissociative anesthesia. Ketamine hydrochloride does not cause muscle relaxation. It is a potent somatic analgesic and is particularly useful for brief minor surgical procedures. Hallucinations, confusion, and disorientation may occur on emergence from anesthesia. See also **dissociative anesthesia.**

keto-, prefix indicating possession of the carbonyl (:C:O) group: *ketoacidosis, ketogenesis, ketonuria.*

ketoacidosis /kē′tōas′idō′sis/ [Gk, *keton,* form of acetone; L, *acidus,* sour, *osis,* condition], acidosis accompanied by an accumulation of ketones in the body, resulting from extensive breakdown of fats because of faulty carbohydrate metabolism. It occurs primarily as a complication of diabetes mellitus. See also **diabetes mellitus, ketosis.** *–ketoacidotic, adj.*
- OBSERVATIONS: Ketoacidosis is characterized by a fruity odor of acetone on the breath, mental confusion, dyspnea, nausea, vomiting, dehydration, weight loss, and, if untreated, coma.
- INTERVENTIONS: Emergency treatment includes the administration of insulin and IV fluids and the evaluation and correction of electrolyte imbalance. Nasogastric intubation and bladder catheterization may be required if the patient is comatose.
- PATIENT CARE CONSIDERATIONS: Before discharge of the patient from the hospital, the nurse carefully reviews the meal plan, activity levels, blood glucose and urine ketone monitoring, and insulin schedule prescribed, emphasizing to the patient that ketoacidosis may be life threatening and is largely avoidable by strict adherence to the patient's diabetic regimen, monitoring, and appropriate action for illness or stress. A referral to a certified diabetes educator and endocrinologist by the primary health care provider is often warranted.

ketoaciduria /-as′idŏŏr″ē·ə/ [Gk, *keton* + L, *acidus,* sour; Gk, *ouron,* urine], presence in the urine of excessive amounts of ketone bodies, occurring as a result of uncontrolled diabetes mellitus, starvation, or any other metabolic condition in which fats are rapidly catabolized. The condition can be diagnosed with a dipstick reagent or acetone test tablet. Also called **ketonuria.** See also **Acetest, ketosis.** *–ketoaciduric, adj.*

17-ketoandrosterone /-andros″tərōn/, a metabolite of a sex hormone secreted by the testes and adrenal glands that may be measured in the urine to assess hormonal and adrenal functions.

ketoconazole /-kō″nəzōl/, an azole antifungal agent.

■ INDICATIONS: It is prescribed for the treatment of candidiasis, coccidioidomycosis, histoplasmosis, and other fungal diseases. Currently, ketoconazole is primarily used topically because there are safer systemic azoles.

■ CONTRAINDICATIONS: Known hypersensitivity to this drug prohibits its use. It should not be used for fungal meningitis. Because it is also an inhibitor of some important drug-metabolizing enzymes and can cause toxic intermediates from other drugs to accumulate, the safe use of ketoconazole with other prescribed medications should be verified.

■ ADVERSE EFFECTS: The most common adverse effects are endocrine in nature—for example, gynecomastia and decreased libido. The most serious adverse effects are liver disorders.

ketogenesis /-jen″əsis/ [Gk, *keton* + Gk, *genein,* to produce], the formation or production of ketone bodies.

ketogenic amino acid /-jen″ik/, an amino acid whose carbon skeleton serves as a precursor for ketone bodies.

ketogenic diet, a diet high in fats (often as medium-chain triglycerides) and proteins and low in carbohydrates, inducing a state that mimics carbohydrate starvation. It may be used in the management of refractory epilepsy and may have some utility in the treatment of other disorders. It has also been used for weight loss.

ketonaemia. See **ketonemia.**

ketone /kē″tōn/ [Fr, *acetone*], an organic chemical compound characterized by having in its structure a carbonyl, or keto, group attached to two alkyl groups. It is produced by oxidation of secondary alcohols.

ketone alcohol [Gk, *keton* + Ar, *alkohl,* essence], an alcohol containing the ketone group.

ketone bodies, two products of lipid pyruvate metabolism, beta-hydroxybutyric acid and aminoacetic acid, from which acetone may arise spontaneously. Ketone bodies are produced from acetyl-CoA in the liver and are oxidized by the muscles. Excessive production leads to their excretion in urine, as in diabetes mellitus. Also called **acetone bodies.**

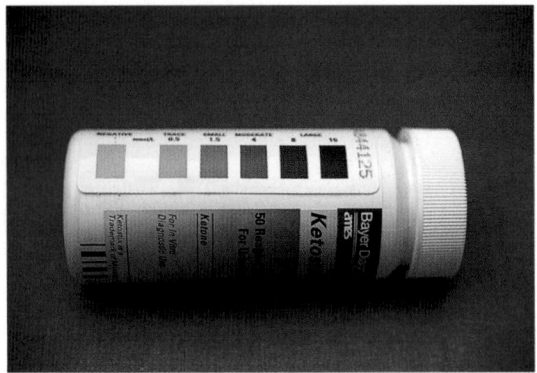

Measurement of ketone bodies
(Belchetz and Hammond, 2003)

ketone group, the chemical carbonyl group of a ketone (i.e., with two alkyl groups attached to it). See also **ketone.**

ketonemia /kē″tōnē″mē·ə/, the presence of ketones, mainly acetone, in the blood. It is characterized by the fruity breath odor of ketoacidosis.

ketonuria. See **ketoaciduria.**

ketoprofen /-prō″fən/, a nonsteroidal antiinflammatory drug with analgesic and antipyretic actions.

■ INDICATIONS: It is prescribed for the treatment of rheumatoid arthritis and osteoarthritis and other conditions causing mild to moderate pain.

■ CONTRAINDICATIONS: Hypersensitivity to ketoprofen or to aspirin or other nonsteroidal antiinflammatory drugs prohibits its use.

■ ADVERSE EFFECTS: Among the more serious adverse effects are GI disturbances, including peptic ulcer and GI bleeding; central nervous system effects of headache, dizziness, and drowsiness; and skin rash.

ketose /kē″tōs/ [Gk, *keton* + *glykys,* sweet], the chemical form of a monosaccharide in which the carbonyl group is a ketone.

ketosis /kitō″sis/ [Gk, *keton* + *glykys,* sweet + *osis,* condition], the abnormal accumulation of ketones in the body as a result of excessive breakdown of fats caused by a deficiency or inadequate use of carbohydrates. Fatty acids are metabolized instead, and the end products, ketones, begin to accumulate. This condition is seen in starvation, occasionally in pregnancy if the intake of protein and carbohydrates is inadequate, and most frequently in diabetes mellitus. See also **diabetes mellitus, ketoacidosis, starvation. –ketotic,** *adj.*

■ OBSERVATIONS: It is characterized by ketonuria, loss of potassium in the urine, and a fruity odor of acetone on the breath.

■ INTERVENTIONS: Frequent blood glucose monitoring by patients with diabetes mellitus facilitates the prompt treatment of high blood glucose levels before ketosis develops.

■ PATIENT CARE CONSIDERATIONS: Untreated, ketosis may progress to ketoacidosis, coma, and death.

ketosis-prone diabetes. See **type 1 diabetes mellitus.**

ketosis-resistant diabetes. See **type 2 diabetes mellitus.**

17-ketosteroid /kē″tōstir″oid, kētō″stəroid/, any of the adrenal cortical hormones, or ketosteroids, that has a ketone group attached to its seventeenth carbon atom. These hormones are commonly measured in the blood and urine to aid the diagnoses of Addison's disease, Cushing syndrome, stress, and endocrine problems associated with precocious puberty, feminization in men, and excessive hair growth. Measured in patients in the morning, the normal concentration in plasma is less than 30 mcg/dL, in the evening, less than 10 mcg/dL. The normal amounts in the urine of men after 24-hour collection are 8 to 15 mg; in women, 6 to 11.5 mg; in children 12 to 15 years of age, 5 to 12 mg; and in children younger than 12 years of age, less than 5 mg. Levels of 17-ketosteroids increase 50% to 100% after an injection of ACTH.

17-ketosteroids (17-KS) test, a rarely used 24-hour urine test that is useful in diagnosing adrenocortical dysfunction. It is used to detect levels of 17-KS, which are metabolites of the testosterone and nontestosterone androgenic sex hormones secreted from the adrenal cortex and the testes.

ketotic /kētot″ik/ [Fr, *acetone*], **1.** pertaining to the presence of ketone in the body. **2.** denoting the presence of a carbonyl group in a chemical compound.

ketotifen /ke″toti′fen/, a noncompetitive H_1-receptor antagonist and mast cell stabilizer used as the fumarate salt, administered orally in the chronic treatment of children with mild atopic asthma and topically to the conjunctiva as an antipruritic in the treatment of allergic conjunctivitis.

keV (kev), an energy unit equivalent to 1000 electron volts. Abbreviation for *kiloelectron volt.*

Kew Gardens spotted fever. See **rickettsialpox.**

keyboard, a computer input device consisting of rows of switches with key tops marked as letters or numbers. Manual pressure on a series or combination of the keys generates an electronic code representing words, data, commands, or other input.

keypad, a numeric keyboard consisting of the numerals 1 to 9 arranged in three ranks of three keys each and an additional key for zero, as on some calculators.

key pinch. See **lateral pinch.**

key points of control, areas of the body, the shoulder and pelvic girdles, that can be handled by a therapist in a specific manner to change an abnormal pattern, to reduce spasticity throughout the body, and to guide the patient's active movements.

key ridge, the lowest point of the zygomaticomaxillary ridge. Also called **zygomaxillare.**

kg, abbreviation for **kilogram.**

kG, abbreviation for *kilogauss.*

kg cal, abbreviation for **kilogram calorie.**

khat, an herbal product taken from a tree found in Africa and the Arabian peninsula.

■ INDICATIONS: It is used for obesity and gastric ulcers, and as a stimulant to offset depression and fatigue. Its efficacy for these indications is unproven because of insufficient reliable data. Khat causes a psychological addicting euphoria and cannot be legally imported into the United States.

■ CONTRAINDICATIONS: It should not be used during pregnancy and lactation, in children, or in those with known hypersensitivity. People with renal, cardiac, or hepatic disease also should avoid its use.

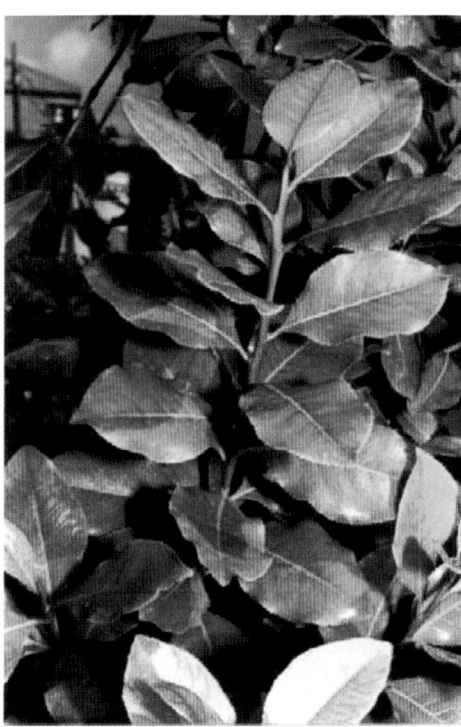

Fresh khat leaves *(Yarom et al, 2010)*

kHz, abbreviation for **kilohertz.**

kidney [ME, *kidnere*], one of a pair of bean-shaped, purplish brown urinary organs in the retroperitoneal abdominal cavity, located on each side of the vertebral column between the twelfth thoracic and third lumbar vertebrae. In most individuals the right kidney is slightly lower than the left. Each kidney is about 11 cm long, 6 cm wide, and 2.5 cm thick. In the newborn the kidneys are about three times as large in proportion to the body weight as in the adult. The kidneys filter the blood and eliminate wastes in the urine through a complex filtration network and resorption system comprising more than 2 million nephrons. The nephrons are composed of glomeruli and renal tubules that filter blood under high pressure, removing urea, salts, and other soluble wastes from blood plasma and returning the purified filtrate to the blood. The average blood flow through the kidney is 1200 mL/min. Blood enters the kidneys through the renal arteries and leaves through the renal veins. The kidneys remove water as urine and return water that has been filtered to the blood plasma, thus helping to maintain the water balance of the body. Hormones produced by the pituitary gland, especially the antidiuretic hormone, control the function of the kidneys in regulating the water-electrolyte balance of the body.

kidney cancer, a malignant neoplasm of the renal parenchyma or renal pelvis. Factors associated with an increased incidence of disease are exposure to aromatic hydrocarbons or tobacco smoke. A long asymptomatic period may precede the onset of the characteristic symptoms, which include hematuria, flank pain, fever, and a palpable mass. Diagnostic measures include urinalysis, excretory urography, nephrotomography, ultrasonography, renal arteriography, and microscopic and cytological studies of cells from the renal pelvis. Adenocarcinoma of the renal parenchyma accounts for 80% of kidney tumors, occurring twice as frequently in men as in women; transitional cell or squamous cell carcinomas in the renal pelvis account for approximately 15% and are equally frequent in both men and women. Radical nephrectomy with lymph node dissection is usually recommended for tumors of the parenchyma. Nephroureterectomy is usually recommended for operable tumors of the renal pelvis. Radiotherapy may be used before or after surgery and as palliation for inoperable tumors. Chemotherapeutic agents may induce temporary remission. See also **renal cell carcinoma, Wilms tumor.**

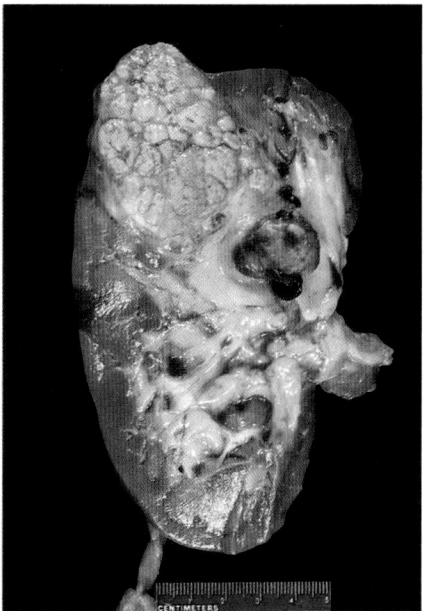

Kidney cancer *(Kumar et al, 2007)*

kidney dialysis. See **hemodialysis.**

kidney disease, any one of a large group of conditions, including infectious, inflammatory, obstructive, vascular, and neoplastic disorders of the kidney. Characteristics of kidney disease are hematuria, persistent proteinuria, pyuria, edema, dysuria, and pain in the flank. Specific symptoms

K

vary with the type of disorder. For example, hematuria with severe, colicky pain suggests obstruction by a kidney stone; hematuria without pain may indicate renal carcinoma; proteinuria is generally a sign of disease in the glomerulus, or filtration unit, of the kidney; pyuria indicates infectious disease; and edema is characteristic of the nephrotic syndrome. Diagnosis of kidney disease is made after laboratory tests and other diagnostic procedures or radiography has been performed. Among the special tests for kidney disorders are excretory urography, IV pyelography, tests of the glomerular filtration rate, biopsy, and ultrasound examination. Treatment depends on the type of disease diagnosed. Some forms of advanced kidney disease may lead to renal failure, coma, and death unless hemodialysis is started. See also **glomerulonephritis, nephrotic syndrome, renal failure, urinary calculus.**

kidney failure. See **renal failure.**

kidney machine. *(Informal)* See **artificial kidney.**

kidney stone. *(Informal)* See **renal calculus.**

Kielhofner, Gary, (1949–2010) occupational therapist, researcher, and scholar who developed the Model of Human Occupation (MOHO), an evidence-based model of practice in occupational therapy. His goal was to assist individuals with chronic health conditions or disabilities in living fulfilling and satisfying lives.

Kielland's forceps. See **obstetric forceps.**

Kielland's rotation /kē″lands/ [Christian Kielland, Norwegian obstetrician, 1871–1941], an obstetric procedure in which Kielland's forceps are used in turning the head of the fetus from an occiput posterior or occiput transverse position to an occiput anterior position. It is performed most commonly to correct an arrest in the active stage of labor. The rotation is done at the midplane of the pelvis. Because it is associated with increased harm to the mother and to the baby, cesarean section is often preferred instead. See also **forceps delivery, obstetric forceps.**

Kiesselbach plexus /kē″səlbäkh′, -bäk′/ [Wilhelm Kiesselbach, German laryngologist, 1839–1902], a convergence of small fragile arteries and veins located superficially on the anterosuperior part of the nasal septum. It is the most common site for septal bleeding.

Kikuchi lymphadenitis /kēkoo′chēz/ [M. Kikuchi, 20th-century Japanese pathologist], a benign, self-limited syndrome of lymphadenopathy, usually in the neck, with a female predominance. Characteristics include patchy necrotizing lesions of the paracortex and proliferation of distinctive histiocytes, plasmacytoid monocytes, and lymphoblasts surrounded by karyorrhectic debris. Some consider it a self-limited form of systemic lupus erythematosus. Also called **histiocytic necrotizing lymphadenitis, subacute necrotizing lymphadenitis,** *Kikuchi disease.* See also **systemic lupus erythematosus.**

killed vaccine [ME, *killen* + L, *vaccinus,* of a cow], a vaccine prepared from dead microorganisms, generally used to provide immunization from organisms that are too virulent to be used in the living attenuated state. The immune system reacts to the presence of the pathogen in the same manner, whether the organism is alive or dead. However, immunity produced by a live, attenuated vaccine is usually more effective.

killer T cells, antigen-stimulated T lymphocytes or cytotoxic T cells that attack foreign antigens directly and destroy cells that bear those antigens. Compare **natural killer cell.** See also **cytoxic T lymphocytes.**

killer yeast, a strain of yeast cells that contains a toxic protein that destroys other yeast strains.

kilo-, prefix meaning "one thousand": *kilocalorie, kilogram, kilometer.*

kilobase (kb), a length of nucleic acid equal to 1000 bases or nucleotides.

kilobase pair (kbp), a length of DNA or double-stranded RNA equal to 1000 base pairs.

kilobyte (K, kb) /kil′ə-bīt/, 1000 bytes (or, more precisely, 1024 bytes).

kilocalorie (kcal) /-kal′ərē/ [Gk, *chilioi,* thousand; L, *calor,* heat], a unit of heat equal to 1000 small calories or 4184 joules. Also called **large calorie.**

kilogram (kg) /-gram/ [Gk, *chilioi,* thousand; Fr, *gramme*], a unit for the measurement of mass in the metric system. One kilogram is equal to 1000 grams or 2.2046 pounds avoirdupois.

kilogram calorie. See **Calorie.**

kilohertz (kHz) /-hurts/ [Gk, *chilioi,* thousand; *hertz,* Heinrich R. Hertz, German physicist, 1857–1894], unit of frequency equal to 1000 (10^3) hertz. See also **hertz.**

kiloliter (kL) /-lē″tər/ [Gk, *chilioi,* thousand; Fr, *litre*], unit of volume equivalent to 1057 quarts, 1000 liters, or 1 cubic meter (1 m^3).

kilometer (km) /-mē″tər/ [Gk, *chilioi,* thousand, *metron,* measure], measure equivalent to 1000 meters (about 0.62 mile).

kilovolt (kV) /-volt/ [Gk, *chilioi,* thousand; *volt,* Count Alessandro Volta, Italian scientist, 1745–1827], measure of electrical potential, 1000 volts.

kilovolt peak (kVp), a measure of the maximum electrical potential in kilovolts across an x-ray tube. Most diagnostic x-ray machines have a kVp of 40 to 150.

Kimmelstiel-Wilson syndrome. See **intercapillary glomerulosclerosis.**

kinaesthesia. See **kinesthesia.**

kinanesthesia /kin′anesthē″zhə/, **1.** an inability to perceive the movement or position of one's body parts. The condition is observed as a sign of ataxia. **2.** a loss of movement sense.

kinase /kī″nās/ [Gk, *kinesis,* motion, *ase,* enzyme], **1.** an enzyme that catalyzes the transfer of a phosphate group or another high-energy molecular group to an acceptor molecule. Each of these kinases is named for its receptor, such as acetate kinase, fructokinase, or hexokinase. **2.** an enzyme that activates a preenzyme (zymogen). Kinds include **bacterial kinase, enterokinase, fibrinokinase, insulin kinase, staphylokinase, streptokinase, streptokinase-streptodornase, urokinase.**

kind firmness, (in psychology) a direct, clear, and confident approach to a patient in which rules and regulations are calmly cited in response to infractions and requests.

kindred /kin″drid/, **1.** a group of genetically related individuals. **2.** families and groups of individuals united by a common bond.

kine-. See **kinesio-, kine-.**

kinematic face-bow /kin′əmat″ik/, an adjustable caliper-like device used for precisely locating the axis of rotation of a mandible through the sagittal plane. Also called **adjustable axis face-bow,** *hinge-bow.*

kinematics /kin′əmat″iks, kī-′/ [Gk, *kinema,* motion], the description, measurement, and recording of body motion without regard to the forces acting to produce the motion. Recordings of body motions are defined in one-plane relationships, although natural motions of the body often occur in more than one plane. Kinematics considers the motions of all body parts relative to the segments of the part involved in the motion and not necessarily in relation to the standard anatomical position. For example, the movements of the fingers are considered in relation to the midline of the hand, not the midline of the body. The most common types of motions studied in kinematics are flexion, extension, adduction, abduction, internal rotation, and external rotation. Kinematics is especially important in orthopedics, rehabilitation medicine, and physical therapy. Also spelled **cinematics.** Compare **kinetics.**

kineplastic amputation. See **kineplasty.**

kineplasty, amputation in which the residual limb is formed in such a way that the muscles are able to produce motion in a prosthesis.

kinesia /kīnē″zhə/ [Gk, *kinein,* to move], a condition caused by erratic or rhythmic motions in any combination of directions, such as in a boat or a car. Severe cases are characterized by nausea, vomiting, vertigo, and headache; mild cases by headache and general discomfort. Various antihistamines are used prophylactically. Motion sickness includes air sickness, car sickness, and seasickness (mal de mer).

-kinesia, suffix meaning "movement": *autokinesia.*

kinesic behavior /kīnē″sik/, nonverbal cues of communication that help to achieve and maintain bonds of attachment between people.

kinesics /kīnē″siks/ [Gk, *kinesis,* motion], the study of body position, posture, movement, and facial expression in relation to communication. The observance of nonverbal interactional behavior is an integral part of health assessment and is used especially in mental health assessment as an objective and measurable tool for diagnosing disturbances of communication and behavioral disorders. See also **body language, communication.**

kinesio-, kine-, prefix meaning "movement": *kinesiology, kinematics, kinesiotherapy.*

kinesiological electromyography /kīnē″sē·əloj″ik/, the study of muscle activity involved in body movements.

kinesiology /-ol″əjē/ [Gk, *kinesis* + *logos,* science], the scientific study of human movement. It includes the study of muscular activity and the mechanics of the movement of body parts.

kinesiotherapist, a health care professional who, under the direction of a physician, treats the effects of disease, injury, and congenital disorders through the use of rehabilitative exercise and education alone. See also **kinesiotherapy.**

kinesiotherapy, a specialized area of health care in which exercise and movement are used as the primary form of rehabilitation. See also **kinesiotherapist.**

kinesis /kīnē″sis, kinē″sis/, physical movement or force, particularly when induced by a stimulus.

-kinesis, -kinesia, suffix meaning an "activation": *chemokinesis, karyokinesis, palikinesia.*

kinesthesia /kin′esthē″zhə/ [Gk, *kinesis,* motion, *aisthesis,* feeling], the perception and awareness of one's own body parts, weight, musculoskeletal activity, and balance. Also spelled **kinaesthesia.**

kinesthetic memory /kin′esthet″ik/, the recollection of movement, weight, resistance, and position of the body or parts of the body essential to everyday functioning. Riding a bike or playing a musical instrument are examples of the use of kinesthetic memory.

kinesthetic sense [Gk, *kinesis,* motion; L, *sentire,* to feel], an ability to be aware of muscular movement and position. By providing information through receptors about muscles, tendons, joints, and other body parts, the kinesthetic

sense helps control and coordinate activities such as walking and talking.

kinetic analysis /kinet″ik/, analysis in which the change of the monitored parameter with time is related to concentration, such as change of absorbance per minute, to determine the rate of a reaction.

kinetic ataxia. See **motor ataxia.**

-kinetic, -cinetic, -cinetical, suffix meaning "movement": *akinetic, biokinetics, cardiokinetic.*

kinetic energy (KE) [Gk, *kinesis,* motion, *energeia*], the energy possessed by an object by virtue of its motion. It is expressed by the formula $KE = (\frac{1}{2})mv^2$, where m represents the mass of the object and v is its velocity.

kinetic hallucination [Gk, *kinesis,* motion + L, *allucinari,* wandering mind], a false perception of body movement. A common form is a dream in which the dreamer senses he or she is falling.

kinetic proofreading, **1.** a molecular activity in which an enzyme distinguishes correct substrates. **2.** a mechanism that permits a ribosome to make correct codon-anticodon interactions.

kinetic reflex [Gk, *kinesis,* motion + L, *reflectere,* to bend back], a postural response resulting from stimulation of the vestibular apparatus. Also called **labyrinthine reflex.**

kinetics /kinet″iks/ [Gk, *kinesis,* motion + L, *icus,* like], **1.** the study of the forces that produce, arrest, or modify the motions of the body. Newton's first and third laws of motion are especially applicable to kinetics. These two laws apply to the forces produced by muscles that act on joints. The reaction forces of the muscles contribute to equilibrium and the motion of the body. Compare **kinematics.** See also **Newton's laws. 2.** the study of the rate of chemical and biochemical reactions as in chemical kinetics and enzyme kinetics. It may also refer to the fate of pharmaceuticals upon administration to an organism in terms of absorption, distribution, metabolism, and excretion. See also **pharmacokinetics.**

kinet(o), kineto- [Gk, *kinesis,* motion], prefix meaning "movable": *kinetochore, kinetoplasm, kinetotherapeutic.*

kinetochore. See **centromere.**

kinetoplasm /kīnet″ōplaz′əm/, the most highly contractile part of a cell.

kinetosis. See **kinesia.**

kinetotherapeutic bath /kinet′ōthur′əpyōō″tik/ [Gk, *kinesis* + *therapeutike,* medical practice + AS, *baeth*], a bath in which underwater exercises are performed to strengthen weak or partially paralyzed muscles.

King airway, a supraglottic airway device designed for placement in the esophagus, providing a direct route for ventilation through the trachea and larynx. Insertion does not require direct laryngoscopy.

King-Devick test /king dev′ik/ [Alan King and Steven Devick, American doctors of optometry], a tool for evaluation of saccade, consisting of a series of charts of numbers. The charts become progressively more difficult to read in a flowing manner because of increasing space between the numbers. Both errors in reading and speed of reading are included in deriving a score. It is a commonly used screening test for oculomotor, visual, and cognitive deficits. See also **saccade.**

King, Imogene, (1923–2007), a nursing theorist who introduced her theory of goal attainment in her book entitled *Toward a Theory for Nursing* (1971). King defines nursing as a process of human interactions between nurses and patients, who communicate to set goals and then agree to meet the goals. King's conceptual framework specifies three interacting systems: personal system, interpersonal system, and social system. She believes that the patient is a personal system within a social system, coexisting through interpersonal processes with other personal systems. The nurse and patient perceive each other and the situation, act and react, interact, and transact. From her major concepts (interaction, perception, communication, transaction, role, stress, growth and development, and time and space), she derives her theory of goal attainment. King describes nursing as a discipline and an applied science, with emphasis on the derivation of nursing knowledge from other disciplines. She suggests that the patient's and nurse's perceptions, judgments, and actions lead to reaction, interaction, and transaction, which she calls the process of nursing.

kin group,   family members who are related genetically, by marriage, or by having legal ties.

kinin /kī″nin/,   any of a group of polypeptides with varying physiological activity, such as contraction of visceral smooth muscle, vascular permeability, and vasodilation. Two principal kinins, bradykinin and lysylbradykinin, are formed in the blood from precursor kininogens by the action of kallikrein and kinases.

kinky hair disease [Du, *kink,* short twist + AS, *haer* + L, *dis* + Fr, *aise,* ease],   an inherited condition characterized by short, sparse, poorly pigmented hair with shafts that are twisted and broken. Other mental and physical disorders are usually associated with the disease. Also called **Menkes kinky hair syndrome.**

kino-, kinesi-, kinesio-,   prefix meaning "movement": *kinematics, kinesiology.*

kinomere.   See **centromere.**

Kinsbourne syndrome /kinz′born/ [Marcel Kinsbourne, Austrian-born physician, b. 1931],   a rare neurological disorder of unknown cause with onset between ages 1 and 3 years. It is characterized by myoclonus of trunk and limbs and by nonrhythmic horizontal and vertical oscillations of the eyes, with ataxia of gait and intention tremor. Some cases have been associated with occult neuroblastoma. Also called **myoclonic encephalopathy of childhood.**

Kinyoun stain,   a modification of the Ziehl-Neelsen acid-fast stain in which organisms are stained cold by using carbol-fuchsin. It is often used for detection of mycobacteria, *Nocardia,* and oocysts of some parasites. See also **carbolfuchsin stain.**

Kirkland knife [Olin Kirkland, American periodontist, 1876–1969; AS, *cnif*],   a surgical knife with a heart-shaped blade that is sharp on all edges. It is used for a primary gingivectomy incision.

Kirklin staging system,   a system for determining the prognosis of colon cancer on the basis of the extent to which the tumor has penetrated the bowel area. See also **cancer staging, Dukes' classification, TNM.**

Kirlian photography,   a photographic technique in which a high-voltage current passed over a subject in contact with photographic film or paper produces an image surrounded by a luminous radiation, or aura, which some assert is a bioenergetic field that can reveal information about the subject's physical health and emotional state.

Kirschner wire /kursh″nər/ [Martin Kirschner, German surgeon, 1879–1942; AS, *wir*],   a threaded or smooth metallic wire 22.86 cm long and available in three diameters. The wire is used in internal fixation of fractures or for skeletal traction. Also called *K-wire.*

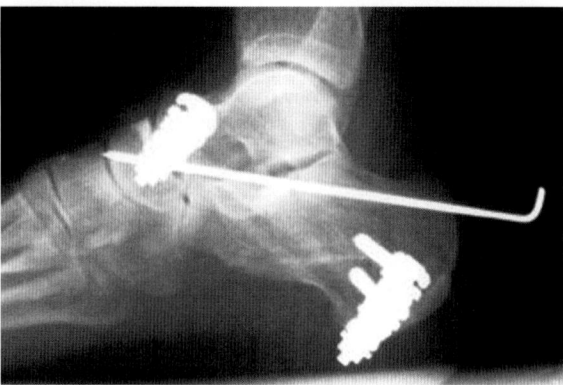

Kirschner wire for internal fixation of calcaneal fracture *(Dayton, Feilmeier, and Hensley, 2014)*

Kite method,   a technique for positioning a patient for radiographic examination of congenital clubfoot. The foot is imaged in two planes and is placed on the image receptor without altering the foot's abnormal alignment.

kiting /kī″ting/,   *(Informal)* the improper and illegal practice of altering a drug prescription to indicate that more of a drug was prescribed than was actually ordered by the physician. Kiting may be done by a patient seeking greater quantities of drugs, especially opioids, than the physician prescribed, or by the pharmacist to increase reimbursement from a third party, such as an insurance company.

KJ,   abbreviation for *knee jerk.*

kL,   abbreviation for **kiloliter.**

klang association.   See **clang association.**

Klebsiella /kleb′zē-el″ə/ [Theodore A.E. Klebs, German bacteriologist, 1834–1913],   a genus of diplococcal bacteria that appear as small, plump rods with rounded ends. Several respiratory diseases, including bronchitis, sinusitis, and some forms of pneumonia, are caused by infection by species of *Klebsiella.*

Klebsiella pneumoniae [Theodore A.E. Klebs; Gk, *pneumon,* lung],   a species of gram-negative, nonmotile bacteria found in soil, water, cereal grains, and the intestinal tract of humans and other animals. It is associated with several pathological conditions, including pneumonia. It is commonly implicated in nosocomial urinary tract infections, especially in immunocompromised patients. Also called **Friedländer's bacillus.**

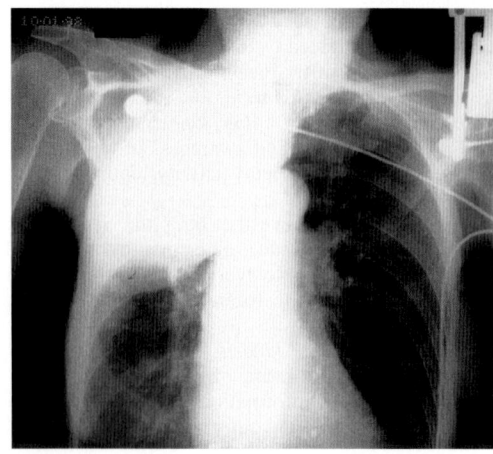

Klebsiella pneumoniae *(Belchetz and Hammond, 2003)*

Klebs-Löeffler bacillus /klebz″ lef″lər/ [Theodore A.E. Klebs, German bacteriologist, 1834–1913; Friederich A.J. Löeffler, German bacteriologist, 1852–1915; L, *bacillum,* small rod], the gram-positive asporogenic bacterium *Corynebacterium diphtheriae,* which has three cultural types according to severity of the cases. See also ***Corynebacterium.***

kleeblattschädel deformity syndrome. See **cloverleaf skull deformity.**

Kleine-Levin syndrome /klīn″ lev″in/ [Willi Kleine, German psychiatrist, 1879–1961; Max Levin, Russian-born American neurologist, 1901–1974], a disorder of unknown cause often associated with periods of abnormal behavior or cognitive abnormalities and characterized by episodic sleep, abnormal hunger, and hyperactivity. The episodes of sleep may last for several hours or days and are followed by confusion on awakening. Symptoms can be interspersed with long periods of normal sleep, cognition, behavior, and mood. There is no specific treatment. Compare **narcolepsy.**

Klein-Waardenburg syndrome. See **Waardenburg syndrome.**

klepto-, prefix meaning "theft" or "stealing": *kleptolagnia, kleptomania.*

kleptolagnia /klep′tōlag″nē·ə/ [Gk, *kleptein,* to steal, *lagneia,* lust], sexual excitement or gratification produced by stealing.

kleptomania /-mā″nē·ə/ [Gk, *kleptein,* to steal, *mania,* madness], a symptom of an impulse control disorder characterized by an abnormal, uncontrollable, and recurrent urge to steal. The objects are taken not for their monetary value, immediate need, or utility but because of a symbolic meaning usually associated with some unconscious emotional conflict; they are usually given away, returned surreptitiously, or kept and hidden. People who have the condition experience an increased sense of tension before committing the theft and intense gratification during the act. Afterward they display signs of depression, guilt, and anxiety over the possibility of being apprehended and losing status in society. In less severe cases the impulse is expressed by continuously borrowing objects and not returning them. Treatment consists of psychotherapy to uncover the underlying emotional problems. See also **impulse control disorder.** *–kleptomaniac, n.*

Klinefelter syndrome /klīn″feltər/ [Harry F. Klinefelter, American physician, 1912–1990], a condition of gonadal defects appearing in males after puberty, caused by an extra X chromosome in at least one cell line. Characteristics are small, firm testes, long legs, gynecomastia, poor social adaptation, subnormal intelligence, chronic pulmonary disease, and varicose veins. The severity of the abnormalities increases with greater numbers of X chromosomes. The most common abnormality is a 47 XXY karyotype. Men with the karyotype XXXXY have marked congenital malformations and cognitive impairment.

Klippel-Feil syndrome /klipel″ fel′, klip″əl fīl′/ [Maurice Klippel, French neurologist, 1858–1942; Andre Feil, French neurologist, b. 1884], a condition of short neck and limited neck movements because of congenital fusion of the cervical vertebrae or reduction in the number of cervical vertebrae. Also called *Klippel-Feil disease, Klippel-Feil malformation, Klippel disease.* See **congenital short neck syndrome.**

Klippel-Trénaunay syndrome /klipel′ trānōnā′/ [Maurice Klippel, French neurologist, 1858–1942; Paul Trénaunay, 20th-century French physician], a rare condition affecting the development of blood vessels, bones, and soft tissues. Large cutaneous hemangiomas, persistent nevus flammeus,

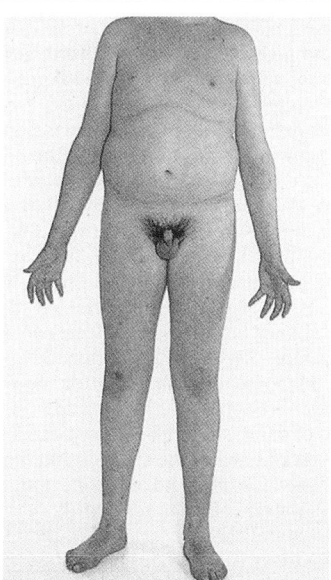

Characteristics associated with Klinefelter syndrome
(Patton and Thibodeau, 2016)

and skin varices are associated with this syndrome. Also called *Klippel–Trénaunay–Weber syndrome.*

Kloehn headgear, an extraoral orthodontic appliance consisting of a cervical strap and a long outer bow, used to retract maxillary teeth or to reinforce tooth anchorage during retraction.

Klonopin, a drug used as an antianxiety, anticonvulsant, or sedative-hypnotic agent, or as a muscle relaxant; it belongs to a class of drugs known as benzodiazepines. Brand name for **clonazepam.**

Klor, an oral electrolyte replacement solution. Brand name for **potassium chloride.**

Klorvess, an oral electrolyte replacement solution. Brand name for **potassium chloride.**

Klumpke palsy /kloomp″kē/ [Augusta Dejerine-Klumpke, French neurologist, 1859–1927], atrophic paralysis of the forearm and hand. It is a rare type of birth injury and involves the seventh and eighth cervical nerves and the first thoracic nerve. The condition may be accompanied by Horner syndrome, ptosis, and miosis because of involvement of sympathetic nerves. Also called **Déjérine-Klumpke paralysis,** *lower brachial plexus palsy.*

K-Lyte/Cl, an oral electrolyte replacement solution. Brand name for **potassium chloride.**

km, abbreviation for **kilometer.**

kneading /nē″ding/ [AS, *cnedan*], a grasping, rolling, and pressing movement, as is used in massaging the muscles. See also **massage.**

knee /nē/ [AS, *cneow*], a joint complex that connects the thigh with the leg. It consists of three condyloid joints, 12 ligaments, 13 bursae, and the patella. The motion of this joint is not a simple gliding motion because the articular surfaces of the bones involved are not mutually adapted to each other. Various orthopedic conditions commonly affect the knee. The knee is relatively unprotected by surrounding muscles and is often injured by blows, sudden stops, and turns, especially those associated with sports. Ligament tears of the knee joint are extremely common in athletes and produce a variety of signs and symptoms, such as effusion, varying degrees of edema, differences in the shape of the knee

K

joint, tenderness on palpation, crepitation, instability of the knee joint, and possible ecchymosis. Torn menisci are very common sports injuries and can cause severe pain, limping, edema, and greatly reduced motion.

knee-ankle interaction, one of the five major kinetic determinants of gait, which helps to minimize the displacement of the body's center of gravity during the walking cycle. The knee and the foot work simultaneously to lower the body's center of gravity. When the heel of the foot is in contact with the ground, the foot is dorsiflexed, and the knee is fully extended so that the associated limb is at its maximum length with the center of gravity at its lower point. Plantar flexion of the foot with the initiation of knee flexion maintains the center of gravity in its forward progression at about the same level, also helping to minimize the vertical displacement of the center of gravity. Knee-ankle interaction is often a factor in the diagnosis and treatment of various orthopedic diseases, deformities, and abnormal conditions and in the analysis and the correction of pathological gaits. Compare **knee-hip flexion, lateral pelvic displacement, pelvic rotation, pelvic tilt.**

kneecap. See **patella.**

knee-chest position. See **genupectoral position.**

knee-elbow position [AS, *cneow* + *elboga*], a position in which a patient being examined rests on the knees and elbows with the head supported on the hands.

knee-hip flexion, one of the five major kinetic determinants of gait, which allows the passage of body weight over the supporting extremity during the walking cycle. Knee-hip flexion occurs during the stance and swing phases of the cycle. The knee first locks into extension as the heel of the weight-bearing limb strikes the ground and is unlocked by final flexion and initiation of the swing phase in the walking cycle. Hip flexion is synchronized with these movements, which help minimize the vertical displacement of the body's center of gravity in the act of walking. Knee-hip flexion is often a factor in the diagnosis and treatment of various orthopedic diseases, deformities, and abnormal conditions and in the analysis and correction of pathological gaits. Compare **knee-ankle interaction, lateral pelvic displacement, pelvic rotation, pelvic tilt.**

knee-jerk reflex. See **patellar reflex.**

knee joint, the complex, hinged joint at the knee, regarded as three articulations in one, comprising condyloid joints connecting the femur and the tibia and a partly arthrodial joint connecting the patella and the femur. The knee joint and its ligaments permit flexion, extension, and, in certain positions, medial and lateral rotation. It is a common site for sprain and dislocation. Also called *articulatio genus.*

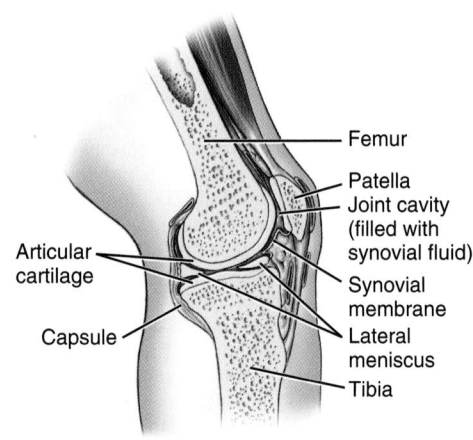

Knee joint (Herlihy, 2014)

knee replacement, the surgical insertion of a hinged prosthesis performed to relieve pain and restore motion to a knee severely affected by osteoarthritis, rheumatoid arthritis, or trauma. With the patient under general or spinal anesthesia, the diseased surfaces are removed and tricompartmental implants are inserted to replace the opposing femorotibial joint and the patellofemoral joint. Physical therapy is prescribed after surgery. Possible complications include infection, hemorrhage, fat embolism, thrombophlebitis, peroneal nerve palsy, loosening of the prosthesis, and flexion contractures. To prevent contractures, the knee is immobilized. The mobility and range of motion of the joint increase slowly. Compare **arthroplasty, hip replacement.**

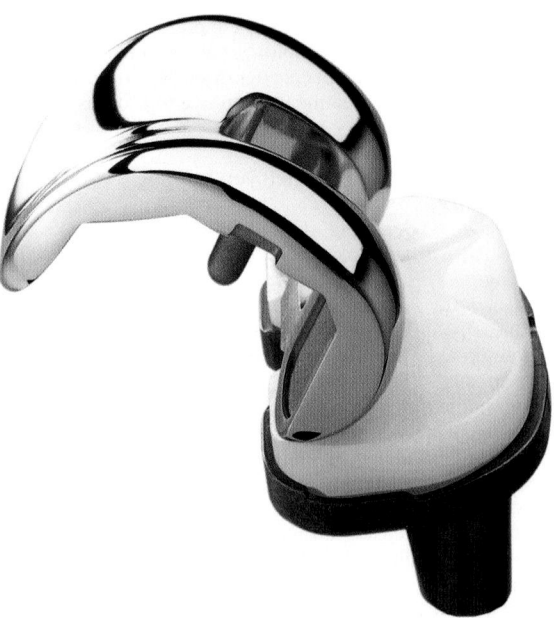

Hinged prosthesis for knee replacement (Scott, 2012)

knee sling, a leg support in sling form used under the knee for Russell traction.

knife needle /nīf/ [AS, *cnif* + *neal*], a slender surgical knife with a needle point, used in the discission of a cataract and other ophthalmic procedures such as goniotomy and goniopuncture.

knock-knee. See **genu valgum.**

knockout mouse, a mouse that has had a specific gene artificially deleted from its genome.

Knoop hardness test /no͞op/ [Frederick Knoop, 20th-century American metallurgist], a method of assessing surface hardness by measuring resistance to the penetration of an indenting tool made of diamond. The test is commonly used for testing the hardness of teeth.

knot /not/ [AS, *cnotta*], **1.** (in surgery) the interlacing of the ends of a ligature or suture so that they remain in place without slipping or becoming detached. The ends of the suture are passed twice around each other before being pulled taut to form a simple surgeon's knot. For additional stability, the ends may be recrossed and a second simple knot made over the first. **2.** *(Informal)* the site of a muscle spasm.

knuckle /nuk′əl/, the dorsal aspect of any interphalangeal joint, but especially of the metacarpophalangeal joints of the flexed fingers. By extension the term is sometimes applied to any anatomical structure of similar appearance, such as an extruded loop of intestine in a hernia.

Kocher's forceps /kō″kərz/ [Emil T. Kocher, Swiss surgeon, 1841–1917], a kind of surgical forceps that has notched jaws, interlocking teeth, and thick curved or straight powerful handles.

Koch's bacillus /kōks/ [Robert Koch, German bacteriologist, 1843–1910; L, *bacillum,* small rod], the *Mycobacterium tuberculosis* microorganism, a gram-positive bacterium.

Koch's phenomenon [Robert Koch; Gk, *phainomenon,* anything seen], a tuberculin reaction that occurs when a culture of tubercle bacilli is injected into the skin of subjects already infected with the disease. In humans a positive tuberculin reaction indicates sensitization resulting from a tuberculosis infection. Also called **Koch's reaction.**

Koch's postulates [Robert Koch; L, *postulare,* to demand], the prerequisites for experimentally establishing that a specific microorganism causes a particular disease. The following conditions must be met: (1) the microorganism must be observed in all cases of the disease; (2) the microorganism must be isolated and grown in pure culture; (3) microorganisms from the pure culture, when inoculated into a susceptible animal, must reproduce the disease; and (4) the microorganism must be observed in and recovered from the experimentally diseased animal.

Koch's reaction. See **Koch's phenomenon.**

Kock pouch. See **continent ileostomy.**

Koebner phenomenon /kōb″nər/ [Heinrich Koebner, Polish dermatologist, 1838–1904; Gk, *phainomenon,* something observed], the development of new skin lesions at areas of superficial injury, such as a scratch, in otherwise healthy skin, occurring in psoriasis, lichen nitidus, lichen planus, and verruca plana.

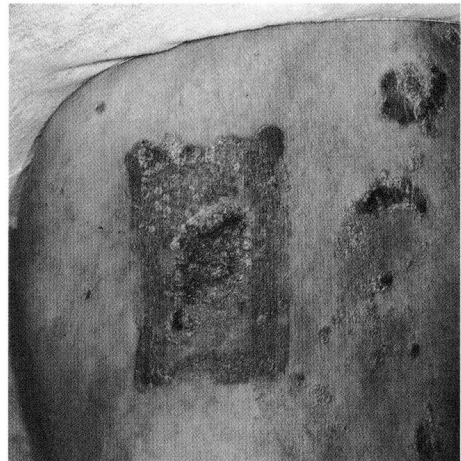

Koebner phenomenon. Psoriasis appearing on the donor site of a skin graft *(Habif, 2009)*

KOH, chemical formula for **potassium hydroxide.**

Kohnstamm phenomenon, an involuntary contraction of a muscle that causes a continued movement of a limb after a strong exertion against resistance has stopped. It is often demonstrated in abduction of the arm.

koilo-, prefix meaning "hollow" or "concave": *koilonychia.*

koilonychia /koi′lōnik″ē·ə/ [Gk, *koilos,* hollow, *onyx,* nail], a condition in which nails are thin and concave from side to side. It is usually familial but may occur with trauma and iron-deficiency anemia.

koinonia [Gk, fellowship or communion], a community or group sharing a common belief, especially a religious belief.

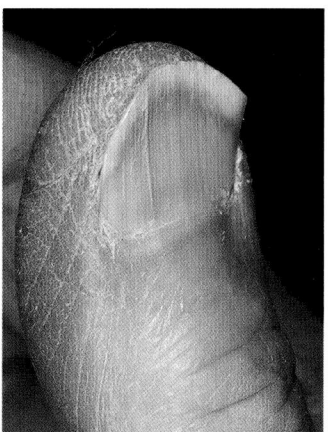

Koilonychia *(Nelson et al, 2016)*

Kolcaba, Katharine, a nursing theorist who developed the Theory of Comfort to help nurses design interventions to increase the physical, psychospiritual, environmental, and social comfort of the patient. Nurses can use the General Comfort Questionnaire to measure outcomes.

kolpo-. See **colpo-, colp-, kolpo-, kysth-, kystho-.**

Konakion, a vitamin K formulation. Brand name for **phytonadione.**

Kopan needle /kō″pən/, a long biopsy needle used to pinpoint the location of a breast tumor on x-ray images. The needle is inserted into the approximate location of the tumor and is left in place during radiography so that it can be repositioned if necessary. In some cases the site is further identified for the surgeon by injecting a colored dye such as methylene blue.

Koplik spots /kop″lik/ [Henry Koplik, American pediatrician, 1858–1927], small red spots with bluish-white centers on the lingual and buccal mucosa, characteristic of measles. The rash of measles usually erupts a day or two after the appearance of Koplik spots.

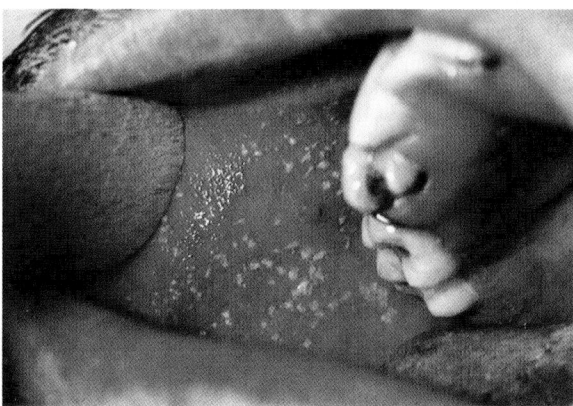

Koplik spots *(Edmond et al, 2003)*

kopr-, kopra-. See **copro-, copr-, kopr-, kopra-.**

Korányi sign /kôr″ənyē/ [Friedrich von Korányi, Hungarian physician, 1828–1913; L, *signum*], a paravertebral area of dullness found posteriorly on the side opposite a pleural effusion. Also called **Grocco sign, Grocco triangle, triangular dullness,** *Korányi-Grocco triangle.*

Korean hand acupuncture, a system of acupuncture in which the hand is considered to be a representation of the entire body and stimulation of specific points on the hand is used to obtain effects in distant areas of the body.

Korean hemorrhagic fever. See **epidemic hemorrhagic fever.**

Korotkoff sounds /kôrot″kôf/ [Nickolai Korotkoff, Russian physician, 1874–1920], sounds heard during the taking of a blood pressure reading using a sphygmomanometer and stethoscope. The sphygmomanometer is inflated enough to collapse an artery. As air is released from the cuff, pressure on the artery is reduced, and the blood is heard pulsing through the collapsed vessel. See also **blood pressure, diastole, sphygmomanometer, systole.**

Korsakoff psychosis /kôr″səkôf/ [Sergei S. Korsakoff, Russian psychiatrist, 1854–1900], a form of amnesia often seen in chronic alcoholics that is characterized by a loss of short-term memory and an inability to learn new skills. The person is usually disoriented, may present with delirium and hallucinations, and confabulates to conceal the condition. The cause of the condition can often be traced to degenerative changes in the thalamus as a result of a deficiency of B complex vitamins, especially thiamine and B_{12}. Deficits are often permanent. Compare **Wernicke encephalopathy.**

kosher [Heb, *kasher,* fit or proper], pertaining to the preparation and serving of foods according to Jewish dietary laws (e.g., keeping dairy and meat separate in cooking and ingesting). Kosher foods include common fruits, vegetables, and cereals, as well as tea and coffee. Foods that are not kosher include pork, birds of prey, and seafood that lacks fins and scales, such as lobster and eels. Most poultry and meat products, excluding pork, are kosher if properly processed.

Kostmann syndrome /kost′mahn/ [Rolf Kostmann, Swedish physician], infantile genetic agranulocytosis. Now called **severe congenital neutropenia.**

K⁺ pump. See **potassium pump.**

Kr, symbol for the element **krypton.**

Krabbe disease. See **galactosyl ceramide lipidosis.**

KRAS gene, a type of oncogene that creates K-ras protein, the activating mutations of which play a key role in neoplastic progression, especially in colorectal, pancreatic, and lung cancer.

Kraske position /kras″kə/ [Paul Kraske, Swiss surgeon, 1851–1930], an anatomical position in which the patient is prone, with hips flexed and elevated, head and feet down. The position is most frequently used for rectal surgery. Also called **jackknife position.**

kraurosis /krôrō″sis/ [Gk, *krauros,* dry, *osis,* condition], a thickening and shriveling of the mucous membranes, particularly the female genitalia. See also **kraurosis vulvae.**

kraurosis vulvae, a skin disease of aged women characterized by dryness, itching, and atrophy of the external genitalia. It is a condition that exhibits a predisposition to leukoplakia and carcinoma of the vulva. See also **lichen sclerosis et atrophicus.**

Krause corpuscles [Wilhelm J.F. Krause, German anatomist, 1833–1910; L, *corpusculum,* little body], any of a number of sensory end organs in the conjunctiva of the eye; mucous membranes of the lips and tongue; epineurium of nerve trunks, the penis, and the clitoris; and synovial membranes of certain joints. Krause corpuscles are tiny cylindric oval bodies with a capsule formed by the expansion of the connective tissue sheath of a medullated fiber. They contain a soft, semifluid core in which the axon terminates either in a bulbous extremity or in a coiled mass. Also called **end bulbs**

of Krause. Compare **Golgi-Mazzoni corpuscles, Pacini corpuscles.**

Krebs cycle, a pathway for the breakdown of metabolites. See **citric acid cycle.**

Krebs-Henseleit cycle. See **urea cycle.**

Krukenberg tumor /kroo″kənbərg/ [Friedrich E. Krukenberg, German pathologist, 1871–1946], a neoplasm of the ovary that is a metastasis of a GI malignancy, usually stomach cancer. Cytological examination often reveals mucoid degeneration and many large cells shaped like signet rings. Also called **carcinoma mucocellulare.**

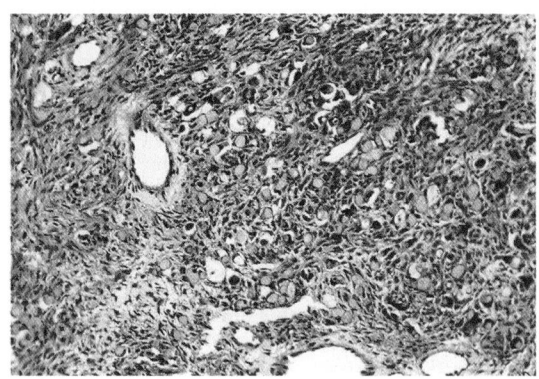

Krukenberg tumor *(Fletcher, 2007)*

krypto-. See **crypto-, crypt-, krypto-.**

krypton (Kr) /krip″ton/, a generally inert, rare, gaseous element present in air. Its atomic number is 36; its atomic mass is 83.80.

KS, ks, abbreviation for **Kaposi sarcoma.**

KUB, a term used in a radiographic examination to determine the location, size, shape, and malformation of the kidneys, ureters, and bladder. Stones and calcified areas may be detected. Abbreviation for *kidney, ureter, and bladder.*

Kuchendorf method /koo″kəndôrf/, (in radiology) a technique for positioning a patient for radiographic examination of the patella. The patella is placed against the image receptor and is moved laterally to reduce superimposition of the femur.

kudzu, an herb that grows in vine form, native to China and Japan and introduced to the United States.

■ INDICATIONS: It is used to reduce alcohol cravings and to treat alcohol hangovers and menopausal symptoms. Its efficacy is unproven.

■ CONTRAINDICATIONS: It should not be used during pregnancy and lactation, in children, or in those with known hypersensitivity. It should be used with caution by people who have heart disease.

Kufs disease /koofs/ [H. Kufs, German psychiatrist, 1871–1955], a rare nervous system disorder characterized by cerebromacular degeneration affecting intellectual function and hypertonicity and by progressive spastic paralysis affecting movement. Also called **adult ceroid lipofuscinosis.**

Kugelberg-Welander syndrome. See **juvenile spinal muscular atrophy.**

Kulchitsky cell carcinoma. See **carcinoid.**

Kulchitsky's cell. See **argentaffin cell.**

Kümmell disease /kim″əl/ [Hermann Kümmell, German surgeon, 1852–1937; L, *dis* + Fr, *aise,* ease], a set of symptoms that develops after a compression fracture of the vertebrae with spinal injury. The symptoms include spinal pain, intercostal neuralgia, kyphosis, and weakness in the legs.

Also called *Kümmell spondylitis,* **posttraumatic spondylitis, traumatic spondylopathy.**

kundalini yoga, a style of yoga whose purpose is the controlled release of latent spiritual energy or life force.

kunecatechins, a topical keratolytic agent.

■ INDICATIONS: This drug is used to treat external genital and perianal warts.

■ CONTRAINDICATIONS: Known hypersensitivity to this drug prohibits its use.

kunitz inhibitor. See **trypsin inhibitor.**

Küntscher nail /koon″chər, kin″chər/ [Gerhard Küntscher, German surgeon, 1902–1972; AS, *naegel*], a stainless steel nail used in orthopedic surgery for the fixation of fractures of the long bones, especially the femur. Also called *Küntscher intramedullary nail.*

Kupffer cells /koop″fər/ [Karl W. von Kupffer, German anatomist, 1829–1902], immobile macrophages that line liver sinusoids. Kupffer cells filter bacteria and other foreign proteins from the blood and initiate immune responses.

kurtosis /kerto′sis/, a statistical measure used to describe the distribution of observed data around the mean.

kuru /koo″roo/ [New Guinea, trembling with fear], a slow, progressive, fatal infection of the central nervous system that was endemic to natives of the New Guinea highlands. The incubation period could be 30 or more years, but death usually occurred within months of the onset of symptoms. It was characterized by ataxia and decreased coordination progressing to paralysis, dementia, slurring of speech, and visual disturbances. Disease was transmitted by ritual cannibalism of brain tissue during funeral rites. The last sufferer of kuru in New Guinea died in 2005. This disease is a model for prion diseases such as BSE and variant CJD.

Kussmaul breathing /koos″moul/ [Adolf Kussmaul, German physician, 1822–1902; AS, *braeth*], abnormally deep, very rapid sighing respirations characteristic of diabetic ketoacidosis and renal failure.

Kussmaul coma [Adolf Kussmaul; Gk, *koma,* deep sleep], a diabetic coma characterized by acidosis and deep breathing or extreme hyperpnea.

Kussmaul sign [Adolf Kussmaul; L, *signum,* mark], **1.** a paradoxic rise in venous pressure with distension of the jugular veins during inspiration, as seen in constrictive pericarditis or mediastinal tumor. **2.** conditions of convulsions and coma associated with a GI disorder caused by absorption of a toxic substance.

kV, abbreviation for **kilovolt.**

Kveim reaction [Morton A. Kveim, Norwegian physician, b. 1892; L, *re,* again, *agere,* to act], a reaction, used in a diagnostic test for sarcoidosis, to an intradermal injection of antigen derived from a lymph node known to be sarcoid. If a noncaseating granuloma appears on the skin at the test site in 4 to 8 weeks, the reaction is said to be positive evidence that the patient has sarcoidosis.

kVp, abbreviation for **kilovolt peak.**

kVp test cassette, (in radiology) a lightproof box containing a copper filter, a series of stepwedges, and an optical attenuator, used to test the accuracy of kVp settings for peak electrical potential across an x-ray tube.

kwashiorkor /kwä′shē·ôr″kôr/ [Afr], a malnutrition disease, primarily of children, caused by severe protein deficiency that usually occurs when the child is weaned from the breast. The child does not lose weight as dramatically and does not look as sick as a marasmic child, who lacks both protein and calories. Some now believe kwashiorkor may relate to bacterial grain contamination and occur when the newly weaned child begins to ingest grain products. Eventually the following symptoms occur: delayed growth, changes in skin and hair pigmentation, diarrhea, loss of appetite, nervous irritability, lethargy, edema, anemia, fatty degeneration of the liver, necrosis, dermatoses, and fibrosis, often accompanied by infection and multivitamin deficiencies. Because dietary fats are poorly tolerated in kwashiorkor, its treatment includes a skimmed milk formula in initial feedings, followed by additional foods until a full, well-balanced diet is achieved. See also **marasmic kwashiorkor, marasmus, protein-energy malnutrition.**

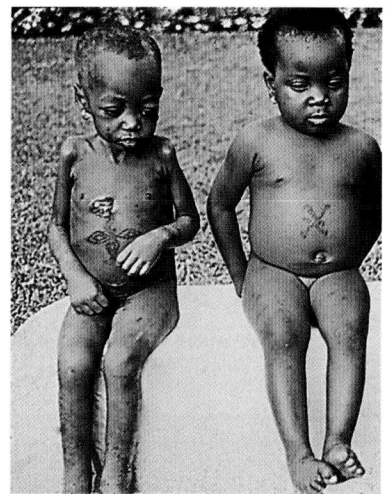

The child on the left has severe muscle wasting with edema, representing marasmic kwashiorkor. The other child pictured does not have a nutritional deficiency. *(Shetty, 2006)*

Kwell, a pediculicide and scabicide. Brand name for **gamma-benzene hexachloride.**

Kyasanur Forest disease, a flavovirus infection transmitted by the bite of a tick, *Haemophysalis spinigera,* that is harbored by shrews and other forest animals in western tropical India. Characteristics of the infection include fever, headache, muscle ache, cough, abdominal and eye pain, and photophobia. Treatment is symptomatic. A vaccine is used in India. Also called **monkey disease.**

kymo-, prefix meaning "waves": *kymography.*

kymography /kēmog″rəfē/ [Gk, *kyma,* wave + *graphein,* to record], a technique for graphically recording motions of body organs, such as the heart and the blood vessels.

kyno-, prefix meaning "dogs." See **cyno-, cyn-.**

kypho-, prefix meaning "hump": *kyphoscoliosis, kyphosis.*

kyphos /kī′fəs/ [Gk, *kyphos,* hunchbacked], the exaggeration or angulation from the normal position of the thoracic vertebral column that is associated with kyphosis. See also **kyphosis.**

kyphoscoliosis /kī′fōskō′lē·ō″sis/ [Gk, *kyphos,* hunchbacked + *skolios* curved + *osis,* condition], an abnormal condition characterized by an anteroposterior and a lateral curvature of the spine. It occurs in children and adults and is often associated with cor pulmonale. Also called **scoliokyphosis.** Compare **kyphosis, scoliosis.** –*kyphoscoliotic, adj.*

K

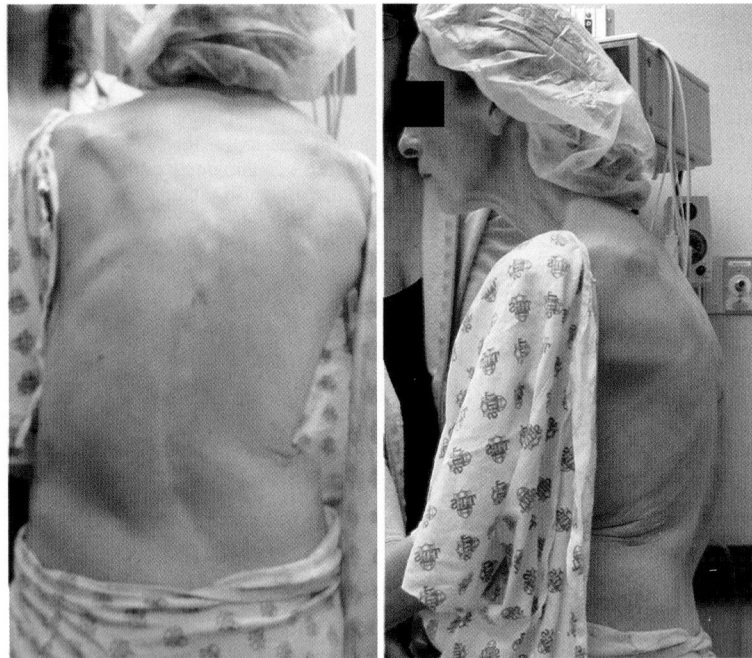

Woman with progressive kyphoscoliosis in adulthood *(Errico et al, 2009)*

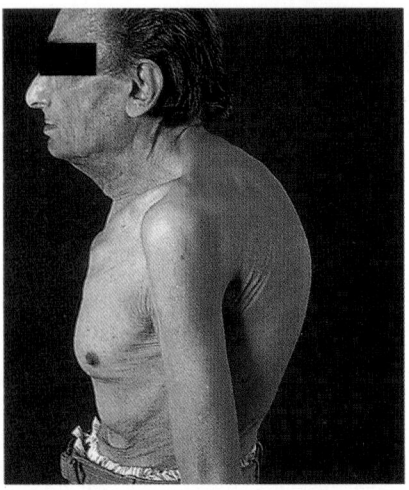

Severe kyphosis of the thoracic spine
(Epstein, Perkin, and Cookson, 2003)

kyphosis /kīfō″sis/ [Gk, *kyphos,* hunchbacked], an abnormal condition of the vertebral column, characterized by increased convexity in the curvature of the thoracic spine as viewed from the side. The spinal sagittal contour ordinarily consists of a lordosis in the lumbar and cervical spinal segments that balances the rounding, or the kyphosis, in the thoracic segment. Kyphosis describes this expected rounding but also is used to describe the abnormal condition of the vertebral column. It may be caused by rickets or tuberculosis of the spine. Adolescent kyphosis is usually self-limiting and often undiagnosed, but if the curvature progresses, there may be moderate back pain. Conservative treatment consists of medication and exercise. A modified Milwaukee brace may be used for severe kyphosis; rarely, spinal fusion may be required. —*kyphotic, adj.*

kysth-, kystho-. See **colpo-, colp-, kolpo-, kysth-, kystho-.**

kyto-. See **cyt-, cyto-.**

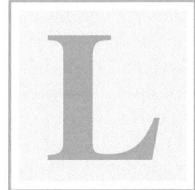

L, 1. symbol for *kinetic potential.* **2.** abbreviation for *Lactobacillus.* **3.** abbreviation for **lambert. 4.** abbreviation for *Latin.* **5.** abbreviation for **liter. 6.** abbreviation for **lung.**

L & A, abbreviation for *reaction of the pupil to light and accommodation.*

La, symbol for the element **lanthanum (La).**

LA, abbreviation for **left atrium.**

lab, abbreviation for **laboratory.**

label [ME, band], **1.** *n.,* a substance with a special affinity for an organ, tissue, cell, or microorganism in which it may become deposited and fixed. **2.** *n.,* an atom or molecule attached to either a ligand or binding protein and capable of generating a signal for monitoring in the binding reaction. **3.** *v.,* to deposit and fix a substance, tissue, cell, or microorganism. **4.** *v.,* to attach a radioisotope to a compound for the purpose of tracing it during a physiological action in the body. **5.** a word or phrase that describes or identifies something or someone.

labeled compound, a chemical substance in which part of the molecules are labeled with a radionuclide or isotope so that observations of the radioactivity or isotopic composition make it possible to follow the compound or its fragments through physical, chemical, or biological processes.

labeling, 1. the providing of information on a drug, food, device, or cosmetic to the purchaser or user. The information may be in any one of various forms, including printing on a carton, adhesive label, package insert, and monograph. Regulations for labeling in the United States are provided by the federal Food and Drug Administration. The label must contain directions for use, unless such directions are exempted by regulation, as well as warnings or contraindications. It must not contain false or misleading information. Health Canada provides guidance for the labeling of pharmaceutical drugs for human use in Canada. **2.** the assignment of a word or term to a form of behavior. It often involves describing what one observes in a client's affect or behavior in order to highlight, clarify, or validate it. **3.** the act of classifying a patient according to a diagnostic category. Labeling can be misleading because not all patients conform to defined characteristics of standard diagnostic categories. Also spelled *labelling.*

la belle indifference /lä bel indifäräNs″/ [Fr, nice indifference], an air of unconcern displayed by some patients toward their physical symptoms. It is no longer considered a clinical sign.

labetalol hydrochloride /ləbet″əlol/, an antihypertensive drug with beta- and alpha-blocking properties.

■ INDICATIONS: It is prescribed for the treatment of moderate to severe hypertension.

■ CONTRAINDICATIONS: The presence of asthma or emphysema prohibits its use. It should be used with caution in patients with diabetes because it may mask symptoms of hypoglycemia, particularly tachycardia.

■ ADVERSE EFFECTS: A common side effect is bradycardia. Among the most serious adverse effects are orthostatic hypotension, fatigue, headache, skin rashes, scalp paresthesia, nausea, and vomiting.

labia /lā″bē·ə/*sing. labium* [L, lip], **1.** the lips. **2.** the fleshy liplike edges of an organ or tissue. **3.** the folds of skin at the opening of the vagina. −**labial,** *adj.*

labial /lā″bē·əl/, pertaining to the lips. See also **bilabial.**

-labial, suffix meaning "lips": *cervicolabial, distolabial.*

labial arch wire, an arch wire of high tensile strength whose arms come through the embrasure between the canine and lateral incisors in the maxillary arch, and between the canines and first premolar in the mandibular arch. It is used primarily for moving teeth in the lingual direction and for retruding the anterior teeth and closing spaces.

labial bar /lā″bē·əl/, (in dentistry) a portion of the metallic substructure that is created to be either labial or buccal to the dental arch and that connects bilateral parts of a mandibular removable partial denture.

labial flange, the part of a denture that occupies the outer vestibule of the mouth.

labial glands [L, *labium,* lip, *glans,* acorn], small mucous or serous glands embedded in the lips.

labial notch, a depression in the border of a denture that accommodates the labial frenum.

labial vestibule, that portion of the facial surface inside the mouth that lies between the lips and the teeth and gingivae or residual alveolar ridges.

labia majora /lā″bē·ə məˈjôrə/*sing. labium majus,* two long lips of skin, one on each side of the vaginal orifice outside the labia minora. They extend from the anterior labial commissure to the posterior labial commissure and form the lateral boundaries of the pudendal cleft. Each labium contains areolar tissue, fat, and a thin layer of nonstriated muscle. In some women the outer surface of each lip may be covered with coarse pubic hair. The embryonic derivations of the labia majora and the scrotum are homologous.

labia minora /lā″bē·ə minˈôrə/*sing. labium minus,* two thin folds of skin between the labia majora, extending from the clitoris backward on both sides of the vaginal orifice, ending between it and the labia majora. Anteriorly each labium divides into an upper and a lower division. The upper divisions pass above the clitoris and meet to form the preputium clitoridis. The lower divisions pass beneath the clitoris and unite to form the frenulum of the clitoris. Opposed surfaces of the labia minora contain sebaceous follicles.

labile /lā″bil/ [L, *labilis,* slipping], **1.** unstable, unpredictable; characterized by a tendency to change or be altered or modified. **2.** (in psychiatry) characterized by rapidly shifting or changing emotions, as in bipolar disorder and certain types of schizophrenia; emotionally unstable.

-labile, suffix meaning "unstable," "subject to change": *thermolabile.*

lability, 1. instability; unpredictability. See **labile. 2.** a sign or symptom characterized by exaggerated changes in mood or affect in rapid succession.

labio-, prefix meaning "lips, particularly the lips of the mouth": *labiodental, labiolingual, labioversion.*

labiodental /lā″bē·ōden″təl/ [L, *labium,* lip, *dens,* tooth], **1.** pertaining to the labial, or lip-facing, surfaces of the 12 anterior teeth. **2.** pertaining to the sounds of speech that require a special coordination of teeth and lips, such as /f/ and /v/.

labioglossolaryngeal paralysis. See **bulbar paralysis.**

labiolingual fixed orthodontic appliance /lā′bē·ōling″-gwəl/ [L, *labium,* lip, *lingua,* tongue], an appliance for correcting or improving malocclusion that is anchored to the maxillary and mandibular first permanent molars. The appliance has labial arches that fit into horizontal buccal tubes attached to anchor bands and lingual arches that are fastened to the lingual side of the anchor bands.

labioversion /lā′bē·ōver′zhən/ [L, *labium,* lip, *vertere,* to turn], displacement of a tooth toward the lips (labially) from the line of occlusion.

labium. See **labia.**

labium majus, *(Obsolete)* now called **labia majora.**

labium minus, *(Obsolete)* now called **labia minora.**

labor [L, work], the physiological processes by which the uterus expels the products of conception, beginning with cervical dilation to the delivery of the placenta. Also spelled **labour.** See also **birth, cardinal movements of labor, station.**

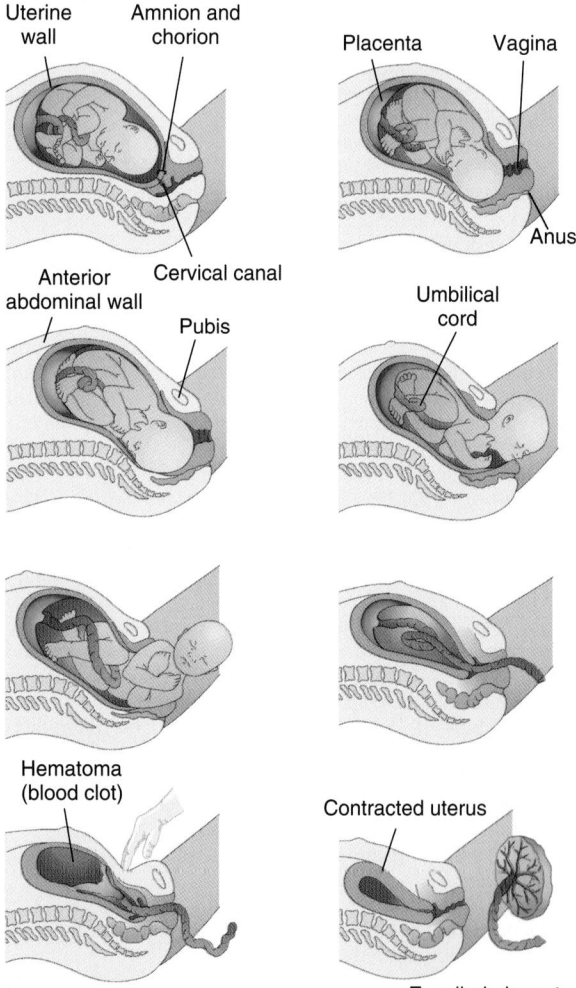

Uterine wall
Amnion and chorion
Placenta
Vagina
Anus
Anterior abdominal wall
Cervical canal
Pubis
Umbilical cord
Hematoma (blood clot)
Contracted uterus
Expelled placenta, membranes, and umbilical cord

Mechanisms of labor *(Moore, Persaud, and Shiota, 2008)*

labor, abnormal. *(Nontechnical)* See **dystocia.**

laboratory (lab) /lab″ərətôr′e/ [L, *laborare,* to labor], **1.** *n.,* a facility, room, building, or part of a building in which scientific research, experimentation, testing, or other investigative activities are carried out. **2.** *adj.,* pertaining to a laboratory. **3.** a specialty area, designed with equipment to facilitate learning for students in the health professions.

laboratory core. See **core,** def. 2.

laboratory diagnosis, a diagnosis arrived at after study of secretions, excretions, or tissue through chemical, microscopic, or bacteriological means or by biopsy. See also **diagnosis.**

laboratory error, any error made by the personnel in a clinical laboratory in performing a test, interpreting data, or reporting or recording the results. Laboratory error must always be considered a possible explanation for findings that are at variance with the composite clinical condition of the patient or are widely divergent from previous laboratory tests. The general procedure is to repeat the test when an abnormal result is found.

laboratory medicine, the branch of medicine in which specimens of tissue, fluid, or other body substances are examined outside the patient, usually in a laboratory. Some fields of laboratory medicine are chemistry, cytology, hematology, histology, and pathology.

Laboratory Response Network (LRN), a network of federal, state, and local laboratories, established in 1999 by the U.S. Centers for Disease Control and Prevention, whose purpose is to provide the laboratory infrastructure and capacity to respond to biological and chemical terrorism and other public health emergencies in the United States.

laboratory test, a procedure, usually conducted in a laboratory, that is intended to detect, identify, or quantify one or more significant substances, evaluate organ functions, or establish the nature of a condition or disease. Laboratory tests range from quite simple to extremely sophisticated. In modern medical practice they are commonly used to help establish or confirm a diagnosis and often aid in the management of disease.

labor coach, a person who assists a woman in labor and delivery by closely attending to her emotional needs and encouraging her to use properly the breathing patterns, concentration techniques, body positions, and massage techniques that were taught in a program of psychophysical preparation for childbirth. The task of a labor coach is to minimize the need for pharmacological pain relief and to decrease or eliminate the use of analgesia or anesthesia. Usually the coach is the father of the baby or a close friend of the mother, but a professional labor coach, often a registered nurse specially trained in a method, may fill the role. Also called **doula, labor support person.** See also **monitrice.**

labored breathing, abnormal respiration characterized by stridor, grunting, nasal flaring, or evidence of increased effort, including the use of accessory muscles of respiration in the chest wall.

labor pains [L, *labor,* work, *poena,* penalty], pain associated with the contraction of the uterus in labor.

labor support person. See **labor coach.**

labour. See **labor.**

labyrinth. See **inner ear.**

labyrinth-, prefix meaning "labyrinth" or "inner ear": *labyrinthitis, labyrinthectomy, labyrinthine.*

labyrinthectomy /lab′ərinthek″təmē/, the destruction of the inner structures of the ear, usually for the management of Ménière disease. Hearing is permanently lost, and balance is affected. Vestibular rehabilitation to regain balance is helpful after the procedure. See also **Ménière disease.**

labyrinthine /lab′ərin″thin/ [Gk, *labyrinthos,* maze], pertaining to or resembling a labyrinth or maze, such as the structure of the inner ear.

labyrinthine reflex. See **kinetic reflex.**

labyrinthine righting, one of the five basic neuromuscular reactions involved in a change of body positions. The change stimulates cells in the semicircular canals of the inner ear, causing neck muscles to respond by automatically adjusting the head to the new position.

labyrinthine vertigo. See **Ménière disease.**

labyrinthitis /lab′ərinthī″tis/ [Gk, *labyrinthos,* maze, *itis*], inflammation or dysfunction of the labyrinthine canals of the inner ear, resulting in vertigo and often accompanied by nausea, vomiting, or malaise.

labyrinthus osseus. See **osseous labyrinth.**

laceration /las′ərā″shən/ [L, *lacerare,* to tear], **1.** an interruption in skin integrity due to tearing or slashing. **2.** a torn, usually jagged wound in soft tissue.

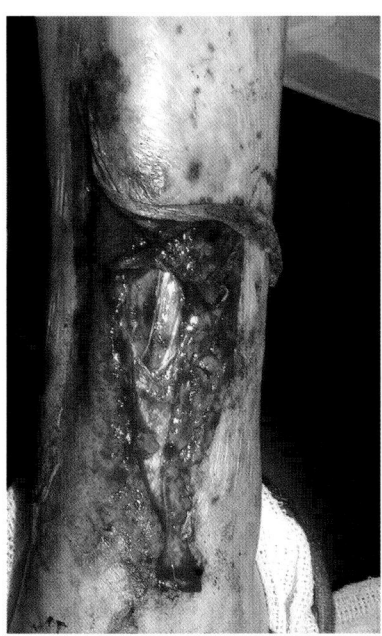

Pretibial laceration *(Lo et al, 2012)*

laceration of cervix [L, *lacerare,* to tear, *cervix,* neck], a wound or irregular tear of the cervix uteri during childbirth.

laceration of the perineum [L, *lacerare,* to tear; Gk, *perineos*], a wound or irregular tear of the perineal tissues during childbirth.

lacertus /ləser′təs/ [L, lizard, because of a fancied resemblance], a general term for certain fibrous attachments of muscles.

lacri-, lachry-, prefix meaning "tears": *lacrimator, lacrimotomy, lacrimal.*

lacrimal /lak″riməl/ [L, *lacrima,* tear], pertaining to tears. Also spelled *lachrymal.*

lacrimal apparatus, a network of structures of the eye that secrete tears and drain them from the surface of the eyeball. These parts include the lacrimal glands, lacrimal ducts, lacrimal canals, lacrimal sacs, and nasolacrimal ducts.

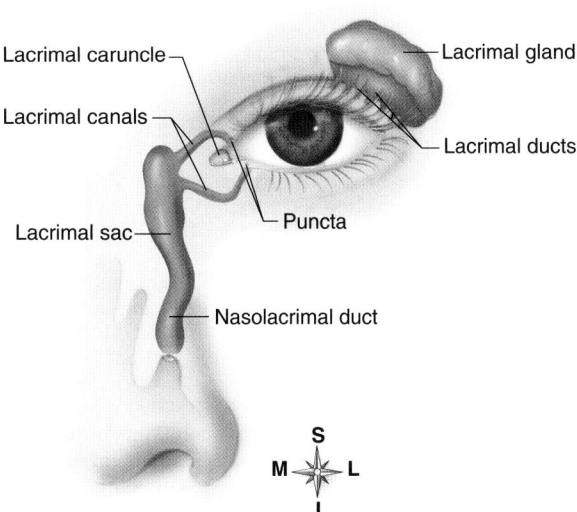

Lacrimal apparatus *(Patton and Thibodeau, 2013)*

lacrimal artery, an artery arising from the ophthalmic artery on the lateral side of the optic nerve that supplies the lacrimal gland, muscles, the anterior ciliary branch to the eyeball, and the lateral sides of the eyelid.

lacrimal bone, one of the smallest and most fragile bones of the face, located at the anterior part of the medial wall of the orbit. It unites with the maxilla to form the groove for the lacrimal sac.

lacrimal canaliculus. See **lacrimal duct.**

lacrimal caruncle, the small, reddish, fleshy protuberance that fills the triangular space between the medial margins of the upper and lower eyelids. It contains sebaceous and sudoriferous glands and secretes a whitish substance that collects and often dries in the corner of the eye.

lacrimal duct, one of a pair of channels through which tears pass from the lacrimal lake to the lacrimal sac of each eye. Also called **lacrimal canaliculus.**

lacrimal fold [L, *lacrima,* tear; AS, *fealdan*], a valvelike fold of mucous membrane at the lower part of the nasolacrimal duct. Also called **Hasner fold.**

lacrimal gland, one of a pair of glands situated superiorly and laterally to the eye bulb in the lacrimal fossa of the frontal bone. It is an oval structure about the size of an almond. The gland has about 10 ducts that run obliquely beneath the conjunctiva and open along the upper and lateral half of the superior conjunctival fornix. The watery secretion from the gland consists of the tears, slightly alkaline and saline, that moisten the conjunctiva.

lacrimal groove, a groove formed by the lacrimal bone and the frontal process of the maxilla that contains the lacrimal sac.

lacrimal lake, an accumulation of fluid secreted by the lacrimal gland. It is drained by the lacrimal canaliculi.

lacrimal papilla, the small conic elevation on the medial margin of each eyelid supporting an apex pierced by the punctum lacrimale through which tears emerge to moisten the conjunctiva.

lacrimal punctum, an opening through which fluid enters each lacrimal canaliculum.

lacrimal reflex [L, *lacrima,* tear, *reflectere,* to bend back], a release of tears in response to stimulation or irritation of the cornea or conjunctiva.

lacrimal sac, the upper end of each of the two nasolacrimal ducts. Each sac is lodged in a deep groove formed by the lacrimal bone and the frontal process of the maxilla. The sac is ovoid and about 13 mm long. Its upper end is closed and rounded, its lower end continuous with the nasolacrimal duct. The lacrimal sacs fill with tears secreted by the lacrimal glands and conveyed through the lacrimal ducts.

lacrimation /lak′rimā″shən/, **1.** the normal continuous secretion of tears by the lacrimal glands. **2.** an excessive amount of tear production, as in crying or weeping.

lacrimator /lak″rimā″tər/, an agent that stimulates the secretion of tears.

lacrimomaxillary suture. See **maxillolacrimal suture.**

lacrimotomy /lak′rimot″əmē/, a surgical incision in the tear duct.

La Crosse encephalitis, encephalitis caused by the La Crosse virus (a California serogroup virus in the family Bunyaviridae), transmitted by *Aedes triseriatus,* seen primarily in children, chiefly in the Midwestern United States. It is one of the most prevalent mosquito-borne diseases recognized in the United States. Most cases result in mild illness.

lact-. See **lacto-, lact-.**

lactalbumin /lak′təlbyoo̅″min/ [L, *lac,* milk, *albus,* white], a simple, highly nutritious protein found in milk. See also **albumin, serum albumin.**

lactam /lak″təm/, a cyclic amide created by the elimination of a molecule of water from aminocarboxylic acid. Lactim is the isomeric form of lactam.

lactase /lak″tās/ [L, *lac* + Fr, *diastase,* enzyme], an enzyme that catalyzes the hydrolysis of lactose to glucose and galactose. Lactase is concentrated in the kidney, liver, and intestinal mucosa. Also called **beta-galactosidase.**

lactase deficiency, an inherited abnormality in which the amount of the digestive enzyme lactase is inadequate for the normal digestion of milk products, resulting in lactose intolerance, the inability to digest lactose (except for the bacterial breakdown of lactose in the large intestine). In adults a relative deficiency may appear as a natural process of aging; it occurs more frequently in persons of Asiatic, Native American, and African heritage. A lactase deficiency also may result from subtotal gastrectomy and may be secondary to any disease of the small intestine in which structural changes occur, such as tropical sprue, ulcerative colitis, infectious hepatitis, and kwashiorkor; severe malnutrition; or some types of antibiotic therapy. See also **lactose intolerance.**

lactate /lak″tāt/, an anion of lactic acid.

lactate dehydrogenase (LDH), an enzyme that is found in the cytoplasm of almost all body tissues, where its main function is to catalyze the oxidation of L-lactate to pyruvate. It is assayed as a measure of anaerobic carbohydrate metabolism and as one of several serum indicators of myocardial infarction and muscular dystrophies. Serum levels of LDH usually rise 12 to 18 hours after myocardial cell necrosis. See also **aspartate aminotransferase, CK isoenzyme fraction, Duchenne muscular dystrophy.**

lactate dehydrogenase (LDH) test, a blood test used to detect levels of lactate dehydrogenase, which is widely distributed throughout the body. Disease or injury to body tissues such as the heart, liver, red blood cells, kidneys, skeletal muscles, brain, and lungs will result in higher-than-normal blood levels. Five separate isoenzymes make up the total LDH, with each body tissue containing a predominance of one or more of these fractions.

lactation /laktā″shən/ [L, *lac,* milk, *atio,* process], the process of synthesis and secretion of milk from the breasts in the nourishment of an infant or child. See also **breastfeeding.**

lactation consultant, a health care professional, often with advanced certification, who provides education and management related to breastfeeding.

lactation mastitis, an accumulation of milk in the secreting ducts of the breast after childbirth, causing all or a part of the breast to become hardened and the tissues to become engorged. Also called **caked breast.**

lactation suppression, measures taken to stop the production of breast milk in the postpartum period. Tight brassieres or the binding of the breasts, restriction of fluids, and the application of ice packs are traditional nondrug approaches.

lacteal /lak″tē·əl/, referring to the tiny vessels in the villi of the wall of the small intestine through which chylomicrons are absorbed and released into the lymphatic system.

lacteal fistula, an abnormal passage opening into a lacteal duct.

lacteal vessel, one of the many central intestinal capillaries in the villi of the small intestine. They open into the lymphatic vessels in the submucosa. The capillary is filled with milky-white chyle caused by the absorption of fat from the lumen (chylomicrons) and passes chyle to the lymph circulation via the thoracic duct to the blood vascular system.

lactic /lak″tik/ [L, *lac* + *icus,* like], referring to milk and milk products. See also **lactic acid, lactose.**

lactic acid, a three-carbon organic acid produced by anaerobic respiration. L-lactic acid in muscle and blood is a product of glucose and glycogen metabolism; D-lactic acid is produced by the fermentation of dextrose by a species of micrococcus; a mixture of both D- and L-isomers is found in the stomach, in sour milk, and in certain foods prepared by bacterial fermentation, such as sauerkraut. Also called **alpha-hydroxypropionic acid,** *2-hydroxypropanoic acid.* See also **glycolysis.**

lactic acid fermentation, **1.** the anaerobic production of lactic acid from glucose. **2.** the souring of milk.

lactic acidosis, a disorder characterized by an accumulation of lactic acid in the blood, resulting in a lowered pH in muscle and serum. The condition occurs most commonly in tissue hypoxia but may also result from liver impairment, respiratory failure, burn trauma, neoplasms, and cardiovascular disease.

lactic acid test, a blood test that measures lactate levels, which are a fairly sensitive and reliable indicator of tissue hypoxia. Lactic acid blood levels are used to document the presence of tissue hypoxia, determine the degree of hypoxia, and monitor the effect of therapy. See also **lactate.**

lactiferous /laktif″ərəs/ [L, *lac* + *ferre,* to carry], pertaining to a structure that produces or conveys milk, such as the tubules of the breasts.

lactiferous duct, one of many channels that carry milk from the lobes of each breast to the nipple.

lactiferous glands [L, *lac,* milk, *ferre,* to carry, *glans,* acorn], glands that secrete or convey milk, such as mammary glands.

lactim. See **lactam.**

lactin. See **lactose.**

Lactinex, a probiotic fixed combination drug used to reestablish normal gastrointestinal flora after antibiotic therapy. Brand name for *Lactobacillus acidophilus, Lactobacillus bulgaricus.*

lactitol /lak′t-tol/, a disaccharide analog of lactulose; it is classified as a sugar alcohol and used as a sweetener. It is also a laxative and is used to treat constipation.

lacto-, lact-, prefix meaning "milk" or "lactic acid": *Lactobacillus, lactation, lactotoxin.*

Lactobacillus /lak′tōbəsil″əs/ [L, *lac* + *bacillum,* small rod], any one of a group of nonpathogenic gram-positive rod-shaped bacteria that produce lactic acid from carbohydrates. Many species are normally found in the human intestinal tract and vagina.

Lactobacillus acidophilus [L, *lac,* milk, *bacillum,* small rod, *acidus,* sour; Gk, *philein,* to love], a bacterium present in the intestinal tract and vagina, as well as in milk and dairy products. The strain is used to manufacture a fermented milk product. Generally considered to be beneficial because it produces vitamin K, lactase, and other antimicrobial substances when ingested. See also **acidophilus milk.**

Lactobacillus bulgaricus, a genus of bacteria used in the production of yogurt.

lactoferrin /lak′tō·fer″in/, an iron-binding protein present in neutrophil granules. By combining with iron, lactoferrin prevents microorganisms from combining with and using iron for their growth and development.

lactoferrin assay, a test of a fecal sample to detect inflammatory white blood cells in the intestinal tract. It is used to help diagnose bacterial enteritis, acute Crohn's disease, and acute ulcerative colitis.

lactogen /lak″təjən/ [L, *lac* + Gk, *genein,* to produce], a drug or other substance that enhances the production and secretion of milk. −*lactogenic, adj.*

lactogenesis /lak″tojen″ēsis/. See **galactopoiesis.**

lactogenic hormone. See **prolactin.**

lacto-ovo-vegetarian /lak′tō ōv′ō vej′əter″ē·ən/, a person whose diet consists primarily of foods of vegetable origin but also includes some animal products, such as eggs *(ovo)* and milk and cheese *(lacto)* but no meat, fish, or poultry. Also called **ovo-lacto-vegetarian.**

lactoperoxidase /-pərok″sidās/, an enzyme found in milk and saliva. It is believed to inhibit a number of microorganisms, functioning in a nonspecific immunity role.

lactose /lak″tos/ [L, *lac* + Gk, *glykys,* sweet], a disaccharide found in the milk of all mammals. On hydrolysis, lactose yields the monosaccharides glucose and galactose. Lactose is used as a laxative, a diuretic, and a component of formulas for infants. Also called **lactin, milk sugar.** See also **lactase deficiency, lactose intolerance, sugar.**

lactose intolerance, a sensitivity disorder resulting in the inability to digest lactose from milk products because of an inadequate production of or defect in the enzyme lactase. Symptoms of the disorder are bloating, flatus, nausea, diarrhea, and abdominal cramps. The diet is adjusted according to the tolerance level; milk-derived foods (milk, cheese, butter, and margarine) and any products containing milk, such as cakes, ice cream, cream soups, and sauces, are restricted. Also called **milk intolerance.** See also **lactase deficiency.**

lactose tolerance test, a diagnostic study utilizing blood samples taken before and after drinking a liquid containing lactose to test how well an individual can process lactose.

lactosuria /lak″təsŏŏr″ē·ə/ [L, *lac* + Gk, *glykys,* sweet, *ouron,* urine], the presence of lactose in the urine, a condition that may occur in late pregnancy or during lactation and in newborns, especially if premature.

lactotoxin /-tok″sin/, any toxic base occurring in milk as a result of decomposition of its proteins.

lactotroph /lak″totrōf″/, a type of acidophil in the adenohypophysis that secretes prolactin. Also called *lactotrope,* **luteotrope, mammotroph.**

lactovegetarian /-vej′əter″ē·ən/, one whose diet consists of milk and milk products *(lacto)* in addition to foods of vegetable origin but does not include eggs, meat, fish, or poultry.

lactulose /lak″tyəlōs/, a nonabsorbable synthetic disaccharide, 4-0-beta-D-galactopyranosyl-D-fructose, $C^{12}H^{22}O^{11}$. It is hydrolyzed in the colon by bacteria primarily to lactic acid and small amounts of formic and acetic acids, which results in increased osmotic pressure and acidification of the colonic contents. It is used as a cathartic in chronic constipation. Because the acidification causes ammonia to be removed from the blood to form ammonium ion, it is also used in the treatment of hepatic coma. Its ability to increase fecal water content, however, may also cause diarrhea.

lacuna /ləkyōō″nə/ *pl. lacunae* [L, pit], **1.** a hollow within a structure, especially bony tissue, in which lie osteoblasts. **2.** a gap, as in the field of vision.

lacunar /lakyōō″nər/ [L, *lacuna,* pit], pertaining to or characterized by the presence of pits, depressions, hollows, or spaces.

lacunar ligament, a crescent-shaped extension of fibers at the medial end of the inguinal ligament that passes backward to attach to the pecten pubis on the superior ramus of the pubic bone.

lacunar state, a pseudobulbar disorder characterized by the appearance of small, smooth-walled cavities in the brain tissue. The condition usually follows a series of small strokes, particularly in older adults with arterial hypertension and arteriosclerosis. Also called **status lacunaris.**

lacus lacrimalis /lā″kəs lak′rimā″ləs/ [L, *lacus,* lake, *lacrimalis,* tears], a triangular space separating the medial ends of the upper and the lower eyelids at the inner canthus where the tears collect. It is an extension of the medial canthus and contains the lacrimal caruncle.

LAD, 1. abbreviation for *left anterior descending.* **2.** abbreviation for **leukocyte adhesion deficiency.**

Ladd's bands, a series of peritoneal folds in patients in whom the cecum ends up in the midabdomen. These folds extend to the right undersurface of the liver and compress the duodenum.

LADME /lad″mē/, an abbreviation for the time course of drug distribution, representing the terms *liberation, absorption, distribution, metabolism,* and *elimination.*

Laënnec catarrh /lā″ənek″/ [René T.H. Laënnec, French physician, 1781–1826; Gk, *kata,* down, *rhoia,* flow], a form of bronchial asthma characterized by the expectoration of small viscous, beadlike bodies of sputum. These bodies, called Laënnec pearls, are formed in the bronchioles.

Laënnec cirrhosis [René T.H. Laënnec; Gk, *kirrhos,* yelloworange, *osis,* condition], a fibrotic form of cirrhosis precipitated by alcohol abuse. Also called **alcoholic cirrhosis.** See also **cirrhosis.**

Laënnec pearls, the small gelatinous casts of the smaller bronchial tubes, expectorated in bronchial asthma. See **Laënnec catarrh.**

Laetrile /lā″ətril/, a substance composed primarily of amygdalin, a cyanogenic glycoside derived from apricot pits. Laetrile has been offered as a cancer medication despite clinical studies by the National Cancer Institute that failed to show benefits from its use. It is claimed that amygdalin is hydrolyzed by enzymes in cancer cells to produce benzaldehyde and hydrogen cyanide, which kill the cancer cells. It is not approved by the U.S. Food and Drug Administration. Also called **vitamin B$_{17}$.**

laevo-. See **levo-.**

laf, abbreviation for **laminar airflow.**

lag, the afterglow of an image on a screen or television camera, caused by phosphorescence.

-lagnia, -lagny, suffix meaning "lust" or "a sexual predilection": *algolagnia, pyrolagnia, urolagnia.*

lag of accommodation, the dioptric value in which the accommodative stimulus exceeds the accommodative response. It occurs when the eyes focus on an object, but instead of focusing directly on the object, the eyes actually focus on a point behind the object.

L

lagophthalmos /lag′ofthal″məs/ [Gk, *lagos,* hare, *ophthalmos,* eye], an abnormal condition in which an eye may not be fully closed because of a neurological, muscular, or mechanical disorder.

lag phase [Dan, *lakke,* go slowly; Gk, *phasis,* appearance], a time span during which bacteria injected into a fresh medium have not begun to multiply, although they may enlarge.

la grippe. *(Obsolete)* See **influenza.**

laissez-faire style, a type of leadership style that allows the group to control decision making and problem solving, using a nonauthoritarian and hands-off approach to group facilitation.

laity /lā′itē/ [Gk, *laikos,* of the people], a nonprofessional segment of the population, as viewed from the perspective of a member of a particular profession. A clergyman may regard a physician as a member of the laity and vice versa.

LAK, abbreviation for *lymphokine-activated killer.* See **lymphokine-activated killer (LAK) cells.**

laked blood /lākt/ [Fr, *laque,* a deep red color], **1.** blood that is clear, red, and homogenous because of hemolysis of the red blood cells, as may occur in poisoning and severe extensive burns. **2.** (in microbiology) an agar medium intended for the isolation, quantitation, and partial identification of obligately anaerobic bacteria that also supports the growth of aerobic and microaerophilic bacteria.

lal-, lalio-, lalo-, prefix meaning "talk, babble": *lallation, lalophobia.*

La Leche League International /lälech″ā/ [Sp, *la leche,* the milk], a nongovernmental organization that coordinates advocacy, education, and training related to breastfeeding.

-lalia, suffix meaning "a disorder of speech": *coprolalia, echolalia, glossolalia.*

lalio-. See **lal-, lalio-, lalo-.**

lallation /lalā″shən/ [L, *lallare,* to babble], **1.** repetitive, unintelligible utterances, such as the babbling of an infant or the mumbled speech of individuals with schizophrenia, alcoholism, or severe cognitive impairments. **2.** a speech disorder characterized by a defective pronunciation of words containing the sound /l/ or by the use of the sound /l/ in place of the sound /r/. Compare **rhotacism.**

lalo-. See **lal-, lalio-, lalo-.**

lalophobia /lal′ōfō″bē·ə/ [Gk, *lalia,* speech, *phobos,* fear], a morbid dread of talking caused by fear and anxiety that one will stammer, mumble, or stutter.

lamarckism /ləmär″kizəm/ [Jean B.P. de Lamarck, French naturalist, 1744–1829; Gk, *ismos,* practice], a theory postulating that organic evolution results from structural changes in plants and animals caused by adaptation to environmental conditions and that these acquired characteristics are transmitted to offspring. Also called *Lamarck's theory, lamarckianism.* Compare **darwinian theory.** −*lamarckian, adj., n.*

Lamaze method /ləmäz″/ [Fernand Lamaze, French obstetrician, 1890–1957], a method of psychophysical preparation for childbirth developed in the 1950s. It requires classes, practice at home, and coaching during labor and delivery. The classes, given during pregnancy, teach the physiology of pregnancy and childbirth, exercises to develop strength in the abdominal muscles and control of isolated muscles of the vagina and perineum, and techniques of breathing and relaxation to promote control and relaxation during labor. The woman is conditioned by repetition and practice to dissociate herself from the source of a stimulus by concentration on a focal point, by consciously relaxing all muscles, and by breathing in a special way at a particular rate—thereby training herself not to pay attention to the stimuli associated with labor. The kind and rate of breathing change with the advancing stages of labor. During the early part of the first

stage of labor, when the uterine cervix is dilated less than 5 cm and the contractions occur every 2 to 4 minutes, last 40 to 60 seconds, and are of mild to moderate strength, the mother does slow chest breathing during contractions. Her fingers may rest lightly on her lower ribs to feel them rise and fall. The abdominal wall does not move with respiration. She may perform an effleurage, or rhythmic fingertip massage, of her lower abdomen during the contractions. The rate of respiration is 10 or fewer breaths a minute, increasing to 12 per minute as labor intensifies. During the active part of the first stage of labor up to the transition to the second stage, the cervix is from 5 cm to nearly fully dilated, the interval between contractions is from 1½ to 4 minutes, and the duration of contractions is from 45 to 90 seconds. (The interval decreases, and the intensity and duration increase as labor progresses.) During contractions the mother breathes quietly and shallowly in her chest. The rate of her breathing varies with the strength of the contractions, increasing during a contraction to as fast as once a second at the peak and slowing to every 6 seconds as the uterus relaxes. She is coached to concentrate on the focal point she has selected, to perform the effleurage of her abdomen, to relax her perineal and vaginal muscles, and to take a cleansing breath at the beginning and end of each contraction. At the end of the first stage of labor, when the cervix is almost completely dilated and the contractions are strong, occurring every 1½ to 2 minutes and lasting 60 to 90 seconds, the mother begins to feel the urge to bear down and push during contractions. She avoids pushing before full dilation by combining several light, shallow breaths in the chest with short puffing exhalations as the urge increases during the contractions. During the second stage of labor the cervix is fully dilated and contractions are strong, frequent, and expulsive. The mother's head and shoulders are supported on pillows. During contractions she is helped to draw her legs back, flexing the thighs against the abdomen, holding them behind the lower thigh with her hands. Her chin is tucked on her chest, the air is blocked from escaping from her lungs, her perineum is relaxed, and she bears down forcibly. Depending on the length of the contraction, several pushes of 10 to 15 or more seconds may be possible during the contraction. As the baby's head crowns, she is asked to pant lightly so that the head may be delivered slowly. The advantages of the method include the need for little or no analgesia for relief of pain and participation in the labor by the mother, giving her a great sense of self-satisfaction at delivery. The father of the baby also benefits by participating in the birth of his child. Compare **Bradley method, Read method.**

lambda /lam″də/, **1.** Λ, λ, the eleventh letter of the Greek alphabet. **2.** a posterior fontanel of the skull marking the point where the sagittal and lambdoidal sutures meet.

lambda chain, a type of light polypeptide chain found in immunoglobulin molecules.

lambda light chain, one of two kinds of smaller polypeptide chains present in an immunoglobulin molecule. See also **kappa light chain.**

lambda wave, a low-voltage occipital wave recorded by electroencephalography during visual activity.

lambdoid /lam″doid/, having the shape of the Greek letter *lambda.*

lambdoidal suture /lamdoi″dəl/, the interdigitating connection between the occipital bone and the parietal bones of the skull. It is continuous with the occipitomastoid suture between the occipital and the mastoid portions of the temporal bones.

lambert (L) /lom″bert, lam″bərt/ [J.H. Lambert, German physicist, 1728–1777], a unit of luminance or brightness of a perfectly diffusing surface, whether emitting or reflecting, equal to a total luminous flux of one lumen per square centimeter.

Lambert-Eaton myasthenic syndrome (LEMS), an autoimmune disorder affecting neuromuscular transmission that causes weakness and fatigue. Also called **Eaton-Lambert syndrome.**

lamella /ləmel″ə/ *pl. lamellae* [L, small plate], **1.** a thin leaf or plate, as of bone. **2.** a medicated disk of glycerin and an alkaloid, for insertion under the eyelid, where it dissolves and is absorbed for local application.

lamellar /ləmel′ər/ [L, *lamella,* small plate], pertaining to or characterized by lamellae.

lamellar exfoliation [L, *lamella + ex,* without, *folium,* leaf], a congenital skin disorder transmitted as an autosomal-recessive trait in which a parchmentlike scaly membrane that covers the infant peels off within 24 hours of birth. Complete healing or a progressively less severe process of reforming and shedding of the scales then occurs. Also called **ichthyosis congenita, ichthyosis fetalis,** *lamellar desquamation of the newborn, lamellar ichthyosis of the newborn.* See also **collodion baby.**

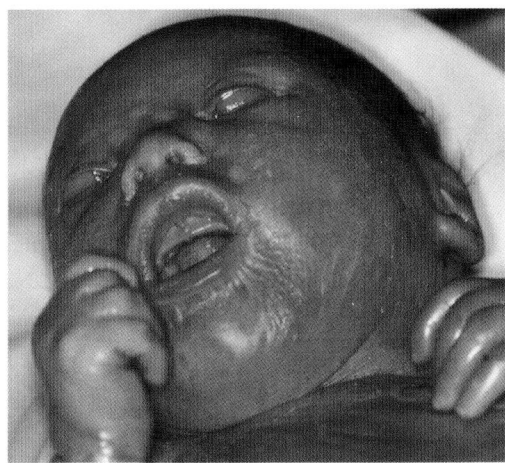

Infant with lamellar exfoliation *(Rodríguez-Pazos et al, 2011)*

lamellar transplant. See **deep lamellar endothelial keratoplasty.**

lameness /lām″nəs/ [ME, *lama,* to break], *(Informal)* a condition of diminished function, particularly because of a foot or leg injury. The term may also be applied to a stiff or painful back that makes walking difficult.

Lamictal, an anticonvulsant drug. Brand name for **lamotrigine.**

lamin-, combining form meaning "layer" or "lamina": *laminated, laminotomy.*

lamina /lam″inə/ *pl. laminae* [L, thin plate], any thin, flat layer of membrane or other bulkier tissue. It may be structureless or part of a structure, as the laminae of the vertebral arch.

lamina densa, a layer of epithelial basal lamina that appears dark in electron micrographs.

lamina dura, **1.** a sheet of compact alveolar bone that lies adjacent to the periodontal membrane, the lining of the alveolus. **2.** a radiographic term used to identify the radiopaque lining of an alveolus.

lamina lucida, an electron-dense layer of the basal lamina lying between the lamina densa and the adjoining cell layer,

divided in the pulmonary alveolus and renal glomerulus into the internal and external laminae rarae.

lamin antibody /lam″in/, a type of immunoglobulin found in the serum of some patients with autoimmune diseases, including systemic lupus erythematosus.

lamina of modiolus. See **modiolus.**

lamina propria, a layer of connective tissue that lies just under the epithelium of a mucous membrane.

laminar airflow (laf) /lam′iner/ [L, *lamina,* plate; Gk, *aer;* AS, *flowan*], a system of circulating filtered air in parallel-flowing planes in hospitals or other health care facilities. The system reduces the risk of airborne contamination and exposure to chemical pollutants in surgical theaters, food-preparation areas, hospital pharmacies, and laboratories.

lamina rara, **1.** in the renal glomerulus and pulmonary alveolus, one of the layers of lamina lucida surrounding the lamina densa. The lamina rara externa is on the epithelial side and the lamina rara interna is on the endothelial side. **2.** a term sometimes used as a synonym for lamina lucida.

laminar flow. See **laminar airlow.**

Laminaria /lam′iner″ē·ə/ [L, *lamina,* plate], a genus of large brown algae that includes seaweed.

laminaria tent, a cone of dried seaweed that swells as it absorbs water. It is used to dilate the cervix nontraumatically in preparation for induced abortion or induced labor.

laminated thrombus /lam″inā′tid/, a blood clot composed of blood platelets, fibrin, clotting factors, and cellular elements arranged in layers, apparently formed at different times.

laminectomy /lam′inek″təmē/ [L, *lamina* + Gk, *ektomē,* excision], surgical removal of the bony arches of one or more vertebrae. It is performed to treat compression fractures, dislocations, herniated nucleus pulposus, and cord tumors and to stimulate the spinal cord. With the patient under general anesthesia and prone to eliminate lordosis, reduce venous congestion, and keep the abdomen free, the laminae are removed, and the underlying problem is corrected. Spinal fusion with cages, rods, screws, and/or bone graft is used to stabilize the spine if several laminae are removed. If the procedure is a cervical laminectomy, the patient is observed for signs of respiratory distress caused by cord edema. Motor function and sensation in the extremities are evaluated every 2 to 4 hours for 48 hours. The dressing is examined frequently for hemorrhage or leakage of cerebrospinal fluid. The patient is taught to logroll without twisting the spine or hips. –*laminectomize, v.*

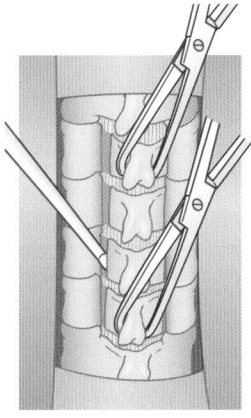

Laminectomy *(Komotar, Mocco, and Kaiser, 2006)*

L

laminin /lam″inin/, any of several large glycoproteins consisting of three polypeptide subunits and found in basement membranes. It facilitates linkage with collagen and other basement membrane components and is involved in neurite regeneration.

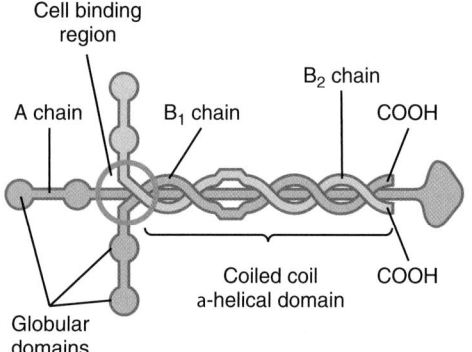

Laminin *(Carlson, 2009)*

laminotomy /-ot″əmē/, the surgical division of the lamina of a vertebral arch. Also called **rachiotomy.**

lamivudine (3TC) /lämiv′udēn/, a nucleoside analog that inhibits reverse transcriptase and is used as an antiviral agent in treatment of hepatitis B infection and, in combination with zidovudine, in treatment of HIV infection and AIDS. Administered orally.

■ INDICATIONS: The Epivir brand name form of this drug is used to treat HIV infection in combination with zidovudine. The Epivir-HBV brand name form is used to treat hepatitis B.

■ CONTRAINDICATIONS: Known hypersensitivity to this drug prohibits its use.

■ ADVERSE EFFECTS: Life-threatening effects are neutropenia, anemia, thrombocytopenia, and pediatric pancreatitis. Other adverse effects are anorexia, cramps, dyspepsia, taste change, hearing loss, and photophobia. Common side effects are fever, headache, malaise, dizziness, insomnia, depression, fatigue, chills, nausea, vomiting, diarrhea, cough, rash, myalgia, arthralgia, and musculoskeletal pain.

lamotrigine /lämo′trijēn/, an anticonvulsive used in treatment of certain forms of epilepsy.

■ INDICATIONS: It is prescribed as adjunct therapy in the treatment of partial seizures in epilepsy patients over the age of 16 and as an adjunct therapy for children under 16 years of age with generalized seizures associated with Lennox-Gastaut syndrome. It is not approved for use in children less than 2 years of age.

■ CONTRAINDICATIONS: Known hypersensitivity to this drug prohibits its use.

■ ADVERSE EFFECTS: The most serious adverse effects include hepatotoxicity, potentially life-threatening rash, and Stevens-Johnson syndrome. When discontinued, the drug should be tapered off gradually over a 2-week period to avoid patient risk-rebound effect.

lampbrush chromosome [Gk, *lampas,* torch; AS, *bryst,* bristle], an excessively large type of chromosome found in the oocytes of many animals. It has long, threadlike, projecting loops, giving it a hairy, brushlike appearance. See also **giant chromosome.**

lampro-, combining form meaning "clear": *lamprophony.*

lamprophony, the clarity and loudness of the spoken voice.

LAN, abbreviation for **local area network.**

lance [L, *lancea,* spear], to incise a furuncle or an abscess to release accumulated pus. A topical anesthetic is applied, the lesion is incised, and the pus is drained. A drain is inserted if the infection is deep. The bacteria involved are most often staphylococci. An antibiotic is given systemically if the boil is facial to prevent infection from spreading into the cranial sinuses. Infected drainage is kept off surrounding skin to prevent a recurrence. Careful handwashing is essential to prevent spread of infection to others.

Lancefield's classification [Rebecca C. Lancefield, American bacteriologist, 1895–1981], a serological classification of streptococci based on their antigenic characteristics. The bacteria are divided into 13 groups by the identification of their pathological action. Group A contains most of the streptococci that cause infection in humans. Groups B to O are less pathogenic and are often present without causing disease. Most are hemolytic; of those, the beta subgroup is the most likely to be the cause of infection.

lancet /lan″sit/ [L, *lancea,* lance], a short, pointed needle-like blade used to obtain a drop of blood for a capillary sample. It has a guard above the blade that prevents deep incision.

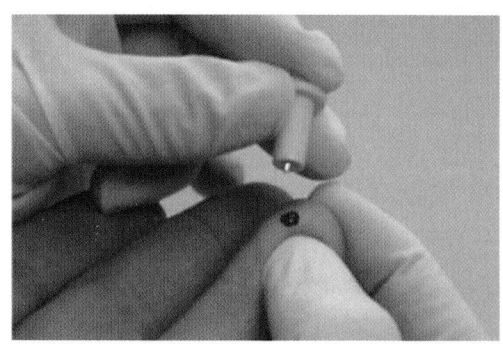

Lancet *(Zakus, 2001)*

lancinating /lan″sinā′ting/ [L, *lancea,* lance], sharply cutting or tearing, such as lancinating pain.

Landau-Kleffner syndrome /län′dou klef′nər/ [William M. Landau, 20th-century American neurologist; F.R. Kleffner, 20th-century American neurologist], an epileptic syndrome of childhood characterized by partial or generalized seizures, psychomotor abnormalities, and language regression that can progress to mutism. The electroencephalogram from bilateral temporal regions is abnormal. Also called **acquired epileptic aphasia.**

Landau reflex /län′dou/, a normal response of infants when held in a horizontal prone position to maintain a convex arc with the head raised and the legs slightly flexed. The reflex is displayed at about 3 months of age. It is poor in those with floppy infant syndrome and exaggerated in hypertonic and opisthotonic infants.

landmark /land′mark/ [AS, *land + meark,* mark], a readily recognizable anatomical structure used as a point of reference in establishing the location of another structure or in determining certain measurements.

landmark position [AS, *land + meark,* mark; L, *positio*], the correct placement of the hands on the chest in cardiopulmonary resuscitation. See also **cardiopulmonary resuscitation.**

Landouzy-Dejerine muscular dystrophy. See **fascioscapulohumeral muscular dystrophy.**

Langer-Giedion syndrome /lang′ər zhēdē·ôN′/ [Leonard O. Langer, Jr., 20th-century American physician; A. Giedion, 20th-century Swiss physician], an inherited disorder characterized by cognitive impairment, microcephaly, multiple outgrowths on the bones, characteristic facies with bulbous nose, sparse hair, cone-shaped epiphyses, loose redundant skin, joint laxity, and other anomalies.

Langerhans cells /lung″ərhuns, lang″ərhans/ [Paul Langerhans, German pathologist, 1847–1888], stellate dendritic cells found mostly in the stratum spinosum of the epidermis. They are believed to have an immune function, with surface markers characteristic of macrophages and monocytes.

Langer line. See **cleavage line.**

Langer's muscle /läng′ərz/ [Carl Ritter von Edenberg von Langer, Austrian anatomist, 1819–1887], a muscle that extends from the insertion of the pectoralis major muscle over the bicipital groove to the insertion of the latissimus dorsi.

Langhans layer. See **cytotrophoblast.**

language /lang″gwij/ [L, *lingua,* tongue], **1.** a defined set of characters that, when used alone or in combinations, forms a meaningful set of words and symbols used for communication. **2.** a unified, related set of commands or instructions that a computer can use to perform work.

language delay, specific language skills that are slow to emerge or develop but that are acquired by the child in the same sequence seen in children without delays. See also **language disorder.**

language disorder, **1.** a partial or complete disruption in the ability to understand and/or produce the conventional symbols or words that comprise one's native language. **2.** a deviation from the usual rate and sequence in which specific language skills emerge.

lano-, prefix meaning "wool": *lanolin.*

lanolin /lan″əlin/ [L, *lana,* wool, *oleum,* oil], a fatlike substance from the wool of sheep. It contains about 25% water as a water-in-oil emulsion and is used as an ointment base and an emollient for the skin. Also called **hydrous wool fat.**

Lanoxin, a cardiac glycoside. Brand name for **digoxin.**

lanreotide, an antigrowth hormone.

■ INDICATIONS: This drug is used to treat acromegaly in patients having an inadequate response to other treatments.

■ CONTRAINDICATIONS: Known hypersensitivity to this drug or latex allergy prohibits its use.

lansoprazole, an antiulcer agent and proton pump inhibitor.

■ INDICATIONS: It is used to treat gastroesophageal reflux disease (GERD), severe erosive esophagitis, poorly responsive systemic GERD, and pathological hypersecretory conditions (Zollinger-Ellison syndrome, systemic mastocytosis, multiple endocrine adenomas). It is also a potentially effective treatment for duodenal and gastric ulcers and for maintenance of healed duodenal ulcers.

■ CONTRAINDICATIONS: Known hypersensitivity to this drug prohibits its use.

■ ADVERSE EFFECTS: Life-threatening effects are cerebrovascular accident, myocardial infarction, shock, hematuria, and hemolysis. Other adverse effects include confusion, agitation, amnesia, depression, diarrhea, vomiting, nausea, acid regurgitation, anorexia, irritable colon, upper respiratory infections, asthma, bronchitis, dyspnea, alopecia, weight gain or loss, gout, deafness, eye pain, otitis media, chest pain, angina, tachycardia, bradycardia, palpitations, hypertension or hypotension, vasodilation, glycosuria, impotence, kidney calculus, breast enlargement, and anemia.

lanthanum (La) /lan″thənəm/ [Gk, *lanthanein,* to escape notice], **1.** a rare earth metallic element. Its atomic number is 57; its atomic mass is 138.91. **2.** a phosphate binder, lanthanum carbonate.

■ INDICATIONS: This drug is used to treat end-stage renal disease.

■ CONTRAINDICATIONS: Hypophosphatemia or known hypersensitivity to this drug prohibits its use.

lanuginous /lənoo″jinəs/ [L, *lanugo,* down], pertaining to lanugo.

lanugo /lanyoo″gō/ [L, down], the soft, downy hair covering a normal fetus beginning in the fifth month of gestation and almost entirely shed by the ninth month.

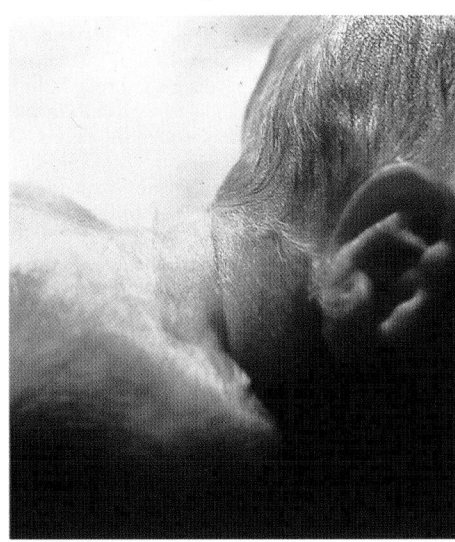

Lanugo *(Eichenfield et al, 2015)*

lanulous /lan″yoolos/ [L, *lana,* wool, *osus,* filled with], downy or covered with short, fine woolly hair, such as the skin of a fetus. See also **lanugo.**

lap, abbreviation for **laparotomy.**

LAP, **1.** abbreviation for *left atrial pressure.* **2.** abbreviation for **leukocyte alkaline phosphatase. 3.** abbreviation for *leucine aminopeptidase.* See **leucine aminopeptidase (LAP) test.**

laparectomy /lap′ərek″təmē/, the surgical removal of tissue from the abdomen wall, usually performed to correct muscle laxity.

laparo- /lap′ərō/, prefix meaning "abdomen" or "abdominal wall": *laparectomy, laparotomy, laparomyitis.*

laparoenterostomy /lap′ərō·en′təros″təmē/ [Gk, *lapara,* loin, *enteron,* bowel, *stoma,* mouth], the surgical installation of a tube through an external opening in the abdomen to drain the bowel. A similar procedure may be used to supply nutrients to a patient with an upper digestive tract obstruction. See also **jejunostomy.**

laparoenterotomy /lap′ərō·en′tərot″əmē/ [Gk, *lapara,* loin, *enteron,* bowel, *temnein,* to cut], a surgical incision in the intestine through the abdominal wall.

laparohysterectomy /-his′tərek″təmē/ [Gk, *lapara,* loin, *hystera,* womb, *ektomē,* excision], a surgical procedure to remove the uterus performed by making an excision through the abdominal wall.

laparohystero-oophorectomy /-his″tərō-/, the surgical removal of the uterus and ovaries through a small incision in the abdominal wall.

laparohysterosalpingo-oophorectomy /-his′tərō′salping″gō-/, the surgical removal of the uterus, ovaries, and fallopian tubes through a small incision in the abdominal wall. Also called **total hysterectomy.**

laparomyitis /-mī-ī″tis/, an inflammation of the abdominal or lumbar muscles.

laparosalpingo-oophorectomy /-salping″gō-/, the surgical removal of the ovaries and fallopian tubes through a small incision in the abdominal wall.

laparoscope /lap″ərəskōp′/ [Gk, *lapara,* loin, *skopein,* to look], a type of endoscope consisting of an illuminated tube with an optical system. It is inserted through the abdominal wall for examining the peritoneal cavity. Also called **celioscope, peritoneoscope.** –*laparoscopic, adj.,* –**laparoscopy,** *n.*

laparoscopic-assisted vaginal hysteroscopy /-skop″ik/, a procedure for viewing the inner surface of the uterus with a specially designed endoscope inserted through the cervix. Before insertion the uterus is inflated with carbon dioxide or a glucose solution administered through the cervix. See also **hysteroscopy, laparoscopy.**

laparoscopic biopsy, biopsy of the abdominal organs performed with instruments introduced through a laparoscope for the removal of tissue.

laparoscopic cholecystectomy. See **cholecystectomy.**

laparoscopic gastric banding (LGB), a surgical procedure for weight loss in which a band is placed around the stomach; the procedure is performed with the use of a fiberoptic instrument.

laparoscopic nephrectomy, a minimally invasive type of nephrectomy performed with laparoscopic techniques.

laparoscopic sterilization [Gk, *lapara,* loin, *skopein,* to view; L, *sterilis,* barren], prevention of pregnancy by inserting a specialized endoscope through a small incision in the abdominal wall and closing off the fallopian tubes with clips or performing electrocoagulation or severance on the tubes.

laparoscopy /lap′ɔros″kɔpē/, a technique to examine the abdominal cavity with a laparoscope through one or more small incisions in the abdominal wall, usually at the umbilicus. The abdominal cavity is filled with gas, usually carbon dioxide, to move the abdominal wall for better inspection. The procedure is used for inspection of the gallbladder, ovaries, and fallopian tubes; diagnosis of endometriosis, intestinal conditions, and hernias; destruction of uterine leiomyomas; and myomectomy. Gynecological sterilization also can be accomplished by fulguration of the oviducts or by tubal ligation. Also called **abdominoscopy.** See also **endoscopy, laparoscope.**

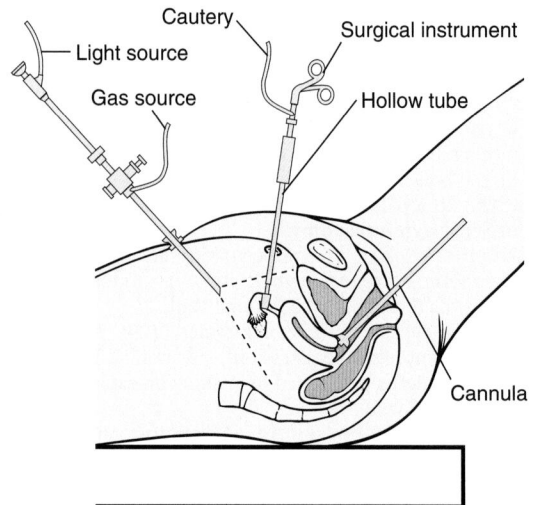

Labeled: Cautery, Light source, Surgical instrument, Gas source, Hollow tube, Cannula

Laparoscopy *(Frazier, 2013)*

laparotomy (lap) /lap′ɔrot″ɔmē/ [Gk, *lapara* + *temnein,* to cut], any surgical incision into the abdominal wall, usually performed under general or regional anesthesia, often on an exploratory basis. –*laparotomize, v.*

laparotomy sponge, a gauze pad with radiopaque thread used as an absorbent and as a covering for the viscera.

lapatinib, a miscellaneous antineoplastic drug.
■ INDICATIONS: This drug is used to treat advanced breast cancer in patients with tumors that overexpress HER2 protein and who have received previous chemotherapy.
■ CONTRAINDICATIONS: Pregnancy, breastfeeding, torsades de pointes, or known hypersensitivity to this drug prohibits its use.
■ ADVERSE EFFECTS: Adverse effects of this drug include fatigue, insomnia, palpitations, anorexia, diarrhea, dyspepsia, mouth ulcerations, nausea, vomiting, xerosis, rash, palmarplantar erythrodysesthesia, and dyspnea. Life-threatening side effects include heart failure, QT prolongation, anemia, neutropenia, and thrombocytopenia.

lapboard [ME, *lappa* + *bord,* plank], **1.** a flat board placed over the lap to serve as a temporary desk or table. Lapboards are sometimes used for individuals with disabilities for writing activities, eating, and preparing food when motor impairments interfere with the ability to use a table or counter. **2.** a padded extension placed on the arm of a wheelchair to support the arm and shoulder.

lapis /lap′is/ [L, stone], any substance that does not easily volatilize, such as lapis dentalis, or tooth tartar.

Laplace's law /läpläs″/ [Pierre S. de Laplace, French physicist, 1749–1827], a principle of physics that the tension on the wall of a sphere is the product of the pressure times the radius of the chamber and that the tension is inversely related to the thickness of the wall.

-lapse, suffix meaning "a slip or fall backward": *collapse, prolapse, relapse.*

large calorie. See **Calorie.**

large for gestational age (LGA) infant, a newborn whose fetal growth was accelerated and whose size and weight at birth fall above the 90th percentile of appropriate for gestational age infants, whether delivered prematurely, at term, or later than term. Factors other than genetic influences that cause accelerated intrauterine growth include maternal diabetes mellitus and Beckwith's syndrome. LGA infants born of diabetic mothers have very pink skin and red, shiny cheeks. They are often listless and limp, feed poorly, and become hypoglycemic within the first few hours. A major problem is that preterm LGA infants, because of their size, are not recognized as high-risk neonates with immature organ system development. Often these infants develop respiratory distress syndrome because pulmonary maturation occurs later in gestation. In cases of Beckwith's syndrome the infant is characterized by gigantism, macroglossia, omphalocele or umbilical hernia. Compare **appropriate for gestational age (AGA) infant, small for gestational age (SGA) infant.**

large intestine [L, *largus,* abundant, *intestinum*], the part of the digestive tract comprising the cecum; appendix; ascending, transverse, descending, and sigmoid colons; and rectum. The ileocecal valve separates the cecum from the ileum.

lariat structure /ler″ē·ɔt/, a ring of intron segments that has been spliced out of a messenger ribonucleic acid molecule by enzymes. Some introns form a long tail attached to the ring, giving the structure the appearance of a microscopic cowboy lariat.

Larmor frequency [Joseph Larmor, Irish physicist, 1857–1942], the frequency of the precession of a charged particle when its motion comes under the influence of an applied magnetic field and a central force.

Larodopa, an antiparkinsonian agent. Brand name for **levodopa.**

Laron dwarfism /lä·rôN′/ [Zvi Laron, Israeli endocrinologist, b. 1927], an autosomal-recessive syndrome of skeletal growth delay resulting from impaired ability to synthesize

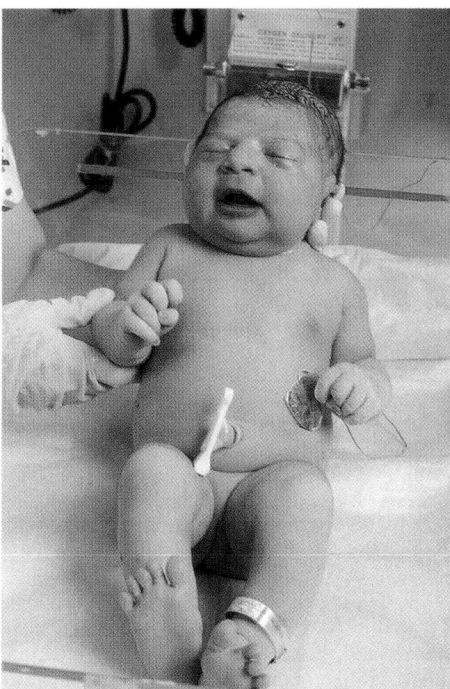

Large for gestational age infant *(Murray and McKinney, 2006)*

insulin-like growth factor I, usually because of growth hormone receptor defects. Also called *Laron syndrome.*

laronidase,   a medication used for enzyme replacement therapy.

■ INDICATIONS: This drug is used to treat mucopolysaccharidosis I.

■ CONTRAINDICATIONS: Known hypersensitivity to this drug prohibits its use.

Larsen syndrome /lär′sən/ [Loren Joseph Larsen, American orthopedic surgeon, b. 1914], a rare genetic disorder characterized by cleft palate, flattened facies, multiple congenital dislocations, and foot deformities.

larva /lär′və/ *pl.* **larvae** [L, specter], the early immature form of an animal, which undergoes metamorphosis to an adult form. It is one of the growth stages for some insects; the state between the egg and the pupolarval stage is the feeding stage in the growth process. −*larval, adj.*

larva migrans.   See **cutaneous larva migrans, visceral larva migrans.**

laryng-.   See **laryngo-, laryng-.**

laryngeal /lerin′jē·əl/ [Gk, *larynx*], pertaining to the larynx.

laryngeal artery,   either of the two arteries, superior and inferior, that are responsible for the major blood supply to the larynx.

laryngeal cancer [Gk, *larynx* + L, *cancer,* crab], a malignant neoplastic disease characterized by a tumor arising from the epithelium of the structures of the larynx. Laryngeal tumors are more common in men than in women and occur most frequently between 50 and 70 years of age. Alcohol intake and tobacco smoking correlate to an increase in the risk of developing the cancer. Persistent hoarseness is usually the first sign. Advanced lesions may cause a sore throat, dyspnea, dysphagia, and cervical adenopathy. Diagnostic measures include direct laryngoscopy, biopsy, MRI, and radiological examination, including tomographic studies and chest films. Malignant tumors of the larynx are usually epidermoid carcinomas. Radiation is generally recommended for small lesions. Total laryngectomy, often combined with radiotherapy, is indicated for extensive lesions. Chemotherapy may be used to try to spare the larynx. After the operation a speech therapist will assist the individual to develop a new sound source for speech. See also **laryngectomy.**

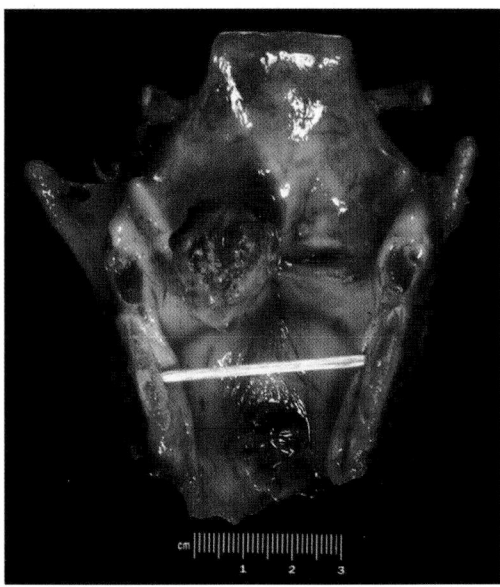

Squamous cell carcinoma of the larynx
(Gattuso et al, 2015)

laryngeal catheterization,   the insertion of a catheter into the larynx for the purpose of removing secretions or introducing gases.

laryngeal diphtheria.   See **diphtheritic laryngitis.**

laryngeal edema,   swelling of the laryngeal mucosa, often due to an allergy. See also **edema of glottis.**

laryngeal inlet,   the opening connecting the larynx and pharynx.

laryngeal mask airway (LMA),   a device for maintaining a patent airway without tracheal intubation, consisting of a tube connected to an oval inflatable cuff that seals the larynx. It was the first effective product to offer significant advantages over traditional methods of airway support during surgical procedures and lifesaving interventions.

laryngeal polyp [Gk, *larynx* + *poly,* many, *pous,* foot], a polyp on the vocal cords that causes hoarseness, resulting from vocal abuse or smoking.

laryngeal pouch.   See **laryngocele.**

laryngeal prominence,   the bulge at the front of the neck produced by the thyroid cartilage of the larynx. Also called **Adam's apple.**

laryngeal reflex [Gk, *larynx* + L, *reflectere,* to bend back], a cough reflex caused by irritation of the arched opening at the back of the throat.

laryngeal vertigo [Gk, *larynx* + L, *vertere,* to turn], a short episode of dizziness or unconsciousness after a paroxysmal attack of coughing or laryngeal spasm. Also called **cough syncope.**

laryngeal web,   a congenital malformation of the larynx that may be thin and translucent or thicker and more fibrotic. It is spread between the vocal folds near the anterior commissure. It may cause hoarseness, aphonia, or respiratory symptoms.

laryngectomy /ler′injek″təmē/ [Gk, *larynx* + *ektomē,* excision], surgical removal of the larynx performed to treat cancer of the larynx. In a partial laryngectomy only the vocal cords are removed. If the malignancy is extensive, the entire larynx is removed, along with the hyoid, epiglottis, false cords, true cords, cricoid cartilage, and two or three rings of the trachea; the trachea is sutured to the skin of the neck, and the patient breathes through his or her neck, not through the mouth. Compare **neck dissection, radical neck dissection.** –*laryngectomize, v.*

■ OBSERVATIONS: After surgery the patient is observed for bleeding. A humidified oxygen vaporizer may decrease coughing and mucous viscosity. IV fluids are given, and liquid feedings may be given via nasogastric tube.

■ INTERVENTIONS: The patient cannot smell, sniff, or blow his or her nose. A Magic Slate and flash cards are useful for communication. Speech loss is permanent after total laryngectomy.

■ PATIENT CARE CONSIDERATIONS: Before complete laryngectomy the patient is referred to a speech pathologist to discuss alaryngeal communication methods. This operation is permanent.

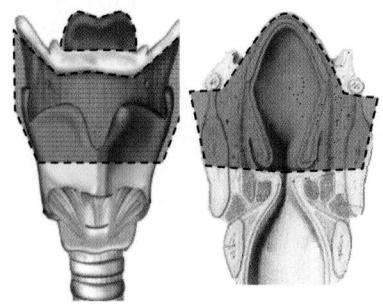

Laryngectomy *(Russi et al, 2012)*

laryngismus stridulus, a sudden laryngeal spasm with cyanosis and inhalation accompanied by a crowing sound, usually seen in children at night. Also called **crowing inspiration, spasmatic croup, spasmodic croup.**

laryngitis /ler′injī″tis/ [Gk, *larynx* + *itis*], inflammation of the mucous membrane lining the larynx, accompanied by edema of the vocal cords with hoarseness or loss of voice, occurring as an acute disorder caused by a cold, irritating fumes, or sudden temperature changes or as a chronic condition resulting from excessive use of the voice, heavy smoking, or exposure to irritating fumes. In acute laryngitis there may be a cough, and the throat usually feels scratchy and painful. The patient is advised to remain in an environment with an even temperature, to avoid talking and exposure to tobacco smoke, and to inhale steam containing aromatic vapors. Acute laryngitis may cause severe respiratory distress in children under 5 years of age because the relatively small larynx of the young child is subject to spasm when irritated or infected and readily becomes partially or totally obstructed. The youngster may develop a hoarse, barking cough and an inspiratory stridor and may become restless, gasping for air. Treatment consists of the administration of copious amounts of vaporized cool mist. Chronic laryngitis may be treated by removal of irritants, avoidance of smoking, voice rest, correction of stressful voice habits, cough medication, steam inhalations, and spraying the throat with an astringent antiseptic, such as hexylresorcinol.

laryngo-, laryng-, prefix meaning "larynx": *laryngocele, laryngography.*

laryngocele /ləring″gōsēl′/, an abnormal air-containing cavity connected to the laryngeal ventricle. It is caused by a protrusion of the mucous membrane of the ventricle and may displace and enlarge the false vocal cord, resulting in hoarseness and airway obstruction. Because a laryngocele is also a potential reservoir of infection, it is usually excised. Also called **laryngeal pouch, saccule of larynx.**

laryngography. See **laryngopharyngography.**

laryngologist /ler′ing·gol″əjist/, a physician who specializes in the diagnosis and treatment of disorders of the throat.

laryngology /ler′ing·gol″əjē/ [Gk, *larynx* + *logos,* science], the branch of medicine that specializes in the causes and treatments of disorders of the larynx.

laryngopharyngeal /-ferin″jē·əl/, pertaining to the larynx and pharynx. See also **laryngopharynx.**

laryngopharyngeal reflux, a complication of gastroesophageal reflux caused by reflux from the esophagus into the pharynx, characterized by a variety of intermittent chronic symptoms, including hoarseness, cough, throat clearing, and dysphagia.

laryngopharyngitis /ləring′gōfer′injī″tis/ [Gk, *larynx* + *pharynx,* throat, *itis*], inflammation of the larynx and pharynx. See also **laryngitis, pharyngitis.**

laryngopharyngography /ləring′gōfer′ing·gog″rəfē/ [Gk, *larynx* + *pharynx* + *graphein,* to record], the radiographic examination of the larynx and pharynx. Also called **laryngography.**

laryngopharynx /ləring′gōfer″ingks/ [Gk, *larynx* + *pharynx,* throat,], one of the three regions of the throat, extending from the hyoid bone to the esophagus. Compare **nasopharynx, oropharynx.** –**laryngopharyngeal,** *adj.*

laryngoplastic phonosurgery, open-neck surgery that restructures the cartilaginous framework of the larynx.

laryngoscope /ləring″gəskōp/, an endoscope for examining the larynx.

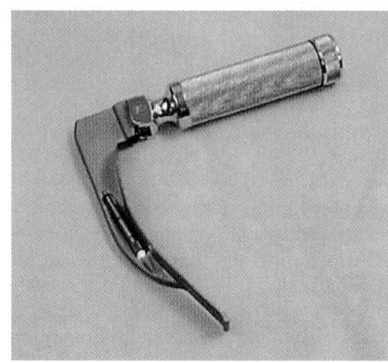

Laryngoscope *(Zakus, 2001)*

laryngoscopy /ler′ing·gos″kəpē/ [Gk, *larynx* + *skopein,* to view], the use of a lighted fiberoptic instrument to view the larynx. See also **indirect laryngoscopy.** –*laryngoscopic, adj.*

laryngospasm /ləring″gōspaz′əm/ [Gk, *larynx* + *spasmos,* spasm], a spasmodic closure of the larynx.

laryngostasis. See **croup.**

laryngotomy /ler′ing·got″əmē/ [Gk, *larynx* + *temnein,* to cut], a surgical incision into the larynx through the cricovocal membrane. It is usually an emergency procedure that is performed when a standard tracheotomy cannot be done.

laryngotracheal tube, the embryonic endodermal tube that is split off from the primordium of the oropharynx and esophagus when the tracheoesophageal septum divides the cranial part of the foregut. It constitutes the primordium of the larynx, trachea, bronchi, and lungs.

laryngotracheitis /-trā′kē·ī″tis/, an inflammation of the larynx and trachea.

laryngotracheobronchitis (LTB) /lering′gōtrā′kē·ō′brong-kī″tis/ [Gk, *larynx* + L, *trachea*; Gk, *bronchos,* windpipe, *itis*], an inflammation of the major respiratory passages, usually causing hoarseness, nonproductive cough, dyspnea, and, in severe cases, significant airway obstruction. Among the causes are infections by coxsackieviruses, echoviruses, *Haemophilus influenzae,* and *Corynebacterium diphtheriae.* Treatment usually includes steam inhalations, cough suppressants, and, for bacterial infections, appropriate antibiotics. See also **croup.**

laryngotracheoesophageal cleft, a cleft between the larynx and the upper trachea resulting from incomplete separation of these structures during embryonic development, with respiratory manifestations including respiratory distress with feeding, flaccid aryepiglottic folds, chronic cough, and increased oral secretions. It is frequently associated with other congenital anomalies of the respiratory system or GI tract. Complications include failure to thrive and recurrent aspiration pneumonia.

laryngotracheotomy /-trā′kē·ot″əmē/, a surgical incision into the larynx and trachea.

larynx /ler″ingks/ [Gk], the organ of voice that is part of the upper air passage connecting the pharynx with the trachea. It accounts for a large bump in the neck called the Adam's apple and is larger in men than in women, although it remains the same size in men and women until puberty. The larynx forms the caudal portion of the anterior wall of the pharynx and is lined with mucous membrane that is continuous with that of the pharynx and the trachea. The larynx extends vertically to the fourth, fifth, and sixth cervical vertebrae and is somewhat higher in women and children. It is composed of three single cartilages and three paired cartilages, all connected by ligaments, moved by various muscles and nerves, and with a blood supply from the common carotid artery and other vessels. The single cartilages are the thyroid, cricoid, and epiglottis. The paired cartilages are the arytenoid, corniculate, and cuneiform, which support the vocal folds. Also called **voice box. –laryngeal,** *adj.*

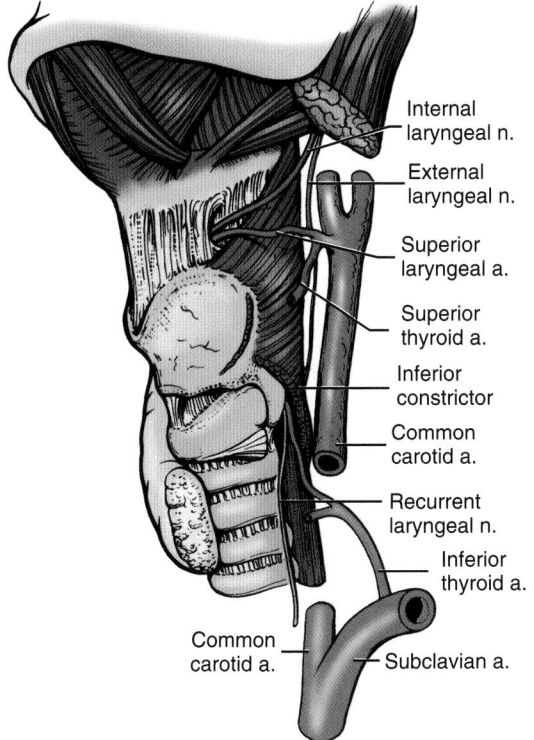

Internal laryngeal n.
External laryngeal n.
Superior laryngeal a.
Superior thyroid a.
Inferior constrictor
Common carotid a.
Recurrent laryngeal n.
Inferior thyroid a.
Common carotid a.
Subclavian a.

Lateral view of larynx and blood supply
(Murray et al, 2015)

LAS, abbreviation for **lymphadenopathy syndrome.**

laser /lā″zər/, a source of intense monochromatic radiation of the visible, ultraviolet, or infrared portions of the spectrum. Lasers are used in surgery to divide or cause adhesions or to destroy or fix tissue in place. Abbreviation for *light amplification by stimulated emission of radiation.* Also called **optic laser, optic maser.**

laser angioplasty, the opening of an occluded artery with laser energy delivered to the site through a fiberoptic probe.

laser bronchoscopy, a procedure to examine the airways performed with the aid of a laser beam directed through fiberoptic equipment. The procedure is used in the diagnosis and treatment of bronchial disorders, tracheobronchial tumors, and subglottic stenosis.

laser iridotomy, a procedure for the treatment of closed-angle glaucoma in which an opening is created in the peripheral iris so that the aqueous fluid is granted access to the trabecular meshwork drainage system. It is usually performed after control of an acute attack when signs of ocular congestion have disappeared. It is also used for prophylaxis against anticipated attacks.

laser pain management, the use of lasers to relieve pain. The laser can be used in place of acupuncture needles at acupuncture points or may be used directly over the source of pain.

laser printer, a high-speed output device for computers using a technique in which laser beams focus images on photosensitive drums. Compare **impact printer.**

laser prostatectomy, removal of the prostate after it has been exposed to a laser either by direct contact with vaporization or by an indirect system that causes coagulation necrosis.

laser trabeculoplasty, an application of argon or selective laser energy to the trabecular meshwork to increase aqueous outflow in the treatment of glaucoma. The procedure may be recommended when intraocular pressure increases despite administration of topical agents. The eye is anesthetized with a topical anesthetic. The trabecular network is viewed through an antireflective-coated four-mirror gonioprism. A power setting and exposure time are selected to blanch the anterior trabecular meshwork with laser energy without causing bubble formation. A potential complication is a temporary increase in intraocular pressure, which is treated with drugs. The effects of laser trabeculoplasty are not always long-lasting.

LASIK /lā′sik/, acronym for laser-assisted in-situ keratomileusis, a refractive surgery on the cornea in which the excimer laser and microkeratome are combined for correction of distance vision. The microkeratome is used to shave a thin slice and create a hinged flap in the cornea, the flap is reflected back, the exposed cornea is reshaped by the laser, and the flap is replaced, without sutures, to heal back into position. Preoperatively, a topical antibiotic and topical anesthesia are instilled in the eye. Postoperatively, the patient receives antibiotic drops and antiinflammatory drops and wears goggles for 24 hours to prevent slippage.

Lasix, a diuretic. Brand name for **furosemide.**

Lassa fever /lä″sə/ [Lassa, Nigeria; L, *febris,* fever], a highly contagious disease of West Africa caused by an arenavirus. It is transmitted by contact with or inhalation of excreta of infected rodents. Person-to-person transmission occurs through contact with infected blood, secretions, or excreta, or transmission may be airborne. See also

Arenavirus, **Argentine hemorrhagic fever, Bolivian hemorrhagic fever.**

■ OBSERVATIONS: Lassa fever is characterized by fever, pharyngitis, dysphagia, and ecchymoses. Varying degrees of deafness occur in one third of cases. Pleural effusion, edema and renal involvement, mental disorientation, confusion, and death from cardiac failure often ensue.

■ INTERVENTIONS: Early treatment with ribavirin and supportive symptomatic care are essential.

■ PATIENT CARE CONSIDERATIONS: Lassa fever is common in West Africa but rarely seen in North America. A case was reported in New Jersey in 2015 following travel to Africa.

last sacraments [ME, *laste* + L, *sacramentum,* solemn oath], a religious ceremony performed by a member of the clergy on behalf of a person about to die. Also called *last rites.*

latanoprost /lah-tan′o-prost″/, an agent applied topically to the conjunctiva for treatment of open-angle glaucoma and ocular hypertension.

latchkey children, *(Informal)* minors who are often at home alone because their parents are at work.

late dyspituitary eunuchism. See **acromegalic eunuchoidism.**

latency period /lā″tənsē/ [L, *latere,* to be concealed; Gk, *peri* + *hodos,* way], **1.** the period between contact with a pathogen and development of symptoms. Also called **incubation period. 2.** the time between stimulus and response. **3.** a stage of psychosocial development. See **latency stage.**

latency stage [L, *latere,* to be concealed; Fr, *estage,* stage], (in psychoanalysis) a period in psychosexual development occurring between 6 years of age and puberty when sexual motivation and expression are repressed or transferred, through sublimation, to the feelings and behavioral patterns expected as typical of the age. In this stage, the child develops same-sex friendships.

latent /lā″tənt/ [L, *latere,* to be concealed], dormant; existing as a potential. For example, tuberculosis may be latent for extended periods of time and become active under certain conditions. —*latency, n.*

latent allergy, an allergy that does not have overt symptoms but that may be detected by tests.

latent carcinoma. See **occult carcinoma.**

latent diabetes. See **impaired glucose tolerance.**

latent energy [L, *latere,* to be concealed; Gk, *energeia*], the energy contained in an object as a result of its position in space, its internal structure, and stresses imposed on it. Also called **potential energy.** Compare **kinetic energy.**

latent heat [L, *latere,* to be concealed; AS, *haetu*], the heat absorbed by a substance when it changes from a solid to a liquid or from a liquid to a gas without an accompanying rise in temperature.

latent learning [L, *latere,* to be concealed; ME, *lernen*], information or knowledge acquired unintentionally. It may remain in the subconscious until a need for the knowledge arises.

latent malaria [L, *latere,* to be concealed; It, *mal* + *aria,* bad air], a continuing infection without clinical symptoms, resulting from a balance established between the parasite and the body's immune system. See also **malaria.**

latent period, the interval between the time of exposure to an injurious dose of radiation and the response.

latent phase, the early stage of labor that is characterized by irregular, infrequent, and mild contractions and little or no dilation of the cervix or descent of the fetus. Also called **prodromal labor.** See also **Friedman curve.**

latent syphilis [L, *latere,* to be concealed; Gk, *syn,* together, *philein,* to love], a stage of syphilis infection in which no clinical symptoms appear, although serological tests indicate the presence of the syphilis spirochete. Latent syphilis occurs in two phases following secondary syphilis. The early phase occurs within 1 year of infection; the late phase occurs after 1 year of infection. Latency can persist for 3 to 30 years and does not always progress to tertiary syphilis. See also **syphilis.**

latent tetany [L, *latere,* to be concealed; Gk, *tetanos,* convulsive tension], a form of tetany that is elicited only by mechanical or electrical stimuli. Symptoms are nonspecific, including generalized weakness and cramping in the hand and foot.

late-phase hypersensitivity reaction, a type I hypersensitivity reaction that occurs after 2 to 4 hours and is mediated by mast cells.

lateral /lat″ərəl/ [L, *latus,* side], **1.** pertaining to the side. **2.** away from the midsagittal plane. **3.** farther from the midsagittal plane. **4.** to the right or left of the midsagittal plane. **5.** pertaining to a speech sound produced by passing air along one or both sides of the tongue, such as /l/. A lateral lisp impacts sounds such as /s/, /z/, /sh/, /ch/, and /j/.

lateral abdominal region. See **lateral region.**

lateral antebrachial cutaneous nerve, a continuation of the musculocutaneous nerve that innervates the skin over the radial side of the forearm and sometimes an area of skin of the back of the hand. Its modality is sensory.

lateral aortic node, a lumbar lymph node in any of three clusters of nodes serving the pelvis and abdomen. The afferent vessels from both sides drain various structures such as the testes, ovaries, kidneys, and lateral abdominal muscles. Most of the efferent vessels from the lateral aortic nodes converge to form the right and left lumbar trunks, which join the cisterna chyli. Compare **preaortic node, retroaortic node.**

lateral aperture of the fourth ventricle, an opening between the end of each lateral recess of the fourth ventricle and the subarachnoid space in the brain.

lateral atlantoaxial joint, either of a pair of joints between the first and second cervical vertebrae, one on each side of the body, formed by the inferior articular surface of the atlas and the superior surface of the axis.

lateral cerebellar nucleus. See **dentate nucleus.**

lateral cerebral sulcus, a deep cleft marking the division of the temporal lobe from the frontal and parietal lobes of the brain. Also called **fissure of Sylvius.**

lateral column. See **lateral horn.**

lateral condensation method, a technique for filling root canals in which a preselected master gutta-percha cone is sealed into the apex of the root and other auxiliary gutta-percha cones are forced laterally and compacted with a spreader hand instrument until the canal is filled. Compare **Johnson method.**

lateral corticospinal tract, a group of nerve fibers in the lateral funiculus of the spinal cord, originating in the cerebral cortex, that controls voluntary movement of the body.

lateral cuneiform bone, one of the three cuneiform bones of the foot. It is located in the center of the front row of tarsal bones between the intermediate cuneiform bone medially, the cuboid bone laterally, the scaphoid bone posteriorly, and the third metatarsal anteriorly. It also articulates with the second and fourth metatarsals. Also called **external cuneiform bone, third cuneiform bone.**

lateral decentering, (in radiology) an error in positioning of the tube head resulting in partial cutoff of the image on the receptor or when a focused grid is in use, also resulting in partial grid cutoff over the entire image.

lateral flexures of rectum, the three lateral bends in the rectum.

lateral geniculate body, one of two elevations of the lateral posterior thalamus receiving visual impulses from the retina via the optic nerves and tracts and relaying the impulses to the calcarine (visual) cortex.

lateral horn, a small hornlike projection of gray matter into the white matter of the spinal cord, located between the anterior and posterior horns or columns. Also called **intermediate column, lateral column.**

lateral humeral epicondylitis, inflammation of the tissue at the lower end of the humerus at the elbow joint, caused by the repetitive flexing of the wrist against resistance. It may result from athletic activity or manual manipulation of tools or other equipment. Pain radiates from the elbow joint. Also called **tennis elbow.** See also **epicondylitis.**

lateral incisal guide angle, the inclination of the incisal guide of a dental articulator in the frontal plane.

lateralis, lateral, a term denoting a structure situated farther from the median plane of the body or the midline of an organ.

laterality. See **handedness.**

lateralization /lat′əral′izā″shən/, the tendency for certain processes to be more highly developed on one side of the brain than the other, such as development of spatial and musical thoughts in the right hemisphere and verbal and logical processes in the left hemisphere in most persons.

lateral ligament of the ankle, one of the three ligaments on the lateral side of the ankle: the anterior talofibular ligament, the posterior talofibular ligament, and the calcaneofibular ligament.

lateral lobes of thyroid gland [L, *latus,* side; Gk, *lobos* + *thyreos,* shield; L, *glans,* acorn], the left and right lobes of the thyroid gland, situated in front of the neck. The two conical lobes lying on either side of and attached to the larynx are connected by a narrow isthmus.

lateral medullary syndrome. See **Wallenberg syndrome.**

lateral nystagmus [L, *latus,* side; Gk, *nystagmos,* nodding], an involuntary jerky movement in which the eyes move from side to side.

lateral pectoral nerve, one of a pair of branches from the brachial plexus that, with the medial pectoral nerve, supplies the pectoral muscles. It lies lateral to the axillary artery, arises from the lateral cord of the plexus or from the anterior divisions of the superior and middle trunks just before they unite into the cord, and ends on the deep surface of the clavicular and the cranial sternocostal parts of the pectoralis major. Compare **medial pectoral nerve.**

lateral pectoral region, the most lateral part of the pectoral region, bounded laterally by the axillary region.

lateral pelvic displacement, one of the five major kinetic determinants of gait. It helps to synchronize the rhythmic movements of walking and is produced by the horizontal shift of the pelvis or relative hip abduction. It is often a factor in the diagnosis and treatment of various orthopedic diseases, deformities, and abnormal conditions and in the analysis and correction of dysfunctional gaits. Compare **knee-ankle interaction, knee-hip flexion, pelvic rotation, pelvic tilt.**

lateral periodontal cyst, a developmental nonkeratinizing odontogenic cyst that arises from the periodontal ligament along the lateral root surface. The appearance is radiolucent with a round or teardrop shape with an opaque lateral margin. If multilocular, it is called a Botryoid odontogenic cyst. See also **Botryoid odontogenic cyst.**

lateral pinch, a grasp in which the thumb is opposed to the middle phalanx of the index finger. Also called **key pinch.**

lateral pivot shift test, a test for integrity of the anterior cruciate ligament. The patient lies prone with the hip flexed and the knee extended. The examiner gradually flexes the knee while pushing the outside of the knee medially and internally rotating the tibia. A thud or jerk at 30 to 40 degrees of flexion indicates deficiency of the anterior cruciate ligament.

lateral plantar nerve, one of the two terminal branches of the tibial nerve that innervates all but three intrinsic muscles in the sole of the foot and a strip of skin on the lateral side of the anterior two thirds of the sole and the adjacent plantar surfaces of the fifth toe and lateral half of the fourth.

lateral prehension, a type of pinch pattern consisting of contact of the thumb pad with the lateral surface of the distal, middle, or proximal phalanx of the index finger. Also called **key pinch, lateral pinch.**

lateral projection, a radiographic representation of the body produced by an x-ray beam that travels from the left to the right side of the body, or vice versa. It is a right lateral projection if the right side of the body is adjacent to the image receptor and a left lateral projection if the left side is adjacent to it.

lateral pubovesical ligament, the lateral branch of the pubovesical ligament in the female, extending from the bladder neck to the tendinous arch of the pelvic fascia.

lateral recumbent position, the posture assumed by the patient lying on the left side with the right thigh and knee drawn up. Also called **English position, obstetric position, semiprone side position.**

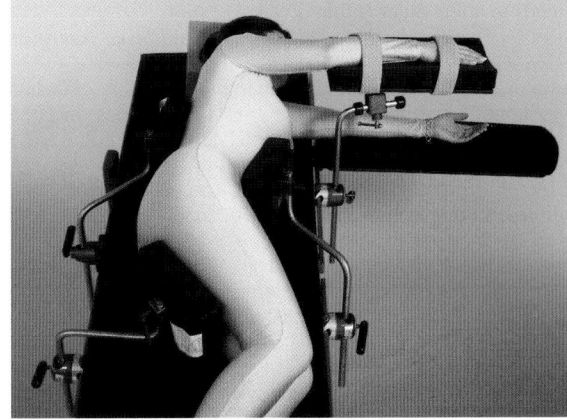

Lateral recumbent position *(Rothrock, 2015)*

lateral region, the part of the abdomen in the middle zone on both sides of the umbilical region. Also called **external abdominal region, lateral abdominal region, lumbar region.** See also **abdominal regions.**

lateral resolution, the resolution of objects in a plane perpendicular to the axis of an ultrasound beam. It is a measure of the ability of the system to detect closely separated objects, such as adjacent blood vessels.

lateral rocking, a sideways rocking of the body used to move the body forward or backward when normal muscle action is not possible. The technique is used by some individuals with disabilities to move the body to or from the edge of a chair or to a different sitting position on a bed. The rocking is performed while leaning the trunk forward with the arms in front and the head in line above the knees and feet, which are pulled back.

lateral rotation, a turning away from the midline of the body. Compare **medial rotation.** See also **rotation.**

lateral sacral artery, one of two arteries that originate from the posterior division of the internal iliac artery and give rise to branches that pass into the anterior sacral foramina to supply related bone and soft tissues, structures in the vertebral canal, and skin and muscle posterior to the sacrum.

lateral sinus [L, *latus,* side, *sinus,* hollow], one of the transverse bilateral sinuses of the dura mater that lie along the attached margin of the tentorium cerebelli. They receive the superior sagittal and straight sinuses and drain into the internal jugular veins.

lateral spinal curvature [L, *latus,* side, *spina,* backbone, *curvatura,* bend], a bending or abnormal curve of the vertebral column to the right or left side. See also **scoliosis.**

lateral sural cutaneous nerve, a branch of the common fibular nerve that innervates skin over the upper lateral leg.

lateral umbilical fold, a fold in the peritoneum produced by a slight protrusion of the inferior epigastric artery and the interfoveolar ligament. The lateral umbilical fold is about 3 cm lateral to the middle umbilical fold. Also called **plica umbilicalis lateralis.**

lateral ventricle [L, *latus,* side, *ventriculus,* little belly], a cavity in each cerebral hemisphere that communicates with the third ventricle through the interventricular foramen.

lateral weight shift, transferring the body's weight away from the midline.

late rickets [Gk, *rhachis,* backbone], a form of rickets in which bones undergo changes because of a kidney defect that results in a vitamin D or calcium deficiency. The disorder tends to affect older children.

latero-, prefix meaning "side": *laterognathism, lateroversion, laterotorsion.*

lateroconal fascia, the lateral part of the renal fascia where its anterior and posterior parts join. This extends on either side posteriorly to the ascending and descending colon and is continuous with the parietal peritoneum.

laterognathism /lat′ərōnath″izəm/, an asymmetric mandible resulting from irregular growth and development, fractures, tumors, or soft tissue atrophy or hypertrophy.

laterotorsion /-tôr″shən/, **1.** displacement of the uterus to one side. **2.** a twisting of the uterus to one side.

lateroversion /-vur″zhən/, the act of turning over or being deflected from one side to the other.

latex /lā″teks/ [L, *liquid*], an emulsion or fluidlike sap produced in special cells or vessels of certain plants. Latex contains resins, proteins, and other substances and is a source of rubber. It can cause allergic reactions in some individuals.

latex allergy, anaphylactic hypersensitivity to soluble proteins in latex, seen most often in patients and health care workers sensitized by repeated exposure to latex.

latex fixation test [L, *latex,* fluid, *figere,* to fasten], a diagnostic study used to detect certain antibodies in body fluids; latex particles are used as passive carriers, and particles clump together following the addition of the antibody. Also called **RA latex test, RF test.** See also **rheumatoid factor.**

Lathrop, Rose Hawthorne [1851–1926], an American nurse who was a daughter of Nathaniel Hawthorne. She established a home in New York for patients with incurable cancer, mostly those who were poor and not accepted in hospitals because of the nature of their disease. Later she became a member of the Third Order of St. Dominic and founded the order of sisters called Servants of Relief for Incurable Cancer, which was received into the Third Order of St. Dominic in 1899. The order founded hospitals wherever there was sufficient need and offered quality care to its patients.

Latin American medical practices, an ethnomedical system representing many healing practices throughout Latin America. In Mexico it is known as *curanderismo.* The etiology of illness is framed in terms of imbalance, which can be between hot and cold in the body, between parts of the body, between patients and the social environment, or between patients and the spiritual realm. These illnesses can be treated by *curanderismo* and biomedicine, but only the *curandero* can treat supernatural ailments. This system has been used to treat *susto* (fear), believed to cause the soul to become dislodged from the body, resulting in illness; *empacho,* a gastrointestinal disorder believed to be caused by blockage in the stomach or intestine; and *mal de ojo* (evil eye), characterized by fever, irritability, headache, and weeping, generally affecting children.

latissimus dorsi /latis″iməs dôr″sī/ [L, widest, *dorsum,* the back], one of a pair of large triangular muscles on the thoracic and lumbar areas of the back. The base of the triangle inserts through lumbar aponeuroses to the spines of lumbar and sacral vertebrae and in the supraspinous ligaments, posterior iliac crest, and the lower four ribs. The fibers of the muscle twist as they pass the scapula and converge at the base of the intertubercular groove of the humerus. The latissimus dorsi extends, adducts, and rotates the arm medially; draws the shoulder back and down; and, with the pectoralis major, draws the body up when climbing. It is innervated by the thoracodorsal nerve. Compare **levator scapulae, rhomboideus major, rhomboideus minor, trapezius.**

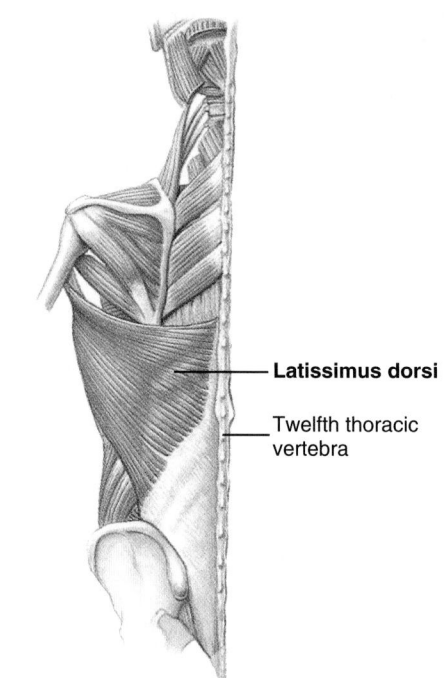

Labels: **Latissimus dorsi** / Twelfth thoracic vertebra

Latissimus dorsi *(Patton and Thibodeau, 2010)*

latitude [L, *latitudio,* breadth], the ability of an x-ray imaging system to produce acceptable images over a range of exposures. If a system has wide latitude, it is possible to image parts of the body that vary in thickness or density with only one exposure. A system of lesser latitude would require a lower exposure over the thin section and a greater exposure where the absorption was greater.

Latrodectus mactans.   See **black widow spider.**

LATS,   abbreviation for **long-acting thyroid stimulator.**

LATS-P,   abbreviation for **long-acting thyroid stimulator protector.**

lattice formation [OFr, *lattis,* geometric design],   a three-dimensional cross-linked structure formed by the reaction of polyvalent antigens with antibodies.

latus /lā′təs/ [L],   broad, wide.

laudanum /lôd″ənəm/ [Gk, *landanon,* gum resin],   a tincture of opium made from a solution of macerated raw opium and 50% alcohol. It is believed to have originated as a secret remedy of Paracelsus, a 16th-century Swiss alchemist and physician.

Lauenstein method,   a technique for positioning a patient for radiographic examination of the hip joint emphasizing the relationship of the femur to the acetabulum. The knee of the affected leg is flexed; then the leg is rotated laterally. The thigh is drawn up to nearly a right angle. Also called **frog leg position.**

laughing gas /laf″ing/,   *(Informal)*   nitrous oxide, a side effect of which is laughter or giggling when administered in low doses.

Launois syndrome /lonwah′/,   pituitary gigantism.

Laurence-Moon-Bardet-Biedl syndrome /lôr″əns mo͞on″ bärdā′ bē′dəl/   [John Zachary Laurence, British ophthalmologist, 1829–1870; Robert C. Moon, American ophthalmologist, 1844–1914; Georges Bardet, French physician, b. 1885; Artur Biedl, Czechoslovakian physician, 1869–1933],   a hereditary condition characterized by obesity, hypogenitalism, cognitive deficits, extra fingers or toes, and retinitis pigmentosa. It is transmitted as an autosomal-recessive trait.

Laurence-Moon syndrome /lô′rəns mo͞on/   [John Zachariah Laurence, British ophthalmologist, 1829-1870; Robert C. Moon, American ophthalmologist, 1844–1914],   an autosomal-recessive disorder characterized by cognitive impairments, pigmentary retinopathy, hypogonadism, and spastic paraplegia.

laureth-9 /law′reth/,   a compound used as a spermicide, surfactant, and sclerosing agent.

lavage /ləväzh″/ [Fr, washing],   **1.** *n.,*   the process of washing out an organ, usually the bladder, bowel, paranasal sinuses, or stomach, for therapeutic purposes. **2.** *v.,*   to perform a lavage. Kinds include *blood lavage,* **gastric lavage, peritoneal dialysis.** See also **irrigation.**

law [AS, *lagu*],   **1.** (in a field of study) a rule, standard, or principle that states a fact or a relationship between factors, such as Dalton's law regarding partial pressures of gas or Koch's law regarding the specificity of a pathogen. **2.** a rule, principle, or regulation established and promulgated by a government to protect or restrict the people affected. **3.** a field of study concerned with such laws. **4.** a collected body of the laws of a people, derived from custom and from legislation.

Law method,   (in radiology) any of several techniques for positioning a patient for radiographic examination of the facial bones, mastoid process, and relationship of the teeth to the maxillary sinuses.

law of definite composition,   (in chemistry) a law stating that a given compound is always made of the same elements present in the same proportion.

law of dominance,   in Mendelian inheritance, the principle that one trait, the dominant allele, will be expressed exclusively in a heterozygote. In modern genetics the law of dominance is incorporated as part of the first Mendelian law, the law of segregation. See also **Mendel's laws.**

law of independent assortment.   See **Mendel's laws.**

law of initial value,   the physiological and psychological principle that states that with a given intensity of stimulation, the degree of change produced tends to be greater when the initial value of baseline functioning is low. The higher the initial level of functioning, the smaller is the change that can be produced.

law of segregation.   See **Mendel's laws.**

law of specific nerve energies.   See **Müller's law.**

law of universal gravitation,   (in physics) the law stating that the force with which bodies are attracted to each other is directly proportional to the masses of the objects and inversely proportional to the square of the distance by which they are separated. See also **gravity, mass.**

lawrencium (Lr) /lôren″sē·əm/ [Ernest O. Lawrence, American physicist, 1901–1958],   a synthetic transuranic metallic element. Its atomic number is 103, and its atomic mass is 262.

laws of cure,   in homeopathy, the four general directions in which cure of a disease moves: from above downward, from inside outward, from more vital to less vital organs, and in reverse order of symptom appearance.

lax,   pertaining to a condition of relaxation or looseness.

laxative (lax) /lak″sətiv/ [L, *laxare,* to loosen],   **1.** *adj.,* pertaining to a substance that causes evacuation of the bowel by a mild action. **2.** *n.,* a laxative agent that promotes bowel evacuation by increasing the bulk of the feces, softening the stool, or lubricating the intestinal wall. Compare **cathartic.**

laxative regimen,   a diet that ensures an adequate intake of high-fiber bulk foods, including fruits and vegetables, to avoid chronic constipation. The regimen is supplemented with fluids and physical exercise.

lay referral system,   an illness referral system through which a person passes from the first recognition of an abnormality to an announcement to the family, to members of the community, to traditional or culturally recognized healers, and then to the regular medical system that includes nurses and physicians. Depending on the culture and the medical care available, some steps may be omitted.

lazy colon.   See **atonic constipation.**

lazy leukocyte syndrome,   an immunodeficiency disease of children characterized by recurrent stomatitis, gingivitis, otitis media, and low-grade fever with severe neutropenia. The condition has been associated with abnormal chemotaxis by leukocytes. It is treated with normal human serum transfusions.

lb [L, *libra*],   abbreviation for **pound.**

lb ap,   equal to 5760 grains or 374.4 g, as opposed to the English pound with 7000 grains or 455 g. Abbreviation for *apothecaries' pound.*

lb avdp,   abbreviation for *avoirdupois pound.*

LBBB,   abbreviation for **left bundle branch block.**

lbf/ft^2,   symbol for *pound-force per square foot.*

lbf/in^2,   symbol for *pound-force per square inch.*

lbm,   abbreviation for **lean body mass.**

LBW,   abbreviation for *low birth weight.* See **low-birth weight (LBW) infant.**

LCAT,   abbreviation for *lecithin-cholesterol acyltransferase.* See **lecithin-cholesterol acetyltransferase (LCAT) deficiency.**

LCBF,   abbreviation for **local cerebral blood flow.**

LCD,   abbreviation for **liquid crystal display.**

L chain,   abbreviation for **light chain.**

LCMRG,   abbreviation for **local cerebral metabolic rate of glucose utilization.**

LD,   abbreviation for **lethal dose.**

LD$_{50}$,   symbol for **median lethal dose.**

LDH, abbreviation for **lactate dehydrogenase.**

LDL, abbreviation for **low-density lipoprotein.**

L**-dopa.** See **levodopa.**

LE, abbreviation for **lupus erythematosus.** See **systemic lupus erythematosus.**

leaching /lē″ching/, removal of the soluble contents of a substance by running water or another liquid through it, leaving the insoluble portion behind.

lead /lēd/ [As, *laedan,* to lead], an electrical connection attached to the body to record electrical activity, especially of the heart or brain. See also **electrocardiograph, electroencephalograph.**

lead (Pb) /led/ [ME, *leed*], a common soft blue-gray metallic element. Its atomic number is 82 and its atomic mass is 207.19. In its metallic form, lead is used as a protective shielding against x-rays. Lead is poisonous, a characteristic that has led to a reduction in the use of lead compounds as pigments for paints and inks. Normal concentrations in whole blood are 0 to 5 mcg/dL. The normal amount in urine after 24-hour collection is less than 100 mcg.

lead apron /led/ [AS, *led* + Fr, *napperon*], a protective shield of lead and rubber that may be worn by the patient and by the radiological technologist or radiologist during exposure to x-rays or other diagnostic radiation. It is intended to guard against excessive exposure of the reproductive and other vital body organs to ionizing radiation. Also called **protective apron.**

lead-containing eyeglasses /led/, glasses that provide radiation shielding for the eyes of radiographic personnel. They are particularly useful during fluoroscopic procedures or angiographic examinations.

lead encephalopathy /led/ [AS, *led* + Gk, *enkephalos,* brain, *pathos,* disease], a condition of brain structure and function resulting from lead poisoning, including exposure to tetraethyl lead. Children are commonly afflicted after eating chips of lead-based paints. The untreated disorder is characterized by delirium, convulsions, mania, cortical blindness, and coma.

lead equivalent /led/, the thickness of a given material required to achieve the same shielding effect against radiation, under specified conditions, as that provided by lead.

leadership [AS, *leadan,* to lead, *scieppan,* to shape], the ability to influence others in the attainment of goals.

lead nephropathy, the kidney damage that accompanies lead poisoning. Lead deposits appear in the epithelium of the proximal tubules and as nuclear inclusions in cells. In time this leads to tubulointerstitial nephritis with chronic renal failure and other symptoms.

lead pipe fracture /led/, a linear fracture that is produced on the side of a bone opposite from the side of impact with a hard object. The point of impact is marked by a compression of bony tissue. Also called **torus fracture.**

lead-pipe rigidity /led/, a state of stiffness and inflexibility that remains uniform throughout the range of passive movement; associated with diseases of the basal ganglia.

lead poisoning /led/, a toxic condition caused by the ingestion or inhalation of lead or lead compounds. Many children develop the condition as a result of eating flaked lead paint. Poisoning also occurs from the ingestion of water from lead pipes and lead salts in certain foods and wines, the use of pewter or earthenware glazed with a lead glaze, and the use of leaded gasoline. Inhalation of lead fumes is common in industry. The acute form of intoxication is characterized by a burning sensation in the mouth and esophagus, colic, constipation or diarrhea, mental disturbances, and paralysis of the extremities, followed in severe cases by convulsions and muscular collapse. Chronic lead poisoning, which is characterized by extreme irritability, anorexia, and anemia, may progress to the acute form. Encephalopathy must be anticipated in children with lead poisoning. See also **plumbism.**

■ OBSERVATIONS: Lead poisoning is frequently asymptomatic, with mild toxicity. Likely initial manifestations include loss of appetite, abdominal discomfort, constipation, fatigue, irritability, headache, insomnia, and myalgia. Toxicity leads to three major clinical syndromes: cerebral (hyperactivity, behavioral problems, learning problems, neurological disability, and/or cognitive impairment); neuromuscular (peripheral neuritis, paresthesias, and poor coordination); and alimentary (anorexia, abdominal cramping, weight loss, intestinal spasm, and rigidity of abdominal wall). Lead exposure in pregnant women can delay fetal development. Diagnosis is made by measuring lead levels in the blood, which will be greater than 10 mcg/dL. Blood studies will also reveal a mild anemia with basophilic stippling. Chronic exposure may lead to renal failure, liver damage, and encephalopathy with blindness, seizures, paralysis, coma, and death. Hearing loss and tooth decay are also associated with lead exposure.

■ INTERVENTIONS: Treatment is dictated by serum lead levels. Children with levels between 10 and 19 mcg/dL are treated conservatively with calcium, iron, zinc, and vitamin C supplements. They are placed on a diet that includes elevated protein and reduced fat levels to reduce lead absorption. For children with blood levels between 20 and 44 mcg/dL, case management with environmental assessment is recommended, with aggressive control and removal of lead hazards. Case reports are made to the local health department for lead levels more than 20 mcg/dL. All occupationally related cases in the United States should be reported to the federal Occupational Safety and Health Administration (OSHA). Chelation with succimer and edetate calcium disodium (EDTA) is used in cases with blood levels greater than 45 mcg/dL or in refractory cases.

■ PATIENT CARE CONSIDERATIONS: All health care providers play an important role in the prevention of and screening for lead poisoning. All children should be screened for lead levels starting at 6 months to 1 year of age. Families should be educated about the risks of exposure to lead and instructed in the detection, removal, or treatment of potential sources of lead in and around the home. When the child has elevated lead levels, the focus is on aggressive reduction of further lead exposure. Education in diet and supplement therapy and the importance of continuing the monitoring of blood levels is also necessary. Families of children undergoing chelation need instructional preparation for the procedure. EMLA (lidocaine/prilocaine) cream should be applied before chelation administration to reduce pain at the injection or infusion site. Seizure precautions should be instituted for children with high lead blood levels. Renal function should be assessed through urinalysis, and lead blood levels rechecked after chelation. If lead exposure is occupationally related, workers should be instructed in the importance and consistent use of proper safety equipment such as respirators.

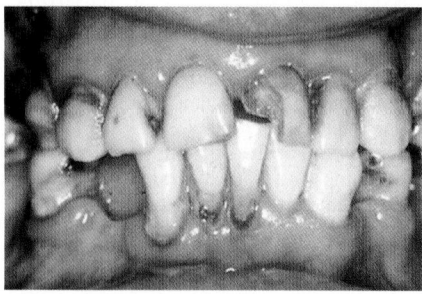

Tooth decay associated with lead poisoning *(Moll, 1997)*

lead shielding /led/,   the use of aprons and other devices containing lead as protective measures against radiation. A layer of lead 1-mm thick can attenuate 99% of x-rays of 50 kVp and 94% of x-rays of 100 kVp.

leakage /le′kaj/,   the escape of something through a break in a barrier or wall.

leakage radiation /lē″kij/   [ONorse, *leka,* to drip; L, *radiare,* to emit rays],   radiation, exclusive of the primary beam, that is emitted through the housing of equipment used in radiation therapy and radiography.

leak point pressure,   as the bladder fills, the pressure at which leakage occurs through the urethra; used as a measure of strength of the urethral sphincters.

leaky gene.   See **hypomorph.**

lean body mass (lbm)   [ME, *lenen,* slender; AS, *bodig* + ME, *massa,* lump],   the combination of cell solids, extracellular and intracellular water, and mineral mass of the body.

learned helplessness /lurnd/,   a behavioral state and personality trait of a person who believes that he or she is ineffectual, his or her responses are futile, and control over the environment has been lost. It may be seen in depression.

learning   [AS, *leornian,* to learn],   **1.** the act or process of acquiring knowledge or some skill by means of study, practice, or experience. **2.** knowledge, wisdom, or a skill acquired through systematic study or instruction. **3.** (in psychology) the modification of behavior through practice, experience, or training. See also **conditioning.**

learning curve,   a graphic presentation of the effects of mastering a performance measure. A learning curve is used to determine how quickly a skill can be mastered by using the combination of the time and number of repetitions it takes to learn a new idea or skill set, combined with the rate at which mastery is achieved. It is often used to measure a person's progress against the average.

learning disability,   an abnormal condition often affecting children of normal or above-average intelligence, characterized by difficulty in learning such fundamental procedures as reading, writing, and numeric calculation. The condition may result from psychological or organic causes and is usually related to slow development of perceptual motor skills. See also **attention deficit disorder, dysgraphia, dyslexia.**

learning-disabled adult,   an adult with a nonspecific difficulty in the learning process, commonly resulting from developmental lag rather than brain damage or demonstrable illness. Research into adult learning disabilities indicates that, as among children, the disability may be expressed throughout the total personality: cognitively, perceptually, and emotionally. Functional difficulties persist, but in adulthood they are expressed in vocational adjustment, work management, and social and family interactions.

learning environment,   the sum of the internal and external circumstances and influences surrounding and affecting a person's learning.

learning theory   [AS, *leornian,* to learn; Gk, *theoria,* speculation],   a group of concepts and principles that attempts to explain the learning process. One concept, Guthrie's contiguous conditioning premise, postulates that each response becomes permanently linked with stimuli present at the time so that contiguity rather than reinforcement is a part of the learning process.

leather-bottle stomach.   See **linitis plastica.**

leave.   See **parole.**

Leber congenital amaurosis /lā″bərz/   [Theodor von Leber, German ophthalmologist, 1840–1917; L, *congenitus,* born with; Gk, *amauroein,* to darken],   a rare kind of blindness or severely impaired vision caused by a defect transmitted as an autosomal-recessive trait and occurring at birth or shortly thereafter. The eyes appear normal externally, but pupillary constriction to light is sluggish or absent, and electroretinographic responses are decreased or absent. Pendular nystagmus, photophobia, cataract, and keratoconus may be present; the ophthalmic disorder may be associated with cognitive impairment and epilepsy. One type of Leber amaurosis results in complete blindness. In a second kind the pathology does not progress, and the patient has very mild vision loss.

Leber plexus /lā′bər/   [Theodor von Leber, German opthamologist, 1840–1917],   a venous plexus in the ciliary region connected with the canal of Schlemm. Also called **Hovius plexus.**

Leboyer method of delivery /ləboiyā″/   [Frederick LeBoyer, French obstetrician, b. 1918],   a psychophysical approach to delivery with the goal of minimizing the trauma of birth by gently and pleasantly introducing the newborn to life outside the womb. It has four aspects: a gentle controlled delivery in a quiet, dimly lighted room, avoidance of pulling on the head, avoidance of overstimulation of the infant's sensorium, and encouragement of maternal-infant bonding. Unnecessary intervention in the process of birth is eschewed. After delivery, the baby is gently laid on the mother's abdomen, the back is massaged as the cord stops pulsating, and, when regular spontaneous respirations are established, the baby is gently supported in a warm tub of water by the father. Many birth centers and obstetric services in the United States have found that no adverse effects result from this method. Some studies in France have suggested superior psychological, social, and intellectual development in young children delivered by this method. Compare **Bradley method, Lamaze method, Read method.**

LE cell,   a neutrophil that has phagocytosed the nucleus of another leukocyte that has already been altered by interacting with the LE factor in the bloodstream. Also called **lupus erythematosus cell.**

lecithin /les″ithin/   [Gk, *lekithos,* yolk],   phosphatidylcholine, a phospholipid common in plants and animals. Lecithin is found in the liver, nerve tissue, semen, and in smaller amounts, in bile and blood. It is essential as a component of all cell membranes and for fat metabolism and is used in the processing of foods, pharmaceutical products, cosmetics, and inks. Rich dietary sources are soybeans, egg yolk, and corn. See also **choline, inositol.**

lecithin-cholesterol acetyltransferase (LCAT) deficiency,   an autosomal-recessive disorder characterized by an accumulation of unesterified cholesterol in the tissues, corneal opacity, hemolytic anemia, proteinuria, renal insufficiency, and premature atherosclerosis. It is caused by a deficiency of LCAT activity.

lecithin/sphingomyelin ratio (L/S ratio),   the ratio of two components of amniotic fluid, used for predicting fetal lung maturity. The normal ratio in amniotic fluid is 2:1 or greater when fetal lungs are mature.

lecitho-,   prefix meaning "yolk of an egg or ovum": *lecithoblast, lecithoprotein.*

lecithoblast /les″ithəblast′/,   an embryonic cell; the primitive endoderm of a two-layered blastodisc.

lecithoprotein /les′ithəprō″tēn/,   a compound formed by lecithin and a protein.

lectin /lek″tin/,   a protein in seeds and other parts of certain plants that binds with glycoproteins and glycolipids on the surface of animal cells, causing agglutination. Some lectins agglutinate erythrocytes in specific blood groups, and others stimulate the production of T lymphocytes.

Ledercillin VK,   a bacterial antibiotic. Brand name for *penicillin V potassium.*

Leeuwenhoekia australiensis   [Anton van Leeuwenhoek, Dutch microscopist, 1632–1723; Australia],   a mite indigenous

L

to New South Wales that burrows into the skin, producing severe irritation. Also called **scrub itch.**

leeway space, the amount by which the space occupied by the primary canine and first and second primary molars exceeds that occupied by the canine and premolar teeth of the secondary dentition, usually averaging 1.7 mm on each side of the dental arch.

Lee-White method [Roger I. Lee, American physician, b. 1881; Paul D. White, American physician, 1886–1973; Gk, *meta,* beyond, *hodos,* way], a method of determining the length of time required for a clot to form in a test tube of venous blood. It is not specific for any coagulation disorder but is often used to monitor coagulation during heparin therapy. See also **clotting time.**

leflunomide, a pyrimidine synthesis inhibitor with antiinflammatory effects.
- INDICATIONS: It is used to treat rheumatoid arthritis.
- CONTRAINDICATIONS: Pregnancy, lactation, hepatic disease, jaundice, positive hepatitis B and C, severe immunosuppression, or known hypersensitivity to this drug prohibits its use.
- ADVERSE EFFECTS: Adverse effects include chest pain, angina pectoris, migraine, bronchitis, cough, respiratory infection, pneumonia, and sinusitis. Common side effects include nausea, anorexia, vomiting, constipation, flatulence, dizziness, insomnia, depression, paresthesia, palpitations, hypertension, rash, pruritus, pharyngitis, and rhinitis.

LeFort I fracture. See **Guérin's fracture.**

left atrioventricular orifice, the opening between the left atrium and ventricle of the heart. Also called *mitral orifice.*

left atrioventricular valve. See **mitral valve.**

left atrium (LA), the uppermost chamber on the left side of the heart. It receives blood from the pulmonary veins.

left brachiocephalic vein [ME, *left,* weak; Gk, *brachys,* short, *kephale,* head], a vessel about 6 cm long that starts in the root of the neck at the junction of the internal jugular and the subclavian veins on the left side and runs obliquely across the thorax to join the right brachiocephalic vein and form the superior vena cava. Also called **left innominate vein.** Compare **right brachiocephalic vein.**

left bundle branch block (LBBB), the failure of the cardiac impulse to propagate down the left bundle branch from the bundle of His, resulting in early activation of the right side of the septum and the right ventricular myocardium. See also **bundle branch block.**

left common carotid artery, the longer of the two common carotid arteries, arising from the aortic arch and having cervical and thoracic parts. The cervical part passes obliquely from the level of the sternoclavicular articulation to the cranial border of the thyroid cartilage, dividing into the left internal and the left external carotid arteries. Compare **right common carotid artery.**

left coronary artery, one of a pair of branches from the ascending aorta, arising in the left posterior aortic sinus, dividing into the left interventricular artery and the circumflex branch, and supplying both ventricles and the left atrium. Compare **right coronary artery.**

left-handedness /left″ han″dĭdnes/, a natural tendency by some persons to favor the use of the left hand in performing certain tasks. Also called **sinistrality.** See also **cerebral dominance, handedness.**

left-heart failure, an abnormal cardiac condition characterized by the impairment of the left side of the heart and elevated pressure and congestion in the pulmonary veins and capillaries. Left-heart failure may be related to right-heart failure, because both sides of the heart are part of a circuit and the impairment of one side will eventually affect the other. Experimentally produced failure of one ventricle may produce significant hemodynamic and biochemical abnormalities of the opposite ventricle, even without the usual signs of failure. In "pure" left-heart failure, the body retains significant amounts of sodium and water and consequently develops peripheral edema without clinical evidence of right-heart failure. It is most commonly caused by coronary artery disease, hypertension, or aortic stenosis. Also called **left-sided failure.** Compare **right-heart failure.** See also **heart failure.**

left hepatic duct, the duct that drains the bile from the left lobe of the liver into the common bile duct.

left innominate vein. See **left brachiocephalic vein.**

left lateral recumbent position [ME, *left* + L, *latus,* side, *recumbere,* to lie down, *positio*], a position in which the patient lies on the left side with the upper knee and thigh drawn upward. See also **semiprone side position.**

left lymphatic duct. See **thoracic duct.**

left pulmonary artery, the shorter and smaller of two arteries conveying venous blood from the heart to the lungs, rising from the pulmonary trunk, connecting to the left lung, and tending to have more separate branches than the right pulmonary artery. In the fetus, it is larger and more important than the right pulmonary artery because it provides the ductus arteriosus that degenerates to become a ligament after birth. Compare **right pulmonary artery.**

left-sided failure. See **left-heart failure.**

left subclavian artery, an artery, divided into three parts, that arises from the aortic arch to supply the vertebral column, spinal cord, ear, and brain. The short second part lies dorsal to the scalenus anterior and forms the arch described by the vessel. The third part runs from the scalenus anterior to the first rib, where it becomes the axillary artery. Compare **right subclavian artery.** See also **subclavian artery.**

left-to-right shunt, **1.** a diversion of blood from the left side of the heart to the right, such as through a septal defect. **2.** a diversion of blood from the systemic to the pulmonary circulation, such as from a patent ductus arteriosus. Pathology results from the inability of the right circulation to compensate for left-sided (systemic) pressures.

left ventricle (LV), the thick-walled chamber of the heart that pumps blood through the aorta and the systemic arteries, the capillaries, and back through the veins to the right atrium. It has walls about three times thicker than those of the right ventricle and contains a mitral valve with two flaps that controls the flow of blood from the left atrium. The left ventricle occupies about half the diaphragmatic surface of the heart and is longer and more conical than the right ventricle, narrowing caudally to form the apex. The chordae tendineae of the left ventricle are thicker, stronger, and less numerous than those in the right ventricle. See also **chordae tendineae.**

left ventricular assist device (LVAD), a mechanical pump that temporarily and artificially aids the natural pumping action of the left ventricle.

left ventricular failure, heart failure in which the left ventricle fails to contract forcefully enough to maintain a normal cardiac output and peripheral perfusion. Pulmonary congestion and edema develop from back pressure of accumulated blood in the left ventricle. Signs include breathlessness, crackles, dyspnea, orthopnea, pallor, sweating, and peripheral vasoconstriction. The heart is usually enlarged, resulting in a displaced point of maximum impulse. A prominent third heart sound (gallop), normal in children and young adults, is a sign of left ventricular failure in older adults with heart disease. Hypertension is common and may be a causative factor or a result of pulmonary edema. Treatment includes meperidine or morphine for sedation, angiotensin-converting enzyme inhibitors or calcium channel blockers to reduce afterload, diuretics, digitalis, and rest. See also **congestive heart failure.**

left ventricular thrust. See **precordial movement.**

left ventricular veins, rarely occurring cardiac veins emptying into the left ventricle of the heart. These are the smallest of all cardiac veins.

leg /leg/ [ONor, *leggr*], **1.** that section of the lower limb between the knee and ankle. **2.** in common usage, the entire lower limb (in which case, the part below the knee is called the lower leg).

legacy /leg″əsē/ [L, *legatum*, bequest], something that is handed down from the past or intended to be bestowed on future generations.

legal [L, *lex*, law], actions or conditions that are permitted or authorized by law.

legal blindness [L, *lex*, law; ME, *blend*, sightless], a state of visual acuity in which no better than 20/200 is measured in the better eye with corrective lenses or a visual field of not more than 20 degrees is obtained.

legal death. See **death.**

leg cylinder cast [ONor, *leggr* + Gk, *kylindros* + ONorse, *kasta*], an orthopedic device of plaster of paris or fiberglass used to immobilize the leg in treating fractures from the ankle to the middle femur. It is used especially for repairing knee fractures and dislocations, for treating soft tissue trauma around the knee, for maintaining postoperative positioning and immobilization of the knee, and for correcting or maintaining correction of knee deformities. The cast extends from the upper thigh to the ankle. The foot is not encased. The long-leg cast may also be used for these purposes because it encases the foot and ensures greater immobilization.

Legg-Calvé-Perthes disease [Arthur T. Legg, American surgeon, 1874–1939; Jacques Calvé, French orthopedist, 1875–1954; Georg C. Perthes, German surgeon, 1869–1927], osteochondrosis of the head of the femur in children, characterized initially by epiphyseal necrosis or degeneration, followed by regeneration or recalcification. Formerly called **Perthes disease, Calvé-Perthes disease.**

legionellosis /lē′jənelō′sis/, infection with a species of *Legionella,* which may cause any of several illnesses, including Legionnaires' disease.

Legionnaires' disease /lē′jənerz″/ [American Legion], an acute bacterial pneumonia caused by infection with *Legionella pneumophila.* It is characterized by an influenza-like illness followed within a week by high fever, chills, muscle aches, and headache. The symptoms may progress to dry cough, pleurisy, and sometimes diarrhea. Usually the disease is self-limited, but mortality has been 15% to 20% in a few localized epidemics. Contaminated air-conditioning cooling towers and warm stagnant water supplies, including water vaporizers, water sonicators, whirlpool spas, and showers, may be sources of organisms. Person-to-person contagion has not occurred. Risk of infection is increased by the presence of other conditions, such as cardiopulmonary diseases. Treatment includes supportive care and antibiotic therapy. Also called **legionellosis.**

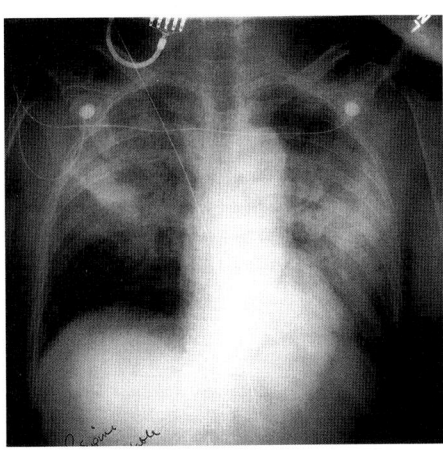

Legionnaires' disease *(Courtesy American College of Radiology)*

Legionnaires' disease antibody test, direct and indirect fluorescent testing for antibodies against *L. pneumophila.*

Leigh disease /lē/ [Archibald Denis Leigh, British neuropathologist, b. 1915], an encephalopathy of unclear clinical and pathological criteria, causing neuropathological damage like that of the Wernicke-Korsakoff syndrome. It occurs in two forms: the infantile form, which may be the same as pyruvate carboxylase deficiency, is characterized by degeneration of gray matter with necrosis and capillary proliferation in the brainstem; hypotonia, seizures, and dementia; anorexia and vomiting; slow or arrested development; and ocular and respiratory disorders. Death usually occurs before age 3. The adult form usually first manifests as bilateral optic atrophy with central scotoma and color blindness; then there is a quiescent period of up to 30 years before late symptoms appear, such as ataxia, spastic paresis, clonic jerks, grand mal seizures, psychic lability, and mild dementia. Also called **subacute necrotizing encephalomyelopathy, subacute necrotizing encephalopathy.** See also **Wernicke-Korsakoff syndrome.**

Leiner disease /lī″nər/ [Karl Leiner, Austrian pediatrician, 1871–1930], a condition in infants of generalized dermatitis, with scaling and erythema, as well as seborrheic dermatitis of the scalp, generalized lymphadenopathy, and diarrhea. Also called **erythroderma desquamativum.**

Leininger, Madeleine [1925–2012], a nursing theorist, author, educator, researcher, and consultant who formulated the foundation of transcultural nursing and the resultant nursing research, education, and practice in this subfield of nursing. The most complete account of transcultural care theory is found in her book titled *Care: The Essence of Nursing and Health* (1984). Some of the major concepts are care, caring, culture, cultural values, and cultural variations. A basic tenet of Leininger's theory is that human beings are inseparable from their cultural background and social structure. She advocates caring as the central theme in nursing care, nursing knowledge, and practice. Caring includes assistive, supportive, or facilitative acts toward an individual or group with evident or anticipated needs. Caring serves to ameliorate or improve human conditions and life ways (life process). Her methodology is borrowed from anthropology, but the concept of caring is an essential characteristic of nursing practice.

leio-, lio-, prefix meaning "smooth": *leiomyoma, leiomyofibroma.*

leiomyofibroma /lī′ōmī′ōfībrō″mə/ *pl. leiomyofibromas, leiomyofibromata* [Gk, *leios,* smooth, *mys,* muscle; L, *fibra,* fiber; Gk, *oma,* tumor], a tumor consisting of smooth muscle cells and fibrous connective tissue, commonly occurring in the uterus in middle-aged women. See also **fibroid.**

leiomyoma /lī′ōmī·ō″mə/ *pl. leiomyomas, leiomyomata,* a benign smooth-muscle tumor occurring most commonly in the uterus, stomach, esophagus, or small intestine. Surgical resection is usually indicated.

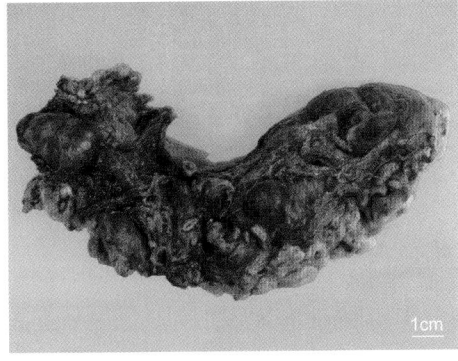

Leiomyoma *(Blake et al, 2014)*

leiomyoma cutis, a neoplasm of the smooth muscles of the skin. The lesion is characterized by many small, tender, red nodules. It may also occur as a solitary genital lesion or a solitary angioleiomyoma arising from the muscle of veins.

leiomyoma uteri, a benign neoplasm of the smooth muscle of the uterus. The tumor is characteristically firm, well-circumscribed, round, and gray-white. Histologically a pattern of whorls is present. Tumors of this kind develop in the myometrium and occur in women between 30 and 50 years of age. They are usually small but may grow quite large and occupy most of the uterine wall. Symptoms vary according to the location and size of the tumors. As they grow, they may cause pressure on neighboring organs, painful menstruation, profuse and irregular menstrual bleeding, vaginal discharge, or frequent urination, as well as enlargement of the uterus. In pregnancy, the tumors may interfere with natural enlargement of the uterus with the growing fetus. Also called **fibroid, fibromyoma uteri, myoma previum.**

leiomyosarcoma /-särkō″mə/ [Gk, *leios,* smooth, *mys,* muscle, *sarx,* flesh, *oma,* tumor], a sarcoma that contains large spindle cells of unstriated muscle.

leipo-. See **lip-.**

Leishman-Donovan body /lēsh″mən don″əvən/ [William B. Leishman, English pathologist, 1865–1926; Charles Donovan, Irish physician, 1863–1951], the resting stage of an intracellular nonflagellated protozoan parasite (*Leishmania donovani*) that causes kala-azar, or visceral leishmaniasis, as it appears in infected tissue specimens.

Leishmania /lēshmä″nē·ə/ [William B. Leishman], a genus of protozoan parasites. These organisms are transmitted to humans by any of several species of sand flies.

leishmaniasis /lēsh′mənī″əsis/ [William B. Leishman], infection with any species of protozoan of the genus *Leishmania.* The diseases caused by these organisms may be cutaneous, mucocutaneous, or visceral. The infection is transmitted to humans by several species of nocturnal *Phlebotomus* sand flies. Other species of the blood-sucking insects infect other animals. Diagnosis is made by microscopic identification of the intracellular nonflagellated protozoan on a Giemsa-stained smear taken from a cutaneous lesion or visceral biopsy. A typical infection may begin with a cutaneous sore and progress to ulceration of the mouth, palate, and nose. Some cases are accompanied by a febrile illness. There are three major types of leishmaniasis: American leishmaniasis, the form found in Central America and South America; kala-azar; and cutaneous leishmaniasis. Kala-azar, also known as visceral leishmaniasis, occurs mainly in the tropical areas of Asia; cutaneous leishmaniasis is encountered most frequently in the Middle East. Also called **kala-azar.** Formerly called *Assam fever.* See also *Leishmania.* −leishmanial, *adj.*

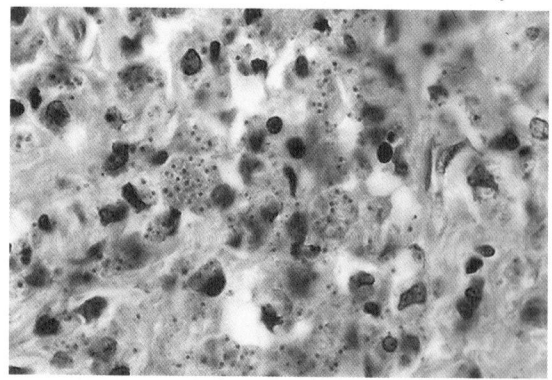

Visceral leishmaniasis *(Kumar, Abbas, and Fausto, 2005)*

leishmanin test. See **Montenegro test.**

leisure, (for health or related reasons) nonobligatory activity that is intrinsically motivated and engaged in during discretionary time, that is, time not committed to obligatory occupations such as work, self-care, or sleep. Occupational therapists, recreational therapists, and leisure therapists have a unique role in assisting clients to participate in meaningful leisure activities. All health professionals should recognize the role of leisure in quality of life, health promotion, and therapeutic bio-psycho-socio-spiritual activities.

-lemma, suffix meaning "a confining membrane": *sarcolemma, oolemma, neurilemma.*

lemniscal system /lemnis″kəl/ [Gk, *lemniskos,* fillet, *systema*], a part of the somatosensory network of large-diameter myelinated A fibers. It includes the dorsal columns and the neospinothalamic tract extending from the spinal cord to the thalamus and cortex.

lemniscus /lemnis″kəs/ [Gk, *lemniskos,* fillet], a band or tract of central nervous system fibers, particularly the ascending axons of secondary sensory neurons leading to the thalamus.

lemon balm, a perennial herb found in the Mediterranean, Asia, Europe, and North America.

■ INDICATIONS: It is used for abdominal gas and cramping and for cold sores. There is evidence of efficacy.

■ CONTRAINDICATIONS: Its use is not recommended during pregnancy and lactation, in children, or in those with known hypersensitivity to this herb. It should not be used in people with hypothyroidism.

lenalidomide, a thalidomide analogue.

■ INDICATIONS: This drug is used to treat transfusion-dependent anemia due to low or intermediate-1-risk myelodysplastic syndrome and to treat multiple myeloma in combination with dexamethasone.

■ CONTRAINDICATIONS: Pregnancy, breastfeeding, and known hypersensitivity to this drug prohibit its use.

■ ADVERSE EFFECTS: Adverse effects of this drug include chest pain, hypotension, palpitations, abdominal pain, anorexia, constipation, diarrhea, nausea and vomiting, dysgeusia, xerosis, anemia, leucopenia, pancytopenia, thrombocytopenia, hypokalemia, hypomagnesia, arthralgia, back pain, myalgia, depression, dizziness, fatigue, fever, headache, sweating, peripheral neuropathy, cough, dyspnea, epistaxis, and rhinitis. A life-threatening side effect is pulmonary embolism.

Lenègre disease /lenāgrā/ [Jean Lenègre, 20th-century French cardiologist, 1904–1972], sclerodegeneration of the conduction system of the heart that eventually results in complete heart block.

length of stay (LOS), the period of time a patient remains in a hospital or other health care facility as an inpatient.

Lennox-Gastaut syndrome (LGS) /len″oks-gästō″/ [William G. Lennox, American neurologist, 1884–1960; Henri Gastaut, French biologist, b. 1914], a condition in which a variety of generalized seizures, such as tonic, atonic, absence, tonic-clonic, akinetic, and myoclonic, begin to appear in the first 5 years of life. Seizures are often intractable and may require multiple antiepileptic medications. Cognitive impairment is often present. Among suggested causes are inherited metabolic abnormalities and perinatal or postnatal disorders. Also called **Gastaut disease.**

lens [L, lentil], **1.** a curved transparent piece of plastic or glass that is shaped, molded, or ground to refract light in a specific way, as in eyeglasses, microscopes, or cameras.

2. *(Informal)* the crystalline lens of the eye. See **crystalline lens.** **–lenticular,** *adj.*

lens capsule, the clear thin elastic capsule that surrounds the lens of the eye. Also called **capsule of the lens.**

lens implant, an artificial lens that is usually implanted at the time of cataract extraction but may also be used for patients with extreme myopia, diplopia, ocular albinism, and certain other abnormalities. The operation is usually performed with a local anesthetic in an outpatient center. Eyedrops containing an antibiotic such as neomycin are instilled before surgery to prevent infection and several times a day for a number of weeks after surgery. After extraction of the cataract, the lens is inserted through a corneal incision. It may be held in place in the anterior chamber by extremely fine sutures to the iris, or, if the lens is implanted into the capsular sac, a miotic agent such as pilocarpine is used to prevent the iris from dilating too widely, which would allow the implant to slip. The implanted lens does not cause the problems with abnormal peripheral vision that are associated with cataract spectacles.

Lente insulin, an intermediate-acting insulin. See also **intermediate-acting insulin.**

lenticonus /len′tikō″nəs/, an abnormal spheric or conic protrusion on the lens of the eye. It is a congenital defect found in Alport syndrome.

lenticular. See **lens.**

lenticular nucleus /lentik″yələr/ [L, *lens,* lentil, *nucleus,* nut], biconvex basal ganglia of the cerebrum, composed of lateral putamen and medial globus pallidus tissue as part of the corpus striatum.

lentiform /len″tifôrm/ [L, *lens + forma*], pertaining to or resembling a lentil shape, such as the lens of the eye.

lentigo /lentī″gō/ *pl. lentigines* [L, freckle], a tan or brown macule on the skin brought on by sun exposure, usually in a middle-aged or older person. It is benign, and no treatment is necessary. However, in some cases it may mimic melanoma and should be biopsied. Compare **freckle.**

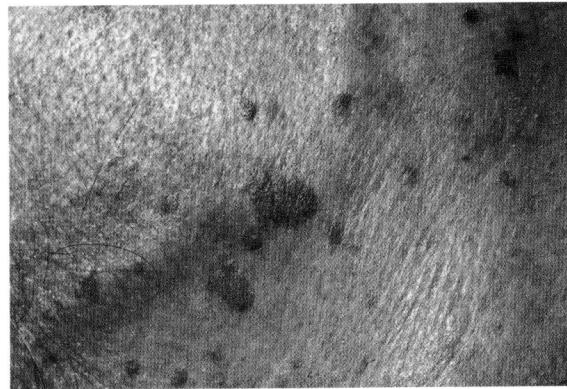

Multiple lentigines (the pleural of lentigo) *(Brinster et. al, 2011)*

lentigo maligna. See **Hutchinson freckle.**

lentigo maligna melanoma, a neoplasm developing from a Hutchinson freckle on the face or other exposed surfaces of the skin in elderly patients. It is asymptomatic, flat, and tan or brown, with irregular darker spots and frequent hypopigmentation. It is one of the major clinical types of melanoma and occurs in 10% to 15% of melanoma patients. See also **nodular melanoma, superficial spreading melanoma.**

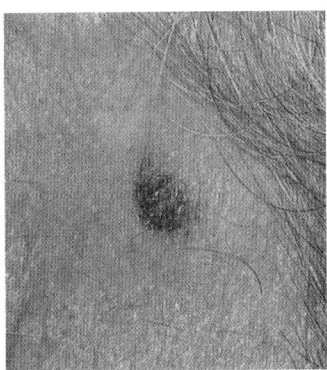

Small facial melanoma in situ (lentigo maligna)
(Bolognia, Jorizzo, and Schaffer, 2012)

lentivirus /len′tivī″rəs/, any member of a genus of retroviruses that have long incubation periods and cause chronic, progressive, usually fatal diseases in humans and other animals and that are capable of infecting both nondividing and actively dividing cells. Species include the types of human immunodeficiency virus.

LEOPARD syndrome, a hereditary syndrome transmitted as an autosomal-dominant trait, consisting of multiple lentigines, asymptomatic cardiac defects, and typical coarse facies. It may also be associated with pulmonary stenosis, sensorineural hearing loss, skeletal changes, ocular hypertelorism, and abnormalities of the genitalia. Also called **multiple lentigines syndrome.**

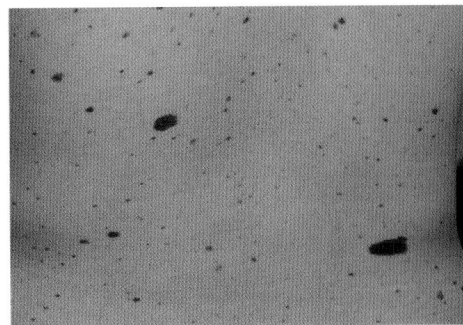

Multiple lentigines associated with LEOPARD syndrome *(Cheng et al, 2013)*

Leopold's maneuver [Christian G. Leopold, German physician, 1846–1911], a series of four steps used in palpating the abdomen of a pregnant woman to determine position and presentation of the fetus.

leper /lep″ər/ [Gk, *lepis,* scaly], *(Obsolete)* a person afflicted with leprosy (Hansen disease).

lepirudin, a direct thrombin inhibitor.
■ INDICATIONS: It is used to treat heparin-induced thrombocytopenia and other thromboembolic conditions.
■ CONTRAINDICATIONS: Known hypersensitivity to hirudins prohibits its use.
■ ADVERSE EFFECTS: Life-threatening effects of lepirudin include heart failure, pericardial effusion, ventricular fibrillation, multiorgan failure, sepsis, hematuria, hemorrhage, intracranial bleeding, and thrombocytopenia. Other adverse effects include GI bleeding, abnormal liver function tests, abnormal kidney function, pneumonia, and allergic skin reactions. Fever is a common side effect. Drug interactions with NSAIDs, aspirin, salicy-

L

lates, and antiplatelets may occur. Use of the herbs feverfew, ginkgo, ginger, and valerian may potentiate bleeding. Caution should be used in its use in patients with cirrhosis of the liver.

leprechaunism /lep′rəkän′izəm/, (Obsolete) now called **Donohue syndrome.**

lepro-, prefix meaning "leprosy": lepromatous, leprosarium.

lepromatous leprosy, a form of leprosy caused by mycobacteria that begins with pale, hairless skin lesions and slowly progresses to involve bones, internal organs, joints, and marrow if left untreated. Long-term antibiotic therapy with clofazimine, dapsone, or rifampin can halt disease progression and cure the disease. See **leprosy.**

lepromin test /leprō″min/, a skin sensitivity test used to distinguish between the lepromatous and tuberculoid forms of leprosy. The test consists of an intradermal injection of lepromin, which is prepared from heat-sterilized Mycobacterium leprae. The appearance of a palpable nodule in 8 to 10 days is indicative of the tuberculoid form of leprosy. As no nodule appears in the lepromatous form, the test is not diagnostic of leprosy. The test is used only to follow the course of the disease. See also **leprosy.**

leprosarium /lep′rōser″ē·əm/ [Gk, lepra, leprosy], a hospital for persons who have leprosy.

leprosy /lep′rəsē/ [Gk, lepra], a chronic communicable disease caused by Mycobacterium leprae that may take either of two forms, depending on the degree of immunity of the host. Tuberculoid leprosy is seen in those with high resistance; lepromatous leprosy is seen in those with little resistance. Also called **Hansen disease.** Kinds include **tuberculoid leprosy, lepromatous leprosy.** See also Mycobacterium. −leprotic, leprous, lepromatous, adj.

■ OBSERVATIONS: Tuberculoid leprosy presents as thickening of cutaneous nerves and anesthetic, saucer-shaped skin lesions. Lepromatous leprosy involves many body systems, with widespread plaques and nodules in the skin, iritis, keratitis, destruction of nasal cartilage and bone, testicular atrophy, peripheral edema, and involvement of the reticuloendothelial system. Blindness may result.

■ INTERVENTIONS: Plastic surgery, physical therapy, and psychotherapy are often necessary. Treatment with sulfones such as dapsone continued for several years usually results in improvement of skin lesions, but recovery from nerve impairment is limited. However, with treatment the disease can be cured.

■ PATIENT CARE CONSIDERATIONS: Contrary to traditional belief, leprosy is not very contagious, and prolonged intimate contact is required for it to be spread between individuals. Children are more susceptible than adults. The disease is found mostly in tropical and subtropical countries.

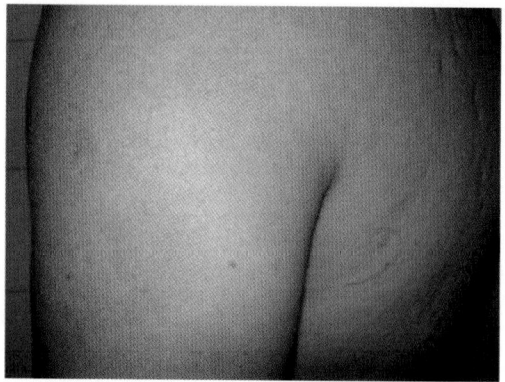

Patient with erythematous plaques associated with lepromatous leprosy (Petiti-Martin et al, 2011)

-lepsy, -lepsia, -lepsis, suffix meaning a "seizure": catalepsy, hemiepilepsy.

-leptic, suffix meaning "a (specified) type of seizure": narcoleptic, epileptic, neuroleptic.

leptin /lep′tin/ [Gk, thin], a peptide secreted by adipose tissue. Leptin inhibits neuropeptide Y and is thought to be an appetite suppressant. It increases expenditure of energy when fat stores increase. Excess leptin has been found in some obese humans, but the majority have normal levels of leptin.

lepto-, prefix meaning "slender, small, thin, or delicate": leptomeninges, leptotene.

leptocyte. See **target cell.**

leptocytosis /lep′tōsītō″sis/ [Gk, leptos, thin, kytos, cell, osis, condition], a hematological disorder in which target cells are present in the blood. Thalassemia, some forms of liver disease, and hemoglobin C disease are associated with leptocytosis.

leptomeningeal cyst. See **arachnoid cyst.**

leptomeninges /lep′tōminin″jēz/ [Gk, leptos + meninx, membrane], the arachnoid membrane and the pia mater, two of the three layers covering the brain and spinal cord. Compare **meninges.**

leptomeningitis /-men′injī″tis/, an inflammation of the arachnoid and pia mater layers of the meninges. See also **meningitis.**

leptonema /lep′tənē″mə/ [Gk, leptos + nema, thread], the threadlike chromosome formation in the leptotene stage in the first meiotic prophase of gametogenesis, before the beginning of synapsis.

leptorrhine, adj., having a long, narrow nasal profile.

Leptospira /-spī′rə/ [Gk, leptos + speira, coil], a genus of the family Leptospiracceae, order Spirochaetales; tightly coiled microorganisms having spirals with hooked ends. The spirochete thrives in the urine of infected animals, especially rodents; is pathogenic to humans and other mammals; and may cause hepatitis, jaundice, skin hemorrhages, fever, renal failure, mental status changes, and muscular illness. See also **leptospirosis.**

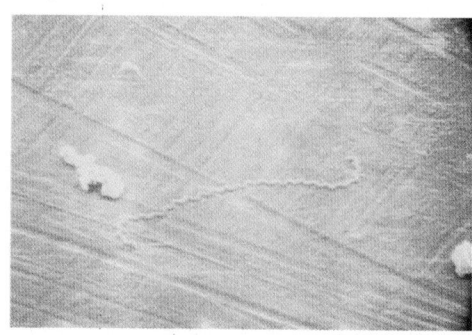

Leptospira interrogans (Courtesy Drs. Abelson and Cameron)

Leptospira **agglutinin,** an agglutinin found in the blood of patients with leptospirosis.

leptospirosis /lep′tōspīrō″sis/ [Gk, leptos + speira + osis, condition], an acute infectious disease caused by several serotypes of the spirochete Leptospira interrogans, considered the most common zoonosis globally. It is transmitted in the urine of infected cattle, horses, pigs, dogs, rodents, or wild animals. Human infections arise directly from bacterial contact with mucous membranes or abraded skin with an infected animal's urine or tissues or indirectly from contact with contaminated water, food, or soil. Occupational contamination accounts for 30% to 50% of the cases. It is increasingly recognized as a disease of recreation. Clinical symptoms may include hepatitis, jaundice, hemorrhage into the skin, fever, chills, renal failure, meningitis with mental status changes, and muscular pain. The spirochete can be isolated from the urine or blood during the acute stage of the disease, and antibodies can be found in the patient's blood during convalescence. Treatment with antibiotics, usually penicillin or doxycycline, may be effective if it is administered during the first few days of the disease. Fluid and electrolyte replacement is essential if jaundice or other signs of severe illness are present. The disease is usually short-lived and mild, but severe infections can damage the kidneys and the liver. Blood pressure and vital signs should be monitored, and the patient's urine should be disposed of carefully to prevent spread of the organism. The most serious form of the disease, Weil disease, makes up 5% to 10% of leptospirosis cases. Also called **autumn fever, mud fever.** See also **nanukayami.**

leptotene /lep″tǝtēn/ [Gk, *leptos* + *tainia,* ribbon], the initial stage in the first meiotic prophase in gametogenesis, in which the chromosomes condense and become visible as single, thin filaments. See also **diakinesis, diplotene, pachytene, zygotene.**

leptotrichosis /lep″totriko′sis/, infection with a species of *Leptotrichia.*

leptotrichosis conjunctivae, name given to Parinaud oculoglandular syndrome when caused by infection with *Leptotrichia.*

Leriche syndrome /lǝrēsh″/ [René Leriche, French surgeon, 1879–1955], a vascular disorder marked by gradual occlusion of the terminal aorta, bilateral iliac arteries, or both; intermittent claudication in the buttocks, thighs, or calves; absence of pulsation in femoral arteries; pallor and coldness of the legs; gangrene of the toes; and, in men, impotence. Symptoms are the result of chronic tissue hypoxia caused by inadequate arterial perfusion of the affected areas. Treatment may include endarterectomy, embolectomy, or synthetic bypass graft at the aortic bifurcation.

lesbian /lez″bē·ǝn/ [Gk, island of Lesbos, home of Sappho], **1.** *n.,* a female homosexual. **2.** *adj.,* pertaining to the sexual preference or desire of one woman for another. –**lesbianism,** *n.*

Lesch-Nyhan syndrome /lesh″ nī″han/ [Michael Lesch, American pediatrician, b. 1939; William L. Nyhan, Jr., American pediatrician, b. 1926], a hereditary disorder of purine metabolism, characterized by cognitive impairment, self-mutilation of the fingers and lips by biting, impaired renal function, and abnormal physical development. It is transmitted as a recessive, sex-linked trait.

Leser-Trélat sign /lā″zǝr trālä″/ [Edmund Leser, German surgeon, 1828–1916; Ulysse Trélat, French surgeon, 1828–1890], a condition of malignant cells present in the skin, characterized by the sudden onset of multiple seborrheic keratoses, with pruritus or enlargement of preexisting keratosis in older adults. It is associated with adenocarcinoma of the stomach, breast cancer, and lung cancer.

lesion /lē″zhen/ [L, *laesus,* an injury], **1.** a wound, injury, or pathological change in body tissue. **2.** any visible local abnormality of the tissues of the skin, such as a wound, sore, rash, or boil. A lesion may be described as benign, cancerous, gross, occult, or primary.

lesser circulation. See **pulmonary circulation.**

lesser multangular bone. See **trapezoid bone.**

lesser occipital nerve [AS, *losian,* to lose; L, *occiput,* back of the head, *nervus,* nerve], one of a pair of cutaneous branches of the cervical plexus, arising from the second cervical nerve and ascending along the side of the head behind the ear to supply the skin. It communicates with the posterior auricular branch of the facial nerve.

lesser omentum [AS, *losian,* to lose; L, *omentum,* entrails], a membranous extension of the peritoneum from the peritoneal layers covering the ventral and the dorsal surfaces of the stomach and the first part of the duodenum. The lesser omentum extends from the portal fissure of the liver to the diaphragm, where the layers separate to enclose the end of the esophagus. It also forms two ligaments, one associated with the liver, the hepatogastric ligament, and the other, the hepatoduodenal ligament, with the duodenum. Also called **gastrohepatic omentum, small omentum.**

lesser petrosal nerve, a small nerve originating in the tympanic plexus that carries preganglionic parasympathetic fibers to the otic ganglion.

lesser sciatic foramen, an opening positioned below the attachment of the pelvic floor formed by the lesser sciatic notch of the pelvic bone, the ischial spine, the sacrospinous ligament, and the sacrotuberous ligament. It acts as a route of communication between the perineum and the gluteal region.

lesser sciatic notch [AS, *losian,* to lose; Gk, *ischiadikos,* hip joint; OFr, *enochier*], a notch on the posterior border of the ischium of the hip bone. It is smooth, is coated with cartilage, and has several ridges corresponding to subdivisions of the obturator internus tendon.

lesser trochanter, one of a pair of conic projections on the shaft of the femur, just below the neck. It is the site of insertion of the psoas major muscle. Also called **trochanter minor.** Compare **greater trochanter.**

LET, abbreviation for **linear energy transfer.**

Letairis, brand name for **ambrisentan.**

let-down, a sensation in the breasts of lactating women that often occurs as the milk flows into the ducts. It may occur when the infant begins to suck or when the mother hears the baby cry or even thinks of giving nourishment to the child.

let-down reflex. See **milk ejection reflex.**

lethal /lē″thǝl/, deadly; capable of causing death.

lethal allele, an allele that produces a phenotypic effect that causes the death of the organism at any stage of life. The allele may be dominant, incompletely dominant, or recessive. Human diseases caused by lethal genes include Huntington disease, which is transmitted as an autosomal-dominant trait, and sickle cell anemia, which shows recessive lethality. Compare **sublethal allele.** See also **lethal equivalent.**

lethal dose (LD), the amount of toxin that produces death in all members of a species population within a specified period of time. See also **median lethal dose.**

lethal equivalent [L, *letum,* death, *aequus,* equal, *valere,* to be strong], a recessive allele carried in the heterozygous state that would be lethal in the homozygous state, or any combination of alleles, each with slightly deleterious effects, that is equivalent to such an allele. It is estimated that a person carries an average of three to eight lethal equivalents. See also **lethal allele.**

L

Primary skin lesions

Description	Examples

Macule

A flat, circumscribed area that is a change in the color of the skin; less than 1 cm in diameter

Freckles, flat moles (nevi), petechiae, measles, scarlet fever

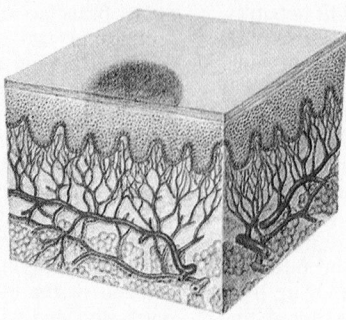

Freckles *(Marks and Miller, 2006)*

Papule

An elevated, firm, circumscribed area less than 1 cm in diameter

Wart (verruca), elevated moles, lichen planus

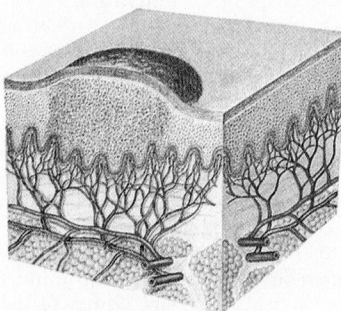

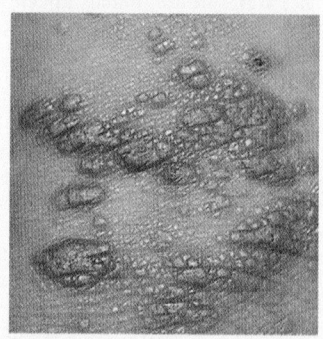

Lichen planus *(Weston, Lane, and Morelli, 2007)*

Patch

A flat, nonpalpable, irregular-shaped macule more than 1 cm in diameter

Vitiligo, port-wine stain, mongolian spots, café-au-lait spots

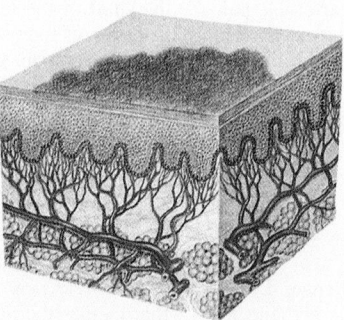

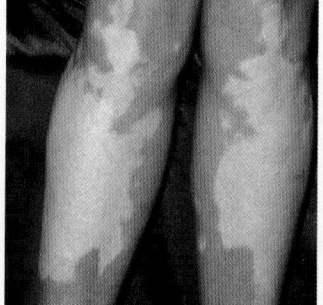

Vitiligo *(White and Cox, 2006)*

Plaque

Elevated, firm, and rough lesion with flat top surface greater than 1 cm in diameter

Psoriasis, seborrheic and actinic keratoses

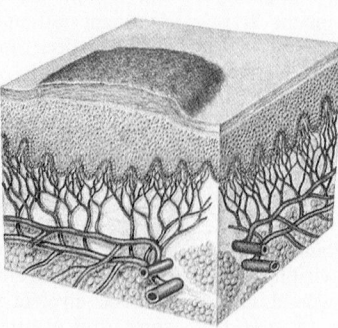

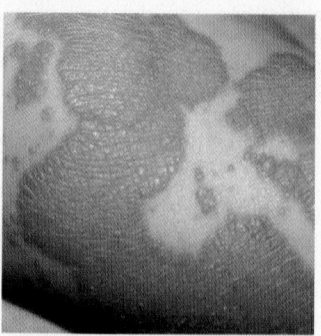

Plaque *(Weston, Lane, and Morelli, 2007)*

Primary skin lesions—cont'd

Description	Examples		

Wheal

Elevated irregular-shaped area of cutaneous edema; solid, transient; variable diameter

Insect bites, urticaria, allergic reaction

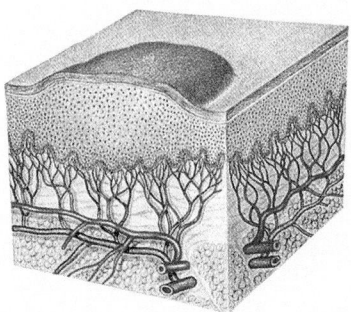

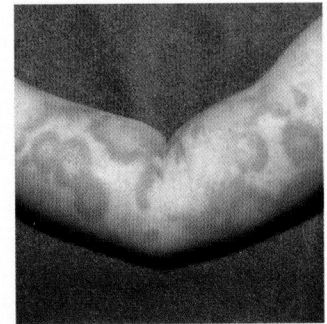

Wheal *(Weston, Lane, and Morelli, 2007)*

Nodule

Elevated, firm, circumscribed lesion; deeper in dermis than a papule; 1 to 2 cm in diameter

Erythema nodosum, lipomas

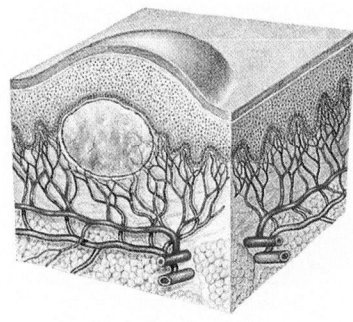

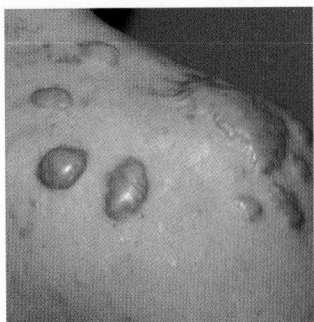

Nodule *(Marks and Miller, 2006)*

Tumor

Elevated and solid lesion; may or may not be clearly demarcated; deeper in dermis; greater than 2 cm in diameter

Neoplasms, benign tumor, lipoma, hemangioma

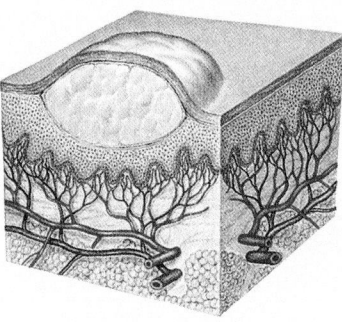

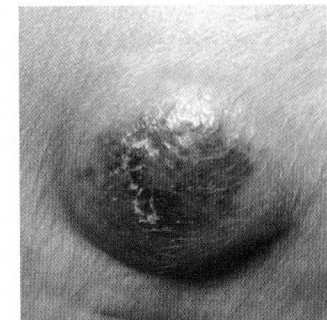

Hemangioma *(Marks and Miller, 2006)*

Vesicle

Elevated, circumscribed, superficial, not into dermis; filled with serous fluid; less than 1 cm in diameter

Varicella (chickenpox), herpes zoster (shingles)

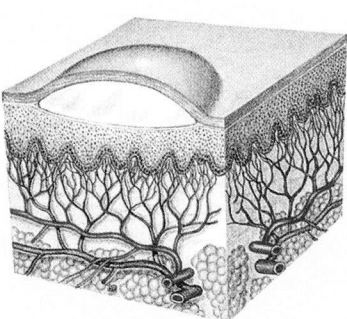

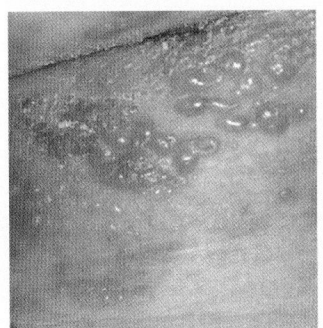

Vesicles caused by zoster *(Weston, Lane, and Morelli, 2007)*

Continued

Primary skin lesions—cont'd

Description	Examples

Bulla

Vesicle greater than 1 cm in diameter

Blister, pemphigus vulgaris

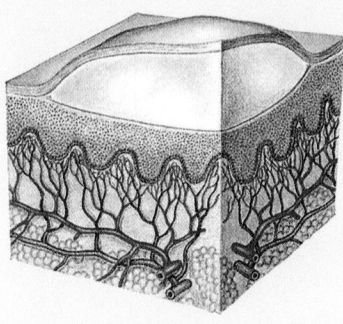

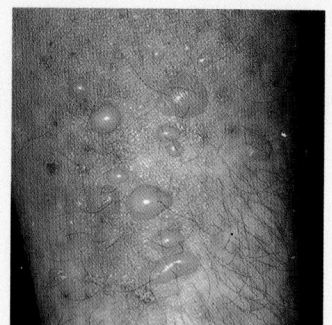

Bullous pemphigoid *(White and Cox, 2006)*

Pustule

Elevated, superficial lesion; similar to a vesicle but filled with purulent fluid

Impetigo, acne

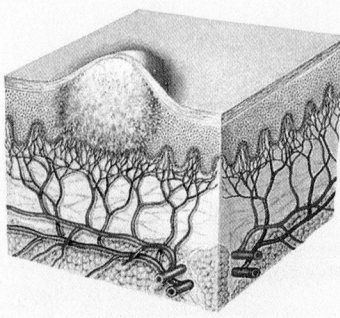

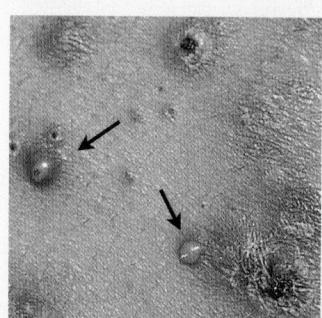

Acne *(Weston, Lane, and Morelli, 2007)*

Cyst

Elevated, circumscribed, encapsulated lesion; in dermis or subcutaneous layer; filled with liquid or semi-solid material

Sebaceous cyst, cystic acne

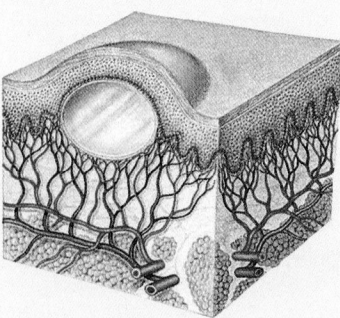

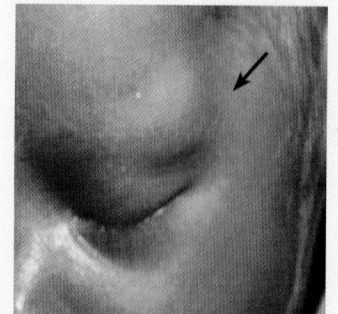

Sebaceous cyst *(Weston, Lane, and Morelli, 2007)*

Telangiectasia

Fine, irregular red lines produced by capillary dilation

Telangiectasia in rosacea

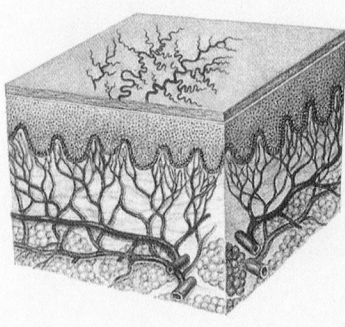

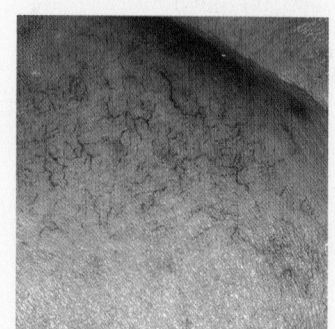

Telangiectasia *(White and Cox, 2006)*

From Seidel et al: *Mosby's guide to physical examination,* ed 7, St. Louis, 2011, Mosby. Modified from Thompson JM, Wilson SF: *Health assessment for nursing practice,* ed 2, St Louis, 2001, Mosby.

Secondary skin lesions

Description	Examples		

Scale

Heaped-up keratinized cells; flaky skin; irregular; thick or thin; dry or oily; variation in size

Flaking of skin with seborrheic dermatitis after scarlet fever, or flaking of skin after a drug reaction; dry skin

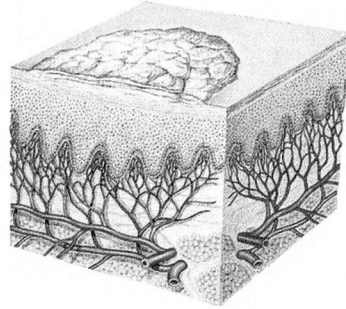

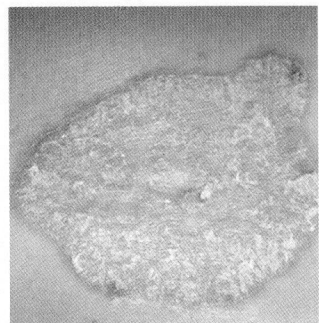

Scale *(Marks and Miller, 2006)*

Lichenification

Rough, thickened epidermis secondary to persistent rubbing, itching, or skin irritation; often involves flexor surface of extremity

Chronic dermatitis

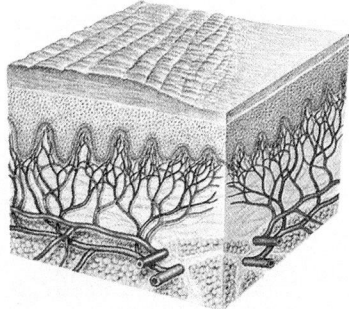

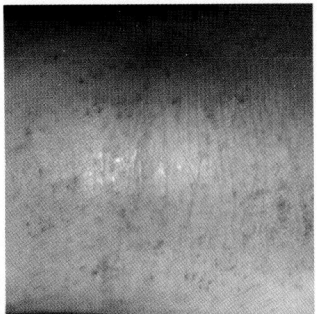

Atopic dermatitis *(Marks and Miller, 2006)*

Keloid

Irregular-shaped, elevated, progressively enlarging scar; grows beyond the boundaries of the wound; caused by excessive collagen formation during healing

Keloid formation after surgery

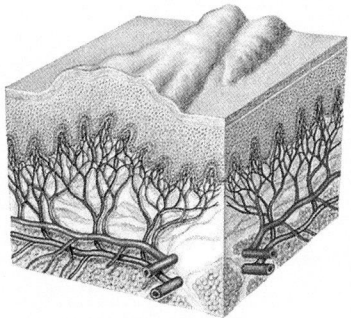

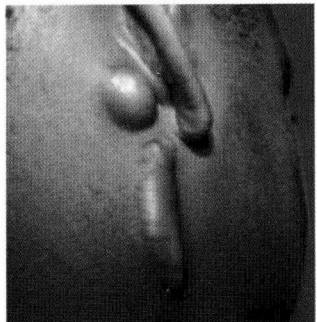

Keloid *(Weston, Lane, and Morelli, 2007)*

Scar

Thin to thick fibrous tissue that replaces normal skin following injury or laceration to the dermis

Healed wound or surgical incision

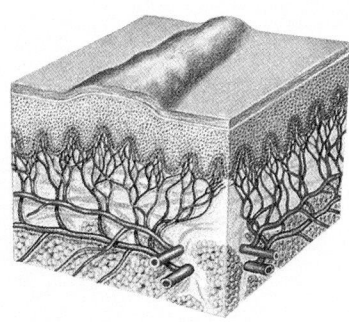

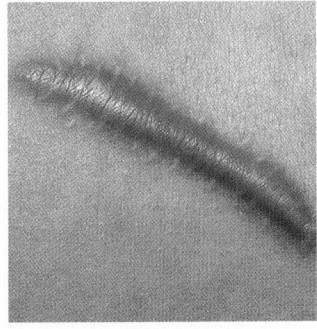

Hypertrophic scar *(White and Cox, 2006)*

L

Continued

Secondary skin lesions—cont'd

Description	Examples		

Excoriation

Loss of the epidermis; linear hollowed-out crusted area

Abrasion or scratch, scabies

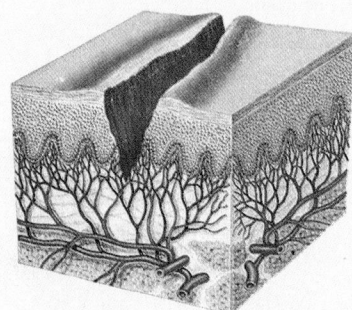

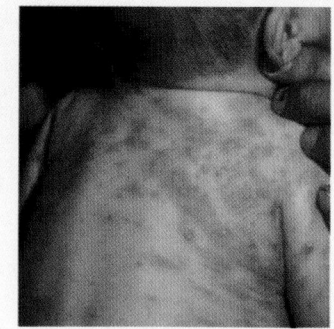

Scabies (Weston, Lane, and Morelli, 2007)

Fissure

Linear crack or break from the epidermis to the dermis; may be moist or dry

Athlete's foot, cracks at the corner of the mouth

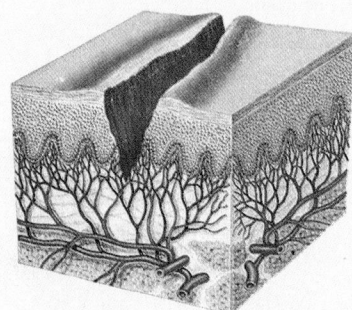

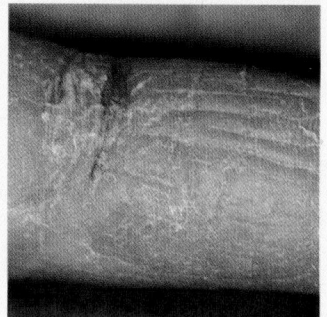

Fissure (Weston, Lane, and Morelli, 2007)

Erosion

Loss of part of the epidermis; depressed, moist, glistening; follows rupture of a vesicle or bulla

Varicella, variola after rupture

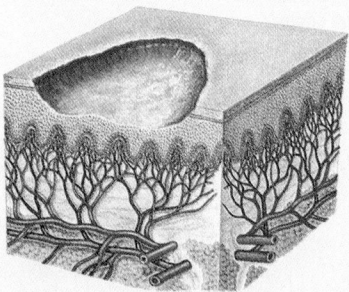

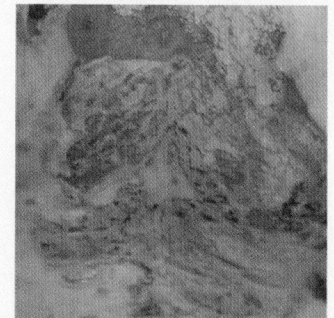

Erosion (Marks and Miller, 2006)

Ulcer

Loss of epidermis and dermis; concave; varies in size

Decubiti, stasis ulcers

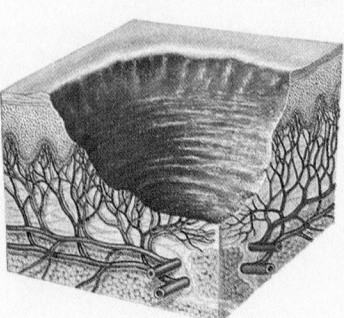

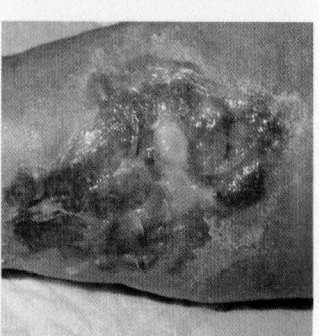

Stasis ulcer (Marks and Miller, 2006)

Secondary skin lesions—cont'd

Description	Examples
Crust	
Dried serum, blood, or purulent exudate; slightly elevated; size varies; brown, red, black, tan, or straw	Scab on abrasion, eczema

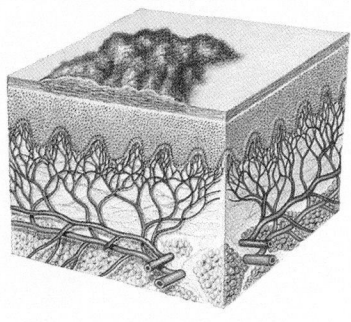
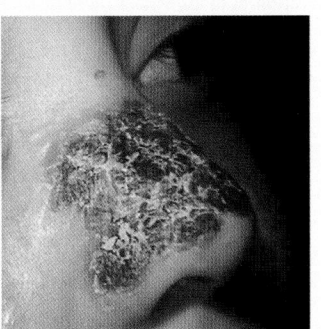

Scab *(Seidel et al, 2011)*

Atrophy	
Thinning of skin surface and loss of skin markings; skin translucent and paperlike	Striae; aged skin

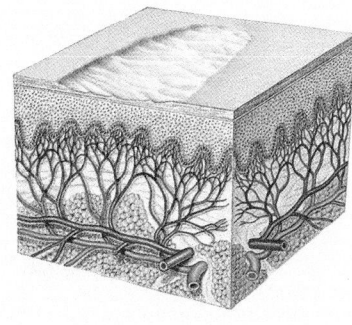
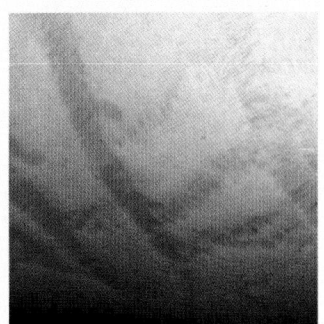

Striae *(Seidel et al, 2011/Courtesy Dr. Antoinette Hood, Department of Dermatology, University of Indiana, Department of Medicine)*

From Ball et al: *Seidel's guide to physical examination*, ed 8, St Louis, 2015, Mosby. Modified from Wilson, SF, Giddens, J: *Health assessment for nursing practice.* ed 4, St. Louis, 2009, Mosby.

lethality /lēthal″itē/, the probability that a person threatening suicide will succeed, based on the method described, the specificity of the plan, and the availability of the means.

lethargic encephalitis. See **epidemic encephalitis.** Also called **encephalitis lethargica.**

lethargy /leth″ərjē/ [Gk, *lethargos,* forgetful], the state or quality of dullness, prolonged sleepiness, sluggishness, or serious drowsiness. Compare **stupor.** –*lethargic, adj.*

letrozole, an antineoplastic nonsteroidal aromatase inhibitor.
- INDICATIONS: It is used to treat metastatic breast cancer in postmenopausal women.
- CONTRAINDICATIONS: Known hypersensitivity or pregnancy prohibits its use.
- ADVERSE EFFECTS: Hepatotoxicity is a life-threatening effect of this drug. Other adverse effects include dyspnea, cough, constipation, heartburn, diarrhea, alopecia, sweating, hot flashes, hypertension, somnolence, dizziness, depression, and anxiety. Common side effects include nausea, vomiting, anorexia, rash, pruritus, headache, and lethargy.

Letterer-Siwe syndrome /let″ərər zē″və/ [Erich Letterer, German pathologist, 1895–1982; Sture A. Siwe, Swedish physician, 1897–1966], any of a group of acquired malignant neoplastic diseases of unknown origin, characterized by histiocytic elements. The syndrome, fatal when untreated, occurs in infancy. Anemia, hemorrhage, splenomegaly, lymphadenopathy, and localized tumorlike swellings over bones are usually present.

Leu, abbreviation for **leucine.**

leucine (Leu) /loo″sēn/ [Gk, *leukos,* white], a white crystalline essential amino acid required for optimal growth in infants and nitrogen equilibrium in adults. It cannot be synthesized by the body and is obtained by the hydrolysis of food protein during digestion. An inherited defect in one of the enzymes involved in the process results in a rare disorder called maple syrup urine disease. See also **amino acid, leucinosis, maple syrup urine disease.**

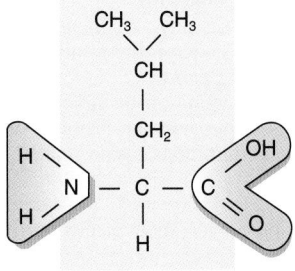

Chemical structure of leucine

leucine aminopeptidase (LAP) test, a blood or 24-hour urine test that detects levels of LAP, used primarily in diagnosing liver, pancreas, and small intestine disorders and in the differential diagnosis of increased levels of alkaline phosphatase.

leucinosis /loo′sinō″sis/ [Gk, *leukos* + *osis,* condition], a condition in which the pathways for the degradation of leucine are blocked and large amounts of the amino acid accumulate in body tissue, producing leucine in the urine. See also **leucine.**

leuco-. See **leuko-, leuco-.**

leucocyte. See **leukocyte.**

leucocyte migration inhibition factor. See **macrophage migration inhibiting factor.**

leucocytopenia. See **leukopenia.**

leucocytosis. See **leukocytosis.**

leucoderma. See **leukoderma.**

leuconychia. See **leukonychia.**

leucopenia. See **leukopenia.**

leucophoresis. See **leukophoresis.**

leucopoiesis. See **leukopoiesis.**

leucorrhoea. See **leukorrhea.**

leucovorin. See **folinic acid.**

leucovorin calcium /loo′kəvôr″in/, a reduced form of folic acid that can be used immediately for nucleic acid synthesis.

■ INDICATIONS: It is prescribed in the treatment of an overdose of a folic acid antagonist and certain cases of megaloblastic anemia. It is also used for leucovorin "rescue" after high-dose methotrexate therapy in osteosarcoma to diminish the toxicity of the methotrexate.

■ CONTRAINDICATIONS: Anemia caused by vitamin B_{12} deficiency or known hypersensitivity to this drug prohibits its use.

■ ADVERSE EFFECTS: Hypersensitivity reactions may occur.

leukaemia, British spelling for leukemia. See **leukemia.**

leukapheresis /loo′kəfərē″sis/ [Gk, *leukos* + *aphairesis,* removal], a donation process by which blood is withdrawn from a vein, white blood cells are selectively removed, and the remaining blood is reinfused into the donor. It is a treatment or supportive care measure in patients with leukocytopenia. Compare **plasmapheresis, plateletpheresis.** See also **apheresis.**

leukemia /lookē″mē·ə/ [Gk, *leukos* + *haima,* blood], a group of malignant neoplasms of hematopoietic tissues characterized by diffuse replacement of bone marrow or lymph nodes with proliferative white blood cell precursors. Peripheral blood WBC counts become elevated, and immature or variant forms appear in the peripheral blood. Leukemia may be chronic or acute, lymphoid, myeloid, or erythroid. In some chronic leukemias, when untreated, the WBC count becomes grossly elevated and can cause retinal hemorrhage, ringing of the ears, mental status changes, prolonged erection, and stroke. Also spelled **leukaemia.** See also **acute childhood leukemia, acute lymphocytic leukemia, acute myeloid leukemia.**

-leukemia, suffix meaning "an increased number of leukocytes in the tissues and/or in the blood": *chloroleukemia, erythroleukemia, aleukemia.*

leukemia cutis, a condition of the skin in which yellowbrown, red, or purple nodular lesions form localized or general diffuse infiltrations. Also called **lymphoderma perniciosa.**

leukemia inhibitory factor (LIF), a cytokine named for its ability to suppress the spontaneous proliferation of lymphoid stem cells.

leukemic. See **leukemia.**

leukemic hiatus, a condition observed in acute myelogenous leukemia in which there are numerous myeloblasts and

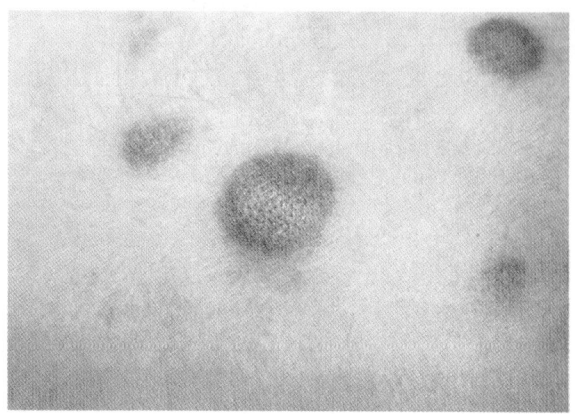

Leukemia cutis *(Weston, Lane, and Morrelli, 2007)*

a number of mature neutrophils in the peripheral blood, with few or no intermediate forms.

leukemic reticuloendotheliosis. See **hairy-cell leukemia.**

leukemoid /lookē″moid/, resembling leukemia.

leukemoid reaction [Gk, *leukos* + *eidos,* form; L, *re,* again, *agere,* to act], a clinical syndrome resembling leukemia in which the white blood cell count is elevated in response to an allergy, inflammatory disease, infection, poison, hemorrhage, burn, or severe physical stress. Compare **leukemia.**

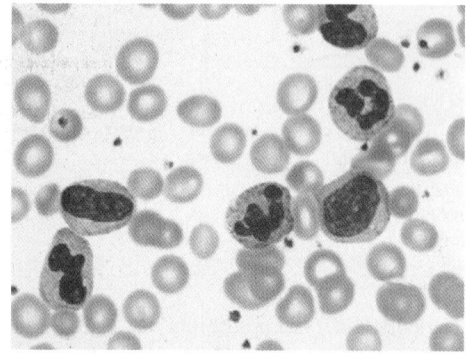

Leukemoid reaction *(Zitelli and Davis, 2007)*

Leukeran, an antineoplastic drug. Brand name for **chlorambucil.**

-leukin, suffix for interleukin-2-type products.

leuko-, leuco-, prefix meaning "white corpuscle" or "white": *leukocytopenia, leukocytosis.*

leukoagglutinin /loo′kō·aglō″tinin/, an antibody that causes white blood cells to adhere to one another.

leukoagglutinin test, a blood test to determine whether WBC incompatibility is the source of transfusion reaction in patients who have undergone complete compatibility testing.

leukoblast /loo′kəblast/ [Gk, *leukos,* white, *blastos,* germ], *(Informal)* an immature leukocyte, or white blood cell. Not in common usage.

leukocoria /loo′kōkor·ē·ə/ [Gk, *leukos,* white + *korē,* pupil]. See **cat's eye amaurosis.**

leukocyte /loo′kəsīt/ [Gk, *leukos* + *kytos,* cell], a blood cell that participates in immunity and inflammation. Five categories of leukocytes are classified by nuclear appearance and the presence or absence of granules in the cytoplasm. Lymphocytes have no granules or a few scattered azurophilic granules. The granulocytes are monocytes, neutrophils,

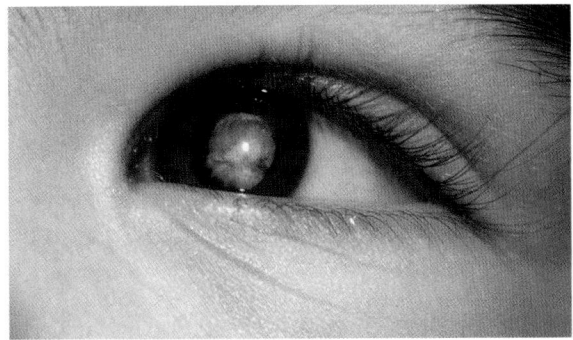

Leukocoria *(Courtesy K. Nischal)*

basophils, and eosinophils. White cells are able to pass through endothelial gap junctions by diapedesis and migrate by ameboid movements. Leukocytes measure 8 to 20 µm in diameter. Normal WBC counts vary from 4500 to 11,500 leukocytes per µL. Leukocytes function as phagocytes of bacteria, fungi, and viruses; detoxifiers of proteins that may result from allergic reactions and cellular injury; and immune system cells. Also called **white blood cell, white corpuscle.** Also spelled **leucocyte.** Compare **erythrocyte, platelets.** See also **complete blood count, differential white blood cell count, leukocytosis, leukopenia.** –**leukocytic,** *adj.*

leukocyte adhesion deficiency (LAD), an autosomal inherited disorder caused by a defective integrin molecule (CD18) that is important for cellular adhesion. This defect causes neutrophils to be immotile and unable to phagocytose. Patients with LAD have recurring bacterial infections and impaired wound healing, which may lead to necrosis and gangrene.

leukocyte alkaline phosphatase (LAP), an enzyme present in lymphocytes that is elevated in various diseases such as cirrhosis and polycythemia and in certain infections. It is measured in the blood to detect these disorders and to differentiate chronic myelogenous (myelocytic) leukemia from leukemoid reactions. Normal amounts of this enzyme in a smear of fresh venous blood are 50 to 150 units. Also called **neutrophil alkaline phosphatase.**

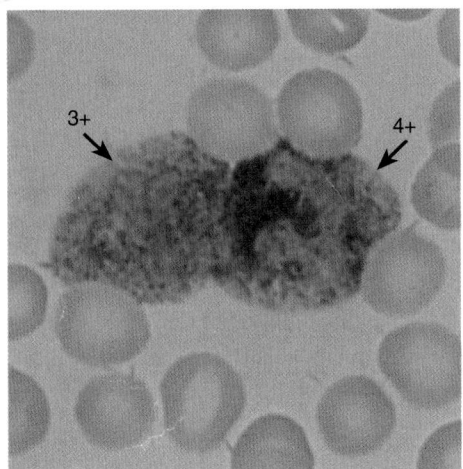

Leukocyte alkaline phosphatase reaction *(Carr and Rodak, 2008)*

leukocyte emigration, the passage (diapedesis) of leukocytes through the endothelial gap junctions of blood vessels in inflammation.

leukocyte migration inhibition factor. See **macrophage migration inhibiting factor.**

leukocytic, pertaining to white blood cells. See **leukocyte.**

leukocytic crystal. See **Charcot-Leyden crystal.**

leukocytoclastic vasculitis /loo′kəsī′təklas″tik/, an allergic inflammation of blood vessels, characterized by deposits of fragmented cells, nuclear dust, necrotic debris, and fibrin staining in the vessels. Many patients develop skin lesions, particularly on the legs, accompanied by arthralgia and fever. The disorder is seen in rheumatoid arthritis and other diseases.

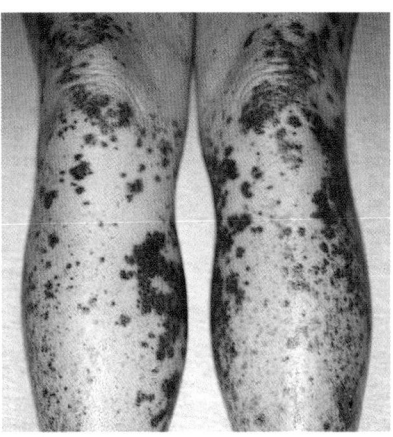

Leukocytoclastic vasculitis: characteristic skin lesions *(Callen et al, 2000)*

leukocytogenesis /-jen″əsis/, the origin and development of leukocytes.

leukocytopenia. See **leukopenia.**

leukocytopoiesis. See **leukopoiesis.**

leukocytosis /loo′kōsītō″sis/ [Gk, *leukos* + *kytos,* cell, *osis,* condition], an abnormally elevated total peripheral white blood cell count, often associated with bacterial infection. Extreme elevations may be associated with leukemia. Also spelled **leucocytosis.** Compare **leukemia, leukemoid reaction, leukopenia.** Kinds include *basophilia,* **eosinophilia, neutrophilia.** See also **leukocyte.**

leukocyturia /loo′kəsītoor″ē-ə/, the presence of white blood cells in the urine.

leukoderma /loo′kōdur″mə/ [Gk, *leukos* + *derma,* skin], a localized loss of skin pigment that can be caused by contact with chemicals that destroy skin pigment cells, a reaction to medication, infection, immune dysfunction, or skin injuries (such as burns). Also spelled **leucoderma.** Compare **vitiligo.**

leukodystrophy /-dis″trəfē/ [Gk, *leukos,* white, *dys* + *trophe,* nourishment], a disease of the white matter of the brain, characterized by demyelination. See also **leukoencephalopathy.**

leukoencephalopathy /loo′kō-ən-sef′əlop′əthē/ [Gk, *leukos,* white + *enkephalos,* brain + *pathos,* disease], any of a group of diseases affecting the white matter of the brain, especially of the cerebral hemispheres, occurring as a rule in infants and children. The term *leukodystrophy* is used to denote such disorders resulting from a defect in the formation and the maintenance of myelin in infants and children.

leukoerythroblastic /loo′kō-erith′rōblas″tik/ [Gk, *leukos* + *erythros,* red, *blastos,* germ, *a* + *haima,* not blood], the presence of immature red blood cells and granulocytes in the peripheral blood and bone marrow, often associated with

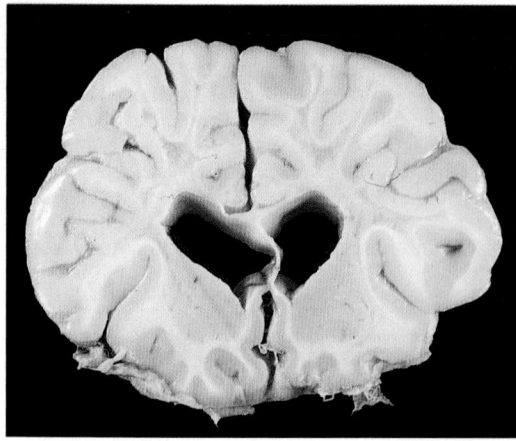

Leukodystrophy *(Kumar, Cotran, and Robbins, 2003)*

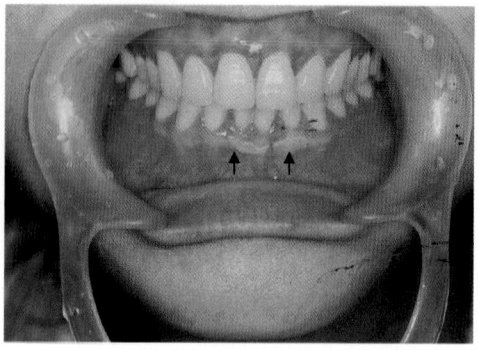

Oral leukoplakia *(Sun et al, 2009)*

primary myelofibrosis and other myeloproliferative neoplasms. See also **myeloid metaplasia.**

leukokoria. See **leukocoria.**

leukonychia /loo'kōnik″ē·ə/ [Gk, *leukos* + *onyx,* nail], a benign condition in which white patches appear under the nails. Trauma, infection, and many disorders can cause white spots or streaks on nails. Also spelled **leuconychia.**

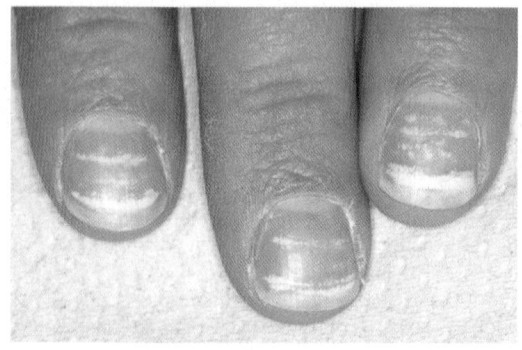

Transverse leukonychia *(Richert et al, 2015)*

leukopenia /loo'kōpē″nē·ə/ [Gk, *leukos* + *penes,* poor], an abnormal decrease in the total peripheral blood white cell count, often associated with chemotherapy or radiation. Leukopenia may result from an idiosyncratic drug reaction and may be seen in acute myeloblastic leukemia. Also called **leucocytopenia.** Also spelled **leucopenia.** Compare **aleukia, leukocytosis.** See also **aplastic anemia, leukocyte.** –*leukopenic, adj.*

leukopenic leukemia. See **aleukemic leukemia.**

leukophlegmasia. See **phlegmasia alba dolens.**

leukophoresis /loo'kōfərē″sis/ [Gk, *leukos* + *phoresis,* being transmitted], a laboratory procedure in which blood is drawn and white blood cells are separated from the blood and the red blood cells are returned to the patient. Also spelled **leucophoresis.**

leukoplakia /loo'kōplā″kē·ə/ [Gk, *leukos* + *plakos,* plate], a precancerous, slowly developing change in a mucous membrane characterized by thickened, white, firmly attached patches that are slightly raised and sharply circumscribed. They may occur on the genitals or in the oral cavity. Those appearing on the lips and buccal mucosa are usually associated with pipe smoking. Malignant potential is evaluated by microscopic study of biopsied tissue. Compare **lichen planus.** See also **lichen sclerosis et atrophicus.**

leukoplakic vulvitis /-plā″kik/ [Gk, *leukos,* white, *plakos,* plate, *vulva* + *itis,* inflammation], a condition in which the skin of the vulva becomes thick and white, develops bleeding fissures, and later becomes atrophic. The condition may progress to cancer.

leukopoiesis /loo'kōpō·ē″sis/ [Gk, *leukos* + *poiein,* to make], the production of white blood cells. Monocytes, neutrophils, basophils, and eosinophils are produced from bone marrow myeloblasts. Lymphocytes develop from lymphoblastic precursors in peripheral lymphoid tissue. Also called **leukocytopoiesis.** Also spelled **leucopoiesis.**

leukorrhea /loo'kôrē″ə/ [Gk, *leukos* + *rhoia,* flow], a white discharge from the vagina. Normally, vaginal discharge occurs in regular variations of amount and consistency during the course of the menstrual cycle. A greater-than-usual amount is normal in pregnancy, and a decrease is to be expected after delivery, during lactation, and after menopause. Leukorrhea is the most common reason for women to seek gynecological care. Also spelled **leucorrhoea.** See also **vaginal discharge.**

leukosarcoma. See **lymphoma.**

leukostasis, a severe elevation of white blood cells, often blast cells. It is typically seen in acute myeloid leukemia, resulting in decreased tissue perfusion due to blockage of blood flow. Also called **symptomatic hyperleukocytosis.**

leukotomy. See **lobotomy.**

leukotoxin /loo'kətok″sin/ [Gk, *leukos* + *toxikon,* poison], a substance that can inactivate or destroy leukocytes. –*leukotoxic, adj.*

leukotrienes /loo'kətrī″ēnz/, a class of biologically active compounds that occur naturally in leukocytes and produce allergic and inflammatory reactions similar to those of histamine. They are thought to play a role in the development of allergic and autoallergic diseases such as asthma, rheumatoid arthritis, inflammatory bowel disease, and psoriasis.

leukovirus /loo'kəvī″rus/ [Gk, *leukos,* white; L, *virus,* poison], a former genus composed of ribonucleic acid tumor viruses, now included in the family Retroviridae.

leuprolide acetate /loo″prōlīd/, an analog of gonadotropin-releasing hormone. It is an agonist administered at levels that desensitize the pituitary gland from responding to it or to endogenous gonadotropin-releasing hormone, thereby preventing pituitary stimulation of sex hormone production by the ovaries or testes.

■ INDICATIONS: It is used for the palliative treatment of advanced prostatic cancer, in the management of endometriosis, and for the treatment of children with central precocious puberty.

■ CONTRAINDICATIONS: Caution should be exercised during the beginning of leuprolide acetate therapy, when symptoms of bone pain, urinary obstruction, and neurological problems may increase. Pregnancy or known hypersensitivity to the drug prohibits its use.

■ ADVERSE EFFECTS: Among adverse effects reported are hot flashes, transient increases in testosterone levels, dizziness, pain, headache, decreased libido, impotence, and injection site irritation.

levalbuterol, an adrenergic β₂-agonist.

■ INDICATIONS: It is used in the treatment and prevention of bronchospasm (reversible obstructive airway disease).

■ CONTRAINDICATIONS: Tachydysrhythmias, severe cardiac disease, or known hypersensitivity to sympathomimetics prohibits its use.

■ ADVERSE EFFECTS: Among adverse effects are insomnia, headache, dizziness, stimulation, hallucinations, flushing, irritability, dry nose, irritation of the nose and throat, palpitations, tachycardia, hypertension, angina, hypotension, arrhythmias, heartburn, nausea, vomiting, and muscle cramps. Common side effects include tremors, anxiety, and restlessness.

levamisole, an immunomodulator used as an adjunct treatment in combination with fluorouracil after surgical resection in patients with Dukes' stage C colon cancer.

levarterenol bitartrate. See **norepinephrine bitartrate.**

levator /livā″tər/ pl. **levatores** [L, levare, to lift up], **1.** a muscle that raises a structure of the body, as the levator ani raises parts of the pelvic diaphragm. **2.** a surgical instrument used to lift depressed bony fragments in fractures of the skull and other bones.

levator anguli oris, a deeply placed oral muscle arising from the maxilla that elevates the corner of the mouth and may help deepen the furrow between the nose and the corner of the mouth during sadness.

levator ani, one of a pair of muscles of the pelvic diaphragm that stretches across the bottom of the pelvic cavity like a hammock, supporting the pelvic organs. It is a broad, thin muscle that separates into the pubococcygeus and the iliococcygeus. It originates from the ramus of the pubic bone, the spine of the ischium, and a band of fascia between the pubis and the ischium; it inserts into the last two segments of the coccyx, the anococcygeal raphe, the sphincter ani externus, and the central tendinous point of the perineum. The left and right levator ani muscles are divided ventrally but converge as a single sheet across the midline dorsally, forming most of the pelvic diaphragm. The levator ani is innervated by branches of the pudendal plexus, which contains fibers from the fourth sacral nerve. It functions to support and slightly raise the pelvic floor. The pubococcygeus draws the anus toward the pubis and constricts it. Compare **coccygeus.**

levatores. See **levator.**

levatores costarum, muscles of the thoracic wall that, together with muscles between the vertebrae and ribs posteriorly, alter the position of the ribs and sternum and so change thoracic volume during breathing.

levator labii superioris, an oral muscle arising from the maxilla just superior to the infraorbital foramen that deepens the furrow between the nose and the corner of the mouth during sadness.

levator labii superioris alaeque nasi, an oral muscle medial to the levator labii superioris that arises from the maxilla next to the nose and inserts into both the alar cartilage of the nose and the skin of the upper lip. It may assist in flaring the nares.

levator palpebrae superioris, one of the three muscles of the eyelid, also considered an extrinsic muscle of the eye. It is thin and flat and rises from the small wing of the sphenoid. It is innervated by the oculomotor nerve. It elevates the upper eyelid and is the antagonist of the orbicularis oculi. Compare **corrugator supercilii, orbicularis oculi.**

levator scapulae, a muscle of the dorsal and lateral aspects of the neck. It arises from the axis and the atlas, and it inserts into the transverse processes of the four upper cervical vertebrae. It is innervated by the third and fourth cervical nerves and acts to raise the scapula and pull it toward the midline.

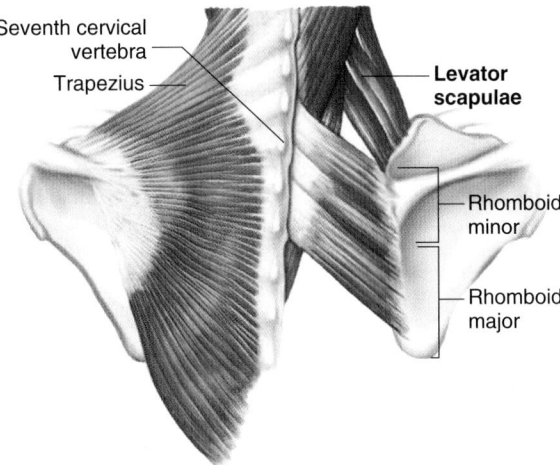

Levator scapulae (Thibodeau and Patton, 2007)

levator veli palatini, one of the muscles originating from the base of the skull that elevate the palate above neutral position and close the pharyngeal isthmus between the nasopharynx and oropharynx.

LeVeen shunt [Harry H. LeVeen, American surgeon, b. 1914], a tube that is surgically implanted to connect the peritoneal cavity and the superior vena cava to drain accumulated fluid from the peritoneal cavity. It is used in cirrhosis of the liver, right-sided heart failure, or abdominal cancer. Before surgery a sodium-restricted diet and diuretics are used to decrease sodium and water retention. With the patient under general anesthesia, a silicone rubber tube is inserted under the subcutaneous tissue from the peritoneal cavity to the superior vena cava. As the patient inhales, the fluid pressure in the peritoneal cavity increases and that in the blood vessel falls, allowing peritoneal fluid to enter the shunt valve. After surgery the patient is closely observed for signs of occlusion of the shunt, GI bleeding, or leakage of peritoneal fluid from the incision. Excessive dilution of the blood may lead to coagulation abnormalities.

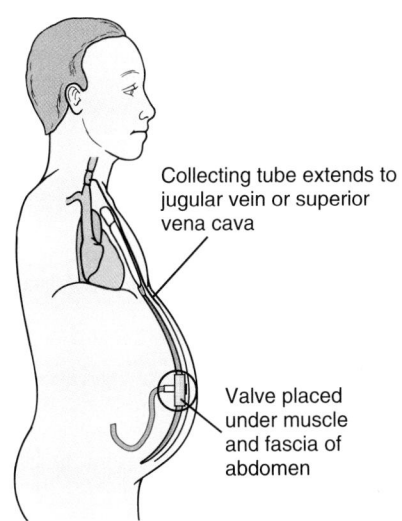

Collecting tube extends to jugular vein or superior vena cava

Valve placed under muscle and fascia of abdomen

LeVeen shunt (Lewis et al, 2007)

level of activities [OFr, *livel* + L, *activus*], pertaining to the hierarchy of nervous system activity that determines the level responsible for certain functions while also being controlled by a higher level, as in the sequence of events in a reflex action.

level of consciousness (LOC) [OFr, *livel* + L, *conscire,* to be aware of], a degree of cognitive function involving arousal mechanisms of the reticular formation of the brain. The stages of response of the mind to stimuli vary from unconsciousness through vague awareness to full attention. The usual standard levels include coma, in which the patient does not appear to be aware of the environment; stupor, in which the patient is vaguely aware of the environment; drowsiness, in which the patient responds to stimuli but may be slow to react; and alert wakefulness. Impaired LOC may be expressed in obtundation or reduced alertness, stupor, syncope, or unresponsiveness. See also **Glasgow Coma Scale, preconscious, subconscious.**

level of inquiry [OFr, *livel* + *inquirere,* to ask about], (in research) one of the levels in a rank-ordered system of classification and organization of the questions to be answered in a research study. The level of inquiry is determined by an analysis of the theory to be developed or tested and the kinds of data to be collected. Studies that describe comprise the first level, whereas those that explain comprise the second level. Those that prescribe or predict are the most difficult to answer or to support.

levels of care, a classification of health care service levels by the kind of care given, the number of people served, and the people providing the care. Kinds include **primary health care, secondary health care, tertiary health care.**

lever /lē″vər, lev″ər/ [L, *levare,* to lift up], any one of the numerous bones and associated joints of the body that act as a simple machine so that force applied to one end of the bone tends to rotate the bone in the direction opposite from that of the applied force. The muscles of the body produce the forces that move the levers. The basic components of a lever are the fulcrum, the force arm, and the weight arm. A first-class lever, such as the joint between the base of the skull and the first cervical vertebra, has a fulcrum between the weight and the applied force. The body contains few second-class levers, which have the weight between the fulcrum and the force. A third-class lever, such as the forearm and elbow, has the force between the fulcrum and the weight. The body uses its third-class levers for speed and its first-class levers for either force or speed, depending on the force applied to the weight arm.

levetiracetam, an anticonvulsant drug.
■ INDICATIONS: It is used to treat partial-onset seizures.
■ CONTRAINDICATIONS: Known hypersensitivity to this drug prohibits its use.
■ ADVERSE EFFECTS: Adverse effects include lowered hematocrit, lowered hemoglobin, infection, dizziness, somnolence, and asthenia.

Lévi-Lorain dwarf. See **pituitary dwarf.**

Levine, Myra Estrin [1920–1996], a nursing theorist who developed a framework for nursing practice with the formulation of Four Conservation Principles: energy, structural integrity, personal integrity, and social integrity. The first edition of her book discussing the conservation principles, *Introduction to Clinical Nursing,* was published in 1969. Levine's emphasis on the ill person in the health care setting reflects the history of health care in the

1960s. Levine's model stresses nursing interventions and interactions based on the scientific background of these principles. Levine viewed people in a holistic manner, as having their own environments, both internal and external. She identified four levels of integration that help a person maintain his or her integrity or wholeness: fight or flight, inflammatory response, response to stress, and perceptual response. The individual's stability is organized by his or her availability of responses and adaptation processes. It is the nurse's task to bring a body of scientific principles on which decisions are based into the situation shared with the patient.

Levin tube /lev″in/ [Abraham L. Levin, American physician, 1880–1940], a plastic catheter introduced through the nose and used in gastric intubation for gastric decompression or gavage feeding. Compare **Miller-Abbott tube.** See also **gastric intubation.**

levitation /lev′itā″shən/ [L, *levitas,* lightness, *atus,* process], (in psychiatry) a hallucinatory sensation of floating or rising in the air. –*levitate, v.*

Levitra, brand name for **vardenafil.**

levo-, prefix meaning "left": *levocardia, levotorsion.*

levobetaxolol /le″vobatak′sälol/, a cardioselective beta-adrenergic blocking agent used in the form of the hydrochloride salt, administered topically to the conjunctiva in treatment of glaucoma and ocular hypertension.

levobunolol /le″vobu′nolol/, a beta-adrenergic blocking agent used in treatment of glaucoma and ocular hypertension, applied topically to the conjunctiva as the hydrochloride salt.

levobunolol hydrochloride /-bun″əlol/, a topical ophthalmic beta-adrenergic blocker drug for glaucoma.
■ INDICATIONS: It is prescribed for the treatment of chronic open-angle glaucoma and ocular hypertension.
■ CONTRAINDICATIONS: It is contraindicated for patients with bronchial asthma, severe chronic obstructive pulmonary disease, sinus bradycardia, second- or third-degree atrioventricular block, overt cardiac failure, or cardiogenic shock.
■ ADVERSE EFFECTS: Adverse effects may include transient ocular burning or stinging, bradycardia, pulmonary edema, and blepharoconjunctivitis.

levobupivacaine, a local anesthetic.
■ INDICATIONS: It is used for local and regional anesthesia for pain management and for continuous epidural analgesia.
■ CONTRAINDICATIONS: Severe liver disease or known hypersensitivity to this drug contraindicates its use. It is also contraindicated in children under 12 years of age and in the elderly.
■ ADVERSE EFFECTS: Life-threatening effects are convulsions, loss of consciousness, myocardial depression, cardiac arrest, arrhythmias, fetal bradycardia, status asthmaticus, respiratory arrest, and anaphylaxis. Other adverse effects include anxiety, restlessness, drowsiness, disorientation, tremors, shivering, bradycardia, hypotension, hypertension, nausea, vomiting, blurred vision, tinnitus, pupil constriction, rash, urticaria, allergic reactions, edema, burning, skin discoloration at the injection site, and tissue necrosis.

levocabastine /le″vokab′ästēn/, an antihistamine applied topically to the conjunctiva as the hydrochloride salt to treat seasonal allergic conjunctivitis.

levocardia /-kär″dē·ə/, a congenital anomaly in which the viscera are transposed to the opposite side of the body, except for the heart, which is in its normal position.

levocarnitine /-kär″nitēn/, an oral drug for carnitine deficiency.

■ INDICATIONS: It is prescribed for the treatment of primary systemic carnitine deficiency.

■ CONTRAINDICATIONS: It should not be given to patients with a known hypersensitivity to carnitine.

■ ADVERSE EFFECTS: Adverse effects include nausea, dizziness, vomiting, abdominal cramps, diarrhea, and body odor.

levocetirizine, a low-sedating antihistamine.

■ INDICATIONS: This drug is used to treat perennial or seasonal rhinitis, allergy symptoms, and chronic idiopathic urticaria.

■ CONTRAINDICATIONS: Breastfeeding, end-stage renal disease, dialysis, and known hypersensitivity to this drug, cetirizine, or hydroxyzine prohibit its use. Children from 6 to 11 years of age with renal disease should not take this drug.

■ ADVERSE EFFECTS: Adverse effects of this drug include asthenia, dry mouth, increased liver function tests, and transient rash. Common side effects include drowsiness and fatigue.

levoclination. See **levotorsion.**

levodopa /lē′vōdō′pə/, an antiparkinsonian agent.

■ INDICATIONS: It is prescribed in the treatment of Parkinson disease, juvenile forms of Huntington disease when rigidity is the main feature, and chronic manganese poisoning (which can lead to Parkinson-like symptoms in welders).

■ CONTRAINDICATIONS: Narrow-angle glaucoma, concomitant use of a monoamine oxidase inhibitor, suspected melanoma, or known hypersensitivity to this drug prohibits its use.

■ ADVERSE EFFECTS: Among the more serious adverse effects are severe GI disturbances, hypotension, various movement disorders, emotional changes, cardiac arrhythmia, and anorexia.

Levo-Dromoran, an opioid analgesic drug. Brand name for **levorphanol tartrate.**

levofloxacin, an antiinfective drug.

■ INDICATIONS: It is used to treat acute sinusitis, acute or chronic bronchitis, community-acquired pneumonia, uncomplicated skin infections, complicated urinary tract infections, and acute pyelonephritis caused by *Streptococcuspneumon iae,Haemophilusinfluenzae,H.parainfluenzae,* and *Moraxellacatarrhalis.*

■ CONTRAINDICATIONS: Known hypersensitivity to quinolones and photosensitivity prohibit its use.

■ ADVERSE EFFECTS: Life-threatening effects are anaphylaxis, multisystem organ failure, hemolytic anemia, pseudomembranous colitis, and Stevens-Johnson syndrome. Other adverse effects include hypoglycemia, hypersensitivity, dizziness, anxiety, encephalopathy, paresthesia, chest pain, palpitations, vasodilation, eosinophilia, lymphopenia, pneumonitis, flatulence, diarrhea, abdominal pain, vaginitis, crystalluria, rash, and pruritus. Common side effects are headache, insomnia, nausea, vomiting, and photosensitivity.

levomethadyl /le″vometh′ädil/, an opioid analgesic used as an adjunct in the treatment of opioid addiction, administered orally as the acetate hydrochloride salt.

Levophed Bitartrate, an adrenergic drug. Brand name for **norepinephrine bitartrate.**

levorphanol tartrate /lē′vôrfā″nol/, an opioid analgesic.

■ INDICATIONS: It is prescribed for the treatment of pain and preoperative analgesia.

■ CONTRAINDICATIONS: Alcoholism, asthma, increased intracranial pressure, respiratory depression, anoxia, or known hypersensitivity to this drug prohibits its use.

■ ADVERSE EFFECTS: Among the more serious adverse effects are drug dependence, orthostatic hypotension, cardiac arrhythmia, and retention of urine.

levothyroxine sodium /-thī′rəksēn/, a thyroid hormone. Also called L-**thyroxine.**

■ INDICATIONS: It is prescribed in the treatment of hypothyroidism.

■ CONTRAINDICATIONS: Recent myocardial infarction or known hypersensitivity to this drug prohibits its use.

■ ADVERSE EFFECTS: The most serious adverse effects are angina, tachycardia, arrhythmias, and tremors.

levotorsion /lev′itôr″shən/, the rotation to the left of the upper pole of the cornea of one or both eyes. Also called **levoclination.**

Lev disease [Maurice Lev, American pathologist, 1908–1994], fibrosis or calcification of the conduction system of the heart that results in varying degrees of heart block in patients with a normal myocardium and coronary arteries.

Levulan Kerastick therapy, a treatment for actinic keratoses and acne that uses topical Levulan ALA activated by a light source to remove lesions and improve the appearance of the skin. See **photochemotherapy.**

levulose. See **fructose.**

levulosuria. See **fructosuria.**

Lewis blood group system, a blood-group system based on antigens present in soluble forms in blood and secretions. The antigens are adsorbed from the plasma onto the red cell membrane. The expressed Lewis phenotype is based on whether the patient is a secretor or nonsecretor of the Lewis gene product.

lewisite /lō″isīt/ [Winford L. Lewis, American chemist, 1878–1943], 2-chlorovinyl arsine, a poisonous blister gas used in World War I that causes irritation of the lungs, dyspnea, damage to the tissues of the respiratory tract, tears, and pain.

Lewy bodies /lā″wē, lō″ē/ [Frederick H. Lewy, German neurologist, 1885–1950], concentric spheres found inside vacuoles in midbrain and brainstem neurons of patients with idiopathic parkinsonism, Alzheimer disease, and other neurodegenerative conditions.

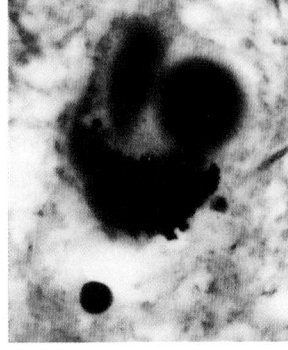

Lewy body in the substantia nigra *(Perkin, 2002)*

-lexia, suffix meaning "reading": *alexia, dyslexia.*

Lexiva, brand name for **fosamprenavir.**

lexor retinaculum of the hand, the thick fibrous band of antebrachial fascia that wraps the carpal canal surrounding the tendons of flexor muscles of the forearm at the distal ends of the radius and the ulna. Also called *retinaculum flexorum manus, volar ligament.*

Leyden-Möbius muscular dystrophy /lī″dənmœ″bē·əs, mē″bē·əs/, a form of limb-girdle muscular dystrophy that begins in the pelvic girdle. Also called **pelvifemoral muscular dystrophy.**

Leydig cells /lī″dig/ [Franz von Leydig, German anatomist, 1821–1908], **1.** cells of the interstitial tissue of the testes

L

that secrete testosterone. **2.** mucous cells that do not pour their secretions out over the surface of the epithelium.

Leydig cell tumor [German anatomist Franz Leydig, 1821-1908], a generally benign neoplasm of interstitial cells of a testis that may cause gynecomastia in adults and precocious sexual development if the lesion occurs before puberty. Less commonly it occurs in the ovary and causes androgenic symptoms. The tumor is usually a circumscribed lobulated palpable mass. Symptoms typically resolve after excision. Compare **Sertoli-Leydig cell tumor.**

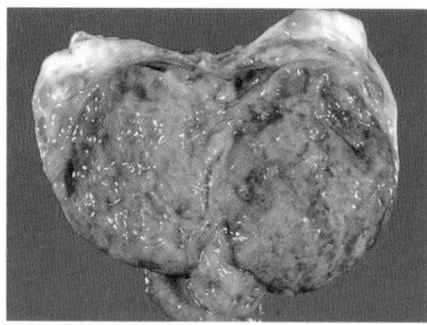

Ovarian Leydig cell tumor *(Olivier et al, 2012)*

LF, abbreviation for *low frequency.*
LFA, abbreviation for *left frontoanterior fetal position.*
LFP, abbreviation for *left frontoposterior fetal position.*
LFT, abbreviation for **liver function test.**
LGA, abbreviation for *large for gestational age.* See **large for gestational age (LGA) infant.**
LGBT, abbreviation for *lesbian, gay, bisexual, or transgender.*
LGBTQ, abbreviation for *lesbian, gay, bisexual, transgender, queer.* The letter *Q* can also represent *questioning.*
LGL syndrome, abbreviation for **Lown-Ganong-Levine (LGL) syndrome.**
LGV, abbreviation for **lymphogranuloma venereum.**
LH, abbreviation for **luteinizing hormone.**
Lhermitte sign /ler″mit/ [Jacques J. Lhermitte, French neurologist, 1877–1959], sudden transient, electric-like shocks spreading down the body when the head is flexed forward, occurring chiefly in multiple sclerosis but also in compression disorders of the cervical spinal cord. The sign is usually elicited by the examiner when the patient is supine.
LH-RH, abbreviation for **luteinizing hormone–releasing hormone.**
Li, symbol for the element **lithium.**
liability /līabil″itē/ [L, *ligare,* to bind], **1.** something one is obligated to do or an obligation required to be fulfilled by law, usually financial in nature. **2.** the amount of money required to fulfill a financial obligation.
Liaison Council on Certification for the Surgical Technologist. See **National Board of Surgical Technology & Surgical Assisting.**
liaison nursing /lē·ā″zən/, a nurse involved in the education of clients, family members, referral sources, and external payers regarding the effective and efficient utilization of program services and available resources.
libel /lī″bəl/ [L, *libellus,* little book], a false accusation written, printed, typewritten, or presented in a picture or a sign that is made with malicious intent to defame the reputation of a person resulting in public embarrassment, contempt, ridicule, or hatred.

liberation /lib′ərā″shən/ [L, *liber,* free], the process of drug release from the dosage form.
libidinal development. See **psychosexual development.**
libido /libē″dō, libī″dō/, **1.** the psychic energy or instinctual drive associated with sexual desire, pleasure, or creativity. **2.** (in psychoanalysis) the instinctual drives of the id. **3.** lustful desire or striving.
Libman-Sacks endocarditis /lib″mən saks″/ [Emanuel Libman, American physician, 1872–1946; Benjamin Sacks, American physician, 1896–1939], the most common manifestation of lupus erythematosus, characterized by warty lesions that develop near the heart valves but rarely affect valvular action. The lesions usually are dry and granular, with a pink or tawny color. They contain basophilic cellular debris and develop in the angle of the atrioventricular valves and at the base of the mitral valve. Also called *Libman-Sacks disease, Libman-Sacks syndrome.*

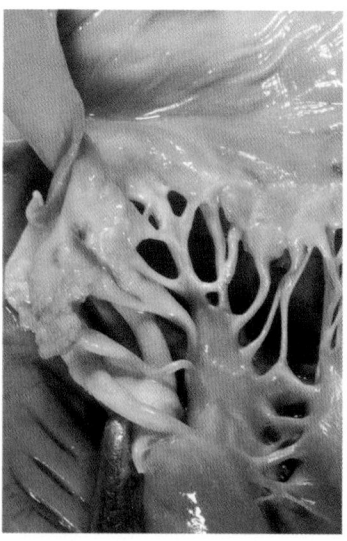

Libman-Sacks endocarditis *(Courtesy Dr. Fred Schoen, Department of Pathology, Brigham and Women's Hospital)*

Librax, a fixed-combination drug containing an anticholinergic and an antianxiety agent. It is used to treat gastric ulcers, irritable bowel syndrome, and gastritis. Brand name for *clidinium bromide, chlordiazepoxide hydrochloride.*
Libritabs, an antianxiety agent. Brand name for *chlordiazepoxide hydrochloride.*
Librium, an antianxiety agent. Brand name for *chlordiazepoxide hydrochloride.*
lice [AS, *lus,*], any of the small wingless insect order of Phthiraptera. This order has been divided into four suborders: Anoplura (sucking lice), Rhyncopthira, Ischnocere, and Amblycer. Lice are ectoparasites of birds and mammals and may spend their entire life cycle on a single host, attaching eggs to the hair shafts or feathers. They transfer to humans by direct contact. Three forms that infect humans are the head louse, *Pediculus humanus capitis*; the body louse, *Pediculus humanus corporis*; and the crab louse, *Phthirus pubis.*
license, an agency- or government-granted permission issued to a health care professional to engage in a given occupation on finding that the applicant has attained the degree of competency and met educational requirements necessary to ensure that the public health, safety, and welfare are reasonably well-protected.

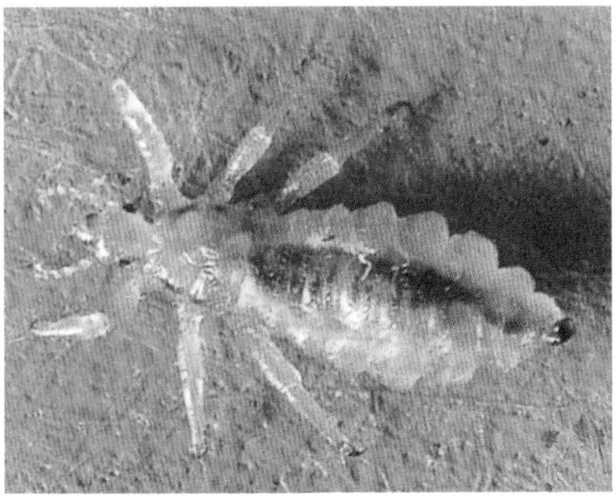

Human body louse *(Courtesy Ken Gray, Oregon State University Extension Services)*

licensed counselor, a mental health provider who has fulfilled certain standards of education and supervised practice and who has passed the National Counselor Examination of the National Board for Certified Counselors.

licensed marriage and family therapist (LMFT), a person who has earned a master's degree or PhD in marriage and family therapy from an accredited graduate program and who has completed at least 1000 hours of supervised clinical practice and scored successfully on the National Certification Examination.

licensed practical nurse (LPN) /lī″sənst/ [L, *licere,* to be allowed; Gk, *praktikos,* fit for action; L, *nutrix,* nurse], **1.** *(in the United States)* a person educated in basic nursing techniques and direct patient care whose qualifications and education have been examined by a state board of nursing and who has legal authorization to practice. The course of education usually lasts 1 year. Once licensed, a licensed practical nurse practices under the supervision of a registered nurse. Also called **licensed vocational nurse.** **2.** *(in Canada)* a person with a diploma from an accredited practical nursing program of 2 to 2½ years who has taken the national practical nursing examination. Each province regulates the practice. The LPN practices under the supervision of an RN or RPN (registered psychiatric nurse).

licensed psychologist, a person who has earned a doctorate in psychology from an accredited graduate school, has completed 2 to 3 years of postgraduate training with special emphasis on the diagnosis and treatment of psychological disorders, and is licensed in the state in which he or she practices. Also called *clinical psychologist.* See also **psychotherapist.**

licensed vocational nurse. See **licensed practical nurse.**

licensure /lī″sənshŏŏr/ [L, *licere,* to be allowed], the granting of permission by a competent authority (usually a governmental agency) to an organization or individual to engage in a practice or activity that would otherwise be illegal. Kinds of licensure include the issuing of licenses for general hospitals or nursing homes, for health professionals such as physicians or nurses, and for the production or distribution of biological products. Licensure is usually granted on the basis of education and examination. It is usually permanent, but a periodic fee, demonstration of competence, or continuing education may be required. Licensure may be revoked by the granting agency for incompetence, criminal acts, or other reasons stipulated in the rules governing the specific area of licensure. Compare **certify.**

lichen amyloidosis /lī″kən/, a common form of amyloidosis characterized by symmetric distribution over the skin of translucent yellowish-brown dome-shaped pruritic papules, most commonly on the lower legs.

lichen aureus, a rare type of chronic pigmented purpura in which the patient has a single red or rust-colored lesion on a lower limb, usually over a perforating vein.

lichenification /līken′ifikā″shən/ [Gk, *leichen,* lichen, *facere,* to make], thickening and hardening of the skin, giving it a leathery, barklike appearance, often resulting from the irritation caused by repeated scratching of a pruritic lesion. *–lichenified, adj.*

lichen nitidus [Gk, *leichen* + L, *nitidus,* bright], a rare skin disorder characterized by numerous flat, glistening, pale, discrete papules measuring 2 to 3 mm in diameter. Lesions are localized in the early stages, chiefly on the lower abdomen, penis, and inner surface of the thighs. Distribution may become more generalized as the disease progresses.

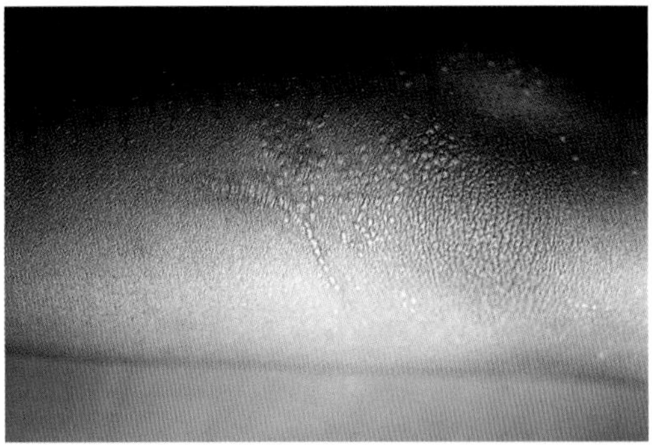

Lichen nitidus *(Callen et al, 2000)*

lichenoid eczema /lī″kənoid/, a chronic inflammatory, cutaneous condition characterized by skin thickening and accentuated skin lesions.

lichen planus, a nonmalignant, chronic, pruritic skin disease of unknown cause that is characterized by small flat purplish polygonal papules or plaques with fine gray lines on the surface. Common sites are flexor surfaces of wrists, forearms, ankles, abdomen, sacrum, and genitalia. On mucous membranes the lesions appear gray and lacy. Nails may have longitudinal ridges. Episodes of disease activity vary but may last for months and may recur. Treatment with topical corticosteroids is common.

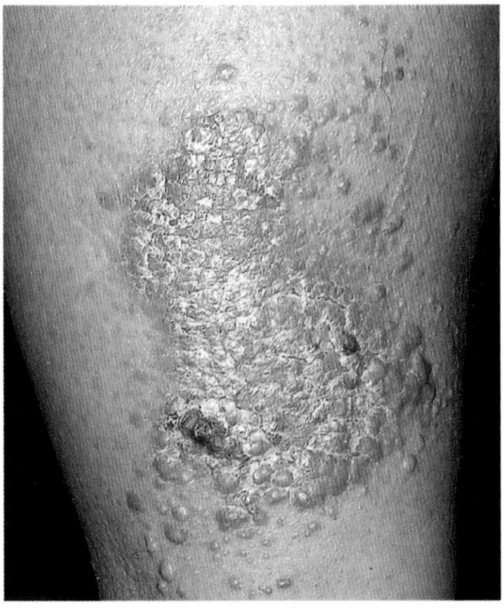

Lichen planus *(Habif, 2010)*

L

lichen sclerosis et atrophicus, a chronic skin disease characterized by white flat papules and black hard follicular plugs. In advanced cases the papules tend to coalesce into large white patches of thin pruritic skin. Lesions often occur on the torso and in the anogenital regions. In the vulvar and perianal area, it occurs as white papules that coalesce into smooth ivory- or porcelain-colored plaque or patches. Also called **white spot disease.** See also **kraurosis vulvae.**

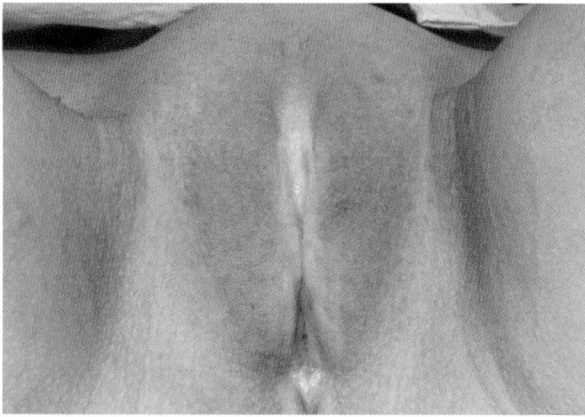

Lichen sclerosis et atrophicus *(Osiecka et al, 2012)*

lichen simplex chronicus, a form of dermatitis characterized by a patch of pruritic confluent papules. Factors such as scratching contribute to its chronicity. Treatment may include topical or intralesional application of corticosteroids to relieve the pruritus.

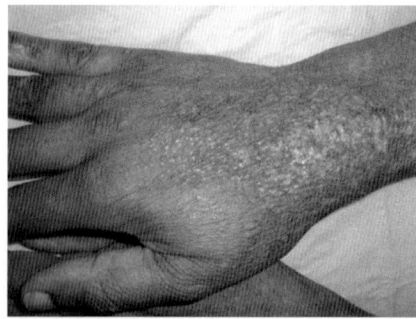

Lichen simplex chronicus *(Ferri and Ferri, 2018)*

lichen urticatus. See **papular urticaria.**

Lichtheimia **sp.,** a fungi present in the environment, usually soil-born or found on decaying plants and baked goods. It is capable of causing mucormycoses, a rare but emerging disease with a poor prognosis, especially in patients who are immunosuppressed. Formerly called *Absidia.*

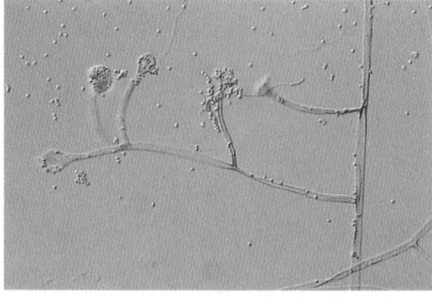

Lichtheimia *(Mahon, Lehman, and Manuselis, 2011)*

licorice, an herb that grows in shrub form in many subtropical areas.

■ INDICATIONS: It is used for allergies, arthritis, asthma, constipation, esophagitis, gastritis, hepatitis, inflammatory conditions, peptic ulcers, poor adrenal function, and poor appetite. Its efficacy for these indications is not proven, but its active ingredients (glycyrrhizin and glycyrrhetinic acid) alter prostaglandin synthesis, are agonists at mineralocorticoid receptors, and prolong the half-life of cortisol.

■ CONTRAINDICATIONS: Licorice should not be used during pregnancy and lactation, in children, or in those with known hypersensitivity. It is also contraindicated in people with liver disease, renal disease, hypokalemia, hypertension, arrhythmias, and congestive heart failure.

lid. See **eyelid.**

Lidex, a glucocorticoid. Brand name for **fluocinonide.**

lidocaine hydrochloride /lī″dəkān/, a local anesthetic agent.

■ INDICATIONS: It is prescribed as a local anesthetic for topical administration or local injection into skin or mucous membranes. It is used parenterally as an antiarrhythmic agent to increase the threshold of electrical stimulation in the ventricles during diastole.

■ CONTRAINDICATIONS: Known hypersensitivity to this drug prohibits its topical use. Adam-Stokes syndrome heart block or known hypersensitivity to this drug prohibits its systemic use.

■ ADVERSE EFFECTS: Among the more serious adverse effects of the systemic administration of the drug are central nervous system disturbances, hypotension, bradycardia, and cardiac arrest. A variety of hypersensitivity reactions may occur from topical administration of this drug. Eating and drinking are avoided for 1 hour after topical application of this drug to the pharynx or the esophagus.

lid poppers. See **amphetamines.**

lie [AS, *licgan,* position], the relationship between the long axis of the fetus and the long axis of the mother. In a longitudinal lie the fetus is lying lengthwise, or vertically, in the uterus, whereas in a transverse lie the fetus is lying crosswise, or horizontally.

Lieberkühn's glands /lē″bərkēnz/ [Johann N. Lieberkühn, German anatomist, 1711–1756; L, *glans,* acorn], tubular glands between the bases of the villi of the small intestine and on the surface of the epithelium of the large intestine. They secrete a watery fluid, not digestive enzymes. Also called *crypts of Lieberkühn,* **follicles of Lieberkühn, intestinal glands.**

lie detector [AS, *leogan,* untruth; L, *detegere,* to uncover], an electronic device or instrument used to detect lying or anxiety in regard to specific questions. A commonly used lie detector is the polygraph recorder that senses and records pulse, respiratory rate, blood pressure, and perspiration. Some experts hold that certain patterns indicate the presence of anxiety, guilt, or fear—emotions that are likely to occur when the subject is lying.

lien. See **spleen.**

lienal vein /lī″ənəl, lē·ē″nəl/ [L, *lien,* spleen, *vena*], a large vein of the lower body that unites with the superior mesenteric vein to form the portal vein. It returns blood from the spleen. Also called **splenic vein.**

lieno-, prefix meaning "spleen": *lienography.*

lienography /lē″ənog″rəfē/, the radiographic examination of the spleen after it has been injected with a contrast medium.

LIF, abbreviation for **leukemia inhibitory factor.**

LiF, symbol for **lithium fluoride.**

life [AS, *lif*], the energy that enables organisms to grow, reproduce, absorb and use nutrients, evolve, and in some organisms to achieve mobility, express consciousness, and demonstrate a voluntary use of the senses.

life costs [AS, *lif* + L, *constare,* constant], the mortality, morbidity, and suffering associated with a given disease or medical procedure.

life cycle, **1.** the interval of time from conception to natural death. **2.** the series of stages from any stage of one generation to the same stage of the next generation.

life expectancy, the probable number of years a person will live after a given age, as determined by mortality in a specific geographic area. It may be individually qualified by the person's condition or race, sex, age, or other demographic factors. Also called **expectation of life.**

life extension [AS, *lif,* life; L, *extenere,* to stretch out], the process of extending the life span of an individual or population by intervention that promotes better use of preventive medicine and use of established diagnostic and therapeutic facilities.

life review, **1.** (in psychiatry) a progressive return to consciousness of past experiences. **2.** reminiscences that occur in old age as a consequence of the realization of the inevitability of death. Also called **reminiscence therapy.**

lifesaving measure, any medical intervention that is implemented when a patient's life is threatened.

life science, the study of the laws and properties of living matter. Compare **physical science.** Kinds include **anatomy, bacteriology, biology.**

life space, a term introduced by American psychologist Kurt Lewin to describe simultaneous influences that may affect individual behavior. The totality of the influences make up the life space.

life span, the length of life of an individual or the average length of life in a population or species.

lifestyle-induced health problems, diseases with natural histories that include conscious exposure to certain health-compromising or risk factors. An example is heart disease associated with cigarette smoking, poor dietary habits, lack of exercise, and sustained unbuffered stress.

life support [AS, *lif,* life; L, *supportare,* to bring up to], the use of any therapeutic technique, device, or technology to maintain physical life functions.

lifetime reserve [AS, *lif* + *tid,* time; L, *re,* again, *servare,* to keep], a lifetime total of days of inpatient hospitalization benefits that may be drawn on by a patient who has exhausted the maximum benefits allowed under Medicare for a single episode of illness.

Li-Fraumeni cancer syndrome /lē′ frômen″ē/ [Frederick P. Li; Joseph F. Fraumeni, Jr.; 20th-century American epidemiologists], a type of familial breast carcinoma affecting young women and associated with soft-tissue sarcomas and other cancers in close relatives.

lift assessment [AS, *lyft,* loft; L, *assidere,* to sit beside], the selection of the most appropriate lift method to use when moving a patient, as from the bed to a chair. The assessment involves consideration of such factors as whether the patient is conscious or unconscious; whether the patient has a visual, hearing, or cognitive impairment; the need for special care in handling patient attachments such as IV lines or monitors; the patient's body weight; and whether the patient has full range of motion or flaccid or spastic limbs.

ligament /lig″əmənt/ [L, *ligare,* to bind], **1.** one of many predominantly white, shiny, flexible bands of fibrous tissue binding joints together and connecting the articular bones and cartilages to facilitate movement. Such ligaments are slightly elastic and composed of parallel collagenous bundles. When part of the synovial membrane of a joint, they are covered with fibroelastic tissue that blends with surrounding connective tissue. Yellow elastic ligaments such as the ligamenta flava connect certain parts of adjoining vertebrae. Compare **tendon. 2.** a layer of serous membrane with little or no tensile strength, extending from one visceral organ to another, such as the ligaments of the peritoneum. See also **broad ligament. –ligamentous,** *adj.*

ligamental tear /lig′əmen″təl/ [L, *ligare,* to bind; AS, *teran,* to destroy], a complete or partial rupture of a ligament caused by an injury to a joint, as by a sudden twisting motion or a forceful blow.

■ OBSERVATIONS: Ligamental tears may occur at any joint but are most common in the knees, where they typically involve the medial, lateral, and posterior ligaments and the anterior and posterior cruciate ligaments. Usually more than one structure is injured because of the way the structures connect with and support each other. The pathological features of knee ligamental tears depend on the location and severity of the injury. A mild tear may cause little damage, with tenderness, swelling, and pain with stress.

■ INTERVENTIONS: Treatment depends on the severity of the injury. Rest, compression, applications of heat and cold, elevation, and early use are usually recommended for mild tears. Injection of an antiinflammatory agent may be desirable. Treatment for a moderate tear in which few fibers have been completely severed is protective. In addition to the above measures, the joint is aspirated and supported. Treatment for a severe, complete tear is restorative and may include immobilization followed by physical therapy or, if necessary, by surgical repair or reconstruction.

■ PATIENT CARE CONSIDERATIONS: Ligamental tears of the knee joint are extremely common in young adults and are often associated with sports injuries. Good physical condition may help prevent many injuries, and proper care during healing is necessary to prevent permanent disability, which is often accompanied by joint instability, stiffness, or pain.

ligament of the head of the femur, a flat band of delicate connective tissue that attaches at one end to the fovea on the head of the femur and at the other end to the acetabular fossa, transverse acetabular ligament, and margins of the acetabular notch. It carries a small branch of the obturator artery, which contributes to the blood supply of the head of the femur.

ligament of the neck of the rib, one of five ligaments of each costotransverse joint, consisting of short, strong fibers passing from the neck of the rib to the transverse process of the adjacent vertebra. Also called **middle costotransverse ligament.**

ligament of the tubercle of the rib, one of the five ligaments of each costotransverse joint, comprising a short, thick fasciculus passing obliquely from the transverse process of a vertebra to the tubercle of the associated rib. Compare **ligament of the neck of the rib.**

ligamentous /lig′əmen″təs/ [L, *ligare,* to bind], pertaining to or having the characteristics of a ligament.

ligamentum arteriosum. See **arterial ligament.**

ligand /lig″ənd, lī″gənd/ [L, *ligare,* to bind], **1.** a molecule, ion, or group bound to the central metal atom of a chemical compound, such as the oxygen molecule in oxyhemoglobin, which is bound to the central iron atom. **2.** an organic molecule attached to a specific site on a cell surface or to a tracer element. The binding is reversible in a competitive binding assay. It may be the analyte or a cross-reactant. Examples include vitamin B_{12}, a ligand with intrinsic factor as the binding protein, and various antigens, which are ligands with antibody-binding proteins.

ligase chain reaction, a type of DNA amplification that uses DNA ligase to link chains and amplify the template containing the sequence in question.

ligases /lī″gāsəz/ [L, *ligare* + Fr, *diastase,* enzyme], a group of enzymes that catalyze the formation of a bond between substrate molecules coupled with the breakdown of a pyrophosphate bond in ATP or a similar donor molecule. Kinds include *synthetase enzymes.*

ligation /līgā″shən/ [L, *ligare,* to bind], *n.,* the procedure of tying off a blood vessel or duct with a suture or wire ligature. It may be performed to stop or prevent bleeding during surgery, to stop spontaneous or traumatic hemorrhage, to prevent passage of material through a duct as in tubal ligation, or to treat varicosities. See also **ligature, tubal ligation, varicose vein.** −*ligate, v.*

ligation clip, a small V-shaped clip made from stainless steel, platinum, titanium, or an absorbable material, used to ligate bleeding vessels.

ligature /lig″əchər/ [L, *ligare,* to bind], **1.** a suture. **2.** a wire, as used in orthodontics.

ligature needle, a long, thin, curved needle used for passing a suture underneath an artery for ligation of the vessel.

ligature wire [L, *ligare,* to bind; AS, *wir*], a soft, thin wire used in dental procedures, particularly to connect brackets or attachments on orthodontic appliances.

light [AS, *leoht*], **1.** electromagnetic radiation of the wavelength and frequency that stimulate visual receptor cells in the retina to produce nerve impulses that are perceived as vision. **2.** electromagnetic radiation with wavelengths longer than ultraviolet light and shorter than infrared light, the range of visible light, generally in the range of 400 to 800 nm.

light-adapted eye [AS, *leoht* + L, *adaptatio* + AS, *eage*], an eye that has been exposed to bright light long enough for chemical and physiological adaptation to take place, such as bleaching of the rhodopsin or visual purple. The loss of cone sensitivity to light may require increased light intensity to obtain the same degree of visual acuity. Also called **photopic eye.**

light bath, the exposure of the patient's uncovered skin to the sun or to actinic light rays from an artificial source for therapeutic purposes.

light chain deficiency, an immunodeficiency disease, such as megaloblastic anemia, that is associated with an alteration in the kappa or lambda light chains of immunoglobulins.

light chain disease, a type of multiple myeloma in which plasma cell tumors produce only monoclonal light chain proteins. Persons with light chain disease may develop lytic bone lesions, hypercalcemia, impaired kidney function, and amyloidosis. See also **gammopathy, heavy chain disease, multiple myeloma.**

light chain (L chain), an immunoglobulin subunit of about 22,000 daltons molecular weight. Compare **heavy chain.**

lightening /līt″əning/ [AS, *leoht,* light], a subjective sensation reported by many women late in pregnancy as the fetus settles lower in the true pelvis, leaving more space in the upper abdomen. The diaphragm, no longer restricted by the fundus of the uterus beneath it, can move down more fully during inspiration, allowing deeper breaths. The stomach, too, is less compressed, so the woman can comfortably eat more food at each meal. Urinary frequency occurs as the fetus drops. The profile of the abdomen changes with lightening because the round, full uterus is visibly lower. The baby is then said to have "dropped."

light-headedness, a condition of feeling giddy, faint, delirious, or slightly dizzy.

light joint compression, a technique to cause approximations of joints; frequently used with patients with hemiplegia to alleviate pain and to offset muscle imbalance temporarily around the shoulder joint.

light microscope [AS, *leoht* + Gk, *mikros,* small, *skopein,* to view], a microscope that uses visible light to view objects too small for the naked eye to see.

light reflex, the mechanism by which the pupil of the eye constricts in response to direct or consensual stimulation with light. Also called **pupillary reflex.** Compare **consensual light reflex.** See also **accommodation reflex, direct light reflex.**

light scatter, light dispersion in any direction by suspended particles in a solution. The degree of scattering depends on the size and shape of the particles.

light therapy [AS, *leoht* + Gk, *therapeia,* treatment], the use of natural light or light of specified wavelengths to treat disease. This may include ultraviolet light, colored light, or low-intensity laser light. The eye is generally the initial entry point for the light because of its direct connection to the brain through the retinal hypothalamic pathway, which affects the autonomic nervous system and endocrine function. Light therapy has been used primarily for attention deficit disorders, seasonal affective disorder, and a variety of other conditions. Light therapy also complements other treatments.

light-touch palpation [AS, *leoht* + Fr, *toucher* + L, *palpare,* to touch gently], a method of examination in which the abdomen is gently depressed 1 to 2 cm to determine the size and position of abdominal organs.

light vaginal bleeding. See **vaginal bleeding.**

lignan, a chemical compound found in plants, especially flax and sesame seeds. Lignans are phytoestrogens and may have antioxidant properties.

ligneous /lig″nē·əs/ [L, *ligum,* wood], woody or resembling wood in texture or other characteristics.

ligneous thyroiditis. See **fibrous thyroiditis.**

lignin /lig″nin/ [L, *lignum,* wood], an insoluble polysaccharide that, with cellulose and hemicellulose, forms the chief part of the skeletal substances of the cell walls of plants. It provides bulk in the diet necessary for proper GI functioning. See also **dietary fiber.**

lignocaine. See **lidocaine hydrochloride.**

limb /lim/ [AS, *lim*], **1.** an appendage or extremity of the body, such as an arm or leg. **2.** a branch of an internal organ, such as a loop of a nephron.

limb-girdle muscular dystrophy [AS, *lim,* limb, *gyrdel*], a form of muscular dystrophy transmitted as an autosomal-recessive trait. The characteristic weakness and degeneration of the muscles begin in the shoulder girdle or in the pelvic girdle. The condition is progressive, regardless of the area in which it is first manifest. Kinds include **Erb muscular dystrophy, Leyden-Möbius muscular dystrophy.**

limbic /lim″bik/ [L, *limbus,* edge], pertaining to something that is marginal or at a junction between structures.

limbic lobe [L, *limbus,* edge; Gk, *lobos,* lobe], the marginal section of the cerebral hemispheres on the medial aspects. It forms a ring of neural tissue around the hypothalamus and some nuclei.

limbic system [L, *limbus,* edge], a group of structures within the rhinencephalon of the brain that are associated with various emotions and feelings such as anger, fear, sexual arousal, pleasure, and sadness. The structures of the limbic system include the cingulate gyrus, the isthmus, the hippocampal gyrus, the uncus, and the amygdala. The structures connect with various other parts of the brain such as the septum and the hypothalamus. Unless the limbic system is modulated by other cortical areas, periodic attacks of uncontrollable rage may occur in some individuals. The function of the system is incompletely understood.

limb kinetic apraxia. See **ideomotor apraxia.**

limb lead /lēd/ [AS, *lim,* limb, *laeden,* lead], an electrocardiographic electrode that is attached to an arm or a leg.

Limbrel, brand name for **flavocoxid.**

limbus /lim″bəs/, an edge or border, such as the corneal limbus at the edge of the cornea bordering the sclera.

lime [AS, *lim*], **1.** any of several oxides and hydroxides of calcium. The various kinds of lime have many uses, including the treatment of sewage, the purification of water and refining of sugar, and the manufacture of materials such as

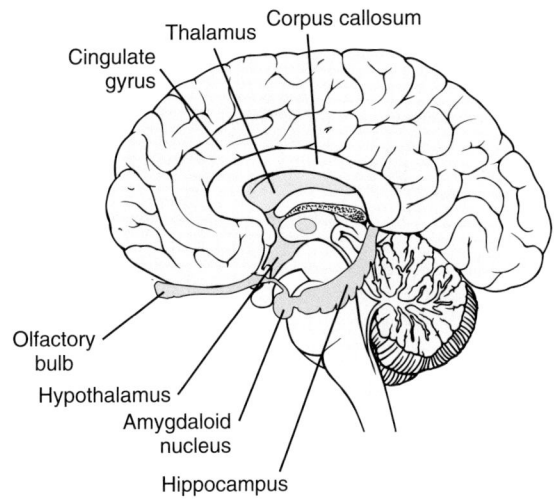

Limbic system *(McKenry and Salerno, 2003)*

plaster and fertilizers. **2.** a citrus fruit yielding a juice with a high ascorbic acid content. Lime juice was one of the first effective agents to be used in the treatment of scurvy. See also **ascorbic acid, scurvy.**

limen.   See **threshold stimulus.**

liminal stimulus.   See **threshold stimulus.**

limitation of motion /lim′itā″shən/   [L, *limes,* limit],   the restriction or reduction of normal range of motion of a body part, caused by disease or injury.

limited fluctuation method of dosing [L, *limes,* limit, *fluctuare,* to wave],   a method of drug administration in which the dose is not allowed to rise or fall beyond specified maximum and minimum limits.

limited scleroderma.   See **CREST syndrome.**

limiting charge,   the maximum amount that can be charged in the United States for the services of a physician who does not accept the restrictions on fees established by Medicare laws. Also called **billing limit.**

limiting resolution,   in computed tomography, the spatial frequency at a modulation transfer function equal to 0.1. The absolute object size that can be resolved by a scanner is equal to the reciprocal of the spatial frequency.

limit of stability,   the greatest distance in any direction a person can lean away from a midline vertical position without falling, stepping, or reaching for support.

limonene,   a chemical derived from citrus peels; it is used as a flavoring agent to enhance the palatability of some medicines and as an additive in food and beverages.

limp [ME, not firm],   an abnormal pattern of ambulation in which the two phases of gait are markedly asymmetric. See also **stance phase of gait, swing phase of gait.**

LINAC,   abbreviation for **linear accelerator.**

Lincocin,   an antibacterial agent. Brand name for **lincomycin hydrochloride.**

lincomycin hydrochloride /lin′kəmī″sin/,   a macrolide antibiotic.
- INDICATIONS: It is prescribed in the treatment of certain infections caused by susceptible bacteria, especially streptococci and staphylococci.
- CONTRAINDICATIONS: Known hypersensitivity to this drug or to clindamycin prohibits its use.
- ADVERSE EFFECTS: Among the more serious adverse effects are blood disorders, diarrhea, and the development of life-threatening pseudomembranous colitis caused by superinfection.

lindane /lin″dān/,   a gamma-benzene hexachloride.
- INDICATIONS: It is prescribed in the treatment of pediculosis and scabies.
- CONTRAINDICATIONS: It is not usually given to infants or pregnant women and is not applied to the face. Known hypersensitivity to this drug prohibits its use.
- ADVERSE EFFECTS: Among the most serious adverse effects are neurological damage and aplastic anemia. Topical administration may result in irritation of eyes, skin, and mucosa.

Lindau–von Hippel disease.   See **von Hippel–Lindau disease.**

line [L, *linea*],   **1.** a connection between two points. **2.** a stripe, streak, or narrow ridge, often imaginary, that serves to connect reference points or to separate various parts of the body, as the hairline or nipple line. **3.** a black absorption line in a continuous spectrum passing through a medium. **4.** an accretion line in the enamel of a tooth marking successive layers of calcification. **5.** a catheter or wire that may be inserted in a vein, such as in an IV line. **6.** the baseline of an electrocardiogram when neither positive nor negative potentials are recorded. **7.** line of sight. Also called **linea.** See also **Frankfurt horizontal plane.**

linea /lin″ē·ə/   [L, line],   a line defining anatomical features, such as the linea alba of the abdomen, the linea albicantes or linea nigra seen on the abdomen during pregnancy, or the linea vitalis curving across the palm at the base of the thumb.

linea alba [L, *linea,* line, *albus,* white],   the white part of the anterior abdominal aponeurosis in the middle line of the abdomen, made of connective tissue representing the fusion of three aponeuroses into a single tendinous band extending from the xiphoid process to the symphysis pubis. It contains the umbilicus. Also called *Hunter line,* **white line.** Compare **linea semilunaris.**

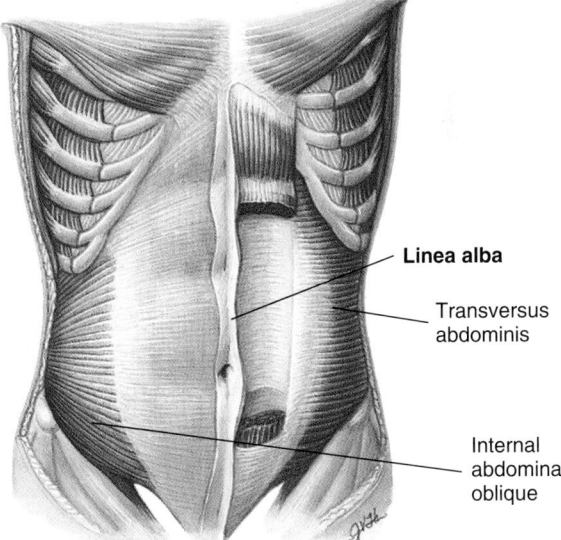

Linea alba *(Thibodeau and Patton, 2003)*

linea arcuata,   the curved tendinous band in the sheath of the rectus abdominis below the umbilicus. It is usually derived from the aponeurosis of the transversus abdominis or the obliquus internus, and sometimes from both of those muscles. It inserts into the linea alba. Compare **linea semilunaris.**

linea aspera, the posterior crest of the femur (thigh bone) that extends proximally into three ridges to which are attached various muscles, including the gluteus maximus, pectineus, and iliacus.

lineae albicantes, lines, white to pink or gray, that occur on the abdomen, buttocks, breasts, and thighs and are caused by the stretching of the skin and weakening or rupturing of the underlying elastic tissue. The condition is usually associated with pregnancy, excessive obesity, rapid growth during adolescence, Cushing syndrome, or prolonged adrenocortical hormone therapy. Also called **stretch mark.**

linea nigra /lin″ē′ənīgrə/, a dark line appearing longitudinally on the abdomen of a pregnant woman during the latter 24 weeks of term. It usually extends from the symphysis pubis midline to the umbilicus and sometimes as far as the sternum.

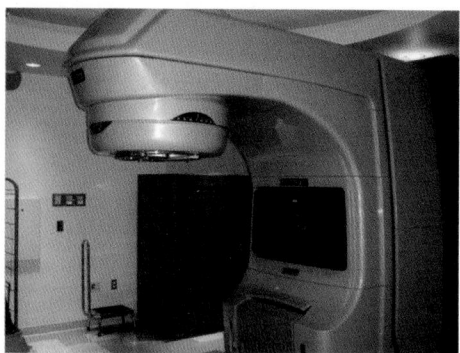

Linear accelerator (Kim et al, 2009)

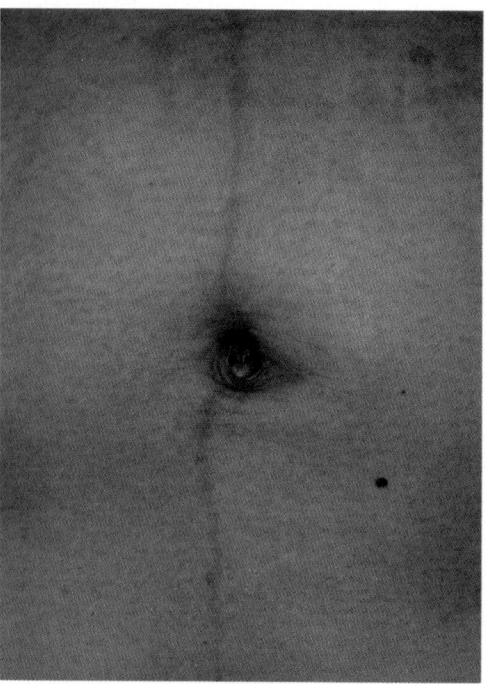

Linea nigra (Bolognia, Jorizzo, and Schaffer, 2012)

linear /lin″ē·ər/ [L, *linea,* line], pertaining to a line or lines, particularly straight lines.

linear accelerator (LINAC) [L, *linea,* line, *accelerare,* to quicken], an apparatus for accelerating charged subatomic particles, used in radiotherapy, physics research, and the production of radionuclides. A pulsed electron beam generated by an electron gun passes through a long, straight vacuum tube containing alternating hollow electrodes. The electrodes are arranged so that when their high-frequency potentials are properly varied, the electrons passing through the tube receive successive increments of energy. The electrons are stopped abruptly by a heavy metal target at the end of the tube and directed by a collimator to deliver supervoltage x-rays to the patient receiving radiotherapy.

linear array, a contiguous sequence of identical discrete detectors, either gas-filled ionization chambers or solid-state semiconductors, used with a fan beam x-ray generator. The detectors read off once for each x-ray pulse. The resulting electronic signal is digitized and stored in a computer memory.

linear energy transfer (LET), the rate at which energy is transferred from ionizing radiation to soft tissue, expressed in terms of kiloelectron volts per micrometer (keV/μm) of track length in soft tissue. The LET of diagnostic x-rays is about 3 keV/μm, whereas the LET of 5 MeV alpha particles is 100 keV/μm.

linear flow velocity, the velocity of a particle carried in a moving stream, usually measured in centimeters per second.

linear fracture, a fracture that extends parallel to the long axis of a bone but does not displace the bone tissue.

linear grid. See **grid.**

linear IgA bullous disease, a condition characterized by linear deposits of immunoglobulin A binding to the area of the lamina lucida. Tense bullae are frequent, and the vesicles are likely to occur on the face, thighs, feet, and flexures. The disease tends to affect women more than men, and half of the patients are under the age of 60. A chronic bullous dermatosis disease of childhood begins in the first 10 years of life with bullae on the trunk, perioral, and pelvic areas but undergoes total remission at adolescence.

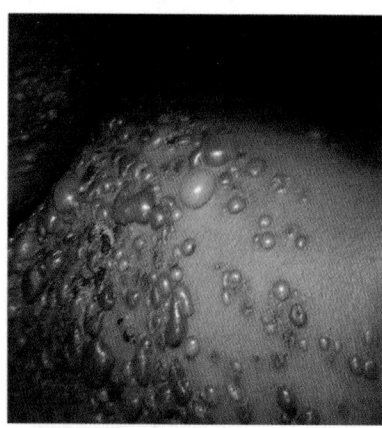

Linear IgA bullous disease (Shah and Laude, 2000)

linearity /lin′ē·er″itē/, the principle that the density of a radiographic exposure is determined by the product of the current and the exposure time.

linear morphea. See **linear scleroderma.**

linear regression, a statistical procedure in which a straight line is established through a data set that best represents a relationship between two subsets or two methods.

linear scan, an ultrasound scan in which the transducer moves at a constant speed along a straight line at right angles to the ultrasound beam.

linear scleroderma, a type of localized scleroderma in which there are bands or lines of thickened skin, especially on the arms and legs, caused by the deposition of collagen. At times it extends into muscle. It often interferes with joint function. Compare **morphea.** See also **localized scleroderma.**

linear staining, the use of fluorescein-labeled goat or rabbit antiimmunoglobulins to produce smooth-staining patterns for study by immunofluorescence microscopy.

linear tomography, tomography that produces a blurring pattern consisting of indistinguishable linear streaks or blurs over the focal-plane image. The pattern is caused by elongation of structures outside the focal plane.

linea semilunaris, the slightly curved line on the ventral abdominal wall, approximately parallel to the median line and lying about halfway between the median line and the side of the body. It marks the lateral border of the rectus abdominis and is visible as a shallow groove when that muscle is tensed. Compare **linea alba.**

linea terminalis, a hypothetic line dividing the upper, or false, pelvis from the lower, or true, pelvis.

linea vitalis. See **linea.**

line compensator, a device that monitors input electric power for medical devices such as x-ray equipment and adjusts for voltage fluctuations.

line density, (in ultrasonography) the number of scan lines used to generate an image.

line focus principle, the principle that viewing a sloped surface at an angle reduces its apparent size. In an x-ray tube the angling of the anode results in the effective focal spot being smaller than the actual focal spot.

line of demarcation [L, *linea* + *de* + *marcare,* to mark], a line that indicates a change in the condition of tissues, such as the boundary between gangrenous and healthy tissues.

line of gravity, an imaginary line that extends from the center of gravity to the base of support.

line pair (lp), a factor that determines the spatial frequency of computed tomography and radiographic images. It consists of multiple parallel lines or bars separated by a space. As the number of line pairs per millimeter decreases, the spatial resolution of the image decreases.

line spread function (LSF), a graph obtained from the image of a narrow line, which quantifies the amount of blur produced by an imaging system.

Lineweaver-Burk transformation /lī″nwēvər burk″/ [Hans Lineweaver, American chemist, b. 1907; Dean Burk, American scientist, 1904–1988; L, *transformare,* to change shape], a method of converting experimental data from studies of enzyme activity so that the data can be displayed on a linear plot. The linear form is derived by using reciprocals of both sides of the equation.

linezolid /lĭnez′olid/, a synthetic antibacterial of the oxazolidinone class, effective against gram-positive organisms and used for the treatment of community-acquired and nosocomial pneumonia, skin and soft tissue infections, and bacteremia. It is administered orally or intravenously.

lingu-, linguo-, prefix meaning "tongue": *lingula, lingualis.*

lingua. See **tongue.**

lingual /ling″gwəl/ [L, *lingua,* tongue], pertaining to or resembling the tongue.

lingual artery [L, *lingua,* tongue], one of a pair of arteries that arises from the external carotid arteries and supplies the tongue and surrounding muscles.

lingual bar, the portion of the metallic base portion of a removable partial denture that is created on the tongue side of the dental arch and that connects bilateral parts of the mandibular removable partial denture.

lingual bone. See **hyoid bone.**

lingual crib, an orthodontic appliance consisting of a wire frame suspended behind the maxillary incisors, used to obstruct undesirable thumb and tongue habits that can produce malocclusions, especially in children.

lingual flange, the part of a mandibular denture that occupies the space adjacent to the residual alveolar ridge and next to the tongue.

lingual frenum. See **frenulum of the tongue.**

lingual gingiva [L, *lingua,* tongue, *gingiva,* gum], the gum tissue covering the teeth on the surfaces facing the tongue.

lingual goiter, a tumor at the back of the tongue formed by an enlargement of the primordial thyrolingual duct.

lingualis leukoplakia [L, *lingua,* tongue; Gk, *leukos,* white, *plax,* plate], a chronic inflammatory lesion characterized by smooth, thick white patches on the surface of the tongue, generally attributed to excessive use of alcohol and tobacco. The lesions may be a precursor of epithelioma.

lingual nerve, a major branch of the mandibular nerve that carries general sensation from the oral part of the tongue, the mucosa on the floor of the oral cavity, and gingiva associated with the lower teeth. It also carries parasympathetic and taste fibers from the oral part of the tongue that are part of the facial nerve.

lingual occlusion. See **linguoocclusion.**

lingual pain, a pain in the tongue, which may be caused by biting the tongue, heavy metal poisoning, Vincent's stomatitis, or infiltration of the lingual muscles by a neoplasm.

lingual papilla. See **papilla.**

lingual rest, a metallic extension attached to the tongue side of an anterior tooth to provide support or indirect retention for a removable partial denture.

lingual thyroid, residual thyroid tissue at the base of the tongue that failed to descend into the neck during embryological development.

lingual tonsil, a mass of lymphoid follicles near the root of the tongue. Each follicle forms a rounded eminence containing a small opening leading into a funnel-shaped cavity surrounded by lymphoid tissue.

lingula /ling″gyələ/ [L, small tongue], any anatomical structure that resembles a tongue.

lingula of the lung [L, *lingula,* small tongue; AS, *lungen*], a tonguelike projection from the costal surface of the upper lobe of the left lung.

lingulectomy /ling′gyəlek″təmē/, a surgical excision of the lingula of the left lung.

linguoocclusal, pertaining to or formed by the tongue side (lingual) and the chewing surface (occlusal) of a posterior tooth or teeth.

linguoocclusion /ling′gwōklō′zhən/ [L, *lingua,* tongue + *occludere,* to close up], malocclusion in which the tooth is leaning toward the tongue from the line of the normal dental arch. Also called **lingual occlusion.**

linguoversion /ling′gwōver′zhən/ [L, *lingua,* tongue + *vertere,* to turn], displacement of a tooth toward the tongue from the line of occlusion.

liniment /lin″imənt/ [L, *linere,* to smear], a preparation, usually containing an alcoholic, oily, or soapy vehicle, that is rubbed on the skin as a counterirritant.

linin /li″nin/ [Gk, *linon,* flax], the faintly staining threads seen in the nuclei of cells, with granules of chromatin attached to the threads. See also **karyolymph.**

linitis /linī″tis/ [Gk, *linon,* flax, *itis,* inflammation], inflammation of cellular tissue of the stomach, as in linitis plastica, seen frequently in adenocarcinoma of the stomach.

linitis plastica, a diffuse fibrosis and thickening of the wall of the stomach, resulting in a rigid, inelastic organ. The layer of connective tissue of the stomach becomes fibrotic and thick, and the stomach wall becomes shrunken and rigid. Causes of this condition include infiltrating undifferentiated carcinoma, syphilis, and Crohn's disease involving the stomach. Also called *leather-bottle stomach.*

linkage /ling″kij/ [Gk, *linke,* connection], **1.** (in genetics) the location of two or more genes on the same chromosome so that they do not segregate independently during meiosis but tend to be transmitted together as a unit. The closer the loci of the genes, the more likely they are to be inherited as a group and associated with a specific trait, whereas the farther apart they are, the greater the chance that they will be separated by crossing over and carried on homologous chromosomes. The concept of linkage, which opposes the independent assortment theory of mendelian genetics, led to the foundation of the modern chromosome theory of genetics. See also **synteny. 2.** (in psychology) the association between a stimulus and the response it elicits. **3.** (in chemistry) the bond between two atoms in a chemical compound or the lines used to designate valency connections between the atoms in structural formulas.

linkage disequilibrium, a nonrandom association of two genes on the same chromosome.

linkage group, a group of genes that tend to be inherited as a unit because they are located on the same chromosome. Without crossing over, all of the genes on a given chromosome constitute a linkage group, and the number of linkage groups in an organism is equal to the number of autosomes in a haploid cell.

linkage map. See **genetic map.**

linked genes [ME, *linke* + Gk, *genein,* to produce], genes that are located so close together on the same chromosome that they tend to be transmitted as a linkage group.

linker [ME, *linke,* connection], a small segment of synthetic DNA used to join DNA fragments in cloning.

linoleic acid /lin′əlē″ik/ [Gk, *linon,* flax, *oleum,* oil], a colorless to straw-colored essential fatty acid with two unsaturated bonds, occurring in many vegetable oils, such as corn, soy, and safflower oils. Commercially produced linoleic acid is used in margarine and animal feeds.

linolenic acid /lin′ōlen″ik/ [Gk, *linon,* flax, *oleum,* oil], an unsaturated essential fatty acid occurring in triglycerides of canola, soy, linseed, and other vegetable oils.

lio-. See **leio-, lio-.**

Lioresal, an antispastic agent. Brand name for **baclofen.**

liothyronine sodium /lī′ōthī″rənēn/, a synthetic thyroid hormone. Also called **triiodothyronine.**

■ INDICATIONS: It is prescribed in the treatment of primary hypothyroidism, myxedema, simple goiter, cretinism, and secondary hypothyroidism.

■ CONTRAINDICATIONS: Hyperthyroidism, thyrotoxicosis, acute myocardial infarction, or known hypersensitivity to this drug prohibits its use. It is used with caution in patients with diabetes mellitus or cardiovascular disease.

■ ADVERSE EFFECTS: Among the serious adverse effects, usually caused by overdosage, are tachycardia, arrhythmias, thyrotoxicosis, nausea, vomiting, hypertension, nervousness, and loss of weight.

liotrix /lī″ətriks/, a uniform mixture of the thyroid hormones T$_3$ and T$_4$.

■ INDICATIONS: It is prescribed in the treatment of hypothyroid conditions.

■ CONTRAINDICATIONS: Most diseases and abnormal conditions of the myocardium or known hypersensitivity to this drug prohibits its use.

■ ADVERSE EFFECTS: Among the more serious adverse effects are symptoms of thyrotoxicosis, including tachycardia, nervousness, insomnia, and fever.

lip [AS, *lippa*], **1.** either the upper or lower fleshy structure surrounding the opening of the oral cavity. **2.** any rimlike structure bordering a cavity or groove. See also **labia.**

LIP, abbreviation for **lymphocytic interstitial pneumonia.**

lip-. See **lipo-, lip-.**

lipase /lī″pās, lip″ās/ [Gk, *lipos,* fat; Fr, *diastase,* enzyme], any of several enzymes produced by the organs of the digestive system that catalyze the breakdown of lipids through the hydrolysis of the linkages between fatty acids and glycerol in triglycerides and phospholipids. Normal blood levels of lipase range from 0 to 110 U/L. See also **fat, fatty acid, glycerol, phospholipid, triglyceride.**

lipase test, a blood test used most often to diagnose acute pancreatitis but that is also useful in helping to diagnose renal failure, intestinal infarction or obstruction, and several other conditions.

lipectomy /lipek″təmē/ [Gk, *lipos* + *ektomē,* excision], an excision of subcutaneous fat, as from the abdominal wall. Also called **adipectomy.**

lipedema /lip′ədē″mə/, a condition in which fat deposits accumulate in the lower extremities from the hips to the ankles, accompanied by symptoms of tenderness in the affected areas. Treatment is dietary.

lipemia /lipē″mē·ə/ [Gk, *lipos* + *haima,* blood], chylomicrons in plasma, causing the plasma to appear cloudy. It occurs after a heavy or fatty meal or the infusion of lipid solutions, or it may indicate a metabolic lipid disorder.

lipid /lip″id, lī″pid/ [Gk, *lipos,* fat, *eidos,* form], any of a structurally diverse group of organic compounds that are insoluble in water but soluble in alcohol, chloroform, ether, and other solvents. Some lipids are stored in the body and serve as an energy reserve but are elevated in various diseases such as atherosclerosis. The normal concentrations of lipids in serum are total, 400 to 800 mg/dL; cholesterol, 150 to 250 mg/dL; fatty acids, 9 to 15 mM/L; phospholipids, 150 to 380 mg/dL; phospholipid as phosphorus, 9 to 16 mg/dL; and triglycerides, 10 to 190 mg/dL. Kinds include **cholesterol, fatty acid, phospholipid, triglyceride.**

lipidosis /lip′idō″sis/ [Gk, *lipos* + *osis,* condition], a general term that includes several rare familial disorders of fat metabolism. The chief characteristic of these disorders is the accumulation of abnormal levels of certain lipids in the body. Kinds include **Gaucher disease, Krabbe disease, Niemann-Pick disease, Tay-Sachs disease.**

lipid pneumonia, an inflammation of the spongy tissue of the lung caused by inhalation of oil droplets into the alveoli. The condition may result from accidentally inhaling oily medications, milk, or other fatty foods or from swimming in petroleum-contaminated water.

lipiduria /lip′idoor″ē·ə/, the presence of lipids (fatty bodies) in the urine.

lipo-, lip-, prefix meaning "fat": *lipase, lipodystrophy, lipoma.*

lipoatrophic diabetes /lip′ō·atrof″ik/, an inherited disease characterized by a total loss of subcutaneous body fat, insulin-resistant diabetes mellitus, acanthosis nigricans, hypermetabolism, hepatomegaly, and hypertrophied musculature. It is associated with a disorder of the hypothalamus that results in excessive blood levels of growth hormone and adrenocorticotropic-releasing hormones. Also called *congenital total lipodystrophy.*

lipoatrophy /lip′ō·at″rəfē/, a breakdown of subcutaneous fat at the site of an insulin injection. It usually occurs after several injections at the same site. Compare **lipohypertrophy.**

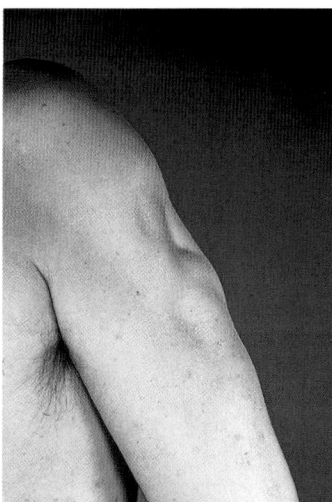

Lipoatrophy at insulin injection site *(Belchetz and Hammond, 2003)*

lipocele. See **adipocele.**

lipochondrodystrophy. See **Hurler syndrome.**

lipochrome /lip″əkrōm/ [Gk, *lipos + chroma,* color], any of the naturally occurring pigments, such as carotene, that contain a lipid and give a yellow color to fats.

lipodystrophia progressiva /-distrō″fē·ə/ [Gk, *lipos + dys,* bad, *trophe,* nourishment; L, *progredior,* to go forth], an abnormal accumulation of fat around the buttocks and thighs and a progressive, symmetric disappearance of subcutaneous fat from areas above the pelvis and on the face. Also called **lipomatosis atrophicans.**

lipodystrophy /lip′ōdis″trəfē/ [Gk, *lipos + dys,* bad, *trophe,* nourishment], any abnormality in the metabolism or deposition of fats. Kinds include *congenital total lipodystrophy, familial partial lipodystrophy,* **insulin lipodystrophy,** *membranous lipodystrophy, progressive lipodystrophy.*

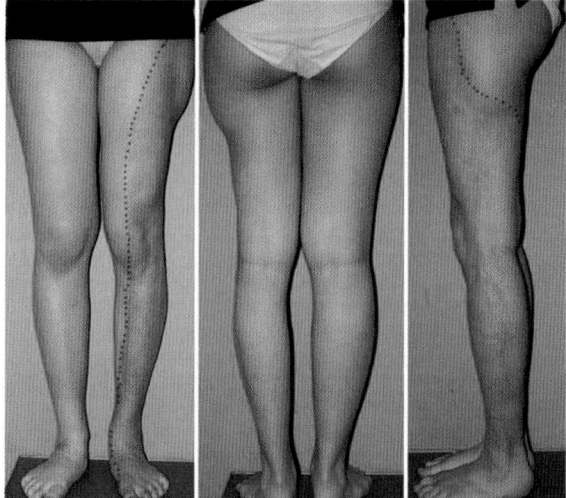

Segmental presentation (gray dotted line) of lipodystrophy in a young woman *(Kim et al, 2008)*

lip of hip fracture, a break in the posterior lip of the acetabulum, often associated with displacement of the hip.

lipofibroma. See **fibrolipoma.**

lipofuscin /lip′əfus″in/, a class of fatty pigments consisting mostly of oxidized fats that are found in abundance in the cells of adults. Lipofuscins accumulate in lysosomes with age.

lipogenesis /-jen″əsis/ [Gk, *lipos,* fat, *genein,* to produce], the production and accumulation of fat.

lipogranuloma /lip′ōgran′yoŏlō″mə/ *pl.* lipogranulomas, lipogranulomata [Gk, *lipos* + L, *granulum,* little grain; Gk, *oma,* tumor], a nodule of necrotic, fatty tissue associated with granulomatous inflammation or a foreign-body reaction around a deposit of injected material containing an oily substance.

lipohypertrophy /lip′ōhīpur″trəfē/, a buildup of subcutaneous fat tissue at a site where insulin has been injected continually. Compare **lipoatrophy.**

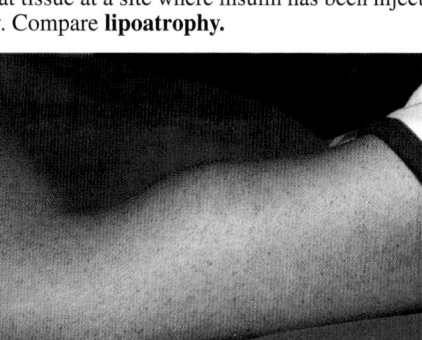
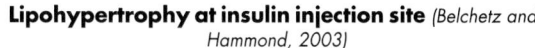

Lipohypertrophy at insulin injection site *(Belchetz and Hammond, 2003)*

lipoic acid /lipō″ik/, a bacterial growth factor found in liver and yeast.

lipoid /lip″oid/, resembling a lipid.

lipoid nephrosis. See **minimal change disease.**

lipolysis /lipol″isis/, the breakdown or destruction of fats.

lipolytic /-lit″ik/, pertaining to the chemical breakdown of fat.

lipolytic digestion, a phase of food digestion in which fat molecules are split into glycerol and fatty acids.

lipoma /lipō″mə/ *pl.* lipomas, lipomata [Gk, *lipos + oma,* tumor], a benign tumor consisting of mature fat cells. Also called **adipose tumor.** See also **multiple lipomatosis.** **–lipomatous,** *adj.*

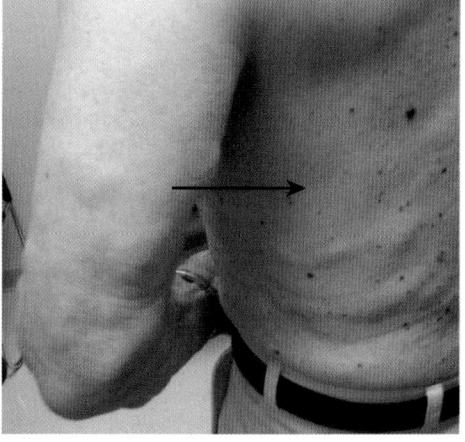

Lipoma *(Wodajo et al, 2010)*

L

-lipoma, suffix meaning "a tumor made up of fatty tissue": *angiolipoma, fibrolipoma, osteolipoma.*

lipoma annulare colli, a diffuse, symmetric accumulation of fat around the neck; not a true lipoma. Also called **Madelung neck.**

lipoma arborescens, a fatty tumor of a joint, characterized by a treelike distribution of fat cells.

lipoma capsulare, a benign neoplasm characterized by the abnormal presence of fat cells in the capsule of an organ.

lipoma cavernosum. See **angiolipoma.**

lipoma diffusum renis. See **lipomatous nephritis.**

lipoma dolorosa. See **lipomatosis dolorosa.**

lipoma fibrosum, a fatty tumor containing masses of fibrous tissue.

lipoma myxomatodes. See **lipomyxoma.**

lipomas. See **lipoma.**

lipoma sarcomatodes. See **liposarcoma.**

lipomata. See **lipoma.**

lipomatosis /lip′ōmətō″sis/ [Gk, *lipos + oma,* tumor, *osis,* condition], a disorder characterized by abnormal tumorlike accumulations of fat in body tissues.

lipomatosis atrophicans. See **lipodystrophia progressiva.**

lipomatosis dolorosa, a disorder characterized by the abnormal accumulation of painful or tender fat deposits. Also called **lipoma dolorosa.**

lipomatosis gigantea, a condition characterized by massive deposits of fat.

lipomatosis renis. See **lipomatous nephritis.**

lipomatous /lipō″mətəs/ [Gk, *lipos,* fat, *oma,* tumor], pertaining to or resembling a benign tumor made up of mature fat cells.

lipomatous myxoma, a tumor containing fatty tissue that arises in connective tissue.

lipomatous nephritis, a rare condition in which the renal nephrons are replaced by fatty tissue. Kidney failure may result. Also called **lipoma diffusum renis, lipomatosis renis.**

lipometabolism /-metab″əliz′əm/ [Gk, *lipos,* fat, *metabole,* change], the chemical processes involved in building up or breaking down fat molecules.

lipomyoma /-mī·ō″mə/ [Gk, *lipos,* fat, *mys,* muscle, *oma,* tumor], a tumor that combines characteristics of a lipoma and a myoma.

lipomyxoma /lip′ōmiksō″mə/ *pl.* lipomyxomas, lipomyxomata [Gk, *lipos + myxa,* mucus, *oma,* tumor], a myxoma that contains fat cells. Also called **lipoma myxomatodes.**

lipophilia /-fil″yə/ [Gk, *lipos,* fat, *philein,* to love], a tendency to attract or absorb fat.

lipoprotein /lip′ōprō″tēn/ [Gk, *lipos + proteios,* first rank], a conjugated protein in which lipids form an integral part of the molecule. They are synthesized primarily in the liver; contain varying amounts of triglycerides, cholesterol, phospholipids, fat-soluble vitamins, and protein; and are classified according to their composition and density. Practically all of the plasma lipids are present as lipoprotein complexes. The elevation of low-density lipoproteins (LDLs) in plasma is associated with an increased risk of atherosclerosis. Normal adult levels of lipoproteins include high-density lipoproteins, greater than 35 mg/dL; LDLs, 60 to 180 mg/dL; and very low-density lipoproteins, 25% to 50%. Kinds include **chylomicron, high-density lipoprotein, low-density lipoprotein, very low–density lipoprotein.**

lipoprotein electrophoresis, a blood test performed on patients with rare lipid profiles to predict coronary arteriosclerotic heart disease.

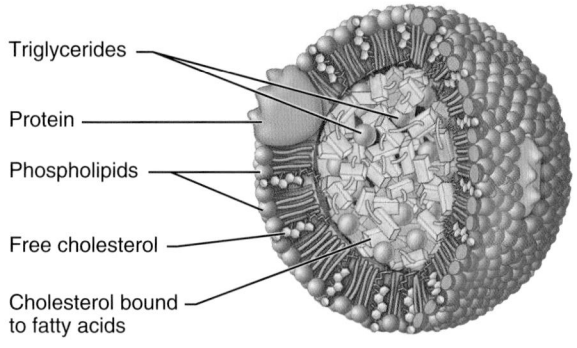

Lipoprotein *(Patton and Thibodeau, 2010)*

lipoprotein lipase (LPL), an enzyme that plays a key role in breaking down triglycerides present in chylomicrons and very low–density lipoprotein particles, releasing their fatty acids for entry into tissue cells.

lipoproteins test (HDL, LDL, and VLDL), a blood test, performed as part of a lipid profile, to identify persons who are at risk for developing heart disease and to monitor therapy if abnormalities are found. Lipoproteins are considered to be an accurate predictor of coronary heart disease.

liposarcoma /lip′ōsärkō″mə/ *pl.* liposarcomas, liposarcomata [Gk, *lipos + sarx,* flesh, *oma,* tumor], a malignant growth of primitive fat cells that occurs in the deep soft tissue of the extremities and retroperitoneum. It is the most common soft tissue sarcoma. Also called **lipoma sarcomatodes.**

liposis. See **lipomatosis.**

liposoluble /-sol″yəbəl/ [Gk, *lipos,* fat; L, *solubilis*], soluble in fats.

liposomal cytarabine, a suspension of cytarabine molecules encapsulated in liposomes. It is a sustained-release preparation that is injected intrathecally in the treatment of meningitis associated with lymphoma.

liposomal daunorubicin, an aqueous solution of the citrate salt of daunorubicin encapsulated within specifically constructed liposomes that shows enhanced selectivity for solid tumors in situ compared with that of the hydrochloride salt. It is administered intravenously in the treatment of advanced Kaposi's sarcoma associated with acquired immunodeficiency syndrome.

liposomal doxorubicin, doxorubicin hydrochloride encapsulated within liposomes, administered intravenously in the treatment of Kaposi's sarcoma associated with acquired immunodeficiency syndrome (AIDS).

liposome /lip′əsōm/ [Gk, *lipos,* fat, *soma,* body], a small, spheric particle consisting of a bilayer of phospholipid molecules surrounding an aqueous solution.

liposuction /-suk″shən/, plastic surgery that removes adipose tissue with a suction pump device. It is used primarily to remove or reduce localized areas of fat around the abdomen, breasts, legs, face, and upper arms where the skin is contractile enough to redrape in a normal manner. Also called **suction lipectomy.**

lip reading. See **speech reading.**

-lipsis, -lipse, suffix meaning "to leave out, fail, omit": *ellipsis, eclipse.*

Liquaemin Sodium, an anticoagulant drug. Brand name for **heparin sodium.**

liquefaction /lik′wəfak″shən/ [L, *liquere,* to flow, *facere,* to make], the process in which a solid or a gas is made liquid.

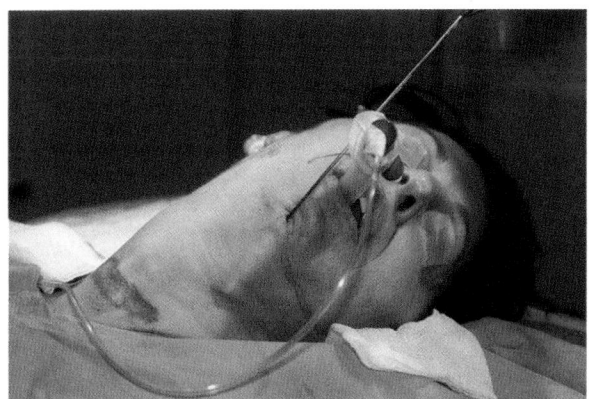

Liposuction (LaTrenta, 2004)

liquefactive degeneration /lik'wəfak″tiv/, dissolution of tissues resulting from hydrolytic enzymes released by leukocytes and tissue cells. It occurs in the skin of patients with lichen planus and lupus erythematosus.

liquid /lik″wid/ [L, *liquere,* to flow], a state of matter, intermediate between solid and gas, in which the molecules move freely among themselves and the substance flows freely with little application of force. Liquids have a fixed volume but assume the shape of the vessel in which they are contained. Compare **fluid.** See also **gas, solid.**

liquid crystal display (LCD), a thin membrane containing liquid crystals, used for displays in computers and monitoring equipment.

liquid diet, a diet consisting of foods that can be served in liquid or strained form but that may include custard, ice cream, pudding, tapioca, and soft-cooked eggs. It is prescribed in acute infections, in acute inflammatory conditions of the GI tract, and for patients unable to consume other soft or semifluid foods, usually after surgery. See also **full-liquid diet.**

liquid glucose, a thick, syrupy, odorless, and colorless or yellowish liquid obtained by the incomplete hydrolysis of starch, primarily consisting of dextrose with dextrins, maltose, and water. It is used as a flavoring agent and may be used as a calorie source, chiefly in treating dehydration.

liquid nitrogen. See **cryogen.**

liquid paraffin. See **mineral oil.**

liquid petrolatum. See **mineral oil.**

liquid scintillation counter, a device for measuring radioactivity, usually beta particles, emitted from a sample dispersed in a liquid scintillation cocktail.

liquor /lik″ər/, **1.** any fluid or liquid, such as liquor amnii, the amniotic fluid. **2.** an alcoholic beverage.

liquorice. See **licorice.**

lisdexamfetamine, a central nervous system stimulant.
- INDICATIONS: This drug is used to treat attention deficit disorder with hyperactivity.
- CONTRAINDICATIONS: Hyperthyroidism, hypertension, glaucoma, severe arteriosclerosis, drug abuse, cardiovascular disease, anxiety, anorexia nervosa, breastfeeding, and known hypersensitivity to sympathomimetic amines prohibit the use of this drug.
- ADVERSE EFFECTS: Adverse effects of this drug include dizziness, headache, dysphoria, irritability, aggressiveness, central nervous system tumor, dependence, addiction, mild euphoria, somnolence, lability, hypertension, decrease in heart rate, MI, growth inhibition, dry mouth, diarrhea, weight loss, impotence, change in libido, and urticaria. Life-threatening

side effects include arrhythmias, cardiomyopathy, angioedema, Stevens-Johnson syndrome, and toxic epidermal necrolysis. Common side effects include hyperactivity, insomnia, restlessness, talkativeness, palpitations, tachycardia, and anorexia.

Lisfranc fracture /lisfrangk″/ [Jacques Lisfranc, French surgeon, 1790–1847], a fracture dislocation of the foot in which one or all of the proximal metatarsals are displaced.

lisinopril, an ACE inhibitor.
- INDICATIONS: Used in the management of high blood pressure and heart failure.
- CONTRAINDICATIONS: Allergy to ACE inhibitors is a contraindication.
- ADVERSE EFFECTS: Dizziness, light-headedness, tiredness, or headache are associated with the administration of lisinopril, especially at the beginning of treatment. Chronic dry cough is a common side effect.

lisp, the mispronunciation of one or more of the sibilant consonant sounds, usually /s/ and /z/. There are two types of lisps—lateral and frontal.

lissencephalia. See **agyria.**

lissencephaly. See **agyria.**

Listeria monocytogenes /lister″ē·ə mon′ōsītoj″inēz/ [Joseph Lister; Gk, *mono,* single, *kytos,* cell, *genein,* to produce], a common species of gram-positive motile bacteria that cause listeriosis and a noninvasive food-borne diarrheal disease.

listeriosis /listir′ē·ō″sis/ [Joseph Lister; Gk, *osis,* condition], an infectious disease caused by a genus of gram-positive motile bacteria that are nonsporulating. *Listeria monocytogenes* infects shellfish, birds, spiders, and mammals in all areas of the world, but infection in humans is uncommon. It is transmitted by direct contact between infected animals and humans, through the ingestion of contaminated meat and dairy products, by inhalation of dust, or by contact with mud, sewage, or soil contaminated with the organism. The disorder is characterized in mild cases by fever, myalgia, nausea, and diarrhea and in severe cases by circulatory collapse, shock, endocarditis, hepatosplenomegaly, and a dark red rash over the trunk and legs. Fever, bacteremia, malaise, and lethargy are commonly seen. Newborns and immunosuppressed debilitated older people are more vulnerable to infection than are immunocompetent children and young or middle-aged adults. The signs of infection and the severity of the disease vary according to the site of infection and the age and condition of the person. Pregnant women characteristically experience a mild brief episode of illness, but fetal infection acquired through the placental circulation in utero is usually fatal. Infection in the newborn apparently results from exposure to the organism in the birth canal of an infected mother. Meningitis and encephalitis occur in 75% of cases. Treatment may include ampicillin, penicillin, tetracycline, or erythromycin given intramuscularly or intravenously. Trimethoprim-sulfamethoxazole is an alternative. If infection is suspected in a pregnant woman, treatment is begun immediately, even before bacteriological culture of the blood, spinal fluid, or vaginal secretions can confirm the diagnosis. All secretions from the patient may contain the organism. Also called *listerosis.*

Lister, Joseph [Scottish surgeon, 1827–1912], the surgeon who introduced the use of antiseptic surgery in hospitals in London in 1867. Lister operations were performed under a spray of diluted carbolic acid, instruments were dipped in carbolic acid, and wounds were dressed with gauze similarly treated.

Liston forceps [Robert Liston, Scottish surgeon, 1794–1847], a kind of bone-cutting forceps.

liter (L) /lē″tər/ [Fr], a derived unit of volume equivalent to 1.057 quarts and defined as the volume occupied by a mass of 1 kg of water at standard temperature and pressure.

lith-. See **litho-, lith-.**

-lith, suffix meaning "a calculus" or "a stone": *choledocholith.*

Lithane, an antimanic drug. Brand name for **lithium carbonate.**

lithiasis /lithī″əsis/ [Gk, *lithos,* stone, *osis,* condition], the formation of calculi in the hollow organs or ducts of the body. Calculi are formed of mineral salts and may irritate, inflame, or obstruct the organ in which they form or lodge. Lithiasis occurs most commonly in the gallbladder, kidney, and lower urinary tract. Lithiasis may be asymptomatic, but more often the condition is extremely painful. Surgery may be necessary if the stones cannot be excreted spontaneously. Lower urinary tract calculi often can be dissolved. See also **biliary calculus, cholelithiasis, renal calculus, urinary calculus.**

-lithiasis, suffix meaning "the presence, condition, or formation of stones": *cholelithiasis, hepatolithiasis, sialolithiasis.*

lithium (Li) /lith″ē-əm/ [Gk, *lithos,* stone], a silver-white alkali metal occurring in various compounds such as petalite and spodumene. Its atomic number is 3; its atomic mass is 6.94. Lithium is the lightest known metal and one of the most reactive elements. Traces of lithium ion occur in animal tissue, and it abounds in many alkaline mineral spring waters. Its salts are used in the treatment of manias, but the mechanisms by which these compounds help to stabilize psychological moods are not understood. Lithium carbonate is a salt commonly used for psychiatric purposes in the United States. It has been effective in the prevention of recurrent attacks of manic-depressive illnesses and has helped correct sleep disorders in manic patients, apparently by suppressing the rapid eye movement phases of sleep. Therapeutic concentrations of lithium have no observable psychotropic effects on normal individuals. In manic patients, lithium salts also produce high-voltage slow waves in the electroencephalograph, often with superimposed beta waves. An important feature of the lithium ion is its relatively small gradient of distribution across biological membranes. Patients suffering severe manic attacks are hospitalized so that they can receive proper medical maintenance. Treatments start with large doses of antipsychotic drugs, which are followed by the gradual and safe introduction of lithium therapy. Ideally lithium treatment is prescribed only for patients with normal sodium intake and normal heart and kidney function.

lithium carbonate, an antimanic agent.

■ INDICATIONS: It is prescribed in the treatment of manic episodes of manic-depressive disorder.

■ CONTRAINDICATIONS: It is used with caution in the presence of renal or cardiovascular disease and is not recommended for children under 12 years of age. Pregnancy or known hypersensitivity to this drug prohibits its use.

■ ADVERSE EFFECTS: Among the most serious adverse effects are renal damage, polydipsia and polyuria, and impairment of mental and physical abilities. Retention of sodium and fluid may occur.

lithium fluoride (LiF), a compound commonly used for thermoluminescent dosimetry.

litho-, lith-, prefix meaning "stone" or "calculus": *lithotripsy, lithotrite.*

Lithobid, an antimanic drug. Brand name for **lithium carbonate.**

lithogenesis /lith″əjen″əsis/ [Gk, *lithos,* stone, *genein,* to produce], the origin of the formation of a calculus.

lithopedion /lith″əpē″dē-ən/ [Gk, *lithos* + *paidion,* child], a fetus that has died during an ectopic pregnancy and has become calcified or ossified. It may remain undiagnosed for decades. Also called **calcified fetus,** *lithopedium,* **ostembryon, osteopedion.**

Lithostat /lith″ostat/, a preparation of a urease inhibitor used in the treatment of kidney stones and urinary tract infections. Brand name for **acetohydroxamic acid.**

Lithotabs, an antimanic drug. Brand name for **lithium carbonate.**

lithotomy /lithot″əmē/ [Gk, *lithos* + *temnein,* to cut], **1.** the surgical excision of a calculus, especially one from the urinary tract. **2.** a position in the operating room in which the patient is supine with legs raised and abducted to expose the perineal region. The legs are placed in stirrups to maintain the position.

lithotomy forceps, a forceps for the extraction of a calculus, usually from the urinary tract.

lithotomy position, the position assumed by the patient lying supine with the hips and the knees flexed and the thighs abducted and rotated externally. Also called **dorsosacral position.**

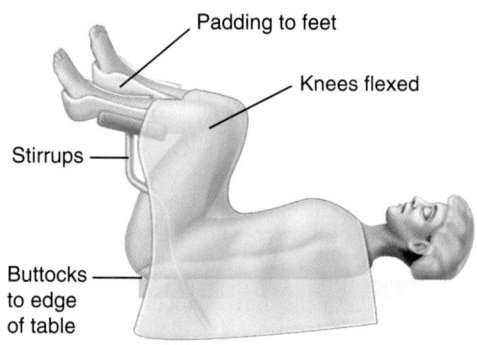

Lithotomy position *(Christensen and Kockrow, 2010)*

lithotripsy /lith″ətrip′sē/ [Gk, *lithos,* stone, *tribein,* to wear away], a procedure for eliminating a calculus in the renal pelvis, ureter, bladder, or gallbladder. It may be crushed surgically or by using a noninvasive method such as a hydraulic, or high-energy, shock wave or a pulsed dye laser. The fragments may then be expelled or washed out.

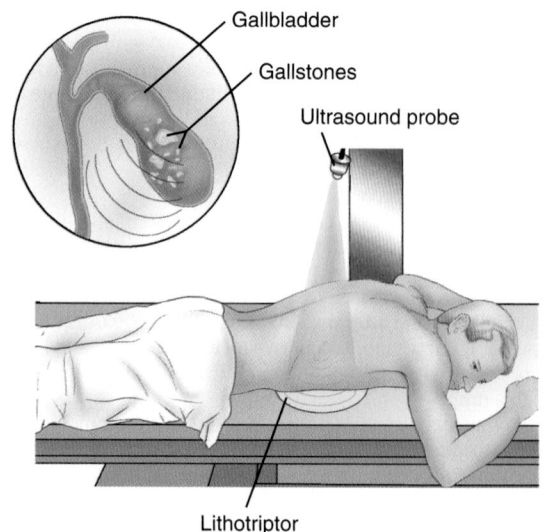

Lithotripsy *(Leonard, 2015)*

lithotrite /lith″ətrīt/ [Gk, *lithos* + L, *terere,* to rub], an instrument for crushing a stone in the urinary bladder. Also called *lithotriptor.* −*lithotrity, n.*

litigant /lit″əgənt/ [L, to go to law], (in law) a party to a lawsuit. See also **defendant, plaintiff.**

litigate /lit″əgāt/, (in law) to carry on a suit or to contest.

litigious paranoia [L, *litigare,* to go to law; Gk, *paranous,* madness], a form of paranoia in which a person seeks legal proof or justification for systematized delusions, such as when a person repeatedly files lawsuits for perceived slights with little or no basis in fact.

litmus paper /lit″məs/ [ONorse, *litmosi,* coloring herb; L, *papyrus,* paper], absorbent paper coated with litmus, a blue dye, that is used to determine pH. Acid substances or solutions turn blue litmus to red. Alkaline substances or solutions do not cause a color change in blue litmus. The pH range is 4.5 (red) to 8.5 (blue).

litter [Fr, *lit,* bed], a stretcher.

Little disease. See **cerebral palsy.**

Litzmann obliquity. See **asynclitism.**

live attenuated measles virus vaccine /əten″yŌŌ·ā′tid/, a vaccine prepared from live strains of measles virus that have been cultured under conditions that cause them to lose their virulence without losing their ability to induce immunity. The vaccine is not recommended for pregnant women or others who may have certain medical conditions that tend to diminish immunity.

live attenuated vaccine, a vaccine prepared from live microorganisms or functional viruses whose disease-producing ability has been weakened but whose immunogenic properties have not.

live birth [AS, *libben,* to be alive; ONorse, *byrth*], the birth of a newborn, irrespective of the duration of gestation, that exhibits any sign of life, such as respiration, heartbeat, umbilical pulsation, or movement of voluntary muscles. A live birth is not always a viable birth.

livedo /livē″dō/ [L, *liveo,* bluish spot], a blue or reddish mottling of the skin that worsens in cold weather and is probably caused by arteriolar spasm. Cutis marmorata is a transient form of livedo. See also **livedo reticularis, cutis marmorata.**

livedo reticularis, a disorder accentuated by exposure to cold and presenting with a characteristic reddish-blue mottling with a typical "fishnet" appearance. The condition involves the entire leg and, less often, the arm. See also **livedo.**

livedo vasculitis. See **segmented hyalinizing vasculitis.**

live measles and mumps virus vaccine, a vaccine prepared from live strains of measles and mumps viruses. The vaccine is commonly combined with live rubella viruses, such as measles, mumps, and rubella vaccine, and administered to normal infants at the age of 15 months. See also **measles, mumps, and rubella virus vaccine live.**

live oral poliovirus vaccine, a vaccine prepared from three strains (trivalent) of live polioviruses. Primary immunization with the vaccine usually begins at the age of 2 months.

liver [AS, *lifer*], the largest gland of the body and one of its most complex organs. It is located in the upper cranial, right part of the abdominal cavity, occupying almost the entire right hypochondrium and the greater part of the epigastrium. In many individuals it extends into the left hypochondrium as far as the mammary line. It has a soft solid consistency, is shaped like an irregular hemisphere, and is dark reddish-brown. The ventral part of the liver is separated by the diaphragm from the sixth to the tenth ribs on the right side and from the seventh and

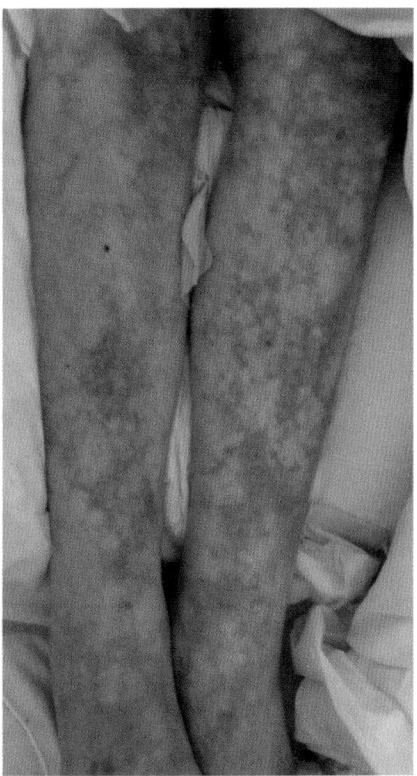

Livedo reticularis of lower extremity *(Lebwohl et al, 2014)*

eighth costal cartilages on the left side. The central section has a deep concavity that fits the vertebral column and the crura of the diaphragm. The liver is divided into four lobes, contains as many as 100,000 lobules, and is served by two distinct blood supplies. The hepatic artery conveys oxygenated blood to the liver, and the hepatic portal vein conveys nutrient-filled blood from the stomach and the intestines. At any given moment the liver holds about 1 pint of blood, or approximately 13% of the total blood supply of the body. The tiny lobules of the organ are composed of polyhedral hepatic cells. These cells communicate with small ducts that connect with larger ducts to form the left and right hepatic ducts that emerge on the caudal surface of the liver. The left and right hepatic ducts converge to form the single hepatic duct, which conveys the bile to the duodenum and gallbladder for storage. More than 500 functions of the liver have been identified. Some of the major functions are the production of bile by hepatic cells; the secretion of glucose, proteins, vitamins, fats, and most of the other compounds used by the body; the processing of hemoglobin for vital use of its iron content; and the conversion of poisonous ammonia to urea. Bile from the liver is stored in the hepatic duct, in numerous blood vessels and in the gallbladder, which is connected to the liver by connective tissue. The liver cells produce about 1 pint of bile daily. The hepatic cells also detoxify numerous ingested substances, such as alcohol, nicotine, and other poisons, as well as various toxic substances produced by the intestine. See also **gallbladder.**

liver abscess [L, *abscedere,* to go away; AS, *lifer*], an abscess in the liver cells, usually caused by an amebic infection, bacterial infection, or trauma. It is characterized by sweats and chills, pain, nausea, and vomiting.

L

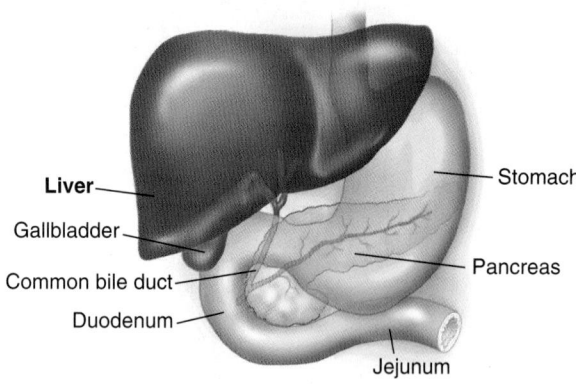

Liver *(Leonard, 2015)*

Labels: Liver, Gallbladder, Common bile duct, Duodenum, Stomach, Pancreas, Jejunum

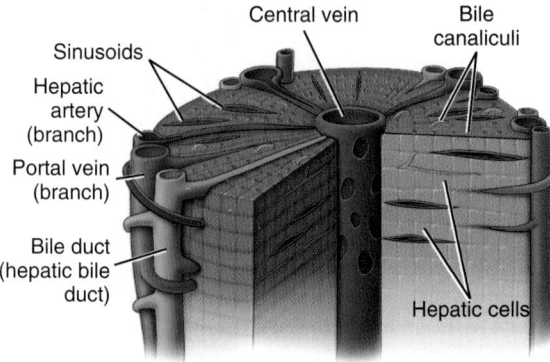

Liver lobule *(Herlihy, 2014)*

Labels: Central vein, Bile canaliculi, Sinusoids, Hepatic artery (branch), Portal vein (branch), Bile duct (hepatic bile duct), Hepatic cells

liver biopsy, a diagnostic procedure in which a special needle is introduced into the liver under local anesthesia to obtain a specimen for pathological examination.

■ METHOD: Before a liver biopsy is performed by a physician, the procedure is explained to the patient, whose baseline vital signs are recorded and who is taught how to inhale and hold the breath during needle insertion. After the patient's possible allergy to the local anesthetic is checked and results of bleeding, clotting, and prothrombin tests are obtained, an analgesic or sedative is administered as ordered. The biopsy is performed with ultrasound visualization. On completion of the biopsy, pressure is applied to the site for 15 minutes. The patient is positioned on the right side for the first 2 hours and remains in a supine position in bed for the next 22 hours. The blood pressure, pulse, and respirations are checked every 15 minutes for the first hour, then every 30 minutes for the next 2 hours, and subsequently every 4 hours or as ordered. The biopsy site is observed every 30 minutes for bleeding, swelling, or increased pain; epigastric or referred shoulder pain may occur. Analgesia and vitamin K are given as ordered, and the recumbent patient is assisted with eating and other activities as needed. A postbiopsy complete blood count is performed.

■ INTERVENTIONS: The health care provider reinforces explanations of the biopsy and its purpose, provides care before and after the procedure, and closely observes the patient for postbiopsy complications such as intraperitoneal hemorrhage, shock, and pneumothorax.

■ OUTCOME CRITERIA: An uneventful liver biopsy is a valuable aid in establishing a diagnosis of hepatic disease, including primary and metastatic malignant neoplastic disease.

liver breath. See **fetor hepaticus.**

liver cancer, a malignant neoplastic disease of the liver. Primary liver cancer is common in Africa and Southeast Asia. Primary tumors are 6 to 10 times more prevalent in men than in women, develop most often in the sixth decade of life, and are associated with cirrhosis of the liver in 70% of the cases. Other risk factors include hemochromatosis, hepatitis, schistosomiasis, exposure to vinyl chloride or arsenic, nonalcoholic fatty liver disease (NAFLD), and possibly nutritional deficiencies. Alcoholism may be a predisposing factor, but nonalcoholic cirrhosis is a greater risk than alcoholic cirrhosis. Aflatoxins in moldy grain and peanuts appear to be linked to high rates of hepatocellular carcinoma in parts of Africa. Characteristics of liver cancer are abdominal bloating, anorexia, weakness, dull upper abdominal pain, ascites, mild jaundice, and a tender enlarged liver; in some cases tumor nodules are palpable on the liver surface. Diagnostic procedures include radioisotope scan, biopsy, and various laboratory studies of liver function. An elevated level of alkaline phosphatase, increased retention of sulfobromophthalein, and the presence of alpha-fetoprotein in the blood suggest liver cancer. Most primary liver tumors are adenocarcinomas, classified as hepatomas when derived from hepatic cells and as cholangiomas if they originate in cells of the bile duct. Systemic chemotherapy may result in temporary tumor regression; it may be administered with a surgically implanted infusion pump. Liver transplantation may also be used to treat eligible individuals. Irradiation is very destructive to liver cells and not very toxic to tumor cells in the liver. See also **hepatoma.**

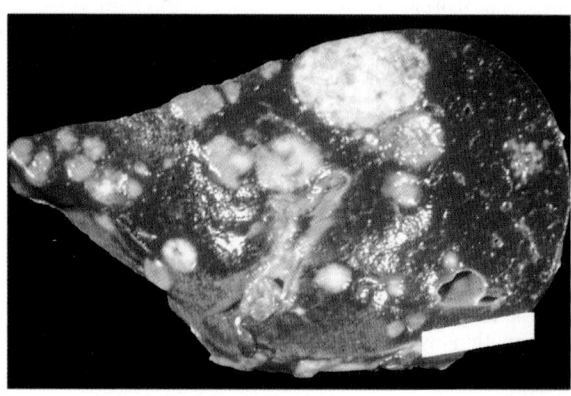

Metastatic liver cancer *(Kumar et al, 2007)*

liver cell carcinoma. See **malignant hepatoma.**

liver disease, any one of a group of disorders of the liver. Characteristics of liver disease are jaundice, anorexia, hepatomegaly, ascites, and impaired consciousness. The exact diagnosis of liver disease is made through a combination of laboratory tests and clinical findings. See also **cholestasis, cirrhosis, hepatitis.**

liver failure [AS, *lifer* + L, *fallere*, to deceive], a condition in which the liver fails to fulfill its function or is unable to meet the demands made on it. Anorexia, fatigue, and weakness are common symptoms of liver cell failure, whereas jaundice indicates a biliary obstruction, and fever may accompany viral or alcoholic liver diseases.

liver flap. See **asterixis.**

liver fluke [AS, *lifer* + *floc*], a parasitic trematode belonging to the class Trematoda, with six genera that may infest the liver. The most important species affecting humans in industrialized countries is *Clonorchis sinensis,* which is usually acquired by eating freshwater fish containing the encysted larvae. The larvae are released in the duodenum, enter the common bile duct, and migrate to other bile ducts, the gallbladder, and pancreatic ducts. The liver fluke may survive for many years in the human biliary tree, releasing eggs into the feces. Infestations are most likely to result from ingestion of raw, dried, salted, or pickled freshwater fish and can be prevented by thorough cooking of such fish.

liver function test (LFT), one of several tests used to evaluate various functions of the liver, including metabolism, storage, filtration, and excretion. Kinds include **alanine aminotransferase (ALT) test, alkaline phosphatase test, prothrombin time,** *serum bilirubin.*

liver scan, a noninvasive technique for visualizing the size, shape, and consistency of the liver and for assessing the liver's functional status. It involves IV injection of a radioactively labeled compound that is readily taken up and trapped in the Kupffer cells of the liver. The radiation emitted by the compound is recorded by a radiation detector and can be recorded with a scintillation camera. Liver scans are useful for diagnosing three-dimensional lesions such as abscesses and tumors, for performing biopsies, and for evaluating hepatomegaly, jaundice, and ascites.

liver segments, the eight regions of the liver based on blood supply and biliary drainage.

liver spot, *(Nontechnical)* a variably pigmented lentigo occurring on the exposed skin of older Caucasians.

liver transplantation, a treatment for end-stage hepatic dysfunction in which a donor liver is matched in size and blood group to the recipient. The transplanted organ may be introduced as an auxiliary liver or as a total replacement. The procedure requires five anastomoses and many units of blood. Because of a shortage of child-size livers, pediatric transplants often are performed with a segment of an adult liver. Common postoperative complications include acute graft rejection, infection, hepatic complications (bile leakage, abscess formation, hepatic thrombosis), acute renal failure, giant emphysematous blebs, and fungal infections.

livid /liv′id/ [L, *lividus,* bluish], pertaining to an injury that is congested and has a bluish discoloration.

lividity /livid′itē/ [L, *lividus,* bluish], a tissue condition of being red or blue because of venous congestion, as in a contusion.

living-in unit. See **rooming-in.**

living related donor, an organ donor who is a close blood relative of the recipient.

living unrelated donor, an organ donor who is not a close blood relative of the recipient.

living will [AS, *libben + willa,* wish], **1.** an advance declaration by a patient that if he or she is determined to be hopelessly and terminally ill, the patient does not want to be connected to life support equipment. See also **durable power of attorney for health care. 2.** a written agreement between a patient and physician to withhold heroic measures if the patient's condition is found to be irreversible. See also **advance directive.**

livor mortis /lī′vər/, a purple discoloration of the skin in dependent body areas following death as a result of blood cell destruction.

lixiviation. See **leaching.**

lizard /liz′ərd/ [L, *lacerta*], a scaly-skinned reptile with a long body and tail and two pairs of legs. The large Gila monster of Arizona, New Mexico, and Utah and the beaded lizard of Mexico are the only North American lizards known to be venomous. The symptoms of their bites and the recommended treatment are similar to those of the bites from poisonous snakes except that antivenin is not available.

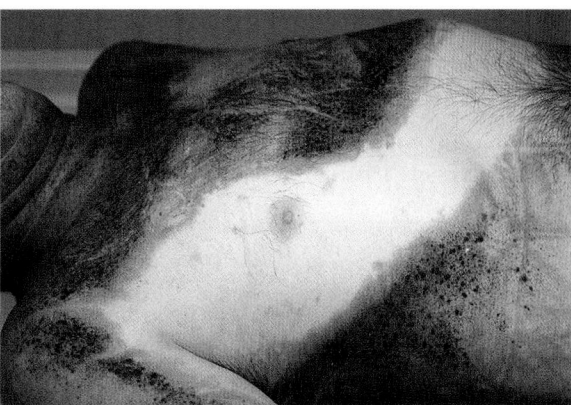

Livor mortis in an individual who expired in the prone position with his arm beneath him preventing lividity
(Connelly et al, 2016)

LLD, abbreviation for **lower level discriminator.**

LLD factor. See **cyanocobalamin.**

LLE, abbreviation for *left lower extremity.*

LLQ, abbreviation for *left lower quadrant of the abdomen.*

LMA, abbreviation for *left mentoanterior fetal position.*

LMD. See **dextran preparation.**

LMFT, abbreviation for **licensed marriage and family therapist.**

LMP, 1. abbreviation for *last menstrual period.* **2.** abbreviation for *left mentoposterior fetal position.*

LMT, abbreviation for *left mentotransverse fetal position.*

LMWH, abbreviation for **low-molecular-weight heparin.**

Loa /lo′ə/, a genus of nematodes of the superfamily Filarioidea. *L. loa* is a threadlike species 2.5 to 5 cm long found in West Africa. It inhabits the subcutaneous connective tissue of the human body and is seen especially as an eye worm about the orbit and under the conjunctiva. It causes itching and occasionally edematous swellings (Calabar swellings). The immature forms or microfilariae are diurnal, being found in the peripheral circulation in greatest concentrations during the day.

LOA, 1. abbreviation for *left occipitoanterior fetal position.* **2.** abbreviation for **looseness of association.**

load, a departure from normal body values for parameters such as water content, salt concentration, and heat. A positive load indicates a higher-than-normal value, whereas a negative load indicates a below-normal value.

loading, 1. the administration of a substance in sufficient quantity to test a patient's ability to metabolize or absorb it. **2.** the exertion of force on a muscle or ligament to increase its strength.

loading response stance stage [AS, *lad,* support; L, *responsum,* reply], one of the five stages of the stance phase of walking or gait, specifically associated with the moment when the leg reacts to and accepts the weight of the body. The loading response stance stage is one of the factors in the diagnoses of many abnormal orthopedic conditions and is often studied in conjunction with analyses of the electromyographic activity of the muscles used in walking. Compare **initial contact stance stage, midstance, preswing stance stage, terminal stance.**

loads [AS, *lad,* support], *(Slang)* a fixed combination of a sedative hypnotic (glutethimide) and a major opioid analgesic (codeine), which is taken orally by drug abusers for a euphoric effect reported to be similar to that produced by heroin but longer lasting. Toxicity may develop, characterized by nystagmus, slurred speech, seizures, coma, pulmonary edema, or sudden apnea and death. Detoxification of an addicted person is managed under close medical supervision with methadone and phenobarbital, as sudden withdrawal can cause death.

Loa loa /lō′ä lō′ä/,   a parasitic worm of western and central Africa that causes loiasis. Also called **eye worm.**

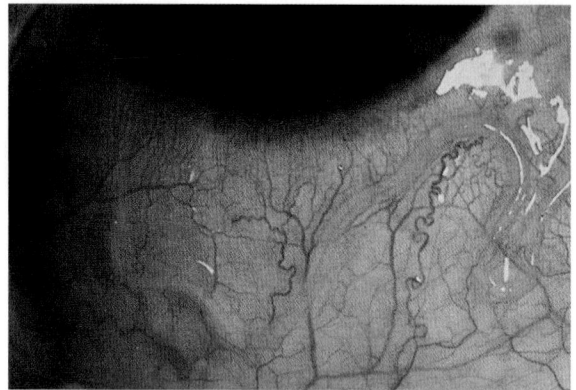

Loa loa *(Conlon and Snydman, 2000)*

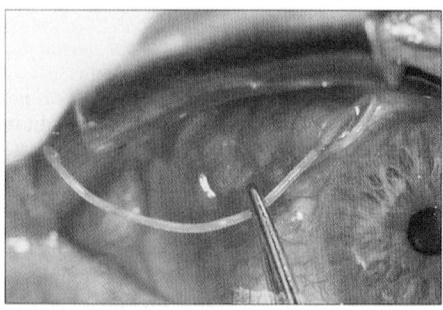

Loa loa being extracted from under the conjunctiva
(Michelson and Friedlaender, 1996/Courtesy Dr. Jonathan Belmont)

lobar.   See **lobe.**

lobar bronchus /lō′bär/   [Gk, *lobos,* lobe, *bronchos,* windpipe],   a bronchus extending from a primary bronchus to a segmental bronchus into one of the lobes of the right or left lung.

lobar buds,   secondary bronchial buds.

lobar nephronia,   acute pyelonephritis.

lobar pneumonia,   a severe infection of one or more of the five major lobes of the lungs that, if untreated, eventually results in consolidation of lung tissue. The disease is characterized by fever, chills, cough, rusty sputum, rapid shallow breathing, cyanosis, nausea, vomiting, and pleurisy. *Streptococcus pneumoniae* is the usual cause; but *Klebsiella pneumoniae, Haemophilus influenzae,* and other streptococci can also produce the disease. If the diagnosis is made early, appropriate antibiotic therapy is highly successful. Complications include lung abscess, atelectasis, empyema, pericarditis, and pleural effusion. Precautions against spread of the contagious disease are important. Because the fatality rate in the elderly and those with underlying systemic illness is high, prophylactic polyvalent pneumococcal vaccine is recommended for them. Compare **bronchopneumonia.**

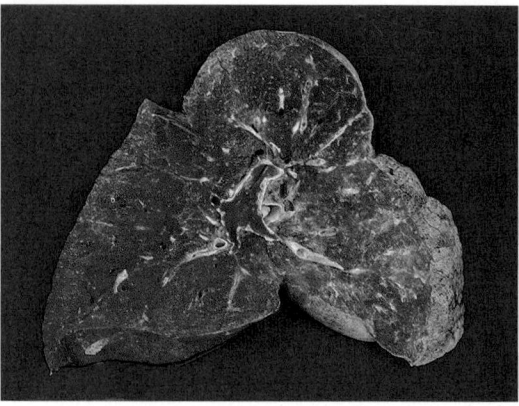

Bacterial lobar pneumonia *(Finkbeiner, Ursell, and Davis, 2009)*

lobate /lō′bāt/,   organized in lobes or rounded divisions. Also called **lobular.**

lobe /lōb/   [Gk, *lobos*],   **1.** a roundish projection of any structure. **2.** a part of any organ demarcated by sulci, fissures, or connective tissue, as the lobes of the brain, liver, and lungs.

lobe-, -lobe,   combining form meaning "a rounded prominence," a lobe: *lobotomy, lobectomy.*

lung lobectomy /lōbek′təmē/   [Gk, *lobos + ektomē,* excision],   the surgical excision of one or more lobes of a lung. It is performed to remove a malignant tumor or large benign tumor and to treat uncontrolled bronchiectasis, trauma with hemorrhage, congenital anomalies, or intractable tuberculosis. Any respiratory infection is cleared before surgery. Administration of antibiotics is begun, and the patient receives a general anesthetic. The chest cavity is entered through a long back-to-front incision (thoracotomy), and the diseased lobe is removed. A large-caliber tube remains in the wound and is connected to a water-sealed drainage system. Oxygen is given after surgery. Vital signs are closely monitored, and deep breathing is encouraged. Blood transfusion may be given, and IV fluids are continued. Pain medication is given. Care is taken that the chest tube remain patent and that the drainage system is sealed and functional. The chest tube is removed 2 to 3 days after surgery. Some compensatory emphysema is expected as the remaining lung tissue overexpands to fill the new space. *–lobectomize, v.*

lobe of ear [Gk, *lobos,* lobe; AS, *eare*],   the lower part of the auricle that contains no cartilage.

lobotomy /lōbot′əmē/   [Gk, *lobos + temnein,* to cut],   a neurosurgical procedure (craniotomy) in which the nerve fibers in the bundle of white matter in the frontal lobe of the brain are severed to interrupt the transmission of various affective responses. Severe intractable depression and pain are among the indications for the operation. It is seldom performed, because it has many unpredictable and undesirable effects, including personality change, aggression, socially unacceptable behavior, incontinence, apathy, and lack of consideration for others. Because lobotomy is simple to perform, it was overused in the treatment of mentally ill patients in the past. A cannula is passed through the bony orbit of the eye, and a wire loop is inserted through the cannula to the cingulum. The nerve fibers are severed with the wire loop. Also called **leukotomy.**

lobster claw deformity.   See **bidactyly.**

lobular.   See **lobate.**

lobular carcinoma /lob″yəlɑr/ [Gk, *lobos* + *karkinos,* crab, *oma,* tumor], a neoplasm that often forms a diffuse mass and accounts for a small percentage of breast tumors. It occurs in the milk lobes of the breast.

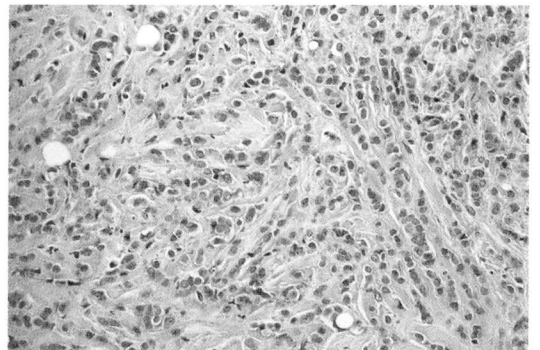

Lobular carcinoma *(Fletcher, 2007)*

lobule /lob″yool/, a small lobe, such as the soft lower pendulous part of the external ear. –**lobular,** *adj.*

loc-, prefix meaning "from a place": *locomotor, locum, locus.*

LOC, **1.** abbreviation for **level of consciousness. 2.** abbreviation for *loss of consciousness.*

local [L, *locus,* place], **1.** *adj.,* pertaining to a small circumscribed area of the body. **2.** *adj.,* pertaining to a treatment or drug applied locally. **3.** *(Informal) n.,* a local anesthetic.

local adaptation syndrome (LAS), the localized response of a tissue, organ, or system that occurs as a reaction to stress. See also **general adaptation syndrome.**

local anesthesia, the infiltration of a local anesthetic medication to induce the absence of sensation into a small area of the body. Brief surgical or dental procedures are the most common indications to avoid general anesthesia. The anesthetic may be applied topically to the surface of the skin or membrane or injected subcutaneously or intradermally. Advantages include low cost, ease of administration, low toxicity, and rapid recovery. A conscious patient can cooperate and does not require respiratory support or intubation. In all cases, the recommended dosage of any agent is the smallest possible to achieve the desired effect because toxicity is directly related to the total amount of drug given. Each local anesthetic agent also has a recommended maximum allowable dose that is not safely exceeded. Compare **general anesthesia, regional anesthesia, topical anesthesia.** See also **anesthesia.**

local anesthetic, a medication used to prevent the transmission of impulses through nerves to eliminate sensation in a defined area of the body. It can also prevent motor and autonomic function in this area. The effect is transient (time limited). Drugs available for local anesthesia are classified as members of the ester or the amide family. Specific preparations are available for topical administration, infiltration, and various kinds of regional administration, including field block, regional block, epidural block, and spinal block. People who are sensitive to local anesthetics of one group often can tolerate those of the other group. The vascularity of the injection site, the speed with which the drug is given, the rapidity of action of the drug, and the presence of epinephrine or Neo-Cobefrin in the solution may affect any adverse response.

local area network (LAN), a system of linking together computers and other electronic office equipment within an office or building, permitting shared use of software and/or peripherals. Compare **wide area network.**

local cerebral blood flow (LCBF), in positron emission tomography, a parametric image of blood flow through the brain expressed as milliliters per minute per 100 g of brain tissue.

local cerebral metabolic rate of glucose utilization (LCMRG), in positron emission tomography, a parametric image of brain activity expressed as milligrams of glucose used per minute per 100 g of brain tissue.

local control, the arrest of cancer growth at the site of origin.

local hypothermia, the cooling of a local area of tissue, particularly brain tissue, to prevent edema development.

local immunity, a state of protection against disease in a particular organ, tissue, or anatomical site, mediated by localized antibodies or lymphoid cells.

local infection [L, *locus,* place, *inficere,* to stain], an infection involving bacteria that invade the body at a specific point and remain there, multiplying, until eliminated.

local infiltration of anesthesia, injection of local anesthetic agents in close proximity to nerve fibers to create a temporary pharmacological loss of sensation in a circumscribed area of the body. Used in dentistry to produce a loss of sensation in and around teeth.

localization /lō′kəlīzā″shən/ [L, *locus,* place], **1.** the designation of a particular site for a lesion or organ function. **2.** the determination of the site of a biological function. **3.** the assignment of a position to an object detected by radiography. –*localize, v.*

localization audiometry. See **audiometry.**

localized scleroderma, thickening and inflammation of the skin from excessive collagen deposition. Compare **systemic sclerosis.** Kinds include **morphea, generalized morphea, linear scleroderma, en coup de sabre.**

localizer image, an image used to localize a specific body part in computed tomography.

localizing symptom. See **symptom.**

local lesion [L, *locus,* place, *laesio,* hurting], **1.** a lesion anywhere on the body that does not spread. **2.** a lesion of the central nervous system characterized by distinctive local symptoms.

local osteolytic hypercalcemia (LOH), a syndrome of malignancy-associated hypercalcemia resulting from the action of locally acting osteolytic factors released in conjunction with tumor deposits adjacent to bone. LOH is frequently caused by cancers such as multiple myeloma; lung, breast, or prostate cancer; or any metastasis of cancer to bone.

local paralysis, a loss of motor control that is confined to a single muscle, muscle group, or part of the body.

local reaction [L, *locus,* place, *re + agere,* to act], a reaction to treatment that occurs at the site at which it was administered.

locant /lō″kənt/, a number or letter code that locates the position of an atom, radical, or compound in the structure of a more complex molecule.

lochia /lō″kē·ə/ [Gk, *lochos,* childbirth], the discharge that flows from the vagina after childbirth. During the first 2 to 4 days after delivery, the lochia is red or brownish red (called lochia rubra) and is made up of blood, endometrial decidua, fetal lanugo, vernix, and sometimes meconium, and it has a fleshy odor. About the third day the amount of blood diminishes. The placental site exudes serous material, erythrocytes, lymph, cervical mucus, and microorganisms from the superficial layer called lochia serosa. During the next 10 to 14 days bacteria appear in large numbers along with mucinous decidual material and epithelial cells, causing the lochia

L

to appear whitish yellow (lochia alba). This may continue for 3 to 6 weeks into the postpartum period.

loci. See **locus.**

locked-in syndrome [ME, *loc* + Gk, *syn,* together, *dromos,* course], a paralytic condition, caused by bilateral destruction of the medulla oblongata or pons, in which a person may be conscious and alert but unable to communicate except by eye movements or blinking (e.g., pseudocoma). The condition renders the individual unable to speak or move any of the limbs. It is most frequently caused by stroke or central pontine myelinolysis.

locked knee [AS, *loc* + *cneow*], a condition in which the knee is fixed in either a flexed or an extended position, often caused by longitudinal splitting of the medial meniscus. Also called **trick knee.**

locked twins. See **interlocked twins.**

lock forceps. See **point forceps.**

locking point [AS, *loc,* lock; L, *punctum,* puncture], a point on the body at which light pressure can be applied to help a weak or debilitated patient maintain a desired posture or position. A basic locking point is the body's center of gravity, at the level of the second sacral vertebra, where mild pressure can assist a patient in standing or walking erect.

lockjaw, (*Informal*) spasm of the masseter muscle of the jaw associated with tetanus. Also called **trismus.** See **tetanus.**

locomotion [L, *locus,* place, *motio,* movement], movement or the ability to move from one place or position to another.

locomotor [L, *locus* + *motio*], pertaining to locomotion.

locomotor ataxia. See **tabes dorsalis.**

loculate /lok″yo͞olāt/ [L, *loculus,* little place], divided into small spaces or cavities.

loculation /lok′yəlā″shən/, the presence of numerous small spaces or cavities.

loculus /lok″yo͞oləs/ [L, little place], a small chamber, pocket, or cavity, such as the interior of a polyp.

locum tenens /lō″kəm ten″ənz/ [L, *locus,* place, *tenere,* to hold], a physician or advanced practice professional who is contracted to work on a temporary basis to fill in for a vacancy, vacation, or extended leave.

locus /lō″kəs/ *pl. loci* [L, place], a specific place or position, such as the locus of a particular gene on a chromosome.

locus ceruleus [L, *locus,* place, *caeruleus,* sky-blue], a deeply pigmented group of several thousand neurons in the floor of the fourth ventricle. It is part of a major norepinephrine pathway of the central nervous system.

locus of control [L, *locus,* place; Fr, *controle*], a center of perceived responsibility for one's behavior. Individuals with an internal locus of control believe that they can control events related to their lives, whereas those with an external locus of control tend to believe that real power resides in forces outside themselves that determine their lives. See also **internal locus of control, external locus of control.**

locus of infection, a site in the body where an infection originates.

lodoxamide /lo-dok′sämīd/, a mast cell stabilizer that inhibits immediate hypersensitivity, applied topically to the eye as the tromethamine salt for treatment of allergen-induced conjunctivitis, keratitis, and keratoconjunctivitis.

Loeffler syndrome. See **Löffler syndrome.**

Loestrin, an oral contraceptive containing a progestin and an estrogen. Brand name for **norethindrone acetate and ethinyl estradiol.**

Löffler syndrome /lef″lər/ [Wilhelm Löffler, Swiss physician, 1887–1972], a benign idiopathic disorder marked by episodes of pulmonary eosinophilia, transient opacities in the lungs, anorexia, breathlessness, fever, and weight loss. Recovery is spontaneous and prompt. Also spelled **Loeffler syndrome.** See also **pulmonary infiltrate with eosinophilia.**

lofstrand crutch, a forearm mobility aid that allows an individual to place his or her weight on the hands and forearms when ambulating.

log-, logo-, -log, -logue, combining form meaning "word, speech, thought": *dialogue, logospasm, logotherapy.*

logad-, prefix meaning "whites of the eyes": *logadectomy.*

logadectomy /log″ah-dek′to-me/ [L, *pro,* logo: whites of the eye], excision of a portion of the conjunctiva.

-logia. See **-logy, -logia.**

login, the process of permitting access to a computer system by identification of the user's credentials.

logo-. See **log-, logo-, -log, -logue.**

logoff, a procedure for terminating interaction between a user and a computer. Also called **sign-off.**

logospasm, spasmodic speech. See also **explosive speech.**

logotherapy /log″ōther″əpē/ [Gk, *logos,* word, *therapeia,* treatment], a treatment modality based on the application of humanistic and existential psychology to assist a patient in finding meaning and purpose in life and unique life experiences.

log roll [ME, *logge* + L, *roto,* turn around], a maneuver used to turn a reclining patient from one side to the other or completely over without flexing the spinal column. The arms of the patient are folded across the chest, and the legs extended. A draw sheet under the patient is manipulated by attending health care team members or nursing personnel to facilitate the procedure.

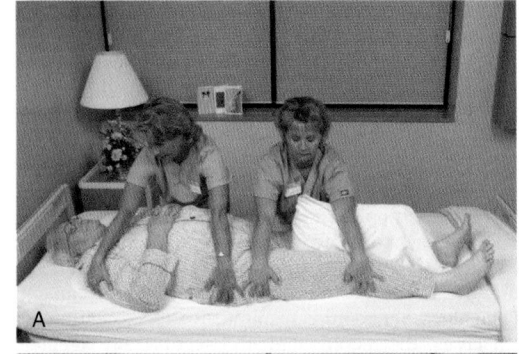
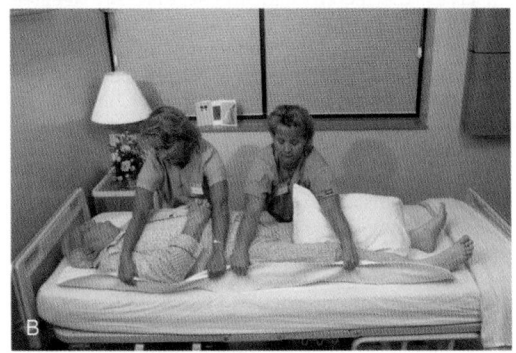

Log roll (Sorrentino, 2012)

-logue. See **log-, logo-, -log, -logue.**

-logy, -logia, a suffix meaning "a science" or "study of": *anthropology, biology, neonatology.*

LOH, abbreviation for **local osteolytic hypercalcemia.**

loiasis /lō-ī″əsis/, a form of filariasis caused by the worm *Loa loa.* The worms may migrate for 10 to 15 years in subcutaneous tissue, producing localized inflammation known as Calabar swellings. Occasionally the migrating worms may be visible beneath the conjunctiva. The disease is acquired through the bite of an infected African deer fly. Treatment with diethylcarbamazine usually results in cure and may also be successful as prophylaxis. See also **filariasis, onchocerciasis.**

loin [ME, *loyn*, flank], a part of the body on each side of the spinal column between the false ribs and the hip bones.

loin pain–hematuria syndrome, a syndrome of intense loin pain, either unilateral or bilateral, lasting from a few days to weeks, followed by hematuria, usually seen in young women; the cause is unknown, but some cases have been linked to treatment with estrogen compounds.

lomefloxacin /lo″mĕflok′säsin/, a broad-spectrum antibiotic effective against a wide range of aerobic gram-negative and gram-positive organisms, used as the hydrochloride salt.

lomefloxacin hydrochloride, the hydrochloride salt of lomefloxacin, administered orally in the treatment of bronchitis and the treatment and prevention of urinary tract infections.

Lomotil, an antidiarrheal fixed-combination drug containing an antiperistaltic agent and an anticholinergic agent. Brand name for **diphenoxylate hydrochloride, atropine sulfate.**

lomustine /lōmus″tēn/, an antineoplastic alkylating agent.
■ INDICATIONS: It is prescribed in the treatment of a variety of malignant neoplastic diseases, including brain tumors and Hodgkin disease.
■ CONTRAINDICATIONS: Known hypersensitivity to this drug prohibits its use.
■ ADVERSE EFFECTS: Among the more serious adverse effects are bone marrow depression, nausea, and vomiting.

Lonalac, brand name for a low-sodium nutritional supplement.

long-acting drug [AS, *lang* + L, *agere*, to do; Fr, *drogue*, drug], a pharmacological agent with a prolonged effect because of a formulation resulting in the slow release of the active principle or the continued absorption of small amounts of the dosage of the drug over an extended period.

long-acting insulin, insulin analogs formulated with recombinant DNA technology. These formulations form microprecipitates when injected into the subcutaneous tissue, delaying absorption from the injection site. They do not have a pronounced peak effect and have a duration of action of approximately 24 hours. Compare **intermediate-acting insulin, short-acting insulin.** See also **insulin.**

long-acting thyroid stimulator (LATS), an immunoglobulin, probably an autoantibody, that exerts a prolonged stimulatory effect on the thyroid gland, causing rapid growth of the gland and excess thyroid function, resulting in hyperthyroidism. It is found circulating in the blood of 50% of people with Graves disease.

long-acting thyroid stimulator protector (LATS-P), an antibody that inhibits the neutralization of long-acting thyroid stimulator and is found in the serum of persons with Graves disease. LATS-P interferes with the binding of thyroid-stimulating hormone to its receptor on the plasma membrane of thyroid cells. See also **long-acting thyroid stimulator.**

long-arm cast [AS, *lang* + *earm*, arm; ONorse, *kasta*], an orthopedic cast applied to immobilize the arm from the hand to the upper arm. It is used in treating fractures of the forearm, elbow, and humerus; for maintaining postoperative positioning of the distal arm, elbow, or upper arm; and for correcting or maintaining the correction of deformities of the distal arm, wrist, or elbow. Compare **short-arm cast.** See also **cast.**

long below-knee (BK) amputation, transtibial amputation in which the division is in the distal third of the tibia. See also **short below-knee (BK) amputation.**

long bone, any of the bones that contribute to the height or length of an extremity, particularly the bones of the legs and arms.

longevity /lonjev″itē/ [L, *longus,* long, *aveum,* age], the number of years an average person of a particular age is expected to continue living. It is determined by statistical tables based on mortality rates of various population groups.

longissimus /lonjis′iməs/ [L, longest, very long], a general term denoting a long structure, as a muscle.

longitudinal /lon′jətoo″dənəl/ [L, *longitudo,* length], 1. pertaining to a measurement in the direction of the long axis of an object, body, or organ, such as the longitudinal arch of the foot. 2. pertaining to a scientific study (nonexperimental research design) that is conducted over a long period of time, such as the Framingham (Massachusetts) Heart Study of heart disease, with data collected from study participants at more than one point in time. Compare **cross-sectional.**

longitudinal diffusion, the diffusion of solute molecules in the direction of flow of the mobile phase.

longitudinal dissociation, the insulation of parallel pathways of cardiac impulses from each other, usually in the atrioventricular junction.

longitudinal fissure [L, *longitudo,* length, *fissura,* cleft], the largest and deepest groove between the medial surfaces of the cerebral hemispheres.

longitudinal presentation [L, *longitudo,* length, *praesentare,* to show], the normal presentation of a fetus, with the long axis of the infant body parallel to that of the mother.

longitudinal sound waves, pressure waves formed by the oscillation of particles or molecules parallel to the axis of wave propagation. The compression and expansion of such waves at high frequencies is the principle on which ultrasonography is based.

long-leg cast, an orthopedic cast applied to immobilize the leg from the toes to the upper thigh. It is used in treating fractures and dislocations of the knee; for maintaining postoperative positioning and immobilization of the knee, distal leg, and ankle; and for correcting or maintaining the correction of the foot, distal leg, and knee. Compare **short-leg cast.** See also **cast.**

long-leg cast with walker, an orthopedic cast applied to immobilize the leg from the toes to the upper thigh in treating certain leg fractures. This type of cast is the same as the long-leg cast but incorporates a rubber walker, enabling the patient to walk while the leg is encased in the cast and when weight-bearing ambulation is allowed. See also **cast.**

long QT syndrome, an inherited cardiac disorder characterized by prolongation of the Q-T interval. The disorder is associated with ventricular tachycardia, cardiac arrhythmias, syncope, and sudden death. Syncopal episodes often occur during physical exercise in young, otherwise healthy persons. This syndrome may also be caused by a variety of drugs.

long-scale contrast, a radiographic image containing a wide range and great number of shades of gray with little difference in the adjacent tones. Also called **low contrast.**

long-term care (LTC), the provision of medical, social, and personal care services on a recurring or continuing basis to persons with chronic physical or mental disorders. The care may be provided in environments ranging from institutions to private homes. Long-term care services usually include symptomatic treatment, maintenance, and rehabilitation for patients of all age groups.

L

long terminal repeats, identical nucleotide sequences occurring at each end of a proviral genome or a transposon and believed to be essential for integration of the molecule into host DNA.

long-term memory, the ability to recall sensations, events, ideas, and other information for long periods of time without apparent effort. It is generally the last memory store to be destroyed in patients with Alzheimer disease. Compare **short-term memory.**

long thoracic nerve, one of a pair of supraclavicular branches from the roots of the brachial plexus. It arises by three roots, from the fifth, the sixth, and the seventh cervical nerves. The fibers from the fifth and the sixth cervical nerves join just after they pierce the scalenus medius and are united with the fibers from the seventh cervical nerve at the level of the first rib. Compare **phrenic nerve.**

long thoracic nerve injury, damage to the nerve (C5-7) that innervates the serratus muscle, which anchors the apex of the scapula to the posterior of the rib cage. Symptoms include an abnormally prominent scapula and difficulty in flexing the outstretched arm above the shoulder level, protracting the shoulder, or performing scapula abduction and adduction. See also **winged scapula.**

long tract signs, neurological signs such as clonus, muscle spasticity, or bladder involvement that usually indicate a lesion in the middle or upper parts of the spinal cord or in the brain.

longus capitis, a muscle that flexes the head.

longus colli, a muscle that flexes the neck anteriorly and laterally, with slight rotation to the opposite side.

Loniten, an antihypertensive drug. Brand name for **minoxidil.**

loop [ME, *loupe*], **1.** a set of instructions in a computer program that causes certain commands to be executed repeatedly if specified criteria are met. **2.** a fine wire that becomes a curved surgical instrument when energized with electricity. It is used in loop excision procedures. **3.** a curve or bend in a tube or tubelike structure. **4.** See **intrauterine device.**

loop colostomy [ME, *loupe* + Gk, *kolon,* colon, *stoma,* mouth], a type of temporary colostomy performed as part of the surgical treatment for repair of some colon diseases. The procedure involves bringing an intact segment of colon proximal to the repair through an abdominal incision and suturing it onto the abdomen. A stoma is created with both proximal and distal lumens opening into it. The colostomy is reversed after resolution of the original pathology. Compare **double-barrel colostomy.** See also **colostomy irrigation, Hirschsprung disease.**

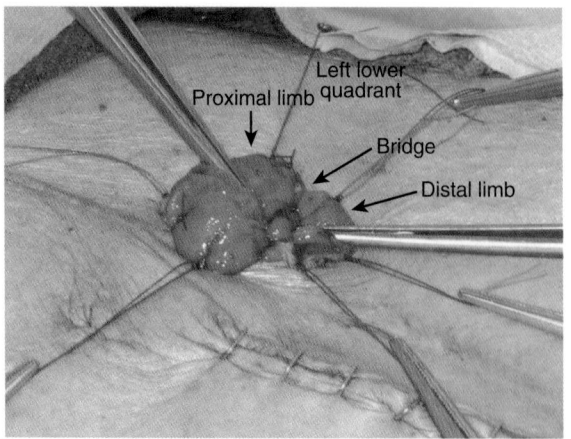

Loop colostomy *(Fleshman et al, 2013)*

loop diuretic. See **diuretic.**

loop excision, the surgical removal of dysplastic tissue cells with a small wire loop. The technique is used in gynecological diagnosis and therapy to remove intraepithelial neoplasms from the uterine cervix. Also called *loop electrical excision procedure.*

loop of Henle /hen′lē/ [ME, *loupe*; Friedrich Gustave Henle, German anatomist, 1809–1885], the U-shaped part of a renal tubule, consisting of a thin descending limb and a thick ascending limb. Also called **Henle's loop.**

loose anagen hair syndrome, a syndrome of unknown cause, usually seen in children, in which scalp hair can be plucked easily and painlessly during the anagen part of the hair cycle, resulting from defective anchorage of the hair shaft to the follicle. There is also slowing of hair growth.

loose associations, a verbal expression of thoughts that are not responsive or logically connected.

loose body, a fragment of solid tissue in a body cavity or joint. Kinds include **joint mouse.**

loose connective tissue. See **connective tissue.**

loose fibrous tissue [ME, *lous,* not fastened], a constrictive, pliable fibrous connective tissue consisting of interwoven elastic and collagenous fibers, interspersed with fluid-filled areolae. It is found in adipose tissue, areolar tissue, reticular tissue, and fibroelastic tissue. Compare **dense fibrous tissue.**

looseness of association (LOA) [ME, *lous,* not fastened], (in psychiatry) a disturbance of thinking in which the association of ideas and thought patterns becomes so vague, fragmented, diffuse, and unfocused as to lack any logical sequences or relationship to any preceding concepts or themes. It is a symptom of schizophrenia. When severe, speech may be incoherent. Also called *associative looseness,* **loosening.**

loosening. See **looseness of association.**

loose-pack joint position, a point in the range of motion of a joint at which articulating surfaces are the least congruent and the supporting structures are the most lax.

Looser zones /lō″zər/ [Emil Looser, Swiss physician, 1877–1936], transverse translucent bands, sometimes symmetric, seen radiographically in the cortex of bones affected with osteomalacia or certain other deficiency diseases.

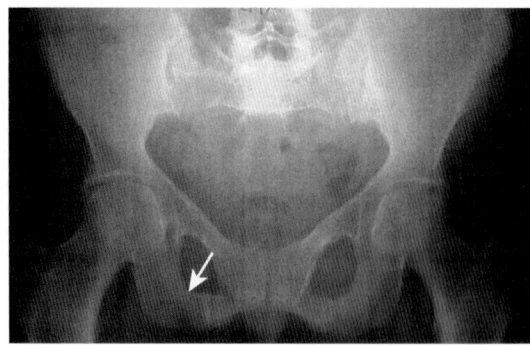

An x-ray of the pelvis showing Looser zones *(Walker et al, 2014)*

Lo/Ovral, an oral contraceptive containing an estrogen and a progestin. Brand name for **ethinyl estradiol, norgestrel.**

LOP, abbreviation for *left occipitoposterior fetal position.*

loperamide hydrochloride /lōper″əmīd/, an antiperistaltic drug.

■ INDICATIONS: It is prescribed in the treatment of diarrhea.

■ CONTRAINDICATIONS: Known hypersensitivity to this drug prohibits its use. It is not given to patients in whom constipation must be avoided.

■ ADVERSE EFFECTS: Among the most serious effects are abdominal pain, constipation, nausea, and vomiting.

loph-, prefix meaning "ridge": *Lophophorata.*

Lophophorata, small aquatic animals with feeding appendages in the shape of a crescent.

Lopid, a lipid-regulating agent. Brand name for **gemfibrozil.**

lopinavir /lopin′ävir/, an HIV protease inhibitor, an orally administered antiviral agent used in combination with ritonavir in the treatment of human immunodeficiency virus infection.

Lopressor, a beta-adrenergic receptor blocking agent used in the treatment of hypertension. Brand name for **metoprolol tartrate.**

Loprox, an antifungal drug. Brand name for *ciclopirox olamine.*

loratadine /lärat′ädēn/, a nonsedating antihistamine (H₁-receptor antagonist) used for treatment of allergic rhinitis and chronic idiopathic urticaria and as a treatment adjunct in asthma; administered orally.

lorazepam /lôrā″zəpam/, a benzodiazepine tranquilizer.

■ INDICATIONS: It is prescribed in the treatment of anxiety, nervous tension, and insomnia and is given intravenously to abort status epilepticus and for preanesthesia.

■ CONTRAINDICATIONS: Acute glaucoma, psychosis, pregnancy, or known hypersensitivity to this drug or to any benzodiazepine prohibits its use.

■ ADVERSE EFFECTS: Among the more serious adverse effects are drowsiness and fatigue. Withdrawal symptoms may occur on discontinuation of the drug, especially after prolonged use or high dosage.

lordoscoliosis /lôr′dōskō′lē·ō″sis/ [Gk, *lordos,* bent, *skoliosis,* curvature], a combination of lordosis and scoliosis.

lordosis /lôrdō″sis/ [Gk, *lordos,* bent forward, *osis,* condition], an abnormal anterior concavity of the lumbar part of the back.

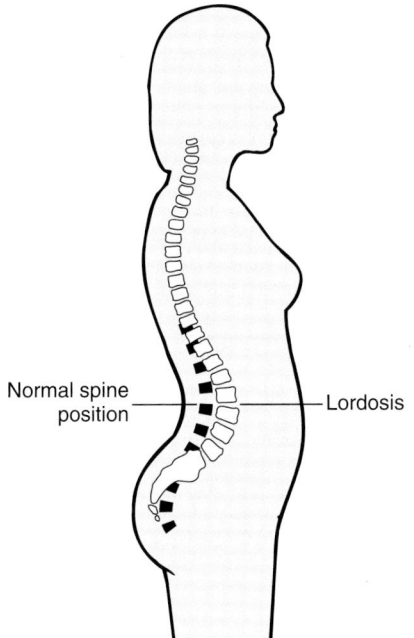

Normal spine position — Lordosis

Lordosis *(Frazier and Drzymkowski, 2009)*

lordotic pelvis /lôrdot″ik/ [Gk, *lordos,* bent forward; L, *pelvis,* basin], a deformed pelvis that bends forward in the lumbar region and is associated with lordosis.

LOS, abbreviation for **length of stay.**

losartan, an antihypertensive drug.

■ INDICATIONS: It is used to treat hypertension, either alone or in combination with other drugs.

■ CONTRAINDICATIONS: Factors that prohibit the use of this drug are known hypersensitivity to tramadol and second- and third-trimester pregnancy.

■ ADVERSE EFFECTS: Life-threatening effects are cerebrovascular accident and myocardial infarction. Other adverse effects are anxiety, confusion, abnormal dreams, migraine, tremor, vertigo, task perversion, angina pectoris, second-degree atrioventricular block, hypotension, blurred vision, burning eyes, conjunctivitis, anorexia, constipation, dry mouth, flatulence, vomiting, impotence, nocturia, urinary frequency, urinary tract infection, anemia, alopecia, dermatitis, dry skin, flushing, photosensitivity, rash, pruritus, sweating, gout, cramps, myalgia, pain, stiffness, congestion, dyspnea, and bronchitis. Common side effects are dizziness, insomnia, arrhythmias, diarrhea, dyspepsia, cough, and upper respiratory infection.

loss of consortium [ME, *lossen,* to lose; L, *consortionis,* companionship], (in law) a claim for damages sought in recompense for the loss of conjugal relations, including society, affection, and assistance, and impairment or loss of sexual relations. Loss of consortium may be charged against a person whose negligence or malfeasance caused injury to the spouse or against a person who caused a marriage to break up.

loss of function, mutations of a gene that cause it to reduce or lose its original function.

LOT, abbreviation for *left occipitotransverse fetal position.*

loteprednol /lo″tĕpred′nol/, a corticosteroid applied topically to the conjunctiva in the treatment of seasonal allergic conjunctivitis, postoperative inflammation, and ocular inflammatory disorders.

lotion [L, *lotio,* a washing], a liquid preparation applied externally to protect the skin or to treat a dermatological disorder.

Lotrimin, an antifungal drug. Brand name for **clotrimazole.**

Lou Gehrig disease. See **amyotrophic lateral sclerosis.**

Louis-Bar syndrome. See **ataxia-telangiectasia syndrome.**

loupe /lo͞op/ [Fr, magnifying glass], a magnifying lens mounted in a frame worn on the head, as used to examine the eyes.

louse. See **lice.**

louse bite, a minute puncture wound produced by a louse. The louse may transmit typhus, trench fever, and relapsing fever. Secondary infection may result from scratching the affected area. Head and body lice are the most common and are frequently found among schoolchildren. Washing and bathing, application of an approved insecticide, and the washing or cleaning of clothes and bed linens are recommended procedures for treatment and prophylaxis against spread of the infestation. See also **pediculosis.**

louse-borne typhus. See **epidemic typhus.**

low back pain (lbp) [ME, low + AS, *baec* + L, *poena,* penalty], local or referred pain at the base of the spine caused by a sprain, a strain, osteoarthritis, ankylosing spondylitis, a neoplasm, or a herniated intervertebral disk. Low back pain is a common complaint and is often associated with poor posture, obesity, sagging abdominal muscles, sitting for prolonged periods of time, or improper body mechanics.

■ OBSERVATIONS: Pain may be localized and static. It may be accompanied by muscle weakness or spasms, or it may radiate down one or both legs, as in sciatica. Pain may be initiated or increased by coughing, sneezing, rising from a seated position, lifting, stretching, bending, or turning. To guard against the pain, the person may decrease the range of motion of the spine. If an intervertebral disk is herniated, deep pressure over the interspace generally causes pain, and flexion of the hip elicits sciatic pain when the knee is extended but not when the knee is flexed (Lasègue's sign).

■ INTERVENTIONS: Specific treatment protocols will be dictated by the cause of the low back pain, the severity of symptoms, and the patient's history. Muscle relaxants, tranquilizers, and antiinflammatory medications may be prescribed. Rest and exercises are frequently a component of treatment. Typically the exercise program is developed and taught by a physical therapist, chiropractor, or physiatrist.

■ PATIENT CARE CONSIDERATIONS: Correct body mechanics, adequate and appropriate exercise, and the elimination of excess weight are emphasized.

low-birth-weight (LBW) infant, a newborn whose weight at birth is less than 2500 g, regardless of gestational age.

low-calcium diet, a diet that restricts the use of calcium and eliminates most dairy foods, all breads made with milk or dry skimmed milk, and deep-green leafy vegetables. It is prescribed for patients with absorptive hypercalciuria. Meats, including beef, lamb, pork, and veal, and poultry, fish, vegetables, legumes, and fruits are recommended.

low-caloric diet, a diet that is prescribed to limit calorie intake, usually to cause a reduction in body weight. It is recommended that women eat at least 1200 calories per day and that men eat at least 1800 calories daily.

low cervical cesarean section, a surgical procedure to deliver a baby through a transverse incision in the thin supracervical part of the lower uterine segment, behind the bladder and the bladder flap. This incision bleeds less during surgery and heals with a stronger scar than the higher vertical scar of the classic cesarean section. Compare **extraperitoneal cesarean section.** See also **cesarean section.**

low-cholesterol diet, a diet that restricts foods containing animal fats and saturated fatty acids, including egg yolk, cream, butter, milk, muscle and organ meats, and shellfish. It concentrates instead on poultry, fish, vegetables, fruits, low-fat dairy products, and polyunsaturated fats. The diet is indicated for persons with high serum cholesterol levels, cardiovascular disorders, obesity, hyperlipidemia, hypercholesterolemia, or hyperlipoproteinemia. Also called **cholesterol-restricted diet, low-saturated-fat diet.**

low contrast. See **long-scale contrast.**

low-density lipoprotein (LDL), a plasma protein provided from very low–density lipoproteins (VLDLs) or by the liver, containing relatively more cholesterol and triglycerides than protein. It is derived in part, if not completely, from the intravascular breakdown of the very low–density lipoproteins and delivers lipids and cholesterol to the body tissues. The high cholesterol content may account for its greater atherogenic potential as compared with the VLDLs.

low-density lipoprotein (LDL) receptor disorder, an inherited disorder transmitted as a dominant trait and characterized by a high level of serum cholesterol, tendinous xanthomas, and early evidence of atherosclerosis, especially of the coronary arteries. Affected individuals at 50 years of age have 3 to 10 times greater risk of ischemic heart disease than the general population. Cholesterol levels are elevated at birth, increase with age, and average 250 to 500 mg/dL in heterozygous adults and 500 to 1000 mg/dL in adults who are homozygous for the gene. Xanthomas begin to appear at 20 years of age and occur most frequently on the Achilles tendon, extensor tendons of the hands, elbows, and tibial tuberosities. In type IIA familial hypercholesterolemia, only low-density lipoprotein (LDL) level is elevated, whereas in type IIB LDL and very low–density lipoprotein levels are increased. The disorder occurs

in Caucasians, African-Americans, and Asian-Americans; the prevalence of the gene in the United States is 1:1000. Treatment includes a diet that is low in cholesterol and saturated fat. Cholestyramine may be given to patients with type IIA familial hypercholesterolemia but not to those with type IIB. Also called **familial hypercholesterolemia, hypercholesterolemic xanthomatosis, hyperlipidemia type IIA, hyperlipidemia type IIB.**

low-dose tolerance, a temporary and incomplete immunosuppression induced by the administration of subimmunogenic doses of soluble antigen. The tolerance is achieved in the neonatal period, when lymphoid cells have not matured enough to activate a response.

lower esophageal sphincter, the terminal few centimeters of the esophagus near the esophagogastric junction, which normally remain constricted except during swallowing and prevent reflux of gastric contents into the esophagus.

lower extremity suspension [ME, low + L, *extremitas + suspendere,* to hang], an orthopedic procedure used in the treatment of bone fractures and the correction of orthopedic abnormalities of the lower limbs. Traction equipment, including metal frames, ropes, and pulleys, is used to relieve the weight of the involved lower limb rather than to exert traction pull. Lower extremity suspension may be either unilateral or bilateral and is used in the postoperative, posttraumatic, or postreduction control of edema. Compare **balanced suspension, upper extremity suspension.**

lower level discriminator (LLD), an electronic device used in nuclear medicine to discriminate against all radionuclide pulses whose heights are below a given level.

lower motor neuron dysarthria, a disorder of articulation caused by weakness or paralysis of the articulatory muscles and marked by a rasping, monotonous voice and, in severe forms, shriveling and flaccidity of the tongue and laxness and tremulousness of the lips, seen in advanced cases of lesions of motor nuclei of the lower pons or medulla oblongata. Also called **flaccid dysarthria.**

lower motor neuron paralysis, paralysis resulting from an injury or lesion that damages the cell bodies or axons, or both, of the lower motor neurons, which are located in the anterior horn cells of the spinal cord and the spinal and peripheral nerves. If complete transection of the spinal cord occurs, voluntary muscle control is totally lost. In partial transection, function is altered in varying degrees, depending on the areas innervated by the nerves involved. In lower motor neuron paralysis the reflex arcs are permanently damaged, causing decreased muscle tone and flaccidity, diminished or absent reflexes, absence of pathological reflexes, local twitching of muscle groups (fasciculations), and progressive atrophy of the atonic muscles. Compare **upper motor neuron paralysis.**

lower pole ureter, the ureter draining the lower pole of a duplex kidney.

lower respiratory tract, one of the two divisions of the respiratory system. The lower respiratory tract includes the left and right bronchi and the alveoli where the exchange of oxygen and carbon dioxide occurs during the respiratory cycle. The bronchi divide into smaller bronchioles in the lungs, the bronchioles into alveolar ducts, the ducts into alveolar sacs, and the sacs into alveoli. The alveolar sacs and the alveoli present a total lung surface of about 850 square feet (79 square meters) for the exchange of oxygen and carbon dioxide, which occurs between the most internal alveolar surface and the tiny capillaries surrounding the external alveolar wall. The lower respiratory tract is a continuation of the upper respiratory tract and is a common site of infections, obstructive conditions, and neoplastic disease. Compare **upper respiratory tract.** See also **lung.**

lower respiratory tract infection. See **respiratory tract infection.**

Lowe syndrome [Charles U. Lowe, American pediatrician, b. 1921], a sex-linked condition in males characterized by progressive mental deterioration, renal tubular dysfunction, and cortical cataracts with or without glaucoma.

low-fat diet [ME, low; AS, *faett*; Gk, *diaita,* lifestyle], a diet containing limited amounts of fat and consisting chiefly of easily digestible foods of high carbohydrate content. It includes all vegetables, lean meats, fish, fowl, pasta, cereals, and whole wheat or enriched bread. Egg yolk and fatty meats are restricted. Meat, eggs, butter and margarine, cream, fried foods, foods prepared in fats, oils, gravy, cheese, peanut butter, nuts, and olives are omitted or restricted. Experts recommend that no more than 30% of one's daily calories should come from fatty foods and that no more than 10% should come from saturated fats. A typical low-fat diet providing approximately 1700 calories per day would contain 85 grams of protein, 220 grams of carbohydrate, and 50 grams of fat. Low-fat diets supply 10% to 15% of total energy as fat. A low-fat diet may be prescribed in the treatment of gallbladder disease, obesity, heart disease, malabsorption syndromes, and hyperlipidemia.

low-fat milk, milk containing 1% to 2% fat, making it an intermediate in fat content between whole and skimmed milk.

low-fiber diet, a diet that restricts the amount of fiber consumed to less than 15 grams a day. See **low-residue diet.**

low-flow oxygen delivery system, respiratory care equipment that allows the patient to inhale some ambient air along with the delivered oxygen. As the patient's ventilatory pattern changes, different amounts of air are mixed with the constant flow of oxygen, thus causing the inspired oxygen concentration to vary. Also called **variable-performance oxygen delivery system.**

low forceps [ME, low + L, *forceps,* pair of tongs], an obstetric operation in which forceps are used to deliver a baby whose head is on the pelvic floor. The procedure is performed most often as an elective procedure to shorten normal labor and to control delivery, usually in conjunction with anesthesia and episiotomy. It is commonly required for the delivery of mothers whose expulsive powers have been weakened by analgesia, anesthesia, or fatigue. Also called **outlet forceps, prophylactic forceps.** Compare **high forceps, mid forceps, natural childbirth, spontaneous delivery.** See also **forceps delivery, obstetric forceps.**

low-grade fever, an oral temperature that is above 98.6° F (37° C) but lower than 100.4° F (38° C) for 24 hours.

low-grade infection [ME, *lah* + L, *gradus,* degree, *inficere,* to stain], a subacute or chronic infection with mild fever and no pus production.

low-lying placenta. *(Nontechnical)* See **placenta previa.**

low-molecular-weight heparin (LMWH), a class of drugs used to prevent potentially fatal blood clots in patients undergoing surgery or patients at risk for blood clots. It has been used to prevent deep vein thrombosis in patients undergoing hip and knee replacements. LMWH has an advantage over regular heparin in that predictable plasma levels are achieved, obviating the need for regular monitoring of prothrombin time and partial thromboplastin time.

Lown-Ganong-Levine (LGL) syndrome /loun″ gənong″ ləvēn″/ [Bernard Lown, American physician, b. 1921; William F. Ganong, American physiologist, b. 1924; S.A. Levine, American physician, 1891–1966], a disorder of the atrioventricular (AV) conduction system marked by ventricular preexcitation. Part or all of the AV nodal connection is bypassed by an abnormal connection between the

atria and the bundle of His. The condition may be discovered by routine electrocardiogram or may be seen in association with paroxysmal atrial arrhythmias, supraventricular tachycardia, atrial flutter, and fibrillation. Treatments include the use of antiarrhythmic drugs such as quinidine sulfate, procainamide, and propranolol; surgical interruption of the abnormal pathway; and implantation of a pacemaker. Also called **short-PR-normal-QRS syndrome.** Compare **Wolff-Parkinson-White syndrome.**

low-power field, the low magnification field of vision under a light microscope.

low-protein diet [ME, *lah,* low; Gk, *proteios,* first rank, *diaita,* way of living], a diet proportionally low in protein, usually designed for persons who must restrict protein intake because of a metabolic abnormality associated with kidney failure or liver disease.

low-purine diet, a diet used as adjunct therapy for gout patients who suffer from a painful accumulation of salts of uric acid in the joints. Purine-rich foods are primary sources of uric acid. They include meat, poultry, fish, and particularly organ meats such as liver, kidney, and sweetbreads. Purine-rich foods are replaced in the diet by dairy products, eggs, and some vegetable sources of proteins. Low-purine diets should be a secondary source of treatment, with weight loss and adequate fluid intake being primary. Also called **purine-restricted diet.**

low-residue diet, a diet that leaves a minimal residue in the lower intestinal tract after digestion and absorption. It consists of tender meats, poultry, fish, eggs, white bread, pasta, simple desserts, clear soups, tea, and coffee. Omitted are highly seasoned or fried foods, all fruits and fruit juices, raw vegetables, whole grain cereals and bread, nuts, jams, and usually milk. The diet is prescribed in cases of diverticulitis and GI irritability or inflammation and before and after GI surgery. Because it is lacking in calcium, iron, and vitamins, it should be used only for a limited time or with nutrient supplementation. The primary care provider's prescription should stipulate low fiber/low residue because low fiber may not always indicate low residue. Compare **low-fiber diet.**

low-salt diet. See **low-sodium diet.**

low-saturated-fat diet, a diet that limits sources of saturated fats from animal meats, egg yolks, butter, and full-fat dairy foods. Two plant sources of saturated fat, coconut oil and palm oil, must also be limited. See also **low-cholesterol diet.**

low-sodium diet, a diet that restricts the use of sodium chloride plus other compounds containing sodium, such as baking powder or soda, monosodium glutamate, sodium citrate, sodium propionate, and sodium sulfate. It is indicated in hypertension, edematous states (especially when associated with cardiovascular disease), renal or liver disease, and therapy with corticosteroids. The degree of sodium restriction depends on the severity of the condition. Foods included in the diet are eggs, skimmed milk, beef, poultry, lamb, pork, veal, fish, potatoes, green beans, broccoli, asparagus, peas, salad ingredients, and fresh fruits. Many flavoring extracts, spices, and herbs can be used to add taste to the diet. Foods to be avoided include fresh or canned shellfish, ham, bacon, frankfurters, luncheon meats, sausage, cheese, salted butter or margarine, any breads or cereals made with salt, beets, carrots, celery, sauerkraut, spinach, and most canned or frozen foods, except those prepared without sodium (for example, frozen fruits and vegetables). Also to be avoided are many drugs that contain sodium, such as laxatives, sedatives, and alkalizers, and drinking water from a source using a water softener that adds sodium. Also called **low-salt diet, salt-free diet, sodium-restricted diet.**

low-vision therapist, a doctor of optometry or ophthalmology who diagnoses and treats ocular and vision problems that cannot be corrected fully by pharmacological means or surgery, conventional eyeglasses, or contact lenses.

loxapine /lok″səpēn/,   an antipsychotic agent.

■ INDICATIONS: It is prescribed in the treatment of schizophrenia.

■ CONTRAINDICATIONS: Parkinson disease, concurrent administration of central nervous system depressants, liver or kidney dysfunction, severe hypotension, or known hypersensitivity to this drug prohibits its use.

■ ADVERSE EFFECTS: Among the more serious adverse effects are hypotension, liver toxicity, a variety of extrapyramidal reactions, and hypersensitivity reactions.

Loxitane,   an antipsychotic drug. Brand name for **loxapine.**

Loxosceles /loksos′ēlēz/,   a genus of six-eyed spiders, some of which have poisonous bites. *L. laeta* is a brown spider of South America, and *L. reclusa* is the brown recluse spider of North America. See **spider bite.**

lozenge.   See **troche.**

lp,   abbreviation for **line pair.**

LP,   abbreviation for **lumbar puncture.**

LPL,   abbreviation for **lipoprotein lipase.**

LPM,   abbreviation for *liters per minute.*

LPN,   abbreviation for **licensed practical nurse.**

LPS Act,   a California law named for sponsors of the legislation (*Lanterman, Petris,* and *Short*) that provides for the protection and treatment of persons judged to be "gravely disabled" and thus unable to provide food, clothing, or shelter for themselves. The legislation was designed to safeguard the constitutional rights of persons threatened with involuntary commitment on the basis of a psychiatric diagnosis. Some other states have similar laws. The updates took effect on January 1, 2014.

Lr,   symbol for the element **lawrencium.**

LRN,   abbreviation for **Laboratory Response Network.**

LSD,   abbreviation for *lysergic acid diethylamide.*   See **lysergide.**

LSF,   abbreviation for **line spread function.**

L-shaped kidney,   a fused kidney in which one renal mass is vertical and the other is inferior to it in a transverse position. This can be either a variety of horseshoe kidney or a type of crossed renal ectopia.

L-spine,   abbreviation for **lumbar spine.**

L/S ratio,   abbreviation for **lecithin/sphingomyelin ratio.**

LTB,   abbreviation for **laryngotracheobronchitis.**

LTC,   abbreviation for **long-term care.**

LTH,   abbreviation for *luteotropic hormone.*

L-thyroxine.   See **levothyroxine sodium.**

L-Trp,   abbreviation for *L-tryptophan.*

Lu,   symbol for the element **lutetium.**

lubb /lub/,   a syllable used to represent the first heart sound in auscultation, which is longer and has a lower pitch than the second heart sound. See also **heart sound.**

lubb-dupp,   an imitation of the two basic sounds heard in the cardiac cycle. *Lubb* represents the first sound (S₁), which is longer and has a lower pitch and is made by the closure of the mitral and tricuspid valves. It is lower in pitch and lasts slightly longer than the second sound, *dupp* (S₂), which is made by the closure of the aortic valve.

lubiprostone,   a miscellaneous GI agent.

■ INDICATIONS: This drug is used to treat chronic idiopathic constipation.

■ CONTRAINDICATIONS: Known hypersensitivity to this drug and GI obstruction prohibit its use.

■ ADVERSE EFFECTS: Adverse effects of this drug include dizziness, depression, fatigue, insomnia, hypertension, chest pain, abdominal distension, constipation, diarrhea, dry mouth, dyspepsia, flatulence, gastroenteritis, viral gastroesophageal reflux

disease, vomiting, fecal incontinence, fecal urgency, urinary tract infection, chest pain, peripheral edema, influenza, pyrexia, viral infection, back pain, arthralgia, muscle cramps, pain in extremities, bronchitis, cough, dyspnea, nasopharyngitis, sinusitis, and upper respiratory infection. Common side effects include headache, nausea, abdominal pain, and eructation.

lubricant /loo″brikənt/   [L, *lubricans,* making slippery],   a fluid, ointment, or other agent capable of diminishing friction and making a surface slippery.

lubricating enema /loo″brəkā′ting/   [L, *lubricans,* making slippery; Gk, *enienai,* to send in],   an enema used to lubricate the anal canal after surgery for hemorrhoids or to prevent fecal impaction. The enema solution may be made with warm olive oil or mineral oil. See also **oil retention enema.**

luc-,   prefix meaning "light": *lucifugal, lucipetal, lucotherapy.*

-lucent,   suffix meaning "light-admitting": *radiolucent, translucent.*

Lucentis,   brand name for **ranibizumab.**

lucid /loo″sid/   [L, *lucidus,* clear],   clear, rational, and able to be understood. See also **lucid interval.**

lucid interval,   a period of relative mental clarity between periods of irrationality, especially in organic mental disorders such as delirium and dementia.

lucidity /loosid′itē/   [L, *lucidus,* clear],   pertaining to clarity of mind, perception, or intelligibility.

lucid lethargy,   a mental state characterized by a loss of will; an inability to act, even though the person is conscious and intellectual function is normal. See also **lethargy.**

lucifugal /loosif″yəgəl/,   repelled by bright light.

Lucio's leprosy phenomenon   [R. Lucio, Mexican physician, 1819–1866],   an acute form of diffuse lepromatous infection of the skin, characterized by intensely red, tender plaques, particularly on the legs. The plaques tend to progress to obstructive vasculitis, ulcers, necrosis, and scarring.

lucipetal /loosip″ətəl/,   attracted to bright light.

lucotherapy.   See **phototherapy.**

Ludiomil,   an antidepressant drug. Brand name for **maprotiline hydrochloride.**

Ludwig angina /lood″vig/   [Wilhelm F. von Ludwig, German surgeon, 1790–1865; L, *angina,* quinsy],   a severe, potentially life-threatening form of cellulitis in the region of the submandibular gland. Inflammatory edema may distort the floor of the mouth and make swallowing difficult. The glottis and tissue fascial planes may swell suddenly, causing respiratory obstruction. Hospitalization, incision, and drainage along with appropriate antibiotic therapy are the usual treatments.

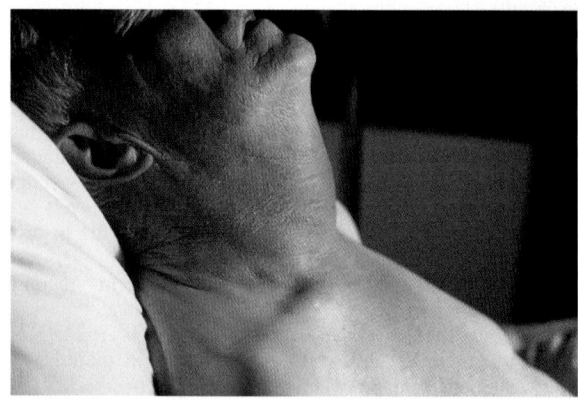

Ludwig angina *(Conlon and Snydman, 2000)*

lue-,   combining form meaning "syphilis": *luetic.*

LUE,   abbreviation for *left upper extremity.*

Luer-Lok connection,   a connection between extracorporeal equipment for peritoneal dialysis and the intraabdominal catheter, using two rigid tubes that screw together.

Luer-Lok syringe /loo″ərlōk″/,   a glass or plastic syringe for injection having a simple screw lock mechanism that securely holds the needle in place. Also called *Luer syringe.*

lues.   See **syphilis.**

luetic.   See **syphilitic.**

-luetic, -luic,   suffix meaning "syphilis": *antiluetic.*

luetic aortitis.   See **syphilitic aortitis.**

Lufyllin,   a respiratory smooth muscle relaxant. Brand name for **dyphylline.**

Lugol's solution [Jean G.A. Lugol, French physician, 1786–1851; L, *solutus,* unbound],   an aqueous solution of iodine (5%) and potassium iodide (10%) that paradoxically suppresses thyroid function, used in preparation for thyroidectomy and during treatment of thyrotoxic crisis.

-luic.   See **-luetic, -luic.**

Lukes-Collins classification [L.J. Lukes; R.D. Collins, 20th-century American pathologists],   a system of identifying non-Hodgkin lymphomas according to B cell, T cell, true, and unclassifiable types. B cell types include lymphocytic, plasmacytic, and follicular cell lymphoma and B cell–derived immunoblastic lymphoma. T cell types include T cell–derived immunoblastic lymphoma and convoluted cell lymphoma. True types are of histiocytic origin.

LUL,   abbreviation for *left upper lobe of lung.*

lumbago /lumbā″gō/   [L, *lumbus,* loin],   pain in the lumbar region caused by a muscle strain, rheumatoid arthritis, osteoarthritis, or a herniated intervertebral disk. Ischemic lumbago, characterized by pain in the lower back and buttocks, is caused by vascular insufficiency, as in terminal aortic occlusion. See also **low back pain.**

lumbar /lum″bər, lum″bär/   [L, *lumbus,* loin],   pertaining to the part of the body between the thorax and the pelvis.

lumbar lordosis,   the dorsally concave curvature of the lumbar spinal column when seen from the side.

lumbar nerves,   the five pairs of spinal nerves rising in the lumbar region of the vertebral column. They become increasingly large the more caudal their origin and pass laterally and downward under the cover of the psoas major or between its fasciculi and form part of the lumbar plexus. The lumbar sympathetic ganglia follow no fixed pattern, and fusions of adjacent ganglia are common. When occurring separately, lumbar ganglia lie on the corresponding vertebra or the intervertebral disk caudally. The ganglion of the second lumbar segment is the largest and the most constant.

lumbar node,   a node in one of the seven groups of parietal lymph nodes serving the abdomen and the pelvis. The lumbar nodes are numerous and are divided into the lateral aortic nodes, preaortic nodes, and retroaortic nodes. They receive the afferent vessels from many different structures, such as the kidneys, the internal reproductive organs, the lateral abdominal muscles, and certain vertebrae, and pass efferents that form lymphatic trunks. Compare **sacral node.** See also **lymph, lymphatic system, lymph node.**

lumbar plexus,   a network of nerves formed by the ventral anterior primary divisions of the first three and the greater part of the fourth lumbar nerves. It is located on the inside of the posterior abdominal wall, either dorsal to the psoas major or among its fibers and ventral to the transverse processes of the lumbar vertebrae. The branches of the lumbar plexus are the iliohypogastric, ilioinguinal, genitofemoral, lateral femoral cutaneous, obturator, accessory obturator, and femoral nerves. The iliohypogastric, ilioinguinal, and genitofemoral nerves supply the caudal part of the abdominal wall. The lateral femoral cutaneous, obturator, accessory obturator, and femoral nerves supply the anterior thigh and the middle of the leg. Only 20% of people have the accessory obturator nerve, which comes from the third and the fourth lumbar nerves. Compare **sacral plexus.** See also **lumbosacral plexus.**

lumbar puncture (LP),   a diagnostic or therapeutic procedure in which a hollow needle and stylet are introduced into the subarachnoid space of the lumbar part of the spinal canal to obtain cerebrospinal fluid (CSF). Strict aseptic technique is used. Diagnostic indications include measuring of CSF pressure; obtaining CSF for laboratory analysis; and injecting oxygen or a radiopaque substance for radiographic visualization of the structures of the nervous system of the spinal canal and meninges and brain. Therapeutic indications for lumbar puncture include removing blood or pus from the subarachnoid space, injecting sera or drugs, withdrawing CSF to reduce intracranial pressure, introducing a local anesthetic to induce spinal anesthesia, and placing a small amount of the patient's blood in the subarachnoid space to form a clot to patch a hole in the dura to prevent leakage of CSF into the epidural space.

■ METHOD: The skin over the interspace of the third and fourth lumbar vertebrae is cleansed. A fenestrated sterile drape is placed over the back, the window over the puncture site. The needle is inserted through the interspace to the subarachnoid space, and the stylet is withdrawn. If the needle is in the proper place, clear, straw-colored CSF will begin to drip out through the needle. Depending on the indication for the procedure, various techniques follow. The pressure of the CSF may be measured with a manometer attached to a catheter and stopcock, or fluid may be withdrawn, visually examined, and sent to the laboratory for chemical or bacteriological analysis.

■ INTERVENTIONS: If the patient is apprehensive, he or she may be given a sedative a half hour before the procedure. The techniques to be used and the treatments to be given or the information to be obtained are explained. The patient is placed in a lateral recumbent position, the back as near the edge of the bed as possible. The legs are flexed on the thighs, the thighs are flexed on the abdomen, and the head and shoulders are bent down, curving the spine convexly to afford the greatest space between the vertebrae. After the procedure, significant signs to be observed by the nurse include pain, change in mentation or alertness, leakage of CSF from the puncture site, fever, and urinary retention. The patient is usually kept flat in bed, often in a prone position, for 1 hour after the procedure.

■ OUTCOME CRITERIA: Lumbar puncture is contraindicated if intracranial tumor is suspected and there is evidence of greatly increased intracranial pressure, if there are signs of infection at the site of puncture, or (to avoid a second puncture) if encephalography or myelography is planned in the near future. Infection, leakage of CSF, headache, nausea, vomiting, dysuria, or signs of meningeal irritation occur in approximately 25% of patients.

L

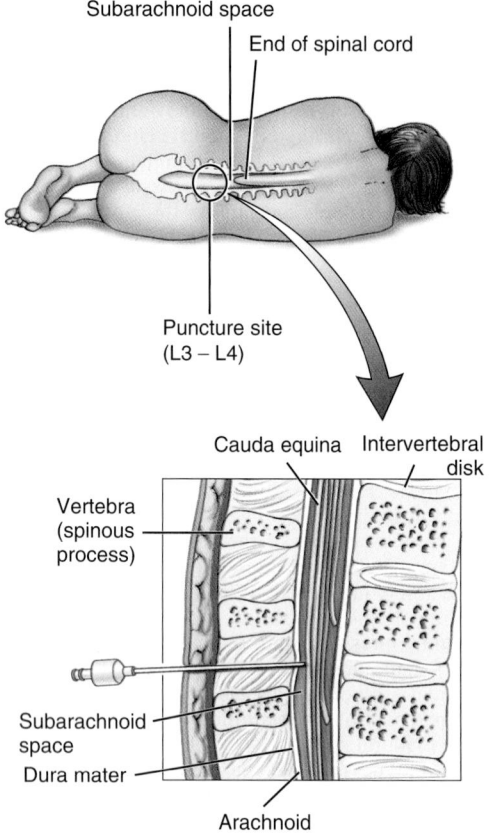

Lumbar puncture *(Herlihy, 2011)*

lumbar radiculopathy, compression and irritation of nerve roots in the lumbar region, with resultant pain in the lower back and lower limbs.

lumbar reflex. See **erector spinae reflex.**

lumbar region. See **lateral region.**

lumbar rib, a rudimentary rib that articulates with the transverse process of the first lumbar vertebra.

lumbar spine (L-spine), that portion of the spine comprising the lumbar vertebrae.

lumbar subarachnoid peritoneostomy, a surgical procedure to drain cerebrospinal fluid in hydrocephalus, usually in the newborn. It spares the kidney but is a slightly less effective method than a lumbar subarachnoid ureterostomy. The procedure may be used when a temporary shunt is needed. A lumbar laminectomy is performed, and then a polyethylene tube is passed from the subarachnoid space around the flank and into the peritoneum. This procedure is performed to correct a communicating type of hydrocephalus.

lumbar subarachnoid ureterostomy, a surgical procedure to drain cerebrospinal fluid through the ureter to the bladder in hydrocephalus, usually in the newborn. A lumbar laminectomy and a left nephrectomy are performed, after which a polyethylene tube is passed from the lumbar subarachnoid space through the paraspinal muscles and into the free ureter. The procedure is performed to correct a communicating type of hydrocephalus.

lumbar veins, four pairs of veins that collect blood by dorsal tributaries from the loins and by abdominal tributaries from the walls of the abdomen. The lumbar veins are connected by the ascending lumbar vein that runs ventral to the transverse processes of the lumbar vertebrae.

lumbar vertebra, one of the five largest segments of the movable part of the vertebral column, distinguished by the absence of a foramen in the transverse process and by vertebral bodies without facets between the sacrum and thoracic vertebrae. The body of each lumbar vertebra is flattened or slightly concave superiorly and inferiorly and is deeply constricted ventrally at the sides. The spinous process of each is thick, broad, and somewhat quadrilateral. The body of the fifth lumbar vertebra is much deeper ventrally than dorsally and in some individuals is defective, tending to weaken the spinal column. Compare **cervical vertebra, coccygeal vertebra, sacral vertebra, thoracic vertebra.**

lumbo-, prefix meaning "loins": *lumbocostal, lumbosacral.*

lumbocostal /lum′bōkos″təl/, pertaining to the lumbar region and ribs.

lumbodorsal fascia, the extensive subdivision of the vertebral fascia that sheaths the sacrospinalis muscle. It spreads caudally to become the glistening white lumbar aponeurosis and the origin of the latissimus dorsi. Medially it attaches to the sacrum, laterally to the ribs and the intercostal fascia, and cranially to the nuchal ligament. See also **thoracolumbar fascia.**

lumbosacral /lum′bōsā″krəl/ [L, *lumbus,* loin, *sacrum,* sacred], pertaining to the lumbar vertebrae and the sacrum. Also called **sacrolumbar.**

lumbosacral plexus [L, *lumbus,* loin, *sacrum,* sacred, *plexus,* braided], the combination of all the ventral anterior primary divisions of the lumbar, the sacral, and the coccygeal nerves. The lumbar and sacral plexuses supply the lower limb. The sacral nerves also supply the perineum through the pudendal plexus and the coccygeal area through the coccygeal plexus. See also **lumbar plexus, sacral plexus.**

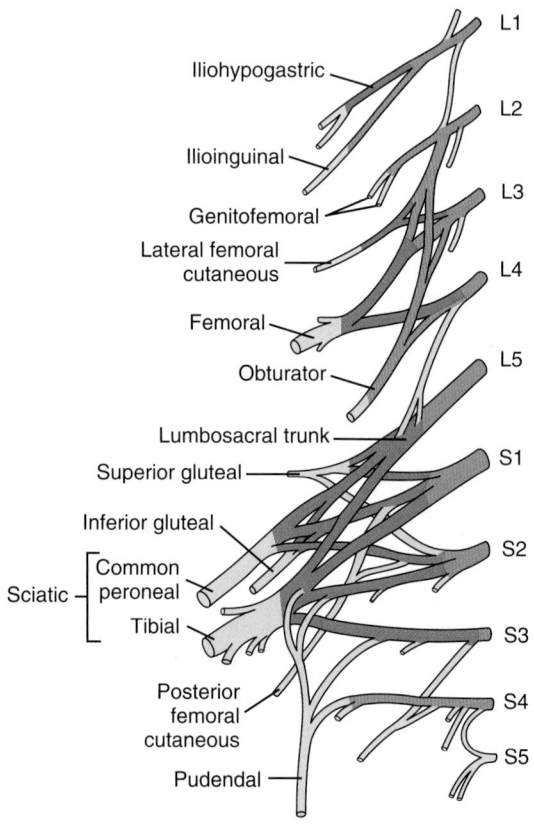

Lumbosacral plexus *(Patton and Thibodeau, 2016)*

lumbrical. See **vermiform.**

lumbrical plus deformity /lum″brikəl/, a complication of rheumatoid arthritis in which the lumbricals (muscles in the hands and feet) become contracted. A main effect of the dysfunction is metacarpophalangeal joint flexion and interphalangeal joint extension. Compare **boutonnière deformity.**

lumen /loo″mən/ *pl. lumina, lumens* [L, light], **1.** a tubular space or the channel within any organ or structure of the body. **2.** a unit of luminous flux that equals the flux emitted in a unit solid angle by a point source of one candle intensity. –*luminal, lumenal, adj.*

lumin-, prefix meaning "light": *luminescence, luminiferous, luminophore.*

lumina, luminal. See **lumen.**

luminance, the brightness of a light-emitting source (e.g., a view box or computer monitor).

luminescence /loo″mines″əns/ [L, *lumen,* light, *escens,* beginning], **1.** the emission of light by a material after excitation by some stimulus. **2.** the emission of light by intensifying-screen phosphors after x-ray interaction. See also **thermoluminescent dosimetry.**

luminiferous /loo′minif″ərəs/ [L, *lumen,* light, *ferre,* to bear], pertaining to a medium that will transmit light.

luminophore /loomin″əfôr/, **1.** an organic compound or chemical grouping that emits light. **2.** a substance that emits light when illuminated.

lumpectomy /lumpek″təmē/ [ME, *lump,* mass, *ektomē,* excision], surgical excision of a tumor without removing large amounts of surrounding tissue. See also **breast cancer.**

lun-, prefix meaning "moon": *lunar, lunacy.*

lunacy, *(Obsolete)* a pejorative term indicating mental illness of some form; the term is no longer used by health and legal professionals.

lunar, crescent-shaped.

lunar month /loo″nər/ [L, *luna,* moon; AS, *monath,* month], a period of 4 weeks or 28 days, approximately the time required for the moon to revolve about the earth.

lunate bone /loo″nāt/ [L, *luna,* moon; AS, *ban*], the carpal bone in the center of the proximal row of carpal bones between the scaphoid and triangular bones. It articulates with five bones, the radius proximally, the capitate and the hamate distally, the scaphoid laterally, and the triangular medially. Also called **os lunatum, semilunar bone.**

Lunesta, brand name for *eszopiclone.*

lung (L) [AS, *lungen*], one of a pair of light, spongy organs in the thorax, constituting the main component of the respiratory system. The two highly elastic lungs are the main mechanisms in the body for inhaling (inspiring) air, from which oxygen is extracted for the arterial blood system, and for exhaling (expiring) carbon dioxide dispersed from the venous system. The right lung is divided into three lobes; the left lung, two lobes. Each lung is conical and has an apex, a base, three borders, and two surfaces. The apex is rounded and extends into the root of the neck about 4 cm above the first rib. The base of the lung is broad and concave, rests on the convex surface of the diaphragm, and with the diaphragm moves up during expiration and down during inspiration. Each lung is composed of an external serous coat, a subserous layer of areolar tissue, and the parenchyma. The serous coat comprises the thin, visceral pleura. The subserous areolar tissue contains many elastic fibers and invests the entire surface of the organ. The parenchyma is composed of secondary lobules divided into primary lobules, each of which consists of blood vessels, lymphatics, nerves, and an alveolar duct connecting with air spaces. The surfaces of the lungs are partially concave, with a cardiac impression that cradles the heart. The bronchial arteries supply blood to nourish the lungs and are derived from the ventral side of the thoracic aorta or from the aortic intercostal arteries.

The bronchial vein is formed at the root of the lung. Most of the blood supplied by the bronchial arteries is returned by the pulmonary veins to the left atrium of the heart. The lungs are pinkish white at birth and darken in later life. The coloring is from carbon granules deposited in the areolar tissue near the surface of the lung. The carbon deposits increase with age. The lungs of men are usually heavier than those of women and usually have a greater capacity. The quantity of air that can be exhaled from the lungs after the deepest inspiration, the vital capacity, averages 3700 cc.

lung abscess [AS, *lungen* + L, *abscedere,* to go away], a complication of an inflammation and infection of the lung, often caused by aspiration of infected material from the mouth. On a chest x-ray, it is characterized by a cavity containing an air-fluid line.

lung agents. See **choking/lung/pulmonary agents.**

lung biopsy, a test to obtain a specimen of pulmonary tissue for histological examination to diagnose pulmonary parenchymal disease, including carcinoma, granuloma, lung diseases caused by toxic exposure, sarcoidosis, and infection.

lung cancer, a pulmonary malignancy attributable in the majority of cases to cigarette smoking. Other predisposing factors are exposure to acronitrile, arsenic, asbestos, beryllium, chloromethyl ether, chromium, coal products, ionizing radiation, iron oxide, mustard gas, nickel, petroleum, uranium, and vinyl chloride. Lung cancer develops most often in scarred or chronically diseased lungs. It is usually far advanced when detected because metastases may precede detection of the primary lesion in the lung. Symptoms of lung cancer include persistent cough, hoarseness, dyspnea, purulent or blood-streaked sputum, chest pain, and repeated attacks of bronchitis or pneumonia. Diagnostic measures include x-ray films, fluoroscopy, tomography, bronchography, angiography, cytological studies of sputum, bronchial washings or brushings, and needle biopsy. Epidermoid cancers and adenocarcinomas each account for approximately 30% of lung tumors; about 25% are small, or oat, cell carcinomas; and 15% are large cell anaplastic cancers. Small cell carcinomas frequently metastasize widely before diagnosis. Surgery is the most effective treatment, but only about 20% are resectable. Lung cancer is essentially incurable unless surgical resection can be accomplished. Thoracotomy is contraindicated if metastases are found in contralateral or scalene lymph nodes. Irradiation is used to treat localized lesions and unresectable intrathoracic tumors and as palliative therapy for metastatic lesions. Radiotherapy may also be administered after surgery to destroy remaining tumor cells and may be combined with chemotherapy. Targeted therapy with drugs such as paclitaxel, carboplatin, irinotecan, and erlotinib has also shown results. Chemotherapy is especially indicated for small cell carcinoma.

lung capacity, a lung volume that is the sum of two or more of the four primary, nonoverlapping lung volumes. Kinds include **functional residual capacity, inspiratory capacity, total lung capacity, vital capacity.**

lung compliance, a measure of the ease of expansion of the lungs and thorax, determined by pulmonary volume and elasticity. A high degree of compliance indicates a loss of elastic recoil of the lungs, as in old age or emphysema. Decreased compliance means that a greater change in pressure is needed for a given change in volume, as in atelectasis, edema, fibrosis, pneumonia, or absence of surfactant. Dyspnea on exertion is the main symptom of diminished lung compliance.

lung fluke [AS, *lungen,* lung, *floc*], a parasitic flatworm of the species *Paragonimus westermani* found throughout Africa, Asia, and Latin America, but rarely in North America. It may enter the body as encysted larvae in crabs and crayfish. Symptoms of infestation include peribronchiolar distress and hemoptysis.

L

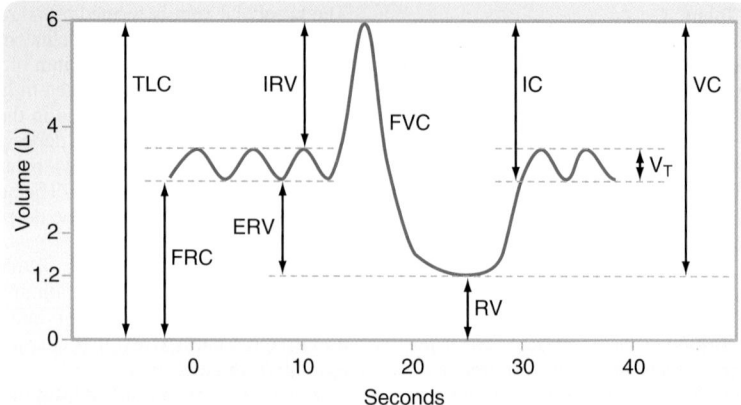

The various lung volumes and capacities. ERV, Expiratory reserve volume; FRC, functional residual capacity; FVC, forced vital capacity; IC, inspiratory capacity; IRV, inspiratory reserve volume; RV, residual volume; TLC, total lung capacity; VC, vital capacity; V$_T$, tidal volume. *(Koeppen and Stanton, 2010)*

lung scan, a radiographic examination of a lung and its function.

lung surfactant, a detergent-like agent that reduces the surface tension of the liquid film covering the inner lining of the pulmonary alveoli. As an alveolus becomes smaller during expiration, the surfactant becomes more concentrated, further reducing the surface tension and preventing alveolar collapse.

lung transplantation, the transfer of an entire pulmonary organ system to a new site. The procedure may be performed as a combined cardiopulmonary transplantation.

lunula /loon″yələ/ *pl.* **lunulae** [L, *luna,* moon], a semilunar structure, such as the crescent-shaped, pale area at the base of a fingernail or toenail.

lupoid, resembling systemic lupus erythematosus.

lupoid hepatitis, an autoimmune form of hepatitis with the histological appearance of chronic active hepatitis. Many patients show lupoid cells in the blood without systemic lupus erythematosus. See also **hepatitis.**

Lupron, a parenteral antineoplastic drug. Brand name for **leuprolide acetate.**

lupus /loo″pəs/ [L, wolf]. *(Nontechnical)* See **systemic lupus erythematosus.**

lupus anticoagulant, an antibody specific for phospho-lipoproteins or phospholipid components of coagulation factors, found in patients with systemic lupus erythematosus. It causes an increase in partial thromboplastin time and is associated with arterial and venous thrombosis, fetal loss, and thrombocytopenia.

lupus band test, a direct immunofluorescent method of visualizing a band of immunoglobulins and complement at the dermal-epidermal junction of involved skin in patients with systemic lupus erythematosus.

lupus erythematosus. See **systemic lupus erythematosus.**

lupus erythematosus cell. See **LE cell.**

lupus pernio, a cutaneous form of sarcoidosis, characterized by smooth, shiny plaques on the face, fingers, and toes, clinically resembling frostbite.

lupus vulgaris, a rare cutaneous form of tuberculosis in which areas of the skin become ulcerated and heal slowly, leaving deeply scarred tissue. The disease is not related to systemic lupus erythematosus.

LUQ, abbreviation for *left upper quadrant of the abdomen.*

Luride, a chemical prophylactic that reduces dental caries. Brand name for *sodium fluoride.*

lusus naturae /loo″səs/ [L, *lusus,* sport, *natura,* nature], a congenital anomaly; teratism.

lute /loot/ [L, *lutum,* mud], **1.** *n.,* a substance such as cement, wax, or clay that coats a surface or joint area to make a tight seal and hold separate pieces together. Also called **luting agent. 2.** *v.,* to coat or seal with such a substance.

lute-, prefix meaning "yellow": *luteinizing.*

luteal /loo″tē-əl/, pertaining to the corpus luteum or its functions or effects.

luteal hormone [L, *luteus,* yellow; Gk, *hormaein,* to set in motion], a hormone produced by the corpus luteum. See also **progesterone.**

luteal phase, the third phase of the human menstrual cycle, when the ovarian follicle that has recently discharged an ovum ruptures and transforms into the corpus luteum, which secretes progesterone. Progesterone acts on the endometrium to build up tissue with a supply of blood for nourishment of the potential embryo. If fertilization and conception do not take place, the estrogen level falls and the menstrual phase begins.

luteal phase deficiency, female infertility or early miscarriage caused by inadequate secretion of progesterone during the luteal phase of the menstrual cycle or poor endometrial lining response to progesterone levels. It is associated with an abnormality in pituitary gland function. Also called *luteal phase defect.*

lutein /loo″tē-in/ [L, *luteus,* yellow], a yellow-red crystalline carotenoid pigment found in plants with carotenes and chlorophylls.

luteinization /loo″tē-in″izā″shən/ [L, *luteus,* yellow], the formation of the corpus luteum from an ovarian follicle that has recently discharged an ovum. The process involves the hypertrophy of the follicular lutein cells and the development of blood vessels and connective tissue at the site.

luteinizing hormone (LH) /loo″tē-ini″zing/ [L, *luteus,* yellow; Gk, *izein,* to cause, *hormein,* to begin activity], a glycoprotein hormone produced by the anterior pituitary gland. It stimulates the secretion of sex hormones by the ovary and the testes and is involved in the maturation of spermatozoa and ova. In men, it induces the secretion of testosterone by the interstitial cells of the testes. Testosterone, together with follicle-stimulating hormone (FSH), induces the maturation of seminiferous tubules and stimulates them to produce sperm. In females, LH, working together with FSH, stimulates the growing follicle in the ovary to secrete estrogen. High concentrations of estrogen stimulate the release of a surge of LH, which stimulates ovulation. LH then induces the development of the ruptured follicle into the corpus luteum, which continues to secrete estrogen and progesterone. The normal

LH concentration in the plasma of men is less than 11 mIU/mL. In premenopausal women it is less than 25 mIU/mL; at midcycle peak it is greater than three times the baseline concentration; in postmenopausal women it is more than 25 mIU/mL. See also **interstitial cell-stimulating hormone, menstrual cycle.**

luteinizing hormone (LH) and follicle-stimulating hormone (FSH) assay, a blood test used in the evaluation of infertility. An LH assay is an easy way to determine if ovulation has occurred. The LH assay and FSH test also are used to determine whether a gonadal insufficiency is primary (a problem with the ovary or testicle) or secondary (caused by pituitary insufficiency resulting in reduced levels of FSH and LH).

luteinizing hormone–releasing hormone (LH-RH), a neurohormone of the hypothalamus that stimulates and regulates the pituitary gland's release of luteinizing hormone.

luteinizing hormone surge, a sharp increase in serum levels of luteinizing hormone seen around the middle of the menstrual cycle about 1 to 2 days before ovulation.

luteoma /lo͞otē·ō′mə/ *pl.* luteomas, luteomata [L, *luteus* + Gk, *oma,* tumor], **1.** a granulosa or theca cell tumor whose cells resemble those of the corpus luteum. **2.** a unilateral or bilateral nodular hyperplasia of ovarian lutein cells, occasionally developing during the last trimester of pregnancy. Also called *pregnancy luteoma.*

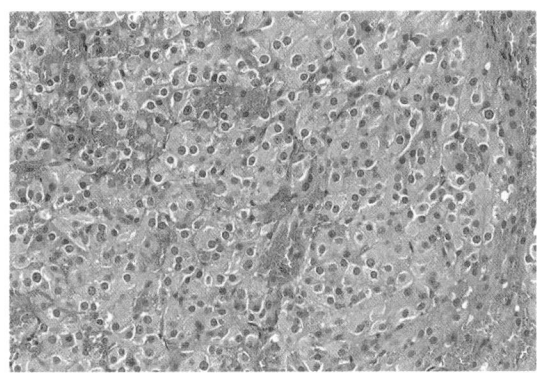

Luteoma of pregnancy *(Fletcher, 2007)*

luteotrope. See **lactotroph.**

luteotropin. See **prolactin.**

lutetium (Lu) /lo͞otē″shē·əm/ [L, *Lutetia,* Paris], a rare earth metallic element. Its atomic number is 71, and its atomic mass is 174.97.

luting agent. See **lute,** def. 1.

Luvox, an antidepressant drug. Brand name for **fluvoxamine maleate.**

lux (lx), a unit of illumination equivalent to one lumen per square meter of surface when measured at right angles to the direction of the light.

luxated joint /luk″sātid/, a dislocated joint in which there is no contact between articular surfaces.

luxation /luksā″shən/ [L, *luxare,* to dislocate], dislocation.

LV, abbreviation for **left ventricle.**

LVAD, abbreviation for **left ventricular assist device.**

LVN, abbreviation for **licensed vocational nurse.** See **licensed practical nurse.**

lx, abbreviation for **lux.**

lyases /lē″āsez/ [Gk, *lyein,* to loosen; Fr, *disastase,* enzyme], a group of enzymes that reversibly split carbon bonds with carbon, nitrogen, or oxygen without hydrolysis

or oxygen reduction reactions. The activity results in two subunits in which one or both may contain a double-bonded carbon. Kinds include **deaminase.**

lyco-, prefix meaning "wolf": *lycomania.*

lycomania, a delusion in which an individual believes he or she can transform into a wolf.

lycopene /lī″kəpēn/ [Gk, *lykopersikon,* tomato], a red crystalline unsaturated hydrocarbon that is the carotenoid pigment in tomatoes and various berries and fruits. It is considered the primary substance from which all natural carotenoid pigments are derived. Numerous studies correlate high intake of lycopene-containing foods with reduced incidence of cancer, cardiovascular disease, and macular degeneration.

lycopenemia /lī″kōpēnē″mē·ə/, a condition characterized by a high concentration of the carotenoid pigment lycopene in the blood, the result of ingesting large amounts of tomato products and other lycopene-rich fruits. Lycopenemia patients may develop a yellowish skin color. This term is not in common usage.

lye poisoning /lī/ [AS, *leah,* lye; L, *potio,* drink], the toxic effects of ingesting caustic soda or sodium hydroxide (NaOH), a powerful alkali. If the chemical has a pH above 11.5, the chemical burn damage to the mouth and throat is usually irreversible. An alkali burn can be more serious than an acid burn because an acid is usually neutralized by the tissues it contacts. See also **alkali poisoning.**

lying-in [AS, *licgan,* lying; L, *in*], **1.** *adj.,* designating the time before, during, and after childbirth. The term is historically associated with the time a woman would spend in bed in the period surrounding childbirth. **2.** *(Obsolete) adj.,* designating a hospital that provided care for women in childbirth and the puerperium. **3.** *n.,* the condition of being in confinement, or childbed.

Lyme disease /līm/ [Lyme, Connecticut, where originally described], an infection caused by the spirochete *Borrelia burgdorferi,* transmitted by the bite of infected *Ixodes* ticks (which are far smaller than dog ticks). In the northeast and north-central United States and Canada, the ticks normally feed on the white-footed mouse, the white-tailed deer, or other mammals and birds. Ticks are most likely to spread infection after 2 or more days of feeding. Most commonly, nymph ticks spread the disease because they are smaller than 2 mm in size and are rarely noticed. In contrast, the larger adult ticks are more likely to be found and removed before they have transmitted infection. See also **erythema migrans.**

■ OBSERVATIONS: The disease first manifests itself as a red skin macule or papule at the bite site with accompanying flu-like symptoms, such as headache, fever, chills, muscle aches, and fatigue. These are often missed or ignored by the individual. In about 50% of cases, other lesions develop soon after onset. Lymphadenopathy, neck pains, and hepatosplenomegaly are also often present in early disease. After weeks or months, neurological abnormalities such as meningitis, meningoencephalitis, neuritis, and radiculopathies appear in about 15% of all cases. Myocardial abnormalities such as atrioventricular block, myopericarditis, and cardiomegaly occur in 8% of cases. Joint inflammation, pain, and arthritis develop in 50% of cases as long as 2 years after transmission. Diagnosis is made through clinical examination with evidence of characteristic lesions and a positive enzyme-linked immunosorbent assay (ELISA). Cultures and biopsy of skin lesions and PCR testing of blood give a definitive diagnosis. However, the lab tests are available only at reference laboratories.

■ INTERVENTIONS: Current treatment centers around the use of oral or intravenous antibiotics. Treatment with appropriate antibiotics in the early stages of Lyme disease usually results in complete recovery. Antibiotics commonly used

L

for oral treatment include doxycycline, amoxicillin, or cefuroxime axetil. Doxycycline is contraindicated in patients younger than 8 years and in pregnant women.

■ PATIENT CARE CONSIDERATIONS: Care for acute disease is focused on rest and monitoring for complications. Education about preventive practices in endemic areas is needed and includes instruction to wear appropriate clothing (long pants tucked in boots) in wooded or grassy areas; use of bug repellent with DEET; keeping grass mowed; keeping woodpiles away from foot-traffic areas and the house; treating pets with tick and flea repellent and keeping pets off furniture; removal of ticks with tweezers; and thorough washing and application of antiseptic to any tick bite. Education is needed about the identification of the *Ixodes* tick and instruction to seek immediate treatment for any *Ixodes* tick bite or bull's-eye–like rash.

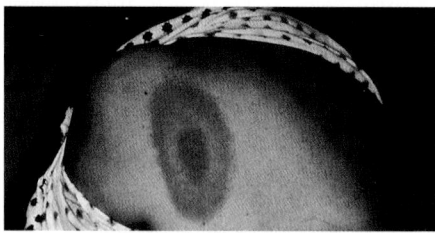

Bull's-eye–like rash associated with Lyme disease
(Stone and Gorbach, 2000)

Lyme disease test, a Western blot–specific blood test to isolate the spirochete *Borrelia burgdorferi,* which causes Lyme disease.

lymph /limf/ [L, *lympha,* water], a thin watery fluid originating in organs and tissues of the body that circulates through the lymphatic vessels and is filtered by the lymph nodes. Lymph enters the bloodstream at the junction of the internal jugular and subclavian veins. Lymph contains chyle, erythrocytes, and leukocytes, most of which are lymphocytes. See also **chyle, lymphatic system, lymphatic vessels.** –lymphatic, *adj.*

lymph-, lympho-, -lymph, combining form meaning "the lymph": *lymphadenectomy, endolymph, perilymph.*

lymphadenectomy, surgical removal of a lymph node or nodes. Also called **lymph node dissection.**

lymphadenitis /limfad´inī˝tis, lim´fəd-/ [L, *lympha* + Gk, *aden,* gland, *itis,* inflammation], an inflammatory condition of the lymph nodes, usually the result of systemic neoplastic disease, bacterial infection, or other inflammatory conditions. The nodes may be enlarged, hard, smooth or irregular, or red and may feel hot. The location of the affected node is indicative of the site or origin of disease.

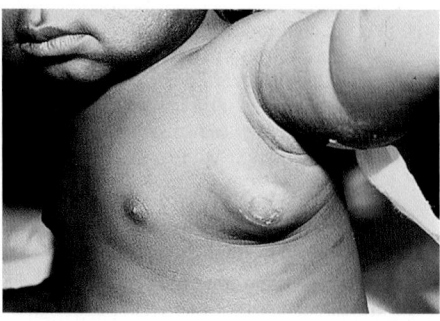

Lymphadenitis *(Cohen, Opal, and Powderly, 2010)*

lymphadenoma, lymphadenoma venereum. See **lymphogranulomatosis.**

lymphadenopathy /limfad´inop˝əthē/, any disorder characterized by a localized or generalized enlargement of the lymph nodes or lymph vessels.

lymphadenopathy syndrome (LAS), a persistent, generalized swelling of the lymph nodes. It may occur as a part of the AIDS wasting syndrome.

lymphangiectasia /limfan´jē-ektā˝zhə/ [L, *lympha* + Gk, *angeion,* vessel, *ektasis,* stretching], dilation of the smaller lymphatic vessels, usually resulting from obstruction in the larger vessels, such as in pelvic tuberculosis, mesenteric node metastases, and certain protozoan diseases.

lymphangiogram /limfan´jē-əgram´/ [L, *lympha,* water; Gk, *angeion,* vessel, *gramma,* record], a radiographic visualization of a part of the lymphatic system.

lymphangiography, an x-ray done with contrast dye that is especially useful in patients suspected of having lymphoma, metastatic tumor, or Hodgkin disease. It is also used to demonstrate the extent and level of lymphatic metastasis, to stage lymphoma patients, to evaluate the results of chemotherapy or radiation therapy, and to evaluate patients with chronic leg swelling.

lymphangioma /limfan´jē-ō˝mə/ *pl.* lymphangiomas, lymphangiomata [L, *lympha* + Gk, *angeion,* vessel, *oma,* tumor], a benign yellowish-tan tumor on the skin, composed of a mass of dilated lymph vessels. The tumor may be removed by excision or electrocoagulation for cosmetic reasons. Also called **angioma lymphaticum.** Compare **hemangioma.**

lymphangioma cavernosum, a tumor formed by dilated lymphatic vessels and filled with lymph mixed with coagulated blood. The lesion, which is often congenital, may cause extensive enlargement of the affected tissue, especially of the tongue and lips. Also called **cavernous lymphangioma.**

lymphangioma circumscriptum, a benign skin lesion that develops from superficial hypertrophic lymph vessels. Most often occurring in children, the lesion is characteristically pigmented and may grow to several centimeters in diameter.

lymphangioma cysticum. See **cystic lymphangioma.**

lymphangiomas. See **lymphangioma.**

lymphangioma simplex, a growth formed by moderately dilated lymph vessels in a circumscribed area of the skin.

lymphangiomata. See **lymphangioma.**

lymphangiosarcoma /limfan´jē-ō´särkō˝mə/ [L, *lympha,* water; Gk, *angeion,* vessel, *sarx,* flesh, *oma,* tumor], a tumor arising from the lymphatic vessels.

lymphangioscintigraphy (LAS) /lim-fan˝je-o-sin-tig´rah-fe/, scintigraphic evaluation of primary and secondary lymphedema by means of radioactive tracers.

lymphangitis /lim´fanjī˝tis/ [L, *lympha* + Gk, *angeion,* vessel, *itis*], an inflammation of one or more lymphatic vessels, usually resulting from an acute streptococcal infection of one of the extremities. It is characterized by fine red streaks extending from the infected area to the axilla or groin and by fever, chills, headache, and myalgia. Oral antibiotics are usually prescribed; analgesics and antiinflammatory agents are also utilized. Warm, moist compresses promote comfort and reduce inflammation. Aseptic technique is important to avoid contagion.

lymphatic /limfat˝ik/ [L, *lympha* + *icus,* form], **1.** pertaining to the lymphatic system of the body, consisting of a vast network of tubes transporting lymph. **2.** pertaining to any of the vessels associated with the lymphatic network.

lymphatic capillary plexus, one of the numerous networks of lymphatic capillaries that collect lymph from the

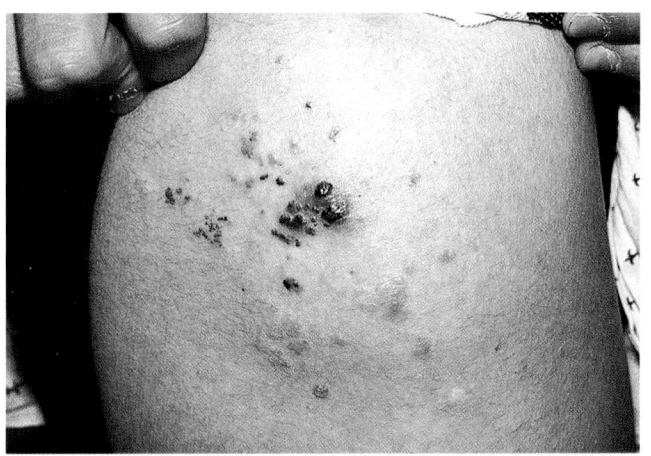

Lymphangioma circumscriptum *(Cohen, 2013)*

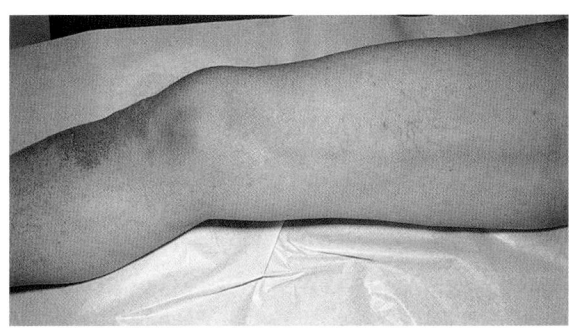

Lymphangitis *(Ferri, 2009)*

intercellular fluid and constitute the beginning of the lymphatic system. The lymphatic vessels arise from the capillary plexuses, which vary in size and number in different regions and organs of the body. The capillary networks do not contain lymphatic valves as do the vessels. The plexuses are especially abundant in the dermis of the skin but also lace many other areas, such as the mucous membranes of the respiratory and digestive systems, testes, ovaries, liver, kidneys, and heart. See also **lymphatic system.**

lymphatic follicles of rectum, concentrations of lymphoid tissue in the tunica mucosa of the rectum.

lymphatic follicles of stomach, small lymphocytic aggregates in the interstitial tissue of the lamina propria of the stomach, especially in the pyloric region.

lymphatic leukemia. See **acute lymphocytic leukemia, chronic lymphocytic leukemia.**

lymphatic nodule. See **malpighian body,** def. 2.

lymphatic organ [L, *lympha,* water; Gk, *organon,* instrument], any body structure composed of lymphatic tissue, such as the thymus, spleen, tonsils, and lymph nodes.

lymphatic system, a vast, complex network of capillaries, thin vessels, valves, ducts, nodes, and organs that helps protect and maintain the internal fluid environment of the entire body by producing, filtering, and conveying lymph and producing various blood cells. The lymphatic network also transports fats, proteins, and other substances to the blood system and restores 60% of the fluid that filters out of the blood capillaries into interstitial spaces during normal metabolism. Small semilunar valves throughout the lymphatic network help to control the flow of lymph and, at the junction with the venous system, prevent venous blood from flowing into the lymphatic vessels. The lymph collected throughout the body drains into the blood through two ducts situated in the neck. The thoracic duct that rises into the left side of the neck is the major vessel of the lymphatic system and conveys lymph from the whole body, except for the right quadrant, which is served by the right lymphatic duct. Lymph flows into the general circulation through the thoracic duct at a rate of about 125 mL per hour during routine exertion. Various body dynamics such as respiratory pressure changes, muscular contractions, and movements of organs surrounding lymphatic vessels combine to pump the lymph through the lymphatic system. The lymphatic capillaries, which are the beginning of the system, abound in the dermis of the skin, forming a continuous network over the entire body, except for the cornea. The system also includes specialized lymphatic organs, such as the tonsils, the thymus, and the spleen. See also **lymph, lymph node, lymph vessels, spleen, thymus,** *Color Atlas of Human Anatomy,* pp. A-20 to A-22.

lymphatic vasculitis, a condition of blood vessel necrosis in which the vessels acquire fibrinoid deposits and are infiltrated by lymphocytes. It is associated with graft-versus-host disease.

lymphatic vessels [L, *lympha,* water, *vascellum,* little vase], fine, thin-walled, transparent valved channels distributed through most tissues. They are often distinguished by their beaded appearance, which is caused by an irregular lumen. The collecting branches form two systems, one generally running with the superficial veins and the other below the deep fascia and including the intestinal lacteals. Lymphatics resemble veins but have more valves, have thinner walls, and contain lymph nodes. They drain through a thoracic duct and a right lymphatic duct into the venous system near the base of the neck. They include three layers: intima, media, and adventitia.

lymph cell. See **lymphocyte.**

lymphedema /lim′fĭdē″mə/ [L, *lympha* + Gk, *oidema,* swelling], a primary or secondary condition characterized by the accumulation of lymph in soft tissue and the resultant swelling caused by inflammation, obstruction, or removal of lymph channels. Lymph drainage from the extremity can be improved with compression and elevation. Light massage in the direction of the lymph flow and thiazide diuretics may be prescribed. Surgery may be performed to remove hypertrophied lymph channels and disfiguring tissue. Kinds include

L

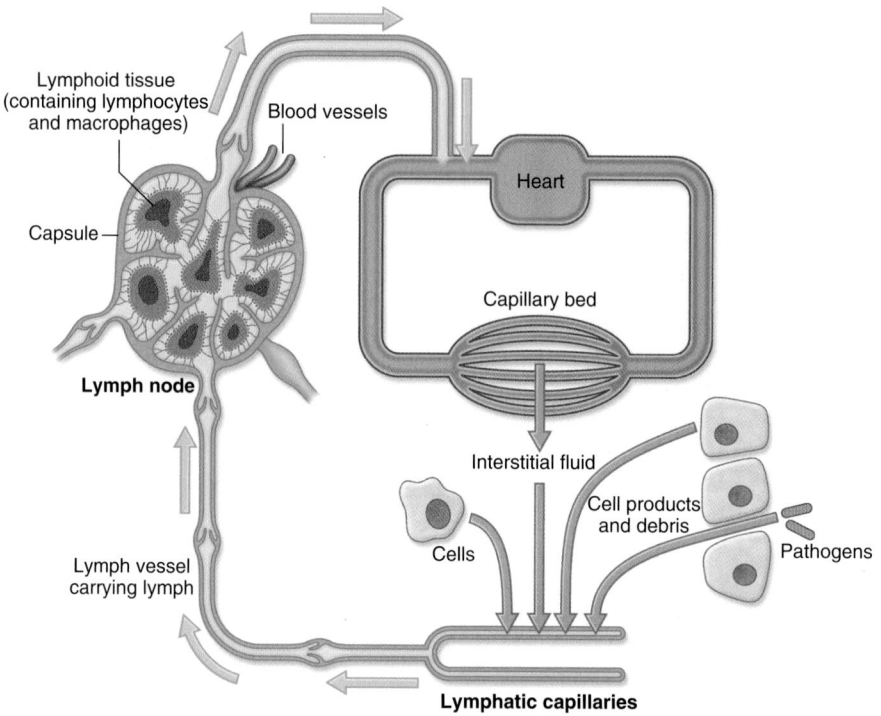

Lymphatic system *(Drake, Vogl, and Mitchell, 2015)*

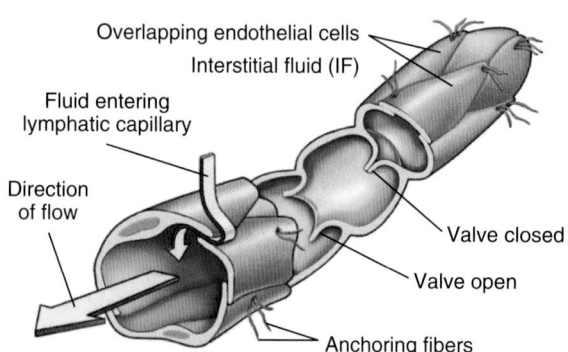

Lymphatic vessel *(Thibodeau and Patton, 2007)*

lymphedema praecox, Milroy disease. See also **secondary lymphedema.** −*lymphedematous, lymphedematose, adj.*

lymphedema praecox, puffiness and swelling of the lower limbs related to an obstruction of the flow of lymph. It is related to abnormalities present from birth, although the swelling is not usually apparent until puberty. The cause is unknown but thought to be genetic. Females are affected more commonly. Also called **Meige disease, Milroy disease.**

lymph node [L, lympha + *nodus,* knot], one of the many small oval structures that filter the lymph and fight infection and in which lymphocytes, monocytes, and plasma cells are formed. The lymph nodes are of different sizes, some as small as pinheads, others as large as lima beans. Each node is enclosed in a capsule, is composed of a lighter-colored cortical part and a darker medullary part, and consists of closely packed lymphocytes, reticular connective tissue laced by trabeculae, and three kinds of sinuses: subcapsular, cortical, and medullary. Lymph flows into the node through afferent lymphatic vessels

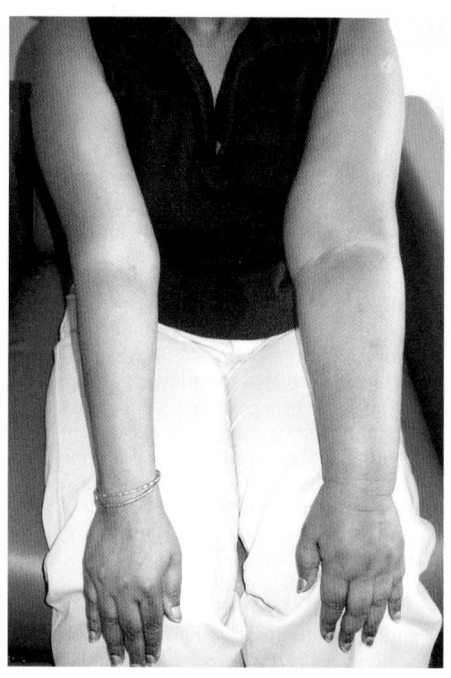

Lymphedema after breast cancer *(Walsh et al, 2009)*

that open into the subcapsular sinuses. Most lymph nodes are clustered in areas such as the mouth, the neck, the lower arm, the axilla, and the groin. The lymphatic network and nodes of the breast are especially crucial in the diagnosis and treatment of breast cancer. Also called *lymph gland.*

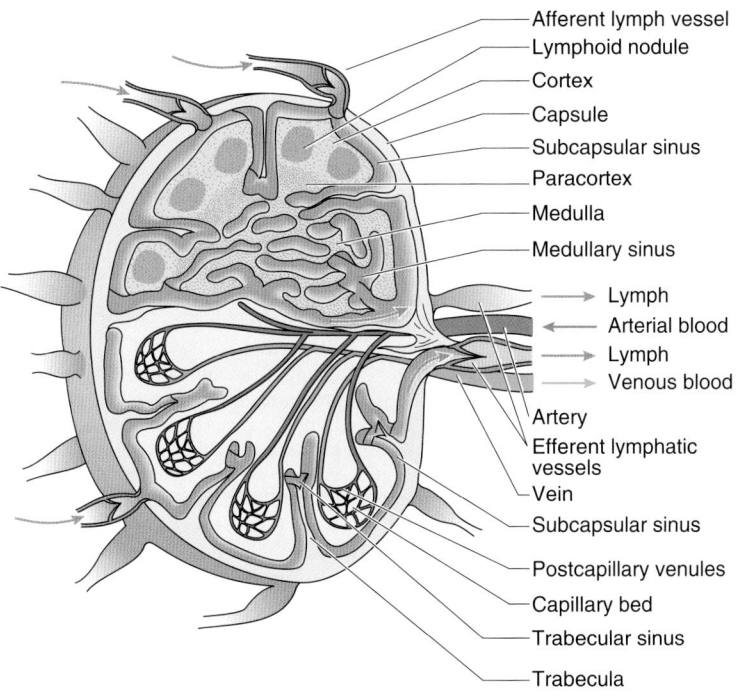

Afferent lymph vessel
Lymphoid nodule
Cortex
Capsule
Subcapsular sinus
Paracortex
Medulla
Medullary sinus

→ Lymph
← Arterial blood
→ Lymph
→ Venous blood

Artery
Efferent lymphatic vessels
Vein
Subcapsular sinus
Postcapillary venules
Capillary bed
Trabecular sinus
Trabecula

A typical lymph node *(Gartner and Hiatt, 2007)*

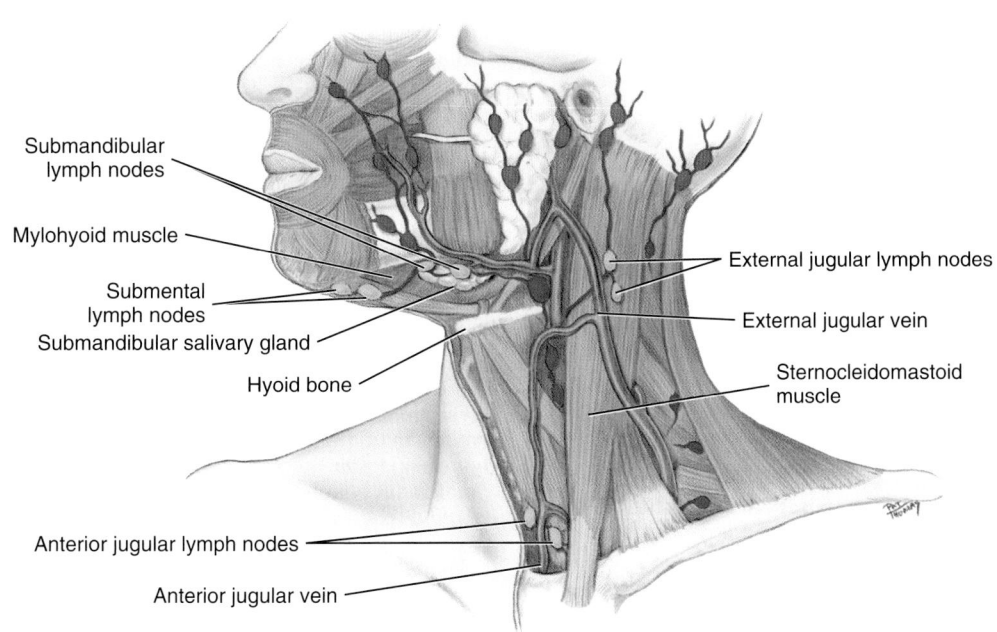

Submandibular lymph nodes
Mylohyoid muscle
Submental lymph nodes
Submandibular salivary gland
Hyoid bone
Anterior jugular lymph nodes
Anterior jugular vein

External jugular lymph nodes
External jugular vein
Sternocleidomastoid muscle

Superficial cervical lymph nodes *(Fehrenbach and Herring, 2012)*

lymph node dissection, surgical removal of a lymph node or chain of lymph nodes. Also called **lymphadenectomy.** Kinds include **sentinel lymph node biopsy.**

lymph nodule [L, *lympha,* water, *nodulus,* small knot], any of the small, densely packed, spheric nodes or aggregations of lymph cells embedded in the reticular meshwork of the lymphatic system, mainly in the tonsils, spleen, and thymus.

lympho-. See **lymph-, lympho-, -lymph.**

lymphoblast /lim″fəblast′/, a large, immature cell that develops into a lymphocyte after an antigenic or mitogenic challenge. *−lymphoblastic, adj.*

lymphoblastic lymphoma, lymphoblastic lymphosarcoma, lymphoblastoma. See **poorly differentiated lymphocytic malignant lymphoma.**

lymphocele /lim″fəsēl/, a circumscribed collection of lymphatic fluid that develops following surgery or interruption of the lymphatic flow. Also called **cystic lymphangioma.**

Lymphocryptovirus /lim″fōkrip′tovi″rus/, a genus of herpesviruses that includes the Epstein-Barr virus and species affecting nonhuman primates.

lymphocyte /lim″fəsīt/ [L, *lympha* + Gk, *kytos,* cell], a family of mononuclear, nonphagocytic white blood cells that circulate in blood, lymph, and peripheral lymphatic tissues. Lymphocytes are categorized as B and T lymphocytes and natural killer cells and are responsible for humoral and cellular immunity and tumor surveillance. Also called **lymph cell.** See also **lymphokine.** –*lymphocytic, adj.*

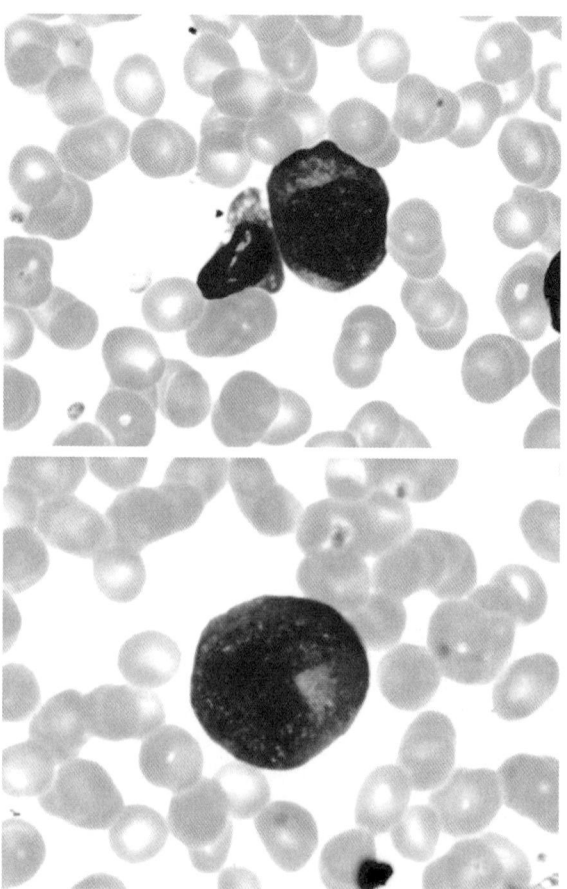

Peripheral blood smear showing reactive lymphocytes from a patient with infectious mononucleosis due to Epstein-Barr virus infection *(Jaffe et al, 2011)*

lymphocyte activation, the stimulation of lymphocytes by antigens or mitogens, rendering them metabolically active and causing them to differentiate into effector cells.

lymphocyte immune globulin, an immunosuppressant. Also called *antithymocyte.*

■ INDICATIONS: It is used to prevent rejection of organ transplants and to treat aplastic anemia.

■ CONTRAINDICATIONS: Known hypersensitivity to this drug prohibits its use.

■ ADVERSE EFFECTS: When this drug is used in renal transplants, life-threatening effects include seizures and anaphylaxis. Other adverse effects include fever, headache, dizziness, weakness, faintness, rash, pruritus, urticaria, wheals, diarrhea, nausea, vomiting, epigastric pain, chest pain, hypertension, and tachycardia. When the drug is used to treat aplastic anemia, seizures are a life-threatening effect. Other adverse effects include fever, chills, headache, light-headedness, encephalitis, postviral encephalopathy, bradycardia, myocarditis, irregularity, nausea, and abnormal liver function tests.

lymphocyte immunophenotyping, a blood test used to detect the progressive depletion of CD4 T lymphocytes, which is associated with an increased likelihood of clinical complications from AIDS. Test results can also indicate if an AIDS patient is at risk for developing opportunistic infections.

lymphocyte transformation, **1.** the morphological changes accompanying lymphocyte activation, in which small, resting lymphocytes are transformed into large, active lymphocytes (lymphoblasts). **2.** an in vitro immunity test process in which a patient's lymphocytes are placed in a culture with an antigen. The rate of transformation, in terms of proliferation and enlargement of T memory cells, is measured by the uptake of radioactive thymidine by the lymphocytes, indicating protein synthesis.

lymphocytic choriomeningitis /lim′fəsit″ik/ [L, *lympha* + Gk, *kytos,* cell, *chorion,* skin, *meninx,* membrane, *itis,* inflammation], an arenavirus infection of the meninges and the cerebrospinal fluid. It is caused by the lymphocytic choriomeningitis virus and characterized by fever, headache, and stiff neck often complicated by aseptic meningitis. The infection occurs primarily in young adults, most often in the fall and winter months. Recovery usually takes place within 2 weeks.

lymphocytic gastritis, chronic gastritis with large numbers of T lymphocytes in the epithelium of the stomach, sometimes associated with celiac disease or *Helicobacter pylori* infection.

lymphocytic hypophysitis, the massive infiltration of the pituitary gland by lymphocytes and plasma cells, with destruction of the normal parenchyma. The disorder is believed to have an autoimmune basis.

lymphocytic interstitial pneumonia (LIP), a diffuse respiratory disorder characterized by fibrosis and accumulation of lymphocytes in the lungs. It is commonly associated with lymphoma and may progress to lymphoma.

lymphocytic leukemia. See **acute lymphocytic leukemia, chronic lymphocytic leukemia.**

lymphocytic lymphoma, lymphocytic lymphosarcoma. See **well-differentiated lymphocytic malignant lymphoma.**

lymphocytic thyroiditis. See **Hashimoto disease.**

lymphocytoma. See **well-differentiated lymphocytic malignant lymphoma.**

lymphocytopenia /lim′fōsī′təpē″nē·ə/ [L, *lympha* + Gk, *kytos,* cell, *penes,* poor], a decreased number of lymphocytes in the peripheral circulation, associated with immunodeficiency, neoplasm, or chemotherapy. Compare **alymphocytosis.** See also **agranulocyte.**

lymphocytosis /lim′fōsītō″sis/, a proliferation of lymphocytes, as occurs in certain chronic diseases and during convalescence from acute infections.

lymphocytotrophic /-trof″ik/, having an affinity for lymphocytes.

lymphoderma perniciosa. See **leukemia cutis.**

lymphoepithelioma /lim′fō·ep′ithē′lē·ō″mə/ [L, *lympha* + Gk, *epi,* above, *thele,* nipple, *oma,* tumor], a poorly differentiated neoplasm developing from the epithelium overlying lymphoid tissue in the nasopharynx. It occurs most frequently in east Asia and Africa. Also called **nasopharyngeal cancer.**

lymphogenesis /-jen″əsis/, the formation of lymph.

lymphogenous leukemia.   See **acute lymphocytic leukemia, chronic lymphocytic leukemia.**

lymphogranulomatosis /-gran′yəlō″mətō″sis/ [L, *lympha*, water, *granulum*, small grain + Gk, *oma*, tumor, *osis*, condition], an infectious granuloma of the lymphatic system. Kinds include **Hodgkin disease, Hodgkin lymphoma, lymphoma, lymphadenoma, lymphadenoma venereum, sarcoidosis.**

lymphogranuloma venereum (LGV) /-gran′yəlō″mə/ [L, *lympha* + *granulum*, small grain; Gk, *oma*, tumor; L, *Venus*, goddess of love], a sexually transmitted disease caused by a strain of the bacterium *Chlamydia trachomatis* that primarily infects the lymphatics. It is characterized by ulcerative genital lesions, marked swelling of the lymph nodes in the groin, headache, fever, and malaise. Ulcerations of the rectal wall occur less commonly. The disease is diagnosed by isolating the organism from an infected node and demonstrating LGV antibodies by serological blood test. Doxycycline is usually prescribed for the patient and any person with whom there has been sexual contact. Also called **lymphopathia venereum.** See also *Chlamydia.*

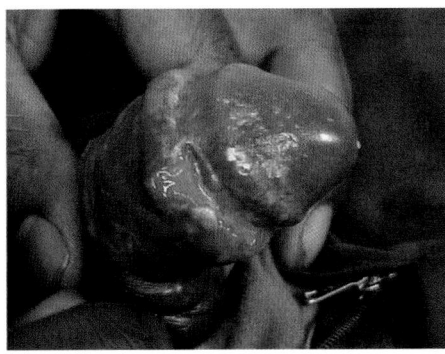

Ulcerative genital lesions of lymphogranuloma venereum *(Cohen, Opal, and Powderly, 2010)*

lymphography.   See **lymphangiography.**

lymphoid /lim″foid/ [L, *lympha*, water; Gk, *eidos*, form], pertaining to lymphocytes or to tissue in which lymphocytes develop.

lymphoid aplasia,   failure of development of lymphoid tissue, as in severe combined immunodeficiency.

lymphoid interstitial pneumonia (LIP),   a form of pneumonia involving the lower lobes with extensive alveolar infiltration by mature lymphocytes, plasma cells, and histiocytes. It is associated with human immunodeficiency virus infection, especially in children; dysproteinemia; and Sjögren's syndrome. This is an AIDS-defining illness in children.

lymphoid leukemia.   See **acute lymphocytic leukemia, chronic lymphocytic leukemia.**

lymphoidocytic leukemia.   See **stem cell leukemia.**

lymphoid ring.   See **Waldeyer's throat ring.**

lymphoid system,   the lymphoid tissue of the body considered collectively. It can be divided into primary (or central) lymphoid tissues—the thymus and bone marrow, where lymphocytes differentiate from stem cells—and secondary (or peripheral) tissues, made up of the lymph nodes, spleen, and gut-associated lymphoid tissue (tonsils, Peyer's patches), where lymphocytes take part in immune responses.

lymphoid tissue [L, *lympha*, water; Gk, *eidos*, form; OFr, *tissu*], tissue that consists of lymphocytes on a framework of reticular cells and fibers, as the tonsils and adenoids.

lymphokine /lim″fōkīn/ [L, *lympha* + Gk, *kinesis*, motion], one of the chemical factors produced and released by T lymphocytes that attracts macrophages to the site of infection or inflammation and prepares them for attack. Kinds include *chemotactic factor,* **cytokine,** *lymphotoxin, migration inhibiting factor,* **mitogenic factor.**

lymphokine-activated killer (LAK) cells, nonspecific cytotoxic cells that are generated in the presence of interleukin-2 and the absence of antigen. They are distinct from human natural killer cells, peripheral T lymphocytes, or memory cytotoxic thymus-derived lymphocytes. LAK cell infusions have been used investigationally for the treatment of cancer.

lympholysis /limfol″əsis/ [L, *lympha* + Gk, *lysein*, to loosen], cellular destruction of target cells by CD8 lymphocytes.

lymphoma /limfō″mə/ [L, *lympha* + Gk, *oma*, tumor], *adj.,* a type of neoplasm of lymphoid tissue that originates in the reticuloendothelial and lymphatic systems. It is usually malignant but in rare cases may be benign. It usually responds to treatment. Kinds include **Burkitt lymphoma, mycosis fungoides, Hodgkin disease, Hodgkin lymphoma, non-Hodgkin lymphoma.**

■ OBSERVATIONS: It is an insidious disorder, beginning as a plaquelike pruritic rash that spreads through the skin and becomes nodular and systemic. The various lymphomas differ in degree of cellular differentiation and content, but the manifestations are similar in all types. Characteristically the appearance of a painless enlarged lymph node or nodes is followed by weakness, fever, weight loss, and anemia. With widespread involvement of lymphoid tissue, the spleen and liver usually enlarge, and GI disturbances, malabsorption, and bone lesions frequently develop.

■ INTERVENTIONS: Treatment for lymphoma includes intensive radiotherapy, chemotherapy, and biological therapies, including interferon and monoclonal antibodies.

■ PATIENT CARE CONSIDERATIONS: Hodgkin disease lymphomas tend to affect young adults but usually respond to recently developed types of therapy. Non-Hodgkin lymphoma (NHL) usually strikes patients around middle age and can be more difficult to treat. Men are more likely than women to develop lymphoid tumors. There has been a dramatic increase in the incidence of acquired immunodeficiency syndrome–related NHL, which is attributed to prolonged survival of such patients related to the availability of antiretroviral agents.

-lymphoma,   suffix meaning "a tumor or neoplastic disorder of lymphoid tissue": *adenolymphoma.*

lymphoma staging,   a system for classifying non-Hodgkin lymphomas according to the extent of the disease for the purpose of treatment and prognosis. The Ann Arbor staging system is commonly used to summarize the extent of the cancer in adults. The stages are described by Roman numerals I through IV, with stage IV indicating the highest level of involvement. Lymphomas that affect an organ outside the lymph system have *E* added to their stage, while those affecting the spleen have an *S* added. The letters *A* or *B* may also be added to a stage, *B* indicating the presence of symptoms associated with advanced disease. An *X* is added to the stage for tumors of the chest with characteristics that suggest the need for more intensive treatment.

lymphomata, lymphomatoid.   See **lymphoma.**

lymphomatoid granulomatosis /limfō″mətoid/, a condition in which lymphocytes and plasma cells infiltrate the blood vessels, producing an angiocentric lesion. It most often affects the lungs, skin, and central nervous system. It is believed to be induced by a combination of Epstein-Barr virus infection, immunosuppressive drugs, and infections such as HIV and/or autoimmune diseases. See also **Wegener granulomatosis.**

lymphopathia venereum.   See **lymphogranuloma venereum.**

lymphopenia.   See **lymphocytopenia.**

lymphopoiesis /-pō·ē'sis/   [L, *lympha,* water; Gk, *poien,* to make],   formation and production of lymphocytes, primarily in peripheral lymphoid tissue. −*lymphopoietic, adj.*

lymphoproliferative /-prōlif"ərativ'/   [L, *lympha,* water, *prolles,* offspring, *ferre,* to bear],   pertaining to the production of excessive quantities of lymphocytes.

lymphoreticular system,   the tissues of the lymphoid and reticuloendothelial systems considered together as one system. See also **lymphoid system.**

lymphoreticulosis /-retik'yəlō"sis/   [L, *lympha* + *reticulum,* little net; Gk, *osis,* condition],   subacute granulomatous inflammation of lymphoid tissue with proliferation of macrophages. The disorder, which can be caused by a cat scratch, is characterized by the formation of an ulcerated papule at the site of the scratch, fever, and tender lymphadenopathy, sometimes progressing to suppuration. Also called **cat-scratch fever.**

lymphorrhagia,   an escape of lymph from a damaged vessel.

lymphorrhoid /limfôr"oid/,   a dilated lymph vessel.

lymphosarcoma.   See **non-Hodgkin lymphoma.**

lymphosarcoma cell leukemia /-särkō"mə/   [L, *lympha* + Gk, *sarx,* flesh, *oma,* tumor],   a malignancy of blood-forming tissues characterized by many lymphosarcoma cells in the peripheral circulation that tend to infiltrate surrounding tissues. These cells are extremely immature and larger and more reticulated than lymphocytes. The disease may accompany lymphoma or exist as a separate entity with bone marrow involvement. Also called **lymphoblastic lymphoma, lymphoblastic lymphosarcoma, lymphoblastoma.**

lymphoscintigraphy /-sintig"rəfē/,   a diagnostic technique using scintillation scanning of technetium-99m antimony trisulfide colloid in a noninvasive test for primary and secondary lymphedema. The radiopharmaceutical is injected subcutaneously in the interdigital space of the hands and feet.

lymphotrophy /limfot"rəfē/,   the nourishment of cells by lymph, particularly in areas lacking adequate blood vessels. This term is not in common usage.

lymph sinuses [L, *lympha,* water, *sinus,* hollow],   continuous small endothelial-lined spaces just below the capsule of the lymph node. The sinuses slow the flow of lymph through the nodes.

lymph vessels.   See **lymphatic system.**

lyo-,   prefix meaning "to loosen or dissolve": *lyophilic.*

Lyon hypothesis /lī"ən/   [Mary L. Lyon, English geneticist, b. 1925],   a hypothesis stating that only one of the two X chromosomes in a female is functional, the other having become inactive early in development. Either the maternal or the paternal X chromosome may be inactivated in any given cell. Therefore an X-linked trait may be expressed by some cells and not by others.

lyonization /lī"ənīzā"shən/   [Mary L. Lyon; Gk, *izein,* to cause],   the process of random inactivation of one of the X chromosomes in the cells of females to compensate for the presence of the double X gene dose. See also **Lyon hypothesis.**

Lyon's ring [Mary L. Lyon],   a type of congenital uropathy in females in which submeatal or distal urethral stenosis causes enuresis, dysuria, and recurring infections. The disorder is treated surgically.

lyophilic /lī'ōfil"ik/   [Gk, *lyein,* to dissolve, *philein,* to love],   pertaining to substances having an affinity for stability in solution. Lyophilic substances are used to stabilize colloids.

lyophilize,   to freeze-dry a substance under vacuum conditions.

Lyrica,   a treatment for fibromyalgia. Brand name for **pregabalin.**

Lys,   abbreviation for **lysine.**

lysate /lī"sāt/,   a product of dissolution of matter by lysis, as in the destruction of proteins by hydrolysis.

lyse,   to cause or produce disintegration of a compound, substance, or cell. See **lysis.**

-lyse.   See **-lyze, -lyse.**

lysemia /līsē"mē·ə/,   *(Obsolete)* the disintegration of red blood cells, accompanied by the release of hemoglobin in the plasma. Now called **hemolysis.**

lysergide /līsur"jīd/   [German: *Lyserg-Säure-Diäthylamid,* (lysergic acid diethylamide).],   a psychotomimetic, semisynthetic medication that is a derivative of ergot that acts at multiple sites in the central nervous system from the cortex to the spinal cord. In susceptible individuals, as little as 20 to 25 mg of the potent drug may cause pupillary dilation, increased blood pressure, hyperreflexia, tremor, muscle weakness, piloerection, and increased body temperature. Larger doses also produce dizziness, drowsiness, paresthesia, euphoria or dysphoria, and synesthesias. Colors may be heard, sounds visualized, and time is felt to pass slowly. Psychological dependence may develop, and use of lysergide is associated with significant hazards, such as panic, serious depression, paranoid behavior, and prolonged psychotic episodes. Also called **acid, LSD.** See also **hallucinogen.**

lysin /lī"sin/,   any protein that causes cell lysis.

-lysin,   suffix meaning "a cell-dissolving antibody": *bacteriolysin, cytolysin. fibrinolysin.*

lysine (Lys) /lī"sēn, lī"sin/,   an essential amino acid needed for proper growth in infants and for maintenance of nitrogen balance in adults. See also **amino acid, protein.**

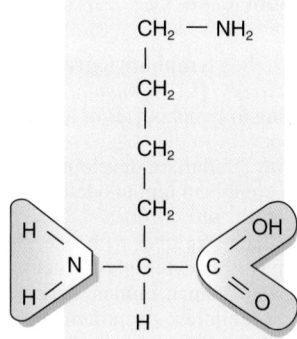

Chemical structure of lysine

lysine intolerance,   a congenital disorder resulting in the inability to hydrolyze the essential amino acid lysine because of an enzyme deficiency or defect. The disorder is characterized by weakness, vomiting, and coma. It is treated by adjusting the protein content of the diet, restricting foods especially high in lysine. See also **lysinemia.**

lysinemia /lī'sinē"mē·ə/,   a condition caused by an inborn error of metabolism and resulting in the inability to hydrolyze the essential amino acid lysine because of an enzyme defect or deficiency. It is characterized by muscle weakness and cognitive impairment. See also **lysine intolerance.**

lysine monohydrochloride, a salt of the amino acid lysine, used as a dietary supplement to increase the use of vegetable proteins such as those of corn, rice, and wheat.

lysinogen /līsin″əjən/, an antigen that stimulates the production of a specific lysin.

lysinurea /lī′sinoo̅r″ē·ə/, the presence of lysine in the urine.

lysinuria /li″snu′re·ä/, an aminoaciduria consisting of excessive lysine in the urine. See also **hyperlysinemia.**

lysis /lī″sis/ [Gk, *lysein*, to loosen], **1.** destruction or dissolution of a cell or molecule through the action of a specific agent. Cell lysis is frequently caused by a lysin. −*lytic, adj.* **2.** gradual diminution in the symptoms of a disease. Compare **crisis. 3.** surgery performed to free adhesions of tissues. See also **adhesiotomy. −lyse,** *v.*

-lysis, suffix meaning "a breaking down" or "detachment": *cytolysis, dialysis, osteolysis.*

lyso-, prefix meaning "dissolution": *lysokinase, lysosome, lysozyme.*

Lysodren, an antineoplastic drug. Brand name for **mitotane.**

lysogenesis /lī″səjen″əsis/ [Gk, *lysein*, loosening, *genein*, to produce], the formation of lysins, antibodies that cause partial or complete dissolution of the target cell.

lysokinase /lī′sōkī″nās/, an enzyme that serves as an activating agent for the production of plasmin.

lysosomal storage disease. See **inborn lysosomal disease.**

lysosome /lī″səsōm/ [Gk, *lysein* + *soma,* body], a cytoplasmic, membrane-bound particle that contains hydrolytic enzymes that function in intracellular digestive processes. The organelles are found in most cells but are particularly prominent in leukocytes and the cells of the liver and kidney. If the hydrolytic enzymes are released into the cytoplasm, they cause self-digestion of the cell. Thus lysosomes may play an important role in certain self-destructive diseases characterized by the wasting of tissue, such as muscular dystrophy. Compare **lysozyme.**

lysotype /lī″sətīp/, a bacterial species type determined by its reaction to certain phages.

lysozyme /lī″səzīm/ [Gk, *lysein* + *en,* within, *zyme,* ferment], an enzyme with antiseptic actions that destroys some foreign organisms. It is found in granulocytic and monocytic blood cells and is normally present in saliva, sweat, breast milk, and tears.

lysso-, prefix meaning "rabies" or "hydrophobia."

lytes /līts/, (*Informal*) a shortened reference to *electrolytes,* especially the levels of potassium, sodium, phosphorus, magnesium, and calcium in the blood, as determined by laboratory testing.

-lytic, suffix meaning "to produce decomposition": *histolytic, lipolytic, oncolytic.*

-lyze, -lyse, combining form meaning "to produce decomposition": *hydrolyze.*

L

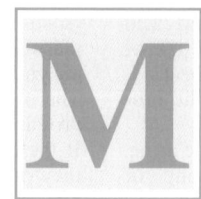

m, **1.** abbreviation for **meter. 2.** symbol for **muscle. 3.** abbreviation for **minim.**

M, **1.** abbreviation for **mega. 2.** abbreviation for **molar. 3.** abbreviation for *distant metastasis* in the tumor, node, metastasis (TNM) system for staging malignant neoplastic disease.

Mr, symbol for **relative molecular mass.**

mA, abbreviation for **milliampere.**

MA, abbreviation for **mental age.**

M.A., a graduate educational level beyond that of the baccalaureate. Abbreviation for *Master of Arts degree.*

MAA, abbreviation for **methacrylic acid.**

Maass, Clara [1876–1901], an American nurse who volunteered for military service at the outbreak of the Spanish-American War, after training and working at the Newark German Hospital, which has since been renamed for her. She worked at army camps where soldiers were dying of yellow fever and then volunteered to go to Havana, Cuba, to participate in experiments to determine the cause of that disease. She was bitten by a mosquito and died 10 days later of yellow fever. She was one of the first nurses to be inducted into the Hall of Fame of the American Nurses Association.

MAB, abbreviation for **monoclonal antibody.**

mabp, abbreviation for *mean arterial blood pressure.*

MAC, **1.** abbreviation for **membrane attack complex. 2.** abbreviation for **mid–upper arm circumference. 3.** abbreviation for **minimum alveolar concentration. 4.** abbreviation for *Mycobacterium avium* **complex (MAC) disease. 5.** abbreviation for **monitored anesthesia care.**

MAC awake, the exhaled (end-tidal) concentration of an inhaled anesthetic agent at which 50% of patients appropriately respond to verbal commands (such as "open your eyes"). It applies only to inhalational agents and is affected by medical comorbidities, age, hypothermia, narcotic administration, and the sedative medications used.

Macdonald triad [J.M. Macdonald, American psychiatrist, 1920–2007]. See **childhood triad.**

mace /mās/, the oil-containing, red, fibrous wrapping of the nutmeg kernel. Dried and ground, it is used as an aromatic spice and flavoring. Historical medicinal uses include the treatment of gastrointestinal disorders and as an analgesic; however, there are no clinical trials supporting its effectiveness. Should not be confused with **Mace.**

Mace, a chemical agent that causes tearing and eye pain. The name is an abbreviation formed by letters in *m*ethylchloroform-2-chloro*ace*tophenone, which is dispersed from a pressurized container to immobilize an attacker.

macerate /mas″ərāt/ [L, *macerare,* to soften], to soften something solid by wetting or soaking.

maceration /-ā″shən/, **1.** the softening and breaking down of skin resulting from prolonged exposure to moisture. **2.** (in histology) the softening of a tissue by soaking, especially in acids, until the connective tissue fibers are dissolved so that the tissue can be teased apart. **3.** (in obstetrics) the degenerative changes with discoloration and softening of tissues and the eventual disintegration of a fetus retained in the uterus after its death.

Machado-Joseph disease /mächä′dō jō′səf/ [Machado and Joseph, afflicted families], a progressive degenerative disease of the central nervous system occurring in families of Portuguese-Azorean descent, having a variety of forms and inherited as an autosomal-dominant trait. There are four major types: Type I, with pyramidal and extrapyramidal deficits; Type II, with cerebellar, pyramidal, and extrapyramidal deficits; Type III, with cerebellar deficits and distal sensorimotor neuropathy; and Type IV, with parkinsonism and distal sensory neuropathy. Also called **Azorean disease, Joseph disease, Portuguese-Azorean disease.**

machinery murmur. See **Gibson murmur.**

machismo /mächis″mō/, (in psychology) a concept of the male that includes both desirable traits of courage and fearlessness and the dysfunctional behaviors of the right to dominate others and to expect respect, regardless of behavior.

Machover Draw-a-Person Test. See **Draw-a-Person (DAP) Test.**

Machupo. See **Bolivian hemorrhagic fever.**

Macleod, John J [1876–1935], Scottish physiologist and co-winner, with Sir Frederick G. Banting, of the 1923 Nobel prize for medicine and physiology for their discovery of insulin. See also **Banting, Sir Frederick G.**

macrencephaly /mak′rənsef′əlē/ [Gk, *makros,* large, *enkephalos,* brain], a congenital anomaly characterized by abnormal largeness of the brain. See also **macrocephaly.** −*macrencephalic, adj.*

macro-, makro-, prefix meaning "large" or "abnormal size": *macrobiosis, macrocytosis, macrophage.*

macroadenoma /mak′rōad′ənō″mə/, a glandular tumor more than 10 mm in diameter.

macroamylase /-am″ilās/, a high-molecular-weight form of amylase. It circulates as a complex with immunoglobulins, usually IgA (70%) or IgG (30%). Because of its size, renal excretion is impaired, causing a persistently raised serum amylase. It is a benign finding that is usually chronic, but may be transient.

macroamylasemia /mak′rō·am′ilāsē″mē·ə/, the presence of macroamylase in the blood.

macrobiosis /-bī·ō″sis/ [Gk, *makros,* long, *bios,* life], a long life.

macrobiotic diet /-bī·ot″ik/, a dietary regimen consisting of whole grains and unprocessed foods. Dairy and animal products, as well as refined foods, are eliminated.

macroblepharia /mak′rōblifer″ē·ə/ [Gk, *makros* + *blepharon,* eyelid], the condition of having abnormally large eyelids.

macrocephaly /mak′rōsef″əlē/ [Gk, *makros* + *kephale,* head], a congenital anomaly characterized by abnormal largeness of the head and brain in relation to the rest of the body, resulting in some degree of cognitive impairment and growth delay. The head is more than two standard deviations above the average circumference size for age, sex, race, and period of gestation, with excessively wide fontanels; the facial features are usually normal. The condition may be caused by some defect in formation during embryonic development, or it may be the result of progressive degeneration processes, such as Schilder disease, Greenfield disease, or congenital lipoidosis. In macrocephaly there is symmetric overgrowth at the head without increased intracranial pressure, as differentiated from hydrocephalus, in which the lateral, asymmetric growth of the head is caused by excessive accumulation of cerebrospinal fluid, usually under increased pressure. Specific diagnostic tests may be necessary to differentiate the two conditions. Treatment is primarily symptomatic, with health care concentrated specifically on helping parents learn to care for a child who experiences developmental and cognitive delays. Also called *macrocephalia,* **megalocephaly.** Compare **microcephaly.** See also **hydrocephalus.** −*macrocephalic, macrocephalous, adj.,* −*macrocephalus, n.*

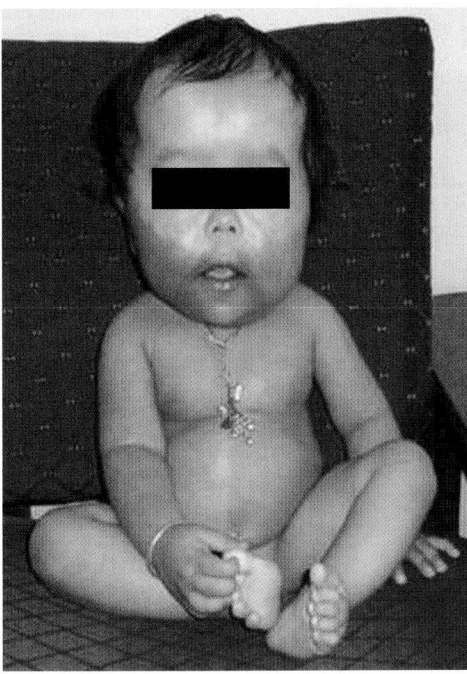

Infant with macrocephaly *(Panigrahi et al, 2012)*

macrocyte /mak′rəsīt/ [Gk, *makros + kytos,* cell], an erythrocyte that exceeds 9 μm in diameter on a peripheral blood film, associated with an MCV greater than 100 fL. Macrocytes are seen in liver disease, alcoholism, megaloblastic anemia with folate or cobalamin deficiency, and in myelodysplastic syndromes. Compare **microcyte.** See also **macrocytic anemia.**

macrocytic /mak′rōsit″ik/ [Gk, *makros + kytos +* L, *icus,* form], (of a cell) larger than normal, such as the erythrocytes in macrocytic anemia.

macrocytic anemia, anemia characterized by impaired erythropoiesis and macrocytes on a peripheral blood film. Macrocytic anemia is seen in liver disease, alcoholism, megaloblastic anemia with folate or cobalamin deficiency, and in myelodysplastic syndromes. Compare **microcytic anemia.**

macrocytosis /mak′rōsītō″sis/ [Gk, *makros + kytos + osis,* condition], abnormal proliferation of macrocytes in the peripheral blood film. See also **anisocytosis.**

Macrodantin, a urinary antibacterial drug. Brand name for **nitrofurantoin.**

Macrodex, a plasma expander. Brand name for **dextran preparation.**

macrodrip /mak″rōdrip/ [Gk, *makros +* AS, *drypan,* to fall in drops], (in IV therapy) an apparatus that is used to deliver measured amounts of IV solutions at specific flow rates based on the size of drops of the solution. The size of the drops is controlled by the fixed diameter of a plastic delivery tube. Different macrodrips deliver 10, 15, or 20 drops per milliliter of solution. Macrodrips are not usually used to deliver a small amount of IV solution or to keep a vein open because the interval between drips is so long that a clot may form at the tip of the IV catheter. Compare **microdrip.**

macroelement, a chemical element required in relatively large quantities for the normal physiological processes of the body. Macroelements include carbon, hydrogen, oxygen, nitrogen, potassium, sodium, calcium, chloride, magnesium, phosphorus, and sulfur. See also **macronutrient.**

macrogamete /-gam′ēt/ [Gk, *makros + gamete,* spouse], a large nonmotile female gamete of certain thallophytes and sporozoa, specifically the malarial parasite *Plasmodium.* It corresponds to the ovum of the higher animals and is fertilized by the smaller, motile male gamete. Compare **microgamete.**

macrogametocyte /-gamē″təsīt/ [Gk, *makros + gamete + kytos,* cell], an enlarged merozoite that undergoes meiosis to form the mature female gamete during the sexual phase of the life cycle of certain thallophytes and sporozoa, specifically the malarial parasite *Plasmodium.* Macrogametocytes are found in the red blood cells of a person infected with the malarial parasite, but they must be ingested by a female *Anopheles* mosquito to complete the maturation process and develop into macrogametes.

macrogenitosomia /mak′rōjen′itōsō″mē-ə/ [Gk, *makros + L, genitalis,* genitalia; Gk, *soma,* body], a congenital condition in which the genitalia are abnormal because of an excess of androgen during fetal development. It is characterized in boys by enlarged external genitalia and in girls by pseudohermaphroditism.

macroglobulin /-glob″yəlin/, a globular serum protein with a molecular mass above 400 kilodaltons, such as the proteinase inhibitor alpha$_2$-macroglobulin. See also **immunoglobulin M.**

macroglobulinemia /mak′rōglob′yo͞olinē″mē-ə/ [Gk, *makros + L, globulus,* small ball; Gk, *haima,* blood], plasma presence of a high-molecular-weight globulin such as alpha$_2$-macroglobulin or an immunoglobulin of the IgM isotype. Macroglobulins raise plasma viscosity and are associated with monoclonal gammopathies of undetermined significance. Also called **Waldenström macroglobulinemia.** Also spelled *macroglobulinaemia.* See also **multiple myeloma.**

M

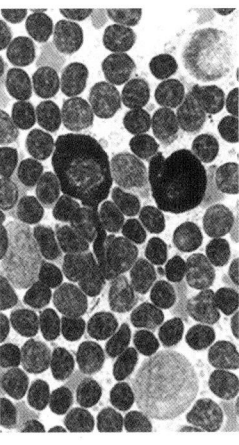

Macroglobulinemia *(Hoffman et al, 2013)*

macroglossia /mak′rōglos″ē·ə/ [Gk, *makros* + *glossa,* tongue], an excessively large tongue. It is seen in certain syndromes of congenital defects, including Down syndrome.

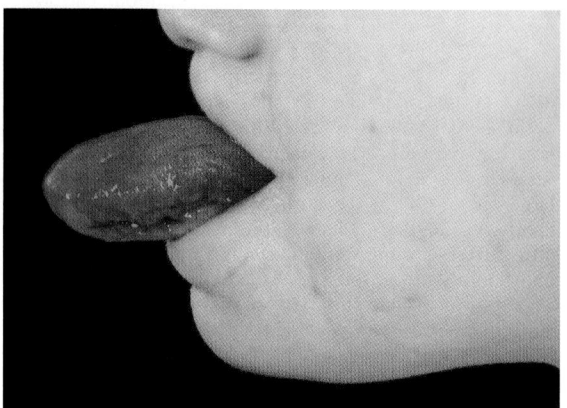

Macroglossia *(Kittur et al, 2012)*

macrognathia /mak′rōnā″thē·ə/ [Gk, *makros* + *gnathos,* jaw], an abnormally large growth of the jaw. Compare **micrognathia.** *–macrognathic, adj.*

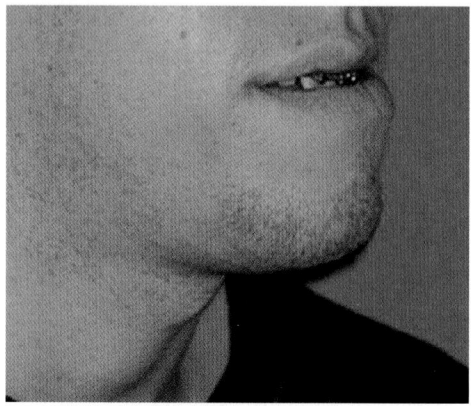

Macrognathia *(O'Ryan, 2012)*

macrolide antibiotic. See **antibiotic.**

macromolecule /-mol″əkyo͞ol/ [Gk, *makros* + L, *moles,* mass], a molecule of colloidal size, such as a protein, nucleic acid, or polysaccharide usually produced via polymerization.

macronodular adrenal disease /-nod″yələr/, a form of Cushing syndrome characterized by massively enlarged adrenal glands.

macronucleus /-no͞o″klē·əs/ [Gk, *makros* + L, *nucleus,* nut], **1.** a large nucleus that occupies a relatively large portion of the cell. **2.** (in protozoa) the larger of two nuclei in each cell, governing cell metabolism and growth as opposed to the micronucleus, which functions in sexual reproduction.

macronutrient /-no͞o″triənt/ [Gk, *makros* + L, *nutriens,* food that nourishes], nutrient required in the greatest amounts: carbohydrate, protein, fat or lipid, and water. See also **macroelement.**

macroovalocyte /mak″rō·o′välosīt/, an enlarged, oval erythrocyte seen in megaloblastic anemia.

macropenis, abnormal largeness of the penis. Also called **macrophallus, megalopenis.**

macrophage /mak″rəfāj/ [Gk, *makros* + *phagein,* to eat], a granular mononuclear phagocyte that circulates as a monocyte in the blood and resides in all tissues. Macrophages recognize and engulf foreign materials and present fragments or epitopes on their membranes to initiate an immune response. Macrophages have many names, including histiocytes, reticuloendothelial cells, Kupffer cells in the liver, and littoral cells in the spleen. Macrophages are the single most abundant cell in the human body, more numerous than skin cells or red blood cells. See also **Kupffer cells, phagocyte, reticuloendothelial system.**

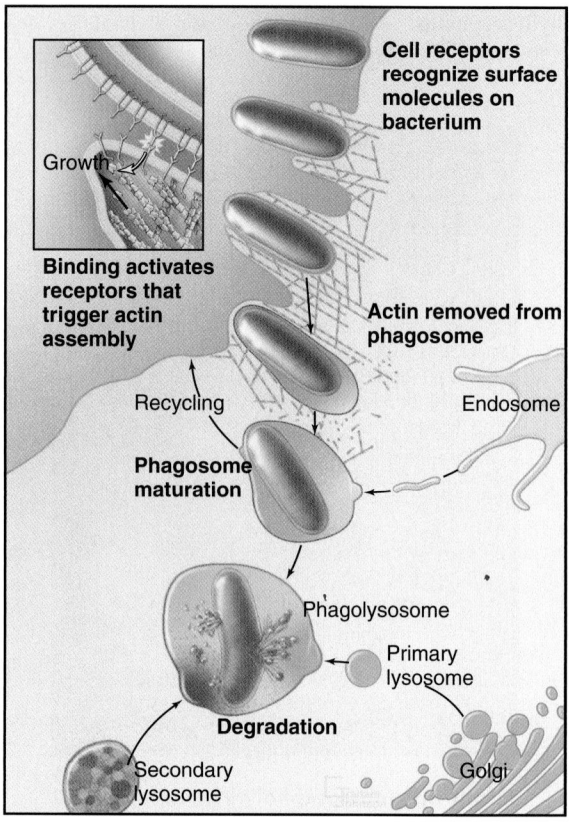

Macrophage ingesting a pathogen *(Pollard and Earnshaw, 2007)*

macrophage activating factor (MAF) [Gk. *makros,* large, *phagein,* to eat; L, *activus,* active, *facere,* to make], a lymphokine released from a sensitized leukocyte that induces changes in the appearance and function of macrophages and makes them active against certain antigens.

macrophage colony–stimulating factor (M-CSF), a glycoprotein growth factor that induces bone marrow stem cells to differentiate into monocytes and macrophages.

macrophage inhibition factor (MIF). See **macrophage migration inhibiting factor.**

macrophage migration inhibiting factor [Gk, *makros,* large, *phagein,* to eat; L, *migrare,* to wander, *inhibere,* to restrain, *facere,* to make], a lymphokine produced by leukocytes that immobilizes macrophages after contact with an antigen. Also called **leucocyte migration inhibition factor, macrophage inhibition factor (MIF).**

macrophallus. See **macropenis.**

macroprolactinoma /-prōlak′tinō″mə/, a prolactin-secreting pituitary tumor more than 10 mm in diameter that causes serum prolactin levels higher than 500 ng/mL. Bromocriptine is used with some success to shrink tumor size before surgery. Frequent monitoring of endocrine status is indicated for the remainder of the patient's life after therapy.

macropsia /makrop″sē·ə/ [Gk, *makros*, large, *opsis*, vision], hallucination in which objects seem larger than they actually are. It may be related to seizure activity, a retinal abnormality, or migraine.

macroreentry circuit /mak′rōrē·en″trē/ [Gk, *makros* + L, *re*, again; Fr, *entree*, entry], a relatively large pathway for the reactivation of myocardial tissue by the same impulse. Examples include a reentry circuit that uses one bundle branch for anterograde conduction and another for retrograde conduction to produce the highly malignant bundle branch reentry ventricular tachycardia. Another circuit runs between the top and bottom of the right atrium and produces atrial flutter.

macroscopic /-skop″ik/ [Gk, *makros*, large, *skopein*, to view], large enough to be examined without magnification. Compare **microscopic.**

macroscopic anatomy. See **gross anatomy.**

macroshock, shock from an electric current of 1 mA or greater. Currents from 1 to 15 mA produce a tingling sensation and some muscle contraction, those from 15 to 100 mA can cause a painful shock, those from 100 to 200 mA can cause cardiac fibrillation or respiratory arrest, and those above 200 mA may produce rapid burning and destruction of tissue.

macrosis /makrō″sis/ [Gk, *makros*, large, *osis*, condition], an increase in the size or volume of an object.

macrosomia. See **gigantism.**

macrostomia. See **cleft cheek.**

macrotear /-ter/, significant damage to soft tissues caused by acute penetrating trauma.

macrothelia, hypertrophy of the nipples.

macula /mak″yələ/ *pl.* **maculae** [L, spot], a small pigmented area or a spot that appears separate or different in color from the surrounding tissue.

macula adherens, a site for cell adhesion. See **desmosome.**

macula albida [L, *macula*, spot, *albidare*, to make white], small white areas in the serous membranes of the pericardium or in the peritoneum or pleura. Also called **milk patch, tache laiteuse.**

macula atrophica, a condition of cutaneous atrophy characterized by the appearance of small glistening white spots on the skin.

macula cerulea. See **blue spot,** def. 1.

macula densa [L, *macula*, spot, *densus*, thick], a thickening in the wall of a distal tubule of the kidney nephron at a point where it is in contact with the afferent glomerulus and in direct opposition to the juxtaglomerular cells. It may be part of a negative-feedback system for sodium.

maculae. See **macula.**

macula folliculi, a spot on the wall of an ovary where a mature follicle will rupture to release an ovum.

macula lutea, an oval yellow spot at the optical "center" of the retina 2 mm from the optic nerve. It contains a pit, no blood vessels, and the fovea centralis, which contains only retinal cones. Central high-acuity vision occurs when an image is focused directly on the fovea centralis of the macula lutea. Also called **macula.**

macular. See **macule.**

macular degeneration (MD) /mak″yələr/ [L, *macula*, spot, *degenerare*, to deviate], a progressive deterioration of the maculae of the retina. Dry macular degeneration is associated with thinning of macular tissues, the deposition of pigment in the macula, or a combination of the two. Wet macular degeneration is the result of new vessel formation that can leak blood and fluid. See also **age-related macular degeneration.**

macular dystrophy, any of a variety of eye disorders that damage the central part of the retina. Several of the disorders are related to gene mutations that affect older adults, including Sorsby's fundus dystrophy, caused by an excessive growth of blood vessels through the basal membrane, which thickens and bleeds. See also **macular degeneration.**

macular rash [L, *macula*, spot; OFr, *rasche*], a skin eruption in which the lesions are flat and less than 1 cm in diameter.

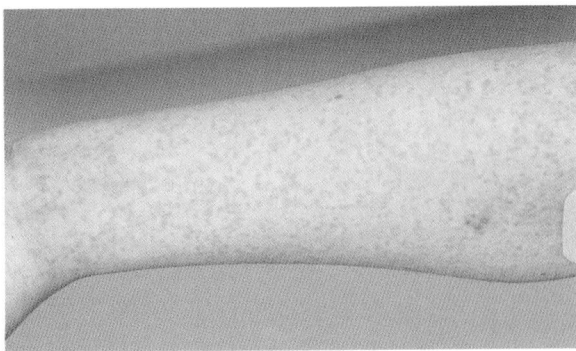

Macular rash in a person with rubella *(Cohen, Opal, and Powderly, 2010)*

macula solaris [L, *macula*, spot, *solaris*, sun], a freckle.

macule /mak″yōōl/ [L, *macula*, spot], **1.** a small flat blemish or discoloration that is level with the skin surface. Examples are freckles and some rashes. Compare **papule.** **2.** a gray scar on the cornea that is visible without magnification. **–macular,** *adj.*

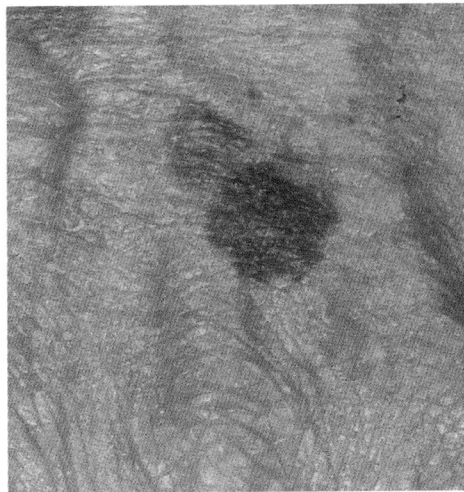

Macule *(du Vivier, 2002/Courtesy Dr. Ellen Wald, University of Wisconsin Children's Hospital)*

maculopapular rash /mak′yəlōpap″yələr/ [L, *macula*, spot, *papula*, pimple; OFr, *rasche*], a skin eruption characterized by distinctive macules and papules.

maculopathy /mak′yəlop″əthē/ [L, *macula*, spot; Gk, *pathos,* disease], a form of macular disease primarily involving the macula lutea.

M

MAD, abbreviation for **multiple autoimmune disorder.**

mad cow disease. See **bovine spongiform encephalopathy.**

Madelung neck [Otto Madelung, German surgeon, 1846–1926], deposits of fatty tissue around the neck and shoulder. Most patients with this condition have a history of alcohol abuse, but it is also associated with diabetes mellitus or hyperlipidemia. Surgical intervention is required if the deposits interfere with breathing. See **lipoma annulare colli.**

mad hatter's disease, occupational exposure to mercury vapors by felt hat workers. See **mercury poisoning.**

Madigan prostatectomy, removal of the prostate gland through an incision between the anus and scrotum.

Madura foot /majˈoorˈe/ [Madura, India; AS, *fot,* foot], a progressive destructive tropical fungal infection of the foot. Also called *maduromycosis.* See also **mycetoma.**

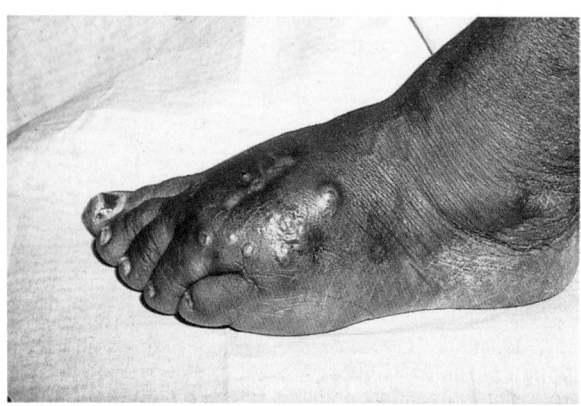

Madura foot *(du Vivier, 2002/Courtesy Dr. Rod Hay)*

MAF, abbreviation for **macrophage activating factor.**

mafenide acetate /mafˈənīd/, a topical antibiotic.
■ INDICATIONS: It is prescribed in the treatment of second- and third-degree burns to prevent infection by microorganisms such as *Pseudomonas aeruginosa.*
■ CONTRAINDICATIONS: Known hypersensitivity to this drug or to sulfonamide prohibits its use.
■ ADVERSE EFFECTS: Among the more serious adverse effects are hypersensitivity reactions and superinfections, particularly by *Candida albicans.*

Maffucci syndrome, a congenital disorder characterized by the proliferation of cartilage at the ends of long bones and by benign, blood-filled tumors of the skin or viscera. See also **cavernous hemangioma, enchondromatosis.**

magaldrate /magˈoldrāte/, an antacid containing a combination of magnesium and aluminum compounds.
■ INDICATIONS: It is prescribed in the treatment of hypersensitivity and stomach upset associated with heartburn, sour stomach, or acid indigestion.
■ CONTRAINDICATIONS: It may alter the absorption of several drugs, such as tetracycline.
■ ADVERSE EFFECTS: A change in bowel function may occur.

Magendie's law. See **Bell's law.**

magical thinking /majˈikəl/, (in psychology) a belief that merely thinking about an event in the external world can cause it to occur. Children ages 4 to 6 sometimes engage in magical thinking. When it occurs later in life, it is regarded as a form of regression to an early phase of development. It may be part of ideas of reference, considered normal in those instances, or may reach delusional proportions when the individual maintains a firm conviction about the belief, despite evidence to the contrary. It may be seen in schizophrenia.

magic-bullet approach [Gk, *magikos,* sorcerer; Fr, *boulette,* small ball; L, *ad,* toward, *prope,* near], **1.** (in traditional diagnostic radiology) the administration of a specific contrast medium to facilitate the radiographic visualization of a given organ, such as the IV injection of a specific dye for renal studies. **2.** (in nuclear medicine) the administration of a specific radionuclide tagged to an appropriate carrier to provide a scintillation camera image of a given organ or structure, such as the use of a substance containing phosphate and technetium for bone scanning.

Magill forceps, angled forceps used to guide a tracheal tube into the larynx or a nasogastric tube into the esophagus under direct vision. It is also used to place pharyngeal packs and remove foreign bodies.

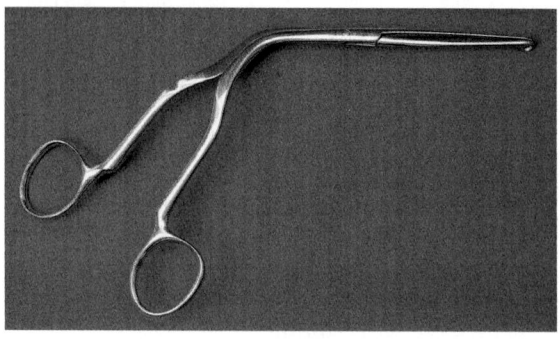

Magill forceps *(Davey and Diba, 2012)*

Maglinte tube [Dean D.T. Maglinte, contemporary American physician], an intestinal tube used in the management of small bowel obstruction. It includes a balloon to prevent reflux of bowel contents into the stomach.

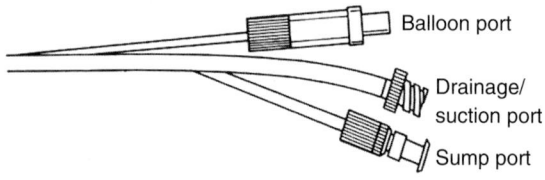

Balloon port
Drainage/suction port
Sump port

Maglinte long tube *(Maglinte, 2013)*

magnesemia /magˈnəsēˈmē·ə/, the presence of magnesium in the blood.

magnesia magma. See **milk of magnesia.**

magnesium (Mg) /magnēˈsē·əm, magnēˈzhəm/ [Gk, magnesia, geographic area in Greece], a silver-white mineral element. Its atomic number is 12; its atomic mass is 24.32. Magnesium occurs abundantly in nature, always in combination with other elements. It is obtained chiefly by the electrolysis of fused salts containing magnesium chloride or by the thermal reduction of magnesia and is used in photography, metallurgy, and various pharmaceuticals such as magnesium sulfate. Magnesium is the second most abundant cation of the intracellular fluids in the body. It is essential for many enzyme activities and the interaction of intracellular particles and binding of macromolecules to subcellular organelles, such as the binding of messenger ribonucleic acid to ribosomes. It also is important to neurochemical transmissions and muscular excitability. The body of the average 145-pound adult contains about 2000 mEq of magnesium, about 50% of which is in the bones, 45% existing as intracellular cations, and about 5% in the extracellular fluid. Absorption of magnesium occurs in the upper small bowel by means of an active process closely related to the transport system for calcium. Magnesium is excreted mainly by the kidney. Renal excretion of magnesium increases during diuresis induced by ammonium chloride, glucose, and organic mercurials. Magnesium affects the central nervous, neuromuscular, and cardiovascular systems. Insufficient magnesium (hypomagnesemia) in extracellular fluid increases the release of acetylcholine and can cause changes in cardiac and skeletal muscle. Some of the conditions that can produce hypomagnesemia are diarrhea, steatorrhea, chronic alcoholism, and diabetes mellitus. Hypomagnesemia may occur in newborns and infants who are fed cow's milk or artificial formulas, apparently because of the high phosphate/magnesium ratio in such diets. Hypomagnesemia is often treated with parenteral fluids containing magnesium sulfate or magnesium chloride. Excess magnesium (hypermagnesemia) in the body can slow the heartbeat, and concentrations greater than 15 mEq/L can produce cardiac arrest in diastole. Excess magnesium also causes vasodilation by direct effects on the blood vessels and by ganglionic blockade. Hypermagnesemia is usually caused by renal insufficiency and is manifested by hypotension, electrocardiographic changes, muscle weakness, sedation, and a confused mental state.

magnesium alginate, the magnesium salt of alginic acid, administered orally as a component of an antacid in the treatment of gastroesophageal reflux disease. It combines with gastric acid to form a viscous gel that floats on top of the gastric contents and acts as a physical barrier to reflux.

magnesium chloride, an electrolyte replenisher and a pharmaceutical necessity for hemodialysis and peritoneal dialysis fluids.

magnesium gluconate, the gluconate salt of magnesium, administered orally in the prevention of hypomagnesemia.

magnesium lactate, the lactate salt of magnesium, administered orally in the prevention of hypomagnesemia.

magnesium salicylate, the magnesium salt of salicylic acid, used as an analgesic, antipyretic, antiinflammatory, and antirheumatic. It is administered orally.

magnesium silicate ($MgSiO_3$), a silicate salt of magnesium. The most common hydrated forms found in nature are asbestos and talc.

magnesium sulfate, a salt of magnesium.

■ INDICATIONS: It is prescribed parenterally to prevent seizures, especially in preeclampsia and acute nephritis in children, and orally to treat constipation and heartburn and to correct magnesium deficiency.

■ CONTRAINDICATIONS: It is used with caution in patients with renal impairment or hypersensitivity to the drug. Respiratory depression, severe cardiac myopathy, heart block, or symptoms of appendicitis or fecal impaction prohibit its use. It is also prohibited in patients in toxemia of pregnancy during the 2 hours before labor.

■ ADVERSE EFFECTS: The most serious adverse effect is circulatory collapse from excessive serum concentrations of magnesium. Respiratory depression, confusion, and muscle weakness also may occur.

■ INDICATIONS: Magnesium sulfate can be used during cardiac arrest primarily to treat torsades de pointes caused by a low serum magnesium level. It can also be used to treat life-threatening ventricular arrhythmias due to digitalis toxicity.

magnesium test, a blood test used to measure levels of magnesium, an electrolyte that is critical in nearly all metabolic processes. Abnormal levels may indicate renal insufficiency,

chronic renal disease, uncontrolled diabetes, diabetic acidosis, Addison disease, hypothyroidism, malnutrition, malabsorption, hypoparathyroidism, and alcoholism.

magnetic field /magnet″ik/ [Gk, *magnesia,* lodestone; AS, *feld*], the region around any magnet in which its effects can be detected.

magnetic field therapy, the placement of magnets directly on the skin, stimulating living cells and increasing blood flow by ionic currents created from polarities on the magnets. Trigger points for magnets are acupuncture points where the action of the magnets serves to activate the tendinomuscular system to readily and widely transmit electrical stimuli. Magnets also increase tissue oxygen perfusion by decreasing vascular resistance, decreasing nerve cell firing, and stimulating various cellular structures. Common physiological responses include vasodilation, analgesia, antiinflammatory action, spasmolytic activity, accelerated healing, and antiedema activity. In addition to the FDA-approved use of pulsed magnetic fields for the treatment of nonunion fractures, it has been tried for a large number of other conditions, usually self-administered by patients.

magnetic flux (N), the product of the average magnetic field times the perpendicular area that it penetrates. It is a quantity of convenience in the statement of Faraday's law and in the discussion of objects such as transformers and solenoids. In the case of an electric generator in which the magnetic field penetrates a rotating coil, the area used in defining the flux is the projection of the coil area onto the plane perpendicular to the magnetic field.

magnetic lines of force [Gk, *magnesia,* lodestone; L, *linea,* line, *fortis,* strong], theoretical lines of magnetism that surround a magnet or fill a magnetic field. The presence of the magnetic force along the imaginary lines can be demonstrated by inserting a sensitive material such as iron filings into the lines of magnetic effect.

magnetic moment [Gk, *magnesia,* lodestone, *momentum,* movement], a measure of the net magnetic field produced by an elementary particle or an atomic nucleus spinning about its own axis. Such fields are similar to the field surrounding a bar magnet and are the basis for magnetic resonance imaging.

magnetic permeability, the measure of the ability of a material to support the formation of a magnetic field within itself. Hence, it is the degree of magnetization that a material obtains in response to an applied magnetic field. Magnetic permeability is typically represented by the Greek letter μ. See also **permeability.**

magnetic resonance (MR), a phenomenon in which the atomic nuclei of certain materials placed in a strong, static magnetic field absorb radio waves supplied by a transmitter at particular frequencies. The energy of the radio waves promotes the nuclei from a low-energy state, in which the nuclear spin is aligned parallel to the magnetic field, to a higher-energy state, in which the nuclear spin has a component transverse or opposed to the field. These nuclei occasionally revert to the lower-energy state by emitting photons at characteristic (resonance) frequencies, providing information about the local magnetic field at the nuclei. The rate at which the nuclei revert, or relax, to the lower-energy state when the source of radio waves is turned off is another important factor. See also **relaxation time.**

magnetic resonance angiography, the use of special MR imaging pulses to visualize the vascular system and identify regions of nonflowing blood. It may be performed with or without contrast agents.

magnetic resonance imaging (MRI) [Gk, *magnesia,* lodestone, *resonare,* to sound again, *imago,* image], medical

M

imaging based on the resonance of atomic nuclei in a strong magnetic field. The field causes those nuclei with an odd number of protons to align and rotate around the axis of the field. Application of a radiofrequency pulse causes the protons to resonate. When the pulse is terminated, the protons "relax" back toward equilibrium. As they do so, they release energy that is detected as a radio signal. Analysis of the amplitude and frequency of the signal yields information about the number and position of nuclei in the tissue, from which the image is produced. MRI is the method of choice for a growing number of disease processes. Among its advantages are its superior soft-tissue contrast resolution, ability to image in multiple planes, and lack of ionizing radiation hazards. MRI is regarded as superior to computed tomography for most central nervous system abnormalities, particularly those of the posterior fossa, brainstem, and spinal cord. It has also become an important tool in musculoskeletal and pelvic imaging. The procedure usually does not require a contrast medium but may use an IV injection of gadolinium. About 15% of patients require an anxiolytic to overcome claustrophobia during MRI, and children may need a sedative as well. Patients must remain motionless for high-quality imaging. Images also may be degraded by motions related to heart contractions, respiration, and bowel peristalsis. Contraindications to MRI are pacemakers, metallic aneurysm clips, and some metallic prostheses and foreign objects. Compare **open magnetic resonance imaging.** Formerly called **zeugmatography.** See also **magnetic resonance.**

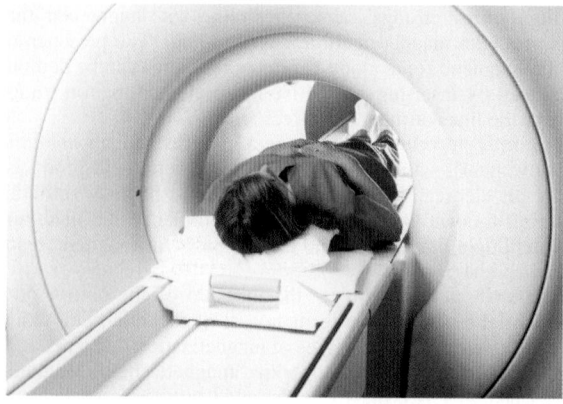

Patient in magnetic resonance imaging machine
(Phillips, 2012)

magnetic resonance urography, imaging of the urinary tract using magnetic resonance imaging, such as to detect obstructions and dilations during pregnancy when other methods are ineffective or undesirable.

magnetic susceptibility, a measure of the ability of a substance to become magnetized.

magnetization /mag′nətīzā″shən/ [Gk, *magnesia,* lodestone, *izein,* to cause], the magnetic polarization of a material produced by a magnetic field (magnetic moment per unit volume).

magnetron /mag″nətron/ [Gk, *magnesia,* lodestone, *trum,* device], a source of microwave energy used in medical linear accelerators to accelerate electrons to the therapeutic energies.

magnification /mag′nifikā″shən/, (in psychology) cognitive distortion in which the effects of one's behavior are magnified. See also **minimization.**

magnification factor, an inherent radiographic degrading of the produced image. A mathematical calculation is used to determine the extent of magnification: the size of a radiographic, photographic, or microscopic image divided by the object size. Magnification factor can be calculated by dividing the distance from the source to the image receptor by the distance from the source to the object.

MAHA, characterized by schistocytes in the peripheral blood film. Abbreviation for **microangiopathic hemolytic anemia.**

Mahaim fiber [I. Mahaim, 20th-century French physician, 1897–1965], one of the conductive tracts in cardiac tissue running between the atrioventricular (AV) node or the AV bundle and the muscle of the ventricular septum. The fibers conduct early excitation impulses.

Mahoney, Mary Eliza [1845–1926], the first African-American nurse. Mahoney did private nursing in the Boston area and was active in furthering intergroup relationships and improving the role of the African-American nurse in the community. A medal in her name, established after her death, was first presented in 1936. It is given to an African-American nurse in recognition of outstanding contribution to the nursing profession.

main en griffe. See **clawhand.**

mainframe computer [OE, *maegen,* strength, *framian,* to progress; L, *computare,* to count], a large general-purpose computer system for high-volume data-processing tasks. It may support large numbers of users simultaneously. Compare **microcomputer, minicomputer.**

mainstreaming /mān″strēming/ [OE, *maegan,* strength; ME, *strem*], **1.** the system of educating children with disabilities in regular classrooms, with special assistance as needed. Also called **inclusion. 2.** the return of persons recovering from mental illness to the community.

maintenance, 1. providing a stable state over a long period as distinguished from a short-term acute effect, as in a drug or treatment plan. **2.** in anesthesia, the surgical or procedural period of anesthesia delivery, in which a combination of inhaled agents and adjunct medications are administered to achieve appropriate surgical and anesthetic conditions.

maintenance dose /mān″tənəns/ [Fr, *maintenir,* to uphold; Gk, *dosis,* giving], the amount of drug required to keep a desired mean steady-state concentration in the tissues.

maintenance roles, social-emotional activities that help maintain involvement in a group and raise personal commitment to the group.

Mainz pouch, any of several continent urinary diversion surgeries using a section of the rectum and sigmoid colon to create a pouch for maintenance of continence.

maitake, a natural product derived from a mushroom that is native to Japan.

■ INDICATIONS: It is used as an immunostimulant and as a treatment for diabetes, hypertension, high cholesterol, and obesity. It is probably safe, but there is no reliable information related to efficacy.

■ CONTRAINDICATIONS: It is not recommended during pregnancy and lactation, in children, or in those with known hypersensitivity until more information is available.

Majocchi granuloma /mäjok″ē/ [Domenico Majocchi, Italian dermatologist, 1849–1929; L, *granulum,* small grain; Gk, *oma,* tumor], a rare type of tinea corporis that involves the follicle and affects the lower legs. It is caused by the fungus *Trichophyton,* which infects the hairs of the affected site and raises spongy granulomas. The lesions persist for 3 to 4 months and are gradually absorbed, or they necrose, often leaving deep scars. Treatment consists of oral antifungal medications. Also called **trichophytic granuloma.**

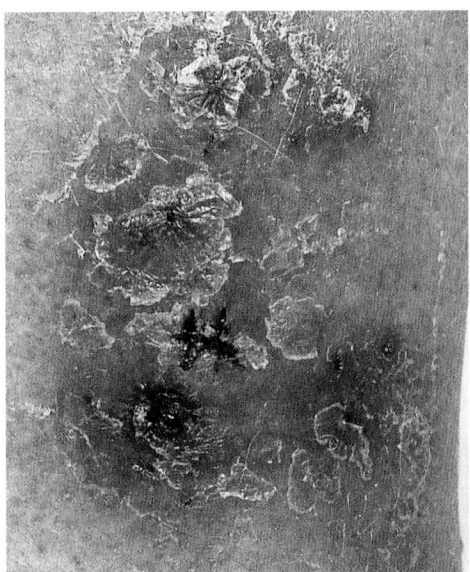

Majocchi granuloma *(du Vivier, 2002)*

major affective disorder.   See **major depressive disorder.**

major connector,   a metal plate or bar used for joining the two halves of a removable partial denture.

major depressive disorder,   a major disorder of mood characterized by a persistent dysphoria, anxiety, irritability, fear, brooding, appetite and sleep disturbances, weight loss, psychomotor agitation or delay, decreased energy, feelings of worthlessness or guilt, difficulty in concentrating or thinking, possible delusions and hallucinations, and thoughts of death or suicide. The disorder, which occurs in children, adolescents, and adults, may develop over a period of days, weeks, or months. Episodes may occur in clusters or singly, separated by several years of normality. The causes of the disorder are multiple and complex and may involve biological, psychological, interpersonal, and sociocultural factors that lead to an unidentifiable intrapsychic conflict. Treatment includes use of antidepressants and electroconvulsive therapy, followed by long-term psychotherapy. Nursing care is needed to ensure adequate nutrition, appropriate balance of fluid intake and output, good personal hygiene, and protection of the patient from self-injury. Occupational therapy practitioners help persons with major depressive disorders engage in daily living tasks (e.g., feeding, dressing, bathing, grooming, and hygiene), education, play, medication management, meal preparation (instrumental activities of daily living), and leisure by developing habits and routines that support participation in life events. Practitioners help clients develop patterns of engagement that provide a healthy balance. Also called **major affective disorder, unipolar disorder.** See also **bipolar disorder, depression, dysthymic disorder.**

Major Diagnostic Category,   a grouping of related diagnoses, such as all those affecting a given organ system of the body; used primarily for billing purposes.

major duodenal papilla,   the common entrance in the duodenum for the bile and pancreatic ducts. See also **minor duodenal papilla.**

major histocompatibility complex,   a molecule that presents antigen peptides to T cells on the surface of cells. Two major classes have been described: major histocompatibility complex (MHC) class I and class II. MHC class I is present on all cells and presents endogenous peptides to CD8 T cells. MHC class II is present only on antigen-presenting cells and presents exogenous peptides to CD4 T cells. MHC, or human leukocyte antigen (HLA) as it is called in humans, also determines the compatibility of tissues or organs transplanted from one individual to another of the same species or from one species to another. See also **HLA complex, human leukocyte antigen, antigen processing.**

major medical insurance,   insurance coverage designed to offset the costs of prolonged or catastrophic illness and injury. Most major medical insurance policies are written to pay a certain percentage of costs up to a predetermined figure, beyond which payment is in full up to a maximum amount, at which point payment ceases. Many require the insured to pay a specified initial, or deductible, amount.

major renal calyx.   See **renal calyx.**

major surgery,   a surgical procedure that is extensive, involving removal or significant repair of organs and/or life-threatening conditions.

major vestibular glands.   See **Bartholin gland.**

making weight,   *(Nontechnical)* (in sports medicine) the practice of rapid weight loss based on the belief that training at a heavier body weight and then dropping weight shortly before competition gives an athlete an advantage.

makro-.   See **macro-, makro-.**

mal /mal, mäl/   [L, *malus,* bad],   an illness or disease, such as grand mal or petit mal seizures.

mal-,   prefix meaning "bad," "poor," or "abnormal": *maladjustment, malalignment.*

malabsorption /mal'əbsôrp″shən/   [L, *malus + absorbere,* to swallow],   impaired absorption of nutrients from the GI tract. It occurs in celiac disease, sprue, dysentery, diarrhea, inflammatory bowel disease, and other disorders. It may result from an inborn error of metabolism, malnutrition, or any chemical or anatomical condition of the digestive system that prevents normal absorption. See also **inborn error of metabolism, malnutrition.**

malabsorption syndrome,   a complex of symptoms resulting from disorders in the intestinal absorption of nutrients, characterized by anorexia, weight loss, abdominal bloating, muscle cramps, bone pain, and steatorrhea. Anemia, weakness, and fatigue occur because iron, folic acid, and vitamin B_{12} are not absorbed in sufficient amounts. Among the many conditions causing this syndrome are gastric or small bowel resection, celiac disease, tropical sprue, Whipple disease, intestinal lymphangiectasia, and cystic fibrosis. Treatment and prognosis are determined by the underlying condition. See also **celiac disease, cystic fibrosis, hypoproteinemia, tropical sprue.**

malacia /məlā″shə/   [Gk, *malakia,* softness],   **1.** a morbid softening or sponginess in any part or any tissue of the body. **2.** a craving for spicy foods, such as mustard, hot peppers, or pickles.

-malacia,   suffix meaning "the softening of tissue": *chondromalacia, keratomalacia, tracheomalacia.*

malacic.   See **malacia.**

maladaptation /mal'adəptā″shən/   [L, *malus + adaptatio*],   faulty intrapersonal adjustment to stress or change. It may involve a failure to make necessary changes in desires, values, needs, and attitudes or an inability to make necessary adjustments in the external world. Illness often provokes maladaptive behavior that worsens the problems accompanying the illness. *—maladaptive, adj.*

maladjusted /mal'adjus″tid/   [L, *malus,* bad, *adjuxtare,* to bring together],   appearing unable to maintain effective relationships needed to fit into the environment and showing irritability, depression, and other psychogenic conditions.

M

maladjustment /mal″ad-just´ment/ [L, *malus* + Fr. *adjuster*], inability to meet the usual challenges of daily life or to successfully adapt to changing situations.

malady /mal″ədē/ [ME, *maladie,* sick], a disease or illness.

malaise /malāz/ [Fr, discomfort], a vague, uneasy feeling of body weakness, distress, or discomfort, often marking the onset of and persisting throughout a disease.

malalignment /mal′əlīn″mənt/ [L, *malus* + *ad,* to, *linea,* line], a failure of parts of the body to align normally, such as the teeth in the dental arch.

malar /mā″lər/ [L, *mala,* cheek], pertaining to the cheek or the cheekbone.

malaria /mələr″ē·ə/ [It, *mal,* bad, *aria,* air], a severe infectious illness caused by one or more of at least four species of the protozoan genus *Plasmodium.* The disease is transmitted from human to human by a bite from an infected *Anopheles* mosquito. Malarial infection can also be spread by blood transfusion from an infected patient or by the use of a contaminated or an infected hypodermic needle. Although the endemic disease is limited largely to tropical areas of South and Central America, Africa, and Asia, a number of new cases are introduced into the United States by refugees, military personnel, and travelers returning from malarial areas. See also **double quartan fever.**
- OBSERVATIONS: Malaria is characterized by chills and fever, anemia, an enlarged spleen, myalgia, arthralgia, weakness, and vomiting. Splenomegaly, anemia, thrombocytopenia, hypoglycemia, pulmonary or renal dysfunction, and neurosis may also occur. *P. falciparum, P. ovale,* or *P. vivax* parasites penetrate the erythrocytes of the human host, where they mature, reproduce, and burst out periodically. Malarial paroxysms occur at regular intervals, coinciding with the development of a new generation of parasites in the body. Because the life cycle of the infecting parasite varies according to species, the clinical patterns of chills and fever vary, as do the course and severity of the disease. Bouts of malaria usually last from 1 to 4 weeks, with attacks occurring less frequently as the disease progresses. Relapse is common, and the disease can persist for years.
- INTERVENTIONS: Malaria prophylaxis involves the administration of chloroquine, tetracycline, doxycycline, or mefloquine. Treatment for active malaria includes the administration of chloroquine, quinine, tetracycline, clindamycin, doxycycline, mefloquine, primaquine, sulfonamides, or pyrimethamine.

malarial hemoglobinuria. See **blackwater fever.**

malarial parasite /mələr″ē·əl/ [It, *mal aria,* bad air; Gk, *parasitos,* guest], one of four known species of *Plasmodium* that may be injected into the human bloodstream by an anopheline mosquito to begin the cycle of malarial disease.

Malarone /mal′ah-rōn/, a combination preparation that acts as an antimalarial agent. Brand name for **proguanil, atovaquone.**

Malassezia /mal′əsē″zē·ə/ [Louis C. Malassez, French physiologist, 1842–1910], a genus of fungi. *Malassezia furfur,* the species normally found on human skin, can cause tinea versicolor in susceptible hosts (previous name: *Pityrosporum oviculare). M. ovalis* is a nonpathogenic organism found in sebaceous areas. Formerly called *Pityrosporum ovale.*

malathion, a widely used organophosphorus insecticide used in dilute topical applications for lice.

malathion poisoning /malā″thē·on, məl′əthī″on/, a toxic condition caused by the ingestion or absorption through the skin of malathion, an organophosphorus insecticide.

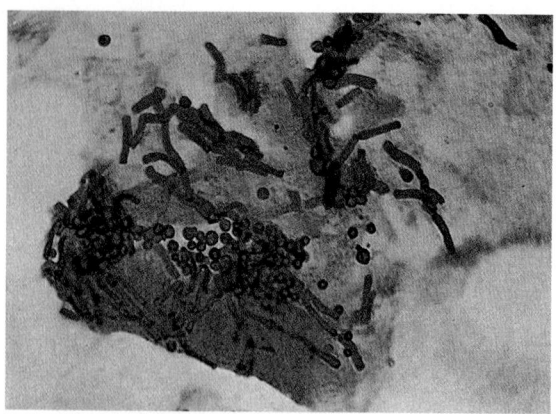

Malassezia furfur (Murray, Rosenthal, and Pfaller, 2002)

Symptoms include vomiting, nausea, salivation, tearing, abdominal cramps, headache, dizziness, weakness, confusion, convulsions, and respiratory difficulties. Malathion is much less toxic than parathion and is the only organophosphorus insecticide approved for household use.

malaxation, the act of manipulating a mass of material. See also **pétrissage.**

Malayan pit viper venom. See **ancrod.**

mal del pinto. See **pinta.**

mal de Meleda /mal·də mel′ədä/ [Fr, *meleda,* sickness], a chronic autosomal-recessive form of keratoderma of the palms and soles of the feet, in which the hyperkeratosis spreads to involve the dorsal aspects of the hands and feet and other areas of the body, with erythematous, scaling, malodorous cutaneous lesions that may cause deep fissuring. Also called **Meleda disease.**

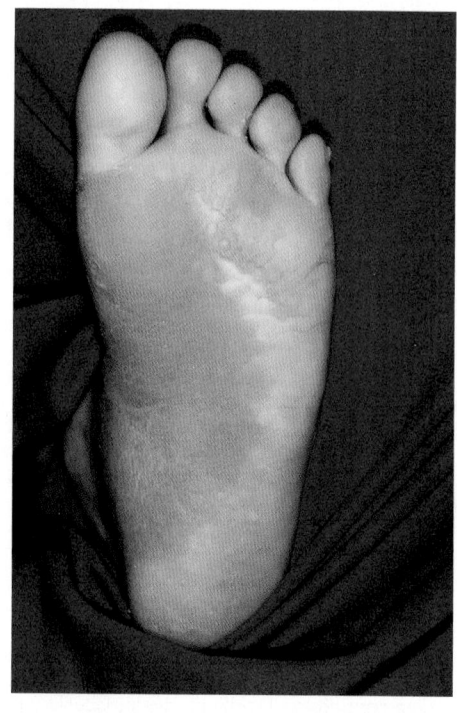

Keratoderma associated with mal de Meleda
(Paller and Mancini, 2011)

mal de mer, seasickness. See also **kinesia.**

male [L, *mas*], **1.** *adj.,* pertaining to the sex that produces sperm cells and fertilizes the female egg to beget offspring; masculine. **2.** *n.,* a male person.

male catheterization, the passage of a catheter through the male urethra for the purpose of draining the urinary bladder or instilling a medication. A French size 14 catheter is usually determined for adult men unless the physician orders a larger size. The male patient is placed in a supine position with the legs extended. The catheter is inserted 17.5 to 22.5 cm or until urine flows. Sterile technique is important throughout the procedure to prevent the introduction of infectious organisms into the bladder.
- OUTCOME CRITERIA: The expected outcome is drainage of urine from the bladder and relief of bladder distension and discomfort. Unexpected outcomes include the absence of urine because of an inability to advance the catheter through the urethra to the bladder. Catheter insertion should never be forced. The male may also experience ongoing discomfort despite catheter patency, which may be a result of urethral spasm, bladder infection, or balloon inflation when the balloon is not entirely in the bladder. Leakage of urine around the catheter may indicate that the catheter size is too small or that the balloon is inadequately inflated.

male climacterium. See **male menopause.**

male factor infertility, infertility of a couple caused by a problem in the male's reproductive system, such as anejaculation, aspermatogenesis, or azoospermia.

male menopause [L, *mas,* male, *men,* month; Gk, *pauein,* to cease], a late middle-age condition affecting some men, who experience anxiety over changes in sexual function and/or desire, increased fatigue, thinning and graying hair, and other signs of aging. Male menopause can stem from actual changes in testosterone levels (over a longer period of time than the more abrupt change in hormone levels typically associated with female menopause). Also called **male climacterium.**

male pattern alopecia [L, *mas,* male; ME, *patron* + Gk, *alopex,* fox mange], a common form of baldness in males, beginning at the frontal scalp and spreading gradually until only a fringe remains around the back of the head. Individual differences are determined by heredity, androgenic stimulation, and aging. Also called *male pattern baldness.*

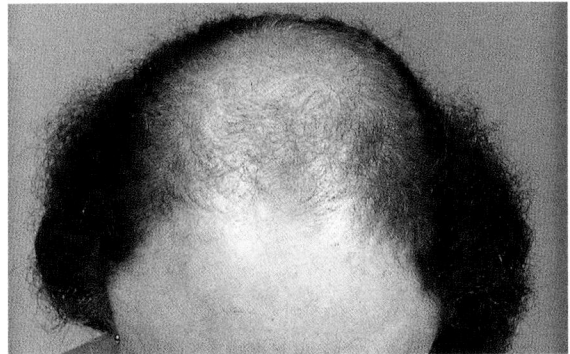

Male pattern alopecia *(du Vivier, 2002)*

male reproductive system assessment, (in medicine and nursing) an evaluation of the condition of the patient's genitalia, reproductive history, and past and present genitourinary infections and disorders.
- METHOD: In a relaxed professional interview the procedures to be conducted are explained and the patient is reassured that his privacy will be scrupulously maintained. He is questioned about his offspring; sexual activity; the existence of nocturia, urgency, frequency, dysuria, urethral discharge, hernia, or genital sores; discomfort or pain in the groin, lower back, or legs; and past treatment for epididymitis, gonorrhea, herpes genitalis, hydrocele, nonspecific urethritis, orchitis, prostatitis, syphilis, and varicocele. The examiner, while inspecting the genitalia, observes universal precautions as indicated by the condition. The penis is examined for swelling, inflammation, and lesions such as herpes vesicles or syphilitic sores, chancres, or scars. Anomalies that may be noted include hypospadias or epispadias, resulting from failed closure of the urethra; elongation of the foreskin constricting the urinary meatus; or swelling of the glans caused by a retracted, tight foreskin. The urethral orifice is inspected for a purulent or bloody discharge, and the scrotum is observed for symmetry and shape; in elderly or debilitated men the scrotum may be elongated and flat. The normally smooth testes, epididymis, and spermatic cords are palpated for the presence of beading and varicosities and the size, location, and consistency of any scrotal mass. Fluid felt around the testes may be seen by darkening the room and illuminating the scrotum with a flashlight. Wrapping the flashlight with clear plastic wrap, which is changed between patients, decreases the risk of bacteria transfer. The patient is asked to cough or bear down to reveal a hernia, and the abdomen is palpated above the symphysis pubis to determine whether the bladder is distended. The inguinal lymph nodes are palpated, and the amount and distribution of pubic hair are observed. The prostate may be examined with the patient in the semiprone side position or lithotomy position but, when possible, the patient should stand bent at a right angle over a table as the examiner's well-lubricated gloved forefinger sweeps the rectal circumference and palpates the lobes and medial sulcus of the gland. The size, consistency, and any localized nodule suggesting a neoplasm of the normally smooth, firm prostate are carefully noted, and the findings are recorded as on a clock dial with the symphysis pubis representing 12 o'clock. When additional studies are indicated, a smear is prepared from the first urine voided after massage of the prostate. Primary screening for prostatic cancer includes the digital rectal examination and a blood test for PSA. Prostatic acid phosphatase is also assessed if prostatic cancer is suspected. Diagnosis is usually established by a biopsy. The assessment includes laboratory studies of any discharge from the penis. A Gram-stained smear usually confirms or rules out a diagnosis of gonorrhea. A fluorescent-tagged antibody method may be required if the result is equivocal. Cultures may be needed to determine whether nonspecific urethritis is caused by *Escherichia coli, Pseudomonas, Staphylococcus, Streptococcus,* or organisms of other pathogenic genera. Syphilis may be diagnosed by the Venereal Disease Research Laboratories serological test, but the fluorescent treponemal antibody-absorption test is the most sensitive and specific diagnostic measure. If infertility is a problem, examinations of multiple semen samples are conducted. Each specimen collected after 3 days of abstinence is inspected in the laboratory to determine whether the volume of the ejaculate approximates the normal 2 to 5 mL average and whether the semen has a pH of 7.7 and a sperm count of 60 to 150 million per milliliter.
- INTERVENTIONS: The health care provider conducts the interview and examination, assembles the results of laboratory studies, and urges the patient to inform his sex partner, or partners, if an infectious disease is diagnosed. Throughout the assessment the health care provider recognizes that the patient may be reluctant to discuss his symptoms and activities and may be sensitive about the necessary procedures.
- OUTCOME CRITERIA: A careful, understanding evaluation of the male patient's reproductive system helps to establish the diagnosis and plan the treatment and aids in allaying the pa-

M

tient's anxiety. The assessment also serves as a public health measure by encouraging the reporting of a sexually transmitted disease to the patient's contacts and proper authorities.

male sexual dysfunction, impaired or inadequate ability of a man to carry on his sex life to his own satisfaction. Symptoms include difficulties in starting and maintaining an erection, premature ejaculation, inability to ejaculate, and loss of desire. Compare **female sexual dysfunction.** See also **impotence, premature ejaculation, sexual dysfunction.**

male sterility [L, *mas* + *sterilis,* barren], the inability of a man to produce sperm. Causes may include environmental factors, such as exposure to heat or radiation, or physiological factors, such as undescended testes, varicocele, prolonged fever, endocrine disorders, cancer chemotherapy, vasectomy, and abuse of alcohol or marijuana. See also **infertility.**

male urethra, a canal extending from the neck of the bladder to the urinary meatus, measuring about 20 cm in length, and presenting a double curve when the penis is flaccid. It is divided into proximal (sphincteric) and distal (conduit) or posterior (prostatic and membranous) and anterior (bulbar and penile).

malfeasance /malfē″zəns/ [Fr, *malfaire,* to do evil], performance of an unlawful, wrongful act. Compare **misfeasance, nonfeasance.**

malformation /mal′fôrmā″shən/ [L, *malus,* bad, *forma,* shape], an anomalous structure in the body. See also **congenital anomaly.**

malfunction /mal′fungk″shən/ [L, *malus,* bad, *functio,* performance], **1.** *n.,* an inability to function normally. **2.** *v.,* not to function normally.

Malgaigne fracture of pelvis /malgā″nyə/ [Joseph F. Malgaigne, French surgeon, 1806–1865], breaks in multiple pelvic bones, including the pubic rami and the wing of the ipsilateral ilium or the sacrum, with associated upper displacement of the hemipelvis.

malicious prosecution /məlish″əs/ [L, *malitia,* wickedness, *prosequi,* to pursue], (in law) a suit begun in malice and pursued without sufficient cause. It is usually an action for damages. Malicious prosecution is a wrongful civil proceeding, and a person who takes an active part in initiating or continuing it is subject to liability.

malign /məlīn/ [ME, *malignen,* deceptive], to show ill will or maliciousness; to act viciously; to harm.

malignant /məlig″nənt/ [L, *malignus,* bad disposition], **1.** tending to become worse and to cause death. See also **virulent. 2.** (describing a cancer) anaplastic, invasive, and metastatic. —*malignancy, n.*

malignant astrocytoma, a high-grade astrocytoma, such as glioblastoma multiforme.

malignant atrophic papulosis, a form of cutaneous lymphocytic vasculitis. The skin disease shows erythematous papules with characteristic porcelain-white centers and elevated borders. The early signs are followed by perforated intestinal ulcers, leading to peritonitis, occluded arterioles, and progressive neurological disability. Also called **Degos disease.**

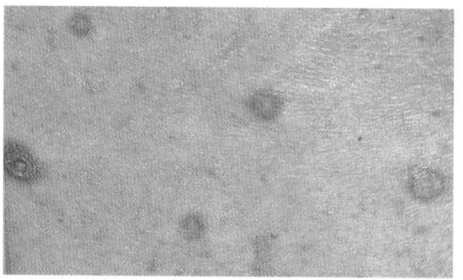

Malignant atrophic papulosis *(Passarini et al, 2010)*

malignant dysentery [L, *malignus,* bad disposition; Gk, *dys,* bad, *enteron,* bowel], a potentially fatal form of dysentery in which symptoms are severe.

malignant edema. See **anthrax.**

malignant endocarditis. See **bacterial endocarditis.**

malignant ependymoma. See **ependymoblastoma.**

malignant granuloma [L, *malignus,* bad disposition, *granulum,* little grain, *oma,* tumor], a malignant lymphoma, such as Hodgkin disease, or a lymphosarcoma.

malignant hemangioendothelioma. See **angiosarcoma.**

malignant hepatoma, a primary liver cancer. Also called **hepatocarcinoma, hepatocellular carcinoma, liver cell carcinoma.** See also **hepatoma, liver cancer.**

malignant hypertension, the most lethal form of hypertension, occurring most often in patients with a history of poorly controlled hypertension. It is a fulminating condition characterized by severely elevated blood pressure that commonly damages the intima of small vessels, the brain, the retina, the heart, and the kidneys. African-American men are at highest risk for the development of malignant hypertension. Also called **accelerated hypertension.** See also **essential hypertension.**

■ OBSERVATIONS: The blood pressure is 180/120 mm Hg or higher, and signs of organ damage are present. Papilledema will be present; changes to the vascular system of the kidneys are noted.

■ INTERVENTIONS: The patient is admitted to the intensive care unit for continuous cardiac monitoring and frequent assessment of neurological status. Urine output is monitored. Intravenous antihypertensive medications and fluids are administered, and care must be taken not to reduce blood pressure too rapidly. The patient's activity is restricted until the blood pressure has stabilized.

■ PATIENT CARE CONSIDERATIONS: At discharge, the health care team should ensure that the patient has appropriate access to follow-up care and is educated in the control of hypertension. Emphasis should be placed on medication adherence, diet, and physical exercise. A weight-loss program may be indicated.

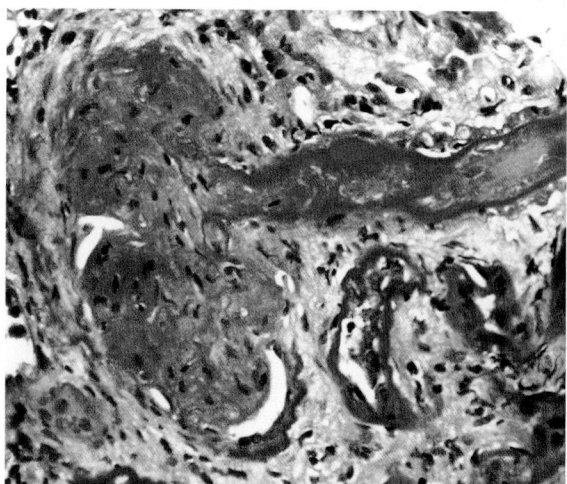

Necrosis of the arteriole in malignant hypertension
(Fogo and Kashgarian, 2012)

malignant hyperthermia (MH), a rare genetic hypermetabolic condition affecting skeletal muscle and occurring in affected people exposed to all halogenated inhalation anesthetics and/or succinylcholine. It is a life-threatening emergency and must be treated immediately. Compare **neuroleptic malignant syndrome.**

■ OBSERVATIONS: MH is characterized by muscle rigidity, rapid heart rate, high body temperature, muscle breakdown, and increased acid content.

■ INTERVENTIONS: Treatment includes discontinuation of the inhalational anesthetic; the administration of dantrolene sodium (Ryanodex®); administration of 100% oxygen; cooling; cessation of surgery; and correction of acidosis and hyperkalemia.

■ PATIENT CARE CONSIDERATIONS: Patients susceptible to malignant hyperthermia must be informed of the condition and susceptible relatives screened. The family is referred to the Malignant Hyperthermia Registry of the Malignant Hyperthermia Association of the United States (MHAUS). Individuals with confirmed malignant hyperthermia should wear a medical alert wristband.

Malignant Hyperthermia Association of the United States (MHAUS), an organization to promote optimum care and scientific understanding of malignant hyperthermia and related disorders. It maintains a hot line for 24-hour assistance and information. MHAUS is available in the United States and Canada at 1-800-MH-HYPER, or 1-800-644-9737, and outside the United States at 001-1-315-464-7079.

malignant malnutrition. See **kwashiorkor.**

malignant melanoma. See **melanoma.**

malignant mesenchymoma, a sarcoma that contains mesenchymal elements.

malignant mole. (Informal) See **melanoma.**

malignant neoplasm, a tumor that tends to grow, invade, and metastasize. The tumor usually has an irregular shape and is composed of poorly differentiated cells. If untreated, it may result in death.

malignant neuroma. See **neurosarcoma.**

malignant pustule. See **anthrax.**

malignant transformation, the changes that a normal cell undergoes as it becomes a cancerous cell. See also **carcinogenesis.**

malignant tumor, a neoplasm that characteristically invades surrounding tissue, metastasizes to distant sites, and contains anaplastic cells. A malignant tumor may cause death if treatment does not intervene.

malingering /məling″gəring/ [Fr, *malingre,* puny, weak], a willful and deliberate feigning of the symptoms of a disease or injury to gain some consciously desired end. *−malingerer, n., −malinger, v.*

malleable /mal″ē·ə·bəl/ [L, to beat], **1.** able to be pressed, hammered, or otherwise forced into a shape without breaking. **2.** a surgical instrument made of metal that can be molded to different shapes to assist in holding back tissues. Also called **ribbon retractor.**

mallei. See **malleus.**

malleolar fold, one of two folds, the anterior and posterior, on the surface of the tympanic membrane. See also **pars flaccida.**

malleolus /məlē″ələs/ *pl. malleoli* [L, little hammer], a rounded bony process, such as the protuberance on each side of the ankle.

malleolus fibulae. See **external malleolus.**

mallet deformity [ME, *maillet,* maul], a loss of the ability to extend the distal joint of a finger or toe. It may be caused by severe damage, such as rupture of the terminal tendon. See also **hammer finger, hammer toe.**

mallet finger. Also called **mallet deformity.** See **hammer finger.**

mallet fracture, a fracture in which the dorsal base fragment of a distal phalanx of a finger or toe is not contiguous with the rest of the phalange. The fracture disrupts the insertion of the distal portion of the extensor mechanism, resulting in a loss of active distal interphalangeal joint extension.

malleus /mal″ē·əs/ *pl. mallei* [L, hammer], one of the three ossicles in the middle ear, resembling a hammer with a head, neck, and three processes. It is connected to the tympanic membrane and transmits sound vibrations to the incus, which communicates with the stapes. Compare **incus, stapes.** See also **middle ear.**

Mallory body /mal″ərē/ [Frank B. Mallory, American pathologist, 1862–1941; AS, *bodig,* body], an eosinophilic cytoplasmic inclusion, alcoholic hyalin, found in the liver cells. It is typically, but not always, associated with acute alcoholic liver injury. See also **cirrhosis.**

Mallory-Weiss syndrome [G. Kenneth Mallory, American pathologist, 1900-1986; Soma Weiss, American physician, 1899-1942], a condition characterized by massive bleeding after a tear in the mucous membrane at the junction of the esophagus and the stomach. The laceration is usually caused by protracted vomiting, most commonly in alcoholics or in people whose pylorus is obstructed. The esophageal tear is located by esophagoscopy or arteriography. Surgery is usually necessary to stop the bleeding.

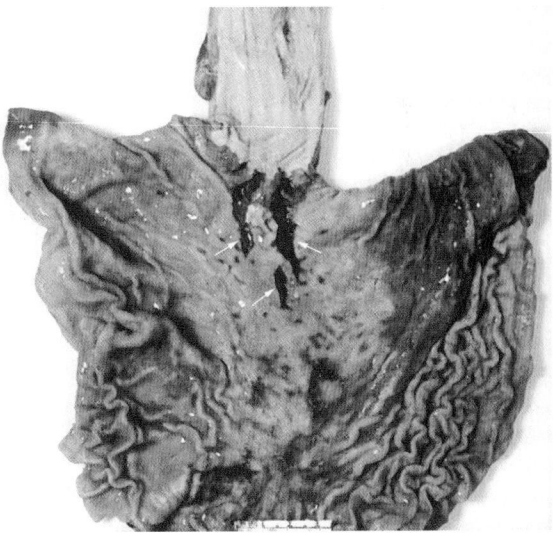

Tear (arrows) associated with Mallory-Weiss syndrome *(Finkbeiner et al, 2009)*

malnutrition /mal′nōōtrish″ən/ [L, *malus,* bad, *nutrire,* to nourish], any disorder of nutrition. It may result from an unbalanced, insufficient, or excessive diet or from impaired absorption, assimilation, or use of foods. Compare **deficiency disease.**

malocclusion /mal′əkloō″zhən/ [L, *malus + occludere,* to shut up], abnormal contact between the teeth of the upper jaw and those of the lower jaw. See also **Angle's classification of malocclusion, occlusion.**

malonic acid (CH₂(COOH)₂) /məlō″nik/, a white, crystalline, highly toxic substance used as an intermediate compound in the production of barbiturates; a dicarboxylic acid.

malpighian body /malpig″ē·ən/[Marcello Malpighi, Italian physician, 1628–1694; AS, *bodig,* body], **1.** the renal corpuscle, which includes a glomerulus with Bowman's capsule. **2.** lymphoid tissue surrounding the arteries of the spleen. Also called **lymphatic nodule.**

malpighian corpuscle [Marcello Malpighi; L, *corpusculum,* little body], one of a number of small, round, deep-red bodies in the cortex of the kidney, each communicating with a renal tubule. Malpighian corpuscles average about 0.2 mm in diameter, with each capsule composed of two parts: a central glomerulus and a glomerular capsule. The corpuscles are part of a filtering system through which nonprotein components of blood plasma enter the tubules for urinary excretion. Also called **malpighian body, renal corpuscle.**

malposition /mal′pəzish″ən/, a wrong or faulty placement of a body part, such as in an untreated fracture.

malpractice /malprak″tis/ [L, *malus* + Gk, *praktikos,* practical], (in law) professional negligence that is the proximate cause of injury or harm to a patient, resulting from a lack of professional knowledge, experience, or skill that can reasonably be expected in others in the profession in similar circumstances or from a failure to exercise reasonable care or judgment in the application of professional knowledge, experience, or skill. The four necessary elements essential to maintain a medical malpractice claim are duty, breach of duty, damages/injury, and causal connection between the breach and the injury. Kinds include **medical abandonment, negligence, omission.**

malpresentation /malpres′əntā″shən/ [L, *malus,* bad, *praesentare,* to show], any presentation in the birth canal other than a vertex presentation.

malrotated kidney, a kidney that failed to rotate properly during its ascent from the pelvis in prenatal development, usually with the hilum facing anteriorly instead of anteromedially.

malrotation /mal′rōtā″shən/, **1.** any abnormal rotation of an organ or body part, such as the vertebral column or a tooth. **2.** a failure of the intestinal tract or other viscera to undergo normal rotation during embryonic development.

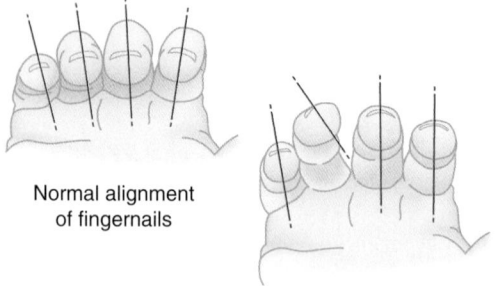

Normal alignment of fingernails

Alignment of fingernails with malrotation of ring finger

Malrotation *(Marx et al/Redrawn from Jobe MT, Calandruccio JH: Fractures, dislocations and ligamentous injuries; In Canale and Beaty, 2008)*

malt /môlt/ [AS, *mealt*], a preparation obtained from germinated grain, such as barley, that contains partially degraded starch and protein with nutritive and digestive properties.

Malta fever. See **brucellosis.**

maltitol /mawl′tītol/, a hydrogenated, partially hydrolyzed starch used as a sweetener.

malt soup extract, an extract of malt from barley grains, containing also a small amount of polymeric carbohydrates, proteins, electrolytes, and vitamins, administered orally as a bulk-forming laxative.

malunion /malyoo͞″nyən/ [L, *malus* + *unus,* one], an imperfect union of previously fragmented bone or other tissue. Causes of bone malunion include osteomyelitis and improper immobilization of a fracture.

malware, malicious codes that affect the security or function of a computer system.

mamillary body /mam″iler′ē/ [L, *mammilla,* nipple; AS, *bodig,* body], either of the two small round masses of gray

matter in the hypothalamus located close to one another in the interpeduncular space. They may be involved with olfactory reflexes.

mamm-, combining form meaning "mammary gland" or "breast": *mammogram, pseudomamma.*

mammary /mam″ərē/ [L, *mamma,* breast], pertaining to the breast.

mammary duct. See **lactiferous duct.**

mammary glands [L, *mamma,* breast, *glans,* acorn], lactiferous glands within the breasts. Glandular tissue forms a radius of lobes containing alveoli, each lobe having a system of ducts for the passage of milk from the alveoli to the nipple. The central part of the breast is filled with glandular tissue. Also called **breast.** See also **lactation.**

mammary papilla. See **nipple.**

mammary region, the part of the pectoral region surrounding the mammary gland.

mammogram /mam″əgram/ [L, *mamma* + Gk, *gramma,* record], radiographic imaging of the soft tissues of the breast.

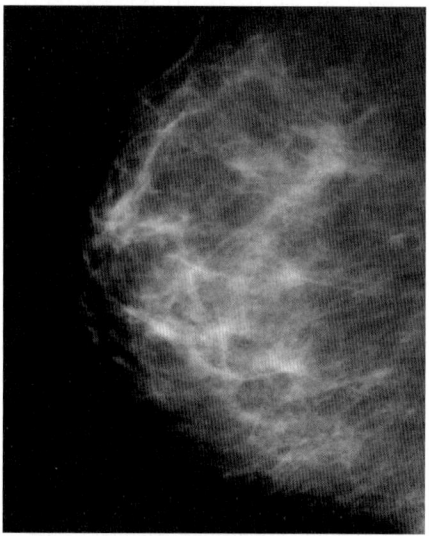

Mammogram

mammography /mamog″rəfē/, the radiographic examination of the soft tissues of the breast. It is used to identify various benign and malignant neoplastic processes.

Mammography Quality Standards Act (MQSA), an act passed into law in the United States in 1992 that requires all mammography facilities to be accredited.

mammoplasty /mam′əplas′tē/ [L, *mamma* + Gk, *plassein,* to mold], plastic reshaping of the breasts, performed to reduce or lift large or sagging breasts, to enlarge small breasts, or to reconstruct a breast after removal of a tumor. To reduce the size of the breasts and raise them, excess tissue is removed from the underside of the breasts. The breast is then lifted, and the nipple drawn through an opening in an overhanging skin flap. To enlarge a breast, a saline-filled or silicone gel prosthesis is inserted in a pocket formed beneath the breast on the chest wall. Potential complications after surgery include infection or rejection by tissues when foreign body implants are used.

MammoSite, brand name for a system for post-lumpectomy breast cancer treatment with targeted radiation. See also **balloon catheter radiation, brachytherapy.**

mammothermography /mam′ōthərmog″rəfē/ [L, *mamma* + Gk, *therme,* heat, *graphein,* to record], a diagnostic procedure in which the breast is examined for abnormal growths by means of a heat-sensitive probe that detects regional differences in blood flow. Compare **mammography.** See also **thermography.**

mammotroph, *(Obsolete)* a cell that produces prolactin. Now called *prolactin-secreting cell.*

man-, combining form meaning "hand": *bimanual, manual.*

managed care, a health care system with administrative control over primary health care services in a medical group practice. The intention is to eliminate redundant facilities and services and to reduce costs. Health education and preventive medicine are emphasized. Patients may pay a flat fee for basic family care but may be charged additional fees for secondary care services. The system of managed care evolved after World War II from the traditional fee for service, in which the patient paid the physician directly for services performed; through a shift toward health insurance organizations, which paid physicians and hospitals from premiums paid by the patients to the insurers; to the advent in the 1960s of government programs, such as Medicare and Medicaid. In the 1980s another economic shift, originating in California, led to the concept of health maintenance organizations (HMOs), with large corporations initially negotiating with groups of health care workers for financing of medical and hospital expenses of the corporation's employees. HMOs also began enrolling individual patients and by the mid-1990s challenged the survival of the traditional insurance systems. See also **health maintenance organization.**

managed care organization (MCO), an organization that combines the functions of health insurance, delivery of care, and administration. Examples include the independent practice association, third-party administrator, management service organization, and physician-hospital organization.

management service organization (MSO), an entity that under contract provides services such as a facility, equipment, staffing, contract negotiation, administration, and marketing. Services may be provided to solo practitioners or groups. Approaches to establishment of the MSO include the hospital-related MSO; the provider-of-care, hospital-related, tax-exempt clinic MSO; and the nonprofit, hospital-sponsored equity MSO.

Mandelamine, an antibacterial agent. Brand name for **methenamine.**

mandible /man″dibəl/ [L, *mandere,* to chew], a large U-shaped bone constituting the lower jaw. It contains the lower teeth and consists of a horizontal part, a body, and two perpendicular rami that join the body at almost right angles. The body of the mandible is curved, somewhat resembling a horseshoe, and has two surfaces and two borders. The superior border of the mandible contains sockets for the 16 lower teeth. It is the only bone in the human body where both condylar joints always have to move congruously. The inferior border provides a groove for the facial artery. Compare **maxilla.**

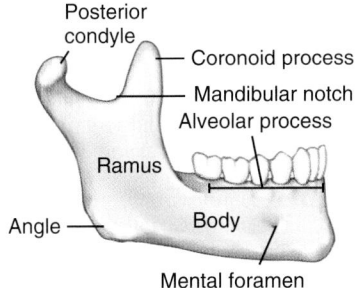

Posterior condyle
Coronoid process
Mandibular notch
Alveolar process
Ramus
Angle
Body
Mental foramen

Mandible

mandibular arch /mandib″yələr/ [L, *mandere,* to chew, *arcus,* bow], the first visceral arch from which the lower jawbone develops.

mandibular block, regional anesthesia of the lower jaw produced by injection of a local anesthetic near the mandibular division of the trigeminal nerve.

mandibular canal [L, *mandere,* to chew, *canalis,* channel], a passage or channel that extends from the mandibular foramen on the medial surface of the ramus of the mandible to the mental foramen. It holds mandibular blood vessels and a part of the mandibular branch of the trigeminal nerve.

mandibular foramen, the opening on the medial surface of the ramus for the transmission of the inferior alveolar nerve and vessels.

mandibular fossa [L, *mandere,* to chew, *fossa,* ditch], a prominent depression in the inferior surface of the squamous part of the temporal bone at the base of the zygomatic process, in which the condyle of the mandible articulates. Also called **glenoid cavity, glenoid fossa.**

mandibular nerve, the largest of the three branches of the trigeminal nerve. Its branches innervate the ear, the cheek, the skin and mucous membrane of the lower lip, the skin of the chin, the teeth and related gingivae, the tongue, and the muscles of the cheek and jaw.

mandibular notch, a depression in the inferior border of the mandible, anterior to the attachments of the masseter muscle, where the external facial muscles cross the inferior border of the mandible. It is a landmark that may be accentuated by arrested condylar growth and other developmental disturbances of the mandible.

mandibular process [L, *mandere,* to chew, *processus*], **1.** the upper alveolar part of the mandible. **2.** the projection of the upper posterior part of the ramus of the mandible bearing the condyle.

mandibular ramus [L, *mandere,* to chew, *ramus,* branch], a broad quadrilateral part of the mandible projecting upward from the posterior end of the body behind the lower teeth. It has two surfaces, four borders, and two processes.

mandibular reflex [L, *mandere,* to chew, *reflectere,* to bend back]. See **jaw jerk.**

mandibular retrusion, mandibular retroposition. See **retrognathia.**

mandibular sling, the connection between the mandible and the maxilla, formed by the masseter and the pterygoideus at the angle of the mandible. When the mouth is opened and closed, the mandible moves around a center of rotation formed by the mandibular sling and the sphenomandibular ligament.

mandibular spine, a protuberance on the mandibular ramus to which the sphenomandibular ligament is attached.

mandibular symphysis, a small vertical ridge that marks the fusion of the left and right parts of the mandible.

mandibular torus, *pl. tori,* a nonneoplastic external bony overgrowth commonly found on the lingual surface of the mandible; it is caused by genetics and environmental conditions such as bruxism. Tori are located bilaterally or unilaterally in the area of the lower canine and first premolar regions. Tori can appear radiopaque in radiographic or dental images. No treatment is necessary unless there is interference with chewing, recurring trauma, or placement of a dental prosthesis. See also **torus palatinus, palatine torus.** Compare **buccal exostosis.**

mandibulofacial dysostosis /mandib′yəlofā″shəl/ [L, *mandere* + *facies,* face; Gk, *dys,* bad, *osteon,* bone], an abnormal hereditary condition characterized by a downward slant of the palpebral fissures, coloboma of the lower lid, an undersized jaw and hypoplasia of the zygomatic arches, and

M

an underdeveloped external ear. Evidence indicates that this disorder is transmitted as an autosomal-dominant trait. The condition occurs in the complete form as Franceschetti syndrome and in the incomplete form as Treacher Collins syndrome. See also **dysostosis.**

Mandol, a cephalosporin antibiotic. Brand name for **cefamandole nafate.**

mandras foot. See **paraactinomycosis.**

mandrel /man″drəl/ [Fr, *mandrin,* boring tool], the shaft of an object, such as a dental polishing disk, cutting device, or sharpening stone, that is inserted into a handpiece or lathe and supports the object while it rotates.

maneuver /mənoo″vər/ [Fr, *manœvre,* action], **1.** an adroit or skillful manipulation or procedure. **2.** (in obstetrics) a manipulation of the fetus, performed to aid in delivery.

mangafodipir /mang″gäfo′dipir/, a contrast-enhancing agent used to improve the images obtained in magnetic resonance imaging of hepatic lesions, administered intravenously as the trisodium salt.

manganese (Mn) /mang″gənēs/ [L, *manganesium,* associated with magnesium], a common metallic element found in trace amounts in tissues of the body, where it aids in the functions of various enzymes. Its atomic number is 25; its atomic mass is 54.938.

manganese nodule, a small node produced by microbial reduction of manganese oxides.

mange /mānj/, a cutaneous disease of domestic and wild animals caused by skin-burrowing mites. See also **scabies.**

mania /mā″nē·ə/ [Gk, madness], a mood characterized by an unstable expansive emotional state; extreme excitement; excessive elation; hyperactivity; agitation; overtalkativeness; flight of ideas; increased psychomotor activity; fleeting attention; and sometimes violent, destructive, and self-destructive behavior, delusions, or hallucinations.

-mania, -manic, 1. suffix meaning a "state of mental disorder." **2.** suffix meaning "a state of psychosis": *megalomania.*

-maniac, 1. suffix meaning "a person exhibiting a type of psychosis": *pyromaniac.* **2.** suffix meaning "a person revealing an inordinate interest in something": *egomaniac, nymphomaniac.*

manic. See **mania.**

manic depressive. See **bipolar disorder.**

manifest deviation. See **eye deviation.**

manifest image, the change on an x-ray image that becomes visible when the latent image undergoes appropriate processing.

manipulation /mənip′yəlā″shən/ [L, *manipulare,* to work with the hands], the skillful use of the hands in therapeutic or diagnostic procedures, such as palpation, reduction of a dislocation, turning a fetus, or various treatments in physical therapy and osteopathy. Kinds include **conjoined manipulation.** See also **massage,** def. 1.

manipulative behavior, deceptive or underhanded efforts to maintain control or have one's own way when interacting with others.

mediate percussion. See **percussion.**

mannitol /man″itol/, a poorly metabolized sugar used as an osmotic diuretic and in kidney function tests.

■ INDICATIONS: It is prescribed to promote diuresis, decrease intraocular and intracranial pressure, promote the excretion of poisons and other toxic wastes, and evaluate renal function.

■ CONTRAINDICATIONS: Pulmonary edema, dehydration, or known hypersensitivity to this drug prohibits its use.

■ ADVERSE EFFECTS: Among the more serious adverse effects are pulmonary edema, heart failure, hyponatremia, headache, vomiting, and confusion.

mannose /man″ōs/, a monosaccharide sugar of the aldose group, found as part of many glycolipids and glycoproteins.

mannosidosis /man′ō·si·dō′sis/, a lysosomal storage disease caused by an enzymatic defect in the metabolism of mannose-containing glycoproteins, resulting in accumulation of oligosaccharides. Characteristics include coarse facies, upper respiratory congestion and infections, profound cognitive deficits, hepatosplenomegaly, cataracts, radiographic signs of skeletal abnormalities, and gibbus deformity. Mannosidosis is divided into type I (infantile onset) and type II (juvenile-adult onset). A severe form manifested as prenatal loss or early death affects the central nervous system (type III). Also called *alpha-mannosidosis.*

■ OBSERVATIONS: Characteristics include coarse facies, upper respiratory congestion and infections, profound cognitive deficits, hepatosplenomegaly, cataracts, radiographic signs of skeletal abnormalities, and gibbus deformity.

■ INTERVENTIONS: Bone marrow transplant has been used with success in some children. Enzymatic treatments are in clinical trials.

■ PATIENT CARE CONSIDERATIONS: Symptoms range from mild to severe. A coordinated approach by the health care team can increase the quality of life for the individual and family.

Mann-Whitney test, Mann-Whitney U test. See **rank sum test.**

manoeuvre. See **maneuver.**

manometer /mənom″ətər/ [Gk, *manos,* thin, *metron,* measure], a device for measuring the pressure of a fluid or gas.

-manometer, suffix meaning "an instrument to measure pressure": *sphygmomanometer.*

manometry /mənom″ətrē/ [Gk, *manos,* thin, *metron,* measure], **1.** the science of pressure movements of liquids or gases. **2.** a technique for measuring changes in the pressure of a gas or liquid that result from a biological or chemical action.

Mansonella /man′sənel″ə/, a genus of nematodes of the superfamily Filarioidea, found in Central and South America and Africa. *M. ozzardi* and *M. perstans* are two species that parasitize humans and cause mild symptoms. See also **mansonellosis.**

Mansonella ozzardi /man′sənel″ə/, a parasitic worm that is indigenous to much of Latin America and the Caribbean islands. It is a relatively benign nematode that infects humans, sometimes causing hydrocele or lymphadenopathy. The larvae live in the bloodstream, and adult worms are found in the visceral mesenteries. The intermediate hosts are biting flies of the genus *Culicoides.*

Mansonella perstans, a long, threadlike worm usually found in Africa. It commonly infects wild and domestic animals and occasionally invades the bloodstream of humans, causing a rash, muscle and joint pains, various neurological disorders, and nodules in the subcutaneous tissues. The larvae are also found in the cerebrospinal fluid of affected patients.

mansonellosis /man′sənelō′sis/, a rare tropical infectious disease caused by nematodes of the genus *Mansonella.* It can cause skin rashes, muscle and joint pains, neurological disorders, and skin lumps. It is mainly found in Africa. The parasite is transmitted through the bite of small flies. Also called **acanthocheilonemiasis.**

mantle cell lymphoma /man″təl/, a rare form of non-Hodgkin lymphoma having a usually diffuse pattern. It mainly affects people over 50 years of age and runs an indolent course, although it may metastasize to the spleen or liver. See also **non-Hodgkin lymphoma.**

Mantoux test /mantoo″/ [Charles Mantoux, French physician, 1877–1947], a tuberculin skin test that consists of intradermal injection of a purified protein derivative of the tubercle bacillus. A hardened, raised red area of 8 to 10 mm, appearing 24 to 72 hours after injection, is a positive reaction. See also **tuberculin test.**

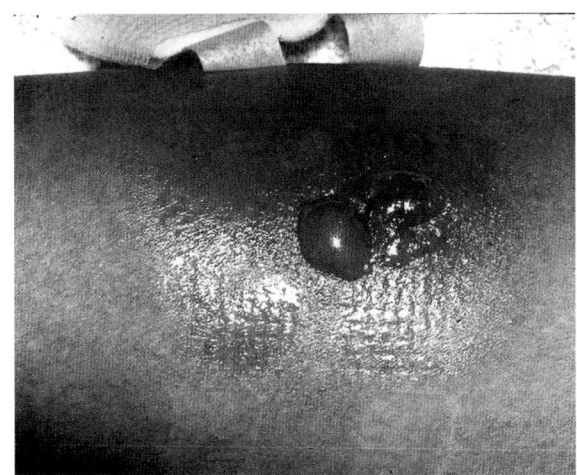

Strongly positive Mantoux test *(Taussig and Landau, 2008)*

manual lymph drainage, the application of light rhythmic strokes, similar to those used in effleurage, to the skin and superficial fascia in the direction of the heart to increase the drainage of lymph from the involved structures. It can be used to reduce edema surrounding fractures. There is no current evidence of efficacy to reduce lymphedema in women with breast cancer.

manual rotation /man″yoo-əl/ [L, *manualis,* hand, *rotare,* to turn], an obstetric maneuver in which a baby's head is turned by hand from a transverse to an anteroposterior position in the birth canal to facilitate delivery. Compare **forceps rotation.**

manubrial, resembling a handle. See **manubrium.**

manubriosternal articulation /mənoo′brē-ōstur″nəl/ [L, *manubrium,* handle; Gk, *sternum,* chest; L, *articularis,* joints], the fibrocartilaginous connection between the manubrium and the body of the sternum. This joint usually closes by 25 years of age. Compare **xiphisternal articulation.**

manubrium /mənoo″brē-əm/ [L, handle], the most anterior of the three bones of the sternum, presenting a broad quadrangular shape that narrows caudally at its articulation with the superior end of the body of the sternum. The pectoralis major and the sternocleidomastoideus are attached to the manubrium. Compare **xiphoid process.** –**manubrial,** *adj.*

manudynamometer /man″oodī′nəmom″ətər/ [L, *manus,* hand; Gk, *dynamis,* force, *metron,* measure], a device for measuring the force or extent of thrust.

manus. See **hand.**

MAO, **1.** abbreviation for **monoamine oxidase. 2.** abbreviation for **maximal acid output.**

MAOI, abbreviation for **monoamine oxidase inhibitor.**

MAO inhibitor, abbreviation for **monoamine oxidase inhibitor.**

MAP, **1.** abbreviation for **mean arterial pressure. 2.** abbreviation for **Miller Assessment of Preschoolers.**

map distance. See **map unit.**

maple bark disease [AS, *mapul* + ONorse, *bark* + L, *dis,* opposite of; Fr, *aise,* ease], a hypersensitivity pneumonitis caused by exposure to the mold *Cryptostroma corticale,* found in the bark of maple trees.

■ OBSERVATIONS: In the susceptible person the condition may be acute, accompanied by fever, cough, dyspnea, and vomiting, or chronic, characterized by fatigue, weight loss, dyspnea on exertion, and a productive cough.

■ INTERVENTIONS: In an acute or severe case a short course of prednisone may be used to control the symptoms; avoiding exposure to the bark prevents further reaction.

■ PATIENT CARE CONSIDERATIONS: Although differential diagnosis may be difficult, a thorough occupational history may reveal the cause and source of exposure.

maple syrup urine disease (MSUD) [AS, *mapul* + Ar, *sharab* + Gk, *ouron,* urine], an inherited metabolic disorder in which an enzyme necessary for the breakdown of the amino acids valine, leucine, and isoleucine is lacking. The disease is usually diagnosed in infancy. It is recognized by the characteristic maple syrup odor of the urine and by hyperreflexia. Stress, fever, and infection aggravate the condition. The long-term treatment team for a child with MSUD should include a metabolic specialist and a dietitian to ensure that the child is provided with the protein and nutrients needed for healthy growth and development with appropriate dietary restrictions. Also called **branched-chain ketoaciduria.**

mapping [L, *mappa,* napkin], the process of locating the relative position of genes on a chromosome through the analysis of genetic recombination. Distances between genes in a linkage group are expressed in map units or morgans. Also called **chromosome mapping.**

maprotiline hydrochloride /maprō″tilēn/, a tetracyclic antidepressant similar to the tricyclics.

■ INDICATIONS: It is prescribed for the treatment of depression.

■ CONTRAINDICATIONS: It is used with caution in conditions in which anticholinergics are contraindicated, in seizure disorders, and in cardiovascular disorders. Concomitant administration of monoamine oxidase inhibitors, recent myocardial infarction, or known hypersensitivity to this drug prohibits its use.

■ ADVERSE EFFECTS: Among the more serious adverse effects are sedation and anticholinergic side effects. A variety of GI, cardiovascular, and neurological reactions (including convulsions) may occur. Like the tricyclics, it is involved in many potential drug interactions.

map unit [L, *mappa,* napkin, *unus,* one], an arbitrary unit of measure used to express the distance between genes on a chromosome. It is calculated from the percentage of recombinations that occur between specific genes so that 1% of crossing over represents one unit on a genetic map, or approximately the number of new combinations that can be detected. The measurement is accurate only for small distances because double crossovers do not appear as new recombinations. Also called **map distance.** See also **morgan.**

marasmic kwashiorkor /məraz″mik/ [Gk, *marasmos,* a wasting; Afr], a malnutrition disease, primarily of children, resulting from the deficiency of both calories and protein. The condition is characterized by severe tissue wasting, dehydration, loss of subcutaneous fat, lethargy, and growth delay. See also **kwashiorkor, marasmus.**

marasmoid /mərāz″moid/, pertaining to severe undernourishment in children. See also **marasmus.**

marasmus /məraz″məs/ [Gk, *marasmos,* a wasting], a condition of extreme malnutrition and emaciation, occurring chiefly in young children. It is characterized by progressive

M

wasting of subcutaneous tissue and muscle. Marasmus results from a lack of adequate calories and proteins and is seen in children with failure to thrive and in individuals in a state of starvation. Less commonly it results from an inability to assimilate or use protein because of a defect in metabolism. Care of the marasmic child involves the reestablishment of fluid and electrolyte balance, followed by the slow and gradual addition of foods as they are tolerated. See also **kwashiorkor.**

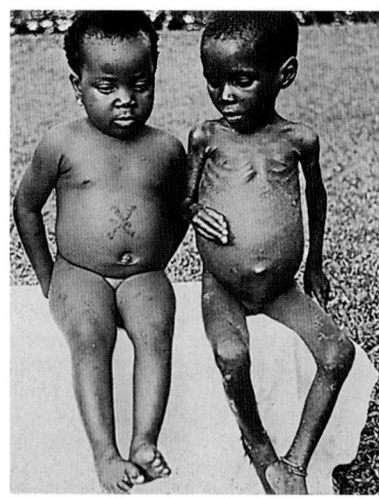

The child on the right exhibits marked muscle wasting with no edema, characteristic of marasmus. The other child pictured does not have a nutritional deficiency
(Shetty, 2006)

marathon encounter group /mer″əthon/ [Marathon, Greece; L, *in,* in, *contra,* against; Fr, *groupe*], an intensive group experience that accelerates self-awareness and promotes personal growth and behavioral change through the continuous interaction of group members for a period ranging from 16 to more than 40 hours. See also **encounter group.**

maraviroc, an antiretroviral drug.
■ INDICATIONS: This drug is used to treat HIV infection in combination with other antiretroviral agents.
■ CONTRAINDICATIONS: Known hypersensitivity to this drug prohibits its use.
■ ADVERSE EFFECTS: Adverse effects of this drug include dizziness, depression, disturbances in consciousness, peripheral neuropathy, paresthesia, dysesthesia, fever, gingival hyperplasia, diarrhea, constipation, dyspepsia, rash, urticaria, pruritus, folliculitis, joint pain, leg pain, muscle cramps, cough, upper respiratory infection, sinusitis, bronchitis, pneumonia, and herpes virus. Life-threatening side effects include MI, cardiac ischemia, bronchospasm, orthostatic hypotension, viral meningitis, pseudomembranous colitis, hepatotoxicity, and respiratory obstruction.

Marax, a fixed-combination respiratory drug containing a smooth muscle relaxant, an adrenergic drug, and an antihistamine. Brand name for **theophylline,** *ephedrine sulfate,* **hydrOXYzine hydrochloride.**

marble bones. See **osteopetrosis.**

Marburg virus disease /mär″bərg/, a severe febrile viral disease characterized by rash, hepatitis, pancreatitis, and severe GI hemorrhages. The disease is caused by the Marburg virus, a member of the Filoviridae family, which also includes the Ebola virus. There is no cure; treatment is supportive. Also called **hemorrhagic fever.** See also **Ebola virus disease.**

Marcaine Hydrochloride, a local anesthetic. Brand name for **bupivacaine hydrochloride.**

march /märch/, the progression of electrical activity through the motor cortex.

Marchesani syndrome. See **Weill-Marchesani syndrome.**

march foot [Fr, *marcher,* to walk; AS, *fot*], an abnormal condition of the foot caused by excessive use, such as in a long march. The forefoot is swollen and painful, and one or more of the metatarsal bones may be broken. See also **stress fracture.**

march fracture. *(Informal)* See **metatarsal stress fracture.**

march hemoglobinuria, a rare abnormal condition, characterized by the presence of hemoglobin in the urine, that occurs after strenuous physical exertion or prolonged exercise, such as marching or distance running.

Marchiafava-Micheli disease /märʹkyəfäʺvə mikāʺlē/ [Ettore Marchiafava, Italian physician, 1847–1935; F. Micheli, Italian physician, 1872–1929], a rare disorder of unknown origin characterized by abnormally high levels of hemoglobin in the urine, occurring episodically, usually (but not always) at night.

Marchi globule /märʺkē/ [Vittoria Marchi, Italian physician, 1851-1908], fragments and particles of broken-up myelin that stain by Marchi's method, seen in degeneration of the spinal cord. See also **globule.**

Marchi's method, a laboratory staining procedure for demonstrating degenerated nerve fibers. The tissue specimen is first fixed in a solution of potassium bichromate (Müller's fluid), which prevents normal nerve fibers from being stained with osmic acid; osmic acid is then applied as a definitive black stain for abnormal nerve fibers.

Marcus Gunn pupil sign [Robert Marcus Gunn, English ophthalmologist, 1850–1909], paradoxic dilation of the pupils in an ophthalmological examination in response to afferent visual stimuli. In a dark room a beam of light is moved from one eye to the other. Normal miosis is caused by the consensual pupil reaction when the normal eye is illuminated, but as the light is moved to the opposite, abnormal eye, the direct reaction to light is weaker than the consensual reaction; hence both pupils dilate.

Marcus Gunn syndrome. See **jaw-winking.**

Marezine, an antiemetic. Brand name for **cyclizine hydrochloride.**

Marfan syndrome /märfäN″/ [Bernard-Jean A. Marfan, French pediatrician, 1858–1942], a hereditary condition that affects the musculoskeletal system and is often associated with abnormalities of the cardiovascular system and the eyes. Inherited as an autosomal-dominant trait, Marfan syndrome affects men and women equally.
■ OBSERVATIONS: Its major musculoskeletal effects include muscular underdevelopment, ligamentous laxity, joint hypermobility, and bone elongation. The extremities of individuals with Marfan syndrome are very long and spiderlike, with arachnodactyly. Most adult patients are over 6 feet (1.8 meters) tall and have asymmetric skulls. Funnel chest is common, and a lateral curvature of the spine may develop and increase during years of rapid vertebral growth, with kyphoscoliosis developing to varying degrees. The severe ligamental laxity and joint hypermobility associated with Marfan syndrome may be seen by radiographic examination and often result in pes valgus and back knee. Pathological alterations of the cardiovascular system appear to produce fragmentation of the elastic fibers in the media of the aorta, which may lead to

aneurysm. Ocular changes include a variety of disorders, including dislocation of the lens. Marfan syndrome does not affect intelligence.

■ INTERVENTIONS: No specific treatment is available, and symptomatic management of the associated problems is the usual alternative. Resulting deformities, such as kyphoscoliosis, may be treated with orthoses or surgery, as indicated.

■ PATIENT CARE CONSIDERATIONS: Health care professionals in schools are in a unique position to both identify students in need of an evaluation for Marfan syndrome and to ensure that students with the syndrome are engaged in appropriate physical and psychosocial activities. Although Marfan syndrome cannot be cured, with proper treatment and management a productive and satisfying life and career are possible.

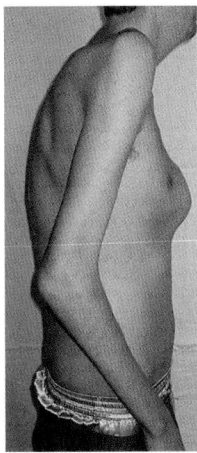

A funnel chest and a lateral curvature of the spine associated with Marfan syndrome *(Demetracopoulos and Sponseller, 2007)*

margin, (in dentistry) the mechanical preparation of a ledge to which a dental restoration meets natural tooth structure. Margins may occur above the gingiva (supragingival) and/or below the gingiva (subgingival). Compare **bevel,** def. 2, **butt, shoulder, chamfer.**

marginal gingiva /mär″jənəl/ [L, *margo,* margin, *gingiva,* gum], the uppermost part of the free gingiva. In health it overlaps the neck and base of the crown of the tooth. During disease states the marginal gingiva can migrate toward the incisal or occlusal portion of the teeth because of edema or swelling; or apical migration or recession may occur.

marginal gyrus [L, *margo,* margin; Gk, *gyros,* turn], the superior frontal convolution on the surface of the cerebral hemispheres.

marginal peptic ulcer [L, *margo,* margin; Gk, *peptein,* to digest; L, *ulcus,* ulcer], an ulcer that develops postoperatively at the surgical anastomosis of the stomach and jejunum. See also **peptic ulcer.**

marginal placenta previa, placenta previa in which the placenta is implanted in the lower uterine segment, with its margin within 2 cm of the internal os of the uterine cervix. During labor as the cervix dilates, bleeding may occur from the separation of the edge of the placenta from the uterus beneath it. Bleeding may be so scant as to pose no clinical problem. In some cases, frank severe hemorrhage may occur, but the pressure of the presenting part of the baby is often sufficient to act as a tamponade, arresting the hemorrhage. Diagnosis of marginal placenta previa may be suggested by the apparent location of the placenta on ultrasonic visualization. Cesarean section is not usually necessary. See also **placenta previa.**

marginal ridge, an elevation of enamel that forms the proximal boundary of the occlusal surface of a tooth.

marginal sinus [L, *margo + sinus,* hollow], a sinus that may encircle the placenta. Also called **placental sinus.**

marginal sinus rupture, a detachment of the placenta from the implantation site. It may be complete, partial, or marginal in abruptio placentae.

margin of safety, an index of a drug's effectiveness and safety. It is calculated as the amount of drug that is lethal to 1% of animals (LD_1) divided by the amount of drug that causes a beneficial effect in 99% of the animals (ED_{99}). See also **dose-response relationship.**

Marie's hypertrophy [Pierre Marie, French neurologist, 1853–1940; Gk, *hyper,* excess, *trophe,* nourishment], chronic enlargement of the joints caused by periostitis. It may be associated with lung cancer. Also called **hypertrophic pulmonary osteopathy.**

Marie-Strümpell arthritis, Marie-Strümpell disease. See **ankylosing spondylitis.**

marijuana. See **cannabis.**

Marin Amat syndrome [Manuel Marin Amat, Spanish ophthalmologist, b. 1879], an involuntary facial movement in which the eyes close when the mouth opens or when the jaws move in mastication. The phenomenon results from a facial nerve paralysis. Also called **inverse Marcus Gunn syndrome.**

Marinesco-Sjögren syndrome /märēnes″kōshur″gren/ [Georges Marinesco, Romanian neurologist, 1863–1938; Karl Gustav Torsten Sjögren, Swedish physician, 1896–1974], a hereditary syndrome transmitted as an autosomal-recessive trait, consisting of cerebellar ataxia; mild to moderate intellectual disability and somatic growth delay; congenital cataracts; inability to chew; thin, brittle fingernails; and sparse, incompletely keratinized hair.

Marinol, an oral antiemetic drug. Brand name for **dronabinol.**

marital rape [L, *rapere,* to seize], forcible sexual intercourse with a spouse.

marital therapy, a type of family therapy aimed at understanding and treating one or both members of a couple in the context of a distressed relationship, but not necessarily addressing the discordant relationship itself. In the past the term has also been used more restrictively as synonymous with marriage therapy, but that is increasingly considered a subset of marital therapy. Also called **couples' therapy.**

mark [AS, *mearc*], any nevus or birthmark.

marker gene. See **genetic marker.**

markers [AS, *mearc*], **1.** body language movements that serve as indicators and punctuation marks in interpersonal communication. **2.** substances associated with some cancers that are detected in higher-than-normal amounts in the blood, urine, or body tissue.

mark:space ratio, (in electronics) the ratio of the duration of the positive-amplitude part of a square wave to that of the negative-amplitude part. See also **duty cycle.**

Maroteaux-Lamy syndrome /märōtō′ lämē′/ [Pierre Maroteaux, French physician, b. 1926; Maurice Emile Joseph Lamy, French physician, 1895–1975], a mucopolysaccharidosis characterized biochemically by the predominance of the mucopolysaccharide dermatan sulfate in the urine and the presence of coarse granules in the leukocytes and clinically by Hurler-like signs with normal intelligence. There are three clinical forms: the severe or classic form shows Hurler-like symptoms; the intermediate form has the same phenotype as pseudo-Hurler polydystrophy; and the mild form is difficult to distinguish from Scheie syndrome. Also called *mucopolysaccharidosis VI.* Compare **Scheie syndrome.** See also **Hurler syndrome, pseudo-Hurler polydystrophy.**

Marplan, an antidepressant drug. Abbreviation for **isocarboxazid.**

marriage therapy, a subset of marital therapy that focuses specifically on enhancing and preserving the bond of marriage between two people.

marrow. See **bone marrow.**

Marseilles fever /märsälz″, märsä″/ [Marseille, France; L, *febris,* fever], a disease endemic around the Mediterranean, in Africa, in the Crimea, and in India, caused by *Rickettsia conorii* transmitted by the brown dog tick *(Rhipicephalus sanguineus).* Characteristic symptoms are chills, fever, an ulcer covered with a black crust at the site of the tick bite, and a rash appearing on the second to fourth day. Also called **boutonneuse fever, Conor disease, escharonodulaire, Indian tick fever, Kenya fever.**

Marshall-Marchetti-Krantz procedure, a surgical procedure performed to correct stress incontinence. The vesicourethropexy involves a retropubic incision and suturing of the urethra, vesicle neck, and bladder to the posterior surface of the pubic bone. Also called *Marshall-Marchetti operation.*

marsupialize /märsoo″pē·əlīz/ [L, *marsupium,* pouch; Gk, *izein,* to cause], to form a pouch surgically to treat a cyst when simple removal would not be effective, such as in a pancreatic or a pilonidal cyst. The cyst sac is opened and emptied. Its edges are sutured to adjacent tissues, and a drain is left in place. Secretions decrease over a period of several months and may eventually cease.

Martinsen, Kari, a nursing theorist who proposed a philosophy of caring in reaction to social and health care inequalities and what she considered nursing's uncritical adoption of science as the basis for nursing. It involves a collectivist vision of humanity in which the individual is dependent upon the community and creation, or nature, and caring rather than control should be the guiding philosophy. As it relates to nursing, caring is simultaneously relational, practical, and moral. Caring involves concrete action based on education and training, without which concern for the patient is mere sentimentality.

Martorell syndrome. See **Takayasu arteritis.**

MAS, abbreviation for **mobile arm support.**

mAs, abbreviation for **milliampere-second.**

masculine /mas″kyəlin/ [L, *masculinus,* male], having the characteristics of a male.

masculinization /mas′kyəlin′izā″shən/ [L, *masculinus* + Gk, *izein,* to cause], the normal development or induction of male sex characteristics. See also **virilization.** −*masculinize, v.*

MASER /mā″sər/, abbreviation for *microwave amplification by stimulated emission of radiation.*

mask [Fr, *masque*], **1.** *v.,* to obscure, as in symptomatic treatment that may conceal the development of a disease. **2.** *v.,* to cover, as does a skin-toned cosmetic that may hide a pigmented nevus. **3.** *n.,* a cover worn over the nose and mouth to prevent inhalation of toxic or irritating materials, to control delivery of oxygen or anesthetic gas, or (by medical personnel) to shield a patient during aseptic procedures from pathogenic organisms normally exhaled from the respiratory tract. Surgical masks are worn by workers to help control the operating room environment during a patient procedure.

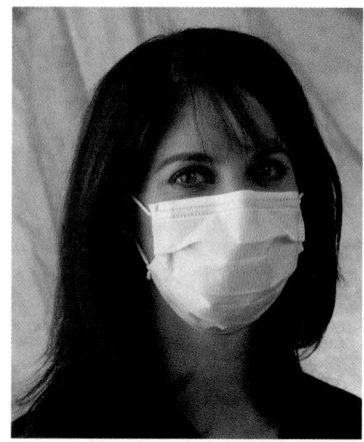

Mask *(Courtesy Medline Industries)*

masked facies. See **parkinsonian facies.**

masked residue, the amino acid part of a peptide that is not accessible for activity after a condensation reaction.

mask image, a radiographic image made either before or immediately after contrast material has been injected but before it reaches the anatomical site being examined. The image thus produced is stored in a computer and displayed on a video monitor. It is then subtracted electronically from a series of additional images. The technique enhances the image of the tissues being studied. See also **remasking.**

masking, **1.** the covering or concealing of a disorder by a second condition. An example is a person's beginning a weight-loss diet while an undiagnosed wasting disease such as cancer has developed. The loss of body weight is attributed to the diet, masking the disease and delaying diagnosis and treatment. **2.** the unconscious display of a personality trait that conceals a behavioral aberration.

masking agent, a cosmetic preparation for covering nevi, surgical scars, and other blemishes. Masking agents are generally composed of a flesh-colored pigment in a lotion or cream base.

masklike facies [Fr, *masque* + L, *facies,* face], an immobile expressionless face with staring eyes and slightly open mouth. It is sometimes associated with parkinsonism or psychiatric conditions.

mask of pregnancy. See **chloasma.**

Maslow's hierarchy of needs /mas″lōz/ [Abraham H. Maslow, American psychiatrist, 1908–1970; Gk, *hierarches,* position of authority; AS, *nied,* obligation], (in psychology) a hierarchic categorization of the basic needs of humans. The most basic needs on the scale are the physiological or biological needs, such as the need for air, food, or water. Of second priority are the safety needs, including protection and freedom from fear and anxiety. The subsequent order of needs in the hierarchic progression are the need to belong, to love, and to be loved; the need for self-esteem; and ultimately the need for self-actualization. To progress from one need to another, the more basic need must first be satisfied.

masochism /mas″ōkiz′əm/ [Leopold von Sacher-Masoch, Austrian author, 1836–1895], pleasure or gratification derived from receiving physical, mental, or emotional abuse. The maltreatment may be inflicted by another person or by oneself. It may involve a need to experience emotional or physical pain, in reality or fantasy, to become sexually aroused. Also called **passive algolagnia.** Compare **sadism.** See also **algolagnia, sadomasochism.** −*masochistic, adj.*

masochist /mas″ōkist/ [Leopold von Sacher-Masoch], a person who derives pleasure or gratification from masochistic acts or abuse. Compare **sadist.** See also **masochism.**

masochistic personality. See **self-defeating personality disorder.**

mass (m) [L, *massa*], **1.** the physical property of matter that gives it weight and inertia. **2.** (in pharmacology) a mixture from which pills are formed. **3.** an aggregate of cells clumped together, such as a tumor. Compare **weight.** See also **inertia.**

mass action law, 1. the mathematical description of reversible reactions that attain equilibrium, generally regarded as applicable to competitive assay. **2.** the rate of a chemical reaction that is proportional to the active masses of the resulting substances.

massage /məsäzh, məsäj″/ [Fr, *masser,* to stroke], the manipulation of the soft tissue of the body through stroking, rubbing, kneading, or tapping to increase circulation, to improve muscle tone, and to relax the patient. The procedure is performed either with the bare hands or through some mechanical means, such as a vibrator. The most common sites for massage are the back, knees, elbows, and heels. Care is taken not to massage inflamed areas, particularly of the extremities, because of the danger of loosening blood clots. Open wounds and areas of rash, tumor, or excessive sensitivity are avoided. Even if the extremities (legs) are not inflamed, they should not be massaged if the client has been immobilized for an extended period of time. The procedure is performed with the patient prone or on the side, comfortably positioned, with an emollient lotion or cream applied to the area to be massaged. The caregiver's hands are warm, and excessive pressure is avoided to prevent pain or injury. Kinds include **cardiac massage, effleurage, flagellation, friction, frôlement, pétrissage, tapotement, vibration.**

-massage, suffix meaning "a therapeutic kneading of the body": *thermomassage.*

massage therapist, a person who performs manipulation of soft tissues or kneading of parts of the body especially to aid circulation, relax the muscles, or relieve pain. Certification and regulation of massage therapists vary greatly by locality.

massage therapy, the manipulation of the soft tissues of the body for the purpose of normalizing them, thereby enhancing health and healing. Kinds include **acupressure, classical Western massage, Shiatsu.**

massed practice, (in occupational therapy) the repetition of a task or skill by a client in the same manner with little rest between trials.

masseter /masē″tər/ [Gk, one who chews], the thick rectangular muscle in the cheek that functions to close the jaw. It is one of the four muscles of mastication. The masseter is innervated by the masseteric nerve from the mandibular division of the trigeminal nerve.

masseteric nerve, a branch of the anterior trunk of the mandibular nerve that penetrates and supplies the masseter muscle.

mass fragment [L, *massa,* lump, *frangere,* to shatter], (in mass spectrometry) a degraded part of a molecule containing one or more charges.

mass hysteria [ME, *maiour,* great; Gk, *hystera,* womb], an episode of psychogenic illness affecting a large group of individuals at the same time. Examples include the witchcraft trials of the 17th century and the irrational mass reaction to the 1938 radio show based on H.G. Wells' science-fiction novel, *War of the Worlds.* Also called **collective hysteria, epidemic hysteria, mass panic, mass psychogenic illness.**

massive lung collapse, a condition in which an entire lung or one of its lobes becomes airless, frequently as a result of an obstruction in a bronchus.

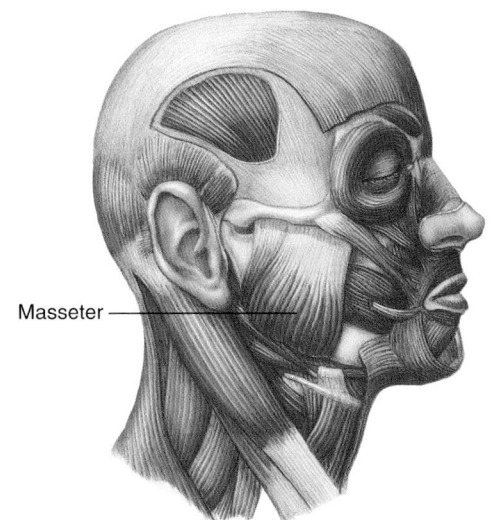

Masseter *(Patton and Thibodeau, 2016)*

massive transfusion syndrome [L, *multus,* many, *plica,* fold, *transfundere,* to pour through; Gk, *syn,* together, *dromos,* course], a hemorrhagic reaction to massive transfusions of platelet-poor stored blood. For an adult, transfusion of 10 units of blood in a 24-hour period is a massive transfusion. Platelet concentrates and/or fresh frozen plasma may be given to correct the deficiency.

mass number (A), the sum of the number of protons and neutrons in the nucleus of an atom or isotope. See also **atomic number.**

mass panic, mass psychogenic illness. See **mass hysteria.**

mass reflex, an abnormal condition, seen in patients with transection of the spinal cord, characterized by a widespread nerve discharge. Stimulation below the level of the lesion results in flexor muscle spasms, incontinence of urine and feces, priapism, hypertension, and profuse sweating.

■ OBSERVATIONS: A mass reflex may be triggered by scratching or other painful stimulus to the skin, overdistension of the bladder or intestines, cold weather, prolonged sitting, or emotional stress. Muscle spasms may be so violent as to propel the patient off a bed or stretcher.

■ INTERVENTIONS: Medications to reduce mass reflexes include diazepam, dantrolene, chlordiazepoxide, and meprobamate. Hubbard baths and exercises in warm water also help. Occasionally chordotomy, rhizotomy, peripheral nerve transection, or tenotomy may be necessary.

■ PATIENT CARE CONSIDERATIONS: Avoid stimulating areas that trigger mass reflexes, and be prepared to accept them when they occur and explain the cause to the patient. It is important to prevent pressure ulcers and bladder infections in paraplegic and tetraplegic patients because they may also serve as triggers to initiate mass reflexes.

mass spectrometer, an analytic instrument for identifying a substance by sorting a stream of charged particles (ions) according to their mass. The sorting is usually accomplished by deflecting a stream of charged particles into a semicircular path as it enters a magnetic field and ultimately strikes a photographic plate or a photomultiplier tube sensor.

mass spectrometry, (in chemistry) a technique for the analysis of a substance in which the molecule is subjected to bombardment by high-energy electrons or atoms to cause ionization and fragmentation to give a series of ions in the gas phase that constitutes the fragmentation pattern observed by using a mass spectrometer. A molecule can frequently be identified just on the basis of its mass spectrum. See also **spectrometry, spectrophotometry.**

mass spectrum, a characteristic pattern obtained from a mass spectrometer.

mass transfer, the movement of mass from one phase to another.

mass transfer-area coefficient (MTAC), the permeability of a dialysis membrane multiplied by the available area of the membrane, calculated as the clearance rate by diffusion when there is no ultrafiltration and when there is not yet any solute in the dialysate.

MAST, abbreviation for **military antishock trousers.**

mast-. See **masto-, mast-.**

mastalgia /mastalˈjə/ [Gk, *mastos,* breast, *algos,* pain], pain in the breast caused by congestion during lactation, an infection, fibrocystic disease, or advanced cancer. The early stages of breast cancer are rarely accompanied by pain. Hormonal changes also may be a factor. –*mastalgic, adj.*

mast cell [Ger, *Mast,* fattening; L, *cella,* storeroom], a constituent of connective tissue containing large basophilic granules that contain heparin, serotonin, bradykinin, and histamine. These substances are released from the mast cell in response to injury, inflammation, and infection.

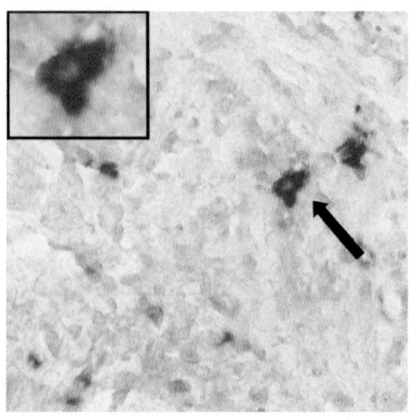

Pulmonary mast cell *(Salamon et al, 2008)*

mast cell leukemia, a malignant neoplasm of leukocytes characterized by connective tissue mast cells in circulating blood.

mast cell tumor [Ger, *Mast,* fattening; L, *cella,* storeroom; L, *tumor*], a connective tissue tumor composed of mast cells. Granules of the cells stain metachromatically with toluidine blue.

mastectomy /mastekˈtəmē/ [Gk, *mastos,* breast, *ektomē,* excision], the surgical removal of one or both breasts, most commonly performed to remove a malignant tumor. In a simple mastectomy the breast is removed without lymph node dissection. In a radical mastectomy some of the muscles of the chest are removed with the breast, together with lymph nodes in the axilla. In a modified radical mastectomy the involved breast and all axillary contents (axillary, pectoral, and superior apical nodes) are removed, but the pectoral muscles are preserved. The tumor is biopsied before the mastectomy. If the specimen shows a malignancy, the tumor and adjacent tissues are removed in one piece. At the end of the surgical procedure a drainage catheter is placed in the wound. The nurse inspects the wound for swelling or excessive bleeding

and encourages the patient to deep breathe. The affected arm is positioned with the hand pointed upward or on pillows so that the hand is higher than the lower arm, with the lower arm above heart level to promote venous return. Hand and wrist movements and elbow flexion and extension are begun within 24 hours and performed regularly. The patient may be fitted with a prosthesis when the wound is completely healed or at the time of the mastectomy. Blood pressures and venipuncture may not be performed on the side of the mastectomy. Emotional support and counseling are essential. See also **breast cancer, modified radical mastectomy, radical mastectomy, simple mastectomy.**

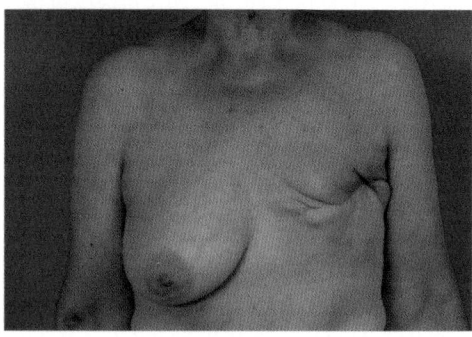

Modified radical mastectomy *(Courtesy Dr. Elizabeth Chabner Thompson)*

master problem list, a list of a patient's problems that serves as an index to his or her record. Each problem, the date when it was first noted, the treatment, and the desired outcome are added to the list as each becomes known. Thus the list provides an ongoing guide for reviewing the health status and planning the care of the patient. See also **SOAP.**

mastery /masˈtərē/ [L, *magister,* chief], command or control of a situation.

-mastia. See **-mazia, -mastia, -masty.**

mastication /masˈtikāˈshən/ [L, *masticare,* to chew], chewing, tearing, or grinding food with the teeth while it becomes mixed with saliva. See also **bolus, digestion, ptyalin.**

masticatory apparatus. See **masticatory system.**

masticatory movement /masˈtikətôrˈē/, motion of the lower jaw in chewing.

masticatory surface. See **occlusal surface.**

masticatory system [L, *masticare,* to chew; Gk, *systema*], the combination of structures involved in chewing, including the jaws, teeth and supporting structures, mandibular and maxillary musculature, temporomandibular joints, tongue, lips, cheeks, oral mucosa, salivary glands, blood supply, and cranial nerves. Also called **masticatory apparatus.** Compare **stomatognathic system.**

mastigophora, protozoa having flagella. See also **protozoon.**

mastigophoran /masˈtigofˈärahn/, any member of the subphylum Mastigophora. Also called *mastigote.*

mastitis /mastīˈtis/ [Gk, *mastos,* breast, *itis,* inflammation], an inflammatory condition of the breast, usually caused by streptococcal or staphylococcal infection. Acute mastitis, most common in the first 2 months of lactation, is characterized by pain, swelling, redness, axillary lymphadenopathy, fever, and malaise. If it is untreated or inadequately treated, abscesses may form. Antibiotics, rest, analgesia, and warm soaks are usually prescribed. Usually breastfeeding may continue. Chronic tuberculous

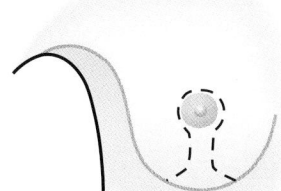

Lateral extension can increase
axillary exposure

Wise pattern

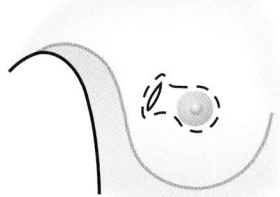

Incision when biopsy site
near areola

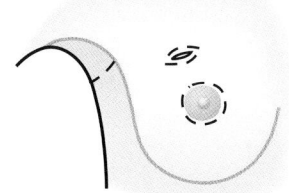

Incision when biopsy site remote from
areola with axillary incision for
lymphadenectomy

Different incisions for patients undergoing mastectomy *(Townsend et al, 2008)*

mastitis is rare; when it occurs, it represents extension of tuberculosis from the lungs and ribs beneath the breast. Granulomatous mastitis is a distinct benign breast condition of unknown etiology occurring in nonlactating women. See also **chronic mastitis.**

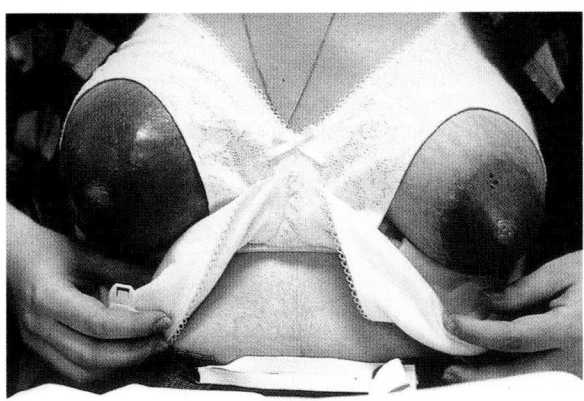

Mastitis *(Courtesy Dr. J. Newman, FRCPC, Hospital for Sick Children)*

masto-, mast-, combining form meaning "breast": *mastitis, mastectomy, mastopexy.*

mastocarcinoma /mas′təkär′sinō″mə/, carcinoma of the mammary gland.

mastocyte. See **mast cell.**

mastocytoma /mas′təsītō″mə/, a tumor that contains mast cells.

mastocytosis /mas′təsītō″sis/ [Ger, *Mast,* fattening; Gk, *kytos,* cell, *osis,* condition], local or systemic overproduction of mast cells, which in rare instances may infiltrate liver, spleen, bones, the GI system, and skin. Systemic mastocytosis may precede mast cell leukemia.

mastoid /mas″toid/ [Gk, *mastos,* breast, *eidos,* form], **1.** pertaining to the mastoid process of the temporal bone. **2.** breast-shaped.

mastoid-, prefix meaning "mastoid process": *mastoidectomy.*

mastoid antrum, a cavity continuous with mastoid cells. It is separated from the middle cranial fossa above by the tegmen tympani.

mastoid cells [Gk, *mastos,* breast, *eidos,* form; L, *cella,* storeroom], air cells in the mastoid process of the temporal bone. Also called *mastoid air cells.*

mastoidectomy /mas′toidek″təmē/ [Gk, *mastos + eidos,* form, *ektomē,* excision], surgical excision of a part of the mastoid part of the temporal bone, frequently performed to treat cholesteatoma. It may also be performed to treat chronic suppurative otitis media or mastoiditis when systemic antibiotics are ineffective. Often done as part of reconstructive procedure and classified as simple modified radical. Entry is made through the ear canal or from behind the ear. In a simple mastoidectomy with the patient under general anesthesia, diseased bones of the mastoid are removed while the ossicles, eardrum, and canal wall are left intact and the eardrum is incised to drain the middle ear. Topical antibiotics are then instilled in the ear. In a radical procedure the eardrum and most middle ear structures are removed. The stapes is left intact so that a hearing aid may be used. The opening to the eustachian tube is plugged. In a modified radical procedure the eardrum and some of the ossicles are saved, and the patient hears better than after a radical mastoidectomy. After surgery any bright red blood on the dressing may indicate hemorrhage. A stiff neck or disorientation may signal the onset of meningitis. Dizziness is usual and may be expected to last for several days.

mastoid fontanel, a posterolateral fontanel that is usually not palpable. See also **fontanel.**

mastoiditis /mas′toidī″tis/ [Gk, *mastos + eidos,* form, *itis,* inflammation], an infection of one of the mastoid bones, usually an extension of a middle ear infection. It is characterized by earache, fever, headache, and malaise. Swelling of the mastoid process often displaces the pinna anteriorly and inferiorly. The infection is difficult to treat, often requiring antibiotic administered intravenously for several days. Children are most often affected. Residual hearing loss may follow the infection.

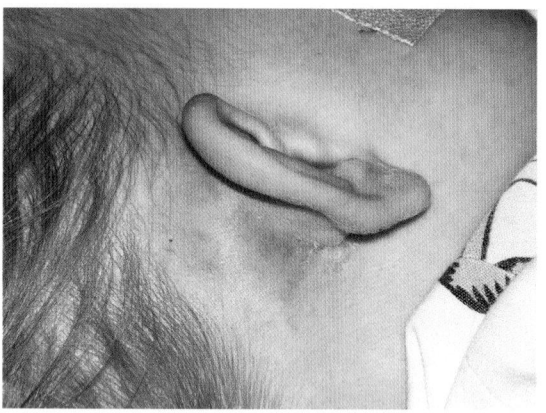

Child with acute mastoiditis *(Glynn and Drake, 2012)*

mastoid process, the irregular conic projection of the caudal, posterior part of the temporal bone, serving as the attachment for various muscles, including the sternocleidomastoideus, splenius capitis, and longissimus capitis. A hollow section of the process contains air cells that are distinguished from a large, irregular tympanic antrum in the superior anterior part of the process. See also **temporal bone.**

mastopathy /mastop″əthē/, any disease of the breast.

mastopexy, a reconstructive procedure in cosmetic surgery to lift the breasts.

masturbation /mas′tərbā″shən/ [L, *masturbari,* to masturbate], sexual activity in which the penis or clitoris is stimulated, usually to orgasm, by means other than coitus. −*masturbatory, masturbatic, adj.,* −*masturbate, v.*

-masty. See **-mazia, -mastia, -masty.**

mat, **1.** abbreviation for **maternity. 2.** abbreviation for **maturity. 3.** abbreviation for **maternal.**

matched group, subjects in a research experiment matched based on a particular variable and then placed into groups. See **group.**

matching layer, a layer of material placed in front of an ultrasound transducer to improve the efficiency of energy transfer into and out of a patient.

materia /mətir″ē·ə/, matter or material, such as materia medica.

materia alba /mətir′ē·ə· al′bə/ [L, white matter], a whitish or cream-colored cheesy mass deposited around the necks of the teeth, composed of food debris, mucin, and dead epithelial cells. It is usually associated with poor oral hygiene.

material fact /mətir″ē·əl/ [L, *materia,* matter, *factum*], **1.** (in law) a fact that establishes or refutes an element essential to the complaint, charge, or defense. The presence of a material fact in a case being tried precludes granting of a summary judgment. **2.** a fact that would be important to a reasonable person in deciding whether to engage in a transaction or not.

materia medica (mat. med.), **1.** the study of the origins, preparation, uses, and effects of drugs and other substances used in medicine. **2.** a substance or a drug used in medical treatment.

matern, abbreviation for **maternity, maternal.**

maternal (mat, matern) /mətur″nəl/ [L, *maternus,* motherhood], **1.** inherited, derived, or received from a mother. **2.** motherly in behavior. **3.** related through the mother's side of the family, such as a maternal grandfather.

maternal and child health (MCH) services, various facilities and programs organized for the purpose of providing medical and social services for mothers and children. Medical services include prenatal and postnatal services, family planning care, and pediatric care in infancy.

maternal antibody, an antibody transmitted from mother to fetus via the placenta. Such antibodies can provide immunity for the fetus and the newborn for up to 6 months after birth. They may also cause hemolytic anemia in newborns in cases of Rh or ABO blood group incompatibility between mother and child.

maternal-child attachment. See **maternal-infant bonding.**

maternal-child separation syndrome. See **separation anxiety.**

maternal death, the death of a woman while pregnant or within 42 days after termination of pregnancy.

maternal deprivation syndrome [L, *maternus,* motherhood, *deprivare,* to deprive; Gk, *syn,* together, *dromos,* course], a condition characterized by developmental delay that occurs as a result of physical or emotional deprivation. It is seen primarily in infants. Typical symptoms include lack of physical growth, with weight below the third percentile for age and size; malnutrition; pronounced withdrawal; silence; apathy; irritability; and a characteristic posture and body language, featuring unnatural stiffness and rigidity with a slow response reaction to others. Causes of the syndrome are usually multiple and complex, involving such factors as parental indifference; emotional instability or insecurity of the mother; lack of or delayed development of the mother-child attachment process; unrealistic expectations or disappointment concerning the sex, appearance, or adaptability of the child; or unfavorable socioeconomic conditions within the family. Treatment often requires hospitalization, especially in cases of severe malnutrition. Care includes assessment of the family situation, and treatment often involves psychotherapy, counseling, or special nursing instruction to help the parents learn to deal with and provide for the child. The nature and extent of the effects of the condition on later physical, emotional, intellectual, and social development vary considerably and depend on the age at which deprivation occurs, the degree and duration of the situation, the child's constitutional makeup, and the substituted care that is provided. Emotionally deprived children often remain below normal in intellectual development, fail to learn acceptable social behavior, and are unable to form trusting, meaningful relationships with others. In severe cases of early and prolonged deprivation, the damage to an infant may be irreversible. See also **failure to thrive.**

maternal effect. See **maternal inheritance.**

maternal immunity, protection against disease acquired by a fetus through the passage of maternal antibodies via the placenta. See also **maternal antibody.**

maternal-infant bonding, the complex process of attachment of a mother to her newborn. Disastrous effects of the disruption or absence of this attachment have long been known. The specific steps in its development and the factors that disturb or encourage it have been identified and described by anthropologists, pediatricians, psychologists, nurses, midwives, and sociologists. The process begins before birth as the parents plan for the pregnancy or discover that the mother is pregnant. The mother feels fetal movement, begins to accept the fetus as an individual, and makes plans for the baby after birth. In the first minutes and hours after birth, a sensitive period occurs during which the baby and the mother become intimately involved with each other through behaviors and stimuli that are complementary and provoke further interactions. The mother touches the baby and holds it en face to achieve eye-to-eye contact. The infant looks back eye to eye. The mother speaks in a quiet high-pitched voice. The mother and the baby move in turn to the voice and sounds of the other, a process known as entrainment, which can be likened to a dance. The infant's movements constitute a response to the mother's voice, and she is encouraged to continue the process. The secretion of oxytocin and prolactin by the maternal pituitary gland is stimulated by the baby's sucking or licking of the mother's breasts; T and B lymphocytes and macrophages are given to the baby in the mother's milk, promoting resistance to infection. The child is also colonized by the normal flora of the mother's skin and nasal passages, improving the baby's ability to fend off infection. Physically the mother provides her body heat for the baby's warmth and comfort. Thus the extended contact in the newborn period satisfies physical and emotional needs of the mother and baby. Experts have made the following recommendations to increase the development of maternal-infant bonding: The special needs of the mother are assessed before delivery; the parents attend classes to prepare them for labor, delivery, and the puerperium; and discussions are held regarding the stresses of pregnancy and the postpartum period. In labor and delivery a companion is encouraged to stay with the mother. After the baby is born, silver nitrate drops or other medications are not placed in the baby's eyes until the mother and the baby have had time to be together en face, with eye contact for an extended period, because the drops cause a film to form over the eyes, dimming vision. During the first hour after birth the parents and the infant are not separated and are given as much privacy as possible. Skin-to-skin contact is encouraged; various methods may be used to maintain an ambient temperature adequate to maintain the baby's temperature.

maternal inheritance, the transmission of traits or conditions controlled by cytoplasmic factors within the ovum that are not self-replicating and are determined by genes within the nucleus. Also called **maternal effect.**

maternal inheritance mendelism. See **inheritance.**

maternal microchimerism, persistence of cells derived from the mother in her offspring. It may play a role in autoimmune disease in the children.

maternal mortality, **1.** the death of a woman as a result of childbearing. **2.** the number of maternal deaths per 100,000 live births. The statistic excludes women who die from ruptured ectopic pregnancy or any other condition in which there was no birth (stillbirth, septic abortion).

maternal placenta [L, *maternus,* motherhood, *placenta,* flat cake], the part of the placenta that develops from the decidua basalis of the uterus and is usually shed along with the fetal elements.

maternal screen testing, a blood or urine screen to determine birth defects and genetic disorders, administered in early pregnancy. It is most important for women over 35 years of age and those who have previously delivered children with birth defects.

maternal serum alpha-fetoprotein (MSAFP) test, a test of a pregnant woman's blood designed to indicate an increased risk for fetal open neural tube defects, such as spina bifida. It may also indicate an increased risk for Down syndrome. See also **alpha-fetoprotein.**

maternity (mat, matern) /mətur″nitē/ [L, *maternus,* motherhood], motherhood; the character and quality of a mother.

maternity cycle [L, *maternus,* motherhood; Gk, *kyklos,* circle], the antepartal, intrapartal, and postpartal periods of pregnancy and the puerperium, from conception to 6 weeks after birth.

maternity nursing, nursing care provided to women and their families during pregnancy and parturition and through the first days of the puerperium. Increasingly postpartum maternity nursing includes the supervision of the mothers' care of their newborns in rooming-in units and may include care of normal newborns in a nursery when they are not with their mother. Maternity nursing includes extensive instruction of mothers in the usual behavior and needs of a newborn, in expected patterns of growth and development of the infant during the first week, and in details of care needed by the mother during the first weeks after birth. Breastfeeding, bottle feeding, baby baths, perineal care, umbilical care, nutrition, and danger signs of the puerperium are usually taught by the maternity nurse. Observation for abnormal conditions, such as thrombophlebitis, mastitis, and other infections, is an ongoing concern in the puerperium. Intrapartum maternity nursing involves the care of mothers in labor and delivery, as well as high-risk nursing, emotional support in labor and delivery, and ongoing observation for the onset of abnormal signs or symptoms. Often pregnant women with medical problems associated with pregnancy are cared for on a special high-risk antepartum unit by specially educated maternity nurses.

mat gold [Fr, *mat,* dull; AS, *geolu,* yellow], a noncohesive form of pure gold. Also called **crystal gold, sponge gold.** See also **gold foil.**

mating /mā″ting/ [D, *mate,* companion], the pairing of individuals of the opposite sex, primarily for purposes of reproduction.

mat. med., abbreviation for **materia medica.**

matrifocal family /mat′rifō″kəl/ [L, *mater,* mother, *focus,* hearth, *familia,* household], a family unit composed of a mother and her children. Biological fathers may have a temporary place in the family.

matrix /mā″triks, mat″riks/ [L, womb], **1.** an intercellular substance. **2.** a basic substance from which a specific organ or kind of tissue develops. Also called **ground substance.** **3.** a form used in shaping a tooth surface in dental procedures. **4.** (in analytical chemistry) material of no interest in an analysis that may have an effect on the analysis. **5.** a rectangular arrangement of elements into rows and columns, often used to display a digital image.

matrix band, a cylindrical copper or stainless steel band or short tube that is seated around a tooth. The band may be filled with impression compound, which flows into a prepared cavity in order to obtain an impression, or it may be used to aid in the placement and contouring of restorative materials. See also **matrix retainer.**

matrix holder, also called *Tofflemire matrix retainer.* See **matrix retainer.**

matrix metalloproteinase, any of a group of endopeptidases that hydrolyze proteins of the extracellular matrix.

matrix retainer, a mechanical device used to secure the ends of a matrix band around a tooth. The band provides a substitute wall where a part of the tooth is missing and helps to compact a restoration into a prepared tooth cavity after the carious lesion has been removed. Also called **matrix holder.** See also **retainer.**

matrix size, the number of pixels allocated to each linear dimension in a digital image.

matrix unguis. See **nailbed.**

matroclinous inheritance /mātrō″klinəs/ [L, *mater,* mother; Gk, *klinein,* to incline], a form of heredity in which the traits of the offspring have been transmitted from the mother.

matter [L, *materia*],   **1.** anything that has mass and occupies space. **2.** any substance not otherwise identified as to its constituents, such as gray matter, pus, or serum exuding from a wound.

Mattis Dementia Rating Scale (DRS-2),   a widely used tool for evaluation of cognitive function dementia in adults over the age of 55 years who have brain dysfunction. It measures overall cognitive functioning on five subscales and can be used at lower ability levels than can be tested by most other methods.

Matulane,   an antineoplastic drug. Brand name for **procarbazine hydrochloride.**

maturation   /mach′ərā″shən/ [L, *maturare,* to ripen],   **1.** the process or condition of attaining complete development. In humans it is the unfolding of full physical, emotional, and intellectual capacities that enable a person to function at a higher level of competency and adaptability within the environment. **2.** the final stages in the meiotic formation of germ cells in which the number of chromosomes in each cell is reduced to the haploid number characteristic of the species. See also **meiosis, oogenesis, spermatogenesis.**

maturational crisis /mach′ərā″shənəl/,   a transitional or developmental period within a person's life, such as puberty, when psychological equilibrium is upset.

mature /məchŏor″/ [L, *maturus,* ripe],   **1.** *v.,* to become fully developed; to ripen. **2.** *adj.,* fully developed or ripened.

mature cataract.   See **ripe cataract.**

mature cell leukemia.   See **polymorphocytic leukemia.**

maturity (mat) /məchŏo″ritē/ [L, *maturus,* ripe],   **1.** a state of complete growth or development, usually designated as the period of life between adolescence and old age. **2.** the stage at which an organism is capable of reproduction.

maturity-onset diabetes.   *(Obsolete)* See **type 2 diabetes mellitus.**

max,   acronym for *maximum.*

maxilla /maksil″ə/ *pl. maxillae* [L, *mala,* jaw],   one of a pair of large bones (often referred to as one bone) that form the upper jaw and teeth, consisting of a pyramidal body and four processes: the zygomatic, frontal, alveolar, and palatine. The maxilla contributes to the hard palate and floor of the nasal cavity.

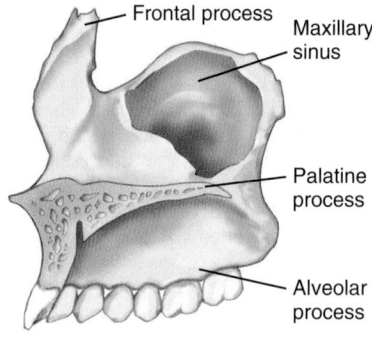

Maxilla

-maxilla,   combining form meaning "upper jaw or the bones composing it": *intermaxilla, submaxilla, palatomaxillary.*

maxillary /mak″səler′ē/ [L, *maxilla,* upper jaw],   pertaining to the upper jaw.

maxillary arch [L, *maxilla,* upper jaw, *arcus,* bow],   the curved bony ridge of the upper jawbone in the shape of a horseshoe, including the dentition and supporting structures.

maxillary artery [L, *maxilla,* upper jaw; Gk, *arteria,* airpipe],   either of two larger terminal branches of the external carotid arteries that rise from the neck of the mandible near the parotid gland and divide into six branches, supplying the deep structures of the face.

maxillary fossa.   See **canine fossa.**

maxillary nerve,   the second division of the trigeminal nerve, a purely sensory nerve that branches into a zygomaticotemporal branch, a zygomaticofacial branch, and the large infraorbital nerve, which in turn has multiple branches that supply the face.

maxillary process [L, *maxilla,* upper jaw, *processus*],   **1.** the alveolar process of the upper jaw that contains the tooth sockets. **2.** the frontal process that extends upward to articulate with the frontal and nasal bones. **3.** the palatine process that helps form the hard palate. **4.** the zygomatic process, or anterior surface, that articulates with the zygomatic bone.

maxillary retroposition, maxillary retrusion.   See **retrognathia.**

maxillary sinus,   one of a pair of large air cells forming a pyramidal cavity in the body of the maxilla. The apex of each sinus extends into the zygomatic arch, and its floor, formed by the alveolar process, is usually 1 to 10 mm below the floor of the nose. In the adult the volume of the sinus averages 14.75 cc. The mucous membrane of the sinus is continuous with that of the nasal cavity. In the fourth month of gestation the embryonic sinus appears as a shallow groove on the medial surface of the bone. It does not reach full size until after the second teething. Also called **antrum of Highmore.** Compare **ethmoidal air cell, frontal sinus, sphenoidal sinus.**

maxillary tuberosity,   a rounded eminence on the posterior surface of the body of the maxilla, behind the root of the third molar through which the posterior superior alveolar nerve enters the maxilla. It becomes prominent after the eruption and growth of the third molars.

maxillary vein,   one of a pair of deep veins of the face, accompanying the maxillary artery and passing between the condyle of the mandible and the sphenomandibular ligament. Each maxillary vein is a tributary of the internal jugular and external jugular veins.

maxillodental /mak′silōden″təl/,   pertaining to or affecting the upper jaw and teeth.

maxillofacial /mak′silōfā″shəl/ [L, *maxilla,* upper jaw, *facies,* face],   pertaining to the maxilla and face.

maxillofacial dysostosis.   See **maxillofacial syndrome.**

maxillofacial prosthesis [L, *maxilla,* upper jaw, *facies,* face],   a prosthetic replacement for part or all of the upper jaw, nose, or cheek. It is applied when surgical repair alone is inadequate.

maxillofacial surgery.   See **oral and maxillofacial surgery.**

maxillofacial syndrome,   a congenital defect of fetal ossification characterized by anteroposterior shortening of the maxilla and various other anomalies, including mandibular prognathism, slanting of the eyes, and malformation of the auricles. Also called **maxillofacial dysostosis.**

maxillofacial trauma,   injury to the jaw and face. Fractures requiring reconstructive surgery tend to occur most frequently in motor vehicle collisions and short falls.

maxillolacrimal suture /-lak″riməl/,   a line of union between the anterior border of the lacrimal bone and the frontal process of the maxilla. Also called **lacrimomaxillary suture.**

maxillomandibular /maksil′ōmandib″yŏolər/,   pertaining to the upper and lower jaws.

maxillomandibular fixation [L, *maxilla,* upper jaw, *mandere,* to chew, *figere,* to fasten],   stabilization of fractures of the face or jaw by temporarily connecting the maxilla and mandible by wires, elastic bands, or metal splints. See also **elastic-band fixation, nasomandibular fixation.**

maxillomandibular relation.   See **jaw relation.**

maxillotomy /mak′silot′əmē/ [L, *maxilla,* upper jaw; Gk, *tomē,* a cutting],   surgical sectioning of the maxilla that allows movement of all or a part of the maxilla into the desired position.

maximal acid output (MAO),   on the pentagastrin test, the output of gastric acid for 1 hour after administration of pentagastrin, expressed as mmol/hr.

maximal breathing capacity.   See **maximum breathing capacity.**

maximal diastolic membrane potential,   the most negative transmembrane potential achieved by a cardiac cell during repolarization. Also called **maximum diastolic potential.**

maximal expiratory flow rate (MEFR),   the rate of the most rapid flow of gas from the lungs during a forced expiration after a full inspiration. Also called *maximal expiratory flow.*

maximal expiratory pressure (MEP),   the greatest pressure of expired air achieved by a person after a full inspiration.

maximal midexpiratory flow rate (MMFR),   the rate of the most rapid flow of gas during the middle half (in terms of volume) of a forced expiration after a full inspiration. It is measured in pulmonary function tests to detect and evaluate chronic obstructive pulmonary diseases, such as bronchitis, emphysema, and asthma.

maximal treadmill test (MTT),   an exercise stress test in which subjects increase their heart rate during exercise to 80% to 90% of the maximal rate, which is estimated from each subject's age and sex. Other methods of stress testing produce the same physiological effect of exercise on the heart without using exercise. These tests use drugs such as dipyridamole to "stress" the heart.

maximum breathing capacity (MBC) /mak″səməm/   [L, *maximus,* greatest; AS, *braeth* + L, *capacitas*],   the maximum volume of gas that a person can inhale and exhale per minute by breathing as quickly and deeply as possible. Also called **maximal breathing capacity.**

maximum diastolic potential.   See **maximal diastolic membrane potential.**

maximum expiratory flow, maximum expiratory flow rate.   See **maximal expiratory flow rate.**

maximum inspiratory pressure (MIP) /mak′səməm/   [L, *maximus,* greatest, *inspirare,* to breathe in, *premere,* to press],   the maximum pressure within the alveoli of the lungs that occurs during a full inspiration.

maximum intensity projection (MIP),   a three-dimensional image processing method used in computed tomography and magnetic resonance.

maximum oxygen uptake,   the greatest volume of oxygen per minute that can be absorbed from the lungs by the blood. Also called **aerobic capacity.**

maximum permissible dose (MPD, M.P.D.).   See **effective dose equivalent limit.**

maximum voluntary isometric contraction (MVIC),   the peak force produced by a muscle as it contracts while pulling against an immovable object, or as it contracts without shortening.

maximum voluntary ventilation (MVV),   the maximum volume of gas that a person can inhale and exhale by voluntary effort per minute by breathing as quickly and deeply as possible. It is measured in pulmonary function tests.

maxofacial surgery,   posttrauma and/or reconstructive and plastic surgery to the jaws and midface region.   Compare **oral and maxillofacial surgery.** See also **dentistry.**

Mayer reflex /mā″ər/ [Karl Mayer, Austrian neurologist, 1862–1932],   a normal reflex elicited by grasping the ring finger and flexing it at the metacarpophalangeal joint of a person whose hand is relaxed with thumb abducted. The normal responses are adduction and apposition of the thumb. The reflex is absent in disease of the pyramidal system.

May-Hegglin anomaly,   a rare autosomal-dominant inherited blood cell disorder characterized by thrombocytopenia and granulocytes with blue ribonucleic acid containing cytopathic inclusions similar to Döhle's bodies.

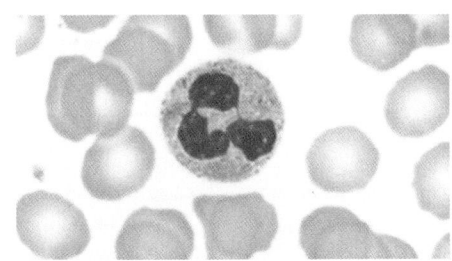

Neutrophils with basophilic inclusions characteristic of May-Hegglin anomaly *(Hoffbrand, Pettit, and Vyas, 2010)*

Mayo scissors.   See **scissors.**

maze procedure.   See **Cox Maze procedure.**

-mazia, -mastia, -masty,   suffix form meaning "(condition of the) breasts": *amazia, gynecomastia, polymastia.*

mazindol /mā″zindōl/,   an anorexiant.

■ INDICATIONS: It is prescribed over a short term to decrease appetite in the treatment of exogenous obesity.

■ CONTRAINDICATIONS: Glaucoma, history of drug abuse, concomitant use of a monoamine oxidase inhibitor, or known hypersensitivity to this drug prohibits its use.

■ ADVERSE EFFECTS: Among the more serious adverse effects are insomnia, palpitation, dizziness, dry mouth, tachycardia, and hypersensitivity reactions.

mb,   abbreviation for *millibar.*

M.B.,   abbreviation for *Bachelor of Medicine.*

mbar,   abbreviation for *millibar.*

MBC,   abbreviation for **maximum breathing capacity.**

MBD, M.B.D.,   abbreviation for **minimal brain dysfunction.** See **attention deficit disorder.**

mbp,   abbreviation for *mean blood pressure.*

mbt,   abbreviation for **mean body temperature.**

mc,   **1.** abbreviation for *millicycle.* **2.**   abbreviation for **millicurie.**

mC,   abbreviation for **millicoulomb.**

Mc,   abbreviation for **megacycle.**

MCAD,   an enzyme involved in degradation of medium-chain fatty acids, medium-chain acyl-CoA dehydrogenase. Deficiency of the enzyme (MCAD deficiency) is characterized by recurring episodes of hypoglycemia, vomiting, and lethargy, with urinary excretion of medium-chain dicarboxylic acids, minimal ketogenesis, and low plasma and tissue levels of carnitine.

McArdle disease /məkär″dəl/ [Brian McArdle, English neurologist, 1911–2002],   an inherited glycolic storage disease marked by an absence of myophosphorylase B and abnormally large amounts of glycogen in skeletal muscle. It is milder than other glycogen storage diseases, characterized by muscle fatigability and stiffness after exercise. The only treatment is avoidance of exercise. Also called

M

glycogen storage disease, type V. See also **glycogen storage disease.**

MCAT,   abbreviation for **Medical College Admission Test.**

McBurney incision /makbur″nē/ [Charles McBurney, American surgeon, 1845–1913], a surgical wound that begins 2 to 5 cm above the anterior superior iliac spine and runs parallel to the external oblique muscle of the abdomen. This incision is used for an appendectomy.

McBurney point [Charles McBurney; L, *pungere,* to puncture], a site of extreme sensitivity in acute appendicitis, situated in the normal area of the appendix midway between the umbilicus and the anterior iliac crest in the right lower quadrant of the abdomen. See also **appendical reflex, appendicitis.**

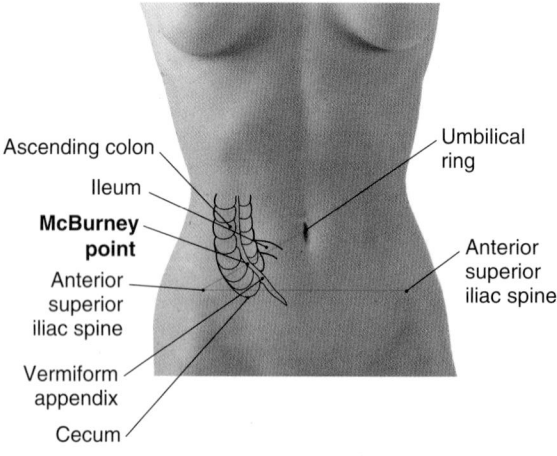

McBurney point *(Paulson, 2013)*

McBurney sign [Charles McBurney, American surgeon, 1845–1913), a reaction of the patient indicating severe pain and extreme tenderness when McBurney point is palpated. Such a reaction indicates appendicitis.

McCall's festoon /məkölz″/, (in dentistry) a ring-shaped enlargement of the gingival margin on the vestibular surface (buccal or labial) of canines and premolars. It may be associated with occlusal trauma.

McCune-Albright syndrome. See **Albright syndrome.**

MCFA,   abbreviation for **medium-chain fatty acid.**

mcg,   abbreviation for **microgram.**

MCH,   1. abbreviation for **maternal and child health (MCH) services. 2.** abbreviation for **mean cell hemoglobin.**

M.Ch.,   abbreviation for *Master of Surgery.*

MCHC,   abbreviation for **mean cell hemoglobin concentration.**

mCi,   abbreviation for **millicurie.**

mCi-hr,   abbreviation for *millicurie-hour.*

McManus, R. Louise [1896–1993], a nurse who established the first national testing service for the nursing profession. She was also instrumental in developing a means of evaluating the nursing programs in community and junior colleges. She established a center for education in nursing research at Teachers College, Columbia University, New York.

McMillan, Mary [1880-1959], early American physical therapist and a founder of the American Physical Therapy Association. She was educated in England and was employed at the Children's Hospital in Liverpool, treating patients with poliomyelitis and spastic paralysis. She returned to America in 1915 and became an influential force in the development of the profession of physical therapy.

McMurray sign /makmur″ē/ [Thomas P. McMurray, English surgeon, 1887–1949], an audible click heard when rotating the tibia on the femur, indicating injury to meniscal structures.

McMurray test, as the patient lies supine with one knee fully flexed, the examiner rotates the patient's foot fully outward while the knee is slowly extended; a painful "click" indicates a tear of the medial meniscus of the knee joint; if the click occurs when the foot is rotated inward, the tear is in the lateral meniscus.

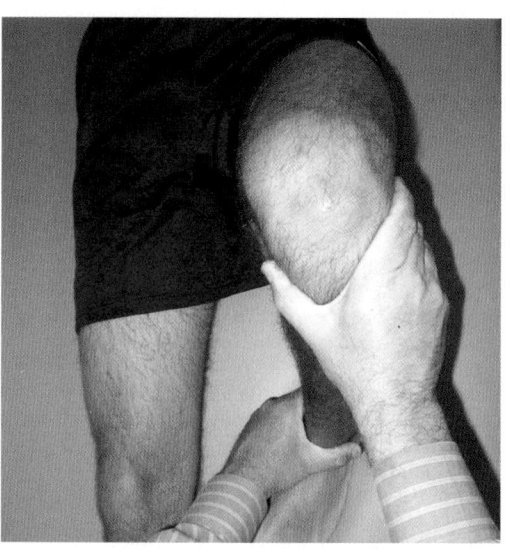

McMurray test *(Waldman, 2011)*

MCO,   abbreviation for **managed care organization.**

medical indigence /in″dijəns/ [L, *indigere,* to need], a condition of having insufficient income to pay for adequate medical care without depriving oneself or one's dependents of food, clothing, shelter, or other living essentials.

M component, an abnormal immunoglobulin fragment that appears in large numbers in patients with macroglobulinemia, heavy chain disease, and multiple myeloma.

MCP,   abbreviation for **metacarpophalangeal.**

M-CSF,   abbreviation for **macrophage colony–stimulating factor.**

MCTD,   abbreviation for **mixed connective tissue disease.**

MCV,   initialism for *mean corpuscular volume.*

Md,   symbol for the element **mendelevium.**

MD,   1. initialism for **muscular dystrophy. 2.** initialism for **macular degeneration.**

M.D.,   abbreviation for *Doctor of Medicine.* See **physician.**

MDA,   initialism for *Muscular Dystrophy Association.*

MDEC tube, a multipurpose diagnostic and enteroclysis triple-lumen intestinal tube used in the management of small bowel disorders. The largest lumen is for suction or fluid instillation, the medium lumen provides access for suction, and the smallest lumen is used to inflate the balloon preventing migration of intestinal fluids. The tip of the tube is weighted. See also **Maglinte tube.**

MDI,   abbreviation for **metered dose inhaler.**

MDMA,   abbreviation for *3,4-methylenedioxymethamphetamine.*

MDR,   initialism for **minimum daily requirement.**

M.D.V.,   abbreviation for *Doctor of Veterinary Medicine.* Also called *DVM.*

Me,   abbreviation for **methyl.**

MEA, abbreviation for **multiple endocrine adenomatosis.**

Meals on Wheels, a program designed to deliver hot meals to the elderly, individuals with disabilities, or others who lack the resources to provide nutritionally adequate meals for themselves on a daily basis.

mean [ME, *mene,* in the middle], occupying a position midway between two extremes of a set of values or data. The arithmetic mean is a value that is derived by dividing the total of a set of values by the number of items in the set. The geometric mean is a value between the first and last of a set of values organized in a geometric progression. Compare **median, mode.**

mean arterial pressure (MAP), the arithmetic mean of the blood pressure in the arterial part of the circulation. It is calculated by adding the systolic pressure reading to two times the diastolic reading and dividing the sum by 3.

mean body temperature, the mass-weighted average temperature of body tissues, indicative of thermal status.

mean cell hemoglobin (MCH), an estimate of the mass of hemoglobin in an average erythrocyte, computed as the ratio of the hemoglobin concentration and the red blood cell count. The MCH reference interval is 28 to 32 picograms. See also **hypochromic anemia, iron-deficiency anemia.**

mean cell hemoglobin concentration (MCHC), the average percentage of hemoglobin per red blood cell computed as the ratio of the hemoglobin to the hematocrit. The MCHC adult reference interval is 32% to 36% in adults.

mean cell volume (MCV), average volume of each red cell, computed as the ratio of hematocrit to the red blood cell count. The MCV reference interval is 80 to 100 fL.

meaningful repetition, (in occupational therapy) the practice needed to fully integrate movements or sequences of steps in a task.

meaningful use, (in patient records) the use of the electronic health record to improve quality of care, increase efficiency, and reduce health disparities.

mean marrow dose (MMD), the estimated average annual somatic radiation received by each person in the United States. It is expressed in terms of bone marrow because irradiation of that tissue is assumed to be a cause of leukemia.

mean platelet volume (MPV) test, a blood test that measures the volume of a large number of platelets as determined by an automated analyzer. The MPV is very useful in the differential diagnosis of thrombocytopenic disorders.

measles /mē″zəlz/ [ME, *meseles,* skin spots], an acute, highly contagious viral disease involving the respiratory tract and characterized by a spreading maculopapular cutaneous rash. It occurs primarily in young children who have not been immunized and in teenagers or young adults who are inadequately immunized. Measles is caused by a paramyxovirus and is transmitted by direct contact with droplets spread from the nose, throat, and mouth of infected people, usually in the prodromal stage of the disease. Indirect transmission by uninfected people or contaminated articles is unusual. Diagnosis is confirmed by the identification of Koplik spots on the buccal mucosa and by serological examination. Also called **morbilli, rubeola.** See also **roseola infantum, rubella.**

■ OBSERVATIONS: An incubation period of 7 to 14 days is followed by the prodromal stage, characterized by fever, malaise, coryza, cough, conjunctivitis, photophobia, anorexia, and the pathognomonic Koplik spots, which appear 1 to 2 days before onset of the rash. Pharyngitis and inflammation of the laryngeal and tracheobronchial mucosa develop, the temperature may rise to 103° F or 104° F (39.4° C to 40° C), and there is marked granulocytic leukopenia. The papules of the rash first appear as irregular brownish pink spots around the hairline, the ears, and the neck, then spread rapidly within 24 to 48 hours to the trunk and extremities, becoming red, maculopapular, and dense and giving a blotchy appearance. Within 3 to 5 days the fever subsides and the lesions flatten, turn a brownish color, and begin to fade, causing a fine desquamation, especially over heavily affected areas.

■ INTERVENTIONS: Routine treatment consists of bed rest, antipyretics, appropriate antimicrobials to control secondary bacterial infection, and, when necessary, application of calamine lotion, cornstarch solution, oatmeal, baking soda, or cool water to relieve itching. Preventive measures include active immunization with measles virus vaccine after the infant is 1 year of age. A booster is recommended at 4 to 6 years of age. Passive immunization with immune serum globulin is recommended for unvaccinated individuals exposed to the disease. One attack of the disease confers lifelong immunity.

■ PATIENT CARE CONSIDERATIONS: Rest, isolation, and quiet activity are recommended as long as fever and rash persist. Acetaminophen, fluids, cool sponge baths, nose drops, and cough medication may be necessary to counteract fever and respiratory symptoms. Bright sunlight may be irritating to the eyes. Special attention is given to the care and cleansing of the eyes and skin, especially in cases of severe papular eruption. An important nursing function is instruction of the parents in the proper home care of the child, because most cases are not serious enough to require hospitalization. The disease is usually benign, and mortality is rare. Complications sometimes occur. The most common are otitis media, pneumonia, bronchiolitis, obstructive laryngitis, laryngotracheitis, and occasionally encephalitis and appendicitis. Rarely, but most gravely, the virus causes subacute sclerosing panencephalitis several years after the acute attack of measles has occurred.

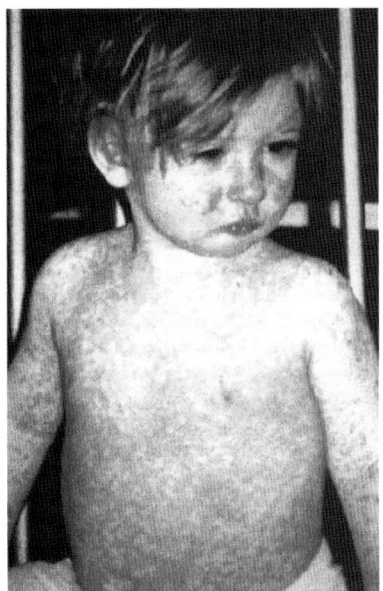

Child with measles *(Marx, Hockenberger, and Walls, 2006)*

measles and rubella virus vaccine live, an active immunizing agent.

■ INDICATIONS: It is prescribed for immunization against measles and rubella.

■ CONTRAINDICATIONS: Immunosuppression, concomitant administration of corticosteroids, tuberculosis, known or suspected pregnancy, hypersensitivity to neomycin (e.g., eggs, chicken, or chicken feathers), neoplasms of the lymphatic system or bone marrow, or active infection prohibits its use. It should not be given for 3 months after the use of whole blood, plasma, or immune serum globulin or for 1 month before or after immunization with other live virus vaccines, except mumps vaccine.

■ ADVERSE EFFECTS: The most serious adverse effect is anaphylaxis.

measles immune globulin. See **immune gamma globulin.**

measles, mumps, and rubella virus vaccine live (MMR), an active immunizing agent.

■ INDICATIONS: It is prescribed for simultaneous immunization against measles, mumps, and rubella.

■ CONTRAINDICATIONS: Immunosuppression, concomitant administration of corticosteroids, tuberculosis, hypersensitivity to neomycin, neoplasms of the lymphatic system or bone marrow, known or suspected pregnancy, or acute infection prohibits its use. It is not given for 3 months after the use of whole blood, plasma, or immune serum globulin, and it is not given for 1 month before or after immunization with other live virus vaccines.

■ ADVERSE EFFECTS: The most serious adverse effect is anaphylaxis.

measles virus, a paramyxovirus (minus sense RNA virus) that is the cause of measles. It is a highly contagious disease that affects mostly children. The measles virus is transmitted by direct contact and respiratory route. Humans are the only target for this virus, and there is no animal reservoir. Symptoms appear 10 to 12 days after the infection and include high fever, bloodshot eyes, runny nose, and body rash. Treatment is supportive; most people recover in 3 to 4 weeks. An effective vaccine is available and is recommended for all children.

measurement /mezh″ərment/ [L, *mensura*], the determination, expressed numerically, of the extent or quantity of a substance, energy, or time. See also **International Unit, metric system.**

measure of central tendency, (in descriptive statistics) an indication of the middle point of distribution for a particular group. Measures include the mean average score, the median or middle score of distribution, and the mode, the most frequently occurring measure.

measure of variability, (in descriptive statistics) a mathematical determination of how much the performance of the group as a whole deviates from the mean or median. The most frequently used measure of variability is the standard deviation.

meatal /mē·ā′təl/ [L, *meatus,* channel], pertaining to a meatus.

meatal stenosis, a constriction or narrowing of the urinary meatus, seen most often in boys or men as a complication of circumcision and meatitis.

meatorrhaphy /mē′ətôr″əfē/ [L, *meatus,* channel; Gk, *rhaphe,* suture], the suturing of the cut end of the urethra to the glans penis after surgery to enlarge the urethral meatus.

meatoscopy /mē′ətos″kəpē/ [L, *meatus* + Gk, *skopein,* to look], the visual examination of any meatus, especially the urethra, usually performed with the aid of a speculum or endoscope.

meatus /mē·ā′təs/ *pl. meatuses* [L, channel], an opening or tunnel through any part of the body, such as the external acoustic meatus that leads from the external ear to the tympanic membrane.

meatus acusticus externus. See **external acoustic meatus.**

meatus acusticus internus. See **internal acoustic meatus.**

meatuses. See **meatus.**

Mebaral, a sedative used as an anticonvulsant drug. Brand name for **mephobarbital.**

mebendazole /məben″dəzōl/, an anthelmintic.

■ INDICATIONS: It is prescribed in the treatment of pinworm, whipworm, roundworm, and hookworm infestations.

■ CONTRAINDICATIONS: Pregnancy or known hypersensitivity to this drug prohibits its use.

■ ADVERSE EFFECTS: Among the most serious adverse effects are abdominal pain and diarrhea.

MEC, the minimum inhibitory concentration that allows a drug to be active. The drug is effective at any level above this threshold value. Abbreviation for *minimum effective concentration.*

mecamylamine hydrochloride /mek′əmil″əmēn/, a ganglionic blocking agent (antihypertensive).

■ INDICATIONS: It is prescribed in the management of severe essential hypertension and uncomplicated malignant hypertension.

■ CONTRAINDICATIONS: Coronary or cerebrovascular insufficiency, recent myocardial infarction, uremia, pyelonephritis, glaucoma, or known hypersensitivity to this drug prohibits its use.

■ ADVERSE EFFECTS: Among the most serious adverse effects are orthostatic hypotension, paralytic ileus, urinary retention, and cycloplegia. The incidence of side effects is very high because the drug reduces all autonomic activity.

mecasermin, a biological response modifier and insulin-like growth factor.

■ INDICATIONS: This drug is used to treat growth failure in children with severe primary insulin-like growth factor–1 deficiency or with growth hormone (GH) gene deletion who have developed neutralizing antibodies to GH.

■ CONTRAINDICATIONS: Known hypersensitivity to this drug or benzyl alcohol, closed epiphyses, active or suspected neoplasia, and IV use prohibit its use.

■ ADVERSE EFFECTS: Adverse effects of this drug include headache, dizziness, cardiac valvulopathy, cardiac murmur, ear pain, otitis media, abnormal tympanometry, papilledema, visual impairment, vomiting, thymus hypertrophy, hypoglycemia, bruising, lipohypertrophy, hypersensitivity reactions, arthralgia, joint pain, snoring, and tonsillar hypertrophy. Life-threatening side effects include seizures, hypoglycemia, ketosis, hypothyroidism, apnea, and antibodies to growth hormone.

mechanical advantage [Gk, *mechane,* machine; L, *abante,* superior position], the ratio of the output force developed by a muscle to the input force applied to the body structure that the muscle moves. Variations in the sizes of muscles and the lengths of bones in different individuals partially account for the differences in mechanical advantage and physical capabilities, such as speed and strength, among body types.

mechanical condenser, a device that delivers automatically controlled impacts for compacting restorative material in the filling of tooth cavities. It may be spring activated, pneumatic, or electrically controlled. Also called **automatic mallet condenser.**

mechanical dead airspace [Gk, *mechane* + AS, *dead* + Gk, *aer* + L, *spatium*], the volume of air that fills the breathing circuits of a mechanical ventilator. The mechanical dead space may be increased if necessary to control hypocapnia and respiratory alkalosis.

mechanical heart-lung, a device connected to the circulatory system to maintain oxygenated blood flow during surgery that requires interruption of normal heart-lung functions, such as open heart surgery. See also **blood pump.**

mechanical lift, a medical device used to transfer clients from one surface to another.

mechanical restraint [Gk, *mechane* + L, *restringere,* to confine], a device made of fabric that hinders a patient's movement, such as a safety vest, hand and wrist straps, mittens, and a stretcher equipped with belts. See also **restraint.**

mechanical vector. See **vector.**

mechanical ventilation, the use of an apparatus designed to intermittently or continuously assist or control pulmonary ventilation. The use of a mechanical ventilator is indicated as a supportive measure in patients affected by respiratory paralysis and in those with ventilatory failure manifested by either alveolar hypoventilation, hypoxemia, or both.

■ METHOD: Many types of ventilators are available. There are two major groups of ventilators: (1) those that generate negative pressure on the exterior surface of the chest, and (2) those that provide intrathoracic positive pressure.

■ INTERVENTIONS: Regardless of the model and capabilities of the mechanical ventilator being used in the treatment of a patient with inadequate ventilation, there are certain general principles that are basic to the competent care of the patient. It is essential that all those who accept responsibility for the care of the patient be fully aware of the physiological effects of mechanical ventilation, particularly in regard to the relationship between the distribution of inspired air in the lung and the status of the blood gases and pH. A second consideration in patient care and assessment of the effects of mechanical ventilation is that of its influence on circulation. An increase in intrathoracic pressure can interfere with the flow of blood through the great vessels and chambers of the heart. The effect can be a pooling of blood in the veins and capillaries of the abdominal organs and a resultant peripheral vascular collapse. Frequent determinations of pulse rate and blood pressure are necessary to detect early development of this complication and ensure prompt treatment. A third consideration is that of the effects of mechanical ventilation on the body fluid–antidiuretic hormone balance. Careful monitoring of the patient's fluid status is required. Finally, a thorough knowledge of the apparatus being used for mechanical ventilation is vital to competent care of the patient. No one should attempt to give patient care without prior instruction in the purpose of the machine and the physiological and physical principles upon which it operates. Patients and/or families who are discharged with a ventilator should also have this knowledge of operation.

■ OUTCOME CRITERIA: Weaning from a ventilator is begun when the clinical evaluation of the patient indicates that full ventilatory support is no longer needed.

mechanism /mek′əniz′əm/, **1.** an instrument or process by which something is done, results, or comes into being. **2.** a machine or machinelike system. **3.** a stimulus-response system. **4.** a habit or drive.

mechanism of injury, the circumstance in which an injury occurs, for example, deceleration in an automobile accident, wounding by a gunshot, or crushing by a heavy object.

mechanism of labor. See **cardinal movements of labor.**

mechano-, prefix meaning "mechanical": *mechanoreceptor.*

mechanoreceptor /mek′ənō′risep″tər/ [Gk, *mechane,* machine; L, *recipere,* to receive], any sensory nerve ending that responds to mechanical stimuli, such as touch, pressure, sound, and muscular contractions. See also **proprioceptor.**

mechlorethamine hydrochloride /mek′lôreth″əmēn/, an antineoplastic alkylating agent. Also called **nitrogen mustard.**

■ INDICATIONS: It is prescribed in the treatment of a variety of neoplasms, especially lymphomas, and of malignant effusions.

■ CONTRAINDICATIONS: Bone marrow depression, pregnancy, infection, or known hypersensitivity to this drug prohibits its use.

■ ADVERSE EFFECTS: Among the most serious adverse effects are bone marrow depression and inflammation caused by extravasation at the site of injection. Nausea, vomiting, and alopecia also may occur.

Meckelian cartilage /mek′elz/ [Johann Friedrich Meckel, German anatomist, 1781–1833], a cartilaginous bar in the embryo. From it or its sheath, the sphenomandibular ligament, the malleus, and the incus develop. Also called *Meckel's rod, Meckel's cartilage.*

Meckel diverticulum [Johann F. Meckel, 1781–1833], an anomalous sac protruding from the wall of the ileum between 30 and 90 cm from the ileocecal sphincter. It is congenital, resulting from the incomplete closure of the yolk stalk, and occurs in 1% to 2% of the population. The diverticulum is usually asymptomatic, but the condition is suggested by signs of appendicitis in infancy; by sudden and painless bleeding in the sac, usually in childhood; or by symptoms of intestinal obstruction. Symptomatic diverticula are most commonly resected. Surgical resection of asymptomatic diverticula is also recommended to prevent potential diverticulitis, obstruction, and blood loss. Many Meckel diverticula are discovered incidentally during surgery for other causes and on postmortem examination.

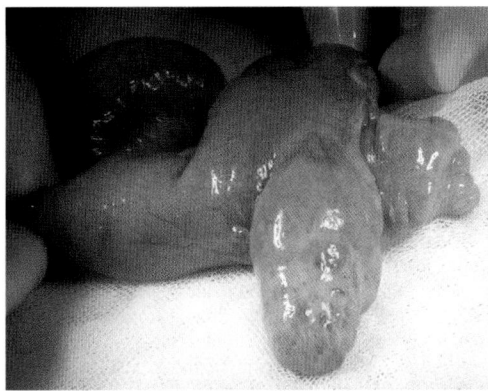

Intraoperative view of double Meckel diverticulum, presenting as acute appendicitis *(Emre et al, 2013)*

Meckel diverticulum nuclear scan, a nuclear scan to detect Meckel diverticulum.

meclizine hydrochloride /mek″lizēn/, an antihistamine.

■ INDICATIONS: It is prescribed in the prevention and treatment of motion sickness.

■ CONTRAINDICATIONS: Newborns and lactating mothers are not given this drug. Asthma or known hypersensitivity to this drug prohibits its use.

■ ADVERSE EFFECTS: Among the more serious adverse effects are drowsiness, skin rash, hypersensitivity reactions, dry mouth, tachycardia, and nervousness.

meclofenamate sodium /mek′lôfen″əmāt/, a nonsteroidal antiinflammatory agent.

■ INDICATIONS: It is prescribed in the treatment of rheumatoid arthritis, osteoarthritis, dysmenorrhea, and other mild to moderate pain.

■ CONTRAINDICATIONS: Known hypersensitivity to aspirin or to nonsteroidal antiinflammatory drugs prohibits its use. It is used with caution in patients who have upper GI disease or impaired renal function.

M

■ ADVERSE EFFECTS: Among the more serious adverse effects are GI distress, peptic ulcers, dizziness, rashes, and tinnitus. This drug interacts with many other drugs.

Meclomen, an antiinflammatory agent. Brand name for **meclofenamate sodium.**

mecocephaly. See **scaphocephaly.**

meconium /mikō″nē·əm/ [Gk, *mekon,* poppy], a material that collects in the intestines of a fetus and forms the first stools of a newborn. It is thick and sticky, usually greenish to black, and composed of secretions of the intestinal glands, some amniotic fluid, and intrauterine debris, such as bile pigments, fatty acids, epithelial cells, mucus, lanugo, and blood. With ingestion of breast milk or formula and proper functioning of the GI tract, the color, consistency, and frequency of the stools change by the third or fourth day after the initiation of feedings. The presence of meconium in the amniotic fluid during labor may indicate fetal distress and may lead to a lack of oxygen and developmental delays.

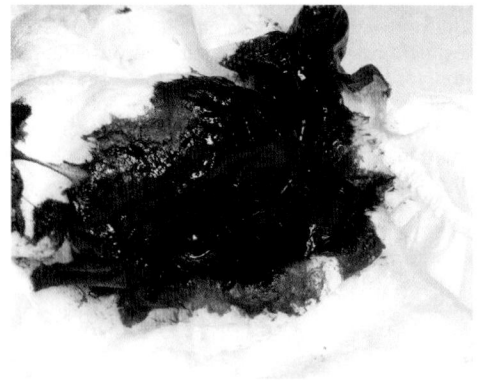

Meconium *(Zitelli and Davis, 2007)*

meconium aspiration, the inhalation of meconium by a fetus or newborn. It can block the air passages and cause failure of the lungs to expand or other pulmonary dysfunction, such as pneumonia or emphysema.

meconium ileus, obstruction of the small intestine in the newborn caused by impaction of thick, dry, tenacious meconium, usually at or near the ileocecal valve. Symptoms include abdominal distension, vomiting, failure to pass meconium within the first 24 to 48 hours after birth, and rapid dehydration with associated electrolyte imbalance. The condition results from a deficiency in pancreatic enzymes and is the earliest manifestation of cystic fibrosis. In uncomplicated cases in which perforation, volvulus, or atresia does not occur, the obstruction may be relieved by giving enemas with a contrast medium, such as a hypertonic solution of meglumine diatrizoate and sodium diatrizoate, under fluoroscopy. Fluid is replaced intravenously to prevent dehydration. If enemas do not dislodge the obstruction, surgery is necessary. See also **meconium plug syndrome.**

meconium periorchitis, a rare condition seen in infant boys after meconium peritonitis has healed, characterized by a hydrocele of meconium in the scrotum that gradually hardens and often resolves spontaneously in time.

meconium peritonitis, peritonitis resulting from perforation of the bowel into the peritoneal cavity in utero or shortly after birth. This causes escape of the meconium into the peritoneal cavity. It occurs most often as a complication of meconium ileus in cystic fibrosis.

meconium plug syndrome, obstruction of the large intestine in the newborn caused by thick, rubbery meconium that may fill the entire colon and part of the terminal ileum. Symptoms include failure to pass meconium within the first 24 to 48 hours after birth, abdominal distension, and vomiting if complete intestinal blockage occurs. A water-soluble contrast enema indicates the presence of a plug and in most cases dislodges it from the bowel wall. Subsequent gentle saline solution enemas may be needed to expel it. The condition may be an indication of Hirschsprung disease or cystic fibrosis. See also **meconium ileus.**

med, abbreviation for **median.**

MED, 1. abbreviation for *minimal effective dose.* 2. abbreviation for **minimal erythema dose.** See **threshold dose.**

medcard /med′kärd/, (in nursing) a small card listing the name, dose, and schedule of administration of each patient's medications, used in dispensing drugs to each patient.

medevac, abbreviation for *medical evacuation.*

medi-, medio-, combining form meaning "middle": *mediocarpal, mediolateral, medialis.*

media, (in occupational therapy) tools used to assist persons in engaging in those occupations they find meaningful; therapeutic media consist of materials used in therapy sessions to help clients meet goals. See also **medium.**

medial /mē″dē·əl/ [L, *medius,* middle], 1. pertaining to, situated in, or oriented toward the midline of the body. Also called **mesial.** 2. pertaining to the tunica media, the middle layer of a blood vessel wall.

medial antebrachial cutaneous nerve, a nerve of the arm that arises from the medial cord of the brachial plexus, medial to the axillary artery. Near the axilla a cutaneous branch emerges to supply the skin over the biceps almost as far as the elbow. It descends on the ulnar side of the arm and divides into the anterior branch and the ulnar branch. The anterior branch is the larger of the two branches, innervating the skin as far as the wrist. The ulnar branch descends as far as the wrist, innervates the skin, and communicates with branches of the ulnar nerve. Compare **medial brachial cutaneous nerve.**

medial arteriosclerosis. See **Mönckeberg arteriosclerosis.**

medial brachial cutaneous nerve, a nerve of the arm arising from the medial cord of the brachial plexus and distributed to the medial side of the arm. It passes through the axilla, pierces the deep fascia in the middle of the arm, and supplies the skin of the arm as far as the olecranon. Compare **medial antebrachial cutaneous nerve.**

medial calcaneal nerve, a nerve that is often multiple and originates from the tibial nerve near the ankle and descends onto the medial side of the heel. It innervates skin on the medial surface and sole of the heel.

medial calcific sclerosis. See **Mönckeberg's arteriosclerosis.**

medial cerebellar nucleus. See **fastigial nucleus.**

medial circumflex femoral artery, an artery that passes medially around the shaft of the femur and near the margin of the adductor brevis, giving off a small branch, which enters the hip joint through the acetabular notch and anastomoses with the acetabular branch of the obturator artery, then divides into two major branches deep to the quadratus femoris muscle. One of these branches ascends to the trochanteric fossa and connects with branches of the gluteal and lateral circumflex femoral arteries. The other branch passes laterally to participate with other arteries to form an anastomotic network of vessels around the hip.

medial cuneiform bone, the largest of three cuneiform bones of the foot, situated on the medial side of the tarsus, between the scaphoid bone and the first metatarsal. It serves as the attachment for various ligaments, the tendons of the tibialis anterior, and the peroneus longus. It articulates with the scaphoid, the intermediate cuneiform, and the first and second metatarsals. Also called **internal cuneiform bone.**

medial fibroplasia, the most common of the various non-atherosclerotic lesions characterized on an angiogram by the string-of-beads sign (areas of the artery wall having protruding aneurysms alternating with stenosis and thinning).

medial geniculate body, one of a pair of areas on the posterior dorsal thalamus that relay auditory impulses from the lateral lemniscus to the auditory cortex.

medialis /mē′dē·ā″lis/ [L, *medius,* middle], pertaining to the middle or to the median plane.

medial labial frenulum, a fold of mucosa on the inner surface of both lips that connects the lip to the adjacent gum.

medial malleolus, the rounded process of the tibia forming the internal surface of the ankle joint. Also called **internal malleolus.**

medial palpebral arteries, small branches of the ophthalmic artery that supply the medial area of the upper and lower eyelids.

medial pectoral nerve, a branch of the brachial plexus that, with the lateral pectoral nerve, supplies the pectoral muscles. It joins the lateral pectoral nerve to form a loop around the artery before ending deep in the pectoralis minor. The loop branches to supply the pectoralis minor and the pectoralis major. Compare **lateral pectoral nerve.**

medial plantar nerve, the major sensory nerve in the sole of the foot. It innervates skin on most of the anterior two thirds of the sole and adjacent surfaces of the medial three and one-half toes, including the great toe. It also innervates three intrinsic muscles: the abductor hallucis, flexor digitorum brevis, and first lumbrical.

medial posterior intertransverse muscles of neck, small muscles passing between the posterior tubercles of adjacent cervical vertebrae, close to the vertebral body, innervated by posterior primary rami of spinal nerves and acting to bend the vertebral column laterally.

medial puboprostatic ligament, a thickening of the superior fascia of the pelvic diaphragm in the male that extends laterally from the prostate to the tendinous arch of the pelvic fascia and continues forward and medially from the tendinous arch to the pubis.

medial pubovesical ligament, the medial branch of the pubovesical ligament in the female, a forward continuation of the tendinous arch of the pelvic fascia to the pubis.

medial rotation, a turning toward the midline of the body. Compare **lateral rotation.** See also **rotation.**

medial umbilical ligament, a remnant of the embryological urachus that continues from the apex of the bladder superiorly up the anterior abdominal wall to the umbilicus.

median (med) /mē′dē·ən/ [L, *medius,* middle], (in statistics) the number representing the middle value of the scores in a sample. In an odd number of scores arrayed in ascending order, it is the middle score. In an even number of scores so arrayed, it is the average of the two central scores.

median antebrachial vein /an′tēbrā″kē·əl/, a superficial vein of the upper limb that drains the venous plexus on the palmar surface of the hand. It ascends on the ulnar side of the anterior forearm and at its terminus joins the median cubital vein. One of the veins of the median cubital complex commonly anastomoses with the deep veins of the forearm. The anastomosis holds the superficial vein in place and makes it a practical choice for venipuncture. Compare **basilic vein, cephalic vein, dorsal digital vein.**

median aperture of fourth ventricle, an opening between the roof of the fourth ventricle and the subarachnoid space.

median arcuate ligament, a tendinous arch that connects the crura of the diaphragm, crossing anteriorly to the aorta at approximately the level of the twelfth thoracic vertebra.

median atlantoaxial joint, one of three points of articulation of the atlas and the axis. The median atlantoaxial joint is a pivot articulation among the dens, the axis, and the ring of the atlas and involves five ligaments. It allows rotation of the axis and the skull, the extent of rotation limited by the alar ligaments.

median basilic vein, one of the superficial veins of the upper limb, often formed as one of two branches from the median cubital vein. The median basilic vein courses across the palmar surface of the forearm near the elbow and is commonly used for venipuncture, phlebotomy, or IV infusion. Compare **basilic vein.**

median cephalic vein, a vein sometimes present as the lateral branch, ending in the cephalic vein, of a bifurcation of the median antebrachial vein.

median cleft facial syndrome. See **frontonasal dysplasia.**

median effective dose (ED$_{50}$), the dose of a drug that may be expected to cause a specific intensity of effect in half of the patients to whom it is given.

median episiotomy, an incision in the perineum in the midline. Although less painful after delivery, it affords less exposure for delivery and may extend into or through the anal sphincter and into the rectum. Also called **midline episiotomy.** Compare **mediolateral episiotomy.** See also **episiotomy.**

median glossitis. See **median rhomboid glossitis.**

median jaw relation, any jaw relation that exists when the mandible is in the median sagittal plane.

median lethal dose (MLD, LD$_{50}$), the amount of a substance or of radiation sufficient to kill one half of a population of organisms within a specified period.

median nerve, one of the terminal branches of the brachial plexus that extends along the radial side of the forearm and the hand, supplying various muscles and the skin of these regions. It arises from the brachial plexus by two large roots, one from the lateral and one from the medial cord. The roots unite to form the trunk of the nerve that courses down the arm with the brachial artery. The median nerve usually has no branches above the elbow. It has a few articular branches to the elbow joint and muscular branches to the forearm; the anterior interosseous nerve; the palmar branch; the muscular branch in the hand; the first, second, and palmar digital nerves; and the proper digital nerves. Compare **musculocutaneous nerve, radial nerve, ulnar nerve.**

median palatine suture, the line of junction between the horizontal parts of the palatine bones that extends from both sides of the skull to form the posterior part of the hard palate.

median plane, a vertical plane that divides the body into right and left halves and passes approximately through the sagittal suture of the skull. Also called **cardinal sagittal plane, midsagittal plane.** Compare **frontal plane, sagittal plane, transverse plane.**

median rhomboid glossitis, a red, depressed, diamond-shaped area on the dorsum of the tongue, frequently irritated by alcohol, hot drinks, or spicy foods. The condition most often occurs in adult men and may be caused by candidiasis. Also called **rhomboid glossitis.**

median sternotomy, a chest surgery technique in which an incision is made from the suprasternal notch to below the xiphoid process. The sternum is then opened with a saw and a sternal retractor is inserted. Closure requires reunion of the sternum with stainless steel sutures. The procedure is used in coronary artery bypass and valve replacement operations.

M

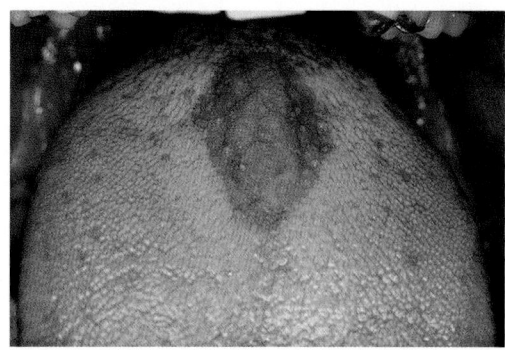

Median rhomboid glossitis *(Regezi, Sciubba, and Jordan, 2008)*

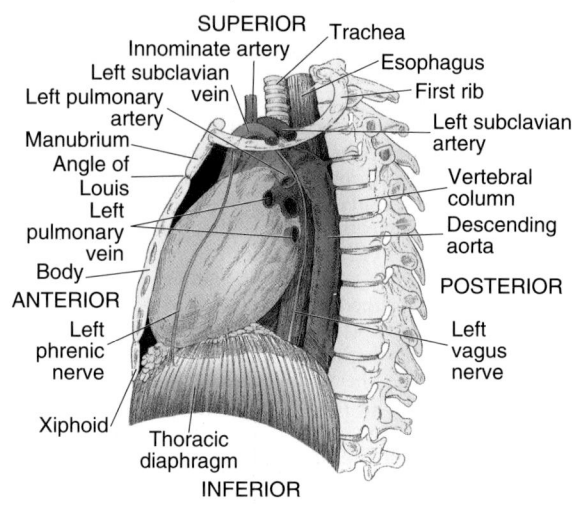

Regions of the mediastinum *(Rothrock, 2015)*

Compare **anterolateral thoracotomy, posterolateral thoracotomy.**

median toxic dose (TD$_{50}$), the dosage that may be expected to cause a toxic effect in half of the patients to whom it is given.

mediastina. See **mediastinum.**

mediastinal /mē′dē·əstī″nəl/ [L, *mediastinus,* midway], pertaining to a median septum or space between two parts of the body, such as the interval between the pleural sacs.

mediastinal cyst, a congenital cyst arising in the mediastinum.

mediastinitis, an inflammation of the mediastinum.

mediastinoscopy /mē′dē·as′tinos″kəpē/ [L, *mediastinus,* midway; Gk, *skopein,* to view], an examination of the space in the chest between the lungs using a mediastinoscope with light, lenses, and biopsy capacity. The mediastinoscope is inserted through a small surgical incision.

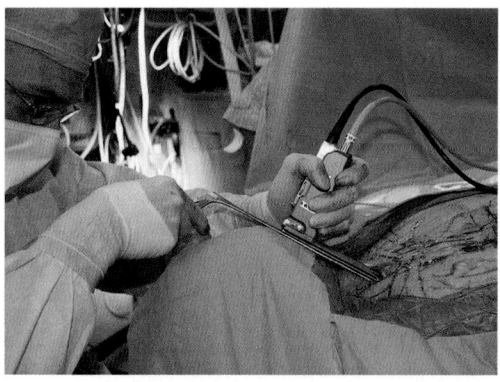

Cervical mediastinoscopy and biopsy *(Schipper and Schoolfield, 2008)*

mediastinum /mē′dē·əstī″nəm/ *pl. mediastina* [L, *mediastinus,* midway], a part of the thoracic cavity in the middle of the thorax, between the pleural sacs containing the two lungs. It extends from the sternum to the vertebral column and contains all the thoracic viscera except the lungs. It is enclosed in a thick extension of the thoracic subserous fascia and is divided into the anterior mediastinum, middle mediastinum, posterior mediastinum, and superior mediastinum. **−mediastinal,** *adj.*

mediate /mē″dē·āt/ [L, *medio,* in the middle], **1.** *v.,* to cause a change, as in stimulation by a hormone. **2.** *v.,* to

settle a dispute, as in collective bargaining. **3.** *adj.,* situated between two places, things, parts, or terms. **4.** *n.,* (in psychology) an event that follows one process or event and precedes another; for example, in the process of cognition, perception follows stimulation and precedes thinking. **−mediating,** *adj.,* **−mediator,** *n.*

mediated transport, the movement of a solute across a membrane with the assistance of a transport agent, such as a protein, that is specific for certain solutes.

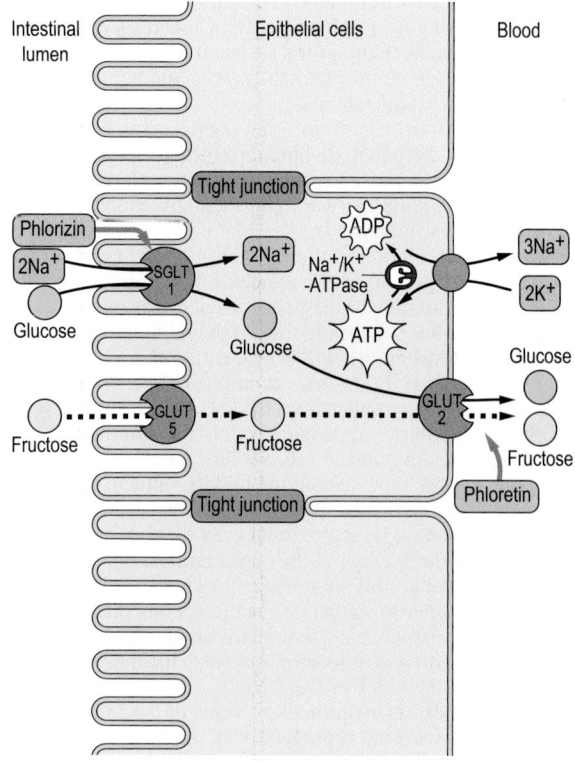

Mediated transport of glucose *(Baynes and Dominiczak, 2015)*

mediate percussion. See **percussion.**

medic, *(Informal)* abbreviation for **paramedic.**

Medicaid /med″ikād/, a U.S. federally funded state-operated program of medical assistance to people with low incomes, authorized by Title XIX of the Social Security Act. Under broad federal guidelines, the individual states determine benefits, eligibility, rates of payment, and methods of administration.

medical. See **medicine.**

medical abandonment, (in law) the unilateral termination of a professional relationship with a patient by a health care provider without proper notice to the patient when care is still required. See also **malpractice.**

medical abortion. See **abortion.**

medical assistant [L, *medicare,* to heal, *assistere,* to stand by], **1.** a person who, under the direction of a licensed supervising clinician, performs various routine administrative and nontechnical clinical tasks in a hospital, clinic, or similar facility. **2.** a category of allied health care personnel whose members help with all aspects of patient care and medical office operations.

medical care, the provision by a physician of services related to the maintenance of health, prevention of illness, and treatment of illness or injury.

medical care plan [L, *medicare,* to heal; OE, *caru,* sorrow, *planus,* floor], a long-range program of professional medical guidance designed to meet specific health objectives. Compare **nursing care plan.**

medical center, **1.** a health care facility. **2.** a hospital, especially one staffed and equipped to care for many patients and for a large number of kinds of diseases and dysfunctions, using sophisticated technology.

Medical College Admission Test (MCAT), an examination taken by persons applying to medical school. The score attained is an important criterion for acceptance. Basic science, intellectual ability, and mathematical and verbal aptitude and knowledge are tested.

medical consultation, a procedure whereby, on request by one physician or health care provider, another physician reviews a patient's medical history, examines the patient, and makes recommendations as to care and treatment. The medical consultant often is a specialist with expertise in a particular field of medicine.

Medical Corps, the branch within each of the armed services comprising the physicians within that service. It is a staff corps (noncombat specialty branch) consisting of physicians who are commissioned medical officers.

medical corpsman /kōr″man/ [L, *medicare,* to heal, *corpus,* body], an enlisted member of the U.S. Navy or U.S. Marine Corps who is trained to provide first aid, supervised medical care, and support.

medical decision level, the concentration of analyte, or body fluid sample being analyzed, at which some medical action is indicated for proper patient care. There may be several medical decision levels for a given analyte.

medical device, a product defined by the U.S. Food and Drug Administration that includes a wide variety of implants, instruments, and other items that affect structure and function but are not metabolized within or on the body. A medical device must also be recognized in the official *National Formulary* or the *United States Pharmacopoeia.* Medical devices are subject to regulation by the FDA. There is a clear distinction between a medical device and drugs, which are subject to a different set of regulations.

medical diagnosis [L, *medicare* + Gk, *dia,* through, *gnosis,* knowledge], the determination of the cause of a patient's illness or suffering by the combined use of physical examination, patient interview, laboratory tests, review of the patient's medical records, knowledge of the cause of observed signs and symptoms, and differential elimination of similar possible causes.

medical diathermy [L, *medicare* + *dia,* through, *therme,* heat], the application of high-frequency electrical currents to generate therapeutic heat in diseased tissues.

medical directive, a general term for documents that provide direction on the type of care a person desires. See also **advance directive, living will.**

medical director, a physician who is usually employed by a hospital to serve in a medical and administrative capacity as head of the organized medical staff. He or she also may serve as liaison for the medical staff with the hospital's administration and governing board.

medical emergency kit, a package of drugs and devices that may be used to deal with life-threatening medical situations. The kit may include positive-pressure ventilation equipment, an oxygen tank, cardiac and other medications, and supplies for airway management, dressings, IV fluids, suction, and splints.

medical engineering, a field of study of biomedical engineering and technological concepts applied to develop equipment and instruments required in health care delivery.

MedicAlert®, a nonprofit U.S. organization that maintains a huge database of information about individuals who are taking one or more medications for a chronic disorder. The database also includes emergency telephone numbers for health professionals treating the patients and provides bracelets or pendants to alert first responders and other health professionals involved in emergency care of the medical condition and prescription drugs taken by the patient, who may be unconscious or confused after an accident or episode of illness. MedicAlert maintains 24-hour access to the database for emergency medical personnel.

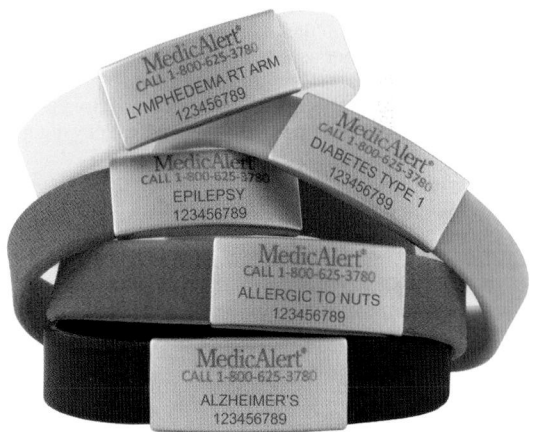

Medic Alert® bracelet *(© 2015 MedicAlert Foundation®.)*

medical doctor. See **physician.**

medical ethics [L, *medicare* + Gk, *ethikos*], the moral conduct and principles that govern members of the medical profession.

Medical Expenditure Panel Survey (MEPS), a set of large-scale surveys of families and individuals, their medical providers, and employers across the United States. It is the most complete source of data on the cost and use of health care and health insurance coverage in the United States.

medical examiner. See **coroner.**

medical futility, **1.** a judgment that further medical treatment of a patient would have no useful result. **2.** a medical treatment whose success is possible although reasoning and experience suggest that it is highly improbable.

medical genetics. See **clinical genetics.**

medical history. See **health history.**

medical home, a setting for the provision of primary health care characterized by a patient-centered philosophy. Members of the health care team collaborate to optimize and coordinate care for patients and their families.

medical illustrator, an artist who creates visual material designed to record and communicate medical, biological, and related knowledge. A medical illustrator requires a strong foundation in biology, anatomy, physiology, pathology, general medicine, and the visual arts. Today most medical illustrators use a computer to create their work.

medical indigency /in″dijen′sē/, the lack of financial reserves adequate to pay for medical care, especially that of a person or family able to manage other basic living expenses.

medical induction of labor. See **induction of labor.**

medical ionization, **1.** an atom that becomes negatively or positively charged that is then used in treatment. See **iontophoresis. 2.** a physical process in which ions flow diffusively in a medium driven by an applied electric field.

medical jurisprudence [L, *medicare* + *jus,* law, *prudentia,* knowledge], the interaction of medicine with civil and criminal law.

medical laboratory technician (MLT), a person who, under the supervision of a medical technologist or physician, performs within the specialty of collection and processing of samples from body fluids, substances, and related matter for testing and evaluation in a lab setting. Medical laboratory technicians are educated in a 2-year associate degree program. Also called **clinical laboratory technician.**

medical marijuana, cannabis or cannabinoids used in the therapeutic management of a disease or to control symptoms of a disease. It is used to reduce nausea and vomiting, improve appetite, and in the management of pain. It is available in many forms, but its use as a medication is not legal in every jurisdiction.

medical model, **1.** the traditional approach to the diagnosis and treatment of illness as practiced by physicians in the Western world since the time of Koch and Pasteur. The physician focuses on the defect, or dysfunction, within the patient, using a problem-solving approach. The medical history, physical examination, and diagnostic tests provide the basis for the identification and treatment of a specific illness. The medical model is thus focused on the physical and biological aspects of specific diseases and conditions. **2.** (in occupational therapy) a focus on the physical, psychological, social, and environmental aspects of a person. Occupational therapists guide clients in the use of their strengths to help them engage in daily activities. Occupational therapists may use a medical model in certain situations but generally combine this model with holistic practice models. **3.** (in nursing) nursing works collaboratively with practitioners using the the medical model. Nursing care is formulated on the basis of a holistic nursing assessment of all dimensions of the person (physical, emotional, mental, and spiritual) that assumes multiple causes for the problems experienced by the patient.

medical necessity, health care services and supplies provided by health care providers and agencies that are appropriate to the evaluation and treatment of a disease, condition, illness, or injury and consistent with the applicable evidence and/or standards of care.

medical nutrition therapy, the assessment of the nutritional status of a patient followed by nutritional therapy, ranging from diet modification to administration of enteral or parenteral nutrition. Compare **diet therapy.**

medical outcomes study, an evaluation of comparable medical care approaches and their relative prognoses.

medical pathology [L, *medicare* + Gk, *pathos,* disease, *logos,* science], the study of diseases not readily treated by surgical procedures.

medical physics, the application of physics concepts, theories, and methods to medicine or health care. See also **health physics.**

medical record [L, *medicare* + ME, *recorden,* to report], that part of a client's health record containing a history of various illnesses or injuries requiring medical care, inoculations, allergies, treatments, prognosis, and frequently health information about parents, siblings, occupation, and military service. See also **chart.**

medical record administrator, a person who oversees the maintenance of records of patients' medical histories, diagnoses, treatments, and outcomes in a manner that meets medical, administrative, legal, ethical, regulatory, and institutional requirements.

medical record technician, a health professional responsible for maintaining components of health information systems consistent with the medical, administrative, ethical, legal, accreditation, and regulatory requirements of the health care delivery system.

medical rounds, bedside visits by physicians, often with medical students, to evaluate, discuss, and plan care for patients in an inpatient facility. Other members of the health care team may participate.

medical secretary, a person who prepares and maintains medical records and performs related secretarial duties.

medical snatch bag, *(Informal)* a light, compact waterproof and shockproof container of emergency medical equipment for advanced prehospital care. It should provide all that is required to relieve an obstructed airway, provide artificial ventilation, arrest hemorrhage from a peripheral site, and establish an IV access for infusion.

medical social worker. See **social worker.**

medical sonographer. See **sonographer.**

medical staff, physicians and dentists who are approved and given privileges to provide health care to patients in a hospital or other health care facility. Medical staff personnel may work full time or part time and may be employed by the facility or granted admitting privileges to practice.

medical staff, courtesy, physicians and dentists who meet certain qualifications of the medical staff of a hospital or other health care facility but who admit patients only occasionally or act as consultants. They do not become part of routine operations or assume permanent responsibilities at those facilities.

medical staff, honorary, physicians and dentists, usually retired, who are recognized by the hospital medical staff for their noteworthy contributions but who may not admit patients to the hospital or participate in medical staff activities.

medical-surgical nursing, the nursing care of adult patients whose conditions or disorders are treated medically, pharmacologically, or surgically.

medical technologist. See **clinical laboratory scientist/ medical technologist.**

medical transcriptionist, a health professional who prepares a written record of patient data dictated by a physician. A certified medical transcriptionist is one who has met the qualifying standards of the American Association of Medical Transcription.

medical vagotomy. See **pharmacological vagotomy.**

medical waste, any discarded biological product, such as blood or tissue removed from operating rooms, morgues, laboratories, or other medical facilities. The term may also be applied to bedding, bandages, syringes, and similar materials that have been used in treating patients and to animal carcasses or body parts used in research. Medical waste is regulated at the state and local levels.

Medical Women's International Association (M.W.I.A.), an international professional organization of women physicians.

medicamentosus /med′ikəmen″tōsəs/ [L, *medicamentum,* drug], pertaining to a drug, particularly to an adverse reaction attributed to a medication.

Medicare /med″iker/, **1.** a federally funded national health insurance program in the United States for people over 65 years of age or who meet other criteria. The program is administered in two parts. Part A provides basic protection against costs of medical, surgical, and psychiatric hospital care. Part B is a voluntary medical insurance program financed in part from federal funds and in part from premiums contributed by enrollees. Medicare enrollment is generally offered to people 65 years of age or older who are entitled to receive Social Security or railroad retirement benefits. Individuals under age 65 can be eligible if they are disabled or have end-stage renal disease. **2.** (in Canada) the unofficial name of the national health insurance program.

medicate /med″ikāt/ [L, *medicare,* to heal], to treat an illness by administering drugs.

medicated bougie /med″ikātid/ [L, *medicare,* to heal; Fr, candle], a bougie containing a medicated agent. See also **bougie.**

medicated enema, a medication administered via an enema. It is usually used preoperatively with patients scheduled for bowel surgery or may be used to treat infections locally.

medicated tub bath, a therapeutic bath in which medication is dispersed in water, usually in the treatment of dermatological disorders.

■ METHOD: The amount of medication and the amount and temperature of the water are specified in the prescription for the bath. The water is run, the medication is added, and the solution is stirred with a bath thermometer to disperse the medication while testing the water temperature, usually between 96° F (35.6° C) and 100° F (37.8° C) but possibly as high as 103° F (39.4° C), as in the treatment of psoriasis vulgaris. Most medicated baths are prescribed as half-hour treatments. A folded towel or waterproof pillow is placed behind the head, and a towel is draped over the shoulders to enhance the patient's comfort. In certain conditions the patient may be asked to scrub affected areas with a brush and washcloth. In others the patient is instructed not to scrub at all. After the bath the skin is patted dry and any ointment, cream, or other topical prescription is applied.

■ INTERVENTIONS: The reason for the treatment is explained to the patient, and instructions are given not to get out of the tub without assistance and not to add water without calling for assistance. If the patient is to scrub the affected areas, the necessary equipment is taken to the bath. The tub is thoroughly scrubbed and rinsed before and after the treatment.

■ OUTCOME CRITERIA: The medicated bath is usually soothing, relaxing, and comforting for the patient. Close attention to instructing the patient fully and to ensuring comfort during the procedure improves compliance with the treatment.

medication /med″ikā″shən/ [L, *medicare,* to heal], **1.** a drug or other substance that is used as a medicine. **2.** the administration of a medicine.

medication error, any incorrect or wrongful administration of a medication, such as a mistake in dosage or route of administration, failure to prescribe or administer the correct drug or formulation for a particular disease or condition, use of outdated drugs, failure to observe the correct time for administration of the drug, or lack of awareness of adverse effects of certain drug combinations. Causes of medication error may include difficulty in reading handwritten orders, confusion about different drugs with similar names, or lack of information about a patient's drug allergies or sensitivities.

medication order, a written order by a physician, dentist, nurse practitioner, or other designated health professional for a medication to be dispensed by a pharmacy for administration to a patient.

medicinal restraint. See **chemical restraint.**

medicinal treatment, therapy of disorders that is based chiefly on the use of appropriate pharmacological agents.

medicine [L, *medicina,* art of healing], **1.** a drug or a remedy for illness. **2.** the art and science of the diagnosis, treatment, and prevention of disease and the maintenance of good health. **–medical,** *adj.* **3.** the art or technique of treating disease without surgery. Two major divisions of medicine are academic medicine and clinical medicine. Kinds include **environmental medicine, family medicine, forensic medicine, internal medicine, physical medicine, physical medicine and rehabilitation.**

medicolegal /med″ikōlē″gəl/ [L, *medicina,* art of healing, *lex,* law], pertaining to both medicine and law. Medicolegal considerations are a significant part of the process of making many patient care decisions and determining definitions and policies for the treatment of mentally incompetent patients and minors, for the performance of sterilization or therapeutic abortion, and for the care of terminally ill patients. Medicolegal considerations, decisions, definitions, and policies provide the framework for informed consent, professional liability, and many other aspects of current practice in the health care field.

Medigap /med″igap/, a health insurance policy sold by a private insurance company to fill gaps in the coverage of an individual's original Medicare plan.

Medihaler-Epi, an adrenergic drug. Brand name for *epinephrine bitartrate.* See **metered dose inhaler.**

mediocarpal /mē″dē-ō-kär″pəl/ [L, *medius,* middle; Gk, *karpos,* wrist], between the two rows of bones of the carpus. Also called **midcarpal.**

mediolateral /mē″dē-ō-lat″ər-əl/ [L. *medius,* middle, *latus,* side], pertaining to the middle and to one side.

mediolateral episiotomy, an episiotomy cut at an angle of approximately 45 degrees with the midline. Although it affords wide exposure for delivery, it is painful after delivery and is prone to hematoma and infection. Compare **median episiotomy.** See also **episiotomy.**

meditation /med″itā″shən/ [L, *meditari,* to consider], a state of consciousness in which the individual eliminates environmental stimuli from awareness so that the mind has a single focus, producing a state of relaxation and relief from stress. A wide variety of techniques are used to clear the mind of stressful outside interference.

meditation therapy, a method of achieving relaxation and consciousness expansion by focusing on a mantra or a key word, sound, or image while eliminating outside stimuli from one's awareness.

Mediterranean fever. See **brucellosis.**

Mediterranean lymphoma. See **immunoproliferative small intestine disease.**

medium /mē″dē-əm/ *pl.* media [L, *medius,* middle], a substance through which something moves or through which it acts. A contrast medium is a substance that has a density different from that of body tissues, permitting visual comparison of structures when used with imaging techniques. A culture medium is a substance that provides a nutritional environment for the growth of microorganisms or cells. A dispersion medium is the substance in which a colloid is dispersed. A refractory medium is the transparent tissues and fluid of the eye that refract light.

medium-chain fatty acid (MCFA),   a fatty acid having a chain length roughly 8 to 12 carbons long. It is absorbed directly into the portal blood, bypassing the lymphatic system.

medium-chain triglyceride (MCT),   a glycerine ester combined with medium-chain triglycerides distinguished from other triglycerides by having 8 to 10 carbon atoms. Once hydrolyzed, these fatty acids can be absorbed directly into the portal system. MCTs in foods are usually high in calories and easily digested.

medius /mē′dē·əs/ [L], in the middle; a term used in reference to a structure lying between two other structures that are anterior and posterior, superior and inferior, or internal and external in position.

MEDLINE /med′līn/, a U.S. National Library of Medicine computer database that covers references to biomedical academic journals covering medicine, nursing, pharmacy, dentistry, veterinary medicine, and health care. It is searchable by a free online search engine, PubMed.

MedRC, specialty units of volunteer health care professionals; the units are designed to meet the need for additional health care support on an as-needed basis. Abbreviation for *medical reserve corps.*

Medrol, a glucocorticoid. Brand name for *methylprednisolone disodium phosphate.*

Medrol Acetate, a glucocorticoid. Brand name for *methylprednisolone acetate.*

medroxyPROGESTERone acetate /medrok′sēprōjes″tə rōn/, a progestin.
- INDICATIONS: It is prescribed in endometrial and renal carcinomas and in the treatment of menstrual disorders caused by hormone imbalance. It is given as a depot injection for contraception (Depo-Provera).
- CONTRAINDICATIONS: Known or suspected pregnancy, thrombophlebitis, embolism, stroke, liver dysfunction, cancer of the breast or genitals, abnormal vaginal bleeding, missed abortion, or known hypersensitivity to this drug prohibits its use.
- ADVERSE EFFECTS: Among the more serious adverse effects are thrombophlebitis, pulmonary embolism, stroke, hepatitis, and cerebral thrombosis.

medrysone /med′risōn/, a glucocorticoid that decreases the infiltration of leukocytes at the site of inflammation. It is used topically in the eye as an antiinflammatory agent.

Med.Sc.D., abbreviation for *Doctor of Medical Science.*

med tech, *(Informal)* abbreviation for **medical technologist.**

medulla /mədul″ə/ *pl.* **medullas, medullae** [L, marrow], 1. the most internal part of a structure or organ, such as the renal medulla. 2. See **medulla oblongata.**

medulla oblongata, a bulbous continuation of the spinal cord just above the foramen magnum and separated from the pons by a horizontal groove. It is one of three parts of the brainstem and primarily contains white matter. The medulla contains the cardiac, vasomotor, and respiratory centers of the brain. Medullary injury or disease often proves fatal. Also called **medulla.** Compare **mesencephalon, pons.**

medulla of the kidney [L, *medulla,* marrow; ME, *kidenei*], a part of the parenchyma of the kidney, beneath the cortex, including the renal pyramids and columns. It

contains few, if any, glomeruli. An inner layer contains the papillae, and the outer part, which extends as far as the arcuate vessels, contains the thick ascending limbs of the loop of Henle.

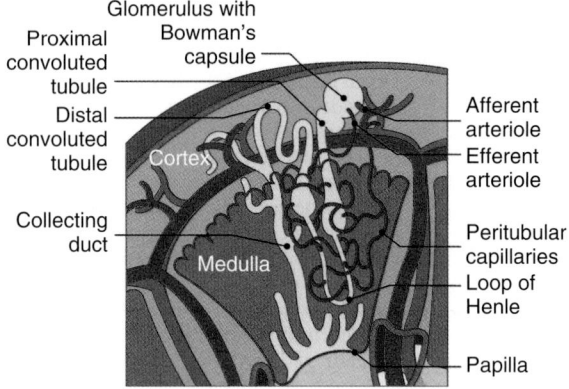

Detailed anatomy of the renal medulla and cortex
(Nikolaidis et al, 2008)

medullary /med″əler·ē, mədul″erē, med″yəler′ē/ [L, *medulla,* marrow], 1. pertaining to the medulla of the brain. 2. pertaining to the bone marrow. 3. pertaining to the spinal cord. See also *medullar.*

medullary carcinoma, a soft malignant neoplasm of the epithelium containing little or no fibrous tissue. Also called **carcinoma medullare, carcinoma molle, encephaloid carcinoma.**

medullary chemoreceptor. See **central chemoreceptor.**

medullary cystic disease, a chronic familial disease of the kidney, characterized by the slow onset of uremia. The disease appears in young children or adolescents, who pass large volumes of dilute urine with greater than normal amounts of sodium. Hemodialysis is the usual treatment for the disease as the uremia progresses and becomes severe. See also **uremia.**

medullary fold. See **neural fold.**

medullary groove. See **neural groove.**

medullary nerve sheath. See **nerve sheath.**

medullary plate. See **neural plate.**

medullary sponge kidney, a congenital defect of the kidney leading to cystic dilation of the collecting tubules. People with this defect often develop a kidney stone or an infection of the kidney caused by urinary stasis. The condition is diagnosed by urographic techniques. Treatment includes drugs to acidify the urine and a diet low in calcium and high in fluids to discourage formation of stones.

medullary tube. See **neural tube.**

medullas. See **medulla.**

medulla spinalis. See **spinal cord.**

medullated /med″yəlā′tid/ [L, *medulla,* marrow], enclosed by a marrowlike substance, such as the myelin sheath of a nerve fiber.

medullated neuroma. See **fascicular neuroma.**

medulloblastoma /mədul′ōblastō″mə/ [L, *medulla* + Gk, *blastos,* germ, *oma,* tumor], a poorly differentiated malignant neoplasm composed of tightly packed cells of spongioblastic and neuroblastic lineage. The tumor usually arises in the cerebellum, occurs most frequently at 5 to 9 years of age, and affects more boys than girls. Medulloblastomas are extremely radiosensitive and grow rapidly. The prognosis is poor.

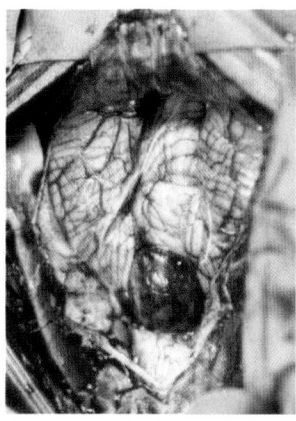

Operative view of medulloblastoma *(Winn, 2011)*

medulloepithelioma.   See **neurocytoma.**

mefenamic acid /mef'ənam″ik/,   a nonsteroidal antiinflammatory agent and analgesic.

■ INDICATIONS: It is prescribed in the treatment of mild to moderate pain, including dysmenorrhea.

■ CONTRAINDICATIONS: GI ulceration or inflammation, impaired renal function, or known hypersensitivity to this drug prohibits its use. It is prescribed with caution for patients with asthma.

■ ADVERSE EFFECTS: Dyspepsia and diarrhea are the most common adverse effects. Other GI symptoms, dizziness, drowsiness, or skin rash occasionally occurs. Severe blood dyscrasias develop rarely.

mefloquine /mef″ləkēn/,   an antimalarial for the prophylaxis and treatment of malaria caused by chloroquine-resistant strains of *Plasmodium falciparum,* or *P. vivax.*

Mefoxin,   a cephalosporin antibiotic. Brand name for **cefoxitin sodium.**

MEFR,   abbreviation for **maximal expiratory flow rate.**

mega-, megalo-, mego-,   **1.** prefix meaning "great" or "huge": *megadose, megalocyte, megacolon.* **2.** a quantity that is 1 million times a given unit: *megahertz.*

megabladder.   See **megalocystis.**

megacaryocyte.   See **megakaryocyte.**

Megace,   an antineoplastic progestational agent. Brand name for **megestrol acetate.**

megacolon /meg″əkōlən/ [Gk, *megas* + *kolon,* colon],   abnormal massive dilation of the colon that may be congenital, toxic, or acquired. Congenital megacolon (Hirschsprung disease) is caused by the absence of autonomic ganglia in the smooth muscle wall of the colon. Toxic megacolon is a grave complication of ulcerative colitis and may cause perforation of the colon, septicemia, and death. Colonoscopy and surgery are the usual treatments for toxic and congenital megacolon. Acquired megacolon is the result of a chronic refusal to defecate, which usually occurs in children who are psychotic or cognitively impaired. The colon becomes dilated by an accumulation of impacted feces. Laxatives, enemas, and psychiatric treatment are often necessary. See also **Hirschsprung disease.**

megacycle.   See **megahertz.**

megacystis,   an abnormally enlarged urinary bladder. Also called **megabladder, megalocystis.**

megacystis-microcolon-intestinal hypoperistalsis,   a rare congenital disorder characterized by a dilated nonobstructive urinary bladder and hypoperistalsis of the gastrointestinal tract.

megadose /meg″ədōs/,   a dose that greatly exceeds the amount usually prescribed or recommended.

megadyne /meg″ədīn/,   a unit of force equal to 1 million dynes.

megaesophagus /meg'ə·isof″əgəs/ [Gk, *megas* + *oisophagos,* gullet],   abnormal dilation of the lower segments of the esophagus caused by distension resulting from the failure of the cardiac sphincter to relax and allow the passage of food into the stomach. See also **achalasia.**

megahertz (MHz) /meg″əhurts/ [Gk, *megas,* large, *hertz,* a number of cycles per second],   a unit of frequency equal to 1 million cycles per second. Also called **megacycle.** See also **hertz.**

megakaryocyte /meg'əker″ē·əsīt′/ [Gk, *megas,* large, *karyon,* nut, *kytos,* cell],   bone marrow cell measuring 35 to 160 μm in diameter and having a multilobed nucleus. Megakaryocytes are platelet precursors. Also spelled **megacaryocyte.** See also **platelets.** *−megakaryocytic, adj.*

megakaryocytic leukemia /meg'əker″ē·ōsit″ik/ [Gk, *megas* + *karyon,* nut, *kytos,* cell],   a rare malignancy of blood-forming tissue in which megakaryocytes proliferate in the bone marrow and circulate in the blood in large numbers.

megalencephaly /meg'əlensef″əlē/ [Gk, *megas* + *enkephalos,* brain],   a condition characterized by pathological parenchymal overgrowth of the brain. In some cases generalized cerebral hyperplasia is associated with cognitive impairment or a brain disorder, such as epilepsy. Also called **macrencephaly.** *−megalencephalic, megalencephalous, adj.*

-megalia.   See **-megaly, -megalia.**

megalo-.   See **mega-, megalo-, mego-.**

megaloblast /meg″əlōblast′/ [Gk, *megas* + *blastos,* germ],   abnormally large nucleated immature erythrocyte that develops in the bone marrow in megaloblastic anemias associated with deficiency of vitamin B_{12}, or folic acid. *−megaloblastic, adj.*

megaloblastic anemia /-blas″tik/,   a hematological disorder characterized by the production of macrocytes in folate and vitamin B_{12} deficiency. See also **nutritional anemia, pernicious anemia.**

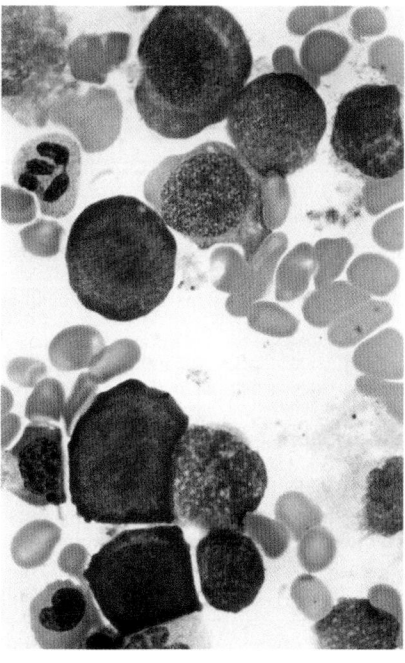

Bone marrow aspirate in megaloblastic anemia
(Winn, 2011)

M

megalocephaly. See **macrocephaly.**

megalocornea, an inherited disorder in which the corneal diameter is enlarged. It may be associated with congenital glaucoma.

megalocystis /meg′əlōsis″tis/ [Gk, *megas + kystis,* bag], an abnormal condition primarily affecting girls, characterized by an enlarged and thin-walled bladder. Surgical reduction of the size of the bladder or diversion of urine through the ileum may correct the condition. Also called **megabladder, megacystis.**

megalocyte /meg″əlōsīt/, an extremely large erythrocyte. This term is not in common usage.

megalocytic interstitial nephritis, an early stage of malacoplakia of the urinary tract in which there are no Michaelis-Gutmann bodies.

megalomania /meg′əlōmā″nē·ə/ [Gk, *megas + mania,* madness], an abnormal mental state characterized by delusions of grandeur in which one believes oneself to be a person of great importance, power, fame, or wealth. Also called **grandiosity.** See also **mania.**

megalopenis. Also called **macrophallus.** See **macropenis.**

megaloureter /meg′əlōyoŏorē″tər/ [Gk, *megas + oureter,* ureter], an abnormal condition characterized by marked dilation of one or both ureters, resulting from dysfunctional peristaltic action of the smooth muscle in the ureters. Treatment may include surgical resection. Also called **megaureter.**

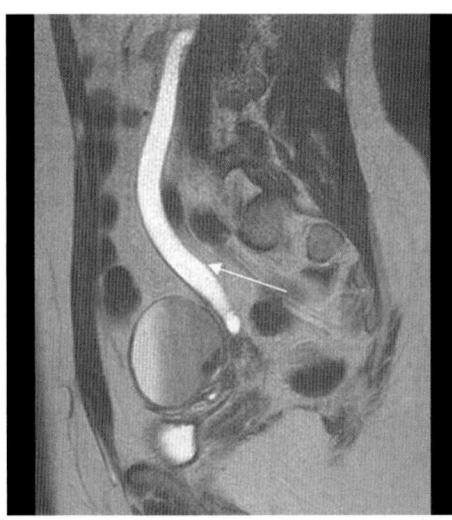

Megaloureter *(Howard and Hamilton, 2013)*

-megaly, -megalia, suffix meaning "an enlargement of a (specified) body part": *cardiomegaly, adrenomegaly, acromegaly.*

megaureter. See **megaloureter.**

megaureter-megacystis syndrome, chronic ureteral dilation associated with hypotonia and dilation of the bladder and gaping of the ureteral orifices, permitting vesicoureteral reflex of urine and resulting in chronic pyelonephritis.

megavitamin therapy /-vī″təmin/, a type of treatment that involves the administration of large doses of certain vitamins and minerals.

megestrol acetate /məjes″trōl/, an antineoplastic progestational agent.

■ INDICATIONS: It is prescribed to treat endometrial cancer and more commonly to palliate advanced endometrial and breast cancer. It is also used to stimulate appetite and to promote weight gain in cachexia patients.

■ CONTRAINDICATIONS: Hypersensitivity to the drug prohibits its use.

■ ADVERSE EFFECTS: Adverse effects include edema and breakthrough bleeding.

mego-. See **mega-, megalo-, mego-.**

meibomian cyst. See **chalazion.**

meibomian gland /mēbō″mē·ən/ [Heinrich Meibom, German physician, 1638–1700], one of several sebaceous glands that secrete sebum from their ducts on the posterior margin of each eyelid. The glands are embedded in the tarsal plate of each eyelid. Also called **palpebral gland, tarsal gland.**

Meige disease /mezh′/ [Henri Meige, French physician, 1866–1940], **1.** dystonia of facial and oromandibular muscles with blepharospasm, grimacing mouth movements, and protrusion of the tongue, usually occurring in older women. Also called **Brueghel syndrome,** *Meige syndrome.* **2.** autosomal-dominant familial form of lymphedema praecox. See **lymphedema praecox.**

Meigs syndrome /megz/ [Joe V. Meigs, American gynecologist, 1892–1963], ascites and hydrothorax associated with a fibroma of the ovaries or other pelvic tumor.

meio-. See **mio-, meio-.**

meiocyte /mī″əsīt/ [Gk, *meiosis,* becoming smaller, *kytos,* cell], any cell undergoing meiosis.

meiogenic /mī′əjen″ik/ [Gk, *meiosis + genein,* to produce], producing or causing meiosis.

meiosis /mī·ō″sis/ [Gk, becoming smaller], the division of a sex cell as it matures into two and then four haploid cells. The nucleus of each receives one half of the number of chromosomes present in the somatic cells of the species. Also called **reduction division.** Compare **mitosis.** See also **anaphase, metaphase, oogenesis, prophase, spermatogenesis, telophase.** *−meiotic, adj.*

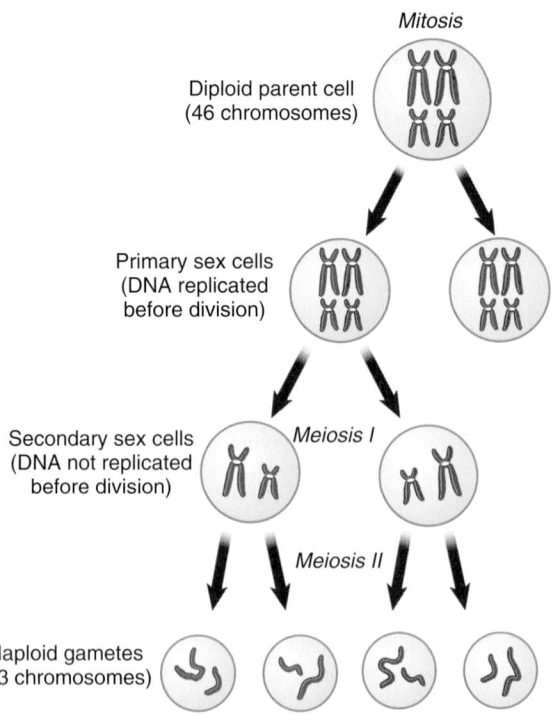

Meiosis *(Patton and Thibodeau, 2016)*

Meissner corpuscle /mīs″nər/ [Georg Meissner, German anatomist, 1829–1905; L, *corpusculum,* little body], any one of a number of small, special pressure-sensitive sensory end organs with a connective tissue capsule and tiny stacked plates in the dermis of the hand and foot, the front of the forearm, the skin of the lips, the mucous membrane of the tongue, the palpebral conjunctiva, and the skin of the mammary papilla. A single nerve fiber penetrates each oval capsule, spirals through the interior, and ends as a globular mass. Also called **tactile corpuscle.** Compare **Golgi-Mazzoni corpuscles, Krause corpuscles.**

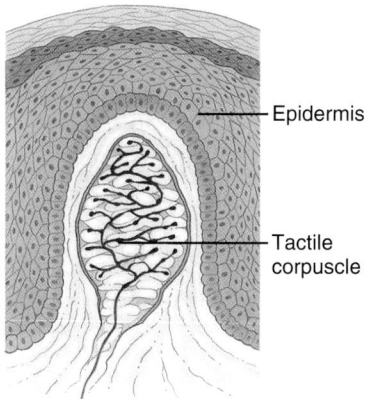

Meissner corpuscle *(Patton and Thibodeau, 2016)*

Meissner's plexus [Georg Meissner; L, *plaited*], small aggregations of ganglion cells located in the submucosa of the intestine.

mel-, melo-, combining form meaning "limb" or "limbs": *erythromelalgia, phocomelia.*

melan-. See **melano-, melan-, mel-.**

melancholia /mel′angkō″lē·ə/ [Gk, *melas,* black, *chole,* bile], a form of severe depression characterized by overwhelming sadness and a lack of interest in normally pleasant activities. See also **depression, major depressive disorder.** —*melancholic, adj.*

melaniferous /mel′ənif″ərəs/ [Gk, *melas,* black; L, *ferre,* to bear], pertaining to a black pigment or imparting a dark coloring.

melanin /mel″ənin/ [Gk, *melas,* black], a black or dark brown pigment that occurs naturally in the hair, skin, and iris and choroid of the eye. See also **melanocyte.**

melanin test, a test for detecting melanin in the urine of patients with malignant melanomas.

melanism /mel″əniz′əm/ [Gk, *melas,* black], an abnormal deposit of dark brown to black melanin pigment in the skin, hair, and other tissues. Also called **melanosis.**

melano-, melan-, mel-, combining form meaning "black": *melanocyte, melancholia, melanoderm.*

melanoameloblastoma /mel′ənō·am′əlōblastō″mə/, a benign neoplasm appearing as a blue-black lesion on the anterior maxilla of infants. The growth is of neuroectodermal origin and consists of small round undifferentiated tumor cells and larger melanin-producing cells. Also called **melanotic neuroectodermal tumor of infancy.**

melanoblast /mel′ənōblast′/ [Gk, *melas,* black, *blastos,* germ], an epithelial tissue cell containing black granules. It develops into a melanocyte from the neural crest and migrates to various parts of the body during the early stages of embryonic life before becoming a mature melanocyte capable of forming melanin.

melanoblastoma /mel′ənō·blastō″mə/, a tumor of poorly differentiated melanin-producing cells.

melanocarcinoma /-kär′sinō″mə/, a malignant melanoma.

melanocyte /mel″ənōsīt′, mələn″ōsīt/ [Gk, *melas* + *kytos,* cell], a body cell capable of producing melanin. Melanocytes are distributed throughout the basal cell layer of the epidermis and form melanin pigment from tyrosine, an amino acid. Melanin granules are then transferred to adjacent basal cells and to hair. Melanocyte-stimulating hormone from the pituitary controls the amount of melanin produced.

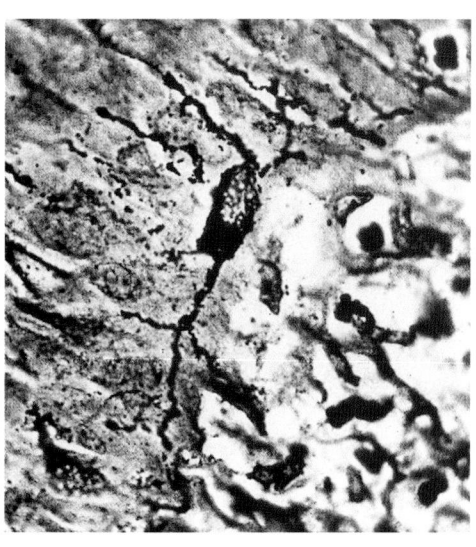

Melanocyte *(du Vivier, 2002)*

melanocyte-stimulating hormone (MSH), a polypeptide hormone, secreted by the pars intermedia of the pituitary gland, that controls the intensity of pigmentation in pigmented cells. It is synthesized on the same large precursor polypeptide as adrenocorticotropic hormone and the enkephalins.

melanocytic nevus /-sit″ik/, a congenital pigmented lesion of the skin caused by a disorder involving melanocytes.

melanoderma /mel′ənōdur″mə/ [Gk, *melas* + *derma,* skin], any abnormal darkening of the skin caused by increased deposits of melanin or the salts of iron or silver.

melanoma /mel′ənō″mə/ *pl.* melanomas, melanomata [Gk, *melas* + *oma,* tumor], any of a group of malignant neoplasms that originate in the skin and that are composed of melanocytes. A melanocytic nevus may be acquired or congenital. The congenital melanocytic nevus is regarded as more likely to develop into a malignant melanoma, primarily because of its larger size. Smaller melanomas tend to develop from a pigmented nevus over several months or years. They may be sporadic and occur most commonly in fair-skinned people having light-colored eyes. A previous sunburn increases a person's risk. Any black or brown spot having an irregular border; pigment appearing to radiate beyond that border; a red, black, and blue coloration observable on close examination; or a nodular surface is suggestive of melanoma and is usually excised for biopsy. Melanomas are most commonly located on the upper back and lower legs of fair-skinned individuals and on the palms of the hands and insoles of the feet of dark-skinned individuals. Melanomas may metastasize and are among the most malignant of all skin cancers. Prognosis depends on the kind of melanoma; its size, depth of invasion, and location; and the age and condition of the patient. Because of the occurrence of

M

melanomas and melanocytic nevi in certain families, a familial atypical mole and melanoma syndrome has been designated. It is defined by the occurrence of melanoma in one or more first- or second-degree relatives, a large number of moles, and moles that demonstrate certain cellular features. Patients with the syndrome have a high lifetime risk of development of melanoma. Compare **blue nevus.** Kinds include **benign juvenile melanoma, lentigo maligna melanoma, primary cutaneous melanoma, superficial spreading melanoma, amelanotic melanoma, nodular melanoma.** See also **Hutchinson freckle.**

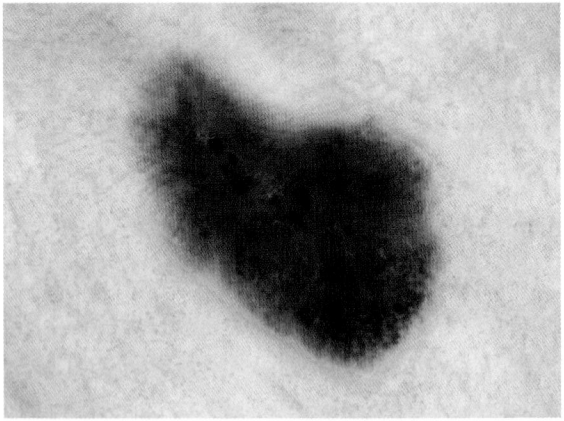

Melanoma (Bolognia et al, 2012)

melanomatosis /-mətō″sis/, **1.** a condition characterized by many widespread melanoma lesions. **2.** the development of melanomas throughout the body.

melanosis. See **melanism.**

melanosis coli /mel′ənō′sis/, an abnormal condition in which the mucous membrane of the colon is pigmented with melanin.

melanosome /mel″ənōsōm′/, one of the oval pigment granules within melanocytes that synthesize melanin.

melanotic carcinoma /mel′ənot″ik/, a malignant pigmented skin cancer.

melanotic neuroectodermal tumor of infancy. See **melanoameloblastoma.**

melanuria /mel′ənŏŏr″ē-ə/, urine that has a dark color caused by the presence of melanin or other pigments.

melasma. See **chloasma.**

melasma gravidarum /mələz′mə/ [Gk, *melas,* black; L, *gravida,* pregnant], a dark pigment or discoloration that may appear on the skin of pregnant women, caused by estrogen and progesterone stimulation of melanin. It is most commonly seen in olive-skinned women.

MELAS syndrome, a familial syndrome of maternal (mitochondrial) inheritance. Abbreviation for *mitochondrial encephalopathy, lactic acidosis, and stroke-like episodes.*

melatonin, a dietary supplement, also known as N-acetyl-5-methoxytryptamine.

■ INDICATIONS: It is used for jet lag and insomnia, for cancer protection, and as an oral contraceptive. Melatonin is effective for treating jet lag and has shown benefit when used in combination therapy for various cancers. It is not very effective for insomnia. There are insufficient data related to its efficacy for other uses.

■ CONTRAINDICATIONS: It is not recommended during pregnancy and lactation, in children, or in those with autoimmune disease or known hypersensitivity to this product.

Meleda disease. See **mal de Meleda.**

melena /məlē″nə, məl″ənə/ [Gk, *melas,* black], abnormal black tarry stool that has a distinctive odor and contains digested blood. It usually results from bleeding in the upper GI tract and is often a sign of peptic ulcer or small bowel disease. See also **gastrointestinal bleeding.**

melena neonatorum [Gk, *melas,* black, *neos,* new; L, *natus,* born], the passage of dark tarry stools by a newborn. The cause is usually the alteration of blood pigment associated with hemorrhage. Normal meconium stools are greenish to black.

meli-, prefix meaning "sweet" or "related to honey": *melicera.*

-melia, suffix meaning "limbs": *dysmelia, ectromelia, phocomelia.*

melicera, *(Obsolete)* a cyst containing thick, viscous fluid.

melioidosis /mel′ē-oidō″sis/ [Gk, *melis,* distemper, *eidos,* form, *osis,* condition], an infection caused by the gram-negative bacillus *Burkholderia pseudomallei.* Acute melioidosis is fulminant and usually characterized by pneumonia, empyema, lung abscess, septicemia, and liver or spleen involvement. Chronic melioidosis is associated with osteomyelitis, multiple abscesses of the internal organs, and development of fistulas from the abscesses. The disease, most commonly seen in China and Southeast Asia, is acquired by direct contact with infected animals. Human-to-human transmission is unlikely. Treatment using chloramphenicol, sulfonamides, or tetracycline for several months is usually successful.

Melkersson-Rosenthal syndrome /mel′kərson rō′zentäl/ [Ernst Gustaf Melkersson, Swedish physician, 1898–1932; Curt Rosenthal, German psychiatrist, 1892–1937], an autosomal-dominant condition usually beginning in childhood or adolescence, characterized chiefly by chronic noninflammatory facial swelling, localized particularly to the lips, with recurrent facial palsy and sometimes fissured tongue. Associated ophthalmic symptoms include lagophthalmos, blepharochalasis, swollen eyelids, burning sensation of the eyes, corneal opacities, retrobulbar neuritis, and exophthalmos. Also called *Melkersson syndrome.*

Mellaril, an antipsychotic agent. Brand name for **thioridazine hydrochloride.**

melon-seed body /mel″ən/, a small, fibrous, loose body in a joint or tendon sheath.

meloxicam /mĕlok′sĭkam/, a nonsteroidal antiinflammatory drug used in the treatment of osteoarthritis. It is administered orally.

melphalan /mel′fəlan/, an antineoplastic alkylating agent.

■ INDICATIONS: It is prescribed in the treatment of malignant neoplastic diseases, including palliative treatment of multiple myeloma and nonresectable ovarian carcinoma.

■ CONTRAINDICATIONS: Pregnancy, recent exposure to antineoplastic medication or to radiation, or known hypersensitivity to this drug prohibits its use.

■ ADVERSE EFFECTS: Among the more serious adverse effects are bone marrow depression, nausea, and vomiting.

melting, **1.** the liquefaction effect of heat. **2.** the thermal denaturation of double-stranded deoxyribonucleic acid into two component strands. **3.** conversion of the solid to the liquid phase.

melting point (mp) [AS, *meltan* + L, *punctus,* pricked], a characteristic temperature at which the solid and liquid forms of a substance are in equilibrium. The melting point of ice is 32° F, or 0° C, at one atmosphere pressure.

memantine, an anti-Alzheimer agent.

■ INDICATIONS: This drug is used to treat moderate to severe dementia in Alzheimer disease.

■ CONTRAINDICATIONS: Known hypersensitivity to this drug prohibits its use.

■ ADVERSE EFFECTS: Adverse effects of this drug include somnolence, headache, hallucinations, hypertension, vomiting, constipation, rash, coughing, dyspnea, back pain, fatigue, and pain. Common side effects include dizziness and confusion.

membrana tectoria /membrā″nə/ [L, *membrana,* thin skin, *tectorium,* a covering], **1.** the broad, strong ligament covering the dens and helping to connect the axis to the occipital bone of the skull. Also called **occipitoaxial ligament. 2.** a spiral membrane projecting from the vestibular lip of the cochlea over the organ of Corti.

membrana tympani.   See **tympanic membrane.**

membrane /mem″brān/ [L, *membrana,* thin skin], a thin layer of tissue composed of epithelial cells and connective tissue that covers a surface, lines a cavity, or divides a space in the body. Kinds include **mucous membrane, serous membrane, skin, synovial membrane.**

membrane attack complex (MAC), a cluster of complement components that creates a pore in the plasma membrane of a cell, leading to the lysis of a cell.

membrane conductance, the degree of permeability of a cellular membrane to certain ions; the reciprocal of the membrane resistance.

membrane diffusion coefficient, a factor that relates the quantitative characteristics of alveolar-capillary membranes to total pulmonary diffusing capacity.

membrane potential [L, *membrana* + *potentia*], the difference in electrical polarization or charge between two sides of a membrane or cell wall. Also called **electric potential gradient.**

membrane responsiveness, the relationship between the membrane potential of a myocardial cell at the time of stimulation and the maximal rate of rise of the action potential.

membranoproliferative glomerulonephritis (MPGN) /mem′brənō′prōlif″ərətiv′/, a chronic form of glomerulonephritis characterized by mesangial cell proliferation, irregular thickening of glomerular capillary walls, thickening of the mesangial matrix, and low serum levels of complement. Also called **mesangiocapillary glomerulonephritis.**

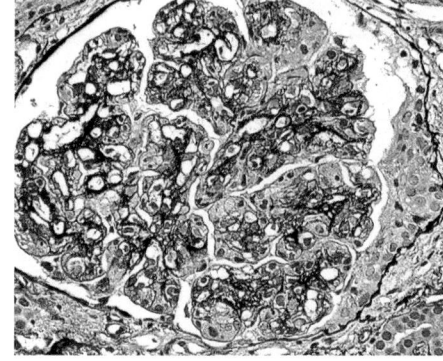

Membranoproliferative glomerulonephritis
(Schena et al, 2015)

membranous /mem′brənəs/ [L, *membrana*], resembling or consisting of a membrane.

membranous dysmenorrhea [L, *membrana* + Gk, *dys,* bad, *men,* month, *rhein,* to flow], a form of spasmodic pain associated with menstruation in which a cast of the uterine cavity is passed.

membranous labyrinth [L, *membrana* + *labyrinthos,* a maze], a network of three fluid-filled membranous semicircular ducts suspended within the bony semicircular canals of the inner ear, associated with the sense of balance. The ducts, which contain endolymph, follow the contours of the bony canals and are about one fourth of the diameter of the canals.

membranous nephropathy.   See **glomerulonephritis.**

membranous pharyngitis [L, *membrana* + Gk, *pharynx,* throat], a diphtheric inflammation of the pharynx with the formation of a false membrane in the throat. See also **diphtheria.**

membranous stomatitis.   See **pseudomembranous stomatitis.**

memory /mem″ərē/ [L, *memoria*], **1.** the mental faculty or power that enables one to retain and to recall, through unconscious associative processes, previously experienced sensations, impressions, ideas, concepts, and all information that has been consciously learned. **2.** the reservoir of all past experiences and knowledge that may be recollected or recalled at will. **3.** the recollection of a past event, idea, sensation, or previously learned knowledge. Kinds include **affect memory, anterograde memory, kinesthetic memory, long-term memory, screen memory, short-term memory, visual memory.** See also **amnesia, déjà vu. 4.** (in occupational therapy) a functional outcome assessed by a variety of standardized tools and therapist expertise related to cognitive capacity, strategy of use of that capacity, and recall of information.

memory cells, 1. See **lymphocyte. 2.** T and B lymphocytes that mediate immunological memory. They are believed to retain information that permits a subsequent antigenic challenge to be followed by a more rapid efficient immunological reaction than that seen with the first exposure.

memory image, a sensation, impression, or sense perception as it is recalled in the memory.

memory training, exercises designed by a variety of health care professionals to enhance cognitive function, especially short-term improvements in working memory for activities of daily living.

mem retinoscopy, a type of dynamic retinoscopy in which the fixation target is a series of letters on the retinoscope or a card with letters at a normal reading distance. It is a common clinical test to assess lag of accommodation.

MEN, abbreviation for **multiple endocrine neoplasia.**

menadione /men′ədi·ōn/, a synthetic fat-soluble provitamin that can be chemically converted in the body to active vitamin K. It is used as a source of vitamin K in the treatment of hypoprothrombinemia associated with vitamin K deficiency, as occurs in hepatic or biliary disease or malabsorption syndromes, or after administration of salicylates, anticoagulants, or certain antibiotics. It is administered orally or intramuscularly. Also called **vitamin K$_3$.** See also **vitamin K.**

menarche /menär″kē/ [Gk, *men,* month, *archaios,* from the beginning], the first menstruation and the commencement of cyclic menstrual function. It usually occurs between 9 and 17 years of age. See also **pubarche.**

menarcheal age /menär″kē·əl/ [Gk, *men,* month, *archaios,* beginning; L, *aetas,* age], the age at which menstruation begins. The normal range is from 9 to 17 years of age. See also **puberty.**

Mendel-Bekhterev reflex.   See **Mendel's reflex.**

mendelevium (Md) /men′dəlē″vē·əm/ [Dimitrii Ivanovich Mendeleev, Russian chemist, 1834–1907], a synthetic element in the actinide group. Its atomic number is 101. The atomic mass of its most stable isotope is 256. It is the ninth transuranic element.

mendelian.   See **mendelism.**

mendelian genetics, mendelian laws.   See **Mendel's laws.**

mendelism /men″dəliz′əm/ [Gregor J. Mendel, Austrian geneticist, 1822–1884], the concept of inheritance derived from the application of Mendel's laws. Also called *mendelianism.* −**mendelian,** *adj.*

Mendel's dorsal reflex of foot. See **Mendel's reflex.**

Mendel's laws [Gregor J. Mendel], the basic principles of inheritance based on breeding experiments on garden peas by the 19th-century Austrian monk Gregor Mendel. These principles are usually stated as the law of segregation and the law of independent assortment. According to the law of segregation, each trait of a species is represented in the somatic cells by a pair of units, now known as genes, which are segregated during meiosis so that each gamete receives only one gene for each trait. In any monohybrid crossing, the possible ratio for the phenotypic expression of a particular dominant trait is 3:1, whereas the genotypic ratio of pure dominants to hybrids to pure recessives is 1:2:1. According to the law of independent assortment, the members of a gene pair on different chromosomes segregate independently from other pairs during meiosis so that the gametes show all possible combinations of genes. Genes on the same chromosome are affected by linkage and segregate in blocks according to the amount of crossing over that occurs, a discovery made after Mendel's work. Also called **mendelian genetics, mendelian laws.** See also **chromosome, crossing over, dominant allele, linkage, meiosis, recessive allele.**

Mendelson syndrome [Curtis L. Mendelson, American obstetrician and cardiologist, 1913-2002], a respiratory condition caused by the aspiration of acidic gastric contents into the lungs. It usually occurs when a person vomits while inebriated, stuporous from anesthesia, or unconscious, as during a seizure. It is marked by bronchoconstriction and destruction of the tracheal mucosa, progressing to a syndrome resembling acute respiratory distress syndrome. Also called **pulmonary acid aspiration syndrome.**

Mendel's reflex /men′dəlz/ [Kurt Mendel, German neurologist, 1874–1946], percussion of the top of the foot normally causing dorsal flexion of the second to fifth toes but in certain organic nervous conditions causing plantar flexion of the toes. Also called **Bekhterev-Mendel reflex, cuboidodigital reflex, dorsocuboidal reflex, Mendel-Bekhterev reflex, Mendel's dorsal reflex of foot, tarsophalangeal reflex.**

Ménétrier disease. See **giant hypertrophic gastritis.**

-menia, suffix meaning "(condition of) menstrual activity": *catamenia.*

Ménière disease /mānē·er″/ [Prosper Ménière, French physician, 1799–1862], a chronic disease of the inner ear characterized by recurrent episodes of vertigo; progressive sensorineural hearing loss, which may be bilateral; and tinnitus.

meningeal /mənin″jē·əl/ [Gk, *meninx,* membrane], pertaining to the meninges, the three layers of membranes covering the brain and spinal cord.

meningeal artery, one of the arteries that supply the dura mater. All are small except the middle meningeal artery, which supplies the greatest part of the dura.

meninges /minin″jēz/ [Gk, *meninx,* membrane], the three membranes enclosing the brain and the spinal cord, comprising the dura mater, the pia mater, and the arachnoid membrane. The pia mater and the arachnoid can become inflamed by bacterial meningitis, causing serious complications that may be life-threatening. −**meningeal,** *adj.*

meningioma /minin′jē·ō″mə/ [Gk, *meninx,* membrane, *oma,* tumor], a mesenchymal fibroblastic tumor of the membranes enveloping the brain and spinal cord. Meningiomas grow slowly, are usually vascular, and occur most commonly near the superior longitudinal transverse and cavernous sinuses of the dura mater of the brain. The tumors may be nodular, plaquelike, or diffuse lesions that invade the skull, causing bone erosion and compression of brain tissue. Meningiomas usually occur in adults.

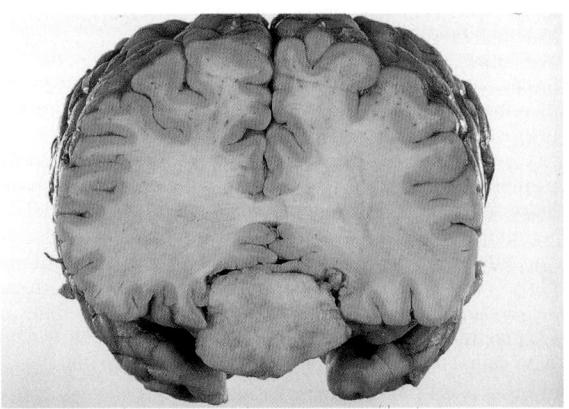

Midline meningioma compressing the frontal lobes
(Ellison et al, 2013)

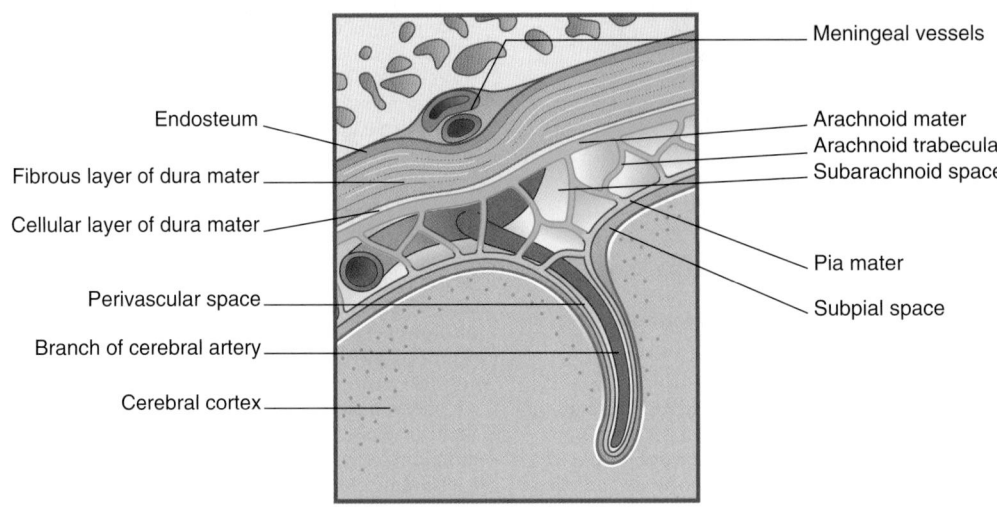

The meninges *(Mtui et al, 2012)*

meningism /minin″jizəm/ [Gk, *meninx* + *ismos,* process], an abnormal condition characterized by irritation of the brain and spinal cord and by symptoms that mimic those of meningitis. In meningism, however, there is no actual inflammation of the meninges.

meningismus /men′injis″məs/ [Gk, *meninx,* membrane], a condition in which the patient shows signs of meningitis but examination reveals no pathological changes in the meninges. The condition is associated with cases of pneumonia in small children. See also **meningism.**

meningitis /min′injī″tis/ *pl.* **meningitides** [Gk, *meninx* + *itis,* inflammation], any infection or inflammation of the membranes covering the brain and spinal cord. It is usually purulent and involves the fluid in the subarachnoid space. The most common causes in adults are bacterial infection with *Streptococcus pneumoniae, Neisseria meningitidis,* or *Haemophilus influenzae.* Aseptic meningitis may be caused by nonbacterial agents such as a high dose of intravenous immunoglobulin, chemicals, neoplasms, or viruses. Many of these diseases are benign and self-limited, such as meningitis caused by strains of coxsackievirus or echovirus. Others are more severe, such as those involving arboviruses, herpesviruses, or poliomyelitis viruses. Yeasts such as *Candida* and *Cryptococcus* may cause a severe, often fatal meningitis. Also called **cerebromeningitis.** Compare **encephalitis.** Kinds include **tuberculous meningitis.**

- OBSERVATIONS: The onset of meningitis is usually sudden and characterized by severe headache, stiffness of the neck, irritability, malaise, and restlessness. Nausea, vomiting, delirium, and complete disorientation may develop quickly. Temperature, pulse rate, and respirations are increased. Residual damage may include deafness, blindness, paralysis, and cognitive impairment. Hydrocephalus also may develop.

- INTERVENTIONS: Bacterial meningitis is treated promptly with antibiotics specific for the causative organism. They are administered intravenously or intrathecally. Antifungal medications, such as amphotericin B, given intravenously or intrathecally for several weeks, may prevent death from fungal meningitis, but serious neurological sequelae may occur.

- PATIENT CARE CONSIDERATIONS: Constant skilled nursing and specialized medical attention is necessary to ensure early recognition of rising intracranial pressure, to prevent aspiration in the event of convulsive seizures, and to prevent airway obstruction. Except for the first day or two of meningococcal disease, strict isolation procedures are unnecessary. IV fluids and nasogastric tube feeding may be necessary for a prolonged period. Sedatives and narcotic analgesics should not be used because they may obscure important neurological signs in addition to depressing vital functions. Upon recovery, a rehabilitation team will play a major role in the development of an individualized treatment plan to redevelop functions lost as a result of meningitis.

meningo-, combining form meaning "membranes covering the brain or spinal cord or other membranes": *meningocele, meningococcus, meningoencephalitis.*

meningocele /mining″gōsēl′/ [Gk, *meninx* + *kele,* hernia], a saclike protrusion of either the cerebral or spinal meninges through a congenital defect in the skull or the vertebral column. It forms a hernial cyst that is filled with cerebrospinal fluid but does not contain neural tissue. The anomaly is designated a cranial meningocele or spinal meningocele, depending on the site of the defect. It can be repaired by surgery. See also **myelomeningocele, neural tube defect.**

meningococcal. See **meningococcus.**

meningococcal meningitis /mining′gōkok′əl/, bacterial meningitis caused by infection with *Neisseria meningitidis,*

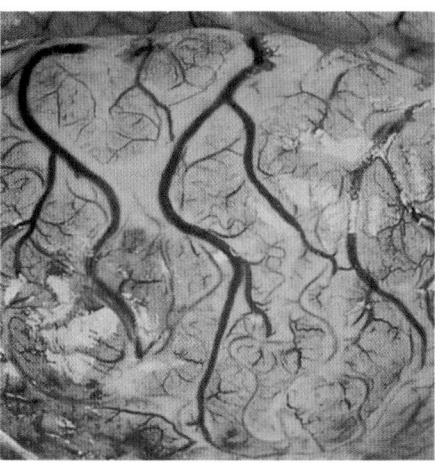

Bacterial meningitis: purulent exudate on surface of cerebral hemisphere *(Perkin et al, 2011)*

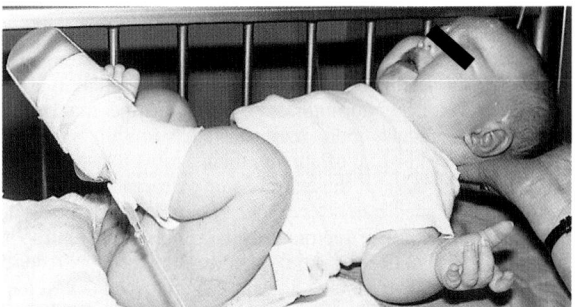

Stiffness of the neck commonly seen in meningitis *(Zitelli and Davis, 2007)*

an acute infectious disease with seropurulent meningeal inflammation. It usually appears in epidemics, and symptoms are those of acute cerebral and spinal meningitis, usually with an eruption of cutaneous erythematous, herpetic, or hemorrhagic spots. The fulminating or malignant form accompanied with bleeding into the adrenal glands is known as Waterhouse-Friderichsen syndrome. Also called **cerebrospinal fever, epidemic cerebrospinal meningitis.** See also **Waterhouse-Friderichsen syndrome.**

meningococcal polysaccharide vaccine /-kok″əl/, one of four active immunizing agents against group A, group C, group Y, or group W-135 meningococcal organisms.

- INDICATIONS: It is prescribed for immunization against meningococcal meningitis, with the serogroup matched according to the local outbreak.

- CONTRAINDICATIONS: Immunosuppression or acute infection prohibits its use.

- ADVERSE EFFECTS: The most serious adverse effect is anaphylaxis.

meningococcemia /mining′gōkoksē″mē·ə/ [Gk, *meninx* + *kokkos,* berry, *haima,* blood], a disease caused by *Neisseria meningitidis* in the bloodstream, subsequently causing vasculitis. Onset is sudden, with chills, pain in the muscles and joints, headache, petechiae, sore throat, and severe prostration. Tachycardia is present, respirations and pulse rate are increased, and fever is intermittent. Treatment of choice is penicillin G. Peripheral circulatory collapse or Waterhouse-Friderichsen syndrome, which is fatal if not aggressively treated, may occur.

M

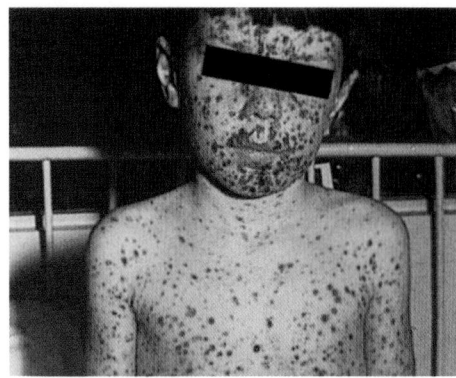

Meningococcemia *(Zitelli and Davis, 2002)*

meningococcus /-kok'əs/ *pl.* **meningococci** [Gk, *meninx* + *kokkos,* berry], a bacterium of the genus *Neisseria meningitidis,* a nonmotile gram-negative diplococcus, frequently found in the nasopharynx of asymptomatic carriers, that may cause septicemia or epidemic cerebrospinal meningitis. Meningococcal infections are not highly communicable. However, crowded conditions, such as may be found in army camps and college dormitories, concentrate the number of carriers and reduce individual resistance to the organism. Hemorrhagic skin lesions are significant clues to the diagnosis. Stained smears of these lesions or of cerebrospinal fluid must be examined quickly because meningococci are fragile and lyse readily. Early treatment with an appropriate antibiotic such as penicillin G is essential for cure. Contacts may receive prophylaxis with rifampin. Several meningococcal vaccines are available. See also **meningitis. –meningococcal,** *adj.*

meningoencephalitis /-ensef'əlī"tis/ [Gk, *meninx,* membrane, *enkephalos,* brain, *itis,* inflammation], an inflammation of both the brain and the meninges, usually caused by a bacterial infection.

meningoencephalocele /mining'gō·ensef"əlōsēl'/ [Gk, *meninx + enkephalos,* brain, *kele,* hernia], a saclike cyst containing brain tissue, cerebrospinal fluid, and meninges that protrudes through a congenital defect in the skull. It may or may not contain parts of the ventricular system and is commonly associated with brain defects. Also called **encephalomeningocele.** See also **neural tube defect.**

meningoencephalomyelitis /mining'gō·ensef'əlōmī'əlī"tis/, a combined inflammation of the brain, spinal cord, and meninges.

meningoencephalopathy /mining'gō·ensef'əlop"əthē/, a noninflammatory disease of the brain and its membranes.

meningomyelitis /-mī'əlī"tis/ [Gk, *meninx,* membrane, *myelos,* marrow, *itis,* inflammation], an inflammation of the spinal cord and its surrounding membranes.

meningomyelocele. See **myelomeningocele.**

meningovascular neurosyphilis /-vas"kyələr/ [Gk, *meninx,* membrane; L, *vasculum,* little vessel; Gk, *neuron,* nerve, *syn,* together, *philein,* to love], a neurosyphilis inflammation of the supporting and nutrient tissues of the central nervous system.

meninx. See **meninges.**

meniscectomy /men'isek"təmē/ [Gk, *meniskos,* crescent, *ektomē,* excision], surgical excision of one of the crescent-shaped cartilages of the knee joint. It is performed when a torn cartilage results in chronic pain and in instability or locking of the joint. After surgery the leg is kept elevated to reduce swelling, and exercises are performed to maintain muscle strength. See also **arthroscopy.**

menisci. See **meniscus.**

meniscocyte. See **erythrocyte.**

meniscocytosis. See **sickle cell anemia.**

meniscus /minis"kəs/ *pl.* **menisci** [Gk, *meniskos,* crescent], **1.** the interface between a liquid and air. **2.** a lens with both convex and concave aspects. **3.** a curved, fibrous cartilage in the knees and other joints. See also **meniscectomy. 4.** the convex or concave upper portion of a liquid in a tube in which the curvature is due to surface tension.

Menkes kinky hair syndrome /men"kēz/ [John H. Menkes, American neurologist, 1928–2008; D, *kinke,* tight twist; AS, *haer*], a familial disorder affecting the normal absorption of copper from the intestine, characterized by the growth of sparse, kinky hair. Infants with the syndrome suffer cerebral degeneration, delayed growth, and early death. Early diagnosis and IV administration of copper may prevent irreversible damage.

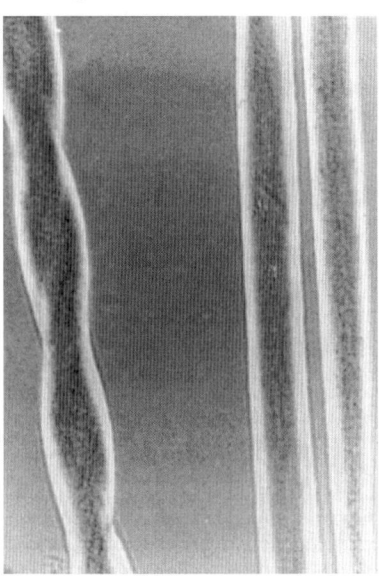

Kinky hair shaft from a patient with Menkes kinky hair syndrome *(left)* compared with two normal hair shafts *(right)* *(Rimoin, 2013)*

meno-, combining form meaning "the menses": *menostasis, menopause, menorrhea.*

menometrorrhagia /men'ōmet'rōrā"jē·ə/ [L, *men,* month; Gk, *metra,* womb, *rhegnyai,* to burst forth], excessive menstrual and uterine bleeding other than that caused by menstruation. It is a combination of metrorrhagia and menorrhagia and may be a sign of a urogenital malignancy.

menopause /men"əpôz/ [L, *men,* month; Gk, *pausis,* to cease], strictly, the cessation of menses, but commonly referring to the period of the female **climacteric.** Menses stop naturally with the decline of cyclic hormonal production and function, usually between 45 and 55 years of age, but may stop earlier in life as a result of illness or surgery or for unknown reasons. As the production of ovarian estrogen and pituitary gonadotropins decreases, ovulation and menstruation become less frequent and eventually stop. Fluctuations in the circulating levels of these hormones occur as the levels decline. Compare **andropause.** See also **artificial menopause.**

■ OBSERVATIONS: Symptoms commonly associated with menopause include hot flashes, night sweats, and sleep disturbances. Vaginal dryness and mood swings are also experienced by some women.

■ INTERVENTIONS: The symptoms of menopause may be relieved by hormone therapy. This can involve the use of either estrogen alone for women who have had a hysterectomy or estrogen with progesterone or progestin in its synthetic form for women who have not had a hysterectomy. Nonhormonal approaches include changes in lifestyle or diet; the use of dietary supplements may also relieve symptoms.

■ PATIENT CARE CONSIDERATIONS: Symptoms associated with menopause vary greatly in severity and the length of time they persist.

menorrhagia /men′ərā″jē·ə/ [L, *men* + *rhegnyai,* to burst forth,], abnormally heavy or long menstrual periods. Menorrhagia occurs occasionally during the reproductive years of most women's lives. If the condition becomes chronic, anemia from recurrent excessive blood loss may result. Abnormal bleeding after menopause always warrants investigation to rule out malignancy. Menorrhagia is a relatively common complication of benign uterine fibromyomata; it may be so severe or intractable as to require hysterectomy. Also called **hypermenorrhea.** Compare **menometrorrhagia, oligomenorrhea.** See also **dysmenorrhea.** –*menorrhagic, adj.*

menorrhea /men′ôrē″ə/ [L, *men* + Gk, *rhoia,* flow], the normal discharge of blood and tissue from the uterus. See also **menorrhagia, menstruation.**

menostasis /minos″təsis/ [L, *men* + Gk, *stasis,* stand still], an abnormal condition in which the products of menstruation cannot escape the uterus or vagina because of stenosis, an occlusion of the cervix, or the introitus of the vagina. An imperforate hymen is a rare cause of menostasis. –*menostatic, adj.*

menotropins /men′ôtrop″inz/ [L, *men* + Gk, *trepein,* to turn], a preparation of gonadotropic hormones from the urine of postmenopausal women.

■ INDICATIONS: It is prescribed with chorionic gonadotropin to induce ovulation or development of multiple ovarian follicles for in vitro fertilization and to stimulate spermatogenesis in males.

■ CONTRAINDICATIONS: Elevated gonadotropin levels in the urine, thyroid or adrenal dysfunction, pituitary tumor, abnormal bleeding, ovarian cyst, pregnancy, or known hypersensitivity to this drug prohibits its use.

■ ADVERSE EFFECTS: Among the more serious adverse effects are ovarian hyperstimulation syndrome, hemoperitoneum, arterial thromboembolism, multiple gestation, and possible birth defects.

menoxenia /men′oksē″nē·ə/ [L, *men* + Gk, *xenos,* strange], any abnormality relating to menstruation.

menses /men″sēz/ [L, *men,* month], the normal flow of blood and decidua that occurs during menstruation. The first day of the flow of the menses is the first day of the menstrual cycle. Also called **catamenia, menstrual period, period.**

menstrual /men″strōō·əl/ [L, *menstrualis,* monthly], pertaining to menstruation.

menstrual age [L, *menstrualis,* monthly, *aetas,* lifetime], the age of an embryo or fetus as calculated from the first day of the last menstrual period.

menstrual colic [L, *menstrualis,* monthly; Gk, *kolikos,* colon pain], a form of dysmenorrhea characterized by abdominal pain during or immediately before menstruation.

menstrual cramps, low abdominal pain that may range from a colicky feeling to a constant dull ache. The pain may radiate to the lower back and legs. Menstrual cramps are often associated with the beginning of menses, reaching a peak in 24 hours and subsiding after 2 days. Treatment may include administration of ibuprofen or other drugs immediately before and after the start of menses. See also **dysmenorrhea.**

menstrual cycle, the recurring cycle of change in the endometrium during which the decidual layer of the endometrium is shed, then regrows, proliferates, is maintained for several days, and is shed again at menstruation. The average length of the cycle from the first day of bleeding of one cycle to the first of another is 28 days. The duration and character vary greatly among women. Normally, menses occur at a frequency of 24 to 38 days, with frequent menses considered to be less than 24 days and infrequent menses greater than 38 days. Cycles begin at menarche and end with menopause. The uterine phases of the cycle are the menstrual phase, proliferative phase, and secretory phase. See also **oogenesis, menses.**

menstrual period. See **menses.**

menstrual phase, the fourth phase of the human menstrual cycle, following the luteal phase and occurring only if fertilization has not taken place. The corpus luteum regresses and is shed through menstruation, and growth begins for the ovarian follicle, leading to the follicular phase of the next menstrual cycle.

menstrual sponge, a small natural sponge or a piece of a synthetic sponge to which a loop of string may be attached. It is inserted into the vagina to absorb the menstrual flow. Once removed, it may be washed, squeezed dry, and reused as necessary throughout menstruation. Menstrual sponges are not commonly used.

menstruation /men′strōō·ā″shən/ [L, *menstruare,* to menstruate], the periodic discharge through the vagina of a bloody secretion containing tissue debris from the shedding of the endometrium from the nonpregnant uterus. The average duration of menstruation is 4 to 5 days, and it recurs at approximately 28-day intervals throughout the reproductive life of nonpregnant women. Kinds include **anovular menstruation, retrograde menstruation, vicarious menstruation.** See also **menstrual cycle.** –*menstruate, v.*

ment-, combining form meaning "mind": *mental, mentality.*

mental[1] /men″təl/ [L, *mens,* mind], **1.** of, relating to, or characteristic of the mind or psyche. **2.** existing in the mind; performed or accomplished by the mind. **3.** of, relating to, or characterized by a disorder of the mind.

mental[2] [L, *mentum,* chin], pertaining to the chin.

mental age (MA), the age level at which one functions intellectually, as determined by standardized psychological and intelligence tests and expressed as the age at which that level is average. Compare **achievement age.** See also **developmental age.**

mental deficiency, (*Obsolete*) now called **intellectual disability.**

mental disorder, any disturbance of emotional equilibrium, as manifested in maladaptive behavior and impaired functioning, caused by genetic, physical, chemical, biological, psychological, or social and cultural factors. Also called **emotional illness, mental illness, psychiatric disorder.**

mental foramen [L, *mentum,* chin], an opening on the lateral part of the body of the mandible, inferior to the second premolar, through which the mental nerve and blood vessels pass.

mental handicap, (*Obsolete*) now called **intellectual disability.**

mental health (MH), a relative state of mind in which a person is able to cope with and adjust to the recurrent stresses of everyday living in an acceptable way.

Mental Health Association, a voluntary nonprofessional agency dedicated to the improvement of mental health facilities and services in community clinics and hospitals,

M

the recruitment and training of volunteers, and the promotion of mental health legislation. Formerly called *National Association for Mental Health.*

mental health consultation, any interaction between two or more health care professionals related to a specific issue of mental health.

mental health nursing. See **psychiatric nursing.**

mental health service, any one of a group of government, professional, or lay organizations operating at a community, state, national, or international level to aid in the prevention and treatment of mental disorders. See also **community mental health center.**

mental hygiene, the study of the development of healthy mental and emotional habits, attitudes, and behavior and the prevention of mental illness. Also called **psychophylaxis.**

mental illness. See **mental disorder.**

mental image, any concept or sensation produced in the mind through memory or imagination.

mentalis, a muscle that arises from the mandible just inferior to the incisor teeth and helps position the lip during pouting or drinking from a cup. It raises and protrudes the lower lip as it wrinkles the skin on the chin.

mentality /mentalʹitē/ [L, *mens,* mind], **1.** the functional power and capacity of the mind. **2.** intellectual character.

mental protuberance, a midline swelling on the base of the mandible on its anterior surface where the two sides of the mandible come together. Just lateral to the mental protuberance, on either side, are the slightly more pronounced mental tubercles.

mental retardation, *(Obsolete)* a term to describe a disorder characterized by subaverage general intellectual function with deficits or impairments in the ability to learn and to adapt socially. The cause may be genetic, biological, psychosocial, or traumatic. Although still in common usage, its use is not consistent with current professional nomenclature. Now called **intellectual disability.**

mental ridge [L, *mentum,* chin; AS, *hyrcg*], a dense elevation that extends from the symphysis menti (the center front of the mandible) to the premolar area on the anterolateral aspect of the body of the mandible.

mental status, the degree of competence shown by a person in intellectual, emotional, psychological, and personality functioning as measured by psychological testing with reference to a statistical norm. See also **mental status examination.**

mental status examination, a diagnostic procedure for determining the mental status of a person. The trained interviewer poses certain questions in a carefully standardized manner and evaluates the verbal responses and behavioral reactions.

mental tubercle [L, *mentum,* chin], one of a bilateral pair of prominences on the lower border of the body of the mandible.

mentation /mentāʹshən/ [L, *mens,* mind, *atus,* process], any mental activity, including conscious and unconscious processes.

menthol /menʹthol/ [L, *menta,* mint], a topical antipruritic with a cooling effect that relieves itching. It is an ingredient in many topical creams and ointments.

mentholated camphor /menʹthəlāʹtid/, a mixture of equal parts of camphor and menthol, used as a local counterirritant.

-mentia, suffix meaning "(condition of the) mind": *dementia, amentia.*

menton /menʹton/ [L, *mentum,* chin], the most inferior point on the chin in the lateral view of a cephalogram. It is a cephalometric landmark used in orthodontic treatment.

mentor /menʹtər/ [Gk, *Mentor,* mythic educator], **1.** a more experienced, trusted adviser or counselor who offers helpful guidance to less experienced colleagues. **2.** a practitioner who enters into a relationship with a client to provide him or her with a source of support and information as he or she learns new roles.

mentum /menʹtəm/ [L, chin], **1.** the chin, especially of the fetus. **2.** a fetal reference point in designating the position of the fetus with respect to the maternal pelvis. For example, left mentum anterior indicates that the fetal chin is presenting in the left anterior quadrant of the pelvis.

menu /menʹyoo/ [Fr, small], a list of choices displayed on a computer screen from which a user selects the next action to be taken, signaling through the keyboard or another device, such as a mouse.

MEP, **1.** abbreviation for **maximal expiratory pressure. 2.** abbreviation for *mean effective pressure.*

mepenzolate bromide /mepenʹzəlāt/, an anticholinergic/antispasmodic agent.

■ INDICATIONS: It is prescribed as an adjunct in treating peptic ulcers and preoperatively to reduce respiratory secretions.

■ CONTRAINDICATIONS: Narrow-angle glaucoma, asthma, obstruction of the genitourinary or GI tract, severe ulcerative colitis, or known hypersensitivity to this drug prohibits its use.

■ ADVERSE EFFECTS: Blurred vision, central nervous system effects, tachycardia, dry mouth, decreased sweating, or hypersensitivity reactions may occur.

Mepergan, a fixed-combination central nervous system drug containing an opioid analgesic and an antihistamine. Brand name for **meperidine hydrochloride, promethazine hydrochloride.**

meperidine hydrochloride /meperʹidēn/, an opioid analgesic.

■ INDICATIONS: It is used to treat moderate to severe pain and to relieve pain and anxiety before or after surgery.

■ CONTRAINDICATIONS: It is used with caution in many conditions, including head injuries, asthma, seizures, impaired renal or hepatic function, or unstable cardiovascular status. Concomitant use of a monoamine oxidase inhibitor or known hypersensitivity to this drug prohibits its use. It is not used if the patient has convulsive disorders.

■ ADVERSE EFFECTS: Among the most serious adverse effects are drowsiness, dizziness, nausea, seizures, constipation, sweating, respiratory and circulatory depression, and drug addiction.

mephobarbital /mefʹōbärʹbitol/, an anticonvulsant and sedative.

■ INDICATIONS: It is prescribed in the treatment of anxiety, nervous tension, insomnia, and epilepsy.

■ CONTRAINDICATIONS: Porphyria or known hypersensitivity to this drug or to barbiturates prohibits its use.

■ ADVERSE EFFECTS: Among the more serious adverse effects are drug dependence, a hangover effect, deficiency in vitamin D, paradoxical excitement, and GI disturbance.

Mephyton, a vitamin K product. Brand name for **phytonadione.**

mepivacaine, carbocaine, a local anesthetic of the amide type with a rapid onset and intermediate duration.

meprobamate /miprōʹbəmāt/, an antianxiety agent.

■ INDICATIONS: It is prescribed in treatment of anxiety and tension.

■ CONTRAINDICATIONS: Intermittent porphyria, CNS depression, narrow-angle glaucoma, pregnancy, or known hypersensitivity to this drug or to the chemically related drug carisoprodol prohibits its use.

■ ADVERSE EFFECTS: Among the most serious adverse effects are exacerbation of intermittent porphyria, augmentation of effects of other central nervous system depressants, and various allergic reactions. Drowsiness and ataxia commonly occur.

mEq,   abbreviation for **milliequivalent.**

mEq/L,   abbreviation for **milliequivalent per liter.**

MEPS,   abbreviation for **Medical Expenditure Panel Survey.**

-mer, -mere, mero-,   **1.** combining form meaning "part, portion": *isomers.* **2.** combining form meaning "polymer": *monomer.*

meradimate /mer-ad′imāt/, an absorber of ultraviolet A radiation, used topically as a sunscreen.

meralgia /miral″jə/ [Gk, *meros,* thigh, *algos,* pain], the presence of pain or discomfort specific to the thigh.

meralgia paresthetica /per′esthet″ikə/, a condition characterized by pain, paresthesia, and numbness on the lateral surface of the thigh in the region supplied by the lateral femoral cutaneous nerve. The cause of the condition is ischemia of the nerve caused by its entrapped position in the inguinal ligament.

mercaptopurine /mərkap′təpyoo″rēn/, an antineoplastic and immunosuppressive drug; a purine antimetabolite. Also called *6-mercaptopurine (6-MP).*

■ INDICATIONS: It is prescribed in the treatment of malignant neoplastic disease, especially as maintenance therapy for acute lymphocytic leukemia.

■ CONTRAINDICATIONS: Known hypersensitivity to this drug prohibits its use.

■ ADVERSE EFFECTS: Among the more severe adverse effects are bone marrow depression and acute GI disturbances, including nausea, vomiting, diarrhea, and stomatitis.

Mercer, Ramona T., a nursing theorist who developed the Maternal Role Attainment model presented in her book *First-Time Motherhood*: *Experiences from Teens to Forties* (1986). Maternal role attainment is an interactional and developmental process. It occurs over a period during which the mother becomes attached to her infant, acquires competence in the care-giving tasks, and expresses pleasure and gratification in her role. The focus of Mercer's work went beyond the concept of the "traditional" mother to encompass a variety of mothering roles, maternal age, health status, family functioning, mother-father relationship, and infant characteristics. Mercer considers a mate's love, support, and nurturance to be important factors in enabling a woman to mother her child.

mercurial /mərkyoor″ē-əl/, **1.** (for health or related reasons) pertaining to mercury, particularly a medicine containing the element mercury. **2.** pertaining to an adverse effect associated with the administration of a mercurial medication, such as a mercurial tremor caused by mercury poisoning.

mercurial diuretic, any one of several diuretic agents that contain mercury in an organic chemical form. The principal use for the drugs is in treating edema of cardiac origin, ascites associated with cirrhosis, or oliguria in the nephrotic stage of glomerulonephritis. Immediate fatal reactions have occurred, usually as a result of ventricular failure after intravascular injection and transient high concentration of mercury in the blood. Flushing, urticaria, fever, and nausea and vomiting are common side effects. Thrombocytopenia, neutropenia, agranulocytosis, systemic mercury poisoning, and severe hypersensitivity reactions are among the more serious adverse effects of the mercurial diuretics. The drugs are contraindicated for use in the presence of renal insufficiency or acute nephritis. Because of the toxicity of these drugs, current practice

usually recommends their replacement with more convenient and less toxic diuretics.

mercurialism. See **mercury poisoning.**

-mercuric, suffix meaning "molecules of bivalent mercury or its compounds."

mercury (Hg) /mur″kyərē/ [L, *Mercurius,* mythic messenger of the gods], a metallic element. Its atomic number is 80; its atomic mass is 200.59. It is the only common metal that is liquid at room temperature, and it occurs in nature almost entirely in the form of its sulfide, cinnabar. Mercury is produced commercially and is used in dental amalgams, thermometers, barometers, and other measuring instruments. It forms many poisonous compounds. The air, soil, and water in many areas of the world have become contaminated by mercury because of the burning of fossil fuels that contain the element and because of the greater use of mercury in industry and agriculture. The major toxic forms of this metal are mercury vapor, mercuric salts, and organic mercurials. Elemental mercury is only mildly toxic when ingested because it is poorly absorbed. The vapor of elemental mercury, however, is readily absorbed through the lungs and enters the brain before it is oxidized. The kidneys retain mercury longer than any of the other body tissues.

mercury bichloride, an extremely poisonous compound formerly used in the treatment of syphilis but now used only as a disinfectant.

mercury nephropathy, acute tubular necrosis caused by mercury poisoning after ingestion of inorganic mercury salts.

mercury poisoning, a toxic condition caused by the ingestion or inhalation of mercury or a mercury compound. The chronic form, resulting from inhalation of the vapors or dust of mercurial compounds or from repeated ingestion of very small amounts, is characterized by irritability, thirst, excessive saliva, loosened teeth, gum disorders, slurred speech, tremors, and staggering. Symptoms of acute mercury poisoning appear in a few minutes to a half hour and include a metallic taste in the mouth, thirst, nausea, vomiting, severe abdominal pain, bloody diarrhea, and renal failure that may result in death. The presence of mercury in the body is determined by a urine test. Free mercury, such as in thermometers, is not absorbed in the GI tract, but because it is very volatile, hazardous vapors may penetrate ordinary toxic dust respirators, causing poisoning by inhalation. Mercury compounds are found in agricultural fungicides and in certain antiseptics and pigments. They are used extensively in industry. Industrial wastes containing mercury have been identified in some areas, and seafood from contaminated waters has caused serious public health problems. Also called **hydrargyrism, mercurialism.** See also **Minamata disease.**

mercury thermometer [L, *Mercurius,* mythic messenger of the gods; Gk, *thermē,* heat, *metron,* measure], a thermometer in which the expandable indicator is mercury. Mercury thermometers are no longer used in clinical practice and have been replaced by digital, chemical dot, and infrared thermometers.

mercy killing. See **euthanasia.**

-meria, suffix meaning "related to parts": *platymeria.*

merisis. See **hyperplasia.**

Merkel cell carcinoma /mer″kəl, mur″kəl/ [Friedrich S. Merkel, German anatomist and physiologist, 1845–1919], a rapidly growing malignant skin tumor that tends to occur on sun-exposed surfaces of older Caucasian individuals. It is composed of small cells in a trabecular pattern that contain dense core granules.

M

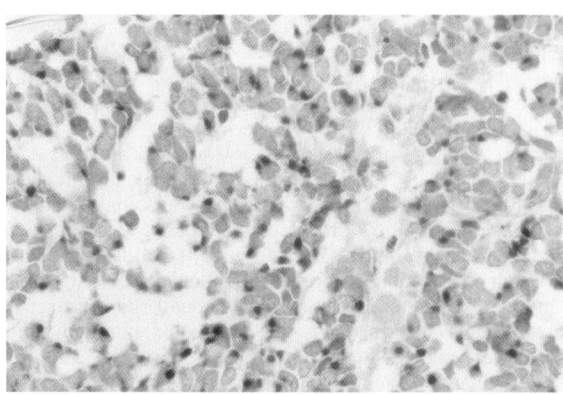

Merkel cell carcinoma *(Skarin, 2003)*

meroanencephaly /mer′ō·an′ənsef′əlē/ [Gk, *meros,* part + *a, enkephalos,* not brain], congenital absence of part of the brain, usually the forebrain and midbrain. Compare **anencephaly.**

meroblastic /mer′əblas″tik/ [Gk, *meros* + *blastos,* germ], pertaining to or characterizing an ovum that contains a large amount of yolk and in which cleavage is restricted to the yolk-free part of the cytoplasm. Compare **holoblastic.**

merocrine gland /mer″əkrin/ [Gk, *meros,* part, *krinein,* to separate; L, *secernere,* to separate], a gland in which the secreting cell remains intact while producing and releasing the secretory product. Compare **apocrine gland, holocrine gland.**

meromelia /mer′əmē″lyə/ [Gk, *meros* + *melos,* limb], **1.** an abnormality of development in which the upper part of the arm or leg is missing so that hands or feet are attached to the body like stumps, generally resulting from the use of thalidomide during pregnancy. **2.** a general designation for the congenital absence of any part of a limb. It is used in reference to such conditions as adactyly, hemimelia, or phocomelia. Compare **amelia,** def. 1.

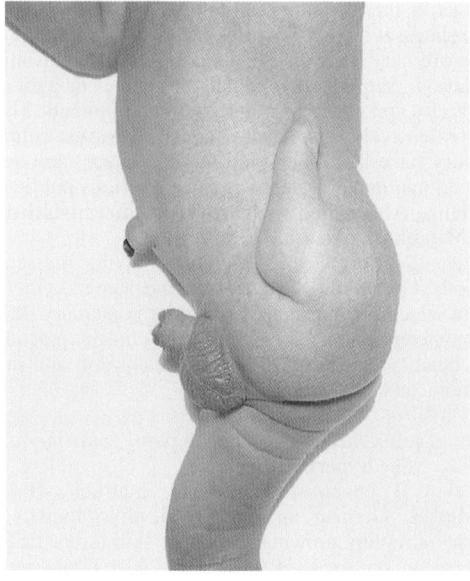

Infant with meromelia *(Schoenwolf et al, 2015)*

meropenem, a miscellaneous antiinfective drug.

■ INDICATIONS: It is used to treat serious infections caused by *Streptococcus pneumoniae,* group A beta-hemolytic streptococci, enterococcus, *Klebsiella, Proteus, Escherichia coli, Pseudomonas aeruginosa, Bacteroides fragilis,* and *B. thetaiotaomicron.* It is also used to treat appendicitis and peritonitis caused by the *viridans* group of streptococci, as well as bacterial meningitis.

■ CONTRAINDICATIONS: Known hypersensitivity to meropenem or imipenem prohibits its use.

■ ADVERSE EFFECTS: Life-threatening effects are seizures, pseudomembranous colitis, hepatitis, eosinophilia, neutropenia, and anaphylaxis. Other adverse effects include fever, somnolence, dizziness, weakness, myoclonia, diarrhea, nausea, vomiting, glossitis, hypotension, palpitations, decreased hemoglobin and hematocrit, urticaria, pain at the injection site, phlebitis, erythema at the injection site, chest discomfort, dyspnea, and hyperventilation. Common side effects are headache, rash, and pruritus.

merozoite /mer′əzō″īt/ [Gk, *meros* + *zoon,* animal], an organism produced from segmentation of a schizont during the asexual reproductive phase of the life cycle of a sporozoon, specifically the malarial parasite *Plasmodium.* Merozoites can either continue the asexual phase of the life cycle by developing into trophozoites and repeating the process of schizogony or differentiate into male and female gametes and enter the sexual stage. See also ***Plasmodium.***

merozygote /mer′əzī″gōt/, an incomplete zygote that contains only part of the genetic material of one of the parents. It occurs during conjugation in bacteria, as part of the donor chromosome is excluded by the transfer mechanism.

MERRF syndrome, a familial syndrome of maternal (mitochondrial) inheritance. Abbreviation for *myoclonus with epilepsy and with ragged red fibers.* Also called **Fukuhara syndrome.**

Merrifield knife, a surgical knife with a long, narrow, triangular blade set into a shank, used for gingivectomy incisions.

Meruvax II, a live virus vaccine that is an active immunizing agent. Brand name for **rubella virus vaccine.**

Merzbacher-Pelizaeus disease. See **Pelizaeus-Merzbacher disease.**

mes-, mesio-, meso-, prefix meaning "middle or median": *mesoderm, mesencephalon, mesiodens.*

mesalamine, an active metabolite of sulfasalazine, used in the prophylaxis and treatment of inflammatory bowel disease and ulcerative proctitis; administered orally or rectally. Also called **5-aminosalicylic acid.**

mesangial /mesan″jē·əl/, pertaining to the mesangium.

mesangial IgA nephropathy. See **Berger disease.**

mesangiocapillary glomerulonephritis. See **membranoproliferative glomerulonephritis.**

mesangium /mesan″jē·əm/, a cellular network in the renal glomerulus that helps support the capillary loops. The mesangial cells are phagocytic and frequently contain macromolecules or inflammatory agents that may aid in diagnosis of a kidney disorder when examined in a laboratory.

mescaline /mes″kəlēn, -lin/ [Mex, *mezcal*], a psychoactive agent with effects similar to LSD, this poisonous alkaloid is derived from a colorless alkaline oil in the flowering heads of the cactus *Lophophora williamsii.* Closely related chemically to epinephrine, mescaline causes heart palpitations, diaphoresis, pupillary dilation, and anxiety. It is a Schedule I substance. The drug, taken in capsules or dissolved in a drink, produces visual hallucinations, such as color patterns and spatial distortions, but it does not ordinarily induce disorientation. Mescaline is used in some religious ceremonies to produce euphoria and a feeling of ecstasy. Also called **peyote.**

mescalism /mes″kəliz′əm/ [Mex, *mezcal*], a type of chemical dependence on the effects of mescal, an intoxicant spirit obtained from a species of cactus (agave).

mesencephalon /mes′ensef″əlon/ [Gk, *mesos,* middle, *enkephalos,* brain], one of the three parts of the brainstem, lying just below the cerebrum and just above the pons. It consists primarily of white matter with some gray matter around the cerebral aqueduct. Deep within the mesencephalon are nuclei of the third and the fourth cranial nerves and the anterior part of the fifth cranial nerve. The mesencephalon also contains nuclei for certain auditory and visual reflexes. Also called **midbrain.** −*mesencephalic, adj.*

mesenchymal chondrosarcoma /meseng″kəməl/ [Gk, *mesos,* middle, *enchyma,* infusion, *chondros,* cartilage, *sarx,* flesh, *oma,* tumor], a rare malignant tumor of soft tissue that develops in many sites. The tumors are highly vascular.

mesenchyme /mes″engkīm/ [Gk, *mesos* + *enchyma,* infusion], a diffuse network of tissue derived from the embryonic mesoderm. It consists of stellate cells embedded in gelatinous ground substance with reticular fibers. −*mesenchymal, adj.*

mesenchymoma /mes′engkimō″mə/ [Gk, *mesos* + *enchyma,* infusion, *oma,* tumor], a mixed mesenchymal neoplasm composed of two or more cellular elements that are not usually associated and fibrous tissue. See also **benign mesenchymoma, malignant mesenchymoma.**

mesenteric /mes′enter″ik/ [Gk, *mesos,* middle, *enteron,* intestine], pertaining to the mesentery, the double layer of peritoneum suspending the intestine from the posterior abdominal wall.

mesenteric adenitis. See **adenitis.**

mesenteric angina, severe pain and discomfort after a heavy meal, resulting from diminished blood supply and concomitant lack of oxygen caused by the narrowing of the celiac and mesenteric artery openings.

mesenteric axis, a line passing transversely between a portion of the GI tract and its adjacent mesentery.

mesenteric ischemia, ischemia in an area of the intestine supplied by a mesenteric artery. Two types are distinguished, occlusive and nonocclusive mesenteric ischemia. It may progress to a mesenteric infarction.

mesenteric node [Gk, *mesos* + *enteron,* intestine; L, *nodus,* knot], a node in one of three groups of superior mesenteric lymph glands serving parts of the intestine. An average of 125 mesenteric nodes in three different groups lie between the layers of the mesentery. The mesenteric nodes receive afferent vessels from the jejunum, ileum, cecum, vermiform appendix, ascending colon, and transverse colon. Compare **ileocolic node, mesocolic node.**

mesenteric panniculitis, inflammation with variable fibrosis of mesenteric fat, usually of the small intestine, causing a solid mass that may displace or obstruct the intestine. Some authorities consider this an inflammatory variant of retractile mesenteritis. Also called *mesenteric lipodystrophy.*

mesenteroaxial volvulus, the less common of the two types of gastric volvulus, in which the stomach twists transversely around its mesenteric axis. This type is more common in children.

mesentery proper /mez″ənter′ē/ [Gk, *mesos* + *enteron,* intestine; L, *propius,* more suitable], a broad fan-shaped fold of peritoneum suspending the jejunum and the ileum from the dorsal wall of the abdomen. The root of the mesentery proper is about 15 cm long and is connected to certain structures ventral to the vertebral column. The intestinal border of the mesentery proper is about 6 m long and separates to enclose the intestine. The cranial part of the mesentery is narrow but widens to about 20 cm and suspends the small intestine and various nerves and arteries. Compare **sigmoid mesocolon, transverse mesocolon.**

MeSH /mesh/, an abbreviation derived from *Medical Subject Headings,* the list of medical terms used by the National Library of Medicine (NLM) for its computerized system of storage and retrieval of published medical reports. The system is also used for indexing medical references.

mesh graft, a partial or split-thickness skin graft that has had multiple slits cut into it. The slits allow the graft to be stretched to several times its original size for coverage of a larger area on the recipient. They also facilitate acceptance of the graft by permitting fluids to escape from beneath the graft.

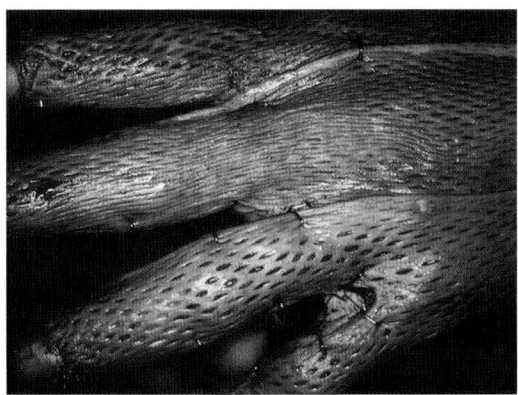

Mesh graft covering burn to the hand *(Hockenberry and Wilson, 2015)*

MeSH terms, subject headings.

mesial. See **medial.**

mesiobuccoocclusal /mē′zē·ōbuk′ō·okloo″zəl/ [Gk, *mesos,* middle; L, *bucca,* cheek; L, *occludere,* to close up], pertaining to the point angle formed by the mesial, buccal, and occlusal surfaces of a tooth. Compare **mesiolinguoocclusal.**

mesiocclusion /mē′zē·okloo″zhən/ [Gk, *mesos* + L, *occludere,* to close up], an occlusal relationship in which the lower teeth are positioned mesially to the upper teeth.

mesiodens /mē″zē·ədenz/ [Gk, *mesos* + L, *dens,* tooth], a supernumerary erupted or unerupted tooth that develops between two maxillary central incisors. Compare **peridens.**

mesiolinguoocclusal, pertaining to the point angle formed by the mesial, lingual, and occlusal surfaces of a tooth. Compare **mesiobuccoocclusal.**

mesioversion /mē′zē·ōvur″zhən/ [Gk, *mesos* + L, *vertere,* to turn], **1.** a condition in which one or more teeth are closer than normal to the midline. **2.** a condition in which the maxilla or mandible is positioned more anteriorly than normal.

mesmerism /mez″məriz′əm/ [Franz A. Mesmer, Austrian physician, 1734–1815], a practice of hypnotism introduced by Mesmer, who believed human health was affected by "celestial magnetic forces." Some patients were reported cured or experienced diminished symptoms by undergoing a "grand crisis," or seizure, while under hypnosis. Mesmer was regarded as a fraud by the medical profession, but his work led to serious studies of the health effects of the power of suggestion.

meso-. See **mes-, mesio-, meso-.**

mesoappendix. See **vermiform appendix.**

mesoblastic nephroma, a renal tumor similar to Wilms tumor but appearing earlier in infancy and with more infiltration of surrounding tissue.

mesocolic node /mes′ōkol″ik/ [Gk, *mesos* + *kolon,* colon; L, *nodus,* knot], a node in one of three groups of superior mesenteric lymph glands, proliferating between the layers of the transverse mesocolon close to the transverse colon. They are best developed near the right and left colic flexures and receive afferents from the jejunum, ileum, cecum, vermiform appendix, ascending colon, and transverse colon. Their efferent vessels pass to the preaortic nodes. Compare **mesenteric node.**

mesoderm /mes″ōdurm/ [Gk, *mesos* + *derma,* skin], (in embryology) the middle of the three cell layers of the developing embryo. It lies between the ectoderm and the endoderm. Bone, connective tissue, muscle, blood, vascular and lymphatic tissue, and the pleurae of the pericardium and peritoneum are all derived from the mesoderm.

mesoduodenum /-dŌō′ədē″nəm/ [Gk, *mesos,* middle; L, *duodeni,* 12 fingers long], a fold of tissue that joins the duodenum to the wall of the abdomen of the fetus. The membrane sometimes persists in later life as the duodenal mesentery.

mesoepididymis /mez′ō·ep′i·did′i·mis/ [Gk, *mesos,* middle + *epi,* above + *didymos,* pair], a fold of tunica vaginalis that sometimes connects the epididymis with the testicle.

mesogastric /-gas″trik/ [Gk, *mesos,* middle, *gaster,* belly], pertaining to the *mesogastrium,* a mesentery of the embryonic stomach.

mesoglia. See **microglia.**

mesogluteus /mez′ō·glŌō′tē·əs/ [Gk, *mesos,* middle + *gloutos,* buttocks], the middle gluteal muscle, which abducts and rotates the thigh medially. Also called *gluteus medius.*

mesojejunum /mez′ō·jə·jŌō′nəm/ [Gk, *mesos,* middle; L, *jejunus,* empty], the mesentery of the jejunum.

mesomere /mez″əmir/ [Gk, *mesos,* middle, *meros,* part], a row of blastomere between the macromere and micromere of the embryo. It develops into the renal tubules.

mesomerism /mĕsom′erizəm/, a quantum superposition of wave functions built from several contributing structures (also called resonance structures or canonical forms) as a way of describing the delocalized electronic structure within certain molecules or polyatomic ions in valence bond theory. The term is used when a chemical structure (molecule, transition state) cannot satisfactorily be described by one single Lewis formula.

mesometritis. See **myometritis.**

mesomorph /mes″əmôrf′/ [Gk, *mesos* + *morphe,* form], a type of body build characterized by a large bone structure, well-developed muscle mass, and an athletic appearance. Compare **ectomorph, endomorph.** See also **athletic habitus.**

mesonephra, mesonephric. See **mesonephros.**

mesonephric duct /-nef″rik/ [Gk, *mesos* + *nephros,* kidney; L, *ducere,* to lead], (in embryology) a duct that in the male gives rise to the ducts of the reproductive system (ductus epididymidis, ductus deferens, seminal vesicle, ejaculatory duct). In the female it persists vestigially as Gartner's duct. Also called **wolffian duct.**

mesonephric tubule, any of the embryonic renal tubules composing the mesonephros. They function as excretory structures during the early embryonic development of humans and other mammals but are later incorporated into the reproductive system. In males the tubules give rise to the efferent and aberrant ductules of the testes, the appendix epididymis, and the paradidymis; in females, to the epoöphoron, paroöphoron, and vesicular appendices. All of the structures are vestigial except the efferent ductules of the testes.

mesonephros /-nef″rəs/ *pl. mesonephra, mesonephroi* [Gk, *mesos* + *nephros,* kidney], the second type of excretory organ to develop in the vertebrate embryo. It consists of a series of twisting tubules that arise from the nephrogenic cord caudal to the pronephros and that at one end form the glomerulus and at the other connect with the excretory mesonephric duct. The organ is the permanent kidney in lower animals, but in humans and various other mammals it is functional only during early embryonic development and is later replaced by the metanephros, although the duct system is retained and incorporated into the male reproductive system. Also called *mesonephron,* **middle kidney, wolffian body.** See also **metanephros, pronephros.** −*mesonephric, mesonephroid, adj.*

mesoridazine /mez′ərid″əzēn/, a phenothiazine antipsychotic drug.

■ INDICATIONS: It is prescribed in the treatment of schizophrenia.

■ CONTRAINDICATIONS: Parkinson disease, concurrent administration of central nervous system depressants, liver or renal dysfunction, severe hypotension, or known hypersensitivity to this drug or to other phenothiazine medications prohibits its use.

■ ADVERSE EFFECTS: Among the more serious adverse effects are prolongation of the QT interval (increases risk of torsades de pointes arrhythmia), hypotension, liver toxicity, a variety of extrapyramidal reactions, persistent tardive dyskinesia, blood dyscrasias, and hypersensitivity reactions.

mesorrhine, a nasal profile of moderate width.

mesosalpinx /mes′ōsal″pingks/ [Gk, *mesos* + *salpinx,* tube], the superior, free border of the broad ligament in which the uterine tubes lie.

mesotaurodontism /mez′ōtô′rōdon′tizəm/ [Gk, *mesos,* middle; L, *taurus,* bull; Gk, *odous,* tooth], (in dentistry) apical displacement of the pulpal floor to the middle of the tooth roots. It is a developmental disturbance of a tooth in which the tooth body is enlarged at the expense of the roots; it is characterized by an enlarged pulp chamber and lack of constriction at the cementoenamel junction. Also called *moderate taurodontism.* See also **hypertaurodontism, taurodontism.**

mesothelial /mez′ōthē″lē·əl/, pertaining to the mesothelium cell layer.

mesothelioma /mes′ōthē′lē·ō″mə/ *pl. mesotheliomas, mesotheliomata* [Gk, *mesos* + *epi,* above, *thele,* nipple, *oma,* tumor], a rare malignant tumor of the mesothelium of the pleura or peritoneum, associated with exposure to asbestos. The lesion, composed of spindle cells or fibrous tissue, may form thick sheets covering the viscera. The prognosis is poor. Also called **celothelioma.**

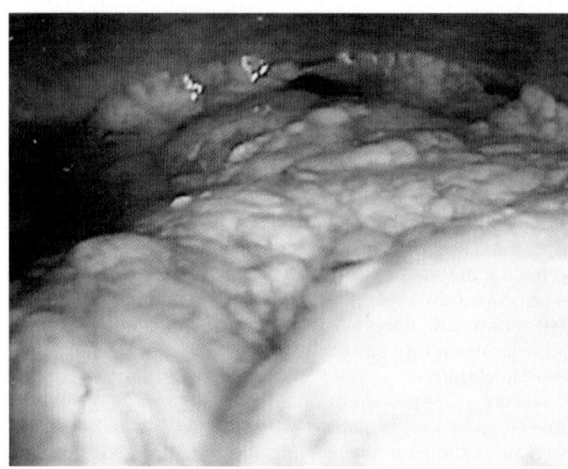

Laparascopic image showing omental deposits of mesothelioma *(Sharma et al, 2010)*

mesothelium /mes′ōthē″lē·əm/ [Gk, *mesos* + *epi,* above, *thele,* nipple], a layer of cells that lines the body cavities of the embryo and continues as a layer of squamous epithelial cells covering the serous membranes of the adult.

messenger RNA (mRNA) /mes″ənjər/ [ME, *messangere,* message bearer; *RNA,* ribonucleic acid], (in molecular genetics) an RNA fraction that carries information from deoxyribonucleic acid to the protein-synthesizing ribosomes of cells. mRNA contains codons that are eventually encoded into amino acids via the translation process.

Mestinon, a neuromuscular blocking agent. Brand name for **pyridostigmine bromide.**

mestranol /mes″trənōl/, an estrogen prescribed in fixed-combination drugs with a progestin as an oral contraceptive.

Met, abbreviation for **methionine.**

MET, abbreviation for **metabolic equivalent of task.**

meta-, **1.** prefix meaning "change" or "exchange": *metabolic, metabolism, metamorphosis.* **2.** prefix meaning "after" or "next": *metabolite, metaphase, metastasis.* **3.** prefix meaning "the 1, 3 position in derivative of benzine."

meta-analysis, a systematic method that takes data from a number of independent studies and integrates them using statistical analysis.

metabiosis /met′əbī·ō″sis/, **1.** a condition in which the growth and metabolism of one organism alter the environment to allow the growth of another organism. **2.** the parasitic dependence of the existence of one organism on that of another.

metabolic /met′əbol″ik/ [Gk, *metabole,* change], pertaining to chemical reactions in the body. See also **metabolism.**

metabolic acidosis, acidosis in which excess acid is added to the body fluids or bicarbonate is lost from them. Acidosis is indicated by a pH of blood below 7.4. In starvation and in uncontrolled diabetes mellitus, glucose is not present or is not available for oxidation for cellular nutrition. This glucose lack causes breakdown of fats for energy, resulting in acidic ketone bodies. The body uses plasma bicarbonate to neutralize these acids. Metabolic acidosis also occurs when oxidation takes place without adequate oxygen, as in heart failure or shock. Severe diarrhea, renal failure, ingestion of toxic substances (e.g., antifreeze or large doses of aspirin), and lactic acidosis also may result in metabolic acidosis. Hyperkalemia may accompany the condition. See also **diabetic ketoacidosis.**

metabolic alkalosis, an abnormal condition characterized by the significant loss of acid in the body or by increased levels of base bicarbonate. Loss of acid may be caused by excessive vomiting, insufficient replacement of electrolytes, hyperadrenocorticism, or Cushing disease. Increased levels of base bicarbonate may have various causes, such as the ingestion of excessive amounts of bicarbonate of soda or other antacids during the treatment of peptic ulcers or the administration of excessive volumes of IV fluids containing high concentrations of bicarbonate. Severe, untreated metabolic alkalosis can lead to coma and death. Compare **respiratory alkalosis.** See also **metabolic acidosis, respiratory acidosis.**

■ OBSERVATIONS: Signs and symptoms of metabolic alkalosis may include apnea, headache, lethargy, muscle cramps, hyperactive reflexes, tetany, shallow and slow respirations, irritability, nausea, vomiting, and atrial tachycardia. Confirmation of the diagnosis is commonly based on laboratory findings that show a blood pH greater than 7.45, a carbonic acid concentration greater than 29 mEq/L, and alkaline urine. The electrocardiogram of a patient with this condition may show atrial tachycardia with a low T wave merging with a P wave.

■ INTERVENTIONS: Treatment seeks to eliminate the underlying cause of alkalosis. Ammonium chloride may be given intravenously to release hydrogen chloride and restore chloride

levels, except in patients with liver or kidney disease. Potassium chloride and normal saline solutions usually replace fluid losses from gastric drainage but are contraindicated in patients with associated congestive heart failure.

■ PATIENT CARE CONSIDERATIONS: Nurses closely monitor the status of the patient and cautiously administer any prescribed IV solutions. Too-rapid infusion of ammonium chloride may hemolyze red blood cells, and an excessive dosage may overcorrect alkalosis and cause acidosis. The fluid intake and output of the patient are carefully noted, and the respiration rate is regularly checked. Decreased respiratory rate indicates an effort to compensate for alkalosis and may cause respiratory acidosis.

metabolic balance [Gk, *metabole,* change; L, *bilanx,* having two scale trays], an equilibrium between the intake of nutrients and their eventual loss through absorption or excretion. In a positive balance the intake of a nutrient exceeds its loss; in a negative balance a nutrient is used or excreted faster than it is consumed in the diet.

metabolic body size, an estimate of the active tissue mass of a person, calculated by the body weight in kilograms to the 0.75 power.

metabolic cirrhosis, cirrhosis of the liver associated with a metabolic disorder such as Wilson disease.

metabolic component, the bicarbonate component of plasma.

metabolic disorder, any pathophysiological dysfunction that results in a loss of metabolic control of homeostasis in the body.

metabolic equivalent of task (MET), a unit of measurement of heat production by the body. One MET is equal to 50 kcal per hour per square meter of body surface of a resting individual.

metabolic failure, the severe and usually rapid failure of mental and physical functions, resulting in death.

metabolic myopathy, myopathy as a result of disordered metabolism, usually caused by genetic defects or hormonal dysfunction.

metabolic pathway, a series of consecutive biochemical reactions or steps through which digested food is transformed into basic nutrients such as amino acids, free fatty acids, and simple carbohydrates.

metabolic rate, the amount of energy liberated or expended in a given unit of time. Energy is stored in the body in energy-rich phosphate compounds (adenosine triphosphate, adenosine monophosphate, and adenosine diphosphate) and in proteins, fats, and complex carbohydrates. See also **basal metabolic rate.**

metabolic respiratory quotient. See **respiratory quotient.**

metabolic syndrome, a combination including at least three of the following: abdominal obesity, hypertriglyceridemia, low level of high-density lipoproteins, hypertension, and high fasting plasma glucose level. It is associated with an increased risk for development of diabetes mellitus and cardiovascular disease.

metabolic tolerance. See **drug tolerance.**

metabolic waste products [Gk, *metabole,* change; L, *vastare,* to destroy, *producere,* to produce], the products of metabolic activity after oxygen and nutrients have been supplied to a cell. These mainly include water and carbon dioxide, along with sodium chloride and soluble nitrogenous salts, which are excreted in urine, feces, and exhaled air.

metabolism /mətab″əliz′əm/ [Gk, *metabole,* change, *ismos,* process], the aggregate of all chemical processes that take place in living organisms, resulting in growth, generation of energy, elimination of wastes, and other body functions as they relate to the distribution of nutrients in the blood after digestion. Metabolism takes place in two steps: anabolism, the constructive phase, in which smaller molecules (such as amino acids) are converted to larger molecules (such as proteins); and catabolism, the destructive phase, in which larger molecules (such as glycogen) are converted to smaller molecules (such as glucose). Exercise, elevated body temperature, hormonal activity, and digestion can increase the metabolic rate, which is the rate determined when a person is at complete rest, physically and mentally. The metabolic rate is customarily expressed (in calories) as the heat liberated in the course of metabolism. See also **acid-base metabolism, anabolism, basal metabolism, catabolism.**

metabolite /mitab″əlīt/ [Gk, *metabole,* change], a substance produced by metabolic action or necessary for a metabolic process. An essential metabolite is one required for a vital metabolic process.

metabolize /mətab″əlīz/ [Gk, *metabole,* change], to undergo metabolism, the breakdown of carbohydrates, proteins, and fats into smaller units; the reorganization of those units as tissue building blocks or as energy sources; and the elimination of waste products of the processes.

metacarpal. See **metacarpus.**

metacarpal phalanx /-kär″pəl/ [Gk, *meta + karpos,* wrist, *phalanx,* line of soldiers], the first portion of the finger that articulates with a carpal bone in the hand.

metacarpophalangeal (MCP) /-kar′pōfəlan″jē·əl/ [Gk, *meta,* beyond, *karpos,* wrist, *phalanx,* line of soldiers], pertaining to the metacarpal bones of the hand and the phalanges of fingers, as in metacarpophalangeal joints.

metacarpophalangeal (MCP) joint dislocation [Gk, *meta + karpos + phalanx* + L, *jungere,* to join, *dis + locare,* to place], the dislocation of a finger at the junction with the metacarpal bone, usually with damage to tendons and other structures.

metacarpus /met′əkär″pəs/ [Gk, *meta,* beyond, *karpos,* wrist], the middle part of the hand, consisting of five slender bones, metacarpals I through V, numbered from the thumb side. Each metacarpal consists of a body and two extremities. **–metacarpal,** *adj., n.*

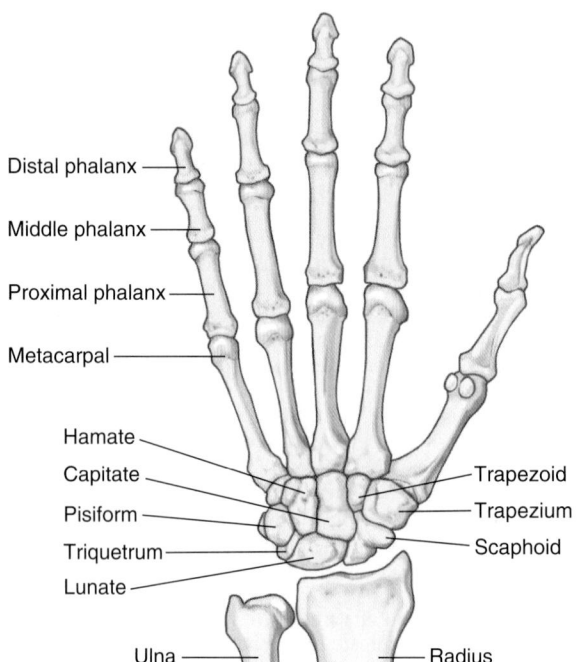

Distal phalanx
Middle phalanx
Proximal phalanx
Metacarpal
Hamate
Capitate
Pisiform
Triquetrum
Lunate
Ulna
Trapezoid
Trapezium
Scaphoid
Radius

Metacarpal bones *(Patton and Thibodeau, 2016)*

metacentric /met′əsen″trik/ [Gk, *meta + kentron,* center], pertaining to a chromosome in which the centromere is located near the center so that the arms of the chromosome are of approximately equal length. Compare **acrocentric, submetacentric, telocentric.**

metachromasia /-krōmā″zhē·ə/ [Gk, *meta,* beyond, *chroma,* color], a tissue-staining phenomenon in which cells being examined acquire a color other than that of the dye used. Cartilage cells, for example, may appear red after being stained with a blue dye. The cause is an interaction between the dye molecules and the acidic radicals of the tissue cells. Also called **metachromism.**

metachromatic leukodystrophy. See **sulfatide lipidosis.**

metachromatic lipids /-krōmat″ik/ [Gk, *meta,* beyond, *chroma,* color, *lipos,* fat], lipid molecules that accumulate in the central nervous system, peripheral nerves, and internal organs of infants who inherit a lipidosis disorder. See also **cerebroside sulfatase.**

metachromatic stain [Gk, *meta + chroma,* color; OFr, *desteindre,* to dye], a basic dye, such as toluidine, that can stain substances a different color than that of the stain.

metachromism. See **metachromasia.**

-metacin, suffix for indomethacin-type antiinflammatory substances.

metacommunication /-kəmyoo′nikā″shən/ [Gk, *meta* + L, *communicare,* to inform], communication that indicates how verbal information should be interpreted; stimuli surrounding the verbal communication that also have meaning, which may or may not be congruent with that of or support the verbal talk. It may support or contradict verbal communication.

metagenesis /met′əjen″əsis/ [Gk, *meta + genein,* to produce], the regular alternation of sexual with asexual methods of reproduction within the same species. **–metagenetic, metagenic,** *adj.*

metal [Gk, *metallon,* a mine], an element that conducts heat and electricity, is malleable and ductile, and forms positively charged ions (cations). About 80% of the known elements are metals.

metal fume fever, an occupational disorder caused by the inhalation of fumes of metallic oxides and characterized by symptoms similar to those of influenza. The condition occurs among workers engaged in welding, metal fabrication, casting, and other occupations dealing with the manipulation of metals. Access to fresh air and treatment of the symptoms usually alleviate the condition. Also called **brass founder's ague, zinc chill, Monday morning fever.** Compare **siderosis.**

metallesthesia /met′əlesthē″zhə/ [Gk, *metallon,* a mine, *aisthesia,* perception], an ability to identify a metal through the sense of touch.

metalloid /met′əloid/, **1.** any element with both metallic and nonmetallic properties, such as silicon, boron, or arsenic. **2.** resembling a metal.

metalloprotein /mətal′ōprō″tēn/, a protein that contains one or more metal atoms.

metallurgy /met″əlur′jē/ [Gk, *metallon,* a mine, *ergein,* to work], the theoretic and applied sciences of the nature and uses of metals.

metals, agents that consist of metallic poisons, such as arsenic, mercury, and thallium. Exposure to metallic poisons can be by inhalation or ingestion. Heavy metals can affect many systems, and large doses or prolonged exposure can lead to death.

metamorphopsia /met′əmôrfop″sē·ə/ [Gk, *meta + morphe,* form, *opsis,* sight], a defect in vision in which objects are seen as distorted in shape, which results from disease of the retina or imperfection of the media.

metamorphosis /met′əmôr″fəsis/ [Gk, *meta + morphe,* form], a change in shape or structure, especially a change from one stage of development to another, such as the transition from the larval to the adult stage.

metamyelocyte /met′əmī″əlōsīt/ [Gk, *meta + myelos,* marrow, *kytos,* cell], a stage in the development of the granulocyte series of leukocytes, between the myelocyte stage and the neutrophilic band. See also **leukocyte, myeloblast, myelocyte.**

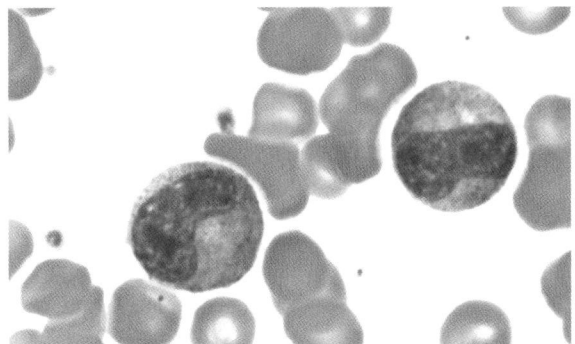

Metamyelocyte *(Young et al, 2014)*

metanephra. See **metanephros.**

metanephric blastema, a mass of intermediate mesodermal cells around the distal end of the ureteric bud that gives rise to nephrons in the permanent kidney. Also called *metanephric cap, metanephric mass.*

metanephrine /met′ənef″rin/, one of the two principal urinary metabolites of epinephrine and norepinephrine in the urine, the other being vanillylmandelic acid. The 24-hour normal adult value for total metanephrine is 1.3 mg.

metanephrogenic /met′ənef′rəjen″ik/ [Gk, *meta + nephros,* kidney, *genein,* to produce], capable of forming the metanephros, or fetal kidney.

metanephros /-nef″rəs/ *pl. metanephra, metanephroi* [Gk, *meta + nephros,* kidney], the third, and permanent, excretory organ to develop in the vertebrate embryo. It consists of a complex structure of secretory and collecting tubules that develop into the kidney. In most mammals there is limited functional use of the metanephric kidney during fetal life because waste materials are transferred across the placenta to the mother for elimination. Also called **hind kidney.** See also **kidney, mesonephros, pronephros.**

metaphase /met″əfāz/ [Gk, *meta + phasis,* appearance], the second of the four stages of nuclear division in mitosis and in each of the two divisions of meiosis, during which the chromosomes become arranged in the equatorial plane of the spindle to form the equatorial plate, with the centromeres attached to the spindle fibers in preparation for separation. See also **anaphase, interphase, meiosis, mitosis, prophase, telophase.**

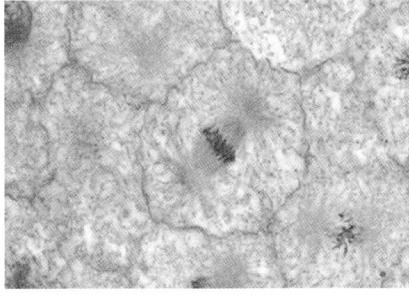

Metaphase *(© Ed Reschke; Used with permission)*

metaphyseal dysostosis /mətaf′izē″əl disostō″sis, met′əfiz″ē·əl disostō″sis/ [Gk, *meta + phyein,* to grow, *dys,* bad, *osteon,* bone], a condition characterized by abnormal mineralization of the metaphyseal area of the bones, resulting in dwarfism. Metaphyseal dysostosis is classified as the Gansen, Schmidt, or Spahar-Hartmann type or as cartilage-hair hypoplasia. The Gansen type is characterized by metaphyseal alterations similar to those of achondroplasia but not involving the skull or the epiphyses of the long bones. The Schmidt type is characterized by developmental changes from the weight-bearing age to approximately 5 years of age. The metaphyseal alterations associated with this type are similar to those of achondroplasia, resulting in moderate dwarfism. The Spahar-Hartmann type is characterized by skeletal changes and severe bowleg. Cartilage-hair hypoplasia is characterized by severe dwarfism and hair that is sparse, short, and brittle. Intellectual disability is not usually associated with metaphyseal dysostosis. Radiographic examination of all types of the disease reveals characteristic widening of the metaphyses of the tubular bones, with normal diaphyseal and epiphyseal ossification centers. Treatment is supportive and symptomatic. No specific modality is used.

metaphyseal dysplasia, a condition characterized by disordered modeling of the long bones, in which the metaphyseal circumference is enlarged and the medullary area is reduced. Metaphyseal dysplasia most often affects the distal femur or the proximal tibia.

metaphysis /mətaf″əsis/ [Gk, *meta + phyein,* to grow], a region of a growing long bone in which diaphysis and epiphysis converge. −metaphyseal, *adj.*

metaplasia /met′əplā″zhə/, the reversible conversion of normal tissue cells into another, less differentiated cell type in response to chronic stress or injury. With prolonged exposure to the inducing stimulus, cancerous transformation can occur.

metaplasm. See **cell inclusion.**

metaprotein. See **acidalbumin.**

metaproterenol sulfate /met′əprōter″inôl/, a beta$_2$ receptor agonist bronchodilator.

■ INDICATIONS: It is prescribed in the treatment of bronchial asthma and chronic obstructive pulmonary disease when a delayed onset but prolonged effect is desired.

■ CONTRAINDICATIONS: Arrhythmias associated with tachycardia or known hypersensitivity to this drug prohibits its use. It should be used with caution in patients with hypertension, hyperthyroidism, congestive heart failure, coronary artery disease, or diabetes.

■ ADVERSE EFFECTS: Among the more serious adverse effects are tachycardia, hypertension, and cardiac arrest.

metaraminol bitartrate /met′äram″inol/, an adrenergic vasopressor.

■ INDICATIONS: It is prescribed in the treatment of hypotension and shock.

■ CONTRAINDICATIONS: Known hypersensitivity to this drug prohibits its use. It is not used with the MAO inhibitors cyclopropane or halothane anesthesia or as the sole drug for hypovolemic hypotension.

■ ADVERSE EFFECTS: Among the more serious adverse effects are cardiac arrhythmia, tissue necrosis at the site of injection, hypertension, tremors, and nausea.

metarubricyte /-roo″brisīt/ [Gk, *meta + L, ruber,* red, *kytos,* cell], a red blood cell precursor, the last nucleated stage of red blood cell production. Metarubricytes are usually confined to the bone marrow but may appear in the peripheral blood in newborns and in uncompensated hemolytic anemia.

metastable solution. See **supersaturate.**

M

metastable state, a transient energy state of an atom with a half-life longer than 10^{-12} seconds (e.g., technetium[99m]).

metastasis /mətas″təsis/ *pl. metastases* [Gk, *meta + stasis,* standing], **1.** an active process by which tumor cells move from the primary location of a cancer by severing connections from the original cell group and establishing remote colonies. Because malignant tumors have no enclosing capsule, cells may escape, become emboli, and be transported by the lymphatic circulation or the bloodstream to implant in lymph nodes and other organs far from the primary tumor. **2.** a tumor that develops away from the site of origin. Compare **anaplasia. –metastatic,** *adj.,* –*metastasize, v.*

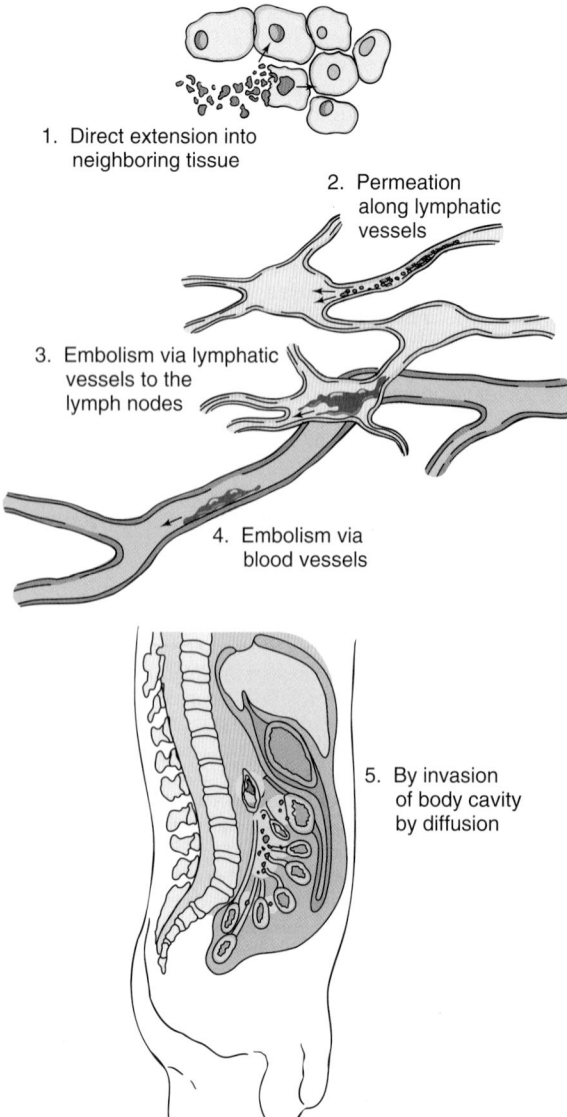

1. Direct extension into neighboring tissue

2. Permeation along lymphatic vessels

3. Embolism via lymphatic vessels to the lymph nodes

4. Embolism via blood vessels

5. By invasion of body cavity by diffusion

Modes of metastasis of cancer *(Monahan and Neighbors, 2007)*

metastasizing mole. See **chorioadenoma destruens.**

metastatic. See **metastasis.**

metastatic abscess /-stat″ik/ [Gk, *meta,* beyond, *stasis,* standing; L, *abscedere,* to go away], any secondary abscess that develops at a point distant from an original infection, resulting from transportation of infectious particles to other locations via the bloodstream.

metastatic calcification [Gk, *meta + stasis,* standing; L, *calx,* lime, *facere,* to make], the pathological process whereby calcium salts accumulate in previously healthy tissues, caused by excessive levels of blood calcium, such as in hyperparathyroidism.

metastatic endometriosis [Gk, *meta,* beyond, *stasis,* standing, *endon,* within, *metra,* womb, *osis,* condition], extraperitoneal lesions that resemble metastases from a carcinoma.

metastatic ophthalmia. See **sympathetic ophthalmia.**

metastatic survey [Gk, *meta,* beyond, *stasis,* standing; OFr, *surveoir,* to examine], a method of monitoring the spread of a cancer by taking a series of periodic x-ray images.

metatarsal /met′ətär″səl/ [Gk, *meta + tarsos,* flat surface], **1.** *adj.,* pertaining to the metatarsus of the foot. **2.** *n.,* any one of the five bones making up the metatarsus.

metatarsal artery. See **arcuate artery of the foot.**

metatarsalgia /met′ətärsal″jə/ [Gk, *meta + tarsos + algos,* pain], a painful condition around the metatarsal bones caused by an abnormality of the foot or by recalcification of degenerated heads of metatarsal bones.

metatarsal phalanx /-tär″səl/ [Gk, *meta + tarsos,* flat surface, *phalanx,* line of soldiers], the bones of the foot and toes.

metatarsal stress fracture, a break or rupture of a metatarsal bone caused by prolonged running or walking. The condition is often difficult to diagnose with x-ray imaging. Also called **march fracture.**

metatarsus /-tär″səs/ [Gk, *meta + tarsos,* flat surface], *n.,* a part of the foot, consisting of five bones, numbered I to V from the medial side. Each bone has a long, slender body; a wedge-shaped proximal end; a convex distal end; and flattened, grooved sides for the attachment of ligaments. The metatarsal bones articulate with the tarsus proximally and the first row of phalanges distally. Deformities of the metatarsus include metatarsus valgus and metatarsus varus.

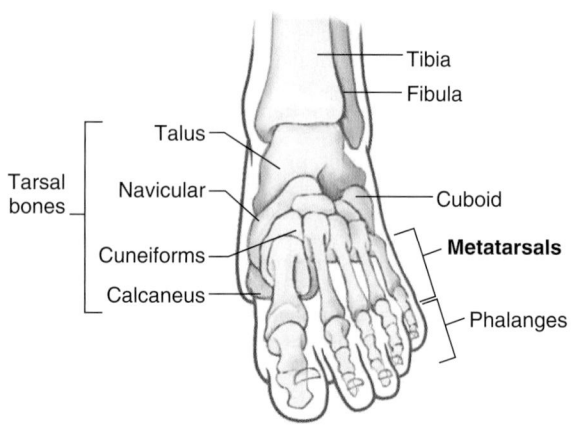

Tibia

Fibula

Talus

Tarsal bones

Navicular

Cuboid

Cuneiforms

Metatarsals

Calcaneus

Phalanges

Metatarsal bones *(Patton and Thibodeau, 2016)*

metatarsus adductus. See **metatarsus varus.**

metatarsus valgus, a congenital deformity of the foot in which the forepart rotates outward away from the midline of the body and the heel remains straight. Also called **duck walk, toeing out.**

metatarsus varus, a congenital deformity of the foot in which the forepart rotates inward toward the midline of the body and the heel remains straight. Also called **intoe, metatarsus adductus, pigeon-toed, toeing in.**

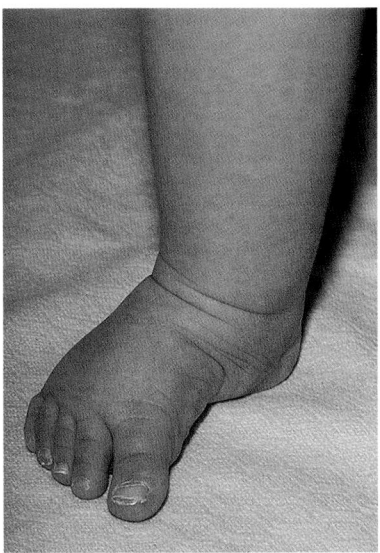

Metatarsus varus *(Courtesy Yvonne Wylie Walston)*

metathalamus /met′əthal″əməs/ [Gk, *meta + thalamos,* chamber], one of five parts of the diencephalon, composed of a medial geniculate body and a lateral geniculate body on each side. The medial geniculate body acts as a relay station for nerve impulses between the inferior brachium and the auditory cortex. The lateral geniculate body is a superficial oval bulge at the posterior end of the thalamus, which accommodates the terminal ends of the fibers of the optic tract. Relay cells project to the visual cortex. Compare **epithalamus, hypothalamus, subthalamus.** *−metathalamic, adj.*

metaxalone /metak″səlōn/, a skeletal muscle relaxant.
■ INDICATIONS: It is prescribed as an adjunct in the treatment of acute skeletal muscle spasm.
■ CONTRAINDICATIONS: Significantly impaired renal or hepatic function, susceptibility to drug-induced hemolytic anemia, or known hypersensitivity to this drug prohibits its use.
■ ADVERSE EFFECTS: Among the more serious adverse effects are hemolytic anemia, leukopenia, and liver dysfunction. GI disturbances, dizziness, and nervousness may occur.

metazoa /-zō″ə/ [Gk, *meta + zoon,* animal], a classification that includes animals that have tissues and organs. All animals except sponges are metazoa.

Metchnikoff's theory /mech″nikofs/ [Elie Metchnikoff, Russian-French biologist, 1845–1916; Gk, *theoria,* speculation], the theory that living cells ingest microorganisms. The theory proved correct, as seen in the process of phagocytosis and the ingestion of injurious microbes by leukocytes.

meteorism [Gk, *meteorizein,* to hold up], accumulation of gas in the abdomen or the intestine, usually with distension.

meteorotropism /mē′tē·ərətrō″pizəm/ [Gk, *meteoros,* high in the air, *trope,* turning], a reaction to meteorological influences shown by various biological occurrences, such as sudden death, attacks of arthritis, and angina. *−meteorotropic, adj.*

meter (m) /mē″tər/ [Gk, metron, measure], a metric unit of length equal to 39.37 inches.

-meter, -metre, 1. suffix meaning "a measuring instrument": *dosimeter, barometer, adipometer.* **2.** suffix meaning "length" or "measure": *centimeter, kilometer, millimeter.*

metered dose inhaler (MDI) /mē″tərd/, a device designed to deliver a measured dose of an inhaled drug. It usually consists of a canister of aerosol spray, mist, or fine powder that releases a specific dose each time it is pushed against a dispensing valve. The device is intended to reduce the risk of overmedication by the patient.

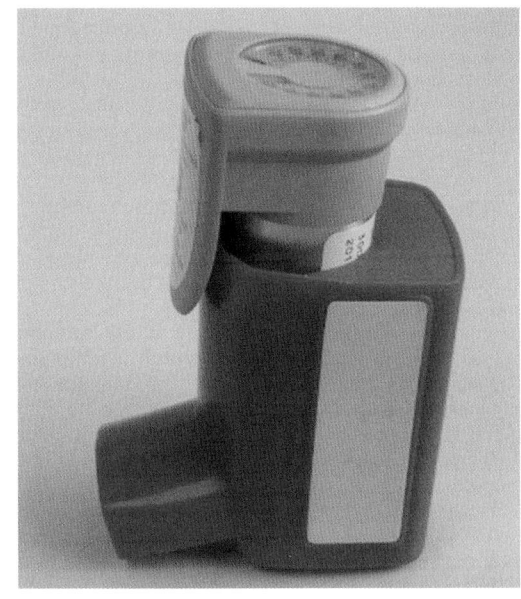

Metered dose inhaler *(Patel et al, 2012)*

metformin /met-for′min/, a hypoglycemic agent that potentiates the action of insulin, used in the treatment of type 2 diabetes mellitus.

metformin hydrochloride, an oral antidiabetic agent.
■ INDICATIONS: It is prescribed in the treatment of type 2 (non–insulin-dependent) diabetes mellitus.
■ CONTRAINDICATIONS: The drug should not be given to patients with allergy to metformin, diabetes associated with high ketone levels, metabolic acidosis, or kidney disease, and it should be discontinued 48 hours before radiology studies using radiopaque materials.
■ ADVERSE EFFECTS: The side effects most often reported include general body discomfort, muscle pain, breathing difficulty, drowsiness, diarrhea, and an unpleasant metallic taste. Metformin may affect vitamin B_{12} absorption.

methacholine /meth″äko′lēn/, a cholinergic agonist, having a longer duration of action than acetylcholine and predominantly muscarinic effects. It has vasodilator and cardiac vagomimetic effects but has largely been replaced by other drugs. It is also used in bronchial challenge tests.

methacholine challenge /meth′əkō″lēn/, a method of measuring airway activity by an inhalation challenge test. The patient inhales a saline aerosol as a control, followed by increasing concentrations of methacholine chloride, a cholinergic drug. The test is used to confirm the diagnosis of asthma when symptoms are not present. This is a potentially dangerous test and should be performed only by qualified personnel, with resuscitation equipment readily available.

methacrylic acid (MAA) /meth′əkril″ik/, an organic acid obtained from Roman chamomile oil that polymerizes into a ceramic-like mass. The methyl ester of methacrylic acid is used in medical and dental products such as enamel sealants. A copolymer is used in tablet coatings.

methadone hydrochloride, an opioid analgesic used for anesthesia or as a substitute for heroin, permitting withdrawal without development of acute abstinence syndrome. Methadone does not produce marked euphoria, sedation, or

M

narcosis. It is not given to pregnant women or to patients with liver disease.

methaemoglobin. See **methemoglobin.**

methaemoglobinuria. See **methemoglobinuria.**

methamphetamine hydrochloride /meth′amfet″əmēn/, a central nervous system stimulant that is easily synthesized and is a major drug of abuse.

■ INDICATIONS: It is prescribed in the treatment of attention deficit hyperactivity disorder and as a short-term treatment for the reduction of appetite in exogenous obesity. An unlabeled use is for the treatment of narcolepsy.

■ CONTRAINDICATIONS: Glaucoma, arteriosclerosis, cardiovascular disease, hypertension, hyperthyroidism, history of drug abuse, concomitant use of a monoamine oxidase inhibitor, or known hypersensitivity to this drug or to other sympathomimetic drugs prohibits its use.

■ ADVERSE EFFECTS: Among the more serious adverse effects are various manifestations of central nervous system excitation, increase in blood pressure, arrhythmia and other cardiovascular effects, nausea, and drug dependence.

methandriol /methan′drē·ol/, an anabolic hormone used as adjunctive therapy in senile and postmenopausal osteoporosis.

methane (CH₄) /meth″ān/, a simple hydrocarbon in the form of colorless gas, produced by the anaerobic decomposition of organic matter. It occurs naturally in the gas from oil wells and coal mines.

methanol (CH₃OH) /meth″ənol/, a clear, colorless, toxic liquid distillate of wood miscible with water, other alcohols, and ether. Methanol is produced industrially from carbon monoxide and hydrogen. It is widely used as a solvent and in the production of formaldehyde. Also called **methyl alcohol, wood alcohol.**

methanol poisoning, a toxic effect of ingestion, inhalation, or absorption through the skin of methanol (methyl alcohol, wood alcohol) that may impair the central nervous system; cause severe acidosis, blindness, and shock; and result in death. Methanol is found in antifreeze, varnish, and deicing agents. Also called **methyl alcohol poisoning.**

methazolamide /meth′əzō″ləmīd/, a carbonic anhydrase inhibitor.

■ INDICATIONS: It is prescribed in the treatment of glaucoma.

■ CONTRAINDICATIONS: Severe kidney or liver dysfunction, hyponatremia, hypokalemia, Addison disease, severe pulmonary obstruction, adrenocortical insufficiency, marked kidney or liver dysfunction, or known hypersensitivity to this drug or many other sulfonamides prohibits its use.

■ ADVERSE EFFECTS: Among the more serious adverse effects are malaise, aplastic anemia, drowsiness, paresthesia, hypersensitivity reactions, and acidosis.

methemoglobin /met′hēməglō″bin, met·he″məglō′bin/, a form of hemoglobin in which the iron component has been oxidized from the ferrous to the ferric state. Methemoglobin cannot carry oxygen. It is a product of various oxidative reactions that constitute normal metabolic activity and is normally present in only trace amounts (about 1%) in the blood, but may increase in chronic inflammation. Maintenance of levels occurs by an active enzymatic reducing capability, the nicotinamide-adenine dinucleotide-methemoglobin reductase system present in normal red blood cells. Also spelled **methaemoglobin.** See also **hemoglobin.**

methemoglobinemia /-ē″mē·ə/, the presence of methemoglobin in the blood.

methemoglobin test, a blood test to detect methemoglobinemia.

methemoglobinuria /-ōōr″ē·ə/ [Gk, *meta,* beyond, *haima,* blood; L, *globus,* ball; Gk, *ouron,* urine], the presence of methemoglobin in the urine. Also spelled **methaemoglobinuria.**

methenamine /methē″nəmēn/, a urinary antibacterial drug.

■ INDICATIONS: It is prescribed in the treatment of urinary tract infections.

■ CONTRAINDICATIONS: Liver or kidney dysfunction or known hypersensitivity to this drug or to mandelic acid prohibits its use. It should not be used by patients receiving sulfonamides.

■ ADVERSE EFFECTS: Among the most serious adverse effects are severe GI disturbances and rashes.

methenamine silver stain, a specialized stain consisting of methenamine and silver nitrate used in histological examinations for the detection of fungi. This stain is the best for detecting fungi in specimens, but it is very time consuming and is used mainly in histology labs.

Methergine, an oxytocic agent. Brand name for **methylergonovine maleate.**

methimazole /məthim″əzōl/, an orally administered antithyroid drug.

■ INDICATIONS: It is prescribed in the treatment of hyperthyroidism.

■ CONTRAINDICATIONS: Use in nursing mothers, because it is excreted in milk, and known hypersensitivity to the drug prohibit its use.

■ ADVERSE EFFECTS: Agranulocytosis, leukopenia, thrombocytopenia, and aplastic anemia may occur.

methionine (Met) /methī″ənēn/, an essential amino acid needed for proper growth in infants and for maintenance of nitrogen balance in adults. It is a source for methyl groups and sulfur in the body. It is also administered as adjunctive treatment in liver diseases. See also **amino acid, protein.**

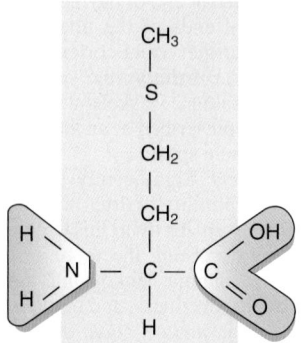

Chemical structure of methionine

methisoprinol. See **inosiplex.**

methocarbamol /meth′əkär″bəmol/, a skeletal muscle relaxant.

■ INDICATIONS: It is prescribed in the relief of skeletal muscle spasm.

■ CONTRAINDICATIONS: Renal dysfunction, central nervous system depression, or known hypersensitivity to this drug prohibits its use. Propylthiouracil is a better choice than methimazole for thyrotoxic crisis.

■ ADVERSE EFFECTS: Among the more serious adverse effects are hypotension and tachycardia. Drowsiness, dizziness, vertigo, and nausea may occur.

method /meth″əd/ [Gk, *meta,* beyond, *hodos,* way], **1.** a technique or procedure for producing a desired effect, such as a surgical procedure, a laboratory test, or a diagnostic technique. **2.** (in occupational therapy) a means or manner of procedure, especially a regular and systematic way of accomplishing a task.

methodology /meth′ədol″əjē/ [Gk, *meta* + *hodos* + *logos*, science], **1.** a system of principles or methods of procedure in any discipline, such as education, research, diagnosis, or treatment. **2.** the section of a research proposal in which the methods to be used are described. The research design, the population to be studied, and the research instruments, or tools, to be used are discussed in the methodology. —*methodological, adj.*

methohexital sodium /meth′ōhek″sitôl/, an IV barbiturate of short duration.
■ INDICATIONS: It is used for the induction of anesthesia in short surgical procedures such as cardioversion.
■ CONTRAINDICATIONS: Porphyria, status asthmaticus, or known hypersensitivity to this drug or to any barbiturate prohibits its use.
■ ADVERSE EFFECTS: Among the more serious adverse effects are respiratory depression, skin rash, muscle tremors, hiccoughs, and cardiovascular dysfunction.

methotrexate /meth′ōtrek″sāt/, an antineoplastic antimetabolite. Also called **amethopterin.**
■ INDICATIONS: It is prescribed in the treatment of a variety of malignant neoplastic diseases of the blood and organs and in the treatment of psoriasis, and it is widely used as an immunosuppressive agent for the treatment of autoimmune diseases such as rheumatoid arthritis.
■ CONTRAINDICATIONS: Blood dyscrasias, severe renal or hepatic impairment, or known hypersensitivity to this drug prohibits its use.
■ ADVERSE EFFECTS: Among the more serious adverse effects are diarrhea, ulcerative stomatitis, bone marrow depression, hepatotoxicity, and skin rash.

methoxsalen /methok″sələn/, a pigmentation agent. Also called **8-MOP.**
■ INDICATIONS: It is used topically for unresponsive psoriasis and enhancement of pigmentation or for repigmentation in vitiligo and is administered orally before long-wave ultraviolet irradiation of severe recalcitrant psoriasis.
■ CONTRAINDICATIONS: Liver impairment, cataracts, age under 12 years, any disease or concomitant use of a drug that may cause photosensitization, squamous cell carcinoma, or known hypersensitivity to this drug prohibits its use.
■ ADVERSE EFFECTS: Among the most serious adverse reactions are central nervous system effects and burns. Gastrointestinal discomfort and allergic reactions also may occur.

methoxyflurane. See **halogenated hydrocarbon.**
3-methoxy-4-hydroxymandelic acid. See **vanillylmandelic acid.**
methscopolamine bromide /meth′skōpō″ləmēn/, an anticholinergic/antispasmodic drug.
■ INDICATIONS: It is prescribed in the treatment of hypermotility of the GI tract and as an adjunct in treatment of peptic ulcer.
■ CONTRAINDICATIONS: Narrow-angle glaucoma, asthma, obstruction of the genitourinary or GI tract, severe ulcerative colitis, or known hypersensitivity to this drug prohibits its use.
■ ADVERSE EFFECTS: Blurred vision, central nervous system effects, tachycardia, dry mouth, decreased sweating, or hypersensitivity reactions may occur.

methsuximide /methsuk″simīd/, an anticonvulsant drug.
■ INDICATIONS: It is prescribed in the treatment of refractory absence seizures.
■ CONTRAINDICATIONS: Known hypersensitivity to this drug or to any succinimide prohibits its use.
■ ADVERSE EFFECTS: Among the more serious adverse effects are blood dyscrasias, liver and kidney damage, and systemic lupus erythematosus.

methyclothiazide /məthī′klōthī″əzīd, meth′əklōthī″əzīd/, a diuretic.
■ INDICATIONS: It is prescribed in the treatment of mild to moderate hypertension and edema.
■ CONTRAINDICATIONS: Anemia, renal or urinary disorders, or known hypersensitivity to this drug, to other thiazide medications, or to sulfonamide derivatives prohibits its use.
■ ADVERSE EFFECTS: Among the more serious adverse effects are hypokalemia, hyperglycemia, hyperuricemia, hypotension, and hypersensitivity reactions.

methyl (Me) /meth″il/, the chemical radical CH_3.
methyl alcohol. See **methanol.**
methyl alcohol poisoning. See **methanol poisoning.**
methylate /meth″ilāt/ [Gk, *methy,* wine, *hyle,* matter], **1.** *n.,* an organic compound in which the hydrogen atom of methanol is replaced by a metal. **2.** *v.,* to add a methyl group, CH_3, to a chemical compound.
methylation /-lā″shən/ [Gk, *methy,* wine, *hyle,* matter], **1.** the introduction of a methyl group, CH_3, to a chemical compound. **2.** the addition of methyl alcohol and naphtha to ethanol to produce denatured alcohol. **3.** attaching a methyl group to segments of DNA to turn off or silence a gene so that no protein is produced from that gene. See also **epigenetics.**
methyl blue, a blue dye of the triarylmethane class, $C_{37}H_{27}N_3O_9S_3Na_2$, used alone or in combination with water blue as a biological stain.
methyldopa /-dō″pə/, an alpha$_2$ receptor agonist that acts in the central nervous system to decrease sympathetic nervous system outflow.
■ INDICATIONS: It is prescribed for the reduction of hypertension in moderate to severe cases.
■ CONTRAINDICATIONS: Use of monoamine oxidase inhibitors, liver dysfunction, or known hypersensitivity to this drug prohibits its use.
■ ADVERSE EFFECTS: Among the more serious adverse effects are liver toxicity and blood dyscrasias. Sedation, dry mouth, nasal stuffiness, and postural hypotension may occur.
methylene blue /meth″əlēn/, a bluish-green crystalline substance used as a histological stain and a laboratory indicator. It is also used in the treatment of cyanide poisoning and methemoglobinemia.
methylergonovine maleate /-ərgon″əvēn/, a synthetic ergot alkaloid.
■ INDICATIONS: It is prescribed as an oxytocic to prevent or to treat postpartum uterine atony, hemorrhage, or subinvolution.
■ CONTRAINDICATIONS: It is not prescribed during pregnancy or given intravenously, except in life-threatening situations. Hypertension, toxemia, or known hypersensitivity to ergot alkaloids prohibits its use.
■ ADVERSE EFFECTS: Among the most serious adverse effects are convulsions and death. Hypertension, nausea, blurred vision, and headaches also may occur. Adverse effects are more common after IV administration.
3-methylfentanyl, a potent heroin substitute and so-called designer drug. It is an analog of fentanyl and reportedly 3000 times as potent as morphine. One ounce represents 25 million doses of a drug with effects equivalent to that of high-grade heroin. A related designer drug is *p*-fluoro fentanyl. See also **designer drugs.**
methylmalonicacidemia /meth′əl·mə·lon′ik·as′i·dē′mē·ə/, **1.** an autosomal-recessive aminoacidopathy characterized by an excess of the carboxylic acid methylmalonic acid in the blood and urine, with metabolic ketoacidosis, hyperammonemia, and excess glycine in the blood and urine, presenting in infancy as failure to thrive, persistent

M

vomiting and dehydration, respiratory distress, and hypotonia. It results from any of several defects that cause deficiency of an enzyme involved in the use of isoleucine, threonine, valine, propionate, and other odd-number chain-length fatty acids for fuel. Treatment consists of dietary supplementation with cobalamin, and carnitine and protein restriction; a diet restricting isoleucine threonine, methionine, and valine may be useful. Also called *methylmalonicaciduria.* **2.** an excess of methylmalonic acid in the blood.

methylphenidate hydrochloride /-fen″idāt/, a central nervous system stimulant.
■ INDICATIONS: It is prescribed in the treatment of attention deficit hyperactivity disorder in children and, more recently, in adults and for narcolepsy in adults.
■ CONTRAINDICATIONS: Glaucoma, severe anxiety, tension, mental depression, or known hypersensitivity to this drug prohibits its use. It is not given to children less than 6 years of age.
■ ADVERSE EFFECTS: Among the more serious adverse effects are nervousness, insomnia, and anorexia. Hypersensitivity reactions and tachycardia may occur.

methylPREDNISolone /-prednis″əlōn/, a glucocorticoid.
■ INDICATIONS: It is prescribed as an antiinflammatory drug and as an immunosuppressant to treat autoimmune disease, cancer, and other disease involving cells of the immune system. It is also administered to suppress graft-versus-host disease after bone marrow transplantation.
■ CONTRAINDICATIONS: Fungal infections or known hypersensitivity to this drug prohibits its systemic use. Viral or fungal infections of the skin, impaired circulation, or known hypersensitivity to this drug prohibits its topical use.
■ ADVERSE EFFECTS: Among the more serious adverse effects of the systemic administration of the drug are upper GI bleeding and endocrine, neurological, fluid, and electrolyte disturbances. Skin reactions may result from topical administration of this drug.

methylrosaniline chloride. See **gentian violet.**
methyl salicylate. See **wintergreen oil.**
methylTESTOSTERone /meth′ïltəstos″tərōn/, an androgen.
■ INDICATIONS: It is prescribed in the treatment of testosterone deficiency and in the palliation of female breast cancer.
■ CONTRAINDICATIONS: Cancer of the male breast or prostate; cardiac, renal, or hepatic disease; hypercalcemia; known or suspected pregnancy; lactation; or known hypersensitivity to this drug prohibits its use.
■ ADVERSE EFFECTS: Among the more serious adverse effects are hypercalcemia, edema, irreversible masculinization of female patients, and jaundice.

methysergide maleate /meth′isur″jïd/, a vasoconstrictor.
■ INDICATIONS: It is prescribed for relief of migraine headache.
■ CONTRAINDICATIONS: Pregnancy, severe infection, liver or kidney dysfunction, cardiovascular or lung disease, or known hypersensitivity to this drug prohibits its use. It is not recommended for use in children.
■ ADVERSE EFFECTS: Among the more serious adverse effects are retroperitoneal fibrosis; hallucinations; abnormally low white cell count; pulmonary and cardiac complications; hemolytic anemia; leg cramps; and pain in the chest, abdomen, back, hands, or feet.

Meticorten, a glucocorticoid. Brand name for **predniSONE.**
metipranolol /met″ipran′älol/, a beta-adrenergic blocking agent, applied topically to the conjunctiva as the hydrochloride salt in the treatment of glaucoma and ocular hypertension.

metoclopramide hydrochloride /met′əklō″prəmīd/, a GI motility agent.
■ INDICATIONS: It is prescribed to stimulate motility of and increase the tone of gastric contractions of the upper GI tract and to prevent emesis.
■ CONTRAINDICATIONS: A history of seizures; concomitant use of drugs that cause extrapyramidal reactions; pheochromocytoma; GI hemorrhage, obstruction, or perforation; or known hypersensitivity to this drug prohibits its use.
■ ADVERSE EFFECTS: Among the more serious adverse effects are extrapyramidal reactions, usually in children, and GI disturbances. Drowsiness and allergic reactions and rash also may occur.

metolazone /mətō″ləzōn/, a diuretic.
■ INDICATIONS: It is prescribed for the treatment of edema and mild to moderate high blood pressure.
■ CONTRAINDICATIONS: Anuria or known hypersensitivity to this drug, to thiazides, or to sulfonamides prohibits its use.
■ ADVERSE EFFECTS: Among the more serious adverse effects are hypokalemia, hyperglycemia, hyperuricemia, and allergic reactions.

"me-too" drug, (*Informal*) a drug product that is similar, identical, or closely related to a drug for which a manufacturer has obtained a new drug application. The drug is placed on the market by a company or companies other than the holder of the new drug application. On the assumption that the new drug has been recognized as safe and effective, clinical trials required of the original manufacturer are not required of the new supplier, but information regarding the manufacture, bioavailability, and labeling of the product is required to complete the abbreviated procedure for approval by the U.S. Food and Drug Administration.

metopic /mətō″pik/, pertaining to the forehead.
metoprolol tartrate /metop″rəlol/, an antiadrenergic; a beta$_1$-receptor antagonist.
■ INDICATIONS: It is prescribed to treat hypertension and angina pectoris and to prevent myocardial infarction and atrial flutter or fibrillation. It also has proven benefits for patients with congestive heart failure when used in combination with other drugs. Unlabeled uses include migraine prophylaxis and treatment of essential tremor and ventricular arrhythmias.
■ CONTRAINDICATIONS: Bradycardia, cardiogenic shock, overt cardiac failure, bronchospastic disease, or known hypersensitivity to this drug prohibits its use.
■ ADVERSE EFFECTS: Among the more serious adverse effects are fatigue, bradycardia, bronchospasms, decreased sexual ability, and GI upset.

metr-, prefix meaning "measure": *metric, metronoscope*
metra-. See **metro-, metra-.**
metralgia /mətral″jə/ [Gk, *metra,* womb, *algos,* pain], tenderness or pain in the uterus. Also called **hysteralgia, hysterodynia, metrodynia, uteralgia.**
metre. See **-meter, -metre.**
-metria, 1. suffix meaning "(condition of the) ability to measure muscular acts": *dysmetria, hypermetria, hypometria.* **2.** suffix meaning "(condition of the) uterus": *parametria.*
metric /met″rik/, pertaining to a system of measurement that uses the meter as a basis. See also **metric system.**
metric equivalent [Gk, *metron,* measure; L, *aequus,* equal, *valare,* to be strong], any value in metric units of measurement that equals the same value in English units (e.g., 2.54 cm equals 1 inch, and 1 L equals 1.0567 quarts).
metric system, a decimal system of measurement based on the meter (39.37 inches) as the unit of length, on the gram (15.432 grains) as the unit of weight or mass, and, as a

derived unit, on the liter (0.908 U.S. dry quart or 1.0567 U.S. liquid quart) as the unit of volume.

metritis /mətrī″tis/ [Gk, *metra,* womb, *itis,* inflammation], inflammation of the walls of the uterus. Also called **uteritis.** Kinds include **endometritis, parametritis.** See also **puerperal fever.**

metro-, metra-, combining form meaning "uterus": *hematometra, metralgia, menometrorrhagia.*

metrocarcinoma /met′rōkär′sinō″mə/ [Gk, *metra,* womb, *karkinos,* crab, *oma,* tumor], a cancer of the uterus.

metrodynia. See **metralgia.**

metromalacia, abnormal softening of the uterus.

metronidazole /met′rənī″dəzōl/, an antimicrobial with activity against anaerobic bacteria and protozoa.

■ INDICATIONS: It is prescribed in the treatment of a variety of infections, including amebiasis, trichomoniasis, anaerobic infections, pseudomembranous colitis, antibiotic-induced infections, and bacterial vaginosis.

■ CONTRAINDICATIONS: First trimester of pregnancy, blood dyscrasias, organic disease, central nervous system disorders, or known hypersensitivity to this drug prohibits its use. It is contraindicated in nursing mothers.

■ ADVERSE EFFECTS: Among the more serious adverse effects are severe GI distress, dizziness, neutropenia, and neurological disturbances. A metallic taste in the mouth is commonly noted.

metronoscope /mətron″əskōp/, **1.** a tachistoscope, a device that exposes a small amount of reading matter to the eyes for brief preset periods. It is used in testing and in aiding individuals to increase reading speed. **2.** an apparatus that exercises the eyes rhythmically to improve binocular coordination.

-metropia, -metropy, suffix meaning "(condition of the) refraction of the eye": *ametropia, emmetropia, anisometropia.*

metroplasty /mē″trəplas′tē/ [Gk, *metra,* womb], reconstructive surgery on the uterus. Also called **uteroplasty.**

metrorrhagia /met′rōrā″jē·ə/ [Gk, *metra,* womb, *rhegnynai,* to burst forth], uterine bleeding other than that caused by menstruation. It may be caused by uterine lesions and may be a sign of a urogenital malignancy, especially cervical cancer.

-metry, -metria, suffix meaning "the process of measuring something specified": *allometry, pelvimetry, symmetry.*

metyrapone /metir″əpōn/, a diagnostic test drug.

■ INDICATIONS: It is used to test hypothalamic and pituitary function.

■ CONTRAINDICATIONS: Adrenocortical insufficiency or hypersensitivity prohibits its use.

■ ADVERSE EFFECTS: Among the most serious adverse effects are nausea, dizziness, and allergic rash.

metyrosine /mətir″əsēn/, an inhibitor of tyrosine hydroxylase, the rate-limiting enzyme for catecholamine synthesis.

■ INDICATIONS: It is prescribed in the treatment of pheochromocytoma before surgery and may be used for long-term therapy if surgery is contraindicated.

■ CONTRAINDICATIONS: Known hypersensitivity to this drug prohibits its use.

■ ADVERSE EFFECTS: Among the more serious adverse effects are extrapyramidal reactions, including tremor and drooling. Sedation is common, and diarrhea and anxiety may occur.

Metzenbaum scissors. See **scissors.**

Meuse fever. See **trench fever.**

mev, MeV, the equivalent of 3.82×10^{-14} small calories, or 1.6×10^{-6} ergs. Abbreviation for *million electron volts.*

mevalonate kinase /məval″ənāt/, an enzyme in the liver and in yeast. It catalyzes the transfer of a phosphate group from adenosine triphosphate to produce adenosine diphosphate and 5-phosphomevalonate.

Mexican bindweed. See *Rivea corymbosa.*

Mexican spotted fever. See **Rocky Mountain spotted fever.**

Mexican typhus [Gk, *typhos,* fever], a form of epidemic typhus carried by lice in Mexico. Also called **tabardillo.**

mexiletine hydrochloride /mek′silē″tin/, an oral antiarrhythmic drug.

■ INDICATIONS: It is prescribed for the treatment of symptomatic ventricular arrhythmias and suppression of premature ventricular contractions.

■ CONTRAINDICATIONS: It is contraindicated in patients with cardiogenic shock or preexisting second- or third-degree atrioventricular block in the absence of a pacemaker.

■ ADVERSE EFFECTS: Among adverse effects reported are upper GI distress, light-headedness, tremor, loss of coordination, diarrhea, sleep disorders, headache, visual disturbances, and palpitations.

Mexitil, an oral antiarrhythmic drug. Brand name for **mexiletine hydrochloride.**

Meyenburg complexes, groups of hamartomas in the bile ducts.

Meyer, Adolf /mi′er/ [1866–1950], Swiss-born psychiatrist in the United States who directed the development of the Henry Phipps Psychiatric Clinic at Johns Hopkins University. His major contributions include propounding the theory of psychobiology, standardizing case histories, and reforming mental health institutions (which were called "insane asylums" at that time).

Meynet node /mānā″/, any of the numerous nodules that may develop within the capsules surrounding joints and in tendons affected by rheumatic diseases, especially in children.

Mezlin, a semisynthetic penicillin antibiotic. Brand name for **mezlocillin sodium.**

mezlocillin sodium /mezlos″ilin/, a semisynthetic penicillin antibiotic.

■ INDICATIONS: It is prescribed for the treatment of lower respiratory tract, intraabdominal, urinary tract, gynecological, and skin infections and bacterial septicemia caused by susceptible strains of multiple microorganisms.

■ CONTRAINDICATIONS: Hypersensitivity to any of the penicillins prohibits its use.

■ ADVERSE EFFECTS: The most serious adverse effects are anaphylaxis, convulsive seizures, epigastric pain, reduction in blood elements, and elevation in hepatic and renal parameters.

mF, abbreviation for *millifarad.* See **farad.**

MFD, abbreviation for *minimum fatal dose.* See **minimum lethal dose.**

mg, abbreviation for **milligram.**

Mg, **1.** symbol for the element **magnesium. 2.** abbreviation for *megagram.*

MH, **1.** abbreviation for **malignant hyperthermia. 2.** abbreviation for **mental health.**

MHC, abbreviation for **major histocompatibility complex.** See **HLA.**

MHD, abbreviation for **minimum hemolytic dose.**

mho. See **siemens.**

MHz, abbreviation for **megahertz.**

MI, initialism for **myocardial infarction.**

miasma /mī·az″mə/ [Gk, *miainein,* defilement], an unwholesome, polluted atmosphere or environment, such as a marsh or swamp containing rotting organic matter. Also called *miasm.*

MIC, abbreviation for **minimal inhibitory concentration.**

M

mica /mī″kə/, an aluminum silicate mineral that occurs in thin laminated scales. Mica is used in paints, plastics, fire protection boards, pigments, and other industrial materials. It is used also as an electric insulator and lubricant.

micafungin, a systemic antifungal drug.
- INDICATIONS: This drug is used in the treatment of esophageal candidiasis and susceptible candida species *(Candida albicans, C. glabrata, C. krusei, C. parapsilosis,* and *C. tropicalis)* and in prophylaxis of candida infections in patients undergoing hepatopoietic stem cell transplantation.
- CONTRAINDICATIONS: Known hypersensitivity to this drug or to other ecinocandins prohibits its use.
- ADVERSE EFFECTS: Adverse effects of this drug include dizziness, flushing, hypertension, phlebitis, abdominal pain, hypokalemia, hypocalcemia, and hypomagnesemia. Life-threatening side effects include seizures, neutropenia, thrombocytopenia, leukopenia, coagulopathy, anemia, and hemolytic anemia. Common side effects include headache; somnolence; nausea; anorexia; vomiting; diarrhea; increased aspartate aminotransferase, alanine aminotransferase, alkaline phosphate, and blood dehydrogenase; hyperbilirubinemia; rash; pruritus; injection site pain; and rigors.

micatosis /mī″kətō″sis/, a form of pneumoconiosis caused by inhalation of mica particles.

micellar chromatography /mīsel″ər/, a method of monitoring minute quantities of drugs in whole body fluids by using micellar or colloidal compounds to keep proteins in solution. The technique eliminates the need to remove proteins that usually interfere with chromatographic analysis of blood serum, urine, or saliva. Micellar chromatography is used to monitor levels of prescribed drugs, as well as illicit drugs.

Michaelis-Menten kinetics [Leonor Michaelis, American biochemist, 1875–1949; Maud L. Menten, Canadian physician in U.S. practice, 1879–1960], a method of transforming drug plasma levels into a linear relationship by using the parameters of drug concentration and a constant, K_m, which is a measure of enzyme-substrate affinity. This is necessary when drug elimination mechanisms are saturable rather than proceeding by first-order kinetics.

-micin, suffix for antibiotics produced by *Micromonospora* strains.

miconazole nitrate /mīkon″əzōl/, an antifungal drug.
- INDICATIONS: It is used topically to treat certain fungal infections of the skin and vagina.
- CONTRAINDICATIONS: Known hypersensitivity to this drug prohibits its use.
- ADVERSE EFFECTS: Among the more serious adverse effects to topical or vaginal application are irritation, burning, and maceration of the skin.

micr-. See **micro-, micr-, mikro-.**

micrencephalia. See **microcephaly.**

micrencephalon /mī″krənsef″əlon/, an abnormally small brain. See also **microcephaly.** *–micrencephalic, adj., n.*

micrencephaly. See **microcephaly.**

micro-, micr-, mikro-, 1. prefix meaning "small": *microanalysis, microglossia.* **2.** prefix meaning "one millionth": *micrometer.*

microabrasion /mi″kro·äbra″zhun/, **1.** (in dentistry) removal of minute amounts of dental enamel by using an abrasive compound delivered under pressure in order to correct enamel defects or remove diseased tooth structure (caries). **2.** should not be confused with **microdermabrasion.**

microabscess /mīkrō·ab″ses/ [Gk, *mikros,* small; L, *abscedere,* to go away], a very small accumulation of pustular material.

microadenoma /mī″krō·ad″ənō″mə/, a pituitary adenoma less than 10 mm in diameter.

microaerophile /mī″krō·er″ōfil/ [Gk, *mikros,* small, *aer,* air, *philein,* to love], a microorganism that requires free oxygen for growth but at a lower concentration than that contained in the atmosphere. Compare **aerobe, anaerobe.** *–microaerophilic, adj.*

microaerotonometer /mī″krō·er″ətonom″ətər/ [Gk, *mikros* + *aer,* air, *tonos,* tension, *metron,* measure], instrument for measuring the volume of gases in blood or other fluids.

microaggregate recipient set /mi″krō·ag″rəgāt/ [Gk, *mikros* + L, *ad,* to, *gregare,* to collect, *recipere,* to receive; AS, *settan*], a device composed of plastic components for the IV delivery of large volumes of stored whole blood or of packed blood cells. The components of the set include the plastic tubing, roller clamp, and special filter that prevents the microaggregates or deteriorated red blood cells from entering the circulatory system of the patient. The plastic tubing of this device has a larger lumen than tubing of most other IV sets, which allows the blood to be delivered more rapidly. Compare **component drip set, component syringe set, straight line blood set.**

microaggression, everyday verbal, nonverbal, or environmental slights or insults communicating negative messages that demean a person or group. They may be unintentional or deliberate. The perpetrator is not always aware of the prejudice underlying the message.

microalbumin test, a urine test to detect a greater than normal albumin concentration in the blood, an early indication of renal disease. Microalbuminuria is indicative of diabetes mellitus, hypertension, cardiovascular disease, nephropathy, urinary bleeding, hemoglobinuria, or myoglobinuria.

microalbuminuria /mī″krō·al′boominoor″ē·ə/, the urinary excretion of small amounts of albumin, below the detection level of routine dipstick analysis. The condition is an early indicator of altered glomerular permeability in diabetes.

microampere /mī″krō·am′pir/, one millionth of an ampere.

microanalysis /mī″krō·anal″isis/, **1.** analysis of minute quantities of material. **2.** identification of substances by examination under a microscope.

microaneurysm /mi″krō·an″yəriz′əm/ [Gk, *mikros* + *aneurysma,* a widening], a microscopic aneurysm characteristic of thrombotic purpura.

microangiopathic hemolytic anemia (MAHA) /mī′krō·anjē·ō·path″ik/, a condition in which narrowing or obstruction of small blood vessels results in distortion and fragmentation of erythrocytes, hemolysis, and anemia.

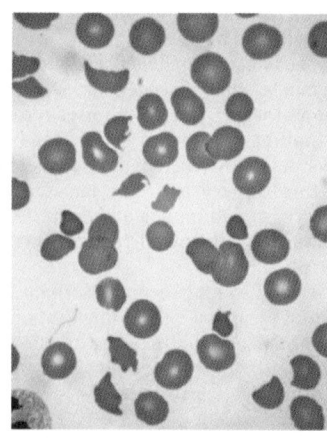

Blood film in microangiopathic hemolytic anemia
(Howard and Hamilton, 2013)

microangiopathy /mī′krō·an′jē·op″əthē/ [Gk, *mikros* + *angeion*, vessel, *pathos*, disease], a disease of the small blood vessels. Examples are diabetic microangiopathy, in which the basement membrane of capillaries thickens, and thrombotic microangiopathy, in which thrombi form in the arterioles and capillaries.

microaspiration, subclinical aspiration of small droplets of saliva, oral fluids, or gastric reflux materials into the lungs.

microbe /mī′krōb/, a microorganism. –*microbial, adj.*

microbial ecology /mīkrō″bē·əl/, the branch of biology that deals with the interaction of microorganisms with their environment.

microbial pesticides, pathogenic microorganisms that are toxic to a particular bacterium, insect, or other pest.

-microbic, suffix meaning "referring to or consisting of microbes": *amicrobic, polymicrobic.*

microbicide /mīkrō″bisīd/ [Gk, *mikros,* small, *bios,* life; L, *cadere,* to kill], any drug, chemical, or other agent that can kill microorganisms.

microbiological assay /-bī·əloj″ik/, **1.** the use of microorganisms for measuring the activity of organic compounds. **2.** the calculation of the purity of nutritional factors such as vitamins by measuring the growth of certain bacteria.

microbiology /mī′krōbī·ol″əjē/ [Gk, *mikros* + *bios,* life, *logos,* science], the branch of biology that is concerned with the study of microorganisms, including bacteria, archaea, viruses, algae, protozoa, and fungi, and their effect on humans. –*microbiologic, microbiological, adj.*

microbiology technologist, a medical technologist who specializes in the identification of bacteria and other microorganisms found in patient tissues and other specimens.

microblast /mī′krōblast′/ [Gk, *mikros,* small, *blastos,* germ], a very small immature red blood cell. This term is not in common usage.

microbody /mī′krōbod′ē/, any of the round membrane-bound granular cytoplasmic particles containing enzymes and other substances, originating in the endoplasmic reticulum of vertebrate liver and kidney cells and other cells and in protozoa, yeast, and many cell types of higher plants. An important type in vertebrates is the peroxisome.

microbrachia /mī′krōbrā″kē·ə/ [Gk, *mikros* + *brachion,* arm], a developmental defect characterized by abnormal smallness of the arms. –*microbrachius, n.*

microcarrier /-ker″ē·ər/, a microscopic bead or sphere that increases the surface area in a tissue culture for the attachment and yield of anchorage-dependent cells.

microcentrum. See **centrosome.**

microcephaly /mī′krōsef″əlē/ [Gk, *mikros* + *kephale,* head], a congenital anomaly characterized by abnormal smallness of the head in relation to the rest of the body and by underdevelopment of the brain, resulting in some degree of intellectual disability. The head is more than two standard deviations below the average circumference size for age, sex, race, and period of gestation. It has a narrow, receding forehead; a flattened occiput; and a pointed vertex. The facial features are generally normal. The condition may be caused by an autosomal-recessive disorder, a chromosomal abnormality, a toxic stimulus such as irradiation or chemical agents, maternal infection during prenatal development, or any trauma, especially during the third trimester of pregnancy or early infancy. There is no treatment, and care is primarily supportive and educational. Also called *microcephalia, microcephalism.* Compare **macrocephaly.** –*microcephalic, microcephalous, adj.,* –*microcephalus, microcephalic, n.*

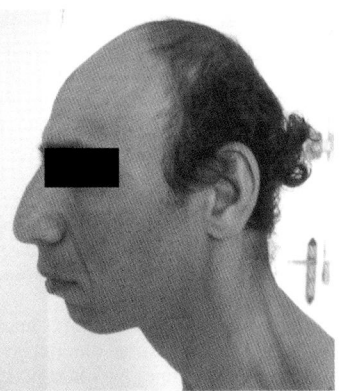

Adult male with microcephaly *(Saadi et al, 2009)*

microcheiria /mī′krōkī″rē·ə/ [Gk, *mikros* + *cheir,* hand], a developmental defect characterized by abnormal smallness of the hands. The condition is usually associated with other congenital malformations or with bone and muscle disorders. Also spelled *microchiria.*

microcide /mī′krəsīd/, an antimicrobial flavoprotein enzyme. It has antibacterial activity only in the presence of glucose and oxygen as it reduces the oxygen to hydrogen peroxide. The enzyme is derived from *Penicillium notatum* and other fungi.

microcirculation /-sur′kyəlē″shən/, the flow of blood throughout the system of smaller vessels of the body, particularly the capillaries.

microcurie (μCi) /mī′krōkyŏŏr″ē/ [Gk, *mikros* + *curie,* Marie Curie], a unit of radioactivity equal to one millionth of a curie, or 3.70×10^4 disintegrations per second. See also **curie.**

microcystic adnexal carcinoma (MAC), a form of adnexal tumor that often appears on the face as a yellow, indurated plaque with ill-defined margins. The patient experiences fullness, pain, burning, anesthesia, or paresthesia in the area of the lesion.

microcyte /mī′krəsīt/ [Gk, *mikros* + *kytos,* cell], an abnormally small erythrocyte with a mean cell volume of less than 80 fL, often occurring in iron-deficiency anemia and thalassemia.

microcythosis [Gk, *mikros,* small, *kytos,* cell], an excessive number of microcytes in the blood.

microcytic /mī′krōsit″ik/ [Gk, *mikros* + *kytos,* cell], (of a cell) pertaining to a smaller-than-normal cell.

microcytic anemia, a hematological disorder characterized by abnormally small erythrocytes, usually associated with iron-deficiency anemia, thalassemia, or anemia of chronic inflammation. Compare **macrocytic anemia.**

microcytosis /mī′krōsītō″sis/ [Gk, *mikros* + *kytos* + *osis,* condition], a hematological condition characterized by erythrocytes that are smaller than normal. Microcytosis is found in iron-deficiency anemia. Compare **poikilocytosis.** See also **anisocytosis.** –**microcytic,** *adj.*

microdactyly /mī′krōdak″təlē/ [Gk, *mikros* + *dactylos,* finger], a developmental defect characterized by abnormal smallness of the fingers and toes. The condition is usually associated with bone and muscle disorders, such as progressive myositis ossificans.

microdermabrasion, a dermatological procedure in which all or part of the stratum corneum is removed by light abrasion, used to improve the appearance of sun-damaged skin, treat hyperpigmentation, and reduce or remove scars. It is more superficial than ordinary dermabrasion, does not require

M

anesthesia, and can be performed in less than an hour. The person may resume ordinary daily activities immediately afterward. Microdermabrasion works best for superficial lesions such as fine lines and age spots; deeper lesions require other treatments.

microdontia, a physically small tooth; an anomaly that may occur in a single tooth, a few teeth (e.g., maxillary peg-shaped lateral incisors), or all teeth.

microdrepanocytic /mī′krōdrep′ənōsit″ik/ [Gk, *mikros* + *drepane,* sickle, *kytos,* cell], pertaining to a blood disorder marked by the presence of both microcytes and drepanocytes, such as occurs in sickle cell thalassemia. This term is not in common usage.

microdrip /mī″krōdrip′/, (in IV therapy) an apparatus for delivering relatively small measured amounts of IV solutions at specific flow rates over time, as when it is necessary to keep a vein open. The size of the drops is controlled by the fixed diameter of the plastic delivery tube. With a microdrip, 60 drops delivers 1 mL of solution.

microelectrode /mī′krō·ilek″trōd/, an electrode with a very small tip for use in brain studies. The device can be inserted without membrane damage into nervous tissue to record the bioelectrical activity of a simple neuron.

microelement. See **micronutrient.**

microencapsulation /mī′krō·enkap′syəlā″shən/ [Gk, *mikros* + *en,* in; L, *capsula,* little box], a laboratory technique used in the bioassay of hormones in which certain antibodies are encapsulated with a perforated membrane. The antibodies cannot escape through the tiny perforations, but hormones that bind with the antibodies may enter the structure to bind with them. Technicians then can measure the amount of hormone present in the specimen. The technique is used for the encapsulation of unstable enzymes and in the preparation of some drugs in slow- or time-release forms.

microencephaly /mī′krō·ensef″əlē/ [Gk, *mikros,* small, *egkephalos,* brain], the condition of being born with an abnormally small brain.

microequivalent /mī′krō·ikwiv″ələnt/, one millionth of an equivalent, the amount of a substance that corresponds to its equivalent mass in micrograms.

microfarad (μF) /mī″krōfer′əd/ [Gk, *mikros* + *farad,* Michael Faraday], a unit of capacitance that equals one millionth of a farad. See also **farad.**

microfilament /-fil″əmənt/, any of the finest of the fibrous cellular filaments, such as the tonofibrils, found in the cytoplasm of most cells, that function primarily as a supportive system. Compare **microtubule.**

microfilaria /mī′krōfiler″ē·ə/ *pl. microfilariae* [Gk, *mikros* + L, *filum,* thread], the prelarval form of any filarial worm. Certain blood-sucking insects ingest these forms from an infected host, and the microfilariae then develop in the body of the insect and become infective larvae. See also **filariasis, loiasis, onchocerciasis,** *Wuchereria.*

microfluorometry. See **cytophotometry.**

microgamete /-gam″ēt/, the small, motile, male gamete of certain thallophytes and sporozoa, specifically the malarial parasite *Plasmodium.* It corresponds to the sperm of higher animals and unites in conjugation with the larger, nonmotile female gamete. Compare **macrogamete.**

microgametocyte /-gamē″təsīt/ [Gk, *mikros* + *gamete,* spouse, *kytos,* cell], an enlarged merozoite that undergoes meiosis to form the mature male gamete during the sexual phase of the life cycle of certain thallophytes and sporozoa, specifically the malarial parasite *Plasmodium.* Microgametocytes are found in the red blood cells of a person infected with the malarial parasite, but they must be ingested by a female *Anopheles* mosquito to complete the maturation process and develop into microgametes.

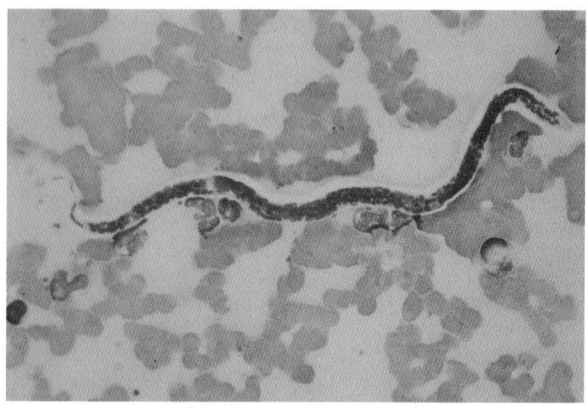

Microfilaria *(Conlon and Snydman, 2000)*

microgastria, a rare disorder in which there is small reservoir capacity of the stomach, leading to megaesophagus, an incompetent gastroesophageal sphincter, reluctance to feed, persistent vomiting, malnutrition, and recurrent respiratory tract infections.

microgenitalia /-jen′itā″lē·ə/, a condition characterized by abnormally small external genitalia.

microglia /mīkrog″lē·ə/ [Gk, *mikros* + *glia,* glue], small, migratory interstitial cells that form part of the central nervous system. They have various forms and slender, branched processes. Microglia serve as phagocytes that collect waste products of the nerve tissue of the body. Also called **Hortega cells, mesoglia.**

microglossia /mī′krō·glos′ē·ə/ [Gk, *mikros,* small + *glōssa,* tongue], undersized tongue.

micrognathia /mī′krōnā″thē·ə/ [Gk, *mikros* + *gnathos,* jaw], underdevelopment of the jaw, especially the mandible. Compare **macrognathia, brachygnathia.** —*micrognathic, adj.*

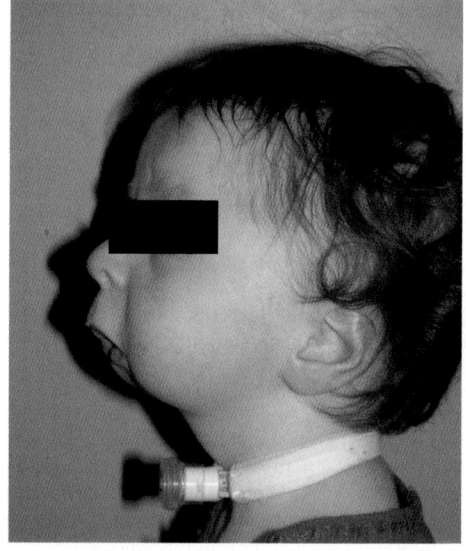

Child with micrognathia *(Kaban, 2009)*

microgram (μg, mcg) /mī″krəgram/, a unit of measurement of mass equal to one millionth (10^{-6}) of a gram. See also **gram.**

microgyri. See **microgyrus.**

microgyria /mī′krōjī″rē·ə/ [Gk, *mikros* + *gyros,* turn], a developmental defect of the brain in which the convolutions are abnormally small, resulting in structural malformation of the cortex. The condition is usually associated with intellectual disability and physical defects. Also called **polymicrogyria.**

microgyrus /mī′krōjī″rəs/ *pl.* **microgyri,** an underdeveloped, malformed convolution of the brain.

microhematocrit, a hematocrit determination performed using less than a milliliter of whole blood in a capillary tube spun by a high-speed centrifuge.

microhm /mī″krōm/ [Gk, *mikros* + *ohm,* George Ohm], a unit of electrical resistance equal to one millionth (10^{-6}) of an ohm. See also **ohm.**

microinjection /mī′krō·injek″shən/, the injection of tiny amounts of a substance into a cell by using micromanipulation instruments.

microinjector /mī′krō·injek″tər/, an instrument that delivers tiny amounts of a substance into a cell.

microinvasive carcinoma /mī′krō·invā″siv/ [Gk, *mikros* + L, *in,* within, *vadere,* to go], a squamous epithelial neoplasm that has penetrated the basement membrane, the first stage in invasive cancer. See also **carcinoma in situ.**

microkeratome /mī′krō·kər′ə·tōm/ [Gk, *mikros* + *keratome*], an instrument for removing a thin slice, or creating a thin hinged flap, on the surface of the cornea.

microleakage /mī′krō·lē′kij/ [Gk, *mikros* + ONorse *leka,* to drip], seepage of minute amounts of salivary fluids, debris, and microorganisms through the microscopic space between a dental restoration or its cement and the adjacent surface of the cavity preparation. It may form a carious lesion and progress through the dentin into the pulp, resulting ultimately in the failure of the restoration and the loss of the tooth.

microlevel interventions /-lev″əl/, health-generating changes performed at the individual level, such as in conditioning or stimulus control therapies.

microliter (μL) /mī″krəlē″tər/, a unit of liquid volume equal to one millionth of a liter, or 1 mm³.

microlith /mī″krəlith/ [Gk, *mikros* + *lithos,* stone], a small rounded mass of mineral matter or calcified stone.

micromanipulation /-mənip′yəlā″shən/, surgical displacement or dissection of very small tissues by using either miniature instruments or mechanical devices that translate large motions into smaller movements.

micromanipulator /-mənip″yəlā′tər/, a guidance accessory to a microscope that performs displacement or dissection of very small tissues.

micromelic dwarf /-mē″lik/ [Gk, *mikros* + *melos,* limb], a person of extremely short stature whose limbs are abnormally short.

micrometer (μm) /mīkrom″ətər/, **1.** an instrument used for measuring small angles or distances on objects being observed through a microscope or telescope. **2.** a unit of measurement, commonly referred to as a micron, that equals one millionth (10^{-6}) of a meter.

micromicron, one millionth of a micron.

micromillimeter. See **nanometer.**

micromyeloblastic leukemia /mī′krōmī′əlōblas″tik/ [Gk, *mikros* + *myelos,* marrow, *blastos,* germ], a malignant neoplasm of blood-forming tissues, characterized by the proliferation of small myeloblasts distinguishable from lymphocytes only by special staining techniques and microscopic examination.

micron (μ, mu) /mī″kron/ [Gk, *mikros,* small], **1.** See **micrometer,** def. 2. **2.** (in physical chemistry) a colloidal particle with a diameter between 0.2 and 10 μm.

Micronase, an oral antidiabetic drug. Brand name for **glyBURIDE.**

microneurography /-nyoo̅org″rəfē/, the recording of impulse conduction in individual nerve fibers by means of a microelectrode. The technique is used in studies of the relationship between body mass and the sympathetic nervous system.

micronodular /-nod″yələr/, characterized by the presence of very small nodules.

micronodular adrenal disease, a rare form of Cushing syndrome caused by multiple bilateral, small, pigmented, autonomous, adrenocorticotropic, hormone–independent, cortisol-secreting adenomas. Also called **primary bilateral micronodular hyperplasia.**

Micronor, an oral contraceptive containing a progestin. Brand name for **norethindrone.**

micronucleus /-noo̅″klē·əs/, **1.** a small nucleus. **2.** the smaller of two nuclei in some protozoa. It functions in sexual reproduction. Compare **macronucleus.**

micronutrient /-noo̅″trē·ənt/, any dietary element essential only in minute amounts for the normal physiological processes of the body, including vitamins and minerals or chemical elements such as zinc or iodine. Also called **microelement, trace element.**

microorganism /-ôr″gəniz′əm/ [Gk, *mikros* + *organon,* instrument], any tiny, usually microscopic entity capable of carrying on living processes. It may be pathogenic. Kinds include **bacteria, fungi, protozoan, virus.**

micropenis. See **microphallus.**

microphage /mī″krəfāj/ [Gk, *mikros* + *phagein,* to eat], a neutrophil capable of ingesting small things, such as bacteria. Compare **macrophage.** −*microphagic, adj.*

microphallus /-fal′əs/ [Gk, *mikros* + *phallos,* penis], an abnormally small penis. When it is observed in the newborn, the health care provider examines the child for other signs of ambiguous genitalia. Also called **micropenis.** See also **ambiguous genitalia.**

microphthalmos /mī″krəfthal″məs/ [Gk, *mikros* + *ophthalmos,* eye], a developmental anomaly characterized by abnormal smallness of one or both eyes. When the condition occurs in the absence of other ocular defects, it is called pure microphthalmos or nanophthalmos. Also called *microphthalmia.* Also spelled *microphthalmus.* −*microphthalmic, adj.*

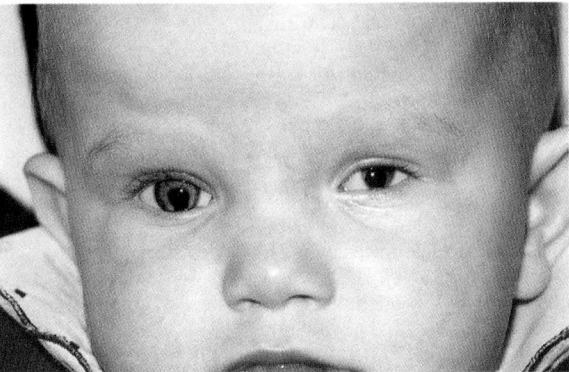

Child with left microphthalmos and bilateral iris colobomas *(Kanski and Bowling, 2011)*

microplasia. See **dwarfism.**

micropodia /-pō″dē·ə/ [Gk, *mikros* + *pous,* foot], a developmental anomaly characterized by abnormal smallness of the feet. The condition is often associated with other congenital malformations or with bone and skeletal disorders.

microprolactinoma /-prōlak″tinō″mə/, a prolactin-secreting pituitary tumor less than 10 mm in diameter, usually associated with menstrual disturbance. Microprolactinomas seldom enlarge, and some resolve spontaneously. Most patients experience a return to ovulatory menstrual cycles and fertility with treatment.

microprosopus /mī′krōprō″səpəs, -prəsō″pəs/ [Gk, *mikros* + *prosopon,* face], a fetus having an abnormally small or underdeveloped face.

micropsia /mīkrop″sē·ə/ [Gk, *mikros* + *opsis,* sight], a condition of vision in which a person perceives objects as smaller than they really are. It may occur during seizure activity. See also **hallucination.** −*microptic, adj.*

micropuncture /mī″krōpunk″cher/, **1.** the creation of minute openings by piercing. **2.** in renal physiology, the process by which nephron segments are pierced.

microreentry /-rē·en″trē/ [Gk, *mikros* + L, *re,* again; Fr, *entree,* entry], the reactivation of myocardial tissue by an impulse transmitted along a very small circuit within the conductive tissue of the heart.

microrrhinia, an extremely small nose.

microscope /mī″krəskōp′/ [Gk, *mikros,* small, *skopein,* to view], an instrument with lenses for viewing very small objects. Kinds include **acoustic microscope, electron microscope.**

microscopic /mī″krəskop″ik/ [Gk, *mikros* + *skopein,* to look], **1.** pertaining to a microscope. **2.** very small; visible only when magnified and illuminated by a microscope. Compare **gross.**

microscopic anatomy, the study of the microscopic structure of the tissues and cells. Kinds include **cytology, histology.**

microscopy /mīkros″kəpē/ [Gk, *mikros* + *skopein,* to look], a technique for observing minute materials with a microscope. Kinds include **darkfield microscopy, electron microscopy, fluorescent microscopy.**

microshock /mī″krəshok/, **1.** shock from an electric current of less than 1 milliampere. It may not be felt. **2.** the passage of current directly into the cardiac tissue.

microsomal enzymes /-sō″məl/, a group of enzymes associated with a certain particulate fraction of liver homogenate that plays a role in the metabolism of many drugs.

microsome /mī″krəsōm/, a fragment of endoplasmic reticulum associated with ribosomes, found in cells that have been homogenized and ultracentrifuged.

microsomia /-sō″mē·ə/ [Gk, *mikros* + *soma,* body], the condition of having an abnormally small and underdeveloped yet otherwise perfectly formed body with normal proportionate relationships of the various parts. See also **primordial dwarf.**

microsphere /mī″krəsfir′/, **1.** a centrosome. **2.** a microscopic globule of radiolabeled material.

microspherocytosis /-sfir″əsītō″sis/, anemia characterized by the presence of microcytes and spherocytes in a peripheral blood film. Spherocytes are red blood cells that are spherical in suspension that lack a central zone of pallor, and whose diameter is reduced on a peripheral blood film. See also **spherocyte.**

Microsporida /mī′krō·spor′i·də/ [Gk, *mikros* + *sporos,* seed], an order of parasitic protozoa found in invertebrates, especially arthropods; in lower vertebrates; and, rarely, in higher vertebrates.

microsporidiosis /mī′krō·spôrid′ē·ō′sis/, infection with protozoa of the order Microsporida, usually seen in immunocompromised patients and usually characterized by diarrhea and wasting.

Microsporum /-spôr″əm/ [Gk, *mikros* + *sporos,* seed], a genus of dermatophytes of the family Moniliaceae. The spores are multiseptate and variable in shape and have thin or thick walls. One species is *M. audouinii,* which causes epidemic tinea capitis in children. Others are *M. canis* and *M. gypseum.*

microstomia /-stō″mē·ə/ [Gk, *mikros,* small, *stoma,* mouth], the condition of having an abnormally small mouth.

microsurgery /-sur″jərē/ [Gk, *mikros,* small, *cheirourgos,* surgery], surgery that involves dissection and manipulation of minute tissue structures under a microscope.

microsurgical epididymal sperm aspiration (MESA), retrieval of sperm from the epididymis by using microsurgical techniques. The procedure is done in men with obstructive azoospermia.

microtear /mī″krəter′/, minor damage to soft tissue.

microthermy /-thur″mē/ [Gk, *mikros* + *therme,* heat], the use of heat generated by radio wave conversion in physical therapy.

microthrombus /mī″krōthrom′bəs/ *pl. microthrombi* [Gk, *mikros,* small + *thrombos,* lump], a small blood clot located in a capillary or other small blood vessel.

microtia /mīkrō′shī·ə/, underdevelopment or complete absence of the auricle of the ear, with a blind or absent external canal. Compare **anotia.**

microtome /mī″krətōm/ [Gk, *mikros* + *temnein,* to cut], a device that cuts specimens of tissue prepared in paraffin blocks into extremely thin slices for microscopic study.

microtrauma /-trô″mə/, a very slight injury or lesion.

microtuboplasty, the surgical repair of an occluded fallopian tube, performed with micro instruments and a microscope.

microtubule, a hollow cylindrical structure (200 to 300 angstroms in diameter and of variable length) that occurs widely within plant and animal cells. Microtubules increase in number during cell division and are associated with the movement of deoxyribonucleic acid material. Compare **microfilament.**

microtubule organizing center (MTOC), region of eukaryotic cells such as a centrosome or basal body from which microtubules grow.

microvascular /-vas″kyələr/, pertaining to the portion of the circulatory system that is composed of the capillary network.

microvilli /-vil″ī/ [Gk, *mikros,* small; L, *villus,* shaggy hair], tiny hairlike folds in the plasma membrane that extend from the surface of many absorptive or secretory cells. They are most clearly visible with an electron microscope but may be seen as a "brush border" with a light microscope.

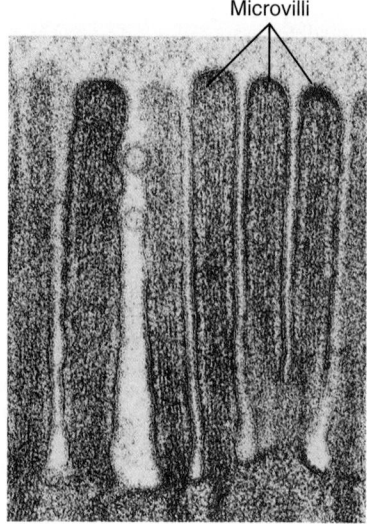

Microvilli *(Courtesy Susumu Ito, Harvard Medical School)*

microwave [Gk, *mikros* + AS, *wafian,* wave], electromagnetic radiation with a wavelength of 1 mm to 30 cm.

microwave interstitial system /mī″krəwāv/, a microwave-generated hyperthermia system that uses up to eight 50-watt applicators to create a heat field in certain accessible tumors no more than 2 inches (5.08 cm) beneath the skin. The microwaves produce a temperature of about 109° F (42.7° C) to destroy the tumor cells. The treatment can be monitored on a video terminal that shows location of the tumor and heat applicators.

microwave thermography, measurement of temperature through the detection of microwave radiation emitted from heated tissue.

Micruroides /mi″krooroi′dēz/, a genus of venomous coral snakes found in Mexico and the southwestern United States. See also **snakebite.**

Micrurus /mikroo′rus/, a genus of venomous coral snakes, including a species found in the southeastern United States and south into Central America. See also **snakebite.**

micturition. See **urination.**

micturition reflex /mik′chərish″ən/ [L, *micturire,* to urinate, *reflectere,* to bend back], a normal reaction to a rise in pressure within the bladder, resulting in contraction of the bladder wall and relaxation of the urethral sphincter, allowing urination. Voluntary inhibition normally prevents incontinence; urination follows withdrawal of the inhibition.

micturition syncope [L, *micturire,* to urinate; Gk, *syn,* together, *koptein,* to cut], a temporary loss of consciousness that tends to affect some adult males after arising from a reclining posture to urinate in an upright posture. The effect is caused by a brief interruption of blood flow to the brain and is often associated with the use of alcohol, which contributes to vasodilation. See also **hypotension, orthostatic hypotension.**

MICU, acronym for *medical intensive care unit.*

MID, abbreviation for **minimal infecting dose.**

mid-, prefix meaning "the middle": *midsagittal.*

Midamor, a diuretic drug. Brand name for **amiloride hydrochloride.**

midarm muscle circumference, **1.** measurement of the left arm with a flexible tape encircling the limb. In children, it is a useful and easily obtained assessment of nutritional status. **2.** a calculation made by subtracting the triceps skin fold from the mid–upper arm circumference measurement. A less than expected circumference may indicate muscle wasting in the upper arm.

midaxillary line /midak″siler′ē/, an imaginary vertical line that passes midway between the anterior and posterior axillary folds.

midazolam hydrochloride /midaz″əlam/, a short-acting central nervous system depressant; a benzodiazepine anxiolytic.

■ INDICATIONS: It is prescribed for preoperative sedation and impairment of memory of preoperative events (retrograde amnesia) and for moderate sedation before short diagnostic endoscopic or dental procedures.

■ CONTRAINDICATIONS: It is contraindicated for patients with acute narrow-angle glaucoma. It should be used with caution in those with open-angle glaucoma.

■ ADVERSE EFFECTS: Possible adverse effects include decreased tidal volume, decreased respiratory rate, apnea, hypotension, hiccups, nausea, vomiting, oversedation, and tenderness at the site of injection.

midbody, **1.** the middle of the body, or the midregion of the trunk. **2.** a mass of granules that appears in the middle of the spindle during mitotic anaphase in a dividing cell.

midbrain. See **mesencephalon.**

midcarpal. See **mediocarpal.**

midclavicular line /mid′kləvik″yoolər/ [AS, *midd* + L, *clavicula,* little key, *linea,* line], (in anatomy) an imaginary line that extends downward over the trunk from the midpoint of the clavicle, dividing each side of the anterior chest into two parts. The left midclavicular line is an important marker in describing the location of various cardiac phenomena, including the point of maximum impulse.

middle adult [AS, *middel* + L, *adultus,* grown up], an individual in the transitional age span between young adult and elderly, approximately 45 to 65 years of age, whose psychological task, according to Erikson, is generativity versus stagnation.

middle cardiac vein, one of the five tributaries of the coronary sinus that drain blood from the capillary bed of the myocardium. It starts at the apex of the heart, rises in the posterior interventricular sulcus, receives tributaries from both ventricles, and ends in the right extremity of the coronary sinus. Compare **great cardiac vein, small cardiac vein.**

middle cerebral artery, the largest of the cerebral arteries and the vessel most commonly affected by cerebrovascular accident.

middle cervical ganglion, a ganglion at the level of the sixth cervical vertebra. Branches from this ganglion pass to spinal nerves C7 to T1, the vertebral artery, and the heart as the middle cardiac nerve.

middle costotransverse ligament. See **ligament of the neck of the rib.**

middle cuneiform bone. See **intermediate cuneiform bone.**

middle ear, the tympanic cavity with the auditory ossicles contained in an irregular space in the temporal bone. It is separated from the external ear by the tympanic membrane and from the inner ear by the oval window. The auditory (eustachian) tube carries air from the posterior nasopharynx into the middle ear. Also called **tympanic cavity.** Compare **external ear, inner ear.**

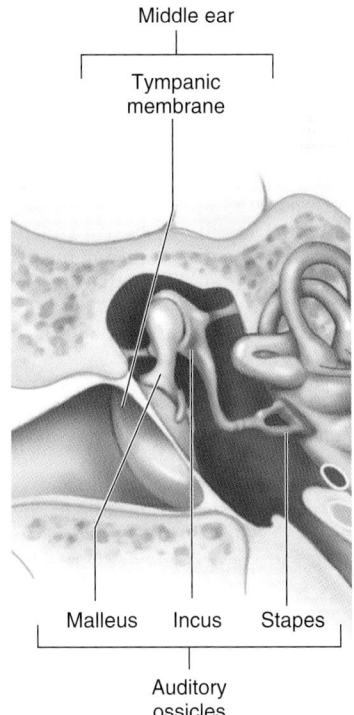

Middle ear *(Mosby, 2013)*

middle kidney.   See **mesonephros.**

middle lobe syndrome,   localized atelectasis of the middle lobe of the right lung, characterized by chronic infection, cough, dyspnea, wheezing, and obstructive pneumonitis. Asymptomatic obstruction of the bronchus may occur. The condition arises when the cuff of lymphatic glands that surrounds the middle lobe bronchus becomes enlarged as a result of nonspecific or tuberculous inflammation during childhood. The bronchus is thus compressed, and bronchiectasis develops in the obstructed part of the lung. Treatment includes antituberculosis chemotherapy, administration of corticosteroids, and surgical excision. See also **atelectasis, bronchiectasis.**

middle mediastinum,   the widest part of the mediastinum, containing the heart, ascending aorta, lower half of the superior vena cava, pulmonary trunk, and phrenic nerves. It is one of three caudal portions of the mediastinum. Compare **anterior mediastinum, posterior mediastinum, superior mediastinum.**

middle molecule,   any molecule with an atomic mass between 350 and 2000 daltons. These molecules accumulate in the body fluids of patients with uremia.

middle-old,   persons from 75 to 84 years of age.

middle plate.   See **nephrotome.**

middle sacral artery,   a small visceral branch of the abdominal aorta, descending to the fourth and fifth lumbar vertebrae, the sacrum, and the coccyx. Minute branches are said to supply the posterior surface of the rectum.

middle suprarenal artery,   one of a pair of small visceral branches of the abdominal aorta, arising opposite the superior mesenteric artery and supplying the suprarenal gland.

middle temporal artery,   one of the branches of the superficial temporal artery on each side of the head. It arises just above the zygomatic arch, pierces the temporal fascia, branches to the temporalis, and anastomoses with the deep temporal branches of the maxillary artery. Compare **deep temporal artery, superficial temporal artery.**

middle temporal gyrus [AS, *middel* + L, *tempus,* time; Gk, *gyros,* turn],   the middle of three gyri of the temporal area of the surface of the brain. It runs horizontally between the inferior and superior temporal sulci of the temporal lobe.

middle umbilical fold,   the fold of peritoneum over the urachal remnant within the abdomen. Approximately 3 cm lateral to the middle umbilical fold is the lateral umbilical fold. Between the lateral and the middle folds is the medial umbilical fold. Also called **plica umbilicalis mediana.**

midface /mid′fās/,   the middle of the face, including the nose, nasion, and glabella.

mid forceps [AS, *midd* + L, *forceps,* pair of tongs],   an obstetric operation in which forceps are applied to the baby's head when it has reached the midplane of the mother's pelvis. An episiotomy is usually performed, and local, regional, or inhalation anesthesia is provided. In some cases, such as severe fetal distress, mid forceps may be the most rapid and the safest means of delivery, but astute selection of cases, skill, and experience are essential. Difficult mid forceps delivery is likely to be more traumatic to the baby and the mother than cesarean section. Compare **high forceps, low forceps.** See also **failed forceps, forceps delivery, obstetric forceps, trial forceps.**

midgut [AS, *midd* + *guttas*],   the central portion of the embryonic alimentary canal, between the foregut and the hindgut. It consists of endodermal tissue, is connected to the yolk sac during early prenatal development, and eventually gives rise to some of the small intestine and part of the large intestine. Compare **foregut, hindgut.**

midgut loop,   a U-shaped loop of intestine that temporarily forms during the period of rapid elongation and rotation of the midgut in embryonic development. It projects into the proximal part of the umbilical cord, to which it is attached via the yolk stalk. With further development, it retracts into the abdomen, rotating further.

midgut volvulus,   volvulus neonatorum involving the entire part of the intestines derived from the midgut.

midlife transition,   a period between early adulthood and middle adulthood that occurs between 40 and 45 years of age. See also **age 30 transition.**

midline /mid′līn/ [AS, *midd* + L, *linea,* line],   an imaginary line that divides the body into right and left halves.

midline episiotomy.   Also called **median episiotomy.**

midoccipital /mid′oksip″itəl/,   pertaining to the center of the occiput.

midodrine,   a vasopressor.

■ INDICATIONS: It is used to treat orthostatic hypotension.

■ CONTRAINDICATIONS: Factors that prohibit its use include known hypersensitivity to midodrine, severe organic heart disease, acute renal disease, urinary retention, pheochromocytoma, thyrotoxicosis, and persistent or excessive supine hypertension.

■ ADVERSE EFFECTS: Adverse effects include drowsiness, restlessness, headache, chills, nausea, anorexia, dry mouth, blurred vision, pruritus, piloerection, rash, urinary urgency, and supine hypertension. Common side effects are paresthesia and pain.

midparental height /-pəren″təl/,   the average height of both parents at 25 to 45 years of age.

midpelvic contraction.   See **contraction.**

midposition /mid′pəzish″ən/,   the end-expiratory or end-tidal level or position of the lung-chest system under any given condition. It determines the functional residual capacity.

Midrin,   a fixed-combination central nervous system drug containing an adrenergic, a hypnotic, and an analgesic, used in the treatment of tension and vascular headaches. Brand name for **isometheptene mucate,** *dichloralphenazone,* **acetaminophen.**

midsagittal plane.   See **median plane.**

midstance /mid′stanz/ [AS, *midd* + L, *stare,* to stand],   one of the five stages in the stance phase of walking, or gait, directly associated with the period of single-leg support of body weight or the period during which the body advances over the stationary foot. During midstance the tibialis posterior and the flexor hallucis longus display their greatest activity. The midstance phase is considered in the diagnosis of many abnormal orthopedic conditions and in the analysis of the associated weaknesses of certain muscles and muscle groups. Compare **initial contact stance stage, loading response stance stage, preswing stance stage, terminal stance.** See also **swing phase of gait.**

midsternum /midstur″nəm/ [AS, *midd* + Gk, *sternon,* chest],   the body of the breast bone (sternum).

midstream catch urine specimen [AS, *midd* + *stream* + L, *captere,* to capture],   a urine specimen collected during the middle of a flow of urine, after the urinary opening has been carefully cleaned. Also called **clean-catch specimen.**

mid–upper arm circumference (MAC),   a measurement of the circumference of the arm at a midpoint between the tip of the acromial process of the scapula and the olecranon process of the ulna. It is an indication of upper arm muscle wasting.

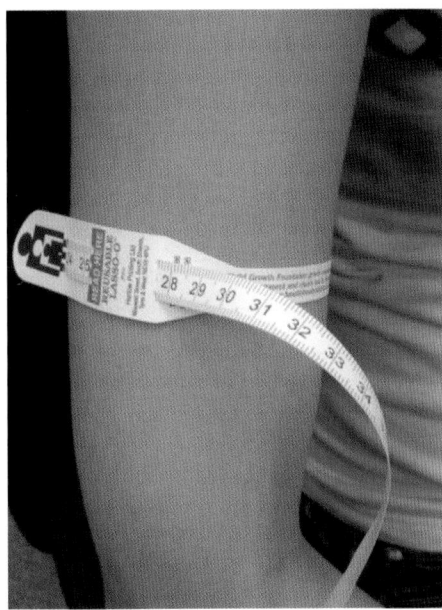

Measurement of mid–upper arm circumference
(Cattermole et al, 2010)

midwife [AS, *midd* + *wif*],   **1.** (in traditional use) a (female) person who assists women in childbirth. Also called **obstetrix. 2.** (according to the International Confederation of Midwives, World Health Organization, and Federation of International Gynecologists and Obstetricians) "a person who, having been regularly admitted to a midwifery educational program fully recognized in the country in which it is located, has successfully completed the prescribed course of studies in midwifery and has acquired the requisite qualifications to be registered and/or legally licensed to practice midwifery." Among the responsibilities of the midwife are supervision of pregnancy, labor, delivery, and puerperium. The midwife conducts the delivery independently, cares for the newborn, procures medical assistance when necessary, executes emergency measures as required, and may practice in a hospital, clinic, maternity home, or private home. The midwife, whose practice may also include well-child care, family planning, and some aspects of gynecology, is often an important source of health counseling in the community. **3.** a nurse midwife or Certified Nurse Midwife.

midwifery /mid″wīf(ə)rē/ [AS, *midd* + *wif*], the employment of a person who is qualified by special training and experience to assist a woman in childbirth. See also **midwife.**

MIF,   abbreviation for **macrophage inhibition factor (MIF).**

mifepristone /mif′əpris″tōn/, an antiprogestin used with misoprostol or other prostaglandins that induces abortion if taken within the first 7 weeks of pregnancy. Two days after taking the drug to end the pregnancy, the woman must take a second drug to cause strong uterine contractions that expel the fetus. Mifepristone is reportedly effective 95.5% of the time, and serious complications are rare. However, the procedure may be somewhat painful, and a small percentage of patients have required blood transfusions. If the drug regimen fails to terminate the pregnancy, the woman must arrange for a surgical abortion to complete the process. Also called **abortion pill, RU-486.**

MIF test,   a test for the production of migration inhibitory factor (MIF) by lymphocytes in response to specific antigens; used for evaluation of cell-mediated immunity. MIF production is absent in certain immunodeficiency disorders, such as Wiskott-Aldrich syndrome and Hodgkin disease. Abbreviation for *migration inhibitory factor test.*

miglitol,   an oral hypoglycemic agent.
■ INDICATIONS: It is used to treat type 2 diabetes mellitus.
■ CONTRAINDICATIONS: Factors that prohibit its use include known hypersensitivity to miglitol, diabetic ketoacidosis, cirrhosis, inflammatory bowel disease, colonic ulceration, partial intestinal obstruction, and chronic intestinal disease.
■ ADVERSE EFFECTS: Hepatotoxicity is a life-threatening side effect. Other adverse effects are low iron and rash. Common side effects are abdominal pain, diarrhea, and flatulence.

miglustat,   a rarely used miscellaneous agent.
■ INDICATIONS: This drug is used to treat adults with mild to moderate type 1 Gaucher disease.
■ CONTRAINDICATIONS: Pregnancy and known hypersensitivity to this drug prohibit its use.

migraine /mī″grān/ [Gk, *hemi,* half, *kranion,* skull], a recurring headache characterized by unilateral onset, severe throbbing pain, photophobia, phonophobia, and autonomic disturbances during the acute phase, which may last for hours or days. The disorder occurs more frequently in women than in men, and a predisposition to migraine may be inherited. The exact mechanism responsible for the disorder is not known, but the head pain may be related to dilation of extracranial blood vessels, which may be the result of chemical changes that cause spasms of intracranial vessels. Allergic reactions, excess carbohydrates, iodine-rich foods, alcohol, bright lights, or loud noises may trigger attacks, which often occur during a period of relaxation after physical or psychic stress. See also **headache.**
■ OBSERVATIONS: An impending attack may be heralded by visual disturbances, such as aura, flashing lights or wavy lines, or by a strange taste or odor, numbness, tingling, vertigo, tinnitus, or a feeling that part of the body is distorted in size or shape. The acute phase may be accompanied by nausea, vomiting, chills, polyuria, sweating, facial edema, irritability, and extreme fatigue. After an attack the individual often has dull head and neck pains and a great need for sleep.
■ INTERVENTIONS: Ergotamine tartrate preparations that constrict cranial arteries can usually prevent the headache from developing if administered early in the onset via injection, suppository, tablet, or nasal spray. Ergotamine tartrate is also available in combination with other drugs, such as caffeine, phenobarbital, and belladonna. Migraine patients unable to tolerate ergot preparations may use other analgesics, including acetaminophen, NSAIDs, triptan, and propoxyphene. If headaches happen frequently, a prophylactic medication may be taken daily.

migrainous cranial neuralgia /mī″grānəs, mīgrā″nəs/ [Gk, *hemi,* half, *kranion,* skull; L, *osus,* having], a variant of migraine, most common in middle-aged men, characterized by closely spaced episodes of excruciating throbbing unilateral headaches often accompanied by dilation of temporal blood vessels, flushing, sweating, lacrimation, nasal congestion or rhinorrhea, ptosis, and facial edema. Repeated episodes usually occur in clusters within a few days or weeks and may be followed by a relatively long remission period. A typical attack begins abruptly, without prodromal signs, as a burning sensation in an orbit or temple, and the resulting radiating intense pain may last 1 or 2 hours. Histamine diphosphate injected subcutaneously in people subject to these headaches produces symptoms identical to those occurring in a spontaneous attack. The pain may be relieved by antihistamines, and ergotamine tartrate preparations may be helpful if administered at the onset of an attack. Oxygen administration and endometracin for prophylaxis may also be used. Also called **cluster headache, histamine headache, Horton's headache.** See also **migraine.**

migrating phlebitis /mī″grāting/ [L, *migrare,* to wander; Gk, *phleps,* vein, *itis,* inflammation], a form of phlebitis characterized by inflammation in one part of a vein and, after remission, in another part of the vein.

migration /mīgrā″shən/ [L, *migrare,* to wander], **1.** (in obstetrics) the passage of the ovum from the ovary into a fallopian tube and then into the uterus. **2.** the movement of cells, as in the migration of endothelial cells in wound healing.

migratory gonorrheal polyarthritis. See **migratory polyarthritis.**

migratory ophthalmia. See **sympathetic ophthalmia.**

migratory polyarthritis /mī″grətôr″ē/, arthritis that progressively affects a number of joints and finally settles in one or more. It occurs in persons with gonorrhea and develops a few days to a few weeks after the onset of gonorrheal urethritis. The patient usually has a moderate fever and 1 to 5 days of migratory polyarthralgia with variable signs of inflammation. In more prolonged episodes initial arthritic sites may clear as new areas are affected, but persistently involved joints are usually severely inflamed and swollen. After the swelling subsides, the overlying skin may peel. Large joints are most affected. Treatment with penicillin or tetracycline generally provides some relief in 24 to 72 hours. Also called **migratory gonorrheal polyarthritis.**

migratory thrombophlebitis, an abnormal condition in which multiple thromboses appear in both superficial and deep veins. It may be associated with malignancy, especially carcinoma of the pancreas, often preceding other evidence of cancer by several months. Pulmonary embolism is uncommon with this condition. Also called **thrombophlebitis migrans.** See also **thrombophlebitis.**

mikro-. See **micro-, micr-, mikro-.**

Mikulicz aphthae. See **Sutton disease.**

Mikulicz syndrome /mik″yŏŏlich′ez/ [Johann von Mikulicz-Radecki, Polish surgeon, 1850–1905], an abnormal bilateral enlargement of the salivary and lacrimal glands. It is found in a variety of diseases, including leukemia, tuberculosis, and sarcoidosis. Also called *Mikulicz disease.* Compare **Sjögren syndrome.**

mild [AS, *milde,* soft], gentle, subtle, or of low intensity, such as a mild infection.

mildew /mil″dyŏŏ/, a visible growth of any of numerous species of saprophytic fungi. Mildew causes discoloration and weakening of fabrics and fibers.

mild fever. See **field fever.**

mild intellectual disability, a category of intellectual disability in which an individual has a below-average IQ (ranging from 55 to 69) and typically requires intermittent support. An individual with this level of impairment is generally able to master academic skills ranging from grades 3 to 7, though more slowly than other students. Compare **moderate intellectual disability.**

milia. See **milium.**

milia neonatorum [L, *milium,* millet; Gk, *neo,* new; L, *natus,* born], a nonpathological dermatological condition characterized by minute epidermal cysts consisting of keratinous debris that occur on the face and occasionally on the trunk of the newborn. They are eliminated by normal desquamation of the skin within a few weeks after birth and leave no scars.

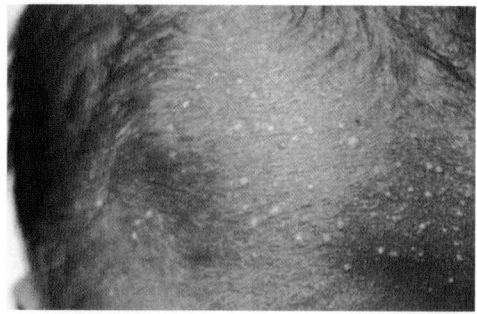

Milia neonatorum *(Weston, Lane, and Morelli, 2007)*

miliaria /mil′ē·er″ē·ə/ [L, *milium,* millet], minute vesicles and papules, often with surrounding erythema, caused by occlusion of sweat ducts during times of exposure to heat and high humidity. Backup pressure may cause sweat to escape into adjacent tissue, producing itching and prickling. Prevention and treatment include cool environment, ventilation, colloidal baths, and dusting powders. Also called **prickly heat.** See also **heat rash.**

miliaria profunda, the deepest type of miliaria, with occlusion of the ducts at the dermoepidermal junction. It occurs following severe, recurrent miliaria rubra and is seen primarily in hot, humid climates. Because large numbers of sweat glands are inactivated, it can lead to heat intolerance or heat stress, as in tropical anhidrotic asthenia.

miliary /mil″ē·er′ē/ [L, *milium,* millet], describing a condition marked by the appearance of very small lesions the size of millet seeds, such as miliary tuberculosis, which is characterized by tiny tubercles throughout the body.

miliary carcinosis, a condition characterized by numerous cancerous nodules resembling miliary tubercles.

miliary fever [L, *milium,* millet; L, *febris*], an elevated temperature associated with excessive sweating and a fine rash.

miliary tuberculosis, extensive dissemination by the bloodstream of tubercle bacilli. In children it is associated with high fever, night sweats, and often meningitis, pleural effusions, or peritonitis. A similar illness may occur in adults but with a less abrupt onset and occasionally with weeks or months of nonspecific symptoms, such as weight loss, weakness, and low-grade fever. Multiple small opacities resembling millet seeds may be evident on chest x-ray films. The liver, spleen, bone marrow, and meninges are often affected. The tuberculin test result may be negative, and diagnosis is made by biopsy of the infected tissue or organ. Combined drug therapy with isoniazid, rifampin, and pyrazinamide is usually successful if the diagnosis is not delayed. Concurrent tuberculous meningitis makes the prognosis less favorable. See also *Mycobacterium,* **tuberculosis.**

milieu /milyœ″, milyŏŏ′/ *pl. milieus, milieux* [Fr, middle], the environment, surroundings, or setting. Kinds include **milieu extérieur, milieu intérieur.**

milieu extérieur /ekstere·œr″/, the external or physical surroundings of an organism, including the social environment, especially the home, school, and recreational facilities, which play a dominant role in personality development.

milieu intérieur /aNtere·œr″/, the basic concept in physiology, originated by Claude Bernard, that multicellular organisms exist in an aqueous internal environment composed of the blood, lymph, and interstitial fluid that bathes all cells and provides a medium for the elementary exchange of nutrients and waste material. All fundamental processes necessary for the maintenance and life of the tissue elements depend on the stability and balance of this environment.

milieus. See **milieu.**

milieu therapy, a type of psychotherapy model in which the total environment is used in treating mental and behavioral disorders. Therapy is primarily conducted in a hospital or other institutional setting, where the entire facility acts as a therapeutic community. The emphasis is on providing pleasant physical surroundings, structured activities, and a stable social environment where behavior modification and personal growth are promoted through patient-group interaction, staff support and understanding, and a humanistic approach. Individual daily routines and treatment modalities, such as drug therapy, occupational therapy, and sensitivity training, are determined by the patient's emotional and interpersonal needs. See also **situational therapy.**

milieux. See **milieu.**

military antishock trousers (MAST) [L, *ante,* opposed; Fr, *choc* + Gael, *triubhas,* trews], a garment designed to produce pressure on the lower part of the body, thereby preventing the pooling of blood in the legs and abdomen. The trousers are used to combat shock and stabilize fractures, promote hemostasis, increase peripheral vascular resistance, and permit autotransfusion of small amounts of blood. They are now rarely used. Also called *medical antishock trousers,* **pneumatic antishock garment.** See **shock trousers.**

military attitude, (in obstetrics) a newborn position in which the head is not flexed and the cervical spine is in extension.

military time. See **24-hour clock system.**

milium /mil″ē·əm/ *pl. milia* [L, millet], a minute white cyst of the epidermis caused by obstruction of hair follicles and eccrine sweat glands. One variety is seen in newborns and disappears within a few weeks. Another type is found primarily on the faces of middle-aged women. Milia may be treated with topical or oral retinoids or by extraction. Compare **comedo.**

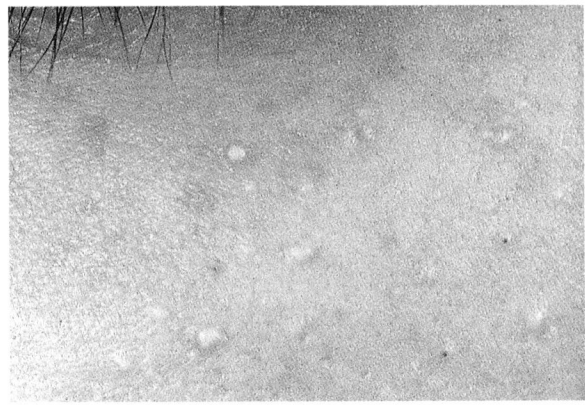

Milia *(du Vivier, 2002)*

milk [AS, *meoluc*], a liquid secreted by the mammary glands or udders of mammalian animals that suckle their young. After weaning, people consume the milk of the cow, as well as that of many other animals, including the goat, camel, mare, reindeer, llama, and yak. Milk is a basic food containing carbohydrate (in the form of lactose); protein (mainly casein, with small amounts of lactalbumin and lactoglobulin); suspended fat; the minerals calcium and phosphorus; and the vitamins A, riboflavin, niacin, thiamine, and, when the milk is fortified, D. Some individuals show a sensitivity reaction to milk caused by a deficiency of the enzyme lactase. See also **breast milk.**

milk-alkali syndrome, a condition of alkalosis caused by the excessive ingestion of milk, antacid medications containing calcium, or other sources of absorbable alkaline substances. The condition results in hypercalcemia, hypocalciuria, and calcium deposits in the kidneys and other tissues. The patient may experience symptoms of nausea, headache, weakness, and kidney damage. This condition occurs most frequently in older adults with peptic ulcers. Also called **Burnett syndrome.**

milk ejection reflex, a normal reflex in a lactating woman elicited by tactile stimulation of the nipple, resulting in release of milk from the glands of the breast. This reflex requires intact nerve connections from nipple to hypothalamus and release of the hormone oxytocin from the posterior pituitary into the bloodstream. Also called **let-down reflex.**

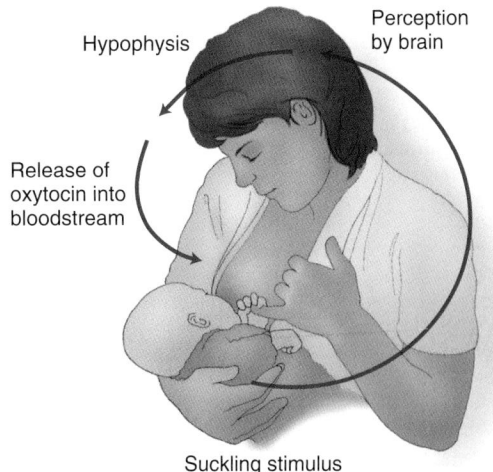

Milk ejection reflex *(Leonard, 2009)*

milker's nodule, a smooth brownish-red papilloma of the fingers or palm that begins as a macule and progresses through a vesicular stage to become a nodule. The disease is acquired from pustular lesions on the udder of a cow infected with poxvirus. No treatment is necessary because immunity is produced after primary infection.

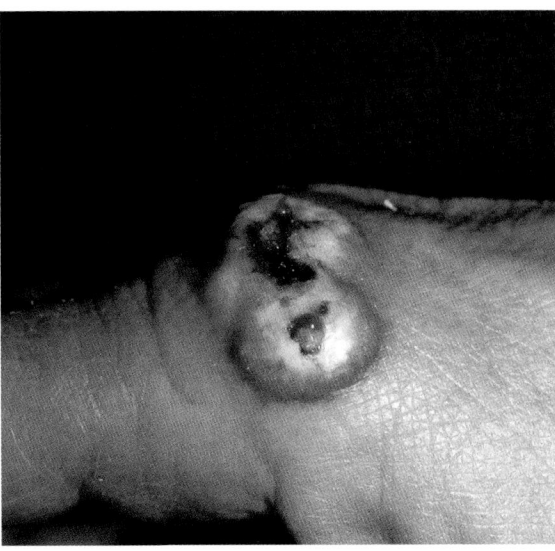

Milker's nodule *(James, Berger, and Eston, 2016)*

milk fever, *(Nontechnical)* postpartum fever that begins with the onset of lactation and lasts only a few hours. It was formerly considered a normal reaction to lactation. Maternal oral temperature during the puerperium does not normally exceed 100.4° F (38° C); continued high readings may indicate infection.

milk globule, a spherical droplet of fat in milk that tends to separate out as cream.

milking, a procedure used to express the contents of a duct or tube, to test for tenderness, or to obtain a specimen for study. The examiner compresses the structure with a finger and moves the finger firmly along the duct or tube to its opening. Also called **stripping.**

milk intolerance. See **lactose intolerance.**

milk leg. See **phlegmasia alba dolens.**

Milkman syndrome [Louis A. Milkman, American radiologist, 1895–1951], a form of osteomalacia characterized by the appearance on the x-ray image of multiple bilateral, symmetric stripes in hypocalcified long bones and in the pelvis and scapula. The stripes indicate pseudofractures.

milk of magnesia, a laxative and antacid containing magnesium hydroxide.

■ INDICATIONS: It is prescribed to relieve constipation and, less commonly, acid indigestion.

■ CONTRAINDICATIONS: Renal impairment, symptoms of appendicitis, or known hypersensitivity to the drug prohibits its use.

■ ADVERSE EFFECTS: Among the most serious adverse effects are diarrhea and hypermagnesemia, which usually occur in patients who have impaired renal function.

milk patch. See **macula albida.**

milkpox. See **alastrim.**

milk sugar. See **lactose.**

milk thistle, an herb that is native to Kashmir but that is also found in North America from Canada to Mexico.

■ INDICATIONS: It is used as protection against alcoholic cirrhosis and hepatitis and as an antiinflammatory. Standardized extracts have shown some efficacy for preventing cirrhosis in clinical trails.

■ CONTRAINDICATIONS: It should not be used during pregnancy and lactation, in children, or in people with hypersensitivity to this herb or other plants in the Asteraceae family.

milky ascites. See **chylous ascites.**

Miller-Abbott tube [Thomas G. Miller, American physician, 1886–1981; William O. Abbott, American physician, 1902–1943], a long, small-caliber double-lumen catheter once widely used in intestinal intubation for decompression and originally containing mercury. One lumen ends in a perforated metal tip and the other in a collapsible balloon. These tubes are radiopaque and can therefore be seen on a radiogram. Similar tubes, such as the Maglinte or MDEC tube have largely replaced the Miller-Abbott tube. Compare **Harris tube.** See also **gastric intubation.**

Miller Assessment of Preschoolers (MAP), a screening assessment of children's sensory and developmental progression that may be used by clinicians to identify preschool children who need further evaluation of sensory and/or motor skills.

Miller syndrome /mil′ər/ [Marvin Miller, 20th-century American pediatrician], a syndrome of extensive facial and limb defects, characterized by malar hypoplasia, downslanting palpebral fissures, micrognathia, cleft lip and palate, cup-shaped ears, lower lid ectropion, postaxial limb deficiencies, and syndactyly. Less frequently present are heart defects and hearing loss. The syndrome is probably an

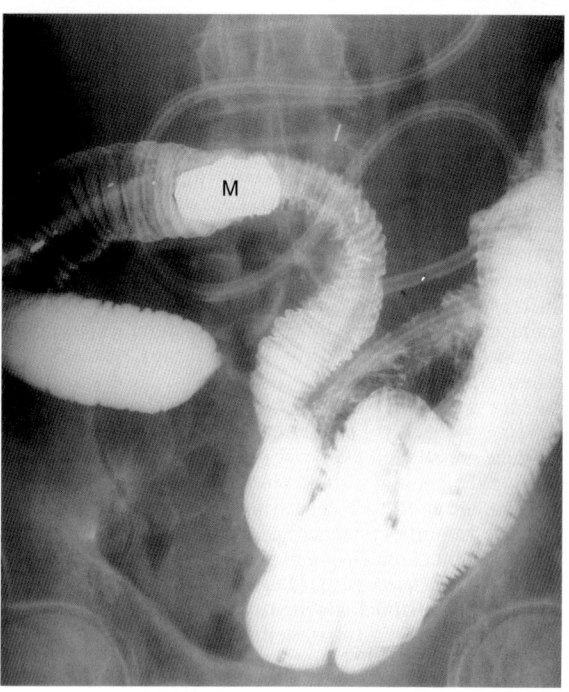

Miller-Abbott tube in patient with small bowel obstruction. The M indicates the mercury filled bag.
(Gore and Levine, 2015)

autosomal-recessive trait. Also called **postaxial acrofacial dysostosis.**

milli-, prefix meaning "1/1000 part": *milliampere, milliliter.*

milliampere (mA) /mil″ēam′pir/ [L, *mille,* thousand; Andre Ampere], a unit of electric current that is one thousandth of an ampere. See also **ampere.**

milliampere-second (mAs), a measure of electric charge obtained by multiplying the electric current in milliamperes by the time in seconds. It is used to describe the exposure setting of a radiography machine and determines the density of the radiographic image.

millicoulomb (mC) /-kyoō′lōm/ [L, *mille,* thousand; Charles A. de Coulomb], a unit of electric charge that is one thousandth of a coulomb. See also **coulomb.**

millicurie (mCi) /-koōr′ē/ [L, *mille,* thousand; Marie Curie], a unit of radioactivity equal to one thousandth of a curie, or 3.70×10^7 disintegrations per second. See also **curie.**

milliequivalent (mEq) /-ikwiv′ələnt/ [L, *mille* + *aequus,* equal, *valere,* to be strong], **1.** the number of grams of solute dissolved in 1 mL of a normal (1 *N*) solution. **2.** one thousandth (10^{-3}) of a gram equivalent.

milliequivalent per liter (mEq/L), one thousandth (10^{-3}) of 1 equivalent of a specific substance dissolved in 1 L of solution or plasma.

milligram (mg) /-gram/ [L, *mille* + Fr, *gramme,* small weight], a metric unit of mass equal to one thousandth (10^{-3}) of a gram.

milliliter (mL) /-lē′tər/ [L, *mille* + Fr, *litre,* a measure], a metric unit of volume that is one thousandth (10^{-3}) of a liter, or 1 cm³.

millimeter (mm) /-mē′tər/, a metric unit of length equal to one thousandth (10^{-3}) of a meter.

millimole (mmol, mM) /-mōl/ [L, *mille* + *moles,* mass], a unit of metric measurement that is equal to one thousandth

(10^{-3}) of a mole. It is the amount of a substance that corresponds to its formula mass in milligrams.

Millin operation, a surgical procedure for treating a large obstructing prostate gland.

milliosmol /mil″ē·oz′mōl/, one thousandth of an osmole. See also **osmole, osmolality, osmolarity.** *−milliosmolar, adj.*

millipede /mil″ipēd′/ [L, *mille* + *pes,* foot], a many-legged wormlike arthropod. Certain species squirt irritating fluids that may cause dermatitis.

millirad (mrad) /-rad/, a unit of absorbed dose of ionizing radiation equal to one thousandth (10^{-3}) of a rad. See also **rad.**

millirem (mrem) a unit of ionizing radiation dose equal to one thousandth (10^{-3}) of a rem. See also **rem.**

milliroentgen (mr, mR) /mil″irent′gən, -jən/ [L, *mille,* thousand; Wilhelm K. Roentgen], a unit of radiation exposure equal to one thousandth (10^{-3}) of a roentgen. See also **roentgen.**

millisecond (msec) /-sek′ənd/ [L, *mille,* thousand; ME, *seconde,* small part], one thousandth (10^{-3}) of a second.

millivolt (mV, mv) /-vōlt/ [L, *mille,* thousand; Alessandro Volta], a unit of electromotive force equal to one thousandth (10^{-3}) of a volt. See also **volt.**

Milroy disease /mil′roiz/ [William Forsyth Milroy, American physician, 1855–1942], congenital hereditary lymphedema of the legs caused by chronic lymphatic obstruction, sometimes involving additional areas, including the arms, trunk, and face. Also called **congenital lymphedema, Meige disease,** *Milroy edema,* **Nonne-Milroy-Meige syndrome.**

Miltown, a sedative drug. Brand name for **meprobamate.**

Milwaukee brace /milwô″kē/ [Milwaukee, Wisconsin; OFr, *bracier,* to embrace], an orthotic device that helps immobilize the torso and neck of a patient in the treatment of scoliosis, lordosis, or kyphosis. It is usually constructed of strong but light metal and fiberglass bars lined with rubber to protect against abrasion. The bars, which commonly connect cervical supports, rib supports, and hip supports, hold the trunk and neck erect while controlling cervical flexion and hip movements.

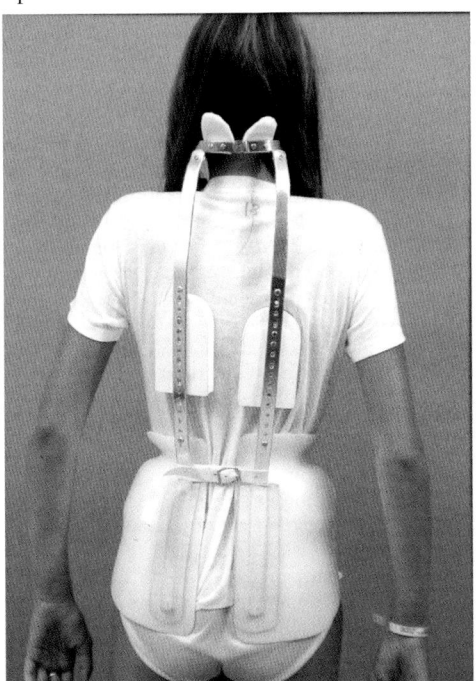

Young girl wearing a Milwaukee brace *(Herring, 2014)*

-mimesis, suffix meaning "simulation" or "imitation": *pathomimesis.*

-mimetic, suffix meaning "simulation of (specified) effects": *adrenomimetic, parasympathomimetic.*

-mimia, suffix meaning "(condition of) ability to express thought through gestures": *hypermimia, paramimia.*

mimicry /mim″ikrē/ [Gk, *mimetikos,* imitation], **1.** the effort of one species or organism to resemble another to obtain an offensive or defensive advantage. **2.** an autonomic nervous system phenomenon in which facial expressions may be the unwilled and largely unconscious expression of feelings and ideas. See also **molecular mimicry.**

mimic spasm /mim″ik/ [Gk, *mimetikos,* imitative, *spasmos,* spasm], involuntary stereotyped movements of a small group of muscles such as of the face. The spasm is usually psychogenic and may be aggravated by stress or anxiety but is generally controllable momentarily. Multiple grimacing and blinking mimic spasms occur in Gilles de la Tourette's syndrome. Also called **tic.**

min, 1. abbreviation for **minim. 2.** abbreviation for *minute.*

Minamata disease /min′əmä″tə/, a severe degenerative neurological disorder caused by the ingestion of seed grain heated with alkyl compounds of mercury or of seafood taken from waters polluted with industrial wastes contaminated by soluble mercuric salts. The term is derived from a tragedy involving Japanese who ate seafood from Minamata Bay. Mercury passes the placental barrier, causing the congenital form of the disease. Symptoms may not appear for several weeks or months; they include paresthesia of the mouth and extremities; tunnel vision; difficulties in speech, hearing, muscular coordination, and concentration; weakness; emotional instability; and stupor. Continued ingestion causes serious damage to the renal tubules and corrosion of the GI tract. Acute cases may result in coma and death. See also **mercury poisoning.**

mind [AS, *gemynd*], **1.** the part of the brain that is the seat of mental activity and that enables one to know, reason, understand, remember, think, feel, react to, and adapt to external and internal stimuli. **2.** the totality of all conscious and unconscious processes of the individual that influence and direct mental and physical behavior. **3.** the faculty of the intellect or understanding, in contrast to emotion and will. See also **brain, intellect, psyche.**

mind-body medicine, a holistic approach to medicine that takes into account the effect of the mind on physical processes, including the effects of psychosocial stressors and conditioning, particularly as they affect the immune system. Many of the therapeutic techniques used have as their purpose increasing the body's natural resistance to disease by managing the stressors.

mindfulness meditation, a technique of meditation in which distracting thoughts and feelings are not ignored but are rather acknowledged and observed nonjudgmentally as they arise to create a detachment from them and gain insight and awareness.

mine damp. See **damp.**

mineral /min″ərəl/ [L, *minera,* mine], **1.** an inorganic substance occurring naturally in the earth's crust, having a characteristic chemical composition and (usually) crystalline structure. **2.** (in nutrition) a compound containing a metal, nonmetal, radical, or phosphate that is needed for proper body function and maintenance of health. The needed substance is usually ingested as a part of such a compound, such as table salt (sodium chloride), instead of as a free element, and the compound is usually referred to by the name of the needed substance.

M

mineral deficiency. See *specific minerals.*

mineralization /-īzā″shən/ [L, *minera* + Gk, *izein,* to cause], the addition of any mineral to the body.

mineral jelly. See **petroleum jelly.**

mineralocorticoid /min′əral′ōkôr″tikoid/ [L, *minera* + *cortex,* bark; Gk, *eidos,* form], a hormone, secreted by the adrenal cortex, that maintains normal blood volume, promotes sodium and water retention, and increases urinary excretion of potassium and hydrogen ions. Aldosterone, the most potent mineralocorticoid with regard to electrolyte balance, acts on the distal tubules of the kidneys to enhance the reabsorption of sodium into the plasma. Trauma and stress increase mineralocorticoid secretion. The synthetic mineralocorticoid fludrocortisone, which has mineralocorticoid and glucocorticoid activity, is used to treat the salt-losing adrenogenital syndrome and the severe corticoid deficiency characteristic of Addison disease. See also **glucocorticoid.**

mineral oil, a laxative, stool softener, emollient, and pharmaceutic aid used as a solvent.

■ INDICATIONS: It is prescribed to prevent constipation, to treat mild constipation, to prepare the bowel for surgery or examination, and to act as a solvent for various preparations.

■ CONTRAINDICATIONS: Appendicitis, fecal impaction, obstruction or perforation of the intestinal tract, pregnancy, or known hypersensitivity to this drug prohibits its use.

■ ADVERSE EFFECTS: Among the more serious adverse effects are laxative dependence, lipid pneumonitis, fat-soluble vitamin deficiency, and abdominal cramps.

mineral soap. See **bentonite.**

miner's cramp. See **heat cramp.**

miner's elbow [L, *minera* + AS, *elboga*], an inflammation of the olecranon bursa, caused by resting the weight of the body on the elbow, as in some coal mining activities. The condition is sometimes seen in schoolchildren who lean on their elbows. Compare **lateral humeral epicondylitis.** See also **bursitis.**

miner's pneumoconiosis. See **anthracosis.**

Minerva cast /minur″və/ [L, *Minerva,* Roman goddess of wisdom; ONorse, *kasta*], an orthopedic cast used to immobilize the cervical and thoracic spine. A Minerva cast is generally made of fiberglass casting material and remains in place for approximately 4 to 12 weeks. The cast is used to immobilize the head and part of the trunk in the treatment of torticollis, cervical and thoracic injuries, and cervical spinal infections. It is not used as frequently as it once was because of advances in the field of orthotics. Also called *Minerva jacket.*

minim (m, min) /min″im/ [L, *minimus,* smallest], a measurement of volume in the apothecaries' system, originally one drop (of water). It is now standardized to 0.06 mL; 60 minims equals 1 fluid dram.

minimal access surgery. See **minimally invasive surgery.**

minimal bactericidal concentration, the lowest concentration of drug that results in a 99.9% reduction in the initial bacterial density. Compare **minimal inhibitory concentration.**

minimal brain dysfunction. See **attention deficit disorder.**

minimal care unit /min′iməl/ [L, *minimus,* smallest], a unit for the treatment of inpatients who are ambulatory and able to meet many of their own daily living needs but require minimal nursing care.

minimal change disease, a kidney disorder characterized by subtle changes in renal function, including albuminuria and presence of lipid droplets in the proximal tubules. It mainly affects small children but also occurs in adults with

idiopathic nephrotic syndrome. It may or may not progress to glomerulonephritis. Also called **lipoid nephrosis, nil disease.** See also **idiopathic nephrotic syndrome.**

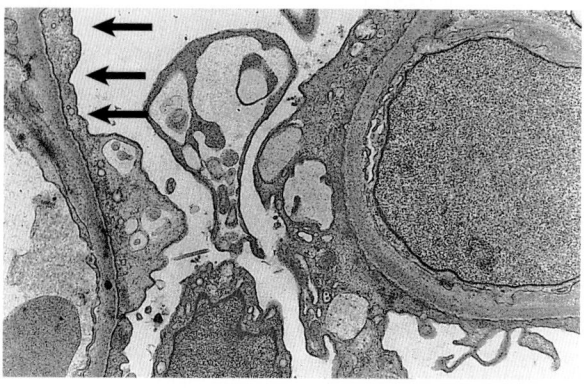

Minimal change disease *(Johnson, Feehally, and Floege, 2015)*

minimal dose. See **minimum dose.**

minimal erythema dose. See **threshold dose.**

minimal infecting dose (MID), the smallest amount of infective material that usually produces infection.

minimal inhibitory concentration (MIC), the lowest concentration of an antibiotic medication in the blood that is effective against a bacterial infection, determined by inoculating the bacteria into a culture medium containing various concentrations of a proposed antibiotic. The lowest antibiotic concentration that stops microbial growth may be used in further treatment of the patient. Also called **minimum inhibitory concentration.** Compare **minimal bactericidal concentration.**

minimally invasive surgery, surgery done with only a small incision or no incision at all, such as through a cannula with a laparoscope or endoscope.

minimal occlusive volume (MOV), the volume to which an endotracheal or tracheostomy tube cuff must be inflated to obliterate an air leak during the inspiratory phase of ventilation. Also called *minimal occlusive pressure.*

minimal residue diet. See **low-residue diet.**

Mini-Mental State Examination (MMSE), a brief psychological test designed to differentiate among dementia, psychosis, and affective disorders. It may include ability to count backward by 7s from 100, to identify common objects such as a pencil and a watch, to write a sentence, to spell simple words backward, and to demonstrate orientation by identifying the day, month, and year, as well as town and country.

minimization /min′imīzā″shən/ [L, *minimum,* smallest; Gk, *izein,* to cause], (in psychology) cognitive distortion in which the effects of one's behavior are underestimated. See also **magnification.**

minimum alveolar concentration (MAC) /min″iməm/, the concentration of inhaled anesthetic within the alveoli at which 50% of people do not move in response to a surgical stimulus. It is the standard measure of potency for volatile anesthetic agents.

minimum daily requirement (MDR) [L, *minimum* + OE, *daeglie* + L, *requirere,* to seek], the daily human requirement of nutrients for health and for prevention of a deficiency disease. The figures, established by the U.S. Food and Drug Administration, are generally extrapolated from experimental animal studies and include an added margin for safety. See also **Estimated Safe and Adequate Daily Dietary Intake.**

minimum dose [L, *minimum,* smallest; Gk, *dosis,* giving], the smallest amount of a drug or other substance needed to produce a desired or specified effect. Because of individual variations in drug response, the minimal dose for one person may be either excessive or insufficient for another patient. Also called **minimal dose.**

minimum hemagglutinating dose, the smallest amount of hemagglutinating agent that causes a complete hemagglutinating reaction in a standard volume of red blood cells.

minimum hemolytic dose (MHD), the smallest amount of a reagent that produces complete lysis of a specified amount of red blood cells. Not in common usage.

minimum inhibitory concentration. See **minimal inhibitory concentration.**

minimum lethal dose (MLD) [L, *minimum,* smallest, *lethum,* death; Gk, *dosis,* giving], the smallest dose of a drug, relative to body weight, that will kill an experimental animal. The MLD may vary with the species of animal tested. Also called *minimum fatal dose.* See also **median lethal dose.**

Minipress, an alpha$_1$ receptor blocking agent used to treat hypertension. Brand name for **prazosin hydrochloride.**

miniprotein /min′iprō″tēn/, a protein that has been reduced in size and complexity without loss of its ability to function.

Minnesota Multiphasic Personality Inventory (MMPI), a commonly used psychological test that includes over 500 statements for interpretation by the subject, used clinically for evaluating personality and detecting various disorders in adults. The current version is the MMPI-2. The adolescent version is the MMPI-A.

Minocin, an antibacterial drug. Brand name for **minocycline hydrochloride.**

minocycline hydrochloride /min′əsī″klēn/, a tetracycline antibiotic.

■ INDICATIONS: It is prescribed for infections caused by gram-positive and gram-negative bacteria, rickettsia, anthrax, and other microorganisms.

■ CONTRAINDICATIONS: It must be used with caution in cases of renal or hepatic dysfunction. Known hypersensitivity to this or other tetracyclines prohibits its use.

■ ADVERSE EFFECTS: Among the more serious adverse effects are GI disturbances, phototoxicity, vestibular toxicity, potentially serious superinfections, and various allergic reactions. Use during pregnancy or in children younger than 8 years of age may result in discoloration of teeth.

minor /mī″nər/ [L, smaller], (in law) a person not of legal age. A person beneath the age of majority. Minors usually cannot consent to their own medical treatment unless they are substantially independent of their parents, are married, support themselves, or satisfy other requirements specified by statute. See also **emancipated minor.**

minor arterial circle of iris, the small artery encircling the outer circumference of the iris.

minor connector, a device that links the major connector or base of a removable partial denture to other denture units, such as rests and direct and indirect retainers.

minor duodenal papilla, the entrance into the duodenum for the accessory pancreatic duct and the junction of the foregut and midgut. It is just below the major duodenal papilla.

minor epilepsy, *(Obsolete)* now called **absence seizure.**

minor hysteria [Gk, *hystera,* womb], a mild disorder that may be expressed in emotional outbursts, repressed anxieties, or conversion of unconscious conflicts into physical symptoms.

minor renal calyx. See **renal calyx.**

minor surgery, a surgical procedure for a minor problem or injury that is not considered life-threatening or hazardous. Compare **major surgery.**

minoxidil /mīnok″sidil/, a vasodilator.

■ INDICATIONS: It is prescribed in the treatment of severe refractory hypertension and as a topical solution for the treatment of androgenic alopecia in both males and females.

■ CONTRAINDICATIONS: Pheochromocytoma, acute myocardial infarctions, dissecting aortic aneurysm, or known hypersensitivity to this drug prohibits its use.

■ ADVERSE EFFECTS: Among the most serious adverse effects are tachycardia, pericardial effusion, cardiac tamponade, salt and water retention, and excessive hair growth. GI disturbances also may occur.

mint, an herb native to Europe that is grown widely throughout the United States and Canada.

■ INDICATIONS: It is used as a flavoring and medicinally for GI disorders. Peppermint oil may exert beneficial effects in irritable bowel syndrome.

■ CONTRAINDICATIONS: Mint should not be used during pregnancy and lactation, in children, or in those with known hypersensitivity to this herb or gastroesophageal reflux disease.

Mintezol, an anthelmintic. Brand name for **thiabendazole.**

minute ventilation /min″it/ [L, *minus,* very small], the total lung ventilation per minute, the product of tidal volume and respiration rate. It is measured by expired gas collection for a period of 1 to 3 minutes. The normal rate is 5 to 10 liters per minute.

mio-, meio-, prefix meaning "less": *miosis, meiosis.*

miosis /mī-ō″sis/ [Gk, *meiosis,* becoming less], **1.** contraction of the sphincter muscle of the iris, causing the pupil to become smaller. Certain drugs and stimulation of the pupillary light reflex result in miosis. **2.** an abnormal condition characterized by excessive constriction of the sphincter muscle of the iris, resulting in pinpoint pupils. Compare **mydriasis.**

miotic /mē-ot″ik/, **1.** *adj.,* pertaining to miosis. **2.** *adj.,* causing constriction of the pupil of the eye. **3.** *n.,* any substance or pharmaceutic, such as pilocarpine, that causes constriction of the pupil of the eye. Such agents are used in the treatment of glaucoma.

MIP, 1. abbreviation for **maximum inspiratory pressure. 2.** abbreviation for **maximum intensity projection.**

miracidium /mir′əsid″ē·əm/ *pl. miracidia* [Gk, *meirakidion,* youthfulness], the ciliated larva of a parasitic trematode that hatches from an egg and can survive only by penetrating and further developing within a host snail into a maternal sporocyte that produces more larvae.

mirage /miräzh″/ [L, *mirari,* to look at], an optical illusion caused by the refraction of light through air layers of different temperatures, such as the illusionary sheets of water that appear to shimmer over stretches of hot sand and pavement. This phenomenon is caused by bending of horizontal light waves upward from the layer of heated air directly over the hot surface. Wind rippling the air layers may produce surprising changes in the shapes and sizes of such mirages. Individuals under severe stress are especially susceptible to interpreting these optic phenomena in bizarre, unrealistic ways.

MIRL, abbreviation for *membrane inhibitor of reactive lysis.* See **protectin.**

mirror image /mir″ər/ [L, *mirare,* to look at, *imago*], **1.** an image formed by a reflection. **2.** a kind of reversed asymmetry of characteristics often found in sets of monozygotic twins. **3.** chemical molecules with the same composition but with asymmetric arrangement of the atoms.

M

mirror speech [L, *mirari,* to look at; AS, *spaec,* speech], an abnormal manner of speaking characterized by the reversal of the order of syllables in a word.

mirtazapine, an antidepressant drug.

■ INDICATIONS: It is used to treat depression, dysthymic disorder, and bipolar disorder with either depression or agitation.

■ CONTRAINDICATIONS: Factors that prohibit its use include known hypersensitivity to tricyclic antidepressants, convulsive disorders, and prostatic hypertrophy. Its use is also contraindicated in patients who are in the recovery phase of a myocardial infarction.

■ ADVERSE EFFECTS: Life-threatening effects are agranulocytosis, thrombocytopenia, eosinophilia, leukopenia, seizures, paralytic ileus, jaundice, hepatitis, acute renal failure, and hypertension. Other adverse effects include confusion, headache, anxiety, tremors, stimulation, nightmares, extrapyramidal symptoms (in the elderly), increased psychiatric symptoms, nausea, vomiting, cramps, epigastric distress, stomatitis, rash, photosensitivity, palpitations, tinnitus, and mydriasis. Common side effects are dizziness, drowsiness, diarrhea, dry mouth, urinary retention, orthostatic hypotension, electrocardiogram changes, tachycardia, and blurred vision.

mis-, prefix meaning "wrong" or "badly": *misfeasance.*

miscarriage. See **spontaneous abortion.**

miscible /mis″ibəl/ [L, *miscere,* to mix], able to be mixed or blended with another substance. Compare **immiscible.**

misdemeanor /mis′dəmē″nər/ [AS, *missan,* to miss; ME, *demenen,* conduct], (in criminal law) an offense that is considered less serious than a felony and carries a lesser penalty, usually a fine or imprisonment for less than 1 year. Conviction for a misdemeanor does not necessarily prohibit practicing a licensed occupation.

misfeasance /misfē″zəns/ [AS, *missan,* to miss; L, *facere,* to make], an improper performance of a lawful act, especially in a way that may cause damage or injury. Compare **malfeasance, nonfeasance.**

Mishel, Merle H., a nursing theorist who developed the Uncertainty in Illness Theory, which asserts that uncertainty is initially a neutral cognitive state representing the inability of the patient with chronic or life-threatening conditions to interpret the outcome of events related to the illness and that nursing interventions must help patients adapt and cope productively with this uncertainty, integrating it into their lives and improving quality of life.

miso-, prefix meaning "hatred of": *misogamy, misogyny.*

misogamy /misog″əmē/ [Gk, *misein,* to hate, *gamos,* marriage], an aversion to marriage. −*misogamic, misogamous, adj.,* −*misogamist, n.*

misogyny /misoj″inē/ [Gk, *misein* to hate, *gyne,* women], an aversion to women. −*misogynistic, adj.,* −*misogynist, n.*

misopedia /mis′ōpē″dē·ə/ [Gk, *misein* + *pais,* children], an aversion to children. −*misopedic, adj.,* −*misopedist, n.*

misophobia, misophobic. See **mysophobia.**

missed abortion [OE, *missan,* to be lacking; L, *ab,* away from, *oriri,* to be born], a condition in which a dead immature embryo or fetus is not expelled from the uterus for 2 months or more. The uterus diminishes in size, and symptoms of pregnancy abate; maternal infection and blood clotting disorders may follow. The fetus and placenta may become necrotic; less commonly the fetus becomes calcified, and the rest of the products of conception are resorbed.

missed period [OE, *missan,* to be lacking; Gk, *peri* + *hodos,* way], an unexplained interruption in the menstrual cycle.

missile fracture [L, *mittere,* to throw], a penetration fracture caused by a projectile, such as a bullet or a piece of shrapnel.

mistura /mistyoo″rə/ [L, mixture], any of a number of mixtures of drugs, usually containing suspensions of insoluble substances intended for internal use. Examples include *mistura kaolini et morphinae,* a mixture of kaolin and morphine, and *mistura cretae pro infantibus,* a mixture of chalk, tragacanth, chloroform water, and other ingredients formulated for the treatment of GI disorders in infants.

mite /mīt/ [AS], a minute arachnid with a flat, almost transparent body and four pairs of legs. Many species of these relatives of ticks and spiders are parasitic, including the chigger and *Sarcoptes scabiei,* which cause localized pruritus and inflammation. Some female mites burrow into the skin and lay eggs that hatch into larvae. The movements of the larvae cause intense itching. See also **chigger, scabies.**

mite typhus. See **scrub typhus.**

Mithracin, an antineoplastic drug. Brand name for **plicamycin.**

mithramycin. See **plicamycin.**

mithridatism. See **tachyphylaxis.**

mitleiden /mit″līdən/ [Ger, *mit,* with, *leiden,* to suffer], psychosomatic symptoms sometimes experienced by expectant fathers.

mito-, prefix meaning "threadlike": *mitochondrion, mitosis.*

mitochondrion /mī″tōkon″drē·on/ *pl.* **mitochondria** [Gk, *mitos,* thread, *chondros,* cartilage], a rodlike, threadlike, or granular organelle that functions in aerobic respiration and occurs in varying numbers in all eukaryotic cells except mature erythrocytes. It is bounded by two sets of membranes, a smooth outer one and an inner one that is arranged in folds, or cristae, that extend into the interior of the mitochondrion, called the matrix. Mitochondria provide the principal source of cellular energy through oxidative phosphorylation and adenosine triphosphate (ATP) synthesis. They also contain the enzymes involved with electron transport and the citric acid and fatty acid cycles. Mitochondria are self-replicating and contain their own DNA, RNA polymerase, transfer RNA, and ribosomes. Also called **chondriosome.** −*mitochondrial, adj.*

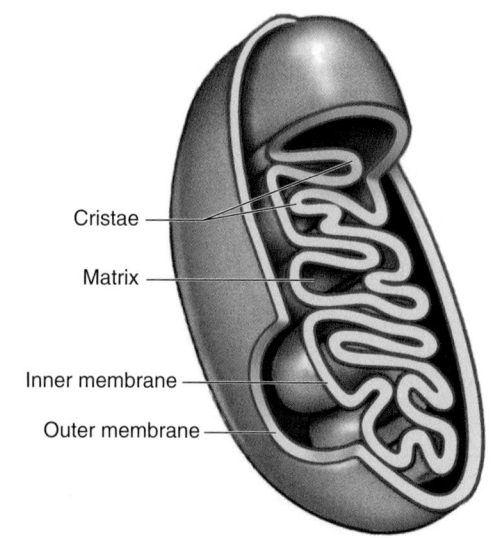

Cristae

Matrix

Inner membrane

Outer membrane

Mitochondrion *(Patton and Thibodeau, 2016)*

mitogen /mī'təjən, mit"-/ [Gk, *mitos* + *genein,* to produce], an agent that triggers mitosis.

mitogenesia /mī'tōjənē"zhə/ [Gk, *mitos* + *genein,* to produce], production resulting from mitosis.

mitogenesis /mī'tōjen"əsis/, the induction of mitosis in a cell. –*mitogenetic, adj.*

mitogenetic radiation /-jənet"ik/, the force or specific energy that is supposedly given off by cells undergoing division. It may in turn stimulate the process of mitosis in other cells. Also called **Gurvich radiation, mitogenic radiation.**

mitogenic factor /-jen"ik/, a lymphokine that is released from activated T lymphocytes and that stimulates the production of normal unsensitized lymphocytes.

mitogenic radiation. See **mitogenetic radiation.**

mitome /mī"tōm/, the reticular network sometimes observed within the cytoplasm and nucleoplasm of fixed cells. See also **cytomitome, karyomitome.**

mitomycin /mītəmī"sin/, an antineoplastic antibiotic.
- INDICATIONS: It is prescribed in the treatment of malignant neoplastic diseases, including disseminated adenocarcinoma of the stomach and pancreas, bladder cancer, and colon cancer.
- CONTRAINDICATIONS: Clotting deficiency, thrombocytopenia, or known hypersensitivity to this drug prohibits its use.
- ADVERSE EFFECTS: The most serious adverse effect is bone marrow depression. GI disturbances, alopecia, and skin reactions commonly occur.

mitosis /mītō"sis, mit-/ [Gk, *mitos,* thread], a type of cell division that occurs in somatic cells and results in the formation of two genetically identical daughter cells containing the diploid number of chromosomes characteristic of the species. It consists of the division of the nucleus followed by the division of the cytoplasm. The former has four stages (prophase, metaphase, anaphase, and telophase), during which the two chromatids of each chromosome separate and migrate to opposite ends of the cell. Mitosis is the process by which the body produces new cells for both growth and repair of injured tissue. Also called **indirect division.** Compare **meiosis.** Kinds include **heterotypic mitosis, homeotypic mitosis, multipolar mitosis, pathological mitosis.** See also **interphase.** –*mitotic, adj.*

mitotane /mī"tətān/, an antineoplastic that destroys normal and neoplastic adrenal cortical cells.
- INDICATIONS: It is prescribed in the treatment of carcinoma of the adrenal cortex and has an unlabeled use for treating Cushing syndrome.
- CONTRAINDICATIONS: Known hypersensitivity to this drug is the only contraindication.
- ADVERSE EFFECTS: Among the more serious adverse effects are GI symptoms, lethargy, and adrenal insufficiency.

mitotic /mītot"ik/ [Gk, *mitos,* thread], pertaining to or characterized by mitosis, the process of cell division in the formation of identical daughter cells.

mitotic figure [Gk, *mitos* + L, *figura,* form], any chromosome or chromosome aggregation during any of the stages of mitosis.

mitotic index, the number of cells per unit (usually 1000 cells) undergoing mitosis during a given time. The ratio is used primarily as an estimation of the rate of tissue growth.

mitotic spindle. See **spindle.**

mitoxantrone, a synthetic antineoplastic antibiotic.
- INDICATIONS: It is prescribed in combination with other approved drugs in the initial treatment of acute nonlymphocytic leukemia in adults and has activity against other leukemias, lymphoma, and breast cancer.
- CONTRAINDICATIONS: It should not be given to patients who are pregnant, have a clinically significant low left ventricular ejection fraction, or have evidence of prior hypersensitivity to this drug. Its use should be accompanied by close and frequent monitoring of hematological and chemical laboratory parameters, as well as frequent patient observation.
- ADVERSE EFFECTS: The side effects most often reported include hypotension, urticaria, dyspnea, rashes, phlebitis, myelosuppression, nausea, and vomiting.

mitral /mī"trəl/ [L, *mitra,* turban], **1.** pertaining to the mitral valve of the heart. **2.** shaped like a miter.

mitral atresia, a congenital absence of the mitral valve associated with transposition of the great vessels or hypoplastic left heart syndrome. See also **valvular heart disease.**

mitral commissurotomy [L, *mitra,* turban, *commissura,* joining together; Gk, *temnein,* to cut], a closed-heart surgical procedure in which the mitral valve is divided at the junction of its cusps for the treatment of mitral valve stenosis.

mitral gradient, the difference in pressure in the left atrium and left ventricle during diastole.

mitral insufficiency. See **mitral regurgitation.**

mitral murmur [L, *mitra,* turban, *murmur,* humming], a high-pitched blowing sound, best heard at the apex of the heart, that is caused by a defective mitral valve.

mitral regurgitation, a backflow of blood from the left ventricle into the left atrium in systole across a diseased mitral valve. The condition may result from congenital valve abnormalities, rheumatic fever, mitral valve prolapse, endocardial fibroelastosis, myocarditis, myocardiopathy, or dilation of the left ventricle as a result of severe anemia. Symptoms include dyspnea, fatigue, intolerance of exercise, systolic murmur, and heart palpitations. Congestive heart failure may ultimately occur. Treatment depends on the severity of the condition. Surgery may be necessary in cases of refractory congestive heart failure, progressive cardiomegaly, and pulmonary hypertension. Also called **mitral insufficiency.** See also **valvular heart disease.**

mitral stenosis. See **mitral valve stenosis.**

mitral valve, a bicuspid valve situated between the left atrium and the left ventricle; the only valve with two, rather than three, cusps. The mitral valve allows blood to flow from the left atrium

M

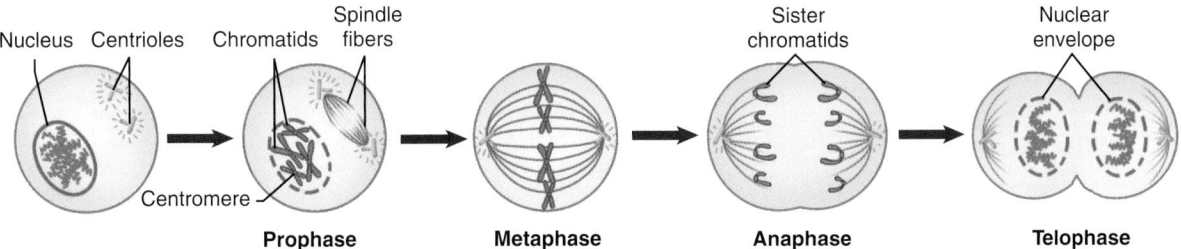

Mitosis *(Patton and Thibodeau, 2010)*

Nucleus Centrioles Chromatids Spindle fibers Centromere **Prophase** **Metaphase** Sister chromatids **Anaphase** Nuclear envelope **Telophase**

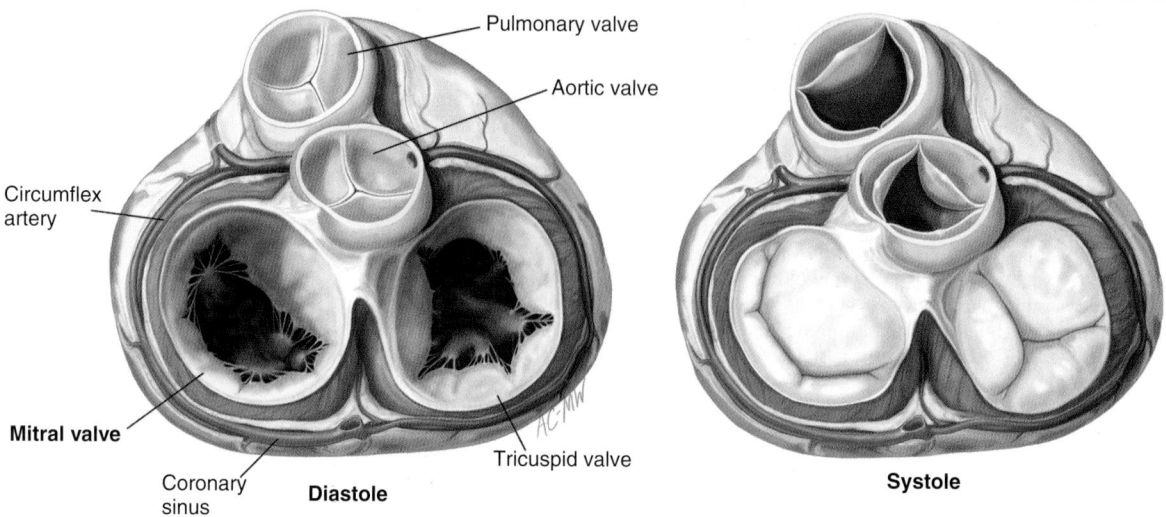

Pulmonary valve

Aortic valve

Circumflex artery

Mitral valve

Coronary sinus   **Diastole**

Tricuspid valve

Systole

Mitral valve in diastole and systole (Carpentier, Adams, and Filsoufi, 2010)

into the left ventricle but prevents blood from flowing back into the atrium. Ventricular contraction in systole forces the blood against the valve, closing the two cusps and assuring the flow of blood from the ventricle into the aorta. The ventral cusp of the mitral valve is longer than the dorsal cusp. Also called **bicuspid valve, left atrioventricular valve.** Compare **aortic valve, pulmonary valve, semilunar valve, tricuspid valve.**

mitral valve prolapse (MVP) syndrome, protrusion of one or both cusps of the mitral valve back into the left atrium during ventricular systole. See also **Barlow syndrome, valvular heart disease.**

mitral valve stenosis, an obstructive lesion in the mitral valve caused by adhesions on the leaflets of the valve, usually the result of recurrent episodes of rheumatic endocarditis or age-related calcification of the valve leaflets. Hypertrophy of the left atrium develops and may be followed by right-sided heart failure and pulmonary edema. Reduced cardiac output characteristically produces fatigue, dyspnea, orthopnea, and cyanosis. Surgical correction of the defective valve may be necessary. The valve may be freed of the adhesions in a mitral commissurotomy, or it may be replaced by a prosthetic valve. See also **atrioventricular (AV) valve, valvular heart disease, valvular stenosis.**

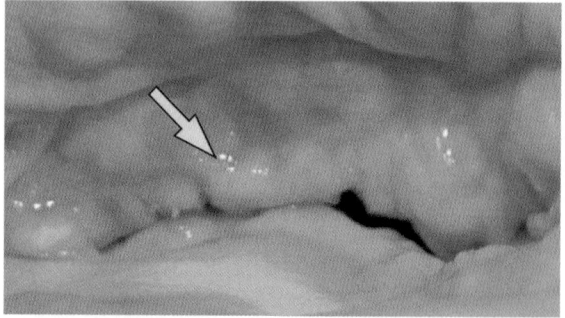

Mitral valve stenosis viewed from the atria
(Chandrashekhar, Westaby, and Narula, 2009)

mittelschmerz /mit″əlshmerts/ [Ger, *Mitte,* middle, *Schmerz,* pain], abdominal pain in the region of an ovary during ovulation, usually occurring midway through the menstrual cycle. Present in many women, mittelschmerz

is useful for identifying ovulation, thus pinpointing the fertile period of the cycle. Also called **intermenstrual pain.**

Mittendorf dot, an eye anomaly characterized by the presence of a small dense floating opacity behind the posterior lens capsule. It is a remnant of the hyaloid artery that was present in the eye during embryonic development. The object usually does not affect vision.

mivacurium, a nondepolarizing neuromuscular blocker.
■ INDICATIONS: This drug is used to facilitate endotracheal intubation and skeletal muscle relaxation during mechanical ventilation, surgery, or general anesthesia.
■ CONTRAINDICATIONS: Known hypersensitivity to this drug prohibits its use.
■ ADVERSE EFFECTS: Adverse effects of this drug include decreased blood pressure, bradycardia, tachycardia, diplopia, rash, urticaria, weakness, and prolonged skeletal muscle relaxation. Life-threatening side effects include paralysis, prolonged apnea, bronchospasm, wheezing, and respiratory depression.

mixed anesthesia. See **balanced anesthesia.**

mixed aneurysm. See **compound aneurysm.**

mixed anxiety-depressive disorder, a mental disorder characterized by symptoms of depression and of anxiety but not meeting the full criteria for either a depressive disorder or an anxiety disorder.

mixed aphasia. See **global aphasia.**

mixed cell malignant lymphoma [L, *miscere,* to mix], a lymphoid neoplasm containing lymphocytes and histiocytes (macrophages).

mixed cell sarcoma, a tumor consisting of two or more cellular elements, excluding fibrous tissue. Also called **malignant mesenchymoma.**

mixed connective tissue disease (MCTD), a systemic disease characterized by the combined symptoms of various collagen diseases, such as synovitis, polymyositis, scleroderma, and systemic lupus erythematosus, with a high concentration of antibodies of ribonucleoprotein. Other symptoms may include arthralgia, muscle inflammation, nondeforming arthritis, swollen hands, esophageal hypomotility, and reduced diffusing capacity of the lungs. Treatment often includes the administration of corticosteroids. Recurrence is common when the steroid medication is discontinued.

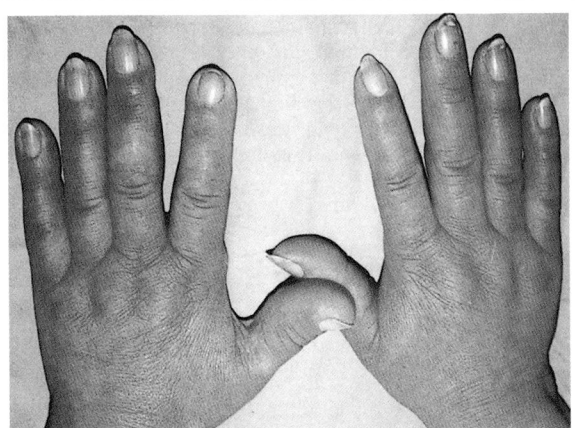

Mixed connective tissue disease affecting the hands
(Ferri, 2009)

mixed culture [L, *miscere*, to mix, *colere*, to cultivate], a laboratory culture that contains two or more different strains of organisms.

mixed dentition, dentition containing both primary and adult secondary teeth. It usually occurs between 6 and 13 years of age. Also called **transitional dentition.**

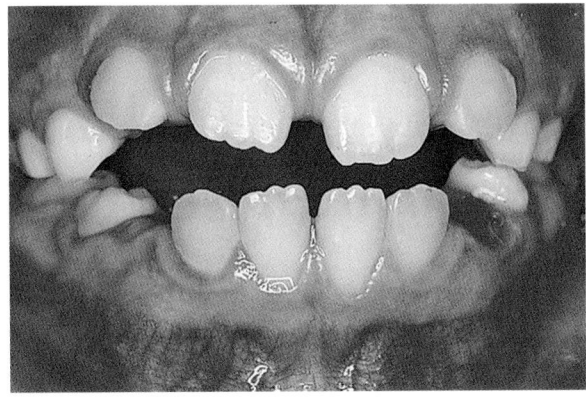

Mixed dentition *(Daniel, Harfst, and Wilder, 2008)*

mixed depression, a severe depressive disorder characterized by severe anxiety accompanied by irritability, racing thoughts, increased or pressured speech, and distractibility. Psychomotor agitation is prominent. Delusions, as well as depression with psychotic features, may also be present.

mixed dust pneumoconiosis, pneumoconiosis that is caused by more than one type of dust.

mixed glioma, a tumor, composed of glial cells, that contains more than one kind of cell, the most common being nonneural cells of ectodermal origin.

mixed hearing loss, deafness that is both conductive and sensorineural in nature.

mixed hyperlipemia, mixed hypertriglyceridemia. See **hyperlipidemia type V.**

mixed infection, an infection by several microorganisms, as in some abscesses, pneumonia, and infections of wounds. Numerous combinations of bacteria, viruses, and fungi may be involved. Compare **endogenous infection, retrograde infection, secondary infection.**

mixed leukemia, a malignancy of blood-forming tissues characterized by the proliferation of more than one predominant cell line.

mixed lymphocyte reaction (MLR), an assay in which lymphocytes from two genetically different individuals are cultured together. T cells from the first individual proliferate in response to allogenic major histocompatibility complex (MHC) molecules expressed on the cell surface of cells of the other individual. It is used primarily for histocompatibility testing before grafting.

mixed neoplasm [L, *miscere*, to mix; Gk, *neos*, new + *plasma*, something formed], a tumor or growth involving two germinal layers of tissue.

mixed nerve [L, *miscere*, to mix, *nervus*], a nerve that contains both sensory and motor fibers.

mixed porphyria. See **variegate porphyria.**

mixed receptive-expressive language disorder, a communication disorder involving both the expression and the comprehension of language, either spoken or signed. Patients have difficulties with language production, such as in selection of words and creation of appropriate sentences, and also have trouble understanding words, sentences, or specific types of words.

mixed sleep apnea, a condition marked by signs and symptoms of both central sleep apnea and obstructive sleep apnea. It often begins as central sleep apnea and develops into the obstructive form. Mixed sleep apnea may also result from obstructive sleep apnea as hypoxia and hypercapnia induce signs and symptoms of the central form. See also **central sleep apnea, obstructive sleep apnea.**

mixed triglyceride breath test, a breath test for pancreatic function, in which a mixture of synthetic triglycerides labeled with carbon 13 is administered to the fasting patient and levels of labeled carbon dioxide in the breath are subsequently measured at regular time intervals. Excessively low carbon dioxide indicates inadequate pancreatic lipase in the intestine.

mixed tumor, a growth composed of more than one kind of neoplastic tissue.

mixed vaccine, an immunizing preparation that protects against more than one kind of pathogen, such as the diphtheria, tetanus, and pertussis vaccine or the measles, mumps, and rubella vaccine.

mixed venous blood, blood that is composed of the venous blood from the heart and all systemic tissues in proportion to their venous returns. In the absence of abnormalities, mixed venous blood is present in the main pulmonary artery.

-mixis, -mixia, -mixie, -mixy, mixo-, combining form meaning "related to intercourse": *amphimixis.*

mixture /miks″chər/ [L, *miscere*, to mix], **1.** a substance composed of ingredients that are not chemically combined and do not necessarily occur in a fixed proportion. **2.** (in pharmacology) a liquid containing one or more medications in suspension. The proportions of the ingredients are specific to each mixture. Compare **compound, solution.** See also **mistura.**

-mixy. See **-mixis, -mixia, -mixie, -mixy, mixo-.**

mL, abbreviation for **milliliter.**

MLD, abbreviation for **minimum lethal dose.**

MLT, abbreviation for **medical laboratory technician.**

MLVA, abbreviation for **multiple-locus variable number of tandem repeat analysis.**

mm, abbreviation for **millimeter.**

mM, abbreviation for **millimole.**

mm³, abbreviation for **cubic millimeter.**

MMFR, abbreviation for **maximal midexpiratory flow rate.**

M

MMIH syndrome, initialism for *megacystis-microcolon-intestinal hypoperistalsis syndrome.*

M-mode, motion modulation in diagnostic ultrasonography. It is a variation of B-mode ultrasound used in echocardiography. See also **B-mode.**

mmol, abbreviation for **millimole.**

MMPI, initialism for **Minnesota Multiphasic Personality Inventory.**

MMR, abbreviation for **measles, mumps, and rubella virus vaccine live.**

MMWR, abbreviation for *Morbidity and Mortality Weekly Report.*

Mn, symbol for the element **manganese.**

mne-, prefix meaning "memory": *mnemonic.*

mnemonics [Gk, *mnemonikos*], a system of memory training that links a new concept or image with one already established in the memory, such as associating the numbers of a combination lock with a birthday or telephone number.

-mnesia, suffix meaning "(condition or type of) memory": *amnesia, hypermnesia.*

-mnestic, -mnesic, suffix meaning "memory": *anamnestic.*

MNL, abbreviation for **mononuclear leukocyte.**

Mo, symbol for the element **molybdenum.**

Moban, an antipsychotic agent. Brand name for **molindone hydrochloride.**

mobile arm support (MAS) /mō″bəl, mōbēl″/, a forearm support device that enables people with upper extremity disabilities to fulfill some activities of daily living, by helping to move the hand into position for self-feeding. It may also be used as a training device and may be mounted on a wheelchair. Also called **balanced forearm orthosis, ball-bearing feeder.**

mobile projection, a radiographic examination performed with a portable x-ray machine outside the radiology department.

mobile unit, an easily transportable radiography unit designed for use outside a radiology department.

mobility /mōbil″itē/ [L, *mobilis*, movable], the velocity a particle or ion attains for a given applied voltage; a relative measure of how quickly an ion may move in an electric field.

-mobility. See **-motility, -mobility.**

Mobitz I heart block /mō″bits/ [Woldemar Mobitz, German physician, 1889–1951; AS, *hoerte*, heart; Fr, *bloc*, block], second-degree or partial atrioventricular (AV) block in which the P-R interval increases progressively until the propagation of an atrial impulse to the ventricles does not occur. Mobitz I heart block is caused by abnormal conduction of the cardiac impulse in the AV node and may be precipitated by increased vagal tone, AV nodal ischemia, or digitalis therapy. It may be a complication of inferior myocardial infarction. Also called **type I AV block, Wenckebach heart block.**

Mobitz II heart block, second-degree or partial atrioventricular block characterized by the sudden nonconduction of an atrial impulse and a periodic dropped beat without prior or subsequent lengthening of the P-R interval. This kind of block usually results from bilateral impaired conduction in the bundle branches. It may be caused by anterior myocardial infarction, myocarditis, drug toxicity, electrolyte disturbances, rheumatoid nodules, and various degenerative diseases. Syncopal attacks, which occur without warning when the patient is upright or recumbent, are common in Mobitz II heart block, which may be transient or suddenly progress to complete block. Long-term therapy may require implantation of a pacemaker. Also called **type II AV block.**

Möbius syndrome /mē″bē·əs/ [Paul J. Möbius, German neurologist, 1853–1902], a rare developmental disorder characterized by congenital bilateral facial palsy, usually associated with oculomotor or other neurological dysfunctions, speech disorders, and various anomalies of the extremities. It is caused by a developmental defect involving the motor nuclei of the cranial nerves. Also called **congenital facial diplegia, congenital oculofacial paralysis, nuclear agenesis.**

moccasin /mok′əsin/, any of several species of snakes of the genus *Agkistrodon.*

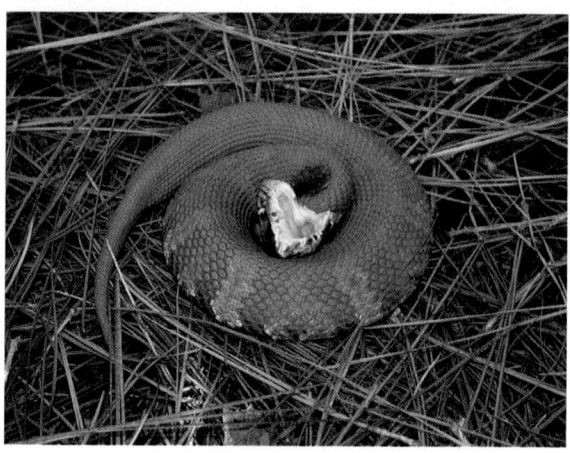

Water moccasin *(John Willson at the Savannah River Ecology Laboratory [SREL])*

Moctanin, a gallstone-dissolving agent. Brand name for **monooctanoin.**

modafinil, a cerebral stimulant.

■ INDICATIONS: It is used to treat narcolepsy.

■ CONTRAINDICATIONS: Factors that prohibit its use include hyperthyroidism, hypertension, glaucoma, severe arteriosclerosis, drug abuse, cardiovascular disease, anxiety, and known hypersensitivity to this drug.

■ ADVERSE EFFECTS: Arrhythmias are a life-threatening effect of this drug. Other adverse effects are hyperglycemia, albuminuria, rhinitis, pharyngitis, lung disorder, dyspnea, asthma, epistaxis, abnormal vision, amblyopia, dizziness, headache, chills, stimulation, anorexia, dry mouth, diarrhea, nausea, vomiting, mouth ulcer, gingivitis, thirst, urinary retention, abnormal ejaculation, hypertension, herpes simplex, and dry skin. Common side effects include hyperactivity, insomnia, restlessness, palpitations, and tachycardia.

modality /mōdal″itē/, **1.** the method of application of a therapeutic agent or regimen. **2.** a sensory entity, such as the sense of vision or taste.

mode /mōd/ [L, *modus*, measure], a value or term in a set or series of data that occurs more frequently than other values or terms.

model /mod″əl/ [L, *modulus*, small measure], (in nursing research) a symbolic representation of the interrelations exhibited by a phenomenon within a system or a process. The model is presented as a conceptual framework or a theory that explains a phenomenon and allows predictions to be made about a patient or a process. A model is analogous to an equation in mathematics. Nursing models usually describe person, environment, health, and nursing.

modeling /mod″əling/, a technique used in behavior therapy in which a person learns a desired response by observing and imitating the behavior.

Modeling and Role Modeling, a theory developed by the nursing theorists Helen C. Erickson, Evelyn M. Tomlin, and Mary Ann P. Swain. Their book, *Modeling and Role Modeling: A Theory and Paradigm for Nursing,* was published in 1983. From a synthesis of multiple concepts related to basic needs, developmental tasks, object attachment, and adaptive coping potential, they developed their highly abstract role-modeling theory. The term *modeling* refers to the development of an understanding of the client's world. Role modeling is the nursing intervention, or nurturance, that requires unconditional acceptance. Erickson, Tomlin, and Swain believe that, although people are alike because of their holism (multiple interacting subsystems), lifetime growth, and development, they are also different because of inherent endowment, adaptation, and self-care knowledge. Role modeling provides a framework for understanding the ways clients structure their worlds. Erickson, Tomlin, and Swain view nursing as a self-care model based on the client's perception of the world and adaptations to stressors.

Model of Human Occupation (MOHO), a model of practice used in occupational therapy designed to understand the complexity of human performance in work, play or leisure, and activities of daily living within specific contexts. MOHO examines interactions among volition, habituation, performance capacity, and environment. This model, used throughout the world, is the life work of Dr. Gary Kielhofner. See also **volition, habituation, performance capacity.**

modem /mō′dəm/, a hardware device for transforming serial binary numbers into an audible tone, and vice versa, for transmission over a telephone, router, radio, or optical system to another computer. Abbreviation for *modulate/ demodulate.*

moderate intellectual disability, a category of intellectual disability in which an individual has a below-average IQ (ranging from 40 to 54) and typically requires some level of support as an adult. This level of impairment generally allows the individual to master academic skills at the level of Grade 2, although significantly more slowly than other students. Compare **mild intellectual disability.**

moderate sedation, the administration of central nervous system depressant drugs and/or analgesics to provide analgesia, relieve anxiety, and/or provide amnesia during surgical, diagnostic, or interventional procedures. Consciousness is depressed, and the patient may fall asleep but is not unresponsive. Oversedation or an adverse patient response to sedation may result in life-threatening complications such as hypotension, loss of airway reflexes, inability to maintain a patent airway, hypoventilation, apnea, or agitation and movement at a critical point in the procedure. Anesthetic monitoring during conscious sedation includes at a minimum the monitoring of blood pressure, electrocardiography, and pulse oximetry. Formerly called **conscious sedation.** See also **anesthesia.**

moderator band /mod′ərā′tər/ [L, *moderari,* to restrain; AS, *bindan,* to bind], a thick bundle of muscle in the central part of the right ventricle of the heart. Missing in some individuals and varying in size in others, it usually contains part of the atrioventricular conduction bundle. Also called **trabecula septomarginalis.**

modesty, propriety of dress, speech, and conduct in relations between patients and health care personnel, including draping and covering of the patient to the greatest extent possible, depending on the type of care or examination.

Modicon, an oral contraceptive containing an estrogen and a progestin. Brand name for **norethindrone acetate and ethinyl estradiol.**

modification /mod′ifikā′shən/, **1.** a process whereby a substance is changed from one form to another. **2.** a change in an organism that is acquired or learned and does not involve inheritance.

modification allele. See **modifying gene.**

modified barium swallow, a radiological examination performed while the patient swallows barium-coated substances, done to assess quality of the swallowing mechanisms of the mouth, pharynx, and esophagus.

modified bed rest, a restriction of activity that varies with the condition. Also called **partial bed rest.**

Modified Interest Checklist, (in occupational therapy) a self-reported inventory of leisure interests; appropriate for adults and adolescents. Its main focus is on avocational interests that influence activity choices. It is especially useful in appreciating the impact of disability on participation in leisure activities.

modified jaw thrust /mod″ifīd/, an upper airway control maneuver to maintain an open airway of an unconscious person in cases of potential spinal injury. In such persons in-line stabilization of the head and neck can be obtained primarily by forward jaw thrust with minimum head extension.

modified milk [L, *modus,* measure, *facere,* to make], cow's milk in an infant formula in which the content has been changed, as when the protein content is reduced and the fat content is increased to correspond to the composition of breast milk. There are other instances of modified milk, as when water is evaporated to manufacture dried whole milk and milk protein concentrates or fat is removed to produce skim milk, or nonfat milk.

modified plantigrade position, a position used in physical therapy to prepare the patient for independent standing and walking. The person stands with feet flat on the ground and the upper limbs leaning on a table or similar structure to support a large part of the weight.

modified radical mastectomy, a surgical procedure in which a breast is completely removed with the underlying pectoralis minor and some of the adjacent lymph nodes. The pectoralis major is not excised. The operation is performed to treat early and well-localized malignant neoplasms of the breast, for which it appears to be as curative as the more extensive radical mastectomy. Care of the individual before and after a modified radical mastectomy is similar to that for a radical mastectomy. Compare **radical mastectomy, simple mastectomy.** See also **lumpectomy, mastectomy, Reach to Recovery.**

modifying gene /mod″ifī′ing/ [L, *modus,* measure; Gk, *genein,* to produce], a gene that alters or influences the expression function of another gene, including the suppression or reduction of the usual function of the modified gene. Also called **modification allele.**

modiolus, a central column of bone around which the cochlea twists. Also called **lamina of modiolus, spiral lamina.**

modulation /mod′yəlā″shən/, an alteration in the magnitude or any variation in the duration of an electrical current. Modulation, which affects physiological responses to various waveforms, may be continuous, interrupted, pulsed, or surging.

modulation transfer function (MTF) [L, *modulus,* small measure; L, *transferre,* to carry, *functio,* performance], a quantitative measure of the ability of an imaging system to reproduce patterns that vary in spatial frequency. The MTF is useful in predicting image degradation in a series of radiographic components.

modulator /mod′ula″ter/, a specific inductor or agent that exerts a moderating or controlling influence on the activity of a molecule or biochemical pathway.

MODY, abbreviation for *maturity-onset diabetes of youth.*

Moeller glossitis /mel″ər/ [Julius O.L. Moeller, German surgeon, 1819–1887], a form of chronic glossitis characterized by burning or pain of the tongue and increased sensitivity to hot or spicy foods. Also called **glossodynia exfoliativa.** See also **glossitis.**

moexipril, an angiotensin-converting enzyme inhibitor.

■ INDICATIONS: It is prescribed in the treatment of high blood pressure alone or in combination with diuretics and in the treatment of left ventricular dysfunction after myocardial infarction.

■ CONTRAINDICATIONS: It should not be given to patients with hypersensitivity reactions to angiotensin-converting enzyme inhibitors or those who are pregnant (especially during second and third trimesters). It should be used with caution in people with renal insufficiency, hypovolemia, or collagen vascular diseases.

■ ADVERSE EFFECTS: The side effects most often reported include digestive tract disorders, depression, headache, dizziness, vertigo, sleeping difficulties, chest pains, and palpitations. There can be pronounced first dose hypotension. Anaphylatic reactions can occur, and angiodema can occur at any time during therapy (but usually with first dose).

mogi-, prefix meaning "difficult" or "with difficulty."

mohel /mō″əl, môhāl″/, in Judaism, ordained to circumcise.

Mohr syndrome /mor/ [Otto Lous Mohr, Norwegian geneticist, 1886–1967], an autosomal-recessive disorder characterized by shortened, fused, and/or extra fingers and toes and bilateral polysyndactyly of the big toe; by cranial, facial, lingual, palatal, and mandibular anomalies; and by episodic neuromuscular disturbances. Also called **orodigitofacial dysostosis, oral-facial-digital (OFD) syndrome, type II.**

moiety /moi″itē/ [L, *medietas,* middle], a part of a molecule that exhibits a particular set of chemical and pharmacological characteristics.

moist cough. See **productive cough.**

moist crackle [OFr, *moiste,* fresh; ME, *krakelen*], an adventitious breathing sound heard on auscultation when air bubbles through fluid or secretions in the bronchi or trachea.

moist gangrene, tissue necrosis that follows a crushing injury or an obstruction of blood flow by an embolism, tight bandages, or a tourniquet. This form of gangrene has an offensive odor, spreads rapidly, and may result in death within days. Compare **dry gangrene.** See **gangrene.**

moist heat [OFr, *moiste* + AS, *haetu*], the use of hot water, towels soaked in hot water, aquathermia pads, hot water bottles, or hot water vapors to reduce inflammation and pain, stimulate circulation, and/or relieve symptoms as directed by a physician. Hot towels should be wrung out to remove surplus moisture and should not be too hot to be held in the hands of the person applying moist heat.

moist rale, a rale heard over fluid in the bronchial tubes.

mol. See **mole².**

molality /mōlal″itē/ [L, *moles,* mass], the number of moles of solute per kilogram of water or other solvent. It refers to the solution concentration.

molal volume. See **mole volume.**

molar (M) /mō″lər/ [L, *moles,* mass], **1.** any of the 12 teeth, six in each dental arch, located posterior to the premolars. The crown of each molar is nearly cubical, convex on its buccal and lingual surfaces, and flattened on its surfaces of contact. Each of the upper molars can have three roots. The roots of each third upper molar are often fused. The lower molars are larger than the upper, and each has two roots. The roots of each third lower molar tend to fuse. Molars are used to crush and grind food. **2.** (M) pertaining to the concentration of a solution, expressed as the number of moles of solute per liter of solution. See also **mole².**

molarity /mōler″itē/ [L, *moles,* mass], the number of moles of solute per liter of solution. It refers to the concentration of the solution.

molar pregnancy, a pregnancy in which a hydatid mole develops from the trophoblastic tissue of the early embryonic stage of development. The signs of pregnancy are all exaggerated: the uterus grows more rapidly than is normal, morning sickness is often severe and constant, blood pressure is likely to be elevated, and blood levels of chorionic gonadotropins are extremely high. The uterus must be evacuated because the mole may develop into a malignant trophoblastic disease, choriocarcinoma. See also **hydatid mole.**

molar solution, a solution that contains 1 mole of solute per liter of solution.

molar volume. See **mole volume.**

mold, **1.** a hollow form for casting or shaping an object, as a prosthesis. **2.** fungi that grow on moist organic matter, breaking it down.

molding /mōl″ding/ [ME, *moulde,* shaping], the natural process by which a baby's head is shaped during labor as it is squeezed into and through the birth passage by the forces of labor. The head often becomes quite elongated, and the bones of the skull may be caused to overlap slightly at the suture lines. The biparietal diameter of the head may be compressed as much as 0.5 cm without intracranial damage. Most of the changes caused by molding resolve themselves during the first few days of life. Compare **caput succedaneum.** See also **cephalhematoma.**

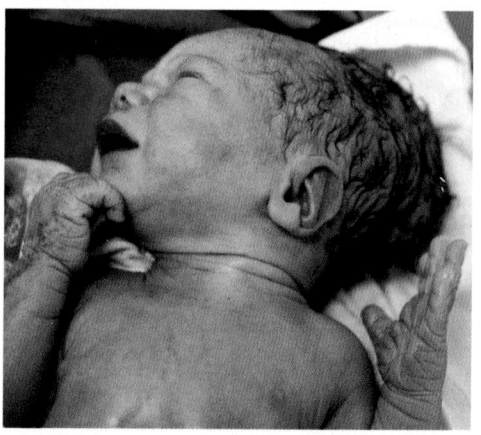

An infant with molding immediately after birth
(Graham and Smith, 2007)

mole¹ [L, mass], **1.** *(Informal)* a pigmented nevus. **2.** (in obstetrics) a hydatid mole.

mole² [L, *molecula,* small mass], the standard unit used to measure the amount of a substance. A mole of a substance is the amount containing the same number of elementary particles as there are atoms in 12 g of carbon-12, typically 6.02 × 10²³ particles. This number is called Avogadro's number. Also spelled **mol.** −*molar, adj.*

molecular biology /məlek″yələr/ [L, *molecula,* small mass; Gk, *bios,* life, *logos,* science], the branch of biology that deals with the physical and chemical interactions of molecules involved in life functions.

molecular genetics [L, *molecula,* small mass; Gk, *genesis,* origin], the branch of genetics that focuses on the chemical structure and the functions, replication, and mutations of the molecules involved in the transmission of genetic information, namely DNA and RNA. Molecular genetics is concerned with the arrangement of genes on DNA, the replication of DNA, the transcription of DNA into RNA, and the translation of RNA into proteins. Also called **biochemical genetics.** See also **recombinant DNA.**

molecular hybridization, (in biochemistry) formation of a partially or wholly complementary nucleic acid duplex by association of single strands, usually between DNA and RNA strands or previously unassociated DNA strands, but also between RNA strands, used to detect and isolate specific sequences, measure homology, or define other characteristics of one or both strands.

molecular lesion. See **point lesion.**

molecular mass, the mass of a molecule of a substance as compared with the mass of an atom of carbon-12. It is equal to the sum of the masses of its constituent atoms and is measured in daltons or grams/mole (g/mol). Formerly called **molecular weight.** See also **atom, atomic mass, molecule.**

molecular mimicry, an occurrence in which sequence similarities between foreign (e.g., pathogens) and self-peptides are sufficient to result in the cross-activation of autoreactive T or B cells. Believed to play a role in the pathogenesis of diseases of the central nervous system and other autoimmune diseases. See also **mimicry.**

molecular pathology [L, *molecula,* small mass; Gk, *pathos,* disease, *logos,* science], the branch of the science of disease that is concerned with the health effects of specific molecules.

molecular sieve, **1.** a crystalline chemical separation device with molecular size pores that adsorbs small but not large molecules. **2.** a cross-linked polymer that forms a porous sieve used as a supporting medium for chromatographic separation of mixtures of solutes.

molecular stutter, a gene defect in which the three-nucleotide code for an amino acid is repeated, missing, or jumbled, causing the gene either to fail to make a specific protein or to make a protein that does not function properly. In Huntington disease, for example, the code for glutamine may be repeated 40 or 50 times in a row in the defective gene. The symptoms of Huntington disease develop in patients with more than 30 glutamine repeats, and the longer the string of repeats, the earlier the symptoms develop.

molecular taxonomy, the classification of organisms on the basis of the distribution and composition of chemical substances in them.

molecular weight (mol wt). See **molecular mass.**

molecule /mol″əkyool/ [L, *molecula,* small mass], the smallest unit that exhibits the properties of an element or compound. A molecule is composed of two or more atoms that are covalently bonded. See also **atom, compound.**

mole percent, a percentage calculation expressed in terms of moles of a substance in a mixture or solution rather than in terms of molecular mass.

mole volume, the volume occupied by one mole of a substance, which may be a solid, liquid, or gas. It is numerically equal to the molecular mass divided by the density. For a gas it is 22.4 L at standard temperature and pressure. Also called **molal volume, molar volume.**

molindone hydrochloride /mol″indōn/, an antipsychotic agent.

■ INDICATIONS: It is prescribed in the treatment of schizophrenia.

■ CONTRAINDICATIONS: Severe central nervous system depression or known hypersensitivity to this drug prohibits its use.

■ ADVERSE EFFECTS: Among the most serious adverse effects are extrapyramidal reactions, hypotension, sedation,

and other reactions characteristic of the phenothiazine antipsychotics.

molluscum contagiosum /məlus′kəm/ [L, *molluscus,* soft], a disease of the skin and mucous membranes caused by a poxvirus, which occurs all over the world. It is characterized by scattered flesh-toned or white papules. Palms of the hands and soles of the feet are not affected. The disease most frequently occurs in children and in adults with an impaired immune response. It is transmitted from person to person by direct or indirect contact and lasts up to 3 years, although individual lesions persist for only 6 to 8 weeks. Diagnosis is easily made by electron microscopy. Curettage or electrical or chemical desiccation helps to clear the lesions, but untreated lesions eventually resolve spontaneously without scarring. Also called *molluscum.*

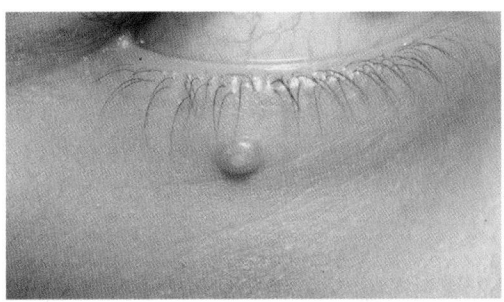

Molluscum contagiosum *(Marks and Miller, 2013)*

Moloney test [Paul J. Moloney, Canadian physician, 1870–1939], *(Obsolete)* a skin test for sensitivity to diphtheria toxoid.

mol wt, abbreviation for **molecular weight.**

molybdenum (Mo) /məlib″dənəm/ [Gk, *molybdos,* lead], a grayish metallic element. Its atomic number is 42; its atomic mass is 95.94. Molybdenum is poisonous if ingested in large quantities. Molybdenum is used as an additive in certain steels.

molybdenum 99, the radionuclide that is the parent of technetium 99 and, as such, is present as a generator in most nuclear medicine departments.

-monab, suffix for monoclonal antibodies.

monad /mon″ad, mō″nəd/, **1.** a unicellular, free-living organism. **2.** a monovalent element or ion. **3.** a haploid set of chromosomes in a spermatid or ootid.

-monam, suffix for monobactam (monocyclic beta-lactam) antibiotics.

monamine. See **monoamine.**

monarthritis /mon′ärthrī″tis/ [Gk, *monos,* single, *arthron,* joint, *itis,* inflammation], arthritis affecting only one joint.

monarticular /mon′ärtik″yələr/ [Gk, *monos,* single; L, *articulus,* joint], pertaining to only one joint.

monascus, a natural product derived from red yeast grown on rice, traditionally used in Chinese medicine and now in more common use as both a medicine and a foodstuff. Commercially prepared supplements are grown under conditions that maximize the production of mevinic acids (statins), primarily lovastatin, agents manufactured and sold by pharmaceutical companies that inhibit cholesterol synthesis. Also called **red yeast.**

■ INDICATIONS: It is used to help maintain acceptable cholesterol levels.

■ CONTRAINDICATIONS: It should not be used during pregnancy and lactation, in children, or in those with known

M

hypersensitivity to monascus or with hepatic disease such as cirrhosis or fatty liver.

monaural /monôr″əl/ [Gk, *monos,* single; L, *auris,* ear], pertaining to one ear.

Mönckeberg arteriosclerosis /meng″kəbərg/ [Johann G. Mönckeberg, German pathologist, 1877–1925], a form of arteriosclerosis in which extensive calcium deposits are found in the tunica media of the artery with little obstruction of the lumen. Also called **medial arteriosclerosis.**

Monday morning fever. See **metal fume fever.**

Monera. See **Procaryotae.**

Monge disease. See **altitude sickness.**

Mongolian spot /mong·gō″lē·ən/ [*Mongol,* Asian ethnic group; ME, *spotte,* stain], a benign bluish-black macule, between 2 and 8 cm, occurring over the sacrum and on the buttocks of some newborns. It is especially common in African-Americans, Native Americans, southern Europeans, and Asian-Americans and usually disappears during early childhood. *Also called slate grey nevus.*

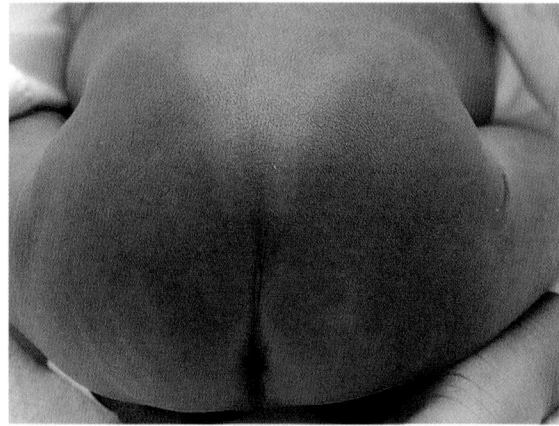

Infant with Mongolian spot *(Douglas, Nicol, and Robertson, 2013)*

mongolism, *(Obsolete)* now called **trisomy 21.** See **Down syndrome.**

monilethrix /mōnil′əthriks/ [L, *monile* necklace; Gk, *thrix,* hair], an autosomal-dominant condition in which the hairs exhibit multiple constrictions, with a beading effect, and are brittle, rarely reaching an inch in length before breaking.

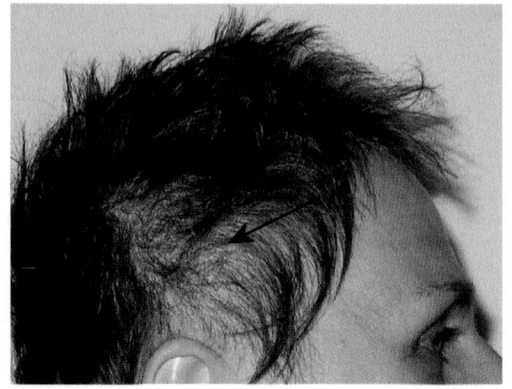

Individual with monilethrix. Arrow highlights the area of constriction *(Rudnicka, Rakowska, and Olszewska, 2013)*

Monilia. See ***Candida albicans.***

monilial vulvovaginitis, moniliasis. See **candidiasis.**

moniliform /mōnil″ifôrm/, resembling a string of beads.

Monistat, an antifungal drug. Brand name for **miconazole nitrate.**

monitor /mon″ətər/ [L, *monere,* to warn], **1.** *v.,* to observe and evaluate a function of the body closely and constantly. **2.** *n.,* a mechanical device that provides a visual or audible signal or a graphic record of a particular function, such as a cardiac monitor or a fetal monitor.

monitored anesthesia care (MAC), a type of anesthesia service where the patient undergoes local anesthesia together with sedation with sedative, anxiolytic, or analgesic medications as needed. The patient is continuously monitored for airway problems, and physiological alterations are anticipated and managed by a qualified anesthesia provider. An essential component of MAC is the periprocedural anesthesia assessment. The provider of MAC must be prepared and qualified to convert to general anesthesia if needed.

monitrice /mon″itris/ [Fr, female instructor], a labor coach, usually a registered nurse, who provides emotional support and leads the mother through labor and delivery.

monkey disease. See **Kyasanur Forest disease.**

monkeypox, an epidemic human disease, caused by exposure to a monkeypox virus, with symptoms resembling those of smallpox. The virus is related antigenically to smallpox and vaccinia organisms.

mono, abbreviation for **mononucleosis.**

mono-, prefix meaning "one": *monochromatic, monoclonal, monoamine.*

monoamine /mon′ō·am″in/, an amine containing one amine group.

monoamine oxidase (MAO), an enzyme that catalyzes the oxidation of amines. See also **monoamine oxidase inhibitor.**

monoamine oxidase inhibitor (MAOI, MAO inhibitor), any of a chemically heterogeneous group of drugs used primarily in the treatment of depression. These drugs also exert an antianxiety effect, especially anxiety associated with phobia. The effects of the drugs vary greatly from patient to patient, and their specific actions leading to clinical benefits are poorly understood. Among the most common adverse effects are drowsiness, dry mouth, orthostatic hypotension, and constipation. Overdosage may cause tremor, euphoria, or manic behavior. MAO inhibitors interact with many drugs and with foods containing large amounts of the amino acid tyramine. Ingestion of these foods by a person taking an MAO inhibitor is likely to cause a severe hypertensive episode associated with headache, palpitations, and nausea. Among these foods are cheeses, red wine, smoked or pickled herring, beer, and yogurt. Among the drugs that interact with MAO inhibitors are dopamine, meperidine, and the indirect acting sympathomimetics, one of which, pseudoephedrine, is an ingredient in many common cold remedies. MAO inhibitors are also sometimes used in the treatment of migraine headache and hypertension. See also **amine pump.**

monobasic acid /mon′ōbā″sik/, an acid with only one replaceable hydrogen atom, such as hydrochloric acid.

monobasic potassium phosphate, the monopotassium salt KH_2PO_4, used as a buffering agent in pharmaceutic preparations and, alone or in combination with other phosphate compounds, as an electrolyte replenisher and urinary acidifier and for prevention of kidney stones.

monobasic sodium phosphate, a monosodium salt of phosphoric acid, used in buffer solutions. Used alone or in combination with other phosphate compounds, it is given intravenously as an electrolyte replenisher, orally or rectally as a laxative, and orally as a urinary acidifier and for prevention of kidney stones.

monobenzone /-ben″zōn/, a depigmenting agent.

■ INDICATIONS: It is prescribed in final depigmentation in extensive vitiligo.

■ CONTRAINDICATIONS: Known hypersensitivity to this drug prohibits its use.

■ ADVERSE EFFECTS: The most serious adverse effect is excessive and irreversible hypopigmentation. Common effects are irritation and allergic reactions of the skin.

monoblast /mon′əblast/ [Gk, *monos,* single, *blastos,* germ], earliest identifiable immature monocyte. Increased production of monoblasts in the marrow and the presence of these forms in the peripheral circulation occur in acute monoblastic leukemias and tuberculosis. Compare **myeloblast.** See also **bone marrow, leukocyte.** –*monoblastic, adj.*

monoblastic leukemia /-blas″tik/, a malignancy of blood-forming organs, characterized by the proliferation of monoblasts and monocytes. The disease develops late in the course of a small but significant number of cases of plasma cell myeloma. Also called **monocytic leukemia, Schilling's leukemia.**

monocarboxylic acid /mon′ō-kär′bok·sil′ik/, a carboxylic acid with a single carboxyl group.

monocarp, *n.,* a plant that bears fruit once and dies.

monocephalus. See **syncephalus.**

monochorial twins, monochorionic twins. See **monozygotic twins.**

monochromatic /-krōmat″ik/, **1.** pertaining to a single color or a single wavelength of light. **2.** describing a person who is totally color blind. **3.** pertaining to a substance that has only one color or stains with only one color.

monochromaticity /-krō′mətis″itē/, the specificity of light in a single defined wavelength. If the specificity is in the visible light spectrum, it is only one color.

Monocid, a cephalosporin-type antibiotic. Brand name for **cefonicid sodium.**

monoclonal /mon′əklō″nəl/ [Gk, *monos* + *klon,* twig], pertaining to or designating a group of identical cells or organisms derived from a single cell or organism. Compare **polyclonal.**

monoclonal antibody (MAB) [Gk, *monos,* single, *klon,* twig; Gk, *anti* + AS, *bodig,* body], an antibody produced in a laboratory from a single clone of B lymphocytes. All MABs produced from the same clone are identical and have the same antigenic specificity.

monoclonal gammopathy. See **gammopathy.**

monocomponent insulin /-kəmpō″nənt/ [Gk, *monos,* single; L, *componere,* to bring together, *insula,* island]. See **single component insulin.**

monocrotic pulse /-krot″ik/ [Gk, *monos,* single, *krotein,* to strike; L, *pulsare,* to beat], a pulse characterized by a single wave.

monoctanoin. See **monooctanoin.**

monocular diplopia /monok″yələr/ [Gk, *monos,* single, *oculus,* eye; Gk, *diploos,* double, *opsis,* vision], a condition in which a double image is perceived with one eye. The cause is a disorder in the refracting medium of the eye, such as a cataract, or partial dislocation of the lens. In rare cases more than two images may be seen with one eye. Also called **uniocular diplopia.**

monocular strabismus [Gk, *monos,* single; L, *oculus,* eye; Gk, *strabismos*], strabismus that is confined to one particular eye. Also called **uniocular squint.**

monocular vision [Gk, *monos,* single; L, *oculus,* eye, *visio,* seeing], a condition of seeing with or using only one eye at a time. Also called **uniocular vision.**

monocutaneous candidiasis, a cellular immunodeficiency disorder associated with fungal *(Candida)* infections of the skin, mucous membranes, nails, and hair. Patients show a lack of immune reaction after intradermal injection of *Candida,* but immunity to other infectious agents is not impaired. About half the patients also exhibit endocrine abnormalities.

monocyte /mon″əsīt/ [Gk, *monos* + *kytos,* cell], a granular peripheral blood mononuclear leukocyte, 13-25 μm in diameter with a lobulated nucleus, containing chromatin material with a lacy pattern and abundant gray-blue cytoplasm filled with fine, bluish granules. See also **monocytosis.** –*monocytic, adj.*

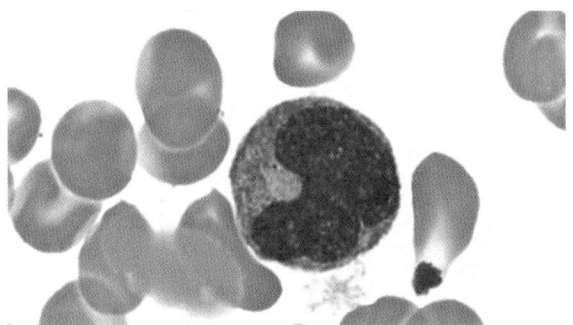

Monocyte micrograph *(Young et al, 2014)*

monocytic leukemia /mon′əsit″ik/, a malignancy of blood-forming tissues in which the predominant cells are monocytes. The disease has an erratic course, characterized by malaise, fatigue, fever, anorexia, weight loss, splenomegaly, bleeding gums, dermal petechiae, anemia, and lack of responsiveness to therapy. There are two forms. In the acute form, more than 20% immature blood cells (blasts) are in the bone marrow, and greater than 80% of those are of the monocytic lineage. In chronic myelomonocytic leukemia there is an increased number of monocytes and blasts in the peripheral blood and bone marrow. Also called **histiocytic leukemia.**

monocytopenia /-sī′təpē″nē·ə/, an abnormally low number of monocytes in the peripheral blood. Also called *monocytic leukopenia.*

monocytosis /mon′ōsītō″sis/, an increased proportion of monocytes in the circulation.

monodactylism /-dak″tiliz′əm/ [Gk, *monos,* single, *daktylos,* finger or toe], a congenital defect in which a person is born with only one finger on the hand or one toe on the foot.

monoethanolamine /mon′ō·eth′ənol″əmēn/. See **ethanolamine.**

monofactorial inheritance /-faktôr″ē·əl/ [Gk, *monos* + L, *factare,* to make], the acquisition or expression of a trait or condition that depends on the transmission of a single specific gene. Compare **multifactorial inheritance.**

monogamy /mənog″əmē/, **1.** the practice of having one long-term sexual partner. **2.** (in biology) the habit of pairing with only one mate.

monohybrid /-hī″brid/ [Gk, *monos* + L, *hybrida,* mixed offspring], pertaining to or describing an individual, organism, or strain that is heterozygous for only one specific trait or that is heterozygous for the single trait or gene locus under consideration.

monohybrid cross, the mating of two individuals, organisms, or strains that have different alleles for only one specific trait or in which only one particular characteristic or gene locus is being followed.

M

monohydric alcohol /-hī″drik/,   an alcohol containing one hydroxyl group.

monoiodotyrosine   /mon′ō-ī-ō′dōtī″rəsin/,   an iodinated amino acid involved in the synthesis of thyroxine (T_4) and triiodothyronine (T_3).

monokaryotic /-ker′ē-ot″ik/,   having a single nucleus.

monolayer /-lā″ər/,   pertaining to or consisting of a single layer of molecules.

monomer /mon″əmər/   [Gk, *monos* + *meros*, part],   **1.** a molecule that repeats itself to form a polymer, such as a molecule of fibrin monomer that polymerizes to form fibrin in the blood-clotting process. –*monomeric, adj.* **2.** a simple molecule of relatively low molecular weight, which is capable of reacting chemically with other molecules to form a dimer, trimer, or polymer. **3.** some basic unit of a molecule, either the molecule itself or functional subunit of it.

monomolecular elimination reaction (E_1) /-məlek″yələr/,   a first-order chemical kinetic reaction in which only one molecule is involved in the slow step reaction. Also called **unimolecular reaction.**

monomphalus /mənom″fələs/   [Gk, *monos* + *omphalos*, navel],   conjoined twins that are united at the umbilicus. Also called **omphalopagus.**

mononeuropathy /-nŏŏrop″əthē/   [Gk, *monos* + *neuron*, nerve, *pathos*, disease],   any disease or disorder that affects a single nerve trunk. Some common causes of disorders involving single nerve trunks are electric shock, radiation, and fractured bones that may compress or lacerate nerve fibers. Casts and tourniquets that are too tight may also damage a nerve by compression or by ischemia. The peripheral nerve trunks are especially vulnerable to compression and entrapment.

mononeuropathy multiplex,   a peripheral nerve disorder characterized by numbness, pain, and weakness in several areas of the body. The symptoms may develop suddenly in the region supplied by one peripheral nerve and days later in the region of another nerve.

mononuclear /-nyŏŏ″klē-ər/   [Gk, *monos*, single; L, *nucleus*, nut kernel],   pertaining to one nucleus, such as a monocyte.

mononuclear leukocyte,   a white blood cell, including lymphocytes and monocytes, with a single nucleus. Also called *mononuclear cell.* Compare **polymorphonuclear.** See also **monocyte.**

mononucleosis (mono) /mon′ōnŏŏ″klē-ō″sis/   [Gk, *monos*, single; L, *nucleus*, nut kernel; Gk, *osis*, condition],   an abnormal increase in the number of mononuclear leukocytes in the blood. See also **infectious mononucleosis.**

mononucleosis spot test,   a rapid slide blood test performed to aid in the diagnosis of infectious mononucleosis, a disease caused by the Epstein-Barr virus (EBV). Abnormal findings may indicate chronic EBV infection, chronic fatigue syndrome, some forms of chronic hepatitis, and Burkitt's lymphoma, which is strongly associated with EBV.

monooctanoin /mon′ō-ok′tənō″in/,   a gallstone-dissolving agent.

■ INDICATIONS: It is used to dissolve cholesterol gallstones.

■ CONTRAINDICATIONS: It is contraindicated in patients with jaundice, severe biliary tract infection, or a history of recent duodenal ulcer or jejunitis.

■ ADVERSE EFFECTS: Adverse effects may include nausea, vomiting, diarrhea, and GI pain.

monoovular twins,   identical twins. Also called **monovular twins, monozygotic twins.**

monophagia /-fā″jə/,   the practice of eating only one kind of food.

monophasic /-fā″sik/,   having one phase, part, aspect, or stage.

monoploid, monoploidic.   See **haploid.**

monopodial symmelia,   a congenital anomaly characterized by the fusion of the lower extremities and the presence of one foot. Compare **dipodial symmelia, sirenomelia, tripodial symmelia.** See also **sympus monopus.**

monopolar electrocautery,   an electrocautery in which current is applied through a handheld active electrode and travels back to the generator through an inactive electrode attached to the patient (the grounding pad), so that the patient is part of the electrical circuit. Also called **unipolar electrocautery.**

Monopril,   an angiotensin-converting enzyme inhibitor. Brand name for **fosinopril.**

monopus /mon″əpəs/   [Gk, *monos* + *pous*, foot],   a fetus or individual with the congenital absence of a foot or leg.

monorchid /monôr″kid/,   a male who has monorchism.

monorchism /mon″ôrkiz′əm/   [Gk, *monos* + *orchis*, testicle, *ismos*, state],   a condition in which only one testicle has descended into the scrotum. Also called *monorchidism.* See also **cryptorchidism.** –*monorchidic, adj.*

monosaccharide /-sak″ərīd/   [Gk, *monos* + *sakcharon*, sugar],   a simple carbohydrate consisting of a single basic sugar unit with the general formula $C_n(H_2O)_n$, with *n* ranging from 3 to 8.

monosodium glutamate (MSG) /-sō″dē·əm/,   a food flavor enhancer derived from naturally occurring salt of glutamic acid and a cause of Chinese restaurant syndrome. It is also used in the treatment of encephalopathies associated with liver disorders. Also called **sodium glutamate.** See also **Chinese restaurant syndrome.**

monosodium urate monohydrate,   the monosodium salt of uric acid, deposited as needle-shaped crystals in the joints and other sites in gout.

monosome /mon″əsōm/   [Gk, *monos* + *soma*, body],   **1.** an unpaired X or Y chromosome, usually X. Also called **accessory chromosome. 2.** the single, unpaired chromosome in monosomy.

monosomy /mon″əsō′mē/   [Gk, *monos* + *soma*, body],   a chromosomal aberration characterized by the absence of one chromosome from the normal diploid complement. In humans the monosomic cell contains 45 chromosomes and is designated 2*n* N 1, such as occurs in the XO condition in Turner syndrome. Compare **trisomy.** See also **aneuploidy.** –*monosomic, adj.*

monosomy X.   See **Turner syndrome.**

monospecific antibody,   pertaining to an antibody that binds to only one type of antigen.

monosymptomatic demyelinating disease,   acute occurrence of any one of a number of symptoms that suggest a diagnosis of multiple sclerosis. Persons who have such an attack may or may not develop multiple sclerosis.

monosynaptic reflex /-sinap″tik/   [Gk, *monos*, single, *synaptein*, to join; L, *reflectere*, to bend back],   a reflex requiring only one afferent and one efferent neuron.

monotherapy /mon′ōther′əpē/   [Gk, *monos*, single + *therapeia*, treatment],   treatment of a condition by means of a single drug.

monotropy /mənot″rəpē/   [Gk, *monos* + *trepein*, to turn],   **1.** a concept, named by J. Bowlby, describing the phenomenon in which an infant appears to be able to bond with only one primary caregiver at a time. –*monotropic, adj.* **2.** (in chemistry) the existence of allotropes of an element, one of which is stable and the other is metastable under all known conditions.

monounsaturated fatty acids.   See **unsaturated fatty acid.**

monovalent /-vā″lənt/, **1.** describing an atom or radical having the valence or combining power of one hydrogen atom. Also called **univalent.** See also **valence. 2.** describing a serum antibody capable of combining with only one antigen or complement.

monovular. See **uniovular.**

monovular twins. See **monoovular twins.**

monovulatory /mənō″vyələtôr′ē/ [Gk, *monos* + L, *ovulum,* small egg, *orius,* characterized by], routinely releasing one ovum during each ovarian cycle. Compare **diovulatory.**

monozygotic (MZ) /-zīgō″tik/ [Gk, *monos* + *zygon,* yoke], pertaining to or developed from a single fertilized ovum, or zygote, such as occurs in identical twins. Compare **dizygotic.** –*monozygous, adj.,* –*monozygosity, n.*

monozygotic twins, two offspring born of the same pregnancy and developed from a single fertilized ovum that splits into equal halves during an early cleavage phase in embryonic development, giving rise to separate fetuses. Such twins are always of the same sex, have the same genetic constitution, possess identical blood groups, and closely resemble each other in physical, psychological, and mental characteristics. Monozygotic twins may have single or separate placentas and membranes, depending on the time during development when division occurs. Monozygotic twinning occurs with relatively uniform frequency in all races, is unaffected by heredity, and represents approximately one third of all twin births. Also called **enzygotic twins, identical twins, true twins, uniovular twins.** Compare **dizygotic twins.** See also **Siamese twins.**

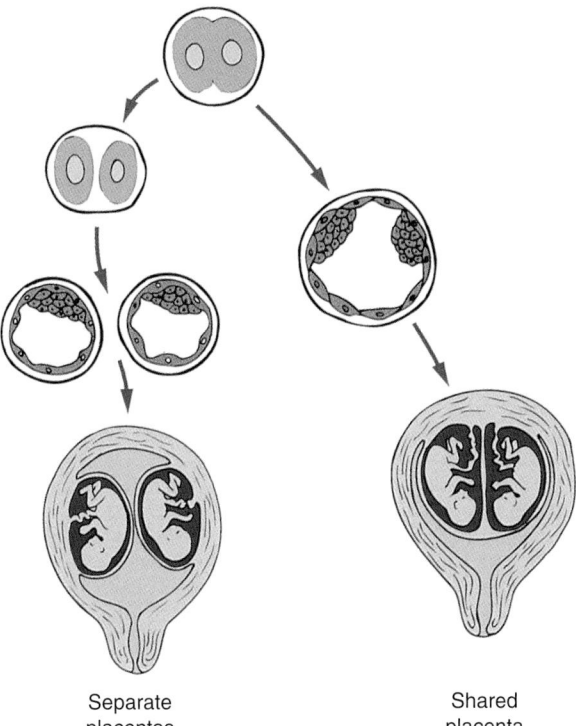

Separate placentas

Shared placenta

Monozygotic twins *(Carlson, 2009)*

Monro-Kellie doctrine /mənrō′ kel′ē/ [Alexander Monro, Scottish anatomist and surgeon, 1733–1817; George Kellie, Scottish anatomist, late 18th century], the doctrine that the central nervous system and its accompanying fluids are enclosed in a rigid container whose total volume tends to remain constant. An increase in volume of one component (e.g., brain, blood, or cerebrospinal fluid) will elevate pressure and decrease the volume of one of the other elements.

mons /mons/ [L, mountain], a mound or slight elevation.

Monsel's solution /monselz′/, a reddish-brown aqueous solution of basic ferric sulfate, prepared from ferrous sulfate and nitric acid and used as an astringent and hemostatic.

Monson curve [George S. Monson, American dentist, 1869–1933; L, *curvus,* a bend], the curve of occlusion in which each tooth cusp and incisal edge lie on the surface of a sphere 8 inches (20 cm) in diameter, with its center in the region of the glabella.

mons pubis. See **mons veneris.**

mons veneris /ven″əris/ [L, *mons,* mountain; *venus,* love], a pad of fatty tissue and thick skin that overlies the symphysis pubis in the woman. After puberty it is covered with pubic hair. Also called **mons pubis, mount of Venus.**

Monteggia fracture /mon-tejxə/ [Giovanni B. Monteggia, Italian physician, 1762–1815], a break in the ulna, associated with radial dislocation or rupture of the annular ligament and resulting in the angulation or overriding of ulnar fragments. Also called *parry fracture.*

montelukast, a leukotriene receptor.

■ INDICATIONS: It is used to treat chronic asthma.

■ CONTRAINDICATIONS: Known hypersensitivity to this drug prohibits its use.

■ ADVERSE EFFECTS: Adverse effects include dizziness, fatigue, headache, abdominal pain, dyspepsia, abnormal liver function tests, rash, asthenia, influenza, cough, and nasal congestion.

Montenegro test /mon′tənā″grō/, a test used in the diagnosis of cutaneous leishmaniasis, in which killed *Leishmania* antigens are injected intradermally. A positive reaction is indicated by the appearance of a palpable nodule in 48 to 72 hours. Also called **leishmanin test.**

Montercaux fracture /monterkō″/, a break in the neck of the fibula associated with the dislocation of the ankle mortise joint.

Montgomery gland. See **areolar gland.**

Montgomery strap /montgom′ərē/, a band of adhesive tape featuring a lace-up design, used to secure dressings that must be changed frequently.

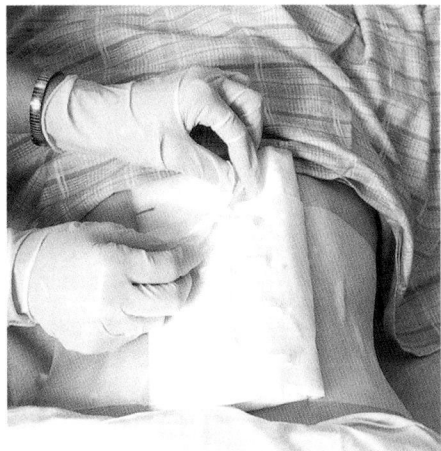

Montgomery strap *(Harkreader, Hogan, and Thobaben, 2007)*

mood, a prolonged subjective emotional state that influences one's whole personality and perception of the world. Examples include sadness, elation, and anger. See also **affect.**

mood-congruent psychotic features /-kon″grōō·ənt/ [AS, *mod,* mind; L, *congruere,* to come together], the characteristics of a psychosis in which the content of hallucinations or delusions is consistent with an elevated, expansive mood or with a depression. Mood congruence is most often noted in mood disorders, whereas schizophrenia is often a mood-incongruent disorder.

mood disorder [AS, *mod,* mind; L, *dis + ordo,* rank], a variety of conditions characterized by a disturbance in mood as the main feature. If mild and occasional, the feelings may be normal. If more severe, they may be a sign of a major depressive disorder or dysthymic reaction or be symptomatic of a bipolar disorder. Other mood disorders may be caused by a general medical condition. Also called **affective disorder.**

mood swing, an oscillation between periods of feelings of well-being and depression. Occasional "blue" periods are not regarded as abnormal. The swings are longer and more intense in persons with manic-depression. See also **bipolar disorder.**

mood theme, a communication theme in which the underlying idea is the emotion communicated by the individual. See **communication theme.**

moon face [AS, *mona,* moon; L, *facies,* face], a condition characterized by a rounded, puffy face. It occurs in people treated with large doses of corticosteroids, such as those with chronic asthma, rheumatoid arthritis, or acute childhood leukemia. The features return to normal when the medication is stopped. Moon face is symptomatic of Cushing disease and Cushing syndrome. Also called *moon facies.* See also **Cushing disease, Cushing syndrome.**

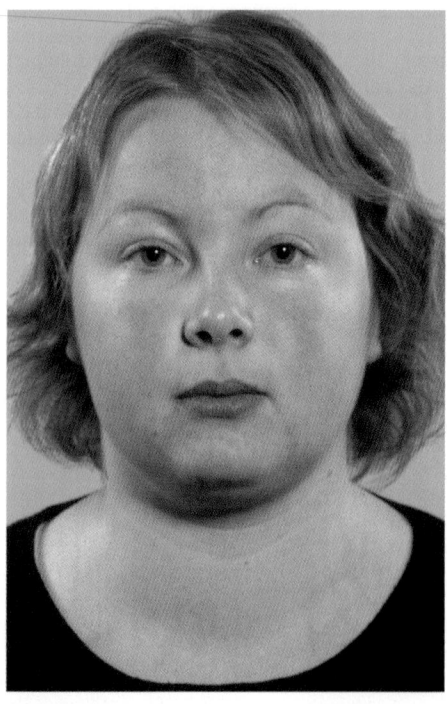

Young woman with a moon face *(Douglas et al, 2013)*

Moore, Ruth Ella /mor/ [1903–1994], the first African-American woman to earn a Ph.D. in bacteriology. Her areas of research were blood groups and the family Enterobacteriaceae.

Moore fracture [Edward M. Moore, American surgeon, 1814–1902], a break in the distal radius with associated dislocation of the ulnar head, which causes the styloid process to be secured under the annular ligaments of the wrist.

Moore, Shirley M., a nursing theorist who, with Cornelia M. Ruland, developed the Peaceful End of Life Theory, which asserts that nurses are integral to the creation of peaceful end-of-life care, which includes freedom from suffering, emotional support, closeness to and participation by significant others, and treatment with empathy and respect. The theory was developed from a standard of care created by expert nurses to manage the care of patients with terminal illness.

8-MOP. See **methoxsalen.**

MOPP /mop/, a combination drug regimen used in the treatment of cancer that contains three antineoplastics, Mustargen (mechlorethamine hydrochloride), Oncovin (vincristine sulfate), and Matulane (procarbazine hydrochloride), plus prednisone (a glucocorticoid). MOPP is prescribed in the treatment of Hodgkin disease. Abbreviation for *Mustargen, Oncovin, procarbazine hydrochloride, prednisone.*

moral distress, an emotional state experienced when an individual recognizes an ethically correct course of action in a situation, yet he or she is unable to follow that course of action.

Moraxella, a genus of the Neisseriaceae family of gram-negative nonmotile cocci. They are found as pathogens and parasites on the mucous membranes of warm-blooded animals.

Moraxella catarrhalis, a species of aerobic nonmotile bacteria found in both the normal and the diseased nasopharynx. It is a cause of otitis media and respiratory diseases. It is a significant pathogen in children and patients with underlying conditions. Formerly called *Neisseria catarrhalis.*

Moraxella lacunata, a species of nonmotile cocci that causes corneal infections and subacute conjunctivitis or angular conjunctivitis in humans.

morbid [L, *morbidus,* diseased], **1.** pertaining to a pathological or diseased condition, either physical or mental. **2.** preoccupied with unwholesome ideas.

morbid anatomy. See **pathological anatomy.**

morbidity /môrbid″itē/ [L, *morbidus,* diseased], **1.** an illness or an abnormal condition or quality. **2.** (in statistics) the rate at which an illness or abnormality occurs, calculated by dividing the number of people who are affected within a group by the entire number of people in that group. **3.** the rate at which an illness occurs in a particular area or population.

Morbidity and Mortality Weekly Report, a weekly epidemiological report on the incidence of communicable diseases and deaths in 120 urban areas of the United States. It is published by the U.S. Centers for Disease Control and Prevention in Atlanta, Georgia. The publication also includes information on accident rates and important international health data.

morbidity rate [L, *morbidus,* diseased, *ratum,* calculation], the number of cases of a particular disease occurring in a single year per a specified population unit, as *x* cases per 1000. It also may be calculated on the basis of age groups, sex, occupation, or other population unit.

morbidity statistics [L, *morbidus,* diseased, *status,* condition], a branch of statistics that is concerned with the disease rate of a population or geographic region.

morbid obesity [L, *morbidus,* diseased, *obesitas,* fatness], an excess of body fat, or weight of 100 pounds over ideal body weight, that increases the risk of developing cardiac and endocrine disturbances, including coronary artery disease and diabetes mellitus, as well as some kinds of cancer.

morbid physiology. See **pathological physiology.**

morbilli. See **measles.**

morbilliform /môrbil″ifôrm/ [L, *morbilli,* little disease, *forma,* form], describing a skin condition that resembles the erythematous maculopapular rash of measles, such as a drug rash.

morcellation, division of solid tissue (as a tumor) into pieces, followed by removal of those pieces.

mordant /môr″dənt/, a substance capable of deepening the reaction of a biological specimen to a stain. The chief mordants are alum, aniline, oil, and phenol.

Morel's syndrome. See **hyperostosis frontalis interna.**

Morgagni globule /môrgan″yē/ [Giovanni B. Morgagni, Italian anatomist, 1682–1771], a minute opaque sphere that may form from fluid coagulation between the eye lens and its capsule, especially in cataract. See also **globule.**

Morgagni's tubercle [Giovanni B. Morgagni], one of several small soft nodules on the surface of each of the areolae in women. The tubercles are produced by large sebaceous glands just below the surface of each areola. They secrete a bacteriostatic lubricating substance during pregnancy and lactation.

morgan /môr″gən/ [Thomas H. Morgan, American biologist, 1866–1945], a unit of measure used in mapping the relative distances between genes on a chromosome. The measurement uses the total crossover value as the basic unit so that 1 morgan equals 100% crossing over or 1 centimorgan equals 1% recombination. One centimorgan is also equal to one map unit. See also **map unit.**

Morganella morganii, urease-producing bacteria found in urinary tract infections and enteric bacteriosis.

morgue /môrg/ [Fr, mortuary], a unit of a hospital with facilities for the storage and autopsy of the dead.

moribund /môr″ibund/ [L, *moribundus,* dying], near death or in the act of dying.

moricizine /morĭ′sĭzēn/, a phenothiazine derivative used as the hydrochloride salt in treatment of ventricular arrhythmias.

morinda, an evergreen shrub that is native to Asia, Australia, and Polynesia.

■ INDICATIONS: This herb is used for headache; arthritis; and digestive, heart, and liver conditions, but there are no reliable data regarding efficacy.

■ CONTRAINDICATIONS: It should not be used during pregnancy and lactation, in children, or in those with known hypersensitivity to this herb or hyperkalemia.

Morita therapy /môrē″tä/ [Shomei Morita, Japanese physician, 1874–1938], an alternative therapy founded between 1910 and 1920 that has as its focus the symptoms of the patient. Its goal is character building, which enables the patient to live responsibly and constructively, even if the symptoms persist.

morning-after pill [AS, *morgen + aefter + pilian,* to peel], *(Informal)* initially, a reference to a large dose of an estrogen given orally over a short period to a woman within 24 to 72 hours after sexual intercourse to prevent conception, most commonly in an emergency such as rape or incest. The woman is warned that the medication may cause the formation of clots, severe nausea and vomiting, and teratogenic and carcinogenic effects on the fetus if pregnancy already exists or if contraception fails. A newer "morning-after" option, mifepristone, provides an effective method of preventing pregnancy with fewer side effects; a single dose prevents pregnancy by interfering with ovulation or preventing implantation.

morning dip, a significant decline in maximal expiratory flow rate (MEFR) observed in some asthmatic patients during the early morning. The MEFR in an asthmatic person tends to follow a circadian rhythm, with a morning dip and a high point in midafternoon.

morning glory. See *Rivea corymbosa.*

morning ptosis, a temporary paralysis of the upper eyelid on awakening from sleep. Also called **waking ptosis.**

morning sickness. See **nausea and vomiting of pregnancy.**

morning stiffness [OE, *morgen + stif*], a period of muscular stiffness after awakening in the morning, a common complaint of patients with arthritis or similar musculoskeletal disorders.

Moro reflex /môr″ō/ [Ernst Moro, German pediatrician, 1874–1951], a normal mass reflex in a young infant (up to 3 to 4 months of age) elicited by a sudden loud noise, such as by striking the table next to the child or by raising the head slightly and allowing it to drop. A normal response consists of flexion of the legs, an embracing posture of the arms, and usually a brief cry. Also called **startle reflex.**

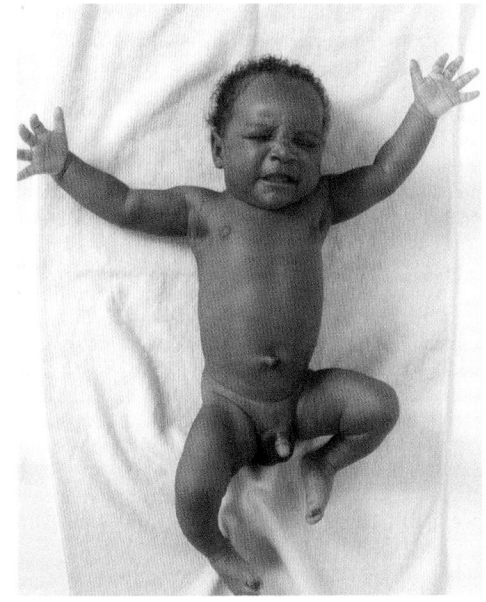

Moro reflex *(Courtesy Paul Vincent Kuntz, Texas Children's Hospital)*

morph-, morpho-, -morph, combining form meaning "form or shape": *endomorph, morphea, morphogenesis.*

morphea /môr″fē·ə/ [Gk, *morphe,* form], the most common type of localized scleroderma. Morphea is characterized by patches of yellowish or ivory-colored hard, dry, smooth skin, usually painless. It is more common in females. Also called **Addison keloid, localized scleroderma.** Also spelled **morphoea.** Formerly called **circumscribed scleroderma.**

-morphia, -morphy, suffix meaning "a condition of form": *pantamorphia.*

morphine /môr″fēn/ [Gk, *Morpheus,* god of sleep], a white crystalline alkaloid derived from the opium poppy, *Papaver somniferum,* the source of its principal pharmacological activity. Morphine acts on the central nervous system to produce both depression and euphoric stimulation, effects that are mediated through its stimulation of mu opioid receptors. Stimulation of mu receptors exerts effects that depress nerve impulse transmission. Even in small amounts morphine depresses the respiratory system. Mu receptors' activation in some instances inhibits the transmission of inhibitory

M

impulses, thereby causing stimulation. Examples of this include the euphoric response and constriction of the pupils by the third cranial nerve. Morphine has a marked analgesic effect because of its stimulation of mu receptors in both the brain and spinal cord, and its principal therapeutic value is for the relief of moderate to severe pain. Morphine rarely provides total relief of pain, but in most cases it reduces the level of suffering. Patients with severe pain may become drowsy and relaxed but seldom achieve the sensation of euphoria associated with use of the drug. Morphine is often given parenterally because its rapid absorption following oral administration is followed by rapid first-pass metabolism to an inactive glucuronide (oral bioavailability ranges from 17% to 33%). Repeated use of morphine leads to tolerance, necessitating increased dosage levels to get the same degree of pain relief. See also **morphine sulfate, morphine tartrate.**

morphine poisoning, adverse effect of injection or ingestion of opioids, marked by symptoms of pinpoint pupils, drowsiness, and shallow respiration. Emergency treatment includes gastric lavage, charcoal, and respiratory support. Naloxone is administered intravenously as needed to arouse the patient, and IV fluid is given to support circulation.

morphine sulfate, an opioid analgesic.
■ INDICATIONS: It is prescribed for relief of moderate to severe pain, including that from myocardial infarction and dyspnea caused by left heart failure, and as a preanesthetic.
■ CONTRAINDICATIONS: Drug dependence or known hypersensitivity to this drug prohibits its use.
■ ADVERSE EFFECTS: Among the more serious adverse effects are increased intracranial pressure, cardiovascular disturbances, respiratory depression, and drug dependence. Nausea, vomiting, constipation, and xerostomia are common.

morphine tartrate, a white crystalline powder used in injections of morphine. It is more soluble in water than morphine itself and is used in various parenteral preparations.

morphinism /môr″finiz′əm/, a pathological state caused by morphine addiction.

-morphism, suffix meaning "the condition of having a (specified) shape": *allomorphism, anthropomorphism, polymorphism.*

morpho-. See **morph-, morpho-, -morph.**

morphoea. See **morphea.**

morphogen /môr″fəjen/, **1.** a soluble substance that controls the embryonic differentiation of a cell or tissue. **2.** a substance secreted by one group of cells that causes a specific change in the growth and differentiation of a different group.

morphogenesis /môr″fəjen″əsis/ [Gk, *morphe* + *genein,* to produce], the development and differentiation of the structures and form of an organism, specifically the changes that occur in the cells and tissue during embryonic development. Also called **morphogeny.**

morphogenetic /-jənet″ik/, (in embryology) pertaining to a substance or hormone that acts as an evocator in differentiation. Also *morphogenic.* See also **differentiation.**

morphogeny. See **morphogenesis.**

morphology /môrfol″əjē/ [Gk, *morphe* + *logos,* science], the study of the physical shape and size of a specimen, plant, or animal. *—morphological, adj.*

morphometry /môrfom″ətrē/, the measurement of the structures and parts of organisms.

-morphosis, suffix meaning "a development or change": *cytomorphosis, metamorphosis.*

Morquio disease /môrkē″ō/ [Luis Morquio, Uruguayan physician, 1867–1935], a familial form of mucopolysaccharidosis that results in abnormal musculoskeletal development in childhood. Dwarfism, hunchback, enlarged sternum, and knock-knees may occur. The disease may first be evident as the child, learning to walk, displays an abnormal, waddling gait. Also called **MPS IV.** See also **mucopolysaccharidosis.**

mortal [L, *mortalis,* perishable], **1.** subject to death. **2.** causing death.

mortality [L, *mortalis,* perishable], **1.** the condition of being subject to death. **2.** the death rate, which reflects the number of deaths per unit of population in any specific region, age group, disease, or other classification, usually expressed as deaths per 1000, 10,000, or 100,000.

mortar /môr″tər/ [L, *mortarium*], a cup-shaped vessel in which materials are ground or crushed by a pestle in the preparation of drugs.

mortinatality /môr″tinātal″itē/ [L, *mors,* death, *natus,* birth], the stillbirth rate. It is calculated by multiplying the number of stillbirths by 1000 and dividing by the total number of births per year. Also called **natimortality.**

mortise joint /môr″tis/ [ME, *mortays,* fixed in, *jungere,* to join], the articulatio talocruralis joint of the ankle.

Morton disease [Thomas G. Morton, American surgeon, 1835–1903; L, *dis* + Fr, *aise,* ease], a form of foot neuralgia caused by a falling metatarsal arch, which puts pressure on the digital branches of the lateral plantar nerve. Also called *Morton foot,* **Morton plantar neuralgia,** *Morton neuroma,* **Morton toe.**

Morton plantar neuralgia [Thomas G. Morton; L, *planta,* foot sole; Gk, *neuron,* nerve, *algos,* pain], a severe throbbing pain that affects the anastomotic nerve branch between the medial and the lateral plantar nerves.

Morton syndrome [Dudley J. Morton, American orthopedist, 1884–1960; Gk, *syn,* together, *dromos,* course], a congenital foreshortening of the first metatarsal segment, causing pain and deformity of the front part of the foot.

Morton toe. See **Morton disease.**

mortuary /môr″chəwer′ē/ [L, *mortuarium,* tomb], a building where the bodies of deceased persons are held for identification, postmortem examination, and preparation for burial or cremation.

morula /môr″ələ/ *pl. morulas, morulae* [L, *morulus,* blackberry], a solid, spherical mass of cells resulting from the cleavage of the fertilized ovum in the early stages of embryonic development. It represents an intermediate stage between the zygote and the blastocyst and consists of blastomeres that are uniform in size, shape, and physiological capabilities. *—morular, adj.*

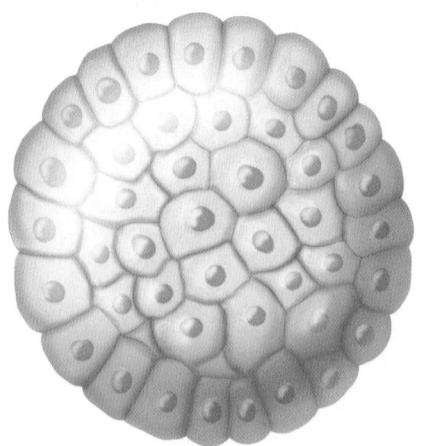

Morula *(Patton and Thibodeau, 2016)*

morulae, morulas. See **morula.**

Morvan disease, a form of syringomyelia with tissue changes in the extremities, such as a paresthesia of the forearms and hands and progressive painless ulceration of the fingertips.

mosaic /mōzā″ik/ [L, *Musa,* goddess of the arts], **1.** an individual or organism that developed from a single zygote but that has two or more kinds of genetically different cell populations. Mosaicism may result from a mutation, crossing over, or, more commonly in humans, nondisjunction of chromosomes during early embryogenesis, which causes a variation in the number of chromosomes in the cells. The type of chromosomal aberration and the fraction of cells that are affected depend on the cleavage stage at which the causative event occurred. Because monosomic cells are nonviable, except in X monosomic conditions, most mosaic conditions caused by nondisjunction in humans represent a mixture of normal and trisomic cells, regardless of whether an autosome or the sex chromosomes are involved. The degree of clinical involvement depends on the type of tissue containing the abnormality and may vary from near normal to full manifestation of a syndrome, such as Down syndrome or Turner syndrome. Compare **chimera.** See also **monosomy, sex chromosome mosaic, trisomy. 2.** a fertilized ovum that undergoes determinate cleavage. See also **mosaic development. −mosaicism,** *n.*

mosaic bone, bone tissue appearing to be made up of many tiny pieces cemented together, as seen on microscopic examination of an x-ray film of the affected bone. It is characteristic of Paget disease. See also **Paget disease.**

mosaic cleavage. See **determinate cleavage.**

mosaic development, a kind of embryonic development occurring in the blastocyst. The fertilized ovum undergoes determinate cleavage, developing according to a precise, unalterable plan in which each blastomere has a characteristic position and limited developmental potency and is a precursor of a specific part of the embryo. Damage to or destruction of these cells results in a defective organism. Compare **regulative development.**

mosaicism /mōzā″isiz′əm/ [L, *Musa,* goddess of the arts], (in genetics) a condition in which an individual or an organism that develops from a single zygote has two or more cell populations that differ in genetic constitution. Most commonly seen in humans is a variation in the number of chromosomes in the cells, which may involve either a particular autosome, such as in Down syndrome, or the sex chromosomes, such as in Turner syndrome and Klinefelter syndrome. See also **mosaic, sex chromosome mosaic.**

mosaic wart, a group of contiguous plantar warts.

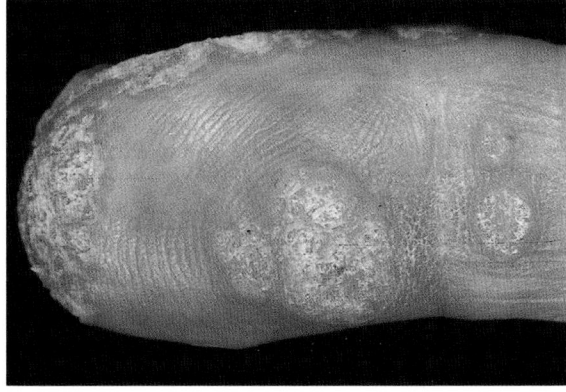

Mosaic wart *(du Vivier, 2002)*

mosquito bite /məskē″tō/ [L, *musca,* a fly; AS, *bitan,* to bite], a bite of a blood-sucking arthropod of the subfamily Culicidae that may result in a systemic allergic reaction in a hypersensitive person, an infection, or, most often, a pruritic wheal. Mosquitoes, which are attracted to hosts by moisture, carbon dioxide, estrogens, sweat, or warmth, are vectors of many infectious diseases.

mosquito forceps, a small hemostatic forceps. See also **Halsted forceps,** def. 1.

Mössbauer spectrometer /mes″bou·ər, mœs″bou·ər/ [Rudolf L. Mössbauer, German physicist, 1929–2011], an instrument that can detect small changes between an atomic nucleus and its environment, such as caused by alterations in temperature, pressure, or chemical state. The device is used in chemical and physical research with applications in medicine.

most probable number, (in bacteriology) a statistical value representing the viable bacterial population in a sample through the use of dilution and multiple tube inoculations.

mot-, prefix meaning "movement": *motoneuron, motivation, motility.*

mother fixation [AS, *modor,* mother; L, *figere,* to fasten], an arrest in psychosexual development characterized by an abnormally persistent, close, and often paralyzing emotional attachment to one's mother. Compare **father fixation.** See also **freudian fixation.**

Mothers Against Drunk Driving (MADD), a nonprofit organization in the United States and Canada dedicated to ending drunk and drugged driving, preventing underage drinking, and supporting victims affected by these crimes.

mother yaw. See **yaw.**

motilin /mōtil″in/, a peptide hormone secreted by enterochromaffin cells of the intestinal tract. It stimulates GI motility and pepsin secretion.

motility /mō″tilitē/ [L, *motare,* to move often], spontaneous but unconscious or involuntary movement. −*motile, adj.*

-motility, -mobility, suffix meaning "the condition of being capable of movement": *hypermotility, hypomotility.*

-motine, suffix for antiviral quinoline derivatives.

motion sickness. See **kinesia.**

motivation /mō′tivā″shən/ [L, *movere,* to move], conscious or unconscious needs, interests, rewards, or other incentives that arouse, channel, or maintain a particular behavior.

motivational conflict /mō′tivā″shənəl/ [L, *movere,* to move, *alis,* relating to, *confluere,* to come together], a conflict resulting from the arousal of two or more motives that direct behavior toward incompatible goals. Kinds include **approach-approach conflict, approach-avoidance conflict, avoidance-avoidance conflict.**

motoneuron /mō′tōnŏŏr″on/ [L, *movere,* to move; Gk, *neuron,* nerve], a motor neuron. Its function is to produce muscle contractions.

motor [L, *movere,* to move], **1.** pertaining to motion, the body apparatus involved in movement, or the brain functions that direct purposeful activities. **2.** pertaining to a muscle, nerve, or brain center that produces or subserves motion.

-motor, suffix meaning "effects of activity in a body part": *nervimotor, psychomotor.*

motor aphasia, the inability to say remembered words, caused by a cerebral lesion in the inferior frontal gyrus (Broca's motor speech area) of the left hemisphere. The condition most commonly is the result of a stroke. The patient knows what to say but cannot articulate the words. Also called **ataxic aphasia, expressive aphasia, frontocortical aphasia, verbal aphasia.**

motor apraxia, the inability to carry out planned movements or to handle small objects, although cognizant of the proper use of the object. The condition results from a lesion in the premotor frontal cortex on the opposite side of the affected limb. Also called **innervation apraxia.** See also **apraxia.**

M

motor area, a portion of the cerebral cortex that includes the precentral gyrus and the posterior part of the frontal gyri and that causes the contraction of the voluntary muscles on stimulation with electrodes. Normal voluntary activity requires associations between the motor area and other parts of the cortex; removal of the motor area from one cerebral hemisphere causes paralysis of voluntary muscles, especially of the opposite side of the body. Various parts of the motor area are associated with different body structures, such as the lower limb, the face, the mouth, and the hand. The parts associated with more delicate, complicated movements, such as those of the hand, are larger than those associated with more general movements.

motor ataxia, an inability to perform coordinated movements. Also called **kinetic ataxia.**

motor control, the systematic transmission of nerve impulses from the motor cortex to motor units, resulting in coordinated contractions of muscles.

motor control frame of reference, (in occupational therapy) a task-oriented approach that encourages the repetition of desired movements in a variety of settings and circumstances. Motor control frame of reference proposes that motor control is best achieved when individuals perform whole tasks that are meaningful to them in the natural environment.

motor coordination, the harmonious functioning of body parts that involve movement, including gross motor movement, fine motor movement, and motor planning.

motor depressant [L, *movere,* to move, *deprimere,* to press down], a drug or agent that reduces the normal functioning level of motor neurons, mainly in voluntary muscles.

motor end plate, a large special synaptic contact between motor axons and each skeletal muscle fiber. Each muscle fiber forms one end plate. See also **end plate.**

motor fiber, one of the fibers (axons) in the cranial and spinal nerves that transmit impulses to and cause contraction of muscle fibers.

motor hallucination [L, *movere,* to move, *alucinari,* wandering mind], the subjective experience of movement when there is no movement.

motor image, a visual concept of one's bodily movements, real or imagined.

motor learning, the process of improving motor skills through practice, with long-lasting changes in the capability for responding. The cerebellum and basal nuclei play a major role in such coordination.

motor nerve, an efferent nerve that conveys impulses to motor end plates or another terminal and is mainly responsible for stimulating muscles and glands.

motor neuron, one of various efferent nerve cells that transmit nerve impulses from the brain or from the spinal cord to muscular or glandular tissue. According to location, some kinds of motor neurons are the peripheral motor neurons and the upper motor neurons. Also called **motoneuron.** Compare **sensory nerve.** See also **nervous system.**

motor neuron disease [L, *movere,* to move, *neuron,* nerve; L, *dis* + Fr, *aise,* ease], any disease of a motor neuron, with degeneration of anterior horn cells, motor cranial nerve nuclei, and pyramidal tracts. Kinds include **amyotrophic lateral sclerosis.**

motor neuron paralysis, an injury to the spinal cord that causes damage to the motor neurons and results in various degrees of functional impairment, depending on the site of the lesion. See also **lower motor neuron paralysis, upper motor neuron paralysis.**

motor nucleus [L, *movere,* to move, *nucleus,* nut kernel], the nucleus of a motor nerve or collection of motor neurons.

motor pathway [L, *movere,* to move; AS, *paeth*], the route of motor nerve impulses from the central neuron to a muscle or gland.

motor planning, the ability to plan and execute skilled, nonhabitual tasks. Also called **motor praxis.**

motor point, 1. a point at which a motor nerve enters a muscle. 2. any point on the skin over a muscle at which electrical stimulation (via electrode) causes contraction of the muscle. See also **motor nerve, nervous system.**

motor praxis. See **motor planning.**

motor protein, protein that moves along a surface, propelled by the energy of adenosine triphosphate hydrolysis.

motor root [L, *movere,* to move; AS, *rot*], the proximal end of a motor nerve at its attachment to the spinal cord.

motor seizure, abnormal electrical activity that arises initially in a localized motor area of the cerebral cortex. The manifestations depend on the site of the abnormal electrical activity, such as tonic contractures of the thumb caused by excessive discharges in the motor area of the cortex controlling the first digit or chewing movements resulting from discharges in the lower part of the motor strip controlling mastication. The disturbance may spread, resulting in generalized convulsion, or it may end in a shower of clonic movements. See also **epilepsy, focal seizure.**

motor sense, the feeling or perception enabling a person to accomplish a purposeful movement, presumably achieved by evoking a sensory engram or memory of the pattern for that specific movement. Proprioceptive signals transmitted by feedback pathways through the cerebellum and sensory areas of the motor cortex are compared with the engram and modify the movement. Experiments with animals show that a movement cannot be performed if the corresponding sensory area of the brain is removed. If the motor area is removed, the movement is accomplished by using a different group of muscles.

motor speech areas [L, *movere,* to move; AS, *spaec* + L, *area,* vacant place], the regions of the cerebral hemispheres that are associated with motor control of speech. For right-handed people the sites are generally located in the left hemisphere. See also **Broca's area.**

motor tract [L, *movere,* to move, *tractus*], an efferent nerve pathway that conveys impulses controlling movement.

motor unit, a functional structure consisting of a motor neuron and the muscle fibers it innervates.

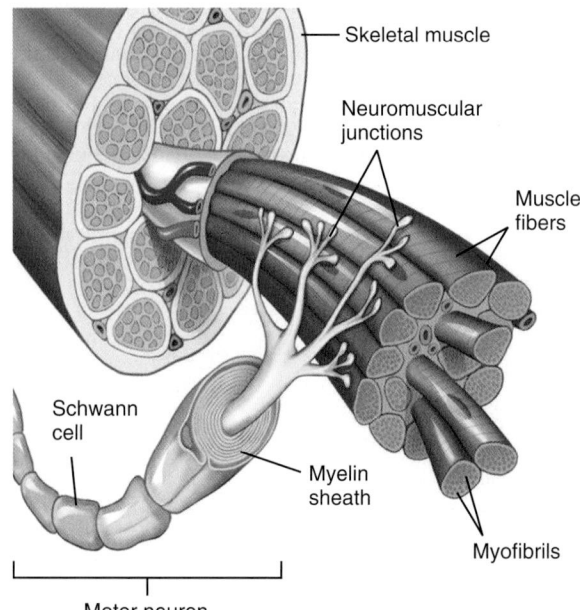

Skeletal muscle

Neuromuscular junctions

Muscle fibers

Schwann cell

Myelin sheath

Myofibrils

Motor neuron

Motor unit

motor unit recruitment, the bringing into activity of additional motor neurons, which causes additional muscle fibers to contract. As more units are recruited and as the frequency of discharge increases, muscle tension increases. The pattern of motor unit recruitment varies, depending on the inherent properties of specific motor neurons.

mottle [ME, *motley,* mixed colors], an effect observed in radiographic imaging when the dose of radiation used is reduced to a level at which individual quantum effects can be seen. At very low doses, the number of photons being produced is so small that the statistical variations in x-ray production can be visualized. Also called **noise, quantum mottle.**

mountain fever. See **Colorado tick fever, Rocky Mountain spotted fever.**

mountain sickness. See **altitude sickness.**

mountain tick fever. See **Colorado tick fever, Rocky Mountain spotted fever.**

mounting /mount′ing/, the preparation of specimens and slides for study.

mount of Venus. See **mons veneris.**

mourning /môr′ning/ [AS, *murnan,* to mourn], a response to the loss of a loved object. It is through mourning that grief is resolved. See also **bereavement, grief.**

mouse [L, *mus*], a hand-controlled computer input device. Moving the device on a flat surface and pushing buttons on its back cause the cursor or pointer to move to target areas or select items on a computer screen. See also **joystick.**

mouse-tooth forceps, a kind of dressing forceps that has one or more fine sharp points on the tip of each blade. The tips turn in, and the delicate teeth interlock.

mouth [AS, *muth*], **1.** the nearly oval oral cavity at the superior, anterior end of the digestive tube, bounded anteriorly by the lips and containing the tongue and the teeth. It consists of the vestibule and the oral cavity proper. The vestibule, situated in front of the teeth, is bounded externally by the lips and the cheeks, internally by the gums and the teeth. The vestibule receives the secretion from the parotid salivary glands. The oral cavity proper is bounded by the alveolar arches and the teeth, communicates with the pharynx, and is roofed by the hard and the soft palates. The tongue forms the greater part of the floor of the cavity. The rest of the floor is formed by the reflection of the mucous membrane from the sides and the bottom of the tongue to the gum lining the inner part of the mandible. The oral cavity proper receives the secretion from the submandibular and sublingual salivary glands. **2.** an orifice.

mouth breathing, breathing through the mouth instead of the nose, usually because of some obstruction of the nasal passages.

mouth guard, a soft, plastic, intraoral appliance that covers the palate and all the occlusal and incisal surfaces of the teeth. It is worn in contact sports to limit damage to tissues of the mouth, lips, and other oral surfaces. Compare **biteguard.**

mouth rinse /mouth′rins/, a solution for cleaning or treating the oral mucosa and controlling dental caries. A typical therapeutic mouth rinse may contain sodium fluoride, glycerine, alcohol, detergents, and other ingredients. Some mouth rinses only remove loose debris and add a fragrance to mask mouth odors.

mouthstick /mouth′stik/, a device that is gripped with the teeth and can be used to type, push buttons, turn pages, operate power wheelchairs, or modify environmental control units and other equipment. It is commonly used by individuals who have a high-level (C4 and up) tetraplegia. Compare **chinstick.**

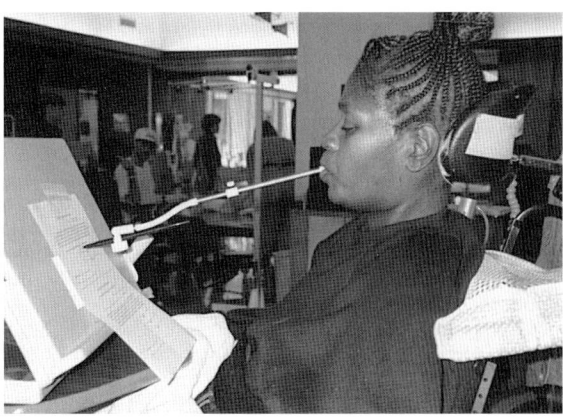

Client using mouthstick for writing *(Umphred et al, 2013)*

mouth-to-mouth resuscitation, a procedure in artificial resuscitation, performed most often with cardiac massage. The victim's nose is sealed by pinching the nostrils closed, the head is extended, and air is breathed by the rescuer through the mouth into the lungs. A mouth-to-mask/rescue shield is often used for rescue breathing. See also **cardiopulmonary resuscitation.**

mouth-to-nose resuscitation, a procedure in artificial resuscitation in which the mouth of the victim is covered and held closed and air is breathed through the victim's nose. See also **mouth-to-mouth resuscitation.**

mouthwash /mouth′wôsh/, a medicated liquid used for cleaning the oral cavity and treating mucous membranes of the mouth. Many over-the-counter mouthwashes contain alcohol, which may contribute to surface softening and increased wear of dental resins and composite materials. See also **mouth rinse.**

MOV, abbreviation for **minimal occlusive volume.**

movement decomposition [L, *movere,* to move, *de,* away, *componere,* to assemble], a distortion in voluntary movement in which motion occurs in a distinct sequence of isolated steps rather than in a normal, smooth, flowing pattern.

movement disorder, any of numerous neurological disorders characterized by disturbances of muscular movement, distinguished as either hyperkinetic (conditions such as chorea, dystonia, hemiballismus, myoclonus, stereotypy, tic, and tremor) or hypokinetic (conditions such as akinetic mutism, psychomotor slowing, and the stiff-man syndrome).

movement therapy, a movement-based therapeutic technique that aids in release of expressions or feelings and aids in promoting feeling and awareness.

moving grid, an x-ray grid that is continuously moved or oscillated throughout the exposure of a radiographic image.

moxibustion /mok″səbus″chən/ [Jpn, *moe kusa,* burning herb; L, *comburere,* to burn up], a method of producing analgesia or altering the function of a body system by igniting moxa, wormwood, or another combustible, slow-burning substance and holding it as near the point on the skin as possible without causing pain or burning. It is also sometimes used with acupuncture.

moxifloxacin, an antiinfective.

■ INDICATIONS: It is used to treat acute bacterial sinusitis caused by *Streptococcus pneumoniae, Haemophilus influenzae,* and *Moraxella catarrhalis;* acute bacterial exacerbation of chronic bronchitis from *S. pneumoniae, H. influenzae, H. parainfluenzae, Klebsiella pneumoniae, Staphylococcus aureus,* and *M. catarrhalis;* and community-acquired

M

pneumonia from *S. pneumoniae, H. influenzae, Mycoplasma pneumoniae, Chlamydia pneumoniae,* and *M. catarrhalis.*

■ CONTRAINDICATIONS: Known hypersensitivity to quinolones prohibits its use.

■ ADVERSE EFFECTS: Seizures are a life-threatening effect of this drug. Other adverse effects include prolonged QT interval, dizziness, fatigue, insomnia, depression, confusion, increased ALT and AST, flatulence, heartburn, oral candidiasis, dysphagia, pruritus, urticaria, photosensitivity, flushing, fever, chills, tremor, arthralgia, and tendon rupture. Common side effects include headache, restlessness, nausea, diarrhea, and rash.

moxifloxacin hydrochloride, the hydrochloride salt of moxifloxacin, administered orally in the treatment of bacterial exacerbation of chronic bronchitis, acute sinusitis, community-acquired pneumonia, and skin and skin structure infections caused by susceptible organisms.

moyamoya disease /moi″əmoi″ə/, a cerebrovascular disorder in which the main cerebral arteries at the base of the brain are replaced by a fine network of vessels. It is caused by progressive stenosis of the large-caliber vessels and development of collateral network. It tends mainly to affect Japanese children and young adults and is characterized by convulsions, hemiplegia, cognitive impairment, and subarachnoid hemorrhage. Patients who survive into adulthood are susceptible to massive intracerebral hemorrhage caused by rupture of the fragile network of new vessels. Few patients live beyond 30 years of age.

6-MP, abbreviation for *6-mercaptopurine.* See **mercaptopurine.**

MPD, M.P.D., abbreviation for **maximum permissible dose.**

MPGN, abbreviation for **membranoproliferative glomerulonephritis.**

M.P.H., abbreviation for *Master of Public Health.*

MPL + PRED, an anticancer drug combination of melphalan and prednisone.

MPO, abbreviation for **myeloperoxidase.**

MPR, abbreviation for **multiplanar reformatting.**

MPS, abbreviation for **mucopolysaccharidosis.**

MPS I, abbreviation for *mucopolysaccharidosis I.* See **Hurler syndrome.**

MPS II, abbreviation for *mucopolysaccharidosis II.* See **Hunter syndrome.**

MPS IV, abbreviation for *mucopolysaccharidosis IV.* See **Morquio disease.**

MPS IV & MPS VII. See **mucopolysaccharidosis.**

MQF, abbreviation for *mobile quarantine facility.*

MQSA, abbreviation for **Mammography Quality Standards Act.**

mr, mR, abbreviation for **milliroentgen.**

mrad, abbreviation for **millirad.**

mrem, abbreviation for **millirem.**

MRI, abbreviation for **magnetic resonance imaging.**

mRNA, abbreviation for **messenger RNA.**

MRSA, initialism for *methicillin-resistant Staphylococcus aureus.*

MS, abbreviation for **multiple sclerosis.**

M.S., **1.** abbreviation for *Master of Science.* **2.** abbreviation for *Master of Surgery.*

MSAFP, abbreviation for *maternal serum alpha-fetoprotein.* See **maternal serum alpha-fetoprotein (MSAFP) test.**

msec, abbreviation for **millisecond.**

MSG, abbreviation for **monosodium glutamate.**

MSH, abbreviation for **melanocyte-stimulating hormone.**

MSLT, abbreviation for **multiple sleep latency test.**

MS/MS, abbreviation for **tandem mass spectrometry.**

MSN, initialism for *Master of Science in Nursing.*

MSO, abbreviation for **management service organization.**

M.T., abbreviation for **medical technologist.** See **clinical laboratory scientist/medical technologist.**

MTOC, abbreviation for **microtubule organizing center.**

MTT, abbreviation for **maximal treadmill test.**

MTX + MP + CTX, an anticancer drug combination of methotrexate, mercaptopurine, and cyclophosphamide.

mu /myo̅o̅, mo̅o̅/, **1.** μ, M, the twelfth letter of the Greek alphabet. **2.** μ. Symbol for **micron.**

muc-, muco-, prefix meaning "mucus": *mucolytic, mucosal.*

Mucha-Habermann disease /mo̅o̅′kä hä′bermän/ [Viktor Mucha, Austrian dermatologist, 1877–1919; Rudolf Habermann, German dermatologist, 1884–1941], an acute or subacute, sometimes relapsing, widespread macular, papular, or vesicular eruption that tends to crusting, necrosis, and hemorrhage, which heals and leaves pigmented depressed scars, followed by the development of a new crop of lesions. Occasionally, progression to a chronic form may occur. Also called **acute lichenoid pityriasis, acute parapsoriasis, Habermann disease, parapsoriasis varioliformis acuta, pityriasis lichenoides et varioliformis acuta.**

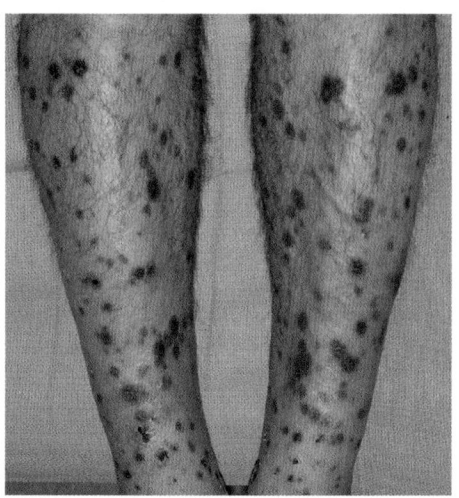

Lesions associated with Mucha-Habermann disease *(Bolognia et al, 2014)*

Much granules /mo̅o̅k, mo̅o̅kh/ [Hans C. Much, German physician, 1880–1932], granules and rods, found in tuberculosis sputum, that stain with Gram stain but not by the usual methods for acid-fast bacilli.

μCi, abbreviation for **microcurie.**

mucilage /m(y)o̅o̅′səlij/, **1.** a sticky mixture of carbohydrates produced by plant cell activity. **2.** a thick aqueous solution of a gum used for suspending insoluble substances and for increasing viscosity.

mucin /myo̅o̅′sin/ [L, *mucus,* slime], a mucopolysaccharide, the chief ingredient in mucus. Mucin is present in most glands that secrete mucus and is the lubricant protecting body surfaces from friction or erosion.

mucinase. See **mucopolysaccharidase.**

mucinoid /myo̅o̅′sinoid/ [L, *mucus* + Gk, *eidos,* form], **1.** resembling mucin. **2.** See **mucoid,** def. 2.

mucinous carcinoma /myo̅o̅′sinəs/, an epithelial neoplasm characterized by a sticky gelatinous consistency caused by copious mucin secretion. Also called *colloid carcinoma,* **gelatiniform carcinoma,** *mucinous adenocarcinoma.* Formerly called **gelatinous carcinoma.**

mucocele /myoo̅′kōsēl/ [L, *mucus,* slime; Gk, *koilia,* cavity], **1.** dilation of a cavity with accumulated mucus secretion. **2.** a dome-shaped mucosal swelling caused by a rupture of a salivary gland duct, which spills mucin into the surrounding tissues. A mucocele is usually caused by trauma. See **mucus extravasation phenomenon, mucus retention cyst.**

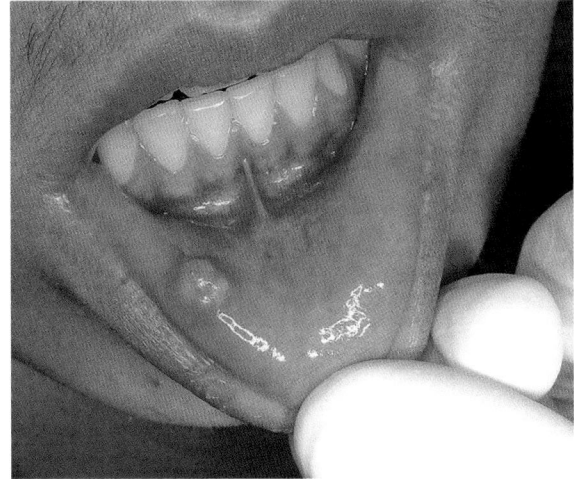

Mucocele *(Wu et al, 2011)*

mucocutaneous /myoo̅′kōkyootā″nē·əs/ [L, *mucus* + *cutis,* skin, *osus,* having], pertaining to the mucous membrane and the skin.

mucocutaneous leishmaniasis. See **American leishmaniasis.**

mucocutaneous lymph node syndrome (MLNS), an acute febrile illness, primarily of young children, characterized by inflamed mucous membranes of the mouth; "strawberry tongue"; cervical lymphadenopathy; polymorphous rash on the trunk; and edema, erythema, and desquamation of the skin on the extremities. Other commonly associated findings include arthralgia, diarrhea, otitis, pneumonia, photophobia, meningitis, and electrocardiographic changes. The cause is unknown. No clear-cut environmental, seasonal, or geographic factors have been discovered, and person-to-person transmission is unproved. A genetic predisposition has been indicated. Treatment includes IV gammaglobulin; aspirin in large doses, which may be prescribed over a long period; and supportive care. Also called **Kawasaki disease.**

■ OBSERVATIONS: The acute stage of the disease begins with a remittent fever (103° F to 105° F) accompanied by extreme irritability, lethargy, and intermittent colicky abdominal pain. The fever typically lasts 7 days to 2 weeks and is unresponsive to antibiotics. After 1 to 2 days, bilateral conjunctivitis occurs. Within 5 days, there is erythema and edema of the hands and feet, a macular rash on the trunk and perineum, strawberry tongue, fissuring of the lips, and reddened pharynx. Cervical lymphadenopathy is present. Ten to 25 days after onset, fever resolves and symptoms diminish. Irritability, anorexia, and conjunctivitis remain. There is peeling of the hands and feet, arthritis, arthralgia, and thrombocytosis. The greatest risk for coronary artery aneurysm occurs during this time. During convalescence, all clinical signs have resolved, but erythrocyte sedimentation rate is still abnormal. ESR blood values return to normal about 6 to 8 weeks after onset. Clinical exam reveals a history of fever with four of five of the following conditions: conjunctivitis, changes in mucosa of oropharynx, edema and erythema of hands and feet, nonvesicular truncal rash, and lymphadenopathy. Blood studies reveal elevated WBCs and platelets; elevated ESR; positive C-reactive protein; and elevated ALT and AST. Chest x-rays may reveal pulmonary infiltrates. An echocardiogram may show depressed left ventricular function. Echocardiograms are also useful to monitor cardiac status during the course of the disease. Complications include coronary arteritis, coronary artery aneurysms, and thrombotic occlusion of an aneurysm leading to a myocardial infarction and possible death. However, prognosis with treatment is excellent, with a mortality rate of less than 0.1%.

■ INTERVENTIONS: Intravenous immunoglobulin is the primary treatment to reduce inflammation in the acute stage. Aspirin therapy is used until temperatures return to normal. Corticosteroids increase possibility of aneurysm and are contraindicated in treatment of MLNS. Anticoagulant and antiplatelet therapy may be used if there is evidence of coronary thrombosis. If the child develops cardiac complications, percutaneous transluminal coronary angioplasty, coronary bypass grafting, or cardiac transplant may be required.

■ PATIENT CARE CONSIDERATIONS: Care is primarily supportive and includes careful monitoring of cardiac status, careful fluid replacement, I & O, comfort measures (lubrication for lips, lotion for skin, and cool cloths), quiet soothing environment, and parental support in attempting to console an irritable child. Parental education is needed about possible cardiac complications. Caregiver instruction in CPR should be provided if cardiac complications are present.

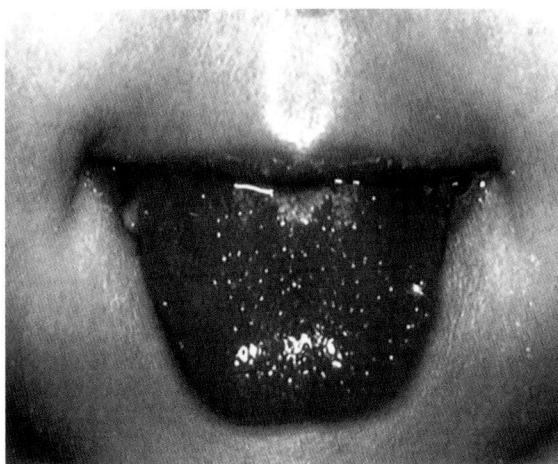

Mucocutaneous lymph node syndrome (Kawasaki disease) *(Hurwitz, 1993/Courtesy Tomisaku Kawasaki, MD)*

mucoderm®, an acellular collagen matrix utilized in autologous soft tissue augmentation for dental implants.

mucoepidermoid carcinoma /myoo̅′kō·ep′idur″moid/ [L, *mucus* + Gk, *epi,* above, *derma,* skin, *eidos,* form], a malignant neoplasm of glandular tissues, especially the ducts of the salivary glands. The tumor contains mucinous and epidermoid squamous cells.

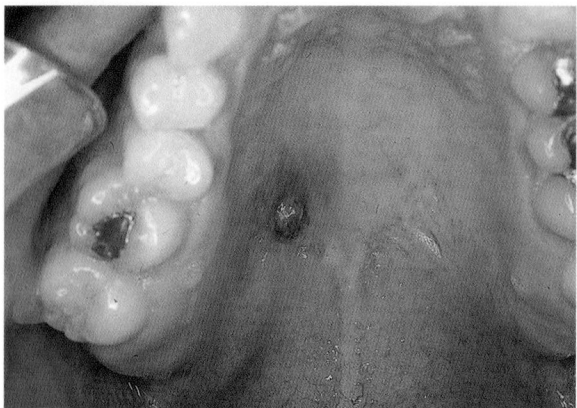

Mucoepidermoid carcinoma *(Regezi, Sciubba, and Pogrel, 2000)*

mucogingival junction /myo͞o′kōjinjī″vəl/ [L, *mucus* + *gingiva,* gum, *jungere,* to join], the scalloped linear area of the gums that separates the free gingiva from the attached gingiva. It can be seen easily by pulling the mandibular lip outward and looking at the labial mucosa of the mandible. Also called *alveolar mucosa.*

mucogingival line. See **free gingival groove.**

mucoid /myo͞o″koid/ [L, *mucus* + Gk, *eidos,* form], **1.** resembling mucus. **2.** pertaining to a group of glycoproteins, including colloid and ovomucoid, similar to the mucins, primarily differing in solubility. Also called **mucinoid.**

mucoid cyst [L, *mucus* + Gk, *eidos,* form, *kytis,* bag], a cyst formed by an overgrowth of a mucous gland or by the spread of mucus into the interstitial tissues. Also called **mucous cyst.**

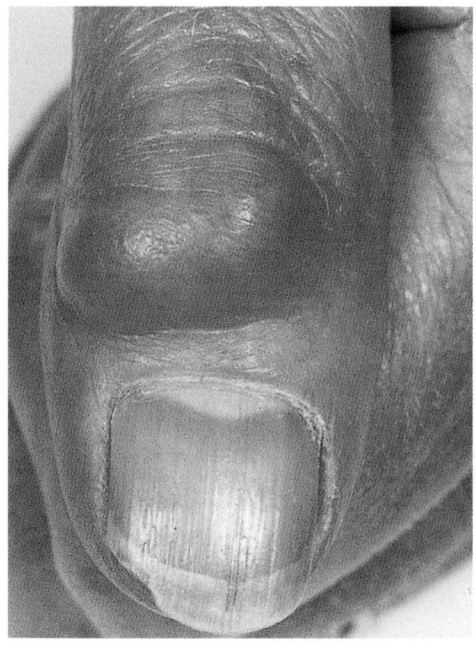

Mucoid cyst *(du Vivier, 2002)*

mucoid tissue. See **embryonic tissue.**

mucolipidosis /myo͞o′kōlip′idō″sis/, any of a group of metabolic disorders characterized by an accumulation of mucopolysaccharides and lipids in the tissues, but without an excess of mucopolysaccharides in the urine. Mucolipidosis includes I cell disease (mucolipidosis II) and pseudo-Hurler polydystrophy (mucolipidosis III).

mucolipidosis II. See **I cell disease.**

mucolipidosis IV, an autosomal-recessive disorder characterized by psychomotor slowing and severe visual impairment, initially manifest in infancy or childhood as corneal clouding. Sialic acid–containing gangliosides are accumulated as a result of deficient ganglioside sialidase activity. However, the deficiency is not believed to be the primary defect.

mucolytic /myo͞o′kəlit″ik/ [L, *mucus* + Gk, *lysis,* loosening], **1.** exerting a destructive effect on mucus. **2.** any agent that dissolves or destroys mucus.

mucomembranous /myo͞o′kəmem″brənəs/ [L, *mucus* + *membrana,* thin skin, *osus,* having], pertaining to a mucous membrane, such as that of the small intestine or the bladder.

Mucomyst, a mucolytic drug; also the antidote for acute acetaminophen poisoning. Brand name for **acetylcysteine.**

mucopolysaccharidase /myo͞o′kōpol′ēsak″əridās′/, an enzyme that breaks down molecules of polysaccharides. Also called **mucinase.**

mucopolysaccharide /myo͞o′kōpol′ēsak″ərīd/ [L, *mucus* + Gk, *polys,* many, *sakcharon,* sugar], a polysaccharide containing hexosamine and sometimes occurring with protein, such as mucins.

mucopolysaccharidosis (MPS) /myo͞o′kōpol′ēsak′əridō″sis/ *pl. mucopolysaccharidoses* [L, *mucus* + Gk, *polys,* many, *sakcharon,* sugar, *osis,* condition], one of a group of genetic disorders characterized by greater-than-normal accumulations of mucopolysaccharides in the tissues, with other symptoms specific to each type. The disorders are numbered MPS I through MPS VII, and each type has a specific eponym. All types are characterized by pronounced skeletal deformity (especially of the face), cognitive impairment and physical slowing, and decreased life expectancy. The disorders may be detected before birth by testing fetal cells present in amniotic fluid. After birth, diagnosis is established through urine testing, skeletal changes observed on radiographic films, and family history. There is no successful treatment. Kinds include **Hunter syndrome, Hurler syndrome, Morquio disease, Sanfilippo syndrome, Sly syndrome.**

mucoprotein /myo͞o′kōprō″tēn, -tē·in/ [L, *mucus* + Gk, *proteios,* first rank], a compound, present in all connective and supporting tissue, that contains polysaccharides combined with protein. It is relatively resistant to denaturation.

mucopurulent /myo͞o′kōpyo͞or″yələnt/ [L, *mucus* + *purulentus,* pus], characteristic of a combination of mucus and pus.

Mucorales, an order of perfect fungi of the class Zygomycetes, made up of bread molds and related fungi. Genera *Absidia, Mucor,* and *Rhizopus* can cause opportunistic mucormycosis in humans.

mucormycosis. See **zygomycosis.**

mucosa /myo͞okō″sə/ *pl. mucosae.* See **mucous membrane.**

mucosal immune system /myo͞okō″səl/, the lymphoid tissues of the mucosal surfaces lining the GI, respiratory, and urogenital tracts.

mucosal neuroma syndrome /mo͞oko″säl no͞oro′mä/. See **multiple endocrine neoplasia, type III.**

mucosal prolapse, prolapse of the mucosa in part of the GI tract. In the colon it sometimes occurs with congenital megacolon.

mucositis /myoo͞′kōsī″tis/, any inflammation of a mucous membrane, such as the lining of the mouth and throat.

mucosulfatidosis. See **multiple sulfatase deficiency.**

mucous. See **mucus.**

-mucous, suffix meaning "containing or composed of or secreting mucus": *submucous.*

mucous colitis. See **irritable bowel syndrome.**

mucous cyst. See **mucoid cyst.**

mucous membrane /myoo͞′kəs/ [L, *mucus + membrana,* thin skin], any one of four major kinds of thin sheets of tissue that cover or line various parts of the body. Mucous membrane lines cavities or canals of the body that open to the outside, such as the linings of the mouth, the digestive tube, the respiratory passages, and the genitourinary tract. It consists of a surface layer of epithelial tissue covering a deeper layer of connective tissue and protects the underlying structure, secretes mucus, and absorbs water, salts, and other solutes. Also called **mucosa.** Compare **serous membrane, skin, synovial membrane.**

mucous plug, (in obstetrics) a collection of thick mucus in the uterine cervix that is often expelled at the onset of dilation of the cervix, just before labor begins or in its early hours. The plug may be dry and firm, following the shape of the endocervical canal, but more often it is semifluid and mucoid, streaked with blood.

mucous shreds. See **shreds.**

mucous tissue. See **embryonic tissue.**

mucous tumor. See **myxoma.**

mucoviscidosis. See **cystic fibrosis.**

mucus /myoo͞′kəs/ [L, slime], the viscous, slippery secretions of mucous membranes and glands, containing mucin, white blood cells, water, inorganic salts, and exfoliated cells. **–mucoid, mucous,** *adj.*

mucus extravasation phenomenon, leakage of mucus into the surrounding connective tissue from a damaged minor salivary gland excretory duct followed by an inflammatory reaction leading to the formation of a pool of macrophages and mucin surrounded by a wall of granulation tissue, visible as a small nodule or vesicle on the oral mucosa. Also called **mucocele.** Compare **mucus retention cyst, ranula.**

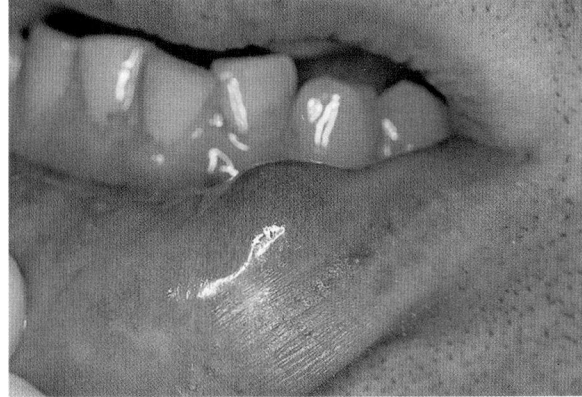

Mucus extravasation phenomenon *(Regezi, Sciubba, and Jordan, 2008)*

mucus retention cyst, a slimy-clear substance that develops an epithelium-lined cavity around itself. It is caused by blockage of a salivary gland duct with mucus, visible as a small nodule on the oral mucosa. Also called **mucocele.** Compare **mucus extravasation phenomenon.**

mucus trap suction apparatus, a catheter containing a trap to prevent mucus being aspirated from the nasopharynx and trachea of a newborn from entering the mouth of the person operating the device. Mucus traps are also found in adult respiratory equipment. Mucus goes into the trap rather than into the suction bottle and can then be sent for analysis.

mud bath, the application of warm mud to the body for therapeutic purposes, especially the relief of pain associated with arthritic disorders.

mud fever, a type of leptospirosis occurring in the summer and autumn in Germany and Russia, caused by *Leptospira interrogans.* It is transmitted to humans by the field mouse *Microtus arvalis* and affects mainly workers in swamps or flooded fields. Also called **autumn fever.**

μF, abbreviation for **microfarad.**

MUGA, acronym for *multigated acquisition scan.*

μg, abbreviation for **microgram.**

mulberry molar, a malformed first adult or secondary molar characterized by dwarfing of the cusps and hypertrophy of the enamel surrounding the cusp with agglomeration of masses of globules, giving it the appearance of a mulberry. It is seen in congenital syphilis and certain other diseases. Also called *mulberry tooth.*

mulibrey nanism /mul′ibrī/, a rare genetic disorder, transmitted as an autosomal-recessive trait, characterized by dwarfism, constrictive pericarditis, muscular hypotonia, anomalies of the skull and face, and characteristic yellow dots in the ocular fundus. The name of the condition is an abbreviation composed of the first two letters of the anatomical sites of the principal defects: *mu*scle, *li*ver, *br*ain, and *ey*es.

müllerian duct /miler″ē-ən, mYl-/ [Johannes P. Müller, German physiologist, 1801–1858], one of a pair of embryonic ducts that become the fallopian tubes, uterus, and vagina in females and that atrophy in males, resulting in formation of the prostatic utricle.

Müller's law /mil′ərz, mYl-/ [Johannes P. Müller], the principle that each type of sensory nerve cell normally responds to only one specific stimulus and gives rise to one sensation. A cell may be excited artificially by other forms of stimuli, but the sensation evoked will be the same. Also called **law of specific nerve energies.**

Müller's maneuver [Johannes P. Müller], an inspiratory effort against a closed airway or glottis. The effort decreases intrapulmonary and intrathoracic pressures and expands pulmonary gas. It is used during fluoroscopic examination to help visualize esophageal varices because it also causes engorgement of intrathoracic vascular structures.

multi- /mul′ti-/, prefix meaning "many": *multipara.*

multiaxial joint. See **ball-and-socket joint.**

multibacillary /mul″tibas′ilare/, having numerous bacilli. See also **leprosy.**

multicellular /-sel″yələr/, **1.** consisting of more than one cell. **2.** containing many cavities.

multicentric mitosis. See **multipolar mitosis.**

multicomponent virus /-kəmpō″nənt/, a virus that occurs in two or more different particles. Each particle contains only one part of the viral genome.

multidisciplinary health care team /-dis″ipliner′ē/, a group of health care workers who are members of different disciplines, each providing specific services to the patient. See also **interprofessional.**

multidrug resistance, **1.** the resistance of tumor cells to more than one chemotherapeutic agent. Resistance may be aided by a P-glycoprotein transmembrane pump that lowers the concentration of drugs in the cell. **2.** the resistance of bacteria, especially *Mycobacterium tuberculosis,* against more than two of the antibiotics that were once effective.

M

multidrug-resistant organisms, antimicrobial resistance, such as in methicillin-resistant *Staphylococcus aureus* and vancomycin-resistant enterococcis.

multifactorial /-faktôr″ē·əl/ [L, *multus,* many, *facere,* to make], pertaining to or characteristic of any condition or disease resulting from the interaction of many factors, specifically the interaction of several genes, usually polygenes, with or without the involvement of environmental factors. Many disorders, such as spina bifida, neural tube defects, and Hirschsprung disease, are considered to be multifactorial.

multifactorial inheritance, the tendency to develop a physical appearance, disease, or condition that is a condition of many genetic and environmental factors, such as stature and blood pressure. See also **polygene.**

multifidus, a group of transversospinales muscles that span the length of the vertebral column. They are best developed in the lumbar region.

multifocal /-fō″kəl/ [L, *multus* + *focus,* hearth], characterized by more than two ectopic foci that pace the heart. The foci may be atrial or ventricular.

multifocal atrial tachycardia, an atrial rhythm with a rate exceeding 100 beats/min caused by multifocal atrial activity and characterized by at least three different shapes of P′ waves on the electrocardiogram. The condition is often associated with chronic obstructive lung disease. Also called **chaotic atrial tachycardia.**

multifocal motor neuropathy, an acquired, autoimmune neuropathy characterized by progressive, asymmetric muscle weakness, affecting especially the arms, with little or no sensory deficit. Electrophysiologically, there is a persistent conduction block in motor nerves.

multiform /mul″tifôrm/ [L, *multus,* many, *forma*], an organ, tissue, or other object that appears in more than one shape.

multigenerational model /-jen′ərā″shənəl/, a model of family therapy that focuses on reciprocal role relationships over a period and thus takes a longitudinal approach. The family is viewed as an emotional system in which patterns of interacting and coping, as well as unresolved issues, can be passed down from one generation to the next and can cause stress to the family members onto whom they are projected.

multigenerational transmission process, the repetition of relationship patterns, including divorce, suicide, and alcoholism, associated with emotional dysfunction that can be traced through several generations of the same family.

multigravida /mul′tigrav″idə/ [L, *multus* + *gravidus,* pregnancy], a woman who has been pregnant more than once. Compare **multipara, primigravida.**

multihospital system /-hos″pitəl/, a group of two or more hospitals owned, sponsored, or managed by a central organization.

multiinfarct dementia /-infärkt″/ [L, *multus* + *infarcire,* to stuff, *de,* away, *mens,* mind], a form of organic brain disease characterized by the rapid deterioration of intellectual functioning, caused by vascular disease. Symptoms include emotional lability; disturbances in memory, abstract thinking, judgment, and impulse control; and focal neurological impairment, such as gait abnormalities, pseudobulbar palsy, and paresthesia.

multilocular cyst /-lok″yələr/ [L, *multus* + *locilus,* little place; Gk, *kystis,* bag], **1.** a cyst containing several loculi or spaces. **2.** a hydatid cyst with many small irregular cavities that may contain tiny parasites with suckers and hooks for attachment but generally little fluid.

multilocular cyst of kidney, a thick-walled cyst in the kidney, found in clusters and usually unilaterally. In children it contains blastema and may develop into a Wilms tumor.

A variety in adults has more fibrous tissue than the juvenile variety.

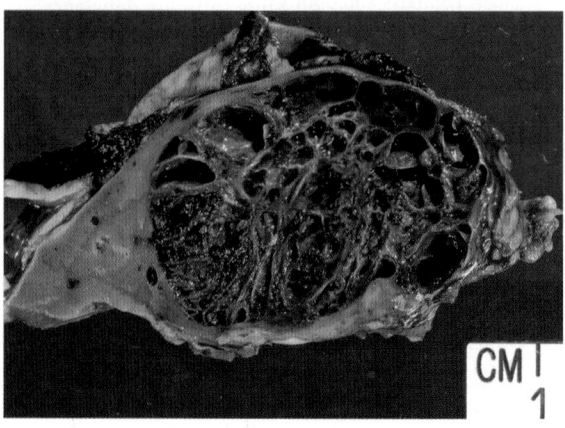

Multilocular cyst of kidney *(Zhou and Netto, 2012)*

multipara /multip″ərə/ *pl. multiparae* [L, *multus* + *parere,* to bear], a woman who has delivered more than one viable infant. Also called **pluripara.** Compare **multigravida, nullipara, primipara.**

multiparity /-per″itē/ [L, *multus,* many, *parere,* to give birth], the status of a mother of more than one child.

multiparous /multip″ərous/ [L, *multus,* many, *parere,* to give birth], having given birth to more than one child.

multipenniform /-pen″ifôrm/ [L, *multus* + *penna,* feather, *forma*], (of a body structure) having a shape resembling a pattern of many feathers, especially the pattern formed by the muscular fasciculi that converge to form several tendons. Compare **bipenniform, penniform.**

multiphase generator /-fāz″/, a generator of x-rays that operates on more than single-phase power. It usually has three phases, which greatly increases the rate at which it produces x-rays.

multiphasic screening /-fā″sik/ [L, *multus* + *phasis,* appearance; ME, *scren*], a technique of screening populations for diseases that combines a battery of screening tests. The technique serves to identify any of several diseases being screened for in a population that is apparently healthy.

multiplanar reformatting (MPR), a technique used in two-dimensional tomographic imaging (computed tomography and magnetic resonance) to generate sagittal, coronal, and oblique views from axial sections.

multiple acyl CoA dehydrogenation deficiency. See **glutaricaciduria.**

multiple autoimmune disorder (MAD) /mul″tipəl/, a condition in which a patient exhibits symptoms of at least two of a group of diseases, including Addison disease, autoimmune thyroid disease, mucocutaneous candidiasis, hypoparathyroiditis, and insulin-dependent diabetes.

multiple benign cystic epithelioma. See **trichoepithelioma.**

multiple carboxylase deficiency, an autosomal-recessive inherited aminoacidopathy correctable by biotin therapy and caused by deficiency of either of two enzymes necessary for activity of several biotin-containing carboxylases. It is characterized by metabolic ketoacidosis, excretion of organic acids in the urine, hyperammonemia, and variable manifestation of breathing difficulties, hypotonia, seizures, ataxia, alopecia, skin rash, and developmental delay. The neonatal form, caused by deficiency of holocaroxylase synthetase, may progress rapidly to coma; the juvenile form, caused by deficiency of biotinase, is characterized additionally by sensorineural deafness and optic atrophy.

multiple cartilaginous exostoses. See **diaphyseal aclasis.**

multiple endocrine adenomatosis (MEA), a condition characterized by functioning tumors in more than one endocrine gland. The disorder is commonly associated with Zollinger-Ellison syndrome and may involve the pituitary, pancreas, and parathyroid glands. It is also seen in multiple endocrine neoplasia (MEN) type I. Also called **familial multiple endocrine.** See also **adenomatosis.**

multiple endocrine deficiency syndrome. See **polyglandular deficiency syndrome.**

multiple endocrine neoplasia (MEN), a hereditary hormonal disorder that occurs in an autosomal-dominant pattern. The endocrine neoplasms may be expressed as hyperplasia, adenoma, or carcinoma and may develop synchronously or metachronously. Kinds include **multiple mucosal neuroma syndrome, Werner syndrome,** See also **multiple endocrine neoplasia, type I, multiple endocrine neoplasia, type II.**

multiple endocrine neoplasia, type I (MEN1), a type of multiple endocrine neoplasia that includes tumors of the pituitary, parathyroid glands, and pancreatic islet cells, often with peptic ulcers and sometimes the Zollinger-Ellison syndrome. See also **multiple endocrine neoplasia.**

multiple endocrine neoplasia, type II, a type of multiple endocrine neoplasia characterized by medullary carcinoma of the thyroid, pheochromocytoma, and hyperplasia of the parathyroid glands. See also **multiple endocrine neoplasia.**

multiple endocrine neoplasia, type III, a type of multiple endocrine neoplasia characterized by a body build similar to that seen in Marfan syndrome as well as mucosal neuromas of the oral and ocular tissues. Other symptoms include thickened eyelids and enlargement of corneal nerves.

multiple exostoses. See **diaphyseal aclasis.**

multiple factor. See **polygene.**

multiple family therapy [L, *multus* + *plica,* fold], psychotherapy in which several families meet weekly to confront and deal with problems or issues that they have in common.

multiple fission, cell division in which the nucleus first divides into several equal parts and then the cytoplasm divides into as many cells as there are nuclei. It is the common form of asexual reproduction in certain acellular organisms. Compare **binary fission.**

multiple fracture, **1.** a fracture break that extends several fracture lines in one bone. **2.** the fracture of several bones at one time or from the same injury.

multiple gene. See **polygene.**

multiple glandular deficiency syndrome. See **polyglandular deficiency syndrome.**

multiple idiopathic hemorrhagic sarcoma. See **Kaposi sarcoma.**

multiple lentigines syndrome. See **LEOPARD syndrome.**

multiple lipomatosis, a rare inherited disorder characterized by discrete localized subcutaneous deposits of fat in the tissues of the body. This fat is not available for metabolic use, even in starvation.

multiple-locus variable number of tandem repeat analysis (MLVA), a laboratory tool designed to recognize tandem repeats and other qualities in the genome of an individual to provide a high-resolution DNA fingerprint for the purpose of identification.

multiple mononeuropathy, an abnormal condition characterized by dysfunction of several individual nerve trunks.

It may be caused by various diseases, such as necrotizing angiopathy, uremia, diabetes mellitus, and some inflammatory immunological disorders.

multiple mucosal neuroma syndrome, a condition of multiple submucosal neuromas or neurofibromas of the lips, tongue, and eyelids. The disease affects young persons and may be associated with tumors of the thyroid or adrenal medulla or with subcutaneous neurofibromatosis. See also **multiple endocrine neoplasia.**

multiple myeloma, a malignant neoplasm of the bone marrow. The tumor, composed of B-lymphocyte plasma cells, disrupts normal bone marrow functions; destroys osseous tissue, especially in flat bones; and causes pain, fractures, hypercalcemia, and skeletal deformities. The onset is insidious, and most people are asymptomatic until the disease is advanced. In addition, the ability of the plasma cells to make functional antibodies decreases, leaving the person immunocompromised. Characteristically abnormal proteins in the plasma and urine, anemia, weight loss, pulmonary complications secondary to rib fractures, and kidney failure are present. The cause is unknown, but radiation and chemical exposure may increase risk. It occurs in people older than 50 years of age and is twice as common among African-Americans as Caucasians. It occurs equally in men and women. Also called **multiple plasmacytoma of bone, myelomatosis, plasma cell myeloma.**

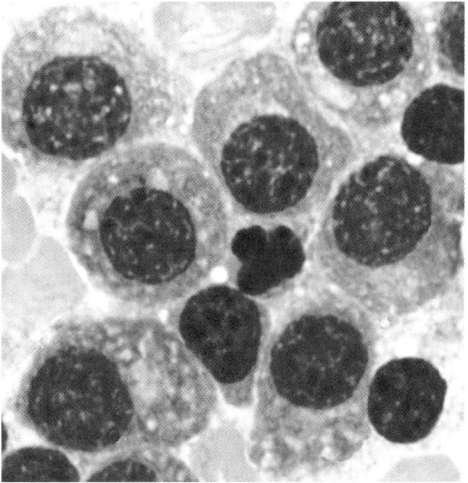

Multiple myeloma *(Carr and Rodak, 2008)*

multiple myositis. See **polymyositis.**

multiple neuroma. See **neuromatosis.**

multiple peripheral neuritis, acute or subacute disseminated inflammation or degeneration of symmetrically distributed peripheral nerves, characterized initially by numbness, tingling in the extremities, hot and cold sensations, and slight fever, progressing to pain, weakness, diminished reflexes, and, in some cases, flaccid paralysis. The disorder may be caused by toxic substances, such as antimony, arsenic, carbon monoxide, copper, lead, mercury, nitrobenzol, organophosphates, and thallium, or by various drugs, including diphenylhydantoin, isoniazid, nitrofurantoin, thalidomide, and vincristine. Multiple peripheral neuritis may occur in alcoholism, arteriosclerosis, beriberi, chronic GI disease, diabetes, leprosy, pellagra, porphyria, rheumatoid arthritis, systemic lupus erythematosus, and many infectious diseases. Therapy consists of removal of the toxic agent or treatment of the causative disease, rest, and medication for pain. See also **Guillain-Barré syndrome.**

multiple personality disorder, *(Obsolete)* now called **dissociative identity disorder.**

multiple plasmacytoma of bone. See **multiple myeloma.**

multiple pregnancy, a pregnancy in which there is more than one fetus in the uterus at the same time.

multiple pterygium syndrome, an autosomal-recessive syndrome characterized by pterygia of the neck, axillae, and popliteal, antecubital, and intercrural areas, accompanied by hypertelorism, cleft palate, micrognathia, ptosis of eyelids, and short stature. Skeletal abnormalities include camptodactyly, syndactyly, clubfoot, and flatfoot, in which the bottom of the foot resembles a rocker, as well as vertebral fusion and rib anomalies. Cryptorchidism is present in males, and labia majora are absent in females. Also called **Escobar syndrome, pterygium syndrome.**

multiple sclerosis (MS) [L, *multus* + *plica,* fold; Gk, *sklerosis,* hardening], a progressive disease characterized by disseminated demyelination of nerve fibers of the brain and spinal cord. Multifocal lesions of plaque destroy the myelin and to a varying degree, oligodendrocytes. It begins slowly, usually in young adulthood, and continues throughout life with periods of exacerbation and remission. The first signs are often paresthesias, or abnormal sensations in the extremities or on one side of the face. Other early signs are muscle weakness, vertigo, and visual disturbances, such as nystagmus, diplopia (double vision), and partial blindness. Later in the course of the disease there may be extreme emotional lability, ataxia, abnormal reflexes, and difficulty in urinating. A history of exacerbation and remission of symptoms and the presence of greater-than-normal amounts of protein in cerebrospinal fluid are characteristic. Most of the brain and spinal cord will show characteristic lesions. As the disease progresses, the intervals between exacerbations grow shorter and disability becomes greater. Treatment involves drugs that affect the function of the immune system; acute episodes, also called exacerbations, are often treated with corticosteroids. Physical therapy may help postpone or prevent specific disabilities. The patient is encouraged to live as normal and active a life as possible. Also called *disseminated multiple sclerosis.*

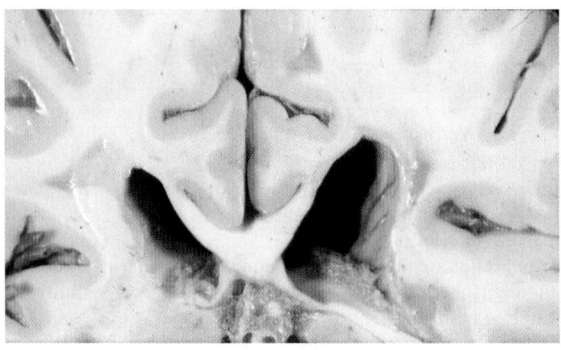

Coronal brain section showing periventricular plaques associated with multiple sclerosis *(Perkin et al, 2011)*

multiple self-healing squamous epithelioma. See **keratoacanthoma.**

multiple sleep latency test (MSLT), a test of the propensity to fall asleep, often used to diagnose narcolepsy. The subject is given five 20-minute nap opportunities at 2-hour intervals, usually after an overnight polysomnogram. The mean latency to sleep onset and the stages of sleep that occur are determined from polygraph records. Well-rested adults have a mean MSLT of 15 minutes. A mean MSLT of less than 5 minutes indicates severe hypersomnia.

multiple sulfatase deficiency, an autosomal-recessive lysosomal storage disease in which a deficiency of at least nine lysosomal and microsomal sulfatases leads to accumulation of sulfate-containing glycolipids, mucopolysaccharides, and steroids. The disorder generally presents as sulfatide lipidosis and later also shows features of mucopolysaccharidoses, variably combining phenotypic features of the specific enzymatic defects. Neurological deterioration is rapid. Also called **mucosulfatidosis.** See also **mucopolysaccharidosis.**

multiplicative growth. See **hyperplasia.**

multipolar mitosis /-pō″lər/ [L, *multus* + *polus,* pole], cell division in which the spindle has three or more poles and results in the formation of a corresponding number of daughter cells. Also called **multicentric mitosis, pluripolar mitosis.** See also **trisomy.**

multiskilled worker, a health team member with at least the education of a nurse assistant who has been trained to perform selected nursing skills and selected skills from the allied health professions under the supervision of a registered nurse. Duties may include, but are not limited to, bedmaking, bathing, assisting with elimination needs, performing phlebotomy, and recording electrocardiograms.

multisource drug /mul″tisôrs/ [L, *multus* + OFr, *sourse,* origin], a pharmaceutic that can be purchased under any of several trademarks from different manufacturers or distributors. See also **generic equivalent, generic name.**

Multispecialty Medical Group. See **Integrated Multispecialty Group.**

multispecific /-spes′ifik/, pertaining to an antibody that binds to more than one type of antigen.

multisynaptic /-sinap″tik/ [L, *multus* + Gk, *synaptein,* to join], pertaining to a nervous process or system of nerve cells requiring a series of synapses.

multitasking, performing two or more tasks with a computer at the same time. The computer actually processes a small part of one task at a time, switching from one to another in a commutative manner, but it can handle so many pieces of data in brief time segments that the operator or operators are not aware of the computer switching. Also called **time-sharing.**

multivalent /mul′tivā″lənt/ [L, *multus* + *valere,* to be strong], **1.** See **polyvalent. 2.** (in immunology) having several sites of attachment for an antibody or antigen.

multivalent vaccine [L, *multus,* many, *valere,* value, *vaccinus,* cow], a vaccine prepared from several antigenic types within a species. Also called **polyvalent vaccine.**

μm, abbreviation for **micrometer.**

mummification /mum′ifikā″shən/ [Per, *mum,* wax; L, *facere,* to make], a dried-up state, such as occurs in dry gangrene or a dead fetus in utero.

mummified fetus /mum″ifīd/, a fetus that has died in utero and has shriveled and dried.

mumps [D, *mompen,* to sulk], an acute viral disease, characterized by a swelling of the parotid glands, caused by a paramyxovirus. It is most likely to affect children between 5 and 15 years of age, but it may occur at any age. In adulthood the infection may be severe. Passive immunity from maternal antibodies usually prevents this disease in children younger than 1 year of age. The incidence of mumps is highest during the late winter and early spring. The mumps paramyxovirus is present in the saliva of the affected individual and is transmitted in droplets or by direct contact. The virus is present in the saliva from 6 days before to 9 days after the onset of the swelling of the parotid gland. The time of maximum communicability is believed to be the 48-hour period immediately before the start of parotid swelling. The prognosis in mumps is good, but the disease sometimes involves complications, such as arthritis, pancreatitis, myocarditis, oophoritis, and nephritis. About half of the men with mumps-induced orchitis suffer some atrophy of the testicles, but, because the condition is usually unilateral, sterility rarely results. Also called **epidemic parotitis, infectious parotitis.**

■ OBSERVATIONS: The common symptoms of mumps usually last for about 24 hours; they include anorexia, headache, malaise, and low-grade fever. These signs are commonly followed by earache, parotid gland swelling, and a temperature of 101° F to 104° F (38.3° C to 40° C). The patient also experiences pain when drinking acidic liquids or when chewing. The salivary glands also may become swollen. Complications, such as epididymoorchitis and mumps meningitis, may develop. In about 25% of the postpubertal men who contract mumps, epididymoorchitis with associated testicular swelling and tenderness that may persist for several weeks develops. Mumps meningitis develops in 10% of patients with mumps and occurs in three to five times as many male as female patients. Diagnosis of mumps is usually based on typical symptoms, especially parotid gland swelling. If the parotid gland is not swollen, confirming diagnosis may be based on serological antibody tests.

■ INTERVENTIONS: The treatment of mumps commonly includes the respiratory isolation of the patient and the administration of analgesics, antipyretics, and fluids adequate to prevent dehydration associated with fever and anorexia. IV fluids may be administered to the patient who cannot swallow as the result of severe parotitis.

■ PATIENT CARE CONSIDERATIONS: The patient is confined to bed and may be given antipyretics and tepid sponge baths to reduce fever. Patients with mumps are also encouraged to drink fluids and to avoid spicy or tart foods and those that require considerable chewing. During the acute phase of the disease, the nurse is especially alert to any signs of central nervous system involvement, such as nuchal rigidity and altered consciousness. All cases of mumps are routinely reported to local health authorities. Nurses aid public health education by stressing the importance of immunization with live attenuated mumps virus for children at 15 months of age and for susceptible people, especially males who are approaching puberty or who are past puberty. Immunization within 24 hours of exposure may prevent the disease or minimize its effects.

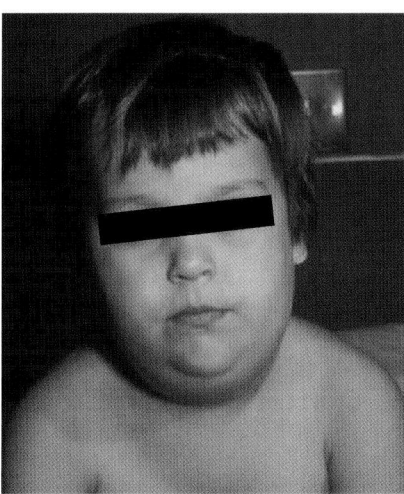

Child with mumps (Centers for Disease Control and Prevention Public Health Image Library ID#4491)

mumps orchitis, an inflammatory disorder of the testis characterized by swelling, with fever, malaise, and acute parotitis. It usually occurs in postpubertal men with a recent history of mumps and may result in testicular atrophy. Also called **orchitis parotidea.**

Mumpsvax, an active immunizing agent. Brand name for **mumps virus vaccine live.**

mumps virus, a paramyxovirus that causes mumps and sometimes tenderness and swelling of the testes, pancreas, ovaries, or other organs.

mumps virus vaccine live, an active immunizing agent.

■ INDICATIONS: It can be prescribed for immunization against mumps. People born before 1957 are considered immune. MMR (mump/measles/rubella) is generally the preferred vaccine for children and adults.

■ CONTRAINDICATIONS: Immunosuppression, concomitant use of corticosteroids, acute infection, pregnancy, or known hypersensitivity to chicken proteins, neomycin, or this drug prohibits its use.

■ ADVERSE EFFECTS: Among the most serious adverse effects are fevers, parotitis, and allergic reactions.

Münchausen syndrome /mun′chousən/ [Baron von Münchausen, German adventurer and confabulator, 1720–1797], an unusual condition characterized by habitual pleas for treatment and hospitalization for a symptomatic but imaginary acute illness. The affected person may logically and convincingly present the symptoms and history of a real disease. Symptoms resolve with treatment, but the person may seek further treatment for another imaginary disease. Also called **pathomimicry.**

Münchausen syndrome by proxy [Baron von Münchausen], a variation of Münchausen syndrome in which the parent persistently fabricates or induces illness in a child with the intent of keeping in contact with hospitals and physicians. The child may endure dozens of surgeries and hospitalizations for illness induced by the parent; nearly 9% of the children die as a result. The mother poses as being a good parent by "saving" the child from medical catastrophe, and the child serves as a manipulative object.

mural /myoo″rəl/ [L, *murus,* wall], **1.** *adj.,* pertaining to something that is found on or against the wall of a cavity, such as a mural thrombus on an interior wall of the heart. **2.** *n.,* a painting on a wall.

mural thrombus [L, *murus,* wall], a thrombus that originates in the wall of a cavity, particularly on a diseased patch of endocardium.

Murchison fever. See **Pel-Ebstein fever.**

muriatic acid /moo″rē·at″ik/ [L, *muria,* brine, *acidus,* sour], hydrochloric acid.

murine typhus /myoo″rēn/ [L, *mus,* mouse; Gk, *typhos,* stupor], an acute arbovirus infection caused by *Rickettsia typhi* and transmitted by the bite of an infected flea. The disease is similar to epidemic typhus but less severe. It is characterized by headache, chills, fever, myalgia, and rash. After an 8- to 16-day incubation period, fever develops and lasts about 12 days. A dull-red maculopapular rash, mainly on the trunk, appears about the fifth day and lasts for 4 to 8 days. Recovery is usually rapid and complete, but death has occurred in elderly or debilitated people. Weil-Felix and complement fixation tests aid in the diagnosis. Chloramphenicol or tetracycline is usually prescribed in treatment. Prevention involves the elimination of the rodents that are the natural host of the organism and the use of appropriate insecticides to control fleas. Also called **endemic typhus, flea-borne typhus, New World typhus, rat typhus, urban typhus.** Compare **epidemic typhus, Rocky Mountain spotted fever.** See also **Brill-Zinsser disease.**

murmur /mur″mər/ [L, a humming], a gentle blowing, fluttering, or humming sound, such as a heart murmur,

M

susceptible to auscultation. Kinds include **systolic murmur, diastolic murmur, continuous murmur.**

muromonab-Cd3 /myoo′rəmon″ab/, a parenteral immunosuppressant drug, a monoclonal antibody that interferes with the function of the T cell antigen recognition receptors.

■ INDICATIONS: It is used to control acute renal transplant rejection, and to control liver or pancreas rejection or graft-versus-host disease when conventional methods are unsuccessful.

■ CONTRAINDICATIONS: Hypersensitivity to muromonab-CD3 or any other murine products; patients experiencing fluid overload or those with greater than 3% weight gain over the past week; uncontrolled hypertension; or uncompensated heart failure.

■ ADVERSE EFFECTS: It causes a first-dose effect within 1 to 3 hours that ranges from mild flu-like symptoms to a life-threatening anaphylaxis. Pulmonary edema, fever, chills, breathing difficulty, chest pain, vomiting, nausea, diarrhea, and tremors are among the adverse effects associated with each administration.

Murphy sign, a test for gallbladder disease in which the patient is asked to inhale while the examiner's fingers are hooked under the liver border at the bottom of the rib cage. The inspiration causes the gallbladder to descend onto the fingers, producing pain if the gallbladder is inflamed. Deep inspiration can be very much limited.

muscarine /mus″kərēn/ [L, *musca,* fly], a choline-related alkaloid present in the poisonous mushroom *Amanita muscaria.* It is similar pharmacologically to acetylcholine, although it is not used in therapeutics.

muscarinic /mus′kərin″ik/ [L, *musca,* fly], **1.** stimulating the postganglionic parasympathetic receptor. **2.** pertaining to the poisonous activity of muscarine.

musca volitans. See **floater.**

muscle (m) /mus″əl/ [L, *musculus*], a kind of tissue composed of fibers or cells that is able to contract, causing movement of body parts and organs. Muscle fibers are richly vascular, excitable, conductive, and elastic. There are two basic kinds—striated muscle and smooth muscle. Striated muscle, which composes all skeletal muscles except the myocardium, is long and voluntary. It responds very quickly to stimulation and is paralyzed by interruption of its innervation. Smooth muscle, of which all visceral muscles are composed, is short and involuntary. It reacts slowly to all stimuli and does not entirely lose its tone if innervation is interrupted. The myocardium is sometimes classified as a third (cardiac) kind of muscle, but it is basically a striated muscle that does not contract as quickly as the striated muscles of the rest of the body. See also **cardiac muscle, striated muscle, smooth muscle.**

muscle albumin, albumin present in muscle.

muscle biopsy [L, *musculus* + Gk, *bios,* life, *opsis,* view], an examination of surgically removed muscle tissue for diagnosis.

muscle bridge, a band of myocardial tissue over one or more of the large epicardial coronary vessels. It may cause constriction of the artery during systole.

muscle cell, any contractile cell peculiar to muscle. Smooth muscle cells are elongated spindle-shaped cells containing a single nucleus and longitudinally arranged myofibrils. Cardiac and skeletal muscle cells are called muscle fibers. Also called **myocyte.** See also **muscle fiber.**

muscle cramp, a sudden intermittent pain in almost any part of the body. It may involve involuntary contractions of variable duration and be accompanied by spasms. Cramps may develop in striated muscle as a result of exertion, high temperature, and excessive loss of sodium, potassium, and magnesium through perspiration. Cramps can also be associated with arthritic conditions and exposure to cold. See also **heat cramp.**

muscle excitability /eksī′təbil″itē/, the ability of a muscle fiber to respond rapidly to a stimulating agent.

muscle fiber, any of the cells of skeletal or cardiac muscle tissue. Skeletal muscle fibers are cylindrical polynuclear cells containing contracting myofibrils, across which run transverse striations, enclosed in a sarcolemma. Cardiac muscle fibers contain one or sometimes two nuclei and myofibrils and are separated from one another by an intercalated disk; although striated, cardiac muscle fibers branch to form an interlacing network.

muscle guarding, a protective response in muscle that results from pain or fear of movement. The condition may be treated through induced relaxation of the muscle by using biofeedback to reduce electromyographic activity.

muscle of expression. See **facial muscle.**

muscle overuse syndrome. See **delayed-onset muscle soreness.**

muscle receptor, a sensory organ that responds to muscle stretch or tension, including muscle spindles and tendon organs. Also called **myoreceptor.**

muscle reeducation, the use of physical therapeutic exercises to restore muscle tone and strength after an injury or disease.

muscle relaxant, an agent that reduces the contractility of muscle fibers. Curare derivatives and succinylcholine compete with acetylcholine and block neural transmission at the myoneural junction. These drugs are used during anesthesia, in the management of patients undergoing mechanical ventilation, and in shock therapy, to reduce muscle contractions in pharmacologically or electrically induced seizures. Several drugs that relieve muscle spasms act at various levels in the central nervous system: baclofen inhibits reflexes at the spinal level; cyclobenzaprine acts primarily in the brainstem; and the benzodiazepines reduce muscle tension, chiefly by acting on mechanisms that control muscle tone. Dantrolene acts directly on muscles in reducing contraction and apparently achieves its effect by interfering with the release of calcium from the sarcoplasmic reticulum.

muscle-setting exercise, a method of maintaining muscle strength and tone by alternately contracting and relaxing a skeletal muscle or group of skeletal muscles without moving the associated body part. Such activity is useful in preventing atrophy of the muscles, especially in patients with conditions involving the joints. See also **isometric exercise.**

muscles of mastication, a group of muscles—the masseter, pterygoideus lateralis, pterygoideus medialis, and temporalis—responsible for movement of the jaws during the process of chewing. All four muscles are innervated by the mandibular division of the trigeminal nerve.

muscles of ventilation [L, *musculus* + *respirare,* to breathe], muscles that provide inspiration, partly by increasing the volume of the chest cavity so that air is drawn into the lungs, including the diaphragm and external intercostal muscles. They are aided during forced breathing by the scalenus muscles, levatores costarum, sternocleidomastoid, pectoralis major, platysma myoides, and serratus superior posterior. Muscles of forced expiration include the external and internal oblique, rectus abdominis, and transverse abdominis.

muscle spindle [L, *musculus* + AS, *spinel*], a specialized proprioceptive sensory organ composed of a bundle of fine striated intrafusal muscle fibers innervated by gamma nerve fibers. Their nuclei are gathered together near the center of each fiber to form a nuclear sac, which is surrounded in turn by sensory, annulospiral nerve endings, all enclosed in a fibrous sheath.

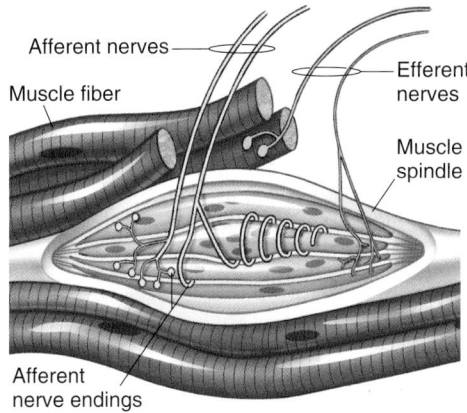

Muscle spindle

muscle testing, a method of evaluating the contractile unit, including the muscle, tendons, and associated tissues, of a moving part of the body by neurological or resistance testing. The tests may include shortened, middle, and lengthened range-of-motion ability; isokinetic measurement of muscle strength, power, and endurance; and functional tests, such as jogging or specific agility drills, as well as radiography, arthroscopy, electromyography, and other medical tests.

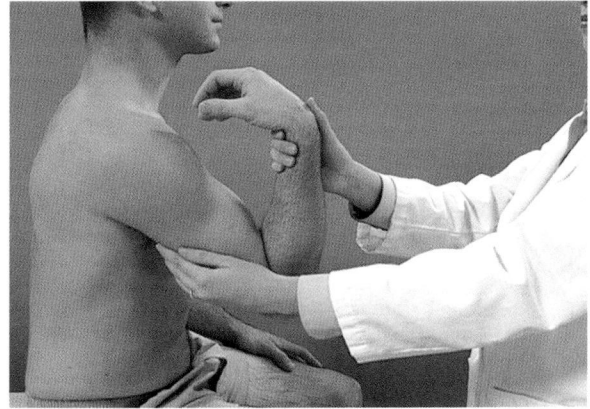

Evaluation of muscle strength (Elsevier, Clinical Skills: Essentials Collection)

muscle tone. See tonus.
muscular /mus″kyələr/ [L, musculus], 1. pertaining to a muscle. 2. characteristic of well-developed musculature.
muscular artery. See distributing artery.
muscular atrophy, a condition of motor unit dysfunction, usually the result of a loss of efferent innervation.
muscular branch of the deep brachial artery, one of several similar branches of the deep brachial artery supplying certain arm muscles, such as the coracobrachialis, biceps brachii, and brachialis.
muscular dystonia /mus″kyələr distō″nē·ə/ [L, musculus + Gk, dys + tonos, tone], a disorder characterized by uncontrollable contractions of muscles, causing repeated unnecessary movements and resulting in distorted body positions.
muscular dystrophy (MD) [L, musculus + Gk, dys, bad, trophe, nourishment], a group of genetically transmitted diseases characterized by progressive atrophy of symmetric groups of skeletal muscles without evidence of involvement or degeneration of neural tissue. In all forms of muscular dystrophy an insidious loss of strength with increasing disability and deformity occurs, although each type differs in the groups of muscles affected, the age of onset, the rate of progression, and the mode of genetic inheritance. The basic cause is unknown but appears to be an inborn error of metabolism. Serum creatine phosphokinase level is increased in affected individuals and acts as a diagnostic aid, especially in asymptomatic children in families at risk. Diagnostic confirmation is made by muscle biopsy, electromyography, and genetic pedigree. Treatment of the muscular dystrophies consists primarily of supportive measures, such as physical therapy and orthopedic procedures to minimize deformity. The main types of the disease are pseudohypertrophic (Duchenne muscular dystrophy), limb-girdle muscular dystrophy, and facioscapulohumeral muscular dystrophy. Rarer forms include Becker muscular dystrophy, distal muscular dystrophy, ocular myopathy, and myotonic muscular dystrophy. Also called **myodystrophy.** See also **myotonic myopathy.**
muscular fatigue, a condition in which a muscle loses its ability to contract as a result of overactivity. It is usually a period after stimulation during which the muscle is unresponsive to a second stimulus.
muscular incompetence [L, musculus + incompetens], a failure of a cardiac valve to close properly because of a dysfunction of the papillary muscles of the heart.
muscular sarcoidosis, the formation of epithelioid tubercles in the skeletal muscles, characterized by interstitial inflammation, fibrosis, atrophy, and damage to the muscle fibers as the tubercles form within and replace normal muscle cells. See also **sarcoidosis.**
muscular system, all of the muscles of the body, including the smooth, cardiac, and striated muscles, considered as an interrelated structural group. See also *Color Atlas of Human Anatomy,* pp. A-8 to A-11.
muscular tone [L, musculus + Gk, tonos, stretching], a normal degree of tension in muscles at rest.
muscular tremor [L, musculus + tremor, shaking], minute regular involuntary contraction of individual muscle fasciculi. If the tremors are mild and occasional, the cause may be physiological. Profuse, persistent, or recurrent widespread muscular twitching often indicates a motor neuron disorder.
muscular triangle. See inferior carotid triangle.
muscular tumor. See myoma.
musculature /mus″kyəlā′chər/, the arrangement and condition of the muscles.
musculi pectinati. See pectinate muscles.
musculo-, prefix meaning "muscle."
musculocutaneous nerve /mus′kyəlōkyo͞otā″nē·əs/ [L, musculus + cutis, skin, osus, having], one of the terminal branches of the brachial plexus. It is formed on each side by division of the lateral cord of the plexus into two branches. Various branches and filaments supply different structures, such as the biceps, the brachialis, the humerus, and the skin of the forearm. Compare **median nerve, radial nerve, ulnar nerve.**
musculophrenic artery, a terminal branch of the internal thoracic artery that passes along the costal margin, goes through the diaphragm, and ends near the last intercostal space. Its branches supply the superior part of the anterolateral abdominal wall.
musculoskeletal /mus′kyo͞olōskel″ətəl/ [L, musculus + Gk, skeletos, dried up], pertaining to the muscles and the skeleton.
musculoskeletal system, all of the muscles, bones, joints, and related structures, such as the tendons and connective

M

tissue, that function in the movement of body parts and organs. See also *Color Atlas of Human Anatomy*, pp. A-8 to A-11.

musculoskeletal system assessment, an evaluation of the condition and functioning of the patient's muscles, joints, and bones and of factors that may contribute to abnormalities in these body structures.

■ METHOD: The patient is questioned about any pain and edema in muscles, joints, and bones; weakness in extremities; limitations in movements and activities; unsteadiness on the feet; fatigability; insomnia; anorexia; and weight loss. The individual's general appearance, age, blood pressure, pulse, respirations, body alignment, ability or inability to move in bed, gait, need for assistance in walking, handgrip, range of motion, and internal and external rotation of extremities are observed. The presence of contractures, deformities, paralysis, contusions, lacerations, wounds, footdrop, wristdrop, paralysis, crutches, brace, cast, prosthesis, cane, walker, pressure ulcers, allergies, skin rash, or tenseness is noted. It is ascertained whether the patient can perform activities of daily living and is able to sit up and turn, whether constipation is a complaint, and whether the individual is independent or dependent. Concurrent diseases or conditions investigated include injury to the spinal cord, nerve impairment, cerebrovascular accident, rheumatoid arthritis, osteoarthritis, bursitis, polyneuritis, multiple sclerosis, muscular dystrophy, myasthenia gravis, fracture, ruptured disk, Ménière disease, and labyrinthitis. It is determined whether the patient previously had orthopedic or spinal surgery, poliomyelitis, hemiplegia, cerebral palsy, parkinsonism, a cerebrovascular accident, ataxia, syphilis, hyperparathyroidism, osteoporosis, rickets, osteomalacia, tuberculosis, alcoholism, and impaired vision or hearing. A family history of carcinoma, diabetes, or tuberculosis and the patient's involvement in a hazardous job or recreation, history of previous accidents, and use of tobacco or medications such as steroids, sedatives, tranquilizers, analgesics, antimalarials, acetylsalicylic acid, or indomethacin are determined. Laboratory studies important for the assessment are assays of serum and urine calcium and phosphorus and of alkaline phosphatase serum level. Diagnostic procedures that may be required include x-ray films of bones, arthrograms, myelograms, arteriograms, arthroscopy, biopsies of bone or muscle, incision and drainage of joints, and electromyograms of muscles.

■ INTERVENTIONS: Health care providers conduct the interview to obtain subjective data, make the necessary observations of the patient, and assemble the information on concurrent and previous disorders, the family history, the patient's social and medication background, and the results of laboratory studies and diagnostic procedures.

■ OUTCOME CRITERIA: A meticulous assessment of the patient's musculoskeletal system is a valuable aid in making the diagnosis, planning the course of therapy, predicting the prognosis, and ensuring the patient's safety.

musculospiral nerve. See **radial nerve.**

musculus trigoni vesicae urinariae superficialis, the superficial layer of the trigonal muscles, continuous proximally with the muscles of the ureteral wall.

musculus uvulae, a muscle that elevates and retracts the uvula, thickening the central part of the soft palate and helping the levator veli palatini muscles close the pharyngeal isthmus between the nasopharynx and oropharynx. It originates from the posterior nasal spine on the posterior margin of the hard palate and is innervated by the vagus nerve through the pharyngeal branch to the pharyngeal plexus.

mush bite, a procedure for making simultaneous tooth impressions used in the construction of study models or full or partial dentures. The patient draws his or her upper and lower jaws together into a block of softened wax, thus indicating the spatial relationship between the maxilla and mandible.

mushroom [ME, *mucheron*], the fruiting body of the fungus of the class Basidomycetes, especially edible members of the order Agaricales, commonly known as field mushrooms or meadow mushrooms. Mushrooms contain some protein and minerals, but they are composed largely of water.

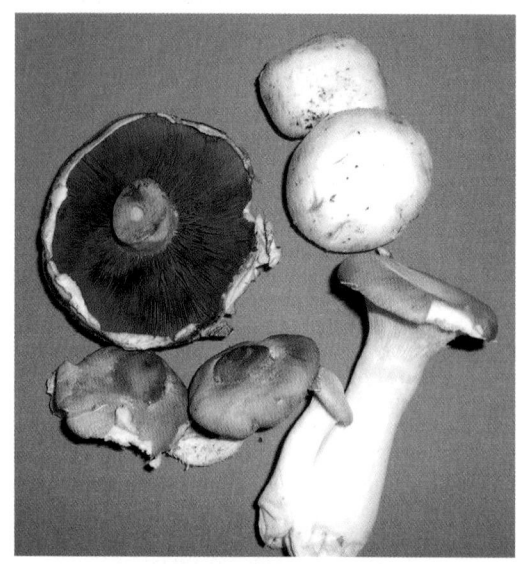

Edible mushrooms

mushroom poisoning, a toxic condition caused by the ingestion of certain mushrooms, particularly species of the genus *Amanita*. Muscarine in *A. muscaria* produces intoxication in a few minutes to 2 hours. Symptoms include lacrimation, salivation, sweating, vomiting, labored breathing, abdominal cramps, diarrhea, and in severe cases convulsions, coma, and circulatory failure. More deadly but slower-acting phalloidin in *A. phalloides* and *A. verna* causes similar symptoms, as well as liver damage, renal failure, and death. Rapid identification of mushroom poisoning and treatment is critical. According to the Center for Food Safety and Applied Nutrition of the U.S. Food and Drug Administration, persons who have ingested poisonous mushrooms and are treated immediately have a mortality rate of 10%, whereas those who are treated 60 or more hours later have a 60% to 90% mortality rate. Also called **phalloidine poisoning.**

mushroom worker's lung, a type of farmer's lung seen in those working on mushroom farms, caused by inhalation of mold spores from mushroom beds.

music therapist, a health professional trained to use music within a therapeutic relationship to address a client's needs, such as facilitating movement and physical rehabilitation, motivating the client to cope with treatment, providing emotional support, and providing an outlet for expressing feelings. A baccalaureate or master's degree and clinical internship are required, after which an individual may take an examination to earn the credential Music Therapist-Board Certified.

music therapy [Gk, *mousike,* music, *therapeia,* treatment], a form of adjunctive psychotherapy in which music is used as a means of recreation and communication, especially with autistic children, and as a means to elevate the mood of depressed and psychotic patients. It is used to effect positive changes in the psychological, physical, cognitive, or social functioning of individuals with health or educational problems and for a wide variety of indications, including mental disorders, developmental and learning disabilities, neurological disabilities, and the management of pain or stress.

Musset sign /mo͞osā″ sīn/ [Alfred de Musset, French poet, 1810–1857], a rhythmic movement of the head and neck synchronous with each ventricular systole. The disorder is named for the patient in whom the condition was first recorded.

mustard gas /mus″tərd/, a poisonous gas used in chemical warfare during World War I. It causes corrosive destruction of the skin and mucous membranes, often resulting in permanent respiratory damage and death.

mustard plaster [L, *mustum* + Gk, *emplastron*], a counterirritant made from dried mustard, flour, and a small amount of water and spread onto a fabric base that is placed on the skin. It must be used with care because it can cause burns.

mustard poultice. See **poultice.**

Mustargen, an antineoplastic drug. Brand name for **mechlorethamine hydrochloride.**

-mustine, suffix for antineoplastic agents, particularly [B-chlorethyl] amine derivatives.

mutacism /myo͞o″təsiz′əm/, mimmation, or the incorrect use of the /m/ sound.

mutagen /myo͞o″təjən/ [L, *mutare,* to change, *genein,* to produce], any chemical or physical environmental agent that induces a genetic mutation or increases the mutation rate. −*mutagenic, adj.,* −*mutagenicity, n.*

mutagenesis /myo͞o″təjen″əsis/, the induction or occurrence of a genetic mutation. See also **teratogenesis.**

Mutamycin, an antineoplastic drug. Brand name for **mitomycin.**

mutant /myo͞o″tənt/ [L, *mutare,* to change], **1.** *n.,* any organism with genetic material that has undergone mutation. **2.** *adj.,* relating to or produced by mutation.

mutant gene, any gene that has undergone a change, such as the loss, gain, or exchange of genetic material, that affects the normal transmission and expression of a trait. Such genes can become inactive or show reduced, increased, or antagonistic activity. Kinds include **amorph, antimorph, hypermorph, hypomorph.**

mutase /myo͞o″tās/, any enzyme that catalyzes the shifting of a chemical group or radical from one position to another within the same molecule or occasionally from one molecule to another.

mutation /myo͞otā″shən/ [L, *mutare,* to change], an unusual change in a gene occurring spontaneously or by induction. The change affects the original expression of the gene. If a mutation occurs in the genome of a gamete, the mutation may be transmitted to later generations. −*mutational, adj.,* −*mutate, v.*

mutein /myo͞o″tē-in, m(y)o͞o″tēn/, a protein molecule that results from a mutation.

mutism /myo͞o″tizəm/ [L, *mutus,* mute], the inability to speak because of a physical defect or emotional problem.

muton /myo͞o″ton/, the smallest DNA segment whose alteration can result in a mutation.

mutually exclusive categories /myo͞o″cho͞o·əlē/, categories on a research instrument that are sufficiently precise to allow each subject, factor, or variable to be classified uniquely, such as male/female.

mutual support group, a type of group in which members organize to solve their own problems. It is led by the group members themselves, who share a common goal and use their own strengths to gain control over their lives.

MV, 1. abbreviation for *megavolt.* **2.** abbreviation for *minute volume.*

mv, mV, abbreviation for **millivolt.**

MVIC, abbreviation for **maximum voluntary isometric contraction.**

mVO₂, symbol for *myocardial oxygen consumption.*

MVP, initialism for *mitral valve prolapse.* See **mitral valve prolapse (MVP) syndrome.**

MVV, abbreviation for **maximum voluntary ventilation.**

M.W.I.A., abbreviation for **Medical Women's International Association.**

MX gene, a human gene that helps the body resist viral infections. When exposed to interferon, the MX gene inhibits the production of viral protein and nucleic acid necessary for the proliferation of new viral particles. The presence of the MX gene helps explain why some individuals are better able to resist certain viral infections, such as influenza, than other people.

my-. See **myo-, my-.**

myalgia /mī·al″jə/ [Gk, *mys,* muscle, *algos,* pain], diffuse muscle pain, usually accompanied by malaise. Also called **myoneuralgia.**

myalgic asthenia /mī·al″jik/ [Gk, *mys* + *algos,* pain, *a* + *sthenos,* without strength], a condition characterized by a general feeling of fatigue and muscular pain, often resulting from or associated with psychological stress.

Myambutol, an antitubercular drug. Brand name for **ethambutol hydrochloride.**

myasthenia /mī′əsthē″nē·ə/ [Gk, *mys* + *a* + *sthenos,* without strength], a condition characterized by an abnormal weakness of a muscle or a group of muscles that may be the result of a systemic myoneural disturbance, such as in myasthenia laryngis, which involves the vocal cord tensor muscles. See also **myasthenia gravis.** −**myasthenic,** *adj.*

myasthenia gravis, an abnormal condition characterized by chronic fatigability and muscle weakness, especially in the face and throat, as a result of a defect in the conduction of nerve impulses at the neuromuscular junction.

■ OBSERVATIONS: Muscular fatigability in myasthenia gravis is caused by the inability of receptors at the myoneural junction to depolarize because of a deficiency of acetylcholine; hence the diagnosis may be made by administering an anticholinesterase drug and observing improved muscle strength and stamina. The onset of symptoms is usually gradual, with ptosis of the upper eyelids, diplopia, and weakness of the facial muscles. The weakness may then extend to other muscles innervated by the cranial nerves, particularly the respiratory muscles. Muscular exertion aggravates the symptoms, which typically vary over the course of the day. The disease occurs in younger women more often than in older women and in men over 60 years of age more often than in younger men.

■ INTERVENTIONS: Anticholinesterase drugs are given. The edrophonium test is used to determine the optimal maintenance dose. Neostigmine or pyridostigmine is the drug most often used.

■ PATIENT CARE CONSIDERATIONS: Physical activity is restricted and rest encouraged. Anticholinesterase drugs are usually administered before meals, and the patient is monitored for toxic side effects. Myasthenic crisis may require emergency respiratory assistance. The patient's diet may have to be adjusted if the ability to chew and swallow is affected.

M

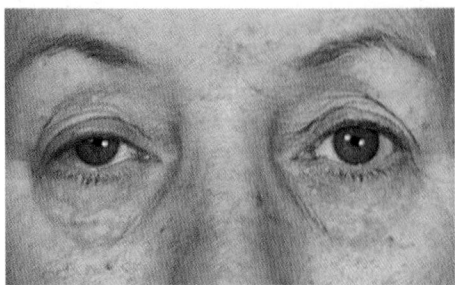

Myasthenia gravis: typical facial expression
(Perkin et al, 2011)

myasthenia gravis crisis, an acute exacerbation of the muscular weakness characterizing the disease, triggered by illness, infection, surgery, emotional stress, or an overdose or insufficiency of anticholinesterase medication.
■ OBSERVATIONS: Typical signs and symptoms include worsening diplopia or muscle weakness that can progress to respiratory distress accompanied by apnea, extreme fatigue, increased muscular weakness, dysphagia, dysarthria, and fever. The patient may be anxious, restless, irritable, and unable to move the jaws or to raise one or both eyelids. If the condition is caused by anticholinesterase toxicity, then anorexia, nausea, vomiting, abdominal cramps, diarrhea, excessive salivation, sweating, lacrimation, blurred vision, vertigo, and muscle cramps and spasms, as well as general weakness, dysarthria, and respiratory distress may occur.
■ INTERVENTIONS: Initial treatment is directed to maintaining airway patency. Oxygen with assisted or controlled ventilation is administered. The patient is placed in a bed in which the head is elevated 30 degrees. The withdrawal or reduction of anticholinergic drugs may be ordered, or they may be given to differentiate the kind of crisis. If the eyelids are affected, the eyes may be covered with a patch and soothing eyedrops may be administered. To enable the patient to communicate, the call bell and a pad and pencil are placed within reach. Nourishment is offered between meals, and a daily intake of up to 2000 mL of fluids is encouraged. Walking as tolerated and other activities are planned at the time of the maximum effect of medication. Active or passive range-of-motion exercises of all extremities are performed several times a day, but rest periods are maintained to prevent fatigue and relapse.
■ PATIENT CARE CONSIDERATIONS: Before discharge the patient is instructed on the importance of taking the prescribed medication with milk, crackers, or bread at the scheduled time and of reporting toxic side effects and symptoms of recurrent or progressive disease. Members of the health care team point out the need to maintain a regular diet, to exercise to tolerance, to rest, and to avoid infections and exposure to hot or cold weather and the use of alcohol and tobacco. Help in planning a schedule that conserves energy for essential activities can enable the patient to be relatively independent and self-sufficient.

myasthenic. See **myasthenia.**

myasthenic crisis /mī'asthen″ik/, an acute episode of muscular weakness. See also **myasthenia gravis crisis.**

myc-. See **myco-, myc-, myceto-, myko-.**

Mycamine, brand name for **micafungin.**

mycelium /mīsē″lē·əm/ *pl. mycelia* [Gk, *mykes,* fungus, *helos,* nail], a mass of interwoven, branched, threadlike filaments that makes up most fungi. Also called **hypha.**

mycetismus /mī'sitiz″məs/. See **mushroom poisoning.**

myceto-. See **myco-, myc-, myceto-, myko-.**

mycetoma /mī'sətō″mə/ [Gk, *mykes + oma,* tumor], a severe fungal infection involving skin, subcutaneous tissue, fascia, and bone. Kinds include **Madura foot.**

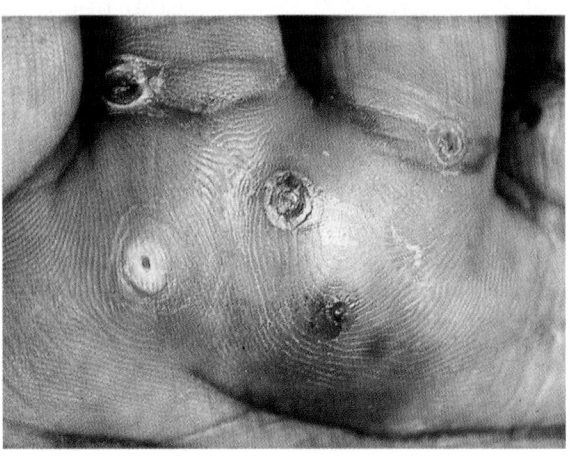

Mycetoma *(du Vivier, 2002/Courtesy Dr. Rod Hay)*

-mycin, suffix for antibiotics produced by *Streptomyces* strains.

Mycitracin, a fixed-combination topical drug containing antibacterial agents. Brand name for **polymyxin B sulfate, bacitracin, neomycin sulfate.**

myco-, myc-, myceto-, myko-, prefix meaning "fungus": *mycobacteriosis.*

mycobacteria /mī'kōbaktir″ē·ə/ [Gk, *mykes + bakterion,* small rod], acid-fast microorganisms belonging to the genus *Mycobacterium.*

mycobacteriosis /mī'kōbak'tirē·ō″sis/ [Gk, *mykes + bakterion + osis,* condition], a tuberculosis-like disease caused by mycobacteria other than *Mycobacterium tuberculosis.*

Mycobacterium /mī'kōbaktir″ē·əm/ [Gk, *mykes + bakterion,* small rod], a genus of rod-shaped acid-fast bacteria having two significant pathogenic species: *Mycobacterium leprae,* which causes leprosy, and *M. tuberculosis,* which causes tuberculosis. *M. avium* complex or *M. avium-intracellulare* disseminated infection may occur in AIDS and cause cervical adenitis in children and pulmonary disease in immunodeficient patients.

Mycobacterium avium **complex (MAC) disease,** systemic disease caused by infection with organisms of the *Mycobacterium avium-intracellulare* complex in patients with human immunodeficiency virus infection. Manifestations include bacteremia, fever, chills, fatigue, night sweats, weight loss, abdominal pain, anemia, and elevated alkaline phosphatase. Also called *MAC disease.* Compare **mycobacteriosis.**

Mycobacterium avium-intracellulare, a complex of slow-growing organisms that cause tuberculosis in birds and swine and that is associated with human pulmonary disease, lymphadenitis in children, and serious systemic disease in immunocompromised patients. See also **mycobacteriosis,** *Mycobacterium avium* **complex (MAC) disease.**

Mycobacterium bovis, a species of bacteria that causes tuberculosis in cattle and other animals and that is transmitted to humans by the ingestion of raw milk contaminated by the microorganism.

Mycobacterium kansasii, a species of slow-growing photochromogenic bacteria that causes tuberculosis-like pulmonary infection in humans. It affects the joints, gonads, spinal fluid, lymph nodes, and viscera. The incidence of this infection has increased with the advent of AIDS.

Mycobacterium leprae, a species of bacteria that causes leprosy. It has not yet been cultivated in vitro. Organisms are isolated from suspect lesions as acid-fast bacilli, typically in intracellular clumps or in groups of bacilli side by side.

Mycobacterium marinum, a species of bacteria that causes a form of tuberculosis in cold-blooded animals, including saltwater fish. The bacterium is also found in swimming pools and aquariums and is associated with skin lesions in humans.

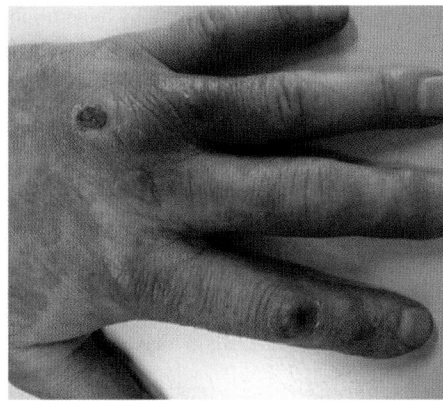

Skin lesions associated with *Mycobacterium marinum*
(Herendael, Dreessen, and Jeurissen, 2012)

Mycolog, a topical fixed-combination drug containing a glucocorticoid. Brand name for *triamcinolone acetonide.*

mycology /mīkol″əjē/ [Gk, *mykes* + *logos,* science], the study of fungi and fungoid diseases. *—mycologic, mycological, adj., —mycologist, n.*

mycomyringitis. See **myringomycosis.**

mycophenolate mofetil, an immunosuppressant used to prevent rejection of allogeneic cardiac, hepatic, and renal transplants. It is administered orally or intravenously.

■ INDICATIONS: It is used to prevent rejection of organ transplants and for prophylaxis of organ rejection in allogenic cardiac transplants.

■ CONTRAINDICATIONS: Known hypersensitivity to this drug or to mycophenolic acid prohibits its use.

■ ADVERSE EFFECTS: Life-threatening effects are leukopenia, thrombocytopenia, anemia, pancytopenia, renal tubular necrosis, and lymphoma. Other adverse effects are arthralgia, muscle wasting, and stomatitis. Common side effects are diarrhea, constipation, nausea, vomiting, rash, dyspnea, respiratory infection, increased cough, pharyngitis, bronchitis, pneumonia, tremor, dizziness, insomnia, headache, fever, peripheral edema, hypercholesterolemia, hypophosphatemia, edema, hyperkalemia, hypokalemia, hyperglycemia, urinary tract infection, hematuria, hypertension, chest pain, and nonmelanoma skin carcinoma.

mycophenolic acid /mī′kōfinō″lik/, a bacteriostatic and fungistatic crystalline immunosuppressant obtained from *Penicillium brevicompactum* and related species.

Mycoplasma /mī′kōplaz″mə/ [Gk, *mykes* + *plassein,* to mold], a genus of ultramicroscopic organisms lacking rigid cell walls and considered to be the smallest free-living organisms. Some are saprophytes, some are parasites, and many are pathogens. One species is a cause of mycoplasma pneumonia, tracheobronchitis, pharyngitis, and bullous myringitis. See also **pleuropneumonia-like organism.**

mycoplasma pneumonia, a contagious disease of children and young adults caused by *Mycoplasma pneumoniae.* It is characterized by a 9- to 12-day incubation period and followed by symptoms of an upper respiratory infection, dry cough, and fever. Also called **Eaton agent pneumonia, primary atypical pneumonia, walking pneumonia.** See also **cold agglutinin.**

■ OBSERVATIONS: Harsh or diminished breath sounds and fine inspiratory rales are frequently heard. Pulmonary infiltrates visible on chest x-ray films may resemble those of bacterial or viral pneumonia and may persist for 3 weeks in untreated cases. Rarely, complications such as sinusitis, pleurisy, polyneuritis, myocarditis, or Stevens-Johnson syndrome may follow the pneumonia. In untreated adults prolonged cough, weakness, and malaise are common. Diagnosis is suggested by physical examination and by observation of the clinical course and elevated cold agglutinin level and is confirmed by a complement fixation test. Prognosis is favorable.

■ INTERVENTIONS: Azithromycin, clarithromycin, or doxycycline; bed rest; a high-protein diet; and an adequate fluid intake are recommended. It is important that infants and people for whom a respiratory illness is particularly hazardous avoid contact with infected individuals.

mycosis /mīkō″sis/ [Gk, *mykes* + *osis,* condition], any disease caused by a fungus. Kinds include **candidiasis, coccidioidomycosis, tinea pedis. –mycotic,** *adj.*

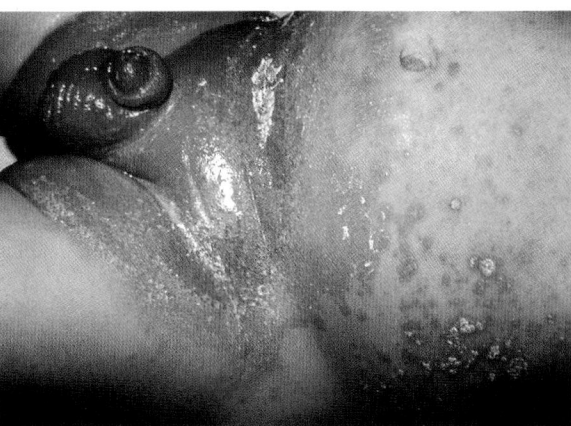

Candidiasis, a kind of mycosis *(Centers for Disease Control and Prevention, Public Health Image Library ID#5143, 1975)*

mycosis fungoides /fung·goi″dēz/, a rare chronic lymphomatous skin malignancy resembling eczema or a cutaneous tumor that is followed by microabscesses in the epidermis and lesions simulating those of Hodgkin disease in lymph nodes and viscera. The condition is considered a distinctive entity by some specialists and a cutaneous manifestation of a malignant lymphoma by others.

Mycostatin, an antifungal drug. Brand name for **nystatin.**

mycotic /mīkot″ik/ [Gk, *mykes,* fungus], pertaining to a disease caused by a fungus.

mycotic aneurysm, a localized dilation in the wall of a blood vessel caused by the growth of a fungus. It usually

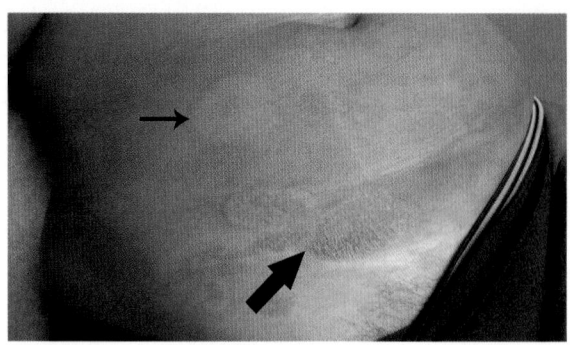

Skin lesions associated with mycosis fungoides
(Pincus, 2014)

occurs as a complication of bacterial endocarditis. See also **bacterial aneurysm.**

mycotic endocarditis /mīkot′ik en′do·kär·dī′tis/ [Gk, *mykes,* fungus; Gk, *endon,* within + *kardia,* heart + *-itis,* inflammatory disease suffix], infectious endocarditis caused by infection by a fungus, most commonly *Candida albicans* and species of *Aspergillus* and *Histoplasma.* Symptoms are usually subacute.

mycotic granuloma of the larynx, a chronic throat condition characterized by white patches on an otherwise bright red mucous membrane. In the southwestern United States it is associated with histoplasmosis of the larynx. It may also be caused by candidiasis as a complication of chemotherapy or an altered immune state.

mycotoxicosis /mī′kōtok′sikō″sis/ [Gk, *mykes* + *toxikon,* poison, *osis,* condition], a systemic poisoning caused by toxins produced by fungal organisms.

mycotoxin /mī′kōtok″sin/, a poison produced by fungi that is harmful to other organisms.

mydriasis /midrī′əsis/ [Gk, *mydros,* hot mass], **1.** dilation of the pupil of the eye caused by contraction of the dilator muscle of the iris, a muscular sheath that radiates outward like the spokes of a wheel from the center of the iris around the pupil. With a decrease in light or the pharmacological action of certain drugs, the dilator acts to pull the iris outward, enlarging the pupil. **2.** an abnormal condition characterized by contraction of the dilator muscle, resulting in widely dilated pupils. Compare **miosis.** See also **alternating mydriasis. –***mydriatic, adj.*

mydriatic and cycloplegic agent /mid′rē·at″ik/ [Gk, *mydros* + *kyklos,* circle, *plege,* stroke], any one of several ophthalmic pharmaceutic preparations that dilate the pupil and paralyze the ocular muscles of accommodation. Mydriatics stimulate alpha adrenergic receptors or block cholinergic muscarinic receptors in the eye, temporarily paralyzing the iris sphincter muscle so that the pupil is maximally dilated. Cycloplegics block cholinergic muscarinic receptors, which temporarily paralyzes accommodation by relaxing the ciliary muscle to focus the lens for far vision. These drugs are used in diagnostic and refractive examination of the eye, before and after various procedures in eye surgery, in some tests for glaucoma, and in the treatment of anterior uveitis and certain kinds of glaucoma. Blurred vision, thirst, flushing, fever, and rash may occur. In children and elderly people ataxia, somnolence, delirium, and hallucination may occur but are rare. Among these drugs are atropine, cyclopentolate, homatropine, scopolamine, and tropicamide. They are prepared in solution for topical ophthalmic application.

myectomy, excision of part of a muscle.

myectomy/myotomy, a surgical method of treating total or near-total intestinal aganglionosis. It combines circular excision of seromuscular tissue from a short segment of bowel and a longitudinal myotomy with creation of a stoma, resulting in a short length of functional intestine that will support increasing amounts of enteral nutrition. Also called *myectomyotomy.*

myel-. See **myelo-, myel-.**

myelacephalus /mī′əlāsef″ələs/ [Gk, *myelos,* marrow, *a* + *kephale,* without head], a fetus, usually a separate monozygotic twin, whose form and parts are barely recognizable. *–myelacephalous, adj.*

myelatelia /mī′ələtē″lē·ə/ [Gk, *myelos* + *atelia,* unfinished], any developmental defect involving the spinal cord.

myelauxe /mī′əlôk″sē/ [Gk, *myelos* + *auxe,* increasing], a developmental anomaly characterized by hypertrophy of the spinal cord.

myelencephalon /mī′əlensef″əlon/, the lower part of the embryonic hindbrain from which the medulla oblongata develops.

-myelia, suffix meaning "(condition of the) spinal cord": *hydromyelia, syringomyelia.*

myelin /mī′əlin/ [Gk, *myelos,* marrow], a lipoproteinaceous substance constituting the sheaths of various nerve fibers throughout the body and enveloping the axis of myelinated nerves. It is largely composed of phospholipids and protein, which gives the fibers a white, creamy color. **–myelinic,** *adj.*

myelinated /mī″əlinā′tid/, (of a nerve) having a myelin sheath.

myelination /mī′əlinā″shən/ [Gk, *myelos* + L, *atio,* process], the process of furnishing or taking on myelin.

myelin globule, a fatlike droplet found in some sputum.

myelinic /mī′əlin″ik/ [Gk, *myelos* + L, *icus,* form of], pertaining to myelin.

myelinic neuroma, a neuroma neoplasm composed of myelinated nerve fibers.

myelinization /mī′əlin″īzā″shən/ [Gk, *myelos* + *izein,* to cause], development of the myelin sheath around a nerve fiber. Also called *myelinogenesis.*

myelinolysis /mī′əlinol″isis/ [Gk, *myelos* + *lysein,* to loosen], a pathological process that dissolves the myelin sheaths around certain nerve fibers, such as those of the pons in alcoholic and undernourished people who are afflicted with central pontine myelinolysis.

myelin sheath, a segmented fatty lamination composed of myelin that wraps the axons of many nerves in the body. The usual thickness of the myelin sheath is between 200 and 800 μm. Various diseases such as multiple sclerosis can destroy myelin wrappings.

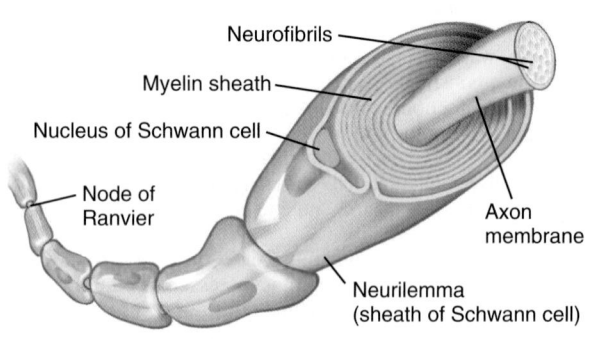

Myelin sheath

myelitis /mī′əlī″tis/, an abnormal condition characterized by inflammation of the spinal cord with associated motor or sensory dysfunction. Kinds include **acute transverse myelitis, poliomyelitis.** –*myelitic, adj.*

myelo-, myel-, prefix meaning "spinal cord" or "bone marrow": *myeloblast, myelocyte, myelomeningocele.*

myeloablation /mī′əlō·ablā′shən/ [Gk, *myelos,* marrow; L, *ab* + *latus,* carried away], severe myelosuppression. See also **bone marrow suppression.**

myeloblast /mī″əlōblast′/ [Gk, *myelos* + *blastos,* germ], earliest recognizable precursor of the granulocytic leukocytes. The cytoplasm appears light blue, scanty, and nongranular when seen in a stained blood film. The nucleus contains distinct chromatin material in strands, together with several nucleoli. In certain leukemias a marked increase in myeloblasts is observed in the marrow and in the peripheral blood. Compare **megaloblast, myelocyte, normoblast.** See also **chronic myelogenous leukemia.** –*myeloblastic, adj.*

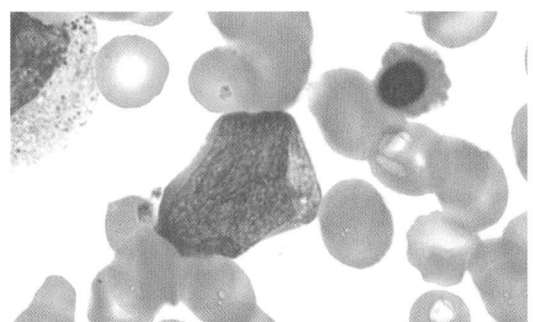

Micrograph of a myeloblast *(Young, O'Dowd, and Woodford, 2014)*

myeloblastemia, Not in common usage. See **myeloblastosis.**

myeloblastic. See **myeloblast.**

myeloblastic leukemia /-blas″tik/, a malignant neoplasm of blood-forming tissues, characterized by many myeloblasts in the circulating blood and tissues. The disease may be a terminal event in the course of chronic granulocytic leukemia, sometimes referred to as "blast crisis."

myeloblastomatosis /mī′əlōblas′tōmətō″sis/ [Gk, *myelos* + *blastos* + *oma,* tumor, *osis,* condition], abnormal localized clusters of myeloblasts in the peripheral circulation.

myeloblastosis /mī′əlōblastō″sis/ [Gk, *myelos* + *blastos* + *osis,* condition], an excess of myeloblasts in the blood.

myelocele /mī″əlōsēl′/ [Gk, *myelos* + *kele,* hernia]. See **myelomeningocele.**

myeloclast /mī″əlōclast′/ [Gk, *myelos* + *klastos,* broken], a cell that breaks down the myelin sheaths of nerves.

myelocyst /mī″əlōsist′/ [Gk, *myelos* + *kystis,* cyst], any benign cyst formed from the rudimentary medullary canals that give rise to the vertebral canal during embryonic development.

myelocystocele /mī″əlōsis″təsēl′/ [Gk, *myelos* + *kystis* + *kele,* hernia]. See **myelomeningocele.**

myelocystomeningocele /mī′əlōsis′tōməning″gōsēl/ [Gk, *myelos* + *kystis* + *menix,* membrane, *kele,* hernia]. See **myelomeningocele.**

myelocyte /mī″əlōsīt′/ [Gk, *myelos* + *kytos,* cell], the third of the maturation stages of the granulocytic leukocytes normally found in the bone marrow. Granules are visible in the cytoplasm. The nuclear material of the myelocyte is denser than that of the myeloblast.

Myelocytes appear on peripheral blood films in chronic myelogenous leukemia or in severe infection. Compare **myeloblast.** See also **chronic myelogenous leukemia.** –*myelocytic, adj.*

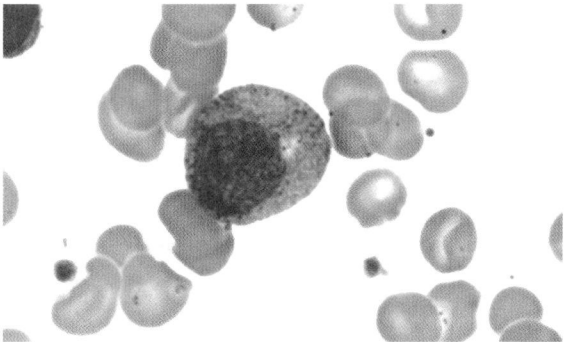

Myelocyte micrograph *(Young, O'Dowd, and Woodford, 2014)*

myelocythemia /mī′əlōsīthē″mē·ə/ [Gk, *myelos* + *kytos* + *haima,* blood], an excessive presence of myelocytes in the circulating blood, such as in myelocytic leukemia. Not in common usage.

myelocytic. See **myelocyte.**

myelocytoma /mī′əlō′sītō″mə/ [Gk, *myelos* + *kytos,* cell, *oma,* tumor], a localized cluster of myelocytes in the peripheral vasculature that may occur in myelocytic leukemia.

myelocytosis. See **myelocythemia.**

myelodiastasis /mī′əlōdī·as″təsis/ [Gk, *myelos* + *diastasis,* separation], disintegration and necrosis of the spinal cord.

myelodysplasia /mī′əlōdisplā″zhə/ [Gk, *myelos* + *dys,* bad, *plassis,* formation], **1.** a general designation for the defective development of any part of the spinal cord. The term is used primarily to describe abnormalities without gross superficial defects, especially of the lower segment, specifically spina bifida occulta. **2.** dysplasia of the myelocytes and other elements in bone marrow.

myelofibrosis /mī′əlōfībrō″sis/, the replacement of bone marrow with fibrous tissue. The condition may be associated with anemia, thrombocytopenia, myeloid metaplasia, new bone formation, polycythemia vera, and other abnormalities. Also called **myelosclerosis.** See also **myeloid metaplasia, primary myelofibrosis.**

myelogenesis /-jen″əsis/ [Gk, *myelos* + *genein,* to produce], **1.** the formation and differentiation of the nervous system, in particular of the brain and spinal cord, during prenatal development. See also **neural tube formation. 2.** the development of the myelin sheath around the nerve fiber. See also **myelinization.**

myelogenous /mī′əloj″ənəs/, pertaining to the cells produced in bone marrow or the tissue from which such cells originate. Also *myelogenetic, myelogenic.*

myelogenous leukemia. See **acute myeloid leukemia.**

myelogeny /mī′əloj″ənē/ [Gk, *myelos* + *genein,* to produce], the formation and differentiation of the myelin sheaths of nerve fibers during the prenatal and postnatal development of the central nervous system.

myelogram /mī″əlōgram′/, **1.** an x-ray film taken after the injection of a radiopaque medium into the subarachnoid space to demonstrate any distortions of the spinal cord, spinal nerve roots, and subarachnoid space. **2.** a graphic representation of a count of the different kinds of cells in a stained preparation of bone marrow.

M

myelography /mī′əlog″rəfē/ [Gk, *myelos* + *graphein,* to record], a radiographic process by which the spinal cord and the spinal subarachnoid space are viewed and photographed after the introduction of a contrast medium. It is used to identify and study spinal lesions caused by trauma or disease. −*myelographic, adj.*

myeloid /mī′əloid/ [Gk, *myelos* + *eidos,* form], **1.** pertaining to the bone marrow. **2.** pertaining to the spinal cord. **3.** pertaining to myelocytic forms that do not necessarily originate in the bone marrow.

myeloid leukemia. See **acute myeloid leukemia, chronic myelocytic leukemia.**

myeloid metaplasia, a disorder in which bone marrow tissue develops in abnormal sites. Characteristics of the condition are anemia, splenomegaly, immature blood cells in the circulation, and hematopoiesis in the liver and spleen. Myeloid metaplasia may be secondary to carcinoma, leukemia, polycythemia vera, or tuberculosis. Kinds include **primary myelofibrosis.**

myeloidosis /mī′əloidō″sis/ [Gk, *myelos* + *eidos,* form, *osis,* condition], an abnormal condition characterized by general hyperplasia of the myeloid tissue. See also **Hodgkin disease, Hodgkin lymphoma, multiple myeloma.**

myeloma /mī′əlō″mə/ [Gk, *myelos* + *oma,* tumor], an osteolytic neoplasm consisting of a profusion of cells typical of the bone marrow that may develop in many sites and cause extensive destruction of the bone. The tumor occurs most frequently in the ribs, vertebrae, pelvic bones, and flat bones of the skull. Intense pain and spontaneous fractures are common. The tumor is radiosensitive, and local lesions are curable. Kinds include **endothelial myeloma, extramedullary myeloma, giant cell myeloma, multiple myeloma, osteogenic myeloma.**

-myeloma, suffix meaning "a tumor composed of cells normally found in bone marrow": *chloromyeloma.*

myeloma cast, a urinary cast containing Bence Jones protein and desquamated cells of the tubular epithelium, seen with multiple myeloma in the condition known as myeloma kidney disease.

myeloma kidney disease, a kidney disorder often characterized by irreversible renal failure. It may involve intratubular coalescence of light chain molecules and obstruction of nephronal flow.

myelomalacia /mī′əlōmələ″shə/ [Gk, *myelos* + *malakia,* softening], an abnormal softening of the spinal cord, caused primarily by inadequate blood supply.

myelomatosis. See **multiple myeloma.**

myelomeningocele /mī′əlō′məning″gōsēl/ [Gk, *myelos* + *menix,* membrane, *kele,* hernia], a developmental defect of the central nervous system in which a hernial sac containing a portion of the spinal cord, its meninges, and cerebrospinal fluid protrudes through a congenital cleft in the vertebral column. The condition is caused primarily by failure of the neural tube to close during embryonic development, although in some instances it may result from the reopening of the tube as a result of an abnormal increase in cerebrospinal fluid pressure. Also called **meningomyelocele, myelocele, myelocystocele, myelocystomeningocele.** Compare **meningocele.** See also **neural tube defect, spina bifida cystica.**

■ OBSERVATIONS: The defect, which occurs in approximately 2 in every 1000 live births, is readily apparent and easily diagnosed at birth. Although the opening may be located at any point along the spinal column, the anomaly characteristically occurs in the lumbar, low thoracic, or sacral region and extends for three to six vertebral segments. The saclike structure may be covered with a thin layer of skin or with a fine membrane that can be easily ruptured, increasing the risk of meningeal infection. The severity of neurological dysfunction is directly related to the amount of neural tissue involved, which can be roughly estimated by the degree of the transillumination of the mass. Usually the condition is accompanied by varying degrees of paralysis of the lower extremities; by musculoskeletal defects such as clubfoot, flexion and joint deformities, or hip dysplasia; and by anal and bladder sphincter dysfunction, which can lead to serious genitourinary disorders. Hydrocephalus, frequently related to the Arnold-Chiari malformation, is the most common anomaly associated with myelomeningocele and occurs in approximately 90% of the cases in which the spinal lesion is located in the lumbosacral region. In most cases, hydrocephalus is apparent at birth, although it may appear shortly afterward. Supplementary diagnostic procedures include x-ray examination of the spine, skull, and chest to determine the extent of the vertebral defect and the presence of other malformations in other organ systems; a computed tomographic scan of the brain to establish the ventricular size and the presence of any structural congenital anomalies; and laboratory examinations, especially urine analysis, culture, blood urea nitrogen evaluation, and creatinine clearance determination. Amniocentesis is recommended for all pregnant women who have had a child with a neural tube defect.

■ INTERVENTIONS: Immediate surgical repair is essential if the defect is leaking cerebrospinal fluid. However, surgical intervention may not be appropriate if neurological involvement is extreme, if the lesion is infected, or if associated problems, such as hydrocephalus, are severe. When surgical repair of the spinal defect is recommended, associated problems are managed by appropriate measures, including shunt procedures for correction of hydrocephalus; antibiotic therapy to reduce the incidence of meningitis, urinary tract infections, and pneumonia; casting, bracing, traction, and surgical techniques for correction of hip, knee, and foot deformities; and prevention and treatment of renal complications. Prognosis is determined by the severity of neurological involvement and the number of associated anomalies. With proper care and long-term maintenance most children can survive and do well. Early death is usually caused by central nervous system infection or by hydrocephalus, whereas mortality in later childhood is caused by urinary tract infection, renal failure, complications from shunt therapy, or pulmonary disease.

■ PATIENT CARE CONSIDERATIONS: Immediate care centers on the prevention of local infection and trauma by carefully handling and positioning the infant, applying sterile moist dressings to the membranous sac, avoiding fecal contamination and breakdown of sensitive skin areas, and maintaining warmth, proper nutrition, and adequate hydration and electrolyte balance. Gentle range-of-motion exercises are carried out to prevent or minimize hip and lower extremity deformity. An important function of all members of the health care team is to involve the parents in the care of the infant as soon as possible and to teach them the essential procedures for adequate home care, including how to observe for signs of complications. The health care team also helps the parents in long-term management by planning activities appropriate to the developmental age and physical limitations of the child and by providing information for teaching all family members about the condition.

myelomere /mī″əlōmir/ [Gk, *myelos* + *meros,* part], any of the embryonic segments of the brain or spinal cord during prenatal development.

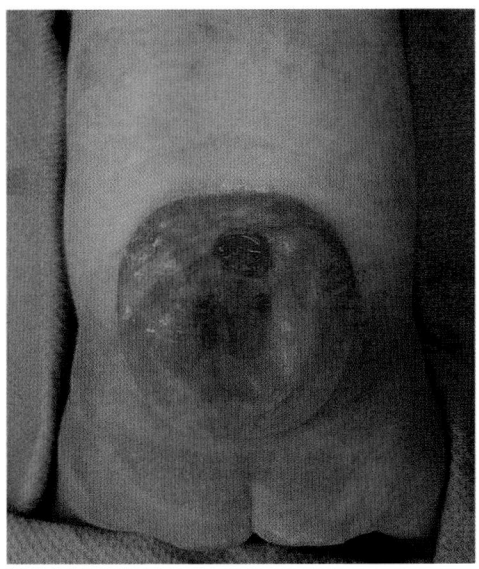

Two-day-old infant with myelomeningocele *(Patel et al, 2012)*

myelomonocytic leukemia.   See **monocytic leukemia.**

myelopathic anemia.   See **myelophthisic anemia.**

myelopathy /mī′əlop″əthē/,   **1.** any disease of the spinal cord. **2.** any disease of the myelopoietic tissues.

myeloperoxidase (MPO) /mī′əlōpərok″sidās/,   a peroxidase enzyme occurring in phagocytic cells that can oxidize halide ions, producing a bactericidal effect.

myelophthisic anemia,   anemia characterized by the presence of immature erythrocytes in the peripheral blood due to the infiltration of the bone marrow by abnormal tissue. Also called **myelopathic anemia.**

myelopoiesis /mī′əlō′pō-ē″sis/ [Gk, *myelos* + *poiein,* to form],   the formation and development of bone marrow or the cells that originate from it. Kinds include **extramedullary myelopoiesis.** −*myelopoietic, adj.*

myeloproliferative neoplasms /mī′əlōprōlif″ərətiv′/,   a family of chronic malignant bone marrow and blood diseases caused by mutations that generate clones of myelocytic or erythrocytic precursors and platelet precursors. Kinds include **chronic myelogenous leukemia, polycythemia vera, essential thrombocythemia, primary myelofibrosis.**

myeloradiculodysplasia   /mī′əlō′rədik′yəlō′dis′plā″zhə/ [Gk, *myelos* + L, *radiculus,* small root; Gk, *dys,* bad, *plassein,* to form],   any developmental abnormality of the spinal cord and spinal nerve roots. See also **myelomeningocele, neural tube defect.**

myeloschisis /mī′əlos″kəsis/ [Gk, *myelos* + *schisis,* cleft],   a developmental defect characterized by a cleft spinal cord that results from the failure of the neural plate to fuse and form a complete neural tube. See also **myelomeningocele, neural tube defect, neural tube formation, rachischisis, spina bifida.**

myelosclerosis.   See **myelofibrosis.**

myelosuppression /-səpresh″ən/.   See **bone marrow suppression.**

myenteric plexus /mī′enter″ik/ [Gk, *mys,* muscle, *enteron,* bowel; L, *plexus,* plaited],   a group of autonomic nerve fibers and ganglion cells in the muscular coat of the intestine.

myesthesia /mī′esthē″zhə/,   perception of any sensation in a muscle, such as touch, direction, proprioception, contraction, relaxation, or extension.

myiasis /mī″yəsis/ [Gk, *myia,* fly, *osis,* condition],   infection or infestation of the body by the larvae of flies, usually through a wound or an ulcer but rarely through intact skin.

myitis.   See **myositis.**

myko-.   See **myco-, myc-, myceto-, myko-.**

Myleran,   an antineoplastic drug. Brand name for **busulfan.**

Mylicon,   an antiflatulent agent. Brand name for **simethicone.**

mylohyoideus /mī′lōhī-oi″dē-əs/ [Gk, *myle,* mill, *hyoeides,* upsilon, U-shaped],   one of a pair of flat triangular muscles that form the floor of the cavity of the mouth. It is innervated by the mylohyoid nerve and acts to raise the hyoid bone and the tongue. Also called *mylohyoid muscle.* Compare **digastricus, geniohyoideus, stylohyoideus.**

myo-, my-,   prefix meaning "muscle": *myocardium, myodiastasis, myoma.*

myocardial.   See **myocardium.**

myocardial infarction (MI) /mī′ōkär″dē-əl/ [Gk, *mys,* muscle, *kardia,* heart; L, *infarcire,* to stuff],   necrosis of a portion of cardiac muscle caused by an obstruction in a coronary artery resulting from atherosclerosis, a thrombus, or a spasm. Also called **heart attack.** See also **acute myocardial infarction.**

■ OBSERVATIONS: The onset of MI is characterized by a crushing, viselike chest pain that may radiate to the left arm, neck, jaw, or epigastrium and sometimes stimulates the sensation of acute indigestion or a gallbladder attack. The patient usually becomes ashen, clammy, short of breath, nauseated, faint, and anxious and often feels that death is imminent. Typical signs are tachycardia, a barely palpable pulse, low blood pressure, mildly elevated temperature, cardiac arrhythmia, and elevation of the S-T segment and Q wave on the electrocardiogram. Laboratory studies usually show an increased sedimentation rate, leukocytosis, and elevated serum levels of creatine kinase and its isoenzyme MB, lactic dehydrogenase and its isoenzymes, and glutamic-oxaloacetic transaminase. Potential complications in MI are pulmonary or systemic embolism, pulmonary edema, acute congestive heart failure, shock, ventricular tachycardia, ventricular fibrillation, and cardiac arrest.

■ INTERVENTIONS: Emergency treatment of MI may require cardiopulmonary resuscitation before the patient reaches the hospital emergency department. Early IV administration of thrombolytic drugs and heparin improves left ventricular function, limits damage, and increases survival rates. Primary percutaneous transvenous coronary angioplasty (PTCA) is being used with increasing frequency and can achieve prompt reperfusion and help prevent the hemorrhagic risks of thrombolysis. Primary PTCA requires a well-staffed, well-equipped cardiac catheterization laboratory that can mobilize within 1 hour and achieve reperfusion within 2 hours.

■ PATIENT CARE CONSIDERATIONS: The patient is admitted to an intensive care unit with continual electrocardiographic monitoring at the acute onset. Blood pressure, temperature, respiration, and apical pulse are checked frequently. Parenteral fluids may be administered, and the patient is usually served a low-sodium, low-cholesterol, low-fat diet. Stool softeners and laxatives may be indicated to prevent straining. The nurse's role in helping the patient and family understand the nature and treatment of the disease is extremely important. Before discharge members of the health care team usually discuss the need to adhere to the prescribed diet and medication, to limit activities, to rest at regular periods, and to avoid caffeine, nicotine, large meals, and emotional stress. A cardiac rehabilitation program is often indicated and can play a major role in improving long-term health.

M

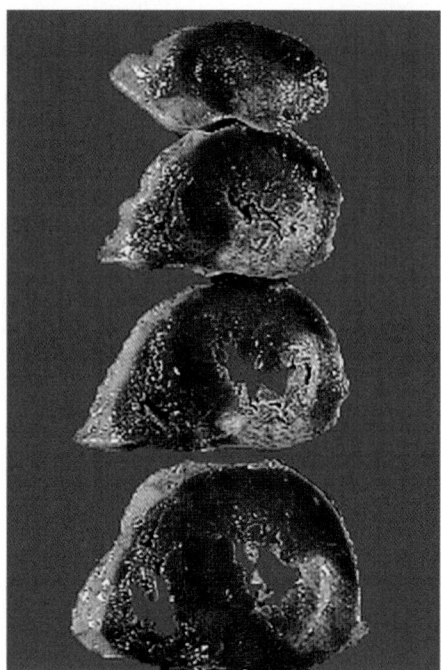

Myocardial infarction. Heart slices demonstrate large extent of an old, scarred infarct along the left ventricular free wall *(Husain, 2012)*

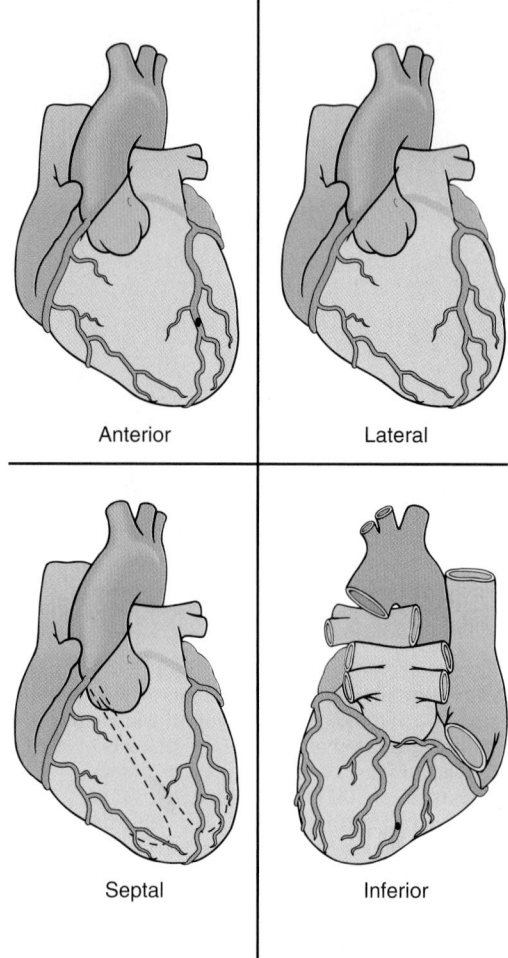

Anterior | Lateral

Septal | Inferior

Common locations of myocardial infarction
(Lewis, Heitkemper, and Dirksen, 2004)

myocardial insufficiency, inadequate functioning of the heart muscle. See also **heart failure.**

myocardial ischemia, a condition of insufficient blood flow to the heart muscle via the coronary arteries, often resulting in chest pain (angina pectoris). In diagnostic imaging, thallium-201 or other substances are injected into the blood to reveal areas of myocardial ischemia.

myocardial perfusion, the flow of blood to the heart muscle.

myocardiograph /mī′ōkär″dē·əgraf′/, a tracing device for recording the activity of heart muscle.

myocardiopathy /mī′ōkär′dē·op″əthē/ [Gk, *mys,* muscle, *kardia,* heart, *pathos,* disease]. See **cardiomyopathy.**

myocarditis /mī′ōkärdī″tis/ [Gk, *mys* + *kardia* + *itis,* inflammation], inflammation of the myocardium. It may be caused by viral, bacterial, or fungal infection; serum sickness; rheumatic fever; or a chemical agent; or it may be a complication of a collagen disease. Myocarditis most frequently occurs in an acute viral form and is self-limited, but it may lead to acute heart failure. Management includes treatment of the cause, analgesia, oxygen, antiinflammatory agents, constant monitoring, and rest to prevent shock or heart failure. See also **acute primary myocarditis, acute secondary myocarditis, acute septic myocarditis.**

myocardium /mī′ōkär″dē·əm/ [Gk, *mys,* muscle, *kardia,* heart], a thick contractile middle layer of uniquely constructed and arranged muscle cells that forms the bulk of the heart wall. The myocardium contains a minimum of other tissue, except blood vessels, and is covered interiorly by the endocardium. The contractile tissue of the myocardium is composed of fibers with the characteristic cross-striations of muscular tissue. The fibers are about one third as large in diameter as those of skeletal muscle and contain more sarcoplasm. They branch frequently and are interconnected to form a network that is continuous except where the bundles and the laminae are attached at their origins and insertions into the fibrous trigone of the heart. Myocardial muscle contains less connective tissue than does skeletal muscle. Specially modified fibers of myocardial muscle constitute the conduction system of the heart, including the sinoatrial node, the atrioventricular (AV) node, the AV bundle, and the Purkinje fibers. Most of the myocardial fibers function to contract the heart. The metabolic processes of the myocardium are almost exclusively aerobic. Many key enzymatic reactions of the heart, such as the citric acid cycle and oxidative phosphorylation, take place in the highly concentrated myocardial sarcosomes. The process of oxidative phosphorylation produces adenosine triphosphate (ATP), the immediate energy source for myocardial contraction. Oxygen, which significantly affects ATP production and contractility, is a critical metabolic component of the myocardium, which consumes from 6.5 to 10 mL/100 g of tissue per minute. Without this oxygen supply, myocardial contractions decrease in a few minutes. The myocardium maintains a relatively constant level of glycogen in the form of sarcoplasmic granules. Compare **epicardium.** See also **cardiac muscle. −myocardial,** *adj.*

myoclonic encephalopathy of childhood. See **Kinsbourne syndrome.**

myoclonic seizure, a seizure characterized by a brief episode of myoclonus (brief lightning-like jerks), with immediate recovery and often without loss of consciousness.

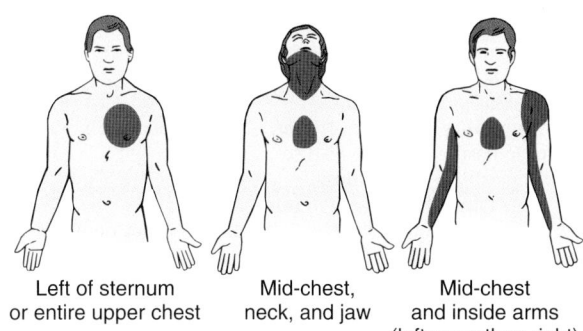

Left of sternum or entire upper chest

Mid-chest, neck, and jaw

Mid-chest and inside arms (left more than right)

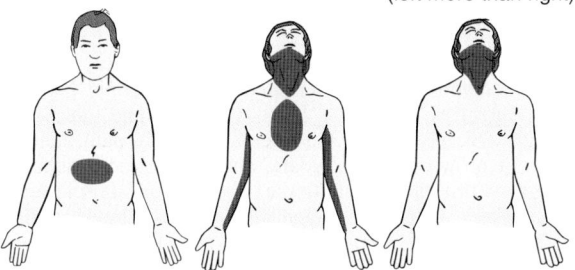

Upper abdomen

Chest, neck, jaw, and inside arms

Center of lower neck to both sides of upper neck and all of jaw

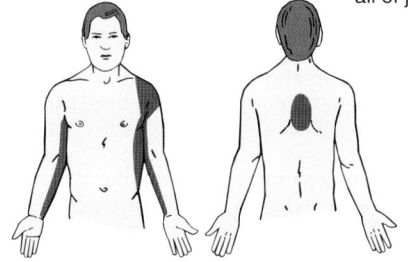

Inside right arm to below elbow, shoulder and inside left arm to waist (left side more often than right)

Between shoulder blades

Locations of pain from myocardial infarction

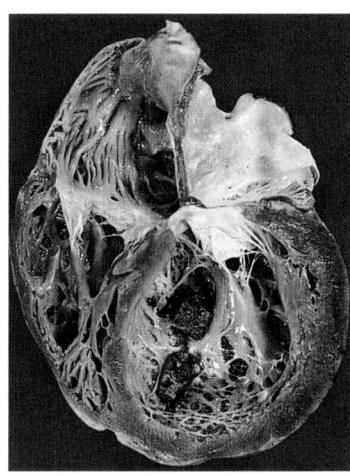

Dilated myocardiopathy *(Damjanov and Linder, 2000)*

myoclonus /mī′ōklō″nəs/ [Gk, *mys* muscle; + *klonos,* contraction], a spasm of a muscle or a group of muscles. —*myoclonic, adj.*

myocutaneous flap /mī′ōkyoo̅·tā′nē·əs/ [Gk, *mys,* muscle; L, *cutis,* skin], a compound flap of skin and muscle with adequate vascularity to permit sufficient tissue to be transferred to the recipient site.

myocyte /mī″əsīt/, a muscle cell.

myodiastasis /mī′ōdī·as″təsis/ [Gk, *mys + diastasis,* separation], an abnormal condition in which there is separation of muscle bundles.

myodystrophy. See **muscular dystrophy.**

myoedema /mī′ō·idē″mə/ *pl. myoedemas, myoedemata,* muscle edema. Compare **myxedema.**

myoelectric, pertaining to the electric property of muscle.

myofascial /mī·ōfa″shē·əl/, pertaining to a muscle and its sheath of connective tissue, or fascia.

myofascial pain, jaw muscle distress associated with chewing or exercise of the masticatory muscles.

myofascial release, a set of massage techniques used to relieve muscle pain resulting from abnormally tight fascia.

myofibril /-fī″bril/ [Gk, *mys + L, fibrilla,* small fiber], a slender striated strand within skeletal and cardiac muscle fibers and composed of bundles of myofilaments. Myofibrils occur in groups of branching threads running parallel to the cellular long axis of the fiber.

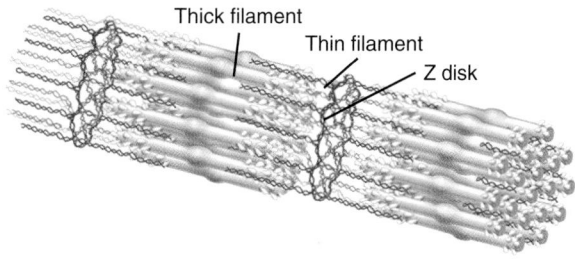

Thick filament

Thin filament

Z disk

Molecular structure of a myofibril
(Patton and Thibodeau, 2016)

myofilament /mī′ōfil′ə·mənt/ [Gk, *mys,* L, *filare,* to spin], any of the numerous ultramicroscopic threadlike structures occurring in bundles in the myofibrils of striated muscle fibers. The thick filaments of myosin and the thin filaments of actin are together responsible for the contractile properties of muscle. Also present are intermediate filaments, of uncertain function. See also **myofibril, actin, myosin.**

myogelosis /mī′ōjəlō″sis/ [Gk, *mys + L, gelare,* to freeze; Gk, *osis*], a condition in which there are hardened areas or nodules within muscles, especially the gluteal muscles. There are no serious consequences of this condition, and no treatment is necessary.

myogenic /mī′ōjen″ik/ [Gk, *mys + genesis,* origin], generated by muscles. The term usually refers to rhythmic activity in cardiac and smooth muscles, which do not require neural input to initiate and maintain contractions.

myoglobin /mī′ōglō″bin/ [Gk, *mys + L, globus,* ball], a ferrous globin complex in muscle consisting of one heme molecule containing one iron molecule attached to a single globin chain. Myoglobin is responsible for the red color of muscle and for its ability to store oxygen. Normal blood levels of myoglobin are 0 to 85 ng/mL. Excessive myoglobin levels may result from burns, muscle-wasting diseases, acute myocardial infarction, or trauma.

myoglobin test, a blood test that detects levels of myoglobin, an oxygen-binding protein found in cardiac and skeletal muscle. Measurement of myoglobin is an index of damage to

M

the myocardium in myocardial infarction or reinfarction and is also an indicator of disease or trauma of the skeletal muscle.

myoglobinuria /-glō′binoŏr″ē·ə/ [Gk, *mys* + L, *globus* + Gk, *ouron,* urine], the presence of myoglobin, an oxygen-storing pigment of muscle tissue, in the urine. The condition usually occurs after massive muscle injury, physical trauma, or electrical injury. The urine has a brown discoloration.

myoglobinuric renal failure /-glō′binoŏr″ik/, a kidney disease in which large amounts of filtered myoglobin coalesce in the tubules, obstructing nephronal flow and producing epithelial cell injury.

myokinase. See **adenylate kinase.**

myoma /mī·ō″mə/ *pl.* myomas, myomata [Gk, *mys* + *oma,* tumor], a common benign fibroid tumor of the uterine muscle. The tumor develops most frequently after 30 years of age in women, especially African-American women, who have never been pregnant. Menorrhagia, backache, constipation, dysmenorrhea, dyspareunia, and other symptoms develop in proportion to the size, location, and rate of growth of the tumor.

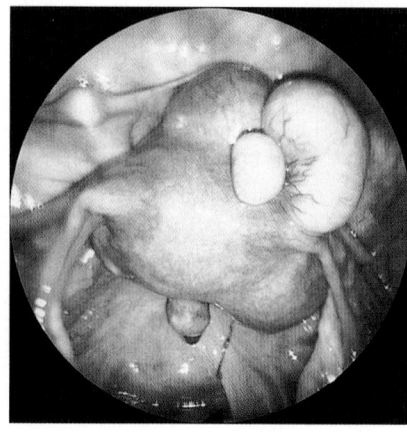

Multiple myomas: laparoscopic view *(Hunt, 1999)*

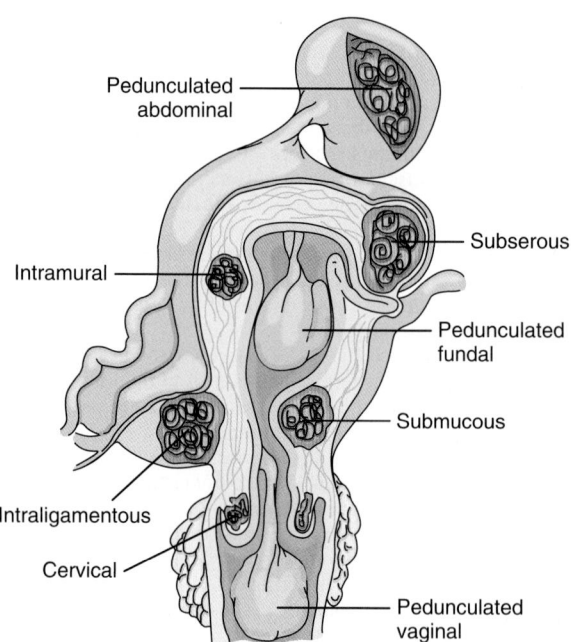

Pedunculated abdominal

Intramural

Subserous

Pedunculated fundal

Submucous

Intraligamentous

Cervical

Pedunculated vaginal

Common locations for myomas of the uterus *(Monahan and Neighbors, 2007)*

myoma previum. See **leiomyoma uteri.**

myomas. See **myoma.**

myoma striocellulare. See **rhabdomyoma.**

myomata. See **myoma.**

myomectomy /mī′ōmek″təmē/, the surgical removal of muscle tissue.

myomere. See **myotome.**

myometria. See **myometrium.**

myometritis /mī′ōmətrī″tis/, an inflammation or infection of the myometrium of the uterus.

myometrium /mī′ōmē″trē·əm/ *pl.* myometria [Gk, *mys* + *metra,* womb], the muscular layer of the wall of the uterus. The smooth muscle fibers of the myometrium course around the uterus horizontally, vertically, and diagonally.

myonecrosis /mī′ōnekrō″sis/ [Gk, *mys* + *necrosis,* death], the death of muscle fibers. Progressive, or clostridial, myonecrosis is caused by the anaerobic bacteria of the genus *Clostridium.* Seen in deep wound infections, progressive myonecrosis is accompanied by pain, tenderness, a brown serous exudate, and a rapid accumulation of gas within the muscle tissue. The affected muscle turns a blackish green. Treatment includes thorough wound debridement, IV administration of penicillin, and hyperbaric oxygen therapy to destroy the anaerobe and to promote healing.

myoneural /mī′ōnoŏr″əl/ [Gk, *mys* + *neuron,* nerve], pertaining to a muscle fiber and the synapse of the motor neuron, especially a nerve ending in a muscle.

myoneuralgia. See **myalgia.**

myoneural junction. See **end plate.**

myopathy /mī·op″əthē/ [Gk, *mys* + *pathos,* disease], an abnormal condition of skeletal muscle characterized by muscle weakness, wasting, and histological changes within muscle tissue, as seen in any of the muscular dystrophies. A myopathy is distinct from a muscle disorder caused by nerve dysfunction. The specific diagnosis is made by using tests of serum enzyme levels, electromyography, and muscle biopsy. See also **muscular dystrophy.** —*myopathic, adj.*

myope /mī″ōp/, an individual who is nearsighted or afflicted with myopia.

myophosphorylase deficiency glycogenosis. See **McArdle disease.**

myopia /mī·ō″pē·ə/ [Gk, *myops,* nearsighted], a condition of nearsightedness caused by the elongation of the eyeball or by an error in refraction so that parallel rays are focused in front of the retina. Also called **nearsightedness, short sight, shortsightedness.** Kinds include **curvature myopia, index myopia, pathological myopia.** —*myopic, adj.*

myopic shift. See **prodromal myopia.**

myoreceptor. See **muscle receptor.**

myorrhaphy /mī·ôr″əfē/ [Gk, *mys* + *rhaphe,* suture], suturing of a wound in a muscle.

myorrhexis /mī′ərek″sis/ [Gk, *mys* + *rhexis,* rupture], the tearing of any muscle. —*myorrhectic, adj.*

myosarcoma /mī′ōsärkō″mə/ [Gk, *mys* + *sarx,* flesh, *oma,* tumor], a malignant tumor of muscular tissue.

myosin /mī″əsin/ [Gk, *mys* + *in,* within], a protein that makes up close to one half of the total protein in muscle tissue. The interaction between myosin and another protein, actin, is essential for muscle contraction. See also **actino-, actin-.**

myositis /mī′əsī″tis/, inflammation of muscle tissue, usually of voluntary muscle. Causes of myositis include infection, trauma, and infestation by parasites. Also called **myitis.** Compare **fibromyalgia.** Kinds include **epidemic myositis, myositis fibrosa, parenchymatous myositis, polymyositis, traumatic myositis.**

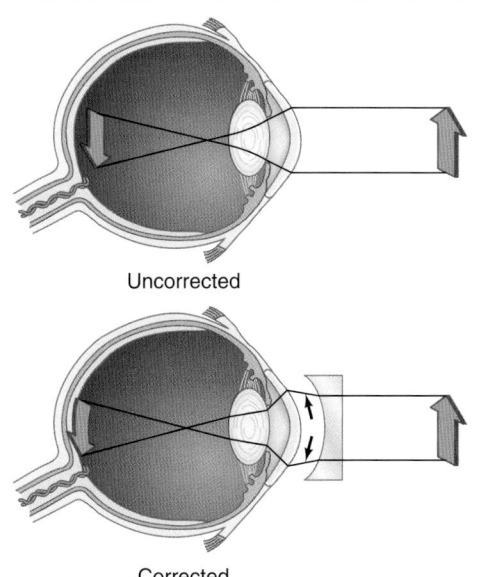

Myopia *(Patton and Thibodeau, 2016)*

myositis fibrosa, an uncommon inflammation of the muscles, characterized by abnormal formation of connective tissue. Also called **interstitial myositis.** See also **myositis.**

myositis ossificans /əsif″əkanz/, a rare inherited disease in which muscle tissue is replaced by bone. It begins in childhood, with stiffness in the neck and back, and progresses to rigidity of the spine, trunk, and limbs. The administration of diphosphonates may prevent the abnormal deposition of bone, but there is no cure after it has occurred. Metabolism of calcium and phosphate remains normal throughout the course of the disease. Compare **myositis.**

myositis ossificans progressiva, a progressive disease, beginning in early life, in which the muscles are gradually converted into bony tissue. Also called **fibrodysplasia ossificans progressiva, progressive ossifying myositis.**

myositis purulenta, any bacterial infection of muscle tissue. This condition may result in the formation of an abscess or multiple abscesses.

myositis trichinosa /trik′ənō″sə/, inflammation of the muscles resulting from infection by the parasite *Trichinella spiralis.*

myostasis /mī′ōstā″sis/ [Gk, *mys* + *stasis,* standing], a condition of muscle weakness in which the resting length of the muscle is shorter than normal, which reduces the maximal tension the muscle can develop when it contracts. In a normal muscle, the force of contraction is greatest at the resting length. −*myostatic, adj.*

myostatic reflex. See **deep tendon reflex.**

myostroma /mī′əstrō″mə/ [Gk, *mys* + *stroma,* covering], the framework of muscle tissue.

myotenotomy /-tenot″əmē/ [Gk, *mys* + *tenon,* tendon, *temnein,* to cut], surgical division of the whole or part of a muscle by cutting through its main tendon.

myotherapy /-ther″əpē/, a technique of corrective muscle exercises involving pressure on fingers and joints to relieve pain or spasms.

myotome /mī′ətōm/ [Gk, *mys* + *temnein,* to cut], **1.** the muscle plate of an embryonic somite that develops into a voluntary muscle. Also called **myomere. 2.** a group of muscles innervated by a single spinal segment. **3.** an instrument for cutting or dissecting a muscle.

myotomic muscle /-tom″ik/, any of the numerous muscles of the trunk of the body, derived from the myotomes and divided into the deep muscles of the back and the thoracoabdominal muscles.

myotomy /mī·ot″əmē/ [Gk, *mys* + *temnein,* to cut], the dissection or cutting of a muscle, performed to gain access to underlying tissues or to relieve constriction in a sphincter, such as in severe esophagitis or pyloric stenosis. With the patient under general anesthesia, a longitudinal cut is made through the sphincter muscle but not through the mucosa lining the stomach. See also **abdominal surgery.**

Myotonachol, a cholinergic drug. Brand name for **bethanechol chloride.**

myotonia /mī′ətō″nē·ə/ [Gk, *mys* + *tonos,* tone], any condition in which a muscle or a group of muscles does not readily relax after contracting. Compare **amyotonia.** −**myotonic,** *adj.*

myotonia atrophica. See **myotonic muscular dystrophy.**

myotonia congenita /konjen″itə/, a rare mild and nonprogressive form of myotonic myopathy evident early in life. The effects of the disorder are hypertrophy and stiffness of the muscles. Also called **Thomsen disease.**

myotonic. See **myotonia.**

myotonic muscular dystrophy /-ton″ik/, a severe form of muscular dystrophy marked by ptosis, facial weakness, and dysarthria. Weakness of the hands and feet precedes that in the shoulders and hips. Myotonia of the hands is usually present. Electromyography is helpful in establishing the diagnosis. Although there is no specific treatment, active and passive exercises are used to alleviate symptoms. Also called **myotonia atrophica, Steinert disease.**

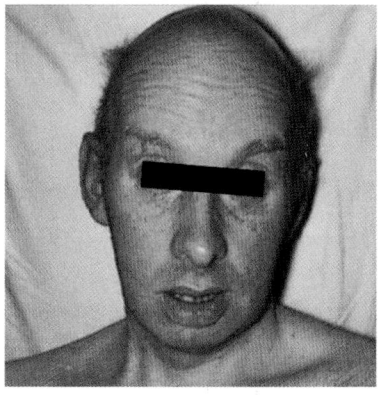

Myotonic muscular dystrophy: characteristic facial expression *(Perkin et al, 2011)*

myotonic myopathy, any of a group of disorders characterized by increased skeletal muscle tone and decreased relaxation of muscle after contraction. Kinds include **myotonia congenita, myotonic muscular dystrophy.**

myotube /mi′otoob/, a developing muscle cell or fiber with a centrally located nucleus.

MyPlate, an icon that replaced the U.S. Department of Agriculture's food pyramid in 2011. It depicts the five food groups to encourage mindful eating habits.

myria-, prefix meaning "a great number."

myringa. See **tympanic membrane.**

myringectomy /mir′injek″təmē/ [L, *myringa,* eardrum; Gk, *ektomē,* excision], excision of the tympanic membrane.

myringitis /mir′injī″tis/ [L, *myringa* + Gk, *itis*], inflammation or infection of the tympanic membrane.

M

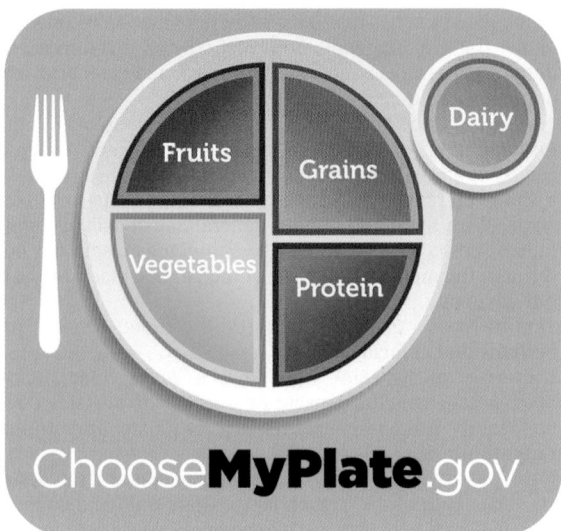

MyPlate *(U.S. Department of Agriculture, 2015)*

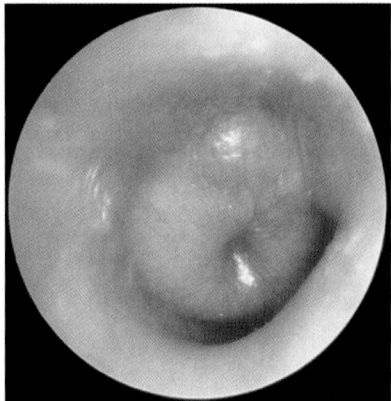

Myringitis *(Raftery, Lim, and Östör, 2014)*

myringo-, combining form meaning "related to the tympanic membrane": *myringoplasty, myringomycosis.*

myringomycosis /miring'gōmīkō"sis/ [L, *myringa* + Gk, *mykes,* fungus, *osis,* condition], a fungal infection of the tympanic membrane. Also called **mycomyringitis.**

myringoplasty /miring"gōplas'tē/ [L, *myringa* + Gk, *plassein,* to mold], surgical repair of perforations of the eardrum with a tissue graft, performed to correct hearing loss. The openings in the eardrum are enlarged, and the grafting material is sutured over them. Topical antibiotics are applied, then a packing of absorbable gelatin sponge to hold the graft in position. After surgery an antihistamine with an ephedrine derivative is given. The patient is instructed to keep the outer ear clean and dry. Debris is removed by gentle suctioning about 12 days after surgery. See also **myringotomy, tympanoplasty.**

myringotomy /mir'ing·got"əmē/ [L, *myringa* + Gk, *temnein,* to cut], surgical incision of the eardrum, performed to relieve pressure and release pus or fluid from the middle ear. Antibiotics are given before surgery and continued afterward. The drum is incised, and cultures may be taken. Fluid is gently suctioned from the middle ear. Eardrops may be instilled, or tubes may be inserted to improve drainage. The patient must be cautioned against putting cotton in the canal because the ear must drain freely. The outer ear is kept clean and dry. If pain increases, the procedure may have to be repeated. Severe headache or disorientation must be reported. Earplugs are required for swimming and showers if tubes are used. Also called **tympanostomy, tympanotomy.** See also **myringoplasty.**

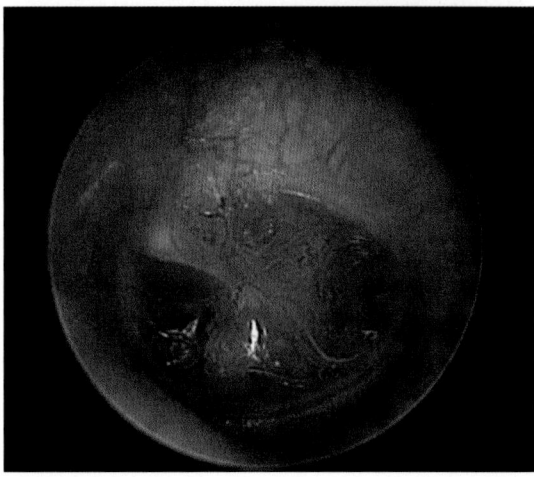

Myringotomy tube in place in the left lower quadrant of the tympanic membrane *(Neuman and Thom, 2008)*

Mysoline, an anticonvulsant drug. Brand name for **primidone.**

mysophobia /mē'sə-/ [Gk, *mysos,* anything disgusting, *phobos,* fear], *adj.,* an anxiety disorder characterized by an overreaction to the slightest uncleanliness or an irrational fear of dirt, contamination, or defilement. Also spelled *misophobia.* —*mysophobic, misophobic, adj.*

myx-, myxo-, prefix meaning "relating to mucus": *myxofibroma, myxoma.*

myxedema /mik'sədē"mə/ [Gk, *myxa,* mucus, *oidema,* swelling], the most severe form of hypothyroidism. It is characterized by swelling of the hands, face, feet, and periorbital tissues and may lead to coma and death. Also spelled *myxoedema.* See also **hypothyroidism.**

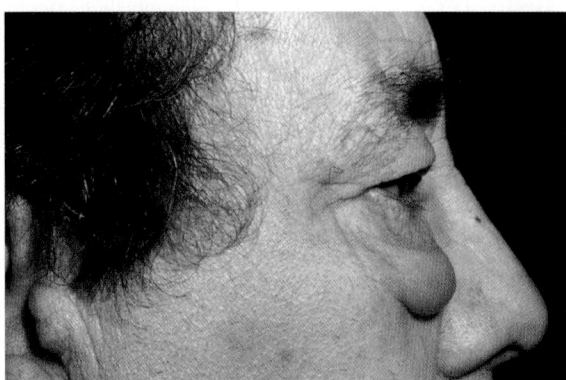

Patient with periorbital swelling associated with myxedema *(Kanski, 2006)*

myxofibroma /mik'sōfībrō"mə/ [Gk, *myxa* + L, *fibra,* fiber; Gk, *oma,* tumor], a fibrous tumor that contains myxomatous tissue. Also called **myxoma fibrosum.**

myxoid. See **mucoid,** def. 1.

myxoma /miksō″mə/ [Gk, *myxa* + *oma,* tumor], a neoplasm of the connective tissue, characteristically composed of stellate cells in a loose mucoid matrix crossed by delicate reticulum fibers. These tumors may grow to enormous size and may occur under the skin but are also found in bones, the genitourinary tract, and the retroperitoneal area. **−myxomatous,** *adj.*

-myxoma, suffix meaning "a soft tumor made up of primitive connective tissues": *lipomyxoma.*

myxoma fibrosum. See **myxofibroma.**

myxoma sarcomatosum. See **myxosarcoma.**

myxomatous. See **myxoma.**

myxopoiesis /mik′sōpō·ē″sis/ [Gk, *myxa* + *poiein,* to make], the production of mucus.

myxosarcoma /mik′sōsärkō″mə/ [Gk, *myxa* + *sarx,* flesh, *oma,* tumor], a sarcoma that contains some connective tissue. Also called **myxoma sarcomatosum.**

myxovirus /mik′sōvī″rəs/ [Gk, *myxa* + L, *virus,* poison], any of a group of medium-size ribonucleic acid viruses that are further divided into orthomyxoviruses and paramyxoviruses. Infection with these viruses is usually caused by transmission of the respiratory secretions of an infected host. The viruses that cause influenza, mumps, and parainfluenza are myxoviruses.

MZ, abbreviation for **monozygotic.**

M

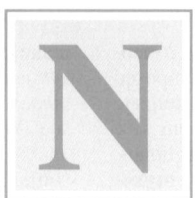

N, 1. symbol for the element **nitrogen. 2.** abbreviation for **normal. 3.** one element of the TNM (tumor, node, metastasis) system for staging malignant neoplastic disease. Abbreviation for **node.** See **cancer staging. 4.** abbreviation for **theoretic plate number. 5.** abbreviation for **asparagine.**

N/1, symbol for **normal solution.**

n, 2n, 3n, 4n, **1.** symbols for the haploid, diploid, triploid, and tetraploid number of chromosomes in a cell, organism, strain, or individual. **2.** symbols used to represent principal quantum numbers of electron shells. The greater the number, the larger the diameter and energy of the electron shell.

NA, abbreviation for **Narcotics Anonymous.**

*N*A, symbol for **Avogadro's number.**

nA, one billionth of an ampere. Abbreviation for *nanoampere.*

n/a, symbol for *not applicable, not available.*

Na, symbol for the element **sodium.**

-nab, combining form for cannabinol derivatives.

nabilone, an antiemetic.

■ INDICATIONS: This drug is used to prevent nausea and vomiting associated with cancer chemotherapy in those who have not responded to other treatment.

■ CONTRAINDICATIONS: Known hypersensitivity to this drug or to cannabinoids prohibits its use.

■ ADVERSE EFFECTS: Adverse effects of this drug include syncope; hallucinations; chest discomfort; orthostatic hypotension; nausea; increased appetite; allergic reactions; rash; photosensitivity; pruritus; and back, joint, muscle, and neck pain. A life-threatening side effect is tachycardia. Common side effects include headache, ataxia, drowsiness, dysphoria, euphoria, sleep disturbance, vertigo, asthenia, concentration difficulties, depression, dry mouth, and anorexia.

nabothian cyst /nabō″thē·ən/ [Martin Naboth, German physician, 1675–1721; Gk, *kystis,* bag], a cyst formed in a nabothian gland of the uterine cervix. It is a common finding on routine pelvic examination of women of reproductive age, especially in women who have borne children. The cyst, which is pearly white and firm, seldom results in adverse or pathological effects. Also called **cervical cyst.**

nabothian gland /nəbō″thē·ən/ [Martin Naboth; L, *glans,* acorn], one of many small, mucus-secreting glands of the uterine cervix.

NAD, 1. abbreviation for **no appreciable disease. 2.** abbreviation for *nicotinamide adenine dinucleotide,* a coenzyme found in all living cells that plays a role in cellular metabolism. The oxidized form is written as NAD+.

NADH, nicotinamide adenine dinucleotide (NAD) + hydrogen (H), a coenzyme found in all living cells and an important driving force behind the electron transport chain within the mitochondrion. Abbreviation for *nicotine adenine dinucleotide, reduced.*

nadir /nā″dər/, the lowest point, as in an individual's blood count after it has been depressed by chemotherapy.

nadolol /nad″ənol/, a beta-adrenergic blocking agent.

■ INDICATIONS: It is prescribed for long-term management of angina pectoris, for hypertension, and for migraine prophylaxis.

■ CONTRAINDICATIONS: Bronchial asthma, sinus bradycardia, greater than first-degree conduction block, cardiogenic shock, overt cardiac failure, or known hypersensitivity to this drug prohibits its use.

■ ADVERSE EFFECTS: Among the more serious adverse effects are bronchospasm, bradycardia, precipitation of heart failure, cardiac arrhythmia, masking of signs of hypoglycemia in diabetics, fatigue, and lethargy. GI disturbances, rashes, and other allergic reactions may also occur.

NADPH, 1. Abbreviation for *nicotine adenine disphosphonucleotide, reduced.* **2.** (in botany and zoology) a molecule that is a plant cell analog of NADH. It plays an important role in the Calvin cycle, where it is used to convert CO_2 to sugar.

NADPH oxidase defect, a disorder in patients with chronic granulomatosis disease. It is caused by an abnormality in the enzyme (nicotinamide adenine dinucleotide phosphate oxidase) that catalyzes the conversion of oxygen to superoxide anions and hydrogen peroxide in phagocytes. Phagocytes with the abnormal enzyme are unable to destroy invading microorganisms.

Naegele's rule, also spelled **Nägele's rule.**

Naegleria /nā·glēr′ē·ə/ [F.P.O. Nägler, 20th-century Austrian bacteriologist], a genus of free-living protozoa, found in freshwater, soil, and sewage, that have both an ameboid and a flagellate stage in their life cycle. Certain species, especially *N. fowleri,* are capable of facultative parasitism, and some strains are highly pathogenic and may cause a highly fatal primary amebic meningoencephalitis. Infection is usually acquired by swimming in water contaminated with the organisms. See also **primary amebic meningoencephalitis.**

naegleriasis /nā′glərī′əsis/, infection with *Naegleria.*

naevus, a visible, circumscribed, long-lasting lesion of the skin or the neighboring mucosa, reflecting genetic mosaicism. See **nevus.**

nafcillin sodium /nafsil″in/, an antibiotic.

■ INDICATIONS: It is prescribed in the treatment of infections caused by penicillinase-producing staphylococci.

■ CONTRAINDICATIONS: Known hypersensitivity to this drug or to other penicillins prohibits its use.

■ ADVERSE EFFECTS: Among the more serious adverse effects are hypersensitivity reactions, nausea, and vomiting.

Naffziger sign /naf″zigər/ [Howard C. Naffziger, American surgeon, 1884–1961], a diagnostic sign for sciatica or a herniated intervertebral disk. Nerve root irritation is produced by the examiner through external jugular venous compression. Also called **Naffziger's test.**

Naffziger syndrome [Howard C. Naffziger], a condition of cervical vertebral muscle spasms secondary to intervertebral disk disease, cervical rib disease, or other disorders. The spasms compress the major nerve plexus of the arm, causing the patient to experience pain in the neck, shoulder, arm, and hand. Also called **scalenus anticus syndrome.** Compare **thoracic outlet syndrome.**

Naffziger's test /naf″zig·ərz/, (for nerve root compression) manual compression of the jugular veins bilaterally. An increase or aggravation of pain or sensory disturbance over the distribution of the involved nerve root confirms the presence of an extruded intervertebral disk or other mass. Also called **Naffziger sign.**

NAFLD, abbreviation for **nonalcoholic fatty liver disease.**

Nägele obliquity [Franz K. Nägele, German obstetrician, 1778–1851], a type of fetal presentation in which the baby presents with the anterior parietal bone in the birth canal, making the biparietal diameter oblique to the pelvic bone. See **asynclitism.**

Nägele's rule /nā″gələz/ [Franz K. Nägele, German obstetrician, 1778–1851; L, *regula,* model], a method for calculating the estimated date of delivery based on a mean length of gestation. Three months are subtracted from the first day of the last normal menstrual period, and 1 year plus 7 days are added to that date.

Nager acrofacial dysostosis /nā″gər/ [Felix R. Nager, Swiss physician, 1877–1959; Gk, *akron,* extremity; L, *facies,* face; Gk, *dys,* bad, *osteon,* bone, *osis,* condition], an abnormal congenital condition characterized by limb deformities such as radioulnar synostosis, hypoplasia, and the absence of the radius or of the thumbs. Also called **dysostosis mandibularis.** Compare **cleidocranial dysostosis, craniofacial dysostosis, mandibulofacial dysostosis.**

Naglazyme, an enzyme replacement. Brand name for *galsulfase.*

nail [AS, *naegel*], **1.** several flattened layers of hard, keratinized epithelial cells with a horny texture at the end of a finger or a toe. Each nail is composed of a root, body, and free edge at the distal extremity. The root fastens the nail to the finger or the toe by fitting into a groove in the skin and is closely molded to the surface of the dermis. The nail matrix beneath the body and the root projects longitudinal vascular ridges, which are easily visible through the translucent tissue of the body. The matrix firmly attaches the body of the nail to the underlying connective tissue. The whitish lunula near the root contains irregularly arranged papillae that are less firmly attached to the connective tissue than the rest of the matrix. The cuticle is attached to the surface of the nail just ahead of the root. Also called **unguis. 2.** any of various metallic nails used in orthopedics to fasten together bones or pieces of bone.

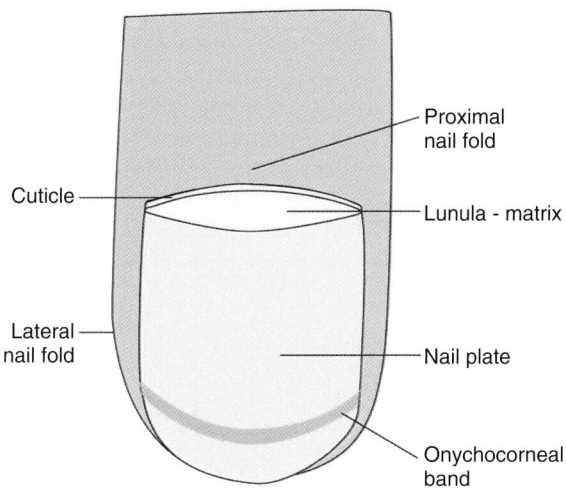

Nail anatomy *(De Berker, 2013)*

- Proximal nail fold
- Cuticle
- Lunula - matrix
- Lateral nail fold
- Nail plate
- Onychocorneal band

nailbed [AS, *naegle,* nail, *bedd,* bed], the dermis beneath the nail. It appears through the clear nail as a series of longitudinal ridges. Also called **matrix unguis.**

nail biting, the habit of excessive biting and chewing one's fingernails and periungual skin, sometimes leading to cutaneous injury. The condition is commonly associated with anxiety. It is also considered a form of motor discharge of inner tension. The recommended treatment includes daily bandaging of injured fingers and frequent applications of a distasteful topical preparation. Also called **onychophagia.**

nail fold, a fold of skin supporting a nail at its base.

nail groove [AS, *naegle* + D, *groeve,* groove], a shallow depression between the nailbed and the nail wall.

nail matrix, the part of the nail apparatus composed of rapidly dividing cells, which give rise to the nail plate. See also **nailbed.**

nail-patella syndrome, a hereditary syndrome consisting of dystrophy of the nails, absence or hypoplasia of the patella, hypoplasia of the lateral side of the elbow joint, and bilateral iliac horns. Also called **hereditary osteoonychodysplasia, onycho-osteodysplasia, osteoonychodysplasia.**

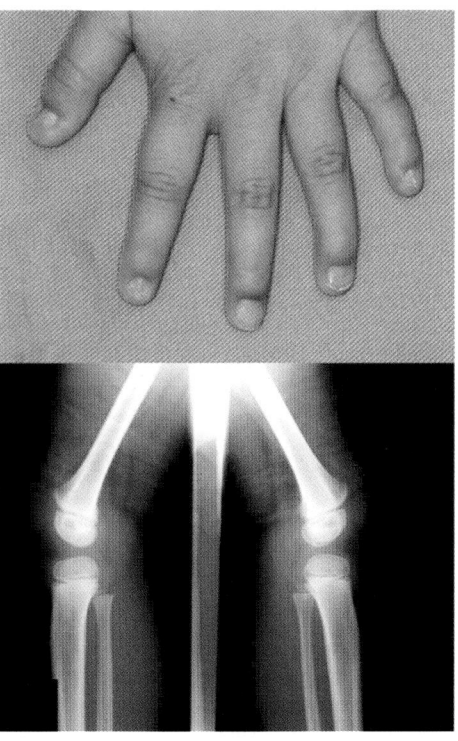

Findings associated with nail-patella syndrome *(Oshimo et al, 2008)*

nail plate, the rigid outer part of a nail. It extends about 8 mm under the nail fold and arises from the nailbed.

nail plate avulsion, a partial or complete removal of the nail plate without disruption of the underlying matrix cells.

nal-, prefix meaning "narcotic agonists or antagonists related to normorphine."

nalbuphine, a synthetic opioid agonist and antagonist.

■ INDICATIONS: This drug is used to treat moderate to severe pain.

■ CONTRAINDICATIONS: Opiate addiction or known hypersensitivity to this drug prohibits its use.

■ ADVERSE EFFECTS: Adverse effects of this drug include dysphoria, hallucinations, dreaming, tolerance, physical dependency, psychological dependency, palpitations, bradycardia, change in blood pressure, orthostatic hypotension,

N

tinnitus, blurred vision, miosis, diplopia, increased urinary output, dysuria, urinary retention, urinary urgency, urticaria, bruising, flushing, diaphoresis, pruritus, and pulmonary edema. Common side effects include drowsiness, dizziness, confusion, headache, sedation, euphoria, nausea, vomiting, anorexia, constipation, cramps, and rash. Respiratory depression is a life-threatening side effect.

Nalfon, an antiinflammatory agent. Brand name for **fenoprofen calcium.**

nalidixic acid /nal′idik″sik/, an antibacterial drug.
- INDICATIONS: It is prescribed in the treatment of certain urinary tract infections.
- CONTRAINDICATIONS: Renal or hepatic insufficiency, a history of convulsive disorders, or known hypersensitivity to this drug prohibits its use. It should not be used in children less than 3 months of age and should be used with care in prepubertal children.
- ADVERSE EFFECTS: Quinolones have caused tendon rupture, especially in prepubertal children, and severe hypersensitivity reactions. Among the more serious effects are increased intracranial pressure, seizures, hemolytic anemia in people affected with glucose-6-phosphate dehydrogenase deficiency, and GI and neurological disturbances.

nalmefene /nal′mĕfēn″/, an opioid antagonist, used as the hydrochloride salt in the treatment of opioid overdose and postoperative opioid depression.

naloxone hydrochloride /nal″əksōn/, an opioid antagonist.
- INDICATIONS: It is prescribed for reversal of respiratory depression and other opioid effects in patients receiving opioid analgesics and in patients who have abused heroin, morphine, or other synthetic opioids.
- CONTRAINDICATIONS: Known hypersensitivity to this drug prohibits its use.
- ADVERSE EFFECTS: Among the most serious adverse effects when given to opioid-dependent patients are side effects associated with opioid withdrawal.

naltrexone hydrochloride /naltrek″sōn/, an oral opioid antagonist.
- INDICATIONS: It is prescribed to block the effects of opioid analgesics, including heroin, morphine, and methadone, in patients recovering from addiction and to treat ethanol dependence.
- CONTRAINDICATIONS: Acute hepatitis or liver failure prohibits its use. Periodic liver function tests are recommended for all patients. Patients must be completely free of opioids before taking naltrexone to prevent severe withdrawal symptoms. Patients must be educated that their tolerance to morphine disappears while they are on naltrexone and that they can be much more sensitive to opioids after discontinuing naltrexone; dosage levels of heroin, morphine, and similar drugs that were previously tolerated could now be fatal.
- ADVERSE EFFECTS: The most serious adverse effects are abdominal pain, cramps, nausea, vomiting, headache, sleep disorders, and joint and muscle pain. Some adverse effects may actually be withdrawal symptoms rather than reactions to naltrexone.

Namaqualand hip dysplasia [Namaqualand region of Africa], an autosomal-dominant genetic defect found in children of African heritage. It is characterized by a growth failure in the femoral epiphysis, resulting in pain and early degenerative arthritis of the hip.

Namenda, a cognitive-enhancing medication used in the treatment of Alzheimer disease. Brand name for **memantine.**

NAMI, abbreviation for **National Alliance on Mental Illness.**

NANB, abbreviation for **non-A, non-B hepatitis.** See **hepatitis C.**

Nance leeway space. See **leeway space.**

NANDA, abbreviation for **North American Nursing Diagnosis Association.**

nandrolone /nan″drəlōn/, an anabolic steroid.
- INDICATIONS: It is prescribed to treat metastatic breast cancer in females and to increase hemoglobin and red cell mass in the management of the anemia of renal insufficiency. It increases hemoglobin and red cell mass.
- CONTRAINDICATIONS: Cancer of the male breast or prostate, liver disease, pregnancy, nephrosis, suspected pregnancy, or known hypersensitivity to this drug prohibits its use.
- ADVERSE EFFECTS: Among the most serious adverse effects are various endocrine disturbances, depending on the patient's age. Hirsutism, acne, liver toxicity, masculinization, and electrolyte imbalances also occur.

nanism /nā″nizəm, nan″-/ [Gk, nanos, dwarf], an abnormal smallness or underdevelopment of the body; growth failure. Also called **nanosomia.** Kinds include **mulibrey nanism, Paltauf nanism, renal nanism, senile nanism, symptomatic nanism.**

nano-, **1.** prefix meaning "small" or "related to smallness or dwarfism": *nanocephaly, nanomelia.* **2.** prefix used in measurement to mean "one billionth (10^{-9})": *nanocurie, nanogram, nanometer.*

nanobots, microscopic materials or mechanisms used to travel within the body. See also **nanotechnology.**

nanocephalia. See **nanocephaly.**

nanocephalic dwarf. See **Seckel syndrome.**

nanocephaly /nā′nōsef″əlē, nan′-/ [Gk, nanos + kephale, head], a developmental anomaly characterized by extreme smallness of the head with an underdeveloped brain. Also called **nanocephalia,** *nanocephalism.*

nanocormia /nā′nōkôr″mē·ə/ [Gk, nanos + kormos, trunk], disproportionate smallness of the trunk of the body in comparison with the head and limbs.

nanocurie (nCi) /nan″əkyŏŏr′ē/ [Gk, dwarf; Marie and Pierre Curie], a unit of radiation equal to one billionth of a curie. See also **curie.**

nanogram (ng) /nan″əgram/ [Gk, nanos + Fr, gramme, small weight], one billionth (10^{-9}) of a gram.

-nanoid, small. See **nanus.**

nanomelia /nā′nōmē′lyə, nan′-/ [Gk, nanos + melos, limb], a developmental defect characterized by abnormally small limbs in comparison with the size of the head and trunk. −*nanomelous, adj.,* −*nanomelus, n.*

nanometer (nm) /nan″əmē″tər/ [Gk, nanos + metron, measure], a unit of measurement equal to one billionth of a meter.

nanophthalmos /nā′nofthal″məs, nan′-/ [Gk, nanos + ophthalmos, eye], the condition in which one or both eyes are abnormally small, although other ocular defects are not present. Also called *nanophthalmia.* See also **microphthalmos.**

nanosecond (ns) /nan″əsek′ənd/ [Gk, nanos, dwarf; L, secundus, second], one billionth (10^{-9}) of a second.

nanosomia. See **nanism.**

nanosomus /nā′nōsō″məs/ [Gk, nanos + soma, body], a person of very short stature.

nanotechnology /-teknol′əjē/, technology at the level of atoms, molecules, and molecular fragments, including their manipulation and the creation of new structures. Nanotechnology holds great promise in health care and is already being used as the basis for new, more effective drug delivery systems.

nanukayami /nä′nŏŏkäyä″mē/ [Jpn], an acute, infectious disease caused by one of the serotypes of the spirochete *Leptospira* that is indigenous to Japan. See also **leptospirosis.**

nanus /nā″nəs/, **1.** See **dwarf. 2.** an individual of abnormally small stature. *−nanoid, adj.*

napalm /nā″päm/, a form of jellied gasoline used in warfare.

napalm burn [AS, *baernan,* burn], a thermal burn caused by contact with flaming napalm. See also **napalm.**

nape [ME], the back of the neck.

naphazoline hydrochloride /nəfaz″əlēn/, an adrenergic vasoconstrictor.

■ INDICATIONS: It is prescribed in the treatment of nasal congestion and as an ophthalmic vasoconstrictor to decrease redness and itching.

■ CONTRAINDICATIONS: Glaucoma or known hypersensitivity to this drug or abnormal sensitivity to sympathomimetic drugs prohibits its use.

■ ADVERSE EFFECTS: Among the most serious adverse effects are those associated with systemic absorption, including sedation and cardiovascular effects. Irritation to mucosa and rebound congestion also may occur.

naphthalene poisoning /naf″thəlēn/ [Gk, *naptha,* flammable liquid; L, *potio,* drink], a toxic condition caused by the ingestion of naphthalene or paradichlorobenzene that may cause increased heart rate, nausea, vomiting, headache, abdominal pain, spasm, and convulsions. Naphthalene and paradichlorobenzene are common ingredients in mothballs, moth crystals, and toilet bowl deodorizers. Paradichlorobenzene is also used as an insecticide in agriculture.

naphthol poisoning. See **phenol poisoning.**

napkin ring tumor [ME, *nappekin,* tablecloth, *hring,* band; L, *tumor,* swelling], a tumor that encircles a tubular structure of the body, usually impairing its function and constricting its lumen to some degree.

NAP-NAP, abbreviation for **National Association of Pediatric Nurse Associates/Practitioners.**

NAPNES, abbreviation for **National Association for Practical Nurse Education and Services.**

napping [ME, *nappen,* to doze], resting for short periods of time, usually during the day, from 15 to 60 minutes without attaining a level of deep sleep.

Naprosyn, a nonsteroidal antiinflammatory, antipyretic, and analgesic agent. Brand name for **naproxen.**

naproxen /naprok″sən/, a nonsteroidal antiinflammatory agent.

■ INDICATIONS: It is prescribed for the relief of fever, migraine headache, inflammatory symptoms of rheumatoid arthritis and osteoarthritis, and mild to moderate pain and for treatment of primary dysmenorrhea, ankylosing spondylitis, tendinitis, bursitis, and acute gout.

■ CONTRAINDICATIONS: Impaired renal function, GI disease, or known hypersensitivity to this drug, to aspirin, or to nonsteroidal antiinflammatory drugs prohibits its use.

■ ADVERSE EFFECTS: Among the more serious adverse effects are GI disorders and peptic ulcers. Dizziness, rashes, and tinnitus commonly occur. This drug interacts with many other drugs.

Naqua, a diuretic and antihypertensive drug. Brand name for **trichlormethiazide.**

naratriptan, a migraine agent.

■ INDICATIONS: It is used in the acute treatment of migraine with or without aura.

■ CONTRAINDICATIONS: The following factors prohibit its use: angina pectoris, a history of myocardial infarction, documented silent ischemia, ischemic heart disease, concurrent use of ergotamine-containing preparations, uncontrolled hypertension, hypersensitivity, severe renal disease (creatinine clearance rate 15 mL/min), and severe hepatic disease in children (Pugh grade C).

■ ADVERSE EFFECTS: Adverse effects include nausea, myalgia, dizziness, sedation, and fatigue. Common side effects include weakness and neck stiffness.

narc, abbreviation for **narcotic.**

Narcan, an opioid antagonist. Brand name for **naloxone hydrochloride.**

narcissism /när″sisiz′əm/ [Gk, *Narcissus,* mythic youth in love with himself], **1.** an abnormal interest in oneself, especially in one's own body and sexual characteristics; self-love. **2.** (in Freudian psychoanalytic theory) sexual self-interest that is a normal characteristic of the phallic stage of psychosexual development, occurring as the infantile ego acquires a libido. Narcissism in the adult is abnormal, representing fixation at this stage of development or regression to it. Compare **egotism.** See also **narcissistic personality, narcissistic personality disorder.**

narcissistic personality, a disposition characterized by behavior and attitudes that indicate an abnormal love of the self. A person with this disposition is self-centered and self-absorbed, is extremely unrealistic concerning attributes and goals, vacillates between overidealizing and devaluing others, and, in general, assumes that he or she is entitled to more than is reasonable in relationships with others. These individuals have a deep fear of abandonment and feel intense shame. Psychotherapy is the treatment of choice. See also **narcissism, egoist.**

narcissistic personality disorder /när′sisis″tik/, a psychiatric diagnosis characterized by an exaggerated sense of self-importance and uniqueness, an abnormal need for attention and admiration, preoccupation with grandiose fantasies concerning the self, and disturbances in interpersonal relationships, usually involving the exploitation of others and a lack of empathy. Compare **antisocial personality disorder.**

narco-, combining form meaning "related to stupor" or "a stuporous state": *narcolepsy, narcotic.*

narcoanalysis /när′kōənal′isis/, an interview conducted while the patient is deeply sedated with medication so that inhibitions are reduced and responses will be more truthful.

narcohypnosis /-hipnō″sis/ [Gk, *narke,* stupor, *hypnos,* sleep], hypnosis induced with the aid of a narcotic drug such as sodium amobarbital or sodium pentothal.

narcolepsy /när″kəlep′sē/ [Gk, *narke,* stupor, *lambanein,* to seize], a syndrome characterized by sudden sleep attacks, cataplexy, sleep paralysis, and visual or auditory hallucinations at the onset of sleep. The syndrome begins in adolescence or young adulthood and persists throughout life. Its cause is unknown, and it is not related to pathological lesions in the brain. Also called **sleep epilepsy.**

■ OBSERVATIONS: Persons with narcolepsy experience an uncontrollable desire to sleep, sometimes many times in one day. Episodes may last from a few minutes to several hours. Momentary loss of muscle tone occurs during waking hours (cataplexy) or while the person is asleep. Narcolepsy may be difficult to diagnose because all people with the disorder do not experience all four symptoms. An electroencephalogram or other brain studies may be used to distinguish narcolepsy from an intracranial mass or encephalitis.

■ INTERVENTIONS: Amphetamines and other stimulant drugs are prescribed effectively to prevent the attacks. Evaluation and treatment by a sleep evaluation center is warranted.

■ PATIENT CARE CONSIDERATIONS: Narcolepsy can negatively affect an individual both socially and professionally.

narcoleptic /när′kəlep″tik/, **1.** *adj.,* pertaining to a condition or substance that causes an uncontrollable desire for sleep. **2.** *n.,* a narcoleptic drug. **3.** *n.,* a person suffering from narcolepsy.

narcosis /närkō″sis/ [Gk, *narkosis,* numbness], a state of insensibility or stupor caused by opioid drugs. See also **narcotic.**

narcotic (narc) /närkot″ik/ [Gk, *narkotikos,* benumbing], **1.** *adj.,* pertaining to a substance that produces insensibility or stupor. **2.** *n.,* a narcotic drug. Narcotic analgesics, derived from opium or produced synthetically, alter perception of pain; induce euphoria, mood changes, mental clouding, and deep sleep; depress respiration and the cough reflex; constrict the pupils and cause smooth muscle spasm, decreased peristalsis, emesis, and nausea. Repeated use of narcotics may result in physical and psychological dependence. Among the narcotic drugs administered clinically for relief of pain are butorphanol tartrate, hydromorphone hydrochloride, morphine sulfate, pentazocine lactate, and meperidine hydrochloride. These drugs act by binding to opiate receptors in the central nervous system; narcotic antagonists such as naloxone hydrochloride, which is used in treating narcotic overdosage, apparently displace opiates from receptor sites. The term is now often used to refer to any illicit drug, and its use is therefore discouraged in medical settings. *Opioid* is now the preferred term.

-narcotic, -narcotical, suffix meaning "analgesic or soporific drugs."

narcotic analgesic. See **analgesic.**

narcotic antagonist. See **opioid antagonist.**

narcotic antitussive. See **antitussive.**

narcotic poisoning [Gk, *narkotikos,* be numbing; L, *potio,* drink], the toxic effects of a narcotic drug that depresses the brain centers, causing unconsciousness or coma. Narcotic drugs are generally derived from opium, but other drugs, including alcohol, can produce similar effects.

Narcotics Anonymous, an international nonprofit organization with the goal of assisting its members to live drug-free.

narcotize /när″kətiz/, to subject to the influence of narcotics.

Nardil, an antidepressant drug. Brand name for **phenelzine sulfate.**

nares /ner″ēz/, the pairs of anterior and posterior openings to the nasal cavity that allow the passage of air to the pharynx and ultimately the lungs during respiration. See also **anterior nares, posterior nares.**

narrow-angle glaucoma. See **glaucoma.**

nas, abbreviation for **nasal.**

nas-. See **naso- nas-.**

nasal (nas) /nā″zəl/ [L, *nasus,* nose], **1.** *adj.,* pertaining to the nose and the nasal cavity. **2.** *n.,* a speech sound produced by having air flow through the nose, such as /n/, /ng/, or /m/. **–nasally,** *adv.*

nasal airway, a flexible, curved piece of rubber or plastic, with one wide, trumpetlike end and one narrow end that can be inserted through the nose into the pharynx. Also called *nasal trumpet.*

nasal balloon tamponade, a procedure for the control of posterior epistaxis in which a nasal balloon is inserted into the nasal cavity and filled with saline solution. Alternatively, a Foley catheter can be placed through the nostril and used in the same manner.

nasal cannula, a device for delivering oxygen by way of two small tubes that are inserted into the nares.

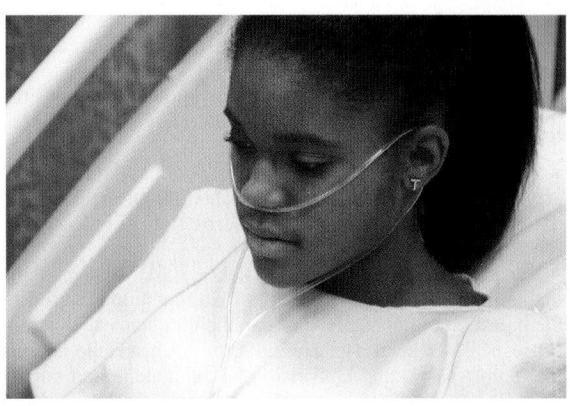

Patient with nasal cannula for oxygen administration

nasal cartilage [L, *nasus,* nose, *cartilago*], a flat plate of cartilage in the lower anterior part of the nasal septum. Also called **septal cartilage.**

nasal cavity, one of a pair of cavities that open on the face through the pear-shaped anterior nares and communicate posteriorly with the pharynx. Each cavity is narrower at the top than at the bottom.

nasal decongestant, a drug that provides temporary relief of nasal symptoms in acute and chronic rhinitis and sinusitis. Most are over-the-counter products compounded with a small amount of vasoconstrictor, such as pseudoephedrine or phenylephrine. An antihistamine may enhance the value of a nasal decongestant in allergic rhinitis, and a corticosteroid may reduce inflammation. Prolonged use or dosage greater than recommended on the package may cause rebound vasodilation and severe congestion (rhinitis medicamentosa). Use is contraindicated in patients with heart disease.

nasal drip, *(Informal)* a method of slowly infusing liquid into a dehydrated infant by means of a catheter inserted through the nose down the esophagus.

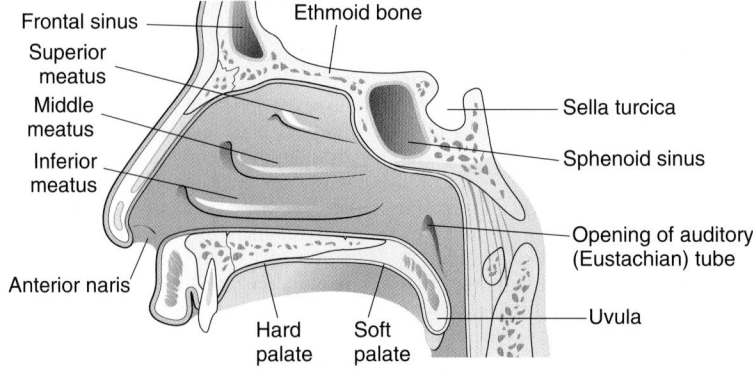

Frontal sinus — Ethmoid bone
Superior meatus
Middle meatus — Sella turcica
Inferior meatus — Sphenoid sinus
Anterior naris — Opening of auditory (Eustachian) tube
Hard palate — Soft palate — Uvula

Nasal cavity *(Salvo, 2012)*

nasal fin, a thickened platelike ectodermal structure between the lateral and medial nasal prominences that thins to form the oronasal membrane.

nasal fossa, one of the pair of approximately equal chambers of the nasal cavity that are separated by the nasal septum and open externally through the nares and internally into the nasopharynx through the internal nares. Each fossa is divided into an olfactory region, consisting of the superior nasal concha and part of the septum, and a respiratory region, constituting the rest of the chamber. Overhanging the three meatuses of each fossa on the lateral wall are the corresponding superior, middle, and inferior nasal conchae. The superior meatus extends obliquely about halfway along the superior border of the middle concha. The middle meatus continues into the atrium and bulges on the lateral wall at the bulla ethmoidalis. The inferior meatus courses below and laterally to the inferior nasal concha and contains the opening of the nasolacrimal duct. The olfactory region is located in the most superior part of the fossa and contains olfactory cells, olfactory nerves, and olfactory hairs. The respiratory region is lined with mucous membrane, numerous glands, nerves, a plexus of dilated veins, and blood spaces. The plexus is easily irritated, causing the membrane to swell, blocking the meatuses and the openings of sinuses.

nasal fracture reduction, repair of the paired nasal bones or cartilage. Reduction can be closed or open. Closed reduction is usually performed by digital and instrumental manipulation with the patient under topical and local anesthesia. When the fracture is severe, open reduction under general anesthesia with interosseous wire fixation of bone fragments may be necessary. Nasal fractures are the most common facial fractures and may lead to obstruction without proper attention. See also **rhinoplasty.**

nasal glioma, a neoplasm characterized by the ectopic growth of neural tissue in the nasal cavity.

nasal instillation of medication, the instillation of a medicated solution into the nostrils by an atomized spray from a squeeze bottle, a dropper, or a nasal inhaler. The patient holds one nostril closed while spraying the medication into the opposite nostril. Nasal spray is administered to the patient in a sitting position. The patient is asked to expectorate any solution that runs down the posterior nares into the throat.

nasalis /nāzal″is/ [L, *nasus,* nose], one of the three muscles of the nose, divided into a transverse part and an alar part. The transverse part arises from the maxilla and covers the bridge of the nose; the alar part attaches at one end to the greater alar cartilage and at the other end to skin at the end of the nose. The transverse part serves to depress the cartilaginous part of the nose and to draw the alar toward the septum. The alar part serves to dilate the nostril. Compare **depressor septi, procerus.**

nasally. See **nasal.**

nasal obstruction [L, *nasus,* nose, *obstruere*], a narrowing of the nasal cavity, thereby reducing the breathing capacity, caused by an irregular or deviated septum, nasal polyps, foreign bodies, or enlarged turbinates. Sinusitis is a common complication of the condition.

nasal placode, an oval area of thickened ectoderm on either ventrolateral surface of the head of the early embryo, constituting the first indication of the olfactory organ.

nasal polyp, a rounded, elongated piece of pulpy, dependent mucosa that projects into the nasal cavity.

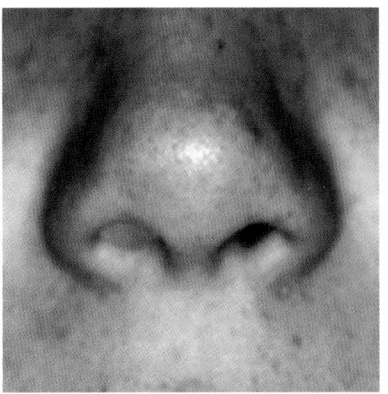

Nasal polyp *(Swartz, 2006)*

nasal septum, the plate of bone and cartilage covered with mucous membrane that divides the nasal cavity.

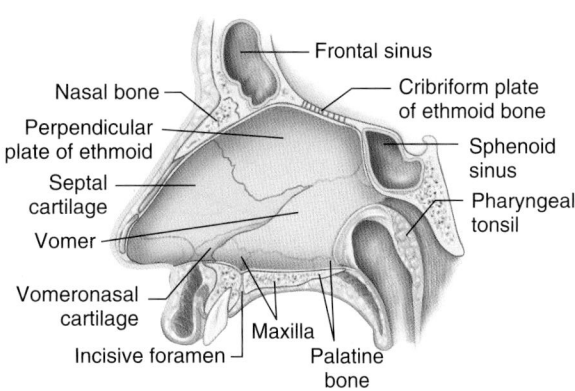

Nasal septum *(Patton and Thibodeau, 2016)*

nasal sinus, any one of the numerous cavities in various bones of the skull, lined with ciliated mucous membrane continuous with that of the nasal cavity. The membrane is very sensitive; easily irritated, it may cause swelling that blocks the sinuses. The nasal sinuses are divided into frontal

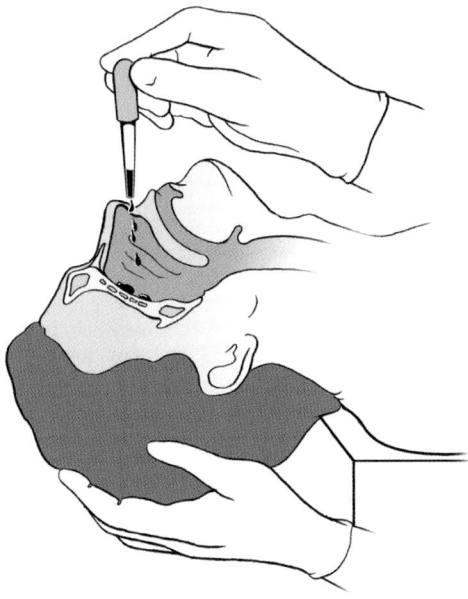

Instillation of nose drops *(deWit and O'Neill, 2014)*

sinuses, ethmoidal air cells, sphenoidal sinuses, and maxillary sinus. See also **sinus.**

Nasarel, an intranasal steroid antiinflammatory agent. Brand name for **flunisolide.**

nascent /nas″ənt, nā″sənt/ [L, *nasci,* to be born], **1.** just born; beginning to exist; incipient. **2.** (in chemistry) pertaining to any substance liberated during a chemical reaction that, because of its uncombined state, is more reactive.

nascent oxygen, oxygen that has just been liberated from a chemical compound.

nasion /nā″zē·on/ [L, *nasus,* nose], **1.** the anthropometric reference point at the front of the skull where the midsagittal plane intersects a horizontal line tangential to the highest points in the superior palpebral sulci. **2.** the depression at the root of the nose that indicates the junction of the intranasal and the frontonasal sutures.

naso- nas-, combining form meaning "nose": *nasociliary, nasolabial, nasolacrimal.*

nasociliary nerve, usually the first branch of the ophthalmic nerve. It branches into the communicating branch with the ciliary ganglion; the long ciliary nerves, which are sensory to the eyeball but may also contain sympathetic fibers for pupillary dilation; the posterior ethmoidal nerve, which supplies the posterior ethmoidal air cells and the sphenoid sinus; the infratrochlear nerve, which distributes to the medial part of the upper and lower eyelids, the lacrimal sac, and the skin of the upper half of the nose; and the anterior ethmoidal nerve, which supplies the anterior cranial fossa, nasal cavity, and skin of the lower half of the nose.

nasogastric /nā″zōgas″trik/ [L, *nasus,* nose; Gk, *gaster,* stomach], pertaining to the nose and stomach, as in nasogastric aspiration of the stomach's contents.

nasogastric back wall echo, (in ultrasonography) an echo from the posterior surface of the nasal cavity.

nasogastric feeding. See **gavage.**

nasogastric intubation, the placement of a nasogastric tube through the nose into the stomach to relieve gastric distension by removing gas, gastric secretions, or food; to instill medication, food, or fluids; or to obtain a specimen for laboratory analysis. After surgery and in any condition in which the patient is able to digest food but not eat it, the tube may be introduced and left in place for tube feeding for a short time.

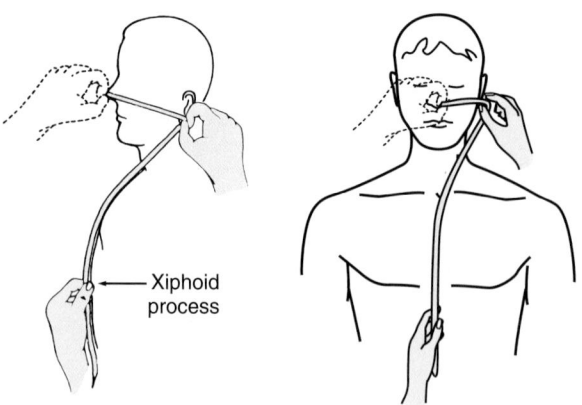

Nasogastric intubation *(Elkin, Perry, and Potter, 2007)*

nasogastric suction, the removal by suction of solids, fluids, or gases from the GI tract through a tube inserted into the stomach or intestines via the nasal cavity. See also **nasogastric intubation.**

nasogastric tube (NG tube), any tube passed into the stomach through the nose. See also **nasogastric intubation.**

nasojejunal tube /nā″zōjijōo″nəl/, a mercury-weighted tube inserted through the nose to allow natural peristaltic movement from the pylorus into the jejunum.

nasolabial /nā″zōlā″bē·əl/ [L, *nasus,* nose, *labium,* lip], pertaining to the nose and lip.

nasolabial reflex [L, *nasus,* nose, *labium,* lip], a sudden backward movement of the head, arching of the back, and extension and stretching of the limbs that occur in infants in response to a light touch to the tip of the nose with an upward sweeping motion. The reflex disappears by about 5 months of age.

nasolacrimal /nā″zōlak″riməl/ [L, *nasus* + *lacrima,* tear], pertaining to the nasal cavity and associated lacrimal ducts.

nasolacrimal duct, a channel that carries tears from the lacrimal sac to the nasal cavity.

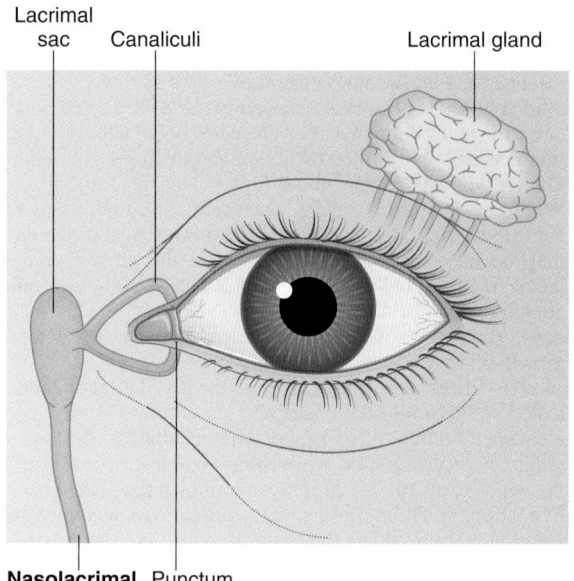

Lacrimal sac   Canaliculi   Lacrimal gland

Nasolacrimal Punctum
duct

Nasolacrimal duct *(Stein, Stein, and Freeman, 2013)*

nasolacrimal groove [L, *nasus,* nose, *lacrima,* tear; D, *groeve,* a shallow depression], a groove on the nasal surface of the upper jaw.

nasomandibular fixation /nā″zōmandib″yōolər/ [L, *nasus* + *mandere,* to chew, *figere,* to fasten], a type of maxillomandibular fixation to stabilize fractures of the jaw by using maxillomandibular splints connected to a wire through a hole drilled in the anterior nasal spine of the maxillary bone. It has been used particularly in patients who have lost all of their natural teeth. See also **maxillomandibular fixation.**

nasomental reflex /-men″təl/ [L, *nasus,* nose, *mentum,* chin, *reflectere,* to bend back], a reflex elicited by tapping the side of the nose, thereby causing contraction of the mentalis muscle with elevation of the lower lip and wrinkling of the skin of the chin.

nasopalatine duct cyst, a nonodontogenic cyst that arises from remnants of the unobliterated nasopalatine duct, presenting as swelling, drainage, and pain in the soft tissue of the incisive papilla, lingual to the maxillary central incisors. See also **incisive canal cyst.**

nasopalatine nerve, the largest of the nasal nerves, which passes across the roof to supply the medial wall of the nasal cavity, then enters the roof of the oral cavity and supplies mucosa, gingiva, and glands adjacent to the incisor teeth.

nasopharyngeal /nā′zōferin″jē·əl/, pertaining to the cavity of the nose and the nasal parts of the pharynx. Also called **rhinopharyngeal.**

nasopharyngeal angiofibroma [L, *nasus* + Gk, *pharynx,* throat], a benign tumor of the nasopharynx consisting of fibrous connective tissue with many vascular spaces. The tumor usually arises in puberty and is more common in boys than in girls. Typical signs are nasal and eustachian tube obstruction, adenoidal speech, and dysphagia. Also called **juvenile angiofibroma, nasopharyngeal fibroangioma.**

nasopharyngeal cancer, a malignant neoplastic disease of the nasopharynx. High titers of antibodies to the Epstein-Barr virus are found in patients of Chinese descent with the cancer; there is evidence of genetic susceptibility, because a certain histocompatibility antigen is associated with the disease and multiple cases occur in some families.
■ OBSERVATIONS: Depending on the site of a nasopharyngeal tumor, there may be nasal obstruction, otitis media, hearing loss, sensory or motor nerve damage, bony destruction of the skull, or deep cervical lymphadenopathy. Diagnostic measures include nasopharyngoscopy, biopsy, and radiological examination of the skull with tomographic studies.
■ INTERVENTIONS: Radiation is the most effective therapy, and chemotherapy is also used.
■ PATIENT CARE CONSIDERATIONS: Squamous cell and undifferentiated carcinomas are the most common lesions. Nasopharyngeal cancer occurs rarely in the United States and frequently in southern China. Exposure to dusts of nickel, chromium, wood, and leather and to isopropyl oil increases the risk of developing nasopharyngeal cancer.

nasopharyngeal fibroangioma. See **nasopharyngeal angiofibroma.**

nasopharyngography /-fer′ingog″rəfē/ [L, *nasus* + Gk, *pharynx,* throat, *graphein,* to record], radiographic imaging and examination of the nasopharynx.

nasopharyngoscopy /nā′zōfer′ing·gos″kəpē/ [L, *nasus* + Gk, *pharynx,* throat, *skopein,* to look], a technique in physical examination in which the nose and throat are visually examined by using a laryngoscope, a fiberoptic device, a flashlight, and a dilator for the nares. −*nasopharyngoscopic, adj.*

nasopharynx /nā′zōfer″ingks/ [L, *nasus* + Gk, *pharynx,* throat], the uppermost of the three regions of the throat (pharynx), situated behind the nasal cavity and extending from the posterior nares to the level above the soft palate. On the posterior wall of the nasopharynx, opposite the posterior nares, are the pharyngeal tonsils. Swollen or enlarged pharyngeal tonsils can fill the space behind the posterior nares and may completely block the passage of air from the nose into the throat. Compare **laryngopharynx, oropharynx.** See also **adenoids, tonsil.** −*nasopharyngeal, adj.*

nasotracheal tube /-trā″kē·əl/ [L, *nasus* + Gk, *tracheia,* rough artery; L, *tubus*], a catheter inserted through the nasal cavity into the trachea. It is commonly attached to a mechanical ventilator or a resuscitator bag to administer oxygen.

Nasu-Hakola disease [T. Nasu, contemporary Japanese physician; H.P.A. Hakola, contemporary Scandinavian physician], a rare autosomal-recessive syndrome of bone cysts with presenile dementia. Also called *polycystic lipomembranous osteodysplasia with sclerosing leucoencephalopathy (PLOSL).*

nat-, combining form meaning "birth": *natal, mortinatality.*

natal /nā′təl/, **1.** [L, *natus*] pertaining to birth. **2.** [L, *nates*] pertaining to the nates, or buttocks.

natalizumab, a multiple sclerosis agent and monoclonal antibody.
■ INDICATIONS: This drug is used to treat ambulatory patients with relapsing-remitting multiple sclerosis who have not responded to other treatments. An unlabeled use is the treatment of Crohn's disease.
■ CONTRAINDICATIONS: Progressive multifocal leukoencephalopathy; murine protein allergy; immunodeficiency (in patients with HIV, AIDS, leukemia, lymphoma, and transplants); and known hypersensitivity to this drug prohibit its use.
■ ADVERSE EFFECTS: Adverse effects of this drug include rigors, syncope, tremors, chest discomfort, hypertension, hypotension, abnormal liver function test, gastroenteritis, amenorrhea, vaginitis, urinary frequency, dermatitis, and pruritus. Life-threatening side effects include progressive multifocal leukoencephalopathy, suicidal ideation, anaphylaxis, and angioedema. Common side effects include headache, fatigue, depression, abdominal discomfort, urinary tract infection, irregular menses, rash, arthralgia, and lower respiratory tract infection.

natamycin /nat″ämi′sin/, a polyene antibiotic used in topical treatment of fungal keratitis, blepharitis, and conjunctivitis.

nateglinide /nāteg′li-nīd/, an antidiabetic agent that lowers blood glucose concentrations by stimulating the release of insulin from pancreatic islet beta cells. It is administered orally in the treatment of type 2 diabetes mellitus, either alone or in combination with metformin.

nates /nā″tēz/ *sing. natis* [L, buttocks]. See **buttocks.**

natimortality. See **mortinatality.**

National Aboriginal Health Organization (NAHO), a Canadian organization with the mission of advancing and promoting the health and well-being of all First Nations, Inuit, and Métis individuals and families through collaborative research, indigenous traditional knowledge, building capacity, and community-led initiatives.

National Alliance on Mental Illness (NAMI), a national nonprofit organization for family members of patients with mental illness; the group is dedicated to education, advocacy, and support.

National Association for Practical Nurse Education and Services (NAPNES), an organization concerned with the education of practical nurses and with the services provided by licensed practical nurses in the United States.

National Association of Pediatric Nurse Associates/ Practitioners (NAP-NAP), an organization of nurses who are prepared by education or experience to give primary care to pediatric patients in the United States. NAP-NAP works in conjunction with the American Academy of Pediatrics.

National Board for Certification in Occupational Therapy (NBCOT), a nonprofit credentialing agency in the United States that regulates the national certification of occupational therapists and occupational therapy assistants through evidence-based practice standards and the validation of knowledge required for competent entry-level practice. Attainment of entry-level certification and recertification allows practitioners to use the credentials of Occupational Therapist Registered (OTR) or Certified Occupational Therapy Assistant (COTA).

National Board of Surgical Technology & Surgical Assisting (NBSTSA), a board, established in 1974, that administers the national certification examinations in the United States for surgical technologists and surgical assistants, and designates the credentials of surgical

N

technologist (CST®) and surgical first assistant (CSFA®) to candidates who successfully pass the exams. Formerly called **Liaison Council on Certification for the Surgical Technologist.**

National Cancer Institute (NCI), an institute of the U.S. National Institutes of Health that leads a national effort to reduce the burden of cancer morbidity and mortality by stimulating and supporting scientific discoveries through basic and clinical biomedical research and training. It conducts and supports programs to understand the causes of cancer; to prevent, detect, diagnose, treat, and control cancer; and to disseminate information to the practitioner, patient, and public in general.

National Center for Chronic Disease Prevention and Health Promotion (NCCDPHP), an organizational component of the U.S. Centers for Disease Control and Prevention charged with preventing premature death and disability from chronic diseases and promoting healthy personal behaviors.

National Center for Devices and Radiological Health (NCDRH), an agency of the U.S. Food and Drug Administration organized in 1982 with the responsibility of providing standards for and regulation of the manufacture and uses of medical devices. Formerly called **Bureau of Medical Devices.**

National Center for Environmental Health (NCEH), an organizational component of the U.S. Centers for Disease Control and Prevention charged with providing national leadership in prevention and control of disease and death resulting from the interaction between people and their environment.

National Center for Health Statistics (NCHS), an organizational component of the U.S. Centers for Disease Control and Prevention charged with providing statistical information that will guide actions and policies to improve the health of the American people.

National Center for HIV/AIDS, Viral Hepatitis, STD, and TB Prevention (HCHHSTP), an organizational component of the U.S. Centers for Disease Control and Prevention charged with providing national leadership in preventing and controlling human immunodeficiency virus infection, sexually transmitted diseases, and tuberculosis. Formerly called **National Center for HIV/AIDS, Viral Hepatitis, STD, and TB Prevention.**

National Center for Infectious Diseases (NCID), an organizational component of the U.S. Centers for Disease Control and Prevention charged with preventing illness, disability, and death caused by infectious diseases in the United States and around the world.

National Center for Injury Prevention and Control (NCIPC), an organizational component of the U.S. Centers for Disease Control and Prevention in the United States charged with preventing death and disability from nonoccupational injuries, including those that are unintentional and those that result from violence.

National Center for Research Resources (NCRR), an institute of the U.S. National Institutes of Health that advances biomedical research and improves human health through research projects and shared resources that create, develop, and provide a comprehensive range of human, animal, technological, and other resources.

National Center on Birth Defects and Developmental Disabilities (NCBDDD), an organizational component of the U.S. Centers for Disease Control and Prevention, charged with providing national leadership in preventing birth defects and developmental disabilities and in improving the health and wellness of people with disabilities.

National Center on Minority Health and Health Disparities (NCMHD), an institute of the U.S. National Institutes of Health whose mission is to reduce and ultimately eliminate health disparities between racial and ethnic minorities (and other groups, such as the urban and rural poor) and society as a whole. It does this by conducting and supporting basic, clinical, and behavioral research and by offering emerging programs, training, and information dissemination in this area.

National Certification Board for Therapeutic Massage and Bodywork, an agency that offers certification in the United States to therapeutic massage and bodywork practitioners who meet eligibility criteria, pass a certification exam, uphold a national code of ethics and standard of practice, and demonstrate continued education in their field.

National Collaborating Centre for the Determinants of Health (NCCDH), six National Collaborating Centres (NCCs) in Canada, established in 2005 to improve the use of scientific research and other knowledge to strengthen public health practices and policies in Canada. The NCCDH identifies knowledge gaps, fosters networks, and translates existing knowledge to produce and exchange relevant, accessible, and evidence-informed products with practitioners, policy makers, and researchers. It aims to improve the response time to health threats within communities and society.

National Committee for Quality Assurance (NCQA), a U.S. independent nonprofit accrediting body for managed health care organizations. Its focus is on improving quality of care in the managed care industry by assessing compliance of health plans to NCQA-developed standards for quality improvement, utilization management, credentialing processes, member rights and responsibilities, preventive services, and record management.

National Council Licensure Examination® (NCLEX®), a comprehensive integrated examination, developed and administered by the National Council of State Boards of Nursing in the United States and Canada, designed to test basic competency for nursing practice. The exam is administered by the individual boards of nursing that are members of the National Council of State Boards of Nursing or by nursing regulatory bodies in Canada. The exam can be offered to candidates for licensure as registered nurses (NCLEX-RN®) or as practical/vocational nurses (NCLEX-PN®).

National Council of State Boards of Nursing, an organization through which boards of nursing from all 50 states, the District of Columbia, Guam, American Samoa, The Commonwealth of the Northern Mariana Islands, Puerto Rico, and the Virgin Islands act and counsel together on matters of common interest and concern related to the safe and effective practice of nursing in the interest of public health, safety, and welfare, including the development of nurse licensure examinations such as the NCLEX-RN® and NCLEX-PN®. See also **NCLEX-RN®, NCLEX-PN®.**

National Eye Institute (NEI), one of several institutes of the U.S. National Institutes of Health. NEI was established in 1968 to support research into the normal functioning of the human eye and visual system, the pathology of visual disorders, and the rehabilitation of the visually handicapped. See also **eye, vision.**

National Formulary, a publication containing the official standards for the preparation of various pharmaceutics not listed in the *United States Pharmacopoeia.* It is revised every 5 years.

national health insurance, a health insurance program in many countries other than the United States that is financed by taxes and administered by the government to provide comprehensive health care that is accessible to all citizens of that nation.

National Health Planning and Resources Development Act of 1974, U.S congressional legislation (PL 93-641) that established a nationwide network of health systems agencies. The act provides for the coordination and direction of national health policy through state and regional regulatory agencies.

National Health Service Corps (NHSC), a program of the U.S. Public Health Service (USPHS) in which health care personnel are placed in areas that are underserved. The corps was established by the Emergency Health Personnel Act of 1970. Nurses, physicians, and dentists serve in rural and urban areas, usually as employees of local health care agencies. The USPHS pays most of the salary of each corps member.

National Heart, Lung, and Blood Institute (NHLBI), an institute of the U.S. National Institutes of Health whose mission is to provide leadership for a national program in diseases of the heart, blood vessels, lungs, and blood, as well as blood resources and sleep disorders. It also has administrative responsibility for the NIH Women's Health Initiative.

National Human Genome Research Institute (NHGRI), an institute of the U.S. National Institutes of Health (NIH) that supports the NIH component of the human genome project.

National Immunization Program (NIP), an organizational component of the U.S. Centers for Disease Control and Prevention charged with preventing disease, disability, and death from vaccine-preventable diseases in children and adults.

National Institute for Occupational Safety and Health (NIOSH), an organizational component of the U.S. Centers for Disease Control and Prevention charged with ensuring safety and health for all people in the workplace through research and prevention.

National Institute of Allergy and Infectious Diseases (NIAID), an institute of the U.S. National Institutes of Health whose mission is to understand, treat, and ultimately prevent infectious, immunological, and allergic disorders affecting human beings.

National Institute of Arthritis and Musculoskeletal and Skin Diseases (NIAMS), an institute of the U.S. National Institutes of Health that supports research into the causes, treatment, and prevention of arthritis, musculoskeletal diseases, and skin diseases.

National Institute of Biomedical Imaging and Bioengineering (NIBIB), an institute of the U.S. National Institutes of Health whose mission is to improve health by promoting fundamental discoveries, design and development, translation, and assessment of technological capabilities in biomedical imaging and bioengineering.

National Institute of Child Health and Human Development (NICHHD), a branch of the U.S. National Institutes of Health that is concerned with all aspects of the growth, development, and health of the children of the United States. It conducts research on fertility, pregnancy, growth, development, and medical rehabilitation, striving to ensure that every child is born healthy and wanted and grows up free from disease and disability.

National Institute of Dental and Craniofacial Research (NIDCR), an institute of the U.S. National Institutes of Health that provides leadership for a national research program designed to understand, treat, and ultimately prevent infectious and inherited craniofacial, oral, and dental diseases and disorders.

National Institute of Diabetes and Digestive and Kidney Diseases (NIDDK), an institute of the U.S. National Institutes of Health that conducts and supports basic and applied research and provides leadership for a national program in diabetes, endocrinology, and metabolic diseases; digestive diseases and nutrition; and kidney, urological, and hematological diseases.

National Institute of Environmental Health Sciences (NIEHS), an institute of the U.S. National Institutes of Health whose mission is to reduce the burden of human illness and dysfunction from environmental causes by defining how environmental exposures, genetic susceptibility, and age interact to affect individuals' health.

National Institute of General Medical Sciences (NIGMS), an institute of the U.S. National Institutes of Health whose mission is to support biomedical research that is not targeted at specific diseases, resulting in an increased understanding of life and a broadened foundation for advances in disease diagnosis, treatment, and prevention.

National Institute of Mental Health (NIMH), **1.** an institute of the U.S. National Institutes of Health whose mission is to provide national leadership in the understanding, treatment, and prevention of mental illnesses through basic research on the brain and behavior, and through clinical, epidemiological, and services research. **2.** a division of the Mental Health Commission of Canada that serves as a catalyst for improving the mental health system and changing the attitudes and behaviors of Canadians surrounding mental health issues. NIMH makes recommendations on how best to improve the systems that are directly related to mental health care.

National Institute of Neurological Disorders and Stroke, an institute of the U.S. National Institutes of Health whose mission is to reduce the burden of neurological diseases by supporting and conducting research (both basic and clinical) on the normal and diseased nervous system, fostering the training of investigators in the neurosciences, and seeking better understanding, diagnosis, treatment, and prevention of neurological disorders.

National Institute of Nursing Research (NINR), an institute of the U.S. National Institutes of Health that supports clinical and basic research to establish a scientific basis for the care of individuals across the life span in a variety of ways.

National Institute of Standards and Technology (NIST), a federal agency in the Department of Commerce that sets accurate measurement standards for commerce, industry, and science in the United States. The NIST compares and coordinates its standards with those of other countries and provides research and technical service to improve computer science, materials technology, building construction, and consumer product safety.

National Institute on Aging (NIA), an institute of the U.S. National Institutes of Health that leads a national program of research on the biomedical, social, and behavioral aspects of the aging process; the prevention of age-related diseases and disabilities; and the promotion of a better quality of life for older Americans.

National Institute on Alcohol Abuse and Alcoholism, an institute of the U.S. National Institutes of Health that conducts research focused on improving the treatment and prevention of alcoholism and alcohol-related problems.

National Institute on Deafness and Other Communication Disorders, an institute of the U.S. National Institutes of Health that conducts and supports biomedical research and research training on normal mechanisms, diseases, and disorders of hearing, balance, smell, taste, voice, speech, and language.

N

National Institute on Drug Abuse (NIDA), an institute of the U.S. National Institutes of Health that seeks to bring the power of science to bear on drug abuse and addiction through support and conduct of research across a broad range of disciplines, with rapid and effective dissemination of results of the research.

National Institutes of Health (NIH), an agency of the U.S. Department of Health and Human Services made up of several institutions and constituent divisions, including the Bureau of Health Manpower Education, the National Library of Medicine, the National Cancer Institute, and several research institutes and divisions. The NIH is divided into two parts: One part is responsible for the funding of biomedical research outside the NIH, and the other conducts research.

National League for Nursing (NLN), an organization concerned with the improvement of nursing education and nursing service and the provision of health care in the United States. Among its many activities are preadmission and achievement tests for nursing students and compilation of statistical data on nursing personnel and trends in health care delivery. The National League for Nursing Commission for Nursing Education Accreditation (CNEA) has the authority and responsibility for accrediting nursing education schools and nursing programs that seek accreditation. A monthly refereed journal, *Nursing Education Perspectives,* is the official publication of the organization.

National League for Nursing Accrediting Commission (NLNAC), a corporation established in 2001 that is a wholly owned subsidiary of the National League for Nursing and is responsible for the accreditation of nursing education schools and programs in the United States.

National Library of Medicine (NLM), a library and information resource center that is part of the National Institutes of Health. It collects, organizes, and makes available biomedical science information to investigators, educators, and practitioners and carries out programs designed to strengthen medical library services in the United States. It offers a free search engine, PubMed, and its electronic databases include MEDLINE and MEDLINEplus.

National Nursing Assessment Services (NNAS), an incorporated national body of member nurse regulatory bodies in Canada that collectively developed a consistent national approach to the initial assessment of internationally educated nurses seeking registration/licensure to practice in Canadian jurisdictions. This includes registered nurses, licensed practical nurses, registered practical nurses in Ontario, and registered psychiatric nurses.

National Marrow Donor Program (NMDP), a coordinating center for bone marrow transplants providing links with national and international registries of prospective volunteer donors of human leukocyte antigen–compatible bone marrow tissue.

National Network for Mental Health (NNMH), an organization in Canada that facilitates networks among consumers of mental health services and their families and friends to provide opportunities for resource sharing, information distribution, and education on mental health issues.

National Organization of Victim Assistance, a private nonprofit organization in the United States of victims and of practitioners who specialize in victims' assistance or witness assistance, criminal justice professionals, researchers, former victims, and others committed to the recognition and implementation of victims' rights and services.

National Quality Registry Network, a voluntary network of organizations that operate registries, as well as others interested in increasing the usefulness of clinical registries to measure and improve patient health outcomes.

natis. See **nates.**

Native American medicine, traditional ways of healing, culturally and spiritually based, used by many Native American Indian tribes, Inuit, and Canadian First Nations and Métis people, often in combination with mainstream or Western medicine.

natremia /nātrē″mē·ə/ [L, *natrium,* sodium; Gk, *haima,* blood], the presence of sodium in the blood.

natriuresis /nā′trēyŏŏrē″sis/ [L, *natrium,* sodium; Gk, *ouresis,* urination], the excretion of greater-than-normal amounts of sodium in the urine. The condition may result from the administration of natriuretic diuretic drugs or from various metabolic or endocrine disorders.

natriuretic /nā′trēyŏŏret″ik/, **1.** *adj.,* pertaining to the process of natriuresis. **2.** *n.,* a substance that inhibits the resorption of sodium ions from the glomerular filtrate in the kidneys, thus allowing more sodium to be excreted with the urine.

natriuretic peptides test, a blood test to predict congestive heart failure, myocardial infarction, systemic hypertension, cor pulmonale, or heart transplant rejection.

natural antibody /nach′(ə)rəl/ [L, *natura,* nature; Gk, *anti* + AS, *bodig,* body], an antibody that is present in serum in the absence of an apparent specific antigen contact.

natural childbirth [L, *natura,* nature; AS, *cild,* child; ME, *bwith,* birth], labor and parturition accomplished by a mother with little or no medical intervention. It is generally considered the optimal way of giving birth and being born, safest for the baby, and most satisfying for the mother. Prerequisites include normal gestation, an adequate birth canal, strong maternal motivation, physical and emotional preparation, and constant and intensive support of the mother during labor and birth. See also **Lamaze method.**

natural dentition, the entire array of inborn elemental teeth in the dental arches at any given time, consisting of primary or secondary dentitions or a mixture of the two. See also **tooth.**

natural family planning method, any of several methods of conception control that do not rely on a medication or a physical device for effectiveness in avoiding pregnancy. Some of the methods are also used to pinpoint the time of ovulation to increase the chance of fertilization when artificial insemination or extraction of an oocyte for in vitro fertilization is to be performed. Kinds include **basal body temperature method of family planning, ovulation method of family planning, symptothermal method of family planning.**

natural foods, foods that have been grown, processed, packaged, and stored without the use of chemical additives. There is no formal U.S. Food and Drug Administration definition of *natural* for food-labeling purposes. See also **organic foods.**

natural immunity, a usually inherent, nonspecific form of immunity to a specific disease. Also called **genetic immunity, innate immunity.** Compare **acquired immunity.** Kinds include **individual immunity, racial immunity, species immunity.** See also **active immunity, passive immunity.**

naturalistic illness /nach′ərəlis′tik/, **1.** a feeling of imbalance, not necessarily disease, thought to be caused by factors such as a disturbance in equilibrium of body systems. Compare **disease. 2.** (in Western medicine) impersonal, mechanistic causes in nature that can be potentially understood and cured. Examples include physical injury and microorganisms as cause of disease.

natural killer cell [L, *natura* + ME, *kullen,* to kill, *cella,* storeroom], a large granular lymphocyte with NK-specific markers, especially CD56. NK cells affect antibody-independent cell-mediated cytotoxicity by recognizing nonself markers on foreign and tumor cells and subsequently killing them.

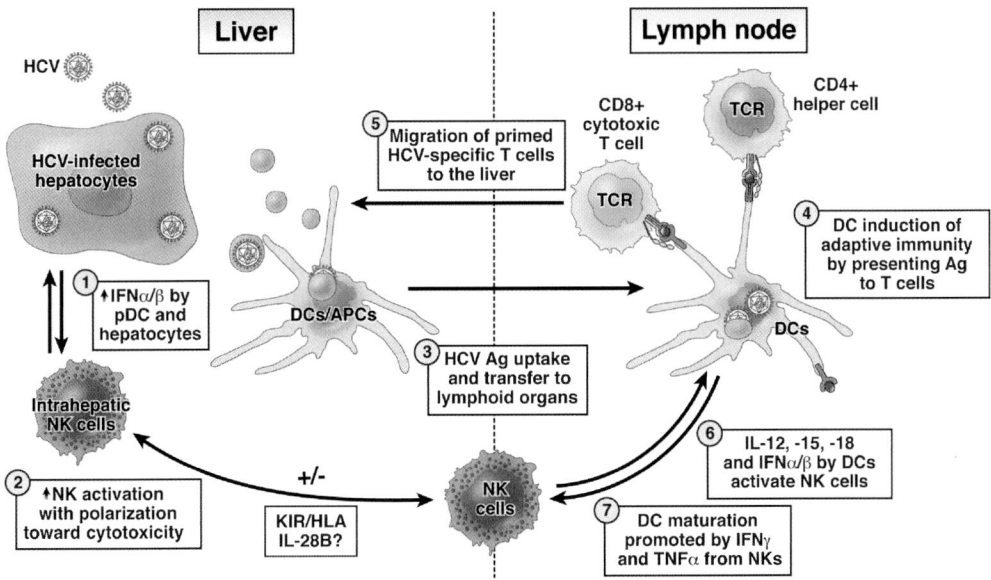

Model of NK cell activation during acute hepatis C infection *(Shoukry, Pelletier, and Chang, 2011)*

natural law, a doctrine that holds that there is a natural moral order or law inherent in the structure of the universe.

naturally acquired immunity. See **acquired immunity.**

natural network, a patient's contacts in the community, including church and social groups, friends, family, and co-workers, who support the patient's function outside the institutional environment.

natural pacemaker, any cardiac pacing site in the heart tissues, as opposed to an artificial pacemaker.

natural radiation, radioactivity that emanates from the soil, groundwater, or cosmic sources. Cosmic radiation includes actinic radiation from the sun and neutrinos from beyond the solar system.

natural selection, the natural evolutionary processes by which the organisms that are best adapted to an environment tend to survive and propagate whereas those that are unfit are less likely to do so. Compare **artificial selection.**

Naturetin, a diuretic drug. Brand name for **bendroflumethiazide.**

nature versus nurture /nur″chər/, a name given to a long-standing controversy as to the relative influences of genetics versus the environment in the development of personality. Nature is represented by instincts and genetic factors and nurture by social influences.

naturopath /nach″ərōpath′/, a person who practices naturopathy.

naturopathic medicine, a philosophy of medicine that presumes that there is an inherent healing power in nature and in every human being. This major health system includes practices that emphasize diet, nutrition, homeopathy, and various mind-body therapies. Emphasis is placed on self-healing, treatment through changes in lifestyle, and the use of prevention techniques that promote health. Currently, 17 states, the District of Columbia, and the U.S. territories of Puerto Rico and the U.S. Virgin Islands have licensing or regulation laws for naturopathic doctors. In Canada, two sets of provincial licensing board exams exist.

naturopathy /nach′ərop″əthē/ [L, *natura* + Gk, *pathos,* disease], a system of therapeutics based on natural foods, light, warmth, massage, fresh air, regular exercise, and the

avoidance of medications. Advocates believe that illness can be healed by the natural processes of the body.

Nauheim bath /nou″hīm/ [Nauheim, Germany; AS, *baeth,* bath], a spa treatment taken in water through which carbon dioxide is bubbled, followed by systematic exercises, once used in the treatment of cardiac conditions. The procedure is named after the natural waters of Bad Nauheim, Germany. Although no longer used for therapy, it may have been an antecedent to the contemporary use of exercise in cardiac rehabilitation. Also called *Nauheim treatment.*

nausea /nô″zē-ə, nô″zhə/ [Gk, *nausia,* seasickness], a sensation accompanying the urge but not always leading to vomiting. Common causes are seasickness and other motion sicknesses, early pregnancy, intense pain, emotional stress, gallbladder disease, food poisoning, central nervous system tumors, and various enteroviruses.

nausea and vomiting of pregnancy (NVP), a common condition of early pregnancy characterized by recurrent or persistent nausea, often in the morning, that may result in vomiting, weight loss, anorexia, general weakness, and malaise. The timing of increased symptoms coincides with an elevation in the level of hCG and shortly after that elevations in estrogen and progesterone, although a causative association is not presently recognized. A severe form is hyperemesis gravidarum, the most common cause of hospital admission in the first half of pregnancy. Also called **morning sickness.** See also **hyperemesis gravidarum.**

■ OBSERVATIONS: It usually does not begin before the sixth week after the last menstrual period and ends by the twelfth to the fourteenth week of pregnancy. Symptoms are seen in 70% to 85% of pregnant women; it is most common in the first trimester.

■ INTERVENTIONS: There are various antiemetic therapies with varying rates of response. Symptomatic relief is often obtained by eating small, easily digested meals frequently and by not allowing the stomach to be empty. In the past, antiemetic drugs were routinely prescribed for this complaint, but this practice is currently reserved for severe cases.

■ PATIENT CARE CONSIDERATIONS: Women with severe NVP may have multiple gestations or molar pregnancy, and evaluation for these problems is indicated in this circumstance.

nauseate. See **nausea.**

nauseous /nô″shəs, nô′zē·əs/ [Gk, *nausia,* seasickness], pertaining to feelings of nausea or reaction to things that may stimulate nausea.

Navane, an antipsychotic agent. Brand name for **thiothixene.**

navel. See **umbilicus.**

Navelbine, a chemotherapeutic mitotic inhibitor. Brand name for **vinorelbine tartrate.**

navicular /navik′yələr/, boat-shaped; sunken.

navicular bone. See **scaphoid bone.**

navicular pads, tarsal supports for flat feet. They are inserted directly under the arch of the foot. Also called **shoe cookies.**

Nb, symbol for the element **niobium.**

n.b., a Latin phrase meaning "note well." Abbreviation for *nota bene.*

NBCOT, abbreviation for **National Board for Certification in Occupational Therapy.**

NBNA, initialism for *National Black Nurses Association.*

NBRC, abbreviation for *National Board for Respiratory Care.*

NBSTSA, abbreviation for **National Board of Surgical Technology & Surgical Assisting.**

NCBDDD, abbreviation for **National Center on Birth Defects and Developmental Disabilities.**

NCCIH, part of the U.S. National Institutes of Health. Abbreviation for *National Center for Complementary and Integrative Health.*

NCCDPHP, abbreviation for **National Center for Chronic Disease Prevention and Health Promotion.**

NCDRH, abbreviation for **National Center for Devices and Radiological Health.**

NCEH, abbreviation for **National Center for Environmental Health.**

NCHS, abbreviation for **National Center for Health Statistics.**

NCI, abbreviation for **National Cancer Institute.**

nCi, abbreviation for **nanocurie.**

NCID, abbreviation for **National Center for Infectious Diseases.**

NCIPC, abbreviation for **National Center for Injury Prevention and Control.**

NCLEX CAT®, administration of National Council Licensure Examination through computerized adaptive testing.

NCLEX-PN®, abbreviation for *National Council Licensure Examination for Practical Nurses.*

NCLEX-RN®, abbreviation for *National Council Licensure Examination for Registered Nurses.*

NCMHD, abbreviation for **National Center on Minority Health and Health Disparities.**

NCQA, abbreviation for **National Committee for Quality Assurance.**

NCRR, abbreviation for **National Center for Research Resources.**

NCSN, a voluntary certification for school nurses offered by the National Association of School Nurses. Abbreviation for *national certified school nurse.*

Nd, symbol for the element **neodymium.**

N.D., abbreviation for *Doctor of Naturopathy.* See also **naturopathic medicine.**

NDA, **1.** abbreviation for *National Dental Association.* **2.** abbreviation for **new drug application.**

NDHA, abbreviation for *National Dental Hygienists' Association.*

Ne, symbol for the element **neon.**

NE, **1.** abbreviation for **niacin equivalent. 2.** abbreviation for **norepinephrine.**

ne-. See **neo-, ne-.**

Neal-Robertson litter, a modified spine board for transporting trauma patients with spinal injuries. It is particularly useful for moving individuals in small spaces. Also spelled *Neil-Robertson litter.*

near-death experience [ME, *nere* + *deth* + L, *experientia,* trial], the subjective observations of people who either have been close to clinical death or have recovered after having been declared dead. Many claim to have witnessed similar episodes of passing through a tunnel toward a bright light and encountering people who preceded them in death. See also **out-of-body experience.**

near drowning [ME, *nere,* almost, *drounen,* to drown], a pathological state in which the victim has survived exposure to circumstances that usually cause drowning. The return of consciousness does not necessarily ensure recovery. Intensive supportive therapy may be required for up to several days. Compare **drowning.** See also **hypothermia.**

nearest neighbor analysis, a biochemical method used to estimate the frequency with which specific pairs of bases are located next to one another.

near field, part of an electromagnetic field. See **Fresnel zone.**

nearsightedness. See **myopia.**

nebivolol, an antihypertensive drug.

■ INDICATIONS: This drug is used to treat hypertension.

■ CONTRAINDICATIONS: Cardiogenic shock, sick sinus syndrome, acute bronchospasm, atrioventricular heart block, and hypersensitivity to this agent or beta blockers prohibit its use. This drug should not be abruptly discontinued.

■ ADVERSE EFFECTS: Adverse effects of this drug include drowsiness, headache, atrioventricular heart block, edema, vomiting, abdominal pain, rash, pruritus, vasculitis, urticaria, psoriasis, hyperuricemia, hypercholesterolemia, and dyspnea. Life-threatening side effects include bradycardia, MI, thrombocytopenia, angioedema, renal failure, pulmonary edema, and bronchospasm. Common side effects include insomnia, fatigue, dizziness, mental changes, nausea, diarrhea, and impotence.

nebula /neb″yələ/ *pl.* **nebulae** [L, cloud], **1.** a slight corneal opacity or scar that seldom obstructs vision and that can be seen only by oblique illumination. **2.** a cloudy appearance in the urine. **3.** an oily concoction that is applied with an atomizer. **4.** mass of interstellate dusts.

nebulization /neb′yəlīzā″shən/ [L, *nebula,* cloud; Gk, *izein,* to cause], a method of administering a drug by spraying it into the respiratory passages of the patient. The medication may be given with or without oxygen to help carry it into the lungs.

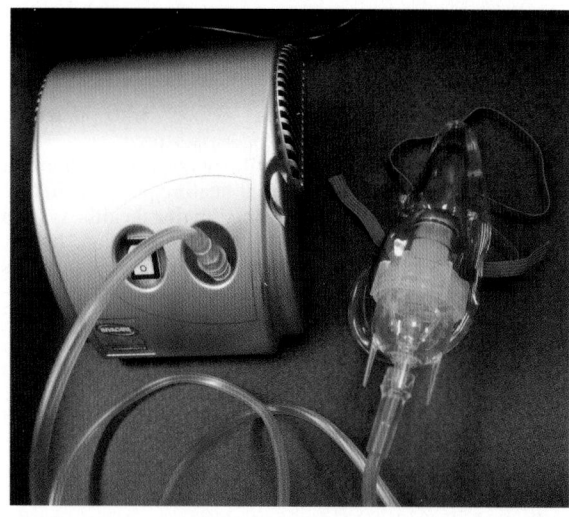

Nebulizer equipment

nebulize /neb″yəlīz/, to vaporize or disperse a liquid in a fine spray.

nebulizer /neb″yəlī′zər/, a device for producing a fine spray. Intranasal medications are often administered by a nebulizer. Also called **atomizer.**

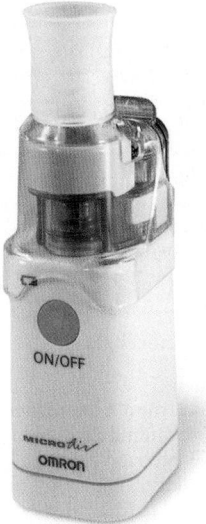

Nebulizer *(Courtesy Omron Healthcare, Inc.)*

NEC, abbreviation for **necrotizing enterocolitis.**

Necator americanus /nekā″tər/ [L, *necare,* to kill], a genus of nematode that is an intestinal parasite and causes hookworm disease. See also *Ancylostoma.*

necatoriasis /nek′ətərī″əsis/ [L, *necare,* to kill; Gk, *osis,* condition], hookworm disease, specifically that caused by *Necator americanus,* the most common North American hookworm. An estimated one third of the world's population is infected with *N. americanus.* The larvae live in the soil; they reach the human digestive tract through contaminated food and water or through the skin of the feet and legs, attach to mucosa in the small bowel, and suck blood from the human host. See also **ancylostomiasis, ground itch, hookworm.**
- OBSERVATIONS: Most infections are asymptomatic. Symptoms include diarrhea, nausea, abdominal pain, and microcytic hypochromic iron-deficiency anemia in the more severe cases.
- INTERVENTIONS: Treatment consists of first correcting the anemia if present and then anthelmintic therapy, usually with pyrantel pamoate or mebendazole.
- PATIENT CARE CONSIDERATIONS: Prevention includes improved sanitation for disposal of human waste to eliminate soil contamination and the avoidance of skin contact with the soil.

necessity /nĕses′te/, something necessary or indispensable. See also **medical necessity, Certificate of Medical Necessity.**

neck [AS, *hnecca*], a constricted section, such as the part of the body that connects the head with the trunk. Other such constrictions are the neck of the humerus and the neck of the uterus.

neck dissection, surgical removal of the cervical lymph nodes, performed to prevent the spread of malignant tumors of the head and neck. With the patient under general anesthesia, the cervical chain of lymph nodes with their lymphatic channels is removed in one mass to prevent the spread of cancer cells. After surgery the patient is observed closely for signs of hemorrhage and difficulty in breathing. Compare **radical neck dissection.**

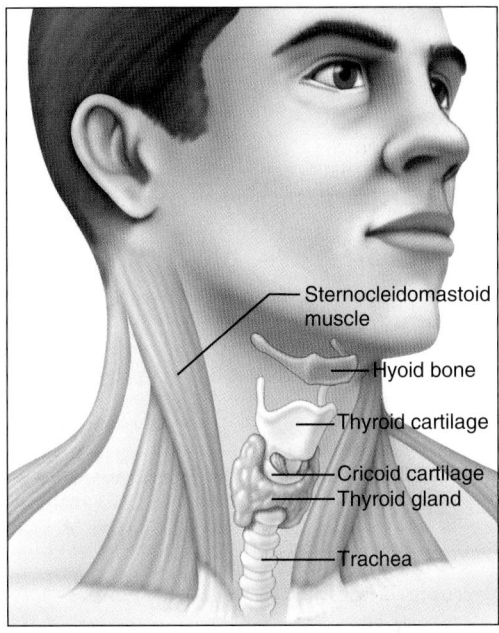

Neck structures *(Harkreader, Hogan, and Thobaben, 2007)*

neck of femur [AS, *hnecca* + L, *femur,* thigh], the part of the long bone of the thigh between the head and the greater and lesser trochanters. The neck of a long bone is often the site of fracture.

neck of gastric gland, a constricted area of a gastric gland just interior to the isthmus.

neck of uterus. See **cervix.**

neck righting reflex, 1. an involuntary response in newborns in which turning the head to one side while the infant is supine causes rotation of the shoulders and trunk in the same direction. The reflex enables the child to roll over from the supine to prone position. Absence of the reflex or persistence beyond about 10 months of age may indicate central nervous system damage. **2.** any tonic reflex associated with the neck that maintains body orientation in relation to the head.

neck ring, a metal ring at the neck of a cervicothoracolumbosacral orthosis. It opens posteriorly for ease in putting on or removing the orthosis and is an attachment for a throat mold and occiput pads. See also **orthosis.**

neck shaft angle, an angle created by the intersection of a line through the femoral shaft and a line through the femoral head and neck. Also called **femoral angle.**

neck sign. *(Informal)* See **Brudzinski sign.**

necro-, combining form meaning "death" or "corpse": *necrophilia, necrosis.*

necrobiosis /nek′rōbī·ō″sis/, **1.** the death of a small area of cells in a large area of living tissue. **2.** the normal death of tissue cells as a result of changes associated with development, aging, atrophy, or degeneration. −*necrobiotic, adj.*

necrobiosis lipoidica /lipoi″dikə/ [Gk, *nekros,* dead, *bios,* life, *lipos,* fat, *eidos,* form], a skin disease characterized by thin, shiny, yellow-to-red plaques on the shins or forearms. Telangiectases and crusting and ulceration of these plaques may occur. Necrobiosis lipoidica is usually associated with diabetes mellitus and occurs most often in women. Treatment includes precise control of the diabetes and, possibly, intralesional application of corticosteroids.

N

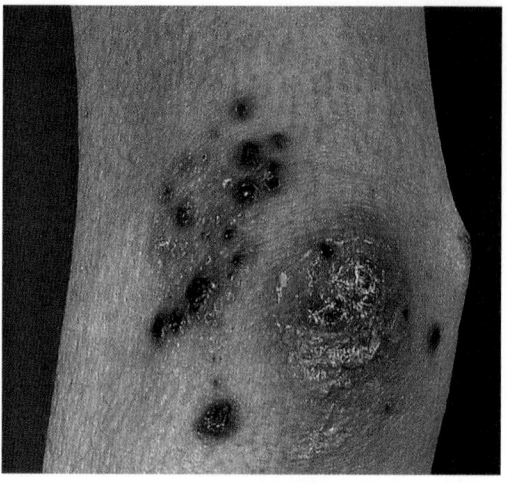

Tissue necrosis *(du Vivier, 2002)*

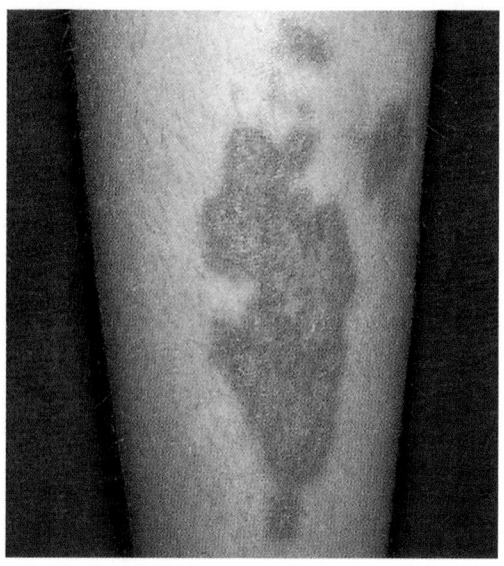

Necrobiosis lipoidica *(Weston, Lane, and Morelli, 2007)*

necrobiotic granulomas, granulomas that share some of the characteristics of both immunological and nonimmunological collections of mononuclear phagocytes. Relatively acellular areas of the skin become necrobiotic, and the col lagen assumes a homogenous, amorphous appearance. See also **granuloma annulare, necrobiosis lipoidica.**

necrogenic /nek′rōjen′ik/ [Gk, *nekros,* dead, *genein,* to produce], **1.** capable of causing death, as of cells or tissue. **2.** originating or caused by infected dead matter. Also called *necrogenous.*

necrology (necrol) /nekrol″əjē/ [Gk, *nekros,* dead, *logos,* science], the study of the causes of death, including the compilation and interpretation of mortality statistics.

necrolysis /nekrol″isis/ [Gk, *nekros* + *lysis,* loosening], disintegration or exfoliation of dead tissue. Compare **necrosis.** −*necrolytic, adj.*

necrophilia /nek′rōfil″yə/ [Gk, *nekros* + *philein,* to love], **1.** a morbid liking for being with dead bodies. **2.** a morbid desire to have sexual contact with a dead body, usually of men to perform a sexual act with a dead woman. −*necrophiliac, necrophile, n.*

necrophobia [Gk, *nekros,* dead, *phobos,* fear], a morbid fear of death and dead bodies. −*necrophobic, adj.*

necropsy, necroscopy. See **autopsy.**

necrosis /nekrō″sis/ [Gk, *nekros* + *osis,* condition], localized tissue death that occurs in groups of cells in response to disease or injury. In coagulation necrosis, blood clots block the flow of blood, causing tissue ischemia distal to the clot. In gangrenous necrosis, ischemia combined with bacterial action causes putrefaction to set in. See also **gangrene, coagulation necrosis, gangrenous necrosis.**

necrotaxis /nek′rōtak″sis/, the attraction of leukocytes to dead or dying cells.

necrotic /nekrot″ik/, pertaining to the death of tissue in response to disease or injury.

necrotic arachnidism, tissue destruction caused by spider venom. See also **spider bite.**

necrotizing /nek′rōtī′zing/ [Gk, *nekros,* death], causing the death of tissues or organisms.

necrotizing angiitis. See **periarteritis nodosa.**

necrotizing enteritis [Gk, *nekros* + *izein,* to cause, *enteron,* intestine, *itis*], acute inflammation of the small and large intestine by the bacterium *Clostridium perfringens,* characterized by severe abdominal pain, bloody diarrhea, and vomiting. Some people recover completely, some survive with chronic bowel obstruction, and some die of perforation of the intestine, dehydration, peritonitis, or septicemia.

necrotizing enterocolitis (NEC), an acute inflammatory bowel disorder that occurs primarily in preterm or low–birth weight neonates, typically within the first 2 weeks of life. It is characterized by ischemic necrosis of the GI mucosa that may lead to perforation and peritonitis. The cause of the disorder is unknown, although it appears to be a defect in host defenses, with infection resulting from normal GI flora rather than from invading organisms. Formula-fed infants are more susceptible to the disorder, possibly because formula lacks the immunoglobulin A antibodies and macrophages found in breast milk that may protect the GI mucosa from damage and bacterial invasion. Also called **pseudomembranous enterocolitis.** See also **enteritis.**

■ OBSERVATIONS: Significant predisposing factors for the condition include prematurity, hypovolemia, respiratory distress syndrome, sepsis, an indwelling umbilical catheter, exchange transfusion, and feeding with hyperosmolar or high-caloric formulas. The condition results from a reflex shunting of blood away from the GI tract, which leads to convulsive vasoconstriction of the mesenteric vessels supplying the intestines. The diminished blood supply interferes with the normal production of mucus and with other bowel functions and results in severe necrosis with bacterial invasion of the bowel wall. Formula-fed infants are more susceptible to the disorder, possibly because formula lacks the immunoglobulin A antibodies and macrophages found in breast milk that may protect the GI mucosa from damage and bacterial invasion. Initial symptoms, which usually develop after several days of life, include temperature instability (usually hypothermia), lethargy, poor feeding, vomiting of bile, abdominal distension, blood in the stools, and decreased or absent bowel sounds. Signs of deterioration are apnea, pallor, hyperbilirubinemia, oliguria, abdominal tenderness, and erythema and edema of the anterior abdominal wall or palpable masses, with eventual respiratory failure leading to death. Diagnosis is confirmed by x-ray visualization of the intestine or by the presence of increased peritoneal fluid or pneumoperitoneum.

■ INTERVENTIONS: Treatment includes discontinuation of oral feeding, IV infusion, abdominal decompression by nasogastric suction, hydration, plasma or whole blood transfusion, and administration of broad-spectrum antibiotics. With routine supportive management, improvement usually occurs within 48 to 72 hours. Oral feedings usually are not resumed for 10 days to 2 weeks. Total parenteral nutrition is necessary during that period. Surgical resection of the affected bowel segment may be necessary, especially if signs of intestinal perforation or peritonitis develop. If a large part of bowel is affected, an ileostomy or colostomy may be necessary. Stenosis of the involved bowel segment may present later complications.

■ PATIENT CARE CONSIDERATIONS: The primary concern of the physician and nurse is to observe high-risk, formula-fed infants for early symptoms of necrotizing enterocolitis, especially for difficulty in feeding, bile-stained regurgitation, bloody stools, temperature fluctuations, or a distended shiny abdomen. After the diagnosis is confirmed, the nurse initiates nasogastric intubation for abdominal decompression and continues to monitor the baby constantly for dehydration and electrolyte balance. Daily weight is taken. Infants who are unable to take fluids by mouth require special oral care. A pacifier helps meet the infant's need to suck. Parents are encouraged to visit and are helped to meet the emotional needs of the infant and to provide tactile, auditory, and visual stimulation. Consultation with an occupational therapist is appropriate. The health care team explains the usual course of the disease and any procedures and keeps the parents informed of the infant's progress. Frequent visits to the care unit facilitate family-infant relationships and provide the health care team with an opportunity to teach proper care techniques before discharge. Most infants who develop NEC recover fully and do not have further feeding problems.

necrotizing fasciitis, a rare bacterial infection causing death of tissue and inflammation of the tissues and structures under the skin. The infection can spread quickly and lead to sepsis, shock, and organ failure.

necrotizing ulcerative gingivitis (NUG), an inflammatory destructive disease of the gingivae primarily caused by the spirochete bacterium *Treponema vincentii*. The disease has a sudden onset with periods of remission and exacerbation. It is usually associated with poor oral hygiene, immunosuppression, smoking, local trauma, poor nutritional status, inadequate sleep, or recent illness and psychological stress. It is most common in conditions in which there is crowding of the teeth and malnutrition. Also called **Vincent angina, Vincent infection, trench mouth.**

■ OBSERVATIONS: It is marked by ulcers of the gingival papillae that become covered by sloughed, necrotic tissue and circumscribed by linear erythema. Foul-smelling breath, increased salivation, bone destruction, lymphadenopathy, and spontaneous gingival hemorrhage are additional features. It may extend to other parts of the oral mucosa, with lesions involving the palate or pharynx.

■ INTERVENTIONS: Treatment includes chlorhexidine, warm saltwater rinses, mouthwashes, antibiotics, analgesics, and dental care to remove and disrupt bacterial flora.

■ PATIENT CARE CONSIDERATIONS: During World War I, this disease was nicknamed trench mouth. Although the disease often occurs in an epidemic pattern, it has not been shown to be contagious.

necrotizing ulcerative periodontitis (NUP), an inflammatory destructive disease of the gingiva that progresses to destruction of the periodontium. Compare **necrotizing ulcerative gingivitis.**

necrotizing vasculitis, an inflammatory condition of blood vessels characterized by necrosis, fibrosis, and proliferation of the inner layer of the vascular wall. Some cases result in occlusion and infarction. Necrotizing vasculitis may occur in rheumatoid arthritis and is common in systemic lupus erythematosus, periarteritis nodosa, and progressive systemic sclerosis. The condition is usually treated with corticosteroids.

nedocromil /ned″okro′mil/, a nonsteroidal antiinflammatory drug administered by inhalation in the treatment of bronchial asthma. It is also administered topically to the conjunctiva as the sodium salt in the treatment of allergic conjunctivitis.

nedocromil sodium, the sodium salt of nedocromil, administered topically to the conjunctiva in the treatment of allergic conjunctivitis.

needle bath [AS, *naedl*, needle], a shower in which fine jets of water are sprayed over the body at acupuncture trigger points, especially to relieve pain.

needle biopsy, the removal of a segment of living tissue for microscopic examination by inserting a hollow needle through the skin or the external surface of an organ or tumor and rotating it within the underlying cellular layers. Also called **fine-needle aspiration.** See also **aspiration biopsy.**

needle filter, a device, usually made of plastic, used for filtering medications that are drawn into a syringe before administration. Some syringe needles have built-in filters; other filters are separate units that are attached to the needle before use. Needle filters commonly are disposable items designed for onetime use.

needle holder, a surgical forceps used to hold and pass a suturing needle through tissue. Also called **suture forceps.**

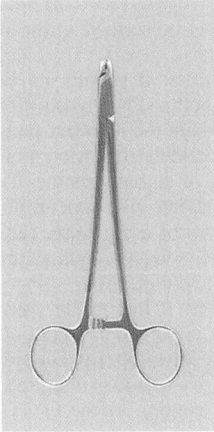

Jarit sternal needle holder *(Tighe, 2015)*

needleless system, equipment that allows the administration of medications through an IV access device with specialized fittings that eliminate the need for a hollow needle.

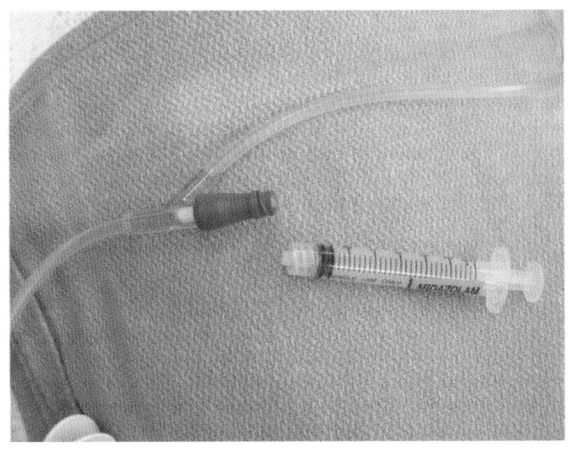

Needleless IV system *(Malamed, 2010)*

N

needlestick injuries, accidental skin punctures resulting from contact with hypodermic syringe needles, IV cannula stylets, needles used to "piggyback" IV infusions, and needles used for drawing blood or administering parenteral injections. The contact may occur accidentally during efforts to inject a patient or as a result of carelessly touching discarded medical waste. Such injuries can be dangerous, particularly if the needle has been used in treatment of a patient with a severe blood-borne infection, such as human immunodeficiency virus. To prevent injuries, used needles are not capped or broken and are disposed of in a rigid puncture-resistant container located near the site of use.

NEEP, abbreviation for **negative end-expiratory pressure.**

Neer and Horowitz classification system [C.S. Neer and B.S. Horowitz, contemporary American orthopedic surgeons], a method of classifying proximal humeral fractures in children on the basis of the degree of separation of the epiphysis from the shaft.

Neer classification system, a method of classifying femoral supracondylar and intercondylar fractures. The system ranges from *type I* for minimal displacement to *type III* for conjoined supracondylar and shaft fractures. The Neer system is also applied to humeral head and neck fractures.

nefazodone hydrochloride /něfa′zodōn/, an antidepressant drug.

- INDICATIONS: It is prescribed in the treatment of mental depression in adults.
- CONTRAINDICATIONS: It should not be given to patients with an allergy to nefazodone hydrochloride or similar antidepressants, patients in the recovery phase of acute myocardial infarction, or patients also using monoamine oxidase inhibitors, pimozide, or carbamazepine. Caution is advised in prescribing it for patients with concurrent use of triazolam or alprazolam, a history of drug abuse, cardiovascular disease, low blood pressure, seizures, benign prostatic hyperplasia, constipation, or suicidal ideation.
- ADVERSE EFFECTS: It has rarely caused life-threatening liver failure, so it should be discontinued immediately if there are signs of hepatic toxicity. The side effects most often reported include dry mouth, impaired vision, eye pain, flulike symptoms, ringing in the ears, swollen limbs, and muscle pain.

negative (neg) /neg′ətiv/ [L, *negare,* to deny], **1.** (of a laboratory test) indicating that a substance or a reaction is not present. **2.** (of a sign) indicating on physical examination that a finding is not present, often meaning that there is no pathological change. **3.** (of a substance) tending to carry or carrying a negative chemical charge.

negative adaptation. See **habituation.**

negative anxiety, (in psychology) an emotional and psychological condition in which anxiety prevents a person's normal functioning and interrupts the person's ability to perform the usual activities of daily living.

negative balance, a state in which the amount of water or an electrolyte excreted from the body is greater than that ingested.

negative catalysis, a decrease in the rate of any chemical reaction caused by a substance that is not consumed and not affected by the reaction. Also called **inhibition.** Compare **catalysis.** See also **catalyst.**

negative electrode [L, *negare,* to deny; Gk, *elektron,* amber, *hodos,* way], an anode, or the negative terminal of a battery or dry cell at which oxidation takes place. It is also the cathode or negative terminal in an electrolytic cell at which reduction takes place.

negative end-expiratory pressure (NEEP), the application of subatmospheric pressure to a patient's airway on exhalation during mechanical ventilation. The technique counterbalances the increase in mean intrathoracic pressure caused by intermittent positive-pressure breathing and is intended to reduce intrathoracic pressure for venous return to the right atrium. Generally the negative pressure is applied by using a jet or Venturi system.

negative feedback, **1.** (in physiology) a decrease in function in response to a stimulus. For example, the secretion of follicle-stimulating hormone decreases as the amount of circulating estrogen increases. **2.** *(Informal)* a critical, derogatory, or otherwise negative response from one person to what another person has communicated. **3.** (in communication theory) patterns of communication and interaction that maintain the status quo.

negative identity, the assumption of a persona that is at odds with the accepted values and expectations of society.

negative pathognomonic symptom /pəthog′nəmon′ik/ [L, *negare,* to deny; Gk, *pathos,* disease, *gnomen,* index, *symptoma,* that which happens], any symptom that is not usually found in a specific condition and that, if present, would not be compatible with the diagnosis.

negative pi meson pion, a form of electromagnetic radiation emitted from a proton linear accelerator.

negative pi meson radiotherapy, a form of radiotherapy using a beam of subatomic particles known as negative pi mesons, or pions, emitted by a proton linear accelerator. When the particles are beamed at a tumor, they cause the atomic nuclei of malignant cells to explode and scatter intensely radioactive subatomic particles through the tumor. Pion radiotherapy requires fewer rad and has a 60% greater biological effect than conventional x-radiation techniques. It also may have less effect on normal tissue near the tumor. Some locally advanced neoplasms, especially those of the prostate, are destroyed. Gliomas and advanced cancers of the head and neck also may be well controlled with pion radiotherapy. Moderate acute toxicity occurs with treatment, but chronic toxicity is minimal. See also **pion.**

negative pressure, a less than ambient atmospheric pressure, as in a vacuum, at an altitude above sea level, or in a hypobaric chamber. Negative pressure may be used in wound healing or to help stimulate or cycle exhalation in intermittent positive-pressure breathing.

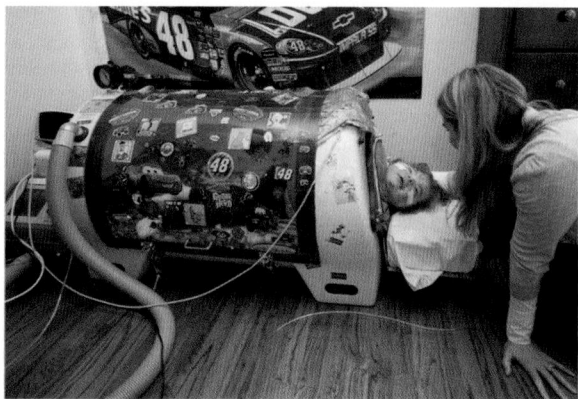

Negative-pressure ventilator *(Courtesy Respironics)*

negative pressure isolation rooms, isolation rooms used for patients with an airborne-transmitted disease. Airflow goes from the corridor into the patient's room. As the patient's room air is exhausted, it is vented to the outside.

negative punishment, a form of behavior modification in which the removal of something after an operant (behavior) decreases the probability of the operant's recurrence.

negative reinforcement, a form of behavior modification in which the removal of something after an operant (behavior) decreases the probability of the operant's recurrence.

negative reinforcer, (in psychology) a stimulus that, when presented immediately after occurrence of a particular behavior, will decrease the rate of occurrence of the behavior.

negative relationship, **1.** (in research) an inverse relationship between two variables. As one variable increases, the other decreases. Also called **inverse relationship.** Compare **positive relationship. 2.** (in psychology) any interpersonal relationship that has an adverse effect on at least one member, making the relationship unhealthy. In its extreme form it is sometimes referred to as a toxic relationship.

negative sequence, the sequence of bases on the strand of a double-stranded nucleic acid that is complementary to the positive-sense strand. In DNA it is the template strand on which the mRNA is synthesized.

negative staining, a technique in which an electron-dense substance is mixed with a specimen, resulting in an electron microscopic image in which the specimen appears translucent against an opaque or dark background.

negative symptom, (in psychiatry) any symptom that takes away from the true character or personality of an individual. The term is used specifically for schizophrenia when flat affect, social withdrawal, and/or a diminished ability to care for the self appear as symptoms. However, negative symptoms can also be seen in psychosis, dementia, and some forms of brain injury. Compare **positive symptom.**

negativism /neg″ətiviz′əm/ [L, *negare,* to deny], a behavioral attitude characterized by opposition, resistance, the refusal to cooperate with even the most reasonable request, and the tendency to act in a contrary manner. The resulting response may be passive, such as the immobile, rigid postures observed in catatonic schizophrenia, or active, as in a belligerent, impulsive, or capricious act, for example, lowering the arms when asked to raise them or sitting down when asked to stand. Negativism can also be seen in oppositional defiant disorder, borderline personality disorder, and attention deficit hyperactivity disorder.

negatron /neg″ətron/, an electron or beta particle with a single negative charge.

NegGram, an antibacterial drug. Brand name for **nalidixic acid.**

neglect /nəglekt″/, **1.** a condition that occurs when a caregiver, parent, or guardian fails to provide minimal physical and emotional care for a child or other dependent person. **2.** (in neurology) a lack of awareness of stimuli on the affected side following a brain injury. Kinds include **unilateral neglect,** *spatial neglect.*

negligence /neg″lijens/ [L, *negligentia,* carelessness], (in law) the commission of an act that a prudent person would not have done or the omission of a duty that a prudent person would have fulfilled, resulting in injury or harm to another person. A professional person is negligent if harm to a client results from such an act or such failure to act, but it must be proved that other prudent members of the same profession would ordinarily have acted differently under the same circumstances. Compare **malpractice.** Kinds include **misfeasance, malfeasance, nonfeasance.**

negligence per se, (in law) a finding of negligence rendered in judgment of a professional action or inaction in violation of a statute or so at odds with common sense that beyond any doubt no prudent person would have been guilty of it.

Negri bodies /nā″grē/ [Adelchi Negri, Italian physician, 1876–1912; AS, *bodig*], intracytoplasmic inclusion bodies found in the brain and central nervous system cells of rabies victims.

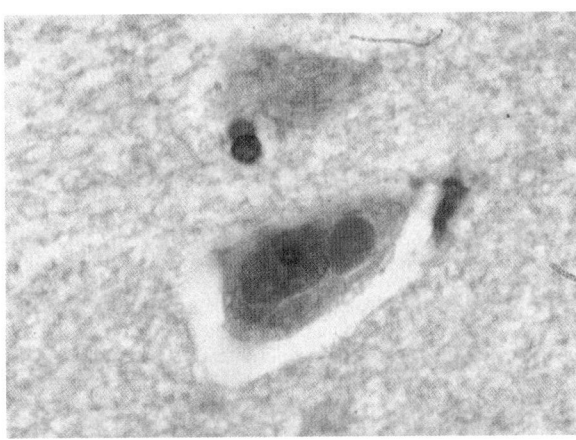

Negri bodies *(Murray, Rosenthal, and Pfaller, 2013)*

NEI, abbreviation for **National Eye Institute.**

Neisseria /nīser″ē·ə/ [Albert L.S. Neisser, Polish dermatologist, 1855–1916], a genus of aerobic to facultatively anaerobic bacteria of the family Neisseriaceae. The gram-negative cocci, which appear in pairs with adjacent sides flattened, are among the normal flora of genitourinary and upper respiratory tracts. Pathogenic species include gonococcus and meningococcus forms.

Neisseria catarrhalis. See *Moraxella catarrhalis.*

Neisseriaceae /nī″serē·ā″si·ē/ [Albert L.S. Neisser], a family of four genera of gram-negative aerobic cocci and rod-shaped bacteria occurring singly or in pairs, chains, or clusters. They are saprophytic or parasitic. The genera are *Actinobacter, Kingella, Moraxella,* and *Neisseria.*

Neisseria gonorrhoeae [Albert L.S. Neisser; Gk, *gone,* seed, *rhoia,* flow], a gram-negative, nonmotile diplococcal bacterium usually seen microscopically as flattened pairs within the cytoplasm of neutrophils. It is the causative organism of gonorrhea. Also called **gonococcus.**

Neisseria meningitidis. See **meningococcus.**

Neisseria sicca [Albert L.S. Neisser], a species of dry or slimy white-to-yellow bacteria normally found in the human nasopharynx and in saliva and sputum.

NEJM, abbreviation for *New England Journal of Medicine.*

nelarabine, an antineoplastic drug.
■ INDICATIONS: This drug is used to treat T cell lymphoblastic leukemia and T cell lymphoblastic lymphoma after relapse or treatment failure with at least two chemotherapeutic agents.
■ CONTRAINDICATIONS: Pregnancy, severe neurotoxicity, and known hypersensitivity to this drug prohibit its use.
■ ADVERSE EFFECTS: Adverse effects of this drug include dizziness; insomnia; rigors; peripheral neuropathy; confusion; headache; edema; leukopenia; anemia; decreased potassium, calcium magnesium, glucose, albumin, bilirubin, aspartate aminotransferase, and alanine aminotransferase; hyperuricemia; increased glucose; myalgia; arthralgia; back pain; weakness; cough; dyspnea; wheezing; and epistaxis. Life-threatening side effects include seizures, paralysis, neutropenia, thrombocytopenia, and pleural effusion. Common side effects include fatigue, nausea, vomiting, anorexia, diarrhea, stomatitis, and constipation.

Nélaton dislocation /nālätôN″/ [Auguste Nélaton, French surgeon, 1807–1873], a dislocation of the ankle in which the distal ends of the tibia and fibula are separated and the talus is forced upward between the tibia and fibula.

N

nelfinavir, an antiviral drug.

■ INDICATIONS: It is used alone or in combination with other drugs to treat HIV.

■ CONTRAINDICATIONS: Known hypersensitivity to protease inhibitors prohibits its use.

■ ADVERSE EFFECTS: Life-threatening effects include anemia, leukopenia, thrombocytopenia, and hemoglobin abnormalities. Other adverse effects include anorexia, dyspepsia, headache, asthenia, poor concentration, dermatitis, pain, bleeding, hypoglycemia, and hyperlipidemia. Common side effects include diarrhea, flatulence, and rash.

Nelson syndrome [Donald H. Nelson, American physician, 1925–2010], a pituitary adenoma that may follow bilateral adrenalectomy for Cushing syndrome. It is characterized by a marked increase in the secretion of adrenocorticotropic hormone and melanocyte-stimulating hormone by the pituitary gland and visual problems because of optic chiasm compression. Treatment includes irradiation to decrease pituitary function and in some cases hypophysectomy. See also **Cushing disease.**

nema-, prefix meaning "thread": *nematode, nematocide.*

-nema, suffix meaning "a threadlike stage in the development of chromosomes": *chromonema.*

nemaline myopathy /nem′əlēn/ [Gk, *nēma,* thread], a nonprogressive disease of muscular tissue of uncertain inheritance, characterized histologically by abnormal threadlike structures in muscle cells and clinically by hypotonia with diffuse weakness of the limbs and trunk, usually beginning in infancy.

nemato-, prefix meaning "nematode" or "threadlike structure": *nematocyst, nematocides, nematodiasis.*

nematocides /nəmat′əsīdz/ [Gk, *nema,* thread, *eidos,* form; L, *caedere,* to kill], chemical pesticides that are used to kill nematode worms.

nematocyst /nem″ətōsist′/ [Gk, *nema,* thread, *eidos,* form, *kystis,* bag], a capsule containing a barbed, threadlike process found in certain cells on the external surface of cnidarians, such as the Portuguese man-of-war and jellyfish. The nematocysts of some cnidarians can penetrate the skin and inject a poison, causing painful and potentially fatal injury.

nematode /nem″ətōd/ [Gk, *nema* + *eidos,* form], a multicellular, parasitic animal of the phylum Nematoda. All roundworms belong to the phylum, including *Ancylostoma duodenale, Ascaris lumbricoides, Enterobius vermicularis, Necator americanus, Strongyloides stercoralis,* and several other species.

nematodiasis /nem′ətōdī″əsis/ [Gk, *nema,* thread, *eidos,* form, *osis,* condition], an infestation of nematode worms.

Nembutal, a barbiturate. Brand name for **pentobarbital.**

-nemia, suffix meaning "blood."

neoadjuvant therapy /nē′ō·ad″jəvənt/, a preliminary cancer treatment, such as chemotherapy or radiation, that usually precedes another phase of treatment.

neoantigen /-an″tijən/ [Gk, *neos,* new, *anti,* against, *genein,* to produce], a new specific antigen that develops in a tumor cell.

neobehaviorism /-bihā″vē·əriz′əm/ [Gk, *neos* + ME, *behaven,* behavior], a school of psychology based on the general principles of behaviorism but broader and more flexible in concept. It stresses experimental research and laboratory analyses in the study of overt behavior and in various subjective phenomena that cannot be directly observed and measured, such as fantasies, love, stress, empathy, trust, and personality. See also **behaviorism.**

neobehaviorist /-ist/, a disciple of the school of neobehaviorism.

neobladder /ne″oblad′er/, a continent urinary reservoir made from a detubularized segment of bowel or stomach, with implantation of ureters and urethra. It is used to replace the bladder after cystectomy.

neoblastic /-blas″tik/ [Gk, *neos* + *blastos,* germ], pertaining to a new tissue or development within a new tissue.

neocerebellum /-ser″əbel′əm/, those parts of the cerebellum that receive input via the corticopontocerebellar pathway.

neocortex /-kôr′teks/ [Gk, *neos,* new; L, *cortex,* bark], the most recently evolved part of the brain. In humans the neocortex includes all of the cerebral cortex except for the hippocampal and piriform areas.

NeoDecadron, a topical fixed-combination drug containing a glucocorticoid and an antibacterial drug. Brand name for *dexamethasone phosphate,* **neomycin sulfate.**

neodymium (Nd), an element with the atomic number of 60. A rare earth metal, neodymium has many industrial uses. Neodymium dust is highly irritating to eyes and mucous membranes.

neogenesis. See **regeneration.**

neoglottis /-glot″is/, a vibrating structure that replaces the glottis in alaryngeal speech, such as after a laryngectomy. Also called **pseudoglottis.**

neologism /nē·ol″əjiz′əm/ [Gk, *neos* + *logos,* word], **1.** a word or term newly coined or used with a new meaning. **2.** (in psychiatry) a word coined by a psychotic or delirious patient that is meaningful only to the patient.

neomycin sulfate /ne′ō-mī″sin/, an aminoglycoside antibiotic.

■ INDICATIONS: It is prescribed orally to treat hepatic coma and infections of the intestine and to prepare the gastrointestinal tract for surgery. It is prescribed topically to treat skin infections.

■ CONTRAINDICATIONS: Renal dysfunction, intestinal obstruction, or known hypersensitivity to this drug or to any aminoglycoside medication prohibits its use. Neomycin is not administered parenterally.

■ ADVERSE EFFECTS: Among the more serious adverse effects are nausea, vomiting, diarrhea, malabsorption, or superinfection. Prolonged treatment in patients with impaired renal function may result in the toxicities of systemic aminoglycosides (e.g., ototoxicity, nephrotoxicity, neuromuscular toxicity). Hypersensitivity reactions may occur with topical administration of this drug.

neon (Ne) /nē′on/ [Gk, *neos,* new], a colorless, odorless, inert gaseous element. Its atomic number is 10; its atomic mass is 20.18. Neon has no compounds and occurs in the atmosphere in the ratio of about 18 parts per million. Some minerals and meteorites contain traces of this element. It is prepared commercially by the fractional distillation of liquefied air and is one of the first components to boil off. Neon is an excellent conductor of electricity, which ionizes the gas and causes it to emit a reddish-orange glow. This characteristic makes neon useful in devices to warn against electric current overload.

neonatal /-nā′təl/ [Gk, *neos* + L, *natus,* born], the period of time covering the first 28 days after birth.

neonatal abstinence syndrome (NAS), a behavioral pattern of irritability, tremulousness, and inconsolability exhibited in newborns exposed to heroin and methadone in the womb. The infant is born addicted to the drugs used by the mother. Symptoms of NAS are associated with withdrawal from those drugs. Following treatment during the neonatal period, the abnormal signs usually resolve. In some infants hypertonicity has persisted for 6 months. See also **infant of chemically dependent mother.**

Neonatal Behavioral Assessment Scale (NBAS), a scale developed by T. Berry Brazelton and colleagues for evaluating the neurological condition and behavior of a newborn by assessing his or her alertness, motor maturity, irritability, consolability, and interaction with people. It consists of a series of 27 reaction tests, including response to inanimate objects, pinprick, light, and the sound of a rattle or bell. The individuality of an infant may be demonstrated for parents by the scale, and some researchers theorize that the quality of the parent-child relationship may be predicted.

neonatal breathing, respiration in newborns. It begins when pulmonary fluid in the lungs is expelled by compression of the thorax during delivery and resorbed from the alveoli into the bloodstream and lymphatics. As air enters the lungs, the chest and lungs recoil to a resting position, but forceful inspirations are necessary to keep the lungs inflated. Such inspirations are triggered by changes in blood gas tension, a strong Hering-Breuer reflex, decrease in body temperature, and tactile stimuli. Irregular fetal breathing movements, which occur during rapid eye movement sleep, may be observed as early as 13 weeks of gestation. At birth the peripheral and central chemoreceptors involved in the control of respiration rate are very active, and newborns are highly sensitive to carbon dioxide during the first weeks. However, the control of rhythm breathing is not fully developed at birth.

neonatal conjunctivitis. See **ophthalmia neonatorum.**

neonatal death, the death of a live-born infant during the first 28 days after birth. Early neonatal death is usually considered to be one that occurs during the first 7 days. Compare **infant death, perinatal death.**

neonatal developmental profile, an evaluation of the developmental status of a newborn based on three examinations: a gestational age inventory, a neurological examination, and a Neonatal Behavioral Assessment score.

neonatal hepatitis, hepatitis of unknown cause with onset in the first few weeks of life. Some cases are associated with viral or bacterial infection; a few are familial. It is characterized by the transformation of hepatocytes into polynuclear giant cells and by conjugated hyperbilirubinemia with jaundice. Most patients recover completely; some develop chronic disease or fatal cirrhosis. Also called **giant cell hepatitis.**

neonatal hyperbilirubinemia. See **hyperbilirubinemia of the newborn.**

neonatal intensive care unit (NICU), a hospital unit containing a variety of sophisticated mechanical devices and special equipment for the management and care of premature and seriously ill newborns. The unit is staffed by a team of nurses and neonatologists who are highly trained in the pathophysiology of the newborn. See also **intensive care unit.**

neonatal jaundice. See **hyperbilirubinemia of the newborn.**

neonatal mortality, the statistical rate of infant death during the first 28 days after live birth, expressed as the number of such deaths per 1000 live births in a specific geographic area or institution in a given time.

neonatal period, the interval from birth to 28 days of age. It represents the period of greatest risk to the infant. Approximately 65% of all deaths that occur in the first year of life happen during this 4-week period.

neonatal pustular melanosis, a transient skin condition of the neonate characterized by vesicles present at birth that become pustular. The lesions contain neutrophils rather than eosinophils as seen in erythema toxicum neonatorum. They disappear within 72 hours, leaving dark spots that gradually fade by about 3 months of age. The cause is unknown. The condition is twice as common in black infants as in white infants.

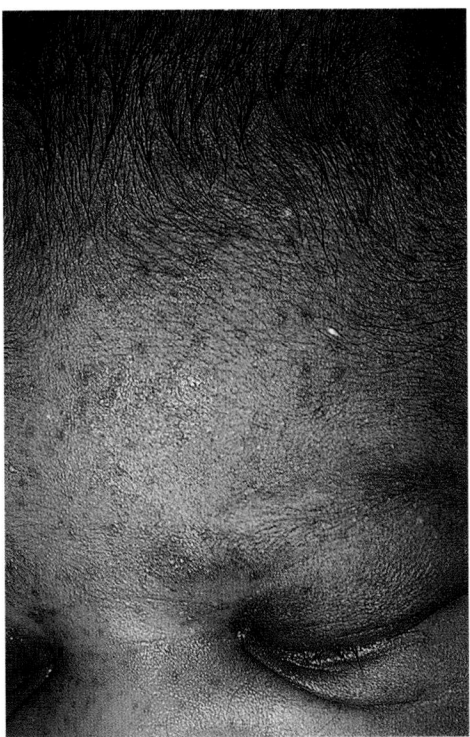

Neonatal pustular melanosis *(Weston, Lane, and Morelli, 2007)*

neonatal thermoregulation, the regulation of the body temperature of a newborn, which may be affected by evaporation, conduction, radiation, and convection.

■ METHOD: To prevent the loss of body heat through evaporation, the infant is patted dry with a warm towel immediately after birth. Loss of heat by conduction is prevented by wrapping the baby in a warm blanket or placing a warm blanket over the baby as the baby lies on the mother's skin and by warming all equipment that is to be used to touch, cover, or examine the infant. Loss of heat by radiation can be minimized by placing the baby under a radiant heater; on a warmed, padded surface; or in skin-to-skin contact with the mother. Loss of body heat by convection is prevented by avoiding drafts, air-conditioning vents, and low ambient temperatures. Infant bassinets have high sides to prevent cross drafts.

■ INTERVENTIONS: The infant is kept covered and protected from any means of heat loss. Because the surface area of the newborn's head is proportionately large when compared with the body, heat loss from the head may be great. Therefore a cap or fold of blanket is placed around the head. Progressive family-centered maternity services, in which the practice after delivery is to place the infant skin-to-skin with the mother, often provide caps made of stockinet. An overhead radiant heater is rolled to the delivery bed to maintain a warm ambient temperature for the infant.

■ OUTCOME CRITERIA: The axillary temperature is normally between 97.7° F (36.5° C) and 99.5° F (37.5° C).

neonatal tyrosinemia. See **tyrosinemia.**

neonatal unit, a unit of a hospital that provides care and treatment of newborns through the age of 28 days, and longer if necessary.

neonatal vital signs monitor, equipment in a specialized neonatal intensive care unit that measures mean blood

N

pressure and mean heart rate from a plastic blood pressure cuff, with values digitally displayed on a monitor. See also **electronic fetal monitor.**

neonatal volvulus, a twisting causing an obstruction in the newborn's gastrointestinal tract, usually cecal or midgut.

neonate /nē″ōnāt/. See **newborn.**

neonatology /nē′ōnātol″əjē/ [Gk, *neos* + L, *natus,* born; Gk, *logos,* science], the branch of medicine that concentrates on the care of the neonate and specializes in the diagnosis and treatment of the disorders of the newborn. –*neonatological, neonatologic, adj.,* –*neonatologist, n.*

neonatorum encephalitis /-nātôr″əm/ [Gk, new; L, born; Gk, brain, inflammation], a brain inflammation that develops in the first 4 weeks of life. Also called **encephalitis neonatorum.**

neo-, ne-, prefix meaning "new": *neoantigen, neoblastic, neonatal.*

neoplasia /nē′ōplā″zhə/ [Gk, *neos* + *plassein,* to mold], the new and abnormal development of cells that may be benign or malignant. –**neoplastic,** *adj.*

neoplasm /nē″ōplaz′əm/ [Gk, *neos* + *plasma,* formation], any abnormal growth of new tissue, benign or malignant. Also called **tumor.** See also **benign, cancer, malignant.** –**neoplastic,** *adj.*

neoplastic /nē′ōplas″tik/ [Gk, *neos,* new, *plassein,* to mold], pertaining to malignancy, neoplasm.

neoplastic fracture, a fracture resulting from a weakness in bone tissue caused by a benign or malignant tumor. Also called **pathological fracture.**

neoplastic pericarditis [Gk, *neos,* new, *plasma,* formation, *peri,* around, *kardia,* heart, *itis,* inflammation], inflammation of the pericardium, usually secondary to a malignant tumor within the area. Also called **carcinomatous pericarditis.**

neoplastic transformation, conversion of a tissue with a normal growth pattern into a malignant tumor.

neoplasty /nē″ōplas′tē/ [Gk, *neos,* new, *plassein,* to mold], a plastic surgery procedure to restore a part or add a new part. –**neoplastic,** *adj.*

Neosporin, a topical, fixed-combination drug containing antibacterial agents. Brand name for **polymyxin B sulfate, neomycin sulfate,** *bacitracin zinc.*

neostigmine bromide /nē′ōstig″mēn/, a reversible acetylcholinesterase inhibitor.

■ INDICATIONS: It is prescribed in situations in which it is desirable to potentiate the effects of neuronally released acetylcholine, such as in the treatment of myasthenia gravis and postoperative urinary retention, and to reverse the effects of nondepolarizing neuromuscular blockers.

■ CONTRAINDICATIONS: Bowel obstruction, urinary tract infection, or known hypersensitivity to this drug or to other bromides prohibits its use. Initial dosages should be administered only in settings equipped for cardiopulmonary resuscitation, and ephinephrine and atropine should be available.

■ ADVERSE EFFECTS: Overdosage causes cholinergic crisis with widespread muscle weakness and paralysis, including the diaphragm, which can cause severe respiratory depression. Excessive salivation and lacrimation, intestinal cramps, urinary urgency, and convulsions are other adverse effects.

neostriatum /-strī-ā″təm/, the most recently evolved part of the corpus striatum, consisting of the caudate nucleus and putamen. The neostriatum receives input from the entire cerebral cortex and other brain areas and provides output to the basal nuclei.

Neo-Synephrine, a vasoconstrictor. Brand name for **phenylephrine hydrochloride.**

neoteny /nē-ot″ənē/ [Gk, *neos,* new, *teinein,* to stretch], the attainment of sexual maturity during the larval stage of development, such as in certain amphibians.

nephelometer /nef′əlom″ətər/ [Gk, *nephele,* cloud, *metron,* measure], a photometric apparatus used to determine the concentration of solids suspended in a liquid or a gas, such as the number of bacteria in a specimen. See also **nephelometry.**

nephelometry /nef′əlom″ətrē/, a technique for detecting proteins in body fluids based on the tendency of proteins to scatter light in identifiable ways. –*nephelometrical, nephelometric, adj.*

nephr-. See **nephro-, nephr-.**

nephrectomy /-ek″təmē/ [Gk, *nephros,* kidney, *ektomē,* excision], the surgical removal of a kidney, performed to remove a tumor or otherwise diseased kidney. In the patient with renal failure, the kidney may be the cause of extreme hypertension, and therefore one or both kidneys are removed. A nephrectomy may also be performed to obtain a kidney for a living donation. Before surgery blood is typed and crossmatched for transfusion. Any testing required for a living donation is completed by both the donor of the kidney and the recipient. During surgery the kidney is approached through either a flank, abdominal, or thoracoabdominal incision and removed. If the thoracic cavity is opened, a chest tube is inserted and connected to water-seal drainage. In the postoperative period respiratory care is critically important as the incision can be painful and interfere with deep breathing.

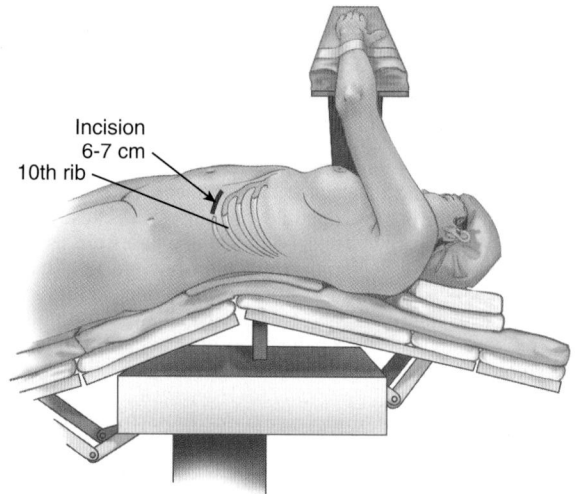

Incision
6-7 cm
10th rib

Patient positioned for a nephrectomy *(Frantzides and Carlson, 2013)*

-nephric, suffix meaning "kidneys": *anephric, mesonephric.*

nephritic /nəfrit″ik/ [Gk, *nephros,* kidney, *itis,* inflammation], pertaining to an inflammation of the kidney.

nephritic calculus. See **renal calculus.**

nephritic factor, a protein found in the serum of patients with membranoproliferative glomerulonephritis. It activates alternative complement pathways.

nephritic gingivitis [Gk, *nephros* + *itis,* inflammation, *gingiva,* gum; Gk, *itis,* inflammation], inflammation of the mouth and gingiva associated with kidney failure, accompanied by pain, the odor of ammonia, and increased salivation. Also called **uremic gingivitis.**

nephritic syndrome, a group of signs and symptoms of a urinary tract disorder, including hematuria, hypertension, and renal failure.

nephritis /nəfrī″tis/ [Gk, *nephros* + *itis,* inflammation], any one of a large group of diseases of the kidney characterized by inflammation and abnormal function. Kinds include **acute nephritis, Alport syndrome, glomerulonephritis,**

Classification of neoplasms

Parent tissue	Benign tumor	Malignant tumor
Epithelium		
Skin and mucous membrane	Papilloma	Squamous cell carcinoma
	Polyp	Basal cell carcinoma
		Transitional cell carcinoma
Glands	Adenoma	Adenocarcinoma
	Cystadenoma	
Endothelium		
Blood vessels	Hemangioma	Hemangiosarcoma
		Angiosarcoma
Lymph vessels	Lymphangioma	Lymphangiosarcoma
Bone marrow		Multiple myeloma
		Ewing sarcoma
		Leukemia
		Lymphosarcoma
		Lymphangioendothelioma
Lymphoid tissue		Reticular cell sarcoma (difficult to classify because of cell embryology)
		Lymphatic leukemia
		Malignant lymphoma
Connective tissue		
Embryonic fibrous tissue	Myxoma	Myxosarcoma
Fibrous tissue	Fibroma	Fibrosarcoma
Adipose tissue	Lipoma	Liposarcoma
Cartilage	Chondroma	Chondrosarcoma
Bone	Osteoma	Osteogenic sarcoma
Synovial membrane	Synovioma	Synovial sarcoma
Muscle tissue		
Smooth muscle	Leiomyoma	Leiomyosarcoma
Striated muscle	Rhabdomyoma	Rhabdomyosarcoma
Nerve tissue		
Nerve fibers and sheaths	Neuroma	Neurogenic sarcoma
	Neurinoma (neurilemmoma)	Neurofibrosarcoma
Ganglion cells	Neurofibroma	Neuroblastoma
Glial cells	Ganglioneuroma	Glioblastoma
	Glioma	Spongioblastoma
Meninges	Meningioma	
Pigmented neoplasms		
Melanoblasts	Pigmented nevus	Malignant melanoma
		Melanocarcinoma
Miscellaneous		
Placenta	Hydatidiform mole	Choriocarcinoma (chorioepithelioma)
	Dermoid cyst	Embryonal carcinoma
		Embryonal sarcoma
		Teratocarcinoma

From Monahan FD et al: *Phipps' medical-surgical nursing: health and illness perspectives,* ed 8, St. Louis, 2007, Mosby.

hereditary nephritis, **interstitial nephritis, parenchymatous nephritis.**

nephro-, nephr-, prefix meaning "kidneys": *nephroblastoma, nephrogram, nephrorrhagia.*

nephroangiosclerosis /nef′rō·an′jē·ō′sklerō″sis/ [Gk, *nephros + angeion,* vessel, *skleros,* hard, *osis,* condition], necrosis of the renal arterioles associated with hypertension. This condition is present in a small number of hypertensive individuals between 30 and 50 years of age. Early signs are headaches, blurring of vision, and a diastolic blood pressure greater than 120 mm Hg. Examination of the retina reveals hemorrhages, vascular exudates, and papilledema. The heart is usually enlarged, especially the left ventricle. Proteins and red blood cells are found in the urine. Heart and kidney failure may occur if the disease remains untreated. Treatment includes measures to lower blood pressure with diet and antihypertensive medications. Hemodialysis is used when preventive measures have failed. Also called **malignant hypertension.** See also **hypertension, renal failure.**

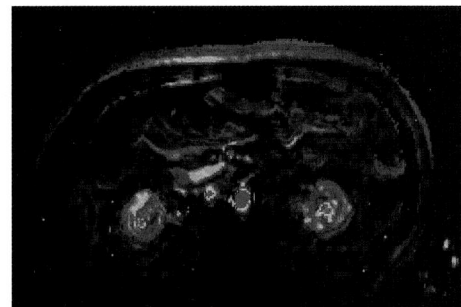

Perfusion MRI of patient with severe bilateral cortical hypoperfusion with known end-stage nephroangiosclerosis *(Dujardin et al, 2007)*

nephroblastoma. See **Wilms tumor.**

nephrocalcinosis /nef′rōkal′sinō″sis/ [Gk, *nephros* + L, *calx,* lime; Gk, *osis,* condition], an abnormal condition of the kidneys in which deposits of calcium form in the parenchyma at the site of previous inflammation or degenerative change. Infection, hematuria, anal colic, and decreased function of the kidney may occur.

nephrocystitis /-sistī″tis/, an inflammation involving both the kidney and the urinary bladder.

nephrocystosis /-sistō″sis/, the formation of cysts in the kidney.

nephrogenic /nef′rōjen″ik/ [Gk, *nephros* + *genein,* to produce], **1.** generating kidney tissue. **2.** originating in the kidney.

nephrogenic ascites, the abnormal presence of fluid in the peritoneal cavity of patients undergoing hemodialysis for renal failure. The cause of this type of ascites is unknown. See also **ascites.**

nephrogenic cord, either of the paired longitudinal ridges of tissue that lie along the dorsal surface of the coelom in the early developing vertebrate embryo. It is formed from the fusion of the nephrotome tissue and gives rise to the structures making up the embryonic urogenital system. See also **mesonephros, metanephros, pronephros.**

nephrogenic diabetes insipidus, an abnormal condition in which the kidneys do not concentrate the urine, resulting in polyuria, polydipsia, and very dilute urine. The secretion of antidiuretic hormone (ADH) by the pituitary is normal, and all kidney function is normal, except the lack of response to ADH. See also **diabetes insipidus.**

nephrogenic rests, remnants of renal blastema tissue found in or around the kidney, which are sometimes precursors of Wilms tumor.

nephrogenous /nəfroj″ənəs/, pertaining to the formation and development of the kidneys.

nephrogram /nef′rōgram/, a radiograph of the kidney.

nephrography /nəfrog″rəfē/, the radiographic examination of the kidney.

nephrohypertrophy /-hīpur″trəfē/ [Gk, *nephros,* kidney, *hyper,* excessive, *trophe,* nourishment], enlargement of the kidney.

nephrolith. See **renal calculus.**

nephrolithiasis /nef′rōlithī″əsis/, a disorder characterized by the presence of calculi in the kidney. See also **renal calculus.**

nephrolithic. See **nephrolith.**

nephrolithotomy /-lithot″əmē/, the surgical removal of renal calculi.

nephrology /nəfrol″əjē/ [Gk, *nephros* + *logos,* science], the study of the anatomy, physiology, and pathology of the kidney. −*nephrological, nephrologic, adj.*

nephrolytic /-lit″ik/ [Gk, *nephros* + *lysis,* loosening], pertaining to the destruction of a kidney.

-nephroma, suffix meaning "a tumor of the kidney or area of the kidney."

nephromere. See **nephrotome.**

nephron /nef″ron/ [Gk, *nephros,* kidney], a structural and functional unit of the kidney resembling a microscopic funnel with a long stem and two convoluted tubular sections. Each kidney contains about 1.25 million nephrons. All nephrons have a renal corpuscle and renal tubules. Juxtamedullary nephrons also have loops of Henle. Each renal corpuscle consists of a glomerulus of renal capillaries enclosed within Bowman's capsule. The renal corpuscles and the convoluted parts of the renal tubules are located in the cortex of the kidney. The loops of Henle and collecting tubules are located in the medulla. Urine is formed in the renal corpuscles and renal tubules by filtration, reabsorption, and secretion. See also **kidney, malpighian corpuscle.**

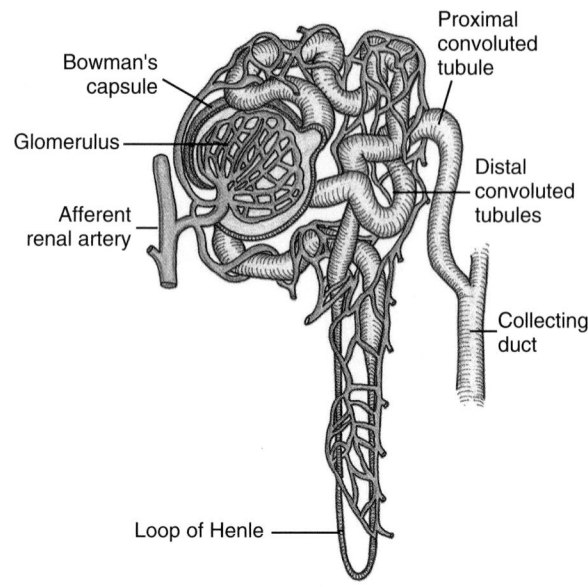

Nephron *(Potter et al, 2013)*

nephronia /nəfrō″nē·ə/, an inflammation of intrarenal connective tissue that occurs in a small percentage of patients with urinary tract infections.

nephronophthisis. See **medullary cystic disease.**

nephroparalysis /-pəral″isis/ [Gk, *nephros,* kidney, *paralyein,* to be palsied], a paralysis of the kidney resulting in a cessation of its functions.

nephropathic cystinosis, one of the types of cystinosis that involves kidney damage and ophthalmic symptoms.

nephropathy /nefrop″əthē/ [Gk, *nephros* + *pathos,* disease], any disorder of the kidney, including inflammatory, degenerative, and sclerotic conditions. See also **kidney disease.**

nephropexy /nef′rəpek′sē/ [Gk, *nephros* + *pexis,* fixation], a surgical operation to fixate a floating or ptotic kidney.

nephroptosis /nef′rəptō″sis/ [Gk, *nephros* + *ptosis,* falling], a downward displacement or dropping of a kidney.

nephrorrhaphy /nəfrôr″əfē/ [Gk, *nephros* + *rhaphe,* suture], an operation that sutures a floating kidney in place.

nephrosclerosis. See **nephroangiosclerosis.**

nephroscope /nef″rəskōp′/ [Gk, *nephros* + *skopein,* to look], a fiberoptic instrument used specifically for visualization of the kidney and the disintegration and removal of renal calculi. The nephroscope is inserted percutaneously.

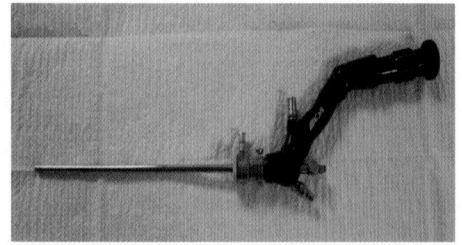

Nephroscope *(Long et al, 2015)*

nephrosis. See **nephrotic syndrome.**

nephrostoma /-stō″mə/ *pl.* **nephrostomas, nephrostomata** [Gk, *nephros* + *stoma,* mouth], the funnel-shaped ciliated opening of the excretory tubules into the coelom of the early developing vertebrate embryo. Also called *nephrostome.* −*nephrostomic, adj.*

nephrostomy /nəfros″təmē/, a surgical procedure in which a flank incision is made so that a catheter can be inserted into the kidney pelvis to drain the kidney, often done to relieve obstruction.

nephrostomy catheter, a catheter used with percutaneous nephrostomy, as for drainage.

nephrotic syndrome /nəfrot″ik/ [Gk, *nephros* + L, *icus,* like], an abnormal condition of the kidney characterized by marked proteinuria, hypoalbuminemia, and edema. It occurs in glomerular disease and thrombosis of a renal vein and as a complication of many systemic diseases, diabetes mellitus, amyloidosis, systemic lupus erythematosus, and multiple myeloma. The nephrotic syndrome occurs in a severe primary form. Also called **nephrosis.** −*nephrotic, adj.*
■ OBSERVATIONS: Presenting symptoms include anorexia, weakness, proteinuria, hypoalbuminuria, and edema.
■ INTERVENTIONS: Treatment and prognosis depend on the underlying cause of disease. Patients with primary nephrotic syndrome usually respond favorably to corticosteroids. Loop diuretics are used to control symptomatic edema, and dialysis may be necessary.
■ PATIENT CARE CONSIDERATIONS: Patients benefit from a comprehensive approach to care that includes diet counseling and exercise.

nephrotome /nef″rətom/ [Gk, *nephros* + *tome,* section], a zone of segmented mesodermal tissue in the developing vertebrate embryo lying along each side of the body dorsal to the abdominal cavity between the somite-forming dorsal mesoderm and the unsegmented lateral plate mesoderm. It is the primordial tissue for the urogenital system and gives rise to the nephrogenic cord. Also called **intermediate cell mass, intermediate mesoderm, middle plate, nephromere.** See also **mesonephros, metanephros, pronephros.**

nephrotomography /-təmog″rəfē/ [Gk, *nephros* + *tome,* section, *graphein,* to record], sectional radiographic examination of the kidneys.

nephrotomy /nəfrot″əmē/ [Gk, *nephros* + *temnein,* to cut], a surgical procedure in which an incision is made in the kidney.

nephrotoxicity, the quality of being destructive to kidney cells. −*nephrotoxic, adj.*

nephrotoxin /-tok″sin/, a toxin with specific destructive properties for the kidneys.

nephroureterolithiasis /nef′rōyo͞orē′tərō′lithī″əsis/, the presence of calculi in the kidneys and ureters.

Neptazane, a carbonic anhydrase inhibitor. Brand name for **methazolamide.**

neptunium (Np) /nept(y)o͞o″nē·əm/ [planet Neptune], a transuranic, metallic element. Its atomic number is 93; its atomic mass is 237. Although neptunium is considered a synthetic element, traces of natural neptunium have been found in uranium ores.

Neri's sign /nā′rēz/ [Vincenzo Neri, Italian neurologist, 1880–1959], a sign of organic hemiplegia, consisting of the spontaneous bending of the knee of the affected side as the leg is passively lifted, the patient being in the dorsal position. With the patient standing, forward bending of the trunk will cause flexion of the knee on the affected side in lumbosacral and iliosacral lesions.

Nernst equation [Hermann W. Nernst, German physicist, 1864–1941; L, *aequare,* to make equal], an expression of the relationship between the electrical potential across a membrane and the ratio between the concentrations of a given species of permeant ion on either side of the membrane.

nerve /nurv/ [L, *nervus*], one or more bundles of impulse-carrying fibers, myelinated or unmyelinated or both, that connect the brain and the spinal cord with other parts of the body. Nerves transmit afferent impulses from receptor organs toward the brain and spinal cord and efferent impulses peripherally to the effector organs. Each nerve consists of an epineurium enclosing fasciculi of nerve fibers; each fasciculus is surrounded by its own sheath of connective tissue, or epineurium. Individual nerve fibers, which are microscopic, consist of formed elements within a matrix of protoplasm enclosed in endoneurium that are enclosed in a neurilemmal sheath. Inside the neurilemma are nerve fibers, also enclosed in a myelin sheath. See also **axon, dendrite, neuroglia, neuron, Schwann cell.**

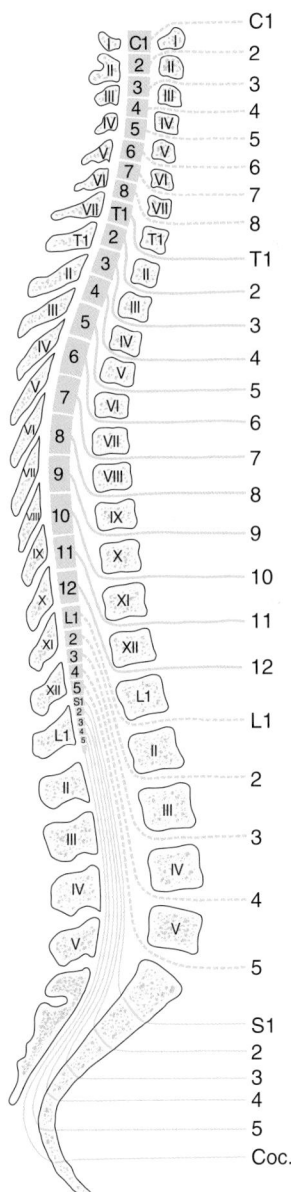

Nerve roots in relation to vertebrae *(Rakel and Rakel, 2011)*

nerve accommodation, the ability of nerve tissue to adjust to a constant source and intensity of stimulation so that some change in either intensity or duration of the stimulus is necessary to elicit a response beyond the initial reaction. Accommodation is probably caused by reduced sodium ion permeability, which results in an increased threshold intensity and subsequent stabilization of the resting membrane potential.

nerve agents, chemicals that interfere with the proper functioning of the nervous system. They are highly potent, and very small amounts can have serious effects. They include sarin, soman, tabun, and VX. Exposure is by inhalation or by skin or eye contact. Nerve agents can also be mixed with water and can be used to poison water supplies so that people can be exposed by drinking contaminated water or getting contaminated water on the skin. These agents act by inhibiting acetylcholinesterase, which allows the muscles to be stimulated constantly, and fatigue of the muscles used for breathing can cause death from respiratory failure. Treatment consists of removing the agent from the body and administration of an antidote (which must be done within minutes of exposure).

nerve block anesthesia. See **conduction anesthesia.**

nerve cable graft, a multistrand free nerve graft taken from elsewhere in the body to bridge a large gap in one of the main nerves in the forearm.

nerve cell. See **neuron.**

nerve compression, a pathological event that causes harmful pressure on one or more nerves, resulting in nerve damage and muscle weakness, atrophy, or paresthesias over time. Any nerve that passes over a rigid prominence is vulnerable, and the degree of damage depends on the magnitude and duration of the compressive force. Various factors may contribute to susceptibility, such as inherited predisposition, malnutrition, trauma, and disease. Various activities associated with routine occupations may unduly compress especially vulnerable nerves, such as the median nerve, radial nerve, femoral nerve, and plantar nerves. Rest and the cessation or modification of causative activities often heal nerve damage caused by compression. Surgery may be required to correct more severe cases. Compare **nerve entrapment.**

nerve conduction test, an electrodiagnostic test of the integrity of the peripheral nerves. It involves placing an electrical stimulator over a nerve and measuring the time required for an impulse to travel over a measured segment of the nerve. The test is used in the diagnosis of nerve entrapment syndrome, radiculopathies, and polyneuropathies.

nerve deafness. See **sensorineural hearing loss.**

nerve endings, the fine branchlike terminations of peripheral neurons. Sensory endings are effectively dendrites lying far from the neuronal cell body, and motor nerve endings are the endings of axons and are called motor end plates. See also **neuron.**

nerve entrapment, an abnormal condition and type of mononeuropathy characterized by nerve damage and muscle weakness or atrophy. The peripheral nerve trunks of the body are especially vulnerable to entrapment in which repeated compression results in significant impairment. Nerves that pass over rigid prominences or through narrow bony and fascial canals are particularly prone to entrapment. The common signs of this disorder are pain and muscular weakness. Nerve damage by entrapment occurs more often when adjacent joints are affected by swelling and inflammation, such as in rheumatoid arthritis, pregnancy, and acromegaly. Signs of nerve entrapment also may develop after repeated bruising of certain nerves by various activities involving repeated motions, such as those associated with knitting and prolonged walking. Compare **nerve compression.** Kinds include **carpal tunnel syndrome.**

nerve excitability [L, *nervus,* nerve, *excitare,* to rouse], the readiness of a nerve cell to respond to a stimulus. See also **all-or-none law.**

nerve fiber, a slender process, the axon of a neuron. Each fiber is classified as myelinated or unmyelinated. Myelinated fibers are further designated as A or B fibers. C fibers are unmyelinated. The A fibers are somatic. A alpha fibers are large fibers and transport impulses at a velocity of 60 to 100 meters per second; A beta fibers are smaller and transmit pressure and temperature impulses at a velocity of 30 to 70 meters per second. A gamma fibers transmit touch and pressure impulses. A delta fibers are the smallest and transmit impulses associated with sharp pain sensation. B fibers are more finely myelinated than A fibers. They are both afferent and efferent and are mainly associated with visceral innervation. The unmyelinated C fibers are efferent postganglionic autonomic and afferent fibers that conduct impulses of prolonged, burning pain sensation from the viscera and periphery.

nerve graft, the transplantation of all or part of a nerve. The procedure may be performed in cases in which the gap in a severed nerve is too large to be repaired by suture alone. The graft provides a pathway that encourages the regrowth of severed axons from the central stump of the damaged nerve. Donor material may consist of heterografts, homografts, or autografts.

nerve growth factor (NGF), a protein whose hormone-like action affects differentiation, growth, and maintenance of neurons.

nerve impulse. See **impulse.**

nerve plexus [L, *nervus,* nerve, *plexus,* plaited], an interwoven network of nerves, such as the lumbar plexus formed by the anterior primary branch of the upper four lumbar nerves.

nerve root, the part of a nerve adjacent to the center to which it is connected.

nerve root impingement, the abnormal protrusion of body tissue into the space occupied by a spinal nerve root. Causes may include disk herniation, tissue prolapse, and inflammation.

nerve sheath [L, *nervus,* nerve; AS, *scaeth*], any of several types of coatings or coverings for nerve fibers and nerve tracts. Kinds include **endoneurial nerve sheath, medullary nerve sheath, myelin sheath, neurilemma.**

nervimotor /ner'vi·mō'tər/ [L, *nervus,* nerve + *motare,* to move], pertaining to a motor nerve.

nervous emesis [L, *nervus* + Gk, *emesis,* vomiting], vomiting that is functional and psychogenic. The condition is regarded as a psychological representation of a desire to reject something.

nervous prostration [L, *nervus* + *prosternere,* to throw down], a condition of irritable weakness and depression, which may be psychogenic or the result of a severe prolonged illness or exhausting experience.

nervous system [L, *nervus,* nerve; Gk, *system*], the extensive, intricate network of structures that activates, coordinates, and controls all the functions of the body. It is divided into the central nervous system, composed of the brain and the spinal cord, and the peripheral nervous system, which includes the cranial nerves and the spinal nerves. These morphological subdivisions combine and communicate to innervate the somatic and visceral parts of the body with the afferent and efferent nerve fibers. Afferent fibers carry sensory impulses to the central nervous system. Efferent fibers carry motor impulses from the central nervous system to the muscles and other organs. The somatic fibers are associated with the bones, muscles, and skin. The visceral fibers are associated with the internal organs, blood vessels, and mucous membranes. Compare **autonomic nervous system.** See also *Color Atlas of Human Anatomy,* pp. A-23 to A-27.

nervous tachypnea [L, *nervus* + Gk, *tachys,* rapid, *pnoia,* breath], a neurotic symptom characterized by quick, shallow breathing.

nervus abducens. See **abducens nerve.**

nervus accessorius. See **accessory nerve.**

nervus facialis. See **facial nerve.**

nervus glossopharyngeus. See **glossopharyngeal nerve.**

nervus hypoglossus. See **hypoglossal nerve.**

nervus oculomotorius. See **oculomotor nerve.**

nervus olfactorius. See **olfactory nerve.**

nervus opticus. See **optic nerve.**

nervus terminalis. See **terminal nerve.**

nervus trigeminus. See **trigeminal nerve.**

nervus trochlearis. See **trochlear nerve.**

nervus vagus. See **vagus nerve.**

Nesacaine, a long-acting local anesthetic. Brand name for **chloroprocaine.**

nesiritide, a vasodilator used to treat acutely decompensated congestive heart failure.

-ness, suffix meaning "a quality or state of being": *illness, fitness.*

nested nails, a pair of nails placed side by side in the medullary canal of long bones during orthopedic surgery.

nested variable, a variable located entirely within another variable, such as the rate of a given disease in one specific city.

net charge, the arithmetic sum of positive and negative charges.

net protein utilization (NPU), a measure of protein quality based on the percentage of ingested nitrogen that is retained by the body. Because NPU does not take into account differences in the digestibility of proteins, it gives a poorly digested but good-quality protein a false low value.

net radiation, the arithmetic difference between solar radiation received and outgoing terrestrial radiation.

nettle, a perennial herb *(Urtica dioica)* that is native to Europe and is now found throughout the United States and parts of Canada. See also **stinging nettle.**

■ INDICATIONS: It is used as a diuretic and as a treatment for hay fever and shows some evidence of efficacy for these indications.

■ CONTRAINDICATIONS: It should not be used during pregnancy and lactation, in children less than 2 years of age, or in people with hypersensitivity to this plant. It should be used only with caution in children and the elderly.

nettle rash [AS, *netele,* nettle; Fr, *rasche,* scurf], a fine urticarial eruption resulting from skin contact with stinging nettle, a common weed with leaves containing histamine. It is characterized by stinging and itching that lasts from a few minutes to several hours.

network [AS, *net* + *wearc*], a system of interconnected computers or CRT terminals and peripheral equipment in which each user has some access to others using the system while sharing data, internal and external storage devices (server), and other capabilities. A local-area network is one in which the computers are interconnected and serve the same facility or corporation.

networking, **1.** the process of developing and using an interaction format with professional colleagues and agencies. **2.** (in psychiatric nursing) the process of developing a set of agencies and professional personnel who are able to create a system of communication and support for psychiatric patients, usually those recently discharged from inpatient psychiatric facilities. Kinds include **natural network, professional network. 3.** a network of supportive contacts or services, such as the Women's Health Network.

network-model HMO, a managed care system analogous to the group-model health maintenance organization (HMO), but with services provided at multiple sites by multiple groups so that a wider geographic area is served.

net wt, abbreviation for *net weight.*

Neufeld nail /nyoo′fəld/ [Alonzo J. Neufeld, American surgeon, 1906–1984], an orthopedic nail with a V-shaped tip and shank used for fixating an intertrochanteric fracture. The nail is driven into the neck of the femur until it reaches a round metal plate screwed onto the side of the femur. It is secured to a receptacle on the plate. Also called *Neufeld angled nail.*

Neufeld roller traction, a traction device for a fractured femur, consisting of a cast for the calf and thigh hinged at the knee. The cast is suspended by a line that passes from the anterior midthigh, around a pulley, to a spring attached to the anterior midleg.

Neuman, Betty, a nursing theorist who developed the Neuman Systems Model, first published in 1972. Her model is influenced by Gestalt theory, which states that the homeostatic process is the process by which an organism maintains its equilibrium. Major concepts include total persons approach, holism, open system, lines of resistance and defense, degree of reaction, interventions, levels of prevention, and reconstitution. A spiritual variable was added to her model later, and created-environment was added to the typology. In the Neuman Systems Model, the client is presented as a whole person, an open system in constant change and in reciprocal interaction with the environment. Neuman believes the nurse should use purposeful interventions and a total-person approach to client care to help individuals, families, and groups reach and maintain a maximum level of total wellness. Nursing intervention is aimed at the reduction of stress and adverse conditions that can affect optimal client functions.

neur-. See **neuro-, neur-.**

neural /noor′əl/ [Gk, *neuron,* nerve], pertaining to nerve cells and their processes.

-neural, -neuric, suffix meaning "nerve" or "nerves": *abneural, myoneural, sensorineural.*

neural canal. See **neurocoele.**

neural cell-adhesion molecule, an immunoglobulin that functions as a molecular recognition molecule, expressed on the surface of neurons, glia, skeletal muscle, and natural killer cells. See also **recognition site.**

neural crest, the ectodermally derived cells along the outer surface of each side of the neural tube in the early stages of embryonic development. The cells migrate laterally throughout the embryo and give rise to spinal, cranial, enteric, and sympathetic ganglia; pigment cells; Schwann cells; and the adrenal medulla. Also called **ganglionic crest, ganglionic ridge.** See also **neural tube formation.**

neural ectoderm, the part of the embryonic ectoderm that develops into the neural tube. See also **neural tube formation.**

neural fold, either of the paired longitudinal elevations resulting from the invagination of the neural plate in the early developing embryo. The folds unite to enclose the neural groove and form the neural tube. Also called **medullary fold.** See also **neural tube formation.**

neuralgia /nooral″jə/ [Gk, *neuron + algos,* pain], an abnormal condition characterized by severe stabbing pain, caused by a variety of disorders affecting the nervous system. –*neuralgic, adj.*

neuralgic amyotrophy /nooral″jik ā′mīot″rəfē/, a brachial plexus disorder characterized by sudden pain and muscle weakness in the upper limbs and sometimes by muscular wasting or atrophy. The cause is unknown. Also called **Parsonage-Turner syndrome.**

neural groove, the longitudinal depression that occurs between the neural folds during the invagination of the neural plate to form the neural tube in the early stages of embryonic development. Also called **medullary groove.** See also **neural tube formation.**

neural impulse. See **impulse.**

neural plate, a thick layer of ectodermal tissue that lies along the central longitudinal axis of the early developing embryo and gives rise to the neural tube and subsequently to the brain, spinal cord, and other tissues of the central nervous system. Also called **medullary plate.** See also **neural tube formation.**

neural tube, the longitudinal tube, lying along the central axis of the early developing embryo, that gives rise to the brain, spinal cord, and other neural tissue of the central nervous system. Also called **cerebromedullary tube, medullary tube.** See also **neural tube defect.**

neural tube defect (NTD), any of a group of congenital malformations involving defects in the skull and spinal column that are caused primarily by the failure of the neural tube to close during embryonic development. In some instances the cleft results from an abnormal increase in cerebrospinal fluid pressure on the closed neural tube during the first trimester of development. The defect may occur at any point along the neural axis or extend the entire length of the spinal column, as in holorachischisis. The amount of deformity and disability depends on the degree of neural involvement, the most severe defect being complete cranioschisis, or the total absence of the skull and defective brain development. Other cerebral dysplasias resulting from the failure of the cranial end of the neural tube to fuse are meningoencephalocele and cranial meningocele. These defects, usually accompanied by severe mental and physical disorders, occur most often in the occipital region of the skull but may also occur in the frontal or basal regions. Most neural tube malformations are caused by incomplete fusion of one or more laminae of the vertebral column, with varying degrees of tissue protrusion and neural involvement. The two most common NTDs are spina bifida and anencephaly. Other NTDs include rachischisis, myelocele, myelomeningocele, and meningocele. In all of these conditions there is constant risk of rupture of the saclike protrusion and danger of meningeal infection. Often immediate surgical repair is necessary. Adequate folate levels during the first month after conception are important in preventing neural tube defects; the U.S. Public Health Service recommends that all women of childbearing age increase their folate intake to 400 mg per day. Many of the major neural tube defects can be determined prenatally by ultrasonic scanning of the uterus and by tests for the presence of elevated concentrations of alpha-fetoprotein levels in the amniotic fluid. Such diagnostic tests are preferably performed during the 14th to 16th week of gestation so that termination of the pregnancy is possible. See also **anencephaly, Arnold-Chiari malformation, spina bifida cystica.**

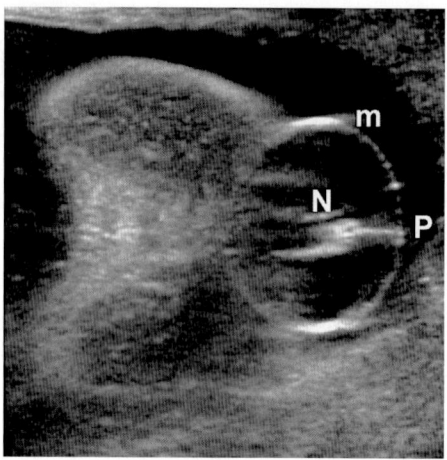

Neural tube defect *(Danzer and Johnson, 2014)*

neural tube formation, the various processes and stages involved in the embryonic development of the neural tube, which subsequently differentiates into the brain, the spinal cord, and other neural tissue of the central nervous system. The primitive tube originates from a flat, single layer of ectodermal tissue that extends longitudinally along the middorsal line of the embryonic disk from the area of the primitive streak forward to the cephalic extremity. This tissue, the neural plate, grows rapidly and becomes thickened, resulting in the invagination and formation of a hollow groove, the neural groove. With continued cell division the groove becomes deeper, and the folds thicken so that they eventually meet and fuse, converting the neural groove into the neural tube. The closing of the neural tube progresses toward both the caudal and the cephalic regions. At the cephalic end the tube expands into a large vesicle with three subdivisions that differentiate into the forebrain (prosencephalon), the midbrain (mesencephalon), and the hindbrain (rhombencephalon). The epithelium of the wall of the tube develops into the various cells of the nervous system. The caudal part of the tube subsequently forms the spinal cord. Failure of any part of the neural tube to close during early embryonic development results in a number of congenital defects. See also **neural tube defect.**

neuraminic acid /noor″ah-min′ik/, a nine-carbon amino acid formed from mannosamine and pyruvate. See also **sialidase.**

neuraminidase /noor′əmē″nədās/, an enzyme that catalyzes the cleavage of *N*-acetyl neuraminic acid from mucopolysaccharides. A hereditary deficiency of the enzyme causes sialidosis and is associated with galactogialidosis; it is characterized by cognitive impairment and skeletal changes, especially dysotosis multiplex. Also called **sialidase.** See also **sialidosis.**

neuraminidase spikes, projections from surfaces of influenza viruses containing neuraminidase that are involved in the release of viruses from infected cells.

neurapraxia /noor′əprak″sē·ə/, the interruption of nerve conduction without loss of continuity of the axon.

neurasthenia /noor′əsthē″nē·ə/ [Gk, *neuron + a + sthenos,* without strength], 1. an abnormal condition that often follows depression, characterized by nervous exhaustion and a vague functional fatigue. 2. (in psychiatry) a stage in the recovery from a schizophrenic experience during which the patient is listless and apparently unable to cope with routine activities and relationships. –*neurasthenic, adj.*

-neure,   suffix meaning "a nerve cell."

neurectomy /noorek′təmē/ [Gk, *neuron*, nerve, *ektomē*, excision],   the surgical excision of a nerve segment.

neurenteric canal /noor′ənter″ik/ [Gk, *neuron* + *enteron*, intestine; L, *canalis*, channel],   a tubular passage between the posterior part of the neural tube and the archenteron in the early embryonic development of lower animals. It corresponds to the notochordal canal of humans and the higher animals. Also called **archenteric canal, blastoporic canal, Braun's canal.**

neuresthenia.   See **fatigue state.**

-neuria,   suffix meaning "a (specified) condition involving nerves": *endoneurial.*

-neuric.   See **-neural, -neuric.**

neurilemma /noor′əlem″ə/ [Gk, *neuron* + *lemma*, sheath],   a layer of cells composed of one or more Schwann cells that forms the segmented myelin sheaths of peripheral nerve fibers. It is necessary for regeneration of peripheral nerves when they have been severed. Also called **Schwann's sheath, sheath of Schwann.** Also spelled **neurolemma.** —**neurilemmatic, neurilemmatous, neurilemmal,** *adj.*

neurilemmoma.   See **schwannoma.**

neurimotor.   See **nervimotor.**

neurinoma /noor′inō″mə/ *pl.* **neurinomas, neurino-mata** [Gk, *neuron* + *oma*, tumor],   **1.** a tumor of the nerve sheath. It is usually benign but may undergo malignant change. Kinds include *acoustic neurinoma.* See also **schwannoma. 2.** a neuroma.

neuritic plaque /noorit′ik/,   an extracellular deposit consisting of beta-amyloid protein mixed with branches of dying nerve cells in the brain of a patient with Alzheimer disease.

neuritis /noorī″tis/ *pl.* **neuritides** [Gk, *neuron* + *itis*, inflammation],   an abnormal condition characterized by inflammation of a nerve. Some of the signs of this condition are neuralgia, hypesthesia, anesthesia, paralysis, muscular atrophy, and defective reflexes.

neuro-, neur-,   prefix meaning "nerves": *neuroclonic, neurohormone, neuromast.*

neuroacanthocytosis   /noor′ō·ə·kan′thō·sī·tō′sis/ [Gk, *neuron*, nerve + *akantha*, thorn + *kytos*, cell + *osis*, condition],   an autosomal-recessive syndrome characterized by tics, chorea, and personality changes, with acanthocytes in the blood.

neuroanatomy /noor′ō·ənat′əmē/,   the branch of biology that is concerned with the structure of the nervous system.

neuroarthropathy /-ärthrop″əthē/ [Gk, *neuron* + *arthron*, joint, *pathos*, disease],   a condition in which a disease of a joint is secondary to a disease of the nervous system.

neurobiology /-bī′ol″əjē/,   a branch of biology that is concerned with the anatomy and physiology of the nervous system.

neuroblast /noor″əblast/ [Gk, *neuron* + *blastos*, germ],   any embryonic cell that develops into a functional neuron; an immature nerve cell. —**neuroblastic,** *adj.*

neuroblastoma /noor′ōblastō″mə/ [Gk, *neuron* + *blastos*, germ, *oma*, tumor],   a highly malignant tumor composed of primitive ectodermal cells derived from the neural plate during embryonic life. The tumor may originate in any part of the sympathetic nervous system but is most common in the adrenal medulla. Neuroblastomas metastasize early and widely to lymph nodes, liver, lungs, and bone. Symptoms may include an abdominal mass, respiratory distress, and anemia. Hormonally active adrenal lesions may cause irritability, flushing, sweating, hypertension, and tachycardia. Before metastasis, treatment with radical surgery, irradiation, and chemotherapy is often successful. Spontaneous remissions may occur, with the tumor undergoing maturation and forming a benign ganglioneuroma. Kinds include **Pepper syndrome.**

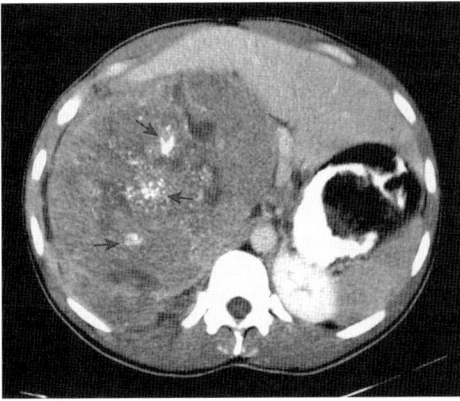

Neuroblastoma *(indicated by arrows)* metastasized to the bone marrow *(Kim and Chung, 2006)*

neurobrucellosis /-broo′səlo″sis/,   a serious complication of a brucellosis infection that affects the nervous system and may cause meningitis, stroke, cranial nerve lesions, or mycotic aneurysms. The condition usually requires treatment with antibiotics that cross the blood-brain barrier.

neurocanal.   See **vertebral canal.**

neurocardiogenic syncope,   a particularly serious type of vasovagal attack, the cause of which is unknown.

neurocele.   See **neurocoele.**

neurocentral /-sen″trəl/ [Gk, *neuron* + *kentron*, center],   pertaining to the neurocentrum and the developing vertebrae in the early stages of embryology.

neurocentrum /-sen″trəm/ [Gk, *neuron* + L, *centrum*, center],   the embryonic mesodermal tissue that subsequently gives rise to the vertebrae. See also **sclerotome.**

neuro check [Gk, *neuron* + ME, *chek*, stop],   *(Nontechnical)* a brief neurological assessment conducted by a member of the health care team, usually the primary care nurse, performed every 4 hours on patients who may have evolving disease, such as stroke. The level of consciousness is evaluated as alert and oriented, lethargic, stuporous, or comatose. The movements of the extremities are determined to be voluntary or involuntary. The pupils of the eyes are observed for equality of dilation, reactivity to light, and ability to accommodate. See also **Glasgow Coma Scale.**

neurochemistry /-kem″istrē/,   a branch of neurology that is concerned with the biochemistry of the nervous system.

neurocirculatory asthenia /-sur′kyələtôr″ē/ [Gk, *neuron* + L, *circulare*, to go around; Gk, *a* + *sthenos*, without strength],   a psychosomatic disorder characterized by nervous and circulatory irregularities, including dyspnea, palpitation, giddiness, vertigo, tremor, precordial pain, and increased susceptibility to fatigue. The symptoms often result from or are associated with psychological stress.

neurocoele /noor″əsēl/ [Gk, *neuron* + *koilos*, hollow],   a system of cavities in the central nervous system of humans and other vertebrate animals. It consists of the ventricles of the brain and the central canal of the spinal cord, which originate from the neural tube during early embryonic development. Also called **neural canal.** Also spelled **neurocele, neurocoel.**

neurocytolysin /-sītol″isin/,   a toxic substance in snake venom that destroys nerve cell membranes.

neurocytolysis /-sītol″isis/,   the destruction of nerve cells.

neurocytoma /noor′ōsītō″mə/ [Gk, *neuron* + *kytos*, cell, *oma*, tumor],   a tumor composed of undifferentiated nerve cells that are usually ganglionic. Also called **neuroma.**

N

neuroderm. See **neuroectoderm.**

neurodermatitis /-dur′mətī″tis/ [Gk, *neuron* + *derma,* skin, *itis,* inflammation], a nonspecific pruritic skin disorder seen in anxious, nervous individuals. Excoriations and lichenification occur on easily accessible, exposed areas of the body such as the forearms and forehead. Sometimes loosely (and incorrectly) referred to as atopic dermatitis. See also **lichen simplex chronicus.**

neurodevelopmental adaptation /-dəvel″əpmen′təl/, the response of the developing brain to sensory, perceptual, and affective stressors during childhood, mediated by neurotransmitters and hormones.

neurodevelopmental treatment (NDT), an evolving neurophysiological rehabilitation approach used to treat persons with central nervous system pathology who have difficulty controlling movements, interfering with function. Originally the focus was on the inhibition of abnormal tone by using reflex-inhibiting patterns and by facilitating basic movement patterns that occur in an automatic fashion. This treatment is sometimes referred to as the Bobath approach although much of the original Bobath intervention techniques are no longer used. This intervention approach continues to evolve with better understanding of how the central nervous system works. The goal of this intervention is to promote motor learning for efficient motor control in various environments. This is done through specific patient-handling skills designed to facilitate the initiation and completion of specific motor tasks.

neuroectoderm /no̅o̅r′ō·ek″tədurm/ [Gk, *neuron* + *ektos,* outside, *derma,* skin], the part of the embryonic ectoderm that gives rise to the central and peripheral nervous systems, including some glial cells. −*neuroectodermal, adj.*

neuroelectric therapy, the use of a low-amperage electrical current to stimulate nerve endings. The action may stimulate endogenous neurotransmitters, such as endorphins that produce symptomatic relief. Kinds include **transcutaneous electrical nerve stimulation (TENS).**

neuroendocrine /no̅o̅r′ō·en′dəkrin/ [Gk, *neuron,* nerve, *endon,* within, *krinein,* to secrete], pertaining to or resembling the effects produced by endocrine glands strongly linked with the nervous system.

neuroendoscope /no̅o̅r″o·en′doskōp″/, an endoscope for examining and performing various interventions in the central nervous system.

neuroendoscopy, the use of a neuroendoscope with the aid of a neuronavigational system to examine the central nervous system and perform minimally invasive neurosurgical procedures.

neuroepithelioma /no̅o̅r′ō·ep′ithē′lē·ō″mə/ [Gk, *neuron* + *epi,* upon, *thele,* nipple, *oma,* tumor], an uncommon neoplasm of neuroepithelium in a sensory nerve. Also called *neuroepithelial tumor.*

neurofibril /-fī″bril/, a threadlike structure found in the cytoplasm of a neuron.

neurofibrillary tangles /-fī″briler′ē/, an intracellular clump of neurofibrils made of insoluble protein in the brain of a patient with Alzheimer disease.

neurofibroma /no̅o̅r′ōfībrō″mə/ *pl. neurofibromas, neurofibromata* [Gk, *neuron* + L, *fibra,* fiber; Gk, *oma,* tumor], a fibrous tumor of nerve tissue resulting from the abnormal proliferation of Schwann cells. Multiple growths in the peripheral nervous system are often associated with abnormalities in other tissues. See also **neurofibromatosis.**

neurofibromatosis /no̅o̅r′ōfī′brōmətō″sis/ [Gk, *neuron* + *fibra,* fiber; Gk, *oma,* tumor, *osis,* condition], a congenital condition transmitted as an autosomal-dominant trait, characterized by numerous neurofibromas of the nerves and skin, café-au-lait spots on the skin, and developmental anomalies of the muscles, bones, and viscera. Many large, pedunculated

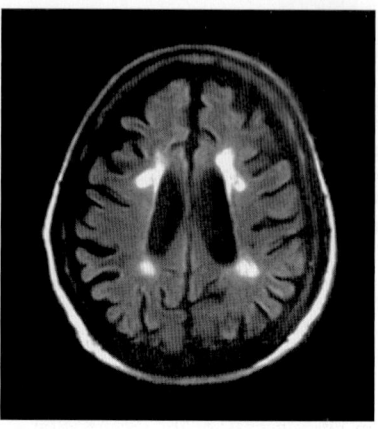

Diffuse neurofibrillary tangles with calcification *(Suda et al, 2009)*

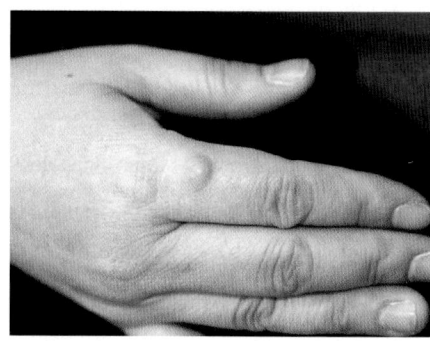

Neurofibroma on right index finger *(Huang, Wu, and Hsieh, 2012)*

soft-tissue tumors may develop. Bone changes may result in skeletal deformities, especially curvature of the spine. Neurofibromas may develop in the alimentary tract, bladder, endocrine glands, and cranial nerves. Also called **multiple neuroma, neuromatosis, Recklinghausen disease, von Recklinghausen disease.**

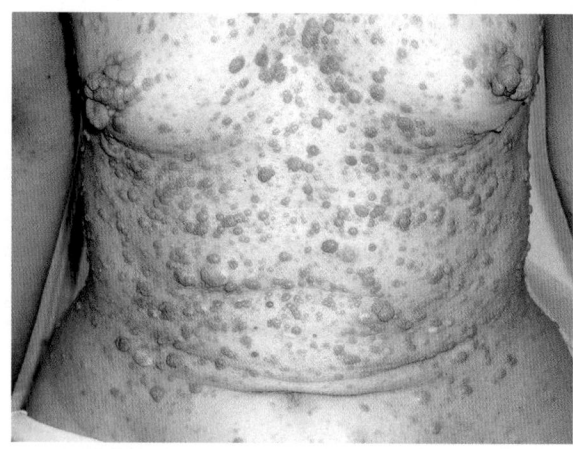

Cutaneous lesions associated with neurofibromatosis *(Levine et al, 2007)*

neurofilament /noŏr′ōfil′əment/ [Gk, *neuron,* nerve + L, *filare,* to spin], a cytoplasmic filament approximately 10 nm in diameter occurring in the neurons. It has a cytoskeletal function and may be involved in the intracellular transport of metabolites.

neurogen /noŏr″əjən/ [Gk, *neuron* + *genein,* to produce], a substance within the early developing embryo that stimulates the primary organizer to initiate the formation of the neural plate, which gives rise to the primary axis of the body. See also **neurotransmitter.**

neurogenesis /-jen″əsis/ [Gk, *neuron* + *genesis,* origin], the formation of the tissue of the nervous system. −*neurogenetic, adj.*

neurogenic /-jen″ik/ [Gk, *neuron* + *genesis,* origin], **1.** pertaining to the formation of nervous tissue. **2.** pertaining to the stimulation of nervous energy. **3.** originating in the nervous system.

neurogenic arthropathy, an abnormal condition associated with neural damage, characterized by the gradual and usually painless degeneration of a joint. One of the major causes of this condition is believed to be a minor injury that is disregarded by the affected individual because of a lack of sensation in the injured tissue. Inadequate rest and care aggravate such injuries and prevent proper healing. See also **neuropathic joint disease.**

neurogenic bladder, dysfunction of the urinary bladder caused by a lesion of the nervous system. Treatment is aimed at preventing infection, controlling incontinence, and preserving kidney function by enabling the bladder to empty completely and regularly. Also called **neuropathic bladder.** Kinds include **flaccid bladder, spastic bladder.**

neurogenic claudication, claudication accompanied by pain and paresthesias in the back, buttocks, and lower limbs that is relieved by stooping, caused by mechanical disturbances resulting from posture or by ischemia of the cauda equina.

neurogenic fracture, a fracture associated with the destruction of the nerve supply to a specific bone.

neurogenic hoarseness, a sign of unilateral vocal cord paralysis. It is asymptomatic, but there may be excessive air escape during speech as a result of incomplete closure of the glottis. Extra effort is required to generate enough airflow to make speech sounds. Untreated, there is a danger of aspiration pneumonia.

neurogenic impotence, penile erectile dysfunction caused by neurological disorders. The disorders may involve the parasympathetic sacral spinal cord or the peripheral efferent autonomic fibers to the penis. See also **impotence, sexual dysfunction.**

neurogenic shock, a form of shock that results from peripheral vascular dilation.

neuroglia /noŏrog″lē·ə/ [Gk, *neuron* + *glia,* glue], the supporting or nonneuronal tissue cells of the central and peripheral nervous system. They perform the less specialized functions of the nerve network. Compare **neuron.** Kinds include **astrocyte, oligodendroglia, microglia.** −*neuroglial, adj.*

neurography /noŏrog″rəfē/, **1.** the study of the action potentials of the nerves. **2.** a technique for visualization of peripheral nerve activity by graphic representation of data obtained by media contrast radiographics or by electric recording.

neurohormone /noŏr″əhôr′mōn/, a hormone produced in neurosecretory cells such as those of the hypothalamus and released into the bloodstream, the cerebrospinal fluid, or intercellular spaces of the nervous system. The product may or may not be a true systemic hormone such as epinephrine.

When the hormone is not a true hormone, it may be a cell product that induces the release of a tropic hormone, which in turn stimulates an endocrine gland to release a systemic hormone. See also **neuromodulator, neurotransmitter.**

neurohypophyseal hormone /-hī′pōfiz″ē·əl/ [Gk, *neuron* + *hypo,* under, *phyein,* to grow], any of the hormones secreted by the posterior pituitary gland. Kinds include **oxytocin, vasopressin.** See also **pituitary gland.**

neurohypophysis /-hīpof″isis/ [Gk, *neuron* + *hypo,* under, *phyein,* to grow], the posterior lobe of the pituitary gland that is the release point of antidiuretic hormone (ADH) and oxytocin. Nervous stimulation from the hypothalamus controls the release of the substances into the blood. When stimulated by the hypothalamus, the neurohypophysis releases ADH by an increase in the osmotic pressure of extracellular fluid in the body. The hormone acts on the cells in the distal and collecting tubules of the kidneys, making them more permeable to water and thus reducing the volume of urine. The neurohypophysis releases oxytocin under appropriate stimulation from the hypothalamus. Oxytocin produces powerful contractions of the pregnant uterus and causes milk to flow from lactating breasts. Stimulation of the nipples of the breast by a nursing infant triggers the release of this hormone. Also called **posterior pituitary gland.** Compare **adenohypophysis.**

neuroimmunology /noŏr′ō·im′yoŏnol″əjē/ [Gk, *neuron* + L, *immunis,* freedom; Gk, *logos,* science], the study of relationships between the immune and nervous systems, such as autoimmune activity in neurological diseases.

neurol, abbreviation for **neurology.**

neurolemma. See **neurilemma.**

neurolepsis /-lep′sis/ [Gk, *neuron* + *lepsis,* seizure], an altered state of consciousness, as induced by a neuroleptic agent, characterized by quiescence, reduced motor activity, decreased anxiety, and indifference to the surroundings. Sleep may occur, but usually the person can be aroused and can respond to commands. Compare **hypnosis,** def. 1. See also **neuroleptic drug.**

neurolepsy /noŏr′əlep′sē/, a mental state characterized by the blocking of autonomic reflexes, as in hypnosis or antipsychotic drug–induced disorders.

neurolept. See **neuroleptic drug.**

neuroleptanalgesia /-lept′anəljē″zē·ə/ [Gk, *neuron* + *lepsis,* seizure, *a* + *algos,* without pain], *(Obsolete)* a form of sedation and analgesia once used that involved the concurrent administration of a neuroleptic such as droperidol and an analgesic such as fentanyl. Anxiety, motor activity, and sensitivity to painful stimuli were reduced; the person was quiet and indifferent to surroundings and was able to respond to commands. If nitrous oxide with oxygen was also administered, neuroleptanalgesia could be converted to neuroleptanesthesia. Adverse reactions, such as a prolonged QT interval produced by a large dose of droperidol, caused this method to be abandoned.

neuroleptanesthesia /-lept′anəsthē″zhə/ [Gk, *neuron* + *lepsis,* seizure, *anaisthesia,* lack of feeling], a form of anesthesia achieved by the administration of a neuroleptic agent, a narcotic analgesic, and nitrous oxide with oxygen. Induction of anesthesia is slow, but consciousness returns quickly after the inhalation of nitrous oxide is stopped.

neuroleptic /-lep″tik/ [Gk, *neuron* + *lepsis,* seizure], **1.** pertaining to neurolepsis. **2.** See **neuroleptic drug.**

neuroleptic anesthesia [Gk, *neuron,* nerve, *lepsis,* seizure, *anaisthesia,* lack of feeling], a form of anesthesia induced by an injection of a butyrophenone derivative with a narcotic analgesic.

neuroleptic drug, a substance that produces a sedating or tranquilizing effect. The term is still used to refer to agents, such as droperidol, used to produce such effects as part of anesthesia or analgesia; however, it is outdated as a synonym for antipsychotic agents because newer agents do not necessarily have such effects. Also called **neurolept, neuroleptic.** Compare **antipsychotic.** See also **tranquilizer.**

neuroleptic malignant syndrome [Gk, *neuron,* nerve, *lepsis,* seizure; L, *malignus,* bad disposition; Gk, *syn,* together, *dromos,* course], a rare, life-threatening condition characterized by hypertonicity, pallor, dyskinesia, fever, incontinence, unstable blood pressure, and pulmonary congestion. It is caused by the administration of neuroleptic drugs at normal or high doses. Reaction to these drugs is idiosyncratic.

neurolinguistic programming (NLP), a complementary therapeutic strategy based on the premise that thought is a representation of sensory experience and that behavior can be modified to achieve a desired result by changing the patient's thought patterns and mental strategies to give the patient more choices in problem solving. It is used for behavior modification and the management of psychosomatic disorders and stress.

neurolinguistics /noor′ō·ling·gwis′tiks/ [Gk, *neuron* + L, *lingua,* tongue], the study of language acquisition, processing, and production at the neurological level.

neurologic, neurological. See **neurology.**

neurological assessment /-loj″ik/ [Gk, *neuron* + *logos,* science; L, *icus,* like, *adsidere,* to approximate], an evaluation of the patient's neurological status and symptoms.

■ METHOD: If alert and oriented, the patient is asked about instances of weakness, numbness, headaches, pain, tremors, nervousness, irritability, or drowsiness. Information is elicited regarding loss of memory, periods of confusion, hallucinations, and episodes of loss of consciousness. The patient's general appearance, facial expression, attention span, responses to verbal and painful stimuli, emotional status, coordination, balance, cognition, and ability to follow commands are noted. Assessment of cranial nerves and deep tendon reflexes is included. If the patient is disoriented, stuporous, or comatose, demonstrated signs of these states are recorded. Observations are made of skin color and temperature; pupillary size, equality, dilation, and reactions to light; respiratory rate, rhythm, and quality; and chest movements and breath sounds. The pulse is checked; ears and nose are examined for possible drainage; strength of the handgrip is tested; and the extremities' sensations and voluntary and involuntary motions are assessed. Urinary output is determined for evidence of polyuria, and the patient's speech is evaluated for signs of slurring and aphasia. Included in the record are concurrent diseases such as hypertension, cancer, and coarctation of the aorta; past illnesses associated with head trauma; seizures; motor, sensory, or emotional disturbances; loss of consciousness; and neurological, medical, or surgical procedures. Pertinent to the assessment are the patient's sleep pattern; medication; personality changes; relationships with family and friends; and a family history of seizures, stroke, mental illness, tumors, or sudden death. Diagnostic aids that may be required for a complete evaluation include a lumbar puncture, complete blood count, myelogram, magnetic resonance imaging, echoencephalogram, brain scan, computerized tomogram, and determinations of glucose, fluid, and electrolyte levels.

■ INTERVENTIONS: A health care professional may conduct the interview to obtain subjective data, examine the patient, and assemble the pertinent background information and results of the diagnostic tests.

■ OUTCOME CRITERIA: A careful neurological assessment is an important aid to the health care team in establishing a diagnosis and the course of treatment.

neurological examination, a systematic examination of the nervous system, including an assessment of mental status, of the function of each of the cranial nerves, of sensory and neuromuscular function, of the reflexes, and of proprioception and other cerebellar functions.

neurologist /nŏōrol″əjist/, a physician who specializes in the nervous system and its disorders.

neurology (neurol) /nŏōrol″əjē/ [Gk, *neuron* + *logos,* science], the field of medicine that deals with the nervous system and its disorders. −*neurological, neurologic, adj.,* −**neurologist,** *n.*

neuroma /nŏōrō″mə/ [Gk, *neuron* + *oma,* tumor], a benign neoplasm composed chiefly of neurons and nerve fibers, usually arising from a nerve tissue. Pain radiating from the lesion to the periphery of the affected nerve is usually intermittent but may become continuous and severe.

-neuroma, suffix meaning "a tumor made up of nerve cells and fibers": *angiomyoneuroma, glioneuroma.*

neuroma cutis, a neoplasm in the skin that contains nerve tissue and may be extremely sensitive to painful stimuli.

neuromas, neuromata. See **neuroma.**

neuroma telangiectodes. See **nevoid neuroma.**

neuromatosis /nŏōr′ōmətō″sis/ [Gk, *neuron* + *oma,* tumor, *osis,* condition], a neoplastic disease characterized by numerous neuromas. Also called **multiple neuroma.** See also **neurofibromatosis.**

neuromechanism /-mek″əniz′əm/, a neurological system whose components work together to produce a central nervous system function.

neuromodulator, a substance that alters nerve impulse transmission.

neuromotor /nŏōr″ōmō′tər/ [Gk, *neuron,* nerve; L, *mover,* to move], pertaining to both the nerves and muscles or to nerve impulses transmitted to muscles.

neuromuscular /nŏōr′ōmus″kyŏōlər/ [Gk, *neuron* + L, *musculus,* muscle], pertaining to the nerves and the muscles.

neuromuscular blockade, the inhibition of a muscular contraction activated by the nervous system, possibly resulting in muscle weakness or paralysis.

neuromuscular blocking agent, a chemical substance that interferes locally with the transmission or reception of impulses from motor nerves to skeletal muscles. Nondepolarizing agents such as metocurine, pancuronium, and tubocurarine competitively block the transmitter action of acetylcholine at the motor end plate. Depolarizing blocking agents such as succinylcholine chloride also compete with acetylcholine for cholinergic receptors of the motor end plate but work by first activating the receptor and then blocking its ability to be reset for subsequent stimulation. Neuromuscular blocking agents are used to induce muscle relaxation in anesthesia, endotracheal intubation, and electroshock therapy and as adjuncts in the treatment of tetanus, encephalitis, and poliomyelitis. Neuromuscular blocking drugs can cause bronchospasm, hyperthermia, hypotension, or respiratory paralysis and are used with caution, especially in patients with myasthenia gravis or with renal, hepatic, or pulmonary impairment and in elderly and debilitated individuals. During surgery, it is important to recognize that these agents prevent muscle movement but do not block the sensation of pain. See also **muscle relaxant.**

neuromuscular electric stimulator (NMES), a device for improving or modulating muscular activation. It may be a portable unit for home treatment of a patient over a long period of time or a large clinical model capable of producing a wider variety of waveforms and modulations of the stimulus. The NMES generates electrical pulses that produce controlled muscle contractions similar to those that occur physiologically. Unless nerve degeneration has occurred, muscles that are weak or paralyzed because of central nervous system involvement should contract when NMES is applied. The procedure may be tested first on an uninvolved muscle on the same or another extremity to establish a normal response.

neuromuscular junction, the area of contact between the ends of a nerve fiber and a fiber of skeletal muscle. Also called **myoneural junction.** See also **motor end plate, myelin, nerve.**

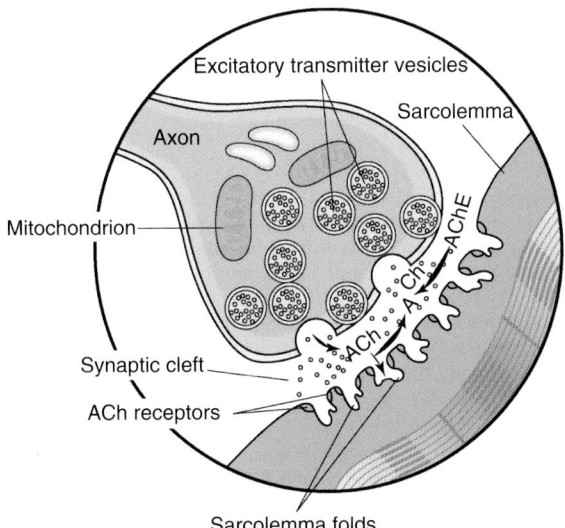

Neuromuscular junction *(AACN, 2008)*

neuromuscular spindle, any one of a number of small bundles of delicate muscular fibers enclosed by a capsule, in which sensory nerve fibers terminate. The spindles vary in length from 0.8 to 5 mm, accommodating as many as four large myelinated nerve fibers that pierce the capsule and lose their myelin sheaths. The nerve fibers end as naked axons encircling the intrafusal fibers with flattened expansions or ovoid disks.

neuromyal transmission /-mī″əl/ [Gk, *neuron + mys,* muscle; L, *transmittere,* to transmit], the passage of excitation from a motor neuron to a muscle fiber at the neuromuscular junction.

neuromyelitis /no͞or′ōmī′əlī″tis/ [Gk, *neuron + myelos,* marrow, *itis,* inflammation], an abnormal condition characterized by inflammation of the spinal cord and peripheral nerves.

neuromyelitis optica (NMO). Also called **Devic disease.**

neuron /no͞or″on/ [Gk, nerve], the basic nerve cell of the nervous system, containing a nucleus within a cell body and extending one or more processes. Neurons can be classified according to the direction in which they conduct impulses or according to the number of processes they extend. Sensory neurons transmit nerve impulses toward the spinal cord and the brain. Motor neurons transmit nerve impulses from the brain and the spinal cord to the muscles and the glandular tissue. Multipolar neurons, bipolar neurons, and unipolar neurons are classified according to the number of processes they extend to the different kinds of neurons. Multipolar neurons have one axon and several dendrites, as do most of the neurons in the brain and the spinal cord. Bipolar neurons, which are less numerous than the other types, have one axon and only one dendrite. Unipolar neurons have one axon and no dendrites. All primary sensory afferents and some autonomic neurons are unipolar. All neurons have one axon, and most have one or more dendrites and have a slightly gray color when clustered, as in the nuclei of the brain and the spinal cord. As the generators and carriers of nerve impulses, neurons function according to electrochemical processes involving positively charged sodium and potassium ions and the changing electrical potential of the extracellular and the intracellular fluid of the neuron. Also spelled **neurone.** *−neuronal, adj.*

neuronal antibody, an antibody found in the cerebrospinal fluid of many systemic lupus erythematosus (SLE) patients with neuropsychiatric manifestations and in some SLE patients without such manifestations.

neuronal ceroid lipofuscinosis. See **Batten disease.**

neuronal sprouting, the growth of axons or dendrites from a damaged neuron or from an intact neuron that projects to an area denervated by damage to other neurons.

neurone. See **neuron.**

neuronitis /no͞or′ənī″tis/ [Gk, *neuron + itis,* inflammation], inflammation of a nerve or a nerve cell, especially the cells and the roots of the spinal nerves.

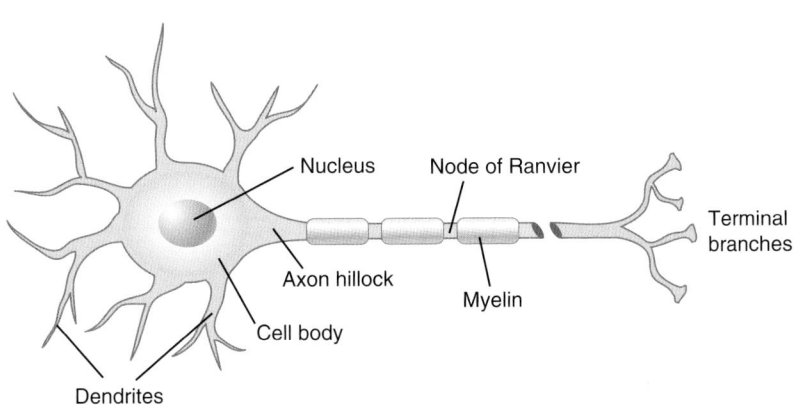

Structure of a myelinated neuron *(Blaustein et al, 2012)*

neuroparalysis /-pəral″isis/, loss of muscle power as a result of a disorder involving the part of the nervous system affecting the muscle.

neuropathic. See **neuropathy.**

neuropathic bladder. See **neurogenic bladder.**

neuropathic joint disease /-path″ik/ [Gk, *neuron* + *pathos,* disease], a chronic progressive degenerative disease of one or more joints, characterized by swelling, joint instability, hemorrhage, heat, and atrophic and hypertrophic changes in the bone. Pain is usually less severe than would be expected by the appearance of the joint on an x-ray film. The disease is the result of an underlying neurological disorder, such as tabes dorsalis from syphilis, diabetic neuropathy, leprosy, or congenital absence or depression of pain sensation. Early recognition of the disease and prophylactic protection of the joint may prevent further damage in some cases. Surgical reconstruction is not usually effective because healing is slow. Amputation may be necessary. Also called **Charcot joint.**

neuropathic pain, pain that results from direct stimulation of the myelin or nervous tissue of the peripheral or central nervous system (except for sensitized C fibers), generally felt as burning or tingling and often occurring in an area of sensory loss. It is seen commonly in patients with uncontrolled diabetes.

neuropathic pain syndrome, a condition of autonomic hyperactivity that results in sharp, stinging, or stabbing pain. The disorder is usually noninflammatory but may result in the destruction of peripheral nerve tissue. It may also be accompanied by changes in skin color, temperature, and edema.

neuropathy /no͞orop″əthē/ [Gk, *neuron* + *pathos,* disease], inflammation or degeneration of the peripheral nerves, such as that associated with lead poisoning. **—neuropathic,** *adj.*

neuropeptide /no͞or·ō·pep′tīd/, any of several types of molecules found in brain tissue, composed of short chains of amino acids including endorphins, enkephalins, vasopressin, and others. They are often localized in axon terminals at synapses and are classified as putative neurotransmitters, although some are also hormones.

neuropeptide Y (NPY), a natural substance that acts on the brain to stimulate eating. Laboratory animals injected with NPY greatly overeat. Substances that block the NPY receptor reduce the appetite. Leptin, a hormone that stimulates weight loss, reduces the output of NPY from the hypothalamus, a major production center. Another natural substance that stimulates the urge to eat is peptide YY. In animal experiments it has appeared to be at least as potent as NPY.

neurophysin /-fiz″in/, one of a group of proteins released from the posterior pituitary gland at the same time as the hormone vasopressin or oxytocin. It is cleared from a larger protein of which vasopressin or oxytocin is a part.

neuroplasticity /-plastis′itē/, the capacity of the nervous system for adaptation or regeneration after trauma.

neuroplasty /no͞or″əplas′tē/ [Gk, *neuron,* nerve, *plassein,* to mold], plastic surgery to repair a nerve.

neuroplegia /no͞or·ōplē″jē·ə/ [Gk, *neuron* + *plege,* stroke], nerve paralysis caused by disease, injury, or the effect of neuroleptic drugs.

neuropore /no͞or″ōpôr/ [Gk, *neuron* + *poros,* pore], the opening at each end of the neural tube during early embryonic development, leading from the central canal of the neural tube to the exterior. The closure of these apertures as the tube grows and differentiates occurs with such precision that they are used to indicate horizons XI and XII in the systematic anatomical charting of human embryonic development. Kinds include **anterior neuropore, posterior neuropore.** See also **horizon, neural tube formation.**

neuropraxia /-prak″sē·ə/ [Gk, *neuron,* nerve, *prassein,* to do], a condition in which a nerve remains in place after a severe injury, although it no longer transmits impulses.

neuroprotection /no͞or·ō·prō·tek′shən/, protection against neurotoxicity. See also **neurotoxicity.**

neuroprotective /no͞or″opro-tek′tiv/, guarding or protecting against neurotoxicity. See also **neurotoxicity.**

neuropsychiatrist /-sīkī″ətrist/, a physician who deals with the relationship between neurological processes and psychiatric disorders.

neuropsychiatry /-sīkī″ətrē/, a branch of medicine that deals with problems of psychiatry as it relates to the neurological function.

neuroradiography /-rā′dē·og″rəfē/, the radiographic examination of the tissues of the nervous system.

neuroradiology /-rā′dē·ol″əjē/, the branch of radiology concerned with diagnosing diseases of the nervous system.

neurorrhaphy /no͞orôr″əfē/ [Gk, *neuron,* nerve, *rhaphe,* suture], a surgical procedure to suture a severed nerve.

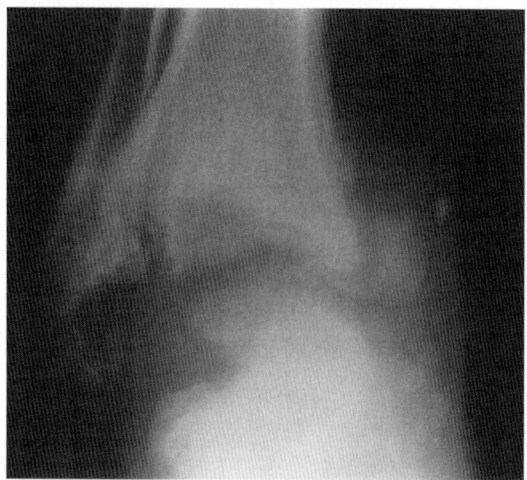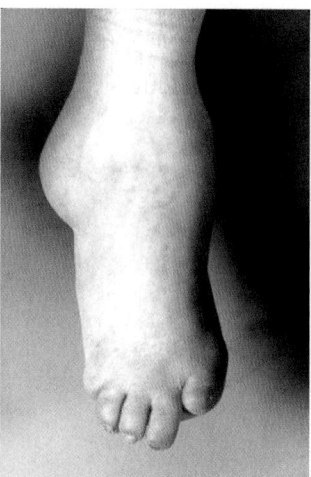

Radiography and image of patient with neuropathic joint disease *(Herring, 2014)*

neurosarcoidosis /-sär′koidō″sis/, a granulomatous disease that may involve any part of the nervous system but most commonly affects the cranial and spinal nerves. Cranial nerve involvement may result in facial paralysis, whereas spinal nerve involvement may manifest as mononeuritis multiplex. If the central nervous system is affected, the vasculature of the brain may be damaged, resulting in stroke.

neurosarcoma /-särkō″mə/ [Gk, *neuron* + *sarx,* flesh, *oma,* tumor], a malignant neoplasm composed of nerve, connective, and vascular tissues. Also called **malignant neuroma.**

neuroscience /noor″ōsī′əns/ [Gk, *neuron,* nerve; L, *scientia*], the study of neurology and related subjects, including neurophysiology, neurosurgery, neuroanatomy, and neuropharmacology.

neurosis /noorō″sis/ *pl. neuroses*, former name for a category of mental disorders in which the symptoms are distressing to the person, reality testing is intact, behavior does not violate gross social norms, and there is no apparent organic cause.

-neurosis, combining form meaning "a disease of the nerves" or "a mental disorder": *psychoneurosis.*

neuroskeleton /-skel″ətən/ [Gk, *neuron,* nerve, *skeletos,* dried up], the parts of the skeleton that surround or otherwise protect the nervous system, particularly the skull and vertebrae.

neurosome /noor″ōsōm/ [Gk, *neuron,* nerve + *soma,* body], **1.** the body of a neuron. **2.** any of the minute particles found in the protoplasm of a neuron.

neurosurgery /-sur″jərē/ [Gk, *neuron* + *cheirourgia,* surgery], any surgery involving the brain, spinal cord, or peripheral nerves. Brain surgery is performed to treat a wound, vascular disorders, or epilepsy; remove a tumor or foreign body; relieve pressure in intracranial hemorrhage or hydrocephaly; excise an abscess; treat parkinsonism; or relieve pain. Before surgery, diagnostic skull x-ray films, a CT, MRI, stereotactic CT or MRI, magnetic resonance angiography, ventriculogram, and/or arteriogram are done; a diagnostic electroencephalogram, lumbar tap, or brain scan may be done. A blood type and crossmatch are done. Parenteral corticosteroids are given if cerebral edema is present, and urea may be given to reduce intracranial pressure. Narcotics and hypnotics are avoided, and the nurse must confirm any that are ordered. After surgery, vital signs and changes in the level of consciousness, speech, and muscle strength are monitored closely. Any yellowish drainage from the wound may be cerebrospinal fluid and is reported immediately. Sterile dressing technique is essential. Surgery of the spine is performed to correct a defect, remove a tumor, repair a ruptured intervertebral disk, or relieve pain. After surgery, vital signs and changes in the level of consciousness, speech, and muscle strength are monitored closely. Any yellowish drainage from the wound may be cerebrospinal fluid and is reported immediately. Sterile dressing technique is essential. Surgery of the spine is performed to correct a defect, remove a tumor, repair a ruptured intervertebral disk, or relieve pain. Before surgery computed tomography or magnetic resonance imaging scans, relevant labs, and perhaps a blood type and crossmatch are done. After surgery the nurse keeps the patient's spine in good alignment. Return of sensation and motor function are monitored carefully. Kinds of spinal surgery include fusion and laminectomy. Surgery on the peripheral nerves is performed to remove a tumor, relieve pain, or reconnect a severed nerve. After surgery the nurse observes closely the return of sensation to the area. Kinds include **sympathectomy.**

neurosyphilis /-sif″ilis/ [Gk, *neuron* + *sys,* hog, *philein,* to love], infection of the central nervous system by *Treponema pallidum,* the causative agent of syphilis, which may invade the meninges and cerebrovascular system. If the brain tissue is affected, general paresis may result. If the spinal cord is infected, tabes dorsalis may result. See also **syphilis.**

neurotendinous /-ten′dinəs/ [Gk, *neuron,* nerve; L, *tendo,* tendon], pertaining to both nerves and tendons.

neurotendinous spindle [Gk, *neuron* + L, *tendo,* tendon; AS, *spinel,* spindle], a capsule containing enlarged tendon fibers, found chiefly near the junctions of tendons and muscles. One or more nerve fibers pierce the side of the capsule and lose their medullary sheaths; the axons subdivide and terminate between the tendon fibers in irregular disks or varicosities. Also called **organ of Golgi.**

neurotensin /-ten″sin/, a peptide neurotransmitter found in various parts of the brain. It is involved in vasodilation, hypotension, and pain perception.

neurotensinoma /-ten′sinō″mə/, a neuroendocrine tumor of the GI tract. Its major secreted product is neurotensin. The tumor originates in nonbeta islet cells, but, unlike other neuroendocrine tumors, it has no distinguishing clinical features.

neurotic /n(y)oorot″ik/ [Gk, *neuron* + *osis,* condition; L, *icus,* like], **1.** *adj.,* pertaining to neurosis. **2.** *adj.,* pertaining to the nerves. **3.** *n.,* one who is afflicted with a neurosis. **4.** *(Informal) n.,* an emotionally unstable person.

-neurotic, **1.** suffix meaning "a (specified) abnormal condition of the nerves": *angioneurotic, aponeurotic, subaponeurotic.* **2.** suffix meaning "an emotional disorder": *psychoneurotic.*

neurotic depression, *(Obsolete)* formerly called **dysthymic disorder.** Now called **persistent depressive disorder.**

neurotmesis /noor′ōtmē″sis/ [Gk, *neuron* + *tmesis,* cutting apart], a peripheral nerve injury in which the nerve is completely disrupted by laceration or traction. It requires surgical approximation, with unpredictable recovery.

neurotological /noor′ōtōloj″ik al/, pertaining to the study of the elements of the ear as they relate to the brain and nervous system. Also called *neurotologic.*

neurotology /noor′ōtol″əjē/, a branch of otology concerned with those parts of the nervous system related to the ear, especially the inner ear and associated brainstem structures. Also called **otoneurology.**

neurotomy /noorot″əmē/, the surgical severing of a nerve or nerves.

neurotoxic /noor′ōtok″sik/, having a poisonous effect on nerves and nerve cells, such as the degenerative effect of ingested lead on peripheral nerves.

neurotoxicity /-toksis″itē/ [Gk, *neuron,* nerve, *toxikon,* poison], the ability of a drug or other agent to destroy or damage nervous tissue.

neurotoxin /noor′ōtok″sin/ [Gk, *neuron* + *toxikon,* poison], a toxin that acts directly on the tissues of the central nervous system, traveling along the axis cylinders of the motor nerves to the brain. The toxin may be secreted in the venom of certain snakes, or it may be present on the spines of a shell or in the flesh of fish or shellfish; it may be produced by certain bacteria or by the cellular disintegration of certain bacteria.

neurotransmitter /-transmit″ər/ [Gk, *neuron* + L, *transmittere,* to transmit], a chemical that modifies or results in the transmission of nerve impulses between synapses. Neurotransmitters are released from synaptic knobs into synaptic clefts and bridge the gap between presynaptic and postsynaptic neurons. Each vesicle within a synaptic knob stores as many as 10,000 neurotransmitter molecules. When a nerve impulse reaches a synaptic knob, thousands of neurotransmitter molecules squirt into the synaptic cleft and bind to specific receptors. This flow allows an associated diffusion of potassium and sodium ions that causes an action potential. Excitatory neurotransmitters decrease the negativity of postsynaptic membrane potentials; inhibitory neurotransmitters increase such potentials. Kinds include **acetylcholine, gamma-aminobutyric acid, norepinephrine.**

N

neurotripsy /-trip′sē/, the surgical crushing of a nerve.

neurotrophic /-trof″ik/, pertaining to the nourishment of nerve cells.

neurotropic viruses /-trop″ik/ [Gk, *neuron,* nerve, *tropein,* to turn, *virus,* poison], viruses with an unexplained attraction to nerve tissue. The predilection also applies to certain toxic chemicals.

neurotropism /nŏŏrot″rəpiz′əm/ [Gk, *neuron,* nerve, *trepein,* to turn], **1.** the tendency for certain microorganisms, poisons, and nutrients to be attracted to nervous tissue. **2.** the tendency of basic dyes to be attracted to nervous tissue.

Neurpro, brand name for **rotigotine.**

neurula /nŏŏr″ələ/ *pl.* **neurulas, neurulae** [Gk, *neuron,* nerve], an early embryo during the period of neurulation when the nervous system tissue begins to differentiate. The embryo at this level of growth represents a third stage in embryonic development, after the morula and blastocyst stages in humans and higher animals and the blastula and gastrula stages in lower animals. In humans the neurula stage occurs from about 19 to 26 days after fertilization.

neurulation /-ā″shən/ [Gk, *neuron* + L, *atus,* process], the development of the neural plate and the processes involved with its subsequent closure to form the neural tube during the early stages of embryonic development. See also **neural tube formation.**

neutral /n(y)ŏŏ″trəl/ [L, *neutralis,* neuter], the state exactly between two opposing values, qualities, or properties. For example, in electricity a neutral state is one in which there is neither a positive nor a negative charge; in chemistry a neutral state is one in which a substance is neither acid nor alkaline. See also **acid, base, pH.**

neutralization /-īzā″shən/ [L, *neutralis* + Gk, *izein,* to cause], the interaction between an acid and a base that produces a solution that is neither acidic nor basic. The usual products of neutralization are a salt and water. —*neutralize, v.*

neutral rotation, the position of a limb that is turned neither toward nor away from the body's midline. When a person is supine and the leg is neutrally rotated, the toes should point straight up.

neutral thermal environment, an environment created by any method or apparatus to maintain the normal body temperature to minimize oxygen consumption and caloric expenditure, such as in an incubator or Isolette for a premature, sick, or low-birth-weight infant. See also **incubator, Isolette.**

neutron /n(y)ŏŏ″tron/ [L, *neuter,* neither; Gk, *elektron,* amber], (in physics) an elementary particle that is a constituent of the nuclei of all elements except the isotopic form of hydrogen [1]H. It has no electric charge and has approximately the same mass as a proton. Compare **electron, proton.** See also **atom.**

neutron activation analysis, the analysis of elements in a specimen, performed by exposing it to neutron irradiation. The irradiation converts many elements in the specimen to radioactive forms that can be identified by their emissions of radiation. The method has limited application to human and animal studies.

neutropenia /nŏŏ′trōpē″nē·ə/ [L, *neuter,* neither; Gk, *penia,* poverty], abnormal decrease in the neutrophil count associated with acute leukemia, chemotherapy, and idiosyncratic drug reactions, predisposing individuals to infection. Compare **leukopenia.** See also **neutrophil.**

neutropenic fever of unknown origin, a fever of at least 38.3° C occurring on several occasions in a patient whose neutrophil level is lower than 500/mm³ or is expected to fall below that level within 1 or 2 days, the cause of which cannot be determined after 3 days of investigation, including 2 days of incubation of cultures.

neutrophil /nŏŏ″trəfil/ [L, *neuter* + Gk, *philein,* to love], polymorphonuclear, granular leukocyte whose cytoplasmic granules stain with neutral dyes. The nucleus stains dark blue and contains three to five segments connected by slender threads of nuclear membrane. The cytoplasm contains fine, inconspicuous neutral granules. Neutrophils are the circulating white blood cells essential for phagocytosis and proteolysis by which bacteria, cellular debris, and solid particles are removed and destroyed. A neutrophil count less than or equal to 500/µL may be life-threatening. See also **basophil, eosinophil, granulocyte.**

neutrophil alkaline phosphatase. See **leukocyte alkaline phosphatase.**

neutrophilia /-fil″yə/, an elevated number of neutrophils in the blood, a common cause of leukocytosis.

neutrophilic leukemia. See **polymorphocytic leukemia.**

Neviaser procedure [T.J. Neviaser, contemporary American orthopedic surgeon], the surgical transfer of a coracoacromial ligament to the clavicle for the repair of an acromioclavicular separation.

nevirapine, an antiretroviral nonnucleoside reverse transcriptase inhibitor.

■ INDICATIONS: It is prescribed in combination for the treatment of human immunodeficiency virus infection.

■ CONTRAINDICATIONS: It should not be given to patients with an allergy or sensitivity to the medication or to patients taking ketoconazole or oral contraceptives. When used alone, there is rapid and uniform appearance of viral resistance.

■ ADVERSE EFFECTS: The side effects most often reported include headache, rash, drug fever, and diarrhea.

nevoid amentia. See **Sturge-Weber syndrome.**

nevoid basal cell carcinoma syndrome (NBCCS) /nē″void/, an inherited form of premalignant skin lesion. It is an autosomal-dominant trait. Multiple basal cell skin cancers and jaw cysts are the most common features.

■ OBSERVATIONS: The condition is diagnosed when there is a combination of major and minor features associated with the disease. Major features include multiple basal cell skin cancers, increased calcium deposits in the head, jaw or bone cysts, pits on the palms of the hands or soles of the feet, and a parent, sibling, or child with the syndrome. Minor features include medulloblastoma, enlarged head size, cleft lip or palate, extra digits, bifid ribs, visual deficits, benign fibrous tumors, and abdominal cysts.

■ INTERVENTIONS: Treatment is symptomatic and individualized to the patient based on presenting features.

■ PATIENT CARE CONSIDERATIONS: The high risk associated with the development of skin cancers mandates that the patient be extremely careful about sun exposure.

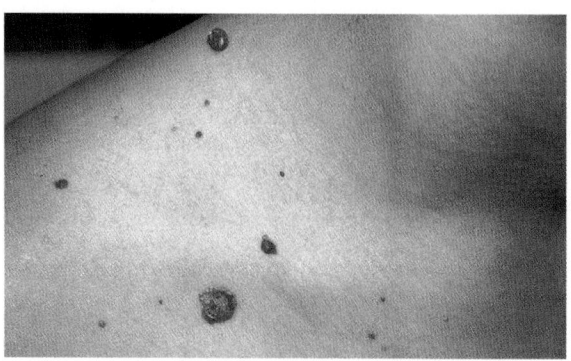

Skin lesions associated with nevoid basal cell carcinoma syndrome *(Cohen, 2013)*

nevoid neuroma [L, *naevus,* birthmark; Gk, *eidos,* form], a tumor of nerve tissue that contains numerous small blood vessels. Also called **neuroma telangiectodes.**

nevus /nē″vəs/ [L, *naevus,* birthmark], a pigmented skin blemish that is usually benign but may become cancerous. Any change in color, size, or texture or any bleeding or itching of a nevus merits investigation. Nevus is a benign tumor composed of nevus cells that are derived from melanocytes. Also called **birthmark, mole**[1]. Also spelled **naevus.** Kinds include **junction nevus,** *compound nevus, congenital nevus,* **epidermal nevus.** See also **blue nevus, nevus flammeus.**

nevus araneus. See **spider telangiectasia.**

nevus flammeus /flam″ē·əs/, a flat capillary hemangioma that is present at birth and that varies from pale red to deep reddish purple. It most commonly occurs on the occiput and rarely causes any problems. If the lesion is on any other part of the body, it tends to be darker colored and, unlike the scalp lesions, does not regress spontaneously. These lesions most often occur on the face. The depth of the color depends on whether the superficial, middle, or deep dermal vessels are involved. On the face the lesion persists and develops a thick, verrucous, nodular surface. Nevus flammeus is usually unilateral, following the distribution of a cutaneous nerve. If the lesion is on the middle of the face, Sturge-Weber syndrome is suspected. Camouflage cosmetics are used to cover the lesion and are the treatment of choice. Also called **port-wine stain.** Compare **Sturge-Weber syndrome.**

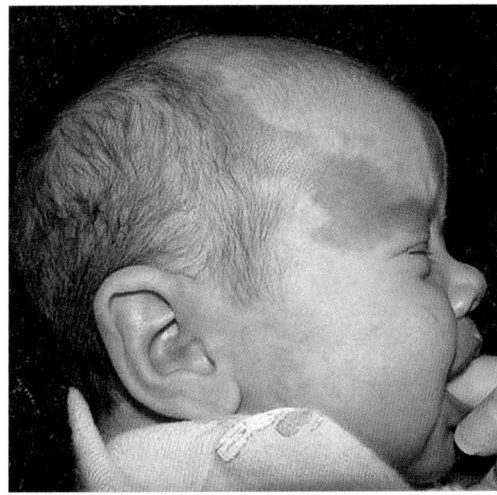

Infant with nevus flammeus *(Maguiness and Liang, 2011)*

nevus sebaceus. Also called **nevus sebaceus of Jadassohn.**

nevus sebaceus of Jadassohn, a congenital skin neoplasm with several cutaneous tissue elements. The most common location is the scalp, face, or neck. It may appear as a yellow or tan waxy patch of alopecia at birth. During puberty the lesion becomes raised, thick, and verrucous. It is usually treated with local excision. Untreated, the lesion may remain benign or become a malignant growth in later life. Also called **nevus sebaceus.**

nevus vascularis. See **capillary hemangioma.**

New Ballard Score [J.L. Ballard, American pediatrician], a system of newborn assessment of gestational maturation. It provides a valid estimation of postnatal maturation for preterm infants with gestational ages greater than 20 weeks and

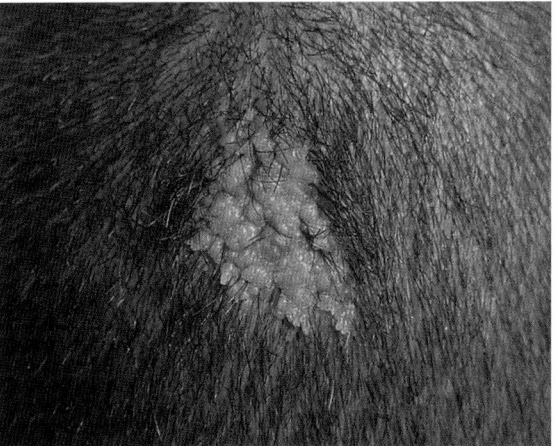

Basal cell carcinoma developing within nevus sebaceus *(Brinster et al, 2011)*

covers a dozen categories, including posture, arm recoil, popliteal angle, skin, plantar surface, and genitals.

newborn [AS, *niwe,* new, *boren,* to bear], a human infant from the time of birth through the 28th day of life. At birth, the gestational age and birth weight are assessed and the newborn is classified accordingly, for example, as large for gestational age, preterm (premature), or low birth weight. Also called **neonate, newborn infant.**

newborn infant. See **newborn.**

newborn intrapartal care, care of the newborn in the delivery area during the time after birth before the mother and infant are transferred to the postpartum unit. See also **intrapartal care, postpartal care.**

■ METHOD: The nasopharynx and mouth may be suctioned to remove excess mucus as the head is born. Depending on the preference and condition of the mother and the policies of the maternity service, the baby may then be placed on the mother's abdomen and covered with a warm, dry blanket or taken by the nurse to an infant warmer. Apgar scores are assigned at 1 minute and 5 minutes of age. Less commonly, another Apgar score is assigned at 10 minutes of age. The baby is handled gently and quietly and may be put to breast if the mother wishes; bright lights are often avoided, and maternal contact is encouraged.

■ INTERVENTIONS: Most newborns are healthy and normal. If abnormal function is observed, expert assistance may be summoned and emergency measures, including tracheal suction with suction equipment and administration of oxygen by ventilator or mask, are initiated. If there are no problems, the nurse may instill erythromycin drops in the conjunctival sacs of the eyes, trim and clamp the umbilical cord, administer an injection of vitamin K, obtain footprints for identification, and diaper and wrap the baby. If the baby needs to be transferred to a nursery or special care facility, the nurse accompanies the infant and acts as the initial liaison for the mother with the nursery.

■ OUTCOME CRITERIA: Most infants born at term are healthy and do not need any medical intervention. Hemorrhage from the umbilical cord, difficult respiration, imperforate anus, endocrine dysfunction, and various other abnormal conditions may occur, but, if a baby has good color; is alert; and can cry, suck, urinate, defecate, and respond to sound and light, the nurse and physician may reassure the mother that the baby is almost invariably healthy and normal. The individuality of each infant is remarkable and may be pointed out to the mother.

N

new drug, a drug for which the U.S. Food and Drug Administration requires premarketing approval.

new drug application, a formal proposal to the U.S. Food and Drug Administration for the approval of a new pharmaceutical for sale and marketing in the United States. Data gathered during animal studies and human clinical trials are a component of the application.

New England Journal of Medicine, a weekly professional medical journal that publishes findings of medical research and articles about controversial political and ethical issues in the practice of medicine.

new growth, an area of increased size, often suspicious for neoplasm or tumor presence or recurrence.

Newman, Margaret A. [b. 1933], a nursing theorist who contributed to the study of nursing theories and models by defining three approaches to the discovery of nursing theory: "borrowing" of theories from related disciplines, analyzing nursing practice situations in search of conceptual relationships, and creating new conceptual systems from which theories can be derived.

new product evaluation committee. See **product evaluation committee.**

newspaper sign, an assessment for ulnar nerve palsy in which an individual is asked to grasp a flat object, such as a newspaper, between his or her thumb and index finger. The examiner then attempts to pull the object out of the subject's hands. Individuals normally are able to maintain a hold on the object without difficulty; the inability to perform this task suggests ulnar nerve palsy. Also called **Froment sign.**

newton /n(y)o͞oʺtən/ [Isaac Newton, English scientist, 1642–1727], a unit of force in the SI system that imparts an acceleration to 1 kilogram of mass of 1 meter per second squared.

Newton's laws [Sir Isaac Newton, English physicist, 1643–1727], laws of motion first published by Isaac Newton. Newton's first law states that bodies at rest stay at rest and bodies in motion keep moving unless they are acted on by an unbalancing force. The second law is that the greater the mass of an object the greater the amount of force needed to accelerate the object. Newton's third law states that every action force has a reaction force that is equal in magnitude but opposite in direction. See also **kinetics,** def. 1.

new tuberculin [ME, *newe* + L, *tuber,* swelling], an extract of the tubercle bacillus from which all soluble material has been removed and glycerin added.

New World leishmaniasis. See **American leishmaniasis.**

New World typhus. See **murine typhus.**

Nexavar, brand name for **sorafenib.**

nexus /nekʹsəs/ *pl. nexus* [L, bond], a bond, especially one between members of a series or group.

Nezelof syndrome /nezʺəlof/ [Christian Nezelof, French physician, 1922-2015], an abnormal condition characterized by absent T cell function, deficient B cell function, fairly normal immunoglobulin levels, and little or no specific antibody production. It affects both male and female siblings, indicating that it may be transmitted as an autosomal-recessive genetic disorder. Another theory is that the disorder is caused by underdevelopment of the thymus gland and the consequent inhibition of T cell development. Still another holds that the disease results from a failure to produce or to secrete thymic humoral factors, especially thymosin. ■ OBSERVATIONS: Patients with Nezelof syndrome have progressively severe, recurrent, and eventually fatal infections. Signs that often appear in infants or in children up to 4 years of age include recurrent pneumonia, otitis media, chronic fungal infections, upper respiratory tract infections, diarrhea, and hepatosplenomegaly. The lymph nodes and tonsils may be enlarged, or they may be totally absent in infants with the disease. Involved patients may develop a tendency toward malignancy. Infection may cause sepsis, which is the usual cause of death. Symptoms that often suggest Nezelof syndrome also include weight loss and poor eating habits. Definite diagnostic evidence of the disease includes defective B cell and T cell immunity despite a normal number of circulating B cells, a moderate-to-high rise in the number of T cells, a deficiency or an increase in one or more classes of immunoglobulins, a nonreactive Schick test after DPT immunization, a reduced or an absent antibody reaction after specific antigen immunization, no thymus shadow on a chest x-ray film, thymus-dependent regions with abnormal lymphoid structure, and a decrease in the number of lymphocytes in the blood. ■ INTERVENTIONS: Initial supportive treatment of Nezelof syndrome may include monthly injections of gamma globulin or monthly infusions of fresh frozen plasma and heavy use of antibiotics to fight infection. The plasma infusions are especially beneficial if the patient cannot produce specific immunoglobulins. Cell-mediated immune function associated with T cells can usually be temporarily restored within weeks by a fetal thymus transplant. Repeated transplants are required to maintain the immunity. Cell-mediated immunity can be only partially restored with either transfer factor therapy or repeated injection of thymosin. Histocompatible bone marrow transplants have been used, but the effectiveness of this treatment method is unclear. ■ PATIENT CARE CONSIDERATIONS: The role of health care providers in treating this condition is essentially supportive. Sites of gamma globulin injection in a large muscle mass are massaged after each injection, and the sites are rotated and recorded to prevent tissue damage. Gamma globulin doses greater than 1.5 mL are divided and injected into more than one site. The nurse also offers support to the parents of children affected by Nezelof syndrome, instructs them on how to recognize the signs of infection, and explains the dangers of allowing affected children to become exposed to infection.

nF, a measurement of the ability to store an electrical charge. Abbreviation for *nanofarad.*

NF1, a gene associated with neurofibromatosis. The gene is normally part of a family that helps regulate the timing of cell divisions. It may become defective, leading to neurofibromatosis expression, when an itinerant sequence of a deoxyribonucleic acid molecule becomes wedged in the NF1 gene.

NF, abbreviation for *National Formulary.*

ng, abbreviation for **nanogram.**

NGF, abbreviation for **nerve growth factor.**

NG tube, abbreviation for **nasogastric tube.**

NGU, abbreviation for **nongonococcal urethritis.**

NHGRI, abbreviation for **National Human Genome Research Institute.**

NHSC, abbreviation for **National Health Service Corps.**

Ni, symbol for the element **nickel.**

NIA, abbreviation for **National Institute on Aging.**

niacin /nīʺəsin/, a white, crystalline, water-soluble vitamin of the B complex, usually occurring in various plant and animal tissues as nicotinamide. It functions as a coenzyme necessary for the breakdown and use of all major nutrients and is essential for healthy skin, normal functioning of the GI tract, maintenance of the nervous system, and synthesis of the sex hormones. It may be used therapeutically to help reduce high blood cholesterol levels. Rich dietary sources of both niacin and its precursor tryptophan are meats, poultry, fish, liver, kidney, eggs, nuts, peanut butter, brewer's yeast, and wheat germ. Symptoms of deficiency include muscular weakness, general fatigue, loss of appetite, various skin eruptions, halitosis, stomatitis, insomnia, irritability, nausea, vomiting, recurring headaches, tender gums, tension, and depression. Severe deficiency results in pellagra. The vitamin is not stored in the body, and daily sources are needed. Niacin toxicity is associated with large doses of nicotinic acid (may occur with a dose as low as 50 to 100 mg). Symptoms include flushing, nausea, dizziness, diarrhea, abdominal pain, and alteration of glucose tolerance. Overdose can also exacerbate preexisting conditions such as cardiac arrhythmias and abnormal liver function. Also called **nicotinic acid.** See also **pellagra.**

niacinamide /nī′əsin″əmīd/, a B complex vitamin. It is closely related to niacin but has no vasodilating action. Also called **nicotinamide.**

niacin equivalent (NE), units used to express niacin content of food. It represents preformed niacin plus tryptophan equivalents (60 mg tryptophan = 1 mg niacin).

NIAMS, abbreviation for **National Institute of Arthritis and Musculoskeletal and Skin Diseases.**

NIB, abbreviation for *National Industries for the Blind.*

NIBIB, abbreviation for **National Institute of Biomedical Imaging and Bioengineering.**

NIC, abbreviation for Nursing Interventions Classification.

niCARdipine /nikär″dipin/, a calcium channel blocker. It causes vasodilation and is prescribed as an antihypertensive and antianginal agent.

niche /nich/ [Fr, recess], a defect in an otherwise even surface, especially a depression or recess in the wall of an organ as seen on a radiograph or by the unaided eye.

NICHHD, abbreviation for **National Institute of Child Health and Human Development.**

Nicholas procedure [J.A. Nicolas, American physician], a surgical method for repairing severe injuries to the ligaments of the knee. It involves five procedures: medial meniscectomy, medial collateral ligament repair, vastus medialis advancement, semitendinosus advancement, and pes anserinus transfer. Also called **five-in-one repair.**

nick [ME, *nyke,* notch], **1.** a split in a single strand of DNA that can be made with the enzyme deoxyribonuclease or with ethidium bromide. **2.** a small cut or superficial wound.

nickel (Ni) [Ger, *Kupfernickel,* copper demon], a silver-white metallic element. Its atomic number is 28; its atomic mass is 58.71. Many people are allergic to nickel. Nickel causes more cases of allergic contact dermatitis than all other metals combined. Many cases occur from exposure to jewelry, coins, buckles, and snaps and from continued use of "carbonless" business forms. Nickel carbonyl, an extremely toxic volatile liquid, may produce serious lung damage if inhaled. Nickel is now a suspected carcinogen.

nickel dermatitis, an allergic contact dermatitis caused by the metal nickel. Exposure usually comes from jewelry, wristwatches, metal clasps, and coins. Sweating increases the degree of rash. Treatment includes avoidance of exposure to nickel and reduction of perspiration. See also **contact dermatitis.**

nick translation, a method of labeling DNA in the laboratory by using the enzyme DNA polymerase.

Nicobid, a water-soluble form of vitamin B$_3$. Brand name for **niacin, niacinamide.**

Nicola procedure, the surgical transfer of the long head of the biceps tendon through the humeral head to correct chronic anterior shoulder dislocation.

Nicorette, a nicotine resin complex. Brand name for **nicotine polacrilex.**

nicotinamide. See **niacinamide.**

nicotine /nik″ətēn/ [Jean Nicot de Villemain, French ambassador to Portugal, 1530–1600], a colorless, rapidly acting toxic and highly addictive substance in plants, most closely associated with tobacco, that is one of the major contributors to the ill effects of smoking.

nicotine adenine disphosphonucleotide, a nonprotein chemical compound utilized in anabolic reactions.

nicotine nasal spray, a product approved by the U.S. Food and Drug Administration for aiding tobacco smoking cessation in adults; not available in Canada. One dose of the nasal spray administers 1 mg of nicotine directly into the nasal membranes. Because of the risk of becoming dependent on the nasal spray, it is recommended that patients not use it for more than 6 months. See also **nicotine replacement therapy.**

nicotine poisoning, poisoning from intake of nicotine, characterized by stimulation of the central and autonomic nervous systems followed by depression of these systems. In fatal cases, death occurs from respiratory failure. See also **acute nicotine poisoning.**

nicotine polacrilex /pōlak″rileks/, a chewing gum (nicotine resin complex) source of nicotine as an adjunct for smoking cessation.

■ INDICATIONS: It may be prescribed as an aid for patients who are trying to quit cigarette smoking.

■ CONTRAINDICATIONS: Use by postmyocardial infarction patients or those with severe or worsening angina pectoris or life-threatening arrhythmias is prohibited. It should be used cautiously in patients with hyperthyroidism, hypertension, type 1 diabetes mellitus, or peptic ulcers. Drug dosages may have to be adjusted in patients taking other drugs with effects that may be increased or decreased when cigarette smoking ceases. Patients should be monitored to ensure that they do not become dependent on the nicotine in the gum.

■ ADVERSE EFFECTS: The most serious adverse effects include burning and soreness of the mouth, lightheadedness, headache, hiccups, nausea, vomiting, and excessive salivation.

nicotine replacement therapy, the use of chewing gum, lozenges, or skin patches as a substitute for tobacco smoke sources to satisfy nicotine cravings.

nicotine stomatitis, oral mucosal changes that are caused by heat and irritation from smoking tobacco. The palatal mucosa may appear intensely red, later to become more keratinized and pale in color with characteristic red dots. Smoking cessation is encouraged.

nicotine withdrawal syndrome, physiological and psychological effects of tobacco dependence that make it difficult for addicted smokers to cease use of nicotine. Withdrawal symptoms in those who quit smoking cigarettes may be diminished by substituting nicotine in the form of chewing gum, lozenges, or transdermal nicotine skin patches.

■ OBSERVATIONS: A wide range of uncomfortable symptoms is associated with nicotine withdrawal. The symptoms include, but are not limited to, nausea, headache, irritability, and difficulty concentrating.

■ INTERVENTIONS: Withdrawal symptoms may be diminished by substituting nicotine in the form of chewing gum, lozenges, or transdermal skin patches.

■ PATIENT CARE CONSIDERATIONS: Smoking cessation programs and support groups can be of benefit to a patient experiencing withdrawal from nicotine.

nicotinic acid. See **niacin.**

NICU /nik″yoo/, abbreviation for **neonatal intensive care unit.**

NID, abbreviation for *National Institute for the Deaf.*

nid-, combining form meaning "to nest" or "a place where an organism can breed": *nidation.*

NIDA, abbreviation for **National Institute on Drug Abuse.**

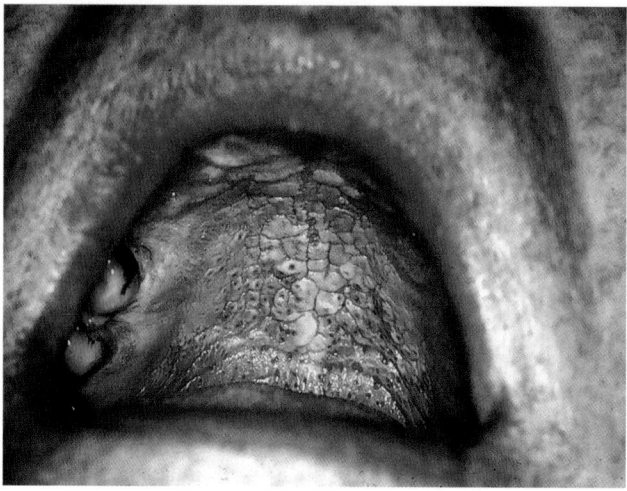

Nicotine stomatitis *(Stefanac and Nesbit, 2017)*

nidation /nīdā″shən/ [L, *nidus,* nest], the process by which an embryo burrows into the endometrium of the uterus. Also called **implantation.** See also **placenta, uterus.**

-nidazole, suffix for metronidazole-type antiprotozoal substances.

NIDCD, abbreviation for **National Institute on Deafness and Other Communication Disorders.**

NIDCR, abbreviation for **National Institute of Dental and Craniofacial Research.**

NIDDM, abbreviation for **non–insulin-dependent diabetes mellitus.** See **type 2 diabetes mellitus.**

nidus /nī″dəs/ [L, nest], a point of origin, focus, or nucleus of a disease process.

Niebauer prosthesis /nē′bou·ər/, a Silastic prosthesis for interphalangeal and thumb joint replacement.

Niemann-Pick disease /nē″mon pik″/ [Albert Niemann, German pediatrician, 1880–1921; Ludwig Pick, German pediatrician, 1868–1935], an inherited group of disorders of lipid metabolism in which there are accumulations of sphingomyelin in the bone marrow, spleen, and lymph nodes. There are several types of Niemann-Pick disease: type A (NPA) and type B (NPB), also called *acid sphingomyelinase deficiency (ASMD);* type C (NPC); and type D (NPD). NPA is seen in all races and ethnicities. In the United States and Canada there is a higher incidence of NPA and NPB among the Ashkenazi Jewish population. Type C is most common in Puerto Rican people of Spanish descent. Type D is seen in French-Canadian people in Nova Scotia. See also **sphingomyelin lipidosis.**

■ OBSERVATIONS: Symptoms vary, depending on the type of disease. Generally, the disease is characterized by enlargement of liver and spleen, anemia, lymphadenopathy, and progressive mental and physical deterioration. Type A symptoms appear in infancy and are manifested by poor feeding, poor motor control, a cherry-red spot in the eye, and abdominal swelling. Type B symptoms are usually milder, occurring in late childhood or adolescence. Type C usually occurs in late adolescence or early adulthood. Blood and bone marrow tests are done to diagnose types A and B; a skin biopsy is the usual test to diagnose types C and D.

■ INTERVENTIONS: There is no effective treatment for type A, and children with the disease usually die within a few years of the onset of symptoms. There are new treatments for types B and C. No specific treatment exists for type D.

A well-balanced diet that is low in cholesterol is recommended.

■ PATIENT CARE CONSIDERATIONS: DNA tests can be done to diagnose carriers of types A and B. In addition to the coordinated support of the health care team, support groups are helpful in assisting parents and children to cope with disease progression.

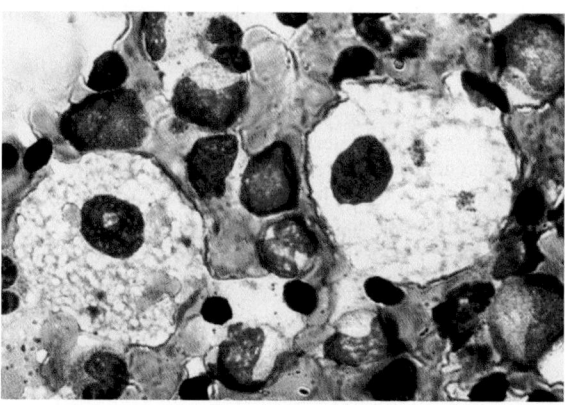

Bone marrow aspirate from a patient with Niemann-Pick disease with large foamy macrophages *(Aster, Poznyakova, and Kutok, 2013)*

NIFEdipine /nifed″ipēn/, a calcium channel blocker.

■ INDICATIONS: It is prescribed for the treatment of vasospastic and effort-associated angina, pulmonary hypertension, and hypertension (sustained-release form only).

■ CONTRAINDICATIONS: Known hypersensitivity to this drug prohibits its use, and immediate-release forms should not be used to treat hypertension. The practice of using short-acting sublingual nifedipine in hypertensive emergencies or pseudoemergencies is dangerous and should be abandoned.

■ ADVERSE EFFECTS: Among the more serious adverse effects are hypotension, peripheral edema, palpitations, dyspnea, nausea, dizziness, flushing, and headache. When given sublingually, stroke, severe hypotension, syncope, heart block, sinus arrest, myocardial infarctions, and fetal distress are among the adverse effects reported.

nifur-, prefix for 5-nitrofuran derivatives.

night blindness.   See **nyctalopia.**

night guard.   See **biteguard.**

Nightingale, Florence [1820–1910], considered the founder of modern nursing. After limited formal training in nursing in Germany and Paris, she became superintendent in 1853 of a small hospital in London. Her outstanding success in reorganizing the hospital led the British government to request that she head a mission to the Crimea, where Britain was fighting a war with Russia. After her return to England in 1856, she wrote *Notes on Hospitals* and *Notes on Nursing* and founded a training school for nurses at St. Thomas' Hospital, where she attracted well-educated, dedicated women. The graduates became matrons of the most important hospitals in Great Britain, thus raising the standards of nursing across the nation and eventually around the world. Although she was, by then, bedridden much of the time, she carried on her work on the sanitary reform of India, conducted a study of midwifery, helped establish visiting nurse services, and worked for the reform of the poor laws in which she proposed separate institutions for the sick, the insane, the incurable, and children. One of Florence Nightingale's outstanding contributions was significantly decreasing the infection-related death rate through cleanliness. After Longfellow wrote *Santa Filomena,* she became known as "The Lady with the Lamp"; the Nightingale Pledge, named after her, embodies her ideals and has inspired thousands of young graduating nurses.

Nightingale pledge, a statement of principles for the nursing profession, formulated by a committee in 1893. It is as follows: "I solemnly pledge myself before God and in the presence of this assembly: To pass my life in purity and to practice my profession faithfully. I will abstain from whatever is deleterious and mischievous, and will not take or knowingly administer any harmful drug. I will do all in my power to elevate the standard of my profession, and will hold in confidence all personal matters committed to my keeping and all family affairs coming to my knowledge in the practice of my profession. With loyalty will I endeavor to aid the physician in his work, and devote myself to the welfare of those committed to my care."

Nightingale ward, a hospital ward designed by Florence Nightingale that revolutionized hospital design. The number of beds allowed in a ward of given size was limited to permit the circulation of air and to enhance general cleanliness and the comfort of patients. Three sides of the ward were windowed to admit light and fresh air. Although multiple-bed wards are now obsolete in hospital design, the concerns and benefits that impelled Miss Nightingale to create them remain central to hospital planning.

nightmare /nīt′mer/ [AS, *niht,* night, *mara,* incubus], a dream occurring during rapid eye movement sleep that arouses feelings of intense inescapable fear, terror, distress, or extreme anxiety and that usually awakens the sleeper. Compare **pavor nocturnus, sleep terror disorder.**

night sight.   See **hemeralopia.**

night splint, any splint or similar device applied to the affected extremity. It is used only at night.

nightstick fracture, an undisplaced fracture of the ulnar shaft caused by a direct blow.

night sweat [AS, *niht* + *swaetan*], **1.** sweating that occurs with a nocturnal fever, as in wasting diseases such as pulmonary tuberculosis or cancer. **2.** nocturnal sweating by a woman as an effect of menopause or perimenopause. The sweating, which may be mild or profuse enough to disrupt sleep, is believed to be caused by fluctuations in estrogen levels. **3.** profuse sweating at night in an environment of normal temperature. It may be associated with medications, hormonal disorders, hypoglycemia or neurological disorders.

night terrors [AS, *niht* + L, *terrour*], a form of dissociated sleep, usually in children, in which there may be repeated episodes of abrupt awakening from sleep with signs of extreme anxiety and panic. The subject may have only fragmentary dream images of a threatening nature. See also **pavor nocturnus, sleep terror disorder.**

night vision [AS, *niht,* night; L, *visio,* seeing], a capacity to see dimly lit objects. It stems from a chemophysical phenomenon associated with the retinal rods. The rods contain the highly light-sensitive chemical rhodopsin, or visual purple, which is essential for the conduction of optic impulses in subdued light. Night vision is sharpest at the periphery of the retina because of the concentration of rods. Night vision may be diminished by a deficiency of vitamin A, an important component of rhodopsin.

nightwalking [AS, *niht* + ME, *walken*], a disorder occurring during nonrapid eye movement sleep in which the subject usually sits up in bed briefly, then gets up and walks around, opening doors, eating, and so on, and eventually returns to bed. The person has no memory of the event the next day. Nightwalking is sometimes associated with the use of sleep medication. Also called **noctambulation, sleepwalking, somnambulism.**

NIGMS, abbreviation for **National Institute of General Medical Sciences.**

nigr-, combining form meaning "black or a variation of the black color": *substantia nigra, acanthosis nigricans.*

NIH, abbreviation for **National Institutes of Health.**

nihilistic delusion /nī′hilis″tik/ [L, *nihil,* nothing, *icus,* form of, *deludere,* to deceive], a persistent denial of the existence of particular things or of everything, including oneself, as seen in various forms of schizophrenia. A person who has such a delusion may believe that he or she lives in a shadow or limbo world or that he or she died several years ago and that only the spirit, in a vaporous form, really exists. See also **delusion.**

Nikolsky sign /nikol″skē/ [Petr V. Nikolsky, Russian dermatologist, 1858–1940], easy separation of the stratum corneum layer of the epidermis from the basal cell layer by rubbing apparently normal skin areas, found in pemphigus and a few other bullous diseases.

nil disease.   See **minimal change disease.**

nilotinib, a miscellaneous antineoplastic drug.
- INDICATIONS: This drug is used to treat chronic- and accelerated-phase Philadelphia chromosome–positive chronic myelogenous leukemia that is resistant to or intolerant of imatinib.
- CONTRAINDICATIONS: Known hypersensitivity to this drug, pregnancy, breastfeeding, hypokalemia, hypomagnesemia, and QT prolongation prohibit its use. This drug should not be used simultaneously with grapefruit products.
- ADVERSE EFFECTS: Adverse effects of this drug include headache, dizziness, fatigue, fever, flushing, paresthesia, palpitations, constipation, diarrhea, alopecia, erythemia, hyperamylasemia, hyperbilirubinemia, hyperglycemia, hyperkalemia, hypocalcemia, hyponatremia, hypomagnesemia, diaphoresis, arthralgia, myalgia, back and bone pain, muscle cramps, cough, and dyspnea. Life-threatening side effects include QT prolongation, torsades de pointes, hepatotoxicity, vomiting, dyspepsia, pancreatitis, neutropenia, thrombocytopenia, anemia, pancytopenia, and bleeding. Common side effects include nausea, anorexia, abdominal pain, and rash.

Nilstat, an antifungal drug. Brand name for **nystatin.**

nilutamide, an antineoplastic hormone.
- INDICATIONS: It is used to treat stage D2 metastatic prostatic carcinoma in combination with surgical castration.
- CONTRAINDICATIONS: Factors that prohibit the use of this drug include known hypersensitivity to nilutamide, severe hepatic impairment, and severe respiratory disease.

N

■ ADVERSE EFFECTS: Hepatotoxicity and interstitial pneumonitis are life-threatening effects. Other adverse effects include hot flashes, drowsiness, insomnia, dizziness, hyperthesia, depression, decreased libido, impotence, testicular atrophy, urinary tract infection, hematuria, nocturia, gynecomastia, diarrhea, nausea, vomiting, increased liver function studies, constipation, dyspepsia, rash, sweating, alopecia, dry skin, dyspnea, upper respiratory infection, pneumonia, anemia, delayed adaption to the dark, and edema.

NIMH, abbreviation for **National Institute of Mental Health.**

nimodipine /ni-mo′dipēn/, a calcium channel blocking agent used as a vasodilator in the treatment of neurological deficits associated with subarachnoid hemorrhage from a ruptured intracranial aneurysm, administered orally.

90–90 traction. See **traction, 90-90.**

NINR, abbreviation for **National Institute of Nursing Research.**

ninth cranial nerve. See **glossopharyngeal nerve.**

niobium (Nb) /nī·ō″bē·əm/ [Gk, *Niobe,* mythic daughter of Tantalus and Amphion], a silver-gray metallic element. Its atomic number is 41; its atomic mass is 92.906. Formerly called **columbium.**

NIOSH, abbreviation for **National Institute for Occupational Safety and Health.**

NIP, abbreviation for **National Immunization Program.**

nipple [ME, *neb,* beak], a small cylindric, pigmented structure that projects just below the center of each breast. The tip of the nipple has about 20 tiny openings to the lactiferous ducts. The skin of the nipple is surrounded by the lighter pigmented skin of the areola. The depth of pigmentation of the nipple and areola in nulliparas varies from rosy pink to brown, depending on the complexion of the individual. In pregnancy the skin of the nipple darkens but loses some of its pigmentation when lactation is completed. Stimulation of the nipple in men and women causes the structure to become erect through the contraction of radiating smooth muscle bundles in the surrounding areola. In women the nipple enlarges somewhat and becomes more sensitive after puberty. Also called **mammary papilla, papilla mammae, papilla mammaria.**

nipple cancer, an inflammatory malignant neoplasm of the nipple and areola that is usually associated with carcinoma in deeper breast structures. It represents only a small percentage of breast cancers and usually begins in the nipple and spreads to the areola. Also called **Paget disease of the nipple.**

nipple discharge, spontaneous exudation of material from the nipple. It may be normal, such as colostrum in pregnancy, or it may be a sign of endocrinological, neoplastic, or infectious disease.

nipple shield, a device to protect the nipples of a lactating woman. The shield is usually made of soft latex, is 4 or 5 cm wide, and has a tab on one side with which the mother may hold it. The baby nurses from an opening at the center of the shield. It is most often used to allow sore or cracked nipples to heal while maintaining lactation. Also called *nipple protector.*

Nipride, a direct-acting vasodilator used for controlled lowering of blood pressure. Brand name for **sodium nitroprusside.**

Nirschl procedure /nur″shəl/, a surgical procedure for treating chronic inflammation of the elbow. It involves excision of a segment from the hypercapsular tendon of the extensor carpi radialis brevis and removal of the head of the anterolateral condyle.

nirvanic state /nirvä″nik, nirvan″ik/, (in Buddhist meditation) a state in which mental processes cease, often leading to a radical alteration of the personality.

NIS, abbreviation for *Nursing Information System.*

nisoldipine, a calcium channel blocker.

■ INDICATIONS: It causes vasodilation and is prescribed, either alone or in combinations, for the management of hypertension.

■ CONTRAINDICATIONS: Factors that prohibit its use include hypersensitivity to nisoldipine or other dihydropyridine calcium channel blockers. High-fat meals and grapefruit juice should be avoided because these foods can cause sudden increases in the blood levels of the drug.

■ ADVERSE EFFECTS: Fluid retention, headache, nausea, dizziness, pharyngitis, shortness of breath, cough, and palpitations are among the more common adverse effects.

Nissl body /nis″əl/ [Franz Nissl, German neurologist, 1860–1919], any one of the large granular structures in the cytoplasm of nerve cells that stains with basic dyes and contains ribonucleoprotein.

NIST, abbreviation for **National Institute of Standards and Technology.**

NIST standard, a radioactive source standardized or certified or both by the National Institute of Standards and Technology.

nit, the egg of a parasitic insect, particularly a louse. It may be found attached to human or animal hair or to clothing fiber. See also **pediculosis.**

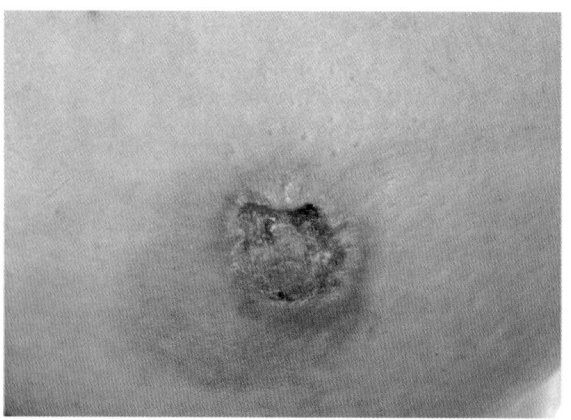

Nipple cancer *(Carty et al, 2007)*

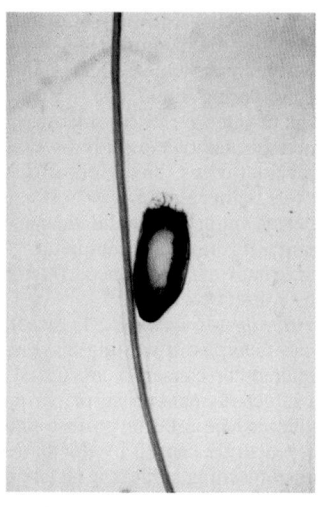

Microscopic view of a nit *(Ko and Elston, 2004)*

nitazoxanide, an antiprotozoal agent used to treat diarrhea caused by *Cryptosporidium parvum* or *Giardia lamblia.*

nitisinone, an orphan drug.

■ INDICATIONS: This drug is used to treat hereditary tyrosinemia type 1.

■ CONTRAINDICATIONS: Tyrosine or phenylalanine intake and known hypersensitivity to this drug prohibit its use.

nitr, 1. abbreviation for **nitrocellulose. 2.** abbreviation for **nitroglycerin.**

nitr-, prefix meaning "related to nitrogen, nitrite, and nitrate."

nitrate /nī″trāt/ [Gk, *nitron,* soda], **1.** the ion NO_3^-. **2.** a salt of nitric acid.

nitric acid (HNO$_3$) /nī″trik/ [Gk, *nitron,* soda; L, *acidus,* sour], a colorless, highly corrosive liquid that may give off suffocating brown fumes of nitrogen dioxide on exposure to air. Traces of nitric acid may be found in rainwater during a thunderstorm. Commercially prepared nitric acid is a powerful oxidizing agent used in photoengraving and metallurgy; in the manufacture of explosives, fertilizers, dyes, and drugs; and occasionally as a cauterizing agent for the removal of warts. Organic nitrates or polyol esters of nitric acid such as nitroglycerin and amyl nitrite are effective vasodilators often used in relieving angina, but exactly how they function in dilating arterial and venous smooth muscle is not yet understood. Historically known as *aqua fortis.*

nitric oxide (NO), 1. a colorless gas and stable free radical commonly found in tissues of humans and other mammals. It is also prepared commercially by passing air through an electric arc. Biologically the effector molecule is commonly synthesized from the amino acid arginine. NO participates in many biological functions, such as neurotransmission, vasodilation, cytotoxicity of macrophages, lipid-lowering therapy, and inhibition of platelet aggregation. NO is involved in smooth muscle action and penile erection. It may improve oxygenation in patients with high-altitude pulmonary edema. NO deprivation may lead to high blood pressure and the formation of atherosclerotic plaque. On contact with air, NO is quickly converted to the very poisonous nitrogen dioxide (NO_2). **2.** a respiratory inhalant.

■ INDICATIONS: It is used in combination with other agents and ventilatory support in the treatment of full-term and near-term (34 weeks) neonates with hypoxic respiratory failure associated with pulmonary hypertension.

■ CONTRAINDICATIONS: Two factors that prohibit its use are dependence on right-to-left shunting of blood and known hypersensitivity.

■ ADVERSE EFFECTS: Life-threatening effects are pulmonary hemorrhage, intracranial hemorrhage, sepsis, stridor, methemoglobinemia, seizures, cerebral infarction, and posttreatment infection. Other adverse effects include atelectasis, hematuria, hyperglycemia, cellulitis, withdrawal syndrome, and hypotension.

nitrite /nī″trīt/ [Gk, *nitron,* soda], an ester or salt of nitrous acid used as a vasodilator and antispasmodic. Among the most widely used nitrites in medicine are amyl, ethyl, potassium, and sodium nitrite.

nitritoid reaction /nī″tritoid/, a group of adverse effects, including hypotension, flushing, light-headedness, and fainting, produced by administration of arsenicals or gold. The reaction is similar to that caused by administration of nitrites.

nitro-, prefix indicating presence of the group -NO$_2$: *nitrobenzene, nitrofuran, nitrocellulose.*

nitrobenzene poisoning /nī″trōben″zēn/, a toxic condition caused by the absorption into the body of nitrobenzene, a pale yellow, oily liquid used in the manufacture of aniline, shoe dyes, soap, perfume, and artificial flavors. Nitrobenzene,

especially its vapors, is extremely toxic. Exposure in industry is usually by inhalation of the fumes or by absorption through the skin. Symptoms of acute poisoning include headache, drowsiness, nausea, ataxia, cyanosis, and, in extreme cases, respiratory failure. Chronic exposure to nitrobenzene may cause headache, fatigue, loss of appetite, and anemia.

Nitro-Bid, a coronary vasodilator. Brand name for **nitroglycerin.**

nitrocellulose (nitr) /-sel″yəlōs/, a mixture of nitrate esters of cellulose made by treating cotton with nitric and sulfuric acids. Solutions in a mixture of ether and alcohol are used as "plastic skin" under the name of collodion. Also called **pyroxylin.** See also **collodion.**

nitrofuran /-fyoo″ran/, one of a group of synthetic antimicrobials used to treat infections caused by protozoa or by certain gram-positive or gram-negative bacteria. The precise mechanism by which nitrofurans exert their antimicrobial effects is not known, but several bacterial and protozoal enzyme systems are inhibited. Two agents commonly prescribed are furazolidone and nitrofurantoin. Furazolidone is used to treat bacterial and protozoal diarrhea and enteritis. Nitrofurantoin is used to treat urinary tract infections caused by *Escherichia coli* and other enteric pathogens of the urinary tract. Systemic administration of nitrofurans is associated with many side effects, the most common being nausea and diarrhea. Serious side effects include polyneuropathies and several hypersensitivity reactions, including pneumonitis and blood dyscrasias. Nitrofurans can cause hemolytic anemia in patients with glucose-6-phosphate dehydrogenase deficiency. Lastly, they cause a harmless brown discoloration of the urine.

nitrofurantoin /nī″trōfyoo͞oran″tō·in, -fyoo͞o′rəntō″in/, a urinary antibacterial drug.

■ INDICATIONS: It is prescribed in the treatment of urinary tract infections caused by some gram-negative bacteria and a few gram-positive bacteria. Some of the more common bacteria that cause urinary tract infections are resistant to nitrofurantoin.

■ CONTRAINDICATIONS: Kidney dysfunction or known hypersensitivity to this drug prohibits its use. It is not given to children under 1 month of age or to pregnant or lactating women. It should be used with caution in people with glucose-6-phosphate dehydrogenase deficiency, vitamin B deficiency, anemia, diabetes mellitus, or electrolyte disturbances.

■ ADVERSE EFFECTS: Among the most serious adverse effects is hypersensitivity pneumonitis, which can lead to fibrosis, neurotoxicity, and hemolytic anemia in patients with glucose-6-phosphate dehydrogenase deficiency. GI disturbances and fever are common.

nitrofurazone /-fyoo͞o″rəzōn/, a topical antibacterial drug.

■ INDICATIONS: It is prescribed in the prophylaxis and treatment of infections in second- and third-degree burns and of the skin and mucous membranes.

■ CONTRAINDICATIONS: Known hypersensitivity to this drug prohibits its use.

■ ADVERSE EFFECTS: Among the most serious adverse effects are severe allergic reactions and superinfections.

nitrogen (N) /nī″trəjən/ [Gk, *nitron,* soda, *genein,* to produce], a gaseous nonmetallic element. Its atomic number is 7; its atomic mass is 14.008. It exists as a diatomic molecule, N_2. Nitrogen constitutes approximately 78% of the atmosphere and is a component of all proteins and a major component of most organic substances in living cells. Nitrogen is essential to the synthesis of necessary proteins, particularly nitrogen-containing compounds or amino acids derived directly or indirectly from plant food. Nitrogen follows a

N

cycle from atmospheric gas into nitrogen-fixing bacteria, into green vascular plants, into humans and animals, and, by decay or in excreted nitrogenous wastes, as urea, back into the soil. Denitrifying bacteria in the soil break down nitrogenous compounds and release gaseous nitrogen. During a 24-hour period in a healthy individual the nitrogen excreted in the urine, feces, and perspiration, together with the nitrogen retained in dermal structures, such as the skin and hair, equals the nitrogen consumed in food and drink. The process of protein metabolism accounts for this nitrogen balance. When protein catabolism exceeds protein anabolism, the amount of nitrogen in the urine exceeds the amount of nitrogen consumed in foods, producing a negative nitrogen balance or a state of tissue wasting. A positive nitrogen balance exists in the body when the nitrogen intake in foods is greater than that excreted in urine. Conditions usually associated with positive nitrogen balance include those related to growth, pregnancy, and convalescence from a tissue-wasting illness. –*nitrogenous, adj.*

nitrogen balance, the relationship between the amount of nitrogen taken into the body, usually as food, and that excreted from the body in urine and feces. Most of the body's nitrogen is incorporated into protein. Positive nitrogen balance, which occurs when the intake of nitrogen is greater than its excretion, implies tissue formation and growth. Negative nitrogen balance, which occurs when more nitrogen is excreted than is taken in, indicates wasting or destruction of tissue.

nitrogen cycle [Gk, *nitron,* soda, *genein,* to produce, *kyklos,* circle], the circulation of nitrogen through natural processes in either of two ways: from the soil to organisms that excrete nitrogen products back into the soil or by bacterial fixation of atmospheric nitrogen through other organisms that decay and release the element back into the atmosphere.

nitrogen dioxide (NO_2), a brownish irritating gas that can be released from silage and the reaction of nitric acid with metals. It may produce symptoms of pulmonary damage in workers who perform ensilage tasks. Some studies indicate that measurable changes in pulmonary function occur when healthy individuals are exposed to NO_2 concentrations of two to three parts per million.

nitrogen fixation, the process by which free nitrogen in the atmosphere is converted by biological or chemical means to ammonia and to other forms usable by plants and animals. Biological nitrogen fixation is the more important process and is accomplished by microorganisms in the soil, either free living or in close association with root nodules of certain plants. In contrast, chemical nitrogen fixation, as is used in industry, requires extremely high temperatures and pressures.

nitrogen mustard. See **mechlorethamine hydrochloride.**

nitrogen narcosis, a condition of depressed central nervous system functions as a result of high partial pressure of nitrogen. See also **decompression sickness.**

nitrogen washout curve, a curve obtained by plotting the concentration of nitrogen in expired alveolar gas during oxygen breathing as a function of time. As a person inhales pure oxygen after breathing ambient air, the nitrogen concentration in exhaled air decreases. In healthy subjects, the concentration is less than 2% after 4 minutes.

nitroglycerin (nitr) /-glis'ərin/, a potent smooth muscle relaxant and vasodilator used in transdermal patches and in a paste as well as in oral and sublingual tablets. Also called **glyceryl trinitrate.**

■ INDICATIONS: It is prescribed for the prevention or relief of angina pectoris. There are recommended limits to the amount of nitroglycerin use before calling for emergency assistance (no more than 3 sublingual tablets at 5-minute intervals). The drug should not be used continuously, because tolerance

develops within 24 to 48 hrs. Nitroglycerin is also used to treat pulmonary hypertension, to help treat congestive heart failure following acute myocardial infarction, and to treat hypertensive emergencies during cardiovascular surgery.

■ CONTRAINDICATIONS: Head trauma, severe anemia, narrow-angle glaucoma, and known hypersensitivity to this drug or other organic nitrates prohibit its use. It should not be used by patients taking sildenafil or similar agents for treating erectile dysfunction.

■ ADVERSE EFFECTS: Among the most serious adverse effects are hypotension, flushing, headache, and syncope.

nitroglycerin tablets, tablets of glyceryl trinitrate, a volatile ester prepared by the action of nitric and sulfuric acids on glycerol, available by prescription. A tablet placed under the tongue provides prompt relief of chest pain from angina, and sustained-release forms (and patches) are available for preventing angina. To derive benefit from these drugs, they must not be used continuously: The body desensitizes to them.

nitromersol /-mur″sol/, an organic mercurial antiseptic that is not a highly effective germicide, sometimes used for the disinfecting of surgical instruments and as an antiseptic on the skin and mucous membranes.

nitroprusside sodium. See **sodium nitroprusside.**

nitrosamines /nīt″rəsam″ēnz/, potentially carcinogenic compounds produced by reactions of nitrites with amines or amides normally present in the body. Nitrites are produced by bacteria in saliva and in the intestine from nitrates normally present in vegetables and in nitrate-treated fish, poultry, and meats. More than 70% of ingested nitrates are from vegetables.

nitroso-, prefix indicating presence of the group —N:O: *nitrosourea.*

nitrosourea /nītrō'sōyo͝oorē″ə/, one of a group of alkylating drugs used as antineoplastic drugs in the chemotherapy of brain tumors, multiple myeloma, Hodgkin disease, adenocarcinomas, hepatomas, chronic leukemias, lymphomas, myelomas, and cancers of the breast and ovaries. They have been less successful in therapy for cancers of the lungs, head, neck, and GI tract. Like other alkylating agents, they have severe toxic effects, including bone marrow depression. Nausea and vomiting are almost always present. These drugs can cause fetal harm and should not be used during pregnancy. Carmustine and lomustine are typical examples of this group. See also **alkylating agent.**

Nitrospan, a coronary vasodilator. Brand name for **nitroglycerin.**

Nitrostat, a coronary vasodilator. Brand name for **nitroglycerin.**

nitrous acid (HNO_2), a weak acid and clinical laboratory reagent formed by the action of strong acids on inorganic nitrites. An aqueous solution of nitrous acid gradually decomposes into nitric oxide and nitric acid.

nitrous oxide (N_2O, NOx) /nī'trəs/, a colorless, odorless gas, first used as an anesthetic agent in 1844; it is the least potent of currently used inhalation anesthetics. It provides analgesia but not complete amnesia or akinesia and is usually supplemented with other drugs. Because high concentrations of nitrous oxide are required, hypoxia is a risk and supplemental oxygen is needed. Nitrous oxide is associated with an increased incidence of nausea and vomiting, environmental pollution, spontaneous abortion in health care workers exposed, and suspected teratogenicity. It has many contraindications to its use. Despite these shortcomings it remains in use in the United States and Canada because of its rapid onset and offset, relative lack of cardiac or respiratory depression, and its low cost. It is most often used to supplement other anesthetic agents, especially during an inhalation induction of children. Nitrous oxide remains a commonly administered dental anesthetic.

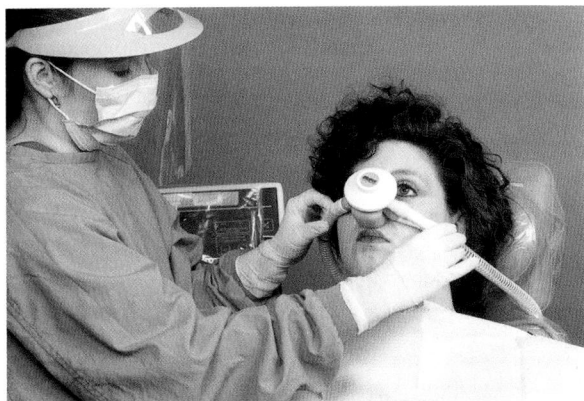

Nitrous oxide administration (Bird and Robinson, 2005)

Nix, a topical pediculicide. Brand name for **permethrin.**

Nizoral, an antifungal agent. Brand name for **ketoconazole.**

NK cell, abbreviation for **natural killer cell.**

NLM, abbreviation for **National Library of Medicine.**

NLN, abbreviation for **National League for Nursing.**

NLNAC, abbreviation for **National League for Nursing Accrediting Commission.**

nm, abbreviation for **nanometer.**

N-m, abbreviation for *newton meter.*

N/m², abbreviation for *newton per square meter.*

NMDP, abbreviation for **National Marrow Donor Program.**

NMDS, abbreviation for **nursing minimum data set.**

NMES, 1. abbreviation for **neuromuscular electric stimulator. 2.** abbreviation for *neuromuscular electrical stimulation.*

NMR, abbreviation for **nuclear magnetic resonance.** See **magnetic resonance.**

NNRTI, abbreviation for **nonnucleoside reverse transcriptase inhibitors.**

No, symbol for the element **nobelium.**

NO, abbreviation for *nitric oxide.*

N₂O, chemical formula for **nitrous oxide.**

Noack syndrome /no′äks/ [Margot Noack, 20th-century German physician], an autosomal-dominant type of anomaly affecting the cranium and digits. Also called **Carpenter syndrome, Sakati-Nyhan syndrome, Goodman syndrome.** See also **acrocephalosyndactyly.**

no appreciable disease (NAD), nothing out of order or identified as wrong.

nobelium (No) /nōbel′ē-əm/ [Alfred Nobel Institute, Stockholm, Sweden], a synthetic, transuranic metallic element. Its atomic number is 102, and the atomic mass of its most stable isotope is 259.

NOC, abbreviation for **Nursing Outcomes Classification.**

Nocardia /nōkär″dē-ə/ [Edmund I.E. Nocard, French veterinarian, 1850–1903], a genus of weakly gram-positive aerobic bacteria, some species of which are pathogenic, such as *Nocardia asteroides.*

nocardiosis /nōkär′dē-ō″sis/ [Edmund I.E. Nocard; Gk, *osis,* condition], infection with *Nocardia* species, most often *N. asteroides,* an aerobic gram-positive species of actinomycetes. It can cause pneumonia, often with cavitation, and chronic abscesses in the brain and subcutaneous tissues, and it can cause cutaneous disease through wounds contaminated with soil. The organism enters via the respiratory tract and spreads by the bloodstream, especially in those who are immunocompromised because of such conditions as HIV infection, organ transplantation, and Cushing syndrome. Surgical drainage of abscesses and sulfonamide therapy for 12 to 18 months cures between 50% and 60% of the cases treated. Combination antibiotic therapy may be required.

nocebo /nose′bo/, an adverse nonspecific side effect occurring in conjunction with a medication but not directly resulting from the pharmacological action of the medication. Compare **placebo.**

noci-, prefix meaning "to cause harm, injury, or pain": *nociceptive, nociceptor.*

nociceptive /nō′sēsep″tiv/ [L, *nocere,* to injure, *capere,* to receive], pertaining to a neural receptor for painful stimuli.

nociceptive reflex [L, *nocere,* to injure, *capere,* to receive, *reflectere,* to bend back], a reflex caused by a painful stimulus.

nociceptive stimulus [L, *nocere,* to injure, *capere,* to receive, *stimulus,* goad], a painful, sometimes detrimental or injurious, stimulus.

nociceptor /nō′sēsep″tər/, a somatic and visceral-free nerve ending of thinly myelinated and unmyelinated fibers. It usually reacts to tissue injury but also may be excited by endogenous chemical substances.

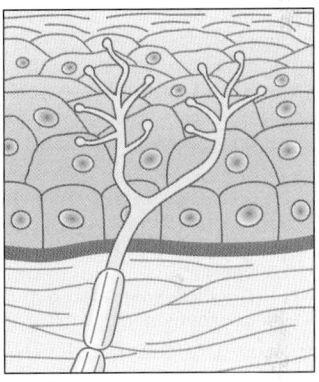

Nociceptors (Patton and Thibodeau, 2016)

no code [AS, *na,* not; L, *caudex,* book], a note written in the patient record and signed by a qualified, usually senior or attending physician instructing the staff of the institution not to attempt to resuscitate a particular patient in the event of cardiac or respiratory failure. This instruction is usually given only when a patient is so gravely ill that death is imminent and inevitable. Also used is DNR ("do not resuscitate"). See also **code,** def. 5.

noct-, prefix meaning "night": *nocturia, nocturnal.*

noctambulation. See **somnambulism.**

nocturia /nokto͞or′ē-ə/ [L, *nocturnus,* by night; Gk, *ouron,* urine], excessive urination at night. It may be a symptom of cardiac, renal, or prostatic disease or bladder outlet obstruction. The condition may also occur in people who drink excessive amounts of fluids, particularly alcohol or coffee, before bedtime or in older patients who have excess body fluids that are mobilized by lying down. Also called **nycturia.** Compare **enuresis.**

nocturnal /noktur′nəl/ [L, *nocturnus,* by night], **1.** pertaining to or occurring during the night. **2.** describing an individual or animal that is active at night and sleeps during the day.

N

nocturnal emission, involuntary emission of semen during sleep, usually in association with an erotic dream. Also called **wet dream.**

nocturnal enuresis [L, *nocturnus,* by night; Gk, *enourein*], involuntary urination while asleep at night.

nocturnal hemoglobinuria. See **hemoglobinuria.**

nocturnal myoclonus, a sleep disorder that usually affects older adults and is marked by thrashing or kicking movements. The condition may be exacerbated by the use of tricyclic depressants used to induce sleep.

nocturnal paroxysmal dyspnea. See **paroxysmal nocturnal dyspnea.**

nocturnal penile tumescence (NPT) [L, *nocturnus,* by night, *penile,* pertaining to the penis, *tumescere,* to begin to swell], a normal condition of penile erection that occurs during sleep throughout most of the lifetime of a male. The occurrence of NPT is important in the diagnosis of impotence because its presence indicates that impotence may be psychogenic.

nod-, prefix meaning "knot": *nodal, nodular, nodule.*

nodal /nō′dəl/ [L, *nodus,* knot], pertaining to a node, particularly the atrioventricular node.

nodal event /nō′dəl/, an occurrence that may cause anxiety, such as birth, death, divorce, marriage, or a child leaving home.

node /nōd/ [L, *nodus,* knot], **1.** a small, rounded mass. **2.** a lymph node. **3.** a single computer terminal in a network of terminals and computers.

nodular /nod″yələr/ [L, *nodus,* knot], (of a structure or mass) small, firm, and knotty. See also **node, nodule.**

nodular circumscribed lipomatosis, a condition in which circumscribed, encapsulated lipomas are distributed around the neck symmetrically, randomly, or like a collar. The adipose deposits may be painful and tender.

nodular cutaneous angiitis, inflammation of small arteries accompanied by skin lesions.

nodular fasciitis, an inflammation of the fascia that causes the formation of nodules.

nodular goiter [L, *nodus,* knot; Gk, *guttur,* throat], an enlarged goiter that contains nodules. It may be toxic and cause hyperthyroidism, or it may be nontoxic. See also **toxic nodular goiter.**

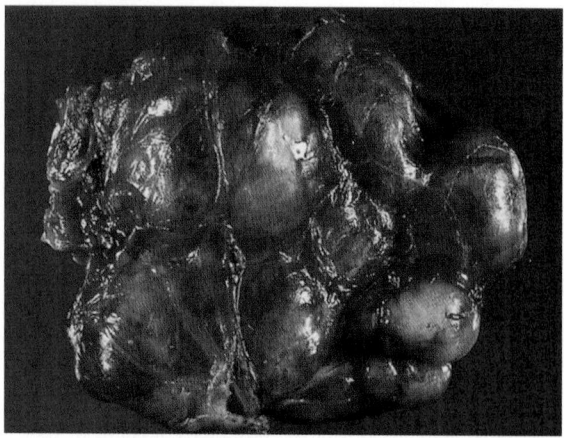

Nodular goiter *(Hagen-Ansert, 2012)*

nodular hyperplasia of the liver, the presence of a regenerative nodule or nodules in the liver.

nodular melanoma, a melanoma that is nodular and uniformly pigmented, usually bluish-black, and sometimes surrounded by an irregular halo of pale, unpigmented skin. The lesion is always raised and may be dome-shaped or polypoid. Most often the tumor is found in middle-aged adults and occurs in 10% to 15% of patients with melanoma. See also **lentigo maligna melanoma, superficial spreading melanoma.**

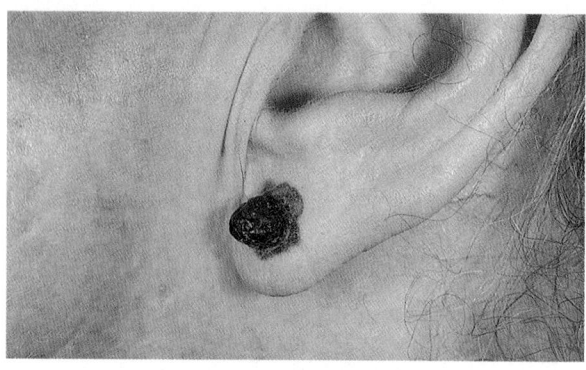

Nodular malignant melanoma *(Courtesy Department of Dermatology, School of Medicine, University of Utah)*

nodule /nod″yo͞ol/ [L, *nodulus,* small knot], **1.** a small node. **2.** a small nodelike structure.

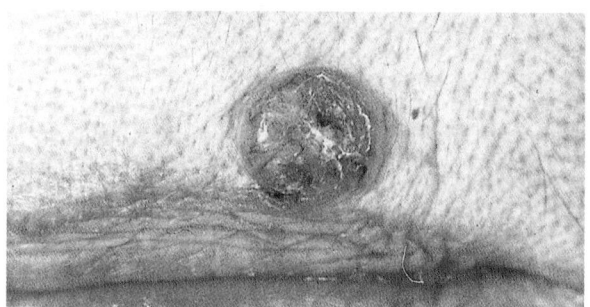

Nodule *(du Vivier, 1993)*

-noia, suffix meaning "(condition of the) mind or will": *paranoia.*

noise, 1. random signals or disturbances that interfere with the normal flow of data through pathways of computers and other electronic devices. **2.** sounds perceived by the auditory system, particularly those that are unpleasant and/or pervasive in the background.

noise-induced hearing loss, a gradual loss of hearing caused by exposure to loud noise over an extended period of time, such as in an individual who works in a noisy environment. The hearing loss is sensorineural in nature and greatest in the higher frequencies. Although an early hearing loss may be temporary, it becomes permanent with increased exposure to noise. Compare **acoustic trauma.**

noise pollution, an unwanted noise level in the environment, causing discomfort and possibly threatening health.

Nolvadex, an antiestrogen drug. Brand name for **tamoxifen.**

noma /nō″mə/ [Gk, *nome,* distribution], an acute, necrotizing ulcerative process involving mucous membranes of the mouth or genitalia. The condition is most commonly seen in severely malnourished, debilitated persons, especially children with poor nutrition and hygiene. There is rapid spreading and painless destruction of bone and soft tissue accompanied by a putrid odor caused by oral anaerobic bacteria, especially *Fusobacterium nucleatum.* Treatment involves high-dose penicillin, debridement, and improved nutrition. Healing eventually occurs, but often with disfiguring defects. Also called **gangrenous stomatitis.**

-noma, suffix meaning "a spreading, invasive gangrene": *adenoma, pelidnoma.*

nomen-, prefix meaning "a name" or "pertaining to names": *nomenclature.*

nomenclature /nō″mənklā′chər, nōmen″-/ [L, *nomen,* name, *clamare,* to call], a consistent, systematic method of naming used in a scientific discipline to denote classifications and avoid ambiguities in names, such as binomial nomenclature in biology and chemical nomenclature in chemistry.

-nomia, suffix meaning "aphasia involving names or naming ability": *anomia, dysautonomia, dysnomia.*

Nomina Anatomica, the book of official international nomenclature for anatomy as designated by the International Congress of Anatomists.

nominal aphasia /nom′inəl/ [L, *nomen* + Gk, *a* + *phasis,* without speech], a type of speech disorder in which the person uses incorrect names in identifying objects. Minor episodes may result from anxiety, fatigue, or senility. Severe cases can indicate a focal lesion on the left side of the brain.

nominal damages, (in law) a very small monetary award, indicating that a plaintiff is correct but has not suffered any substantial injury or loss requiring compensation. See **damages.**

nominal data. See **categoric data.**

nomo-, prefix meaning "usage or law": *nomogram.*

nomogram /nom″əgram, nō″mə-/ [Gk, *nomos,* law, *gramma,* a record], **1.** a graphic representation, by any of various systems, of a numeric relationship. **2.** a graph on which a number of variables are plotted so that the value of a dependent variable can be read on the appropriate line when the values of the other variables are given.

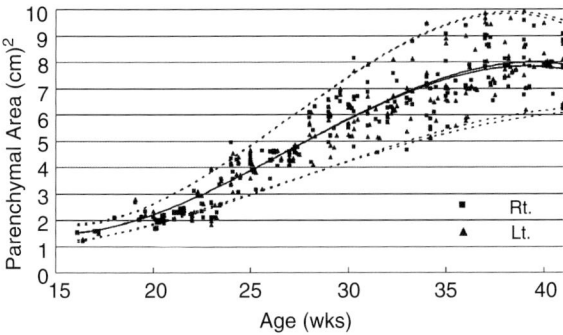

Nomogram of parenchymal area growth *(Shin et al, 2007)*

-nomy, suffix meaning "received knowledge in a field": *physiognomy.*

non-, prefix meaning "not": *noninvasive, noncompliant.*

nona-, noni-, prefix meaning "nine": *nonigravida, nonipara.*

nonabsorbable surgical sutures /nonəbsôr″bəbəl/ [L, *non,* not, *absorbere* + Gk, *cheirourgos,* surgeon; L, *sutura*], sutures of silk, nylon, steel, or other materials that resist absorption. They are used mainly in deep tissues, where it is important for them to remain in place.

nonadherent cell /-ədhir″ənt/, a cell such as a lymphocyte that will not adhere to a smooth surface of laboratory equipment.

nonadherent dressing [L, *non* + *adhesio,* sticking to; OFr, *dresser,* to arrange], a dressing designed specifically not to stick to the dried secretions of a wound.

nonadhesive skin traction /-ədhē″siv/ [L, *non,* not, *adhesio,* sticking to], a type of skin traction in which the therapeutic pull of traction weights is applied over the body structure involved with foam-backed traction straps that do not stick to the skin. Nonadhesive skin traction straps may be easily removed to facilitate skin care and are usually used when continuous traction is not required. The straps decrease the patient's vulnerability to skin breakdown by spreading the traction pull over a wide area of skin surface. Compare **adhesive skin traction.**

nonalcoholic fatty liver disease (NAFLD), the accumulation of excess fat in the liver cells of individuals who do not have a history of alcohol abuse. It is most common in people over 50 with obesity, diabetes, or both. In early stages there are usually no symptoms other than abnormal liver function tests. As the disease progresses, physical symptoms are variable and include fatigue, memory loss, and fluid retention. Also called **hepatic steatosis.**

non-A, non-B hepatitis. See **hepatitis C.**

nonbacterial prostatitis, prostatitis with pain and increased numbers of inflammatory cells but without history of urinary tract infection.

nonbacterial thrombotic endocarditis /-baktir″ē·əl/ [L, *non* + *bakerion,* small rod], one of the three main types of endocarditis, characterized by various kinds of lesions affecting the heart valves, most often on the left side of the heart. The disease may be the first step in the development of bacterial endocarditis, and the lesions may cause peripheral arterial embolisms, resulting in death. The disease equally affects men and women between 18 and 90 years of age and causes heart murmurs in about 30% of cases. There is no successful treatment, but anticoagulation therapy may be used to reduce the incidence of peripheral arterial embolism. See also **Libman-Sacks endocarditis.**

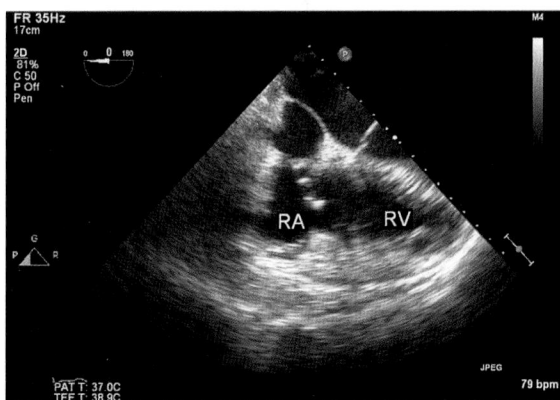

Transesophageal echocardiogram showing thickening of the tricuspid leaflets associated with nonbacterial thrombotic endocarditis *(© 2010 American Society of Echocardiography)*

nonbinary, an individual whose gender identity is neither exclusively male nor female.

noncardiogenic pulmonary edema. See **adult respiratory distress syndrome.**

noncellulose polysaccharides /-sel″yəlōs/, food substances such as hemicellulose, pectins, gums, mucilages, and algal products that absorb water and swell to a larger bulk. They slow emptying of food from the stomach, bind bile acids, provide fermentation material for the colon, and prevent spastic colon pressure.

noncommunicating hydrocephalus. See **hydrocephalus.**

noncompetitive inhibition /-kəmpet″itiv/, (in pharmacology) a form of inhibition in which a substance (drug) occupying a receptor cannot be displaced from the receptor by increasing the number of other molecules through the principle of mass action. The drug is irreversibly bound to the receptor.

noncompliant, *adj.,* describing an unwillingness to adhere to a prescribed plan of care. Causes are multifactorial and often related to an unrealistic or inappropriate prescription by the health care provider.

non compos mentis /non″ kom′pos men″tis/ [L, not of sound mind], a legal term applied to a person declared to be mentally incompetent.

noncontact (air-puff) tonometry, an eye test that uses a puff of air to estimate intraocular pressure. No anesthesia is required to administer the test.

nondepolarizing blocking agent, a compound that causes paralysis of skeletal muscle by blocking neural transmission at the neuromuscular junction. It acts by competitive binding to and inactivation of the cholinergic receptors of the motor end plate without depolarizing the postsynaptic membrane.

nondirective therapy /-direk″tiv/ [L, *non + digere,* to direct], a psychotherapeutic approach in which the psychotherapist refrains from giving advice or interpretation as the client is helped to identify conflicts and to clarify and understand feelings and values. Compare **directive therapy.** See also **client-centered therapy.**

nondisjunction /-disjungk″chən/ [L, *non + disjungere,* to disjoint], failure of homologous pairs of chromosomes to separate during the first meiotic division or of the two chromatids of a chromosome to split during anaphase of mitosis or the second meiotic division. The result is an abnormal number of chromosomes in the daughter cells. Compare **disjunction.** See also **monosomy, trisomy.**

nonessential amino acid /-esen″shəl/, any amino acids that are not essential to the diet because the body can synthesize their molecules from other amino acids. See also **amino acid, essential amino acid.**

nonfat milk. See **skimmed milk.**

nonfeasance /nonfē″zəns/ [L, *non + facere,* to do], a failure to perform a task, duty, or undertaking that one has agreed to perform or has a legal duty to perform. Compare **malfeasance, misfeasance.** See also **negligence.**

nonfluent aphasia, difficulty in communicating orally and with written words. Also called **motor aphasia.**

nongonococcal urethritis (NGU) /-gon′əkok″əl/ [L, *non + Gk, gone,* seed, *kokkos,* berry], an infectious condition of the urethra in males that is characterized by mild dysuria and a small to moderate amount of penile discharge. The discharge may be white or clear, thin or mucoid, or, less often, purulent. The infection is often caused by the obligate intracellular parasite *Chlamydia trachomatis.* Untreated NGU may result in urethral stricture, epididymitis, proctitis, and chronic inflammation of the urethra. Women exposed to the exudate during coitus may develop a hypertrophic erosion of the cervix and purulent cervical mucus. An infant passing through the cervix and vagina of a mother infected with *C. trachomatis* may develop conjunctivitis and nasopharyngeal infection in the first few days after birth and pneumonia at 3 to 4 months. Diagnosis of NGU is made by excluding gonococcal urethritis through microscopic examination and bacteriological culture of the exudate. Nearly 50% of all cases of urethritis are nongonococcal. Most cases of

NGU are successfully treated with tetracycline or erythromycin. Sexual contacts are treated whether or not they are symptomatic.

nonheme iron /non″hēm/, one of two forms of dietary iron. It is less efficiently absorbed than heme iron. All plant food sources and 60% of animal food sources contain nonheme iron.

nonhemolytic jaundice /-hē′məlit″ik/ [L, *non* + Gk, *haima,* blood, *lysein,* to loosen; Fr, *jaune,* yellow], a form of jaundice that is caused by a liver disease rather than the destruction of red blood cells.

non-Hodgkin lymphoma (NHL) /- hoj″kən/, a diverse group of malignant solid tumors of peripheral lymphoid tissue, distinguished from Hodgkin lymphoma by the absence of Reed-Sternberg cells. The most common manifestation is a painless enlargement of one or more peripheral lymph nodes. The prevalence of Hodgkin lymphoma peaks at 50 years of age and may be mild or aggressively malignant, depending upon cell category.

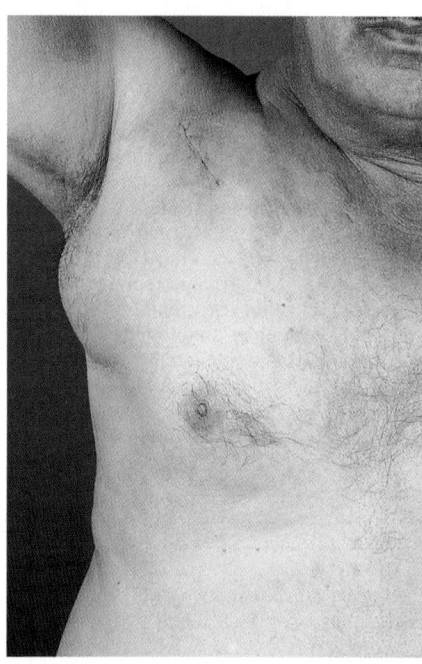

Enlargement of axillary nodes associated with non-Hodgkin lymphoma *(Hoffbrand, Pettit, and Vyas, 2010)*

nonigravida /nō′nigrav″idə/ [L, *nonus,* nine, *gravidus,* pregnancy], a woman pregnant for the ninth time.

noni juice, the juice of *Morinda citrifolia.* Although the juice is often promoted for health benefits, there is no evidence of effectiveness in preventing or treating disease.

noninfective valvular mass /-infek″tiv/, a growth or swelling on one of the heart valves associated with autoimmune diseases or with cardiac or extracardiac malignancies. Such masses are frequently asymptomatic and are discovered only at autopsy.

noninflammatory diarrhea /-inflam″ətôr″ē/, a profuse watery diarrhea without fever or vomiting that begins 6 to 24 hours after ingesting food contaminated by bacterial toxins produced by either *Clostridium perfringens* or *Bacillus cereus.* The food poisoning usually involves raw meat or other proteinaceous foods exposed to warm temperatures for several hours.

non–insulin-dependent diabetes mellitus. See **type 2 diabetes mellitus.**

noninvasive /-invā″siv/ [L, *non* + *in,* into, *vadere,* to go], pertaining to a diagnostic or therapeutic technique that does not require the skin to be broken or a cavity or organ of the body to be entered, for obtaining a blood pressure reading by auscultation with a stethoscope and sphygmomanometer.

noninvasive ventilation, mechanical ventilation that does not use an artificial airway, such as positive pressure ventilation with a nasal or face mask.

nonionic /-ī·on′ik/, pertaining to compounds without a net negative or positive charge.

nonionizing radiation /-ī″ənī′zing/ [L, *non* + Gk, *ion,* going, *izein,* to cause], radiation for which the mechanism of action in tissue does not directly ionize atomic or molecular systems through a single interaction.

nonipara /nōnip″ərə/ [L, *nonus,* nine, *parere,* to bear], a woman who has given birth to nine offspring.

nonketotic hyperglycinemia /nonkētot′ik/, a usually fatal autosomal-recessive aminoacidopathy with accumulation of glycine in body fluids, particularly the blood, urine, and cerebrospinal fluid. It has neonatal onset and is characterized by lethargy, metabolic acidosis with ketosis, absence of cerebral development, seizures, myoclonic jerks, and frequently coma and respiratory failure. It is caused by a defect in one or more of the enzymes involved in the cleavage of glycine. Also called **methylmalonicacidemia, propionicacidemia.**

nonmyelinated nerve fiber /-mī″əlinā′tid/ [L, *non* + Gk, *myelos,* marrow; L, *nervus,* nerve, *fibra,* fiber], a nerve fiber that lacks the fatty myelin insulating sheath. Such fibers form the gray matter of the nervous system, as distinguished from the white matter of myelinated fibers. Also called *nonmedullated nerve fiber.*

Nonne-Milroy-Meige syndrome. See **Milroy disease.**

nonnucleoside reverse transcriptase inhibitors (NNRTI), a class of antiretroviral drugs that inhibit human immunodeficiency virus replication by blocking the reverse transcriptase enzyme essential for viral replication. These drugs have a different mechanism of action and side-effect profile from other reverse transcriptase inhibitors. See also **nucleoside reverse transcriptase inhibitors.**

nonnutritive sucking, an infant contracting the muscles of the lip and mouth to make a partial vacuum with a thumb, fingers, hand, a pacifier, or other inanimate object for comfort.

nonnutritive sweetener /-nōō″tritiv/, a chemical additive such as saccharin, aspartame, acesulfame, or sucralose that gives a sweet taste to foods without contributing significant calories. The sugar substitute is either not metabolized or so intensely sweet that the calorie count is negligible.

nonorganic hearing loss. See **functional hearing loss.**

nonossifying fibroma /-os″ifī′ing/, a sharply circumscribed, eccentrically located lesion in the metaphyses of long bones in children. Microscopic examination reveals whorl patterns of spindle cells, fibrous tissue, numerous xanthoma cells, and occasional giant cells.

nonosteogenic fibroma /-non′ostē·əjen″ik/, a common bone lesion characterized by degeneration and proliferation of the medullary and cortical tissue near the ends of the diaphyses of the large long bones of the lower extremities. Frequently the lesion causes no symptoms and is only discovered during radiographic examination of the skeleton for other reasons.

nonpalpable testis /-pal″pəbəl/, a testis that cannot be felt and may be intraabdominal or absent.

nonparametric test of significance /-per′əmet″rik/ [L, *non* + Gk, *para,* beside, *metron,* measure], (in statistics) one of several tests that uses a qualitative approach to analyze rank order data and incidence data that cannot be assumed to have a normal distribution. Kinds include **chi square, Spearman's rho.**

nonparous /-per″əs/ [L, *non* + *parere,* to bear], indicating a woman who has never given birth to a child. Also called **nulliparous.**

nonpenetrating wound /-pen″ətrā′ting/ [L, *non,* not, *penetrare,* to penetrate; AS, *wund*], a wound that does not break the surface of the skin. Also spelled *non-penetrating wound.*

nonpermissive host /-pərmis″iv/, an animal or cell that resists the replication of an infectious agent.

nonpneumatic antishock garment, a multisectioned garment for the lower half of the body, fashioned from flexible materials and Velcro. It is used to treat shock and to stabilize and prevent further bleeding in women with obstetric hemorrhage who do not have access to a hospital.

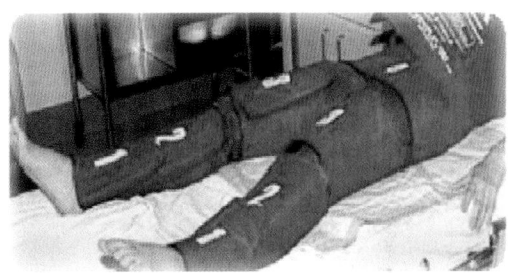

Full application of the nonpneumatic antishock garment *(Lester et al, 2011)*

nonpolar /-pō″lər/ [L, *non* + *polus,* pole], pertaining to molecules that have low polarity and have a hydrophobic affinity, tending to exclude or avoid water. Nonpolar substances tend to dissolve in nonpolar solvents. Compare **polar.**

nonpolar solvent /-pō″lər/, a liquid solvent without significant partial charges on any atoms, as in the hydrocarbons, or where the polar bonds are arranged in such a way that the effects of their partial charges cancel out, as in carbon tetrachloride. Liquid hydrocarbons are the most common examples. Also called **fat solvent.**

nonproductive cough /-prəduk″tiv/ [L, *non* + *producere,* to produce], a sudden, noisy expulsion of air from the lungs that may be caused by irritation or inflammation and does not remove sputum from the respiratory tract. In patients with respiratory tract infections, the condition may be treated by administering expectorants such as ammonium chloride, ammonium carbonate, sodium iodide, potassium iodide, ipecac, or terpin hydrate, which "liquefy" respiratory tract secretions and may result in productive coughing. If suppression of coughing is required (when there is no sputum to be expelled), antitussives that depress the cough reflex may be prescribed, including codeine or dextromethorphan. Intratracheal suctioning may be necessary when secretions cause severe respiratory difficulty and coughing is unproductive. Compare **productive cough.**

nonproductive infection. See **abortive infection.**

nonproprietary name /-prəprī″əter′ē/ [L, *non* + *proprietas,* owner, *nomen,* name], the chemical or generic name of a drug or device, as distinguished from a brand name or trademark. A nonproprietary name may be indicated by the letters *USAN,* for United States Adopted Names, or by *INN,* for International Nonproprietary Names, used in Canada and elsewhere. See also *USAN.*

nonprotein nitrogen (NPN) /-prō′tēn/ [L, *non* + Gk, *proteios,* first rank, *nitron,* soda, *genein,* to produce], the

N

nitrogen in the blood that is not a constituent of protein, such as the nitrogen associated with urea, uric acid, creatine, and polypeptides. Approximately one half of the nonprotein nitrogen in the blood is associated with urea.

nonrapid eye movement, the position of the eyes during sleep with the eyes closed and the body at rest but not in deep sleep. Compare **rapid eye movement. See also sleep.**

nonreassuring fetal status (NRFS), indirect measurements of intrauterine fetal status (such as fetal heart rate, fetal blood gas determinations, amniotic fluid volume estimations, and intrauterine fetal response to external stimulation) that are suggestive of fetal oxygenation that could result in serious neonatal complications.

nonrebreather /non′rēbrēth′ər/, (Informal) a breathing system having one-way valves so that exhaled carbon dioxide is expelled from the system and not inhaled again.

nonreflex bladder. See **flaccid bladder.**

nonresponse bias, (in epidemiology) errors that may develop when a part of those selected and identified as study subjects cannot or will not participate in the study. The bias may occur when the group of nonrespondents differs systematically from respondents with respect to exposure or disease status. To minimize this bias, a high participation rate is necessary, or a survey is made of nonresponders to determine whether or how they might differ with regard to the risk of disease or exposure.

nonreversible inhibitor /-rivur″səbəl/ [L, non + revertere, to turn back, inhibere, to restrain], an effector substance that binds permanently to an active site of an enzyme, inhibiting the normal catalytic activity of the enzyme.

nonsecretor /-səkrē′tər/ [L, non + secernere, to separate], a person who does not secrete ABO blood group substances in mucous secretions of the saliva or gastric juice. The condition is genetically determined.

nonseg, abbreviation for *nonsegmented.*

nonseminomatous testicular tumors /-sem′inom″ətəs/, any of a variety of histological types of testicular carcinoma, including embryonal cell carcinoma, teratocarcinoma, and tumors with mixed elements. Treatment for most cases depends on the stage of the cancer at the time of diagnosis.

nonsense mutation, a mutation in which one of the three terminator codons in the mRNA used to signal the end of a polypeptide appears in the middle of a genetic message and causes premature termination of transcription and release of incomplete, generally nonfunctional polypeptides from the ribosome. Kinds include **amber mutation, ochre mutation, opal mutation.**

nonsexual generation. See **asexual reproduction.**

nonshivering thermogenesis /-shiv′əring/, a natural method by which newborns can produce body heat by increasing their metabolic rate.

non–small cell carcinoma, a general term comprising all lung carcinomas except small cell carcinoma, including adenocarcinoma of the lung, large cell carcinoma, and squamous cell carcinoma.

non–small cell carcinoma of lung, a major category of histological types of lung carcinomas, including adenocarcinoma of the lung, large cell carcinoma, and squamous cell carcinoma. Treatment depends on the stage of development of the cancer at the time of initial presentation. The treatment of choice for otherwise physically fit patients with early stages of disease is resection.

nonspecific binding (NSB) /-spəsif″ik/, in ligand binding assay, the part of a tracer used in a competitive-binding assay that is found in the bound fraction, independent of the binding reaction.

nonspecific immunosuppression, a therapy, including the use of immunosuppressive drugs and high doses of radiation, that blunts or abolishes the response of the immune system to all antigens.

nonspecific urethritis (NSU) [L, non, not, species, form], inflammation of the urethra of unknown origin. Onset of symptoms is often related to sexual intercourse. The acute phase of NSU is seldom seen in women, but the chronic phase is a common urological difficulty among women. The condition is noted by urethral discharge in men and by reddening of the urethral mucosa in women. Treatment with antibiotics is not always successful. See also **nongonococcal urethritis.**

nonspecific vaginitis [L, non, not, species, form, facere, to make, vagina, sheath; Gk, itis, inflammation], a term formerly used for any vaginal inflammation for which no specific pathogen could be identified. Most cases of vaginitis today are found to be caused by infections of *Gardnerella vaginalis* in combination with anaerobic bacteria, although nearly one third of all cases are caused by a protozoa, *Trichomonas vaginalis.*

nonspecular reflection, diffuse ultrasound reflections (scatter) at rough surfaces or irregular boundaries.

nonspherocytic hemolytic anemia. See **congenital nonspherocytic hemolytic anemia.**

nonsteroidal antiinflammatory drug (NSAID) /-stir″oidəl/, any of a group of drugs having antipyretic, analgesic, and antiinflammatory effects. They counteract or reduce inflammation by inhibiting cyclooxygenase, the enzyme responsible for prostaglandin synthesis. NSAIDs may be indicated in the treatment of mild-to-moderate pain, rheumatoid arthritis, osteoarthritis, ankylosing spondylosis, gouty arthritis, fever, nonrheumatic inflammation, and dysmenorrhea. Classic examples include aspirin, ibuprofen, and ketoprofen. Drugs such as celecoxib, refecoxib, and valdecoxib selectively block only the inductible form of cyclooxygenase (COX-2), the form of the enzyme that appears in cells at sites of inflammation.

nonstress test (NST) /non″stres/, an evaluation of the fetal heart rate response to natural contractile activity or to an increase in fetal activity. Also called *fetal activity determination.*

nonsuppurative osteomyelitis /-sup″yərā′tiv/, tuberculosis of the bone.

nonthrombocytopenic purpura /-throm′bōsī″təpē′nik/, a disorder characterized by purplish or reddish skin areas. The condition does not involve a decrease in the number of platelets.

nontoxic /-tok′sik/, not poisonous. See also **atoxic.**

nontreponemal antigen test, any of various tests detecting serum antibodies to reagin (cardiolipin and lecithin) derived from host tissue in the diagnosis of the *Treponema pallidum* infection of syphilis.

nontropical sprue /-trop′ikəl/ [L, non, not; Gk, tropikos, of the solstice; D, sprouw], a malabsorption syndrome resulting from an inborn inability to digest foods that contain gluten. See also **celiac disease, tropical sprue.**

nonulcerative blepharitis /-ul″sərətiv′/ [L, non + ilcus, ulcer; Gk, blepharon, eyelid, itis, inflammation], a form of blepharitis characterized by greasy scales on the margins of the eyelids around the lashes and hyperemia and thickening of the skin. Nonulcerative blepharitis is often associated with seborrheic dermatitis.

nonunion /-yoo̅′nyən/, pertaining to a fractured bone that fails to heal properly. See also **false joint.**

nonvascularized graft, a graft in which the blood supply to the grafted tissue is not maintained.

nonvenereal syphilis.   See **endemic syphilis.**

nonverbal communication /-vur″bəl/,   the transmission of a message without the use of words. It may involve any or all of the five senses. See also **body language.**

nonviable /-vī″əbəl/   [L, *non* + *vita,* life],   unable to exist independently after birth.

nonvital bleaching,   a procedure in which an oxidizing agent is placed directly within the pulp chamber of a nonvital tooth and sealed closed for a short period of time. This results in lightening the shade of tooth color of a nonvital tooth.

nonvital pulp   [L, *non,* not, *vita,* life, *pulpa,* flesh],   dead dental pulp caused by a disease or trauma that interferes with the blood supply. Also called **dead pulp.**

nonvital tooth.   See **pulpless tooth.**

Noonan syndrome,   the phenotype of Turner syndrome (webbed neck, ptosis, hypogonadism, congenital heart disease, and short stature) without gonadal dysgenesis. Formerly called male Turner syndrome until the female counterpart was identified.

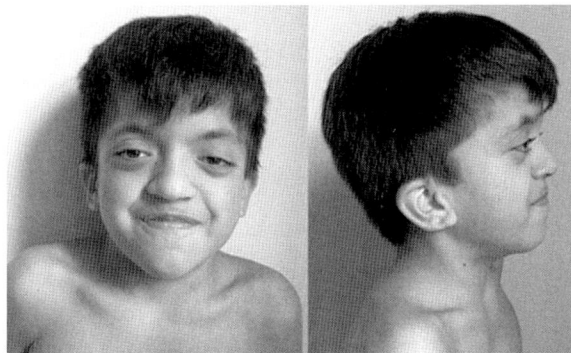

Young boy with the characteristic appearance of Noonan syndrome (Courtesy of M.A. Patton)

nootropic /nō·ətrop″ik/,   a chemical designed to increase brain metabolism.

Norcuron,   an IV neuromuscular blocking drug. Brand name for **vecuronium bromide.**

norepinephrine (NE) /nôr′epinef″rin/,   an adrenergic hormone (catecholamine) that acts to increase blood pressure by vasoconstriction but does not affect cardiac output. It is synthesized by the adrenal medulla, the peripheral sympathetic nerves, and the central nervous system. It is available as a drug, levarterenol, which is used to maintain the blood pressure in acute hypotension secondary to trauma, heart disease, or vascular collapse.

norepinephrine bitartrate,   a commercial preparation of an endogenous agonist of alpha$_1$, alpha$_2$, and beta$_1$ adrenergic.
- INDICATIONS: It is prescribed in the treatment of shock that persists after hypovolemia has been corrected.
- CONTRAINDICATIONS: Known hypersensitivity to this drug or bisulfite preservatives prohibits its use. Hypovolemia and vascular thrombosis are contraindications unless it is used as a short-term lifesaving procedure to maintain perfusion of vital organs. It is not used in conjunction with cyclopropane or halothane anesthesia because of the increased risk of arrhythmia.
- ADVERSE EFFECTS: Among the more serious adverse effects are local tissue necrosis at the site of injection, bradycardia, and headache. Overdosage can cause hypertension, periph-

eral or cardiac ischemia or infarctions, hemorrhagic strokes, and convulsions.

no response (NR),   the condition in which the maximum decrease in treated tumor volume is less than 50%.

norethindrone /nôreth″indrōn/,   a progestin.
- INDICATIONS: It is prescribed in the treatment of abnormal uterine bleeding and endometriosis and is used alone or as a component in oral contraceptive medications.
- CONTRAINDICATIONS: Thrombophlebitis, liver dysfunction, unusual vaginal bleeding, breast cancer, or known hypersensitivity to this drug prohibits its use. It is not recommended for use during pregnancy and should be used with caution in patients with asthma, diabetes, cardiac or renal dysfunction, hyperlipidemia, migraines, seizure disorders, or psychic depression.
- ADVERSE EFFECTS: Among the more serious adverse effects are breakthrough bleeding, amenorrhea, GI disturbances, breast changes, and masculinization of the female fetus. The drug should be discontinued immediately if vision problems (e.g., double vision, complete or partial loss of vision) or migraine headaches appear. Progestin-only contraceptives have a higher rate of failure.

norethindrone acetate and ethinyl estradiol,   a combination oral contraceptive containing a progestin (norethindrone) and an estrogen (ethinyl estradiol).
- INDICATIONS: It is prescribed for contraception, for the treatment of acne, for moderate to severe vasomotor symptoms in menopause, and for the prevention of osteoporosis in postmenopausal women at high risk. Unlabeled uses include hypermenorrhea, endometriosis, and female hypogonadism.
- CONTRAINDICATIONS: Thrombophlebitis, severe hypertension, coronary artery disease, diabetes with vascular complications, migraine headaches, breast or reproductive organ cancer, unusual vaginal bleeding, gallbladder disease, liver dysfunction or tumor, or known hypersensitivity to this drug prohibits its use. It is not given during lactation, pregnancy, or suspected pregnancy or to women over the age of 35 who smoke more than 15 cigarettes per day.
- ADVERSE EFFECTS: Among the more serious adverse effects are thrombophlebitis, embolism, hypertension, myocardial infarction, cerebrovascular accident, depression, headache, premenstrual syndrome, cramps, breakthrough bleeding, porphyria, embolism, jaundice, and gallbladder disease.

Norflex,   a skeletal muscle relaxant with anticholinergic properties. Brand name for **orphenadrine citrate.**

norfloxacin /nôrflok″səsin/,   an oral antibacterial drug.
- INDICATIONS: It is prescribed for the treatment of bacterial urinary tract infections, sexually transmitted gonorrhea, and proctitis.
- CONTRAINDICATIONS: Hypersensitivity to quinolones or pregnancy or lactation prohibits its use. It should be used with caution in patients younger than 18 years because of arthropathy. Concomitant use of nitrofurantoin drugs is not recommended, and concomitant use of corticosteroids can increase the risk of arthropathy in the elderly.
- ADVERSE EFFECTS: Typical side effects include nausea, dizziness, and headache. Severe hypersensitivity reactions, tendon rupture, and numerous other effects have been reported with relatively low incidence.

Norgesic Forte,   a fixed-combination drug that includes muscle relaxant with anticholinergic activity. The drug is used for the relief of mild or moderate pain from acute musculoskeletal disorders. Brand name for **orphenadrine citrate, aspirin, caffeine.**

norgestimate /nor-jes′t-māt/, a synthetic progestational agent used in combination with an estrogen component as an oral contraceptive.

norgestrel /nôrjes″trəl/, a progestin.

■ INDICATIONS: It is prescribed alone or in combination with estrogen as a contraceptive.

■ CONTRAINDICATIONS: Thrombophlebitis, liver dysfunction, unusual vaginal bleeding, breast cancer, or known hypersensitivity to this drug prohibits its use. The drug should be used with caution in patients with a history of depression.

■ ADVERSE EFFECTS: Among the more serious adverse effects are thrombophlebitis, embolism, depression, amenorrhea, dysfunctional uterine bleeding, breast changes, and masculinization of a female fetus. It should be discontinued immediately if vision changes, such as a complete or partial loss of vision or double vision, occur.

Norinyl, several formulations of oral contraceptives containing a progestin (norethindrone) and an estrogen (mestranol or ethinyl estradiol). Brand name for **norethindrone, mestranol, ethinyl estradiol.**

norm [L, *norma*, rule], **1.** a measure of a phenomenon generally accepted as the ideal standard performance against which other measures of the phenomenon may be measured. **2.** abbreviation for **normal.**

norma basalis /nôr″mə basā″lis/ [L, rule; Gk, *basis*, foundation], the inferior surface of the base of the skull with the mandible removed, formed by the palatine bones, the vomer, the pterygoid processes, and parts of the sphenoid and temporal bones.

normal (N, norm) /nôr′məl/ [L, *norma*, rule], **1.** describing a standard, average, or typical example of a set of objects or values. **2.** describing a chemical solution in which 1 L contains 1 g of a substance or the equivalent in replaceable hydrogen ions. **3.** describing people in a nondiseased population. **4.** a gaussian distribution.

-normal, suffix meaning "relating to a norm": *paranormal.*

normal curve. See **bell-shaped curve.**

normal dental function, the correct and healthy action of opposing teeth during chewing. Compare **occlusion.**

normal diet. See **regular diet.**

normal distribution, (in statistics) a theoretic distribution frequency of variable data usually represented graphically by a bell-shaped curve that reaches a peak about the mean.

normal dwarf. See **primordial dwarf.**

normal flora. See **flora.**

normal human serum albumin, an isotonic preparation of pooled human serum albumin for treating hypoproteinemia, hypovolemia, and threatened or existing shock.

normal hydrogen electrode. See **standard hydrogen electrode.**

normal last shoes, orthopedic shoes for infants and children constructed with a normal sole.

normal phase, a chromatographic mode in which the mobile phase is less polar than the stationary phase.

normal pressure hydrocephalus [L, *norma*, rule, *premere*, to press; Gk, *hydor*, water, *kephale*, head], a condition in which there is dilation of the ventricles without an increase in intracranial pressure. Classic symptoms are gait disturbance, memory/cognitive problems, and urinary incontinence. Diagnosis is made by lumbar puncture to remove cerebrospinal fluid and by watching to see if any of the symptoms improve.

normal saline, 9 grams of sodium chloride dissolved in water to a total volume of 1000 mL. The percentage of sodium chloride is 0.9%. Also called **physiological saline.**

normal saline solution [L, *norma*, rule, *sal* + *solutus,* dissolved], a 0.9% w/v (grams of solute per milliliter of solution) sterile solution of sodium chloride in water that is isotonic with blood and injectable intravenously.

normal salt solution. See **normal saline solution.**

normal sinus rhythm (NSR) [L, *norma*, rule, *sinus,* hollow; Gk, *rhythmos*], the normal heartbeat initiated by the pacemaker in the sinus node, with a heart rate of 60 to 100 beats/min.

normal solution (N/I, N) [L, *norma*, rule, *solutus,* dissolved], a solution that contains the gram-equivalent weight of a reagent per liter.

normal strain, a quantity described by the quotient of the change of length of a line and its original length.

normal stress, (in physics) a quantity described by the quotient of distributed force and area when the force is perpendicular to the area.

normal temperature [L, *norma*, rule, *temperatura*], for a normal person at rest, an oral clinical temperature of 98.6° F or 37° C. Actual "normal" temperatures may range a fraction of a degree or increments of a whole degree higher or lower because of effects of sleep, exercise, eating, sleeping, metabolism, and the ambient temperature. Rectal temperature average a fraction of a degree higher than oral temperatures. Axillary and temporal readings are usually lower than oral temperatures.

normo-, prefix meaning "normal": *normoblast, normotensive.*

normoblast /nôr″məblast/ [L, *norma* + Gk, *blastos,* germ], nucleated bone marrow red blood cell precursor. Developmental stages include the pronormoblast, the basophilic normoblast, the polychromatophilic normoblast, and the orthochromic normoblast. After the extrusion of the nucleus of the normoblast, the young erythrocyte becomes known as a reticulocyte and enters the circulating blood. Compare **erythrocyte.** See also **reticulocyte.**

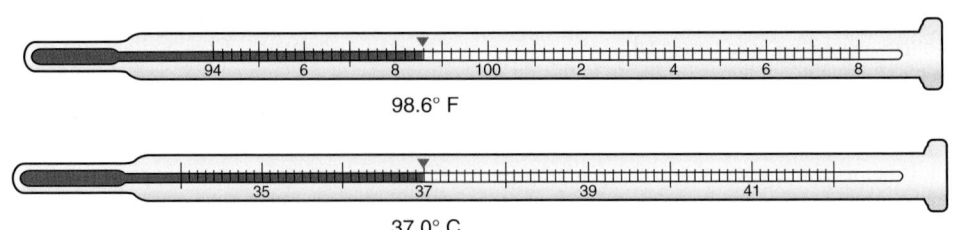

Normal temperature readings (Sorrentino and Remmert, 2012)

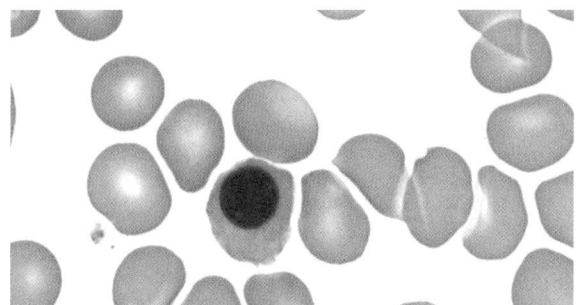

Normoblast from bone marrow smear *(Young, O'Dowd, and Woodford, 2014)*

normochromic /nôr′məkrō″mik/ [L, + Gk, color], pertaining to a blood cell having normal color resulting from the presence of an adequate amount of hemoglobin. Compare **hypochromic.** See also **red cell indexes.**

normocyte /nôr″məsīt/ [L, *norma* + Gk, *kytos,* cell], an ordinary, normal adult red blood cell of average size having a diameter of 7 μm. Compare **macrocyte, microcyte.**

Normodyne, an antihypertensive drug. Brand name for **labetalol hydrochloride.**

normoglycemic /-glīsē″mik/, pertaining to a normal blood glucose level.

normotensive /-ten″siv/, pertaining to the condition of having normal blood pressure. Normal blood pressure is typically 120/80 but may be lower in younger individuals or athletes.

normoventilation /-ven′tilā″shən/, the alveolar ventilation rate that produces an alveolar carbon dioxide pressure of about 40 mm Hg at any metabolic rate.

normoxia /nôrmok″sē·ə/, an ambient oxygen pressure of about 150 (plus or minus 10) torr or the partial pressure of oxygen in atmospheric air at sea level.

Noroxin, an oral antibacterial drug. Brand name for **norfloxacin.**

Norpace, an antidysrhythmic cardiac depressant. Brand name for **disopyramide phosphate.**

Norpramin, an antidepressant drug. Brand name for **desipramine hydrochloride.**

Nor-QD, an oral contraceptive containing a progestin but no estrogen. Brand name for **norethindrone.**

North American blastomycosis, an infection caused by inhaling the fungus *Blastomyces dermatitidis.* It may resemble bacterial pneumonia, and x-ray films of the chest may show cavities. Painless, well-demarcated verrucous or ulcerated skin lesions occur on the face and hands. Occasionally lesions of the oral mucous membrane may be mistaken for squamous cell carcinoma. The disease may progress to involve bones and the brain; many viscera are infected in fatal cases. Diagnosis is made by microscopic examination of body secretions. Treatment is ketoconazole/itraconazole or amphotericin B given intravenously, depending on the severity, or in the most severe cases a combination of amphotericin B and sulfonamides. Also called **Gilchrist disease.** Compare **paracoccidioidomycosis.**

North American coral snake antivenin, antivenin to *Micrurus fulvius.*

North American Nursing Diagnosis Association (NANDA), a professional organization of registered nurses created in 1982. The purpose of the organization is "to develop, refine, and promote a taxonomy of nursing diagnostic terminology of general use to the professional."

North Asian tick-borne rickettsiosis, an infection, acquired in the Eastern Hemisphere, caused by *Rickettsia*

sibirica, transmitted by ticks. It resembles Rocky Mountain spotted fever. Usual findings include a generalized maculopapular rash involving palms and soles, fever, and lymph node enlargement. It is rarely fatal and responds quickly to treatment with chloramphenicol. No vaccine is available. Compare **Rocky Mountain spotted fever.** See also **boutonneuse fever, relapsing fever.**

North Asian tick typhus. See **Siberian tick typhus.**

Northern blot test, an electrophoretic test for identifying the presence or absence of particular mRNA molecules and nucleic acid hybridization. See also **Southern blot test.**

Norton risk scale /nor′tən/, a tool for estimating a patient's risk for developing pressure ulcers. The patient is rated from 1 to 4 on five different factors, with a score of 14 or more indicating high risk.

nortriptyline hydrochloride /nôrtrip″tilēn/, a tricyclic antidepressant.

■ INDICATIONS: It is prescribed in the treatment of mental depression. Unlabeled uses include chronic pain, anxiety, enuresis, and attention-deficit/hyperactivity disorder.

■ CONTRAINDICATIONS: Concomitant administration of monoamine oxidase inhibitors, recent myocardial infarction, pregnancy or known hypersensitivity to this drug or to other tricyclic medications prohibits its use. It is used with caution in patients who have a seizure disorder or a cardiovascular disease.

■ ADVERSE EFFECTS: Among the more serious adverse effects are sedation and GI, cardiovascular, and neurological reactions. It interacts with many other drugs.

Norvir, a protease inhibitor. Brand name for **ritonavir.**

Norwalk agent [Norwalk, Ohio, site where first identified], a norovirus that produces gastroenteritis symptoms. The infection is transmitted from one person to another and is involved in 40% of the nonbacterial diarrhea cases in children and adults. It contains a single strand + sense RNA genome.

Norwegian scabies [Norway; L, *scabere,* to scratch], a severe infestation of human skin by an itch mite, *Sarcoptes scabiei.* The condition is associated with intense itching, crusting and scaling of the skin, and insect egg burrows that appear as discolored lines in the affected skin areas. The infestation is so named because it was first described in Norway, but it can occur anywhere in the world. Compare **scabies.**

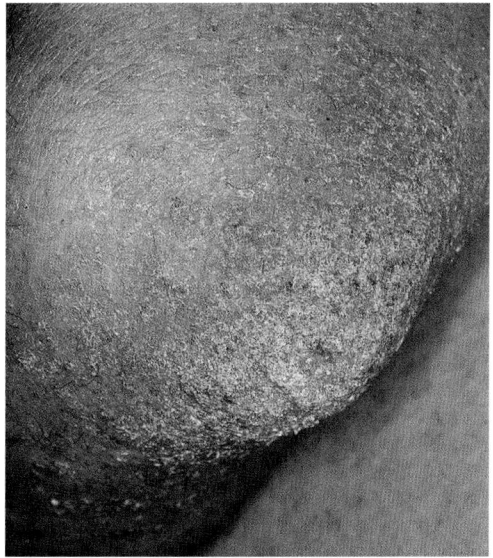

Norwegian scabies on elbow *(Bolognia, Jorizzo, and Schaffer, 2012)*

N

nose [AS, *nosu*], the structure that protrudes from the anterior part of the face and serves as a passageway for air to and from the lungs. The nose filters the air, warming, moistening, and chemically examining it for impurities that might irritate the mucous lining of the respiratory tract. The nose also contains receptor cells for smell, and it aids the faculty of speech. It consists of an internal and an external part. The external part, which protrudes from the face, is considerably smaller than the internal part, which lies over the roof of the mouth. The hollow interior part is separated into a right and a left cavity by a septum. Each cavity is divided into the superior, middle, and inferior meati by the projection of nasal conchae. The external part of the nose is perforated by two nostrils (anterior nares), and the internal part by two posterior nares. The pairs of sinuses that drain into the nose are the frontal, maxillary, ethmoidal, and sphenoidal sinuses. Ciliated mucous membrane lines the nose, closely adhering to the periosteum. The mucous membrane is continuous with the skin through the nares and with the mucous membrane of the nasal part of the pharynx through the choanae. The mucous membrane contains the olfactory cells that form the olfactory nerve that enters the cranium.

nosebleed [AS, *nosu* + ME, *blod,* blood], *(Informal)* abnormal hemorrhage from the nose. Emergency responses to nosebleed include seating the patient upright with the head thrust forward to prevent swallowing of blood. Asking the patient to apply pressure with both thumbs directly under the nostril and above the lips may block the main artery supplying blood to the nose. Alternatively, pressure with both forefingers on each side of the nostril often slows bleeding by blocking the main arteries and their branches. Continued bleeding may require the insertion within the nostril of cotton or another absorbent material saturated with local anesthesia and vasoconstricting agents, followed by the reapplication of pressure. Continued bleeding may require cautery. Also called **epistaxis.**

nose drops, a medicated solution to be dropped into the nose.

NOSIE, abbreviation for **nurses' observation scale for inpatient evaluation.**

noso-, prefix meaning "disease": *nosocomial, nosology.*

nosocomial /nos′əkō″mē·əl/ [Gk, *nosokomeian,* hospital], **1.** pertaining to a hospital. **2.** pertaining to a secondary disorder associated with hospitalization but unrelated to the primary condition of the patient.

nosocomial fever of unknown origin, a fever of at least 38.3° C occurring on several occasions in a hospitalized patient in whom neither fever nor infection was present on admission and for which a cause cannot be determined after 3 days of investigation, including 2 days of incubation of cultures.

nosocomial infection, an infection acquired at least 72 hours after hospitalization, often caused by *Candida albicans, Escherichia coli,* hepatitis viruses, herpes zoster virus, *Pseudomonas,* or *Staphylococcus.*

nosology /nōsol″əjē/ [Gk, *nosos,* disease, *logos,* science], the science of classifying diseases. See also **nomenclature.**

nostrils. See **anterior nares.**

notch [Fr, *noche*], an indentation or a depression in a bone or other organ, such as the auricular notch or the cardiac notch.

not criminally responsible due to a mental disorder (NCRMD), a fundamental principle of the criminal justice system in Canada, asserting that an accused must possess the capacity to understand that his or her behavior was wrong in order to be found guilty of an offense.

nothing by mouth (NPO) [L, *nil per os,* nothing by mouth], a patient care instruction advising that the patient is prohibited from ingesting food, beverage, or medicine. It is usually posted above the bed of a patient who is about to undergo surgery or special diagnostic procedures requiring that the digestive tract be empty or who is unable to tolerate food and fluids by mouth for some reason.

no-threshold curve, a linear dose-response curve that assumes that there is no detectable threshold below which there is no harm. As applied in nuclear medicine, there is no identifiable concentration of radiation below which no response curve occurs.

notifiable [L, *nota,* mark, *facere,* to make], pertaining to certain conditions, diseases, and events that must, by law, be reported to a governmental agency, such as birth, death, smallpox, certain other communicable diseases, and certain violations of public health regulations.

notifiable diseases, diseases that are classified as reportable by each state and territorial health department, which also prescribes the manner and time of reporting.

noto-, prefix meaning "the back": *notochord, notogenesis, notomelus.*

notochord /nō″tōkôrd/ [Gk, *noton,* back, *chorde,* cord], an elongated strip of mesodermal tissue that originates from the primitive node and extends along the dorsal surface of the developing embryo beneath the neural tube, forming the primary longitudinal skeletal axis of the body of all chordates. In humans and other higher vertebrates, the structure is replaced by vertebrae, although a remnant of it remains as part of the nucleus pulposus of the intervertebral disks. See also **neural tube.** −*notochordal, adj.*

notochordal canal /nō′tōkôr″dəl/ [Gk, *noton* + *chorde,* cord; L, *canalis,* channel], a tubular passage that extends from the primitive pit into the head process during the early stages of embryonic development in mammals. It perforates the splanchnopleure layer so that the yolk sac and the amnion are connected temporarily. Also called **chordal canal.**

notochordal plate. See **head process.**

notogenesis /nō′tōjen″əsis/ [Gk, *noton* + *genein,* to produce], the formation of the notochord. −*notogenetic, adj.*

notomelus /nətom″ələs/ [Gk, *noton* + *melos,* limb], a congenital malformation in which one or more accessory limbs are attached to the back.

Nott retinoscopy, a type of dynamic retinoscopy in which the fixation target is 40 cm from the eye. The test is first done with the object farther away than the target distance and then continued while the target is moved toward the patient until neutrality is observed.

nourish /nur″ish/ [L, *nutrire,* to suckle], to furnish the essential foods or nutrients for maintaining life.

nourishment /nur″ishmənt/, **1.** the act or process of nourishing or being nourished. **2.** any substance that nourishes and supports the life and growth of living organisms.

Novahistine, a fixed-combination drug containing an antihistamine and an adrenergic decongestant. Brand name for **chlorpheniramine maleate,** *pseudoephedrine.*

Novantrone, a synthetic antineoplastic anthracenedione. Brand name for **mitoxantrone.**

Novocain, a local anesthetic. Brand name for **procaine hydrochloride.**

NOx, abbreviation for a mixture of oxides of nitrogen, including nitric oxide, nitrogen dioxide, and nitrous oxide. See also **nitric oxide, nitrogen dioxide, nitrous oxide.**

Noxafil, brand name for **posaconazole.**

noxious /nok″shəs/ [L, *noxius,* harm], harmful, injurious, or detrimental to health.

Noyes test /noiz/, an orthopedic knee test performed with the knee extended and the thigh relaxed. The knee is partially dislocated anterolaterally. As the knee is gradually flexed, the dislocation is reduced at about 30 degrees of flexion.

Np, symbol for the element **neptunium.**

NP, abbreviation for **nurse practitioner.**

NPH insulin, an intermediate-acting insulin suspension. Abbreviation for *neutral protamine Hagedorn.*

NPN, abbreviation for **nonprotein nitrogen.**

NPO, abbreviation for **nothing by mouth.**

n-**propyl alcohol (C$_3$H$_7$OH)** /en″prō″pil/, a clear, colorless liquid used as a solvent for resins.

NPT, abbreviation for **nocturnal penile tumescence.**

NPU, abbreviation for **net protein utilization.**

NPY, abbreviation for **neuropeptide Y.**

NR, **1.** abbreviation for **no response. 2.** abbreviation for *nodal rhythm.*

NREM, abbreviation for **nonrapid eye movement.** See **sleep.**

NRTI, abbreviation for **nucleoside reverse transcriptase inhibitors.**

NSAID, acronym for **nonsteroidal antiinflammatory drug.**

NSB, abbreviation for **nonspecific binding.**

NSCCN, initialism for *National Society of Critical Care Nurses of Canada.*

N-s/m^2, abbreviation for *newton second per square meter.*

NSNA, initialism for *National Student Nurses Association.*

NSR, abbreviation for **normal sinus rhythm.**

NSU, abbreviation for **nonspecific urethritis.**

N-telopeptide test (NTx), a urine test that detects levels of N-telopeptide, a biochemical marker of bone metabolism and the most sensitive and specific indicator of bone resorption. It is used primarily to monitor the effect of antiresorptive therapy in women with osteoporosis.

NTP, ntp, abbreviation for *normal temperature and pressure.*

n-type semiconductor. See **semiconductor.**

nu /n(y)oo̅/, N, ν, the thirteenth letter of the Greek alphabet.

Nubain, a synthetic opioid analgesic used as an adjunct to anesthesia. Brand name for *nalbuphine hydrochloride.*

nuc, abbreviation for *nuclear.*

nucha /noo̅′kə/ *pl.* **nuchae** [Fr, *nuque,* nape], the nape, or back of the neck. −**nuchal,** *adj.*

nucha-, prefix meaning "the neck": *nuchal cord.*

nuchal cord /noo̅′kəl/ [Fr, *nuque,* nape; Gk, *chorde*], an abnormal but common condition in which the umbilical cord is wrapped around the neck of the fetus in utero or of the baby as it is being born. It is usually possible to slip the loop or loops of cord gently over the child's head. Sometimes it is a single loose loop, and the shoulders may deliver through it. If it is tight, it may be clamped in two places and cut with sterile, blunt-tipped scissors. The condition occurs in more than 25% of deliveries, more often with long cords than with short ones.

nuchal ligament, the fibrous membrane that reaches from the external occipital protuberance and median nuchal line to the spinous process of the seventh vertebra. A fibrous lamina from the ligament attaches to the posterior tubercle of the atlas and the spinous processes of the cervical vertebrae, forming a septum between muscles on either side of the neck.

nuchal line, one of the curved lines that extend laterally from the external occipital protuberance, a midline projection visible on the occipital bone.

nuchal rigidity, a resistance to flexion of the neck, a condition seen in patients with meningitis.

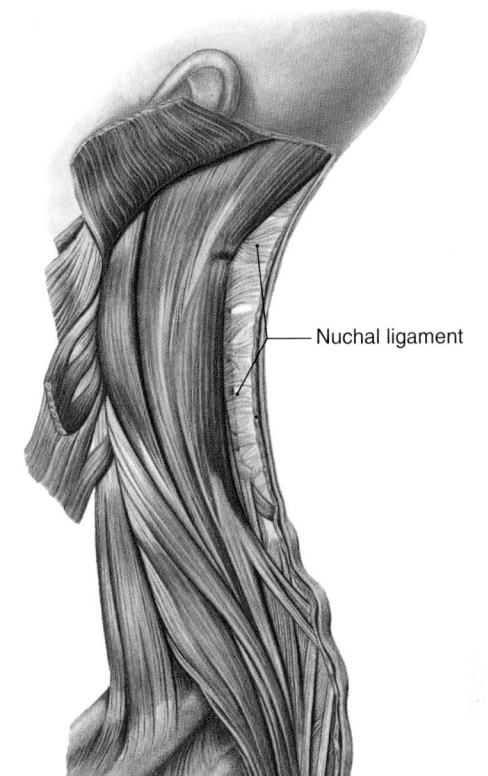

Nuchal ligament *(Modified from Paulsen and Waschke, 2013)*

nuchocephalic reflex /noo̅′kəsefal″ik/, a test for diffuse cerebral dysfunction, such as in senility. When the shoulders are turned to the left or the right, the head fails to turn in the same direction within a half-second.

Nuck's canal, Nuck's diverticulum. See **processus vaginalis peritonei.**

nucle-. See **nucleo-, nucle-.**

-nuclear, suffix meaning "nucleus": *mononuclear, polynuclear.*

nuclear agenesis. See **Möbius syndrome.**

nuclear envelope, a double membrane that surrounds the nucleus of a eukaryotic cell. Also called **karyotheca.**

nuclear family /n(y)oo̅′klē-ər/ [L, *nucleus,* nut kernel, *familia,* household], a family unit consisting of two parents and their children. Compare **extended family, matrifocal family.**

nuclear fission. See **fission.**

nuclear hyaloplasm. See **karyolymph.**

nuclear isomer, one of two or more nuclides with the same number of neutrons and protons in the nucleus (the same atomic number, or Z, and the same atomic mass, or A) but existing in different energy states.

nuclear magnetic resonance. See **magnetic resonance.**

nuclear medicine, a medical discipline that uses radiation emitted by radioactive isotopes in the diagnosis and treatment of disease. Forms of radiation important in nuclear medicine include alpha and beta particles, gamma rays, and x-rays. Radioactive elements used in nuclear medicine, called radionuclides or radiopharmaceuticals, are produced artificially. Radiopharmaceuticals are used as tracers for assessing the structure, function, secretion, excretion, and volume of a particular organ or tissue. They are also used to analyze biological specimens and to treat specific diseases

N

such as thyroid cancer. An important component of nuclear medicine is imaging, which involves administering radiopharmaceuticals to a patient orally, intravenously, or by inhalation to localize a specific organ or system and its structure and function. Scanning instruments convert the radioactive emissions into an image of the organ or system.

nuclear medicine technologist, an allied health professional who uses radioactive and stable nuclides to make diagnostic evaluations of the anatomical or physiological conditions of the body and who provides therapy with unsealed radioactive sources. Responsibilities include application of a special knowledge of radiation physics and safety regulations to limit radiation exposure; preparation and administration of radiopharmaceuticals; use of radiation detection devices and other kinds of laboratory equipment that measure the quantity and distribution of radionuclides deposited in a patient specimen; and performance of in vivo and in vitro diagnostic procedures. The Nuclear Medicine Technology Certification Board, along with the American Registry of Radiologic Technologists, creates and maintains examinations for nuclear medicine technologists.

nuclear physics, the study of atomic nuclei and their reactions.

nuclear problem, (in psychology) an underlying reason for an individual's reaction to a precipitating event.

nuclear radiology, the branch of radiology that uses radioactive materials in the diagnosis and treatment of health disorders.

nuclear sap. See **karyolymph.**

nuclear scanning, a diagnostic technique that uses an injected, ingested, or inhaled radioactive material and a scanning device to determine the size, shape, location, and function of various body parts and systems. Also called **radionuclide organ imaging.**

nuclear spin, an intrinsic form of angular momentum possessed by atomic nuclei containing an odd number of nucleons (protons or neutrons).

nuclear transplantation, the transfer of the nucleus of one cell into the cytoplasm of another.

nucleic acid /nōōklē′ik/ [L, *nucleus + acidus,* sour], a high–molecular-weight polymeric compound composed of nucleotides, each consisting of a purine or pyrimidine base, a ribose or deoxyribose sugar, and a phosphate group. Nucleic acids are involved in the determination and transmission of genetic characteristics. Kinds include **deoxyribonucleic acid, ribonucleic acid.** See also **nucleotide.**

nucleic acid amplification, amplification of a specific nucleic acid sequence, such as to test for the presence of a given virus or bacteria in a sample. Kinds include **DNA amplification, ligase chain reaction, polymerase chain reaction.**

nucleic acid amplification technique, any of various in vitro methods by which a DNA or RNA sequence is amplified, making it more readily detectable for various procedures or tests. The original, and still most commonly used, is the polymerase chain reaction.

nucleic acid test, any of various tests that use molecular biology techniques to detect and identify microorganisms, including viruses, on the basis of their nucleic acids. It includes culture confirmation tests, which identify organisms grown in culture, and direct tests, which can identify the organisms directly in a specimen. Direct tests can be further subdivided on the basis of whether their target nucleic acids are nonamplified or amplified for the test; the former are based on identification of a unique target sequence by using a labeled probe; the latter are classified as nucleic acid amplification tests.

nucleocapsid /nōō′klē·ōkap″sid/ [L, *nucleus + capsa,* box], a viral enclosure consisting of a capsid or protein coat and a nucleic acid that it surrounds. Some viruses consist solely of bare nucleocapsids; others have more complex enclosures.

nucleochylema /nōō′klē·ōkīlē″mə/ [L, *nucleus +* Gk, *chylos,* juice, *haima,* blood], the ground substance of the nucleus, as distinguished from that of the cytoplasm.

nucleochyme. See **karyolymph.**

nucleocytoplasmic /nōō′klē·ōsī′tōplas″mik/ [L, *nucleus +* Gk, *kytos,* cell, *plasma,* something formed], of or relating to the nucleus and cytoplasm of a cell.

nucleocytoplasmic ratio, the ratio of the volume of a nucleus of a cell to the volume of the cytoplasm. The proportion is usually constant for a specific cell type, and an increase is indicative of malignant neoplasms. Also called **karyoplasmic ratio, nucleoplasmic ratio.**

nucleohistone /nōō′klē·ōhis″tōn/ [L, *nucleus +* Gk, *histos,* tissue], a complex consisting of DNA and a histone protein that is the basic constituent of the chromatin in a cell nucleus.

nucleolar organizer /nōōklē″ələr/ [L, *nucleolus,* little nut kernel; Gk, *organon,* instrument, *izein,* to cause], a part of the nucleus of the cell, thought to consist of heterochromatin, that is responsible for the formation of the nucleolus. Also called *nucleolar zone,* **nucleolus organizer.**

nucleolus /nōōklē″ələs/ *pl. nucleoli* [L, little nut kernel], any one of the small, dense structures composed largely of ribonucleic acid that are situated within the cytoplasm of cells. Nucleoli are essential in the formation of ribosomes that synthesize cell proteins.

nucleolus organizer. See **nucleolar organizer.**

nucleon /n(y)ōō″klē·on/, a collective term applied to protons and neutrons within the nucleus.

nucleo-, nucle-, prefix meaning "nucleus": *nucleochylema, nucleohistone, nucleolus.*

nucleophilic /-fil″ik/, pertaining to some molecules, particularly nucleic acids and proteins, having electrons that can be shared and thus form bonds with alkylating agents.

nucleoplasm /nōō″klē·əplaz′əm/ [L, *nucleus +* Gk, *plasma,* something formed], the protoplasm of the nucleus as contrasted with that of the cell. Also called **karyoplasm.** Compare **cytoplasm.** *−nucleoplasmic, adj.*

nucleoplasmic ratio. See **nucleocytoplasmic ratio.**

nucleoplasmin, an acidic protein found in the nucleus that binds to histone and participates in nucleosome assembly.

nucleoprotein /-prō″tēn/ [L, *nucleus +* Gk, *proteios,* first rank], a molecule in which protein is combined with nucleic acid in a cell nucleus.

nucleoside /nōō″klē·əsīd′/, a component of a nucleotide that consists of a nitrogenous base linked to a pentose sugar.

nucleoside analog, a structural analog of a nucleoside, a category that includes both purine analogs and pyrimidine analogs.

nucleoside monophosphate kinase, a liver enzyme that catalyzes the reversible transfer of a phosphate group from adenosine triphosphate, producing adenosine diphosphate and a nucleoside diphosphate.

nucleoside reverse transcriptase inhibitors (NRTI), a class of antiretroviral drugs that mimic one or more of the components of deoxyribonucleic acid (DNA) or ribonucleic acid and interrupt the viral replication process. The drugs (nucleoside analogs) work by being incorporated into the DNA made by the viral reverse transcriptase enzyme that is essential for viral replication. Inserting a nucleoside analog into the new viral DNA strand terminates the viral chain, halting the replication process before it is completed. Examples of nucleoside analogs include zidovudine (AZT), didanosine (ddI), zalcitabine (ddC), stavudine (d4T), and lamivudine (3TC). See also **nonnucleoside reverse transcriptase inhibitors.**

nucleosome /noo″klē·əsōm′/ [L, *nucleus* + Gk, *soma,* body], any one of the repeating DNA-histone complexes that appear as beadlike structures at distinct intervals along a chromosome.

5′-nucleotidase /noo″klē·ot″idās/, an enzyme, elevated in some liver disorders and cancer of the pancreas. It is infrequently measured in the blood to diagnose certain liver and bone diseases. This enzyme is widely distributed throughout the body but is found in high concentrations in the liver and pancreas. The normal accumulation in serum is 0.1 to 6 units.

5′-nucleotidase test, an infrequently performed blood test used to help diagnose liver disease, particularly cholestasis. It provides information similar to that from the alkaline phosphatase (ALP) test. However, unlike ALP, 5′-nucleotidase is specific to the liver, so this test is used to confirm liver disease when ALP results are uncertain.

nucleotide /noo″klē·ətīd′/, a compound consisting of one or more phosphate groups, a pentose sugar, and a nitrogenous base. Chains of nucleotides form DNA and RNA; free nucleotides, such as adenosine triphosphate and guanosine triphosphate, are important energy carriers in all cells.

nucleus /n(y)oo″klē·əs/ [L, nut kernel], **1.** the central controlling body within a living cell, usually a spheric unit enclosed in a membrane and containing genetic codes for maintaining life systems of the organism and for issuing commands for growth and reproduction. −*nuclear, adj.* **2.** a group of nerve cells of the central nervous system having a common function, such as supporting the sense of hearing or smell. **3.** the center of an atom consisting of an element-specific number of protons and neutrons. A probability cloud of electrons exists around the atomic nucleus. **4.** *adj.,* the central element in an organic chemical compound or class of compounds. Formerly called **cytoblast.**

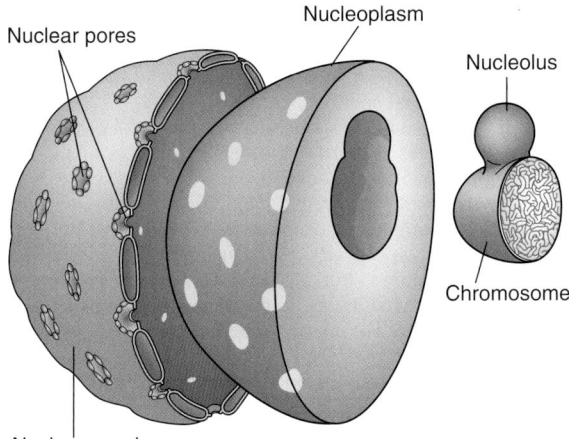

Nucleus *(Huether and McCance, 2012)*

nucleus pulposus, the gelatinous center of a vertebral disk. See **pulpy nucleus.**

nuclide /noo″klīd/ [L, *nucleus,* nut kernel], a species of atom characterized by the constitution of its nucleus, in particular by the number of protons and neutrons. Thus Co-59 and Co-60 are both isotopes of cobalt and are each nuclides. Co-60 is a radionuclide because it undergoes radioactive decay.

nudge control, a mechanical device on a prosthesis that can be pressed by the chin to lock or unlock one or more joints of the prosthesis.

NUG, abbreviation for **necrotizing ulcerative gingivitis.**

Nuhn gland /noon/ [Anton Nuhn, German anatomist, 1814–1889], a gland on the inferior surface and near the apex and midline of the tongue.

nuke, *(Slang)* a nucleoside analog. See also **nucleoside reverse transcriptase inhibitors.**

null cell [L, *nullus,* not one, *cella,* storeroom], a lymphocyte that develops in the bone marrow and lacks the characteristic surface markers of the B and T cells (surface immunoglobulin or the pan-T antigen). Null cells represent a small proportion of the lymphocyte population. Stimulated by the presence of an antibody, null cells can attack certain cellular targets directly. They kill tumor or viral-infected cells, although not with the specificity of cytotoxic T cells. A null cell is a type of natural killer cell. The term *null cell* is no longer in common use. Compare **B cell, T cell.** See also **cytotoxin, immune gamma globulin, natural killer cell.**

null hypothesis (H₀), (in research) a type of hypothesis used in statistics that proposes that no statistical significance exists between the variables being studied.

nulli-, prefix meaning "none": *nullipara, nulligravida.*

nulligravida /nul′igrav″ədə/, a woman who has never been pregnant.

nullipara /nulip′ərə/ *pl. nulliparae* [L, *nullus,* not one, *parere,* to bear], a woman who has not given birth to a viable infant. The designation "para 0" indicates nulliparity. Compare **multipara, primipara.**

nulliparity /nul″iper′itē/ [L, *nullus,* none, *parere,* to bear], the status of a woman who has never borne a child.

nulliparous /nulip′ərəs/ [L, *nullus,* none, *parere,* to bear], never having given birth.

num, abbreviation for *number, numeral.*

numbness /num′nəs/ [ME, *nomen,* loss of feeling], a partial or total lack of sensation in a body part resulting from any factor that interrupts the transmission of impulses from the sensory nerve fibers. Numbness is often accompanied by tingling.

numeric pain scale /n(y)oo″mer″ik/, a pain assessment system in which patients are asked to rate their pain on a scale from 1 to 10, with 10 representing the worst pain they have experienced or could imagine.

numeric taxonomy, a system of classifying organisms on the basis of the overall similarities of the measurable phenotypic characters they share. The system is used to classify strains of bacteria, as well as to separate closely related species of plants and animals.

nummular dermatitis /num′yələr/ [L, *nummuli,* petty cash; Gk, *derma,* skin, *itis,* inflammation], a skin disease characterized by coin-shaped, vesicular, or scaling eczema-like lesions, commonly on the forearms and front of the calves. The cause is unknown. Keeping the skin hydrated is important. A health care provider should be consulted as the lesions can be difficult to treat.

nummular psoriasis. See **psoriasis.**

Numorphan, an opioid analgesic. Brand name for **oxymorphone hydrochloride.**

Nupercainal, a local anesthetic. Brand name for *dibucaine hydrochloride.*

Nuremberg tribunal [Nuremberg, Germany; L, *tribunus,* platform for administration of justice], an international tribunal planned and implemented by the United Nations War Crimes Commission to detect, apprehend, try, and punish people accused of war crimes. In preparation for

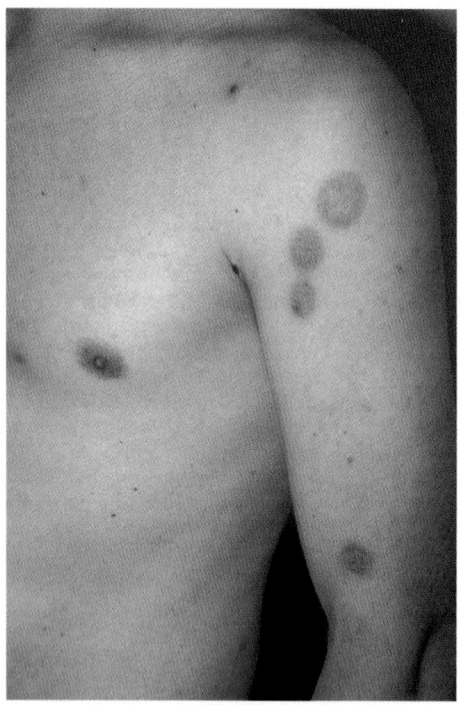

Nummular dermatitis *(Halberg, 2012)*

the prosecution of World War II criminals, the U.S. War Department assigned Andrew Ivy, M.D., to devise a set of principles to govern the participation of human beings in medical research, which became known as the Nuremberg code. The principle and practice of informed consent were reinforced by the precedent set in the trials in which Nazi physicians were declared guilty of crimes against humanity in performing experiments on human beings who were not volunteers and did not consent. See also **Helsinki Accords.**

nurse [L, *nutrix*], **1.** *n.,* a person educated and licensed in the practice of nursing; one who is concerned with "the diagnosis and treatment of human responses to actual or potential health problems" (American Nurses Association). The practice of the nurse includes data collection, diagnosis, planning, treatment, and evaluation within the framework of the nurse's singular concern with the patient's response to the problem, rather than to the problem itself. In a cooperative participatory relationship with the client or patient, the nurse acts to promote, maintain, or restore the health of the person; wellness is the goal. A collegial collaborative relationship with other health professionals who share a mission and a common database furthers the practice of nursing. The nurse may be a generalist or a specialist and, as a professional, is ethically and legally accountable for the nursing activities performed and for the actions of others to whom the nurse has delegated responsibility. **2.** *v.,* to provide nursing care. See also **five-step nursing process, nursing, registered nurse.**

nurse anesthetist,   a registered nurse qualified by advanced study in an accredited program in the specialty of nurse anesthesia to manage patient care during the administration of all types of anesthesia in selected surgical situations. Nurse anesthetists are primarily involved in the direct administration of anesthesia to a single patient but often have other duties such as airway management in emergency situations. See also **certified registered nurse anesthetist.**

nurse cell,   a cell that transfers nutrients to an oocyte via a cytoplasmic bridge. Compare **Sertoli cell.**

nurse-client interaction,   any process in which a nurse and a client exchange or share information, verbally or nonverbally. It is fundamental to communication and is an essential component of the nursing assessment.

nurse clinician,   a nurse who is prepared to identify and diagnose problems of clients by using increased knowledge and skills gained through advanced study in a specific area of nursing practice. The specialist may function independently within standing orders or protocols and collaborates with associates to implement a care plan that is focused on the client.

nurse coordinator,   a registered nurse who coordinates and manages the activities of nursing personnel engaged in specific nursing services, such as obstetrics or surgery, for two or more patient care units.

Nurse Corps,   the branch within each of the armed services comprising the nurses within that service, such as the Army Nurse Corps. In each of the armed services, the members of the Nurse Corps have the rank, title, responsibilities, and status of commissioned officer.

nurse educator,   a registered nurse in the United States whose primary area of interest, competence, and professional practice is the education of nurses. Minimum education required is a master's of science in nursing. The National League for Nursing offers certification for nurse educators.

nurse manager,   the individual responsible for nursing practice and quality of care, usually on a single unit or department, working in collaboration with staff nurses. The nurse manager usually assumes responsibility for personnel and budget matters related to nursing. See also **head nurse.**

nurse midwife,   a registered nurse qualified by advanced education and clinical experience in obstetric and neonatal care and certified by the American College of Nurse Midwives. The nurse midwife manages the perinatal care of women having a normal pregnancy, labor, and childbirth. Compare **doula.** See also **certified nurse-midwife.**

nurse navigator,   a registered nurse who coordinates, advocates, and assists patients to cope successfully with the complexity of a specific hospital, physician's office, hospital service, or hospital area.

nurse practice act,   a statute enacted by the legislature of each of the states or by the appropriate officers of the districts or possessions. The act delineates the legal scope of the practice of nursing within the geographic boundaries of the jurisdiction. The purpose of the act is to protect the public.

nurse practitioner (NP),   a registered nurse who has advanced education in nursing (a master's of science in nursing or a doctorate in nursing practice) and clinical experience in a specialized area of nursing practice. NPs are certified by passing an examination administered by a professional organization such as the American Nurses' Credentialing Center. They collaborate with other health care providers to deliver primary care to patients with common acute or stable chronic medical conditions in ambulatory care settings. Some NPs also function in a specialty, tertiary, or long-term care setting. NPs may offer a variety of services, such as complete physical examinations, health assessments, and patient education. Specialty certification is required. The scope of all advanced nursing practice is influenced by state laws, federal laws, insurance practices, and regional acceptance. Some insurance organizations recognize NPs as primary health care providers and allow direct reimbursement for their services.

nursery diarrhea /nur′sərē/ [L, *nutrix,* nurse; Gk, *dia,* through, *rhein,* to flow], diarrhea of the newborn. In nurseries outbreaks of diarrhea caused by *Escherichia coli,*

Salmonella, echoviruses, or adenoviruses are potentially life-threatening to the infant. The neonate may be infected at the time of birth by organisms from the mother's stool or infected later by organisms spread by the hands of hospital personnel. The most serious aspect of the disease is fluid loss, leading to dehydration and electrolyte imbalance. Care includes maintaining fluid and electrolyte balance and administering antibiotics, if appropriate. Good handwashing technique, use of disposable nursing bottles and nipples, and early isolation of infected infants reduce the possibility of such outbreaks.

nurse's aide, a person who is employed to carry out basic nonspecialized tasks in the care of patients, such as bathing and feeding, making beds, and transporting patients, under the supervision and direction of a registered nurse. Many hospitals offer education and orientation programs for newly hired nurse's aides and inservice education for continued training.

Nurses' Association of the American College of Obstetrics and Gynecology. See **Association of Women's Health, Obstetric, and Neonatal Nurses.**

nurses' observation scale for inpatient evaluation (NOSIE) [developed by G. Honigfeld and C.J. Klett,], a 30-item scale designed to assess the behavior of patients on an inpatient unit. NOSIE is quick, simple to administer, and may be used to assess patients who may be too ill to participate in more interactive rating scales, including nonverbal individuals.

nurses' registry, an employment agency that provides nurses to work in temporary positions at facilities. See also **float nurse.**

nurses' station, an area in a clinic, unit, or ward in a health care facility that serves as the administrative center for nursing care for a particular group of patients. It is usually centrally located and may be staffed by a unit secretary or clerk who assists with paperwork, telephone, and other communication. Before going on duty, nurses usually meet there to receive daily assignments, review the patients' charts, and update the files. In a critical care unit, the nurses' station may also contain panels of visual display terminals that allow centralized monitoring of many patients and computer terminals that allow access to information in the patients' records or to a data bank of clinical information. In other parts of a hospital, the nurses' station is equipped in any of various ways appropriate to the care of the patients in that area or unit.

nursing, **1.** the practice in which a nurse assists "the individual, sick or well, in the performance of those activities contributing to health or its recovery (or to a peaceful death) that he would perform unaided if he had the necessary strength, will or knowledge. And to do this in such a way as to help him gain independence as rapidly as possible" (Virginia Henderson). **2.** "the diagnosis and treatment of human responses to actual or potential health problems" (American Nurses Association). There are four principal characteristics that further define nursing care: the phenomena that concern nurses; the use of theories to observe the need for nursing intervention and to plan nursing action; the nursing action taken; and an evaluation of the effects of the actions relative to the phenomena. This definition of nursing provides a framework for the nursing process, including data collection, diagnosis, planning, treatment, and evaluation. The nursing process is supported by standards of nursing practice that are congruent with the definition and that provide more specific guidelines for practice. These standards include systematic, continuous collection of data concerning the health status of the client in recorded form that is accessible and that may be communicated. A nursing diagnosis is derived from the data collected. A plan for nursing care incorporates goals derived from the nursing diagnosis and the priorities and approaches to achieve the goals as indicated by the nursing diagnosis. Nursing actions, which are selected and performed with the client's participation, provide for promotion, maintenance, or restoration of the client's health and serve to maximize the client's health care abilities. The progress or lack of progress toward the goal is mutually determined by the client and the nurse, resulting in reassessment, reordering of priorities, establishment of new goals, and revision of the plan for nursing care. Nursing touches on, intersects with, and complements other professional roles in health care, addressing itself to a wide range of health-related responses in people who are well and in those who are not. Nursing seeks to diagnose and treat the response to the problem; thus the concerns of nursing are less circumscribed and discrete than those of other health-related professions. These concerns include the following: limitations of the client's self-care ability; impaired ability to function in any fundamental area such as sleeping, breathing, eating, maintaining circulation; pain, anxiety, fear, loneliness, grief, or other physical or emotional problems related to health, illness, or treatment; impaired social or intellectual processes; impaired ability to make decisions and choices; alteration of self-image as required by the change in health; dysfunctional perception of health or health care activities; extra demands posed by such normal life processes as birth, growth, or death; and difficulty in affiliative relationships. Various concepts, principles, processes, and actions developed and examined in nursing research guide the steps in the nursing process from initial observation and diagnosis through evaluation, based on intrapersonal, interpersonal, and systems theories. The boundary for nursing practice is not static; it tends to move outward as the needs and capacities of society change. Collegial, collaborative practice with members of other health care professions further softens the boundaries of nursing practice. All health care professionals share a mission and a scientific database, and to some degree their practices overlap. At its core, nursing is nurturative, generative, and protective; preventive care is a part of every nurse's practice. Nurses value independence and self-respect. They are guided by an ethical and humanitarian philosophy in which every human being deserves respect, regardless of racial, social, cultural, sexual, economic, religious, or other factors. The nurse practices in the context of a relationship with the client, family, or group that is professional and yet close, in an interpersonal sense. The function of a nurse involves the physical intimacy of laying on of hands; compassion and constant recognition of the person's dignity are essential. Nursing is practiced by specialists and generalists. Generalists provide most nursing care; specialists, having added to their basic knowledge an organized and systematized body of knowledge and competencies, practice in specialized areas of nursing. Nursing care is given to people at all stages of life in the home, hospital, place of employment, school, or any environment where nursing care is needed. Nurses are ethically and legally accountable for their practice and for delegation of responsibilities to others. **3.** the professional practice of a nurse. **4.** the process of acting as a nurse, of providing care that encourages and promotes the health of the person or persons being served. See also **nursing process. 5.** See **breastfeeding.**

nursing assessment, an identification by a nurse of the needs, preferences, and abilities of a patient. Assessment includes an interview with and observation of a patient by the nurse and considers the symptoms and signs of the condition, the patient's verbal and nonverbal communication, the

N

patient's medical and social history, and any other information available. Among the physical aspects assessed are vital signs, skin color and condition, motor and sensory nerve function, nutrition, rest, sleep, activity, elimination, and consciousness. Among the social and emotional factors included in assessment are religion, occupation, attitude toward hospital and health care, mood, emotional tone, and family ties and responsibilities. Assessment is extremely important because it provides the scientific basis for a complete nursing care plan.

nursing assistant, a person trained in basic nursing techniques and direct patient care who practices under the supervision of a registered nurse. The qualifications to become a certified nursing assistant vary from state to state.

nursing audit, a review of the patient record designed to identify, examine, or verify the performance of certain specified aspects of nursing care by using established criteria. A concurrent nursing audit is performed during ongoing nursing care. A retrospective nursing audit is performed after discharge from the care facility, using the patient's record. Often a nursing audit and a medical audit are performed collaboratively, resulting in a joint audit.

nursing bottle caries. (Informal) See **early childhood caries.**

nursing care plan, a plan, based on a nursing assessment and a nursing diagnosis, carried out by a nurse. It has four essential components: identification of the nursing care problems or nursing diagnoses and statement of the nursing approach to solve those problems; statement of the expected benefit to the patient; statement of the specific actions by the nurse that reflect the nursing approach and achieve the goals specified; and evaluation of the patient's response to nursing care and readjustment of that care as required. The nursing care plan is begun when the patient is admitted to the health service, and, after the initial nursing assessment, a diagnosis is formulated and nursing orders are developed. The goal of the process is to ensure that nursing care is consistent with the patient's needs and progress toward self-care. A written nursing care plan should be a part of every patient's chart. See also **diagnosis, nursing assessment, nursing diagnosis, nursing orders, problem-solving approach to patient-centered care.**

nursing diagnosis, a statement of a health problem or of a potential problem in the client's health status that a nurse is licensed and competent to treat. Four steps are required in the formulation of a nursing diagnosis. A database is established by collecting information from all available sources, including interviews with the client and the client's family, a review of any existing records of the client's health, observation of the client's response to any alterations in health status, a physical assessment, and a conference or consultation with others concerned in the client's care. The database is continually updated. The second step includes analysis of the client's responses to the problems, healthy or unhealthy, and classification of those responses as psychological, physiological, spiritual, or sociological. The third step is the organization of the data so that a tentative diagnostic statement can be made that summarizes the pattern of problems discovered. The last step is confirmation of the sufficiency and accuracy of the database by evaluation of the appropriateness of the diagnosis to nursing intervention and by the assurance that, given the same information, most other qualified practitioners would arrive at the same nursing diagnosis. In use, each diagnostic category has three parts: the term that concisely describes the problem, the probable cause of the problem, and the defining characteristics of the problem. A number of nursing diagnoses have been identified and are listed as accepted by the North American Nursing Diagnosis Association, and they are updated and refined at periodic meetings of the group.

nursing differential, an allowance added to payments to hospitals for services rendered to Medicaid patients in recognition that the cost of providing nursing services to such patients is greater than the cost to the general patient population.

nursing director, a nurse whose function is the administrative and clinical leadership of the nursing service of a division of a health care facility. Also called **nursing supervisor.**

nursing ethics [L, *nutrix,* nurse; Gk, *ethikos,* character], the values or moral principles governing relationships between the nurse and patient, the patient's family, other members of the health professions, and the public. See also **Code for Nurses.**

nursing goal, a general goal of nursing involving activities that are desirable but difficult to measure, such as self-care, good nutrition, and relaxation. Compare **nursing objective.**

nursing health history, data collected about a patient's level of wellness, changes in life patterns, sociocultural role, and mental and emotional reactions to illness.

nursing home. See **extended care facility.**

nursing intervention, any act by a nurse that implements the nursing care plan or any specific objective of that plan, such as turning a comatose patient to avoid the development of decubitus ulcers or teaching insulin injection technique to a patient with diabetes before discharge from the hospital. The patient may require intervention in the form of support, limitation, medication, or treatment for the current condition or to prevent the development of further stress. See also **nursing process.**

nursing intervention model, (in nursing research) a conceptual framework used to determine appropriate nursing interventions. The model is a holistic representation of the patient and the health care system. The patient's physiological, psychological, sociocultural, and developmental status; the patient's stressors and ability to react to them; and the levels and patterns of available health care are observed. The goal is to learn what nursing interventions would be most effective for the particular problem within the particular health care system.

Nursing Interventions Classification (NIC), a comprehensive, standardized system to classify treatments performed by nurses. It is a clinical tool developed by a research team at the University of Iowa that describes and defines the knowledge base for nursing curricula and practice. There are at present 554 nursing interventions that describe the treatments nurses perform. Each intervention has been labeled, defined, and given a list of appropriate activities. The full range of activities that nurses perform on behalf of patients is included, both independent and collaborative interventions and both direct and indirect care. A taxonomy is provided to help the nurse find what is most relevant to her or his practice area. NIC interventions have been linked to NANDA diagnoses. It is considered part of the clinical decision making of the nurse to decide and document the nursing diagnoses, desired outcomes, interventions used, and outcomes achieved. The NIC system provides a standardized language to document interventions.

nursing licensure compact, an agreement between two or more states or other jurisdictions that the licensing of a type of nursing or a nursing specialty in one place will be valid in the other.

nursing minimum data set (NMDS), a minimum set of items of information with uniform definitions and categories concerning the specific dimension of nursing, which meets the information needs of multiple data users in the health care system. It is the first attempt to standardize the collection of essential nursing data.

nursing objective, a specific aim planned by a nurse to decrease a person's stress, to improve the ability to adapt, or both. A nursing objective may be physical, emotional, social, or cultural and may involve the person's family, friends, and other patients. It is the purpose of any specific nursing order or nursing intervention. Some common nursing objectives are adequate understanding by the patient of certain details of the condition, adequate and comfortable daily elimination, a certain amount of rest, a balanced diet, and participation in specific items of self-care. Compare **nursing goal.**

nursing observation, an objective evaluation made by a nurse of the various aspects of a client's condition. It includes the person's general appearance, emotional affect, nutritional status, habits, and preferences, as well as body temperature, skin condition, and any abnormal processes, including those of which the client complains. The client's religious preference, ethnic background, and familial relationships are also noted. Compare **nursing assessment, nursing intervention.**

nursing orders, specific instructions for implementing the nursing care plan, including the patient's preferences, timing of activities, details of health education necessary for the particular patient, role of the family, and plans for care after discharge. Nursing orders must be signed by the professional nurse who writes them. They should not duplicate the orders of the medical staff or of other members of the health team.

Nursing Outcomes Classification (NOC), a comprehensive, standardized system to classify outcomes of nursing interventions. It is a clinical tool developed by a research team at the University of Iowa that describes and defines the knowledge base for nursing curricula and practice. At present, NOC includes 490 nursing outcomes for use for individual patients or individual family caregivers in the home. NOC outcomes have been linked to NANDA diagnoses. It is considered part of the clinical decision making of the nurse to decide and document the nursing diagnoses, desired outcomes, interventions used, and outcomes achieved.

nursing process, the process that serves as an organizational framework for the practice of nursing. It encompasses all of the steps taken by the nurse in caring for a patient: assessment, nursing diagnosis, planning, implementation, and evaluation. The rationale for each step is founded in nursing theory. The process requires a systematic approach to the person's situation, beginning with assessment and including an evaluation and reconciliation of the perceptions by the person, the person's family, and the nurse. A plan for the nursing actions to be taken may then be made, and, with the participation of the person and the person's family, the plan may be set. The plan developed with the person and the person's family is then implemented. The outcome is evaluated with the person and the person's family. The steps follow each other at the start of the process but may need to be taken concurrently in some situations. The process does not reach completion with evaluation. The steps are begun again, allowing recurrent evaluation of the assessment, plan, goals, and actions. See also **five-step nursing process, nursing.**

nursing process model, a conceptual framework in which the nurse-patient relationship is the basis of the nursing process. The nursing process is represented as dynamic and interpersonal, the nurse and the patient being affected by each other's behavior and by the environment around them. Each successful two-way communication is termed a "transaction" and can be analyzed to discover the factors that promote transactions. The constraints that the various systems in the environment (personal, interpersonal, and social) place on the development of the relationship are also examined. The nurse views the patient as a person with whom to have transactions that achieve defined adaptive objectives toward the goal of health.

nursing research, a detailed systematic study of a problem in the field of nursing. Nursing research is practice- or discipline-oriented and is essential for the continued development of the scientific base of professional nursing practice.

Nursing Research, a bimonthly refereed journal containing papers and other materials concerning nursing research. The goal of the journal is to stimulate research in nursing and disseminate research findings.

nursing rounds, chart rounds, walking rounds, teaching rounds, or grand rounds that are held specifically for nurses and that focus on nursing care. See also **rounds.**

nursing specialty, a nurse's selected professional field of practice, such as surgical, pediatric, obstetric, or psychiatric nursing. Compare **subspecialty.**

nursing supervisor. See **nursing director.**

nursing theorist, a person who develops integrated concepts or frameworks of nursing roles, functions, objectives, and activities and their relationships to clients and the roles of other health professionals.

nursing theory, an organized framework of concepts and purposes designed to guide the practice of nursing.

nursology /nursol″əjē/ [L, *nutrix,* nurse; Gk, *logos,* science], a conceptual framework for the study and practice of nursing. The nurse and the patient have the opportunity to grow, and the science of nursing may emerge from investigations and syntheses.

Nursoy, a hypoallergenic nutritional supplement for infants.

nurture /nur′chər/, to feed, rear, foster, or care for, such as in the nourishment, care, and training of growing children.

nutation /nootā′shən/ [L, *nutare,* to nod], the act of nodding, especially involuntary nodding as occurs in some neurological disorders.

nutcracker esophagus. See **symptomatic esophageal peristalsis.**

nutcracker phenomenon, compression of the left renal vein between the aorta and the superior mesenteric artery, causing hypertension in the kidney with flank pain and sometimes fever and gross hematuria. Also called *nutcracker syndrome.*

nutmeg poisoning, the toxic effect of ingesting large amounts of the dried kernels of the seeds of nutmeg *(Myristica fragrans)* or its volatile oils. The oils contain terpenes and myristicin, which can cause tachycardia, nausea, vomiting, agitation, and hallucinations.

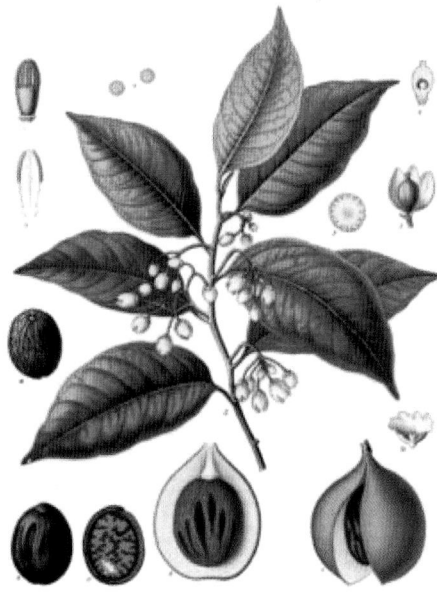

Nutmeg *(Farrar et al, 2014)*

nutraceuticals /noo″träsoo′tĭkalz/, **1.** functional foods. **2.** foods thought to have a beneficial effect on human health.

Nutramigen, a milk-substitute formula that is prepared from a soy isolate base and is lactose free. It is prescribed for infants with galactosemia and as a protein supplement for people with lactose intolerance.

nutri-, prefix meaning "nourishment": *nutrient, nutritional.*

nutrient /noo″trē·ənt/ [L, *nutriens,* food that nourishes], a chemical substance that provides nourishment and affects the nutritive and metabolic processes of the body. Nutrients are essential for growth, reproduction, and maintenance of health.

nutrient artery of the humerus, one of a pair of branches of the deep brachial arteries, arising near the middle of the arm and entering the nutrient canal of the humerus.

nutrient canal. See **interdental canal.**

nutrient density, the relative ratio obtained by dividing a food's contribution to the needs for a nutrient by its contribution to calorie needs.

nutrient enema [L, *nutriens* + Gk, *enienai,* injection], the introduction of saline or glucose into the body via the rectum. Its use is extremely rare in clinical practice. See also **enteral nutrition.**

nutrient supplements, vitamins and other nutrients that may not be necessary for healthy adults with an adequate intake of proper nutrients but that may be needed under certain circumstances for elderly adults or persons in a debilitated or undernourished state.

nutriment /noo″trimənt/ [L, *nutriens,* food that nourishes], any substance that nourishes and aids the growth and the development of the body. See also **food.**

nutrition /n(y)ootrish″ən/ [L, *nutriens*], **1.** nourishment. **2.** the sum of the processes involved in the taking in of nutrients and their assimilation and use for proper body functioning and maintenance of health. The successive stages include ingestion, digestion, absorption, assimilation, and excretion. **3.** the study of food and drink as related to the growth and maintenance of living organisms.

nutritional /n(y)ootrish″ənəl/ [L, *nutrire,* to nourish], pertaining to the quality of food or eating behavior that provides nourishment through assimilation of food to tissues.

nutritional-alcoholic cerebellar degeneration. See **alcoholic-nutritional cerebellar degeneration.**

nutritional anemia [L, *nutrire,* to nourish; Gk, *a* + *haima,* without blood], a disorder characterized by the inadequate production of hemoglobin or erythrocytes caused by a nutritional deficiency of iron, folic acid, or vitamin B_{12}. See also **iron-deficiency anemia, megaloblastic anemia, pernicious anemia.**

nutritional care, the substances, procedures, and setting involved in ensuring the proper intake and assimilation of nutriments, especially for the hospitalized patient.

■ METHOD: Depending on the patient's condition, nutritional requirements may be provided by regular meals with menus selected from the prescribed diet, by tube feeding, or by parenteral hyperalimentation. Meals are served on attractive trays in an environment conducive to eating. Distasteful procedures are avoided before and after mealtime. Patients who are unable to feed themselves are assisted, and abnormal intake of food is recorded and reported. Supplemental nourishment is supplied when indicated, and fluids are offered between meals. The nutritional assessment includes observations of the patient's appetite; food preferences; allergies; height; intake and output; weight; measurements of the head, arms, abdomen, and skinfold thickness; skin color and turgor; and condition of the mouth, eyes, nails, and hair. Any cutaneous lesions, thyroid enlargement, dental caries, loose teeth, ill-fitting dentures, gum problems, nausea, vomiting, dehydration, diarrhea, or constipation is noted.

nutritional science, a body of science that relates to the processes involved in nutrition.

nutrition base, a person's normal nutritional requirements before modification to accommodate a specific condition.

nutritionist /n(y)ootrish″ənist/ [L, *nutrire,* to nourish], a licensed nutritionist has earned credentials from a nationally recognized nutrition licensing body, such as the Commission on Dietetic Registration of the Academy of Nutrition and Dietetics, the Certification Board for Nutrition Specialists, or the Clinical Nutrition Certification Board. Some states require licensure of nutritionists while others do not. Licensed nutritionists are regulated by their certification boards, as well as by the states in which they practice. Once licensed to practice in a particular state, a licensed nutritionist may legally provide nutrition counseling, nutrition services, and advice. Settings in which licensed nutritionists may work include hospitals, long-term care facilities, schools, community programs, and nonprofit organizations. A registered dietitian may be considered a licensed nutritionist, depending upon a state's licensing laws, but not all licensed nutritionists are registered dietitians.

Nutting, Mary Adelaide [1858–1947], a Canadian-born American nursing educator and reformer. As head of Johns Hopkins School of Nursing in Baltimore beginning in 1894, she improved course content and teaching facilities, instituted a 6-month preparatory course, reduced the 12-hour day to 8 hours, and abolished the monthly payment system to students. At Teachers College, Columbia University, she created and developed the Department of Nursing and Health and became the first professor of nursing in the world. With Lavinia Dock she wrote *History of Nursing* (published in 1907), a classic in nursing literature.

Nuvigil, brand name for *armodafinil.*

nux vomica /nuks′ vom′ikə/ [L, *nux,* nut, *vomere,* to vomit], the dried ripe seeds of a small Asian tree, *Strychnos nux vomica,* a source of the alkaloids strychnine and brucine. The seeds are powdered, and the strychnine content is reduced to a little more than 1% by the addition of lactose for use as a bitter tonic and nerve stimulant. It is unsafe at this concentration. Homeopathic remedies of nux vomica are much more diluted and are considered safe.

nV, abbreviation for *nanovolt.*

nyctalopia /nik′təlō″pē·ə/ [Gk, *nyx,* night, *alaos,* obscure, *ops,* eye], poor vision at night or in dim light resulting from decreased synthesis of rhodopsin, vitamin A deficiency, retinal degeneration, or a congenital defect. Also called *day sight,* **night blindness.** −*nyctalopic, adj.*

nycto-, combining form meaning "night" or "darkness": *nyctophobia.*

nyctophobia /nik′tō-/ [Gk, *nyx* + *phobos,* fear], an anxiety reaction characterized by an obsessive, irrational fear of darkness.

nycturia. See **nocturia.**

nympho-, *(Slang)* prefix indicating a relationship to the female gender: *nymphomaniac.*

nymphomaniac /-mā′nē·ak/, *(Obsolete)* a term once used to describe a woman thought to display characteristics of insatiable desire for sexual satisfaction. See also **sexual deviance.**

nystagmus /nĭstag″məs/ [Gk, *nystagmos,* nodding], involuntary, rhythmic movements of the eyes. The oscillations may be horizontal, vertical, rotary, or mixed. Jerking nystagmus, characterized by faster movements in one direction than in the opposite direction, is more common than pendular nystagmus, in which the oscillations are approximately equal in rate in both directions. Jerking nystagmus occurs normally when an individual observes a moving object, but on other occasions it may be a sign of barbiturate intoxication or of labyrinthine vestibular, vascular, or neurological disease. Labyrinthine vestibular nystagmus, most frequently rotary, is usually accompanied by vertigo and nausea. Vertical nystagmus is considered pathognomonic of disease of the tegmentum of the brainstem; nystagmus occurring only in the abducting eye is said to be a sign of multiple sclerosis. Seesaw nystagmus, in which one eye moves up and the other down, may be observed in bilateral hemianopia. Pendular nystagmus occurs in albinism, in various diseases of the retina and refractive media, and in miners after many years of working in darkness. In miners the eye movements are very rapid, increase on upward gaze, and are often associated with vertigo, head tremor, and photophobia. Electronystagmography, used in testing for vestibular disease and evaluating patients with vertigo, hearing loss, or tinnitus, records changes in the electrical field around the eyes. Nystagmus is measured as the person gazes at various objects and is placed in various positions and when cold or warm water or air is introduced into the external auditory canal. This final test causes nystagmus of equal intensity in normal individuals. In patients with an inner ear or neural disorder, nystagmus may be more intense, diminished, or absent. Also called **nystaxis.** −*nystagmic, adj.*

nystatin /nis″tətin/, an antifungal antibiotic.

■ INDICATIONS: It is prescribed in oral, topical, and vaginal formulations for the treatment of fungal infections of the GI tract, skin, and vagina.

■ CONTRAINDICATIONS: Known hypersensitivity to this drug is the only contraindication.

■ ADVERSE EFFECTS: There are no known serious adverse effects. Mild GI distress and mild skin reactions may occur.

nystaxis. See **nystagmus.**

N

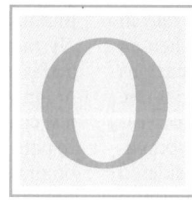

O, symbol for the element **oxygen.**

Ω, symbol for **ohm.**

O₂, symbol for an *oxygen molecule.*

oario-. See **ovario-, ovari-, oario-, ootheco-.**

OASDHI, abbreviation for **Old Age, Survivors, Disability and Health Insurance Program.**

oat cell carcinoma [AS, *ate,* oat; L, *cella,* storeroom; Gk, *karkinos,* crab, *oma,* tumor], a malignant, usually bronchogenic epithelial neoplasm consisting of small, tightly packed round, oval, or spindle-shaped epithelial cells that stain darkly and contain neurosecretory granules and little or no cytoplasm. Tumors produced by these cells do not form bulky masses but usually spread along submucosal lymphatics. Many malignant tumors of the lung are of this type. Surgical resection usually is not possible, and chemotherapy and radiation therapy are not effective in treatment; thus the long-term prognosis is poor. Also called **small cell carcinoma.**

oatmeal bath, a colloid treatment for pruritus and other skin disorders. The procedure consists of placing plain, unflavored oatmeal in a muslin bag or thin sock to infuse into bathwater or of adding special colloidal oatmeal preparations directly to tub water. The bath has a soothing effect on irritated skin.

OAV syndrome. See **Goldenhar syndrome.**

OAWO, abbreviation for **opening abductory wedge osteotomy.**

ob-, prefix meaning "against, in the way, oppose": *obliteration, obsolescence, obtuse.*

OB, 1. *(Informal)* abbreviation for **obstetrician. 2.** abbreviation for **obstetrics.**

obduction /əbdukʺshən/ [L, *obductio,* a covering], a forensic medical autopsy.

Ober and Barr procedure, a surgical method for treating weak biceps muscles by transfer of the brachioradialis muscle.

Ober procedure, a surgical method for treating paralytic clubfoot by transfer of the posterior tibial tendon to the third cuneiform or metatarsal.

Obersteiner-Redlich zone /ōʺbərshtīʺnər rädʺlish, ōʺbərstēʺnər redʺlik/ [H. Obersteiner, Austrian neurologist, 1847–1942; Emil Redlich, Austrian neurologist, 1866–1930], a thin line of demarcation between fibers of the peripheral nervous system and the spinal cord or brainstem. It is produced by a basal lamina separating the Schwann cells and collagen of the peripheral nervous system from the neuroglia of the central nervous system.

Ober test [Frank R. Ober, American surgeon, 1861–1925], an examination for tightness in the tensor fasciae latae, a muscle that flexes and rotates the thigh. The patient lies on one side with the lower hip and knee flexed on the table and the upper hip extended while the knee is flexed. Inability to place the upper knee on the table indicates tightness in the muscle.

obese /ōbēsʹ/ [L, *obesus,* swollen], pertaining to an excessive accumulation of body fat. A body mass index of greater than or equal to 30.0 indicates obesity. See also **body mass index.**

obesity /ōbēʺsitē/ [L, *obesitas,* fatness], an abnormal increase in the proportion of fat cells, mainly in the viscera and subcutaneous tissues of the body. Obesity may be exogenous or endogenous. Hyperplastic obesity is caused by an increase in the number of fat cells in the increased adipose tissue mass. Hypertrophic obesity results from an increase in the size of the fat cells in the increased adipose tissue mass.

■ OBSERVATIONS: Obesity is manifested as excess body weight for height. Overweight is determined by a body mass index (BMI) of 25 to 29.9 kg/m², and obesity is a BMI = 30 kg/m². Body fat distribution can be assessed by waist-to-hip ratios, with a ratio of greater than 1.0 for men and greater than 0.8 for women signaling increased risk of obesity. Morbidity and mortality are increased in the obese. Complications include predisposition to diabetes mellitus, hypertension, hyperlipidemia, coronary artery disease, cerebrovascular disease, osteoarthritis, sleep apnea, and certain cancers.

■ INTERVENTIONS: Treatment is aimed at weight reduction and modification of risk factors such as diabetes, hypertension, and elevated lipid levels. There are three major components in weight-loss therapy: diet therapy, physical activity, and lifestyle and behavioral modifications. Any number of approaches have been espoused that incorporate one or all of the three components. None has proved consistently successful for losing weight and maintaining weight loss. These include pharmacological drugs that suppress appetite or limit nutrient absorption; nutritional consult and diets that limit calories, fat, and carbohydrates; behavioral counseling and support networks; and surgery, such as gastroplasty, gastric partitioning, gastric bypass, and lipectomy. Blood pressure, glucose, and lipid levels are regularly monitored, and persistent elevations are treated pharmacologically.

■ PATIENT CARE CONSIDERATIONS: Obesity is an epidemic that requires a coordinated effort involving prevention and treatment by many members of the health care team. Efforts are aimed at reinforcement of long-term lifestyle changes, including a balanced diet and regular exercise. Instruction is aimed at developing mutually agreed-on diet and exercise goals and successful management of blood pressure, lipid levels, and glucose levels.

obex /ōʺbeks/, a small triangular membrane formed at the caudal angle of the rhomboid fossa or fourth ventricle of the brain.

obfuscation /obʹfəskāʺshən/ [L, *obfuscare,* to darken], the act of making becoming confused, clouded, or obscure.

OBGYN, initialism for *obstetrics and gynecology.*

OB-Gyn, *(Informal)* initialism for *obstetrics and gynecology.*

object /obʺjəkt/, **1.** (in psychology) something through which an instinct can achieve its goal. **2.** in psychoanalytic terms, a person other than self. See also **object relations. 3.** (in occupational therapy) tools, materials, and equipment used in the process of carrying out an activity. **4.** to refute or refuse.

object blindness, an inability to recognize objects or analyze spatial relationships. The condition is associated with lesions of the right cerebral hemisphere in right-handed

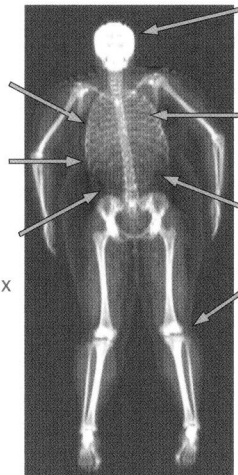

CNS/psychosocial
    Pseudotumour cerebri
    Decreased quality of life
Cardiovascular
    Raised blood pressure
    Dyslipidemia
    Atherosclerosis
    Chronic inflammation
    Coagulopathy
Renal
    Hyperfiltration
    Glomerulopathy
Orthopedic
    Lower-limb malalignment
    SCFE
    Osteoarthritis

Pulmonary
    Obstructive sleep apnea
    Asthma
    Exercise intolerance
Endocrine
    Insulin resistance
    PCOS
    Pubertal advancement
Gastrointestinal/nutrition
    Fatty liver disease
    Gastro-esophageal reflux
    Cholelithiasis
    Iron deficiency
    Vitamin D deficiency

Dual energy x-ray absorptiometry in a young, obese girl with a BMI of 38 *(Han, Lawlor, and Kimm, 2010)*

Classification of overweight and obesity by BMI, waist circumference, and associated disease risks

	BMI (kg/m²)	Obesity class	Disease risk^a relative to normal weight and waist circumference	
			Men 102 cm (40 in) or less Women 88 cm (35 in) or less	Men >102 cm (40 in) Women >88 cm (35 in)
Underweight	< 18.5		—	—
Normal^b	18.5–24.9		—	—
Overweight	25.0–29.9		Increased	High
Obesity	30.0–34.9	I	High	Very high
	35.0–39.9	II	Very high	Very high
Extreme obesity	40.0+	III	Extremely high	Extremely high

Source: National Heart, Lung, and Blood Institute, National Institutes of Health, 2015.
^aDisease risk for type 2 diabetes, hypertension, and cardiovascular disease.
^bIncreased waist circumference also can be a marker for increased risk, even in persons of normal weight.

patients. Also called **visual agnosia. See also psychic blindness, hysteric blindness.**

object constancy,   **1.** the ability to perceive an object as unchanging even under different conditions of observation. Lack of object constancy is a primary symptom of borderline personality disorder, adversely affecting the ability to bond with and trust others. **2.** (in child development) a step in development, usually achieved before the age of 2, in which a child gains the understanding that just because someone or something is out of sight, it is not gone. Regarding caregivers, the infant learns that the caregiver will return and builds trust and faith in others. See also **object permanence.**

objective /əbjek″tiv/ [L, *objectare,* to set against], **1.** *n.,* a goal and/or statement of outcomes for an educational program. **2.** *adj.,* pertaining to a phenomenon or clinical finding that is observed; not subjective. An objective finding is often described in health care as a sign that can be seen, heard, felt, or measured.

objective data collection, the process in which data relating to the client's problem are obtained through direct physical examination, including observation, palpation, percussion, and auscultation, and by laboratory analyses and radiological and other studies. Compare **subjective data collection.**

objective lens, a lens that accepts light from the output phosphor of a radiographic image-intensifier tube and converts the light into a parallel beam for recording an image.

objective sign [L, *objectum,* something cast before, *signum,* sign], a clinical observation that can be seen, heard, measured, or otherwise recorded by an examining physician, nurse, or other health care provider.

objective symptom [L, *objectum,* something cast before; Gk, *symptoma,* that which happens], a symptom accompanied by signs that tend to confirm the patient's physical complaint and enable the examining physician, nurse, or other health care provider to deduce the cause.

objective tinnitus, a noise produced in the ear that can be heard by another person, particularly someone using a stethoscope. Compare **subjective tinnitus**. See also **tinnitus.**

object permanence, a capacity to perceive that something exists even when it is not seen. See also **object constancy,** def. 2.

object relations, an emotional bond between one person and another, as contrasted with interest in and love for the self. It is usually described in terms of capacity for loving and reacting appropriately to others. An object relation is delayed or not achieved in borderline personality disorders. See also **object constancy,** def. 1.

obligate /ob″ligit, -gāt/ [L, *obligare,* to bind], characterized by the ability to survive only in a particular set of environmental conditions, such as an obligate parasite, which can survive only within the host organism. Compare **facultative.**

obligate aerobe, an organism that cannot grow in the absence of oxygen. Compare **facultative aerobe.** See also **aerobe.**

obligate anaerobe, an organism that cannot grow in the presence of oxygen, such as *Clostridium tetani, C. botulinum,* and *C. perfringens.*

obligate parasite. See **parasite.**

obligatory water loss /oblig″ətôr′ē/, the volume of water required for daily urinary excretion of metabolic waste products. This amount of water loss is necessary to maintain normal health. See also **optional water loss.**

oblique /oblēk″/ [L, *obliquus,* slanted], a slanting direction or any variation from the perpendicular or the horizontal.

oblique bandage, a circular bandage applied spirally in slanting turns, usually to a limb.

oblique fiber, any of the bundled collagenous filaments, extending from the alveolar bone to the cementum of the tooth in an apical direction on lateral view. Oblique fibers constitute approximately two thirds of the periodontal fibers and help the tooth resist vertical pressure, driving it into the socket.

oblique fissure of the lung, 1. the groove marking the division of the lower and the middle lobes in the right lung. **2.** the groove marking the division of the upper and the lower lobes in the left lung.

oblique fracture, a slanted fracture of the shaft along the bone's long axis.

oblique illumination. See **illumination.**

oblique lie, a presentation of a fetus in which the long axis of the fetal body crosses that of the maternal body at an angle close to 45 degrees. The shoulder will usually present first, but the arm or part of the trunk may also present first.

oblique popliteal ligament, an extension of the tendon of semimembranosus that reinforces the fibrous membrane of the knee joint posteromedially.

oblique presentation [L, *obliquus,* slanted, *praesentare,* to show], a presentation in which the long axis of the fetus is oblique to the long axis of the mother. Also called **oblique lie.**

obliquity of pelvis /oblik″witē/ [L, *obliquus,* aslant], an abnormal tilt of the pelvis with respect to the spinal column.

obliquus externus abdominis. See **external abdominal oblique muscle.**

obliquus internus abdominis. See **internal abdominal oblique muscle.**

obliteration /oblit′ərā″shən/ [L, *obliterare,* to efface], the removal or loss of function of a body part by surgery, disease, or degeneration.

obliterative phlebitis /oblit″ərətiv′/ [L, *obliterare,* to efface; Gk, *phleps,* vein, *itis,* inflammation], a form of phlebitis in which the inflammation results in permanent closure of the vessel. Also called **adhesive phlebitis.**

OBS, 1. abbreviation for **organic brain syndrome. 2.** abbreviation for **obstetrics. 3.** abbreviation for **observation.**

observation [L, *observare,* to watch], **1.** the act of watching carefully and attentively. **2.** a report of what is seen or noticed, such as a nursing or occupational therapy observation.

observation hip, a condition in which a child experiences a limp, pain in the hip, and limited hip motion. So called because it must be "observed" by the clinician, as there is no definitive x-ray or blood test for diagnosis. It resolves spontaneously in approximately 3 to 6 weeks. Also called **transient synovitis.**

obsession [L, *obsidere,* to haunt], a persistent and recurrent thought or idea with which the mind is continually and involuntarily preoccupied and that cannot be expunged by logic or reasoning.

obsessive-compulsive /obses″iv/ [L, *obsidere,* to haunt, *compellere,* to impel], a type of thought disturbance characterized by unwanted repetitive thoughts that lead to an overt need to act upon these thoughts for relief. The relief is generally short-lived. The cause of this disturbance is anxiety-based but not always clearly identifiable.

obsessive-compulsive disorder (OCD), an anxiety disorder characterized by recurrent and persistent thoughts, ideas, and feelings or repetitive acts sufficiently severe to cause marked distress, consume considerable time, or significantly interfere with the patient's occupational, social, or interpersonal functioning. See also **compulsive ritual.**

obsolescence /ob′səles″əns/ [L, *obsolescere,* to decay], **1.** a falling into disuse because of age or loss of function. **2.** a state of being useless.

obstetric anesthesia [L, *obstetrix,* midwife; Gk, *anaisthesia,* lack of feeling], **1.** any of various procedures used to provide anesthesia for childbirth, including local anesthesia for episiotomy or episiotomy repair; regional anesthesia for labor or delivery, such as by paracervical block or pudendal block; or, for a wider block, epidural, subdural (spinal), caudal, or saddle block. Anesthesia for cesarean section may be achieved with an epidural or subdural (spinal) block or by general anesthesia. **2.** a field of study of the science related to the delivery of anesthetic care to pregnant and postpartum patients.

obstetric forceps, forceps used to assist delivery of the fetal head. They vary in weight, length, shape, and mechanism of action, but all consist of a pair of instruments comprising a handle, a shank, and a blade. The blade is curved and sometimes has openings. The shank is long enough to allow the blade to reach the fetal head. The several styles of forceps are designed to assist in various clinical situations. The station of the fetus in the pelvis, the position of the head in relation to the pelvis, the size of the fetus, and the preference of the operator all affect the choice of forceps. Kinds include **Barton forceps, Elliot forceps, Kielland's forceps, Piper forceps, Simpson forceps.** See also **forceps delivery.**

obstetrician (OB) /ob′stətrish″ən/, a physician who specializes in the branch of medicine concerned with pregnancy and childbirth.

obstetric, obstetrical. See **obstetrics.**

obstetric position. See **lateral recumbent position.**

obstetrics (OB) /obstet″riks/ [L, *obstetrix,* midwife], the branch of medicine concerned with pregnancy and childbirth, including the study of the physiological and pathological function of the female reproductive tract and the care of the mother and fetus throughout pregnancy, childbirth, and the immediate postpartum period.

obstetrix, *(Obsolete)* now called **midwife.**

obstipation /ob′stipā″shən/ [L, *obstipare,* to press], **1.** a condition of extreme and persistent constipation caused by obstruction in the intestinal system. See also **constipation. 2.** a process of blocking. −*obstipant, n.,* −*obstipate, v.*

obstruction /obstruk″shən/ [L, *obstruere,* to build against], **1.** something that blocks or clogs. **2.** the act of blocking or preventing passage. **3.** the condition of being obstructed or clogged. −**obstructive,** *adj.,* −*obstruct, v.*

obstruction series, a test, consisting of a series of x-ray films, performed on the abdomen of patients with suspected bowel obstruction, paralytic ileus, perforated viscus,

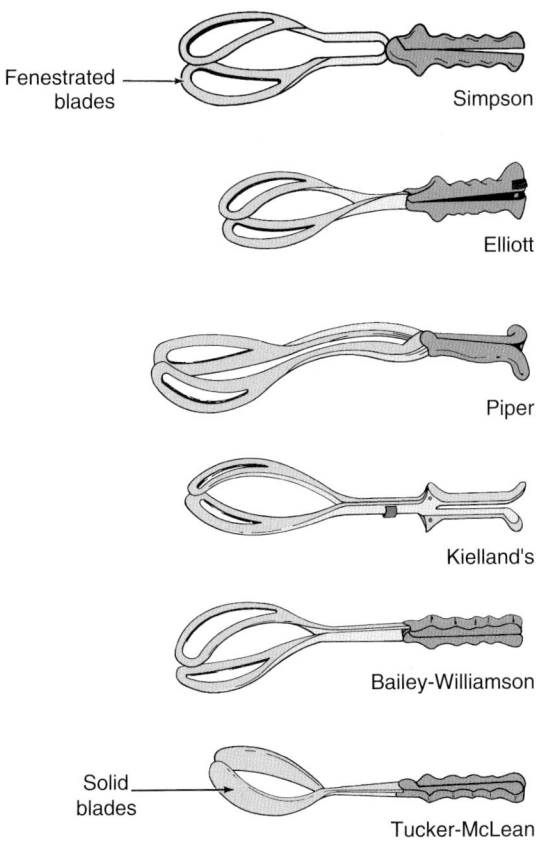

Fenestrated blades — Simpson

Elliott

Piper

Kielland's

Bailey-Williamson

Solid blades — Tucker-McLean

Obstetric forceps *(Lowdermilk et al, 2016)*

abdominal abscess, kidney stones, appendicitis, or foreign body ingestion.

obstructive, **1.** the act of blocking or clogging. See **obstruction. 2.** the state of being closed off.

obstructive airway disease /əbstruk″tiv/, any respiratory disease characterized by air trapping that is caused by decreased airway diameter or increased airway secretions or both. Kinds include **chronic bronchitis, emphysema.** See also **chronic obstructive pulmonary disease, cystic fibrosis.**

obstructive anuria [L, *obstruere,* to build against; Gk, *a + ouron,* without urine], an almost complete absence of urination caused by blockage of the urinary tract. See also **obstructive uropathy.**

obstructive biliary cirrhosis [L, *obstruere,* to build against, *bilis,* bile; Gk, *kirrhos,* yellow-orange, *osis,* condition], a form of secondary cirrhosis in which a stricture develops in the bile ducts. The condition may develop after cholecystectomy, gallstones, or a tumor.

obstructive constipation [L, *obstruere,* to build against, *constipare,* to crowd together], a condition in which feces are retained in the intestine because of a blockage in the lumen.

obstructive hydroureter, megaureter in the segment proximal to an obstruction, such as that caused by aperistalsis that interferes with passage of urine.

obstructive jaundice. See **cholestasis.**

obstructive nephropathy, nephropathy caused by obstruction of the urinary tract (usually the ureter), with hydronephrosis, slowing of the glomerular filtration rate, and tubular abnormalities.

obstructive sleep apnea, a form of sleep apnea involving a physical obstruction in the upper airways, most commonly the glottis. While often described as occuring mainly in obese patients, it in fact is also seen routinely in patients with a norml body mass index (BMI). It is also often associated with patients with secondary pulmonary insufficiency or a constitutional defect. A nonobese person with a congenital abnormality of the upper airways also may experience obstructive sleep apnea. See also **pickwickian syndrome, continuous positive airway pressure.**

■ OBSERVATIONS: The condition is usually marked by recurrent sleep interruptions, snoring, choking and gasping spells on awakening, and drowsiness caused by loss of normal sleep.

■ INTERVENTIONS: Treatment is with continuous positive airway pressure (CPAP) using a mask at night attached to a respirator. These devices also often include a heated humidifier so that the air provided is not drying to the nasal surfaces.

■ PATIENT CARE CONSIDERATIONS: Uncorrected, the disorder often leads to central sleep apnea, pulmonary failure, and cardiac abnormalities, as well as loss of deep or REM sleep.

obstructive uropathy, any pathological condition that blocks the flow of urine. Causes of the condition include prostate enlargement, renal calculi, and congenital stenosis. The condition may lead to impairment of kidney function and an increased risk of urinary infection.

obtund /obtund″/ [L, *obtundere,* to blunt], **1.** to deaden pain. **2.** to render insensitive to unpleasant or painful stimuli by reducing the level of consciousness, such as by anesthesia or a strong opioid analgesic.

obtundation /ob′tundā″shən/ [L, *obtundere,* to blunt, *atus,* process], a greatly reduced level of consciousness. The patient is not yet comatose but is close, arousing only with very strong stimulus.

obtunded, obtundent, obtundity. See **obtund.**

obturation /ob′t(y)ərā″shən/ [L, *obturare,* to stop up], an obstruction of an opening, such as an intestinal blockage.

obturator /ob″tərā′tər, ob″tyərā′tər/ [L, *obturare,* to close], **1.** a device used to block a passage or a canal or to fill in a space, such as a prosthesis implanted to bridge the gap in the roof of the mouth in a cleft palate. **2.** *(Nontechnical)* an obturator muscle or membrane. **3.** a device that is placed into a large-bore cannula during insertion to prevent potential blockage by residual tissues.

obturator artery, an artery that supplies the adductor region of the thigh.

obturator canal, a passageway between the pelvic cavity and the adductor region of the thigh formed in the superior aspect of the obturator foramen between bone, a connective tissue membrane, and muscles that fill the foramen. The upper margin of the canal is marked by the obturator groove.

obturator dislocation. See **dislocation of the hip.**

obturator externus, the flat, triangular muscle covering the outer surface of the anterior wall of the pelvis. It arises in several pelvic structures, including the rami of the pubis and the ramus of each ischium, and inserts into the trochanteric fossa of the femur. It functions to rotate the thigh laterally. Compare **obturator internus.**

obturator foramen, a large opening on each side of the lower part of the hip bone, formed posteriorly by the ischium, superiorly by the ilium, and anteriorly by the pubis.

O

obturator internus, a muscle that covers a large area of the inferior aspect of the lesser pelvis, where it surrounds the obturator foramen. It functions to rotate the thigh laterally and to extend and abduct the thigh when it is flexed. Compare **obturator externus, piriformis.**

obturator membrane, a tough fibrous membrane that covers the obturator foramen of each side of the pelvis.

obturator muscles [L, *obturare,* to close, *musculus*], a pair of thigh muscles, the external and internal obturators. The external obturator flexes and rotates the thigh laterally, and the internal obturator abducts and rotates the thigh laterally.

obturator nerve, a branch of the lumbar plexus that supplies the adductor region of the thigh.

obturator sign [L, *obturare,* to close, *signus,* sign], a sign of appendicitis or other peritoneal inflammation. The internal rotation of the right leg with the leg flexed to 90 degrees at the hip and knee and a resultant tightening of the internal obturator muscle may cause abdominal discomfort indicative of, for example, appendicitis.

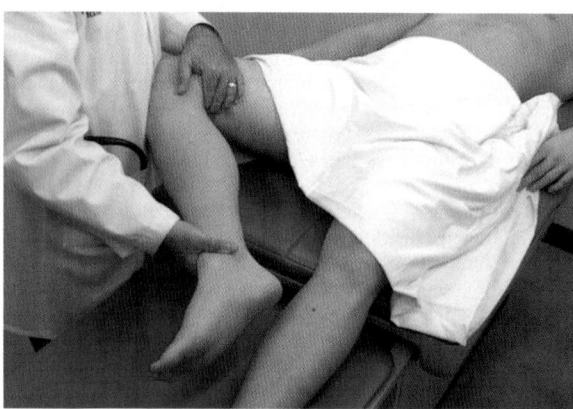

Obturator sign *(Swartz, 2009)*

obtuse, **1.** *adj.,* describing an angle that is greater than 90 degrees and less than 180 degrees. **2.** *adj.,* showing slowness or difficulty in ascertaining the meaning of others.

obv, abbreviation for **obverse.**

obverse, the position of facing the examiner during a health assessment.

oc-, prefix meaning "against" or "in the way." See also **ob-.**

OC, abbreviation for **oral contraceptive.**

OCA, abbreviation for **oculocutaneous albinism.**

occ, abbreviation for **occipital.**

occipit-, occipito-, combining form meaning "back of the head": *occipital, occipitofrontal.*

occipita. See **occiput.**

occipital (occ) /oksip″itəl/, **1.** pertaining to the back of the head. **2.** situated near the occipital bone, such as the occipital lobe of the brain.

occipital anchorage, an orthodontic anchorage in which the resistance is borne by the top and back of the head and the force is transmitted to the teeth by means of the headgear and heavy elastics connected with attachment on the teeth.

occipital artery, one of a pair of tortuous branches from the external carotid arteries that divides into six branches and supplies parts of the head and scalp. Each terminal part at the vertex of the skull is accompanied by the greater occipital nerve.

occipital bone, the cuplike bone at the back of the skull, marked by a large opening, the foramen magnum, that communicates with the vertebral canal. The occipital bone articulates with the two parietal bones, the two temporal bones, the sphenoid, and the atlas.

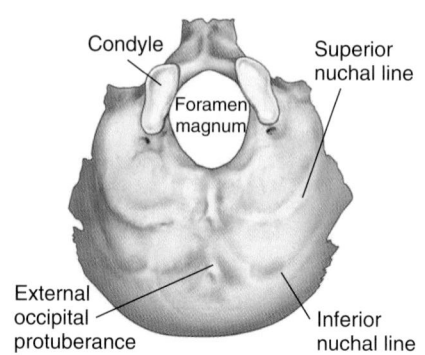

Occipital bone

occipital condyles, paired structures on each anterolateral border of the foramen magnum that articulate with the atlas.

occipital condyle syndrome, a condition characterized by a stiff neck and severe localized occipital pain that intensifies with neck flexion. It is associated with unilateral involvement of the twelfth cranial nerve, difficulty in articulating words, and difficulty in swallowing.

occipitalization /oksip′italīzā″shən/, a process of bony ankylosis of the atlas with the occipital bone.

occipital lobe, one of the five lobes of each cerebral hemisphere, occupying a relatively small pyramidal part of the occipital pole. The occipital lobe lies beneath the occipital bone and presents medial, lateral, and inferior surfaces. Compare **central lobe, frontal lobe, parietal lobe, temporal lobe.**

occipital sinus, the smallest of the cranial sinuses and one of six posterior superior venous channels associated with the dura mater. Compare **inferior sagittal sinus, straight sinus, superior sagittal sinus.**

occipito-. See **occipit-, occipito-.**

occipitoaxial ligament. See **membrana tectoria.**

occipitobregmatic /oksip′itōbregmat″ik/ [L, *occiput,* back of the head; Gk, *bregma,* front of the head], pertaining to the occiput and the bregma.

occipitofrontal /oksip′itōfrun″təl/ [L, *occiput + frons,* forehead], pertaining to the occiput and the frontal bone of the skull.

occipitofrontalis /oksip′itōfrəntal″is/, one of a pair of thin, broad muscles covering the top of the skull, consisting of an occipital belly and a frontal belly connected by an extensive aponeurosis. It is the muscle that draws the scalp and raises the eyebrows. Compare **temporoparietalis.**

occipitomastoid suture, the articulation across the lower part of the calvaria between the temporal bone and the occipital bone.

occipitoparietal fissure. See **parietooccipital sulcus.**

occiput /oksip″ət′/ *pl. occipita,* the back part of the head.

occlude. See **occlusion.**

occluded /əkloo″did/ [L, *occludere,* to close up], closed, plugged, blocked, or obstructed.

occlusal /əkloo″səl/ [L, *occludere,* to close up], pertaining to a closure, such as the contact between the teeth of the upper and lower jaws.

occlusal adjustment, the intentional mechanical modification of selected biting surfaces of teeth to improve the contact of or relationship between opposing tooth surfaces, their supporting structures, the muscles of mastication, and the temporomandibular joints. See also **bite.**

occlusal contouring, the modification by grinding of occlusal tooth irregularities, such as uneven marginal ridges and extruded or malpositioned teeth. See also **bite.**

occlusal form, the shape of the occluding surfaces of a tooth, a row of teeth, or any dentition.

occlusal harmony, a combination of healthy and nondisruptive occlusal relationships between the teeth and their supporting structures, the associated neuromuscular mechanisms, and the temporomandibular joints.

occlusal lug. See **occlusal rest.**

occlusal plane [L, *occludere,* to close up, *planum,* level ground], an imaginary flat regular surface passing through the occlusal or biting surfaces of the teeth. It represents the mean of the curvature of the occlusal (biting) surface. Also called **biteplane.** See also **curve of Spee.**

occlusal radiograph, an intraoral radiograph or dental image made with the film or image receptor placed on the occlusal biting surfaces of one of the arches. It shows the relationship of teeth to underlying structures in the alveolar process, such as cysts and abscesses.

occlusal recontouring, the reshaping of a biting (occlusal) surface of a natural or artificial tooth.

occlusal relationship, the relationship of the mandibular teeth to the maxillary teeth when they are in a defined contact position. See also **Angle's classification of malocclusion.**

occlusal rest, an indent created on the top surface of a posterior tooth to support a removable partial denture. Also called **occlusal lug.**

occlusal rest angle, the slant formed by an occlusal rest with its upright minor connector of a removable partial denture framework. Also called **rest angle.**

occlusal spillway, a natural groove that crosses a cusp ridge or a marginal ridge of a tooth.

occlusal surface [L, *occludere,* to close up, *superficies,* surface], the chewing surface of a primary or secondary posterior tooth in one arch that makes contact or near contact with the corresponding surface of a tooth in the opposite arch. Also called **masticatory surface.**

occlusal trauma, injury to a tooth and surrounding structures caused by improper biting (malocclusive) stresses, including trauma, temporomandibular joint dysfunction, and bruxism.

occlusion /əkloo″zhən/ [L, *occludere,* to close up], **1.** (in anatomy) a blockage in a canal, vessel, or passage of the body; the state of being closed. **2.** (in dentistry) any contact between the incising or masticating surfaces of the maxillary and mandibular teeth. –**occlusive,** *adj.,* –**occlude,** *v.*

occlusion rim, an artificial dental structure with biting surfaces attached to temporary or permanent denture bases, used for recording the relation of the maxilla to the mandible and for positioning the teeth. Also called **bite block.**

occlusive /əkloo″siv/, **1.** pertaining to something that effects an occlusion or closure, such as an occlusive dressing. **2.** See **occlusion.**

occlusive dressing, a dressing that prevents air from reaching a wound or lesion and that retains moisture, heat, body fluids, and medication. It may consist of a sheet of thin plastic affixed with transparent tape.

occlusive mesenteric infarction, mesenteric infarction caused by occlusion of one of the mesenteric arteries, such as by a thrombus or mechanical compression.

occlusive mesenteric ischemia, mesenteric ischemia caused by occlusion of one of the mesenteric arteries, such as by a thrombus or mechanical compression.

occlusometer. See **gnathodynamometer.**

occult /əkult″/ [L, *occultare,* to hide], hidden, not visible, or difficult to observe directly, such as occult prolapse of the umbilical cord or occult blood.

occult blood, blood that is not obvious on examination and is from a nonspecific source, with obscure signs and symptoms. It may be detected by means of a chemical test or by microscopic or spectroscopic examination. Occult blood is often present in the stools of patients with GI lesions.

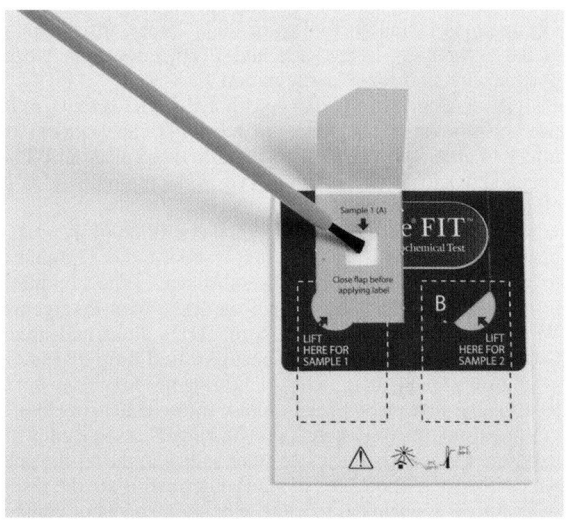

Occult blood test *(© 2015 Enterix Inc. All rights reserved.)*

occult blood test [L, *occultare,* to hide; AS, *blod* + L, *testum,* crucible], a test for the presence of microscopic amounts of blood in the feces secondary to bleeding in the digestive tract. The fecal immunochemical test (FIT) is a newer kind of stool test to detect hidden blood in the stool. It is more specific than other kinds of occult blood tests as it identifies only human blood and does not require special dietary preparation. Kinds include **gFOBT, guaiac test.**

occult carcinoma, a small carcinoma that does not cause overt symptoms. The carcinoma may remain localized, be discovered only incidentally at autopsy after death resulting from another cause, or metastasize and be discovered as a result of metastatic disease. Also called **latent carcinoma.**

occult ectopic ACTH syndrome, a medical condition that mimics the clinical and biochemical picture of Cushing disease. The cause is usually a tumor that secretes adrenocorticotropic hormone in the lungs, thymus, pancreas, adrenal medulla, or thyroid gland.

occult fracture, a fracture that cannot be detected by radiographic standard examination until several weeks after injury. The break is most likely to occur in the ribs, tibia, metatarsals, hip, or navicular. It is accompanied by the usual signs of pain and trauma and may produce soft tissue edema. Magnetic resonance imaging or a bone scan may be used to confirm a suspected occult fracture.

occupancy /ok″yəpənsē/ [L, *occupare,* to take possession of], the ratio of average daily hospital census to the total number of beds maintained during the reporting period.

occupancy factor (T), a classification used to refer to the level of human occupancy of an area adjacent to a source of radiation. The classification level is used to determine the amount of shielding required in the walls. Examples of classification levels include the following: T, rated as full, for an office or laboratory next to an x-ray facility; partial, for corridors and restrooms; or occasional, for stairways, elevators, closets, and outside areas.

occupation, activities of daily life in which people engage. Occupations occur in context and are influenced by the interplay among client factors, performance skills, and performance patterns. Occupations occur over time; have purpose, meaning, and perceived utility to the client; and can be observed by others (e.g., preparing a meal) or be known to the person involved (e.g., learning through reading a textbook). Occupations can involve the execution of multiple activities for completion and can result in various outcomes. Occupations include activities of daily living, instrumental activities of daily living, rest and sleep, education, work, play, leisure, and social participation.

occupational accident /ok′yəpā″shənəl/ [L, *occupare*, to take possession of, *accidere*, to happen], an accident or injury to an employee that occurs in the workplace or while engaged in a job activity. In most cases the injured worker is eligible for compensation.

occupational asthma, an abnormal condition of the respiratory system resulting from exposure in the workplace to allergenic or other irritating substances. The condition is most common among people working with detergents, Western red cedar, cotton, flax, hemp, grain, flour, and stone. See also **asthma, byssinosis, occupational lung disease.**

occupational deafness, a loss of hearing resulting from noise levels in the workplace. See also **noise-induced hearing loss.**

occupational dermatoses, skin disorders associated with exposure to toxic chemicals or other agents in the workplace. An estimated 80% of cases of contact dermatitis are the result of exposure to chemical irritants. Common agents of contact dermatitis in the workplace are glass fibers, cutting fluids, chemical stains, and polyhalogenated aromatic compounds such as phenol, naphthalene, and aniline herbicide intermediates. Factors influencing development of dermatoses include skin thickness, skin permeability, anatomical site, concentration of chemical, surface area of exposure, and type of substance in which the toxic chemical is dissolved or mixed.

occupational disability, a condition in which a worker is unable to perform regular duties and carry out the functions required to complete a job satisfactorily because of an occupational disease or an occupational accident.

occupational disease, a disease that results from a particular type of employment, usually from the effects of long-term exposure to specific substances or continuous or repetitive physical acts.

occupational health, the ability of a worker to function at an optimum level of well-being at a worksite as reflected in terms of productivity, work attendance, disability compensation claims, and employment longevity.

occupational history, a component of the health history in which questions are asked about the person's occupation, source of income, effects of the work on the worker's health or the worker's health on the job, the duration of the job, and to what degree the occupation satisfies the person. Any adverse effects known to be associated with the work or the place of work are investigated by further questions by the interviewer; for example, a tennis player might be asked about musculoskeletal problems.

occupational lung disease, any of a group of abnormal conditions of the lungs caused by the inhalation of dusts, fumes, gases, or vapors in an environment where a person works. See also **chronic obstructive pulmonary disease, metal fume fever, occupational asthma, silo filler's disease.**

occupational medicine, a field of preventive medicine concerned with the medical problems and practices relating to occupations and especially to the health of workers in various industries.

occupational neurosis. See **occupational stress.**

occupational performance, (in occupational therapy) the act of doing and accomplishing a selected action (performance skill), activity, or occupation that results from a dynamic interaction among the client, the context, and the activity.

occupational performance tasks, activities that can be used to measure the potential ability or actual proficiency in the handling of certain objects and the use of skills related to a given occupation.

occupational socialization, the adaptation of an individual to a given set of job-related behaviors, particularly the expected behavior that accompanies a specific job.

occupational stress, a disorder associated with a job or work. The anxiety may be expressed in the form of extreme tension and anxiety and the development of physical symptoms such as headache or cramps. Also called **occupational neurosis.** See also **burnout.**

occupational therapist (OT), an allied health professional who is nationally certified to practice occupational therapy. The OT uses purposeful activity and interventions designed to maximize the independence and health of any client who is limited by physical injury or illness, cognitive impairment, psychosocial dysfunction, mental illness, or a developmental or learning disability. During assessment, an OT works with a client to determine how the onset of disease or impairment adversely impacts the client's prioritized daily occupations. Services include the education of the client and the client's family and community; interventions directed toward developing daily living skills, work readiness, or work/school performance; remediation of sensory-motor, perceptual, or neuromuscular impairments; and adaptation of the contextual or physical environment to facilitate the performance of chosen occupations.

occupational therapy (OT), the therapeutic use of everyday life activities (occupations) with individuals or groups for the purpose of enhancing or enabling participation in roles, habits, routines, and rituals in home, school, workplace, community, and other settings. Occupational therapy practitioners use their knowledge of the transactional relationship among the person, his or her engagement in valued occupations, and the context to design occupation-based intervention plans that facilitate change or growth in client factors and performance skills needed for successful participation. See also **occupational therapist.**

occupational therapy aide, a person who, under the supervision of an occupational therapist (OT) or OT assistant, performs clerical and other treatment-related tasks necessary for the implementation of occupational therapy programs.

occupational therapy assistant. See **certified occupational therapy assistant.**

occupational therapy practice framework, an official document of the American Occupational Therapy Association, intended for internal and external audiences, that presents a summary of interrelated constructs that define and guide occupational therapy practice. It outlines occupational therapy's contribution in promoting the health and participation of people, organizations, and populations through engagement in occupation.

occurrence policy /əkur″əns/ [L, *occurere*, to run, *politica*, pertaining to the state], a professional liability insurance policy that covers the holder during the period an alleged act of malpractice occurred. Occurrence policies are said to have a "long tail" because the statute of limitations on malpractice allegations is unlimited. Thus an individual could be sued years after an event took place. If the individual held an occurrence type of malpractice policy, there would be protection under that policy. Under a claims-made policy there would not be protection unless the policy was current.

OCD, abbreviation for **obsessive-compulsive disorder.**

ochre mutation, a genetic alteration that causes the synthesis of polypeptide chain to terminate prematurely because the triplet of nucleotides in mRNA that normally codes for the next amino acid in the chain becomes uracil-adenine-guanine (UAG), the sequence that signals the end of the chain. It is one of three possible nonsense mutations. See also **amber mutation, opal mutation, nonsense mutation.**

ochronosis /ō′krənō″sis/ [Gk, *ochros,* yellow, *osis*], an inherited error of protein metabolism characterized by an accumulation of homogentisic acid, resulting in degenerative arthritis and brown-black pigment deposited in connective tissue and cartilage. It is often caused by alkaptonuria or poisoning with phenol. Bluish macules may be noted on the sclera, fingers, ears, nose, genitalia, buccal mucosa, and axillae. Urine color may be dark. See also **alkaptonuria.**

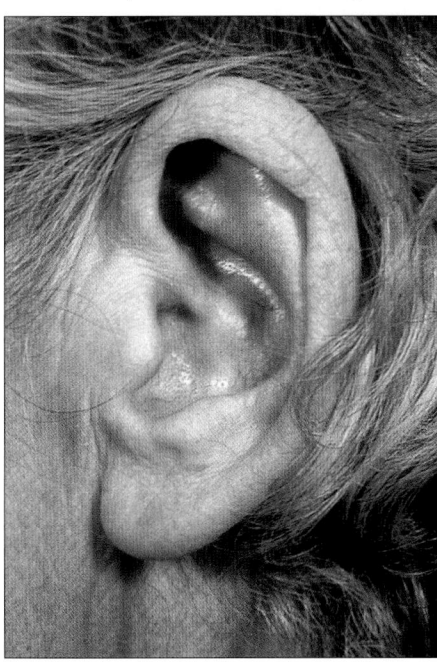

Blue-gray pigmentation of the ear cartilage in a patient with ochronosis (Hochberg et al, 2015)

OCN, initialism for *Oncology Certified Nurse.*

oncotic pressure. See **colloid osmotic pressure.**

OCT, **1.** abbreviation for **oxytocin challenge test.** **2.** abbreviation for **ornithine carbamoyltransferase.** See **ornithine carbamoyltransferase (OCT) deficiency.**

octacosanol, a dietary supplement. Also called *1-octacosanol.*
■ INDICATIONS: It may be used for herpes, inflammation of the skin, amyotrophic lateral sclerosis (ALS), and physical endurance. There are insufficient data to support routine use.
■ CONTRAINDICATIONS: Octacosanol should not be used during pregnancy and lactation or in children.

octan /ok″tan/, occurring at 7-day intervals, or every 8th day.

octanoic acid breath test, a breath test for gastric emptying. The patient is administered a test meal containing octanoic acid labeled with carbon 13, and the breath is assessed at intervals for levels of labeled carbon dioxide; excessive carbon dioxide is seen when gastric emptying is inadequate. The test is not universally accepted as valid.

octa-, octi-, octo-, prefix meaning "the number eight" or "series of eight": *octigravida, octan, octagenarian.*

octaploid, octaploidic. See **polyploid.**

octigravida /ok′tigrav″ədə/ [L, *octo,* eight, *gravidus,* pregnancy], a woman who is pregnant for the eighth time.

octinoxate /oktin′ok-sāt/, an absorber of ultraviolet B radiation, used topically as a sunscreen. Also called **octyl methoxycinnamate.**

octisalate /ok″tĭsal′āt/, a substituted salicylate that absorbs ultraviolet light in the UVB range, used as a sunscreen.

octo-. See **octa-, octi-, octo-.**

octocrylene /ok′to-kril″ēn/, a sunscreen that absorbs ultraviolet rays in the UVB range.

octogenarian, an individual whose age is 80 to 89.

octopus /ok′təpəs/, any of numerous carnivorous marine mollusks having eight tentacles and venom.

octreotide, an antidiarrheal and hormone that mimics natural somatostatin.
■ INDICATIONS: The two brand names of this drug are used for different purposes. Sandostatin is used to treat acromegaly, carcinoid tumors, and vasoactive intestinal peptide tumors (VIPomas). Sandostatin LAR Depot is used for long-term maintenance of acromegaly, carcinoid tumors, and VIPomas. Octreotide is also used for refractory hypoglycemia.
■ CONTRAINDICATIONS: Known hypersensitivity to this drug prohibits its use.
■ ADVERSE EFFECTS: Common side effects include headache, dizziness, fatigue, weakness, sinus bradycardia, conduction abnormalities, hyperglycemia, ketosis, hypothyroidism, diarrhea, nausea, abdominal pain, vomiting, flatulence, distension, and joint and muscle pain. Life-threatening effects include seizure, arrhythmias, congestive heart failure, hepatitis, GI bleeding, and pancreatitis.

octreotide scan, a nuclear scan performed to detect neuroendocrine tumors, both primary and metastatic.

octyl methoxycinnamate /ok′til mĕthok″sesin′āmāt/, an organic compound found in sunscreens. See also **octinoxate.**

ocul, short for a Latin word that means "pertaining to the eyes." Acronym for *oculis.*

ocular /ok″yəlǝr/ [L, *oculus,* eye], **1.** *adj.,* pertaining to the eye. **2.** *n.,* an eyepiece of an optic instrument.

ocular dysmetria, a visual disorder in which the eyes are unable to fix the gaze on an object or follow a moving object with accuracy. It is often characterized by overshooting, in which the eyes move farther than the intended object of fixation. It is a sign of cerebellar disease.

ocular herpes [L, *oculus,* eye; Gk, *herpein,* to creep], a herpesvirus infection of the eye that usually resolves with no treatment. When treatment is implemented, the purpose is to minimize scarring. See also **herpes simplex keratitis, herpes zoster ophthalmicus.**

ocular hypertelorism, a developmental defect involving the frontal region of the cranium, characterized by an abnormally widened bridge of the nose and increased distance between the eyes. The condition is often associated with other cranial and facial deformities and some degree of intellectual disability. Also called **orbital hypertelorism.**

ocular hypertension, a condition of intraocular pressure that is higher than normal but that has not resulted in a constricted visual field or increased cupping of the optic nerve head. See also **glaucoma.**

ocular hypotelorism, a developmental defect involving the frontal region of the cranium, characterized by an abnormal narrowing of the bridge of the nose and decreased distance between the eyes with resulting convergent strabismus.

O

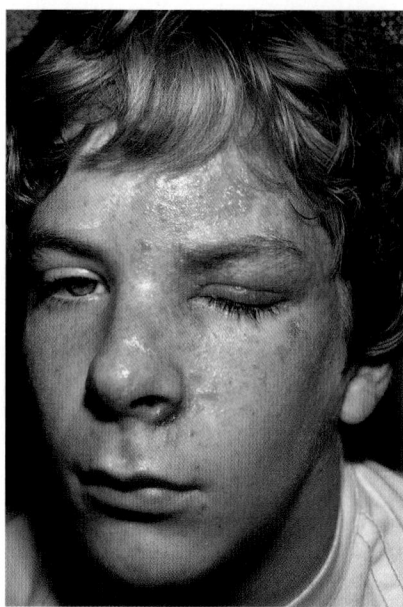

Young boy with ocular herpes *(Habif, 2010)*

The condition is often associated with other cranial and facial deformities, primarily microcephaly, trigonocephaly, and some degree of intellectual disability. Also called **orbital hypotelorism.**

ocular melanoma, malignant melanoma arising from the structures of the eye, usually the choroid, ciliary body, or iris, and occurring most often in the fourth and fifth decades of life; the most common site of metastasis is the liver, and such metastasis is often fatal.

ocular myopathy, slowly progressive weakness of ocular muscles, characterized by decreased mobility of the eye and drooping of the upper lid. The disorder may be unilateral or bilateral and may be caused by damage to the oculomotor nerve, an intracranial tumor, or a neuromuscular disease.

ocular refraction [L, *oculus,* eye, *refringere,* to break apart], an examination of vision to determine the need for corrective lenses.

oculo-, combining form meaning "eye": *oculomotor, oculocephalic reflex, oculogyric crisis.*

oculoauriculovertebral dysplasia. See **Goldenhar syndrome.**

oculocephalic reflex /ok′yəlō′səfal″ik/ [L, *oculus* + Gk, *kephale,* head; L, *reflectere,* to bend backward], a test of the integrity of brainstem function. When the patient's head is quickly moved to one side and then to the other, the eyes will normally lag behind the head movement and then slowly assume the midline position. Failure of the eyes to either lag properly or revert back to the midline in an adult indicates a lesion on the ipsilateral side at the brainstem level. Also called **doll's head maneuver.**

oculocerebral-hypopigmentation syndrome /ok′yəlō′-sərē′brəl/ [L, *oculus,* eye + *cerebrum,* brain], an autosomal-recessive syndrome marked by cutaneous hypopigmentation, microphthalmos, small opaque corneas, gingival hypertrophy, and cerebral defect manifested by spasticity, mental and physical disabilities, and athetoid movements. Also called **Cross syndrome.**

oculocerebrorenal syndrome. See **Lowe syndrome.**

oculocutaneous albinism (OCA) /ok′yo͞olōkyo͞otā′-nē·əs/, a human albinism occurring in 10 types, all distinguished in their incidence and genetic, biochemical, and clinical characteristics but having in common varying degrees of decreased melanotic pigment of the skin, hair, and eyes; hypoplastic foveas; photophobia; nystagmus; and decreased visual acuity.

oculoglandular syndrome /ok′yəlōglan″dyələr/, a granulomatous form of conjunctivitis affecting one eye, associated with a visibly enlarged and tender lymph node on the same side. The most common causes are cat-scratch disease and tularemia.

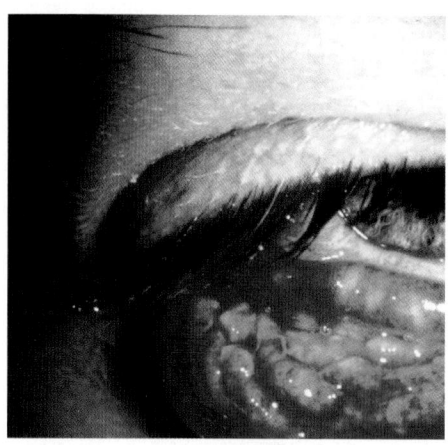

Oculoglandular syndrome *(Kliegman et al, 2016)*

oculogyric crisis /ok′yəlōjī″rik/ [L, *oculus* + *gyrare,* to turn around], a paroxysm in which the eyes are held in a fixed position, usually up and sideways, for minutes or several hours, often occurring in postencephalitic patients with signs of parkinsonism. In some cases the eyes are held down or sideways, and there may be spasm or closing of the lids. Oculogyric crises may be precipitated by emotional stress and neuroleptic overdose, and patients with the disorder frequently show psychiatric symptoms.

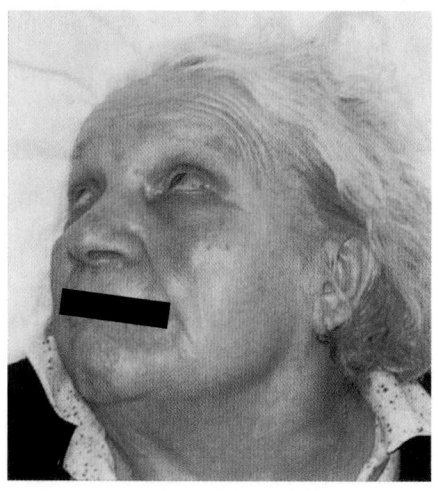

Woman with oculogyric crisis *(Perkin et al, 2011)*

oculomotor /-mō″tər/ [L, *oculus,* eye, *motor,* mover], pertaining to movements of the eyeballs.

oculomotor apraxia, Cogan type (COMA) [David Glendenning Cogan, American ophthalmologist,

1908–1993], an absence or defect of horizontal eye movements so that when the patient tries to look at an object off to one side, the head must turn to bring the eyes into line with the object, and the eyes exhibit nystagmus.

oculomotor nerve [L, *oculus* + *motor,* mover], one of a pair of cranial nerves essential for eye movements, supplying certain extrinsic and intrinsic eye muscles. They pass through the superior orbital fissure, connecting to the brain in nucleus III. Also called **nervus oculomotorius, third cranial nerve.**

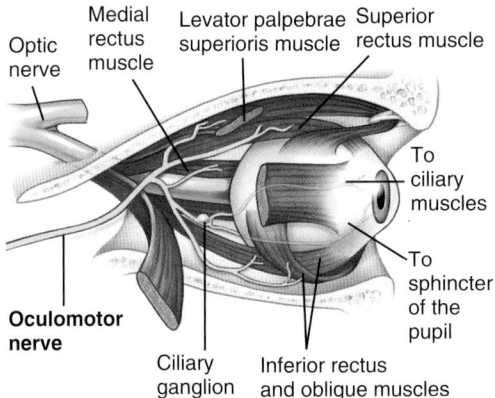

Oculomotor nerve

oculomotor nucleus [L, *oculus,* eye, *motor,* mover, *nucleus,* nut kernel], a nucleus of a third cranial nerve arising in the midbrain.

oculus. See **eye.**

Ocusert Pilo, a cholinergic agonist used topically to treat glaucoma. Brand name for **pilocarpine hydrochloride.**

OD, 1. a notation for the Latin phrase *oculus dexter,* meaning *right eye. OD* should no longer be used as an abbreviation for *right eye* because of the potential for error. **2.** abbreviation for *Doctor of Optometry.* **3.** initialism for **overdose.**

odaxetic /ō′dakset″ik/ [Gk, *odaxein,* a biting pain], causing a tactile sensation of itching or biting.

OD'd /ōdēd″/, (*Slang*) overdosed; usually referring to a person who has suffered adverse effects from an excessively large dose of a drug of abuse.

Oddi's sphincter [Ruggero Oddi, Italian surgeon, 1864–1913; Gk, *sphigein,* to bind], a band of circular muscle fibers around the lower part of the common bile duct and pancreatic duct, near the common duct junction with the duodenum.

-ode, suffix meaning "a type of pathway": *anode, cathode, electrode.*

odont-. See **odonto-, odont-.**

odontalgia. See **toothache.**

odontectomy /ōdontek″təmē/ [Gk, *odous,* tooth, *ektomē,* cut out], the extraction of a tooth by removal of the bone from around the roots before force is applied.

-odontia, -odontic, suffix meaning "teeth": *gerodontics, endodontics.*

odontiasis /ō′dontī″əsis/, the process of teething.

-odontie. See **-odontia, -odontic.**

odontitis /ō′dontī″tis/ [Gk, *odous* + *itis,* inflammation], abnormal enlargement of a tooth pulp, usually resulting from inflammation of the odontoblasts (cells responsible for dentin formation) rather than of the mature, or erupted, tooth. It may be caused by infection, tumor, or trauma. See also **pulpitis.**

odonto-, odont-, combining form meaning "teeth": *odontoblast, odontectomy.*

odontoblast /ōdon″təblast′/ [Gk, *odous,* tooth, *blastos,* germ], one of the connective tissue cells in the periphery of the dental pulp that develops into the primary and secondary dentin of a tooth. Also called *dentinoblast.*

odontodynia. See **toothache.**

odontodysplasia /-displā″zhə/ [Gk, *odous* + *dys,* bad, *plasis,* forming], an abnormality in the development of the teeth, characterized by deficient formation of enamel and dentin. The teeth have a marked reduction in radiodensity in a radiograph of the teeth, giving them a ghostlike appearance due to the presence of thin amounts of enamel and dentin. It most often affects the maxillary central and lateral incisors, usually on one side of the midline. The cause is unknown, and extraction is the treatment of choice. Also called **ghost teeth.** See also **shell teeth.**

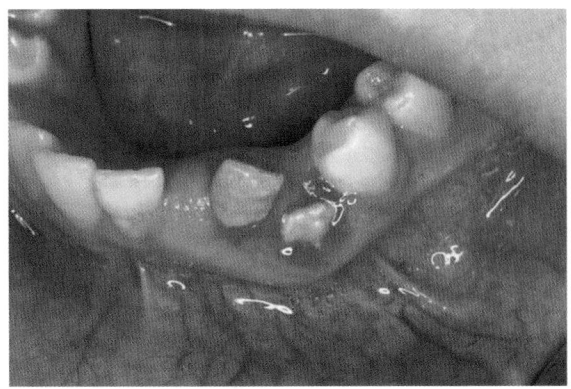

Regional odontodysplasia *(Sapp, 2004)*

odontogenesis /-jen″əsis/ [Gk, *odous,* tooth, *genein,* to produce], the origin and formation of developing teeth. Also called **odontogeny.**

odontogenesis imperfecta. See **dentinogenesis imperfecta.**

odontogenic /ōdon′tōjen″ik/ [Gk, *odous* + *genein,* to produce], **1.** pertaining to the generation of teeth. **2.** developing in tissues that produce teeth.

odontogenic cyst, 1. a cyst derived from epithelium related to tooth development, usually containing fluid or semisolid material, that develops along lines of embryonic fusion or during various stages of tooth formation and development and is nearly always enclosed within bone. Odontogenic cysts are subclassified as developmental or inflammatory in origin. Kinds include **dentigerous cyst, primordial cyst, odontogenic keratocyst,** *gingival cyst of the newborn, eruption cyst.* **2.** any of a variety of lesions of mouth tissues, including the relatively common dentigerous cyst, which is associated with the crown of an unerupted third molar or maxillary cuspid.

odontogenic fibroma, a benign neoplasm of the jaw derived from the embryonic part of the tooth germ, dental follicle, or dental papilla or from the periodontal membrane.

odontogenic fibrosarcoma, a malignant neoplasm of the jaw that develops in a mesenchymal component of a tooth or tooth germ.

odontogenic keratocyst (OKC), a distinctive developmental odontogenic cyst that arises from the dental lamina, containing clear fluid or a semisolid material. This usually asymptomatic lesion can occur at any age and is found upon radiographic or dental imaging. Large lesions may present

O

with pain, swelling, or drainage. OKC may exhibit aggressive clinical behavior, and it has a relatively high recurrence rate. It is associated with nevoid basal cell carcinoma syndrome.

odontogenic myxoma, a rare tumor of the jaw that may develop from the mesenchyme of the tooth germ.

odontogeny. See **odontogenesis.**

odontoid ligament. See **alar ligament.**

odontoid process [Gk, *odous* + *eidos,* form; L, *processus*], the toothlike projection that rises perpendicularly from the upper surface of the body of the second cervical vertebra (axis) and that serves as a pivot point for the rotation of the atlas (first cervical vertebra), enabling the head to turn. Also called **dens.**

odontoid vertebra. See **axis.**

odontology /ō′dontol″əjē/ [Gk, *odous* + *logos,* science], the scientific study of the anatomy and physiology of the teeth and of the surrounding structures of the oral cavity.

odontoma /ō′dontō″mə/ [Gk, *odous* + *oma,* tumor], the most common of odontogenic tumors, a benign tumor consisting of cementum, dentin, enamel, and pulp tissue that may be arranged in the form of teeth (compound odontoma) or as an unrecognizable mass of enamel and dentin (complex odontoma). Also called **gestant anomaly.**

odontoperiosteum. See **periodontium,** def. 1.

odor /ō″dər/ [L, a smell], a scent or smell. The sense of smell is activated when airborne molecules stimulate receptors of the first cranial nerve.

odoriferous /ō′dərif″ərəs/ [L, *odor,* smell, *ferre,* to bear], pertaining to something that produces a smell, particularly one that is strong or offensive.

odorous /ō″dərəs/ [L, *odor,* smell], pertaining to something that has an odor, smell, or fragrance.

ODTS, abbreviation for **organic dust toxic syndrome.**

odynacusis [Gk, *odyne,* pain, *akouein,* to hear], a painful sensitivity to noise.

-odyna, -odyne, -odynia, odyno-, combining form meaning "pain": *anodyne, odynacusis.*

odynophagia /od′inōfā″jə/ [Gk, *odyne,* pain, *phagein,* to swallow], a severe sensation of burning, squeezing pain while swallowing caused by irritation of the mucosa or a muscular disorder of the esophagus, such as gastroesophageal reflux; bacterial or fungal infection; tumor; achalasia; or chemical irritation.

oedema. See **edema.**

Oedipus complex /ed″ipəs, ē″dəpəs/ [Gk, *Oedipus,* mythic king who slew his father and married his mother], **1.** (in Freudian psychoanalytic theory) a child's desire for a sexual relationship with the parent of the opposite sex, usually with strong negative feelings for the parent of the same sex. **2.** a son's desire for a sexual relationship with his mother. Compare **Electra complex.** See also **phallic stage.**

OEM, abbreviation for *optical electron microscope.*

OER, abbreviation for **oxygen enhancement ratio.**

oesophagectomy. See **esophagectomy.**

oesophagitis. See **esophagitis.**

oesophagoscopy. See **esophagoscopy.**

oesophagus. See **esophagus.**

oestriol. See **estriol.**

oestrogen. See **estrogen.**

oestrone. See **estrone.**

o/f, abbreviation for *oxidation/fermentation.*

OFD, abbreviation for *oral-facial-digital.*

off-center grid, (in radiology) a focused grid that is perpendicular to the central-axis x-ray beam but is shifted laterally. This positioning error results in grid cutoff across the entire x-ray image.

off-cycle time, (in managed care) a time during which open enrollment in a health plan is usually not permitted.

off-focus radiation, (in radiology) x-rays produced by stray electrons that interact at points on the anode other than the focal spot.

Office of the Inspector General (OIG) of the United States, an agency within the U.S. Department of Health and Human Services that enforces Medicare regulations and investigates and prosecutes charges of Medicare fraud and abuse.

off-level grid, (in radiology) a grid that is not perpendicular to the central-axis x-ray beam. The cause is either a malpositioned x-ray tube or an improperly positioned grid.

off-line, pertaining to access to computer information not directly connected to a computer. Compare **online.**

ofloxacin /oflak″səsin/, a fluoroquinolone antibiotic.

■ INDICATIONS: It is used to treat complicated systemic infections when first-line agents are not an option; it is applied topically for local eye infections.

■ CONTRAINDICATIONS: Its use is contraindicated during pregnancy and in children. A known hypersensitivity to quinolones also prohibits its use.

■ ADVERSE EFFECTS: Adverse effects include acute tendinopathy, QT interval prolongation, dizziness, headache, and GI upset. Usage of the drug also carries a warning for permanent neurotoxicity ranging from peripheral neuropathy to seizures.

Ogden classification system, a system for categorizing different kinds of epiphyseal fractures.

Ogden plate, a long metal plate used for fixing long bone fractures. It is designed to accommodate preexisting intramedullary devices, such as rods or the stem of a prosthesis, and has slots that can accept encircling bands.

Ogen, an estrogen. Brand name for **estropipate.**

Ogsten line [Sir Alexander Ogsten, Scottish surgeon, 1844–1929], a line drawn through the knee from the adduction tubercle to the intercondylar notch, used as a guide for transection of the condyle in the surgical repair of knock-knee.

OH, symbol for **hydroxyl.**

o.h., short for a Latin phrase meaning "hourly." Abbreviation for *omni hora.*

OHF, abbreviation for **Omsk hemorrhagic fever.**

ohm (Ω) [Georg S. Ohm, German physicist, 1787–1854], a unit of measurement of electric resistance. One ohm is the resistance of a conductor in which an electrical potential of 1 volt produces a current of 1 ampere. See also **ampere, Ohm's law, volt, watt.**

Ohm's law [Georg S. Ohm], the principle that the strength or intensity of an unvarying electric current is directly proportional to the electromotive force and inversely proportional to the resistance of the circuit.

-oi, a plural-forming suffix in borrowings from Greek.

-oid, suffix meaning "resembling or having the appearance of" something specified: *alkaloid, amyloid, ceroid.*

OIG, initialism for *Office of the Inspector General.* See **Office of the Inspector General (OIG) of the United States.**

oiko-, eco-, prefix meaning "house": *ecology, ecosystem.*

oil [L, *oleum*], any of a large number of greasy liquid substances not miscible in water. Oil may be fixed or volatile and is derived from animal, vegetable, or mineral matter.

oil-in-water emulsion, an emulsion in which oil is the dispersed liquid and an aqueous solution is the continuous phase. Water can be used to dilute such an emulsion or to remove it, as from skin or clothing.

oil retention enema, an enema containing about 200 to 250 mL of an oil-based solution given to soften a fecal mass.

The patient is asked to retain the solution for 30 minutes to several hours. See also **lubricating enema.**

ointment [L, *unguentum,* a salve], a semisolid, externally applied preparation, usually containing a drug. Various ointments are used as local analgesic, anesthetic, antibiotic, astringent, depigmenting, irritant, and keratolytic agents. Also called **salve, unction, unguent.**

ointment base, a vehicle for the medicinal substances carried in an ointment.

-ol, **1.** suffix designating a member of the alcohol group: *ethanol, methanol, phenol.* **2.** suffix meaning "an oil": cholesterol.

olanzapine, an atypical antipsychotic and neuroleptic.

■ INDICATIONS: It is used to treat schizophrenia and related disorders.

■ CONTRAINDICATIONS: Known hypersensitivity to this drug prohibits its use.

■ ADVERSE EFFECTS: The most common side effects are weight gain, hyperglycemia, and other endocrine-like effects. Orthostatic hypotension, GI disturbances, and dry mouth have been reported. Movement disorders, extrapyramidal symptoms, and neuroleptic malignant syndrome are possible but less likely.

Old Age Security, the government of Canada's largest pension program, funded out of the country's general revenue.

Old Age, Survivors, Disability and Health Insurance Program (OASDHI), a benefit program, administered by the U.S. Social Security Administration, that provides cash benefits to workers who are retired or disabled, their dependents, and survivors; it is commonly referred to as Social Security. The program also provides health insurance benefits for people over 65 and for people under 65 who are disabled. The health insurance benefits are commonly referred to as Medicare. See also **Medicare.**

old dislocation, a dislocation in which inflammatory changes have occurred.

Older Americans Act Amendment of 1987, U.S. federal legislation authorizing support of Title III nutritional services for state and county programs on aging. The services include both congregate and home-delivered meals, with related nutritional education.

Older Americans Resources and Services Scale, a scale of instrumental activities of daily living, consisting of eight questions designed to assess a person's degree of involvement with family and society.

old-old, pertaining to persons 85 years of age and older. This term is increasingly used in demographics, statistics, and research to define a new large group of much older adults, adults who are living longer because of advances in medicine, technology, and lifestyle.

old tuberculin [ME, *ald* + L, *tubercle*], the original formula for an extract of the tubercle bacillus used in the treatment of tuberculosis by Koch, using a glycerin-broth culture of *Mycobacterium tuberculosis* after filtration and concentration of the liquid. Compare **tuberculin purified protein derivative.**

Old World leishmaniasis. See **cutaneous leishmaniasis.**

-ole, suffix meaning "a small or little example of the noun named": *arteriole.*

oleandrism /ō′lē·an″drizəm/, a toxic effect of ingesting or inhaling the cardiac glycoside contained in the roots, bark, flowers, and seeds of oleander *(Nerium oleander),* an evergreen ornamental shrub. Symptoms range from nausea and vomiting to bradycardia and cardiac arrest.

olecranon /ōlek″rənon/ [Gk, *olekranon,* tip of the elbow], a proximal projection of the ulna that forms the tip of the elbow and fits into the olecranon fossa of the humerus

when the forearm is extended. The anterior surface of the olecranon forms part of the trochlear notch that articulates with the trochlea of the humerus. Also called **olecranon process.**

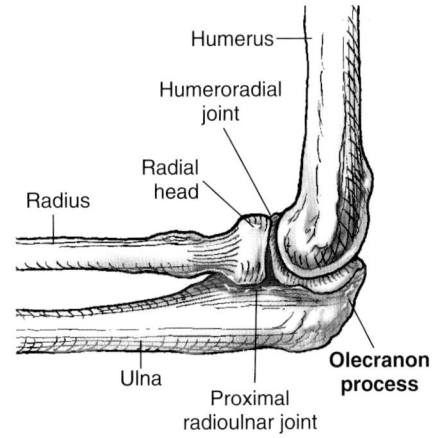

Olecranon process *(Frank, Long, and Smith, 2012)*

olecranon bursa, the bursa of the elbow.

olecranon fossa, the depression in the posterior surface of the humerus that receives the olecranon of the ulna when the forearm is extended. Compare **coronoid fossa.**

olecranon process. See **olecranon.**

olefiant gas. See **ethylene.**

olefin /ō″ləfin/ [L, *oleum,* oil, *facere,* to make], any of a group of unsaturated aliphatic hydrocarbons containing one or more double bonds in the carbon chain. Also called **alkene.**

oleic acid /ōlē″ik/ [L, *oleum,* oil, *acidus,* sour], a colorless, monounsaturated omega-9 fatty acid occurring in almost all natural fats. It is a liquid at room temperature. Commercial oleic acid is used in soaps, cosmetics, ointments, lubricants, and food additives.

oleo-, eleo-, prefix meaning "oil": *oleoresin, oleovitamin.*

oleoresin /ō′lē·ōrez′in/ [L, *oleum,* oil + *resin*], **1.** any natural combination of a resin and a volatile oil, such as exudes from pines and other plants. **2.** a compound prepared by exhausting a drug by percolation with a volatile solvent, such as acetone, alcohol, or ether, and evaporating the solvent.

oleovitamin /ō′lē·ōvī″təmin/, a preparation of fish-liver oil or edible vegetable oil that contains one or more of the fat-soluble vitamins or their derivatives.

oleovitamin A, an oily preparation, usually fish-liver oil or fish-liver oil diluted with an edible vegetable oil, containing the natural or synthetic form of vitamin A.

oleovitamin D₂. See **calciferol.**

Olestra, a synthetic fat substitute derived from sucrose and eight acids of vegetable oils. Olestra adds no calories or fats to the food into which it is incorporated. Because the molecules of Olestra are larger and more tightly packed than those of ordinary fats, they cannot be broken down by digestive enzymes and cannot enter the bloodstream. Adverse effects reported include cramping and loose stools in some people and inhibition of absorption of some vitamins. A newer formulation is fortified with certain fat-soluble vitamins.

olfaction /olfak″shən/ [L, *olfacere,* to smell], **1.** the act of smelling. **2.** the sense of smell, which involves the detection and perception of airborne chemicals that enter the nose and dissolve in mucus within a membrane called the olfactory epithelium.

O

olfactory bulb [L, *olfactus,* sense of smell, *bulbus,* swollen root], the area of the forebrain where the olfactory nerves terminate and the olfactory tracts arise.

olfactory center [L, *olfactus,* sense of smell; Gk, *kentron*], the part of the brain responsible for the subjective appreciation of odors, a complex group of neurons located near the junction of the temporal and parietal lobes.

olfactory cortex [L, *olfactus,* sense of smell, *cortex,* bark], the part of the cerebral cortex, including the pyriform lobe and the hippocampus formation, that is concerned with the sense of smell. Also called **archeocortex.**

olfactory foramen, one of several openings in the cribriform plate of the ethmoid bone.

olfactory hallucination [L, *olfactus,* sense of smell, *alucinari,* to wander mentally], a condition in which an individual has false perceptions of odors, which are usually repugnant or offensive. The hallucinations are sometimes associated with guilt feelings.

olfactory lobe [L, *olfactus,* sense of smell; Gk, *lobos,* lobe], a structure involved in the sense of smell in lower animals. Vestiges of the tissue are found in the cerebral hemispheres of humans.

olfactory nerve, one of a pair of nerves associated with the sense of smell. They are composed of numerous fine filaments that ramify in the mucous membrane of the olfactory area. The fibers of the olfactory nerve are nonmedullated and unite into fasciculi that form a plexus under the mucous membrane and rise in grooves or canals in the ethmoid bone. The fibers pass into the skull and form synapses with the dendrites of the mitral cells. The area in which the olfactory nerves arise is situated in the most superior part of the mucous membrane that covers the superior nasal concha. The olfactory sensory endings are modified epithelial cells and are the least specialized of the special senses. The olfactory nerves connect with the olfactory bulb and the olfactory tract, which are components of the part of the brain associated with the sense of smell. Also called **first cranial nerve, nervus olfactorius.**

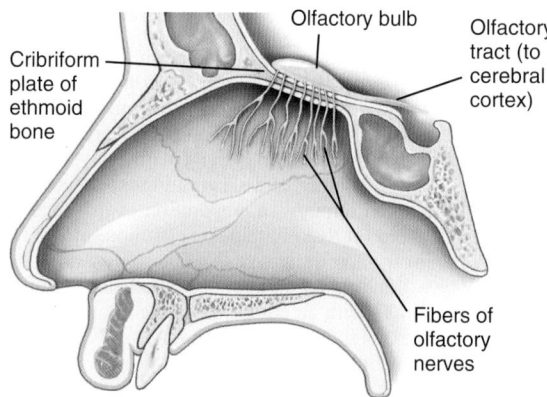

Olfactory nerve (Seidel et al, 2011)

olfactory organ [L, *olfactus,* sense of smell], the apparatus in the mucous membrane of the nose responsible for the sense of smell. It includes the sensory nerve endings and the olfactory bulb of the brain.

olfactory receptors [L, *olfactus,* sense of smell, *recipere,* to receive], bipolar nerve cells located in the nasal epithelium. Axons of the cells are receptors of the olfactory nerve.

olig-. See **oligo-.**

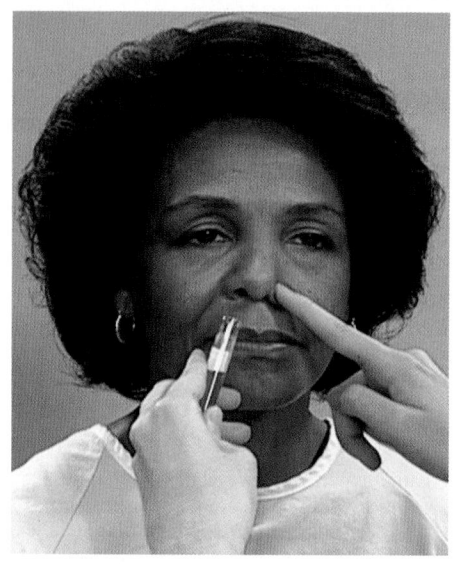

Olfactory nerve assessment (Seidel et al, 2011)

oligemia /ol′ijē″mē·ə/ [Gk, *oligos,* little, *haima,* blood], a condition of hypovolemia or reduced circulating intravascular volume. Also spelled *oligaemia.*

oligo-, prefix meaning "few, little": *oligodactyly, oligodontia, oligogenic.*

oligoclonal banding /ol′igōklō″nəl/, a process by which cerebrospinal fluid IgG is distributed, after electrophoresis, in discrete bands. Approximately 90% of multiple sclerosis patients show oligoclonal banding.

oligodactyly /ol′igōdak″tilē/ [Gk, *oligos* + *dactylos,* finger], a congenital anomaly characterized by the absence of one or more of the fingers or toes. Also called *oligodactylia, oligodactylism.* −*oligodactylic, adj.*

oligodendroblastoma. See **oligodendroglioma.**

oligodendrocyte /ol′igōden″drəsīt/ [Gk, *oligos* + *dendron,* tree, *kytos,* cell], a type of neuroglial cell with dendritic projections that coil around axons of neural cells. The projections continue as myelin sheaths over the axons.

oligodendroglia /ol′igōdendrog″lē·ə/, one of three types of glia cells that, with the nerve cells, compose the central nervous system and are characterized by sheetlike processes that wrap around individual axons to form a myelin sheath of nerve fibers.

oligodendroglioma /ol′igōden′drōglī·ō″ mə/ *pl. oligodendrogliomas, oligodendrogliomata* [Gk, *oligos* + *dendron,* tree, *glia,* glue, *oma,* tumor], an uncommon brain tumor composed of nonneural ectodermal cells that form part of the supporting connective tissue around nerve cells. The lesion, a firm reddish-gray mass with calcified spots and a distinct margin, may be large. The tumor develops most often in frontal, parietal, and paraventricular sites but also may occur in the cerebellum. Also called **oligodendroblastoma.**

oligodontia /ol′igōdon″shə/ [Gk, *oligos* + *odous,* tooth], a genetically determined dental defect characterized by the development of fewer than the normal number of teeth.

oligogalactia /ol′ī-go-gah-lak´shah/ [Gk, *oligo,* scant, *gala,* milk], extremely low milk production.

oligogenic /ol′igōjen″ik/ [Gk, *oligos* + *genein,* to produce], pertaining to hereditary characteristics produced by one or only a few genes.

oligohydramnios /-hidram″nē·əs/ [Gk, *oligos* + *hydor,* water, *amnion,* fetal membrane], an abnormally small amount or absence of amniotic fluid.

oligomeganephronia /ol′igōmeg′ənefrō″nē·ə/ [Gk, *oligos* + *megas,* large, *nephros,* kidney], a type of congenital renal hypoplasia associated with chronic renal failure in children. The condition is characterized by a decreased number of functioning nephrons and hypertrophy of other renal elements without the presence of aberrant tissue. Also called *oligomeganephronic renal hypoplasia.* —oligomeganephronic, adj.

oligomenorrhea /-men′ôrē″ə/ [Gk, *oligos* + L, *men,* month, *rhoia,* flow], abnormally light or reduced menstruation. Also spelled *oligomenorrhoea.*

oligonucleotide /-noo″klē·ətīd′/, a compound formed by linking a small number of nucleotides.

oligopeptide /-pep″tīd/, a peptide composed of fewer than 20 amino acids.

oligopnea, oligopnoea, slow breathing. See **bradypnea.**

oligosaccharide /-sak″ərīd/, a compound formed by a small number of monosaccharide units.

oligospermia /ol′igōspur″mē·ə/ [Gk, *oligos* + *sperma,* seed], a low number of spermatozoa in the semen. Also called **oligozoospermatism.** Compare **azoospermia.**

oligotroph /ol′igətrof′/, an organism that can survive in a nutrient-poor environment.

oligozoospermatism. See **oligospermia.**

oliguria /ol′igyoor″ē·ə/ [Gk, *oligos* + *ouron,* urine], a diminished capacity to form and pass urine—less than 500 mL in every 24 hours—so that the end products of metabolism cannot be excreted efficiently. It is usually caused by imbalances in body fluids and electrolytes, renal lesions, or urinary tract obstruction. Also called *oliguresis.* Compare **anuria.** —oliguric, adj.

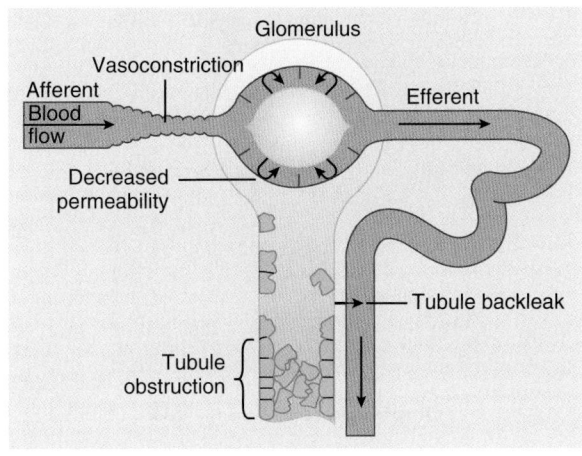

Oliguria (Goldman et al, 2008)

olisthetic /ōlisthet″ik/, pertaining to olisthy, or bone slippage.

olisthy /ōlis″thē/ [Gk, *olisthanein,* to slip], the slippage of a bone from its normal anatomical site, as in a slipped disk.

olivary body /ol″iver′ē/ [L, *oliva* + AS, *bodig*], an olivary nucleus on the medulla oblongata, part of an aggregate of small, densely packed nerve cells.

olivopontocerebellar /ol′ivōpon′tōser′ibel″ər/ [L, *oliva,* olive, *pons,* bridge, *cerebellum,* small brain], pertaining to the olivae, the middle peduncles, and the cerebellum.

olivopontocerebellar atrophy (OPCA), a group of hereditary ataxias characterized by mixed clinical features of pure cerebellar ataxia, dementia, Parkinson-like symptoms, spasticity, choreoathetosis, retinal degeneration, myelopathy,

and peripheral neuropathy. Various forms of OPCA are transmitted by autosomal-dominant or autosomal-recessive inheritance.

Ollier disease. See **enchondromatosis.**

Ollier dyschondroplasia /ol′ē-ā″/ [Louis X.E.L. Ollier, French surgeon, 1830–1900; Gk, *dys,* bad, *chondros,* cartilage, *plasis,* formation], a rare disorder of bone development in which the epiphyseal tissue responsible for growth spreads through the bones, causing abnormal irregular growth and deformity. The long bones and the ilia are most often affected. Orthopedic procedures to correct deformities may be necessary and helpful, but progressive disability is the usual prognosis. See also **hereditary multiple exostoses.**

olmesartan medoxomil, an angiotensin receptor blocker used in the treatment of hypertension and heart failure.

-ology, suffix meaning "the study or science of": *biology, pathology, physiology.*

-olol, suffix meaning "beta-blocker."

olopatadine /o″lopat′ahdēn/, a histamine H₁ receptor antagonist used as the hydrochloride salt in the topical treatment of allergic conjunctivitis.

o.m., a notation for a Latin phrase meaning "every morning." Abbreviation for *omni mane.*

oma-. See **omo-, oma-.**

-oma, suffix meaning "a tumor": *capsuloma, glioma, neurinoma.*

Omaha System, a research-based standardized terminology for practice documentation and data management for use by multiple health care disciplines. It incorporates three standardized schemes: the problem classification scheme, the intervention scheme, and the problem rating scale for outcomes.

omalgia /ōmal″jə/ [Gk, *omos,* shoulder, *algos,* pain], pain in the shoulder.

omalizumab, a monoclonal antibody.

■ INDICATIONS: This drug is used to treat moderate to severe persistent asthma in patients who have severe symptoms despite therapy with the standard of care.

■ CONTRAINDICATIONS: Known hypersensitivity to this drug prohibits its use.

■ ADVERSE EFFECTS: Adverse effects of this drug include earache, dizziness, fatigue, pain, viral infections, upper respiratory infections, pruritus, dermatitis, injection site reactions, arthralgia, fracture, and leg and arm pain. A life-threatening side effect is malignancy.

omarthritis /ō′märthrī″tis/, inflammation of the shoulder joint.

ombudsman /om″bədzmən/ [ONorse, *umbothsmathr,* commission man], (for health or related reasons) a person who investigates and mediates patients' problems and complaints in relation to a hospital's services. Also called **patient representative.**

omega /ōmē″gə, ōmā″gə, om″əgə/, Ω, ω, the 24th letter of the Greek alphabet.

omega-3 fatty acid, a fatty acid with a double bond located at the third carbon atom away from the omega (methyl) end of the molecule. Major sources are cold-water fish and vegetable oils. Omega-3 fatty acids, such as eicosapentaenoic acid and docosahexaenoic acid, appear to have protective functions in preventing the formation of blood clots and reducing the risk of coronary heart disease. See also **essential fatty acid.**

omega-6 fatty acid, an unsaturated fatty acid in which the double bond closest to the omega (methyl) end of the molecule occurs at the sixth carbon from that end. Major sources are vegetable and seed oils.

O

omega-9 fatty acid, a polyunsaturated fatty acid found in animal and vegetable fats.

omega-oxidation, a metabolic pathway of fatty acid oxidation involving the carbon atom farthest removed from the original carboxyl group.

omenta. See **omentum.**

omental /ōmen″təl/ [L, *omentum,* membrane of the bowels], relating to the omentum.

omental appendix, a peritoneal accumulation of fat associated with the colon.

omental bursa, a cavity in the peritoneum behind the stomach, the lesser omentum, and the lower border of the liver and in front of the pancreas and duodenum.

omental foramen, a restricted opening connecting the two sacs of the peritoneum. Also called **epiploic foramen.**

omentectomy /ō′mentek″təmē/, the surgical excision of all or part of the fold of peritoneum connecting the stomach with other abdominal organs.

omentum /ōmen″təm/ *pl. omenta, omentums* [L, membrane of the bowels], an extension of the peritoneum that enfolds one or more organs adjacent to the stomach. See also **greater omentum, lesser omentum. –omental,** *adj.*

omicron /ōm″ikron/, O, o, the 15th letter of the Greek alphabet.

omission /ōmish″ən/ [L, *omittere,* to neglect], **1.** (in law) intentional or unintentional neglect to fulfill a duty required by law. **2.** (in pharmacology) a drug error in which a requisite dose is wrongly missed.

Ommaya reservoir [A.K. Ommaya, contemporary Pakistani neurosurgeon], a device placed under the scalp and used to deliver medications to the cerebrospinal fluid.

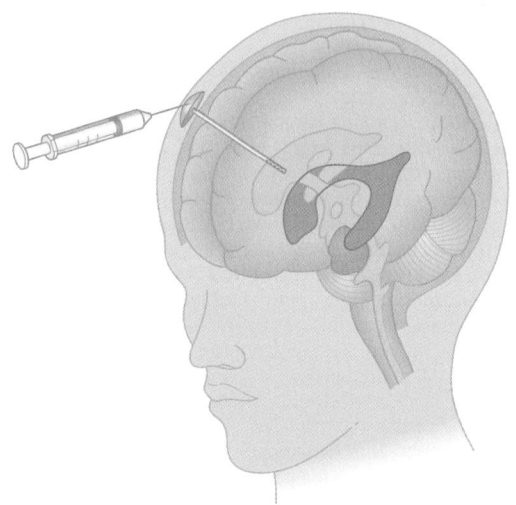

Ommaya reservoir *(Cibas and Ducatman, 2014)*

omni-, combining form meaning "all": *omnipotence, omnivorous.*

omnifocal lens /om′nēfō″kəl/ [L, *omnis,* all, *focus,* hearth, *lentil*], an eyeglass lens designed for both near and far vision with the reading part in a variable curve.

Omnipen, a penicillin antibacterial agent. Brand name for **ampicillin.**

omnipotence /omnip″ətəns/, (in psychology) an infantile perception that the outside world is part of the organism and within it, which leads to a primitive feeling of all-powerfulness.

omnivorous /omniv″ərəs/ [L, *omnis,* all, *vorare,* to devour], eating both plants and animals.

omn. noct., *(Obsolete)* short for a Latin phrase meaning "every night." Abbreviation for *omni nocte.*

omn. quad. hor., *(Obsolete)* short for a Latin phrase meaning "every quarter of an hour." Abbreviation for *omni quadrante hora.*

omo-, oma-, prefix meaning "shoulder": *omalgia, omohyoid.*

omohyoid, a muscle that depresses and fixes the hyoid bone.

omophagia /om′ōfā″jē·ə/ [Gk, *ōmos,* raw, *phagein,* to eat], the eating of raw foods, particularly raw meat or fish.

omphal-. See **omphalo-, omphal-.**

omphalic /omfal″ik/ [Gk, *omphalos,* navel], pertaining to the umbilicus.

omphalitis /om′fəlī″tis/, an inflammation of the umbilical stump marked by redness, swelling, and purulent exudate in severe cases. This condition is rare in developed countries.

omphalo-, omphal-, combining form meaning "the navel": *omphalocele, omphalosite.*

omphaloangiopagus. See **allantoidoangiopagus.**

omphalocele /om″fəlōsēl′/ [Gk, *omphalos* + *kele,* hernia], congenital herniation of intraabdominal viscera through a defect in the abdominal wall around the umbilicus. The defect is usually closed surgically soon after birth. Compare **gastroschisis.**

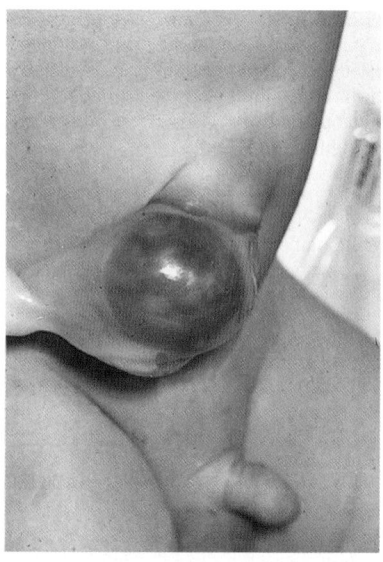

Omphalocele *(O'Doherty, 1986)*

omphalodidymus. See **gastrodidymus.**

omphalogenesis /-jen″əsis/ [Gk, *omphalos* + *genesis,* origin], the formation of the umbilicus or yolk sac during embryonic development. –*omphalogenetic, adj.*

omphalomesenteric artery. See **vitelline artery.**

omphalomesenteric circulation. See **vitelline circulation.**

omphalomesenteric duct. See **yolk stalk.**

omphalomesenteric fistula, an abnormal passageway between the umbilicus and the terminal ileum, formed by persistence of the intraembryonic part of the yolk stalk.

omphalomesenteric vein. See **vitelline vein.**

omphalopagus. See **monomphalus.**

omphalosite /om″fəlōsīt′/ [Gk, *omphalos* + *sitos,* food], the underdeveloped parasitic member of unequal conjoined twins united by the vessels of the umbilical cord. The omphalosite has no heart, derives its blood supply from the placenta of the autosite, and is incapable of independent existence after birth. See also **allantoidoangiopagus.**

OMS, abbreviation for **Organisation Mondiale de la Santé.** See **World Health Organization.**

Omsk hemorrhagic fever (OHF) /ômsk/ [Omsk, Russia], an acute infection seen in the western Siberian regions of Omsk, Novosibirsk, Kurgan, and Tyumen caused by a flavivirus transmitted by the bite of an infected tick or by handling infected rodents, especially muskrats. It is characterized by fever, headache, epistaxis, GI and uterine bleeding, and other hemorrhagic manifestations. Treatment is supportive; recovery usually occurs.

-on, **1.** suffix meaning "an elementary atomic particle": *electron, nucleon, proton.* **2.** suffix meaning "a unit": *photon.* **3.** suffix meaning "a (nonmetallic) chemical element": *carbon, krypton, silicon.*

o.n., *(Obsolete)* a notation for a Latin phrase meaning "every night." Abbreviation for *omni nocte.*

onanism /ō″nəniz′əm/, ejaculation outside the vagina. See also **masturbation, coitus interruptus.**

Oncaspar, an oncolytic agent. Brand name for **pegaspargase.**

Onchocerca /ong′kōsər′kə/ [Gk, *onkos,* tumor + *kerkos,* tail], a genus of nematode parasites of the superfamily Filarioidea that infects humans and ruminants. The adults live and breed in subcutaneous fibroid nodules. The young (the microfilariae) are carried by the lymph and are found chiefly in the skin, subcutaneous connective tissues, and eyes. *O. volvulus* is a common parasite of humans that breeds in fast-flowing rivers and streams in tropical regions of the Americas and Africa, particularly West Africa. It is the cause of human onchocerciasis and is transmitted by the bites of buffalo gnats.

onchocerciasis /ong′kōsərkī″əsis, sī″əsis/ [Gk, *onkos,* swelling, *kerkos,* tail, *osis,* condition], a form of filariasis common in Central and South America and Africa, characterized by subcutaneous nodules, pruritic rash, and eye lesions. It is transmitted by the bites of black flies that deposit *Onchocerca volvulus* microfilariae under the skin. Also called **river blindness.**

■ OBSERVATIONS: The microfilariae migrate to the subcutaneous tissue and eyes, and fibrous nodules form around the developing adult worms. Hypersensitive reactions to the dying microfilariae include extreme pruritus, a cellulitis-like rash, lichenification, depigmentation, and rarely, elephantiasis. Involvement of the eye may include keratitis, iridocyclitis, and rarely, blindness from choroidoretinitis. Diagnosis is made by demonstrating microfilariae by skin biopsy or in the eye by slit lamp.

■ INTERVENTIONS: Treatment is diethylcarbamazine for the microfilariae and surgical excision of nodules to remove adult worms. The broad-spectrum antiparasitic drug ivermectin is also used for treatment.

■ PATIENT CARE CONSIDERATIONS: Protective clothing and control of black flies are the best preventives.

onco-, prefix meaning "swelling, mass, or tumor": *oncology.*

oncofetal protein /-fē″təl/ [Gk, *onkos* + L, *fetus,* pregnant; Gk, *proteios,* first rank], a protein normally produced by fetal tissue and also by cancerous tissues in adult life.

oncogene /ong″kōjēn/ [Gk, *onkos* + *genein,* to produce], a potentially cancer-inducing gene. Under normal conditions such genes play a role in the growth and proliferation of cells, but, when altered in some way by a cancer-causing agent such as radiation, a carcinogenic chemical, or an oncogenic virus, they may cause the cell to be transformed to a malignant state.

oncogenesis /ong′kōjen″əsis/ [Gk, *onkos* + *genesis,* origin], the process initiating and promoting the development

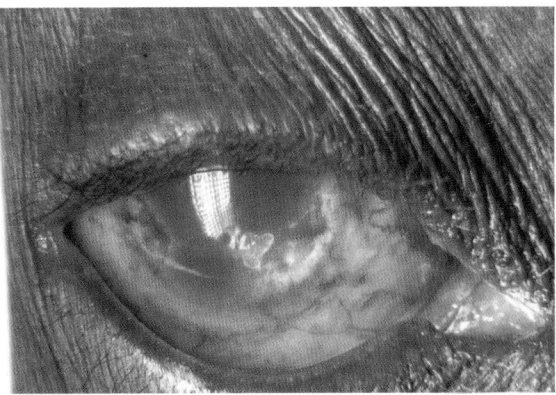

Ocular changes in onchocerciasis *(Magill et al, 2013)*

of a neoplasm through the action of biological, chemical, or physical agents. Compare **carcinogenesis, sarcomagenesis, tumorigenesis.**

oncogenic /ong′kōjen″ik/ [Gk, *onkos,* swelling, *genein,* to produce], pertaining to the origin and development of tumors or cancer.

oncogenic viruses, an epidemiological class of viruses that are acquired by close contact or injection. The viruses may induce cell transformation and malignancy.

oncogenous osteomalacia /ongkoj″ənəs/, a bone disorder caused by mesenchymal tumors. Patients may have normal-to-low serum calcium levels, a low serum phosphorus level, and an elevated serum alkaline phosphatase level.

oncological emergencies /ong′kōloj″ik/, cancer-related disorders that require emergency medical or surgical care. Kinds include **superior vena cava syndrome, cardiac tamponade, hypercalcemia of malignancy, spinal cord compression.**

oncologist /ongkol″əjist/, a physician who specializes in the study and treatment of neoplastic diseases, particularly cancer.

oncology /ongkol″əjē/ [Gk, *onkos,* swelling, *logos,* science], **1.** the branch of medicine concerned with the study of malignancy. **2.** the study of cancerous growths.

Oncology Nursing Society (ONS), an organization of nurses interested in or specializing in cancer patient nursing. The national publication of the ONS is *Oncology Nursing Forum.*

oncolysis /ongkol″isis/, **1.** the destruction of or disposal of neoplastic cells. **2.** the reduction of a swelling or mass.

oncolytic /ong′kōlit″ik/, pertaining to the destruction of tumor cells.

oncornaviruses. See **Oncovirinae.**

oncoscint scan, a nuclear scan used to detect recurrent metastatic colorectal or ovarian cancer.

oncotic /ongkot″ik/ [Gk, *onkos,* a swelling], pertaining to or resulting from the presence of a swelling.

oncotic pressure [Gk, *onkos,* a swelling; L, *premere,* to press], the osmotic pressure of a colloid in solution, such as when there is a higher concentration of protein in the plasma on one side of a cell membrane than in the neighboring interstitial fluid. Also called **colloid osmotic pressure.**

oncotic pressure gradient, the difference between the osmotic pressure of blood and that of tissue fluid or lymph. It is an important force in maintaining fluid balance between the vascular space and the interstitium.

Oncovin, an antineoplastic drug. Brand name for **vinCRIStine sulfate.**

O

Oncovirinae /ong′kōvir″inē/, a subfamily of ribonucleic acid viruses, including types A, B, C, and D genera of oncoviruses. They are classified on the basis of morphology and type of host. Also called **oncornaviruses.** See also **oncovirus.**

oncovirus /ong′kōvī″rəs/ [Gk, *onkos* + L, *virus,* poison], a member of a family of viruses associated with leukemia and sarcoma in animals and, possibly, in humans.

Ondine curse syndrome /ondēn′/ [L, *Undine,* mythic water nymph; ME, *curs,* invocation], See **congenital central hypoventilation syndrome.**

-one, suffix for organic compounds: *acetone, ketone.*

one-and-a-half spica cast, an orthopedic cast that covers the trunk cranially to the nipple line, one leg caudally as far as the toes, and the other leg caudally as far as the knee. For stability, there is often a diagonal crossbar to connect the parts of the cast encasing the legs. This type of cast is used for immobilization during healing of a fractured femur or after surgical hip repair or for correction and maintenance of the correction of a hip deformity. Compare **bilateral long-leg spica cast, unilateral long-leg spica cast.**

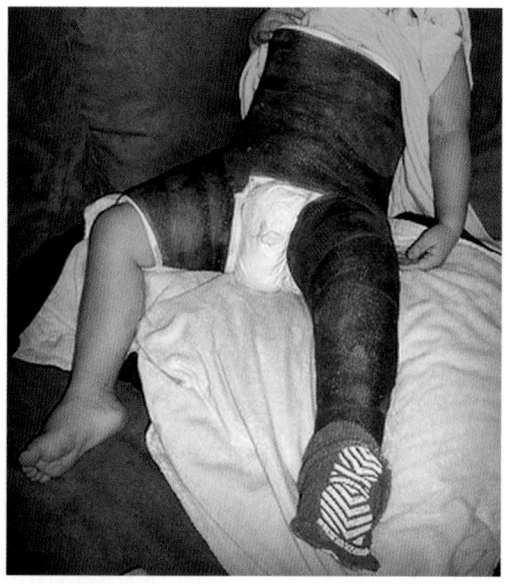

One-and-a-half-leg hip spica cast *(Flynn et al, 2011)*

one-child sterility. See **acquired sterility.**

one gene/one enzyme hypothesis, a general rule, proposed in 1941 by G. Beadle and E. Tatum, that each gene in a chromosome controls the synthesis of one enzyme. A modification of this idea, the one gene/one polypeptide hypothesis, accommodates the fact that all gene products are polypeptides but not all polypeptides are enzymes. A further modification, the one cistron/one polypeptide concept, accommodates alternate splicing and alternative promoter sequences.

one gene/one polypeptide, a hypothesis that each gene in a chromosome determines a particular polypeptide. It is now known that some genes also code for various types of RNA involved in protein synthesis.

oneiro-, prefix meaning "dream."

one-to-one care, **1.** a method of organizing nursing services in an inpatient care unit in which one registered nurse assumes responsibility for all nursing care provided to one patient for the duration of one shift. The patient requiring

1:1 nursing care is a patient who is in a critical health state, is a suicidal risk, or who may be on medical equipment/devices requiring constant supervision and care. **2.** physical and/or occupational therapy and/or speech rehabilitation provided by therapists, who work individually with a single patient in their homes, in schools, in assisted-living facilities, or in senior residences.

one-to-one relationship, **1.** (in psychotherapy) a mutually defined, collaborative, goal-directed client-therapist connection. **2.** (in computer processing) a relational database in which one parent entry has either no or only one child entry.

one-way speaking valve, a valve, placed on the end of a tracheostomy tube, that opens during inhalation and closes during exhalation so that the exhaled air is directed through the vocal cords and out the mouth and nose, allowing a person who has had a tracheostomy to speak. See also **Passy-Muir valve.**

-onide, suffix for acetal-derived topical steroids.

-onium, suffix for quaternary ammonium derivatives.

onlay [AS, *ana,* up, *licagan,* to lie], **1.** (in dentistry) a cast type of metal restoration retained by friction, dental luting cement, and mechanical forces in a prepared tooth, used for restoring one or more of the tooth's cusps and adjoining occlusal surfaces. Compare **inlay,** def. 2. **2.** (in dentistry) an occlusal rest part of a removable partial denture, extended to cover the entire occlusal surface of a tooth.

onlay graft, a bone graft in which the transplanted tissue is laid directly onto the surface of the recipient bone.

online, access to information directly connected with and accessible to a computer. Compare **off-line.**

on/off phenomenon, a periodic loss of the efficacy of levodopa in the treatment of Parkinson disease, without obvious relationship to the timing of levodopa administration. Also called **random off.**

ONS, abbreviation for **Oncology Nursing Society.**

onset of action, the amount of time required after the administration of a medication for its effects to be observed.

ontogenesis. See **ontogeny.**

ontogenetic /on′tōjənet″ik/, **1.** of, relating to, or acquired during the development of an organism. **2.** describing an association based on visible morphological characteristics and not necessarily indicative of a natural evolutionary relationship. Also called *ontogenic.*

ontogeny /ontoj″ənē/ [Gk, *ontos,* being, *genein,* to produce], the development of one organism from a single-celled ovum to the time of birth, including all phases of differentiation and growth. Compare **phylogeny.** See also **comparative anatomy.**

onych-. See **onycho-, onych-.**

onychia /ōnik″ē·ə/ [Gk, *onyx,* nail], inflammation of the nailbed. Compare **paronychia.**

-onychia, suffix meaning "a condition of the fingernails or toenails": *anonychia, koilonychia, pachyonychia.*

onycho-, onych-, combining form meaning "the nails": *onychomycosis, eponychium, onychodystrophy onychogryphosis.*

onychodystrophy [Gk, *onyx,* nail, *dys,* bad, *trophe,* nourishment], a condition of malformed or discolored fingernails or toenails.

onychogryphosis /on′ikōgrifō″sis/ [Gk, *onyx* + *gryphein,* to curve, *osis,* condition], thickened, curved, clawlike overgrowth of fingernails or toenails.

onycholysis /on′ikol″isis/ [Gk, *onyx* + *lysein,* to loosen], separation of a nail from its bed, beginning at the free margin. The separation may be associated with psoriasis, dermatitis of the hand, fungal infection, *Pseudomonas* infection, or many other conditions.

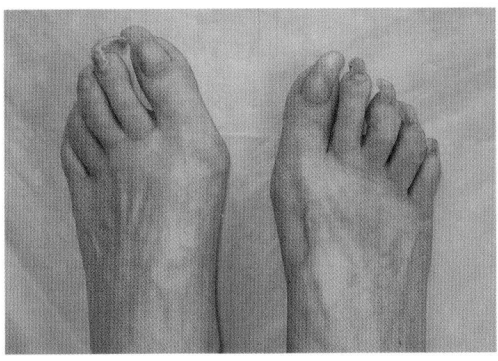

Onychogryphosis *(Miller et al, 2009)*

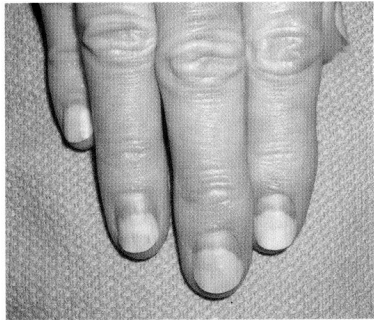

Onycholysis *(Velez and Jellinek, 2013)*

onychomycosis /on′ikō′mīkō″sis/ [Gk, *onyx* + *mykes*, fungus, *osis*, condition], any fungal infection of the nails.

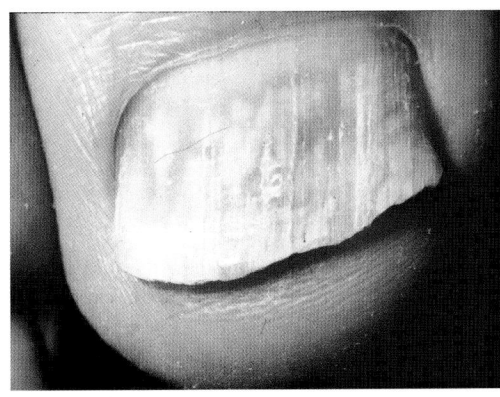

Onychomycosis *(Coleman, Fleckman, and Huang, 2014)*

onycho-osteodysplasia. See **nail-patella syndrome, osteoonychodysplasia.**

onychophagia. See **nail biting.**

onychosis [Gk, *onyx,* nail, *osis,* condition], a condition of atrophy or dystrophy of the nails, usually caused by a dermatosis such as a fungal infection.

onychotillomania /on′ikōtil′əmā″nē·ə/ [Gk, *onyx,* nail, *tillein,* to pluck, *mania,* madness], a nervous habit of picking at the nails to the point of tissue damage (i.e., bleeding).

onychotomy /on′ikot″əmē/, a surgical incision into a nailbed.

oo-, combining form meaning "egg" or "ovum": *ooblast, oocyesis, ootid.*

oob, abbreviation for *out of bed.*

ooblast /ō″əblast/ [Gk, *oon,* egg, *blastos,* germ], a female germ cell from which a mature ovum is developed.

oocenter. See **ovocenter.**

oocyesis /ō′əsī·ē″sis/ [Gk, *oon* + *kyesis,* pregnancy], an ectopic ovarian pregnancy.

oocyst /ō″əsist/ [Gk, *oon* + *kystis,* bag], a stage in the development of sporozoa consisting of a zygote enclosed by cyst wall. Oocysts of malarial parasites are found in the stomachs of infected mosquitoes. Oocysts of toxoplasma organisms are contained in the feces of infected cats. Compare **oocyte.**

oocyte /ō″əsīt/ [Gk, *oon* + *kytos,* cell], a primordial or incompletely developed ovum.

oocyte donation, a method of assisted reproductive technology in which an oocyte from a fertile woman is aspirated for incubation in the uterus of a woman who has female factor infertility, such as after oophorectomy or premature menopause. Fertilization may be either in vitro or in utero.

oocytin /ō′əsī″tin/, the substance in a spermatozoon that stimulates the formation of the fertilization membrane after penetration of an ovum.

oogamy /ō·og″əmē/ [Gk, *oon* + *gamos,* marriage], **1.** sexual reproduction by the fertilization of a large nonmotile female gamete by a smaller, actively motile male gamete, such as occurs in certain algae and the malarial parasite *Plasmodium.* **2.** (in biology) heterogamy. Compare **isogamy.** −*oogamous, adj.*

oogenesis /ō′əjen″əsis/ [Gk, *oon* + *genesis,* origin], the formation of the female gametes, or ova. The female infant is born with the entire number of primary oocytes that will function throughout reproductive life. Only a fraction of these survive until puberty, and only a small percentage will be ovulated. Follicles containing the primary oocytes are found in varying stages of development in the ovary of the sexually mature woman. Egg and sperm formation differ considerably in the number and size of gametes resulting from gametogenesis, the total number of gametes produced in a lifetime, and the time sequence for the initiation of the meiotic divisions and the completion of the cycle. Also called **ovogenesis.** Compare **spermatogenesis.** See also **gametogenesis, meiosis, menstrual cycle, ovulation.** −*oogenetic, adj.*

oogonium /ō′əgō″nē·əm/ [Gk, *oon* + *gonos,* offspring], the precursor cell from which an oocyte develops in the fetus during intrauterine life. Also called **ovogonium.** See also **oogenesis.**

ookinesis /ō′əkinē″sis/ [Gk, *oon* + *kinesis,* movement], the chromosomal movement occurring in the nucleus of the egg cell during maturation and fertilization. Also called *ookinesia.* See also **oogenesis.**

ookinete /ō′əkinēt″/ [Gk, *oon* + *kinein,* to move], the motile elongated zygote that is formed by the fertilization of the macrogamete during the sexual reproductive phase of the life cycle of a sporozoan, specifically the malarial parasite *Plasmodium.* It penetrates the lining of the stomach of the female *Anopheles* mosquito and attaches to the outer wall, where it forms an oocyst and gives rise to sporozoites.

ookinetic. See **ookinesis.**

oolemma. See **zona pellucida.**

oophor-. See **oophoro-, oophor-, ootheco-.**

oophoralgia /ō′əfôral″jə/ [Gk, *oophoron,* ovary, *algos,* pain], a pain in an ovary.

oophorectomy /ō′əfərek″təmē/ [Gk, *oophoron,* ovary, *ektomē,* excision], the surgical removal of one or both ovaries. It is performed to remove a cyst or tumor, excise an

O

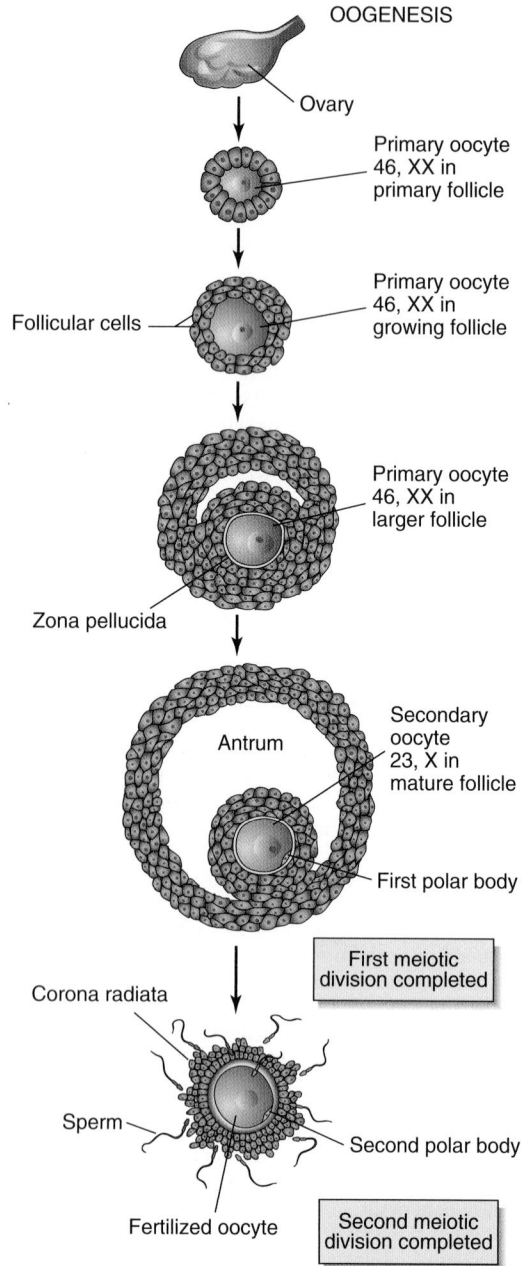

OOGENESIS

Ovary

Primary oocyte 46, XX in primary follicle

Follicular cells

Primary oocyte 46, XX in growing follicle

Primary oocyte 46, XX in larger follicle

Zona pellucida

Antrum

Secondary oocyte 23, X in mature follicle

First polar body

First meiotic division completed

Corona radiata

Sperm

Second polar body

Fertilized oocyte

Second meiotic division completed

Oogenesis *(Moore, Persaud, and Shiota, 2008)*

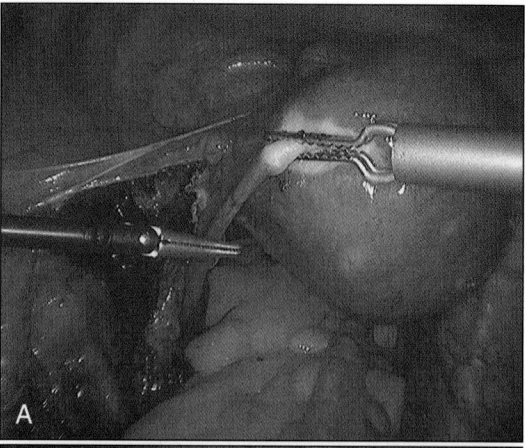

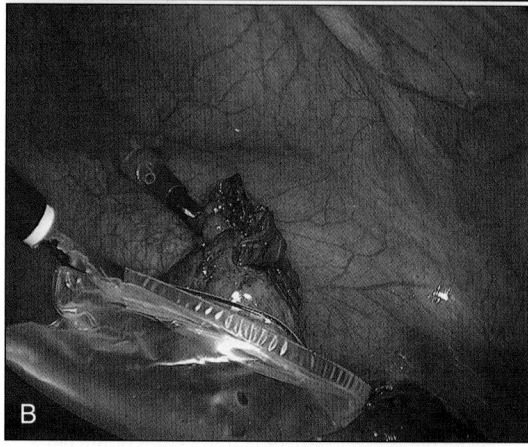

Ooophorectomy. A, The fallopian tube and utervarian ligament are ligated close to the uterus. B, The specimen is removed in an Endocatch bag
(Bristow and Armstrong, 2010)

abscess, treat endometriosis, or in breast cancer to remove the source of estrogen, which stimulates some types of cancer. If both ovaries are removed, sterility results, and menopause is abruptly induced; in premenopausal women one ovary or a part of one ovary may be left intact unless a malignancy is present. The operation routinely accompanies a hysterectomy in menopausal or postmenopausal women. Regional or general anesthesia is used. Unless a malignancy is present, estrogen may be given to treat the unpleasant side effects of the abrupt onset of menopause. Also called **ovariectomy.**

oophoritis /ō′əferī″tis/, an inflammatory condition of one or both ovaries, usually occurring with salpingitis or another infection.

oophoro-, oophor-, ootheco-, combining form meaning "ovary": *epoophoron, oophorectomy, oophorosalpingitis.*

oophorosalpingectomy /ō′əfôr′əsal′pinjek″təmē/ [Gk, *oophoron + salpinx,* tube, *ektomē,* excision], the surgical removal of one or both ovaries and the corresponding fallopian tubes, performed to remove a cyst or tumor, excise an abscess, or treat endometriosis. A bilateral procedure causes sterility and induces menopause, unless a malignancy is present; estrogen therapy may be started to relieve the unpleasant side effects of the abrupt onset of menopause.

oophorosalpingitis /ō′əfôr′əsal′pinjī″tis/ [Gk, *oophoron,* ovary, *salpinx,* tube, *itis,* inflammation], an inflammation involving both the ovary and the fallopian tube.

ooplasm /ō′əplaz′əm/ [Gk, *oon + plasma,* something formed], the cytoplasm of the egg, or ovum, including the yolk in lower animals. Also called **ovoplasm.**

oosperm /ō′əspurm/ [Gk, *oon + sperma,* seed], a fertilized ovum; the cell resulting from the union of the pronuclei of the spermatozoon and the ovum after fertilization; a zygote.

ootheco-. See **oophoro-, oophor-, ootheco-.**

ootid /ō″ətid/ [Gk, *ootidion,* small egg], the nearly mature ovum after penetration by the spermatozoon and completion of the second meiotic division but before the fusion of the pronuclei to form the zygote. It is one of the four cells resulting from oogenesis. See also **meiosis, oogenesis.**

OP,   **1.** abbreviation for *operative procedure.* **2.** initialism for **outpatient facilities.**

opacity /ōpas″itē/ [L, *opacitus,* shadiness], pertaining to an opaque quality of a substance or object, such as cataract opacity.

opalescent /ō′pəl·es′ənt/, showing a milky iridescence, like an opal.

opal mutation, a genetic alteration that causes the synthesis of a polypeptide chain to terminate prematurely because the triplet of nucleotides that normally codes for the next amino acid in the chain becomes uracil-adenine-guanine, the sequence that signals the end of the chain. An opal mutation is one of the three possible nonsense mutations. See also **amber mutation, ochre mutation, nonsense mutation.**

opaque /ōpāk″/ [L, *opacus,* obscure], **1.** pertaining to a substance or surface that neither transmits nor allows the passage of light. **2.** neither transparent nor translucent.

OPCA, abbreviation for **olivopontocerebellar atrophy.**

OPD, abbreviation for **outpatient department.**

-ope, suffix meaning "pertaining to the eye": *myope.*

open amputation [AS, *offan,* open; L, *amputare,* to cut away], a kind of amputation in which a straight, guillotine cut is made without skin flaps. Open amputation is performed if an infection is probable, developing, or recurrent. The cross section is left open for drainage, and skin traction is applied to prevent retraction. Antibiotic therapy is begun, and surgical closure is completed when the infection clears. Compare **closed amputation.** See also **gangrene.**

open-angle glaucoma. See **glaucoma.**

open bite, an abnormal dental condition in which the anterior teeth in the maxilla do not occlude those in the mandible in any mandibular position. Compare **closed bite.**

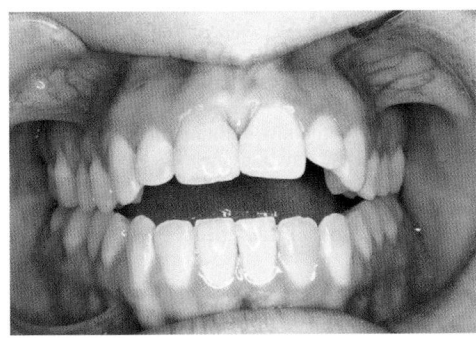

Open bite *(Proffit, Fields, and Sarver, 2013)*

open-cavity tympanomastoidectomy, a tympanomastoidectomy with removal of the posterior wall of the ear canal, such as radical mastoidectomy and modified radical mastoidectomy. See also **mastoidectomy.**

open-chain exercise, exercise in which the distal aspect of the extremity is free in space and not in contact with the ground.

open circuit, an electric circuit in which current flow ceases.

open-circuit breathing system, a breathing apparatus used in cardiopulmonary therapy in which rebreathing does not occur. Gas is inspired through a breathing branch or limb that is connected to a gas source or open to the ambient atmosphere. Expired gas flows through a directional valve into a collecting reservoir or into the ambient atmosphere.

open dislocation, a joint displacement accompanied by a break in the skin. Formerly called **compound dislocation.**

open drainage. See **drainage.**

open-drop anesthesia, the oldest and simplest anesthetic technique. It is no longer used in the United States. A volatile liquid anesthetic agent such as ether is dripped, one drop at a time, onto a porous cloth or mask held over the patient's face. The liquid then vaporizes and is inhaled by the spontaneously breathing patient. With this method, it is difficult to control the anesthetic depth and the pollution of the operating room. Chloroform and ether were the major general anesthetics adaptable to open-drop administration.

open-enrollment period, a time during which individuals can enroll in a health care plan.

open fracture. See **compound fracture.**

open fracture grading system, a system for dividing open fractures into five categories, ranging from a clean wound that communicates to the fracture site and measures less than 1 cm (grade I) to a fracture requiring repair of arteries (grade V).

open heart surgery, any heart surgery in which the chest is opened, including minimally invasive surgery. Conventional open heart surgery uses a cardiopulmonary bypass machine. Minimally invasive techniques may not.

open kinetic chain exercise. Also called **open-chain exercise.** Compare **closed-chain exercise.**

opening abductory wedge osteotomy (OAWO), a procedure for treating a bunion deformity in which a bone graft is used to open the wedge cut into the bone and bring the first metatarsal closer to the second.

opening of ileocecal valve, the slitlike or oval orifice in the ileocecal valve, seen in a cadaver. It has two flaps or lips, one above and one below, that form the valve and project at thickened folds into the lumen of the large intestine. In the living individual this structure is the ostium ileale.

opening pressure, the amount of pressure measured in a manometer after insertion of a spinal needle into the subarachnoid space.

opening wedge osteotomy, a procedure for treating bunion deformity in which a proximal cut is made in the metatarsal to reduce the deformity. It is performed with or without tendon transfers.

open magnetic resonance imaging (open MRI), a procedure that allows visualization of soft-tissue structures of the body. Because the patient is not enclosed within the magnetic resonance unit, claustrophobic reactions do not occur with open magnetic resonance imaging, but the scan does take substantially longer to complete. As with traditional magnetic resonance imaging, patients must remain motionless, and images may be degraded by motions related to heart contractions, respiration, and bowel peristalsis. Contraindications to MRI are pacemakers, metallic aneurysm clips, and some metallic prostheses and foreign objects. Compare **magnetic resonance imaging.** See also **magnetic resonance.**

open medical staff, (in managed care) the opening of hospital medical staff membership to all physicians in the community who meet membership and clinical privilege requirements.

open MRI, abbreviation for **open magnetic resonance imaging.**

open operation, a surgical procedure that provides a full view of the structures or organs involved through membranous or cutaneous incisions. Compare **laparoscopy, minimally invasive surgery.**

open-panel HMO, a health maintenance organization (HMO) in which physicians treat both HMO and private patients.

open PHO, a physician-hospital organization in which all physicians on the hospital medical staff can participate.

open pneumothorax [AS, *open* + Gk, *pneuma,* air, *thorax,* chest], the presence of air or gas in the chest as a result of an open wound in the chest wall.

open reduction [AS, *open* + L, *reducere,* to lead back], a surgical procedure for reducing a fracture or dislocation by exposing the skeletal parts involved.

open rhinolalia. See **hypernasality.**

open system, a system that interacts with its environment.

open-wedge osteotomy, a straight cut made across a bone, leaving a wedge-shaped gap in the bone.

open wound [AS, *open* + *wund*], a wound that disrupts the integrity of the skin.

operable /op″ərəbəl/ [L, *operare,* to work], amenable to surgical intervention, as a disease or injury may be.

operant /op″ərənt/ [L, *operare,* to work], any act or response occurring without an identifiable stimulus. The result of the act or response determines whether or not it is repeated.

operant conditioning, a form of learning used in behavioral therapy in which the person undergoing therapy is rewarded for the correct response and punished for the incorrect response. Also called **instrumental conditioning, shaping.**

operant level, the frequency or form of a performance under baseline conditions before any systematic conditioning procedures are introduced.

operating field, an isolated area where surgery is performed; it must be kept sterile by aseptic techniques. Also called *operative field.* See also **surgical asepsis.**

operating microscope /op″ərā′ting/ [L, *operare* + Gk, *mikros,* small, *skopein,* to look], a binocular microscope used in delicate surgery, especially surgery of the eye or ear. The standing type of operating microscope has a motorized zoom system operated by a foot pedal that quickly changes the magnification. The operating microscope that attaches to a surgeon's head has interchangeable lenses for different magnifications. Also called **surgical microscope.**

operating room (OR, O.R.), **1.** a room in a health care facility in which surgical procedures requiring anesthesia are performed. **2.** *(Informal)* a suite of rooms or an area in a health care facility in which patients are prepared for surgery and undergo surgical procedures.

operating room technician. See **Certified Surgical Technologist,** def. 2.

operating system (OS), the main system programs of a computer that manage the hardware and application resources, including data input and output. Applications require an operating system to support and enable their function.

operating telescope, a magnifying lens that gives low magnification and a wide field of vision.

operation /op″ərā″shən/, any surgical procedure, such as an appendectomy or a hysterectomy.

operationalization of behavior /op″ərā″shənal″īzā″shən/, (in psychology) the stating of a patient's complaints or problems in specific, observable behavioral terms.

operative cholangiography /op″ərətiv′/ [L, *operare* + Gk, *chole,* bile, *angeion,* vessel, *graphein,* to record], a procedure for radiographically outlining the major bile ducts during surgery. It involves the injection of a radiopaque contrast medium directly into the ducts. The procedure is usually performed to detect residual calculi in the biliary tract. See also **cholangiography.**

operative dental surgeon. See **dental surgeon.**

operative dentistry, that phase of dentistry concerned with restoration of parts of the teeth that are defective through disease, trauma, or abnormal development to a state of normal

function, health, and aesthetics, including preventive, diagnostic, biological, mechanical, and therapeutic techniques.

operator gene /op″ərā″tər/ [L, *operare* + Gk, *genein,* to produce], a section of bacterial DNA that regulates the transcription of structural genes in an operon by interacting with a repressor protein. The operator gene serves as the starting point in the coding sequence.

operatory /op″ərətor″ē/ [L, *operare,* to work], the dental surgical working area of a dental office, in which treatment is provided to patients.

operculitis, inflammation of the gums around a partially erupted tooth. Also called **pericoronitis.**

operculum /ōpur″kyo͞oləm/ *pl.* **opercula, operculums** [L, lid], a lid or covering, such as the mucous plug that blocks the cervix of the gravid uterus or the temporal operculum of the cerebral temporal hemisphere that overlaps the insula as an extension of the superior surface of the temporal lobe.

operon /op″əron/ [L, *operare,* to work], a section of bacterial DNA consisting of an operator gene and one or more structural genes with related functions. Transcription of the structural genes is controlled by the operator gene in conjunction with a regulator gene. See also **operator gene, regulator gene.**

ophid-, prefix meaning "snake or snakelike": *ophidiophobia.*

-ophidia, suffix meaning "venomous snakes."

ophidiophobia, fear of snakes.

ophth, abbreviation for **ophthalmology.**

ophthalm-. See **ophthalmo-.**

ophthalmia /ofthal″mē-ə/ [Gk, *ophthalmos,* eye], severe inflammation of the conjunctiva or the deeper parts of the eye. Kinds include **ophthalmia neonatorum, sympathetic ophthalmia, trachoma.**

-ophthalmia, suffix meaning "a pathological or anatomical condition of the eye": *exophthalmia, synophthalmia, xerophthalmia.*

ophthalmia neonatorum /nē″ōnətôr″əm/, a purulent conjunctivitis and keratitis of the newborn resulting from exposure of the eyes to chemical, chlamydial, bacterial, or viral agents. Chemical conjunctivitis usually occurs as a result of the instillation of silver nitrate in the eyes of a newborn to prevent a gonococcal infection. Also called **neonatal conjunctivitis.** See also **conjunctivitis.**

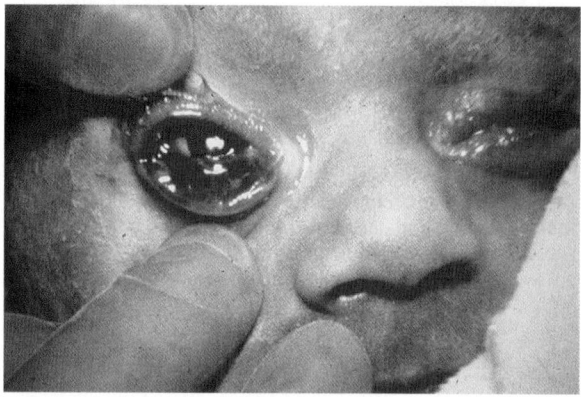

Ophthalmia neonatorum *(Cohen and Powderly, 2004/Courtesy Dr. M. Puolakkainne)*

ophthalmic /ofthal″mik/ [Gk, *ophthalmos,* eye], pertaining to the eye.

ophthalmic administration of medication, the administration of a drug by instillation of a cream, an ointment, or a liquid drop preparation in the conjunctival sac. The correct strength and amount of the drug are selected, and the medication is instilled into the eye or eyes as directed. The prescription is written in full, specifying *right eye, left eye,* or *both eyes;* abbreviations should not be used. Ophthalmic preparations are often refrigerated for storage but are given at room temperature. For administration the patient is positioned comfortably, lying back on a bed or examining table or sitting up with the neck hyperextended. The cul-de-sac of the conjunctival sac is exposed by gentle traction on the tissue just below the lower eyelid. The medication is placed into the sac as the patient is instructed to look away from the point of instillation. The dispenser is not allowed to touch the eye, and the medication is not placed directly on the cornea. The eyelid is slowly released, and the patient is asked to roll the eye around a few times to spread the medication over the entire surface of the eye. Applying pressure with the finger at the inner canthus may decrease systemic absorption.

ophthalmic dispensing optician, an allied health professional who adapts and fits corrective eyewear, including eyeglasses and contact lenses, as prescribed by an ophthalmologist or optometrist. Degree programs are usually 2 years.

ophthalmic herpes zoster. See **herpes zoster ophthalmicus.**

ophthalmic laboratory technician, a person who, working from a prescription written by an ophthalmologist or optometrist, cuts, grinds, edges, and finishes lenses and fabricates eyewear.

ophthalmic medical technician, an allied health professional who assists ophthalmologists by collecting data and administering treatment ordered by the ophthalmologist. These specialists are qualified to take medical histories; administer diagnostic tests; make anatomical and functional ocular measurements; test ocular functions, including visual acuity, visual fields, and sensorimotor functions; administer topical ophthalmic medications; and instruct the patient in home care and the use of contact lenses. Ophthalmic medical technologists perform all duties performed by technicians but are expected to do so at a higher level of expertise.

ophthalmic nerve [Gk, *ophthalmos,* eye; L, *nervus,* nerve], the first division of the trigeminal nerve (CN V), supplying sensory innervation to the forehead, scalp, lacrimal gland, eye, and side of the nose.

ophthalmic solution, a specially prepared sterile preparation free of foreign particles for instillation of a medication into the eye.

ophthalmic vein, one of two venous channels in the orbit, the superior ophthalmic vein and the inferior ophthalmic vein, that communicate with the cavernous sinus. This communication can be a route by which infections spread from outside to inside the cranial cavity.

ophthalmic vesicle. See **optic vesicle.**

ophthalmitis /of′thalmī″tis/ [Gk, *ophthalmos,* eye, *itis,* inflammation], an inflammation of the eye.

ophthalmo-, ophthalm- /ofthal′mō-/, prefix meaning "eye": *ophthalmodynia, ophthalmoplegia, ophthalmospasm.*

ophthalmodynamometer /-din′əmom″ətər/ [Gk, *ophthalmos,* eye, *dynamis,* force, *metron,* measure], an instrument for measuring pressure on the sclera while the fundus is studied with an ophthalmoscope. It may be used to measure blood pressures in the ophthalmic artery.

ophthalmodynia /-din″ē·ə/ [Gk, *ophthalmos,* eye, *odyne,* pain], a pain in the eye.

ophthalmologic, opthalmological. See **ophthalmology.**

ophthalmologist /of′thalmol″əjist/, a physician who specializes in ophthalmology.

ophthalmology (ophth) /of′thalmol″əjē/ [Gk, *ophthalmos* + *logos,* science], the branch of medicine concerned with the study of the physiology, anatomy, and pathology of the eye and the diagnosis and treatment of disorders of the eye. −*ophthalmologic, ophthalmological, adj.*

ophthalmopathy /of′thəlmop′ə·thē/ [Gk, *ophthalmos,* eye + *pathos,* disease], any disease of the eye.

ophthalmoplasty /ofthal″mōplas′tē/ [Gk, *ophthalmos,* eye, *plassein,* to mold], plastic surgery of the eye or the area around the eye.

ophthalmoplegia /ofthal′maplē″jē·ə/ [Gk, *ophthalmos* + *plege,* stroke], an abnormal condition characterized by paralysis of the motor nerves of the eye. Bilateral ophthalmoplegia of rapid onset is associated with acute myasthenia gravis, acute thiamine deficiency, botulism, and acute inflammatory cranial polyneuropathy. These diseases are potentially very destructive and require prompt attention. In some patients with myopathic ophthalmoplegia, structural abnormalities and biochemical disorders may be evident in limb muscles. Ophthalmoplegia is also associated with ocular dystrophy.

ophthalmoplegia plus. See **Kearns-Sayre syndrome.**

ophthalmoscope /ofthal″məskōp/ [Gk, *ophthalmos* + *skopein,* to look], a device for examining the interior of the eye. It includes a light, a mirror with a single aperture through which the examiner views, and a dial holding several lenses of varying strengths. The lenses are selected to allow clear visualization of the structures of the eye at any depth. If the patient or the examiner ordinarily requires extensive correction of a refractive error, the examination may require that the corrective lenses should be worn for the examination. Also called **funduscope.**

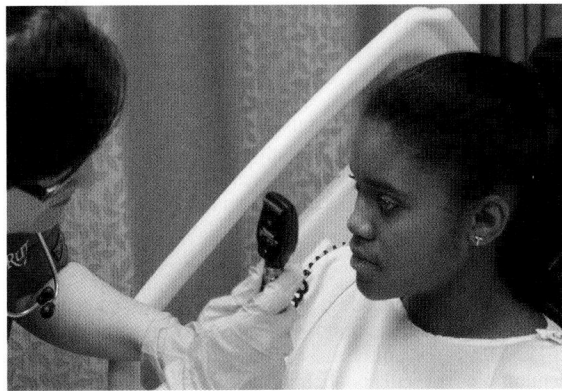

Preparing for an exam with an ophthalmoscope
(Courtesy Rutgers School of Nursing—Camden. All rights reserved.)

ophthalmoscopy /of′thalmos″kəpē/, the technique of using an ophthalmoscope to examine the eye. Also called **funduscopy.** See also **fundus microscopy.**

ophthalmospasm /ofthal″mōspaz′əm/ [Gk, *ophthalmos,* eye, *spasmos*], a sudden involuntary contraction of the eyeball.

-opia, -opic, -opical, -ops, -opsia, -opsy, -opy, suffix meaning "a (specified) visual condition": *myopia, chromatopsia, senopia.*

opiate /ō″pē·it/ [Gk, *opion,* poppy juice], **1.** a drug that contains opium, derivatives of opium, or any of several semisynthetic or synthetic drugs with opium-like activity. **2.** *(Informal)* any soporific or opioid drug. **3.** pertaining to a substance that causes sleep or relief of pain. Morphine and related opiates may produce unwanted side effects such as respiratory depression, nausea, vomiting, dizziness, and constipation. Patients with reduced blood volume are more susceptible to the hypotensive effect of morphine and related drugs. Opiates are used with extreme caution in obese patients and in those with head injuries, emphysema, or other problems associated with decreased respiratory function. In patients with prostatic hypertrophy, morphine may cause acute urinary retention, requiring repeated catheterization. Also called **opioid.**

opiate poisoning [Gk, *opion,* poppy juice; L, *potio,* drink], toxic effects of a potent opioid, including depression of the brain centers, causing unconsciousness and diminished respirations. Acute intoxication is characterized by euphoria, flushing, itching, and constriction of pupils, followed by decreased respiratory rate, hypotension, lowered body temperature, and abnormally slow heartbeat. Withdrawal is marked by effects generally the opposite of opiate poisoning, depending on the type of opioid, the size of the dose, and the duration of opioid use.

opiate receptor [Gk, *opion,* poppy juice; L, *recipere,* to receive], transmembrane proteins that bind to endogenous opioid neuropeptides and exogenous morphine and similar natural or synthetic compounds. The three major classes of these receptors are designated mu, kappa, and delta. Morphine preferentially stimulates mu receptors to produce analgesia, euphoria, respiratory depression, constipation, and pinpoint pupils. Some other drugs (e.g., butorphanol) can selectively block mu receptors while stimulating kappa receptors; this provides moderate to high pain relief with low abuse potential. Stimulation of delta receptors can also contribute to analgesia. The receptors are found in high concentrations in the dorsal horn of the spinal cord and in the brain regions involved with pain modulation or pain transmission (e.g., periaqueductal gray matter). Endogenous agonists at these receptors include endorphins, enkephalins, and dynorphins.

-opic, -opical. See **-opia, -opic, -opical, -ops, -opsia, -opsy, -opy.**

opinion /əpin″yən/ [L, *opinari,* to suppose], **1.** (in law) a statement by the court, usually in writing, of the reasoning behind its decision or judgment in a particular case. **2.** a statement prepared for a client by an attorney that represents the attorney's understanding of the law as it pertains to a legal question posed by the client.

opioid /ō″pē-oid/ [Gk, *opion,* poppy juice, *eidos,* form], strictly speaking, pertaining to natural and synthetic chemicals that have opium-like effects similar to morphine, though they are not derived from opium. Examples include endorphins or enkephalins produced by body tissues or synthetic methadone. Morphine and related drugs are often included in this category because the term narcotic has lost its original meaning.

opioid antagonist, a drug that blocks mu, kappa, or delta opioid receptors. It is used primarily in the treatment of opioid-induced, mu receptor–mediated respiratory depression. The opioid antagonist naloxone may be administered intravenously, subcutaneously, or intranasally. Naltrexone may be administered orally, as well as by a depot injection intramuscularly.

opioid receptor, any of a number of types of receptors for opiates and opioids. At least seven different types are postulated at different locations in the body, grouped into three major classes (delta, kappa, and mu) according to the specific substances they bind to and the specific physiological effect or effects that binding causes or inhibits.

opisthion /ō·pis′thē·on/ [Gk, *opisthion,* rear, posterior], a landmark located at the midpoint of the posterior border of the foramen magnum.

opistho-, prefix meaning "backward" or "relating to the back": *opisthorchiasis, opisthotonos.*

opisthorchiasis /ō′pisthôrkī″əsis/ [Gk, *opisthen,* behind, *orchis,* testicle, *osis,* condition], infection with one of the species of *Opisthorchis* liver flukes commonly found in the Philippines, India, Thailand, and Laos. Carcinoma of the intrahepatic bile ducts may be a late complication. Adequate cooking of freshwater fish prevents the disease.

Opisthorchis sinensis. See *Clonorchis sinensis.*

opisthotonos /ō′pisthot″ənəs/ [Gk, *opisthios,* posterior, *tonos,* straining], a prolonged severe spasm of the muscles causing the back to arch acutely, the head to bend back on the neck, the heels to bend back on the legs, and the arms and hands to flex rigidly at the joints. It is related to meningitis.

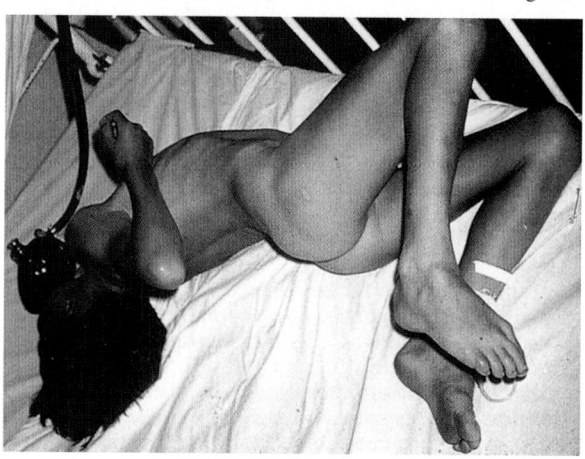

Opisthotonos *(Farrar, 1992)*

opium /ō″pē·əm/ [Gk, *opion,* poppy juice], a milky exudate from the unripe capsules of *Papaver somniferum* and *Papaver album* yielding 9.5% or more of anhydrous morphine. It is an opioid analgesic, a hypnotic, and an astringent. Opium contains several alkaloids, including codeine, morphine, and papaverine. See also **codeine sulfate, morphine sulfate, opium tincture, papaverine hydrochloride, paregoric, codeine phosphate.**

opium alkaloid, one of several alkaloids isolated from the milky exudate of the unripe seed pods of *Papaver somniferum,* a species of poppy indigenous to the Near East. Two of the alkaloids, codeine and morphine, are used clinically for the relief of pain, but their use entails the risk of physical or psychological dependence. Morphine is the standard against which the analgesic effect of newer drugs for relief of pain is measured. The opium alkaloids and their semisynthetic derivatives, including heroin, act on the central nervous system, producing analgesia, change in mood, drowsiness, and mental slowness. The effects in a person who has pain are usually pleasant. Euphoria and pain-free sleep are not uncommon, but nausea and vomiting sometimes occur. In usual doses the analgesic effects are achieved without loss of consciousness. The opium alkaloids have several other effects on the various systems of the body: coughing is suppressed; the electrical activity pattern of the brain resembles that of sleep; the pupils constrict; respiration is depressed in rate, minute volume, and tidal exchange; the secretory activity and motility of the GI tract are diminished; and biliary and pancreatic secretions are reduced. The use of morphine as an antidiarrheal preceded its use as an analgesic by hundreds of years. Prepared in a tincture, it remains the most effective constipating agent available. Papaverine, another opium alkaloid, does not cause analgesia but is used clinically as a vasodilator.

opium tincture, an analgesic and antidiarrheal drug.
- INDICATIONS: It is prescribed in the treatment of intestinal hyperactivity, cramping, and diarrhea.
- CONTRAINDICATIONS: Drug dependence, the presence of toxic matter in the bowel, or known hypersensitivity to this drug prohibits its use.
- ADVERSE EFFECTS: Among the more serious adverse effects are drug dependence, toxic megacolon, and central nervous system depression.

Oppenheim reflex /op″ənhīm/ [Herman Oppenheim, German neurologist, 1858–1919], a variation of Babinski reflex elicited by firmly stroking downward on the anterior and medial surfaces of the tibia, characterized by extension of the great toe and fanning of other toes. It is a sign of pyramidal tract disease. Compare **Chaddock reflex, Gordon reflex.** See also **Babinski reflex.**

opponens digiti minimi, a muscle that originates from the hook of the hamate and from the adjacent flexor retinaculum and inserts into the medial margin and palmar surface of the fifth metacarpal, rotating it toward the palm.

opponens pollicis, the largest of the three thenar muscles. It rotates and flexes the first metacarpal on the trapezium, bringing the pad of the thumb into a position facing the pads of the fingers.

opportunistic infection [L, *opportunus,* convenient, *icus,* form], **1.** an infection caused by normally nonpathogenic organisms in a host whose resistance has been decreased by disorders such as diabetes mellitus, human immunodeficiency virus (HIV) infection, or cancer; a surgical procedure such as a cerebrospinal fluid shunt or a cardiac or urinary tract catheterization; or immunosuppressive drugs. Long-term use of antibiotics or other drugs may also affect the immune system, creating an opportunity for microorganisms not usually pathogenic to become pathogens. People with HIV are particularly susceptible to such infections. **2.** an unusual infection with a common pathogen, such as cellulitis, meningitis, or otitis media.

opportunistic pathogen, an organism that exists harmlessly as part of the normal human body environment and does not become a health threat until the body's immune system fails.

opposition [L, *opponere,* to oppose], the relation between the thumb and the other digits of the hand for the purpose of grasping objects between the thumb and fingers.

oppositional defiant disorder (ODD), a behavioral disorder most often diagnosed in childhood. It is characterized by uncooperative, defiant, and hostile behavior toward peers and authority figures.

oprelvekin /o-prel′vĕ-kin″/, recombinant interleukin-11, used as a stimulator of platelet production to prevent prolonged thrombocytopenia after myelosuppressive chemotherapy.

ops-, opto-, opti-, optico-, prefix meaning "visible" or "vision" or "sight": *optokinetic, optic, optometrist.*

-ops, -opsia. See **-opia, -opic, -opical, -ops, -opsia, -opsy, -opy.**

opscan, acronym for *optical scanning.*

opsin, a protein that combines with retinal rods to form visual pigments (rhodopsin and iodopsin) in the photoreceptor cells of the retina.

opsonin /op″sənin/ [Gk, *opsonein,* to supply food], an antibody or complement split product that, on attaching to foreign material, microorganisms, or other antigens, enhances phagocytosis of that substance by leukocytes and other macrophages. **—opsonize,** *v.*

opsonization /op″sənizā″shən/ [Gk, *opsonein* + *izein,* to cause], the action of opsonin. Also called *opsonification.*

opsonize. See **opsonin.**

-opsy. See **-opia, -opic, -opical, -ops, -opsia, -opsy, -opy.**

opti-. See **ops-, opto-, opti-, optico-.**

optic [Gk, *optikos,* sight], pertaining to the eyes or to sight. Also **optical.**

-optic, -optical, suffix meaning "vision": *bioptic, panoptic, orthoptic.*

optic activity /op″tik/, the rotation of the plane of polarized light clockwise or counterclockwise. Substances that rotate the plane of polarized light to the right are dextrorotatory; those that rotate the plane to the left are levorotatory.

optical. See **optic.**

optical biopsy, any technique that uses the interaction of light and tissue to provide information about the tissue.

optical disk, a large-capacity digital data-storage device used to store digital images.

optically stimulated luminescence dosimeter (OSL dosimeter), a personal radiation monitoring device similar to the thermoluminescence dosimeter but using aluminum oxide to absorb the energy of x-rays and a laser rather than heat to release the stored energy and measure the dose of ionizing radiation received. See also **thermoluminescent dosimetry.**

optic angle. See **visual angle.**

optic atrophy, wasting of the optic disc resulting from degeneration of fibers of the optic nerve and optic tract. In primary optic atrophy the disc is white and sharply margined, the central depression (physiological cup) is enlarged, and the optic foramen of the sclera is clearly visible. In secondary atrophy the disc is gray, its margins are blurred, the depression is filled in, and the foramen is difficult to detect. Optic atrophy may be caused by a congenital defect, inflammation, occlusion of the central retinal artery or internal carotid artery, alcohol, arsenic, lead, tobacco, or other toxic substances. Degeneration of the disc may also accompany arteriosclerosis, diabetes, glaucoma, hydrocephalus, pernicious anemia, and various neurological disorders.

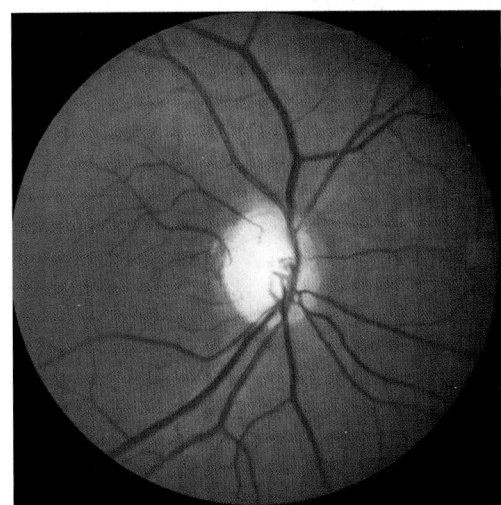

Optic atrophy *(Willis, 2008)*

optic brightener, a compound that absorbs ultraviolet light and emits visible light.

optic chiasm [Gk, *optikos,* sight, *chiasma,* crossed lines], a point near the thalamus and hypothalamus where parts of each optic nerve cross over.

optic coupling, the attachment of the crystal window of a scintillator to the window of a photomultiplier tube. It maximizes the transmission of light from the scintillator to the interior of the photomultiplier tube.

optic cup, a two-layered embryonic cavity that develops in early pregnancy. The optic cup is completed by the seventh week with the closing of the choroidal fissure. The cup initially develops from the infolding of the optic vesicle after the vesicle separates from the embryonic ectoderm. The cells of the optic cup differentiate to form the retina that first develops its layers of rods and cones in the central part of the cup, growing as the layer gradually spreads toward the cup margin. The outer layer of the cup persists as the pigmented layer of the retina; the inner layer develops the nervous elements and the supporting fibers of the retina. Compare **optic stalk.**

optic density, a number describing the blackening of an x-ray film in any specified location. In general, the optic density is the logarithm of the ratio of incident light intensity to the intensity of light transmitted through that area and is measured with a densitometer.

optic disc, the small blind spot on the surface of the retina, located about 3 mm to the nasal side of the macula. It is the point where the fibers of the retina leave the eye and become part of the optic nerve. It is the only part of the retina that is insensitive to light. At its center the porus opticus marks the point of entrance of the central artery of the retina. Also called **blind spot, discus nervi optici.**

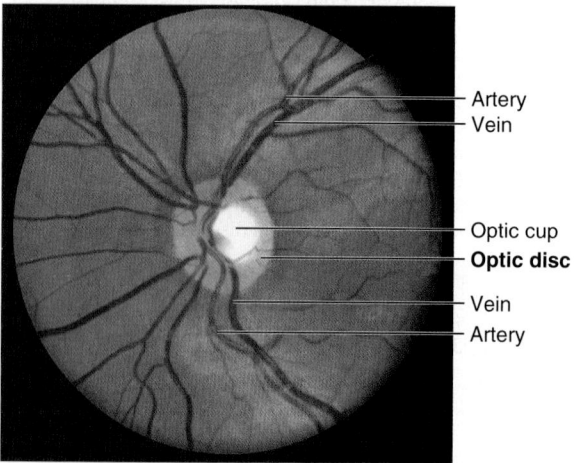

Artery
Vein
Optic cup
Optic disc
Vein
Artery

Optic disc *(Courtesy Karen Ann Klima, BA, CRA, COMT, The Johns Hopkins Center for Hereditary Eye Diseases, The Wilmer Eye Institute)*

optic fissure. See **retinal fissure.**

optic foramen [Gk, *optikos,* sight, *foramen,* hole], an aperture in the root of the lesser wing of the sphenoid bone transmitting the optic nerve.

optic glioma, a slow-growing tumor on the optic nerve or in the chiasm, composed of glial cells. Symptoms may include loss of vision, secondary strabismus, exophthalmos, and ocular paralysis.

optician /optish´ən/ [Gk, *optikos,* sight], a person who grinds and fits eyeglasses and contact lenses by prescription. To become an optician, a person must graduate from high school and complete a 4- or 5-year apprenticeship. In some states licensure is required.

optic illusion [Gk, *optikos,* sight; L, *illudere,* to mock], a false visual image derived from a misinterpretation of sensory stimuli caused by physical or psychological factors or

both. A common optic illusion is the appearance of railroad tracks merging in the distance.

optic laser, optic maser. See **laser.**

optic nerve, one of a pair of nerves that transmit visual impulses. The optic nerve is not a true cranial nerve but is rather an extension of the brain. It consists mainly of coarse myelinated fibers that arise in the retinal ganglionic layer, traverse the thalamus, and connect with the visual cortex. At the optic chiasm the fibers from the inner or nasal half of the retina cross to the optic tract of the opposite side. The remaining fibers from the temporal or outer half of each retina are uncrossed and pass to the visual cortex on the same side. The visual cortex functions in the perception of light, shade, and objects. The optic nerve fibers correspond to a tract of fibers within the brain. Also called **nervus opticus, second cranial nerve.**

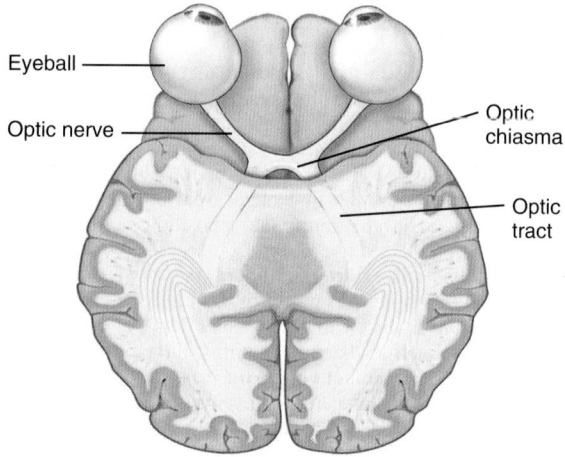

Eyeball
Optic nerve
Optic chiasma
Optic tract

Optic nerve

optic neuritis [Gk, *optikos,* sight, *neuron,* nerve, *itis,* inflammation], inflammation, degeneration, or demyelinization of the optic nerve or optic disc caused by a wide variety of diseases. Loss of vision is the cardinal symptom. Also called **retrobulbar neuritis.**

optic neuropathy [Gk, *optikos,* sight, *neuron,* nerve, *pathos,* disease], a disease, generally noninflammatory, of the eye, characterized by dysfunction or destruction of the optic nerve tissues. Causes include an interruption in the blood supply, compression by a tumor or aneurysm, a nutritional deficiency, and toxic effects of a chemical. The disorder, which can lead to blindness, usually affects only one eye.

optico-. See **ops-, opto-, opti-, optico-.**

opticokinetic. See **optokinetic.**

optic papilla. See **papilla.**

optic radiation [Gk, *optikos,* sight; L, *radiare,* to shine], a system of fibers from the lateral geniculate body of the thalamus that passes through the sublenticular part of the internal capsule to the striate area.

optic righting, one of the five basic neuromuscular reactions that enable a person to change body positions. It involves a reflex that automatically orients the head to a new optical or visual fixation point, depending on the body position change.

optic righting reflex [Gk, *optikos,* sight; AS, *riht* + L, *reflectere,* to bend back], a reflex that restores normal posture and head position with the help of visual clues.

optics /op´tiks/ [Gk, *optikos,* sight], **1.** (in physics) a field of study that deals with the electromagnetic radiation of wavelengths shorter than radio waves but longer than x-rays. **2.** (in physiology) a field of study that deals with vision and the process by which the functions of the eye and the brain are integrated in the perception of shapes, patterns, movements, spatial relationships, and color.

optic stalk, one of a pair of slender embryonic structures that becomes the optic nerve. In the embryo the optic stalk develops during the second week and attaches the optic vesicle to the wall of the brain. The stalk becomes complete during the seventh week of pregnancy when the choroidal fissure closes and is later converted into the optic nerve when retinal nerve fibers fill the cavity of the stalk. A few fibers grow into the stalk from the brain. About the tenth week after birth, the fibers of the optic nerve receive their myelin sheaths. Compare **optic cup.**

optic system assessment, an evaluation of the patient's eyes, vision, and current and past disorders or injuries that may be responsible for abnormalities in the individual's optic system.

■ METHOD: The patient is interviewed to determine if vision is blurred, double, decreased, or absent in one or both eyes or diminished peripherally at night or in bright light. The interviewer asks if halos or lights are seen and if the patient collides with unfamiliar objects or is unable to distinguish objects held too close or too far; if the eyes water, itch, or feel tender, painful, or fatigued; and if an injury to the eye, face, or head has occurred. Observations are made of the patient's general appearance, vital signs, kind of eyeglasses or contact lenses worn, the amount of tearing, ability to blink, tendency to rub the eyes, and visual acuity. Evidence is recorded of conjunctivitis, drainage, optic hemorrhage, edema or ptosis of the eyelids, exophthalmos, strabismus, nystagmus, scleral edema, chalazion, lacerations, contusions, or a foreign body in the eye. Carefully noted are signs of aging; glaucoma; cataract; retinal detachment; and the presence of multiple sclerosis, diabetes mellitus, myasthenia gravis, gonorrhea, thyroid dysfunction, sinus problems, or cerebral trauma or tumors. The patient's report of previous eye operations or treatments, head or face trauma, arteriosclerosis, glomerulonephritis, retinal degeneration, episodes of coma, therapy with oxygen, and drug misuse are investigated, as well as a family history of glaucoma or diabetes. Also explored are the possibility that the patient has a hazardous job or recreation (and note is made of any safety precautions taken); the individual's misuse of alcohol; and use of medication, especially antibiotics, antiemetics, miotics, mydriatics, and acetazolamide. Diagnostic aids available for the evaluation include a test of visual fields, an x-ray film of the orbit and skull, an ophthalmoscopic examination, tonometry, a brain scan, and microscopic studies of conjunctival scrapings.

■ INTERVENTIONS: A health care provider conducts the interview, observes the patient, and assembles pertinent background data and the results of the diagnostic procedures.

■ OUTCOME CRITERIA: A careful assessment of the patient's eyes and vision and of certain aspects of the medical, family, and social history is a significant aid in establishing the diagnosis of an optic system disorder.

optic thermometer, a temperature-measuring device in which the properties of transmission and reflection of visible light are temperature dependent, the detection of which can be related to tissue temperature.

optic tract [Gk, *optikos,* sight; L, *tractus*], a flat band of nerve fibers running backward and laterally around each cerebral peduncle from the optic chiasma to the lateral geniculate body. Each tract carries information from the two eyes.

optic vesicle, an early embryonic outgrowth from the ventrolateral wall of the forebrain. Its cells develop into the retina and optic nerve of the eye. Also called **ophthalmic vesicle.**

Optimine, an antihistamine. Brand name for **azatadine maleate.**

optional water loss /op″shənəl/, a volume of average daily water loss, in addition to obligatory water loss, depending on physical activities, climate, and other factors. See also **obligatory water loss.**

opto-. See **-ops, -opsia.**

optokinetic /op′tōkinet″ik/ [Gk, *optikos,* sight, *kinesis,* motion], pertaining to movement of the eyeballs in response to the movement of objects across the visual field, as in optokinetic nystagmus. Also called **opticokinetic.**

optometric vision therapy, a treatment plan prescribed to correct or improve specific dysfunctions of the vision system. It includes, but is not limited to, the treatment of strabismus (turned eye), other dysfunctions of binocularity (eye teaming), amblyopia (lazy eye), accommodation (eye focusing), ocular motor function (general eye movement ability), and visual-motor and visual-perceptual abilities.

optometric vision therapy technician (OVTT), an allied health professional, supervised by an optometrist, who participates in evaluating clients and in planning and implementing optometric vision therapy programs.

optometrist /optom″ətrist/ [Gk, *optikos,* sight, *metron,* measure], a person who practices optometry. An optometrist is awarded the degree of Doctor of Optometry (O.D.) after completion of at least 3 years of college followed by 4 years in an approved college of optometry. A state examination and license are also required. See also **optician, optometry.**

optometry /optom″ətrē/ [Gk, *optikos,* sight, *metron,* measure], the practice of primary eye care, including testing the eyes for visual acuity, prescribing corrective spectacles or contact lenses and topical medications, and managing binocular vision disorders. See also **optician.**

OPV, abbreviation for **oral poliovirus vaccine.**

-opy. See **-opia, -opic, -opical, -ops, -opsia, -opsy, -opy.**

OR, O.R., abbreviation for **operating room.**

ora /ō′rə/ *pl.* **orae** [L], an edge or margin.

oral /ôr″əl/ [L, *oralis,* pertaining to the mouth], pertaining to the mouth. Compare **buccal, parenteral.**

oral administration of medication, the administration of a tablet, a capsule, an elixir, or a solution or other liquid form of medication by mouth. An adequate amount of water should be given to lubricate or dissolve the solid medications or to dilute the liquid forms for swallowing. Preparations with a disagreeable taste may be given with something of sufficient flavor to disguise the bad taste. Substances that are harmful to the teeth are given through a straw. People who have difficulty swallowing pills or capsules may find it easier to swallow the medication if they look up as they swallow. Looking up while swallowing opens the esophagus. With patients who have difficulty swallowing, the oral cavity is always checked for pocketing the medication. Research shows that sitting up for 15 to 30 minutes after oral medications promotes dissolution of the medication and decreases gastric irritation. Kinds include **buccal administration of medication, sublingual administration of a medication.**

oral airway, a curved tubular device of rubber, plastic, or metal placed in the oropharynx during general anesthesia and other situations in which the level of consciousness is impaired. Its purpose is to maintain free passage of air and keep the tongue from obstructing the trachea. The artificial airway is not removed until the patient begins to awaken and regains pharyngeal, cough, and swallowing reflexes.

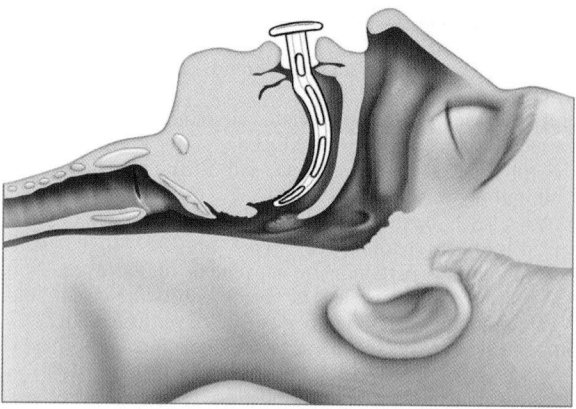

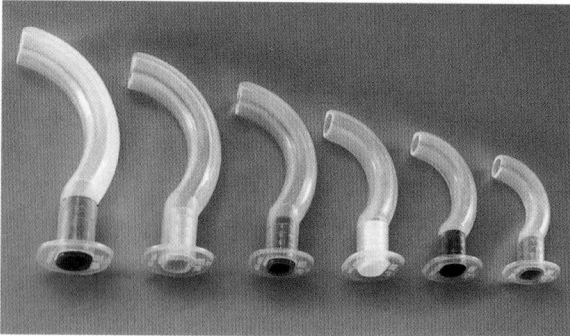

Oral airways *(Courtesy Rusch, Inc.)*

oral and maxillofacial surgeon, a dental specialist who addresses the diagnoses and surgical and adjunctive treatments of hard and soft tissue diseases, injuries, and defects of the oral cavity and structures and the facial region. One of the ten dental specialties.

oral and maxillofacial surgery [L, *oralis,* pertaining to the mouth; Gk, *cheirourgos,* surgeon], one of the 10 recognized dental specialties. Oral and maxillofacial surgery is the specialty that includes the diagnosis and surgical and adjunctive treatment of diseases, injuries, and defects involving both the functional and aesthetic aspects of the hard and soft tissues of the oral and maxillofacial region. Also called **maxillofacial surgery, oral surgery.** See also **dental surgeon.**

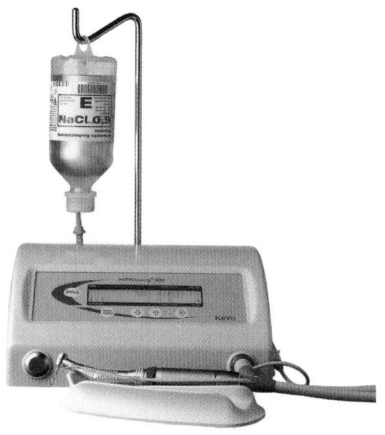

Surgical handpiece for oral surgery *(Courtesy KaVo Dental)*

oral cancer, a malignant neoplasm on the lip or in the mouth that occurs at an average age of 60, with a frequency eight times higher in men than in women. Predisposing factors are alcoholism; heavy use of tobacco; poor oral hygiene; ill-fitting dentures; syphilis; Plummer-Vinson syndrome; betel nut chewing; and, in lip cancer, pipe smoking and overexposure to sun and wind. Premalignant leukoplakia or erythroplasia or a painless nonhealing ulcer may be the first sign of oral cancer; localized pain usually occurs later, but lymph nodes may be involved early in the course. Diagnostic measures include digital examination, biopsy, exfoliative cytology, x-ray film of the mandible, and chest films to detect metastatic lung lesions. Almost all oral tumors are epidermoid carcinomas. Adenocarcinomas occur occasionally, whereas sarcomas and metastatic lesions from other sites are rare. Small primary lesions may be treated by excision or irradiation, and more extensive oral tumors may be treated by surgery, with removal of involved lymph nodes and preoperative or postoperative radiotherapy. Among chemotherapeutic agents administered are cisplatin, methotrexate, 5-fluorouracil, bleomycin, and Adriamycin. Postoperative nursing care involves maintenance of airway patency, relieving pain, promoting adequate nutrition, and health teaching regarding follow-up care and psychosocial adjustment if body image has been affected.

oral cavity [L, *oralis,* pertaining to the mouth, *cavum,* cavity], the space within the mouth that contains the tongue and teeth. See also **mouth.**

oral cavity proper. See **mouth.**

oral character, (in psychoanalysis) a kind of personality that exhibits patterns of behavior originating in the first phase of infancy, the oral stage. This personality is characterized by optimism, self-confidence, and carefree generosity, reflecting the pleasurable aspects of the stage, or by pessimism, futility, anxiety, and sadism as manifestations of frustrations or conflicts occurring during the period. See also **oral eroticism, psychosexual development.**

oral contraceptive (OC), oral hormone medication for contraception. The two major sex hormones in females are estrogens and progestins. When synthetic forms of these hormones are taken, they inhibit the production of gonadotropin-releasing hormone by the hypothalamus; the pituitary therefore does not secrete gonadotropins to stimulate follicular maturation and ovulation. Depending on the formulation, cyclical changes in the uterus, vagina, and breasts may be similar to a normal menstrual cycle. Progestin-only oral contraceptives generally do not block ovulation. Instead they cause the cervical mucus to remain thick, which prevents the entry of sperm into the uterus and fallopian tubes. Seasonale, an extended-cycle method of contraception with menstrual periods every three months, was recently approved by the FDA. Contraindications to the oral contraceptives include pregnancy, diabetes mellitus, liver disease, hyperlipidemia, thrombotic complications, coronary artery disease, and sickle cell disease. Patients with depression and migraine headaches and those who are heavy cigarette smokers need to be followed up more often. The pregnancy rate when oral contraceptives are used correctly is less than 0.2% a year. See also **contraception.**

oral decongestant, a sympathomimetic, alpha agonist drug such as pseudoephedrine, prescribed for the relief of nasal congestion. Oral decongestants do not appear to cause nasal swelling after long periods of use. They are commonly combined with antihistamines for the treatment of allergic rhinitis. Abuse may cause constipation.

oral dosage, the administration of a medicine by mouth.

oral eroticism, (in psychoanalysis) a libidinal fixation at, or regression to, the oral stage of psychosexual development, often reflected as an oral character. Also called *oral erotism.* Compare **anal eroticism.**

oral examination [L, *oralis,* pertaining to the mouth, *examinatio,* weighing], a clinical, visual, and tactile inspection and investigation of the hard and soft structures of the oral cavity for purposes of assessment, diagnosis, planning, treatment, and evaluation. Before the examination, the client's full medical and dental health histories are obtained. Radiographs or dental images are used in conjunction with an oral examination to help visualize the underlying bony and soft tissue structures.

oral-facial-digital (OFD) syndrome, type I, an X-linked dominant disorder lethal in males characterized by camptodactyly, polydactyly, and syndactyly; cranial, facial, lingual, and dental anomalies; and intellectual disability, familial trembling, alopecia, and seborrhea of the face and milia. Also called **orodigitofacial dysostosis,** *orofaciodigital syndrome, type I.*

oral-facial-digital (OFD) syndrome, type II. See **Mohr syndrome.**

oral-facial-digital (OFD) syndrome, type III, an autosomal-recessive disorder characterized by postaxial hexadactyly of the hands and feet; ocular, lingual, and dental anomalies; and profound intellectual disability. Also called **orodigitofacial dysostosis,** *orofaciodigital syndrome, type III.*

oral hairy leukoplakia. See **hairy leukoplakia.**

oral herpes. See **herpes simplex.**

oral hygiene, the condition or practice of maintaining the tissues and structures of the mouth. Oral hygiene includes brushing the tongue and teeth to remove food particles and residue, bacteria, and plaque; massaging the gums with a toothbrush, dental floss, or water irrigator to stimulate circulation and remove foreign matter; and cleansing dentures and ensuring their proper fit to prevent irritation. Dependent or unconscious patients are assisted in maintaining a healthy oral condition. Such care includes lubricating the lips and cleaning the inside of the cheeks, the roof of the mouth, and the tongue as well as the teeth and gingiva. In addition, the health care provider checks for carious teeth, broken teeth, and loose teeth that might be swallowed or aspirated.

oral hypoglycemic agent, an oral antidiabetic agent commonly used in the treatment of type 2 diabetes mellitus. Oral hypoglycemic agents are not prescribed as a substitute for diet and exercise but rather as adjunctive therapy. An oral hypoglycemic agent cannot be used as monotherapy in patients with type 1 diabetes mellitus because these patients lack sufficient insulin.

oral mucosa, the mucous membrane of the cavity of the mouth, including the gingiva (gums).

oral pathology, the branch of pathology that deals with the structural and functional changes in cells, tissues, and organs of the oral cavity that cause or are caused by disease.

oral poliovirus vaccine (OPV), an attenuated preparation of live poliovirus that confers immunity to poliomyelitis. Also called **Sabin vaccine.**

■ INDICATIONS: Replaced by inactivated poliovirus vaccine (IPV), OPV supplies in the United States will be limited once existing supplies are depleted. It was routinely prescribed for immunization against poliomyelitis, but its use is now limited to treatment in areas with outbreaks of paralytic polio.

■ CONTRAINDICATIONS: Immunosuppression, concomitant use of corticosteroids, cancer, immunoglobulin abnormalities, or acute infection prohibits its use.

■ ADVERSE EFFECTS: Adverse effects are uncommon. Cases of vaccine-induced paralytic disease have occurred but are very rare. Nonetheless, it is because of the risk of vaccine-induced paralytic poliomyelitis that an all-IPV immunization schedule is recommended for children in the United States.

oral prophylaxis [L, *oralis,* pertaining to the mouth; Gk, *prophylax,* advance guard], (in dentistry) the science and practice of preventing the onset of diseases of the teeth and adjoining mouth tissues. It involves removing bacterial plaque, food debris, stains, and calculus from the crowns and roots with hand scaling or ultrasonic scaling instruments and hand or electric polishers.

oral rehydration solutions (ORS) [L, *oralis,* pertaining to the mouth, *re + hydor,* water, *solutus,* dissolved], solutions of electrolytes and glucose used in oral rehydration therapy. The recommended electrolytes include NaCl, KCl, and trisodium citrate.

oral rehydration therapy (ORT), the adjustment of water, glucose, and electrolyte balance in a dehydrated patient by giving fluids with measured amounts of essential ingredients by mouth.

oral sadism, (in psychoanalysis) a sadistic form of oral eroticism manifested by such behavior as biting, chewing, and other aggressive impulses associated with eating habits. Compare **anal sadism.**

oral stage, (in psychoanalysis) according to Freud, the initial stage of psychosexual development occurring in the first 12 to 18 months of life, when the feeding experience and other oral activities are the predominant source of pleasurable stimulation. Adult patterns of behavior associated with this stage include overeating, loquaciousness, alcoholism, smoking addictions, and a sarcastic personality. See also **oral character, psychosexual development.**

oral surgeon. See **dental surgeon, oral and maxillofacial surgeon.**

oral surgery. See **oral and maxillofacial surgery.**

oral temperature [L, *oralis,* pertaining to the mouth, *temperatura*], the body temperature as recorded by a clinical thermometer placed in the mouth. It is normally around 98.6° F (37° C), but it may vary within a fraction of a degree, depending on the individual and such factors as time of day, sleep, and exercise and whether measured before or after a meal. See also **normal temperature.**

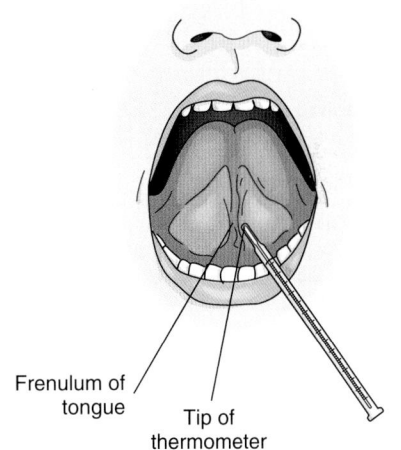

Frenulum of tongue

Tip of thermometer

Placement of thermometer for oral temperature measurement *(Sorrentino, 2008)*

oral tolerance therapy, a treatment in which a patient ingests a foreign protein in an attempt to develop tolerance to that protein when it is encountered as an antigen. In addition to inhibiting allergic reactions, the therapy may suppress immune responses in general.

Orap, an oral neuroleptic drug. Brand name for **pimozide.**

ora serrata retinae, the irregular, serrated demarcation between the retina and the ciliary body. It is the most anterior peripheral part of the retina.

orb /ôrb/ [L, *orbis,* circle], describing something spheric or globelike.

orbicular /ôrbik″yəl/ər/ [L, *orbiculus,* little circle], pertaining to something round or circular.

orbicular bone [L, *orbiculus,* little circle; AS, *ban*], a knob on the end of the long process of the incus that articulates with the stapes.

orbicularis ciliaris /ôrbik′yōōlär″is/ [L, *orbiculus,* little circle; *cilium,* eyelash], one of the two zones of the ciliary body of the eye, extending from the ora serrata of the retina to the ciliary processes at the margin of the iris. The orbicularis ciliaris is about 4 mm wide and increases in thickness as it approaches the ciliary processes.

orbicularis oculi, the muscular body of the eyelid, encircling the eye and comprising the palpebral, orbital, and lacrimal muscles. It arises from the nasal part of the frontal bone, the frontal process of the maxilla in front of the lacrimal groove, and the anterior surface of the medial palpebral ligament. The palpebral muscle functions to close the eyelid gently; the orbital muscle functions to close it more energetically, such as in winking. Also called **orbicularis palpebrarum.** Compare **corrugator supercilii, levator palpebrae superioris.**

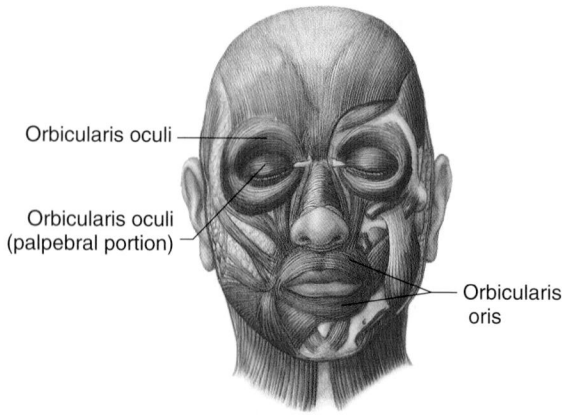

Muscles of the face: orbicularis oculi and orbicularis oris *(Patton and Thibodeau, 2016)*

orbicularis oris, the muscle surrounding the mouth. It consists partly of fibers derived from other facial muscles such as the buccinator that are inserted into the lips and partly of fibers proper to the lips. It serves to close and purse the lips.

orbicularis palpebrarum. See **orbicularis oculi.**

orbicularis pupillary reflex, a normal phenomenon elicited by forceful closure of the eyelids or attempting to close them while they are held apart, resulting first in constriction and then dilation of the pupil.

orbit /ôr″bit/ [L, *orbita,* wheel track], one of a pair of bony, conical cavities in the skull that accommodate the eyeballs and associated structures, such as the eye muscles, nerves, and blood vessels. The medial walls of the orbits are approximately parallel with each other and with the middle line, but the lateral walls diverge widely. The roof of each orbit is formed by the orbital plate of the frontal bone and the small wing of the sphenoid bones. The openings that communicate with each orbit are the optic foramen, the superior and the inferior orbital fissures, the supraorbital foramen, the infraorbital canal, the anterior and posterior ethmoidal foramina, the zygomatic foramen, and the canal for the nasolacrimal duct. *–orbital, adj.*

orbital aperture /ôr″bitəl/, an opening in the cranium to the orbit of the eye.

orbitale /ôrbitā′lē/ [L, *orbitalis,* pertaining to the orbit], an anthropometric landmark, the lowest point on the inferior margin of the orbit.

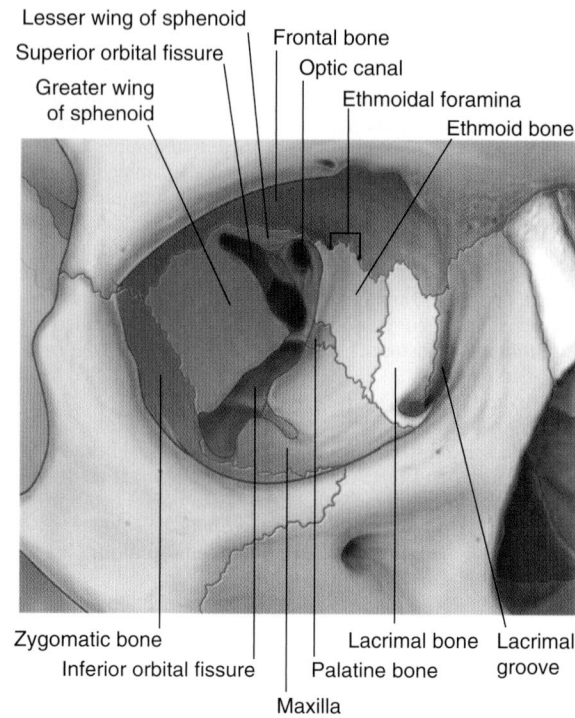

Lesser wing of sphenoid
Superior orbital fissure
Greater wing of sphenoid
Frontal bone
Optic canal
Ethmoidal foramina
Ethmoid bone
Zygomatic bone
Inferior orbital fissure
Maxilla
Palatine bone
Lacrimal bone
Lacrimal groove

. **Bones of the orbit** *(Drake, Vogl, and Mitchell, 2015)*

orbital fat, a semifluid adipose cushion that lines the bony orbit supporting the eye. Selective loss of fatty tissue caused by hormonal imbalances may produce "bulging" of the eye. Traumatic loss of the fat causes a sunken appearance of the eye. Replacement of the fat by tumor or abnormal tissue may be discovered on ophthalmological examination. The examiner gently presses on the front of the eyes through the eyelids. Normally each eye may be displaced 0.5 cm into the socket.

orbital fissure [L, *orbita,* wheel track, *fissura,* cleft], the space between the floor and lateral wall of the orbit, serving as a conduit for nerves and blood vessels.

orbital hypertelorism. See **ocular hypertelorism.**

orbital hypotelorism. See **ocular hypotelorism.**

orbital myositis, an inflammation of the external ocular muscles. The process, which is generally autoimmune, may be associated with pain, forward displacement of the eyeball, and paralysis of the ocular muscles. It can be part of orbital inflammatory syndrome.

orbital optic neuritis. See **optic neuritis.**

orbital pseudotumor, a specific inflammatory reaction of the orbital tissues of the eye, characterized by exophthalmos and edematous congestion of the eyelids.

orbitography /ôr′bitog″rəfē/, the radiographic examination of the bony cavity containing the eye.

orbitomeatal line /ôr′bitō′mē·ā″təl/ [L, *orbita,* wheel track, *meatus,* passage], (in radiology) a skull positioning line that passes through the outer canthus of the eye and the center of the external auditory meatus.

orbitopathy /orbitop′əthē/ [L, *orbita,* wheel track + Gk, *pathos,* disease], disease affecting the orbit and its contents.

Orbivirus /ôr″bivī′rəs/ [L, *orbis,* ring], a genus of the Reoviridae family of viruses that contains double-stranded ribonucleic acid. It is characterized by an outer layer of rings of capsomeres. Insects are hosts for orbiviruses. Colorado tick fever and African horse sickness are among infections caused by species of these viruses. Orbiviruses are primarily

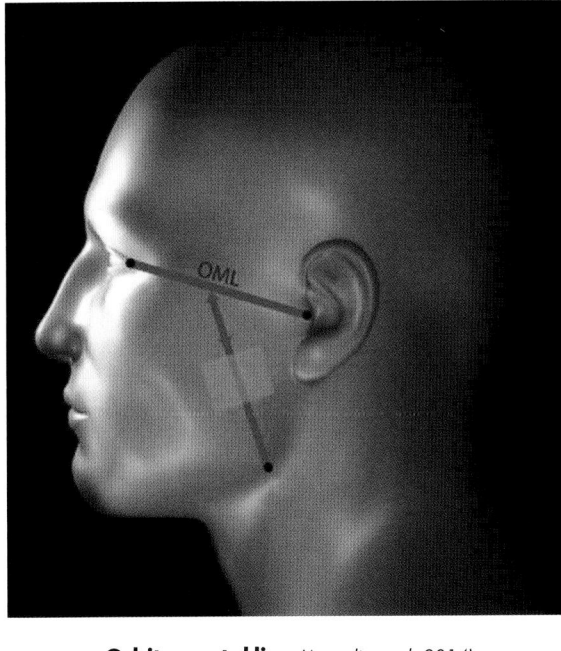

Orbitomeatal line *(Apaydin et al, 2014)*

animal pathogens; only 7 out of 100 of these are linked to clinical human disease.

orcheoplasty. See **orchioplasty.**

orchi-. See **orchio-, orchi-, orchido-.**

orchidectomy /ôr′kidek″təmē/ [Gk, *orchis,* testis, *ektomē,* excision], surgical removal of one or both testes. It may be indicated for serious disease or injury to the testis or to control cancer of the prostate by removing a source of androgenic hormones. Also called **orchiectomy.**

orchiditis. See **orchitis.**

orchido-. See **orchio-, orchi-, orchido-.**

orchidoplasty. See **orchioplasty.**

orchiectomy. See **orchidectomy.**

orchio-, orchi-, orchido-, prefix meaning "testes": *orchiopexy, orchitis.*

orchiopexy /ôr″kē·ōpek′sē/ [Gk, *orchis* + *pexis,* fixation], an operation to mobilize an undescended testis, bring it into the scrotum, and attach it so that it will not retract.

orchioplasty /ôr″kē·ōplas′tē/ [Gk, *orchis,* testis, *plassein,* to mold], a surgical procedure involving a testis. Also called **orcheoplasty, orchidoplasty.**

orchis. See **testis.**

orchitis /ôrkī″tis/ [Gk, *orchis* + *itis,* inflammation], inflammation of one or both of the testes, characterized by swelling and pain. The condition is often caused by mumps, syphilis, or tuberculosis. Symptomatic treatment includes support and elevation of the scrotum, cold packs, and analgesics. Also called **didymitis, orchiditis.**

orchitis parotidea. See **mumps orchitis.**

orciprenaline sulfate. See **metaproterenol sulfate.**

ordered pairs [L, *ordo,* series, *par,* equal], pertaining to graph coordinates in which the first number of the pair represents a distance along the *x* (horizontal) axis and the second number is plotted along the *y* (vertical) axis.

orderly /ôr″dərlē/, **1.** *n.,* an attendant who assists in the care of hospital patients. **2.** *adj.,* in order; with regular arrangements, method, or system. −*orderliness, adj.*

order of procedure, the sequence in which the required steps are taken to complete an operation, such as preparation of the patient and preparation of the cavity and restoration of a tooth.

ordinate, the vertical line in a graph along which is plotted one of the variables considered in a study, such as temperature in a time-temperature study. Compare **abscissa.**

Orem, Dorothea E. [1914-2007], author of the Self-Care Nursing Model, a nursing theory introduced in 1959. The Orem theory describes the role of the nurse in helping a person experiencing inabilities in self-care. The goal of the Orem system is to meet the patient's self-care demands until the family and/or patient is capable of providing care. The process is divided into three categories: *universal,* which consists of self-care to meet physiological and psychosocial needs; *developmental,* the self-care required when one goes through developmental stages; and *health deviation,* the self-care required when one has a deviation from a healthy status. Assessment is made of therapeutic self-care demand, the self-care agency, and self-care deficits in the areas of knowledge, skills, motivation, and orientation. There are three systems for meeting the patient's self-care deficits. They are *wholly compensatory,* in which the patient has no active role; *partly compensatory,* in which the patient and nurse have active roles; and *educative development,* in which patients can meet their need for self-care with some assistance from the nurse.

Orencia, a modified antibody, fusion protein. Brand name for **abatacept.**

Oretic, a thiazide diuretic drug. Brand name for **hydrochlorothiazide.**

-orexia, suffix meaning "(condition of the) appetite": *anorexia, pseudoanorexia, dysorexia.*

orexigenic /ôrek′sijen″ik/ [Gk, *orexis,* longing, *genein,* to produce], a substance that increases or stimulates the appetite.

oreximania /ôrek′simā″nē·ə/ [Gk, *orexis* + *mania,* madness], a condition characterized by a greatly increased appetite and excessive eating resulting from an unrealistic or exaggerated fear of becoming thin. Compare **anorexia nervosa.**

orexis /ôrek″sis/ [Gk, longing], **1.** desire; appetite. **2.** the aspect of the mind involving feeling and striving as contrasted with the intellectual aspect.

orf [AS], a contagious viral skin disease acquired from infected sheep and goats, characterized by painless vesicles that may progress to red, weeping nodules and finally to crusting and healing. Fingers, hands, wrist, and face are common sites. Treatment is not necessary because the condition is self-limited, and active infection results in immunity. Also called **contagious pustular dermatitis.**

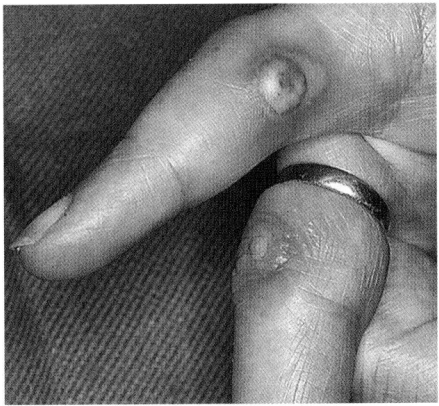

Orf *(Gawkrodger and Ardern-Jones, 2012)*

Orfadin, adjunct to dietary treatment of hereditary tyrosinemia. Brand name for **nitisinone.**

organ [Gk, *organon,* instrument], a structural part of a system of the body that is composed of tissues and cells that enable it to perform a particular function, such as the liver, spleen, digestive organs, reproductive organs, or organs of special sense. Each one of the paired organs can function independently of the other. The liver, pancreas, spleen, and brain may maintain normal or near-normal function with over 30% of the organ damaged, destroyed, or excised. Also called **organon, organum.**

organ albumin, albumin characteristic of a particular organ.

organelle /ôrgənel′/ [Gk, *organon,* instrument], **1.** any one of various specialized macromolecular structures bound within most cells, such as the mitochondria, the Golgi apparatus, the endoplastic reticulum, the lysosomes, and the centrioles. **2.** any one of the tiny structures of protozoa associated with locomotion, metabolism, and other processes. Also called *organella.*

organic /ôrgan″ik/ [Gk, *organikos*], **1.** *n.,* any chemical compound containing carbon, other than simple metal carbonate, hydrogen carbonate, or cyanides. Compare **inorganic. 2.** *adj.,* pertaining to an organ.

-organic, suffix meaning "related to the internal organs of the body."

organic brain syndrome. See **organic mental disorder.**

organic chemistry, the branch of chemistry concerned with the composition, properties, and reactions of chemical compounds containing carbon. Specifically, the study of the hydrocarbons and their derivatives.

organic disease [Gk, *organikos* + L, *dis* + Fr, *aise,* ease], any disease associated with detectable or observable changes in one or more body organs.

organic dust, dried particles of plants, animals, fungi, or bacteria that are fine enough to be wind-borne. Many kinds of organic dust cause various respiratory disorders if inhaled. See also **asthma, bagassosis, byssinosis, hay fever.**

organic dust toxic syndrome (ODTS), any nonallergic, noninfectious respiratory illness caused by inhalation of organic dust, as from moldy silage, hay, or other agricultural products. Symptoms include shaking chills or sweats, cough or shortness of breath, headache, anorexia, and myalgia. See also **farmer's lung, hypersensitivity pneumonitis.**

organic evolution, 1. the theory that all existing forms of animal and plant life have descended with modification from previous simpler forms or from a single cell. **2.** the origin and perpetuation of species.

organic foods, foods that have been produced and processed without the use of commercial chemicals such as fertilizers or pesticides or synthetic substances that enhance color or flavor. Organic foods must meet legally regulated production standards in order to use the term *organic.*

organic headache, a headache caused by any of a wide variety of intracranial disorders, including sinus or ear infections, brain tumors, and subdural hematomas. See also **headache.**

organic mental disorder (OMD), any of a *DSM-IV* class of psychiatric disorders characterized by progressive deterioration of the mental processes and caused by permanent brain damage or temporary brain dysfunction.

organic mental syndrome, former term for a constellation of psychological or behavioral signs and symptoms associated with brain dysfunction of unknown or unspecified cause and grouped according to symptoms. Designating certain conditions as having an organic basis, possibly implying that others do not, is currently discouraged. Compare **organic mental disorder.**

organic mood syndrome, a term used in a former system of classification, denoting an organic mental syndrome characterized by the presence of manic or depressive mood disturbance caused by a specific organic factor and not associated with delirium. Such disorders are now mainly classified as *substance-induced mood disorders* and *mood disorders due to a general medical condition.*

organic motivation. See **physiological motivation.**

organic murmur, an abnormal cardiac sound caused by congenital or acquired heart disease.

organic personality syndrome, a term used in a former system of classification, denoting an organic mental syndrome characterized by a marked change in behavior or personality, caused by a specific organic factor and not associated with delirium or dementia. The most common causes are space-occupying lesions of the brain, head trauma, and cerebrovascular disease. See also **organic mental syndrome.**

organic psychosis [Gk, *organikos* + *psyche,* mind, *osis,* condition], a condition characterized by a loss of contact with reality caused by an alteration in brain tissue function.

organic solvents, chemicals that dissolve other chemicals. Organic solvents are commonly encountered and affect a wide variety of systems. Organic solvents are used in the synthesis of many different types of organic compounds, including pharmaceuticals. The signs and symptoms of exposure depend on the organ involved and duration of contact.

organic vertigo [Gk, *organikos* + L, *vertigo,* dizziness], vertigo that is associated with a central nervous system disorder such as cerebellar lesions or tabes dorsalis.

organification /ôrgan′ifikā″shən/, a process in the thyroid gland whereby iodide is oxidized and incorporated into tyrosyl residues (tyrosine) of thyroglobulin. Organification is catalyzed by the enzyme thyroid peroxidase.

Organisation Mondiale de la Santé. See **World Health Organization.**

organism /ôr″gəniz′əm/ [Gk, *organon,* instrument], an entity capable of carrying on life functions. All organisms are composed of cells.

organization center /ôr′gənīzā″shən/ [Gk, *organon* + *izein,* to cause], a focal point within the developing embryo from which the organism grows and differentiates. In vertebrates this point is the chorda-mesoderm of the dorsal lip of the blastopore.

organizer /ôr″gənī′zər/ [Gk, *organon* + *izein,* to cause], (in embryology) any part of the embryo that induces morphological differentiation in some other part. Those parts that are formed and in turn give rise to other parts are classified as organizers of the second degree, third degree, and so on as the embryo develops in complexity. Kinds include **nucleolar organizer, primary organizer.**

organo-, prefix meaning "organ or organs": *organotherapy, organogenesis, organomegaly.*

organoaxial volvulus, the more common of the two types of gastric volvulus, in which the stomach twists around its longitudinal axis. This type is more common in the elderly.

organocarbamate insecticide poisoning /ôr′gənōkär″bəmāt/, an adverse reaction to pesticides derived from esters of carbonic acid. Some of these insecticides are formulated in methyl alcohol, acquiring its added toxicity. The effects are similar to those of organophosphate insecticides, but the toxicity is less, and the duration of effects is shorter. The organocarbamate insecticides rarely produce overt central nervous system effects. See also **organophosphate insecticide poisoning.**

organochlorine insecticide poisoning /-klôr″ēn/, an adverse reaction to DDT-like pesticides such as chlordane and methoxychlor. Symptoms include central nervous system disorders, convulsions, increased myocardial irritability, and depressed respiration.

organ of Corti [Gk, *organon*; Alfonso Corti, Italian anatomist, 1822–1888], the true organ of hearing, a spiral structure within the cochlea containing hair cells that are stimulated by sound vibrations. The hair cells convert the vibrations into nerve impulses that are transmitted by the cochlear part of the vestibulocochlear nerve to the brain. Also called **spiral organ of Corti.** See also **basilar membrane.**

Receptors for hearing

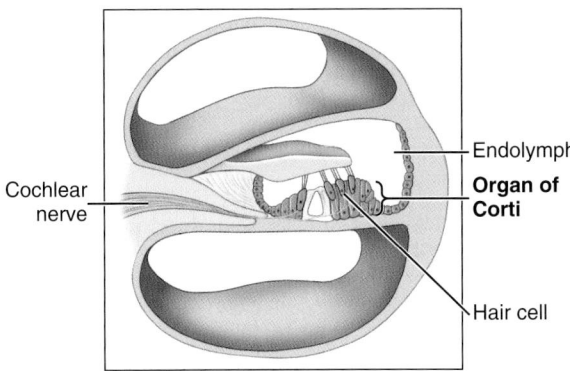

Organ of Corti *(Herlihy, 2014)*

organ of Giraldés. See **paradidymis.**

organ of Golgi. See **neurotendinous spindle.**

organogenesis /-jen″əsis/ [Gk, *organon* + *genesis*, origin], (in embryology) the formation and differentiation of organs and organ systems during embryonic development. In humans the period extends from approximately the end of the second week through the eighth week of gestation. During this time the embryo undergoes rapid growth and differentiation and is extremely vulnerable to environmental hazards and toxic substances. Any interference with the sequential processes involved with organogenesis causes an arrest in development and results in one or more congenital anomalies. Also called *organogeny.* See also **embryological development, prenatal development.** *−organogenetic, adj.*

organoid /ôr″gənoid/ [Gk, *organon* + *eidos*, form], **1.** *adj.,* resembling an organ. **2.** *n.,* any structure that resembles an organ in appearance or function, specifically an abnormal tumor mass. See also **organelle.**

organoid neoplasm, a growth that resembles a body organ. Compare **heterologous tumor.**

organoid tumor. See **teratoma.**

organomegaly /-meg″əlē/ [Gk, *organon*, instrument, *megas,* large], abnormal enlargement of an organ, particularly an organ of the abdominal cavity.

organon. See **organ.**

organophosphate, any of a class of anticholinesterase chemicals used in certain pesticides and war gases. Organophosphates act by causing irreversible inhibition of cholinesterase.

organophosphate insecticide poisoning /-fos″fāt/, an adverse reaction to organophosphate pesticides such as malathion and chlorothion, as well as nerve gas agents. Symptoms include nausea, vomiting, abdominal cramping, headache, blurred vision, and excessive salivation.

organophosphorus /or″gäno-fos″färus/, a compound containing phosphorus bound to an organic molecule. Some are used as insecticides and others are nerve gases; they are highly toxic acetylcholinesterase inhibitors.

organophosphorus compound poisoning, poisoning, often fatal, by excessive exposure to an organophosphorus compound. There are usually neurological symptoms, such as axonopathy and paralysis.

organotherapy /-ther″əpē/ [Gk, *organon* + *therapeia,* treatment], the treatment of disease by administering animal endocrine glands or their extracts. Whole glands are no longer implanted, but substances derived from animal organs are widely used. Also called *biological mRNA therapy.* *−organotherapeutic, adj.*

organotypic growth /ôr″gənōtip″ik/ [Gk, *organon* + *typos,* mark], the controlled reproduction of cells, such as that which occurs in the normal growth of tissues and organs. Compare **histiotypic growth.**

organ specificity, a term describing a substance or activity that is identified with a specific organ, commonly applied to enzymes that function in particular organ systems.

organum. See **organ.**

orgasm /ôr″gasəm/ [Gk, *orgein,* to be lustful], the sexual climax, a series of strong involuntary contractions of the muscles of the genitalia, accompanied in males by ejaculation of semen, experienced as exceedingly pleasurable, and set off by sexual excitation of critical intensity. *−orgasmic, adj.*

orgasmic maturity /ôrgas″mik/, the physiological maturity of the reproductive system that enables the individual to complete the adult sexual response cycle.

orgasmic platform [Gk, *orgein* + Fr, *plate-forme,* a flat form], congestion of the lower vagina during sexual intercourse.

orient /ôr″ē-ənt/ [L, *oriens,* rising sun], **1.** to make someone aware of new surroundings, including people and their roles; the layout of a facility; and its routines, rules, and services. New patients are oriented to a hospital, as are new staff to a hospital unit. **2.** to help a person become aware of a situation or simply of reality, such as when a patient recovers from anesthesia. *−oriented, adj., −orientation, n.*

Oriental medical practices, a term referring to ancient forms of medicine that focus on prevention and secondarily treat disease with an emphasis on maintaining balance through the body by stimulating a constant, smooth-flowing Qi energy. Herbs, acupuncture, massage, diet, and exercise are also used.

oriental sore. *(Obsolete)* Also called **Aleppo boil, Delhi boil.** See **cutaneous leishmaniasis.**

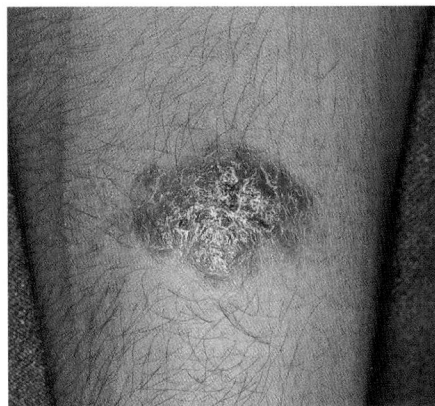

Cutaneous leishmaniasis sore *(James, Berger, and Eston, 2016)*

orientation /ôr″ē-əntā″shən/ [L, *oriens* + *itio,* process], **1.** the direction of a fragment of nucleic acid inserted into a vector. The orientation of the fragment may be the same as that of the genetic map of the vector (the *n* orientation) or opposite (the *u* orientation). **2.** the awareness of one's physical environment with regard to time, place, and the identity of other people; the ability to adapt to such an existing or new environment. Disorientation is usually a symptom of organic brain disease and most psychoses.

orientation and mobility specialist, a human services professional who specializes in helping the visually impaired and legally blind to acclimate to their physical environments.

oriented. See **orient.**

Orientia tsutsugamushi /ôr′e·enshe′ə tso͞otso͞ogəmo͞o′she/ [L, *oriens,* east; Jpn, *tsutsuga,* illness + *mushi,* tick], a species of organisms, formerly known as *Rickettsia tsutsugamushi,* that causes scrub typhus. It is widespread throughout southern and eastern Asia, northern Australia, Indonesia, and the Pacific islands and is transmitted from infected rodents to humans by mites of the family Trombiculidae.

orifice /ôr′ifis/ [L, *orificium,* opening], the entrance or outlet of any body cavity. Also called **ostium.** *–orificial, adj.*

ori gene /ôr′ē/, (in molecular genetics) the site or region in which deoxyribonucleic acid replication starts.

origin /ôr′ijin/ [L, *origo,* source], the more fixed or most proximal attachment of two points of a muscle. Compare **insertion.**

Orimune, an active immunizing agent. Brand name for **live oral poliovirus vaccine.**

Orinase, an oral sulfonylurea antidiabetic drug. Brand name for **TOLBUTamide.**

Orlando (Pelletier), Ida Jean [1926–2007], a nursing theorist who first described her nursing process theory in *The Dynamic Nurse-Patient Relationship* (1972). Her theory stresses the reciprocal relationship between the nurse and patient and the use of the nursing process to meet the patient's needs and thus alleviate distress. Three elements—patient behavior, nurse reaction, and nursing actions—comprise a nursing situation. Orlando divided actions into those that are either automatic or deliberate. Perceptions, thoughts, and feelings are not explored in automatic actions. Deliberate actions are those that may yield solutions to problems and also prevent problems. She focused on the patient's verbal and nonverbal expressions of needs. The nurse reacts to the patient's behavior by discerning both the meaning of the distress and what would alleviate the distress. Orlando's contribution as a theorist has advanced nursing from personal and automatic responses to disciplined and professional practice responses.

orlistat, a lipase inhibitor.
■ INDICATIONS: It is used to manage obesity.
■ CONTRAINDICATIONS: Malabsorption syndrome, cholestasis, and known hypersensitivity to this drug prohibit its use.
■ ADVERSE EFFECTS: Adverse effects include back pain, arthritis, myalgia, tendinitis, depression, anxiety, dizziness, headache, fatigue, nausea, vomiting, abdominal pain, infectious diarrhea, rectal pain, tooth disorder, urinary tract infection, vaginitis, menstrual irregularity, influenza, upper respiratory infection, eye-ear-nose-throat symptoms, dry skin, and rash. Common side effects include insomnia, oily spotting, flatus with discharge, fecal urgency, fatty/oily stool, oily evacuation, and fecal incontinence.

Ornish diet, a vegetarian diet containing 10% of calories from fat, 20% from protein, and 70% from carbohydrates, used in combination with stress reduction techniques and moderate exercise for the prevention and treatment of cardiovascular disease.

ornithine /ôr′nithēn/, an amino acid, not a constituent of proteins, that is produced as an important intermediate substance in the urea cycle. It is formed by the hydrolization of arginine by arginase and is subsequently converted into citrulline. It decomposes by losing carbon dioxide, producing putrescine and a strong foul odor characteristic of decaying animal tissue. Also called **diaminovaleric acid.**

ornithine carbamoyltransferase, an enzyme in the blood that increases in patients with liver and other diseases. Its normal concentration in serum is 8 to 20 mIU/mL. Also called **ornithine transcarbamoylase.**

ornithine carbamoyltransferase (OCT) deficiency, an X-linked aminoacidopathy involving the biosynthesis of urea. Most hemizygous males show complete deficiency and do not survive the neonatal period. Heterozygous females show varying degrees of deficiency and age of onset. Characteristic signs include hyperammonemia, neurological abnormalities, and orotic aciduria.

ornithine cycle. See **urea cycle.**

ornithine transcarbamoylase. See **ornithine carbamoyltransferase.**

Ornithodoros /ôr′nithod″ərəs/ [Gk, *ornis,* bird, *doros,* leather bag], a genus of ticks, some species of which are vectors for the spirochetes of relapsing fevers.

ornithosis. See **psittacosis.**

oro-, prefix meaning "mouth": *orolingual, oromaxillary, oropharynx.*

orodigitofacial dysostosis. See **oral-facial-digital (OFD) syndrome, type I; oral-facial-digital (OFD) syndrome, type II; oral-facial-digital (OFD) syndrome, type III.**

orofacial /ôr′ōfā″shəl/ [L, *os, oris,* mouth, *facies,* face], pertaining to the mouth and face.

orofaciodigital syndrome. See **oral-facial-digital (OFD) syndrome, type I, oral-facial-digital (OFD) syndrome, type II, oral-facial-digital (OFD) syndrome, type III.**

oropharyngeal dysphagia /ôr′ōfərin″jē·əl/, difficulty in either the oral or pharyngeal phases of swallowing, such as in chewing, initiating the swallow, or propelling the bolus through the pharynx to the esophagus. It is caused by multiple neurological, structural, or other medical conditions.

oropharyngeal isthmus. See **faucial isthmus.**

oropharynx /ôr′ōfer″ingks/ [L, *oris,* mouth; Gk, *pharynx,* throat], one of the three anatomical divisions of the pharynx that lies posterior to the mouth and is continuous above with the nasopharynx and below with the laryngopharynx. It extends behind the mouth from the soft palate above to the level of the hyoid bone below and contains the palatine and lingual tonsils. Compare **laryngopharynx, nasopharynx.**

orotic acid /ôrot″ik/, a pyrimidine synthesized in the cell from carboxyl phosphate and aspartic acid by means of condensation, dehydration, and oxidation.

orotic aciduria, a rare autosomal-recessive inherited disorder of pyrimidine metabolism. It includes signs and symptoms of macrocytic hypochromic anemia with megaloblastic changes in bone marrow, leukopenia, delayed growth, and urinary excretion of large amounts of orotic acid.

Oroya fever. See **bartonellosis.**

-orphan, suffix for morphine-derived opioid agonists or antagonists.

orphan disease /ôr′fən/, any rare health disorder for which no treatment has been developed. See also **orphan drug.**

orphan drug /ôr″fən/ [Gk, *orphanos,* without parents; ME, *drogge*], a term that generally refers to drugs needed to treat rare diseases but can encompass any pharmaceutic product available to physicians and patients in countries other than the United States that has not been "adopted" by a domestic pharmaceutic manufacturer or distributor. An orphan drug may not be available in the United States because total sales would not justify the expense of research and development or because the medication may be a natural substance that cannot be effectively protected by patent laws against competition from a similar form of the product. The U.S. Orphan Drug Act of 1983 offers federal financial incentives to commercial and nonprofit organizations to develop and market drugs previously unavailable in the United States for rare diseases affecting fewer than 200,000 people. The FDA assists in the process with its office of Orphan Product Development.

orphan virus [Gk, *orphanos*, without parents; L, *virus*, poison], a virus that has been isolated and identified, although it has not been associated with any particular disease.

orphenadrine citrate /ôrfen″ədrēn/, a skeletal muscle relaxant with anticholinergic and antihistaminic activity.

■ INDICATIONS: It is prescribed in the treatment of severe muscle strain.

■ CONTRAINDICATIONS: Myasthenia gravis, glaucoma or other contraindications to anticholinergic agents, or known hypersensitivity to this drug prohibits its use.

■ ADVERSE EFFECTS: Among the most serious adverse effects are those associated with anticholinergic activity, such as dry mouth and tachycardia, and allergic reactions.

-orrhagia, -rrhagia, -rrhage, suffix meaning "excessive flow": *hemorrhage, metrorrhagia.*

-orrhea, -rrhea, suffix meaning "flow" or "discharge": *galactorrhea, rhinorrhea.*

-orrhexis, -rrhexis, suffix meaning "to rupture": *acanthorrhexis, myorrhexis.*

ORS, abbreviation for **oral rehydration solutions.**

ORT, abbreviation for **oral rehydration therapy.**

orthetist. See **orthotist.**

ortho, abbreviation for **orthopedics.**

ortho- /ôr′thə-/, prefix meaning "straight, normal, correct": *orthogenesis, orthodontist, orthotopic.*

orthoboric acid. See **boric acid.**

orthochromatic /or′thō·krō·mat′ik/, denoting a photographic emulsion sensitive to all colors except red.

orthoclase ceramic feldspar /ôr″thəklās/ [Gk, *orthos,* straight, *klassis,* breaking, *keramikos,* pottery], a plentiful clay in the solid crust of the earth, used to fill space and give body to fused dental porcelain. Compare **feldspar.**

Orthoclone OKT3, an immunosuppressant drug. Brand name for **muromonab-Cd3.**

orthodontic appliance /-don″tik/ [Gk, *orthos* + *odous,* tooth], any device used to modify tooth position. Kinds include **extraoral anchorage, intraoral orthodontic appliance, retainer.**

orthodontic attachment. See **bracket.**

orthodontic band, a thin metal ring, usually made of stainless steel, that is fitted over a tooth and bonded or cemented to it for securing orthodontic attachments to the tooth. See also **adjustable orthodontic band.**

orthodontics and dentofacial orthopedics /ôr′thədon″tiks/ [Gk, *orthos* + *odous,* tooth], the specialty of dentistry concerned with the diagnosis and treatment of malocclusion and irregularities of the teeth.

orthodontic wire. See **arch wire.**

orthodontist /-don″tist/, one of the ten dental specialties. Orthodontists practice the diagnosis, prevention, and correction of malocclusion along with neuromuscular and skeletal abnormalities of the developing or mature oral structures of the teeth.

orthodromic conduction /ôr′thədrom″ik/ [Gk, *orthos* + *dromos,* course; L, *conducere,* to connect], the conduction of a neural impulse in the normal direction, from a synaptic junction or a receptor forward along an axon to its termination with depolarization. Compare **antidromic conduction.**

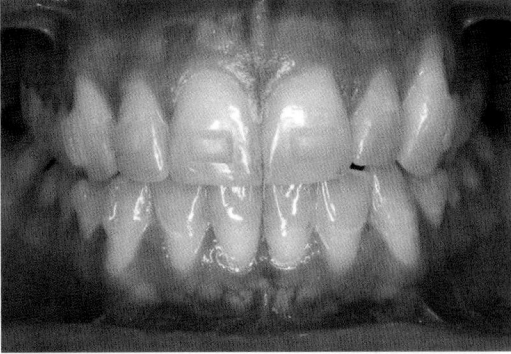
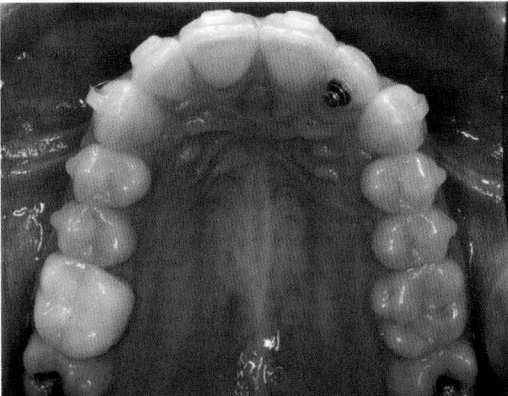
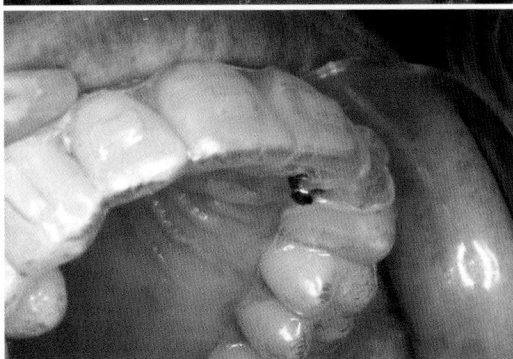

Invisalign orthodontic appliance *(Proffit, Fields, and Sarver, 2013)*

orthogenesis /ôr′thəjen″əsis/ [Gk, *orthos* + *genesis,* origin], the theory that evolution is controlled by intrinsic factors within the organism and progresses according to a predetermined course rather than in several directions as a result of natural selection and other environmental factors. −*orthogenetic, adj.*

orthogenic /-jen″ik/ [Gk, *orthos* + *genein,* to produce], **1.** pertaining to orthogenesis; orthogenetic. **2.** pertaining to the treatment and rehabilitation of children who are mentally or emotionally disturbed. See also **orthopsychiatry.**

orthogenic evolution, change within an animal or plant induced solely by an intrinsic factor and independent of any environmental elements. Also called **bathmic evolution.**

orthognathic surgery, reconstruction of the mandible, the maxilla, or both, performed to repair acquired or congenital facial defects like cleft palate. Surgery is usually not performed until the patient has enough permanent teeth to permit postoperative immobilization. Although an oral and maxillofacial surgeon performs the surgery, an ortho-dontist and sometimes a speech and language therapist are involved in the planning. Root canal surgery is a common complication.

Orthohepadnavirus /or″thohepad′nahvi″rus/, a genus of hepadnaviruses that includes the hepatitis B virus infecting humans.

orthokinetic cuff /-kinet″ik/ [Gk, *orthos,* straight, *kinesis,* movement; ME, *cuffe*], an elastic covering for a muscle that provides tactile stimulation sufficient to induce contraction and that restricts contraction of an opposing muscle.

orthokinetics /-kinet″iks/ [Gk, *orthos,* straight, *kinesis,* movement], **1.** a therapy for hypertrophic osteoarthritis in which an effort is made to change muscular action from one group to another to protect a joint. **2.** a therapy for spasticity that uses an orthotic device to enable contraction of one muscle while inhibiting its antagonist. **3.** the movement of microscopic particles in the same direction during sedimentation as a result of the effect of gravity on Brownian motion.

orthologous genes /ôrthol″əgəs/, genes in different species that are similar in their nucleotide sequences, suggesting that they originated from a common ancestral gene.

orthomolecular medicine, a system for the prevention and treatment of disease based on the theory that each person's biochemical environment is genetically determined and specific to the individual. Therapy is provided by supplementation with substances naturally present in the body, such as vitamins, minerals, trace elements, and amino acids, in amounts that are optimized for each individual to correct nutritional deficiencies and the resulting biochemical abnormalities.

orthomyxovirus /ôr′thəmik′sōvī″rəs/ [Gk, *orthos* + *mykes,* fungus; L, *virus,* poison], a member of a family of viruses that includes several organisms responsible for human influenza infection.

Ortho-Novum, oral contraceptives containing a progestin and an estrogen. Brand name for *norethindrone acetate,* **ethinyl estradiol, mestranol.**

orthopaedics. See **orthopedics.**

orthopantogram /ôr′thəpan′təgram/ [Gk, *orthos* + *pan,* all, *gramma,* record], a radiograph that is taken extraorally and shows a panoramic view of the entire dentition, alveolar bone, structure of the maxilla and mandible, and other adjacent structures on a single image.

orthopedic nurse /-pē″dik/ [Gk, *orthos* + *pais,* child], a nurse whose primary area of interest, competence, and professional practice is concerned with the prevention and correction of disorders of the locomotor system, including the skeleton, muscles, joints, and related tissues.

orthopedic oxford, a hard leather shoe with a leather or rubber sole, sometimes with a steel shank between the floor of the shoe and the sole, and with firmly constructed sides that support the foot in an upright position. The shoe is constructed so that assistive devices can be added. It is used to relieve pain and improve function in foot disabilities.

orthopedics /-pē″diks/ [Gk, *orthos,* straight, *pais,* child], a branch of health care that is concerned with the prevention and correction of disorders of the musculoskeletal system of the body. Also spelled **orthopaedics.**

orthopedic surgery [Gk, *orthos,* straight, *pais,* child, *cheirourgia,* surgery], the branch of medicine that is concerned with the treatment of the musculoskeletal system, including the skeleton, muscles, joints, and related tissues, mainly by manipulative and operative methods.

orthopedic traction, a procedure in which a patient is maintained in a device attached by ropes and pulleys to weights that pull on an extremity or body part while countertraction

is maintained. Traction is applied most often to reduce and immobilize fractures, but it also is used to overcome muscle spasm, stretch adhesions, correct certain deformities, and help release arthritic contractures. Side arm traction is a kind of skin traction used to align a fractured humerus after open reduction. Skeletal traction is exerted directly on a bone by means of a wire or pin inserted under anesthesia during the open reduction of a fracture; the ends of the pin protruding through the skin on both sides of the bone are sometimes covered with corks and are attached to a metal U-shaped spreader or bow, which in turn is attached to the traction rope. Skin or skeletal traction applied to a lower extremity by a balanced suspension apparatus, such as the Thomas splint and Pearson's attachment, permits the patient to move more freely in bed. The leg is balanced with countertraction, and any slack in traction caused by the patient's movements is taken up by the suspension apparatus. Bryant's traction, for treating fractures of the femur shaft in young children, uses a suspension apparatus to hold the legs at right angles to the body. A girdle that fits over the iliac crests and pelvis is used to apply traction for the relief of low back pain, and a cervical halter is used in applying traction to reduce neck pain. Cervical traction also may be used when a fracture of the cervical spine is suspected. Traction may be applied directly to the skin if the rope-pulley-weight system is attached to bands of adhesive, moleskin, or foam rubber or to a splint affixed to the affected limb.

■ METHOD: To maintain the required constant pull, the traction ropes are kept taut, free to ride over the pulleys, and securely tied to the weights, which must hang free—away from the bed and off the floor. Countertraction is maintained by elevating the patient's bed under the body part to which traction is applied. A chest restraint sheet may be applied to the patient in side arm traction for countertraction if necessary. During the initial stages of traction, the involved extremity is checked every 2 hours for quality of the distal pulse, color, warmth, motion, sensation, pain, and swelling. Blood pressure, temperature, pulse, and respirations are recorded every 4 hours until stable. Pain is controlled, and the patient is positioned as ordered. If the patient is in balanced suspension, abduction of the leg and a 20-degree angle between the thigh and bed are maintained; the heel is kept free of the sling under the calf. A harness restraint is used to prevent a child in Bryant's traction from turning over, and the child's buttocks are raised slightly from the mattress. Bed linen is changed only as necessary, and an air mattress is used when required. Every 2 hours the patient is helped with deep breathing and coughing exercises. Bony prominences are massaged, but vigorous rubbing is avoided. Lotion is applied to the skin, which is periodically inspected for signs of redness, abrasions, blisters, dryness, itching, excoriation, and pressure areas. For patients in skeletal traction, the pin insertion sites are inspected for signs of infection. The patient is observed every 4 hours for neurological signs, such as tingling, numbness, and loss of sensation or motion; for thrombophlebitis in the involved extremity; and for evidence of a pulmonary blood clot or fat embolus, as indicated by decreased breath sounds, fever, tachypnea, diaphoresis, anxiety, pallor, bloody or purulent sputum, tachycardia, or acute, severe chest pain. Oral hygiene is administered every 4 hours, and, unless contraindicated, a daily intake of 2 to 3 L of fluids is encouraged. As the patient's condition improves, his or her position is changed every 4 hours; if the kind of traction permits and if the upper extremities are not involved, a trapeze is added to the bed. The patient is taught to perform range-of-motion exercises with the uninvolved extremities, dorsiflexion and plantar flexion of the ankles, and isometric exercises, such as gluteal and abdominal contraction. A high-protein, low-carbohydrate diet is served, and vitamin and iron therapy may be ordered. The immobilized patient uses a flat, fracture bedpan and usually requires stool softeners or a mild laxative.

■ INTERVENTIONS: The patient in traction often needs extensive physical care and emotional support. The patient is encouraged to verbalize feelings and concerns about prolonged hospitalization and absence from work or school. To the greatest degree possible, the nurse encourages the patient to participate in self-care and to engage in diversions, such as handicrafts, reading, watching television, and listening to the radio. If the patient is not allowed to elevate to the head of the bed, specialized glasses called prism glasses aid in the ability to watch television.

■ OUTCOME CRITERIA: Diligent attention and nursing care are necessary to prevent pressure ulcers, infection, constipation, kidney stones, and other sequelae of immobility.

orthopedist /-pē″dist/, a physician with additional training as an orthopedic surgeon who specializes in the assessment and correction of conditions of the musculoskeletal system, which includes the skeleton, muscles, joints, and related tissues. Also called **orthopod.**

orthopnea /ôrthop″nē·ə/ [Gk, *orthos* + *pnoia,* breath], an abnormal condition in which a person must sit or stand to breathe deeply or comfortably. It occurs in many disorders of the cardiac and respiratory systems, such as asthma, pulmonary edema, emphysema, pneumonia, congestive heart failure, and angina pectoris. Assessment includes noting the number of pillows used by the patient. Patients with orthopnea also report sleeping in recliners. Also spelled *orthopnoea.* See also **dyspnea.** *−orthopneic, adj.*

orthopneic position /ôr′thopnē″ik/ [Gk, *orthos,* straight, *pnoia,* breath; L, *positio*], a body position that enables a patient to breathe comfortably. Usually it is one in which the patient is sitting up and bent forward with the arms supported on a table or chair arms. Also called *orthopnea posture.*

orthopod. See **orthopedist.**

orthopoxvirus /or′thopoksvi″rus/, any member of a genus of poxviruses, including the viruses that cause human smallpox and vaccinia.

orthopsychiatry /-sīkī″ətrē/ [Gk, *orthos* + *psyche,* mind, *iatreia,* treatment], the branch of psychiatry that specializes in correcting incipient and borderline mental and behavioral disorders, especially in children, and in developing preventive techniques to promote mental health and emotional growth and development. It involves a collaborative approach from psychology, psychiatry, and psychiatric social work. See also **mental hygiene.**

orthoptic /ôrthop″tik/ [Gk, *orthos* + *ops,* eye], **1.** pertaining to normal binocular vision. **2.** pertaining to a procedure or technique for correcting the visual axes of eyes improperly coordinated for binocular vision.

orthoptic examination, an ophthalmoscopic examination of the binocular function of the eyes, typically performed by an orthoptist. A stereoscopic instrument presents a slightly different picture to each eye. The examiner notes the degree to which the pictures are combined by the normal process of fusion. If the person has diplopia, separate pictures are seen. If the person has suppression amblyopia, only one picture is seen. Vision training may improve binocular vision in some conditions.

orthoptic training [Gk, *orthos,* straight; *ops,* eye; ME, *trainen*], a type of therapy for correction of squint or other ocular muscle disorders by the use of eye exercises.

orthoptist /ôrthop″tist/ [Gk, *orthos* + *ops,* eye], an allied health professional qualified by postsecondary training and successful completion of an examination by the American Orthoptist Council who, under the supervision of an ophthalmologist, tests

eye muscles and teaches exercise programs designed to correct eye coordination defects.

orthorexia, obsessive behavior associated with the pursuit of a healthful diet.

orthoroentgenography /ôr′thōrent′gənog″rəfē/, a radiographic method for measuring disparity of limb length. Three separate radiographs are made of the hip, knee, and ankle (for the leg) or the shoulder, elbow, and wrist (for the arm) to produce an image of the whole limb.

orthoscopy /ôrthos″kəpē/ [Gk, *orthos,* straight, *skopein,* to view], the use of an orthoscope for examining the fundus of the eye.

orthosis /ôrthō″sis/ [Gk, *orthos,* straight], an externally applied device designed to control, correct, or compensate for a deformity, deforming forces, or impaired function. Orthosis often involves the use of special braces. Formerly called **splint. −orthotic,** *adj., n.*

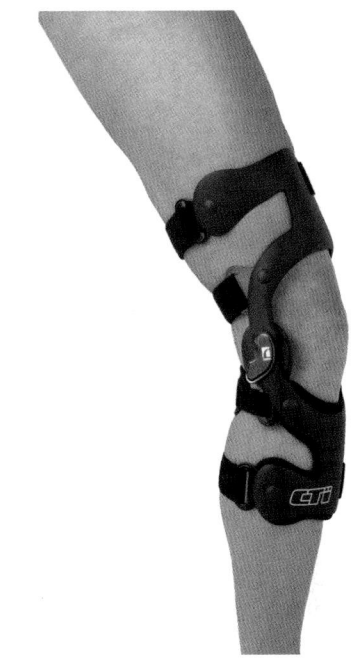

Knee orthosis *(Courtesy Truform Orthotics and Prosthetics)*

orthostasis /-stā″sis/, a normal physiological response of the sympathetic system to counteract a fall in blood pressure when a person who is lying down assumes the upright position.

orthostatic /-stat″ik/ [Gk, *orthos* + *statikos,* standing], pertaining to an erect or standing position.

orthostatic albuminuria. See **orthostatic proteinuria.**

orthostatic hypotension, a fall in systolic blood pressure >20 mm Hg or in diastolic blood pressure >10 mm Hg within 3 minutes of standing. It can produce dizziness and fainting. Also called **postural hypotension.**

orthostatic intolerance, an abnormal response to standing upright that results from decreased blood pressure and inadequate blood flow to the brain, characterized by a variety of symptoms, including light-headedness, palpitations, tremulousness, visual disturbances, and syncope. It occurs in both acute and chronic forms and is frequently seen as a transient condition in space travelers returning from microgravity. The cause is unknown but may be related to abnormalities in the autonomic regulation of cardiovascular function.

orthostatic proteinuria, presence of protein in the urine, especially in teenagers who have been standing for a long period. It disappears when they recline and is of no pathological significance. Also called **orthostatic albuminuria, postural albuminuria, postural proteinuria.**

orthotic /ôrthot″ik/ [Gk, *orthos,* straight], pertaining to orthosis. See also **orthosis.**

orthotics /ôrthot″iks/ [Gk, *orthos,* straight], the design and use of external appliances to support a paralyzed muscle, promote a specific motion, or correct a musculoskeletal deformity.

orthotist /ôr″thətist/ [Gk, *orthos,* straight], a person who designs, fabricates, and fits braces or other orthopedic appliances prescribed by physicians. A certified orthotist is one who passed the examination of the American Orthotist and Prosthetic Association. Also spelled **orthetist.**

orthotonos /ôrthot″ənəs/ [Gk, *orthos* + *tonos,* tension], a straight, rigid posture of the body caused by physiological tetanus, resulting from strychnine poisoning or tetanus infection. The neck and all other parts of the body are in a position of extension but not as severely as in opisthotonos. Compare **emprosthotonos.**

orthotopic liver transplantation [Gk, *orthos,* straight, *topos,* place], a graft of donor liver tissue placed in the same anatomical location as the original, removed organ in the recipient.

orthotopic neobladder, a urinary reservoir fashioned from a bowel segment that is in the normal anatomical position of the bladder and attached directly to the urethra, with discharge of urine through the urethra.

orthotopic ureterocele, a ureterocele occurring in a ureter in the proper position in the trigone of the bladder. It may be small and asymptomatic or large and extending deeply into the bladder.

orthovoltage /-vōl″tij/ [Gk, *orthos,* straight; Count Alessandro Volta], the energy range of 100 to 350 kiloelectron volts supplied by some x-ray generators used for radiation therapy. Such generators have largely been replaced by equipment that operates in the megaelectron volt range. See also **volt.**

Ortolani sign /ôr″təlä″nē/ [Marius Ortolani, 20th-century Italian surgeon], a click heard in a test for a congenital dislocated hip. It is noted in infancy when the hip slips into or out of the socket. Also called *Ortolani click.*

Ortolani test [Marius Ortolani; L, *testum,* crucible], a procedure used to evaluate the stability of the hip joints in newborns and infants. The baby is placed on his or her back, and the hips and knees are flexed at right angles and abducted until the lateral aspects of the knees are touching the table. The examiner's fingers are extended along the outside of the thighs, with the thumbs grasping the insides of the knees. Internal and external rotation are attempted, and symmetry of mobility is evaluated. A click or a popping sensation (Ortolani's sign) may be felt if the joint is unstable, caused by the head of the femur moving out of the acetabulum under pressure from the examiner's hands during rotation and abduction. See also **congenital dislocation of the hip.**

Orudis, a nonsteroidal antiinflammatory agent. Brand name for **ketoprofen.**

-ory, suffix meaning "pertaining to, function of, process of": *sensory.*

os. See **bone.**

Os, symbol for the element **osmium.**

OS, **1.** a notation for a Latin phrase meaning "left eye." Abbreviation for *oculus sinister.* **2.** initialism for *computer operating system.*

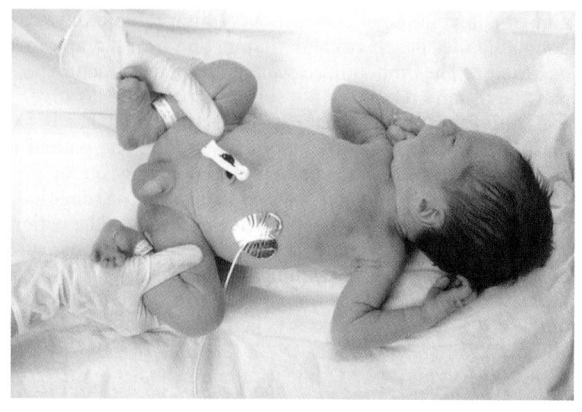

Ortolani test *(McKinney et al, 2013)*

Osborne and Cotterill procedure, the surgical correction of a chronic dislocated elbow by means of capsular reefing, the folding in or overlapping of soft tissue followed by surgical suture to make the joint tighter.

Osborn wave, an abnormal upward deflection in the electrocardiogram (ECG) occurring at the junction of the QRS complex and the S-T segment. It is often found in ECGs of patients with moderate hypothermia and becomes more pronounced as body temperature declines. Also called **J wave.**

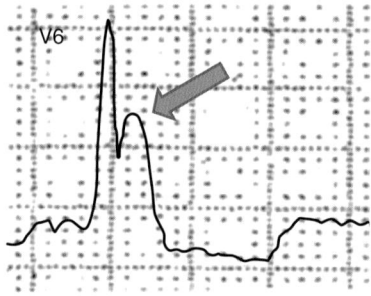

Osborn wave *(Chhabra and Spodick, 2013)*

osc, **1.** abbreviation for **oscillator. 2.** abbreviation for **oscilloscope.**

os calcis. See **calcaneum, calcaneus.**

os capitatum. See **capitate bone.**

oscheitis /os″kē-ī″tis/, an inflammation of the scrotum.

oscheo-, prefix meaning "scrotum": *oscheocele.*

oscheocele, swelling of the scrotum.

oscillation /os′ilā″shən/ [L, *oscillare,* to swing], **1.** a back-and-forth motion. **2.** vibration or the effects of a mechanical or electric vibrator.

oscillator (osc) /os″ilā′tər/ [L, *oscillare,* to swing], an electric or other device that produces oscillations, vibrations, or fluctuations, such as an alternating electric current generator.

oscillopsia /os′silop″sē-ə/, abnormal jerky eye movements that are commonly associated with multiple sclerosis but can also result from head injury. They create a subjective sensation that the environment is oscillating.

oscilloscope (osc) /osil″əskōp/ [L, *oscillare,* to swing; Gk, *skopein,* to look], an instrument that displays a visual representation of electric variations on the fluorescent screen of a cathode ray tube. The graphic representation is produced by a beam of electrons on the screen. The beam is focused or directed by a magnetic field that is influenced in turn by a source such as an amplified current produced by heart contractions. As used in cardiology, the oscilloscope can function as a continuous electrocardiogram.

os coxae. See **innominate bone.**

os cuboideum. See **cuboid bone.**

-ose, **1.** suffix meaning "a carbohydrate": *cellulose, lactose, sucrose.* **2.** suffix meaning "a primary product of hydrolysis."

oseltamivir, an antiviral drug.

■ INDICATIONS: It is used to treat type A influenza.

■ CONTRAINDICATIONS: Known hypersensitivity to this drug prohibits its use.

■ ADVERSE EFFECTS: Adverse effects include fatigue, diarrhea, abdominal pain, and cough. Common side effects include headache, dizziness, insomnia, nausea, and vomiting.

Osgood osteotomy /oz″go͞od/, a surgical procedure for correcting the malrotation of a femur.

Osgood-Schlatter disease /-shlat″ər/ [Robert B. Osgood, American surgeon, 1873–1956; Carl Schlatter, Swiss surgeon, 1864–1934], inflammation or partial separation of the tibial tubercle caused by chronic irritation, usually as a result of overuse of the quadriceps muscle. The condition is seen primarily in muscular, athletic adolescent boys and is characterized by swelling and tenderness over the tibial tubercle that increase with exercise or any activity that extends the leg. Treatment consists primarily of antiinflammatory medications and exercises to stretch the thigh's quadriceps. A patellar tendon strap may also be of value. Also called *Osgood's disease,* **Schlatter-Osgood disease, Schlatter's disease.**

OSHA /ō″shä/, the U.S. federal agency that regulates worker safety. Acronym for *Occupational Safety and Health Administration.*

os hamatum. See **hamate bone.**

os hyoideum. See **hyoid bone.**

-osis, **1.** suffix meaning "a (specified) action, process, or result": *narcosis, zygosis.* **2.** suffix meaning "increase in a pathological condition": *psittacosis, varicosis.*

OSL dosimeter, abbreviation for **optically stimulated luminescence dosimeter.**

Osler disease. See **Osler-Weber-Rendu syndrome, polycythemia.**

Osler nodes /ōs″lər/ [William Osler, American-British physician, 1849–1919], tender reddish or purplish subcutaneous nodules of the soft tissue on the ends of fingers or toes, seen in subacute bacterial endocarditis and usually lasting only 1 or 2 days. The nodes represent bacterial embolisms from the infected heart valve.

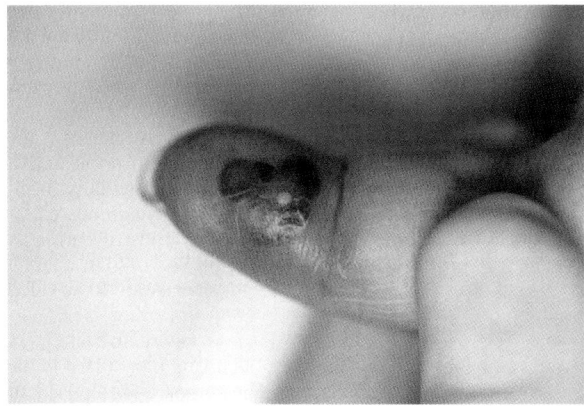

Osler nodes *(Nguyen and Maartens, 2004)*

Osler-Weber-Rendu syndrome /ōs″lər web″ər randōō″/ [William Osler; Frederick P. Weber, British physician, 1863–1962; Henri J.L.M. Rendu, French physician, 1844–1902]. See **hereditary hemorrhagic telangiectasia.**

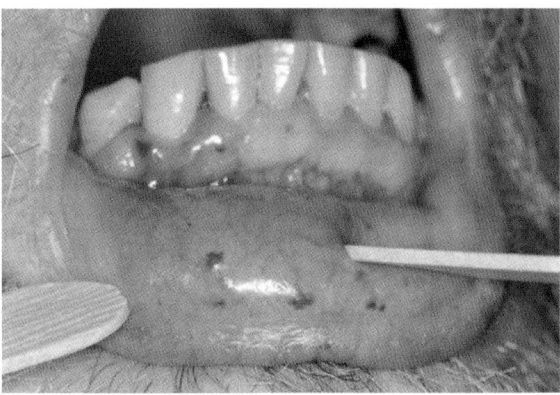

Small telangiectatic lesions on the lip and gingiva associated with Osler-Weber-Rendu syndrome
(Haarmann et al, 2007)

os lunatum. See **lunate bone.**

osm, **1.** abbreviation for **osmosis.** **2.** abbreviation for *osmotic.*

os magnum. See **capitate bone.**

osmesthesia /os′məthē″zhə/ [Gk, *osme,* odor, *aisthesis,* feeling], the ability to perceive and distinguish odors; the sense of smell.

-osmia, suffix meaning "(condition of the) sense of smell": *autosmia, hyperosmia, parosmia.*

osmium (Os) /oz″mē-əm/ [Gk, *osme,* odor], a hard, grayish, pungent-smelling metallic element. Its atomic number is 76; its atomic mass is 190.2. Used to produce alloys of extreme hardness, it is highly toxic and is slowly converted to the highly volatile, pungent-smelling, extremely toxic osmium tetroxide (OsO_4) in air.

osmo-, **1.** prefix meaning "odor": *osmology, osmometer.* **2.** prefix meaning "impulse" or "osmosis": *osmoceptors, osmolality, osmoregulation.*

osmoceptors /oz″mōsep″tərz/ [Gk, *osme* + L, *recipere,* to receive], receptors in the anterior hypothalamus that respond to osmotic pressure, thereby regulating thirst and production of the antidiuretic hormone.

osmol, osmolal. See **osmole.**

osmolal gap /ozmōl″əl/, a difference between the observed and calculated osmolalities in serum analysis. The calculated osmolar values include sodium concentration multiplied by 2, plus glucose and blood urea nitrogen.

osmolality /oz′mōlal″itē/, the osmotic pressure of a solution expressed in osmols or milliosmols per kilogram of water. Normal adult blood osmolality is 285 to 295 mOsm/kg H_2O. Compare **osmolarity.**

osmolal solution, the solute concentration expressed in the number of osmoles per kilogram of solvent.

osmolar /osmō″lər/, pertaining to the osmotic characteristics of a solution of one or more molecular substances, ionic substances, or both, expressed in osmoles or milliosmoles.

osmolarity /oz′mōler″itē/, the osmotic pressure of a solution expressed in osmoles or milliosmoles per liter of the solution. Compare **osmolality.**

osmolar solution, the solute concentration expressed in the number of osmoles per liter of solution.

osmole /os″mōl/ [Gk, *osmos,* impulse, *osis,* condition + mole (molecule)], *adj.,* the quantity of a substance in solution in the form of molecules, ions, or both (usually expressed in grams) that has the same osmotic pressure as one mole of an ideal nonelectrolyte. Also spelled *osmol.* −*osmolal, adj.*

osmology /ozmol″əjē/ [Gk, *osme,* odor, *ōsmos,* impulse, *logos,* science], **1.** the science of the sense of smell and the production and composition of odors. **2.** the branch of science that is concerned with osmosis.

osmometer /ozmom′ə·tər/ [Gk, *ōsmos,* impulse + *metron,* measure], **1.** a device for measuring the acuity of the sense of smell. **2.** a device for measuring osmotic pressure either directly or indirectly. It was formerly used to assess the extent of dehydration or blood loss.

osmometry /ozmom″ətrē/ [Gk, *ōsmos,* impulse, *metron,* measure], the field of study that deals with the phenomenon of osmosis and the measurement of osmotic forces. −*osmometric, adj.*

Osmone-Clarke procedure, a surgical method for correcting splayfoot. It involves soft tissue release of the medial and lateral foot with peroneus brevis tendon transfer.

osmoreceptor /-risep″tər/ [Gk, *ōsmos,* impulse; L, *recipere,* to receive], **1.** a neuron in the hypothalamus that is sensitive to the relative fluid/solute concentration in the blood plasma and that regulates the secretion of antidiuretic hormone. **2.** a receptor of smell stimuli.

osmoreceptor cell, a cell that recognizes changes in extracellular fluid osmolality.

osmoregulation /-reg′yəlā″shən/ [Gk, *ōsmos,* impulse; L, *regula,* rule], the act of influencing or controlling the speed and extent of osmosis.

osmosis (osm) /ozmō″sis, os-/ [Gk, *ōsmos,* impulse, *osis,* condition], the movement of a pure solvent such as water through a differentially permeable membrane from a solution that has a lower solute concentration to one that has a higher solute concentration. The membrane is impermeable to the solute but is permeable to the solvent. The rate of osmosis depends on the concentration of solute, the temperature of the solution, the electrical charge of the solute, and the difference between the osmotic pressures exerted by the solutions. Movement across the membrane continues until the concentrations of the solutions equalize. −*osmotic (osm), adj.*

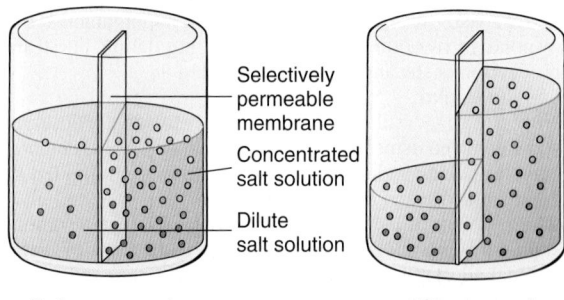

Osmosis *(Rothrock, 2015)*

osmotic diarrhea, a form of diarrhea associated with water retention in the bowel resulting from an accumulation of nonabsorbable water-soluble substances. An excessive intake of hexitols, sorbitol, and mannitol (used as sugar substitutes in candies, chewing gum, and dietetic foods) can result in slow absorption and rapid small intestine motility, leading to osmotic diarrhea. It may also occur in infants if they intake an undiluted concentrated form of formula. The severity of the condition varies directly with the amount of such sugar substitutes consumed and diminishes when intake is reduced. Also called *chewing gum diarrhea,* **dietetic food diarrhea.**

osmotic diuresis, diuresis resulting from the presence of certain nonabsorbable substances in tubules of the kidney, such as mannitol, urea, or glucose.

osmotic fragility, an assay in which whole blood is pipetted to each of a series of saline solutions of graduated concentration. The series begins with water and increases in concentration to normal (0.85%) saline. The osmotic fragility test is used to detect spherocytosis because spherocytes rupture (lyse) in saline concentrations near the normal level. The assay also detects target cells, which, owing to their reduced hemoglobin content, are able to withstand osmotic stress and rupture only at very dilute saline concentrations. Also called *erythrocyte fragility.*

osmotic pressure, the pressure exerted on a differentially permeable membrane by a solution containing one or more solutes that cannot penetrate the membrane, which is permeable only by the solvent surrounding it. See also **osmosis.**

osmotic transfection, a method of inserting foreign deoxyribonucleic acid (DNA) molecules into cells by putting cells into a dilute solution that causes them to rupture. The cell membranes quickly repair themselves without irreversible injury to the cells. During the rupture period the alien DNA is added to the fluid and is absorbed into the cell nuclei. The foreign DNA can be detected in the cells as a transfection marker.

os naviculare pedis. See **scaphoid bone.**

osphresis /osfrē″sis/ [Gk, smell], olfaction; the sense of smell.

oss-, prefix meaning "bone": *osseous, ossicle, ossification.*

osseointegrated implant /os′ē·ō·in′tegrātəd/ [Gk, *osteon,* bone; L, *integrare,* to make whole], an endosteal implant containing pores into which osteoblasts and supporting connective tissue can migrate, made of metallic, ceramic, or polymeric materials. Also called *osteointegrated implant.*

osseous /os″ē·əs/ [L, *os,* bone], bony; consisting of or resembling bone.

osseous labyrinth [L, *os,* bone; Gk, *labyrinthos,* maze], the bony part of the internal ear, which transmits sound vibrations from the middle ear to the eighth cranial nerve. It is composed of three cavities: the vestibule, the semicircular canals, and the cochlea, all of which contain perilymph, in which a membranous labyrinth is suspended. Also called **labyrinthus osseus.** Compare **membranous labyrinth.**

ossicle /os″ikəl/ [L, *ossiculum,* little bone], a small bone such as the malleus, the incus, or the stapes, all of which are ossicles of the middle ear. −*ossicular, adj.*

ossiferous /osif″ərəs/ [L, *os,* bone, *ferre,* to bear], pertaining to the formation of bone or bone tissue.

ossification /os′ifikā″shən/ [L, *os + facere,* to make], the development of bone. Intramembranous ossification is that preceded by membrane, such as in the process initially forming the roof and sides of the skull. Intracartilaginous endochondral ossification is that preceded by rods of cartilage, such as that forming the bones of the limbs.

ossify /os″ifī/ [L, *os,* bone, *facere,* to make], to develop into bone.

ossifying fibroma /os″ifī′ing/ [L, *os + facere,* to make], a slow-growing, benign neoplasm, occurring most often in the jaws, especially the mandible. The tumor is composed of bone that develops within fibrous connective tissue.

oste-. See **osteo-, oste-.**

Ossification *(McCance and Huether, 2014)*

ostealgia /os′tē·al″jə/ [Gk, *osteon,* bone, *algos,* pain], any pain that is associated with an abnormal condition within a bone, such as osteomyelitis. −*ostealgic, adj.*

osteanagenesis. See **osteoanagenesis.**

osteitis /os′tē·ī″tis/ [Gk, *osteon + itis,* inflammation], an inflammation of bone caused by infection, degeneration, or trauma. Symptoms include swelling; tenderness; dull, aching pain; and redness in the skin over the affected bone. Kinds include **osteitis deformans, osteitis fibrosa cystica.** See also **osteomyelitis, Paget disease.**

osteitis deformans. See **Paget disease.**

osteitis fibrosa cystica, an inflammatory degenerative condition in which normal bone is replaced by cysts and fibrous tissue. It is usually associated with hyperparathyroidism.

osteitis fibrosa disseminata. See **Albright syndrome.**

ostembryon. See **lithopedion.**

ostemia /ostē″mē·ə/, an abnormal congestion of blood in a bone.

ostempyesis /os′təmpī·ē″sis/, an accumulation of pus within a bone.

osteo /os″tē·ō/, **1.** abbreviation for **osteopath. 2.** abbreviation for **osteopathy. 3.** pertaining to bone osteology, the study of bones.

osteo-, oste-, prefix meaning "bone": *osteoblast, osteoclastoma, osteopathy.*

osteoanagenesis /os′tē·ō·an′ə·jen″ə·sis/ [Gk, *osteon + ana,* again, *genesis,* origin], the regeneration or formation of bone tissue. Also called **osteanagenesis.**

osteoaneurysm /-an″yəriz′əm/, a dilation of the wall of a blood vessel within a bone.

osteoarthritis /os′tē·ō′ärthrī″tis/ [Gk, *osteon + arthron,* joint, *itis,* inflammation], a form of arthritis in which one or many joints undergo degenerative changes, including subchondral bony sclerosis, loss of articular cartilage, and proliferation of bone spurs (osteophytes) and cartilage in the joint. Inflammation of the synovial membrane of the joint is common late in the disease. Osteoarthritis is the most common form of arthritis. Its cause is unknown but may include chemical, mechanical, genetic, metabolic, and endocrine factors. Emotional stress often aggravates the condition. The disease usually begins with pain after exercise or use of the joint. Stiffness, tenderness to the touch, crepitus, and enlargement develop. Deformity, incomplete dislocation, and synovial effusion may eventually occur. Involvement of the hip, knee, or spine causes more disability than osteoarthritis of other areas. Treatment includes rest of the involved joints; use of a cane, a walker, or crutches to decrease weight-bearing; heat; and antiinflammatory drugs. Overweight patients may be advised to lose weight. Systemic corticosteroids are contraindicated, but intraarticular injections of corticosteroids may give relief. Surgical treatment is sometimes necessary and may reduce pain and greatly improve the function of a joint. Hip replacement, joint debridement, fusion, and decompression laminectomy are some of the surgical procedures used in treating advanced osteoarthritis. Also called **degenerative joint disease.** Compare **rheumatoid arthritis.**

■ OBSERVATIONS: Early symptoms include deep, aching joint pain that is aggravated by exercise and that worsens as the day progresses. Inactivity contributes to stiffness. Midcourse of the disease is marked by reduced joint motion, tenderness, crepitus, grating sensation, flexion contractures, and joint enlargement. Manifestations late in the disease include tenderness on palpation, pain with passive ROM, increase in degree and duration of pain, joint deformity, and subluxation. Diagnosis is made by using clinical exam, with presence of usual manifestations plus possible Heberden or Bouchard nodes of the finger joints. Gait analysis may reveal altered motion patterns. Radiology may reveal narrowed joint space, increased density of subchondral bone, pseudocysts in subchondral marrow, and/or osteophytes at joint periphery. Analysis of synovial fluid typically shows high-viscosity fluid that is yellow or transparent in color. Cultures of fluid are negative; WBC count is 200 to 2000/μL, with less than 25 polymorphonuclear leukocytes. Osteoarthritis of the spine can cause compression of the spinal cord, leading to weakness in the extremities, incontinence of bowel and bladder, and impotence.

■ INTERVENTIONS: Treatment is aimed at pain reduction, slowing the degenerative process, and increasing joint mobility. Oral analgesics are used for pain; NSAIDs are used for inflammation; muscle relaxants and intraarticular steroid injections provide some transient relief.

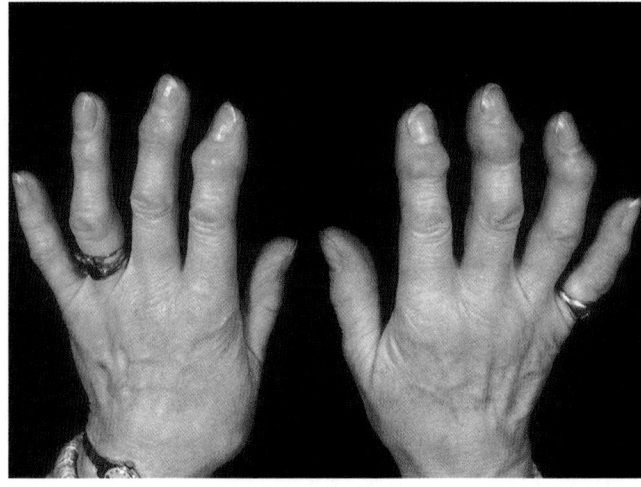

Bouchard nodes in proximal interphalangeal joints with osteoarthritis
(Waldman, 2012)

Topical agents (capsaicin) may provide temporary pain relief. Dietary supplements glucosamine and chondroitin sulfate are used for pain relief and improvement in joint mobility. Arthroscopy, osteotomy, laminectomy, fusion, or total joint replacement may be considered if conservative therapy fails.

■ PATIENT CARE CONSIDERATIONS: Goals of the health care team include pain management, maintenance of joint function, increasing activity tolerance, and maintaining independence in self-care activities. Pain management makes use of a combination of pharmacological (analgesics, muscle relaxants, and steroids) and nonpharmacological (moist heat, massage, and rest) methods. Joint function is maintained by a judicious balance of rest and activity and use of a regular exercise program (isometric, isotonic, isokinetic, strengthening, stretching, ROM, and balance exercises). Joint protection measures, such as losing weight to reduce joint load, using assistive devices to aid mobility, avoiding forceful or repetitive movement, using good body mechanics and erect posture, and developing pacing techniques for daily routines can improve activity tolerance. Joint stability can be enhanced by actions such as avoiding soft chairs, using recliners, and placing pillows under knees; wearing sturdy, low-heeled shoes; removing environmental hazards; and using mobility aids and joint support devices. Decreasing pain and increasing joint flexibility lead to a prolonged ability to perform activities of daily living.

osteoarthritis deformans endemica. See **Kashin-Bek disease.**

osteoarthropathy /-ärthrop′əthē/ [Gk, *osteon + arthron,* joint, *pathos,* disease], any disorder affecting bones and joints.

osteoarthrosis /-arthrō″sis/, a condition of chronic arthritis, usually mechanical, without inflammation.

osteoarticular /-artik″yələr/, pertaining to or affecting bones and joints.

osteoarticular brucellosis, a form of brucellosis that affects mainly the weight-bearing joints.

osteoarticular graft, a transplant of bone that contains a joint surface.

osteoblast /os″tē·ə·blast′/ [Gk, *osteon + blastos,* germ], a bone-forming cell that is derived from the embryonic mesenchyme and, during the early development of the skeleton, differentiates from a fibroblast to function in the formation of bone tissue. Osteoblasts synthesize the collagen and glycoproteins to form the osteoid matrix and, with growth, develop into osteocytes. See also **ossification.** —*osteoblastic, adj.*

osteoblastic sarcoma. See **giant cell myeloma.**

osteoblastoma /-blastō″mə/ *pl. osteoblastomas, osteoblastomata,* a small, benign, fairly vascular tumor of poorly formed bone and fibrous tissue, occurring most frequently in the vertebrae, femur, tibia, or bones of the upper extremities in children and young adults. The tumor may cause pain, erosion, and resorption of native bone. Excision is the preferred treatment. Also called **osteoid osteoma.**

osteocachexia /-kəkek″sē·ə/, a chronic disease that causes bone wasting, usually resulting from malnutrition.

osteocalcin /-kal″sin/, a protein found in the extracellular matrix of bone and dentin and involved in regulating mineralization in the bones and teeth.

osteocarcinoma /-kär′sinō″mə/ [Gk, *osteon,* bone, *karkinos,* crab, *oma,* tumor], cancer of the bone.

osteochondral graft /-kon″drəl/, a transplant containing both bone and cartilage.

osteochondritis /-kəndrī″tis/ [Gk, *osteon,* bone, *chondros,* cartilage, *itis,* inflammation], a disease of the epiphyses, or bone-forming centers of the skeleton, that begins with necrosis and tissue fragmentation and is followed by repair and regeneration. Kinds include *osteochondritis deformans juvenilis,* **osteochondritis dissecans,** *osteochondritis ischiopubica, osteochondritis juvenilis, osteochondritis necroticans.*

osteochondritis dissecans [Gk, *osteon,* bone, *chondros,* cartilage; L, *dissecare,* to cut apart], a joint disorder in which a piece of cartilage and neighboring bone tissue become detached from an articular surface.

osteochondrodystrophy. See **Morquio disease.**

osteochondrofibroma /-kon′drōfībrō″mə/, a tumor containing tissues of osteoma, chondroma, and fibroma.

osteochondrolysis. See **osteochondrosis dissecans.**

osteochondroma /os′tē·ōkondrō″mə/ [Gk, *osteon + chondros,* cartilage, *oma,* tumor], a benign tumor composed of bone and cartilage. The onset is usually in childhood. It affects more males than females.

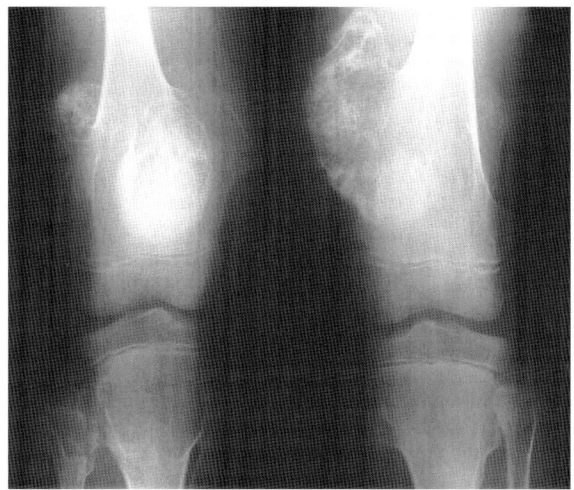

Osteochrondromas on the bone surface
(Pannier and Legeai-Mallet, 2008)

osteochondromatosis /-kon′drōmətō″sis/, the transformation of synovial villi into bone and cartilage masses, causing loose bodies in the joints. It usually develops in joints affected by injury or degenerative disease.

osteochondropathy /-kəndrop″əthē/, a condition affecting both bone and cartilage and characterized by abnormal enchondral ossification.

osteochondrosarcoma /-kon′drōsärkō″mə/ [Gk, *osteon,* bone, *chondros,* cartilage, *karkinos,* crab, *oma,* tumor], a cancer of the bone and cartilage.

osteochondrosis /-kondrō″sis/ [Gk, *osteon + chondros,* cartilage, *osis,* condition], a disease affecting the ossification centers of bone in children. It is initially characterized by degeneration and necrosis, followed by regeneration and recalcification. Kinds include **Legg-Calvé-Perthes disease, Osgood-Schlatter disease, Scheuermann disease.**

osteochondrosis dissecans /dis″əkənz/, the formation of a separate center of bone and cartilage on an epiphyseal surface. The stray fragment may remain in place, be absorbed, or break off and become a loose body.

osteoclasia /-klä″zhə/ [Gk, *osteon + klasis,* breaking], **1.** the destruction and absorption of bony tissue by osteoclasts, such as during growth or the healing of fractures. **2.** the degeneration of bone through disease. See also **osteolysis.**

osteoclasis /os′tē-ōk″ləsis/, the intentional surgical fracture of a bone to correct a deformity. Also called **osteoclasty.**

osteoclast /os′tē-əklast′/ [Gk, *osteon + klasis,* breaking], **1.** a large type of multinucleated bone cell with a large amount of acidophilic cytoplasm that functions to absorb and remove osseous tissue. During bone healing of fractures, or during certain disease processes, osteoclasts excavate passages through the surrounding tissue by enzymatic action. Osteoclasts become activated in the presence of parathyroid hormone and also in a lymphokine substance produced by lymphocytes in such diseases as multiple myeloma and malignant lymphomas. Also called **osteophage.** See also **ossification. 2.** a surgical instrument used in the fracturing or refracturing of bones for therapeutic purposes, such as correction of a deformity.

osteoclast activating factor, a lymphokine that promotes the resorption of bone.

osteoclastic /-klas″tik/, **1.** pertaining to osteoclasts. **2.** destructive to bone.

osteoclastoma /os′tē-ōklastō″mə/ *pl.* osteoclastomas, osteoclastomata [Gk, *osteon + klasis,* breaking, *oma,* tumor], a giant cell tumor of the bone that occurs most frequently at the end of a long bone and appears as a mass surrounded by a thin shell of new periosteal bone. The lesion may be malignant and may cause local pain, loss of function, weakness, and pathological fracture. Also called **giant cell myeloma, giant cell tumor of bone.**

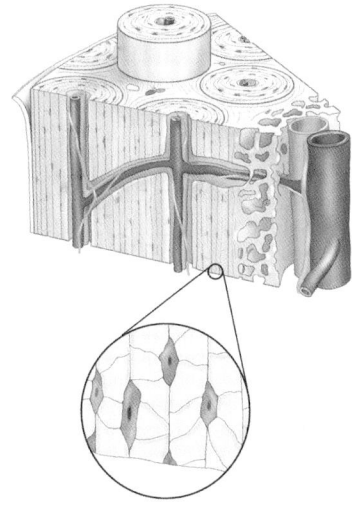

Osteoclastoma *(Courtesy American College of Radiology)*

osteoclasty. See **osteoclasis.**

osteocope /os′tē-əkōp/, a painful, syphilitic bone disease.

osteocystoma /-sistō″mə/, a cystic tumor in a bone.

osteocyte /os′tē-əsīt/ [Gk, *osteon + kytos,* cell], a bone cell; a mature osteoblast that has become embedded in the bone matrix. It occupies a small cavity and sends out protoplasmic projections that anastomose with those of other osteocytes to form a system of minute canals within the bone matrix. −*osteocytic, adj.*

osteodensitometer /-den′sitom″ətər/ [Gk, *osteon,* bone; L, *densus,* thick; Gk, *metron,* measure], an apparatus for measuring the density of bone tissue.

osteodentin /-den″tin/, dentin that resembles bone. It is found chiefly in the teeth of fish and certain other animals but also occurs occasionally in humans when odontoblasts are entrapped by rapidly developing secondary dentin.

osteodermia /-dur″mēə/, a condition in which skeletal changes occur in the skin, such as a bony tumor of the skin. Also called **osteoma cutis.**

osteodiastasis /-dī·as″təsis/, an abnormal separation of bones.

osteodynia /-din″ē·ə/, bone pain.

osteodystrophy /-dis″trəfē/ [Gk, *osteon + dys,* bad, *trophe,* nourishment], any generalized defect in bone development, usually associated with disturbances in calcium and phosphorus metabolism and renal insufficiency, such as in renal osteodystrophy. Also called *osteodystrophia.*

osteoenchondroma /os′tē-ō-en′kəndrō″mə/, a benign bone and cartilage tumor within a bone.

osteofibrochondrosarcoma /-fī′brokon″drōsärkō″mə/, a malignant tumor containing bone, cartilage, and fibrous tissues.

osteofibroma /-fibrō″mə/ [Gk, *osteon,* bone; L, *fibra,* fiber; Gk, *oma,* tumor], a tumor composed of both bony and fibrous tissues.

O

osteogenesis /-jen″əsis/ [Gk, *osteon* + *genesis,* origin], the origin and development of bone tissue. Also called **osteogeny.** See also **ossification.** −**osteogenous, osteogenetic, osteogenic,** *adj.*

osteogenesis imperfecta, a genetic disorder involving defective development of the connective tissue. It is inherited as an autosomal-dominant trait and is characterized by abnormally brittle and fragile bones that are easily fractured by the slightest trauma. In its most severe form, the disease may be apparent at birth, when it is known as osteogenesis imperfecta type II. The newborn has multiple fractures that have occurred in utero and is usually severely deformed because of imperfect formation and mineralization of bone. Most infants die shortly after birth, although a few survive as deformed dwarfs with normal mental development if no head trauma has occurred. If the disease has a later onset, it is called osteogenesis imperfecta type I and usually runs a milder course. Symptoms generally appear when the child begins to walk, but they become less severe with age, and the tendency to fracture decreases and often disappears after puberty. Other manifestations of the condition include blue sclerae, translucent skin, hyperextensibility of ligaments, hypoplasia of the teeth, recurrent epistaxis, excess diaphoresis, mild hyperpyrexia, and a tendency to bruise easily and develop otosclerosis with hearing loss. There is a broad expressivity of the disease so that the number and extent of pathological features may range from minimal to severe involvement. Also called *Adair-Dighton syndrome, brittle bones,* **fragilitas ossium, hypoplasia of the mesenchyme, osteopsathyrosis.**

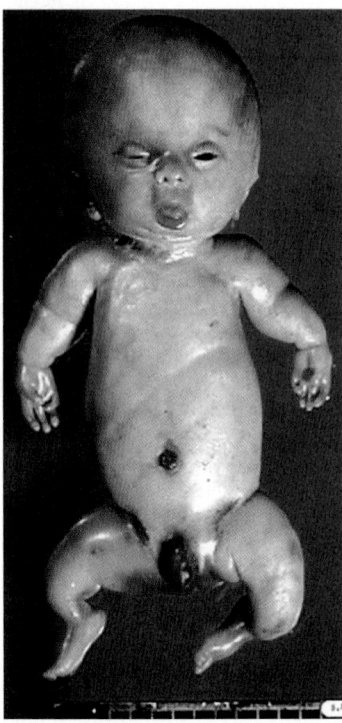

Infant with osteogenesis imperfecta *(Lipson, 2005)*

osteogenetic. See **osteogenesis.**

osteogenic, composed of or originating from any tissue involved in the development, growth, or repair of bone. Also **osteogenous.**

osteogenic myeloma. See **myeloma.**

osteogenic sarcoma. See **osteosarcoma.**

osteogenous. See **osteogenic.**

osteogeny. See **osteogenesis.**

osteohalisteresis /-hal′istərē″sis/, a condition of soft bones caused by a loss or deficiency of mineral elements.

osteoid /os″tē·oid/ [Gk, *osteon* + *eidos,* form], pertaining to or resembling bone.

osteoid osteoma. See **osteoblastoma.**

osteolipochondroma /-līp′ōkəndrō″mə/, a cartilage tumor with bone and fat elements.

osteolipoma /-līpō″mə/, a fatty tumor containing bone elements.

osteology /os′tē·ol″əgē/ [Gk, *osteon,* bone, *logos,* science], the branch of medicine concerned with the development and diseases of bone tissue.

osteolysis /os′tē·ol″isis/ [Gk, *osteon* + *lysis,* loosening], the degeneration and dissolution of bone caused by disease, infection, or ischemia. The condition commonly affects the terminal bones of the hands and feet, such as in acro-osteolysis, and is seen in disorders involving blood vessels, such as Raynaud disease, scleroderma, and systemic lupus erythematosus. −*osteolytic, adj.*

osteolytic hypercalcemia /-lit″ik/, a malignancy associated with excess calcium in the blood. It may be caused by either widespread skeletal metastases or extensive bone marrow involvement by a primary hematological tumor.

osteoma /os′tē·ō″mə/ *pl. osteomas, osteomata,* a tumor of bone tissue.

-osteoma, combining form meaning "a tumor composed of bone tissue, usually benign."

osteoma cutis. See **osteodermia.**

osteomalacia /-məlā″shə/ [Gk, *osteon* + *malakia,* softening], an abnormal condition of lamellar bone, characterized by a loss of calcification of the matrix and resulting in softening of the bone. It is accompanied by weakness, fracture, pain, anorexia, and weight loss. The condition is the result of an inadequate amount of phosphorus and calcium available in the blood for mineralization of the bones. This deficiency may be caused by a diet lacking these minerals or vitamin D, by a lack of exposure to sunlight and hence an inability to synthesize vitamin D, or by a metabolic disorder causing malabsorption of minerals. Osteomalacia results from and also complicates many other diseases and conditions. Treatment usually includes administration of the necessary vitamins and minerals and therapy appropriate for the underlying disorder. Also called **adult rickets.** See also **hyperparathyroidism, Paget disease, rickets.**

osteomas, osteomata. See **osteoma.**

osteomesopyknosis /-mez′ōpiknō″sis/, a genetic disorder transmitted as an autosomal trait, characterized by osteosclerosis of the axial spine, pelvis, and proximal areas of long bones.

osteomyelitis /-mī·əlī″tis/ [Gk, *osteon* + *myelos,* marrow, *itis,* inflammation], local or generalized infection of bone and bone marrow, usually caused by bacteria introduced by trauma or surgery, by direct extension from a nearby infection, or via the bloodstream. Staphylococci are the most common causative agents.

■ OBSERVATIONS: The long bones in children and the vertebrae in adults are the most common sites of infection as a result of hematogenous spread. Persistent, severe, and increasing bone pain; tenderness; guarding on movement; regional muscle spasm; and fever suggest this diagnosis. Draining sinus tracts may accompany posttraumatic osteomyelitis or osteomyelitis from a contiguous infection. Specific diagnosis and selection of therapy depend on bacterial examination of bone, tissue, or pus.

■ INTERVENTIONS: Treatment includes bed rest and parenteral antibiotics for several weeks. Surgery may be necessary to remove necrotic bone and tissue, obliterate cavities, remove infected prosthetic appliances, and apply prostheses to stabilize affected parts. Chronic osteomyelitis may persist for years with exacerbations and remissions despite treatment.

■ PATIENT CARE CONSIDERATIONS: Normal precautions are used in disposing of any drainage. Absolute rest of the affected part may be necessary, with a careful positioning using pillows and sandbags for good alignment. During the early phase of infection, pain is extremely severe, and extraordinary gentleness in moving and manipulating the infected part is essential.

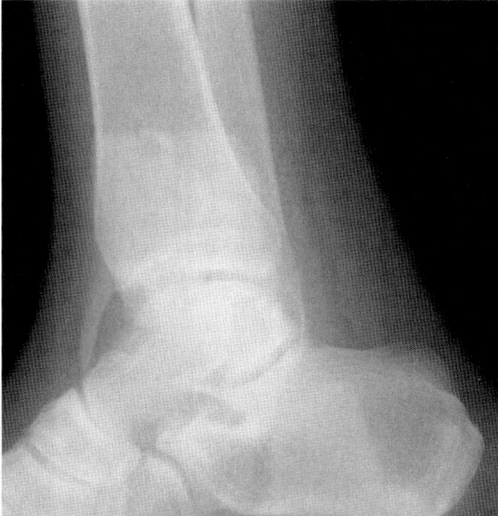

Acute osteomyelitis of the distal tibia *(Pretorius and Solomon, 2011)*

osteomyelodysplasia /os′tē·ōmī′əlō′displā″zhə/ [Gk, *osteon,* bone, *myelos,* marrow, *dys + plasis,* forming], a loss of bone tissue through absorption of minerals, usually associated with leukopenia and sometimes with fever. It may result from an excess of parathyroid hormone.

osteon /os′tē·on/ [Gk, bone], the basic central structural unit of compact bone, consisting of the haversian canal and its concentric rings of 4 to 20 lamellae. Most of the units run with the long axis of the bone. Also called **haversian system.**

-osteon, -osteum, suffix meaning "bone."

osteonal bone /os′tē·ō′nəl/, bone tissue composed of tiny chalky tubes with an arteriole running down the middle and circular laminations of bone concentric with an artery. It is seen in mature adults.

osteonecrosis /os′tē·ō′nəkrō″sis/ [Gk, *osteon + nekros,* dead, *osis* condition], the destruction and death of bone tissue, such as from ischemia, infection, malignant neoplastic disease, or trauma. **–osteonecrotic,** *adj.*

osteoonychodysplasia /os′tē·ō·on′i·kō·dis·plā′zhə/ [Gk, *osteon,* bone, *onyx,* nail, *dys,* bad, *plassein,* to form], **1.** abnormal development of nails and bones. Also called **onycho-osteodysplasia. 2.** See **nail-patella syndrome.**

osteopath (osteo) /os′tē·ōpath′/, a physician who specializes in osteopathy. Also called **osteopathist.**

osteopathic. See **osteopathy.**

osteopathic scoliosis. See **congenital scoliosis.**

osteopathist. See **osteopath.**

osteopathology /-pathol″əjē/ [Gk, *osteon,* bone, *pathos,* disease, *logos,* science], the study of bone diseases.

osteopathy (osteo) /os′tē·op″əthē/ [Gk, *osteon + pathos,* disease], a therapeutic approach to the practice of medicine that uses all the usual forms of medical diagnosis and therapy, including drugs, surgery, and radiation, but that places greater emphasis on the relationship between the organs and the musculoskeletal system than traditional medicine does. Osteopathic physicians recognize and correct structural problems using manipulation. See also **physician. –osteopathic,** *adj.*

osteopedion. See **lithopedion.**

osteopenia /-pē″nē·ə/ [Gk, *osteon + penes,* poverty], **1.** reduced bone mass due to a decrease in the rate of osteoid synthesis to a level insufficient to compensate normal bone lysis. See also **osteoporosis. 2.** any decrease in bone mass below the normal.

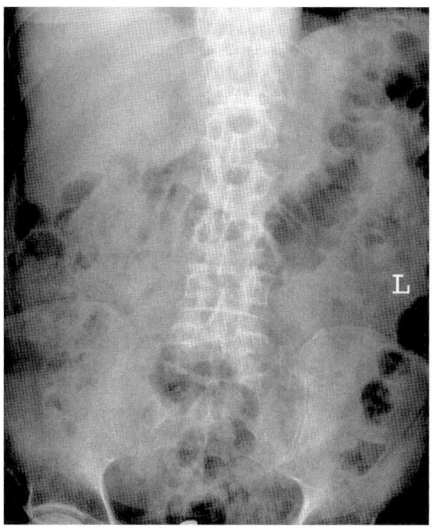

Osteopenia *(Courtesy Ohio State University Medical Center)*

osteoperiosteal graft /-per′ē·os″tē·əl/, a bone graft that includes the periosteal membrane covering the bone.

osteopetrosis /os′tē·ōpētrō″sis/ [Gk, *osteon + petra,* stone, *osis,* condition], an inherited disorder characterized by a generalized increase in bone density, probably caused by faulty bone resorption resulting from a deficiency of osteoclasts. In its most severe form, transmitted as an autosomal-recessive condition, the bone marrow cavity is obliterated, causing severe anemia, marked deformities of the skull, and compression of the cranial nerves, which may result in deafness and blindness and lead to an early death. A milder, benign form, transmitted as an autosomal-dominant trait, is characterized by short stature, fragile bones that fracture easily, and a tendency to develop osteomyelitis. Also called **ivory bones, marble bones, osteosclerosis fragilis.** See also **Albers-Schönberg disease. –osteopetrotic,** *adj.*

osteophage. See **osteoclast.**

osteophlebitis /-fləbī″tis/, an inflammation of the veins that are a part of the vascular system of bones.

osteophyte /os″tē·əfīt/, a bony outgrowth, usually found around a joint. It is commonly seen in degenerative joint disease.

osteoplast. See **osteoblast.**

osteoplastica /-plas″tikə/, a form of bone inflammation associated with cystic fibrosis.

O

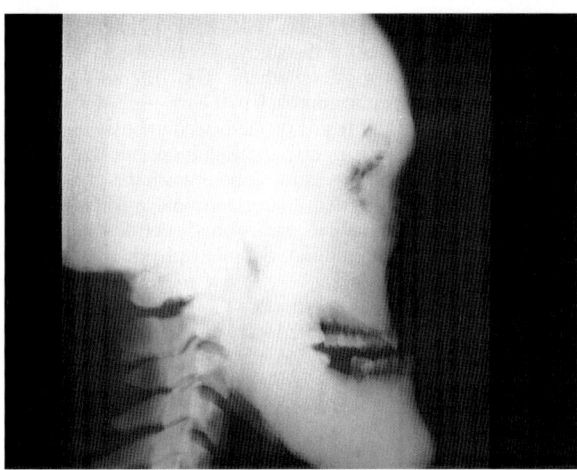

Osteopetrosis *(Regezi, Sciubba, and Jordan, 2012)*

osteoplasty /o'stē·əplas'tē/ [Gk, *osteon*, bone, *plassein*, to mold], plastic surgery performed on bone tissue.

osteopoikilosis /os'tē·ōpoi'kilō"sis/ [Gk, *osteon* + *poikilos*, mottled, *osis*, condition], an inherited condition of the bones, transmitted as an autosomal-dominant trait, characterized by multiple areas of dense calcification throughout the osseous tissue, producing a mottled appearance on x-ray examination. It is a benign condition, usually without symptoms and of unknown cause. Also called **osteosclerosis fragilis congenita.** *—osteopoikilotic, adj.*

osteoporosis /os"tē·ōpərō"sis/ [Gk, *osteon* + *poros*, passage, *osis*, condition], a disorder characterized by abnormal loss of bone density and deterioration of bone tissue, with an increased fracture risk. It occurs most frequently in postmenopausal women, sedentary or immobilized individuals, and patients on long-term steroid therapy. Osteoporosis may be without a known cause or secondary to other disorders, such as thyrotoxicosis or the bone demineralization caused by hyperparathyroidism. **–osteoporotic,** *adj.*

■ OBSERVATIONS: Individuals are typically asymptomatic early in the disease. The first symptom is usually a dull, aching, constant pain in the bones, particularly the back and chest. The pain may radiate down the leg, and muscle spasms may be present. As the spinal column mass diminishes, dorsal kyphosis and cervical lordosis increase, leading to multiple compression fractures of the spine and a reduction in height. Other fractures occur with minimal or no trauma. Clinical evaluation reveals a complex of risk factors such as estrogen deficiency, androgen deficiency, hyperthyroidism, nulliparity, chronic malnutrition, long-term lack of calcium intake, long history of tobacco use, ethanol abuse, steroid use or abuse, sedentary lifestyle, immobility, familial history, and underlying skeletal disease. Bone mineral density (BMD) tests reveal loss of bone density. X-rays show decreased radiodensity after 25% to 40% loss of bone calcium. Immobility from increased fractures and deformity from spinal crushing are common complications.

■ INTERVENTIONS: Treatment focuses on calcium and vitamin D supplementation; the use of calcitonin, bisphosphonates (etidronate, alendronate, pamidronate), selective estrogen receptor modulators (raloxifene), or human monoclonal antibody (denosumab) to prevent bone resorption; nonsteroidal antiinflammatory drugs for pain; and the use of estrogen-progestin supplements, which is controversial. Calcium levels are monitored regularly.

■ PATIENT CARE CONSIDERATIONS: Nursing care is aimed at prevention and early detection. Prevention is centered around proper nutrition with a balanced diet rich in calcium and vitamin D; regular exercise that emphasizes strengthening and weight bearing; cessation of tobacco use and ethanol abuse; and adequate fluoride ingestion. Bone density surveys should be encouraged every 1 to 3 years after age 49 for early detection. Acute care stresses good nutrition with calcium and vitamin D supplementation; a consistent exercise regimen, including moderate, weight-bearing hyperextension and resistance exercises to slow calcium loss and strengthen musculature; heat and massage for muscle spasm; orthopedic supports for back and neck to prevent stress fractures; and canes to aid in walking. Instruction in fall and fracture prevention measures is important to help the individual decrease fracture risk and maintain independence in activities of daily living. Education about medication effects and side effects is needed.

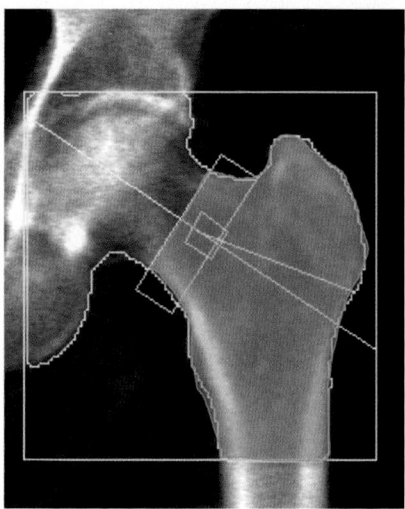

Dual-energy x-ray absorptiometry of proximal femur of a woman with osteoporosis *(© 2015 Canadian Association of Radiologists)*

osteoporosis of disuse [Gk, *osteon*, bone, *poros*, passage, *osis*, condition; L, *dis*, not; ME, *usen*, to act], a decrease in bone mass that occurs in sedentary individuals. It is seen in patients who do not put loading forces on their bones, as in individuals who are paralyzed or confined to a bed or wheelchair.

osteoporotic /-pərot"ik/ [Gk, *osteon*, bone, *poros*, passage, *osis*, condition], pertaining to osteoporosis.

osteopsathyrosis. See **osteogenesis imperfecta.**

osteorrhaphy. See **osteosuture.**

osteosarcoma /os'tē·ō'särkō"mə/ [Gk, *osteon* + *sarx*, flesh, *oma*], a malignant tumor of the bone, composed of anaplastic cells derived from mesenchyme. It is the most common type of primary malignant bone tumor, accounting for 35% of such malignancies. It occurs most often in the distal femur. Metastasis to the lung occurs more often in males than in females. It occurs most frequently between the second and fourth decade of life. Also called **osteogenic sarcoma.**

osteosclerosis /os'tē·ōsklerō"sis/ [Gk, *osteon* + *skleros*, hard, *osis*, condition], an abnormal increase in the density of bone tissue. The condition occurs in a variety of disease states and is commonly associated with ischemia, chronic infection, and tumor formation. It also may be caused by faulty bone resorption as a result of some abnormality

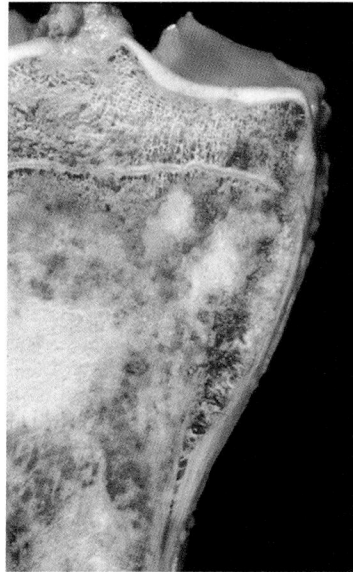

Intramedullary osteosarcoma of the proximal tibial metaphysis *(Gonzalez and Cates, 2012)*

involving osteoclasts. See also **achondroplasia, osteopetrosis, osteopoikilosis. −osteosclerotic,** *adj.*

osteosclerosis fragilis.   See **osteopetrosis.**

osteosclerosis fragilis congenita.   See **osteopoikilosis.**

osteosclerotic.   See **osteosclerosis.**

osteosuture /-sōo″chər/,   the surgical repair of a fractured bone by wiring or suturing the fragments together. Also called **osteorrhaphy.**

osteosynovitis /-sin′ōvī″tis/ [Gk, *osteon,* bone; Gk, *syn,* together; L, *ovum,* egg; Gk, *itis,* inflammation],   an inflammation of the synovial membrane of a joint and the surrounding bone tissue.

osteosynthesis /-sin″thəsis/,   the surgical fixation of a bone by any internal mechanical means. It is usually performed in the treatment of fractures.

osteotabes /-tā″bēz/,   a condition usually affecting infants in which bone marrow cells are destroyed and the marrow disappears.

osteotelangiectasia /-telan′jē·əktā″zhə/,   a sarcoma of the bone characterized by dilated capillaries.

osteothrombophlebitis /-throm′bōfləbī″tis/,   a progressive inflammation of small venules and intact bone often accompanied by clot formation.

osteothrombosis /-thrəmbō″sis/,   a blockage of blood vessels in bone tissue.

osteotome /os″tē·ətōm′/ [Gk, *osteon* + *temnein,* to cut],   a surgical instrument for cutting through bone.

osteotomy /os′tē·ot″əmē/ [Gk, *osteon* + *temnein,* to cut],   the sawing or cutting of a bone. Kinds of osteotomy include block osteotomy, in which a section of bone is excised; cuneiform osteotomy to remove a bone wedge; and displacement osteotomy, in which a bone is redesigned surgically to alter the alignment or weight-bearing stress areas.

osteotripsy /-trip′sē/,   any percutaneous reduction of a bony prominence or callus.

-osteum.   See **-osteon, -osteum.**

ostium.   See **orifice.**

ostium primum defect, ostium secundum defect.   See **atrial septal defect.**

ostomate /os″təmāt/ [L, *ostium,* mouth],   a person who has undergone an ostomy.

ostomy /os″təmē/   [L, *ostium,* mouth,],   *(Informal)* a surgical procedure in which an incision or stoma is surgically created in the wall of the abdomen to allow the passage of urine from the bladder or of intestinal contents from the bowel. An ostomy procedure may be performed to correct an anatomic defect, relieve an obstruction, or permit treatment of a severe infection or injury of the urinary or intestinal tract. Each procedure is named for the anatomic location of the ostomy, such as a colostomy, ureterostomy, cecostomy, or cystostomy.

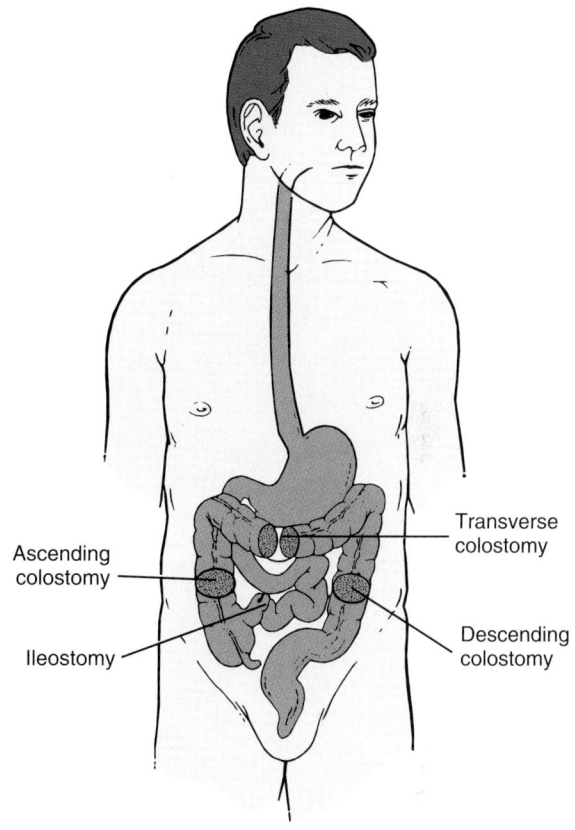

Ascending colostomy

Transverse colostomy

Descending colostomy

Ileostomy

Ostomy sites

O

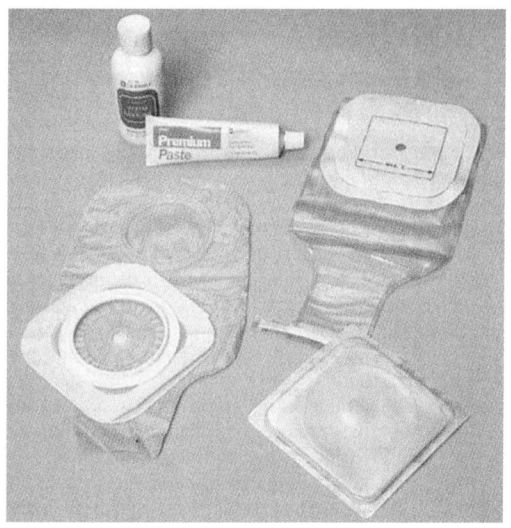

Ostomy pouches *(Potter and Perry, 2007)*

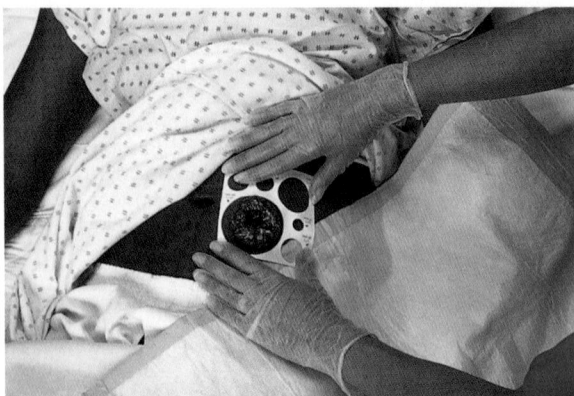

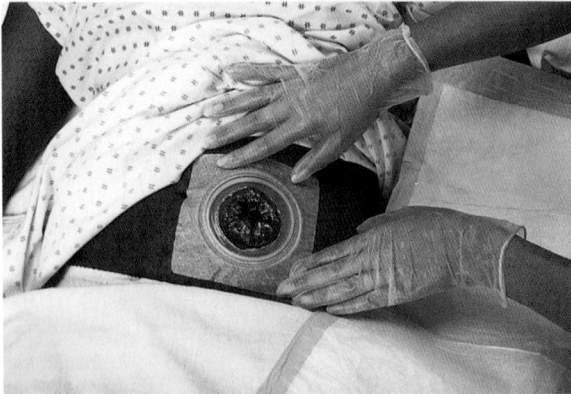

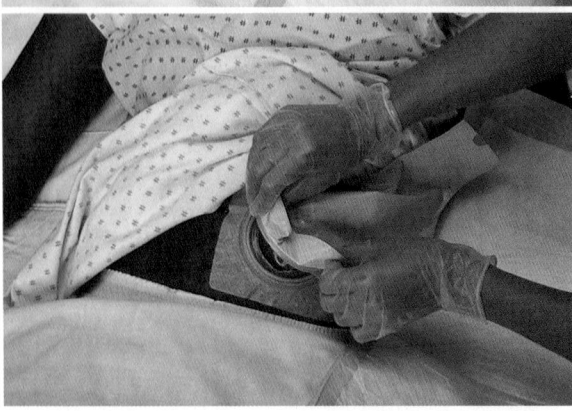

Ostomy care *(Harkreader, Hogan, and Thobaben, 2007)*

-ostomy, suffix meaning "to form a new opening" or "pertaining to a mouthlike opening": *colostomy, ileostomy, tracheostomy.*

ostomy care, the management and support of a patient with a surgical opening created in the bladder, ileum, or colon for the temporary or permanent passage of urine or feces, necessitated by carcinoma, intestinal obstruction, trauma, or severe ulceration distal to the site of the incision. In most cases the opening is covered with a temporary disposable bag in the operating room.

■ METHOD: The patient with a colostomy or an ileostomy is helped to accept the stoma and the change in body image that frequently causes grief or in some instances denial. Discussions of the person's feelings are encouraged, and questions regarding the procedure and possible changes in the person's lifestyle are answered in a positive manner. The disposable bag, called an appliance, is changed when necessary, and the character, color, and amount of odor and drainage are observed. Mucus secretion from the stoma usually begins within 48 hours after the surgery, fecal drainage within 72 hours. The stoma is inspected periodically for color, bleeding, stricture, retraction, and infection and is measured periodically to determine the size of the appliance that is to be used. There is mild to moderate swelling of the stoma the first 2 to 3 weeks postoperatively. Size of the stoma is determined with a stoma measuring card. Each time the temporary or permanent appliance is changed, the skin around the stoma is washed with soap and water, rinsed thoroughly, and patted dry with a clean towel. If the skin is irritated or excoriated, karaya powder, alone or mixed with an ointment, is spread over the area before the appliance is reinstalled. A pouch should never be placed directly on irritated skin without the use of a skin barrier. An adhesive substance may be used to maintain a tight seal with the appliance. Deodorant drops, aspirin, or various bismuth or chlorophyll preparations or mouthwash solutions are added to the ostomy bag to control odor. The diet is planned according to the kind of ostomy. Ileostomates require food high in sodium and potassium, such as bananas, citrus juices, molasses, and cola, and are advised to avoid fried, highly seasoned, and rich foods, nuts, raisins, raw fruits other than bananas, and anything that produces gas or causes diarrhea. Gas-producing foods such as cabbage, beans, broccoli, cauliflower, and corn; foods causing disturbing odors such as onions, eggs, and fish; and sharp condiments are contraindicated. A low-residue diet is ordered for most ostomates. The fluid intake is carefully maintained.

■ INTERVENTIONS: Before discharge, each step in the care of the stoma and surrounding skin is rehearsed with the patient; the equipment that will be available at home is used during this rehearsal. The patient is urged to establish a regular pattern of evacuation and to report any signs of wound infection or obstruction, such as nausea, vomiting, decreased drainage from the stoma, abdominal distension, and cramps. Normal daily activity is encouraged.

■ OUTCOME CRITERIA: Visiting nurse referrals may be indicated for client assessment and education. Referrals to support groups are also encouraged. Clients are encouraged to keep appointments with care providers. The ability of the patient to adjust to the ostomy procedures and equipment is greatly affected by the nursing care received in the days after surgery. A positive patient, matter-of-fact approach; sensitive emotional support; and thorough teaching of self-care measures are essential aspects of ostomy nursing care.

ostomy irrigation, a procedure for cleansing, stimulating, and regulating the evacuation from an artificially created orifice. Fluids used in irrigation include tap water and saline or medicated solutions. Necessary equipment includes properly sized irrigator tips, catheters, drainage bags that allow for insertion of the catheter, water-soluble lubricants, gloves, an irrigation container, and shields to prevent leakage. Loop and double-barrel colostomies require a sequential irrigation of the proximal loop, distal loop, and rectum to prevent the accumulation of discharge.

os trapezium. See **trapezium.**

os trapezoideum. See **trapezoid bone.**

os trigonum /os′trigō″nəm/, a small foot bone just posterior to the talus. It is sometimes confused with a fracture of the posterior tubercle of the talus.

os triquetrum. See **triangular bone.**

OT, 1. abbreviation for **occupational therapist. 2.** abbreviation for **occupational therapy.**

ot-. See **oto-, ot-, -otic.**

Comparison of ileostomy and colostomy

| | Ileostomy | Colostomy | | |
		Ascending	Transverse	Sigmoid
Stool consistency	Liquid to semiliquid	Semiliquid	Semiliquid to semiformed	Formed
Fluid requirement	Increased	Increased	Possibly increased	No change
Bowel regulation	No	No	No	Yes (if there is a history of a regular bowel pattern)
Pouch and skin barriers	Yes	Yes	Yes	Dependent on regulation
Irrigation	No	No	No	Possibly every 24-48 hr (if patient meets criteria)
Indications for surgery	Ulcerative colitis, Crohn's disease, diseased or injured colon, birth defect, familial polyposis, trauma, cancer	Perforating diverticulitis in lower colon; trauma; inoperable tumors of colon, rectum, or pelvis; rectovaginal fistula	Same as for ascending; birth defect	Cancer of the rectum or rectosigmoidal area; perforating diverticulum; trauma

otalgia /ōtal″jə/, a pain in the ear. Also called **otodynia, otoneuralgia.**

OTC, abbreviation for **over the counter.**

OTC drug, an over-the-counter medication. See **patent medicine.**

Othello syndrome /ōthel″ō/ [Othello, jealous Shakespearean character], a psychopathological condition characterized by suspicion of a spouse's infidelity and morbid jealousy. This condition may be accompanied by rage and violence and is frequently associated with paranoia.

-otia, suffix meaning "(condition of the) ear": *microtia, synotia.*

otic /ō″tik, ot″ik/ [Gk, *ous,* ear], pertaining to the ear. Also called **auricular.**

-otic. See **oto-, ot-, -otic.**

otics /ō″tiks, ot″iks/, a group of drugs used locally to treat inflammation of the external ear canal or to remove excess cerumen.

otic vertigo, a sensation of rotation motion caused by an inner ear disease. Its subcategories are Ménière disease, inner ear dysfunction, fistula or other pressure sensitivity, unilateral paresis, and benign paroxysmal positional vertigo.

otitic /ōtit″ik/ [Gk, *ous,* ear], pertaining to otitis.

otitic barotrauma. See **barotrauma.**

otitis /ōtī″tis/ [Gk, *ous + itis,* inflammation], inflammation or infection of the ear. Kinds include **otitis externa, otitis media.**

otitis externa, inflammation or infection of the external canal or the auricle of the external ear. Major causes are allergy, bacteria, fungi, viruses, and trauma. Allergy to nickel or chromium in earrings and to chemicals in hair sprays, cosmetics, hearing aids, and medications, particularly sulfonamides and neomycin, is common. *Staphylococcus aureus, Pseudomonas aeruginosa,* and *Streptococcus pyogenes* are common bacterial causes. Herpes simplex and herpes zoster viruses are frequently implicated. Eczema, psoriasis, and seborrheic dermatitis also may affect the external ear. Abrasions of the ear canal may become infected, and excessive swimming may wash out protective cerumen, remove skin lipids, and lead to secondary infection. Otitis externa is more prevalent during hot, humid weather. Folliculitis is particularly painful in the external auditory meatus and is a common occupational hazard in nurses, caused by irritation from the earpieces of stethoscopes. Treatment includes oral analgesics, thorough local cleansing, topical antimicrobials to treat infection, and topical corticosteroids to reduce inflammation. Prevention includes measures to avoid trauma and to reduce maceration of the skin. Malignant otitis externa is a complication of external otitis externa that occurs in immunocompromised patients.

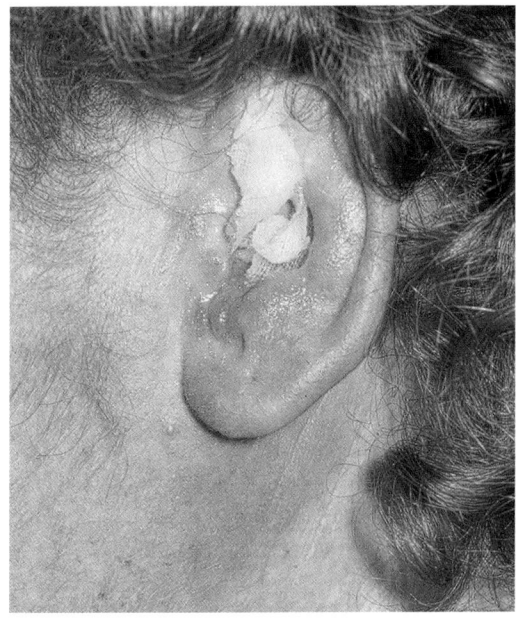

Malignant otitis externa *(White and Cox, 2006)*

otitis interna. See **labyrinthitis.**

otitis mastoidea [Gk, *ous,* ear, *itis,* inflammation, *mastos,* breast, *eidos,* form], an inflammation of the middle ear associated with a mastoid infection.

otitis media, an inflammation or infection of the middle ear, common in early childhood. Acute otitis media is most often caused by *Haemophilus influenzae, Moraxella catarrhalis,* or *Streptococcus pneumoniae.* Chronic otitis media is usually caused by gram-negative bacteria such as *Proteus, Klebsiella,* and *Pseudomonas.* Allergy, *Mycoplasma,* and several viruses also may be causative factors. Otitis media is often preceded by an upper respiratory infection.

■ OBSERVATIONS: Organisms gain entry to the middle ear through the eustachian tube. The small diameter and horizontal orientation of the tube in infants predisposes them to infection. Obstruction of the eustachian tube and accumulation of exudate may increase pressure within the middle ear, forcing infection into the mastoid bone or rupturing the tympanic membrane. Symptoms of acute otitis media include a sense of fullness in the ear, diminished hearing,

O

pain, and fever. Usually only one ear is affected. Squamous epithelium may grow in the middle ear through a rupture in the tympanic membrane; development of a cholesteatoma and hearing loss may occur if repeated infections cause an opening to persist. Pneumococcal otitis media may spread to the meninges.

■ INTERVENTIONS: Treatment includes antibiotics, analgesics, local heat, nasal decongestants, needle aspiration of secretions collected behind the membrane, and myringotomy.

■ PATIENT CARE CONSIDERATIONS: Parents are taught to recognize and watch for early warning signs of otitis media. The use of vaporizers and decongestants is often recommended during an upper respiratory tract infection as prophylaxis against otitis media. Chronic otitis media may result in hearing loss and delays in speech development.

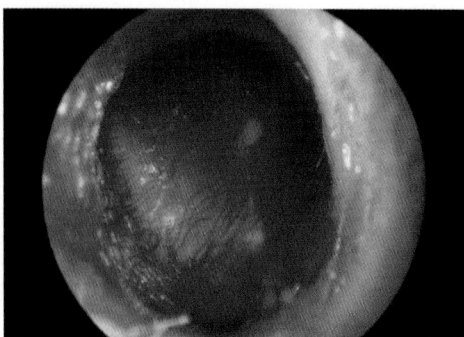

Otitis media *(Mir, 2003)*

otitis sclerotica [Gk, *ous*, ear, *itis*, inflammation, *sclerosis*, hardening], a sclerosing type of inflammation of the middle ear.

oto-, ot-, -otic, combining form meaning "ear": *otocephaly, otoacoustic emissions, otolith.*

otoacoustic emissions, echoes emitted by the outer hair cells of the inner ear. These echoes are used to evaluate the integrity of the inner ear and to screen hearing in newborns.

otocephalic, otocephalous. See **otocephaly.**

otocephalus /ō′tōsef″ələs/, a fetus with otocephaly.

otocephaly /ō′tōsef″əlē/ [Gk, *ous* + *kephale*, head], a congenital malformation characterized by the absence of the lower jaw, defective formation of the mouth, and union or close approximation of the ears on the front of the neck. See also **agnathocephaly.** −*otocephalic, otocephalous, adj.*

otoconia, small crystals in the inner ear that play an important role in balance. Abnormalities are a common cause of vertigo and imbalance. Also called **statoconia.**

otocranial debris, otoliths that have been dislodged by trauma and may move about in the semicircular canals when the head changes position.

otodynia. See **otalgia.**

otolaryngologist /-ler′ing·gol″əjist/ [Gk, *ous* + *larynx* + *logos*, science], a physician who specializes in the diagnosis and treatment of diseases and injuries of the ears, nose, and throat. Also called **ENT specialist.** Compare **otologist.**

otolaryngology /-ler′ing·gol″əjē/ [Gk, *ous* + *larynx* + *logos*, science], a branch of medicine dealing with the diagnosis and treatment of diseases and disorders of the ears, nose, throat, and adjacent structures of the head and neck.

otolith /ō″təlith/ [Gk, *ous*, ear, *lithos*, stone], **1.** a calculus in the middle ear. **2.** any of the crystals of calcium carbonate attached to the hair cells of the inner ear as gravity orientation receptors.

otolith righting reflex [Gk, *ous* + *lithos*, stone], an involuntary response in newborns in which tilting of the body when the infant is in an erect position causes the head to return to the upright position. The reflex enables the infant to raise the head and is important for development of later gross motor skills. Absence of the reflex may indicate central nervous system damage.

otologist /ōtol″əjist/, a physician trained in the diagnosis and treatment of diseases and other disorders of the ear. Compare **otolaryngologist.**

otology /ōtol″əjē/ [Gk, *ous* + *logos*, science], the study of the ear, including the diagnosis and treatment of its diseases and disorders.

-otomy, suffix meaning "to make an incision or cut into": *phlebotomy, tracheotomy.*

otomycosis /ō′tōmīkō″sis/, a lesion of the external ear caused by a fungus infection.

otoneuralgia. See **otalgia.**

otoneurology. See **neurotology.**

otoplasty /ō″təplas′tē/ [Gk, *ous* + *plassein*, to mold], a common procedure in reconstructive plastic surgery in which, for cosmetic reasons, some of the cartilage in the ears is removed to bring the auricle and pinna closer to the head.

otopyosis /ō′təpi·ō″sis/, a pus-producing inflammation of the ear, occurring either in the tympanic cavity or the external auditory meatus.

otorrhea /ō′tərē″ə/ [Gk, *ous* + *rhoia*, flow], any discharge from the external ear. Otorrhea may be serous, sanguinous, or purulent or contain cerebrospinal fluid.

otosclerosis /ō′tōsklərō″sis/ [Gk, *ous* + *skleros*, hard, *osis*, condition], a hereditary condition of unknown cause in which irregular ossification occurs in the ossicles of the middle ear, especially of the stapes, causing hearing loss. It is usually first noticed between 11 and 30 years of age. Women are affected twice as often as men. The condition may worsen during pregnancy. Stapedectomy or stapedotomy is usually successful in restoring hearing.

otoscope /ō″təskōp′/ [Gk, *ous* + *skopein*, to look], an instrument used to examine the external ear, the eardrum, and, through the eardrum, the ossicles of the middle ear. It consists of a light, a magnifying lens, a speculum, and sometimes a device for insufflation.

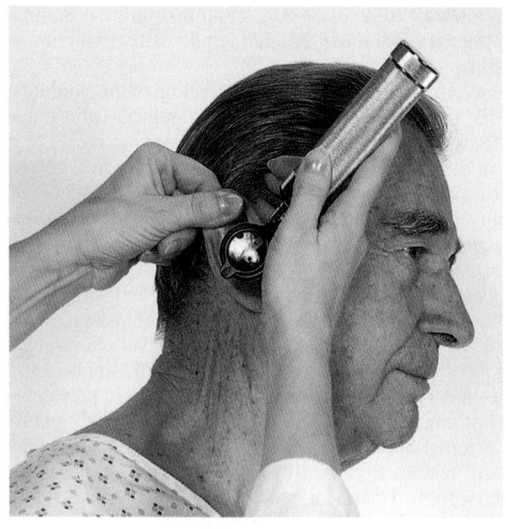

Assessment with an otoscope *(deWit and O'Neill, 2014)*

otoscopy /ōtos″kəpē/ [Gk, *ous,* ear, *skopein,* to view], an inspection of the tympanic membrane and other parts of the outer ear with an otoscope, an instrument for examining the drum membrane.

otospongiosus. See **otosclerosis.**

ototoxic hearing loss, hearing loss caused by ingestion of toxic substances. Also called **toxic deafness.**

ototoxicity /ō′tōtok″sisitē/ [Gk, *ous* + *toxikon,* poison], the harmful effects of certain substances on the eighth cranial nerve or the organs of hearing and balance. Common ototoxic drugs include the aminoglycoside antibiotics, aspirin, furosemide, and quinine. −ototoxic, *adj.*

OTR, initialism for *occupational therapist registered.*

Otrivin, a nasal adrenergic vasoconstrictor. Brand name for **xylometazoline hydrochloride.**

Otto pelvis /ot″ō/ [Adolph W. Otto, German surgeon, 1786–1845], a type of hip dislocation that involves a gradual central displacement of the femur. The cause is unknown.

O.U., *(Obsolete)* notation for a Latin phrase meaning "either eye." Identified as an error-prone abbreviation that should not be used. Abbreviation for *oculus uterque.*

oubain /wäbā″in/, a crystalline glycoside derived from the seeds of *Strophanthus gratus* and the wood of *Acocanthera oubaio.* It blocks Na+K+ATPase similarly to strophanthin-K and the digitalis glycosides and is often used in pharmacological studies because of its greater solubility in water. It is also used as an arrow poison.

Ouchterlony double diffusion [Orjan T.G. Ouchterlony, Swedish bacteriologist, b. 1914], a form of gel diffusion technique in which antigen and antibody in separate cells are allowed to diffuse toward each other.

ounce (oz) /ouns/ [L, *uncia,* one twelfth], a unit of mass equal to 1/16 of a pound avoirdupois or 28.349 grams. Also called *ounce avoirdupois.*

-ous, -eous, suffix meaning "an element or compound with a valence lower than the corresponding one ending in *-ic*": *ferrous, hypochlorous acid.*

outbreak /out′brāk/, (in epidemiology) the occurrence of infection with a particular disease in a small, localized group, such as the population of a village. The term is sometimes used more broadly to refer to an epidemic or a pandemic.

outbreeding [AS, *ut,* out, *bredan,* to breed], the production of offspring by the mating of unrelated individuals, which can lead to superior hybrid traits or strains. Compare **inbreeding.** See also **heterosis.**

outcome [AS, *ut* + *couman,* to come], the condition of a patient at the end of therapy or a disease process, including the degree of wellness and the need for continuing care, medication, support, counseling, or education.

outcome criteria, standards that focus on observable or measurable results of nursing and other health service activities.

outcome data, information collected to evaluate the capacity of a client to function at a level described in the outcome statement of a nursing care plan or in standards for patient care.

outcome measure, a measure of the quality of medical care, the standard against which the end result of the intervention is assessed.

outer zone of renal medulla, the part of the renal medulla nearest to the cortex. It contains part of the distal straight tubule and the medullary collecting tubule and is subdivided into the inner stripe and the outer stripe.

outlet [AS, *ut* + *laetan,* to permit], an opening through which something can exit, such as the pelvic outlet.

outlet contraction, a pelvis in which one or more of its diameters is reduced so that it interferes with the normal mechanism of childbirth. Also called **outlet contracture.** See **contraction,** def. 4.

outlet contracture, an abnormally small pelvic outlet. It may be anteroposterior or transverse and is of significance in childbirth because it may impede or prevent passage of a baby through the birth canal. Anteroposterior contracture caused by fixation of the coccyx may sometimes be overcome by the force of labor, freeing the bones and allowing them to move back. Significant narrowing of the space between the ischial tuberosities is unlikely to be overcome and is most commonly associated with a heavy, android type of pelvis.

outlet forceps. See **low forceps.**

outlier, **1.** (in managed care) a case in which costs exceed the allowable amount for the specific diagnosis or treatment. The outlier amount is typically specified in advance in the contract between the provider and payer. **2.** (in research) an observation that differs from all others, suggesting that a gross error has occurred in sampling, measurement, or analysis.

outline form [AS, *ut* + *lin,* thread], the shape of the cavosurface of a prepared tooth cavity before the tooth surface or surfaces are restored.

out-of-body experience (oobe), a sensation that the mind has separated temporarily from the body. The feeling tends to occur when the patient is asleep, in a trance, or unconscious as during surgery. The person visualizes his or her body as an impersonal observer might. In some cases the person visualizes objects or persons who are beyond the range of normal senses. Occasionally a patient near death learns after awakening that he or she has been declared clinically dead during the moments of the experience. See also **near-death experience.**

out of phase, a series of events or actions that are not synchronous with a previously established periodic process or phenomenon. An oscillation or periodic process that runs in an opposite direction or pattern is sometimes described as 180 degrees out of phase.

out-of-plan services, services given to a patient by a provider outside the managed care system. The patient may be responsible for a larger copayment than if the services were received within the plan.

out-of-pocket limit, the most an individual or family pays for services covered by an insurance policy.

outpatient anesthesia. See **ambulatory anesthesia.**

outpatient department, a unit of a hospital or clinic that cares for patients who need brief therapy or evaluation, or surgical procedures that do not require an overnight stay.

outpatient facilities [AS, *ut* + L, *patientia,* endurance], pertaining to a health care facility for patients who are not hospitalized or to the treatment or care of such a patient. Compare **inpatient.** Kinds include **day hospital, community mental health center.**

output [AS, *ut* + *putian,* to put], **1.** the total of any and all measurable liquids lost from the body, including urine, vomitus, and diarrhea; drainage from wounds and fistulas; and those removed by suction equipment. The output is recorded as a means of monitoring a patient's fluid and electrolyte balance. **2.** the end product of a system.

output amplifier, an apparatus used to increase the amplitude of the voltage output of a generator and control it at a specific level.

output device, any device that converts information from a computer into a form that is readable by humans or another machine, such as a printer or monitor display.

outreach program, a system of delivery of services to patients who are not likely to access treatment independently, particularly mentally ill older adults in rural environments.

O

They are considered most at risk because mental health and social services are usually not readily available. Outreach programs can diagnose and treat homebound clients with physical limitations or major psychiatric illnesses who are socially isolated.

ova.   See **ovum.**

ova and parasites test /ō″va/,   a microscopic examination of feces for parasites, such as amebas or worms and their ova, which are indicators of parasitic disorders.

ovale malaria.   See **tertian malaria.**

oval foramen,   **1.** an opening in the septum between the right and the left atria in the fetal heart. This opening provides a bypass for blood that would otherwise flow to the fetal lungs. Most of the blood from the inferior vena cava in the fetus flows through the foramen ovale into the left atrium. After birth the foramen ovale functionally closes when the newborn takes the first breath and full circulation through the lungs begins. Also called **foramen ovale.** See also **ductus arteriosus. 2.** an oval foramen situated laterally to the foramen rotundum of the sphenoid bone.

ovalocytes /ō″vəlōsīts′/   [L, *ovalis,* egg-shaped; Gk, *kytos,* cell],   elliptical or oval-shaped red blood cells with pale centers occasionally found in patients with hereditary elliptocytosis. See also **elliptocytosis.**

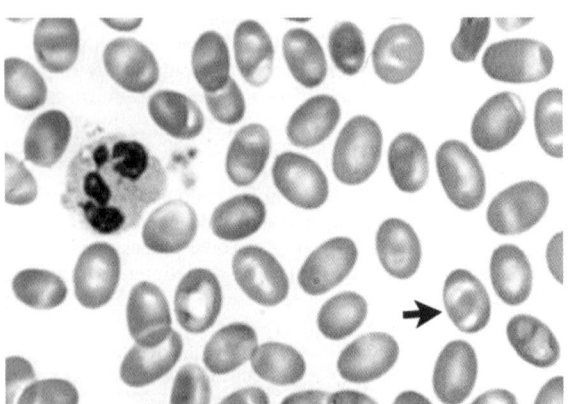

Ovalocytes *(Orkin et al, 2015)*

ovalocytosis.   See **elliptocytosis.**

oval window /ō″vəl/   [L, *ovum*; ME, *windoge*],   an aperture in the wall of the middle ear, leading to the inner ear. The footplate of the stapes vibrates in the oval window, transmitting sound waves to the cochlea. Also called **vestibular window.**

ovari-.   See **ovario-, ovari-, oario-, ootheco-.**

-ovaria,   suffix meaning "(condition of the) ovary or ovarial activity": *paraovarian.*

ovarian /ōver′ē·ən/   [L, *ovum,* egg],   pertaining to the female reproductive organ in which eggs are produced.

ovarian artery,   a slender branch of the abdominal aorta arising caudal to the renal arteries and supplying an ovary. Compare **testicular artery.**

ovarian carcinoma,   a malignant neoplasm of the ovaries rarely detected in the early stage and usually far advanced when diagnosed. It occurs frequently in the fifth decade of life. Ovarian cancer appears to be increasing in the United States. Risk factors of the disease are infertility, nulliparity or low parity, delayed childbearing, repeated spontaneous abortion, endometriosis, group A blood type, family history, previous history of breast or colorectal cancer, previous irradiation of pelvic organs, and exposure to chemical carcinogens such as asbestos and talc. Characteristics of the disease as it advances are abdominal swelling and discomfort, abnormal vaginal bleeding, weight loss, dysuria or abnormal frequency of urination, constipation, and a palpable ovarian mass, especially in postmenopausal women. Most ovarian carcinomas are papillary or serous, followed in frequency by mucinous, endometrial, and undifferentiated cancers. In many cases the cancer spreads over the surface of the peritoneum, and, early in the course of the lesion, tumor cells invade the lymphatic vessels under the diaphragm and the paraaortic nodes. Also called *ovarian cancer.*

■ OBSERVATIONS: After an insidious onset and asymptomatic period, the tumor may become evident as a palpable abdominal or pelvic mass accompanied by irregular or excessive menses or postmenopausal bleeding. In advanced cases the patient may have ascites, edema of the legs, and pain in the abdomen and the backs of the legs. Papanicolaou smear may show malignant cells if the tumor is advanced; CA-125 may be elevated; an ultrasonic examination can demonstrate an ovarian mass but does not distinguish between a benign and malignant lesion. A computed tomographic scan may be useful in detecting ovarian cancer, but a definitive diagnosis requires surgical exploration.

■ INTERVENTIONS: Approximately half of the tumors diagnosed are unresectable. Treatment of resectable lesions consists of total abdominal hysterectomy, removal of both ovaries and tubes, omentectomy, and biopsies of any suspicious sites, especially in the liver and diaphragm. Chemotherapeutic agents that may be administered after surgery include chlorambucil, cisplatin, cyclophosphamide, melphalan, taxol, docetaxel, and thiotepa. Radiation therapy may be used alone or in conjunction with chemotherapy. "Second-look" surgery is usually performed 1 year after chemotherapy to confirm the eradication of the tumor.

■ PATIENT CARE CONSIDERATIONS: Regular yearly pelvic examinations after 40 years of age contribute significantly to early diagnosis and the possibility of curative treatment.

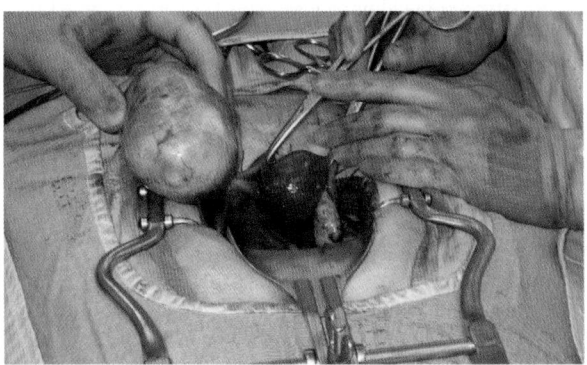

Carcinoma in the left ovary *(Baggish and Karram, 2011)*

ovarian cyst,   a globular sac filled with fluid or semisolid material that develops in or on an ovary, the female reproductive organ that produces eggs. It may be transient and physiological or pathological. Kinds include **chocolate cyst, dermoid cyst,** *corpus luteum cyst.*

ovarian fimbria,   the longest of the processes that make up the uterine fimbria tube, extending along the free border of the mesosalpinx. It is fused to the ovary so that the ostium of the tube relates to the ovary. Also called *fimbriated extremity of fallopian tube.*

ovarian follicle [L, *ovum* + *folliculus*, small bag], a cavity or recess in an ovary containing a liquor that divides the follicular cells into layers and surrounds an ovum.

ovarian hormone. See **relaxin.**

ovarian hyperstimulation syndrome (OHSS), a rare complication associated with in vitro fertilization.
- OBSERVATIONS: Pain in the left lower quadrant of the abdomen is usually noted. Ultrasonography of the pelvis is appropriate and will often reveal a cyst on the ovary. Hypercoagulability, ascites, pleural effusions, and thrombosis can occur.
- INTERVENTIONS: Conservative management is based on symptoms.
- PATIENT CARE CONSIDERATIONS: The syndrome is usually self-limited.

ovarian pregnancy, a rare type of ectopic pregnancy in which the conceptus is implanted within the ovary.

ovarian reserve, the number and quality of oocytes in the ovaries of a woman of childbearing age.

ovarian seminoma. See **dysgerminoma.**

ovarian varicocele, a varicose swelling of the veins of the uterine broad ligament. Also called **pelvic varicocele.**

ovarian vein, one of a pair of veins that emerge from convoluted plexuses in the broad ligament near the ovaries and the uterine tubes. The veins from each plexus ascend and unite to form single veins. The right ovarian vein opens into the inferior vena cava and the left ovarian vein into the renal vein. In some individuals the ovarian veins contain valves and greatly enlarge during pregnancy. Compare **testicular vein.**

ovariectomy. See **oophorectomy.**

ovario-, ovari-, oario-, ootheco-, prefix meaning "ovary": *ovariocentesis, ovariectomy.*

ovariocele /ōver″ē·əsēl/, a hernia of an ovary or protrusion of an ovary through the vaginal wall.

ovariocentesis /ōver′ē·ōsente″sis/, surgical puncture of an ovary and drainage of an ovarian cyst.

ovariohysterectomy /-his′tərek″təmē/, the surgical removal of the uterus and ovaries.

ovary /ō″vərē/ [L, *ovum,* egg], one of the paired female gonads found on each side of the lower abdomen, beside the uterus in a fold of the broad ligament. At ovulation, an egg is expelled from a follicle on the surface of the ovary under the stimulation of the gonadotrophic hormones follicle-stimulating hormone (FSH) and luteinizing hormone (LH). The remainder of the follicle (corpus luteum) secretes the hormones estrogen and progesterone, which regulate the menstrual cycle by a negative-feedback system in which an increase in estrogen decreases the secretion of FSH by the pituitary gland and an increase in progesterone decreases the secretion of LH. Each ovary is normally firm and smooth and resembles an almond in size and shape. The ovaries generally are homologous to the testes.

Ovcon, an oral contraceptive containing a progestin and an estrogen. Brand name for **norethindrone acetate and ethinyl estradiol.**

overactive bladder, a condition characterized by a nearly constant urge to urinate. Also called **irritable bladder.** See also **urgency, urinary incontinence.**
- OBSERVATIONS: The urge to urinate is difficult to control and can result in embarrassing episodes of incontinence.
- INTERVENTIONS: Bladder training and pelvic floor exercises are two common and effective treatments for overactive bladder. There are also a number of pharmacological agents that increase bladder capacity and/or help to coordinate the urinary musculature.
- PATIENT CARE CONSIDERATIONS: The need to urinate can be disruptive to the quality of life. Although common in older adults, it is not a normal component of aging. There

are physiological causes of this disorder, and those should be explored.

overbite /ō″vərbīt/ [AS, *ofer,* over, *bitan,* to bite], increased vertical overlapping of the mandibular anterior (lower front) teeth by the maxillary anterior (upper front) teeth, usually measured perpendicular to the occlusal plane. Compare **overclosure, overjet.**

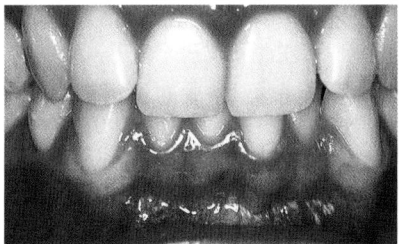

Overbite *(Nanda, 2005)*

overclosure /-klō″zhər/ [AS, *ofer* + L, *claudere,* to close], an abnormal condition in which the mandible rises beyond the point of normal occlusal contact, caused by drifting of teeth, loss of occlusal vertical dimension, change in tooth shapes through grinding, or loss of teeth.

overcoat /ō″vər-kōt/, See *abrasion layer.*

overcompensation /-kom′pənsā″shən/ [AS, *ofer* + L, *compensare,* to weigh together], an exaggerated attempt to overcome a real or imagined physical or psychological deficit. The attempt may be conscious or unconscious. See also **compensation.**

overdenture /-den″chər/ [AS, *ofer* + L, *dens,* tooth], a complete or partial removable denture supported by retained roots or teeth to provide improved support, stability, and tactile and proprioceptive sensation and to reduce bone resorption.

overdose (OD) /-dōs/, an excessive use of a drug, resulting in adverse reactions ranging from mania or hysteria to coma or death.

overdrive suppression /-drīv/ [AS, *ofer* + *drifan,* to drive], the inhibitory effect of a faster cardiac pacemaker on a slower one.

overeruption /-irup″shən/, the projection of a tooth beyond the normal occlusal plane. Also called **supereruption, supraclusion, supraocclusion.**

overflow /-flō/ [AS, *ofer* + *flowan*], the flooding or excessive discharge of a fluid, such as urine, saliva, or bile.

overflow incontinence [AS, *ofer* + *flowan* + L, *incontinentia,* inability to retain], an overflow of urine from a distended paralyzed bladder. See also **incontinence, urinary incontinence.**

overgrafting /-graf″ting/, placing an additional transplant over a previously healed tissue graft. It is sometimes performed to strengthen a split-thickness graft or to replace epithelium that may have been lost.

overgrowth [AS, *ofer* + ME, *growen*], an excessive growth, usually referring to organ or tissue development. Also called **hypertrophy.**

overhang /-hang/ [AS, *ofer* + *hangian,* to hang], an excess of dental filling material that projects beyond the margin of a tooth cavity preparation. It can trigger gingivitis, periodontitis, or caries by providing a harbor for bacteria.

overhydration /-hīdrā″shən/, an excess of water in the body. Also called **hyperhydration.**

overinclusiveness /-inkloo″sivnəs/ [AS, *ofer* + L, *includere,* to include], a type of association disorder observed in some schizophrenia patients. The individual is unable to think in a precise manner because of an inability to keep irrelevant elements outside perceptual boundaries.

overjet /-jet/ [AS, *ofer* + Fr, *jeter,* to throw], increased projection of the upper teeth in front of the lower teeth, usually measured parallel to the occlusal plane. Also called **horizontal overlap.** Compare **overbite, overclosure.**

overlap /-lap″/, to extend over and cover part of an existing surface or structure.

overlay /ō″vərlā/, to add to an existing condition or structure; to lay on top of something.

overlearning /-lur″ning/, the practice of a task that continues beyond the point where performance meets a specified standard so that the task becomes automatic.

overload /-lōd/, **1.** a burden greater than the capacity of the system designed to move or process it. **2.** (in physiology) any factor or influence that stresses the body beyond its natural limits and may impair its health.

overnutrition /-nŌotrish″ən/, a condition of excess nutrient and energy intake over time. Overnutrition may be regarded as a form of malnutrition when it leads to morbid obesity.

overoxygenation /-ok″sijənā″shən/ [AS, *ofer* + Gk, *oxys,* sharp, *genein,* to produce; L, *atio,* process], an abnormal condition in which the oxygen concentration in the blood and other tissues of the body is greater than normal. The condition is characterized by a fall in blood pressure, decreased vital capacity, fatigue, errors in judgment, paresthesia of the hands and feet, anorexia, nausea, vomiting, and hyperemia.

overresponse /-rispons″/, an abnormally strong reaction to a stimulus.

overriding /-rī″ding/ [AS, *ofer* + *ridan*], **1.** *n.,* the slipping of either part of a fractured bone past the other. **2.** *adj.,* extending beyond the usual position.

overripe cataract /-rīp/ [AS, *ofer* + OE, *reap*], a cataract in which a completely opaque lens solidifies and shrinks.

oversensing /-sen″sing/, the sensation of stimuli, such as magnetism or static electricity, that are not normally detected by the sense organs.

overshoot /ō″vərshŌot″/, **1.** *v.,* to go beyond or exceed a target or goal. **2.** *n.,* an upper part of a structure that extends beyond the lower part.

over the counter (OTC), (in pharmacology) medications and agents available to the consumer without a prescription.

overtone, 1. any tone produced by voice or a musical instrument that is of a higher frequency than the lowest or fundamental tone of a sound. **2.** a harmonic.

overweight /-wāt/ [AS, *ofer* + *gewiht,* weight], **1.** more than normal in body weight after adjustment for height, body build, and age, or 10% to 20% above the person's "desirable" body weight. **2.** a body mass index between 25.0 and 29.9. See also **body mass index.**

overwintering /-win″təring/, persistence of seasonal infectious agents beyond their normal period of activity, particularly warm weather pathogen vectors that remain operative into the winter months.

ovi-, ovo-, combining form meaning "ovum" or "egg": *ovicide, ovipositor, ovoplasm.*

ovicidal /ō′visī″dəl/, causing destruction of an ovum.

ovicide /ō″visīd/, an agent that destroys ova.

oviduct. See **fallopian tube.**

oviferous /ōvif″ərəs/ [L, *ovum,* egg, *ferre,* to bear], bearing or capable of producing ova (egg cells).

oviparous /ōvip″ərəs/ [L, *ovum* + *parere,* to bring forth], giving birth to young by laying eggs. Compare **ovoviviparous, viviparous.**

oviposition /ō′vipəsish″ən/ [L, *ovum* + *ponere,* to place], the act of laying or depositing eggs by a female oviparous animal.

ovipositor /ō′vipos″itər/ [L, *ovum* + *ponere,* to place], a specialized organ, found primarily in insects, for depositing eggs on plants or in the soil. It may be modified into a stinger, as in worker bees and wasps.

ovo-. See **ovi-, ovo-.**

ovocenter /ō′vəsen″tər/ [L, *ovum* + *centrum,* center], the centrosome of a fertilized ovum. Also called **oocenter.**

ovoflavin /ō′vəflā″vin/ [L, *ovum* + *flavus,* yellow], a riboflavin derived from the yolk of eggs.

ovogenesis. See **oogenesis.**

ovoglobulin /ō′vəglob″yŌolin/ [L, *ovum* + *globulus,* small sphere], a globulin protein derived from the white of eggs.

ovogonium. See **oogonium.**

ovoid /ō″void/, egg-shaped; oval.

ovoid arch [L, *ovum* + Gk, *eidos,* form; L, *arcus,* bow], a dental arch that curves smoothly from the molars on one side to those on the opposite side to form half an oval.

ovo-lacto-vegetarian. See **lacto-ovo-vegetarian.**

ovomucin /ō′vəmyŌo″sin/ [L, *ovum* + *mucus,* slime], a glycoprotein derived from the white of eggs.

ovomucoid /ō′vəmyŌo″koid/ [L, *ovum* + *mucus,* slime; Gk, *eidos,* form], pertaining to a glycoprotein, similar to mucin, derived from the white of eggs.

ovoplasm. See **ooplasm.**

ovotestis /ō′vətes″tis/ [L, *ovum* + *testis,* testicle], a gonad that contains both ovarian and testicular tissue; a hermaphroditic gonad. −*ovotesticular, adj.*

ovo-vegetarian. See **vegetarian.**

ovovitellin. See **vitellin.**

ovoviviparous /ō′vəvivip″ərəs/ [L, *ovum* + *vivus,* living, *parere,* to bring forth], bearing young in eggs that are hatched within the body, as in some reptiles and fishes. Compare **oviparous, viviparous.**

Ovral, an oral contraceptive containing a progestin and an estrogen. Brand name for **norgestrel, ethinyl estradiol.**

Ovrette, an oral contraceptive containing a progestin. Brand name for **norgestrel.**

OVTT, abbreviation for **optometric vision therapy technician.**

ovulation /ov′yəlā″shən/ [L, *ovum* + *atio,* process], expulsion of an ovum from the ovary on spontaneous rupture of a mature follicle as a result of cyclic ovarian and pituitary endocrine function. It usually occurs on or about the eleventh to the fourteenth day before the next menstrual period and may cause brief, sharp lower abdominal pain on the side of the ovulating ovary. See also **oogenesis.** −*ovulate, v.*

ovulation method of family planning, a natural method of family planning that uses observation of changes in the character and quantity of cervical mucus to determine the time of ovulation during the menstrual cycle. Because pregnancy occurs with fertilization of an ovum extruded from the ovary at ovulation, the method is used to increase or decrease the woman's chance of becoming pregnant by causing or avoiding insemination by spontaneous or artificial means during the fertile period associated with ovulation. The cyclic changes in gonadotropic hormones, especially estrogen, cause changes in the quantity and character of cervical mucus. In the first days after menstruation, scant thick mucus is secreted by the cervix. These "dry days" are "safe days," with ovulation several days away. The quantity of mucus then increases; it is pearly white and sticky, becoming clearer and less sticky as ovulation approaches; these "wet days" are "unsafe days." During and just after ovulation the mucus is clear, slippery, and elastic; it resembles the uncooked white of an egg. The day on which this sign is most apparent is the "peak day," probably the day before ovulation. The 4 days after the "peak day" are "unsafe"; fertilization might occur. By the end of the 4 days, the mucus becomes pearly white and sticky again and progressively decreases in quantity until menstruation supervenes to begin a new cycle. Essential to the effectiveness of this method are thorough instruction by a family planning counselor and strong self-motivation in the couple. During the first cycle, abstinence may be necessary to allow observation of the mucus without the confusing addition of semen or contraceptive foam, cream, or jelly, if being used. Daily close monitoring of the mucus is necessary even after several cycles because the length of the "safe" and "unsafe" periods and the time of ovulation vary from cycle to cycle, as they do from woman to woman. After delivery and during lactation the method is not effective until the menses have become regular. Effectiveness of the method in identifying the most fertile days of the cycle is augmented by using the basal body temperature method. This combined method is called the symptothermal method of planning. Proponents of the ovulation method claim the benefits of low cost, naturalness, and effectiveness. Detractors emphasize a limited public health application of the method, stating that it requires extensive teaching and self-motivation and that its effectiveness is limited by the ability of the user to observe correctly and diligently the changes in the cervical mucus. Abstinence may be necessary for up to 10 days by a woman whose menstrual cycles are long or are of irregular length. Also called **Billings method, cervical mucus method of family planning.**

ovulatory /ov″yələtôr′ē/ [L, *ovum*], pertaining to ovulation.

ovulatory phase, the second phase of the human menstrual cycle, during which the luteinizing hormone surge, the follicle-stimulating hormone surge, and ovulation occur. It is followed by the luteal phase.

ovulocyclic /ov′yəlōsī″klik/, pertaining to recurrent events associated with the ovulatory cycle.

ovulocyclic porphyria, episodes of acute abnormalities of porphyrin metabolism that tend to recur in the premenstrual period.

ovum /ō″vəm/ *pl. ova* [L, egg], **1.** an egg. **2.** the secondary oocyte (female germ cell) extruded from the ovary at ovulation.

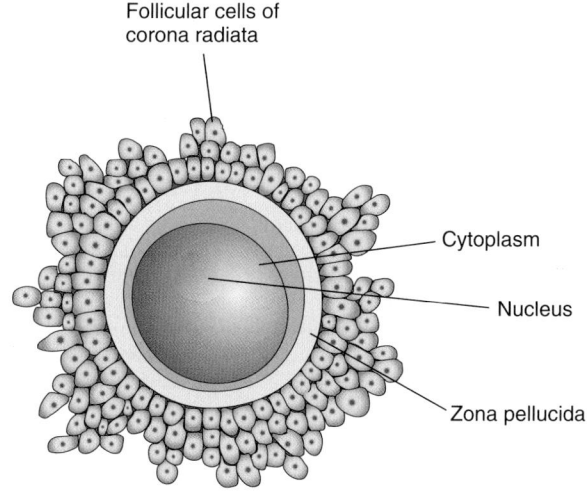

Follicular cells of corona radiata

Cytoplasm

Nucleus

Zona pellucida

Ovum *(Moore, Persaud, and Torchia, 2016)*

owl-eye cell, an enlarged cell infected by cytomegalovirus and containing large inclusion bodies, found mainly in the renal epithelium.

Owren disease [Paul A. Owren, Norwegian hematologist, 1905–1990], a rare autosomal-recessive congenital bleeding disorder caused by a deficiency of coagulation factor V. It is characterized by easy bruising at an early age and other hemophilia-like symptoms. Also called **parahemophilia.**

ox-, oxi-, combining form meaning "presence of oxygen": *oxidize.*

oxacillin sodium /ok′səsil″in/, a semisynthetic, penicillinase-resistant penicillin antibiotic.

■ INDICATIONS: It is prescribed in the treatment of severe bacterial infections caused by penicillinase-producing staphylococci.

■ CONTRAINDICATIONS: Known hypersensitivity to this drug or to any other penicillin prohibits its use.

■ ADVERSE EFFECTS: Among the most serious effects are anaphylaxis and other less severe allergic reactions, GI disturbances, and pruritus ani and vulvae.

-oxacin, suffix for nalidixic acid–type antibacterial agents.

oxal-, oxalo-, combining form indicating molecules derived from oxalic acid: *oxalate.*

oxalate $(C_2O_4{}^{2-})$ /ok″səlāt/, an anion of oxalic acid.

oxalated blood /ok″səlā′tid/, blood to which a soluble ester of oxalic acid has been added to prevent coagulation.

oxalemia /ok′səlē″mē·ə/, elevated levels of oxalates in the blood.

oxalic acid $(H_2C_2O_4)$ /oksal″ik/, a member of a family of dibasic acids found in many common plants, such as buckwheat, wood sorrel, and rhubarb. It is an important reagent and is used in bleaching and drying. Poisonous if ingested in excessive amounts, oxalic acid is used in veterinary medicine as a hemostatic. In dietary intake of foods containing oxalic acid, the substance binds with calcium and is sometimes found in renal calculi and the urine of patients with hyperoxaluria. Also called **ethanedioic acid.**

oxaliplatin, an antineoplastic agent used to treat metastatic carcinoma of the colon or rectum in combination with 5-FU/leucovorin.

oxalosis /ok′səlō″sis/, a condition in which calcium oxalate crystals accumulate in the kidneys, heart, and other organs and urinary excretion of oxalate increases. Oxalosis-inducing agents include oxalic acid, methoxyflurane, ethylene glycol, and ascorbic acid.

oxaluric acid /ok′səloor″ik/, a compound derived from uric acid or from parabanic acid, which occurs in normal urine.

-oxan, suffix for benzodioxan-derived alpha-adrenoceptor antagonists.

oxandrolone /oksan″drəlōn/, an androgen.

■ INDICATIONS: It is prescribed in the treatment of bone pain accompanying osteoporosis and for the stimulation of weight gain after extensive surgery or trauma or when a pathophysiological reason exists for failure to maintain normal weight.

■ CONTRAINDICATIONS: Cancer of the male breast or prostate, liver disease, pregnancy or suspected pregnancy, or known hypersensitivity to this drug prohibits its use.

■ ADVERSE EFFECTS: Among the more serious adverse reactions are hirsutism, acne, liver toxicity, electrolyte imbalances, and various endocrine effects in some patients.

oxaprozin /ok″säpro′zin/, a nonsteroidal antiinflammatory drug, used in treatment of arthritis.

oxazepam /oksā″zəpam/, a benzodiazepine tranquilizer.

■ INDICATIONS: It is prescribed to relieve anxiety and nervous tension and manage ethanol withdrawal, and it has unlabeled use for treatment of simple partial seizures.

O

■ CONTRAINDICATIONS: Acute narrow-angle glaucoma, psychotic disorders, or known hypersensitivity to this drug prohibits its use.

■ ADVERSE EFFECTS: Among the more serious adverse effects are withdrawal symptoms resulting from discontinuation of treatment. Dizziness and fatigue commonly occur.

oxazolidinone /ok″säzo-lid′ĭ-nōn/, any of a class of synthetic antibacterial agents effective against gram-positive organisms.

oxcarbazepine /oks″kär-baz′ĕ-pēn/, an anticonvulsant used in the treatment of partial seizures. It is administered orally.

-oxef, suffix for oxacefalosporanic acid–derived antibiotics.

-oxemia, suffix meaning a "(specified) state of oxygen in the blood": *anoxemia, hyperoxemia, hypoxemia.*

-oxia, suffix meaning "(condition of) oxygenation": *anoxia, normoxia, hypoxia.*

oxiconazole /ok″sĭ-kon′äzōl/, a topical antifungal agent used as the nitrate salt in the treatment of athlete's foot and ringworm.

oxidant /ok″sidənt/ [Gk, *oxys,* sharp], an oxidizing agent.

oxidase /ok″sidās/ [Gk, *oxys,* sharp], an enzyme that induces biological oxidation by activating the oxygen in molecules containing the element, such as hydrogen peroxide.

oxidation /ok′sidā″shən/ [Gk, *oxys,* sharp, *genein,* to produce, L, *atio,* process], **1.** any process in which the oxygen content in a compound or the number of bonds to oxygen (or another electronegative element, such as a halogen) is increased. **2.** any reaction in which the positive valence of a compound or a radical is increased because of a loss of electrons. **3.** any process in which the hydrogen content in a compound or the number of bonds to hydrogen (or another element of low electronegativity, such as a metal) is decreased. *–oxidative, n.,* **–oxidize,** *v.*

oxidation-reduction reaction, a chemical change in which electrons are removed (oxidation) from an atom, ion, or molecule, accompanied by a simultaneous transfer of electrons (reduction) to another. The reaction may also involve the transfer of electronegative atoms (e.g., oxygen) or atoms of low electronegativity (e.g., hydrogen or metal) from one molecule to another. Also called **redox.**

oxidative phosphorylation /ok″sidā′tiv/, an ATP-generating process in which oxygen serves as the final electron acceptor. The process occurs in mitochondria and is the major source of adenosine triphosphate generation in aerobic organisms.

oxidative stress, **1.** any of various pathological changes seen in living organisms in response to excessive levels of cytotoxic oxidants and free radicals in the environment. **2.** use of antioxidant intake in the diet to provide both preventive and therapeutic advantage and reduce the damaging effects of free radicals on cellular constituents.

oxidative water [Gk, *oxys,* sharp, *genein,* to produce; L, *ativus,* related to], water produced by the oxidation of molecules of food substances, such as the conversion of glucose to water and carbon dioxide.

oxide /ok″sīd/, **1.** a compound of oxygen and another element or radical. **2.** a dianion of oxygen, O^{2-}.

oxidize /ok″sidīz/ [Gk, *oxys,* sharp, *genein,* to produce, *izein,* to cause], (of an element or compound) to combine or cause to combine with oxygen, to remove hydrogen, or to increase the valence of an element through the loss of electrons. *–oxidizing, adj.,* **–oxidation,** *n.*

oxidizing agent, a compound that readily gives up oxygen or accepts hydrogen or electrons from another compound. In chemical reactions an oxidizing agent acts as an acceptor of electrons, thereby increasing the valence of an element.

oxidoreductase /ok′sidō′riduk″tās/, an enzyme that catalyzes a reaction in which one substance is oxidized while another is reduced. Kinds include *alcohol dehydrogenase.*

oximeter /oksim″ətər/, a device used to measure oxyhemoglobin in arterial blood. See also **pulse oximeter.**

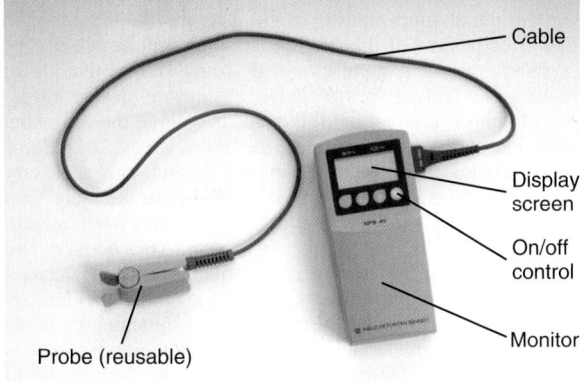

Labels: Cable, Display screen, On/off control, Monitor, Probe (reusable)

Pulse oximeter *(Bonewit-West, 2013)*

oximetry, a photodiagnostic method of monitoring arterial blood oxygen saturation (SaO_2). Oximetry is commonly used to titrate levels of oxygen in hospitalized patients. It is used for monitoring the patient's oxygenation status during the perioperative period or any other time of heavy sedation, during mechanical ventilation, and in many clinical situations, such as pulmonary rehabilitation programs and stress testing. See also **pulse oximeter.**

oxprenolol /oks-pren′älol/, a nonselective beta-adrenergic blocking agent, administered orally as the hydrochloride salt in the treatment of hypertension, hypertrophic cardiomyopathy, cardiac arrhythmias, and myocardial infarction.

Oxsoralen, a pigmentation agent. Brand name for **methoxsalen.**

oxtriphylline /oks′trəfil″ēn/, a bronchodilator.

■ INDICATIONS: It is prescribed in the treatment of bronchial asthma, bronchitis, and emphysema.

■ CONTRAINDICATIONS: Known hypersensitivity to this drug or other xanthine derivatives prohibits its use. It is used with caution in patients with ulcer or coronary disease for whom cardiac stimulation might be harmful.

■ ADVERSE EFFECTS: Among the more common adverse effects are GI distress, palpitations, nervousness, and insomnia.

oxy-, **1.** prefix meaning "sharp," "quick," or "sour": *oxyacoia.* **2.** prefix indicating the presence of oxygen in a compound: *oxyhemoglobin.*

oxyacoia, an abnormal hearing acuity. Increased sensitivity to sound is sometimes associated with paralysis of the stapedius muscle.

oxybenzene. See **carbolic acid.**

oxybutynin chloride /ok′sibo͞o″tinin/, an anticholinergic drug.

■ INDICATIONS: It is prescribed in the treatment of neurogenic bladder.

■ CONTRAINDICATIONS: Glaucoma, obstruction of the GI or urinary tract, ulcerative colitis, paralytic ileus, toxic megacolon, or known hypersensitivity to this drug or to other anticholinergics prohibits its use.

■ ADVERSE EFFECTS: Among the more serious adverse effects are decreased sweating, urinary retention, blurred vision, tachycardia, and severe allergic reactions.

oxycalorimeter /ok′sēkal′ôrim″ətər/, an apparatus that measures the heat of combustion of organic materials in terms of oxygen consumed. Each liter of oxygen is roughly equivalent to 5 calories.

oxycellulose /ok′sēsel″yəlōs/, **1.** cellulose that has been oxidized so that all or most of the glucose residues have been converted to glucuronic acid residues for use as an absorbent in chromatography. **2.** cellulose that has been partially oxidized for use as a local hemostatic.

oxycephaly /ok′sisef″əlē/ [Gk, *oxys* + *kephale,* head], a congenital malformation of the skull in which premature closure of the coronal and sagittal sutures results in accelerated upward growth of the head, giving it a long, narrow appearance with the top pointed or conic. Also called **acrocephaly, hypsicephaly,** *oxycephalia,* **steeple head, tower head, tower skull, turricephaly.** See also **craniostenosis.** −*oxycephalous, oxycephalus, n.*

oxycodone hydrochloride /ok″sikōdōn/, an opioid agonist.

■ INDICATIONS: It is used to treat moderate to severe pain, often in combination with nonopioid analgesics. OxyContin is a formulation that should be used only when severe persistent pain is anticipated.

■ CONTRAINDICATIONS: It is used with caution in many conditions, including head injuries, asthma, impaired renal or hepatic function, or unstable cardiovascular status. Known hypersensitivity to this drug prohibits its use.

■ ADVERSE EFFECTS: Among the most serious adverse effects are drowsiness, dizziness, nausea, constipation, respiratory and circulatory depression, and drug addiction.

oxygen (O) /ok″səjən/ [Gk, *oxys,* sharp, *genein,* to produce], a tasteless, odorless, colorless gas essential for human respiration and metabolism. Its atomic number is 8; its atomic mass is 15.9994. Oxygen makes up approximately 21% of the gases in the atmosphere. In anesthesia, oxygen functions as a carrier gas for the delivery of anesthetic agents to tissues. In respiratory therapy, oxygen is administered to increase the amount circulating in the blood. Overdose of oxygen can cause irreversible toxicity in people with pulmonary abnormalities, especially when complicated by chronic carbon dioxide retention. Prolonged administration of high concentrations of oxygen may cause irreversible retinal damage to infants' eyes. An oxygen-rich environment is favorable to fire and explosion. Thus smoking, open flame, or electric spark must be avoided when oxygen is being administered. See also **oxygen toxicity.**

oxygenation /ok′səjənā″shən/, **1.** the process of combining or treating with oxygen. **2.** the passive diffusion of oxygen from the alveolus to the pulmonary capillary, where it binds to hemoglobin in red blood cells or dissolves into the plasma. −*oxygenate, v.*

oxygen capacity of blood, the maximum amount of oxygen that can combine chemically with a given amount of hemoglobin in blood. It does not include oxygen dissolved in plasma. Although 1 g of hemoglobin theoretically can bind a maximum of 1.34 mL of oxygen at standard temperature and pressure, this value is never actually achieved in vivo because of factors such as the formation of carboxyhemoglobin and the presence of methemoglobin or other inactive hemoglobins.

oxygen concentration in blood, the concentration of oxygen in a blood sample, including both oxygen combined with hemoglobin and oxygen dissolved in the plasma.

oxygen consumption, the amount of oxygen used by the body per minute. For normal aerobic metabolism, it is about 250 mL/min. Also called **oxygen uptake.**

oxygen cost of breathing, the rate at which the respiratory muscles consume oxygen as they ventilate the lungs.

oxygen debt, the quantity of oxygen that the lungs take up during recovery from exercise or apnea that is in excess of the quantity needed for resting metabolism before the exercise or apnea. Oxygen debt represents replenishment of the oxygen store that was depleted during the time that oxygen uptake from the air was inadequate for aerobic metabolism. See also **oxygen consumption.**

oxygen delivery system, a device that delivers oxygen through the upper airways to the lungs at concentrations above that of ambient air. There are two general types: the high-flow oxygen delivery system, which can supply all of the needs of a patient for inspired gas at a given fractional inspired oxygen, and the low-flow oxygen delivery system, which cannot supply all of the patient's needs for oxygen and delivers fractional inspired oxygen that varies with ventilatory demand.

oxygen dissociation curve, graphic expression of the affinity of hemoglobin for oxygen as a function of the partial pressure of oxygen. Dissociation is influenced by pH, temperature, and carbon dioxide pressure. Formerly called *oxyhemoglobin dissociation curve.*

oxygen enhancement ratio (OER), a measure of tumor sensitivity to the presence or absence of oxygen, expressed as the ratio of radiation dose required to produce a given effect with no oxygen present to the dose required to produce the same effect in 1 atmosphere of air.

oxygen hood, a device placed over the head of a patient to deliver high concentrations of oxygen.

oxygen mask, a device used to administer oxygen, shaped to fit snugly over the mouth and nose and secured in place with a strap or held with the hand. The mask has inspiratory and expiratory valves allowing oxygen to be inhaled or pumped into the respiratory tract and carbon dioxide to be exhaled into the environment. Oxygen flows at a prescribed rate through a catheter to the mask. See also **Ambu bag.**

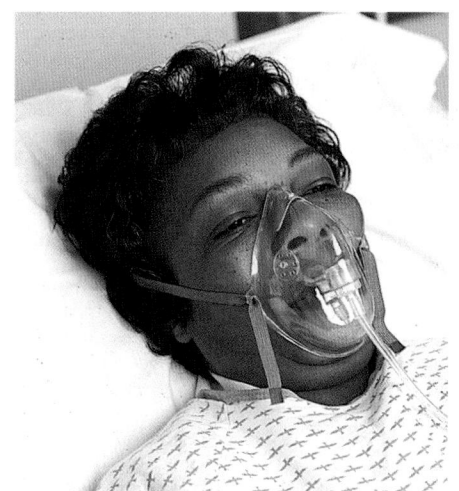

Oxygen mask *(Potter et al, 2011)*

oxygen P50, the oxygen pressure necessary for 50% saturation of hemoglobin at body temperature and at pH 7.4 or for 40 mm Hg of carbon dioxide pressure. The P50 is used as a measure of hemoglobin affinity for oxygen.

oxygen radicals [Gk, *oxys,* sharp; L, *radix,* root], a substituent group of chemical elements rich in oxygen but incapable of prolonged existence in a free state. Oxygen radicals are used in some types of therapy.

oxygen saturation,   **1.** the fraction of the hemoglobin molecules in a blood sample that are saturated with oxygen at a given partial pressure of oxygen. Normal saturation is 95% to 100%. **2.** percentage of hemoglobin-bound oxygen compared to total capacity of the hemoglobin.

oxygen store,   the total quantity of oxygen stored in various body compartments, including the lungs, arterial and venous blood, and tissues. In a human weighing 70 kg, blood contains about 800 mL of oxygen as oxyhemoglobin, muscles contain about 150 mL as oxymyoglobin, alveolar gas contains a few hundred milliliters, and about 50 mL is dissolved in the tissues.

oxygen tension,   the partial pressure of oxygen molecules dissolved in a liquid, such as blood plasma.

oxygen tent [Gk, *oxys*, sharp; ME, *tente*],   a canopy that encloses the head and neck of a patient and provides humidified oxygen. See also **Croupette.**

oxygen therapy,   any procedure in which oxygen is administered to a patient to relieve hypoxia.

■ METHOD: Of the many methods for providing oxygen therapy, the one selected depends on the condition of the patient and the cause of hypoxia. Low or moderate amounts of oxygen may be supplied to postoperative patients by a nasal catheter or cannula. A precise amount of oxygen may be delivered by a Venturi mask. Patients with chronic obstructive lung disease must receive low-flow oxygen to prevent the elimination of their stimulus to breathe (low O_2 levels). If hypoxia is the result of impaired cardiac function, a high concentration of oxygen may be delivered by a nonrebreathing or partial rebreathing mask. Humidity and drugs in aerosol form may be given with oxygen through a variety of devices, such as an aerosol face mask, Croupette, or T-piece.

■ INTERVENTIONS: Thorough and careful observation of the patient's need for oxygen and response to therapy are important. The concentration of oxygen received by the patient must not be assumed by the rate and concentration at which it is delivered; a person whose respirations are rapid and shallow receives more oxygen than does a person breathing deeply and slowly. Many clinical situations require frequent laboratory evaluations of the levels of arterial blood gases or oxygen saturation levels by means of pulse oximetry. Thorough knowledge of the equipment used and the condition being treated enables the health care professional to care safely and effectively for the patient who requires oxygen.

■ OUTCOME CRITERIA: Oxygen therapy may be used in the treatment of any condition that results in hypoxia. Although there are several kinds of hypoxia, all result in hypoxemia. Oxygen administration may relieve hypotension, cardiac arrhythmias, tachypnea, headache, disorientation, nausea, and agitation characteristic of hypoxia, as well as restore the ability of the cells of the body to carry on normal metabolic function.

oxygen tolerance,   an increased capacity to withstand the toxic effects of abnormally high oxygen tension as a result of any adaptive change occurring within an organism.

oxygen toxicity,   a condition of oxygen overdosage that can result in pathological tissue changes, such as retinopathy of prematurity or bronchopulmonary dysplasia. It can also decrease the hypoxic drive to breathe.

oxygen transport,   the process by which oxygen is absorbed by red blood cell hemoglobin in the lungs and carried to the peripheral tissues. Hemoglobin combines with oxygen when present at a high concentration, such as in the lungs, and releases oxygen when the concentration is low, such as in the peripheral tissues. See also **hemoglobin.**

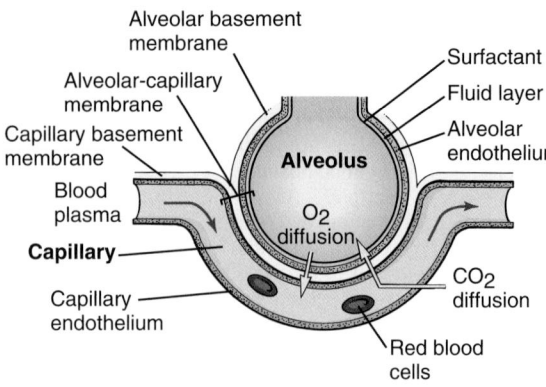

Oxygen transport *(Beare and Myers, 1998)*

oxygen uptake (VO_2).   See **oxygen consumption.**

oxygen-utilization coefficient,   the extraction coefficient for oxygen in any given tissue. See also **coefficient.**

oxyhemoglobin   /ok′sēhē″məglō′bin, -hem″-/   [Gk, *oxys + genein,* to produce, *haima,* blood; L, *globus,* ball],   the product of combining hemoglobin with oxygen. The loosely bound complex dissociates easily when the concentration of oxygen is low. Also spelled *oxyhaemoglobin.*

oxymesterone /ok′sēmes″tərōn/,   an androgen and anabolic steroid involved in tissue building.

oxymetazoline hydrochloride   /ok′sēmətaz″əlēn/,   an adrenergic vasoconstrictor.

■ INDICATIONS: It is prescribed topically in the treatment of nasal congestion and for the relief of eye redness caused by minor eye irritation.

■ CONTRAINDICATIONS: Hyperthyroidism, diabetes, use of a monoamine oxidase inhibitor within 14 days, or known hypersensitivity to this drug prohibits its use.

■ ADVERSE EFFECTS: Among the more serious adverse effects are rebound congestion, central nervous system stimulation, hypertension, and transient stinging.

oxymetholone /ok′sēmeth″əlōn/,   an anabolic steroid.

■ INDICATIONS: It is prescribed in the treatment of anemias caused by antineoplastic drugs.

■ CONTRAINDICATIONS: Cancer of the male breast or prostate, liver disease, pregnancy or suspected pregnancy, or known hypersensitivity to this drug prohibits its use.

■ ADVERSE EFFECTS: Among the more serious adverse effects are hirsutism, acne, liver toxicity, electrolyte imbalances, and, depending on the patient's age, various endocrine effects.

oxymorphone hydrochloride /ok′sēmôr″fōn/,   an opioid analgesic.

■ INDICATIONS: It is prescribed for relief of moderate to severe pain, as a preoperative medication, and to support anesthesia.

■ CONTRAINDICATIONS: Drug dependence, increased intracranial pressure, respiratory depression, or known hypersensitivity to this drug prohibits its use. It should not be used for extended periods during pregnancy.

■ ADVERSE EFFECTS: Among the more serious adverse effects are drug dependence, urinary retention, and respiratory or circulatory depression.

oxyntic cells,   hydrochloric acid–producing cells of the stomach. Also called **parietal cells.**

oxyopia /ok′sē·ō″pē·ə/   [Gk, *oxys + opsis* vision],   unusual acuteness of vision. A person with normal (20/20) vision when standing 20 feet (approximately 6 meters) from the standard Snellen eye chart can read the seventh line of letters, each of which is an eighth of an inch high. An individual with oxyopia can read smaller letters at that distance. Also called *oxyopy.*

oxyphil cell /ok″səfil/, a cell of the parathyroid glands that takes up acidic stains and has a dark nucleus and fine, granular cytoplasm. Such cells occur singly or in small groups and increase in number with age. Also called *oxyphilic cell.*

oxytalan /ok′sētal″ən, oksit′ələn/, a type of connective tissue fiber particular to the periodontal membrane. These fine, elastic-like fibers bend to attach to the tooth surface.

oxytetracycline /ok′sētet′rəsī″klēn/, a tetracycline antibiotic.

■ INDICATIONS: It is prescribed in the treatment of bacterial and rickettsial infections.

■ CONTRAINDICATIONS: Pregnancy, early childhood, or known hypersensitivity to this or other tetracyclines prohibits its use. It is used with caution in patients who have renal or liver dysfunction.

■ ADVERSE EFFECTS: Among the more serious adverse effects are GI disturbances, phototoxicity, potentially serious superinfections, and various hypersensitivity reactions. Discoloration of teeth may occur in children exposed to the drug in utero or before 8 years of age.

oxytetracycline calcium, a tetracycline antibiotic.

oxytocia /ok′sētō″shə/, rapid childbirth.

oxytocic /ok′sitō″sik/ [Gk, *oxys* + *tokos,* birth], **1.** pertaining to a substance that is similar to the hormone oxytocin. **2.** any one of numerous drugs that stimulates the smooth muscle of the uterus to contract. The administration of an oxytocic can initiate and enhance rhythmic uterine contraction at any time, but relatively high doses are required for such responses in early pregnancy. Oxytocic agents commonly used include oxytocin, certain prostaglandins, and the ergot alkaloids. These drugs are used to induce or augment labor at term, control postpartum hemorrhage, correct postpartum uterine atony, produce uterine contractions after cesarean section or other uterine surgery, and induce therapeutic abortion. These drugs are used with extreme caution in parturients with severe hypotension and hypertension, partial placenta previa, cephalopelvic disproportion, or grand multiparity. The risk of using these agents is much higher in mothers who have undergone recent uterine surgery or who have suffered recent sepsis or trauma. The most serious adverse reaction is sustained tetanic contraction of the uterus, resulting in fetal hypoxia or rupture of the uterus.

oxytocin /ok′sitō″sin/, **1.** a polypeptide secreted by magnocellular neurons in the hypothalamus and stored as a posterior pituitary hormone along with vasopressin. It promotes uterine contractions and milk ejection and contributes to the second stage of labor. **2.** a uterotonic.

■ INDICATIONS: It is prescribed to stimulate contractions in inducing or augmenting labor and to contract the uterus to control postpartum bleeding.

■ CONTRAINDICATIONS: Cephalopelvic disproportion, unfavorable fetal position, or known hypersensitivity to this drug prohibits its use.

■ ADVERSE EFFECTS: Among the more serious adverse effects are tetanic contraction, jaundice, uterine rupture, and fetal anoxia.

oxytocin challenge test, a stress test for the assessment of intrauterine function of the fetus and the placenta. It is performed to evaluate the ability of the fetus to tolerate continuation of pregnancy or the anticipated stress of labor and delivery. A dilute IV infusion of oxytocin is begun, regulated by an infusion pump. The uterine activity is monitored with a tocodynamometer, and the fetal heart rate is monitored with an ultrasonic sensor as the uterus is stimulated to contract by the oxytocin. The amount of solution infused is increased as necessary to cause the uterus to contract for 30 to 40 seconds three times every 10 minutes. The fetal heart rate is observed for variability and for the timing of any marked variation from the normal in relation to uterine contractions. Decelerations of the fetal heart rate in certain repeating patterns may indicate fetal distress. One quarter of the infants diagnosed by this method as being in distress are normal. Therefore, other tests of fetal well-being are recommended before performing an emergency cesarean section or induction of labor.

oxyuriasis. See **enterobiasis.**

oxyuricide /ok′sē-o͞o′risīd/, an agent that destroys pinworms.

Oxyuris vermicularis. See *Enterobius vermicularis.*

oz, abbreviation for **ounce.**

oz ap [L, *uncia*], a unit of weight equal to 31.1035 grams. Abbreviation for *apothecary ounce.*

ozena /ōzē″nə/ [Gk, *ozein,* to have an odor], a condition of the nose characterized by atrophy of the nasal conchae and mucous membranes. Symptoms include crusting of nasal secretions, discharge, and, especially, a very offensive odor. Ozena may follow chronic inflammation of the nasal mucosa.

ozone (O_3) [Gk, *ozein,* to have an odor], an allotropic form of oxygen consisting of molecules containing three oxygen atoms. Ozone is formed when oxygen is present in an electric discharge, as might occur in a lightning storm. Ozone is used as a bleaching, cleaning, and oxidizing agent and has a faint, chlorinelike odor.

ozone hole, a seasonal depletion of the steady-state ozone concentration in the stratosphere, particularly over Antarctica. Depletion of the ozone level has significant impact on health and the environment.

ozone shield, the layer of ozone that hangs in the atmosphere from 20 to 40 miles above the surface of the earth and protects the earth from excessive ultraviolet radiation. Some experts claim that the manufacture of various chemicals, such as chlorofluorocarbons used as propellants in aerosol sprays, and the effects of high-flying jet aircraft are destroying this protective layer and allowing excessive amounts of ultraviolet radiation to penetrate the earth's atmosphere, thus subjecting humans to increased dangers of skin cancer and other health problems. Some chemistry experts and federal health officials also claim that an additional threat comes from nitrous oxide in nitrogenous fertilizers rising into the atmosphere and reacting unfavorably with the ozone shield. The ozone shield is implicated in certain health problems that affect some air travelers. See also **ozone sickness.**

ozone sickness, an abnormal condition caused by the inhalation of ozone that may seep into jet aircraft at altitudes over 40,000 feet. It is characterized by headaches, chest pains, itchy eyes, and sleepiness. Exactly why and how ozone causes this condition is not known. It is more prevalent early in the year and occurs more often over the Pacific Ocean.

oz t [L, *uncia*], a unit of weight equal to 31.103 grams. Abbreviation for *troy ounce.*

O

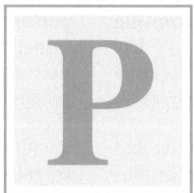

P, 1. abbreviation for *power.* **2.** abbreviation for **pressure.**
P, 1. symbol for the element **phosphorus. 2.** symbol for *after,* **post. 3.** symbol for *first parental generation.* **4.** symbol for *first pulmonic sound.*

p. See **partial pressure.** Symbol for *gas partial pressure.*

p17, symbol for a protein that lines the interior of the human immunodeficiency virus envelope.

P1E1, P2E1, P3E1, P4E1, P6E1, brand names for fixed-combination ophthalmic drugs containing a cholinergic (pilocarpine hydrochloride) and an adrenergic (epinephrine bitartrate). The numbers indicate the percentage of each ingredient in the solution; for example, P2E1 contains 2% pilocarpine hydrochloride and 1% epinephrine bitartrate. Brand name for **pilocarpine hydrochloride,** *epinephrine bitartrate.*

P$_2$, symbol for *second pulmonic sound.*

p24, symbol for a protein that surrounds the ribonucleic acid and reverse transcriptase of the human immunodeficiency virus.

P$_{50}$, the partial pressure of oxygen at which hemoglobin is half saturated with bound oxygen.

P & A, 1. abbreviation for *percussion and auscultation.* **2.** abbreviation for *posterior and anterior.*

pA, abbreviation for **picoampere.**

Pa, 1. symbol for **pascal. 2.** symbol for the element **protactinium.**

PA, 1. abbreviation for **physician assistant. 2.** abbreviation for **pulmonary artery.**

P-A, p-a, abbreviation for **posteroanterior.**

PABA, a topical sunscreen. See also **paraaminobenzoic acid (H$_2$NC$_6$H$_4$COOH) (PABA).**

pabulin /pab″yəlin/ [L, *pabulum,* food], products of fat and protein digestion found in the blood after a meal.

pabulum /pab″yələm/ [L, food], a substance that is food or nutrient.

PAC, abbreviation for **premature atrial complex.**

pacchionian foramen /pak′ē·ō″nē·ən/ [Antonio Pacchioni, Italian anatomist, 1665–1720], a thick opening in the center of the diaphragm of sella through which the infundibulum passes. Also called **foramen diaphragmatis.**

pacchionian granulations. See **arachnoid villi.**

PACE /pās/, abbreviation for **Program of All-inclusive Care of the Elderly.**

pacemaker [L, *passus,* step; AS, *macian,* to make], **1.** the sinoatrial node composed of specialized nervous tissue and located at the junction of the superior vena cava and the right atrium. It initiates the contractions of the atria, which transmit the impulse onto the atrioventricular (AV) node, thereby initiating the contraction of the ventricles. An ectopic or idioventricular pacemaker, originating in the atria, AV node, or ventricle, may cause contractions in cases of abnormal heart functioning. Also called **cardiac pacemaker. 2.** an electric apparatus used in most cases to increase the heart rate in severe bradycardia by electrically stimulating the heart muscle. A pacemaker may be permanent or temporary, emit the stimulus at a constant and fixed rate, or fire only on demand.

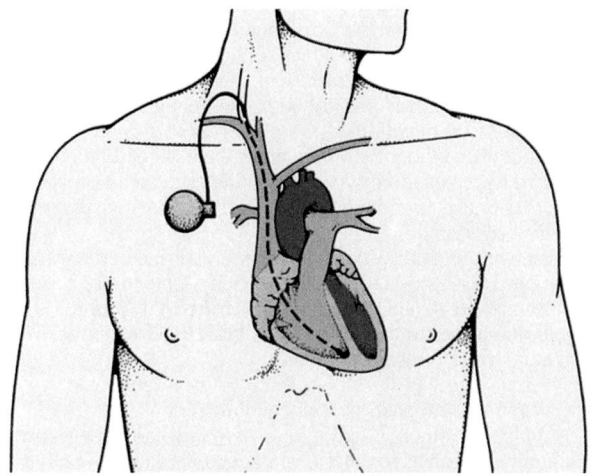

Pacemaker *(Thibodeau and Patton, 2007)*

pachometer, equipment used to measure the thickness of an object. See **pachymeter.**

pachy- /pak′i-/, prefix meaning "thick": *pachycheilia, pachyderma.*

pachyblepharon /-blef″əron/ [Gk, *pachy,* thick], a thickening of the tarsal border of the eyelid.

pachycheilia /-kī″lē·ə/, an abnormal thickening or swelling of the lips.

pachycholia /-kō″lē·ə/, a thickening of the bile.

pachychromatic /-krōmat″ik/, characterized by coarse chromatin filaments.

pachychymia /-kī″mē·ə/, thickness of the partially digested food moving from the stomach into the duodenum.

pachydactyly /pak′ēdak″tilē/ [Gk, *pachy* + *daktylos,* finger], an abnormal thickening of the fingers or toes. –*pachydactylous, pachydactylic, adj.*

pachyderma /-dur″mə/, an overgrowth or thickening of the skin and subcutaneous tissues.

pachyderma alba /-dur′mə/ [Gk, *pachy* + *derma,* skin; L, *albus,* white], an abnormal state in which the buccal mucosa has an appearance suggestive of whitened elephant hide. Also called **pachyderma oralis.**

pachyderma laryngis, an overgrowth of epithelium in the posterior glottis, sometimes affecting the vocal cords.

pachyderma oralis. See **pachyderma alba.**

pachyderma vesicae, a potentially malignant condition of white plaques in the mucous membrane at the base of the bladder.

pachydermoperiostosis /-dur′moper′ē·ostō″sis/, a syndrome characterized by a thickening and folding of the facial skin, clubbing of the fingers, and new bone formation over the ends of the long bones.

pachyglossia /-glos″ē·ə/, an abnormal thickening of the tongue.

pachygnathy /-gnoth″ē/, an abnormal thickening of the mandible. See also **macrognathia.**

pachygyria /-jī″rē·ə/, a broadening and flattening of the gyri of the brain.

pachyleptomeningitis /-lep′təmin′injī″tis/, an inflammation of all the membranes of the brain and spinal cord.

pachylosis /-lō″sis/, a condition of rough, dry, and thickened skin.

pachymenia /-mē″nē·ə/, an abnormal thickness of the skin or other membranes.

pachymeninges. See **pachymeninx.**

pachymeningitis /-min′injī″tis/, an inflammation of the dura mater.

pachymeningopathy /-mining″gōpath′ē/, an abnormality, other than inflammation, involving the dura mater.

pachymeninx /-mē″niks/ *pl. pachymeninges* [Gk, *pachys,* thick, *meninx,* membrane]. See **dura mater.**

pachymeter /pakim″ətər/ [Gk, *pachy* + *metron,* measure], an instrument used to measure thickness, especially of a thin structure, such as a membrane or a tissue. Also called **pachometer.**

pachynema /pak′inē″mə/ [Gk, *pachy* + *nema,* thread], the postsynaptic tetradic chromosome formation that occurs in the pachytene stage of the first meiotic prophase of gametogenesis.

pachynsis /pakin″sis/, any thickening of tissues having a pathological cause.

pachyonychia /pak′ē-ōnik″ē-ə/, an abnormal thickness of the fingernails or toenails.

pachyonychia congenita [Gk, *pachy* + *onyx,* nail; L, *congenitus,* born with], a congenital deformity characterized by abnormal thickening and raising of the nails on the fingers and the toes and thickening of skin on the palms of the hands and the soles of the feet. The papillae of the tongue also atrophy, causing a whitish coating over the lingual surface.

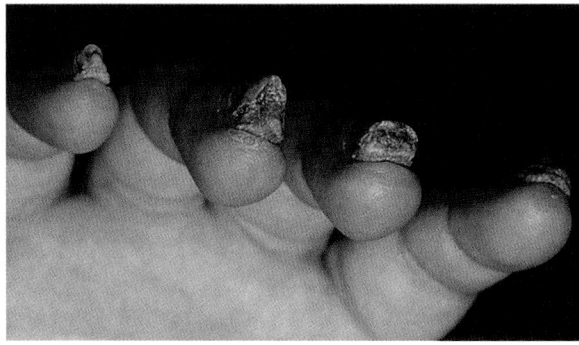

Pachyonychia congenita *(Hordinsky, Sawaya, and Scher, 2000)*

pachyotia /pak′ē-ō″shə/, an abnormal thickness of the auricle of the ears. Also called **boxer's ear.** See also **cauliflower ear.**

pachypelviperitonitis /-pel′vēper′itənī″tis/, pelvic peritonitis associated with a thickening of the tissues.

pachyperitonitis /-per′itənī″tis/, an inflammation and abnormal thickening of the tissues of the peritoneum.

pachypleuritis /-plo͞orī″tis/, an inflammation and thickening of the pleural membranes.

pachysalpingitis. See **parenchymatous salpingitis.**

pachysalpingoovaritis /-salping′gō-ō′verī″tis/, an inflammation and thickening of the tissues of the ovaries and fallopian tubes.

pachysomia /-sō″mē·ə/ [Gk, *pachys,* thick, *soma,* body], an abnormal thickening of the soft tissues of the body.

pachytene /pak″itēn/ [Gk, *pachy* + *tainia,* ribbon], the third stage in the first meiotic prophase of gametogenesis,

in which the paired homologous chromosomes form tetrads. The bivalent pairs become short and thick and intertwine so that four chromatids are visible. See also **diakinesis, diplotene, leptotene, zygotene.**

pachyvaginalitis /-vaj′inəlī″tis/, an inflammation and thickening of the membrane covering the testis and epididymis.

pachyvaginitis /-vaj′inī″tis/, chronic inflammation and thickening of the walls of the vagina.

pacifier /pas″ifī′ər/ [L, *pacificare,* to bring peace], **1.** an agent that soothes or comforts. **2.** a nipple-shaped object used by infants and children for sucking. The safest pacifiers are constructed in one piece, are large enough that only the nipple fits into the mouth, and have a handle that can be easily grasped. The American Academy of Pediatrics recommends waiting to introduce a pacifier until a baby is 1 month old and breastfeeding is well established.

pacing [L, *passus,* step], setting of the heart's rhythm by the sinus node, by another site in the heart, or by an artificial electrical stimulator. Also called **atrial pacing, endocardial pacing, sequential pacing, ventricular pacing.** See also **programmable pacemaker.**

pacing wire [L, *passus,* step; AS, *wir*], the electrical connection between a pulse generator and a pacing electrode in a cardiac pacemaker.

Pacini corpuscles /päsē″nē/ [Filippo Pacini, Italian anatomist, 1812–1883; L, *corpusculum,* little body], special sensory end organs resembling tiny white bulbs. Each is attached to the end of a single nerve fiber in the subcutaneous, submucous, and subserous connective tissue of many parts of the body, especially the palm of the hand, sole of the foot, genital organs, joints, and pancreas. They average about 3 mm in diameter, are pressure sensitive and vibration sensitive, contain numerous concentric layers around a central core, and in cross section resemble an onion. Also called *pacinian corpuscles.* Compare **Golgi-Mazzoni corpuscles, Krause corpuscles.**

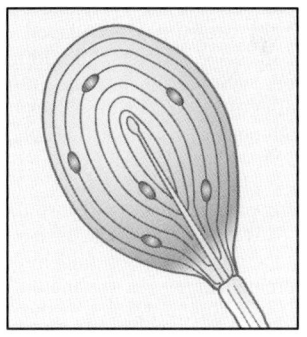

Pacini corpuscle *(Patton and Thibodeau, 2016)*

pacinitis /pas′inī″tis/, an inflammation of the Pacini corpuscles.

pack [ME, *pakke,* bundle], **1.** a treatment in which the entire body or a portion of it is wrapped in wet or dry towels or in ice for various therapeutic purposes, as with cold packs for relieving swelling, reducing a high temperature associated with malignant hyperthermia, or inducing hypothermia during certain surgical procedures, especially heart surgery and organ transplantation. **2.** a tampon. **3.** the act of applying a dressing or dental cement to a surgical wound. **4.** a surgical dressing to cover a wound or to fill the cavity left from extraction of a tooth, especially a wisdom tooth.

package insert (P.I.), a leaflet that, by order of the U.S. Food and Drug Administration, must be placed inside the

P

package of every prescription drug. The leaflet must include the brand name for the drug, its generic name, and its mechanism of action; state its indications, contraindications, warnings, precautions, adverse effects, and dosage forms; and include instructions for the recommended dose, time, and route of administration.

packed cells [ME, *pakke,* bundle; L, *cella,* storeroom], a preparation of blood cells separated from liquid plasma, often administered in severe anemia to restore adequate levels of hemoglobin and red blood cells without overloading the vascular system with excess fluids. Also called *packed red blood cells.* See also **component therapy, pooled plasma.**

packed cell volume (PCV) [ME, *pakke* + L, *cella,* storeroom, *volumen,* paper roll], percentage of packed red blood cells in a centrifuged column of whole blood. Also called **hematocrit reading.**

packer, an instrument for tamponing or introducing a pack of gauze into a wound. See also **plugger.**

packing [ME, *pakke*], **1.** material used to fill a wound or cavity. **2.** the act of inserting material into a wound or cavity, especially a wound with tunneling.

paclitaxel, an anticancer drug derived from the bark of the rare, slow-growing Pacific yew tree. It is used in the treatment of ovarian cancer. Paclitaxel prevents cancer cells from dividing; it arrests cell division by attaching to microtubules that regulate the formation of spindles necessary for cell division. The anticancer effect of paclitaxel was discovered by the National Cancer Institute in 1963 during a routine investigation of thousands of plant compounds. It takes about 60 pounds of yew bark to produce enough paclitaxel to treat a single patient for several weeks. Semisynthetic and synthetic methods of production have reduced, but not eliminated, the use of yew bark.

PaCO₂, abbreviation for **partial pressure of carbon dioxide in arterial blood.**

PACS, abbreviation for *picture archiving and communications system,* a medical imaging technology consisting of a network of computers used to replace conventional film with electronically stored and displayed digital images. It provides archives for storage of multimodality images, integrates images with patient database information, facilitates laser printing of images, and displays both images and patient information at work stations throughout the network. See also **DICOM.**

pad [D, *paden,* cushion], **1.** a mass of soft material used to cushion shock, prevent wear, or absorb moisture, such as the abdominal pads used to absorb discharges from abdominal wounds or to separate viscera and improve accessibility during abdominal surgery. **2.** (in anatomy) a mass of fat that cushions various structures, such as the infrapatellar pad lying below the patella among the patellar ligament, the head of the tibia, and the femoral condyles.

PAD, **1.** abbreviation for **peripheral arterial disease. 2.** abbreviation for **pulsatile assist device.**

p. ae. [L, *partes* + *aequales*], symbol for *equal parts.*

paed-, paedo-. See **ped-, pedo-.**

paediatrician. See **pediatrician.**

paediatrics. See **pediatrics.**

paedogenesis. See **pedogenesis.**

paedophilia. See **pedophilia.**

pagetoid /paj″ətoid/, resembling Paget disease.

Paget-Schroetter syndrome, Paget-von Schroetter syndrome. See **effort thrombosis.**

Paget disease /paj″ət/ [James Paget, English surgeon, 1814–1899], a common nonmetabolic disease of bone of unknown cause, usually affecting middle-aged and elderly people and characterized by excessive bone destruction and unorganized bone repair. Also called **osteitis deformans.**

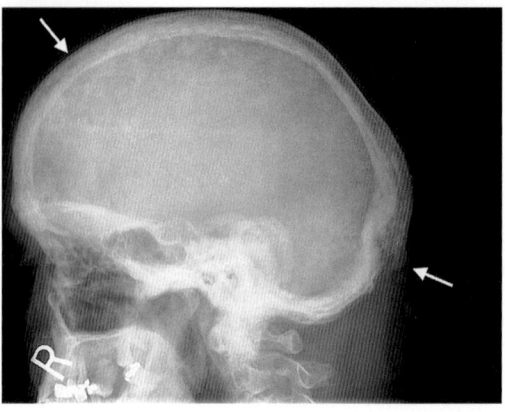

Paget disease: skull radiograph *(Courtesy Ohio State University Medical Center)*

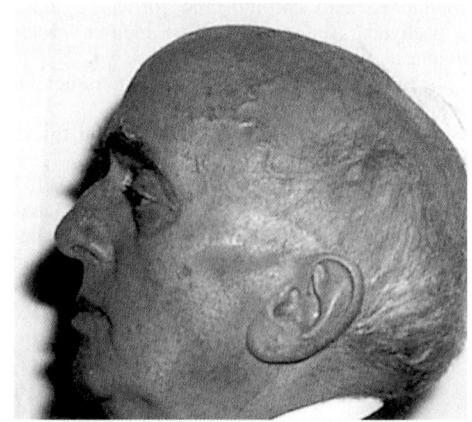

Individual with enlarged skull due to Paget disease *(Moll, 1997)*

Paget disease of the nipple. See **nipple cancer.**

Pagliaro combined modality treatment [L. Pagliaro, contemporary American physician], the use of chemotherapy in combination with surgery or irradiation or both in the treatment of cancer.

pagophagia /pā′gōfā″jē·ə/ [Gk, *pagos,* frost, *phagein,* to eat], an abnormal condition characterized by a craving to eat enormous quantities of ice. It is associated with a lack of the nutrient iron. −*pagophagous, pagophagic, adj.*

-pagus, suffix meaning "conjoined twins": *craniopagus, pygopagus, gastrothoracopagus.*

PAHA, abbreviation for **paraaminohippuric acid.**

PAHA sodium clearance test, a procedure formerly used for detecting kidney damage or certain muscle diseases that determined the rate at which the kidneys removed the sodium salt of paraaminohippuric acid from the blood and urine.

PAHO, abbreviation for *Pan American Health Organization.*

PAI, abbreviation for *plasminogen activator inhibitor.*

PAI-1, abbreviation for **plasminogen activator inhibitor 1 test.**

pain [L, *poena,* punishment], an unpleasant sensation caused by noxious stimulation of the sensory nerve endings. It is a subjective feeling and an individual response to the cause. Pain is a cardinal symptom of inflammation and is valuable in the diagnosis of many disorders and conditions. It may be mild or severe, chronic or acute, lancinating, burning, dull or sharp,

Factors that influence pain tolerance

Increase tolerance	Decrease tolerance
Alcohol	Fatigue
Drugs	Anger
Hypnosis	Boredom
Warmth	Anxiety
Rubbing	Persistent pain
Distraction	Stress
Faith	Depression
Strong beliefs	

From Monahan FD et al: *Phipps' medical-surgical nursing: health and illness perspectives,* ed 8, St Louis, 2007, Mosby.

precisely or poorly localized, or referred. The experience of pain is influenced by physical, mental, biochemical, psychological, physiological, social, cultural, and emotional factors. See also **referred pain, acute pain, chronic pain.**

pain and suffering, (in law) an element in a claim for damages that allows recovery for the mental and physical pain, suffering, distress, and trauma that an individual has endured as a result of injury.

pain assessment, an evaluation of the reported pain and the factors that alleviate or exacerbate it, as well as the response to treatment of pain. Responses to pain vary widely among individuals, depending on many different physical and psychological factors, such as specific diseases and injuries and the health, pain threshold, fear, anxiety, and cultural background of the individual involved, as well as the way the person expresses pain experiences. See also **pain intervention, pain mechanism.**
■ METHOD: The patient is asked to describe the cause of the pain, if known; its intensity, location, and duration; the events preceding it; the pattern usually followed for handling pain; previous treatments and effectiveness; allergies; and ways in which the pain has affected the activities of daily living. Intensity of pain is often assessed by using pain scales (numeric or face scales). Severe pain causes pallor; cold perspiration; piloerection; dilated pupils; and increases in the pulse, respiratory rate, blood pressure, and muscle tension. When brief, intense pain subsides, the pulse may be slower and the blood pressure lower than before the pain began. If pain occurs frequently or is prolonged, the pulse rate and blood pressure may not increase markedly, and, if pain persists for many days, there may be an increased production of eosinophils and 17-ketosteroids and greater susceptibility to infections. The patient's statements regarding pain; tone of voice, speed of speech, cries, groans, or other vocalizations; facial expressions; body movements; or tendency to withdraw are all noted. Pertinent background information in the assessment includes a record of the patient's chronic conditions, previous surgery, and any illnesses that caused pain; the patient's experiences with relatives and friends in pain; the role or position of the patient in the family structure; and the patient's use of alcohol and drugs, including use of OTC and illicit drugs. Key aspects in evaluating pain intensity are the size of the area, the tenderness within the pain area, and the effects of movement and pressure on the pain. Duration of pain is considered in terms of hours, days, weeks, months, or years. Pain patterns are associated with various sensations such as burning, pricking, aching, rhythmic throbbing, and effects on the sympathetic and the parasympathetic nervous systems. Evaluation includes the meanings the individual may attach to pain, such as a test of character, a penance, or a sign of worsening illness. Such interpretations may affect the intensity of pain and mask its significance.

■ INTERVENTIONS: Health care providers must establish a relationship with the patient; they often use individual or group counseling to teach patients about pain and how to modify the anxiety associated with it. Analgesics are usually prescribed and should be administered before the pain becomes intense. In addition to rest and relaxation, approaches to pain relief may include the reduction of noxious stimuli, the provision of pleasant sensory input, and the distraction of the patient by using guided imagery. A referral of the patient to a pain clinic is appropriate for chronic pain.
■ OUTCOME CRITERIA: Dramatic relief of intense or chronic pain is often difficult to accomplish, but the patient can be helped to learn to handle pain effectively and to function fairly normally.

painful bladder syndrome. See **interstitial cystitis.**

pain intervention, the attempt to relieve pain by various measures, such as administration of NSAIDs and opiates. The psychological effects of pain must be considered. Effective pain intervention depends on proper evaluation of the type of pain the patient is experiencing, the physical and psychological origins of the pain, and the behavioral patterns commonly associated with different kinds of pain. The most common method of pain intervention is the administration of narcotics, such as morphine, but many authorities believe that the exclusive use of pain-killing drugs without consideration and implementation of psychological aids is too narrow an approach. There are few patients without a psychogenic overlay on the physical experience of pain, and comprehensive pain intervention uses methods and procedures that incorporate both psychological and physical measures. Methods of pain intervention for acute pain are different from those for chronic pain. Acute pain, occurring in the first 24 to 48 hours after surgery, is often difficult to relieve, and narcotics seldom alleviate it completely. Some authorities believe that the individual who has undergone repeated surgical operations has a decreased tolerance for pain. The type of pain intervention usually depends on the description of the pain by the individual experiencing it. Mild pain may best be relieved by comfort measures and the distraction afforded by television, visitors, reading, and other passive activities. Moderate pain may best be relieved by a combination of comfort measures and drugs. Cognitive dissonance, often used to ameliorate moderate pain, encourages the patient to reflect on pleasant experiences and describe them to health care personnel. Intervention to relieve severe pain often includes the administration of narcotics, purposeful interaction between the patient and attending hospital personnel, reduction of environmental stimuli, increased comfort measures, and "waking imagined analgesia," in which the patient is encouraged to concentrate on and become distracted by former pleasant experiences, such as relaxing on a beach surrounded by cool ocean water. In the alleviation of all types of pain, dampening or decreasing stimuli that create pain is the chief goal. Pain often increases in a cold room because the muscles of the patient tend to contract, but the local application of cold, such as with an ice pack, often alleviates pain by reducing swelling. Pain intervention seeks to reduce the effects of other factors that compound pain, such as fatigue and anxiety. Coping with pain becomes increasingly difficult as the patient becomes more tired. Sensory restriction may increase pain because it blocks otherwise effective distraction; overstimulation may cause fatigue and anxiety, thus increasing pain. Pain intervention by the use of drugs includes the administration of mild nonnarcotic analgesics and of much more potent and potentially addictive opioids, such as morphine. Opioid analgesics administered for the relief of pain, cough, or diarrhea provide only symptomatic treatment and are used cautiously in the care of patients with acute or chronic diseases. They may obscure the symptoms or the progress of the disease, and repeated daily administration of any opioid eventually produces some tolerance to the therapeutic effects of the drug and some physical dependence on the dosage. The risk of development of psychological and physical dependency on any drug is always present, especially with opioids. In usual doses opioids relieve suffering by altering the emotional component of the painful experience and by effecting analgesia. Some caregivers are so concerned about the addictive dangers of opioids that they tend to prescribe initial doses that are too low or too infrequent to alleviate pain. Some other patients with more rapid metabolisms may require such drugs at shorter intervals. Many drugs are appropriate substitutes for the potent opioids morphine and codeine. Some of the effective semisynthetic substitutes are hydrocodone, dihydrocodeine, and meperidine. The narcotic analgesics act on the central nervous system, but the salicylates and other nonnarcotic drugs act at the site of origin of the pain. Some nonnarcotic drugs, such as aspirin, indomethacin, ibuprofen, or naproxen, also have antiinflammatory and antipyretic activity. In patients who are sensitive to or are unable to take aspirin, acetaminophen is an acceptable substitute, as are the nonsteroidal antiinflammatory drugs. Pain intervention in the treatment of terminal illnesses uses numerous drugs that relieve pain and produce euphoria and tranquility in patients who would otherwise suffer greatly. Nerve block by the injection of alcohol, chordotomy, and other neurosurgical interventions may sometimes be used. Other techniques include acupuncture; hypnosis; behavior modification, in which treatment consists of reducing medication and gradually increasing mobility through exercise and any other appropriate modality; biofeedback; and transcutaneous electrical nerve stimulation. See also **pain assessment.**

pain mechanism, the network that communicates unpleasant sensations and the perceptions of noxious stimuli throughout the body in association with physical disease and trauma involving tissue damage. The gate control theory of pain is an attempt to explain the role of the nervous system in the pain response. It states that pain signals that reach the nervous system excite a group of small neurons that form a "pain pool." When the total activity of these neurons reaches a minimum level, a theoretic gate opens up and allows the pain signals to proceed to higher brain centers. The areas in which the gates operate are considered to be in the spinal cord dorsal horn and the brainstem. The pattern theory holds that the intensity of a stimulus evokes a specific pattern, which is interpreted by the brain as pain. This perception is the result of the intensity and frequency of stimulation of a nonspecific end organ. Some authorities believe that bradykinin and histamine, two chemical substances produced by the body, cause pain. Pain killers produced naturally by the body are the enkephalins and the endorphins. Some studies indicate that the enkephalins are 10 times as potent as morphine in reducing pain. It is known that after histamine and some other naturally occurring chemical substances are released in the body, pain sensations travel along fast-conducting and slow-conducting nerve fibers. These pain-transmitting neuropathways communicate the pain sensation to the dorsal root ganglia of the spinal cord and synapse with certain neurons in the posterior horns of the gray matter. The pain sensation is then transmitted to the reticular formation and the thalamus by neurons that form the anterolateral spinothalamic tract. It is then conveyed to various areas of the brain, such as the cortex and the hypothalamus, by synapses at the thalamus. The immediate reaction to pain is transmitted over the reflex arc by sensory fibers in the dorsal horn of the spinal cord and by synapsing motor neurons in the anterior horn. This anatomical pattern of sensory and motor neurons allows the individual to move quickly at the touch of some harmful stimulus, such as extreme heat or cold. Nerve impulses alerting the individual to move away from such stimuli are simultaneously sent along efferent nerve fibers from the brain. Also called *gate theory of pain, pain pathway.*

pain receptor, any one of the many free nerve endings throughout the body that warn of potentially harmful changes in the environment, such as excessive pressure or temperature. The free nerve endings constituting most of the pain receptors are located chiefly in the epidermis and in the epithelial covering of certain mucous membranes. They also appear in the stratified squamous epithelium of the cornea, in the root sheaths and the papillae of the hairs, and around the bodies of sudoriferous glands. The terminal ends of pain receptors consist of unmyelinated nerve fibers that often anastomose into small knobs between the epithelial cells. Any kind of stimulus, if it is intense enough, can stimulate the pain receptors in the skin and the mucosa, but only radical changes in pressure and certain chemicals can stimulate the pain receptors in the viscera. Referred pain results only from stimulation of pain receptors located in deep structures, such as the viscera, the joints, and the skeletal muscles, and never from pain receptors in the skin.

paint [Fr, *peindre*], **1.** *v.,* to apply a medicated solution to the skin, usually over a wide area. **2.** *n.,* a medicated solution that is applied in this way. Kinds include **antiseptic, germicide, sporicide.**

pain threshold, the point at which a stimulus, usually one associated with pressure or temperature, activates pain receptors and produces a sensation of pain. Individuals with low pain thresholds experience pain much sooner and faster than those with higher thresholds; individuals' reactions to stimulation of pain receptors vary.

pair, 1. two corresponding items similar in form and function. **2.** one object composed of two joined interdependent parts. See also **base pair.**

PAL, abbreviation for *posterior axillary line.*

palatable /pal″ətəbəl/ [L, *palatum,* palate], pleasant to the taste.

palatal /pal″ətəl/ [L, *palatum,* palate], **1.** pertaining to the palate or palate bone. **2.** pertaining to the lingual surface of a maxillary tooth.

palatal cyst of the newborn, a common finding in newborns in which small cysts form during embryological development or during development of the minor salivary glands of the hard palate, each of which entrap epithelium to form tiny cysts. Epstein pearls form along the median palatal raphe, while Bohn nodules are scattered over the hard palate near its junction with the soft palate.

palatal shelf, lateral palatine process.

palate /pal″it/ [L, *palatum*], the bony muscular partition between the oral and nasal cavities that forms the roof of the mouth. It is divided into the hard palate and the soft palate. Also called **uraniscus. –palatine, palatal,** *adj.*

palatine [L, palate], pertaining to or belonging to the palate.

palatine aponeurosis, the major structural element of the soft palate to which other muscles of the palate attach. It is attached anteriorly to the margin of the hard palate, but it is unattached posteriorly, where it ends in a free margin.

palatine arch [L, *palatum + arcus,* bow], the vault-shaped muscular structure forming the soft palate between the mouth and the nasopharynx. An opening in the arch connects the mouth with the oropharynx; the uvula is suspended from the middle of the posterior border of the arch.

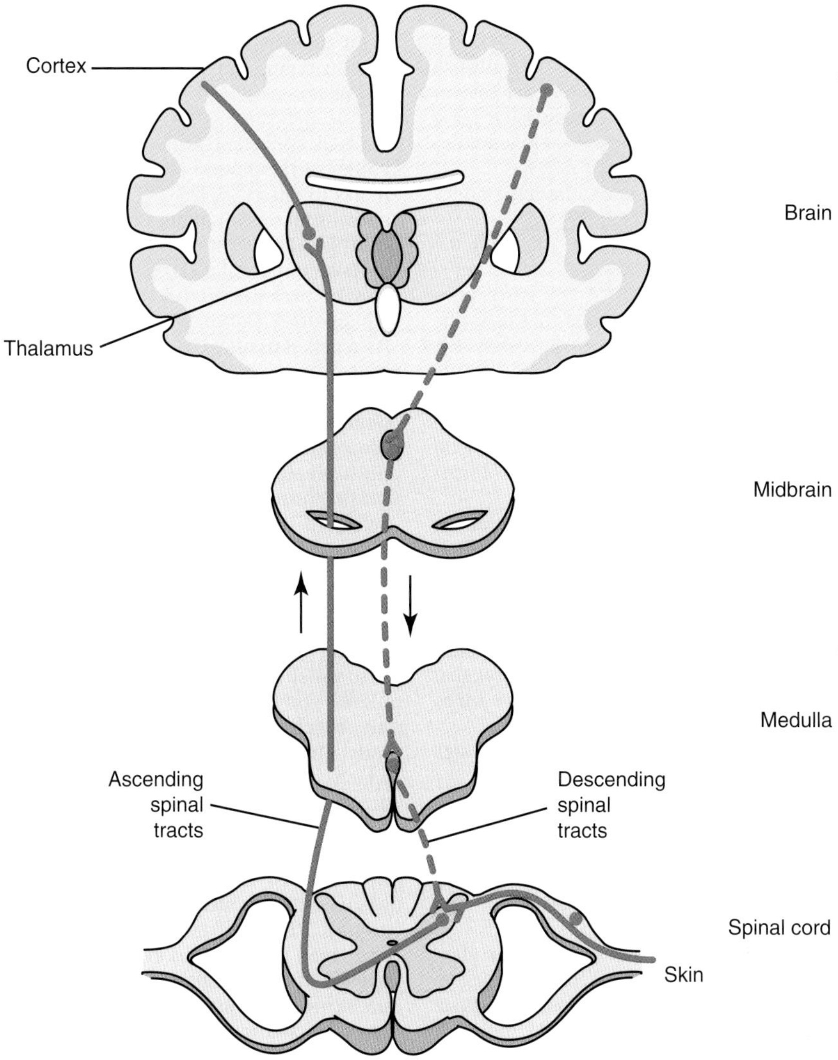

Pain reception pathway *(Monahan et al, 2007)*

palatine bone, one of a pair of bones of the skull forming the posterior part of the hard palate, part of the nasal cavity, and the floor of the orbit of the eye. It resembles the letter *L* and consists of horizontal and vertical parts and three processes.

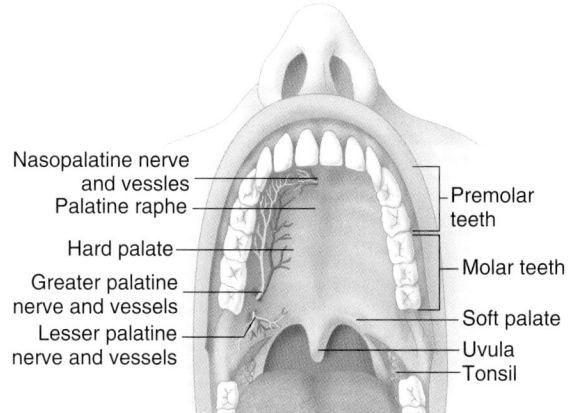

Anatomy of the palate *(Tyers and Collin, 2008)*

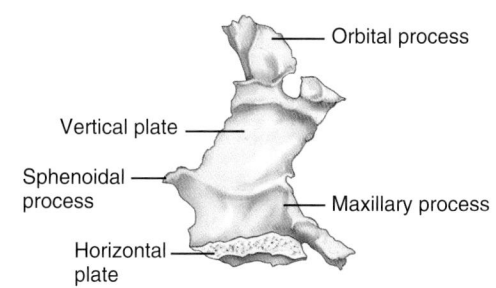

Palatine bone

palatine foramina, the openings in the palatine canal. The greater palatine foramina transmit the greater palatine nerve and vessels to the hard palate. The lesser palatine foramina distribute the lesser palatine nerve and vessels to the soft palate.

palatine raphe, a medial longitudinal ridge of the mucosa of the hard palate that ends anteriorly in a small oval elevation, the incisive papilla, which overlies the incisive fossa formed between the horizontal plates of the maxillae immediately behind the incisor teeth.

palatine ridge, any one of the four to six transverse ridges on the anterior surface of the hard palate.

palatine rugae, the numerous transverse folds of the mucosa of the hard palate.

palatine suture, any one of a number of thin wavy lines marking the joining of the palatine processes that form the hard palate. See also **median palatine suture, transverse palatine suture.**

palatine tonsil, one of a pair of almond-shaped masses of lymphoid tissue between the palatoglossal and palatopharyngeal arches on each side of the fauces. They are covered with mucous membrane and contain numerous lymph follicles and various crypts.

palatine torus, a bony ridge along the hard palate at the line of fusion of the left and right jawbone segments. It is believed to be caused by inheritance or environmental influences such as bruxism. There is no treatment unless the overlying tissue is traumatized or interferes with the placement of a denture prosthesis. A large torus can interfere with intubation with an endotracheal tube or insertion of a laryngeal mask airway. Also called **torus palatinus. Compare torus mandibularis.**

palatine uvula, an elongated mucosal process that hangs from the middle of the back edge of the soft palate.

palatitis, an inflammation of the hard palate.

palato-, combining form meaning "palate": *palatoglossal, electropalatography, palatomaxillary.*

palatoglossal /pal′ətoglos″əl/ [L, *palatum,* palate; Gk, *glossa,* tongue], pertaining to both the palate and the tongue.

palatoglossus /-glos″əs/, the muscle that underlies the glossopalatine arch. The palatoglossus muscles depress the palate, move the arches toward the midline like curtains, and elevate the back of the tongue. These actions help close the fauces. It is innervated by the vagus nerve, or cranial nerve X.

palatognathous /pal′ətog″nəthəs/, pertaining to a cleft palate.

palatograph /pal′ətōgraf′/, a device that records the movement of the palate while the person is speaking.

palatomaxillary /-mak″siler′ē/ [L, *palatum + maxilla,* jaw], pertaining to the palate and the maxilla.

palatonasal /-nā″zəl/ [L, *palatum + nasus,* nose], pertaining to the palate and the nose.

palatopharyngeal /-ferin″jē·əl/, pertaining to the palate and pharynx.

palatopharyngeus /-ferin″jē·əs/, a muscle with an origin at the back of the soft palate and an insertion on the posterior border of the thyroid cartilage and the wall of the pharynx. It acts to raise the pharynx. The muscle is innervated by the pharyngeal branch of the vagus nerve, cranial nerve X.

palatopharyngoplasty /-fering″gōplas′tē/, the surgical excision of palatal and oropharyngeal tissues. The procedure may be performed to treat cases of snoring or sleep apnea thought to be caused by obstructions in the nose or pharynx. Also called **uvulopalatopharyngoplasty.**

palatopharyngorrhaphy, surgical repair of defects in the uvula, soft palate, and pharynx. See also **staphylopharyngorrhaphy.**

palatoplasty /pal′ətōplas′tē/, plastic surgery of the palate.

palatoplegia /-plē″jē·ə/, paralysis of the soft palate.

palatorrhaphy /pal′ətôr″əfē/, the surgical repair of a cleft palate.

palatosalpingeus /-salpin″jē·əs/, the tensor muscle of the soft palate. It arises from the scaphoid fossa of the sphenoid bone.

palatoschisis /pal′ətos″kisis/, See **cleft palate.**

pale infarct [L, *pallidus,* pallid, *infarcire,* to stuff], a wedge of dead tissue that is white because of an absence of blood. Also called **anemic infarct, white infarct.**

paleo-, prefix meaning "old": *paleogenesis, paleocortex.*

paleocerebellum /pal′ē-ōser′əbel″əm/, the phylogenetically oldest part of the cerebellum, including the vermis, which connects the cerebellar hemispheres, and the flocculus, or lobule, on the posterior lobe. Also called *spinocerebellum.*

paleocortex /-kôr″teks/, the phylogenetically oldest part of the cerebral cortex, particularly the olfactory bulb.

paleogenesis. See **palingenesis.**

paleogenetic /-jənet″ik/ [Gk, *palaios,* long ago, *genesis,* origin], **1.** a trait or structure of an organism or species that originated in a previous generation. **2.** relating to the development of such a trait or structure.

paleokinetic /-kinet″ik/, pertaining to primitive reflexes and other automatic muscular movements.

paleolithic diet, the consumption of foods that would have been available to ancient ancestors and the elimination of processed foods, sugar, soft drinks, and bread. Also called *paleo diet.*

paleontology. See **biology.**

paleopathology /-pathol″əjē/, the science of disease in ancient eras based on the condition of remains of mummies, skeletons, and other archeological findings.

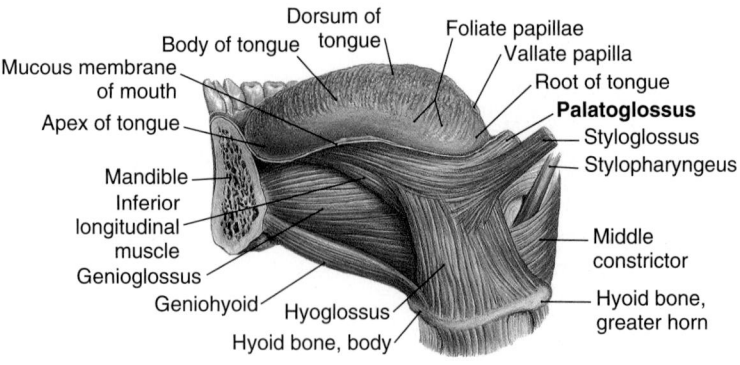

Palatoglossus muscle *(Paulsen, 2013)*

pali-. See **palin-, pali-.**

palikinesia /pal'ikīnē"zhə/, a condition in which involuntary movements are constantly repeated.

palilalia /pal'ilā"lyə/ [Gk, *palin,* again, *lalein,* to babble], an abnormal condition characterized by the increasingly rapid repetition of the same word or phrase, usually at the end of a sentence.

palin-, pali-, prefix meaning "again": *palindromia, palikinesia, palingenesis.*

palindrome /pal"indrōm'/ [Gk, *palin + dromos,* course], a segment of DNA in which identical or almost identical sequences of bases run in opposite directions of the complementary strands. Palindromes are often sites for attack by restriction endonucleases.

palindromia /pal'indrō"mē·ə/, the recurrence of a disease.

palingenesis /pal'injen"əsis/ [Gk, *palin + genesis,* origin], **1.** the regeneration of a lost part. **2.** the hereditary transmission of ancestral structural characteristics, especially abnormalities, in successive generations. Also called **paleogenesis.** Compare **cenogenesis.** –*palingenic, palingenetic, adj.*

paliperidone, an antipsychotic drug.

■ INDICATIONS: This drug is used to treat schizophrenia.

■ CONTRAINDICATIONS: Lactation, seizure disorders, AV block, QT prolongation, torsades de pointes, and known hypersensitivity to this drug or to risperidone prohibit its use. Geriatric patients should not use this drug.

■ ADVERSE EFFECTS: Adverse effects of this drug include dizziness, orthostatic hypotension, blurred vision, vomiting, and weight gain. Life-threatening side effects include seizures, neuroleptic malignant syndrome, tachycardia, heart failure, and QT prolongation. Common side effects include EPS, pseudoparkinsonism, akathisia, dystonia, tardive dyskinesia, drowsiness, insomnia, agitation, anxiety, headache, nausea, anorexia, and constipation.

palivizumab, a monoclonal antibody.

■ INDICATIONS: It is used to prevent serious lower respiratory tract disease caused by respiratory syncytial virus in pediatric patients.

■ CONTRAINDICATIONS: Use is prohibited in adults, in patients with cyanotic congenital heart disease, and in patients with known hypersensitivity to this drug.

■ ADVERSE EFFECTS: Adverse effects include nausea, vomiting, diarrhea, increased AST, upper respiratory infection, otitis media, rhinitis, pharyngitis, rash, and injection site reaction.

palladium (Pd) /pəlā"dē·əm/ [Gk, *Pallas Athena,* mythic goddess and protector of Troy], a hard silvery metallic element. Its atomic number is 46; its atomic mass is 106.42. Highly resistant to tarnish and corrosion, palladium is used in high-grade surgical instruments; in dental inlays, bridgework, and orthodontic appliances; and in catalytic converters.

pallanesthesia /pal'anesthē"zhə/, a condition characterized by an inability to sense vibrations.

pallesthesia /pal'esthē"zhə/ [Gk, *pallein,* to quiver], hypersensitivity to vibration, particularly that caused by a tuning fork placed on a bony prominence.

palliate /pal"ē·āt/ [L, *palliare,* to cloak], to soothe or relieve. –*palliative, adj.,* –*palliation, n.*

palliative treatment /pal"ē·ətiv'/ [L, *palliare,* to cloak, *tractare,* to handle], therapy designed to relieve or reduce intensity of uncomfortable symptoms but not to produce a cure. Some kinds of palliative treatment are the use of narcotics to relieve pain in a patient with advanced cancer, the creation of a colostomy to bypass an inoperable obstructing lesion of the bowel, and the debridement of necrotic tissue in a patient with metastatic malignancy. Compare **definitive treatment, expectant treatment.**

pallid /pal'id/ [L, *pallidus,* pale], lacking color; pale.

pallidectomy /pal'idek"təmē/ [L, *pallidus,* pale; Gk, *exome,* cutting out], the destruction of all or part of the globus pallidus by chemicals or freezing.

pallidotomy /pal'idot"əmē/, the surgical production of lesions in the globus pallidus for the treatment of extrapyramidal disorders.

pallidum. See **globus pallidus.**

pallium. See **cerebral cortex.**

pallor /pal"ər/ [L, *paleness*], an unnatural paleness or absence of color in the skin.

palm /päm/ [L, *palma*], the flexor anterior surface of the hand, beyond the wrist to the base of the fingers, exclusive of the thumb and fingers.

palm and sole system of identification, a method of identifying individuals by the patterns of ridges in the skin of the palms of the hands and soles of the feet. Like fingerprints, the patterns are helpful in identification of infants and others.

palmar /pal"mər/ [L, *palma*], pertaining to the palm.

palmar aponeurosis [L, *palma* + Gk, *apo,* from, *neuron,* nerve], a sheet of fascia under the skin of the palm and surrounding the muscles. Also called **palmar fascia.**

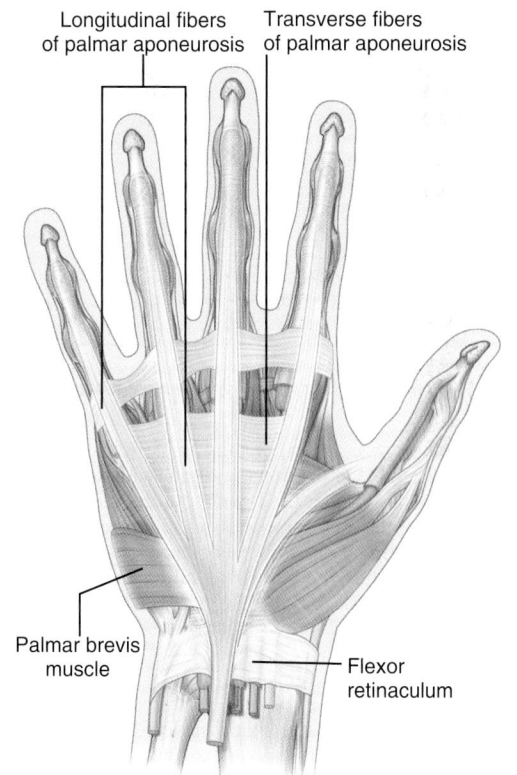

Longitudinal fibers of palmar aponeurosis   Transverse fibers of palmar aponeurosis

Palmar brevis muscle

Flexor retinaculum

Palmar aponeurosis *(Drake, Vogl, and Mitchell, 2015)*

palmar crease, a normal groove across the palm of the hand.

palmar erythema, an inflammatory redness of the palms of the hands. The condition is frequently associated with cardiac disease, pregnancy, cirrhosis of the liver, and rheumatoid arthritis.

palmar fascia. See **palmar aponeurosis.**

palmar grasp reflex [L, *palma,* palm; ONorse, *grapa,* grab], a flexion of the fingers caused by stimulation of the palm of the hand. The reflex is present at birth and usually disappears by 6 months of age.

P

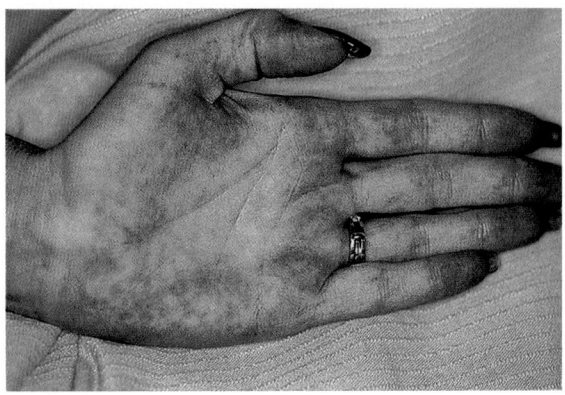

Palmar erythema *(Bolognia, Jorizzo, and Schaffer, 2012)*

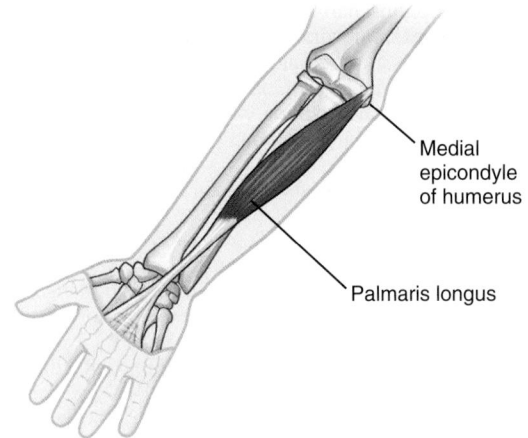

Palmaris longus

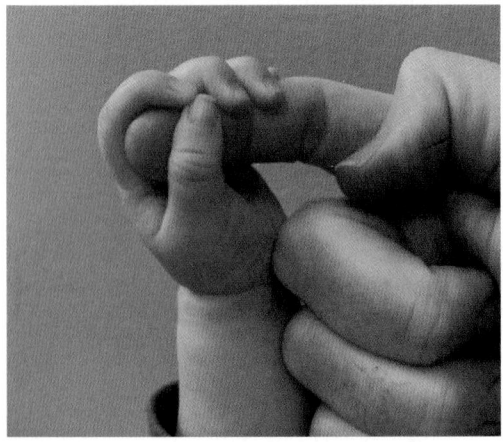

Palmar grasp reflex in the newborn

palmar interossei, the four unipennate muscles originating from the metacarpals of the digits with which each is associated. They adduct the thumb and the index, ring, and little fingers at the metacarpophalangeal joints.

palmaris brevis, a small intrinsic muscle of the hand that deepens the cup of the palm by pulling on skin over the hypothenar eminence and forming a distinct ridge. This may improve grip. Palmaris brevis is innervated by the superficial branch of the ulnar nerve.

palmaris longus /pəlmer′is/, a long, slender, superficial fusiform muscle of the forearm, lying on the medial side of the flexor carpi radialis that functions to flex the hand. Compare **flexor carpi radialis, flexor carpi ulnaris.**

palmar metacarpal artery, any one of several arteries arising from the deep palmar arch that supply the fingers.

palmar pinch, a thumbless grasp in which the tips of the other fingers are pressed against the palm of the hand. See also **pinch, tip pinch.**

palmar reflex, a reflex that curls the fingers when the palm of the hand is stroked.

palmature /pal″məchər/ [L, *palma*], an abnormal condition in which the fingers are webbed.

palm-chin reflex. See **palmomental reflex.**

Palmer notation, a system for designating teeth in which the mouth is divided into quadrants indicated by a right-angle symbol oriented right or left and up or down. The teeth in each quadrant are numbered from 1 to 8, starting with the central incisor and ending with the third molar. The system is no longer in general use. See also **FDI numbering system, universal tooth coding system.**

palmitic acid ($CH_3[CH_2]_{14}COOH$) /palmit″ik/ [L, *palma*], a saturated fatty acid that commonly occurs in animal and vegetable fats and oils. It is a carboxylic acid used in the production of soaps and candles. Also called **hexadecanoic acid.**

palmitin /pal″mitin/, a triglyceride consisting of palmitic acid present in palm oil and other vegetable and animal fats.

palmityl alcohol. See **cetyl alcohol.**

palmomental reflex /pal′məmen″təl/ [L, *palma* + *mentum*, chin, *reflectere,* to bend back], an abnormal neurological sign, elicited by scratching the palm of the hand at the base of the thumb, characterized by contraction of the muscles of the chin and corner of the mouth on the same side of the body as the stimulus. It is occasionally seen in normal individuals, but an exaggerated reflex may occur in patients with pyramidal tract disease, latent tetany, increased intracranial pressure, central facial paresis, and dementia. Also called **palm-chin reflex.**

palmoplantar erythrodysesthesia (PPE), a dermatological toxicity associated with some chemotherapeutic medications; it is characterized by tingling and tenderness on the palm of the hand and sole of the foot that progresses to symmetrical redness, swelling, and pain. Also called **hand-foot syndrome.**

palonosetron, an antiemetic.
■ INDICATIONS: This drug is used to prevent nausea and vomiting associated with cancer chemotherapy.
■ CONTRAINDICATIONS: Known hypersensitivity to this drug prohibits its use.
■ ADVERSE EFFECTS: Adverse effects of this drug include abdominal pain, weakness, hyperkalemia, anxiety, rash, and arthralgia. A rare life-threatening side effect is bronchospasm. Common side effects include diarrhea, constipation, headache, dizziness, drowsiness, fatigue, insomnia, fever, and urinary retention.

palpable /pal″pəbəl/ [L, *palpare,* to touch gently], perceivable by touch.

palpation /palpā″shən/ [L, *palpare,* to touch gently], a technique used in physical examination in which the examiner feels the texture, size, consistency, and location of certain body parts with the hands.

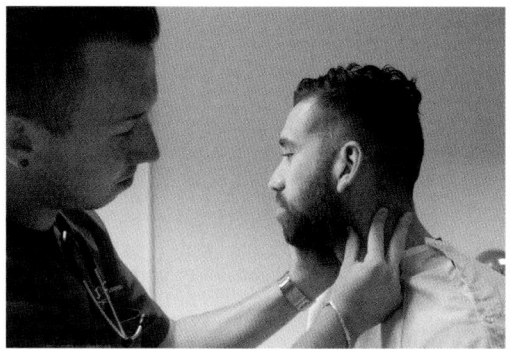

Palpation *(Courtesy Rutgers School of Nursing—Camden. All rights reserved.)*

palpatory percussion /pal″pətôr′ē/ [L, *palpare,* to touch gently, *percutere,* to strike hard], a technique in physical examination in which the vibrations produced by percussion are evaluated by using light pressure of the flat of the examiner's hand.

palpebra. See **eyelid.**

palpebral commissure. See **canthus.**

palpebral conjunctiva. See **conjunctiva.**

palpebral fissure /pal″pəbrəl/ [L, *palpebra,* eyelid, *fissura,* cleft], the opening between the margins of the upper and lower eyelids.

palpebral gland. See **meibomian gland.**

palpebra superior /pal″pəbrə/ pl. *palpebrae superiores,* the upper eyelid, larger and more movable than the lower eyelid and furnished with an elevator muscle.

palpebrate /pal″pəbrāt/, **1.** *v.,* to wink or blink. **2.** *adj.,* having eyelids.

palpitate /pal″pitāt/ [L, *palpitare,* to flutter], to pulsate rapidly, as in the unusually fast beating of the heart under various conditions of stress and in certain heart problems.

palpitation /pal″pitā″shən/ [L, *palpitare,* to flutter], a pounding or racing of the heart. It is associated with normal emotional responses and with heart disorders. Some people may complain of pounding heart and display no evidence of heart disease, whereas others with serious heart disorders may not detect associated abnormal palpitations. Some patients complain of palpitations after receiving digitalis because it increases the force of heart contractions. **–palpitate,** *v.*

PALS, abbreviation for **pediatric advanced life support.**

palsy /pôl″zē/ [Gk, *para,* beyond, *lysis,* loosening], an abnormal condition characterized by paralysis. Kinds include **Bell palsy, cerebral palsy, Erb palsy.**

Paltauf nanism /päl″touf/ [Arnold Paltauf, Czechoslovakian physician, 1860–1893; Gk, *nanos,* dwarf], dwarfism associated with excessive production or growth of lymphoid tissue.

Pamelor /pam′ĕ-lor/, a tricyclic antidepressant drug. Brand name for **nortriptyline hydrochloride.**

-pamide, suffix for sulfamoylbenzoic acid–derived diuretics.

pamidronate disodium, the disodium salt of pamidronate, used in the treatment of malignancy-associated hypercalcemia, osteitis deformans, and osteolytic bone metastases associated with breast cancer and myeloma. It is administered intravenously.

-pamil, suffix for verapamil-type coronary vasodilators.

Pamine, an anticholinergic drug. Brand name for **methscopolamine bromide.**

p-aminohippurate /ah-me″no-hip′u-rāt/, a salt, conjugate base, or ester of *p*-aminohippuric acid. The sodium salt is used to measure effective renal plasma flow and to determine the functional capacity of the tubular excretory mechanism.

pampiniform /pampin″ifôrm/ [L, *pampinus,* vine tendril, *plexus,* plaited], having the shape of a tendril.

pampiniform body. See **epoophoron.**

pampiniform plexus [L, *pampinus,* vine tendril, *plexus,* plaited], a network of veins in the spermatic cord that drains the testes into the testicular vein in the lower abdomen.

pan- /pan-/, prefix meaning "all": *panacea, pancarditis, pandemic.*

panacea /pan′əsē″ə/ [Gk, *pan,* all, *akeia,* remedy], **1.** a universal remedy. **2.** an ancient name for an herb or a liquid potion with healing properties. **3.** a remedy for all disease; a cure-all.

panacinar emphysema /pan′əsin′ər/ [Gk, *pan,* all + L, *acinus,* grape], one of the principal types of emphysema, characterized by relatively uniform enlargement of air spaces throughout the terminal bronchioles and alveoli. It is an inherited condition. Also called **chronic hypertrophic emphysema, diffuse emphysema, ectatic emphysema, generalized emphysema, panlobular emphysema, vesicular emphysema.**

panagglutinable /pan′əglo͞o″tinəbəl/, pertaining to red blood cells that are agglutinable by the sera of all blood groups of the same species.

panagglutinin /pan′əglo͞o″tinin/, an antibody that causes clumping (agglutination) of red blood cells of all blood groups of a species.

Panama fever. See **Chagres fever.**

pananencephaly /panan′ensef″əlē/, pain that affects all parts of the body.

panangiitis /panan′jē-ī′tis/, an inflammation that affects all layers of a blood vessel.

panarteritis /-är′tərī″tis/ [Gk, *pan,* all, *arteria,* artery, *itis,* inflammation], an inflammation that involves all the tissue layers of an artery.

panarthritis /-ärthrī″tis/ [Gk, *pan* + *arthron,* joint], an abnormal condition characterized by the inflammation of many joints in the body. **–panarthritic,** *adj.*

panatrophy /panat″rəfē/, **1.** a general atrophy of all parts of a body or structure. **2.** a rare disorder associated with atrophy of cutaneous and subcutaneous tissue, characterized by prominence of underlying body structures as all levels of skin and subcutaneous tissue are reduced in thickness.

panbronchiolitis /panbrong″kē-əlī″tis/, chronic inflammation and obstruction of the bronchioles caused by the accumulation of foam cells. It usually leads to bronchiectasis.

pancake kidney /pan″kāk/ [ME, *panne,* pan, *kaka,* cake, *kidnere*], a congenital anomaly in which the left and right kidneys are fused into a single mass in the pelvis. The fused kidney has two collecting systems and two ureters and frequently becomes obstructed because of its abnormal position.

pancarditis /-kärdī″tis/ [Gk, *pan* + *kardia,* heart, *itis,* inflammation], an abnormal condition characterized by inflammation of the entire heart, including the endocardium, myocardium, and pericardium.

Pancoast syndrome /pan″cōst/ [Henry K. Pancoast, American radiologist, 1875–1939], **1.** a combination of signs associated with a tumor in the apex of the lung. The signs include neuritic pain in the arm, atrophy of the muscles

P

of the arm and the hand, and Horner syndrome and are caused by the damaging effects of the tumor on the brachial plexus and sympathetic ganglia. **2.** an abnormal condition caused by osteolysis in the posterior part of one or more ribs, sometimes involving associated vertebrae.

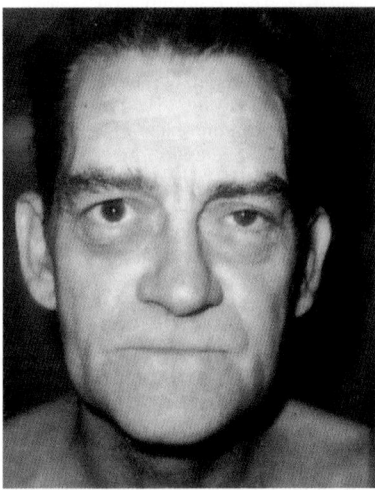

Individual with characteristic facial appearance associated with Horner syndrome in a patient with Pancoast syndrome *(Skarin, 2010)*

Pancoast tumor. See **pulmonary sulcus tumor.**

pancolectomy /-kōlek″təmē/ [Gk, *pan* + *kolon*, colon, *ektomē*, excision], the excision of the entire colon, necessitating an ileostomy.

pancreas /pan″krē·əs/ [Gk, *pan*, all, *kreas*, flesh], an elongated grayish pink lobulated gland that stretches transversely across the posterior abdominal wall in the epigastric and hypochondriac regions of the body and secretes various substances, such as digestive enzymes, insulin, and glucagon. It is divided into a head; a flattened, elongated body; and a tail in contact with the spleen. The head of the gland, divided from the body by a small constriction, is tucked into the curve of the duodenum. The tapered left extremity of the organ forms the tail. In adults the pancreas is about 13 cm long. A compound, mixed gland composed of exocrine and endocrine tissue, it contains a main duct that runs the length of the organ, draining smaller ducts and emptying into the duodenum at the major duodenal papilla, the same site that accommodates the entrance of the common bile duct.

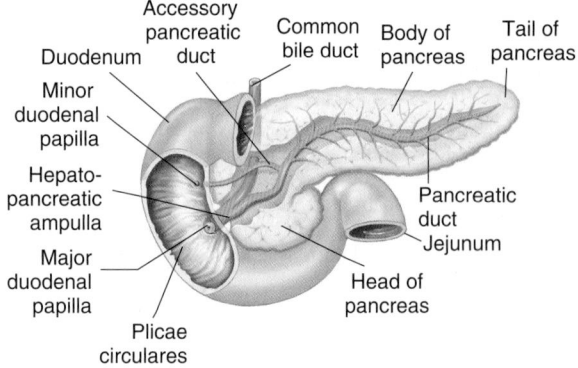

Pancreas *(Patton and Thibodeau, 2016)*

pancreas scan, a computed tomography scan of the pancreas after the IV injection of a radiopaque contrast medium; it is used for detecting various abnormalities, such as tumors, cysts, and infections.

-pancreat, suffix meaning "pancreas": *bilopancreatic, hepatopancreatic.*

pancreatalgia /pan′krē·ətal″jə/, pain in or near the pancreas.

pancreatectomy /pan′krē·ətek″təmē/ [Gk, *pan* + *kreas* + *ektomē*, excision], the surgical removal of all or part of the pancreas, performed to excise a cyst or tumor, treat pancreatitis, or repair trauma. The GI tract is reconstructed, usually with an anastomosis between the pancreatic duct and the upper jejunum. Drains are left in the wound. After surgery the patient is given a low-sugar, low-fat diet. If the entire pancreas is removed, pancreatic insufficiency develops, requiring precise management of both diet and enzyme replacement therapy as well as insulin injections or the use of an insulin pump. A frequent complication is the formation of a fistula in the pancreatic bile duct, allowing digestive enzymes to contact adjacent tissues.

pancreatemphraxis /pan′krē·at′emfrak″sis/, hypertrophy or congestion of the pancreas caused by an obstruction in the pancreatic duct.

pancreatic abscess, an infection characterized by a collection of pus in or around the pancreas.

pancreatic autodigestion, premature breakdown of pancreatic zymogens into digestive enzymes that digest pancreatic tissue, causing acute pancreatitis.

pancreatic buds, two outgrowths, one dorsal and one ventral, from the endodermal lining of the caudal part of the embryonic foregut that fuse and develop into the pancreas.

pancreatic cancer [Gk, *pan* + *kreas* + L, *cancer,* crab], a malignant neoplastic disease of the pancreas characterized by anorexia, flatulence, weakness, dramatic weight loss, epigastric or back pain, jaundice, pruritus, a palpable abdominal mass, recent onset of diabetes, and clay-colored stools if the pancreatic and biliary ducts are obstructed. Symptoms depend on the location of the tumor within the pancreas or in metastatic sites. Diagnostic measures include barium radiographic studies of the stomach and duodenum, transhepatic cholangiography (endoscopic retrograde cholangiopancreatography), laboratory evaluation of liver function, celiac arteriography, computed axial tomography, and magnetic resonance imaging. Exploratory laparotomy is often required for a definitive diagnosis. About 90% of pancreatic tumors are adenocarcinomas; two thirds are in the head of the pancreas. Most tumors are not resectable at the time of diagnosis, but localized cancers in the pancreas may be treated by partial pancreatectomy with excision of the common bile duct, duodenum, and distal part of the stomach. Functioning islet cell lesions may be excised or treated with streptozocin, an antibiotic toxic to beta cells of the pancreas. Total gastrectomy is recommended for gastrin-producing islet cell tumors that are resectable and accompanied by severe peptic ulcer disease. Radiotherapy or chemotherapy with docetaxel, cisplatin, femocitabine, or mitomycin C may offer temporary palliation, but cancer of the pancreas has a poor prognosis. Few people live for more than 1 year after diagnosis. Most nursing care is of a palliative nature. Pancreatic cancer occurs three to four times more often in men than in women. Though uncommon, it is increasing in incidence in the industrialized areas of the world. People who smoke more than 10 to 20 cigarettes a day, have diabetes mellitus, or have been exposed to polychlorinated biphenyl compounds are at increased risk of development of pancreatic cancer.

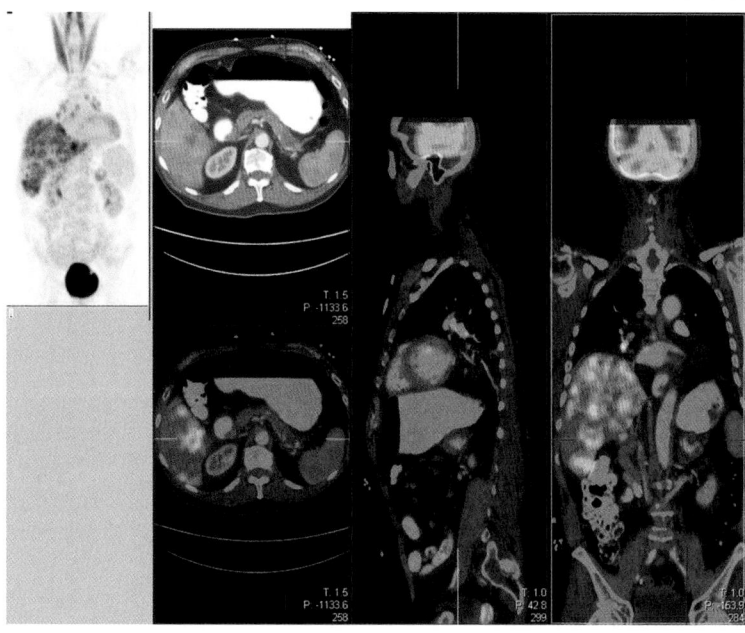

Axial CT scan showing enlargement of the tail of the pancreas associated with pancreatic cancer
(Mettler and Guiberteau, 2012)

pancreatic collum, neck of pancreas: a constricted portion marking the junction of the head and body of the pancreas.

pancreatic diabetes [Gk, *pan,* all, *kreas,* flesh, *diabainein,* to pass through], a unique clinical and metabolic form of diabetes mellitus caused by chronic pancreatitis. See also **diabetes mellitus.**

pancreatic diarrhea. See **Verner-Morrison syndrome.**

pancreatic diverticulum, one of a pair of membranous pouches arising from the embryonic duodenum. These two diverticula later form the pancreas and its ducts.

pancreatic dornase, an enzyme from beef pancreas that has been used as a mucolytic for upper respiratory infections and cystic fibrosis.

pancreatic duct, the primary secretory channel of the pancreas. Also called **duct of Wirsung.** Compare **accessory pancreatic duct.**

pancreatic enzyme, any one of the enzymes secreted by the pancreas in the process of digestion. The most important are trypsin, chymotrypsin, steapsin, and amylopsin. See also **pancreatic juice.**

pancreatic enzyme digestion, the action of pancreatic enzymes in the process of breaking down food into its constituents.

pancreatic enzyme therapy, replacement therapy for conditions of pancreatic insufficiency with malabsorption, such as cystic fibrosis.

pancreatic hormone, any one of several chemical compounds secreted by the pancreas and associated with the regulation of cellular metabolism. Major hormones secreted by the pancreas are insulin amylin, glucagon, somatostatin, and pancreatic polypeptide. Somatostatin is secreted by the delta cells, and pancreatic polypeptide is secreted by a group of glandular cells arranged in a halo around each islet of Langerhans. Insulin is secreted by beta cells of the islets of Langerhans; glucagon is secreted by alpha cells of the islets of Langerhans.

pancreatic insufficiency, a condition characterized by inadequate production and secretion of pancreatic hormones or enzymes. It usually occurs secondary to a disease process destructive to pancreatic tissue. Nutritional malabsorption, anorexia, poorly localized upper abdominal or epigastric pain, malaise, and severe weight loss often occur. Alcohol-induced pancreatitis is the most common form of the condition. Supportive care, specific treatment of the cause, and replacement or augmentation of the absent or lacking substances are usually recommended as therapy for pancreatic insufficiency.

pancreatic juice, the fluid secretion of the pancreas, produced by the stimulation of food in the duodenum. It contains water, protein, inorganic salts, and enzymes. The juice is essential in breaking down proteins into their amino acid components, reducing dietary fats to glycerol and fatty acids, and converting starch to simple sugars.

pancreatic lithiasis. See **pancreatolithiasis.**

pancreaticoduodenal /pan′krē·at′ikōdoo′ədē″nəl/, pertaining to the pancreas and duodenum.

pancreaticoduodenectomy /pan′krē·ətōdoo′ədənek″t əmē/ [Gk, *pan + kreas* + L, *duodeni,* twelve fingers; Gk, *ektomē,* excision], a surgical procedure in which the head of the pancreas, the entire duodenum, a portion of the jejunum, the distal third of the stomach, and the lower half of the common bile duct are excised, usually to relieve obstruction caused by tumors, often malignant. Continuity is reestablished among the biliary, pancreatic, and GI systems. The operation is performed to remove the periampullary masses that occur in certain forms of biliary tract cancer. Also called **Whipple procedure.**

pancreaticolienal node /pan′krē·at′ikō′lī·ē″nəl/ [Gk, *pan + kreas* + L, *lien,* spleen, *nodus,* knot], a node in one of three groups of lymph glands associated with branches of the abdominal and pelvic viscera that are supplied by branches of the celiac artery. The pancreaticolienal nodes accompany the splenic artery along the posterior surface and the upper border of the pancreas. Their afferent vessels, which originate from the stomach, the spleen, and the pancreas, join the celiac group of preaortic nodes. Also called **splenic gland.** Compare **gastric node, hepatic node.**

P

pancreatic rest, ectopic pancreatic tissue, usually in the stomach or small intestine, forming a polyplike lesion.

pancreatin /pan″krē·ətin′, -krē·ā″tin/, a concentrate of pancreatic enzymes from swine or beef cattle.

- INDICATIONS: It is prescribed as an aid to digestion to replace endogenous pancreatic enzymes in cystic fibrosis and after pancreatectomy.
- CONTRAINDICATIONS: Known hypersensitivity to this drug or to pork or beef protein, acute pancreatitis, or a flare in chronic pancreatitis prohibits its use.
- ADVERSE EFFECTS: There are no known serious adverse effects. High doses may cause nausea or diarrhea.

pancreatitis /pan″krē·ətī″tis/ [Gk, *pan* + *kreas* + *itis,* inflammation], an inflammatory condition of the pancreas that may be acute or chronic. Acute pancreatitis is generally the result of damage to the biliary tract, as by alcohol, trauma, infectious disease, or certain drugs. It is characterized by severe abdominal pain (generally epigastric or upper left) radiating to the back, fever, anorexia, nausea, and vomiting. There may be jaundice if the common bile duct is obstructed. The development of pseudocysts or abscesses in pancreatic tissue is a serious complication. Treatment includes nasogastric suction to remove gastric secretions. To prevent any stimulation of the pancreas, nothing is given by mouth. The client may be given antacids to decrease the acid, which stimulates the pancreas. IV fluids and electrolytes are administered, and nonmorphine derivatives are given to relieve pain. The causes of chronic pancreatitis are similar to those of the acute form. When the cause is alcohol abuse, there may be calcification and scarring of the smaller pancreatic ducts. Abdominal pain, nausea, and vomiting occur, as well as steatorrhea and creatorrhea, caused by the diminished output of pancreatic enzymes. Pancreatic insulin production may be diminished, and diabetes mellitus develops in some patients. Treatment includes analgesics for pain and subtotal pancreatectomy when pain is intractable. A pancreatic extract is given orally to replace the missing enzymes; vitamin supplements are essential; and calcium supplements may be needed. Both forms of pancreatitis are diagnosed by history, physical examination, radiological studies, endoscopy, and laboratory analysis of the amount of pancreatic enzymes in the blood.

pancreatoduodenostomy /-doo′ədənos″təmē/, a surgical procedure to establish a fistula or duct from the pancreas into the duodenum.

pancreatogastrostomy /-gastros″təmē/, the surgical establishment of a fistula or duct from the pancreas to the stomach.

pancreatogenic /-jen″ik/, originating in the pancreas.

pancreatography /pan″krē·ətog″rəfē/ [Gk, *pan* + *kreas* + *graphein,* to record], visualization of the pancreas or its ducts by radiography, ultrasonography, computed tomography, or radionuclide imaging following injection of a contrast medium into the ducts during surgery or via an endoscope.

pancreatojejunostomy /-jij′oonos″təmē/, the surgical establishment of a fistula or duct from the pancreas to the jejunum to relieve the pain associated with chronic pancreatitis.

pancreatolith /pan″krē·at″əlith/, a stone or calculus in the pancreas.

pancreatolithiasis /pan″kre·ətolithī″əsis/, the presence of calculi in the pancreas or pancreatic duct.

pancreatolithotomy /lithot″əmē/, the surgical removal of pancreatic calculi.

pancreatolysis /pan″krē·ətol″isis/, destruction of the pancreas by pancreatic enzymes.

pancreatomegaly /-meg″əlē/, an abnormal enlargement of the pancreas.

pancreatopathy /pan″krē·ətop″əthē/, any disease of the pancreas.

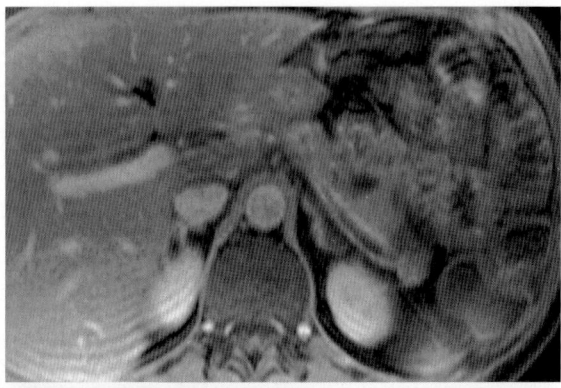
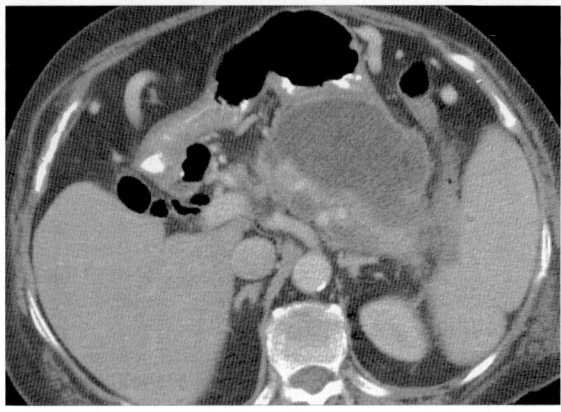

MRI of acute pancreatitis *(Gore and Levine, 2015)*

pancreatotomy /pan″krē·ətot″əmē/, a surgical incision in the pancreas.

pancreatropic /pan″krē·ətrop″ik/, exerting an influence on the pancreas. Also called *pancreatotropic.*

pancreolauryl test, (for pancreatic function) the oral administration of fluorescein dilaurate and the monitoring of its cleavage to yield lauric acid as a measure of pancreatic esterase activity.

pancuronium bromide /pan″kyərō″nē·əm/, a skeletal muscle relaxant; a nondepolarizing neuromuscular blocker.

- INDICATIONS: It is prescribed as an adjunct to anesthesia and mechanical ventilation.
- CONTRAINDICATIONS: Known hypersensitivity to this drug or to other bromides prohibits its use. Ventilation always must be supported during the use of neuromuscular blockers. Patients with renal and hepatic disease require dosage adjustments, and pancuronium is not recommended during pregnancy. Some diseases (e.g., myasthenia gravis) can potentiate the effects of pancuronium, whereas others (e.g., diabetes mellitus) can antagonize the drug's effects.
- ADVERSE EFFECTS: The most serious adverse effects are prolonged muscle relaxation and respiratory depression.

pancytopenia /pan″sītəpē″nē·ə/ [Gk, *pan* + *kytos,* cell, *penia,* poverty], simultaneous reduction in red blood cell, white blood cell, and platelet counts. See also **anemia, aplasia, neutropenia. –pancytopenic,** *adj.*

pancytopenia-dysmelia. See **Fanconi anemia.**

pancytopenic. See **pancytopenia.**

p and a, a notation in the patient's chart after physical examination of the chest. Abbreviation for *percussion and auscultation.*

pandemia /-dē″mē·ə/ [Gk, *pan,* all, *demos,* people], a disease epidemic that affects all or most of a population group.

pandemic /-dē″mik/ [Gk, *pan* + *demos,* people], (of a disease) occurring throughout the population of a country, a people, or the world.

pandiastolic /-dī′əstol″ik/ [Gk, *pan* + *dia,* through, *stellein,* to set], pertaining to the complete diastole. Also called **holodiastolic.**

panencephalitis /pan′ənsef′əlī″tis/ [Gk, *pan* + *enkephale,* brain, *itis*], inflammation of the entire brain characterized by an insidious onset, a progressive course with deterioration of motor and mental functions, and evidence of a viral cause. One example is subacute sclerosing panencephalitis, an uncommon childhood disease thought to be caused by a "slow" latent measles virus after recovery from a previous infection. Most of the patients are younger than 11 years of age, and many more boys than girls are affected. The disease results in ataxia, myoclonus, atrophy, cortical blindness, and mental deterioration. Antiviral drugs, immunosuppressants, and interferon inducers are sometimes administered, but the disease is usually unremitting and fatal.

panendoscope /-en″dəskōp′/ [Gk, *pan* + *endon,* within, *skopein,* to look], a cystoscope that allows a wide view of the interior of the bladder and urethra with a specialized lens system.

panesthesia /-esthē″zhə/ [Gk, *pan* + *aisthesis,* feeling], the total of all sensations experienced by an individual at one time. Compare **cenesthesia.**

pang, a sudden severe but temporary pain.

pangenesis /-jen″əsis/ [Gk, *pan* + *genesis,* origin], an idea that each cell and particle of a parent reproduces itself in progeny.

panhidrosis, perspiration over the entire body.

panhypopituitarism /panhī′pōpitoo̅″itəriz′əm/ [Gk, *pan* + *hypo,* under, *pituita,* phlegm], generalized insufficiency of pituitary hormones, resulting from damage to or deficiency of the gland. Prepubertal panhypopituitarism, a rare disorder usually associated with a suprasellar cyst or craniopharyngioma, is characterized by dwarfism with normal body proportions, subnormal sexual development, and insufficient thyroid and adrenal function. Diabetes insipidus is frequently present, bitemporal hemianopia or complete blindness may occur, and skin is often yellow and wrinkled, but mentality is usually unimpaired. X-ray films show delayed fusion of the epiphyses, suprasellar calcification, and, frequently, destruction of the sella turcica. The condition is treated with cortisone, thyroid and sex hormone replacement, and human growth hormone. Postpubertal panhypopituitarism may be caused by postpartum pituitary necrosis (Sheehan syndrome), resulting from thrombosis of pituitary circulation during or after delivery or other trauma to the pituitary. Characteristic signs of the disorder are failure to lactate, amenorrhea (in females), weakness, cold intolerance, lethargy, and loss of libido and of axillary and pubic hair. There may be bradycardia or hypotension, and progression of the disorder leads to premature wrinkling of the skin and atrophy of the thyroid and adrenal glands. Treatment consists of the administration of the hormones of the target organs. Panhypopituitarism may also be caused by pituitary apoplexy, hemorrhage, or head trauma. Also called **hypophyseal cachexia, pituitary cachexia, Simmonds disease.**

panhysterectomy /pan′histərek″təmē/ [Gk, *pan* + *hystera,* uterus, *ektomē,* excision], complete surgical removal of the uterus and cervix. See also **hysterectomy.**

panic /pan″ik/, an intense, sudden, and overwhelming fear or feeling of anxiety that produces terror and immediate physiological changes that result in paralyzed immobility or senseless, hysteric behavior.

panic attack [Gk, *panikos,* of the god Pan; Fr, *attaquer*], an episode of acute anxiety that occurs unpredictably, with feelings of intense apprehension or terror accompanied by dyspnea, dizziness, sweating, trembling, and chest pain or palpitations. The attack may last several minutes and may occur again in certain situations. Compare **anxiety attack.**

panic disorder. See **anxiety attack.**

panitumumab, a miscellaneous antineoplastic drug.

■ INDICATIONS: This drug is used to treat metastatic colon cancer expressing epidermal growth factor receptor.

■ CONTRAINDICATIONS: Known hypersensitivity to this drug prohibits its use.

■ ADVERSE EFFECTS: Adverse effects of this drug include fatigue, ocular toxicity, peripheral edema, anorexia, mouth ulceration, abdominal pain, constipation, thrombophlebitis, pruritus, skin fissure, hypocalcemia, hypomagnesemia, antibody formation, dyspnea, pneumonitis, and wheezing. Life-threatening side effects include exfoliative dermatitis, bronchospasm, cough, hypoxia, and pulmonary fibrosis. Common side effects include nausea, diarrhea, vomiting, and rash.

panivorous /paniv″ərəs/ [L, *panis,* bread, *vorare,* to devour], pertaining to the practice of subsisting exclusively on bread. *–panivore, n.*

panlobular emphysema. See **panacinar emphysema.**

panmyelosis /panmī′əlō″sis/, a pathological condition characterized by a proliferation of bone marrow cells of all types. This term is not in common usage.

Panner disease, a rare form of osteochondrosis in which abnormal bony growth occurs in the capitulum of the humerus.

panniculitis /pənik′yəlī″tis/ [L, *panniculus,* piece of cloth; Gk, *itis,* inflammation], a chronic inflammation of subcutaneous fat in which the skin becomes hardened, particularly over the abdomen and thorax. Small subcutaneous masses of hard tissue are found in the affected areas. Some forms of the inflammation may be marked by the appearance of painless subcutaneous nodules on the lower extremities.

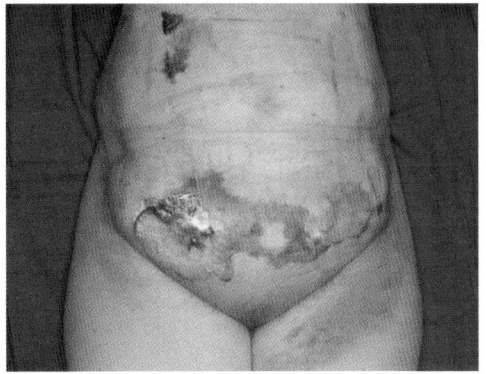

Panniculitis *(Larcher et al, 2011)*

panniculus /pənik″yələs/ *pl. panniculi* [L, small garment], **1.** a membranous layer. **2.** the many sheets of fascia covering various structures in the body.

pannus /pan″əs/ [L, *cloth*], **1.** an abnormal condition of the cornea, which becomes vascularized and infiltrated with granular tissue just beneath the surface. Pannus may develop in the inflammatory stage of trachoma or after a detached retina, glaucoma, iridocyclitis, or other degenerative eye disorder. **2.** abnormal tissue growth caused by thickening of the synovial membrane lining the joints.

panography /pənog″rəfē/, a method of tomography that visualizes curved surfaces of the body at any depth. In dentistry it is accomplished by simultaneous radiography or dental imaging of the maxillary and mandibular dental arches and associated structures along two axes of rotation. A panoramic image is recorded on an intensifying screen that rotates with the radiation source around the patient's head. The image is converted to digital form to be viewed on a computer screen. See also **panoramic radiograph.**

panophobia. See **panphobia.**

panophthalmitis /pan′ofthalmī″tis/ [Gk, *pan* + *ophthalmos,* eye, *itis*], an inflammation of the entire eye, usually caused by virulent pyogenic organisms, such as strains of meningococci, pneumococci, streptococci, anthrax bacilli, and clostridia. Initial symptoms are pain, fever, headache, drowsiness, edema, and swelling. As the infection progresses, the iris appears muddy and gray, the aqueous humor becomes turbid, and precipitates form on the posterior surface of the cornea. Treatment consists of intensive systemic and local antibiotic therapy. Evisceration of the globe or excision of the eye may be required, but excision is contraindicated if surrounding tissues are infected.

panoptic /panop″tik/ [Gk, *pan,* all, *opsis,* vision], pertaining to the enhanced visual effect produced by stains applied to microscopic specimens.

panoramic radiograph /pan′ôram″ik/ [Gk, *pan* + *horama,* view; L, *radiare,* to emit rays; Gk, *graphein,* to record], an x-ray image of a curved body surface, such as the upper and lower jaws, on a single film. Also called **pantomograph,** *panoramic radiography.*

panotitis /pan′ōtī″tis/, a general inflammation of the ear, including the middle ear.

PanOxyl, a keratolytic agent. Brand name for **benzoyl peroxide.**

panphobia /-fō″bē·ə/ [Gk, *pan* + *phobos,* fear], an anxiety disorder characterized by an irrational fear of everything. Also called **panophobia, pantophobia.** *–panphobic, adj.*

panplegia /panplē″jē·ə/, paralysis of all four extremities.

pansclerosis /pan′sklirō″sis/, a general hardening of a tissue or body part.

pansystolic /-sistol″ik/, pertaining to the entire systole. Also called **holosystolic.**

pansystolic murmur. See **systolic murmur.**

pant-. See **panto-, pant-.**

pantothenic acid, a vitamin of the B complex present in all living tissues, almost entirely in the form of a coenzyme A (CoA). This coenzyme has many metabolic roles in the cell, and a lack of pantothenic acid can lead to depressed metabolism of both carbohydrates and fats. The daily requirement for this vitamin has not been established and no definite deficiency syndrome has been recognized in humans, perhaps due to its wide occurrence in almost all foods.

panthenol /pan″thənôl/, **1.** an alcohol converted in the body to pantothenic acid, a vitamin in the B complex. Also called **pantothenyl alcohol. 2.** a viscous liquid derived from pantothenic acid, a member of the vitamin B_{12} group.

panting [Fr, *panteler,* to gasp], a ventilatory pattern characterized by rapid, shallow breathing commonly used during labor. Panting usually moves gas back and forth in the anatomical dead space at a high flow rate, which evaporates water and removes heat but produces little or no alveolar ventilation. It does not usually cause carbon dioxide levels to be affected. Compare **hyperventilation.**

panto-, pant-, prefix meaning "all, the whole": *pantophobia, pantoscopic, pantograph.*

pantograph /pan″təgraf′/, **1.** a jointed device for copying a plane figure to any desired scale. **2.** a device that

incorporates a pair of face bows fixed to the jaws, used for inscribing centrically related points and arcs leading to the points on segments relatable to the three craniofacial planes.

pantomograph /pantom″əgraf/. See **panoramic radiograph.**

pantomography /-mog″rəfē/ [Gk, *pan* + *graphein,* to record], panoramic radiography or dental imaging for obtaining simultaneous radiographs or images of the maxillary and mandibular dental arches and related structures.

pantophobia. See **panphobia.**

pantoprazole /panto′prah-zōl/, a gastric acid pump inhibitor with properties similar to those of omeprazole. It is administered orally and intravenously as the sodium salt in the treatment of erosive esophagitis associated with gastroesophageal reflux disease and intravenously as the sodium salt in the treatment of hypersecretion associated with Zollinger-Ellison syndrome or other neoplastic conditions.

pantoscopic /pan′təskop″ik/, pertaining to bifocal eyeglasses designed for both reading and distance viewing. The bottom half is for close vision, and the top half is for far vision.

pantamorphia, *(Obsolete)* shapeless.

pantanencephaly /pantan′ensef″əlē/, a congenital absence of all or nearly all brain tissue.

pantothenic acid /pan′təthen″ik/, a member of the vitamin B complex. It is widely distributed in plant and animal tissues, almost entirely in the form of coenzyme A (CoA). This coenzyme has many metabolic roles in the cell, and a lack of pantothenic acid can lead to depressed metabolism of both carbohydrates and fats. No definite deficiency syndrome has been recognized in humans, perhaps due to its wide occurrence in almost all foods.

pantothenyl alcohol. See **panthenol.**

pantropic virus, a virus that affects or has an affinity for many different kinds of tissue or organs.

panzootic, occurring among animals over a wide geographic area.

PaO$_2$, symbol for **partial pressure of oxygen in arterial blood.**

PAO$_2$, symbol for *partial pressure of alveolar oxygen.*

pap, **1.** any soft, soggy food. **2.** porridge or gruel.

papain /pəpā″ēn/, a proteolytic enzyme from the fruit of *Carica papaya,* a tropical melon tree. It is prescribed for enzymatic debridement of wounds and promotion of healing.

Papanicolaou (Pap) test /pap′ənik′əlou″/ [George N. Papanicolaou, Greek physician in U.S. practice, 1883–1962], a simple smear method of examining stained exfoliative cells. It is used most commonly to detect cancers of the cervix, but it may be used for tissue specimens from any organ. A smear, the Papanicolaou's (Pap) smear, is usually obtained during a routine pelvic examination annually beginning at 21 years of age. The technique permits early diagnosis of cancer and has contributed to a lower death rate from cervical cancer. The findings are usually reported descriptively. Also called **Pap smear, Pap test.**

papaverine hydrochloride /papav″ərēn/, a smooth muscle relaxant and vasodilator.

■ INDICATIONS: It is prescribed in the treatment of cardiovascular or visceral spasms.

■ CONTRAINDICATIONS: Known hypersensitivity to this drug prohibits its use, and it must be used with caution in patients with glaucoma. It must be administered slowly because it can cause apnea and arrhythmias. Larger dosages can cause AV block.

■ ADVERSE EFFECTS: The most serious adverse effects include jaundice, tachycardia, arrhythmias, drowsiness, headache, weakness, nausea, and vomiting.

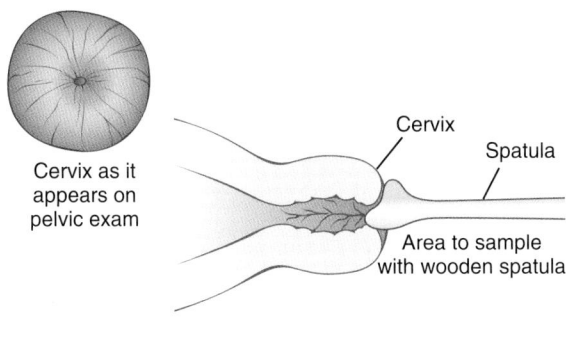

Cervix as it appears on pelvic exam

Cervix

Spatula

Area to sample with wooden spatula

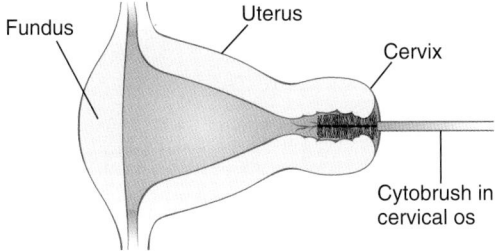

Fundus

Uterus

Cervix

Cytobrush in cervical os

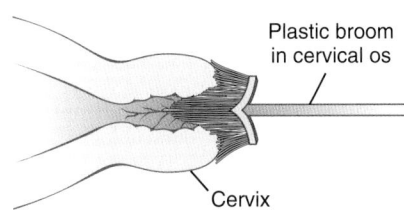

Plastic broom in cervical os

Cervix

Collecting a Pap smear sample *(Dehn and Asprey, 2013)*

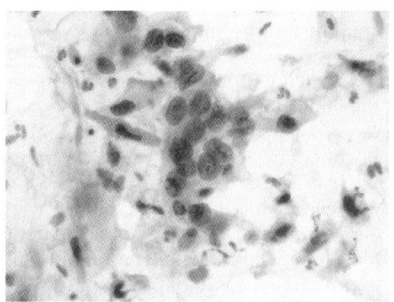

Positive Pap smear indicative of cervical cancer
(Courtesy Dr. Edmund Cibas, Department of Pathology, Brigham and Women's Hospital)

papaya /pəpī″ə/, the fruit of the tropical *Carica papaya* tree and the source of the proteolytic enzyme papain used in blood group serological evaluation. Papain is also used to prevent adhesions. A common nonmedicinal use is as a meat tenderizer.

paper, a material produced in sheets, usually from wood pulp or other cellulose products. It can be adapted for many purposes, such as litmus paper for testing acidity, filter paper, and articulating carbon paper used to record points of contact between teeth of the upper and lower jaws.

paper chromatography [Gk, *papyros,* papyrus], the separation of a mixture into its components by filtering it through a strip of special paper.

paper-doll fetus. See **fetus papyraceus.**

paper point, in root canal therapy, a cone of variable width and taper, usually made of paper or a paper product, used to dry or maintain a liquid disinfectant in the canal. Also called **absorbent point.**

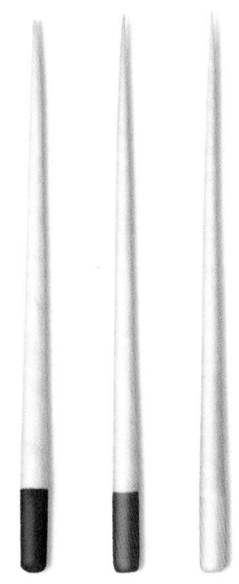

Paper points color coded for size *(Courtesy Pac-Dent, Inc.)*

paper radioimmunosorbent test (PRIST), a technique for determining total immunoglobulin E levels in patients with type I hypersensitivity reactions.

papill-, prefix meaning "resembling a nipple": *papillate, papilledema, papilloma.*

papilla /pəpil″ə/ *pl. papillae* [L, nipple], **1.** a small nipple-shaped projection, such as the conoid papillae of the tongue and the papillae of the dermis that extend from collagen fibers, the capillary blood vessels, and sometimes the nerves of the dermis. **2.** the optic papilla, a round white disc in the fundus oculi, which corresponds to the entrance of the optic nerve. Also called **optic disc.**

papilla duodeni major. See **hepatopancreatic ampulla.**

papillae. See **papilla.**

papilla mammae, papilla mammaria. See **nipple.**

papilla of Vater. See **hepatopancreatic ampulla.**

papillary /pap″əle′rē/ [L, *papilla,* nipple], pertaining to a papilla.

papillary adenocarcinoma, a malignant neoplasm characterized by small papillae of vascular connective tissue covered by neoplastic epithelium that projects into follicles, glands, or cysts. The tumor is most common in the ovaries and thyroid gland. Also called *polyploid adenocarcinoma.*

papillary adenocystoma lymphomatosum, a unique tumor, consisting of epithelial and lymphoid tissues, that develops in the area of the parotid and submaxillary glands. Also called **adenolymphoma, Warthin tumor.** See also **adenocyst.**

papillary adenoma, a benign epithelial tumor in which the membrane lining the glandular tissue forms papillary

P

processes that project into the alveoli or grow out of a cavity's surface.

papillary carcinoma, a malignant neoplasm characterized by fingerlike projections.

papillary duct, any one of the thousands of straight collecting renal tubules that descend through the medulla of the kidney and join with others to form the common ducts opening into the renal papillae. Compare **loop of Henle.** See also **kidney.**

papillary muscle, any one of the rounded or conical muscular projections attached to the chordae tendineae in the ventricles of the heart. The papillary muscles vary in number. The two main muscles are the anterior papillary muscle and the posterior papillary muscle. The papillary muscles are associated with the atrioventricular valves that they help open and close. Compare **chordae tendineae, trabecula carnea.**

papillary tumor. See **papilloma.**

papillate /pap″ilit/, marked by papillae or nipplelike prominences.

papilledema /pap′ilədē″mə/ *pl. papilledemas, papilledemata* [L, *papilla* + Gk, *oidema,* swelling], swelling of the optic disc, visible on ophthalmoscopic examination of the fundus of the eye, caused by increase in intracranial pressure. The meningeal sheaths that surround the optic nerves from the optic disc are continuous with the meninges of the brain; therefore increased intracranial pressure is transmitted forward from the brain to the optic disc in the eye to cause swelling. Also spelled *papilloedema.*

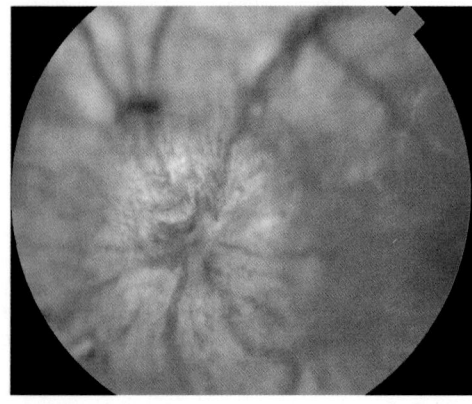

Papilledema *(Roy, Fraunfelder, and Fraunfelder, 2008)*

papilliform /pəpil″ifôrm/, shaped like a nipple.

papillitis /pap′ilī″tis/ [L, *papilla* + Gk, *itis,* inflammation], **1.** inflammation of a papilla, such as the lacrimal papilla. **2.** inflammation of the optic disc.

papilloadenocystoma /pap′ilō·ad′ənō′sistō″mə/, a benign epithelial tumor in which the lining develops in numerous small folds.

papillocarcinoma [L, *papilla,* nipple; Gk, *oma,* tumor, *karkinos,* crab, *oma,* tumor], a malignant tumor in which there are papillary outgrowths.

papilloma /pap′ilō″mə/ [L, *papilla* + Gk, *oma,* tumor], a benign epithelial neoplasm characterized by a branching or lobular tumor. Also called **papillary tumor.**

papilloma papovavirus. See **papovavirus.**

papillomatosis /pap′ilōmətō″sis/ [L, *papilla* + Gk, *oma,* tumor, *osis,* condition], an abnormal condition characterized by widespread development of nipplelike growths.

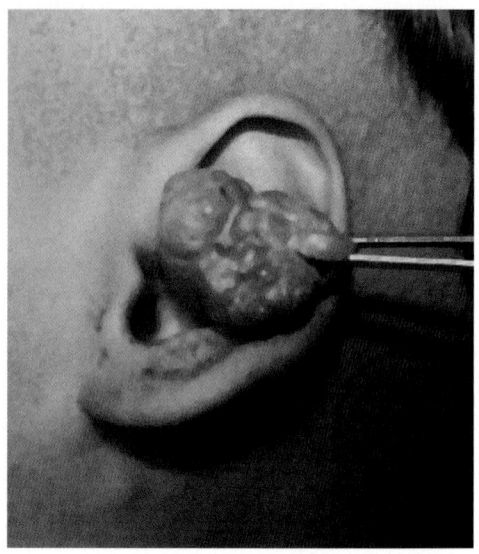

Papilloma of the ear *(Biswas et al, 2007)*

papillomatosis coronae penis. See **hirsutoid papilloma of the penis.**

papillomavirus /pap′ilō′məvī″rəs/ [L, *papilla* + Gk, *oma,* tumor; L, *virus,* poison], the virus that causes warts in humans.

Papillon-Lefèvre syndrome /pä′pēyôN′ lə·fev′rə/ [M.M. Papillon, 20th-century French dermatologist; Paul Lefèvre, 20th-century French dermatologist], an autosomal-recessive disorder occurring between the first and fifth years of life, characterized by palmoplantar keratoderma resembling psoriasis, which may also involve the elbows, knees, tibias, external malleoli, and other areas; ectopic calcifications of the skull; and periodontitis and premature shedding of both the primary and secondary teeth.

papilloretinitis /pap′ilōret′inī″tis/ [L, *papilla* + *rete,* net; Gk, *itis,* inflammation], an inflammatory occlusion of a retinal vein.

papillotomy /pap′ilot″əmē/, a surgical incision in the papilla of the duodenum.

papovavirus /pap′əvəvī″rəs/ [(abbreviation) *pa*pilloma *po*lyoma *va*cuolating *virus*], one of a group of small deoxyribonucleic acid (DNA) viruses, some of which may be potentially cancer-producing. The human wart is caused by a kind of papovavirus, but it very rarely undergoes malignant transformation. Kinds include **papilloma papovavirus, polyoma papovavirus, SV40 papovavirus.**

pappataci fever. See **phlebotomus fever.**

Pappenheimer bodies [A.M. Pappenheimer, U.S. pathologist, 1878–1955], red blood cell inclusions composed of ferric iron. On Prussian blue iron stain preparations, they appear as multiple dark blood irregular granules at the periphery of the cell. On Wright stain blood films they appear as pale blue clusters. Also called **siderotic granules.**

pappus /pap″əs/ [Gk, *pappos,* down], the first growth of beard, characterized by downy hairs.

Pap smear, Pap test. See **Papanicolaou (Pap) test.**

papula /pap″yələ/ [L, *papula,* pimple], a small superficial elevation of the skin.

papular /pap″yələr/, pertaining to or resembling a papule.

papular acrodermatitis of childhood. See **Gianotti-Crosti syndrome.**

papular scaling disease [L, *papula,* pimple; AS, *scealu*], any of a group of skin disorders characterized by discrete, raised, dry, scaling lesions. Also called **papulosquamous disease.** Kinds include **lichen planus, pityriasis rosea, psoriasis.**

papular urticaria [L, *papula,* pimple + *urtica,* nettle], a persistent cutaneous eruption representing a hypersensitivity reaction to insect bites (e.g., mites, fleas, bedbugs, gnats, mosquitoes, animal lice), seen primarily in atopic children and characterized by crops of small urticarial papules and wheals and transitional forms of these lesions, which may become secondarily infected or lichenified as a result of rubbing and scratching. Also called **lichen urticatus, strophulus.**

papulation /pap'yəlā″shən/ [L, *papula,* pimple, *atus,* process], the development of papules.

papule /pap″yool/ [L, *papula,* pimple], a small, solid, raised skin lesion less than 1 cm in diameter, such as that found in lichen planus and nonpustular acne. Compare **macule.** –**papular,** *adj.*

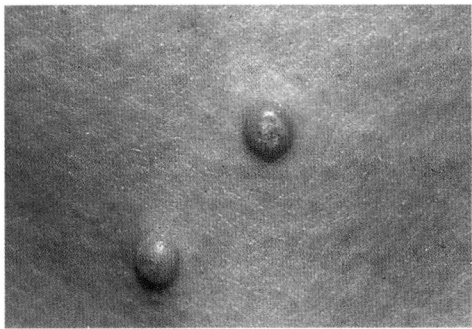

Papules *(du Vivier, 2002)*

papulo-, prefix meaning "papules" or "pimples": *papular, papulosis.*

papuloerythematous /pap'yəlō·er'ithem″ətəs/, pertaining to an eruption of solid circumscribed elevations on reddened skin.

papulopustular /pap'yəlōpus″tyələr/, pertaining to a skin eruption of both raised areas of skin containing pustular material and circumscribed, solid elevations of skin with no visible fluid.

papulosis /pap'yəlō″sis/, a widespread occurrence of papules over the body.

papulosquamous /pap'yəlōskwā″məs/ [L, *papula,* pimple, *squama,* scale], pertaining to a skin eruption that is both papular and scaly.

papulosquamous disease. See **papular scaling disease.**

papulovesicular /pap'yəlō'vesik″yələr/, pertaining to a skin rash characterized by both papules and small fluid-filled sacs.

papyraceous /pap'irā″shəs/ [Gk, *papyros,* paper], having a paperlike quality. Also spelled *papyraceus.*

papyraceous fetus. See **fetus papyraceus.**

Paquin technique, a type of reimplantation of the ureter in which the ureter is excised from its attachment to the bladder and reattached in a more posteromedial position.

par, a pair, specifically a pair of cranial nerves, such as the *par nonum,* or ninth pair.

PAR, abbreviation for **pulmonary arteriolar resistance.**

par-, **1.** prefix meaning "aside," "beyond," "apart from," "against": *parotid, paranoia.* **2.** See **para-, par-.**

para /par″ə/ [L, *parere,* to bear], a woman who has produced an infant, regardless of whether the child was alive or stillborn. The term is used with numerals to indicate the number of pregnancies carried to more than 20 weeks' gestation, such as para 2, indicating two pregnancies. See also **nullipara, parity.**

para-, par-, prefix meaning "similar," "beside," "beyond," "supplementary to," "disordered": *parabiosis, paraplegia.*

-para, -parous, suffix meaning "to bear or give birth": *gemmipara, oviparous, primipara.*

paraactinomycosis /per'ə·ak'tinō'mīkō″sis/, a chronic pulmonary infection similar to actinomycosis. The infection is caused by bacteria of the genus *Nocardia.*

para-aminobenzenesulfonic acid. See **sulfanilic acid.**

para-aminobenzoic acid ($H_2NC_6H_4COOH$) **(PABA)** /per'ə·amē'nōbenzō″ik/, a substance, often associated with the vitamin B complex, found in cereals, eggs, milk, and meat, and present in detectable amounts in blood, urine, spinal fluid, and sweat. It is widely used as a sunscreen that forms a partial chemical conjugation with constituents of the horny layer and resists removal by water and sweat. PABA is a sulfonamide antagonist and may be an effective agent for the treatment of scleroderma, dermatomyositis, and pemphigus.

para-aminohippuric acid (PAHA, PHA) /per'ə·amē'nōhipoor″ik/, the *p*-aminobenzamide derivative of glycerin. Its sodium salt is used for measuring effective renal plasma flow and determining kidney function.

para-aminosalicylic acid (PAS, PASA) /per'ə·amē'nōsal'isil″ik/, a bacteriostatic agent. Also called **aminosalicylic acid.**

■ INDICATIONS: It is prescribed for the treatment of pulmonary and extrapulmonary tuberculosis and has unlabeled indications for Crohn's disease.

■ CONTRAINDICATIONS: Known hypersensitivity to this drug prohibits its use. It may interact with other drugs such as digoxin.

■ ADVERSE EFFECTS: Among the most serious effects are nausea, vomiting, diarrhea, and abdominal pain. Fever, skin eruptions and other kinds of hypersensitivity reactions, goiter, hypokalemia, and acidosis may occur.

paraballism /per'əbôl″izəm/ [Gk, *ballismos,* jumping about], involuntary jerking movements of the legs.

parabiosis /-bī·ō″sis/, the fusion of two eggs or embryos, resulting in conjoined twins.

parabolic /-bol″ik/, (in ultrasonics) pertaining to flow conditions in blood vessels. Under parabolic flow, blood cells in the middle of the vessels move the fastest, with a gradual decrease in flow velocity for points farther away from the center.

paracanthoma /-kənthō″mə/, a tumor that develops from the abnormal overgrowth of the prickle cell layer of the skin.

paracellular transport, transport of molecules around cells and through tight junctions in an epithelial cell layer.

paracelsian method /-sel″sē·ən/ [Philippus Aureolus Paracelsus, Swiss alchemist and physician, 1493–1541], the use of chemical agents, such as sulfur, iron, lead, and arsenic, in the treatment of disease.

paracenesthesia /-sen'esthē″zhə/, any abnormality in the general sense of well-being.

paracentesis /per'əsentē″sis/ [Gk, *para* + *kentesis,* puncturing], a procedure in which fluid is withdrawn from a body cavity. An incision is made in the skin, and a hollow trocar, cannula, or catheter is passed through the incision into the cavity to allow outflow of fluid into a collecting device. Paracentesis is most commonly performed to remove excessive accumulations of ascitic fluid from the abdomen. Strict asepsis is followed. The patient needs to empty the bladder before this procedure to decrease the risk of bladder trauma. The patient is assessed for any adverse reaction.

P

paracentesis thoracis [Gk, *para* + *kentesis,* puncturing, *thorax,* chest], the aspiration of fluid or air or both through a needle inserted into the pleural cavity.

paracentesis tympani. See **myringotomy.**

paracentral /-sen′trəl/ [Gk, *para* + *kentron*], close to a center or a central part.

paracervical /-sur′vikəl/ [Gk, *para* + L, *cervix,* neck], pertaining to the area adjacent to the cervix.

paracervical block, a form of regional anesthesia in which a local anesthetic is injected into each side of the uterine cervix to block nerves innervating the uterine cervix. Paracervical block is not the anesthesia of choice for labor and delivery, given the high incidence of fetal bradycardia and its efficacy in only the first stage of labor, but it is an option during abortion and other gynecological procedures.

paracervix /-sur′viks/, the connective tissue of the pelvic floor, extending from the uterine cervix.

paracetamol. See **acetaminophen.**

paracholera /-kol′ərə/, an infectious disease with symptoms similar to those of cholera but not caused by the true infectious agent, *Vibrio cholerae.*

parachute reflex /per′əshōōt/, a variation of the Moro reflex whereby an infant is tested for motor nerve development by suspending him or her in the prone position and then dropping him or her a short distance onto a soft surface. If the motor nerve development is normal, the infant at 4 to 6 months will extend the arms, hands, and fingers on both sides of the body in a protective movement. Also called **startle reflex.**

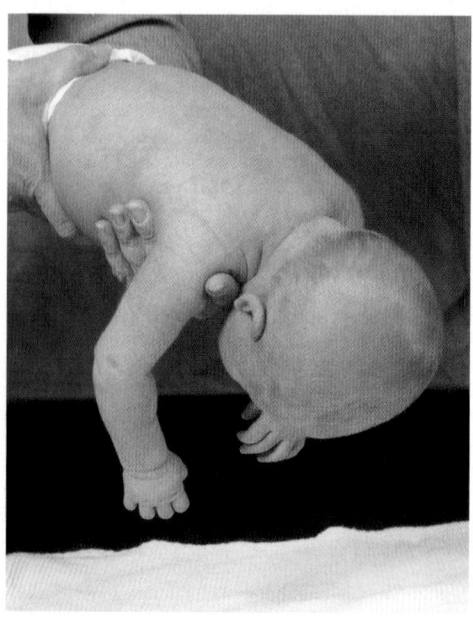

Parachute reflex *(Courtesy Paul Vincent Kuntz, Texas Children's Hospital, Houston, Texas)*

paracinesia. See **parakinesia.**

paracme /perak′mē/, **1.** the phase of a fever or disease marked by a subsidence of symptoms. **2.** the point of involution, beyond the prime of life. Also called *paracmasis.*

paracoccidioidomycosis /per′əkoksid′ē·oi′dōmīkō′sis/ [Gk, *para* + *kokkos,* berry, *eidos,* form, *mykes,* fungus, *osis,* condition], a chronic, occasionally fatal fungal infection caused by *Paracoccidioides brasiliensis.* It is characterized by ulcers of the oral cavity, larynx, and

nose. Other effects include large, draining lymph nodes; cough; dyspnea; weight loss; and skin, genital, and intestinal lesions. The disease occurs in Mexico and Central and South America and is acquired by inhalation of spores of the fungus. Diagnosis is by microscopic examination of a smear prepared from a lesion. This infection is sensitive to the use of sulfonamides, amphotericin B, and the azole antifungals. Azoles are preferred over sulfonamides and amphotericin B because they are less toxic, more effective, and require a shorter duration of treatment. Azoles are available in an oral form. Also called *paracoccidioidal granuloma,* **South American blastomycosis.** Compare **North American blastomycosis.**

paracolic gutters, depressions formed between the lateral margins of the ascending and descending colon and the posterolateral abdominal wall through which material can pass from one region of the peritoneal cavity to another.

paracolitis /-kōlī′tis/, an inflammation of the outer peritoneal coat of the colon.

paracolpium /-kol″pē·əm/, the connective and other tissues around the vagina.

paracortex /-kôr″teks/, the thymus-dependent area of a lymph node between the subscapular cortex and the medullary cord.

paracrine /per′əkrēn/, an endocrine function in which effects of a hormone are localized to adjacent or nearby cells.

paracusis /per′əkōō″sis/, a disorder involving the sense of hearing, including distortions of pitch.

paracystitis /-sistī′tis/, an inflammation of the connective tissues around the urinary bladder.

paradenitis /-dēnī″tis/, an inflammation of tissues around a gland.

paradentium. See **periodontium,** def. 1.

paradichlorobenzene poisoning. See **naphthalene poisoning.**

paradidymal /-did″iməl/ [Gk, *para,* beside, *didymos,* twin], **1.** pertaining to the paradidymis. **2.** beside the testis.

paradidymis /per′ədid″imis/ *pl. paradidymides* [Gk, *para* + *epi,* above, *didymos,* twin], a rudimentary structure in the male, situated on the spermatic cord of the epididymis, that consists of vestigial remains of the caudal part of the embryonic mesonephric tubules. A similar vestigial structure, the paroophoron, is found in the female. Also called **organ of Giraldés, parepididymis.** See also **appendix epididymidis.**

paradigm /per″ədīm, -dim/, a pattern that may serve as a model or example.

paradipsia /-dip″sē·ə/, an abnormal desire for fluids unrelated to body needs.

paradoxic /-dok″sik/ [Gk, *paradoxos,* strange], pertaining to a person, situation, statement, or act that may appear to have inconsistent or contradictory qualities or that may be true but appears to be absurd or unbelievable. Also **paradoxical.**

paradoxic aciduria, a metabolic alkalosis condition that may involve an exchange of sodium and hydrogen ions for potassium. It may occur with prolonged nasogastric suctioning or repeated vomiting.

paradoxical. See **paradoxic.**

paradoxic breathing [Gk, *paradoxos* + AS, *braeth*], a condition in which a part of the lung deflates during inspiration and inflates during expiration. The condition usually is associated with a chest trauma, such as an open chest wound or rib cage damage as in flail chest. In such cases the condition is sometimes called internal paradoxic breathing. External paradoxic breathing may be observed during deep general anesthesia.

paradoxic bronchospasm, a constriction of the airways after treatment with a sympathomimetic bronchodilator.

paradoxic incontinence. See **retention with overflow.**

paradoxic intention, a logotherapeutic technique that encourages a patient to do what he or she fears and if possible to exaggerate it to the point of humor. The technique is used in the treatment of phobias.

paradoxic pulse. See **pulsus paradoxus.**

paradoxic pupillary reflex, the response of a pupil to light that is the reverse of a normal reflex, as when the pupil contracts in a darkened room. It can be a sign of severe congenital visual deficit.

paradoxic thrombosis syndrome. See **heparin-induced thrombocytopenia with thrombosis.**

paraffin /per″əfin/ [L, *parum*, little + *affinis*, related], any of a group of hydrocarbons or hydrocarbon mixtures of the paraffin series as indicated by the formula, $C_nH_{(2n+2)}$. Examples include methane gas, kerosene, and paraffin wax. Also called **alkane.**

paraffin bath [L, *parum*, little, *affinis*, related], the application of heat to a specific area of the body through the use of paraffin. The part is quickly immersed in heated liquid wax and then withdrawn so that the wax solidifies to form an insulating layer. The procedure is repeated until the layer is 5 to 10 mm thick, and then the entire area is wrapped in an insulating material, such as a loose-fitting plastic bag or paper towels. The technique is effective for heating traumatized or inflamed areas, especially the hands, feet, and wrists, and is used primarily for patients with arthritis and rheumatism or any joint condition. Also called **wax bath.**

paraffin method, (in surgical pathology) a method used in preparing a selected portion of tissue for pathological examination. The tissue is fixed, dehydrated, and infiltrated by and embedded in paraffin, forming a block that is cut with a microtome into slices 8 μm thick. This method, which is more commonly used than the frozen section method, is slower and therefore not used during surgery.

paraffinoma /per″əfinō″mə/, a tumor caused by the prosthetic or therapeutic injection of paraffin beneath the skin.

paraffin section [L, *parum*, little + *affinis*, related, *sectio*], a histological section cut from tissue that has been embedded in paraffin wax.

Paraflex, a skeletal muscle relaxant. Brand name for **chlorzoxazone.**

parafollicular C cell /-folik″yələr/, a calcitonin-secreting cell located between follicles.

Parafon Forte, a skeletal muscle relaxant used for the relief of painful musculoskeletal conditions. Brand name for **chlorzoxazone.**

paraganglioma /-gang′glē-ō″mə/, a tumor derived from the chromoreceptor tissue of a paraganglion.

paraganglion /-gang″glē-on/ *pl.* **paraganglia** [Gk, *para* + *ganglion*, knot], any one of the small groups of chromaffin cells associated with the ganglia of the sympathetic nerve trunk and situated outside the adrenal medulla, most often near the sympathetic ganglia along the aorta and its branches. The paraganglia are also connected with the ganglia of the celiac, renal, suprarenal, aortic, and hypogastric plexuses. The paraganglia secrete the hormones epinephrine and norepinephrine. Also called **chromaffin body.** See also **chromaffin cell.**

parageusia /-joo″sē-ə/, a disorder involving the sense of taste.

paragonimiasis /per″əgon′imī″əsis/ [Gk, *para* + *gonimos*, generative, *iasis*, condition], chronic infection by the lung fluke *Paragonimus westermani*, occurring most commonly in Asia. The disease is acquired by ingesting cysts in infected freshwater crabs or crayfish, the intermediate hosts.

■ OBSERVATIONS: It is characterized by hemoptysis, bronchitis, pain, diarrhea, and occasionally abdominal masses. There may also be ocular pathological conditions, cerebral involvement with paralysis, or seizures.

■ INTERVENTIONS: Praziquantel given orally is the usual treatment.

■ PATIENT CARE CONSIDERATIONS: Adequate cooking of shellfish prevents the disease.

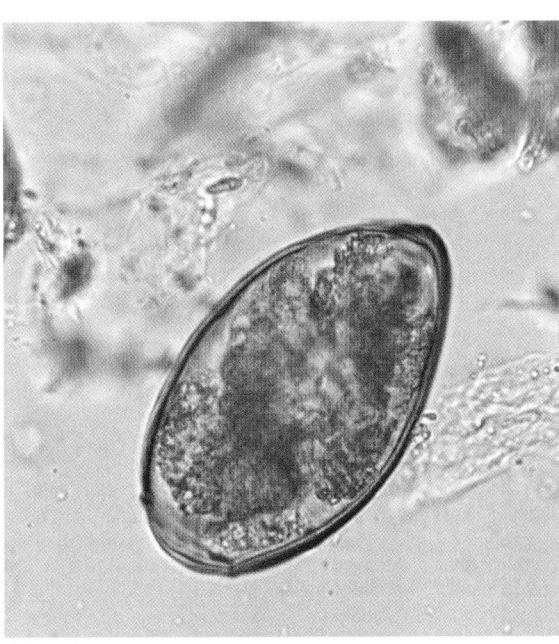

Photomicrograph of a stool specimen mount revealing the presence of a *Paragonimus westermani* termatode egg *(CDC/Dr. Mae Melvin)*

parahemophilia. See **Owren disease.**

parahippocampal gyrus, a convolution on the inferior surface of each cerebral hemisphere, lying between the hippocampal and collateral sulci.

parahormone /-hôr″mōn/, a substance produced through normal metabolism that may exert an influence on a remote organ even though it is not a true hormone. Carbon dioxide is a parahormone because of its effects on respiration.

parahypnosis /-hipnō″sis/ [Gk, *para* + *hypnos*, sleep], a form of disordered sleep that is observed in hypnosis and narcosis.

parainfectious /par″ah-in-fek′shus/, pertaining to manifestations of infectious disease that are caused by the immune response to the infectious agent.

parainfluenza virus /per″ə-in′floo-en″zə/ [Gk, *para* + It, *influenza*, influence], a myxovirus with four serotypes, causing respiratory infections in infants, young children, and, less commonly, adults. Type 1 and 2 parainfluenza viruses may cause laryngotracheobronchitis or croup; type 3 is a cause of croup, tracheobronchitis, bronchiolitis, and bronchopneumonia in children; and types 1, 3, and 4 are associated with pharyngitis and the common cold. Compare **influenza, rhinovirus.**

parakeratosis /-ker′ətō″sis/, an abnormal formation of horn cells of the epidermis caused by the persistence of nuclei, incomplete formation of keratin, and moistness and swelling of the horn cells. It is observed as scaling in many conditions such as psoriasis.

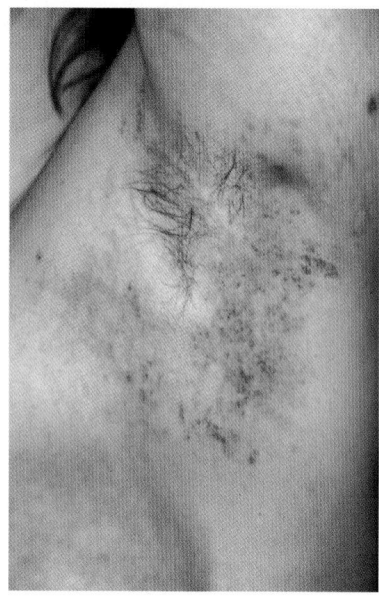

Parakeratosis in axilla *(Calonje et al, 2012)*

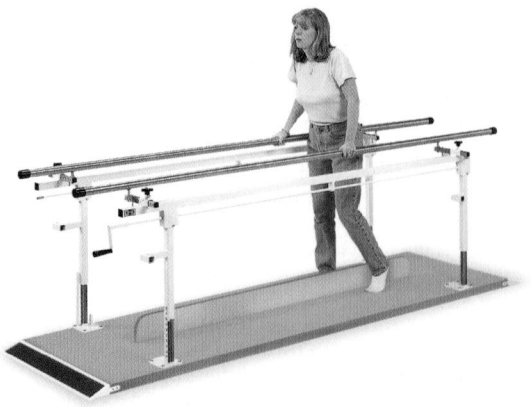

Parallel bars *(© 2014 Housmann Industries Inc.)*

parakinesia /-kinē″zhə/ [Gk, *para* + *kinesis,* movement], an abnormality of movement resulting from a nerve disorder in a muscle, such as an irregularity of one of the ocular muscles. Also called **paracinesia.**

parakinesis. See **telekinesis.**

paraldehyde /peral″dəhīd/, a clear, colorless, strong-smelling liquid obtained by the polymerization of acetaldehyde with a small amount of sulfuric acid. It is used as a solvent and was historically administered orally, intravenously, intramuscularly, or rectally to induce hypnotic states or sedation. It is still available but has widely been replaced by newer and safer barbiturates, sleeping pills, and benzodiazepines.

paralinguistic cues, nonverbal elements, such as intonation, body posture, gestures, and facial expression, that modify the meaning of verbal communication.

parallax /per″əlaks/ [Gk, *parallelos,* side-by-side], the apparent displacement of an object at different distances from the eyes when viewed by both eyes together. It is the basis of stereoscopic vision and depth perception.

parallel grid /per″əlel/ [Gk, *parallelos,* side-by-side; ME, *gredire*], (in radiography) an x-ray grid that has lead strips oriented parallel to each other.

parallelogram condenser /per″əlel″əgram′/ [Gk, *parallelos* + *gramma,* record; L, *condensare,* to make thick], an instrument with an end shaped like a parallelogram (a four-sided plane rectilinear figure with opposite sides parallel), used for compacting amalgams in restoring teeth.

parallel bars, an apparatus with two narrow side-by-side long rods of wood, metal, or similar rigid material with a space between the rods that allows for ambulation or other weight-bearing exercises. The height of the bars is often adjustable to allow easy gripping of the rods by individuals of different heights.

parallel play [Gk, *parallelos* + AS, *plegan,* to play], a form of play among a group of children, primarily toddlers, in which each engages in an independent activity that is similar to but not influenced by or shared with the others. Compare **cooperative play.** See also **associative play, solitary play.**

parallel processing, the use of multiple processors for the simultaneous execution of steps of a computer program that would normally run sequentially, done in order to shorten the time necessary to run the program.

parallel talk, a form of speech used during children's play therapy in which the clinician verbalizes activities of the child without requiring answers to questions. The parallel talk may take a form such as, "I'm making a cake. You are making a cake, too." The clinician repeats utterances of the child correctly and may parallel the child's actions.

parallergic /per″alur″jik/, having a nonspecific sensitivity to allergens as a result of a prior sensitization with a specific allergen.

Paralympics /per″əlim′piks/ [Gk, *para* + *plege,* stroke, + Gk, *Olympia,* ancient location of athletic contests], an international competitive wheelchair sports event, usually held in association with the official quadrennial Olympic Games. Also called **ParaOlympics.**

paralysis /pəral″isis/ *pl. paralyses* [Gk, *paralyein,* to be palsied], the loss of muscle function, sensation, or both. It may be caused by a variety of problems, such as trauma, disease, and poisoning. Paralyses may be classified according to the cause, muscle tone, distribution, or body part affected. See also **flaccid paralysis, spastic paralysis.**

paralysis agitans. See **Parkinson disease.**

paralytic /per″əlit″ik/ [Gk, *paralyein,* to be palsied], pertaining to the characteristics of paralysis.

paralytic dementia. See **paresis,** def. 2.

paralytic ileus [Gk, *paralyein,* to be paralyzed, *eilein,* to twist], a decrease in or absence of intestinal peristalsis. It may occur after abdominal surgery or peritoneal injury or be associated with severe pyelonephritis; ureteral stone; fractured ribs; myocardial infarction; extensive intestinal ulceration; heavy metal poisoning; porphyria; retroperitoneal hematomas, especially those associated with fractured vertebrae; or any severe metabolic disease. The most common overall cause of intestinal obstruction, paralytic ileus is mediated by a hormonal component of the sympathoadrenal system. Also called **adynamic ileus.**

■ OBSERVATIONS: Paralytic ileus is characterized by abdominal tenderness and distension, absence of bowel sounds, lack of flatus, and nausea and vomiting. There may be fever, decreased urinary output, electrolyte imbalance, dehydration, and respiratory distress. Loss of fluids and electrolytes may be extreme, and, unless they are replaced, the condition may lead to hemoconcentration, hypovolemia, renal insufficiency, shock, and death.

■ INTERVENTIONS: Typically, computed tomography of the abdomen and pelvis is performed with PO and IV contrast to rule out anatomical obstruction. The patient is kept in bed in a low Fowler's position, and nothing is given by mouth. A nasogastric tube may be inserted into the stomach and connected to intermittent suction and the patient is positioned to facilitate the advancement of the tube, which is checked at intervals, usually every 30 to 60 minutes. The character of GI drainage is monitored at intervals, usually every 2 to 4 hours, and any increase or decrease in the amount or changes in the color or consistency is reported. Bowel sounds, blood pressure, pulse, and respirations are checked every 2 to 4 hours, or as indicated in a particular circumstance, and rectal temperature usually every 4 hours. Abdominal girth is measured at least every 2 hours, and any increase is reported. Parenteral fluids with electrolytes and medication to promote peristalsis are administered as ordered; intake and output are measured, and, if less than about 30 mL of urine is excreted per hour, the physician is informed. The patient is helped to turn and deep breathe every 2 to 4 hours and is given oral hygiene every 1 to 2 hours. Active or passive range-of-motion exercises are performed every 4 hours. Walking is helpful as gravity is a useful force. When intestinal output increases and bowel sounds return, the intestinal tube may be clamped and small amounts of warm tea may be given. If pain, distension, or cramps do not recur, the intestinal tube may be removed, but a rectal tube or an enema may be ordered to relieve distension.

■ PATIENT CARE CONSIDERATIONS: The concerns of the health care providers include monitoring and reporting the signs of paralytic ileus and its potential complications, ensuring that the patient is as comfortable as possible, explaining the purpose of the intestinal tube, and walking with the patient, encouraging ambulation. The patient is instructed to try to avoid mouth breathing because swallowed air can increase distension. Before surgery, patients need reassurance that the sutures are strong and the distended abdomen will not burst.

paralytic incontinence [Gk, *paralyein,* to be palsied; L, *incontinentia,* inability to retain], urinary or fecal incontinence resulting from loss or impaired motor nerve control of the sphincter muscles.

paralytic mydriasis [Gk, *paralyein,* to be palsied, *mydriasis,* pupil enlargement], an area of depressed vision that is on the periphery of the visual field.

paralytic poliomyelitis [Gk, *paralyein,* to be palsied, *polios,* gray, *myelos,* marrow, *itis,* inflammation], a flaccid paralysis of the limbs resulting from damaged lower motor neurons. Progressive bulbar paralysis with respiratory and vasomotor failure may result when the brainstem nuclei are involved.

paralytic shellfish poisoning. See **shellfish poisoning.**

paralytic stroke [Gk, *paralyein,* to be palsied; AS, *strac*], a sudden attack of paralysis caused by disease or injury to the brain or spinal cord.

paralyze /per′əlīz/ [Gk, *paralyein,* to be palsied], **1.** to produce or enter into a state of paralysis. **2.** to cause loss of muscle power.

paramagnetic /pär″amagnet′ik/, being attracted by a magnet and assuming a position parallel to that of a magnetic force, but not becoming permanently magnetized. Paramagnetism is due to the presence of unpaired electrons in the material.

paramagnetic substance, a substance with positive magnetic susceptibility resulting from the presence of unpaired atomic electrons (e.g., gadolinium chelates). These substances enhance magnetic relaxation and are often used as contrast agents in magnetic resonance imaging.

paramedic (medic) /-med′ik/ [Gk, *para* + L, *medicina,* art of healing], an allied health professional with specialized training who responds to emergencies to stabilize a patient until hospital care is available. –*paramedical, adj.*

paramesonephric duct /per′əmēz′ōnef″rik/ [Gk, *para* + *mesos,* middle, *nephros,* kidney], one of a pair of embryonic ducts that develops into the uterus and the uterine tubes. Also called **müllerian duct.**

parameter /pəram″ətər/ [Gk, *para* + *metron,* measure], **1.** a value or constant used to describe or measure a set of data representing a physiological function or system, as in the use of acid-base relationships of the blood as parameters for evaluating the function of a patient's respiratory system. **2.** a statistical value of a population group. **3.** *(Informal)* limit or boundary.

parametria. See **parametrium.**

parametric imaging /-met″rik/ [Gk, *para* + *metron,* measure; L, *imago,* image], **1.** a diagnostic procedure in which an image of an administered radioactive tracer is derived mathematically, such as by dividing one image by another. **2.** in positron emission tomography, a procedure in which a physiological parameter such as blood flow is mapped according to anatomical position.

parametric statistics, statistics that assume that a population has a symmetric, such as a gaussian or normal, distribution.

parametritis /per′əmetrī″tis/ [Gk, *para* + *metra,* womb, *itis*], an inflammatory condition of the tissue of the structures around the uterus. See also **pelvic inflammatory disease.**

parametrium /per′əmē″trē·əm/ *pl. parametria* [Gk, *para* + *metra,* womb], the lateral extension of the uterine subserous connective tissue into the broad ligament. Compare **endometrium, myometrium.**

paramimia, the use of gestures that do not match the underlying feelings of an individual.

paramitome. See **hyaloplasm.**

paramnesia /per′amnē″zhə/ [Gk, *para* + *amnesia,* forgetfulness], **1.** a perversion of memory in which one believes that one remembers events and circumstances that never actually occurred. Compare **déjà vu. 2.** a condition in which words are remembered and used without comprehension of their meaning.

paramyloidosis /peram′iloidō″sis/, **1.** an accumulation of amyloid-like protein in the tissues. **2.** any of several hereditary forms of amyloidosis characterized by sensory changes and muscle atrophy caused by amyloid deposits in somatic and visceral nerves.

paramyxovirus /-mik′sōvī″rəs/ [Gk, *para* + *myxa,* mucus; L, *virus,* poison], a member of a family of viruses that includes the organisms that cause parainfluenza, mumps, and some respiratory infections.

paranasal /-nā″zəl/ [Gk, *para* + L, *nasus,* nose], pertaining to an area near or alongside the nose, such as the paranasal sinuses.

paranasal sinus, any one of the air cavities in various bones around the nose, such as the frontal sinus in the frontal bone lying deep to the medial part of the superciliary ridge and the maxillary sinus within the maxilla between the orbit, the nasal cavity, and the upper teeth. Compare **confluence of the sinuses, occipital sinus.** See also **accessory nasal sinuses.**

paraneoplastic cerebellar degeneration, the most common paraneoplastic syndrome affecting the brain, occurring most commonly with ovarian and breast carcinoma and Hodgkin disease, characterized pathologically by severe loss of Purkinje cells and clinically by insidious and progressive truncal and appendicular ataxia, dysarthria, nystagmus, and, occasionally, dementia. In some women with gynecological or breast carcinoma, it is associated with an autoantibody (anti-Yo).

P

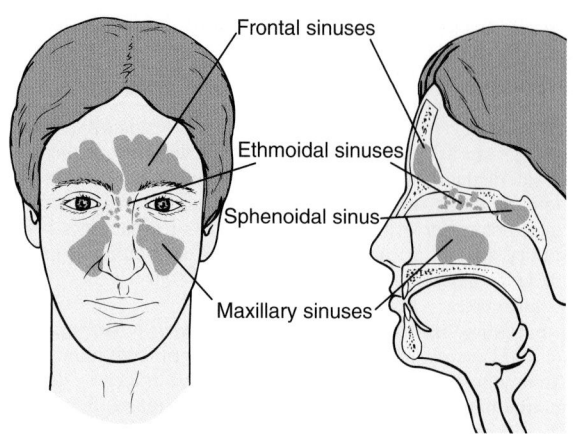

Paranasal sinuses *(Lewis et al, 2011)*

paraneoplastic syndromes /-nē'əplas″tik/ [Gk, *para* + *neos,* new, *plassein,* to mold, *syn,* together, *dromos,* course], the indirect effects of a tumor that occur distant to the tumor or metastatic site. They may result from the production of active proteins, polypeptides, or inactive hormones by the tumor.

paranephric fat. See **pararenal fat.**

paranesthesia /peran'esthē″zhə/, anesthesia affecting the lower half of the body.

parangi. See **yaws.**

paranoia /per'ənoi″ə/ [Gk, *para* + *nous,* mind], (in psychiatry) a condition characterized by an elaborate, overly suspicious system of thinking. It often includes delusions of persecution and grandeur usually centered on one major theme, such as a financial matter, a job situation, an unfaithful spouse, or another problem, such as being followed or monitored by the CIA, FBI, or outer space aliens; being the victim of computer tampering; or being poisoned. Also spelled *paranoea.* Compare **paranoid schizophrenia.** *–paranoiac, n.*

paranoia querulans. See **querulous paranoia.**

paranoid /per″ənoid/ [Gk, *para* + *nous,* mind, *eidos,* form], **1.** *adj.,* pertaining to or resembling paranoia. **2.** *n.,* a person afflicted with a paranoid disorder. **3.** *(Informal)* a person, or pertaining to a person, who is overly suspicious or exhibits persecutory trends or attitudes.

paranoid disorder, a mental disorder characterized by an impaired sense of reality and persistent delusions. Kinds include **paranoia, shared paranoid disorder.**

paranoid ideation, an exaggerated, sometimes grandiose, belief or suspicion, usually not of a delusional nature, that one is being harassed, persecuted, or treated unfairly.

paranoid personality, a personality characterized by paranoia.

paranoid personality disorder, a psychiatric disorder characterized by extreme suspiciousness and distrust of others to the degree that one blames them for one's mistakes and failures and goes to abnormal lengths to validate prejudices, attitudes, or biases.

paranoid reaction, a psychopathological condition that may be associated with delirium or dementia and characterized by the gradual formation of delusions, usually of a persecutory nature and often accompanied by related hallucinations. Other manifestations of senile degeneration, such as memory loss and confusion, may not accompany the reaction.

paranoid schizophrenia, a form of schizophrenia characterized by persistent preoccupation with illogical, absurd, and changeable delusions, usually of a persecutory, grandiose, or

jealous nature, accompanied by related hallucinations. The symptoms include extreme anxiety, exaggerated suspiciousness, aggressiveness, anger, argumentativeness, and hostility, which may lead to violence. Compare **paranoia.** Formerly called **heboid paranoia.** See also **schizophrenia.**

paranoid state, a transitory abnormal mental condition characterized by illogical thought processes and generalized suspicion and distrust, with a tendency toward persecutory ideas or delusions.

paranormal /-nôr″məl/ [Gk, *para* + L, *normalis,* rule], pertaining to phenomena that cannot be explained by normal scientific investigation.

paranuclear body. See **centrosome.**

ParaOlympics. See **Paralympics.**

paraoperative, pertaining to the accessories essential to operative surgery, such as sterilization and the care of instruments and gloves.

paraparesis /-pərē″sis/ [Gk, *para* + *paresis,* paralysis], a partial paralysis, usually affecting only the lower extremities.

parapedesis /-pedē″sis/, any secretion or excretion through an abnormal passageway.

paraperitoneal /-per'itənē″əl/, near or beside the peritoneum.

paraperitoneal nephrectomy [Gk, *para* + *peri* + *tenein,* to stretch, *nephros,* kidney, *ektome,* excision], the surgical removal of a kidney through an extraperitoneal incision.

parapertussis /per'əpərtus″is/ [Gk, *para* + L, *per,* very, *tussis,* cough], an acute bacterial respiratory infection caused by *Bordetella parapertussis,* having symptoms closely resembling those of pertussis. It is usually milder than pertussis, although it can be fatal. It is possible to be infected with both *B. parapertussis* and *B. pertussis* at the same time. There is no effective vaccine for *B. parapertussis.*

parapharyngeal abscess /per'əfərin″jē-əl/ [Gk, *para* + *pharynx,* throat; L, *abscedere,* to go away], a suppurative infection of tissues adjacent to the pharynx, usually a complication of acute pharyngitis or tonsillitis. Infection may spread to the jugular vein, where it may cause thrombophlebitis and septic emboli. Systemic antibiotics and surgical drainage may be required. Also called *parapharyngeal space abscess.* Compare **peritonsillar abscess, retropharyngeal abscess.** See also **tonsillitis.**

paraphasia /-fā″zhə/ [Gk, *para* + *phrasein,* to utter], **1.** a condition in which a person hears and comprehends words but is unable to speak correctly. Incoherent words are substituted for intended words, thereby creating sentences that are unintelligible. **2.** speech that is incoherent, unintelligible, and apparently incomprehensible but may be meaningful when carefully interpreted by a psychotherapist. Also called **jargon aphasia, word salad.**

paraphia /pə-rā'fē-ə/ [Gk, *para,* apart from or against + *haphē,* touch], a disorder of the sense of touch. Also called **dysaphia.**

paraphilia /per'əfil″yə/ [Gk, *para* + *philein,* to love], sexual perversion or deviation. A condition in which the sexual instinct is expressed in ways that are socially prohibited or unacceptable or are biologically undesirable, such as the use of a nonhuman object for sexual arousal, sexual activity with another person that involves real or simulated suffering or humiliation, or sexual relations with a nonconsenting partner. Kinds include **exhibitionism, pedophilia, transvestism, voyeurism, zoophilia.** *–paraphiliac, adj., n.*

paraphimosis /per'əfimō″sis/ [Gk, *para* + *phimoein,* to muzzle], a condition characterized by an inability to replace the foreskin in its normal position after it has been retracted behind the glans penis. Caused by a narrow or inflamed foreskin, the condition may lead to gangrene. Circumcision may be required. Compare **phimosis.**

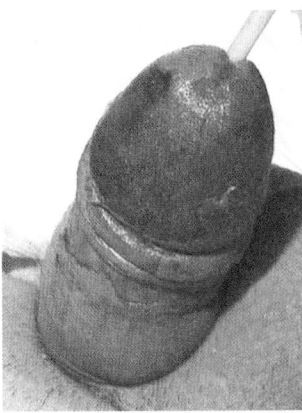

Paraphimosis *(Courtesy Dr. Patrick C. Walsh, The Johns Hopkins University School of Medicine)*

paraphrenia /-frē″nē·ə/, a psychiatric condition that is primary to an affective illness or organic mental disorder. Gross disturbances of affect, volition, and function, which are characteristic of schizophrenia, are not prominent, but paranoid delusions and hallucinations are always present.

paraplasm /per″əplaz′əm/ [Gk, *para* + *plassein,* to mold], any abnormal growth or malformation. Compare **hyaloplasm.** –*paraplasmic, adj.*

paraplastic /-plas″tik/ [Gk, *para* + *plassein,* to mold], **1.** misshapen or malformed. **2.** showing abnormal formative power; of the nature of a paraplasm.

paraplectic. See **paraplegic.**

paraplegia /per′əplē″jē·ə/ [Gk, *para* + *plege,* stroke], paralysis characterized by motor or sensory loss in the lower limbs and trunk. Approximately 11,000 spinal cord injuries reported each year in the United States involve paraplegia. Such injuries commonly result from automobile and motorcycle accidents, sporting accidents, falls, and gunshot wounds. Paraplegia less commonly results from nontraumatic lesions, such as scoliosis, spina bifida, or neoplasms. Compare **hemiplegia, quadriplegia.** –*paraplegic, adj., n.*

■ OBSERVATIONS: The signs and symptoms of paraplegia may develop immediately from trauma and include the loss of sensation, motion, and reflexes below the level of the lesion. Depending on the level of the lesion and whether damage to the spinal cord is complete or incomplete, the patient may lose bladder and bowel control, and sexual dysfunctions may develop. An incomplete spinal cord injury does not usually inhibit circumanal sensation, voluntary toe flexion, or sphincter control. A complete spinal cord injury destroys sensation and voluntary muscle control and usually causes the permanent loss of muscle function distal to the injury.

■ INTERVENTIONS: The treatment of paraplegia seeks to restore proper spine alignment, stabilize the injured spinal area, decompress any involved neurological structures, and rehabilitate the patient as quickly as possible. At the accident scene when spinal cord injury is suspected, the patient must not be moved until strapped and stabilized on a board. Such stabilization helps to prevent permanent damage to any injured spinal structures. Drugs such as baclofen may be administered to relieve any muscle spasms associated with dysfunction of the upper motor neurons.

■ PATIENT CARE CONSIDERATIONS: When the paraplegic patient progresses from bed rest to use of a wheelchair, the nurse is alert to any signs of orthostatic hypotension. Special binders and antiembolism hose are used to help the patient adjust to the transition from bed to wheelchair. Prevention of pressure sores is an important priority. Other treatment may include a high-bulk diet and the administration of suppositories to prevent constipation.

paraplegic /-plē″jik/ [Gk, *para* + *plege,* stroke], pertaining to a person affected by paraplegia or a condition resembling paraplegia. Also called **paraplectic.**

parapneumonic empyema, thoracic empyema occurring as a complication of pneumonia.

parapraxia /-prak″sē·ə/ [Gk, *para* + *praxis,* doing], **1.** the abnormal performance of purposive actions, such as performance of one movement occurring in place of another intended movement. **2.** forgetfulness with a tendency to misplace things.

parapraxis, an error of speech or action thought to represent an unconscious wish. Also called **freudian slip.**

paraproctitis /-proktī″tis/, an inflammation affecting the tissues around the rectum and anus.

paraprostatitis /-pros′tətī″tis/, an inflammation of the tissues around the prostate gland.

paraprotein /-prō″tēn/, an abnormal protein similar to an antibody. Paraproteins are produced in certain conditions, such as myeloma, and their presence in blood can represent a biomarker of disease.

parapsoriasis /per′əsərī″əsis/ [Gk, *para* + *psorian,* to itch], a group of chronic skin diseases resembling psoriasis, characterized by maculopapular, erythematous, scaly eruptions without systemic symptoms. Parapsoriasis is resistant to all treatment.

Parapsoriasis *(Bolognia et al, 2012)*

P

parapsoriasis varioliformis acuta. See **Mucha-Habermann disease.**

parapsychology /-sīkol″əjē/ [Gk, *para* + *psyche,* mind, *logos,* science], a branch of psychology concerned with the study of alleged psychic phenomena, such as clairvoyance, extrasensory perception, and telepathy.

paraquat poisoning /per″əkwot′/ [Gk, *para* + L, *quaterni,* four each, *potio,* drink], a toxic condition caused by the ingestion of paraquat dichloride, a highly poisonous herbicide. Characteristically, progressive pulmonary fibrosis and damage to the esophagus, kidneys, and liver develop several days after ingestion. After fibrosis begins, death is inevitable, usually within 3 weeks. The mechanism of action of the poison is unknown. Most often poisoning results from accidental occupational exposure. There is considerable concern that the inhalation of the smoke of marijuana treated with the herbicide may cause intoxication, but no clinical syndrome resulting from such exposure has been documented.

pararectal fossa, either of two cavities formed by folds of the peritoneum, one on either side of the rectum, varying in size according to distension of the rectum. In males this is continuous with the rectovesical pouch, and in females it is continuous with the rectouterine pouch.

parareflexia /-riflex″sē·ə/, any abnormal condition of the reflexes.

pararenal fat, a layer of fat that accumulates posteriorly and posterolaterally to each kidney. It is the final layer of fat and fascias associated with the kidney. Also called **paranephric fat.** See also **perirenal fat.**

pararhotacism. See **rhotacism.**

parasacral /-sā″krəl/ [Gk, *para* + *sacrum*], pertaining to the area around the sacrum.

parasalpingitis /-sal′pinjī″tis/, an inflammation of the tissues around the fallopian tubes.

paraseptal emphysema. See **distal acinar emphysema.**

parasite /per″əsīt/ [Gk, *parasitos,* guest], **1.** an organism living in or on and obtaining nourishment from another organism. A facultative parasite may live on a host but is capable of living independently. An obligate parasite is one that depends entirely on its host for survival. **2.** See **parasitic fetus.** –*parasitic, adj.*

parasitemia /per′əsītē″mē·ə/ [Gk, *parasitos* + *haima,* blood], the presence of parasites in the blood. Compare **bacteremia, fungemia, viremia.**

parasitic fetus /-sit″ik/ [Gk, *parasitos* + L, *icus,* like, *fetus,* pregnant], the smaller, usually malformed member of conjoined, unequal, or asymmetric twins that is attached to and dependent on the more normal fetus for growth and development. Compare **autosite.**

parasitic fibroma, a pedunculated uterine fibroid deriving part of its blood supply from the omentum.

parasitic glossitis, a mycosis of the tongue, characterized by a black or brown furry patch on the posterior dorsal surface. The patch is composed of hypertrophied filiform papillae that measure about 1 cm in length and are easily broken. This condition may occur as the result of poor oral hygiene, the use of broad-spectrum antibiotics, or radiation treatment of the neck and head. The condition, caused by *Cryptococcus linguae-pilosasae* in symbiosis with *Nocardia lingualis,* produces no discomfort and may be treated with a simple mouthwash. The patch may disappear spontaneously and later reappear. Also called **black hairy tongue, glossitis parasitica, glossophytia.**

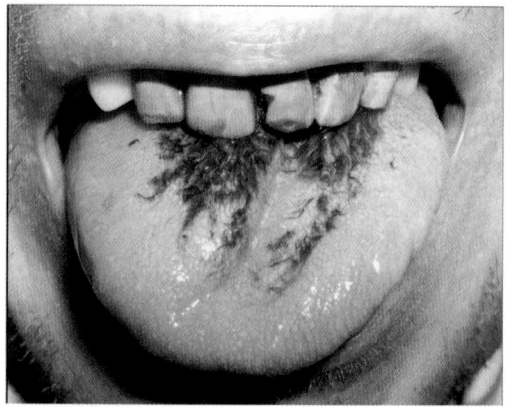

Parasitic glossitis *(Nisa and Giger, 2011)*

parasitic hemoptysis [Gk, *parasitos,* guest, *haima,* blood + *ptyein,* to spit], the spitting of bright red blood caused by a parasitic infection. The condition usually involves the lung fluke *(Paragonimus)* or tapeworms *(Echinococcus).*

parasitism /per″əsitiz′əm/ [Gk, *parasitos,* guest], the relationship between two different organism types whereby one organism (the parasite) receives benefits from the other organism (the host) by inducing damage to it.

parasternal line. See **costoclavicular line.**

parasympathetic /-sim′pəthet″ik/ [Gk, *para* + *sympathein,* to feel with], pertaining to the craniosacral division of the autonomic nervous system, consisting of the oculomotor, facial, glossopharyngeal, vagus, and pelvic nerves. The actions of the parasympathetic division are mediated by the release of acetylcholine and primarily involve the protection, conservation, and restoration of body resources. Preganglionic parasympathetic fibers, which emerge from the hypothalamus, other brain areas, and sacral segments of the spinal cord, form synapses in ganglia located near or in the walls of the organs to be innervated. Reactions to parasympathetic stimulation are highly localized and tend to counteract the adrenergic effects of sympathetic nerves. Parasympathetic fibers slow the heart; stimulate peristalsis; promote the secretion of lacrimal, salivary, and digestive glands; induce bile and insulin release; dilate peripheral and visceral blood vessels; constrict the pupils, esophagus, and bronchioles; and relax sphincters during micturition and defecation. Postganglionic parasympathetic fibers extend to the uterus, vagina, oviducts, and ovaries in females and to the prostate, seminal vesicles, and external genitalia in males, innervating blood vessels of pelvic organs in both sexes; stimulation of these nerves causes vasodilation in the clitoris and labia minora and erection of the penis.

parasympathetic ganglion [Gk, *para* + *sympathein,* to feel with, *ganglion,* knot], a cluster of nerve cell bodies of the parasympathetic division of the autonomic nervous system. The nerves are functionally antagonistic to those of the sympathetic division.

parasympathetic nervous system. See **autonomic nervous system.**

parasympatholytic. See **anticholinergic.**

parasympathomimetic /per′əsim′pəthō′mimet″ik/ [Gk, *para* + *sympathein,* to feel with, *mimesis,* imitation],

1. *adj.,* pertaining to a substance producing effects similar to those caused by stimulation of a parasympathetic nerve. **2.** *n.,* an agent whose effects mimic those resulting from stimulation of parasympathetic nerves, especially those produced by acetylcholine. Also called **cholinergic.**

parasympathomimetic drug. See **cholinergic.**

parasynovitis /-sinəvī″tis/, an inflammation of the tissues around a joint.

parasystole [Gk, *para + systole,* contraction], an independent ectopic rhythm whose pacemaker cannot be discharged by impulses of the dominant (usually the sinus) rhythm because an area of depressed conduction surrounds the parasystolic focus. In the classic parasystole, the interectopic intervals are exact multiples of a common denominator reflecting the protected status of the parasystolic focus; however, the ectopic focus is usually influenced by the phasic events around its protection zone (modulated parasystole). Thus the sinus rhythm may modulate the parasystolic rhythm so that criteria for absolute, undisturbed regularity are not fulfilled. Fusion beats are common because of the simultaneous discharge of the ventricles by both the sinus and the parasystolic impulses.

parataxic distortion /per′ətak″sik/ [Gk, *para + taxis,* arrangement], **1.** a defense mechanism in which current interpersonal relationships are perceived and judged according to a mode of reference established by an earlier experience. **2.** Harry S. Sullivan's term for inaccuracies in judgment and perception. See also **transference.**

parataxic mode, a term introduced by H.S. Sullivan to identify a childhood perception of the physical and social environment as being illogical, disjointed, and inconsistent. The parataxic mode may persist into adulthood in some individuals.

parathion poisoning /per′əthī″on/ [Gk, *para + thio,* phosphate, *on +* L, *potio,* drink], a toxic condition caused by the ingestion, inhalation, or absorption through the skin of the highly toxic organophosphorus insecticide parathion. Symptoms include nausea, vomiting, abdominal cramps, confusion, headache, lack of muscular control, convulsions, and dyspnea.

parathyroid-, parathyro-, prefix meaning "parathyroid glands": *parathyroidectomy.*

parathyroidectomy /-thī′roidek″təmē/ [Gk, *para + thyreos,* shield, *eidos,* form, *ektomē,* excision], the surgical removal of a parathyroid gland.

parathyroid gland /-thī′roid/ [Gk, *para + thyreos,* shield, *eidos,* form; L, *glans,* acorn], any one of several small structures, usually four, attached to the dorsal surfaces of the lateral lobes of the thyroid gland. The parathyroid glands secrete parathyroid hormone, which helps maintain the blood calcium concentration and ensures normal neuromuscular irritability, blood clotting, and cell membrane permeability. Each parathyroid gland is an oval brownish red disk measuring about 6 by 4 mm. The parathyroids are divided, according to their location, into the superior parathyroids and the inferior parathyroids. The superior parathyroids, usually two, are commonly situated, one on each side, on the caudal border of the cricoid cartilage beside the junction of the pharynx and the esophagus. The inferior parathyroids, also usually two, may be situated on the caudal edge of the lateral lobes of the thyroid gland or adjacent to one of the inferior thyroid veins. These glands are composed of intercommunicating columns of cells bound by connective tissue with a rich supply of capillaries. Parathyroid hypofunction usually causes tetany, which can be treated by the administration of calcium salts or parathyroid extracts.

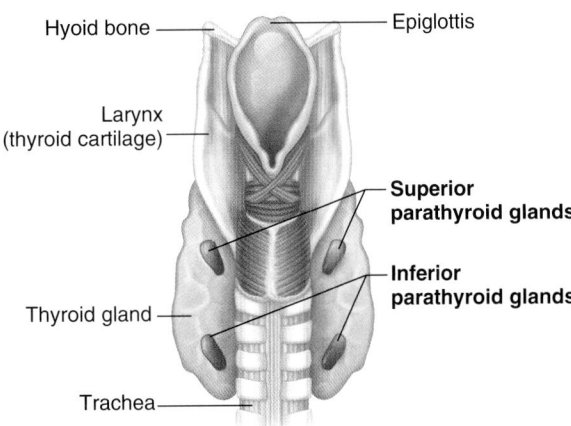

Parathyroid glands *(Patton and Thibodeau, 2016)*

parathyroid hormone (PTH), a hormone secreted by the parathyroid glands that acts to maintain a constant concentration of calcium in the extracellular fluid. The hormone regulates absorption of calcium from the GI tract; mobilization of calcium from the bones; deposition of calcium in the bones; and excretion of calcium in the breast milk, feces, sweat, and urine. Surgical removal of the parathyroid glands, as may inadvertently occur in thyroidectomy, results in hypocalcemia, leading to anorexia, tetany, seizures, and death if not corrected. Normal parathyroid laboratory findings are less than 2000 pg/mL. See also **hypoparathyroidism.**

parathyroid hormone (PTH) test, a blood test that is useful in establishing a diagnosis of hyperparathyroidism and distinguishing nonparathyroid from parathyroid causes of hypercalcemia. PTH is secreted by the parathyroid gland in response to hypocalcemia.

parathyroid scan, a nuclear scan used to determine the number of parathyroid glands involved in hyperparathyroidism. Enlargement of all four glands indicates parathyroid hyperplasia. Enlargement of only one indicates adenoma or cancer.

parathyroid tetany [Gk, *para + thyreos,* shield, *tetanos,* convulsive tension], a form of tetany (hypocalcemia) that is caused by a deficiency of parathyroid secretion.

parathyrotropic /-thī′rōtrop″ik/, stimulating the growth or rate of activity of the parathyroid glands.

paratonia. See **gegenhalten.**

paratrichosis /-trikō″sis/, an abnormality in the distribution, growth, and quantity of scalp hair.

paratriptic /-trip″tik/, pertaining to an agent that causes chafing.

paratrooper fracture /-troo″pər/ [Fr, *parasol + troupe,* company; L, *fractura,* break], a break in the distal tibia and its malleolus, commonly occurring when an individual jumps from an elevated platform and lands feet first on the ground, subjecting the ankles to extreme force. The fracture may be bilateral.

paratyphlitis /-tiflī″tis/ [Gk, *para + typhlos,* blind, *itis,* inflammation], an inflammation of the tissues around the cecum and vermiform appendix. Also called **perityphlitis.**

paratyphoid fever /-tī″foid/ [Gk, *para + typhos,* stupor, *eidos,* form; L, *febris,* fever], a bacterial infection, caused by any *Salmonella* species other than *S. typhi* and characterized by symptoms resembling typhoid fever, although somewhat milder. See also **rose spots,** *Salmonella,* **salmonellosis, typhoid fever.**

paraurethral duct /per′əyŏorē″thrəl/ [Gk, *para* + *oure-thra*, urethra; L, *ducere*, to lead], one of a pair of ducts that drain the bulbourethral glands into the vestibule of the vagina. Also called **Skene's duct.**

paravaccinia virus /-vaksin″ē·ə/, a member of a subgroup of poxviruses that can infect humans through direct contact with infected livestock. It is related to the smallpox virus and is the cause of pseudocowpox, which produces milker's nodules. See also **milker's nodule.**

paravaginitis /-vaj′ini″tis/, an inflammation of the tissues around the vagina.

paravertebral /-vur″təbrəl/ [Gk, *para* + L, *vertebra,* joint], pertaining to the area alongside the spinal column or near a vertebra.

paravertebral block [Gk, *para* + L, *vertebra* + OFr, *bloc*], **1.** the blocking of transmission of somatic impulses by the spinal nerves by injection of a local analgesic solution near the point of their emergence. **2.** the blocking of the paravertebral sympathetic chain of nerves anterolateral to the vertebral bodies.

paravertebral sympathetic trunk, the trunk formed by ascending and descending postganglionic fibers, together with all the ganglia, that extends the entire length of the vertebral column on each side and enables the visceral motor fibers of the sympathetic part of the autonomic division of the peripheral nervous system to be distributed to peripheral regions innervated by all spinal nerves.

paravesical fossa, the fossa formed by the peritoneum on each side of the urinary bladder, into which the obturator canal opens. In females it is the lateral part of the vesicouterine pouch.

paravesical spaces, a pair of subdivisions of the extraperitoneal space found lateral to the prevesical space.

paraxial /perak″sē·əl/, pertaining to an organ or other structure located near the axis of the body.

parchment skin /pärch″mənt/ [Fr, *parchemin* + AS, *scinn*], thin, wrinkled, or stretched skin that is exceptionally fragile.

paregoric /per′əgôr″ik/, a camphorated tincture of opium.

■ INDICATIONS: It is prescribed in the treatment of diarrhea and as an analgesic.

■ CONTRAINDICATIONS: Known hypersensitivity to this drug or to any opium derivative prohibits its use. It should not be used when diarrhea is caused by a toxic substance.

■ ADVERSE EFFECTS: Drowsiness and dizziness are common. When used as directed, nausea and constipation may occur. Other adverse effects include respiratory depression, hypotension, miosis and, with continued use, psychological dependence.

parencephalitis /per′ensef′əli″tis/, an inflammation of the cerebellum.

parencephalocele /per′ensef″əlōsēl′/, a protrusion of the cerebellum through a hole in the cranium.

parenchyma /pəreng″kimə/ [Gk, *para* + *enchyma,* infusion], the functional tissue or cells of an organ or gland, as distinguished from supporting or connective tissue.

parenchymal. See **parenchymatous.**

parenchymal cell /pəreng″kiməl/, any cell that is a functional element of an organ, such as a hepatocyte.

parenchyma of prostate, glandular substance consisting of small compound tubulosaccular or tubuloalveolar glands that makes up the bulk of the prostate. It is surrounded by muscular substance and permeated by muscular strands.

parenchymatous /per′əngkim″ətəs/ [Gk, *para* + *enchyma,* infusion], pertaining to or resembling the functional tissues of an organ or gland. Also **parenchymal.**

parenchymatous myositis. See **myositis.**

parenchymatous nephritis. See **nephritis.**

parenchymatous neuritis [Gk, *para* + *enchyma,* infusion; L, *osus,* like], any inflammation affecting the substance, axons, or myelin of the nerve. Also called **axial neuritis.** See also **neuritis.**

parenchymatous salpingitis, an inflammation and thickening of the fallopian tubes. Also called **pachysalpingitis.**

parent [L, *parens*], a mother or father; one who bears offspring. –*parental, adj.*

parental generation (P_1) /pəren″təl/, the initial cross between two varieties in a genetic sequence. The parents of any individual belonging to a first filial generation.

parental grief, the behavioral reactions that characterize the grieving process and result in the resolution of grief at the loss of a child from expected or unexpected death. All people who survive the loss of a loved one normally experience symptoms of both somatic and psychological distress, such as feelings of guilt and hostility accompanied by changes in usual patterns of conduct. When the death of a child with a terminal illness is expected, there is time for anticipatory grieving, so that parents can evaluate their relationship with the child, set priorities for the duration of time involved, and prepare for the actual death of the child. In such cases, parental grieving begins with the discovery of the diagnosis of a life-threatening condition. Parents' adjustment to the diagnosis involves a complete cycle of reactions that extends over an indefinite period, depending on the severity and nature of the disease. The immediate reactions are shock and disbelief, followed by acute grief at the anticipation of losing the child. Periods of depression, anger, hope, fear, and anxiety alternate during induction therapy, remission, and maintenance of the disease as parents learn to accept and cope with the situation. Heightened anticipatory grieving recurs during episodes of relapse, and the parents experience increased fear, depression, and final acceptance of death during the terminal stages of the illness. Although families can prepare themselves for the expected loss, at the time of death there is a period of acute grief, during which parents need to express their deep sorrow and anger. An extended phase of mourning follows, with the eventual resolution of grief and reintegration into society. In sudden, unexpected death, parents are denied the advantages of anticipatory grief and, because of the lack of time to prepare, usually have extreme feelings of guilt and remorse. Each member of the health care team can play an important role in helping such parents assess their feelings so that they can work through them and progress through the resolution of grief and the mourning process, which in unexpected death take a much longer time. The function of the health care providers during all phases of parental grief is primarily supportive, and the degree of intervention depends on the family's strengths and weaknesses in coping with the crisis. Health care team members can act directly, or they can help find other potential sources of support for the parents, such as extended family members, other parents who have lost children, or specific community services or agencies. A large part of the support involves helping families explore new ways of coping, not only to meet the present crisis but to grow and change. Always an important nursing consideration is the education of the parents about all aspects of the child's illness, especially in terminal conditions. See also **death, grief reaction.**

parental leave. See **family care leave.**

parent-child relationship. See **maternal-infant bonding.**

parent education, thoughtful conveyance of information enabling the parent to provide high-quality child rearing.

parent ego state, (in transactional analysis) an ego state that incorporates the feelings and behavior learned from parents or other authority figures; a part of the self that offers advice like that of one's own parents, containing messages that emphasize what one "ought to" or "should not" do.

parenteral /pəren″tərəl/ [Gk, *para + enteron,* bowel], pertaining to treatment other than through the digestive system. **–parenterally,** *adv.*

parenteral absorption, the taking up of substances within the body by structures other than the digestive tract.

parenteral dosage, pertaining to a medication administered by a route that bypasses the GI tract, such as a drug given by injection.

parenteral hyperalimentation. See **total parenteral nutrition.**

parenterally. See **parenteral.**

parenteral nutrition, the administration of nutrients by a route other than the alimentary canal, most often through a central intravenous line. The nutrients may not be nutritionally complete but maintain fluid and electrolyte balance during the immediate postoperative period and in other conditions, such as shock, coma, malnutrition, and chronic renal and hepatic failures. Increasingly, long-term outpatient use of parenteral nutrition for conditions interfering with gastrointestinal absorption such as Crohn's disease and ischemic bowel disease is employed. See also **total parenteral nutrition.**

■ METHOD: The nutrients, or parenteral fluids, usually consist of physiological saline solution with glucose, amino acids, electrolytes, vitamins, and medications. Lipids can be added as a supplementary infusion for individuals requiring long-term nutritional supplementation.

■ PATIENT CARE CONSIDERATIONS: Nutritional needs may change with time; careful monitoring is required. Patient education on care for long-term use is imperative.

■ OUTCOME CRITERIA: Maintenance of a healthy weight, the provision of sufficient energy to participate in activities of daily living, and appropriate fluid and electrolyte balance are expected outcomes.

parent figure [L, *parens + figura,* form], **1.** a parent or a substitute parent or guardian who cares for a child, providing the physical, social, and emotional requirements necessary for normal growth and development. **2.** a person who symbolically represents an ideal parent, having those attributes that one conceptualizes as necessary for forming the perfect parent-child relationship.

parent image, a conscious and unconscious concept that a child forms concerning the roles and characteristics of the personality of the mother and father. See also **imago, primordial image.**

Parents Anonymous, a self-help group for parents who have abused their children or who feel that they are prone to maltreat them. The organization offers support and guidance, provides a forum for discussing mutual problems, and furnishes a distressed parent with a positive mechanism for coping with anger by talking to another member rather than by releasing his or her emotions on the child. See also **child abuse.**

Parents Without Partners, a self-help group for single parents, including those who are separated, divorced, or widowed.

parepididymis. See **paradidymis.**

paresis /pərē″sis, per″isis/ [Gk, *paralyein,* to be palsied], **1.** motor weakness or partial paralysis related in some cases to local neuritis. Also called **dementia paralytica, general paresis, paralytic dementia. 2.** a late manifestation of neurosyphilis, characterized by generalized paralysis, tremulous incoordination, transient seizures, Argyll Robertson pupils, and progressive dementia caused by degeneration of cortical neurons. Paresis resulting from untreated syphilis usually develops in the third to fifth decade but may occur at an early age in patients with congenital syphilis. **–paretic,** *adj.*

-paresis, suffix meaning "incomplete or partial paralysis": *hemiparesis.*

paresthesia /per′esthē″zhə/ [Gk, *para + erethizein,* to excite], any subjective sensation, experienced as numbness, tingling, or a "pins and needles" feeling. Paresthesias often fluctuate according to such influences as posture, activity, rest, edema, congestion, or underlying disease. It can be transient or chronic in nature. When experienced in the extremities, it is sometimes identified as acroparesthesia. Also spelled *paraesthesia.* See also **acanthesia.**

paresthetic pain. See **paresthesia.**

paretic /peret″ik/ [Gk, *paresis,* paralysis], pertaining to or resembling partial paralysis.

paretic dementia. See **general paresis.**

pareunia. See **coitus.**

paricalcitol, a vitamin D analog.

■ INDICATIONS: It is used to treat hypoparathyroidism.

■ CONTRAINDICATIONS: Known hypersensitivity to this drug and hypercalcemia prohibit its use.

■ ADVERSE EFFECTS: Sepsis is a life-threatening effect. Other adverse effects include nausea, vomiting, anorexia, dry mouth, light-headedness, palpitations, pneumonia, edema, chills, fever, and flu.

paries /per″i·ēz/ *pl. parietes,* the wall of a hollow organ or cavity in the body.

parietal /pərī″ətəl/ [L, *paries,* wall], **1.** pertaining to the outer wall of a cavity or organ. **2.** pertaining to the parietal bone of the skull or the parietal lobe of the cerebrum.

parietal abdominal fascia, the fascia lining the wall of the abdominal cavity.

parietal bone, one of a pair of bones forming the sides of the cranium. Each parietal bone has two surfaces, four borders, and four angles and articulates with five bones: the opposite parietal, occipital, frontal, temporal, and sphenoid.

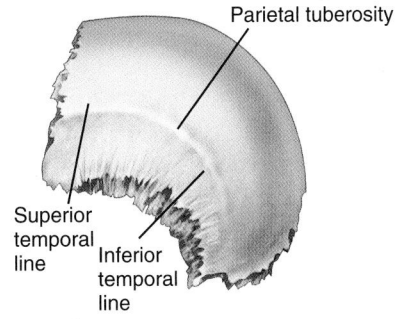

Parietal tuberosity

Superior temporal line

Inferior temporal line

Parietal bone

parietal cells [L, *paries,* wall, *cella,* storeroom], the cells on the periphery of the gastric glands of the stomach. They are located on the basement membrane beneath the chief cells and secrete hydrochloric acid.

parietal endopelvic fascia. See **parietal pelvic fascia.**

parietal hernia. See **Richter hernia.**

parietal layer of glomerular capsule, the layer of the glomerular capsule opposite the visceral layer, with the urinary space in between. It is composed of simple squamous epithelium.

parietal lobe, a portion of each cerebral hemisphere that occupies the parts of the lateral and medial surfaces that are covered by the parietal bone. On the lateral surface of the hemisphere the parietal lobe is separated from the frontal lobe by the central sulcus and from the temporal lobe by an imaginary line that extends from the posterior ramus of the lateral sulcus toward the occipital pole. It is concerned with language mechanisms and general sensory functions. Compare **central lobe, frontal lobe, occipital lobe, temporal lobe.**

parietal lymph node, any one of the small oval glands that filter the lymph coursing through the lymphatic vessels in the walls of the thorax or through the lymphatic vessels associated with the larger blood vessels of the abdomen and the pelvis. The parietal lymph nodes of the thorax include the sternal nodes, intercostal nodes, and diaphragmatic nodes. The parietal lymph nodes of the abdomen and pelvis include the common iliac nodes, epigastric nodes, external iliac nodes, iliac circumflex nodes, internal iliac nodes, lumbar nodes, and sacral nodes. See also **lymph, lymphatic system, lymph node.**

parietal pain, a sharp sensation of distress in the parietal pleura, aggravated by respiration and thoracic movements and caused by pneumonia; empyema; pneumothorax; asbestosis; tuberculosis; neoplasm; or the accumulation of fluid resulting from heart, liver, or kidney disease. Pain arising from the parietal pleura lining the chest wall is perceived over the involved area, but that arising from the central part of the diaphragm is referred to the posterior shoulder area; pain from the costal portions of the diaphragm is referred to the adjacent thoracic wall.

parietal pelvic fascia, the layer of fascia surrounding the abdominal cavity, composed of transversalis fascia, the fascia covering muscle associated with the upper regions of the pelvic bones, and similar fascia covering the muscles of the pelvic cavity. Also called **parietal endopelvic fascia.**

parietal pericardium [L, *paries,* wall; Gk, *peri + kardia,* heart], an outer layer of the serous pericardium that is not in direct contact with the heart muscle.

parietal peritoneum, the portion of the largest serous membrane in the body that lines the abdominal wall. Compare **visceral peritoneum.** See also **peritoneal cavity.**

parietal pleura, the outer layer of the pleura, lining the walls of the thoracic cavity.

parietes. See **paries.**

parietoacanthial projection, a technique for producing a radiographic image of the facial bones and maxillary sinuses. The patient faces the image receptor (IR) and tilts the forehead away from the IR, with the nose barely touching and the chin resting on the surface of the IR. The orbitomeatal line forms a 37-degree angle with the plane of the IR. The x-ray beam is perpendicular and passes through the parietal bones and exits at the junction of the patient's nose and upper lip or at the location of the anterior nasal spine. Formerly called *Waters method.* See also **orbitomeatal line.**

parietomastoid suture, the suture at which the mastoid part of the temporal bone articulates superiorly with the parietal bone.

parietooccipital /pərī′ətō·oksip″itəl/ [L, *paries + occiput,* back of the head], pertaining to the parietal and occipital bones or cerebral lobes.

parietooccipital sulcus, a groove on each cerebral hemisphere marking the division of the parietal and occipital lobes of the cerebrum. Also called **occipitoparietal fissure.**

parietotemporal /-tem″pərəl/ [L, *paries,* wall, *tempus,* temple], pertaining to the temporal and parietal bones of the cranium. Also called **temporoparietal.**

parietovisceral /-vis″ərəl/, pertaining to the abdominal wall and abdominal organs.

-parin, suffix for heparin derivatives.

Parinaud oculoglandular syndrome /per″ōnō/ [Henri Parinaud, French ophthalmologist, 1844–1905], a term often used to refer to conjunctivitis that is usually unilateral, follicular, and followed by enlargement of the preauricular lymph nodes and tenderness. The syndrome has a wide range of causes, including tularemia, cat-scratch fever, and lymphogranuloma venereum. Also called *Parinaud ophthalmoplegia.*

paring board. See **spikeboard.**

pari passu /per″ē pas″ōō/ [L, *par,* equal, *passus,* step], at the same time or in equal proportions.

paritonsillar abscess. See **parapharyngeal abscess.**

parity /per″itē/ [L, *parere,* to give birth], **1.** (in obstetrics) the classification of a woman by the number of liveborn children and stillbirths she has delivered at more than 20 weeks of gestation. Commonly parity is noted with the total number of pregnancies and represented by the letter *P* or the word *para.* A para 4 (P4) gravida 5 (G5) has had four deliveries after 20 weeks and one abortion or miscarriage before 20 weeks. Currently a more complete system is in use: the total number of term infants (T) is followed by the number of premature infants (P), the number of abortions or miscarriages before 20 weeks' gestation (A), and the number of children living at present (L). This system may be abbreviated as *TPAL.* **2.** (in epidemiology) the classification of a woman by the number of live-born children she has delivered. **3.** (in computer processing) the condition of a set of items, either even or odd in number, used as a means for checking errors, such as in the transmission of information between various elements of the same computer.

parkinsonian. See **Parkinson disease.**

parkinsonian facies [James Parkinson, English physician, 1755–1824; L, *facies,* face], a masklike and immobile facial expression, usually occurring with Parkinson disease. Infrequent blinking also occurs. Also called **masked facies.**

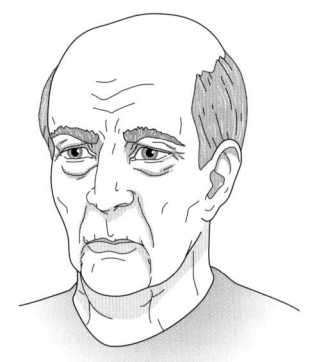

Parkinsonian facies *(Kaufman, 2007)*

parkinsonian tremor [James Parkinson; L, *tremor,* shaking], a mild resting tremor with slow, regular oscillations of three to six per second, exacerbated by fatigue, cold, or emotion. The tremors usually, but not always, cease during voluntary movement of the affected part and during sleep. Also called **pill-rolling tremor.**

parkinsonism /pär″kənsəniz′əm/ [James Parkinson], a neurological disorder characterized by tremor; muscle rigidity; hypokinesia; a slow, shuffling gait; and difficulty in chewing, swallowing, and speaking. It is caused by various lesions in the extrapyramidal motor system. Signs and symptoms of parkinsonism resemble those of idiopathic Parkinson disease and may develop during or after acute encephalitis and in syphilis, malaria, poliomyelitis, and carbon monoxide poisoning. Parkinsonism may occur in patients treated with antipsychotic drugs. Also called **shaking palsy.** See also **Parkinson disease.**

Parkinson disease [James Parkinson], a slowly progressive degenerative neurological disorder characterized by resting tremor, pill rolling of the fingers, a masklike facies, shuffling gait, forward flexion of the trunk, loss of postural reflexes, and muscle rigidity and weakness. It is usually an idiopathic disease of people over 60 years of age; it may occur in younger people, however, especially after acute encephalitis or carbon monoxide or metallic poisoning, particularly by reserpine or phenothiazine drugs. Typical pathological changes are destruction of neurons in basal ganglia; loss of pigmented cells in the substantia nigra; and depletion of dopamine in the caudate nucleus, putamen, and pallidum, structures in the neostriatum that normally contain high levels of the neurotransmitter dopamine. Signs and symptoms of Parkinson disease, which include resting tremor, bradykinesias, drooling, increased appetite, intolerance to heat, oily skin, emotional instability, and impaired judgment, are increased by fatigue, excitement, and frustration. Palliative and symptomatic treatment of the disease focuses on correcting the imbalance between depleted dopamine and abundant acetylcholine in the striatum because dopamine normally appears to inhibit excitatory cholinergic activity in this brain area. Levodopa, a dopamine precursor that crosses the blood-brain barrier, may be used, but many patients experience side effects, such as nausea, vomiting, insomnia, orthostatic hypotension, and mental confusion. Carbidopa-levodopa, which contains an inhibitor of the enzyme dopa decarboxylase, limits peripheral metabolism of levodopa and thus causes fewer side effects. Anticholinergic drugs, such as benztropine mesylate, biperiden, procyclidine, and trihexyphenidyl, may be used as therapeutic agents but often cause ataxia, blurred vision, constipation, dryness of the mouth, mental disturbances, slurred speech, and urinary urgency or retention. Amantadine hydrochloride, an antiviral drug with antiparkinsonian activity, promotes the accumulation of dopamine in extracellular or synaptic sites, but the therapeutic effectiveness may not last more than 3 months in some patients; side effects, such as mental confusion, visual disturbances, and seizures, occur infrequently. Also called **paralysis agitans.**

Parkinson mask [James Parkinson; Fr, *masque*], an expressionless face with eyebrows raised and smoothing but immobility of facial muscles.

Parlodel, a dopamine receptor agonist. Brand name for **bromocriptine mesylate.**

Parnate, an antidepressant. Brand name for **tranylcypromine sulfate.**

parole /pərōl′/, (in psychiatry) a system of supervision of a patient who has been physically released from a hospital setting but is still listed as an inpatient and may be returned to the hospital without further court action. Also called **leave.**

paromomycin sulfate /per′əmōmī″sin/, an oral antiamebic aminoglycoside antibiotic.

■ INDICATIONS: It is prescribed in the treatment of intestinal amebiasis, tapeworms, and Cryptosporidium and is used preoperatively to suppress intestinal flora.

■ CONTRAINDICATIONS: Intestinal inflammation, intestinal obstruction, or known hypersensitivity to this drug prohibits its use.

■ ADVERSE EFFECTS: Among the most serious effects are GI distress and diarrhea. Less common adverse effects include headache, vertigo, and pruritus.

paronychia /per′ənik″ē·ə/ [Gk, *para* + *onyx,* nail], an infection of the fold of skin at the margin of a nail. Treatment includes hot compresses or soaks, antibiotics, and possibly surgical incision and drainage. Compare **onychia.**

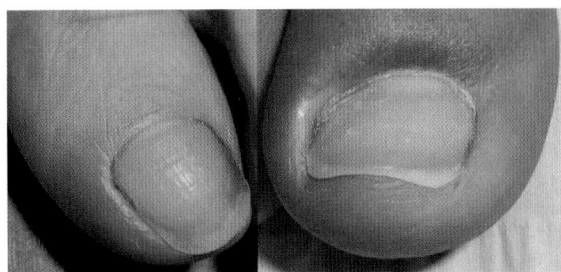

Paronychia *(Chang, 2015)*

paroophoritis /per′ō·of′ərī″tis/ [Gk, *para* + *oon,* egg, *pherein,* to bear, *itis*], inflammation of the paroophoron, the tissues surrounding the ovary.

paroophoron /per′ō·of″əron/ [Gk, *para* + *oon,* egg, *pherein,* to bear], a small vestigial remnant of the mesonephros, consisting of a few rudimentary tubules lying in the broad ligament between the epoophoron and the uterus. It is most evident in very young girls. A similar vestigial structure, the aberrant ductule, is found in the male. Also called **parovarium.** Compare **epoophoron.**

parosmia /pəroz″mē·ə/ [Gk, *para* + *osme,* smell], any dysfunction or distortion concerning the sense of smell. See also **anosmia, cacosmia.**

parosteitis /per′ostē·ī″tis/, an inflammation of the tissues adjacent to or associated with a bone.

parosteosis /per′ostē·ō″sis/, the development of bone in an abnormal location, such as in the area of the periosteum or in the skin.

parotid /pərot″id/ [Gk, *para* + *ous,* ear], near the ear.

parotid abscess, a collection of pus in a parotid salivary gland.

parotid duct [Gk, *para* + *ous,* ear; L, *ducere,* to lead], a tubular canal, about 7 cm long, that extends from the anterior part of the parotid gland near the ear to the mouth. It crosses the masseter after leaving the parotid gland, pierces the buccinator, runs for a short distance obliquely forward between the buccinator and the mucous membrane of the mouth, and opens on the oral surface of the cheek through a small opening opposite the second upper molar tooth. Also called **Stensen's duct.** See also **parotid gland, salivary gland.**

parotidectomy /pərot′idek″təmē/ [Gk, *para* + *ous* + *ektomē,* excision], the surgical removal of the parotid gland.

parotid gland [Gk, *para* + *ous,* ear; L, *glans,* acorn], one of the largest pairs of salivary glands that lies at the side of the face just below and in front of the external ear. The main part of the gland is superficial, somewhat flattened, and quadrilateral. It is enclosed in a capsule continuous with the deep cervical fascia. The parotid duct starts at the anterior part of the gland and opens on the inside of the cheek opposite the second upper molar. Compare **sublingual gland, submandibular gland.** See also **salivary gland.**

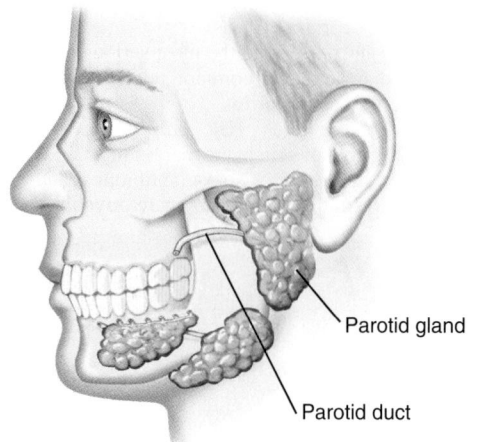

Parotid duct and parotid gland

parotitis /per′ətī″tis/ [Gk, *para* + *ous,* ear, *itis,* inflammation], inflammation or infection of one or both parotid salivary glands. See also **mumps.**

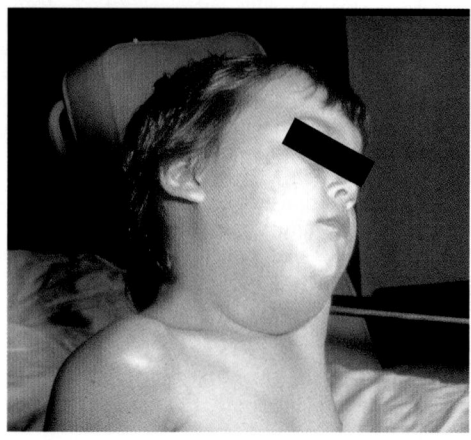

Child with parotitis *(Plotkin, 2008/Courtesy Centers for Disease Control and Prevention)*

parous /per″əs/, having borne one or more viable offspring.

-parous, suffix meaning "pertaining to the quantity of offspring produced simultaneously or to the method of gestation": *multiparous, fissiparous.*

parovarian /per′ōver″ē·ən/ [Gk, *para* + L, *ovum,* egg], pertaining to residual tissues in the area near the fallopian tubes and the ovary.

parovarium. See **epoophoron.**

paroxetine, a selective serotonin reuptake inhibitor.

■ INDICATIONS: It is prescribed in the treatment of mental depression, obsessive-compulsive disorder, panic disorders, and anxiety disorders, including social anxiety and general anxiety. Unlabeled uses include treatment of impulse control disorders, premenstrual syndrome, and vasomotor symptoms of menopause.

■ CONTRAINDICATIONS: It should not be given to patients taking monoamine oxidase inhibitors. Caution is advised in administering the drug to patients with a history of drug abuse, mania, seizures, suicidal tendencies, or kidney or liver disease.

■ ADVERSE EFFECTS: The side effects most often reported include decreased libido and ejaculatory disturbances, nausea, diarrhea, vomiting, constipation, abdominal pain, flatulence, changes in appetite, and muscle weakness. Paroxetine may also cause SIADH and/or hyponatremia and lead to or exacerbate coagulation disturbances because of impairment of platelet aggregation.

paroxysm /per″əksiz′əm/ [Gk, *paroxynein,* to stimulate], **1.** a marked, usually episodic increase in symptoms. **2.** a convulsion, fit, seizure, or spasm. −*paroxysmal, adj.*

paroxysmal atrial tachycardia. See **paroxysmal supraventricular tachycardia.**

paroxysmal AV nodal reentry tachycardia [Gk, *paroxysmos,* irritation; L, *nodus,* knot; Gk, *tachys,* fast, *kardia,* heart], a type of paroxysmal supraventricular tachycardia usually initiated by a premature atrial complex and sustained by an atrioventricular nodal reentry mechanism. A vagal maneuver is usually successful in restoring sinus rhythm. If it is not, adenosine or verapamil, procainamide, and cardioversion are tried, in succession.

paroxysmal cold hemoglobinuria (PCH), a rare autoimmune hemolytic anemia disorder marked by hemolysis minutes or hours after exposure to cold. Characterized by the presence of a biphasic hemolysin, called the Donath-Landsteiner antibody, which hemolyzes red cells after exposure to cool temperatures and then warming back to 37° C. Systemic symptoms include the passage of dark urine, severe pain in the back and legs, headache, vomiting, diarrhea, and moderate reticulocytosis. Temporary hepatosplenomegaly and mild hyperbilirubinemia may follow the onset of an attack.

paroxysmal cough [Gk, *paroxysmos,* irritation; AS, *cohhetan,* cough], a severe attack of coughing, as may accompany whooping cough, bronchiectasis, or a lung injury.

paroxysmal hemoglobinuria, the sudden passage of hemoglobin in urine, occurring after local or general exposure to low temperatures, as in paroxysmal cold hemoglobinuria.

paroxysmal junctional tachycardia. See **paroxysmal supraventricular tachycardia.**

paroxysmal labyrinthine vertigo. See **Ménière disease.**

paroxysmal nocturnal dyspnea (PND), a disorder characterized by sudden attacks of respiratory distress that awaken the person, usually after several hours of sleep in a reclining position. This occurs because of increased fluid central circulation with reclining position. It is most commonly caused by pulmonary edema resulting from congestive heart failure. The attacks are often accompanied by coughing, a feeling of suffocation, cold sweat, and tachycardia with a gallop rhythm. Sleeping with the head propped up on pillows may prevent PND, but treatment of the underlying cause is required to prevent fluid from accumulating in the lungs. Also called **nocturnal paroxysmal dyspnea.** See also **dyspnea.**

paroxysmal nocturnal hemoglobinuria (PNH), an acquired hemolytic anemia caused by a clonal stem cell mutation that results in an absence of glycosylphosphatidylinositol-anchored proteins, including decay-accelerating factor (DAF) and CD55. Red cells lacking DAF and CD55 have an increased susceptibility to complement activation and lysis, resulting in intravascular hemolysis and hemoglobinuria, especially during sleep.

paroxysmal supraventricular tachycardia, an ectopic heart rhythm with a rate of 170 to 250 beats/min. It begins abruptly with a premature atrial or ventricular beat and is supported by an atrioventricular (AV) nodal reentry mechanism or by an AV reentry mechanism involving an accessory pathway. Formerly called **paroxysmal atrial tachycardia, paroxysmal junctional tachycardia.**

paroxysmal ventricular tachycardia [Gk, *paroxysmos,* irritation; L, *ventriculus,* little belly; Gk, *tachys + kardia*], a rapid heartbeat of sudden onset and termination caused by a quick succession of discharges from an ectopic site in a ventricle.

parrot fever. See **psittacosis.**

parry fracture. See **Monteggia fracture.**

pars /pärs/ *pl. partis* [L, part], a part, such as the pars abdominalis esophagi. See also **part.**

Parse, Rosemarie Rizzo, a nursing theorist who, in her *Man-Living-Health: A Theory of Nursing* (1981), synthesized Martha E. Rogers' principles and concepts (Science of Unitary Human Beings) and the work of existential phenomenologists. Parse's view of nursing is based on humanism as opposed to positivism. Her theory addresses the unity of humans' lived experience, the lived experience of health. She used the term *man* to express male and female. Man chooses from options and bears responsibility for choices. Parse deduces three principles of Man-Living-Health, each interrelated with three concepts: (1) meaning (ultimate meaning and the meaningful moments of life) with the concepts of imaging, valuing, and languaging; (2) rhythmicity (rhythmic patterns of living) with the concepts of revealing-concealing, enabling-limiting, and connecting-separating; and (3) cotranscendence (reaching out beyond self) with the concepts of powering, originating, and transforming. Parse proposes that nursing is a human science and rejects the traditional view of nursing as an emerging natural science. See also **Rogers, Martha E.**

pars fetalis. See **fetal placenta.**

pars flaccida, the thin and slack part of the tympanic membrane superior to the anterior and posterior malleolar folds. See also **pars tensa.**

pars interarticularis, a region of the vertebra between the superior and inferior facet joints that is susceptible to trauma.

Parsonage-Turner syndrome. See **neuralgic amyotrophy.**

pars planitis /pärz plä·nī′tis/, **1.** a granulomatous uveitis of the ciliary disk (pars plana of the ciliary body). **2.** intermediate uveitis.

pars tensa, the thick and taut part of the tympanic membrane. See also **pars flaccida.**

part [L, *pars*], a part of a larger area, such as the condylar part of the occipital bone. See also **pars.**

part-, prefix meaning "related to childbirth": *parturient, parturition.*

part. aeq., a notation for a Latin phrase meaning "in equal parts." Abbreviation for *partes aequales.*

parthenogenesis /pär′thənōjen″əsis/ [Gk, *parthenos,* virgin, *genesis,* origin], a type of nonsexual reproduction in which an organism develops from an unfertilized ovum, as in many simpler animals. The development of the unfertilized ovum may be artificially induced through mechanical or chemical stimulation. Also called **unicellular reproduction.** *–parthenogenic, parthenogenetic, adj.*

partial anodontia, partial absence of the teeth. It is a relatively common congenital condition characterized by the absence of one or more teeth because of the absence of their anlage (or primordium), which is seldom associated with other anomalies. Acquired partial anodontia relates to the extraction of specific teeth to gain space for orthodontic therapy. Also called **hypodontia.**

partial bed rest a restriction of activities; the degree of restriction varies with the condition. Also called **modified bed rest.**

partial breech extraction. See **assisted breech.**

partial cleavage /pär″shəl/, mitotic division of only part of a fertilized ovum, usually the activated cytoplasmic part surrounding the nucleus. Compare **total cleavage.** See also **meroblastic.**

partial crown, a restoration that replaces some but not all surfaces of a tooth. Also called *three-quarter crown.*

partial denture [L, *pars,* part, *dens,* tooth], a dental prosthesis, either fixed or removable, used to replace one or more missing teeth. Kinds include **articulated partial denture, bridgework, extension partial denture, fixed cantilever, fixed partial denture, removable partial denture, sectional denture, unilateral denture.**

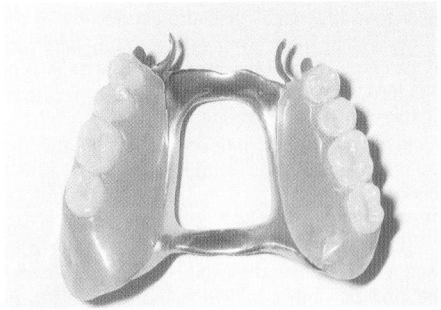

Removable partial denture *(Christensen, 2002)*

partial dislocation [L, *pars + dis + locare,* to place], the partial, abnormal separation of the articular surfaces of a joint. Also called **incomplete dislocation, subluxation.**

partial hospitalization program, an organizational entity that provides therapeutic services to patients who use only day or night hospital services or adult day health services rather than regular inpatient hospitalization services.

partial involution. See **uterine subinvolution.**

partial liquid ventilation, ventilatory support in which the lungs are filled to the level of the functional residual capacity with a liquid perfluorocarbon. Mechanical ventilation is then superimposed, and oxygen and carbon dioxide are transferred through the liquid.

partially acid-fast /pär″shəlē/, capable of retaining the stain carbolfuchsin during mild acid decolorization. This ability is found in bacteria of the genus *Nocardia* because of the presence of unusual long-chain fatty acids in their cell walls.

partially edentulous arch, a dental arch in which one or more but not all natural teeth are missing.

partial placenta previa, placenta previa in which the placenta is implanted in the lower uterine segment and partially covers the internal os of the uterine cervix. As the cervix dilates in labor, the part of the placenta that lies over the cervix is separated, causing bleeding from the villous spaces of the uterine wall. Depending on the degree of separation, the bleeding may be scant or severe, resulting in hemorrhage that is life-threatening to the mother and the baby. Treatment may require cesarean section if the pressure of the presenting part of the baby is not sufficient to tamponade the bleeding site, stopping the hemorrhage. Diagnosis of partial placenta previa may be made before bleeding occurs by ultrasonic visualization or digital palpation in the course of prenatal examination. See also **marginal placenta previa, placenta previa.**

partial pressure, the pressure exerted by any one gas in a mixture of gases or in a liquid, with the pressure directly related to the concentration of that gas to the total pressure of the mixture. The concentration of oxygen in the atmosphere represents approximately 21% of the total atmospheric pressure, calculated at 760 mm Hg under standard conditions. Therefore, the partial pressure of atmospheric oxygen is about 160 mm Hg (760 mm Hg × 0.21).

partial pressure of carbon dioxide in arterial blood (PaCO$_2$), the portion of total blood gas pressure exerted by carbon dioxide. It decreases during heavy exercise, during rapid breathing, or in association with severe diarrhea, uncontrolled diabetes, or diseases of the liver or kidneys. It increases with chest injuries or respiratory disorders. The reference interval is 35 to 45 mm Hg in arterial blood and 40 to 45 mm Hg in venous blood.

partial pressure of oxygen in arterial blood (PaO$_2$), the portion of total blood gas pressure exerted by oxygen. It is lower than normal in patients with asthma, obstructive lung disease, or certain blood diseases and in healthy individuals during vigorous exercise. The normal PaO$_2$ in arterial blood is 95 to 100 mm Hg.

partial response, the condition in which the maximum decrease in treated tumor volume is at least 50% but less than 100%.

partial root amputation. See **apicoectomy.**

partial shadowing, (in ultrasonics) a manifestation of decreased echo signal amplitudes returning from regions lying beyond an object in which the attenuation is higher than the average attenuation in adjacent overlying regions.

partial thromboplastin time (PTT), a test for detecting coagulation defects of the intrinsic system by adding activated partial thromboplastin to a sample of test plasma and to a control sample of normal plasma. The time required for the formation of a clot in test plasma is compared with that in the normal plasma. A delayed clotting time suggests an abnormality in one or more factors of the intrinsic system. If indicated, specific factor abnormalities can be identified by exposing the test plasma to a series of plasma samples with known factor deficiencies and observing for coagulation, which occurs only if the test plasma provides the missing clotting factors. PTT is one of the basic tests used to measure specific factor activity and to detect hemophilias. It can be used to monitor liver function and to monitor the activity of the anticoagulant heparin. The normal activated PTT in plasma is 25 to 45 seconds after the addition to the plasma sample of partial thromboplastin reagent and ionized calcium. Also called **activated partial thromboplastin time.** Compare **prothrombin time.** See also **hemostasis.**

partial volume artifact, an artifact caused by a mixture of tissues with different attenuation coefficients within any given voxel.

partial zona dissection (PZD), an older micromanipulation technique used in male factor infertility. A cut is made into the zona pellucida and spermatozoa are inserted.

participant, 1. a subject in a research project. **2.** See **enrollee.**

particle /pär″tikəl/ [L, *particula,* small part], **1.** any fundamental unit of matter. **2.** a minute fragment or speck.

particulate /pärtik″yəlit/, pertaining to a minute discrete particle or fragment of a substance or material.

-partite, suffix meaning "having the (specified) number of parts": *bipartite.*

parts per million (PPM, ppm), the ratio of the amount of one substance to the amount of another, expressed as a unit of solute dissolved in one million units of solution. It denotes the number of units of one substance relative to one million units of another substance. It may be further expressed in terms of mass-to-mass, volume-to-volume, or another relationship of units of measure.

parturient /pärt(y)o̅o̅″rē·ənt/ [L, *parturire,* to desire to bring forth], pertaining to the act of childbirth.

parturition /pär′t(y)o̅o̅rish″ən/ [L, *parturire,* to desire to bring forth], the process of giving birth.

parulis. See **gumboil.**

paruresis, the inhibition of urination as a result of psychological or other reasons.

paruria /pəro̅o̅r″ē·ə/, any defect of the urination process.

parvovirus B19 /pär″vo̅vī″rəs/, a small single-stranded deoxyribonucleic acid virus of the Parvoviridae family that infects humans, causing erythema infectiosum, aplastic crisis in hemolytic anemia, and other disorders. Another strain of the Parvoviridae, canine P2, causes acute enteritis and myocarditis in dogs.

parvovirus B19 antibody test, a blood test used to detect the presence of antibodies to the B19 parvovirus, a known human pathogen. The B19 virus is associated most commonly with erythema infectiosum (also called fifth disease), but also with joint inflammation, purpura, hydrops fetalis, and aplastic anemia.

parvule /pär″vyo̅o̅l/, a very small pill. Also called **pilule.**

PAS, PASA, abbreviation for **paraaminosalicylic acid.**

pascal (Pa), a unit of measurement of pressure in the SI system.

Pascal's principle /poskuls′, paskals″/ [Blaise Pascal], (in physics) a law stating that a confined liquid transmits pressure applied to it from an external source equally in all directions. Pascal's principle provides the basis for all hydraulic devices.

PASG, abbreviation for **pneumatic antishock garment.** See **military antishock trousers.**

Pasqualini syndrome [C. Pasqualini, Argentinian physician]. See **fertile eunuch syndrome.**

pass. See **conditional discharge.**

passage /pas″ij/, **1.** an opening, channel, route, or gap. **2.** the movement of something from one place to another, as in evacuation of the bowels.

passiflora /pas′iflôr″ə/, the passion flower, *Passiflora incarnata,* a climbing herb. It has flowers and fruiting tops that are the source of medications used as antispasmodics and sedatives and for the treatment of burns, dysmenorrhea, hemorrhoids, and insomnia.

passion flower, an herbal product derived from a perennial climbing vine that is native to tropical and subtropical areas of the Americas and is also found in the southeastern United States.

■ INDICATIONS: It is used orally for the treatment of insomnia and restlessness and gastrointestinal disturbances associated with nervousness. It is used topically for the treatment of hemorrhoids, burns, and inflammation. Other traditional uses include treatment of menopause, pain, palpitations, arrhythmias, and hypertension. It may be effective in relieving nervousness; there are insufficient reliable data regarding its effectiveness for other indications.

■ CONTRAINDICATIONS: It should not be used during pregnancy and lactation, in children, or in those with known hypersensitivity.

passive [L *passivus*], **1.** pertaining to behavior that subordinates the individual's own interests to the demands of others. **2.** pertaining to an action that is initiated and sustained by an external agent.

passive-aggressive personality [L, *passivus* + *aggressus,* combative, *persona,* character], a personality characterized by a chronically negativistic disposition with passive resistance and aggression manifested by forceful actions or attitudes expressed in an indirect, nonviolent manner, such as pouting, obstructionism, procrastination, inefficiency, stubbornness, and forgetfulness. Compare **aggressive personality, passive-dependent personality.** See also **passive-aggressive personality disorder.**

passive-aggressive personality disorder, a psychiatric disorder characterized by the indirect expression of resistance to occupational or social demands. It results in persistent pervasive ineffectiveness, lack of self-confidence, poor interpersonal relationships, and pessimism that can lead in severe cases to major depression, alcoholism, or drug dependence. The behavior often reflects an unexpressed hostility or resentment stemming from a frustrating interpersonal or institutional relationship on which an individual is overly dependent. Treatment may consist of behavior therapy or any of the various psychotherapeutic procedures, depending on the individual and the severity of the condition.

passive algolagnia. See **masochism.**

passive anaphylaxis. See **antiserum anaphylaxis.**

passive carrier [L, *passivus* + OFr, *carier*], **1.** a healthy person whose body carries the causal organisms of an infectious disease although the person has not contracted the disease and remains symptomless. **2.** a person who carries a gene associated with a hereditary trait although the trait is not expressed in the person. Also called **symptomless carrier.**

passive clot, a clot that forms in an aneurysm when circulation is interrupted.

passive congestion [L, *passivus* + *congerere,* to heap together], an excessive amount of blood accumulation in an organ as a result of increased venous pressure.

passive-dependent personality [L, *passivus* + Fr, *dependre,* to depend; L, *persona,* character], a personality characterized by helplessness, indecisiveness, and a tendency to cling to and seek support from others. Compare **passive-aggressive personality.**

passive euthanasia, the ending of life by the deliberate withholding of drugs or other life-sustaining treatment.

passive exercise, repetitive movement of a part of the body as a result of an externally applied force or a voluntary effort to move another part of the body. Passive exercise can be used to prevent contractures and maintain joint mobility but does not promote muscle maintenance. Compare **active exercise.** See also **aerobic exercise, anaerobic exercise.**

passive expiration [L, *passivus* + *expirare,* to breathe out], normal exhalation that occurs without direct muscular effort, as during normal tidal breathing. Air is expelled from the lungs as a result of the recoil effect of elastic tissues in the chest, lungs, and diaphragm.

passive immunity, a form of acquired immunity resulting from antibodies that are transmitted naturally through the placenta to a fetus, through the colostrum to an infant, or artificially by injection of antiserum for treatment or prophylaxis. Passive immunity is not permanent and does not last as long as active immunity. Compare **active immunity.** See also **immune response, natural immunity.**

passive incontinence [L, *passivus* + *incontinentia*], urine overflow that may occur when the bladder (musculus detrusor vesicae) is paralyzed and greatly distended. See also **incontinence.**

passive lingual arch, an orthodontic appliance that may help maintain tooth space and dental arch length when bilateral primary molars are prematurely lost.

passive lung collapse [L, *passivus* + AS, *lungen* + L, *collabi*], a condition of dyspnea, cough, and hemoptysis with pigmented cells caused by an obstructed blood flow from the lungs to the heart.

passive motion [L, *passivus* + *motio*], involuntary motion caused by an external force rather than by voluntary muscular effort. See also **passive exercise.**

passive movement, the moving of parts of the body by an outside force without voluntary action or resistance by the individual. Also called **passive exercise.** Compare **active movement.**

passive play, play in which a person does not participate actively. For younger children such activity may include watching and listening to others, observing other children or animals, listening to stories, or looking at pictures. Older children are passively entertained by games and toys that require concentration and intellectual skill, such as chess, reading, listening to music, or watching television. Compare **active play.**

passive range of motion (PROM), the moving of a joint through its range of motion with no effort from the individual—for example, the movement of a knee joint through its range of motion by a therapist or equipment after surgery.

passive recoil, the return of elastic tissue to its normal length and position when applied tension on the tissue is released.

passive sensitization [L, *passivus* + *sentire,* to feel], a temporary form of sensitization induced by injecting serum from a sensitized individual. See also **passive immunity.**

passive smoking, the inhalation by nonsmokers of the smoke from other people's cigarettes, pipes, or cigars. The amount of such smoke inhaled by a nonsmoker is small compared with that inhaled by tobacco users. However, passive smoking can aggravate respiratory illnesses and contribute to serious diseases, including cancer. Infants, fetuses, and individuals with chronic heart and lung diseases or allergies to tobacco can be adversely affected by passive smoking. See also **secondhand smoke.**

passive stretching, stretching that involves only noncontractile elements, such as ligaments, fascia, bursae, dura mater, and nerve roots. Examples include manipulation of a muscle, such as during therapeutic massage or during isometric exercises in which there is no range of motion of the body part involved.

passive symptom [L, *passivus* + Gk, *symptoma,* that which happens], a symptom that attracts little or no attention. Also called **static symptom.**

passive transfer, the conferring of immunity to a nonimmune host by injection of antibodies or lymphocytes from an immune or sensitized donor.

passive transfer test. See **Prausnitz-Küstner test.**

passive transport, the movement of small molecules across the membrane of a cell by diffusion. Passive transport occurs when the chemicals outside a cell become concentrated and start moving into the cell, changing the intracellular equilibrium. Passive transport is essential to various processes of metabolism, such as the intake of digestive products by the cells lining the intestines. Compare **active transport, osmosis.**

passive tremor. See **resting tremor.**

passivity /pəsiv″itē/ [L, *passivus*], a maladaptive mental state of submission, dependence, or inactivity.

Passy-Muir valve, a one-way speaking valve for use with tracheostomy tubes. Its normal position at rest is closed, so that it is open only during inhalation and closes during exhalation, allowing air to pass through the vocal folds for phonation.

paste /pāst/, a topical semisolid formulation containing a pharmacologically active ingredient in a fatty base, a viscous or mucilaginous base, or a mixture of starch and petrolatum. Typically it is used externally only.

Pasteur effect /pastŏor´, pästœr´/ [Louis Pasteur, French chemist, 1822–1895], the inhibiting effect of oxygen on carbohydrate fermentation by living cells.

Pasteurella /pas´tərel´ə/ [Louis Pasteur], a genus of gram-negative bacilli or coccobacilli, including species pathogenic to humans and domestic animals. *Pasteurella* infections may be transmitted to humans by animal bites or scratches. The plague bacillus, *Pasteurella pestis,* is now called *Yersinia pestis*; *P. tularensis,* which causes tularemia, has been reclassified as *Francisella tularensis.*

Pasteurella pestis. *(Obsolete)* See *Yersinia pestis.*

pasteurellosis /pas´tərelō´sis/ [Louis Pasteur], a local wound infection, caused by the gram-negative bacillus *Pasteurella multicide,* which may be acquired through the bite or scratch of an infected animal, usually a cat.

pasteurization /pas´tərīzā´shən/ [Louis Pasteur; Gk, *izein,* to cause], the process of applying heat, usually to milk or cheese, for a specified period for the purpose of killing or slowing the development of pathogenic bacteria. *–pasteurize, v.*

pasteurized milk /pas´tərīzd/ [Louis Pasteur; Gk, *izein,* to cause; AS, *moluc,* milk], milk that has been treated by heat to destroy pathogenic bacteria.

Pasteur, Louis [French chemist, 1822–1895], promoter of the germ theory of infection and developer of the pasteurization process to kill pathogenic organisms in milk. Pasteur also developed several vaccines and pioneered the development of stereochemistry by separating mirror image isomers.

Pasteur treatment [Louis Pasteur], a method of preventing rabies by daily injections of attenuated cultures of rabies virus cultured in the central nervous system tissues of rabbits. The treatment, developed by Pasteur, is no longer used. See also **human diploid cell rabies vaccine.**

past health [ME, *passen,* to pass; AS, *hoelth,* sound body], (in a health history) an overall summary of the person's general health to date, including past injuries, allergies, surgical procedures, immunizations, hospitalizations, and obstetric and psychiatric history. The past health information is obtained from the person or the person's family at the initial interview and becomes part of the permanent record. See also **health history.**

Pastia's lines /pas´te·əz/ [Chessec Pastia, 20th-century Romanian physician], lines of hyperpigmentation seen in the body folds in scarlet fever.

pastille /pastēl´, pas´til/, **1.** a gelatin-based sweetened and molded medication impregnated with a therapeutic substance intended to be sucked. See also **troche. 2.** a chemically treated paper disk that undergoes color changes when exposed to radiation. **3.** a small mass containing aromatic substances and benzoic acid that is burned for fumigation. Also spelled *pastil.*

pastoral counseling department /pas´tərəl/ [L, *pastor,* shepherd], the hospital chaplaincy service.

past pointing [OFr, *passer* + L, *punctus,* pricked], the inability to place a finger on another part of the body accurately, indicating a lack of coordination in voluntary movements.

Patau syndrome. See **trisomy 13.**

patch [ME, *pacche*], **1.** *n.,* a small spot of surface tissue that differs from the surrounding area in color or texture or both and is not elevated above it. **2.** *n.,* a small, thin piece of material that adheres to the skin and is impregnated with medication, as in a nicotine patch. **3.** *v.,* to correct a defect, as with skin or mesh.

patch test, a skin test for identifying allergens, especially those causing contact dermatitis. The suspected substance (food, pollen, animal fur) is applied to an adhesive patch that is placed on the patient's skin. Another patch, with nothing on it, serves as a control. After a certain period (usually 24 to 48 hours) both patches are removed. If the skin under the suspect patch is red and swollen and the skin under the control area is not, the test result is said to be positive, and the person is probably allergic to that substance. Compare **radio-allergosorbent test.**

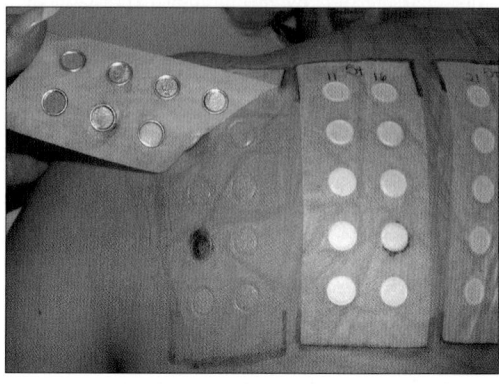

Removing patch tests *(Marks and Miller, 2013)*

patella /pətel´ə/ [L, small dish], a flat, large sesamoid bone at the front of the knee joint, having a pointed apex that attaches to the patellar ligament. The convex anterior surface of the bone is perforated for the passage of nutrient vessels and covered by an expansion from the tendon of the quadriceps femoris. Also called **kneecap.**

patellar /pətel´ər/ [L, *patella,* small dish], pertaining to the patella.

patellar-bearing supracondylar/suprapatellar (PTBSC/SP) socket, a type of patellar-tendon below-the-knee bearing prosthesis with a socket that extends in front, medially, and laterally to accommodate both the patella and the femoral condyles. The higher socket increases knee stability, and a suspension strap is not required.

patellar bursa [L, *patella,* small dish; Gk, *byrsa,* wineskin], any of the fluid-filled connective tissue sacs around the kneecap. Kinds include **prepatellar bursa, suprapatellar bursa.**

patellar ligament [L, *patella* + *ligare,* to bind], the central part of the common tendon of the quadriceps femoris. The ligament is a strong flat ligamentous band, about 8 cm long, attached proximally to the apex and the adjoining margins of the patella and distally to the tuberosity of the tibia. Its superficial fibers are continuous with the front of the patella with those of the tendon of the quadriceps femoris.

patellar reflex, a deep tendon reflex, elicited by a sharp tap on the tendon just distal to the patella, normally characterized by contraction of the quadriceps muscle and extension of the leg at the knee. The reflex is hyperactive in disease of the pyramidal tract above the level of the second lumbar vertebra. Also called **knee-jerk reflex, quadriceps reflex.** See also **deep tendon reflex.**

patellar-tendon bearing (PTB) prosthesis, an ankle-foot orthosis that provides prolonged stretch to the posterior leg musculature and may create extension force at the knee joint.

patellar-tendon bearing supracondylar (PTB/SC) socket, a lower-leg prosthesis with supracondylar (above a condyle) and suprapatellar (above the patella) suspension.

patellectomy /pat´əlek´təmē/ [L, *patella,* small dish; Gk, *ektomē,* excision], the surgical removal of the patella.

patellofemoral chondrosis, the softening or loss of smooth cartilage covering the back of the kneecap.

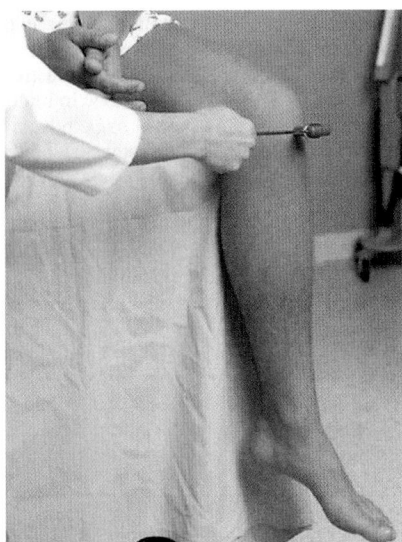

Elicitation of the patellar reflex *(Elkin, Perry, and Potter, 2007)*

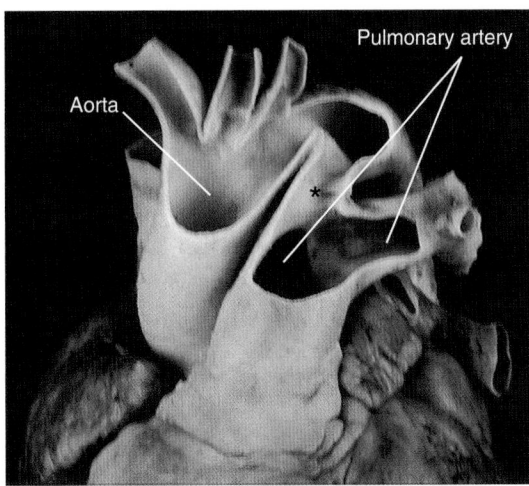

Patent ductus arteriosus (asterisk) *(Damjanov and Linder, 2000)*

patency /pā″tənsē/ [L, *patens,* open], a state of being open or exposed.

patent /pā″tənt/ [L, *patens,* open], open and unblocked, such as a patent airway or a patent anus.

patent ductus arteriosus (PDA), an abnormal opening between the pulmonary artery and the aorta caused by failure of the fetal ductus arteriosus to close after birth. It is seen primarily in premature infants. The defect allows blood from the aorta to flow into the pulmonary artery and recirculate through the lungs, where it is reoxygenated and returned to the left atrium and left ventricle, placing an increased workload on the left side of the heart and causing increased pulmonary vascular congestion and resistance. Clinical manifestations include cardiomegaly, especially of the left atrium and left ventricle; dilated ascending aorta; bounding pulses resulting from increased systolic pressure; tachycardia; and a typical machinery-like murmur that is heard during all of systole and most of diastole. Characteristic auscultatory and radiological findings are sufficient to confirm diagnosis so that cardiac catheterization is not necessary. Correction is delayed until the child is old enough to tolerate surgery and until spontaneous closure, which sometimes occurs. Untreated complications include congestive heart failure, pulmonary vascular disease, calcification of the ductal site, and infective endocarditis. See also **congenital cardiac anomaly.**

patent medicine [L, *patens,* open, *medicina*], a drug available to the general public without a prescription. The ingredients and contraindications are usually listed on the label or wrapper. Also called **OTC drug, proprietary drug.**

patent urachus, a congenital anomaly in which the urachus remains patent from the bladder to the umbilicus, with a channel that may be small or large and leakage of urine at the umbilicus.

paternal /pətur″nəl/ [L, *pater,* father], pertaining to fatherhood, characteristic of a father, or related through a father.

paternal engrossment. See **bonding.**

paternity test /pətur″nitē/ [L, *pater* + *testum,* crucible], a test to establish proof that a man is the biological father of an individual. The use of a DNA profile to determine if two individuals are biologically parent and child is the most accurate method; samples can be easily obtained by using buccal cells found on the inside of the father's and child's cheek. Another method still in use includes a test based on genetic blood groups that is used mainly to exclude the possibility that a particular man could be the father of a specific child.

Paterson-Kelly syndrome. See **Plummer-Vinson syndrome.**

Paterson-Parker dosage system [James R.K. Paterson, English radiologist; H.M. Parker, 20th-century American-English physicist], a radiotherapy system that uses sources of specific relative loadings arranged according to defined rules, which lead to a homogenous dose in the implanted region.

path [AS, *paeth*], a route or course along which something moves, such as a circuit of the nervous system that is followed by sensory or motor nerve impulses. See also **pathway.**

path-. See **patho-, path-.**

path, 1. *(Informal)* abbreviation for **pathological. 2.** abbreviation for **pathology.**

-path, -pathic, -pathy, suffix meaning "disease" or "suffering": *cardiopathy, naturopathic, osteopathy.*

pathetic /pəthet″ik/, pertaining to something that engenders emotions of sympathy, pity, and sadness.

-pathetic, -pathetical /pəthet″ik/, combining form meaning "emotions": *parasympathetic, sympathetic.*

pathfinder, a thin, flexible, cylindrical instrument containing a series of filiform guides, used to locate strictures.

-pathic. See **-path, -pathic, -pathy.**

patho-, path-, prefix meaning "disease": *pathogen, pathogenic, pathology.*

pathodontia. See **dental pathology.**

pathogen /path″əjən/ [Gk, *pathos,* disease, *genein,* to produce], any microorganism capable of producing disease. **–pathogenic,** *adj.*

pathogenesis /-jen″əsis/ [Gk, *pathos* + *genesis,* origin], the source or cause of an illness or abnormal condition.

pathogenic /-jen″ik/ [Gk, *pathos,* disease, *genein,* to produce], capable of causing or producing a disease. Also called *pathogenetic.*

pathogenicity /-jənis″itē/, the ability of a pathogenic agent to produce a disease.

P

pathogenic occlusion, an abnormal closure of the teeth, capable of producing unhealthy changes in the teeth, supporting tissues, and related structures.

pathogenic theory of medicine. See **germ theory.**

pathognomonic /pəthog′nəmon″ik/ [Gk, *pathos* + *gnomon,* index], (of a sign or symptom) specific to a disease or condition, such as Koplik spots on the buccal and lingual mucosa, which are indicative of measles.

pathognomonic symptom. See **symptom.**

pathological (path.) /-loj″ikəl/ [Gk, *pathos* + *logos,* science], pertaining to a condition that is caused by or involves a disease process.

pathological absorption, the assimilation of excremental liquids or bacterial substances within the bloodstream.

pathological amenorrhea [Gk, *pathos,* disease, *logos,* science, *a* + *men,* month, *rhoia,* to flow], a stoppage or absence of menstrual discharge from the uterus as a result of a disease.

pathological anatomy, (in applied anatomy) the study of the structure and morphological characteristics of the tissues and cells of the body as related to disease.

pathological diagnosis, a diagnosis arrived at by an examination of the substance and function of the tissues of the body, especially of the abnormal developmental changes in the tissues by histological techniques of tissue examination.

pathological fracture. See **neoplastic fracture.**

pathological histology [Gk, *pathos,* disease, *logos,* science, *histos,* tissue, *logos,* science], the study of the effects of disease on the structure, composition, and function of tissues.

pathological microorganisms [Gk, *pathos,* disease, *logos,* science, *mikros,* small, *organon,* instrument, *ismos,* condition], any microscopic life form, from a virus to a nematode, that has the potential to cause disease.

pathological mitosis, any cell division that is atypical, asymmetric, or multipolar and results in an unequal number of chromosomes in the nuclei of the daughter cells. It is indicative of malignancy, as occurs in cancer and the genetic anomalies.

pathological myopia, a type of severe, progressive nearsightedness characterized by changes in the fundus of the eye, posterior staphyloma, and deficient corrected acuity. Refractive error is greater than −8.00 diopters, and axial length is greater than 32.5 mm. Pathological myopia increases the risk of retinal detachment by affecting the curvature of the crystalline lens.

pathological physiology, 1. the study of the physical and chemical processes involved in the functioning of diseased tissues. 2. the study of the modification of the normal functioning processes of an organism caused by disease. Also called **morbid physiology.** See also **pathophysiology.**

pathological reflex [Gk, *pathos,* disease, *logos,* science; L, *reflectere,* to bend back], any abnormal reflex that is caused by a lesion in or an organic disease of the nervous system.

pathological retraction ring, a ridge that may form around the uterus at the junction of the upper and lower uterine segments during the prolonged second stage of an obstructed labor. The lower segment is abnormally distended and thin, and the upper segment is abnormally thick. The ring, which may be seen and felt abdominally, is a warning of impending uterine rupture. Also called **Bandl's ring.** Compare **constriction ring, physiological retraction ring.**

pathological sleep [Gk, *pathos,* disease, *logos,* science; AS, *slaep*], excessive sleep associated with a neurological disorder such as encephalitis lethargica, or sleeping sickness.

pathological triad, the combination of three respiratory disease conditions: bronchospasm, retained secretions, and mucosal edema. This triad is typically found in chronic bronchitis and asthma. It is treated with bronchodilators, hydration, mucolytics, and decongestants.

pathologist /pəthol″əjist/, a physician specializing in the study of disease. A pathologist usually specializes in autopsy or in clinical or surgical pathology.

pathologists' assistant, an allied health professional who, under the direct supervision of a licensed pathologist, participates in autopsies and in the examination, dissection, and processing of tissue specimens. Baccalaureate and master's degree programs are available.

pathology (path.) /pəthol″əjē/ [Gk, *pathos,* disease, *logos,* science], the study of the characteristics, causes, and effects of disease, as observed in the structure and function of the body. Cellular pathology is the study of cellular changes in disease. Clinical pathology is the study of disease by the use of laboratory tests and methods.

pathomimesis /path′ō-mi-mē′sis/ [Gk, *patho,* disease, *mimesis,* imitate], the imitation of a disease or disorder, which may be intentional or subconscious.

pathomimicry. See **Münchausen syndrome.**

pathophysiology /-fiz′ē-ol″əjē/ [Gk, *pathos,* disease, *physis,* nature, *logos,* science], the study of the biological and physical manifestations of disease as they correlate with the underlying abnormalities and physiological disturbances. Pathophysiology does not deal directly with the treatment of disease. Rather, it explains the processes within the body that result in the signs and symptoms of a disease.

pathosis, a disease condition.

pathway [AS, *paeth* + *weg*], 1. a network of neurons that provides a transmission route for nerve impulses from any part of the body to the spinal cord and the cerebral cortex or from the central nervous system to the muscles and organs. 2. a chain of chemical reactions that produces various compounds in critical sequence, such as the Embden-Meyerhof pathway.

-pathy. See **-path, -pathic, -pathy.**

patient (pt.) /pā″shənt/ [L, *pati,* to suffer], 1. a recipient of a health care service. 2. a health care recipient who is ill or hospitalized. 3. a client in a health care service.

patient advocate. See **ombudsman.**

patient assignment, a specialty capitation method in which patients choose a provider in each specialty represented. Capitation payments are then distributed accordingly to the providers selected.

patient care committee, a hospital staff organization, composed of medical, nursing, and other health professionals, with responsibility for monitoring all patient care practices to ensure that predetermined standards are met.

patient care technician, a health technician working under the supervision of a registered nurse, physician, or other health professional to provide basic patient care. Duties may include taking vital signs, obtaining blood and urine samples, performing basic diagnostic tests, and assisting the patient as needed.

patient compensation fund, a fund usually established by state law, commonly financed by a surcharge on malpractice premiums and used to pay malpractice claims.

patient-controlled analgesia (PCA), a drug-delivery system that dispenses a preset dose of an analgesic agent, typically to an intravenous or epidural catheter, when the patient pushes a button on an electric cord. The device consists of a computerized pump with a chamber containing the drug. The patient administers a dose when the need for pain relief arises. A lockout interval automatically inactivates the system if a patient tries to increase the number of doses within a preset period.

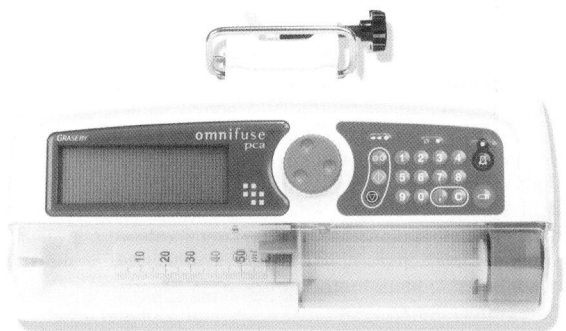

Patient-controlled analgesia pump (Al-Shaikh and Stacey, 2013)

patient day (P.D.), a unit in a system of accounting used by health care facilities and health care planners. Each day represents a unit of time during which the services of the institution or facility are used by a patient; thus 50 patients in a hospital for 1 day would represent 50 patient days.

patient dumping, the premature discharge of Medicare or indigent patients from hospitals for economic reasons. A 1986 U.S. federal rule requires hospitals to advise Medicare patients on admission for treatment of their right to challenge what they consider as premature discharge after treatment. The regulation was adopted after initiation of a Medicare policy of paying hospitals according to a particular illness, regardless of the length of hospitalization, as an incentive for hospitals to reduce the period of inpatient care.

patient interview, a systematic interview of a patient, the purpose of which is to obtain information that can be used to develop an individualized plan for care. Also called *client interview.*

patient mix, **1.** the distribution of demographic variables in a patient population, often represented by the percentage of a given race, age, sex, or ethnic derivation. **2.** the distribution of indications for admission in a patient population, such as surgical, maternity, or trauma.

patient plan of care, a document developed after the patient assessment that identifies the nursing diagnoses to be addressed in the hospital or clinic. The plan of care includes the objectives, nursing interventions, and time frame for accomplishment and evaluation. It should be formulated with input from the patient and the patient's family.

Patient Protection and Affordable Care Act, a federal statute enacted by the 111th U.S. Congress and signed into law by President Barack Obama on March 23, 2010. The act is often referred to with a shortened form of its name, the Affordable Care Act (ACA), or by its nickname, Obamacare.

patient record, a collection of documents that provides an account of each episode in which a patient visited or sought treatment and received care or a referral for care from a health care facility. The record is confidential and is usually held by the facility, and the information in it is released only to the patient or with the patient's written permission. It contains the initial assessment of the patient's health status, the health history, laboratory and radiological reports of tests performed, notes by nurses, physicians, and other health care professionals regarding the daily condition of the patient, and notes by consultants, as well as order sheets, medication sheets, admission records, discharge summaries, and other pertinent data. A problem-oriented medical record also contains a master problem list. The patient record is increasingly maintained in an electronic format. Also called **chart.** See also **medical record.**

patient representative. See **ombudsman.**

patient representative services, hospital services provided by designated staff members relating to the investigation and mediation of patients' complaints and the promotion and protection of patients' rights. See also **ombudsman.**

Patient's Bill of Rights, a list of the patient's rights promulgated by the American Hospital Association. It offers some guidance and protection to patients by stating the responsibilities that a hospital and its staff have toward them and their families during hospitalization, but it is not a legally binding document.

Patient Self-Determination Act, an act mandating that individuals enrolled in health care facilities are informed on admission in writing of their rights to formulate advance directives and to consent to or refuse treatment.

Patient Zero, the initial patient in the population of an epidemiological investigation.

Patrick test, a test for pain or dysfunction in the hip and sacroiliac joints in which overpressure is applied at the knee during flexion, abduction, and external rotation of the hip. While applying pressure on the knee, the examiner also applies counterpressure at the opposite anterior superior iliac spine. Also called **fabere sign, figure-four test.**

patrilineal /pat'rilin″ē·əl/ [L, *pater,* father, *linea,* line], pertaining to a line of descent through the male members of the family.

patten /pat″ən/, a metal support worn on a shoe to prevent weight-bearing on the opposite leg.

patterning /pat″ərning/ [ME, *patron*], a method of treatment or act of establishing a system or pattern of stimuli to enhance development in individuals who have suffered a brain injury or disorder that disrupts normal sensory-motor activities.

patulous /pat′yələs/ [L, *patulus,* open], pertaining to something that is open or spread apart.

paucibacillary /paw″səbas′əlā-re/, containing just a few bacilli. See also **leprosy.**

pau d'arco, an herbal product harvested from the inner bark of an evergreen flowering tree native to Florida, the West Indies, Mexico, and Central and South America. Also called *taheebo, lapacho.*

Paul-Bunnell test [John R. Paul, American physician, 1893–1971; Walls W. Bunnell, American physician, 1902–1966], an old term for a blood test for heterophil antibodies, used for confirming a diagnosis of infectious mononucleosis. See also **heterophil antibody test.**

pauresis /pôrē″sis/, the inhibition of urination for psychological or other reasons.

Pautrier microabscess /pôtrēyā″/ [Lucien M.A. Pautrier, French dermatologist, 1876–1959; Gk, *mikros,* small; L, *abscedere,* to go away], an accumulation of intensely staining mononuclear cells in the epidermis characterizing malignant lymphoma of the skin, especially mycosis fungoides. See also **mycosis fungoides.**

Pauwels fracture /pou″əlz/ [Friedrich Pauwels, 20th-century German surgeon; L, *fractura,* break], a break in the proximal femoral neck with varying degrees of angulation.

Pavabid, a smooth muscle relaxant. Brand name for **papaverine hydrochloride.**

pavement epithelium. See **squamous epithelium.**

Pavlik harness, a device used to correct hip dislocations in infants with developmental dysplasia of the hip, consisting of a set of straps that holds the hips in flexion and abduction.

Pavlov, Ivan Petrovich /pav″lôv, pä″vlôf/ [1849–1936], a Russian physiologist who discovered a pattern of conditioned stimulus-reflex learning, the manner in which the physiological mechanism of digestion is controlled by the nervous system, and a theory of the causes and treatment of human neuroses.

pavor /pā″vôr/ [L, quaking], a reaction to a frightening stimulus, characterized by excessive terror.

pavor diurnus /dī·ur″nəs/, a sleep disorder occurring in children during daytime sleep in which they cry out in alarm and awaken in fear and panic. See also **sleep terror disorder.**

pavor nocturnus /noktur″nəs/, a sleep disorder occurring in children during nighttime sleep in which they cry out in alarm and awaken in fear and panic. See also **nightmare, sleep terror disorder.**

Pavulon, a neuromuscular blocking agent. Brand name for **pancuronium bromide.**

PAWP, abbreviation for **pulmonary artery wedge pressure.** See **pulmonary wedge pressure.**

Paxil, a selective serotonin reuptake inhibitor. Brand name for **paroxetine.**

Payr's clamp /pī″ərz/ [Erwin Payr, German surgeon, 1871–1946; AS, *clam,* fastener], a heavy clamp used in GI surgery.

Pb, symbol for the element **lead.**

PBL, abbreviation for *peripheral blood lymphocytes.*

PC, **1.** abbreviation for **professional corporation. 2.** abbreviation for **personal computer. 3.** a notation for a Latin phrase meaning "after meals." Abbreviation for *post cibum.*

PCB, abbreviation for **polychlorinated biphenyls.**

pcc, abbreviation for *precipitated calcium carbonate.*

PCC, abbreviation for **prothrombin complex concentrate.**

PCCM, abbreviation for **primary care case management.**

PCH, abbreviation for **paroxysmal cold hemoglobinuria.**

PCI, abbreviation for **percutaneous coronary intervention.**

PCIS, an online computer system that contains full medical care data on all the residents or the patients at the point of care. Abbreviation for *Patient Care Information System.*

PCLN, abbreviation for **psychiatric consultation liaison nurse.**

PCOS, abbreviation for **polycystic ovary syndrome.**

P.C.P., abbreviation for **primary care physician.**

PCP, **1.** abbreviation for **phencyclidine hydrochloride. 2.** abbreviation for *Pneumocystis* **pneumonia.**

PCR, **1.** abbreviation for **polymerase chain reaction. 2.** abbreviation for **protein catabolic rate.**

PCT, abbreviation for **porphyria cutanea tarda.**

PCWP, abbreviation for **pulmonary capillary wedge pressure.** See **pulmonary wedge pressure.**

PD, abbreviation for **peritoneal dialysis.**

Pd, symbol for the element **palladium.**

PD, P.D., **1.** abbreviation for **patient day. 2.** abbreviation for *pupil diameter.* **3.** abbreviation for **pupillary distance. 4.** abbreviation for **pulse duration.**

PDA, **1.** abbreviation for **patent ductus arteriosus. 2.** abbreviation for **personal digital assistant.**

PDL, abbreviation for **periodontal ligament.**

PDR, initialism for *Physicians' Desk Reference.*

PE, abbreviation for **pulmonary embolism.**

PEA, abbreviation for **pulseless electrical activity.**

Peaceful End of Life Theory. See **Ruland, Cornelia M., Moore, Shirley M.**

peak [ME, *pec*], the amount of medication in the blood that represents the highest level during a drug administration cycle.

peak acid output (PAO), on the pentagastrin test, after administration of pentagastrin, the sum of the two highest 15-minute outputs of gastric acid multiplied by 2; expressed as millimoles per hour.

peak and trough specimens, serum samples collected to determine the level of an antibiotic or other pharmaceutic agent in the blood. Peak specimens, which represent the highest level, are generally collected ½ hour after the dose is given intravenously or 1 hour after it is given intramuscularly. Trough specimens, representing the lowest level, are generally collected approximately ½ hour before the next dose. See also **peak method of dosing.**

peak compressional pressure, (in ultrasonics) the temporal maximum positive pressure in a medium during the passage of a pulsed sound wave. It is expressed in pascals or megapascals.

peak concentration, the maximum amount of a substance or force, such as the highest concentration of a drug measured after it is administered.

peak expiratory flow, the greatest rate of airflow that can be achieved during forced expiration, beginning with the lungs fully inflated. Also called *peak expiratory flow rate.*

peak flow meter, an instrument for measuring the flow of air in the early part of forced expiration.

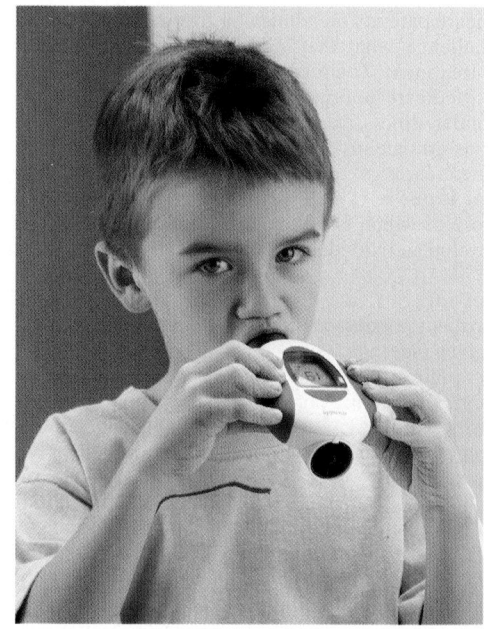

Child using peak flow meter *(Courtesy HealthScan Products, Inc.)*

peak height velocity, a point in pubescence in which the tempo of growth is the greatest.

peak level, the highest concentration, usually in the blood, that a substance reaches during the period under consideration, after which it declines, such as the highest blood glucose level attained during a glucose tolerance test.

peak method of dosing, the administration of a drug dosage so that a specified maximum level is reached to produce a desired effect, such as lowering the blood pressure.

peak mucus sign, a lubricative, cloudy-to-clear, white cervical mucus that occurs during periods of high estrogen levels, particularly at the time of ovulation. See also **spinnbarkeit.**

peak refractional pressure, (in ultrasonics) the temporal maximum negative pressure in a medium occurring during the passage of a pulsed ultrasound wave. It is expressed in pascals or megapascals.

Pean clamp, a curved or straight hemostatic clamp with serrations along the entire length of the jaw.

pearly penile papules. See **hirsutoid papilloma of the penis.**

pearly tumor. See **cholesteatoma.**

pear-shaped bladder, a urinary bladder with widening of the inferior section, seen in conditions such as pelvic lipomatosis, perivesical hematoma or urinoma, and lymphoma or lymphocyst.

Pearson's product movement correlation [Karl Pearson, English mathematician, 1857–1936], (in statistics) a statistical test of the relationship between two variables measured in interval or ratio scales. Correlations computed fall between +1.00 and −1.00. The closer to 1 (positive or negative), the higher the correlation.

peau d'orange /pō″dôräNzh″/ [Fr, skin of orange], a dimpling of the skin that gives it the appearance of the skin of an orange. It is common in advanced breast cancer.

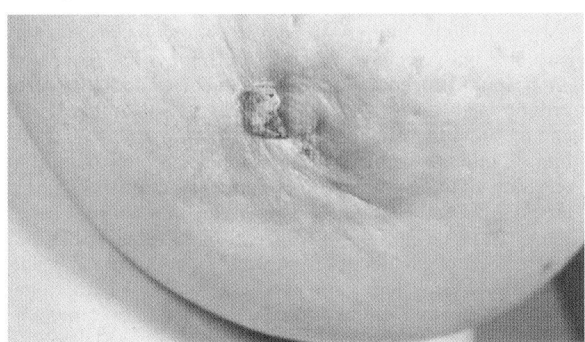

Peau d'orange *(Skarin, 2010)*

pecilo-. See **poikilo-, pecilo-, poecil-.**

Pecquet's cistern. See **chyle cistern.**

pecten /pek″tən/, **1.** a ridge extending laterally from the pubic tubercle to which the pectineal part of the inguinal ligament is attached. **2.** a vascular pleated membrane that extends from the optic disc to the vitreous humor in some animals.

pectenitis /pek″tənī″tis/, an inflammation of the anal canal, causing interference with the anal sphincter muscle.

pecten pubis. See **pectineal line.**

pectin /pek″tin/ [Gk, *pektos,* congealed], a gelatinous carbohydrate substance found in fruits and succulent vegetables and used as the setting agent for jams and jellies and as an emulsifier and stabilizer in many foods. It also adds to the diet bulk necessary for proper GI functioning. See also **dietary fiber.**

pectinate muscles, the ridges that cover the walls of the atrium proper and the right auricle. Also called **musculi pectinati.**

pectineal ligament, the fibers that extend from the lacunar ligament along the pectineal line of the pelvic brim. Also called **Cooper's ligament.**

pectineal line, a ridge on the superior ramus of the pubic bone. Also called **pecten pubis.**

pectineus /pektin″ē·əs/ [L, *pecten,* comb], the most anterior of the five medial femoral muscles. It functions to flex and adduct the thigh and to rotate it medially. Compare **adductor brevis, adductor longus, adductor magnus, gracilis.**

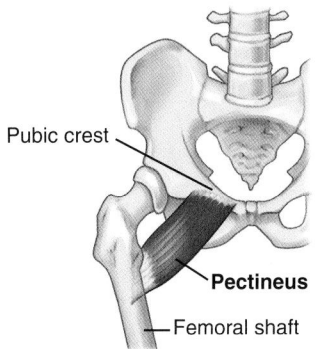

Pectineus muscle

pector-, prefix meaning "breast": *pectoralgia, pectoriloquy.*

pectoral /pek″tərəl/ [L, *pectus,* breast], pertaining to the thorax or chest.

pectoralgia /pek″tôral″jə/, a pain in the thorax.

pectoralis major /pek″tərā″lis, pek″tərəlis′/ [L, *pectus,* breast], a large muscle of the upper chest wall that acts on the joint of the shoulder. Thick and fan-shaped, it arises from the clavicle, the sternum, the cartilages of the second to the sixth ribs, and the aponeurosis of the obliquus externus abdominis. It serves to flex, adduct, and medially rotate the arm in the shoulder joint.

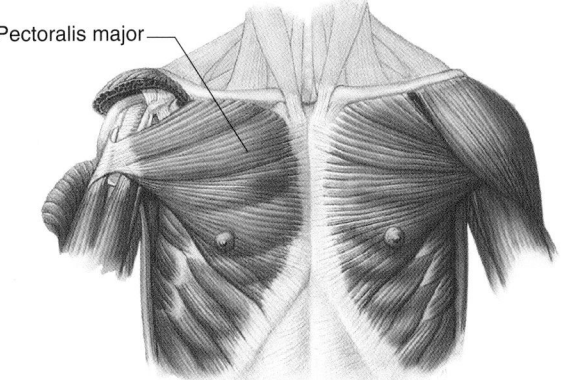

Pectoralis major *(Patton and Thibodeau, 2016)*

pectoralis minor, a thin triangular muscle of the upper chest wall beneath the pectoralis major. The base arises from the third, fourth, and fifth ribs on their upper outer surfaces. It inserts as a flat tendon into the coracoid process of the scapula. It functions to rotate the scapula, to draw it down and forward, and to raise the third, the fourth, and fifth ribs in forced inspiration. Compare **pectoralis major, subclavius.**

pectoriloquy /pek″təril″əkwē/, a phenomenon in which voice sounds, including whispers, are transmitted clearly through the pulmonary structures and are clearly audible through a stethoscope. It is often a sign of lung consolidation.

P

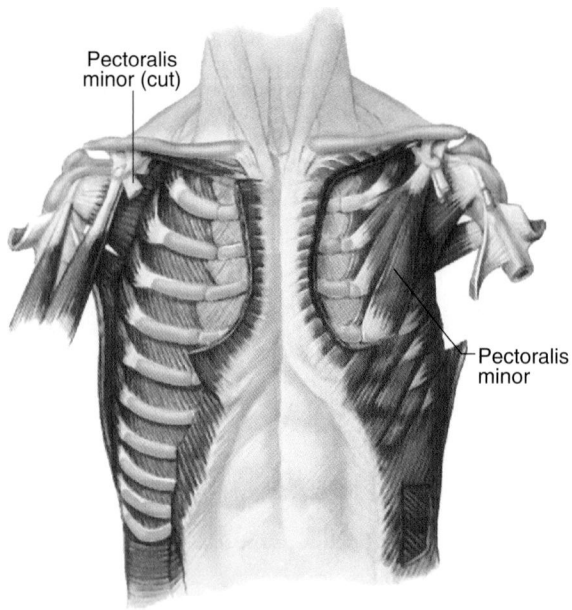

Pectoralis minor *(Patton and Thibodeau, 2016)*

pectus carinatum. See **pigeon breast.**

pectus excavatum. See **funnel chest.**

ped-. See **pedia-, ped-, pedo-.**

pedagogy /ped″əgōj′ē/ [Gk, *pais,* child, *agogos,* leader], the art and science of teaching children based on a belief that the purpose of education is the transmittal of knowledge.

pedal /ped″əl/ [L, *pes,* foot], pertaining to the foot.

-pedal. See **-pedic, -pedal.**

-pede. See **-ped, -pede.**

pederosis. See **pedophilia.**

pedes. See **pes.**

-pedia, -paedia, -peia, suffix meaning "to educate" or "a compendium of knowledge": *pharmacopeia.*

Pediaflor, a dental preparation used in prophylaxis against dental caries in children. Brand name for *sodium fluoride.*

Pedialyte, a balanced solution containing various electrolytes.

pedia-, ped-, pedo-, prefix meaning "child": *pediatrician, pedodontics, pedophilia.*

pediatric /pē′dē·at″rik/ [Gk, *pais,* child, *iatreia,* treatment], pertaining to preventive and primary health care and treatment of children and the study of childhood diseases.

pediatric advanced life support (PALS), a system of critical care procedures and facilities, such as the intensive care nursery, for the basic and advanced treatment of seriously ill or injured infants and children. It includes the neonatal resuscitation program as recommended by the American Academy of Pediatrics and the American Heart Association.

pediatric anesthesia [Gk, *pais,* child, *iatreia,* treatment], a subspecialty of anesthesiology dealing with the anesthesia of neonates, infants, special needs patients, and children.

pediatric dentistry, one of the 10 recognized specialties of dentistry. Pediatric dentistry is devoted to the diagnosis and treatment of dental problems affecting children. Also called **pedodontics.**

pediatric dosage, the determination of the correct amount, frequency, and total number of doses of a medication to be administered to a child or infant. Such variables as the age, weight, body surface area, and ability of the child to absorb, metabolize, and excrete the medication must be considered, as well as the expected action of the drug, possible side effects, and potential toxicity. Various formulas have been devised to calculate pediatric dosage from a standard adult dose, although the most reliable method is to use one of the formulas to calculate the proportional amount of body surface area to body weight. See also **Clarks rule.**

pediatric hospitalization, the confinement of a child or infant in a hospital for diagnostic testing or therapeutic treatment. Regardless of age or the degree of illness or injury, hospitalization constitutes a major crisis in the life of a child, and the emotional trauma may elicit various behavioral reactions that the nurse must recognize and be prepared to cope with to facilitate recovery. The dominant factors influencing stress, which vary according to the child's developmental age, his or her previous experience with illness, and the seriousness of the condition, include separation from the parents and familiar environment, disruption of routine patterns of daily life, loss of independence, and worry about bodily injury or painful experiences. The nurse can minimize stress by preparing the child and family through prehospital counseling; by encouraging active parental participation in the child's care through rooming-in facilities or frequent visits; by maintaining as normal a daily routine as possible, especially with eating, sleeping, hygiene, and play activities; by explaining all hospital procedures and the immediate and long-term prognosis in terms that the child can easily understand; and by providing support and guidance for parents and siblings. Child life specialists can also be extremely helpful in teaching coping strategies to children and families during a hospitalization. The nurse also may use the hospital experience to foster an improved parent-child relationship and to teach other members of the family about proper health care. Emergency admission greatly increases the emotional trauma of hospitalization, making the nurse's role in counteracting negative reactions even more significant.

pediatrician /pē′dē·ətrish″ən/ [Gk, *pais,* child, *iatreia,* treatment], a physician who specializes in the development and care of infants and children and in the treatment of their diseases. Also called **pediatrist.** Also spelled **paediatrician.**

pediatric nurse practitioner (PNP), a nurse practitioner who, by advanced study and clinical practice, such as in a master's degree program or certificate program in pediatric nursing, has gained advanced knowledge in the nursing care of infants and children. See also **pediatric nursing.**

pediatric nursing, the branch of nursing concerned with the care of infants and children. Pediatric nursing requires knowledge of normal psychomotor, psychosocial, and cognitive growth and development, as well as of the health problems and needs of people in this age group. Preventive care and anticipatory guidance are integral to the practice of pediatric nursing. See also **pediatric nurse practitioner.**

pediatric nutrition, the maintenance of a proper wellbalanced diet consisting of the essential nutrients and the adequate caloric intake necessary to promote growth and sustain the physiological requirements at the various stages of a child's development. Nutritional needs vary considerably with age, level of activity, and environmental conditions, and they are directly related to the rate of growth. In the prenatal period growth totally depends on adequate maternal nutrition. During infancy the need for calories, especially in the form of protein, is greater than at any postnatal period because of the rapid increase in both height and weight. From toddlerhood through the preschool and middle childhood years, growth is uneven and occurs in spurts, with a resulting fluctuation in appetite and calorie consumption. In general, the average child expends 55% of energy on metabolic maintenance, 25% on activity, 12% on growth, and 8% on excretion. The accelerated growth phase during adolescence has greater nutritional requirements, although food habits are often influenced by emotional factors, peer pressure, and fad diets. Inadequate nutrition, especially during critical periods of growth, results in delayed development or illness, such as anemia from deficiency of iron or scurvy from deficiency of vitamin C. The role of the nurse is to educate and give nutritional guidance for good eating habits. A special problem is overfeeding in the early childhood years, which may lead to obesity or hypervitaminosis. See also **recommended dietary allowances,** *specific vitamins.*

pediatrics /pē′dē·at″triks/, a branch of medicine concerned with the development and care of infants and children. Its specialties are the particular diseases of children and their treatment and prevention. Also called **peds.** Also spelled **paediatrics. –pediatric,** *adj.*

pediatric surgery, the special preparation and care of the child undergoing surgical procedures for injuries, deformities, or disease. In addition to the usual fears and emotional trauma of illness and hospitalization, the child is especially concerned about being anesthetized. Younger children worry more about what will happen to them and how they will feel after awakening from anesthesia, whereas older children fear the operation itself and possible death, the loss of control while under anesthesia, and any change in body image or mutilation of parts. The role of the nurse is to prepare the child psychologically and physically for the particular surgical procedure and any postoperative reactions; to offer support to the parents and involve them as much as possible in the care, both before and after surgery; and to explain immediate and long-term prognoses. See also **pediatric hospitalization.**

pediatrist. See **pediatrician.**

-pedic, -pedal, suffix meaning "feet": *bipedal, carpopedal.*

pedicle [L, *pediculus,* little foot], a narrow stalk, stem, or tube of tissue attached to a tumor, skin flap, bone, or organ.

pedicle clamp /ped″ikəl/ [L, *pediculus,* little foot; ME, *clam,* fastener], a locking surgical forceps used for compressing blood vessels or pedicles of tumors during surgery. Also called **clamp forceps.**

pedicle flap operation, a surgical procedure for grafting gingival tissue from a donor site to the site of an isolated defect, usually a tooth surface denuded of attached gingiva.

pedicle of vertebral arch, one of the paired parts of the vertebral arch that connect a lamina to the vertebral body.

pediculicide /pədik″yo͞olisīd′/ [L, *pediculus,* little foot, *caedere,* to kill], any of a group of drugs that kill lice.

pediculosis /pədik′yo͞olō″sis/ [L, *pediculus* + *osis,* condition], an infestation with blood-sucking lice. *Pediculosis capitis* is infestation of the scalp with lice. *Pediculosis corporis* is infestation of the skin of the body with lice. *Pediculosis palpebrarum* is infestation of the eyelids and eyelashes with lice. *Pthirus pubis* (formerly called *pediculosis pubis*) is infestation of the pubic hair region with lice. An over-the-counter treatment is pyrethrin or permethrin containing topical agents. Malathion and lindane are other treatments, although misuse can result in neurotoxicity. See also **crab louse, lice.**

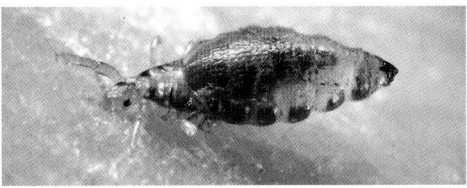

Blood sucking louse in pediculosis *(CDC/ Frank Collins, Ph.D.)*

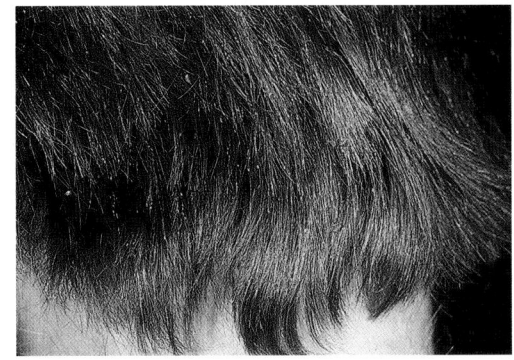

Pediculosis capitis (Courtesy Dr. Robert Zax)

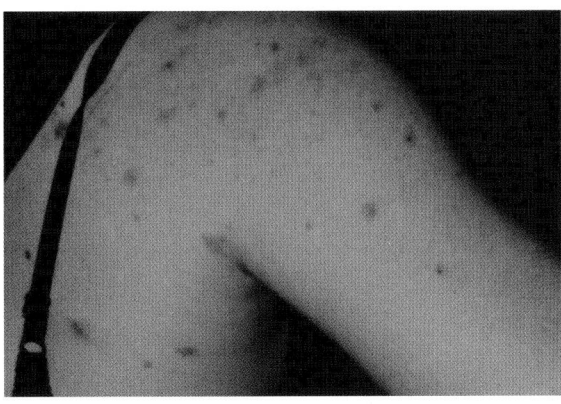

Pediculosis corporis (Lemmi and Lemmi, 2000)

pediculous /pədik″yələs/ [L, *pediculus*], infested with sucking lice.

Pediculus humanus capitis, a species of head lice.

Pediculus humanus corporis, a species of body lice.

pedicure /ped″ikyo͞or/, care of the feet, especially trimming of the toenails.

pedigree /ped″əgrē/ [Fr, *pied de grue,* crane's foot pattern], **1.** line of descent; lineage; ancestry. **2.** a chart that shows the genetic makeup of a person's ancestors, used in the mendelian analysis of an inherited characteristic or disease in a particular family. It typically uses squares to represent males and circles to represent females. The figures may be unshaded, shaded, or partially shaded to designate normal individuals, those affected by the disease or trait, and those who are carriers. The generations are numbered with roman numerals at the left, with the most recent at the bottom, and members within each generation are designated by arabic numerals from left to right according to age, with the oldest at the left. The inquiry begins with the siblings of the affected

P

person and proceeds to the parents and grandparents and any of their immediate relatives. See also **Punnett square.**

pedo-. See **pedia-, ped-, pedo-.**

pedodontics. See **pediatric dentistry.**

pedogenesis /pē′dōjen′əsis/ [Gk, *pais,* child, *genesis,* origin], *adj.,* the production of offspring by young or larval forms of animals, often by parthenogenesis, as in certain amphibians. Also spelled **paedogenesis.** –*pedogenetic, adj.*

pedophilia /ped′əfil′ē·ə/ [Gk, *pais,* child, *philein,* to love], **1.** an abnormal interest in children. **2.** (in psychiatry) a psychosexual disorder in which the fantasy or act of engaging in sexual activity with prepubertal children is the preferred or exclusive means of achieving sexual excitement and gratification. It may be heterosexual or homosexual. Also called **pederosis.** Also spelled **paedophilia.** See also **paraphilia.** –*pedophilic, adj.*

-ped, -pede, suffix meaning "foot" or "feet": *biped, dorsalis pedis.*

peds. See **pediatrics.**

peduncle /pədung″kəl/ [L, *pes,* foot], a stemlike connecting part, such as the pineal peduncle or a peduncle graft. –*pedunculate, peduncular, adj.*

pedunculated /pədung″kyəlā′tid/ [L, foot], pertaining to a structure with a stalk or peduncle.

pedunculotomy /pədung″kyəlot″əmē/, a surgical incision in a cerebral peduncle.

pedunculus /pədung″kyələs/ [L, *pes,* foot], a stalk, stem, or stalklike anatomical structure.

peeling, the loss of all or part of the epidermis, as may occur after a sunburn or exposure to a chemical.

PEEP, abbreviation for **positive end-expiratory pressure.**

peeping testis, an undescended testis in the peritoneal cavity that moves slightly across the internal inguinal ring.

Peeping Tom. See **voyeur.**

peer [L, *par,* equal], a person deemed an equal for the purpose at hand. A peer is usually a colleague or associate of roughly the same age or level of mental endowment.

peer review, an appraisal by professional coworkers of equal status of the way an individual health professional conducts practice, education, or research. The appraisal uses accepted standards as measures against which performance is weighed. See also **Professional Standards Review Organization.**

Peganone, an anticonvulsant drug. Brand name for **ethotoin.**

pegaptanib, a miscellaneous ophthalmic agent that binds to vascular endothelial growth factor, thereby inhibiting angiogenesis.

■ INDICATIONS: This drug is used in the treatment of neovascular age-related macular degeneration. It may be used alone or with photodynamic therapy.

■ CONTRAINDICATIONS: Ocular or periocular infections and known hypersensitivity to this drug prohibit its use.

■ ADVERSE EFFECTS: Adverse effects of this drug include retinal detachment and traumatic cataract. Common side effects include anterior chamber inflammation, blurred vision, conjunctival hemorrhage, corneal edema, cataract, eye discharge, eye pain, increased intraocular pressure, punctuate keratitis, reduced visual acuity, vitreous floaters, vitreous opacities, blepharitis, conjunctivitis, and photophobia.

pegaspargase, a modified version of the enzyme L-asparaginase used in cancer chemotherapy.

■ INDICATIONS: It is prescribed in the treatment of acute lymphoblastic leukemia, during a blast crisis of chronic lymphocytic leukemia, and during salvage therapy in non-Hodgkin lymphoma. It may also be effective in those who are hypersensitive to other forms of the enzyme.

■ CONTRAINDICATIONS: It should not be given to patients with pancreatitis, those who have had significant hemorrhagic events associated with prior use of the enzyme, or those who have experienced serious allergic reactions to the product.

■ ADVERSE EFFECTS: The side effects most often reported include chills, fever, nausea and vomiting, edema, pain, chemical hepatotoxicities, and coagulopathies.

pegfilgrastim /peg-fil-gras′tim/, a long-acting colony-stimulating factor produced by recombinant technology and used as an adjunct in patients with bone marrow suppression caused by antineoplastic therapy.

peginterferon alfa-2a, a covalent conjugate of recombinant interferon alfa-2a and polyethylene glycol, used in the treatment of chronic infection by hepatitis C virus. It is administered subcutaneously.

peginterferon alfa-2b, a covalent conjugate of recombinant interferon alfa-2b and polyethylene glycol, used in the treatment of chronic infection by hepatitis C virus. It is administered subcutaneously.

PEL, abbreviation for **permissible exposure limit.**

Pel-Ebstein fever /pel″ eb″stēn/ [Pieter K. Pel, Dutch physician, 1852–1919; Wilhelm Ebstein, German physician, 1836–1912], a fever recurring in cycles of several days or weeks, characteristic of Hodgkin disease or other malignant lymphomas. Also called **Murchison fever.**

Pelger-Huët anomaly /pel″gər hyoo″ət/ [Karel Pelger, Dutch physician, 1885–1931; G.J. Huët, Dutch physician, 1879–1970; Gk, *anomalia,* irregular], an inherited disorder characterized by granulocytes with unusually coarse nuclear material and dumbbell-shaped or peanut-shaped nuclei. Normal nuclear segmentation does not occur, but there are no clinical consequences.

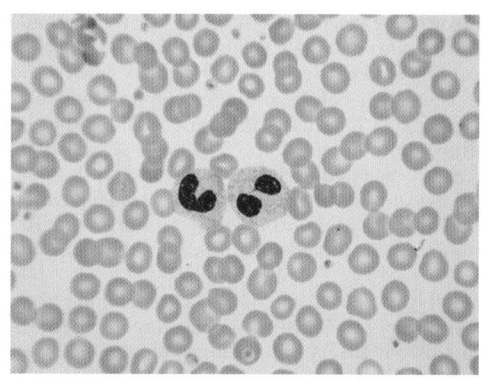

Pelger-Huët anomaly *(Goldman et al, 2016)*

pelidnoma /pel′idnō″mə/, a circumscribed elevated dark patch on the skin. Also called *pelioma.*

peliosis hepatitis /pel′ē·ō″sis/, the presence of blood-filled cavities in the liver. The cavities may become lined by endothelium and may be found in patients who are infected with human immunodeficiency virus or who use oral contraceptives or anabolic steroids.

Pelizaeus-Merzbacher disease /pā′lētsā′oos·merts′bäkər/ [Friedrich Pelizaeus, German physician, 1850–1917; Ludwig Merzbacher, German physician, 1875–1942], an X-linked leukoencephalopathy occurring in early life and running a slowly progressive course into adolescence or adulthood. It is marked by nystagmus, ataxia, tremor, choreoathetoid movements, parkinsonian facies, dysarthria, and mental deterioration. Pathologically, there is diffuse demyelination in the white substance of the brain that may involve

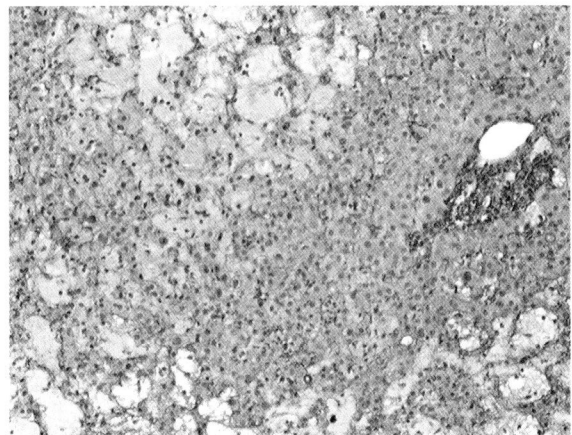

Peliosis hepatitis with lobular blood cysts
(Feldman et al, 2016)

the brainstem, cerebellum, and spinal cord. There is no cure. Treatment is symptomatic and supportive. Also called **familial centrolobar sclerosis, Merzbacher-Pelizaeus disease,** *Pelizaeus-Merzbacher sclerosis.*

pell-, prefix meaning "skin": *pellagra, pellicle.*

pellagra /pəlā″grə, pəlag″rə/ [It, *pelle,* skin, *agra,* rough], a disease resulting from a deficiency of niacin or tryptophan or a metabolic defect that interferes with the conversion of the precursor tryptophan to niacin. It once was commonly seen in individuals whose diet consisted primarily of corn, which is low in tryptophan. Compare **kwashiorkor.** Kinds include **pellagra sine pellagra, typhoid pellagra.** **–pellagrous,** *adj.*

■ OBSERVATIONS: It is characterized by scaly dermatitis, especially of the skin exposed to the sun; glossitis; inflammation of the mucous membranes; diarrhea; and mental disturbances, including depression, confusion, disorientation, hallucination, and delirium.

■ INTERVENTIONS: Treatment and prophylaxis consist of the administration of niacin and tryptophan, usually in conjunction with other vitamins, particularly thiamine and riboflavin, and a well-balanced diet containing foods rich in these nutrients, such as liver, eggs, milk, and meat.

■ PATIENT CARE CONSIDERATIONS: Patients usually do well following the correction of niacin levels.

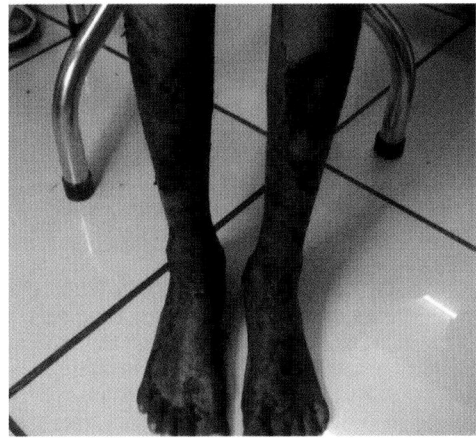

Pellagra lesions on legs *(Naveen et al, 2013)*

pellagra sine pellagra /sī″nē, sē″nə/, a form of pellagra in which the characteristic dermatitis is not present. See **pellagra.**

pellagrous. See **pellagra.**

Pellegrini disease /pel′əgrē″nēz/ [Augusto Pellegrini, Italian surgeon, b. 1877], ossification of the upper part of the medial collateral ligament, sometimes accompanied by bony growth at the internal condyle of the femur. The condition usually follows a leg injury. Also called *Pelligrini-Stieda disease.*

pellet /pel″it/, a pilule or very small pill.

pellicle /pel″ikəl/, 1. a thin film or skin. 2. a scum or crust on a solution.

pelo-, prefix meaning "mud": *pelotherapy.*

pelotherapy /pē′lōther″əpē/, the treatment of certain conditions with baths or packs of mud, peat, or earth on part or all of the body surface.

pelves. See **pelvis.**

pelvi-, prefix meaning "pelvis": *pelvimetry, pelvisacral.*

pelvic abscess [L, *pelvis,* basin, *abscedere,* to go away], a pus-producing lesion in the pelvic peritoneum, usually originating in the rectouterine pouch.

pelvic axis, an imaginary curved line that passes through the centers of the various anteroposterior diameters of the pelvis.

pelvic bones [L, *pelvis,* basin; AS, *ban*], a combination of the ilium, ischium, and pubis. Compare **innominate bone.**

pelvic brim, the curved top of the bones of the hip extending from the anterosuperior iliac crest in front on one side around and past the sacrum to the crest on the other side. Below the brim is the pelvis.

pelvic cellulitis, bacterial infection of the parametrium, occurring after childbirth or spontaneous or therapeutic abortion. It represents an extension of infection via the blood vessels and lymphatics from a primary wound infection in the external genitalia, perineum, vagina, cervix, or uterus. It is characterized by fever, uterine subinvolution, chills and sweats, abdominal pain that spreads laterally, and, if untreated, the formation of a large abscess and signs of peritonitis. It occurs most commonly between the third and the ninth days after delivery or abortion. Treatment includes an antibiotic, bed rest, IV fluids, and drainage of any abscess that forms. Oxytocics may be given to augment involution.

pelvic classification, 1. a process in which the anatomical and spatial relationships of the bones of the pelvis are evaluated, usually to assess the adequacy of the pelvic structures for vaginal delivery. Caldwell-Moloy's system of classification is the one most commonly used. 2. one of the types in a classification system of the pelvis. See also **Caldwell-Moloy pelvic classification.**

pelvic congestion syndrome, an abnormal gynecological condition characterized by chronic low back pain, dysuria, dysmenorrhea, vague lower abdominal pain, vaginal discharge, and dyspareunia. The cause of the symptoms is not understood; formerly it was thought that the vascular bed of the area was distended with blood, but this has not been demonstrated. Women between 25 and 45 years of age are most often affected.

pelvic diameter [L, *pelvis,* basin; Gk, *diametros,* measuring across], 1. at the rim of the pelvis, a line from the lumbosacral angle to the symphysis pubis. 2. at the pelvic outlet, a line from the tip of the coccyx to the lower border of the symphysis pubis.

pelvic diaphragm, the inferior aspect of the body wall, stretched like a hammock across the pelvic cavity and comprising the levator ani and the coccygeus muscles. It holds the abdominal contents, supports the pelvic viscera, and is pierced by the anal canal, the urethra, and the vagina. It

P

is reinforced by fasciae and muscles associated with these structures and with the perineum.

pelvic examination, a diagnostic procedure in which the external and internal genitalia are physically examined by inspection, palpation, percussion, and auscultation. It should be performed regularly throughout a woman's life. See also **female reproductive system assessment.**

■ METHOD: The woman empties her bladder, disrobes, and puts on an examining gown. Breast examination is often carried out before the pelvic examination. The woman is made as comfortable as possible in the dorsal lithotomy position, her feet in stirrups and her buttocks at the very edge of the foot of the examining table, and is then draped. Particular attention is paid to the suprapubic area to detect any masses extending from the pelvis above the symphysis and to the groin to detect inguinal lymphadenopathy or hernia. If a mass is felt, percussion may be performed to delineate it. If pregnancy is suspected, palpation and percussion of the uterus and auscultation of fetal heart tones are attempted. The examiner then moves to the stool at the foot of the table between the patient's legs. The labia majora are spread apart to permit inspection of the clitoris, the urethral meatus, the labia minora, and the vaginal vestibule. Any swelling, discoloration, lesion, scar, cyst, discharge, or bleeding is noted. Skene's and Bartholin glands and ducts are palpated and milked, and any secretions expressed are evaluated and a specimen is spread on culture medium. The urethra is assessed for color and shape. The tone of the perineal and paravaginal musculature is assessed. Cystocele, rectocele, or varying degrees of uterine descensus may be observed as the woman is asked to bear down. The speculum is warmed, lubricated with warm water, and introduced gradually. The examiner is careful to direct the speculum along the axis of the vagina, which is at an angle of approximately 45 degrees to the axis of the table if the woman is lying flat. The speculum may need to be moved lightly from side to side to slip it over the vaginal rugae. The woman is advised that she may feel a stretching sensation. The speculum is gently opened and its position is adjusted to hold the vaginal folds out of the way to reveal the cervix. The color and condition of the vaginal epithelium are observed, and the position, size, and quality of the superficial epithelium are evaluated. Specimens for bacteriological study are obtained before the Papanicolaou (Pap) test. For the Pap test, scrapings of the endocervix and the cervix and a sample of the vaginal secretions may be secured on a Pap stick and an applicator and lightly spread on labeled glass slides. The slides are immediately sprayed or dipped into a fixative. Another method is a liquid-based Pap test, in which the endocervical and cervical secretions are sampled with a collection device and then deposited into a solution. The slide is made at the laboratory. This liquid may also be tested for human papillomavirus, which is known to be a causative factor for cervical cancer. The speculum is then closed, rotated slightly, removed from the vagina, and, if not disposable, rinsed or placed directly into a germicidal solution. In the bimanual part of the examination, two gloved fingers are well lubricated and inserted slowly and gently into the vagina. The examiner uses the opposite hand to apply pressure to the lower abdomen in several positions and directions to move the uterus, tubes, and ovaries into positions in which they may be felt. The size, shape, position, mobility, and consistency of the organs and tissues are evaluated, and any tenderness or discomfort is noted. Rectal or rectovaginal examination is then performed. Before the insertion of a finger in the anus, lateral pressure is applied to the sphincter, and the woman is urged to bear down lightly to relax the muscle and minimize discomfort.

■ INTERVENTIONS: Minor thoughtlessness or inadvertent movement may cause tension and make the examination more difficult for the woman and for the examiner. Instruments, culture materials, a light, drapes, and a gown are all made ready beforehand. The table, instruments, and drapes are clean and warm. Materials from previous examinations are not in evidence. The woman is forewarned of what to expect at each step of the examination. Gentleness and quietness are exercised at all times. On completion of the examination the woman is helped to slide well back on the table before sitting up. Syncope after pelvic examination is uncommon but not rare; there is risk of injury should the patient faint and fall from the examining table. The woman is observed briefly after sitting up before being left alone. She is then given tissues, a sanitary napkin or tampon, and a private area in which to dress.

■ OUTCOME CRITERIA: Pelvic examination may demonstrate many pelvic abnormalities and diseases. Cytological and bacteriological specimens are conveniently obtained. A pelvic examination cannot be satisfactorily performed without the cooperation of the woman being examined. Inadequate relaxation, obesity, extensive scarring, pelvic tenderness, and heavy vaginal discharge also may preclude an adequate examination.

pelvic exenteration /eksen′tərā″shən/, the surgical removal of all reproductive organs and their lymph nodes and en bloc removal of the rectum, distal sigmoid colon, urinary bladder, distal ureters, internal iliac vessels, entire pelvic floor with accompanying pelvic peritoneum, levator muscles, and perineum. Pelvic exenteration is the preferred treatment for recurrent or persistent carcinoma of the cervix after radiation therapy.

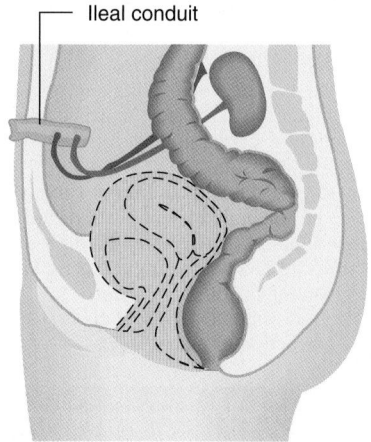

Ileal conduit

Anterior pelvic exenteration *(Black and Hawks, 2009)*

pelvic floor, the soft tissues enclosing the pelvic outlet.

pelvic floor electrical stimulation (PFES), functional electrical stimulation of the muscles of the pelvic floor, delivered through a vaginal or rectal probe, used in the treatment of stress incontinence.

pelvic girdle [L, *pelvis,* basin; AS, *gyrdel*], a bony ring formed by the hip bones, the sacrum, and the coccyx.

pelvic hematoma, an accumulation of blood in the soft tissues of the pelvis, as may occur during childbirth.

pelvic inferior aperture. See **pelvic outlet.**

pelvic inflammatory disease (PID), any inflammatory condition of the female pelvic organs, especially one caused by bacterial infection. Characteristics of the condition include fever; foul-smelling vaginal discharge; pain in the lower abdomen; abnormal uterine bleeding; pain with coitus; and tenderness or pain in the uterus, affected ovary, or fallopian tube on bimanual pelvic examination. If an abscess has already developed, a soft, tender fluid-filled mass may be palpated. Bed rest and antibiotics are usually prescribed, but surgical drainage of an abscess may be required. Severe, fulminating PID may necessitate hysterectomy to prevent fatal septicemia. If the cause is infection by gonococci or chlamydiae, the woman's sexual partners are also treated with antibiotics. Severe PID is usually very painful. The woman may be prostrate and require narcotic analgesia. Recurrent or severe PID often results in scarring of the fallopian tubes, obstruction, and infertility.

■ OBSERVATIONS: PID may be either acute or chronic. Acute onset typically occurs after onset of menses. Symptoms typically include progressive lower abdominal pain with guarding and rebound tenderness, fever, copious purulent cervical discharge, nausea and vomiting, malaise, urinary urgency and frequency, vaginal itching, and maceration. Chronic PID is manifested as chronic pain, menstrual irregularities, and recurrence and exacerbation of acute symptoms. Diagnosis is made through a clinical exam that reveals typical symptomatology coupled with elevated WBCs and erythrocyte sedimentation rate plus a positive culture of secretions. On pelvic examination, moving of the cervix causes severe pain and rebound tenderness that is present in the abdomen. Transvaginal ultrasound may show thickened fluid-filled fallopian tubes or adnexal mass. MRI and laparoscopy may be used to detect pelvic abnormalities. Common complications include general peritonitis, sterility, and ectopic pregnancy.

■ INTERVENTIONS: Acute treatment is aimed at control and alleviation of infection with combinations of antiinfective drugs. Laparoscopy may be used to drain antibiotic-resistant abscesses, salpingolysis to remove adhesions, salpingostomy to reopen blocked fallopian tubes, and salpingo-oophorectomy for ruptured fallopian tubes or ectopic pregnancy. In vitro fertilization may be used in women with PID-induced sterility who wish to have children.

■ PATIENT CARE CONSIDERATIONS: Nursing plays a key role in prevention, early recognition, and prompt treatment. Education is aimed at reducing factors that place women at increased risk, such as unprotected sex, multiple sex partners, exposure to urethritis, or STDs, and frequent vaginal douching; recognizing conditions that make one more susceptible to PID, such as IUD insertion, recent abortion, or pelvic surgery, and improper use of antibiotics; and seeking treatment for any signs of vaginal infection, such as any evidence of abnormal vaginal odor or discharge. Acute care is supportive and aimed at adequate rest in a semi-Fowler's position and adequate hydration. IUDs require removal during treatment. Instruction is given about the proper use of antibiotics. Education stresses sexual abstinence and avoidance of tampons and douching during treatment. Sexual partners need to be tracked and treated if PID was associated with an STD.

pelvic inlet, (in obstetrics) the inlet to the true pelvis, bounded by the sacral promontory, the horizontal rami of the pubic bones, and the top of the symphysis pubis. Because the infant must pass through the inlet to enter the true pelvis and to be born vaginally, the anteroposterior, transverse, and oblique dimensions of the inlet are important measurements to be made in assessing the pelvis in pregnancy. There are three anteroposterior diameters: the true conjugate, the obstetric conjugate, and the diagonal conjugate. The true conjugate can be measured only on radiographic films because it extends from the sacral promontory to the top of the symphysis pubis. Its normal measurement is 11 cm or more. The obstetric conjugate is the shortest of the three. It extends from

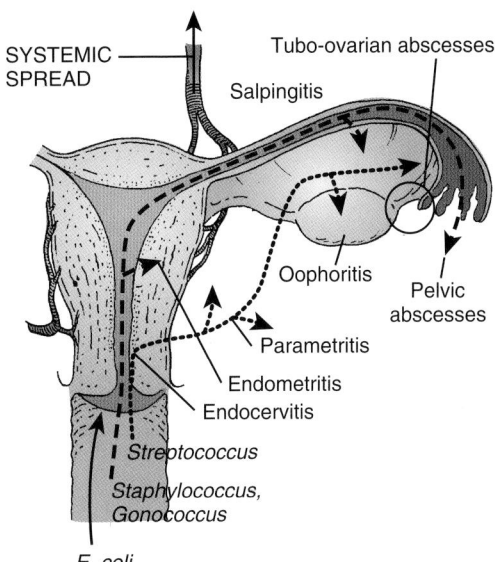

Routes of spread of pelvic inflammatory disease
(Black and Hawks, 2005)

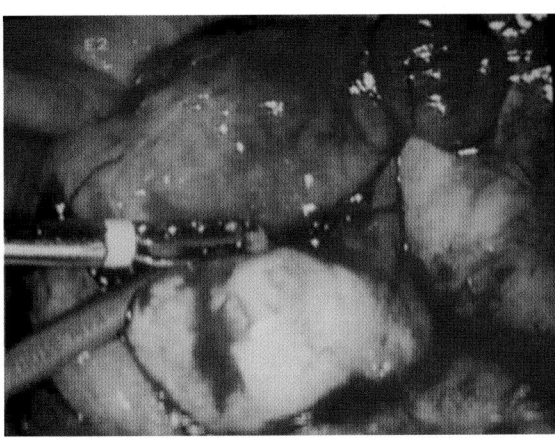

Laparoscopic view of severe pelvic inflammatory disease *(Shaw et al, 2011)*

the sacral promontory to the thickest part of the pubic bone and measures 10 cm or more. The diagonal conjugate is the most easily and commonly assessed because it extends from the lower border of the symphysis pubis to the sacral promontory. It normally measures 11.5 cm or more. The inlet is said to be contracted when any of these diameters is smaller than normal. The anteroposterior diameters are shorter than normal in the small gynecoid and platypelloid pelvis. The transverse diameter of the inlet is bounded by the inferior border of the walls of the iliac bones and is measured at the widest point. It is normally close to 13.5 cm but may be less in the small gynecoid pelvis and anthropoid pelvis. The oblique diameters of the pelvis extend from the juncture of the sacrum and ilium to the eminence on the ilium on the opposite side of the pelvis. Each oblique diameter measures nearly 13 cm. This dimension is smaller than normal in the small gynecoid and platypelloid pelves. See also **android pelvis, anthropoid pelvis, gynecoid pelvis, platypelloid pelvis.**

P

pelvic kidney. See **ptotic kidney.**

pelvic lipomatosis, deposition of fat around the pelvic cavity, a disorder of unknown cause. As it progresses the fat may compress the pelvic organs, causing urinary tract, kidney, or other symptoms.

pelvic minilaparotomy /min′ēlap′ərot″əmē/, a surgical operation in which the lower abdomen is entered through a small suprapubic incision. It is performed most often for tubal sterilization but also for diagnosis and treatment of ectopic pregnancy, ovarian cyst, endometriosis, and infertility. It may be performed as an alternative to laparoscopy, often on an outpatient basis. The patient is placed in the supine position, and the abdomen is prepared with antiseptic solution and covered with sterile drapes. An incision a few centimeters long is made, usually transversely, in the suprapubic fold of skin in the midline and is then carried down through the fat and fascia, between the rectus abdominis muscles, and into the peritoneal cavity. Bleeding is ligated, and a small self-retaining retractor is placed in the incision. A laparoscope may be used for visualization. The sterilization or other procedure is performed. After hemostasis is ensured, each tube is replaced in its anatomical position, and the incision is closed in layers. Because incisional pain in the postoperative period may mask the pain of intraperitoneal bleeding, vital signs are monitored frequently. Tachycardia and hypotension not alleviated by analgesia may be signs of hemorrhage or injury to the bowel. Before discharge, outpatients are carefully instructed in postoperative danger signs and proper care of the incision at home. Arrangements are made for follow-up examination. Often minilaparotomy may be performed faster and less expensively than laparoscopy. Though small, the minilaparotomy incision is considerably larger than is the usual laparoscopy incision. It is therefore less pleasing cosmetically, as well as more painful in the postoperative period. Compare **laparoscopy.**

pelvic outlet, the space surrounded by the bones of the lower part of the true pelvis. In men the shape of the pelvic outlet is narrower than that in women, but this is of no clinical significance. In women the shape and size of the pelvis vary and are of importance in childbirth. The shapes are classified by the length of the diameters as compared with each other and by the thickness of the bones. The diameters of the outlet are the anteroposterior, from the symphysis pubis to the coccyx, and the intertuberous, laterally from one to the other ischial tuberosity. See also **pelvic classification.**

pelvic pain, pain in the pelvis, as occurs in appendicitis, oophoritis, and endometritis. The character and onset of pelvic pain and any factors that alleviate or aggravate it are significant in making a diagnosis.

pelvic part of ductus deferens, the distal part of the ductus deferens, where it is within the pelvic cavity and terminates at the ampulla ductus deferentis.

pelvic pole, the end of the axis at which the breech of the fetus is located.

pelvic presentation [L, *pelvis,* basin, *praesentare,* to show], a breech presentation.

pelvic rotation, one of the five major kinematic determinants of gait, involving the alternate rotation of the pelvis to the right and the left of the body's central axis. The usual pelvic rotation occurring at each hip joint in most healthy individuals is approximately 4 degrees to each side of the central axis. Pelvic rotation occurs during the stance phase of gait and involves a medial to lateral circular motion. During normal locomotion or walking, considered a progressive sinusoidal movement, pelvic rotation serves to minimize the vertical displacement of the body's center of gravity. Analysis of pelvic rotation is often a factor in diagnosis of various orthopedic diseases, deformities, and abnormal bone conditions and in the correction of pathological gaits. Compare **knee-ankle interaction, knee-hip flexion, lateral pelvic displacement, pelvic tilt.**

pelvic rotunda [L, *pelvis,* basin, *rotundus,* wheel], a part of the ear appearing as a funnel-shaped depression of the tympanum above the fenestra cochlea.

pelvic tilt, one of the five major kinematic determinants of gait that lowers the pelvis on the side of the swinging lower limb during the walking cycle. Through the action of the hip joint the pelvis tilts laterally downward, adducting the lower limb in the stance phase of gait and abducting the opposite extremity in the swing phase of gait. The knee joint of the non-weight-bearing limb flexes during its swing phase to allow the pelvic tilt. Pelvic tilt helps minimize the vertical displacement of the body's center of gravity, thus conserving energy during walking. It is often a factor in the diagnosis and treatment of various orthopedic diseases, deformities, and abnormal conditions and in the analysis and correction of pathological gaits. Compare **knee-ankle interaction, knee-hip flexion, lateral pelvic displacement, pelvic rotation.**

pelvic ultrasonography, an ultrasound examination of a woman performed to identify paracervical, endometrial, or ovarian pathology or the risk of fetal abnormalities.

pelvic varicocele. See **ovarian varicocele.**

pelvifemoral /pel′vēfem″ərəl/ [L, *pelvis,* basin, *femur,* thigh], pertaining to the structures of the hip joint, especially the muscles and the area around the bony pelvis and the head of the femur that make up the pelvic girdle.

pelvifemoral muscular dystrophy. See **Leyden-Möbius muscular dystrophy.**

pelvimeter /pelvim″ətər/ [L, *pelvis,* basin; Gk, *metron,* measure], a device for measuring the diameter and capacity of the pelvis.

pelvimetry /pelvim″ətrē/, the act or process of determining the dimensions of the bony birth canal. Kinds include **clinical pelvimetry, x-ray pelvimetry.**

pelviotomy. See **pubiotomy.**

pelvis /pel′viz/ *pl.* **pelves** [L, basin], the lower part of the trunk of the body, composed of four bones, the two innominate bones laterally and ventrally and the sacrum and coccyx posteriorly. It is divided into the greater, or false, pelvis and the lesser, or true, pelvis by an oblique plane passing through the sacrum and the pubic symphysis. The greater pelvis is the expanded part of the cavity situated cranially and ventrally to the pelvic brim. The lesser pelvis is situated distally to the pelvic brim, and its bony walls are more complete than those of the greater pelvis. The inlet and outlet of the pelvis have three important diameters: anteroposterior, oblique, and transverse. The pelvis of a woman is usually smaller but wider and more circular than that of a man. Also called **true pelvis.**

pelvisacral /pel′visā″krəl/, pertaining to the pelvis and sacrum.

pelvospondylitis ossificans /pel′vōspon′dilī″tis/, inflammation of the pelvic part of the spine with deposits of bony material between the sacral vertebrae.

PEM, abbreviation for **protein-energy malnutrition.**

pemetrexed, an antineoplastic-antimetabolite.

■ INDICATIONS: This drug is used in combination with cisplatin in the treatment of malignant pleural mesothelioma and as a single agent in the treatment of non–small cell lung cancer.

■ CONTRAINDICATIONS: Pregnancy, an absolute neutrophil count less than 1500 cells/mm³, a creatinine clearance count of less than 45 mL/min, thrombocytopenia (less than 100,000/mm³), anemia, and known hypersensitivity to this drug prohibit its use.

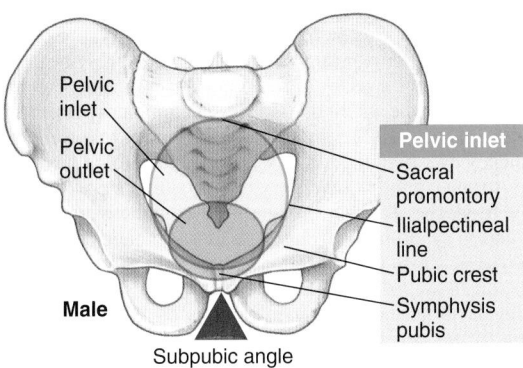

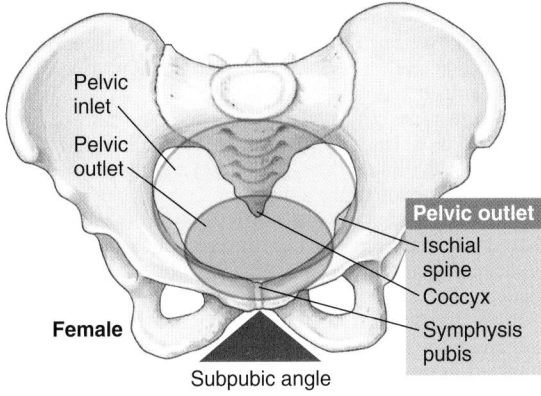

Comparison of male and female bony pelvis *(Patton and Thibodeau, 2016)*

■ ADVERSE EFFECTS: Adverse effects of this drug include creatinine elevation. Life-threatening effects include thrombosis and embolism, renal failure, neutropenia, leukopenia, thrombocytopenia, myelosuppression, anemia, and infection with or without neutropenia. Common side effects include fatigue, fever, mood alteration, neuropathy, chest pain, nausea, vomiting, anorexia, diarrhea, ulcerative stomatitis, constipation, dysphagia, dehydration, rash, desquamation, and dyspnea.

pemirolast /pĕ-mir′o-last″/, a mast cell stabilizer that inhibits type I hypersensitivity reactions, administered topically to the conjunctiva as the potassium salt to prevent pruritus associated with allergic conjunctivitis.

pemphigoid /pem″figoid/ [Gk, *pemphix,* bubble, *eidos,* form], a bullous disease resembling pemphigus, distinguished by thicker-walled bullae arising from erythematous macules or urticarial bases. Oral lesions are uncommon. It may rarely be associated with an internal malignancy. Spontaneous remission occasionally occurs after several years. Treatment usually includes oral corticosteroids. Compare **pemphigus.**

pemphigus /pem″figəs, pemfi″gəs/ [Gk, *pemphix,* bubble], an uncommon, severe disease of the skin and mucous membranes, characterized by thin-walled bullae arising from apparently normal skin or mucous membrane. The bullae rupture readily, leaving raw patches. The person loses weight, becomes weak, and is subject to major infections. Treatment with corticosteroids and other immunosuppressive medications has changed the prognosis of this disease from almost certain fatality to a controllable problem compatible

with a nearly normal life. The cause is unknown. Compare **pemphigoid.**

pemphigus chronicus. See **pemphigus vulgaris.**

pemphigus erythematosus. See **erythematous pemphigus.**

pemphigus vulgaris [Gk, *pemphix,* bubble; L, *vulgus,* common], a chronic, progressive autoimmune disease that is often fatal, characterized by the formation of bullae on otherwise normal oral mucosal membrane. Also called **pemphigus chronicus.**

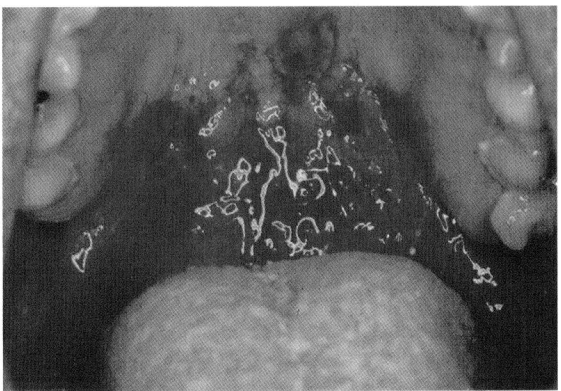

Hemorrhagic ulcers on the soft palate associated with pemphigus vulgaris *(Brinster et al, 2011)*

penbutolol /pen-bu′tah-lol/, a beta-adrenergic blocking agent with intrinsic sympathomimetic activity. It is used as an antihypertensive in the form of the sulfate salt.

penciclovir /pen-si′klo-vir/, a compound that inhibits viral DNA synthesis in herpesviruses 1 and 2, used in the treatment of recurrent herpes labialis. It is applied topically.

Pender, Nola J. [b. 1941], a nursing theorist who first presented her Health Promotion Model for nursing in her book *Health Promotion in Nursing Practice* (1982). She developed the idea that promoting optimal health supersedes preventing disease. Pender's theory identifies cognitive-perceptual factors in the individual, such as importance of health, perceived benefits of health-promoting behaviors, and perceived barriers to health-promoting behaviors. These factors are modified by demographic and biological characteristics and interpersonal influences, as well as situational and behavioral factors. They help predict participation in health-promoting behavior. The individual's definition of health for himself or herself has more importance than a general statement about health. A major assumption in Pender's theory is that health, as a positive high-level state, is assumed to be a goal toward which an individual strives.

pendular nystagmus [L, *pendulus,* hanging down; Gk, *nystagmos,* nodding], an undulating involuntary movement of the eyeball.

pendulous /pen″dələs/, hanging loose or lacking proper support.

pendulous abdomen [L, *pendulus,* hanging down, *abdomen*], an abnormal condition in which the anterior abdominal wall becomes relaxed and allows the abdomen to hang down over the pubic region.

pendulum exercises. See **Codman exercises.**

-penem, suffix for certain antibiotics, including analogs of penicillanic acid.

penetrance /pen″ətrəns/ [L, *penetrare,* to penetrate], the regularity with which an allele is expressed in a person who carries it. If an allele always produces its effect on the phenotype, it is fully penetrant. Achondroplasia is caused by a fully penetrant allele; if the allele is present, achondroplasia results. If an allele produces its effect less frequently than 100% of the time, it is not fully penetrant. Retinoblastoma develops in 90% of the children carrying the allele for the disease; in 10% of children the allele is nonpenetrant. –*penetrant, adj.*

penetrate /pen′ətrāt/ [L, *penetrare*], **1.** *v.,* to enter or pierce a barrier. **2.** *adj.,* pertaining to the degree to which x-rays pass through matter.

penetrating wound /pen′ətrā″ting/ [L, *penetrare* + AS, *wund*], a wound that breaks the skin and enters into a body area, organ, or cavity.

penetration /pen′ətrā″shən/, **1.** a piercing or entering. **2.** intellectual discernment. **3.** a stage in establishment of a viral infection in which the viral genetic material enters the host cell through fusion, phagocytosis, or injection.

penetrometer. See **stepwedge.**

-penia, suffix meaning "a (specified) deficiency": *glycopenia, neutropenia.*

penicillamine /pen′isil″əmēn/, a chelating agent.

■ INDICATIONS: It is prescribed for the treatment of Wilson disease and cystinuria and can be prescribed to bind with and remove heavy metals from the blood when there is poisoning resulting from metals such as copper, lead, mercury, arsenic, and gold (succimer is preferred for lead and mercury toxicity). It is also prescribed as a palliative in the treatment of systemic sclerosis (scleroderma) and rheumatoid arthritis when other medications have failed.

■ CONTRAINDICATIONS: Known hypersensitivity to this drug or penicillamine-related aplastic anemia prohibits its use. It is not given to patients who are pregnant or who have kidney dysfunction.

■ ADVERSE EFFECTS: Among the more serious adverse effects are fever, rashes, and blood dyscrasias. Severe bone marrow depression and immune disorders have been associated with long-term use of this drug. D-penicillamine is less toxic than the L form, and much of the reported toxicity is caused by the use of the L or DL form.

penicillic acid /pen′isil″ik/, an antibiotic compound isolated from various species of the fungus *Penicillium.*

penicillin /pen′isil″in/ [L, *penicillus,* paintbrush], any one of a group of antibiotics derived from cultures of species of the fungus *Penicillium* or produced semisynthetically. Various penicillins administered orally or parenterally for the treatment of bacterial infections exert their antimicrobial action by inhibiting the biosynthesis of cell-wall mucopeptides during active multiplication of the organisms. Penicillin G is a widely-used therapeutic agent for meningococcal, pneumococcal and streptococcal infections; syphilis; and other diseases. It is rapidly absorbed when injected intramuscularly or subcutaneously, but it is inactivated by gastric acid and hydrolyzed by penicillinase produced by most strains of *Staphylococcus aureus.* Penicillin V is also active against gram-positive cocci, with the exception of penicillinase-producing staphylococci, and, because it is resistant to gastric acid, it is effective when administered orally. Penicillins resistant to the action of the enzyme penicillinase (beta-lactamase) are cloxacillin, dicloxacillin, methicillin, nafcillin, and oxacillin. Ampicillin and amoxicillin are broad-spectrum aminopenicillins active against gram-negative organisms, including *Escherichia coli, Haemophilus influenzae, Neisseria gonorrhoeae, Salmonella, Shigella,* and *Proteus mirabilis.* Extended-spectrum penicillins include carbenicillin, piperacillin, and ticarcillin. These drugs are effective against the same bacteria killed by the aminopenicillins and are also effective against a number of additional bacteria, including species of *Pseudomonas, Enterobacter, Klebsiella,*

Proteus, and *Bacteroides.* Hypersensitivity reactions are common in patients receiving penicillin and may appear in the absence of prior exposure to the drug, presumably because of unrecognized exposure to a food or other substance containing traces of the antibiotic. The most common hypersensitivity reactions are rash, fever, and bronchospasm, followed in frequency by vasculitis, serum sickness, and exfoliative dermatitis. In some patients severe erythema multiforme accompanied by headache, fever, arthralgia, and conjunctivitis (Stevens-Johnson syndrome) develop. The most frequent cause of anaphylactic shock is an injection of penicillin.

penicillinase /pen′əsil″ənās/, an enzyme elaborated by certain bacteria, including many strains of staphylococci, that inactivates penicillin and thereby promotes resistance to the antibiotic. A purified preparation of penicillinase, derived from cultures of saprophytic spore-forming *Bacillus cereus,* is used in the treatment of adverse reactions to penicillin. Also called **beta-lactamase.**

penicillinase-producing *Neisseria gonorrhoeae,* those strains of *Neisseria gonorrhoeae* that are resistant to the effects of penicillin because of the production of penicillinase (beta-lactamase).

penicillinase-producing staphylococci, strains of staphylococcal organisms that elaborate the penicillin-inactivating enzyme penicillinase (beta-lactamase) and thereby resist the bactericidal action of the antibiotic.

penicillinase-resistant antibiotic, an antimicrobial agent that is not rendered inactive by penicillinase, an enzyme produced by certain bacteria, especially by strains of staphylococci. The semisynthetic penicillins cloxacillin sodium, dicloxacillin sodium, methicillin sodium, nafcillin sodium, and oxacillin sodium resist the action of penicillinase and are used in treating infections caused by staphylococci that elaborate the enzyme.

penicillin G benzathine, a long-acting depot form of penicillin.

■ INDICATIONS: It is used primarily for the treatment of syphilitic infection outside the central nervous system. It is given by deep intramuscular injection to achieve steady concentrations in the plasma and to slow systemic absorption from the repository in the muscle. Absorption occurs in a period that ranges from 12 hours to several days. It may be administered as prophylaxis against susceptible strains of bacteria, primarily gram-positive bacteria.

■ CONTRAINDICATIONS: Hypersensitivity to this drug or to other penicillins prohibits its use.

■ ADVERSE EFFECTS: The most serious adverse effect is anaphylaxis. The most common side effects are diarrhea, maculopapular rash, urticarial rash, fever, bronchospasm, vasculitis, serum sickness, and exfoliative dermatitis.

penicillin G potassium, a narrow-spectrum antibiotic for parenteral use.

■ INDICATIONS: It is prescribed in the treatment of many gram-positive bacterial infections (generally excluding *Staphylococcus),* some gram-negative infections (e.g., *Neisseria),* syphilis, and some anaerobes.

■ CONTRAINDICATIONS: Known hypersensitivity to this drug or to any penicillin prohibits its use.

■ ADVERSE EFFECTS: Among the more serious adverse effects are allergic reactions that vary from minor skin rashes to anaphylaxis. Nausea and diarrhea occur frequently.

penicillin V, a narrow spectrum bacterial antibiotic for oral administration. Also called *penicillin phenoxymethyl.*

■ INDICATIONS: It is prescribed for prophylaxis against rheumatic fever and in the treatment of ear, nose, throat, skin, and urinary tract infections caused by susceptible bacterial strains (primarily gram-positive bacteria).

■ CONTRAINDICATIONS: Known hypersensitivity to this drug or to any penicillin prohibits its use.

■ ADVERSE EFFECTS: Among the more serious adverse effects are anaphylaxis and urticaria.

penicilliosis /pen′isil′ē·ō″sis/ [L, *penicillus,* paintbrush; Gk, *osis,* condition], pulmonary infection caused by fungi of the genus *Penicillium.*

Penicillium /pen′isil″ē·əm/ [L, *penicillus,* paintbrush], a genus of imperfect fungi, some species of which have been tentatively linked to disease in humans, most notably in immunocompromised patients. Many species are commonly found in the human environment. Penicillin G is obtained from *Penicillium chrysogenum* and *P. notatum.*

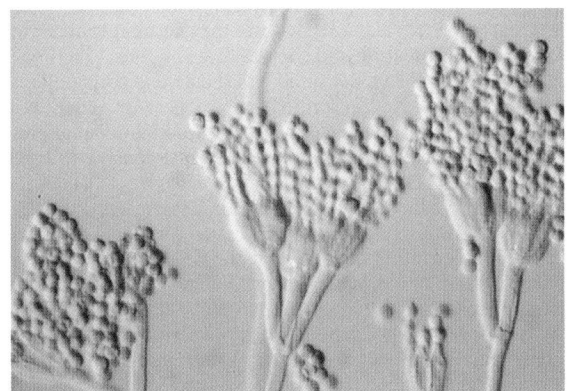

Penicillium species *(Mahon, Lehman, and Manuselis, 2015)*

penile /pē″nīl/ [L, penis], pertaining to the penis.

penile cancer /pē″nīl/ [L, *penis,* penis, *cancer,* crab], a rare malignancy of the penis generally occurring in uncircumcised men and associated with genital herpesvirus infection and poor hygiene. It is often mistaken for a venereal wart. Smegma may be a causative factor, but the specific substance and mechanism are unknown. Leukoplakia or the flat-topped papules of balanitis xerotica obliterans may be premalignant lesions, and the velvety red painful papules of Queyrat's erythroplasia are penile squamous cell carcinoma in situ. Cancer of the penis usually presents as a local mass or a bleeding ulcer and metastasizes early in its course. Surgical treatment involves partial or total amputation of the penis and excision of inguinal nodes and adjacent tissue when necessary. Radiotherapy is often used preoperatively and postoperatively. Methotrexate or bleomycin also may be administered, especially in metastatic disease. Postoperative interventions include observation and assessment for depression caused by body image change.

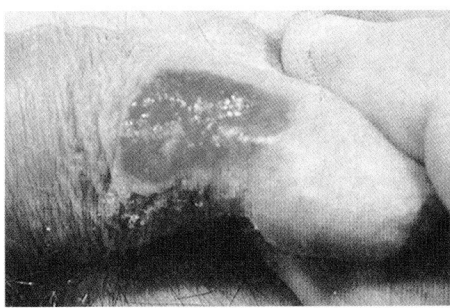

Penile cancer *(Courtesy Dr. Patrick C. Walsh, The Johns Hopkins University School of Medicine)*

penile curvature, abnormal curving of the penis to one side when erect. Also called *clubbed penis.*

penile prosthesis [L, *penis* + Gk, *prosthesis,* addition], a device that can be surgically implanted in the penis to treat erectile dysfunction. Some such devices have mechanisms that control production of an erection. Penile prostheses can be semirigid (maintaining a continuous state of erection) or inflatable plastic cavernosal cylinders attached to a pump that forces fluid from a reservoir into the cylinders, producing an erection.

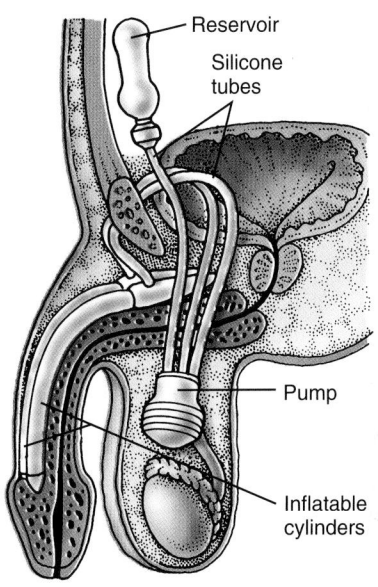

Inflatable penile prosthesis *(Ignatavicius, Workman, and Mishler, 2002)*

penile reflex. See **bulbocavernosus reflex, bulbospongiosus reflex.**

penis /pē″nis/ [L, male sex organ], the external reproductive organ of a man, homologous with the clitoris of a woman. It is attached with ligaments to the front and sides of the pubic arch and is composed of three cylindrical masses of cavernous tissue covered with skin. The corpora cavernosa penis surrounds a median mass called the corpus spongiosum penis, which contains the greater part of the urethra. The subcutaneous fascia of the penis is directly continuous with that of the scrotum, which contains the testes.

penis envy, literally, female envy of the male penis, but generally a female wish for male attributes, position, and advantages. It is believed by some psychologists to be a significant factor in female personality development. Compare **castration anxiety.**

-pennate, suffix meaning "having feathers."

penniform /pen″ifôrm/ [L, *penna,* feather, *forma,* form], pertaining to the shape of a feather, especially the patterns of muscular fasciculi that correlate with the range of motion and the power of muscles. Penniform fasciculi converge on one side of certain tendons. Muscles with more fasciculi have greater power but less range of motion than muscles with fewer fasciculi. Compare **bipenniform, multipenniform.**

penoscrotal fusion, a developmental anomaly in which the penis is fused to the scrotum.

penoscrotal transposition, a developmental anomaly in which the two halves of the scrotum are found lateral to the shaft of the penis or sometimes higher, often accompanied by hypospadias.

Penrose drain [Charles B. Penrose, American surgeon, 1862–1925; AS, *draehen,* teardrop], a thin rubber tube used as a surgical drain device.

pent-, penta-, prefix meaning "five": *pentose, pentadactyl.*

pentachlorophenol poisoning /pen′təklôr′ōfē″nol/, a toxic effect of skin absorption of sodium pentachlorophenate, an antimildew agent sometimes used in laundering. The condition has affected newborns with occasionally fatal symptoms of fever and profuse sweating, caused by skin contact with pentachlorophenate residue on diapers and nursery linens.

pentad /pen′tad/, **1.** a pentavalent chemical element. **2.** a relationship among five things.

pentadactyl /pen′tədak″til/ [Gk, *pente,* five, *daktylos,* fingers or toes], having five fingers per hand and five toes per foot.

pentagastrin test, a test of gastric function comparing basal acid output with a peak acid output. After the patient fasts overnight, a basal acid output and its pH are obtained for secretion of stomach acid. Then pentagastrin is administered into the stomach through a nasogastric tube and maximal acid output and peak acid output values are obtained. Also called *pentagastrin stimulation test.*

pentalogy of Cantrell /pen·tal′ə·jē kan-trel/ [Gk, *pente,* five + *logos,* word; James R. Cantrell, 20th-century American physician], a cleft in the inferior part of the sternum associated with midline abdominal defects such as omphalocele and defective pericardium and diaphragm with communication between the pericardial and peritoneal cavities and with cardiac anomalies such as ventricular septal defect or, less often, atrial septal defect, tetralogy of Fallot, or left ventricular diverticulum.

Pentam 300, an antiprotozoal agent. Brand name for **pentamidine isethionate.**

pentamidine isethionate, a parenteral antiprotozoal drug.

■ INDICATIONS: It is prescribed in the treatment and prevention of pneumonia caused by *Pneumocystis jiroveci,* particularly in patients who have human immunodeficiency syndrome. It can also be used to treat trypanosomiasis and visceral leishmaniasis.

■ CONTRAINDICATIONS: To reduce the risk of toxicity, the following tests must be carried out before, during, and after therapy: blood urea nitrogen, serum creatinine, blood glucose, complete blood and platelet counts, liver function, serum calcium, and electrocardiogram.

■ ADVERSE EFFECTS: Among adverse reactions to the injectable form of pentamidine are hypotension, hypoglycemia, leukopenia, thrombocytopenia, cardiac arrhythmias, acute renal failure, hypocalcemia, Stevens-Johnson syndrome, elevated serum creatinine level, elevated liver function results, pain or induration at the injection site, nausea, anorexia, fever, and rash. Some of these side effects are reduced by an aerosol formulation of pentamidine, but the aerosol causes other adverse effects, including fatigue, dizziness, and dyspnea.

pentaploid. See **polyploid.**

Pentatrichomonas hominis /pen′tətrik′əmō″nəs/, a species of parasitic protozoan flagellate, formerly part of the genus *Trichomonas,* that lives symbiotically in the colon of humans. Formerly called *Trichomonas hominis.*

pentavalent /pəntav″ələnt/ [Gk, *pente,* five; L, *valere,* to have worth], **1.** *n.,* a chemical radical or element that has a valency of 5. **2.** *adj.,* pertaining to a body formed by the association of five chromosomes held together by chiasmata at the first division of meiosis.

pentazocine hydrochloride /pentā″zəsēn/, an agonist/ antagonist opioid analgesic that stimulates kappa opioid receptors and blocks the mu opioid receptors. Also called *pentazocine lactate.*

■ INDICATIONS: It is prescribed for the relief of moderate to severe pain.

■ CONTRAINDICATIONS: Known hypersensitivity to this drug prohibits its use. It is administered with caution to patients with head injury, seizures, acute myocardial infarction, or kidney or liver dysfunction and to those undergoing biliary surgery. Pentazocine can cause withdrawal symptoms in patients with a history of opioid drug abuse and dependency.

■ ADVERSE EFFECTS: Nausea and dizziness commonly occur. Other minor problems include constipation, malaise, headache, restlessness, urinary tract spasms, blurred vision, miosis, and drowsiness. High doses may cause respiratory or circulatory depression and coma.

pentobarbital /pen′təbär″bitol/, a sedative and hypnotic.

■ INDICATIONS: It is prescribed as a preoperative sedative, to induce coma during treatment of increased intracranial pressure, and to abort status epilepticus unresponsive to other medications.

■ CONTRAINDICATIONS: Porphyria or known hypersensitivity to this drug or to other barbiturates prohibits its use. It is used with caution in patients with impaired respiratory or liver function or a history of dependence on sedative or hypnotic drugs.

■ ADVERSE EFFECTS: Among the more serious adverse reactions are respiratory or circulatory depression, paradoxical excitement, jaundice, or various hypersensitivity reactions. Nausea and hangover-like symptoms may occur.

pentosan /pen′to-san″/, a carbohydrate derivative used as an antiinflammatory, in the form of pentosan polysulfate sodium, in the treatment of interstitial cystitis. It is administered orally. See also **pentosan polysulfate sodium.**

pentosan polysulfate sodium, a polysulfate derivative of a xylose-containing, glucuronate-substituted pentosan, with an average molecular weight between 4000 and 6000 Da and having fibrinolytic and anticoagulant actions. It is used as an antiinflammatory in the treatment of interstitial cystitis; it is administered orally.

pentose /pen″tōs/ [Gk, *pente,* five; L, *osus,* having], a monosaccharide made of carbohydrate molecules, each containing five carbon atoms. It is produced by the body and is elevated after the ingestion of certain fruits, such as plums and cherries, and in certain rare diseases.

Pentothal Sodium, a barbiturate drug. Brand name for **thiopental sodium.**

pentoxifylline /pentok″sēfil′ēn/, a drug that lowers blood viscosity by making red blood cells even more flexible.

■ INDICATIONS: It is prescribed for the treatment of intermittent claudication associated with chronic occlusive arterial limb disease but should not be used as a replacement for other types of medications used for peripheral vascular disease because its efficacy is marginal. There are several unlabeled uses for the drug for which decreased blood viscosity could be advantageous, including cerebrovascular disease and diabetic neuropathy.

■ CONTRAINDICATIONS: It should not be administered to patients who are allergic to xanthines or who have had recent episodes of bleeding, especially in the brain or retina, and should be used with caution if renal impairment is present.

■ ADVERSE EFFECTS: Among the most serious adverse effects are nausea, dyspepsia, dizziness, angina, arrhythmia, and hypotension.

Pen-Vee K, an antibiotic. Brand name for *penicillin V potassium.*

Pepcid, an H₂ receptor antagonist used as antiulcer medication. Brand name for **famotidine.**

Peplau, Hildegard E. [1909–1999], a pioneer in nursing theory development and a proponent in the 1950s of the concept that nursing is an interpersonal process. Borrowing heavily from the knowledge base of psychology, Peplau proposed hypotheses based on the premise of the interpersonal process. From the early work evolved a nursing goal to foster the assumption that humans value, strive for, and have a right to independence. In a 1952 work, Peplau wrote that the nurse-patient relationship occurs in phases during which the nurse functions as a resource person, a counselor, and a surrogate. The four phases of the process are orientation, identification, exploitation, and resolution. The nurse assists in orientation when a patient with a need seeks help. Identification assures the patient that the nurse can understand his or her situation. Exploitation begins when the patient uses the services available. Resolution is marked as old needs are met and newer ones emerge.

peplos /pep″los/, a lipoprotein coat that may surround a virion.

peppermint, the dried leaves and flowering tops of the herb *Mentha piperita.* A source of a volatile oil, it is used as a carminative and antiemetic.

peppermint oil, a volatile oil from fresh aboveground parts of the flowering plant of peppermint *(Mentha piperita),* used as a flavoring agent for drugs and as a gastric stimulant and carminative.

pepper spray, an aerosolized form of oleoresins from capsicum, highly irritant to the skin and mucous membranes. It is used similarly to tear gas.

Pepper syndrome [William Pepper, American physician, 1874–1947], **1.** *(Obsolete)* a neuroblastoma of the adrenal glands that usually metastasizes to the liver. **2.** a rare genetic disorder. See **Cohen syndrome.**

pep pills, *(Slang)* amphetamines, diet pills, or any other stimulants.

peps-, pept-, prefix meaning "digestion": *pepsin, peptidase, peptone.*

-pepsia, -pepsy, -peptic, suffix meaning "a state of the digestion": *apepsia, dyspepsia.*

pepsin /pep″sin/ [Gk, *pepsis,* digestion], an enzyme secreted in the stomach that catalyzes the hydrolysis of protein. Preparations of pepsin obtained from pork and beef stomachs are sometimes used as digestive aids. See also **enzyme, hydrolysis.**

pepsinogen /pəpsin″əjən/ [Gk, *pepsis + genein,* to produce], a zymogenic substance secreted by pyloric and gastric chief cells. It is converted to the enzyme pepsin in an acidic environment, as in the presence of hydrochloric acid produced in the stomach.

pepsinuria /pep′sinoor″ē-ə/ [Gk, *pepsis,* digestion + *ouron,* urine], the presence of pepsin in urine.

-pepsy. See **-pepsia, -pepsy, -peptic.**

PEP syndrome. See **POEMS syndrome.**

pept-. See **peps-, pept-.**

peptic /pep″tik/ [Gk, *peptein,* to digest], pertaining to digestion or to the enzymes and secretions essential to digestion.

-peptic. See **-pepsia, -pepsy, -peptic.**

peptic ulcer, a sharply circumscribed loss of the mucous membrane of the stomach, duodenum, or any other part of the GI system exposed to gastric juices containing acid and pepsin. Also called **gastric ulcer.**

■ OBSERVATIONS: Peptic ulcers may be acute or chronic. Acute lesions are almost always multiple and superficial. They may be totally asymptomatic and usually heal without scarring or other sequelae. Chronic ulcers are true ulcers. They are deep, single, persistent, and symptomatic; the muscular coat of the wall of the organ does not regenerate; a scar forms, marking the site, and the mucosa may heal completely. Peptic ulcers are caused by a combination of factors, including an excessive secretion of gastric acid, inadequate protection of the mucous membrane, stress, heredity, and the use of certain drugs, including the corticosteroids, certain antihypertensives, and antiinflammatory medications (especially acetylsalicylic acid and nonsteroidal antiinflammatory drugs). A bacterium present in the gut—*Helicobacter pylori*—is a common cause of peptic ulcer disease. Characteristically ulcers cause a gnawing pain in the epigastrium that does not radiate to the back, is not aggravated by a change in position, and has a temporal pattern that mimics the diurnal rhythm of gastric acidity.

■ INTERVENTIONS: Symptomatic relief is provided with drugs that either neutralize or block secretion of acid and frequent small bland meals. The underlying cause is treated if known. If *H. pylori* is present, a 2-week triple therapy regimen of tetracycline, metronidazole, and bismuth may be given. Hemorrhage caused by perforation of the muscle and blood vessels may require surgical resection of the damaged area. The diagnosis and evaluation of peptic ulcers involve serial radiographic studies using a contrast medium and endoscopy. A definitive diagnosis is important because the early signs of cancer of the stomach and duodenum resemble those of peptic ulcers.

■ PATIENT CARE CONSIDERATIONS: The patient is reassured that in most cases the ulcers heal completely and that the pain may be controlled with simple measures. The nurse emphasizes the correct use of antacids and the other medications prescribed. Usually the patient is instructed to eat frequent small meals consisting of foods known to be nonirritating. For many but not all patients, fatty, highly spiced, heavy, or fibrous foods are likely to provoke pain. The use of tobacco and alcohol is discouraged.

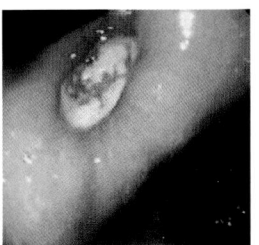

Peptic ulcer *(Courtesy Dr. Pankaj Jay Pasricha)*

peptidase /pep″tidās/ [Gk, *peptein,* to digest, *ase,* enzyme suffix], a protein-splitting enzyme that breaks peptides into amino acids. It occurs naturally in plants, yeasts, certain microorganisms, and digestive juices.

peptide /pep″tīd/ [Gk, *peptein,* to digest], a molecular chain compound composed of two or more amino acids joined by peptide bonds. See also **amino acid, polypeptide, protein.**

peptidergic /pep′tidur″jik/, using small peptides as neurotransmitters.

peptide YY. See **neuropeptide Y.**

peptidyl-dipeptidase A. See **angiotensin-converting enzyme.**

peptogenic /pep′təjen″ik/, pertaining to an agent that produces peptones or pepsin.

peptone /pep″tōn/, a derived protein, which may be produced by hydrolysis of a native protein with an acid or enzyme.

Peptostreptococcus /pep′təstrep′təkok″əs/, a genus of gram-positive anaerobic chemoorganotrophic bacteria that occur in pairs or chains. The potentially pathogenic organisms are found in normal and pathological female genital tracts and in the intestinal and respiratory tracts of normal humans. They have been associated with a variety of disorders ranging from appendicitis to putrefactive wounds.

Peptostreptococcus anaerobius, a potentially pathogenic species of anaerobic bacterium found throughout the body, including the mouth, the intestinal and respiratory tracts, and body cavities, particularly the vagina.

per-, **1.** prefix meaning "throughout, or completely": *peracephalus, perfuse, permeable.* **2.** prefix meaning "a large amount (in chemical terms)" or designating a combination of an element in its highest valence: *peracetate, peracid, perhydride.* **3.** prefix meaning "around, near, enclosing": *periapical, pericardium.*

peracephalus /pur′əsef″ələs/ *pl. peracephali* [L, *per,* completely; Gk, *a + kephale,* not head], a fetus or individual with a malformed head.

peracetic acid /per″ah-se′tik/, peroxyacetic acid, CH_3COOOH, a strong oxidizing agent sometimes used for sterilization.

perceived severity /pərsēvd″/ [L, *percipere,* to perceive, *severus,* serious], (in health belief model) a person's perception of the seriousness of the consequences of contracting a disease. Compare **perceived susceptibility.**

perceived susceptibility, (in health belief model) a person's perception of the likelihood of contracting a disease. Compare **perceived severity.**

percentage depth dose /pərsen″tij/ [L, *per,* completely, *centum,* hundred; ME, *dep,* deep; L, *dosis,* something given], the amount of therapeutic radiation delivered at a specified dose, expressed as a percentage of the skin dose.

percentile, each of the 100 equal groups of a statistical distribution. A percentile rank of 80 indicates that 20% of the total number of cases scored above and 80% scored below in whatever characteristics were being studied.

percent solution, a relationship of a quantity of solute to the quantity of solution, multiplied by 100, expressed in terms of mass of solute per mass of solution. It can be expressed in terms of mass solute per mass solution, volume solute per volume solution, or mass solute (g) per volume (mL) solution. An example of a 5% by mass solution is 5 g of glucose dissolved in 95 g of water, forming 100 g of solution.

percent systole [L, *per + centum* + Gk, *systole,* contraction], the fraction of the duration of each heartbeat that is devoted to the contraction of the ventricles.

percept /pur″sept/ [L, *percipere,* to perceive], the mental impression of an object that is gained through the use of the senses.

perception /pərsep″shən/ [L, *percipere,* to perceive], **1.** the conscious recognition and interpretation of sensory stimuli that serve as a basis for understanding, learning, and knowing or for motivating a particular action or reaction. **2.** the result or product of the act of perceiving. Kinds include **depth perception, extrasensory perception, facial perception, stereognostic perception. –perceptual,** *perceptive, adj.*

perceptivity /pur′səptiv″itē/, the ability to receive sense impressions.

perceptual. See **perception.**

perceptual constancy /pərsep″choo·əl/ [L, *percipere,* to perceive, *cum,* together with, *stare,* to stand], (in Gestalt psychology) the phenomenon in which an object is seen in the same way under varying circumstances.

perceptual defect, any of a broad group of disorders or dysfunctions of the central nervous system that interfere with the conscious mental recognition of sensory stimuli. Such conditions are caused by lesions at specific sites in the cerebral cortex that may result from any illness or trauma affecting the brain at any age or stage of development. Impairment of mental activity, cognitive processes, and emotional responses may be diffuse, as occurs in organic mental disorders, such as the psychoses, delirium, and dementia, and in attention deficit disorder, or they may be manifested focally, as in aphasia, apraxia, epilepsy, disorders of memory, cerebrovascular disorders, and various intercranial neoplasms.

perceptual deprivation, the absence of or decrease in meaningful groupings of stimuli, which may result from a constant background noise or constant inadequate illumination.

perceptual monotony, a mental state characterized by a lack of variety in the normal pattern of everyday stimuli.

perchloromethane. See **carbon tetrachloride.**

Percodan, a fixed-combination medication containing aspirin and an opioid analgesic, used to treat moderate to severe pain. Brand name for **aspirin, oxycodone hydrochloride.**

Percogesic, a fixed-combination drug containing an antihistamine and an analgesic, used to treat mild to moderate pain. Brand name for **phenyltoloxamine citrate, acetaminophen.**

percolation /pur′kəlā″shən/ [L, *percolare,* to strain], **1.** the act of filtering any liquid through a porous medium. **2.** (in pharmacology) the removal of the soluble parts of a crude drug by passing a liquid solvent through it.

per contiguum, spreading from one body structure to a contiguous area.

per continuum, describing the spread of an inflammation or other disease process from one body part to another through continuous tissue.

percuss /pərkus″/ [L, *percutere,* to strike hard], to perform percussion by striking, for example, the thoracic or abdominal wall, thereby producing sound vibrations that aid in diagnosis.

percussion /pərkush″ən/ [L, *percutere,* to strike hard], **1.** a technique in physical examination of tapping the body with the fingertips or fist to evaluate the size, borders, and consistency of some of the internal organs and to discover the presence of and evaluate the amount of fluid in a body cavity. Immediate or direct percussion is percussion performed by striking the fingers directly on the body surface. Indirect, mediate, or finger percussion involves striking a finger of one hand on a finger of the other hand (normally the second phalanx of the third digit) as it is placed over the organ. See also **percussor, pleximeter. 2.** See **cupping and vibrating.**

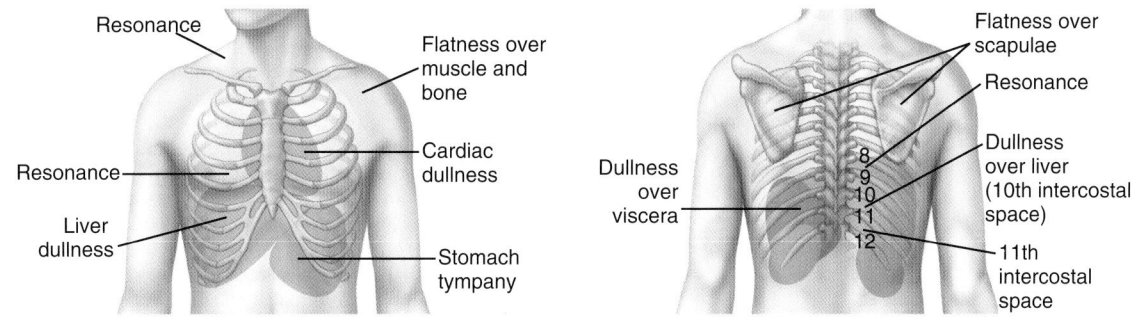

Percussion: normal notes over the anterior *(left)* and posterior *(right)* chest and upper abdomen
(Harkreader, Hogan, and Thobaben, 2007)

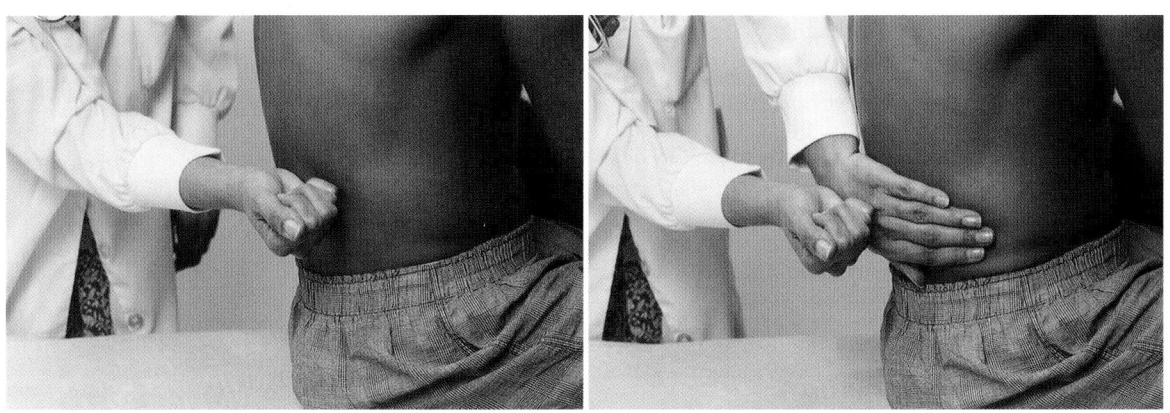

Percussion: direct and indirect *(Wilson and Giddens, 2001)*

percussor /pərkus″ər/ [L, a striker], a small hammerlike diagnostic tool having a rubber head that is used to tap the body lightly in percussion. Also called **plexor, reflex hammer.** See also **percussion.**

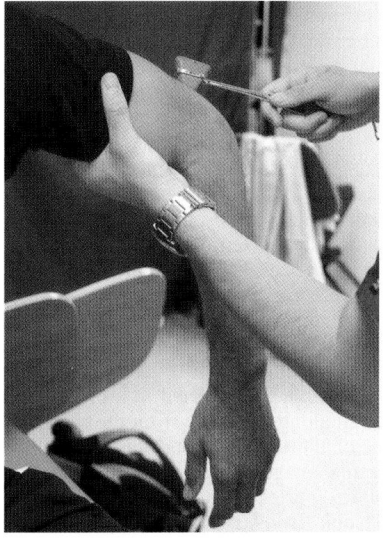

Eliciting reflex with percussor *(Courtesy Rutgers School of Nursing—Camden. All rights reserved.)*

percutaneous /pur′kyo͞otā″nē·əs/ [L, *per* + *cutis*, skin], performed through the skin, such as a biopsy; aspiration of fluid from a space below the skin with a needle, catheter, and syringe; or instillation of a fluid in a cavity or space by similar means.

percutaneous absorption, the process of absorption through the skin from topical application.

percutaneous catheter, a catheter inserted through the skin rather than through an orifice, such as a central venous catheter or one used for hemodialysis or peritoneal dialysis.

percutaneous catheter placement, a technique in which an intracatheter is introduced through the skin into an artery and placed at a site or structure to be studied by selective angiography and other diagnostic procedures. The puncture site is infiltrated with a local anesthetic before insertion of the catheter. A special needle is inserted into the artery, and a long, flexible, spring guide is passed through the needle for approximately 15 cm. The needle is then removed, the catheter is advanced to the desired position, and the guide is withdrawn. The catheter is withdrawn at the end of the procedure.

percutaneous coronary intervention (PCI), the management of coronary artery occlusion by any of various catheter-based techniques, such as percutaneous transluminal coronary angioplasty, atherectomy, angioplasty using the excimer laser, and implantation of coronary stents and related devices.

percutaneous endoscopic gastrostomy (PEG), the creation of a new opening in the stomach for enteral tube feedings. It can also be used for gastric decompression. PEG is accomplished by puncturing the abdominal wall after the stomach has been distended. A tube is then inserted through the abdominal wall into the stomach under endoscopic guidance. It can be performed with the patient under local anesthesia or moderate sedation or analgesia in the endoscopic suite, in the operating room, or at bedside in the critical care unit.

P

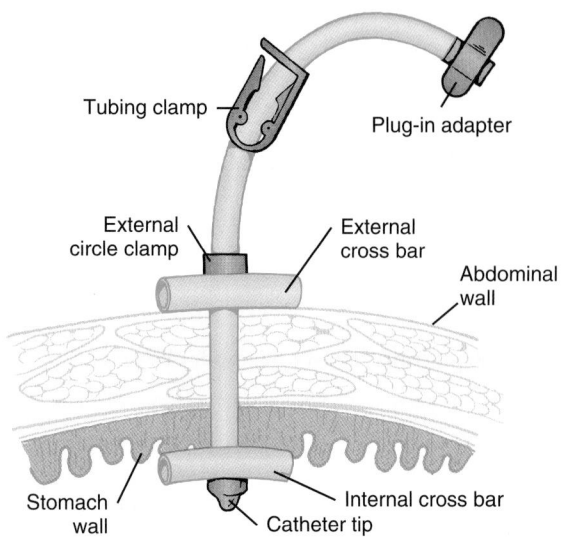

Percutaneous endoscopic gastrostomy tube *(Black and Hawks, 2009)*

percutaneous epididymal sperm aspiration, retrieval of sperm from the epididymis by using fine-needle aspiration, performed in men with obstructive azoospermia.

percutaneous nephrolithotomy, a uroradiological procedure performed to extract stones from within the kidney or proximal ureter by percutaneous surgery after the stones have been visualized radiologically.

percutaneous nephroscope, a thin fiberoptic probe that can be inserted into the kidney through an incision in the skin. Light transmitted along the fibers allows visualization of the inside of the kidney. The device is equipped with a tool that can be used to grasp and remove small kidney stones.

percutaneous transhepatic biliary drainage, drainage of the biliary tree by the introduction of a catheter through the liver and into the biliary tree under radiological guidance. Also called *percutaneous transhepatic cholangiodrainage.*

percutaneous transhepatic cholangiography (PTC), the radiographic examination of the structure of the bile ducts. A contrast medium is injected through a needle passed directly into a hepatic duct.

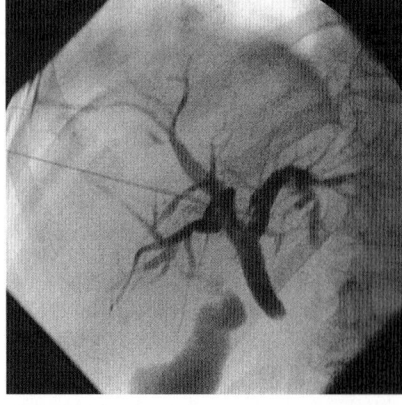

Percutaneous transhepatic cholangiogram showing the biliary system *(Courtesy Ohio State University Medical Center)*

percutaneous transluminal angioplasty (PTA), a procedure for dilating blood vessels in the treatment of peripheral artery disease. Under fluoroscopic guidance a balloon-tipped catheter is inserted into a stenotic artery and the balloon is inflated. The inflated balloon may dilate the artery by stretching its elastic fibers or by flattening accumulation of plaque. See also **percutaneous transluminal coronary angioplasty.**

percutaneous transluminal coronary angioplasty (PTCA), a technique in the treatment of atherosclerotic coronary heart disease and angina pectoris in which some plaques in the arteries of the heart are flattened against the arterial walls, resulting in improved circulation. The procedure involves threading a catheter through the vessel to the atherosclerotic plaque, inflating and deflating a small balloon at the tip of the catheter several times, and then removing the catheter. The procedure is performed under radiographic or ultrasonic visualization. When it is successful, the plaques remain compressed and the symptoms of heart disease, including the pain of angina, are decreased. An alternative is coronary bypass surgery which may be necessary if arteries are narrowed or blocked in several areas, or there is a blockage in one of the larger main arteries,

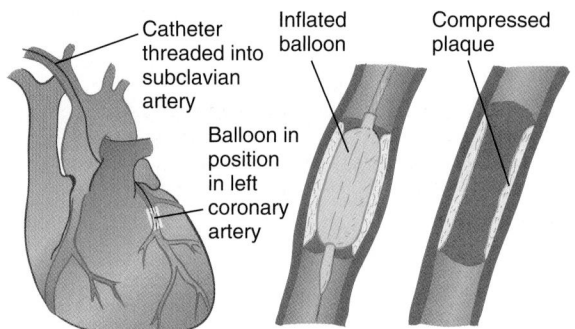

Percutaneous transluminal coronary angioplasty *(Black and Hawks, 2009)*

percutaneous transluminal renal angioplasty (PTRA), percutaneous transluminal angioplasty to enlarge the lumen of a sclerotic renal artery, preserve renal function, and treat renovascular hypertension.

per diem rate /pər dē″əm, dī″əm/ [L, *per diem,* daily, *ratus,* reckoned], an established rate of payment for hospital services.

per discharge payment, a payment method in which costs of resources used for the entire hospital stay are the responsibility of the hospital. The hospital is then compensated according to a contractually determined amount per discharge.

perencephaly /per′ensef″əlē/, a condition characterized by one or more cerebral cysts.

Perez reflex /pərez″, per″ez/ [Bernard Perez, French physician, 1836–1903; L, *reflectere,* to bend back], the normal response of an infant to cry, flex the limbs, and elevate the head and pelvis when supported in a prone position with a finger pressed along the spine from the sacrum to the neck. Persistence of the reflex beyond the 6 months of age may indicate brain damage.

perfectionism /pərfek″shəniz′əm/ [L, *perficere,* to complete], a subjective state in which a person pursues an extremely high standard of performance and, in many cases, demands the same standards of others. Failure to attain the goals may lead to feelings of defeat and other adverse psychological consequences.

perflation /pərflā″shən/, a method of opening a passage or cavity entrance with air pressure.

perfluorocarbon /pərfloor′ōkär″bən/, any of a group of chemicals with limited capacity for transporting oxygen through the circulatory system. They can be used for certain blood substitute purposes, regardless of the blood type of the patient. They are stable at room temperatures, have a pH of 7.4, and are free of infectious pathogens. Also called **artificial blood, blood substitute.**

perforans /pur″fôrənz/ [L, *perforare,* to pierce], penetrating. The term applies mainly to nerves, muscles, or other anatomical features that penetrate other structures, such as perforans gasseri, or nerves of the musculocutaneous tissues.

perforate [L, *perforare,* to pierce], **1.** *v.,* to pierce, punch, puncture, or otherwise make a hole. **2.** *adj.,* riddled with small holes. **3.** *adj.,* (of the anus) having a normal opening; not imperforate. **–perforation,** *n.*

perforating arteries, three arteries that branch from the deep artery of the thigh as it descends anterior to the adductor brevis muscle. All three penetrate through the adductor magnus near its attachment to the linea aspera to enter and supply the posterior compartment of thigh. The ascending and descending branches of the vessels interconnect to form a longitudinal channel that participates in forming an anastomotic network of vessels around the hip and inferiorly anastomoses with branches of the popliteal artery behind the knee.

perforating capsular plexus, a vascular plexus around the renal capsule, supplied by the perforating radiate, inferior, suprarenal, renal, and testicular or ovarian arteries.

perforating cutaneous nerve, a nerve that originates in the sacral plexus and penetrates directly through the sacrotuberous ligament to course to the skin over the inferior aspect of the buttocks.

perforating fracture, an open fracture caused by a projectile, making a small surface wound.

perforating radiate arteries, small arteries that are continuations of the cortical radiate arteries and perforate the renal capsule.

perforating ulcer /pur″fôrā′ting/ [L, *perforare,* to pierce, *ilcus*], **1.** an ulcer that penetrates the thickness of a wall or membrane, such as a peptic ulcer of the digestive tract. **2.** a deep, painless ulcer, often on the sole of the foot, of a person whose skin is insensitive because of a disease such as diabetes.

perforation /pur″fôrā″shən/ [L, *perforare,* to pierce], a hole or opening made through the entire thickness of a membrane or other tissue or material.

perforation of stomach or intestines, a condition in which disease or injury has resulted in a leakage of digestive tract contents into the peritoneal cavity. A common cause is a ruptured appendix or perforating peptic ulcer. Immediate surgical intervention is needed to prevent peritonitis.

perforation of the uterus, a puncture of the uterus, as may be caused by a curet or by an intrauterine contraceptive device.

performance capacity, (in occupational therapy) the ability of a person to accomplish a task or complete an activity as supported by the status of his or her physical and mental abilities; performance capacity is also influenced by the person's subjective experience (the lived body). See also **Model of Human Occupation.**

perfusion /pərfyoo″zhən/ [L, *perfundere,* to pour over], **1.** the passage of a fluid through a specific organ or an area of the body. **2.** a therapeutic measure whereby a drug intended for an isolated part of the body is introduced via the bloodstream.

perfusionist /pərfyoo″zhənist/ [L, *perfundere,* to pour over], an allied health professional who assists in performing procedures that involve extracorporeal circulation, such as during open-heart surgery or hypothermia.

perfusion lung scan, a radiographic examination of the lungs and their function performed after an IV injection of a radioactive material. It is performed to detect areas of lung perfusion as an aid in the diagnosis of pulmonary embolism. The procedure is usually done in conjunction with a ventilation scan, in which the patient inhales radioactive material and the lung is scanned to detect lung areas receiving ventilation. Also called **perfusion scan.**

perfusion rate, the rate of blood flow through the capillaries per unit mass of tissue, expressed in milliliters per minute per 100 g.

perfusion scan. See **perfusion lung scan.**

perfusion technologist, a person who, under the supervision of a physician, operates a heart-lung machine used for cardiopulmonary bypass during surgery.

per gene, a gene that is associated with circadian rhythms of some animal species. Mutations of the per gene locus result in alterations of their biorhythms. A similar DNA sequence occurs in the human genome, but its effect on human circadian rhythms is unknown.

pergolide /per′golīd/, a long-acting ergot derivative with dopaminergic properties, used as the mesylate salt in treatment of parkinsonism. It is administered orally.

Pergonal, a human menopausal gonadotropin used to treat anovulation and infertility.

peri-, prefix meaning "around": *pericardial, pericolitis.*

periacinous /per″e·as′inus/, near or around a small saclike dilation, particularly in the lung or a gland.

Periactin, an antihistamine and antipruritic drug used to treat rash and other symptoms of allergies. Brand name for **cyproheptadine hydrochloride.**

periadenitis /per′i·ad′ənī″tis/, an inflammation of tissues around a gland.

periadenitis mucosa necrotica recurrens. See **Sutton disease.**

perianal /per′i·ā″nəl/ [Gk, *peri,* around; L, *anus*], pertaining to the area around the anus.

perianal abscess [Gk, *peri,* around; L, *anus + abscedere,* to go away], a focal, purulent subcutaneous infection in the region of the anus. Treatment includes hot soaks, antibiotics, and possibly incision and drainage. If a rectal fistula or perianal space is found to be the cause of recurrent perianal abscesses, surgical excision is usually performed.

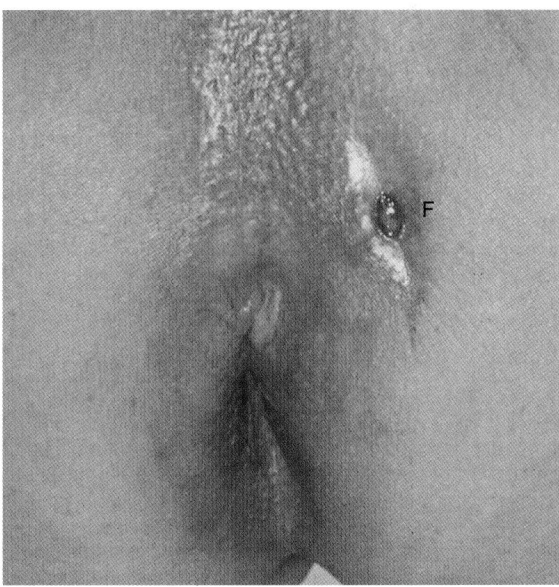

Perianal abscess *(Quick, 2014)*

periangitis. See **periarteritis.**

periaortic /per′i·ā·ôr″tik/ [Gk, *peri,* around, *aerein,* to raise], pertaining to the area around the aorta.

periaortitis /per′i·ā′ôrtī′tis/, an inflammation of the adventitia or surrounding tissues of the aorta.

periapical /per′i·ap″ikəl/ [Gk, *peri* + L, *apex,* top], pertaining to the tissues surrounding the apex of a tooth root, including the periodontal membrane and the alveolar bone.

periapical abscess, an infection around the root of a tooth, usually a result of the bacterial spread of dental caries into the root canal, leading to pulpal necrosis. Radiographically, the infection will appear radiolucent around the apex of the tooth. The abscess may perforate, following the path of least resistance into the oral cavity or maxillary sinus; extend into nearby bone, causing osteomyelitis; or, more often, spread to soft tissues, causing cellulitis and a swollen face. There may be associated fever, redness, pain, malaise, and nausea. Treatment includes access into the pulp chamber of the tooth to establish drainage and relieve pain, followed by antibiotics and late root canal therapy or tooth extraction. Also called **dental abscess, tooth abscess.**

periapical cyst. See **radicular cyst.**

periapical fibroma, a mass of benign connective tissue that may form at the apex of a tooth with normal pulp.

periapical infection, infection surrounding the root of a tooth, often accompanied by toothache.

periapical radiograph, a dental x-ray film or dental imaging used to detect changes in the bone surrounding the roots of the teeth. Also called *periapical image.*

periappendicitis decidualis /per′i·apen′disī″tis/, an inflammation of the vermiform appendix, with the presence of decidual cells in the peritoneum of the appendix. It occurs in cases of right tubal pregnancy with adhesions between the appendix and the fallopian tubes.

periappendicular /per′i·ap′əndik″yələr/ [Gk, *peri,* around; L, *appendere,* to hang upon], pertaining to the area around the appendix.

periarterial /per′i·ärtir″ē·əl/ [Gk, *peri,* around, *arteria,* airpipe], pertaining to the area around an artery.

periarteritis /per′i·är′tərī″tis/ [Gk, *peri* + *arteria,* airpipe, *itis*], inflammation of the outer coat of one or more arteries and the tissue surrounding them. Also called **periangitis.** Kinds include **periarteritis nodosa, syphilitic periarteritis.**

periarteritis gummosa. See **syphilitic periarteritis.**

periarteritis nodosa, a progressive polymorphic disease of the connective tissue that is characterized by numerous large and palpable nodules or clusters of visible nodules along segments of middle-sized arteries, particularly near points of bifurcation. The disease causes occlusion of vessels, resulting in regional ischemia, hemorrhage, necrosis, and pain. Early signs of the disease include tachycardia, fever, weight loss, and pain in the viscera. Kidney, lung, and intestinal involvement is common. Other systems and organs of the body may also be affected. Periarteritis nodosa is treated with corticosteroids and cytotoxic drugs. Also called **necrotizing angiitis.**

periarthritis /per′i·ärthrī″tis/, inflammation of tissues around a joint.

periarticular /per′i·ärtik″yələr/ [Gk, *peri,* around; L, *articulus,* joint], pertaining to the area around a joint.

peribronchial /-brong″kē·əl/, surrounding a bronchus.

peribronchiolar /-brong″kē·ō′lər/ [Gk, *peri,* around, *bronchiolus*], pertaining to the area around the bronchioles.

pericalyceal /per″ikal″isē′al/, near or around a renal calyx.

pericardia. See **pericardium.**

pericardiac /-kär″dē·ak/ [Gk, *peri,* around, *kardia,* heart], **1.** pertaining to the pericardium. **2.** pertaining to the area around the heart.

pericardial. See **pericardium.**

pericardial adhesion /-kär″dē·əl/ [Gk, *peri,* around, *kardia,* heart; L, *adhesio,* sticking to], an attachment of the pericardium to the heart muscle, sometimes restricting the muscle's action. In some cases a previous inflammation or surgery may result in dense fibrous adhesions that obliterate the pericardium. The condition may be general or localized and may involve adhesion between the two layers of pericardium (internal adhesive pericarditis), obstructing the pericardial cavity, or between one layer and surrounding tissues such as the diaphragm, mediastinum, or chest wall (external adhesive pericarditis) as a result of an inflammatory process. Also called **adherent pericardium.**

pericardial artery [Gk, *peri* + *kardia,* heart, *arteria,* airpipe], one of several small vessels branching from the thoracic aorta, supplying the dorsal surface of the pericardium.

pericardial effusion [Gk, *peri,* around, *kardia,* heart; L, *effundere,* to pour out], an abnormal accumulation of blood or fluids in the sac surrounding the heart. Also called **hydropericardium.**

pericardial friction rub [Gk, *peri,* around, *kardia,* heart; L, *fricare,* to rub; ME, *rubben*], the rubbing together of inflamed membranes of the pericardium, as may occur in pericarditis or after a myocardial infarction. It produces a sound audible on auscultation. Also called *pericardial murmur, pericardial rub.*

pericardial tamponade. See **cardiac tamponade.**

pericardiectomy /per′i·kär′dē·ek′tə·mē/ [Gk, *peri,* around + *kardia,* heart + *ektomē,* excision], excision of the pericardium.

pericardiocentesis /per′ikär′dē·ō′sintē″sis/ [Gk, *peri* + *kardia,* heart, *kentesis,* pricking], a procedure for drawing fluid in the pericardial space between the serous membranes by surgical puncture and aspiration of the pericardial sac. Also called *pericardicentesis.*

pericardioperitoneal canals, a pair of passages in the embryo connecting the primordial pericardial and peritoneal cavities.

pericardiotomy /-kär′di·ot″əmē/, a surgical incision in the pericardium.

pericarditis /per′ikärdī″tis/ [Gk, *peri* + *kardia,* heart, *itis*], inflammation of the pericardium associated with trauma, malignant neoplastic disease, infection, uremia, myocardial infarction, collagen disease, or unknown causes. See also **acute nonspecific pericarditis.**

■ OBSERVATIONS: Two stages are observed if treatment in the first stage does not halt progress of the condition to the extremely grave second stage. The first stage is characterized by fever; substernal chest pain that radiates to the shoulder or neck; dyspnea; a dry, nonproductive cough; a rapid and forcible pulse; a pericardial friction rub; and a muffled heartbeat over the apex. The patient becomes increasingly anxious, tired, and orthopneic. During the second stage a serofibrinous effusion develops within the pericardium, restricting cardiac activity. If the effusion is purulent (caused by bacterial infection), a high fever, sweat, chills, and prostration also occur. The heart sounds become muffled, weak, and distant on auscultation, and a bulge is visible on the chest over the precordial area.

■ INTERVENTIONS: The patient is kept in bed, and the head of the bed is elevated 45 degrees to decrease dyspnea. Hypothermia treatment may be necessary to reduce the body temperature. An antibiotic or antifungal and analgesic may be ordered. Oxygen and parenteral fluids are usually given, vital signs are evaluated, and the chest is auscultated frequently. Pericardiocentesis or pericardiotomy may be performed to remove accumulated fluid or to make a diagnosis.

■ PATIENT CARE CONSIDERATIONS: Emotional support of a patient being treated for pericarditis requires remaining with the person if he or she is anxious and explaining all procedures thoroughly. During recovery, rest periods are planned and the person is urged to avoid fatigue and exposure to upper respiratory infections. The patient is told to report symptoms of recurrence, including fever, chest pain, and dyspnea.

pericardium /per′ikär″dē·əm/ *pl.* **pericardia** [Gk, *peri* + *kardia,* heart], a fibroserous sac that surrounds the heart and the roots of the great vessels. It consists of the serous pericardium and the fibrous pericardium. The serous pericardium consists of the parietal layer, which lines the inside of the fibrous pericardium, and the visceral layer, which adheres to the surface of the heart. Between the two layers is the pericardial space, which contains a few drops of pericardial fluid to lubricate opposing surfaces of the space and allow the heart to move easily during contraction. Injury or disease may cause fluid to accumulate in the space, causing a wide separation between the heart and the outer pericardium. The fibrous pericardium, which constitutes the outermost sac and is composed of tough, white fibrous tissue lined by the parietal layer of the serous pericardium, fits loosely around the heart and attaches to large blood vessels emerging from the top of the heart but not to the heart itself. It is relatively inelastic and protects the heart and the serous membranes. If pericardial fluid or pus accumulates in the pericardial space, the fibrous pericardium cannot stretch, causing a rapid increase of pressure around the heart. –**pericardial,** *adj.*

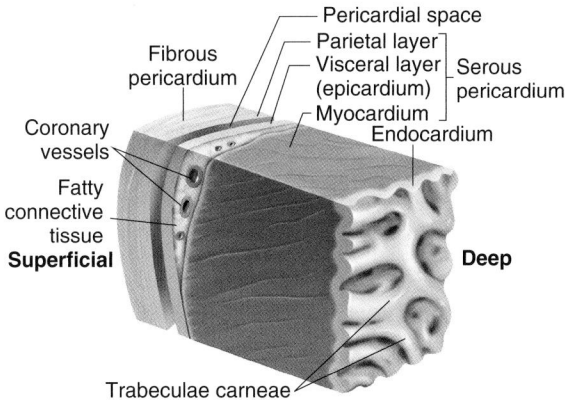

Pericardium *(Patton and Thibodeau, 2016)*

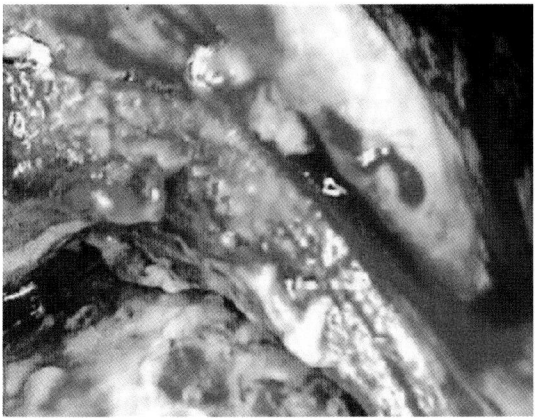

Intraoperative view of the exposed pericardium
(Vindas-Cordero et al, 2008)

pericarp, *n.,* the part of a plant that develops from the ovary wall and surrounds the seeds.

pericholangitis /per′əkō′lanjī″tis/ [Gk, *peri* + *chole,* bile, *angeion,* vessel, *itis,* inflammation], an inflammatory condition of the tissues surrounding the bile ducts in the liver. Pericholangitis is a complication of ulcerative colitis and portal hypertension. Treatment of the ulcerative colitis has little effect on the liver disease. See also **ulcerative colitis.**

perichondrial bone /-kon″drē·əl/ [Gk, *peri,* around, *chondros,* cartilage; AS, *ban*], bone that forms in the perichondrium of the cartilaginous template. Also called **chondrial bone, periosteal bone.**

perichondrium /-kon″drē·əm/, a fibrous, irregular connective tissue sheath and membrane surrounding both hyaline and elastic cartilages.

perichrome /per″ikrōm/, a nerve cell in which the stainable chromophil substance is scattered throughout the cytoplasm.

pericolic abscess, an abscess just outside the colon as a result of perforation, complicating diverticulitis. Also called **peridiverticular abscess.**

pericolitis /-kōlī″tis/, an inflammation of the connective tissue around the colon. Also called *pericolonitis.*

pericoronitis /-kôr′ənī″tis/, inflammation of the gum tissue around the crown of a tooth, usually associated with the eruption of a third molar. Treatment depends on the severity of the condition and may include the use of antibiotics, lavage with a copious amount of fluid, removal of the inflamed tissue, or extraction of the tooth. In most cases the inflammation subsides after the tooth has fully erupted.

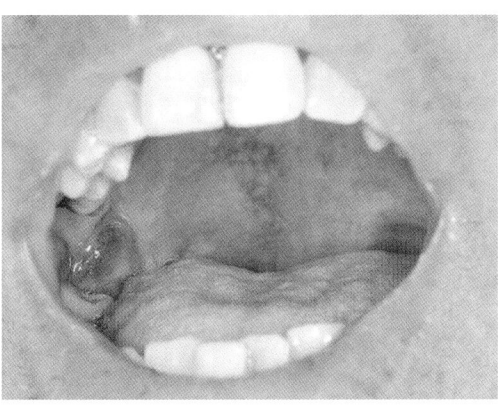

Pericoronitis *(Palmason, Marty, and Treister, 2011)*

pericranium /-krā″nē·əm/, the connective tissue membrane that surrounds the skull.

pericystium /-sis″tē·əm/, the tissues around a gallbladder or urinary bladder.

peridens, a supernumerary tooth found other than in the midline of the dental arch. Compare **mesiodens.**

periderm /per″idurm/, the outermost layer of flattened epidermis on an embryo or fetus during the first 6 months of gestation.

perididymitis /-did′imī″tis/, an inflammation of the tunica vaginalis testis.

peridiverticular abscess. See **pericolic abscess.**

peridontium. See **periodontium,** def. 1.

peridural anesthesia. See **epidural anesthesia/ analgesia.**

periencephalitis /per′i·ensef′əlī″tis/, an inflammation of the membranes and surface of the brain, including the cortex.

perifocal /-fō″kəl/, pertaining to tissues situated around a focus of infection.

perifollicular /-folik″yələr/ [Gk, *peri,* around; L, *folliculus,* small bag], pertaining to the area around a follicle.

perifolliculitis /-folik″yəlī″tis/ [Gk, *peri* + L, *folliculus,* small bag; Gk, *itis*], inflammation of the tissue surrounding a hair follicle. Compare **folliculitis.**

periglottic /-glot″ik/, around the tongue, particularly the base of the tongue.

periglottis /-glot″is/, the mucous membrane of the tongue.

perihepatitis /per′i-hep′ə-ti′tis/, inflammation of the peritoneal capsule of the liver and other nearby tissues.

periimplantoclasia /per′i-implan′tōklā″zhə/, a pathological tissue reaction surrounding implanted foreign material, characterized by local inflammation.

perikaryon /per′iker″ē-on/ [Gk, *peri* + *karyon,* nut], the cytoplasm of a cell body exclusive of the nucleus and any processes, specifically the cell body of a neuron. Also called **cyton.** –*perikaryontic, adj.*

perilymph /per′ilimf/ [Gk, *peri* + L, *lympha,* water], the clear fluid separating the osseous labyrinth from the membranous labyrinth in the internal ear. Compare **endolymph.**

perimenopause /-men″əpôs/, a span of 4 to 6 years preceding menopause when menstrual cycles and blood flow may be irregular. As estrogen levels decline, osteoporosis begins, and women are at increased risk for cardiovascular disease.

perimeter /pərim″ətər/ [Gk, *peri,* around, *metron,* measure], **1.** the circumference, outer edge, or periphery of an object. **2.** an instrument for measuring visual fields. **3.** an instrument for measuring the circumference of teeth.

perimetrium /per′imē″trē-əm/ [Gk, *peri* + *metra,* womb], the serous membrane enveloping the uterus.

perimetry /pərim″ətrē/, the determination and mapping of the limits of the visual field.

perimolysis /-mol″isis/, decalcification of the teeth caused by exposure to gastric acid in patients with chronic vomiting, as may occur in anorexia or bulimia. See **erosion.**

perinatal /per′inā″təl/ [Gk, *peri* + L, *natus,* birth], pertaining to the time and process of giving birth or being born.

perinatal AIDS, acquired immunodeficiency syndrome acquired by infants and children from their mothers during pregnancy, during delivery, or from ingesting infected breast milk. See **acquired immunodeficiency syndrome.**

perinatal asphyxia. See **asphyxia neonatorum.**

perinatal death, 1. the death of a fetus weighing 500 g or more at 22 or more weeks of gestation. **2.** the death of an infant between birth and the end of the neonatal period.

perinatal mortality, the statistical rate of fetal and infant death, including stillbirth, from 28 weeks of gestation to the end of the neonatal period of 4 weeks after birth. Perinatal mortality is usually expressed as the number of deaths in a given period per 1000 live births in a specific geographic area or program.

perinatal period, an interval extending approximately from the 28th week of gestation to the 28th day after birth.

perinatal physiology, the physiology of the process of giving birth or being born.

perinatologic, perinatological. See **perinatology.**

perinatologist /-nātol″əjəst/, a physician who specializes in the diagnosis and treatment of disorders of pregnancy, childbirth, and the puerperium in the mother and child.

perinatology /-nātol″əjē/ [Gk, *peri* + L, *natus,* birth; Gk, *logos,* science], a branch of medicine concerned with the study of the anatomical and physiological characteristics of mothers and their unborn and newborns, with diagnosis and treatment of disorders occurring in them during pregnancy, childbirth, and the puerperium.

perindopril, an antihypertensive.

■ INDICATIONS: It is used to treat hypertension.

■ CONTRAINDICATIONS: A history of angioedema and known hypersensitivity to this drug prohibit its use.

■ ADVERSE EFFECTS: Life-threatening effects are agranulocytosis, neutropenia, proteinuria, and renal failure. Other adverse effects include chest pain, tachycardia, arrhythmias, syncope, anxiety, nausea, vomiting, colitis, diarrhea, constipation, flatulence, rash, purpura, alopecia, hyperhidrosis, visual changes, double vision, dry burning eyes, increased frequency of polyuria or oliguria, rales, angioedema, and hyperkalemia. Common side effects include hypotension, insomnia, dizziness, and tinnitus.

perineal. See **perineum.**

perineal artery, an artery that originates near the anterior end of the pudendal canal and gives off a transverse perineal branch and a posterior scrotal or labial artery to surrounding skin and tissue.

perineal body [Gk, *perineos,* perineum; AS, *bodig*], a mass of tissue composed of muscle and fascia between the vagina and rectum in females and between the scrotum and rectum in males.

perineal care [Gk, *perineos,* perineum], a cleansing procedure prescribed for the perineum after various obstetric and gynecological procedures. Sterile or clean perineal care may be prescribed. It is done also after elimination and as a routine part of hygiene care (bed bath) using clean technique rather than sterile.

■ METHOD: In the sterile procedure the cleansing strokes always move from the vulva toward the anus and from the midline out. After each stroke, the disposable washcloth or pledget is discarded, and a new one is used for the next stroke. A sterile basin, gloves, forceps, pledgets, and pitcher or measure containing sterile solution are used. The draped patient is assisted into position on her back with a bedpan or a disposable pad beneath her buttocks, and 200 to 300 mL of solution is poured over the vulva. Then pledgets moistened with the solution are used to cleanse the area more thoroughly. The pledgets are held with sterile forceps or a sterile gloved hand. The area is dried using sterile pledgets, and the bedpan is removed. The patient then rolls to one side for cleansing and drying of the posterior area. Strokes should always move away from the perineal area. In providing clean perineal care disposable washcloths and a basin or a squeeze bottle of warm water are used. A fresh disposable washcloth is used for each cleansing stroke and each drying stroke. The strokes are always from anterior to posterior. Soap may be used.

■ INTERVENTIONS: Perineal care is given at prescribed intervals and after urination and defecation.

■ OUTCOME CRITERIA: Sterile and clean perineal care is practiced to remove secretions or dried blood from a wound and to prevent contamination of the urethral and vaginal areas or perineal wounds with fecal matter or urine.

perineal dislocation. See **dislocation of the hip.**

perineal membrane, a thick triangular fascial sheet that fills the space between the arms of the pubic arch and has a free posterior border.

perineal pad [Gk, *perineos,* perineum], a cushion of soft material used to cover the perineum to absorb the menstrual flow or to protect a wound or incision.

perineal raphe, a ridge along the median line of the perineum that runs forward from the anus. In the male, it is continuous with the raphe of the scrotum and the raphe of the penis.

perineo-, prefix meaning "related to the perineum": *perineostomy.*

perineocele /per′inē″əsēl′/, a hernia in the perineal area, around the rectum.

perineorrhaphy /per′inē·ôr″əfē/ [Gk, *perineos* + *rhaphe*, suture], a surgical procedure in which an incision, tear, or defect in the perineum is repaired by suturing.

perineostomy /per′inē·os″təmē/, the surgical creation of an opening between the urethra and the skin of the perineal region.

perineotomy /per′inē·ot″əmē/ [Gk, *perineos* + *temnein,* to cut], a surgical incision into the perineum. See also **episiotomy.**

perinephric abscess /-nef″rik/ [Gk, *peri,* around, *nephros,* kidney; L, *abscedere,* to go away], an abscess that develops in the fatty tissue around a kidney. It is usually secondary to an abscess originating earlier in the cortex of the organ. Also called *perinephritic abscess.*

perinephric fat. See **perirenal fat.**

perinephrium /-nef″rē·əm/, the connective tissue around the kidneys.

perineum /per′inē″əm/ [Gk, *perineos*], the part of the body situated dorsal to the pubic arch and the arcuate ligaments, ventral to the tip of the coccyx, and lateral to the inferior rami of the pubis and the ischium and the sacrotuberous ligaments. The perineum supports and surrounds the distal parts of the urogenital and GI tracts of the body. In the female the central fibrous perineal body is larger than in the male; the bulbospongiosus, which is a sphincter around the orifice of the vagina and a cover over the clitoris, does not exist in the male perineum. In men and women the muscles are innervated by the perineal branch of the pudendal nerve. −**perineal,** *adj.*

perinocele, a hernia in the perineum.

perinodal fiber /-nō″dəl/ [Gk, *peri* + L, *nodus,* knot], any of the atrial fibers surrounding the atrioventricular or sinus node.

period /pir″ē·od/, **1.** an interval of time. **2.** one of the stages of a disease. **3.** (in physics) the duration of a single cycle of a periodic wave or event. **4.** See **menses.**

periodic /pir′ē·od″ik/ [Gk, *peri* + *hodos,* way], (of an event or phenomenon) recurring at regular or irregular intervals. −**periodicity,** *n.*

periodic apnea of the newborn, a normal condition in the full-term newborn, characterized by an irregular pattern of rapid breathing followed by a brief period of apnea, usually associated with rapid eye movement (REM) sleep. Apnea in the newborn not associated with REM sleep or with periodic breathing is ominous because it is symptomatic of intracranial bleeding, seizure activity, infection, pneumonia, hypoglycemia, drug depression, or various cardiac defects. See also **sudden infant death syndrome.**

periodic breathing. See **Cheyne-Stokes respiration.**

periodic deep inspiration, an occasional deep breath that may be 1.5 times the normal tidal volume. Many mechanical ventilators can be set to provide a selected number of deep inspirations each hour. The process helps prevent atelectasis. Also called **sigh.**

periodic fever [Gk, *peri,* around, *hodos,* way; L, *febris*], **1.** a hereditary illness with intermittent episodes of fever accompanied by abdominal or pleuritic pain. It affects mainly Sephardic Jews, Armenians, and Arabs. Onset occurs between 10 and 20 years of age. Some cases are complicated by symptoms of arthritis, splenomegaly, and renal amyloidosis that may progress to a fatal kidney disorder. **2.** See **familial Mediterranean fever.**

periodic hyperinflation, a normal phenomenon of unconscious sighing or deep breathing. It tends to occur most frequently during periods of physical inactivity. Because of the apparent need for periodic hyperinflation, an artificial sigh is often programmed into mechanical ventilators. See also **periodic deep inspiration.**

periodicity /pir″ē·ədis″itē/ [Gk, *periodikos,* periodical], events or episodes that tend to repeat at predictable intervals. For example, filarial worms may appear in cutaneous blood vessels at night but not in daylight hours, and malaria may cause paroxysms at 24-, 48-, or 72-hour intervals, depending on the species of pathogen.

periodic peritonitis, periodic polyserositis. See **familial Mediterranean fever.**

periodic table, a systematic arrangement of the chemical elements. An earlier version was devised in 1869 by Dmitri Ivanovich Mendeleev (Russian chemist, 1834–1907). By arranging the elements in order of their atomic weights, he was able to show relationships, such as valency, that occurred at regular intervals and was able to predict the properties of elements still undiscovered in the 19th century. The elements in the modern periodic table are arranged according to atomic number.

periodontal /per′ē·ōdon″təl/ [Gk, *peri* + *odous,* tooth], pertaining to the supporting structures of a tooth, including the fibrous connective tissue (periodontal membrane), cementum, alveolar bone, and gingiva.

periodontal abscess [Gk, *peri,* around, *odous,* tooth; L, *abscedere,* to go away], a localized acute bacterial infection in the area around a tooth. It usually occurs in a site with preexisting periodontal pockets and usually affects the deeper structures of the periodontium. It does not arise from the pulp of the tooth. The infection is classified according to its location in the periodontal tissues, such as lateral, lateral alveolar, parietal, or peridental.

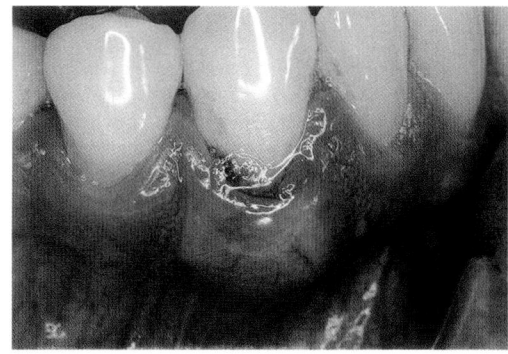

Periodontal abscess *(Newman et al, 2015)*

periodontal disease, a pathological condition of the tissues that support and surround a tooth or teeth, such as inflammation of the periodontal membrane or periodontal ligament or the bony hard tissues surrounding the tooth or teeth. Compare **gingivitis.**

periodontal disease index, a measure developed by Siguard Ramfjord in 1959 based on Russell's Periodontal Index. The index utilizes objective measures of plaque, calculus, and observed physical characteristics of the gingiva and periodontium. Six teeth (3, 9, 12, 19, 25, 28) called Ramfjord's teeth are selected and evaluated. Gingiva is evaluated first with the observation of changes in color, form or shape, presence or absence of stippling, and consistency, followed by measurement of gingival crevice depth.

periodontal index, a measure of an individual's periodontal condition. It is determined by adding scores based on the condition of the gingiva and dividing the sum by the number of teeth present. Individuals with clinically normal gingiva have an index of 0 to 0.2. The index reaches a maximum of 8.0 in persons with severe terminal destructive periodontitis.

periodontal ligament (PDL), the fibrous connective tissue that surrounds a tooth and attaches the tooth to the alveolus. It is composed of many bundles of collagenous tissue arranged in groups, which lie at differing angles relative to the root of the tooth, the alveolus, and the gingiva due to the forces of mastication, between which lies loose connective tissue interwoven with blood vessels, lymphatic vessels, and nerves. Also called **periodontium.**

periodontal pocket [Gk, *peri,* around, *odous,* tooth; Fr, *pochette*], a pathological increase in the depth of the gingival crevice or sulcus surrounding a tooth at the gingival margin. Kinds include **gingival pocket, infrabony pocket, intraalveolar pocket, intrabony pocket, relative pocket, simple periodontal pocket, suprabony periodontal pocket, supracrestal periodontal pocket.**

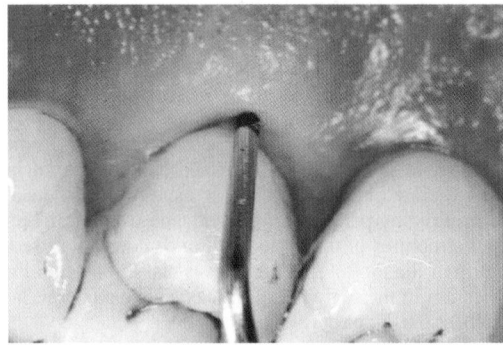

Deep periodontal pocket *(Newman et al, 2015)*

periodontal probe [Gk, *peri,* around, *odous,* tooth; L, *probare,* to test], **1.** a slender, tapered, flat or cylindric instrument with indentations spaced in millimeters, designed for introduction into the gingival sulcus for the purpose of measuring its depth. **2.** a slender tapered instrument with or without millimeter indentations or contrasting colors for measuring furcations of the roots of premolars and molars. Also called **furcation probe.**

periodontics /-don″tiks/ [Gk, *peri,* around, *odous,* tooth], one of the 10 specialties of dentistry; concerned with the diagnosis, treatment, and prevention of diseases of the periodontium. Also called *periodontia,* **periodontology.**

periodontist /-don″tist/, a dentist who specializes in treating the supporting structures of the teeth.

periodontitis /per′ē·ō′dontī″tis/, inflammation of the periodontium caused by a complex reaction initiated when subgingival plaque bacteria are in close contact with the epithelium of the gingival sulcus. Injury arises from toxins and enzymes produced by the bacteria and from host-mediated defense responses. Apical movement of the junctional epithelium, which indicates attachment loss and alveolar bone loss, is diagnostic of periodontitis. See also **periodontal disease.**

periodontium /per′ē·ō·don′shē·əm/ *pl. periodontia* [Gk, *peri,* around + *odous,* tooth], **1.** the tissues that invest or help invest and support the teeth, including the periodontal ligament, gingivae, cementum, and alveolar and supporting bone. Also called **odontoperiosteum, paradentium, periodontium. 2.** See **periodontal ligament.**

periodontoclasia [Gk, *peri* + *odous,* tooth, *klasis,* breaking], the loosening of secondary teeth caused by breakdown and absorption of the supporting bone.

periodontology. See **periodontics.**

perioperative /per′i·op″ərativ/ [Gk, *peri,* around; L, *operari,* to work], pertaining to the time before (preoperative), during (intraoperative), and after (postoperative) surgery.

perioperative nursing [Gk, *peri* + L, *operari,* to work, *nutrix,* nurse], nursing care provided to surgery patients before and during the procedure and in the recovery room.

perioperative nursing data set, a nursing language specialized for vocabulary that addresses the perioperative patient experience from preadmission until discharge. See also **perioperative nursing.**

periorbita /per′i·ôr″bitə/ [Gk, *peri* + L, *orbita,* wheel mark], the periosteum of the orbit of the eye. It is continuous with the dura mater and the sheath of the optic nerve and extends a process at the margin of the orbit to form the orbital septum. The periorbita is loosely connected to the bones of the orbit, from which it can be easily detached.

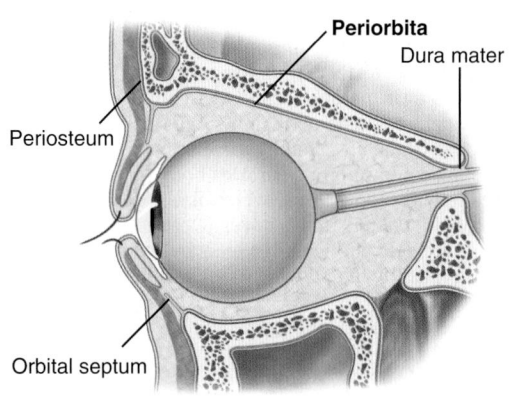

Periorbita *(Drake, Vogl, and Mitchell, 2015)*

periorbital /per′i·ôr″bitəl/, pertaining to the area surrounding the socket of the eye.

periorbital ecchymosis. See **raccoon eyes.**

periosteal /per′i·os″tē·əl/ [Gk, *peri,* around, *osteon,* bone], pertaining to the periosteum, the membrane covering the bones.

periosteal bone. See **perichondrial bone.**

periosteal layer, the outer layer of the dura mater; the periosteum of the cranial cavity. It is firmly attached to the skull and is continuous with the periosteum on the outer surface of the skull at the foramen magnum and other intracranial foramina. See also **dura mater.**

periosteum /per′i·os″tē·əm/ [Gk, *peri* + *osteon,* bone], a thick, fibrous vascular membrane covering the bones, except at their extremities. It consists of an outer layer of collagenous tissue containing a few fat cells and an inner layer of fine elastic fibers. Periosteum is permeated with the nerves and blood vessels that innervate and nourish underlying bone. The membrane is thick and markedly vascular over young bones but thinner and less vascular in later life. Bones that lose periosteum through injury or disease usually scale or die.

periostitis /per′i·ostī″tis/ [Gk, *peri* + *osteon,* bone, *itis*], inflammation of the periosteum. The condition is caused by chronic or acute infection or trauma and is characterized by tenderness and swelling of the affected bone, pain, fever, and chills. In severe cases blood or an albuminous serous exudate forms under the membrane. In syphilitic infections periostitis may occur as an early symptom.

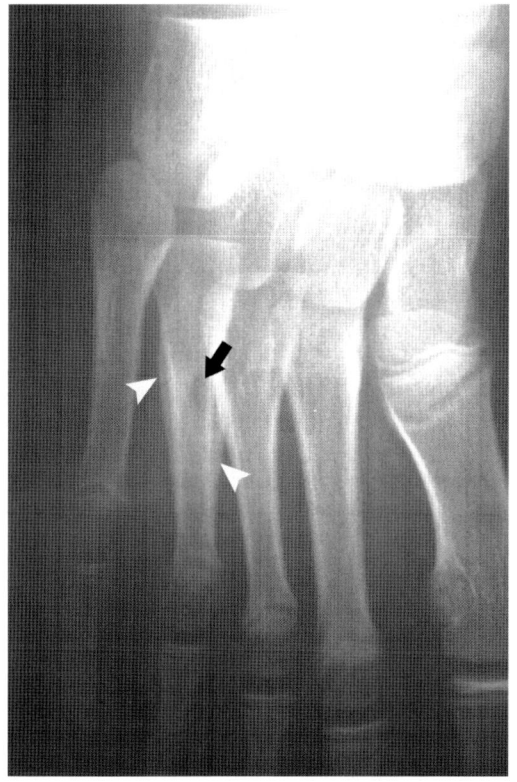

Periostitis *(Suresh, 2011)*

peripatetic /-pətet″ik/ [Gk, *peripatein,* to walk about], pertaining to an ambulatory person, particularly one who travels frequently.

peripelvic cyst. See **renal sinus cyst.**

peripelvic extravasation, extravasation of urine into the area around the renal pelvis.

peripheral /pərif″ərəl/ [Gk, *periphereia,* circumference], pertaining to the outside, surface, or surrounding area of an organ, other structure, or field of vision.

peripheral acrocyanosis of the newborn, a normal transient condition of the newborn characterized by pale cyanotic discoloration of the hands and feet, especially the fingers and toes. The blueness fades as the baby begins to breathe easily but returns if the baby is allowed to become chilled.

peripheral angiography [Gk, *peri,* around, *phereia,* boundary, *angeion,* vessel, *graphein,* to record], the study of the peripheral blood vessels by radiography after radiopaque dye is injected into the circulation.

peripheral arterial disease (PAD), a systemic form of atherosclerosis producing symptoms in the cardiac, cerebral, and renal vascular systems. It affects up to 2% of individuals between 37 and 69 years of age and about 10% of persons over 70 years of age. The incidence is highest among males with diabetes mellitus. Other risk factors include obesity and stress. Blood flow is restricted by an intraarterial accumulation of soft deposits of lipids and fibrin that harden over time, particularly at bends or bifurcations of the arterial walls. Patients generally are not aware of the changes until the diameter of the arterial lumen has been reduced by half. Early symptoms include intermittent claudication and ischemic rest pain. See also **arterial insufficiency.**

peripheral arteriovenography, the radiographic examination of the blood vessels in the peripheral parts of the body, such as the arms and legs, after the injection of a contrast medium into these vessels.

peripheral blood stem cells, stem cells that circulate in the peripheral blood rather than the bone marrow. Their numbers can be artificially increased by exposure to hematopoietic growth factors so that they can be harvested for peripheral blood stem cell transplantation. Also called *peripheral blood progenitor cells.*

peripheral device, any hardware device that may be attached to a computer's central processing unit via a cable or Wi-Fi signal, such as a printer, monitor, or external backup drive.

peripheral giant cell granuloma, a relatively uncommon oral hyperplastic growth in response to gingival injury; it consists of multinucleated giant cells. The cells resemble osteoclasts; some researchers believe the granuloma is a formation of mononuclear phagocytes. The lesion can be sessile or pedunculated and can develop at any age, occurring along the gingiva or the alveolar mucosa, typically anterior to the molars. It is caused by local irritation or trauma but is not thought to be a reparative reaction for the body. A similar lesion located within bone is called a central giant cell granuloma. Compare **peripheral ossifying fibroma, cementifying fibroma.**

peripheral glioma. See **schwannoma.**

peripheral lesion [Gk, *perphereia* + L, *laesio,* hurting], an injury to any tissues distal to the main organ systems. A peripheral nerve lesion is usually traumatic and interrupts the flow of impulses between the site of the lesion and the nerve root or plexus.

peripherally inserted central catheter (PICC), a long catheter introduced through a vein in the arm, then through the subclavian vein into the superior vena cava or right atrium to administer parenteral fluids (as in hyperalimentation) or medications or to measure central venous pressure.

peripheral motor neuron [Gk, *peripheria* + L, *motor,* mover; Gk, *neuron,* nerve], an effector neuron located outside the central nervous system, usually in a ganglion of the sympathetic or parasympathetic nervous system.

peripheral nervous system, the motor and sensory nerves and ganglia outside the brain and spinal cord. The system consists of 12 pairs of cranial nerves, 31 pairs of spinal nerves, and their various branches in body organs. Sensory, or afferent, peripheral nerves transmitting information to the central nervous system and motor, or efferent, peripheral nerves carrying impulses from the brain usually travel together but separate at the cord level into a posterior sensory root and an anterior motor root. Fibers innervating the body wall are designated somatic. Those supplying internal organs are termed visceral. The autonomic system includes the peripheral nerves involved in regulating cardiovascular, respiratory, endocrine, and other automatic body functions. Nerves in the sympathetic or thoracolumbar division of the autonomic system secrete norepinephrine and cause peripheral vasoconstriction, cardiac acceleration, coronary artery dilation, bronchodilation, and inhibition of peristalsis. Parasympathetic nerves, which constitute the craniosacral division of the autonomic system, secrete acetylcholine; cause peripheral vasodilation, cardiac inhibition, and bronchoconstriction; and stimulate peristalsis. Injury to a peripheral nerve results in loss of movement and sensation in the area innervated distal to the lesion.

P

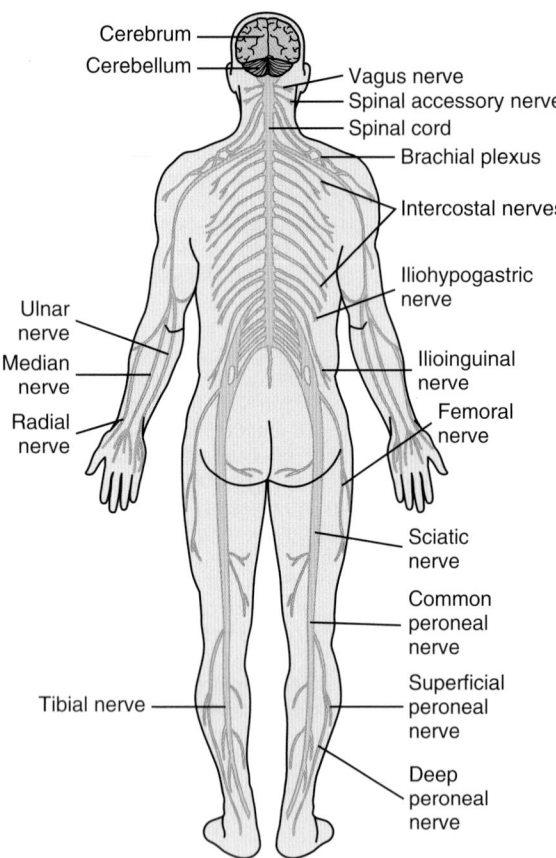

Peripheral nervous system *(Sorrentino, 2015)*

Labels: Cerebrum, Cerebellum, Vagus nerve, Spinal accessory nerve, Spinal cord, Brachial plexus, Intercostal nerves, Iliohypogastric nerve, Ulnar nerve, Median nerve, Radial nerve, Ilioinguinal nerve, Femoral nerve, Sciatic nerve, Common peroneal nerve, Superficial peroneal nerve, Tibial nerve, Deep peroneal nerve

peripheral neuropathy, any functional or organic disorder of the peripheral nervous system. Kinds include **paresthesia.**

peripheral ossifying fibroma, a relatively uncommon benign gingival growth of mesenchymal cells from the periosteum or the periodontal ligament. It is a sessile or pedunculated lesion, containing fibroblastic mineralized tissue surrounded by a fibropurulent membrane. It may resemble a cementifying fibroma. This type of lesion differs from peripheral odontogenic fibromas and central ossifying fibromas.

peripheral plasma cell myeloma. See **plasmacytoma.**

peripheral polyneuritis. See **multiple peripheral neuritis.**

peripheral polyneuropathy. See **multiple peripheral neuritis.**

peripheral pulse [Gk, *periphereia* + L, *pulsare,* to beat], the series of waves of arterial pressure caused by left ventricular systoles as measured in the limbs.

peripheral scotoma [Gk, *periphereia* + *skotos,* darkness, *oma,* tumor], a lost area of the visual field that is located peripherally and does not involve the central 30 degrees of vision.

peripheral vascular disease (PVD), any abnormal condition that affects the blood vessels and lymphatic vessels, except those that supply the heart. Different kinds and degrees of PVD are characterized by a variety of signs and symptoms, such as numbness, pain, pallor, elevated blood pressure, and impaired arterial pulsations. Causative factors include obesity, cigarette smoking, stress, sedentary occupations, and numerous metabolic disorders. PVD in association with bacterial endocarditis may involve emboli in terminal

arterioles and produce gangrenous infarctions of distal parts of the body, such as the tip of the nose, the pinna of the ear, the fingers, and the toes. Large emboli may occlude peripheral vessels and cause atherosclerotic occlusive disease. Treatment of severe cases may require amputation of gangrenous body parts. Less severe peripheral vascular problems may be treated by eliminating causative factors, especially cigarette smoking, and by administering various drugs, such as salicylates and anticoagulants. Kinds include **atherosclerosis, arteriosclerosis.**

peripheral vascular resistance, a resistance to the flow of blood determined by the tone of the vascular musculature and the diameter of the blood vessels. It is responsible for blood pressure when coupled with stroke volume.

peripheral vision, a capacity to see objects in the outer aspects of the field of view caused by reflected light waves that fall on areas of the retina distant from the macula.

peripheral zone, a large area of the prostate, just beneath the capsule, covering the posterior and lateral aspects and composed mainly of acinar glandular tissue. Its ducts drain into the prostatic urethra along most of its length.

periphery /pərif″ərē/ [Gk, *peri,* around, *phereia,* boundary], **1.** parts or areas near or outside a perimeter or boundary. **2.** the outer body parts, such as the skin or limbs.

perirectal /-rek″təl/ [Gk, *peri,* around; L, *rectus,* straight], pertaining to the area around the rectum.

perirenal fat, an accumulation of extraperitoneal fat that completely surrounds the kidney. Enclosing this fat is a membranous condensation of extraperitoneal fascia, the renal fascia. Also called **perinephric fat.** See also **pararenal fat.**

perirenal hematoma, a hematoma resulting from a perirenal hemorrhage.

perirenal hemorrhage, hemorrhage from the kidney into the perirenal space, such as from trauma, vasculitis, aneurysm, tumor, renal infarct, or cyst.

perirenal space, the part of the retroperitoneal space that is within the renal fascia and contains the kidney, perirenal fat, adrenal gland, and proximal ureter. Also called *perinephric space.*

perisinusitis /-sī′nəsī·tis/ [Gk, *peri,* around; L, *sinus,* hollow], an inflammation of the structures around a sinus.

peristalsis /-stal″sis, -stôl″sis/ [Gk, *peri* + *stalsis,* contraction], the coordinated, rhythmic, serial contraction of smooth muscle that forces food through the digestive tract, bile through the bile duct, and urine through the ureters.

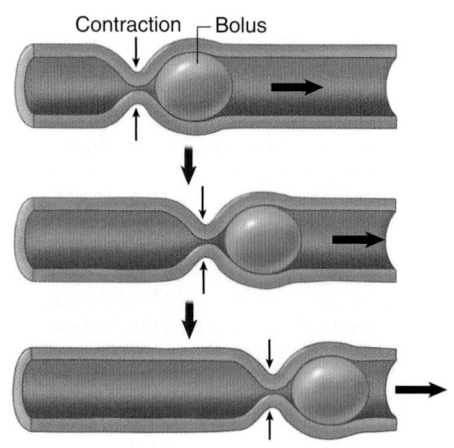

Peristalsis *(Patton and Thibodeau, 2016)*

Labels: Contraction, Bolus

peristaltic /-stal″tik, -stôl″tik/ [Gk, *peri* + *stalsis,* contraction], pertaining to peristalsis.

peristaltic rush, a powerful wave of contractile activity that travels long distances down the small intestine, caused by intense irritation or unusual distension. Also called *peristaltic reflex.*

peristomal /per′istō″məl/, pertaining to the area of skin surrounding a stoma in the abdominal wall.

peritoneal /-tənē″əl/ [Gk, *peri* + *teinein,* to stretch], pertaining to the peritoneum.

peritoneal abscess [Gk, *peri* + *teinein* + L, *abscedere,* to go away], an abscess in the peritoneal cavity, the result of peritonitis and usually complicated by adhesions.

peritoneal cavity [Gk, *peri* + *teinein,* to stretch], the potential space between the parietal and visceral layers of the peritoneum, which are normally in contact. The peritoneal cavity is divided into the greater and lesser sac. The greater sac is the peritoneal cavity, and the lesser sac is the omental bursa. The omental bursa is associated with the dorsal surface of the stomach and the surrounding structures. See also **omental foramen.**

peritoneal dialysis (PD), a dialysis procedure performed to correct an imbalance of fluid or of electrolytes in the blood or to remove toxins, drugs, or other wastes normally excreted by the kidney. The peritoneum is used as a diffusible membrane. Peritoneal dialysis may be performed nightly for chronically ill children while they sleep and also may be carried out regularly at home. It is contraindicated in patients with extensive intraabdominal adhesions, localized peritoneal infection, and gangrenous or perforated bowels, although peritonitis may itself sometimes be treated by peritoneal lavage and antibiotics administered during peritoneal dialysis.

■ METHOD: Under local anesthesia a many-eyed catheter is sutured in place in the peritoneum and a sterile dressing is applied. The catheter is connected to the inflow and outflow tubing with a Y connector, and the air in the tubing is displaced by the dialysate to prevent introduction of air into the peritoneal cavity. The amount and the kind of dialysate and the length of time for each exchange cycle vary with the age, size, and condition of the patient. There are three phases in each cycle. During inflow the dialysate is introduced into the peritoneal cavity. During equilibration (swell) the dialysate remains in the peritoneal cavity. By means of osmosis, diffusion, and filtration, the needed electrolytes pass via the vascular peritoneum to the blood vessels of the abdominal cavity, and the waste products pass from the blood vessels through the vascular peritoneum into the dialysate. During the third phase (drain) the dialysate is allowed to drain from the peritoneal cavity by gravity.

■ INTERVENTIONS: The fluid is warmed to body temperature before instillation, and heparin, antibiotics, or other substances may be added to the dialysate. The patient's fluid balance, respirations, pulse, blood pressure, temperature, and mental state are frequently evaluated, and blood glucose and electrolyte levels are tested regularly. The amount of fluid instilled and the amount and character of the fluid drained are noted. Bacteriological cultures of the drainage are performed regularly. A daily diet that is low in sodium, high in fat and carbohydrates, and that includes 20 to 40 g of protein is usually offered. Medication for pain may be necessary. Most peritoneal dialysis is now done in the home, not in facility. A visiting nurse referral is done for appropriate teaching and assessment with follow-up in dialysis centers. The need for dialysis and the techniques, dangers, and advantages of peritoneal dialysis are explained to the patient and the family.

■ OUTCOME CRITERIA: Peritoneal dialysis may result in several complications, including perforation of the bowel, peritonitis, atelectasis, pneumonia, pulmonary edema, hyperglycemia, hypovolemia, hypervolemia, and adhesions. Peritonitis, the most common problem, is usually caused by failure to use aseptic technique and is characterized by fever, cloudy dialysate, leukocytosis, and abdominal discomfort. Dialysis may usually be continued while the infection is treated with antibiotics, which are given systemically or intraperitoneally. Atelectasis and pneumonia may result from compression of the thoracic cavity, with decreased respiratory excursion and blood flow to the bases of the lungs caused by an excessive volume of dialysate in the peritoneal cavity. Dyspnea, tachypnea, rales, and tachycardia require reevaluating the amount of dialysate, raising the head of the bed, and administering respiratory therapy to prevent atelectasis and pneumonia. Because patients with diabetes are at risk of developing hyperglycemia, serum and urine glucose levels are monitored, and, if necessary, sorbitol may be substituted for glucose in the dialysate. If dialysate fluid is retained in the peritoneal cavity, hypervolemia may occur, predisposing the patient to pulmonary edema and congestive heart failure. If the dialysate is removed too rapidly or if the dialysate used is a hypotonic glucose solution, hypovolemia may result. Adhesions often develop as a result of local irritation to the surrounding tissues caused by the intraperitoneal catheter.

peritoneal dialysis solution, a solution of electrolytes and other substances that is introduced into the peritoneum to remove toxic substances from the body in some patients with renal failure.

peritoneal endometriosis [Gk, *peri* + *teinein,* to stretch, *endon,* within, *metra,* womb], ectopic endometrial tissue found in the pelvic cavity. See also **implantation endometriosis.**

peritoneal equilibration test, the calculation of the ratio of plasma to dialysis solution concentrations of solutes, such as creatinine and glucose, after a certain specific dwell time.

peritoneal fluid, a naturally produced fluid in the abdominal cavity that lubricates surfaces, thereby preventing friction between the peritoneal membrane and internal organs.

peritoneo-, prefix meaning "peritoneum": *peritoneal, peritonitis.*

peritoneoscope. See **laparoscope.**

peritoneoscopy /-tō′nē-os″kəpē/ [Gk, *peri* + *teinein* + *skopein,* to view], the use of an endoscope to inspect the peritoneum through a stab incision in the abdominal wall.

peritoneum /per′itōnē″əm/ [Gk, *peri* + *teinein,* to stretch], an extensive serous membrane that lines the entire abdominal wall of the body and is reflected over the contained viscera. It is divided into the parietal peritoneum and the visceral peritoneum. In men the peritoneum is a closed membranous sac. In women it is perforated by the free ends of the uterine tubes. The free surface of the peritoneum is smooth mesothelium, lubricated by serous fluid that permits the viscera to glide easily against the abdominal wall and against one another. The mesentery of the peritoneum fans out from the main membrane to suspend the small intestine. Other parts of the peritoneum are the transverse mesocolon, the greater omentum, and the lesser omentum.

peritonitis /per′itəni″tis/ [Gk, *peri* + *teinein,* to stretch, *itis*], an inflammation of the peritoneum. It is produced by bacteria or irritating substances introduced into the abdominal cavity by a penetrating wound or perforation of an organ in the GI tract or the reproductive tract. Peritonitis is caused most commonly by rupture of the appendix but also occurs after perforations of intestinal diverticula, peptic ulcers, gangrenous gallbladders, gangrenous obstructions of the small

P

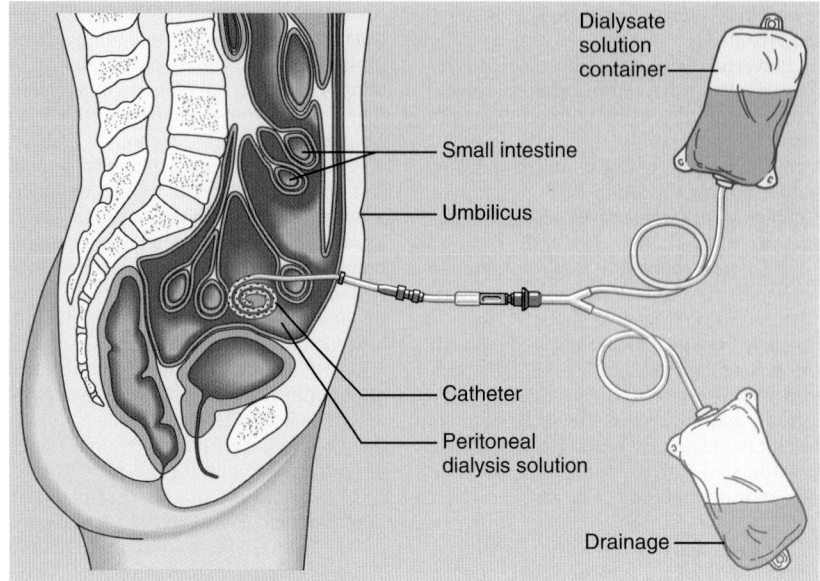

Peritoneal dialysis (Goldman et al, 2004)

bowel, or incarcerated hernias, as well as ruptures of the spleen, liver, ovarian cyst, or fallopian tube, especially in ectopic pregnancy. In some cases, peritonitis is secondary to the release of pancreatic enzymes, bile, or digestive juices of the upper GI tract, and there are reports of postoperative peritonitis caused by cornstarch used to powder surgical gloves. The bacteria most frequently identified as causative agents in peritonitis are *Escherichia coli, Bacteroides, Fusobacterium,* and anaerobic and aerobic streptococci. Pneumococci occasionally found in peritonitis in girls are thought to enter the abdominal cavity via the vagina and fallopian tubes. See also **acute diffuse peritonitis, adhesive peritonitis.**
■ OBSERVATIONS: Characteristic signs and symptoms include abdominal distension, rigidity and pain, rebound tenderness, decreased or absent bowel sounds, nausea, vomiting, and tachycardia. The patient has chills and fever; breathes rapidly and shallowly; is anxious, dehydrated, and unable to defecate; and may vomit fecal material. Leukocytosis, an electrolyte imbalance, and hypovolemia are usually present, and shock and heart failure may ensue.

peritonitis meconium [Gk, *peri* + *teinein,* to stretch, *itis,* inflammation, *mekon,* poppy], a condition of peritonitis in a newborn resulting from rupture of the digestive tract. The inflammation is caused by leakage of meconium, or fecal contents, into the peritoneal cavity.

peritonsillar /-ton″silər/ [Gk, *peri* + L, *tonsilla*], pertaining to the area around a tonsil.

peritonsillar abscess [Gk, *peri* + L, *tonsilla,* tonsil, *abscedere,* to go away], an infection of tissue between the tonsil and pharynx, usually after acute follicular tonsillitis. The symptoms include dysphagia, pain radiating to the ear, and fever. Redness and swelling of the tonsil and adjacent soft palate are present. Treatment includes antibiotics, warm saline solution irrigation, incision and drainage with suction if there is no spontaneous rupture of the abscess, and sometimes tonsillectomy. Also called **quinsy.** Compare **parapharyngeal abscess, retropharyngeal abscess.** See also **tonsillitis.**

peritubular capillary, any of the capillaries around the proximal and distal convoluted tubules of the kidney.

perityphlitis. See **paratyphlitis.**

periumbilical /per′i·umbil″ikəl/ [Gk, *peri,* around, *umbilicus,* navel], pertaining to the area around the umbilicus.

periungual /per′i·ung″gwəl/ [Gk, *peri* + L, *unguis,* nail], pertaining to the area around the fingernails or the toenails.

periurethral zone, a narrow area of the prostate consisting of the short ducts adjacent to the prostatic urethra. It is sometimes a site of benign prostatic hyperplasia, but not as commonly as the transitional zone.

periurethritis /per″-u″rĕ-thri′tis/, inflammation of the tissue around the urethra. Also called **spongiositis.**

perivascular goiter /per′ivas″kyōōlər/ [Gk, *peri* + L, *vasculum,* little vessel, *guttur,* throat], an enlargement of the thyroid gland surrounding a large blood vessel.

perivascular spaces [Gk, *peri,* around; L, *vasculum,* little vessel, *spatium,* space], spaces that surround blood vessels as they enter the brain. They communicate with the subarachnoid space. Also called **Virchow-Robin spaces, Virchow's spaces.**

perivertebral /-vur′təbrəl/ [Gk, *peri,* around, *vertebra,* joint], pertaining to the area around a vertebra.

perivesical spaces, subdivisions of the extraperitoneal space found anterior to the urinary bladder.

perivitelline /-vitel″ēn/ [Gk, *peri* + L, *vitellus,* yolk], surrounding the vitellus or yolk mass.

perivitelline space, the space between a mammalian ovum and the zona pellucida, into which the polar bodies are released at the time of maturation. In some animals it is a fluid-filled space that separates the fertilization membrane from the vitelline membrane surrounding the ovum after the penetration of a spermatozoon.

Perkin's line, a line through the anterior inferior iliac spine, perpendicular to Hilgenreiner's line, used in radiographic assessment of the hip joint.

perle /purl, perl/ [Fr, pearl], a soft gelatin capsule filled with liquid medicine.

perlèche, single or multiple fissures and cracks at the corner of the mouth on one side or both sides, which in advanced stages may spread to the lips and cheeks. Causes include primary or superimposed infection with microorganisms, such as *Candida albicans,* staphylococci, or streptococci; poor hygiene; drooling of saliva; overclosure of the jaws in patients without teeth or with ill-fitting dentures; or riboflavin deficiency. Also called **angular cheilitis, angular cheilosis, angular stomatitis.** See also **cheilitis, cheilosis.**

perlingual /pərling′gwəl/ [L, *per + lingua,* tongue], pertaining to the administration of drugs through the tongue, which absorbs substances through its surface. See also **sublingual administration of a medication.**

permanent dentition, adult teeth. See **secondary dentition.**

permanent pacemaker [L, *permanere,* to remain, *passus,* step; ME, *maken*], any electric pacemaker implanted inside a patient's body for permanent use.

permanent teeth. See **secondary dentition.**

permeability /pur″mē·əbil′itē/ [L, *permeare,* to pass through], the degree to which one substance allows another substance to pass through it. See also **capillary permeability, magnetic permeability, osmosis. –permeable,** *adj.*

permeable /pur′mē·əbəl/ [L, to pass through], a condition of allowing fluids and certain other substances to pass through, such as a permeable membrane. See also **osmosis.**

per member per month (PMPM), usual unit of measure for capitation payments that payers provide to providers, both hospitals and physicians. These payments also include ancillary service use.

permethrin /pərmeth″rin/, a topical pediculicide and scabicide.
- INDICATIONS: It is used for the treatment of head lice and their nits, for the treatment of scabies, and as prophylaxis when there are epidemics of lice.
- CONTRAINDICATIONS: Allergies to pyrethrin, pyrethroids, or chrysanthemum flowers prohibit its use.
- ADVERSE EFFECTS: Among reported adverse effects are itching, mild burning or stinging, numbness, discomfort, mild erythema, and scalp rash.

permissible dose /pərmis″ibəl/ [L, *permittere,* to permit, *dosis,* something given], the maximum amount of radiation that may be expected to produce no significantly harmful results if given to an individual over a specific amount of time.

permissible exposure limit (PEL), an occupational health standard instituted to safeguard workers against exposure to toxic material in the workplace. PELs are the result of the 1970 U.S. Occupational Safety and Health Act, which established the Occupational Safety and Health Administration (OSHA), the policing and enforcing arm of the act, and the National Institute for Occupational Safety and Health (NIOSH), which represents the research arm. OSHA publishes PELs and short-term exposure limits based on recommendations of NIOSH. Also called *permissible exposure level.*

permissive hypercapnia, ventilation that allows $PaCO_2$ to rise slowly over time as the pH becomes normalized. The goal is to reduce tidal volume and rate while preventing volutrauma during mechanical ventilation. Patients may need to be sedated during this.

Permitil, a tranquilizer. Brand name for **fluphenazine hydrochloride.**

pernicious /pərnish″əs/ [L, *perniciosus,* destructive], potentially injurious, destructive, or fatal unless treated, such as pernicious anemia.

pernicious anemia [L, *perniciosus,* destructive; Gk, *a + haima,* not blood], a rare autoimmune form of megaloblastic anemia that results from autoantibodies to parietal cells and intrinsic factor essential for the absorption of cyanocobalamin (vitamin B_{12}). The maturation of red blood cells in bone marrow becomes disordered, the white blood cell count is reduced, and the polymorphonuclear neutrophils become hypersegmented. Weakness, numbness and tingling in the extremities, fever, pallor, anorexia, and weight loss may occur. The condition is usually treated with cyanocobalamin injection and with folic acid and iron therapy. Also called *Addison anemia.* See also **atrophic gastritis, intrinsic factor, nutritional anemia.**

pernicious vomiting [L, *perniciosus,* destructive, *vomere,* to vomit], a severe life-threatening episode of vomiting that may occur during pregnancy. Also called **incoercible vomiting.** See also **hyperemesis gravidarum.**

pernio. See **chilblain.**

pero-, prefix meaning "maimed" or "deformed": *perobrachius, perodactylus.*

perobrachius /pē′rōbrā″kē·əs/ [Gk, *peros,* damaged, *brachion,* arm], a fetus or individual with malformed arms.

perochirus /pē′rōkī″rəs/ [Gk, *peros + cheir,* hand], a fetus or individual with malformed hands.

perocormus. See **perosomus.**

perodactylia. See **perodactyly.**

perodactylus /pē′rōdak″tiləs/, a fetus or an individual with a deformity of the fingers or the toes, especially the absence of one or more digits.

perodactyly /pē′rōdak″tilē/ [Gk, *peros + daktylos,* finger], a congenital anomaly characterized by a deformity of the digits, primarily the complete or partial absence of one or more of the fingers or toes. Also called **perodactylia.**

peromelia /pē′rōmē″lyə/ [Gk, *peros + melos,* limb], a congenital anomaly characterized by the malformation of one or more of the limbs. Also called *peromely.* **–peromelus,** *n.*

-perone, suffix for certain neuroleptics or antianxiety agents.

peroneal /per′ənē″əl/ [Gk, *perone,* brooch], pertaining to the outer part of the leg, over the fibula and the peroneal nerve.

peroneal muscular atrophy, a condition characterized by symmetric weakening or atrophy of the foot and ankle muscles and the development of hammertoes. This disease is a dominantly inherited condition that occurs in a hypertrophic neuropathy form or in a neuronal form. The hypertrophic neuropathy form results in demyelination of nerve fibers and characteristic onion bulb formations. Affected individuals usually have high plantar arches and an awkward gait caused by weak ankle muscles. In the neuronal form this condition usually starts in the second decade of life and causes muscle weaknesses similar to those associated with the hypertrophic neuronal form. Both forms of the disease may also involve mild sensory loss in the lower limbs. Affected individuals may be helped by corrective surgery and leg braces that stabilize weak ankle joints.

peroneo-, combining form meaning "related to the fibula or surrounding area."

peroneus brevis /per′ənē″əs/ [Gk, *perone + L, brevis,* short], the smaller of the two lateral muscles of the leg lying under the peroneus longus. It pronates and plantar flexes the foot. Compare **peroneus longus.**

peroneus longus, the more superficial of the two lateral muscles of the leg. The muscle pronates and plantar flexes the foot. Compare **peroneus brevis.**

peronia /pərō″nē·ə/ [Gk, *peros,* damaged], a congenital malformation or developmental anomaly.

P

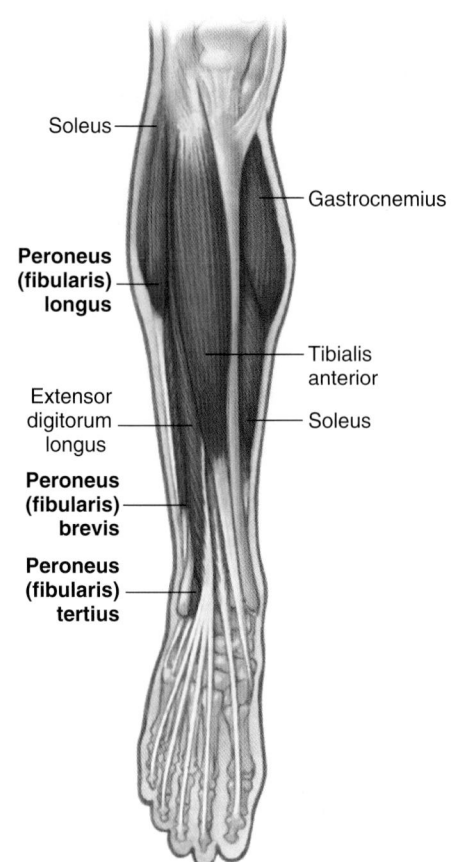

Soleus

Gastrocnemius

Peroneus (fibularis) longus

Tibialis anterior

Extensor digitorum longus

Soleus

Peroneus (fibularis) brevis

Peroneus (fibularis) tertius

Peroneus brevis and peroneus longus *(Patton and Thibodeau, 2016)*

peropus /pərō″pəs/ [Gk, *peros* + *pous,* foot], a fetus or individual with malformed feet, often in association with some defect of the legs.

per os /pər os″/ [L], by mouth.

perosomus /pē′rōsō″məs/ [Gk, *peros* + *soma,* body], a fetus or individual whose body, especially the trunk, is severely malformed.

perosplanchnia /pē′rōsplangk″nē-ə/ [Gk, *peros* + *splanch-non,* viscera], a congenital anomaly characterized by the malformation of the viscera.

peroxide. See **hydrogen peroxide.**

peroxisome /pər-ok′si-sōm/, any of the microbodies present in vertebrate animal cells, especially liver and kidney cells, that are rich in the enzymes peroxidase, catalase, D-amino acid oxidase, and, to a lesser extent, urate oxidase. Their functions are not fully understood, but they participate in metabolic oxidations involving hydrogen peroxide, purine metabolism, cellular lipid metabolism, and gluconeogenesis. See **microbody.**

perphenazine /pərfen″əzēn/, a phenothiazine derivative used as an antipsychotic and antiemetic/antivertigo agent.

■ INDICATIONS: It is prescribed in the treatment of schizophrenia and in the control of severe nausea and vomiting in adults. Unlabeled uses include treatment of ethanol withdrawal, Huntington's chorea, Tourette's syndrome, spasmodic torticollis, and dementia in the elderly.

■ CONTRAINDICATIONS: Parkinson disease, the concurrent administration of central nervous system depressants, liver

or renal dysfunction, severe hypotension, bone marrow depression, blood dyscrasias, or known hypersensitivity to any phenothiazine prohibits its use.

■ ADVERSE EFFECTS: Among the more serious adverse effects are hypotension, liver toxicity, extrapyramidal reactions, blood dyscrasias, and hypersensitivity reactions.

per primam intentionem [L], a notation for a Latin phrase meaning "by primary (first) intention."

per rectum [L], by rectum.

PERRLA /pur″lə/, abbreviation for *p*upils *e*qual, *r*ound, *r*eact to *l*ight, *a*ccommodation. While performing an assessment of the eyes, one evaluates the size and shape of the pupils, their reaction to light, and their ability to accommodate. If all findings are normal, the abbreviation is noted in the account of the physical examination.

Persantine, an inhibitor of platelet aggregation. Brand name for **dipyridamole.**

per se [L], by itself, or of itself.

per secundum intentionem [L], by second intention.

perseveration /pur′səvərā″shən/ [L, *persevero,* to persist], the involuntary and pathological persistence of the same verbal response or motor activity regardless of the stimulus or its duration. The condition occurs primarily in patients with brain damage or organic mental disorders, although it may also appear in schizophrenia as an association disturbance. It is caused by a neurological deficit.

Persian Gulf syndrome, a diffuse collection of symptoms reported by many veterans of the 1991 Persian Gulf war. Symptoms vary widely, but include fatigue, joint pain, headache, and sleep disturbances. Musculoskeletal and connective tissue diseases are also common. The specific cause is unknown, but explanations include exposure to chemicals from burning oil wells, insecticides, and poisons linked to inoculations against biological warfare or to chemical weapons used by the Iraqi army.

persistent depressive disorder, chronic depression lasting at least 2 years in adults and 1 year in children. At least two of the following symptoms are also present: appetite disturbance, sleep disturbance, low energy, low self-esteem, poor concentration or difficulty making decisions, and feelings of hopelessness. Formerly called **dysthymia.**

persistent cloaca /pərsis″tənt/ [L, *persistere,* to persist, *cloaca,* sewer], a congenital anomaly in which the intestinal, urinary, and reproductive ducts open into a common cavity, a result of the failure of the urorectal septum to form during prenatal development. Also called **congenital cloaca.**

persistent vegetative state, a state of wakefulness accompanied by an apparent complete lack of cognitive function, experienced by some patients in an irreversible coma. Vegetative functions and brainstem reflexes are intact, but the cortex is permanently damaged. It is considered by some to be a pejorative term. Also called **unresponsive wakefulness syndrome.**

persona /pərsō″nə/ *pl. personae* [L, mask], (in analytic psychology) the personality façade or role that a person assumes and presents to the outer world to satisfy the demands of the environment or society or to express some intrapsychic conflict. The persona masks the person's inner being or unconscious self. Compare **anima.** See also **archetype.**

personal and social history /pur″sənəl/, (in a health history) an account of the personal and social details of a person's life that serves to identify the person. Place of birth, religion, race, marital status, number of children, military status, occupational history, and place of residence are the usual components of this part of the history, but it may often include other information, such as education; current living situation; and smoking, alcohol, and drug habits. The personal and social history is obtained at the initial interview and becomes a part of the permanent record.

personal assistance. See **custodial care.**

personal care services, the services performed by health care workers to assist patients in meeting the requirements of daily living.

personality /pur′sənal″itē/ [L, *personalis,* role], **1.** the composite of the behavioral traits and attitudinal characteristics by which one is recognized as an individual. **2.** the behavior pattern each person develops, both consciously and unconsciously, as a means of adapting to a particular environment and its cultural, ethnic, national, and provincial standards.

personality disorder, a psychiatric diagnosis characterized by disruption in relatedness. It is manifested in any of a large group of mental disorders characterized by rigid, inflexible, and maladaptive behavior patterns and traits that impair a person's ability to function in society by severely limiting adaptive potential. Kinds include **antisocial personality disorder, borderline personality, passive-aggressive personality disorder.** See also **character disorder.**

personality test, any of a variety of standardized tests used in the evaluation or assessment of various facets of personality structure, emotional status, and behavioral traits. Compare **achievement test, aptitude test, intelligence test, psychological test.** See also **Minnesota Multiphasic Personality Inventory.**

personal orientation, **1.** a continually evolving process in which a person determines and evaluates the relationships that appear to exist between him or her and other people. **2.** the assessment of those relationships derived by a person.

personal protective equipment (PPE), a part of standard precautions for all health care workers to prevent skin and mucous membrane exposure when in contact with blood and body fluid of any patient. Personal equipment includes protective laboratory clothing, disposable gloves, eye protection, and face masks. See also **Standard Precautions.**

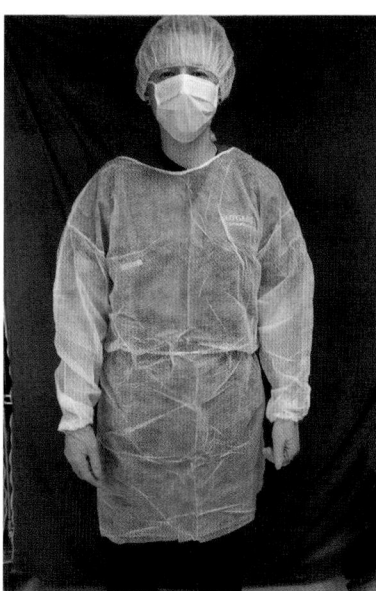

Personal protective equipment: mask, protective clothing, and gloves *(Courtesy Rutgers School of Nursing— Camden. All rights reserved.)*

personal space, the area surrounding an individual that is perceived as private by the individual, who may regard a movement into the space by another person as intrusive. Personal space boundaries vary somewhat in different cultures, but in general they are regarded as a distance of about 1 meter (3 feet) around the individual.

personal unconscious, (in analytic psychology) the thoughts, ideas, emotions, and other mental phenomena acquired and repressed during one's lifetime. Compare **collective unconscious.**

personal zone, an individual protective zone in which the boundaries may contract or expand according to contextual characteristics, usually between 18 inches and 4 feet. Also called **personal space.**

person year, a statistical measure representing one person at risk of development of a disease during a period of 1 year.

perspiration /pur′spirā″shən/ [L, *per* + *spirare,* to breathe], **1.** the act or process of perspiring; the excretion of fluid by the sweat glands through pores in the skin. **2.** the fluid excreted by the sweat glands, consisting of water containing sodium chloride, phosphate, urea, ammonia, and other waste products. Perspiration serves as a mechanism for excretion and for regulation of body temperature. Abnormal amounts of perspiration usually result from organic causes but may also be precipitated by severe emotional stress. Also called **sweat.** Kinds include **insensible perspiration, sensible perspiration.** See also **diaphoresis.** −*perspire, v.*

per tertiam intentionem [L], a Latin notation meaning "by tertiary (third) intention."

Perthes disease, now called **Legg-Calvé-Perthes disease.**

Pertofrane, an antidepressant. Brand name for **desipramine hydrochloride.**

perturbation /pur′tərbā″shən/ [L, *per* + *tubare,* to disturb], a cause or a condition of disturbance, disorder, or confusion.

pertussis /pərtus″is/ [L, *per* + *tussis,* cough], an acute, highly contagious respiratory disease characterized by paroxysmal coughing that ends in a loud whooping inspiration. It occurs primarily in infants and in children less than 4 years of age who have not been immunized. The causative organism, *Bordetella pertussis,* is a small, nonmotile gram-negative coccobacillus. A similar organism, *B. parapertussis,* causes a less severe form of the disease called parapertussis. Also called **whooping cough.**

■ OBSERVATIONS: Transmission occurs directly by contact or inhalation of infectious particles, usually spread by coughing and sneezing, and indirectly by contact with freshly contaminated articles. Diagnosis consists of positive identification of the organism in nasopharyngeal secretions. The initial stages of the disease are difficult to distinguish from bronchitis or influenza. A fluorescent antibody staining technique specific for *B. pertussis* provides an accurate means of early diagnosis. The incubation period averages 7 to 14 days, followed by 6 to 8 weeks of illness divided into three distinct stages: catarrhal, paroxysmal, and convalescent. Onset of the catarrhal stage is gradual, usually beginning with coryza, sneezing, a dry cough, a slight fever, listlessness, irritability, and anorexia. The cough becomes paroxysmal after 10 to 14 days; it occurs as a series of short rapid bursts during expiration followed by the characteristic whoop, caused by a spasm of the epiglottis, a hurried, deep inhalation that has a high-pitched crowing sound. There is usually no fever, and the respiratory rate between paroxysms is normal. During the paroxysm there is marked facial redness or cyanosis and vein distension, the eyes may bulge, the tongue may protrude, and the facial expression usually indicates severe anxiety and distress. Large amounts of a viscid mucus may be expelled during or after paroxysms, which occur from 4 to 5 times a day in mild cases and as many as 40 to 50 times a day in severe cases. Vomiting frequently occurs after the paroxysms as a result of gagging or choking on the mucus. In infants, choking may be more common than the characteristic whoop. This stage lasts from 4 to 6 weeks, with the attacks being most frequent and severe during the first 1 to 2 weeks, then gradually declining and disappearing. During the convalescent stage a simple persistent cough is usual. For a period of up to 2 years after the initial attack, paroxysmal coughing may accompany respiratory infections.

■ INTERVENTIONS: Routine treatment consists of bed rest, adequate nutrition, and adequate amounts of fluid. Erythromycin or another antibacterial may be prescribed to reduce transmission or to control secondary infection. Hospitalization may be necessary for infants and children with severe or prolonged paroxysms and for those with dehydration or other complications. Oxygen may be needed to relieve dyspnea and cyanosis. IV therapy may be necessary when prolonged vomiting interferes with adequate nutrition. Intubation is rarely necessary but may be lifesaving in infants if the thick mucus cannot be easily suctioned from the air passages. Pertussis immune globulin is available, but its efficacy has not been established and its use is not recommended. Active immunization is recommended with pertussis vaccine, usually in combination with diphtheria and tetanus toxoids in a series of injections at 2, 4, and 6 months of age and boosters at 12 to 18 months and 4 years of age. One attack of the disease usually confers immunity, although some second, usually mild, episodes have occurred.

■ PATIENT CARE CONSIDERATIONS: Severe paroxysms in an infant may require oxygen, suction, and intubation. The child needs to be kept calm and protected from respiratory irritants such as dirt, smoke, or dust. Overstimulation, noise, or excitement may precipitate paroxysms. Adequate nutrition and adequate fluids are encouraged through frequent small feedings. Common complications of the disease include bronchopneumonia; atelectasis; bronchiectasis; emphysema; otitis media; convulsions; hemorrhage, including subarachnoid and subconjunctival hemorrhage and epistaxis; weight loss; dehydration; hernia; prolapsed rectum; and asphyxia, especially in infants. Paroxysms can be fatal.

pertussis immune globulin, a passive immunizing agent against whooping cough. See also **pertussis.**

■ INDICATIONS: It is prescribed for immediate, but short-lived, immunization against whooping cough.

■ CONTRAINDICATIONS: Known hypersensitivity to this drug prohibits its use.

■ ADVERSE EFFECTS: Among the more serious adverse effects is anaphylaxis.

pertussis vaccine, an active immunizing agent.

■ INDICATIONS: It is prescribed for immunization against pertussis when the administration of diphtheria, pertussis, and tetanus vaccine is contraindicated.

■ CONTRAINDICATIONS: Thrombocytopenia or known hypersensitivity to the vaccine prohibits its use.

■ ADVERSE EFFECTS: Among the most serious adverse reactions are severe allergic reactions, pain and induration at the site of injection, and fever.

per vaginam [L], via the vagina.

pervasive developmental disorders, 1. a collection of disorders marked by delays in communication and social development; difficulty in understanding language relating to events, objects, or people; atypical play skills and transitions; and repetitive movements or maladaptive behavioral patterns. See also **autism spectrum disorders. 2.** a group

of pediatric health conditions affecting a variety of bodily functions and structures with a wide range of severity.

perversion /pərvur″shən/ [L, *pervertere,* to turn about], 1. any deviation from what is considered normal or natural. 2. the act of causing a change from what is normal or natural. 3. *(Informal)* (in psychiatry) any of a number of sexual practices that deviate from what is considered normal adult behavior. See also **paraphilia.**

pervert /pur″vərt/ [L, *pervertere*], 1. *(Informal)* a person whose sexual pleasure is derived from stimuli almost universally regarded as unnatural, such as a fetishist or sadomasochist; a paraphiliac. 2. one whose sexual behavior deviates from a social or statistical norm but is not necessarily pathological.

pes /pēz, pās/ *pl. pedes* [L, foot], the foot or a footlike structure.

pes cavus. See **clawfoot.**

pes equinus [L, *pes* foot, *equinus,* pertaining to a horse], a deformity of the foot in which the toes are extremely flexed, walking is done on the dorsal surface of the toes, and the heel does not touch the ground. Treatment is by splinting, serial casts, or surgery. Also called **talipes equinus.**

pes planus. See **flatfoot.**

pessary /pes″ərē/ [Gk, *pessos,* oval stone], a device inserted in the vagina to treat uterine prolapse, uterine retroversion, or cervical incompetence. It is used in the treatment of women whose advanced age or poor general condition precludes surgical repair. Pessaries are also used in younger women in evaluating symptomatic uterine retroversion and in managing cervical incompetence in pregnancy. A pessary must be removed, usually daily, for cleaning. A Smith-Hodge pessary is a rubber- or vinyl-covered wire rectangle that fits between the pubic bone and the posterior vaginal fornix, supporting the uterus and holding the cervix in a posterior position. A Gellhorn pessary is an inflexible device made of acrylic resin or plastic (Lucite) in the form of a large collar button. It has a canal through the stem that allows drainage of vaginal secretions. The large end of the pessary is placed deep in the vagina, the small end of the stem protruding at the introitus. A doughnut pessary is a permanently inflated flexible rubber doughnut that is inserted to support the uterus by blocking the canal of the vagina. An inflatable pessary is a collapsible rubber doughnut to which a flexible stem containing a rubber valve is attached. The collapsed pessary is inserted, inflated with a bulb similar to that of a sphygmomanometer, and deflated for removal. A bee cell pessary is a soft rubber cube. In each face of the cube is a conical depression that acts as a suction cup when the pessary is in the vagina. A diaphragm pessary is a contraceptive diaphragm used for uterovaginal support. A similar device of somewhat heavier construction is sometimes used. A stem pessary is a slim curved rod that can be fitted into the cervical canal for uterine positioning. It is rarely used today.

pessimism /pes″imiz′əm/ [L, *pessimus,* worst], the inclination to anticipate the worst possible results from any action or situation or to emphasize unfavorable conditions, even when progress or gain might reasonably be expected. *−pessimist, n.*

pesticide poisoning /pes″tisīd/ [L, *pestis,* plague, *caedere,* to kill, *potio,* drink], a toxic condition caused by the ingestion or inhalation of a substance used for the eradication of pests. Kinds include **malathion poisoning, parathion poisoning.** See also **herbicide poisoning, rodenticide poisoning.**

pestilence /pes″tiləns/ [L, *pestilentia,* infectious disease], any epidemic of a virulent infectious or contagious disease.

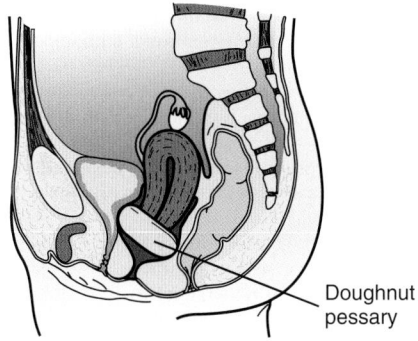

Doughnut pessary to correct uterine prolapse
(Phillips, 2007)

pestis.   See **bubonic plague.**

pes valgus [L, *pes,* foot, *valgus,* bent outward],   deviation of the foot outward at the talocalcanean joint.

PET /pet/,   abbreviation for **positron emission tomography.**

peta-,   prefix indicating a number in the range of 10^{15}.

petaling /pet″əling/,   a process of smoothing the raw or ragged edges of a plaster cast to prevent skin irritation.

petalo-,   prefix meaning "leaf."

petechiae /pētē″kē·ē/*sing.* petechia* [It, *petecchie,* flea-bites],   numerous tiny purple or red spots appearing on the skin as a result of tiny hemorrhages within the dermal or submucosal layers. Petechiae range from pinpoint to pinhead size and are flush with the surface. Compare **ecchymosis.**

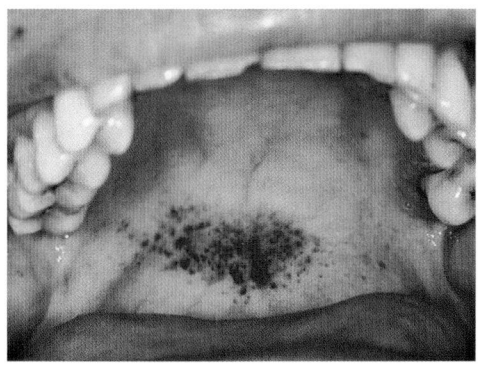

Palatal petechiae *(Eisen and Lynch, 1998)*

petechial [It, *petecchie*],   pertaining to tiny red or purple spots caused by an extravasation of blood into the skin. Compare **ecchymosis.**

petechial fever /pitē″kē·əl/ [It, *petecchie* + L, *febris,* fever],   any febrile illness accompanied by small petechiae on the skin, such as seen in meningococcemia or in the late stage of typhoid fever.

petechial hemorrhage [It, *petecchie* + Gk, *haima,* blood, *rhegnynei,* to gush],   a small discrete hemorrhage under the skin.

pethidine.   See **meperidine hydrochloride.**

petit mal epilepsy.   See **absence seizure.**

petit mal seizure.   See **absence seizure.**

petit pas gait /pet″ē pä, ptē″pä″/,   a manner of walking with short, mincing steps and shuffling with loss of associated movements. It is seen in cases of parkinsonism as well as in diffuse cerebral disease resulting from multiple small infarcts.

Petit's sinus.   See **aortic sinus.**

Petren's gait /pet″rənz/,   a hesitant form of walking in which a patient takes a few steps, halts, and then takes a few more steps. In some cases the patient must be encouraged to begin the next brief walking period. The condition is seen in elderly people and those with paretic disease.

Petri dish /pē″trē, pā″trē/   [Julius R. Petri, German bacteriologist, 1852–1921],   a shallow circular glass dish used to hold solid culture media.

petrification /pet″rifikā″shən/,   the process of becoming calcified or stonelike.

pétrissage /pā″trisäzh″/   [Fr, *petrir,* to knead],   a technique in massage in which the skin is gently lifted and squeezed. Pétrissage promotes circulation and relaxes muscles. Compare **effleurage, rolling effleurage.**

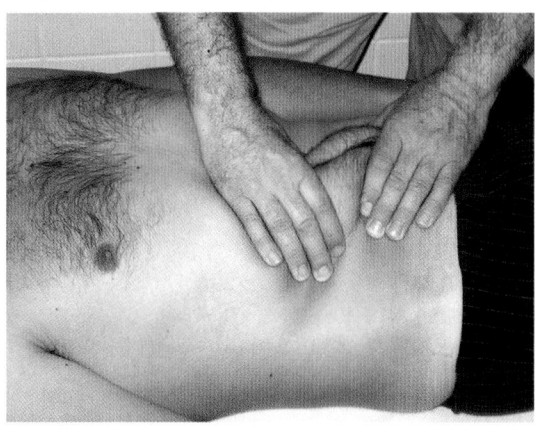

Pétrissage *(Harkreader, Hogan, and Thobaben, 2007)*

petrolatum /pet″rəlā″təm/   [L, *petra,* rock, *oleum,* oil],   a purified mixture of semisolid hydrocarbons obtained from petroleum and commonly used as an ointment base or skin emollient. The common trade name is Vaseline.

petrolatum gauze,   absorbent gauze permeated with white petrolatum.

petroleum distillate poisoning /pətrō″lē·əm/,   a toxic condition caused by the ingestion or inhalation of a petroleum distillate, such as fuel oil, lubricating oil, glue used in making model airplanes or the like, and various solvents. Nausea, vomiting, chest pain, dizziness, and severe depression of the central nervous system characterize the condition. Severe or fatal pneumonitis may occur if the substance is aspirated. Therefore induced emesis is contraindicated. See also **kerosene poisoning.**

petroleum jelly,   a nonliquid colloidal solution or gel of soft paraffin. It is an intermediate product of the distillation of petroleum and is used as a topical soothing medication for burns and abrasions. Also called **mineral jelly.** See also **petrolatum.**

petrosal sinuses,   channels, superior and inferior, that drain the cavernous sinuses into the transverse sinuses. The superior petrosal sinuses receive cerebral and cerebellar veins, whereas the inferior petrosal sinuses receive cerebellar veins and veins from the internal ear and brainstem. Basilar sinuses connect the inferior petrosal sinuses to each other and to the vertebral plexus of veins.

petrosphenoidal fissure /pet″rōsfēnoi″dəl/   [L, *petra,* rock; Gk, *sphen,* wedge, *eidos,* form],   a fissure on the floor of the cranial fossa between the posterior edge of the great wing of the sphenoid bone and the petrous part of the temporal bone.

petrous /pet″rəs/   [L, *petra,* rock],   resembling a rock or stone.

petr-, petro-,   prefix meaning "stone" or "the petrous region of the temporal bone": *petrifaction, petrous.*

P

PET scan, positron emission tomography, or the image obtained from it.

Peutz-Jeghers syndrome /poits′ jeg′ərz/ [J.L.A. Peutz, Dutch physician, 1886–1957; Harold J. Jeghers, American physician, b. 1904], an inherited disorder transmitted as an autosomal-dominant trait, characterized by multiple intestinal polyps and abnormal mucocutaneous pigmentation, usually over the lips and buccal mucosa. If obstruction or bleeding occurs, surgical removal of the polyps may be indicated.

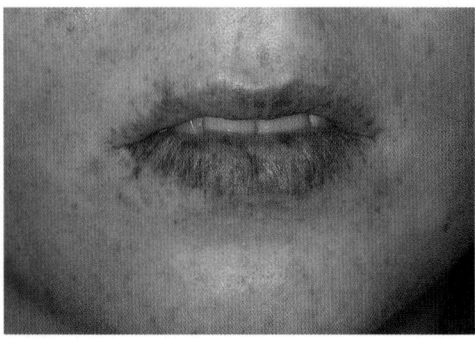

Peutz-Jeghers syndrome *(Regezi, Sciubba, and Jordan, 2012)*

-pexis, -pexia, -pexy, suffix meaning "a fixation of something specified": *cardiomyopexy, mastopexy, retinopexy.*

Peyer's patches, a group of solitary nodules or groups of lymph nodes forming a single layer in the mucous membrane of the ileum opposite the mesenteric attachment. They are oval patches about 1 cm wide that extend for about 4 cm along the intestine. In most individuals they appear in the distal ileum, but they also appear in the jejunum of a few individuals.

peyote /pā·ō″tē/ [Aztec, *peyotl*], **1.** a cactus from which a hallucinogenic drug, mescaline, is derived. **2.** See **mescaline.**

Peyronie disease /pārōnē/ [François de la Peyronie, French physician, 1678–1747], a disease of unknown cause resulting in fibrous induration of the corpora cavernosa of the penis. An association with Dupuytren contracture of the palm has been recognized. The chief symptom of Peyronie disease is painful erection. Palliative treatment includes radiation therapy and intralesional corticosteroid injections. There is no known cure.

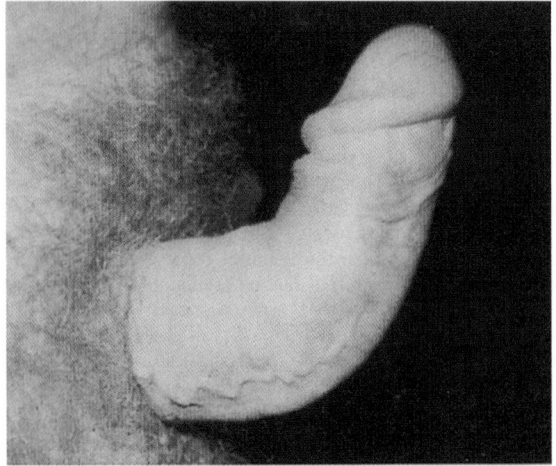

Peyronie disease *(Courtesy Dr. Patrick C. Walsh, The Johns Hopkins University School of Medicine)*

Pezzer catheter /pezā/ [Oscar M. de Pezzer, French surgeon, 1853–1917], a self-retaining catheter with a bulbous tip.

pF, abbreviation for *picofarad.*

Pfizerpen-AS, an antibacterial agent. Brand name for *penicillin G procaine.*

Pflex, an inspiratory muscle trainer designed to increase respiratory muscle strength. See **inspiratory resistance muscle training.**

PFT, abbreviation for **pulmonary function test.**

PG, abbreviation for **prostaglandin.**

PGI₂, abbreviation for **prostacyclin.**

PGY, abbreviation for *postgraduate year,* describing medical school graduates during their postgraduate training as interns (PGY-1, first year), residents (PGY-2, -3, -4), or fellows (PGY-4, -5).

pH, a scale representing the relative acidity (or alkalinity) of a solution, in which a value of 7.0 is neutral, below 7.0 is acid, and above 7.0 is alkaline. The numeric pH value indicates the relative concentration of hydrogen ions in the solution compared with that of a standard (1 molar) solution. It is equal to the negative log of the hydrogen ion concentration expressed in moles per liter. Abbreviation for *potential hydrogen.* See also **acid, acid-base balance.**

Ph, symbol for **phenyl.**

Ph¹, symbol for **Philadelphia chromosome.**

PHA, 1. abbreviation for **paraaminohippuric acid. 2.** abbreviation for **phytohemagglutinin.**

phaco-, phako-, prefix meaning "lens": *phacocele, phacocyst, phacoglaucoma.*

phacolytic glaucoma, an abnormal condition characterized by an acute autoimmune reaction of the eye. It is caused by hypersensitivity of the eye to the protein of the crystalline lens and commonly follows trauma to the crystalline lens or cataract surgery. Associated symptoms include swelling and inflammation of the eye, severe pain, and blurred vision. The substance of the lens is invaded by polymorphonuclear cells and mononuclear phagocytes. Accurate diagnosis must differentiate between this condition and infectious endophthalmitis. Therapy is supportive and commonly includes the administration of corticosteroids and atropine. Refractory cases may require surgical removal of the lens. Also called **endophthalmitis phacoanaphylactica.** Compare **uveitis.**

phacomalacia /fak″ōməlā″shə/ [Gk, *phalos,* lens, *malkia,* softness], an abnormal condition of the eye in which the lens becomes soft as a result of the presence of a soft cataract.

phacomatosis. See **phakomatosis.**

phaeohyphomycosis /fē′ōhī′fōmīkō″sis/, an opportunistic fungal infection, other than mycetoma and chromoblastomycosis, caused by the dematiaceous, or darkly pigmented, molds.

phage. See **bacteriophage.**

-phage, -phag, -phagia, -phagy, suffix meaning "to eat or consume": *bacteriophage, dysphagia.*

phage typing /fāj/ [Gk, *phagein,* to eat, *typos,* mark], the identification of bacteria by testing their vulnerability to bacterial viruses.

-phagia. See **-phage, -phag, -phagia, -phagy.**

phago-, prefix meaning "eating" or "ingestion": *phagocyte, phagocytize.*

phagocyte /fag″əsīt/ [Gk, *phagein* + *kytos,* cell], a cell that is able to surround, engulf, and digest microorganisms and cellular debris. Fixed noncirculating phagocytes include the fixed macrophages. Free circulating phagocytes include the polymorphonuclear neutrophils.

phagocytic /-sit′ik/ [Gk, *phagein,* to eat, *kytos,* cell], pertaining to phagocytes or phagocytosis.

phagocytic vacuole.   See **phagosome.**

phagocytize /fag′əsitīz′/ [Gk, *phagein,* to eat, *kytos,* cell], to engulf and destroy bacteria or other foreign materials. Also called *phagocytose.*

phagocytosis /fag′əsītō″sis/ [Gk, *phagein* + *kytos* + *osis,* condition], the process by which certain cells engulf and destroy microorganisms and cellular debris. The process includes multiple steps: (a) activation when cells move toward a foreign particle, (b) binding of surface receptors on the phagocyte to the surface of the particle, (c) engulfment of the particle, (d) fusing of lysosomes to digest the phagocytosed material with formation of a phagosome, (e) formation of phagolysosomes for the intracellular destruction of microorganisms and pathogens, and (f) eventual expulsion of the residual body from the cell. −**phagocytize,** *v.*

phagolysosome, a cytoplasmic body formed by the fusion of a phagosome, or ingested particle, with a lysosome containing hydrolytic enzymes. The enzymes digest most of the material within the phagosome.

phagosome /fag″əsōm/, a membrane-bound cytoplasmic vesicle within the phagocyte that engulfs it. The vesicle contains phagocytized materials and may fuse with a lysosome, forming a phagolysosome within which the lysosome digests the phagocytized material. Also called **phagocytic vacuole.**

-phagy.   See **-phage, -phag, -phagia, -phagy.**

-phakia, suffix meaning "a lens": *aphakia, keratophakia, pseudophakia.*

phako-.   See **phaco-, phako-.**

phakomatosis /fak′ōmətō″sis/ *pl. phakomatoses* [Gk, *phako,* lens, *oma,* tumor, *osis,* condition], (in ophthalmology) any of several hereditary syndromes characterized by benign tumorlike nodules of the eye, skin, and brain. The four disorders designated phakomatoses are neurofibromatosis (Recklinghausen disease), tuberous sclerosis (Bourneville disease), encephalotrigeminal angiomatosis (Sturge-Weber syndrome), and cerebroretinal angiomatosis (von Hippel-Lindau disease). Also spelled **phacomatosis.**

phal, **1.** abbreviation for **phalanges. 2.** abbreviation for **phalanx.**

phalangeal /fəlan″jē·al/ [Gk, *phalanx,* line of soldiers], pertaining to a phalanx.

phalanges (phal).   See **phalanx.**

-phalangia, suffix meaning "a condition of the bones of the fingers or toes": *symphalangia.*

phalanx /phal/ *pl. phalanges* [Gk, line of soldiers], any of the 14 tapering bones composing the fingers of each hand and the toes of each foot. They are arranged in three rows at the distal end of the metacarpus and the metatarsus. The fingers each have three phalanges (proximal, middle, and distal); the thumb has two. Toes 2 through 5 each have three phalanges; the great toe has two (proximal and distal). The phalanges of the foot are smaller and less flexible than those of the hand.

phall-.   See **phallo-, phall-.**

phallic /fal″ik/ [Gk, *phallos,* penis], pertaining to the penis or penis-shaped.

phallic stage [L, *phallos,* penis, *stare,* to stand], (in psychoanalysis) the period in psychosexual development occurring between 3 and 6 years of age, when emerging awareness and

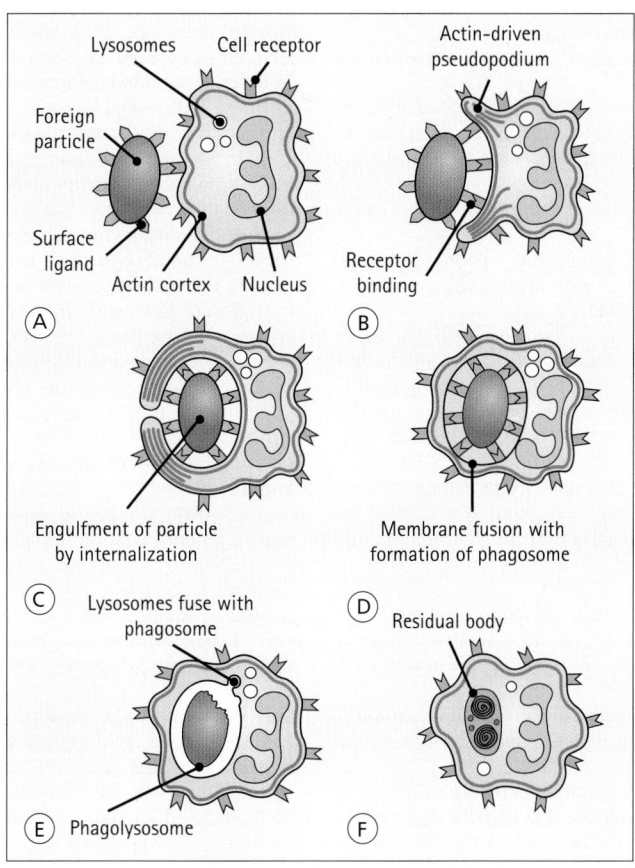

Phagocytosis steps *(Lowe and Anderson, 2015)*

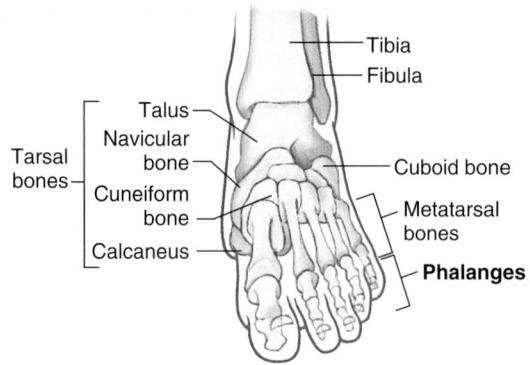

Phalanges of the foot *(Courtesy Yvonne Wylie Walston)*

self-manipulation of the genitals are a predominant source of pleasurable experience. Fixation at this stage may lead to extreme aggressiveness in adulthood, or it may be a precipitating factor in the development of psychosexual disorders. The Oedipus complex and Electra complex develop at this stage. See also **psychosexual development.**

phallic symbol [Gk, *phallos*, penis, *symbolon*, sign], (in psychoanalysis) any object that may be thought to resemble a penis.

phallo-, phall-, prefix meaning "penis": *phallic, phalloplasty.*

phalloidin /faloi″din/, a poison present in the mushroom *Amanita phalloides.* Ingestion of phalloidin results in bloody diarrhea, vomiting, severe abdominal pain, kidney failure, and liver damage. Approximately 50% of phalloidin poisonings are fatal. Also spelled *phalloidine.*

phalloidine poisoning. See **food poisoning, mushroom poisoning.**

phalloplasty /fal″ōplas′tē/, a surgical procedure to lengthen, thicken, reconstruct, or otherwise reshape the penis. It may be performed to correct congenital defects, such as epispadias.

phallus. See **penis.**

-phane, -phan, suffix meaning "a thing with a (specified) appearance."

phantasm /fan″taz′əm/ [Gk, *phantasma*, vision], an illusory image, such as an optical illusion of something that does not exist. See also **phantom vision.**

phantom /fan′təm/ [Gk, *phantasma*, vision], a mass of material similar to human tissue used to investigate the effect of radiation beams on human beings. Phantom materials can range from water to complex chemical mixtures that faithfully mimic the human body as it would interact with radiation.

phantom image, an image that appears in a tomographic image that is not actually in the focal plane. It is created by the incomplete blurring or fusion of the blurred margins of some structures characteristic of the type of tomographic motion used.

phantom limb syndrome, a phenomenon common after amputation of a limb in which sensation or discomfort is experienced in the missing limb. In some people severe pain persists. See also **pseudesthesia.**

phantom tumor, a swelling resembling a tumor, usually caused by muscle contraction or gaseous distension of the intestines.

phantom vision, a sense perception occurring in the form of a visual illusion or hallucination. It is usually regarded as a pseudohallucination in that the person sensing the perception is aware that the phenomenon is illusory. Also called **phantasm, pseudohallucination.**

phao-. See **pheo-, phao-.**

phar, 1. abbreviation for **pharmacy. 2.** abbreviation for **pharmacology. 3.** abbreviation for **pharmaceutic.**

Pharm.B., abbreviation for *Bachelor of Pharmacy.*

Pharm.D., abbreviation for *Doctor of Pharmacy.*

pharmaceutic (phar) /fär′məsoo″tik/ [Gk, *pharmakeuein*, to give drugs], 1. *adj.,* pertaining to pharmacy or drugs. 2. *n.,* a drug.

pharmaceutical chemistry (pharm chem), the science dealing with the composition and preparation of chemical compounds used in medical diagnoses and therapies.

pharmaceutic necessity, a substance having slight or no value therapeutically but used in the preparation of various pharmaceutics, including preservatives; solvents; ointment bases; and flavoring, coloring, diluting, emulsifying, and suspending agents.

pharmacist /fär′məsist/ [Gk, *pharmakon*, drug], a person prepared to formulate, dispense, and provide clinical information on drugs or medications to health professionals and patients, through completion of a university program in pharmacy of at least 4 years' duration and passing state and federal licensure exams.

pharmacodynamics /-dīnam′iks/ [Gk, *pharmakon*, drug, *dynamis*, power], the study of how a drug acts on a living organism, including the pharmacological response and the duration and magnitude of response observed relative to the concentration of the drug at an active site in the organism.

pharmacogenetics /-jənet″iks/ [Gk, *pharmakon*, drug, *genesis*, origin], the study of the effect of the genetic factors belonging to a group or to an individual on the response of the group or the individual to certain drugs.

pharmacognosy, the study of chemicals taken from natural sources to be used as drugs or in the preparation of drugs. Sources may include plants, animals, or other life forms such as fungi, molds, and yeasts.

pharmacokinetics /fär′məkōkinet″iks/ [Gk, *pharmakon* + *kinesis*, motion], the study of the action of drugs within the body, which can, in many respects, be envisioned more accurately as the actions of the body on an administered drug. It includes studies of the mechanisms of drug absorption, distribution, metabolism, and excretion; onset of action; duration of effect; biotransformation; and effects and routes of excretion of the metabolites of the drug.

pharmacological agent /-loj′ik/, any oral, parenteral, or topical substance used to alleviate symptoms and treat or control a disease process or aid recovery from an injury.

pharmacological treatment. See **treatment.**

pharmacological vagotomy, the use of medications to curtail functions of the vagus nerve. Also called **medical vagotomy.**

pharmacologist /fär′məkol′əjist/, a specialist in the preparation, properties, uses, and actions of drugs.

pharmacology (phar) /-kol′əjē/ [Gk, *pharmakon* + *logos*, science], the study of the preparation, properties, uses, and actions of drugs.

pharmaco-, pharmo-, prefix meaning "drugs" or "medicine": *pharmacodynamics, pharmacogenetics, pharmacologist.*

pharmacopoeia /fär′məkəpē″ə/ [Gk, *pharmakon* + *poiein*, to make], 1. a compendium containing descriptions, recipes, strengths, standards of purity, and dosage forms for selected drugs. 2. the available stock of drugs in a pharmacy. 3. the total of all authorized drugs available within the jurisdiction of a given geographic or political area. Also spelled *pharmacopeia.* See also **British Pharmacopoeia, United States Pharmacopoeia.**

pharmacotherapy /-ther′əpē/ [Gk, *pharmakon,* drug, *therapeia*], the use of drugs to treat diseases.

pharmacy (phar) /fär′məsē/ [Gk, *pharmakon*], **1.** the study of preparing and dispensing drugs. **2.** a place for preparing and dispensing drugs.

pharmacy technician, a person who prepares and dispenses prescriptions under the supervision of a pharmacist.

pharm chem, *(Informal)* abbreviation for **pharmaceutical chemistry.**

-pharmic, combining form meaning "drugs" or "medicinal remedies."

pharmo-. See **pharmaco-, pharmo-.**

pharyng-. See **pharyngo-, pharyng-.**

pharyngeal /ferin′jē-əl/ [Gk, *pharynx,* throat], pertaining to the pharynx.

pharyngeal aponeurosis [Gk, *pharynx,* throat, *apo,* from, *neuron,* sinew], a sheet of connective tissue immediately beneath the mucosa of the pharynx.

pharyngeal bursa, a blind sac at the base of the pharyngeal tonsil.

pharyngeal membrane, a thin fold of ectoderm and endoderm that separates the pharyngeal pouches from the branchial clefts in a developing embryo.

pharyngeal nerve, a nerve that passes posteriorly from the pterygopalatine ganglion and through the palatovaginal canal to supply the mucosa and glands of the nasopharynx.

pharyngeal recess. See **torus tubarius.**

pharyngeal reflex. See **gag reflex.**

pharyngeal tonsil. See **adenoid.**

pharynges. See **pharynx.**

pharyngitis /fer′injī″tis/ [Gk, *pharynx* + *itis*], inflammation or infection of the pharynx, usually causing a sore throat. Some causes of pharyngitis are diphtheria, herpes simplex virus, infectious mononucleosis, and streptococcal infection. Acute pharyngitis is a sudden, severe inflammation of the pharynx. Chronic pharyngitis is a persistent throat inflammation that may be associated with the lymphoid granules in the pharyngeal mucosa. Specific treatment depends on the cause. The appearance of the mouth, nose, and throat and throat culture aid in differential diagnosis of a bacterial or viral cause. Symptoms may be relieved by analgesic medication, drinking of warm or cold liquids, or saline solution irrigation of the throat. See also **strep throat.**

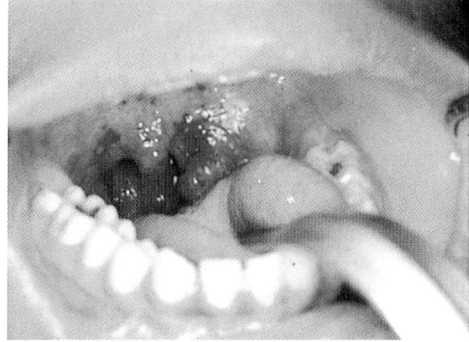

Acute viral pharyngitis *(Courtesy Dr. Edward Applebaum, Head, Department of Otolaryngology, University of Illinois Medical Center)*

pharyngobasilar fascia, a thick layer of fascia that lines the inner surface of the pharyngeal wall and, with the buccopharyngeal fascia, reinforces the pharyngeal wall where muscle is deficient, particularly above the level of the superior constrictor where the pharyngeal wall is formed almost entirely of fascia.

pharyngoconjunctival fever /fəring′gōkon′jungktī″vəl/ [Gk, *pharnyx* + L, *conjunctivus,* connecting, *febris,* fever], an adenovirus infection characterized by fever, sore throat, and conjunctivitis. This epidemic illness is particularly prevalent in the summer, and it is spread by droplet infection and direct contact. Contaminated water in lakes and swimming pools is a common source of infection. See also **adenovirus.**

pharyngoesophageal constriction, the narrowing where the pharynx ends and the cervical esophagus begins, the site of the pharyngoesophageal sphincter.

pharyngo-, pharyng-, prefix meaning "pharynx": *pharyngoplasty, pharyngoscope, pharyngotonsillitis.*

pharyngoplasty /fəring′gōplas″tē/ [Gk, *pharynx,* throat, *plassein,* to mold], surgical repair of the pharynx.

pharyngoscope /fəring′gəskōp/ [Gk, *pharynx* + *skopein,* to view], an endoscopic device for examining the lining of the pharynx.

pharyngoscopy /fer′ing·gos″kəpē/ [Gk, *pharynx,* throat, *skopein,* to view], the examination of the throat with a pharyngoscope.

pharyngotonsillitis /-ton′silī″tis/ [Gk, *pharynx* + L, *tonsilla* + Gk, *itis,* inflammation], an inflammation involving the pharynx and the tonsils.

pharynx /fer″inks/ *pl. pharynxes, pharynges* [Gk], the throat, a tubular structure about 13 cm long that extends from the base of the skull to the esophagus and is situated immediately in front of the cervical vertebrae. The pharynx serves as a passageway for the respiratory and digestive tracts and changes shape to allow the formation of various vowel sounds. The pharynx is composed of muscle, is lined with mucous membrane, and is divided into the nasopharynx, the oropharynx, and the laryngopharynx. It contains the openings of the right and left auditory tubes, the openings of the two posterior nares, the fauces, the opening into the larynx, and the opening into the esophagus. It also contains the pharyngeal tonsils, the palatine tonsils, and the lingual tonsils. Also called **throat.** See also **larynx.**

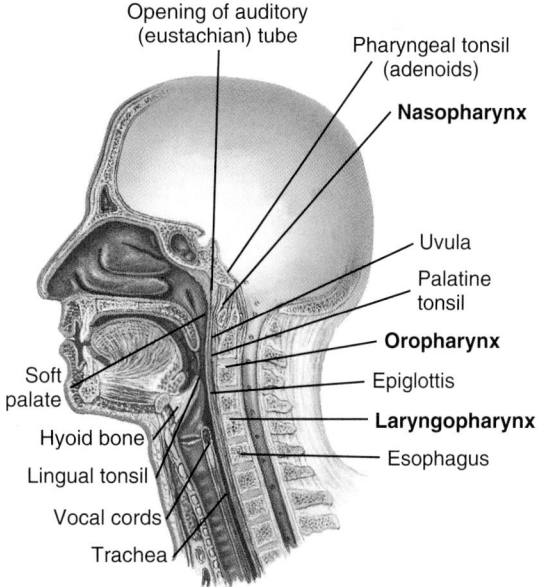

Pharynx *(Thibodeau and Patton, 2007)*

phase /fāz/ [Gk, *phasis,* appearance], in a periodic function, such as rotational or sinusoidal motion, the position relative to a particular part of the cycle.

phase 0, (in cardiology) the upstroke of the action potential.

phase 1, (in cardiology) the initial rapid repolarization phase of the action potential, seen in ventricular and His-Purkinje action potentials.

phase 2, (in cardiology) the plateau of the action potential, occurring during repolarization.

phase 3, (in cardiology) the terminal rapid repolarization phase of the action potential.

phase 4, (in cardiology) the period of electrical diastole. A graph of phase 4 shows a gradual upward slope in a pacemaker cell, whereas phase 4 in a nonpacemaker cell is flat.

phase-contrast microscopy, a type of light microscopy in which a special condenser and objective with a phase-shifting ring are used to visualize small differences in refractive index as differences in intensity or contrast. It is useful in viewing unstained specimens that appear transparent.

phased array /fāzd/, an array transducer assembly that has very thin rectangular elements arranged side by side. It relies on electronic beam steering to sweep sound beams over a sector-shaped scanned region. Beam steering is done by using electronic time delays in the transmitting and receiving circuits.

phase microscope, a microscope with a special condenser and objective containing a phase-shifting ring that allows the viewer to see small differences in refraction indexes as differences in image intensity or contrast. The phase microscope is used especially for examining transparent specimens, such as living or unstained cells and tissues.

phase of maximum slope, the time of rapid cervical dilation and rapid fetal descent in the active phase of labor. See also **Friedman curve.**

phase one study, a clinical trial to assess the risk that may arise from administering a new treatment modality. A phase two study evaluates the clinical effectiveness of the new modality, and a phase three study compares its effectiveness with that of the best existing treatment.

phasic /fā″zik/ [Gk, *phasis*], **1.** pertaining to a process proceeding in stages or phases. **2.** pertaining to a type of afferent or sensory nerve receptor of the proprioceptive system that responds to rate versus length changes in a muscle spindle. It is triggered by such stimuli as quick stretching, vibrations, and tapping.

-phasis, -phasia, -phasic, -phasy, suffix meaning "speech, utterance": *aphasia, bradyphasia.*

Ph.D., abbreviation for *Doctor of Philosophy.*

Phe, abbreviation for **phenylalanine.**

-phemia, a combining form meaning "a (specified) disorder of speech": *aphemia.*

phen-, prefix indicating derivation from benzene: *phenol.*

phenacetin /fənas″itin/, an analgesic no longer marketed because of its carcinogenic properties. Also called **acetophenetidin.**

Phenaphen with Codeine, an analgesic-antipyretic. Also called **acetaminophen, codeine sulfate.**

phenazopyridine hydrochloride /fen′əzōpī″ridēn/, a urinary tract analgesic.

■ INDICATIONS: It is prescribed to reduce the pain of cystitis or other urinary tract infections or to relieve the pain following clinical procedures of the urinary tract.

■ CONTRAINDICATIONS: Renal or hepatic insufficiency or known hypersensitivity to this drug prohibits its use.

■ ADVERSE EFFECTS: Among the more serious adverse effects are headache and GI disturbances.

phencyclidine hydrochloride (PCP) /fensī″klidēn/, a piperidine derivative administered parenterally to achieve neuroleptic anesthesia. Because of its marked hallucinogenic properties, it is not used therapeutically in the United States. Its reported use as an abused substance has declined in recent years. Also called **angel dust.**

phendimetrazine tartrate /fen′dīmet″rəsēn/, a sympathomimetic amine used as an anorectic agent.

■ INDICATIONS: It is prescribed to reduce appetite during the first few weeks of dieting during treatment of exogenous obesity. Its beneficial effects slowly disappear over 3 to 12 weeks.

■ CONTRAINDICATIONS: Cardiovascular disease, hypertension, hyperthyroidism, glaucoma, nervousness, a history of drug abuse, concomitant administration of central nervous system stimulants or monoamine oxidase inhibitors, or known hypersensitivity to this drug prohibits its use.

■ ADVERSE EFFECTS: Among the more serious adverse effects are central nervous system stimulation, elevated blood pressure, insomnia, dry mouth, and tolerance to the drug.

-phene, -phen, suffix denoting members of the phenol group.

phenelzine sulfate /fē′nəlzēn/, a monoamine oxidase inhibitor.

■ INDICATIONS: It is prescribed in the treatment of depression, especially atypical endogenous depression and depression associated with adverse life events.

■ CONTRAINDICATIONS: Liver dysfunction, congestive heart failure, pheochromocytoma, concomitant use of sympathomimetic drugs or foods high in tryptophan or tyramine, or known hypersensitivity to this drug prohibits its use.

■ ADVERSE EFFECTS: Among the most serious adverse effects are orthostatic hypotension, vertigo, constipation, blurred vision, headache, overactivity, and dryness of the mouth. Monoamine oxidase inhibitors produce many adverse drug interactions.

Phenergan, a phenothiazine derivative. Brand name for **promethazine hydrochloride.**

phenic acid. See **carbolic acid, phenol.**

phenobarbital /fē′nəbär″bital/, a barbiturate anticonvulsant and sedative-hypnotic. Also called **sodium phenobarbital.**

■ INDICATIONS: It is prescribed in the treatment of seizure disorders and as a long-acting sedative.

■ CONTRAINDICATIONS: Porphyria, severe pain, respiratory problems, or known hypersensitivity to this drug or other barbiturates prohibits its use.

■ ADVERSE EFFECTS: Among the most serious adverse reactions are ataxia, porphyria, paradoxic excitement, drowsiness, occasional rashes, and, rarely, blood dyscrasias. It is involved in many drug interactions.

phenobarbital-phenytoin serum levels /-fen′itō″in/, the concentration of phenobarbital and phenytoin in the serum, monitored to maintain concentrations sufficient to control seizures but not high enough to cause toxic reactions. The control of seizures is commonly obtained in adults with plasma concentrations of phenobarbital that average 10 mcg/mL per daily dose of 1 mcg/kg; in children, 5 to 7 mcg/mL per daily dose of 1 mcg/kg. The control of seizures is commonly obtained with plasma concentrations of phenytoin that average 10 mcg/mL, whereas toxic effects, such as nystagmus, typically develop with a concentration of 20 mcg/mL. Ataxia may develop at a concentration of 30 mcg/mL and lethargy at a concentration of 40 mcg/mL.

phenocopy /fē′nōkop′ē/ [Gk, *phainein,* to appear; L, *copia,* plenty], a phenotypic trait or condition that is induced by environmental factors but closely resembles a phenotype usually produced by a specific genotype. The trait is neither inherited nor transmitted to offspring. Such conditions as deafness, cretinism, cognitive impairment, and congenital cataracts are caused by mutant genes but can also result from a number of different agents, such as the rubella virus in the case of congenital cataracts. Because phenocopies may present problems in genetic screening and genetic counseling, all exogenous factors must be ruled out before any congenital trait or defect is labeled hereditary.

phenol /fē′nol/ [Gk, *phainein,* to appear; L, *oleum,* oil], **1.** See **carbolic acid. 2.** any of a large number and variety of chemical products closely related in structure to the alcohols and containing a hydroxyl group attached to a benzene ring. The phenols are components of dyes, plastics, disinfectants, antimicrobials, and other drugs, including salicylic acid.

phenol block, neurolytic block using hydroxybenzene (phenol), intended to anesthetize a particular nerve permanently. The technique is sometimes used to control spasticity in specific muscle groups or to block transmission of nerve impulses in chronic pain conditions such as cancers. Morbidity can be high, and pain frequently recurs.

phenol camphor, an oily mixture of camphor and phenol, used as an antiseptic and toothache remedy.

phenol coefficient, a measure of the disinfectant activity of a given chemical in relation to carbolic acid. The activity is expressed as the ratio of a dilution of the chemical that kills in 10 minutes but not in 5 minutes to the 1:90 dilution of carbolic acid, which kills in 10 minutes but not in 5 minutes.

phenolphthalein /fē′nolthal″ē-in, -thā′lēn/, **1.** a cathartic and pH indicator with a range of 8.5 (colorless) to 9.0 (red). **2.** an indicator of hydrogen ion in urine and gastric juice.

phenol poisoning, corrosive poisoning caused by the ingestion of compounds containing phenol, such as carbolic acid, creosote, cresol, guaiacol, and naphthol. Characteristic of phenol poisoning are burns of the mucous membranes; weakness; pallor; pulmonary edema; seizures; and respiratory, circulatory, cardiac, and renal failure. Rarely, esophageal stricture may develop as a complication of extensive tissue damage. Also called **carbolic acid poisoning, carbolism.**

phenolsulfonphthalein /fē′nolsul′fōnfthal″ē-in/, a bright red water-soluble triphenylmethane dye used as an indicator at pH 7.7. Also called *phenol red.* See also **cystochromoscopy.**

phenomenon /finom″ənən/ *pl.* **phenomena** [Gk, *phainomenon,* something seen], a sign that is often associated with a specific illness or condition and is therefore diagnostically important.

phenothiazine /fē′nōthī″əzēn/, a yellow to green crystalline compound that is a source of dyes and is used in veterinary medicine to treat infestations of threadworms and roundworms. It is too toxic for human use, but derivatives of phenothiazine are used in antipsychotic and antihistamine medications. See also **phenothiazine derivatives.**

phenothiazine derivatives, any of a group of drugs that have a three-ring structure in which two benzene rings are linked by a nitrogen and a sulfur. They represent the largest and oldest group of antipsychotic compounds in clinical medicine. Chlorpromazine and prochlorperazine can be viewed as the prototypes of the many phenothiazines and their congeners that are used as adjuncts to general anesthesia and as antiemetics, antipsychotic agents (major tranquilizers), and antihistamines. This group of drugs largely revolutionized the practice of psychiatric medicine, a process that is now continuing with the introduction of the newer atypical antipsychotics such as risperidone and olanzapine. Unlike the barbiturates, which act exclusively on the central nervous system (CNS), the phenothiazines exert significant influence on many organ systems of the body at once. For example, they exert antiadrenergic, anticholinergic, and antihistaminic activity. The effects on the CNS differ according to individual drug and patient status. All phenothiazine tranquilizers are withheld from patients with severe CNS depression or epilepsy and are given with caution to those with liver disease.

phenotype /fē′nətīp/ [Gk, *phainein,* to appear, *typos,* mark], **1.** the complete observable characteristics of an organism or group, including anatomical, physiological, biochemical, and behavioral traits, as determined by the interaction of genetic makeup and environmental factors. **2.** a group of organisms that resemble each other in appearance. Compare **genotype.**

phenoxy-, prefix indicating the presence of a chemical group composed of phenyl and an atom of oxygen: *phenoxybenzamine.*

phenoxybenzamine hydrochloride /fēnok′sēben′zə mēn/, an irreversible (noncompetitive) alpha$_1$-adrenergic receptor blocker producing long-lasting blockade.
■ INDICATIONS: It is prescribed in the control of pheochromocytoma and other instances of hypertensive crisis. If tachycardia is excessive, concomitant administration of propranolol may be necessary.
■ CONTRAINDICATIONS: Hypotension or known hypersensitivity to this drug prohibits its use.
■ ADVERSE EFFECTS: Among the more serious adverse effects are severe hypotension, tachycardia, and GI irritation.

phenoxymethyl penicillin. See **penicillin V.**

phentermine hydrochloride /fen″tərmēn/, a sympathomimetic amine used as an anorectic agent.
■ INDICATIONS: It is prescribed as a short-term adjunct to decrease appetite during treatment of obesity with a regimen of caloric reduction, exercise, and behavioral modification.
■ CONTRAINDICATIONS: Arteriosclerosis, cardiovascular disease, hypertension, glaucoma, hyperthyroidism, or known hypersensitivity to this drug or to other sympathomimetic drugs prohibits its use.
■ ADVERSE EFFECTS: Among the more serious adverse effects are restlessness, insomnia, tachycardia, increased blood pressure, and dry mouth. The combination of phentermine with fenfluramine or dexfenfluramine has been linked to cases of primary pulmonary hypertension, which can be fatal.

phentolamine /fentol″əmēn/, an alpha$_1$-adrenergic receptor blocker.
■ INDICATIONS: It is prescribed in the control of symptoms of pheochromocytoma before and during surgery and for dermal necrosis and sloughing after extravasation of parenteral drugs with alpha-adrenergic effects (e.g., norepinephrine, epinephrine, dopamine).
■ CONTRAINDICATIONS: History of myocardial infarction, angina, coronary artery disease, cerebrovascular disease, renal impairment, or known hypersensitivity to this drug prohibits its use.
■ ADVERSE EFFECTS: Among the more serious adverse effects are tachycardia, cardiac arrhythmias, anginal pain, and hypotension.

phenyl (Ph) /fē′nil, fen′il/, a monovalent organic radical, C_6H_5, derived from benzene.

phenylacetic acid /fen′iləsē″tik/, a catabolite of phenylalanine, excessively formed and excreted (sometimes conjugated with glutamine) in phenylketonuria.

phenylalanine (Phe) /fen′ilal″ənēn/, an essential amino acid necessary for the normal growth and development of infants and children and for normal protein metabolism throughout life. The normal value of this amino acid in serum is less than 3 mg/dL in adults and 1.2 to 3.5 mg/dL in newborns. It is abundant in milk, eggs, and other common foods. See also **amino acid, phenylketonuria, protein.**

P

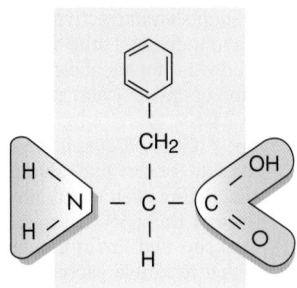

Chemical structure of phenylalanine

phenylalaninemia /fen′il′aləninē″mē·ə/, the presence of phenylalanine in the blood. See also **hyperphenylalaninemia.**

phenyl carbinol. See **benzyl alcohol.**

phenylephrine hydrochloride /-ef′rēn/, an alpha-adrenergic agonist.

■ INDICATIONS: It is prescribed for maintenance of blood pressure and is used locally as a nasal or ophthalmic vasoconstrictor.

■ CONTRAINDICATIONS: Narrow-angle glaucoma, concomitant administration of monoamine oxidase inhibitors, or known hypersensitivity to this drug prohibits its use.

■ ADVERSE EFFECTS: Among the more serious adverse effects to the systemic administration of this drug are arrhythmias and an excessive rise in blood pressure. Anxiety, congestion, and hypersensitivity reactions may result from local administration.

phenylethyl alcohol ($C_6H_5CH_2CH_2OH$) /-eth′il/, a colorless fragrant liquid with a burning taste, used as a bacteriostatic agent and preservative in medicinal solutions. Also called **benzyl carbinol,** *2-phenylethanol.*

phenylic acid, phenylic alcohol. See **carbolic acid.**

phenylketonuria (PKU) /fen′əlkē′tōnyoor″ē·ə, fē′nəl-/, abnormal presence of phenylketone and other metabolites of phenylalanine in the urine, characteristic of an inborn metabolic disorder caused by the absence or a deficiency of phenylalanine hydroxylase, the enzyme responsible for the conversion of the amino acid phenylalanine into tyrosine. Accumulation of phenylalanine is toxic to brain tissue. Untreated individuals have very fair hair, eczema, a mousy odor of the urine and skin, and progressive cognitive impairment. Treatment consists of a diet low in phenylalanine. All babies in the United States and Canada are tested for PKU. See also **Guthrie bacterial inhibition assay.** *—phenylketonuric, adj.*

phenylketonuria (PKU) test, a blood or urine test performed to determine the presence of the enzyme required to utilize phenylalanine, an amino acid that is needed for normal growth and development. The blood sample is usually taken from the baby's heel (called a heel stick).

phenyl methanol. See **benzyl alcohol.**

phenylpyruvic acid /fen′ilpīroo″vik/, a product of the metabolism of phenylalanine. The presence of phenylpyruvic acid in the urine is indicative of phenylketonuria.

phenylpyruvic amentia. See **phenylketonuria.**

phenyl salicylate, the salicylic ester of phenol. Also called *salol.* See also **salol camphor.**

phenyltoloxamine citrate /fen′iltəlok″səmēn/, an antihistamine usually used in a fixed-combination drug with an analgesic.

phenytoin /fen′ətō″in/, a drug that alters cell membrane conduction of Na^+, thereby blocking sodium-dependent action potentials in nerve, heart, and muscle tissues.

■ INDICATIONS: It is prescribed as an anticonvulsant for the treatment and prevention of tonic-clonic seizures, complex partial seizures, and seizures resulting from head trauma or surgery. It has an unlabeled use as an antiarrhythmic agent, particularly in digitalis-induced ventricular arrhythmias. Establishing and maintaining the desired plasma concentration can be difficult because phenytoin has a high but variable amount of protein binding (typically 80%) and undergoes capacity-limited metabolism (Michaelis-Menten kinetics), with a half-life ranging from approximately 7 to 42 hrs.

■ CONTRAINDICATIONS: Known hypersensitivity to this drug or to other hydantoins prohibits its use. It is used with caution in patients with a history of hepatic or hematologic abnormalities and in the presence of certain arrhythmias. Phenytoin has been shown to cause fetal malformations, but the benefit to risk ratio can often justify continued use during pregnancy.

■ ADVERSE EFFECTS: Among the more serious adverse effects are ataxia, nystagmus, hypersensitivity reactions, and gingival hyperplasia. Rarely, a variety of severe reactions occurs. This drug interacts with many other drugs.

pheo-, phao-, prefix meaning "dusky": *pheochromocytoma.*

pheochromocytoma /fē′ōkrō′mōsītō″mə/ *pl. pheochromocytomas, pheochromocytomata* [Gk, *phaios,* dark, *chroma,* color, *kytos,* cell, *oma,* tumor], a vascular tumor of chromaffin tissue of the adrenal medulla or sympathetic paraganglia, characterized by hypersecretion of epinephrine and norepinephrine, causing persistent or intermittent hypertension. Typical signs include headache, flushing, palpitation, sweating, nervousness, hyperglycemia, nausea, vomiting, and syncope. Weight loss, myocarditis, cardiac arrhythmia, and heart failure may occur. The tumor occurs most commonly at 40 to 60 years of age, and only a small percentage of the lesions are malignant. The cause is unknown. The diagnosis may be established by laboratory assays showing increased catecholamines and their metabolites in urine and by pressor tests; intravenously injected histamine causes a sharp increase in blood pressure, and the administration of phentolamine produces a marked decrease. Surgical excision is the usual treatment; patients with nonresectable tumors may be treated with adrenergic blocking agents or with methyl tyrosine, a drug that reduces norepinephrine production. Also spelled *phaeochromocytoma.*

■ OBSERVATIONS: The most prominent sign is severe sustained or episodic hypertension. This is accompanied by a classic symptom triad of severe, pounding paroxysmal headache, palpitations, and profuse sweating. Visual disturbances, dilated pupils, lower extremity paresthesia, nausea and vomiting, dizziness, tremors, and tachycardia are also seen during paroxysm. An elevated plasma concentration of normetanephrine or metanephrine from a 24-hour urine collection is a 100% sensitive test for pheochromocytoma. A clonidine suppression test reveals persistent elevations in plasma norepinephrine. CT scans and MRIs are useful for tumor location. Complications that typically result from nontreatment or advanced disease include uncontrolled hypertension, diabetes, cardiomyopathy, cardiac arrhythmias, and heart failure.

■ INTERVENTIONS: The primary treatment for pheochromocytoma is surgical removal of the tumor via laparoscopic adrenalectomy. Individuals are stabilized, starting about 2 weeks preoperatively, with a combination of sympathetic blocking agents and liberal salt and fluid intake. Preoperative palpation of the abdomen is contraindicated because it could cause sudden release of catecholamine and severe hypertension. Any persistent hypertension or postoperative hypertension after surgery is managed with conventional antihypertensive drug therapy. Individuals with nonresectable tumors are treated with alpha blockers or methyl tyrosine.

■ PATIENT CARE CONSIDERATIONS: Careful monitoring of blood pressure is crucial in preoperative and postoperative periods to detect abrupt and severe fluctuations. Cardiac monitoring is done to detect cardiac complications, such as arrhythmia. Rest, nourishment, hydration, and emotional support are also needed. Nursing plays a crucial role in screening and case finding. Screening should be done for anyone who exhibits signs of malignant or paradoxical hypertension or displays a poor response to antihypertensive drug therapy. Individuals with neurofibromatosis are also at increased risk for pheochromocytoma.

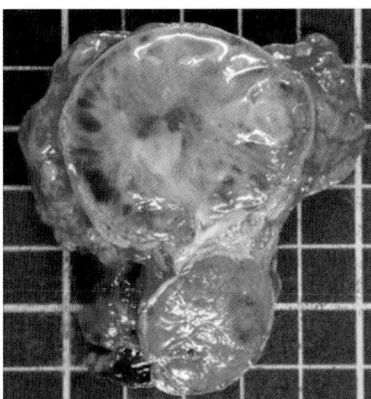

Gross appearance of the left adrenal gland showing an upper grey-red pheochromocytoma with a cystic area *(Ghander et al, 2012)*

pheochromocytoma suppression and provocative testing, a blood test to diagnose pheochromocytoma, consisting of either the administration of glucagon to provoke a rise in catecholamine levels or the administration of clonidine to suppress catecholamine levels.

pheresis. See **apheresis.**

pheromone /fer″əmōn′/ [Gk, *pherein,* to carry, *hormaein,* to stimulate], a substance secreted by an organism that elicits a particular response from another individual of the same species, usually of the opposite sex. Pheromones may be sexual stimulants or attractants or alarm or trail-making substances; in social insects they have a role in the determination of castes.

phi /fī/, Φ, φ, the twenty-first letter of the Greek alphabet.

Phialophora /fī″älof′ərə/, a genus of imperfect fungi. *P. verrucosi* is a cause of chromoblastomycosis, and *P. jeanselmei* is a cause of maduromycosis.

phil-, prefix meaning "having an affinity for" or "having a love for": *philanthropist.*

-phil, -phile, 1. combining form meaning "a lover or admirer" of something specified: *pedophilia.* 2. suffix meaning "having an affinity for or being strongly attracted to a specified thing": *acidophil, argyrophil.*

-phil, -philic, -philous, suffix meaning "of that which has an attraction to or is stained by": *chromaphil, hydrophilic, lipophilia.*

Philadelphia chromosome (Ph¹) [Philadelphia, Pennsylvania], a translocation of the long arm of chromosome 22, often seen in the abnormal myeloblasts, erythroblasts, and megakaryoblasts of patients who have chronic myelocytic leukemia.

philanthropist, an individual who provides money or gifts to charities to accomplish the mission of assisting others.

-philia, -phily, -philous, suffix meaning "having a love, craving, affinity for": *paraphilia, necrophilia.*

philtrum /fil′trəm/, the vertical groove in the center of the upper lip.

-phily. See **-philia, -phily, -philous.**

phimosis /fīmō″sis/ [Gk, muzzle], tightness of the prepuce of the penis that prevents the retraction of the foreskin over the glans. The condition is usually congenital but may be the result of infection. Circumcision is the usual treatment. An analogous condition of the clitoris occurs rarely. Compare **paraphimosis.** See also **phimosis vaginalis.**

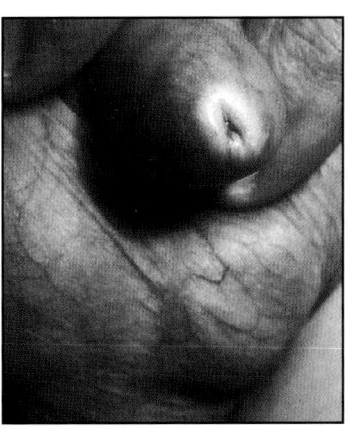

Phimosis *(Lissauer et al, 2012)*

phimosis vaginalis /vaj′inā″lis/, congenital narrowness or closure of the vaginal opening.

pHisoHex, a sudsing antibacterial skin cleanser. Brand name for **hexachlorophene.**

phleb-. See **phlebo-, phleb-.**

phlebectomy /fləbek′təmē/ [Gk, *phleps,* vein, *ektomē,* excision], the surgical removal of a vein or part of a vein.

phlebitis. See **thrombophlebitis.**

phlebo-, phleb- /fleb′ō-/, prefix meaning "vein" or "veins": *phlebitis, phlebograph, phlebostasis.*

phlebogram /fleb′əgram/ [Gk, *phleps,* vein, *gramma,* record], 1. a radiograph obtained by phlebography. 2. a graphic representation of the venous pulse obtained by phlebography. Also called **venogram.**

phlebograph /fleb′əgraf′/, a device for producing a graphic record of the venous pulse.

phlebography /fləbog″rəfē/ [Gk, *phleps* + *graphein,* to record], 1. the radiographic examination of veins injected with a radiopaque contrast medium. 2. the graphic recording of the venous pulse. Also called **venography.**

phlebography of the lower extremities, an x-ray study with contrast dye designed to identify and locate thrombi within the venous system of the lower extremities.

phlebostasis /-stā″sis/, an abnormally slow flow of blood in the veins, which are usually distended. Also called **venostasis.**

phlebostatic axis /-stat′ik/ [Gk, *phleps* + *stasis,* standing still], the approximate location of the right atrium, found at the intersection of the midaxillary and a line drawn from the fourth intercostal space at the right side of the sternum. The phlebostatic axis is used extensively in hemodynamics.

phlebothrombosis /fleb′ōthrombō″sis/ [Gk, *phleps* + *thrombos,* lump, *osis,* condition], an abnormal condition in which a clot forms within a vein. It is usually caused by hemostasis, hypercoagulability, or occlusion. In contrast to that in thrombophlebitis, the wall of the vein is not inflamed. Also called **venous thrombosis.** Compare **thrombophlebitis.**

phlebotomist /fləbot″əmist/ [Gk, *phleps,* vein + *ektomē*], a person with special training in the practice of drawing blood.

phlebotomize /fləbot′əmīz/ [Gk, *phleps,* vein, *ektomē,* excision], to open a vein to remove blood.

phlebotomus fever /fləbot″əməs/ [Gk, *phleps* + *tomos,* cutting; L, *febris,* fever], an acute mild infection caused by one of five distinct arboviruses transmitted to humans by the bite of an infected sandfly. It is characterized by rapidly developing fever, headache, eye pain, conjunctivitis, myalgia, and occasionally a macular or urticarial rash. Aseptic meningitis also may occur. The disease is widespread in hot, dry areas where sandflies abound, and it has been seen in Panama and Brazil. Phlebotomus fever is self-limited. Supportive therapy, including fluids and aspirin, is recommended. A second attack may occur a few weeks after the first. Also called *ephemeral fever,* **pappataci fever, sandfly fever, three-day fever.**

phlebotomy /fləbot″əmē/ [Gk, *phleps* + *temnein,* to cut], the incision of a vein for the letting of blood, as in collecting blood from a donor. Phlebotomy is the chief treatment for polycythemia vera and may be performed every 2 to 3 months or more frequently if required. The procedure is sometimes used to decrease the amount of circulating blood and pulmonary engorgement in acute pulmonary edema. At one time phlebotomy was practiced for almost every disorder. Also called **venesection.**

phleg-. See **phlogo-, phleg-.**

phlegm /flem/ [Gk, *phlegma,* mucus, sluggishness], thick mucus secreted by the tissues lining the airways of the lungs.

phlegmasia alba dolens [Gk, *phlegmone,* inflammation; L, *albus,* white, *dolens,* painful], thrombophlebitis of the femoral vein, resulting in pain and edema of the leg. It may occur after childbirth or a severe febrile illness. Also called **thrombotic phlegmasia.**

phlegmasia cerulea dolens. See **blue phlebitis.**

phlegmatic /flegmat′ik/ [Gk, *phlegma,* mucus, sluggishness], pertaining to a person who appears dull or apathetic, or calm and composed to an extent that excitation is difficult.

phlegmon /fleg′mon/ [Gk, *phlegmone,* inflammation], an inflammation of connective tissue.

phlegmonous gastritis /fleg″mənəs/ [Gk, *phlegmone* + *osis,* condition], a rare but severe form of gastritis involving the connective tissue layer of the stomach wall. It occurs as a complication of systemic infection, peptic ulcer, cancer, surgery, or other severe stress and represents an acute abdominal emergency. Treatment includes surgery, antibiotics, and analgesics.

phlegm-, prefix meaning "mucus": *phlegmatic.*

phlogo-, phleg-, rarely used prefix meaning "inflammation": *phlegmon, phlegmasia.*

phlyctenular keratoconjunctivitis /fliktə′yələr/ [Gk, *phlyktaina,* blister], an inflammatory condition of the cornea, characterized by tiny ulcerating nodules. It is seen most often in children as a response to allergens found in *Mycobacterium tuberculosis,* gonococci, *Candida albicans,* or various parasites. Vitamin deficiency may be a factor. The condition responds to topical corticosteroids, but corneal scars may remain. Also called *phlyctenulosis, scrofulous keratitis.* See also **eczematous conjunctivitis.**

PHO, abbreviation for **physician-hospital organization.**

phob-, combining form meaning "fear," "panic," or "morbid dread": *phobia, phobic, photophobia.*

-phobe, -phobiac, -phobist, suffix meaning "one who fears" something specified: *chromophobe.*

phobia /fō″bē·ə/ [Gk, *phobos,* fear], an obsessive, irrational, and intense fear of a specific object, such as an animal or dirt; of an activity, such as meeting strangers or leaving the familiar setting of the home; or of a physical situation, such as heights and open or closed spaces. Typical manifestations of phobia include faintness, fatigue, palpitations, perspiration, nausea, tremor, and panic. Also called **phobic anxiety, phobic disorder, phobic reaction.** Compare **compulsion.** Kinds include **agoraphobia, algophobia, claustrophobia, erythrophobia, gynephobia, lalophobia, mysophobia, nyctophobia, photophobia, xenophobia, zoophobia.** See also **simple phobia, social phobia.** −**phobic,** *adj.*

-phobia, suffix meaning "abnormal fear" of the object, experience, or place specified: *agoraphobia, claustrophobia, nyctophobia.*

phobiac /fō″bē·ak/, a person who exhibits or is afflicted with a phobia.

-phobiac. See **-phobe, -phobiac, -phobist.**

phobic /fō″bik/ [Gk, *phobos,* fear], pertaining to or resembling phobia.

-phobic, -phobous, **1.** suffix meaning "exhibiting or possessing an aversion to or fear of (something)": *necrophobic.* **2.** suffix meaning "the absence of a strong affinity": *chromophobic, hydrophobic.*

phobic anxiety. See **phobia.**

phobic desensitization [Gk, *phobos,* fear; L, *de* + *sentire,* to feel], a method of resolving an ego dystonic or uncomfortable behavior pattern by gradual reentry into the emotionally upsetting life situation in stages, first in fantasy and then in real life. It is similar to the psychotherapeutic techniques of flooding. See also **flooding,** def. 2.

phobic disorder. See **anxiety disorder, phobia.**

phobic neurosis. See **phobia.**

phobic reaction. See **phobia.**

phobic state, a condition characterized by extreme anxiety resulting from the excessive, irrational fear of a particular object, situation, or activity. See also **phobia.**

-phobist. See **-phobe, -phobiac, -phobist.**

-phobous. See **-phobic, -phobous.**

phocomelia /fō″kəmē″lyə/ [Gk, *phoke,* seal, *melos,* limb], a developmental anomaly characterized by absence of the upper part of one or more of the limbs so that the feet or hands or both are attached to the trunk of the body by short, irregularly shaped stumps, resembling the fins of a seal. The condition, caused by interference with the embryonic development of the long bones, is rare and is seen primarily as a side effect of the drug thalidomide taken during early pregnancy. Also called **seal limbs.** Compare **amelia.** −*phocomelic, adj.*

phocomelic dwarf /fō″kəmē″lik/, a dwarf in whom the long bones of any or all of the extremities are abnormally short.

phocomelus /fōkom″ələs/, an individual who has phocomelia.

phon-. See **phono-, phon-.**

phonation /fōnā″shən/ [Gk, *phone,* sound; L, *atio,* process], the production of voice through the vibration of the vocal folds of the larynx coupled with airflow directed upward from the lungs.

-phone, suffix meaning "sound" or "voice": *telephone.*

phonetics /fōnet″iks/ [Gk, *phone,* voice], **1.** the science of speech sounds used in language. **2.** a written code used by speech-language pathologists and linguists to represent speech sounds. Speech-language pathologists use the International Phonetic Alphabet (IPA).

-phonia. See **-phony, -phonia, -phonic.**

phonic, pertaining to voice, sounds, or speech.

-phonic. See **-phony, -phonia, -phonic.**

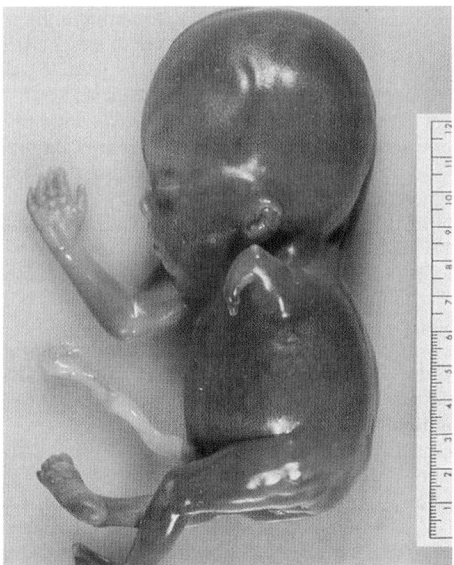

Phocomelia of the left upper limb *(Courtesy Dr. D.K. Kalousek, Department of Pathology, University of British Columbia, Children's Hospital)*

phono-, phon-, prefix meaning "sound, often specifically the sound of the voice": *phonocardiograph, phonology, phonation.*

phonocardiogram /fō′nōkär″dē·əgram′/, a graphic recording obtained from a phonocardiograph.

phonocardiograph /-kär″dē·əgraf′/ [Gk, *phone,* sound, *kardia,* heart, *graphein,* to record], an electroacoustic device that produces graphic heart sound recordings using a system of microphones and associated recording equipment. One microphone is usually placed on the chest near the base of the heart. It records the timing of the aortic and pulmonary components of the second heart sound and the loudest murmurs. Another microphone is positioned on the chest over the apex of the heart. It is connected to filters that allow the recording of low-frequency sounds, such as those associated with atrial and ventricular gallops, as well as higher-frequency sounds, such as those associated with mitral regurgitation and ventricular septal defect. To ensure an accurate recording, the examiner also uses audiophones to monitor the sounds and an oscilloscope to monitor cardiac impulses. Phonocardiographs are used in the diagnosis and monitoring of heart disorders. Also called **electrocardiophonograph.** *−phonocardiographic, adj.*

phonocardiography /-kär′dē·og″rəfē/ [Gk, *phone + kardia + graphein,* to record], the recording of heart sounds and murmurs by a phonocardiograph.

phonological disorder /fō′nə·loj′i·k/, a communication disorder of unknown cause, characterized by failure to use age- and dialect-appropriate sounds in speaking, with errors in the selection, production, or articulation of sounds. The most common errors are omissions, substitutions, and distortions of speech sounds.

phonology /fōnol′əjē/, the study of speech sounds, particularly the principles governing the way speech sounds are used in a given language.

phonophoresis /fō′nōfərē″sis/, a therapeutic technique in which ultrasound waves are used to force topical medicines, such as hydrocortisone, aspirin, and lidocaine, into subcutaneous tissues. Continuous phonophoresis for up to 10 minutes can drive a drug applied to the skin surface about 5 cm into muscle tissue. Because of the risk that the patient may be hypersensitive to the medication, the technique is used with caution.

phonoreceptor /-risep′tər/ [Gk, *phone,* sound; L, *recipere,* to receive], a device for receiving sound impulses.

-phony, -phonia, -phonic, suffix meaning "sound or a type of speech": *autophony, aphonia, organophonic.*

phor-, prefix meaning "bearing, carrying": *phoresis.*

-phore, -phor, suffix meaning a "bearer" or "possessor": *iodophor, camphor, luminophore.*

phoresis, a symbiotic relationship in which one organism attaches to another for the purpose of transport.

-phoresis, suffix meaning "a movement in a (specified) manner or medium": *anaphoresis, electrophoresis, diaphoresis.*

-phoria, **1.** suffix meaning "(condition of the) visual axes of the eye": *esophoria, exophoria.* **2.** suffix meaning an "emotional state": *euphoria, dysphoria.*

phoropter /for-op′ter/, an instrument for evaluation of vision, with lenses placed on dials in a unit that is positioned in front of the patient.

phosphatase /fos″fətāz/, an enzyme that acts as a catalyst in chemical reactions involving phosphorus. It is present in serum, semen, the kidney, and the prostate. It is essential in the calcification of bone. See also **catalyst, enzyme.**

phosphate (PO_4^{3-}) /fos′fāt/, **1.** an anion of phosphoric acid. **2.** a salt of phosphoric acid. Phosphates are extremely important in living cells, particularly in the storage and use of energy and the transmission of genetic information within a cell and from one cell to another. See also **adenosine diphosphate, adenosine triphosphate, phosphorus.**

phosphate binder, a substance, such as aluminum hydroxide, calcium acetate, or calcium carbonate, that binds phosphate in the blood, removing it from circulation. It is used in treatment of hyperphosphatemia in patients with end-stage renal disease or hypoparathyroidism.

phosphate-bond energy, **1.** the Gibbs energy for hydrolysis of a phosphate compound. **2.** a measure of relative phosphorylation power.

phosphatemia /fos′fətē″mē·ə/ [Gk, *phosphoros,* bringer of light; Gk, *haima,* blood], a condition of excessive levels of phosphates in the blood.

phosphate (PO_4) test, a blood test used to detect hyperphosphatemia and hypophosphatemia. Abnormal phosphate levels are associated with renal failure, acromegaly, hyperparathyroidism or hypoparathyroidism, liver disease, advanced lymphoma or myeloma, hemolytic anemia, hypercalcemia, chronic alcoholism, vitamin D deficiency, diabetic acidosis, hyperinsulinism, and sepsis, among other conditions.

phosphatide /fos′fətīd/, phosphatidic acid or any of its esters. Phosphatidic acid (diacylglycerol phosphate) consists of glycerol esterified to phosphoric acid and to two fatty acids. Phosphatides are major components of cell membranes. Also called **phosphoglyceride, phosphotidate.**

phosphaturia /fos′fətoor″ē·ə/ [Gk, *phosphoros,* bringer of light, *ouron,* urine], an excessive level of phosphates in the urine. Also called **phosphuria.**

phosphoglycerate kinase /fos′fōglis″ərāt/, an enzyme that catalyzes the reversible transfer of a phosphate group from adenosine triphosphate to D-3-phosphoglycerate, forming d-1,3-biphosphoglycerate. The reaction is one of the steps in gluconeogenesis.

phosphoglyceride. See **phosphatide.**

Phospholine Iodide, a cholinergic drug. Brand name for **echothiophate iodide.**

phospholipase /fos′fōli″pās/, any of a group of enzymes that catalyze the hydrolysis of phospholipids. Various phospholipases digest cell membranes, aid in the synthesis of prostaglandins, and help produce arachidonic acid, one of the essential fatty acids.

phospholipid /fos′fōlip″id/ [Gk, *phos,* light, *pherein,* to bear, *lipos* fat], a phosphorus-containing lipid. Kinds include **phosphatide, sphingomyelin.**

phospholipid as phosphorus. See **lipid.**

phospholipid transfer protein (PLTP), a ubiquitous protein having multiple functions in lipoprotein metabolism. In plasma, it plays an important role in high-density lipoprotein (HDL) metabolism by mediating the transfer of phospholipids from triglyceride-rich lipoproteins to HDL and the transfer of phospholipids between HDL molecules.

phosphomevalonate kinase /fos′fōməval″ənāt/, an enzyme that catalyzes the transfer of a phosphate group from adenosine triphosphate to produce adenosine diphosphate and 5-pyrophosphomevalonate.

phosphorescence /fos′fôres″əns/ [Gk, *phos,* light, *pherein,* to bear], **1.** a glow of yellow phosphorus caused by slow oxidation. **2.** the emission of visible light without accompanying heat as observed in phosphorus that has been exposed to radiation, which continues beyond a few nanoseconds after radiation has ceased.

phosphoric acid (H_3PO_4) /fosfôr′ik/, a clear, colorless, odorless liquid that is irritating to the skin and eyes and moderately toxic if ingested. It is used in the production of fertilizers, soaps, detergents, animal feeds, and certain drugs.

phosphorus (P) /fos′fərəs/ [Gk, *phos,* light, *pherein,* to bear], a nonmetallic chemical element occurring extensively in nature as a component of phosphate rock. Its atomic number is 15; its atomic mass is 30.975. Phosphorus forms a series of sulfides used commercially in the manufacture of matches. It can be prepared in yellow or white, red, and black allotropic forms. Phosphorus is essential for the metabolism of protein, calcium, and glucose. The body uses phosphorus in its combined forms, which are obtained from such nutritional sources as milk, cheese, meat, egg yolk, whole grains, legumes, and nuts. A nutritional deficiency of phosphorus can cause weight loss, anemia, and abnormal growth. Phosphorus is essential to the body for the production of adenosine triphosphate and for the process of glycolysis. Elemental white or yellow phosphorus is extremely poisonous and produces severe GI irritation. If ingested, it can produce hemorrhage, cardiovascular failure, and death. Chronic poisoning by phosphorus is characterized by anemia, cachexia, bronchitis, and necrosis of the mandible. Normal adult blood levels of phosphorus are 3 to 4.5 mg/dL or 0.97 to 1.45 mmol/L (SI units).

phosphorus poisoning, a toxic condition caused by the ingestion of white or yellow phosphorus, sometimes found in rat poisons, certain fertilizers, and fireworks. Intoxication is characterized initially by nausea, throat and stomach pain, vomiting, diarrhea, and an odor of garlic on the breath. After a few days of apparent recovery, nausea, vomiting, and diarrhea recur with renal and hepatic dysfunction. Physical contact with the vomitus and feces of the patient is avoided.

phosphorylase /fosfôr′ilās/ [Gk, *phosphoros,* bringer of light + *ase,* enzyme suffix], any of a group of physiologically important enzymes that catalyze reactions between phosphates and glycogen or other starch components, yielding glucose-1-phosphate.

phosphorylation /fosfôr′ilā″shən/, the process of attaching a phosphate group to a protein, sugar, or other compound.

phosphotidate. See **phosphatide.**

phosphuria. See **phosphaturia.**

phot /fot/ [Gk, *phos,* light], the centimeter-gram-second unit of illumination, being one lumen per square centimeter.

phot-. See **photo-, phot-.**

photic /fō′tik/ [Gk, *phos,* light], pertaining to light.

-photic, suffix meaning "ability to see at a (specified) light level."

photic epilepsy [Gk, *phos,* light, *epilepsia,* seizure], a condition in which epileptic attacks may be triggered by flickering light. During an electroencephalogram, a bright light is flashed to try to stimulate this kind of epilepsy. Also called **photogenic epilepsy.**

photoablation /fō″to·ah·bla′shun/, volatilization of tissue by ultraviolet rays emitted by a laser.

photoaging /fō″to·āj′ing/, premature aging of the skin caused by long-term exposure to sunlight or other ultraviolet radiation.

photoallergic /-əlur′gik/ [Gk, *phos,* light, *allos,* other, *ergein,* to work], exhibiting a delayed hypersensitivity reaction after exposure to light. Compare **phototoxic.** See also **photoallergic contact dermatitis.**

photoallergic contact dermatitis, a papulovesicular, eczematous, or exudative skin reaction that occurs 24 to 48 hours after exposure to light in a previously sensitized person. The sensitizing substance concentrates in the skin and requires chemical alteration by light to become an active antigen. Among common photosensitizers are phenothiazines, hexachlorophene, oral hypoglycemic agents, and sulfanilamide. Prevention requires avoidance of the photosensitizer and of sunlight. Treatment is the same as that for any other inflammatory dermatitis.

photoallergy /-al′ərjē/ [Gk, *phos,* light, *allos,* other + *ergein,* to work], a sensitivity to light that causes allergic reactions.

photobiology /-bī·ol″əjē/, the study of the effects of light on organisms.

photocatalytic, *adj.,* causing, involving, or relating to the acceleration of a chemical reaction by a material that absorbs light.

photochemistry /fō″tōkem′istrē/ [Gk, *phos,* light, *chemeia,* alchemy], the branch of chemistry that deals with the chemical properties or effects of light.

photochemotherapy /-kē′mōther″əpē/ [Gk, *phos + chemeia,* alchemy, *therapeia,* treatment], a kind of chemotherapy in which the effect of the administered drug is enhanced by exposing the patient to light. Also called **photodynamic therapy.** See also **chemotherapy.**

photochromogen /-krō″məjen/, **1.** a pigment that develops as a result of exposure to light. **2.** a type of mycobacterium that is nonpigmented in the dark but produces a yellow pigment on constant exposure to light.

photodisintegration /-disin′təgrā″shən/, the emission of a nuclear fragment caused by the interaction of a high-energy x-ray with an atomic nucleus. It may occur when an x-ray photon with energy greater than 10 MeV escapes interaction with the electron cloud or nuclear force field of an atom and is absorbed directly by the nucleus.

photodynamic therapy. Also called **Levulan Kerastick therapy.** See **photochemotherapy.**

photoelectron /-ilek″tron/ [Gk, *phos,* light + *elektron,* amber], any electron that is discharged when light strikes a metal surface.

photogenic epilepsy. See **photic epilepsy.**

photokinetic /-kinet′ik/ [Gk, *phos,* light, *kinesis,* movement], pertaining to any movement that is stimulated by light rays.

photometer /fōtom″ətər/ [Gk, *phos + metron,* measure], an instrument that measures light intensity. It usually is composed of a source of radiant energy, a filter for wavelength selection, a cuvette holder, a detector, and a readout device.

photomultiplier /-mul′tiplī″ər/ [Gk, *phos,* light; L, *multiplex,* many folds], a device used in many radiation detection applications that converts low levels of light into electrical pulses. A bank of such tubes is used in gamma cameras to view a crystal.

photon /fō′ton/ [Gk, *phos,* light], the smallest quantity of electromagnetic energy. It has no mass and no charge but travels at the speed of light. Photons may occur in the form of x-rays, gamma rays, or quanta of light. The energy *(E)* of a photon is expressed as the product of its frequency *(v)* and Planck constant *(h),* as in the equation $E = hv$. X-ray photons occur in frequencies of 10^{18} to 10^{21} Hz and energies that range upward from 1 KeV.

photophobia /-fō″bē·ə/ [Gk, *phos* + *phobos,* fear], **1.** abnormal sensitivity to light, especially of the eyes. The condition is prevalent in albinism and various diseases of the conjunctiva and cornea and may be a symptom of such disorders as measles, psittacosis, encephalitis, Rocky Mountain spotted fever, and Reiter's syndrome. **2.** (in psychiatry) a morbid fear of light with an irrational need to avoid light places. The anxiety disorder is seen more often in women than in men and is usually caused by a repressed intrapsychic conflict symbolically related to light. −*photophobic, adj.*

photo-, phot-, prefix meaning "light": *photoablation, photoreceptor, photophobia.*

photopic eye. See **light-adapted eye.**

photopic vision /fōtop′ik/, daylight vision, which depends primarily on the function of the retinal cone cells.

photoprotective /-prətek′tiv/, protective against the potential adverse effects of ultraviolet light.

photoreaction /-rē·ak′shən/ [Gk, *phos* + L, *re,* again, *agere,* to act], any chemical reaction that is stimulated by the influence of light.

photoreceptor /-risep′tər/ [Gk, *phos,* light; L, *recipere,* to receive], a nerve cell that is receptive to light stimuli.

photoreceptor layer [L, *columna,* column; AS, *lecgan*], the layer of rods and cones in the retina.

photorefractive /fo″to-re-frak′tiv/, pertaining to the refraction of light. See also **photorefractive keratectomy.**

photorefractive keratectomy (PRK) /-refrak″tiv/, a surgical procedure in which an excimer laser is used to reshape the human cornea to improve the refractive properties of the eye and reduce or eliminate the need for eyeglasses. The excimer laser does not require that incisions be made in the cornea. Rather than cutting, the laser shaves off preprogrammed outer layers of corneal tissue. The excimer laser is programmed to emit a measured and concentrated light beam to reshape a small part of the central cornea. It allows for correction of myopia of up to −10.0 diopters. Compare **radial keratotomy.** See also **refractive keratotomy.**

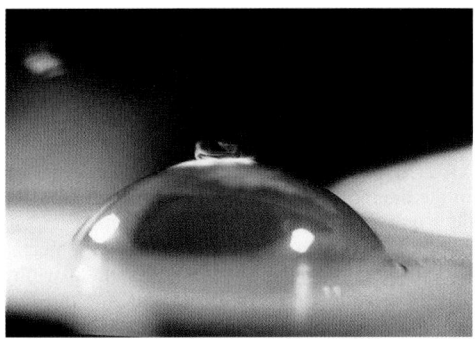

Photorefractive keratectomy *(Kanski and Bowling, 2011/ Courtesy C. Barry)*

photoscan /fō′tōskan′/, a radiograph that shows the distribution of a radiopharmaceutical in the body.

photosensitive /-sen″sitiv/ [Gk, *phos* + L, *sentire,* to feel], pertaining to increased reactivity of the skin to sunlight caused by a disorder such as albinism or porphyria, or, more frequently, by the use of certain drugs. Relatively brief exposure to sunlight or to an ultraviolet lamp may cause edema, papules, urticaria, or acute burns in individuals with endogenous or acquired photosensitivity. Treatment involves avoidance of exposure to sunlight or the photosensitizing agent.

photosensitivity /-sen′sitiv″itē/, **1.** sensitivity of a cell to light. **2.** any abnormal response to exposure to light, specifically, a skin reaction requiring the presence of a sensitizing agent and exposure to sunlight or its equivalent. Photosensitivity includes photoallergic and phototoxic reactions and is common in systemic lupus erythematosus.

photosensitization /-sen′sitīzā′shən/ [Gk, *phos,* light; L, *sentire,* to feel], the process of rendering an organism sensitive to the effects of light. −*photosensitizer, n.*

photostimulable phosphor, a material used to capture radiographic images in computed radiography systems.

photosynthesis /fōtōsin″thəsis/ [Gk, *phos* + *synthesis,* putting together], a process by which plants, algae, and some bacteria containing chlorophyll synthesize organic compounds, chiefly carbohydrates, from atmospheric carbon dioxide and water, using light for energy and liberating oxygen in the process. −*photosynthetic, adj.*

phototherapy /-ther′əpē/ [Gk, *phos* + *therapeia,* treatment], the treatment of disorders by the use of light, especially ultraviolet light. Ultraviolet light may be used in the therapy of acne, pressure ulcers and other indolent ulcers, psoriasis, and hyperbilirubinemia. Also called **lucotherapy.** See also **photochemotherapy.** −*phototherapeutic, adj.*

phototherapy in the newborn, a treatment for hyperbilirubinemia and jaundice in the newborn that involves the exposure of an infant's bare skin to intense fluorescent light. The blue range of light accelerates the excretion of bilirubin in the skin, decomposing it by photooxidation.

■ METHOD: The infant is placed nude under the fluorescent lights with the eyes and genitalia covered. The baby is turned frequently, and the body temperature is monitored, using a skin thermistor. All vital signs are carefully noted, and details regarding position of the bulbs, time and duration of treatment, and the infant's response are charted. Adverse effects of phototherapy include dehydration: An infant may need 25% more fluid during treatment. Loose stools and "bronze baby" syndrome may occur.

■ INTERVENTIONS: The nurse performs phototherapy and may be responsible for collecting specimens for serial tests for bilirubin level in the blood. Breastfeeding may be discontinued during treatment but often is not. Additional water may be given. The family is encouraged to visit and to participate in caring for the infant. They may be told that the eye shields are necessary but do not seem to bother the infant.

■ OUTCOME CRITERIA: Bilirubin levels usually decrease by 3 to 4 mg/dL in the first 8 to 12 hours of therapy. Thus simple jaundice clears rapidly. Excess bilirubin and jaundice that are the result of hemolytic disease or infection may be controlled with phototherapy, but the underlying cause is treated separately. Recovery is usually complete. The long-term safety of phototherapy has not been established. Short-term efficacy and practicality of use are certain.

phototoxic /-tok′sik/ [Gk, *phos* + *toxikon,* poison], characterized by a rapidly developing nonimmunological reaction of the skin when it is exposed to a photosensitizing substance and light. Compare **photoallergic.** See also **phototoxic contact dermatitis.**

phototoxic contact dermatitis, a rapidly appearing, sunburnlike response of areas of skin that have been exposed to the sun after contact with a photosensitizing substance. Hyperpigmentation may follow the acute reaction. Coal tar derivatives, oil of bergamot (often used in cosmetics and beverages), and many plants containing furocoumarin (cowslip, buttercup, carrot, parsnip, mustard, and yarrow) are known photosensitizing materials. Treatment includes Burrow's solution, emollient creams such as Acid Mantle, and topical corticosteroids.

-phragma, -phragm, suffix meaning "a septum or musculomembranous barrier between cavities": *diaphragm, hemidiaphragm.*

-phrasia, suffix meaning "an abnormal condition of speech": *aphrasia.*

phren /fren/ [Gk, mind], **1.** the diaphragm. **2.** the mind.

phrenetic /frənet′ik/ [Gk, *phren*], frenzied, delirious, maniacal.

phreni-, phrenico-, phreno-, prefix meaning "mind or the diaphragm": *phrenology.*

-phrenia, suffix meaning "a disordered condition of mental activity": *hebephrenia, paraphrenia, schizophrenia.*

phrenic /fren′ik/ [Gk, *phren*, mind], **1.** pertaining to the diaphragm. **2.** pertaining to the mind.

-phrenic, 1. suffix meaning "the diaphragm or adjacent regions of the body": *costophrenic, subphrenic.* **2.** suffix meaning "characteristic of a disorder of the mind": *schizophrenic.*

phrenic nerve, one of a pair of branches of the cervical plexus, arising from the first four cervical nerves and passing to the diaphragm. It contains about half as many sensory as motor fibers and is generally known as the motor nerve to the diaphragm, although the lower thoracic nerves also help innervate the diaphragm. The pleural branches of the phrenic nerve are very fine filaments supplying the mediastinal pleura. The pericardial branches are delicate filaments passing to the upper pericardium. The terminal branches diverge after passing separately through the diaphragm and are distributed on the abdominal surface of the diaphragm. On the right side, a branch near the inferior vena cava communicates with the phrenic plexus in association with a phrenic ganglion. There is no phrenic ganglion on the left side. Also called **internal respiratory nerve of Bell.** Compare **accessory phrenic nerve.**

phrenicoceliac part of suspensory muscle of duodenum, a band of skeletal muscle that passes from the right crus of the diaphragm to join the celiacoduodenal part (pars coeliacoduodenalis) and attach to the celiac trunk.

phreno-. See **phreni-, phrenico-, phreno-.**

phrenology [Gk, *phren*, mind], the study of the conformation of the skull based on the assumption that mental faculties are localized in particular sites on the surface of the brain. According to phrenologists, intelligence or other faculties of a person may be mirrored through elevations in the skull overlying the particular area of the brain.

PHSP, abbreviation for **physician health service plan.**

Phthirus /thī′rəs/ [Gk, *phtheir*, louse], a genus of bloodsucking lice that includes the species *P. pubis*, the crab louse.

phthisis /tis′is, thī′sis/ [Gk, *phthisis*, wasting away], any wasting disease involving all or part of the body, such as pulmonary tuberculosis.

phyco-, prefix meaning "seaweed": *phycology.*

phycologist /fēkol′əjist/, a person who specializes in the study of algae. Also called **algologist.**

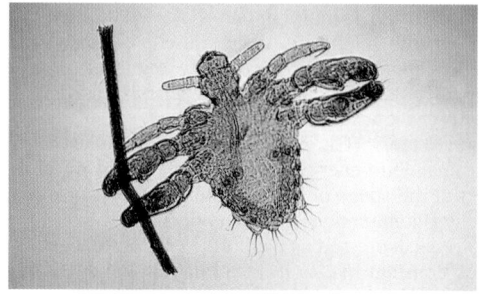

***Phthirus pubis* grasping a hair** *(Auerbach, 2007)*

phycology /fēkol′əjē/ [Gk, *phykos,* seaweed, *logos,* science], the branch of science that is concerned with algae. Also called **algology.**

phycomycosis /fī′kōmīkō′sis/ [Gk, *phykos* + *mykes,* fungus, *osis,* condition], a fungal infection caused by a species of the order Phycomycetes. These organisms are common in the soil and are not usually pathogenic. Severe nosocomial pulmonary phycomycosis sometimes occurs with advanced diabetes mellitus that is untreated or out of control and complicated by ketoacidosis. See also **zygomycosis.**

phyl-, prefix meaning "guarding" or "preservation": *phylactic.*

phylactic /filak′tik/ [Gk, *phylax,* guard], **1.** serving to protect. **2.** something that produces phylaxis.

-phylaxis, suffix meaning "protection": *anaphylaxis, prophylaxis.*

-phyll, -phyl, suffix meaning "a leaf": *chlorophyll.*

phyllo- /fil′ō-/, prefix meaning "leaves": *phyllodes, podophyllotoxin.*

phylloquinone. See **vitamin K₁.**

phylo- /fī′lō-/, prefix meaning "type, kind, race, or tribe": *phylogenesis, phylogeny.*

phylogenesis. See **phylogeny.**

phylogenetic /fī′lōgənet″ik/ [Gk, *phylon,* tribe, *genesis,* origin], **1.** relating to or acquired during phylogeny. **2.** based on a natural evolutionary relationship, such as a system of classification. Also called *phylogenic.*

phylogeny /filoj″ənē/ [Gk, *phylon* + *genesis*], the development of the structure of a particular race or species as it evolved from earlier forms of life. Also called **phylogenesis.** Compare **ontogeny.** See also **comparative anatomy.**

phylum /fī′ləm/ [Gk, *phylon,* tribe], a major subdivision of a kingdom of organisms, representing one or more classes.

-phyma, suffix meaning "a swelling or tumor": *rhinophyma.*

Physalia /fisā′lēə/, a genus of marine invertebrates of the phylum Cnidaria. See **Portuguese man-of-war.**

physi-. See **physio-, physi-.**

physiatrics. See **physiatry.**

physiatrist /fiz′ē-at″rist/, a physician specializing in physical medicine and rehabilitation who has been certified by the American Board of Physical Medicine and Rehabilitation after completing residency and other requirements.

physiatry /fizī″ətrē/, a branch of medicine that specializes in the diagnosis, treatment, and management of disease or injury and the rehabilitation from resultant impairments and disabilities primarily by using "physical" means, such as physical therapy and medications. Essentially, physiatry emphasizes a wide range of treatments for the musculoskeletal system (the muscles, bones, and associated nerves, ligaments, tendons, and other structures) and the musculoskeletal disorders that cause pain or difficulty with functioning. The treatment focuses on helping the patient become as functional and pain-free as possible for the best quality of life achievable. Also called **physiatrics, physical medicine, physical medicine and rehabilitation.**

-physical, suffix meaning "natural": *psychophysical.*

physical abuse /fiz'ikəl/ [Gk, *physikos,* natural; L, *abuti,* to abuse], one or more episodes of aggressive behavior, usually resulting in physical injury with possible damage to internal organs, sense organs, the central nervous system, or the musculoskeletal system of another person.

physical allergy, a hypersensitive reaction to physical factors, such as cold, heat, light, or trauma. Common characteristics include pruritus, urticaria, and angioedema. Usually specific antibodies are found in people having physical allergies. Photosensitivity may be caused by the use of certain cosmetics or drugs. Prophylaxis typically includes an attempt to remove the stimulus, and treatment involves the use of antihistamines or steroids. Compare **contact dermatitis.** See also **atopic dermatitis.**

physical assessment, the part of the health assessment representing a synthesis of the information obtained in a physical examination. It involves the detailed examination of the body from head to toe using the techniques of observation/inspection, palpation, percussion, and auscultation.

physical chemistry, the natural science dealing with the relationship between chemical and physical properties of matter.

physical dependence, substance dependence in which there is evidence of tolerance, withdrawal, or both.

physical diagnosis, the diagnostic process accomplished by the study of the physical manifestations of health, disease, and illness revealed in the physical examination, as guided by the patient's complete history and supported by various laboratory tests. Physical diagnosis is to medicine what the health assessment is to nursing.

physical examination, an investigation of the body to determine its state of health, using any or all of the techniques of inspection, palpation, percussion, auscultation, and smell. The physical examination, history, and initial laboratory tests constitute the database on which a diagnosis is made and on which a plan of treatment is developed.

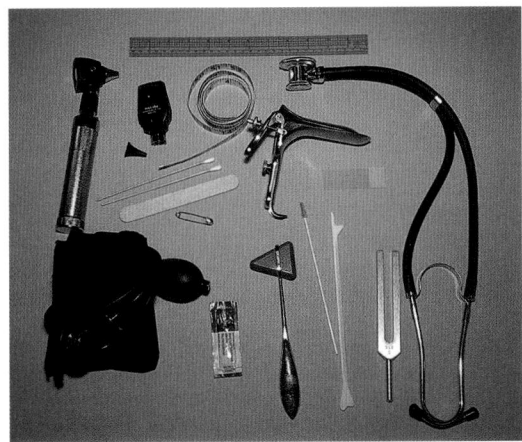

Equipment used during a physical examination *(Potter and Perry, 2005)*

physical fitness, the ability to carry out daily tasks with alertness and vigor, without undue fatigue, and with enough energy reserve to meet emergencies or to enjoy leisure time pursuits.

physical medicine, physical medicine and rehabilitation. See **physiatry.**

physical science, the study of the properties and behavior of nonliving matter. Compare **life science.** Kinds include **chemistry,** *geology,* **physics.**

physical sign [Gk, *physikos,* natural; L, *signum*], an objective indicator found during physical diagnosis or detected by inspection, palpation, percussion, or auscultation.

physical therapist (PT), a person who is licensed in the examination, evaluation, and treatment of physical impairments through the use of special exercise, application of heat or cold, and other physical modalities. The goal is to assist persons who are physically challenged to maximize independence and improve mobility, self-care, and other functional skills necessary for daily living. A physical therapist becomes qualified by studying an accredited curriculum leading to a Doctor of Physical Therapy degree (DPT).

physical therapy (PT), the treatment of disorders with physical agents and methods, such as massage, manipulation, therapeutic exercises, cold, heat (including paraffin, shortwave and microwave diathermy, and ultrasonic heat), hydrotherapy, electrical stimulation, and light to assist in habilitating or rehabilitating patients and restoring function after an illness or injury. Also called **physiotherapy.**

physical therapy assistant (PTA), a person who, under the supervision of a physical therapist, assists in carrying out patient treatment programs, providing treatment that improves mobility, relieves pain, and prevents or lessens physical disabilities of patients. An assistant usually has an associate's degree and in some states is licensed.

physician /fizish'ən/ [Gk, *physikos,* natural], a health professional who has earned a degree of Doctor of Medicine (M.D.) or Doctor of Osteopathic Medicine (D.O.) after completing an approved course of study at an approved medical school. Satisfactory completion of National Board Examinations, usually given during both the second and the final years of medical school and after graduation, is also required. An M.D. or D.O. usually enters a hospital internship or residency program for at least 2 years of postgraduate training before beginning practice or further training in a specialty. To practice medicine, an M.D. or D.O. is required to obtain a license from the state in which professional services will be performed. See also **osteopath.**

physician assistant (PA), a person academically and clinically prepared to practice medicine under the supervision of a licensed doctor of medicine or osteopathy. Within the physician/PA relationship, PAs exercise autonomy in medical decisions and provide a wide range of diagnostic and therapeutic services. Training programs average 25 to 27 months. National certification is available to graduates of approved training programs, a master's degree level in most states.

physician extender, a health care provider who is not a physician but who performs medical activities typically performed by a physician. It is most commonly a nurse practitioner or physician assistant.

physician health service plan (PHSP), (in the United States) a general term relating to an arrangement for provision of professional (physician) services only.

physician-hospital organization (PHO), (in the United States) a management service organization in which the partners are physicians and hospitals. The PHO organization contracts for physician and hospital services.

Physician's Desk Reference, a compendium compiled annually, containing information supplied by their manufacturers about drugs, primarily prescription drugs and products used in diagnostic procedures in the United States.

physicist /fis"isist/, a scientist who specializes in physics.

physico-, combining form meaning "natural" or "knowledge of nature."

physics /fiz'iks/ [Gk, *physikos,* natural], the study of matter and energy, particularly as related to motion and force.

-physics, suffix meaning "the science of the nature of": *biophysics, psychophysics.*

physio-, physi-, prefix meaning "related to nature or to physiology": *physiological, physiopathological, physiotherapy.*

physiognomy /fiz'ē·og″nəmē/ [Gk, *physis,* nature, *gnosis,* knowledge], a discredited method of judging the personality and other characteristics of a client by studying the face and general carriage of the body.

physiological /fiz'ē·əloj″ikəl/ [Gk, *physis,* nature, *logos,* science], pertaining to physiology, particularly normal functions as opposed to the pathological.

physiological age [Gk, *physis,* nature, *logos,* science; L, *aetas,* age], the age of the body as determined by its stage of development in terms of functional norms for various systems.

physiological albuminuria [Gk, *physis,* nature, *logos,* science; L, *albus,* white; Gk, *ouron,* urine], the presence of albumin in the urine in the absence of any disease.

physiological amenorrhea [Gk, *physis,* nature, *logos,* science, *a + men,* month, *rhoia,* to flow], an absence of menstruation having a nonpathological cause, such as pregnancy, lactation, menopause, or a prepubertal state of maturity.

physiological antidote [Gk, *physis + logos + anti,* against, *dotos,* that which is given], a drug that has the opposite effect on the body from that caused by a poisonous or toxic substance.

physiological chemistry. See **biochemistry.**

physiological contracture [Gk, *physis + logos,* science; L, *contractio,* drawing together], a temporary condition in which muscles may contract and shorten for a considerable period. Drugs, temperature extremes, and local accumulation of lactic acid are possible causes.

physiological dead space. See **dead space,** def. 2.

physiological dwarf. See **primordial dwarf.**

physiological flexion, an excessive amount of flexor tone that is normally present at birth because of the existing level of central nervous system maturation and fetal positioning in the uterus.

physiological fourth heart sound. See **S₄.**

physiological hypertrophy, a temporary increase in the size of an organ or part caused by normal physiological functions, such as occurs in the walls of the uterus and in the breasts during pregnancy.

physiological incompatibility, a condition in which substances, such as drugs, may have mutually antagonistic effects on the body.

physiological jaundice [Gk, *physis,* nature, *logos,* science; Fr, *jaune,* yellow], a simple jaundice of newborns that involves the breaking down of the excessive number of red blood cells that may be present at birth.

physiological motivation, a body need, such as for food or water, that initiates behavior directed toward satisfying the particular need. Also called **organic motivation.** Compare **social motivation.**

physiological murmur. See **functional murmur.**

physiological occlusion, 1. a closure of the teeth that complements and enhances the functions of the masticatory system. 2. a closure of the teeth that produces no pathological effects on the stomatognathic system, normally dissipating the stresses placed on the teeth and creating a balance between the stresses and the adaptive capacity of the supporting tissues. 3. an acceptable occlusion in a healthy gnathic system.

physiological psychology, the study of the interrelationship of physiological and psychological processes, especially the effects of a change from normal to abnormal.

physiological retraction ring, a ridge around the inside of the uterus that forms during the second stage of normal labor at the junction of the thinned lower uterine segment and thickened upper segment. It forms as a result of progressive lengthening of the muscle fibers of the lower segment and concomitant shortening of the muscle fibers of the upper segment. Compare **constriction ring, pathological retraction ring.**

physiological saline, a 0.9% sodium chloride solution that is isotonic with tissue fluids or blood. Also called **normal saline.** See also **saline solution.**

physiological salt solution, a normal saline solution, usually consisting of a sterile 0.9% weight/volume solution of sodium chloride in distilled water. It is isotonic with normal body fluids.

physiological tetanus, a state of sustained muscular contraction without periods of relaxation caused by repetitive stimulation of the motor nerve trunk at frequencies so high that individual muscle twitches are fused and cannot be distinguished from one another. Also called **tetanic spasm, tonic spasm.** See also **tetanic contraction, tonic convulsion.**

physiological third heart sound. See **S₃.**

physiological tremor [Gk, *physis + logos*; L, *tremor,* shaking], any shaking or trembling caused by physiological factors, such as fatigue, fear, or cold.

physiologist /fiz'ē·ol″əjist/ [Gk, *physis,* nature, *logos,* science], a person who specializes in the science of living organisms.

physiology /fiz'ē·ol″əjē/ [Gk, *physis + logos,* science], 1. the study of the processes and function of the human body. 2. the study of the physical and chemical processes involved in the functioning of organisms and their parts. Compare **anatomy.** Kinds include **comparative physiology, developmental physiology, hominal physiology, pathological physiology.**

physiopathological /fiz'ē·əpath'əloj″ikəl/ [Gk, *physis,* nature, *pathos,* disease, *logos,* science], pertaining to the physiological approach to disease.

physiotherapy. See **physical therapy.**

physique /fizēk″/, the body structure and development of a person.

-physis, suffix meaning "a growth" or "growing": *metaphysis, apophysis, epiphysis.*

physo-, prefix meaning "air" or "gas."

physostigmine salicylate, an acetylcholinesterase inhibitor.

■ INDICATIONS: It is an ophthalmic preparation prescribed as a miotic agent for the treatment of glaucoma, and it is administered systemically for treating the toxic effects of excessive cholinergic receptors blockade (e.g., resulting from atropine poisoning).

■ CONTRAINDICATIONS: Asthma, gangrene, diabetes, cardiovascular disease, or mechanical obstruction of the intestines or urinary tract prohibits its use. It is also not administered to patients in any vagotonic state or to those receiving choline esters or depolarizing neuromuscular blocking agents.

■ ADVERSE EFFECTS: Among the adverse effects are hypersalivation, diaphoresis, lacrimation, miosis, bradycardia, palpitations, nervousness, and convulsions.

phytanic acid, a branched-chain fatty acid derived from the enzymatic degradation of phytol; it is consumed in red meats, dairy products, and fatty fish.

phytanic acid storage disease /fītan″ik/, a rare genetic disorder of lipid metabolism in which phytanic acid accumulates in the plasma and tissues. The condition is characterized by ataxia, peripheral neuropathy, retinitis pigmentosa, and abnormalities of the bone and skin. Also called **Refsum syndrome.**

phyte-. See **phyto-, phyt-, phyte-.**

-phyte, a suffix meaning "that which grows in or on or produces": *chrodrophyte, saphrophyte, osteophyte.*

phytochemical, the active chemical components, or constituents, present in a plant that account for its medicinal properties.

phytoestrogens, an estrogen-like compound found in soybeans and soy products.

phytogenesis /fī'tōjen"əsis/ [Gk, *phyton,* plant, *genein,* to produce], the origin and evolution of algae and plants.

phytogenous /fītoj"ənəs/ [Gk, *phyton,* plant, *genein,* to produce], **1.** produced by or originating in algae or plants. **2.** pertaining to phytogenesis.

phytohemagglutinin (PHA) /fī'tōhem"əgloo̅"tinin/ [Gk, *phyton,* plant, *haima,* blood; L, *agglutinare,* to glue], a hemagglutinin that is derived from a plant, specifically the lectin obtained from the red kidney bean. Also called **phytolectin.**

phytohemagglutinin test, a test to identify genetic carriers of cystic fibrosis, performed by exposing white blood cells to phytohemagglutinin. A normal reaction involves a noticeable increase in cell protein. Molecular genetic markers are now available for the diagnosis of cystic fibrosis.

phytolectin. See **phytohemagglutinin.**

phytonadione, **1.** See **vitamin K₁. 2.** an agent used to promote the production of prothrombin to treat hypoprothrombinemia. It is administered via the oral and parenteral routes.

phyto-, phyt-, phyte-, prefix meaning "plant or plants": *phytochemical, phytoestrogens, phytotherapy.*

phytotherapy. See **herbal medicine.**

pi /pī/, **1.** Π, π, the sixteenth letter of the Greek alphabet. **2.** (in mathematics) the ratio of a circle's circumference to its diameter.

P.I., **1.** (in patient records) abbreviation for *present illness.* **2.** abbreviation for *International Pharmacopeia.* **3.** (in research) abbreviation for *principal investigator.* **4.** (in pharmacology) abbreviation for **package insert.**

pia, abbreviation for **pia mater.**

pia-arachnoid /pī'ə·arak'noid/ [L, *pia,* tender; Gk, *arachne,* spider, *eidos,* form], pertaining to both the pia mater and arachnoid layers of the meninges covering the brain and spinal cord.

piagetian /pī'äzhe"tē·ən/, pertaining to the theories and viewpoints of Jean Piaget. See also **Piaget, Jean.**

Piaget, Jean /zhän pē·äzhā"/ [1896–1980], a Swiss psychologist and genetic epistemologist who established the Genevan school of developmental psychology. From his original training in zoology and his early work in testing schoolchildren in the laboratory, Piaget developed a premise that human intelligence is an extension of biological adaptation. He assumed that human intelligence evolves in a series of stages that are related to age. At each successive stage, intellectual adaptation is more general and shows a higher level of logical organization.

pia mater (pia) /pē"ə mā"tər, pī"ə/ [L, *pia,* tender, *mater,* mother], the innermost of the three meninges covering the brain and the spinal cord. It is closely applied to both structures and carries a rich supply of blood vessels, which nourish the nervous tissue. The cranial pia mater covers the surface of the brain and dips into the fissures and sulci of the cerebral hemispheres. The spinal pia mater is thicker, firmer, and less vascular than the cranial pia mater and consists of two layers. The outer layer is composed of longitudinal collagenous fibers. The inner layer wraps the entire spinal cord and, at the end of the cord, is prolonged into the filum terminale. The pia mater also forms the denticulate ligament, which extends the entire length of the spinal cord on both sides. Compare **arachnoid, dura mater.** See also **meninges.**

pian. See **yaws.**

pian bois. See **forest yaws.**

pica /pī"kə/ [L, magpie], a craving to eat nonfood substances, such as dirt, clay, chalk, glue, ice, starch, or hair. The appetite disorder may occur with some nutritional deficiency states (particularly iron deficiency), with pregnancy, and in some forms of mental illness.

Pick disease [Arnold Pick, Czech neurologist, 1851–1924], a form of dementia that may occur in middle age. This disorder mainly affects the frontal and temporal lobes of the brain and characteristically produces slow disintegration of intellect, personality, and emotions and degeneration of cognitive abilities. See also **dementia.**

pickwickian syndrome /pikwik"ē·ən/ [*Pickwick Papers* by Charles Dickens], an abnormal condition characterized by obesity, decreased pulmonary function, somnolence, and polycythemia.

pico-, prefix meaning "one trillionth" (10^{-12}) of the unit designated: *picogram, picoampere, picosecond.*

picoampere, a measure of electrical current, equal to one millionth of one millionth (10^{-12}) of an ampere.

picogram (pg) /pī"kəgram/, a unit of measure equal to one trillionth of a gram, or 10^{-12} gram.

picornavirus /pīkôr"nəvī"rəs/ [It, *pico,* small; *RNA,* ribonucleic acid; L, *virus,* poison], a member of a group of small ribonucleic acid (RNA) viruses that are ether-resistant. The two main genera are *Enterovirus* and *Rhinovirus.* These viruses cause poliomyelitis, herpangina, aseptic meningitis, encephalomyocarditis, and foot-and-mouth disease.

picosecond (ps), a unit of measure equal to one trillionth of a second (10^{-12} second).

picro-, prefix meaning "bitter": *picrotoxin.*

picrotoxin /pik"rōtok"sin/ [Gk, *pikros,* bitter, *toxikon,* poison], a central nervous system stimulant obtained from the seeds of *Anamirta cocculus,* formerly used as an antidote for acute barbiturate poisoning.

PID, abbreviation for **pelvic inflammatory disease.**

PIE, abbreviation for **pulmonary infiltrate with eosinophilia.**

piebald /pī"bôld/ [L, *pica,* magpie; ME, *balled,* smooth], **1.** having patches of white hair or skin caused by an absence of melanocytes in those nonpigmented areas. It is a hereditary condition. Compare **albinism, vitiligo. 2.** having two colors: black and white or brown and white; mottled. *−piebaldism, n.*

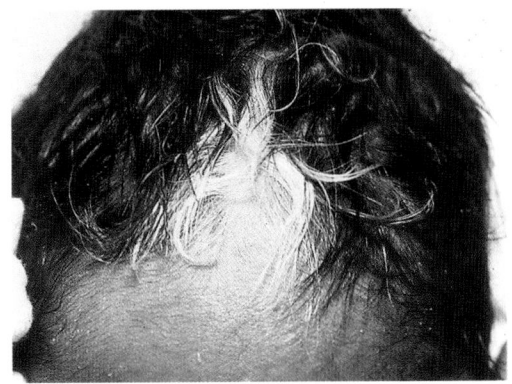

Piebaldism *(Zitelli, Davis, and Nowalk, 2012)*

P

Piedmont fracture /pēd′mənt/, an oblique break in the distal radius, with fragments of bone pulled into the ulna.

piedra /pē·ā″drə/, fungal disease of the hair shaft characterized by the presence of small black or white nodules. Black piedra is caused by *Piedria bortae*. White piedra (called trichosporosis) is caused by *Trichosporon beigelii*.

Pierre Robin syndrome /pyer rob″in, pyer rōban″/ [Pierre Robin, French histologist, 1867–1950], a complex of congenital anomalies including a small mandible, cleft lip, cleft palate, other craniofacial abnormalities, and defects of the eyes and ears, including glaucoma. Intelligence is usually normal. Plastic surgery may achieve satisfactory cosmetic repair, but speech therapy, orthodontia, and psychological counseling and support are often necessary.

-piesis, a suffix for certain terms relating to pressure; for example, anisopiesis.

piez-, prefix meaning "pressure": *piezochemistry, piezelectric.*

piezochemistry /pī·ē′zōkem″istrē/ [Gk, *piezein*, to press, *chemeia* alchemy], a branch of chemistry concerned with reactions that occur under pressure.

piezoelectric activity, the changing of electric surface charges of a structure that force the structure to change shape. Also called **electropiezo activity.**

piezoelectric effect /pī·ē′zō·ilek″trik/ [Gk, *piezein*, to press, *elektron* amber; L *effectus*], **1.** the generation of a voltage across a solid when a mechanical stress is applied. **2.** the dimensional change resulting from the application of a voltage. **3.** (in ultrasound) the conversion of one form of energy into another, such as the conversion of electrical energy into mechanical energy.

pigeon breast /pij′ən/ [L, *pipio*, young bird; AS, *broest*, breast], a congenital structural defect characterized by a prominent anterior projection of the xiphoid and the lower part of the sternum and by a lengthening of the costal cartilages. It may cause cardiorespiratory complications but rarely warrants surgical correction. Also called **pectus carinatum, pigeon chest.** *–pigeon-breasted, adj.*

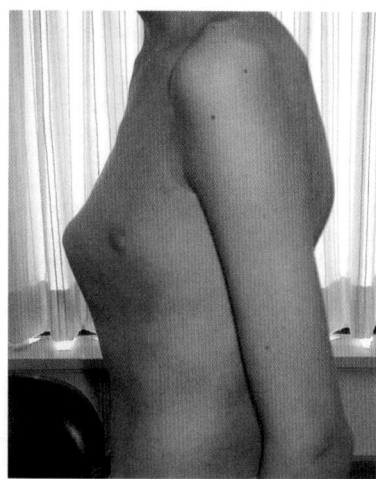

Pigeon breast *(Townsend et al, 2008)*

pigeon breeder's lung, a respiratory disorder caused by acquired hypersensitivity to antigens in bird droppings. It is characterized by chills, fever, and difficult breathing. The symptoms subside when exposure to the allergen ceases. Also called **bird breeder's lung, hen worker's lung.**

pigeon chest. See **pigeon breast.**

pigeon-toed. See **metatarsus varus.**

piggyback port [AS, *piken*, pick; ME, *pakke*, pack; L, *portus*, haven], a special coupling in the primary IV tubing that allows a supplementary, or piggyback, solution to run into the IV system. The piggyback port includes a back check valve that automatically prevents the primary IV solution from flowing while the piggyback solution is flowing. When the piggyback solution stops flowing, the back check valve allows the flow of the primary IV solution. Piggyback ports are part of piggyback IV sets, which are used for intermittent drug administration.

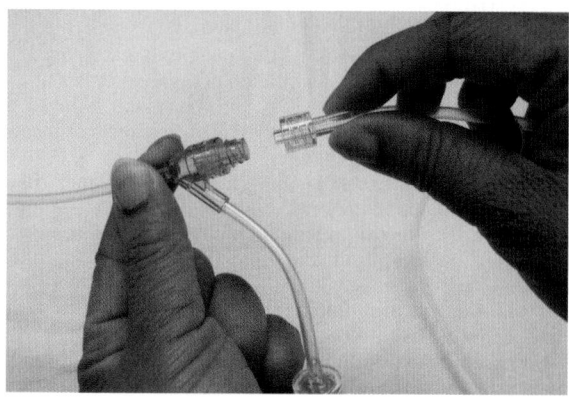

Piggyback port *(Courtesy the University of Medicine and Dentistry of New Jersey, School of Nursing)*

pigment /pig″mənt/ [L, *pigmentum*, paint], **1.** any organic coloring material produced in the body, such as melanin. **2.** any colored, paintlike medicinal preparation applied to the skin surface. *–pigmented, pigmentary, adj., –pigmentation, n.*

pigmentary retinopathy /pig″mənter′ē/, a disorder of the retina characterized by deposits of pigment and increasing loss of vision.

pigmentation, pigmented. See **pigment.**

pigmented villonodular synovitis /pig′məntid/, a disease of the joints characterized by fingerlike proliferative growths of synovial tissue, with hemosiderin deposition within the synovial tissue. The cause of the disorder is unknown.

pigment layers, the parts of the eye comprising the pigmented strata of the ciliary body, iris, and retina.

pigmy. See **pygmy.**

pigtail stent, a ureteral stent with a curl near the end like that of a pig's tail to maintain it in place.

pil, a shortened form for the Latin words for "pill" and "pills." Abbreviation for *pilula, pilulae.*

pilar cyst /pī′lər/ [L, *pilus*, hair; Gk, *kystis*, bag], an epidermoid cyst of the scalp. Its keratinized contents are firmer and less cheesy than the material in epidermoid cysts found elsewhere. The cyst originates from the middle part of the epithelium of a hair follicle. Treatment is surgical excision. Also called **wen.** Compare **epidermoid cyst.**

Pilates method, a gentle but focused exercise-based system that tones, stretches, and strengthens the body in a nonimpact, balanced system of body-mind exercise and mobilizes the body to move with maximum efficiency and minimum effort. Classes include mat work and use of equipment designed to provide resistance against tensioned springs to isolate and develop specific muscle groups. This method can achieve an improvement of body alignment and breathing, increased body awareness, and efficient and graceful movement.

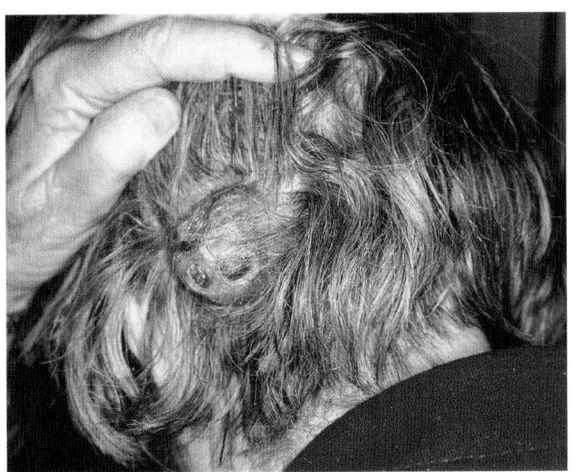

Pilar cyst *(James et al, 2016)*

piles. See **hemorrhoid.**

pili. See **pilus.**

pili annulati [L, *pilus,* hair + *annulus,* ring], a condition in which the individual hairs appear to be marked by alternating bands of white as a result of some barrier in the hair that prevents passage of light and causes the rays to be reflected back, giving the appearance of white bands.

piliform /pī′lifôrm/ [L, *pilus,* hair], having the appearance of hair.

pi lines /pī/, radiograph artifacts that result from dirt or chemical stains on a processing roller. They occur at intervals of pi (3.14) times the diameter of the roller.

pill. See **tablet.**

pillion fracture /pil′yən/ [Gael, *pillean,* couch; L, *fractura,* break], a T-shaped break in the distal femur with displacement of the condyles posterior to the femoral shaft, caused by a severe blow to the knee.

pill-rolling tremor. See **parkinsonian tremor.**

pilo-, prefix meaning "resembling or composed of hair": *pilonidal, pilomotor, pilosebaceous.*

pilocarpine and epinephrine /pī′lōkär″pēn/, a fixed-combination drug used in the treatment of glaucoma, containing a cholinergic (pilocarpine hydrochloride) and an adrenergic vasoconstrictor (epinephrine bitartrate).

pilocarpine and physostigmine, a fixed-combination drug used in the treatment of glaucoma, containing a cholinergic (pilocarpine hydrochloride) and a short-acting cholinesterase inhibitor (physostigmine salicylate). Both ingredients reduce intraocular pressure.

pilocarpine hydrochloride, a cholinergic derived from the leaves of the jaborandi tree and other species of *Pilocarpus.* It is used mainly in a topical ophthalmic preparation as a miotic to contract the pupil in cases of glaucoma. Pilocarpine is administered orally to increase saliva production in patients with xerostomia. Other consequences of cholinergic receptor stimulation include diaphoresis, bronchoconstriction, urinary urgency, nausea, and diarrhea.

pilomotor reflex /pī′lōmō″tər/ [L, *pilus,* hair, *motor,* mover, *reflectere,* to bend back], erection of the hairs of the skin caused by contraction of small involuntary arrector muscles (arrectores pilorum) in response to a chilly environment, emotional stimulus, or skin irritation. This normal reaction is abolished below the level of a transverse spinal cord lesion and may be exaggerated on the affected side in a patient with hemiplegia. Also called **gooseflesh, horripilation,** *piloerection.*

pilonidal /pī′lənī″dəl/ [L, *pilus,* hair, *nidus,* nest], a growth of hair in a cyst or other internal structure.

pilonidal cyst [L, *pilus* + *nidus,* nest], a cyst that often develops in the sacral region of the skin. Pilonidal cysts may sometimes be recognized at birth by a depression, sometimes by a hairy dimple in the midline of the back in the sacrococcygeal area. Usually these cysts do not cause any problems, but occasionally a sinus or fistula develops in early adulthood that communicates with the skin, resulting in infection. A fistula also may develop to the spinal tract from a pilonidal cyst. If a cyst becomes infected or inflamed, it is excised, and the space is surgically closed after the infection or inflammation has been effectively treated. A pilonidal cyst is not a true cyst but a poorly drained anaerobic abscess.

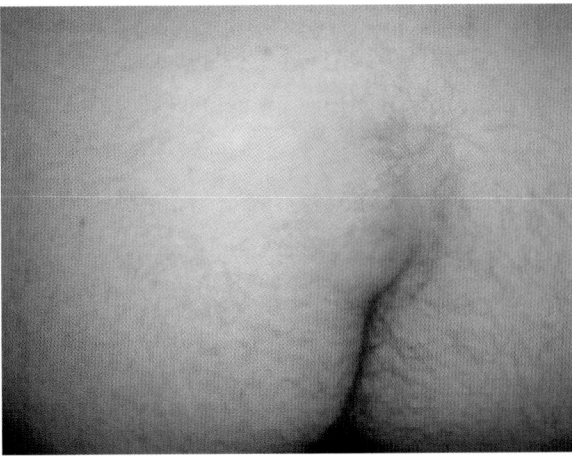

Pilonidal cyst *(Courtesy of Pilonidal Support Alliance, Long Beach, California)*

pilonidal cystectomy, a procedure performed to remove an abscessed pilonidal cyst with sinus tracts. Most common in young men, abscesses are drained during the acute stage and surgically excised during remission.

pilonidal fistula, an abnormal channel containing a tuft of hair, situated most frequently over or close to the tip of the coccyx but also occurring in other regions of the body. Treatment is surgical. Also called **pilonidal sinus.**

pilonidal sinus [L, *pilus* + *nidus* + *sinus,* curve], a cavity or sinus containing hair, in a dermoid cyst or the deepest layers of the skin. In most instances the hair originates in another area and becomes lodged in the sinus.

pilosebaceous /pī′lōsibā″shəs/ [L, *pilus* + *sebum,* fat], pertaining to a hair follicle and its oil gland.

pilot study, a small preliminary version of a proposed research study, conducted to refine the methodology of subsequent studies.

pilule. See **parvule.**

pilus /pē″ləs/ *pl.* **pili** [L, hair], **1.** a hair or hairlike structure. **2.** (in microbiology) a fine filamentous appendage found on certain bacteria and similar to flagellum except that it is shorter, straighter, and found in greater quantities in the organism. Pili consist solely of protein and are associated with antigenic properties of the cell surface.

Pima, an expectorant. Brand name for **potassium iodide.**

pimelo-, prefix meaning "fat": *pimelorrhea.*

pimelorrhea. See **fatty diarrhea.**

pimozide /pim′əzīd/, an antipsychotic agent from the diphenylbutylpiperidine class.

■ INDICATIONS: It is prescribed for the suppression of motor and phonic tics associated with Gilles de la Tourette's syndrome.

■ CONTRAINDICATIONS: It may cause electrocardiography changes, including a prolonged QT interval, and should not be given to patients with a congenital prolonged QT interval or a history of cardiac arrhythmias. It also may lower the seizure threshold of patients who are also taking an anticonvulsant drug. It should not be taken concurrently with drugs that are inhibitors of CYP3a4 (e.g., ketoconazole, erythromycin).

■ ADVERSE EFFECTS: Among the more serious adverse effects are extrapyramidal effects, persistent tardive dyskinesia, sedation, drowsiness, constipation, dry mouth, visual disturbances, and electrocardiograph changes.

pimple [ME, *pinple*], a small papule, pustule, or furuncle.

pin [AS, *pinn*], **1.** *v.,* (in orthopedics) to secure and immobilize fragments of bone with a nail. **2.** See **nail,** def. 2. **3.** *n.,* (in dentistry) a small metal rod or peg, used as a support in rebuilding a tooth.

pinch, a compression or squeezing of the end of the thumb in opposition to the end of one or more of the fingers. An example is the pulp pinch, a type of grasp in which the pulp, or fleshy mass at the end of the fingers, is pressed against the pulp at the end of the thumb. See also **lateral pinch, palmar pinch, tip pinch.**

pinch graft [Fr, *pince* + Gk, *graphion,* stylus], a small circular deep graft of skin only a few millimeters in diameter. It is cut so that the center is of whole skin but the edges consist of only epidermis.

pinch grip. See **tip pinch.**

pinch meter, a type of dynamometer that measures the strength of a finger pinch.

pincushion distortion, **1.** inward bowing of gridded straight lines in an image as a result of lens distortion. **2.** the image of a square object thus resembling a pincushion or pillow. **3.** a distortion of a fluoroscopic image associated with the use of image intensifier tubes. See also **barrel distortion.**

pindolol /pin′dəlol/, a beta-adrenergic blocker with intrinsic sympathomimetic activity.

■ INDICATIONS: It is prescribed in the treatment of hypertension, alone or concomitantly with a diuretic.

■ CONTRAINDICATIONS: Bronchial asthma, overt cardiac failure, cardiogenic shock, second- and third-degree heart block, or severe bradycardia prohibits its use. It must be used with caution in patients with diabetes.

■ ADVERSE EFFECTS: Among the most serious adverse effects are bradycardia, hypotension, syncope, tachycardia, aggravation of bronchospasm, and GI disturbances.

pineal /pin′ē·əl/ [L, *pineus,* pine cone], **1.** pertaining to the pineal body. **2.** resembling a pine cone.

pineal body [L, *pineas,* pine cone; AS, *bodig,* body], a cone-shaped structure in the brain, situated between the superior colliculi, the pulvinar, and the splenicum of the corpus callosum. Its precise function has not been established. It may secrete the hormone melatonin, which appears to inhibit the secretion of luteinizing hormone. Also called **epiphysis cerebri, pineal gland.**

pinealectomy /pin′ē·əlek″təme/ [L, *pineus* + Gk, *ektomē,* excision], the surgical removal of the pineal body.

pineal gland. See **pineal body.**

pineal hyperplasia syndrome, an abnormal condition caused by overgrowth of the pineal gland. It is characterized by severe insulin resistance, dry skin, thick nails, hirsutism, early dentition, and sexual precocity. Teeth develop prematurely and are malformed. External genitalia may reach adult size by 4 years of age. Ketoacidosis may occur despite high levels of endogenous insulin. Similar abnormalities are associated with some pineal tumors.

pinealoma /pin′ē·əlō″mə/ *pl.* pinealomas, pinealomata [L, *pineas* + Gk, *oma,* tumor], a rare neoplasm of the pineal body in the brain, characterized by hydrocephalus, pupillary changes, gait disturbances, headache, nausea, and vomiting.

pineal peduncle [L, *pineus,* pine cone, *peduncle,* small foot], the stalk of the pineal body.

pineal tumor, a neoplasm of the pineal body. See also **pinealoma.**

pine tar [L, *pinus,* pine; AS, *teoru,* tar], a topical antieczematic and a rubefacient. It is a common ingredient in creams, soaps, and lotions used in the treatment of chronic skin conditions, such as eczema or psoriasis.

pinguecula /ping·gwe′kyoo·lə/ *pl.* pingueculae [L, somewhat fatty], a yellowish spot of proliferation on the bulbar conjunctiva near the junction of the sclera and cornea, usually on the nasal side, likely related to ultraviolet light exposure and chronic environmental irritation. It is seen in elderly people with an extensive history of sun exposure.

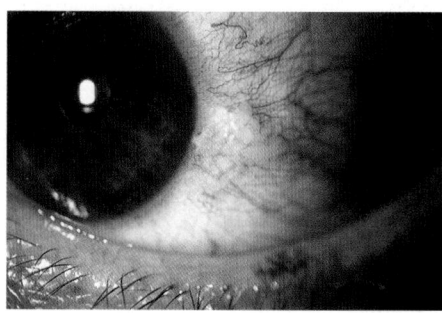

Pinguecula *(Kanski and Bowling, 2011)*

pinhole pupil [ME, *pyn* + *hol* + L, *pupilla,* little girl], a very small pupil, which may be a congenital condition, an effect of the use of miotics, or the result of an inflamed iris.

pinhole retention [ME, *pyn* + *hol* + L, *retinere,* to hold], retention developed by drilling one or more holes, 2 to 3 mm in depth, in suitable areas of a cavity preparation to supplement resistance and retention form.

pinhole test, **1.** a test performed on a person who has diminished visual acuity to distinguish a refractive error from organic disease. A refractive error may be corrected with glasses, whereas organic disease may signal the development of preventable blindness. Several pinholes, 0.5 to 2 mm in diameter, are punched in a card. The patient selects one and looks through it with one eye at a time, without wearing corrective lenses. If visual acuity is improved, the defect is refractive; if not, it is organic. The pinhole effect results from blocking peripheral light waves, which are most distorted by refractive error. **2.** a test to determine the size of the focal spot of an x-ray tube. **3.** a test to trace the path of x-ray tube movement.

Pin-Index Safety System (PISS), a system for identifying connectors for certain small cylinders of medical gases that have flush valve outlets rather than threaded outlets. The identifying code consists of a specific combination of two holes in the face of the valve into which connecting pins for a particular type of gas must fit in perfect alignment. For example, the index hole position for a cylinder of oxygen is 2–5, for nitrous oxide it is 3–5, and so on. See also **Diameter-Index Safety System.**

pink disease. See **acrodynia.**

pinkeye. See **conjunctivitis.**

Pink or Blue Test™, a blood test that can determine the sex of a fetus as early as seven weeks' gestation.

Pinkus' disease. See **lichen nitidus.**

pinna. See **auricle.**

pinocyte /pī′nəsīt′/ [Gk, *pinein,* to drink, *kytos,* cell], a cell that can absorb liquids by pinocytosis. *–pinocytic, adj.*

pinocytosis /pī′nōsītō″sis/ [Gk, *pinein + kytos + osis,* condition], the process by which extracellular fluid is taken into a cell. The plasma membrane develops a saccular indentation filled with extracellular fluid and then pinches off the indentation, forming a vesicle or vacuole of fluid within the cell.

pinprick test, a test of a person's ability to detect a cutaneous pain sensation and to differentiate such sensations from pressure stimuli. The test is performed with a pin or needle gently applied to a skin area where it cannot be observed by the subject. The application of the pin is alternated with the pressing of a dull object against the skin. Care is taken to prevent penetration of the dermis, and the sharp object used should be sterilized or discarded after the test.

pinta /pēn″tə/ [Sp, spot], an infection of the skin caused by *Treponema carateum,* a common organism in South and Central America. The bacterium gains entry into the body through a break in the skin. Prolonged exposure and close contact appear to be necessary for transmission. The primary lesion is a slowly enlarging papule with regional lymph node enlargement, followed in 1 to 12 months by a generalized red to slate-blue macular rash. Eventually these lesions become depigmented. Diagnosis is based on serological tests and dark-field microscopic examination of scrapings from skin lesions. Treatment with penicillin G is effective. Also called *azul, azula,* **carate, mal del pinto.** Compare **yaws.**

pin track infection [ME, *pyn + trak,* trace; L, *inficere,* to taint], an abnormal condition associated with skeletal traction or external fixation devices and characterized by infection of superficial, deeper, or soft tissues or by osteomyelitis. These infections may develop at skeletal traction pin sites. Some of the signs of pin track infection are erythema at the pin sites, drainage and odor, pin slippage, elevated temperature, and pain. Superficial infection at the pin site is treated with antibiotics administered topically or orally. Deeper infection at the pin sites usually requires removal of the pins and antibiotic therapy.

pinworm. See *Enterobius vermicularis.*

PIO₂, symbol for *partial pressure of inspired oxygen.*

pioglitazone, an oral antidiabetic.

■ INDICATIONS: It is used to treat stable type 2 diabetes mellitus.

■ CONTRAINDICATIONS: Lactation, diabetic ketoacidosis, and known hypersensitivity to this drug prohibit its use. It is also contraindicated in children.

■ ADVERSE EFFECTS: Common adverse effects include myalgia, sinusitis, upper respiratory infection, pharyngitis, headache, and aggravated diabetes mellitus.

pion /pī″on/ [Gk, *pi,* 16th letter of Greek alphabet, *meson,* nuclear particle], any of a family of subatomic particles that can be created in nuclear reactions. Pions are unstable but can exist long enough to be formed into beams and used in certain types of medical therapy, such as the treatment of brain tumors. Pions of suitable energy can penetrate the skull and deliver most of their energy to a tumor while sparing overlying normal tissue. See also **negative pi meson pion.**

pipecuronium /pip″ě-ku-ro′ne-um/, a nondepolarizing neuromuscular blocking agent used as an adjunct to anesthesia, inducing skeletal muscle relaxation and facilitating management of patients on mechanical ventilation. It is administered intravenously.

Piper forceps. See **obstetric forceps.**

pipestem ureter, stenosis and calcification of a ureter, seen as a complication of renal tuberculosis that has spread into the ureter.

pipette /pīpet′, pipet″/ [Fr, little pipe], **1.** a calibrated transparent open-ended tube of glass or plastic used for measuring or transferring small quantities of a liquid or gas. **2.** use of a pipette to dispense liquid.

Pipracil, an antibiotic. Brand name for *piperacillin sodium.*

piriform /pir′ifôrm/ [L, *pirum,* pear, *forma*], pear-shaped. Also spelled **pyriform.**

piriform aperture [L, *pirum,* pear, *forma,* form, *apertura,* opening], the pear-shaped anterior nasal opening in the skull.

piriform fascia. See **fascia of piriform muscle.**

piriformis /pir′ifôr″mis/ [L, *pirum + forma*], a flat pyramidal muscle lying almost parallel to the posterior margin of the gluteus medius. It is partly within the pelvis and partly at the back of the hip joint. It is innervated by branches of the first and second sacral nerves and functions to rotate the thigh laterally and to abduct and to help extend it. Compare **obturator externus, obturator internus.**

Pirogoff's amputation [Nikolai I. Pirogoff, Russian surgeon, 1810–1881], an ankle joint amputation in which the posterior process of the calcaneum is retained at the skin flap and opposed to the cut end of the tibia.

Pirquet test /pir ketx/ [Clemens P. von Pirquet, Austrian physician, 1874–1929], a tuberculin skin test that consisted of scratching the tuberculin material onto the skin. Also called **von Pirquet test.** See also **tuberculin test.**

pisiform /pī″sifôrm, pē″-/ [L, *pisum,* pea, *forma*], pea-shaped.

pisiform bone [L, *pisa,* pea, *forma,* form; AS, *ban,* bone], a small pea-shaped spheroidal carpal bone in the proximal row of carpal bones. It articulates with the triangular bone and is attached to the flexor retinaculum, the flexor carpi ulnaris, and the abductor digiti minimi.

Piskacek's sign /pis′kə·cheks/ [Ludwig Piskacek, Austrian obstetrician, 1854–1933], asymmetric enlargement of the body of the pregnant uterus as a result of its enlargement in the cornual region, usually over the site of implantation. Piskacek's sign is an indication of pregnancy.

pisohamate ligament, the ligament that connects the pisiform bone to the hamate. It is an extension of the flexor carpi ulnaris.

pisometacarpal ligament, the ligament that connects the pisiform bone to the fifth metacarpal.

PISS, abbreviation for **Pin-Index Safety System.**

pistol-shot sound, a sharp slapping sound heard by auscultation over the femoral pulse of a patient with aortic incompetence. It is caused by a large-volume pulse with a sharp rise in pressure.

pit and fissure cavity [AS, *pytt* + L, *fissura,* cleft, *cavum,* cavity], a cavity or area of decay that starts in a tiny groove or fault in tooth enamel, usually on an occlusal surface of a molar or premolar. In the classification of caries, it represents class I caries.

pit and fissure sealant. See **dental sealant.**

pitch [ME, *picchen*], **1.** the highness or lowness of a tone or sound depending on the rate of vibration of the sound source. **2.** (in helical computed tomography) the ratio of table advancement per 360-degree rotation of the x-ray tube to the detector collimator.

P

pithing /pith'ing/ [AS, *pitha*], the destruction of the central nervous system of an experimental animal in preparation for physiological research. It is usually done by inserting a blunt probe through a foramen.

Pitocin, an oxytocic. Brand name for **oxytocin.**

Pitressin, an antidiuretic hormone. Brand name for **vasopressin.**

pitting [AS, *pytt*], **1.** small, punctate indentations in fingernails or toenails, often a result of psoriasis. **2.** an indentation that remains for a short time after pressing edematous skin with a finger. **3.** small depressed scars in the skin or other organ of the body. **4.** the removal by the spleen of material from within erythrocytes without damage to the cells.

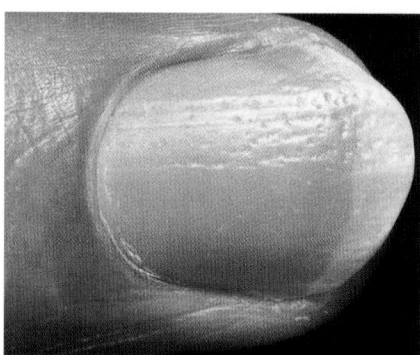

Pitting of the fingernails (du Vivier, 2002)

pitting edema [AS, *pytt* + Gk, *oidema*, swelling], an edema characterized by a condition in which a finger pressed into the skin over an accumulation of fluid will result in a temporary depression in the skin. Normal skin and subcutaneous tissues quickly rebound when the pressure is released.

pituicyte /pit(y)oo'isīt/ [L, *pituita*, phlegm; Gk, *kytos*, cell], a primary cell of the posterior lobe of the pituitary gland.

pituit-, prefix meaning "phlegm": *pituitary.*

pituitarism /pit(y)oo'itəriz″əm/ [L, *pituita*, phlegm], any condition caused by a defect or failure of the pituitary gland.

pituitary /pit(y)oo'iter'ē/, pertaining to the pituitary gland.

pituitary adamantinoma. See **craniopharyngioma.**

pituitary cachexia. See **panhypopituitarism, postpubertal panhypopituitarism.**

pituitary dwarf [L, *pituita*, phlegm; AS, *dweorge*], a individual whose impaired growth development is caused by a deficiency of growth hormone resulting from hypofunction of the anterior lobe of the pituitary. In most cases the cause is unknown and the defect is limited to a lack of somatotropin, although in some instances gonadotropins, adrenocorticotropic hormone, and thyroid stimulating hormone also may be deficient. The body is properly proportioned, with no facial or skeletal deformities, and mental and sexual development is normal. The condition is usually diagnosed in childhood by radiographic examination of the bones and radioimmunoassay of levels of plasma growth hormone. Also called **hypophyseal dwarf, Lévi-Lorain dwarf,** *Paltauf's dwarf.*

pituitary eunuchism, a form of failure of sexual development and impotence resulting from disease or dysfunction of the pituitary gland.

pituitary gland [L, *pituita*, phlegm], an endocrine gland suspended beneath the brain in the pituitary fossa of the sphenoid bone, supplying numerous hormones that govern many vital processes. It is divided into an anterior adenohypophysis and a smaller posterior neurohypophysis. The anterior lobe of the gland is composed of polygonal cells related to the production of seven hormones. The hormones, controlled by hypothalamic releasing factors, include growth hormone (somatotropin), prolactin, thyroid-stimulating hormone, follicle-stimulating hormone, luteinizing hormone, adrenocorticotropic hormone, and melanocyte-stimulating hormone. The posterior lobe is morphologically an extension of the hypothalamus and the source of vasopressin (antidiuretic hormone) and oxytocin. Vasopressin inhibits diuresis by promoting nephron water reabsorption and raises blood pressure. Oxytocin stimulates the contraction of smooth muscle, especially in the uterus. Also called **hypophysis, hypophysis cerebri.** See also **adenohypophysis, neurohypophysis.**

pituitary myxedema [L, *pituita* + Gk, *myxa*, mucus, *oidema*, swelling], a type of hypothyroid condition secondary to an anterior pituitary disease.

pituitary nanism, a type of dwarfism associated with hypophyseal infantilism. See also **pituitary dwarf.**

pituitary snuff lung, a type of hypersensitivity pneumonitis that sometimes occurs among users of pituitary snuff. The antigens to which the hypersensitivity reaction occurs are found in serum proteins of cows and pigs and in pituitary tissue. Symptoms of the acute form of the disease include chills, cough, fever, dyspnea, anorexia, nausea, and vomiting. The chronic form of the disease is characterized by fatigue, chronic cough, weight loss, and dyspnea on exercise. Also called *pituitary snuff takers' disease.*

pituitary stalk, a structure that connects the pituitary gland with the hypothalamus.

pit viper [AS, *pytt* + L, *vipera*, snake], any one of a family of venomous snakes found in the Western Hemisphere and Asia, characterized by a heat-sensitive pit between the eye and nostril on each side of the head and hollow perforated fangs that are usually folded back in the roof of the mouth. With the exception of coral snakes, all indigenous poisonous snakes in the United States are pit vipers. See also **copperhead, cottonmouth, rattlesnake.**

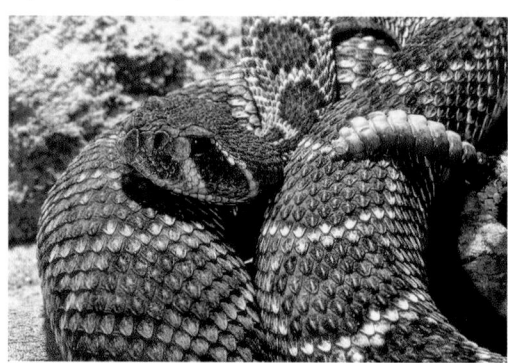

Pit viper (Courtesy St. Louis Zoo)

pityriasis /pitərī'əsis/ [Gk, *pityron*, bran], any of a number of skin diseases that have in common lesions that resemble dandrufflike scales without obvious signs of inflammation.

pityriasis alba [Gk, *pityron*, bran; L, *albus*, white], a common idiopathic dermatosis characterized by round or oval finely scaling patches of hypopigmentation, usually on the cheeks. The lesions are sharply demarcated and occasionally pruritic and are found primarily in children and adolescents. The condition may recur, but spontaneous clearing is the usual prognosis. Treatment includes lubricating creams and topical corticosteroids. Compare **pityriasis rosea.**

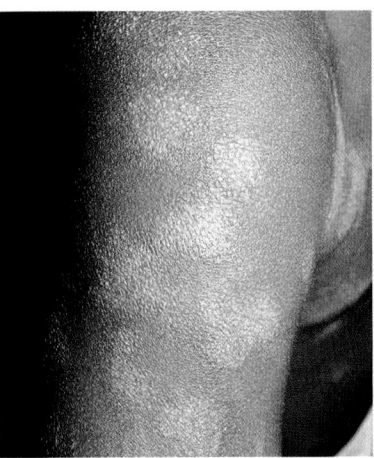

Pityriasis alba *(Cohen, 2013)*

pityriasis lichenoides, a rare, self-limited skin disease with discolored papular lesions, encompassing a spectrum from pityriasis lichenoides et varioliformis acuta to pityriasis lichenoides chronica.

pityriasis lichenoides et varioliformis acuta. See **Mucha-Habermann disease.**

pityriasis nigra. See **tinea nigra.**

pityriasis rosea, a self-limited skin disease in which a slightly scaling pink macular rash spreads over the trunk and other unexposed areas of the body. A characteristic feature is the herald patch, a larger, more scaly lesion that precedes the diffuse rash by several days. The smaller lesions tend to line up with the long axis parallel to normal lines of cleavage of the skin. Mild itching is the only symptom. The disease lasts 4 to 8 weeks and rarely recurs. Compare **pityriasis alba.**

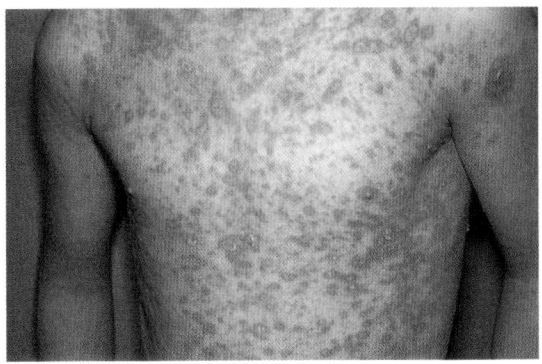

Pityriasis rosea: macular rash *(Cohen, 1993)*

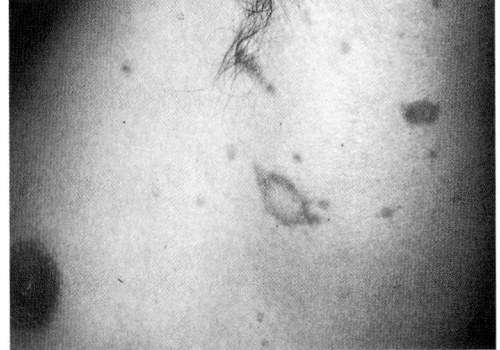

Pityriasis rosea: herald patch *(Swartz, 2009)*

pityriasis rubra pilaris [Gk, *pityron,* bran; L, *ruber* red, *pilus,* hair], a chronic inflammatory cutaneous disease characterized by tiny acuminate, reddish brown follicular papules topped by central horny plugs in which are embedded hairs; disseminated yellowish pink scaling patches; and often solid confluent hyperkeratosis of the palms and soles with a tendency to fissuring.

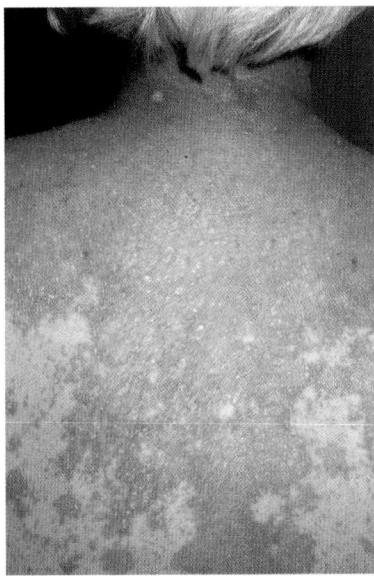

Pityriasis rubra pilaris *(Lebwohl, 2014)*

Pityrosporum ovale. See *Malassezia.*

pivot joint /piv′ət/ [Fr, hinge; L, *jungere,* to join], a synovial joint in which movement is limited to rotation. The joint is formed by a pivotlike process that may turn within a ring composed partly of bone and partly of ligament. The proximal radioulnar articulation is a pivot joint in which the head of the radius rotates within the ring formed by the radial notch of the ulna and the annular ligament. Also called **trochoid joint.** Compare **ball-and-socket joint, condyloid joint, gliding joint, hinge joint, saddle joint.**

pivot transfer, the movement of a person from one site to another, such as from a bed to a wheelchair, when there is a loss of control of one side of the body or when one side of the body is immobile. The person is helped to a position on the strong side of the body, either left or right, with both feet on the floor, heels behind the knees, and knees lower than the hips. The person stands with the weight on the strong leg, pivots on it, and carefully lowers the body into the wheelchair.

pixels, small cells of information that make up the matrix of a digital image on a computer monitor screen. Acronym for *picture elements.*

PJC, abbreviation for *premature junctional complex.*

PK, abbreviation for **psychokinesis.**

pK$_a$, the negative logarithm of the ionization constant of an acid, a measure of the strength of an acid. The lower the pK$_a$, the stronger the acid.

PKA, abbreviation for **protein kinase.**

PKD, abbreviation for **polycystic kidney disease.**

PK test, abbreviation for **Prausnitz-Küstner test.**

PKU, abbreviation for **phenylketonuria.**

placebo /pləsē″bō/ [L, shall please], an inactive substance, such as saline solution, distilled water, or sugar, or

P

a less than effective dose of a harmless substance, such as a water-soluble vitamin, prescribed as if it were an effective dose of a needed medication. Placebos are used in experimental drug studies to compare the effects of the inactive substance with those of the experimental drug. They are also prescribed for patients who cannot be given the medication they request or who, in the judgment of the health care provider, do not need that medication.

placebo effect, a physical or emotional change occurring after a substance is taken or administered that is not the result of any special property of the substance. The change may be beneficial, reflecting the expectations of the patient and often those of the person giving the substance.

placement /plās′mənt/ [Fr, *placer,* to place], (in dentistry) the positioning of a dental prosthesis, such as a removable denture, in its planned site on the dental arch.

placement path, (in dentistry) the direction of insertion and removal of a removable partial denture on its supporting oral structures. The path can be varied by altering the plane to which the guiding abutment surfaces of the denture are made parallel. The choice of a placement path is considered a compromise that best fulfills five requirements: minimal torque on abutment teeth, minimal interference, maximum retention, establishment of adequate guide plane surfaces, and acceptable aesthetic qualities. Also called *path of insertion.*

placent-, combining form meaning "a cakelike mass": *placenta.*

placenta /pləsen′tə/ [L, flat cake], a highly vascular fetal organ that exchanges with the maternal circulation, mainly by diffusion of oxygen, carbon dioxide, and other substances. It begins to form on approximately the eighth day of gestation when the blastocyst touches the wall of the uterus and adheres to it. Placentation begins as the trophoblast is able to digest cells of the endometrium, causing a small erosion on the uterine wall in which an embryo nidates. Human chorionic gonadotropin (HCG), which is chemically identical to luteinizing hormone, is secreted by the developing placenta and promotes survival and hormone production of the corpus luteum. The presence of HCG in the maternal blood and urine is an indicator of early pregnancy. The trophoblastic layer continues to infiltrate the maternal tissues with fingerlike projections, called chorionic villi. By the third month of pregnancy the placenta is able to secrete large amounts of progesterone, enough to relieve the corpus luteum of that function. At term the normal placenta is one seventh to one fifth of the weight of the infant. The maternal surface is lobulated and has a dark red rough, liverlike appearance. The fetal surface is smooth and shiny, covered with the fetal membranes, and marked by large white blood vessels beneath the membranes that fan out from the centrally inserted umbilical cord. The time between the infant's birth and the expulsion of the placenta is the third and last stage of labor.

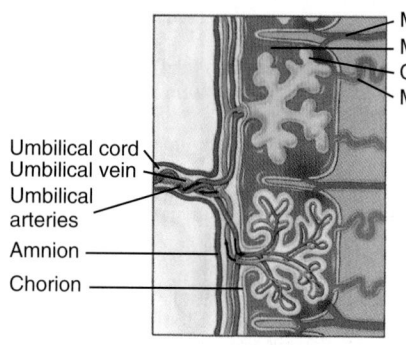

Cross section of the placenta *(Applegate, 2011)*

-placenta, -placental, suffix meaning "an organ shaped like a flat cake": *fetoplacental, retroplacental, transplacental.*

placenta abruptio. See **abruptio placentae.**

placenta accreta, a placenta that invades the uterine muscle, making separation from the muscle difficult. See also **adherent placenta.**

placenta battledore. See **battledore placenta.**

placenta bipartitia. See **bilobate placenta.**

placental /pləsen′təl/ [L, *placenta,* flat cake], pertaining to the placenta.

placental abruption. See **abruptio placentae.**

placental bruit [L, *placenta,* flat cake; Fr, *bruit,* noise], a humming noise caused by fetal circulation, heard in the pregnant uterus. It is synchronized with the mother's pulse.

placental dysfunction. See **placental insufficiency.**

placental dystocia, a prolonged or otherwise difficult delivery of the placenta. See also **dystocia.**

placental hormone, one of the hormones produced by the placenta, including human placental lactogen, chorionic gonadotropin, estrogen, progesterone, and a thyrotropin-like hormone.

placental infarct, a localized ischemic hard area on the fetal or maternal side of the placenta.

placental insufficiency, an abnormal condition of pregnancy, manifested clinically by a decreased rate of fetal and uterine growth. One or more placental abnormalities cause dysfunction of maternal-placental or fetal-placental circulation sufficient to compromise fetal nutrition and oxygenation. Some of the abnormalities that can result in placental insufficiency are abnormal implantation of the placenta, multiple pregnancies, abnormal attachments of the umbilical cord or anomalies of the cord itself, and abnormalities of the placental membranes. Histopathological abnormalities that can cause placental insufficiency include intervillous thrombi, placental infarction, and breaks in the placental membrane that result in fetal bleeding into the maternal circulation. Placental insufficiency also may result from placental senescence in postmaturity; systemic diseases, such as erythroblastosis fetalis and diabetes mellitus; or bacterial, viral, parasitic, or fungal infections. Also called **placental dysfunction.** See also **intrauterine growth retardation, postmature infant.**

placental membrane, a layer of tissue in the placenta between the fetal and maternal blood systems. The membrane regulates the diffusion of materials between the two systems.

placental presentation [L, *placenta,* flat cake, *praesentare,* to show]. See **placenta previa.**

placental scan, a scan of the uterus of a pregnant woman, performed after an IV injection of a contrast medium, used for locating the fetus and placenta and for detecting intrauterine bleeding.

placental sinus. See **marginal sinus.**

placental stage of labor, the third stage of labor, when the placenta and membranes are expelled from the uterus after the birth of the child.

placental thrombosis [L, *placenta,* flat cake; Gk, *thrombos,* lump, *osis,* condition], intravascular coagulation that occurs in the placenta and veins of the uterus.

placental transmission [L, *placenta,* flat cake; L, *transmittere,* to transmit], the transference of a drug or other substance across the placenta.

placenta previa /prē′vē·ə/, (Informal) a condition of pregnancy in which the placenta is implanted abnormally in the uterus so that it impinges on or covers the internal os of the uterine cervix. It is the most common cause of painless bleeding in the third trimester of pregnancy. Its cause is unknown. The incidence of the condition increases with increased parity from approximately 1 in 1500 primiparas to approximately 1 in 20 grand multiparas. Even slight dilation of the internal os can cause enough local separation of an abnormally implanted placenta to result in bleeding. If severe hemorrhage occurs, immediate cesarean section is usually required to stop the bleeding and to save the mother's life; it is performed regardless of the stage of fetal maturity. Before hemorrhage, placenta previa may be diagnosed by ultrasonography and treated with complete bed rest under close observation. Even at rest sudden massive hemorrhage can occur without warning. Vaginal examination is usually contraindicated if placenta previa is present or suspected because palpation can cause local placental separation and precipitate hemorrhage. Cautious and very gentle intracervical palpation may be performed to determine the existence and exact extent of placenta previa. Before this examination an IV infusion is begun, the woman's blood is typed and crossmatched, and preparations for immediate cesarean section are made. If the placenta is next to or near, rather than touching or covering, the cervical os, labor and vaginal delivery may be attempted. Central placenta previa refers to a placenta that has grown to cover the internal cervical os completely; low-lying placenta identifies a placenta that is just within the lower uterine segment; and partial or marginal placenta previa is a condition in which the placenta partially covers the internal cervical os. Also called **previa, placental presentation.** Compare **abruptio placentae.**

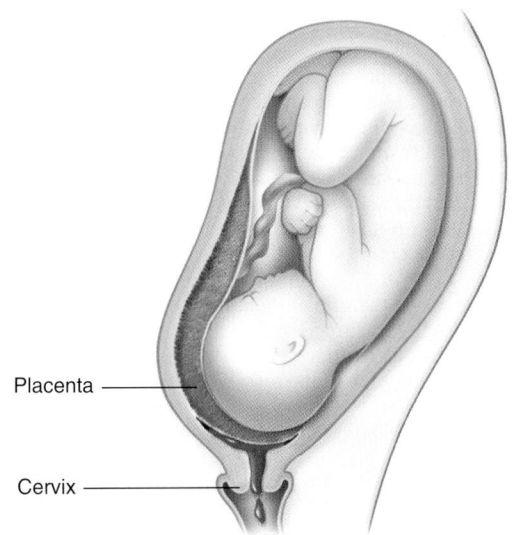

Placenta

Cervix

Placenta previa *(Patton and Thibodeau, 2010)*

placenta previa partialis, a placenta that partially obstructs the internal cervical os.

placenta souffle [L, *placenta,* flat cake; Fr, *souffle,* puff], a soft blowing or humming sound produced by fetal circulation at the placenta.

placenta succenturiate, an accessory placenta.

plafond fracture, a fracture that involves the buttress part of the malleolus of a bone.

plagiocephaly /plā′jē-ōsef″əlē/ [Gk, *plagios,* askew, *kephale,* head], a congenital malformation of the skull in which premature or irregular closure of the coronal or lambdoidal sutures results in asymmetric growth of the head, giving it a twisted, lopsided appearance so that the maximum

length is not along the midline but on a diagonal. Also called *plagiocephalism.* See also **craniostenosis.** *–plagiocephalous, plagiocephalic, adj.*

plague /plāg/ [L, *plaga,* blow], an infectious disease transmitted by the bite of a flea from a rodent infected with the bacillus *Yersinia pestis.* Plague is primarily an infectious disease of rats: The rat fleas feed on humans only when their preferred rodent hosts, usually rats, have been killed by the plague in a rat epizootic. Therefore epidemics occur after rat epizootics. Aerosolized *Y. pestis* could be used to cause the pneumonic form in a bioterrorism attack. Kinds include **bubonic plague, pneumonic plague, septicemic plague.** See also *Yersinia pestis.*

plague vaccine, an active immunizing agent prepared with killed plague bacilli.

■ INDICATIONS: It is prescribed for immunization against plague after probable exposure or as protection for travelers in endemic areas, such as Southeast Asia.

■ CONTRAINDICATIONS: Immunosuppression or acute infection prohibits its use.

■ ADVERSE EFFECTS: Among the most serious adverse effects are allergic reactions, inflammation at the site of injection, headache, and malaise.

plaintiff /plān′tif/ [ME, *plaintif,* one who complains], (in law) a person who files a lawsuit initiating a legal action. The plaintiff complains or sues for remedial relief and names a complainant in various civil actions. In criminal actions the prosecution is the plaintiff, acting on behalf of the people of the jurisdiction.

-plakia, suffix meaning "a plate or flat plane, usually on a mucous membrane": *leukoplakia.*

planar, 1. See **plane. 2.** a method for representing pixel colors on a computer screen.

planar view, a two-dimensional view of a process or function.

planar xanthoma /plā′nər/ [L, *planum,* level; Gk, *xanthos,* yellow, *oma,* tumor], a yellow or orange flat macule or slightly raised papule containing foam cells and occurring in clusters in localized areas, such as the eyelids. These lesions may be widely distributed over the body. Also called **plane xanthoma, xanthoma planum.** See also **xanthelasmatosis.**

Planck constant (h) /plangk/ [Max Planck, German physicist, 1858–1947], a fundamental physical constant that relates the energy of radiation to its frequency. It is expressed as 6.63×10^{-27} erg-seconds or 6.63×10^{-34} joule-seconds. See also **photon.**

plane [L, *planum,* level], **1.** *n.,* a flat surface determined by three points in space. **2.** *n.,* an extension of a longitudinal section through an axis, such as the coronal, horizontal, transverse, frontal, and sagittal planes, used to identify the position of various parts of the body in the study of anatomy. **3.** *v.,* the act of paring or of rubbing away. **4.** *n.,* a superficial incision in the wall of a cavity or between tissue layers, especially in plastic surgery.

plane xanthoma. See **planar xanthoma.**

planigraphic principle /plan′igraf″ik/, a rule of tomography in which the fulcrum or axis of rotation is raised or lowered to alter the level of the focal plane but the tabletop height remains constant.

plankton /plangk′tən/ [Gk, *planktos,* wandering], nearly microscopic floating or weakly swimming organisms (both photosynthetic and nonphotosynthetic) found in lakes and oceans that provide the initial level in the food chain for aquatic animals.

planktonic bacteria, drifting or floating single-cell microorganisms lacking a true nucleus and organelles.

planned change, an alteration of the status quo by means of a carefully formulated program that follows four steps: unfreezing the present level, establishing a change relationship, moving to a new level, and freezing at the new level. The program can be implemented by collaborative, coercive, or emulative means.

planned parenthood, a philosophical framework central to the development of contraceptive methods, contraceptive counseling, and family planning programs and clinics. Advocates hold that each woman has the right to decide when to conceive and bear children and that contraceptive and gynecological care and information should be available to help her become or prevent becoming pregnant. See also **contraception.**

planning [L, *planum*], (in five-step nursing process) a category of nursing behavior in which a strategy is designed to achieve the goals of care for an individual patient, as established in assessing and analyzing. Planning includes developing and modifying a care plan for the patient, collaborating with other personnel, and recording relevant information. To develop the plan the nurse anticipates the patient's needs according to established priorities; involves the patient and the patient's family and significant others in designing the plan; uses all information necessary for managing the patient's care, including recorded information from other health professionals and the age, sex, culture, ethnicity, and religion; plans for the patient's comfort, activity, and function; and chooses nursing measures that are necessary to deliver care as planned. With the cooperation of other health personnel, the nurse coordinates care for the benefit of the patient and identifies resources in the health care facility or community for social or health assistance as needed by the client or the patient's family. All information relevant to the management of the patient's care plan is recorded. Planning follows analyzing and precedes implementing in the five-step nursing process. See also **analyzing, assessing, evaluating, implementing, nursing process.**

plano-, prefix meaning "wandering": *planoconcave, planoconvex.*

planoconcave lens, a lens with one plane and one concave side.

planoconvex lens, a lens with one plane and one convex side.

plant /plant/, any multicellular eukaryotic organism that performs photosynthesis to obtain its nutrition. Plants comprise one of the five kingdoms in the most widely used classification of living organisms.

plantago seed /plantă″gō/, a bulk-forming laxative derived from *Plantago psyllium* seeds.

■ INDICATIONS: It is prescribed in the treatment of constipation and nonspecific diarrhea.

■ CONTRAINDICATIONS: Symptoms of appendicitis, intestinal obstruction, or GI ulceration prohibit its use.

■ ADVERSE EFFECTS: Among the more serious adverse effects are intestinal obstruction and allergic reactions.

plantar /plan″tər/ [L, *planta*, sole], pertaining to the sole of the foot. See also **volar.**

plantar aponeurosis, the tough fascia surrounding the muscles of the soles of the feet. Also called **plantar fascia.**

plantar arch [L, *planta*, sole, *arcus*, bow], the hollow on the sole of the foot.

plantar calcaneocuboid joint, a synovial joint between the facet on the anterior surface of the calcaneus and the corresponding facet on the posterior surface of the cuboid that allows sliding and rotating movements involved with inversion and eversion of the foot. It also contributes to pronation and supination of the forefoot on the hindfoot.

plantar calcaneonavicular ligament, a broad, thick ligament of the foot that spans the space between the

sustentaculum tali and the navicular bones, supports the head of the talus, and resists depression of the medial arch of the foot.

plantar fascia. See **plantar aponeurosis.**

plantar fasciitis, painful inflammation of the thick fibrous band on the sole of the foot.

plantar flexion [L, *planta*, sole, *flectere*, to bend], a toe-down motion of the foot at the ankle. It is measured in degrees from the 0-degree position of the foot at rest on the ground with the body in a standing position.

plantar grasp reflex, a reflex characterized by the flexion of the toes when the sole of the foot is stroked gently. It is present in infants at birth but should disappear after 6 weeks.

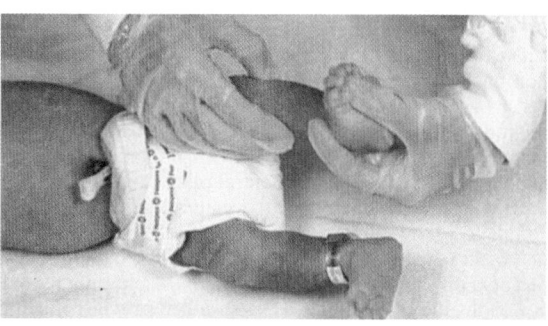

Plantar grasp reflex in the newborn *(Ball et al, 2015)*

plantaris /planter″is, plantä″ris/ [L, *planta*], one of three superficial muscles at the back of the leg, between the soleus and the gastrocnemius. The plantaris is a small muscle that arises from the distal part of the linea aspera of the femur and from the oblique popliteal ligament of the knee joint. It has a small fusiform belly, ending in a long, slender tendon that inserts into the calcaneus. The plantaris is innervated by a branch of the tibial nerve containing fibers from the fourth and the fifth lumbar and the first sacral nerves. It plantar-flexes the foot and the leg. Compare **gastrocnemius, soleus.**

plantar neuroma, a tumor or growth of nerve cells and nerve fibers on the sole of the foot.

plantar reflex, the normal response elicited by firmly stroking the outer surface of the sole from heel to toes, characterized by flexion of the toes. Compare **Babinski reflex.**

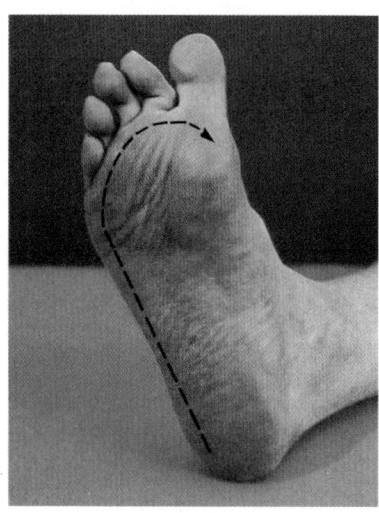

Plantar reflex *(Seidel et al, 2015)*

plantar wart, a painful verrucous lesion on the sole of the foot, primarily at points of pressure, such as over the metatarsal heads and the heel. Caused by the common wart virus, it appears as a soft central core and is surrounded by a firm hyperkeratotic ring resembling a callus. Multiple tiny black spots on the surface represent bits of coagulated blood. It is distinguished from a callus in that skin markings are interrupted by a plantar wart. Treatment methods include excision, electrodesiccation, cryotherapy, laser treatment, and use of topical acids and blistering agents. See also **mosaic wart.**

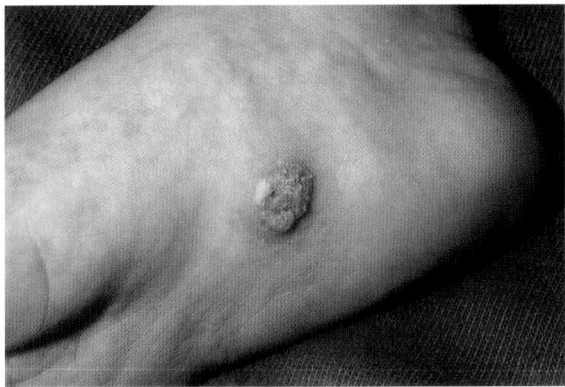

Plantar wart *(Weston, Lane, and Morelli, 2007)*

plantigrade /plan″tigrād′/ [L, *planta,* sole, *gradi,* to walk], **1.** *adj.,* pertaining to or characterizing the human gait; walking on the sole of the foot with the heel touching the ground. **2.** *n.,* a position in which an individual is standing flexed at the hips and bearing some weight through the upper extremities.

plant toxin [ME, *plante* + Gk, *toxikon,* poison], any poisonous substance derived from a plant, such as ricin, which is produced by castor-oil seeds.

plaque /plak/ [Fr, plate], **1.** a flat, often raised patch on the skin or any other organ of the body. **2.** a patch of atherosclerosis. **3.** a usually thin film on the teeth. It is made up of mucin and colloidal material found in saliva and often secondarily invaded by bacteria. Also called **bacterial plaque.**

Plaquenil Sulfate, an antimalarial, antiarthritic, and lupus erythematosus suppressant agent. Brand name for **hydroxychloroquine sulfate.**

-plasia, -plastia, suffix meaning "(condition of) formation or development": *anaplasia, dysplasia, hypoplasia.*

-plasm, -plasma, suffix meaning "cell or tissue substance": *deutoplasm, axoplasm, ectoplasm.*

plasma /plaz′mə/ [Gk, something formed], the watery light yellow fluid part of the lymph and the blood in which leukocytes, erythrocytes, and platelets are suspended. Plasma is made up of water, electrolytes, proteins, glucose, fats, bilirubin, and gases and is essential for carrying the cellular elements of the blood through the circulation, transporting nutrients, maintaining the acid-base balance of the body, and transporting wastes from the tissues. Plasma and interstitial fluid correspond closely in content and concentration of proteins. Therefore plasma is important in maintaining the osmotic pressure and the exchange of fluids and electrolytes between the capillaries and the tissues. Compare **serum.**

plasma-, combining form meaning "the liquid part of the blood": *plasmapheresis, plasmosome.*

plasma cell, a lymphoid or lymphocyte-like cell normally found in the bone marrow, the end stage of B lymphocyte maturation. On a Wright-stain marrow smear, plasma cells possess an eccentric nucleus with dark blue-staining chromatin arranged in a pattern like the spokes of a wheel. Plasma cells secrete immunoglobulins. Malignant plasma cells, called myeloma cells, are seen in bone marrow sheets and often in peripheral blood in multiple myeloma. See also **B cell, multiple myeloma.**

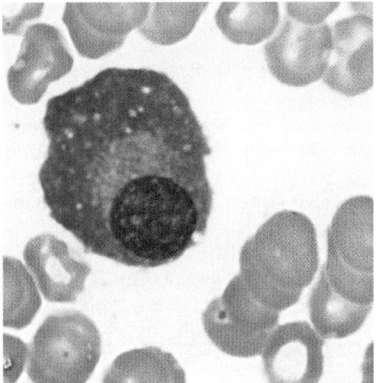

Plasma cell *(Carr and Rodak, 2008)*

plasma cell leukemia, an unusual neoplasm of blood-forming tissues in which the predominant cells are plasmacytes. The disease may develop with multiple myeloma or arise independently. Bence Jones proteinuria, abnormal serum globulins, hepatomegaly, and splenomegaly are usual in plasma cell leukemia. In most cases plasma cell leukemia is fatal, but some patients respond to treatment with alkylating agents and glucocorticoids.

plasma cell myeloma. See **multiple myeloma.**

plasma cell tumor, 1. a plasma cell dyscrasia. **2.** See **extramedullary myeloma.**

plasmacytoma /plaz′məsītō″mə/ *pl. plasmacytomas, plasmacytomata,* a focal neoplasm containing plasma cells that may develop in the bone marrow, as in multiple myeloma, or outside the bone marrow, as in tumors of the viscera and the mucosa of the nasal, oral, and pharyngeal areas. Also called **peripheral plasma cell myeloma, plasma cell tumor.**

plasma exchange [Gk, *plassein,* to mold; L, *ex + cambire,* to change; Gk, *therapeia,* treatment], a method of treating certain diseases by removing a part of the patient's plasma and replacing it with albumin, plasma, or other fluids. The goal may be to reduce a pathogenic molecule, protein, autoantibody, alloantibody, immune-complex, drug, toxin, or inhibitor, or to replace deficient plasma with normal plasma. Also called **therapeutic plasmapheresis.**

plasma expander, a 5% glucose solution that is administered intravenously to increase the plasma volume and oncotic pressure of a patient. See **volume expander.**

plasma membrane, the outer covering of a cell, often having projecting microvilli and containing the cellular cytoplasm. The plasma membrane is so thin and delicate that it is barely visible with a light microscope and can be studied in detail only with an electron microscope. The membrane controls the exchange of materials between the cell and its environment by various processes, such as osmosis, phagocytosis, pinocytosis, and secretion. Also called **cell membrane.**

plasmapheresis /plaz′məfərē″sis/, the removal of plasma from previously withdrawn blood by centrifugation, reconstitution of the cellular elements in an isotonic solution, and reinfusion of this solution into the donor or another client who needs red blood cells rather than whole blood. Compare **leukapheresis, plateletpheresis.** See also **apheresis.**

P

plasma protein, albumin, fibrinogen, prothrombin, and the gamma globulins, which constitute 6% to 7% of the blood plasma. Proteins maintain osmotic pressure, increase blood viscosity, and help maintain blood pressure. All the plasma proteins except the gamma globulins are synthesized in the liver. See also **antibody, serum.**

plasma refilling rate, in hemodialysis, the rate at which plasma that has been withdrawn and dialyzed flows back into the patient's circulatory system.

plasma renin activity, the action of the enzyme renin (produced by the kidney), measured in plasma to aid in the diagnosis of adrenal disease associated with hypertension. The normal adult value in plasma is 0.2 to 4 ng/mL/hr, depending on salt intake and the time the patient is in an upright position before a renin activity test. An upright position raises production of renin, and a high salt intake lowers it.

plasma renin assay (PRA), a blood test that measures the rate of generation of angiotensin. The most commonly used renin assay, it is a screening procedure for detecting essential, renal, or renovascular hypertension, and it is also performed to diagnose and separate primary from secondary hyperaldosteronism.

plasmasome. See **plasmosome.**

plasma thromboplastin component deficiency. See **hemophilia.**

plasma thromboplastin antecedent (PTA). *(Obsolete)* See **factor XI.**

plasma volume, the total volume of plasma in the body, elevated in diseases of the liver and spleen and in vitamin C deficiency and lowered in Addison disease, dehydration, and shock. The normal plasma volume in males is 39 mL/kg of body weight; in females, 40 mL/kg.

plasma volume extender [Gk, *plassein* + L, *volumen,* paper roll, *extendere,* to stretch], an IV solution of dextran, proteins, or other substances used to treat shock caused by blood volume loss.

plasmid /plaz′mid/ [Gk, *plasma,* something formed], in a bacterium, a small, circular molecule of DNA that is separate from the bacterial genome. Plasmids often carry genes that affect the ability of bacteria to respond to environmental challenges. For example, a bacterium containing the R (resistance) plasmid is able to resist many antibacterial drugs that act in different ways. Plasmids may be passed from one bacterium to another and are replicated in later generations of any bacterium carrying them. Molecular geneticists often use plasmids to insert specific genes into genomes of bacteria and other organisms.

plasmidotrophoblast. See **syncytiotrophoblast.**

plasmin. See **fibrinolysin.**

plasminogen, inactive precursor of plasmin, the enzyme that digests fibrinogen during fibrinolysis. See **fibrinogen.**

plasminogen activator, the enzyme that converts plasminogen to plasmin. Also called **tissue activator.**

plasminogen activator inhibitor 1, a protein produced by the endothelium that is a risk factor for atherosclerosis.

plasminogen activator inhibitor 1 test, a blood test to determine the level of PAI-1. Increased levels are indicative of acute coronary syndrome, coronary artery disease, restenosis after coronary angioplasty, infection, inflammation, trauma, type 1 diabetes, insulin resistance syndrome, or pregnancy. Decreased levels are indicative of bleeding disorders.

plasminogen test, a blood test used to diagnose suspected plasminogen deficiency in patients who present with multiple thromboembolic episodes. Abnormal levels of plasminogen are also characteristic of disseminated intravascular coagulation, primary fibrinolysis, cirrhosis and other severe liver diseases, pregnancy, eclampsia, and some inflammatory conditions.

plasmo-, prefix meaning "of or related to plasma, or to the substance of a cell": *plasmodesma.*

plasmodesma *pl. plasmodesmata,* small channels connecting the cytoplasm in plant and algal cells.

Plasmodium /plazmō″dē·əm/ *pl. plasmodia* [Gk, *plasma* + *eidos,* form], a genus of protozoa, several species of which cause malaria, transmitted to humans by the bite of an infected *Anopheles* mosquito. *Plasmodium falciparum* causes falciparum malaria, the most severe form of the disease; *P. malariae* causes quartan malaria; *P. ovale* causes mild tertian malaria with oval red blood cells; and *P. vivax* causes common tertian malaria. See also *Anopheles,* **blackwater fever.**

plasmosome /plaz″məsōm/ [Gk, *plasma* + *soma,* body], the true nucleolus of a cell as distinguished from the karyosomes in the nucleus. Also spelled **plasmasome.**

plast-, prefix meaning "to form, mold, or develop": *plaster cast, plastic, plasticity.*

-plast, -plastia, -plasia, -plastic, suffix meaning "pertaining to the formation or development of": *anaplastic, alloplast.*

plaster [Gk, *emplastron*], **1.** any composition of a liquid and a powder that hardens when it dries, such as plaster of paris; it is used in shaping a cast to support a fractured bone as it heals. **2.** *(Informal)* a home remedy, such as a mustard plaster, consisting of a semisolid mixture applied to a part of the body as a counterirritant or for other therapeutic reasons.

plaster cast [Gk, *emplastron,* plaster; ONorse, *kasta*], a traditional cast used to encase and immobilize a part of the body, made from a gauze roll impregnated with plaster of paris. The gauze is dipped in warm water and wrapped around the body part. Modern casts are often made of materials such as fiberglass or plastic instead of plaster of paris.

plaster of paris [Gk, *emplastron,* plaster; Paris, France], a white powder, calcium sulfate hemihydrate, that is mixed with water to make a paste that can be molded to encase a body part.

-plastia. See **-plasia, -plastia, -plast, -plastia, -plastic.**

plastic /plas′tik/ [Gk, *plastikos*], **1.** *adj.,* tending to build up tissues or to restore a lost part. **2.** *adj.,* conformable; capable of being molded. **3.** *n.,* a high-molecular-weight polymeric material, usually organic, capable of being molded, extruded, drawn, or otherwise shaped and then hardened into a form. **4.** *n.,* material that can be molded.

plasticity /plastis′itē/ [Gk, *plassein,* to mold], the quality of being plastic or formative.

plastic surgery [Gk, *plassein,* to mold, *cheirourgia,* surgery], surgery to heal, reconstruct, restore function, and correct disfigurement or scarring resulting from trauma or acquired or congenital lesions or defects. In performing corrective plastic surgery, the surgeon may use tissue from the patient or from another person or an inert material that is nonirritating, has a consistency appropriate to the use, and is able to hold its shape and form indefinitely. Implants are commonly used in mammoplasty for breast augmentation. Skin grafting is the most common procedure in plastic surgery. Z-plasty and Y-plasty are simpler techniques often performed instead of grafting in areas of the body covered by skin that is loose and elastic, such as the neck, axilla, throat, and inner aspect of the elbow. Dermabrasion is used to remove pockmarks, acne scars, or signs of traumatic skin damage. Chemical peeling is another technique in corrective plastic surgery. It is used primarily for removing fine wrinkles on the face. Tattooing, in which a pigment is tattooed into the skin of a graft, is performed to change the color of the graft to resemble more closely the surrounding skin. Reconstructive plastic surgery is performed to correct birth defects, to repair structures destroyed by trauma, and to replace tissue removed in other surgical procedures. Cleft lip and cleft palate repair and other maxillofacial surgical procedures, including rhinoplasty, otoplasty, and rhytidoplasty, are among these reconstructive procedures. Care of the patient before and after plastic surgery may require considerable sensitivity and tact. The patient may be exceedingly uncomfortable about the real or perceived appearance of the defect. An accepting, nonjudgmental attitude of all staff members is to the patient's benefit. Optimal nutritional status helps a graft to "take" and speeds healing. Each procedure and technique involves particular kinds of care in the preoperative and postoperative periods. Instructions and assistance in self-care activities are also specific to the procedure. Success of most of the procedures depends greatly on the patient's cooperation and on fastidious nursing care. The correction of a visible abnormality may be of inestimable benefit to the patient's assurance, self-esteem, and function in society. Also called **cosmetic surgery, reconstructive surgery.** See also *specific procedures.*

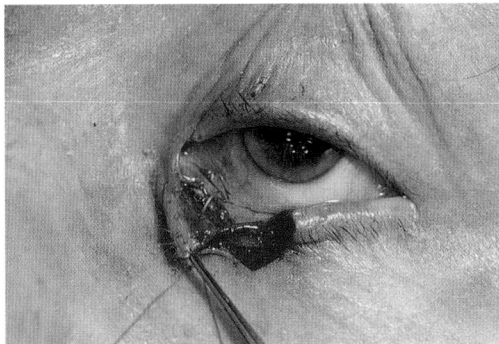

Plastic surgery: excision of excess lid tissue *(Tyers and Collin, 2007)*

-plasty, suffix meaning "molding, formation, or surgical repair on a (specified) body part or by (specified) means": *angioplasty, cervicoplasty, neoplasty.*

plate [Fr, *plat,* flat dish], **1.** a flat structure or layer, such as a thin layer of bone or the frontal plate between the sides of the ethmoid cartilage and the sphenoid bone in the fetus. **2.** a single partitioning unit of a chromatographic system.

platelet aggregation, platelet cohesion, mediated by glycoprotein membrane receptors and fibrinogen, part of a sequential mechanism leading to the initiation and formation of a thrombus or hemostatic plug. Aggregation is used as an in vitro platelet function assay, and is induced by adenosine diphosphate, arachidonic acid, thrombin, and collagen.

platelet aggregation test, a blood test that can detect diseases that affect either platelet number or function, thereby prolonging bleeding time. This test can provide information about prolonged platelet aggregation times, connective tissue disorders such as lupus erythematosus, recent cardiopulmonary or dialysis bypass, various myeloproliferative diseases, primary protein disease, von Willebrand's disease, uremia, and congenital disorders such as Wiskott-Aldrich syndrome, Bernard-Soulier syndrome, and glycogen storage disorders.

platelet antibody detection test, a blood test used to detect immune-mediated destruction of platelets. Such destruction can cause paroxysmal hemoglobinuria as well as immunological thrombocytopenia, which includes idiopathic thrombocytopenia purpura, posttransfusion purpura, neonatal thrombocytopenia, and drug-induced thrombocytopenia.

platelet count, a blood test that is performed on all patients who develop petechiae, spontaneous bleeding, or increasingly heavy menses. It is also used to monitor the course of the disease or therapy for thrombocytopenia or bone marrow failure.

plateletpheresis /plat′litfer′əsis/ [Fr, *platelet* + Gk, *aphairesis,* to carry away], collection of platelets from a donor using the apheresis technique. Also called **thrombapheresis, thrombotapheresis.** Compare **leukapheresis, plasmapheresis.** See also **apheresis.**

platelets /plat′lits/ [Fr, small plate], anucleate blood cells, 1 to 3 μm in diameter. Platelets are formed from bone marrow megakaryocytes. Approximately one third of circulating platelets become temporarily sequestered in the spleen. Platelets are disk-shaped, contain no hemoglobin, and are essential for coagulation and in maintenance of hemostasis. The platelet count reference interval is 150,000 to 450,000/μL. Also called **thrombocyte.** Compare **erythrocyte, leukocyte.** See also **thrombocytopenia, thrombocytosis.**

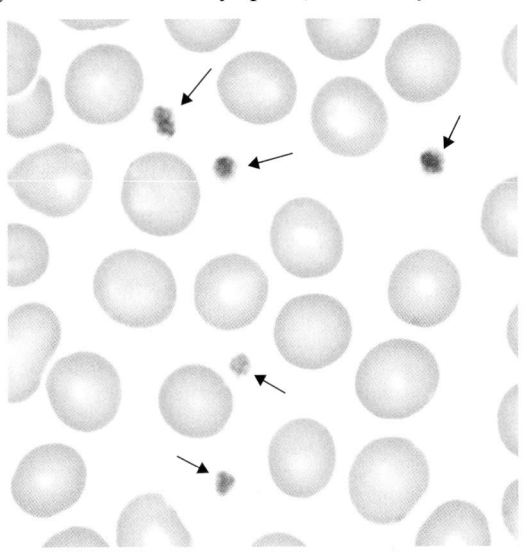

Platelets *(Carr and Rodak, 2008)*

platform, a collective term for computer hardware and software components of a particular system.

-platin, suffix for platinum-based antineoplastics.

platinized gold foil /plat″inīzd/ [Sp, *plata,* silver; AS, *geolu,* gold; L, *folium,* leaf], (in dentistry) a thin sheet of platinum sandwiched between two sheets of gold, used for making parts of dental restorations requiring greater hardness than that obtained with other materials, such as copper amalgam.

Platinol, an antineoplastic drug. Brand name for **cisplatin.**

platinum (Pt) /plat″ənəm/ [Sp, *plata,* silver], a silverwhite soft metallic element. Its atomic number is 78; its atomic mass (weight) is 195.09. Platinum is used in dentistry, jewelry, and manufacture of chemical apparatus that must withstand high temperatures. Platinum is a good catalyst for a variety of chemical reactions.

platinum foil, (in dentistry) a very thin sheet of pure platinum that has a high fusing point, making it an ideal matrix in various soldering procedures for fabricating orthodontic appliances and dentures. It is also commonly used as the internal form of porcelain dental restorations during fabrication.

platy-, prefix meaning "broad" or "flat": *platyabdominalgia, platypelloid, platycoria.*

platyabdominalgia [Gk, *platys,* flat], a symptom of abdominal pain that is aggravated when the patient is in a standing or upright position and resolves when the patient lies flat and converts to a supine position.

platycoria /plat″ĭ-kor′e-ah/, a dilated condition of the pupil of the eye.

platyhelminth /plat′ihelmin″thēz/ [Gk, *platys,* broad, *helmins,* worm], an invertebrate of the phylum Platyhelminthes that includes parasitic tapeworms (class Cestoda) and flukes (classes Monogenea and Trematoda) as well as mostly free-living species, such as planarians (class Turbellaria).

platymeria, flattening of bones in the lower extremities.

platypelloid pelvis /plat′əpel″oid/ [Gk, *platys,* broad, *pella,* bowl, *eidos,* form; L, *pelvis,* basin], a rare type of pelvis in which the inlet is round like the gynecoid type in the anterior section, but the posterior section is foreshortened by its flat and heavy border. The sacrum is hollow and inclines posteriorly, and the sidewalls are convergent. In the midplane the transverse diameter is much wider than the narrowed anteroposterior diameter. Vaginal delivery is not usually possible in the 3% of women who have platypelloid pelves.

platyrrhine, a broad, flat nasal profile.

platysma /plətiz″mə/ [Gk, *platys,* broad], one of a pair of platelike, wide muscles at the side of the neck. It arises from the fascia covering the superior parts of the pectoralis major and the deltoideus, crosses the clavicle, and rises obliquely and medially along the side of the neck. The platysma covers the external jugular vein as the vein descends from the angle of the mandible to the clavicle. The platysma is innervated by the cervical branch of the facial nerve and serves to draw down the lower lip and the corner of the mouth. When the platysma fully contracts, the skin over the clavicle is drawn toward the mandible, increasing the diameter of the neck.

play [AS, *plegan,* sport], any spontaneous or organized activity that provides enjoyment, entertainment, amusement, or diversion. It is essential in childhood for the development of personality and as a means for physical, intellectual, and social development. Play provides an outlet for releasing tension and stress, as well as a means for testing and experimenting with new or fearful roles or situations. Play is the primary role of childhood and a key part of occupational therapy and nursing care of children. In hospital settings, play helps relieve the tension and anxiety of being in unfamiliar surroundings and separated from parents, and it gives the child a sense of security and a means of expressing fears and fantasies. Play also offers health professionals one of the most effective methods of communicating with and gaining the trust of the child and helping him or her to understand treatments and procedures. Kinds include **active play, associative play, cooperative play, dramatic play, parallel play, passive play, skill play, solitary play.** See also **play therapy.**

play therapy, a form of psychotherapy in which a child plays in a protected and structured environment with games and toys provided by a therapist, who observes the behavior, affect, and conversation of the child to gain insight into thoughts, feelings, and fantasies. As conflicts are discovered, the therapist often helps the child understand and work through them.

pleasure principle /plezh′ər/ [Fr, *plaisir,* pleasure; L, *principium*], (in psychoanalysis) the need for immediate gratification of instinctual drives. Compare **reality principle.**

pledget /plej″ət/, a small, flat compress made of cotton gauze, or a tuft of cotton wool, lint, or a similar synthetic material, used to wipe the skin, absorb drainage, or clean a small surface.

-plegia, -plegic, suffix meaning "a (specified) paralysis": *cycloplegia, paraplegic.*

Plegine, an anorexiant. Brand name for **phendimetrazine tartrate.**

pleio-. See **pleo-, pleio-.**

pleiotropic gene /plī′ətrop″ik/, a gene that produces many effects in the phenotype.

pleiotropy /plī·ot″rəpē/ [Gk, *pleion,* more, *trepein,* to turn], the production by a single gene of a complex of unrelated phenotypic effects. The effects may be a manifestation of a particular disorder, such as the cluster of symptoms in Marfan's syndrome: aortic aneurysm, dislocation of the optic lens, skeletal deformities, and arachnodactyly, any or all of which may be present.

Plenaxis, brand name for **abarelix.**

pleo-, pleio-, prefix meaning "more": *pleocytosis, pleotrophy.*

pleocytosis /plē″ōsītō′sis/, presence of a greater-than-normal number of cells in the cerebrospinal fluid.

plerocercoid /plir′ōsur″koid/, the second larval stage of the cestode *Diphyllobothrium latum.* It develops in the second intermediate host, a freshwater fish, and is infective to humans if ingested.

plessimeter. See **pleximeter.**

plethora /pleth′ərə/ [Gk, *plethore,* fullness], a term applied to the beefy red coloration of a newborn. The "boiled lobster" hue of the infant's skin is caused by an unusually high proportion of erythrocytes per volume of blood. The term formerly was used to describe any red-faced person. *–plethoric, adj.*

plethysmogram /pləthiz″məgram′/ [Gk, *plethynein,* to increase, *gramma,* to record], a tracing produced by a plethysmograph.

plethysmograph /pləthiz″məgraf′/, an instrument for measuring and recording changes in the size and volume of extremities and organs by measuring changes in their blood volume. *–plethysmographic, adj.*

plethysmography /pleth′izmog″rəfē/ [Gk, *plethynein,* to increase, *graphein,* to record], the measurement of changes in the volume of organs or other body parts, particularly those changes resulting from blood flow.

pleur-. See **pleuro-, pleur-.**

pleura /plo͞or″ə/ *pl. pleurae* [Gk, rib], a delicate serous membrane enclosing the lung, composed of a single layer of flattened mesothelial cells resting on a delicate membrane of connective tissue. Beneath the membrane is a stroma of collagenous tissue containing yellow elastic fibers. The pleura divides into the visceral pleura, which covers the lung, dipping into the fissures between the lobes, and the parietal pleura, which lines the chest wall, covers the diaphragm, and reflects over the structures in the mediastinum. The parietal and visceral pleurae are separated from each other by a small amount of fluid that acts as a lubricant as the lungs expand and contract during respiration. See also **pleural cavity, pleural space.** *–pleural, adj.*

pleural biopsy, the removal of pleural tissue for histological examination after exudative fluid indicative of infection, neoplasm, or tuberculosis is obtained by thoracentesis or when a pleural-based tumor, reaction, or thickening is indicated by a chest x-ray.

pleural cavity [Gk, *pleura,* rib; L, *cavum,* cavity], the space within the thorax that contains the lungs. Between the ribs and the lungs are the visceral and parietal pleurae.

pleural cupola. See **cervical pleura.**

pleural effusion, an abnormal accumulation of fluid in the intrapleural spaces of the lungs. It is characterized by chest pain, dyspnea, adventitious lung sounds, and nonproductive cough. The fluid is an exudate or a transudate from inflamed pleural surfaces and may be aspirated or surgically drained. An exudate may result from pulmonary infarction, trauma, tumor, or infection, such as tuberculosis. The specific cause of the exudate is treated. Treatment of the effusion may include the administration of corticosteroids, diuretics, or vasodilators; oxygen therapy; intermittent positive-pressure breathing; or thoracentesis or use of a mobile system such as the Pleurx catheter.

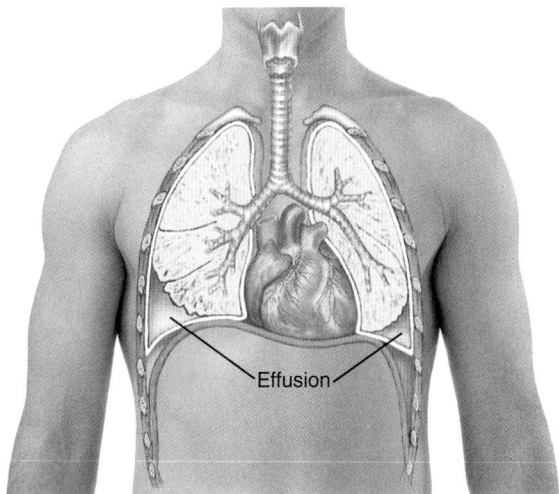

Pleural effusion *(Wilson and Giddens, 2013)*

pleural friction rub.   See **pleuropericardial rub.**

pleural space, the potential space between the visceral and parietal layers of the pleurae. The space contains a small amount of fluid that acts as a lubricant, allowing the pleurae to slide smoothly over each other as the lungs expand and contract with respiration.

pleurisy /plŏŏr″əsē/ [Gk, *pleura + itis,* inflammation], inflammation of the parietal pleura of the lungs. It is characterized by dyspnea and stabbing pain, leading to restriction of ordinary breathing with spasm of the chest on the affected side. A pleural friction rub may be heard on auscultation. Simple pleurisy with undetectable exudate is called fibrinous or dry pleurisy. Pleural effusion indicates extensive inflammation with considerable amounts of exudate in the pleural spaces. Common causes of pleurisy include bronchial carcinoma, lung or chest wall abscess, pneumonia, pulmonary infarction, and tuberculosis. The condition may result in permanent adhesions between the pleura and adjacent surfaces. Treatment consists of pain relief and therapy for the primary disease. See also **acute pleurisy, adhesive pleurisy, pleural effusion, pleurodynia, pulmonary edema.** –**pleuritic,** *adj.*

pleurisy with effusion [Gk, *pleura + itis,* inflammation; L, *effundere,* to pour out], pleurisy in which there is an accumulation of fluid in the intrapleural space. The fluid has a high specific gravity as a result of a high concentration of fibrin and clots.

pleuritic /plŏŏrit″ik/ [Gk, *pleura,* rib], pertaining to a condition of pleurisy.

pleuritis.   See **pleurisy.**

pleuro-, pleur-, prefix meaning "the pleura or side": *pleurisy, pleurodynia, pleuropneumonia.*

pleurodynia /plŏŏr″ōdin″ē·ə/ [Gk, *pleura + odyne,* pain], acute inflammation of the intercostal muscles and the muscular attachment of the diaphragm to the chest wall. It is characterized by sudden, severe pain and tenderness, fever, headache, and anorexia. These symptoms are aggravated by movement and breathing. The lungs are not affected, and

characteristically there is no cough or pleural effusion. See also **epidemic pleurodynia.**

pleuropericardial folds, a pair of small ridges that originate along the lateral body walls in the fifth week of embryonic development and project into the cranial ends of the pericardioperitoneal canals to divide the pleural cavities from the pericardial cavity. They later develop into the pleuropericardial membranes.

pleuropericardial rub /-per′ikär″dē·əl/ [Gk, *pleura + peri,* around, *kardia,* heart; ME, *rubben,* to scrape], an abnormal coarse, grating sound heard on auscultation of the lungs during late inspiration and early expiration. It occurs when the visceral and parietal pleural surfaces rub against each other. The sound is not affected by coughing. A pleuropericardial rub indicates primary inflammatory, neoplastic, or traumatic pleural disease or inflammation secondary to infection or neoplasm. Also called **pleural friction rub.** See also **breath sound, Kussmaul breathing, rhonchus, wheeze.**

pleuroperitoneal cavity.   See **splanchnocoele.**

pleuroperitoneal hiatus, a posterolateral opening in the fetal diaphragm. Its failure to close leaves a congenital posterolateral defect that may become a site for a congenital diaphragmatic hernia. Also called *foramen of Bochdalek.*

pleuropneumonia /plŏŏr″ōnŏŏmō″nē·ə/ [Gk, *pleura + pneumon,* lung], **1.** a combination of pleurisy and pneumonia. **2.** an infection of cattle resulting in inflammation of both the pleura and lungs, caused by microorganisms of the *Mycoplasma* group. See also **pleuropneumonia-like organism.**

pleuropneumonia-like organism (PPLO), a group of filterable organisms of the genus *Mycoplasma* similar to *M. mycoides,* the cause of pleuropneumonia in cattle.

pleurothotonos /plŏŏr″əthot″ənəs/ [Gk, *pleurothen,* side of the body, *tonos,* tension], an involuntary, severe, prolonged contraction of the muscles of one side of the body, resulting in an acute arch to that side. It is usually associated with tetanus infection or strychnine poisoning. Compare **emprosthotonos, opisthotonos, orthotonos.**

plex-, prefix meaning "a stroke" or "to strike": *pleximeter, plexor.*

-plex, -plexus, suffix meaning "a braid, nerve, network": *complex, heteroduplex.*

-plexia, -plexy, suffix meaning "condition resulting from a crippling or serious occurrence": *apoplexy, cataplexy.*

plexiform neuroma /plek′sifôrm/ [L, *plexus,* braided, *forma,* form; Gk, *neuron,* nerve, *oma,* tumor], a neoplasm composed of twisted bundles of nerves. Also called **Verneuil neuroma.**

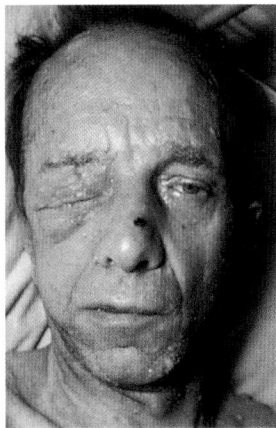

Individual with a plexiform neuroma affecting the face *(Moll, 1997)*

P

pleximeter /pleksim″ətər/ [Gk, *plessein,* to strike, *metron,* measure], a mediating device, such as a percussor or finger, used to receive light taps in percussion. Also called **plessimeter.** See also **percussion.**

plexor. See **percussor.**

plexus /plek′səs/ *pl.* **plexuses** [L, braided], a network of intersecting nerves and blood vessels or of lymphatic vessels. The body contains many plexuses, such as the brachial plexus, the cardiac plexus, the cervical plexus, and the solar plexus.

-plexus. See **-plex, -plexus.**

plexuses. See **plexus.**

-plexy. See **-plexia, -plexy.**

plic-, prefix meaning "a fold or ridge": *plica, plication.*

plica /plī″kə/ *pl.* **plicae** [L, *plicare,* to fold], a fold of tissue within the body, such as the plicae transversales of the rectum and the plicae circulares of the small intestine.

plica circularis. See **circular fold.**

plicae. See **plica.**

plical. See **plica.**

plicamycin /plī″kəmī′sin/, an antineoplastic agent. Formerly called **mithramycin.**

■ INDICATIONS: It is prescribed primarily in the treatment of malignant tumors of the testis. It is also prescribed in the treatment of hypercalcemia and hypercalciuria associated with cancer.

■ CONTRAINDICATIONS: Clotting disorders, thrombocytopenia, kidney or liver dysfunction, bone marrow depression, or known hypersensitivity to this drug prohibits its use.

■ ADVERSE EFFECTS: Among the more serious adverse effects are thrombocytopenia and clotting defects. Nausea and stomatitis commonly occur.

plica semilunaris conjunctivae. See **semilunar fold of the conjunctiva.**

plication /plīkā′shən/, any operation that involves folding, shortening, or decreasing the size of a muscle or hollow organ, such as the stomach, by taking in tucks.

plication of stomach [L, *plicare,* to fold; Gk, *stomakhos,* gullet], a surgical treatment for obesity in which tucks are created in the wall of the stomach.

plica umbilicalis lateralis. See **lateral umbilical fold.**

plica umbilicalis mediana. See **middle umbilical fold.**

pliers /plī′ərz/, small tong-jawed pincers for bending metals or holding small objects. Various forms are often used in dentistry.

Plimmer's bodies [Henry G. Plimmer, English biologist, 1857–1918], small round encapsulated bodies found in cancers and once thought to be the causative parasites. Also called *Behla's bodies.*

-ploid, -ploidy, suffix meaning "having a (specified) number of chromosome sets": *heptaploid, octaploid, polyploid.*

ploidy /ploi′dē/ [Gk, *eidos,* form], the status of a cell nucleus in regard to the number of complete chromosome sets it contains.

plosive. See **stop.**

plug [D, *plugge,* stopper], a mass of tissue cells, mucus, or other matter that blocks a normal opening or passage of the body, such as a cervical plug.

plugger, (in dentistry) an instrument for condensing or consolidating a filling material, such as a dental amalgam into a tooth restoration or gutta-percha into a root canal. **See also packer; amalgam condenser; automatic mallet condenser; back action condenser; condenser; electromallet condenser; hand condenser; Hollenback condenser; mechanical condenser; parallelogram condenser; pneumatic condenser.**

plumbism /plum′izəm/ [L, *plumbum,* lead], a chronic form of lead poisoning caused by absorption of lead or lead salts. See also **lead poisoning.**

Plummer's disease [Henry S. Plummer, American physician, 1874–1937], goiter characterized by a hyperfunctioning nodule or adenoma and thyrotoxicosis. Also called **toxic nodular goiter.**

Plummer-Vinson syndrome /plum′ər vin″sən/ [Henry S. Plummer; Porter P. Vinson, American physician, 1890–1959], a rare disorder associated with severe and chronic iron deficiency anemia, characterized by glossitis, koilonychia, and dysphagia caused by esophageal webs at the level of the cricoid cartilage. Also called **Paterson-Kelly syndrome, sideropenic dysphagia.**

plunging goiter. See **diving goiter.**

pluri-, prefix meaning "more": *pluripara, pluricentric, pluripotential.*

pluricentric blastoma. See **blastoma.**

pluripara /plŏŏrip″ərə/ [L, *plus,* more, *parere,* to bear], a woman who has borne three or more children.

pluripolar mitosis. See **multipolar mitosis.**

pluripotential stem cell. See **stem cell.**

plutonium (Pu) /plŏŏtō′nē·əm/ [planet *Pluto*], a synthetic transuranic metallic element. Its atomic number is 94; the atomic mass of its longest-lived isotope is 242. A highly toxic heavy metal, plutonium is used in nuclear power plants, and was used in the assembly of early nuclear weapons.

plyometrics, bounding or high-velocity exercise that entails eccentric and rapid concentric contractions, such as jumping or weighted ball throwing and catching. Also called *plyometric training.*

pm, abbreviation for *picometer.*

Pm, symbol for the element **promethium.**

PMDD, abbreviation for **premenstrual dysphoric disorder.**

pmh, abbreviation for *past medical history.*

PMI, abbreviation for **point of maximum impulse.**

PMN, abbreviation for **polymorphonuclear.**

PMS, pms, abbreviation for **premenstrual syndrome.**

PMT, abbreviation for *premenstrual tension.* See **premenstrual syndrome.**

PND, 1. abbreviation for **paroxysmal nocturnal dyspnea. 2.** abbreviation for **postnasal drip.**

-pnea, -pnoea, pneo-, combining form meaning "breath" or "breathing": *eupnea, dyspnea, pneopneic.*

pneopneic reflex /nē′ōnē″ik/ [Gk, *pnoe,* breath; L, *reflectere,* to bend back], a change in the normal breathing rhythm when an irritating gas is introduced into the lungs.

pneuma-. See **pneumato-, pneuma-.**

pneumatic /nŏŏmat″ik/ [Gk, *pneuma,* air], pertaining to air or gas.

pneumatic antishock garment. See **shock trousers.**

pneumatic condenser [Gk, *pneuma,* air; L, *condensare,* to thicken], a pneumatic device that delivers compacting blows of variable force to restorative material used in filling tooth cavities. The frequency of the blows may be up to 360 per minute. Also called **Hollenback condenser.**

pneumatic heart driver, a mechanical device that regulates compressed air delivery to an artificial heart, controlling heart rate, percent systole, and delay in systole.

pneumatic lithotripsy, lithotripsy in which a rigid probe is inserted through the ureter and pneumatic pressure is applied directly to the calculus.

pneumatic retinopexy, a treatment for retinal detachment involving injection of gas into the posterior vitreous cavity in such a way that the gas bubble presses against the area of torn retina, forcing it back into place.

pneumatic splint. See **inflatable splint.**

pneumato-, pneuma-, prefix meaning "air," "gas," "respiration": *pneumatocele, pneumatogram, pneumatic.*

pneumatocele /noōmat″əsēl′/, **1.** a thin-walled cavity in the lung parenchyma caused by partial airway obstruction. **2.** a hernial protrusion of lung tissue. **3.** a tumor or sac containing gas, especially of the scrotum. Also called **pneumonocele.**

pneumatocephalus. See **pneumocephalus.**

pneumatogram /noōmat″əgram′/ [Gk, *pneuma,* air, *gramma,* to record], a tracing made by a pneumograph of chest movements during breathing. Also called **pneumogram.**

pneumo-, pneumono-, prefix meaning "lungs," "air," or "the breath": *pneumocentesis, pneumonia, pneumoperitoneum.*

pneumobelt /noō′mōbelt/, a corset with an inflatable bladder that fits over the abdominal area. The bladder is connected by a hose to a ventilator that delivers positive pressure at an adjustable rate and pressure. It is used to assist in the respiratory rehabilitation of patients with high cervical injuries to alleviate strain.

pneumocentesis /-sentē′sis/ [Gk, *pneumon,* lung, *kentesis,* pricking], a procedure in which a lung is punctured to drain fluid contents.

pneumocephalus /noō′mō·sef′ə·ləs/ [Gk, *pneuma* air + *kephalē,* head], the presence of air in the intracranial cavity. Also called **intracranial pneumatocele, pneumatocephalus, pneumocrania, pneumoencephalocele.**

pneumococcal /noō′mōkok″əl/ [Gk, *pneumon,* lung, *kokkos,* berry], pertaining to bacteria of the genus *Pneumococcus.*

pneumococcal heptavalent conjugate vaccine, a preparation of capsular polysaccharides from the seven serotypes of *Streptococcus pneumoniae* most commonly isolated from children 6 years of age or younger coupled with a nontoxic variant of diphtheria toxin, used as an active immunizing agent for infants and children at risk for pneumococcal disease. It is administered intramuscularly.

pneumococcal meningitis [Gk, *pneumon,* lung, *kokkos,* berry, *meninx,* membrane, *itis,* inflammation], meningitis caused by pneumococcal infection. See also ***Streptococcus pneumoniae.***

pneumococcal nephritis, nephritis or glomerulonephritis from infection with *Streptococcus pneumoniae,* usually as a complication of pneumonia or empyema.

pneumococcal pneumonitis, inflammation of the lungs caused by an infection with pneumococcal bacteria.

pneumococcal vaccine, an active immunizing agent containing antigens of the 23 types of *Pneumococcus* associated with more than 98% of the cases of pneumococcal pneumonia in the United States and Europe.

■ INDICATIONS: It is prescribed for persons over 2 years of age who are at high risk of development of severe pneumococcal pneumonia, all adults over 65 years of age, and immunocompromised adults.

■ CONTRAINDICATIONS: Pregnancy, early childhood (less than 2 years of age), or known hypersensitivity to the vaccine prohibits its use.

■ ADVERSE EFFECTS: Among the more serious adverse effects are inflammation at the site of injection, fever, and hypersensitivity.

pneumococcal vaccine polyvalent, a preparation of purified capsular polysaccharides from the 23 serotypes of *Streptococcus pneumoniae* causing the majority of pneumococcal disease, used as an active immunizing agent in persons more than 2 years of age. It is administered intramuscularly.

pneumococcus /noō′mōkok″əs/ [Gk, *pneumon* + *kokkos,* berry], a gram-positive diplococcal bacterium of the species *Streptococcus pneumoniae,* the most common cause of bacterial pneumonia. More than 85 subtypes of this organism are known. A vaccine protective against 35 serotypes has been developed and is recommended for those over 65 years of age, those with a chronic lung disease, or those with human immunodeficiency virus infection. See also **lobar pneumonia, pneumonia,** *Streptococcus pneumoniae.*

pneumoconiosis /noō′mōkō′nē·ō″sis/ [Gk, *pneumon* + *konis,* dust, *osis,* condition], any disease of the lung caused by chronic inhalation of dust, usually mineral dust of occupational or environmental origin. Kinds include **anthracosis, asbestosis, silicosis.**

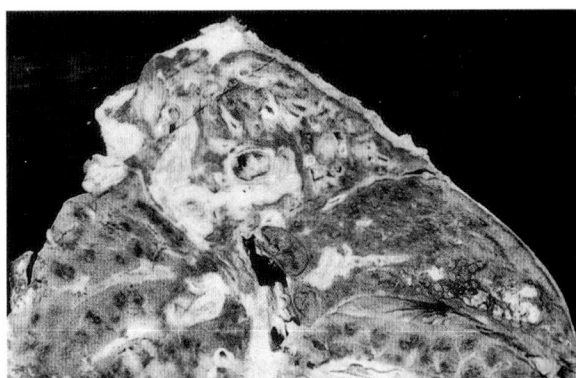

Hematite pneumoconiosis *(Skarin, 2010)*

pneumoconstriction /noō′mōkənstrik″shən/, an area of collapsed lung tissue that results from mechanical stimulation of an exposed part of the lung. It is produced by local reflex muscular closure of alveolar ducts and alveoli.

pneumocrania. See **pneumocephalus.**

Pneumocystis jiroveci /noō′mōsis′tis/, a microorganism that causes pneumocystosis, a type of interstitial cell pneumonitis.

Pneumocystis **pneumonia (PCP)** [Gk, *pneuma,* air, *kystis,* bag, *pneumon,* lung], a type of interstitial plasma cell pneumonia in which the alveoli become honeycombed with an acidophilic material. The patient may or may not be febrile but usually is weak, dyspneic, and cyanotic.

pneumocystosis /noō′mōsistō″sis/ [Gk, *pneuma,* air, *kystis,* bag, *osis,* condition], infection with the fungus *Pneumocystis jiroveci,* usually seen in patients with human immunodeficiency virus infection; premature, malnourished infants; or debilitated or immunosuppressed people, particularly those with hematologic malignancies. It is characterized by fever, cough, tachypnea, and frequently cyanosis. The diagnosis is difficult to make and usually requires obtaining a specimen by an induced sputum procedure or bronchoalveolar lavage and special staining techniques. Mortality rates are near 100% in untreated patients. Treatment with pentamidine isethionate or a combination of trimethoprim and sulfamethoxazole, trimetrexate plus folic acid, trimethoprim plus dapsone, atovaquone, or primaquine plus clindamycin is effective. Patients at risk should receive prophylaxis against acute infection. Also called **interstitial plasma cell pneumonia.**

pneumoencephalocele. See **pneumocephalus.**

pneumogastric nerve. See **vagus nerve.**

pneumogram. See **pneumatogram.**

pneumograph /noō′məgraf/, a device that records breathing movements by means of an inflated coil around the chest. It mainly measures the ventilatory cycle rather than the amplitude of breathing movements.

pneumohemopericardium. See **hemopneumopericardium.**

pneumohemothorax /-hem'ōthôr″aks/ [Gk, *pneuma,* air, *haima,* blood, *thorax,* chest], an accumulation of air and blood in the pleural cavity.

pneumolysin /nōomol″isin/, virulence factor produced by *Streptococcus pneumoniae* associated with cytolysis.

pneumomediastinum /nōo'mōmē′dē·əstī″nəm/ [Gk, *pneuma,* air, *mediastinus,* midway], the presence of air or gas in the mediastinal tissues. In infants it may lead to pneumothorax or pneumopericardium, especially in those with respiratory distress syndrome or aspiration pneumonitis. In older children the condition may result from bronchitis, acute asthma, pertussis, cystic fibrosis, or bronchial rupture from cough or trauma. Also called **Hamman disease.**

pneumonectomy /nōo'mənek′təmē/ [Gk, *pneumon,* lung, *ektomē,* excision], the surgical removal of all or part of a lung. See also **lobectomy.**

pneumonia /nōomō″nē·ə/ [Gk, *pneumon,* lung], an acute inflammation of the lungs, often caused by inhaled pneumococci of the species *Streptococcus pneumoniae.* The alveoli and bronchioles of the lungs become plugged with a fibrous exudate. Pneumonia may also be caused by other bacteria, as well as by viruses, rickettsiae, and fungi. Kinds include **aspiration pneumonia, interstitial pneumonia, bronchopneumonia, eosinophilic pneumonia, lobar pneumonia, mycoplasma pneumonia, viral pneumonia.** See also **acute lobar pneumonia, atypical pneumonia.**

Factors predisposing to pneumonia

- Aging
- Air pollution
- Altered consciousness: alcoholism, head injury, seizures, anesthesia, drug overdose, stroke
- Altered oropharyngeal flora secondary to antibiotics
- Bed rest and prolonged immobility
- Chronic diseases: chronic lung disease, diabetes mellitus, heart disease, cancer, end-stage renal disease
- Debilitating illness
- Human immunodeficiency virus (HIV) infection
- Immunosuppressive drugs (corticosteroids, cancer chemotherapy, immunosuppressive therapy after organ transplant)
- Inhalation or aspiration of noxious substances
- Intestinal and gastric feedings via nasogastric or nasointestinal tubes
- Malnutrition
- Smoking
- Tracheal intubation (endotracheal intubation, tracheostomy)
- Upper respiratory tract infection
- Resident of a long-term care facility

From Lewis SL et al: *Medical-surgical nursing: assessment and management of clinical problems,* ed 8, St. Louis, 2011, Mosby.

-pneumonia, suffix meaning "an inflammation of the lungs": *pleuropneumonia, bronchopneumonia.*

-pneumonic, **1.** suffix meaning "related to pneumonia": *parapneumonic.* **2.** suffix meaning "related to the lungs."

pneumonic plague /nōomon′ik/ [Gk, *pneumon,* lung; L, *plaga,* stroke], a highly virulent and rapidly fatal form of plague characterized by bronchopneumonia. There are two forms: primary pneumonic plague, which results from involvement of the lungs in the course of bubonic plague, and secondary pneumonic plague, which results from the inhalation of infected particles of sputum from a person having pneumonic plague. Aerosolized *Yersinia pestis* could be used to cause pneumonic plague in a bioterrorism attack.

Compare **bubonic plague, septicemic plague.** See also **plague,** *Yersinia pestis.*

pneumonitis /nōo'mənī″tis/ *pl. pneumonitides* [Gk, *pneumon + itis*], inflammation of the lung. Pneumonitis may be caused by a virus or may be a hypersensitivity reaction to chemicals or organic dusts, such as bacteria, bird droppings, or molds. It is usually an interstitial, granulomatous, fibrosing inflammation of the lung, especially of the bronchioles and alveoli. Dry cough is a common symptom. Treatment depends on the cause but includes removal of any offending agents and administration of corticosteroids to reduce inflammation. Compare **pneumonia.**

pneumono-. See **pneumo-, pneumono-.**

pneumonocele. See **pneumatocele.**

pneumonopathy /nōo'mənop″əthē/, any disease or disorder involving the lungs.

pneumonopleuritis /-plōorī″tis/, a combined disorder of pneumonia and pleurisy.

pneumonotherapy /-ther″əpē/, the treatment of lung disease.

pneumopericardium /-per'ikär″dē·əm/, the presence of air or gas in the pericardial sac.

pneumoperitoneum /nōo'mōper'itənē″əm, -per'itənē″əm/ [Gk, *pneuma,* air, *peri,* around, *teinein,* to stretch], the presence of air or gas within the peritoneal cavity of the abdomen. It may be spontaneous, such as from rupture of a hollow, gas-containing organ, or induced for diagnostic or therapeutic purposes.

pneumoperitonitis /nōo'mōper'itənī″tis/, an acute inflammation of the peritoneal cavity accompanied by the presence of air or gas.

pneumotachometer /-takom′ətər/, a device that measures the flow of respiratory gases. The pressure gradient is directly related to flow, thus allowing a computer to derive a flow curve measured in liters per minute.

pneumothorax /nōo'mōthôr″aks/ [Gk, *pneuma,* air, *thorax,* chest], the presence of air or gas in the pleural space, causing a lung to collapse. Pneumothorax may be the result of an open chest wound that permits the entrance of air, the rupture of an emphysematous vesicle on the surface of the lung, or a severe bout of coughing. It may also occur spontaneously without apparent cause.

■ OBSERVATIONS: The onset of pneumothorax is accompanied by a sudden sharp chest pain, followed by difficult, rapid breathing; decreased breath sounds and cessation of normal chest movements on the affected side; tachycardia; a weak pulse; hypotension; diaphoresis; an elevated temperature; pallor; dizziness; and anxiety.

■ INTERVENTIONS: The patient is assured that the condition can be treated, is urged to remain still, and is placed in bed in Fowler's position. Oxygen is administered through a nasal cannula, unless contraindicated, and the air in the pleural space is immediately aspirated. A chest tube is inserted and attached to an underwater seal; a waterless, disposable system; or a mobile chest drain; the tube is not removed until air is no longer expelled through the seal and a radiographic examination shows that the lung is completely expanded. Pain may be controlled by administering appropriate analgesics, but the use of respiratory depressants is avoided. Intermittent positive-pressure breathing may be administered.

■ PATIENT CARE CONSIDERATIONS: The patient is taught how to turn, cough, breathe deeply, and perform passive exercises and is told to avoid stretching, reaching, or making sudden movements. The patient is advised not to smoke but to drink fluids copiously, to exercise, to avoid fatigue and strenuous activity, and to report any symptoms of recurrence, such as chest pain, difficult breathing, fever, or respiratory infection.

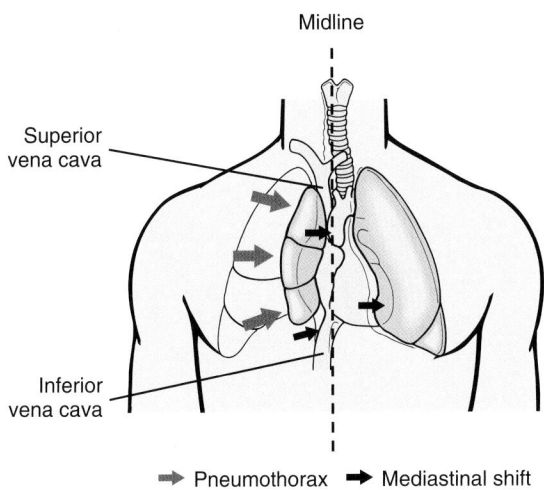

Midline

Superior
vena cava

Inferior
vena cava

➡ Pneumothorax ➡ Mediastinal shift

Pneumothorax *(Lewis et al, 2011)*

PNF, abbreviation for **proprioceptive neuromuscular facilitation.**

PNH, abbreviation for **paroxysmal nocturnal hemoglobinuria.**

-pnoea. See **-pnea, -pnoea, pneo-.**

PNP, abbreviation for **pediatric nurse practitioner.**

Po, symbol for the element **polonium.**

PO, p.o., a route for administration of medications, from the Latin phrase *per os,* meaning "by mouth." Abbreviation for **per os.**

PO₂. See **partial pressure.** Symbol for *partial pressure of oxygen.*

pocket /pok′ət/, a saclike space. See also **cavity, pouch, recess.**

pockmark [AS, *pocc + meark*], a pitted scar on the skin, usually the result of acne or a smallpox or chickenpox pustule at the site.

pod-. See **podo-, pod-.**

podagra, inflammation involving the great toe caused by gout.

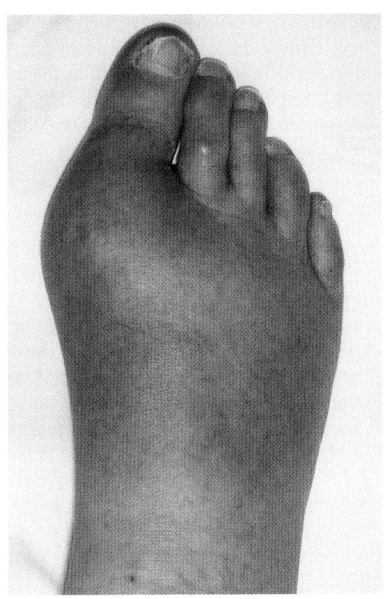

Podagra *(Hochberg et al, 2015)*

podalgia, foot pain.

podalic /pōdal′ik/ [Gk, *pous,* foot], pertaining to the feet.

podalic version, the shifting of the position of a fetus to position the feet at the outlet during labor.

podiatrist /pədī″ətrist/, a health professional who diagnoses and treats disorders of the feet. Podiatrists complete a 4-year postgraduate educational program leading to a degree of Doctor of Podiatric Medicine (D.P.M.). Also called **chiropodist.**

podiatry /pədī″ətrē/ [Gk, *pous + iatros,* healer], the diagnosis and treatment of diseases and other disorders of the feet. Also called **chiropody.**

-podium, suffix meaning "something footlike": *autopodium, zygopodium.*

podo-, pod-, prefix meaning "foot": *podogra, podalic, podiatry.*

podofilox /po-dof′-iloks/, a corrosive preparation that inhibits cell mitosis and is used for topical treatment of venereal warts.

podophyllotoxin /pō′dōfil′ətok″sin/ [Gk, *pous + phyllon,* leaf, *toxikon,* poison], any one of a group of substances derived from the roots of *Podophyllum peltatum,* a common plant species known as mayapple or American mandrake. Podofilox, a derivative, is prescribed in the topical treatment of condyloma acuminatum and other types of warts. Several podophyllotoxin derivatives have been used as purgatives and studied for their antineoplastic effects, including the inhibition of mitosis. Podophyllotoxins are not recommended for use in early pregnancy.

poecil-. See **poikilo-, pecilo-, poecil-.**

POEMS syndrome, a multisystem syndrome combining *p*olyneuropathy, *o*rganomegaly, *e*ndocrinopathy, *m*onoclonal gammopathy, and *s*kin changes. It may be linked to a dysproteinemia such as the presence of unusual monoclonal proteins and light chains. Also called **Crow-Fukase syndrome, PEP syndrome.**

-poesis, -poiesis, suffix meaning "formation or production of": *cholesterolopoiesis, erythropoiesis, hemopoiesis.*

-poetic, -poietic, suffix meaning "production of something specified": *hematopoetic, erythropoietic.*

poetry therapy, a form of bibliotherapy in which a selected poem is used to evoke feelings and responses for discussion in a therapeutic setting. The poem may be a published work or one created by the patient, and poetic devices, such as rhythm, image, and metaphor contribute to the therapeutic effect.

pogonion /pō·gō′nē·on/ [Gk, diminutive of *pōgōn,* beard], the most anterior point in the contour of the chin in the sagittal plane.

-poiesis. See **-poesis, -poiesis.**

-poietic. See **-poetic, -poietic.**

poikilo-, pecilo-, poecil-, prefix meaning "varied" or "irregular": *poikilocytosis, poikiloderma, poikilothermic.*

poikilocytosis /poi′kilō′sītō″sis/ [Gk, *poikilos,* variation, *kytos,* cell, *osis,* condition], abnormal variation of red blood cell shape in a Wright-stained peripheral blood film. The term *poikilocytosis* is used only when the red blood cell shape cannot be more specifically defined. Compare **sickle cell, target cell, ovalocytes, schistocyte.**

poikiloderma atrophicans vasculare /-dur′mə/ [Gk, *poikilos,* variation, *derma,* skin, *a + trophe,* not nourishment; L, *vasculum,* little vessel], an abnormal skin condition characterized by hyperpigmentation or hypopigmentation, telangiectasia, and atrophy of the epidermis. It may be symmetric or patchy, localized, or widespread. It tends to be permanent.

P

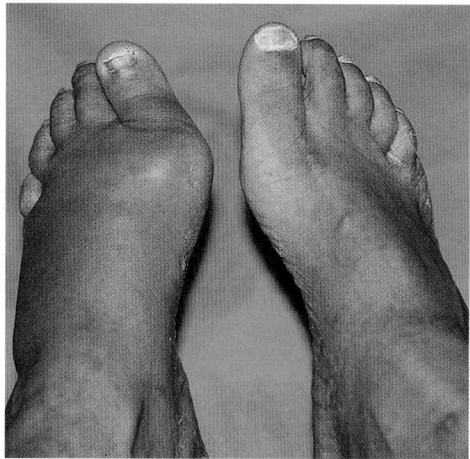

Poikiloderma atrophicans vasculare *(du Vivier, 2002/ Courtesy St. Mary's Hospital)*

poikiloderma congenitale. See **Rothmund-Thomson syndrome.**

poikiloderma of Civatte, a common benign progressive dermatitis characterized by erythematous patches on the face and neck that become dry and scaly. As the condition progresses, pigment is deposited around the hair follicles, extending down the lateral aspects of the neck. Photosensitivity is sometimes associated with this dermatitis. Also called **reticulated pigmented poikiloderma.**

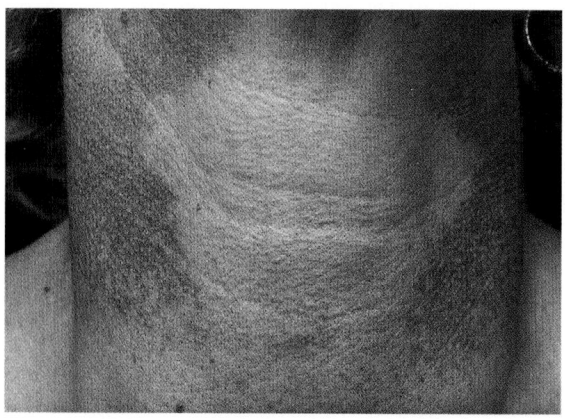

Poikiloderma of Civatte *(du Vivier, 2002)*

poikilothermic. See **cold-blooded.**

point [L, *punctus,* pricked], a small spot or designated area.

point A. See **subspinale.**

point behavior [L, *punctus,* pricked; AS, *bihabban,* to behave], the orientation of body parts in a certain direction within a quantum of space.

point forceps, a dental hand instrument with a flexible metal quick-release lock used to hold filling cones during their placement in root canal filling. Also called **insertion forceps, lock forceps,** *locking forceps.*

point lesion, a disruption of single chemical bonds caused by effects of ionizing radiation on a macromolecule. Also called **molecular lesion.**

point mutation [L, *punctus,* pricked, *mutare,* to change], a mutation in which only a single nucleotide of DNA is changed.

point of maximum impulse (PMI), the place where the apical pulse is palpated as strongest, often in the fifth intercostal space of the thorax, just medial to the left midclavicular line.

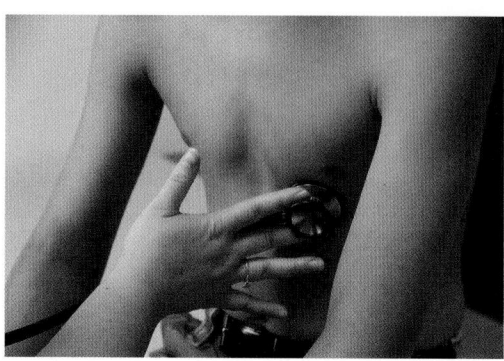

Auscultation at the point of maximum impulse *(Courtesy Rutgers School of Nursing—Camden. All rights reserved.)*

point-of-service plan, (in the United States) a plan in which the member may seek care outside the network or directly from preferred providers with initial evaluation by a primary care provider but must pay a deductible and/or copayment.

point Po. See **porion.**

point system, (in the United States) a specialty capitation method in which points are assigned for each patient seen in specific diagnostic or service categories. Periodically points are totaled and income is distributed proportionally.

poise /poiz/ [Jean L.M. Poiseuille, French physiologist, 1799–1869], a unit of liquid or gas (fluid) viscosity expressed in terms of grams per centimeter per second (g × cm^{-1} × sec^{-1}). The centipoise, or 1/100 of a poise, is more commonly used.

poison /ˈpoizən/ [L, *potio,* drink], any substance that impairs health or destroys life when ingested, inhaled, or absorbed by the body in relatively small amounts. Some toxicologists suggest that, depending on the dose, all substances are poisons. Many experts state that it is impossible to categorize any chemical as either safe or toxic and that the real concern is the risk or hazard associated with the use of any substance. Clinically all poisons are divided into those that respond to specific treatments or antidotes and those for which there is no specific treatment. Research continues to develop effective antitoxins for poisons, but there are relatively few effective antidotes. Maintaining respiration and circulation is the most important aspect of treatment. See also **poisoning treatment. –poisonous,** *adj.*

poison center, a telephone service with toxicology experts providing emergency treatment advice for all kinds of poisonings 24 hours a day. Poison control centers also provide poison prevention information to the community and education about recognition and treatment of poison exposures for health care providers. By gathering data about the outcomes of poison exposures, they also identify new or unexpected toxic hazards, allowing for product recalls, reformulations, or repackaging. Their staffs include physicians, nurses, and pharmacists with training in toxicology. Poison centers can be reached by calling 1-800-222-1222. Also called *poison control center.*

poisoning, **1.** the act of administering a toxic substance. **2.** the condition or physical state produced by the ingestion of, injection of, inhalation of, or exposure to a poisonous substance. Identification of the poison ingredients and presentation of a container label are critical to expeditious diagnosis and treatment.

Poisonous plants

Plant	Toxic Parts
Apple	Leaves, seeds
Apricot	Leaves, stem, seed pits
Azalea	All parts
Buttercup	All parts
Castor	Bean or seeds—extremely toxic
Cherry (wild or cultivated)	Twigs, seeds, foliage
Daffodil	Bulbs
Dumbcane (dieffenbachia)	All parts
Elephant ear	All parts
English ivy	All parts
Foxglove	Leaves, seeds, flowers
Holly	Berries, leaves
Hyacinth	Bulbs
Ivy	Leaves
Mistletoe*	Berries, leaves
Oak tree	Acorn, foliage
Philodendron	All parts
Plum	Pit
Poinsettia†	Leaves
Poison ivy, poison oak	Leaves, fruit, stems, smoke from burning plants
Pokeweed, pokeberry	Roots, berries, leaves [when eaten raw]
Pothos	All parts
Rhubarb	Leaves
Tulip	Bulbs
Water hemlock	All parts
Wisteria	Seeds, pods
Yew	All parts

*Eating one or two berries or leaves is probably nontoxic.
†Toxic if ingested in massive quantities.
Modified from Hockenberry MJ, Wilson D: *Wong's nursing care of infants and children,* ed 9, St Louis, 2011, Mosby.

poisoning treatment, the symptomatic and supportive care given a patient who has been exposed to or who has ingested a toxic drug, commercial chemical, or other dangerous substance. In the case of oral poisoning a primary effort should be directed toward recovery of the toxic substance before it can be absorbed into the body tissues. A poison control center should be called immediately.

poison ivy, any of several species of climbing vine of the genus *Rhus,* characterized by shiny three-pointed leaves. It is common in North America and causes severe allergic contact dermatitis in many people. Localized vesicular eruption with itching and burning results and may be treated with antipruritic lotions, cool compresses, or topical corticosteroid ointment or cream. Severe cases may require corticosteroids given intramuscularly or orally. See also **rhus dermatitis, urushiol.**

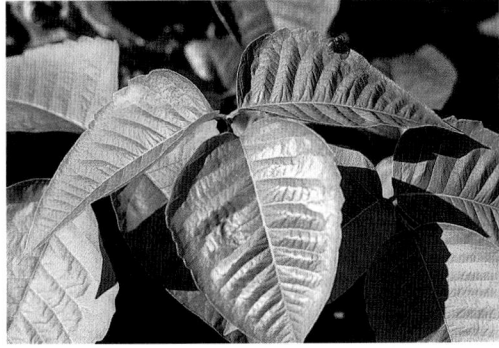

Poison ivy (Sasseville, 2009)

poison ivy dermatitis [L, *potio,* drink; ME, *ivi* + Gk, *derma,* skin, *itis,* inflammation], an allergic contact dermatitis caused by exposure to a nonvolatile skin-irritating oil, urushiol, present in the leaves and other plant parts of poison ivy, a member of the *Rhus toxicodendron* species. Other *Rhus* species producing the same kind of contact dermatitis are poison oak and poison sumac. Also called **rhus dermatitis.**

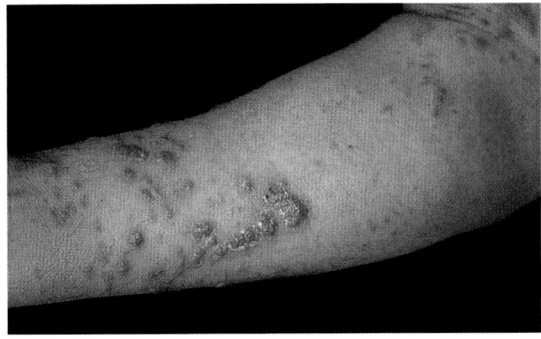

Poison ivy dermatitis (Sasseville, 2009)

poison oak, any of several species of shrub of the genus *Rhus,* common in North America. Skin contact results in allergic dermatitis in many people. The characteristics and treatment of the condition are similar to those of poison ivy. See also **poison ivy, rhus dermatitis, urushiol.**

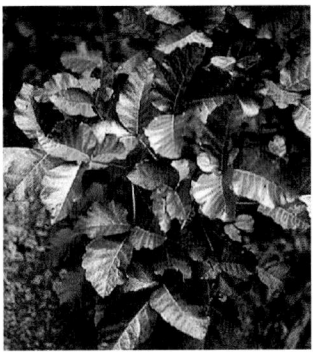

Poison oak (Froberg, Ibrahim, and Furbee, 2007)

poisonous. See **poison.**

poison sumac /sōo″mak/, a shrub of the genus *Rhus,* common in North America. Skin contact results in allergic dermatitis in many people. The characteristics and treatment of the condition are similar to those of poison ivy. See also **poison ivy, rhus dermatitis, urushiol.**

poker spine. See **bamboo spine.**

Poland syndrome /pō′lənd/ [Alfred Poland, British physician, 1820–1872], unilateral absence of the sternocostal head of the pectoralis major muscle and ipsilateral syndactyly. Also called *Poland anomaly.*

polar [L, *polus,* pole], pertaining to molecules that have atoms bearing substantial partial electric charges that are not distributed symmetrically. These molecules are hydrophilic, tending to attract or aggregate with water. Polar substances tend to dissolve in polar solvents. Compare **nonpolar.** See also **pole, polus.**

Polaramine, an antihistaminic. Brand name for **dexchlorpheniramine maleate.**

polar body, one of the small cells produced during the two meiotic divisions in the maturation of a female gamete, or ovum. Polar bodies are nonfunctional and incapable of being fertilized. See also **oogenesis.**

polarity /pōler″itē/ [L, *polus*], **1.** the existence or manifestation of opposing qualities, tendencies, or emotions, such as pleasure and pain, love and hate, strength and weakness, dependence and independence, and masculinity and femininity. The concept is central to various psychotherapeutic approaches, such as client-centered therapy, in which the key to self-actualization lies in accepting polarity within oneself. **2.** (in physics) the distinction between a negative and a positive electric charge.

polarity therapy, a bodywork technique that combines tissue manipulation with theories of vital energy derived from ayurveda and acupuncture. It is believed that energy blockages within the body result in imbalances, which in turn manifest as pain. Manipulation, using light touch and medium and deep pressure, is used to release these energy blockages and restore balance. Exercise and nutritional and lifestyle counseling may also be included in the therapy.

polarization /pō′lərīzā′shən/ [L, *polus* + Gk, *izein,* to cause], the concentration, within a population or group, of members' interests, beliefs, and allegiances around two conflicting positions.

polarization microscope [L, *polus,* pole; Gk, *mikros,* small, *skopein,* to view], a microscope that uses polarized light for special diagnostic purposes, such as examining crystals of chemicals found in patients with gout and related disorders.

polarized light /po′lərīzd/ [L, *polus* + AS, *leoht*], light that is propagated in such a way that the radiation waves occur in only one direction in the vibration plane and not at random.

polarographic oxygen analyzer /pō′lərōgraf″ik/, an electrochemical device used to analyze the proportion of oxygen molecules in respiratory care systems. The oxygen is measured in terms of an electron current produced after it acquires electrons from a negative electrode in a hydroxide bath. Batteries are used to polarize the electrodes in the bath.

pole [L, *polus*], **1.** (in biology) an end of an imaginary axis drawn through the symmetrically arranged parts of a cell, organ, ovum, or nucleus. **2.** one of a pair of opposite forces or attractants, as in magnetism or electricity. **3.** (in anatomy) the point on a nerve cell at which a dendrite originates. –**polar,** *adj.*

poles of kidney, either end of an axis through the length of a kidney. They are designated as the upper pole of kidney (extremitas superior renis) and the inferior pole of kidney (extremitas inferior renis).

pol gene, a segment of a retrovirus, such as the human immunodeficiency virus, that encodes its reverse transcriptase enzyme.

policy /pol″isē/ [Gk, *politeia,* the state], a principle or guideline that governs activities in a facility that employees or members of the institution or organization are expected to follow.

polio. See **poliomyelitis.**

polio-, prefix meaning "gray matter in the nervous system": *polioencephalitis, poliomyelitis.*

polioencephalitis /pō′lē·ō′ensef′əlī″tis/ [Gk, *polios,* gray, *enkephalos,* brain, *itis*], an inflammation of the gray matter of the brain caused by infection of the brain by a poliovirus.

polioencephalomeningomyelitis /pō′lē·ō′ensef′əlō- məning″gōmī′əlī″tis/ [Gk, *polios,* gray, *enkephalos,* brain, *meninx,* membrane, *myelos,* marrow, *itis,* inflammation], an inflammation that involves the gray matter of the brain and spinal cord and also the meninges.

polioencephalomyelitis /pō′lē·ō′ensef′əlōmī′əlī″tis/ [Gk, *polios* + *enkephalos* + *myelos,* marrow, *itis*], inflammation of the gray matter of the brain and the spinal cord, caused by infection by a poliovirus.

polioencephalopathy /pō′lē·ō′ensef′əlop″əthē/ [Gk, *polios,* gray, *enkephalos,* brain, *pathos,* disease], a pathological condition affecting the gray matter of the brain.

poliomyelitis /pō′lē·ōmī′əlī″tis/ [Gk, *polios* + *myelos,* marrow, *itis*], an infectious disease caused by one of the three polioviruses. Asymptomatic, mild, and paralytic forms of the disease occur. Several factors influence susceptibility to the virus and the course of the disease: More boys than girls are severely affected, stress increases susceptibility, more pregnant than nonpregnant women acquire the paralytic form of the disease, and the severity of the infection increases with age. It is transmitted from person to person through fecal contamination or oropharyngeal secretions. The disease is prevented by vaccination. Also called **polio.** See also **acute atrophic paralysis, poliovirus.**

■ OBSERVATIONS: Asymptomatic infection has no clinical features, but it confers immunity. Abortive poliomyelitis lasts only a few hours and is characterized by minor illness with fever, malaise, headache, nausea, vomiting, and slight abdominal discomfort. Nonparalytic poliomyelitis is longer lasting and is marked by meningeal irritation with pain and stiffness in the back and by all the signs of abortive poliomyelitis. Paralytic poliomyelitis begins as abortive poliomyelitis. The symptoms abate, and for several days the person seems well. Malaise, headache, and fever recur; pain, weakness, and paralysis develop. The peak of paralysis is reached within the first week. In spinal poliomyelitis, viral replication occurs in the anterior horn cells of the spine, causing inflammation, swelling, and, if severe, destruction of the neurons. The large proximal muscles of the limbs are most often affected. Bulbar poliomyelitis results from viral multiplication in the brainstem. Bulbar and spinal poliomyelitis often occur together.

poliomyelitis vaccine. See **poliovirus vaccine.**

poliomyelitis virus. See **poliovirus.**

poliosis /pō′lē·ō″sis/ [Gk, *polios* + *osis,* condition], depigmentation of the hair on the scalp, eyebrows, eyelashes, mustache, beard, or body. The condition may be inherited and generalized or acquired and localized in patches. Acquired localized poliosis often occurs in alopecia areata.

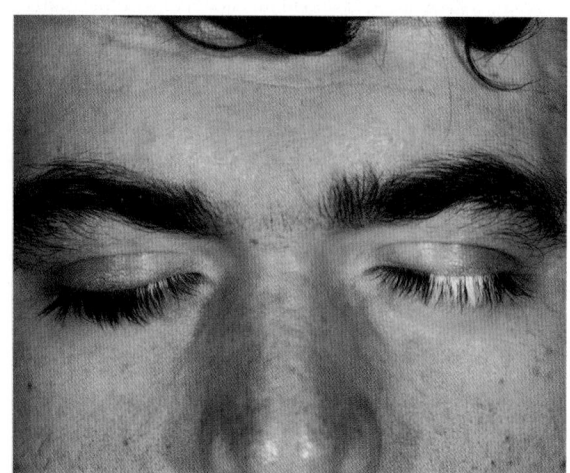

Poliosis *(Hordinsky, Sawaya, and Scher, 2000)*

poliovirus /-vī′rəs/ [Gk, *polios* + L, *virus,* poison], a member of the family Picornaviridae and the causative organism of poliomyelitis. This very small ribonucleic acid virus has three serologically distinct types. Infection or immunization with one type does not protect against the others. Also called **poliomyelitis virus.**

poliovirus vaccine, a vaccine prepared from poliovirus to confer immunity to it. The inactivated poliovirus vaccine (IPV) is a suspension of three strains of polioviruses that have been inactivated in formalin so that normal activity of the organisms has been destroyed. IPV is given subcutaneously at 2 mo, 4 mo, between 6 and 18 mo, and between 4 and 6 yr, and is the form of vaccination recommended in the United States. A trivalent live oral form of vaccine, TOPV, rarely causes vaccine-associated paralysis after administration. This reaction has not occurred with IPV and is the reason that use of TOPV is being discontinued in the United States. TOPV is, nevertheless, the treatment of choice in areas of the world where polio is still endemic. Also called **poliomyelitis vaccine; Salk vaccine; poliovirus vaccine, inactivated.**

poliovirus vaccine, inactivated. See **poliovirus vaccine.**

polishing [L, *polire,* to make smooth], **1.** creation of a smooth and glossy finish on a surface, as of a tooth, dental restoration, or denture. **2.** a tendency of patients with right temporal lobe lesions to deny dysphoric affect and minimize socially disapproved behavior while exaggerating other qualities.

Politano-Leadbetter technique, a type of ureteroneocystostomy in which the ureter is excised from its attachment to the bladder and reattached in a more medial and superior position.

political nursing /pəlit′ikəl/ [Gk, *politia,* the state, *nutrix,* nurse], the use of knowledge about power processes and strategies to influence the nature and direction of health care and professional nursing. The constituency of political nursing is patients, both diagnosed and potential, as communities, groups, or individuals.

pollen allergy. See **hay fever.**

pollen coryza. See **hay fever.**

pollenogenic, pertaining to a plant that produces pollen or something that is produced by pollen.

pollex /pol′eks/ *pl. pollices* [L], **1.** the thumb. **2.** the big toe.

pollinosis. See **hay fever.**

pollutant /pəloo′tənt/ [L, *polluere,* to defoul], an unwanted substance that occurs in the environment, usually with health-threatening effects. Pollutants may exist in the atmosphere as gases or fine particles that may be irritating to the lungs, eyes, and skin; in drinking water as dissolved or suspended substances; and in foods or beverages as carcinogens or mutagens.

polonium (Po) /pəlō′nē-əm/ [Polonia, Poland], a radioactive element that is one of the disintegration products of uranium. Its atomic number is 84; its atomic mass is approximately 210.

polus /pō′ləs/ *pl. poli* [L, pole] **1.** either of the opposite ends of any axis. **2.** the official anatomical designation for the extremity of an organ. See also **pole.**

poly-, prefix meaning "many" or "much": *polyamine, polycystic, polydactyly,*

polyacrylamide /-akril′əmīd/, a polymer of acrylamide and, usually, some cross-linking derivative.

polyamine /pol′ē-am′ēn/, any compound that contains two or more amine groups, such as spermidine, spermine, and putrescine, that are normally found in human tissue. Many polyamines function as essential growth factors in microorganisms, such as in DNA synthesis and gene expression.

polyanionic /pol′ē-an′ī-on″ik/ [Gk, *polys,* many, *ana,* against, *jenai,* to go], pertaining to multiple negative electric charges.

polyarteritis /pol′ē-är′tərī″tis/ [Gk, *polys + arteria,* airpipe, *itis,* inflammation], an abnormal inflammatory condition of several arteries.

polyarteritis nodosa, a severe and poorly understood collagen vascular disease characterized by widespread inflammation and necrosis of small and medium-sized arteries and

ischemia of the tissues they serve. Any organ or organ system may be affected. The disease attacks men and women between 20 and 50 years of age. Its cause is unknown, although immunological factors are suspected. Polyarteritis nodosa may be acute and rapidly fatal or chronic and wasting. It is characterized by fever, abdominal pain, weight loss, neuropathy, and, if the kidneys are affected, hypertension, edema, and uremia. Some symptoms may mimic those of GI or cardiac disorders. Diagnosis is based on the clinical signs, results of laboratory tests, and findings of biopsy of sites affected by the disease. Aggressive treatment includes massive doses of corticosteroids and immunosuppressive drugs. Physical therapy helps the patient to maintain muscle tone and prevents or slows the development of disability.

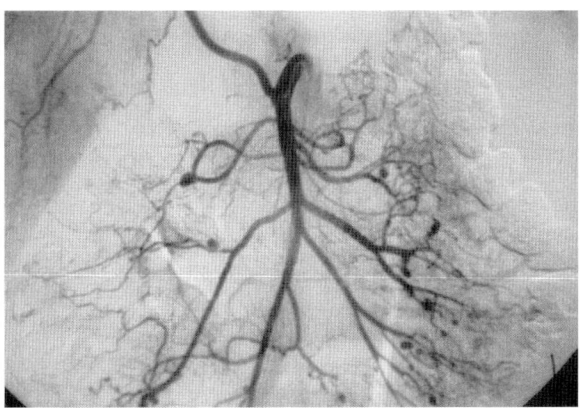

Polyarteritis nodosa *(Goldman et al, 2016)*

polyarthralgia /pol′ē-ärthral″jə/ [Gk, *polys + arthron,* joint, *algos,* pain], pain in several joints simultaneously.

polyarthritis /-ärthrī′tis/, an inflammation that involves more than one joint. The inflammation may migrate from one joint to another, or there may be simultaneous involvement of two or more joints.

polyarticular /-ärtik′yələr/ [Gk, *polys,* many, *articulus,* joint], pertaining to many joints.

polycarbonate glasses, clear, impact-resistant lenses. See also **safety glasses.**

polycarboxylate cement /pol′ēkär·bok′si·lāt/, a dental cement used as a luting agent for cementing restorations and as a cavity lining.

polychlorinated biphenyls (PCBs) /-klôr″inā′tid/, a group of more than 30 isomeric compounds used in plastics, insulation, and flame retardants and varying in physical form from oily liquids to crystals and resins. All are potentially toxic and carcinogenic. The toxicity varies with the type of PCB and concurrent exposure to other substances, such as carbon tetrachloride. Mild exposure may cause chloracne; severe exposure may result in hepatic damage.

polychondritis /pol′ēkon·drī′tis/ [Gk, *polys,* many + *chondros,* cartilage + *itis,* inflammation], inflammation involving many cartilages of the body.

polychromasia, **1.** variation in the hemoglobin content of erythrocytes. **2.** See **polychromatophilia.**

polychromatic /-krōmatik/ [Gk, *polys + chroma,* color], a light of many colors or wavelengths. The term is usually applied to white light, although it may also refer to a defined part of the spectrum.

polychromatophil /pol′ēkrōmat″əfil/, any cell or structure that may be stained by several different dyes.

polychromatophilia /pol'ēkrō'matəfil″yə/ [Gk, *polys* + *chroma* + *philein,* to love], an elevated reticulocyte count on a peripheral blood film stained with new methylene blue dye or an increase in the number of polychromatophilic red blood cells on a Wright-stained blood film. Reticulocytosis or polychromatophilia indicates bone marrow regeneration in hemolytic anemia or chronic blood loss. Also called **polychromasia.**

Polycillin, an antibacterial. Brand name for **ampicillin.**

polyclinic, **1.** a hospital affiliated with a school that does not limit practice to a specific specialty. It is usually a component of a hospital's name in the United States. **2.** an institution providing a wide range of health services that does not require an overnight stay. Polyclinics are more numerous in the European Union, Russia, and India than in the United States.

polyclonal /pol'ēklō″nəl/ [Gk, *polys* + *klon,* cutting], pertaining to or designating a group of cells or organisms derived from several cells. Compare **monoclonal.**

polyclonal gammopathy. See **gammopathy.**

Polycose, brand name for an easily digestible and rapidly absorbed nutritional supplement for oral and tube feeding containing glucose polymers. It is not formulated for use as the sole source of nutrition.

polycystic /-sis'tik/ [Gk, *polys* + *kystis,* bag], characterized by the presence of many cysts.

polycystic kidney disease (PKD), an abnormal condition in which the kidneys are enlarged and contain many cysts. There are two unrelated hereditary diseases in which there is massive enlargement of the kidney with cyst formation: Autosomal dominant polycystic kidney disease (ADPKD), formerly called adult polycystic kidney disease, is the most common type of cystic disease of the kidneys. It is usually manifested during the third decade of life. Renal failure may appear by the fifth decade, with terminal failure occurring in the next 10 years, although in some cases it never appears. Although there is rarely any liver dysfunction accompanying this disorder, cyst formation in the liver does occur. Autosomal recessive polycystic kidney disease (ARPKD), formerly called childhood polycystic kidney disease, is diagnosed at birth or in the first 10 years of life and is much less common than the autosomal dominant form. Both the kidney and the liver are involved, causing renal failure and liver failure with portal hypertension. Characteristic symptoms early in the process include pain, hematuria, urinary tract infection, kidney stones, and obstructive uropathy with anuria.

■ INTERVENTIONS: Treatment of both types of polycystic kidney disease is largely symptomatic. Renal dialysis and kidney transplantation during end-stage renal disease can prolong life but offer no cure. Families with histories of polycystic kidney disease benefit from genetic counseling and may need help in coping with the prospect of future offspring affected with the disease.

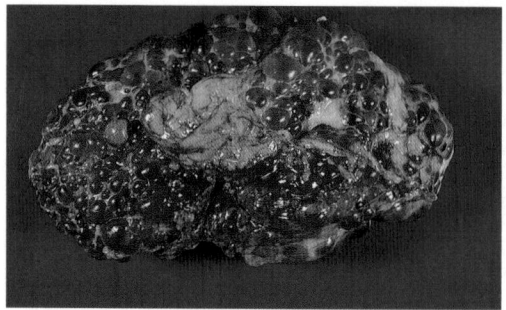

Polycystic kidney disease *(Damjanov, 2012)*

polycystic liver, congenital cystic disease of the liver. Also called *polycystic liver disease.*

polycystic ovary syndrome (PCOS), an endocrine disturbance characterized by anovulation, amenorrhea, hirsutism, and infertility. It is caused by increased levels of testosterone, estrogen, and luteinizing hormone (LH) and decreased secretion of follicle-stimulating hormone (FSH). The increased level of LH associated with this disorder may be the result of an increased sensitivity of the pituitary to stimulation by releasing hormone or of excessive stimulation by the adrenal gland. It may also be associated with a variety of problems in the hypothalamic-pituitary-ovarian axis, with extragonadal sources of androgens, or with androgen-producing tumors. This condition is transmitted as an X-linked dominant or autosomal-dominant trait. The depressed but continuous production of FSH associated with this disorder causes continuous partial development of ovarian follicles. Numerous follicular cysts, 2 to 6 mm in diameter, may develop. The affected ovary commonly doubles in size and is invested by a smooth pearly white capsule. The increased level of estrogen associated with this abnormality raises the risk of cancers of the breast and endometrium. Depending on the severity of symptoms and the patient's desire to become pregnant, treatment involves suppression of hormonal stimulation of the ovary, usually by use of female hormones or resection of part of one or both ovaries. Also called *hyperandrogenic chronic anovulations,* **Stein-Leventhal syndrome.**

polycythemia /pol'ēsīthē″mē·ə/ [Gk, *polys* + *kytos,* cell, *haima,* blood], an increase in the red blood cell count and circulating red blood cell mass that may be primary or secondary to pulmonary disease, heart disease, or prolonged exposure to high altitudes. Also called **Osler disease, polycythemia vera.** Compare **hypoplastic anemia, leukemia.** See also **altitude sickness, erythrocytosis.**

■ OBSERVATIONS: Clinical manifestations for polycythemia include weakness and fatigue; headache and vertigo; visual disturbances (scotoma, double or blurred vision); dyspnea; nosebleeds; night sweats; and epigastric and joint pain. Later signs include pruritus, clubbing of digits, a reddened face with engorged retinal veins, and hepatosplenomegaly. Secondary polycythemia may display hypoxemia in the absence of hepatosplenomegaly and hypertension. Lab results in primary polycythemia include elevated red blood cell counts; elevated white blood cell counts with basophilia; elevated hemoglobin; thrombocytosis; elevated alkaline phosphatase, uric acid, and albumin; and elevated histamine levels with low serum erythropoietin levels. Bone marrow aspiration shows panmyelosis. Thrombosis, cerebrovascular accident, peptic ulcers, myeloid metaplasia, leukemia, and hemorrhage are common complications in primary polycythemia and result in the death of about 50% of untreated individuals within 18 months of the appearance of symptoms. The median survival rate in treated individuals is 7 to 15 years.

■ INTERVENTIONS: Management of secondary polycythemia is directed at treating the underlying causes. The treatment for primary polycythemia is directed at reducing blood volume and viscosity and inhibiting bone marrow activity. The treatment mainstay is serial phlebotomy and is used to reduce RBC mass. Hydration therapy is used to reduce blood viscosity. Chemotherapeutic agents may be used to induce myelosuppression. Adjunctive therapy includes allopurinol to treat hyperuricemia, antihistamines to reduce pruritus, analgesics for joint pain, and antacids for gastric hyperacidity. A splenectomy may be indicated to treat resistant splenomegaly.

■ PATIENT CARE CONSIDERATIONS: Nursing during the acute phase includes careful monitoring of intake and output during hydration therapy and phlebotomy to avoid overhydration or underhydration. Comfort measures are instituted to relieve joint pain, itching, and heartburn. Passive and active range of motion and ambulation are used to promote circulation and prevent thrombus formation. If chemotherapeutic agents are used, education is needed about effects and side effects. Education is also important, and stress is placed on the chronic nature of the disease, the need for long-term phlebotomy treatment, and the impending complications that will occur if the disease is left untreated.

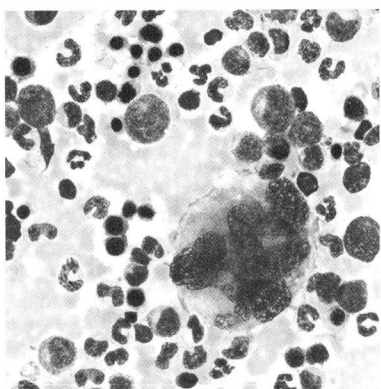

Polycythemia *(Carr and Rodak, 2008)*

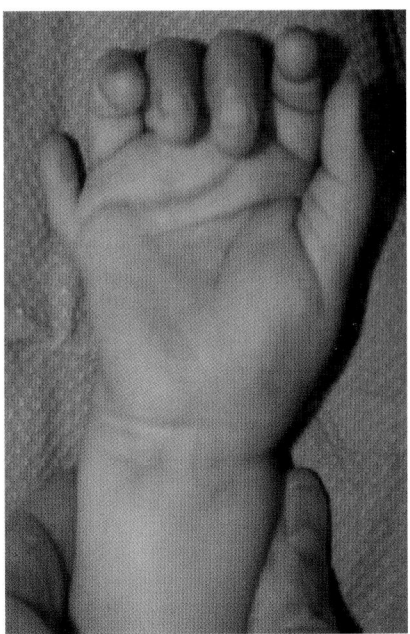

Polydactyly *(Chung, 2009)*

polycythemia rubra vera (PV) [Gk, *polys,* many, *kytos,* cell, *haima,* blood; L, *ruber,* red, *verus,* true], a myeloproliferative neoplasm characterized by an elevation in the red blood cell count, hematocrit, hemoglobin level, and number of leukocytes and by thrombocytosis. The skin and mucous membranes acquire a maroon or plum color, and hepatomegaly, splenomegaly, hypertension, and neurological symptoms develop. The condition is associated with the JAK2 mutation. Also called **primary polycythemia.**

polycythemia vera. See **polycythemia.**

polydactyly /-dak′tilē/ [Gk, *polys* + *daktylos,* finger], a congenital anomaly characterized by the presence of more than the normal number of fingers or toes. The condition is usually inherited as an autosomal-dominant characteristic and can usually be corrected by surgery shortly after birth. Also called **hyperdactyly,** *polydactylia, polydactylism.*

polydipsia /pol′ēdip″sē·ə/ [Gk, *polys* + *dipsa,* thirst], **1.** excessive thirst. It is characteristic of several different conditions, including diabetes mellitus, in which an excessive concentration of glucose in the blood osmotically pulls intracellular fluid into the bloodstream and increases the excretion of fluid via increased urination, which leads to hypovolemia and thirst. In diabetes insipidus the deficiency of the pituitary antidiuretic hormone results in excretion of copious amounts of dilute urine, reduced fluid volume in the body, and polydipsia. In nephrogenic diabetes insipidus there is also copious excretion of urine with consequent polydipsia. Polyuria resulting from other forms of renal dysfunction also leads to polydipsia. The condition also may be psychogenic in origin. **2.** *(Informal)* alcoholism.

polyelectrolyte /pol′ē·ilek″trəlīt/ [Gk, *polys* + *elektron,* amber, *lytos,* soluble], a substance with many charged or potentially charged groups.

polyendocrine deficiency syndromes. See **polyglandular autoimmune syndromes.**

polyene, **1.** a chemical compound with a carbon chain of four or more atoms and several conjugated double bonds. **2.** any of a group of antibiotic, antifungal agents with similar structure, such as Amphotericin B or Nystatin; they are produced by a species of *Streptomyces* that damage cell membranes by forming complexes with sterols.

polyesthesia /pol′ē-esthē″zhə/ [Gk, *polys* + *aisthesis,* feeling], a sensory disorder involving the sense of touch in which a stimulus to one area of the skin is also felt at nonstimulated sites.

polyestradiol phosphate /-es′trədī″ôl/, a polymer of estradiol phosphate having estrogenic activity similar to that of estradiol. Among the more serious adverse effects are loss of libido, impotence, gynecomastia, fluid retention and edema, and, rarely, cholestatic jaundice.

polyethylene /pol′ē-eth″ilēn/, a strong but flexible synthetic resin produced by the polymerization of ethylene. Polyethylene materials have been used in surgery.

polyethylene glycol, a polymer of ethylene oxide and water, available in liquid form or as waxy solids used in various pharmaceutical preparations as a water-soluble ointment base. Polyethylene glycol is also used as a laxative.

polygene /pol′ējēn′/ [Gk, *polys* + *genein,* to produce], any of a group of nonallelic genes that individually exert a small effect but interact in a cumulative manner to produce a particular characteristic, usually of a quantitative nature, such as size, weight, skin pigmentation, or degree of intelligence. Also called **cumulative gene, multiple factor, multiple gene.** See also **multifactorial inheritance.**

polygenic inheritance. See **multifactorial inheritance.**

polyglactin, a filamentous material that is used for absorbable sutures.

polyglandular autoimmune syndromes, a group of rare disorders manifested by subnormal functioning of more than one endocrine gland. Type I is characterized by the appearance of mucocutaneous candidiasis, often occurring in childhood, and is associated with hypoparathyroidism and adrenal insufficiency. It occurs in siblings, without involvement of other generations in the family. Type II (also called Schmidt syndrome) involves primary adrenal insufficiency and primary thyroid failure occurring in the same patient for unclear reasons. Many of these patients have an autoimmune disorder and

P

form antibodies against cellular fractions of many endocrine glands. See also **Schmidt syndrome, polyendocrine deficiency syndromes,** *polyglandular autoimmune diseases.*

polyglandular deficiency syndrome, primary failure of any combination of endocrine glands, including the adrenals, thyroid, gonads, parathyroids, and endocrine pancreas. It is often accompanied by autoimmune abnormalities that affect systems other than the endocrine system. Also called **multiple endocrine deficiency syndrome, multiple glandular deficiency syndrome.**

polyglucosan /-glōō′kəsan/ [Gk, *polys* + *glykys,* sweet], a large molecule consisting of many anhydrous polysaccharides.

polygraph /pol′ē·graf/ [Gk, *polys* + *graphein,* to write], an apparatus for simultaneously recording several mechanical or electrical impulses, such as blood pressure, pulse, and respiration, and variations in electrical resistance of the skin. Also called **lie detector.**

polyhedral, having many sides or surfaces.

polyhidrosis. See **hyperhidrosis.**

polyhybrid /-hī′brid/ [Gk, *polys* + L, *hybrida,* offspring of mixed parents], pertaining to or describing an individual, organism, or strain that is heterozygous for more than three specific traits or gene pairs or that is the offspring of parents differing in more than three specific gene pairs.

polyhybrid cross, the mating of two polyhybrid individuals, organisms, or strains.

polyhydramnios, an excessive amount of amniotic fluid (more than 2000 mL). See **hydramnios.**

polyidrosis. See **hyperhidrosis.**

polyleptic /pol′ēlep″tik/ [Gk, *polys* + *lambanein,* to seize], describing any disease or condition marked by numerous remissions and exacerbations.

polymastia, the presence of supernumerary mammary glands or nipples.

polymenorrhea, an abnormally frequent recurrence of the menstrual cycle. Also called *polymenia.*

polymer /pol″imər/ [Gk, *polys* + *meros,* part], a compound formed by combining or linking a number of monomers, or small molecules. A polymer may be composed of many units of more than one type of monomer (a copolymer) or of many units of the same monomer (a homopolymer).

polymerase /pə·lim′ər·ās/, any enzyme that catalyzes polymerization, especially of nucleotides to polynucleotides.

polymerase chain reaction (PCR), a rapid technique for in vitro amplification of specific DNA or RNA sequences, allowing small quantities of short sequences to be analyzed without cloning. The process can be used to make prenatal diagnoses of genetic diseases and to identify an individual by analysis of a single tissue cell.

polymerization /pə·lim′ər·i·zā′shən/, the act or process of forming a compound (polymer), usually of high molecular weight, by the combination of simpler molecules (monomers).

polymerize /pol′əmərīz″/ [Gk, *polys,* many, *meros,* parts], to convert two or more molecules into a polymer.

polymethacrylate cement, a cement used in dentistry and in surgery, especially orthopedic surgery, consisting of an acrylic resin formed by the polymerization of methyl methacrylate monomers.

polymicrobial /-mīkrō′bē·əl/ [Gk, *polys,* many, *mikros,* small, *bios,* life], pertaining to a number of species of microbes.

polymicrobial necrotizing fasciitis. See **Fournier gangrene.**

polymicrobic infection /-mīkrō′bik/ [Gk, *polys,* many, *mikros,* small, *bios,* life; L, *inficere,* to stain], an infection involving more than one species of pathogen. Also called **mixed infection.**

polymicrogyria. See **microgyria.**

polymorphic /-môr′fik/ [Gk, *polys,* many, *morphe,* form], pertaining to the ability to assume two or more distinct forms, such as the existence of two or more forms of chromosomes or hemoglobins in a population.

polymorphism /pol′ēmôr″fizəm/ [Gk, *polys* + *morphe,* form], **1.** the state or quality of existing or occurring in several different forms. **2.** the state or quality of appearing in different forms at different stages of development. Kinds include **balanced polymorphism, genetic polymorphism. –polymorphic,** *adj.*

polymorphocytic leukemia /pol′ēmôr′fəsit″ik/ [Gk, *polys* + *morphe* + *kytos,* cell, *leukos,* white, *haima,* blood], a neoplasm of blood-forming tissues in which mature segmented granulocytes are predominant. Also called **mature cell leukemia, neutrophilic leukemia.**

polymorphonuclear /pol′ēmôr′fōnōō″klē·ər/ [Gk, *polys* + *morphe* + L, *nucleus,* nut kernel], having a nucleus with a number of segments connected by fine threads of nuclear membrane.

polymorphonuclear neutrophil, a neutrophil with a segmented nucleus.

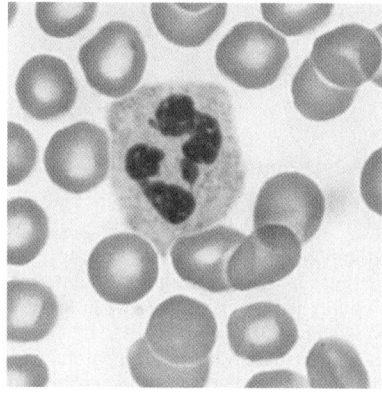

Polymorphonuclear cell *(Carr and Rodak, 2008)*

polymorphous /pol′ēmôr″fəs/ [Gk, *polys* + *morphe,* form], occurring in many varying forms, possibly changing in structure or appearance at different stages.

polymorphous light eruption, a common recurrent superficial vascular reaction to sunlight or ultraviolet light in susceptible individuals. Within 1 to 4 days after exposure to the light, small erythematous papules and vesicles appear on otherwise normal skin; they then disappear within 2 weeks. A delayed allergic response is a possible cause.

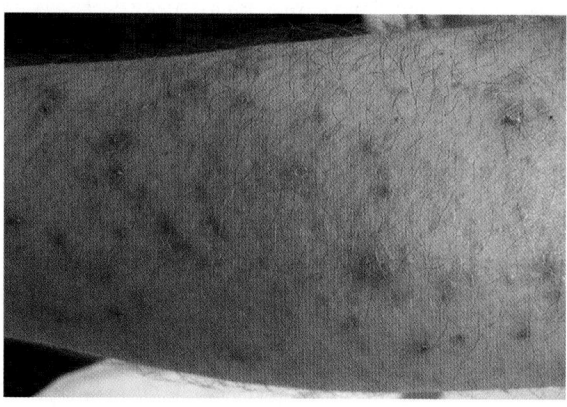

Polymorphous light eruption *(Brinster et al, 2011)*

polymyalgia rheumatica /-mī·al′jə/ [Gk, *polys + mys,* muscle, *algos,* pain, *rheuma,* flux], a chronic, episodic inflammatory disease of the large arteries that usually develops in people over 60 years of age. The disease primarily affects the arteries in muscles. It is characterized by pain and stiffness of the back, shoulder, or neck that is usually more severe on rising in the morning. There may also be a cranial headache, which affects the temporal and occipital arteries, causing a severe throbbing headache. Serious complications of polymyalgia rheumatica include arterial insufficiency, coronary occlusion, stroke, and blindness. Patients with the disease usually have a high erythrocyte sedimentation rate. The disease may follow a self-limited course. However, adrenocorticosteroids have proved highly effective in reducing inflammation and in speeding recovery.

polymyositis /pol′ēmī′ōsī″tis/ [Gk, *polys + mys,* muscle, *itis*], inflammation of many muscles, usually accompanied by deformity, edema, insomnia, pain, sweating, and tension. Some forms of polymyositis are associated with malignancy. See also **dermatomyositis.**

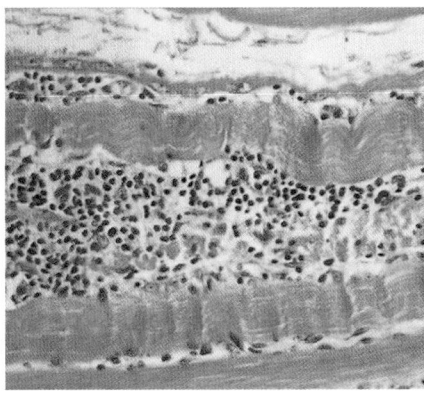

Polymyositis: muscle biopsy *(Perkin, 2002)*

polymyxin B sulfate, an antibiotic.
- INDICATIONS: It is commonly prescribed for infections of the eye and urinary tract.
- CONTRAINDICATIONS: Known hypersensitivity to this drug prohibits its use.
- ADVERSE EFFECTS: When it is given topically, allergies are the most common problem.

polyneuralgia /-nooral′jə/ [Gk, *polys,* many, *neuron,* nerve, *algos,* pain], a type of neuralgia that affects several nerves at the same time.

polyneuritis /-noorī′tis/ [Gk, *polys,* many, *neuron,* nerve, *itis,* inflammation], an inflammation involving many nerves.

polyneuropathy /-noorop′əthē/ [Gk, *polys,* many, *neuron,* nerve, *pathos,* disease], a condition in which many peripheral nerves are afflicted with a disorder.

polynuclear, having many nuclei.

polyoma papovavirus. See **papillocarcinoma.**

polyopia /pol′ē·ō″pē·ə/ [Gk, *polys + ops,* eye], a defect of sight in which one object is perceived as many images; multiple vision. The condition can occur in one or both eyes. See also **diplopia.**

polyp /pol′ip/ [Gk, *polys + pous,* foot], a small tumorlike growth that projects from a mucous membrane surface.

polypapilloma /-pap′ilō″mə/ [Gk, *polys,* many; L, *papilla,* nipple; Gk, *oma*], multiple papillomas or stalked tumors.

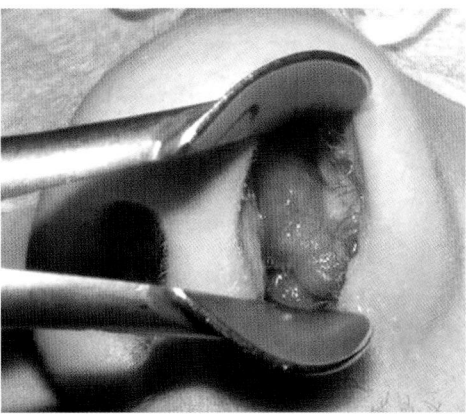

Nasal polyp *(Swartz, 2009)*

polypeptide /pol′ēpep″tīd/, a long chain of amino acids joined by peptide bonds. Very long polypeptides are usually called proteins. Polypeptides may be formed by partial hydrolysis of proteins or synthesized from free amino acids.

polyphagia /pol′ēfā″jē·ə/ [Gk, *polys + phagein,* to eat], excessive, uncontrolled eating. Also called **hyperphagia.** See also **bulimia.**

polypharmacy /-fär′məsē/, the use of a number of different drugs, possibly prescribed by different health care providers and filled in different pharmacies, by a patient who may have one or several health problems.

polyploid /pol″əploid/ [Gk, *polys + plous,* times], **1.** *n.,* an individual, organism, strain, or cell that has more than twice the haploid number of chromosomes characteristic of the species. The multiple of the haploid number is denoted by the appropriate prefix, as in triploid, tetraploid, pentaploid, hexaploid, heptaploid, octaploid, and so on. Polyploidy is rare in animals, producing individuals that are abnormal in appearance and usually infertile. It is common in plants, however; such plants generally are larger, have larger cells, and are hardier than diploid plants. **2.** *adj.,* pertaining to such an individual, organism, strain, or cell. Also called **polyploidic.** Compare **aneuploid.** –**polyploidy,** *n.*

polyploidic. See **polyploid.**

polyploidy /pol′iploi′dē/, the state or condition of having more than two complete sets of chromosomes.

polypoid [Gk, *polys,* many, *pous,* foot, *eidos,* form], like a polyp or tumor on a stalk.

polyposis /-pōsis/ [Gk, *polys + pous,* foot, *osis,* condition], an abnormal condition characterized by the presence of numerous polyps. See also **familial polyposis.**

polyposis coli [Gk, *polys,* many, *pous,* foot, *osis,* condition, *kolikos* colon], a condition of multiple polyps in the large intestine.

polyradiculitis /pol′ērədik′yoolī″tis/ [Gk, *polys + L, radicula,* rootlet; Gk, *itis*], inflammation of many nerve roots, such as found in Guillain-Barré syndrome.

polyribosome. See **polysome.**

polysaccharide /-sak″ərīd/ [Gk, *polys + sakcharon,* sugar], a carbohydrate polymer that is formed from three or more molecules of simple carbohydrates. Kinds include **dextrin, starch, glycogen, cellulose, gum.**

polysaccharide-iron complex, ferric iron complexed to a low-molecular-weight polysaccharide prepared by extensive hydrolysis of starch and used as an oral medication to increase iron levels.

P

polysome /pol″isōm/ [Gk, *polys* + *soma,* body], a group of ribosomes joined by a molecule of messenger RNA containing a portion of the genetic code that is to be translated. Polysomes are found in the cytoplasm during protein synthesis. Also called **ergosome, polyribosome.** See also **translation.**

polysomnographic technologist, a person who monitors sleep studies and records the relevant physiological variables. Also called **sleep technologist.**

polysomnography /pol′ē-som·nog′rə-fē/ [Gk, *polys,* many + L, *somnus,* sleep + Gk, *graphein,* to write or record], the polygraphic recording during sleep of multiple physiological variables, both directly and indirectly related to the state and stages of sleep, to assess possible biological causes of sleep disorders.

polysomy /pol″isō′mē/, the presence of more than two copies of a chromosome in an otherwise diploid somatic cell as the result of chromosomal nondisjunction during meiosis. The chromosome may be duplicated three (trisomy), four (tetrasomy), or more times. Males with Klinefelter syndrome may have a genotype of XXY, XXXY, or XXXXY. Polysomic females with three, four, or five X chromosomes may have a higher frequency of intellectual disability.

Polysporin, an ophthalmic and topical fixed-combination antibiotic ointment containing two antibacterials. Brand name for **polymyxin B sulfate, bacitracin.**

polystichia /pol″e-stik′e-ah/, two or more rows of eyelashes on an eyelid.

polysulfide polymer /pol′əsul′fīd/, an elastomeric synthetic rubber used in dentistry as an impression material for fixed partial prosthodontic structures, inlays for single quadrants, and dental impressions. Also called *polysulfide rubber.*

polysynaptic /-sinap″tik/ [Gk, *polys,* many, *synaptein,* to join], pertaining to nerve cells that end in synapses.

polysyndactyly /-sindak″tilē/ [Gk, *polys,* many, *syn,* together, *daktylos,* finger or toe], multiple webbing or fusion between fingers or toes. Also called **synpolydactyly.**

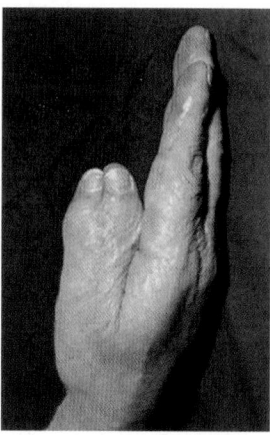

Polysyndactyly *(Moll, 1997)*

polytene chromosome /pol′itēn/ [Gk, *polys* + *tainia,* band], an excessively large type of chromosome consisting of a large number of copies of the chromosome bundled side by side. Polytene chromosomes are produced by repeated rounds of DNA synthesis without mitosis and are bundles of unseparated chromonemata filaments found primarily in the salivary glands of certain insects. See also **giant chromosome.**

polythiazide /-thī·az″īd/, a thiazide diuretic.

■ INDICATIONS: It is prescribed as adjunctive therapy in the treatment of hypertension and edema.

■ CONTRAINDICATIONS: Anuria or known hypersensitivity to this drug, other thiazides, or sulfonamide derivatives prohibits its use.

■ ADVERSE EFFECTS: Among the more serious adverse effects are hypokalemia, hyperglycemia, hyperuricemia, and various hypersensitivity reactions.

polyunsaturated /-unsach″ərā′tid/ [Gk, *polys,* many; AS, *un,* not; L, *saturare,* to fill], pertaining to a chemical compound containing more than one double or triple bond that can be opened to accept more atoms into the molecule, thereby making the compound saturated. A polyunsaturated fatty acid is one in which there are two or more double bonds in the chain of carbon atoms that can be opened to accept hydrogen atoms.

polyunsaturated fatty acid. See **unsaturated fatty acid.**

polyuria /pol′ēyŏŏr″ē·ə/ [Gk, *polys* + *ouron,* urine], the excretion of an abnormally large quantity of urine. Some causes of polyuria are diabetes insipidus, diabetes mellitus, use of diuretics, excessive fluid intake, and hypercalcemia.

polyvalent, denoting the capacity of an element to combine with two or more atoms.

polyvalent antiserum. See **antiserum.**

polyvalent vaccine /-vā″lənt/ [Gk, *polys,* many; L, *valere,* worth, *vaccinus,* cow], a vaccine prepared from several different antigens of a species. Also called **multivalent vaccine.**

Poly-Vi-Flor, an oral fixed-combination pediatric drug containing several vitamins and sodium fluoride.

polyvinyl chloride (PVC) /-vī′nil/, a tasteless, odorless, clear hard resin with many industrial uses, including packaging, clothing, and insulation of pipes and wires. Workers in its manufacture are at risk primarily because of the toxicity of its parent compound, vinyl chloride. It releases hydrochloric acid when burned. Excessive inhalation of its dust can cause pneumoconiosis.

polyvinylidene fluoride (PVF₂) /-vīnil″idēn/, a commonly used piezoelectric material in a hydrophone. It is also used in imaging transducers.

Pomeroy technique, a method of tubal ligation in which a loop of fallopian tube is picked up and ligated at its base with an absorbable suture, about 5 cm from the uterine cornua, and the tied loop is then resected. Also called *Pomeroy operation.*

POMP /pomp/, an abbreviation for a combination drug regimen used in the treatment of cancer, containing three antineoplastics: *P*urinethol (mercaptopurine), *O*ncovin (vincristine sulfate), and *m*ethotrexate, and *p*rednisone (a glucocorticoid).

Pompe disease [J.C. Pompe, 20th-century Dutch physician; L, *dis,* opposite of; Fr, *aise,* ease], a rare genetic disorder that is a form of muscle glycogen storage disease, characterized by a generalized accumulation of glycogen resulting from a deficiency of acid maltase (alpha-1,4-glucosidase). It is usually fatal in infants, causing cardiac or respiratory failure. Children with Pompe disease appear cognitively impaired and hypotonic, seldom living beyond 20 years of age. In adults, muscle weakness is progressive, but the disease is not fatal. Also called **glycogen storage disease, type II.** See also **glycogen storage disease.**

POMR, abbreviation for **problem-oriented medical record.**

ponos. See **kala-azar.**

pons /ponz/ *pl. pontes* [L, bridge], **1.** a prominence on the ventral surface of the brainstem, between the medulla oblongata and the cerebral peduncles of the midbrain. The pons consists of white matter and a few nuclei and is divided

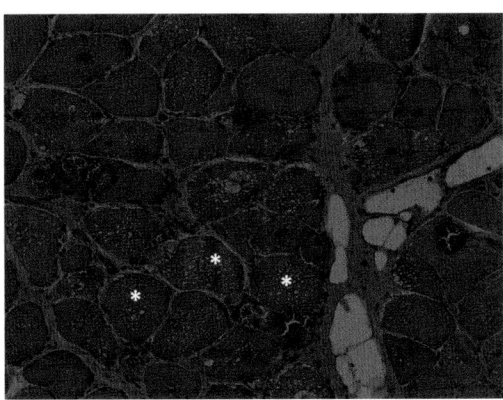

Muscle biopsy stained with hematoxylin-eosin shows extensive vacuolar changes (*asterisk*) associated with Pompe disease (Dasouki et al, 2014)

into a ventral part and a dorsal part. The ventral part consists of transverse fibers separated by longitudinal bundles and small nuclei. The dorsal part comprises the tegmentum, which is a continuation of the reticular formation of the medulla containing the nucleus of the abducens nerve, the nucleus of the facial nerve, the motor nucleus of the trigeminal nerve, the sensory nuclei of the trigeminal nerve, the nucleus of the cochlear division of the eighth nerve, the superior olive, and the nuclei of the vestibular division of the eighth nerve. Also called **bridge of Varolius. 2.** any slip of tissue connecting two parts of a structure or an organ of the body. –*pontile, pontine, adj.*

Ponstel, an antiinflammatory and analgesic. Brand name for **mefenamic acid.**

pont-, combining form meaning "bridge": *pontic, pontine.*

pontes. See **pons.**

Pontiac fever. See **Legionnaires' disease.**

pontic /pon″tik/ [L, *pons*, bridge], the suspended member of a removable partial denture or fixed bridge, such as an artificial tooth, usually occupying the space previously occupied by the natural tooth crown.

pontile, pontine. See **pons.**

pontine micturition center, a center in the pons that contributes to control of the bladder and inhibition of tension of the urethral sphincters.

pontine nucleus [L, *pons*, bridge, *nucleus*, nut kernel], nerve cells in the basilar part of the pons where impulses are relayed between the cerebrum and cerebellum.

pontine respiratory center. See **apneustic center.**

Pontocaine, a local anesthetic. Brand name for **tetracaine hydrochloride.**

PONV, abbreviation for **postoperative nausea and vomiting.**

pooled plasma [AS, *pol* + Gk, *plasma,* something formed], plasma pooled from many donors and used to prepare plasma protein derivatives. Source plasma is plasma collected specifically for the manufacture of derivatives; recovered plasma is plasma separated from whole blood donations.

poorly differentiated lymphocytic malignant lymphoma, a lymphoid neoplasm containing cells resembling lymphoblasts that have a fine nuclear structure and one or more nucleoli. Also called **lymphoblastic lymphoma, lymphoblastic lymphosarcoma, lymphoblastoma.**

popliteal /poplit″ē-əl, pop′litē″əl/ [L, *poples*, ham of the knee], pertaining to the area behind the knee.

popliteal artery [L, *poples,* ham of the knee; Gk, *arteria,* airpipe], a continuation of the femoral artery, extending from the opening in the abductor magnus, passing through the popliteal fossa at the knee, dividing into 10 branches, and supplying various muscles of the thigh, leg, and foot. Its branches are the anterior tibial, posterior tibial, patellar rete, genicular articular, sural, medial superior genicular, lateral superior genicular, middle genicular, medial inferior genicular, and lateral inferior genicular.

popliteal fossa, the hollow at the posterior part of the knee.

popliteal node, a node in one of the groups of lymph glands in the leg. Approximately seven small popliteal nodes are embedded in the fat of the popliteal fossa at the back of the knee. Compare **anterior tibial node, inguinal node.**

popliteal pterygium syndrome, 1. a congenital syndrome consisting chiefly of popliteal webs, cleft palate, lower lip pits, and dysplasia of the toenails. A wide variety of other abnormalities may be associated. Also called **popliteal web syndrome. 2.** popliteal webbing associated with cleft lip and palate, fistula of the lower lip, syndactyly, nail dysplasia, and clubfoot. Also called **Fèvre-Languepin syndrome.**

popliteal pulse, the pulsation of the popliteal artery, behind the knee, best palpated with the patient lying prone with the knee flexed.

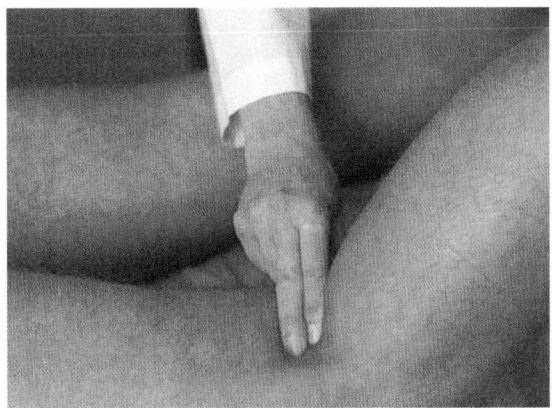

Assessment of the popliteal pulse (Potter et al, 2011)

popliteal web syndrome. See **popliteal pterygium syndrome,** def. 1.

population /pop′yəlā″shən/ [L, *populus,* the people], **1.** an interbreeding group of individuals characterized by genetic continuity through several generations. **2.** a group of individuals collectively occupying a particular geographic locale. **3.** any group that is distinguished by a particular trait or situation. **4.** any group from which samples may be measured for some variable characteristic for statistical purposes.

population at risk, a group of people who share a characteristic that causes each member to be susceptible to a particular event, such as nonimmunized children who are exposed to poliovirus or immunosuppressed people who are exposed to herpesvirus. Also called **vulnerable population.**

population genetics, a branch of genetics that applies mendelian inheritance to groups and studies the frequency of alleles and genotypes in breeding populations. See also **Hardy-Weinberg equilibrium principle.**

population health, the mental, physical, and psychosocial outcomes related to the health and well-being of specific groups of individuals.

por-, poro-, prefix meaning "a cavity, opening, passage, or pore": *porous, porion, porosis.*

P

poractant alfa, a lung surfactant extract.

- INDICATIONS: It is used in the treatment (rescue) of respiratory distress syndrome in premature infants.
- CONTRAINDICATIONS: None is currently known.
- ADVERSE EFFECTS: Concurrent illnesses that have occurred during treatment with this drug include pulmonary air leaks, pulmonary interstitial emphysema, apnea, pulmonary hemorrhage, patent ductus arteriosus, intracranial hemorrhage, severe intracranial hemorrhage, necrotizing enterocolitis, posttreatment sepsis, and posttreatment infection. Adverse effects include bradycardia, oxygen desaturation, pallor, vasoconstriction, hypotension, and hypertension.

porcelain /por'sə·lən/, a white, translucent, dense ceramic material produced by fusing under high temperature a mixture of feldspar, kaolin, quartz, whiting, and other substances. See **dental porcelain.**

porcine /pôr'sīn/ [L, *porcinus,* piglike], obtained from or related to hogs, such as porcine insulin.

porcine graft [L, *porcinus,* piglike; Gk, *graphion,* plant stylus], a temporary biological heterograft made from the skin of a pig.

-pore, suffix meaning "an opening or passageway": *blastopore, gastropore, neuropore.*

porfimer, a miscellaneous antineoplastic.
- INDICATIONS: It is used to treat completely obstructing esophageal cancer and endobronchial non–small cell lung cancer.
- CONTRAINDICATIONS: Factors that prohibit the use of this drug include porphyria, porphyrin allergy (porfimer), tracheoesophageal or bronchoesophageal fistula, and major blood vessels with eroding tumors.
- ADVERSE EFFECTS: Life-threatening effects of this drug are cardiac failure, pleural effusion, and tracheoesophageal fistula. Other adverse effects are pneumonia, dyspnea, respiratory insufficiency, dehydration, weight decrease, anemia, photosensitivity reaction, urinary tract infection, and moniliasis. Common side effects include hypotension, hypertension, atrial fibrillation, tachycardia, abdominal pain, constipation, diarrhea, dyspepsia, dysphagia, eructation, esophageal edema and/or bleeding, hematemesis, melena, nausea, vomiting, anorexia, anxiety, confusion, and insomnia.

poriomania /pôr'ē·ōmā"nē·ə/, a tendency to leave home impulsively or to be a vagabond.

porion /por'ē·on/ [Gk, *poros,* passage], the most lateral point on the roof of the bony external acoustic meatus, vertically over the middle of the meatus. Also called **point Po.**

pork tapeworm. See *Taenia solium.*

pork tapeworm infection [L, *porcus,* pig, hog (male); AS, *taeppe,* tape, *wyrm,* worm; L, *inficere,* to stain], an infection of the intestine or other tissues caused by adult and larval forms of the tapeworm *Taenia solium.* The pork tapeworm is unique in that it can use humans as both intermediate hosts for larvae and definitive hosts for the adult worm. Humans are usually infected with the adult worm after eating contaminated undercooked pork. The infection is rare in the United States and Canada but relatively common in South America, Asia, and Russia. See also **cysticercosis, tapeworm infection.**

poro-. See **por-, poro-.**

porosis /pərō"sis/ [Gk, *poros,* passage], a condition of thinning bone tissue, particularly its supporting connective tissue, as in osteoporosis.

porous /pôr"əs/ [Gk, *poros,* passage], pertaining to something with pores or openings allowing air or fluid to readily pass.

porphobilinogen /pôr'fōbilin"əjən/, a chromogen substance that is an intermediate in the biosynthesis of heme

and porphyrins. It appears in the urine of people with porphyria, representing an error of metabolism. See also **heme, porphyria.**

porphyria /pôrfir"ē·ə/ [Gk, *porphyros,* purple], a group of inherited disorders in which there is abnormally increased production of substances called porphyrins. Two major classifications of porphyria are erythropoietic porphyria, characterized by the production of large quantities of porphyrins in the blood-forming tissue of the bone marrow, and hepatic porphyria, in which large amounts of porphyrins are produced in the liver. Clinical signs common to both classifications of porphyria are photosensitivity, abdominal pain, and neuropathy. See also **acute intermittent porphyria, uroporphyria.**

porphyria cutanea tarda (PCT), the most common form of porphyria, characterized by cutaneous photosensitivity that causes scarring bullae, hyperpigmentation, facial hypertrichosis, and sometimes sclerodermatous thickenings and alopecia. It is frequently associated with alcohol abuse, liver disease, or hepatic siderosis. Urinary levels of uroporphyrin and coproporphyrin are increased, and activity of a specific enzyme involved in heme biosynthesis is decreased. The cause is debated, but two types are generally recognized: an autosomal-dominant (or familial) form in which activity of the affected enzyme is reduced to half normal in liver, erythrocytes, and fibroblasts, and a sporadic (but probably also familial) form in which the reduction is confined to the liver. Both types are believed to be heterozygous, with clinical expression occurring in adulthood, precipitated by disease or environmental factors. A more severe homozygous form begins in childhood and is called hepatoerythropoietic porphyria. See also **porphyria, hepatoerythropoietic porphyria.**

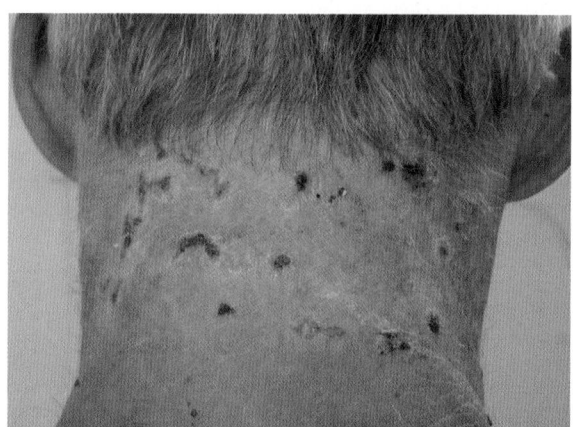

Porphyria cutanea tarda *(Mikula et al, 2012)*

porphyrin /pôr"fərin/ [Gk, *porphyros,* purple], any iron- or magnesium-free pyrrole derivative occurring in many plant and animal tissues. Normal findings of porphyrins in urine are 50 to 300 mg/24 hours.

porphyrinogen /por"f-rin'o-jen/, the reduced form of a porphyrin. The porphyrinogens are the functional intermediates in the biosynthesis of heme. If oxidized to their corresponding porphyrins, such as occurs in porphyrias, they are irreversibly removed from the biosynthetic pathway and accumulate in tissue. Their nomenclature corresponds to that of the porphyrins.

porphyrins and porphobilinogens test, a quantitative analysis of urinary porphyrins and porphobilinogens to screen for porphyria.

portability /pôr′təbil″itē/ [L, *portare,* to carry], a property of computer software that permits its use in a variety of compatible operating systems.

portacaval shunt /pôr′təkā″vəl/ [L, *porta,* gateway, *cavus,* cavity; ME, *shunten*], a shunt created surgically to increase blood flow from the portal circulation by carrying it into the vena cava.

Portagen, a nutritional supplement containing protein, carbohydrate, and fat.

porta hepatis. See **portal fissure.**

portal /pôr″təl/ [L, *porta,* gateway], *n.,* an entrance.

portal circulation [L, *porta,* gateway, *circulare,* to go around], the pathway of blood flow from the GI tract and spleen to the liver via the portal vein and its tributaries. Also called **hepatic portal circulation.**

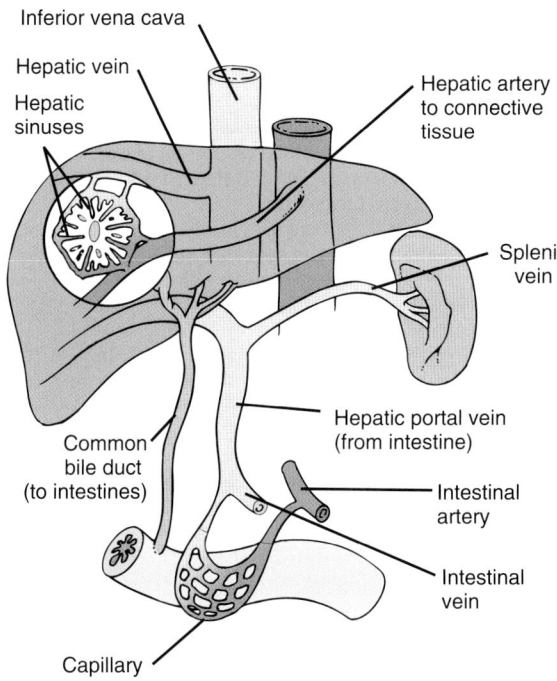

Portal circulation *(Mosby, 2003)*

portal fissure [L, *porta* + *fissura,* cleft], a fissure on the visceral surface of the liver along which the portal vein, the hepatic artery, and the hepatic ducts pass. Also called **porta hepatis.**

portal hypertension, an increased venous pressure in the portal circulation caused by compression or occlusion in the portal or hepatic vascular system. It results in splenomegaly, large collateral veins, ascites, and, in severe cases, systemic hypertension and esophageal varices. Portal hypertension is frequently associated with cirrhosis.

portal of entry, the route by which an infectious agent enters the body, such as through nonintact skin.

portal system, arrangement of blood vessels in which blood exiting one tissue is immediately carried to a second tissue before being returned to the heart and lungs for oxygenation and redistribution.

portal-systemic encephalopathy. See **hepatic coma.**

portal vein, a vein from the small intestine that ramifies in the liver and ends in capillary-like sinusoids that convey the blood to the inferior vena cava through the hepatic veins. The portal vein passes behind the duodenum and ascends through the lesser omentum to the porta hepatis, where it divides into the right and left branches. The vein is surrounded by the hepatic plexus of nerves and is accompanied by numerous lymphatic vessels, some lymph nodes, and corresponding branches of the hepatic artery. The right branch of the portal vein enters the right lobe of the liver, and the left branch enters the left lobe.

portal venous shunt. See **postcaval shunt.**

Porter-Silber reaction [Curt C. Porter, American biochemist, b. 1914; Robert H. Silber, American biochemist, b. 1915], a reaction, visible as a change in color to yellow, that indicates the amount of adrenal steroids (the 17-hydroxycorticosteroids) excreted per day in the urine. The test is used to evaluate adrenocortical function but is now largely supplanted by immunoassay techniques.

portoenterostomy /pôr′tō·en′təros″təmē/ [L, *porta* + Gk, *enteron,* bowel, *stoma,* mouth, *temnein,* to cut], construction of a bile drainage system with an intestinal conduit to correct biliary atresia. There are several procedural approaches, such as anastomosis of the jejunum by a Roux-en-Y loop to the portal fissure region to establish bile flow from the bile ducts to the intestine. The procedure is indicated in patients younger than 3 months of age. The operation is successful in most cases, but in a significant number of patients late mortality occurs because of chronic medical problems. Without the operation, biliary cirrhosis develops with an attendant early death. Also called **Kasai operation.**

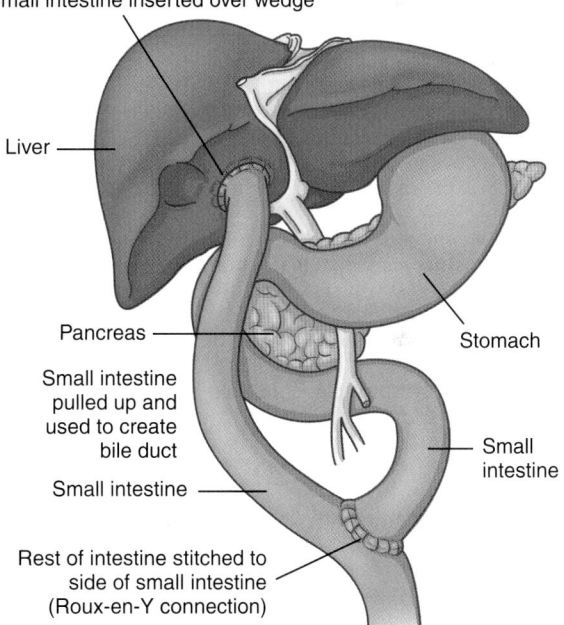

Portoenterostomy *(McCance and Huether, 2014)*

Portuguese-Azorean disease. See **Machado-Joseph disease.**

Portuguese man-of-war /por′chəgēs/, any member of the genus *Physalia,* in the phylum Cnidaria. All species have a large purple air sac that allows them to float on the surface of the water, and from which many long tentacles of stinging polyps hang. The tentacles are equipped with nematocysts that are able to penetrate the skin of humans, causing intense pain. Paralysis can result from numerous stings.

port-wine stain. See **nevus flammeus.**

posaconazole, a systemic antifungal.

■ INDICATIONS: This drug is used for prevention of aspergillus, *Candida* infection, and oropharyngeal candidiasis in the immunocompromised.

■ CONTRAINDICATIONS: Fungal meningitis, onychomycosis or dermatomycosis in cardiac dysfunction, and hypersensitivity to this drug or other systemic antifungals or azoles prohibit its use.

■ ADVERSE EFFECTS: Adverse effects of this drug include insomnia, fever, rigors, weakness, anxiety, hypertension, hypotension, tachycardia, anemia, cramps, abdominal pain, flatulence, gynecomastia, impotence, decreased libido, malaise, hypokalemia, and tinnitus. Life-threatening side effects include GI bleeding, hepatotoxicity, toxic epidermal necrolysis, and rhabdomyolysis. Common side effects include headache, dizziness, nausea, vomiting, anorexia, diarrhea, pruritus, edema, and fatigue.

position /pəzish″ən/ [L, *positio*], **1.** any one of many postures of the body, such as the anatomical position, lateral recumbent position, or semi-Fowler's position. See specific positions. **2.** (in obstetrics) the relationship of an arbitrarily chosen fetal reference point, such as the occiput, sacrum, chin, or scapula, on the presenting part of the fetus to its location in the maternal pelvis.

-position, combining form meaning "the putting or setting in place": *juxtaposition.*

positional behavior /pəzish′ənəl/, the orientation and movement of a primate's body.

positional vertigo, a severe but brief episode of vertigo associated with a change of body position, as when a patient lies down. It may be caused by an injury or disease of the utricle. Also called **postural vertigo. See also cupulolithiasis.**

positioner /pə·zish′ənər/, a resilient rubbery and plastic removable appliance fitted over the occlusal surfaces of the teeth to obtain limited tooth movement and stabilization, usually at the end of orthodontic treatment.

position sense, a variety of muscular senses by which the position or attitude of the body or its parts is perceived. Also called **posture sense, proprioception.**

positive /poz′itiv/ [L, *positivus,*], **1.** (of a laboratory test result) indicating that a substance or a reaction is present. **2.** (of a sign) indicating on physical examination that a finding is present, often meaning that there is pathological change. **3.** (of a substance) tending to carry or carrying a positive chemical charge.

positive balance, a state in which the amount of water or an electrolyte excreted from the body is less than that ingested.

positive end-expiratory pressure (PEEP), positive airway pressure applied at the end of the exhalation phase during mechanical ventilation. Each successive breath begins from a new baseline. Air is delivered in cycles of constant pressure through the respiratory cycle. The patient is usually but not always intubated, and a ventilator cycles the air through an endotracheal tube. PEEP is used for the relief of respiratory distress secondary to prematurity, pancreatitis, shock, pulmonary edema, trauma, surgery, or other conditions in which spontaneous respiratory efforts are inadequate and arterial levels of oxygen are deficient. Close observation is necessary during PEEP therapy because excessive PEEP may decrease venous return to the heart. Blood gases and vital signs are monitored closely. If PEEP does not significantly improve the patient's condition, its level is increased or it may be discontinued. Compare **continuous positive airway pressure.**

positive feedback, **1.** (in physiology) an increase in function in response to a stimulus. For example, micturition increases after the flow of urine has started, and the uterus

contracts more frequently and with greater strength after it has begun to contract in labor. **2.** *(Informal)* an encouraging, favorable, or otherwise positive response from one person to what another person has communicated.

positive identification, the unconscious modeling of one's personality on that of another who is admired and esteemed. See also **identification.**

positive mask. See **reversal film.**

positive pressure, **1.** a greater-than-ambient atmospheric pressure. **2.** any technique in which compressed gas or air is delivered to the airways at greater-than-ambient pressure. Positive-pressure techniques in respiratory therapy require a flow-regulating device and a delivery system, such as a cannula, mouthpiece, endotracheal tube, or tracheostomy tube.

positive pressure breathing unit. See **IPPB unit.**

positive pressure ventilation (PPV), any of numerous types of mechanical ventilation in which gas is delivered into the airways and lungs under positive pressure, producing positive airway pressure during inspiration. It may be done via either an endotracheal tube or a nasal mask.

positive relationship, (in research) a direct relationship between two variables in which as one increases, the other can be expected to increase. Also called **direct relationship.** Compare **negative relationship.**

positive sequence, the sequence of the bases on the strand of a double-stranded nucleic acid that encodes the product. In DNA it is the strand that encodes the RNA, having thus the same base sequence except changing T for U in the RNA.

positive signs of pregnancy, three unmistakable signs of pregnancy: fetal heart tones, heard on auscultation; fetal skeleton, seen on x-ray film or ultrasonogram; and fetal parts, felt on palpation.

positive symptom, a symptom of the acute phase of schizophrenia. Compare **negative symptom.**

positron /pos′itron/, a positively charged particle emitted from neutron-deficient radioactive nuclei; the antiparticle of an electron.

positron emission tomography (PET) [L, *positivus* + Gk, *elektron,* amber; L, *emittere,* to send out; Gk, *tome,* section, *graphein,* to record], a computerized radiographic technique that uses radioactive substances to examine the metabolic activity of various body structures. The patient either inhales or is injected with a metabolically important substance such as glucose, carrying a radioactive element that emits positively charged particles, or positrons. When the positrons combine with electrons normally found in the cells of the body, gamma rays are emitted. The electronic circuitry and computers of the PET device detect the gamma rays and construct color-coded images that indicate the intensity of metabolic activity throughout the organ involved. The radioactive isotopes used in PET are very short-lived, so that patients undergoing a PET scan are exposed to very small amounts of radiation. Researchers use PET to examine blood flow and the metabolism of the heart and blood vessels, to study and diagnose cancer, and to investigate the biochemical activity of the brain.

Posner-Schlossman syndrome. See **glaucomatocyclitic crisis.**

post. See **dowel.**

post-, prefix meaning "after" or "behind": *postcoital, postganglionic, posthumous.*

postanesthesia care unit (PACU), an area adjoining the operating room to which patients who have received sedative, general, and regional anesthetics are taken for nursing assessment and care while recovering from anesthesia. Vital signs, adequacy of ventilation, level of consciousness, surgical site, and levels of pain are carefully

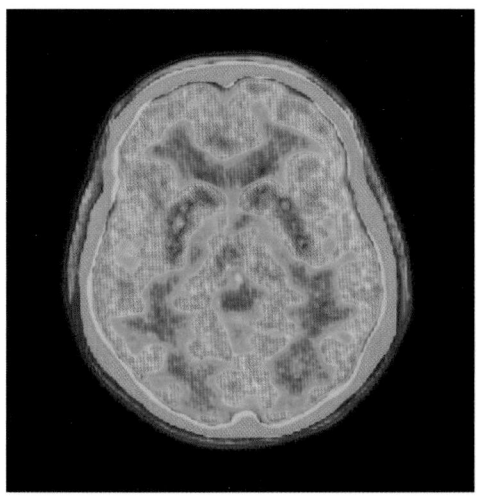

Image of brain produced by positron emission tomography *(Patel et al, 2017)*

monitored as the patient recovers consciousness. The PACU has nursing staff with specific skills to care for patients, and a certified registered nurse anesthetist or anesthesiologist is available. Formerly called **recovery room.** See also **postoperative care.**

postaxial /pōst·ak′sē·əl/ [L, *post,* after; Gk, *axon,* axis], posterior to an axis. In anatomical usage, this refers to the medial (ulnar) aspect of the upper limb and the lateral (fibular) aspect of the lower limb.

postaxial acrofacial dysostosis. See **Miller syndrome.**

postcaval shunt /-kā′vəl/ [L, *post,* after, *vena cava* + ME, *shunten*], any of several surgical anastomoses of the portal and systemic circulations to relieve symptoms of portal hypertension. Also called **portacaval shunt, portal venous shunt.**

postcentral gyrus /-sen′trəl/ [L, *post,* after; Gk, *kentron,* center, *gyros,* turn], a convolution of the brain immediately posterior to the central sulcus of the cerebrum. It is the location of the sensory strip for the contralateral side of the body.

postcoital /-kō′itəl/ [L, *post,* after, *coire,* to come together], after sexual intercourse.

postcoital contraceptive, a contraceptive that blocks or terminates pregnancy after sexual intercourse. Also called **emergency contraceptive.**

postcoital test, (for infertility) examination of secretions aspirated from the vaginal fornix and endocervical canal after coitus to determine the number and condition of spermatozoa present and the extent to which they have penetrated the cervical mucus. See also **Huhner test.**

postcommissurotomy syndrome /-kəmis′yərot″əmē/ [L, *post,* after, *commissura,* a union; Gk, *temnein,* to cut], a condition of unknown cause occurring within the first few weeks after cardiac valvular surgery, characterized by intermittent episodes of pain and fever, which may last weeks or months and then resolve spontaneously.

postconcussional syndrome /-kənkush″ənəl/ [L, *post* + *concussio,* shake violently], a condition that follows head trauma, characterized by dizziness, poor concentration, headache, hypersensitivity, and anxiety. It usually resolves itself without treatment. Also called **posttraumatic syndrome.**

postdate pregnancy /-dāt″/ [L, *post,* after, *data* + *praegnans,* bearing child], a pregnancy that lasts more than 42 weeks. Also called **postterm pregnancy.**

postdural puncture headache (PDPH). See **spinal headache.**

posterior /postir″ē·ər/ [L, behind], **1.** *adj.,* in the back part of a structure, such as the dorsal surface of the human body. **2.** *n.,* the back part of something. **3.** *adj.,* toward the back. Compare **anterior.**

posterior Achilles bursitis, a painful heel condition caused by inflammation of the bursa between the Achilles tendon and the calcaneus. It is commonly associated with Haglund deformity.

posterior antebrachial cutaneous nerve, a nerve that branches off from the radial nerve, innervates the skin of the dorsal aspect of the forearm, and has a general sensory modality.

posterior asynclitism. See **asynclitism.**

posterior atlantoaxial ligament, one of five ligaments connecting the atlas to the axis. It is broad, thin, and fixed to the inferior border of the anterior arch of the atlas and to the ventral surface of the body of the axis. Compare **anterior atlantoaxial ligament.**

posterior atlantooccipital membrane, one of a pair of thin, broad fibrous sheets that form part of the atlantooccipital joint between the atlas and the occipital bone and contain an opening for the vertebral artery and the suboccipital nerve. Also called *posterior atlantooccipital ligament.* Compare **anterior atlantooccipital membrane.**

posterior auricular artery, one of a pair of small branches from the external carotid arteries, dividing into auricular and occipital branches and supplying parts of the ear, scalp, and other structures in the head.

posterior circumflex humeral artery, an artery that originates from the third part of the axillary artery, leaves the axilla through the quadrangular space in the posterior wall, and enters the posterior scapular region where it supplies related muscles and the glenohumeral joint.

posterior column. See **posterior horn.**

posterior common ligament. See **posterior longitudinal ligament.**

posterior costotransverse ligament, one of the five ligaments of each costotransverse joint, comprising a fibrous band passing from the neck of each rib to the base of the vertebra above. Compare **superior costotransverse ligament.**

posterior drawer sign, an orthopedic test used to determine laxity of the posterior cruciate ligament of the knee. The patient is positioned with hips at 45 degrees and knees flexed at 90 degrees while the examiner stabilizes the foot and pushes the tibia backward. Also, with both the hips and knees flexed at 90 degrees, the examiner holds the heels together and observes the knees to compare the relative posterior sag of the tibia.

posterior ethmoidal artery, an artery that supplies the ethmoidal air cells and the nasal cavity.

posterior ethmoidal nerve, a nerve that supplies the posterior ethmoidal air cells and the sphenoid sinus.

posterior fontanel, a small triangular area between the occipital and parietal bones at the junction of the sagittal and lambdoidal sutures. See also **fontanel.**

posterior fossa, a depression on the posterior surface of the humerus, above the trochlea, that lodges the olecranon of the ulna when the elbow is extended.

posterior horn [L, behind, *cornu,* horn], the horn-shaped projection of gray matter in the posterior region of the spinal cord. It relays information related to touch and pressure from muscles and regulates precise movement and unconscious proprioception. Also called **dorsal column, dorsal horn, posterior column.**

P

posterior inferior cerebellar artery syndrome. See **Wallenberg syndrome.**

posterior kidney, posterior segment of kidney; the renal segment located most posteriorly.

posterior ligament. See **rectovaginal ligament.**

posterior liver, a term used to refer to the posterior region that is not part of either the left part or the right part of the liver but is coextensive with the caudate lobe.

posterior longitudinal ligament, a thick strong ligament attached to the dorsal surfaces of the vertebral bodies, extending from the occipital bone to the coccyx. Also called **posterior common ligament.** Compare **anterior longitudinal ligament.**

posterior median fissure, a narrow groove in the closed part of the medulla oblongata.

posterior mediastinal node, a node in one of three groups of thoracic visceral nodes, connected to the part of the lymphatic system that serves the esophagus, pericardium, diaphragm, and convex surface of the liver. Most of the efferent vessels of the posterior mediastinal nodes end in the thoracic duct, but some join the tracheobronchial nodes. Compare **thoracic visceral node.**

posterior mediastinum, the irregularly shaped lower part of the mediastinum parallel with the vertebral column. It is bounded ventrally by the pericardium, inferiorly by the diaphragm, dorsally by the vertebral column from the fourth to the twelfth thoracic vertebra, and laterally by the mediastinal pleurae. It contains the bifurcation of the trachea, two primary bronchi, the esophagus, the thoracic duct, many large lymph nodes, and various vessels, such as the thoracic part of the aortic arch. Compare **anterior mediastinum, middle mediastinum, superior mediastinum.**

posterior nares, a pair of posterior internal openings in the nasal cavity connecting it with the nasopharynx and allowing the inhalation and exhalation of air. Each is an oval aperture that measures about 2.5 cm vertically and is about 1.5 cm in diameter. Also called **choana.** Compare **anterior nares.**

posterior neuropore, the embryonic opening at the inferior end of the neural tube from neural canal to exterior. It closes at about the 25 somite stage, which indicates the end of horizon XII in the numeric anatomical charting of human embryonic development. Compare **anterior neuropore.** See also **horizon.**

posterior occlusion. See **distoclusion.**

posterior palatal seal area, the area of soft tissues along the junction of the hard and soft palates on which displacement, within the physiological tolerance of the tissues, can be applied by a maxillary full or partial denture to aid its retention. Also called *post dam.*

posterior parietal artery, an artery that originates at the terminal part of the middle cerebral artery and serves the posterior parietal lobe of the brain.

posterior pituitary gland. See **neurohypophysis.**

posterior ramus, a branch of each spinal nerve. Collectively, the posterior rami innervate the back.

posterior rhizotomy [L, behind; Gk, *rhiza,* root, *temnein,* to cut], a surgical procedure for cutting the posterior, or sensory, nerve root to relieve intractable pain or to relieve spasms from neurological causes such as cerebral palsy.

posterior sagittal anorectoplasty, plastic surgery to create a functional anus and rectum in children with imperforate anus or other anorectal malformations. Also called *Peña procedure.*

posterior spinal arteries, one of two arteries that originate in the cranial cavity, usually arising directly from a terminal branch of each vertebral artery, and descend along the spinal cord, each as two branches that bracket the posterolateral

sulcus and the connection of posterior roots with the spinal cord. They are reinforced along their length by 8 to 10 segmental medullary arteries, the largest of which is the artery of Adamkiewicz.

posterior subcapsular cataract [L, *capsula* + Gk, *katarrhaktes,* waterfall], a visual opacity caused by a thickening of the epithelial cells lining the capsule. The condition is frequently the result of the aging process or a disease that involves surrounding eye tissues.

posterior temporal artery, the posterior temporal branch of the middle cerebral artery, originating in the middle cerebral artery and supplying the cortex of the posterior temporal lobe. It has no branches.

posterior tibial artery, one of the divisions of the popliteal artery, supplying various muscles of the lower leg, foot, and toes. Compare **anterior tibial artery.**

posterior tibialis pulse, the pulse of the posterior tibialis artery palpated on the medial aspect of the ankle, just posterior to the prominence of the malleolus.

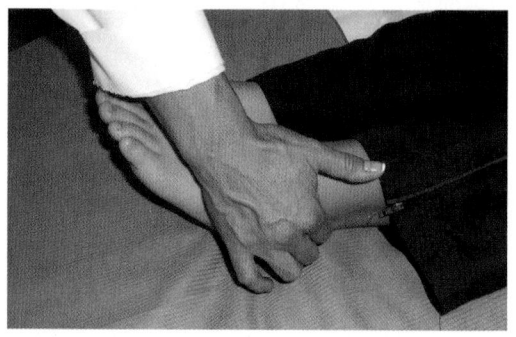

Palpation of the posterior tibialis pulse *(Courtesy Rutgers School of Nursing—Camden. All rights reserved.)*

posterior tooth, any of the maxillary and mandibular molars of the primary dentition or the premolars and molars of the secondary dentition or of prostheses. Compare **anterior tooth.**

posterior uveitis, uveitis involving the posterior segment of the eye. See also **choroiditis, chorioretinitis.**

posterior vaginal hernia. See **vaginal hernia.**

posterior vein of left ventricle, one of the five tributaries of the coronary sinus that drain blood from the capillary bed of the myocardium. It courses along the diaphragmatic surface of the left ventricle, accompanying the circumflex branch of the left coronary artery. In some individuals it ends in the great cardiac vein. Compare **great cardiac vein, middle cardiac vein, small cardiac vein.**

postero-, prefix meaning "posterior part": *posteroanterior, posteroexternal, posterosuperior.*

posteroanterior (P-A, p-a) /pos″tərō-antir″ē-ər/ [L, *posterus,* coming after, *anterior,* before], the direction from back to front.

posteroexternal /pos″tər-ō-ek-ster′nəl/ [L, *posterus,* coming after, *externus,* outward], situated on the outer side of a posterior aspect.

posteroinferior /-infir″ē-ər/ [L, *posterus,* coming after, *inferior,* lower], pertaining to a position that is both lower and behind.

posterolateral /-lat″ərəl/ [L, *posterus,* coming after, *latus,* side], pertaining to a position behind and to the side.

posterolateral sulcus, a shallow depression on each side of the posterior surface of the spinal cord that marks where the posterior rootlets of the spinal nerve enter the cord.

posterolateral thoracotomy, a chest surgery technique in which an incision is made in the submammary fold, below the tip of the scapula. The incision is continued posteriorly along the course of the ribs and upward as far as the spine of the scapula. It requires division of the trapezius, rhomboideus, latissimus dorsi, and serratus anterior muscles. Compare **anterolateral thoracotomy, median sternotomy.**

posteromedial /pos′tər·ō·mē′dē·əl/ [L, *posterus,* coming after, *medius,* middle], situated toward the middle of the posterior surface.

posteromedial central arteries of posterior communicating artery, branches of the posterior communicating artery that supply the medial surface of the thalamus and the walls of the third ventricle.

posteroparietal /pos′tər·ō·pə·rī′ə·təl/ [L, *posterus,* coming after, *paries,* wall], situated at the posterior part of the parietal bone.

posterosuperior /pos′tər·ō·sōō·pēr′ē·ər/ [L, *posterus,* coming after, *superior,* higher], situated posteriorly and superiorly.

postganglionic /-gang′glē·on″ik/ [L, *post,* after; Gk, *ganglion,* knot], distal to a ganglion.

postganglionic fiber, the axon of a nerve cell whose cell body is situated in a ganglion.

postganglionic neuron [L, *post,* after; Gk, *ganglion,* knot, *neuron,* nerve], a neuron that is distal to or beyond a ganglion.

posthepatic cirrhosis. See **postnecrotic cirrhosis.**

posthepatic jaundice /pōst′hepat″ik/ [L, *post,* after; Gk, *hepar,* liver; Fr, *jaune,* yellow], jaundice caused by obstruction of the bile ducts.

posthumous /pos″chəməs/ [L, *post,* after, *humare,* to bury], after a person's death.

posthypnotic suggestion /-hipnot′ik/ [L, *post,* after; Gk, *hypnos,* sleep; L, *suggerere,* to suggest], an action suggested to a hypnotized subject during a trance that the subject carries out on awakening from the trance. The action is in response to a cue, and the subject usually does not know why he or she is performing it.

postictal /pōst′iktəl/ [L, *post* + L, *ictus,* blow or stroke], **1.** after a seizure. **2.** confused. *–postictus, n.*

postinfectious /-infek″shəs/ [L, *post* + *inficere,* to stain], after an infection.

postinfectious encephalitis. See **encephalitis.**

postinfectious glomerulonephritis, the acute form of glomerulonephritis, which may follow 1 to 6 weeks after a streptococcal infection, most often in childhood. Characteristics of the disease are hematuria, oliguria, edema, and proteinuria, especially in the form of granular casts. There may be slight impairment of renal function in adults, but most patients recover fully in 1 to 3 months. There is no specific treatment for this form of glomerulonephritis. Restriction of dietary protein and the prescription of diuretics may be necessary until kidney function returns to normal. Also called **acute glomerulonephritis.** See also **chronic glomerulonephritis, subacute glomerulonephritis.**

■ OBSERVATIONS: Onset of symptoms occurs 1 to 6 weeks after a streptococcal infection. Symptoms include hypertension, headache, edema, oliguria, dark urine, reduced urine output, flank pain, weight gain, fever, chills, nausea, and vomiting; about half of cases are asymptomatic. Diagnosis is made through a series of lab tests. Hematuria (microscopic or gross), proteinuria, sediment, and RBC casts are seen on urinalysis. Blood chemistries reveal increased blood urea nitrogen, increased serum creatinine, increased serum lipids, and decreased serum albumin. ASO titers are positive. Complications include congestive heart failure, acute or chronic renal failure, and end-stage renal disease.

■ INTERVENTIONS: Treatment focuses on treating symptoms and preventing complications. Antihypertensives are administered for hypertension, diuretics are given for edema, and antiinfective drugs are administered if an infection is still present. Electrolytes are monitored and abnormalities corrected. Diet therapy focuses on restricted sodium, restricted potassium, and low protein to combat electrolyte abnormalities and uremia. Hemodialysis or peritoneal dialysis may be used to treat renal failure.

■ PATIENT CARE CONSIDERATIONS: Management in acute care focuses on supportive measures. Rest, fluid, and electrolyte restrictions and dietary reduction of protein are necessary until signs of inflammation (e.g., proteinuria and hematuria) subside. Instruction centers on restrictions and proper administration of a full course of antibiotics. Prevention is also key and involves encouraging individuals to seek early diagnosis and treatment of sore throats and skin lesions, particularly in children.

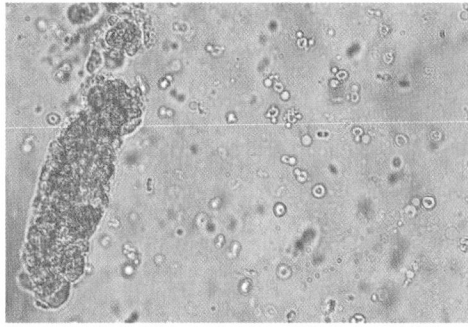

Postinfectious glomerulonephritis: red blood cell cast
(Campbell, Walsh, and Retik, 2002)

postinfectious psychosis [L, *post,* after, *inficere,* to stain; Gk, *psyche,* mind, *osis,* condition], psychotic behavior that follows a severe infection, such as pneumonia, scarlet fever, malaria, uremia, or typhoid fever.

post–lumbar puncture headache /-lum″bar/ [L, *post,* after, *lumbus,* loin, *punctura;* AS, *heafod* + *acan*], a headache that occurs within a few hours after a lumbar puncture and usually lasts 1 or 2 days to several weeks. It may be accompanied by nausea and vomiting and improves when the patient lies down.

postmastectomy exercises /-məstek″təmē/ [L, *post* + Gk, *mastos,* breast, *ektomē,* excision], exercises essential to the prevention of shortening of the muscles, prevention of contracture of the joints, and improvement in lymph and blood circulation after mastectomy.

■ METHOD: The woman is asked to flex and extend the fingers of the affected arm in the recovery room and to pronate and supinate the forearm immediately on return to her room after recovery from anesthesia and surgery. The postoperative mastectomy exercises are begun gradually at the surgeon's discretion. Brushing her teeth and hair is encouraged as effective exercise. Other exercises are usually taught, including four specific exercises: climbing the wall, arm swinging, rope pulling, and elbow spreading. They are performed as follows: *Climbing the wall:* The patient stands facing a wall, toes close to the wall. The elbows are bent, and the palms of the hands are placed on the wall at shoulder height. The hands are moved up the wall together until the woman feels pain or pulling on the incision, then returned

P

to the starting position. *Arm swinging*: While standing, the patient bends forward from the waist, allowing both arms to relax and hang naturally. The arms are swung together from the shoulders from left to right and then in circles parallel to the floor, clockwise and counterclockwise. She straightens up slowly. *Rope pulling*: A rope is attached over a shower rod or a hook. Each end of the rope is grasped, and the patient alternately pulls each end, raising one arm after the other to the height at which incisional pain or pulling is felt. The rope is shortened until the affected arm is raised almost directly overhead. *Elbow spreading*: The hands are clasped behind the neck, and the elbows are slowly raised to chin level while the head is held erect. Gradually the elbows are spread apart to the point at which incisional pain or pulling is felt.

■ INTERVENTIONS: Specific exercises may be ordered. The patient is shown how to do them and is encouraged to continue them at home.

■ OUTCOME CRITERIA: With proper exercise, full range of motion returns; both arms can be extended fully and equally high over the head. The woman benefits from having something active to do to help herself during the difficult period of adjustment after mastectomy. Many activities of daily life provide good exercise, such as reaching high shelves, hanging clothes, and gardening.

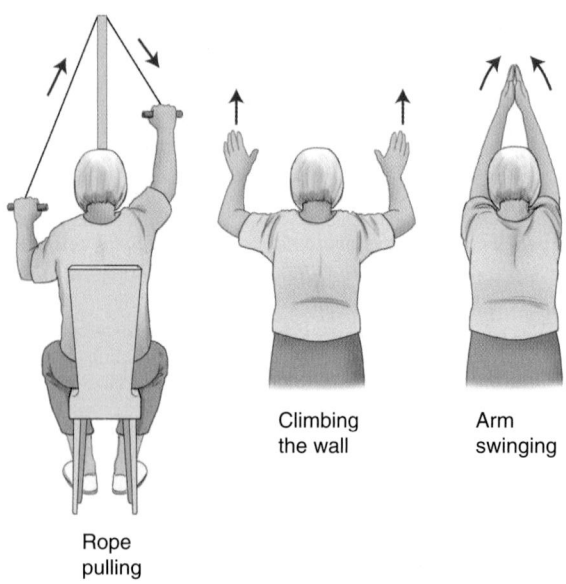

Rope pulling

Climbing the wall

Arm swinging

Postmastectomy exercises *(Lewis et al, 2014)*

postmature infant, an infant born after the end of the 42nd week (288 days) of gestation, bearing the physical signs of placental insufficiency. Characteristically the baby has dry, peeling skin; long fingernails and toenails; and folds of skin on the thighs and sometimes on the arms and buttocks. Hypoglycemia and hypokalemia are common. Postmature infants often look as if they have lost weight in utero. The newborn is fed early, and the calcium and potassium levels in the blood are monitored and corrected, if necessary, to prevent seizures and neurological damage. To prevent the syndrome, labor may be induced as gestation approaches 42 weeks. To anticipate the problems associated with the syndrome, the fetus and the mother may be electronically monitored through labor. Also called *postmature newborn,* **postterm infant.**

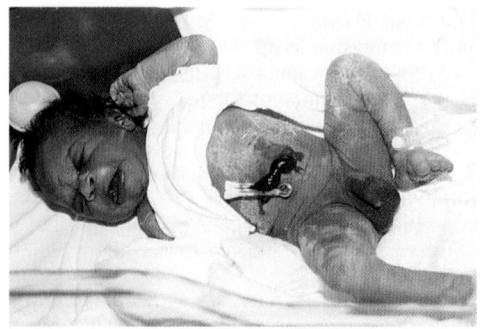

Dry skin of postmature infant *(Murray and McKinney, 2006)*

postmaturity /-məchoo̅″ritē/ [L, *post* + *maturare,* to become ripe], **1.** overdevelopment or maturity. **2.** beyond the normal date for maturity, as in a postmature infant. See also **dysmaturity, postmature infant.** –*postmature, adj.*

postmenopausal /-men′əpô″səl/ [L, *post* + *men,* month; Gk, *pauein,* to cease], pertaining to the period of life after menopause.

postmenopausal hemorrhage, bleeding from the uterus after menopause.

postmenopausal vaginitis [L, *post,* after, *men,* month; Gk, *pauein,* to cease; L, *vagina,* sheath; Gk, *itis,* inflammation], an inflammation caused by degenerative changes in the vaginal mucosa after menopause. Also called **atrophic vaginitis.**

postmortem /môr′təm/ [L, *post* + *mors,* death], *adj.,* after death. See **postmortem examination.**

postmortem cesarean section [L, *post,* after, *mors,* death, *secare,* to cut, *sectio*], delivery of a fetus by incision into the uterus after death of a woman. Also called *postmortem delivery.*

postmortem examination [L, *post,* after, *mors,* death, *examinatio*], an examination of a body after death by a person trained in pathology. Also called **autopsy,** *(Informal)* **postmortem.**

postmortem graft [L, *post,* after, *mors,* death; Gk, *graphion,* stylus], the transplanting of a cornea, artery, or other body part from a deceased person to repair a defect in a living body. Also called **cadaver graft.**

postmortem lividity, the black and blue discoloration of the skin of a cadaver, resulting from an accumulation of deoxygenated blood in subcutaneous vessels.

postmyocardial infarction syndrome /-mī·əkär″dē·əl/ [L, *post* + Gk, *mys,* muscle, *kardia,* heart; L, *infarcire,* to stuff], a condition that may occur days or weeks after an acute myocardial infarction. It is characterized by chest pain, fever, pericarditis with a friction rub, pleurisy, pleural effusion, joint pain, and elevated white blood cell count and sedimentation rate. It tends to recur and often provokes severe anxiety, depression, and fear that another heart attack is occurring. Treatment includes aspirin, reassurance, and a short course of corticosteroids. Care includes close observation and emotional support, especially when debilitating anxiety and depression are present. Also called **Dressler syndrome.**

postnasal /-nā″zəl/ [L, *post,* after, *nasus,* nose], pertaining to the region posterior to the nasal cavity.

postnasal drip (PND) [L, *post* + *nasus,* nose; AS, *dryppan*], a drop-by-drop discharge of nasal mucus into the posterior pharynx caused by rhinitis, chronic sinusitis, or hypersecretion by the nasopharyngeal mucosa. It is often accompanied by a feeling of obstruction, an unpleasant taste, and fetid breath. Methods of treatment include the application of drops or sprays of phenylephrine or ephedrine sulfate to constrict blood vessels and reduce hyperemia, sinus irrigation to improve drainage, and use of appropriate antibiotics. Therapy for allergies may be indicated in some cases, and surgery may be required if the nasal passages are obstructed by polyps or a deviated septum.

postnecrotic cirrhosis /-nekrot′ik/ [L, *post* + Gk, *nekros,* dead; *kirrhos,* yellowish, *osis,* condition], a nodular form of cirrhosis that may follow hepatitis or other inflammation of the liver. Also called **posthepatic cirrhosis.** See also **cirrhosis.**

postoperative (post-op) /-op″ərətiv′/ [L, *post* + *operari,* to work], pertaining to the period of time after surgery. It begins with the patient's emergence from anesthesia and continues through the time required for the acute effects of the anesthetic and surgical procedures to abate.

postoperative atelectasis, a form of atelectasis in which collapse of lung tissue is caused by the depressant effects of anesthetic drugs or the inability to breathe deeply or cough effectively because of pain. Deep breathing and coughing are encouraged at frequent postoperative intervals to prevent this condition.

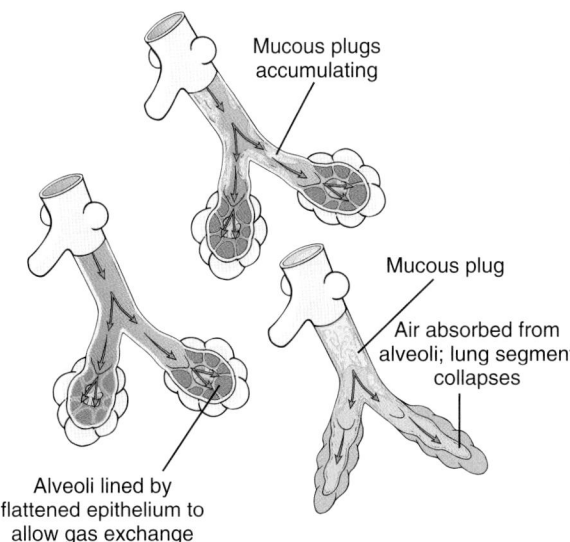

Mucous plugs accumulating

Mucous plug

Air absorbed from alveoli; lung segment collapses

Alveoli lined by flattened epithelium to allow gas exchange

Postoperative atelectasis *(Lewis et al, 2014)*

postoperative bed, a surface prepared for a patient who is weak or unconscious, as when recovering from anesthesia. The bed is in the flat position. The bottom sheet may be covered with a cotton bath blanket that is tucked tightly beneath the mattress. The top linen is fan-folded to the far side of the bed and not tucked in. The bed is made in this way to simplify transferring a patient from a stretcher into the bed.

postoperative care, the management of a patient after surgery. See also **preoperative care.**
■ METHOD: Before the patient's discharge from the operating room to the postanesthesia care unit, the surgical drapes, ground plate, and restraints are removed and a sterile dressing may be applied to the incision. The patency and connections of all drainage tubes and the flow rate of parenteral infusions are checked. The patient's cleanliness and dryness are given attention, and the gown is changed, avoiding exposing the individual. The patient is transferred slowly and cautiously to a stretcher or bed, maintaining body alignment

and protecting the limbs. When indicated, an oral or nasal airway is inserted or a previously inserted endotracheal tube is suctioned. Respiration may be assessed with a pulse oximeter; if respiration remains impaired, the anesthetist is notified. The blood pressure, pulse, and respirations are initially reported to the anesthetist and are then checked at least every 15 minutes or as ordered. At similar intervals the level of consciousness, reflexes, and movements of extremities are observed, and the incision, drainage tubes, and IV infusion site are inspected. Medication, blood or blood components, and oxygen are administered as ordered, and fluid intake and output are measured. Pain is controlled with analgesics. The patient is kept warm and dry and positioned for optimal ventilation and comfort. At the first sign of vomiting, the head or body is turned to one side and suction is applied to prevent aspiration. Oral hygiene is administered to keep the mouth and tongue moist. The chest is auscultated for breath sounds every 30 minutes, and the patient, when reactive, is helped to turn and deep breathe. The tympanic or axillary temperature is taken every 1 to 4 hours. When rested and able to move the extremities well, and after having exhibited stable vital signs, the patient may be transferred to the assigned room, if the drainage tubes are functioning, the dressings show no bleeding or excessive drainage, and the anesthesiologist approves the move. The family is informed of the patient's progress and expectations for the postoperative period. The airway patency; rate, depth, and character of respirations; pulse; blood pressure; temperature; skin color; level of consciousness; and condition of dressings and drainage tubes are assessed. If respirations are noisy, the patient is assisted in coughing. A rapid, weak, thready pulse may indicate increased bleeding and is reported, especially if other signs of impending shock, such as hypotension or changes in level of consciousness, are evident. The dressing is examined at frequent intervals, and excessive drainage is reported immediately. The side rails of the bed are raised for safety and the head is slightly elevated, unless contraindicated. A cardiac monitor may be connected. Parenteral fluids and pain medication are administered as ordered. Fluid intake and output are measured; range-of-motion exercises to extremities are performed, and ambulation, when ordered, is assisted.
■ INTERVENTIONS: The postanesthesia care nurse performs the immediate postoperative procedures, and the clinical unit nurse provides ongoing care, emotional support, and instructions for the patient and family. Special attention is given to preventing trauma postoperatively, as may occur when confused or elderly patients fall when getting out of bed.
■ OUTCOME CRITERIA: Meticulous postoperative care prevents falls, infections, and other complications and promotes the healing of the incision and restoration of the patient to health.

postoperative cholangiography, (in diagnostic radiology) a procedure for outlining the major bile ducts. A radiopaque contrast material is injected into the common bile duct via a T-tube inserted during surgery. It is usually performed after a cholecystectomy to discover any residual calculi. See also **cholangiography.**

postoperative ileus [L, *post* + *operari,* to work; Gk, *eilein,* to twist], an absence of normal intestinal function caused by a loss of peristaltic muscular action of the intestine after surgery.

postoperative nausea and vomiting (PONV), nausea and vomiting occurring after a surgical procedure.

postoperative paresthesia, prolonged dysfunction of a nerve after surgery, typically because of a mechanical injury or prolonged duration of a local anesthetic.

P

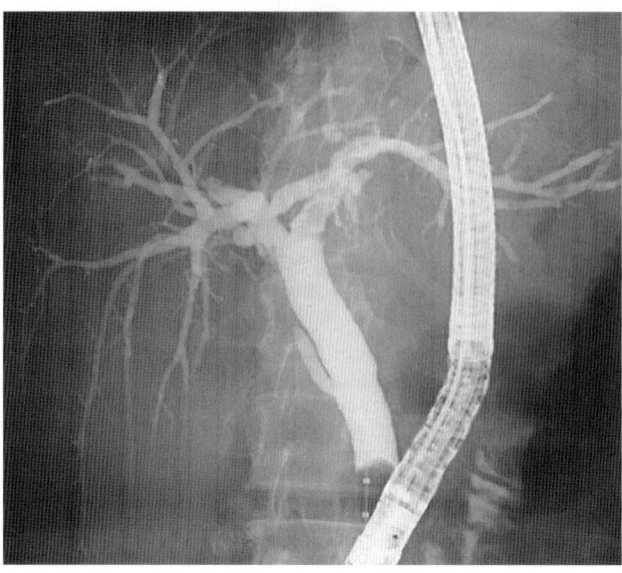

Postoperative cholangiography *(Chandrasekhara, et al, 2019)*

postparalytic /-per′əlit″ik/ [L, *post* + Gk, *paralyein,* to be palsied], pertaining to the period after a loss of muscle function.

postpartal care /-pär″təl/ [L, *post* + *partus,* birth], care of the mother and her newborn during the first few days of the puerperium. See also **antepartal care, intrapartal care, newborn intrapartal care.**

postpartum /pōstpär″təm/, after childbirth.

postpartum blues [L, *post,* after, *partus,* birth; ME, *bleu*], an emotional effect of childbirth experienced by mothers, consisting mainly of transient feelings of sadness for a period of about 72 hours. If the symptom persists for a longer period, the diagnosis of depression may apply. The condition may require psychotherapy, use of antidepressant medications, or both. It may occur more than once in the same person after subsequent pregnancies and may have serious consequences if untreated. See also **postpartum depression.**

postpartum depression [L, *post* + *partus* + *deprimere,* to press down], an abnormal psychiatric condition that occurs after childbirth, typically from 3 days to 6 weeks after birth. It is characterized by symptoms that range from mild "postpartum blues" to an intense suicidal depressive psychosis. Severe postpartum depression occurs approximately once in every 2000 to 3000 pregnancies. The cause is not proved; neurochemical and psychological influences have been implicated. Approximately one third of patients are found to have had some degree of psychiatric abnormality predating the pregnancy. The disorder recurs in subsequent pregnancies in 25% of cases. Some women at risk for postpartum depression may be identified during the prenatal period: those who have made no preparations for the expected baby, expressed unrealistic plans for postpartum work or travel, or denied the reality of the responsibilities of parenthood. Depending on the severity of the disorder, psychoactive medication or psychiatric hospitalization may be necessary.

Postpartum Depression Theory. See **Beck, Cheryl Tatano.**

postpartum hemorrhage [L, *post,* after, *partus,* birth; Gk, *haima,* blood, *rhegnynai,* to burst forth], excessive bleeding (a loss of more than 500 mL of blood) after childbirth.

postpartum iliofemoral thrombophlebitis [L, *post,* after, *parturs,* birth, *ilia,* flank, *femur,* thigh; Gk, *thrombos,* lump, *phleps,* vein, *itis,* inflammation], thrombophlebitis involving the iliofemoral artery after childbirth.

postpartum pituitary necrosis [L, *post* + *partus* + *pituita,* phlegm; Gk, *nekros,* dead, *osis,* condition], an infarct of the pituitary resulting from hypovolemia and shock in the immediate postpartum period. The condition causes a state of hypopituitarism; lactation may not develop, pubic and axillary hair may be lost, and symptoms of hypoglycemia and amenorrhea are experienced. See also **Sheehan syndrome.**

postpartum psychosis [L, *post,* after, *partus,* birth; Gk, *psyche,* mind], an episode of psychosis, which may be depressive, after childbirth. Because the condition usually develops in the month after childbirth, endocrinological factors are believed to be a cause.

postperfusion syndrome /-pərfyoo″zhən/ [L, *post* + *perfundere,* to pour over], a cytomegalovirus (CMV) infection occurring between 2 and 4 weeks after the transfusion of fresh blood containing CMV. It is characterized by prolonged fever, hepatitis, rash, atypical lymphocytosis, and occasionally jaundice. No specific treatment is available.

postpericardiotomy syndrome /pōst′perikär′dē·ot″ əmē/ [L, *post* + Gk, *peri,* around, *kardia,* heart, *temnein,* to cut], a condition that sometimes occurs days or weeks after pericardiotomy, characterized by symptoms of pericarditis, often without any fever. It appears to be an autoimmune response to damaged cells of the myocardium and pericardium. See also **pericarditis.**

postpill amenorrhea /-pill´/ [L, *post* + *pilla,* ball; Gk, *a,* not, *men,* month, *rhoia,* flow], failure of normal menstrual cycles to resume within 3 months after discontinuation of oral contraception. The pathophysiological characteristics of this uncommon condition are poorly understood. Postpill amenorrhea is rarely permanent. See also **amenorrhea.**

postpoliomyelitis muscular atrophy (PPMA) /-pō´lē-ōmī´əlī˝tis/ [L, *post,* after; Gk, *polios,* gray, *myelos,* marrow, *itis,* inflammation; L, *musculus* + Gk, *a,* not, *trophe,* nourishment], a recurrence of muscular weakness and other neuromuscular symptoms in people who recovered from acute paralytic polio many years earlier. The condition may or may not affect the same muscles that were damaged in the earlier polio attack.

postpolycythemic myeloid metaplasia /-pol´isīthē˝mik/ [L, *post* + Gk, *polys,* many, *kytos,* cell, *haima,* blood, *myelos,* marrow, *eidos,* form, *meta,* with, *plassein,* to mold], a late-developing anemia in polycythemia vera, caused by bone marrow fibrosis. The production of red blood cells occurs only in the liver and spleen. This condition is frequently complicated by leukemia, especially if the patient has been treated with ionizing radiation. See also **myelofibrosis, myeloid metaplasia, polycythemia.**

postprandial, after a meal.

postprandial glucose test, a blood test in which a meal acts as a glucose challenge to the body's metabolism. It is an easily performed screening test for diabetes mellitus. A 1-hour glucose screen, using a 50-g oral glucose load, is used to detect gestational diabetes mellitus.

postprandial pain [L, *post,* after, *prandium,* meal, *poena,* penalty], pain that occurs after a meal.

postprocessing /-pros˝əsing/, (in ultrasonics) manipulation and conditioning of signals and image data after they emerge from the scan converter and before they are displayed. Postprocessing is used to change the assignment of image brightness versus echo signal amplitude in memory.

postpuberal, postpubertal. See **postpuberty.**

postpubertal panhypopituitarism /-pyoo˝bərtəl/ [L, *post* + *pubertas,* maturation; Gk, *pan,* all, *hypo,* below, *pituita,* phlegm], insufficiency of pituitary hormones, caused by pituitary necrosis resulting from a blood clot in the artery supplying the gland or trauma to the gland. The disorder is characterized initially by weakness, lethargy, loss of libido, intolerance to cold and, in females, by failure to lactate and amenorrhea. It leads eventually to loss of axillary and pubic hair, bradycardia, hypotension, premature wrinkling of the skin, and atrophy of the thyroid and adrenal glands. Treatment consists of the administration of thyroid hormone, corticosteroids, and sex hormones. Also called **hypophyseal cachexia, pituitary cachexia, Simmonds disease.** Compare **prepubertal panhypopituitarism.**

postpuberty /-pyoo˝bərtē/ [L, *post* + *pubertas,* maturation], a period of approximately 1 to 2 years after puberty during which skeletal growth slows and the physiological functions of the reproductive years are established. Also called *postpubescence.*

postrenal anuria /-rē´nəl/ [L, *post* + *renes,* kidney; Gk, *a* + *ouron,* not urine], cessation of urine production caused by obstruction of the ureters or urethra.

postresection filling. See **retrograde filling.**

poststeroid lobular panniculitis [L, *panniculus,* piece of cloth], subcutaneous nodules that may develop in a layer of fatty connective tissue in children 1 to 13 days after discontinuation of steroid therapy. The condition resolves spontaneously with or without readministration of the medication. Compare **poststeroid panniculitis.**

poststeroid panniculitis /pos˝təroid pənik´yəlī˝tis/ [L, *panniculus,* piece of cloth], subcutaneous nodules that may develop in children after withdrawal of corticosteroid treatment for rheumatic fever or nephrotic syndrome. The condition resolves spontaneously or with readministration of the medication. Compare **poststeroid lobular panniculitis.**

postsynaptic /-sinap˝tik/ [L, *post* + Gk, *synaptein,* to join], **1.** situated after a synapse. **2.** occurring after a synapse has been crossed.

postterm infant. See **postmature infant.**

postterm pregnancy. See **postdate pregnancy.**

posttetanic potentiation (PTP), an increase in neurotransmitter release after a brief high-frequency train of action potentials.

posttransfusion syndrome /-transfyoo˝zhən/ [L, *post,* after, *transfundere,* to pour through; Gk, *syn,* together, *dromos,* course], a complex of adverse reactions that may accompany or follow IV administration of blood or blood components. Reactions may include hemolytic effects, headache and back pain, allergies to an unknown component in donor blood, circulatory overloading, effects of cold blood that chill the patient's cardiovascular system, and effects of microaggregates in stored blood.

posttransplant diabetes, glucose intolerance or overt hypoglycemia that first appears after an organ transplant. Some cases are steroid diabetes caused by use of steroid immunosuppressive agents.

posttraumatic /-trômat˝ik/ [L, *post,* after; Gk, *trauma,* wounded], pertaining to any emotional, mental, or physiological consequences after a major illness or injury.

posttraumatic amnesia [L, *post* + Gk, *trauma,* wound], a period of amnesia between a brain injury resulting in memory loss and the point at which the functions concerned with memory are restored.

posttraumatic epilepsy. See **traumatic epilepsy.**

posttraumatic osteoporosis [L, *post,* after; Gk, *trauma,* wound, *osteon,* bone, *poros,* passage, *osis,* condition], a loss of bone density that develops after an injury or other severe health episode. It may occur as a result of disease.

posttraumatic spondylitis. See **Kümmell disease.**

posttraumatic stress disorder (PTSD), a *DSM-V* psychiatric disorder characterized by an acute emotional response to a traumatic event or situation involving severe environmental stress, such as a natural disaster, airplane crash, serious automobile accident, military combat, or physical torture.

posttraumatic syndrome. See **postconcussional syndrome.**

postulate /pos˝chəlāt/ [L, *postulare,* to demand], a hypothesis that is offered as true without proof or as a basis for argument or debate.

postural albuminuria. See **orthostatic proteinuria.**

postural background movements /pos˝chərəl/ [L, *ponere,* to place], the spontaneous body adjustments, requiring vestibular and proprioceptive integration, that maintain the center of gravity, keep the head and body in alignment, and stabilize body parts, such as the shoulder girdle when the hand reaches for a distant object.

postural drainage, the use of positioning to drain secretions from specific segments of the bronchi and the lungs into the trachea. Coughing usually expels secretions from the trachea. Also called **bronchial drainage.** See also **cupping and vibrating.**

P

Positions for postural drainage

Lung segment	Position of client	Lung segment	Position of client

Adult

Bilateral — High-Fowler position

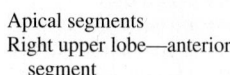

Left lower lobe—lateral segment — Left lateral in Trendelenburg position

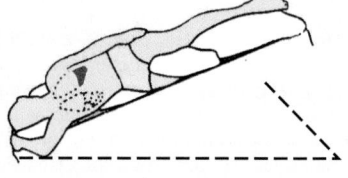

Apical segments
Right upper lobe—anterior segment — Supine with head of bed elevated 15 to 30 degrees

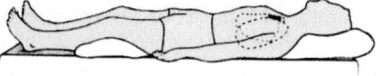

Right lower lobe—lateral segment — Right side-lying in Trendelenburg position

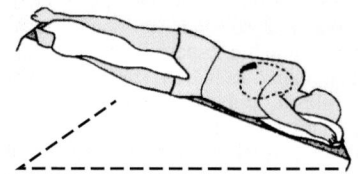

Left upper lobe—anterior segment — Supine with head elevated

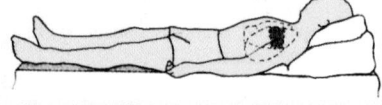

Right lower lobe—posterior segment — Prone in Trendelenburg position with abdomen and thorax elevated

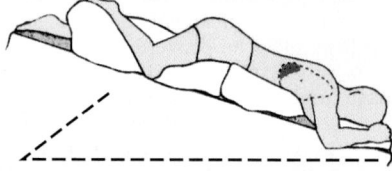

Right upper lobe—posterior segment — Side lying with right side of chest elevated on pillows

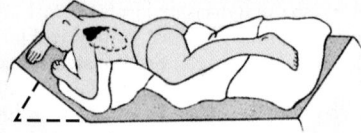

Right middle lobe—posterior segment — Prone with thorax and abdomen elevated

Left upper lobe—posterior segment — Side lying with left side of chest elevated on pillows

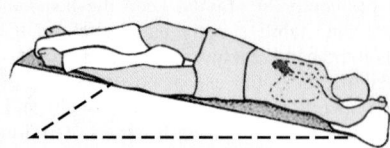

Both lower lobes—anterior segment — Supine in Trendelenburg position

Right middle lobe—anterior segment — Three-fourths supine position with dependent lung in Trendelenburg position

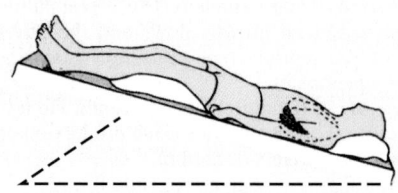

Positions for postural drainage—cont'd

Lung segment	Position of client	Lung segment	Position of client
Both lower lobes—posterior segment	Prone in Trendelenburg position with abdomen and thorax elevated	Bilateral—middle anterior segments	Sitting on nurse's lap, leaning against nurse

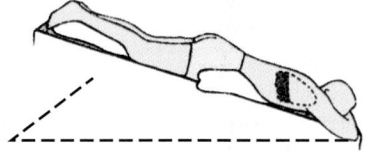
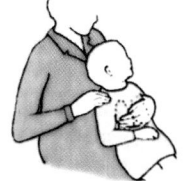

Child

Bilateral— apical segments	Sitting on nurse's lap, leaning slightly forward, flexed over pillow	Bilateral lobes— anterior segments	Lying supine on nurse's lap, back supported with pillow

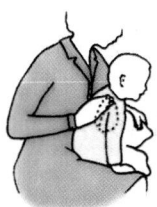
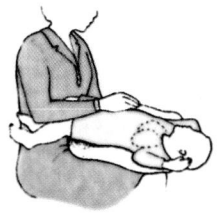

From Potter PA, Perry AG: *Fundamentals of nursing,* ed 7, St Louis, 2009, Mosby.

■ METHOD: Positions that promote drainage from the affected parts of the lungs are selected. Pillows and raised sections of the hospital bed are used to support or elevate parts of the body. The procedure is begun with the patient level, and the head is gradually lowered to a full Trendelenburg position. Inhalation through the nose and exhalation through the mouth are encouraged. Simultaneously the nurse or other health care provider may use cupping and vibration over the affected area of the lungs to dislodge and mobilize secretions. The person is then helped to a position conducive to coughing and is asked to breathe deeply at least three times and to cough at least twice.
■ INTERVENTIONS: A patient who is dyspneic or who has hemoptysis or signs of cerebral hemorrhage, increased intracerebral pressure, or lung abscess is not placed in a head-down position without caution and a specific medical order. Suction is kept available in all cases in which the patient may not be able to expel the secretions that have drained into the trachea. The patient's tolerance for the procedure and the position is carefully observed. Fatigue is prevented.
■ OUTCOME CRITERIA: Effectiveness of the procedure depends on positioning that allows drainage by gravity and on liquefaction, ciliary action, and effective breathing. As the secretions are cleared, the patient becomes better able to breathe, is more comfortable, and may move about more freely; thus the respiratory passages may remain freer of obstructing secretions and resume their expected function.

postural hypotension.   See **orthostatic hypotension.**

postural mechanism,   a term used to encompass muscle tone, postural tone, equilibrium, and righting responses, as well as protective extension reactions.

postural proteinuria.   See **orthostatic proteinuria.**

postural reflex [L, *ponere,* to place, *reflectere,* to turn back],   any of several reflexes associated with maintaining normal body posture.

postural vertigo.   See **positional vertigo.**

posture /pos″chər/ [L, *ponere,* to place],   the position of the body with respect to the surrounding space. A posture is determined and maintained by coordination of the various muscles that move the limbs, by proprioception, and by the sense of balance.

posture sense.   See **position sense.**

postvaccinal encephalitis /-vak″sinəl/ [L, *post,* after, *vaccinus,* of a cow; Gk, *enkephalos,* brain, *itis,* inflammation],   acute encephalitis after vaccination, especially with vaccinia (smallpox vaccine) or the Semple rabies vaccine.

postvaccinal encephalomyelitis [L, *post,* after, *vaccinus,* of a cow; Gk, *enkephalos,* brain, *myelos,* marrow, *itis,* inflammation],   acute encephalomyelitis after vaccination.

postviral fatigue syndrome /-vīrəl/ [L, *post,* after, *virus,* poison, *fatigare,* to tire; Gk, *syn,* together, *dromos,* course],   a condition after a viral infection of chronic muscle fatigue unrelieved by rest. Other symptoms may include visual and hearing difficulties, low-grade fever, stiff neck, urinary frequency, and insomnia. Also called **benign myalgic encephalomyelitis, Iceland disease, Royal Free disease.**

pot-, combining form meaning "related to drinking": *potable.*

potable water /pō"təbəl/ [L, *potare,* to drink], water that can be consumed without concern for adverse health effects. Potable water does not have to taste good. Likewise, water may be palatable but not necessarily safe to drink.

potassemia /pōt'əsē"meiə/ [D, *potasschen,* potash; Gk, *haima,* blood], an excess of potassium in the blood.

potassium (K) /pətas"ē-əm/ [D, *potasschen,* potash], an alkali metal element, the seventh most abundant element in the earth's crust. Its atomic number is 19; its atomic mass is 39.10. Potassium salts are necessary to the life of all plants and animals. Potassium in the body constitutes the predominant intracellular cation, helping to regulate neuromuscular excitability and muscle contraction. Sources of potassium in the diet are whole grains, meat, legumes, fruit, and vegetables. The average adequate daily intake for most adults is 2 to 4 g. Normal adult levels of blood potassium are 3.5 to 5 mEq/L or 3.5 to 5 mmol/L (SI units). Potassium is important in glycogen formation, protein synthesis, and correction of imbalances of acid-base metabolism, especially in association with the action of sodium and hydrogen ions. Potassium salts are very important as therapeutic agents but are extremely dangerous if used improperly. The kidneys play an important role in controlling the secretion and absorption. Aldosterone stimulates sodium reabsorption and potassium secretion by the kidneys. The major extrarenal adaptation to this process involves the absorption of potassium by the body tissues, especially the tissues of the muscles and the liver. Potassium is most commonly depleted in the body by an increased rate of excretion by the kidneys or the GI tract. Increased renal excretion may be caused by diuretic therapy, large doses of anionic drugs, or renal disorders. Increased GI excretion of potassium may occur with the loss of GI fluid through vomiting, diarrhea, surgical drainage, or chronic use of laxatives. Potassium loss through the skin is rare but can result from perspiring during excessive exercise in a hot environment.

potassium and sodium phosphate, any of various preparations containing both sodium and potassium phosphate in some combination of the monobasic and dibasic salts of each. It is used as an electrolyte replenisher, urinary acidifier, and antiurolithic.

potassium channel blocking agent, any of a class of antiarrhythmic agents that inhibit the movement of potassium ions through potassium channels, thus prolonging repolarization of the cell membrane. Also called *potassium channel blocker.*

potassium chloride (KCl), a white crystalline salt used as a substitute for table salt in the diet of people with cardiovascular disorders, in administration of the potassium ion, and as a constituent of Ringer's solution.

■ INDICATIONS: It is prescribed in the treatment of hypokalemia resulting from a variety of causes and of digitalis intoxication.

■ CONTRAINDICATIONS: Hyperkalemia; concomitant use of spironolactone, amiloride, or triamterene; Addison disease; renal impairment; or known hypersensitivity to this drug prohibits its use.

■ ADVERSE EFFECTS: Among the most serious adverse effects are hyperkalemia and, when the drug is given orally, ulceration of the small bowel.

potassium hydroxide (KOH), a white, soluble, highly caustic compound. Occasionally used in solution as an escharotic for bites of rabid animals, KOH has many laboratory uses as an alkalinizing agent, including the preparation of clinical specimens for examination for fungi under the microscope.

potassium indoxyl sulfate. See **indican.**

potassium iodide, an expectorant.

■ INDICATIONS: It is prescribed in the treatment of chronic bronchitis, bronchiectasis, asthma, and other pulmonary disease with excess mucus formation and of various thyroid disorders.

■ CONTRAINDICATIONS: Acute bronchitis, known or suspected pregnancy, or known hypersensitivity to this drug or to any iodide prohibits its use.

■ ADVERSE EFFECTS: Among the more serious adverse effects are hypersensitivity, goiter, myxedema, GI disturbance, and skin lesions.

potassium penicillin V. See **penicillin V.**

potassium phosphates, a combination of monobasic and dibasic potassium phosphates used as an electrolyte replenisher.

potassium pump, a mechanism that involves energy-dependent pumping of potassium or the active transport of the potassium ion (K^+) across a biological membrane using the energy of K^+-activated adenosine triphosphatase. Also called **K^+ pump.** See also **calcium pump, sodium-potassium pump.**

potassium-sparing diuretic. See **diuretic.**

potency /pō"tənsē/ [L, *potentia,* power], **1.** (in embryology) the range of developmental possibilities of which an embryonic cell or part is capable, regardless of whether the stimulus for growth or differentiation is natural, artificial, or experimental. See also **competence,** def. 1. **2.** a measure of the strength of the active chemical components contained in an herb or herbal preparation. Standardized products ensure the consumer of receiving a dosage containing a consistent potency. Compare **concentration.**

potent /pō"tənt/ [L, *potentia,* power], powerful or strong.

-potent, -potential, combining form meaning "powerful" or "able to do" something specified: *pluripotential, equipotential.*

potential /pəten"shəl/ [L, *potentia*], an expression of the energy involved in transferring a unit of electric charge. The gradient or slope of a potential causes the charge to move. The movement of 1 coulomb of charge from a potential of *V* to a potential of *V*-1 volts requires 1 joule of energy.

potential abnormality of glucose tolerance, Individuals who have never had abnormal glucose tolerance but who have an increased risk of diabetes or impaired glucose tolerance. Factors associated with an increased risk of type 1 diabetes mellitus include having circulating islet cell antibodies, being a monozygotic twin or sibling of a type 1 diabetes patient, and being the offspring of a type 1 diabetes patient. Factors associated with an increased risk of type 2 diabetes mellitus include being a first-degree relative of a type 2 diabetes patient (particularly in a family in which there are several generations with type 2 diabetes); giving birth to a neonate weighing more than 9 pounds (4.086 kilograms); being a member of a racial or ethnic group with a high prevalence of diabetes, such as some Native American groups; and being an obese adult.. See also **diabetes mellitus.**

potential difference, the difference in electric potential between two points. It represents the work involved in the release of energy by the transfer of a unit quantity of electricity from one point to another.

potential energy [L, *potentia,* power; Gk, *energeia*], the energy contained in a body as a result of its position in space, internal structure, and stresses imposed on it. Also called **latent energy.**

potential life, a criterion used by the U.S. Centers for Disease Control and Prevention to gauge premature death rates. Among younger individuals, it is based on an assumption that the person would have lived to 65 years of age if life had not been interrupted by a particular disease or injury. The leading cause of loss of potential life in young people is accidents, followed by cancer and heart disease. For older people the system is based on years of potential life lost before 85 years of age, in which case cancer and heart disease rank first and second.

potential trauma, (in dentistry) a change in tissue that may occur because of existing malocclusion or dental disharmony.

potentiate /pōten′shē·āt/, to increase the strength or degree of activity of something.

potentiation /pōten′shē·ā″shən/ [L, *potentia*], a synergistic action in which the effect of two drugs given simultaneously is greater than the sum of the effects of each drug given separately.

potentiometer /pōten′shē·om″ətər/ [L, *potentia* + Gk, *metron,* measure], a voltage-measuring device.

Potter-Bucky grid [Hollis E. Potter; Gustav Bucky; 20th-century American radiologists; ME, *gredire,* grate], an x-ray grid that oscillates during the exposure of a radiographic image, blurring the grid lines. Also called *Potter-Bucky diaphragm.* See also **grid.**

Pott's disease. See **tuberculous spondylitis.**

Pott's fracture [Percival Pott, English physician, 1713–1788], a break in the fibula near the ankle, often accompanied by a break in the malleolus of the tibia or a rupture of the internal lateral ligament. Also called **Dupuytren fracture.**

potty chair [AS, *pott* + ME, *chaire*], a small chair that has an open seat over a removable pot; it is used for the toilet training of young children.

pouch [OFr, *pouche*], any small saclike appendage or pocket, such as Rathke pouch in the embryonic roof cavity. See also **cul-de-sac.**

pouch of Douglas. See **cul-de-sac of Douglas.**

poultice /pōl″tis/ [L, *puls,* porridge], **1.** a soft, moist pulp spread between layers of gauze or cloth and applied hot to a surface to provide heat or to counter irritation. Kinds include **mustard plaster. 2.** plant material (such as crushed fresh herbs) that has been wrapped in gauze or similar soft cloth, moistened, and applied topically.

pound (lb) [L, *pondus,* weight], a unit of measure equal to 16 ounces, avoirdupois; 0.45359 kg; 7000 grains.

P. ovale, abbreviation for *Plasmodium ovale.*

poverty /pov′ərtē/ [L, *paupertas*], **1.** a lack of material wealth needed to maintain existence. **2.** a loss of emotional capacity to feel love or sympathy.

povidone /pō″vidōn/, a polymerized form of vinylpyrrolidone, a white hygroscopic powder readily soluble in water, used as a dispersing and suspending agent in drugs. It also has been used as a blood volume extender and, in a complex with iodine, as a topical antiseptic.

povidone-iodine /pō′vidōn ī″ədīn/, an antiseptic microbicide.

■ INDICATIONS: It is prescribed as a topical microbicide for disinfection of wounds, as a preoperative surgical scrub, for vaginal infections, and for antiseptic treatment of burns. A drop is also often placed into the eyes of neonates to prevent ophthalmia neonatorum.

■ CONTRAINDICATIONS: Known hypersensitivity to this drug or to iodine prohibits its use.

■ ADVERSE EFFECTS: Among the more serious adverse effects are local skin irritation, redness, and swelling.

Powassan virus infection [Powassan, Ontario], an uncommon form of encephalitis caused by a tick-borne arbovirus found in eastern Canada and the northern United States.

powder, the dried product of an extraction process in which a substance is first mixed with a solvent such as alcohol or water. Then, the solvent is removed completely. The dry solid that remains either is already in powder form or may be ground into it.

power centric, the position of the mandible during a forceful bite.

power mode, a method of color flow processing and display in which the Doppler signal amplitude or the signal intensity, averaged over a small interval, is displayed rather than the average Doppler frequency. Velocity and flow direction are not displayed, and artifacts do not affect the image.

power of attorney [Fr, *pouvoir* + OFr, *atorne,* legal agent], a document authorizing one person to take legal actions on behalf of another, to act as an agent for the grantor. The legality of a power of attorney may be challenged if the grantor can be found to have been mentally incompetent at the time the authority was granted.

power stroke, a working movement of a dental scaling instrument, used for splitting or dislodging calculus from the surface of a tooth or tooth root.

pox [ME, *pokkes,* pustules], **1.** any of several vesicular or pustular exanthematous diseases terminating in scars. **2.** the pitlike scars of smallpox or chicken pox. **3.** *(Obsolete)* syphilis. Now called **syphilis.**

poxvirus /poksvī″rəs/ [ME, *pokkes* + L, *virus,* poison], a member of a family of viruses that includes the organisms that cause molluscum contagiosum, smallpox, and vaccinia.

PPD, abbreviation for **purified protein derivative.**

PPE, abbreviation for **personal protective equipment.**

PPLO, abbreviation for **pleuropneumonia-like organism.**

PPM, ppm, abbreviation for **parts per million.**

PPMA, abbreviation for **postpoliomyelitis muscular atrophy.**

PPNG, abbreviation for **penicillinase-producing** *Neisseria gonorrhoeae.*

PPO, abbreviation for **preferred provider organization.**

PPS, abbreviation for **prospective payment system.**

PPV, **1.** abbreviation for **positive pressure ventilation. 2.** abbreviation for **pulse pressure variation.**

Pr, symbol for the element **praseodymium.**

PR, abbreviation for **prosthion.**

practical anatomy. See **applied anatomy.**

practical nurse. See **licensed practical nurse.**

practice guideline, a detailed description of a process of patient care management that will facilitate improvement or maintenance of health status or slow the decline in health status in certain chronic clinical conditions. The purpose of a practice guideline is to assist health care providers to identify preferred treatment by providing links among diagnoses, treatments, and outcomes and by describing alternatives available for each patient. Practice guidelines provide a basis for evaluation of care and allocation of resources. See also **clinical pathway.**

practice models /prak″tis/ [Gk, *praktikos,* practical], the patterns by which health care services are made available to people in different settings.

practice setting, the context or environment within which nursing care is given.

practice theory, (in nursing research) a theory that describes, explains, and prescribes nursing practice in general. It serves as the basis for specific items in the curriculum of nursing education and for the development of theories in the administration of nursing and nursing education.

P

practicing /prak″tising/,   the second subphase of the separation-individuation phase in Mahler's system of preoedipal development, when the child is able to move away from the mother and return to her for emotional nurturing. The child may feel elation in response to this investigation of the environment and through practicing locomotor skills.

practicing medicine without a license,   (in law) practicing activities defined under state law in the medical practice act without physician supervision, direction, or control.

practitioner /praktish″ənər/ [Gk, praktikos],   a person qualified to practice in a special professional field, such as a nurse practitioner.

Prader-Willi syndrome /prä″dər wil″ē/ [A. Prader, 20th-century Swiss physician; H. Willi; Gk, syn, together, dromos, course],   a congenital metabolic condition characterized by hypotonia, hyperphagia, marked obesity, hypogonadism, and cognitive impairment. When diabetes mellitus occurs with the other symptoms, the condition is called Royer syndrome. Administration of growth hormones may accelerate growth and improve strength. Testosterone may increase penis size, and puberty can be accomplished with hormone replacement. See also Angelman syndrome.

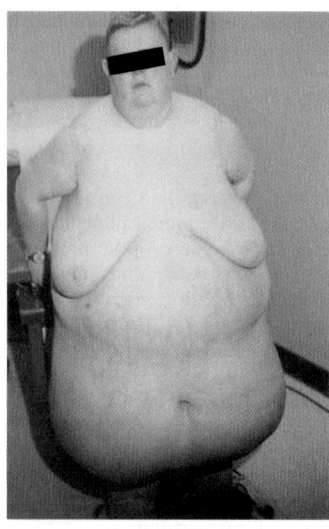

Individual with characteristic appearance of Prader-Willi syndrome (Morgan and Weinsier, 1998)

prae-.   See pre-, prae-.

praecox [L, premature],   pertaining to something that occurred at an earlier stage of life or development.

praevia /prē″vē·ə/ [L],   having occurred at an earlier time or in front of a place. Also called praevius.

pragmatic /pragmat″ik/,   pertaining to a belief that ideas are valuable only in terms of their consequences.

pragmatism /prag″mətiz″əm/ [Gk, pragma, deed],   a philosophy concerned with actual practice and practical results as opposed to theory and speculation.

pralidoxime chloride /pral″ədok′sēm/,   a cholinesterase reactivator.

■ INDICATIONS: It is prescribed as an antidote for organophosphate poisoning and drug overdosage in the treatment of myasthenia gravis.

■ CONTRAINDICATIONS: Known hypersensitivity to this drug prohibits its use. It is contraindicated in poisoning by carbamate insecticides that react with pralidoxime.

■ ADVERSE EFFECTS: Among the most serious adverse effects are dizziness, tachycardia, hyperventilation, and muscle weakness. These reactions are most common when the drug is injected too rapidly.

-pramine,   suffix for imipramine-type compounds.

pramipexole,   an antiparkinson agent.

■ INDICATIONS: It is used to treat parkinsonism.

■ CONTRAINDICATIONS: Known hypersensitivity prohibits its use.

■ ADVERSE EFFECTS: Life-threatening effects are hemolytic anemia, leukopenia, and agranulocytosis. Other adverse effects include psychosis, hallucination, depression, dizziness, constipation, impotence, and blurred vision. Common side effects include agitation, insomnia, nausea, anorexia, and orthostatic hypotension.

pramlintide,   an antidiabetic that modulates and slows stomach emptying, prevents postprandial rise in plasma glucagon, decreases appetite, and leads to decreased caloric intake and weight loss.

■ INDICATIONS: This drug is used as an adjunct to insulin therapy to treat uncontrolled type 1 or type 2 diabetes.

■ CONTRAINDICATIONS: Gastroparesis and known hypersensitivity to this drug or to metacresol prohibit its use.

■ ADVERSE EFFECTS: Adverse effects of this drug include headache, fatigue, dizziness, nausea, vomiting, anorexia, abdominal pain, injection site reactions, hypoglycemia (while used with insulin), arthralgia, cough, pharyngitis, and systemic allergy.

Pramosone,   a fixed-combination topical drug containing a glucocorticoid and a topical anesthetic that is used to treat perianal pain and swelling. Brand name for hydrocortisone acetate, pramoxine hydrochloride.

pramoxine hydrochloride /prəmok″sēn/,   a local anesthetic for the relief of pain and itching associated with dermatoses, anogenital pruritus, hemorrhoids, anal fissure, and minor burns.

prandial /pran″dē·əl/ [L, prandium, meal],   pertaining to a meal. The term is used in relation to timing, such as postprandial or preprandial.

praseodymium (Pr) /prā′sē·ōdīm″ē·əm/ [Gk, prasaios, light-green, didymos, twin],   a rare earth metallic element. Its atomic number is 59, and its atomic mass is 140.91.

portable chest x-ray,   a radiographic examination of the chest performed with a portable x-ray machine. The image receptor is placed against the patient's back, and the x-ray tube is positioned in front of the patient. The patient is positioned as upright as possible to allow for visualization of fluid levels in the lungs.

Prausnitz-Küstner test (PK test) /prous″nits kist″nər/ [Otto C. Prausnitz, German hygienist, 1876–1963; Heinz Küstner, German gynecologist, 1897–1963],   a skin test formerly used to measure the presence of immunoglobulin E. An allergic response was transferred to a nonallergic person who acted as a surrogate to permit identification of the allergen. It is no longer used because of the high risk of transfer of hepatitis or blood-borne diseases such as acquired immunodeficiency syndrome. Also, serum IgE can now be measured by in vitro assays, such as the radioallergosorbent test and radioimmunosorbent test. Also called passive transfer test. Compare patch test, radioallergosorbent test. See also anaphylaxis.

pravastatin /prav′ahstat″in/,   an antihyperlipidemic agent that acts by inhibiting cholesterol synthesis, used as the sodium salt in the treatment of hypercholesterolemia and other forms of dyslipidemia and to lower the risks associated with atherosclerosis and coronary heart disease. It is administered orally.

-praxia, combining form meaning "to achieve" or "to do (perform)": *dyspraxia, echopraxia, neuropraxia.*

praxis [Gk, action], **1.** a concept that deals with actions and overt behavior or the performance of an action to the exclusion of metaphysical thought. **2.** the ability to plan and then execute movement.

-praxis, -praxia /prak′sis/, combining form meaning "to achieve, do, act, or treat based on theory": *echopraxia, parapraxis.*

prazepam /praz″əpam/, a benzodiazepine derivative used to treat anxiety.
■ INDICATIONS: It is not available in the United States, but it is prescribed elsewhere for the treatment of anxiety disorders or the short-term relief of symptoms of anxiety and has several unlabeled uses, including alcohol and opiate withdrawal, spasticity, and partial seizures.
■ CONTRAINDICATIONS: Acute narrow-angle glaucoma or known sensitivity to this drug or other benzodiazepines prohibits its use.
■ ADVERSE EFFECTS: Among the more serious, but rare, adverse effects are confusion, tremor, palpitations, and diaphoresis.

-prazole, suffix for antiulcerative benzimidazole derivatives.

prazosin hydrochloride /prä″zəsin/, an antihypertensive, peripherally acting alpha$_1$-adrenergic blocker.
■ INDICATIONS: It is prescribed to treat hypertension and to decrease afterload in congestive heart disease. Unlabeled uses include treatment of benign prostatic hyperplasia and Raynaud phenomenon.
■ CONTRAINDICATIONS: Known hypersensitivity to this or similar drugs (e.g., terazosin, doxazosin) prohibits its use.
■ ADVERSE EFFECTS: The initial dose of the medication can cause a large drop in blood pressure and syncope, especially in patients who are volume depleted or are concurrently using beta blockers. Common ongoing adverse effects include tachycardia, palpations, orthostatic hypotension, fainting, dizziness, headache, drowsiness, urinary urgency, weakness, and nausea. Rarely cataracts have appeared or worsened with the use of prazosin.

PRE, abbreviation for **progressive resistance exercise.**

preadmission certification /prē′ədmish″ən/, a system whereby physicians are required to obtain advance approval for nonemergency hospital admissions for patients covered by Medicare, Medicaid, and managed health care plans, as well as most third-party payers. The system is intended to determine whether the patient can be treated as an outpatient or in another, less expensive manner than hospitalization. Emergency admissions require post hoc approval. Also called **precertification.**

preagonal ascites /prē·ag″ənəl/ [L, *prae,* before; Gk, *agon,* struggle, *askos,* bag], a rapid accumulation of fluid within the peritoneal cavity, representing the transudation of serum from the circulatory system. Preagonal ascites immediately precedes death in some cases. See also **ascites.**

prealbumin test (PAB, TBPA), a blood, 24-hour urine, or cerebrospinal fluid analysis. It is useful as a marker of nutritional status and is a sensitive indicator of protein synthesis and catabolism. This test is done frequently on patients receiving total parenteral nutrition.

preanal /prē·ā″nəl/, located anterior to the anus.

preanesthetic medication. See **premedication.**

preaortic node /prē′ā·ôr″tik/ [L, *prae* + Gk, *aerein,* to raise; L, *nodus,* knot], a node in one of the three sets of lumbar lymph nodes that serve various abdominal viscera supplied by the celiac, superior mesenteric, and inferior mesenteric arteries. The preaortic nodes lie ventral to the aorta and are divided into the celiac nodes, superior mesenteric nodes, and inferior mesenteric nodes. Most of the efferent vessels from the preaortic nodes unite to form the lymphatic intestinal trunk that enters the cisterna chyli. Compare **lateral aortic node, retroaortic node.**

preauricular /prē′ôrik″yələr/, located anterior to the auricle of the ear.

preauthorization, a decision made by a health insurer or plan that services, prescriptions, and/or durable medical equipment are medically necessary.

precancerous /-kan″sərəs/ [L, *prae* + *cancer,* crab], pertaining to a stage of abnormal tissue growth that is likely to develop into a malignant tumor.

precancerous dermatitis. See **intraepidermal carcinoma.**

precautionary labels /prikô″shəner′ē/, information and identification that must be applied to the containers of all hazardous chemicals, including flammables, combustibles, corrosives, carcinogens, and potential carcinogens.

prececocolic fascia, an extension sometimes found in the parietal abdominal fascia, crossing anterior to the cecum, adjacent to the ascending colon.

precedent /pres′ədənt/ [L, *praecedere,* to go before], a previously adjudged decision that serves as an authority in a similar case.

precentral gyrus /-sen″trəl/ [L, *prae* + Gk, *kentron,* center, *gyros,* turn], a convolution of the cerebral hemisphere immediately anterior to the central sulcus of the cerebrum in each hemisphere. It is the location of the motor strip that controls voluntary movements of the contralateral side of the body. Also called **anterior central gyrus.**

preceptorship /-sep″tərship′/ [L, *prae* + *capere,* to take up], **1.** the position of teacher or instructor. **2.** a defined period of time in which two people (a nurse with a student nurse or an experienced nurse with a new graduate) work together so that the less experienced person can learn and apply knowledge and skills in the practice setting with the help of the more experienced person.

precertification, authorization for a specific medical procedure before it is done or for admission to an institution for care. It is required for payment by most U.S. managed care organizations.

precession /-sesh″ən/ [L, *praecedere,* to go before], a comparatively slow gyration of the axis of a spinning body such that the axis traces out a cone, caused by the application of a torque. The magnetic moment of a nucleus with spin experiences such a torque when inclined at an angle to an applied magnetic field, resulting in precession at the Larmor frequency.

precipitant /-sip″ətənt/ [L, *praecipitare,* to cast down], a substance that causes another to settle, separate, or deposit from a solution, such as a reagent that causes certain metals to precipitate.

precipitate /prəsip″itāt, -it/ [L, *praecipitare,* to cast down], **1.** *v.,* to cause a substance to separate or settle out of solution. **2.** *n.,* a substance that has separated from or settled out of a solution. **3.** *adj.,* occurring hastily or unexpectedly.

P

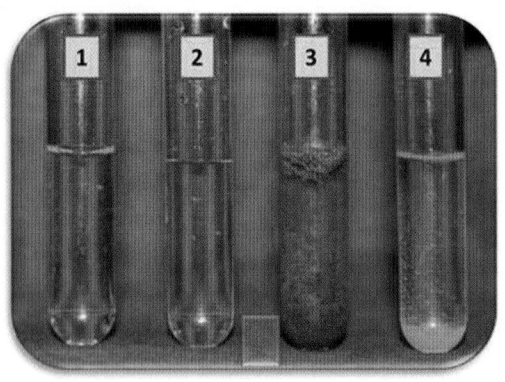

Test tubes with varying amounts of precipitate *(Thaha et al, 2017)*

precipitate delivery /-sip″itit/, childbirth that occurs with such speed or in such a situation that the usual preparations cannot be made. See also **emergency childbirth.**

precipitating factor /-sip′itā′ting/, an element that causes or contributes to the occurrence of a disorder.

precipitation /-sip′itā′shən/ [L, *praecipitare,* to cast down], a process whereby solid particles are made to settle out of a solution so that they can be separated from other dissolved substances.

precipitin /prəsip″itin/ [L, *praecipitare* + Gk, *anti,* against; AS, *bodig,* body; Gk, *genein,* to produce], an antibody that causes the formation of an insoluble complex when combined with a specific soluble antigen. Compare **agglutinin.** See also **agglutination, antiglobulin.**

precision attachment /pri·sish′ən/ [L, *praecidere,* to cut short], (in dentistry) a device using a close-fitting male and female portion to adjoin fixed or removable partial dentures to the crown of an abutment tooth or a restoration. Also called *precision anchorage.* See also **precision rest, intracoronal retainer.**

precision rest /prisish″ən/ [L, *praecidere,* to cut short; AS, *rest*], (in dentistry) a rigid denture support consisting of two tightly fitting parts, the insert of which rests firmly against the gingival part of the device.

preclinical /-klin″ikəl/ [L, *prae* + Gk, *kline,* bed], a stage in a disease when a specific diagnosis cannot be made because adequate signs and symptoms have not yet developed.

precocious /-kō″shəs/ [L, *praecoquere,* to mature early], pertaining to the early, often premature, development of physical or mental qualities.

precocious carrier. See **amebic carrier state.**

precocious dentition, an abnormal acceleration of the eruption of the primary or secondary teeth, usually associated with an endocrine imbalance, such as excess growth hormone or hyperthyroidism. Compare **retarded dentition.**

precocious puberty [L, *praecoquere,* to mature early, *pubertas*], abnormally early development of sexual maturity. It is usually marked by early breast development and ovulation in girls before 8 years of age and the production of mature sperm in boys before 10 years of age.

precognition /-kognish″ən/, the alleged intuitive foreknowledge of events. Compare **premonition.**

preconscious /-kon″shəs/ [L, *prae,* before, *conscire,* to be aware], **1.** *adj.,* before the development of self-consciousness and self-awareness. **2.** *n.,* (in psychiatry) the mental function in which thoughts, ideas, emotions, or memories not in immediate awareness can be brought into the consciousness, usually through associations, without encountering any intrapsychic resistance or repression. **3.** *n.,* the mental phenomena capable of being recalled, although not present in the conscious mind.

precordial. See **precordium.**

precordial lead. See **chest lead.**

precordial movement, any motion of the anterior wall of the thorax localized in the area over the heart. Variations of precordial movements include apical impulse, left ventricular thrust, and right ventricular thrust.

precordial pain [L, *prae,* before, *cor,* heart; *poena,* penalty], pain in the chest wall over the heart.

precordium /-kôr″dē·əm/ [L, *prae,* before, *cor,* heart], the part of the front of the chest wall that overlays the heart and the epigastrium. **–precordial,** *adj.*

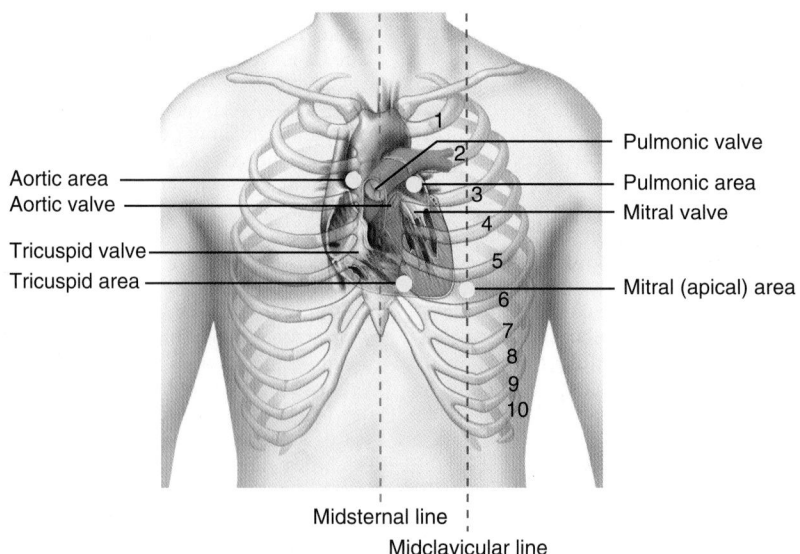

Aortic area
Aortic valve
Tricuspid valve
Tricuspid area
Pulmonic valve
Pulmonic area
Mitral valve
Mitral (apical) area
Midsternal line
Midclavicular line

Precordium *(Harkreader and Hogan, 2007)*

precordial thump, a sharp, quick blow to the sternum for patients with witnessed, monitored, unstable ventricular tachycardia, including pulseless ventricular tachycardia, if a defibrillator is not immediately ready for use. Its use should not delay the initiation of cardiopulmonary resuscitation (CPR). Once taught as part of the CPR procedure, it is no longer recommended for unwitnessed cardiac arrest.

Precose, an antidiabetic agent. Brand name for **acarbose.**

precursor /-kur″sər/ [L, *prae + currere,* to run], **1.** something preceding, or coming before, another. **2.** a prognostic characteristic or feature of a patient's health data, such as a radiographic or laboratory finding, that is associated with a higher or lower risk of death than the average.

precursor therapy, a type of treatment involving the use of nutrients that may influence neurological clinical conditions. An example is the use of choline, a B complex vitamin precursor of acetylcholine, in the treatment of tardive dyskinesia.

pred-, combining form for prednisone or prednisolone derivatives.

predeciduous dentition /-disid″yoo·əs/ [L, *prae + decidere,* to fall off], the epithelial structures in the mouth of the infant before the eruption of the primary teeth. See also **primary dentition, teething.**

prediabetes. See **potential abnormality of glucose tolerance, impaired glucose tolerance.**

prediastole /-dī·as″təlē/ [L, *prae,* before; Gk, *dia + stellein,* to set], the part of the cardiac cycle between late systole and early diastole.

prediastolic murmur /-dī·əstol″ik/ [L, *prae + Gk, dia + stellein,* to set; L, *murmur,* humming], a murmur heard during cardiac systole.

predictive hypothesis /-dik″tiv/ [L, *prae + dicere,* to say; Gk, foundation], (in research) a hypothesis that predicts the nature of a relationship among the variables to be studied. Also called **research hypothesis.** Compare **null hypothesis.**

predictive validity, validity of a test or a measurement tool that is established by demonstrating the ability of a test or measure to predict the results of an analysis of the same data made with another test instrument or measurement tool. See also **validity.**

predictor variable. See **independent variable.**

predisposing cause /-dispō″sing/ [L, *prae + disponere,* to arrange, *causa*], any condition that enhances the specific cause of a disease, such as susceptibility caused by hereditary or lifestyle factors.

predisposing factor [L, *prae + disponere,* to dispose], any conditioning factor that influences both the type and the amount of resources that the individual can elicit to cope with stress. It may be biological, psychological, genetic, or sociocultural.

predisposition /-dis′pəzish″ən/ [L, *prae + disponere,* to dispose], a state of being particularly susceptible.

prednicarbate /pred″n-kahr′bāt/, a synthetic corticosteroid used topically for the relief of inflammation and pruritus in certain dermatoses.

prednisoLONE /prednis″əlōn/, a glucocorticoid.
- INDICATIONS: It is prescribed as treatment for inflammation of the skin, conjunctiva, and cornea and for immunosuppression.
- CONTRAINDICATIONS: Fungal infections or known hypersensitivity to this drug prohibits its systemic use. Viral or fungal infections of the skin, impaired circulation, or known hypersensitivity to this drug prohibits its topical use.
- ADVERSE EFFECTS: Among the more serious adverse effects to the systemic administration of this drug are GI,

endocrine, neurological, fluid, and electrolyte disturbances. Skin reactions may result from topical administration of this drug.

predniSONE /pred″nisōn/, a glucocorticoid.
- INDICATIONS: It is prescribed in the treatment of severe inflammation and for immunosuppression.
- CONTRAINDICATIONS: Viral or fungal infections of the skin, impaired circulation, or known hypersensitivity to this drug prohibits its use.
- ADVERSE EFFECTS: Among the more serious adverse effects to the systemic administration of the drug are GI, endocrine, neurological, fluid, and electrolyte disturbances. Skin reactions may occur from topical administration of this drug.

predonated autologous blood, blood donated before surgery or another invasive procedure for use in a possible autologous transfusion.

preeclampsia /prē′iklamp″sē·ə/ [L, *prae + Gk, ek,* out, *lampein,* to flash], an abnormal condition of pregnancy characterized by the onset of acute hypertension after the 24th week of gestation. The classic triad of preeclampsia is hypertension, proteinuria, and edema. The cause of the disease remains unknown despite 100 years of research by thousands of investigators. It occurs in 5% to 7% of pregnancies, most often in primigravidas, and is more common in some areas of the world than others. The incidence is particularly high in the southeastern part of the United States. The incidence increases with increasing gestational age, and it is more common in cases of multiple gestation, hydatidiform mole, or hydramnios. A typical lesion in the kidneys, glomeruloendotheliosis, is pathognomonic. Termination of the pregnancy results in resolution of the signs and symptoms of the disease and in healing of the renal lesion. Preeclampsia is classified as mild or severe. Mild preeclampsia is diagnosed if one or more of the following signs develop after the 24th week of gestation: systolic blood pressure of 140 mm Hg or more or a rise of 30 mm Hg or more above the woman's usual systolic blood pressure; diastolic blood pressure of 90 mm Hg or more or a rise of 15 mm Hg or more above the woman's usual diastolic blood pressure; proteinuria; and edema. Severe preeclampsia is diagnosed if one or more of the following is present: systolic blood pressure of 160 mm Hg or more or a diastolic blood pressure of 110 mm Hg or more on two occasions 6 hours apart with the woman at bed rest; proteinuria of 5 g or more in 24 hours; oliguria of less than 400 mL in 24 hours; ocular or cerebrovascular disorders; and cyanosis or pulmonary edema. Preeclampsia commonly causes abnormal metabolic function, including negative nitrogen balance, increased central nervous system irritability, hyperactive reflexes, compromised renal function, hemoconcentration, and alterations of fluid and electrolyte balance. Complications include premature separation of the placenta, hypofibrinogenemia, hemolysis, cerebral hemorrhage, ophthalmological damage, pulmonary edema, hepatocellular changes, fetal malnutrition, and lowered birth weight. The most serious complication is eclampsia, which can result in maternal and fetal death. Healthy living conditions, including a diet high in protein, calories, and essential nutritional elements, and rest and exercise are associated with a decreased incidence of preeclampsia. Treatment includes rest, sedation, magnesium sulfate, and antihypertensives. Ultimately, if eclampsia threatens, delivery by induction of labor or cesarean section may be necessary. Formerly called **toxemia of pregnancy.** See also **eclampsia.**

preemie. See **premature infant.**

preexcitation /prē′eksitā″shən/ [L, *prae* + *excitare,* to arouse], activation of part of the ventricular myocardium earlier than would be expected if the activating impulses traveled only down the normal routes and had experienced a normal delay within the atrioventricular (AV) node. Preexcitation may be a result of either an AV accessory pathway (Wolff-Parkinson-White syndrome), which is reflected on the electrocardiogram by a short P-R interval and a broad QRS complex, or an excessively fast intranodal pathway (Lown-Ganong-Levine syndrome), which manifests with a short P-R interval and a normal QRS complex. The degree of preexcitation is determined by the speed at which the impulse traverses the atrial tissue and the accessory pathway or the AV node. See also **accessory pathway.**

preexisting condition /prē′iksis″ting/ [L, *prae* + *existere,* to have reality, *conditio*], any injury, disease, or disability that may have occurred at some time in the past and may predispose an individual to limited health in the future.

preexposure prophylaxis (PrEP), medication taken by individuals at risk for HIV. When taken daily, it is highly effective for preventing HIV from sex or injection drug use.

preferential anosmia /pref′əren″shəl/ [L, *praeferens,* being preferred; Gk, *a* + *osme,* not smell], the inability to smell certain odors. The condition is often caused by psychological factors concerning either a particular smell or the situation in which the smell occurs.

preferred provider organization (PPO) /-furd″/ [L, *praeferre,* to put before], an organization of physicians, hospitals, and pharmacists whose members discount their health care services to subscriber patients. A PPO may be organized by a group of physicians, an outside entrepreneur, an insurance company, or a company with a self-insurance plan. See also **health maintenance organization.**

preformation /-fôrmā″shən/ [L, *prae* + *formatio,* formation], an early theory in embryology in which the organism is contained in minute and complete form within the germ cell and, after fertilization, grows from microscopic to normal size. Compare **epigenesis.**

preformed water /-fôrmd″/ [L, *prae* + *forma,* form; AS, *waeter*], the water that is contained in foods.

prefrontal lobotomy /-frôn″təl/ [L, *prae* + *frons,* forehead; Gk, *lobos,* lobe, *temnein,* to cut], a surgical procedure in which connecting fibers between the prefrontal lobes of the brain and the thalamus are severed. An archaic technique, it is rarely used today but formerly was an accepted procedure for treating schizophrenic patients with uncontrollable, destructive behavior. After surgery patients were often apathetic, docile, and lacking social graces and decision-making abilities of even the simplest kind. If only the white fibers are severed, the procedure is called a prefrontal leukotomy.

preg, abbreviation for **pregnancy.**

pregabalin, an anticonvulsant.
- INDICATIONS: This drug is used to treat neuropathic pain associated with diabetic peripheral neuropathy, partial-onset seizures, and postherpetic neuralgia.
- CONTRAINDICATIONS: Known hypersensitivity to this drug prohibits its use. This drug should not be abruptly discontinued.
- ADVERSE EFFECTS: Adverse effects of this drug include dizziness, fatigue, confusion, euphoria, incoordination, nervousness, neuropathy, tremor, vertigo, somnolence, ataxia, amnesia, abnormal thinking, dry mouth, blurred vision, nystagmus, amblyopia, constipation, flatulence, abdominal pain, weight gain, ecchymosis, back pain, pruritus, impotence, and dyspnea.

preganglionic neuron /-gang′glē·on″·ik/ [L, *prae* + Gk, *gagglion,* knot, *neurom,* nerve], a neuron whose axon terminates in contact with another nerve cell located in a peripheral ganglion.

Pregestimil, a hypoallergenic nutritional supplement for infants.

pregnancy (preg) /preg′nənsē/ [L, *praegnans,* pregnant], the gestational process, comprising the growth and development within a woman of a new individual from conception through the embryonic and fetal periods to birth. Pregnancy lasts approximately 266 days (38 weeks) from the day of fertilization, but it is clinically considered to last 280 days (40 weeks; 10 lunar months; $9\frac{1}{3}$ calendar months) from the first day of the last menstrual period. The expected date of delivery (EDD) is calculated on the latter basis even if a woman's periods are irregular. If a woman is certain that coitus occurred only once during the month of conception and if she knows the date on which coitus occurred, the EDD may be calculated as 266 days from that date. Pregnancy begins after coitus at or near the time of ovulation (usually about 14 days before a woman's next expected menstrual period). Of the millions of ejaculated sperm cells, thousands reach the female ovum in the outer end of the fallopian tube, but usually only one penetrates the egg for union of the male and female pronuclei and conception. The zygote, genetically a unique entity, begins cell division as it is transported to the uterine cavity, where it implants in the uterine wall. Maternal and embryological elements together form the beginnings of the placenta, which grows into the substance of the uterus. The placenta functions in maternal-fetal exchange of nutrients and waste products, although the maternal and fetal bloods do not normally mix. The conceptus is in some aspects like a foreign graft or transplant in the mother. Although an immune response is normally activated in the mother, all of her tissues and organs undergo change, many of them profound and some of them permanent. Cardiac output increases 30% to 50% in pregnancy. The increase begins at about the sixth week, reaches a maximum about the sixteenth week, declines slightly after the thirtieth week, and rapidly falls off after delivery. It returns to prepregnancy level about the sixth week after delivery. The stroke volume of the heart increases, and the pulse rate becomes more rapid: Normal pulse rate in pregnancy is approximately 80 to 90 beats/min. Blood pressure may drop slightly after the twelfth week of gestation and return to its usual level after the twenty-sixth week. The circulation of blood to the pregnant uterus near term is about 1 L/min, requiring about 20% of the total cardiac output. Total blood volume also increases in pregnancy; plasma volume increases more than red cell volume, and this results in a drop in the hematocrit, caused by dilution. The number of white blood cells increases: The normal white blood cell count in pregnancy is often above 15,000/mL.
- PATIENT CARE CONSIDERATIONS: The emotional experiences of pregnancy, as reported by pregnant women, are normal and healthy, but extraordinary. A pregnant woman is "herself," but in a very unfamiliar way. She has a sense of heightened function and expectancy. Being keenly aware of the rapid and inevitable changes her body is undergoing, she is more intensely interested in herself. Her concern for the perfection of her baby, her anticipation of the exertion of labor, and her contemplation of the new or expanded responsibilities of motherhood all serve to intensify her emotional tone.

Pregnancy table for expected date of delivery

Find the date of the last menstrual period in the top line (light-face type) of the pair of lines.
The dark number (bold-face type) in the line below will be the expected day of delivery.

	1	2	3	4	5	6	7	8	9	10	11	12	13	14	15	16	17	18	19	20	21	22	23	24	25	26	27	28	29	30	31	
Jan.	1	2	3	4	5	6	7	8	9	10	11	12	13	14	15	16	17	18	19	20	21	22	23	24	25	26	27	28	29	30	31	
Oct.	**8**	**9**	**10**	**11**	**12**	**13**	**14**	**15**	**16**	**17**	**18**	**19**	**20**	**21**	**22**	**23**	**24**	**25**	**26**	**27**	**28**	**29**	**30**	**31**	**1**	**2**	**3**	**4**	**5**	**6**	**7**	**Nov.**
Feb.	1	2	3	4	5	6	7	8	9	10	11	12	13	14	15	16	17	18	19	20	21	22	23	24	25	26	27	28				
Nov.	**8**	**9**	**10**	**11**	**12**	**13**	**14**	**15**	**16**	**17**	**18**	**19**	**20**	**21**	**22**	**23**	**24**	**25**	**26**	**27**	**28**	**29**	**30**	**1**	**2**	**3**	**4**	**5**				**Dec.**
Mar.	1	2	3	4	5	6	7	8	9	10	11	12	13	14	15	16	17	18	19	20	21	22	23	24	25	26	27	28	29	30	31	
Dec.	**6**	**7**	**8**	**9**	**10**	**11**	**12**	**13**	**14**	**15**	**16**	**17**	**18**	**19**	**20**	**21**	**22**	**23**	**24**	**25**	**26**	**27**	**28**	**29**	**30**	**31**	**1**	**2**	**3**	**4**	**5**	**Jan.**
April	1	2	3	4	5	6	7	8	9	10	11	12	13	14	15	16	17	18	19	20	21	22	23	24	25	26	27	28	29	30		
Jan.	**6**	**7**	**8**	**9**	**10**	**11**	**12**	**13**	**14**	**15**	**16**	**17**	**18**	**19**	**20**	**21**	**22**	**23**	**24**	**25**	**26**	**27**	**28**	**29**	**30**	**31**	**1**	**2**	**3**	**4**		**Feb.**
May	1	2	3	4	5	6	7	8	9	10	11	12	13	14	15	16	17	18	19	20	21	22	23	24	25	26	27	28	29	30	31	
Feb.	**5**	**6**	**7**	**8**	**9**	**10**	**11**	**12**	**13**	**14**	**15**	**16**	**17**	**18**	**19**	**20**	**21**	**22**	**23**	**24**	**25**	**26**	**27**	**28**	**1**	**2**	**3**	**4**	**5**	**6**	**7**	**Mar.**
June	1	2	3	4	5	6	7	8	9	10	11	12	13	14	15	16	17	18	19	20	21	22	23	24	25	26	27	28	29	30		
Mar.	**8**	**9**	**10**	**11**	**12**	**13**	**14**	**15**	**16**	**17**	**18**	**19**	**20**	**21**	**22**	**23**	**24**	**25**	**26**	**27**	**28**	**29**	**30**	**31**	**1**	**2**	**3**	**4**	**5**	**6**		**April**
July	1	2	3	4	5	6	7	8	9	10	11	12	13	14	15	16	17	18	19	20	21	22	23	24	25	26	27	28	29	30	31	
April	**7**	**8**	**9**	**10**	**11**	**12**	**13**	**14**	**15**	**16**	**17**	**18**	**19**	**20**	**21**	**22**	**23**	**24**	**25**	**26**	**27**	**28**	**29**	**30**	**1**	**2**	**3**	**4**	**5**	**6**	**7**	**May**
Aug.	1	2	3	4	5	6	7	8	9	10	11	12	13	14	15	16	17	18	19	20	21	22	23	24	25	26	27	28	29	30	31	
May	**8**	**9**	**10**	**11**	**12**	**13**	**14**	**15**	**16**	**17**	**18**	**19**	**20**	**21**	**22**	**23**	**24**	**25**	**26**	**27**	**28**	**29**	**30**	**31**	**1**	**2**	**3**	**4**	**5**	**6**	**7**	**June**
Sept.	1	2	3	4	5	6	7	8	9	10	11	12	13	14	15	16	17	18	19	20	21	22	23	24	25	26	27	28	29	30		
June	**8**	**9**	**10**	**11**	**12**	**13**	**14**	**15**	**16**	**17**	**18**	**19**	**20**	**21**	**22**	**23**	**24**	**25**	**26**	**27**	**28**	**29**	**30**	**1**	**2**	**3**	**4**	**5**	**6**	**7**		**July**
Oct.	1	2	3	4	5	6	7	8	9	10	11	12	13	14	15	16	17	18	19	20	21	22	23	24	25	26	27	28	29	30	31	
July	**8**	**9**	**10**	**11**	**12**	**13**	**14**	**15**	**16**	**17**	**18**	**19**	**20**	**21**	**22**	**23**	**24**	**25**	**26**	**27**	**28**	**29**	**30**	**31**	**1**	**2**	**3**	**4**	**5**	**6**	**7**	**Aug.**
Nov.	1	2	3	4	5	6	7	8	9	10	11	12	13	14	15	16	17	18	19	20	21	22	23	24	25	26	27	28	29	30		
Aug.	**8**	**9**	**10**	**11**	**12**	**13**	**14**	**15**	**16**	**17**	**18**	**19**	**20**	**21**	**22**	**23**	**24**	**25**	**26**	**27**	**28**	**29**	**30**	**31**	**1**	**2**	**3**	**4**	**5**	**6**		**Sept.**
Dec.	1	2	3	4	5	6	7	8	9	10	11	12	13	14	15	16	17	18	19	20	21	22	23	24	25	26	27	28	29	30	31	
Sept.	**7**	**8**	**9**	**10**	**11**	**12**	**13**	**14**	**15**	**16**	**17**	**18**	**19**	**20**	**21**	**22**	**23**	**24**	**25**	**26**	**27**	**28**	**29**	**30**	**1**	**2**	**3**	**4**	**5**	**6**	**7**	**Oct.**

P

pregnancy epulis. See **gingival hormonal enlargement.**

pregnancy gingivitis, an enlargement or hyperplasia of the gingivae caused by plaque, poor oral hygiene, and hormonal imbalance during pregnancy. It is usually limited to the interdental papillae. See **gingival hormonal enlargement.**

pregnancy-induced hypertension. See **gestational hypertension.**

pregnancy luteoma. See **luteoma.**

pregnancy rate, (in statistics) the ratio of pregnancies per 100 woman-years, calculated as the product of the number of pregnancies in the women observed multiplied by 12 (months), divided by the product of the number of women observed multiplied by the number of months observed. For example, if 50 women used one contraceptive method for 12 months and 5 of them became pregnant, the pregnancy rate would be 10 per 100 woman-years.

pregnanediol /pregnān″dē·ol/, a crystalline, biologically inactive compound in the urine of women during pregnancy or during the secretory phase of the menstrual cycle. A dihydroxy derivative of the saturated steroid pregnane, pregnanediol is the end product of metabolism of progesterone in the urine.

pregnanediol test, an infrequently used 24-hour urine test that evaluates progesterone production by the ovaries and placenta. It is useful in documenting whether ovulation has occurred, and if so, when. The test is used primarily to monitor progesterone supplementation in patients with an inadequate luteal phase.

pregnant /preg″nənt/ [L, praegnans], gravid; with child.

prehensile /-hen″sil/ [L, prehendre, to seize], able to grasp.

prehension /-hen′shən/, the use of the hands and fingers to grasp, pick up objects, or pinch.

prehospital care, any initial medical care given an ill or injured patient by a paramedic or other person before the patient reaches the hospital emergency department.

preimplantation genetic diagnosis (PGD), in assisted reproductive technology, the determination of chromosomal abnormalities in the embryo before it is transferred to the uterus.

preinfarction angina /pre′infärc″shən/ [L, prae + infarcire, to stuff; angina, quinsy], angina pectoris before a myocardial infarction.

preinvasive carcinoma. See **carcinoma in situ.**

prekallikrein /prekal″ikre′in/, a plasma protein that is the proenzyme of plasma kallikrein. It is cleaved to its active enzyme form by activated coagulation factor XII.

preload /prē″lōd/ [L, prae + AS, lad], the stretch of ventricular muscle fibers at end diastole. It is reflected by the ventricular pressure and volume at that part of the cardiac cycle. Cardiac output increases with preload. Also called **preload filling pressure.**

preload filling pressure, the load on the ventricular muscle fibers at the end of diastole or just before contraction. The preload on the heart is estimated by the left ventricular filling pressure. Cardiac performance increases with preload.

premalignant fibroepithelioma /-məlig″nənt/ [L, prae + malignus, bad disposition, fibra, fiber; Gk, epi, above, thele, nipple, oma, tumor], an elevated white- or flesh-colored sessile neoplasm formed of interlacing ribbons of epithelial cells on a hyperplastic mesodermal stroma. The tumor occurs most often on the lower trunk of older people and may be found in association with or develop into superficial basal cell carcinoma.

Premarin, conjugated estrogens for treating low estrogen levels. Brand name for **conjugated estrogen.**

Premarin with Methyltestosterone, a fixed-combination hormonal drug containing Premarin and an androgen. Brand name for **Premarin, methylTESTOSTERone.**

premarket approval (PMA) /-mar″kit/, permission given by the federal government to equipment manufacturers to sell their devices to the medical profession.

premature /-məchoor″/ [L, praematurus, too soon], **1.** not fully developed or mature. **2.** occurring before the appropriate or usual time. –**prematurity,** n.

premature alopecia [L, praematurus, too soon; Gk, alopex, fox mange], acquired baldness in a person who is not old.

premature atrial complex (PAC), an atrial depolarization that occurs earlier than expected. It is indicated electrocardiographically by an early P′ wave followed by a normal QRS complex. PACs may be the result of atrial enlargement or ischemia or may be caused by stress, caffeine, or nicotine. They may occur occasionally or in a regular pattern. Occasional PACs usually have no significance, but frequent PACs may lead to atrial fibrillation or to paroxysmal supraventricular tachycardia. Also called **atrial extrasystole, atrial premature complex,** atrial premature beat.

premature beat [L, praematurus, too soon; AS, beatan], an electrocardiogram deflection or complex that occurs earlier than expected in the ongoing rhythm pattern. Also called **premature complex, premature impulse.**

premature complex, any electrocardiogram deflection representing either the ventricles or atria that occurs early with respect to the dominant rhythm.

premature ejaculation, uncontrollable, untimely ejaculation of semen often caused by anxiety during sexual intercourse. Behavioral techniques can be learned by the man and his partner, or medication may be used to extend the length of time between erection and ejaculation. See also **ejaculation, erection.**

premature impulse. See **premature beat.**

premature infant, any neonate, regardless of birth weight, born before 37 weeks of gestation. Because exact gestational age is often difficult to determine, low birth weight is a significant criterion for identifying the high-risk infant with incomplete organ system development. Predisposing factors associated with prematurity include multiple pregnancy, toxemia, chronic disease, acute infection, sensitization to blood incompatibility, any severe trauma that may interfere with normal fetal development, substance abuse, and teenage pregnancy. In most instances the cause is unknown. The incidence of prematurity is highest among women from low socioeconomic circumstances, for whom poor nutrition and lack of prenatal medical care are often precipitating factors. The premature infant usually appears small and scrawny, with a large head in relation to body size, and weighs less than 2500 g. The skin is thin, smooth, shiny, and translucent, with the underlying vessels clearly visible. The arms and legs are extended, not flexed, as in the full-term infant. There is little subcutaneous fat, sparse hair, few creases on the soles and palms, and poorly developed ear cartilage. In boys the scrotum has few rugae, and the testes may be undescended; in girls the labia gape and the clitoris is prominent. Among the common problems of the premature infant are variations in thermoregulation, chilling, apnea, respiratory distress, sepsis, poor sucking and swallowing reflexes, small stomach capacity, lowered tolerance of the alimentary tract that may lead to necrotizing enterocolitis, immature renal function, hepatic dysfunction often associated with hyperbilirubinemia, incomplete enzyme systems, and susceptibility to various metabolic upsets, such as hypoglycemia, hyperglycemia, and hypocalcemia. The degree of complications and the rate of survival of premature infants are directly related to the state of physiological and anatomical maturity of the various organ systems at the time of birth, the condition of the infant other than prematurity, and the quality of postnatal care. With treatment in a neonatal intensive care unit, survival rates improve yearly. In increasing numbers of very small babies, development is normal, and those who do not have seizures or apneic spells in the first few days are unlikely to suffer neurological or physical sequelae of their prematurity. Of primary concern for the nurse caring for the premature infant are the stabilization of body temperature by maintaining a neutral thermal environment, the maintenance of respiration, the prevention of infection, the provision of adequate nutrition and hydration, and the conservation of energy. Important functions of the health care team are to involve the parents in the care of the infant, to explain therapeutic procedures, and to facilitate attachment between the infant and family. Also called **preemie, preterm infant.** Compare **postmature infant.**

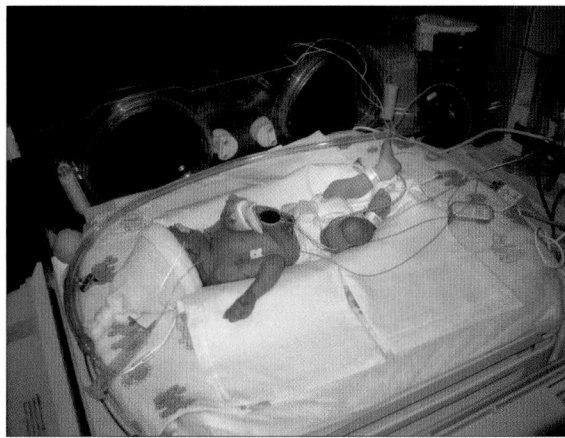

Premature infant *(Courtesy Eric S. Patrick, M.D.)*

premature labor.   See **preterm labor.**

premature newborn, preterm newborn.   See **premature infant.**

premature rupture of membranes, the spontaneous rupture of the amniotic sac before the onset of labor.

premature systole [L, *praematurus* + Gk, *systole,* contraction], a ventricular contraction that occurs too early as a result of a discharge of an ectopic focus in the atria, atrioventricular junction, or ventricle.

premature thelarche.   See **thelarche.**

premature ventricular complex (PVC), a ventricular depolarization that occurs earlier than expected. It appears on the electrocardiogram as an early, wide QRS complex without a preceding related P wave. PVCs may be idiopathic or caused by stress, electrolyte imbalance, ischemia, hypoxemia, hypercapnia, ventricular enlargement, or a toxic reaction to drugs. They may occur occasionally, in a regular pattern, or as several in sequence. Occasional PVCs are not clinically significant in healthy individuals, but they may produce decreased cardiac output in people with heart disease. Frequent PVCs may be a precursor to ventricular tachycardia or fibrillation.

prematurity /-məchoo̅′ritē/ [L, *praematurus,* too soon], pertaining to an event that occurs before the usual or expected time, such as a premature birth.

premedication /-med′ikā″shən/ [L, *prae* + *medicare,* to heal], **1.** any sedative, tranquilizer, hypnotic, antinausea, or anticholinergic medication administered before anesthesia to relieve anxiety, prevent nausea, reduce oral secretions, and decrease pain. The choice of drug depends on such variables as the patient's age and physical condition and the specific operative procedure. **2.** the administration of such medications. *–premedicate, v.*

premenarchal /-mənär″kəl/ [L, *prae,* before; Gk, *men,* month, *archaios,* from the beginning], before the start of the first menstrual period.

premenopausal /-men″ə·pô″səl/ [L, *prae* + Gk, *men,* month, *pauein,* to cease], before the start of menopause.

premenstrual /-men″stroo̅·əl/ [L, *prae,* before, *menstrualis,* monthly], before the start of menstruation each month.

premenstrual dysphoric disorder (PMDD), a mental health condition in women that begins 1 or 2 weeks before menstrual flow. Symptoms include depression, tension, mood swings, irritability, decreased interest, difficulty in concentrating, fatigue, changes in appetite or sleep, physical symptoms, and a sense of being overwhelmed. The condition affects 3% of menstruating women, usually between 25 and 30 years of age. Compare **premenstrual syndrome.**

premenstrual syndrome (PMS, pms) [L, *prae* + *menstrualis,* monthly, *tendere,* to stretch], a syndrome of nervous tension, irritability, weight gain, edema, headache, mastalgia, dysphoria, sleep changes, and lack of coordination occurring during the last few days of the menstrual cycle before the onset of menstruation. Several theories attempt to explain the cause of the syndrome, including nutritional deficiency, stress, hormonal imbalance, and various emotional disorders.

premise /prem″is/ [L, *prae* + *mittere,* to send], a proposition that is presented as the basis of an argument and is usually established beforehand.

premolar /prēmō″lər/ [L, *prae* + *mola,* mill], one of eight teeth, four in each dental arch, located lateral and posterior to the canine teeth and anterior to the molars. They are smaller and shorter than the canine teeth. The crown of each premolar is compressed anteroposteriorly and surmounted by two cusps, and the neck is oval. The root is single and compressed in all premolars except the upper first, which usually has two roots. Usually an anterior and a posterior groove are also present. The upper premolars are larger than the lower premolars. Also called **bicuspid.** Compare **canine tooth, incisor, molar.**

premonition /-mənish″ən/, a sense of an impending event without prior knowledge of it.

premonitory /-mon″iter′ē/ [L, *prae* + *monere,* to warn], an early symptom or sign of a disease. The term is commonly used to describe minor symptoms that precede a major health problem.

premorbid personality /-môr″bid/, a personality characterized by early signs or symptoms of a mental disorder. The specific defects may indicate whether the condition will progress to schizophrenia, a bipolar disorder, or another type of condition.

prenatal /-nā″təl/ [L, *prae* + *natus,* birth], occurring or existing before birth, referring to both the care of the woman during pregnancy and the growth and development of the fetus. Also called **antenatal.** See also **antepartal care.**

prenatal care.   See **antepartal care.**

prenatal cocaine exposure, exposure to cocaine in utero, which can cause birth defects and long-range health problems. Contributing causes may include poor sperm quality of a male cocaine user, poor nutritional habits and/or alcohol or tobacco abuse by the mother during pregnancy, or the direct effect of the drug itself, which can cross the placental barrier. See also **neonatal abstinence syndrome.**

prenatal development, the entire process of growth, maturation, differentiation, and development that occurs between conception and birth. On approximately the 14th day before the next expected menstrual period ovulation usually occurs. If the egg is fertilized, it immediately begins the course to fetal maturity and birth. During the first 14 days the fertilized ovum undergoes cell division several times, becoming a morula and then a blastocyst that is able to implant in the

P

uterine wall. From the beginning of the third to the end of the seventh week of embryonic development, implantation deepens and completes. Primitive uteroplacental circulation originates between the enlarging trophoblast and the maternal endometrial tissue of the uterus. The amniotic cavity appears as an opening between the inner cell mass and the invading trophoblast. A thin lining in the cavity becomes the amnion. At this point the embryo is a two-layered embryonic disk composed of an ectoderm and an endoderm. As the disk thickens in the middle, giving rise to the third cell layer, or mesoderm, the basic structural systems of the body begin to form. The neural tube develops as a precursor of the central nervous system in the midline of the cranial part of the ectoderm. Primitive blood vessels and blood cells, a heart tube, and umbilical vessels are formed and begin to function. Arm and leg buds may appear, and rudimentary gut, lungs, and kidneys form. By the fifth week the brain has begun to grow rapidly, the heart tube is divided into chambers, the palate and the upper lip are forming, and the urogenital system is developing. By the end of the seventh week all essential systems are present. The period from the eighth week to birth is called the fetal stage. From the 8th to the 10th week the fetus continues to grow and development is rapid. The head is almost half of its total length, and arms, legs, and face are clearly recognizable. The fetus floats in the amniotic fluid of the amniotic sac within the uterus; the umbilical vessels in the cord extend to a rapidly growing placenta. By the twelfth week the facial features are formed and the eyelids are present but not yet closed because they have not divided into upper and lower eyelids. The palate is fusing, a neck connects the large head and the body, and tooth buds and nailbeds have begun to form. Identification of the external genitalia is possible for the first time. From the 13th to the 16th week the arms, legs, and trunk grow rapidly, and the fetus is active. Scalp hair develops. The skeleton of the fetus is calcified and may be seen on an x-ray film. A sonogram sometimes detects respiratory movements. Between the 17th and the 20th week of pregnancy the mother usually first feels the baby move. The fetus looks like a very small baby at this time. There are eyebrows and tiny nipples; during fetoscopic examination the fetus has been seen and photographed sucking its thumb and grasping its own umbilical cord. At the 24th week the external ears are smooth and soft and the skin is wrinkled and translucent. The body is covered with lanugo and vernix and weighs a little more than 1 pound. At 28 weeks subcutaneous fat begins to develop, fingernails and toenails are present, the eyelids are separate, the eyes may open, scalp hair is well developed, and in males the testes are at the internal inguinal ring or below. In a modern neonatal intensive care unit most of the babies born at 28 weeks survive. By the 32nd week the fetus weighs between 3 and 4 pounds. The hair is fine and woolly, the fingernails and toenails have grown to the tips of the fingers and toes, and there are one or two creases on the anterior part of the soles of the feet. The areolae of the breasts are visible but flat. In females the clitoris is prominent and the labia majora are small and separated. At 36 weeks the body and the limbs are fuller and more rounded, creases involve the anterior two thirds of the soles, and the skin is thicker and less translucent. As the fetus reaches term, between 38 and 42 weeks, the vernix decreases, and the ear cartilage is developed. In males the testes are in the scrotum. In females the labia majora meet in the midline and cover the labia minora and the clitoris. At 40 weeks the average fetus weighs 7 ¼ pounds and is between 19 and 22 inches long. Prenatal development may be adversely affected by several factors. Between 2 and 14 weeks of gestation, ionizing radiation and some drugs may have profound effects on morphological and functional development. During the first 10 days of development, any damage usually kills the conceptus. Various viruses, malnutrition, trauma, or maternal disease may also affect the morphological development of a rapidly differentiating structure or organ during the embryological or early fetal stage. After 14 weeks, when all of the organs, systems, and body parts have formed, any adverse effects are largely functional; major morphological damage does not occur.

prenatal diagnosis   any of various diagnostic techniques to determine whether a developing fetus is affected with a genetic disorder or other abnormality. Such procedures as radiographic examination and ultrasound scanning can be used to follow fetal growth and detect structural abnormalities; amniocentesis enables fetal cells to be obtained from the amniotic fluid for culture and biochemical assay for detection of metabolic disorders and chromosomal analysis; fetoscopy enables fetal blood to be withdrawn from a blood vessel of the placenta and examined for disorders such as thalassemia, sickle cell anemia, and Duchenne muscular dystrophy. If any of the test results are positive and the child is likely to be born with a severe defect or disease, the parents need support and advice from genetic counselors on whether to terminate the pregnancy. If the parents decide to have the baby, the members of the health care team can help educate them about the specific disorder and prepare them for the special care required of a child with a disabilty or genetic abnormality. Also called **antenatal diagnosis.** See also **chorionic villus sampling, genetic counseling, genetic screening.**

prenatal surgery,   any surgical procedure that is performed on a fetus. The technique has been used to correct hydrocephalus, urinary tract obstructions, and many other conditions.

preoccupation /prē·ok′yəpā″shən/,   a state of being self-absorbed or engrossed in one's own thoughts to a degree that hinders effective contact with or relationship to external reality.

pre-op /prē·op″/,   abbreviation for **preoperative.**

preoperational thought phase /prē·op′ərā″shənəl/   [L, *prae* + *operari,* to work; AS, *thot* + Gk, *phainein,* to show],   a Piagetian phase of child development, during the period of 2 to 7 years of age, when the child focuses on the use of language as a tool to meet his or her needs.

preoperative (pre-op) /prē·op″ər·ativ′/   [L, *prae* + *operari,* to work],   pertaining to the period before a surgical procedure. Commonly the preoperative period begins with the first preparation of the patient for surgery, such as when the surgery is scheduled. Within 1 week, the preoperative patient has relevant studies, labs, x-ray, and a history and physical examination. It ends with the induction of anesthesia in the operating suite.

preoperative care,   the preparation and management of a patient before surgery. The patient's nothing-by-mouth (NPO) status, nutritional state, medical and surgical history, allergies, current medication, physical handicaps, signs of infection, and elimination habits are recorded. The patient's understanding of the operative, preoperative, and postoperative procedures; the patient's ability to verbalize anxieties; and the family's knowledge of the planned surgery are ascertained and education provided. The accuracy of patient's signed informed consent is verified, requests in the physician's preoperative orders are fulfilled, and the patient's identification bands and blood type are checked. Vital signs are recorded, and any abnormalities of the electrocardiogram, chest x-ray, or laboratory tests are reported to the surgeon and anesthesiologist. If needed, the number of matched blood units required to be held for a possible blood transfusion is determined. When ordered, an enema is given, a bowel preparation is completed, a nasogastric tube or indwelling catheter is inserted, and parenteral fluids are administered. If preoperative sedation is administered, the side rails of the bed are raised. Before transfer to the operating

Timetable of Human Prenatal Development
1 to 6 Weeks

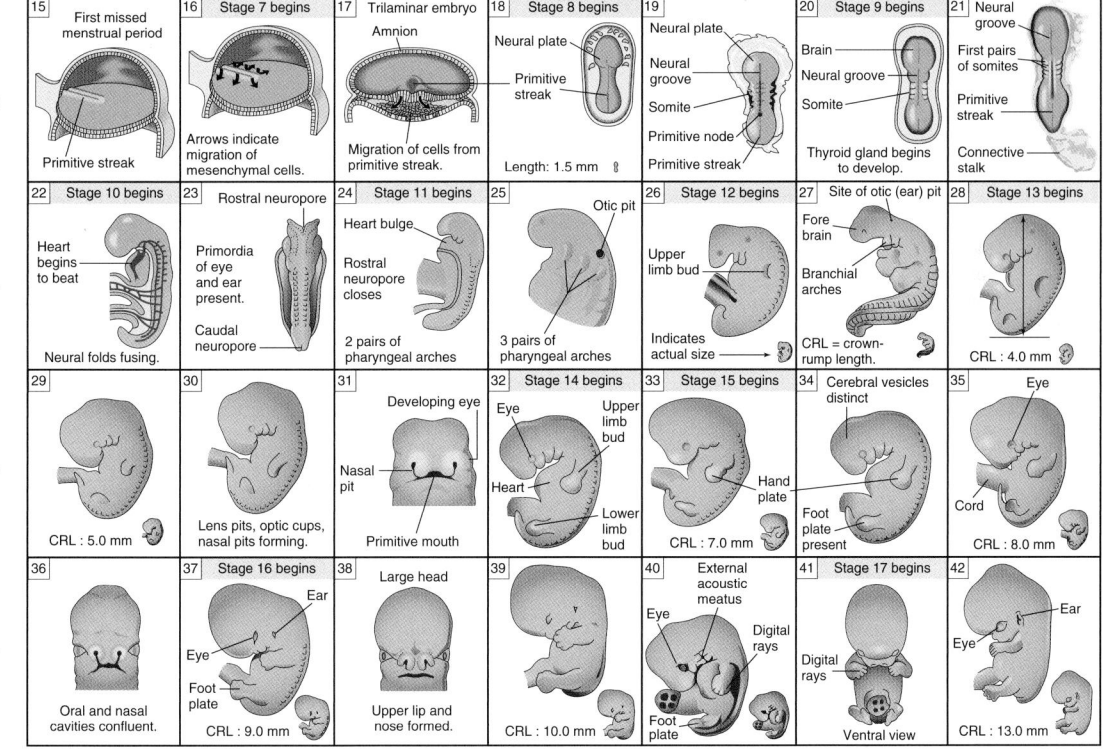

Timetable of prenatal development *(Moore and Persaud, 2008)*

Continued

Timetable of Human Prenatal Development
7 to 10 Weeks

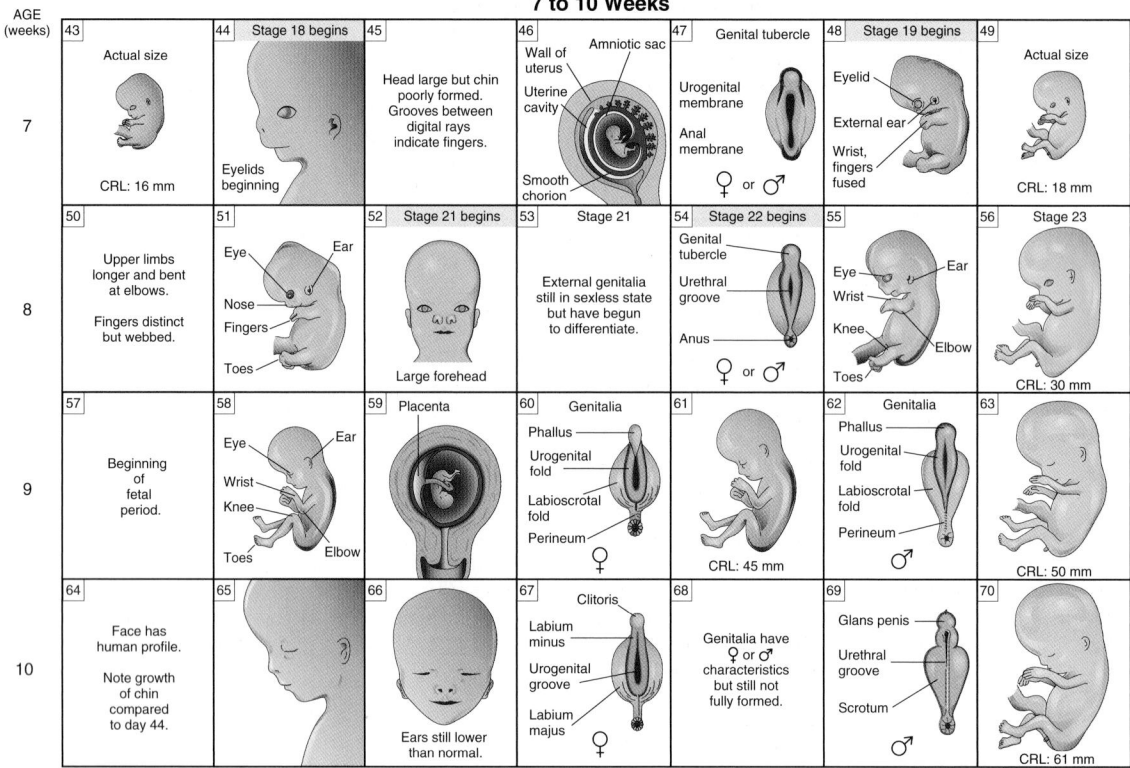

AGE (weeks)

7

43 — Actual size — CRL: 16 mm

44 — Stage 18 begins — Eyelids beginning

45 — Head large but chin poorly formed. Grooves between digital rays indicate fingers.

46 — Wall of uterus, Amniotic sac, Uterine cavity, Smooth chorion

47 — Genital tubercle, Urogenital membrane, Anal membrane — ♀ or ♂

48 — Stage 19 begins — Eyelid, External ear, Wrist, fingers fused

49 — Actual size — CRL: 18 mm

8

50 — Upper limbs longer and bent at elbows. Fingers distinct but webbed.

51 — Eye, Ear, Nose, Fingers, Toes

52 — Stage 21 begins

53 — Stage 21 — External genitalia still in sexless state but have begun to differentiate. Large forehead

54 — Stage 22 begins — Genital tubercle, Urethral groove, Anus — ♀ or ♂

55 — Eye, Ear, Wrist, Knee, Elbow, Toes

56 — Stage 23 — CRL: 30 mm

9

57 — Beginning of fetal period.

58 — Eye, Ear, Wrist, Knee, Toes, Elbow

59 — Placenta

60 — Genitalia — Phallus, Urogenital fold, Labioscrotal fold, Perineum — ♀

61 — CRL: 45 mm

62 — Genitalia — Phallus, Urogenital fold, Labioscrotal fold, Perineum — ♂

63 — CRL: 50 mm

10

64 — Face has human profile. Note growth of chin compared to day 44.

65

66 — Ears still lower than normal.

67 — Clitoris, Labium minus, Urogenital groove, Labium majus — ♀

68 — Genitalia have ♀ or ♂ characteristics but still not fully formed.

69 — Glans penis, Urethral groove, Scrotum — ♂

70 — CRL: 61 mm

Eleventh Week to Full Term

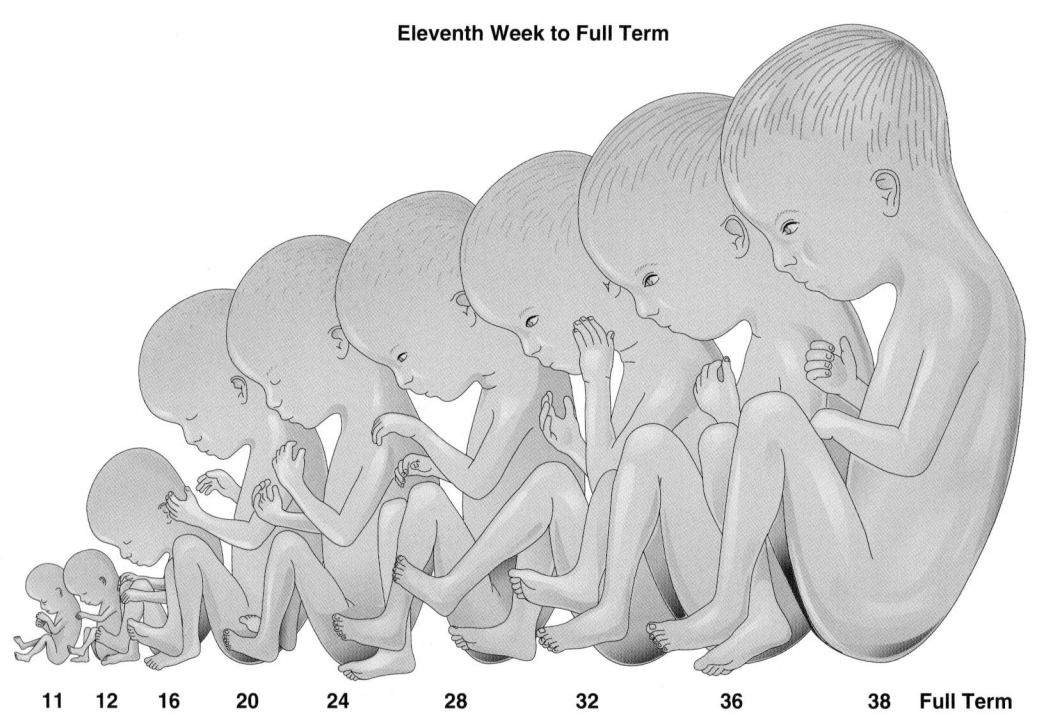

11 12 16 20 24 28 32 36 38 Full Term

Timetable of prenatal development—cont'd *(Moore, Persaud, and Torchia, 2016)*

room with the completed chart, the patient voids, and any dentures, contact lenses, jewelry, and valuables are removed for safekeeping.

■ INTERVENTIONS: The nurse performs and explains the preoperative procedures; reinforces the physician's explanation of the operation; provides instruction and emotional support; answers the patient's questions as honestly as possible, avoiding standard cliches in responding to any anxiety; and reassures the patient that medication will be available to relieve postoperative pain. Depending on the surgical procedure, the nurse shows the patient how to turn, cough, deep breathe, and support the incision during coughing. Instructions on leg exercises are also given. The nurse informs the patient and the patient's family about the postoperative period in the postanesthesia care unit or the intensive care unit, if indicated.

■ OUTCOME CRITERIA: The patient who is carefully prepared for an operation, psychologically and physically, experiences less anxiety and is more likely to make an uneventful recovery.

prep,   **1.** abbreviation for *prepare.* **2.** a term often used in relation to surgery. Abbreviation for *preparation.*

PrEP,   abbreviation for **preexposure prophylaxis.**

preparatory prosthesis /prep″ərətôr′ē/,   a temporary artificial limb that is fitted to the residual limb soon after amputation. It permits ambulation and biomechanical adaptation during the first several weeks after surgery. A rigid removable dressing is usually applied, which allows for inspection of the residual limb for signs of hemorrhage or tissue deterioration before a permanent or definitive prosthesis is fitted. Also called **temporary prosthesis.**

prepared childbirth.   See **natural childbirth.**

preparedness /prepār′ed-nes/,   the state of being ready beforehand for a given event.

prepared tooth cavity /priperd″/   [L, *praeparare,* to make ready, *cavum,* cavity],   a tooth space that has been carved or shaped with a compressed-air or electric dental handpiece and other hand instruments to receive and retain a restoration. Also called **cavity prep.**

prepartal /prepahr′tal/.   See **antepartal.**

prepartum /-pär″təm/,   before childbirth.

prepatellar /-pətel″ər/   [L, *prae,* before, *patella,* small dish],   pertaining to the area in front of the patella.

prepatellar bursa [L, *prae + patella,* small dish; Gk, *byrsa,* wineskin],   a bursa between the tendon of the quadriceps muscle group and the lower part of the femur continuous with the cavity of the knee joint.

prepatellar bursitis [L, *prae,* before, *patella* + Gk, *byrsa,* wineskin, *itis,* inflammation],   an inflammation of the bursa in front of the patella and beneath the skin over the site.

prepayment /-pā″mənt/   [L, *prae + pacere,* to pacify],   the payment in advance for health care services by subscribers to a third-party insurance program.

preperitoneal hernia,   an interstitial hernia located between the parietal peritoneum and the transversalis fascia.

pre-, prae-,   prefix meaning "before" or "in front of": *precursor, preload, praecox.*

preprandial /-pran″dē·əl/   [L, *prae + prandium,* meal],   before a meal.

preprocessing /prēpros″əsing/,   (in ultrasonics) conditioning and manipulation of echo signals before their storage in the scan memory.

prepubertal, prepubertal.   See **prepuberty.**

prepubertal panhypopituitarism /-pyoo″bərtəl/   [L, *prae, + pubertas,* maturity; Gk, *pan,* all, *hypo,* under, *pituita,* phlegm],   insufficiency of pituitary hormones, caused by damage to the gland usually associated with a suprasellar cyst or craniopharyngioma occurring in childhood. The disorder is characterized by extremely small stature with normal body proportions; subnormal sexual development; impaired thyroid and adrenal function; and yellow, wrinkled

skin. Diabetes insipidus is frequently present, and there may be bitemporal hemianopia or complete blindness, but the patient's mentality is usually normal. Radiographic pictures show delayed fusion of the epiphyses and suprasellar calcification, and the sella turcica is often destroyed. The condition is treated with cortisone, thyroid and gonadotrophic hormones, and human growth hormone.

prepuberty /-pyoo″bərtē/   [L, *prae + pubertas,* maturity],   the period immediately before puberty, lasting approximately 2 years. It is characterized by preliminary physical changes, such as accelerated growth and appearance of secondary sex characteristics, that lead to sexual maturity.

prepubescence /prē′pyoobes″əns/,   the state of being prepubertal. —**prepubescent,** *adj.*

prepuce /prē′pyoos/   [L, *praeputium,* foreskin],   a fold of skin that forms a retractable cover, such as the foreskin of the penis or the fold around the clitoris. —**preputial,** *prepucial, adj.*

preputial /prē-pyoo′shəl/,   pertaining to the prepuce.

prerenal /-rē″nəl/   [L, *prae,* before, *ren,* kidney],   **1.** pertaining to the area in front of the kidney. **2.** pertaining to events occurring before reaching the kidney.

prerenal anuria [L, *prae + renes,* kidneys; Gk, *a + ouron,* not urine],   cessation of urine production that results when the blood pressure in the kidney is too low to maintain glomerular filtration pressure.

prerenal uremia [L, *prae,* before, *ren,* kidney; Gk, *ouron,* urine, *haima,* blood],   a condition of kidney failure in which the primary cause may be outside the kidney, as in congestive heart failure or some severe cases of alkalosis.

presacral fascia,   a layer of parietal pelvic fascia between the sacrum and the rectum in which the superior and inferior hypogastric plexuses are embedded.

presacral space,   a subdivision of the extraperitoneal space found between the urinary bladder and the sacrum.

presby-,   prefix meaning "aging" or "being elderly": *presbycusis, presbyopia, presbycardia.*

presbycardia /prez′bēkär″dē·ə/   [Gk, *presbys,* old man, *kardia,* heart],   an abnormal cardiac condition that especially affects elderly individuals and may be associated with heart failure in the presence of other complications, such as heart disease, fever, anemia, mild hyperthyroidism, and excess fluid administration. Presbycardia may be associated with decreased myocardial elasticity and mild fibrotic changes of the heart valves, but the basis for these changes and the associated pigmentation of the heart is not known.

presbycusis /-koo″sis/   [Gk, *presbys + akousis,* hearing],   hearing loss associated with aging. It usually involves both a loss of hearing sensitivity and a reduction in the clarity of speech.

presbyopia /prez′bē·ō″pē·ə/   [Gk, *presbys + ops,* eye],   a refractive condition in which the accommodative ability of the eye cannot meet the accommodative demand for near work. It results from a loss of elasticity of the lens of the eye. The condition commonly develops with advancing age, with the first symptoms appearing about age 40. Compare **visual accommodation.** —**presbyopic,** *adj.*

presbyopic /prez′bē·op″ik/   [Gk, *presbys,* old man, *ops,* eye],   pertaining to a decrease in accommodation of the lens as one grows older and resulting in a shift toward hyperopia or farsightedness.

preschizophrenic state /prēskit′səfren″ik, prē′-/   [L, *prae* + Gk, *schizein,* to split, *phren,* mind],   a period before psychosis is evident when the patient deviates from normal behavior but does not demonstrate psychotic symptoms of delusions, hallucinations, or stupor.

prescreen /-skrēn/   [L, *prae* + ME, *screen*],   **1.** *v.,* to evaluate a person or a group of people to identify those who are at greater risk of development of a specific condition in order to select those who are in particular need of special diagnostic procedures or health care. **2.** *(Informal) n.,* a rapid, superficial examination of a person who does not appear to be acutely ill. It may include taking a medical history.

prescribe /priskrīb″/ [L, *prae* + *scribere,* to write], **1.** to write an order for a drug, treatment, or procedure. **2.** to recommend or encourage a course of action.

prescription /priskrip″shən/, an order for medication, therapy, or therapeutic device given by a properly authorized person, which ultimately goes to a person properly authorized to dispense or perform the order. A prescription is usually in written form; can be e-mailed from a secure encrypted computer system, written, phoned, or faxed; and includes the patient's name and address, the date, the R symbol (superscription), the medication prescribed (inscription), directions to the pharmacist or other dispenser (subscription), the acceptability of dispensing a generic, directions to the patient that must appear on the label, prescriber's signature, and in some instances, an identifying number.

prescription drug [L, *prae* + *scribere* + Fr, *drogue*], a drug that can be dispensed to the public only with an order given by a properly authorized person. The designation of a medication as a prescription drug is made by the U.S. Food and Drug Administration.

prescriptive intervention mode /priskrip″tiv/ [L, *praescriptus,* prescribed, *intervenire,* to come between, *modus,* measure], a therapeutic situation in which the health professional tells the patient explicitly how to solve a problem so that less collaboration between the consultant and patient is needed.

prescriptive theory, a theory that comprises a description of a specific activity, a statement of the goal of the activity, and an analysis of the elements of the activity, which together constitute a prescription for reaching the goal.

presence /prez′əns/, a mode of being available in a situation with the wholeness of one's individual being; a gift of self that can be given freely, invoked, or evoked.

presenile /-sē″nīl/ [L, *prae,* before, *senex,* aged], pertaining to a condition in which a person manifests signs of aging in early or middle life.

presenile dementia, dementia occurring in younger persons, usually in persons age 65 or younger. Because most cases are the result of Alzheimer disease, the term is sometimes used to denote the early-onset form of dementia of the Alzheimer type; it has also been used more generally to denote Alzheimer disease.

presentation. See **fetal presentation.**

presentation of the cord. See **funic presentation.**

present health [L, *praesentare,* to show; AS, *haelth*], (in a health history) a succinct chronological account of any recent changes in the health of the patient and of the circumstances or symptoms that prompted the person to seek health care.

presenting part /prəsən″ting/ [L, *praesentare* + *pars,* part], the part of the fetus that lies closest to the internal os of the cervix.

presenting symptom. See **symptom.**

preservative /prisur″vətiv/ [L, *praeservare,* to keep], a chemical or other agent that reduces the rate of decomposition of a substance.

presomite embryo /prēsō″mīt/ [L, *prae* + Gk, *soma,* body, *en,* in, *bryein,* to grow], an embryo in any stage of development before the appearance of the first pair of somites (segments), which in humans usually occurs around 19 to 21 days after fertilization of the ovum. See also **somite.**

-pressin, suffix for vasoconstrictors, particularly vasopressin derivatives.

pressor /pres″ər/ [L, *premere,* to press], describing a substance that tends to cause a rise in blood pressure.

pressoreceptor. See **baroreceptor.**

pressure (P) /presh′ər/ [L, *premere,* to press], a force, or stress, applied to a surface by a fluid or an object, usually measured in units of force per unit of area, such as pounds per square inch. Other units are mm Hg, bar, atm.

pressure acupuncture, a system of acupuncture involving the application of pressure, such as by the tip of a finger, to certain specified points of the body. See also **acupuncture.**

pressure area, (in dentistry) an oral area that is subject to excessive displacement of soft tissue by a prosthesis.

pressure control ventilation, positive pressure ventilation in which breaths are augmented by air at a rate and fixed amount of pressure, with tidal volume not being fixed. It is used particularly for patients with acute respiratory distress syndrome.

pressure cycling, the delivery of gas under positive pressure during inspiration until an adjustable, preselected pressure has been reached.

pressure diuresis, increased urinary excretion of water when there is an increase of arterial pressure, a compensatory mechanism to maintain blood pressure within the normal range.

pressure dressing, **1.** a bandage or cloth material firmly applied to exert pressure to stop bleeding. **2.** a constricting bandage to prevent edema or provide support for varicose veins. It also is commonly used in the treatment of burns and after skin grafting.

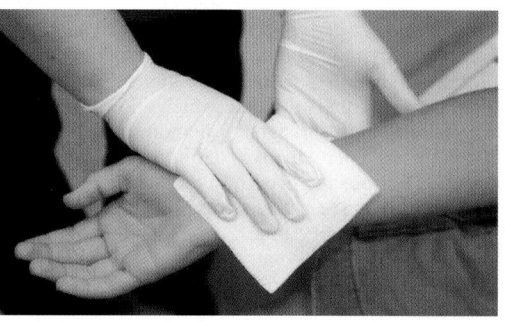

Pressure dressing *(Courtesy Rutgers School of Nursing—Camden. All rights reserved.)*

pressure edema, **1.** edema of the lower extremities caused by pressure of a pregnant uterus against the large veins of the area. **2.** edema of the fetal scalp after cephalic presentation.

pressure natriuresis, increased urinary excretion of sodium along with water when there is an increase of arterial pressure, a compensatory mechanism to maintain blood pressure within the normal range.

pressure necrosis. See **pressure ulcer.**

pressure point, **1.** a point over an artery where the pulse may be felt. Pressure on the point may be helpful in stopping the flow of blood from a wound distal to it. **2.** a site that is extremely sensitive to pressure, such as the phrenic pressure point along the phrenic nerve between the sternocleidomastoid and the scalenus anticus on the right side. Pressure at this site may be symptomatic of gallbladder dysfunction.

pressure-sensitive adhesive (PSA), a transdermal drug-delivery device that uses polymers that are permanently tacky at room temperature and adhere to the skin when slight pressure is applied.

pressure sore. See **pressure ulcer.**

pressure support ventilation (PSV), the augmentation of spontaneous breathing effort with a specific amount of positive airway pressure. The patient initiates the inspiratory flow and sets his or her own respiration rate and tidal volume. PSV can be used to decrease the work of breathing in a patient being weaned from mechanical ventilation.

pressure transducer, an electronic device that converts pressure (such as blood pressure) into electrical signals that can be recorded graphically and monitored.

pressure trigger, a trigger for initiating assisted ventilation, consisting of a mechanism for measuring pressure and starting assisted ventilation when pressure reaches a given level.

pressure ulcer, an inflammation, sore, or ulcer in the skin over a bony prominence, most frequently the sacrum, elbows, heels, outer ankles, inner knees, hips, shoulder blades, and occipital bone of high-risk patients, especially those who are obese, elderly, or suffering from chronic diseases, infections, injuries, or a poor nutritional state. It results from ischemic hypoxia of the tissues caused by prolonged pressure on them. Pressure ulcers are most often seen in aged, debilitated, immobilized, or cachectic patients. The sores are graded by stages of severity. Prevention of pressure ulcers is a cardinal aspect of nursing care. Treatment specific to the location and the extent of the condition is planned. Also called **bedsore, decubitus ulcer, pressure necrosis, pressure sore.**

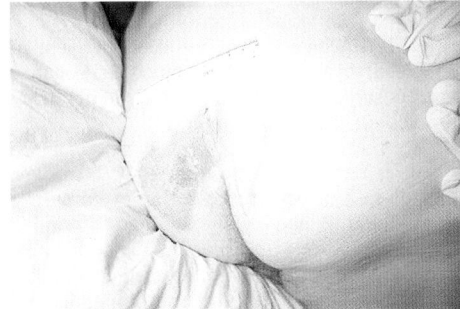

Stage I pressure ulcer *(Courtesy Laurel Wiersma, RN, MSN, CNS, Barnes-Jewish Hospital)*

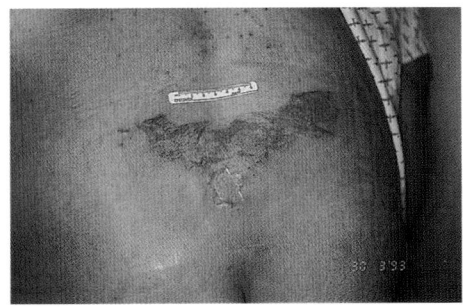

Stage II pressure ulcer *(Courtesy Laurel Wiersma, RN, MSN, CNS, Barnes-Jewish Hospital)*

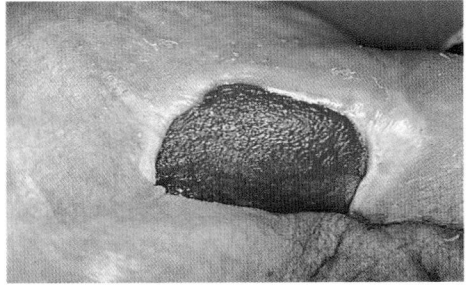

Stage III pressure ulcer *(Courtesy Laurel Wiersma, RN, MSN, CNS, Barnes-Jewish Hospital)*

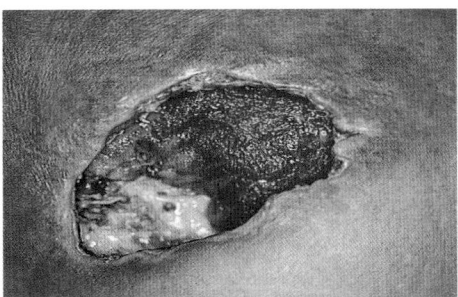

Stage IV pressure ulcer *(Courtesy Laurel Wiersma, RN, MSN, CNS, Barnes-Jewish Hospital)*

pressure injury care, the management and prevention of pressure injury. Also called *decubitus ulcer care, pressure ulcer care.*

■ METHOD: The prevention of pressure injuries, or pressure ulcers, begins with an understanding of proper body positioning, the importance of turning and repositioning, and the need for suitable support surfaces for sleeping and sitting. Support surfaces include overlays, mattress replacements, specialty beds, and special chair cushions. "Donut" rings should not be used to relieve pressure because they reduce blood supply. Bedfast patients should be repositioned at least every 2 hours, and chairfast patients should be repositioned every 15 minutes. Bed linen should be kept dry and wrinkle free. To avoid shear, a sheet or mechanical lift is used to move a patient. Skin should be inspected at least once daily for redness or discoloration, and each time the patient is repositioned the bony areas should be inspected. Dark skin will not show redness; close observation is needed to detect changes in color. A prophylactic measure is daily skin care, in which all areas are washed, rinsed, and dried thoroughly, and lotion is gently applied to bony prominences. The perineal and perianal areas are washed with mild soap and warm water after defecation and urination. A high-protein diet with vitamin and mineral supplements is usually required. One method of classifying pressure injuries/ulcers is staging. If necrotic material exists in the pressure injury, staging is not possible until it has been removed. Necrotic material can be eschar or slough. Topical wound management involves debridement, wound cleansing, the application of dressings, and possibly adjunct therapy (electrical stimulation, hyperbaric oxygen, ultrasound). Clinical Practice Guidelines for Treatment of Pressure Injury may be obtained from the U.S. Department of Health and Human Services, Agency for Health Care Policy and Research. Normal saline is recommended for cleaning most pressure injuries/ulcers. An ideal dressing for a pressure injury/ulcer should protect the wound and provide ideal hydration. The pressure injury/ulcer wound bed should be moist. Devices such as heat lamps and hair dryers should not be used. Dead space within a wound should be eliminated by loosely filling all cavities with dressing materials.

■ INTERVENTIONS: All members of the health care team play a major role in the prevention of pressure injuries/ulcers and in their treatment if they occur. Turning the patient at frequent intervals, applying prescribed medications and dressings to the lesions, practicing meticulous daily skin care, and encouraging good nutrition are all important. Active or passive exercises and, when indicated, debridement of advanced injuries/ulcers are all measures that play a role in prevention and healing.

■ OUTCOME CRITERIA: Pressure injuries/ulcers are often resistant to treatment, and large areas of ulceration can be life-threatening and costly, especially in a debilitated patient.

Prompt and continued care of early lesions can prevent invasion of underlying tissue and promote healing. The health care team should elicit the cooperation and participation of the patient in a plan that includes all preventive measures. The importance of frequent change of position, pressure, friction, moisture, shear, and good nutrition is emphasized.

pressure ventilator, a mechanical ventilator in which gas delivery is limited by a predetermined pressure.

presternal region, the region of the thorax overlying the sternum, bounded laterally by the pectoral regions.

presumptive signs /prē-sump″tiv/ [L, *praesumere,* to take beforehand, *signum,* mark], manifestations that indicate a pregnancy, although they are not necessarily positive. Presumptive signs may include cessation of menses and morning sickness. See also **Chadwick's sign.**

preswing stance stage/prē″swing/ [L, *prae* + AS, *swingan,* to fling; L, *stare,* to stand; OFr, *estage,* stage], one of the five stages in the stance phase of walking or gait, a brief transitional period of double-limb support during which one leg is rapidly relieved of body-bearing weight and prepared for the swing forward. The type of preswing used by an individual is a factor in the diagnosis of many abnormal orthopedic conditions. Compare **initial contact stance stage, loading response stance stage, midstance, terminal stance.** See also **swing phase of gait.**

presymptomatic disease /-simp″təmat″ik/ [L, *prae* + Gk, *symptoma,* a happening], an early stage of disease when physiological changes have begun but no signs or symptoms are observed.

presynaptic/-sinap″tik/ [L,*prae*+*synaptein,*to join], **1.** situated near or before a synapse. **2.** before a synapse is crossed.

presystole /-sis″təlē/ [L, *prae,* before; Gk, *systole,* contraction], the interval in the cardiac cycle immediately before systole. **–presystolic,** *adj.*

presystolic /-sistol″ik/ [L, *prae* + Gk, *systole,* contraction], pertaining to the period before systole.

presystolic murmur (psm) [L, *prae,* before; Gk, *systole,* contraction; L, *murmur,* humming], a heart murmur heard immediately before systole in cases of mitral valve stenosis.

preterm /prē′turm″/ [L, *prae,* before; Gk, *terma,* limit], **1.** *n.,* events before a specific date. **2.** *adj.,* pertaining to a shorter-than-normal period of gestation.

preterm birth, any birth that occurs before the 37th week of gestation. See also **premature infant.**

preterm contractions, irregular tightening of the pregnant uterus that begins in the first trimester and increases in frequency, duration, and intensity as pregnancy progresses. Contractility of uterine muscle increases in pregnancy. Near-term, strong preterm contractions are often difficult to distinguish from the contractions of true labor. Also called **Braxton Hicks contractions, false labor.**

preterm infant. See **premature infant.**

preterm labor, labor that occurs earlier in pregnancy than normal, either before the fetus has reached a weight of 2000 to 2500 g or before the 37th or 38th week of gestation. No single measure of fetal weight or gestational age is used universally to designate preterm birth; local or institutional policy dictates which of several standards is applied. Prematurity is a concomitant of 75% of births that result in neonatal mortality. It may occur spontaneously, or it may be iatrogenic. The incidence of preterm labor increases in inverse proportion to maternal age, weight, and socioeconomic status. Incidence is higher for African-American women, women who have not had adequate prenatal care or have an abnormal obstetric history, and women who smoke or whose diet is deficient in protein or calories. Predisposing conditions include maternal infection, low weight gain, uterine bleeding, multiple gestation, polyhydramnios, uterine abnormalities, incompetent

cervix, premature rupture of membranes, and intrauterine fetal growth delay. The cause of preterm labor is poorly understood; in some cases there may be several contributing causes. In some pregnancies preterm labor may be homeostatic, resulting in the best possible outcome under the particular abnormal conditions. If preterm labor itself constitutes a threat to the fetus, the outcome of pregnancy may be improved if labor can be inhibited. Determining accurately which pregnancies are likely to benefit from the inhibition of labor and which are not is difficult. Medications used to stop labor are not always effective. Misdiagnosis of gestational age and fetal condition may lead to induction of labor that is inadvertently premature; preterm babies whose birth has been brought about inappropriately early account for 15% of admissions to newborn intensive care nurseries. Also called **premature labor.** See also **small for gestational age (SGA) infant.**

pretibial /prētib″ē-əl/ [L, *prae* + *tibia,* shinbone], pertaining to the area of the leg in front of the tibia.

pretibial fever, an acute infection caused by *Leptospira autumnalis.* It is characterized by headache, chills, fever, enlarged spleen, myalgia, low white blood cell count, and rash on the anterior surface of the legs. Also called **Fort Bragg fever.**

pretrial discovery. See **discovery.**

prevalence /prev″ələns/ [L, *praevalentia,* a powerful force], (in epidemiology) the number of all new and old cases of a disease or occurrences of an event during a particular period. Prevalence is expressed as a ratio in which the number of events is the numerator and the population at risk is the denominator. See also **rate.** **–prevalent,** *adj.*

prevention /-ven″shən/ [L, *praevenire,* to anticipate], (in nursing care) actions directed to preventing illness and promoting health to reduce the need for secondary or tertiary health care. Prevention includes such nursing actions as assessment, including disease risk; application of prescribed measures, such as immunization; health teaching; early diagnosis and treatment; and recognition of disability limitations and rehabilitation potential. In acute care nursing many interventions are simultaneously therapeutic and preventive.

preventive /-ven″tiv/ [L, *praevenire,* to anticipate], pertaining to hindering the occurrence of an illness or decreasing the incidence of a disease.

preventive care, a pattern of nursing and medical care that focuses on disease prevention and health maintenance. It includes early diagnosis of disease, discovery and identification of people at risk of development of specific problems, counseling, and other necessary intervention to avert a health problem. Screening tests, health education, and immunization programs are common examples of preventive care.

preventive dentistry [L, *praevenire,* to anticipate, *dens,* tooth], the science of the care required to prevent disease of the teeth and supporting structures. Most important is the daily practice of oral hygiene, proper diet, and regular professional care. There are three levels of preventive dentistry: the use of a topical fluoride gel to prevent caries is an example of primary prevention; a dental restoration is an example of secondary prevention; and a fixed bridge is an example of tertiary prevention.

preventive health care. See **preventive care.**

preventive medicine [L, *praevenire,* to anticipate, *medicina*], the branch of medicine that is concerned with the prevention of disease and methods for increasing the power of the patient and community to resist disease and prolong life.

preventive nursing [L, *praevenire,* to anticipate, *nutrix,* nurse], the branch of nursing concerned with general health promotion, teaching of early recognition and treatment of disease, encouragement of lifestyle modification, and prevention of further deterioration of the disabled.

preventive psychiatry, the use of theoretic knowledge and skills to plan and implement programs designed to achieve primary, secondary, and tertiary prevention of the onset of psychiatric disorders.

preventive treatment, a procedure, measure, substance, or program designed to prevent a disease from occurring or a mild disorder from becoming more severe. Various diseases are prevented by immunizations with vaccines, antiseptic measures, the avoidance of smoking, regular exercise, prudent diet, adequate rest, correction of congenital anomalies, and screening programs for the detection of preclinical signs of disorders. Also called **prophylactic treatment.**

prevertebral ganglia, collections of postganglionic sympathetic neuronal cell bodies in recognizable aggregations along the abdominal prevertebral plexus. They include the celiac, superior mesenteric, aorticorenal, and inferior mesenteric ganglia and play a critical role in the innervations of the abdominal viscera.

previa. See **placenta previa.**

previllous embryo /prēvil″əs/ [L, *prae* + *villus,* hairy; Gk, *en,* in, *bryein,* to grow], an embryo of a placental mammal at any stage before the development of the chorionic villi, which in humans occurs between the first and second months after fertilization.

previtamin. See **provitamin.**

prevocational evaluation /-vōkā″shənəl/, an evaluation of the abilities and limitations of a patient undergoing rehabilitation for a disabling disorder. The goal is to find eventual employment in a sheltered workshop or in the general community. The evaluation usually leads to selective placement of the patient in an appropriate business or industry.

prevocational training, a rehabilitation program designed to prepare a patient for the performance of useful paid work in a sheltered setting or community. It may involve training in basic work skills and counseling as required for a typical employment setting.

Prezista, a protease inhibitor medication used in the treatment of HIV infections. Brand name for **darunavir.**

PRF, abbreviation for **pulse repetition frequency.**

priapism /prī″əpiz′əm/ [Gk, *priapos,* phallus], an abnormal condition of prolonged or constant penile erection, often painful and seldom associated with sexual arousal. It may result from localized infection, a lesion in the penis or the central nervous system, or the use of medications or recreational drugs such as cocaine. It sometimes occurs in men who have acute leukemia or sickle cell anemia.

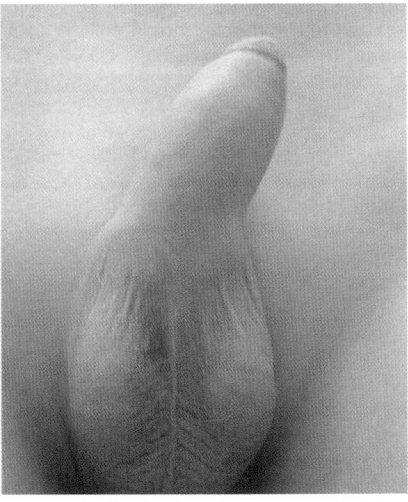

Priapism *(Kiss et al, 2007)*

priapitis /prī′əpī″tis/, inflammation of the penis.

priapus. See **penis.**

prickle cell layer. See **stratum spinosum.**

prickly heat. See **miliaria.**

-pride, suffix for sulpiride derivatives.

-pril, suffix for captopril-type antihypertensive agents.

prilocaine hydrochloride /pril″ōkān/, a local anesthetic agent of the amide family, used for nerve block, epidural, and regional anesthesia. It is not used for spinal or topical anesthesia. Prilocaine hydrochloride is about half as toxic as lidocaine but, because methemoglobinemia is a possible reaction to its administration, is not used for patients with hypoxic conditions of any kind.

prim-, primi-, prefix meaning "first": *primary, primigravida, primer.*

-prim, suffix for trimethoprim-type antibacterials.

prima facie rights /prī″mə fā″shē·ə/, rights on the surface, or face, that may be overridden by stronger conflicting rights or by other values.

primal scream therapy /prī″məl/, a nonmainstream form of psychotherapy developed by Arthur Janov that focuses on repressed pain of infancy or childhood. The goal of the therapy is to enable the patient to surrender his or her anxiety defenses and "become real."

primaquine phosphate /prī″məkwin/, an antimalarial.

■ INDICATIONS: It is prescribed in the treatment of malaria and prevention of relapse during recovery from the disease; it eradicates the tissue schizonts of *Plasmodium vivax* and *P. ovale* infections.

■ CONTRAINDICATIONS: Lupus erythematosus, rheumatoid arthritis, concomitant use of bone marrow depressants or hemolytic drugs, or known hypersensitivity to this drug prohibits its use. It must be used with caution in patients with glucose-6-phosphate dehydrogenase deficiency.

■ ADVERSE EFFECTS: Among the more serious adverse effects are hemolytic anemia, agranulocytosis, and abdominal distress.

primary /prī″mərē/ [L, *primus,* first], **1.** first in order of time, place, development, or importance. **2.** not derived from any other source or cause, specifically the original condition or set of symptoms in disease processes, such as a primary infection or a primary tumor. **3.** (in organic chemistry) referring to the first and simplest compound in a related series, formed by the substitution of one of two or more atoms or of a group in a molecule. Compare **secondary, tertiary.**

primary abscess [L, *primus* + *abscedere,* to go away], an abscess that develops at the original point of infection by a pus-producing microorganism.

primary afferent fiber. See **gamma efferent fiber.**

primary alveolar hypoventilation. See **Ondine curse syndrome.**

primary amebic meningoencephalitis (PAM), a rare and often fatal acute, febrile, purulent meningoencephalitis caused by free-living soil and water amebas of the genera *Naegleria* and *Acanthamoeba.* Infection caused by *Naegleria* is generally seen in young persons who swim or bathe in contaminated freshwater, the pathogens gaining access to the central nervous system by penetrating the nasal mucosa and cribriform plate and then following the olfactory bulbs and nerves to the brain and meninges. By contrast, *Acanthamoeba* infections tend to be more benign, are more often seen in older or immunocompromised persons, and are sometimes associated with spontaneous recovery; the mode of transmission of these infections is not known, but hematogenous spread from amebic infection at distant sites has been reported.

primary amenorrhea. See **amenorrhea.**

primary amputation, amputation performed after severe trauma, after the patient has recovered from shock and before infection occurs. Compare **secondary amputation.**

primary amyloidosis.   See **amyloidosis.**

primary apnea,   a self-limited condition characterized by an absence of respiration. It may follow a blow to the head and is common immediately after birth in the newborn who breathes spontaneously when the carbon dioxide level in the circulation reaches a certain value. Reflexes are present and the heart is beating, but the skin may be pale or blue and muscle tone is diminished. No treatment is necessary, but careful observation, maintenance of body temperature, and oral pharyngeal aspiration are usually performed. Within seconds the newborn usually begins breathing, becomes pinker, moves the arms and legs, and cries. Compare **periodic apnea of the newborn, secondary apnea.**

primary atelectasis,   failure of the lungs to expand fully at birth, most commonly seen in premature infants or those narcotized by maternal anesthesia. The infant is usually cared for in an incubator in which the temperature and humidity may be closely monitored. Nursing care includes changing the infant's position frequently to assist respiration, suctioning to remove bronchial secretions, and feeding very slowly to prevent abdominal distension.

primary atypical pneumonia.   See **mycoplasma pneumonia.**

primary bilateral micronodular hyperplasia.   See **micronodular adrenal disease.**

primary biliary cholangitis,   an inflammatory condition in which the flow of bile through the ductules of the liver is obstructed. Primary biliary cirrhosis most commonly affects women in their middle years and is often associated with antimitochondrial antibodies. Its cause is unknown. It is characterized by itching, jaundice, steatorrhea, and enlargement of the liver and spleen. The disease is slowly progressive. Care must be taken to rule out secondary biliary cirrhosis caused by obstruction of the biliary structures outside the liver, because the latter condition can be treated more successfully. Compare **biliary calculus, biliary obstruction.**

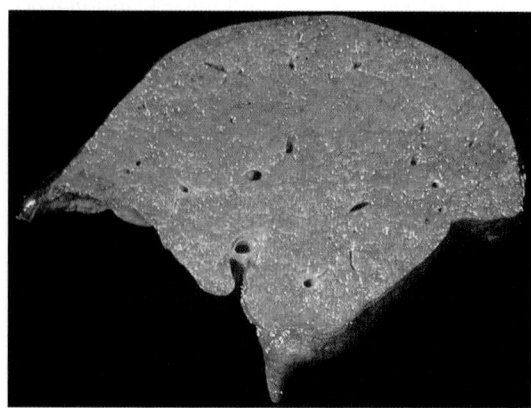

Primary biliary cholangitis *(Kumar, Abbas, and Aster, 2013)*

primary biliary cirrhosis,   a chronic inflammatory condition of the liver. It is characterized by generalized pruritus; enlargement and hardening of the liver; weight loss; and diarrhea with pale, bulky stools. Petechiae, epistaxis, or hemorrhage resulting from hypoprothrombinemia may also be evident. Pathological fractures and collapsed vertebrae may develop as the result of the associated malabsorption of vitamin D and calcium. Xanthomas commonly develop when the serum cholesterol level exceeds 450 mg/dL. The cause of primary biliary cirrhosis is unknown, although it is associated with autoimmune disorders. The condition most

often affects women 40 to 60 years of age. The diagnosis is confirmed by liver biopsy and cholangiography. Antibody is nearly always present. Jaundice, dark urine, pale stools, and cutaneous xanthosis may occur in the later stages of this disease. Treatment commonly includes the administration of fat-soluble vitamins A, D, E, and K to prevent and correct deficiencies caused by malabsorption. Life expectancy is about 5 years for symptomatic patients after the onset of jaundice. Compare **secondary biliary cirrhosis.**

primary bronchial buds,   two outgrowths from the respiratory diverticulum, which ultimately become the right and left primary bronchi and also give rise to the secondary bronchial buds.

primary bronchus,   one of the two main air passages that branch from the trachea and convey air to the lungs as part of the respiratory system. The right primary bronchus enters the right lung nearly opposite the fifth thoracic vertebra. The left primary bronchus divides into bronchi for the superior and anterior lobes of the lung. The bronchi, like the trachea, are composed of rings of hyaline cartilage, fibrous tissue, mucous membrane, and glands. The right primary bronchus has a more direct extension of the trachea than the left. Hence foreign objects entering the trachea usually drop into the right bronchus rather than the left. See also **bronchial tree.**

primary carcinoma,   a neoplasm at the site of origin.

primary care,   the first contact in a given episode of illness, which leads to a decision regarding a course of action to resolve the health problem.

primary care case management (PCCM),   (in the United States) a situation in which primary care receives concurrent utilization management review, and discharge planning is used to minimize resource consumption while maintaining quality of care.

primary care physician (PCP, P.C.P.) [L, *primus* + ME, *caru,* sorrow; Gk, *physikos,* natural],   a physician who usually is the first health professional to examine a patient and who recommends secondary care physicians, medical or surgical specialists with expertise in the patient's specific health problem, if further treatment is needed.

primary caries.   See **dental caries.**

primary cell,   an irreversible (nonrechargeable) electromotive force cell, such as a standard 1.5-volt alkaline battery.

primary cell culture,   a cell line derived directly from the parent tissue. Cells in primary culture have the same karyotype and chromosome number as those in the original tissue.

primary colors,   a small number of fundamental colors. In visual science these are red, green, and blue, the colors specifically picked up by the retinal cones. Mixtures of varying proportions of the primary colors will yield white light in addition to the 150 discriminable hues of normal human vision. In painting and printing, the primary colors are red, blue, and yellow. When combined properly, these colors yield black and all other visible hues. See also **prismatic colors.**

primary constriction.   See **centromere.**

primary curvature of vertebral column,   a dorsally convex part of the spinal (vertebral) column.

primary cutaneous melanoma,   a malignant neoplasm on the skin at the site of origin.

primary dementia.   See **Alzheimer disease.**

primary dental caries,   dental caries developing in a tooth that was previously unaffected. Compare **secondary dental caries.**

primary dentition,   the set of 20 teeth that appears normally during infancy, consisting of four incisors, two canines, and four molars in each jaw. The teeth start developing at about the sixth week of fetal life as a thickening of the epithelium along the line of the future jaw. During the seventh week the epithelium splits longitudinally into labial and lingual strands. The former becomes the labiodental lamina, and the latter forms the dental lamina, which develops 10 enlargements in each jaw. The enlargements appear at about the ninth week and correspond to the future teeth. In most individuals, the first tooth erupts through the gum about 6 months after birth. Thereafter one or more teeth erupt about every month until all 20 have appeared. The primary teeth are usually shed between the ages of 6 and 13 years, although the timing varies greatly from person to person. Also called **deciduous dentition, first dentition, primary teeth.** Compare **secondary dentition.** See also **predeciduous dentition, teething, tooth.**

primary dermatitis [L, *primus* + Gk, *derma,* skin, *itis,* inflammation], skin eruption caused by a substance that can produce cell damage on initial contact, as opposed to that which develops as a sensitivity reaction to an allergen.

primary distal RTA. See **distal renal tubular acidosis.**

primary drive. See **drive.**

primary dysmenorrhea. See **dysmenorrhea.**

primary effusion lymphoma, a B cell lymphoma associated with human herpesvirus 8 infection, characterized by the occurrence of lymphomatous effusions in body cavities without the presence of a solid tumor.

primary endometriosis [L, *primus* + Gk, *endon,* within, *metra,* womb, *osis,* condition], an ingrowth of the muscle walls of the uterus by the mucous membrane lining of the organ. Also called **adenomyosis, endometriosis interna.**

primary fissure, a fissure that marks the division of the anterior and posterior lobes of the cerebellum.

primary gain, a benefit, primarily relief from emotional conflict and freedom from anxiety, attained through the use of a defense mechanism or other psychological process. Compare **secondary gain.**

primary gangrene [L, *primus* + Gk, *gangraina*], a form of gangrene that occurs without preceding inflammation.

primary health care, a basic level of health care that includes programs directed at the promotion of health, early diagnosis of disease or disability, and prevention of disease. Primary health care is provided in an ambulatory facility to limited numbers of people, often those living in a particular geographic area. It includes continuing health care, as provided by a family nurse practitioner.

primary hemorrhage [L, *primus* + Gk, *haima,* blood, *rhegnynei,* to burst forth], a hemorrhage immediately after an injury.

primary host. See **definitive host.**

primary hypertension. See **essential hypertension.**

primary intention. See **intention.**

primary iritis [L, *primus* + Gk, *iris,* rainbow, *itis,* inflammation], an inflammation of the iris that results from a source within the body, such as a systemic disease. Also called **endogenous iritis.**

primary lateral sclerosis, a slowly progressing degenerative brain disease characterized by weakness, spasticity, hyperreflexia, and a positive Babinski sign. It involves neurons of the motor cortex but not the brainstem or spinal cord neurons. Also called **spastic primary paraplegia.**

primary lesion [L, *primus* + *laesio,* hurting], a sore or wound that develops at the point of inoculation of the disease, usually referring to a syphilis chancre. Also called **initial lesion.**

primary myelofibrosis, chronic, eventually fatal myeloproliferative neoplasm in which normal bone marrow hematopoietic tissue is replaced by reticulin fibers and blood cell production moves to other organs, called myeloid metaplasia. The peripheral blood film presents all stages of myelocytic

and erythrocytic maturation and teardrop-shaped red blood cells called dacryocytes.

primary nurse, a nurse who is responsible for the planning, implementation, and evaluation of the nursing care of one or more clients 24 hours a day for the duration of the hospital stay. See also **primary nursing.**

primary nursing, a system for the distribution of nursing care in which care of one patient is managed for the entire 24-hour day by one nurse who directs and coordinates other nurses and personnel caring for the patient; schedules all tests, procedures, and daily activities for that patient; and cares for that patient personally when on duty. In acute care the primary care nurse may be responsible for only one patient; in intermediate care the primary care nurse may be responsible for three or more patients. Nurse midwives and other nurse practitioners practice primary nursing. Some advantages are continuity of care for the patient; accountability of the nurse for that care; patient-centered care that is comprehensive, individualized, and coordinated; and the professional satisfaction of the nurse. Compare **team nursing.**

primary oocyte, an oocyte that has begun but not completed the first maturation division. It is derived from an oogonium by differentiation near the time of birth.

primary organizer, the part of the dorsal lip of the blastopore that is self-differentiating and induces the formation of the neural plate that gives rise to the main axis of the embryo.

primary palate, a shelf formed from the medial nasal process of an embryo that separates the primitive nasal cavity from the oral cavity.

primary physician, **1.** the physician who usually takes care of a patient. **2.** the physician who first sees a patient for the care of a given health problem. **3.** a family practice physician or general practitioner. See also **family medicine.**

primary pneumonic plague. See **pneumonic plague.**

primary polycythemia. See **polycythemia rubra vera.**

primary prevention, a program of activities directed at improving general well-being while also involving specific protection for selected diseases, such as immunization against measles.

primary processes, (in psychoanalytic theory) unconscious processes, originating in the id, that obey laws different from those of the ego. These processes occur in the least disguised form in infancy and in the dreams of the adult.

primary progressive aphasia, a speech disorder seen with certain degenerative brain diseases, consisting of deterioration of speech and language ability over a period of years without significant loss of memory or ability to understand language.

primary progressive apraxia of speech, a speech disorder similar to primary progressive aphasia except that a prominent feature is the inability of the patient to produce the sequence of muscle movements necessary to produce understandable speech, although comprehension of speech remains intact. See also **primary progressive aphasia.**

primary proximal RTA. See **proximal renal tubular acidosis.**

primary relationships, relationships with intimates, close friends, and family.

primary sclerosing cholangitis, a progressive, chronic, fibrosing inflammation of the bile ducts of unknown cause, occurring most commonly in young men and frequently in association with chronic ulcerative colitis. It also occurs as a complication of HIV infection. See also **AIDS cholangiopathy.**

P

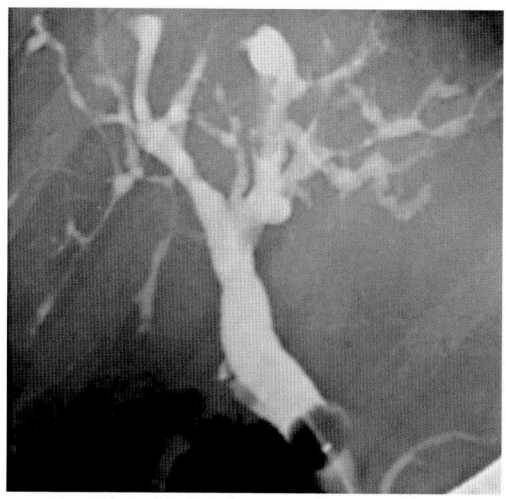

Primary sclerosing cholangitis *(Feldman, Friedman, and Brandt, 2010)*

primary sensation, a feeling or impression resulting directly from a particular stimulus. See also **sensation,** def. 1.

primary sequestrum, a piece of dead bone that completely separates from sound bone during the process of necrosis. Compare **secondary sequestrum.**

primary sex character, an inherited trait directly concerned with the reproductive function of the primary sex organs of the individual.

primary shock, a state of physical collapse comparable to fainting. It may be the result of slight pain, such as that produced by venipuncture, or may be caused by fright. Primary shock is usually mild, self-limited, and of short duration. Severe injury may prolong and merge primary shock with secondary shock. Compare **hemorrhagic shock.**

primary sterility [L, *primus* + *sterilis,* barren], the inability to produce offspring caused by a functional failure of the ovaries or the testes.

primary symptoms. See **symptom.**

primary syphilis. See **syphilis.**

primary teeth. See **primary dentition.**

primary triad, in A.T. Beck's theory of depression, the three major cognitive patterns that force the individual to view self, environment, and future in a negative manner.

primary tuberculosis, the childhood form of tuberculosis, most commonly occurring in the lungs, the posterior pharynx, or, rarely, the skin. Infants lack resistance to the disease and are readily infected and especially vulnerable to rapid and extensive spread of infection through the body. In childhood the disease is usually brief and benign, characterized by regional lymphadenopathy, calcification of the tubercles, and residual immunity. The disease may reactivate later in life. The tuberculin test result will be positive for life. See also **tuberculosis.**

primate /prī″māt, prī″mit/ [L, *primus,* first], a member of the order of mammals that includes lemurs, monkeys, apes, and humans. Most primates have large brains, stereoscopic vision, and hands and feet developed for grasping.

Primaxin, a broad-spectrum parenteral antibiotic. Brand name for **imipenem-cilastatin sodium.**

prime mover /prīm/ [L, *primus* + *movere,* to move], a muscle that acts directly to produce a desired movement amid other muscles acting simultaneously to produce the same movement indirectly. Most movements of the body require the combined action of numerous muscles. Compare **antagonist, fixation muscle, synergist.**

primer /prī″mər/, **1.** a short piece of DNA or RNA complementary to a given DNA sequence that acts as a point at which replication can proceed, as in a polymerase chain reaction. **2.** a molecule, such as a small polymer, that induces the synthesis of a larger molecule.

primidone /prī″mədōn/, an anticonvulsant.

■ INDICATIONS: It is prescribed in the treatment of seizure disorders, including tonic-clonic, psychomotor, and focal epilepsy-like seizures, and has an unlabeled use for treating familial (essential) tremor.

■ CONTRAINDICATIONS: Porphyria, pregnancy, or known hypersensitivity to this drug or to phenobarbital, a metabolite of primidone, prohibits its use. The drug must be used with caution in those having renal, hepatic, or pulmonary insufficiency.

■ ADVERSE EFFECTS: The most serious adverse effect, seen on rare occasions, is megaloblastic anemia. Drowsiness, ataxia, and dizziness are common. Drug dependency and other adverse effects of phenobarbital may occur.

primigravida /prim″igrav″idə/ [L, *primus* + *gravidus,* pregnancy], a woman pregnant for the first time. Also called **gravida.** Compare **multigravida, primipara.** –**primigravid,** *adj.*

primipara /primip″ərə/ [L, *primus* + *parere,* to bear], a woman who has given birth to one viable infant, indicated by the notation *para 1* on the patient's chart. Compare **multipara, nullipara, primigravida.**

primiparity /prim″iper″itē/ [L, *primus* + *parere,* to bear], the condition of having borne one child.

primiparous /primip″ərəs/ [L, *primus* + *parere,* to bear], pertaining to a woman who has borne one child.

primitive /prim″itiv/ [L, *primivus*], **1.** undeveloped; undifferentiated; rudimentary; showing little or no evolution. **2.** embryonic; formed early in the course of development; existing in an early or simple form. Compare **definitive.**

primitive fold. See **primitive ridge.**

primitive groove, a furrow in the posterior region of the embryonic (primordial) disk. It indicates the cephalocaudal axis that results from the active involution of cells forming the primitive streak.

primitive gut. See **archenteron.**

primitive heart tube, the primordium of the heart, formed by fusion of the two lateral endocardial tubes.

primitive line. See **primitive streak.**

primitive node, a knoblike accumulation of cells at the cephalic end of the primitive streak in the early stages of embryonic development in humans and higher animals. It consists of mesoderm cells that give rise to the notochord, and it corresponds to the dorsal lip of the blastopore in lower animals. Also called **Hensen's knot, Hensen's node.**

primitive pit, a minute indentation at the anterior end of the primitive groove in the early developing embryo. It lies posterior to the primitive node and probably functions as an opening into the notochordal canal in humans and higher animals and into the neurenteric canal in lower animals.

primitive reflex, any reflex normal in an infant or fetus. Its presence in an adult usually indicates serious neurological disease, such as dementia. Kinds include **grasp reflex, Moro reflex, sucking reflex.**

primitive ridge, a ridge that bounds the primitive groove in the early stages of embryonic development. Also called **primitive fold.** See also **primitive streak.**

primitive streak, a dense area on the central posterior region of the embryonic disk. It is formed by the morphogenetic movement of a rapidly proliferating mass of cells that spreads between the ectoderm and endoderm, giving rise to the mesoderm layer. This seamlike elongation indicates the cephalocaudal axis along which the embryo develops, and it corresponds to the blastopore of lower animal groups. Also called **primitive line.**

primordia. See **primordium.**

primordial /primôr″dē·əl/ [L, *primordium,* origin], **1.** characteristic of the most undeveloped or earliest state, specifically those cells or tissues that are formed in the early stages of embryonic development. **2.** first or original; primitive.

primordial cyst, a developmental odontogenic cyst that forms in place of a tooth. One of three kinds of follicular cysts, consisting of an epithelium-lined sac that contains fluid and appears radiographically as a light area in the affected jaw. It develops from a dental enamel organ before the formation of hard tissue. See **odontogenic keratocyst.**

primordial dwarf, a person of extremely short stature who is otherwise perfectly formed, with the usual proportions of body parts and normal mental and sexual development. The condition may be genetically related, involving some defect in the ability to use growth hormone, or it may occur sporadically within a particular population. Also called **hypoplastic dwarf, normal dwarf, physiological dwarf, pure dwarf, true dwarf.** See also **pituitary dwarf, pygmy.**

primordial germ cell, any of the large spheric diploid cells that are formed in the early stages of embryonic development and are precursors of the oogonia and spermatogonia. They are formed outside the gonads and migrate to the embryonic ovaries and testes for maturation. See also **oogenesis, spermatogenesis.**

primordial image, (in analytic psychology) the archetype or original parent, representing the source of all life. It occurs in the memory as a stage preceding the differentiation of the actual mother and father. See also **collective unconscious.**

primordial oocyte, an oocyte very early in its development.

primordial sex cords. See **gonadal cords.**

primordium /primôr″dē·əm/ *pl.* **primordia** [L, origin], the first recognizable stage in the embryonic development and differentiation of a particular organ, tissue, or structure. Also called **anlage, rudiment.**

principal /prin′sipəl/ [L, *principalis,* first in rank], first in authority or importance.

principal cell. See **chief cell.**

Principen, an antibacterial. Brand name for **ampicillin.**

principle /prin″sipəl/ [L, *principium,* foundation], **1.** a general truth or established rule of action. **2.** a prime source or element from which anything proceeds. **3.** a law on which others are founded or from which others are derived.

principle of infinitesimal dose, one of the fundamental principles of homeopathy, a system of medical practice based on the tenet that the body can heal itself; the principle states othat the more a remedy is diluted (even to the point that none of the medicinal substance is likely to be present), the more powerful and longer lasting will be its effect.

principles of instrumentation, (in dentistry)six rules for the use of mirrors and other hand-driven and motor-driven devices in dentistry and dental hygiene: (1) grasp, (2) fulcrum, (3) insertion, (4) adaptation and angulation, (5) activation (lateral pressure and working stroke), and (6) rest.

Prinivil, an angiotensin-converting enzyme inhibitor used for hypertension. Brand name for **lisinopril.**

P-R interval, the interval from the beginning of the P wave to the beginning of the QRS complex on an electrocardiogram. It represents the atrioventricular conduction time, which normally is between 0.12 and 0.20 second.

Prinzmetal angina [Myron Prinzmetal, American cardiologist, 1908–1994], chest pain caused by severe reversible coronary artery spasm. It is associated with S-T segment elevation that reverts to normal within minutes. The S-T segment elevation indicates total occlusion of the epicardial coronary artery. Also called **variant angina.**

prion /prī″on/, one of several kinds of proteinaceous particles believed to be responsible for transmissible neurodegenerative diseases, including scrapie in sheep and kuru and Creutzfeldt-Jakob disease in humans. Because prions lack detectable nucleic acid, they are not inactivated by the usual procedures for destroying viruses. They also do not trigger an immune response.

prion disease, any of a group of fatal degenerative diseases of the nervous system caused by abnormalities in the metabolism of prion protein. These diseases are unique in that they may be transmitted genetically as an autosomal-dominant trait or by infection with abnormal forms of the protein (prions). Inherited forms result from mutations in the gene that codes for prion protein; such mutations may occur sporadically. Hereditary forms include some forms of Creutzfeldt-Jakob disease, Gerstmann-Sträussler syndrome, and fatal familial insomnia. Infectious forms of the disease result from ingestion of infected tissue or the introduction of infected tissue into the body (kuru and some forms of Creutzfeldt-Jakob disease). The latter has occasionally occurred during surgical procedures. It has also occurred as the result of injection of human growth hormone prepared from infected pituitary glands. Prion diseases also occur in animals. Also called **subacute spongiform encephalopathy, transmissible neurodegenerative disease, transmissible spongiform encephalopathy.**

priority /prī·ôr″itē/ [L, *prius,* previously], actions established in order of importance or urgency to the welfare or purposes of the organization, patient, or other person at a given time.

Priscoline, a peripheral vasodilator. Brand name for **tolazoline hydrochloride.**

prism /priz″əm/ [Gk, *prisma,* that which is seen through], **1.** a solid of glass, plastic, or a similar substance with a triangular or polygonal cross section, which splits up a ray of light into its constituent colors and turns or deflects light rays toward its base. Prisms are used to correct deviations of the eyes because they alter the apparent situation of objects. **2.** enamel prism, or calcified rods, surrounded by organic prism cuticle joined together to form tooth enamel. **3.** an adverse prism or verger prism used to test and train ocular muscles.

prismatic colors /prizmat″ik/, the seven rainbow hues (red, orange, yellow, green, blue, indigo, and violet) produced from white light when it is reduced to its component wavelengths by the dispersion effect of a prism.

privacy /prī″vəsē/, a culturally specific concept defining the degree of one's personal responsibility to others in regulating behavior that is regarded as intrusive. Some privacy-regulating mechanisms are physical barriers (closed doors or drawn curtains, such as around a hospital bed) and interpersonal types (lowered voices or refraining from social media posts).

P

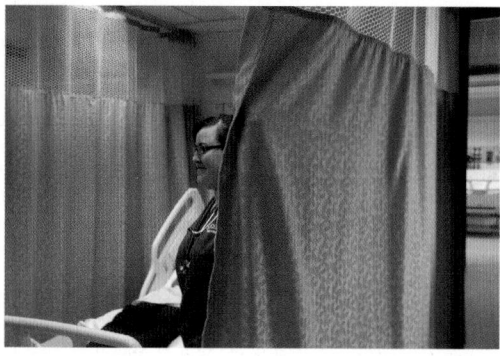

Privacy curtain *(Courtesy Rutgers School of Nursing—Camden. All rights reserved.)*

private duty nurse /prī″vit/, a nurse who may work in an institution, caring for a patient on a fee-for-service basis. The private duty nurse is not a member of the institution staff. Private duty care also occurs in the home.

private practice, the work of a professional health care provider who is independent of economic or policy control by professional peers except for licensing and other legal restrictions.

-privia, suffix meaning "a (specified) condition of loss or deprivation."

privileged communication /priv″ilijd/, a legal term used in court-related proceedings concerning the right to reveal information that belongs to the person who spoke. It may prevent the listener from disclosing the information without the permission of the speaker. Privileged communication may exist between a patient and a health professional only if the law specifically establishes it.

privileges /priv″ilij′əs/ [L, *privilegium,* private law], authority granted to a physician or dentist by a hospital governing board to provide patient care in the hospital. Clinical privileges are limited by the individual's professional license, experience, and competence. Emergency privileges may be granted by a hospital governing board or chief executive officer in an emergency and without regard to the physician's or dentist's regular service assignment or status. Temporary privileges may be granted a physician or dentist to provide health care to patients for a limited period or to a specific patient.

Privine, an alpha₁-adrenergic agonist. Brand name for **naph-azoline hydrochloride.**

PRK, abbreviation for **photorefractive keratectomy.**

PRL, abbreviation for **prolactin.**

prn, p.r.n., (in prescriptions) a notation for a Latin phrase meaning "as needed." The administration times are determined by the patient's needs. Abbreviation for **pro re nata.**

Pro, abbreviation for **proline.**

pro-, prefix meaning "first" or "in front of": *procerus, prodromal, progravid.*

proaccelerin. See **factor V.**

probability /prob′əbil′itē/ [L, *probabilitas*], **1.** a measure of the likelihood that something will occur. **2.** a mathematic ratio of the number of times something will occur to the total number of possible occurrences.

probable signs /prob′əbəl/ [L, *probabalis,* credible, *signum,* mark], clinical signs that there is a definite likelihood

of pregnancy. Examples include enlargement of the abdomen, Goodell's sign, Hegar sign, Braxton Hicks sign, and positive hormonal test results. Compare **presumptive signs.**

proband. See **propositus.**

Pro-Banthine, an anticholinergic. Brand name for **propantheline bromide.**

probe, **1.** any device used to explore an opening such as a sinus or wound. Common types of probes include a probe with a blunt leading end, a drum probe with a sounding device for the detection of metallic foreign particles, and an eyed probe with a small opening at one end for introducing a guiding thread along a fistula. **2.** any device or agent, such as a radioactively tagged isotope or a molecular deoxyribonucleic acid fragment probe, inserted into a medium to obtain information about a structure or substance. **3.** a Doppler probe used to detect blood flow in a vessel. **4.** the act of exploring or investigating an action or unfamiliar matter.

probenecid /prōben″əsid/, a uricosuric and adjunct to antibiotics.

■ INDICATIONS: It is prescribed in the treatment of gout and as an adjunct to prolong the activity of penicillin or cephalosporins in some infections, such as gonorrhea.

■ CONTRAINDICATIONS: Uric acid kidney stones, blood dyscrasias, or known hypersensitivity to this drug prohibits its use. It is not initiated during an acute attack of gout but is continued if an attack occurs during treatment. It is not given to children less than 2 years of age. Concomitant administration of salicylates decreases the effect of probenecid.

■ ADVERSE EFFECTS: Among the most serious adverse reactions are hemolytic anemia, GI disturbances, headache, urinary frequency, and minor allergic reactions. It is involved in many drug interactions, particularly with salicylate drugs.

probiotics, microorganisms present in food or supplements that confer health benefits.

problem /prob″ləm/ [Gk, *proballein,* to throw forward], any health care condition that requires diagnostic, therapeutic, or educational action. It also refers, in nursing, to any unmet or partially met basic human need.

problem-based learning, an instructional strategy designed to develop critical thinking skills through the presentation of real-life clinical situations assessed and explored by students working in collaborative groups with faculty, other clinician experts, and their peer group.

problem-oriented medical record (POMR), a method of recording data about the health status of a patient in a problem-solving system. The POMR preserves the data in an easily accessible way that encourages ongoing assessment and revision of the health care plan by all members of the health care team. The particular format of the system used varies from setting to setting, but the components of the method are similar. A database is collected before beginning the process of identifying the patient's problems. The database consists of all information available that contributes to this end, such as that collected in an interview with the patient and family or others, that from a health assessment or physical examination of the patient, and that from various laboratory and radiological tests. It is recommended that the database be as complete as possible, limited only by potential hazard, pain or discomfort to the patient, or excessive assumed expense of the diagnostic procedure. The interview, augmented by prior records, provides the patient's history, including the reason for contact; an identifying statement that is a descriptive profile of the person; a family illness history; a history of the current illness; a history of past illness; an account of the patient's current health practices; and a review of systems.

The physical examination or health assessment makes up the second major part of the database. The extent and depth of the examination vary from setting to setting and depend on the services offered and the condition of the patient. The next section of the POMR is the master problem list. The formulation of the problems on the list is similar to the assessment phase of the nursing process. Each problem as identified represents a conclusion or a decision resulting from examination, investigation, and analysis of the database. *A* problem is defined as anything that causes concern to the patient or to the caregiver, including physical abnormalities, psychological disturbance, and socioeconomic problems. The master problem list usually includes active, inactive, temporary, and potential problems. The list serves as an index to the rest of the record and is arranged in five columns: a chronological list of problems, the date of each problem's onset, the action taken, the outcome (often its resolution), and the date of the outcome. Problems may be added, and intervention or plans for intervention may be changed; thus the status of each problem is available for the information of all members of the various professions involved in caring for the patient. The third major section of the POMR is the initial plan, in which each separate problem is named and described, usually on the progress note in a SOAP format: *S,* subjective data from the patient's point of view; *O,* the objective data acquired by inspection, percussion, auscultation, and palpation and from laboratory and radiological tests; *A,* assessment of the problem that is an analysis of the subjective and objective data; and *P,* the plan, including further diagnostic work, therapy, and education or counseling. After an initial plan for each problem is formulated and recorded, the problems are followed in the progress notes by narrative notes in the SOAP format or by flow sheets showing the significant data in a tabular manner. A discharge summary is formulated and written, relating the overall assessment of progress during treatment and the plans for follow-up or referral. The summary allows a review of all the problems initially identified and encourages continuity of care for the patient.

problem-solving approach to patient-centered care, (in nursing) a conceptual framework that incorporates the overt physical needs of a patient with covert psychological, emotional, and social needs. It provides a model for caring for the whole person as an individual, not as an example of a disease or a medical diagnosis. Nursing is defined within this model as a problem-solving process. The patient is viewed as a person who is in an impaired state, less than usually able to perform self-care activities. Nursing problems are conditions experienced by the patient or the patient's family for which the nurse may provide professional service. The nurse makes a nursing diagnosis that identifies the impaired state and determines the care needed to augment the patient's ability to perform self-care. The requirements for care are classified in four levels: care given to sustain life is sustenal care; care given to assist the patient in self-care is remedial care; care that helps the patient develop new skills and goals in self-care is restorative care; and care given to guide the patient to a level of self-help beyond the normal level is preventive care. The approach identifies 21 nursing problems and sorts them into four groups: problems relating to comfort, hygiene, and safety; physiological balance; psychological and social factors; and sociological and community factors. See also **nursing care plan.**

problem-solving interview. See **interview.**

procainamide hydrochloride /prōkăn″əmīd/, an antiarrhythmic agent.

■ INDICATIONS: It is prescribed in the treatment of a variety of cardiac arrhythmias, including premature ventricular contractions, ventricular tachycardia, and atrial fibrillation.

■ CONTRAINDICATIONS: Myasthenia gravis, heart block, or known hypersensitivity to this drug, to procaine, or to related local anesthetics prohibits its use.

■ ADVERSE EFFECTS: Among the more serious adverse effects are GI disturbances, hypersensitivity reactions, agranulocytosis, and a syndrome resembling lupus erythematosus.

procaine hydrochloride /prō″kān/, a local anesthetic of the ester family.

■ INDICATIONS: It is administered for local anesthesia by infiltration and injection and for caudal, epidural, and other regional anesthetic procedures. It is not used for topical anesthesia.

■ CONTRAINDICATIONS: Known hypersensitivity to anesthetics of the ester group prohibits its use. It is not injected into inflamed or infected tissue, and large doses are not given to patients with heart block.

■ ADVERSE EFFECTS: Among the most serious adverse effects are potentially serious neurological and cardiovascular reactions that result from inadvertent intravascular administration. Allergic reactions also may occur.

procarbazine hydrochloride /prōkär″bəzēn/, an antineoplastic.

■ INDICATIONS: It is prescribed in the treatment of a variety of neoplasms, including Hodgkin disease, lymphomas, brain tumors, and lung cancer.

■ CONTRAINDICATIONS: Bone marrow depression or known hypersensitivity to this drug prohibits its use.

■ ADVERSE EFFECTS: Among the most serious adverse effects are bone marrow depression and GI disturbances, particularly nausea and vomiting.

Procardia, a calcium channel blocker. Brand name for **NIFEdipine.**

procaryocyte. See **prokaryocyte.**

procaryon. See **prokaryon.**

procaryosis. See **prokaryosis.**

Procaryotae /prōker″ē-ō″tē/, (in bacteriology) a kingdom of bacteria, viruses, and blue-green algae that includes all microorganisms in which the nucleoplasm has no basic protein and is not surrounded by a nuclear membrane. The kingdom has two divisions: cyanobacteria, which includes the blue-green bacteria, and bacteria. Also called **Monera.** See also **prokaryocyte.**

procaryote. See **prokaryote.**

procedural knowledge, the type of knowledge involved in performing a task (e.g., riding a bike). Procedural knowledge involves implicit learning, which a learner may be unaware of or unable to explain. Compare **declarative knowledge.**

procedure /prəsē″jər/ [L, *procedere,* to proceed], the sequence of steps to be followed in establishing some course of action.

procercoid /prōsur″koid/, the first stage in the life cycle of certain tapeworms that develop from the coracidium stage of *Diphyllobothrium latum.* The tapeworm develops in the body of the first intermediate host, either a crustacean or a copepod of the genus *Diaptomus.*

procerus /prəsir″əs/ [L, stretched], one of three muscles of the nose. It is a small pyramidal muscle that arises from the fascia of the nasal bone and the lateral nasal cartilage and inserts into the skin over the lower part of the forehead between the eyebrows. It is innervated by buccal branches of the facial nerve. The procerus functions to draw down the eyebrows and wrinkle the nose. Compare **depressor septi, nasalis.**

process /pros″əs/ [L, *processus*], **1.** *n.,* a series of related events that follow in sequence from a particular state or condition to a conclusion or resolution. **2.** *n.,* a natural growth that projects from a bone or other part. **3.** *v.,* to put through a particular series of interdependent steps, as in preparing a chemical compound.

processor. See **central processing unit.**

process recording, (in nursing education) a system used for teaching nursing students to understand and analyze verbal and nonverbal interaction. The conversation between nurse and patient is written on special forms or in a special format. The student nurse is instructed to record observations, perceptions, thoughts, and feelings, as well as conversations. The student also is asked to analyze his or her communication, determining and naming both therapeutic and nontherapeutic techniques used within an interaction. The process recording is then studied by the nursing instructor to discover patterns of difficulty in communicating with the patient and to help the student nurse identify them.

processus vaginalis peritonei /prəses″əs/ [L, *processus,* process, *vagina,* sheath; Gk, *peri,* around, *teinein,* to stretch], a diverticulum of the peritoneal membrane that during embryonic development extends through the inguinal canal. In males it descends into the scrotum to form the processus vaginalis testis; in females it is usually completely obliterated. Also called **Nuck's canal, Nuck's diverticulum.**

prochlorperazine /-klôrper″əzēn/, a phenothiazine antipsychotic and antiemetic.

■ INDICATIONS: It is prescribed in the treatment of psychotic disorders, and it may be used in the control of nausea and vomiting.

■ CONTRAINDICATIONS: Parkinson disease, the concurrent administration of central nervous system depressants, liver or renal dysfunction, severe hypotension, or known hypersensitivity to any phenothiazine prohibits its use.

■ ADVERSE EFFECTS: Among the more serious adverse effects are hypotension, liver toxicity, extrapyramidal reactions, blood dyscrasias, and hypersensitivity reactions.

prochlorperazine maleate. See **prochlorperazine.**

prochromosome. See **karyosome.**

procidentia /-siden″shə/ [L, *procidere,* to fall forward], the prolapse of an organ. The term is usually applied to a prolapsed uterus.

procoagulant /-kō·ag″yələnt/, an inactive coagulation protein that becomes activated during the coagulation process to form a serine protease or cofactor and produce a fibrin clot. Prothrombin is an example.

proconvertin. See **factor VII.**

procreate /prō″krē·āt/ [L, *procreare,* to create], to produce offspring.

procreation /-krē·ā″shən/ [L, *procreare,* to create], the entire reproductive process of producing offspring. –**procreate,** *v.*

proct-. See **procto-.**

proctalgia /proktal″jə/ [Gk, *proktos,* anus, *algos,* pain], a neurological pain in the anus or lower rectum.

proctalgia fugax [Gk, *proktos + algos,* pain; L, *fugax,* fleeting], periodic pain in the anus, possibly muscular in origin, that follows a pattern and is sometimes relieved by food and drink.

-proctia, suffix meaning "anus" or "rectum."

proctitis /proktī″tis/ [Gk, *proktos,* anus, *itis*], inflammation of the rectum and anus caused by infection, trauma, drugs, allergy, or radiation injury. Acute or chronic, it is accompanied by rectal discomfort and the repeated urge to pass feces and inability to do so. Pus, blood, or mucus may be present in the stools, and tenesmus may occur. Also called **rectitis.**

procto-, prefix meaning "anus" or "rectum": *proctocele, proctodeum, proctoscopy.*

proctocele. See **rectocele.**

proctocolectomy /prok′tōkəlek″təmē/, a surgical procedure in which the anus, rectum, and colon are removed. An ileostomy is created for the removal of digestive tract wastes.

The procedure treats severe, intractable ulcerative colitis or Crohn's disease. See also **ileoanal anastomosis.**

Proctocort, an anorectal preparation containing a glucocorticoid. Brand name for **hydrocortisone.**

proctodeum /proktō″dē·əm/ *pl. proctodea* [Gk, *proktos + hodiaos,* a route], a depression of the ectoderm, behind the urorectal septum of the developing embryo, that forms the anus and anal canal when the cloacal membrane ruptures. Also spelled *proctodaeum.* Compare **stomodeum.** –*proctodeal, proctodaeal, adj.*

proctodynia /-din′ē·ə/ [Gk, *proktos + odyne,* pain], pain in or around the anus.

proctologist /proktol″əjist/, a physician who specializes in proctology.

proctology /proktol″əjē/ [Gk, *proktos + logos,* science], the branch of medicine concerned with treating disorders of the colon, rectum, and anus.

proctoplasty /prok″təplas′tē/ [Gk, *proktos,* anus, *plassein,* to mold], a plastic surgery procedure performed on the anus and rectum.

proctoscope /prok′təskōp′/ [Gk, *proktos + skopein,* to look], an instrument used to examine the rectum and the distal part of the colon. It consists of a light mounted on a tube or speculum. Compare **sigmoidoscope.**

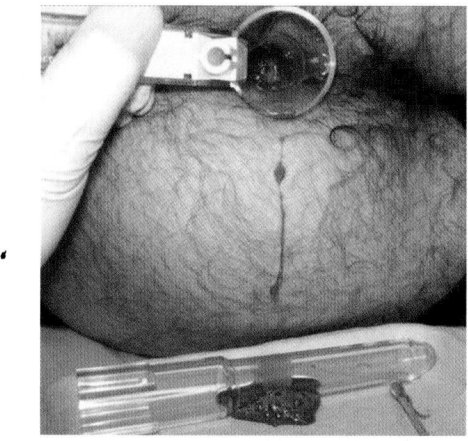

Proctoscope *(White, 2014)*

proctoscopy /proktos″kəpē/, the examination of the rectum with an endoscope inserted through the anus.

proctosigmoidoscopy /prok′tōsig′moidos″kəpē/ [Gk, *proktos + sigmoid + skopein,* to view], the use of a sigmoidoscope to examine the internal lumen of the rectum and pelvic colon.

procumbency /prōkum′bensē/ [L, *procumbere,* to lean forward], excessive inclination of the incisor teeth toward the lips.

procyclidine hydrochloride /prōsī″klədēn/, an anticholinergic.

■ INDICATIONS: It is prescribed in the treatment of parkinsonism and drug-induced extrapyramidal dysfunction and controls sialorrhea resulting from neuroleptic medication.

■ CONTRAINDICATIONS: Narrow-angle glaucoma, asthma, obstruction of the genitourinary or GI tract, severe ulcerative colitis, or known hypersensitivity to this drug prohibits its use.

■ ADVERSE EFFECTS: Among the more serious adverse effects are confusion, disorientation, blurred vision, central nervous system effects, tachycardia, dry mouth, decreased sweating, and hypersensitivity reactions.

prodromal /-drō″məl/ [Gk, *pro,* before, *dromos,* course], pertaining to early symptoms that may mark the onset of a disease.

prodromal labor [Gk, *prodromos,* running before; L, *labor,* work], the early period in parturition before uterine contractions become forceful and frequent enough to result in progressive dilation of the uterine cervix.

prodromal myopia, an optical condition in which the ability to do close work without eyeglasses returns, but usually as a symptom of developing cataracts. Also called **myopic shift.**

prodromal phase, a clear deterioration in function before the active phase of a mental disturbance. It is not caused by a disorder in mood or a psychoactive substance and includes some residual phase symptoms.

prodromal rash, a rash that precedes a potentially more serious skin eruption caused by an infectious disease.

prodromal symptom [Gk, *pro + dromos,* course, *symptoma,* that which happens], a symptom that may be the first indication of the onset of a disease.

prodrome /prō″drōm/ [Gk, *prodromos,* running before], **1.** an early sign of a developing condition or disease. **2.** the earliest phase of a developing condition or disease. Many infectious diseases such as chickenpox or measles are most contagious during the prodromal period. **–prodromal,** *adj.*

prodrug /prō′drug/, an inactive or partially active drug that is metabolically changed in the body to an active drug.

product evaluation committee /prod′əkt/, a hospital committee composed of medical, nursing, purchasing, and administrative staff members whose purpose is to evaluate health care–related products and advise on their procurement. Also called **new product evaluation committee.**

productive cough /prəduk′tiv/ [L, *producere* + AS, *cohhetan,* to cough], a sudden, noisy expulsion of air from the lungs that effectively removes sputum from the respiratory tract and helps clear the airways, permitting air to reach the alveoli. Coughing is stimulated by irritation or inflammation of the respiratory tract, which is caused most frequently by infection or sinus drainage secondary to rhinitis. Deep breathing, with contraction of the diaphragm and intercostal muscles and forceful exhalation, promotes productive coughing in patients with respiratory infections. Mucolytic agents liquefy mucus in the respiratory tract so that it can be raised and expectorated more easily. Atropine and other anticholinergic drugs decrease pulmonary secretions. Also called **moist cough, wet cough.** See also **nonproductive cough.**

-profen, suffix for ibuprofen-type antiinflammatory or analgesic substances.

Profenal, an oral nonsteroidal antiinflammatory analgesic. Brand name for **suprofen.**

professional corporation (PC) /prəfesh″ənəl/ [L, *professio,* profession], a corporation formed according to the law of a particular state for the purpose of delivering a professional service. In some states corporations may not practice law, medicine, surgery, or dentistry; in some states nurses may form or be partners in a professional corporation. According to the laws of the various states, professional corporations may offer legal and tax benefits to the members of the corporation.

professional liability, the legal obligation of health care professionals or their insurers to compensate patients for injury or suffering caused by acts of omission or commission by the professionals. Professional liability is a better characterization of the responsibility of all professionals to their patients than is the concept of malpractice, but the idea of professional liability is central to malpractice.

professional network, (in psychiatric nursing) the network of professional resources available to support the psychiatric outpatient in the community. The network may include a therapist, hospital day treatment program, social work agency, and other agencies.

professional organization, an organization whose members share a professional status, created to deal with issues of concern to the professional group or groups involved.

Professional Standards Review Organization (PSRO), an organization formed under the U.S. Social Security Act Amendments of 1972 to review the services provided under Medicare, Medicaid, and Maternal Child Health programs. Review is conducted by physicians to ascertain the need for the program and to ensure that it is carried out in accord with certain criteria, norms, and standards and, in institutional situations, in a proper setting.

profibrinolysin. See **fibrinogen.**

profile /prō′fīl/ [L, *profilare,* to outline], a short sketch, diagram, or summary relating to a person or thing.

profunda /prōfun″də/ [L, *profundus,* deep], pertaining to structures, mainly blood vessels, that are deeply embedded in tissues.

profunda femoris artery. See **deep artery of the thigh.**

profuse sweat /prəfyoos″/ [L, *profundere,* to pour out; AS, *swaetan*], excessive perspiration. Also called **diaphoresis.**

progenital herpes, herpes genitalis.

progenitive /-jen″itiv/ [Gk, *pro,* before, *genein,* to produce], capable of producing offspring; reproductive.

progenitor /-jen″itər/ [Gk, *pro + genein*], **1.** a parent or ancestor. **2.** someone or something that begets or creates.

progeny /proj″ənē/ [L, *progenies*], **1.** offspring; an individual or organism resulting from a particular mating. **2.** the descendants of a known or common ancestor.

progeria /prōjir″ē·ə/ [Gk, *pro + geras,* old age], an abnormal congenital condition characterized by premature aging, appearance in childhood of gray hair and wrinkled skin, small stature, absence of pubic and facial hair, and posture and habitus of an aged person. Death usually occurs before 20 years of age. Also called **Hutchinson-Gilford syndrome.** Compare **infantilism.**

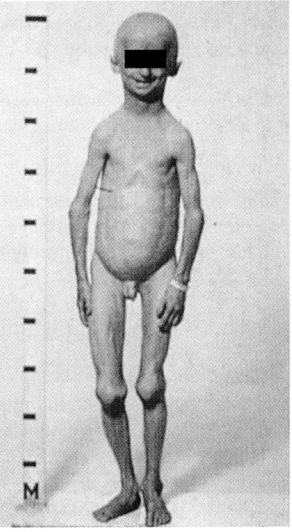

Individual with characteristic appearance of progeria
(Patton and Thibodeau, 2010)

progestagen. See **progestogen.**

progestagen-only contraceptive, an oral contraceptive consisting only of a small dose of a progestational agent to be taken every day.

progestational /prō′jestā″shənəl/ [Gk, *pro* + L, *gestare,* to bear], pertaining to a drug with effects similar to those of progesterone, the hormone produced by the corpus luteum and adrenal cortex during the luteal phase of the menstrual cycle that prepares the uterus for reception of the fertilized ovum. Natural and synthetic preparations of progesterone and its derivative medroxyprogesterone acetate are used in the treatment of secondary amenorrhea and abnormal uterine bleeding. Progestational compounds, such as norethindrone and norgestrel, are constituents of oral contraceptives. The use of progestins to prevent habitual or threatened abortion is no longer recommended.

progestational agent [L, *pro* + *gestare,* to bear, *agere,* to do], any chemical having the same action as progesterone produced by the corpus luteum and the placenta.

progestational phase. See **secretory phase.**

progesterone /prəjes″tərōn/, a natural progestational hormone.

■ INDICATIONS: It is used to prevent endometrial hyperplasia in nonhysterectomized, postmenopausal women who are receiving conjugated estrogen tablets; to treat dysfunctional uterine bleeding caused by hormonal imbalances; as a contraceptive in intrauterine devices; and in intravaginal gel for women using assisted reproductive technology.

■ CONTRAINDICATIONS: Thrombophlebitis, liver dysfunction, breast cancer, undiagnosed uterine bleeding, pregnancy, previous stroke, or hypersensitivity to this drug prohibits its use.

■ ADVERSE EFFECTS: Among the more serious adverse reactions are pain at the site of injection, breast pain, dizziness, headache, fatigue, emotional lability, abdominal pain, muscle weakness, catabolic effects, and electrolyte disturbances.

progesterone assay, a blood test that is useful in documenting whether ovulation has occurred and, if so, when. This information may be used to help women with difficulty becoming pregnant. Repeated assays may also be used to monitor the status of the placenta in high-risk pregnancy and progesterone supplementation in patients with an inadequate luteal phase.

progesterone receptor assay, a tumor-specimen analysis used primarily to determine the prognosis and treatment of breast cancer.

progestin /-jes″tin/, **1.** progesterone. **2.** any of a group of hormones, natural or synthetic, secreted by the corpus luteum, placenta, or adrenal cortex that have a progesterone-like effect on the uterine endometrial lining to prepare it for implantation of the blastocyst.

progestogen /-jes″təjən/, any natural or synthetic progestational hormone. Also called **progestin.** Also spelled **progestagen.**

proglottid /prōglot″id/ [Gk, *pro* + *glossa,* tongue], a sexual segment of an adult tapeworm, containing both male and female reproductive organs. Each mature segment is shed and produces additional tapeworms.

prognathism /prog″nəthiz′əm/ [Gk, *pro* + *gnathos,* jaw], an abnormal facial configuration in which one or both jaws project forward. It may be real or imaginary, depending on anatomical and developmental factors. Real prognathism may exist when both the mandible and the maxilla increase in length or when the maxillary length is normal and the mandibular length increases excessively. Imaginary prognathism may exist when the maxilla is underdeveloped and the mandibular length is normal. See **Angle's classification of malocclusion,** class III. *−prognathic, adj.*

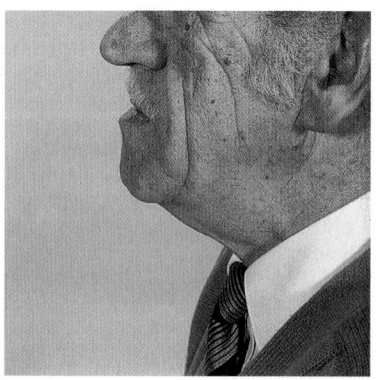

Prognathism *(Belchetz and Hammond, 2003)*

prognosis /prognō″sis/ [Gk, *pro* + *gnosis,* knowledge], a prediction of the probable outcome of a disease based on the condition of the person and the usual course of the disease as observed in similar situations.

prognostic /prognos″tik/ [Gk, *pro* + *gnosis,* knowledge], pertaining to signs and symptoms that may indicate the outcome of an illness or injury.

prognosticate /prognos″tikāt/ [Gk, *pro,* before, *gnosis,* knowledge], to forecast or predict from facts, present indications, or signs, such as the course a disease may take and the final outcome.

prognostic indicators, factors, such as staging, tumor type, and laboratory studies, that may indicate treatment effectiveness and outcomes.

Prograf, an immunosuppressive drug. Brand name for **tacrolimus.**

program /prō″grəm/ [Gk, *pro* + *gramma,* record], a sequence of instructions, written in a computer programming language, that controls the functions of a computer.

program documentation. See **documentation.**

programmable pacemaker /-gram″əbəl/ [Gk, *pro* + *graphein,* to record; L, *passus,* step; ME, *maken*], an electronic pacemaker with multiple settings that can be modified after implantation.

programmed aging theory, 1. a theory of aging that states that life expectancy is predetermined and timed for individual species, with cells programmed to divide a certain number of times. Functional changes in the cells cause aging of the cells and thus the organism. **2.** any of various theories of aging based on timed functional changes. See **theories of aging.**

programmed pacing, control of the heart rate by a programmable pacemaker. See also **pacing.**

programmer /prō″grəmər/, a person skilled in writing or coding computer programs.

programming language. See **language.**

Program of All-inclusive Care of the Elderly (PACE) /pās/, a U.S. federally supported program of comprehensive care with a primary objective of keeping clients in the community as long as medically, socially, and financially possible. It uses a team approach in which professionals assess client needs, develop a care plan, integrate primary care and other services, and arrange for implementation of services. PACE is sponsored by one or more facilities and community groups and receives funds from Medicare, Medicaid, and private donations. A forerunner of PACE is the San Francisco On Lok program, which provides comprehensive adult day care, custodial or personal care, drug treatment, dentistry, and housekeeping for older persons who have a level of impairment that usually requires admission to a nursing facility.

progravid /-grav″id/ [L, *pro* + *gravid,* pregnant], before pregnancy.

progression /-gresh″ən/, a carcinogenic process whereby cells genetically altered by initiators undergo a second (nongenetic) cell expansion that allows uncontrollable growth.

progressive /-gres″iv/ [L, *progredi,* to advance], describing the course of a disease or condition in which the characteristic signs and symptoms become more prominent and severe, such as progressive muscular atrophy.

progressive assistive exercise, an exercise designed to improve the strength of a muscle group progressively by gradually decreasing assistance required of a therapist for an active motion, thereby increasing the patient's active effort. See also **progressive resistance exercise.**

progressive bulbar atrophy. See **progressive bulbar palsy.**

progressive bulbar palsy [L, *progredi,* to advance], a motor neuron disease affecting the brainstem, characterized by weakness of the laryngeal, pharyngeal, tongue, and facial muscles. The patient experiences progressive dysarthria and dysphagia. The muscular weaknesses increase the risk for choking and aspiration pneumonia. Emotional lability is a component of the disease. Also called **progressive bulbar atrophy.**

progressive bulbar paralysis, now called **progressive bulbar palsy.**

progressive diaphyseal dysplasia. Also called **Camurati-Engelmann disease.**

progressive familial intrahepatic cholestasis, an autosomal-recessive type of intrahepatic cholestasis of hepatocellular origin. Affected children often develop cirrhosis by age 10 and die during adolescence. At least three different genetic defects cause varieties of the disease. Also called **Byler disease.**

progressive histoplasmosis. See **histoplasmosis.**

progressive interstitial hypertrophic neuropathy. See **Déjérine-Sottas disease.**

progressive myonecrosis. See **myonecrosis.**

progressive myopia [L, *progredi* + Gk, *myops,* nearsighted], a condition in which myopia increases, continuing into adulthood.

progressive ophthalmoplegia [L, *progredi*], a form of ocular muscle paralysis that usually begins with ptosis and gradually involves all of the extraocular muscles.

progressive osseous heteroplasia. See **osteodermia.**

progressive ossifying myositis. See **myositis ossificans progressiva.**

progressive patient care, a system of care in which patients are placed in units on the basis of their needs for care as determined by the degree of illness rather than on the basis of a medical specialty. The usual levels or stages of progressive patient care are intensive care, intermediate care, and minimal care.

progressive relaxation, a technique for combating tension and anxiety by systematically tensing and relaxing muscle groups.

progressive resistance exercise (PRE), a method of increasing the strength of a weak or injured muscle by gradually increasing the resistance against which the muscle works, such as by using graduated weights. Also called **graduated resistance exercise.** See also **active resistance exercise, DeLorme technique, progressive assistive exercise.**

progressive scan mode, a method of cathode ray tube scanning in which all of the lines are scanned successively (in interlaced scanning, the odd lines are scanned first and then the even lines).

progressive spinal muscular atrophy of infants. See **Werdnig-Hoffmann disease.**

progressive subcortical encephalopathy. See **Schilder disease.**

progressive supranuclear palsy [L, *supra,* above, *nucleus,* nut kernel; Gk, *paralyein*], a rare progressive neurological disorder of unknown cause occurring in middle age, more often in men. It is characterized by paralysis of eye muscles, ataxia, neck and trunk rigidity, pseudobulbar palsy, and parkinsonian facies. Dementia and inappropriate emotional responses also are common. Treatment usually includes the antiparkinsonian drug levodopa for control of extrapyramidal symptoms. Also called **Steele-Richardson-Olszewski syndrome.** See also **Parkinson disease.**

progressive systemic sclerosis. See **scleroderma.**

progress notes [L, *progredi* + *nota,* mark], (in the patient record) notes made by a nurse, physician, social worker, physical therapist, and other health care professionals that describe the patient's condition and the treatment given or planned. Progress notes may follow the problem-oriented medical record format. The physician's progress notes usually focus on the medical or therapeutic aspects of the patient's condition and care. The nurse's progress notes, although recording the medical conditions of the patient, usually focus on the objectives stated in the nursing care plan. These objectives may include responses to prescribed treatments, the ability to perform activities of daily living, and acceptance or understanding of a particular condition or treatment. Progress notes in an in-hospital setting are recorded daily; those in a clinic or office setting are usually preceded by an episodic or interval history and are recorded as accounts of each visit.

proguanil /progwahn″il/, an antimalarial agent. Its use in the United States is limited because of the development of drug-resistant malarial parasites. The drug is still used effectively, however, in combination with atovaquone in the prevention of *Plasmodium falciparum* malaria.

proinsulin /prō·in″s(y)əlin/ [L, *pro* + *insula,* island], a single-chain peptide molecule that is a precursor of insulin.

projectile vomiting /-jek″til/, expulsive vomiting that is extremely forceful, with vomitus expelled some distance.

projection /-jek″shən/ [L, *projectio,* thrown forward], **1.** a protuberance; anything that thrusts or juts outward. **2.** the act of perceiving an idea or thought as an objective reality. **3.** (in psychology) an unconscious defense mechanism by which an individual attributes his or her own unacceptable traits, ideas, or impulses to another. It is noted in some stages of schizophrenia.

projection reconstruction imaging, the techniques used in magnetic resonance (MR) imaging to obtain a cross-sectional image of an object. Such an image is computer-reconstructed from a series of MR profiles recorded all around an object by rotating the gradient field superimposed on the static magnetic field.

projective test /-jek″tiv/ [L, *projectio,* thrown forward], a kind of diagnostic, psychological, or personality test that uses unstructured or ambiguous stimuli, such as inkblots, a series of pictures, abstract patterns, or incomplete sentences, to elicit responses that reflect a projection of various aspects of the individual's personality. See also **Rorschach test.**

prokaryocyte /prōker″ē·əsīt′/ [Gk, *protos,* first, *karyon,* nut, *kytos,* cell], a cell without a true nucleus and with nuclear material scattered throughout the cytoplasm. Prokaryocytic organisms (Procaryotae) include bacteria, mycoplasmas, actinomycetes, and blue-green algae. Also spelled **procaryocyte.** Compare **eukaryocyte.**

prokaryon /prōker″ē·on/ [Gk, *protos* + *karyon,* nut], a region within a bacterial cell that contains most of the bacterial DNA. It is not separated from the rest of the cell by a membrane. Also spelled **procaryon.** Compare **eukaryon.**

prokaryosis /-ker′ē·ō″sis/ [Gk, *protos + karyon + osis,* condition], the condition of having a prokaryon. Also spelled **procaryosis.** Compare **eukaryosis.**

prokaryote /prōker″ē·ōt/ [Gk, *protos + karyon*], *adj.,* a unicellular organism that does not contain a true nucleus surrounded by a double membrane; a bacterium. Division usually occurs through simple fission. Also spelled **procaryote.** Compare **eukaryote.** –*prokaryotic, adj.*

prokaryotic cell, a cell without a true nucleus. See also **cell.**

prokinetic /pro″kinet′ik/, stimulating movement or motility, such as a drug that promotes GI motility. See **gastrokinetic drugs.**

prolactin (PRL) /prōlak″tin/ [Gk, *pro,* before, *lac,* milk], a hormone produced and secreted into the bloodstream by the anterior pituitary gland. Prolactin stimulates the development and growth of the mammary glands after the glands have been prepared by estrogen, progesterone, thyroxine, insulin, growth hormone, glucocorticoids, and human placental lactogen. After parturition, prolactin, together with glucocorticoids, is essential for the initiation and maintenance of milk production. Prolactin synthesis and release from the pituitary are mediated by the central nervous system in response to suckling by the infant. When suckling or its mechanical equivalent ceases, prolactin secretion slows and milk production ceases. Prolactin has no known function in human males. Prolactin is similar to growth hormone in its chemical structure. Prolactin excess is seen with prolactin-secreting pituitary tumors in both sexes. Also called **lactogenic hormone.**

prolactin levels test, a blood test that is helpful for monitoring the disease activity of pituitary adenomas.

prolapse /prō″laps, prōlaps″/ [L, *prolapsus,* falling], the dropping, falling, sinking, or sliding of an organ from its normal position or location in the body, such as a prolapsed uterus or rectum.

prolapsed cord /prōlapst/, an umbilical cord that protrudes beside or ahead of the presenting part of the fetus.

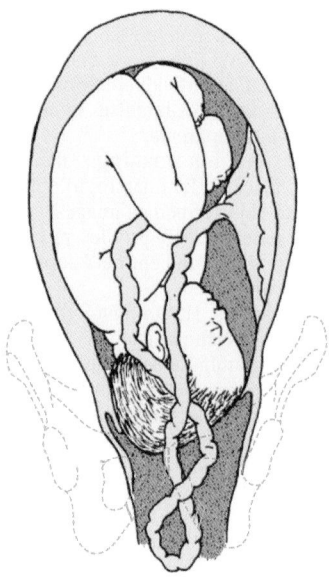

Prolapsed cord *(Silvestri, 2011)*

prolapsed hemorrhoid [L, *prolapsus,* falling; Gk, *haimorrhois,* a vein that loses blood], an internal hemorrhoid that protrudes through the anal orifice.

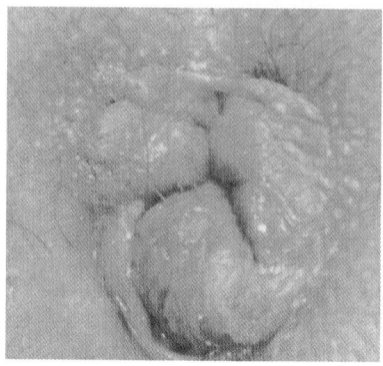

Prolapsed hemorrhoids *(Courtesy Gershon Efron, M.D., Sinai Hospital of Baltimore)*

prolapsed ureterocele, an intravesical ureterocele that extends beyond the bladder neck down into the urethra, usually seen in females.

prolapse of anus [L, *prolapsus,* falling, *anus*], the protrusion of the mucous membrane of the anus through the external sphincter.

prolapse of rectum [L, *prolapsus,* falling, *rectus,* straight], a protrusion of the mucous membrane of the lower part of the rectum through the anal orifice.

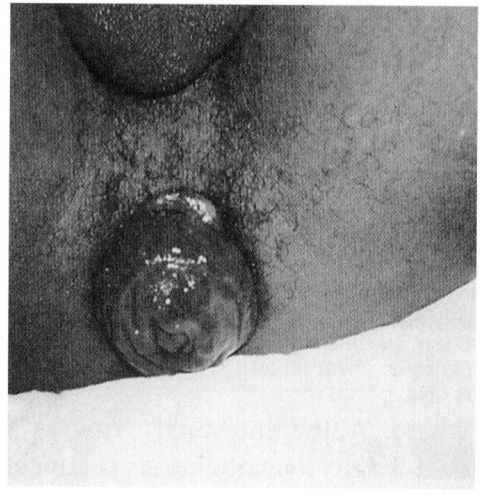

Prolapse of the rectum *(Seidel, 2003/Courtesy Gershon Efron, M.D., Sinai Hospital of Baltimore)*

prolapse of uterus [L, *prolapsus,* falling, *uterus,* womb], the descent of the uterine cervix into the vagina, partly into the vagina, or outside the vagina.

Prolastin, alpha₁-antitrypsin. Brand name for *alpha₁-proteinase inhibitor, human.*

proliferation /-lif′ərā″shən/ [L, *proles,* offspring, *ferre,* to bear], the reproduction or multiplication of similar forms. The term is usually applied to increases of cells or cysts. –*proliferative,* **prolific,** *adj.,* –*proliferate, v.*

proliferation inhibiting factor, a lymphokine that restricts cell division in tissue cultures.

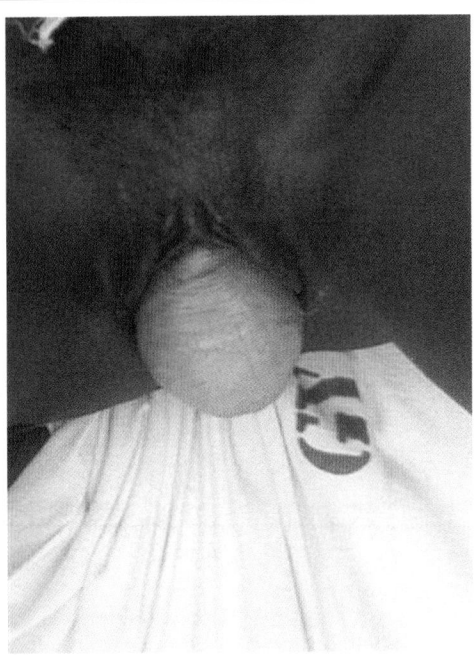

Uterine prolapse *(Dim et al, 2008)*

proliferative-follicular phase.   See **proliferative phase.**

proliferative glomerulonephritis,   any of various types of glomerulonephritis accompanied by proliferation of endothelial or mesangial cells in the glomeruli. Kinds include **acute glomerulonephritis,** *diffuse glomerulonephritis,* **membranoproliferative glomerulonephritis,** *mesangial proliferative glomerulonephritis, rapidly progressive glomerulonephritis.*

proliferative phase /-lif″ərətiv/,   the phase of the menstrual cycle after menstruation. Under the influence of follicle-stimulating hormone from the pituitary, the ovary produces increasing amounts of estrogen, causing the lining of the uterus to become dense and richly vascular. The phase is terminated by rupture of a mature follicle and subsequent ovulation. Also called **proliferative-follicular phase.** Compare **menstrual phase, secretory phase.**

prolific /lif″ik/   [L, *proles,* offspring, *ferre,* to bear],   highly productive.

proline (Pro) /prō″lēn/,   a nonessential amino acid found in many proteins of the body, particularly collagen. See also **amino acid, protein.**

prolonged gestation /-longd″/   [L, *prolongare,* to lengthen, *gestare,* to bear],   a pregnancy that lasts longer than the usual period of 41 weeks.

prolonged release   [Gk, *pro,* before, *longus,* long],   a term applied to a drug that is designed to deliver a dose of a medication over an extended period. The most common device for this purpose is a soft, soluble capsule containing minute pellets of the drug for release at different rates in the GI tract, depending on the thickness and nature of the oil, fat, wax, or resin coating on the pellets. Another system consists of a porous plastic carrier impregnated with the drug and a surfactant to facilitate the entry of GI fluids that slowly leach out of the drug. Ion exchange resins that bind to drugs and liquids containing suspensions of slow-release drug granules are also used to provide medication over an extended period. Various mechanisms and vehicles have also been developed to prolong the release of drugs after injection. Also called **timed release.**

Proloprim,   an antibacterial. Brand name for **trimethoprim.**

PROM,   abbreviation for **passive range of motion.**

promastigote /prōmas″tigōt/,   the flagellate stage of a trypanosome. It is found in the insect intermediate host or in culture.

promethazine hydrochloride /-meth″əzēn/,   a phenothiazine antiemetic, antihistamine, and sedative.

■ INDICATIONS: It is prescribed in the treatment of motion sickness, nausea, rhinitis, itching, and skin rash and as an adjunct to anesthesia and pain control.

■ CONTRAINDICATIONS: Known hypersensitivity to this drug or to other phenothiazines or severe central nervous system depression or coma prohibits its use.

■ ADVERSE EFFECTS: Drowsiness, hypotension, and dry mouth are the most common adverse effects.

promethium (Pm) /-mē″thē·əm/   [L, *Prometheus,* mythic character who gave fire to humans],   a radioactive rare earth metallic element. Its atomic number is 61; its atomic mass is 145.

prominence /prom″inəns/   [L, *prominentia,* sticking out],   any protuberance or projection of a structural feature.

promontory of the sacrum /prom″əntôr′ē/   [L, *promontorium,* headland],   the superior projecting part of the sacrum at its junction with the L5 vertebra.

promoter /-mō″tər/   [L, *promovere,* to move forward],   **1.** a DNA sequence that initiates transcription of the genetic code. **2.** a cocarcinogen that encourages cells altered by initiators to reproduce more rapidly than normal, increasing the probability of malignant transformation. Examples include chlorophenothane (DDT), phenobarbital, saccharin, sunlight, and some chemicals in cigarette smoke. The effects of promoters are sometimes reversible.

prompt insulin zinc suspension   [L, *promptus,* ready],   a fast-acting noncrystalline semilente insulin prescribed in the treatment of diabetes mellitus when a prompt, intense, and short-acting response is desired. It is only slightly slower-acting than insulin injection. See also **short-acting insulin.**

promyelocyte /prōmī″ələsīt′/,   precursor in the bone marrow myelocytic series that is intermediate in development between a myeloblast and a myelocyte. The cytoplasm contains prominent primary granules. Promyelocytes appear in peripheral blood in acute promyelocytic leukemia.

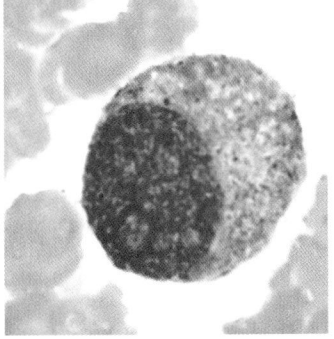

Promyelocyte *(Carr and Rodak, 2008)*

pronation /prōnā″shən/   [L, *pronare,* to bend forward],   **1.** assumption of a prone position, one in which the ventral surface of the body faces downward. **2.** (of the arm) the rotation of the forearm so that the palm of the hand faces downward or backward. **3.** (of the foot) the lowering of the medial edge of the foot by turning it outward and through abduction in the tarsal and metatarsal joints. –*pronate, v.*

P

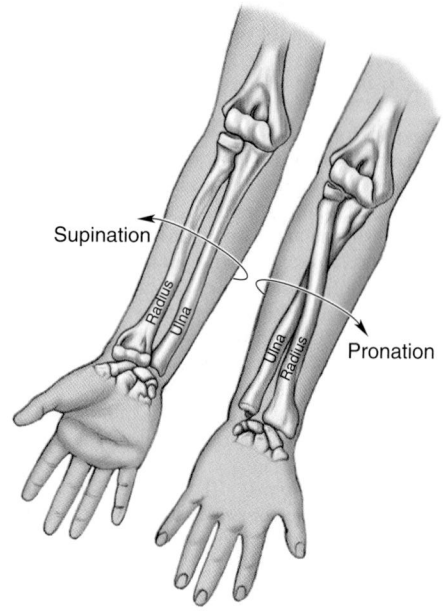

Pronation *(Herlihy, 2014)*

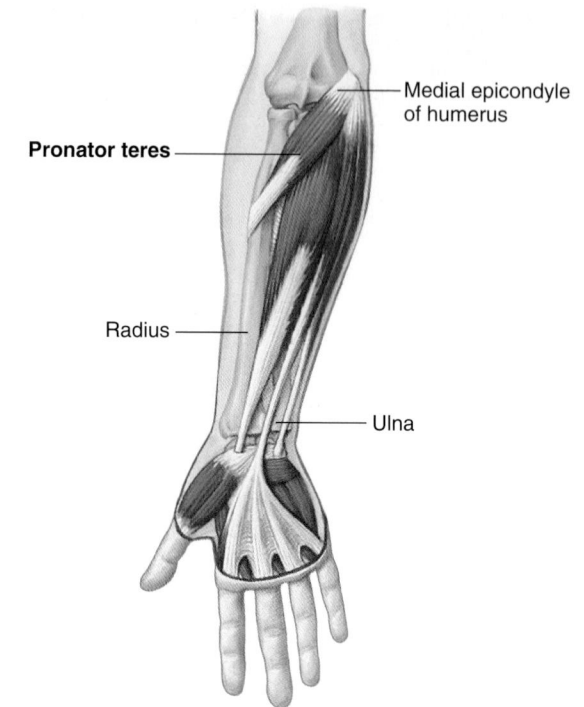

Pronator teres *(Patton and Thibodeau, 2016)*

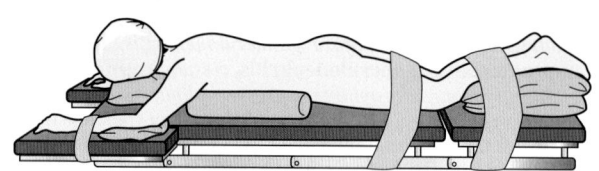

Prone position *(Phillips, 2013)*

pronator quadratus /prōnā″tər/,   a muscle of the forearm. It originates on the distal fourth of the anterior surface and border of the ulna and inserts onto the distal fourth of the anterior surface of the radius. It functions to pronate the forearm and hand.

pronator reflex [L, *pronare* + *reflectere,* to bend back],   a reflex elicited by holding the patient's hand vertically and tapping the distal end of the radius or ulna, resulting in pronation of the forearm. Hyperactivity of the reflex may be seen with lesions of the pyramidal system above the level of the sixth cervical nerve root. Also called **ulnar reflex.**

pronator syndrome [L, *pronare,* to bend forward; Gk, *syn,* together, *dromos,* course],   the compression of the median nerve in the forearm between the two heads of the pronator teres muscle.

pronator teres /ter″əs/,   a superficial muscle of the forearm, arising from a humeral and an ulnar head and ending in a flat tendon that inserts into the radius. It functions to pronate the hand. Compare **flexor carpi radialis, flexor carpi ulnaris, flexor digitorum superficialis, palmaris longus.**

prone /prōn/   [L, *pronare,* to bend forward],   **1.** having a tendency or inclination. **2.** (of the body) being in horizontal position when lying face downward. Also called **ventral recumbent.** Compare **supine.**

proneness profile /prōn″nəs/   [L, *pronare,* to bend forward, *profilare,* to outline],   a screening process that evaluates the probability of developmental problems in the early years of a child's life. Screening ideally begins during prenatal care and continues after birth. Several of the variables in the proneness profile that appear to be significant in selecting the infants who are at risk are the indicators of perinatal health of the mother and infant, especially complications of pregnancy, delivery, the neonatal period, and the puerperium; characteristics of the mother, especially her temperament, educational level, perception of the life situation, and perception of the infant; characteristics of the infant, including alertness, activity pattern, and responsiveness; and behaviors of the infant and caregiver as they interact. The proneness profile is followed by a developmental profile that assesses the current status of the infant and caregiver. Three areas to be considered are characteristics of the infant, including adaptation and response to the environment, the ability to give interpretable cues, and the developmental progress as compared with established norms; characteristics of the caregiver, including adaptation to the new infant, sensitivity to cues from the infant, and techniques for relieving distress; and the healthful quality of the environment, including health, safety, comfort, and stimulation.

prone-on-elbows,   a body position in which the person rests the upper part of the body on the elbows while lying face down. The position is used as an initial rehabilitation exercise in training a person with a cerebellar dysfunction to achieve various goals. In this position, the person can practice weight shifting through the hips to a quadruped position without the risk of falling from a standing position.

pronephric.   See **pronephros.**

pronephric duct /-nef″rik/   [Gk, *pro,* before, *nephros,* kidney; L, *ducere,* to lead],   one of the paired ducts that connect the tubules of each of the pronephros with the cloaca in the early developing vertebrate embryo. They later become the functional mesonephric ducts. Also called **archinephric canal, archinephric duct.**

pronephric tubule, any of the segmentally arranged excretory units of the pronephros in the early developing vertebrate embryo. The tubules open into the pronephric duct and communicate with the coelom through a nephrostoma. In humans and the higher vertebrates, the tubules are present only in vestigial form; in lower animals they are functional.

pronephros /-nef″rəs/ *pl.* *pronephroi* [Gk, *pro* + *nephros,* kidney], the earliest and simplest kind of excretory organ in the developing vertebrate embryo. In humans and other mammals the structure is nonfunctional. Also called **archinephron, head kidney,** *pronephron.* See also **mesonephros, metanephros.** –**pronephric,** *adj.*

prone posture [L, *pronare,* to bend forward, *ponere,* to place], a posture assumed by lying flat with the face forward in response to certain disorders of the spine or viscera.

pronucleus /-noo″klē·əs/ *pl.* *pronuclei* [Gk, *pro* + L, *nucleus,* nut kernel], the nucleus of an ovum or a spermatozoon after fertilization but before fusion of the chromosomes to form the nucleus of the zygote. Each pronucleus contains the haploid number of chromosomes, is larger than the normal nucleus, and is diffuse in appearance. The pronucleus of the ovum is formed only after it has completed its second meiotic division and the second polar body has formed, which occur after the spermatozoon has penetrated. It then loses its nuclear envelope, releasing the chromosomes so that synapsis with the chromosomes of the male pronucleus, which is contained in the head of the spermatozoon, can occur. Also called **germinal nucleus, germ nucleus.** See also **oogenesis, spermatogenesis.**

propagation /prop′əgā″shən/ [L, *propagare,* to generate], the process of increasing or causing to increase.

propanoic acid. See **propionic acid.**

2-propanol. See **isopropyl alcohol.**

2-propanone. See **acetone.**

propantheline bromide /-pan″thəlēn/, an anticholinergic/antispasmodic.

■ INDICATIONS: It is prescribed as an adjunct in peptic ulcer therapy, irritable bowel syndrome, and pancreatitis and for spasm of the ureters or urinary bladder.

■ CONTRAINDICATIONS: Narrow-angle glaucoma, asthma, obstruction of the genitourinary or GI tract, severe ulcerative colitis, megacolon, myasthenia gravis, or known hypersensitivity to this drug prohibits its use.

■ ADVERSE EFFECTS: Among the more serious adverse effects are blurred vision, central nervous system effects, tachycardia, dry mouth, decreased sweating, and hypersensitivity reactions.

proparacaine hydrochloride /prōper″əkān/, a rapid-acting topical anesthetic of the amide family. Also called **proxymetacaine.**

■ INDICATIONS: It is used for tonometry, gonioscopy, removal of foreign objects from the eye, and other minor ophthalmological procedures and preoperatively for major eye surgery. One drop gives 15 minutes of optic anesthesia.

■ CONTRAINDICATIONS: Proparacaine hydrochloride is not administered to individuals with cardiac disease, hyperthyroidism, or multiple allergies. People given the drug should be warned not to touch their eyes until the anesthetic has worn off.

■ ADVERSE EFFECTS: Adverse optic effects may occur with proparacaine, but systemic reactions are rare. Prolonged use may injure the eye.

properidin system. See **alternative pathway of complement activation.**

prophase /prō″fāz/ [Gk, *pro* + *phasis,* appearance], the first of four stages of nuclear division in mitosis and in each of the two divisions of meiosis. In mitosis the chromosomes progressively shorten and thicken to form individually recognizable elongated double structures composed of two chromatids held together by a centromere. The nucleolus and nuclear membrane disappear, the spindle and polar bodies are formed, and the chromosomes begin to migrate toward the midplane of the developing spindle. In the first meiotic division, prophase is complex and subdivided into five stages: leptotene, zygotene, pachytene, diplotene, and diakinesis. In the second meiotic division the same processes occur as in mitotic prophase. See also **anaphase, interphase, meiosis, metaphase, mitosis, telophase.**

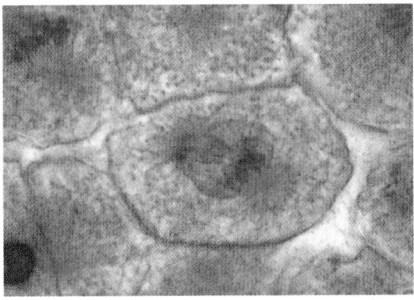

Prophase (© Ed Reschke; Used with permission)

prophylactic /prō′filak″tik/ [Gk, *prophylax,* advance guard], **1.** *adj.,* preventing the spread of disease. –*prophylactically, adv.* **2.** *n.,* an agent that prevents the spread of disease. **3.** *n.,* a popular name for a condom. See also **condom.**

prophylactic forceps. See **low forceps.**

prophylactic odontomy, (in dentistry) the surgical removal of harmful pits and fissures in the posterior primary and secondary molars to prevent the formation of caries in those areas.

prophylactic treatment. See **preventive treatment.**

prophylaxis /prō′filak″sis/ [Gk, *prophylax,* advance guard], prevention of or protection against disease, often involving the use of a biological, chemical, or mechanical agent to destroy or prevent the entry of infectious organisms.

Propionibacterium /prō′pē·on′ēbaktir′ē·əm/ [Gk, *pro* + *pion,* fat, *bakterion,* small rod], a genus of nonmotile, anaerobic, gram-positive bacteria found on the skin of humans, in the intestinal tract of humans and animals, and in dairy products. *Propionibacterium acnes* is common in acne pustules. Formerly called *Corynebacterium acnes.*

propionic acid /prō′pē·on′ik/, an aliphatic carboxylic acid that is a chemical component of sweat. It can be formed by fermentation of sugars by several species of bacteria. Also called **propanoic acid.**

propionic acidemia /prō′pē·on′ikas′idē″mē·ə/ [Gk, *pro* + *pion,* fat; L, *acidus,* sour; Gk, *haima,* blood], a rare inherited metabolic defect caused by the failure of the body to metabolize the amino acids valine, isoleucine, and methionine, characterized by lethargy, cognitive impairment, and delayed motor development. Acidosis results from the accumulation of propionic acid in the body.

propionic fermentation [Gk, *pro* + *pion* + L, *fermentare,* to cause to ferment], the production of propionic acid by the action of certain bacteria on sugars or lactic acid.

P

Proplex T, brand name for the human clotting factor IX complex.

propofol /pro′pah-fol/, a short-acting sedative and hypnotic used as a general anesthetic or sedative agent; it is administered intravenously.

proportional /prəpôr″shənəl/, pertaining to the relationship between two quantities when a fractional variation of one is always accompanied by the same fractional change in the other.

proportional gas detector, a device for measuring alpha and beta forms of radioactivity.

proportional mortality [L, *pro* + *portio,* part, *mortalis,* subject to death], a statistical method of relating the number of deaths from a particular condition to all deaths within the same population group for the same period.

proposition /prop′əzish″ən/ [L, *proponere,* to place forward], **1.** *n.,* a statement of a truth to be demonstrated or an operation to be performed. **2.** *v.,* to bring forward or offer for consideration, acceptance, or adoption.

propositus /prōpoz″itəs/ [L, *proponere,* to place forward], a person from whom a genealogical lineage is traced, as is done to discover the pattern of inheritance of a familial disease or a physical trait. Also called **proband.**

propoxyphene hydrochloride, an analgesic removed from the worldwide market because of serious adverse effects.

propranolol hydrochloride /-pran″əlol/, a nonselective beta-adrenergic receptor blocking agent.
- INDICATIONS: It is prescribed in the treatment of hypertension, angina pectoris, catecholamine-induced cardiac arrhythmias, pheochromocytoma, essential tremor, and migraine headache and for various unlabeled uses such as treatment of anxiety and aggressive behavior.
- CONTRAINDICATIONS: Asthma, COPD, pulmonary edema, bradycardia, second or third degree heart block, congestive heart failure unless secondary to a tachyarrhythmia treatable with beta-blockers, pregnancy (especially second and third trimester), or known hypersensitivity to this drug prohibits its use.
- ADVERSE EFFECTS: Among the more serious adverse effects are heart failure, heart block, increased airway resistance, augmentation of hypoglycemic response, GI disturbances, and hypersensitivity reactions. Withdrawal syndrome has been observed in some patients.

proprietary /-prī′əter′ē/ [L, *proprietas,* property], **1.** pertaining to an institution or other organization that is operated for profit. **2.** pertaining to a product, such as a drug or device, that is made for profit.

proprietary drug. See **patent medicine, proprietary medicine.**

proprietary hospital, a hospital operated as a profit-making organization. Many proprietary hospitals are owned by physicians who operate them primarily for their own patients but also accept patients from other physicians. Some proprietary hospitals are owned by investor groups or large corporations.

proprietary medicine, any pharmaceutic preparation or medicinal substance that is protected from commercial competition because its ingredients or method of manufacture is kept secret or is protected by trademark or copyright.

proprioception /prō′prē-əsep″shən/ [L, *proprius,* one's own, *capere,* to take], sensation pertaining to stimuli originating from within the body related to spatial position and muscular activity or to the sensory receptors that they activate. Compare **exteroceptive, interoceptive.** See also **autotopagnosia.**

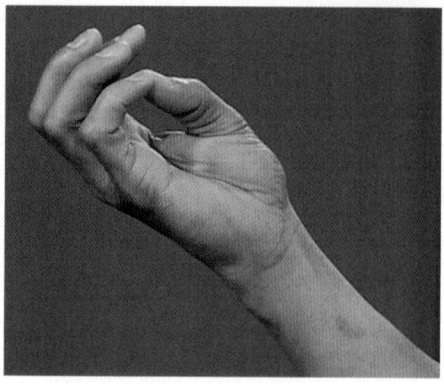

Assessment of proprioception *(Seidel et al, 2011)*

proprioceptive /prō′prē-əsep″tiv/ [L, *proprius,* one's own, *capere,* to take], pertaining to the sensations of body movements and awareness of posture, enabling the body to orient itself in space without visual clues.

proprioceptive feedback, muscle-joint input that provides information regarding one's body position.

proprioceptive impulse, a nerve impulse that originates with a sensory ending in muscle, joint, or tendon. Such impulses provide information to the central nervous system about the relative position of body parts.

proprioceptive neuromuscular facilitation (PNF), an activity, such as a therapeutic technique, that helps initiate a proprioceptive response in a person. An example is a slow rocking movement that relaxes an anxious person by stimulating vestibular and proprioceptive nerve receptors. Techniques are used to facilitate total body responses or selective postural extensors.

proprioceptive receptor. See **proprioceptor.**

proprioceptive reflex [L, *proprius* + *capere,* to take, *reflectere,* to bend back], any reflex initiated by stimulation of proprioceptors, such as the increase in respiratory rate and volume induced by impulses arising from muscles and joints during exercise.

proprioceptive sensation [L, *proprius* + *capere* + *sentire,* to feel], the feeling of body movement and position, including motion of the arms and legs, resulting from stimuli received by special sense organs in the muscles, tendons, joints, and inner ear. The stimuli may be produced by changes in muscle tension or stretching and reaction to the pull of gravity on the body.

proprioceptor /prō′prē-əsep″tər/ [L, *proprius* + *capere*], any sensory nerve ending, such as those located in muscles, tendons, joints, and the vestibular apparatus, that responds to stimuli originating from within the body related to movement and spatial position. Also called **proprioceptive receptor.** Compare **exteroceptor, interoceptor.** See also **mechanoreceptor.**

proptosis /proptō″sis/ [L, *pro* + *ptosis,* falling], a bulging, protrusion, or forward displacement of a body organ or area.

propulsion /-pul″shən/ [L, *propellere,* to drive forward], **1.** the process of pushing forward. **2.** the tendency of some patients, particularly those afflicted with nervous disorders, to push or fall forward while walking as their center of gravity is displaced.

propylene glycol (CH₃CHOHCH₂OH) /prop″ilēn/, a colorless viscous liquid used as a solvent in the preparation of certain medications. It also inhibits the growth of fungi and microorganisms and is used commercially as an antifreeze.

propylformic acid. See **butyric acid.**

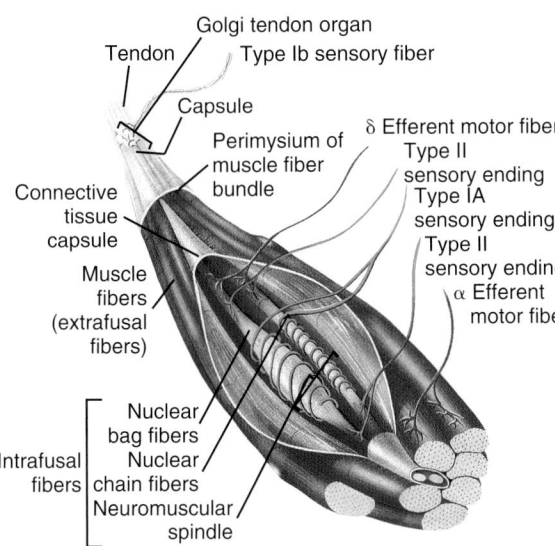

Proprioceptor *(Patton and Thibodeau, 2016)*

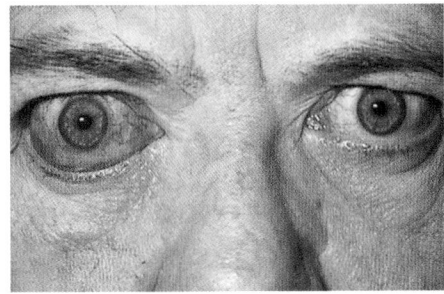

Proptosis of the right eye *(Kanski and Nischal, 1999)*

propylthiouracil /prō'pilthī"əyoor"əsil/, an inhibitor of thyroid hormone biosynthesis.

■ INDICATIONS: It is prescribed in treatment of hyperthyroidism and thyrotoxic crisis and in preparation for thyroidectomy.

■ CONTRAINDICATIONS: Mental depression, cold intolerance, or known hypersensitivity to this drug prohibits its use. Caution is recommended in pregnancy, in patients older than 40 years of age (can cause hypoprothrombinemia and bleeding), and in use in combination with other drugs that can cause agranulocytosis.

■ ADVERSE EFFECTS: Among the more serious adverse effects are GI distress, pruritus, and rashes. Rarely blood dyscrasia occurs.

pro re nata. See **prn, p.r.n..**

prorenin /prōren'in/, the inactive precursor of renin, stored in the juxtaglomerular cells of the kidney and activated by cleavage to renin. Also called *big renin.*

pros-. See **proso-, pros-.**

proscribe /prōskrīb"/, to forbid. −*proscriptive, adj.*

prosector /-sek"tər/ [L, *prosecare,* to cut off], a person who, under the supervision of a pathologist, performs gross dissections and prepares autopsy specimens for pathological examination.

prosencephalon /pros'ensef"əlon/ [Gk, *pro* + *enkephalon,* brain], the anterior primitive cerebral vesicle, comprising the diencephalon and telencephalon. Also called **forebrain.** Compare **mesencephalon.**

proso-, pros-, prefix meaning "forward, or anterior": *prosencephalon.*

Pro Sobee, a commercial milk-substitute formula that is prepared from a soy isolate base and is lactose free. It is prescribed for infants with galactosemia and people with lactose intolerance. It is supplemented with other nutrients, is fortified with vitamins and minerals, and is available in both powder and liquid forms. See also **Nutramigen.**

prosopalgia. See **trigeminal neuralgia.**

-prosopia, suffix meaning "(condition of the) face": *aprosopia.*

prosopo-, prefix meaning "face": *prosopopilary, prosopospasm, prosoposternodidymus.*

prosopopilary virilism /pros'əpōpī"lərē/, a heavy growth of facial hair.

prosopospasm /pros"əpōspaz'əm/ [Gk, *prosopon,* face, *spasmos*], a spasm of the facial muscles, such as may occur in tetanus.

prosoposternodidymus /pros'əpōstur'nədid"əməs/ [Gk, *prosopon,* face, *sternon,* chest, *didymos,* twin], a fetus consisting of conjoined twins united laterally from the head through the sternum.

prosopothoracopagus /pros'əpōthôr'əkop"əgəs/ [Gk, *prosopon* + *thorax,* chest, *pagos,* fixed], conjoined symmetric twins who are united laterally in the frontal plane from the thorax through most of the head region.

prospective medicine /-spek"tiv/ [L, *proscipere,* to look forward, *medicina,* art of healing], the early identification of pathological or potentially pathological processes and the prescription of intervention to stop them.

prospective payment system (PPS), a payment mechanism for reimbursing hospitals for inpatient health care services in which a predetermined rate is set for treatment of specific illnesses. The system was originally developed by the U.S. federal government for use in treatment of Medicare recipients. See also **diagnosis-related group.**

prospective reimbursement, a method of payment to an agency for health care services to be delivered that is based on predictions of what the agency's costs will be for the coming year.

prospective study, an analytic study designed to determine the relationship between a condition and a characteristic shared by some members of a group. The population selected is healthy at the beginning of the study. Some of the members of the group share a particular characteristic, such as cigarette smoking. The researcher follows the population group over a period of time, noting the rate at which a condition, such as lung cancer, occurs in the smokers and in the nonsmokers. A prospective study may involve many variables or only two; it may seek to demonstrate a relationship that is an association or one that is causal. Prospective studies produce a direct measure of risk called the relative risk. Compare **retrospective study.** See also **relative risk.**

prost-, -prost, combining form for prostaglandin derivatives.

prostacyclin (PGI₂) /pros'təsī"klin/, a prostaglandin. It is a biologically active product of arachidonic acid metabolism in human vascular walls and a potent inhibitor of platelet aggregation. It inhibits the vasoconstrictor effect of angiotensin and stimulates renin release and has been used to treat pulmonary hypertension.

prostaglandin (PG) /pros'təglan"din/ [Gk, *prostates,* standing before; L, *glans,* acorn], one of several potent unsaturated fatty acids that act in exceedingly low concentrations on local target organs. Prostaglandins are produced in small amounts and have a large array of significant effects. Those given in tablets or in solutions for oral or IV use effect changes in vasomotor tone, capillary permeability, smooth muscle tone, aggregation of platelets, endocrine and exocrine functions, and the autonomic and central nervous systems. Some of the pharmacological uses of the prostaglandins are termination of pregnancy and treatment of asthma and gastric hyperacidity.

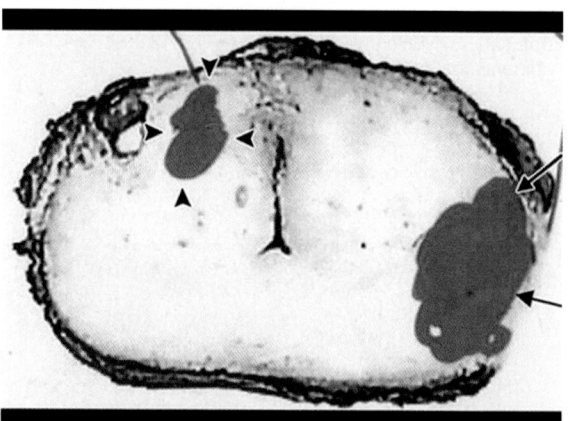

Prostaglandin
(PGE)

Prostaglandin E *(Thibodeau and Patton, 2007)*

prostaglandin endoperoxide synthase /pros″tah·glan′din en″doperok′sīd sin′thās/, an enzyme of the oxidoreductase class that has both cyclooxygenase and peroxidase activities, which together catalyze part of the synthesis of prostaglandins and thromboxanes from arachidonic acid.

prostaglandin inhibitor, an agent that prevents the production of prostaglandins. Kinds include **nonsteroidal anti-inflammatory drug.**

prostanoic acid /pros′tənō″ik/, a 20-carbon aliphatic carboxylic acid that is the basic framework for prostaglandin molecules, which differ according to the location of hydroxyl and keto substitutions at various positions along the molecule.

prostate /pros″tāt/ [Gk, *prostates,* standing before], a gland in men that surrounds the neck of the bladder and the proximal part of the urethra and produces a fluid that becomes part of semen. A firm structure normally about the size of a chestnut, the prostate is located in the pelvic cavity, below the inferior part of the symphysis pubis and ventral to the rectum, through which it can be felt, especially when it is enlarged. A depression on its cranial border accommodates the entry of the two ejaculatory ducts from the seminal vesicles. The prostate is composed of glandular and muscular tissue and contracts during ejaculation of seminal fluid. The prostatic secretion contains alkaline phosphatase, citric acid, prostate-specific antigen, and various proteolytic enzymes. **–prostatic,** *adj.*

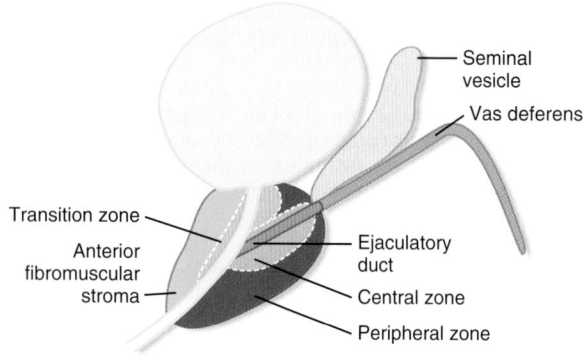

Prostate *(Darlymple, Leyendecker, and Oliphant, 2009)*

prostate cancer, the most common invasive cancer among American males, rarely occurring before the age of 39 and most often affecting men between the ages of 60 and 79. Ninety-five percent are adenocarcinomas; the remaining types are transitional cell carcinoma, squamous cell carcinoma, sarcoma, and ductal carcinoma. The cause is unknown, but it is believed to be hormone-related. The disease may cause no direct symptoms but can be detected in the course of diagnosing bladder or ureteral obstruction, hematuria, or pyuria. The cancer can spread to cause bone pain in the pelvis, ribs, or vertebrae. It is commonly detected by prostate-specific antigen testing and digital rectal examination, with confirmation by core-needle biopsy. Treatment is by surgery, radiation therapy, or hormones, depending on the age of the patient, extent of disease, and other individual factors.

Photomicrograph of prostate cancer showing prostate capsule penetration in the left peripheral zone *(arrows)* and a prostate tumor lesion *(red)* in the right central gland *(arrowheads)* [Talab et al, 2012]

prostatectomy /pros′tətek″təmē/ [Gk, *prostates* + *ektomē,* excision], surgical removal of a part of the prostate gland, such as that performed for benign prostatic hypertrophy, or the total excision of the gland, as performed for malignancy. Type and crossmatching of blood are done to prepare for possible transfusion. In the transurethral approach, the most common approach, a resectoscope is inserted into the urethra, and through it shavings of prostatic tissue are cut off at the bladder opening. The perineal approach is used for biopsy when early cancer is suspected or for the removal of calculi. In the suprapubic approach a large catheter is positioned into the bladder through the abdomen. Wound drains are placed in both the perineal and the suprapubic approaches. After surgery hematuria is expected for several days. Bleeding may be controlled by increasing the pressure at the balloon end of the urethral catheter. If arterial the bleeding is bright red with clots and increased viscosity and may lead to hemorrhagic shock, requiring transfusion and surgical intervention. The bladder catheter is connected to a closed system of irrigation with drainage. Meticulous aseptic technique is required to prevent infection when tending catheters, tubings, and collection bags, as well as when changing the dressing. Catheter patency is ensured, as well as care to prevent blockage or kinking of the drainage tubes. Accidental removal or dislodging of catheters is prevented. Bladder spasm may occur if a catheter becomes blocked or result from the irritation of the balloon of the catheter in the bladder. Antispasmodic drugs may prevent spasm but are not given in severe cardiac

Labels on Prostate diagram: Seminal vesicle, Vas deferens, Transition zone, Anterior fibromuscular stroma, Ejaculatory duct, Central zone, Peripheral zone

disease or if glaucoma is present. The nurse also assesses the patient's ability to void in adequate amounts when the urethral catheter is removed. Complications of prostatectomy include urethral stricture, especially with the transurethral approach; urinary incontinence; and impotence, especially with the perineal approach.

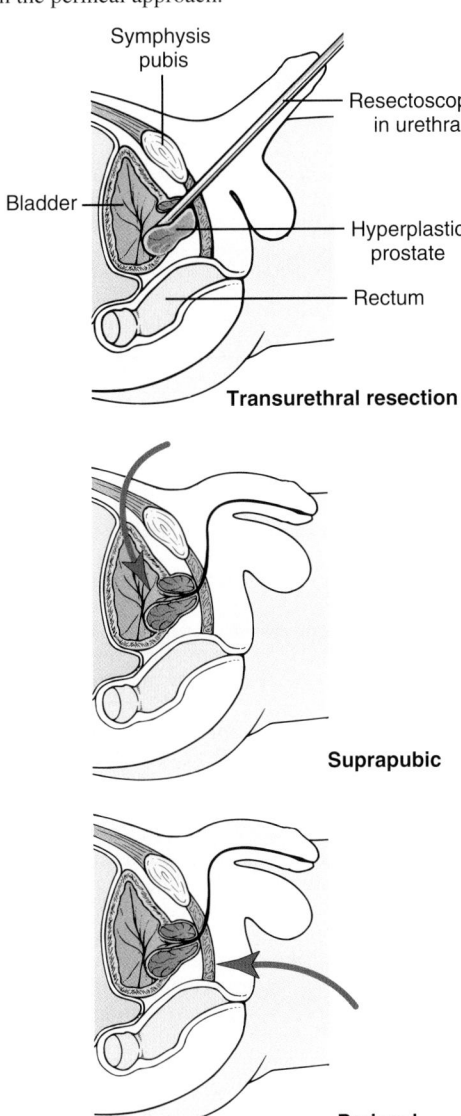

Transurethral resection

Suprapubic

Perineal

Prostatectomy *(Lewis et al, 2007)*

prostate-specific antigen (PSA), a protein produced by the prostate that may be present at elevated levels in patients with cancer or other disease of the prostate. It can also be elevated with any stimulation of the prostate, including digital rectal exam (DRE) or ejaculation.

prostate-specific antigen (PSA) test, a blood test used to detect prostatic cancer and to monitor the patient's response to therapy. The PSA velocity monitors the change in PSA with time, and the percent-free PSA is assessed as an independent predictor of prostate cancer risk. Currently, PSA is considered the most sensitive tumor marker for this type of cancer.

prostatic /prostat″ik/, pertaining to the prostate.

prostatic acid phosphatase (PAP), the first major serum marker for prostate cancer, widely used for screening, staging, and posttreatment monitoring. Also called *prostatic specific acid phosphatase.* See also **acid phosphatase.**

prostatic calculus [Gk, *prostates,* standing before; L, *calculus,* pebble], a solid calcification formed in the prostate. Typically small and multiple, prostatic calculi are often the product of chronic prostatitis and are usually composed of calcium carbonate and/or calcium phosphate. They are not clinically significant and do not require treatment.

prostatic catheter, a catheter that is approximately 16 inches (41 cm) long and has an angled tip. It is used in male urinary bladder catheterization to bypass an enlarged prostate gland obstructing the urethra. Also called **coudé catheter.**

prostatic ductule /duk″tyŏŏl/ [Gk, *prostates* + L, *ductulus,* little duct], any of 12 to 20 tiny excretory tubes that convey the alkaline secretion of the prostate and open into the floor of the prostatic part of the urethra. The ductules are joined together by areolar tissue, supported by extensions of the fibrous capsule of the prostate and its muscular stroma, and wrapped in a delicate network of capillaries.

prostatic fascia, a condensation of fascia around the anterior and lateral region of the prostate that contains and surrounds the prostatic plexus of veins and is continuous posteriorly with the rectovesical septum, which separates the posterior surface of the prostate and the base of the bladder from the rectum.

prostatic fluid, the secretion of the prostate gland, which contributes to formation of the semen.

prostatic hypertrophy. See **benign prostatic hyperplasia, prostatomegaly.**

prostatic syncope [Gk, *prostates,* standing before, *syn,* together, *koptein,* to cut], a temporary loss of consciousness caused by restricted cerebral blood flow that may occur during a digital rectal examination of the prostate.

prostatic urethral polyps, presence of numerous polyps in the prostatic urethra, sometimes causing obstruction, seen in male children as a developmental anomaly and in older males in some inflammatory reactions.

prostatic utricle, the part of the urethra in men that forms a cul-de-sac about 6 mm long behind the middle lobe of the prostate. It is composed of fibrous tissue, muscular fibers, and mucous membrane. Numerous small glands open on its inner surface. It is homologous with the uterus in women. Also called **uterus masculinus.** See also **prostate.**

prostatism /pros″tətiz′əm/ [Gk, *prostates,* standing before], an abnormal condition of the prostate, particularly an enlargement of the gland, resulting in obstructed urinary flow.

prostatitis /pros″təti″tis/ [Gk, *prostates* + *itis,* inflammation], an inflammation of the prostate gland, usually the result of infection. The patient complains of burning, urinary frequency, and urgency. Acute prostatitis is a sudden, severe inflammation of the prostate, whereas chronic prostatitis is a persistent inflammation of the prostate characterized by dull, aching pain in the lower back or perineal area and dysuria; other symptoms may include fever and discharge from the penis. Treatment consists of antibiotics, sitz baths, bed rest, and fluids. Also called **chronic bacterial prostatitis.** Compare **benign prostatic hyperplasia.**

prostatomegaly /pros″tətōmeg″əlē/ [Gk, *prostates* + *megas,* large], hypertrophy, or enlargement, of the prostate.

prosthesis /prosthē″sis/ *pl. prostheses* [Gk, addition], **1.** an artificial replacement for a missing body part, such as an artificial limb or total joint replacement. **2.** a device designed and applied to improve function, such as a hearing aid. See also **maxillofacial prosthesis, Starr-Edwards prosthesis.** —*prosthetic, adj.*

P

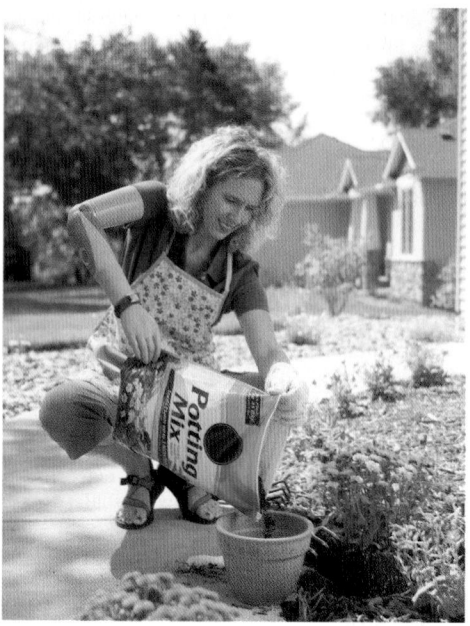

Woman with an upper extremity prosthesis (*Courtesy Otto Bock Orthopedic Industry, Inc*)

prosthetic heart valve /prosthet″ik/ [Gk, *prosthesis,* addition; AS, *hoerte* + L, *valva,* door, leaf], an artificial heart valve.

prosthetic restoration. See **restoration.**

prosthetics /prosthet″iks/ [Gk, *prosthesis,* addition], the design, construction, and attachment of artificial limbs or other systems to assume the function of missing body parts. See also **orthotics.**

prosthetist /pros″thətist/, a person who fabricates and fits artificial limbs and similar devices prescribed by a physician. A certified prosthetist is one who has successfully completed the examination of the American Orthotic and Prosthetic Association.

prosthion **(PR)** /pros′thē·on/ [Gk, *prosthios,* foremost], the point of the maxillary alveolar process that projects most anteriorly in the midline of the maxilla, used for measuring upper facial height and determining the gnathic index.

prosthodontics /pros′thədon″tiks/ [Gk, *prosthesis* + *odous,* tooth], one of the ten specialties of dentistry; devoted to the construction of artificial appliances that replace missing teeth or restore parts of the face.

Prostigmin, a cholinergic drug. Brand name for **neostigmine bromide.**

Prostin VR Pediatric, a proprietary form of prostaglandin. Brand name for **alprostadil.**

prostration /prostrā″shən/ [L, *prosternere,* to throw down], **1.** a condition of extreme exhaustion and inability to exert oneself further, as in heat prostration or nervous prostration. **2.** lying face down in front of something or someone to show reverence. –*prostrate, adj.*

prot-. See **proto-, prot-.**

protactinium (Pa) /-taktin″ē·əm/ [Gk, *protos,* first, *aktis,* ray], a radioactive element. Its atomic number is 91, and its atomic mass is 231.04. Its decay products are actinium and an alpha particle. See also **actinium.**

protamine **sulfate** /prō″təmēn/, a heparin antagonist derived from fish sperm.

■ INDICATIONS: It is prescribed to diminish or reverse the anticoagulant effect of heparin, particularly in cases of heparin overdosage.

■ CONTRAINDICATIONS: Pregnancy, allergy to fish, or known hypersensitivity to this drug prohibits its use.

■ ADVERSE EFFECTS: Among the more serious adverse effects are hypotension, dyspnea, and bradycardia. Dosage greater than needed to neutralize heparin causes the toxic and anticoagulant effects of protamine.

protamine zinc insulin (PZI) suspension, a long-acting insulin that is absorbed slowly at a steady rate and is used to maintain baseline levels of insulin. Combination therapy with regular insulin may be necessary for adequate control.

protanopia /-tənō″pē·ə/, a form of color blindness in which the person is unable to distinguish shades of red. Also called **red blindness.**

protaxic mode of experience /-tak″sik/, (in psychology), a type of primitive experience characterized by sensations, feelings, and fragmented images of short duration that are not logically connected.

protease /prō″tē·ās/, an enzyme that is a catalyst in the breakdown of peptide bonds that join the amino acids in a protein. See also **proteolysis.**

protease inhibitor, a substance that blocks activity of endopeptidase (protease), such as in a virus. See also **HIV protease inhibitor.**

protectin /protek″tin/, a membrane-bound protein, CD59, that protects normal bystander cells from lysis after complement activation in nearby bacteria or immune complexes.

protective /-tek″tiv/ [L, *protegere,* to cover], guarding another person from danger or injury and providing a safe environment.

protective apron. See **lead apron.**

protective isolation [L, *protegere,* to cover in front; It, *isolare,* detached], **1.** the practice of confining a patient with a virulent infectious disease in a separate area so that contact with other people can be minimized. **2.** the practice of placing a highly susceptible person, such as an immunodeficient patient, in a separate area where the risk of contact with pathogenic microorganisms can be controlled.

protein /prō″tē·in, prō″tēn/ [Gk, *proteios,* first rank], any of a large group of naturally occurring complex organic nitrogenous compounds. Each is composed of large combinations of amino acids (usually 50 or more) containing the elements carbon, hydrogen, nitrogen, oxygen, and occasionally sulfur, phosphorus, iron, iodine, or other essential constituents of living cells. Twenty-two amino acids have been identified as vital for proper growth, development, and maintenance of health. The body can synthesize 13 of these, the nonessential amino acids, whereas the remaining 9 must be obtained from dietary sources and are termed *essential.* Protein is the major source of building material for muscles, blood, skin, hair, nails, and the internal organs. It is necessary for the formation of many hormones, enzymes, and antibodies and may act as a source of energy. Rich dietary sources are meat, poultry, fish, eggs, milk, and cheese, which are classified as complete proteins because they contain the nine essential amino acids. Nuts and legumes, including navy beans, chickpeas, soybeans, and split peas, are also good sources but are incomplete proteins because they do not contain all the essential amino acids in adequate amounts. Protein deficiency causes abnormal growth and tissue development in children, leading to kwashiorkor, whereas in adults it results in lack of vigor and stamina, weakness, mental depression, poor resistance to infection, impaired healing of wounds, and slow recovery from disease. Excessive intake of protein may in some conditions result in fluid imbalance.

protein antibiotic.   See **bacteriocin.**

proteinase /prō′tē·inās/ [Gk, *proteios,* first rank, *ase,* enzyme suffix],   a proteolytic enzyme that splits protein molecules at central linkages. Also called **tryptase.**

protein C,   plasma coagulation control protein that, when activated, inactivates coagulation factors Va and VIIIa.

protein calorie malnutrition.   See **protein-energy malnutrition.**

protein catabolic rate (PCR),   a calculation derived by multiplying 6.25 times the amount of nitrogen in grams excreted in the urine over a given time period, which represents the amount of protein catabolized by the body in excess of protein synthesis. In a healthy steady state of nitrogen balance, it approximates the amount of protein in the diet.

protein C–protein S test,   a blood test performed to determine the activity of proteins C and S. Deficient activity of one or both of these proteins is associated with liver disease, severe malnutrition, hypercoagulability, autoimmune diseases, and intervascular thrombosis.

protein/creatinine ratio,   the ratio of protein to creatinine in the urine, calculated as a measure of proteinuria.

proteinemia /prō′tē·inē″mē·ə/ [Gk, *proteios,* first rank, *haima,* blood],   an excessive level of protein in the blood. Also called **hyperproteinemia.**

protein-energy malnutrition (PEM),   a wasting condition resulting from a diet inadequate in either protein or energy (calories) or both. These inadequacies are major problems for children in developing countries. Also called **energy-protein malnutrition,   protein calorie malnutrition.** See also **kwashiorkor,   marasmic kwashiorkor, marasmus.**

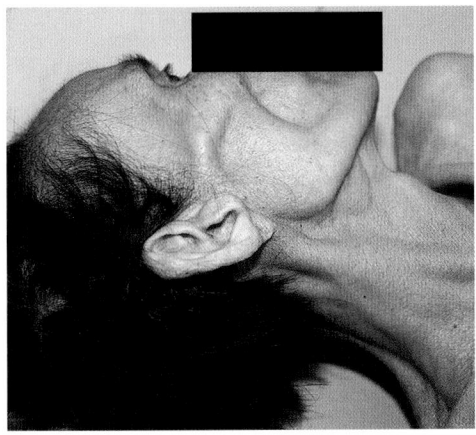

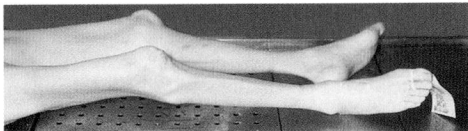

Protein-energy malnutrition *(Finkbeiner, Ursell, and Davis, 2009)*

protein hydrolysate injection,   a fluid and nutrient replenisher.

■ INDICATIONS: It is prescribed to correct a negative nitrogen balance and to provide parenteral nutrition in other clinical situations.

■ CONTRAINDICATIONS: Renal failure, anuria, severe liver disease, hepatic coma, or known hypersensitivity to one or more of the amino acids prohibits its use.

■ ADVERSE EFFECTS: Among the more serious adverse effects are hypotension, abdominal pain, convulsions, phlebitis, thrombosis, and edema.

protein kinase (PKA),   a protein that catalyzes the transfer of a phosphate group from adenosine triphosphate to produce a phosphoprotein.

protein metabolism,   the processes whereby protein foods are used by the body to make tissue proteins, together with the processes of breakdown of tissue proteins in the production of energy. Food proteins are first broken down into amino acids, then absorbed into the bloodstream, and finally used in body cells to form new proteins. Amino acids in excess of the body's needs may be converted by liver enzymes into keto acids and urea. The keto acids may be used as sources of energy via the citric acid cycle, or they may be converted into glucose or fat for storage. Urea is excreted in urine and sweat. Growth hormone, insulin, and androgens stimulate protein formation, and adrenal cortical hormones tend to cause breakdown of body proteins. Diseases affecting protein metabolism include homocystinuria, liver disease, maple sugar urine disease, and phenylketonuria.

protein sensitization [Gk, *proteios,* first rank; L, *sentire,* to feel],   a reaction that follows parenteral introduction of a foreign protein into the body. Symptoms of varying severity, including serum sickness, occur when the same foreign protein is reintroduced into the body at a later date.

protein truncation test,   a method for detection of one or more translation termination mutations in a gene that cause a truncated, usually inactive, protein to be synthesized. The appropriate genomic DNA or mRNA is isolated, amplified by polymerase chain reaction, and used as a template for in vitro transcription and translation. The size of the resulting protein is compared with that of a wild type protein by means of SDS-polyacrylamide gel electrophoresis.

proteinuria /prō′tēnyoor″ē·ə/ [Gk, *proteios + ouron,* urine],   the presence in the urine of abnormally large quantities of protein, usually albumin. Healthy adults excrete less than 250 mg of protein per day. Persistent proteinuria is usually a sign of renal disease or renal complications of another disease, such as hypertension or heart failure. However, proteinuria can result from heavy exercise or fever. Also called **albuminuria.**

proteo-,   prefix meaning "protein": *proteoglycans, proteolysis, proteolipid.*

proteoglycans,   glycosylated proteins present in virtually all extracellular matrices of connective tissues. The major biological function of proteoglycans is to provide hydration and swelling pressure to the tissue, enabling it to withstand compressional forces. Other biological functions are being studied.

proteolipid /prō′tē·ōlip″id/ [Gk, *proteios + lipos,* fat],   a type of lipoprotein in which lipid material forms more than half of the molecule. It is insoluble in water and occurs primarily in the brain.

proteolysis /prō′tē·ol″isis/ [Gk, *proteios + lysis,* loosening],   a process in which water added to the peptide bonds of proteins breaks down the protein molecule into simpler substances. Numerous enzymes may catalyze this process. The action of mineral acids and heat also may induce proteolysis. *–proteolytic, adj.*

Proteus /prō′tē·əs/ [Gk, *Proteus,* mythic god who changed shapes],   a genus of motile, gram-negative bacilli often associated with nosocomial infections, normally found in feces, water, and soil. *Proteus* may cause urinary tract infections, pyelonephritis, wound infections, diarrhea, bacteremia, and endotoxic shock. Some species are sensitive to penicillin; most respond to the aminoglycoside antibiotics and cephalosporins.

Proteus mirabilis, a species of anaerobic, motile, rod-shaped bacteria found in putrid meat, abscesses, and fecal material. It is a leading cause of urinary tract infections.

Proteus morganii, a species of bacteria associated with infectious diarrhea in infants.

Proteus syndrome /prō'tē·us/, a rare congenital disorder with highly variable manifestations, including partial gigantism of the hands and feet with hypertrophy of the palms and soles, nevi, hemihypertrophy, subcutaneous tumors, macrocephaly and other skull abnormalities, and abdominal or pelvic lipomatosis. The cause is unknown, although a genetic origin, possibly of autosomal-dominant transmission, has been conjectured. Although symptoms can be treated, there is no known cure.

Proteus vulgaris, a species of bacteria that is a frequent cause of urinary tract infections. The bacteria are found in feces, water, and soil.

prothrombin, a plasma protein that is converted to the active form, factor IIa, or thrombin, when cleaved by factor Xa bound to factor Va. Thrombin then cleaves fibrinogen to fibrin, which forms the fibrin clot. Also called **factor II.**

prothrombin complex concentrate (PCC). See **factor IX complex.**

prothrombinemia /-ē″mē·ə/ [L, *pro,* before; Gk, *thrombos,* lump, *haima,* blood], the presence of prothrombin in the blood.

prothrombin time (PT), a one-stage test for detecting certain plasma coagulation defects caused by a deficiency of factors V, VII, or X. Thromboplastin and calcium are added to a sample of the patient's plasma and simultaneously to a sample from a normal control. The amount of time required for clot formation in both samples is observed. Thrombin is formed from prothrombin in the presence of adequate calcium, thromboplastin, and the essential tissue coagulation factors. A prolonged PT therefore indicates deficiency in one of the factors, as in liver disease, vitamin K deficiency, or anticoagulation therapy with the drug warfarin sodium. Normal findings of prothrombin time are 11 to 12.5 seconds. Compare **partial thromboplastin time, International Normalized Ratio.** See also **blood clotting.**

protist, a member of the kingdom Protista, which includes eukaryotic, mostly unicellular organisms with animal-like (protozoa), plantlike (algae), or funguslike (slime molds) modes of nutrition.

protium (^{1}H) /prō'tēəm/, ordinary, or light, hydrogen, as opposed to deuterium (^{2}H) or tritium (^{3}H). See also **deuterium, tritium.**

proto-, prot-, prefix meaning "first": *protoTease, protocol, protoblast.*

protocol /prō'təkôl/ [Gk, *protos,* first, *kolla,* glued page], a written plan specifying the procedures to be followed in giving a particular examination, conducting research, or providing care for a particular condition. See also **standing orders.**

proton /prō'ton/ [Gk, *protos,* first], a positively charged particle that is a fundamental component of the nucleus of all atoms. The number of protons in the nucleus of an atom equals the atomic number of the element. Compare **electron, neutron.** See also **atomic mass.**

proton density, a measure of proton concentration, or the number of atomic nuclei per given volume. It is one of the

major determinants of magnetic resonance signal strength in hydrogen imaging.

proton pump inhibitor, an agent that inhibits gastric acid secretion by blocking the action of hydrogen ions, potassium ions, and adenosine triphosphatase at the secretory surface of gastric parietal cells. Also called **gastric acid pump inhibitor.**

Protopam Chloride, a cholinesterase reactivator. Brand name for **pralidoxime chloride.**

protopathic sensibility /prō'təpath″ik/, pertaining to the somatic sensations of fast localized pain; slow, poorly localized pain; and temperature.

protoplasm. See **cytoplasm.**

protoplasmic /-plaz″mik/ [Gk, *protos,* first, *plasma,* something formed], pertaining to or composed of protoplasm, the substance of which animal and vegetable cells are formed.

protoplast /prō'təplast/ [Gk, *protos* + *plassein,* to mold], **1.** (in biology) the protoplasm of a cell without its containing membrane. **2.** a first entity or an original. *–protoplastic, adj.*

protoporphyria /prō'tōpôrfir″ē·ə/ [Gk, *protos* + *porphyros,* purple, *haima,* blood], increased levels of protoporphyrin in the blood and feces.

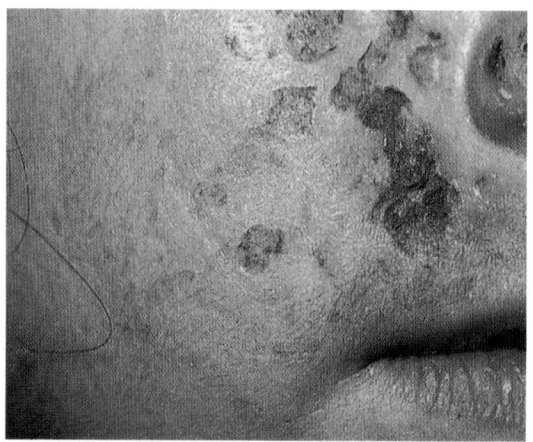

Erythropoietic protoporphyria *(Weston, Lane, and Morelli, 2007)*

protoporphyrin /prō'tōpôr″firin/ [Gk, *protos* + *porphyros*], a kind of porphyrin that combines with iron and protein to form various important organic molecules, including catalase, hemoglobin, and myoglobin. See also **heme.**

protostoma. See **blastopore.**

prototaxic mode /prōtətak″sik/ [Gk, *protos* + *taxis,* arrangement, *modus,* measure], a stage in infancy, according to H.S. Sullivan's theory, characterized by a lack of differentiation between the self and the environment.

prototype /prō'tətīp/ [Gk, *protos,* first, *typos,* mark], the primary or original form of an object or organism.

protozoal infection /-zō′əl/, any disease caused by single-celled organisms of the subkingdom Protozoa. Kinds include **amebic dysentery, malaria, schistosomiasis, trichomoniasis, trypanosomiasis.**

protozoan /-zō″ən/ [Gk, *protos,* first, *zoon,* animal], pertaining to or caused by protozoa.

protozoon /prō'təzō″ən/ *pl.* **protozoa** [Gk, *protos* + *zoon,* animal], a unicellular protist that ingests food. Protozoa include free-living forms, such as amebas and paramecia, as well as parasites. Approximately 30 protozoa are pathogenic to humans, including *Plasmodium,* which causes malaria, and *Trypanosoma,* which causes sleeping sickness. See also **mastigophora.**

protracted dose /prōtrak″tid/ [L, *pro,* before, *trahere,* to draw, *dosis,* something given], a low amount of therapeutic radiation delivered continuously over a relatively long period.

protriptyline hydrochloride /-trip″tilēn/, a tricyclic antidepressant.

■ INDICATIONS: It is prescribed in the treatment of endogenous depression marked by withdrawal and anergy.

■ CONTRAINDICATIONS: Concomitant administration of monoamine oxidase inhibitors, recent myocardial infarction, or known hypersensitivity to any tricyclic medication prohibits its use. It is used with caution when anticholinergics are contraindicated, in seizure disorders, and in cardiovascular disease.

■ ADVERSE EFFECTS: Among the more serious adverse effects are sedation and anticholinergic side effects. A variety of GI, cardiovascular, and neurological reactions may occur. It interacts with many other drugs.

Protropin, a synthetic human growth hormone. Brand name for **somatrem.**

protrusio bulbi. See **exophthalmia.**

protrusion /-troo″zhən/ [L, *protrudere,* to push forward], a state or condition of being forward or projecting.

protrusive incisal guide angle /-troo″siv/, the inclination of the incisal guide of a dental articulator in the sagittal plane.

protrypsin. See **trypsinogen.**

protuberance /-t(y)oo″bərəns/ [L, *pro* + *tuberare,* to swell], an anatomical landmark that appears as a blunt projection, eminence, or swelling, such as the chin, buttock, or bulge of the frontal bone above the eyebrow.

proud flesh [AS, *prud* + *flaesc*], excessive granulation tissue. See also **cicatrices, keloid, scar.**

Proventil, a bronchodilator. Brand name for **albuterol.**

Provera, a progestin. Brand name for **medroxyPROGESTERone acetate.**

provider, a hospital, clinic, health care professional, or group of health care professionals who provide a service to patients.

Provincial/Territorial Nurses Association (PTNA), an association of Canadian nurses organized at the provincial or territorial level. The Canadian Nurses' Association is a federation of the 11 PTNAs.

provirus /-vī″rəs/, a stage of viral replication in which the viral genetic information has been integrated into the genome of the host cell. It may be activated spontaneously or by a specific stimulus to direct the cell to produce new virions to progress to a complete virus.

provitamin /prōvī″təmin/, a precursor of a vitamin; a substance found in certain foods that in the body may be converted into a vitamin. Also called **previtamin.**

provocative diagnosis /-vok″ətiv/ [L, *provocare,* to call forth; Gk, *dia,* through, *gnosis,* knowledge], a diagnosis in which the identity and cause of an illness are discovered by inducing an episode of the condition. For example, in immunology, an allergen causing an allergic response is shown to be a causative factor in the patient's allergic condition.

prox, abbreviation for **proximal.**

proxemics /proksē″miks/ [L, *proximus,* nearest], the study of spatial distances between people and their effect on interpersonal behavior, especially in relation to population density, placement of people within an area, territoriality, personal space, and the opportunity for privacy.

proximal (prox) /prok″siməl/ [L, *proximus*], nearer to a point of reference or attachment, usually the trunk of the body, than other parts of the body. Proximal interphalangeal joints are those closest to the hand or the surface of a tooth in relation to the abutting tooth nearer or farther from the anteroposterior median plane. Compare **distal.**

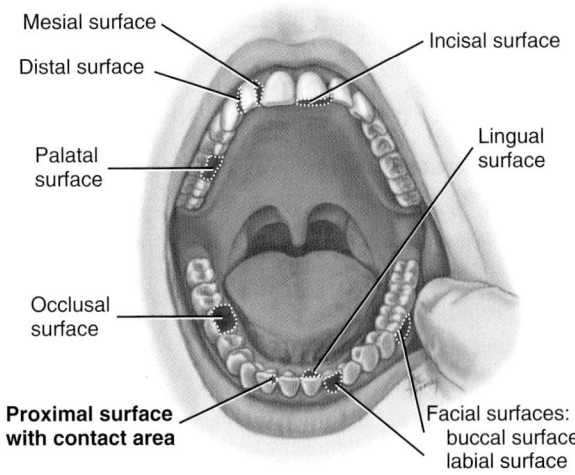

Proximal surface of the tooth *(Bath-Balogh and Fehrenbach, 2011)*

proximal cavity, a cavity that occurs on the mesial or distal surface of a tooth.

proximal contact [L, *proximus,* nearest, *contingere,* to touch], an area of touch between the distal surface of one tooth and the mesial surface of an adjacent tooth.

proximal contour, the shape or form of the mesial or the distal surface of a tooth.

proximal dental caries, decay that may occur in the mesial or distal surface of a tooth.

proximal part of prostatic urethra, the first portion of the prostatic urethra, up to and including the seminal colliculus.

proximal radioulnar articulation, the pivot joint between the circumference of the head of the radius and the ring formed by the radial notch of the ulna and the annular ligament. The joint allows the rotary movements of the head of the radius in pronation and supination. Also called **superior radioulnar joint.** Compare **distal radioulnar articulation.**

proximal renal tubular acidosis (RTA), an abnormal condition characterized by excessive acid accumulation and bicarbonate excretion. It is caused by the defective reabsorption of bicarbonate in the proximal tubules of the kidney and the resulting flow of excessive bicarbonate into the distal tubules, which normally secrete hydrogen ions. This disruption impedes the formation of titratable acids and ammonium for excretion and ultimately leads to metabolic

P

acidosis. Treatment is the same as for renal tubular acidosis. In primary proximal RTA the defective reabsorption of bicarbonate is the sole causative factor. In secondary proximal RTA the resorptive defect is one of several causative factors and may result from tubular cell damage produced by various disorders, such as Fanconi's syndrome. Compare **distal renal tubular acidosis.**

proximate /prok″simit/ [L, *proximus,* nearest], the nearest to a point of origin or attachment.

proximate cause [L, *proximus,* nearest], a legal concept of cause-and-effect relationships in determining, for example, whether an injury would have resulted from a particular cause.

proximity principle /proksim″itē/ [L, *proximus + principium,* origin], a rule that when two or more objects are close to each other, they may be seen as a perceptual unit.

proxi-, proximo-, prefix meaning "near or opposite of distal, central, or a point of attachment": *proximal, proximity, proximate.*

proxymetacaine. See **proparacaine hydrochloride.**

Prozac, an oral antidepressant. Brand name for **fluoxetine hydrochloride.**

PrP, a viruslike infectious agent associated with Creutzfeldt-Jakob disease. Abbreviation for *prion protein.*

prune-belly syndrome, a syndrome, occurring almost exclusively in males, in which the lower part of the rectus abdominis muscle and the lower and medial parts of the oblique muscles are absent, the bladder and ureters are usually greatly dilated, the kidneys are small and dysplastic with hydronephrosis, and the testes are undescended. The abdomen is protruding and thin-walled with wrinkled skin, giving the syndrome its name.

prurigo /prŏŏrī″gō/ [L, an itch], any of a group of chronic inflammatory conditions of the skin characterized by severe itching and multiple dome-shaped small papules capped by tiny vesicles. As a result of repeated scratching, crusting and lichenification may occur. Some causes of prurigo are allergies, drugs, endocrine abnormalities, malignancies, and parasites. Specific treatment depends on the cause. Symptomatic therapy is the same as for pruritus. A mild form of the disease is called *prurigo mitis,* a more severe form, *prurigo agria, prurigo ferox, or nodular prurigo.*

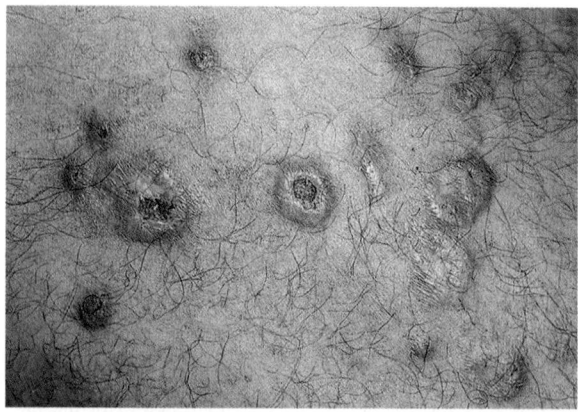

Nodular prurigo *(Callen et al, 2000)*

pruritic. See **pruritus.**

pruritic urticarial papules and plaques of pregnancy (PUPPP) /prŏŏrit″ik/, small, semisolid, intensely itching blisters that may appear on the abdomen of a pregnant woman and spread peripherally. They begin in the third trimester and resolve spontaneously after delivery.

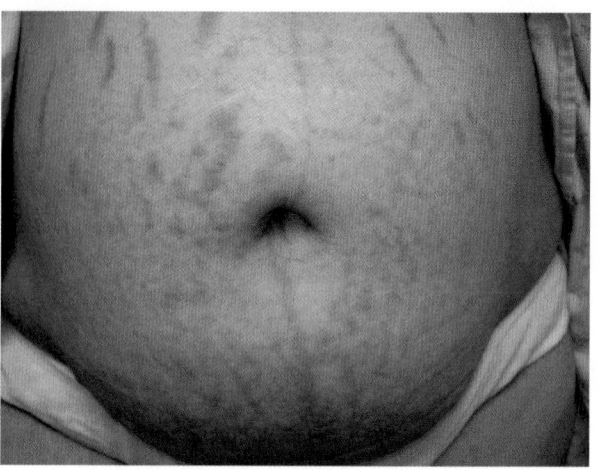

Pruritic urticarial papules and plaques of pregnancy (PUPPP) *(Taylor, Pappo, and Aronson, 2016)*

pruritus /prŏŏrī″təs/ [L, *prurire,* to itch], the symptom of itching, an uncomfortable sensation leading to the urge to scratch. Scratching may result in secondary infection. Some causes of pruritus are allergy, infection, jaundice, chronic renal disease, lymphoma, and skin irritation. Treatment is best directed at the cause. Symptomatic relief may be obtained with antihistamines, starch baths, topical corticosteroids, cool water, or alcohol applications. **–pruritic,** *adj.*

pruritus ani, a common chronic condition of itching of the skin around the anus. Some causes are candidal infection, contact dermatitis, external hemorrhoids, pinworms, psoriasis, and psychogenic illness. Treatment is best directed at the specific cause. However, symptomatic relief may be obtained with careful cleansing, soothing creams or lotions, topical corticosteroids, antihistamines, and tranquilizers.

pruritus hiemalis. See **winter itch.**

pruritus vulvae, itching of the external genitalia of a female. The condition may become chronic and result in lichenification, atrophy, and occasionally malignancy. Some causes of pruritus vulvae are contact dermatitis, lichen sclerosus et atrophicus, psychogenic pruritus, trichomoniasis, and vaginal candidiasis. Treatment of the condition depends on its cause.

Prussian blue /prush″ən/ [Prussia, Germany; ME, *blew*], a chemical stain used on microscopic preparations. It demonstrates the presence of copper by developing a bright blue color.

ps, abbreviation for **picosecond.**

PSA, 1. abbreviation for **pressure-sensitive adhesive.** 2. abbreviation for **prostate-specific antigen.**

PSA failure. See **biochemical relapse.**

psammo-, prefix meaning "sand" or "sandlike material": *psammoma, psammoma body.*

psammoma /samō″mə/ *pl. psammomas, psammomata* [Gk, *psammos,* sand, *oma,* tumor], a neoplasm containing small calcified granules (psammoma bodies) that occurs in the meninges, choroid plexus, pineal body, and ovaries. Also called **sand tumor.**

psammoma body, a round layered mass of calcareous material occurring in benign and malignant epithelial and connective tissue neoplasms and in some chronically inflamed tissue.

psammomas, psammomata. See **psammoma.**

-pselaphesia, -pselaphesis, suffix meaning "(condition of the) tactile sense": *apselaphesia.*

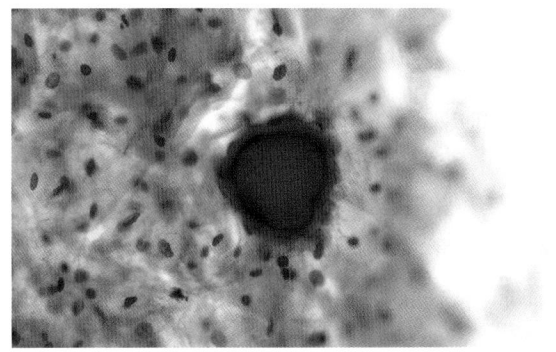

Psammoma body *(McKee, 1997)*

pseud-. See **pseudo-, pscud-.**

pseudarthritis /sŏŏ′därthrī″tis/ [Gk, *pseudes,* false, *arthron,* joint, *itis,* inflammation], musculoskeletal pain that does not involve the joints.

pseudesthesia /sŏŏ′desthē″zhə/ [Gk, *pseudes,* false, *aisthesis,* feeling], a sensation experienced without an external stimulus or a sensation that does not correspond to the causative stimulus, such as phantom limb pain occurring after an amputation.

pseudo-, pseud-, prefix meaning "false": *pseudoesthesia, pseudocyst, pseudorubella.*

pseudoacanthosis nigricans /-ak′ənthō″sis/, a condition of pigmented velvety thickening of the flexural skin, often with skin tags. It occurs most commonly in obese persons with dark complexions or in persons with endocrine disorders and is secondary to maceration of the skin from sweating. Compare **acanthosis nigricans.**

pseudoactinomycosis. See **paraactinomycosis.**

pseudoagraphia /sŏŏ′dō-ə-graf′ē-ə/ [Gk, *pseudes,* false + *a, graphein,* not to write], a type of dysgraphia in which the patient can copy writing but cannot write to express ideas. Also called **echographia.**

pseudoainhum /sŏŏ″do-in′yoom/, ringlike constrictions around the digits, limbs, or trunk, occurring both congenitally and in association with a wide variety of hereditary and nonhereditary disorders. The most severe cases of congenital pseudoainhum result in autoamputation in utero.

pseudoallele /-əlēl″/ [Gk, *pseudes* + *allelon,* of one another], one of two or more closely linked genes on a chromosome that appear to function as a single allelic pair but occupy distinct, nearly corresponding loci on homologous chromosomes. Such gene pairs produce a mutant effect in the diploid state when located on homologous chromosomes but are capable of being separated by crossing over during meiosis to produce a wild-type effect when recombined on either of the homologues. *–pseudoallelic, adj., –pseudoallelism, n.*

pseudoaneurysm /-an″yəriz′əm/, **1.** a dilation of an artery caused by damage to one or more layers of the artery as a result of arterial trauma or rupture of a true aneurysm. **2.** a tortuosity of a blood vessel or cavity resulting from a herniated infarction. Also called **pulsatile hematoma.**

pseudoankylosis /-ang′kilō″sis/ [Gk, *pseudes,* false, *ankylosis,* joint stiffness], fixation of a joint caused by inflexibility of body structures outside the joint. Compare **true ankylosis.**

pseudoanodontia /-an′ōdon″shə/, an absence of teeth caused by failure of the teeth to erupt.

pseudoanorexia /-an′ərek″sē-ə/ [Gk, *pseudes* + *a* + *orexis,* without appetite], a condition in which an individual eats secretly while claiming a lack of appetite and inability to eat. Also called **false anorexia.** Compare **anorexia.**

pseudoarthrosis. See **false joint.**

pseudoataxia /-ətak″sē-ə/ [Gk, *pseudes,* false, *ataxia,* without order], a loss of control over voluntary movements that does not involve an organic lesion.

pseudobulbar affect (PBA), uncontrollable episodes of laughing or crying not in proportion to the precipitating event. It is associated with neurological conditions and movement disorders.

pseudobulbar paralysis /-bul″bər/ [Gk, *pseudes,* false; L, *bulbus,* swollen root, *paralyein,* to be palsied], a condition resembling progressive bulbar paralysis, with dysarthria and dysphagia, but in which weakness of the bulbar muscles is of the upper motor neuron type. It may result from multiple bilateral infarcts of the cerebral cortex.

pseudocephalocele /-sef″əlōsēl′/, a noncongenital cerebral hernia resulting from a skull injury or disease.

pseudochancre /-shang″kər/, an indurated genital sore resembling or simulating a chancre.

pseudocholinesterase. See **cholinesterase.**

pseudochondroplasia /-əkon′drōplā″zhə/, a hereditary condition resembling achondroplasia but developing after birth.

pseudochylous ascites /-kī″ləs/ [Gk, *pseudes* + *chylos,* juice, *askos,* bag], the abnormal accumulation in the peritoneal cavity of a milky fluid that resembles chyle. The turbidity of the fluid is caused by cellular debris in the fluid. Pseudochylous ascites is indicative of an abdominal tumor or infection. Compare **chylous ascites.** See also **ascites.**

pseudoclaudication /-klô′dikā″shən/, painful cramps that are not caused by peripheral artery disease but rather by spinal, neurological, or orthopedic disorders, such as spinal stenosis, diabetic neuropathy, or arthritis.

pseudocoxalgia. See **Perthes disease.**

pseudocyesis /-sī-ē″sis/ [Gk, *pseudes* + *kyesis,* pregnancy], a condition in which a woman believes that she is pregnant when she is not. Certain signs and symptoms suggest pregnancy, such as the absence of the menses, although conception has not occurred and therefore there is no embryonic development. The condition may be psychogenic in origin or caused by a tumor or endocrine dysfunction. Also called **false pregnancy, pseudopregnancy, spurious pregnancy.**

pseudocyst /sŏŏ″dəsist/ [Gk, *pseudes* + *kystis,* bag], a space or cavity containing gas or liquid but without a lining membrane. Pseudocysts commonly occur after pancreatitis when digestive juices break through the normal ducts of the pancreas and collect in spaces lined by fibroblasts and surfaces of adjacent organs. Symptoms are caused by displacement of abdominal structures or fluid or by atelectasis at the base of the left lung. Ultrasound and computed tomography are useful in diagnosis; surgical drainage is the best therapy. Also called **adventitious cyst, false cyst.** See also **pancreatitis.**

pseudodementia /-dimen″shə/, a syndrome that mimics dementia. It needs to be differentiated from depression.

pseudoephedrine hydrochloride /-ef″ədrēn/, an adrenergic agonist that acts as a vasoconstrictor and decongestant. Also called *pseudoephedrine sulfate.*

■ INDICATIONS: It is prescribed for the relief of nasal congestion.

■ CONTRAINDICATIONS: Known hypersensitivity to sympathomimetic drugs prohibits its use. Interaction with monoamine oxidase inhibitors may cause hypertensive crisis. It is prescribed with caution in patients who have hypertension, glaucoma, heart disease, diabetes, or urinary retention.

P

■ ADVERSE EFFECTS: Among the more serious adverse effects are central nervous system stimulation, headache, tachycardia, and increased blood pressure.

pseudoepitheliomatous keratotic and micaceous balanitis, rare, white, plaquelike, hyperkeratotic lesion of the glans penis that may be premalignant and progress to a verrucous type of carcinoma.

pseudofracture /-frak″chər/ [Gk, *pseudes,* false; L, *fractura*], radiological evidence of a thickened periosteum and new bone formation over what looks like an incomplete fracture.

pseudogene /soo″dōjēn′/ [Gk, *pseudes* + *genein,* to produce], a DNA sequence that resembles a gene and may be derived from one but lacks a genetic function.

pseudoglandular period, the period or phase of prenatal lung development lasting from about the 6th to 16th week, and followed by the canalicular period. Repeated branching of bronchi and bronchioles takes place to form primordial conductive airways, and the lungs resemble exocrine glands. Fetuses delivered during this phase are not viable because the lungs are not capable of respiration until the 24th to 26th week. Also called *pseudoglandular phase.*

pseudoglottis. See **neoglottis.**

pseudogout. See **chondrocalcinosis.**

pseudo-Graefe's sign, slow descent of the upper eyelid on looking down, and quick ascent on looking up. It is associated with recovery from paralysis of the third cranial nerve.

pseudogynecomastia /-gī′nəcōmas″tē·ə/, enlarged breasts in a male caused by fat accumulation.

pseudohallucination. See **phantom vision.**

pseudohermaphrodism. See **pseudohermaphroditism.**

pseudohermaphrodite /-hərmaf″redīt/ [Gk, *pseudes,* false, *Hermaphroditos,* son of Hermes and Aphrodite], a person who has male gonads but female external genitalia or a person who has female gonads but male external genitalia.

pseudohermaphroditism /-hərmaf″rəditiz′əm/ [Gk, *pseudes* + *Hermaphroditos,* son of Hermes and Aphrodite], a condition in which a person exhibits the somatic characteristics of both sexes though possessing the physical characteristics of either males (testes) or females (ovaries). Also spelled **pseudohermaphrodism.** See also **ambiguous genitalia, feminization,** def. 2, **hermaphroditism.** −*pseudohermaphroditic, adj.*

pseudo-Hurler polydystrophy, a disorder similar to but milder than I cell disease and thought to result from the same enzyme deficiency as Hurler disease, but to a lesser extent. See also **I cell disease.**

pseudohyperkalemia /-hī′pərkəlē″mē·ə/, a laboratory artifact indicating an elevated blood potassium level caused by potassium released in vitro from cells in the blood sample.

pseudohyperparathyroidism /-hī′pərper′əthī″roidiz′əm/, signs of hypercalcemia in a cancer patent in the absence of primary hyperparathyroidism or skeletal metastases.

pseudohypertension /-hī′pərten″shən/, a blood pressure reading that erroneously appears elevated as a result of arterial compliance. The condition occurs most often in elderly patients.

pseudohypertrophic muscular dystrophy. See **Duchenne muscular dystrophy.**

pseudohypertrophy /-hīpur″trəfē/, abnormal enlargement of an organ or body structure caused by an overgrowth of fatty and fibrous tissues.

pseudohypoaldosteronism /-hī′pōaldos′tərōn′izəm/, **1.** a hereditary disorder of infancy characterized by severe salt and water depletion and other signs of aldosterone deficiency, even though normal or elevated amounts of aldosterone are secreted. Causes include aldosterone receptor defects and renal dysfunction. Some affected infants outgrow the need for dietary salt supplements in early childhood. **2.** the endocrine abnormality associated with sodium-losing nephropathy, usually resulting from chronic pyelonephritis, seen primarily in adults. See also **Gordon syndrome.**

pseudohyponatremia /-hī′pōnātrē″mē·ə/, a decreased sodium concentration that does not correspond to a true hypotonic disorder. It may result instead from volume displacement by massive hyperlipidemia or hyperproteinemia.

pseudohypoparathyroidism /-hī′pōper′əthī″roidiz′əm/, a condition of end-organ resistance characterized by hypocalcemia, growth failure, and skeletal abnormalities such as short fingers. See also **Albright hereditary osteodystrophy.**

pseudoileus /soo′dō·il″ē·əs/, **1.** a condition resembling an intestinal obstruction caused by paralysis of a part of the bowel wall. **2.** an adynamic bowel obstruction.

pseudoisochromatic /soo′dō·ī′sōkrōmat″ik/, pertaining to visual test materials in which dots that differ in color appear to be a similar color to a person with color blindness. See also **Ishihara color test.**

pseudojaundice /-jôn″dis/ [Gk, *pseudes* + Fr, *jaune,* yellow], a yellow discoloration of the skin that is not caused by hyperbilirubinemia. The excessive ingestion of carotene results in a form of pseudojaundice.

pseudolymphoma /-limfō″mə/, a benign disorder of lymphoid cells or histiocytes that produces clinical features of a malignant lymphoma.

pseudolysogeny /-līsoj″ənē/, a condition in which a bacteriophage is carried in a culture of a bacterial strain by infecting susceptible variants of the strain.

pseudomamma /-mam″ə/, a glandular structure resembling a nipple or mammary gland, sometimes found in a dermoid ovarian cyst.

pseudomania /-mā″nē·ə/, **1.** a condition in which a person claims to have committed crimes of which he or she is really innocent. **2.** a deliberately pretended condition of mental illness.

pseudomegacolon /-meg″əkō′lon/, a dilation of the colon in an adult patient.

pseudomembrane /-mem″brān/ [Gk, *pseudes,* false; L, *membrana*], a membrane consisting of coagulated fibrin, bacteria, and leukocytes that forms in the throats of diphtheria patients.

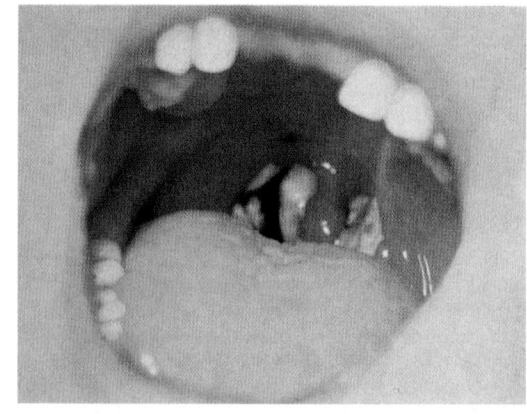

Diphtheria pseudomembrane *(Courtesy Dr. Norman Begg)*

pseudomembranous /-mem″brənəs/, describing a false membrane, as occurs in diphtheria.

pseudomembranous colitis /-mem″brənəs/ [Gk, *pseudes* + L, *membrana,* thin skin], a diarrheal disease frequently found in hospitalized patients who have received antibiotics that caused overgrowth of the anaerobic spore-forming toxin *Clostridium difficile.* Patients have profuse watery diarrhea, fever, and cramping and are found to have exudates of the colon on endoscopy. Diagnosis is made by identifying the offending toxin in the stool of the affected patient. Antidiarrheals are strictly contraindicated because a life-threatening dilation of the bowel called toxic megacolon may result. The bacterium is passed from patient to patient by health care workers who fail to wash their hands adequately. Strict isolation of infected stools is necessary to prevent outbreaks of epidemics. Treatment with oral vancomycin or parenteral metronidazole usually will result in abatement of symptoms within 3 to 5 days. In mild to moderate cases, supportive therapy alone is required.

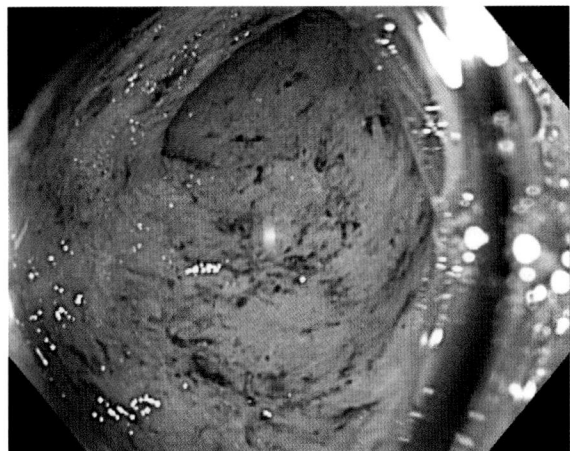

Colonoscopic examination image showing pseudomembranous colitis *(Fons et al, 2013)*

pseudomembranous enterocolitis. See **necrotizing enterocolitis.**

pseudomembranous stomatitis, a severe inflammation of the mouth that produces a membranelike exudate. The inflammation may be caused by various bacteria or by chemical irritants. It may produce dysphagia, pain, fever, and swelling of the lymph glands, or it may remain localized and mild.

pseudomenstruation /-men′stroo·ā″shən/, bleeding from the uterus that resembles menstruation but is not associated with the usual changes in endometrial tissues.

pseudomnesia /soo′dōmnē″zhə/, a memory aberration in which a client claims to remember events that actually have not taken place.

pseudomonad /soo′dōmō″nad, soodom″ənad/, a bacterium of the genus *Pseudomonas.*

Pseudomonas /soodom″ənas/ [Gk, *pseudes* + *monas,* unit], a genus of gram-negative bacteria isolated from wounds, burns, and infections of the urinary tract that includes several free-living species in soil and water and some opportunistic pathogens, such as *Pseudomonas aeruginosa.* Pseudomonads are notable for their fluorescent pigments and their resistance to disinfectants and antibiotics.

Pseudomonas aeruginosa [Gk, *pseudes,* false, *monas,* unity], a species of gram-negative, nonspore-forming, motile bacteria that may cause various human diseases ranging from purulent meningitis to nosocomial infected wounds. Also called ***Pseudomonas pyocyanea.***

Pseudomonas maltophilia. See ***Xanthomonas maltophilia.***

Pseudomonas pyocyanea. See ***Pseudomonas aeruginosa.***

pseudomutuality /-moo′tyoo·al″itē/ [Gk, *pseudes* + L, *mutuus,* reciprocal], (in psychotherapy) an atmosphere maintained by family members in which surface harmony and a high degree of agreement with one another hide deep and destructive intrapsychic and interpersonal conflicts. The family acts as if it is close and happy when in fact it is not.

pseudomyopia /-mī·ō″pē·ə/, overaccommodation during distance viewing that results in distance blur.

pseudomyxoma /-miksō″mə/, a mucus-rich tumor.

pseudomyxoma peritonei, the presence in the peritoneal cavity of mucoid matter from a ruptured ovarian cyst or a ruptured mucocele of the appendix.

pseudonystagmus. See **end-positional nystagmus.**

pseudopapilledema /-pap′ilēdē″mə/, a congenitally swollen optic disc that resembles papilledema but with no retinal hemorrhages or exudates or any systemic signs of increased intraocular pressure.

pseudoparalysis /-pəral″isis/, a condition in which a person appears to be unable to move the arms or legs but has no "true" paralysis. In infants, the condition may be caused by pain in joints resulting from a disease such as rickets or scurvy.

pseudoparaplegia /-per′əplē″jə/, a form of psychogenic paralysis.

pseudoparesis /-pərē″sis/, a form of psychogenic paralysis.

pseudopelade /-pelād″, -pē″lād/, a scarring type of alopecia, preceded by folliculitis, in which one or more areas of baldness may appear and spread to become joined, forming an area of smooth fingerlike projections that are slightly depressed in the skin.

pseudopericarditis /-per′ikärdī″tis/, an auscultation sound resembling a friction rub when the diaphragm of a stethoscope is over the apex beat. It is actually caused by the movement of tissue in the intercostal space.

pseudophakia /-fā″kē·ə/, artificial lens implantation after cataract surgery.

pseudophakodonesis /-fā″kōdənē″sis/, excessive movement by an intraocular lens implant.

Pseudophyllidea /-filid″ē·ə/, an order of tapeworms with an aquatic life cycle. The scolex usually has two opposing sucking organs.

pseudopod /soo″dəpod/ [Gk, *pseudes,* false, *pous,* foot], a temporary cytoplasmic process of an ameba that can be extended to propel the organism or to engulf food. Also called *pseudopodium.*

pseudopolyp /-pol″ip/, a projecting mass of granulation tissue that may develop in ulcerative colitis and become covered by regenerating epithelium.

pseudopregnancy. See **pseudocyesis.**

pseudoprognathism /-prog″nəthiz′əm/, a condition in which the mandible is forced forward from its normal position by an occlusal disorder.

pseudopseudohypoparathyroidism /soo′dōsoo′dōhī′pō par′əthī″roidizəm/, an incomplete form of pseudohypoparathyroidism characterized by the same constitutional features but by normal levels of calcium and phosphorus in the serum. See also **pseudohypoparathyroidism.**

pseudopsychosis /-sīkō″sis/, a condition such as malingering that may resemble a true mental and behavioral disorder.

pseudopterygium /soo′dopterij″ē·əm/, a fold of conjunctiva that has become attached to the cornea after an injury or disease.

pseudoptosis /soo′doptō″sis/, an abnormally small palpebral fissure.

pseudopuberty /-p(y)oo″bərtē/, the appearance of somatic and functional changes in an individual before the chronological age of puberty.

pseudorabies. See **infectious bulbar paralysis.**

pseudoretinitis pigmentosa /-ret′inī″tis/, a pigmentary mottling of the retina that may follow an eye injury.

pseudorubella. See **roseola infantum.**

pseudosarcoma /-särkō″mə/, a spindle cell epithelioma on skin that has been exposed to irradiation.

pseudosclerema. See **adiponecrosis subcutanea neonatorum.**

pseudosmallpox. See **alastrim.**

pseudostrabismus /-strəbiz″məs/, an appearance of strabismus caused by an epicanthal fold of skin, which narrows the visible width of the sclera medial to the iris.

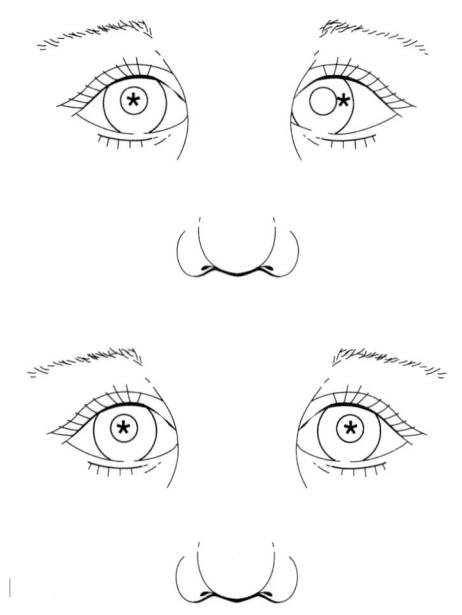

Pseudostrabismus *(Goldbloom, 2011)*

pseudostratified /-stra″tifīd/ [Gk, *pseudes,* false, *stratum,* cover], pertaining to a type of layered epithelium in which the nuclei of adjacent cells are at different levels.

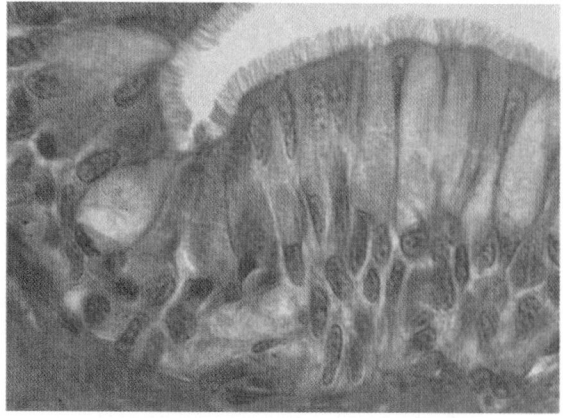

Pseudostratified columnar epithelium
(© Ed Reschke; Used with permission)

pseudotabes /-tā″bēz/, any neuropathy with symptoms like those of tabes dorsalis.

pseudotruncus arteriosus /-trung″kəs/, a condition in which blood is carried to the pulmonary arteries by collateral vessels.

pseudotubercle /-t(y)oo″bərkəl/, a nodule that resembles a tuberculosis granule but is caused by a microorganism other than *Mycobacterium tuberculosis.*

pseudotuberculosis /-t(y)oobur′kyəlō″sis/, a pulmonary condition with symptoms resembling those of tuberculosis but not caused by *Mycobacterium tuberculosis.*

pseudotumor /-t(y)oo″mər/ [Gk, *pseudes* + L, *tumor,* swelling], a false tumor.

pseudotumor cerebri, a condition characterized by increased intracranial pressure, headache, blurring of the optic disc margins, vomiting, and papilledema without neurological signs, except palsy of the sixth cranial nerve. Also called **benign intracranial hypertension, meningeal hydrops.**

pseudovariola. See **alastrim.**

pseudovitamin /-vī″təmin/, a substance that has a chemical structure similar to that of a vitamin but lacks the physiological effects.

pseudoxanthoma elasticum. See **Grönblad-Strandberg syndrome.**

psi /sī/, Ψ, ψ, the twenty-third letter of the Greek alphabet.

p.s.i., abbreviation for *pounds per square inch.*

psia, abbreviation for *pounds per square inch, absolute.*

psig, abbreviation for *pounds per square inch, gauge.*

psilocin /sī″ləsin/, one of several indole-derived psychomimetic drugs. It is related chemically to psilocybin.

psilocybin /sī′lōsī″bin, -sib″in/, a psychedelic drug and an active ingredient of various Mexican hallucinogenic mushrooms of the genus *Psilocybe mexicana.* It can produce altered states of mood and consciousness and has no acceptable medical use in the United States. Psilocybin is controlled under Schedule I of the Controlled Substances Act of 1970, which bans the prescription of psilocybin and numerous other drugs and allows their procurement and use only for special research projects authorized by the Drug Enforcement Administration of the U.S. Department of Justice.

psittacosis /sit′əkō″sis/ [Gk, *psittakos,* parrot], an infectious illness caused by the bacterium *Chlamydia psittaci,* characterized by respiratory pneumonia–like symptoms and transmitted to humans inhaling dried secretions from infected birds, especially pet birds and poultry. The clinical manifestations of the disease are extremely variable and resemble those of a great number of infectious diseases, but fever, cough, anorexia, and severe headache are almost always present. All chlamydiae are difficult to isolate and culture, but a history of exposure to birds is highly suggestive. A demonstrated rise in antibody titer confirms a diagnosis. Tetracycline or doxycycline is usually used to treat psittacosis. Isolation is advised. Also called **ornithosis, parrot fever.** See also *Chlamydia.*

psm, abbreviation for **presystolic murmur.**

psoas major /sō″əs/ [Gk, *psoa,* loin], a long muscle originating from the transverse processes of the lumbar vertebrae and the fibrocartilages and sides of the vertebral bodies of the lower thoracic vertebrae and the lumbar vertebrae. It joins the iliacus to form the iliopsoas deep in the pelvis as it passes under the inguinal ligament and inserts in the lesser trochanter. It acts to flex and rotate the thigh and to flex and laterally bend the spine. Compare **psoas minor.**

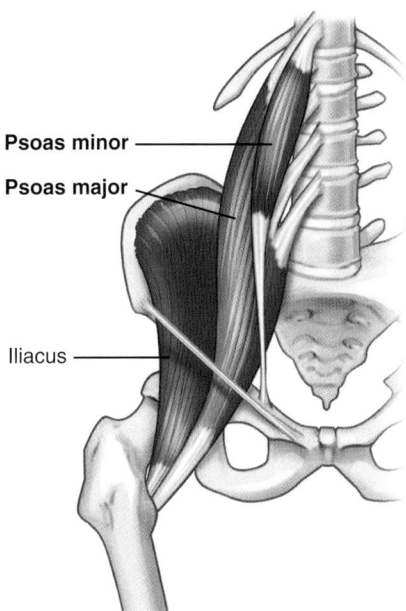

Psoas major and minor

psoas minor, a long, slender muscle of the pelvis, ventral to the psoas major. Many individuals do not have this muscle. The psoas minor functions to flex the spine. Compare **psoas major.**

psoas part of iliopsoas fascia, the part of the fascia that invests the psoas major muscle.

psomophagia /sō′mōfā″jē·ə/, the swallowing of food that has not been chewed properly.

psor-, prefix meaning "itching": *psoralen-type photosensitizer, psorelcosis.*

psoralen-type photosensitizer /sôr″ələn/, any one chemical compound that contains photosensitizing psoralen and reacts on exposure to ultraviolet light to increase the melanin in the skin. Naturally occurring psoralen photosynthesizers, such as 5- and 8-methoxypsoralen, are found in buttercups, carrot greens, celery, clover, cockleburs, dill, figs, limes, parsley, and meadow grass. Some psoralen-type photosensitizers produced as pharmaceutics are methoxsalen and trioxsalen; both are used to enhance skin pigmentation or tanning in the treatment of skin diseases, such as psoriasis and vitiligo. Such drugs are carefully administered to prevent oversensitization of the skin and other complications. Psoralen-type photosensitizers are also used in the manufacture of some perfumes, colognes, and pomades. Such chemicals cause unique skin reactions, such as berlock dermatitis, in some individuals. Oil of bergamot, extracted from the peels of small oranges grown in southern France and Italy, is a photosensitizing psoralen used as a tea flavoring and in perfumes.

psorelcosis /sôr′əlkō″sis/, an ulceration of the skin caused by scabies.

psorenteritis /sôr′enterī″tis/, an inflammation of the intestines.

psoriasis /sərī″əsis/ [Gk, itch], a chronic skin disorder characterized by circumscribed red patches covered by thick, dry, silvery adherent scales. Exacerbations and remissions are typical. Kinds include **guttate psoriasis, pustular psoriasis,** *universe psoriasis.* See also **psoriatic arthritis.** −*psoriatic, adj.*

■ OBSERVATIONS: The onset of symptoms is gradual, and the disorder is characterized by periods of chronic exacerbation and remission. The scalp, elbows, knees, back, and buttocks are the most common sites. The nails, eyebrows, axillae, and anal and genital regions may also be affected. The lesions are well-defined dry, nonpruritic papules or plaques overlaid with shiny silver scales, and they heal without scarring. The skin may be reddened and hot to touch. Affected nails are pitted, discolored, thickened, and crumbly. Diagnosis is based on evaluation of characteristic lesions. Common complications include psoriatic arthritis and exfoliative psoriatic dermatitis, which can lead to crippling and general debility.
■ INTERVENTIONS: Limited disease is treated with topical corticosteroids. Calcipotriene, tar products, and other keratolytics are used in lotion, cream, ointment, or shampoo form to treat lesions. Lubricants are used to soften skin. Exposure to sunlight and short-wave or long-wave ultraviolet light therapy may be useful to treat generalized disease. Antineoplastic agents such as methotrexate may used for severe recalcitrant disease. A number of new medications target the immune system.
■ PATIENT CARE CONSIDERATIONS: Psoriasis is often emotionally disabling due to changes in appearance. The focus is on helping individuals adapt to the chronic relapsing nature of the disease and adjust to body image challenges. Support groups and stress-reduction programs can be helpful. Instruction is needed to prevent mechanical injury to skin and to reinforce the fact that lesions are not communicable.

psoriasis universalis [Gk, *psoriasis,* itch; L, *universus,* on the whole], a severe attack of psoriasis in which most or all of the skin is involved.

psoriatic arthritis /sôr′e·at″ik/, a form of arthritis associated with psoriatic lesions of the skin and nails, particularly at the distal interphalangeal joints of the fingers and toes.
■ OBSERVATIONS: Stiffness and swelling, as well as joint pain, are the main symptoms of psoriatic arthritis.
■ INTERVENTIONS: There is no cure; control of symptoms is the goal. Medications used to manage symptoms include nonsteroidal antiinflammatory drugs (NSAIDs), disease-modifying antirheumatic drugs (DMARDs), immunosuppressant medications, and TNF-alpha inhibitors. Members of the health care team should emphasize the importance of joint protection, maintenance of a healthy weight, and appropriate exercise. The control of stress is also an important intervention.
■ PATIENT CARE CONSIDERATIONS: Psoriatic arthritis can occur in people without psoriatic skin lesions. Activity is important, and the medications used to control symptoms can cause fatigue. The patient should be encouraged to remain active.

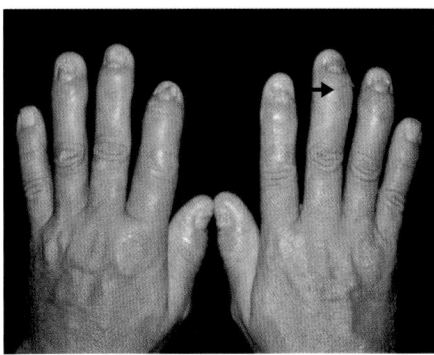

Psoriatic arthritis in distal interphalangeal joints
(Scott, 2012)

PSRO, abbreviation for **Professional Standards Review Organization.**

PSS, abbreviation for **progressive systemic sclerosis.** See **scleroderma.**

PSSO, 1. abbreviation for *peer specialist second opinion.* **2.** abbreviation for *physician support services organization.*

PSV, abbreviation for **pressure support ventilation.**

PSW, abbreviation for **psychiatric social worker.**

psych, abbreviation for **psychology.**

psych-. See **psycho-, psych-.**

psychalgia. See **psychic pain.**

psychataxia /sī′kətak″sē·ə/, a condition of mental confusion and inability to concentrate or fix attention.

psyche /sī′kē/ [Gk, mind], **1.** the aspect of one's mental faculty that encompasses the conscious and unconscious processes. **2.** the vital mental or spiritual entity of the individual as opposed to the body or soma. **3.** (in psychoanalysis) the total components of the id, ego, and superego, including all conscious and unconscious aspects. Compare **soma.**

psychedelic /sī′kədel″ik/ [coined in 1956 by Humphry Osmond from Gk, *psyche* + *deloun,* to reveal], **1.** describing a mental state characterized by altered sensory perception and hallucination accompanied by euphoria or fear, usually caused by the deliberate ingestion of drugs or other substances known to produce this effect. **2.** describing any drug or substance that causes this state, such as mescaline or psilocybin.

psychiatric /sī′kē·at″rik/ [Gk, *psyche,* mind, *iatreia,* treatment], pertaining to psychiatry.

psychiatric consultation liaison nurse (PCLN), an advanced practice nurse with a master's degree in psychiatric nursing. The practice focuses on emotional, spiritual, developmental, cognitive, and behavioral responses of patients with actual or potential physical dysfunction.

psychiatric disorder. See **mental disorder.**

psychiatric emergency service [Gk, *psyche* + *iatreia,* treatment], a hospital service that provides immediate initial evaluation and treatment to mentally ill patients on a 24-hour-a-day basis.

psychiatric foster care, a service for discharged psychiatric patients who receive observation and care in an approved foster home.

psychiatric home care, a service whereby a discharged psychiatric patient is provided observation and care in his or her place of residence. Many state laws require that the client be homebound.

psychiatric hospital, a health care facility providing inpatient and outpatient therapeutic services to clients with behavioral or emotional illnesses.

psychiatric inpatient unit, a hospital ward or similar area used for the treatment of inpatients who require psychiatric care.

psychiatric nurse practitioner, a nurse practitioner who, by advanced study and clinical practice, has gained expert knowledge in the care and prevention of mental disorders. See also **psychiatric nursing.**

psychiatric nursing, the branch of nursing concerned with the prevention, care, and cure of mental disorders and their sequelae. It uses theories of human behavior as its scientific framework and requires the use of the self as its art or expression in nursing practice. Some of the activities of the psychiatric nurse include providing a safe therapeutic milieu; working with patients or clients on the real day-to-day problems they face; identifying and caring for the physical aspects of the patient's problems, including drug therapy reactions; assuming the role of social agent or parent for the patient in various recreational, occupational, and

social situations; conducting psychotherapy; and providing leadership and clinical assistance for other nurses and health care workers. Psychiatric nurses work in many settings; their responsibilities vary with the setting and with the level of expertise, experience, and training of the individual nurse. Also called **mental health nursing.**

psychiatric social worker (PSW), a social worker who specializes in or works exclusively with the mentally ill.

psychiatrist /sīkī″ətrist/ [Gk, *psyche,* mind, *iatreia,* treatment], a physician with additional medical training and experience in the diagnosis, prevention, and treatment of mental disorders.

psychiatry /sīkī″ətrē/ [Gk, *psyche* + *iatreia,* treatment], the branch of medical science that deals with the causes, treatment, and prevention of mental, emotional, and behavioral disorders. Kinds include **community psychiatry, descriptive psychiatry, dynamic psychiatry, existential psychiatry, forensic psychiatry, orthopsychiatry. –psychiatric,** *adj.*

psychic /sī′kik/ [Gk, *psyche,* mind], a practitioner of the systematic study of parapsychology, a category of alleged psychological phenomena that cannot be explained by scientific thinking.

-psychic, suffix meaning "relation between mind and body": *biopsychic, extrapsychic, intrapsychic.*

psychic blindness [Gk, *psyche,* mind; AS, *blind*], a somatoform disorder that is manifested by the total or partial loss of vision in eyes that are organically normal. Despite the symptoms claimed, the patient usually reacts to light and avoids objects that might cause injury. The condition is frequently the result of an inner conflict or psychological stress, such as an unconscious effort to avoid a threatening or guilt-inducing situation. See also **conversion disorder.**

psychic contagion. See **psychic infection.**

psychic energy, mental energy such as thinking, perceiving, and remembering. See also **libido.**

psychic impotence [Gk, *psyche,* mind; L, *in* + *potentia,* power], a functional disorder of the male who is unable to perform sexual intercourse despite normal genitalia and sexual desire. The term generally applies to an inability to achieve and maintain an erection, but the disorder may be manifested in other forms, such as premature ejaculation or the need for certain conditions.

psychic infection [Gk, *psyche* + L, *inficere,* to stain], the spread of psychic effects or influences on others on a small scale, as in folie à deux, or on a large scale, as in the dance and witch manias of the Middle Ages or the spread of hysteria or panic in a crowd. Also called **psychic contagion.** See also **sympathy.**

psychic pain [Gk, *psyche,* mind; L, *poena,* penalty], a functional pain that, in the absence of any organic cause, is usually associated with feelings of acute anxiety. In some cases, the person may experience hallucinations or obsessions. Also called **psychalgia.**

psychic suicide, the termination of one's own life without the use of physical means or agents, such as by an older person, widowed after many years of marriage, who becomes sufficiently depressed to lose "the will to live."

psychic trauma, an emotional shock or injury or a distressful situation that produces a lasting impression, especially on the subconscious mind. Some causes of psychic trauma may include abuse or neglect in childhood, rape, and loss of a loved one. Psychotherapeutic sessions in which the injured person can ventilate feelings can help alleviate psychic trauma.

psychoacoustics /sī′kō·əkōōs″tiks/, the branch of science concerned with the physical features of sound as it relates to the psychological and physiological aspects of the sense of hearing in the unimpaired ear.

psychoactive /sī′kō·ak″tiv/ [Gk, *psyche,* mind; L, *activus*], pertaining to a drug or other agent that affects such normal mental functioning as mood, behavior, or thinking processes, such as stimulants, sedatives, or hallucinogens.

psychoanalysis /sī′kō·ənal″isis/ [Gk, *psyche + analyein,* to separate parts], a branch of psychiatry founded by Sigmund Freud, devoted to the study of the psychology of human development and behavior. From its systematized method for investigating the processes of the mind evolved a system of psychotherapy based on the concepts of a dynamic unconscious. By using such techniques as free association, dream interpretation, and analysis of defense mechanisms, emotions and behavior are traced to the influence of repressed instinctual drives in the unconscious. Treatment consists of helping the individual become aware of the existence of repressed emotional conflicts, analyzing their origin and through the process of insight bringing them into the consciousness so that irrational and maladaptive behavior can be altered. See also **psychosexual development.**

psychoanalyst /sī′kō·an′əlist/, a psychotherapist, usually a psychiatrist, who has had special training in psychoanalysis and who applies the techniques of psychoanalytic theory.

psychoanalytic /sī′kō·an′əlit′ik/, **1.** pertaining to psychoanalysis. **2.** using the techniques or principles of psychoanalysis (e.g., the study of the unconscious processes) in an attempt to examine causality.

psychobiology /-bī′ol″əjē/ [Gk, *psyche + bios,* life, *logos,* science], **1.** the study of biochemical foundations of thought, mood, emotion, affect, and behavior. **2.** personality development and functioning in terms of the interaction of the body and the mind. **3.** a school of psychiatric thought introduced by Adolf Meyer that stresses total life experience, including biological, emotional, and sociocultural factors, in assessing the psychological makeup or mental status of an individual.

psychocatharsis. See **catharsis.**

psychodiagnosis /-dī′agnō″sis/ [Gk, *psyche,* mind, *dia + gnosis,* knowledge], the study of a personality through observations of behavior and mannerisms combined with various tests.

psychodrama /-dram″ə/, a form of group psychotherapy, originated by J.L. Moreno, in which people act out their emotional problems through improvisational dramatizations.

psychodynamics /-dīnam″iks/ [Gk, *psyche + dynamis,* power], the study of the forces that motivate behavior. It may include the influence of past experiences on present behavior and the influence of mental and emotional forces on development and behavior.

psychoendocrinology /sī′kō·en′dōkrinol″əjē/, the study of the relationship between endocrinology and psychology.

psychoesthesia, a sensation of cold perceived although the body is warm.

psychogalvanic /-galvan″ik/, pertaining to the effects of psychological influences on the electrical properties of skin.

psychogender /-jen″dər/, the psychological sex as expressed in gender attitudes of a person, as distinguished from biological or somatic sex.

psychogenesis /sī′kōjen″əsis/ [Gk, *psyche + genesis,* origin], **1.** the development of the mind or of a mental function or process. **2.** the development or production of a physical symptom or disease having a mental or psychic origin rather than an organic cause. **3.** the development of emotional states, either normal or abnormal, from the interaction of conscious and unconscious psychological forces. Compare **somatogenesis.**

psychogenic /sī′kōjen″ik/ [Gk, *psyche + genein,* to produce], **1.** originating within the mind. **2.** referring to any physical symptom, disease process, or emotional state that is of psychological rather than physical origin. Also *psychogenetic.* See also **psychosomatic.**

psychogenic pain [Gk, *psyche,* mind; L, *poena,* penalty], a functional pain that does not have any known organic cause.

psychogenic pain disorder, a disorder characterized by persistent pain for which there is no apparent organic cause. The condition is often accompanied by other sensory or motor dysfunction, such as paresthesia or muscle spasm.

psychogenic polydipsia. See **compulsive polydipsia.**

psychogenic vomiting, vomiting that is stimulated by anxiety and emotional distress.

psychogeusic /-jōō″sik/, pertaining to the psychological influences on taste.

psychograph /si′kōgraf/, **1.** a chart for graphically recording the personality traits of an individual. **2.** a written description of the mental functioning of an individual.

psychokinesia /sī′kōkinē″zhə, -kīnē″zhə/ [Gk, *psyche + kinesis,* motion], impulsive behavior resulting from deficient or defective inhibitions without benefit of processing between the stimulus and the response.

psychokinesis (PK) /sī′kōkinē″sis, -kīnē″sis/ [Gk, *psyche + kinesis,* motion], the alleged direct influence of the mind or will on matter to produce motion in objects without the intervention of the physical senses or a physical force.

psychokinetics /sī′kōkinet″iks, -kīnet″iks/, the study of psychokinesis.

psycholinguistics /-ling·gwis″tiks/, the study of language as a form of behavior, including language development, speech, and personality.

psychological miscarriage, an absence or deficiency of a mother's love for her infant or absence of mother-child bonding.

psychological test [Gk, *psyche + logos,* science; L, *testum,* crucible], any of a group of standardized tests designed to measure or ascertain such characteristics of an individual as intellectual capacity, motivation, perception, role behavior, values, level of anxiety or depression, coping mechanisms, and general personality integration. Compare **achievement test, aptitude test, intelligence test, personality test.**

psychologist /sīkol″əjist/, a person who specializes in the study of the structure and function of the brain and related mental processes of animals and humans. A clinical psychologist is one who is qualified by graduate study in psychology and training in clinical psychology and who provides testing and counseling services to patients with mental and emotional disorders.

psychology (psych) /sīkol″əjē/ [Gk, *psyche + logos,* science], **1.** the study of behavior and of the functions and processes of the mind, especially as related to the social and physical environment. **2.** a profession that involves the practical applications of knowledge, skills, and techniques in the understanding of, prevention of, or solution to individual or social problems, especially in regard to the interaction between the individual and the physical and social environment. **3.** the mental, motivational, and behavioral characteristics and attitudes of an individual or group of individuals. Kinds include **analytic psychology,** *animal psychology,* **behaviorism, clinical psychology, cognitive psychology, educational psychology, experimental psychology, humanistic psychology,** *phenomenology,* **social psychology.** –*psychological, psychologic, adj.*

psychometrician /sī′kōmətrish″ən/ [Gk, *psyche,* mind, *metron,* measure], a specialist who performs quantitative estimation or measurement of personality and intelligence. The testing is not treatment-oriented.

psychometrics /sī'kōmet″riks/ [Gk, *psyche* + *metron*, measure], the development, administration, or interpretation of psychological and intelligence tests. Also called *psychometry*.

psychomotor /-mō'tər/ [Gk, *psyche* + L, *motare*, to move about], pertaining to or causing voluntary movements usually associated with neural activity.

psychomotor and physical development of infants, a branch of pediatric psychiatry that is concerned with the development of skills requiring coordination of sensory processes and motor activities, including infant reflexes, developmental timetables, and emotional and behavioral disorders.

psychomotor development, the progressive attainment by the child of skills that involve both mental and muscular activity, such as the ability of the infant to turn over, sit, or crawl at will and of the toddler to walk, talk, control bladder and bowel functions, and begin solving cognitive problems. The mean chronological ages at which certain psychomotor skills are attained by most children follow.

12 weeks	Looks at own hand
20 weeks	Able to grasp objects voluntarily
24 weeks	Able to roll from back to front at will
11 months	Creeps with abdomen off the floor and imitates speech sounds
15 months	Able to walk without help
24 months	Has a vocabulary of 300 or more words and uses pronouns
30 months	Able to jump with both feet
3 years	Able to ride a tricycle and to feed self well
4 years	Able to hop and skip on one foot, catch and throw a ball; is independent, boasts, tattles, and shows off
5 years	Able to tie shoelaces and cut with scissors, tries to please, interested in facts about world, gets along more easily with parents

psychomotor domain, the area of observable performance of skills that require some degree of neuromuscular coordination.

psychomotor epilepsy. See **psychomotor seizure.**

psychomotor learning, acquisition of the ability to perform motor skills.

psychomotor retardation, a generalized slowing of motor activity related to a state of severe depression or dementia.

psychomotor seizure, a temporary impairment of consciousness characterized by psychic symptoms, loss of judgment, automatic behavior, and abnormal acts. It is often associated with temporal lobe disease. No apparent convulsions occur, but there may be loss of consciousness or amnesia for the episode. During the seizure the individual may appear drowsy, intoxicated, or violent and may commit asocial acts or crimes, but normal activities, such as driving a car, typing, or eating, may continue at an automatic level. Psychic symptoms, including visual and auditory hallucinations, a sense of unreality, and déjà vu, may be present and may be accompanied by visceral symptoms, such as chest pain, transient respiratory arrest, tachycardia, and GI discomfort, and by abnormal sensations of smell and taste. Also called **psychomotor epilepsy.**

psychoneuroimmunology /-nŏŏr'ō·imyŏŏnol″əjē/, a discipline that studies the relationships between psychological states and the immune response.

psychoneurosis. See **neurosis.**

psychoneurotic. See **neurotic.**

psychoneurotic disorder. See **neurosis.**

psychooncology /sī'kō·ongkol″əjē/, the psychological effects of cancer, particularly the psychosocial needs of the patient and the patient's family.

psychopath /sī'kōpath/ [Gk, *psyche* + *pathos*, disease], a person who has an antisocial personality disorder. Also called **sociopath.** See also **antisocial personality, antisocial personality disorder.** –**psychopathic,** *adj.*

psychopathia. See **psychopathy.**

psychopathia sexualis /sī'kōpā″thē·ə sek'shŏŏ·al″is/ [Gk, *psyche* + *pathos,* disease; L, *sexus,* male or female], a mental disease characterized by sexual perversion.

psychopathic. See **psychopath.**

psychopathic personality. See **antisocial personality.**

psychopathologist /-pəthol″əjist/, one who specializes in the study and treatment of mental disorders. See also **psychiatrist.**

psychopathology /-pəthol″əjē/, **1.** the study of the causes, processes, and manifestations of mental disorders. **2.** the behavioral manifestation of any mental disorder. See also **psychiatry.**

psychopathy /sīkop″əthē/, any disease of the mind, congenital or acquired, not necessarily associated with subnormal intelligence. Also called **psychopathia.**

psychopharmaceutical /-fär′məsŏŏ″tikəl/, a drug used in the treatment of mental health disorders.

psychopharmacology /-fär′məkol″əjē/ [Gk, *psyche* + *pharmakon,* drug, *logos,* science], **1.** the scientific study of the effects of drugs on behavior and normal and abnormal mental functions. **2.** the use of these drugs in the treatment of mental illness.

psychophylaxis. See **mental hygiene.**

psychophysical /-fiz″ikəl/, pertaining to the psychosocial and physical aspects of a client's health and illness.

psychophysical preparation for childbirth, a program that prepares women for giving birth by teaching them the physiological characteristics of the process, exercises to improve muscle tone and physical stamina, and various techniques of breathing and relaxation to promote control and comfort during labor and delivery. There are several methods of psychophysical preparation for childbirth. Among the goals of all of the methods are a decrease in the mother's fear and pain, a decrease in or elimination of the use of analgesia and anesthesia in childbirth, and an increase in the mother's participation and cooperation, resulting in a reduced need for obstetric intervention. Kinds include **Bradley method, Lamaze method, Leboyer method of delivery, Read method.**

psychophysics /-fiz″iks/ [Gk, *psyche* + *physikos,* natural], the branch of psychology concerned with the relationships between physical stimuli and sensory responses.

psychophysiological /-fiz″ē·əloj″ikəl/ [Gk, *psyche* + *physikos,* natural], pertaining to physical symptoms, usually under the control of the autonomic nervous system, with emotional origins and involving a single organ system; psychosomatic.

psychophysiological disorder, any of a large group of mental disorders that are characterized by the dysfunction of an organ or organ system controlled by the autonomic nervous system and that may be caused or aggravated by emotional factors. The disorders are named and classified according to the organ system involved, such as cardiovascular, respiratory, musculoskeletal, and GI. Also called **psychosomatic illness, psychosomatic reaction.**

psychophysiology /-fiz″ē·ol″əjē/, **1.** the study of physiology as it relates to various aspects of psychological or behavioral function. See also **psychophysiological disorder. 2.** the study of mental activity by physical examination and observation.

psychoprophylactic preparation for childbirth /-prō′-filak″tik/, a system of prenatal education for giving birth using the Lamaze method of natural childbirth. See also **psychophysical preparation for childbirth.**

psychoprophylaxis /-prō′filak″sis/, a type of psychotherapy that is directed to prevention of emotional disorders. For example, it is used in the preparation for childbirth to reduce a woman's anxiety about pain and birth of a normal child.

psycho-, psych-, prefix meaning "the mind": *psychedelic, psychodynamics, psychogenic.*

psychorelaxation /-ri′laksā″shən/, the systematic desensitization to stress and anxiety by the practice of general body relaxation.

psychosensory /-sen″sərē/, pertaining to the perception and interpretation of sensory stimuli.

psychoses. See **psychosis.**

psychosexual /-sek″shoo̅-əl/ [Gk, *psyche* + L, *sexus,* male or female], pertaining to the psychological and emotional aspects of of sex. See also **psychosexual development, sexual disorder.**

psychosexual development, (in psychoanalysis) the emergence of the personality through a series of stages from infancy to adulthood. Each stage is relatively fixed in time and characterized by a dominant mode of achieving libidinal pleasure through the interaction of the person's biological drives and the environmental restraints. The stages of psychosocial development, as developed by Sigmund Freud, are the oral stage, anal stage, phallic stage, latency stage, and genital stage.

psychosexual disorder. See **sexual disorder.**

psychosexual dysfunction. See **sexual disorder.**

psychosexuality. See **psychosexual.**

psychosis /sīkō′sis/ *pl. psychoses* [Gk, *psyche* + *osis,* condition], any major mental disorder of organic or emotional origin characterized by a gross impairment in reality testing, in which the individual incorrectly evaluates the accuracy of his or her perceptions and thoughts and makes incorrect references about external reality, even in the face of contrary evidence. It is often characterized by regressive behavior, inappropriate mood and affect, and diminished impulse control. Symptoms of psychoses include hallucinations and delusions. See also **acute psychosis, ambulatory schizophrenia.**

-psychosis, suffix meaning "a serious mental disorder": *pseudopsychosis.*

psychosocial /-sō″shəl/ [Gk, *psyche* + L, *socialis,* partners], pertaining to a combination of psychological and social factors.

psychosocial assessment, an evaluation of a person's mental health, social status, and functional capacity within the community, generally conducted by psychiatric social workers.

psychosocial development, (in child development) a description devised by Erik Erikson of the normal serial development of trust (birth to 12 months), autonomy (1 to 2 years), initiative (3 to 5 years), industry, identity (12 to 18 years), intimacy, generativity, and ego integrity (60s and above). The development begins in infancy and progresses as the infantile ego interacts with the environment. For the child to reach a new stage successfully, the tasks of the preceding one should be fully mastered.

psychosomatic /sī′kōsəmat″ik/ [Gk, *psyche* + *soma,* body], **1.** pertaining to psychosomatic medicine. **2.** relating to, characterized by, or resulting from the interaction of the mind or psyche and the body. **3.** relating to the expression of an emotional conflict through physical symptoms. See also **conversion disorder, psychogenic, psychophysiological disorder.**

psychosomatic approach, the interdisciplinary or holistic study of physical and mental disease from a biological, psychosocial, and sociocultural point of view.

psychosomatic illness. See **psychophysiological disorder.**

psychosomatic medicine, the branch of medicine concerned with the interrelationships between mental and emotional reactions and somatic processes, in particular the manner in which intrapsychic conflicts influence physical symptoms. It maintains that the body and mind are one inseparable entity and that both physiological and psychological techniques should be applied in the study and treatment of illness. Also called **psychosomatics.**

psychosomatic pain [Gk, *psyche,* mind, *soma,* body; L, *poena,* penalty], pain that is caused in part by psychological factors.

psychosomatic reaction. See **psychophysiological disorder.**

psychosomatics. See **psychosomatic medicine.**

psychosomatogenic /-sōmat′əjen″ik/, pertaining to factors that cause or lead to the development of psychophysiological coping measures as learned responses to stressors.

psychostimulant /-stim″yələnt/, an agent that increases psychomotor activity in most patients. It improves concentration and impulse control in attention deficit hyperactivity disorder.

psychosurgery /-sur″jərē/ [Gk, *psyche* + *cheirourgia*], surgical interruption of certain nerve pathways in the brain, performed to treat selected cases of chronic unremitting anxiety, agitation, or obsessional neuroses. Modern psychotherapeutic drugs have replaced psychosurgery in most cases. Psychosurgery is performed when the condition is severe and when alternative treatments, such as psychotherapy, drugs, and electroshock, have proved ineffective. The procedure may be a limited prefrontal lobotomy, in which connecting fibers in the frontal region are cut, or a modified bifrontal tractotomy, in which nerve tracts of the brainstem are severed. Light general anesthesia is given. Postoperative nursing care includes observation for signs of leakage of cerebrospinal fluid. A marked alteration of personality is unavoidable. Various cognitive and affective functions also are affected, depending on the location of the induced lesion, the extent of destruction of nerve tissue, and the age, sex, and condition of the patient.

psychosynthesis /-sin″thəsis/, a form of psychotherapy that focuses on three levels of the unconscious—lower, middle, and higher unconscious, or superconscious. The goal of the treatment is the re-creation or integration of the personality.

psychotherapeutic drugs /-ther′əp(y)oo̅″tik/ [Gk, *psyche,* mind, *therapeutike,* medical practice; Fr, *drogue*], drugs that are prescribed for their effects in relieving symptoms of anxiety, depression, or other mental disorders.

psychotherapeutics /-tiks/ [Gk, *psyche* + *therapeia,* treatment], the treatment of mental disorders by means of psychotherapy.

psychotherapist /-ther″əpist/, one who practices psychotherapy, including psychiatrists, licensed psychologists, psychiatric nurses, psychiatric social workers, and individuals trained in counseling. The specific requirements for education and training differ markedly in content, breadth, and duration, depending on the form of psychotherapy practiced. Licensing procedures and definitions of practice vary from state to state. Compare **psychoanalyst.**

psychotherapy /-ther″əpē/ [Gk, *psyche* + *therapeia,* treatment], any of a large number of related methods of treating mental and emotional disorders by psychological techniques rather than by physical means.

P

psychotic /sīkot″ik/ [Gk, *psyche* + *osis,* condition], **1.** *adj.,* pertaining to psychosis. **2.** *n.,* a person exhibiting the characteristics of a psychosis. **3.** *adj.,* not in contact with reality.

psychotic disorder. See **psychosis.**

psychotic insight, a stage in the development of a psychosis that follows an initial experience of confusion, bizarreness, and apprehension, characterized by an insight that enables the patient to interpret the external world in terms of a delusional system of thinking. With the new insight, the factors that had previously been confusing become a part of the systematized pattern of the delusion, which, although irrational to an observer, is perceived by the patient as the attainment of exceptionally lucid thinking.

psychotic reaction. See **psychosis.**

psychotogenic /sīkot′əjen″ik/, pertaining to an agent that is capable of inducing symptoms of psychosis.

psychotomimetic /sīkot′ōmimet″ik/, a drug or other substance whose effects mimic the symptoms of psychosis, such as hallucinations.

psychotropic /-trop″ik/ [Gk, *psyche* + *trepein,* to turn], exerting an effect on the mind or modifying mental activity, as in psychotropic medications.

psychotropic drugs, drugs that affect the psychic functions, behavior, or experience of a person using them.

psychro-, prefix meaning "cold": *psychrometer, psychrophore, psychroesthesia.*

psychroesthesia /si′krō-esthē″zhə/, **1.** a chill. **2.** a sensation of cold although the body is warm.

psychrometer /sīkrom″ətər/, an instrument for calculating the degree of humidity in the atmosphere by comparing the temperatures of two thermometers, one with a wet bulb and one with a dry bulb. The difference in temperature between the two thermometers indicates the relative humidity.

psychrometry /sīkrom″ətrē/, the calculation of relative humidity and water vapor pressure from psychrometer data and barometric pressure.

psychrophore /sī″krəfôr/, a double-lumen catheter through which cold water is circulated.

psyllium husk, the cleaned, dried seed coat from the seeds of *Plantago* species, used as a bulk-forming laxative.

psyllium seed. See **plantago seed.**

Pt, symbol for the element **platinum.**

PT, 1. abbreviation for **physical therapist. 2.** abbreviation for **physical therapy. 3.** abbreviation for **prothrombin time.**

pt, abbreviation for **patient.**

PTA, 1. abbreviation for **percutaneous transluminal angioplasty. 2.** abbreviation for **plasma thromboplastin antecedent. 3.** abbreviation for **physical therapy assistant.**

PTB, abbreviation for *patellar-tendon bearing.* See **patellar-tendon bearing (PTB) prosthesis.**

PTB/SC, abbreviation for **patellar-tendon bearing supracondylar (PTB/SC) socket.**

PTCA, abbreviation for **percutaneous transluminal coronary angioplasty.**

pterion /tir″ē-on/, a point near the sphenoid fontanel of the skull, at the junction of the greater wing of the sphenoid, squamous, temporal, frontal, and parietal bones. It also intersects the course of the anterior division of the middle meningeal artery.

pteroylglutamic acid. See **folic acid.**

pterygium /tərij″ē-əm/ [Gk, *pterygion,* wing], a thick triangular patch of pale hypertrophied tissue that extends medially from the nasal border of the cornea to the inner canthus of the eye.

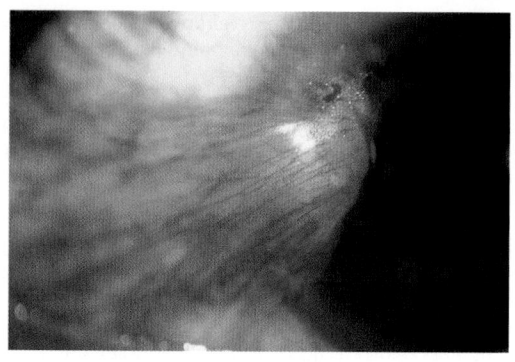

Pterygium *(Courtesy Ben Serar, MA, CRA)*

-pterygium, suffix meaning "a (specified) abnormality of the conjunctiva": *pseudopterygium.*

pterygium colli. See **webbed neck.**

pterygium syndrome. See **multiple pterygium syndrome.**

pterygoid /ter″igoid/ [Gk, *pteryx,* wing, *eidos,* form], pertaining to a winglike structure.

pterygoideus lateralis. See **external pterygoid muscle.**

pterygoideus medialis. See **internal pterygoid muscle.**

pterygoid fossa, a depression that separates the medial and lateral plates of each pterygoid process.

pterygoid hamulus, a hooklike projection at the inferior end of each medial plate of the pterygoid process.

pterygoid plexus, one of a pair of extensive networks of veins between the temporalis and the pterygoideus lateralis muscles, extending between surrounding structures in the infratemporal fossa. It communicates with the facial vein through the deep facial and angular veins. Compare **maxillary vein.**

pterygoid process [Gk, *pteryx,* wing, *eidos,* form; L, *processus*], any one of the paired processes of the sphenoid bone.

pterygomandibular /ter′igōmandib″yəlar/ [Gk, *pteryx,* wing, *eidos,* form; L, *mandere,* to chew], pertaining to the pterygoid process and the mandible.

pterygomandibular raphe, a tendinous band between the pterygoid hamulus superiorly and the mandible inferiorly. It is the point of attachment for the buccinators and superior pharyngeal constrictor muscles.

pterygomaxillary /-mak″siler′ē/ [Gk, *pteryx,* wing, *eidos,* form; L, *maxilla,* jaw], pertaining to the sphenoid bone and the maxilla.

pterygomaxillary notch, a fissure at the junction of the maxilla and the pterygoid process of the sphenoid bone. Also called **hamular notch.**

pterygopalatine fossa, a space shaped like a teardrop between the bones on the lateral side of the skull immediately posterior to the maxilla. It is a major site of distribution for the maxillary nerve and for the terminal part of the maxillary artery.

PTH, abbreviation for **parathyroid hormone.**

Pthirus pubis. See **crab louse.**

PTNA, abbreviation for **Provincial/Territorial Nurses Association.**

ptoma-, prefix meaning "corpse": *ptomaine, ptomainemia.*

ptomaine /tō″mān/ [Gk, *ptoma,* corpse], an imprecise term introduced in the 19th century to identify a group of nitrogenous substances found in putrefied proteins. Because injection of the substances produced toxic reactions, the ptomaines were once regarded as poisonous. Later studies showed that the same substances were produced by the normal digestion of proteins in the human intestine without toxic effects.

ptomainemia /tō'mānē″mē·ə/, a condition caused by the presence of a ptomaine, a potentially toxic amine, in the blood.

ptosis /tō″sis/ [Gk, *falling*], an abnormal condition of one or both upper eyelids in which the eyelid droops because of a congenital or acquired weakness of the levator muscle or paralysis of the third cranial nerve. The condition may be treated surgically by shortening the levator muscle. **−ptotic,** *adj.*

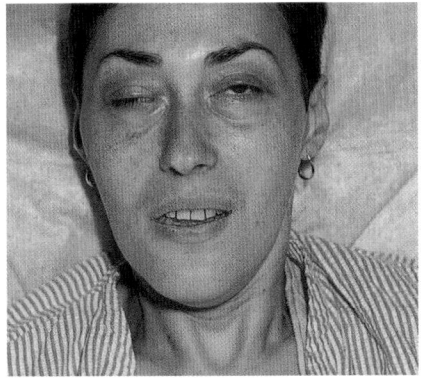

Woman with ptosis *(Swartz, 2009)*

-ptosis, suffix meaning "a falling, drooping, or prolapse of an organ": *coloptosis, nephrotosis, glossoptosis.*

ptotic. See **ptosis.**

ptotic kidney /tot″ik/, a kidney that is abnormally situated in the pelvis, usually over the sacral promontory behind the peritoneum. The condition may be either congenital or secondary to trauma. It is usually asymptomatic, but during pregnancy the flow of urine from a ptotic kidney may be obstructed.

PTSD, abbreviation for **posttraumatic stress disorder.**

PTT, abbreviation for **partial thromboplastin time.**

ptyalin /tī″əlin/ [Gk, *ptyalon,* spittle], a starch-digesting enzyme present in saliva. It hydrolyzes starch and glycogen. Its optimal pH is 6.9. Also called **amylase.**

ptyalism /tī″əliz′əm/ [Gk, *ptyalon,* spittle], excessive salivation, such as sometimes occurs in the early months of pregnancy. It is also a clinical sign of mercury poisoning. Also called **hyperptyalism.** See also **sialorrhea.**

ptyalo-, prefix meaning "saliva": *ptyalocele.*

ptyalocele /tī-al′o-sēl/, a cystic tumor containing saliva.

ptyocrinous /tī·ok″rinəs/, pertaining to the secretion of the contents of a unicellular gland in the form of extruded granules.

p-type semiconductor. See **semiconductor.**

-ptysis, suffix meaning "a spitting of matter": *hemoptysis.*

Pu, symbol for the element **plutonium.**

pub-, pubo-, prefix meaning "grown up" or "adult": *pubarche, puberty, pubescence.*

pubarche /pyoōbär″kē, pyoō″bärkē/ [L, *puber,* ripe, *arch,* beginning], onset of puberty. It is marked by the beginning of the development of secondary sexual characteristics.

pubertal /p(y)oō″bərtəl/ [L, *pubertas,* age of maturity], pertaining to puberty.

puberty /p(y)oō″bərtē/ [L, *pubertas,* age of maturity], the period of life at which the ability to reproduce begins. It is a stage of development when genitalia reach maturity and secondary sex characteristics appear. The onset normally occurs in females between 9 and 13 years of age with the development of breasts and menarche. In males, puberty usually occurs between 12 and 14 years of age and is characterized by the ejaculation of sperm.

puberulic acid /pyoōber″yoōlik/, an antibiotic isolated from the mold *Penicillium puberulum* that prevents the replication of gram-positive bacteria.

pubes. See **pubis.**

pubescent /p(y)oōbes″ənt/ [L, *pubescere,* to reach puberty], pertaining to the beginning of puberty.

pubescent uterus [L, *pubescere,* to reach puberty, *uterus,* womb], a uterus in which the cervix and body of the uterus remain of equal size in adult life, similar to that of an adolescent prior to menstruation.

pubic /p(y)oō″bik/ [L, *pubis*], pertaining to or involving the region of the pubic symphysis.

-pubic, suffix meaning "the frontal part of the pelvis": *iliopubic, retropubic, suprapubic.*

pubic bone. See **pubis.**

pubic dislocation. See **dislocation of the hip.**

pubic hair /p(y)oō″bik/ [L, *pubis* + AS, *haer*], hair of the pubic region.

pubic ligament, either of the two ligaments, superior and inferior, associated with the pubic symphysis.

pubic region [L, *pubes,* signs of maturity, *regio,* territory], the most inferior part of the abdomen in the lower zone between the right and left inguinal regions and below the umbilical region. Also called **hypogastric region, hypogastrium.** See also **abdominal regions.**

pubic symphysis, the slightly movable interpubic joint of the pelvis, consisting of two pubic bones separated by a disk of fibrocartilage and connected by two ligaments. Also called **symphysis pubis.**

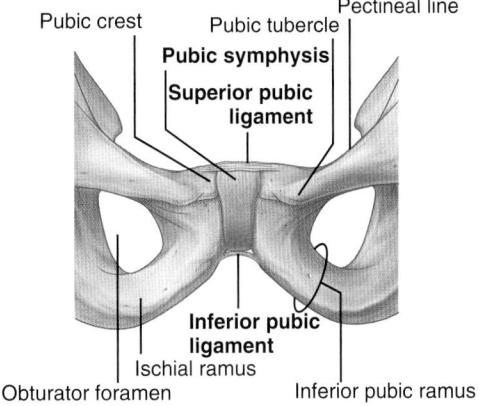

Pubic symphysis *(Drake, Vogl, and Mitchell, 2015)*

pubiotomy /p(y)oō′bi·ot″əmē/, the separation of the pubic bone, performed to increase the capacity of the pelvis to permit passage of a fetus. Also called **pelviotomy.**

pubis /pyoō″bis/ *pl. pubes* [L, *pubes*], one of a pair of pubic bones that join at the pubic symphysis and, with the ischium and the ilium, form the hip bone. The pubis forms one fifth of the acetabulum and is divisible into the body, the superior ramus, and the inferior ramus. The external surface of the pubis serves as the origin of the adductor longus, the obturator externus, the adductor brevis, and the proximal part of the gracilis. The internal surface of the pubis forms part of the anterior wall of the pelvis, giving origin to the levator ani and the obturator internus. The pubic crest affords attachment to the rectus abdominis, the pyramidalis, and the inguinal falx. The lateral part of the superior ramus of the pubis presents the superior, the inferior, and the dorsal surfaces. The superior surface presents the iliopectineal line. The inferior ramus gives origin to the gracilis, a part of the obturator externus, the adductor brevis, the adductor magnus, the obturator internus, and the constrictor urethrae. Compare **ilium, ischium.**

public health [L, *publicus,* of the people; AS, *haelth*], a field of medicine that deals with the physical and mental health of the community, particularly in such areas as water supply, waste disposal, air pollution, and food safety. In the United States there are more than 3000 state, county, or city public health agencies. The U.S. Public Health Service was organized in 1798 to provide hospital care for American merchant seamen. Subsequent legislation has expanded the role of the federal agency to include such services as the Food and Drug Administration; the National Library of Medicine; health care for Native Americans and Alaska Natives; protection against impure and unsafe foods, drugs, cosmetics, and medical devices; control of alcohol and drug abuse; and protection against unsafe radiation-producing projects.

public health dentistry. See **dental public health.**

public health nursing, a field of nursing that is concerned with the health needs of the community as a whole. Public health nurses may work with families in the home, in schools, at the workplace, in government agencies, and at major health facilities. A home care nursing service is provided by nurses who have special education in public health and are employed by such voluntary agencies as the Visiting Nurses Association or Visiting Nurse Service, or Victorian Order of Nurses for Canada. Public health nurses enter practice through a baccalaureate program accredited in the United States by the Accreditation Commission for Education in Nursing or the Commission on Collegiate Nursing Education, which prepares them to work as generalists. Additional recognition is offered through a certification program administered by the American Nurses Credentialing Center.

public sector, (in health care) typically, government at the federal, state, provincial, and local levels. It may refer to other community organizations and lobbying groups.

publish or perish [L, *publicare,* to make public, *perire,* to come to naught], *(Informal)* a practice followed in many academic institutions in which a contract for employment is renewed only if a candidate has demonstrated scholarship by having work published in a book or in a reputable refereed professional or scientific journal. This work is required in addition to whatever obligations for teaching or professional practice are entailed in the position.

pubo-. See **pub-, pubo-.**

pubocapsular /p(y)o͞o′bōkap″sələr/, pertaining to the pubis and articular capsule of the hip joint.

pubocervical ligament, a condensation of fascia that extends from the cervix to the anterior pelvic wall. It is thought to help stabilize the uterus in the pelvic cavity. See also **cardinal ligament, levator ani, uterosacral ligament.**

pubococcygeal /p(y)o͞o′bōkoksij″ē·əl/ [L, *pubis* + Gk, *kokkyx,* cuckoo's beak], pertaining to the pubis and the coccyx.

pubococcygeus exercises /pyo͞o′bōkoksij″ē·əs/ [L, *pubes* + Gk, *kokkyx,* cuckoo's beak; L, *exercere,* to make strong], a regimen of isometric exercises in which a woman executes a series of voluntary contractions of the muscles of her pelvic diaphragm and perineum in an effort to increase the contractility of her vaginal introitus or to improve retention of urine. Also called **Kegel exercises.**

■ METHOD: The exercise involves the familiar muscular squeezing action that is required to stop the urinary stream while voiding; that action is performed in an intensive, repetitive, and systematic way throughout each day.

■ INTERVENTIONS: The woman is instructed in how to duplicate the squeezing, pulling-up action. A woman whose mus-

cles are particularly attenuated may have difficulty understanding or feeling the muscular action involved. It is often helpful for her to be told that the action is exactly the same as that required to stop the flow of urine. When the woman can effect the contraction required, she is asked to hold the contraction for 6 to 10 seconds, allowing the muscles to relax completely between contractions. She is then advised to perform 10 to 15 repetitions of the contraction in a series and to repeat the series three to four times each day. She is further advised that the physiological nature of muscular exercise is such that weakened muscles may gain strength during the early phases of an exercise program and that, with diligence, she can expect to notice significant improvement in control that will continue as she maintains the regimen of exercise.

■ OUTCOME CRITERIA: Laxity and weakness of the pubococcygeus muscles, often a result of childbirth, may predispose certain women to looseness of the vaginal introitus and to stress incontinence. These problems may be ameliorated as the strength and tone of the muscles are increased through exercise. The rapidity with which a woman can, during voiding, close off the urinary stream is taken as a measure of the strength and tone of her pubococcygeus muscles. Ideally she should be able to perform the action completely and almost instantly.

pubofemoral ligament, a triangular ligament anteroinferior to the hip joint. Its base is attached medially to the iliopubic eminence, adjacent bone, and obturator membrane.

puboprostatic /p(y)o͞o′bōprostat″ik/, relating to the pubis and prostate gland.

pubovaginal sling, a support constructed of rectoabdominal fascia or synthetic mesh used to stabilize the bladder in treatment of stress incontinence.

pudenda, pudendal. See **pudendum.**

pudendal /pu-den′dal/, pertaining to or supplying the pudendum, such as pudendal nerves or a pudendal block.

pudendal block /p(y)o͞oden″təl/ [L, *pudendus,* shameful; Fr, *bloc,* lump], a form of regional anesthetic block administered to provide anesthesia of the perineum, which is particularly useful during the expulsive second stage of labor. The pudendal nerves are anesthetized by the injection of a local anesthetic near the trunk of each nerve as it passes over the sacrospinous ligament, just below the ischial spine. A 10-mL syringe, a long needle, and a guide are used in the procedure. The injection is most easily performed transvaginally. Pudendal block anesthetizes the perineum, vulva, and perirectal area without affecting the muscular contractions of the uterus. When the block is properly administered, the risk is minimal. However, modern obstetric anesthesia most often utilizes epidural analgesia.

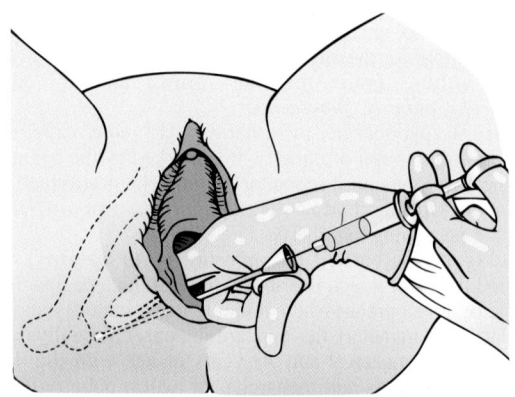

Pudendal block *(Lowdermilk et al, 2016)*

pudendal canal. See **Alcock's canal.**

pudendal nerve, one of the branches of the pudendal plexus that arises from the second, third, and fourth sacral nerves; passes between the piriformis and coccygeus; and leaves the pelvis through the greater sciatic foramen. It divides into five branches supplying the external genital structures and the pelvic region. The branches of the pudendal nerve are the inferior rectal nerve, perineal nerve, and dorsal nerve of the penis or of the clitoris. See also **pudendal plexus.**

pudendal plexus, a network of motor and sensory nerves formed by the anterior branches of the second and the third and all of the fourth sacral nerves. It is often considered part of the sacral plexus. The pudendal plexus lies in the posterior hollow of the pelvis. The branches of the plexus are the visceral branches, the muscular branches, and the pudendal nerve. The visceral branches arise from the second, third, and fourth sacral nerves and supply the bladder, prostate, seminal vesicles, uterus, external genitalia, and some of the intestinal tract. The muscular branches arise from the fourth and sometimes the third and fifth sacral nerves and supply the levator ani, sphincter ani, and coccygeus. Compare **lumbar plexus, sacral plexus.** See also **pudendal nerve.**

pudendum /p(y) oōden″dəm/ *pl. pudenda* [L, *pudendus,* shameful], the external genitalia, especially of women. In a woman it comprises the mons veneris, the labia majora, the labia minora, the vestibule of the vagina, and the vestibular glands. In a man it comprises the penis, scrotum, and testes.

puer-, prefix meaning "child": *puericulture, puerilism, puerperium, puerperal.*

puericulture /pyoō″ərikul′chər/ [L, *pueri,* children, *colere,* to cultivate], the rearing and training of children. *–puericulturist, n.*

puerile /pyoō″əril, -īl/ [L, childish], pertaining to children or childhood; juvenile. *–puerility, n.*

puerilism /pyoō″əriliz′əm/ [L, *puerilis,* childish], childishness, particularly when manifested in an older adult.

puerility. See **puerile.**

puerpera /pyoō·er″pərə/ [L, *puerpus,* childbirth], a woman who has just given birth.

puerperal /pyoō·er″pərəl/ [L, *puerpus,* childbirth], **1.** pertaining to the period immediately after childbirth. **2.** pertaining to a woman (a puerpera) who has just given birth to an infant.

puerperal eclampsia [L, *puerpus,* childbirth; Gk, *ek,* out, *lampein,* to flash], a condition of coma and convulsive seizures occurring after childbirth. It is associated with hypertension, edema, and proteinuria. See also **puerperal fever.**

puerperal fever, a syndrome associated with systemic bacterial infection and septicemia that occurs after childbirth, usually as a result of unsterile obstetric technique. It is characterized by endometritis, fever, tachycardia, uterine tenderness, and foul lochia. If it is untreated, prostration, renal failure, bacteremic shock, and death may occur. The causative organism is most often one of the hemolytic streptococci. Puerperal fever was little known before hospital childbirth became common, early in the 19th century; then it became an endemic and frequently epidemic scourge that resulted in the deaths of many thousands of mothers and infants. Maternal mortality rates of 20% and higher were common in parts of the world where childbirth occurred in hospitals. Ignaz Philipp Semmelweis, in Vienna, noted that women attended by midwives were much less likely to contract the disease than those attended by physicians and medical students. Midwives did not perform frequent vaginal examinations during labor and did not participate in autopsies. Although the germ theory of disease had not yet been elaborated, Semmelweis deduced that the causative agent of the disease was being transmitted by doctors and students from the infected cadavers in the autopsy room to women in labor on the maternity wards. After institution of a policy requiring that the hands and instruments of obstetric attendants be disinfected, the maternal mortality rate in his clinic dropped dramatically. His work was widely ignored or discredited for almost half a century because physicians were unwilling to believe that they were the agents of transmission. Late in the 19th century, after Pasteur's discovery of microbes, Semmelweis was posthumously vindicated. Sterile techniques were gradually instituted, but not until the fourth decade of the 20th century did puerperal fever cease to be the leading cause of maternal death. Postpartum uterine infection is common but is effectively treated with massive parenteral doses of antibiotics before it becomes a systemic illness. Also called **childbed fever, puerperal sepsis.**

puerperal mania, a rare acute mood disorder that sometimes occurs in women after childbirth, characterized by a severe manic reaction. Compare **postpartum depression, postpartum psychosis.** See also **mania.**

puerperal mastitis [L, *puerpus,* childbirth; Gk, *mastos,* breast, *itis,* inflammation], a form of acute mastitis in a nursing mother.

puerperal metritis. See **puerperal fever.**

puerperal phlebitis [L, *puerpus,* childbirth; Gk, *phleps,* vein, *itis,* inflammation], an inflammation that begins in a uterine vein after childbirth and spreads to other veins, particularly the iliac and femoral veins.

puerperal psychosis. See **postpartum psychosis.**

puerperal sepsis, an infection acquired during the puerperium.

puerperium /pyoō″ərpir″ē·əm/ [L, *puerperus*], the time after childbirth, lasting approximately 6 weeks, during which the anatomical and physiological changes brought about by pregnancy resolve and a woman adjusts to the new or expanded responsibilities of motherhood and nonpregnant life.

PUFA, abbreviation for **polyunsaturated fatty acid.** See **unsaturated fatty acid.**

puff [ME *puf*], a short, soft, blowing sound heard on auscultation.

puffer fish /puf′ər fish/, any of several species of marine fish of genera *Fugu, Sphaeroides, Tetraodon,* and others, which when disturbed can inflate themselves to a spherical shape. The flesh of puffer fish contains tetrodoxin, and if the fish is ingested, it can cause fatal tetrodotoxism unless it has been properly prepared by trained chefs.

Pulex /pyoō″leks/ [L, flea], a genus of fleas, some species of which transmit arthropod-borne infections, such as plague and epidemic typhus.

pulmo-, pulmon-, prefix meaning "the lungs": *pulmoaortic, pulmonologist, pulmonary.*

pulmoaortic /pool′mō·ā·ôr″tik/, pertaining to the lungs and aorta.

pulmon-. See **pulmo-, pulmon-.**

pulmonary /pool″məner′ē/ [L, *pulmo,* lungs], pertaining to the lungs or the respiratory system. Also **pulmonic.**

pulmonary acid aspiration syndrome. See **Mendelson syndrome.**

pulmonary agents. See **choking/lung/pulmonary agents.**

pulmonary alveolar proteinosis [L, *pulmoneus,* lungs, *alveolus,* little hollow; Gk, *proteios,* first rank, *osis,* condition], a condition in which the air sacs of the lungs become filled with protein and lipids, progressing to respiratory failure. The cause is unknown.

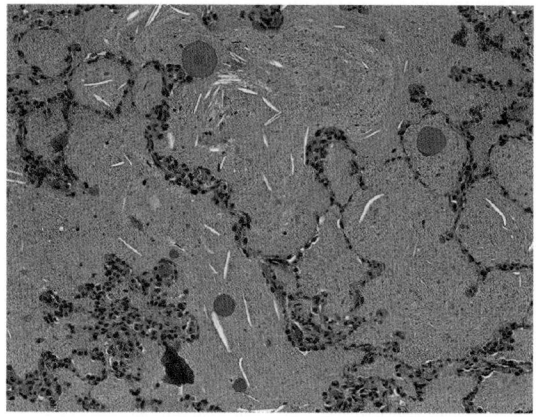

Sputum specimen of patient with pulmonary alveolar proteinosis *(Broaddus et al, 2016)*

pulmonary alveolus. See **alveolus.**

pulmonary angiography [L, *pulmoneus,* lungs; Gk, *angeion,* vessel, *graphein,* to record], the radiographic examination of the blood vessels of the lungs after the injection of radiopaque contrast medium into the pulmonary circulation. It is used to detect pulmonary emboli.

pulmonary anthrax. See **woolsorter's disease.**

pulmonary arteriolar resistance (PAR), pressure loss per unit of blood flow from the pulmonary artery to a pulmonary vein.

pulmonary artery (PA) [L, *pulmoneus,* lungs; Gk, *arteria,* airpipe], one of two arteries, the left one supplying the left lung and the right one supplying the right lung. The lobar branches are named according to the lobe they supply, such as apical *(ramus apicalis).*

pulmonary artery catheter [L, *pulmoneus,* lungs; Gk, *arteria + katheter,* a thing lowered], any of various cardiac catheters for measuring pulmonary arterial pressures, introduced into the venous system through a large vein and guided by blood flow into the superior vena cava, the right atrium and ventricle, and the pulmonary artery.

pulmonary artery wedge pressure. See **pulmonary wedge pressure.**

pulmonary atresia [L, *pulmoneus,* lungs; Gk, *a + tresis,* without perforation], a congenital heart defect of the right ventricular outflow tract. One form consists of an intact ventricular septum with an interatrial communication and a persistent patent ductus arteriosus. A more extreme form is the four-defect tetralogy of Fallot.

pulmonary atrium, any of the spaces at the end of an alveolar duct into which alveoli open.

pulmonary candidiasis [L, *pulmones,* lungs; L, *candidus,* white + Gk, *-iasis,* disease suffix], a type of fungal pneumonia caused by infection with *Candida* species, seen especially in immunocompromised patients or those with malignancies. Also called ***Candida* pneumonia.**

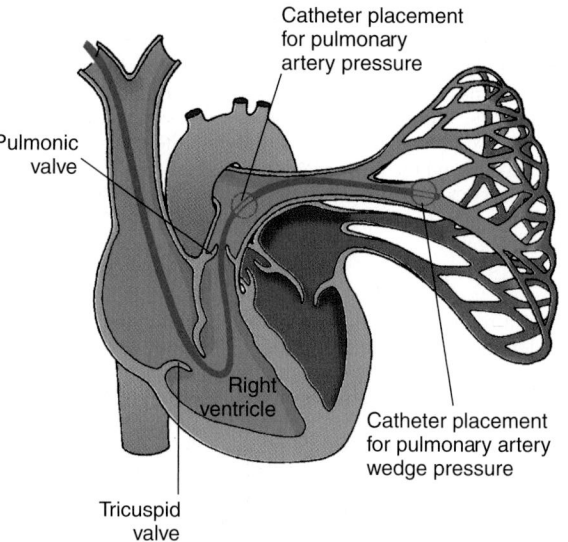

Placement of pulmonary artery catheter *(Ignatavicius and Workman, 2010)*

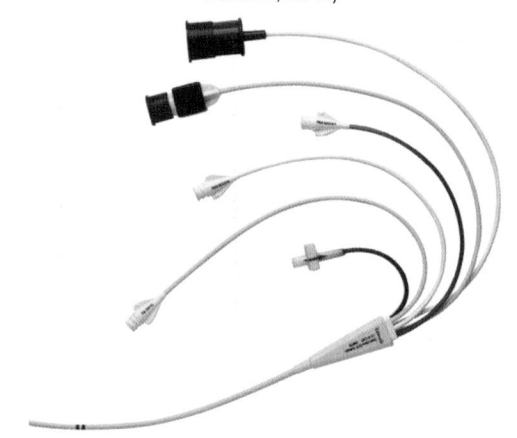

Pulmonary artery catheter *(Courtesy Edwards Critical Care Division, Baxter Healthcare Corporation)*

pulmonary capillary wedge pressure. See **pulmonary wedge pressure.**

pulmonary carcinosis. See **alveolar cell carcinoma.**

pulmonary circulation [L, *pulmoneus,* lungs, *circulare*], the blood flow through the network of vessels between the heart and the lungs for the oxygenation of blood and removal of carbon dioxide. Also called **lesser circulation.**

pulmonary compliance. See **compliance,** def. 2.

pulmonary congestion [L, *pulmoneus,* lungs, *congerere,* to heap together], an excessive accumulation of fluid in the lungs, usually associated with either an inflammation or congestive heart failure.

pulmonary disease, any abnormal condition of the respiratory system, characterized by cough, chest pain, dyspnea, hemoptysis, sputum production, stridor, or adventitious sounds. Less common symptoms include anxiety, arm and shoulder pain, tenderness in the calf of the leg, erythema nodosum, swelling of the face, headache, hoarseness, joint pain, and somnolence. Diagnostic procedures for pulmonary diseases include bronchoscopy; cytological, serological, and biochemical examination of bronchial secretions; laryngoscopy; pulmonary function tests; and radiography. Obstructive respiratory disease is the result of a reduction of airway size that impedes airflow. The obstruction may result from bronchospasm, edema of the bronchial mucosa, or excessive bronchial secretions. Obstructive disease is characterized by reduced expiratory flow rates and increased total lung capacity. Acute obstructive respiratory diseases include asthma, bronchitis, and bronchiectasis; chronic obstructive diseases include emphysema, chronic bronchitis, or combined emphysema and chronic bronchitis. Patients with obstructive diseases may have acute respiratory failure from any respiratory stress, such as infections or general anesthesia. Restrictive respiratory disease is caused by conditions that limit lung expansion, such as fibrothorax, obesity, a neuromuscular disorder, kyphosis, scoliosis, spondylitis, or surgical removal of lung tissue. Pregnancy causes a self-limiting restrictive disease in the third trimester. Characteristics of restrictive respiratory disease are decreased forced expired vital capacity and total lung capacity, with increased work of breathing and inefficient exchange of gases. Acute restrictive conditions are the most common pulmonary cause of acute respiratory failure. Infectious diseases include pneumonia and tuberculosis.

pulmonary dysmaturity syndrome, a respiratory disorder of premature infants in which the lungs contain focal emphysematous blebs and thickened alveolar walls. The infants commonly die of hypoxia.

pulmonary edema, the accumulation of extravascular fluid in lung tissues and alveoli, caused most commonly by congestive heart failure. Serous fluid is pushed through the pulmonary capillaries into alveoli and quickly enters bronchioles and bronchi. The condition also may occur in barbiturate and opiate poisoning, diffuse infections, hemorrhagic pancreatitis, and renal failure and after a stroke, skull fracture, near-drowning, inhalation of irritating gases, and rapid administration of whole blood, plasma, serum albumin, or IV fluids. See also **pleural effusion.**

■ OBSERVATIONS: Signs and symptoms of pulmonary edema include tachypnea; labored, shallow respirations; restlessness; apprehensiveness; air hunger; cyanosis; and blood-tinged or frothy pink sputum. The peripheral and neck veins are usually engorged, blood pressure and heart rate are increased, and the pulse may be full and pounding or weak and thready. There may be edema of the extremities, adventitious breath sounds in the lungs, respiratory acidosis, and profuse diaphoresis.

■ INTERVENTIONS: Acute pulmonary edema is an emergency condition requiring prompt treatment. The patient is given oxygen and placed in bed in a high Fowler's position, and IV morphine sulfate is usually administered immediately to relieve pain, to quiet breathing, and to allay apprehension. Morphine also acts as a pulmonary vasodilator. A cardiotonic, such as digitalis or dobutamine, and a fast-acting diuretic, such as furosemide or bumetanide, may be given. Oxygen may be ordered. While the patient is acutely ill, the blood pressure, respiration, apical pulse, and breath sounds are checked frequently or continually monitored. Parenteral fluids, if indicated, are infused slowly in limited quantities. A low-sodium diet is served, and the patient's intake and output of fluids are measured. The patient is weighed daily, and any sudden weight gain is noted and reported.

■ PATIENT CARE CONSIDERATIONS: The nurse provides continued care and emotional support. The physical therapist and occupational therapist direct the patient to exercise to tolerance with frequent rest periods. All health care providers should educate the patient to report any symptoms, to avoid smoking, and to follow the regimen ordered for medication, diet, and return checkups.

pulmonary embolism (PE), the blockage of a pulmonary artery by fat, air, tumor tissue, or a thrombus that usually arises from a peripheral vein (most frequently one of the deep veins of the legs). Predisposing factors include an alteration of blood constituents with increased coagulation, damage to blood vessel walls, and stagnation or immobilization, especially when associated with pregnancy and childbirth, congestive heart failure, polycythemia, or surgery. Pulmonary embolism is difficult to distinguish from myocardial infarction and pneumonia. It is characterized by dyspnea, anxiety, sudden chest pain, shock, and cyanosis. Pulmonary infarction, which often occurs within 24 hours after the formation of a pulmonary embolus, is further characterized by pleural effusion, hemoptysis, leukocytosis, fever, tachycardia, atrial arrhythmias, and striking distension of the neck veins. Analysis of blood gases reveals arterial hypoxia and hypocapnia. Pulmonary embolism is detected by chest radiographic films, pulmonary angiography, and radioscanning of the lung fields. Two thirds of patients with a massive pulmonary embolus die within 2 hours. Initial resuscitative measures include external cardiac massage, oxygen, vasopressor drugs, embolectomy, and correction of acidosis. The formation of further emboli is prevented by the use of anticoagulants, sometimes the use of streptokinase or urokinase, and also surgical intervention. Ambulation, exercise, and use of sequential compression devices on the lower extremities also are recommended for prevention. A vena cava filter may be inserted if pulmonary emboli recur.

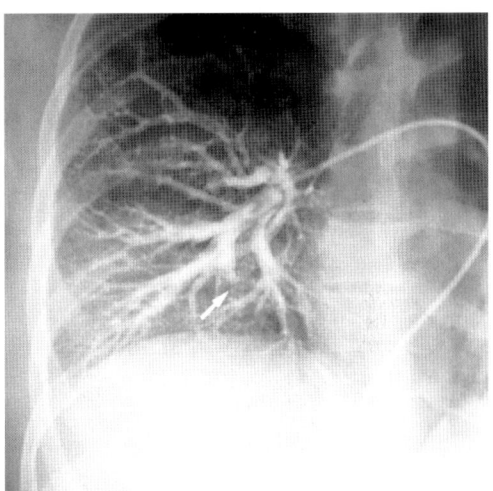

Pulmonary embolism *(Black and Hawks, 2009)*

pulmonary emphysema, a chronic obstructive disease of the lungs, marked by an overdistension of the alveoli and destruction of the supporting alveolar structure. See also **emphysema.**

pulmonary fibrosis. See **fibrosis of the lungs.**

pulmonary function laboratory, an area of a hospital or other health facility used for examination and evaluation of patients' respiratory function.

pulmonary function test (PFT), a procedure for determining the capacity of the lungs to exchange oxygen and carbon dioxide efficiently. There are two general kinds of respiratory function tests. One measures ventilation, or the ability of the bellows action of the chest and lungs to move gas in and out of alveoli; the other kind measures the diffusion of gas across the alveolar capillary membrane and the perfusion of the lungs by blood. Efficient gas exchange in the lungs requires a balanced ventilation-perfusion ratio, with areas receiving ventilation well perfused and areas receiving blood flow capable of ventilation. Basic ventilation studies are performed with a spirometer and recording device as the patient breathes through a mouthpiece and connecting tube; a nose clip prevents nasal breathing. Measurements or calculations are made of the tidal volume (TV), or gas inspired and expired in a normal breath; the inspiratory reserve volume (IRV), or the maximal volume that can be inspired after a normal respiration; the expiratory reserve volume (ERV), or the maximal volume that can be expired forcefully after a normal expiration; the residual volume (RV), or the gas remaining in the lungs after maximal expiration; and the minute volume, or the gas inspired and expired in 1 minute of normal breathing. The vital capacity of the lungs is equal to TV + IRV + ERV, and the total lung capacity to TV + IRV + ERV + RV. Bronchospirometric measurements of the ventilation and oxygen consumption of each lung separately are performed by using a specially constructed double-lumen catheter with two balloons. One balloon is inflated to seal off the contralateral lung when the other lung is tested. Arterial blood gas studies, including determinations of the acidity, partial pressure of carbon dioxide and of oxygen, and oxyhemoglobin saturation, provide information on the diffusion of gas across the alveolar capillary membrane and the adequacy of oxygenation of tissues. See also **blood gas determination, forced expiratory volume, maximum breathing capacity.**

pulmonary groove, a depression on each side of the vertebral bodies that accommodates the posterior part of the lung.

pulmonary hypertension, abnormally high blood pressure within the pulmonary circulation. See also **cor pulmonale.**

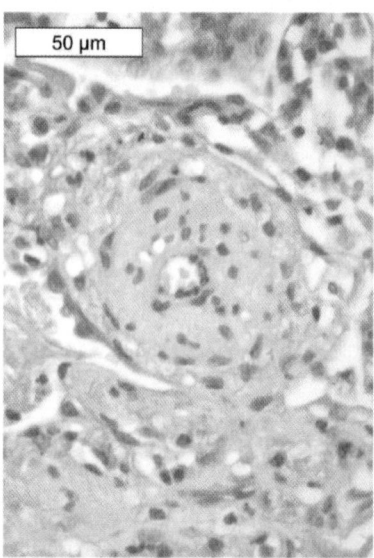

Pulmonary hypertension from COPD showing cellular intimal proliferation in small muscular arteries
(Broaddus et al, 2016)

pulmonary infarction (PI) [L, *pulmoneus,* lungs, *infarcire,* to stuff], necrosis in a part of a lung caused by an obstruction in a branch of a pulmonary artery. See also **pulmonary embolism.**

pulmonary infiltrate with eosinophilia (PIE), a hypersensitivity reaction characterized by infiltration of alveoli with eosinophils and large mononuclear cells, edema, and inflammation of the lungs. The simplest form of the condition, in which patchy, migratory infiltrates cause minimal symptoms, is a self-limited reaction elicited by helminthic infections and by certain drugs, such as paraaminosalicylic acid, sulfonamides, and chlorpropamide. A more prolonged illness, characterized by fever, night sweats, cough, dyspnea, weight loss, and more severe tissue reaction, occurs in certain drug allergies and in bacterial, fungal, and parasitic infections. Tropical eosinophilia with paroxysmal nocturnal asthma, dyspnea, cough, low-grade fever, and malaise is related to filarial infection and may occur in long-standing asthma and periarteritis nodosa. See also **Löffler syndrome.**

pulmonary insufficiency [L, *pulmoneus,* lungs, *in + sufficere,* to suffice], a failure of the pulmonary valve to close properly.

pulmonary ligament, a thin bladelike fold of pleura extending from the hilum to the mediastinum that may stabilize the position of the inferior lobe of the lung and may also accommodate the down-and-up translocation of structures in the root during breathing.

pulmonary opening, opening of pulmonary trunk, pulmonary orifice.

pulmonary orifice, orifice of pulmonary trunk, the opening between the pulmonary trunk and the right ventricle of the heart. Also called **pulmonary opening, opening of pulmonary trunk.**

pulmonary oxygen toxicity [L, *pulmoneus,* lungs; Gk, *toxikon,* poison], a form of oxygen poisoning caused by breathing air having an oxygen concentration of 50% or higher for 12 to 24 hours. Pathophysiological effects include pulmonary capillary endothelial damage and alveolar epithelial cell destruction. Clinical manifestations include cough, substernal pain, nausea, vomiting, and atelectasis.

pulmonary pleura, the part of the pleural membrane that covers the lungs, as distinguished from the parietal layer of pleura that lines the inner aspect of the thoracic cavity. Also called **visceral pleura.**

pulmonary renal syndrome, antiglioblastoma multiforma nephritis.

pulmonary stenosis, an abnormal cardiac condition generally characterized by concentric hypertrophy of the right ventricle with relatively little increase in diastolic volume. When the ventricular septum is intact, this condition may be caused by valvular stenosis, infundibular stenosis, or both; it produces a pressure difference during systole between the right ventricular cavity and the pulmonary artery. Pulmonary stenosis is most often congenital but also may be produced after birth by any of a number of types of lesions. Severe pulmonary stenosis may result in heart failure and death, but mild to moderate forms of this disorder are relatively well tolerated. Also called **pulmonic stenosis.** See also **congenital cardiac anomaly, valvular heart disease, valvular stenosis.**

pulmonary sulcus tumor, a destructive, invasive neoplasm that develops at the apex of the lung and infiltrates the ribs, vertebrae, and brachial plexus. Also called **Pancoast tumor.**

pulmonary surfactant. See **surfactant,** def. 2.

pulmonary trunk, the short, wide vessel that conveys venous blood from the right ventricle of the heart to the lungs. It is approximately 5 cm long and 3 cm in diameter, and it ascends obliquely, dividing into right and left branches.

pulmonary tuberculosis, infection of the lungs by *Mycobacterium tuberculosis.* The first infection is usually quiescent but may develop later into tuberculous pneumonia and other conditions. See also **tuberculosis.**

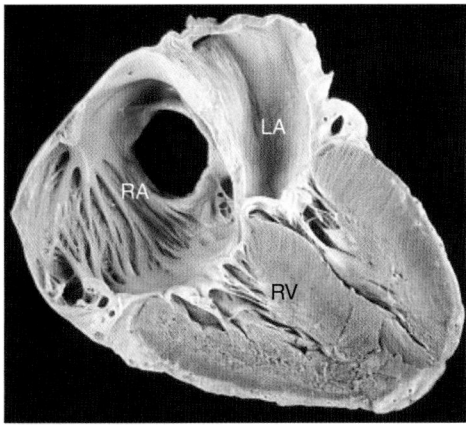

Pulmonary stenosis *(Damjanov and Linder, 2000)*

pulmonary valve, a cardiac structure composed of three semilunar cusps that close during each heartbeat to prevent blood from flowing back into the right ventricle from the pulmonary trunk. The cusps are separated by sinuses that resemble tiny buckets when they are closed and filled with blood. These flaps grow from the lining of the pulmonary trunk. When they collapse from the ejection of ventricular blood, they open the valve and allow deoxygenated blood to flow through the pulmonary artery and on to the lungs. Compare **aortic valve, mitral valve, tricuspid valve.**

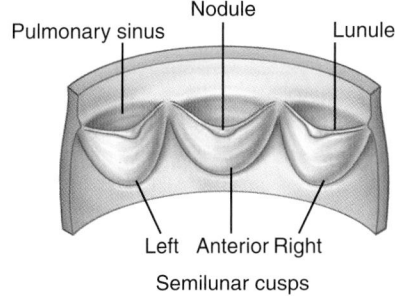

Pulmonary valve *(Drake, Vogl, and Mitchell, 2015)*

pulmonary vascular resistance (PVR), the resistance in the pulmonary vascular bed against which the right ventricle must eject blood.

pulmonary vein, one of two pairs of large vessels that return oxygenated blood from each lung to the left atrium of the heart. The right pulmonary veins pass dorsal to the right atrium and the superior vena cava. The left pulmonary veins pass ventral to the descending thoracic aorta. Compare **pulmonary trunk.**

pulmonary ventilation. See **respiration,** def. 2.

pulmonary wedge pressure (PWP), the pressure produced by an inflated latex balloon against the inner wall of a pulmonary artery. A pulmonary artery catheter or similar balloon-tipped catheter is inserted through a subclavian, jugular, or femoral vein to the vena cava and on through the right atrium and ventricle to the pulmonary artery. The balloon is inflated briefly, during which time it measures left ventricular diastolic pressure. The procedure is used in the diagnosis of congestive heart failure, myocardial infarction, and other conditions. Also called **pulmonary artery wedge pressure.**

pulmonary Wegener granulomatosis, a rare fatal disease of young or middle-aged men, characterized by granulomatous lesions of the respiratory tract, focal necrotizing arteritis, and finally widespread inflammation of body organs. Pulmonary infarction and glomerulonephritis may occur.

pulmonic. See **pulmonary.**

-pulmonic, suffix meaning "the lungs."

pulmonic stenosis. See **pulmonary stenosis.**

pulmonologist /pŏŏl′mə·nol′ə·jist/ [L, *pulmo,* lung], an individual skilled in pulmonology.

pulmonology /pŏŏl′mōnol′ə·jē/ [L, *pulmo,* lung], the science concerned with the anatomy, physiology, and pathology of the lungs.

pulp [L, *pulpa,* flesh], **1.** any soft, coherent, solid, spongy tissue, such as that contained within the spleen, the pulp chamber of the tooth, or the distal subcutaneous pads of the fingers and the toes. **2.** (in dentistry) the contents of the pulp chamber of a tooth, composed of soft connective tissue and cells called odontoblasts, along with vascular, lymphatic, and nervous elements. **−pulpy,** *adj.*

pulp abscess [L, *pulpa,* flesh + *abscedere,* to go away], a bacterial infection that develops in the pulp cavity of a tooth and usually exits at the apex of the tooth root.

pulpaceous /pulpā″shəs/, pertaining to a substance that is pulpy or macerated.

pulpal /pul″pəl/, pertaining to pulp.

pulp amputation. See **pulpotomy.**

pulp canal, the space occupied by the nerves, blood vessels, and lymphatic vessels in the radicular part of the tooth. The internal anatomy of the tooth progresses apically from the pulp chamber to pulp canal to the apex. Also called **root canal.**

pulp canal therapy. See **root canal therapy.**

pulp cavity, the space in a tooth bounded by the dentin and containing the dental pulp. It is divided into the pulp chamber and the pulp canal and is collectively called the root canal.

pulp chamber, the space occupied by the nerves, blood vessels, and lymphatic vessels deep within the crown of the tooth. Internal anatomy of the tooth progresses from pulp chamber to pulp canal to apex.

pulpectomy /pulpek″təmē/ [L, *pulpa,* flesh; Gk, *ektomē,* excision], the surgical removal of all or part of the pulp of a tooth.

pulpifaction /pul″pifak″shən/, the act of reducing something to a pulp.

pulpitis /pulpī″tis/, infection or inflammation of the dental pulp.

pulpless tooth /pulp″ləs/, a tooth in which the dental pulp is necrotic or has been removed. Also called **devitalized tooth, nonvital tooth.**

pulpodontia. See **endodontics.**

pulpotomy /pul·pot′ə·mē/, pediatric pulp therapy consisting of partial excision of the dental pulp and application of a medicated dressing into the tooth, allowing the root portion of the pulp to remain vital. Secondary tooth root canal therapy is not performed, as the primary tooth root(s) must resorb for succession of the secondary tooth. Also called **pulp amputation.**

pulp pinch. See **pinch.**

pulp stone. See **denticle.**

pulp test. See **vitality test.**

pulpy. See **pulp.**

pulpy nucleus, the central part of each intervertebral disk, consisting of a pulpy elastic substance that loses some of its resiliency with age. The nucleus pulposus may be suddenly compressed and squeeze out through the annular fibrocartilage, causing a herniated disk and extreme pain. Also called **nucleus pulposus.**

pulsate /pul″sāt/ [L, *pulsare,* to beat], to throb or vibrate rhythmically, as does the heart during its contraction-relaxation cycle.

pulsatile /pul″sətil/ [L, *pulsare,* to beat], pertaining to an activity characterized by a rhythmic pulsation.

pulsatile assist device (PAD), a flexible, valveless balloon conduit contained within a rigid, plastic cylinder that is inserted into the arterial circulation to provide pulsatile perfusion during a cardiopulmonary bypass.

pulsatile hematoma. See **pseudoaneurysm.**

pulsatility index /pul′sətil″itē/, a measure of the variability of blood velocity in a vessel, equal to the difference between the peak systolic and minimum diastolic velocities divided by the mean velocity during the cardiac cycle.

pulsating exophthalmos /pul″sāting/ [L, *pulsare,* to beat; Gk, *ex + ophthalmos,* eye], an eye disorder characterized by a bulging, pulsating eyeball, caused by an arteriovenous aneurysm involving the internal carotid artery and the cavernous sinus of the orbit.

pulsation /pəl·sā′shən/ [L, *pulsatio*], a throb or rhythmical beat, as of the heart.

pulse [L, *pulsare,* to beat], **1.** a rhythmic beating or vibrating movement. **2.** a brief electromagnetic wave. **3.** the regular, recurrent expansion and contraction of an artery, produced by waves of pressure caused by the ejection of blood from the left ventricle of the heart as it contracts. The pulse is easily detected on superficial arteries, such as the radial and carotid arteries, and corresponds to each beat of the heart.

pulse curve. See **sphygmogram.**

pulsed Doppler, a type of Doppler device that transmits a short-duration burst of sound into the region to be examined. The Doppler-shifted signals are processed from a limited depth range. The depth range is determined by a sample gate whose position and size usually can be selected by the instrument operator.

pulse deficit, a condition in which a peripheral pulse rate is less than the ventricular contraction rate as auscultated at the apex of the heart or seen on the electrocardiogram, indicating a lack of peripheral perfusion.

pulsed laser, a laser that emits short bursts of energy at fixed intervals rather than a continuous stream of energy.

pulse duration (P.D., PD), (in ultrasonics) a measure of the time a transducer oscillates for each pulse. The shorter the pulse duration, the better the axial resolution.

pulse-echo response profile, a graph of the amplitude of an ultrasound echo from a small reflector versus the distance from the reflector beam axis. The reflector is scanned perpendicular to the axis of the ultrasound transducer beam.

pulse-echo ultrasound, a diagnostic technique in which short-duration ultrasound pulses are transmitted into the region to be studied, and echo signals resulting from scattering and reflection are detected and displayed. The depth of a reflective structure is inferred from the delay between pulse transmission and echo reception.

pulse generator, the power source for a cardiac pacemaker system, usually fueled by lithium, supplying impulses to the implanted electrodes either at a fixed rate or in some programmed pattern.

pulse height analyzer, a device that accepts or rejects electronic pulses according to their amplitude or energy, commonly used to select certain gamma radiation energies.

pulseless disease. See **Takayasu arteritis.**

pulseless electrical activity (PEA), continued electrical rhythmicity of the heart in the absence of effective mechanical function. It may be caused by the uncoupling of ventricular muscle contraction from electrical activity or may be a result of cardiac damage with respiratory failure and cessation of cardiac venous return. Also called **electromechanical dissociation.**

pulse MR, a magnetic resonance (MR) technique that uses radiofrequency pulses and Fourier transformation of the MR signal. Pulse MR has largely replaced older, continuous-wave techniques.

pulse oximeter, an optical device that measures the amount of oxygen-saturated hemoglobin in the tissue capillaries by transmitting a beam of light through the tissue to a receiver. This noninvasive method of measuring the saturated hemoglobin is a useful screening tool for determining basic respiratory and cardiovascular function. This cliplike device may be used on an earlobe, across the bridge of the nose, in the mouth, on a toe, or on a fingertip. As the amount of saturated hemoglobin alters the wavelengths of the transmitted light, analysis of the received light is translated into a percentage of oxygen saturation (SO_2) of the blood. Also called *pulse ox.* Compare **blood gas determination.**

pulse point, one of the sites on the surface of the body where arterial pulsations can be easily palpated. The most commonly used pulse point is over the radial artery at the wrist. Other pulse points include the temporal artery in front of the ear; the common carotid artery at the lower level of the thyroid cartilage; the facial artery at the lower margin of the jaw; and the femoral, popliteal, posterior tibialis, and dorsalis pedis pulse points.

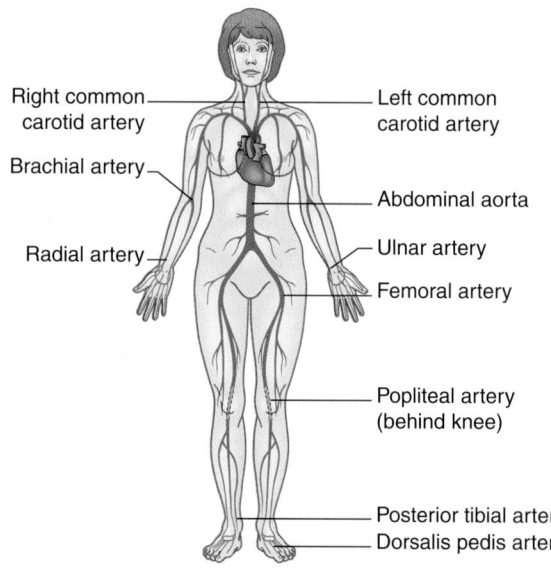

Right common carotid artery
Left common carotid artery
Brachial artery
Abdominal aorta
Radial artery
Ulnar artery
Femoral artery
Popliteal artery (behind knee)
Posterior tibial artery
Dorsalis pedis artery

Pulse points *(Naish and Court, 2015)*

pulse pressure, the difference between the systolic and diastolic blood pressures, normally 30 to 50 mm Hg.

pulse pressure variation (PPV), a measure of cardiac and pulmonary interactions in a ventilated patient.

pulser /pul″sər/, a component of an ultrasound instrument that provides signals for exciting the piezoelectric transducer in order to transmit an ultrasound beam.

pulse rate [L, *pulsare + reri,* to calculate], the number of pulse beats per minute, normally the same as the heart rate. The normal pulse rate in an average adult varies from 60 to 80 beats/min, with fluctuations occurring with exercise, injury, illness, and emotional reactions. The average pulse rate for a newborn is 120 beats/min, which slows throughout childhood and adolescence. At about 12 years of age, females begin to have a higher pulse rate than males.

pulse repetition frequency (PRF), (in ultrasonics) the number of acoustic pulses transmitted per second.

pulse sequence, the sequence of radiofrequency pulses and magnetic gradients used to generate a magnetic resonance image.

PULSES profile, an assessment tool that measures six functions and factors to evaluate the degree of independence possessed by a disabled individual. The score is used in the assessment of progress made in rehabilitation as well as to help identify the severity of disability. The six are: *P*hysical condition (i.e., general health), *U*pper limb function, *L*ower limb function, *S*ensory function, *E*xcretory function, and *S*upport (e.g., social, psychological, financial support).

pulse-synchronous tinnitus, a whooshing, whistling, or humming noise heard in one or both ears that is synchronous with an individual's pulse rate. It is only audible to the person experiencing it. It is an important indicator of intracranial hypertension.

pulse wave [L, *pulsare,* to beat; AS, *wafian*], a transient increase in blood pressure that spreads like a wave through the arterial system. It begins with the ejection of blood by the ventricles during systole.

pulse width. See **duration.**

-pulsion, combining form meaning "the action or condition of pushing forward": *compulsion, propulsion, repulsion.*

pulsus alternans /pul″səs ôl″tərnanz/ [L, *pulsare + alternare,* to alternate], a pulse characterized by a regular alternation of weak and strong beats without changes in the pulse rate. Also called *alternans,* **alternating pulse.**

pulsus magnus. See **full pulse.**

pulsus paradoxus, an abnormally large decrease in systolic blood pressure and pulse wave amplitude during inspiration. The normal fall in pressure is less than 10 mm Hg. An excessive decline may be a sign of tamponade, adhesive pericarditis, severe lung disease, advanced heart failure, or other conditions. Also called **paradoxic pulse.**

pulsus parvus et tardus [L, *pulsus,* beat, *parvus,* small, *tardus,* slow], a small pulse with low pressure that rises and falls gradually. The condition occurs in aortic stenosis.

pulsus tardus [L, *pulsus,* beat, *tardus,* slow], a pulse with a gradual rise and fall in amplitude.

pultaceous, pertaining to a substance that is pulpy or macerated.

pulverize /pul″vəriz/ [L, *pulvis,* dust], to reduce to a fine powder.

pulverulent /pulver″ələnt/, having the form of a fine powder.

pulvule /pul″vyo͞ol/ [L, *pulvis,* dust], a proprietary type of capsule containing a dose of a drug in powder form.

pumice /pum″is/ [L, *pumex*], a finely divided volcanic rock used in powdered or solid form for smoothing or polishing surfaces.

pump [ME, *pumpe*], **1.** *n.,* an apparatus used to move fluids or gases by suction or positive pressure, such as an infusion pump or stomach pump. **2.** *n.,* a physiological mechanism by which a substance is moved, usually by active transport across a cell membrane, such as a sodium-potassium pump. **3.** *v.,* to move a liquid or gas by suction or positive pressure.

pump lung. See **adult respiratory distress syndrome.**

pump oxygenator [ME, *pumpe + Gk, oxys,* sharp, *genein,* to produce], a device that pumps oxygenated blood through the body during cardiopulmonary surgery.

punch biopsy [L, *pungere,* to prick; Gk, *bios,* life, *opsis,* view], the removal of living tissue for microscopic examination, usually bone marrow aspirates from the sternum, by

means of a punch. Compare **exfoliative cytology, needle biopsy.**

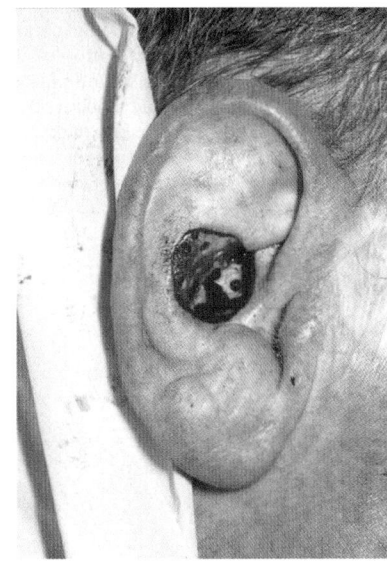

Punch biopsy on the ear *(White and Cox, 2006)*

punchdrunk syndrome, a condition resulting from repeated cerebral concussions, characterized by an abnormal gait, slow movement, tremor, and slurred or halting speech.

punch forceps, a surgical instrument used to cut out a disk of dense or resistant tissue, such as bone and cartilage. The ends of the blades of the punch forceps are perforated to grip the involved tissue. There are several varieties of this instrument, with blades and tips specially designed for different surgical needs.

punct-, prefix meaning "a point" or "like a point": *punctate, punctiform, puncture.*

punctate /pungk″tāt/ [L, *punctum,* point], marked with elevated or colored dots or punctures.

punctiform /pungk″tifôrm/, of very small size, as is a bacterial colony in a solid medium.

punctum /pungk″təm/, a physiological area or point.

punctum caecum, blind spot.

punctum lacrimale /lak″rimā″lē/ *pl. puncta lacrimalia* [L, *punctum,* prick, *lacrima,* tear], a minute circular aperture in the medial opening into the nasolacrimal sac. The puncta drain the tears that travel from the lacrimal glands through the lacrimal ducts to the conjunctiva. Puncta clogged with mucus or dirt cause irritation and discomfort.

puncture /pungk″chər/ [L, *punctura*], **1.** *v.,* to prick or pierce a surface, as with a needle or knife. **2.** *n.,* a wound or opening made by piercing.

puncture of the antrum [L, *punctura + Gk, antron,* cave], a cavity or hollow, as is made in piercing the wall of the maxillary sinus to drain pus.

puncture wound [L, *punctura + AS, wund*], a traumatic injury caused by skin penetration by an object, such as a knife, nail, or slender fragment of metal, wood, glass, or other material. In such an injury to the eye, a lung, or a visceral organ, the object or implement is not removed until the person has been transported to a medical facility. Minor puncture wounds are treated with thorough cleansing. If a puncture wound is allowed to close at the skin before deeper healing has occurred, suppuration often results. A tetanus toxoid immunization is usually given for such wounds.

P

punitive damages.   See **damages.**

Punnett square [Reginald C. Punnett, English geneticist, 1875–1967; OFr, *esquarre*], a matrix that shows all of the possible combinations of male and female gametes when one or more pairs of independent alleles are crossed. Letters representing the male and female gametes are placed along the left side and the top of the matrix, respectively. The genotypes of the offspring produced by each pairing of gametes occupy the cells in the matrix. See also **pedigree.**

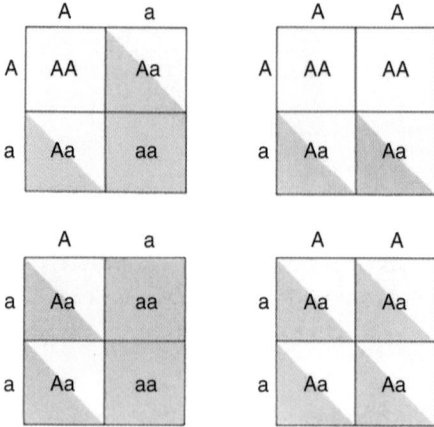

Punnett square *(Thibodeau and Patton, 2007)*

pupa /pyoo″pə/ [L, doll], a stage between the larval and adult stages in the life cycle of many insects, including flies, butterflies, and beetles. It has the basic external features of the adult form but without expanded wings.

pupil /pyoo″pəl/ [L, *pupa*, doll], a circular opening in the iris of the eye, located slightly to the nasal side of the center of the iris. Like the iris, the pupil lies posterior to the cornea and the anterior chamber of the eye and is anterior to the lens. Its diameter changes with contraction and relaxation of the muscular fibers of the iris as the eye responds to changes in light, emotional states, and autonomic stimulation. The pupil is the window of the eye through which light passes to the lens and the retina. See also **dilator pupillae, sphincter pupillae. –pupillary,** *adj.*

pupill-.   See **pupillo-, pupill-.**

pupillary /pyoo″piler′ē/ [L, *pupilla*], pertaining to the pupil.

pupillary distance (PD), a measurement of the space between the centers of the pupils and the bridge of the nose.

pupillary reflex.   See **accommodation reflex, light reflex.**

pupillary ruff, a brown wrinkled rim on the edge of the pupil, derived from posterior pigment epithelium of the iris.

pupillary skin reflex.   See **ciliospinal reflex.**

pupillo-, pupill-, prefix meaning "the pupil": *pupillary, pupillometry, pupillomotor.*

pupillometry /pyoo′pilom″ətrē/, the measurement of the pupil.

pupillomotor /pyoo′pilōmō″tər/, pertaining to the autonomic nerve fibers of the smooth muscles of the iris.

PUPPP /pup/, abbreviation for **pruritic urticarial papules and plaques of pregnancy.**

PUPs, refers to individuals participating in clinical trials. Abbreviation for *previously untreated patients.*

pur-, prefix meaning "pus": *purulent, purulence.*

pure /pyoor/, **1.** free of contamination by extraneous matter. **2.** a state in which a substance contains nothing other than itself.

pure dwarf.   See **primordial dwarf.**

pure science.   See **science.**

pure tone audiometry.   See **audiometry.**

purgation.   See **catharsis.**

purgative /pur″gətiv/ [L, *purgare,* to purge], a strong medication usually administered by mouth to promote evacuation of the bowel or to produce several bowel movements.

purge /purj/ [L, *purgare*], **1.** *v.,* to evacuate the bowels, as with a cathartic. **2.** *n.,* a cathartic. **3.** *v.,* to make free of an unwanted substance. **–purgative,** *adj., n.*

purified cotton, cotton freed from impurities, bleached, and sterilized. It is used as a surgical dressing.

purified protein derivative (PPD) /pyoo″rifīd/, a dried form of tuberculin used in testing for past or present infection with tubercle bacilli. This product is usually introduced into the skin during such tests and may produce a tuberculin reaction (wheal) within 48 to 72 hours. See also **tuberculin test, tuberculosis.**

purine /pyoo″rēn/ [L, *purus,* pure, *urina,* urine], any one of a large group of nitrogenous compounds. Purines are produced as end products in the digestion of certain proteins in the diet, but some are synthesized in the body. Purines are also present in many medications and other substances, including caffeine, theophylline, and various diuretics, muscle relaxants, and myocardial stimulants. Hyperuricemia may develop in some people as a result of an inability to metabolize and excrete purines. A low-purine diet or a purine-free diet may be required. Foods that are high in purines include anchovies and sardines; sweetbreads, liver, kidneys, and other organ meats; legumes; and poultry. The foods lowest in purine content include eggs, fruit, cheese, nuts, sugar, gelatin, and vegetables other than legumes.

purine base [L, *purus,* pure], any of the purine derivatives found in animal waste products or in nucleic acids. They include hypoxanthine, xanthine, and uric acid (waste products), and adenine and guanine (nucleic acids).

purine-free diet, a diet that excludes foods that are rich sources of purines. Foods particularly high in purines include organ meats, such as liver, kidney, and sweetbreads, as well as red meats, poultry, and fish. Those items can be replaced by milk, eggs, cheese, and some vegetable sources of protein. See also **purine.**

purine-low diet, a diet that excludes some foods rich in purines, such as certain meat products, fish, and poultry, and particularly anchovies, meat extracts, sardines, and organ meats. Also called **low-purine diet.**

purine-restricted diet.   See **low-purine diet.**

Purinethol, an antineoplastic drug. Brand name for **mercaptopurine.**

Purkinje cells /pərkin″jē, pur″kinjē, -jā/ [Johannes E. Purkinje, Czech physiologist, 1787–1869], large neurons with dendrites that extend to the molecular lay and provide the only output from the cerebellar cortex after the cortex processes sensory and motor impulses from the rest of the nervous system.

Purkinje fiber [Johannes E. Purkinje], one of the myocardial fibers that are the termination of the bundle branches. The fibers comprise part of the conduction system of the heart. See also **Purkinje network.**

Purkinje network [Johannes E. Purkinje], a complex fibrous network of large muscle cells that spread through the right and the left ventricles of the heart and carry the impulses that contract those chambers almost simultaneously. The fibers that connect with Purkinje fibers start in the atrioventricular (AV) node in the right atrium of the heart, along the lower part of the interatrial septum. Impulses generated in the sinoatrial node travel through the muscle fibers

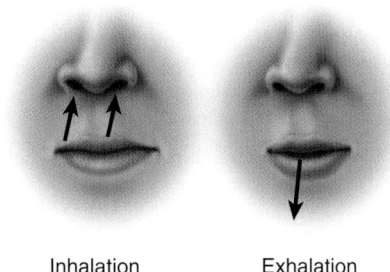

Purkinje network *(Phillips, 2012)*

of both atria of the heart, starting atrial contraction. As the impulse enters the AV node from the right atrium, it allows both atria to contract completely before the impulse spreads into the ventricles. The velocity of the impulse increases after the impulse leaves the AV node and spreads via the atrioventricular bundle (bundle of His) to the bundle branches, and finally to Purkinje fibers. Purkinje fibers are larger in diameter than ordinary cardiac muscle fibers and contain relatively few peripheral myofibrillae. They have abundant sarcoplasm and larger central nuclei than ordinary cardiac muscle. See also **cardiac cycle, intraventricular block.**

purposeful activity /pur″pəsfool/, activity that depends on consciously planned and directed involvement of the person. It is believed that conscious involvement in body movements enhances the development of sensorimotor control and coordination during therapeutic or rehabilitative exercises.

purpur-, prefix meaning "purple": *purpura.*

purpura /pur″pyərə/ [L, purple], any of several bleeding disorders characterized by hemorrhage into the tissues, particularly beneath the skin or mucous membranes, producing ecchymoses or petechiae. Compare **petechiae, ecchymosis.** Kinds include **nonthrombocytopenic purpura,** *thrombocytopenic purpura.* **–petechiae, purpuric,** *adj.*

purpura rheumatica [L, *purpura,* purple; Gk, *rheum,* flow], a distinctive clinical sign associated with hemorrhages of the skin and other tissues. The lesions are red or purple and do not blanch on pressure. Purpura is related to either a disorder of the blood or an abnormality affecting the blood vessels.

purpura senilis /senē″lis/ [L, *purpura,* purple, *senilis,* aged], a skin condition affecting older people and characterized by fragile blood vessel walls that rupture on minimal trauma. Also called **senile purpura.**

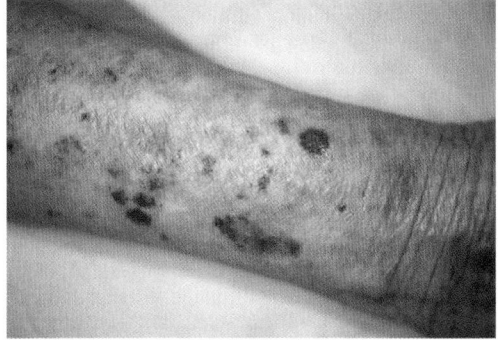

Purpura senilis *(Swartz, 2009)*

purpuric. See **purpura.**

pursed-lip breathing /purst-/, respiration characterized by deep inspirations followed by prolonged expirations through pursed lips. It is done to increase expiratory airway pressure, improve oxygenation of the blood, and help prevent early airway closure.

Inhalation   Exhalation

Pursed-lip breathing *(Harkreader, Hogan, and Thobaben, 2007)*

purse-string suture [L, *sutura*], a continuous suture placed in a circle about a round wound. The opening is closed by tightly drawing the ends of the suture together.

purulence /pyoor″(y)ələns/ [L, *purulentus,* pus formation], the condition of producing or discharging pus. Also called *purulency.*

purulent /pyoor″(y)ələnt/ [L, containing pus], producing or containing pus.

purulent conjunctivitis [L, *purulentus,* pus formation, *conjunctivus,* connecting; Gk, *itis,* inflammation], an inflammation of the conjunctiva caused by suppurative microorganisms, including species of *streptococci, gonococci,* and *pneumococci.*

purulent diarrhea [L, *purulentus,* pus formation; Gk, *dia + rhein,* to flow], diarrhea in which stools contain pus, a sign of a purulent GI tract infection.

purulent inflammation [L, *purulentus,* pus formation, *inflammare,* to set afire], an inflammation that is accompanied by the formation of pus.

purulent iritis [L, *purulentus,* pus formation; Gk, *iris,* rainbow, *itis,* inflammation], an inflammation of the iris accompanied by the formation of pus.

purulent keratitis [L, *purulentus,* pus formation; Gk, *keras,* horn, *itis,* inflammation], a severe form of keratitis leading to disintegration of the cornea if untreated. The condition commonly begins with a bacterial infection of the lacrimal sac, occurs frequently in elderly patients who have poor nutrition, and spreads into a pus-producing ulcer.

purulent pancreatitis [L, *purulentus,* pus formation; Gk, *pan,* all, *kreas,* flesh, *itis,* inflammation], inflammation of the pancreas accompanied by pus formation.

purulent rhinitis [L, *purulentus,* pus formation; Gk, *rhis,* nose, *itis,* inflammation], an infection of the nasal mucosa that is accompanied by pus formation. The condition is often secondary to a systemic infection, such as measles.

purulent synovitis [L, *purulentus,* pus formation; Gk, *syn,* together; L, *ovum,* egg], an inflammation of the synovial membrane of a joint with pus formation in the cavity.

pus [L, corrupt matter], a creamy, viscous fluid exudate that is the result of fluid remains of necrosis of tissues. It is usually pale yellow to yellow green, sometimes whitish, and sometimes bloody. Its main constituent is an abundance of polymorphonuclear leukocytes. Bacterial infection is its most common cause. The character of the pus, including its color, consistency, quantity, or odor, may be of diagnostic significance.

pus cell, a necrotic polymorphonuclear leukocyte, a major component of pus. Also called *pus corpuscle.*

push-up block. See **handblock.**

pustular psoriasis [L, *pustula,* blister; Gk, *psoriasis,* itch], a severe form of psoriasis consisting of bright red patches and sterile pustules all over the body. Crops of lesions lasting 4 to 7 days occur every few days in cycles over weeks or months. Recurrences are inevitable. Fever, leukocytosis, and hypoalbuminemia are associated. In rare cases, hypovolemia and kidney failure occur. Hospitalization may be necessary for fluid replacement, steroid therapy, and sedation. Compare **guttate psoriasis.** See also **psoriasis.**

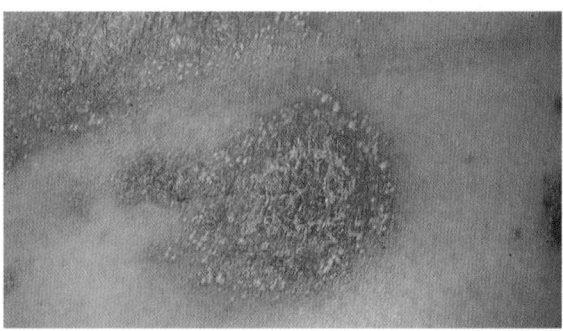

Pustular psoriasis *(Beth-Jones, 2013)*

pustule /pus″chool/ [L, *pustula*], a small circumscribed elevation of the skin containing fluid that is usually purulent. *−pustular, adj.*

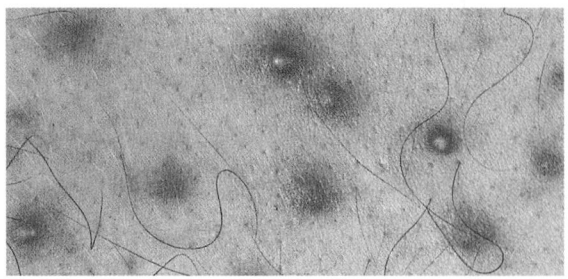

Pustule *(du Vivier, 2002)*

putamen /pyoōtā″mən/ [L, husk], a part of the lentiform nucleus that is lateral to the globus pallidus. It is associated with the corpus striatum and receives connections from the suppressor centers of the cortex.

putrefaction /pyoō′trəfak″shən/ [L, *puter,* rotten, *facere,* to make], the decay of enzymes, especially proteins, that produces foul-smelling compounds, such as ammonia, hydrogen sulfide, and mercaptans.

putrefactive /-fak′tiv/ [L, *puter,* rotten, *facere,* to make], causing, promoting, or relating to putrefaction.

putrefy /pyoō″trəfī/ [L, *puter,* rotten, *facere,* to make], to decay, with the production of foul-smelling substances, especially putrescine and mercaptans, which are associated with the decomposition of animal tissues and proteins.

putrescine /pyoō″tresēn/, a foul-smelling toxic ptomaine produced by the decomposition of the amino acid ornithine during the decay of animal tissues, bacillus cultures, and fecal bacteria.

putrid /pyoō″trid/ [L, *putridus,* rotten], decomposed.

putromaine /pyoōtrō″mān/, any toxin produced by the decay of food within a living body.

PUVA, an abbreviation for a psoriatic photochemotherapy treatment consisting of a medication called *p*soralen plus *u*ltraviolet light of *A* (long) wavelength.

P value, (in research) the statistical probability of the occurrence of a given finding by chance alone in comparison with the known distribution of possible findings, considering the kinds of data, the technique of analysis, and the number of observations. The P value may be noted as a decimal: P <.01 means that the likelihood that the phenomena tested occurred by chance alone is less than 1%. The lower the P value, the less likely the finding would occur by chance alone.

PVB. See **VBP.**

PVC, **1.** abbreviation for **polyvinyl chloride. 2.** abbreviation for **premature ventricular complex.**

PVP-I, abbreviation for **povidone-iodine.**

PVR, abbreviation for **pulmonary vascular resistance.**

pW, abbreviation for *picowatt.*

P wave, the component of the cardiac cycle shown on an electrocardiogram as an inverted U-shaped curve that follows the T wave and precedes the QRS complex. It represents atrial depolarization.

P′ wave (P prime wave), a P wave that is generated from a site other than the sinus node; an ectopic P wave.

PWP, abbreviation for **pulmonary wedge pressure.**

pyaemic embolism. See **pyemic embolism.**

pycno-, pykno-, prefix meaning "density" or "thickness": *pyknometer.*

pyel-. See **pyelo-, pyel-.**

pyelitis /pī′əlī″tis/, an inflammation of the renal pelvis, often accompanied by symptoms such as pain and tenderness in the loins, irritability of the bladder, bloody or purulent urine, and a peculiar pain on flexion of the thigh. See also **pyelonephritis.**

pyelo-, pyel-, prefix meaning "pelvis or kidney": *pyelography, pyelolithotomy.*

pyelogram /pī′əlōgram′/ [Gk, *pyelos,* pelvis, *gramma,* record], a radiographic image of the kidneys and ureters taken after the IV or intraureteral injection of a radiopaque contrast medium. It shows the size and location of the kidneys, the outline of the ureters and bladder, the filling of the renal pelves, the patency of the urinary tract, and any cysts or tumors within the kidneys. Retrograde pyelograms, which demonstrate filling of the renal collecting structures, are taken after the contrast medium is injected into the ureters by means of catheters in a cystoscope introduced through the urethra into the bladder. Also called **urogram.**

pyelography. See **intravenous pyelography.**

pyelointerstitial backflow, backflow of fluid from the renal pelvis into interstitial tissue under certain conditions of back pressure.

pyelolithotomy /pī′əlō′lithot″əmē/, a surgical procedure in which renal calculi are removed from the pelvis of the ureter.

pyelonephritis /pī′əlōnəfrī″tis/ [Gk, *pyelos* + *nephros,* kidney, *itis,* inflammation], a diffuse pyogenic infection of the pelvis and parenchyma of the kidney. Acute pyelonephritis usually results from an infection that ascends from the lower urinary tract to the kidney. *Escherichia coli* contamination of the urethral meatus is a common cause in females. Infection may spread to the kidney from other locations in the body. The onset of acute pyelonephritis is rapid and characterized by fever, chills, pain in the flank, nausea, and urinary frequency. Urinalysis reveals the presence of bacteria and white blood cells (WBCs). Antimicrobial treatment is continued for 10 days to 2 weeks. Relapse or reinfection is common. Chronic pyelonephritis develops slowly after bacterial infection of the kidney and may progress to renal failure. Most cases are associated with some form of obstruction, such as a stone or a stricture of the ureter. Treatment includes removal of the cause of obstruction and long-term antimicrobial therapy.

■ OBSERVATIONS: The onset of symptoms is fairly rapid and is characterized by dull, constant flank pain, chills, and fever. Concomitant signs of a lower urinary tract infection (e.g., urinary frequency and dysuria) occur in about one third of individuals. Clinical symptoms are confirmed by urinalysis, which shows antibody-coated bacteria, bacteriuria, WBC casts, and pyuria; a CBC shows an increase in WBCs. Renal function studies may assist in the diagnosis of chronic disease. The most common complication of acute disease is septic shock and/or chronic pyelonephritis. With chronic disease, there is a 2% to 3% chance of developing end-stage renal failure.

■ INTERVENTIONS: Oral or parenteral antiinfective drugs are used to combat infection. Continuous suppression antiinfective therapy may be used to treat recurrent or chronic infection. Antipyretics are used for fever. Hydration is managed by forcing oral fluids or using IV fluids for those unable to take in adequate oral fluids. Follow-up urine cultures are used to track effectiveness of antiinfective drugs. Surgery is used to drain large collections of pus and to correct underlying obstructions. Placement of a nephrostomy tube may be necessary to promote drainage of urine.

■ PATIENT CARE CONSIDERATIONS: Key goals for acute pyelonephritis are to reduce fever, relieve pain, promote comfort, and prevent complications. Individuals should be encouraged to drink at least 8 glasses of fluids daily even after acute infection subsides. Input and output should be closely monitored and urine should be checked for frequency, consistency, color, and odor. Rest is indicated to reduce fatigue, increase comfort, and allow the body to combat the infection. Education is aimed at teaching the individual about the disease, with a focus on the necessity to continue the full course of antibiotic therapy and to get follow-up urine cultures to ensure that infection is gone. Instruction is also necessary in preventing infection (cleansing perineum, proper wiping technique, adequate fluid intake, and cleansing after sexual activity) and in recognizing and treating early signs of urinary tract infection.

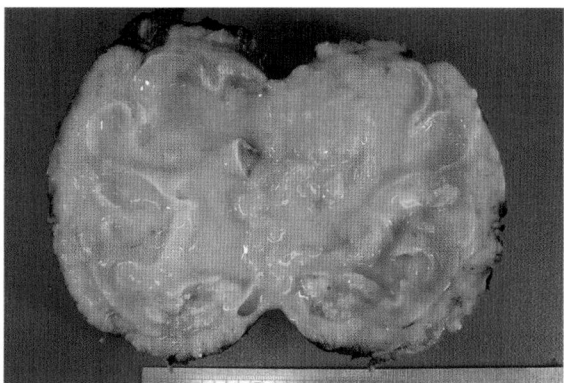

Acute pyelonephritis *(Zhou, Netto, and Epstein, 2012)*

pyelonephritis of pregnancy, a renal infection during pregnancy characterized by dilation of the renal pelvis and the ureters. Some degree of ureteric obstruction may be caused by the gravid uterus.

pyeloplasty /pī′əlōplas′tē/, the surgical reconstruction of the kidney pelvis.

pyelosinus backflow, backflow of fluid from the renal pelvis into the renal sinus under certain conditions of back pressure.

pyelovenous backflow, backflow of fluid from the renal pelvis into the venous system under certain conditions of back pressure.

pyemesis /pī·em″əsis/, the action of vomiting purulent material.

pyemic embolism /pī·ē″mik/ [Gk, *pyon,* pus, *haima,* blood, *embolos,* plug], an infective embolus producing an abscess. Also spelled **pyaemic embolism.**

pygeum, an herbal product derived from an evergreen tree native to Africa.

■ INDICATIONS: This herb is used for benign prostate hypertrophy, for which there is some evidence of efficacy, and as an antiinflammatory medication, for which there are insufficient reliable data regarding efficacy.

■ CONTRAINDICATIONS: Pygeum is not recommended during pregnancy and lactation, in children, or in those with known hypersensitivity to this plant.

pygmalianism /pigmā″lē·əniz′əm/ [Gk, *Pygmalion,* mythic sculptor who fell in love with his statue], a psychosexual abnormality in which the individual directs erotic fantasies to an object that he or she has created.

pygmy /pig″mē/ [L, *pygmaeus,* dwarf], an extremely small person whose body parts are proportioned accordingly. Also spelled **pigmy.** See also **primordial dwarf.**

pygo-, prefix meaning "buttocks": *pygoamorphus, pygodidymus, pygopagus.*

pygoamorphus /pī′gō·əmôr″fəs/ [Gk, *pyge,* buttocks, *a* + *morphe,* not form], asymmetric, conjoined twins in which the parasitic member is represented by an undifferentiated amorphous mass attached to the autosite in the sacral region.

pygodidymus /pī′gōdid″əməs/ [Gk, *pyge,* buttocks, *didymos,* twin], **1.** a malformed fetus that has a double pelvis and hips. **2.** conjoined twins who are fused in the cephalothoracic region but separated at the pelvis.

pygomelus /pīgom″ələs/ [Gk, *pyge* + *melos,* limb], a malformed fetus that has an extra limb or limbs attached to the buttock. Also called **epipygus.**

pygopagus /pīgop″əgəs/ [Gk, *pyge* + *pegos,* fixed], conjoined twins consisting of two fully formed or nearly formed fetuses united in the sacral region so that they are positioned back to back.

pyknic /pik″nik/ [Gk, *pyknos*, thick], describing a body structure characterized by short, round limbs; a full face with a broad head and thick shoulders; a short neck; stockiness; and a tendency to obesity. Compare **asthenic habitus, athletic habitus.** See also **endomorph.**

pykno-. See **pycno-, pykno-.**

pyknodysostosis /pik″nō·dis′os·tō′sis/ [Gk, *pyknos*, thick + *dys,* bad + *osteon,* bone + *osis,* condition], an autosomal-recessive symptom complex consisting of dwarfism, osteopetrosis, partial agenesis of terminal digits of hands and feet, cranial anomalies, frontal and occipital bossing, and hypoplasia of the angle of the mandible.

pyknometer /pik-nom′ĕ-ter/, an instrument for determining the specific gravity of fluids.

pyknosis /piknō″sis/, the condensation of nuclear material into a solid, darkly staining mass in a dying cell. It is characterized by the clumping of chromatin and shrinking of the nucleus of the cell. The cell itself may enlarge in response to cell necrosis.

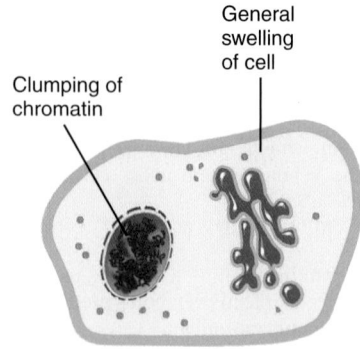

Pyknosis *(Huether and McCance, 2008)*

pyla /pī″lə/, the opening between the third ventricle and the cerebral aqueduct.

pyle-, prefix meaning "portal vein": *pylethrombophlebitis.*

pylethrombophlebitis /pī′ləthrom′bōfləbī″tis/, inflammation of the portal vein with formation of a thrombus.

pylon /pī″lon/ [Gk, gate], an artificial lower limb, often a narrow vertical support consisting of a socket with wooden side supports and a rubber-clad peg end. It may be used as a temporary prosthesis.

pylori. See **pylorus.**

pyloric /pīlôr″ik/ [Gk, *pyle,* gate, *ouros,* guard], pertaining to the pylorus, the opening between the stomach and duodenum.

pyloric antrum, that part of the stomach between the pyloric canal and the body of the stomach.

pyloric canal, the narrow, constricted region of the pyloric part of the stomach.

pyloric constriction, the constriction at the distal end of the pylorus, overlying the pyloric orifice, marking the junction of the stomach and duodenum.

pyloric obstruction and dilation /pīlôr″ik/ [Gk, *pyle,* gate, *ouros,* guard; L, *obstruere,* to build against, *dilatare,* to widen], a reaction of the stomach to pyloric obstruction, which increases the resistance to the expulsion of partly digested food from the stomach. As a result, the stomach may become hypertrophied, then dilated. Excessive consumption of food and beverages contributes to the condition.

pyloric orifice [Gk, *pyle,* gate, *ouros,* guard; L, *orificium,* opening], the opening of, or passage between, the stomach into the duodenum, lying to the right of the midline at the level of the upper border of the first lumbar vertebra. The orifice is usually indicated on the surface of the stomach by the circular duodenopyloric constriction.

pyloric spasm. See **pylorospasm.**

pyloric sphincter, a sphincter at the opening from the stomach into the duodenum. It is usually closed, opening only for a moment when a peristaltic wave passes over it. Also called **pyloric valve.**

pyloric stenosis, a narrowing of the pyloric sphincter at the outlet of the stomach, causing an obstruction that blocks the flow of food into the small intestine. The condition occurs as a congenital defect in 1 of 200 newborns and occasionally in older adults secondary to an ulcer or fibrosis at the outlet. Diagnosis is made in infants by the presence of forceful projectile vomiting and palpation of a hard, prominent pylorus and in adults by x-ray examinations after a barium meal. Surgical correction is done with the patient under light general anesthesia after the stomach is emptied. The muscle fibers of the outlet are cut, without severing the mucosa, to widen the opening. After surgery in adults, a stomach tube remains in place and observation is maintained for signs of hemorrhage or of blockage of the tube. See also **pyloromyotomy.**

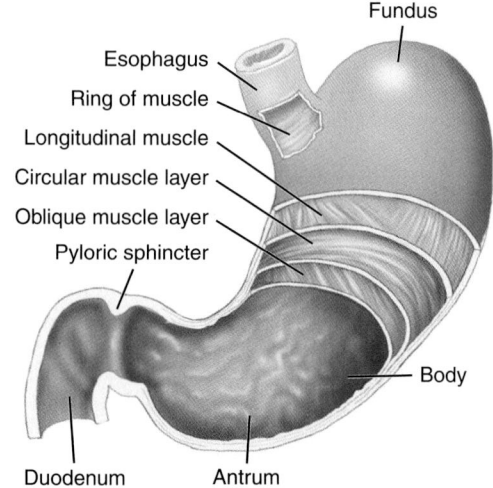

Hypertrophic pyloric stenosis *(Hagen-Ansert, 2006)*

pyloric ulcer. See **peptic ulcer.**

pyloric valve. See **pyloric sphincter.**

pyloro-, prefix meaning "the pylorus": *pyloroplasty, pylorospasm.*

pyloroduodenitis /pilôr′ōdoo′ədənī″tis/, an inflammation of the pylorus and the duodenum.

pyloromyotomy /pīlôr′ōmī·ot″əmē/ [Gk, *pyle + ouros + mys,* muscle, *temnein,* to cut], the incision of the longitudinal and circular muscle of the pylorus, which leaves the mucosa intact but separates the incised muscle fibers. It is the treatment of choice for hypertrophic pyloric stenosis, a congenital condition that obstructs the stomach. Also called **Fredet-Ramstedt operation, Ramstedt-Fredet operation.** See also **pyloric stenosis.**

pyloroplasty /pīlôr″əplas′tē/ [Gk, *pyle + ouros + plassein,* to mold], a surgical procedure performed to relieve pyloric stenosis by widening the pyloric outlet. Before surgery any electrolyte imbalances or fluid deficiencies are corrected; sodium chloride and potassium chloride solutions may be given to correct ion losses from vomiting, which is characteristic of pyloric stenosis. With the patient under anesthesia the pyloric opening is dilated. Diarrhea is a common postoperative complication.

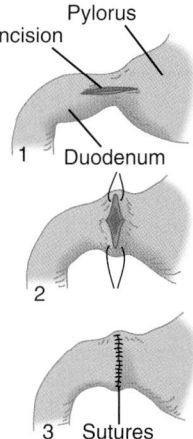

Pyloroplasty *(Black and Hawks, 2009)*

pylorospasm /pīlôr″əspaz′əm/ [Gk, *pyle* + *ouros* + *spasmos*], a spasm of the pyloric sphincter of the stomach, as occurs in pyloric stenosis.

pylorostomy /pī′lôros″təmē/, the surgical establishment of a fistula from the abdominal surface to the stomach at a point near the pylorus.

pylorotomy /pī′lôrot″əmē/ [Gk, *pyle*, gate, *ouros*, guard, *temnein*, to cut], a surgical incision of the pylorus, usually performed to remove an obstruction.

pylorus /pīlôr″əs/ *pl.* **pylori, pyloruses** [Gk, *pyle*, gate, *ouros*, guard], a narrow, nearly tubular part of the stomach that angles to the right from the body of the stomach toward the duodenum. The most common position of the pylorus is about 3 cm to the right of the sagittal axis. It is distinctively marked by the thickening of the pyloric sphincter, and its lining is composed of an intestinal kind of epithelium rather than the gastric kind common to the body of the stomach. **−pyloric,** *adj.*

pyo- /pī′ō-/, prefix meaning "pus": *pyocele.*

pyocele, an accumulation of pus in the scrotum.

pyocolpos, an accumulation of pus in the vagina.

pyocyanic /pī′ōsī·an″ik/, pertaining to pus that is blue or to an organism that produces blue pus, such as *Pseudomonas pyocyanea.*

pyocyanin /pī′ōsī″ənin/, a blue or blue-green pigment that may be extracted from *Pseudomonas aeruginosa* with chloroform.

pyocyst /pī′əsist/ [Gk, *pyon*, pus, *kytos*, cell], a pus-filled cyst.

pyocystitis /-sistī″tis/, an inflammation involving a pus-filled cyst within the urinary bladder.

pyoderma /pī′ōdur″mə/ [Gk, *pyon*, pus, *derma*, skin], any purulent skin disease, such as impetigo. Also called **pyodermia.**

pyoderma gangrenosum, a rapidly evolving, idiopathic, chronic, debilitating skin disease that usually accompanies a systemic disease, especially chronic ulcerative colitis, and is characterized by irregular, boggy, blue-red ulcers with undermined borders surrounding purulent necrotic bases.

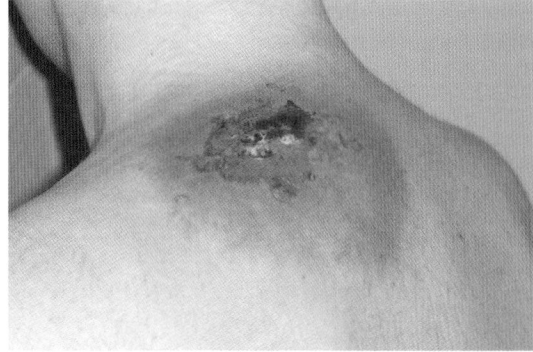

Pyoderma gangrenosum *(Kalu and Williams, 2007)*

pyodermia. See **pyoderma.**

pyogenic /pī′əjen″ik/ [Gk, *pyon* + *genein*, to produce], pus-producing.

pyogenic exotoxin, extracellular toxin secreted by *Streptococcus pyogenes* that may be associated with fever and the development of renal failure, respiratory distress, and necrosis.

pyogenic granuloma, a small nonmalignant mass of excessive granulation tissue, usually found at the site of an injury. This condition is most often seen in pregnant women, children, and patients taking Indinavir, Soriatane, Accutane, and oral contraceptives. Most often a dull red, it contains numerous capillaries, bleeds readily, and is very tender. It may be attached by a narrow stalk. Treatment is with electrocautery or topical silver nitrate. Also called **telangiectatic granuloma.** See also **granuloma.**

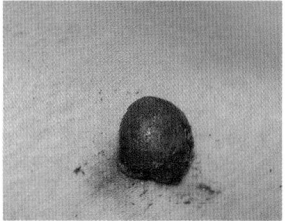

Pyogenic granuloma *(Johns Hopkins Hospital, 2015)*

pyogenic infection [Gk, *pyon*, pus, *genein*, to produce; L, *inficere*, to stain], any infection that results in pus production.

pyogenic microorganisms [Gk, *pyon*, pus, *genein*, to produce, *mikros*, small, *organon*, instrument], microorganisms that produce pus. Kinds include *Bacillus, Clostridium,* **gonococcus,** *Staphylococcus, Streptococcus.*

pyohemothorax /-hem′ōthôr″aks/ [Gk, *pyon*, pus, *haima*, blood, *thorax*, chest], an accumulation of pus and blood in the pleural cavity.

pyonephrolithiasis /-nef′rōlithī″əsis/, an accumulation of pus and calculi in the kidney.

pyophylactic /-filak″tik/ [Gk, *pyon*, pus, *phylax*, protector], providing protection against purulent infections, such as administering an antibiotic before the onset of an infection.

pyophysometra /-fī′sōmē″trə/, an accumulation of pus and gas in the uterus.

pyopneumopericardium /pī′ōnoo′mōper′ikär″dē·əm/, the presence of pus and air or gas in the pericardial sac.

P

pyopneumoperitonitis /pī′ōnoo̅′mōper′itənī″tis/, inflammation of the peritoneal cavity caused by an accumulation of air and pus in the cavity.

pyopyelectasis /-pī′əlek″təsis/, a dilation of the renal pelvis of the kidney resulting from an accumulation of pus.

pyorrhea /pī′ərē″ə/ [Gk, *pyon + rhoia,* flow], **1.** a discharge of pus. **2.** a purulent inflammation of the tissues surrounding the teeth. Also spelled *pyorrhoea. −pyorrheal, adj.*

-pyorrhea, suffix meaning "the flowing or discharge of pus": *pyorrhea.*

pyosalpinx /pī′ōsal″pingks/ [Gk, *pyon + salpinx,* tube], an accumulation of pus in a fallopian tube. See also **salpingitis.**

pyospermia, a complication of chronic prostatitis marked by pus in the seminal fluid. Also called *pyosemia.*

pyostatic /-stat″ik/, arresting the formation of pus.

pyostomatitis /-stō′mətī″tis/, an inflammation of the mouth.

pyothorax /-thôr″aks/, **1.** a collection of pus in the pleural cavity. **2.** purulent pleurisy.

pyoureter /pī′ōyoo̅r″ətər, -yoo̅rē″tər/, the presence of pus in the ureter.

pyoverdin /-vur″din/, a yellow pigment produced by some strains of *Pseudomonas aeruginosa.*

pyramid /pir″əmid/ [Gk, *pyramis*], a mass of tissue rising to an apex, such as the pyramids of the cerebellum and kidneys.

pyramidal /piram″idəl/ [Gk, *pyramis*], pertaining to the shape of a pyramid.

pyramidal cell [Gk, *pyramis* + L, *cella,* storeroom], a neuron with a pyramid-shaped cell body in the gray matter of the cerebral cortex.

pyramidalis /piram′idā″lis/, one of a pair of anterolateral muscles of the abdomen, contained in the lower end of the sheath of the rectus abdominis, which arises from the crest of the pubis and is inserted into the linea alba upward about halfway to the navel. It is innervated by a branch of the twelfth thoracic nerve and functions to tense the linea alba. Compare **rectus abdominis, transversus abdominis.**

pyramidal nucleus [Gk, *pyramis* + L, *nucleus,* nut kernel], a band of gray matter lying between the olivary nucleus and the midline that projects fibers contralaterally to the vermis part of the cerebellum.

pyramidal tract, a pathway composed of groups of nerve fibers in the white matter of the spinal cord through which motor impulses are conducted to the anterior horn cells from the opposite side of the brain. These descending fibers, the nerve cell bodies of which are found in the precentral cortex, regulate the voluntary and reflex activity of the muscles through the anterior horn cells.

pyramidotomy /piram′idot″əmē/, the surgical severance of pyramidal tracts in the treatment of disorders associated with involuntary muscle contractions.

pyrantel pamoate /pīran″təl/, an anthelmintic.
- INDICATIONS: It is prescribed in the treatment of infestation by roundworms or pinworms.
- CONTRAINDICATIONS: Known hypersensitivity to this drug prohibits its use. Caution should be used in patients with anemia or severe malnutrition.
- ADVERSE EFFECTS: Among the more serious adverse effects are nausea, abdominal cramps, diarrhea, dizziness, and skin rash.

pyrazinamide /pī′rəzin″əmīd/, an antimycobacterial.
- INDICATIONS: It is prescribed in combination chemotherapy in the treatment of tuberculosis in hospitalized patients who fail to respond to other medications.
- CONTRAINDICATIONS: Severe liver damage, acute gout, or known hypersensitivity to this drug prohibits its use. Use

with caution in patients with renal failure, chronic gout, diabetes mellitus, or porphyria.
- ADVERSE EFFECTS: Common side effects include malaise, nausea, GI upset, and arthralgia and myalgia. Among the more serious adverse reactions are hepatotoxicity and hyperuricemia.

pyrenemia /pī′rənē″mē·ə/, a condition in which nucleated erythrocytes are present in the blood.

pyrethrin and piperonyl butoxide /pī″rəthrin, piper″ənil/, a fixed-combination scabicide and pediculicide.
- INDICATIONS: It is prescribed in the treatment of infestations of head, body, and pubic lice.
- CONTRAINDICATIONS: Known hypersensitivity to chrysanthemums, ragweed, or this drug prohibits its use.
- ADVERSE EFFECTS: Among the more serious adverse effects are irritation of the skin and the mucous membranes.

pyretic /pīrek″tik/ [Gk, *pyretos,* fever], pertaining to or characterized by fever. Also called *pyrectic.*

pyreto-, prefix meaning "fever": *pyretogenic, pyretotherapy.*

pyretogenic /pī′rətojen″ik/ [Gk, *pyretos,* fever, *genein,* to produce], inducing, causing, or resulting from a fever.

pyrexia. See **fever.**

-pyrexia, suffix meaning "a febrile condition": *apyrexia, hyperpyrexia.*

Pyridium, a urinary tract analgesic. Brand name for **phenazopyridine hydrochloride.**

pyridostigmine bromide /pir′idōstig″mēn/, an acetylcholinesterase inhibitor that prolongs the effects of neuronally released acetylcholine.
- INDICATIONS: It is prescribed in the treatment of myasthenia gravis and is used as an antagonist to nondepolarizing muscle relaxants, such as curare.
- CONTRAINDICATIONS: Intestinal or urinary obstruction, bradycardia, hypotension, or known hypersensitivity to this drug or to other anticholinesterases prohibits its use.
- ADVERSE EFFECTS: Among the more serious adverse effects are nausea, diarrhea, abdominal cramps, muscle cramps, and weakness.

pyridoxal phosphate /pir′ədok″səl/, an enzyme that acts with pyridoxamine phosphate and transaminase to catalyze the reversible transfer of an amino group from an alpha-amino acid to an alpha-keto acid, especially alpha-ketoglutaric acid. Such processes are essential to metabolism.

pyridoxamine phosphate /pir′ədok″səmēn/, an enzyme that participates with pyridoxal phosphate and transaminase in the reversible transfer of an amino group from an alpha-amino acid to an alpha-keto acid.

pyridoxine /pir′ədok″sēn/, a water-soluble white crystalline vitamin that is part of the B complex. It is derived from pyridine and converted in the body to pyridoxal and pyridoxamine for synthesis. It functions as a coenzyme essential for the synthesis and breakdown of amino acids, the conversion of tryptophan to niacin, the breakdown of glycogen to glucose 1-phosphate, the production of antibodies, the formation of heme in hemoglobin, the formation of hormones important in brain function, the proper absorption of vitamin B_{12}, the production of hydrochloric acid and magnesium, and the maintenance of the balance of sodium and potassium, which regulates body fluids and the functioning of the nervous and musculoskeletal systems. Rich dietary sources are meats, especially organ meats; whole-grain cereals; soybeans; peanuts; wheat germ; and brewer's yeast. Milk and green vegetables supply smaller amounts. The most common symptoms of deficiency are seborrheic dermatitis about the eyes, nose, and mouth and behind the ears; cheilosis; glossitis and stomatitis; nervousness; depression; peripheral neuropathy; and lymphopenia, leading to convulsions in infants and anemia in adults. Treatment and prophylaxis consist of administration of the vitamin and a diet rich in foods containing it. Several drugs interfere with the use of pyridoxine, notably isoniazid and penicillamine, and supplements of the vitamin are recommended with the use of these drugs. The need for increased amounts of pyridoxine is related to protein intake and occurs during pregnancy, lactation, exposure to radiation, cardiac failure, aging, and use of oral contraceptives. Also called *pyridoxine hydrochloride,* **vitamin B**$_6$.

pyriform. See **piriform.**

pyrimethamine /pir′imeth″əmēn/, an antimalarial.

■ INDICATIONS: It is prescribed in the treatment of malaria and toxoplasmosis.

■ CONTRAINDICATIONS: Use is contraindicated in chloroguanide-resistant malaria, in patients with megaloblastic anemia resulting from folate deficiency, and in patients who are hypersensitive to the drug. Caution is recommended in use of the drug to treat toxoplasmosis because dosages needed may be at a toxic level.

■ ADVERSE EFFECTS: Among the more serious adverse effects, primarily with large doses, are megaloblastic anemia, atrophic glossitis, leukopenia, and convulsions.

pyrimidine /pərim″ədēn/, an organic compound of heterocyclic nitrogen found in nucleic acids and in many drugs, including the antiviral drugs acyclovir, ribavirin, and trifluridine.

pyro-, combining form meaning "fire," "heat," or "produced by heating": *pyrogen, pyrolagnia, pyromania.*

pyrogen /pī″rəjən/ [Gk, *pyr,* fire, *genein,* to produce], any substance or agent that tends to cause a rise in body temperature, such as some bacterial toxins. See also **fever.** −*pyrogenic, adj.*

pyroglobulin /pī′rōglob″yəlin/, an immunoglobulin that precipitates irreversibly when heated. Pyroglobulins are often present in the blood of patients with diseases such as multiple myeloma.

pyroglutamic acid /pi″roglootam′ik/, an uncommon amino acid derivative.

pyrolagnia /pī′rōlag″nē-ə/ [Gk, *pyr* + *lagneia,* lust], sexual stimulation or gratification from watching or setting fires.

pyrolysis /pirol″isis/, the decomposition of a chemical compound by the application of heat.

pyromania /pī′rōmā″nē-ə/ [Gk, *pyr* + *mania,* madness], an impulse-control disorder characterized by an uncontrollable urge to set fires. The disorder presents itself in terms of a tension phase along with increased mental arousal before the act, which is followed by a feeling of self-fulfillment after the act.

pyromaniac /pī′rōmā″nē-ak/, **1.** *n.,* a person having or displaying characteristics of pyromania. **2.** *adj.,* pertaining to or exhibiting pyromania. −*pyromaniacal, adj.*

pyropoikilocytosis /pī′rōpoi′kilō′sītō″sis/, a recessive inherited disorder characterized by severe hemolysis, irregular shapes of red blood cells, and sensitivity of blood cells to fragmentation in vitro after minor temperature variations.

pyrosis. See **heartburn.**

pyroxylin. See **nitrocellulose.**

pyrrole (C$_4$H$_4$NH) /pirōl″, pir″ōl/ [Gk, *pyrrhos,* red], a five-membered heterocyclic aromatic substance occurring naturally in many compounds in the body. Bridged pyrrole rings surround the Fe^{2+} ion in the hemoglobin molecule.

pyruvate carboxylase /pī′roo·vāt kär·bok′sə·lās/, an enzyme that catalyzes the irreversible carboxylation of pyruvate, a reaction necessary for gluconeogenesis from lactate or amino acids forming pyruvate and also providing four-carbon compounds for the citric acid cycle. The enzyme is a mitochondrial protein occurring in liver but not in muscle. Deficiency of the enzyme, an autosomal-recessive trait, causes severe psychomotor slowing and lactic acidosis in infants. There is a particularly severe, rapidly fatal form in which hyperammonemia, citrullinemia, and an excess of lysine in the blood are also present.

pyruvate dehydrogenase complex /pī′roo·vāt dē·hī′drō·jən·ās/, a multienzyme complex consisting of at least three distinct enzymes; it catalyzes the formation of acetyl coenzyme A from pyruvate and coenzyme A. The acetyl coenzyme A is used in fatty acid synthesis, for acetylations, and for oxidation by means of the citric acid cycle. Deficiency of any component of the complex results in excess of lactic acid in the blood, ataxia, and psychomotor slowing.

pyruvate kinase /pī′rəvāt/, an enzyme essential for anaerobic glycolysis in red blood cells. It catalyzes the transfer of a phosphate group from adenosine triphosphate to produce adenosine diphosphate.

pyruvate kinase deficiency, a congenital hemolytic anemia transmitted as an autosomal-recessive trait. The homozygous condition is characterized by severe chronic hemolysis. The heterozygous form is usually asymptomatic and of no clinical significance, although mild to severe anemia may occur.

pyruvic acid /pīroo″vik/, a compound formed as an end product of glycolysis, the anaerobic stage of glucose metabolism. It may enter the citric acid cycle if oxygen is present. Under anaerobic conditions it may be converted to lactic acid, which accumulates in muscle tissue.

pyuria /pīyoor″ē-ə/, the presence of an excessive number of white blood cells in the urine, typically more than four leukocytes per high-power field count. It is generally a sign of an infection in the urinary tract but can reflect inflammation from chemical or radiation causes. Bacterial pyuria usually is caused by infection of the bladder and urethra. See also **bacteriuria.**

PZI, abbreviation for *protamine zinc insulin.* See **protamine zinc insulin (PZI) suspension.** □

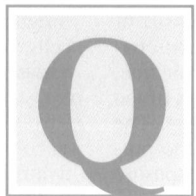

Q

Q, symbol for *volumetric flow rate.*

q.2h. [L, *quaque,* every, *secunda,* two, *hora,* hours], notation for a Latin phrase meaning "every 2 hours." Abbreviation for *quaque secunda hora.*

q.3h. [L, *quaque,* every, *tertia,* three, *hora,* hours], notation for a Latin phrase meaning "every 3 hours." Abbreviation for *quaque tertia hora.*

q.4h. [L, *quaque,* every, *quarta,* four, *hora,* hours], notation for a Latin phrase meaning "every 4 hours." Abbreviation for *quaque quarta hora.*

q.6h. [L, *quaque,* every, *sex,* six, *hora,* hours], notation for a Latin phrase meaning "every 6 hours." Abbreviation for *quaque sexta hora.*

q.8h. [L, *quaque,* every, *octa,* eight, *hora,* hours], notation for a Latin phrase meaning "every 8 hours." Abbreviation for *quaque octa hora.*

Q angle, the angle of incidence of the quadriceps muscle relative to the patella. The Q angle determines the tracking of the patella through the trochlea of the femur. As the angle increases, the chance of patellar compression problems increases. See also **angle of incidence.**

QCT, abbreviation for **quantitative computed tomography.**

q.d. [L, *quaque,* every, *die,* day], **1.** *(Obsolete)* an abbreviation formerly used to indicate "every day." Because of the danger of misinterpretation, *q.d.* is on The Joint Commission's "Official 'Do Not Use' List of Abbreviations." It is also identified on the Institute for Safe Medication's "List of Error-Prone Abbreviations, Symbols, and Dose Designations." Now written out as *daily.* **2.** abbreviation for *quartile deviation.*

22q11.2 deletion syndrome, a disorder caused by a microdeletion of chromosome 22 with a wide variety of presenting signs and symptoms. Formerly called **DiGeorge syndrome.**

■ OBSERVATIONS: Symptoms frequently noted include attention deficit hyperactivity disorder, autism, or other behavioral problems. Cleft palate is often present, as are heart defects. Cognitive and speech delays may be present. The missing section of chromosome 22 can affect every body system.

■ INTERVENTIONS: There is no cure for the syndrome, but there are numerous treatments and therapies that can help the individual have a good quality of life. The earlier treatment is initiated, the more effective it will be.

■ PATIENT CARE CONSIDERATIONS: Most individuals with the deletion syndrome do well, especially if appropriate treatment is initiated promptly.

qdrnt, abbreviation for **quadrant.**

Q fever [L, *febris*], an acute febrile illness, usually respiratory, caused by the rickettsia *Coxiella burnetii (Rickettsia burnetii).* The disease is spread through contact with infected domestic animals, by inhaling the rickettsiae from their hides or drinking their contaminated milk, or by being bitten by a tick harboring the organism. Illness is especially common among those who work with sheep, goats, and cattle. The organism can survive for long periods in the environment as

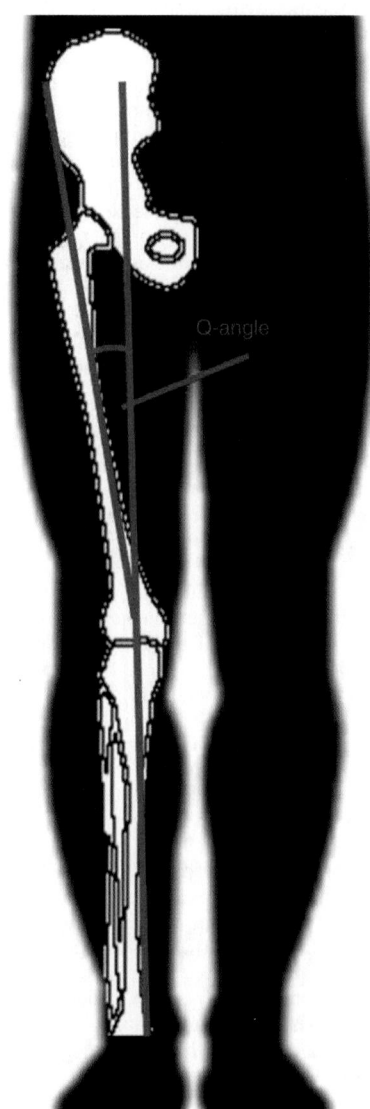

Q angle *(Lester, Watson, and Hutchinson, 2014)*

it is resistant to heat and drying. Compare **scrub typhus.** See also **Australian Q fever, typhus.**

■ OBSERVATIONS: Onset is abrupt, and high fever may persist for 3 weeks or more. Symptoms are variable and may include a severe headache, nonproductive cough, diarrhea, abdominal pain, and chest pain.

■ INTERVENTIONS: Treatment with tetracycline is usually effective in 36 to 48 hours.

■ PATIENT CARE CONSIDERATIONS: People who are regularly exposed to domestic animals can be vaccinated against Q fever; however, the vaccine is not commercially available in the United States. A single airborne organism can infect a susceptible individual. Q fever has a history of use in biological warfare and is considered a potential terrorist threat.

q.h. [L, *quaque,* every, *hora,* hour], a notation for a Latin phrase meaning "every hour." Abbreviation for *quaque hora.*

Qi /chē/, in traditional Chinese medicine, the vital energy of the human body.

qid, q.i.d. [L, *quater,* four, *in die,* daily], a notation for a Latin phrase meaning "four times a day." Abbreviation for *quater in die.*

Qi Gong /ˈchē-ˈgŭŋ/, a practice designed to promote well-being and the relief of mental and physical symptoms through a process of mental exercises and focus, based on the belief that the body can adjust itself through a series of intentional mental relaxation processes.

Q-R interval, the period from the start of the QRS complex to the peak of the R wave on an electrocardiogram.

QRS complex, a series of waveforms on an electrocardiogram that represents both normal and abnormal depolarization of ventricular muscle cells. It is composed of Q, R, and S waves: a Q wave is the negative deflection before the first R wave, an R wave is any positive deflection, and an S wave is the negative deflection after an R wave. If there is no R wave, the totally negative complex is designated QS. A combination of uppercase and lowercase letters is used to describe the amplitude of each wave. Some variations of the QRS complex are qR, QR, qRs, rS, RS, and rSR. Also called **QRS wave.**

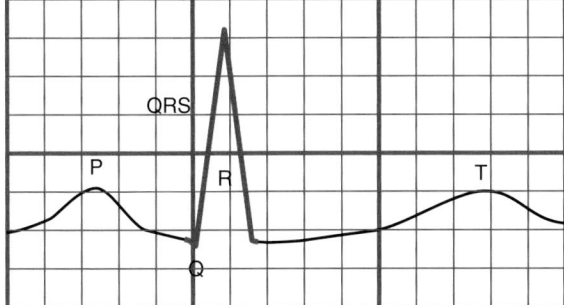

Normal QRS complex *(Wesley, 2012)*

QRST complex [L, *complexus*], a series of waveforms on an electrocardiogram consisting of the QRS complex, the S-T segment, and the T wave. It represents depolarization and repolarization of the ventriclular muscle cells.

QRS wave. See **QRS complex.**

q.s. [L, *quantum,* quantity, *sufficit,* sufficient], (in prescriptions) a notation for a Latin phrase meaning "quantity required." Abbreviation for *quantum sufficit.*

Q test, (in statistics) a statistical test used to identify outliers in a dataset.

Q-switched laser, a laser containing a switching device that causes the laser to produce very high intensity impulses of very short duration.

Q-switching, a laser technique that achieves high peak power in nanosecond pulses of energy. It is most often used in health care to remove unwanted brown spots, sun freckles, or tattoos. The laser energy pulse releases the pigment into the skin so that it can be reabsorbed.

qt, abbreviation for **quart.**

Q-T interval, the period from the beginning of the QRS complex to the end of the T wave on an electrocardiogram. It reflects the refractory period of the heart. A long Q-T interval

is associated with the life-threatening ventricular tachycardia known as torsades de pointes. Quinidine, procainamide, and disopyramide can lengthen the Q-T interval.

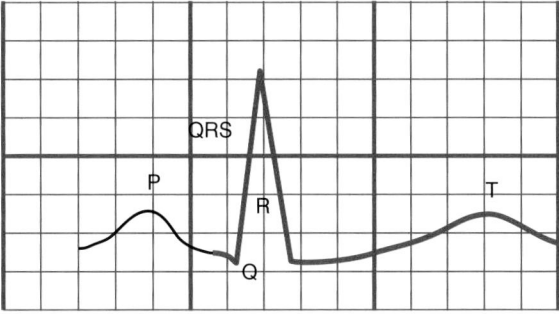

Q-T interval *(Wesley, 2012)*

Quaalude, a sedative-hypnotic. It is no longer distributed in the United States and is a Schedule III controlled substance in Canada. Brand name for *methaqualone.*

quack. *(Slang)* See **charlatan.**

quackery, the practice or methods of misrepresentation in the diagnosis and treatment of disease.

quad, **1.** abbreviation for **quadriceps femoris. 2.** abbreviation for **quadrilateral. 3.** abbreviation for **quadrant. 4.** abbreviation for **quadriplegia.**

quad cane, a cane adapted for increased stability by providing a four-legged rectangular base of support.

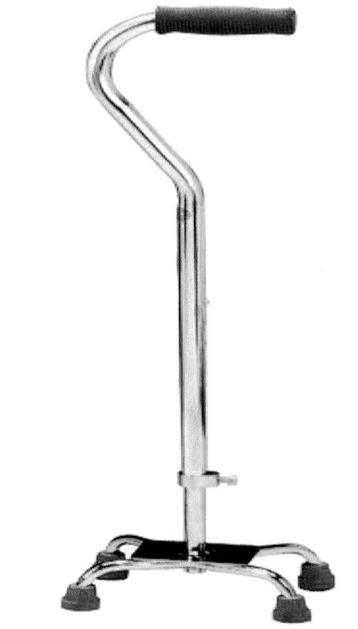

Quad (four-legged) cane *(Constantinescu, Leonard, and Kurlan, 2006)*

quad coughing /kwod/, a form of assisted coughing for patients with central nervous system disorders such as spinal cord injury who are unable to generate sufficient force to clear respiratory secretions. After a maximal inspiration, the patient coughs while a qualified health or allied health professional exerts gentle upward and inward pressure with both hands on the abdomen. The patient's family and support

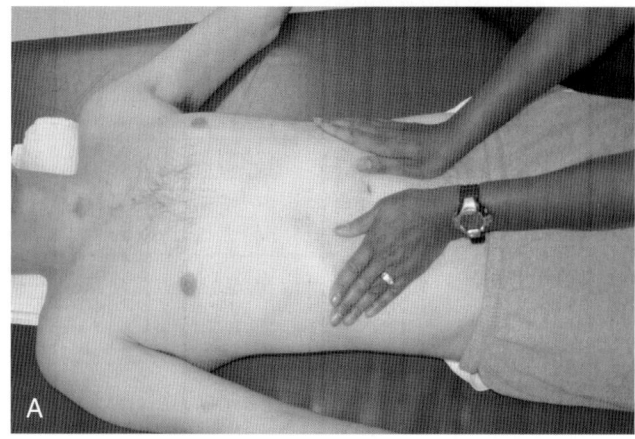

Hand placement in quad coughing *(Umphred et al, 2013)*

system can also be taught the procedure. The increased intraabdominal pressure produces a more forceful cough.

quadr-, quadri-, combining form meaning "four": *quadrangular, quadrilateral, quadrivalent.*

quadrangular bandage /kwodrang″gələr/, a towel or other large rectangular sheet of cloth folded over for use as a wrapping for a wound of the abdomen, chest, or head. Also called **cravat bandage.**

quadrant (qdrnt, quad) /kwod″rənt/ [L, *quadrans,* a fourth part], **1.** one quarter of a circle. **2.** one quarter of an anatomical area formed by the division of the area by imaginary vertical and horizontal lines bisecting each other. See **abdominal quadrant.**

quadrantanopsia /kwodran′tənop″sē·ə/, a loss of vision in a quarter section of the visual field of one or both eyes. The cause may vary with the quadrant affected.

quadrantectomy /kwod′rantek″təmē/, a partial mastectomy in which a tumor and at least a 1-inch margin of surrounding tissue along with the pectoralis muscle fascia are excised in one quadrant of a breast.

quadrant streak, a technique for microbial inoculation in which a single colony is isolated on a culture plate divided into four sections.

quadratus labii superioris. See **zygomaticus minor.**

quadratus lumborum, a muscle that connects the pelvis to the spine.

quadri-. See **quadr-, quadri-.**

quadriceps femoris /kwod″riseps/ [L, *quattuor,* four, *caput,* head, *femur,* thigh], the large extensor muscle of the anterior thigh, composed of the rectus femoris, the vastus lateralis, the vastus medialis, and the vastus intermedius. The quadriceps forms a large dense mass covering the front and sides of the femur. Tendons of the four parts of the muscle unite at the distal part of the thigh, forming a single strong tendon that embeds the patella and inserts onto the tibial tuberosity. The muscle functions to extend at the knee and flex the thigh.

quadriceps reflex. See **patellar reflex.**

quadridigitate. See **tetradactyly.**

quadrigeminal /kwod′rijem″inəl/ [L, *quadrigeminum,* fourfold], **1.** in four parts. **2.** a fourfold increase in size or frequency. **3.** having four symmetric parts.

quadrigeminal pulse, a pulse in which a pause occurs after every fourth beat.

quadrilateral, a shape having four sides and four angles.

quadrilateral socket /kwod′rilat″ərəl/, a four-sided prosthetic socket design for people with above-the-knee amputations.

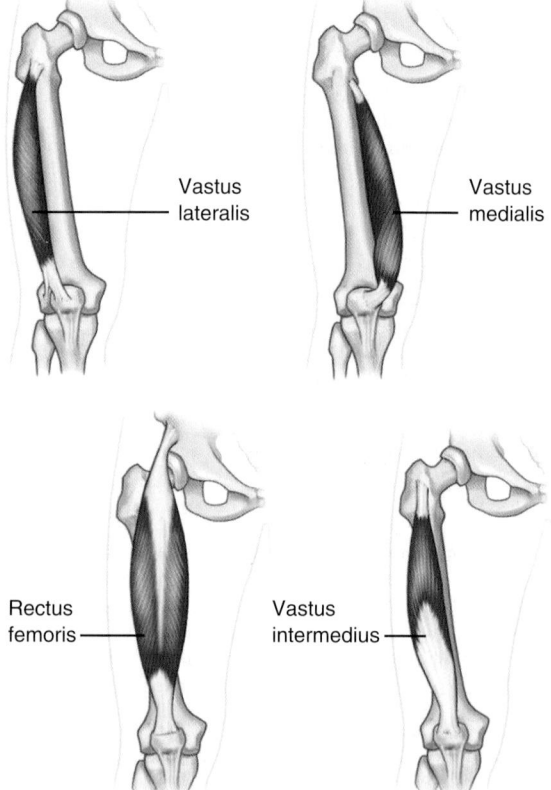

Vastus lateralis

Vastus medialis

Rectus femoris

Vastus intermedius

Quadriceps femoris group of thigh muscles

The posterior brim is designed to fit directly beneath the ischial tuberosity so that the person literally sits on it.

quadripedal extensor reflex. See **Brain's reflex.**

quadriplegia (quad) /kwod′rəplē″jē·ə/ [L, *quattuor,* four; Gk, *plege,* stroke], a condition in which there is impairment in movement or muscle tone involving all four extremities. See also **tetraplegia.**

quadrivalent /kwod′rivā″lənt/, a chemical element or radical with a valence of four.

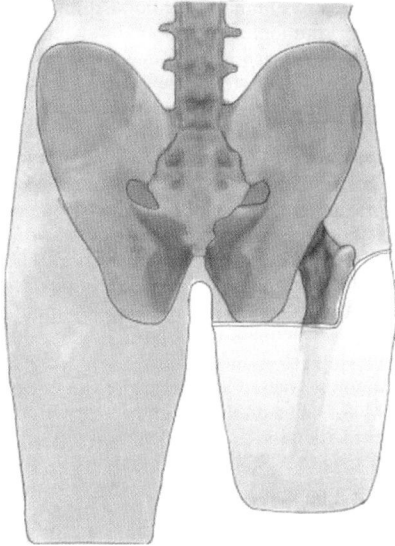

Quadrilateral socket *(Lusardi et al, 2013)*

quadruped /kwod″rŏoped′/ [L, *quattuor,* four, *pes,* foot], **1.** any four-footed animal. **2.** a position involving weight bearing on all fours (hands and knees).

quadruplet /kwod″rŏoplit, kwodrō″plit/ [L, *quadruplex,* fourfold], any one of four offspring born after the same gestation period during a single pregnancy. See also **Hellin's law.**

quadrupole mass filter, a four-pole magnet system used to separate charged mass fragments in a mass spectrometer.

qual anal, abbreviation for **qualitative analysis.**

quale /kwā″lē/ *pl. qualia* [L, *qualis,* what kind], **1.** the quality of a particular thing. **2.** a quality considered as an independent entity, e.g., the chest pain experienced with a myocardial infarction. **3.** (in psychology) a feeling, sensation, or other conscious process that has its unique particular quality regardless of its external meaning or frame of reference.

qualified /kwol″ifīd/ [L, *qualis*], (for health or related reasons) pertaining to a health professional or health facility that is formally recognized by an appropriate agency or organization as meeting certain standards of performance related to the professional competence of an individual or the eligibility of an institution to participate in an approved health care program.

qualitative /kwol″itā′tiv/ [L, *qualis*], pertaining to the quality, value, or nature of something.

qualitative analysis (qual anal) [L, *qualis,* what kind; Gk, *analysis,* a loosening], **1.** (in chemistry) the study of a sample of material to determine what chemical substances are present. **2.** (in research) the analysis and interpretation of data that cannot be analyzed by statistical methods. Compare **quantitative analysis.**

qualitative test, a test that determines the presence or absence of a substance.

quality /kwol″itē/ [L, *qualis*], **1.** a descriptive specification of the penetrating nature of an x-ray beam. It is influenced by kilovoltage and filtration: a higher kilovoltage produces more penetration, and filtration removes selected wavelengths and "hardens" the beam. **2.** (in speech therapy) refers to the nature of phonation produced by the vocal folds. Disorders of voice quality include hoarseness, harshness, breathiness, and glottal fry.

quality assessment measures, formal systematic organizational evaluation of overall patterns or programs of care, including clinical, consumer, and systems evaluation.

quality assurance, (for health or related reasons) a pledge to the public by those within the various health disciplines that they will work toward the goal of an optimally achievable degree of excellence in the services rendered to every patient. See also **quality management.**

■ METHOD: A quality assurance program takes into account the need to define that which is to be measured. Quality assurance implies a clear understanding of what is meant by quality and a valid and reliable method for evaluating the care that is provided. Implementation of a quality assurance program involves the development of criteria based on acceptable standards of care and norms of professional behavior. The norms are established by members of the profession or professions who are expert in the care of a specific patient population. Evaluation is conducted by a review committee and may be retrospective or concurrent.

■ PATIENT CARE CONSIDERATIONS: The ultimate goal of both retrospective and concurrent review is improvement of patient care. Individual members of the health care team hold themselves accountable to the public and patient for the caliber of care they provide.

■ OUTCOME CRITERIA: *Outcome* represents a measurable change in the health/illness status of the patient that is the end result of the care the patient received. *Cost-benefit* refers to the expenditure of money, time, and effort in providing health care and the relationship this cost bears to the actual benefits to the recipient of care. It is the promise to evaluate outcomes thoroughly and to employ the results of the evaluation for continuous improvement of patient care that is the essence of quality assurance.

quality assurance program. See **quality assurance.**

quality control, a method of repeated assay of known standard materials and the monitoring of reaction parameters to ensure precision and accuracy.

quality factor, a term that expresses the biological damage that radiation can produce. Doses of different types of radiation can be set equal to one another if the actual absorbed dose is multiplied by the quality factor. The product is called the dose equivalent and is measured in sieverts or rem.

quality management, systems designed to improve the effectiveness of treatments, therapies, and services while increasing satisfaction. See also **quality assurance.**

quality of life [L, *qualis,* what kind; AS, *lif*], a measure of the optimum energy or force that endows a person with the power to cope successfully with the full range of challenges encountered in the real world. The term applies to all individuals, regardless of illness or disability, on the job, at home, or in leisure activities. Quality enrichment methods can include activities that reduce boredom and allow a maximum amount of freedom in choosing and performing various tasks. Although assessment tools are available to evaluate physical and social dimensions of quality of life, an individual's general sense of well-being or satisfaction with the attributes of life is often more difficult to evaluate.

quantitative /kwon″titā′tiv/ [L, *quantus,* how much], capable of being measured or counted.

quantitative analysis [L, *quantum,* how much; Gk, *analysis,* a loosening], **1.** (in chemistry) the determination of the amounts of constituents in a sample of material. Kinds include **gravimetric analysis, volumetric analysis, spectrophotometric analysis. 2.** (in research) the use of statistical methods to analyze data. Compare **qualitative analysis.**

quantitative computed tomography (QCT), a type of computed tomography that calculates and displays bone density in three dimensions. QCT is used mainly for lumbar spine studies but can also be applied in hip and peripheral bone mineral evaluations.

quantitative inheritance. See **multifactorial inheritance.**

quantitative test [L, *quantum,* how much, *testum,* crucible], a test that determines the amount of a substance per unit volume or unit weight.

quantitative ultrasound, an ultrasound technique for assessing bone mineral density. Its main advantage is the complete absence of radiation; a disadvantage is the confounding influence of soft tissue.

quantum dots, nanocrystals with semiconductor properties whose diameter is smaller than 10 nm. They are used in research related to nanoprobes for tumor-targeted, dual-modal, in vivo imaging.

quantum mechanics. See **quantum theory.**

quantum mottle. See **mottle.**

quantum theory /kwon″təm/ [L, *quantum,* how much; Gk, *theoria,* speculation], (in physics) the theory dealing with the interaction of matter and electromagnetic radiation, particularly at the atomic and subatomic levels, according to which radiation consists of small units of energy called quanta. Radiation can be absorbed only in whole quanta, and the energy content of a quantum is inversely proportional to its wavelength. Also called **quantum mechanics.** See also **Planck constant.**

quarantine /kwor″əntēn/ [It, *quarantina,* forty], **1.** isolation of people with communicable disease or those exposed to communicable disease during the contagious period in an attempt to prevent spread of the illness. **2.** the practice of detaining travelers or vessels coming from places of epidemic disease, originally for 40 days, for the purpose of inspection or disinfection.

quart (qt) /kwôrt/ [L, *quartus,* fourth], a unit of volume fluid measure equivalent to ¼ gallon, 2 pints, 32 ounces, or 946.24 mL. The British Imperial quart is equal to 40 ounces, or 1.136 L, and the American quart for dry measure is 1.101 L.

quartan /kwôr″tən/ [L, *quartanus,* relating to the fourth], recurring on the fourth day, or at about 72-hour intervals. See also **quartan malaria.**

quartan malaria, a form of malaria caused by the protozoan *Plasmodium malariae* and characterized by febrile paroxysms that occur every 72 hours. Also called *quartan fever.* Compare **falciparum malaria, tertian malaria.** See also **malaria.**

quarti-, prefix meaning "fourth": *quartile.*

quartile /kwôr″təl, kwôr″tīl/ [L, *quartus,* fourth], (in statistics) one fourth of the distribution of scores. The first quartile would be the lowest 25% of scores, the second quartile would represent scores in the range of 26% to 50%, and so on.

quartz crystal therapy, an alternative therapy that involves placement of a four- or six-sided quartz crystal over a chakra, or major energy station, of the body, such as the brow, throat, heart, stomach, abdomen, base of the spine, or near the skull, to act as a destressor and to support the immune system. No scientific evidence currently exists to support the efficacy of crystal therapy.

quartz silicosis. See **silicosis.**

quasispecies /quah″z-spe′sēz/, a swarm of viruses with similar genetic structure sharing a host with other quasispecies of different genetic makeup. Usually all quasispecies in one host are descended from a single ancestor strain.

quaternary /kwot″əner′ē, kwətur″nərē/ [L, *quattuor,* four], **1.** *adj.,* pertaining to a chemical compound in which four atoms or groups of elements are bonded to one atom, such as a quaternary ammonium compound in which four organic radicals are substituted for the four hydrogen molecules on an ammonium ion. **2.** *n.,* fourth-level structure in proteins, as in the structure of hemoglobin made up of two alpha-globulins and two beta-globulins.

quaternary ammonium derivative, a substance whose chemical structure has four carbon groups attached to a positively charged nitrogen atom. When the quaternary ammonium ion has more than about 16 carbon atoms, it is usually a strong emulsifying agent, highly water soluble but relatively insoluble in lipids.

quazepam /kwah′zĕ-pam/, a long-acting benzodiazepine administered orally for the treatment of insomnia.

■ INDICATIONS: It is used when an individual has difficulty falling or staying asleep.

■ CONTRAINDICATIONS: Contraindicated in pregnancy. The drug should not be taken if there is a history of allergic reactions to this medication or other benzodiazepines.

■ ADVERSE EFFECTS: Some individuals using this medicine have engaged in activity such as driving or eating while not fully awake and with no memory of the activity.

Queckenstedt test /kwek″ənstet/ [Hans H.G. Queckenstedt, German physician, 1876–1918], a test for an obstruction in the spinal canal in which the jugular veins on each side of the neck are compressed alternately. The pressure of the spinal fluid is measured by a manometer connected to a lumbar puncture needle or catheter. Normally, occlusion of the veins of the neck causes an immediate rise in spinal fluid pressure. If the vertebral canal is blocked, no rise occurs. If increased intracranial pressure is suspected, this test should not be performed. The Queckenstedt test has now largely been replaced by imaging, most often magnetic resonance imaging. See also **spinal canal.**

Queensland tick typhus, an infection caused by *Rickettsia australis* occurring in Australia, transmitted by ticks, and resembling mild Rocky Mountain spotted fever. Treatment includes the administration of chloramphenicol or tetracycline. Prevention depends on avoiding tick bites and on the prompt removal of attached ticks. Compare **boutonneuse fever, North Asian tick-borne rickettsiosis, Rocky Mountain spotted fever.**

Quelidrine, a fixed-combination respiratory medication containing adrenergics, an antihistaminic, an antitussive, and an expectorant. Brand name for **phenylephrine hydrochloride,** *epHEDrine hydrochloride, ammonium chloride,* **dextromethorphan hydrobromide, chlorpheniramine maleate.**

quellung reaction /kwel″ung/ [Ger, *Quellung,* swelling; L, *re,* again, *agere,* to act], the swelling of the capsule of a bacterium, seen in the laboratory when the organism is exposed to specific antisera. This phenomenon is used to identify the genera, species, or subspecies of the bacteria causing a disease, including *Haemophilus influenzae, Neisseria meningitidis,* and many kinds of streptococci.

quenching /kwen″ching/, **1.** a process of removing or reducing an energy source, such as heat or light. **2.** stopping or diminishing a chemical or enzymatic reaction. **3.** decreasing counting efficiency in beta liquid scintillation caused by interfering materials. **4.** preventing emission of light from fluorescent compounds. **5.** satisfying or slaking a craving or need.

Quengel cast /kwen″gəl/, a two-section orthopedic cast for immobilizing the lower extremity from the foot or ankle to below the knee and the upper thigh to just above the knee. The two parts of the cast are connected by hinges at knee level, medially and laterally. The Quengle cast is used for the gradual correction of knee contractures.

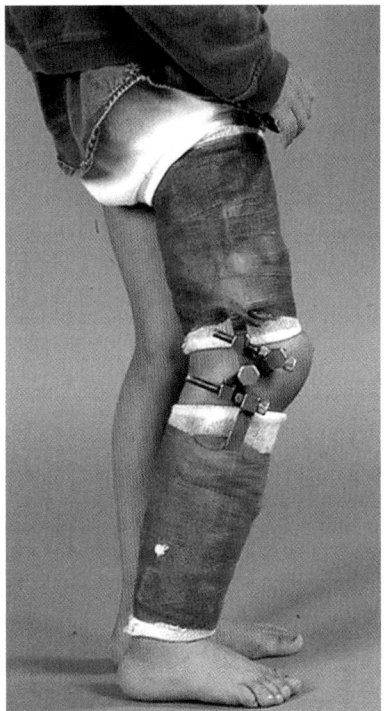

Quengel cast *(Herring, 2008)*

quercetin /kwur″sitin/, a yellow, crystalline, flavonoid pigment found in oak bark, the juice of lemons, asparagus, and other plants. It is used to reduce abnormal capillary fragility.

querulous paranoia /kwer″(y)ələs/ [L, *queri,* to complain; Gk, *para,* beside, *nous,* mind], a form of paranoia characterized by extreme discontent and habitual complaining, usually about imagined slights by others. Also called **paranoia querulans.**

Quervain disease /kervānz″, kerveNz″/ [Fritz de Quervain, Swiss surgeon, 1868–1940; L, *dis*; Fr, *aise,* ease], chronic tenosynovitis of the abductor pollicis longus and extensor pollicis brevis tendons of the thumb. Also called *de Quervain disease, de Quervain syndrome.* See also **tenosynovitis.**

Questran, an ion-exchange resin used to lower blood cholesterol levels. Brand name for **cholestyramine resin.**

quetiapine, an atypical antipsychotic.

■ INDICATIONS: It is used in the treatment of schizophrenia and similar disorders, as well as bipolar disorder.

■ CONTRAINDICATIONS: Known hypersensitivity to this drug prohibits its use.

■ ADVERSE EFFECTS: Life-threatening effects are seizures, neuroleptic malignant syndrome, and tachycardia. Other adverse effects include extrapyramidal symptoms, pseudoparkinsonism, akathisia, dystonia, tardive dyskinesia, drowsiness, insomnia, agitation, anxiety, orthostatic hypotension, abdominal pain, dry mouth, rhinitis, rash, asthenia, back pain, fever, and ear pain. Common side effects include headache, dizziness, nausea, anorexia, and constipation.

quick connect [ME, *quic,* living; L, *connectere,* to bind], a plastic or similar connecting device that is attached to or implanted in a patient who will be joined to an electromechanical or other apparatus. A patient whose circulatory system is supported by an artificial heart, for example, may have a push-fit connector sewn to the natural atria, aorta, and pulmonary artery; a plastic lip on the artificial ventricle then can be securely snapped onto the quick-connect device.

quick-cure resin. See **self-curing resin.**

quickening /kwik″(ə)ning/ [ME, *quic,* living], the first feeling by a pregnant woman of movement of her baby in utero, usually occurring between 16 and 20 weeks of gestation.

quick pulse, a pulse that strikes the finger smartly and leaves it quickly. Also called *pulsus celer.*

quiescent /kwī·es″ənt/, **1.** inactive, quiet, or at rest. **2.** latent. **3.** dormant.

quiet alert /kwī″ət/, a period when a neonate is calm and attentive, with eyes open, ready to become acquainted with an adult person. Newborns spend about 10% of their time in this state.

Quigley traction /kwig″lē/, a type of traction for lateral malleolar and trimalleolar fractures in which a stockinette is placed around the leg and ankle and attached to an overhead frame, thus suspending the leg by the ankle.

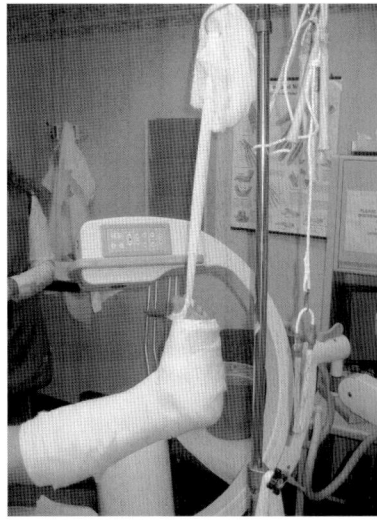

Quigley traction *(Miller, Hart, and MacKnight, 2010)*

quin-, prefix meaning "quinine": *quinoline, quinidine.*

-quin, -quine, suffix naming antimalarial medicinal compounds from quinine: *chloroquine.*

Quinaglute, a class I antiarrhythmic drug. Brand name for **quinidine gluconate.**

Quincke disease /kwing″kē/ [Heinrich I. Quincke, German physician, 1842–1922; L, *dis* + Fr, *aise,* ease], a potentially fatal chronic condition of subcutaneous edema, abdominal pain, urticaria, and laryngeal edema. Among its causes is anaphylactic reaction. Also called **angioedema,** *Quincke edema.*

Quincke pulse [Heinrich I. Quincke], an abnormal alternate blanching and reddening of the skin or nails that may be observed in several ways, such as by pressing the front edge of the fingernail and watching the blood in the nailbed recede and return. This pulsation is characteristic of aortic insufficiency and other abnormal conditions but may also occur in otherwise normal individuals. Formerly it was thought to be caused by pulsation of the capillaries; it is now known to be caused by pulsation of subpapillary arteriolar and venous plexuses. Also called **capillary pulse,** *Quincke sign.*

Quinidex, a class I antiarrhythmic medication. Brand name for **quinidine.**

quinidine /kwin″ədēn, -din/, an antiarrhythmic agent administered as a bisulfate, gluconate, or polygalacturonate or as sulfate salts.

■ INDICATIONS: It is prescribed in the treatment of atrial flutter, atrial fibrillation, premature ventricular contractions, and tachycardias. It is also used in the treatment of malaria.

■ CONTRAINDICATIONS: Known hypersensitivity to this drug prohibits its use. It is contraindicated in thrombocytopenia, myasthenia gravis, and some arrhythmias, particularly those associated with heart block.

■ ADVERSE EFFECTS: Among the most serious adverse effects are cardiac arrhythmia, hypertension, and cinchonism. Rare but potentially fatal hypersensitivity reactions such as anaphylaxis and thrombocytopenia may occur. Diarrhea, nausea, and vomiting are common.

quinidine gluconate. See **quinidine.**

quinine /kwī″nīn/ [Sp, *quina,* bark], a white, bitter, crystalline alkaloid made from cinchona bark. It was formerly used in antimalarial medications and replaced when chloroquine became available. However, in the form of one of its soluble salts it is used to treat chloroquine-resistant malaria in South America and Africa. Very dilute amounts of quinine are found in some beverages. See also **antimalarial.**

quinoa, a gluten-free, high-protein grain.

quinoline /kwin′o-lēn/, an amine or alkaloid with antiseptic, antipyretic, and antimalarial properties. It is derivable from quinine, coal tar, and various other sources.

quinolone /kwin″əlōn/, any of a class of antibiotics that act by interrupting the replication of deoxyribonucleic acid (DNA) molecules in bacteria. The action involves inhibition of the bacteria's gyrase so that positively supercoiled DNA cannot be relaxed for DNA transcription and replication. Also called *fluoroquinolones.* Kinds include *ciprofloxacin (Cipro), levofloxacin (Levaquin).*

quinque-, prefix meaning "five."

quinsy, a collection of pustular material beside the tonsil. See also **peritonsillar abscess.**

quint-, prefix meaning "fifth" or "fivefold": *quintessence, quintuplet.*

quintan /kwin″tən/ [L, *quintanus,* relating to the fifth], recurring on the fifth day, or at about 96-hour intervals. See also **trench fever.**

quintana fever. See **trench fever.**

quintessence /kwintes″əns/ [L, *quinta + essentia,* the fifth essence], **1.** a highly concentrated extract of any substance.

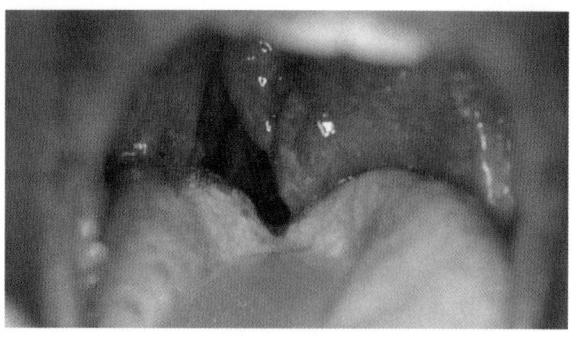

Quinsy *(Pfenninger, 2011)*

2. a tincture or extract containing the most essential components of plant materials.

quintuplet /kwin′tooplit, kwintō″plit/ [L, *quintuplex,* fivefold], any one of five offspring born after the same gestation period during a single pregnancy. See also **Hellin's law.**

quinupristin /kwinu′pris-tin/, a semisynthetic streptogramin antibacterial agent effective against a variety of grampositive organisms. It is used in conjunction with dalfopristin in the treatment of serious bacteremia caused by vancomycin-resistant *Enterococcus faecium* and complicated skin and skin structure infections caused by *Streptococcus pyogenes* or methicillin-sensitive *Staphylococcus aureus.* It is administered intravenously.

quotidian /kwōtid″ē·ən/ [L, *quotidianus,* daily], occurring every day; for example, a malarial fever with daily attacks.

quotient /kwō″shənt/, the number obtained by dividing one number by another. See also **achievement quotient, intelligence quotient, respiratory quotient.**

quot. op. sit [L, *quoties,* as often as, *op. sit,* if necessary], notation for a Latin phrase meaning "as often as necessary." Abbreviation for *quoties opus sit.*

q.v. [L, *quantum,* quantity, *volo,* wish], notation for a Latin phrase meaning "quantity as desired." Abbreviation for *quad vide.*

Q wave, the first negative component of the QRS complex on an electrocardiogram. Lengthening of the wave indicates myocardial infarction. If an R wave is not present, the totally negative complex is called QS. See also **QRS complex.**

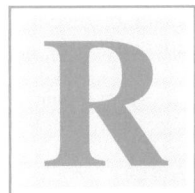

r, abbreviation for *right.*

R, 1. abbreviation for **resolution. 2.** abbreviation for **respiration. 3.** abbreviation for **respiratory exchange ratio. 4.** abbreviation for **roentgen. 5.** symbol for **arginine.**

R$_f$, symbol for a ratio used in paper and thin-layer chromatography, representing the distance from the origin to the center of the separated zone divided by the distance from the origin to the solvent front.

R$_i$, symbol for *inhibitory receptor molecule.*

R$_s$, symbol for *stimulatory receptor molecule.*

R$_x$, 1. a notation for the Latin *recipe,* meaning "take." **2.** (in pharmacology) symbol for **prescription.**

Ra, symbol for the element **radium.**

RA, 1. abbreviation for **rheumatoid arthritis. 2.** abbreviation for *right atrium.*

rabbit fever. See **tularemia.**

rabbit test. See **Friedman's test.**

rabeprazole, a proton pump inhibitor.

■ INDICATIONS: Rabeprazole is used to treat gastroesophageal reflux disease (GERD), severe erosive esophagitis, poorly responsive systemic GERD, pathological hypersecretory conditions such as Zollinger-Ellison syndrome, systemic mastocytosis, multiple endocrine adenomas, and active duodenal ulcers.

■ CONTRAINDICATIONS: Known hypersensitivity to this drug prohibits its use.

■ ADVERSE EFFECTS: Life-threatening effects are proteinuria, hematuria, pancytopenia, thrombocytopenia, neutropenia, and leukocytosis. Other adverse effects include abdominal swelling, anorexia, irritable colon, esophageal candidiasis, epistaxis, urticaria, alopecia, hypoglycemia, increased hepatic enzymes, weight gain, tinnitus, angina, tachycardia, bradycardia, palpitations, peripheral edema, urinary tract infection, increased creatinine, testicular pain, glycosuria, and fever. Common side effects include headache, dizziness, asthenia, diarrhea, abdominal pain, vomiting, nausea, constipation, flatulence, acid regurgitation, upper respiratory infections, cough, rash, and back pain.

rabid /rab″id/ [L, *rabidus,* raving], **1.** pertaining to or suffering from rabies. **2.** displaying signs of madness, agitation, delirium, hallucinations, and bizarre behavior.

rabies /rā″bēz/ [L, *rabere,* to rave], an acute, usually fatal viral disease of the central nervous system of mammals. It is transmitted from animals to people through infected saliva. *−rabid* /rab′id/, *adj.*

■ OBSERVATIONS: The reservoir of the virus is chiefly wild animals, including skunks, bats, foxes, and raccoons, and unvaccinated dogs and cats. After introduction into the human body, often by a bite of an infected animal, the virus travels along nerve pathways to the brain and later to other organs. An incubation period ranges from 10 days to 1 year and is followed by a prodromal period characterized by fever, malaise, headache, paresthesia, and myalgia. After several days severe encephalitis, delirium, agonizingly painful muscular spasms, seizures, paralysis, coma, and death ensue.

■ INTERVENTIONS: Few nonfatal cases have been documented in humans; survival in those cases has been the result of intensive supportive care by the health care team. There is no treatment once the virus has reached the tissue of the nervous system. Local treatment of wounds inflicted by rabid animals may prevent the disease. The wound is cleansed with soap, water, and a disinfectant. A deep wound may be cauterized and rabies immune globulin injected directly into the base of the wound. For active immunization a series of three intramuscular injections with adsorbed vaccine (RVA), purified chick embryo cell vaccine, or human diploid cell rabies vaccine is begun. If vaccine is administered, intramuscular injection is given on days 0, 7, and 21 or 28. Great effort is made to locate and examine the animal. The animal that is suspected of being rabid is not immediately killed but put in isolation and carefully observed. If the animal is well in 10 days, there is little danger of rabies developing from the bite. Tissue from the animal's brain may be examined microscopically or by fluorescent antibody screening techniques.

■ PATIENT CARE CONSIDERATIONS: Rabies virus infection can be eradicated from most communities by prophylactic immunization of domestic animals, stringent measures for the control of domestic animals, and elimination of any wild animals acting as reservoirs of infection. A preexposure vaccination is advised for those at risk, such as veterinarians, animal handlers, and some laboratory workers. Health care professionals may encourage compliance with such efforts and teach the necessity of avoiding direct contact with wild animals and the importance of immediate first aid for any animal bite and reporting such contact to health care providers.

rabies immune globulin (RIG), a solution of antirabies immune globulin.

■ INDICATIONS: It is used in conjunction with human diploid cell culture rabies vaccine for possible protection against rabies in persons suspected of exposure to rabies.

■ CONTRAINDICATIONS: Previous administration of this preparation or known hypersensitivity to this solution, to gamma globulin, or to thimerosal prohibits its use.

■ ADVERSE EFFECTS: Among the more serious adverse effects are soreness at the site of injection, fever, and hypersensitivity reactions.

rabies-neutralizing antibody test, a blood test performed on those who work with animals and have received the human diploid cell rabies vaccine and on those who may have been exposed to the rabies virus.

rabies vaccine, one of the sterile suspensions of killed rabies virus.

■ INDICATIONS: It is prescribed for immunization and postexposure prophylaxis against rabies.

■ CONTRAINDICATIONS: A history of allergic reaction to components of the vaccine prohibits its use. Several preparations of the vaccine are available in North America, and contraindications vary among brands.

■ ADVERSE EFFECTS: Among the most serious adverse effects are severe hypersensitivity reactions. Pain and inflammation at the site of injection were once common but are now rare.

rabies virus group [L, *rabere,* to rave, *virus,* poison; It, *gruppo,* knot], the genus of viruses that includes the organism that causes rabies in humans, the *lyssa* virus. See also **rhabdovirus.**

raccoon eyes, *(Informal)* ecchymotic areas surrounding both eyes, suggestive of a basilar skull fracture or childhood neuroblastoma. Also called *periorbital ecchymosis.*

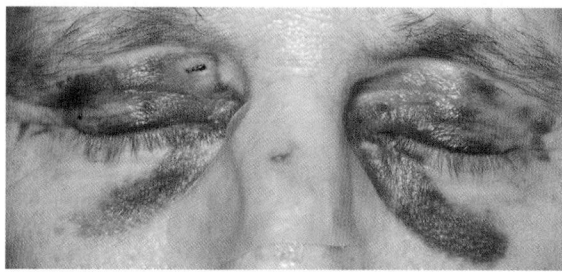

Patient with periorbital ecchymosis (raccoon eyes)
(Sprung and Weingarten, 2014)

race [It, *razza*], a term often used for a group of genetically related people who share certain physical characteristics. The U.S. Census Bureau data identify six ethnic and racial categories: White American, Black or African American, Native American and Alaska Native, Asian American, Native Hawaiian and Other Pacific Islander, and people of two or more races.

racemic /rāsē″mik/ [L, *racemus,* bunch of grapes], pertaining to a compound made up of equal amounts of dextrorotatory and levorotatory isomers, rendering it optically inactive under polarized light.

racemic epinephrine. See **epinephrine.**

racemose /ras″əmōs′/ [L, *racemus*], like a bunch of grapes. The term is used in describing a structure, such as pulmonary alveoli, in which many branches terminate in nodular cystlike forms.

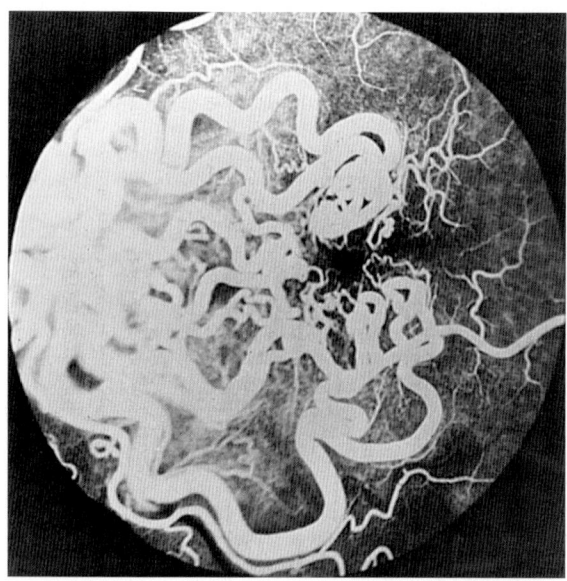

Fluorescein angiogram racemose arteriovenous malformation in the retina *(Daroff et al, 2012)*

racemose aneurysm, a pronounced dilation of lengthened and tortuous blood vessels, which may form a tumor. Also called **cirsoid aneurysm.**

-racetam, suffix for piracetam-type nootropic substances.

rachial /rā′kē·əl/ [Gk, *rhachis,* backbone], pertaining to the spinal column. Also **rachidial.**

rachialgia /rā′kē·al′jə/ [Gk, *rhachis,* backbone + *algos,* pain], pain in the vertebral column. Formerly called **rachiodynia.**

rachidial. See **rachial.**

rachio-, rachi-, rhachi-, prefix meaning "the spine": *rachiopagus, rachial, rachiotomy.*

rachiodynia. *(Obsolete)* See **rachialgia.**

rachiopagus /rā′kē·op″əgəs/ [Gk, *rachis,* backbone, *pagos,* fixed], conjoined symmetric twins united back to back along the spinal column. Also called **rachipagus.**

rachiotomy, *(Obsolete)* now called **laminotomy.**

rachipagus, conjoined twins united back to back. See **rachiopagus.**

rachiresistance /rā′kēresis″təns/ [Gk, *rachis,* backbone], a failure to respond adequately to spinal anesthesia.

rachischisis /rəkis″kəsis/ [Gk, *rachis* + *schizein,* to split], a congenital fissure of one or more vertebrae. See also **neural tube defect, spina bifida.**

rachischisis totalis. See **complete rachischisis.**

rachitic. See **rickets.**

rachitis /rəkī″tis/ [Gk, *rachis* + *itis,* inflammation], **1.** rickets. **2.** an inflammatory disease of the vertebral column.

rachitis fetalis annularis, congenital enlargement of the epiphyses of the long bones, which can lead to growth disorders.

rachitis fetalis micromelia, congenital shortening of the long bones.

racial unconscious. See **collective unconscious.**

rad /rad/, abbreviation for **radiation absorbed dose.**

radappertization /rad′apur′tizā″shən/, the irradiation of food for the destruction of *Clostridium botulinum.*

radarkymography /rā′därkīmog″rəfē/ [radar + Gk, *kyma,* wave, *graphein,* to record], a technique for showing the size and outline of the heart that uses a radar tracking device and a fluoroscopic screen to display images produced by electrical impulses passed over the chest surface.

Radford nomogram [Edward P. Radford, Jr., American physiologist, b. 1922], a mathematical chart device used in respiratory therapy to estimate combined tidal volumes and rates for mechanical ventilation. It is based on the three parameters of body weight, sex, and respiratory rate.

radi-, combining form meaning "root": *radiculitis, radiculopathy.*

radial /rā″dē·əl/ [L, *radius,* ray], pertaining to the radius.

radial artery [L, *radius,* ray], an artery in the forearm, starting at the bifurcation of the brachial artery and passing in 12 branches to the forearm, wrist, and hand. In the forearm it extends from the neck of the radius to the forepart of the styloid process; in the wrist, from the styloid process to the carpus; in the hand, from the carpus, across the palm, to the little finger. In the forearm the branches of the radial artery are the radial recurrent, muscular, palmar carpal, and superficial palmar; in the wrist the branches are the dorsal carpal and the first dorsal metacarpal. In the hand the branches are the princeps pollicis, radialis indicis, deep palmar arch, palmar metacarpal, perforating, and recurrent.

radialis. See **radial.**

radial keratotomy (RK), a surgical procedure in which a series of tiny shallow incisions is made in the cornea to flatten it, thereby reducing refractive error. The operation is performed using local anesthesia and requires only 10 minutes. Hospitalization is not necessary. Radial keratotomy usually corrects mild to moderate myopia. Compare **photorefractive keratectomy.** See also **refractive keratotomy.**

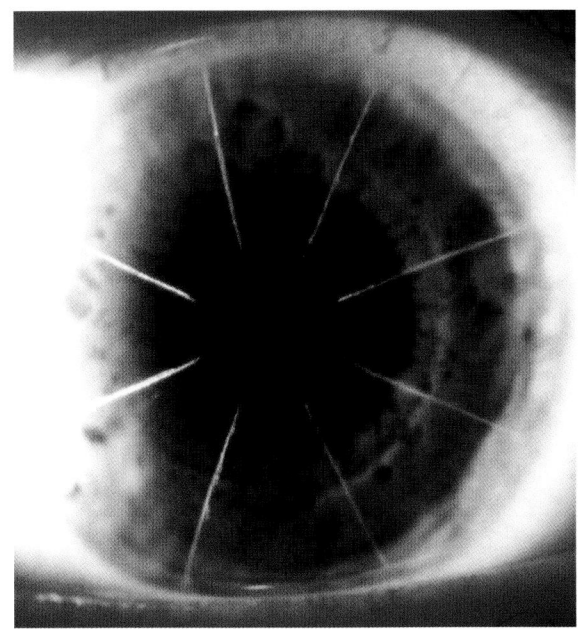

Radial keratotomy incisions *(Krachmer and Palay, 2014)*

radial nerve, the largest branch of the brachial plexus, arising on each side as a continuation of the posterior cord. It supplies the skin of the arm and forearm and their extensor muscles. The branches of the radial nerve are the medial muscular branches, the posterior brachial cutaneous nerve, the posterior muscular branches, the posterior antebrachial cutaneous nerve, the lateral muscular branches, the superficial branch, and the deep branch. Also called **musculospiral nerve.** Compare **median nerve, musculocutaneous nerve, ulnar nerve.**

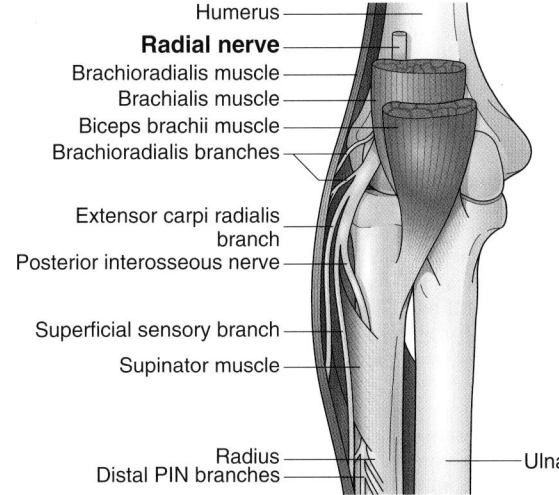

Humerus
Radial nerve
Brachioradialis muscle
Brachialis muscle
Biceps brachii muscle
Brachioradialis branches
Extensor carpi radialis branch
Posterior interosseous nerve
Superficial sensory branch
Supinator muscle
Radius
Distal PIN branches
Ulna

Radial nerve and surrounding structures *(Kim et al, 2008)*

radial nerve palsy, a type of mononeuropathy characterized by radial nerve damage with symptoms of forearm muscle weakness and sensory loss. It may be caused by excessive compression of the radial nerve against a hard surface in individuals insensitized by the intake of alcohol or sedatives. It may also be caused by the repeated compression of the nerve by various

weights. Time and the withdrawal of causative compression usually ensure full recovery. Also called **Saturday night palsy.**

radial notch of ulna, the narrow lateral depression in the coronoid process of the ulna that receives the head of the radius.

radial paralysis [L, *radius* + Gk, *paralyein*], paralysis of muscles supplied by the radial nerve, mainly the wrist and finger extensors. See **dropped wrist.**

radial pulse, the pulse of the radial artery palpated at the wrist over the radius. The radial pulse is the one most often taken because of the ease with which it is palpated.

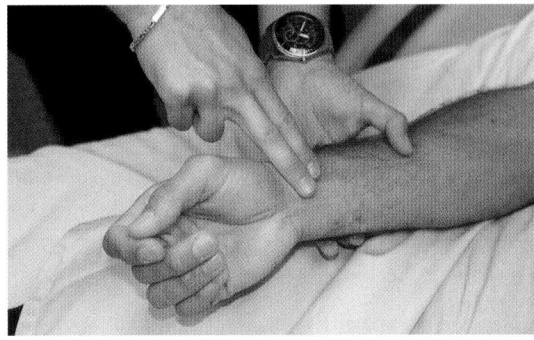

Palpation of the radial pulse *(Courtesy Rutgers School of Nursing—Camden. All rights reserved.)*

radial recurrent artery, a branch of the radial artery arising just distal to the elbow, ascending between the branches of the radial nerve, and supplying several muscles of the arm and the elbow.

radial reflex, a normal reflex elicited by tapping over the distal radius, with the response being flexion of the forearm. Flexion of the fingers may also occur if the reflex is hyperactive.

radial symmetry, a form of symmetry in which body parts are arranged around a central axis, as found in animals such as jellyfish and sea urchins.

radial tuberosity, a large blunt projection on the medial surface of the radius for the attachment of the biceps brachii tendon.

radiant /rā″dē·ənt/ [L, *radiare,* to emit rays], pertaining to any object that emits rays or is the center of rays that spread outward.

radiant energy [L, *radiare,* to emit rays; Gk, *energeia*], energy emitted as electromagnetic radiation, such as radio waves, infrared radiation, visible light, ultraviolet light, x-rays, and gamma rays.

radiant heat, a form of infrared energy that is emitted in electromagnetic waves from a central source. It proceeds outward in wavelengths greater than those of visible light. Objects absorbing the energy experience a rise in temperature.

radiate /rā″dē·āt/ [L, *radiare,* to emit rays], to diverge or spread from a common point or center.

radiate crown, 1. a network of fibers that weaves through the internal capsule of the cerebral cortex and intermingles with the fibers of the corpus callosum. **2.** an aggregate of cells that surrounds the zona pellucida of the ovum.

radiate ligament, a ligament that connects the head of a rib with a vertebra and an associated intervertebral disk.

radiation /rā″dē·ā″shən/ [L, *radiatio*], **1.** the emission of energy, rays, or waves. **2.** the use of a radioactive substance in the diagnosis or treatment of disease.

radiation absorbed dose (rad), the amount of energy from any type of ionizing radiation deposited in tissue. One rad is equal to 0.01 J/kg of matter. The international system unit is the gray (Gy), in which 1 Gy is equivalent to 100 rad. Compare **roentgen.** See also **absorbed dose, rem.**

radiation burn, a burn resulting from exposure to radiant energy in the form of sunlight, x-rays, or nuclear emissions or explosion. Ionizing radiation can produce tissue damage directly by striking a vital molecule such as deoxyribonucleic acid. See also **ionizing radiation injury.**

radiation caries, tooth decay triggered by exposure of the head to ionizing radiation. It especially affects the cementoenamel junction and the coronal root area. Radiation makes the teeth more susceptible to caries by decreasing salivation, which with swallowing washes the teeth. Radiation reduces the vitality of dental tissues and alters oral bacteria. Radiation caries is often a side effect of radiation therapy for oral malignancies. See also **dental caries.**

radiation cataract [L, *radiare,* to emit rays; Gk, *katarrhaktes,* portcullis], a cataract that is caused by excessive exposure of the eye to x-rays or other types of radiation that cause a change in the protein molecules of the lens.

radiation cystitis, inflammatory changes in the urinary bladder caused by ionizing radiation. Also called *radiocystitis.*

radiation dermatitis [L, *radiare,* to emit rays; Gk, *derma,* skin, *itis,* inflammation], an acute or chronic inflammation of the skin caused by exposure to ionizing radiation, as in cancer radiation therapy. There are four levels of involvement, which are graded from 1-4. Also called **radiodermatitis.**

■ OBSERVATIONS: Symptoms may not appear until 3 weeks after exposure. Grade 1 includes mild erythema; grade 2, moderate to brisk erythema with patchy, moist desquamation. Grade 3 includes moist desquamation and bleeding induced by minor trauma or abrasions. Grade 4 is characterized by skin necrosis and ulceration. In severe cases the condition can progress to scarring, fibrosis, and atrophy. There may also be changes in skin pigmentation.

■ INTERVENTIONS: Skin reactions should be assessed at least once a week. Washing and drying of the skin is recommended for all patients receiving radiotherapy. Topical applications can be considered on an individual basis and are prescribed for individuals with grade 2 and 3 dermatitis. This level of involvement mandates that care should be managed by a team that includes a radiation oncologist, a medical oncologist, a nurse, and a dermatologist. A wound specialist should be involved for grade 4 dermatitis.

■ PATIENT CARE CONSIDERATIONS: Patients should be advised to avoid sun exposure, the use of irritants such as perfume and alcohol-based products, and to avoid scratching the area.

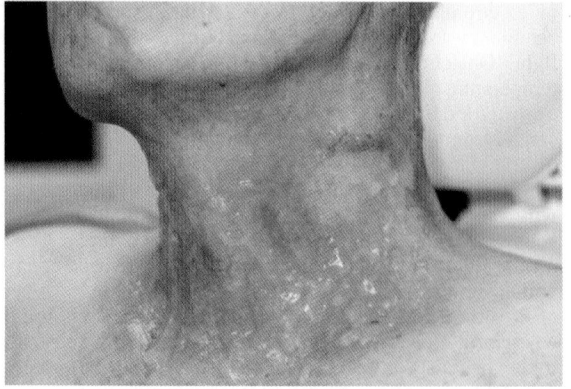

Grade 2 radiation dermatitis *(Miyazaki et al, 2014)*

radiation detector, a device for detecting the presence and sometimes the amount of radiation. It counts the number of radioactive particles reaching it and can be designed to detect cosmic radiation. An ionization chamber collects the ion pairs formed by the passage of radiation through the device. Also called **Geiger-Müller (GM) counter,** *Geiger counter.*

Radiation Effects Research Foundation (RERF), an organization that studies the long-term effects of the atomic bombings of Hiroshima and Nagasaki during World War II on survivors. The RERF has focused on the incidence of leukemia, which reached a plateau around 1950 before beginning to decline, and has examined the varied effects related to the different types of radiation produced by the two bombs, one fueled with uranium and the other with plutonium. The RERF is the successor to the Atomic Bomb Casualty Commission.

radiation exposure, a measure of the ionization produced in air by x-rays or gamma rays. It is the sum of the electric charges on all ions of one sign that are produced when all electrons liberated by the radiation in a volume of air are completely stopped, divided by the mass of air in that volume. The conventional unit of exposure is the roentgen; the SI unit, which has largely replaced the roentgen, is the coulomb per kilogram (C/kg). Acute radiation exposure is exposure of short duration to intense ionizing radiation, usually occurring as the result of an accidental spill of radioactive material. Exposure of the whole body to approximately 10,000 rad (100 Gy) causes neurological and cardiovascular breakdown and is fatal within 24 hours. A dose between 500 and 1200 rad (5 and 12 Gy) destroys GI mucosa, produces bloody diarrhea, and may cause death in several days. A dose of 200 to 500 rad (2 to 5 Gy) destroys the blood-forming organs and may cause death in a few weeks.

radiation exposure, emergency procedures, first-aid treatment of a person who has received external body radiation through exposure to radioactive material or internal radiation contamination by inhaling or ingesting radioactive material. External radiation exposure is treated initially by cleansing and surgical isolation to protect others. One who has inhaled or ingested radioactive material should be given emergency treatment similar to a person who has been exposed to chemical poisons. Body wastes should be collected and checked for radiation levels. If the victim has also suffered a wound, care must be taken to avoid cross-contamination of exposed surfaces. In general, except for taking special precautions to control the spread of radiation effects, the patient should be given any lifesaving emergency treatment needed, and personnel handling the patient should wear surgical gowns, caps, and gloves. Also called **emergency handling of radiation accidents.**

radiation force, **1.** (in sonography) a small, steady force that is produced when a sound beam strikes a reflecting or absorbing surface. It is proportional to the acoustic power. **2.** (in radiology) the force generated by radiation pressure. Generally, radiation force is too small to be detected under everyday circumstances; however, it does play a crucial role in some settings, such as astronomy and astrodynamics.

radiation hygiene, the art and science of protecting human beings from injury by radiation. It reduces clinical exposure from external radiation through protective barriers of radiation-absorbing material, ensures safe distances between people and radiation sources, reduces radiation exposure times, or uses combinations of all these measures. To protect against the dangers of internal radiation, precautions seek to restrict inhalation, ingestion, and other modes of entry of radioactive substances into the body.

radiation leakage, radiation that exits the x-ray tube housing anywhere other than through the port window as part of the useful beam.

radiation nephritis, kidney damage caused by ionizing radiation. Symptoms include glomerular and tubular damage, hypertension, and proteinuria, sometimes leading to renal failure. It may be acute or chronic, and some varieties do not manifest until years after the radiation exposure.

radiation oncologist, a physician with special training in the use of ionizing radiation in the treatment of cancers.

radiation oncology, the study of the treatment of cancer with ionizing radiation.

radiation protection, the use of devices, equipment, distance, and barriers to reduce the risk of exposure to ionizing radiation in a health care facility, research center, or industrial site where radiation-emitting devices are operated.

radiation risk, a hazard to health resulting from exposure to natural and synthetic radioactive materials. Radiation sources include cosmic rays, radon, radium, and other radionuclides in the soil; nuclear reactors, accelerators, and weapons; uranium mining and milling; and diagnostic and therapeutic x-ray devices.

radiation safety committee, an organization responsible for monitoring and maintaining a safe radiation environment in institutions where radiation is produced and/or used.

radiation sensitivity, a measure of the response of tissue to ionizing radiation.

radiation sickness, an abnormal condition resulting from exposure to ionizing radiation. The severity of the condition is determined by the intensity of radiation, the length of time of exposure, and the area of the body affected. Moderate exposure may cause headache, nausea, vomiting, anorexia, and diarrhea; long-term exposure may result in sterility, leukemia or other forms of cancer, alopecia, and cataracts.

radiation symbol, a universal symbol consisting of three red wedges arranged at positions 120 degrees apart around a central red circle on a yellow background. The symbol identifies sources or containers of radioactive materials and areas of potential radiation exposure.

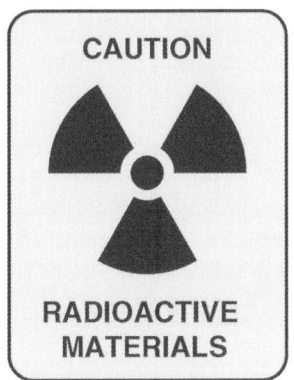

International radiation symbol *(Harkreader and Hogan, 2007)*

radiation syndrome. See **radiation sickness.**

radiation therapist, a radiological technologist who administers radiation therapy services to patients and observes patients during treatment. Preparation includes completion of an accredited program in radiation therapy and a minimum of an associate's degree; however, some jurisdictions require a bachelor's degree. Certification by the American Registry of Radiologic Technologists is required by most employers in the United States. Duties may include tumor localization, dosimetry, patient follow-up, patient education, and record keeping. The radiation therapist often works as a member of a cancer treatment team.

radiation therapy. See **radiotherapy.**

radiation therapy technologist. See **radiation therapist.**

radiation toxicity, the degree of virulence of a given exposure or dose of ionizing radiation. Also called **radiotoxicity.**

radical /rad″ikəl/ [L, *radix,* root], **1.** *n.,* an atom or group of atoms that contains an unpaired electron. A radical does not exist freely in nature except for O_2, NO, and NO_2. **2.** *adj.,* pertaining to drastic therapy, such as the surgical removal of an organ, limb, or other part of the body.

radical dissection, the surgical removal of tissue in an extensive area surrounding the operative site. Most often it is performed to identify and excise all tissue that may possibly be malignant to decrease the chance of recurrence and usually includes adjacent lymph nodes.

radical hysterectomy, surgical removal of the uterus, uterine ligaments, cervix, and an inch or two of the deep vagina around the cervix. See also **hysterectomy.**

radical lymphadenectomy, removal of lymph nodes in the area of the peritoneum. See also **retroperitoneal lymph node dissection.**

radical mastectomy, surgical removal of an entire breast; pectoral muscles; axillary lymph nodes; and all fat, fascia, and adjacent tissues as one surgical treatment for breast cancer. Edema of the arm on the affected side is the rule because the axillary lymphatic structures that drain the lymph from the arm are removed during surgery. A pressure dressing is usually applied and left in place until bleeding and drainage have decreased. A drain is usually left in the wound for several days. Compare **modified radical mastectomy, simple mastectomy.** See also **lumpectomy, mastectomy.**

radical neck dissection, dissection and removal of all lymph nodes and removable tissues under the skin of the neck, performed to prevent the spread of malignant tumors of the head and neck that have a reasonable chance of being controlled. Thorough mouth hygiene is given, and antibiotics are begun. A tracheostomy may be done.

radical nephrectomy, the surgical removal of a kidney, usually performed in the treatment of cancer of the kidney.

radical retropubic prostatectomy, radical prostatectomy through the retropubic space via a suprapubic incision for the treatment of malignancy.

radical surgery [L, *radix,* root; Gk, *cheirourgia,* surgery], surgery that is usually extensive and complex and intended to correct a severe health threat such as a rapidly growing cancer. See also **radical dissection.**

radical therapy, 1. a treatment intended to cure, not palliate. **2.** a definitive extreme treatment, not a conservative treatment (e.g., a radical mastectomy rather than a simple or partial mastectomy).

radical vulvectomy, extensive removal of tissue in the external area of the vagina that may include lymph nodes and additional tissue. See also **vulvectomy.**

radicidation /rā′disidā″shən/, the irradiation of food to inactivate nonsporing pathogens of *Salmonella* and other microorganisms.

radicular /rədik″yələr/ [L, *radix,* root], **1.** pertaining to a root, such as a spinal nerve root or radical. **2.** (in dentistry) pertaining to the root of a tooth.

radicular artery, arteries arising from the segmental spinal arteries at every vertebral level. They supply the anterior and posterior roots of the spine.

radicular cyst [L, *radix,* root; Gk, *kystis,* bag], a cyst with a wall of fibrous connective tissue and a lining of stratified

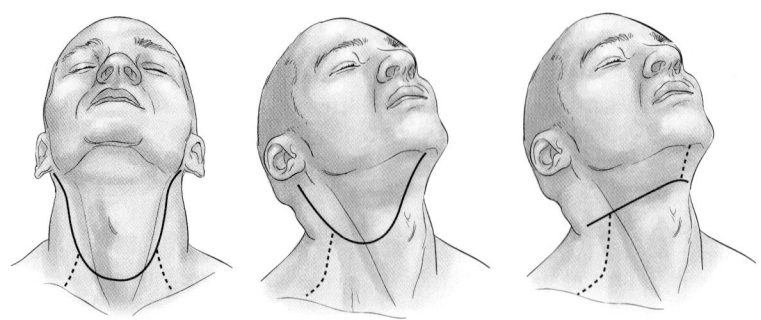

Neck incisions for radical neck dissection *(Phillips, 2012)*

squamous epithelium that is attached to the root apex of a tooth with dead pulp or a defective root canal filling. Also called **periapical cyst, root end cyst.**

radicular retainer, (in dentistry) a type of anchor, such as a dowel crown, that lies within the body of a tooth, usually in the root. Resistance to displacement and shear is developed by extending an attached dowel into the root canal of the tooth. Compare **dowel.**

radicular retention, (in dentistry) resistance to displacement of a dental prosthesis developed by placing a metal projection into the treated root canal of a pulpless tooth. See also **radicular retainer.**

radiculitis /rədik′yəlī″tis/ [L, *radix,* root; Gk, *itis,* inflammation], an inflammation involving a spinal nerve root, resulting in pain and hyperesthesia.

radiculopathy /rədik′yəlop″əthē/ [L, *radix,* root; Gk, *pathos,* disease], a disease involving a spinal nerve root.

radii. See **radius.**

radio- /rā′dē·ō-/, combining form meaning "radiation," sometimes referring specifically to emission of radiant energy, to radium, or to the radius: *radioactive, radiobiology, radiohumeral.*

radioactive /rā′dē·ōak″tiv/ [L, *radius,* ray, *activus,* active], giving off radiation as the result of the disintegration of atomic nuclei.

radioactive carbon. See **tracer.**

radioactive contamination, the undesirable addition of radioactive material to the body or part of the environment, such as clothing or equipment. Contamination of the body may occur through ingestion, inhalation, or absorption. Instruments, drapes, surgical gloves, or clothing that come in contact with the serous fluids, blood, or urine of patients containing radiation emitters may become contaminated. If items are found to be contaminated, they must be disposed of according to institutional and federal standards for the disposal of radioactive waste.

radioactive contrast medium, a solution or colloid containing radioactive material used for visualizing soft tissue structures. Such contrast media indicate their positions or distribution in the body by their gamma ray emissions.

radioactive decay, the disintegration of the nucleus of an unstable nuclide by the spontaneous emission of charged particles, photons, or both.

radioactive element, an element subject to spontaneous degeneration of its nucleus accompanied by the emission of alpha particles, beta particles, or gamma rays. All elements with atomic numbers greater than 83 are radioactive. Naturally occurring radioactive elements include radium,

thorium, and uranium. Several radioactive elements not found in nature have been produced by the bombardment of stable elements with subatomic particles in a cyclotron. Compare **stable element.** See also **radioactivity.**

radioactive half-life. See **half-life.**

radioactive implant, a small container holding a radioactive isotope that is embedded in tissues for purposes of interstitial radiotherapy.

radioactive iodine (RAI), a radioactive isotope of iodine used in diagnostic radiology and radiotherapy, especially in the treatment of some thyroid conditions. A common form is ^{131}I. Also called **radioiodine.**

radioactive iodine excretion, the elimination by the body of radioactive iodine (RAI) administered in a test of thyroid function and in the treatment of hyperthyroidism. Most RAI is excreted in urine, but small amounts may be found in sputum, perspiration, feces, and vomitus.

radioactive iodine excretion test, a method of evaluating thyroid function that entails measuring the amount of radioactive iodine (RAI) in urine after the patient is given an oral tracer dose of RAI in the form of the isotope ^{131}I. Normally, 5% to 35% of the dose is absorbed by the thyroid; absorption is increased in hyperthyroidism and decreased in hypothyroidism, and the amount excreted in urine is inversely proportional to the uptake of RAI. After administration of the tracer, a scintillation detector is placed over the patient's neck at 2, 6, and 24 hours to measure the amount of RAI accumulated by the thyroid; the amount excreted is assayed in urine collected for 24 hours after the oral dose. See also **radioactive iodine uptake.**

radioactive iodine uptake (RAIU), the absorption and incorporation by the thyroid of radioactive iodine (RAI), administered orally as a tracer dose in a test of thyroid function and in larger doses for the treatment of hyperthyroidism. The radioisotope ^{131}I is rapidly absorbed in the stomach and concentrated in the thyroid. Normal findings are 4% to 12% absorbed in 2 hours, 6% to 15% absorbed in 6 hours, and 8% to 30% absorbed in 24 hours. Patients receiving a large therapeutic dose of RAI may require hospitalization for several days. See also **radioactive iodine excretion test.**

radioactive tracer, a molecule containing a radioactive atom, which can be followed through a physiological system with radiation detectors.

radioactivity /-activ″itē/, the emission of alpha or beta particles or gamma radiation as a consequence of nuclear disintegration. Natural radioactivity is a property exhibited by all chemical elements with an atomic number greater than

83; artificial or induced radioactivity is created through the bombardment of stable elements with subatomic particles or high levels of gamma radiation or x-radiation.

radioallergosorbent test (RAST) /rā′dē·ō′alur′gōsôr″bənt/ [L, *radius* + Gk, *allos,* other, *ergein,* to work; L, *absorbere,* to swallow], a test in which a technique of radioimmunoassay is used to identify and quantify IgE in serum that has been mixed with known allergens. If an atopic allergy to a substance exists, an antigen-antibody reaction occurs with characteristic conjugation and clumping. The test is an in vitro method of demonstrating allergic reactions. Compare **patch test, Prausnitz-Küstner test.**

radiobiology /-bī·ol″əjē/ [L, *radius* + Gk, *bios,* life, *logos,* science], the branch of the natural sciences dealing with the effects of radiation on biological systems.

radiocarcinogenesis /-kär′sinəjen″əsis/, the production of cancer by exposure to ionizing radiation.

radiocarpal articulation /-kär″pəl/ [L, *radius* + Gk, *karpos,* wrist], the condyloid joint at the wrist that connects the radius and distal surface of an articular disk with the scaphoid, lunate, and triangular bones. The joint involves four ligaments and allows all movements but rotation. The capsule of the wrist joint is reinforced by palmar radiocarpal, palmar ulnocarpal, and dorsal radiocarpal ligaments. In addition, radial and ulnar collateral ligaments of the joint span the distance between the styloid processes of the radius and ulna and the adjacent carpal bones. Also called **wrist joint.**

radiochemistry /-kem″istrē/ [L, *radius* + Gk, *chemiea,* alchemy], the branch of chemistry that deals with the properties and behavior of radioactive materials and the use of radionuclides in the study of chemical and biological problems.

radiocolloids /rā″dē·ōkol′oidz/, radioisotopes in pure form in solution, which tend to act more like colloids than solutes.

radiocurable /-kyoo″rəbəl/, pertaining to the susceptibility of tumor cells to destruction by ionizing radiation.

radiodensity. See **radiopacity.**

radiodermatitis /-dur′mətī″tis/. See **radiation dermatitis.**

radiofrequency (rf) /-frē″kwənsē/ [L, *radius* + *frequens*], the part of the electromagnetic spectrum with frequencies lower than about 10^{10} Hz, used to produce magnetic resonance images.

radiofrequency ablation, unmodulated, high-frequency, alternating current flow that is applied to heart tissue to raise its temperature and injure cells for the purpose of destroying ectopic foci and accessory pathways. Radiofrequency ablation of accessory pathways is a cure for the arrhythmias associated with Wolfe-Parkinson-White syndrome and is successfully used in atrial flutter and idiopathic ventricular tachycardia. It has replaced surgical ablation.

radiofrequency pulse, a short burst of electromagnetic radiation in the radiofrequency range, used in combination with magnetic gradients to generate a magnetic resonance image.

radiofrequency (rf) signal, **1.** an electrical signal whose frequency is in the rf range. **2.** a signal within an ultrasound instrument between the transducer terminals and components where rectification and filtering occur.

radiofrequency therapy, the use of radiofrequency energy to disrupt nerve function for therapeutic purposes, such as the treatment of pain syndromes and arrhythmias.

radiograph /rā″dē·əgraf′/, an x-ray image. Also called *radiogram.*

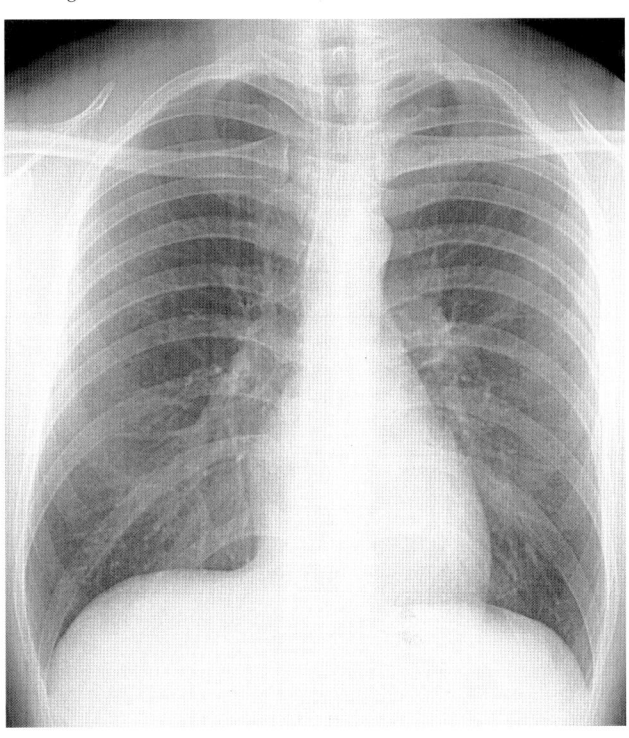

Normal chest radiograph *(Muller and Silva, 2008)*

radiographer /rā′dē·og″rəfər/. See **radiologic technologist.**

radiographic. See **radiography.**

radiographic contrast medium, *(Obsolete)* now called **radiopaque contrast medium.**

radiographic grid /-graf″ik/, a device used to reduce the amount of scatter radiation reaching an image receptor. Grids consist of strips of radiopaque materials alternating with strips of radiolucent materials. See also **grid.**

radiographic image, a representation of body images generated by imaging modalities such as ultrasonography, CT, MRI, nuclear imaging, and radiography.

radiographic magnification, a procedure used to improve visualization of fine blood vessels and small bony structures during x-ray imaging. Magnification is achieved by increasing the distance of the object from the radiographic image receptor or by decreasing the distance of the x-ray source from the image receptor.

radiographic position, the specific position of the body or a body part in relation to the image receptor during radiographic imaging.

radiographic projection, the path taken by an x-ray beam as it passes through the body. For example, an anteroposterior projection refers to a beam that enters the anterior (front) of the body and exits the posterior (back).

radiographic view, the image as seen by the image receptor of a radiographic imaging system. It is the opposite of the radiographic projection.

radiography /rā′dē·og″rəfē/ [L, *radius* + Gk, *graphein,* to record], the production of shadow images on an image receptor through the action of ionizing radiation. The image is the result of the differential attenuation of the radiation in its passage through the object being radiographed. **–radiographic,** *adj.*

radiohumeral /rā′dē·ōhyoo̅′mərəl/ [L, *radius* + *humerus,* shoulder], pertaining to the radius and humerus.

radioimmunoassay (RIA) /rā′dē·ō·im′yənō·as″ā/ [L, *radius* + *immunis,* free; Fr, *essayer,* to try], a technique in radiology used to determine the concentration of an antigen, antibody, or other protein in the serum. The technique involves the injection of a known amount of a radioactively labeled substance that reacts with the protein in question.

radioimmunofluorescence assay (RIFA) /rā′dē·ō·im′yən ō′floores″əns/, a test for the presence of antibodies sometimes used to confirm the results of ELISA or other methods.

radioimmunosorbent test (RIST) /rā′dē·ō·im′yənōsôr′bənt/ [L, *radius* + *immunis* + *absorbere,* to swallow], a test that uses serum immunoglobulin E to detect allergies to various substances such as certain cosmetics, animal fur, dust, and grasses.

radioimmunotherapy /ra′dē·ōim-mu″no-ther′ah-pe/, use of radionuclides to deliver monoclonal antibodies to targeted cancer cells.

radioiodine /rā′dē·ō·ī′ədīn/. See **radioactive iodine.**

radioiodine uptake, uptake of radioiodine from the blood by the thyroid gland. See also **radioiodine uptake test.**

radioiodine uptake test, one of the most common thyroid function tests. A known quantity of radioiodine is administered, and 6 and 24 hours later the percent that has been absorbed by the thyroid gland is calculated. An increased uptake indicates hyperthyroidism, and a decreased uptake indicates hypothyroidism. Patients who have recently been exposed to iodine compounds, such as in dietary supplements, contrast media, medications, or antiseptics, may not be good candidates for this test.

radioisotope /rā′dē·ō·ī′sətōp/ [L, *radius* + Gk, *isos,* equal, *topos,* place], a radioactive form of an element, which may be used for therapeutic and diagnostic purposes.

radioisotope scan, a two-dimensional representation of the gamma rays emitted by a radioisotope showing its concentration in a body site, such as the thyroid gland, brain, or kidney. Radioisotopes used in diagnostic scanning may be administered intravenously or orally.

radiological. See **radiology.**

radiological anatomy /-loj″ik/ [L, *radius* + Gk, *logos,* science], (in applied anatomy) the study of the structure and morphology of the tissues and organs of the body based on their x-ray visualization.

Radiological Society of North America (RSNA), an international organization of radiologists, medical physicists, and other medical professionals.

radiologic technologist, an allied health professional who, under the supervision of a physician radiologist, operates radiographic equipment and assists radiologists and other health professionals and whose competence has been tested and approved by the American Registry of Radiologic Technologists. The Canadian Association of Medical Radiation Technologists (CAMRT) is Canada's national professional association and certifying body for medical radiation technologists and therapists. Also called **radiographer, x-ray technologist.**

radiologic units, units used to measure radiation. Kinds include **SI: becquerel, gray, sievert, coulomb/kilogram (C/kg); conventional: curie, rad, roentgen, rem.**

radiologist /rā′dē·ol′əjist/, a physician who specializes in radiology. A certified radiologist in the United States is one whose competence has been tested and approved by the American Board of Radiology. Also called **roentgenologist.**

radiology /-ol″əjē/ [L, *radius* + *logos,* science], the branch of medicine concerned with radioactive substances and with the diagnosis and treatment of disease by visualizing through the use of various sources of radiant energy. Formerly called **roentgenology.**

radiolucency /-loo̅″sənsē/ [L, *radiare* + *lucere,* to shine], the ability of materials of relatively low atomic number to allow most x-rays to pass through them, producing dark areas on images.

radiolucent /-loo̅″sənt/ [L, *radiare,* to emit rays, *lucere,* to shine], pertaining to materials that allow x-rays to penetrate with a minimum of absorption.

radionecrosis /-nəkrō″sis/, tissue death caused by radiation.

radionuclide /-noo̅″klīd/ [L, *radiare* + *nucleus,* nut kernel], an isotope that undergoes radioactive decay. Any element with an excess of either neutrons or protons in the nucleus is unstable and tends toward radioactive decay, with the emission of energy that may be measurable with a detector. The processes of radioactive decay include beta particle emission, electron capture, isomeric transition, and positron emission. Positron-emitting radionuclides are important in positron emission tomography and in medical research. Radionuclides used in scintigraphy include ^{123}I, ^{131}I, ^{111}In, ^{75}Se, ^{99m}Tc, and ^{201}Tl. Radionuclides of cobalt, iodine, phosphorus, strontium, and other elements are used for treatment of tumors and cancers and for nuclear imaging of internal parts of the body. See also **nuclear scanning.**

radionuclide angiocardiography, the radiographic examination of cardiac blood vessels after an IV injection of a radiopharmaceutical.

radionuclide imaging, the noninvasive examination of various parts of the body, especially the heart, using a radiopharmaceutical such as thallium-201 and a detection device such as a gamma camera, rectilinear scanner, or positron camera. See also **cardiac radionuclide imaging.**

radionuclide organ imaging. See **nuclear scanning.**

radiopacity /-pas″itē/ [L, *radiare,* to emit rays, *opacus,* obscure], the ability to stop or reduce the passage of x-rays. Bones have relative radiopacity and therefore display as white areas on an x-ray image. Lead has marked radiopacity and therefore is widely used to shield x-ray equipment and atomic power sources. Also called **radiodensity. –radiopaque,** *adj.*

radiopaque /-pāk″/ [L, *radiare* + *opacus,* obscure], not permitting the passage of x-rays or other radiant energy. See also **radioactive element, radioactivity. –radiopacity,** *n.*

radiopaque contrast medium, a substance that stops the passage of x-rays and is used to outline the interior of hollow structures, such as heart chambers, blood vessels, the GI tract, and joint spaces, in x-ray or fluoroscopic images. Formerly called **radiographic contrast medium.** Compare **radiolucency.**

radiopathology /-pəthol″əjē/, a branch of medicine involving both pathology and radiology and concerned with the effects of ionizing radiation on body tissues.

radiopharmaceutical /-fär′məsoo̅″tikəl/ [L, *radiare* + Gk, *pharmakeuein,* to give a drug], a drug that contains radioactive atoms. Kinds include **diagnostic radiopharmaceutical, research radiopharmaceutical, therapeutic radiopharmaceutical.**

radiopharmacist /-fär″məsist/, a person responsible for formulating and dispensing prescribed radioactive tracers and for the clinical aspects of radiopharmacy. Radiopharmacists are required to receive training in radioactive tracer techniques, the safe handling of radioactive materials, the preparation and quality control of drugs for administration to humans, and the basic principles of nuclear medicine. Institutional, state, and federal regulations require completion of a program in nuclear pharmacy, including coursework in radiation safety, radiopharmacy techniques, health physics, and instrumentation. Some jurisdictions require licensure as a pharmacist.

radiopharmacy /-fär″məsē/ [L, *radiare* + Gk, *pharmakeuein,* to give a drug], a facility for the preparation and dispensing of radioactive drugs and for the storage of radioactive materials, inventory records, and prescriptions of radioactive substances. The radiopharmacy is usually the correlation point for radioactive wastes, the unit responsible for waste disposal or storage, and a center for clinical investigations using radioactive tracers. It may also be a center for research and for the training of students and residents in radiology and nuclear medicine.

radioprotectant /rā″dē·opro-tek′tant/, **1.** *adj.,* providing protection against the toxic effects of ionizing radiation. **2.** See **radioprotector.**

radioprotective drugs /-prətek″tiv/ [L, *radiare,* to emit rays, *protegere,* to cover; Fr, *drogue*], pharmaceuticals that protect the body against ionizing radiation. An example is Lugol's solution, an aqueous solution of iodine used to supply iodine internally, thereby blocking the uptake of radioactive iodine.

radioprotector /rā″dē·ōpro-tek″ter/, an agent that provides protection against the toxic effects of ionizing radiation.

radioresistance /-risis″təns/ [L, *radiare* + *resistare,* to withstand], the ability of cells, tissues, organs, organisms, chemical compounds, or any other substances to remain unchanged by radiation. Compare **radiosensitivity. –radioresistant,** *adj.*

radioresistant /-risis″tənt/, unchanged by or protected against damage by radioactive emissions such as x-rays, alpha particles, or gamma rays. Compare **radiosensitive.** See also **radioactivity.**

radioresponsive /-rispon″siv/, responding to radiation, either positively or negatively.

radiosensitive /-sen″sitiv/ [L, *radiare* + *sentire,* to feel], **1.** capable of being changed by or reacting to radioactive emissions such as x-rays, alpha particles, or gamma rays. Compare **radioresistant.** See also **radioactivity. 2.** a cell characteristic indicating the degree of susceptibility to changes produced by ionizing radiation. For example, immature cells are said to be more radiosensitive than mature cells; cells of the nervous system are less radiosensitive than blood cells.

radiosensitivity /-sen′sitiv″itē/, the relative susceptibility of cells, tissues, organs, organisms, or any other substances to the effects of radiation. Cells of self-renewing tissues, such as those in the crypts of the intestine, are the most radiosensitive. Cells that divide regularly but mature between divisions, such as spermatogonia and spermatocytes, are somewhat less radiosensitive. Long-lived cells that usually do not divide unless there is a suitable stimulus, such as liver, kidney, and thyroid cells, are even less radiosensitive. Least radiosensitive are cells that have lost the ability to divide, such as neurons. Compare **radioresistance. –radiosensitive,** *adj.*

radiosensitizers /-sen′sitī″zərs/ [L, *radiare,* + *sentire* + Gk, *izein,* to cause], drugs that enhance the killing effect of radiation on cells.

radiotherapist /-ther″əpist/, a health professional who specializes in the use of radiation, including the application of radiopharmaceuticals, in the treatment of disease. See also **radiation oncologist.**

radiotherapy /-ther″əpē/ [L, *radiare,* to emit rays; Gk, *therapeia,* treatment], the treatment of neoplastic disease by using x-rays or gamma rays to deter the proliferation of malignant cells by decreasing the rate of mitosis or impairing DNA synthesis. Compare **radium therapy.**

radiotoxicity. See **radiation toxicity.**

radioulnar articulation /-ul″nər/ [L, *radius,* ray, *ulna,* elbow, arm], the articulation of the radius and the ulna, consisting of a proximal articulation, a distal articulation, and three sets of ligaments.

radium (Ra) /rā″dē·əm/ [L, *radius,* ray], a radioactive metallic element of the alkaline earth group. Its atomic number is 88. Four radium isotopes occur naturally and have different atomic masses: 223, 224, 226, and 228. The isotope with atomic mass 226 is the most abundant. It is formed by the disintegration of uranium 238, has a half-life of 1620 years, and decays by alpha emission to form radon 222. Radium occurs in the uranium minerals carnotite and pitchblende, which contain about 3×10^{-7} g of radium per gram of uranium. Radium has been used extensively as a radiation source in the treatment of cancer but is gradually being replaced in such therapy by cobalt and cesium.

radium-226, a radioactive isotope historically used for brachytherapy. It is now being replaced by cesium-137 and cobalt-60, which have similar energy characteristics but are not subject to hazardous leakage as radium sources sometimes are.

radium insertion, the introduction of metallic radium into a body cavity, such as the uterus or cervix, to treat cancer.

radium therapy [L, *radius,* ray; Gk, *therapeia,* treatment], the use of radium and its radioactive emissions to treat disease. Compare **radiotherapy.**

radius /rā″dē·əs/ *pl. radii* [L, ray], the lateral bone of the forearm lying parallel to the ulna and partially revolving around it. Its proximal end is small and forms a part of the elbow joint. The distal end is large and forms a part of the wrist joint. The radius receives the insertions of various muscles and articulates with the humerus, ulna, scaphoid, lunate, and triangular bones.

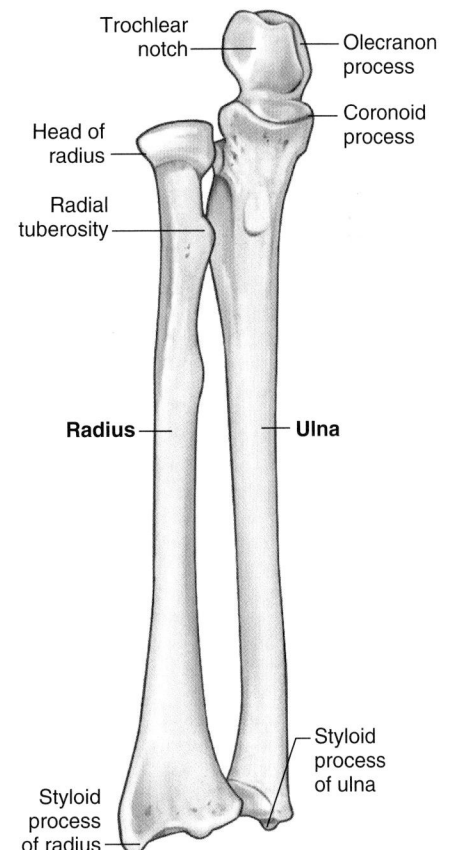

Radius and ulna *(Patton and Thibodeau, 2010)*

radix. See **root.**

radon (Rn) /rā″don/ [L, *radiare*, to emit rays], a radioactive, chemically inert, gaseous element. Its atomic number is 86, and its atomic mass is 222. A decay product of radium, radon is used in radiation cancer therapy. Radon is also released by rocks, soil, and groundwater and is a common source of background radiation, with an intensity that varies in different geographic areas.

radon-222, a radioactive decay product of radium-226 that has been used to fill permanent implants in tumors. It is being replaced by the more manageable radionuclide iodine-125.

radon daughters, ions that are decay products of radon. They are regarded as a potential health hazard by the U.S. Environmental Protection Agency because they tend to adhere to surfaces, such as the alveoli of the lungs, where they can cause ionizing radiation damage.

radon seed, a small, sealed tube of glass or gold containing radon for insertion into body tissues in the treatment of malignancies. It is visible radiographically.

ragpicker disease, *(Slang)* now called **anthrax.**

ragweed /rag′wēd/ [ME, *ragge*, rag + AS, *weod*, herb, grass, weed], any of various species of plants of the genus *Ambrosia* whose pollen can cause hay fever.

RAI, abbreviation for **radioactive iodine.**

RAIU, abbreviation for **radioactive iodine uptake.**

RA latex test, *(Obsolete)* now called **latex fixation test.**

rale. See **crackle.**

raloxifene, a selective estrogen receptor modulator.
- INDICATIONS: It is used to prevent osteoporosis in postmenopausal women.
- CONTRAINDICATIONS: Pregnancy, lactation, and known hypersensitivity to raloxifene prohibit its use.
- ADVERSE EFFECTS: Adverse effects include insomnia, migraines, depression, hot flashes, diarrhea, anorexia, cramps, vaginitis, urinary tract infection, leukorrhea, endometrial disorder, breast pain, rash, sweating, weight gain, peripheral edema, arthralgia, myalgia, leg cramps, arthritis, sinusitis, pharyngitis, increased cough, pneumonia, and laryngitis. Nausea is a common side effect.

raltegravir, an antiretroviral.
- INDICATIONS: This drug is used to treat HIV in combination with other retrovirals.
- CONTRAINDICATIONS: Breastfeeding and known hypersensitivity to this drug prohibit its use.
- ADVERSE EFFECTS: Adverse effects of this drug include fatigue, fever, dizziness, nausea, vomiting, diarrhea, abdominal pain, asthenia, gastritis, rash, urticaria, pruritus, pain or phlebitis at IV site, unusual sweating, alopecia, hyperamylasia, hyperglycemia, and myopathy. Life-threatening side effects include hepatitis, oliguria, proteinuria, hematuria, glomerulonephritis, acute renal failure, renal tubular necrosis, anemia, neutropenia, and rhabdomyolysis.

RAM, abbreviation for **random-access memory.**

ramelteon, a sedative-hypnotic with antianxiety properties.
- INDICATIONS: This drug is used to treat insomnia.
- CONTRAINDICATIONS: Alcohol intoxication, hepatic encephalopathy, lactation, and known hypersensitivity to this drug prohibit its use. This drug should not be administered to infants or children.
- ADVERSE EFFECTS: Adverse effects of this drug include dizziness, somnolence, fatigue, headache, insomnia, depression, nausea, diarrhea, dysgeusia, vomiting, myalgia, arthralgia, decreased blood cortisol, influenza, and upper respiratory infection.

rami-, combining form meaning "branch": *ramification.*

ramification /ram′ifikā″shən/ [L, *ramus*, branch, *facere*, to make], **1.** (in anatomy and physiology) a branching, distribution. **2.** the consequences or results of an action.

ramify. See **ramus.**

rampant dental caries, dental caries that involves several teeth, appears suddenly, and often progresses rapidly.

Ramsay Hunt syndrome [James Ramsay Hunt, American neurologist, 1872–1937], a neurological condition resulting from invasion of the seventh nerve ganglia and the geniculate ganglion by varicella zoster virus, characterized by severe ear pain, facial nerve paralysis, vertigo, hearing loss, and often mild generalized encephalitis. The vertigo may last days or weeks but usually resolves itself. The facial paralysis may be permanent, and the hearing loss, which is rarely permanent, may be partial or total. Treatment usually includes the prescription of corticosteroid drugs. Also called **herpes zoster oticus.**

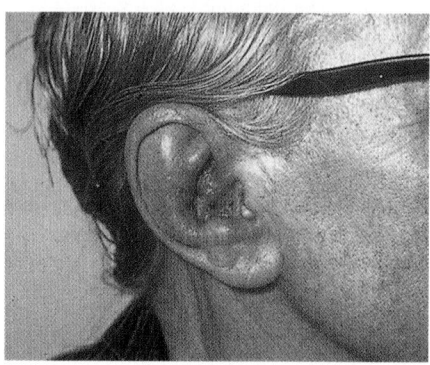

Varicella zoster virus infection in Ramsay Hunt syndrome *(Perkin et al, 2011)*

Ramstedt-Fredet operation, now called **pyloromyotomy.**

ramus /rā″məs/ *pl. rami* [L, branch], a small branchlike structure extending from a larger one or dividing into two or more parts, such as a branch of a nerve or artery or one of the rami of the blood vessel or nerve.

ramus of mandible, a quadrilateral process projecting upward from the posterior part of either side of the mandible.

Ranchos Los Amigos Scale [Rancho Los Amigos National Rehabilitation Center, California], a scale of cognitive functioning developed as a behavioral rating scale to aid in assessment and treatment of head-injured persons. Eight levels of cognitive functioning are identified, from I (no response) to VIII (purposeful and appropriate behavioral response).

rancidity /ransid″itē/, the unpleasant taste and smell of fatty foods that have undergone decomposition, liberating butyric acid and other volatile lipids.

random-access memory (RAM) /ran″dəm/, (in computer processing) the part of a computer's memory available to execute programs and temporarily store data. It can usually be used for both reading and writing. RAM data is automatically erased when the computer is turned off unless the file has been saved. Compare **read-only memory.**

random controlled trial [ME, *randoun*, run violently; Fr, *contrôle*, check, *trier*, to grind], a study plan for a proposed new treatment in which subjects are assigned on a random basis to participate either in an experimental group receiving the new treatment or in a control group that does not.

random genetic drift. See **genetic drift.**

randomization [ME, *randoun*, run violently], the process of assigning subjects or objects to a control or experimental group that gives each item of a set an equal probability of being chosen for the group.

random mating [ME, *randoun*, run violently, *gemate*], a pairing of subjects when each individual has an equal chance of mating with those of other genetic backgrounds.

random off. See **on/off phenomenon.**

random sampling [ME, *randoun,* run violently; L, *exemplum*], a method of sampling for a study in which each individual has an equal chance of being selected and the choice of a particular individual does not affect the chances of the others.

random selection, a method of choosing subjects for a research study in which all members of a particular group have an equal chance of being selected.

random voided specimen, a voided urine specimen obtained at any point in a 24-hour period.

Ranexa, a medication used in the management of angina. Brand name for **ranolazine.**

range /rānj/ [OFr, *ranger,* to arrange in a row], the interval between the lowest and highest values in a series of data.

range abnormalities, uncertainties in the actual range from which Doppler signals or echo signals originate. In pulsed Doppler instruments a high pulse repetition frequency can result in range ambiguities.

range equation, a relationship between the distance to a reflector and the time it takes for a pulse of ultrasound to propagate to the reflector and return to the transducer.

range of accommodation [OFr, *ranger* + L, *accommodatio*], (in ophthalmology) the distance between the farthest point at which an object can be seen clearly with accommodation fully relaxed and the nearest distance at which an object can be observed with full accommodation, measured in meters or centimeters.

range of motion (ROM) [OFr, *ranger* + L, *motio*], the extent of movement of a joint, measured in degrees of a circle. Compare **proprioceptive neuromuscular facilitation. See also active range of motion, passive range of motion.**

range-of-motion exercise [OFr, *ranger,* to arrange in a row; L, *motio,* movement], any body action involving the muscles, joints, and natural movements, such as abduction, adduction, extension, flexion, pronation, supination, and rotation. Such exercises are usually applied actively or passively in the prevention and treatment of orthopedic deformities, in the assessment of injuries and deformities, and in athletic conditioning. They are important for joint mobility. See also **active range of motion, passive range of motion.**

ranibizumab, an ophthalmic drug that binds to the receptor binding site of active forms of vascular endothelial growth factor A.

■ INDICATIONS: This drug is used in the treatment of neovascular macular degeneration.

■ CONTRAINDICATIONS: Ocular infections and known hypersensitivity to this drug prohibit its use.

■ ADVERSE EFFECTS: Adverse effects of this drug include dizziness; headache; blepharitis; cataract; conjunctival hem-

Range-of-motion exercises

Body part	Type of joint		Type of movement
Neck, cervical spine	Pivotal		Flexion: bring chin to rest on chest Extension: return head to erect position Extension: bend head back as far as possible
			Lateral flexion: tilt head as far as possible toward each shoulder
			Rotation: turn head as far as possible in circular movement
Shoulder	Ball and socket		Flexion: raise arm from side position forward to position above head Extension: return arm to position at side of body Extension: move arm behind body, keeping elbow straight

Continued

Range-of-motion exercises–cont'd

Body part	Type of joint	Type of movement
		Abduction: raise arm to side to position above head with palm away from head Adduction: lower arm sideways and across body as far as possible
		Internal rotation: with elbow flexed and shoulder at side, rotate shoulder by moving arm until thumb is turned inward and toward back External rotation: with elbow flexed and shoulder at side, move arm until thumb is upward and lateral to head
		Circumduction: move arm in full circle (Circumduction is combination of all movements of ball-and-socket joint.)
Elbow	Hinge	Flexion: bend elbow so that lower arm moves toward its shoulder joint and hand is level with shoulder Extension: straighten elbow by lowering hand
Forearm	Pivotal	Supination: turn lower arm and hand so that palm is up Pronation: turn lower arm so that palm is down
Wrist	Condyloid	Flexion: move palm toward inner aspect of forearm Extension: move fingers and hand posterior to midline

Range-of-motion exercises–cont'd

Body part	Type of joint	Type of movement
	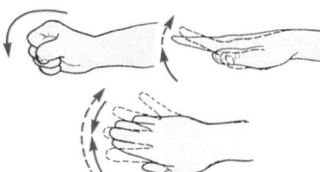	Hyperextension: bring dorsal surface of hand back as far as possible Abduction: Place hand with palm down and extend wrist laterally toward fifth finger Adduction: Place hand with palm down and extend wrist medially toward thumb
Fingers	Condyloid hinge 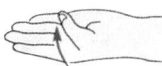 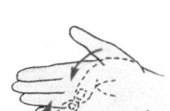	Flexion: make fist Extension: straighten fingers Hyperextension: bend fingers back as far as possible Abduction: spread fingers apart Adduction: bring fingers together
Thumb	Saddle 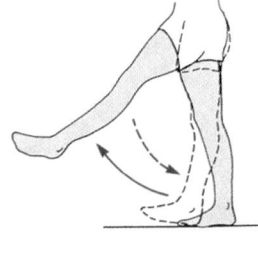	Flexion: move thumb across palmar surface of hand Extension: move thumb straight away from hand Abduction: extend thumb laterally (usually done when placing fingers in abduction and adduction) Adduction: move thumb back toward hand Opposition: touch thumb to each finger of same hand
Hip	Ball and socket 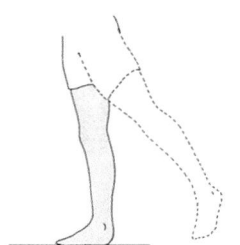	Flexion: move leg forward and up Extension: move back beside other leg Extension: move leg behind body

Continued

Range-of-motion exercises–cont'd

Body part	Type of joint	Type of movement
		Abduction: move leg laterally away from body Adduction: move leg back toward medial position and beyond if possible Internal rotation: turn foot and leg toward other leg at the hip External rotation: turn foot and leg away from other leg at the hip
		Circumduction: move leg in circle
Knee	Hinge	Flexion: bring heel back toward back of thigh Extension: return leg to the floor
Ankle	Hinge	Dorsal flexion: move foot so that toes are pointed upward Plantar flexion: move foot so that toes are pointed downward
Foot	Gliding	Inversion: turn sole of foot medially Eversion: turn sole of foot laterally
Toes	Condyloid	Flexion: curl toes downward Extension: straighten toes Abduction: spread toes apart Adduction: bring toes together

Modified from Potter PA, Perry AG: *Fundamentals of nursing,* ed 7, St. Louis, 2009, Mosby.

orrhage and hyperemia; detachment of the retinal pigment epithelium; dryness, irritation, and pain in the eye; visual impairment; vitreous floaters; ocular infection; constipation; nausea; hypertension; urinary tract infection; thromboembolism; bronchitis; cough; sinusitis; and upper respiratory infection.

ranitidine /ranit″idēn/, a histamine H_2 receptor antagonist.

■ INDICATIONS: It is prescribed in the treatment of gastroesophageal reflux disease and gastric hypersecretory conditions.

■ CONTRAINDICATIONS: Known sensitivity to this drug prohibits its use. The drug should be used in pregnancy only if clearly needed and with caution in those with severe hepatic or renal impairment.

■ ADVERSE EFFECTS: Among the most serious adverse effects are acquired hemolytic anemia, agranulocytosis, atrioventricular block, agitation, dizziness, headaches, rashes, gynecomastia, and loss of libido.

Rankine scale [William J.M. Rankine, Scottish physicist, 1820–1870], an absolute temperature scale calculated in degrees Fahrenheit. Absolute zero on the Rankine scale is −460° F, equivalent to −273° C. See also **Kelvin scale.**

rank sum test, a nonparametric statistical test for ordinal data, testing the null hypothesis that two samples are drawn from the same population against the alternative hypothesis that the two samples are drawn from two populations having probability distributions of the same shape but different locations. It is based on the value of the rank sum statistic, which is calculated as the sum of the ranks of each sample after the observations in both samples are jointly ranked in ascending order; if and only if the null hypothesis is true, the average ranks of the two samples will be similar. Also called **Mann-Whitney test, Mann-Whitney U test.**

ranolazine, an antianginal drug.

■ INDICATIONS: This drug is used in combination with other antianginals (such as amlodipine, beta-blockers, or nitrates) to treat chronic stable angina pectoris in those who have not responded to other treatment options.

■ CONTRAINDICATIONS: Preexisting Q-T prolongation, hepatic disease (Child-Pugh class A, B, or C), hypokalemia, renal failure, torsades de pointes, ventricular arrhythmia, ventricular tachycardia, and known hypersensitivity to this drug prohibit its use.

■ ADVERSE EFFECTS: Adverse effects of this drug include headache, dizziness, palpitations, nausea, vomiting, constipation, dry mouth, peripheral edema, and dyspnea. A life-threatening side effect of this drug is Q-T prolongation.

ranula /ran″yoolə/ pl. ranulae [L, rana, frog], a large mucocele in the floor of the mouth, usually caused by obstruction of the ducts of the sublingual salivary glands and less commonly caused by obstruction of the ducts of the submandibular salivary glands. Also called **hydroglossa.**

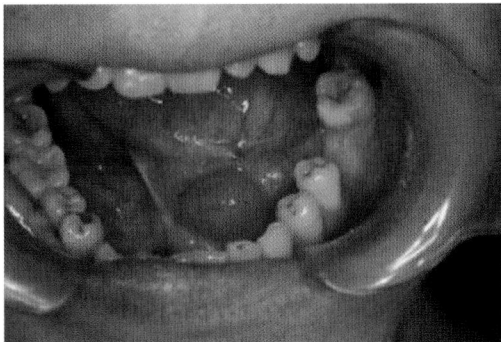

Ranula (Regezi, Sciubba, and Jordan, 2008)

Ranvier's nodes /ränvē-āz′, räN-/ [Louis A. Ranvier, French pathologist, 1835–1922], constrictions in the medullary substance of a nerve fiber at more or less regular intervals.

rape [L, rapere, to seize], a sexual assault, homosexual or heterosexual, the legal definitions for which vary from state to state. Rape is a crime of violence or one committed under the threat of violence, and its victims are treated for medical and psychological trauma. Kinds include **statutory rape.** See also **sexual assault.**

■ OBSERVATIONS: Characteristically the victim is frightened and feels vulnerable, humiliated, and personally violated. General physical examination may reveal cuts, bruises, and other injuries. Pelvic or genital examination may show traumatic injury to the internal or external genitalia or anus.

■ INTERVENTIONS: Careful physical examination should be conducted by specially trained health care personnel, and a detailed history obtained. Evidence and medical specimens are collected as indicated. Ideally counseling is available and offered immediately to all victims of rape. In the case of a woman who has been raped by a man, a pregnancy test may be performed to document current pregnancy status. Prophylaxis against conception may be administered. Medications may be given to prevent the development of sexually transmitted disease. Arrangements for ongoing emotional support are made.

■ PATIENT CARE CONSIDERATIONS: A trained empathetic caregiver of the same gender is assigned to stay with the victim. Privacy for the history, examination, and police interview is ensured. The victim may or may not choose to report the incident to the police. The victim must sign a special form to allow specimens to be released to a law enforcement agency. In general, it is the role of the caregiver and other specially trained medical workers to examine, treat, and collect specimens as necessary but not to decide that rape has occurred. Before discharge it should be ascertained that someone can be with the victim, since depression, anger, guilt, and fear may occur after rape.

rape counseling, counseling by a trained person provided to a victim of rape. Rape counseling ideally begins at the time the crime is first reported, as in an emergency department. Initially the counselor offers sensitive support for the victim by accepting the victim in a nonprejudicial, noncritical way. The victim's response to the trauma of the assault is empathetically elicited, and three basic statements are made: the counselor is sorry that the rape happened, is glad that the injuries are not worse, and does not think that the victim was wrong or did anything wrong. Counseling personnel may provide supportive services and advocacy and liaison between the victim and medical, legal, and law enforcement authorities. This involves staying with the

Rape prevention measures

Prevention of attack

Set house lights to go on and off by timer.
Keep light on at all entrances.
Install safety locks on windows and doors.
Have key ready before reaching door of house or car.
Look in car before entering.
Never let strangers enter the house; insist on identification from all service personnel; check identity with agency if suspicious.
Do not list first name on mailbox or in telephone directory.
Be alert when walking; stay in lighted areas.
Walk down center of street if possible.
Avoid lonely or enclosed areas.

From Monahan FD et al: *Phipps' medical-surgical nursing: health and illness perspectives,* ed 8, St. Louis, 2007, Mosby.

R

victim during medical examination, during police or district attorney's questioning, and throughout the criminal justice process.

raphe /rā″fē/ [Gk, *rhaphe,* seam], a crease, ridge, or seam of the halves of various symmetric parts, such as the abdominal raphe of the linea alba or the raphe penis, which appears as a narrow dark streak on the inferior surface of the penis. Also spelled **rhaphe.**

raphe nuclei, a subgroup of the reticular nuclei of the brainstem found in narrow longitudinal sheets along the raphae of the medulla oblongata, pons, and mesencephalon. They include many neurons that synthesize serotonin. Their ascending fibers project to parts of the limbic system, and their descending fibers project to other brainstem nuclei, the medulla oblongata, and the pons. In the group are the magnus raphe nucleus, median raphe nucleus, obscurus raphe nucleus, pallidal raphe nucleus, pontine raphe nucleus, posterior raphe nucleus, inferior linear nucleus, intermediate linear nucleus, and superior linear nucleus.

raphe of tongue [Gk, *rhaphe,* seam; AS, *tunge*], a fibrous wall that forms a line of union between the right and left sides of the tongue.

rapid-acting insulin, insulin with an onset of action of 15 minutes.

rapid eye movement (REM), a phase of sleep in which there is rapid movement of the eyes and vivid dreams. See also **sleep.**

rapid grower /rap″id/, a saprophytic mycobacterium in group IV of the Runyon classification system that grows within 3 to 5 days. See also **Runyon classification system, saprophyte.**

rapid plasma reagin test (RPR test), an agglutination examination used in screening for syphilis. The test detects two groups of antibodies. The first is a nontreponemal antibody (reagin) directed against a lipoidal agent resulting from a *Treponema pallidum* infection. The second is an antibody directed against the *T. pallidum* organism itself.

rapid pulse [L, *rapidus,* rush, *pulsare,* to beat], a pulse faster than normal. Also called **tachycardia.**

rapport /rapôr″/ [Fr, agreement], **1.** a sense of mutuality and understanding. **2.** harmony, accord, confidence, and respect underlying a relationship between two persons, which is an essential bond between a therapist and patient. It should be distinguished from transference, which is unconscious.

rapprochement /räprôshmäN″/ [Fr, *rapprocher,* to bring together], (in child development) a subphase of the separation-individuation phase of Mahler's system of child development. This subphase occurs from approximately 14 months to 2 years or more. This stage is characterized by a rediscovery of and reestablishment with the mother or a significant nurturer in an attempt to have needs met.

Raptiva, a drug voluntarily withdrawn from the U.S. market in 2009. Brand name for *efalizumab.*

raptus /rap″təs/ [L, *rapere,* to seize], **1.** a state of intense emotional or mental excitement, often characterized by uncontrollable activity or behavior resulting from an irresistible impulse; ecstasy; rapture. **2.** any sudden or violent seizure or attack.

rare-earth element [L, *rarus,* thin; AS, *earthe* + L, *elementum*], a metallic element having an atomic number between 57 and 71, inclusively. Also called *rare-earth metal.* See also **rare-earth screen.**

rare-earth screen, (*Obsolete*) an x-ray-intensifying screen made of rare-earth elements, such as yttrium and gadolinium. These screens enable lower radiation doses to be used while producing acceptable film densities.

rarefaction /rer′əfak″shən/, **1.** reductions in density of a tissue. **2.** reduction in the density of a medium, such as air, which is denser close to the earth and the pull of gravity and has a reduced density at higher stratospheric levels. **3.** (in physical science) reductions in density of a medium (air, pressure, wave motion) at a location in the medium accompanying cyclical pressure reductions during the passage of a sound wave. For example, the prong of a tuning fork vibrates in the air, and air adjacent to the prong is compressed. When the prong springs back in the opposite direction, it leaves an area of reduced air pressure.

RAS, abbreviation for **reticular activating system.**

rasagiline, an antiparkinson agent.

■ INDICATIONS: This drug is used alone or with levodopa to treat idiopathic Parkinson disease.

■ CONTRAINDICATIONS: Lactation, pheochromocytoma, and known hypersensitivity to this drug or monoamine oxidase inhibitors prohibit its use.

■ ADVERSE EFFECTS: Adverse effects of this drug include drowsiness, hallucinations, depression, headache, malaise, paresthesia, vertigo, syncope, angina, orthostatic hypotension, diarrhea, dry mouth, dyspepsia, impotence, decreased libido, conjunctivitis, fever, flu syndrome, neck pain, allergic reaction, alopecia, arthralgia, arthritis, dyskinesia, and rhinitis. A life-threatening side effect is hypertensive crisis (after ingestion of tyramine products).

rasburicase, an antineoplastic antimetabolite used to reduce uric acid levels in children with leukemia or lymphoma and in chemotherapy patients with solid tumor malignancies.

rash [OFr, *rasche,* scurf], a skin eruption. Kinds include **butterfly rash, diaper rash, drug rash, heat rash.**

Rashkind procedure /rash″kind/ [William J. Rashkind, American physician, 1922–1986; L, *procedere,* to go forth], the enlargement of an opening in the cardiac septum between the right and left atria. It is performed to relieve congestive heart failure in newborns with certain congenital heart defects by improving the oxygenation of the blood. The procedure allows more mixing between oxygenated blood from the lungs and systemic blood without the risk of surgery, sustaining life until the child is 2 to 3 years of age and a shunt can be created to carry systemic blood to the lungs. Also called **balloon septostomy.**

■ METHOD: Before surgery a cardiac catheterization is done to pinpoint the defect. Under light general anesthesia, a deflated balloon is passed pervenously through the foramen ovale into the left atrium. The balloon is inflated and pulled across the septum to enlarge the opening.

■ PATIENT CARE CONSIDERATIONS: After surgery the infant is observed carefully for respiratory difficulty, signs of hypoxia, or decreasing cardiac output. Humidified oxygen is administered. Fluids and electrolytes are closely monitored.

■ OUTCOME CRITERIA: Stable arterial oxygen saturations can be achieved with this procedure.

Rasmussen's aneurysm /rahs′moosənz/ [Fritz Waldemar Rasmussen, Danish physician, 1834–1877], dilation of a pulmonary artery in a tuberculous cavity. Rupture causes hemorrhage and hemoptysis.

raspberry leaves, an herbal product harvested from the raspberry plant; found worldwide.

■ INDICATIONS: It is used to facilitate childbirth, as a uterine tonic, and as a treatment for dysmenorrhea, fever, and vomiting, but there are insufficient reliable data regarding effectiveness.

■ CONTRAINDICATIONS: It should not be used medicinally during pregnancy and lactation and is contraindicated in those with known hypersensitivity to this plant.

raspberry tongue /raz″berē/, a dark red tongue with a smooth surface and prominent papillae, seen after shedding of the white coating characteristic of the early stage of scarlet fever. See also **strawberry tongue.**

RAST, abbreviation for **radioallergosorbent test.**

rat-bite fever [AS, *raet + bitan,* to bite], either of two distinct infections transmitted to humans, commonly by the bite of a rat or mouse but also by contact with excretions of the mouth, nose, or urine of an infected animal. Kinds include **Haverhill fever, sodoku.**

■ OBSERVATIONS: It is characterized by fever, headache, malaise, nausea, vomiting, and rash. In the United States and Canada the disease is more commonly caused by *Streptobacillusmoniliformis.* Its unique features are a rash on palms and soles, painful joints, prompt healing of the wound, and a duration of 2 weeks. In the Far East, rat-bite fever is usually caused by *Spirillumminus* and is associated with an asymmetric rash on the extremities, no joint symptoms, a relapsing fever, swelling at the site of the wound, regional lymphadenopathy, and a duration of 4 to 8 weeks. Relapse is common.

■ INTERVENTIONS: Penicillin administered intramuscularly is effective in treating either form of the disease.

■ PATIENT CARE CONSIDERATIONS: If left untreated, severe complications, such as infection of the heart valves, may occur.

rate [L, *ratus,* reckoned], a numeric ratio, often used in the compilation of data concerning the prevalence and incidence of events, in which the number of actual occurrences appears as the numerator and the number of possible occurrences appears as the denominator. When 1 person in 15 fails an examination, the failure rate is said to be 1/15 (or "one in fifteen"). Standard rates are stated in conventional units of population such as neonatal mortality per 1000 or maternal mortality per 100,000.

rate-pressure product, the heart rate multiplied by the systolic blood pressure. It is a clinical indicator of myocardial oxygen demand.

rate-responsive pacer, an electronic pacemaker whose rate can be adjusted as required to meet physiological demands.

Rathke bundles. See **trabecula carnea.**

Rathke pouch /rät″kē/ [Martin H. Rathke, German anatomist, 1793–1860; OFr, *pouche*], a depression that forms in the roof of the mouth of an embryo, anterior to the buccopharyngeal membrane, around the fourth week of gestation. The walls of the diverticulum develop into the anterior lobe of the pituitary gland.

Rathke pouch tumor. See **craniopharyngioma.**

rating of perceived exertion (RPE), a scale for quantifying perceived exertion, with 6 being extremely light exertion and 20 being extremely hard. The American College of Sports Medicine (ACSM) has recalibrated the scale from 1 to 10. The ACSM has also established minimal guidelines pertaining to the frequency, intensity, and duration of exercise needed to produce a training effect.

ratio /rā″shō/ [L, a reckoning], the relationship of one quantity to one or more other quantities, expressed as a proportion of one to the others and written either as a fraction (8/3) or linearly (8:3).

rational /rash″ənəl/ [L, *rationalis,* reasonable], **1.** pertaining to a measure, method, or procedure based on reason. **2.** pertaining to a therapeutic method based on an understanding of the cause and mechanisms of a specific disease and the potential effects of the drugs or procedures used in treating the disorder. **3.** sane; capable of normal reasoning or behavior.

rationale /rash″ənal″/ [L, *rationalis,* reasonable], a system of reasoning or a statement of the reasons used in explaining data or phenomena.

rational emotive behavior therapy, (in psychotherapy) a cognitive behavioral therapy based on the premise that people's beliefs strongly affect their emotional functioning and that the beliefs can be modified to allow individuals to lead happy and productive lives.

rational emotive therapy (RET), *(Obsolete)* a form of cognitive therapy. Now called **rational emotive behavior therapy.**

rationalization /rash″ənal′īzā″shən/, the most commonly used defense mechanism, in which an individual justifies ideas, actions, or feelings with seemingly acceptable reasons or explanations. It is often used to preserve self-respect, reduce guilt feelings, or obtain social approval or acceptance.

rational treatment. See **treatment.**

ratio solution, the relationship of a solute to a solution expressed as a proportion, such as 1:1000, or parts per thousand.

rat tapeworm infection. See **hymenolepiasis.**

rattle [ME, *ratelen*], an abnormal sound heard by auscultation of the lungs in some forms of pulmonary disease. It consists of a coarse vibration more intense than a crackle, very much like a rhonchus, caused by the movement of moisture and the separation of the walls of small air passages during respiration.

rattlesnake [ME, *ratelen* + AS, *snacan,* to creep], a poisonous pit viper with a series of loosely connected, horny segments at the end of the tail that make a noise like a rattle when shaken. More than 25 species of rattlesnakes are found in the Americas, including most parts of the United States and Canada. They have a hematoxin in their venom, and they are responsible for most of the poisonous snake bites in the United States. Immediate treatment includes keeping the victim quiet and immobilizing the bite area at the level of the heart. Antivenin is available. Also called *rattler.* See also **snakebite.**

rat typhus. See **murine typhus.**

rauwolfia alkaloid [Leonhard Rauwolf, German botanist, 1535–1596], any one of more than 20 alkaloids derived from the root of a climbing shrub, *Rauwolfia serpentina,* indigenous to India and the surrounding area. Formerly used as an antipsychotic agent, it is today confined to the treatment of hypertension and usage in tranquilizing alkaloid drugs such as reserpine. Numerous brand name formulations of the principal alkaloid reserpine are available.

rauwolfia serpentina, the dried root from *Rauwolfia serpentina.*

■ INDICATIONS: It is prescribed in the treatment of mild hypertension and agitation due to psychosis.

■ CONTRAINDICATIONS: Mental depression, peptic ulcer, ulcerative colitis, electroconvulsive therapy, or known hypersensitivity to this drug prohibits its use. It can interact adversely with monoamine oxidase inhibitors.

■ ADVERSE EFFECTS: Among the more serious adverse effects are symptoms resembling parkinsonism, glaucoma, cardiac arrhythmias, and GI bleeding.

Rauzide, a diuretic medication. Brand name for **bendroflumethiazide, rauwolfia serpentina.**

raw data, **1.** (in radiology) the information obtained by radio reception of a magnetic resonance signal as stored by a computer. Specific computer manipulation of the data is

R

required to construct an image. **2.** (in research) information that has not been analyzed and is as collected and recorded.

ray [L, *radius*],   a beam of radiation, such as heat or light, moving away from a source.

rayl /rāl/   [John W.S. Rayleigh],   the unit for characteristic acoustic impedance. Its fundamental units are $kg/m^2/s$.

Rayleigh scatterer /rā″lē/   [John W.S. Rayleigh, English physicist, 1842–1919],   reflecting objects whose dimensions are much smaller than the ultrasonic wavelength. The scattered intensity from a volume of Rayleigh scatterers increases rapidly with increasing frequency, being related to frequency raised to the fourth power.

Ray, Marilyn Anne,   a nursing theorist who introduced the Theory of Bureaucratic Caring, which emphasizes the interconnectedness of nursing care and health care organizations. The theory emphasizes the holistic nature of an organization rather than simple cause-effect relationships of individual actions. Spiritual-ethical caring by nurses, the ultimate goal of which is the promotion of well-being through caring, has a positive effect on health care organizations and can become an economic resource.

Raynaud phenomenon /rānō″/   [Maurice Raynaud, French physician, 1834–1881],   intermittent attacks of ischemia of the extremities of the body, especially the fingers, toes, ears, and nose, caused by exposure to cold or by emotional stimuli. ▪ OBSERVATIONS: The attacks are characterized by severe blanching of the extremities, followed by cyanosis, then redness; they are usually accompanied by numbness, tingling, burning, and often pain. Normal color and sensation are restored by heat. The attacks usually occur secondary to such conditions as scleroderma, rheumatoid arthritis, systemic lupus erythematosus, thoracic outlet syndrome, drug intoxications, dysproteinemia, myxedema, primary pulmonary hypertension, and trauma. ▪ INTERVENTIONS: Therapy for the secondary form depends on recognition and treatment of the underlying disease. Idiopathic forms, which occur most frequently in young women 18 to 30 years of age, may be controlled by protecting the body and extremities from the cold, by the use of mild sedatives and vasodilators, and by avoiding smoking. Biofeedback techniques are useful in training the client to increase the temperature of the affected extremity, ears, or nose. Drug therapy can also relieve symptoms. ▪ PATIENT CARE CONSIDERATIONS: The condition is called Raynaud disease when there is a history of symptoms for at least 2 years with no progression of symptoms and no evidence of an underlying cause.

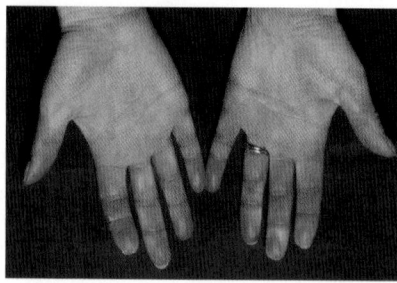

Raynaud phenomenon *(Lebwohl et al, 2014)*

Raynaud sign.   See **acrocyanosis.**

Rb,   symbol for the element **rubidium.**

RBBB,   abbreviation for **right bundle branch block.**

RBC,   abbreviation for **red blood cell.** See **erythrocyte.**

RBE,   abbreviation for **relative biological effectiveness.**

RBRVS,   abbreviation for **resource-based relative value scale.**

RCEEM,   abbreviation for **Recognized Continuing Education Evaluation Mechanism.**

R.C.P.,   abbreviation for **Royal College of Physicians.**

RCPSC,   abbreviation for **Royal College of Physicians and Surgeons of Canada.**

R.C.S.,   abbreviation for **Royal College of Surgeons.**

RD,   abbreviation for **registered dietitian.**

RDAs,   abbreviation for **recommended dietary allowances.**

RDH,   abbreviation for **registered dental hygienist.**

rdi,   abbreviation for **recommended daily intake.**

RDS,   abbreviation for **respiratory distress syndrome of the newborn.**

Re,   symbol for the element **rhenium.**

re-,   prefix meaning "back," "again," "contrary": *reaction, recombination, recurrent.*

reabsorption /rē′əbsôrp″shən/,   the process of something being absorbed again, such as the removal of calcium from the bone back into the blood. Also called **resorption.**

reacher /rē″chər/,   an assistive device with a pincer-type claw and an extended handle that can be used to reach and grasp objects overhead or on the floor by persons with upper extremity disabilities or those who lose the ability to bend and stoop. Also called **extended arm.**

Reach to Recovery [AS, *reacan,* to reach; ME, *recoveren,* to get back],   a national volunteer organization that offers counseling and support to women with breast cancer and their families. Many of the members have had mastectomies themselves.

reaction /rē-ak″shən/   [L, *re,* again, *agere,* to act],   a response to a substance, treatment, or other stimulus, such as an antigen-antibody reaction, an allergic reaction, or an adverse pharmacological reaction.

reaction formation,   an unconscious defense mechanism in which a person expresses toward another person or situation feelings, attitudes, or behaviors that are the opposite of what would normally be expected. An example is an alcoholic who criticizes social drinking.

reaction time [L, *re,* again, *agere,* to act; AS, *tima*],   the interval between the application of a stimulus and the beginning of a response. Compare **lag phase.**

reactivate /rē-ak″tivāt/   [L, *re + activus*],   to make active again, as in adding fresh serum to restore the potency of an original supply of the serum.

reactivation /rē-ak′tivā″shən/,   the restoration of impaired biological activity caused by chemical reaction, thermal application, genetic recombination, or helper elements.

reactivation tuberculosis,   a form of secondary tuberculosis that recurs as a result of the activation of a dormant endogenous infection. Causes of the reactivation may include loss of immunity, hormonal changes, or poor nutrition.

reactive.   See **reaction.**

reactive airways disease,   any of several conditions characterized by wheezing and allergic reactions. Kinds include **asthma, bronchiolitis, chronic obstructive lung disease.**

reactive arthritis /rē-ak′tiv/   [L, *re + activus,* active],   arthritis after an infection, such as urethritis caused by *Chlamydia trachomatis* or enteritis caused by *Campylobacter, Salmonella, Shigella,* or *Yersinia.*

reactive decision /rē-ak′tiv/   [L, *re + activus*],   (in psychology) a decision made by an individual in response to the influence or goals of others.

reactive depression,   *(Obsolete)* an emotional condition characterized by an acute feeling of despondency, sadness, and depressive dysphoria; it varies in intensity and duration. The condition is caused by some identifiable external situation or environmental stress and is generally relieved when the circumstance is altered or the conflict understood and resolved. Now called **situational depression.** See also **depression.**

reactive gastritis, gastric inflammation caused by the presence of a harmful substance, such as an NSAID, bile refluxing from the duodenum, or a toxic chemical. It may be either acute or chronic. See also **chemical gastritis.**

reactive hypoglycemia, low levels of glucose in the circulating blood (45 to 50 mg/dL) in an arterialized specimen after ingestion of carbohydrates. Patients who have had stomach surgery, causing food to travel quickly into the intestine, frequently experience this symptom.

Revised Hearing Handicap Inventory and Revised Hearing Handicap Inventory—Screening, measures of the impact of hearing loss, including psychosocial impact, on everyday experiences. The inventory and screening measures can be used for adults of all ages.

reactive inflammation [L, *re* + *activus* + *inflammare*, to set afire], an inflammation that develops as a reaction to an antigen.

reactive psychosis, (in psychiatry) a psychotic episode that results from a specific set of external circumstances. See also **brief reactive psychosis.**

reactor /rē·ak″tər/, **1.** (in psychology) a family therapist who lets a family in therapy take the lead and then follows in that direction. **2.** (in radiology) a cubicle in which radioisotopes are artificially produced.

read [AS, *raedan*, to advise], **1.** (in computer processing) to retrieve or transfer data from some storage location or medium, such as a disk. **2.** to comprehend the written word.

reading [AS, *raedan*], **1.** (in genetics) the linear process in which the genetic information contained in a nucleotide sequence is decoded, as in the translation of the messenger RNA into a sequence of amino acids in a polypeptide. **2.** the graphic representation produced by medical equipment, such as an ECG reading.

reading disorder, a language disorder in which one's reading ability is significantly below intellectual capacity. The disorder is marked by faulty oral reading, slow reading, or reduced comprehension.

Read method [Grantley Dick-Read, English obstetrician, 1890–1959], a method of psychophysical preparation for childbirth. It was the first "natural childbirth" program, a term coined by Dr. Read in the 1930s. Read held that childbirth is a normal, physiological procedure and that the pain of labor and delivery is of psychological origin—the fear-tension-pain syndrome. He countered women's fears with education about the physiological process, encouraged a positive welcoming attitude, corrected false information, and led tours of the hospital. To decrease tension he developed a series of breathing exercises for use during the various stages of labor. To foster relaxation and optimal physical function in labor and recovery after delivery, he incorporated a series of physical exercises to be performed regularly in classes and in practice at home during pregnancy. Currently many authorities who advocate use of other aspects of the Read method strongly recommend that a woman in labor not lie on her back. Supine hypotension is frequently the result of this position, because the uterus can fall back, occluding the vena cava and decreasing the volume of blood returned to the heart, thus reducing the volume of the cardiac output. Maternal hypotension follows, resulting in decreased placental perfusion and an inadequate supply of oxygen to the fetus. Today the woman using the Read method spends most of labor lying on her side or in a semisitting position with her knees, back, and head well supported. Compare **Bradley method, Lamaze method.**

read-only memory (ROM), (in computer processing) the part of a computer's memory in which information is permanently stored on specialized processors. The operator may have access to the memory, but only for purposes of reading the contents. ROM also executes automatically when the computer is started. Special equipment or programming is required to write, erase, or alter the contents of read-only memory. Compare **random-access memory.**

readthrough [AS, *raedan* + *thurh*, through], transcription beyond the normal termination sequence in a DNA template, caused by the occasional failure of RNA polymerase to respond to the end-point signal.

reagent /rē·ā″jənt/ [L, *re*, again, *agere*, to act], a chemical substance known to react in a specific way. A reagent is used to detect or synthesize another substance in a chemical reaction. Examples include Benedict's reagent, used to test for glucose, and Biuret reagent, used to test for protein.

reagent strip, a strip of paper impregnated with a reagent to a given substance, used in testing for that substance in a body fluid or other secretion.

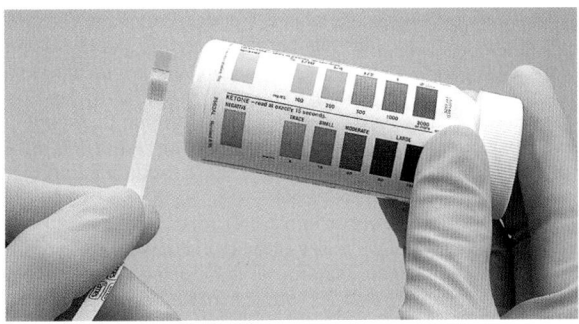

Reagent strip *(Sorrentino, 2008)*

reagin /rē″ājin/ [L, *re* + *agere*], **1.** an antibody associated with human atopy, such as asthma and hay fever. It attaches to mast cells and basophils and sensitizes the skin and other tissues. In antigen-antibody reactions it triggers the release of histamine and other mediators that cause atopic symptoms. **2.** a nonspecific, nontreponemal antibody-like substance found in the serum of individuals with syphilis. It can combine with an antigen prepared as a lipid extract of normal tissue, a phenomenon that constitutes the basis of the serological tests for syphilis. See also **nontreponemal antigen test.** –*reaginic, adj.*

REAL classification [Revised European-American Lymphoma classification], a categorization of lymphomas based on histological criteria. It incorporates all nodal and extranodal lymphoid tumors, including Hodgkin disease.

reality /rē·al″itē/ [L, *res*, factual], the culturally constructed world of perception, meaning, and behavior that members of a culture regard as true.

reality orientation, a formal activity that uses specific approaches to assist confused or disoriented persons toward an awareness of reality, or the "here and now," as by emphasizing the time, day, month, year, situation, and weather.

reality principle, an awareness of the demands of the environment and the need for an adjustment of behavior to meet those demands, expressed primarily by the renunciation of immediate gratification of instinctual pleasures to obtain long-term and future goals. In psychoanalysis this function is held to be performed by the ego. Compare **pleasure principle.**

reality testing, **1.** (in psychoanalysis) an ego function that enables one to differentiate between external reality and an inner imaginative world and to behave in a manner that exhibits an awareness of accepted norms and customs. Impairment of reality testing is indicative of a disturbance in ego functioning that may lead to psychosis. **2.** techniques used to distinguish between reality and fantasy.

reality therapy, a form of psychotherapy developed by William Glasser (1925-2013), an American psychiatrist. Its aims are to help define and assess basic values within the framework of a current situation and to evaluate the person's present behavior and future plans in relation to those values. The emphasis in treatment is on the present rather than the past and on behavior rather than feelings; it focuses on responsible behavior as a means of personal fulfillment.

real time [L, *res,* factual; AS, *tid,* tide], an application of computerized equipment that allows data to be processed with relation to ongoing external events, so that the operators can make immediate diagnostic or other decisions based on the current data output. Ultrasound scanning uses real-time control systems, making results available almost simultaneously with the generation of the input data.

real-time imaging. See **dynamic imaging.**

real-time scanning, the imaging of an entire object, or a cross-sectional slice of the object, at a single moment. To produce such an image, the data must be recorded quickly over a very short time rather than by accumulation over a longer period.

reamer [AS, *ryman,* to make room], **1.** a tool with a straight or spiral cutting edge, used in a rotating motion to enlarge a hole or clear an opening. **2.** (in dentistry) an instrument with a tapered and loosely spiraled metal shaft, used for enlarging, shaping, and cleaning root canals.

reapproximate /rē′əprok″simāt/ [L, *re,* again, *approximare,* to come near], to rejoin tissues separated by surgery or trauma so that their anatomical relationship is restored.

reasonable accommodation /rē″zənəbəl/, an interpretation of the U.S. Americans With Disabilities Act regarding responsibility of an employer to provide an adequate work environment for a disabled but otherwise competent employee. The rule may apply to making facilities accessible, restructuring jobs, reassigning disabled employees to vacant positions, modifying work schedules, acquiring or modifying equipment, and adjusting training materials and examinations. The employer may not be required to provide reasonable accommodation if it can be shown to impose an "undue hardship" on the business operation.

reasonable care [L, *rationalis*], the degree of skill and knowledge used by a competent health practitioner in treating and caring for the sick and injured.

reasonable charge, **1.** (in Medicare) the lowest customary charge by a physician for a service. **2.** the prevailing charge by a group of physicians in the area for a particular service.

reasonable cost, the amount a medical insurer will reimburse for a particular health service based on the cost to the provider for delivering that service.

reasonable person, (in law) a hypothetical person who possesses the qualities that are used as an objective standard on which to judge a defendant's action in a negligence suit. In such suits it must be decided whether or not a reasonable person, under the same circumstances, would have acted in the same way as the defendant.

reasonably prudent person doctrine /rē″zənəblē′/, (in law) the concept that a person of ordinary sense will exercise sound judgment in meeting the needs of another person. It is used as a legal standard in the evaluation of negligence. The conduct of the accused is compared to the reasonably prudent person.

reattachment /rē′ətach″mənt/ [L, *re,* again; OFr, *attachier*], **1.** the rejoining of accidentally severed body parts. **2.** the rejoining of periodontal membrane fibers to the cementum of a tooth and the alveolar bone to restore a loosened tooth.

rebase /rēbās′/ [L, *re,* again, *basis,* base], a process of refitting a denture by replacing or adding to its base material without changing the occlusal relationships of the teeth.

rebirthing /rēbur″thing/, a form of psychotherapy developed by Leonard Orr that focuses on the breath and breathing apparatus. Orr believes the premature severing of the umbilical cord deprives the newborn of oxygen and forces him or her to suddenly learn to breathe through fluid-filled lungs, resulting in panic and terror with every breath taken. The goal of treatment is to overcome the trauma of the birth-damaged breathing apparatus so that the person is able to use the breath as a supportive and creative part of life.

rebound /rē″bound/ [Fr, *rebondir,* to bounce], **1.** recovery from illness. **2.** a sudden contraction of muscle after a period of relaxation, often seen in conditions in which inhibitory reflexes are lost.

rebound congestion, swelling and congestion of the nasal mucosa that follows the vasodilator effects of decongestant medications.

rebound effect. See **aftermovement.**

rebound phenomenon [OFr, *rebondir* + Gk, *phainomenon,* anything seen], a renewal of reflex activity after the stimulus that triggered the original action has been removed. It may be indicative of a lesion of the cerebellum.

rebound tenderness, a sign of inflammation of the peritoneum in which increased pain is elicited by the sudden release of the fingertips pressing on the abdomen. Most examiners check for rebound tenderness in the quadrant opposite the area of pain. One hand is used, with the fingers placed perpendicular to the plane of the abdomen. The area of pain may be diffuse or relatively sharply circumscribed. See also **appendical reflex, peritonitis.**

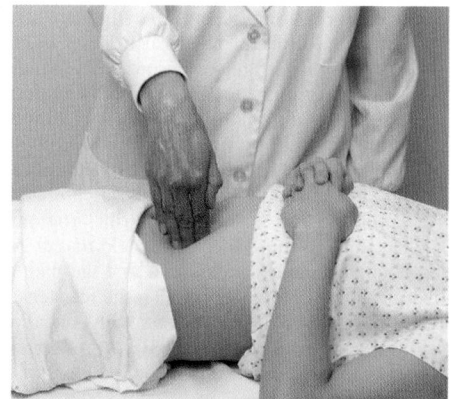
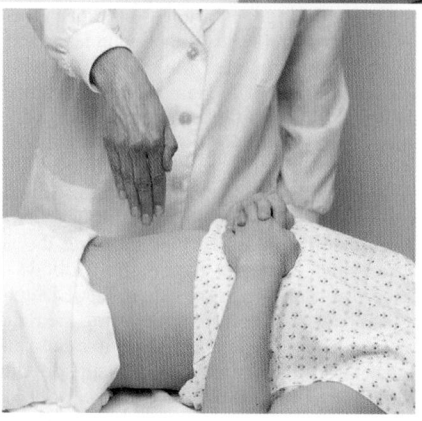

Testing for rebound tenderness *(Wilson and Giddens, 2009)*

rebreather, **1.** a breathing apparatus that allows the breathing of a combination of supplied oxygen and exhaled or room air. **2.** a reservoir mask that allows room air to flow in through ports so that it is mixed with supplied oxygen.

rebreathing /rēbrē'thing/ [L, *re* + AS, *braeth,* breath], breathing in a closed system. Exhaled gas mixes with the gas in the system, and some of this mixture is then reinhaled. Rebreathing, which may result in progressively decreasing concentrations of oxygen and progressively increasing concentrations of carbon dioxide in the blood, can occur in poorly ventilated environments.

rebreathing bag, (in anesthesia) a flexible bag attached to a mask. It may function as a reservoir for anesthetic gases during surgery or for oxygen during resuscitation.

recalcification /rēkal'sifikā"shən/ [L, *re* + *calx,* lime, *facere,* to make], the restoration of lost calcium salts in the body needed for normal neuromuscular excitability, excitation-coupling contraction in cardiac and smooth muscle stimulus-secretion coupling, maintenance of tight junctions between cells, blood clotting, and compressional strength of bone.

recannulate /rēkan'yəlāt/ [L, *re* + *cannula,* small reed], to make a new opening through an organ or tissue, such as opening a passage through an occluded blood vessel.

recapitulation concept /rē'kəpit'yəlā"shən/ [L, *re* + *capitulum,* small head], the notion, formulated by German naturalist Ernst Heinrich Haeckel (1834–1919), that an organism during the course of embryonic development passes through stages that resemble the structural form of species from which it evolved. It is summarized by the statement "ontogeny recapitulates phylogeny." The concept is now regarded as an oversimplification. Also called **biogenetic law, Haeckel law.**

receiver /risē'vər/ [L, *recipere,* to receive], **1.** (in communication theory) the person or persons to whom a message is sent. **2.** the part of a hearing aid that converts electric signals to acoustic signals.

receiver operating characteristic (ROC) curve, a curve that plots the true-positive fraction versus false-positive fraction in diagnostic studies.

receiving sensitivity pattern /risē'ving/, the spatial response of an ultrasound transducer as an echo detector. For a single-element transducer it is essentially the same as the transmitted beam. For transducer arrays it can be quite different from the transmitted beam.

receptive aphasia /risep"tiv/, a form of sensory aphasia marked by impaired comprehension of language. It is generally precipitated by organic impairment such as stroke. Also called **Wernicke aphasia, Wernicke encephalopathy.**

receptor /risep"tər/ [L, *recipere,* to receive], **1.** a chemical structure, usually of protein or carbohydrate, on the surface of a cell that combines with an antigen to produce a discrete immunological component. **2.** a sensory nerve ending that responds to various kinds of stimulation. **3.** a specific cellular protein that must first bind a hormone before cellular response can be elicited. The protein may be in the cytoplasm or in the cell membrane and has a special affinity for toxins and complement-fixing antibodies.

receptor editing, the process in which the light chain of a self-reactive antigen receptor expressed on immature B cells is replaced with another light chain that will not confer autoreactivity.

receptor site [L, *recipere,* to receive, *situs*], a location on a cell surface where certain molecules, such as enzymes, neurotransmitters, or viruses, attach to interact with cellular components.

receptor theory of drug action, the concept that certain drugs produce their effects by acting specifically at a receptor site within the cell or its membrane.

recess /rē"ses, rises"/ [L, *recedere,* to retreat], a small hollow cavity, such as the epitympanic recess in the middle ear or the retrocecal recess extending as a small pocket behind the cecum.

recessive /rises"iv/ [L, *recedere*], pertaining to or describing a gene, the effect of which is masked or hidden if there is a dominant gene at the same locus. If both genes are recessive and produce the same trait, the trait is expressed in the individual.

recessive allele, the member of a pair of alleles that lacks the ability to express itself in the presence of a dominant allele at the same locus. It is expressed only in the homozygous state. Compare **dominant allele.** See also **autosomal-recessive inheritance.**

recessive trait, an inherited characteristic that is determined by a recessive allele.

recidivism (recid) /risid"iviz'əm/ [L, *recidivus,* falling back], a tendency by an ill person to relapse or return to a hospital.

recipient /risip"ē·ənt/ [L, *recipere,* to receive], a person who receives a blood transfusion, tissue graft, or organ.

reciprocal beat /risip"rəkəl/, an atrial or ventricular complex on an electrocardiogram resulting from return of an impulse to its chamber of origin. Also called **echo beat.**

reciprocal change, a change detected electrocardiographically in a wall of the heart opposite the site of a myocardial infarction. In acute inferior wall infarction, reciprocal changes are considered a sign of more extensive myocardial damage.

reciprocal force, (in dentistry) a force applied by an orthodontic anchorage in which the resistance of one or more teeth and their adnexa is used to move one or more opposing teeth and their adnexa.

reciprocal gene. See **complementary gene.**

reciprocal inhibition, **1.** the theory in behavior therapy that, if an anxiety-producing stimulus occurs simultaneously with a response that diminishes anxiety, the stimulus may cause less anxiety. For example, deep chest or abdominal breathing and relaxation of the deep muscles appear to diminish anxiety and pain in childbirth. See also **systemic desensitization. 2.** an early mobility phase that serves a protective function. The muscle acting on one side of a joint (agonist) quickly contracts while its opposite (antagonist) relaxes. An example is seen in infants who randomly flex and extend their arms and legs.

reciprocal translocation, the mutual exchange of genetic material between two nonhomologous chromosomes. Also called **interchange.** Compare **balanced translocation, robertsonian translocation.**

reciprocation /risip"roka'shən/, **1.** (in dentistry) the means by which one part of a removable partial denture framework is made to counter the effect created by another part of the framework. **2.** (in psychology) the giving and receiving that take place in a relationship.

reciprocity /res'ipros"itē/ [Fr, *réciprocité*], a mutual agreement to exchange privileges, dependence, or relationships. An example is an agreement between two governing bodies to accept the medical credentials of nurses or physicians licensed in either community.

Recklinghausen canal /rek"linghou'sən/ [Friedrich D. von Recklinghausen, German pathologist, 1833–1910], the small lymph space in the connective tissues of the body. Also called **von Recklinghausen canal.**

Recklinghausen disease. See **neurofibromatosis.**

Recklinghausen tumor [Friedrich D. von Recklinghausen], a benign tumor, derived from smooth muscle containing connective tissue and epithelial elements, that occurs in the wall of the oviduct or posterior uterine wall. Also called **adenomyosis, von Recklinghausen tumor.**

R

reclining /riklī″ning/, leaning backward. −*recline, v.*

recluse spider. See **brown recluse spider.**

recognition site /rek′əgnish″ən/, a location on a nucleic acid or protein to which a specific ligand binds.

Recognized Continuing Education Evaluation Mechanism (RCEEM), (in radiation therapy) a control process for checking that educational activities meet certain standards and for establishing programs for evaluating educational opportunities and activities.

recombinant /rēkom″binənt/ [L, *re,* again, *combinare,* to combine], **1.** *n.,* a molecule, a cell, or an organism that results from the recombination of genes, regardless of whether naturally or artificially induced. **2.** *adj.,* pertaining to such a molecule, a cell, or an organism. See also **recombinant DNA.**

recombinant DNA, a DNA molecule in which rearrangement of the genes has been experimentally induced. Enzymes are used to break isolated DNA molecules into fragments that are then rearranged in the desired sequence. DNA sequences from another organism of the same or a different species may also be introduced into the molecule, which is then replicated, resulting in both genotypic and phenotypic alterations in the organism that carries the recombinant DNA. See also **genetic engineering.**

recombinant factor VIII concentrate, a concentrate of factor VIII prepared by recombinant DNA technology used to treat bleeding in hemophilia A patients (factor VIII deficiency). See **FVIII.**

recombinant FVIIa concentrate, a concentrate of activated factor VII developed to treat bleeding in hemophilia patients with inhibitors. Activated factor VII acts directly on factor X and bypasses factor VIII or IX activity in the coagulation process.

recombinant human erythropoietin, a glycoprotein that controls red blood cell production. It is produced by recombinant DNA technology.

recombinant tPA. See **tissue plasminogen activator.**

recombinant vaccine, a suspension of attenuated viruses or killed microorganisms developed through recombinant DNA techniques.

recombination /rē′kombinā″shən/ [L, *re* + *combinare*], **1.** the formation of new arrangements of genes within the chromosomes as a result of independent assortment of unlinked genes, crossing over of linked genes, or intracistronic crossing over of nucleotides. See also **recombinant DNA. 2.** the coupling of oppositely charged ions liberated by ionizing radiation. Ionic recombination lowers the total number of charges collected by a dosimeter, thus causing the radiation dose to be underestimated. A technique for determining the magnitude of ionic recombination is routinely applied in accurate dosimetry.

Recombivax HB, brand name for *hepatitis B vaccine (recombinant).*

recommended daily intake (RDI), the daily amount of a nutrient that has been identified as an acceptable level for ingestion for the majority of the population in the United States. See also **recommended dietary allowances.**

recommended dietary allowances (RDAs) /rek′əmen″did/ [L, *re* + *commendere,* to commend], levels of daily intake of essential nutrients judged by the Food and Nutrition Board of the National Research Council to be adequate to meet the known nutrient needs of practically all healthy people.

recon /rē″kon/ [L, *re* + *combinare* + Gk, *ion,* going], the smallest genetic unit that is capable of recombination, thought to be a triplet of nucleotides.

reconstitution /rē′konstit(y)oo″shən/ [L, *re* + *constituere,* to establish], **1.** the continuous repair of tissue damage.

2. the act of mixing or diluting medications or other substances; adding liquid to powdered drugs.

reconstruction time /rē′kənstruk″shən/, the period between the end of a scan and the appearance of an image.

reconstructive mammaplasty, breast reconstruction after mastectomy.

reconstructive surgery. See **plastic surgery.**

record /rek″ərd/, a written form of communication that permanently documents information relevant to the care of a patient. See also **medical record, documentation,** def. 1, **charting, patient record.**

recorded detail /rikôr″did/, the accuracy of structural lines as recorded on a radiographic image.

Recovery, Inc /rikuv″əry/, (Obsolete) now called **Recovery International.**

Recovery International, a self-help group that provides support for persons with mental illness. Formerly called **Recovery, Inc.**

recovery room. See **postanesthesia care unit.**

recreational drug, any substance with pharmacological effects that is taken voluntarily for personal pleasure or satisfaction rather than for medicinal purposes. The term is generally applied to alcohol, barbiturates, amphetamines, THC, PCP, cocaine, and heroin, but it also includes caffeine.

recreational therapist, a person who uses recreational activities to reduce the effects of disability or illness so that patients can function more effectively in their families and communities. A baccalaureate degree is required. The American Therapeutic Recreation Association (ATRA) and the Canadian Therapeutic Recreation Association (CTRA) provide mechanisms for certification.

recreational therapy /rē′krē·ā″shənəl/ [L, *recreare,* to renew], a form of adjunctive treatment in which games or other group activities are used as a means of modifying maladaptive behavior, awakening social interests, or improving the ability to interact and function in socially acceptable ways.

recrudescence /rē′kroodes″əns/ [L, *re* + *crudescere,* to become hard], a return of symptoms of a disease during a period of recovery.

recrudescent /-ənt/ [L, *re* + *crudescere,* to become hard], the return of disease symptoms after a period of remission.

recrudescent hepatitis, a form of acute viral hepatitis marked by a relapse during the period of recovery. A minority of patients experience it, and the prognosis for ultimate recovery is rarely affected.

recrudescent typhus. See **Brill-Zinsser disease.**

recruitment /rikroot″mənt/, **1.** the perception of a rapid growth of loudness, commonly seen in sensorineural hearing losses that are cochlear in nature. The impaired ear cannot hear faint sounds but hears intense sounds as loudly as a normal ear. **2.** in muscle contractions, the ability to recruit additional motor units into action as the need to overcome resistance increases and/or the ability to limit muscle fatigue during prolonged contractions. **3.** (in research) the activities associated with attracting suitable candidates for participation in a study.

rect-, combining form meaning "rectum": *rectal, rectocele, rectovesical.*

recta, rectal. See **rectum.**

rectal abscess /rek″təl/ [L, *rectus,* straight, *abscedere,* to go away], a tender mass of pustular material in the perianal area.

rectal alimentation [L, *rectus,* straight, *alimentum,* nourishment], (Obsolete) the delivery of nourishment in concentrated form by injection or instillation through the rectum. Also called **rectal feeding.**

rectal anesthesia [L, *rectus,* straight], sedation anesthesia achieved by the insertion, injection, or infusion of an anesthetic agent into the rectum. This procedure is sometimes used in children and other patients who may be uncooperative or unable to tolerate medications. Absorption is unpredictable. Once an intravenous catheter can be inserted, the anesthetic is quickly converted to parenteral sedation or a general anesthetic.

rectal cancer. See **colorectal cancer.**

rectal feeding. See **rectal alimentation.**

rectal instillation of medication, the instillation of a medicated suppository, cream, or gel into the rectum. Some conditions treated by this method are constipation, pruritus ani, and hemorrhoids. See also **enema.**

■ METHOD: The patient lies on the left side, with the lower leg extended and the upper leg flexed. The health care provider unwraps the suppository and, wearing a glove, raises the upper buttock, exposing the anus. The suppository may be self-lubricating, or it may need to be lubricated with a water-soluble lubricant. The suppository is then gently inserted past the anal sphincter. The health care provider then wipes the anus with a tissue or piece of toilet paper. Occasionally a drug may be given in a medicated enema.

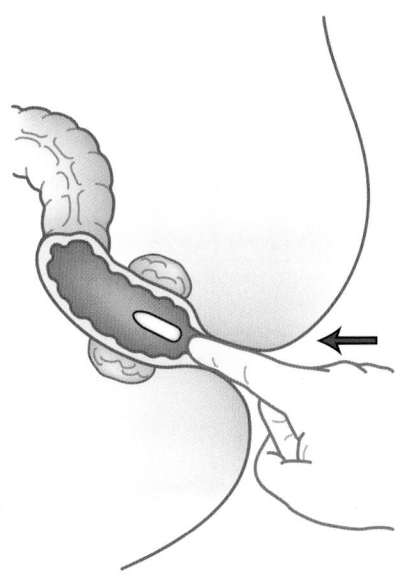

Rectal instillation of medicine *(Harkreader and Hogan, 2007)*

rectal reflex, the normal response (defecation) to the presence of an accumulation of feces in the rectum. Also called **defecation reflex.**

rectal speculum, a medical instrument that enlarges the diameter of the rectum for examination.

rectal stenosis, stenosis or stricture of the rectum. Also called *proctostenosis, rectostenosis.*

rectal temperature [L, *rectus,* straight, *temperatura*], body temperature as measured by a clinical thermometer placed in the rectum. Rectal temperatures average 0.5° F to 0.75° F (0.3° C to 0.4° C) higher than oral temperatures.

rectal thermometer [L, *rectus* + Gk, *thermē,* heat, *metron,* measure], a clinical thermometer suitable for measuring body temperature in the rectum.

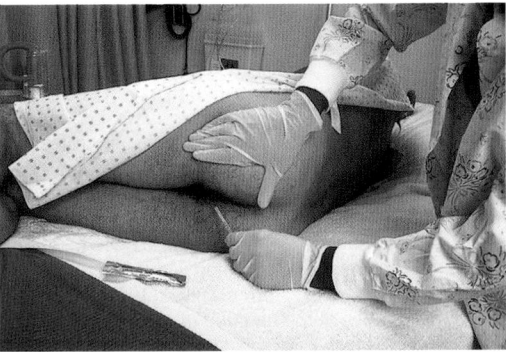

Placement of thermometer for rectal temperature measurement *(Harkreader and Hogan, 2007)*

rectal ultrasound of the prostate, an ultrasound used to diagnose cancer and to help stage rectal cancers.

rectification /rek′tifikā″shən/, **1.** the conversion of alternating current into direct current. **2.** a step in echo signal processing in a pulse-echo ultrasound instrument in which radiofrequency signals, which oscillate both above and below zero volts, are converted.

rectifier /rek′tifī″ər/, an electric device that converts alternating current into pulsating direct current (DC).

rectilinear scanner /rek′tilin″ē·ər/, a device that generates an image of an anatomical structure by detecting radioactivity within the structure.

rectitis. See **proctitis.**

recto-, prefix meaning "straight" or "rectum": *rectoscope, rectosigmoidoscopy.*

rectocele /rek″təsēl′/ [L, *rectus* + Gk, *koilos,* hollow], a protrusion of the rectum and posterior wall of the vagina into the vagina. The condition, which occurs after the muscles of the vagina and pelvic floor have been weakened by childbearing, old age, or surgery, may reflect a congenital weakness in the wall and may, if severe, result in dyspareunia and difficulty in evacuating the bowel. Also called **proctocele.** Compare **cystocele.**

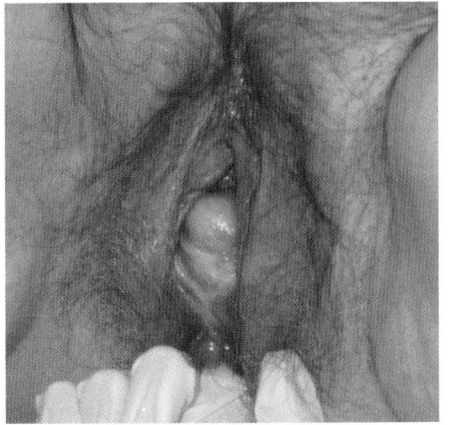

Rectocele protruding from the vaginal introitus *(Townsend et al, 2008)*

rectocolitis, inflammation of the rectum and colon. Also called **coloproctitis.**

rectoplasty. See **proctoplasty.**

R

rectosacral fascia, the fusion of the inferior part of the presacral fascia with the visceral fascia on the posterior aspect of the rectum.

rectoscope, *(Obsolete)* now called **proctoscope.**

rectosigmoid /rek′tōsig″moid/ [L, *rectus* + Gk, *sigma,* the letter S, *eidos,* form], pertaining to the part of the large intestine that includes the lower part of the sigmoid and the upper part of the rectum.

rectosigmoidoscopy /-sig′moidəs″kəpē/ [L, *rectus,* straight; Gk, *sigma,* the letter S, *eidos,* form, *skopein,* to view], the examination of the rectum and pelvic colon with a sigmoidoscope.

rectosigmoid sphincter, circular muscle fibers in the wall of the large intestine at the junction of the sigmoid colon and rectum. Also called *O'Beirne sphincter.*

rectouterine excavation, rectouterine pouch. See **cul-de-sac of Douglas.**

rectovaginal fistula /-vaj″ənəl/ [L, *rectus,* straight, *vagina,* sheath, *fistula,* pipe], an abnormal passage or opening between the rectum and the vagina.

rectovaginal ligament, one of the four main uterine support ligaments. It helps hold the uterus in position by maintaining traction on the cervix. Also called **posterior ligament.**

rectovaginal septum, a band of loose connective tissue between the vagina and the ampulla of the rectum.

rectovesical /-ves″ikəl/ [L, *rectus,* straight, *vesica,* bladder], pertaining to the rectum and bladder.

rectovesical septum, a partition that separates the posterior surface of the vagina from the rectum.

rectum /rek″təm/ *pl.* rectums, recta [L, *rectus*], the lower part of the large intestine, about 12 cm long, continuous with the descending sigmoid colon, proximal to the anal canal. It follows the sacrococcygeal curve, ends in the anal canal, and usually contains three transverse semilunar folds: one situated proximally on the right side, a second one extending inward from the left side, and the third and largest fold projecting caudally. Each fold is about 12 mm wide. The folds overlap when the intestine is empty or defecation occurs. —*rectal, adj.*

rectus abdominis /rek″təs/, one of a pair of anterolateral muscles of the abdomen, extending the whole length of the ventral aspect of the abdomen. The pair is separated by the linea alba. Each rectus arises in a lateral tendon from the crest of the pubis and is interlaced by a medial tendon with the muscle of the opposite side. The rectus abdominis inserts into the fifth, sixth, and seventh ribs. It functions to flex the vertebral column, tense the anterior abdominal wall, and assist in compressing the abdominal contents. Compare **external abdominal oblique muscle, internal abdominal oblique muscle, pyramidalis, transversus abdominis.**

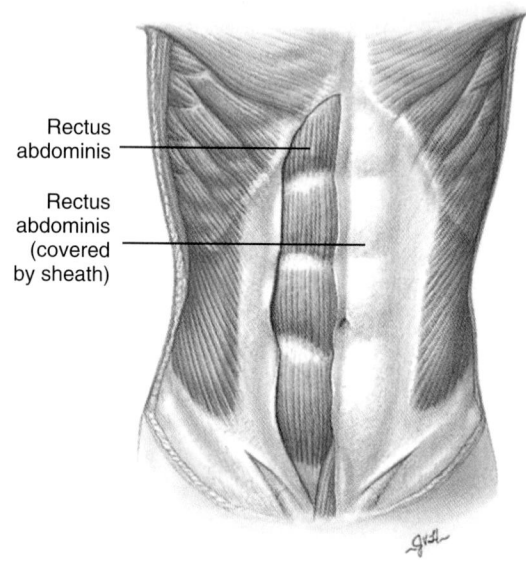

Rectus
abdominis

Rectus
abdominis
(covered
by sheath)

Rectus abdominis muscles *(Thibodeau and Patton, 2003)*

rectus capitis anterior, rectus capitis lateralis. See **rectus muscle.**

rectus capitus posterior. See **rectus muscle.**

rectus femoris, a fusiform muscle of the anterior thigh, one of the four parts of the quadriceps femoris. With the quadriceps group, it functions to extend the lower leg. Compare **vastus intermedius, vastus lateralis, vastus medialis.** See also **quadriceps femoris.**

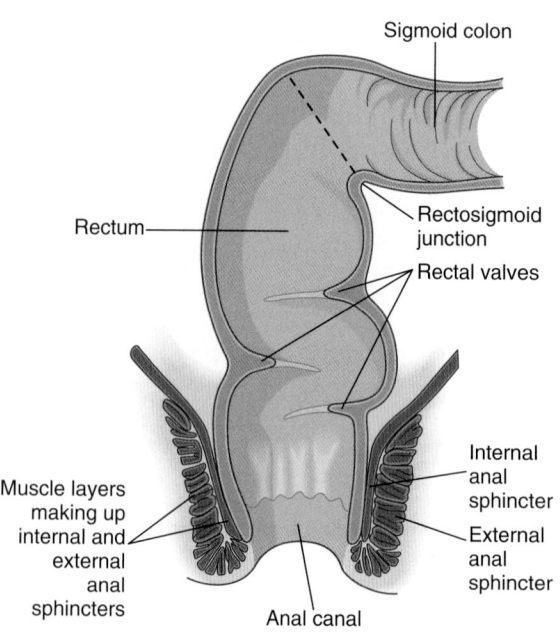

Sigmoid colon

Rectum

Rectosigmoid
junction

Rectal valves

Internal
anal
sphincter

External
anal
sphincter

Muscle layers
making up
internal and
external
anal
sphincters

Anal canal

Rectum *(Leonard, 2009)*

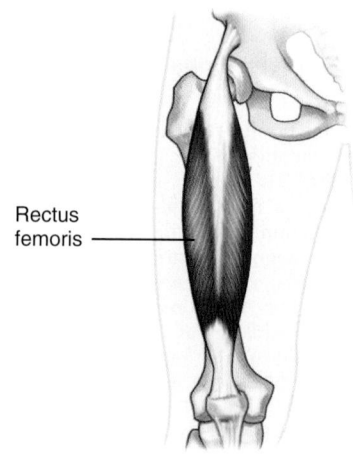

Rectus
femoris

Rectus femoris

rectus muscle [L, straight, *musculus*], a muscle of the body that has a relatively straight form. Also called **rectus capitus posterior.** Kinds include **rectus capitis anterior, rectus capitis lateralis.** See also **rectus abdominis.**

recumbency /rikum″bənsē/ [L, *recumbere,* to lie down], the state of lying down or leaning against something.

recumbent /rikum″bənt/ [L, *recumbere,* to lie down], lying down or leaning backward. See also **reclining. –recumbency,** *n.*

recuperate /rikoo″pərāt/ [L, *recupare,* to regain], to recover one's health and strength.

recuperation /rikoo″pərā″shən/ [L, *recupare,* to regain], the process of recovering health and strength.

recurrence /rikur″əns/ [L, *recurrere,* to run back], the reappearance of a sign or symptom of a disease after a period of remission.

recurrence risk, the chance that a disease first identified in one member of a family will appear in other members of the same genetic lineage.

recurrent /rikur″ənt/ [L, *recurrere,* to run back], returning periodically, as in a *recurrent* sign or symptom of disease.

recurrent bandage [L, *recurrere,* to run back], a strip of cloth that is wrapped several times around itself, usually applied to the head or to a residual limb after amputation.

recurrent caries, an acidic destruction of dental tissues that have previously experienced such destruction and that have previously undergone dental restoration.

recurrent fever. See **relapsing fever.**

recurrent inhibition, central nervous system inhibition of muscle fibers of the same muscle that is contracting, providing more control over movement. Compare **reciprocal inhibition,** def. 2. See also **Renshaw cells.**

recurrent polyserositis. See **familial Mediterranean fever.**

recurrent pregnancy loss, the loss of two or more consecutive pregnancies.

recurrent respiratory papillomatosis, the recurrent growth of benign squamous cell papillomas in the larynx and trachea, caused by the human papillomavirus and leading to a severe narrowing of the airway, which may require frequent treatments. Onset is in childhood or early adulthood.

recurring scarring aphthae. See **Sutton disease.**

recurvatum /rē″kərvā″təm/ [L, *recurvare,* to bend back], backward thrust or bending, for example, of the knee caused by weakness of the quadriceps or a joint disorder.

red blindness, (Nontechnical) a color vision deficiency. See also **protanopia.**

red blood cell. See **erythrocyte.**

red blood cell cast, a urine sediment cast that contains red blood cells, signifying bleeding in the kidney, seen in glomerulonephritis.

red blood cell (RBC) count [AS, *read* + *blod* + L, *cella,* storeroom; Fr, *conter,* to count], a count of the erythrocytes in a specimen of whole blood, commonly made with an electronic counting device. The normal concentrations of RBCs in the whole blood of males are 4.6 to 6.2 million/mm³. In females the concentrations are 4.2 to 5.4 million/mm³.

red blood cell indices. See **red cell indexes.**

red blood cells, a preparation of red blood cells separated from a donor unit of whole blood. It is administered to patients to restore adequate levels of hemoglobin and oxygen-carrying capability without overloading the vascular system with excess fluid.

red blood cell (RBC) survival study, a nuclear scan that is often performed on patients with hemolytic anemia. The test is carried out in two parts. The first determines the half-life of the RBC within the circulation, and the second images the spleen, liver, and pericardium.

Red Book, a book published by the American Academy of Pediatrics, Inc., updated approximately every 3 years, providing evidence-based guidance regarding infectious diseases and immunization practices for infants, children, and adolescents.

red bug. (Nontechnical) See **chigger.**

red cell. See **erythrocyte.**

red cell indexes, a series of relationships that characterize the red cell population in terms of size, hemoglobin content, and hemoglobin concentration. Derived mathematically from the red cell count and hemoglobin and hematocrit values, the indexes are useful in making differential diagnoses of several kinds of anemia. The values reported are the mean corpuscular hemoglobin, the mean corpuscular hemoglobin concentration, and the mean corpuscular volume. Also called *red cell indices,* **red blood cell indices.** See also **iron-deficiency anemia.**

red clover, a preparation of the flower heads of *Trifolium pratense,* used internally for coughs and respiratory symptoms and externally for chronic skin conditions, such as psoriasis and eczema. It is also used in traditional Chinese medicine.

red corpuscle. See **erythrocyte.**

Red Cross. (Informal) See **American Red Cross, International Federation of Red Cross and Red Crescent Societies (IFRC).**

redeye. (Informal) See **allergic conjunctivitis.**

red fever. See **dengue fever.**

red-green blindness, red-green color blindness, (Nontechnical) popular names for any imperfect perception of red and green tints, including all of the most common types of color vision deficiency. See **deuteranomaly, deuteranopsia, protanopia.**

red hepatization. See **hepatization.**

redia /rē″dē·ə/, an elongated second or third larval stage of a fluke of the class Trematoda that develops in a sporocyst and matures into numerous daughter redia (cercariae). See also **cercaria.**

red infarct [AS, *read* + L, *infarcire,* to stuff], a pathological change that occurs in brain tissue that has been rendered ischemic by lack of blood. With restricted blood flow, diapedesis of red blood cells occurs into the parenchyma of the brain without actually producing a well-formed hematoma, producing only infiltration of erythrocytes.

red man syndrome. See **red neck syndrome.** See also **vancomycin.**

red marrow [AS, *read* + AS, *mearh,* marrow], the red vascular substance consisting of connective tissue and blood vessels containing primitive blood cells, macrophages, megakaryocytes, and fat cells. It is found in the cavities of many bones, including flat and short bones, bodies of the vertebrae, sternum, ribs, and articulating ends of long bones. Red marrow manufactures and releases leukocytes, erythrocytes, and thrombocytes into the bloodstream. Compare **yellow marrow.**

red mite. See **chigger.**

red neck syndrome, an allergic reaction to a rapid infusion of the antimicrobial agent vancomycin. It is characterized by flushing, pruritus, and erythema of the head and upper body resulting from histamine release. Also called **red man syndrome.**

redon /rē″don/, the smallest unit of DNA capable of recombination, which may be as small as one base pair. Compare **cistron, muton.**

redox, abbreviation for *reduction-oxidation (reaction).* See **oxidation-reduction reaction.**

red tide. See ***Gonyaulax catenella,*** **shellfish poisoning.**

reduce /rid(y)oos″/ [L, *reducere,* to lead back], **1.** (in surgery) to restore a part to its original position after displacement, as in the reduction of a fractured bone by bringing ends or fragments back into alignment or of a hernia by returning the bowel to its normal position. A fracture may be reduced under local or general anesthesia. If performed by external manipulation alone, the reduction is said to be closed; if surgery is necessary, it is said to be open. See also **fracture, hernia, invagination, traction. 2.** to decrease the amount, size, extent, or number of something, as of body weight.

reducible hernia /rid(y)o͞o″səbəl/ [L, *reducere,* to lead back, *hernia,* rupture], a hernia in which the protruding tissues can be manipulated into a normal position.

reducing agent /rid(y)o͞o″sing/ [L, *reducere,* to lead back, *agere,* to do], a substance that donates electrons to another substance in a chemical reaction.

reducing diet. See **weight-reduction diet.**

reduction /riduk″shən/ [L, *reducere*], **1.** the addition of hydrogen to a substance. Also called **hydrogenation. 2.** the removal of oxygen from a substance. **3.** the decrease in the valence of the electronegative part of a compound. **4.** the addition of one or more electrons to a chemical substance. **5.** the correction of a fracture, hernia, or luxation. **6.** the reduction of data, as in converting interval data to an ordinal or nominal scale of measurement.

reduction division. See **meiosis.**

reductionism /riduk″shəniz′əm/, **1.** an approach that tries to explain a behavior, concept, scientific event, or theory in terms of the simplest facts that are known to be accurate. **2.** (in biology) a belief that knowledge from one area of scientific study (for example, genetics) can be explained by knowledge from another area of study (molecular biology).

reduction ureteroplasty, surgical tapering or plication of the ureter for treatment of megaureter.

red yeast, a eukaryotic fungus used in the production of fermented foods. See **monascus.**

Reed, Pamela G., a nursing theorist who developed the Self-Transcendence Theory. Self-transcendence is the expansion of a person's concept of self through introspection, interaction with other people and the surrounding environment, integration of the past and future, and spirituality. See also **Self-Transcendence Theory.**

Reed-Sternberg cell [Dorothy M. Reed, American pathologist, 1874–1964; Karl Sternberg, Austrian pathologist, 1872–1935], one of a number of large, abnormal, multinucleated reticuloendothelial cells in the lymphatic system found in Hodgkin disease. The number and proportion of Reed-Sternberg cells identified are the basis for the histopathological classification of Hodgkin disease.

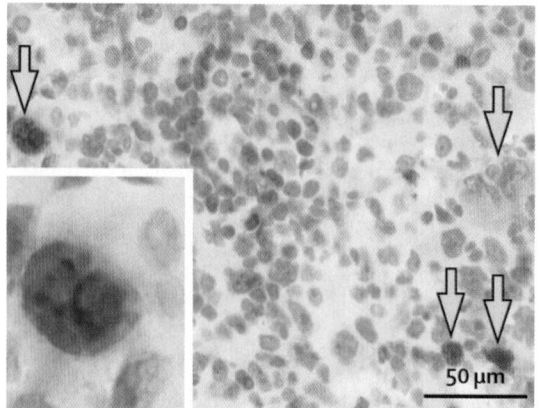

Reed-Sternberg cell *(Courtesy Dr. Robert W. McKenna, Department of Pathology, University of Texas Southwestern Medical School)*

reefer, *(Informal)* marijuana leaves rolled into cigarette paper for smoking. See also **cannabis.**

reentry /rē·en″trē/ [L, *re,* again; Fr, *entrée*], (in cardiology) the reactivation of myocardial tissue for the second or subsequent time by the same impulse. Reentry is one of the most common causes of arrhythmias. For example, paroxysmal supraventricular tachycardia may be caused by sinus nodal reentry, atrioventricular (AV) nodal reentry, or AV reentry by way of the AV node and an accessory pathway; atrial flutter is caused by an atrial macroreentry circuit. Reentry also underlies some forms of ventricular tachycardia and extrasystoles. AV and AV nodal reentry mechanisms may be terminated by a vagal maneuver, adenosine, or procainamide.

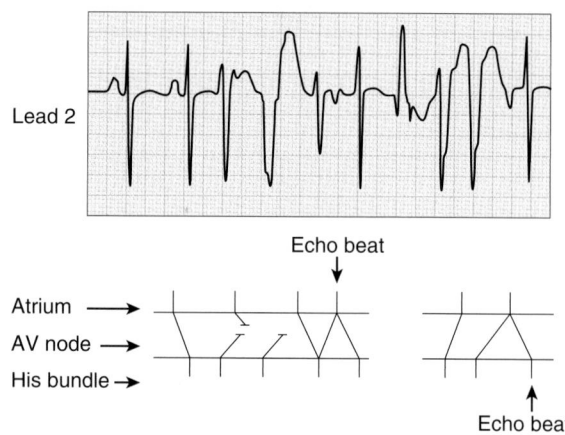

Antegrade and retrograde echo beats caused by AV node reentry *(Mithilesh and Zipes, 2012)*

refeeding /re-fēd′ing/, restoration of normal nutrition after a period of fasting or starvation.

refeeding syndrome, moderate to severe electrolyte and fluid shifts occurring when there is a resumption of nutritional intake after a period of starvation. Hypophosphatemia is common, and heart failure sometimes occurs.

refereed journal /ref′ərēd″/ [L, *referre,* to bring back, *diurnalis,* daily record], a professional or literary journal in which articles or papers are selected for publication by a panel of peers who are experts in the field. They read and evaluate each of the articles submitted for publication. The important national professional journals in health care are refereed.

reference electrode /ref″ərəns/ [L, *referre,* to bring back; Gk, *elektron,* amber, *hodos,* way], an electrode that has an established potential and is used as a reference against which other potentials may be measured.

reference group, a group with which a person identifies or wishes to belong.

reference interval, distribution of test results that are normal for a selected population of healthy persons. Reference intervals are interpreted according to age, sex, and race. Also called *normal range,* **reference range.**

reference intervals, ranges of the normal concentration or activity of blood analytes determined by measuring the analyte in selected healthy subjects. Reference intervals vary by age and ethnicity. Because laboratories use various measurement methods and instruments, reference intervals vary from laboratory to laboratory.

reference range. See **reference interval.**

Liver — Heart — Liver

Stomach

Gallbladder

Small intestine — Ovary

Colon

Appendix — Kidney

Right ureter — Bladder

Typical areas of referred pain *(Lewis et al, 2011)*

referential idea. See **idea of reference.**

referential index deletion /ref′ərən″shəl/, a neurolinguistic programming term that pertains to the omission of the specific person being discussed, such as when a person states "they are responsible" but does not indicate who "they" represents.

referral /rifur′əl/ [L, *referre,* to bring back], a process whereby a patient or the patient's family is introduced to additional health resources in the community, as in helping a patient find an appropriate community health nurse after discharge from a hospital.

referred pain /rifurd″/ [L, *referre + poena,* punishment], pain felt at a site different from that of an injured or diseased organ or body part. For example, angina, the pain of coronary artery insufficiency, may be felt in the left shoulder, arm, or jaw.

referred sensation, a feeling or impression that occurs at a site other than where the stimulus is initiated. Also called **reflex sensation.** See also **sensation,** def. 1.

refined birth rate /rifīnd/ [L, *re + finire,* to finish], (in epidemiology) the ratio of total births to the total female population, considered during a period of 1 year. Compare **birth rate, crude birth rate, true birth rate.**

reflecting /riflek″ting/, a communication technique in which the listener picks up the feeling or tone of the patient's message and repeats it back to the patient. This often includes restatement of selected patient words. It encourages the patient to continue with clarifying comments. It is a means of assisting patients to better understand their own thoughts and feelings.

reflection /riflek″shən/ [L, *reflectere,* to bend back], **1.** a form of reentry in myocardial tissue in which, after encountering delay in one fiber, an impulse enters a parallel fiber and returns retrogradely to its source. **2.** the return or reentry of ultrasound waves where there is a discontinuity in the characteristic acoustic impedance along the propagation path. The intensity of the reflection is related to the difference in the characteristic acoustic impedance across the interface. **3.** the ability of a practitioner to consider factors and to think about process, procedures, intervention, and outcome to learn from experiences. **4.** (in communication theory) a technique in which the listener picks up the feeling or tone of the patient's message and repeats it back to the patient. This often includes restatement of selected patient words. It encourages the patient to continue with clarifying comments. It is a means of assisting patients to better understand their own thoughts and feelings.

reflex /rē″fleks/ [L, *reflectere,* to bend back], **1.** a backward or return flow of energy or of an image, as a reflection. **2.** a reflected action, particularly an involuntary action or movement.

reflex action, the involuntary functioning or movement of any organ or body part in response to a particular stimulus. The function or action occurs immediately, without the involvement of the will or consciousness.

reflex ankle clonus. See **ankle clonus.**

reflex apnea, involuntary cessation of respiration caused by irritating noxious vapors or gases.

reflex arc [L, *reflectere,* to bend back, *arcus,* bow], a simple neurological unit of a sensory neuron that carries a stimulus impulse to the spinal cord, where it connects with a motor neuron that carries the reflex impulse back to an appropriate muscle or gland.

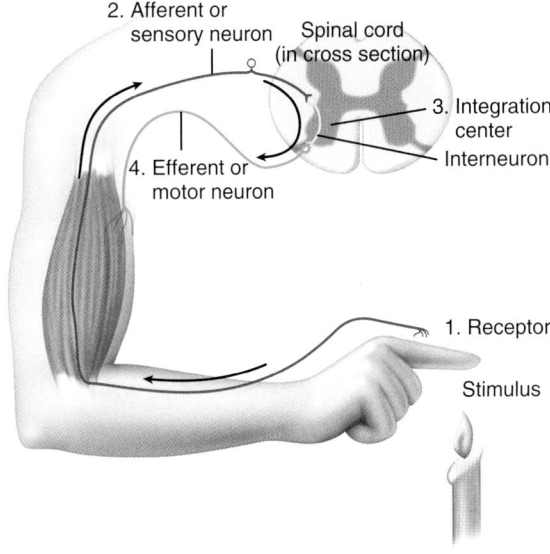

2. Afferent or sensory neuron   Spinal cord (in cross section)

3. Integration center

Interneuron

4. Efferent or motor neuron

1. Receptor

Stimulus

Reflex arc *(Harkreader and Hogan, 2007)*

reflex bladder, contraction of the detrusor muscles not mediated by the brain, causing incontinence. Reflex bladder is common in patients with spinal cord lesions above the sacral area and intact spinal cord segments. Also called **automatic bladder.**

reflex center [L, *reflectere,* to bend back; Gk, *kentron*], any part of the nervous system in which reception of afferent impulses results in a discharge of efferent impulses leading to some change in a muscle or gland.

reflex dyspepsia, an abnormal condition characterized by impaired digestion associated with the disease of an organ not directly involved with digestion. See also **dyspepsia.**

reflex emesis [L, *reflectere,* to bend back; Gk, *emesis,* vomiting], vomiting or gagging that is induced by touching the mucous membrane of the throat or is a result of other noxious stimuli. Also called **gag reflex, vomiting reflex.**

R

reflex hammer [L, *reflectere,* to bend back; AS, *hamer*], a percussion mallet with a rubber head used to tap tendons, nerves, or muscles to elicit reflex reactions.

reflex incontinence, the urinary incontinence that accompanies detrusor muscle hyperreflexia.

reflex inhibiting pattern (RIP), **1.** a conscious set of neuromuscular actions directed toward inhibition of a natural reflex. Examples include actions taken to suppress a sneeze and the learned inhibitions of toilet training. **2.** a set or positions that inhibit abnormal muscle tone. See also **Bobath, Karel and Berta, neurodevelopmental treatment.**

reflexology /rē′fleksol″əjē/, an alternative medicine technique that uses reflex points on the hands and feet. Pressure is applied at points that correspond to various body parts with the intention of eliminating blockages thought to produce pain or disease. The goal is to bring the body into balance.

reflex seizure, a seizure, which may be partial or generalized, triggered by a sensory stimulus, which may be tactile, visual, auditory, or musical.

reflex sensation. See **referred sensation.**

reflex sympathetic dystrophy (RSD), a diffuse, persistent pain involving central reorganization of sensory processing. It is characterized by vasomotor disorders, limited joint mobility, and trophic changes. The condition usually follows an injury to an afferent pathway and affects an extremity. Also called **complex regional pain syndrome.**

reflex tachycardia [L, *reflectere,* to bend back; Gk, *tachys,* fast, *kardia,* heart], a rapid heart sinus rhythm caused by a variety of autonomic nervous system effects, such as blood pressure changes, fever, or emotional stress.

reflex vasodilation [L, *reflectere,* to bend back, *vas,* vessel, *dilatare,* to spread out], any blood vessel dilation that results from stimulation of vasodilator nerves or inhibition of vasoconstrictors of the sympathetic nervous system, including by epinephrine-type drugs.

reflux /rē″fluks/ [L, *refluere,* to flow back], an abnormal backward or return flow of a fluid. Kinds include **gastroesophageal reflux, hepatojugular reflux, vesicoureteral reflux.**

reflux esophagitis, esophageal irritation and inflammation that result from reflux of the stomach contents into the esophagus. See also **gastroesophageal reflux.**

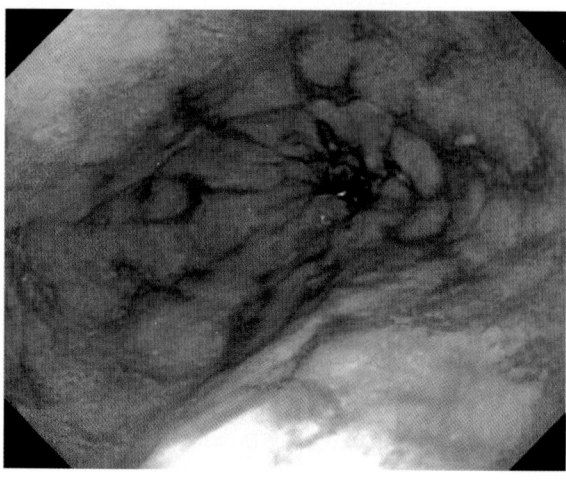

Reflux esophagitis: endoscopic view *(Goldman et al, 2012)*

reflux laryngitis, a burning sensation in the hypopharynx and larynx caused by nocturnal gastric reflux. It occurs most commonly in older patients who sleep in the recumbent position.

refracting angle. See **angle of refraction.**

refracting medium, the transparent tissues and fluid of the eye that refract light.

refraction /rifrak″shən/ [L, *refringere,* to break apart], **1.** *n.,* the change of direction of energy as it passes from one medium to another of different density. **2.** *n.,* an examination to determine and correct refractive errors of the eye. **3.** *n.,* (in ultrasonography) the phenomenon of bending wave fronts as the acoustic energy propagates from the medium of one acoustic velocity to a second medium of differing acoustic velocity. **4.** *adj.,* pertaining to the recovery period after an action potential either in muscular or nervous tissue. —*refractive, adj.*

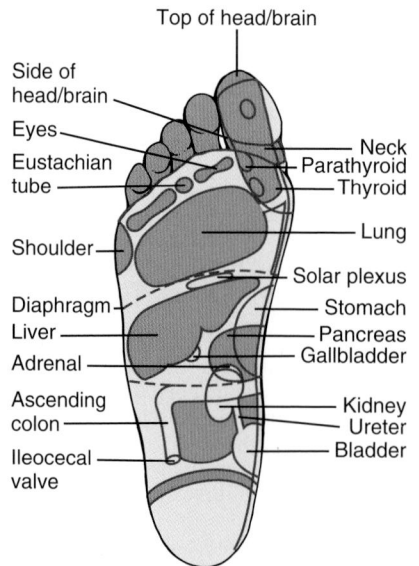
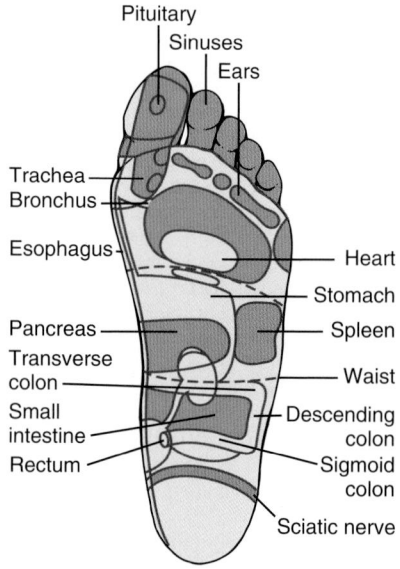

Reflexology foot maps *(Swartz, 2009)*

refraction of eye [L, *refringere*, to break apart; AS, *eage*], the deflection of light from a straight path through the eye by various ocular tissues, including the cornea, lens, aqueous humor, and vitreous body.

refractive error /rifrak″tiv/, a defect in the ability of the lens of the eye to focus an image accurately, as occurs in nearsightedness and farsightedness.

refractive index, a numeric expression of the refractive power of a medium as compared with that of air, which has a refractive index value of 1. The refractive index is related to the number, charge, and mass of vibrating particles in the material through which light is passing and may be used as a measure of the total solids in a solution.

refractive keratotomy (RK), a surgical procedure in which a varying number of radial or perpendicular incisions are made to flatten the cornea, resulting in the elimination or reduction of myopia or astigmatism. Incisions are made partially through the cornea sparing the central cornea. This type of refractive surgery has been largely replaced by newer methods using lasers. See also **radial keratotomy.**

refractometer /rē′frəktom″ətər/ [L, *refringere*, to break apart; Gk, *metron*, measure], an instrument for measuring the refractive index of a substance, used primarily for measuring the refractivity of solutions. See also **refractive index.**

refractoriness /rifrak″tôrines′/, the property of excitable tissue that determines how closely together two action potentials can occur.

refractory /rifrak″tərē/ [L, *refringere*], **1.** pertaining to a disorder that is resistant to treatment. **2.** pertaining to a property of conductive tissue to return to its original state in preparation for a second stimulus.

refractory medium. See **medium.**

refractory period, the time from phase 0 to the end of phase 3 of the action potential, divided into effective and relative. In pacing terminology, the period during which a pulse generator is unresponsive to an input signal of specified amplitude. The effective refractory period is from phase 0 to approximately −60 mV during phase 3 of the action potential, a time during which it is impossible for the myocardium to respond with a propagated action potential, or even to a strong stimulus. The relative refractory period is from approximately −60 mV during phase 3 to the end of phase 3 of the action potential, the time during which a depressed response is possible to a strong stimulus. Also called *refractory phase, refractory state.*

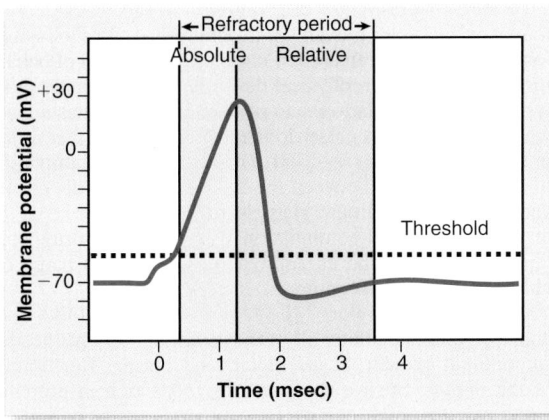

Refractory period *(Patton and Thibodeau, 2010)*

reframing /rēfrā″ming/, changing the conceptual and/or emotional viewpoint in relation to which a situation is experienced and placing it in a different frame that fits the "facts" of a concrete situation equally well, thereby changing its entire meaning.

Refsum syndrome /ref″sŏŏm/ [Sigvald Refsum, Norwegian physician, 1907–1991], a rare hereditary disorder of lipid metabolism in which phytanic acid cannot be broken down. It is characterized by ataxia, abnormalities of the bones and skin, peripheral neuropathy, cardiomyopathy, deafness, and retinitis pigmentosa. Foods containing phytanic acid must be avoided to prevent progressive deterioration. Also called **phytanic acid storage disease.**

refusal of treatment, the right of a patient to refuse treatment after the physician has informed the patient of the diagnosis, prognosis, available alternative interventions, risks and benefits of those options, and risk and probable outcome of no intervention.

regeneration /rijen′ərā″shən/, the process of repair, reproduction, or replacement of lost or injured cells, tissues, or organs. Also called **neogenesis.**

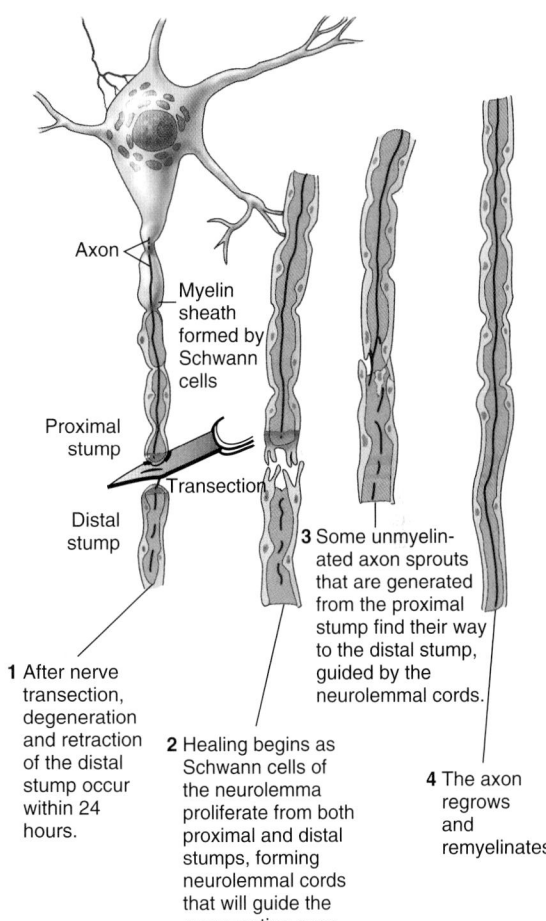

Regeneration of a nerve *(Ignatavicius and Workman, 2010)*

regimen /rej″imən/ [L, guidance], a strictly regulated and/or organized therapeutic program such as a diet or exercise schedule.

regional /rē″jənəl/ [L, *regio*, territory], pertaining to a geographic area, such as a regional medical facility, or to a part of the body, such as regional anesthesia.

regional anatomy, the study of the structural relationships among the organs and the parts of the body. Kinds include **surface anatomy, cross-sectional anatomy.**

regional anesthesia, 1. anesthesia provided by injecting a local anesthetic to block a group of sensory nerve fibers. The tissues are anesthetized layer by layer, as the surgeon approaches the deeper structures of the body. Regional anesthesia has largely replaced local anesthesia for major procedures. Compare **general anesthesia, local anesthesia, topical anesthesia.** Kinds include **Bier block, brachial plexus anesthesia, caudal anesthesia, conduction anesthesia, epidural anesthesia/analgesia, paracervical block, pudendal block, spinal anesthesia.** See also **anesthesia.** 2. (in dentistry) the loss of sensation to pain, temperature, and pressure of a tooth, teeth, jaw, and soft tissue caused by deposit of a local anesthetic agent in close proximity to a nerve or nerves. Compare **block anesthesia,** def. 2, **local infiltration of anesthesia.** Kinds include *posterior superior alveolar block, middle superior alveolar block, anterior superior alveolar block.*

regional control, the control of cancer in sites that represent the first stages of spread from the local origin.

regional enteritis. See **Crohn's disease.**

regional hyperthermia, the elevation of temperature over an extended volume of tissue.

regionalization /rē′jənal′īzā″shən/, (in health care planning) the organization of a system for the delivery of health care within a region to avoid costly duplication of services and to ensure availability of essential services.

region of interest (ROI), (in radiography) an area on a digital image that circumscribes a desired anatomical location. Image processing systems permit drawing of ROIs on images. The average parametric value is computed for all pixels within the ROI and returned to the operator.

region of recombination, (in radioassay) the first stage of amplitude of an electric signal in a gas-filled radiation detector when the voltage is very low. No electrons are attracted to the central electrode, and ion pairs produced in the chamber will recombine.

regiospecific, pertaining to a chemical reaction favoring a single positional or structural isomer.

register /rej″istər/ [L, *regerere,* to bring back], in computed tomography, a device in the central processing unit that stores information for future use.

registered dental hygienist. See **dental hygienist.**

registered dietitian (RD) /rej″istərd/, a professional trained in foods and the management of diets (dietetics). In the United States, registered dietitians are credentialed by the Commission on Dietetic Registration of the American Dietetic Association; in Canada, by the provincial regulatory body. Credentialing is based on completion of a B.S. or M.S. degree program and an approved dietetic internship; dietitians must also pass a registration examination.

registered health information administrator (RHIA®), an expert in managing patient health information and medical records. The RHIA is also responsible for the administration of computer information systems.

registered nurse (RN), 1. (in the United States) a nurse who has completed a course of study at a state-approved school of nursing and passed the National Council Licensure Examination® (NCLEX®). A registered nurse may use the initials RN after the signature. RNs are licensed to practice by individual states; however, the Nursing Licensure Compact (NLC) is an agreement among states that allows nurses to have one license but the ability to practice in other states that are part of the agreement. 2. (in Canada) a nurse who has completed a course of study (now a baccalaureate degree) at an approved school of nursing and passed the NCLEX®-Canada, administered by the Canadian Nurses Association (CNA). See also **nurse, nursing.**

registered record administrator (RRA), *(Obsolete)* now called **registered health information administrator.**

registered respiratory therapist (RRT), an allied health professional with expertise in the scientific knowledge and theory of clinical problems of respiratory care. Duties include the collection and evaluation of patient data to determine an appropriate care plan, selection and assembly of equipment, conduction of therapeutic procedures, and modification of prescribed plans to achieve one or more specific objectives. In the United States, the National Board for Respiratory Care certifies the RRT. In Canada, RRT certification is granted by the Canadian Society of Respiratory Therapists.

registered technologist (RT), 1. (in radiology) a medical imaging or radiation therapy professional who is certified by the American Registry of Radiologic Technologists or equivalent or holds an unrestricted license in medical imaging or radiation therapy under state statute in one or more radiological specialties. See also **radiologic technologist.** 2. *(Informal)* (in a health care facility) an allied health professional who specializes in a particular health care field and qualifies for registration and/or certification in that specialty. Kinds include **medical technologist, cardiovascular technologist, sleep technologist.**

registered trademark®, a designation that a product has been legally recorded in an official government record as being owned by an entity. Companies that manufacture medications and durable medical products register a trademark to indicate they have exclusive rights to use a particular name. See also **trademark.**

registrar /rej″isträr/, an administrative officer whose responsibility is to maintain the records of an institution.

registration /rej′istrā″shən/ [L, *registratio*], 1. a learning or memory recorded in the central nervous system of an impression resulting from a stimulus. 2. the recording of vital personal information such as health data. 3. the recording of professional qualification information relevant to government licensing regulations.

registry /rej″istrē/ [L, *regerere,* to bring back], 1. an office or agency in which lists and records pertaining to employment are maintained for nurses, occupational and physical therapists, and other health care professionals. 2. (in epidemiology) a listing service for incidence data pertaining to the occurrence of specific diseases or disorders, such as a tumor registry.

Regitine, an alpha-adrenergic blocking agent. Brand name for **phentolamine.**

regression /rigresh″ən/ [L, *regredi,* to go back], 1. a retreat or backward movement in conditions, signs, or symptoms. 2. a return to an earlier, more primitive form of behavior. 3. a tendency in physical development to become more typical of the population than of the parents, such as a child who attains a height closer to the average than to that of tall or short parents. −*regress, v.* 4. (in statistics) an examination of the relationship between the independent and dependent variables. See also **linear regression.**

Regroton, a fixed-combination cardiovascular drug containing a diuretic and an antihypertensive. Brand name for **chlorthalidone, reserpine.**

regular diet /reg″yələr/ [L, *regula,* rule], a full, well-balanced diet containing all of the essential nutrients needed for optimal growth, tissue repair, and normal functioning of the organs. Such a diet contains foods rich in proteins, carbohydrates, high-quality fats, minerals, and vitamins in proportions that meet the specific caloric requirements of the individual. Also called **normal diet.**

regular insulin, a short-acting insulin prescribed in the treatment of diabetes mellitus when the desired action is relatively prompt, intense, and short-acting. The onset of action is between 30 and 60 minutes. The peak is in 2 to 3 hours, and the duration of action is approximately 8 to 10 hours. Regular insulin can be mixed with long-acting forms of insulin. Compare **intermediate-acting insulin, long-acting insulin, rapid-acting insulin.**

regulative cleavage. See **indeterminate cleavage.**

regulative development /reg″yəlā′tiv/ [L, *regula,* rule], a type of embryonic development in which the fertilized ovum undergoes indeterminate cleavage, producing blastomeres that have similar developmental potencies and are each capable of giving rise to a single embryo. Determination of the particular organs and parts of the embryo occurs during later stages of development and is influenced by inductors and intercellular interaction. Damage or destruction of various cells during the early stages of development results in readjustments and substitutions so that a normal organism is formed. Compare **mosaic development.**

regulator /reg′yəlā′tər/, (in genetics) the part of a DNA molecule undergoing replication that controls the replication and coordinates with cell division.

regulator gene /reg″yəlā′tər/, a gene that regulates or suppresses the activity of one or more structural genes. Also called **repressor gene.**

regulatory CD4 T cell (Treg), a subset of CD4 T cells that can inhibit inflammatory immune responses. Tregs can suppress the immune response either via secretion of anti-inflammatory cytokines, such as IL-10 or TGF beta, or via direct interaction with other immune cells, such as dendritic cells.

regulatory HIV gene, one of a set of genes in the genome of the human immunodeficiency virus (HIV) that influences the expression of other HIV genes. One regulatory gene (tat) stimulates expression, a second (nef) may inhibit expression, and a third (rev) provides feedback to the others.

regulatory sequence /reg″yələtôr′ē/ [L, *regula + sequi,* to follow], a series of DNA nucleotides that regulate the expression of a gene.

regurgitant menstruation. See **retrograde menstruation.**

regurgitant murmur /rigur″jitənt/ [L, *re + gurgitare,* to flow back, *murmur,* humming], a heart murmur caused by the backflow of blood through the partly closed cusps of a defective valve. Kinds include **diastolic murmur, systolic murmur.**

regurgitation /rēgur′jitā″shən/ [L, *re,* again, *gurgitare,* to flow back], **1.** the backward flow from the normal direction, as the return of swallowed food into the mouth. **2.** the backward flow of blood through a defective heart valve, named for the affected valve, as in aortic regurgitation. See also **reflux.**

regurgitation jaundice [L, *re + gurgitare,* again to flow back; Fr, *jaune,* yellow], jaundice caused by bile pigment entering the blood and lymphatic systems as a result of biliary obstruction.

rehabilitation (rehab) /rē′habil′itā″shən/ [L, *re + habitalas,* aptitude], the restoration of an individual or a part to the previous level of function or the highest level of function possible after a disabling disease, injury, addiction, or incarceration. Compare **habilitation.**

rehabilitation center, a facility providing therapy, counseling, mental health care, and other services for rehabilitation. The center may offer occupational therapy, physical therapy, speech therapy, specialized nursing care, vocational education, and individualized therapies to promote the achievement of the goals established with the patient, his or her family, and the rehabilitation team. See also **rehabilitation.**

rehabilitation counselor, a human services professional who helps clients with emotional or physical disabilities. Rehabilitation counselors work with clients to overcome or manage the personal, social, and physical effects of disabilities on employment or independent living. Rehabilitation counselors may earn certification from the Commission on Rehabilitation Counselor Certification and are eligible for licensure by nearly all states that regulate counselors. Most certified rehabilitation counselors practice in the United States; those who practice in Canada are known as Canadian Certified Rehabilitation Counselors (CCRCs).

rehabilitation teacher, a specialized, university-educated, and certified professional who teaches independent living skills to individuals who are blind or visually impaired, as well as communication skills using Braille and the use of assistive technology. Rehabilitation teachers are integral members of multidisciplinary service teams, providing consultations and referrals to community services that are unique to visual impairments. The National Blindness Professional Certification Board (NBPCB) offers the National Certification in Rehabilitation Teaching for the Blind (NCRTB) as a five-year renewable certification, awarded to those who successfully meet all established requirements.

Rehfuss stomach tube /rā″fəs/ [Martin E. Rehfuss, American physician, 1887–1964], a specially designed gastric tube with a graduated syringe, used for withdrawing specimens of the contents of the stomach for study after a test meal.

rehydration /rē′hīdrā″shən/ [L, *re* + Gk, *hydor,* water], restoration of normal water balance in a patient by giving fluids orally or intravenously.

Reid's baseline [Robert W. Reid, Scottish anatomist, 1851–1939], the baseline of the skull, a hypothetic line extending from the inferior orbital ridge to the center of the aperture of the external auditory meatus. Also called **Frankfurt line.**

Reifenstein's syndrome /rī″fənstīnz/ [Edward C. Reifenstein, Jr., American physician, 1908–1975], male hypogonadism of unknown origin marked by azoospermia, undescended testes, gynecomastia, testosterone deficiency, and elevated gonadotropin titers. The condition appears to be inherited as an X-linked recessive trait, but no chromosomal abnormality has been identified.

reiki /ra′ke/, a Japanese healing tradition with the goal of rebalancing the complex energy systems that compose the body when they have become out of balance.

reiki therapy /rī″kē/, a complementary therapy in which a practitioner places his or her hands on or above a specific body area and transfers what is called "universal life energy" to the patient. That energy, it is claimed, provides the strength, harmony, and balance necessary to treat health disturbances. Reiki sessions are generally held in a quiet setting in comfortable surroundings and may be as short as 5 minutes for treatment of a specific part of the body or as long as an hour for a full-body treatment.

reimbursement /rē′imburs″mənt/ [L, *re + im,* in; Fr, *bourse,* purse], a method of payment, usually by a third-party payer, for medical treatment, therapies, or hospital costs.

reimplantation /rē′im·plan·tā′shən/, the reinsertion of tissue or a structure, such as a tooth, into the site from which it was previously lost or removed.

reinfection /rē′infek″shən/, a second infection by the same microorganism either after recovery or during the original infection.

reinforcement /rē′infôrs″mənt/ [L, *re* + Fr, *enforcir,* to strengthen], (in psychology) a process in which a response is strengthened by the fear of punishment or the anticipation of reward.

R

reinforcement-extinction, (in psychology) a process of socialization in which one learns to engage in certain behaviors (reinforcement) or to avoid certain behaviors (extinction). The anticipated result is that the reinforced behaviors become habitual and those that undergo extinction disappear.

reinforcer /rē'infôr″sər/, (in psychology) a stimulus that increases the probability that a behavior will recur.

Reiter syndrome /rī'tər/ [Hans Reiter, German physician, 1881–1969], an arthritic disorder predominantly of adult males resulting from infection with *Shigella flexneri, Salmonella, Yersinia,* or *Chlamydia* or from enterocolitis. See also **dactylitis, reactive arthritis.**
■ OBSERVATIONS: Reiter syndrome most often affects the ankles, feet, and sacroiliac joints and is usually associated with conjunctivitis and urethritis. The onset may be marked by unexplained diarrhea and low-grade fever, followed in 2 to 4 weeks by conjunctivitis. Superficial ulcers may form lesions on the palms and the soles. Arthritis usually persists after the conjunctivitis and urethritis subside, but it may become episodic.
■ INTERVENTIONS: Treatment includes a short course of tetracycline to treat the infection and phenylbutazone to relieve pain and inflammation in the joint.
■ PATIENT CARE CONSIDERATIONS: Sexual partners should be tested. Recovery is expected, but recurrent arthritic symptoms may continue for several years.

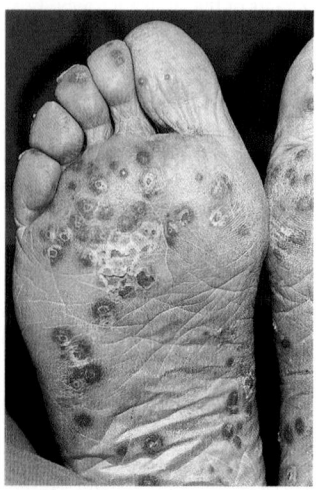

Superficial ulcers associated with Reiter syndrome
(Moll, 1997)

reject analysis /rē'jekt/, (in radiology) a quality assurance protocol; the study of rejected radiographic images to determine the cause for their being discarded.

rejection /rijek″shən/ [L, *re + jacere,* to throw], **1.** an immunological attack against organisms or substances that the immune system recognizes as foreign, including grafts and transplants. See also **acute rejection, chronic rejection. 2.** the act of excluding or denying affection to another person.

rejunctive /rijungk″tiv/, (in psychotherapy) pertaining to a relationship that is characterized by moves toward trustworthy relatedness.

rejuvenation /rējoo′vənā″shən/ [L, *re + juvenis,* youth], the restoration of youthful health and vitality.

relapse /rilaps″/ [L, *relabi,* to slide back], **1.** *v.,* to exhibit again the symptoms of a disease from which a patient appears to have recovered. **2.** *n.,* the recurrence of a disease after apparent recovery.

relapsing [L, *relabi,* to slide back], pertaining to the return of disease after a period of apparent recovery.

relapsing fever, any one of several acute infectious diseases marked by recurrent febrile episodes, caused by various strains of the spirochete *Borrelia.* The disease is transmitted by both lice and ticks and is often seen during wars and famines. It has occurred in several western states of the United States but is more commonly found in South America, Asia, and Africa. See also ***Borrelia duttonii.***
■ OBSERVATIONS: The first episode usually starts with a sudden high fever (104° F to 105° F, or 40° C to 40.56° C), accompanied by chills, headache, neuromuscular pains, and nausea. A rash may appear over the trunk and extremities, and jaundice is common during the later stages. Each attack lasts 2 or 3 days and culminates in a crisis of high fever, profuse sweating, and a rise in heart and respiratory rate. This is followed by an abrupt drop in temperature and a return to normal blood pressure.
■ INTERVENTIONS: Penicillins and tetracycline have been the treatment of choice in relapsing fever. A number of other antibiotics are also employed. Other interventions are supportive.
■ PATIENT CARE CONSIDERATIONS: People typically relapse after 7 to 10 days of normal temperature. Mortality rates can be high; however, survivors eventually recover completely. In louse-borne disease there is usually only a single relapse; in tick-borne disease several successively milder relapses may occur.

relapsing polychondritis, a rare disease of unknown cause resulting in inflammation and destruction of cartilage with replacement by fibrous tissue. Autoimmunity may be involved in this condition. Most commonly the ears and noses of middle-aged people are affected with episodes of tender swelling, often accompanied by fever, arthralgias, and episcleritis. Consequences include floppy ears, collapsed nose, hearing loss, or hoarseness and airway obstruction because of laryngeal and tracheal cartilage involvement. Corticosteroids suppress the activity of the disease.

relation searching /rilā″shən/ [L, *relatio*], a research strategy used to discover and describe relationships between and among variables. For example, it may be used to describe various nursing situations to examine the efficacy of certain aspects of nursing care.

relative biological effectiveness (RBE) /rel″ətiv/ [L, *relatio*], a measure of the cell-killing ability of a particular radiation compared with that of 250 keV x-rays. The ratio of the number of cells killed with the test radiation over the number killed with the 250 keV radiation is the RBE.

relative centrifugal force (RCF), a method of comparing the force generated by various centrifuges on the basis of the speeds of rotation and distances from the center of rotation.

relative cephalopelvic disproportion. See **cephalopelvic disproportion.**

relative growth, the comparison of the various increases in size of similar organisms, tissues, or structures at different time intervals.

relative humidity (r/h), the amount of moisture in the air compared with the maximum the air could contain at the same temperature.

relative molecular mass. See **molecular mass.**

relative periodontal pocket. See **periodontal pocket.**

relative pocket. See **periodontal pocket.**

relative refractory period. See **refractory period.**

relative risk, the ratio of the chance of a disease developing among members of a population exposed to a factor compared with a similar population not exposed to the factor. In many cases the relative risk is modified by the duration or intensity of exposure to the causative factors.

relative sterility [L, *relatio + sterilis,* barren], a condition of infertility in which one or more factors tend to reduce the chances of becoming pregnant. See also **sterility.**

relative value unit (RVU), a comparable service measure used by hospitals to permit comparison of the amounts of resources required to perform various services within a single department or between departments. It is determined by assigning weight to such factors as personnel time, level of skill, and sophistication of equipment required to render patient services. RVUs are a common method used with bonus plans based partially on productivity.

relativism. See **cultural relativism.**

relax /rilaks′/ [L, *relaxare,* to ease], to reduce tension or anxiety.

relaxant /rilak″sənt/ [L, *relaxare,* to ease], a drug or other agent that tends to reduce tension, as a muscle relaxant or bowel relaxant.

relaxation /rē′laksā″shən/ [L, *relaxare,* to ease], **1.** a reducing of tension, as when a muscle relaxes between contractions. **2.** (in magnetic resonance imaging) the return of excited nuclei to their normal unexcited state by the release of energy.

relaxation response, a protective mechanism against stress that brings about decreased heart rate, lower metabolism, and decreased respiratory rate. It is the physiological opposite of the "fight or flight," or stress, response.

relaxation therapy, treatment in which patients are taught to perform breathing and relaxation exercises and to concentrate on a pleasant situation. An integral part of the Lamaze method of childbirth, relaxation therapy is also used to relieve various kinds of pain and physical manifestations of stress. Various yoga exercises and aspects of hypnotherapy may be included in the treatment program, and biofeedback techniques may be used to demonstrate actions that induce relaxation. Some patients learn through relaxation therapy to relax taut muscles at will, to abort migraine attacks, or to reduce their blood pressure. See also **Lamaze method.**

relaxation time, (in magnetic resonance imaging) the characteristic time it takes for a sample of atoms, whose nuclei have first been aligned along a static magnetic field and then excited to a higher-energy state by a radiofrequency (rf) signal, to return to a lower-energy equilibrium state. Two time parameters are used to describe the return, or relaxation, to the equilibrium state once the rf signal is turned off: T_1 describes the relaxation of the system of spins into a condition of thermal equilibrium with its surroundings. T_2 describes the relaxation of the energy that is traded within the system itself. Maps of the values of T_1 or T_2 as a function of position in the cross-sectional view constitute magnetic resonance images. Also called **transverse relaxation time.**

relaxin /rilak″sin/, a polypeptide hormone used to relax the pelvic ligaments and dilate the cervix during labor.

releasing hormone (RH), one of several peptides produced by the hypothalamus and secreted directly into the anterior pituitary gland via a connecting vein. Each of the releasing hormones stimulates the pituitary to secrete a specific tropic hormone. Thus corticotropic-releasing hormone stimulates the pituitary to secrete adrenocorticotropic hormone, whereas growth hormone–releasing hormone stimulates the secretion of growth hormone. Formerly called *releasing factor.*

releasing stimulus, (in psychology) an action or behavior by one individual that serves as a cue to trigger a response in others. An example is yawning by one person, which results in yawning by others in the group.

reliability /rilī′əbil″itē/ [L, *religare,* to fasten behind], (in research) the extent to which a test measurement or device produces the same results with different investigators, observers, or administration of the test over time. If repeated use of the same measurement tool on the same sample produces the same consistent results, the measurement is considered reliable. Compare **validity.**

relief area [L, *relevare,* to lighten], the part of the tissue surface under a prosthesis on which pressure is reduced or eliminated.

relieve /rē·lēv′/ [L, *relevare,* to lighten], to mitigate or remove pain or distress.

relieving factor /rilē″ving/, an agent that alleviates a symptom.

religiosity /rilij′ē·os″itē/ [L, *religiosus*], a psychiatric symptom characterized by the demonstration of excessive or affected piety.

-relin, suffix for prehormones or hormone-release stimulating peptides: *sermorelin.*

reline /rēlīn′/ [L, *re + linea*], the resurfacing of the tissue side of a denture with new base material. Compare **rebase.**

-relix, suffix for hormone release–inhibiting peptides: *cetrorelix.*

rem /rem, är″ē′em′/, conventional unit for a dose of ionizing radiation that produces in humans the same effect as one roentgen of x-radiation or gamma radiation. A rem is equal to 0.01 sievert in the International System of Units (SI). An acronym for *roentgen equivalent man.* See also **sievert.**

REM /rem, är″ē′em′/, a dream state. Abbreviation for **rapid eye movement.** See **sleep,** def. 1.

remasking /rēmas″king/, in digital fluoroscopy, the production of one or more additional mask images if the first is inadequate because of patient motion, noise, or other factors. See also **mask image.**

remdesivir, a nucleoside analogue prodrug. In 2020 the FDA issued an emergency use authorization for remdesivir in the treatment of hospitalized patients with a suspected or confirmed case of COVID-19 caused by the coronavirus SARS-CoV-2.

remedial /rimē″dē·əl/ [L, *remediare,* to cure], **1.** designed to improve or cure. **2.** describing measures taken to help get back on track or to enhance or refresh learning, such as remedial steps taken after a medication error to improve knowledge and safety.

remifentanil, an opiate agonist analgesic.

■ INDICATIONS: It is used in combination with other drugs in general anesthesia and as a primary anesthetic in general surgery.

■ CONTRAINDICATIONS: Use is prohibited in people with hypersensitivity to remifentanil and in children less than 12 years of age.

■ ADVERSE EFFECTS: Life-threatening effects are asystole, respiratory depression, and apnea. Other adverse effects include drowsiness, confusion, sedation, euphoria, delirium, agitation, anxiety, anorexia, constipation, cramps, dry mouth, urinary retention, dysuria, rash, urticaria, bruising, flushing, diaphoresis, pruritus, tinnitus, blurred vision, miosis, diplopia, palpitations, change in blood pressure, facial flushing, syncope, and rigidity. Common side effects are dizziness, headache, nausea, vomiting, and bradycardia.

reminiscence /rem′inis″əns/ [L, *reminisci,* to remember], the recollection of past personal experiences and significant events.

reminiscence therapy, a psychotherapeutic technique in which self-esteem and personal satisfaction are restored, particularly in older persons, by encouraging patients to review past experiences of a pleasant nature. It is used in Alzheimer disease when initially long-term memory stores are more intact than short-term and in other forms of dementia. Compare **life review.**

remission /rimish″ən/ [L, *remittere,* to abate], the partial or complete disappearance of the clinical and subjective characteristics of a chronic or malignant disease. Remission may be spontaneous or the result of therapy. In some cases remission is permanent, and the disease is cured. Compare **cure.**

R

remittent fever /rimit″ənt/ [L, *remittere* + *febris,* fever], daily variations of an elevated temperature, with exacerbations and remissions but never a return to normal.

remnant radiation /rem″nənt/ [L, *remanere,* to remain], the radiation that passes through an object and that can produce an image on a radiographic image receptor.

remodeling /rēmod″əling/ [L, *re* + *modus,* to copy again], the process of changing a body part or area, as in reconstructive surgery.

remote afterloading /rimōt″/ [L, *removere,* to remove], a radiotherapy technique in which an applicator, such as an acrylic mold of an area to be irradiated, is placed in or on the patient and then loaded from a safe source with a high-activity radioisotope. The applicator contains grooves for the insertion of nylon tubes into which the radioactive material can be introduced. Remote afterloading is used in the treatment of head, neck, vaginal, and cervical tumors. See also **afterloading.**

remotivation /rē′mōtivā″shən/ [L, *re* + *motus,* movement], the use of special techniques to stimulate individuals to become motivated to learn and interact.

remotivation group, a treatment group that is organized with the purpose of stimulating the interest, awareness, and communication of withdrawn and institutionalized patients with mental health problems.

removable lingual arch /rimoo″vəbəl/ [L, *removere,* to remove], an orthodontic arch wire designed to fit the lingual surface of the teeth and aid their orthodontic movement. Two posts soldered to each end of the wire fit snugly into the vertical tubes of molar anchor bands.

removable orthodontic appliance, a device placed inside the mouth to correct or alleviate malocclusion and designed to be removed or replaced by the patient.

removable partial denture, a prosthesis that replaces one or more missing teeth, made so that it can readily be removed from the mouth. Compare **fixed partial denture.** See also **partial denture.**

removable rigid dressing, a dressing similar to a cast used to encase the stump of an amputated limb. It is usually applied to permit the fitting of a temporary prosthesis so that ambulation can begin soon after surgery.

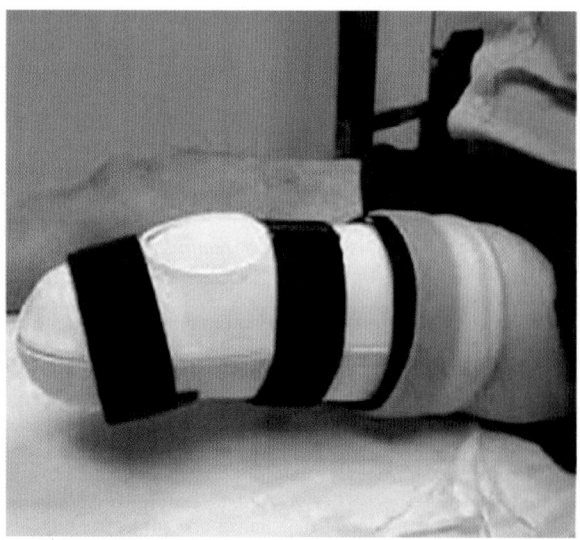

Removable rigid dressing *(Cameron, 2020)*

ren-, -reno, combining form meaning "kidney": *renal, renin, renoprotective.*

renal /rē″nəl/ [L, *ren,* kidney], pertaining to the kidney.

renal acidosis [L, *ren,* kidney, *acidus,* sour; Gk, *osis,* condition], an excessive increase in the H⁺ ions in body fluids because of impaired kidney function. The acidosis can result from excessive loss of bicarbonate or from the inability to excrete phosphoric and sulfuric acid.

renal adenocarcinoma. See **renal cell carcinoma.**

renal aminoaciduria, aminoaciduria caused by defective transport mechanisms for amino acids in the renal tubules. See also **aminoaciduria.**

renal anemia, anemia occurring as a complication of chronic kidney disease, mainly caused by deficiency of erythropoietin in the blood.

renal angiography, a radiographic examination of the renal artery and associated blood vessels after the injection of a contrast medium.

renal anuria. See **anuria.**

renal artery, one of a pair of large, visceral branches of the abdominal aorta, arising inferior to the superior mesenteric artery at the level of the disk between the first and second lumbar vertebrae. The left renal artery is somewhat more superior than the right. Before reaching the kidney, each divides into four branches. The renal arteries supply the kidneys, suprarenal glands, and the ureters.

renal biopsy, the removal of kidney tissue for microscopic examination. It is conducted to establish the diagnosis of a renal disorder and to aid in determining the stage of the disease, the appropriate therapy, and the prognosis. An open biopsy involves an incision, permits better visualization of the kidney, and carries a lower risk of hemorrhage. A closed or percutaneous biopsy performed by aspirating a specimen of tissue with a needle requires a shorter period of recovery and is less likely to cause infection. Contraindications to percutaneous biopsy include bleeding disorders, uncontrolled hypertension, and presence of a single kidney.
■ METHOD: Before biopsy, the procedure is explained and the patient is medically evaluated and tested for bleeding or coagulation time. Aspirin or coumadin therapy is discontinued for a period of time determined by the primary care provider. Informed consent is obtained. The patient's blood is usually typed and crossmatched with two units of donor blood that are held for a possible transfusion until there is no threat of bleeding after the procedure. An open biopsy is generally carried out in the operating room, but the percutaneous procedure may be performed in the radiology department or the patient's room. The location of the kidney, determined by a plain x-ray image, dye contrast study, or fluoroscopic or ultrasound examination, is marked on the patient's skin in ink for a needle biopsy. The patient is then placed prone over a sandbag and soft pillow with the body bent at the level of the diaphragm, the shoulders on the bed, and the spine in straight alignment. A local anesthetic is injected, and the physician inserts the biopsy needle in the lower pole of the kidney, because this area contains the smallest number of large renal vessels. The needle is quickly withdrawn, and, after pressure is applied to the site for 30 to 60 minutes, a pressure bandage is applied. The patient is turned and kept supine and motionless for the next 4 hours. The dressing, blood pressure, and pulse are checked every 5 to 10 minutes for the first hour, then at frequency determined by institutional protocols. Excessive drainage, decreased blood pressure, tachycardia, or elevated temperature is reported to the physician. Fluids are forced to the maximum allotted for the patient's condition. The amount and character of urinary output are noted, and the physician is informed if hematuria occurs. The patient is kept in bed for at least 24 hours and is cautioned not to lift

any heavy objects for 10 days or to take any anticoagulants until the primary care provider gives permission.

■ INTERVENTIONS: The nurse offers an explanation of the procedure, prepares and positions the patient for the percutaneous procedure, and, on its completion, provides care and emotional support.

■ OUTCOME CRITERIA: A biopsy is the most accurate measure for determining the nature and stage of a renal pathological condition.

renal calculus, a concretion occurring in the kidney. If the stone is large enough to block the ureter and stop the flow of urine from the kidney, it must be removed by either major surgical or radiological fluoroscopy procedures. Also called **kidney stone, nephritic calculus, nephrolith.** See also **nephroscope.**

renal calyx, the first unit in the system of ducts in the kidney carrying urine from the renal pyramid of the medulla to the renal pelvis for excretion through the ureters. There are two divisions: the minor renal calyx, with several others, drains into a larger major renal calyx, which in turn joins other major calyces to form the renal pelvis.

renal capsule [L, *ren,* kidney, *capsula,* little box], the investing tissue around the kidney, divided into the fibrous renal capsule and the adipose renal capsule.

renal cast, a cast formed from gelled protein precipitated in the renal tubules and molded to the tubular lumen. Pieces of these casts break off and are washed out with the urine. In renal disease, casts may be seen containing red or white blood cells. Also called **urinary casts.** Kinds include **granular cast, hyaline cast,** *waxy cast, epithelial cast.*

renal cell carcinoma, a malignant neoplasm of the kidney. Also called *adenocarcinoma of the kidney,* **clear cell carcinoma of the kidney.** See also **kidney cancer, Wilms' tumor.**

renal colic, sharp, severe pain in the lower back over the kidney, radiating forward into the groin. Renal colic usually accompanies forcible dilation of a ureter, followed by spasm as a stone is lodged or passed through it. See also **urinary calculus.**

renal corpuscle. See **malpighian corpuscle.**

renal cortex, the highly vascularized granular outer layer of the kidney, containing approximately 1.25 million glomeruli and convoluted tubules, which filter body wastes from the blood, reclaim useful materials, and dispose of the remainder as urine.

renal cortical necrosis, necrosis of the renal cortex caused by ischemia, often following acute tubular necrosis. It is usually seen as a complication of an obstetric condition, such as abruptio placentae, septic abortion, preeclampsia, retained fetus, or amniotic fluid embolism.

renal diabetes mellitus. See **renal glycosuria.**

renal dialysis [L, *ren,* kidney; Gk, *dia* + *lysis,* loosening], a process of diffusing blood across a semipermeable membrane to remove substances that a normal kidney would eliminate, including poisons, drugs, urea, uric acid, and creatinine. Renal dialysis may restore electrolytes and acid-base imbalances. See also **continuous ambulatory peritoneal dialysis, hemodialysis.**

renal diet, a diet prescribed in chronic renal failure and designed to control intake of protein, potassium, sodium, phosphorus, and fluids, depending on individual conditions. Carbohydrates and fats are the principal sources of energy. Protein is limited; the amount is determined by the patient's condition and is usually supplied from milk, eggs, and meat. Cereals, bread, rice, and pasta are the primary sources of calories. Some vegetables and fruits are included, depending on the degree of restriction of potassium and phosphorus. Special commercial flours and breads have been developed that are protein-free and low in potassium and sodium. The low potassium level of the diet also makes it useful in hyperkalemia. The diet may be nutritionally inadequate and should be supplemented with vitamins and electrolytes. See also **Giordano-Giovannetti diet.**

renal failure, inability of the kidneys to excrete wastes, concentrate urine, and conserve electrolytes. The condition may be acute or chronic. See also **acute tubular necrosis.**

■ OBSERVATIONS: Acute renal failure is characterized by oliguria and the rapid accumulation of nitrogenous wastes in the blood (azotemia). It results from hemorrhage, trauma, burn, toxic injury to the kidney, acute pyelonephritis or glomerulonephritis, or lower urinary tract obstruction. Many forms of acute renal failure are reversible after the underlying cause has been identified. Acute renal failure may have three typical phases: prodromal, oliguric, and postoliguric. Chronic renal failure may result from many other diseases. The early signs include sluggishness, fatigue, and mental dullness. Later, anuria, convulsions, GI bleeding, malnutrition, and various neuropathies may occur. The skin may turn yellow-brown. Congestive heart failure and hypertension are frequent complications, the results of hypervolemia. Urinalysis reveals greater-than-normal amounts of urea and creatinine, waxy casts, and a constant volume of urine regardless of variations in water intake. Anemia frequently occurs.

■ INTERVENTIONS: Treatment includes restricted intake of fluids and of all substances that require excretion by the kidney. Antibiotics and diuretics are also used.

■ PATIENT CARE CONSIDERATIONS: The prognosis depends on the underlying cause. When medical measures have been exhausted, long-term hemodialysis or peritoneal dialysis is often begun, and kidney transplantation is considered.

renal failure index (RFI), an assessment of acute renal failure that compares the sodium clearance with the creatinine clearance: RFI |m = $U_{Na} U_{Cr}/P_{Cr}$, where P_{Cr} |m = plasma concentration of creatinine, U_{Cr} |m = urinary concentration of creatinine, and U_{Na} |m = urinary concentration of sodium. A value below 1.0 indicates renal failure because of prerenal azotemia, and a value above 2.0 suggests that it is caused by acute tubular necrosis.

renal fascia, a membranous condensation of extraperitoneal fascia that encloses the perirenal fat surrounding the kidney.

renal fat. See **adipose capsule.**

renal glycosuria [L, *ren,* kidney; Gk, *glykys,* sweet, *ouron,* urine], a familial condition characterized by lowered renal threshold to sugar. Blood glucose levels may be normal, although sugar is excreted in the urine. Also called **renal diabetes mellitus.**

renal hematuria [L, *ren,* kidney; Gk, *haima,* blood, *ouron,* urine], presence of blood in the urine because of a kidney disorder.

renal hypercalciuria, hypercalciuria caused by primary renal wasting of calcium, which stimulates production of parathyroid hormone to increase calcium resorption in the intestine. This type is not linked to formation of renal calculi.

renal hypertension, hypertension resulting from aortic or renal artery atherosclerosis or from kidney disease, including chronic glomerulonephritis, chronic pyelonephritis, renal carcinoma, and renal calculi. Analgesic abuse and certain drug reactions may also result in renal hypertension. Therapy depends on the cause and may include antibiotics, diuretics, or surgery. Untreated renal hypertension is likely to result in kidney damage and cardiovascular disease.

R

renal insufficiency [L, *ren,* kidney, *in* + *sufficere,* to suffice], partial kidney function failure characterized by less-than-normal urine excretion.

renal lithiasis. See **nephrolithiasis.**

renal nanism, dwarfism associated with infantile renal osteodystrophy.

renal osteodystrophy, a condition resulting from chronic renal failure and characterized by uneven bone growth and demineralization. See also **renal nanism, renal rickets.**

renal papilla. See **papilla.**

renal parenchyma, the functional tissue of the kidney, consisting of the nephrons.

renal pelvis [L, *ren* + *pelvis,* basin], a funnel-shaped dilation that drains urine from the kidney into the ureter.

renal plasma flow (RPF), the amount of plasma that perfuses the kidneys per unit time. Approximately 90% of the total constitutes the *effective renal plasma flow,* the portion that perfuses functional renal tissue, such as the glomeruli.

renal pseudotumor, any mass in the kidney that is normal tissue but mimics something abnormal, such as in Bertin's column hypertrophy or a dromedary hump.

renal pyramid [L, *ren,* kidney; Gk, *pyramis*], any one of several conical masses of tissue that form the kidney medulla. The base of each pyramid adjoins the kidney's cortex; the apex terminates at a renal calyx. The pyramids consist of the loops of Henle and the collecting tubules of the nephrons.

renal replacement lipomatosis, asymmetric fatty change in the kidney where renal parenchyma has become replaced by fatty tissue, such as with an infection or presence of a calculus. Symptoms include decreased renal function with inflammation, pain, pyuria, and sometimes pyelonephritis.

renal revascularization, surgical correction of occlusion of a renal artery through a technique such as renal artery endarterectomy or a bypass procedure.

renal rickets, a condition characterized by rachitic changes in the skeleton and caused by chronic nephritis. See also **renal osteodystrophy.**

renal scan, a nuclear medicine scan of the kidneys performed after the IV injection of a radioactive substance. It is used to assess renal perfusion and function, particularly in renal failure, renovascular hypertension, and following kidney transplantation.

renal sclerosis [L, *ren,* kidney; Gk, *skerosis,* hardening], arteriosclerosis or fibrosis of the arterioles of the kidney. See also **nephroangiosclerosis.**

renal sinus cyst, a cyst in a renal sinus, usually derived from aberrant lymphatic vessels, occurring either alone or in groups. Most appear after the fifth decade of life in association with inflammation, obstruction, or a calculus. They may be asymptomatic or may expand to cause pelvic compression and local deformity with pain, hematuria, infection, and pyuria.

renal sinus lipomatosis, increased fat in the renal sinuses. A symmetric, usually asymptomatic, increase is seen in obesity, steroid therapy, and the atrophy that accompanies the aging process. An asymmetric increase known as renal replacement lipomatosis, which can have severe symptoms, occurs when infection destroys part of the renal parenchyma. See also **renal replacement lipomatosis.**

renal transplantation [L, *ren,* kidney, *transplantare*], the surgical transfer of a complete kidney from a donor to a recipient. Also called *kidney transplant.*

renal tuberculosis, disease of the kidney caused by *Mycobacterium tuberculosis,* usually from bacillemia in cases of pulmonary tuberculosis. Pathological changes include granulomatous inflammation and caseous necrosis of kidney tissue. Also called *nephrotuberculosis.*

renal tubular acidosis (RTA), an abnormal condition associated with persistent dehydration, metabolic acidosis, hypokalemia, hyperchloremia, and nephrocalcinosis. It is caused by the kidney's inability to conserve bicarbonate and to adequately acidify the urine. Some forms of RTA are more prevalent in women, older children, and young adults. Prolonged RTA can cause hypercalciuria and the formation of kidney stones. Prognosis depends on treatment and the extent of renal damage but is usually good. Compare **distal renal tubular acidosis, ketoacidosis, metabolic acidosis, proximal renal tubular acidosis, respiratory acidosis.**

■ OBSERVATIONS: Common signs and symptoms of RTA, especially in children, include anorexia, vomiting, constipation, delayed growth, excessive urination, nephrocalcinosis, and rickets. RTA can also cause urinary tract infections and pyelonephritis. Confirming diagnosis of distal RTA is based on laboratory tests that show impaired urine acidification in association with systemic metabolic acidosis. Confirming diagnosis of proximal RTA is based on tests that show bicarbonate wasting as a result of impaired reabsorption. Other significant laboratory findings may include decreased sodium bicarbonate, pH, potassium, and phosphorus; increased serum chloride, alkaline phosphatase, urinary bicarbonate, and potassium; and urine with low specific gravity.

■ INTERVENTIONS: Treatment includes the replacement of excessively secreted substances, especially bicarbonate, and may include the administration of sodium bicarbonate tablets, potassium, vitamin D to preserve calcium metabolism, and antibiotics to counter pyelonephritis. Surgery may be required to remove renal calculi.

■ PATIENT CARE CONSIDERATIONS: The health care team carefully monitors the results of altered laboratory tests, especially those involving potassium levels and urine pH. The patient's urine is strained to capture any kidney stones for analysis, and the nurse is alert to any signs of hematuria. A patient with a low potassium level is usually advised to eat potassium-rich foods such as bananas, oranges, and baked potatoes. The patient and family are encouraged to seek genetic counseling and RTA screening.

renal tubule [L, *ren,* kidney, *tubulus,* small tube], the part of the kidney's nephron that leads from the glomerulus to the collecting tubules. It consists of a looping segment and two convoluted sections. These canals resorb selected materials back into the blood and secrete, collect, and conduct urine.

renal vein renin assay, a blood test used to diagnose renovascular hypertension. It is helpful in determining whether a stenosis seen on a renal angiogram is significantly contributing to hypertension.

Rendu-Osler-Weber syndrome. See **hereditary hemorrhagic telangiectasia.**

Renese, a thiazide diuretic. Brand name for **polythiazide.**

renin /rē″nin/ [L, *ren,* kidney], a renal proteolytic enzyme, produced by and stored in the juxtaglomerular apparatus that surrounds each arteriole as it enters a glomerulus. The enzyme affects the blood pressure by catalyzing the change of angiotensinogen to angiotensin I, which is then converted to angiotensin II, strong pressor. Normal findings of adult plasma renin, measured in an upright position and sodium depleted, are 2.9 to 10.8 ng/mL/hr. Should not be confused with **rennin.**

renin-angiotensin system, the regulation of sodium balance, fluid volume, and blood pressure. In response to reduced perfusion, renin is secreted, which hydrolyzes a plasma globulin to release angiotensin I, which is rapidly hydrolyzed to angiotensin II, a powerful vasoconstrictor; angiotension II also stimulates aldosterone secretion, which causes sodium retention, an increase in blood pressure, and restoration of renal perfusion, which shuts off the signal for renin release (negative feedback). Angiotensin-converting enzyme also deactivates bradykinin, a vasodilator. Also called *renin-angiotensin-aldosterone system.*

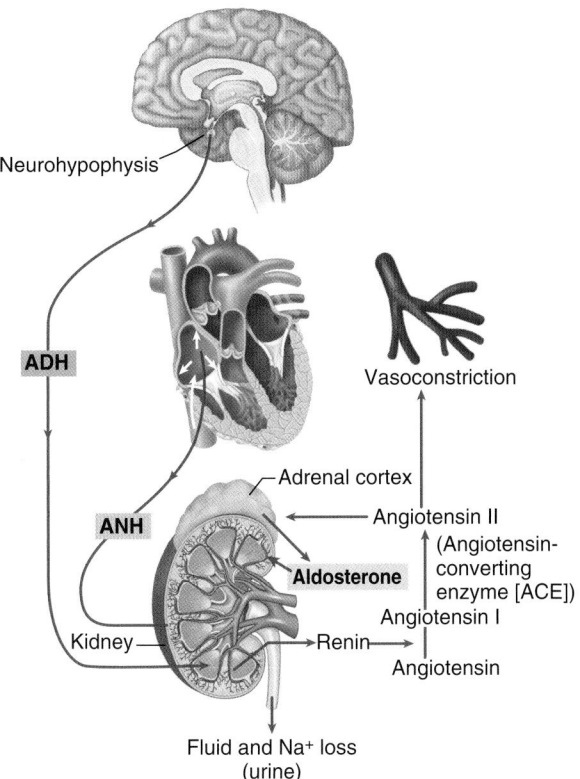

Renin-angiotensin system *(Patton and Thibodeau, 2010)*

renin test.   See **plasma renin activity.**

rennin /ren″in/ [ME, *rennen,* to run], a milk-curdling enzyme that occurs in the gastric juices of infants and is also contained in the rennet produced in the stomach of calves and other ruminants. It is an endopeptidase that converts casein to paracasein and was formerly used extensively as a curdling agent by the cheese industry. An artificially produced microbial rennet rather than the enzyme extracted from rennet in calves is used in half of the cheese produced in the United States and Canada today. Also called **chymosin.** Should not be confused with **renin.**

renogram /rē″nəgram/, an image resulting from a renal scan.

-renone, suffix for spironolactone-type aldosterone antagonists.

renoprotective /re″no-pro-tek′tiv/, protecting the kidney against harmful effects, such as of a drug or other chemical.

Renshaw cells /ren″shô/ [B. Renshaw, American neurologist, 1911–1948; L, *cella,* storeroom], small cells that reduce motor neuron discharge through a feedback circuit involving axon collaterals that excite interneurons. The system prevents rapid repeated firing of motor neurons.

ReoPro, an antithrombotic agent. Brand name for **abciximab.**

reovirus /rē′ōvī″rəs/ [*r*espiratory *e*nteric *o*rphan + L, *virus*], any one of three ubiquitous, double-stranded ribonucleic acid viruses found in the respiratory and alimentary tracts of both healthy and sick people. Reoviruses have been implicated in some cases of upper respiratory tract disease and infantile gastroenteritis.

repaglinide, an antidiabetic medication.

■ INDICATIONS: It is used to treat stable type 2 diabetes mellitus.

■ CONTRAINDICATIONS: Known hypersensitivity to meglitinides, diabetic ketoacidosis, and type 1 diabetes mellitus prohibit its use.

■ ADVERSE EFFECTS: Hypoglycemia is a life-threatening effect. Other adverse effects include paresthesia, nausea, vomiting, diarrhea, constipation, dyspepsia, rash, allergic reactions, back pain, arthralgia, upper respiratory infection, sinusitis, rhinitis, and bronchitis. Headache and weakness are common side effects.

repeat /rĕ-pēt′/, **1.** *n.,* something occurring more than once, particularly over and over. **2.** *v.,* to replicate an action more than once.

repercussion /rē′pərkush″ən/ [L, *repercussio,* rebounding], **1.** (in obstetrics) ballottement. **2.** being driven back by a powerful resistance. **3.** the reduction of a swelling or tumor.

reperfusion /rē′pərfyoo̅″zhən/, blocked arteries that are opened to reestablish blood flow. It may be accomplished through thrombolytic therapy or percutaneous transluminal angioplasty.

repetition compulsion /rep′ətish″ən/ [L, *repetere,* to repeat], an unconscious and maladaptive need to revert to and repeat earlier situations, behavior patterns, and acts to experience previously felt emotions or relationships. See also **compulsion.**

repetition time (TR), in magnetic resonance pulse sequences, the time interval before the basic pulse sequence is repeated.

repetitive stress injury /ripet″ətiv/, tissue damage associated with tasks that require repeated movements of the hands, legs, or trunk, such as meat cutting, computer keyboarding, or playing musical instruments. Effects include chronic nerve and joint pain, spine damage, and carpal tunnel syndrome. Among recommended preventive measures are frequent rest breaks and ergonomic improvements for the workplace.

replacement /riplās″mənt/ [Fr, *replacer,* to put in place again], the substitution of a missing part or substance with a similar structure or substance, such as the replacement of an amputated limb with a prosthesis or the replacement of lost blood with donor blood.

replacement therapy, **1.** the use of a medicinal product to replace a natural hormone or enzyme that the body is no longer able to produce in sufficient amounts. **2.** a psychotherapeutic technique of replacing abnormal behavior with healthy, constructive activities.

replication /rep′likā″shən/ [L, *replicare,* to fold back], **1.** a process of duplicating, reproducing, or copying; literally, a folding back of a part to form a duplicate. **2.** (in research) the exact repetition of an experiment, performed to confirm the initial findings. **3.** (in genetics) the duplication of the polynucleotide strands of DNA or the synthesis of DNA. The process involves the unwinding of the double helix molecule to form two single strands, each of which acts as a template for the synthesis of a complementary strand. The two resulting molecules of DNA each contain one new and one parental strand, which coil to form the double helix. −*replicate, v.*

R

replicator /rep″likā′tər/ [L, *replicare*], a segment of DNA that initiates and controls the replication of the molecule.

replicon /rep′ləkon/ [L, *replicare*], a segment of DNA that is undergoing replication. It is regulated by a section of the molecule called the regulator, which controls replication and coordinates it with cell division.

repolarization /rēpō′lərīzā″shən/ [L, *re + polus,* pole; Gk, *izein,* to cause], the process by which the membrane potential of a neuron or muscle cell is restored to the cell's resting potential. In a cardiac muscle cell, the repolarization process begins after phase 0 of the action potential and is completed by the end of phase 3. It encompasses the effective and relative refractory periods and correlates with the Q-T interval on the electrocardiogram. See also **cardiac action potential.**

report /ripôrt′/ [L, *re + portare,* to carry], **1.** (in nursing) the transfer of information from the nurses on one shift to the nurses on the following shift or before the transfer of a patient from one unit to another. Report is given systematically at the time of change of shift. The nurse manager, team leader, or primary nurse conducts the report, summarizing the progress and status of each patient for the nurses who will next assume responsibility for the care. The provider of the information is said to "give report," and the oncoming staff to "take report." Report may be given to the assembled oncoming staff, or it may be tape recorded so that staff members can listen to it individually or in a group on their own schedule. **2.** (in occupational and physical therapy) the documentation of the evaluation, intervention, or outcome of therapy. Reports are provided to team members, family members, or agencies (e.g., schools or hospitals).

reportable diseases /ripôr′təbəl/, diseases that must be reported by the health care provider to public health authorities, given their contagious nature. They include but are not limited to malaria, poliomyelitis, typhus, yellow fever, cholera, bubonic plague, STDs, and AIDS.

repositioning /rē′pəzish″əning/ [L, *reponere,* to put back], **1.** the restoration of an organ or body part to its natural position, as repositioning an inverted uterus or changing the position of the jaws. **2.** changing the position of a client to prevent complications associated with immobility.

representative group /rep′rəsen″tətiv/, a group of individuals whose members represent all the various sectors of a community.

repression /ripresh″ən/ [L, *reprimere,* to press back], **1.** the act of restraining, inhibiting, or suppressing. **2.** (in psychoanalysis) an unconscious defense mechanism that also underlies all defense mechanisms, whereby unacceptable thoughts, feelings, ideas, impulses, or memories, especially those concerning some traumatic past event, are pushed from the consciousness because of their painful guilt association or disagreeable content and are submerged in the unconscious, where they remain dormant but operant. Such repressed emotional conflicts are the source of anxiety that may lead to any of the anxiety disorders. Compare **suppression.** −*repressive, adj.,* −*repress, v.*

repressive-inspirational approach /ripres″iv/, a psychotherapeutic approach used in some groups to discourage the breaking down of defense mechanisms. Members are encouraged to focus on positive feelings and group strengths. This approach is commonly used in groups of patients with chronic mental illness.

repressor /ripres″ər/ [L, *reprimere,* to press back], a protein produced by a regulator gene. It binds to a sequence of nucleotides in an operator gene, blocking the transcription of one or more structural genes.

repressor gene. See **regulator gene.**

reproduction /rē′prəduk″shən/ [L, *re + producere,* to produce], **1.** the sum of the cellular and genetic phenomena by which organisms produce offspring similar to themselves so that the species is perpetuated. In humans the germ cells, spermatozoa in the male and ova in the female, unite during fertilization to form the new individual. Kinds include **asexual reproduction, cytogenic reproduction, sexual reproduction. 2.** the creation of a similar structure, situation, or phenomenon; duplication; replication. **3.** the recalling of a former idea or impression or of something previously learned. −**reproductive,** *adj.*

reproductive /rē′prəduk″tiv/ [L, *re + producere,* to produce], pertaining to the process of reproduction.

reproductive endocrinology, the study of the maternal female hormone system, including the activities of the hypothalamus, pituitary, and ovaries from puberty through menopause.

reproductive system, the male and female gonads, associated ducts and glands, and external genitalia that function in the procreation of offspring. In women these include the ovaries, fallopian tubes, uterus, vagina, clitoris, and vulva. In men they include the testes, epididymis, vas deferens, seminal vesicles, ejaculatory duct, prostate, and penis. Also called **genital tract, genitourinary system, urogenital system.**

repulsion /ripul″shən/ [L, *repellere,* to drive away], **1.** the act of repelling, disjoining. **2.** a force that separates two bodies or things. **3.** (in genetics) the situation in linked inheritance in which the alleles of two or more mutant genes are located on homologous chromosomes so that each chromosome of the pair carries one or more mutant and wild-type genes, which are located close enough to be inherited together. Compare **coupling.** See also **trans configuration.**

request for proposal (RFP) /rikwest″/ [L, *requaerere,* to require, *propronere,* to propound], a solicitation by a funding agency for proposals to accomplish a particular goal. The RFP lists the requirements a project must meet to receive funding.

required arch length /rikwī″ərd/ [L, *requaerere,* to require], the sum of the mesiodistal widths of all the natural teeth in a dental arch. It represents the minimum arch length that can accommodate all of the teeth in the arch.

RES, abbreviation for **reticuloendothelial system.**

Rescriptor, an antiretroviral nonnucleoside reverse transcriptase inhibitor agent. Brand name for **delavirdine.**

rescue dose. See **breakthrough dose.**

Rescue Remedy, the essences of five flowers (cherry plum, clematis, impatiens, rock rose, and star of Bethlehem) in a spray, drop, or lozenge formulation, used for the acute treatment of stress. Brand name for **Bach remedies.**

research /risurch′, rē″surch/ [Fr, *rechercher,* to investigate], the diligent inquiry or examination of data, reports, and observations in a search for facts or principles.

research hypothesis, a statement created to predict the outcome of a study. See **predictive hypothesis.**

research instrument, a testing device for measuring a given phenomenon, such as a paper and pencil test, a questionnaire, an interview, a research tool, or a set of guidelines for observation.

research measurement, an evaluation of the quantity or incidence of a given variable obtained by using a research instrument.

research radiopharmaceutical, a drug that is labeled with a small quantity of a radioactive tracer to allow its biodistribution to be studied. It may later be used in a nonradioactive form.

resection /risek″shən/, the excision of a significant part of an organ or structure. Resection of an organ may be partial or complete. Kinds include **wedge resection, bladder neck resection, segmental resection.**

reserpine /res″ərpēn/, a depleter of biogenic amines (e.g., norepinephrine, dopamine) from nerve terminals.

■ INDICATIONS: It is prescribed in the treatment of mild to moderate high blood pressure and has unlabeled uses for tardive dyskinesia and certain neuropsychiatric disorders.

■ CONTRAINDICATIONS: Mental depression, peptic ulcer, ulcerative colitis, or known hypersensitivity to this drug prohibits its use.

■ ADVERSE EFFECTS: Among the more serious adverse effects are mental depression, extrapyramidal effects, impotence, aggravation of peptic ulcer, and paradoxical excitement.

reserve /rizurv″/ [L, *reservare*, to save], a potential capacity to maintain vital body functions in homeostasis by adjusting to increased need, such as cardiac reserve, pulmonary reserve, and alkali reserve. See also **homeostasis.**

reserve capacity [L, *reservare*, to save; Gk, *aer*], the volume of air that can be exhaled with maximum effort after completion of a normal expiration. Also called *reserve air,* **supplemental air.**

reserve cell carcinoma. See **oat cell carcinoma.**

reservoir /rez″ərvwär/ [Fr, *réservoir*], a chamber or receptacle for holding or storing a fluid.

reservoir bag, a component of an anesthesia machine in which gas accumulates, forming a contained supply of gas for use during manual control of ventilation. It serves as a visible monitor of respiratory rate and depth during spontaneous respiration.

reservoir host, a nonhuman host that serves as a means of sustaining an infectious organism as a potential source of human infection. Wild monkeys are reservoir hosts for the yellow fever virus, which can spread from the jungle to infect humans.

reservoir of infection, a continuous source of infectious disease. People, animals, and plants may be reservoirs of infection.

resident /rez″idənt/ [L, *residere*, to remain], **1.** a physician in one of the postgraduate years of clinical training after the first, or internship, year. The length of residency varies according to the specialty. See also **PGY. 2.** a person who receives inpatient care in a long-term care facility.

resident bacteria, bacteria living in a specific area of the body.

residential care facility /rez′iden″shəl/, a facility that provides custodial care to persons who, because of physical, mental, or emotional disorders, are not able to live independently.

residual /rizij″oo·əl/ [L, *residuum*, remainder], **1.** *adj.,* pertaining to the part of something that remains after an activity that removes the bulk of the substance. **2.** *n.,* (in psychology) an aftereffect of an experience that influences latent behavior.

residual air. See **residual volume.**

residual cyst, an odontogenic cyst that remains in the jaw after the removal of a tooth or by incomplete removal of all cystic material from the cystic area.

residual dental caries, any decayed material remaining in a prepared tooth cavity.

residual function [L, *residuum*, remainder, *functio,* performance], the remaining ability to function after a serious illness or injury.

residual limb, the portion of a limb remaining after an amputation.

residual ridge, the part of the alveolar ridge that remains after the alveolar process has disappeared after extraction of the teeth.

residual schizophrenia [L, *residuum*], *(Obsolete)* a form of schizophrenia in which the essential features of delusions, hallucinations, incoherence, or gross disorganization are much less prominent. See also **schizophrenia.**

residual urine, urine that remains in the bladder after urination.

residual volume (RV) [L, *residuum,* remainder, *volumen,* papyrus roll], the amount of air remaining in the lungs at the end of a maximum expiration.

residue-free diet /rez″id(y)oo/ [L, *residuum,* remainder; AS, *freo* + Gk, *diaita,* way of life], a diet free of nondigestible cellulose or fiber, such as found in semisolid bland food.

resilience /rizil″yəns/ [L, *resilere,* to spring back], **1.** a concept that proposes a recurrent human need to weather periods of stress and change successfully throughout life. The ability to weather each period of disruption and reintegration leaves the person better able to deal with the next change. **2.** the ability of a body to return to its original form after being stretched or compressed.

resin /rez″in/ [L, *resina*], **1.** a mixture of carboxylic acids, essential oils, and terpenes (hydrocarbons of the formula $C_{10}H_{16}$), occurring as exudations on various trees and shrubs or produced synthetically. Resins are highly combustible semisolids or amorphous solids that are insoluble in water, although some are soluble in ethanol and others in carbon tetrachloride, ether, and volatile oils. Most are soft and sticky but harden after exposure to cold. **2.** any of a variety of solid or semisolid amorphous substances that are insoluble in organic solvents but not in water. Orally administered bile-acid binding resins such as cholestyramine and colestipol interrupt the normal enterohepatic circulation of bile acids and increase their excretion in the stool. Since bile acids are synthesized by the liver from cholesterol, the liver extracts more LDL cholesterol from the plasma to replace them, and, as a consequence, circulating levels of LDL cholesterol decrease.

res ipsa loquitur /rās″ ip″sə lok″witoor/ [L, the thing speaks for itself], a legal concept, important in many malpractice suits, describing a situation in which an injury occurred when the defendant was solely and exclusively in control and in which the injury would not have occurred had due care been exercised. Classic examples of res ipsa loquitur are a sponge left in the abdomen after abdominal surgery or the amputation of the wrong extremity.

resistance /rizis″təns/ [L, *resistere,* to withstand], **1.** an opposition to a force, such as the resistance offered by the constriction of peripheral vessels to the blood flow in the circulatory system. **2.** the frictional force that opposes the flow of an electric charge, as measured in ohms. **3.** (in respiratory therapy) the process or power of acting against a force placed on it, pertaining to thoracic resistance, tissue resistance, and airway resistance.

resistance form, the shape given to a prepared tooth cavity imparting strength and durability to the masticatory dislodging forces of a dental restoration and remaining tooth structure.

resistance-inducing factor (RIF), an agent that interferes with multiplication of a virus or other pathogen.

resistance to flow, the pressure differential required to produce a given rate of flow of a gas or liquid through a vessel.

resistance training, any method or form of strength training used to resist, overcome, or bear force.

resistance transfer factor. See **R factor.**

resistance vessels, the blood vessels that form the major part of the total peripheral resistance to blood flow. Resistance vessels include small arteries, arterioles, and metarterioles.

R

resistant /rizis″tənt/, **1.** pertaining to the ability of a microorganism to remain unaffected by an antimicrobial agent. **2.** pertaining to a phenomenon that exists when a disease is not susceptible or cured by the standard treatment regimen.

resistive magnet /resis″tiv/, a simple electromagnet in which electricity passing through coils of wire produces a magnetic field.

resocialization /rēsō′shəlīzā″shən/ [L, *re + socialis,* partners; Gk, *izein,* to cause], the reintegration of a client into family and community life after critical or long-term hospitalization.

resolution (R) [L, *re + solvere,* to solve], **1.** the state of having made a firm determination or decision on a course of action. **2.** the ability of an imaging process to distinguish adjacent structures in an object. It is an important measure of image quality. **3.** the ability of a chromatographic system to separate two adjacent peaks. The degree of separation between two peaks is represented by the symbol **R.**

resolving power /rizol″ving/, **1.** the ability to separate closely migrating substances, as in electrophoresis. **2.** the ability to distinguish closely positioned objects as distinct entities.

resolving time, the minimum time between radiation-induced ionizations that can be detected by a Geiger-Müller–type scintillation device.

resonance [L, *vocalis + resonare,* to sound again], **1.** an echo or other sound produced by percussion of an organ or cavity of the body during a physical exam. **2.** the process of energy absorption by an object that is tuned to absorb energy of a specific frequency. Other frequencies have no effect. **3.** modification of the laryngeal tone as it passes through the pharynx and oral cavity to produce an increase in the intensity and quality of the sound.

resonance frequency, **1.** in an ultrasound transducer, the frequency for which the response of a transducer to an ultrasound beam is a maximum. **2.** the frequency at which the transducer most efficiently converts electric signals to mechanical vibrations. **3.** (in magnetic resonance) the frequency at which a nucleus absorbs radio energy when placed in a magnetic field.

resonant /rez″ənənt/ [L, *resonare,* to sound again], pertaining to a sound that vibrates on percussion or is amplified by sympathetic vibrations in another medium.

resonating /rez″ənā′ting/ [L, *resonare,* to sound again], pertaining to vibrations or pulsations that are synchronous with a source of sound waves or electromagnetic oscillations.

resorb /risôrb″/ [L, *resorbere,* to swallow again], to absorb again.

resorbent /risôr″bənt/ [L, *resorbere*], a material or agent that is used to absorb blood or other substances.

resorcinol /rizôr″sinol/, an antiseptic substance used as a keratolytic agent in the dermatoses. It is also used in dyes and pharmaceutics and as a chemical intermediate.

resorption /risôrp″shən/ [L, *resorbere,* to swallow again], **1.** the loss of substance or bone by physiological or pathological means, such as the reduction of the volume and size of the residual ridge of the mandible or maxillae. **2.** the cementoclastic and dentinoclastic action that may occur on a tooth root. Also called **external resorption, internal resorption.**

resource-based relative value scale (RBRVS), a system for a Medicare fee schedule designed to address the promise of compensation to a physician for the time involved in giving physical and mental status examinations and obtaining patient history from family members.

Respbid, a smooth muscle relaxant. Brand name for **theophylline.**

respiration **(R)** /res′pirā″shən/ [L, *respirare,* to breathe], **1.** the molecular exchange of oxygen and carbon dioxide within the body's tissues. **2.** the process of moving air into and out of the lungs. The rate varies with the age and condition of the person. Also called **breathing, pulmonary ventilation, ventilation. –respiratory,** *adj.*

External Respiration

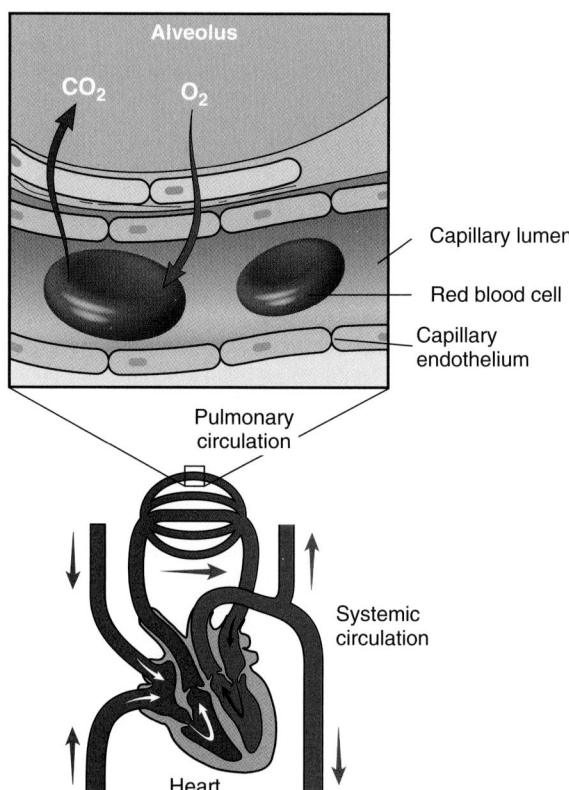

Mechanism of respiration *(Bonewit-West, 2012)*

respiration of infants [L, *respirare,* to breathe, *infans,* unable to speak], a rate of breathing at birth that averages 40 to 50 breaths per minute. The rate declines to 15 to 20 breaths per minute at puberty.

respiration rate [L, *respirare,* to breathe, *ratum,* rate], the rate of breathing. It is typically from 40 to 50 breaths per minute for newborns, 20 to 25 breaths per minute for older children, and 12 to 20 breaths per minute for teenagers and adults. An adult rate of 25 breaths per minute may be regarded as accelerated, whereas a rate of less than 12 breaths per minute is abnormally low. The rate may be more rapid in fever, acute pulmonary infection, diffuse pulmonary fibrosis, gas gangrene, left ventricular failure, thyrotoxicosis, and states of tension. Slower breathing rates may result from head injury, coma, or narcotic overdose. Also called **breathing frequency, respiratory rate.** See also **bradypnea, hyperpnea, hypopnea.**

Patterns of respiration

Pattern		Description
Normal (eupnea)		Regular and comfortable at a rate of 12-20 breaths per minute
Bradypnea		Slower than 12 breaths per minute
Tachypnea		Faster than 20 breaths per minute
Hyperventilation (hyperpnea)		Faster than 20 breaths per minute, deep breathing
Sighing		Frequently interspersed deeper breath
Air trapping		Increasing difficulty in getting breath out
Cheyne-Stokes		Varying periods of increasing depth interspersed with apnea
Kussmaul		Rapid, deep, labored
Biot		Irregularly interspersed periods of apnea in a disorganized sequence of breaths
Ataxic		Significant disorganization with irregular and varying depths of respiration

From Mosby: *Mosby's PDQ for RN,* ed 3, St. Louis, 2013, Mosby.

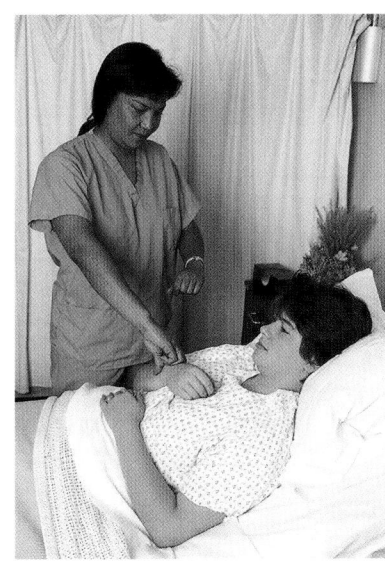

Assessment of respiration rate *(Elkin, Perry, and Potter, 2007)*

respirator /res″pirā′tər/ [L, *respirare*], an apparatus used to modify air for inspiration or to improve pulmonary ventilation. The term is commonly used to mean a ventilator. See also **IPPB unit, nebulizer.**

respiratory, **1.** pertaining to structures and function related to breathing. See also **respiration. 2.** pertaining to cellular metabolic processes.

respiratory acidosis, an abnormal condition characterized by a low plasma pH resulting from reduced alveolar ventilation. The hypoventilation inhibits the excretion of carbon dioxide, which consequently combines with water in the body to produce carbonic acid, thus reducing plasma pH. Respiratory acidosis can result from disorders such as airway obstruction, medullary trauma, neuromuscular disease, chest injury, pneumonia, pulmonary edema, emphysema, and cardiopulmonary arrest. It may also be caused by the suppression of respiratory reflexes with narcotics, sedatives, hypnotics, or anesthetics. Also called **carbon dioxide acidosis.** Compare **metabolic acidosis.** See also **metabolic alkalosis, respiratory alkalosis.**

■ OBSERVATIONS: Some common signs and symptoms of respiratory acidosis are headache, dyspnea, fine tremors, tachycardia, hypertension, and vasodilation. Confirming diagnosis is usually based on a $PaCO_2$ over the normal 45 mm Hg and an arterial pH below 7.35.

■ INTERVENTIONS: Ineffective treatment of acute respiratory acidosis can lead to coma and death. Treatment seeks to remove or inhibit the underlying causes of associated hypoventilation. Any airway obstructions are immediately removed. Mechanical ventilation and oxygen therapy may be used, and IV bronchodilators and sodium bicarbonate may be administered.

■ PATIENT CARE CONSIDERATIONS: The patient with respiratory acidosis is carefully monitored for any changes in arterial blood gas pressures, electrolyte concentrations, and respiratory, cardiovascular, and central nervous system functions. In patients requiring mechanical ventilation, patent airways are maintained and tracheal tubes are suctioned as needed. Adequate hydration is also important.

respiratory alkalosis, an abnormal condition characterized by a high plasma pH resulting from increased alveolar ventilation. The consequent acceleration of carbon dioxide excretion lowers the plasma level of carbonic acid, thus raising plasma pH. The hyperventilation may be caused by pulmonary and nonpulmonary problems. Some pulmonary causes are acute asthma, pulmonary vascular disease, and pneumonia. Some nonpulmonary causes are aspirin toxicity, anxiety, fever, metabolic acidosis, inflammation of the central nervous system, gram-negative septicemia, and hepatic failure. Compare **metabolic alkalosis.** See also **metabolic acidosis, respiratory acidosis.**

■ OBSERVATIONS: Deep and rapid breathing at rates as high as 40 breaths per minute is a major sign of respiratory alkalosis. Other symptoms are light-headedness, dizziness, peripheral paresthesia, tingling of the hands and feet, muscle weakness, tetany, and cardiac arrhythmia. Confirming diagnosis is often based on a $PaCO_2$ below 35 mm Hg and a pH greater than 7.45. PaO_2 may be higher than 100. In the acute stage, blood pH rises in proportion to the fall in $PaCO_2$, but in the chronic stage it remains within the normal range of 7.35 to 7.45. The carbonic acid concentration is normal in the acute stage of this condition but below normal in the chronic stage.

■ INTERVENTIONS: Treatment of respiratory alkalosis concentrates on removing the underlying causes. Severe cases, especially those caused by extreme anxiety, may be treated by having the patient breathe into a paper bag and inhale exhaled carbon dioxide to compensate for the deficit being created by hyperventilation. Sedatives may also be administered to decrease the ventilation rate.

■ PATIENT CARE CONSIDERATIONS: The nurse monitors neurological, neuromuscular, and cardiovascular functions; arterial blood gases; and serum electrolyte levels. The patient benefits from explanations of laboratory tests and treatment.

respiratory arrest, the cessation of breathing.

respiratory assessment, an evaluation of the condition and function of a person's respiratory system.

■ OUTCOME CRITERIA: An accurate and thorough assessment of respiratory function is an essential component of the physical examination and is vital to the diagnosis or ongoing care of a respiratory illness.

respiratory bronchiole. See **bronchiole.**

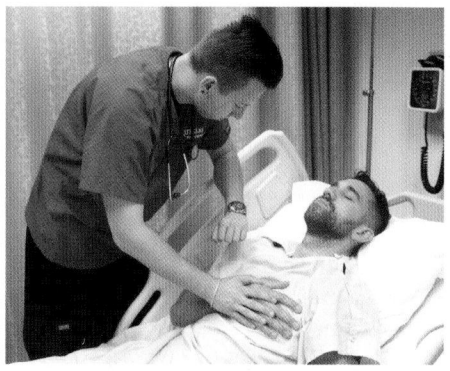

Assessment of the respiratory system *(Courtesy Rutgers School of Nursing—Camden. All rights reserved.)*

respiratory burn, tissue damage to the respiratory system resulting from the inhalation of a hot gas or burning particles, as may occur in a fire or explosion. Immediate hospitalization and oxygen therapy are recommended. Compare **smoke inhalation.**

respiratory center, a group of nerve cells in the pons and medulla of the brain that controls the rhythm of breathing in response to changes in levels of oxygen, carbon dioxide, and hydrogen ions in the blood and cerebrospinal fluid. Such changes activate central and peripheral chemoreceptors, which send impulses to the respiratory center, triggering an increase or a decrease in the breathing rate. In patients with retention of carbon dioxide, the respiratory center becomes insensitive to carbon dioxide, and the main stimulus to ventilation is hypoxemia. This effect often occurs in chronic lung disease, requiring careful monitoring of oxygen administration and oxygen levels. The respiratory center is inhibited by barbiturates, anesthetics, tranquilizing agents, and morphine. See also **hyperventilation, hypoventilation, hypoxia.**

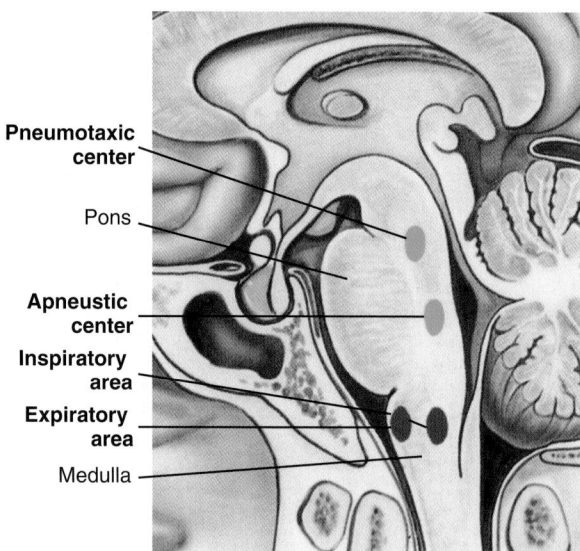

Pneumotaxic center

Pons

Apneustic center

Inspiratory area

Expiratory area

Medulla

Respiratory centers of the brainstem *(Thibodeau and Patton, 2007)*

respiratory component (αPCO₂), the acid component of an acid-base control system that is modified by the respiratory status.

respiratory cycle. See **breathing cycle.**

respiratory depressant [L, *respirare,* to breathe, *depremere,* to press down], a drug or other agent that diminishes normal breathing functions. Most respiratory depressants, such as alcohol and opiates, act by depressing the central nervous system.

respiratory depression [L, *respirare,* to breathe, *depremere,* to press down], respiration that has a rate below 12 breaths per minute or that fails to provide full ventilation and perfusion of the lungs. Also called **respiratory insufficiency.**

respiratory distress syndrome of the newborn (RDS), an acute lung disease of the newborn, characterized by airless alveoli, inelastic lungs, a respiration rate greater than 60 breaths per minute, nasal flaring, intercostal and subcostal retractions, grunting on expiration, and peripheral edema. The condition occurs most often in premature babies. It is caused by a deficiency of pulmonary surfactant, resulting in overdistended alveoli and, at times, hyaline membrane formation, alveolar hemorrhage, severe right-to-left shunting of blood, increased pulmonary resistance, decreased cardiac output, and severe hypoxemia. Treatment includes measures to correct shock, acidosis, and hypoxemia and use of continuous positive airway pressure to prevent alveolar collapse. Also called **hyaline membrane, idiopathic respiratory distress syndrome.** Compare **adult respiratory distress syndrome.**

■ OBSERVATIONS: Signs and symptoms usually appear within 6 hours of birth and include rapid respirations, nostril flaring, expiratory grunting, chest retractions, labored breathing, frothing at lips, inspiratory crackles, cyanosis, and weak cry. These manifestations progress to apnea, flaccidity, unresponsiveness, mottling, peripheral edema, oliguria, hypotension, and bradycardia. Diagnosis is made by clinical exam, chest x-rays that display a diffuse granular pattern in bilateral lung fields indicating atelectasis, and bronchograms representing dilated air-filled bronchioles. Pulmonary function studies are run to differentiate a pulmonary from extrapulmonary illness. Blood gases are taken to determine the extent of respiratory function and acid-base imbalances. Possible complications include intraventricular hemorrhage, tension pneumothorax, retinopathy of prematurity, bronchopulmonary dysplasia, apnea, patent ductus arteriosus, congestive heart failure, neurological sequelae, necrotizing enterocolitis, pneumonia, sepsis, and/or death.

■ INTERVENTIONS: Treatment is largely supportive. Exogenous surfactant is administered as soon as possible after birth and the infant is transported to the intensive care unit. Ventilation is started by continuous positive airway pressure. Warm, humidified oxygen therapy is used. Nutrition is managed by parenteral therapy (nipple and gavage feeding are contraindicated). Continued and aggressive laboratory monitoring of respiratory, circulatory, acid-base, and electrolyte status is performed. Blood transfusions may be necessary to replace blood lost during aggressive monitoring. Preventive measures are instituted with pregnant women by administering betamethasone injections to those mothers 24 to 48 hours before the delivery of any premature infant 24 to 34 weeks in gestation.

■ PATIENT CARE CONSIDERATIONS: Acute nursing and respiratory care is focused on adequate ventilation, oxygenation, maintenance of fluid and nutrition, and prevention of complications. Positioning aids in ventilation; use of blanket rolls and warmers reduces heat loss and lowers oxygen and glucose consumption and metabolic requirements. Careful intake and output, daily weights, and hydration assessments are used to monitor fluids and nutrition. Care clustering helps provide rest between the multiple interventions, such as suctioning, blood sticks, arterial blood gas draws, medication administration, and assessments. Parental support and education about infant treatments and monitoring are necessary. Parents should be educated about the self-limiting nature of the disease. The need for long-term medical follow-up should be stressed to monitor for and detect potential neurological and respiratory sequelae.

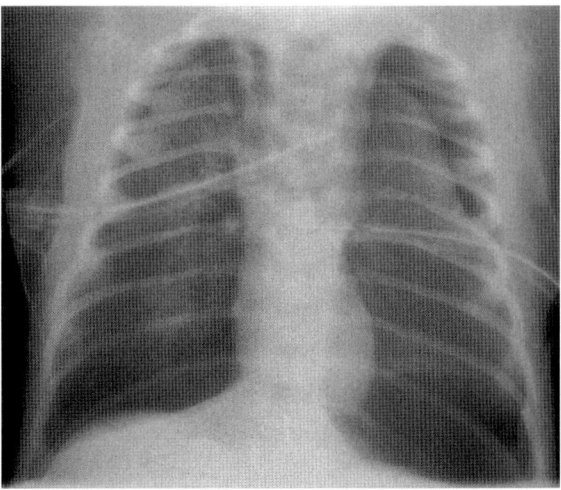

Respiratory distress syndrome in a newborn *(Adam et al, 2008)*

respiratory diverticulum, a pouchlike protrusion from the foregut that gives rise to the trachea, bronchi, and the branches that form the tracheobronchial tree.

respiratory exchange ratio (R), the ratio of the amount of carbon dioxide produced to the amount of oxygen consumed or taken up.

respiratory failure, the inability of the cardiovascular and pulmonary systems to maintain an adequate exchange of oxygen and carbon dioxide in the lungs. Respiratory failure may be caused by a failure in oxygenation or in ventilation. Oxygenation failure is characterized by refractory hypoxemia and occurs in diseases that affect the alveoli or interstitial tissues of the lungs, such as alveolar edema, emphysema, fungal infections, leukemia, lobar pneumonia, lung carcinoma, various pneumoconioses, pulmonary eosinophilia, sarcoidosis, or tuberculosis. Ventilatory failure, characterized by increased arterial tension of carbon dioxide, occurs in acute conditions in which retained pulmonary secretions cause increased airway resistance and decreased lung compliance, as in bronchitis. Ventilation may also be reduced by depression of the respiratory center by barbiturates or opiates, hypoxia, hypercapnia, intracranial diseases, trauma, or lesions of the neuromuscular system or thoracic cage. Respiratory failure in preexisting chronic lung diseases may be precipitated by added stress, as with cardiac failure, surgery, anesthesia, or respiratory tract infections. Treatment of respiratory failure includes clearing the airways by suction, bronchodilators, or tracheostomy or endotracheal tube with ventilator support; antibiotics for infections that are usually present; anticoagulants for pulmonary thromboemboli; and electrolyte replacement in fluid imbalance. Oxygen may be administered in some cases; in others it may further decrease the respiratory reflex by removing the stimulus of a decreased

R

level of oxygen. Chronic respiratory failure may result in cor pulmonale with congestive heart failure and respiratory acidosis. See also **acute respiratory failure, airway obstruction, carbon dioxide, hypercapnia, hyperventilation, hypoxemia, hypoxia, respiratory acidosis.**

respiratory insufficiency. See **respiratory depression.**

respiratory muscles, the muscles that produce volume changes of the thorax during breathing. The inspiratory muscles include the hemidiaphragms, external intercostals, scaleni, sternomastoids, trapezius, pectoralis major, pectoralis minor, subclavius, latissimus dorsi, serratus anterior, and muscles that extend the back. The expiratory muscles are the internal intercostals, the abdominals, and the muscles that flex the back.

respiratory quotient (RQ), the ratio of the volume of carbon dioxide produced to the volume of oxygen consumed per unit of time by the body under steady-state conditions. Depending on the net metabolic needs of all parts of the body at a given moment, the ratio ranges from 0.7 to 1 and averages around 0.8. The RQ varies for different metabolic fuels: the RQ of fat is lower than that of protein, which is lower than that of glucose. Also called **metabolic respiratory quotient.**

respiratory rate. See **respiration rate.**

respiratory rhythm, a regular, oscillating cycle of inspiration and expiration, controlled by neuronal impulses transmitted between the respiratory centers in the brain and the muscles of inspiration in the chest and diaphragm. The normal breathing pattern may be altered by a variety of conditions. See also **apnea, apneustic breathing, Biot respiration, Cheyne-Stokes respiration, chronic obstructive pulmonary disease, Hering-Breuer reflex, hyperventilation, hypoventilation, Kussmaul breathing, tachypnea.**

respiratory standstill, the cessation of respiratory movements.

respiratory syncytial virus (RSV, RS virus), a member of a subgroup of myxoviruses that, in tissue culture, causes formation of giant cells or syncytia. It is a common cause of epidemics of acute bronchiolitis, bronchopneumonia, and the common cold in young children and sporadic acute bronchitis and mild upper respiratory tract infections in adults. Symptoms of infection with this virus include fever, cough, and severe malaise. The virus occasionally is fatal in infants. Systemic invasion by the virus does not happen, and secondary bacterial invasion is uncommon. Treatment includes rest, high humidity, adequate fluid intake, and, in severe cases, oxygen and ribavirin aerosol. Compare **rhinovirus.** See also **bronchiolitis, bronchitis, bronchopneumonia, cold.**

respiratory syncytial virus immune globulin (RSV-IGIV), an immune serum.

■ INDICATIONS: It is used in children less than 2 years of age with bronchopulmonary dysplasia or in those born prematurely to prevent serious lower respiratory tract infection caused by respiratory syncytial virus.

■ CONTRAINDICATIONS: Factors that prohibit its use are hypersensitivity to this drug or to other human immunoglobulin preparations and IgA deficiency.

■ ADVERSE EFFECTS: Life-threatening effects are respiratory distress, hypoxia, anaphylaxis, and angioneurotic edema. Other adverse effects are tachypnea, rales, wheezing, fever, hypertension, tachycardia, fluid overload, diarrhea, gastroenteritis, vomiting, rash, overdose effect, and inflammation at the injection site.

respiratory syncytial virus immune globulin intravenous, a preparation of immunoglobulin G from pooled adult human plasma selected for high titers of antibodies against respiratory syncytial virus. It is used for passive immunization of infants and children less than 24 months of age; administered by IV infusion.

respiratory system. See **respiratory tract.**

respiratory therapist, a graduate of a program approved by the Commission on Accreditation of Allied Health Education Programs, designed to qualify the person for the registry examination of the National Board for Respiratory Care. See also **registered respiratory therapist.**

respiratory therapy (RT), **1.** any treatment that maintains or improves the ventilatory function of the respiratory tract. RT uses scientific applications of technology to assist in the diagnosis, treatment, management, and care of patients with cardiopulmonary and associated disorders. **2.** *(Informal)* the department in a health care facility that provides respiratory therapy for the patients of the facility.

respiratory therapy technician, a graduate of a program in the United States approved by the Commission on Accreditation of Allied Health Education Programs, designed to qualify the person for the technician certification examination of the National Board for Respiratory Care. The program requires a special curriculum of basic sciences with supervised clinical experience.

respiratory therapy technician, certified (CRTT), an allied health professional who administers general respiratory care. Duties can include collection and review of clinical data; examination of the patient by inspection, palpation, percussion, and auscultation; and assembling and maintaining equipment used in respiratory care.

respiratory tract, the complex of organs and structures that performs the pulmonary ventilation of the body and the exchange of oxygen and carbon dioxide between ambient air and blood circulating through the lungs. It also warms the air passing into the body and assists in the speech function by providing air for the larynx and the vocal cords. Every 24 hours about 500 cubic feet of air (150 m³) passes through the respiratory tract of the average adult, who breathes in and out between 12 and 18 times a minute. The respiratory tract is divided into the upper respiratory tract and the lower respiratory tract. Also called **respiratory system.** See also *Color Atlas of Human Anatomy,* pp. A-28 to A-31.

respiratory tract infection, any infectious disease of the upper or lower respiratory tract. Upper respiratory tract infections (URIs) include the common cold, laryngitis, pharyngitis, rhinitis, sinusitis, and tonsillitis. Lower respiratory tract infections include bronchitis, bronchiolitis, pneumonia, and tracheitis.

respiratory zone, structures deep in the lungs that are directly involved in gas exchange, beginning where the terminal bronchioles join a respiratory bronchiole, leading to an alveolar duct, and opening into a cluster of alveoli. Compare **conducting zone.**

respirometer /res′pirom″ətər/ [L, *respirare,* to breathe; Gk, *metron,* measure], an instrument used to analyze the quality of a patient's respirations.

respite care /res″pit/ [L, *respicere,* to look back], **1.** short-term health services for the dependent older adult, either at home or in an institutional setting. **2.** the provision of temporary care for a patient who requires specialized or intensive care or supervision that is normally provided by his or her family at home. Respite care provides the family with relief from demands of the patient's care.

respite time /res″pit/, relief time from responsibilities for the care of a patient, an individual, or a family member.

respondeat superior /respon″dē·at/ [L, let the master answer], the concept that an employer may be held liable for torts committed by employees acting within the scope of their employment.

respondent conditioning.   See **classical conditioning.**

responder /rispon″dər/ [L, *respondere,* to promise in return], a person whose tumor shrinks in volume by at least 50% as a result of chemotherapy, radiation, or other treatment.

response /rispons″/ [L, *responsum,* reply], **1.** a reaction of an organism to a stimulus. **2.** (in psychology) a category of negative punishment in which the reinforcer is lost or withdrawn after an operant.

response time, **1.** the period between the input of information into a computer, central processing unit, or other processor and the response or output, measured in milliseconds or nanoseconds or fractions thereof. **2.** the period between the application of a stimulus and the response of a cell or cells.

rest [AS, *restan,* to rest], (in dentistry) an extension from a prosthesis that provides vertical support for a dental restoration.

rest angle. See **occlusal rest angle.**

rest area, a prepared surface on a tooth or fixed restoration into which an arm or a removable partial denture fits. Also called **rest seat, occlusal rest,** *incisal rest.*

resting cell, a cell that is not undergoing division. See also **interphase.**

resting membrane potential, the transmembrane voltage that exists when a neuron or muscle cell is not producing an action potential.

resting potential [AS, *rest* + L, *potentia,* power], the electric potential across a nerve cell membrane before it is stimulated to release the charge. The resting potential for a neuron is between 50 and 100 mV, with the excess of negatively charged ions inside the cell membrane.

resting splint, *(Informal)* a static orthotic device designed to support an extremity for the relief of pain and inflammation. It is also used to restrict motion and maintain the extremity in a position of function.

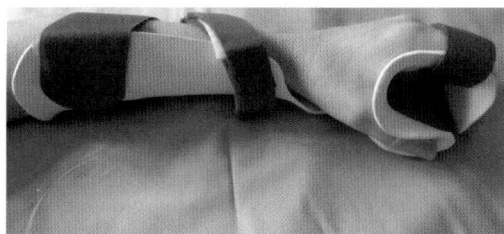

Resting splint

resting tremor, an involuntary trembling or shaking movements that happen when a person is at rest. It is one of the signs of Parkinson disease. Also called **passive tremor.** See also **action tremor, tremor.**

restitution /res′tit(y)o͞o″shən/, the spontaneous turning of the fetal head to the right or left after it has extended through the vulva.

rest jaw relation, the postural relation of the mandible to the maxilla when the patient is resting comfortably in the upright position. The condyles are in a neutral, unstrained position in the mandibular fossae, and the mandibular musculature is in a state of minimum tonic contraction necessary to maintain the posture.

rest joint position, the position of a joint where the joint surfaces are relatively incongruent and the support structures are relatively lax. The position is used extensively in passive mobilization procedures.

restless legs syndrome [AS, *restlaes* + ONorse, *leggr*], a benign condition of unknown origin accompanied by an irresistible urge to move the legs. It is often characterized by an irritating sensation of uneasiness, tiredness, and itching deep within the muscles of the leg, especially the lower part of the limb, and sometimes by pain. Also called **anxietas tibiarum, Ekbom syndrome, Wittmaack-Ekbom syndrome.**

restoration /res′tôrā″shən/ [L, *restaurare,* to restore], any tooth filling, inlay, onlay, crown, partial or complete denture, or prosthesis that restores or replaces missing tooth structure, entire teeth, or oral tissues. Also called **dental restoration, prosthetic restoration.**

restoration contour, the profile of the surfaces of teeth that have been restored.

restoration of cusps, a reduction and inclusion of tooth cusps within a tooth cavity preparation and their restoration to functional occlusion with an artificial dental material.

restorative /ristôr″ətiv/ [L, *restaurare*], pertaining to the power or ability to restore or renew a person to a normal state of health or consciousness.

Restoril, a hypnotic agent. Brand name for **temazepam.**

restraint /ristrānt″/ [L, *restringere,* to confine], any one of numerous mechanical devices or chemical agents used to hinder or restrict a patient's movement. Examples of mechanical restraints are specially designed slings, jackets, or diapers. Restraints that are too tight may cause skin irritation; those that fit too loosely do not serve their purpose. When a restraining device needs to be used, it should be correctly sized for the patient and allow enough space for two fingers to fit between the patient's skin and the restraint. Restraints are usually removed every 4 hours or more frequently to assess skin integrity and provide skin care. Release of restraints at least every 2 hours is recommended to allow range-of-motion exercises and assistance with activities of daily living. Throughout the period of restraint, it is important to continue recording all physical and psychosocial assessments in accordance with hospital protocol. The least restrictive restraint that promotes patient safety or positioning is required. See also **mechanical restraint.**

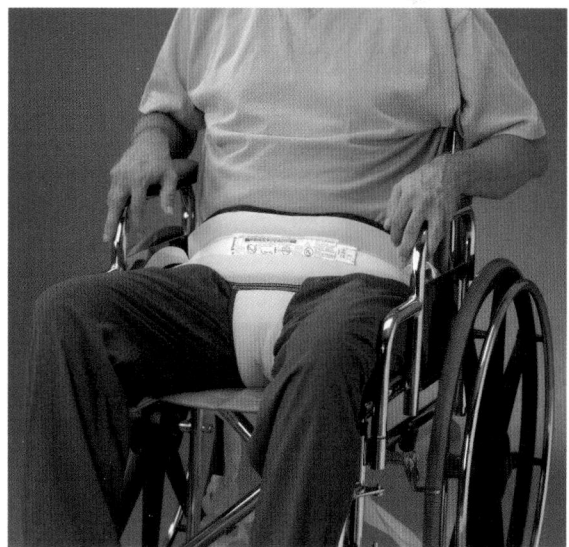

A restraint belt helps prevent forward sliding in wheelchairs *(Courtesy Posey)*

restraint in bed [L, *restringere,* to confine; AS, *bedd*], the confinement of a person to bed rest by the use of mechanical, physical, or chemical means, if needed.

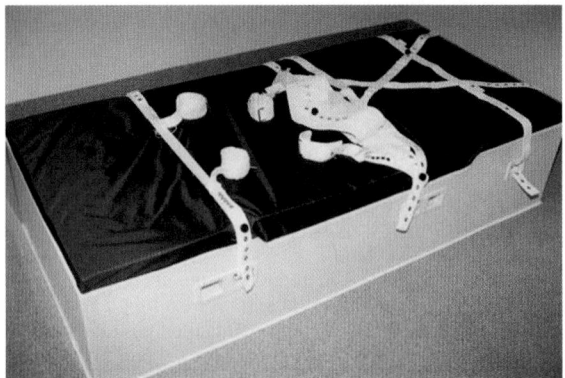

Restraint bed *(Courtesy Max-Secure Systems, Inc. Williamsville, New York)*

restraint of trade, an illegal act that interferes with free competition in a commercial or business transaction so as to restrict the production of a product or the provision of a service, affect the cost of a product or a service, or control the market in any way to the detriment of the consumers or purchasers of the service or product. The Clayton Act and the Sherman Antitrust Act are U.S. federal statutes that embody the basic concepts of the definition and the illegal nature of restraint of trade.

restriction endonuclease /ristrik″shən en′dōnoo″klē·ās/ [L, *restringere* + Gk, *endon,* within; L, *nucleus,* nut kernel; Fr, *diastase,* enzyme], an enzyme that cleaves DNA at a specific site. Each of the many endonucleases isolated from various bacteria acts at a different site, making it possible for researchers to divide DNA molecules at selected locations. See also **restriction fragment length polymorphism.**

restriction fragment, a fragment of DNA produced by cleavage by a specific endonuclease.

restriction fragment length polymorphism (RFLP), a difference in the DNA sequences of homologous chromosomes as revealed by different lengths of the restriction fragments produced by enzymatic digestion of a selected region of chromosomes. RFLPs are believed to be inherited according to mendelian laws and have been used to locate the genes associated with several inherited disorders, including Huntington disease.

restrictive cardiomyopathy. See **constrictive cardiomyopathy.**

restrictive disease, a respiratory disorder characterized by restriction of expansion of the lungs or chest wall, resulting in diminished lung volumes and capacities. Causes include impaired neuromuscular contraction, impaired lung expansion, thoracic deformities, and pleural-based diseases.

rest seat. See **rest area.**

resume, résumé. See **curriculum vitae.**

resuscitation /risus′itā″shən/ [L, *resuscitare,* to revive], the process of sustaining the vital functions of a person in respiratory or cardiac failure while reviving him or her by using techniques of artificial respiration and cardiac massage, correcting acid-base imbalance, and treating the cause of failure. See also **cardiopulmonary resuscitation.**

resuscitator /risus″itā′tər/, an apparatus for pumping air into the lungs. It consists of a mask snugly applied over the mouth and nose, a reservoir for air, and a manually or electrically powered pump. Often oxygen may be added to the air in the reservoir. See also **Ambu bag, bag-valve-mask resuscitator.**

RET, abbreviation for **rational emotive therapy.**

retail dentistry /rē″tāl/ [ME, *retailen,* to divide into pieces], the practice of fee-for-service dentistry in an exclusively retail environment, such as a shopping center or a department store, with the specific intention of attracting the customers of that retail environment by using the marketing techniques of the retailers involved.

retain. See **retention.**

retained placenta /ritānd″/ [L, *retinere,* to hold, *placenta,* flat cake], the failure of the placenta to be delivered during an appropriate period, usually 30 minutes, following birth of the infant. A retained placenta can lead to excessive bleeding.

retainer [L, *retinere,* to hold], **1.** the part of a dental prosthesis that is cemented to an abutment tooth to which the suspended part of a bridge (called the pontic) is attached. It may be an inlay, a partial crown, or a complete crown. **2.** an appliance for maintaining teeth positions and jaw relations gained by orthodontic procedures. Also called *retaining orthodontic appliance.* **3.** the part of a fixed prosthesis that attaches a pontic to the abutment teeth. **4.** any clasp, attachment, or device for fixing or stabilizing a dental prosthesis.

retake /rē″tāk/, the repeat of a radiograph because of inadequate technical quality, patient motion, mispositioning of the body part, or equipment malfunction.

retard, to slow.

retardation /rē′tärdā″shən/ [L, *retardare,* to check], the slowing down of any mental or physical activity. Psychomotor retardation may occur in depression, as when the person walks and talks slowly or is unable to get out of bed in the morning.

retarded dentition, an abnormal delay in the eruption of the primary or secondary teeth, resulting from malnutrition, malposition of the teeth, a hereditary factor, or a metabolic imbalance, such as hypothyroidism. Also called **delayed dentition.** Compare **precocious dentition.**

retarded depression, the depressive phase of bipolar disorder.

retarded ejaculation, the inability of a male to ejaculate after having achieved an erection. This often accompanies the aging process. Also called *delayed ejaculation.*

retch [AS, *hraecan,* to spit], a strong, wrenching attempt to vomit that does not bring up anything. Compare **eructation, vomit.**

rete /rē″tē/ [L, net], a network, especially of arteries or veins. –**retial,** *adj.*

rete arteriosum. See **arterial network.**

retention /riten″shən/, **1.** a resistance to movement or displacement. **2.** the ability of the digestive system to hold food and fluid. **3.** the inability to urinate or defecate. **4.** the ability of the mind to remember information acquired from reading, observation, or other processes. **5.** the inherent property of a dental restoration to maintain its position without displacement under axial stress. **6.** a characteristic of proper tooth cavity preparation in which provision is made for preventing vertical displacement of the cavity filling. **7.** a period of treatment during which an individual wears an appliance to maintain teeth in positions to which they have been moved by orthodontic procedures. –**retain,** *v.*

retention cyst [L, *retinere,* to hold; Gk, *kystis,* bag], a cyst caused by blockage of the excretory duct of a gland so that glandular secretions are retained. Also called **secretory cyst.**

retention enema [L, *retinere,* to hold; Gk, *enienai,* to send in], a medicinal or nutrient enema specially formulated so that it will remain in the bowel without stimulating the nerve endings that would ordinarily result in evacuation. See also **oil retention enema.**

retention form, (in dentistry) the provision made in a prepared tooth cavity to hold in place a restoration and to prevent its displacement.

retention groove, (in dentistry) a depression formed by preparing vertical constrictions in a prepared tooth cavity, which improves the holding ability (retention form) of a restoration. Compare **resistance form.**

retention of urine, an abnormal, involuntary accumulation of urine in the bladder as a result of a loss of muscle tone in the bladder, neurological dysfunction or damage to the bladder, obstruction of the urethra, or administration of a narcotic analgesic, especially morphine.

retention pin, (in dentistry) a small metal pin that extends from the dentin into a tooth restoration to improve the stability of a tooth restoration.

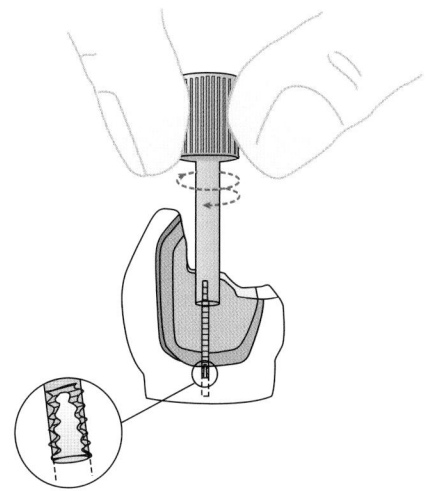

Placement of a retention pin *(Bird and Robinson, 2012)*

retention procedure, a method established by state laws or mental health codes for committing a person to a psychiatric institution. In the United States, most states recognize four types of retention: emergency, informal, involuntary, and voluntary admission. In Canada, patients/clients can be retained under the Mental Health Acts of the various provinces and territories.

retention time (ta), **1.** (in chromatography) the amount of time elapsed from the injection of a sample into the chromatographic system to the recording of the peak (band) maximum of the component in the chromatogram. **2.** the length of time a compound is retained on a chromatography column.

retention with overflow [L, *retinere,* to hold; AS, *ofer + flowan*], a complication of bladder outlet obstruction in which the bladder is full but is not emptied completely. Urine dribbles out with a sense of urgency, or uncontrollable intermittent leakage occurs. Also called **paradoxic incontinence.**

rete peg. See **epithelial peg.**

reteplase /ret′ĕ-plās/, a recombinant form of tissue plasminogen activator used intravenously as a thrombolytic agent in treatment of myocardial infarction.

retial. See **rete.**

reticul-, prefix meaning "netlike": *reticular, reticulocyte, reticuloendothelioma.*

reticular /ritik″yələr/ [L, *reticulum,* little net], (of a tissue or surface) having a netlike pattern or structure.

reticular activating system (RAS), a functional (rather than morphological) system in the brain essential for wakefulness, attention, concentration, and introspection. A network of nerve fibers in the thalamus, hypothalamus, brainstem, and cerebral cortex contributes to the system.

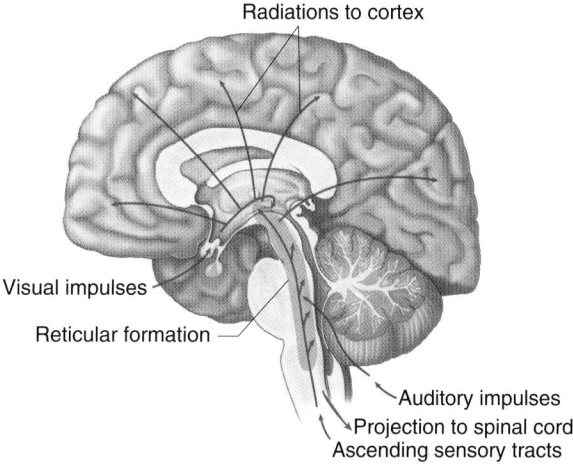

Reticular activating system *(Patton and Thibodeau, 2010)*

reticular formation, a small, thick cluster of neurons nestled within the brainstem, including the medulla that controls the level of consciousness and other vital functions of the body. The reticular formation constantly monitors the state of the body through connections with the sensory and motor tracts. Certain nerve cells in the formation regulate the flow of hydrochloric acid in the stomach. Other cells regulate swallowing, tongue movements, and movements of the face, eyes, and tongue.

reticular membrane, a netlike membrane over the organ of Corti; the free ends of the outer acoustic hair cells pass through its apertures. Also called *reticular lamina.*

reticular nuclei, nuclei found in the reticular formation of the brainstem, primarily in longitudinal columns in three groups: the median column reticular nuclei (which include the raphe nuclei), the medial column reticular nuclei, and the lateral column reticular nuclei. The term also encompasses several other nuclei that are not in any of the three columns, such as the reticular nucleus of the thalamus.

reticulated pigmented poikiloderma, a red coloration in the cheeks and neck. See **poikiloderma of Civatte.**

reticulin /ritik″yəlin/ [L, *reticulum,*], an albuminoid substance found in the connective fibers of reticular tissue.

reticulocyte /ritik″yələsīt′/ [L, *reticulum* + Gk, *kytos,* cell], an immature erythrocyte characterized by a meshlike pattern of nucleic acids when stained using new methylene blue dye. Reticulocytes normally account for less than 2% of the circulating erythrocytes. A greater proportion reflects increased bone marrow generation of red blood cells. Also called *polychromatophilic erythrocyte* when seen in a Wright-stained peripheral blood film. Compare **erythrocyte.** See also **normoblast.**

reticulocyte count, a count of the number of reticulocytes in a whole blood specimen, used in determining bone marrow activity. The reticulocyte count is lowered in hemolytic diseases and chronic infection; it is elevated after hemorrhage or during recovery from anemia. The normal concentration of

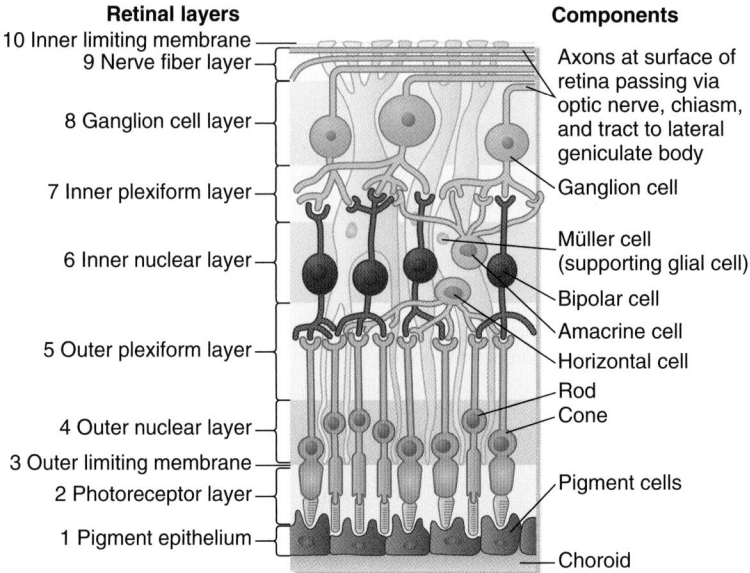

Retinal layers

10 Inner limiting membrane
9 Nerve fiber layer
8 Ganglion cell layer
7 Inner plexiform layer
6 Inner nuclear layer
5 Outer plexiform layer
4 Outer nuclear layer
3 Outer limiting membrane
2 Photoreceptor layer
1 Pigment epithelium

Components

Axons at surface of retina passing via optic nerve, chiasm, and tract to lateral geniculate body
Ganglion cell
Müller cell (supporting glial cell)
Bipolar cell
Amacrine cell
Horizontal cell
Rod
Cone
Pigment cells
Choroid

Layers of the retina (Koeppen and Stanton, 2010)

reticulocytes in whole blood in adults is 0.5% to 1.5% of total red blood cells.

reticulocytopenia /ritik′yəlōsī′təpē″nē·ə/ [L, *reticulum* + Gk, *kytos,* cell, *penia,* poverty], a decrease below the reference interval lower limit of 0.5% in the number of reticulocytes in a blood sample.

reticulocytosis /-sītō″sis/, an increase over the reference interval upper limit of 2.0% in the number of reticulocytes in the circulating blood that may represent a normal increase in activity of the bone marrow in response to blood loss.

reticuloendothelial cells /ritik′yəlō·en′dōthē″lē·əl/ [L, *reticulum* + Gk, *endon,* within, *thele,* nipple], albuminoid or scleroprotein cells lining vascular and lymph vessels and capable of phagocytosing bacteria, viruses, and colloidal particles or of forming immune bodies against foreign particles.

reticuloendothelial system (RES), a functional rather than anatomical system of the body involved primarily in defense against infection and in disposal of the products of the breakdown of cells. It is made up of macrophages; the Kupffer cells of the liver; and the reticulum cells of the lungs, bone marrow, spleen, and lymph nodes. Disorders of this system include eosinophilic granuloma, Gaucher's disease, Hand's disease, and Niemann-Pick disease.

reticuloendothelioma /-thē″lē·ō′mə/, a tumor consisting of cells of the reticuloendothelial system.

reticuloendotheliosis /ritik′yəlō·en′dōthē′lē·ō″sis/, an abnormal condition characterized by increased growth and proliferation of the cells of the reticuloendothelial system. See also **reticuloendothelial system.**

reticulogranular /-gran′yələr/ [L, *reticulum* + *granulum,* little grain], pertaining to a cloudy appearance of the lungs on a chest radiograph of a patient with respiratory distress syndrome.

reticulosarcoma. See **undifferentiated malignant lymphoma.**

reticulum cell sarcoma. See **histiocytic malignant lymphoma.**

retin-, prefix meaning "retina": *retinol, retinopathy.*

-retin, suffix for retinol derivatives.

retina /ret″inə/ [L, *rete,* net], a 10-layered, delicate nervous tissue membrane of the eye, continuous with the optic nerve, that receives images of external objects and transmits visual impulses through the optic nerve to the brain. The retina is soft and semitransparent and contains rhodopsin. It consists of the outer pigmented layer and the nine-layered retina proper. These nine layers, starting with the most internal, are the internal limiting membrane, the stratum opticum, the ganglion cell layer, the inner plexiform layer, the inner nuclear layer, the outer plexiform layer, the outer nuclear layer, the external limiting membrane, and the layer of rods and cones. The outer surface of the retina is in contact with the choroid, the inner surface with the vitreous body. The retina is thinner anteriorly, where it extends nearly as far as the ciliary body, and thicker posteriorly, except for a thin spot in the exact center of the posterior surface where focus is best. The photoreceptors end anteriorly in the jagged ora serrata at the ciliary body, but the membrane of the retina extends over the back of the ciliary processes and the iris. The retina becomes clouded and opaque if exposed to direct sunlight. See also **Jacob x membrane, macula, optic disc.**

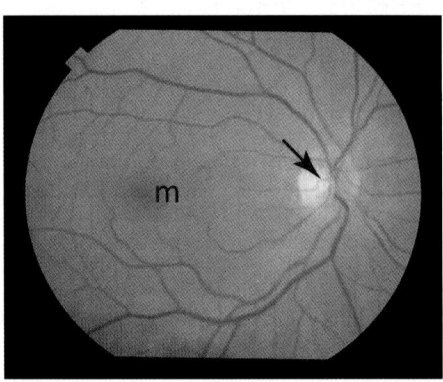

Normal retina illustrating the optic disc (arrow) and macula region (m) (Shepherd et al, 2013)

Retin-A, an antiacne medication. Brand name for **tretinoin.**

retinaculum /ret′inak″yələm/ *pl.* *retinacula* [L, halter], **1.** a structure that retains an organ or tissue. **2.** an instrument for retracting tissues during surgery.

retinaculum extensorum manus. See **extensor retinaculum of the hand.**

retinal /ret″inəl, ret′inal″/ [L, *rete*], **1.** *n.,* an aldehyde precursor of vitamin A produced by the enzymatic dehydration of retinol. It is the active form of the vitamin necessary for night, day, and color vision. See also **retinene, vitamin A. 2.** *adj.,* pertaining to the retina.

retinal detachment, a separation of the retina from the retinal pigment epithelium in the back of the eye. It usually results from a hole or tear in the retina that allows the vitreous humor to leak between the choroid and the retina. Severe trauma to the eye, such as a contusion or penetrating wound, may be the proximate cause, but in the great majority of cases retinal detachment is the result of internal changes in the vitreous chamber associated with aging or, less frequently, inflammation of the interior of the eye.

■ OBSERVATIONS: In most cases, retinal detachment develops slowly. The first symptom is often the sudden appearance of a large number of floating spots loosely suspended in front of the affected eye. The person may not seek help because the number of spots tends to decrease during the days and weeks after the detachment. The person may also notice a curious sensation of flashing lights as the eye is moved. Because the retina does not contain sensory nerves that relay sensations of pain, the condition is painless. Detachment usually begins at the thin peripheral edge of the retina and extends gradually beneath the thicker, more central areas. The person perceives a shadow that begins laterally and grows in size, slowly encroaching on central vision. As long as the center of the retina is unaffected, the vision, when the person is looking straight ahead, is normal. When the center becomes affected, the eyesight is distorted, wavy, and indistinct. If the process of detachment is not halted, total blindness of the eye ultimately results. The condition does not spontaneously resolve itself.

■ INTERVENTIONS: Surgery is usually required to repair the hole and prevent leakage of vitreous humor that separates the retina from its source of nourishment, the choroid. If the condition is discovered early when the hole is small and the volume of vitreous humor lost is not large, the retinal hole may be closed by causing a scar to form on the choroid and to adhere to the retina around the hole. The scar may be produced by heat, laser energy, or cold. The scar is held against the retina by local pressure achieved by a variety of surgical techniques.

■ PATIENT CARE CONSIDERATIONS: Retinal detachment requires treatment. The degree of restoration of sight depends on the extent and duration of separation. Unless replaced, a detached retina slowly dies after several years of detachment. Blindness resulting from retinal detachment is irreversible.

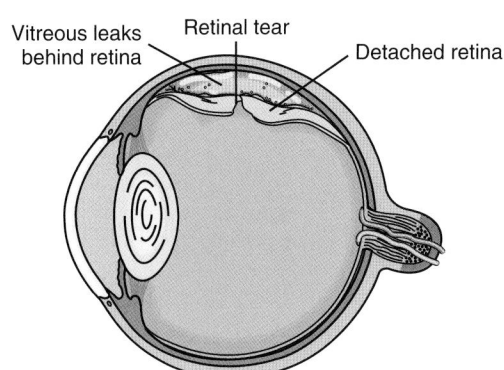

Retinal detachment: tear in retina *(Monahan et al, 2007)*

retinal fissure, a ventral groove formed by invagination of the optic cup and its stalk by vascular mesenchyme from which the hyaloid vessels develop. Also called **optic fissure.**

retinene /ret″inin/ [L, *rete*], either of the two carotenoid pigments found in the rods of the retina that are precursors of vitamin A and are activated by light. See also **retinal, retinol.**

retinitis /ret′inī″tis/ [L, *rete*, net; Gk, *itis,* inflammation], an inflammation of the retina.

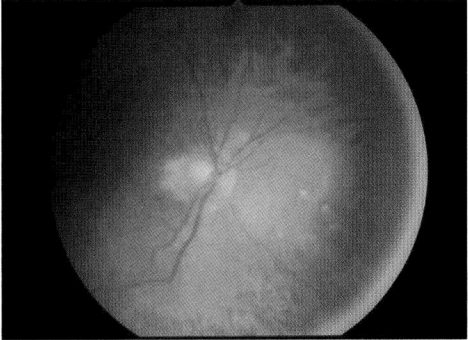

Retinitis secondary to cytomegalovirus infection
(Goldman et al, 2008)

retinitis pigmentosa [L, *rete*, net; Gk, *itis,* inflammation; L, *pigmentum,* paint], a group of diseases, often hereditary, characterized by bilateral primary degeneration of the retina beginning in childhood and progressing to blindness by middle age. Clinical signs include night blindness, reduced visual fields, depigmentation of the retinal pigment epithelium, and macular degeneration. Length of time to legal blindness varies widely.

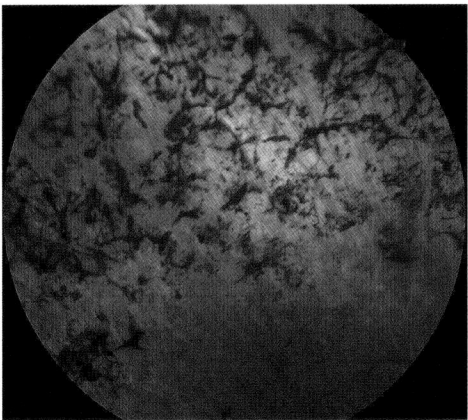

Retinitis pigmentosa *(Kanski, 2006)*

retinoblastoma /ret′inōblastō″mə/ *pl.* *retinoblastomas, retinoblastomata* [L, *rete* + Gk, *blastos,* germ, *oma,* tumor], a congenital hereditary neoplasm developing from retinal germ cells. Characteristic signs are diminished vision, strabismus, retinal detachment, and an abnormal pupillary reflex. The rapidly growing tumor may invade the brain and metastasize to distant sites. Treatment includes removal of the eye and as much of the optic nerve as possible, followed by radiation and chemotherapy. It is bilateral in about 30% of the cases. The more affected eye is enucleated, and the other eye is treated with radiation, antibiotics, cryotherapy, or photocoagulation, singly or in combination. Because many of the cases are transmitted as an autosomal-dominant trait with incomplete penetration, genetic counseling is advisable.

R

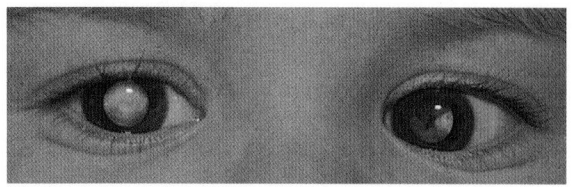

Retinoblastoma *(Skarin, 2010)*

retinocerebral angiomatosis. See **von Hippel–Lindau disease.**

retinochoroiditis /-kôr′oidī″tis/ [L, *rete*, net; Gk, *chorion*, skin, *itis*, inflammation], an inflammation of the retina and choroid coat of the eye. Compare **chorioretinopathy.**

retinodialysis /ret′inō′dī·al″isis/ [L, *rete* + Gk, *dia*, through, *lysis*, loosening], a separation or tear in the retina in its anterior part, in the area of the ora serrata, just behind the ciliary body.

retinoid /ret″inoid/ [L, *rete*, net; Gk, *eidos*, form], **1.** resembling the retina. **2.** pertaining to any of a group of compounds whose molecules contain 20 carbon atoms structurally related to retinal, retinol, and other substances, some of which exhibit vitamin A activity. Retinoid analogs have been used in the prevention and treatment of various skin cancers and treatment of the digestive and respiratory tracts. **3.** resinlike or having a resemblance to resin.

retinol /ret″inol/ [L, *rete*], one form of vitamin A. It is found in the retinas of mammals. See also **vitamin A.**

retinol equivalent (RE), a unit used for quantifying the vitamin A value of sources of vitamin A, including both preformed retinoids in animal foods and precursor carotenoids in plant foods. RE is defined as 3.3 International Units of vitamin A.

retinopathy /ret′inop″əthē/ [L, *rete* + Gk, *pathos*, disease], a group of noninflammatory eye disorders. Major contributing conditions include diabetes, hypertension, and atherosclerotic vascular disease.

retinopexy /ret′inopek″se/, restoration of the retina to its proper anatomical location.

retinoschisis /ret′i·nos′ki·sis/ [L, *rete*, net + *schisis*, cleavage], splitting of the retina. In the juvenile form the splitting occurs in the nerve fiber layer (stratum opticum), and in the adult form it occurs in the outer plexiform layer. The disorder is usually more benign and slowly progressive than retinal detachment. Compare **retinal detachment.**

retinoscope /ret″inəskōp′/ [L, *rete*, net; Gk, *skopein*, to view], an instrument used in retinoscopy to determine errors of refraction.

retinoscopy /ret′inos″kəpē/ [L, *rete*, net; Gk, *skopein*, to view], a procedure for examining the eyes for possible errors of refraction. The examiner shines a light into the eye through the pupillary opening and notes the movements of reflex from the fundus, which will vary with the type of refractive error. The movements indicate the types of lenses needed to neutralize the refractive errors. Also called **shadow test.**

retirement center /ritī″ərmənt/ [Fr, *retirer*, to withdraw; Gk, *kentron*, center], a facility or organized program to provide social services and activities for senior citizens who generally do not require ongoing health care.

retract /ritrakt″/ [L, *retractare*, to draw back], to shrink, make shorter, or pull back.

retracted nipple [L, *retractare*, to draw back; ME, *neb*], a nipple drawn inward, resulting from cancer or adhesions below the skin surface or a natural condition present at birth.

retractile mesenteritis /rē·trak′tīl/ [L, *retractare*, to draw back; Gk, *mesos*, middle, *enteron*, intestine, *itis*, inflammation], inflammation of the mesentery, producing thickening, sclerosis, and retraction and occasionally resulting in distortion of intestinal loops.

retraction /ritrak″shən/ [L, *retractare*, to draw back], **1.** the displacement of tissues to expose a part or structure of the body. **2.** a distal movement of the teeth. **3.** a distal or retrusive position of the teeth, dental arch, or jaw.

retraction of the chest, the visible sinking in of the soft tissues of the chest between and around the firmer tissue of the cartilaginous and bony ribs, as occurs with increased inspiratory effort or obstruction at some level of the respiratory tract. The extent of retraction depends on the level of an obstruction. Retraction begins in the intercostal spaces. If increased effort is needed to fill the lungs, supraclavicular and infraclavicular retraction may be seen. In infants, sternal retraction occurs with only a slight increase in respiratory effort, the result of the pliability of their chests. Compare **intercostal bulging.**

retractor /ritrak″tər/ [L, *retractare*], an instrument for holding back the edges of tissues and organs to maintain exposure of the underlying anatomical parts, particularly during surgery.

retro-, prefix meaning "backward" or "located behind": *retrobulbar, retroperitoneal, retroversion.*

retroanterograde amnesia /ret′rō·anter″ōgrād/ [L, *retro*, backward, *antero*, foremost, *gradus*, step; Gk, *amnesia*, forgetfulness], a memory disorder in which current events may be assigned to the past and past events may be regarded as current.

retroaortic node /ret′rō·ā·ôr″tik/ [L, *retro*, backward; Gk, *aerein*, to raise], a node in one of three sets of lumbar lymph nodes that serve various structures in the abdomen and pelvis. They lie below the cisterna chyli on the bodies of the third and the fourth lumbar vertebrae and receive the lymphatic trunks from the lateral aortic nodes and preaortic nodes. The efferent vessels from the retroaortic nodes end in the cisterna chyli. Compare **lateral aortic node, preaortic node.**

retroauricular /ret′rō·ôrik″yələr/ [L, *retro*, backward, *auricula*, little ear], pertaining to a location behind the ear.

retrobulbar /-bul″bər/ [L, *retro*, backward, *bulbus*, swollen root], **1.** pertaining to the area behind the pons (posterior to the medulla oblongata). **2.** pertaining to the area behind the eyeball.

retrobulbar block, a block performed by injection of a local anesthetic into the retrobulbar space to anesthetize and immobilize the eye.

retrobulbar neuritis [L, *retro*, backward, *bulbus*, swollen root; Gk, *neuron* + *itis*, inflammation]. See **optic neuritis.**

retrobulbar pupillary reflex, an abnormal response of a pupil to light. After initial constriction of the pupil, dilation occurs as the stimulus continues. It is a sign of retrobulbar neuritis.

retrocaecal. See **retrocecal.**

retrocalcaneal space, the space between the posterior calcaneus and the calcaneal tendon, occupied by the calcaneal bursa.

retrocecal /-sē″kəl/ [L, *retro*, backward, *caecus*, blind], pertaining to the region behind the cecum. Also spelled **retrocaecal.**

retroclusion /ret′rōkloo̅″zhən/, a method of controlling hemorrhage from an artery by compressing it between tissues on either side. A needle is inserted through the tissues above the bleeding vessel, then turned around and down so that it also passes through the tissues beneath the artery.

retrofilling /ret′rofil″ing/, a method of root canal therapy in which the canal is filled from the apex, which has been surgically exposed.

retroflexion /-flek″shən/ [L, *retro* + *flectere*, to bend], an abnormal position of an organ, such as the uterus, in which the organ is tilted back acutely and folded over on itself.

retroflexion of the uterus, a condition in which the body of the uterus is bent backward at an angle with the cervix, the position of which usually remains unchanged. Causes of a retroflexed uterus include pregnancy and complications from endometriosis or fibroids.

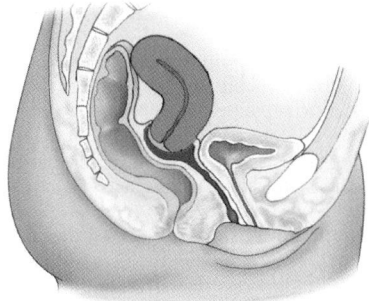

Retroflexion of the uterus *(Leonard, 2009)*

retrognathia /ret′rōnā″thē·ə/ [L, *retro*, backward; Gk, *gnathos*, jaw], a condition in which either or both jaws recede with respect to the frontal plane of the forehead. According to Angle's classification of malocclusion, the facial profile of a person with a Class II malocclusion is retrognathic. Also called **mandibular retrusion, mandibular retroposition, maxillary retroposition, maxillary retrusion.** See also **Angle's classification of malocclusion.**

retrognathism /ret′rōnā″thizəm/ [L, *retro* + Gk, *gnathos*, jaw], a facial abnormality in which a jaw, usually the mandible, or both jaws are posterior to their normal facial positions. Also called **bird face retrognathism.**

retrograde /ret′rəgrād/ [L, *retro* + *gradus*, step], **1.** moving backward; moving in the opposite direction to that which is considered normal. **2.** degenerating; reverting to an earlier state or worse condition. **3.** catabolic.

retrograde amnesia, the loss of memory for events occurring before a particular time in a person's life, usually before the event that precipitated the amnesia. The condition may result from disease, brain injury or damage, or a traumatic emotional incident. Compare **anterograde amnesia.**

retrograde cystoscopy, a technique for radiographically examining the bladder in which a catheter is inserted through the urethra into the bladder, allowing the urine present in the bladder to pass through the catheter. A radiopaque medium is introduced, filling the bladder, and the contour of the bladder is observed, using serial x-ray imaging or fluoroscopy. Also called **cystoscopic urography.** See also **cystogram, retrograde pyelography.**

retrograde ejaculation [L, *retro*, backward, *gradus*, step, *ejaculari*, to throw out], an ejaculation of semen in a reverse direction into the urinary bladder. It may result from surgery or medication.

retrograde filling, a restoration placed in the apical part of a tooth root to seal the apex of a previously treated root canal. Also called **postresection filling.**

retrograde flow [L, *retro*, backward; AS, *flowan*], the flow of fluid in a direction other than normal, as in regurgitation.

retrograde infantilism. See **acromegalic eunuchoidism.**

retrograde infection, an infection that spreads along a tubule or duct against the flow of secretions or excretions, as in the urinary and lymphatic systems.

retrograde menstruation, a backflow of menstrual discharge through the uterine cavity and fallopian tubes into the peritoneal cavity. Fragments of endometrium may attach to the ovaries or other organs, causing endometriosis. Also called **regurgitant menstruation.**

retrograde pyelography, a radiographic technique for examining the structures of the collecting system of the kidneys that is especially useful in locating a urinary tract obstruction. A radiopaque contrast medium is injected through a urinary catheter into the ureters and the calyces of the pelves of the kidneys.

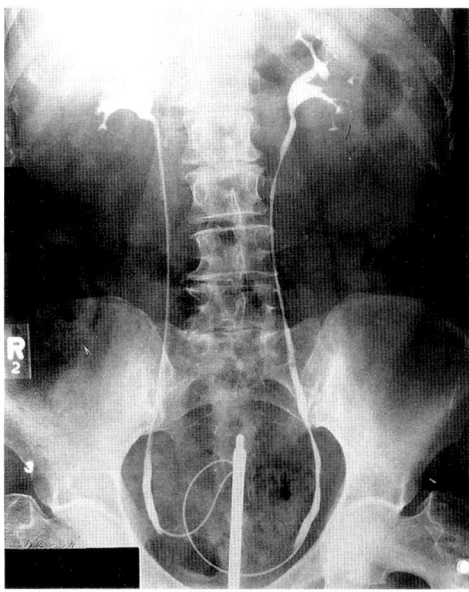

Normal retrograde pyelography *(Wein et al, 2007)*

retrograde urethrography, radiographic examination of the urethra after suspicion of obstruction of its external orifice and injection of contrast material that travels in a retrograde direction toward the bladder. It is used for evaluation of strictures, diverticula, and trauma.

retrograde urography. See **retrograde pyelography.**

retrograde Wenckebach /veng″kəbäk, -bäkh/ [Karel F. Wenckebach, Dutch-Austrian physician, 1864–1940], a delay in the conduction of impulses from the ventricles or atrioventricular junction to the atria. The delay increases progressively until an impulse fails to reach the atria.

retrogression /-gresh″ən/ [L, *retro* + *gradi*, to step], a return to a less complex state, condition, or behavioral adaptation; degeneration; deterioration. See also **regression.**

retroinguinal space, the subdivision of the extraperitoneal space bounded by the peritoneum above and the fascia transversalis below.

retrolental fibroplasia /-len″təl/ [L, *retro* + *lentil*, lens, *fibra*, fiber; Gk, *plassein*, to mold], **1.** a formation of fibrous tissue behind the lens of the eye, resulting in blindness. **2.** a severe form of retinopathy in premature infants associated with complete retinal detachment. It can be prevented by timely administration of retinal laser therapy.

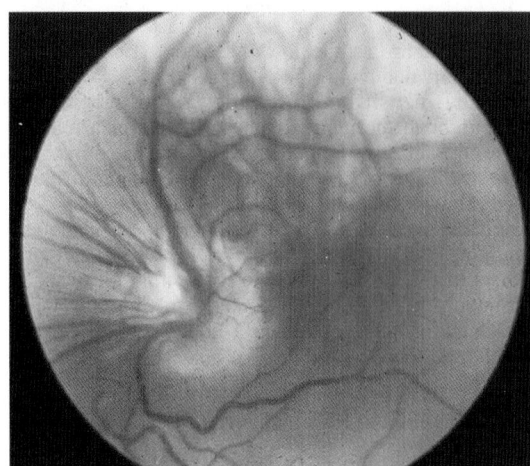

Retrolental fibroplasia *(Zitelli and Davis, 2007)*

retromammary space, a layer of loose connective tissue separating the breast from the deep fascia, providing some degree of movement over underlying surfaces.

retromolar pad /-mō″lər/ [L, *retro* + *mola,* mill; D, *paden,* cushion], a mass of soft tissue, usually pear-shaped, that marks the distal termination of the mandibular residual ridge. It is composed of mucous glands and fibers of the buccinator muscle, the pterygomandibular raphe, the superior constrictor muscle, and the temporal tendon.

retromylohyoid space /ret′rōmī′lōhī″oid/ [L, *retro* + Gk, *myle,* mill, *hyoeides,* U-shaped; L, *spatium*], the part of the alveolingual sulcus that is distal to the distal end of the mylohyoid ridge.

retroperitoneal /-per′itənē″əl/ [L, *retro* + Gk, *peri,* around, *teinein,* to stretch], pertaining to organs closely attached to the posterior abdominal wall and partly covered by peritoneum, rather than suspended by that membrane.

retroperitoneal abscess, a collection of pus between the peritoneum and the posterior abdominal wall.

retroperitoneal fibrosis, a chronic inflammatory process, usually of unknown cause, in which fibrous tissue surrounds the large blood vessels in the lower lumbar area. It frequently causes constriction of the midportion of the ureters, which may lead to hydronephrosis and azotemia. Occasionally the fibrosis spreads upward to involve the duodenum, bile ducts, and superior vena cava. Symptoms include low-back and abdominal pain; weakness; weight loss; fever; and, with urinary tract involvement, frequency of urination, hematuria, polyuria, or anuria. Methysergide, taken to prevent migraine headaches, is one known cause of this condition. Treatment includes stopping methysergide and instituting surgical release of the ureters from the fibrosis with transplantation laterally or intraperitoneally.

retroperitoneal hematoma, hematoma resulting from a retroperitoneal hemorrhage.

retroperitoneal hemorrhage, hemorrhage from the kidney into the retroperitoneal space, such as from trauma, vasculitis, an aneurysm, a tumor, a renal infarct, or a cyst.

retroperitoneal lymph node dissection, surgical removal of lymph nodes bilaterally behind the peritoneum, and the lymph channels and fat around both renal pedicles, the vena cava, and the aorta, including the bifurcation of the aorta. The dissection is usually performed in an attempt to eliminate sites of lymphoma or metastases from malignancies

originating in pelvic organs or genitalia. Also called **radical lymphadenectomy.**

retroperitoneum /-per′itənē″əm/ [L, *retro,* backward; Gk, *peri* + *teinein,* to stretch], the space behind the peritoneum.

retropharyngeal abscess /-fərin″jē-əl/ [L, *retro* + Gk, *pharynx,* throat], a collection of pus in the tissues behind the pharynx accompanied by difficulty in swallowing, fever, and pain. Occasionally the airway becomes obstructed. Treatment includes appropriate parenteral antibiotics and surgical drainage. Tracheostomy may be necessary. Compare **parapharyngeal abscess, peritonsillar abscess.**

retroplacental /-pləsen″təl/, behind the placenta.

retrospective chart audit /-spek″tiv/ [L, *retro* + *spicere,* to look], a format for an audit developed by the Joint Commission on Accreditation of Healthcare Organizations. The audit involves several steps that outline a procedure for evaluating the effectiveness of the care given at a particular institution and for correcting any deficiencies found by reviewing the patient's records after discharge and comparing the data with standards held to be adequate by the Commission.

retrospective nursing audit. See **nursing audit.**

retrospective study, a study in which a search is made for a relationship between one (usually current) phenomenon or condition and another that occurred in the past. An example is a study of the family histories of young women diagnosed as having clear cell adenomas of the vagina, which yielded a relationship between the administration of diethylstilbestrol to the mothers of the women during pregnancy and the development of the condition in the daughters. See also **case-control study.**

retrosternal /-stur″nəl/ [L, *retro,* backward; Gk, *sternon,* chest], behind the sternum.

retrouterine /re′trōyoo″tərin/, behind the uterus.

retroversion /-vur″zhən/ [L, *retro* + *vertere,* to turn], **1.** a common condition in which an organ is tipped backward, usually without flexion or other distortion. The uterus may be retroverted in as many as one fourth of normal women. Uterine retroversion is measured as first-, second-, or third-degree, depending on the angle of tilt with respect to the vagina. Compare **anteversion.** See also **anteflexion, retroflexion. 2.** an abnormal condition in which the teeth or other maxillary and mandibular structures are posterior to their normal positions. Also called **retrusion.** —*retrovert, v.*

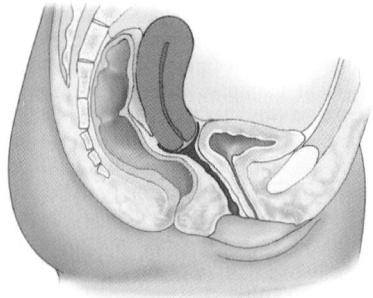

Retroversion of the uterus *(Leonard, 2009)*

Retrovir, an antiretroviral medication. Brand name for **zidovudine.**

retrovirus /-vī″rəs/ [L, *retro* + *virus*], any of a family of ribonucleic acid (RNA) viruses containing the enzyme reverse transcriptase in the virion. The genetic information of the virus is stored in a molecule of single-stranded ribonucleic acid. After entering the target cell, the virus uses reverse transcriptase to direct the cell to make viral deoxyribonucleic acid (DNA). The DNA becomes integrated into the DNA of the host cell. Retroviruses are enveloped and assemble their capsids in the cytoplasm of the host cell. Retroviruses are used in laboratory research to import foreign DNA into a cell. They are transmitted by sexual contact with an infected person, through exposure to infected blood or blood products, and perinatally from an infected mother to the child. Human immunodeficiency virus (HIV1, HIV2), which causes acquired immunodeficiency syndrome, is a retrovirus. Other retroviruses include members of the Oncornaviridae family, such as human T cell lymphotropic virus type 1 (HTLV-1) and human T cell lymphotropic virus type 2, which cause adult T cell leukemia, hairy cell leukemia, tropical spastic paresis, and HTLV-1-associated myelopathy.

retrusion. See **retroversion,** def. 2.

Rett's syndrome /ret/ [Andreas Rett, 20th-century Austrian physician], a pervasive developmental disorder affecting the gray matter of the brain, occurring exclusively in females and present from birth. It is progressive and is characterized by autistic behavior, ataxia, dementia, seizures, and loss of purposeful use of the hands, with cerebral atrophy, mild hyperammonemia, and decreased levels of biogenic amines. Also called **cerebroatrophic hyperammonemia.**

reuptake /re·up′tāk/, reabsorption of a previously secreted substance.

revaccination /rēvak′sinā″shən/, an immunization that is repeated, although the original was successful. In the United States the CDC publishes a schedule for revaccinations; in Canada the Public Health Agency of Canada publishes the schedule.

revascularization /rēvas′kyələr′īzā″shən/ [L, *re* + *vasculum,* small vessel; Gk, *izein,* to cause], the restoration by surgical means of blood flow to an organ or a tissue, as in bypass surgery.

reverberation /rivur′bərā″shən/, **1.** the phenomenon of multiple reflections within a closed system. **2.** an artifact in ultrasound caused by multiple echoes from parallel tissue interfaces.

Reverdin's needle /reverdaNz″/ [Jaques L. Reverdin, Swiss surgeon, 1842–1929], a surgical needle with an eye that can be opened and closed with a slide.

reversal film /rivur″səl/, (in radiology) a reverse-tone duplicate of an x-ray image showing black changed to white and white to black. Also called **diapositive, positive mask.**

reverse Barton's fracture /rivurs″/ [L, *revertere,* to turn back; John R. Barton, American surgeon, 1794–1871], a break in the volar articular surface of the radius, with associated displacement of the carpal bones and radius.

reverse bevel. See **contra bevel,** def. 1.

reverse Colles' fracture. See **Smith fracture.**

reverse curve, a convex curve of dental occlusion, as viewed in the frontal plane.

reversed bandage /rivurst″/, a roller bandage that is reversed on itself with a half twist so that it lies smoothly, conforming to the contour of the extremity. See also **roller bandage.**

reversed coarctation. See **Takayasu arteritis.**

reversed I:E ratio. See **inverse I:E ratio.**

reversed phase, a chromatographic mode in which the mobile phase is more polar than the stationary phase.

reverse isolation, isolation procedures designed to protect a patient from infectious organisms that might be carried by the staff, other patients, or visitors or on droplets in the air or on equipment or materials. Absolute reverse isolation is rarely necessary and requires elaborate specialized equipment. Protective modified reverse isolation is less restrictive but is not prolonged needlessly because the patient usually feels lonely and sensorially deprived. Handwashing, gowning, gloving, sterilization or disinfection of materials brought into the area, and other details of housekeeping vary with the reason for the isolation and the usual practices of the hospital.

reverse peristalsis. See **antiperistalsis.**

reverse transcriptase (RT) /revers′tran-skrip′tās/, an enzyme of RNA viruses that catalyzes the transcription of RNA to DNA, which is then incorporated into the genome of the host cell. This is the reverse of the usual mechanism for replication of genetic information; in the presence of this enzyme, it is the RNA that serves as the template for DNA copies. It is one mechanism by which reproduction of cancer cells is facilitated. Also called **RNA-dependent DNA polymerase.** See also **retrovirus.**

reverse transcriptase inhibitor, a compound that inhibits the enzyme used by retroviruses to synthesize complementary DNA from viral RNA inside host cells.

reverse Trendelenburg [Friedrich Trendelenburg], a position in which the lower extremities are placed lower than the body and head, which are elevated on an inclined plane.

reversible /rivur′sibəl/, able to return to its original state or condition, as in a chemical reaction.

reversible brain syndrome, any of a group of acute brain disorders characterized by a disruption of cognition, as in delirium. The symptoms widely vary. The disorder is related to a variety of biological stressors. Recovery is likely.

reversible obstructive airway disease, a condition characterized by bronchospasm that is reversible by intervention. Kinds include **asthma.**

reversible vascular hyperplasia, a variation of Kaposi sarcoma in which human immunodeficiency virus may induce cells to produce a chemical growth factor. The growth factor, in turn, makes lymphatic endothelial cells proliferate. The process may cascade as each new Kaposi sarcoma cell produces more growth factor.

reversion /rivur″zhən/, **1.** the appearance in offspring of traits expressed in previous but not recent generations. **2.** a return to an original phenotype by mutation or reinstatement of the original genotype.

review of systems (ROS), a detailed assessment of each body system, performed to ascertain the presence of deviations from normal. See **health assessment.**

Revised Trauma Score, a system of combining cardiopulmonary assessment with the Glasgow Coma Score in estimating the degree of injury and the prognosis in a trauma patient. The cardiopulmonary factors included are respiratory rate and systolic blood pressure.

Revlimid, a chemotherapeutic agent. Brand name for **lenalidomide.**

Reyataz, a protease inhibitor medication. Brand name for **atazanavir.**

Reye syndrome /rā″/ [Ralph D.K. Reye, Australian pathologist, 1912–1978], a combination of acute encephalopathy and fatty infiltration of the internal organs that may follow acute viral infections. This syndrome has been associated with influenza B, chickenpox (varicella), the enteroviruses, and the Epstein-Barr virus. It usually affects people under 18 years of age, characteristically causing an exanthematous rash, vomiting, and confusion about 1 week after the onset of a viral illness. In the late stage there may be extreme disorientation followed by coma, seizures, and respiratory arrest. Laboratory tests reveal greater-than-normal amounts of SGOT and SGPT, bilirubin, and ammonia in the blood. A specimen obtained by liver biopsy shows fatty degeneration and confirms the diagnosis. Mortality varies between 20% and 80%, depending on the severity of symptoms. The cause of Reye syndrome is unknown; however, there appears to be an association with the administration of aspirin. Therefore aspirin is given only if prescribed by a physician for any condition in infants or children. Aspirin should not be given in cases of chickenpox or suspected influenza. No specific treatment is available. Insulin, antibiotics, and mannitol may be given. Blood gases, blood pH, and blood pressure are monitored frequently. Intensive supportive nursing care with meticulous monitoring of all vital functions and prompt correction of any imbalance are of extreme significance in the outcome of this syndrome.

■ OBSERVATIONS: Reye syndrome is staged by the characteristics manifested. In stage I, the child is usually quiet, lethargic, and drowsy, with episodes of vomiting. Pupil reactions are brisk, and commands are followed. Serum lab values show evidence of liver dysfunction; EEG is type 1. In stage 2, there is evidence of deep lethargy, confusion, delirium, and combativeness. Reflexes are hyperreflexic, and hyperventilation is present. Pupillary reactions are sluggish. In stage 3, senses are obtunded, and light coma is present with seizure activity and decorticate rigidity. Pupillary light reaction is still intact. EEG is type II. In stage 4, the coma deepens with seizure activity and decerebrate rigidity. There is loss of oculocephalic reflexes, and pupils are fixed. EEG is type III or IV, and there is evidence of brain dysfunction. In stage 5, there is deep coma, loss of deep tendon reflexes, respiratory arrest, fixed and dilated pupils, and type IV EEG. Definitive diagnosis is established by liver biopsy or by a threefold rise in levels of serum aspartate aminotransferase, serum alanine aminotransferase, or serum ammonia. Survivors may exhibit a neuropsychological deficit.

■ INTERVENTIONS: Deterioration is generally rapid and requires early diagnosis and aggressive treatment. Care in stages 1 and 2 is largely supportive, with frequent monitoring and evaluation of neurological status. Management of cerebral edema and increased intracranial pressure is a key focus in stages 3 through 5 and is monitored with an ICP monitor and treated by administration of mannitol, glycerol, and/or hyperventilation via endotracheal tube and ventilator. Pancuronium bromide is used to immobilize the child on a ventilator. Seizures are managed by IV phenytoin. NG tubes, urinary catheters, and peripheral IVs are placed to manage fluids. An arterial catheter is placed to permit continuous blood pressure measurement and to monitor blood gases. A central venous catheter permits monitoring of blood volume and cardiac function and administration of hypertonic solutions. A pulmonary artery catheter may be inserted to monitor pulmonary artery pressure and cardiac output. A cooling blanket may be indicated to manage temperature. If increased intracranial pressure fails to respond to treatment, a decompressive craniotomy may be indicated. Prevention is targeted around routine vaccinations for influenza and varicella and avoidance of aspirin in children.

■ PATIENT CARE CONSIDERATIONS: Interventions during acute disease are continuous and intensive. Careful evaluation is required for neurological, cardiac, and respiratory systems. Management is required for multiple lines and tubes, including peripheral and central IV lines, arterial lines, CVP lines, ICP monitors, retention catheters, NG tubes, and endotracheal tubes. Management of ventilator settings is required. Careful fluid management and intake and output is required to reduce cerebral edema and prevent dehydration. Careful supportive care, including careful hygiene, positioning, and passive range of motion, is required to maintain skin integrity and prevent sequelae of immobility. Sensory stimulation is needed for the unconscious child. Emotional support for parents is essential because the sudden severity and intensity of the disease and its aggressive treatment are sources of extreme anxiety and fear. Prevention is targeted around education about maintaining routine vaccinations for influenza and varicella and the avoidance of aspirin in children.

rf, 1. abbreviation for **radiofrequency.** 2. abbreviation for **rheumatic fever.**

Rf, 1. symbol for the element **rutherfordium.** 2. (in chromatography) abbreviation for *retardation factor* or *ratio to (solvent) front.*

RF, abbreviation for **rheumatoid factor.**

R factor, an episome in bacteria that is responsible for drug resistance and is transmissible to progeny and to other bacterial cells by conjugation. The part of the episome involved in replication and transmission is called *resistance transfer factor.*

RFP, abbreviation for **request for proposal.**

RF test. See **latex fixation test.**

RGP, abbreviation for *rigid gas permeable.* See **rigid gas permeable (RGP) contact lens.**

Rh, 1. abbreviation for *rhesus.* See **Rh factor.** 2. symbol for the element **rhodium.**

r/h, 1. abbreviation for **relative humidity.** 2. abbreviation for *roentgens per hour.*

rhabdo-, rhabdi-, prefix meaning "rod-shaped" or "pertaining to a rod": *rhabdomyoblast, rhabdomyoma, rhabdosphincter.*

rhabdomyo-, prefix meaning "striated or skeletal muscle": *rhabdomyolysis.*

rhabdomyoblast /rab′dōmī″əblast′/ [Gk, *rhabdos,* rod, *mys,* muscle, *blastos,* germ], large, round, spindle-shaped cells with cross striations, found in some rhabdomyosarcomas.

rhabdomyoblastoma. See **rhabdomyosarcoma.**

rhabdomyolysis /rab′dōmī·ol″isis/, a paroxysmal, potentially fatal syndrome caused by the breakdown of skeletal muscle fibers. It is characterized by the presence of myoglobin in the urine. It may result from untreated compartment syndrome. It is also associated with acute renal failure.

rhabdomyoma /rab′dōmī·ō″mə/ *pl. rhabdomyomas, rhabdomyomata* [Gk, *rhabdos,* rod, *mys,* muscle, *oma*], a tumor of striated muscle that may occur in the uterus, vagina, pharynx, tongue, or heart. Also called **myoma striocellulare.**

rhabdomyosarcoma /rab′dōmī′ō·särkō″mə/ *pl. rhabdomyosarcomas, rhabdomyosarcomata* [Gk, *rhabdos* + *mys,* muscle, *sarx,* flesh, *oma*], a highly malignant tumor derived from primitive striated muscle cells that occurs most frequently in the head and neck and is also found in the genitourinary tract, extremities, body wall, and retroperitoneum. In some cases the onset is associated with trauma. Also called **rhabdomyoblastoma,** *rhabdosarcoma.*

■ OBSERVATIONS: The initial symptoms depend on the site of tumor development and indicate local tissue or organ destruction, such as dysphagia, vaginal bleeding, hematuria, or obstructed flow of urine. Diagnostic measures may include barium x-ray studies, angiography, or tomography. Embryonal rhabdomyosarcoma occurs in the head, neck, or trunk of young children; alveolar rhabdomyosarcoma is usually seen in the extremities of adolescents; and the pleomorphic form is most common in the legs of adults.

■ INTERVENTIONS: Treatment for rhabdomyosarcoma depends on the site and the presence of metastasis. Surgical excision is rarely possible because the tumor is poorly encapsulated and tends to spread. Amputation of an affected limb or extremity may be curative. Radiotherapy and chemotherapy with combinations of medications increase the rate of survival.

■ PATIENT CARE CONSIDERATIONS: An interdisciplinary approach to meeting the individual needs of patients and caregivers is important. Immediately after diagnosis, during treatment, and in recovery, patients receive care from health care professionals who specialize in exercise, stress management, nutrition, and activities of daily living. Support groups can also assist the family and patient to deal with the disease.

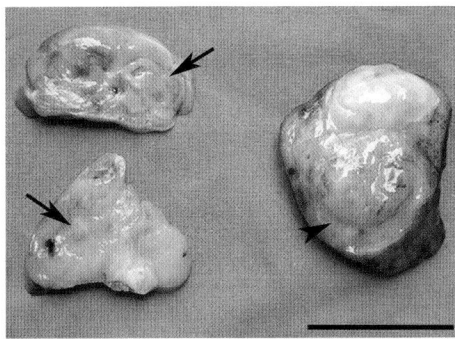

Rhabdomyosarcoma — gross transverse sections of the sarcoma *(Corradi et al, 2012)*

rhabdosphincter /rab′dōsfingk″tər/, a sphincter composed of striated muscle fibers.

rhabdovirus /rab′dōvī″rəs/ [Gk, *rhabdos* + L, *virus,* poison], a member of a family of viruses that includes the organism causing rabies.

rhachi-. See **rachio-, rachi-, rhachi-.**

rhagades /rag″ədēz/ [Gk, chinks], cracks or fissures in skin that has lost its elasticity, especially common around the mouth. See also **cheilosis.**

-rhage, -rrhage, -rhagia, -rrhagia, combining form meaning "excessive flow": *hemorrhage, metrorrhagia.*

Rh antiserum [Rh, rhesus; Gk, *anti,* against; L, *serum,* whey], a serum that contains Rh antibodies.

rhaphe. See **raphe.**

-rhaphy, -rrhaphy, combining form meaning "suturing in place": *colporrhaphy, glossorrhaphy.*

Rh blood group. See **Rh factor.**

rhd, 1. abbreviation for *radioactive health data.* **2.** abbreviation for **rheumatic heart disease.**

rhe /rē/, **1.** an absolute unit of fluidity in the centimeter-gram-second system. **2.** the reciprocal of the unit of viscosity expressed as 1/poise or 1/centipoise.

-rhea, -rrhea, suffix meaning "flow" or "discharge": *galactorrhea, rhinorrhea.*

rhegmatogenous /reg′mətoj″ənəs/ [Gk, *rhegma,* breakage, *gen,* producing], arising from a tear or rupture in an organ.

rhegmatogenous retinal detachment, a separation of the retina associated with a hole, break, or tear in the sensory layer of the retina. The detachment occurs secondary to the passage of vitreous fluid through the break.

rhenium (Re) /rē″nē·əm/ [L, *Rhenus,* Rhine], a hard, brittle, metallic element. Its atomic number is 75; its atomic mass is 186.21. Rhenium has a high melting point and is used in x-ray tube anodes and thermometers for measuring high temperatures.

rheo-, prefix meaning "electric current, stream, flow": *rheobase, rheogram, rheostosis.*

rheobase /rē″əbās/, the least amount of electricity that will produce a stimulated response.

rheoencephalogram /rē′ō·ensef″əlōgram′/, a graphic representation of the changes in electric conductivity of the head caused by blood flowing through vessels in the head.

rheogram /rē″əgram/, a plot of shear stress versus the shear flow of a fluid.

rheology /rē·ol″əjē/, the study of the flow and deformation of matter.

Rheomacrodex, a plasma expander. Brand name for *dextran 40.*

rheometry /rē·om″ətrē/ [Gk, *rheos,* current, *metron,* measure], a technique for measuring the velocity of blood flow.

rheostat /rē″əstat/ [Gk, *rheos,* current, *statikos,* causing to stand], a variable resistance electric device that can be adjusted to control the strength of a current.

rheostosis /rē′ostō″sis/, a condition of bone overgrowth marked by streaks in the bones.

rhestocythemia /res′tōsīthē″mē·ə/, the presence of damaged red blood cells in the peripheral circulation.

Rhesus factor. See **Rh factor.**

rheum / room̅/ [Gk, *rheuma,* flow], a watery or mucous discharge from the skin or mucous membranes.

Rheum palmatum, an herb known as Chinese rhubarb, Turkish rhubarb, or wild rhubarb, used in herbal therapies. In large quantities it is poisonous. It is contraindicated in pregnancy because it may cause uterine contractions.

rheumatic. See **rheumatism.**

-rheumatic, suffix meaning "relating to or exhibiting traits of rheumatism": *antirheumatic.*

rheumatic aortitis, an inflammatory condition of the aorta occurring in rheumatic fever. It is characterized by disseminated focal lesions that may progressively form patches of fibrosis.

rheumatic arteritis, a complication of rheumatic fever characterized by generalized inflammation of arteries and arterioles. Fibrin mixed with cellular debris may invade, thicken, and stiffen vessel walls, and the affected vessels may be surrounded by hemorrhage and exudate.

rheumatic carditis [Gk, *rheuma,* flux, *kardia,* heart, *itis,* inflammation], pericarditis, myocarditis, and endocarditis that may be associated with acute rheumatic fever.

rheumatic chorea. See **Sydenham chorea.**

rheumatic endocarditis [Gk, *rheuma,* flux, *endon,* within, *kardia,* heart, *itis,* inflammation], inflammation of the endocardium in association with acute rheumatic fever.

rheumatic fever (rf), a systemic inflammatory disease that may develop as a delayed reaction to an inadequately treated infection of the upper respiratory tract by group A beta-hemolytic streptococci. The disease usually occurs in young school-age children and may affect the brain, heart, joints, skin, or subcutaneous tissues. Also called **acute articular rheumatism.** See also **rheumatic heart disease.**

■ OBSERVATIONS: The onset of rheumatic fever is usually sudden, often occurring 1 to 5 symptom-free weeks after recovery from a sore throat or scarlet fever. Early symptoms generally include fever, joint pain, nosebleeds, abdominal pain, and vomiting. The major manifestations of this disease include migratory polyarthritis affecting numerous joints and carditis, which causes palpitations, chest pain, and, in severe cases, symptoms of cardiac failure. Sydenham's chorea is usually the sole late sign of rheumatic fever and may initially be manifested as an increased awkwardness and tendency to drop objects. As the chorea progresses, irregular body movements may become extensive, occasionally involving the tongue and facial muscles, resulting in incapacitation. Other developments may include transient erythema marginatum with circular lesions and subcutaneous rheumatic nodules on various joints and tendons, the spine, and the back of the head. There is no specific diagnostic test for rheumatic fever. The development of serum antibodies to streptococcal antigens is a positive diagnostic sign. Affected individuals may also develop leukocytosis, moderate anemia, and proteinuria. C-reactive protein, evaluated in a specimen of blood, is abnormally high in concentration. Recurrences of rheumatic fever are common. Except for carditis, all the manifestations of the disease usually subside without any permanent effects. Mild cases may last 3 to 4 weeks. Severe cases with associated arthritis and carditis may last 2 to 3 months.

■ INTERVENTIONS: Management of rheumatic fever includes bed rest and severe restriction of normal activity. Penicillin is often administered, even if throat cultures are negative, and steroids or salicylates may be used, depending on the severity of any associated carditis and arthritis.

■ PATIENT CARE CONSIDERATIONS: Symptoms largely determine the type of nursing care. The nurse is alert to signs of toxicity associated with salicylate, steroid, and antibiotic therapies. The nurse also monitors the patient's fluid status with regard to cardiac function, helps minimize joint pains by properly positioning the patient, and gives emotional support.

rheumatic heart disease (rhd), damage to heart muscle and heart valves caused by episodes of rheumatic fever. When a susceptible person acquires a group A beta-hemolytic streptococcal infection, an autoimmune reaction may occur in heart tissue, resulting in permanent deformities of heart valves or chordae tendineae. See also **aortic stenosis, mitral valve stenosis, rheumatic fever.**

■ OBSERVATIONS: Symptoms are associated with damage to cardiac valves and may include shortness of breath and edema. A cardiac murmur may be present.

■ INTERVENTIONS: Prevention is a priority. Prompt treatment of streptococcal infections and close follow-up for those who have experienced rheumatic fever may prevent further damage. Surgery is often required to repair or replace heart valves in patients with severely damaged valves,

■ PATIENT CARE CONSIDERATIONS: Involvement of the heart may be evident during acute rheumatic fever, or it may be discovered long after the acute disease has subsided.

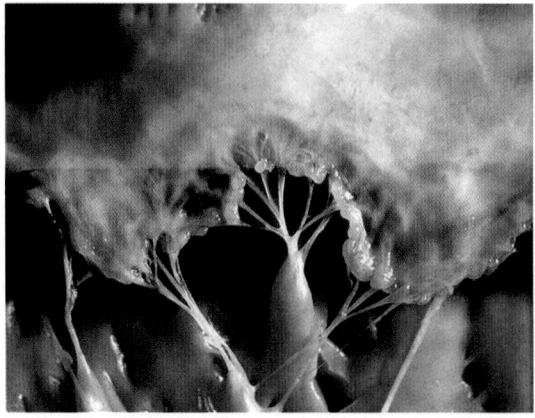

Rheumatic heart disease *(Kumar et al, 2007)*

rheumatic nodules [Gk, *rheuma,* flux; L, *nodulus,* small knot], aggregations of fibroblasts and lymphoid cells that

may accumulate in soft tissues and over bony prominences of patients afflicted with rheumatoid arthritis and rheumatic fever.

rheumatic scoliosis [Gk, *rheuma,* flux, *skoliosis,* curvature], a form of scoliosis associated with muscle spasms and acute inflammation. Also called **inflammatory scoliosis.**

rheumatid /rōo″mətid/ [Gk, *rheuma,* flux], a skin eruption that sometimes occurs with rheumatic disorders.

rheumatism /rōo″mətiz′əm/ [Gk, *rheuma,* flux], **1.** *(Nontechnical)* any of a large number of inflammatory conditions of the bursae, joints, ligaments, or muscles characterized by pain, limitation of movement, and structural degeneration of one or more parts of the musculoskeletal system. **2.** the syndrome of pain, limitation of movement, and structural degeneration of elements in the musculoskeletal system, as may occur in gout, rheumatoid arthritis, systemic lupus erythematosus, ankylosing spondylitis, and many other diseases.

rheumatoid arteritis /rōo″mətoid/ [Gk, *rheuma,* flux, *arteria,* airpipe, *itis,* inflammation], inflammation of the arterial walls associated with a rheumatic disorder. See also **rheumatoid coronary arteritis.**

rheumatoid arthritis (RA) [Gk, *rheuma,* flux, *eidos,* form, *arthron,* joint, *itis,* inflammation], a chronic, inflammatory, destructive, and sometimes deforming collagen disease that has an autoimmune component. It is characterized by symmetric inflammation of synovial membranes and increased synovial exudate, leading to thickening of the membranes and swelling of the joints. Rheumatoid arthritis usually first appears when patients, most often women, are between 36 and 50 years of age. The course of the disease is variable but is most frequently marked by alternating periods of remission and exacerbation. Also called **arthritis deformans,** *atrophic arthritis.* See also **ankylosing spondylitis, juvenile rheumatoid arthritis.**

■ OBSERVATIONS: The medical diagnosis and prognosis of rheumatoid arthritis are based on a variety of clinical and laboratory findings. The disease may first be present with fatigue, weakness, poor appetite, low-grade fever, anemia, and an increased erythrocyte sedimentation rate. The diagnostic criteria listed by the American Rheumatism Association include morning stiffness, joint pain or tenderness, swelling of at least two joints, subcutaneous nodules (called arthritic nodules and usually found at pressure points such as the elbows), structural changes in joints seen on x-ray film, a positive rheumatoid factor agglutination test, decreased precipitation of mucin from synovial fluid, and characteristic histological changes on pathological examination of the fluid. Higher titers of rheumatoid factor are correlated with more severe forms of the disease, especially forms with extraarticular manifestations, such as cardiac involvement, vasculitis, pulmonary disease, and proteinuria. There may also be a thickening of synovial membranes, called pannus formation. In long-term, severe, chronic rheumatoid arthritis, Felty's syndrome may be present. Rheumatoid arthritis is not always progressive, deforming, or debilitating; most patients may continue in their jobs.

■ INTERVENTIONS: Treatment includes sufficient rest, range-of-motion exercises to maintain joint function, medication for the relief of pain and reduction of inflammation, orthopedic intervention to prevent or correct deformities, proper nutrition, and weight loss, if necessary. Salicylates are usually given. If improvement is not achieved, other antiinflammatory agents may be used, such as indomethacin, phenylbutazone, antimalarials, gold salts, or some antineoplastic drugs. Corticosteroids are prescribed with caution because of their side effects, including gastric ulcer, adrenal suppression, and osteoporosis. Disease-modifying antirheumatic drugs (DMARDs) and biological response modifiers can slow the progression of the disease and prevent permanent damage to the joints and other tissues. Other treatments, including diathermy, ultrasound, warm paraffin applications, underwater exercise, and applications of heat, are occasionally used.

■ PATIENT CARE CONSIDERATIONS: The health care team monitors drug treatment and notes its effects. Health care providers also encourage the patient to get sufficient sleep and to rest both small and weight-bearing joints. The involvement of occupational and physical therapy is important to ensure that measures to protect the joints are implemented. The most effective use of heat or cold; instruction in muscle-strengthening exercises and in methods for easing pain and preventing deformities, such as the proper use of pillows, splints, or molds; and offers of emotional support should also be addressed.

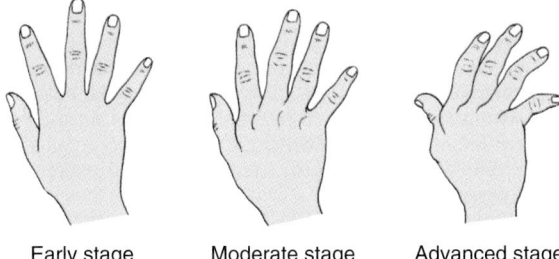

Early stage   Moderate stage   Advanced stage

Stages of rheumatoid arthritis *(Monahan and Neighbors, 1998)*

rheumatoid coronary arteritis, an abnormal condition characterized by a thickening of the tunica intima of the coronary arteries, which may produce coronary insufficiency. Rheumatoid coronary arteritis is a collagen disease that causes inflammation and fibrinoid degeneration of connective tissue. It is commonly treated with glucocorticoids.

rheumatoid factor (RF), antiglobulin antibodies often found in the serum of patients with a clinical diagnosis of rheumatoid arthritis. Rheumatoid factors are present in about 70% of such cases, but they may also be found in such widely divergent diseases as tuberculosis, parasitic infections, leukemia, and connective tissue disorders. See also **latex fixation test.**

rheumatoid factor (RF) test, a blood test whose results are positive in approximately 80% of patients with rheumatoid arthritis. Abnormal levels of RF that are lower than those characteristic of rheumatoid arthritis may indicate systemic lupus erythematosus, Sjögren's syndrome, scleroderma, and other autoimmune conditions. RF is not a useful disease marker because its presence does not disappear in patients who are experiencing a remission from the disease symptoms.

rheumatoid pneumoconiosis. See **Caplan syndrome.**

rheumatoid spondylitis. See **Strümpell-Marie disease.**

rheumatologist /roo̅o̅'mətol'ə″jist/, a specialist in the treatment of disorders of the connective tissue.

rheumatology /-ol″əjē/ [Gk, *rheuma,* flux, *logos,* science], the study of disorders characterized by inflammation, degeneration, or metabolic derangement of connective tissue and related structures of the body. These disorders are sometimes referred to collectively as rheumatism.

Rh factor, refers to the D antigen found on the erythrocytes of 85% of the Caucasian population and varying frequencies in other populations. Rh-positive or Rh-negative refers to the presence or absence of the D antigen, but many other antigens are also part of this system, most notably C, c, E, and e. D is the most immunogenic antigen outside the ABO system; therefore D-negative recipients should receive only D-negative donor blood to avoid exposure and immunization to D. D-negative mothers who carry D-positive infants should receive Rh immune globulin to prevent immunization during pregnancy and delivery. Also called **Rhesus factor.** See also **anti-Rh agglutinin, erythroblastosis fetalis, Rh$_O$(D) immunoglobulin.**

Rh genes [Rh, rhesus; Gk, *genein,* to produce], Rh antigens on the red cell membrane produced by allelic genes at two closely linked loci on chromosome 1, RhD and RhCE.

rhigo-, combining form meaning "shivering" or "cold."

Rh immune globulin. See **Rh$_O$(D) immunoglobulin.**

rhin-. See **rhino-.**

rhinalgia /rīnal″jə/, pain involving the nose.

Rh incompatibility, the agglutination (clumping together) of red blood cells as a result of mixing different antigens (agglutinogens) present on the surface of the cells. This agglutination is an immune reaction and depends on the formation of antibodies against the specific agglutinogen (Rh factor) present on the red blood cells and in blood from a transfusion or fetal tissues. The immune reaction does not occur immediately, but depends on the gradual formation of antibodies. For example, a D-negative (Rh negative) person who has been previously exposed to D-positive red cells through transfusion or pregnancy may produce anti-D, and therefore be incompatible with all D-positive (Rh positive) red cells. See also **Rh factor.**

rhinedema /rī′nedē″mə/, a fluid accumulation in the mucous membrane of the nose.

rhinencephalon /rī′nensef″əlon/ *pl. rhinencephala* [Gk, *rhis,* nose, *encephalon,* brain], the part of each cerebral hemisphere that contains the limbic system, which is associated with the emotions. See also **limbic system.**

rhinenchysis /rī′nenkī″sis, rīnen″kisis/, douching of the nasal cavity.

rhinitis /rīnī″tis/ [Gk, *rhis* + *itis,* inflammation], inflammation of the mucous membranes of the nose, usually accompanied by swelling of the mucosa and a nasal discharge. It may be complicated by sinusitis. Also called **coryza.** Kinds include *acute rhinitis,* **allergic rhinitis, atrophic rhinitis, vasomotor rhinitis.**

rhino- /rī″nō-/, combining form meaning "nose" or "nose-like structure": *rhinolith, rhinolalia, rhinoplasty.*

Rhinocort, a nasal corticosteroid. Brand name for **budesonide.**

rhinoentomophthoromycosis /rī′no-en″to-mof″tho-ro-mi-ko′sis/, the usual form of an infection by *Conidiobolus coronatus,* marked by development of large polyps in the subcutaneous tissues of the nose and paranasal sinuses. Orbital involvement with unilateral blindness may follow. Sometimes, especially in weak or immunocompromised patients, it can spread to the central nervous system and cause fatal rhinocerebral zygomycosis.

rhinolaryngitis /-ler′inji″tis/ [Gk, *rhis,* nose, *larynx,* throat, *itis,* inflammation], an inflammation of the mucous membranes of the nose and throat.

rhinolith /rī″nəlith/, a concretion in the nasal cavity.

rhinolithiasis /rī′nəlithī″əsis/, the formation of concretions in the nasal cavity.

R

rhinologist /rīnol″əjist/, a physician who specializes in the diagnosis and treatment of disorders of the nose.

rhinology /rīnol″əjē/, a branch of medicine specializing in the diagnosis and treatment of disorders involving the nose.

rhinomanometer /rī′nōmənom″ətər/, a device for measuring the air pressure in the nose. It is used in the diagnosis of nasal obstruction.

rhinomycosis /rī′nōmīkō″sis/, a fungal infection of the mucous membrane of the nose.

rhinopathy /rīnop″əthē/ [Gk, *rhis* + *pathos,* disease], any disease or malformation of the nose.

rhinopharyngeal. See **nasopharyngeal.**

rhinophycomycosis /rī′nōfī′kōmīkō″sis/, an infection of the nasal and paranasal sinuses caused by the phycomycete *Entomophthora coronata.* The infection often spreads to surrounding tissues, including the eye and brain.

rhinophyma /rī′nōfī″mə/ [Gk, *rhis* + *phyma,* tumor], a form of rosacea in which there is sebaceous hyperplasia. See also **rosacea.**

- OBSERVATIONS: Redness, prominent vascularity, swelling, and distortion of the skin of the nose can cause significant disfigurement.

- INTERVENTIONS: Treatment includes dermabrasion, electrosurgery, plastic surgery, and laser resurfacing. The changes in appearance can cause emotional stress that the health care provider should address.

- PATIENT CARE CONSIDERATIONS: There is no known cause for rhinophyma. At one time, it was attributed to excessive alcohol use. There is no clinical evidence or research to support this attribution.

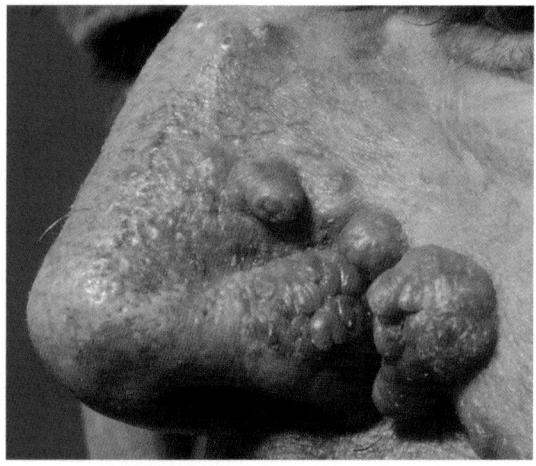

Rhinophyma *(Regezi, Sciubba, and Jordan, 2008)*

rhinoplasty /rī″nəplas′tē/ [Gk, *rhis* + *plassein,* to mold], a procedure in plastic surgery in which the structure of the nose is changed or shaped. Bone or cartilage may be removed, tissue grafted from another part of the body, or synthetic material implanted to alter the shape. After surgery any respiratory difficulty is reported immediately. The head of the bed should be elevated postoperatively. Frequent oral care is given, and ice compresses are applied to decrease the pain and edema that usually occur. Edema and discoloration around the eyes are expected to last for several days. The procedure is most frequently performed for cosmetic reasons.

rhinorrhagia /rī′nôrā″jə/ [Gk, *rhis,* nose, *rhegnynein,* to gush forth], a profuse nosebleed. Compare **epistaxis.**

rhinorrhea /rī′nôrē″ə/ [Gk, *rhis* + *rhoia,* flow], **1.** the free discharge of a thin, watery nasal fluid. **2.** the flow of cerebrospinal fluid from the nose after an injury to the head.

rhinosalpingitis /rī′nōsal′pinji″tis/, an inflammation of the mucous membranes of the nose and eustachian tube.

rhinoscleroma /rī′nosklirō″mə/, a chronic inflammation in the nose spreading to the larynx and pharynx. The cause is an infection of *Klebsiella rhinoscleromatis.*

rhinoscope /rī″nəskōp/, an instrument for examining the nasal passages through the anterior nares or through the nasopharynx.

rhinoscopy /rīnos″kəpē/ [Gk, *rhis* + *skopein,* to look], an examination of the nasal passages to inspect the mucosa and detect inflammation, deformities, or asymmetry, as in deviation of the septum. The nasal passages may be examined anteriorly by introducing a speculum into the anterior nares or posteriorly by introducing a rhinoscope through the nasopharynx. −*rhinoscopic, adj.*

rhinosporidiosis /rī′nōspərid′ē-ō″sis/ [Gk, *rhis* + *sporo,* seed, *osis,* condition], an infection caused by the fungus *Rhinosporidium seeberi.* It is characterized by fleshy red polyps on the mucous membranes of the nose, conjunctiva, nasopharynx, and soft palate. The disease may be acquired by swimming or bathing in infected water. The most effective treatment is electrocautery.

rhinostenosis /rī′nōstənō″sis/, an abnormal narrowing of a nasal passage.

rhinotomy /rīnot″əmē/ [Gk, *rhis* + *temnein,* to cut], a surgical procedure in which an incision is made along one side of the nose, performed to drain accumulated pus from an abscess or a sinus infection. Under local anesthesia the flap of skin and lining of the nose are turned back to provide a full view of the nasal passages for radical sinus surgery.

rhinovirus /rī′nōvī″rəs/ [Gk, *rhis* + L, *virus,* poison], any of about 100 serologically distinct, small ribonucleic acid viruses that cause about 40% of acute respiratory illnesses. Infection is characterized by dry scratchy throat, nasal congestion, malaise, and headache. Fever is minimal. Nasal discharge lasts 2 or 3 days. Children may also develop a cough. Type-specific antibodies may last for 2 to 4 years. The treatment is nonspecific and may include rest, analgesics, antihistamines, and nasal decongestants. Complete recovery is usual. Also called **coryza virus.** Compare **adenovirus, parainfluenza virus, respiratory syncytial virus.** See also **cold.**

rhitid-. See **rhytid-, rhitid-.**

rhitidoplasty. See **rhytidoplasty.**

rhitidosis. See **rhytidosis.**

rhizo-, combining form meaning "root": *rhizome, rhizoid.*

rhizoid /rī″zoid/, resembling a root or serving to anchor.

rhizome, an underground plant stem, growing more or less horizontally, that usually has roots on its underside and bears buds.

rhizomelia /rī′zōmē″lyə/ [Gk, *rhizo,* root, *melos,* limb], **1.** a disorder of the hips and shoulders. **2.** an anomaly in the length of the arms and legs of an individual.

rhizomelic /rī′zəmel″ik/ [Gk, *rhizo,* root, *melos,* limb], pertaining to the hips and shoulder.

rhizomeningomyelitis /rī′zōmining′gōmī′əlī″tis/, an inflammation of the nerve roots, meninges, and spinal cord.

Rhizopus /rī″zōpəs/, a genus of fungi having a sexual phase and an asexual phase and reproducing by both sexually and asexually produced spores. It includes some species identified as a cause of zygomycosis in humans. Several species are molds and saprobes on fruits, vegetables, or baked goods and can cause mucormycosis.

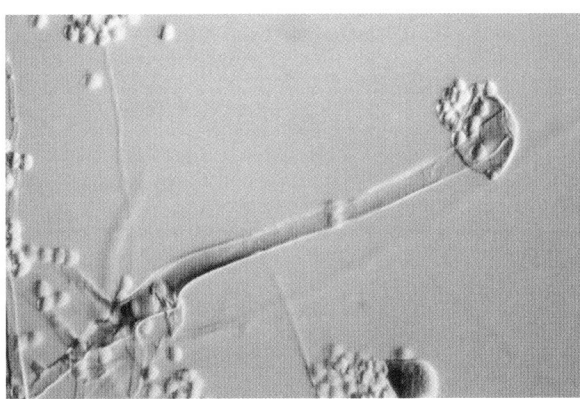

Rhizopus *(Mahon, Lehman, and Manuselis, 2011)*

rhizotomy /rīzot″əmē/, the surgical resection of the dorsal root of a spinal nerve, performed to relieve pain and sometimes to decrease spasms.

Rh negative. See **Rh factor.**

rho /rō/, P, ϱ, the seventeenth letter of the Greek alphabet.

Rhodesian trypanosomiasis /rōdē″zhən/, an acute form of African trypanosomiasis, caused by the parasite *Trypanosoma brucei rhodesiense.* The disease may progress rapidly, causing encephalitis, coma, and death in only a few weeks. Also called **kaodzera,** *Trypanosoma brucei rhodesiense.* Compare **Gambian trypanosomiasis.** See also **African trypanosomiasis.**

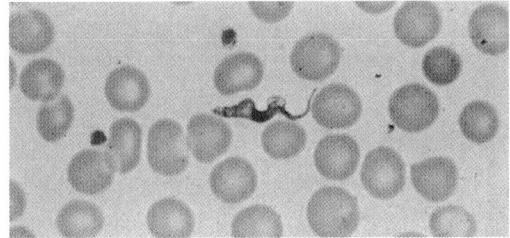

***Trypanosoma rhodesiense,* the parasite that causes Rhodesian trypanosomiasis** *(Goldman et al, 2012)*

Rh₀(D) immunoglobulin, a passive immunizing agent. Also called **Rh immune globulin.**

■ INDICATIONS: It is prescribed to prevent Rh sensitization after abortion, miscarriage, ectopic pregnancy, or normal birth to an Rh-negative mother of an Rh-positive infant or fetus.

■ CONTRAINDICATIONS: It is not given to an Rh₀(D)-positive patient or to the infant or those previously sensitized to Rh.

■ ADVERSE EFFECTS: The most serious adverse effect is anaphylaxis.

rhodium (Rh) /rō″dē·əm/ [Gk, *rhodon,* rose], a grayish-white metallic element. Its atomic number is 45; its atomic mass is 102.91. Rhodium is used for providing a hard lustrous coating on other metals and in the making of mirrors.

rhodo-, a combining form meaning "red": *rhodopsin.*

rhodopsin /rōdop″sin/ [Gk, *rhodon,* rose, *opsis,* vision], the purple pigmented compound in the rods of the retina, formed by a protein, opsin, and a derivative of vitamin A, retinal. Rhodopsin gives the outer segments of the rods a purple color and adapts the eye to low-density light. The compound breaks down when struck by light, and this chemical change triggers the conduction of nerve impulses. Brief periods of darkness allow the opsin and the retinal to reconstitute the rhodopsin, which accounts for the short delay a person experiences in adapting to sudden or drastic changes in lighting, as when moving out of bright sunlight into a darkened room or from darkness into bright light. Closing the eyes is a natural reflex that allows reconstitution of rhodopsin. Compare **iodopsin.** See also **visual purple.**

Rhodotorula /rō′dətôr″yələ/, a genus of yeasts, including species such as *R. rubra,* that has been identified as the cause of endocarditis and septicemia, particularly in immunocompromised patients.

rhoencephalography, a technique for monitoring blood flow in the brain by recording pulsatile changes in the electric impedance of the brain.

RhoGAM, an immune globulin. Brand name for **Rh₀(D) immunoglobulin.**

rhombencephalon /rom′bensef″əlon/ [Gk, *rhombos,* parallelogram, *enkephalos,* brain], the most caudal of the three primary vesicles of the embryonic brain.

rhomboid /rom″boid/ [Gk, *rhombos,* rhombus, *eidos,* form], resembling the shape of an oblique equilateral parallelogram, as a rhomboid muscle.

rhomboidal sinus /rom″boidəl/, an opening in the central canal of the lumbar spinal cord.

rhomboideus major /romboi″dē·əs/ [Gk, *rhombos,* rhombus, *eidos,* form], a muscle of the upper back below and parallel to the rhomboideus minor. It inserts into the lower half of the medial border of the scapula. With the rhomboideus minor, it functions to draw the scapula toward the vertebral column while supporting it and drawing it slightly upward. Compare **latissimus dorsi, levator scapulae, rhomboideus minor, trapezius.**

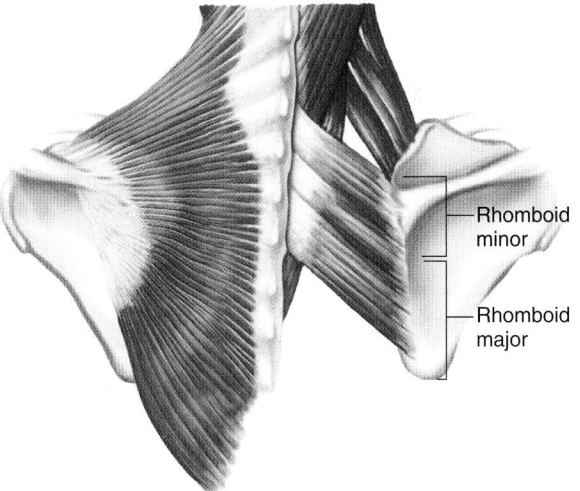

Rhomboid minor

Rhomboid major

Rhomboideus major and rhomboideus minor *(Patton and Thibodeau, 2010)*

rhomboideus minor, a muscle of the upper back, above and parallel to the rhomboideus major. It arises from the nuchal ligament and from the spinous processes of the seventh cervical and first thoracic vertebrae. It inserts into the upper part of the medial border at the root of the spine of

R

the scapula. With the rhomboideus major, it acts to draw the scapula toward the vertebral column while supporting the scapula and drawing it slightly upward. Compare **latissimus dorsi, levator scapulae, rhomboideus major, trapezius.**

rhomboid glossitis. See **median rhomboid glossitis.**

rhombomere /rom″bəmir/, any of the nine segments of the embryonic neural tube.

rhonchus /rong″kəs/ *pl.* *rhonchi* [Gk, *rhonchos,* snore], an abnormal sound heard on auscultation of an airway obstructed by thick secretions, muscular spasm, neoplasm, or external pressure. The continuous rumbling sound is more pronounced during expiration and characteristically clears on coughing, whereas gurgles do not.

rhotacism /rō″təsizm/, a speech disorder consisting of imperfect pronunciation of the /r/ sound. Also called **pararhotacism.** Compare **lallation.**

Rh positive. See **Rh factor.**

r-HuEPO, abbreviation for **recombinant human erythropoietin.**

rhus /rus/, any member of the genus *Rhus.*

Rhus, a genus of vines and shrubs of the family Anacardiaceae, many of which are poisonous. Some species contain urushiol, a highly allergenic oleoresin mixture, and contact with them produces a severe dermatitis (rhus dermatitis) in sensitive persons. The most important toxic species are *Rhus radicans* L. (poison ivy), *R. diversiloba* L. (western poison oak), *R. quercifolia* (eastern poison oak), and *R. vernix* L. (poison sumac).

rhus dermatitis /rōōs/ [Gk, *rhous,* sumac], a form of contact dermatitis caused by exposure to an allergenic oil, toxicodendrol, present in any part of a plant of the genus *Rhus* such as poison ivy, poison oak, or poison sumac. Contact with a rhus plant can result in severe itching, rashes, and blistering. Even the smoke of burning rhus plants may be toxic. See also **contact dermatitis.**

rhyp-, combining form meaning "filth."

rhythm /rith′əm/ [Gk, *rhythmos*], the relationship of one impulse to neighboring impulses as measured in time, movement, or regularity of action.

rhythmic nystagmus, oscillatory movement of the eyeballs. See **nystagmus.**

rhythm method. *(Informal)* See **natural family planning method.**

rhytid /ri′tid/, skin wrinkle.

rhytid-, rhitid-, combining from meaning "wrinkle" or "wrinkled": *rhytidectomy, rhytidosis.*

rhytidectomy. See **face lift.**

rhytidoplasty /ritid″ōplas′tē/ [Gk, *rhytis,* wrinkle, *plassein,* to mold], a procedure in reconstructive plastic surgery in which the skin of the face is tightened, wrinkles are removed, and the skin is made to appear firm and smooth. An incision is made at the hairline, and excess skin is separated from the supporting tissue and excised. The edges of the remaining skin are pulled up and back and sutured at the hairline. A pressure dressing is applied and left in place for 24 to 48 hours. Postoperative medication for pain is often necessary. The sutures are removed several days after discharge in an outpatient facility or in the surgeon's office. Also called **face lift.** Also spelled **rhitidoplasty.**

rhytidosis /rit′idō″sis/ [Gk, *rhytis,* wrinkle, *osis,* condition], a wrinkling, especially of the cornea. Also spelled **rhitidosis.**

RIA, abbreviation for **radioimmunoassay.**

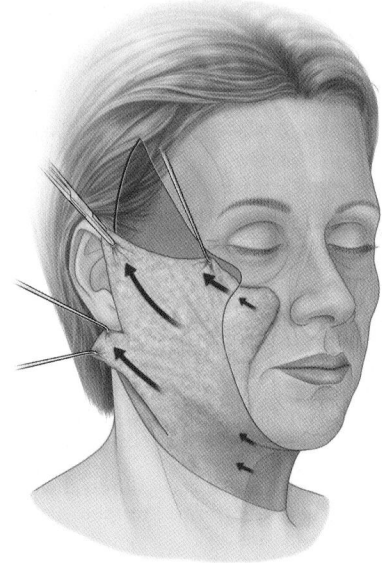

Rhytidoplasty *(Black and Hawks, 2009)*

rib [AS, roof], one of the 12 pairs of arches of bone forming a large part of the thoracic skeleton. The first seven ribs on each side are called *true ribs* because they articulate directly with the sternum and vertebrae. The remaining five ribs are called *false ribs.* The first three attach ventrally to ribs above; the last two are free at their ventral extremities and are called *floating ribs.* True ribs are also known as vertebrosternal ribs; false ribs as vertebrocostal ribs; and floating ribs as vertebral ribs. See also **thorax.**

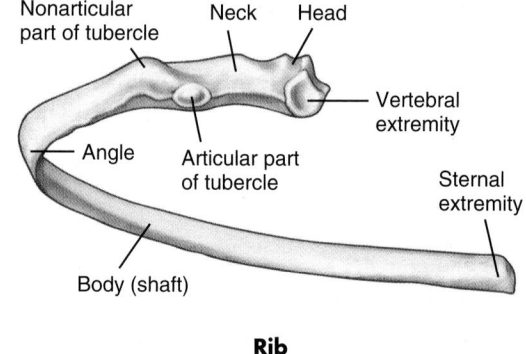

Rib

ribavirin /rī′bəvir″in/, an aerosol antiviral drug.

■ INDICATIONS: It is prescribed for the treatment of respiratory syncytial virus infections for the lower respiratory tract in infants and small children.

■ CONTRAINDICATIONS: It is not recommended for infants requiring assisted ventilation.

■ ADVERSE EFFECTS: Reported side effects include bacterial pneumonia, pneumothorax, apnea, hypotension, and cardiac arrest, conditions that may also have resulted from the patient's underlying disease; deteriorated respiratory function; rash; conjunctivitis; and reticulocytosis.

ribbon retractor, a malleable surgical instrument that can be bent into different shapes to position and hold back body tissues during a surgical procedure.

rib fracture, a break in a bone of the thoracic skeleton caused by a blow or crushing injury or by violent coughing or sneezing. It may also be a pathological fracture secondary to metastatic disease. The ribs most commonly broken are the fourth to eighth ribs; if the bone is splintered or the fracture is displaced, sharp fragments may pierce the lung, causing hemothorax or pneumothorax.

■ OBSERVATIONS: The patient with a fractured rib suffers pain, especially on inspiration, and usually breathes rapidly and shallowly. The site of the break is generally very tender to the touch, and the crackling of bone fragments rubbing together may be heard on auscultation. Breath sounds may be absent, decreased, or accompanied by rales and rhonchi. The location and nature of the fracture are determined by chest x-ray studies. The patient is observed for signs of hemoptysis, hemothorax, flail chest, atelectasis, pneumothorax, and pneumonia.

■ INTERVENTIONS: Fractured ribs may be splinted with an elastic belt or bandage or adhesive strapping. To prevent irritation, the area may be shaved and painted with tincture of benzoin before the adhesive tape is applied. Increasingly, however, no splints are used, because they compromise chest expansion and predispose the patient to pulmonary complications. If hospitalization is required, the patient is placed in a semi-Fowler's position, and the blood pressure, pulse, temperature, respirations, and breath sounds are checked every 2 to 4 hours. An analgesic may be ordered, but morphine sulfate is avoided because it depresses respiration. If strapping and analgesic medication fail to relieve pain, the physician may perform a regional nerve block by infiltrating the intercostal spaces above and below the fracture site with 1% procaine.

■ PATIENT CARE CONSIDERATIONS: The nurse assists in splinting the chest, administers the ordered medication, helps the patient to turn, and instructs the patient in how to perform deep breathing, coughing, and range-of-motion exercises of the extremities.

riboflavin /ri′bōflā″vin/ [*ribose* + L, *flavus,* yellow], a yellow, crystalline, water-soluble pigment, one of the heat-stable components of the B vitamin complex. It combines with specific flavoproteins and functions as a coenzyme in the oxidative processes of carbohydrates, fats, and proteins. Small amounts of riboflavin are found in the liver and kidneys, but it is not stored to any great degree in the body and must be supplied regularly in the diet. Common sources are organ meats, milk, cheese, eggs, green leafy vegetables, meat, whole grains, and legumes. Deficiency of riboflavin is rare and produces cheilosis; local inflammation; desquamation; encrustation; glossitis; photophobia; corneal opacities; proliferation of corneal vessels; seborrheic dermatitis about the nose, mouth, forehead, ears, and scrotum; trembling; sluggishness; dizziness; edema; inability to urinate; and vaginal itching. Also called **vitamin B$_2$.** See also **ariboflavinosis.**

ribonuclear protein (RNP) /ri′bōnoo″klē·ər/ [*ribose*; L, *nucleus,* nut kernel; Gk, *proteios,* first rank], a conjugated protein consisting of a protein molecule and a nucleic acid.

ribonuclease (RNase) /-noo″klē·ās/, a class of endonucleases that hydrolyzes ribonucleic acids.

ribonucleic acid (RNA) /ri′bōnoo͞oklē″ik/ [*ribose* + L, *nucleus,* nut kernel, *acidus,* sour], a nucleic acid, found in both the nucleus and cytoplasm of cells, that plays several roles in the translation of the genetic code and the assembly of proteins. Kinds include **messenger RNA, ribosomal RNA, transfer RNA.** See also **deoxyribonucleic acid.**

ribonucleoside /ri′bōnoo͞o″klē·əsīd′/, a nucleoside in which the sugar component is ribose. The ribonucleosides of RNA are adenosine, cytidine, guanosine, and uridine.

ribonucleotide /-noo͞o″klē·ətīd′/, a class of nucleotides in which the pentose is D-ribose.

ribose /ri′bōs/, a 5-carbon sugar that occurs as a component of RNA.

ribosomal RNA (rRNA) /ri′bōsō″məl/, the ribonucleic acid of ribosomes and polyribosomes.

ribosome /ri′bəsōm/ [*ribose* + Gk, *soma,* body], an organelle composed of RNA and protein that functions in the synthesis of protein. Ribosomes interact with messenger RNA and transfer RNA to link amino acid into a polypeptide chain in a sequence determined by the sequence of nucleotides in the messenger RNA. Ribosomes may exist singly, in clusters as polysomes, or attached to the "rough" endoplasmic reticulum. See also **translation.**

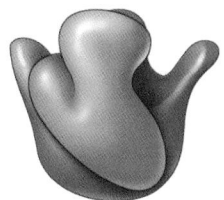

Ribosome *(Patton and Thibodeau, 2010)*

ribosome-inactivating protein (RIP), one of a variety of enzymes that cleave the *N*-glycosidic bond of adenine in a specific ribosomal RNA sequence. Type 1 RIPs are single-chain proteins. Some type 2 RIPs, such as ricin, possess a galactose-specific lectin domain that binds to cell surfaces, making them potent toxins.

ribosuria /ri′bəsoo͞or″ē·ə/, the presence of ribose in the urine, usually a sign of muscular dystrophy.

ribovirus. See **RNA virus.**

rib shaking, a procedure in physiotherapy in which constant, downward pressure is applied with an intermittent shaking motion of the hands on the rib cage over the area being drained. It is done with the flat part of the palm of the hand over the lung segment being drained during 4 to 12 prolonged exhalations by the patient through pursed lips.

rib vibration, a procedure in physiotherapy similar to rib shaking but done with a downward vibrating pressure with the flat part of the palm during exhalations.

RICE, an acronym for *r*est, *i*ce, *c*ompression, *e*levation, referring to the treatment for sprains and strains.

rice diet [Gk, *oryza,* rice, *diaita,* way of living], a diet consisting only of rice, fruit, fruit juices, and sugar, supplemented with vitamins and iron. Salt is forbidden. It is prescribed for the treatment of hypertension, chronic renal disease, and obesity. It should not be followed for any length of time because the severe dietary restrictions may lead to nutritional deficiencies or imbalance. Also called **Kempner rice-fruit diet.**

Richards, Linda [1841–1930], a nurse considered to be the first American-trained nurse, and a graduate of the first class of the New England Hospital for Women and Children. She then studied at the Nightingale Training School in London and in 1873 organized the Massachusetts General Hospital Training School. In 1885 she was sent to Japan to develop a training school at the Charity Hospital. In 1891 she took charge of the Philadelphia Visiting Nurse Society. She is credited with being the first to keep written records on patients, a practice she started when she worked as night superintendent at Bellevue Hospital in New York City.

Richet's aneurysm. See **fusiform aneurysm.**

Richter hernia /rik″tər, rish″tər/ [August G. Richter, German surgeon, 1742–1812], a small nonpalpable

R

visceral protrusion involving only a part of the intestinal wall. Also called **parietal hernia.**

ricin /rī″sin/, a poison made from waste produced in processing castor beans. It can take the form of a powder, mist, or pellet or can be dissolved in water or weak acid and can be used as a poison by ingestion, inhalation, or injection. As little as 500 micrograms can be a fatal dose. It cannot be spread by person-to-person contact. Poisoning is treated by minimizing exposure and by supportive care. There is no antidote. Also called *ricinine.* See also **ribosome-inactivating protein.**

rickets /rik″əts/ [Gk, *rachis,* backbone, *itis,* inflammation], a condition caused by a deficiency of vitamin D, seen primarily in infancy and childhood and characterized by abnormal bone formation. See also **osteodystrophy, osteomalacia, vitamin D. −rachitic,** *adj.*

■ OBSERVATIONS: Characteristic manifestations in infants and children include soft, pliable bones; softening of skull bones; enlargement of ribs at costochondral junctions; limb deformities; epiphyseal swelling (bowed legs and knock-knees); pigeon breast deformity; Harrison's groove; spinal deformities; and possible decrease in thoracic volume. The spleen and liver may be enlarged, and the body is generally tender to touch. Bone deformities are seen on radiographic images. Adults may have bone pain, fractures, weakness, weight loss, and malaise.

■ INTERVENTIONS: Prevention and treatment are the same and include a diet rich in calcium, phosphorus, and vitamin D and adequate exposure to sunlight. Surgical intervention may be indicated for correction of a slipped femoral epiphysis in infants and young children. Deformities may need correction through bracing. The health care team should focus on prevention, with education about the importance of calcium and vitamin D in the diet and the prevention of complications associated with existing disease.

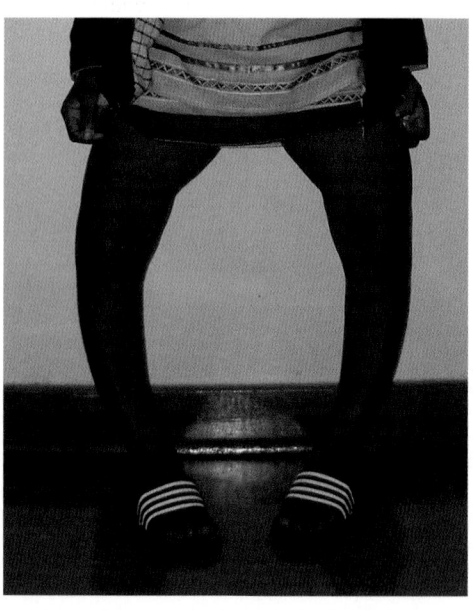

Child with deformity characteristic of rickets *(Kumar et al, 2007)*

Rickettsia /riket′sē·ə/ [Howard T. Ricketts, American pathologist, 1871–1910], a genus of microorganisms that combines aspects of both bacteria and viruses. They can be observed with a light microscope, divide by fission, and may be controlled with antibiotics. They also exist as viruslike

intracellular parasites, living in the intestinal tracts of insects such as lice. Thus a human infested with lice is also likely to be infected with a form of typhus transmitted by *Rickettsia prowazeki.* Rickettsial diseases have been responsible for many of history's worst epidemics. The various species are distinguished on the basis of similarities in the diseases they cause. The spotted fever group includes diseases such as Rocky Mountain spotted fever and rickettsialpox; the typhus group includes epidemic typhus and murine typhus; and a miscellaneous group includes Q fever and trench fever. Rickettsial diseases are uncommon in parts of the world where insect and rodent populations are well controlled. −*rickettsial, adj.*

Rickettsia burnetii. See *Coxiella burnetii.*

rickettsial disease [Howard T. Ricketts; L, *dis* + Fr, *aise,* ease], an infection caused by a species of *Rickettsia.*

rickettsialpox /riket″sē·əlpoks′/ [Howard T. Ricketts; ME, *pokkes,* pustules], a mild, acute infectious disease caused by *Rickettsia akari* and transmitted from mice to humans by mites *(Allo dermanyssus sanguineus).* It is characterized by an asymptomatic crusted primary lesion, chills, fever, headache, malaise, myalgia, and a rash resembling chickenpox. About 1 week after onset of symptoms, small, discrete, maculopapular lesions appear on any part of the body, but rarely on palms or soles. These lesions become vesicular and dry and form scabs. Eventually the scabs fall off, leaving no scars. Chloramphenicol or tetracycline hastens recovery. Prevention involves the elimination of house mice. Also called **Kew Gardens spotted fever.** Compare **Rocky Mountain spotted fever.** See also *Rickettsia.*

rickettsiosis /riket′sē·ō″sis/ *pl.* **rickettsioses** [Howard T. Ricketts; Gk, *osis,* condition], any of a group of infectious diseases caused by microorganisms of the genus *Rickettsia.* Kinds of rickettsioses include a spotted fever group (boutonneuse fever, rickettsialpox, Rocky Mountain spotted fever), a typhus group (epidemic typhus, murine typhus, scrub typhus), and a miscellaneous group (Q fever, trench fever). See also *Rickettsia,* **boutonneuse fever, rickettsialpox, Rocky Mountain spotted fever, epidemic typhus, murine typhus, scrub typhus, Q fever, trench fever.**

Ridaura, an oral disease-modifying antirheumatoid drug. Brand name for **auranofin.**

rider's bone [AS, *ridan,* to ride, *ban,* bone], a bony deposit that sometimes develops in horseback riders on the inner side of the lower end of the tendon of the adductor muscle of the thigh. Also called **cavalry bone.**

rider's sprain [OFr, *espreindre,* to force out], a sprain of the adductor muscles of the thigh resulting from horseback riding.

ridge /rij/ [AS, *hyrcg*], a projection or projecting structure, such as the gastrocnemial ridge or crest on the posterior surface of the femur giving attachment to the gastrocnemius muscle.

ridge extension, an intraoral surgical operation for deepening the labial, buccal, or lingual sulci.

ridge lap, the part of an artificial tooth that is adjacent to or approximates the residual ridge. Proper ridge lap can give the appearance of a natural tooth.

Riedel's struma, Riedel's thyroiditis. See **fibrous thyroiditis.**

Rieder's cell leukemia /rē″dərz/ [Hermann Rieder, German pathologist, 1858–1932], a malignant neoplasm of blood-forming tissues characterized by the presence in blood of large numbers of atypical myeloblasts with immature cytoplasm and relatively mature lobulated, indented nuclei.

RIF, abbreviation for **resistance-inducing factor.**

rifa-, prefix for rifamycin-derived antibiotics.

rifabutin /rif″ah-bu′tin/, an antibacterial used for the prevention of disseminated *Mycobacterium avium* complex disease in patients with advanced HIV infection. It is administered orally.

Rifadin, an antibacterial agent. Brand name for **rifampin.**

rifampin /rif″əmpin/, an antibacterial.

■ INDICATIONS: It is prescribed in combination for the treatment of tuberculosis, staphylococcal infections, and *Legionella* pneumonia, and in meningococcal meningitis and *Hemophilus influenzae* prophylaxis.

■ CONTRAINDICATIONS: Liver dysfunction or disease or known hypersensitivity to this drug or to rifamycin prohibits its use.

■ ADVERSE EFFECTS: Among the more serious adverse effects are liver toxicity and a syndrome resembling influenza. GI distress; aches and cramps; and discoloration of urine, saliva, and sweat commonly occur. This drug interacts with many other drugs.

rifamycin /rif″ah-mi′sin/, any of a family of antibiotics biosynthesized from a strain of *Streptomyces mediterranei,* effective against a broad spectrum of bacteria. The five components are designated A, B, C, D, and E; rifamycins O, S, and SV are derivatives of the B component, and AG and X are derivatives of the O component. It is used for the initial treatment and retreatment of pulmonary tuberculosis and for prevention of meningococcal infections in close contacts of patients with *Neisseria meningitidis* infections.

rifapentine, an antitubercular.

■ INDICATIONS: Rifapentine is used to treat pulmonary tuberculosis. It must be used in combination with at least one other antitubercular.

■ CONTRAINDICATIONS: Known hypersensitivity to rifamycin prohibits its use.

■ ADVERSE EFFECTS: Life-threatening effects include pancreatitis, hematuria, proteinuria, thrombocytopenia, leukopenia, neutropenia, lymphopenia, and leukocytosis. Other adverse effects include rash, pruritus, urticaria, acne, visual disturbances, gout, arthrosis, edema, aggressive reaction, bilirubinemia, hepatitis, increased AST/ALT, pyuria, urinary casts, headache, fatigue, anxiety, dizziness, anemia, purpura, and hematoma. Common side effects include nausea, vomiting, anorexia, diarrhea, and heartburn.

rifaximin, a miscellaneous antiinfective.

■ INDICATIONS: This drug is used to treat traveler's diarrhea caused by *Escherichia coli* in adults and children older than 12 years of age.

■ CONTRAINDICATIONS: Known hypersensitivity to this drug prohibits its use.

■ ADVERSE EFFECTS: Adverse effects of this drug include abnormal dreams, dizziness, insomnia, and vomiting. Common side effects include abdominal pain, constipation, defecation urgency, flatulence, nausea, rectal tenesmus, headache, and pyrexia.

Rift Valley fever, a bunyavirus infection of Egypt and east Africa spread by mosquitoes or by handling infected sheep, buffalo, goats, camels, and cattle. Those individuals infected with RVF virus typically exhibit no symptoms or a mild illness that involves fever and abnormalities of the liver. It is characterized by abrupt fever, chills, headache, and generalized aching, followed by epigastric pain, anorexia, loss of taste, and photophobia. Retinitis may cause vision loss in 1% to 10% of cases. The disease is of short duration; recovery occurs typically after 2 days to a week and is usually complete. There is no specific treatment. A killed virus vaccine that provides protection for 2 years is available in the United States for those at risk, such as laboratory workers and veterinarians.

RIG, abbreviation for **rabies immune globulin.**

Riga-Fede disease /rē′gä fā′dä/ [Antonio Riga, Italian physician, 1832–1919; Francesco Fede, Italian pediatrician, 1832–1913], an ulceration of the lingual frenum in some infants, caused by abrasion of the frenum by natal or neonatal teeth. Also called **Fede disease.**

right atrial catheter, an indwelling IV catheter inserted centrally or peripherally and threaded into the superior vena cava and right atrium.

right atrioventricular orifice, the opening between the right atrium and ventricle of the heart. Also called *tricuspid orifice.*

right atrioventricular valve. See **tricuspid valve.**

right brachiocephalic vein [AS, *riht* + Gk, *brachion,* arm, *kephale,* head], a vessel, about 2.5 cm long, that starts in the root of the neck at the junction of the internal jugular and the subclavian veins on the right side and descends vertically from behind the sternal end of the clavicle to join the left brachiocephalic vein and form the superior vena cava. The right brachiocephalic vein, like the left, receives various tributaries, such as the vertebral vein, the internal thoracic vein, and the inferior thyroid vein. Compare **left brachiocephalic vein.**

right bundle branch block (RBBB), impaired transmission or absence of transmission of electric impulses from the atrioventricular (AV) bundle of His to the right ventricle. The block may be complete or incomplete and may be caused by a lesion in the right bundle branch or a small, focal lesion in the AV bundle. RBBB is often associated with right ventricular hypertrophy, especially in athletes and individuals under 40 years of age. In older individuals RBBB is commonly caused by coronary artery disease. A complete RBBB commonly occurs after surgical closure of a ventricular septal defect.

right common carotid artery, the shorter of the two common carotid arteries, arising from the brachiocephalic trunk, passing obliquely from the level of the sternoclavicular articulation to the upper border of the thyroid cartilage, and dividing into the right internal and external carotids. Compare **left common carotid artery.**

right coronary artery, one of a pair of branches of the ascending aorta, arising in the right posterior aortic sinus, passing along the right side of the coronary sulcus, and dividing into the right interventricular artery and a large marginal branch. It supplies both ventricles, the right atrium, and the sinoatrial node. Compare **left coronary artery.**

right coronary vein. See **small cardiac vein.**

right-handedness, a natural tendency to favor the use of the right hand. Also called **dextrality.** See also **cerebral dominance, handedness.**

right-hand rule, a principle of physics in which the direction of current flow in a wire is related to the position of the imaginary lines of force of the magnetic field about the wire. Thus, if the fingers of the right hand are flexed to represent the magnetic field and the thumb is extended, the thumb points in the direction of current flow.

right-heart failure, an abnormal cardiac condition characterized by the impairment of the right side of the heart and congestion and elevated pressure in the systemic veins and capillaries. The most common cause of right-heart failure is left-heart failure because both sides of the heart are part of a circuit and what affects one side will eventually affect the other. Right ventricular infarction, pulmonic stenosis, and pulmonary hypertension can also result in right-heart failure. In failure associated with either side of the heart, cardiac output is usually decreased. Also called **right-sided failure.** Compare **left-heart failure.** See also **heart failure.**

R

right hepatic duct, the duct that drains bile from the right lobe of the liver into the common bile duct.

righting reflex [AS, *riht* + L, *reflectere,* to bend back], any one of the neuromuscular responses to restore the body to its normal upright position when it has been displaced. The righting reflexes involve complicated mechanisms and processes associated with the structures of the internal ear, such as the utricle, the saccule, the macula, and the semicircular canals. Any change in the position of the head produces a change in the pressure on the gelatinous membrane of the macula. The fibers of the nerve (vestibular branch of the eighth cranial nerve) transmit impulses to the brain, producing a sense of position. The head and trunk are thus kept in alignment. Also activating righting reflexes are proprioceptors in muscles and tendons and visual nerve impulses. Also called **body righting reflex.**

right interventricular artery. See **dorsal interventricular artery.**

right lymphatic duct, a vessel that conveys lymph from the right upper quadrant of the body into the bloodstream in the neck at the junction of the right internal jugular and the right subclavian veins. About 1.25 cm long, the duct courses over the medial border of the scalenus anterior. At its orifice are two semilunar valves that prevent venous blood from flowing backward into the duct. Lymph drains into the right lymphatic duct from numerous capillaries and vessels and from three lymphatic trunks in the right quadrant. Compare **thoracic duct.** See also **lymphatic system.**

right part of liver, the part of the liver that receives blood from the right branches of the hepatic portal vein and hepatic artery proper and whose bile flows out through the right hepatic duct. Also called *right liver.*

right pulmonary artery, the longer and slightly larger of the two arteries conveying venous blood from the heart to the lungs. It arises from the pulmonary trunk, bends to the right behind the aorta, and divides into two branches at the root of the right lung. Compare **left pulmonary artery.**

right-sided failure. See **right-heart failure.**

right subclavian artery, a large artery that arises from the brachiocephalic artery. It has several important branches: the axillary, vertebral thoracic, and internal thoracic arteries and the cervical and costocervical trunks, which perfuse the right side of the upper body.

right-to-know laws, laws that require employers to inform workers regarding health effects of materials they must handle, including toxic chemicals and radioactive substances. Under the authority of the U.S. Occupational Safety and Health Act of 1970, the National Institute for Occupational Safety and Health periodically revises recommendations or limits of exposure to potentially hazardous substances in the workplace. It also recommends appropriate preventive measures designed to reduce or eliminate adverse health effects of these hazards and publishes its recommendations in a variety of public documents.

right-to-left shunt [ME, *shunten*], a shunt in which unoxygenated venous blood bypasses the lungs and directly enters the arterial system, as in the tetralogy of Fallot and other conditions.

right umbilical vein, the right of the two veins in the umbilical cord that carry blood from the placenta to the sinus venosus of the heart in the early embryo. It degenerates during the seventh week.

right ventricle, the relatively thin-walled chamber of the heart that pumps blood received from the right atrium into the pulmonary arteries to the lungs for oxygenation. The right ventricle is shorter and rounder than the long conical left ventricle. The chordae tendineae of the tricuspid valve of the right ventricle are finer than the coarse strands of the chordae tendineae of the left ventricle. See also **heart.**

right ventricular thrust. See **precordial movement.**

rigid. See **rigidity.**

rigid gas permeable (RGP) contact lens, a contact lens made of rigid plastic that transmits oxygen to the cornea, which makes the lens more comfortable to wear. In comparison with soft lenses, RGP lenses hold their shape better and offer clearer vision, are more durable, and are less prone to harbor bacteria and protein deposits. However, they cause discomfort on initial wearing and require a short adaptation period. Also called **gas permeable contact lens.**

rigidity /rijid″itē/ [L, *rigere,* to be stiff], a condition of hardness, stiffness, or inflexibility. **–rigid,** *adj.*

rigidus /rij″idəs/ [L, stiff], a deformity characterized by limited motion, especially dorsiflexion of the great toe. This condition causes pain and may ultimately produce degenerative changes of the involved joints.

rigor /rig″ər/ [L, stiffness], **1.** a rigid condition of the body tissues, as in rigor mortis. **2.** a violent attack of shivering that may be associated with chills and fever.

rigor mortis /môr″tis/, the rigid stiffening of skeletal and cardiac muscle shortly after death.

Riley-Day syndrome. See **dysautonomia.**

riluzole, a glutamate antagonist.

■ INDICATIONS: This drug is used to treat amyotropic lateral sclerosis.

■ CONTRAINDICATIONS: Known hypersensitivity to this drug prohibits its use.

■ ADVERSE EFFECTS: Neutropenia and exfoliative dermatitis are life-threatening effects. Other adverse effects are nausea, vomiting, dyspepsia, anorexia, diarrhea, flatulence, stomatitis, dry mouth, hypertonia, depression, dizziness, insomnia, somnolence, vertigo, pruritus, eczema, alopecia, decreased lung function, rhinitis, increased cough, hypertension, tachycardia, phlebitis, palpitations, postural hypertension, urinary tract infection, and dysuria.

rim [OE, *rima,* edge], an outer edge, which may be curved or circular, as on an occluding surface built on a temporary or permanent denture base.

rima /rī″mə/, a cleft or fissure.

Rimactane, an antibacterial. Brand name for **rifampin.**

rima glottidis. See **glottis.**

rimantadine /ri-man′tah-dēn/, an antiviral agent used in prophylaxis and treatment of influenza A.

rima respitoria, rima vestibule. See **false glottis.**

rimexolone /r-mek′sah-lōn″/, a corticosteroid used in topical treatment of inflammation after eye surgery and of uveitis affecting the anterior structures of the eye.

rimose /rī″mōs/, having many clefts or fissures.

Rimso-50, a urinary tract antiinflammatory agent. Brand name for **dimethyl sulfoxide.**

rimula /rim″yələ/ [L, small cleft], a very small fissure in the brain or spinal cord.

ring [AS, *hring*], **1.** a circular band surrounding a central opening. **2.** a closed chainlike linkage of atoms.

ring centriole, a common misnomer for the anulus of the spermatozoon, which is not actually a centriole.

ring chromosome [AS, *hring*], a circular chromosome formed by the fusion of the two ends. It is the primary type of chromosome found in bacteria.

ring-down artifact, (in sonography) an echo pattern caused by reverberation in a bubble or other soft tissue entity.

ring-down time, (in ultrasonics) the time required for vibration of the transducer element at its resonance frequency to decrease to a negligible level following excitation. See also **pulse duration.**

ringed sideroblast /sid″ərōblast′/ [Gk, *sideros,* iron, *blastos,* germ], an iron-rich nucleated red blood cell precursor in the bone marrow characterized by a perinuclear ring of siderotic granules.

Ringer's lactate solution, a fluid and electrolyte replenisher. Also called **Hartmann's solution.**

■ INDICATIONS: It is prescribed for correction of extracellular volume and electrolyte depletion.

■ CONTRAINDICATIONS: Kidney failure, congestive heart failure, or hypoproteinemia prohibits its use.

■ ADVERSE EFFECTS: Among the more serious adverse effects are sodium excess and fluid overload, which may lead to pulmonary and peripheral edema.

ring removal from swollen finger, a technique for taking off a tightly fitting ring. It consists of slipping the end of a string under the ring while moving the ring toward the hand. The rest of the string is then wound around the swollen part of the finger a number of times, after which the string is unwound from the hand side, gradually easing the ring toward the fingertip. The process may need to be repeated to complete the removal.

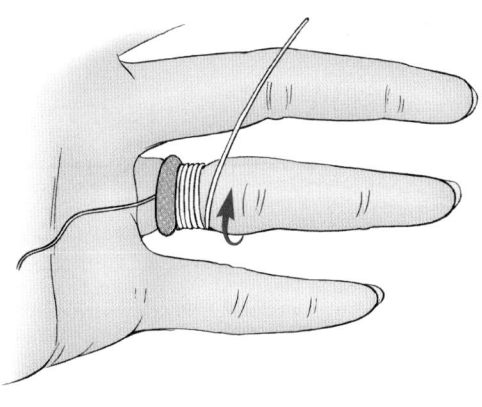

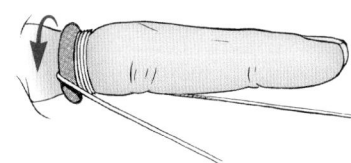

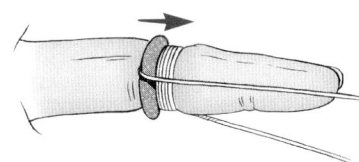

Ring removal from swollen finger using the string technique *(Auerbach, 2012)*

ringworm. See **tinea.**

Rinne tuning fork test /rin″ə/ [Heinrich A. Rinne, German otologist, 1819–1868], a method of distinguishing conductive from sensorineural hearing loss. The base of a vibrating tuning fork is placed against the patient's mastoid bone.

While one ear is tested, the other is masked. When the patient no longer hears the sound, the time in seconds is noted, and the fork is positioned about ½ inch from the external auditory meatus on the same side. The time the sound is heard is noted. Air-conducted sound should be heard twice as long as bone-conducted sound after bone conduction stops. In sensorineural loss the sound is heard relatively longer by air conduction; in conductive hearing loss the sound is heard longer by bone conduction. The test may be performed with tuning forks of 256, 512, and 1024 cycles.

-rinone, suffix for inamrinone-type cardiotonic agents.

Rio Grande fever. See **abortus fever.**

Riopan, a fixed-combination medication containing an antacid and an antiflatulent. Brand name for **magaldrate, simethicone.**

riot control agents, agents normally used for crowd control; including the compounds chloroacetophenone, chlorobenzylidenemalononitrile, chloropicrin, bromobenzylcyanide, and benzoxazepine. They are used as liquids or aerosols and exposure is by inhalation or by contact with the eyes or skin. They incapacitate by irritating the area of contact and cause irritation of the skin and mucous membranes and respiratory distress. High doses can cause blindness and death. Treatment is by removal of clothing and removing the agent from the skin and eyes. Effects cease shortly after the agent is removed. Also called **tear gas.**

RIP, **1.** abbreviation for **reflex inhibiting pattern. 2.** abbreviation for **ribosome-inactivating protein.**

ripe cataract [OE, *ripan* + Gk, *katarrhaktes,* portcullis], a mature cataract that produces swelling and opacity of the entire lens. Also called **mature cataract.**

risedronate, a bone-resorption inhibitor.

■ INDICATIONS: It is used to treat Paget disease.

■ CONTRAINDICATIONS: Hypersensitivity to biphosphonates prohibits its use.

■ ADVERSE EFFECTS: Dizziness and headache are adverse effects. Common side effects include abdominal pain, anorexia, diarrhea, nausea, bone pain, arthralgia, and chest pain.

risk-benefit analysis, the consideration of whether a medical or surgical procedure, particularly a radical approach, is worth the risk to the patient as compared with possible benefits if the procedure is successful.

risk factor [Fr, *risque,* hazard; L, *factor,* maker], a factor that causes a person or a group of people to be particularly susceptible to an unwanted, unpleasant, or unhealthful event, such as immunosuppression, which increases the incidence and severity of infection, or cigarette smoking, which increases the risk of developing a respiratory or cardiovascular disease.

risk management, a function of administration of a hospital or other health facility directed toward identification, evaluation, and correction of potential risks that could lead to injury to patients, staff members, or visitors and result in property loss or damage.

risorius /risôr″ē·əs/ [L, *ridere,* to laugh], one of the 12 muscles of the mouth. A muscular fibrous band, it arises in the fascia over the masseter and inserts into the skin at the corner of the mouth. It acts to retract the angle of the mouth, as in a smile.

Risser cast /ris″ər/ [Joseph C. Risser, American surgeon, 1892–1942], an orthopedic device for encasing the entire trunk of the body, extending over the cervical area to the chin. In rare cases it extends over the hips to the knees. The Risser cast is made of plaster of paris or fiberglass and is used to immobilize the trunk in the treatment of scoliosis and in the preoperative or postoperative correction or maintenance of correction of scoliosis. Compare **body jacket, turnbuckle cast.**

RIST, abbreviation for **radioimmunosorbent test.**

risus caninus /rī″səs/ [L, *risus,* laughter, *caninus,* doglike], a grinning facial distortion caused by tension in the occipitofrontalis and other facial muscles as a result of tetanus.

risus sardonicus /särdon″ikəs/ [L, *risus,* laughter; Gk, *sardonius,* mocking], a wry, masklike grin caused by spasm of the facial muscles, as seen in tetanus.

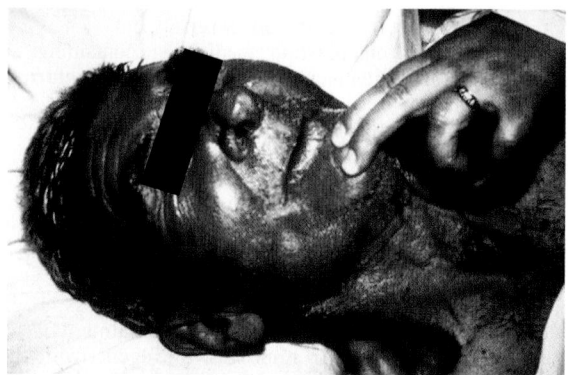

Grin associated with risus sardonicus *(Stone and Gorbach, 2000)*

Ritalin, a central nervous system stimulant. Brand name for **methylphenidate hydrochloride.**

Ritgen maneuver, an obstetric procedure used to control delivery of the fetal head. It involves applying upward pressure from the coccygeal region to extend the head during actual delivery, thereby protecting the musculature of the perineum.

ritodrine hydrochloride /rit″ədrēn/, a uterine relaxant.

■ INDICATIONS: It is prescribed in pregnancy management to stop the uterus from contracting in preterm labor.

■ CONTRAINDICATIONS: It is not given before the twentieth week of gestation. Known hypersensitivity to this drug prohibits its use.

■ ADVERSE EFFECTS: Among the more serious adverse reactions are tachycardia, palpitations, headache, nausea, and alterations in blood pressure. Pulmonary edema and death have occurred when it has been given concomitantly with corticosteroids to prevent the development of respiratory distress syndrome in the premature neonate.

ritonavir, a protease inhibitor.

■ INDICATIONS: It is prescribed in the treatment of acquired immunodeficiency syndrome as part of a multidrug regimen including at least three antiretroviral drugs.

■ CONTRAINDICATIONS: Hypersensitivity to ritonavir precludes its use. Concurrent use of any of several other drugs is either contraindicated or warrants caution, including ergot derivatives, benzodiazepine sedative-hypnotics, some antiarrhythmic medications, some HMG-CoA reductase inhibitors (statins), some erectile dysfunction medicines, and some analgesics.

■ ADVERSE EFFECTS: Protease inhibitors cause problems with lipid metabolism and lead to hyperlipidemia, hyperglycemia and redistribution of body fat (e.g., buffalo hump), central obesity, breast enlargement, and facial atrophy. Additional side effects often reported include nausea, vomiting, diarrhea, and numbness about the lips.

Ritter disease [Gottfried Ritter von Rittershain, German physician, 1820–1883], a rare staphylococcal infection of newborns that begins with red spots about the mouth and chin, gradually spreading over the entire body, and is followed by generalized exfoliation. Vesicles and yellow crusts may also be present. Ritter disease is potentially fatal; the prevention of dehydration and treatment with intravenous antibiotics are essential. Also called **dermatitis exfoliativa neonatorum, staphylococcal scalded skin syndrome.** Compare **toxic epidermal necrolysis.**

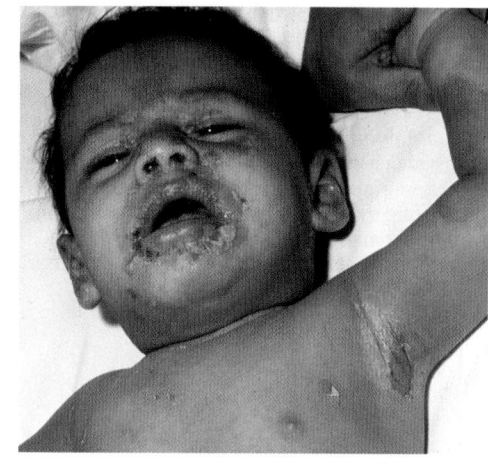

Child with Ritter disease *(Weston, Lane, and Morelli, 2007)*

ritual /rich″oо̄wəl/, 1. a mental health disorder characterized by repetitive sequences of stereotyped daily life routines, such as repeated handwashing, that interferes with an individual's level of functioning. 2. a prescribed order of ceremonial acts or series of acts. 3. a detailed procedure followed faithfully or regularly.

ritual circumcision, a surgical procedure with religious significance for removing the prepuce of the male in Jewish communities and to a lesser extent in other societies. In Jewish families the male circumcision is usually performed on the eighth day after birth. The practice dates back thousands of years. See also **circumcision.**

rituximab, a miscellaneous antineoplastic.

■ INDICATIONS: It is used to treat non-Hodgkin lymphoma (CD20 positive, B cell).

■ CONTRAINDICATIONS: Known hypersensitivity to this drug or to murine proteins prohibits its use.

■ ADVERSE EFFECTS: Life-threatening effects include leukopenia, neutropenia, thrombocytopenia, and bronchospasm. Other adverse effects include fever, chills, asthenia, headache, angioedema, hypotension, and myalgia. Common side effects include nausea, vomiting, anorexia, irritation at the injection site, and rash.

rivastigmine /riv″ah-stig′mēn/, a reversible inhibitor of cholinesterase, believed to increase the level of acetylcholine available in the central nervous system. It is administered orally as the tartrate salt as an adjunct in the treatment of mild to moderate dementia of the Alzheimer type.

Rivea corymbosa, a twining vine of the botanical family of Convolvulaceae. The seeds contain indole alkaloids, a source of lysergic acid diethylamide, which have an effect of altered perception when ingested in large quantities. The seeds have been used in religious ceremonies of indigenous

Latin American cultures since the era of the Aztecs. Also called **Mexican bindweed, morning glory.**

river blindness. See **onchocerciasis.**

Rivinus notch, tympanic notch /rēvē″nəs/ [Augustus Q. Rivinus, German anatomist, 1652–1723], a deficiency in the tympanic sulcus of the ear that forms an attachment for the flaccid part of the tympanic membrane and the malleolar folds. Also called *Rivinus incisure, tympanic incisure.*

rivus lacrimalis /rī′vəs/ [L, stream of tears], a channel between the eyelids and the surface of the eye that normally allows a flow of moisture when the eyes are closed.

rizatriptan, a migraine agent.

- INDICATIONS: It is used in the acute treatment of migraine.
- CONTRAINDICATIONS: Factors prohibiting its use include angina pectoris, a history of myocardial infarction, documented silent ischemia, Prinzmetal's angina, ischemic heart disease, concurrent use of ergotamine-containing preparations, uncontrolled hypertension, basilar or hemiplegic migraine, and known hypersensitivity.
- ADVERSE EFFECTS: Adverse effects include chest tightness, chest pressure, nausea, and dry mouth. Common side effects include dizziness, headache, and fatigue.

RK, **1.** abbreviation for **radial keratotomy. 2.** abbreviation for **refractive keratotomy.**

R.L.E., abbreviation for *right lower extremity.*

R.L.L., abbreviation for *right lower lobe of lung.*

r-loop, (in molecular genetics) a distinctive loop formation seen under an electron microscope. It is composed of a single helical strand of deoxyribonucleic acid (DNA) wound with a hybrid strand containing another single strand of DNA with a strand of ribonucleic acid.

RLQ, abbreviation for *right lower quadrant.*

RMP, abbreviation for *right mentoposterior fetal position.*

RMSF, abbreviation for **Rocky Mountain spotted fever.**

RMT, abbreviation for *right mentotransverse fetal position.*

Rn, symbol for the element **radon.**

RN, abbreviation for **registered nurse.**

RNA, abbreviation for **ribonucleic acid.**

RNA amplification, an in vitro technique used to increase the number of copies of a specific segment of RNA to aid in its detection.

RNA-dependent DNA polymerase, also called *RNA-directed DNA polymerase.* See **reverse transcriptase.**

RNA polymerase, an enzyme that catalyzes the assembly of ribonucleoside triphosphates into RNA, with single-stranded DNA serving as the template. Also called *RNA nucleotidyltransferase.*

RNase, abbreviation for **ribonuclease.**

RNA splicing, (in molecular genetics) the process by which base pairs that interrupt the continuity of genetic information in deoxyribonucleic acid are removed from the precursors of messenger ribonucleic acid.

RNA virus, any of a group of viruses whose genome is composed of RNA, including most viruses that infect animal cells. Also called **ribovirus.** Kinds include *Arenavirus,* **coronavirus, orthomyxovirus, picornavirus, rhabdovirus, Toga virus.**

RN, BC, abbreviation for *registered nurse, board certified.*

RNP, abbreviation for **ribonuclear protein.**

ROA, abbreviation for *right occipitoanterior fetal position.*

Robaxin, a skeletal muscle relaxant. Brand name for **methocarbamol.**

Robb, Isabel Hampton [1860–1910], a Canadian-born American nursing educator and writer. She was the first to institute a systematic, step-by-step course for nursing students that integrated clinical experience and classwork and the first educator to arrange for the affiliation of her students at other hospitals for specialized training. She also helped establish university affiliation for nursing education and postgraduate courses. When the Johns Hopkins School of Nursing was established in Baltimore in 1889, she became its first director, establishing the high standards for both the practical and theoretic aspects of nursing education that became the base from which she worked to establish national standards. She was one of the founders of *The American Journal of Nursing* and one of the forerunners of the American Nurses Association.

robertsonian translocation /rob′ərtsō″nē·ən/ [William R.B. Robertson, 1881–1941, American biologist], the exchange of entire chromosome arms, with the break occurring at the centromere, usually between two nonhomologous acrocentric chromosomes. It produces one large, metacentric chromosome and one extremely small chromosome. The latter carries little genetic material and may be lost through successive cell divisions, leading to a reduction in total chromosome number. Compare **balanced translocation, reciprocal translocation.**

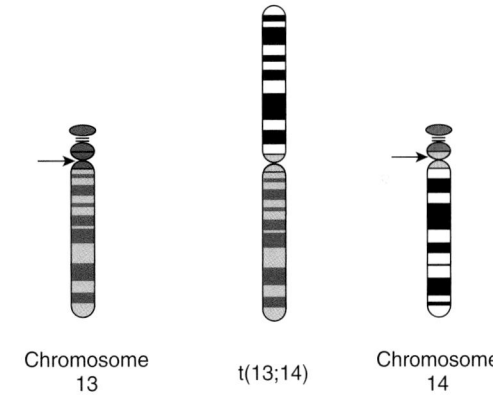

Chromosome 13   t(13;14)   Chromosome 14

Robertsonian translocation (Jorde et al, 2006)

Roberts syndrome /rob′ərts/ [John Bingham Roberts, American surgeon, 1852–1924], a hereditary syndrome, transmitted as an autosomal-recessive trait, consisting of imperfect development of the long bones of the limbs and associated with cleft palate and lip and other anomalies.

Robinow syndrome /rob′inou/ [Meinhard Robinow, American physician, 1909–1997], dwarfism associated with increased interorbital distance, malaligned teeth, bulging forehead, depressed nasal bridge, and short limbs. Also called **fetal face syndrome,** *Robinow dwarfism.*

Robinul, an anticholinergic medication. Brand name for **glycopyrrolate.**

Robitussin, an expectorant; also available in various fixed-combination preparations with an antihistamine, with a decongestant, or with a cough suppressant. Brand name for **guaifenesin.**

robotic /rōbot″ik/, pertaining to a robot, a mechanical or electronic device that resembles a human being, operating automatically or by remote control with the ability to perform a variety of complex tasks.

robotic surgery, the performance of operative procedures with the assistance of robotic technology. It allows great precision and is used for remote-control, minimally invasive procedures. Current systems consist of computer-controlled electromechanical devices that work in response to controls manipulated by the surgeon.

Rocaltrol, a synthetic vitamin D analog. Brand name for **calcitriol.**

Rocephin, a cephalosporin antibiotic. Brand name for **ceftriaxone sodium.**

Rochalimaea /rosh'əlimē″ə/, a genus of bacteria resembling *Rickettsia* but found extracellularly in an arthropod host. The species, *R. quintana* (now called *Bartonella quintana),* is a cause of trench fever as transmitted by the body louse. A related bacterium, *R. henselae,* is a cause of bacillary angiomatosis in immunocompromised humans, including those with human immunodeficiency virus infection.

rocker knife, a knife with a curved blade at the tip that cuts with a rocking motion. It is designed to help individuals who have the functional use of only one hand or limited arm function in performing cutting motions.

rock fever. See **brucellosis.**

rocking bed, 1. (in respiratory care) a device that rocks a patient from 30 degrees head up to 15 degrees head down several times a minute. The rocking moves the abdominal contents, and the resulting diaphragmatic movement assists ventilation of the lungs. The device is no longer in common use. **2.** a mattress mounted on a slowly moving platform with a rhythmic motion that may play a role in promoting sleep.

Rocky Mountain spotted fever (RMSF), a serious tickborne infectious disease occurring throughout the temperate zones of North and South America, caused by *Rickettsia rickettsii.* Also called **Mexican spotted fever, mountain fever, mountain tick fever, spotted fever.** Compare **murine typhus, rickettsialpox.** See also **boutonneuse fever, scrub typhus, typhus.**

■ OBSERVATIONS: It is characterized by chills, fever, severe headache, myalgia, mental confusion, and rash. Erythematous macules first appear on wrists and ankles, spreading rapidly over the extremities, trunk, and face and usually on the palms and soles. Hemorrhagic lesions, constipation, and abdominal distension are also common. The diagnosis is based on clinical examination and confirmed by laboratory analyses, including immunofluorescent antibody screens, complement fixation test, and Weil-Felix test.

■ INTERVENTIONS: Individuals treated with doxycycline within 5 days typically recover. Those treated after 5 days may experience a more severe illness, requiring hospitalization or intensive care. If left untreated, RMSF can be fatal. Prevention and early treatment are critically important.

■ PATIENT CARE CONSIDERATIONS: Prevention includes the use of insect repellents, the wearing of protective clothing, frequent inspection of the body, and careful removal of wood or dog ticks. No vaccine is available. Care must be taken not to crush ticks, because infection may be acquired through skin abrasions.

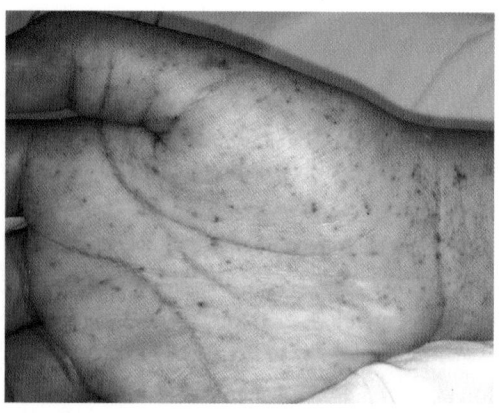

Rocky Mountain spotted fever *(Long, Prober, and Fischer, 2018)*

rocuronium /ro″ku-ro′ne-um/, a neuromuscular blocking agent used as an adjunct in general anesthesia to facilitate endotracheal intubation and as a skeletal muscle relaxant during surgery or mechanical ventilation. It is administered intravenously.

rocuronium bromide, a nondepolarizing neuromuscular blocking agent.

■ INDICATIONS: It is prescribed as an adjunct to general anesthesia in providing skeletal muscle relaxation.

■ CONTRAINDICATIONS: It should not be given to patients with a known hypersensitivity to the product.

■ ADVERSE EFFECTS: The side effects most often reported include nausea, vomiting, respiratory problems, arrhythmias, hiccups, injection site edema, and rash.

rod [AS, *rodd*], **1.** a straight cylindric structure. **2.** one of the tiny cylindric elements arranged perpendicular to the surface of the retina. Rods contain the chemical rhodopsin, which adapts the eye to detect low-intensity light and gives the rods a purple color. Each rod is 40 to 60 μm in length and about 2 μm thick and consists of a slender reactive outer segment and an inner granular segment. When bright light strikes a rod, rhodopsin rapidly breaks down; it reforms gradually in low-intensity light. Compare **cone.** See also **iodopsin, Jacob x membrane, rhodopsin.**

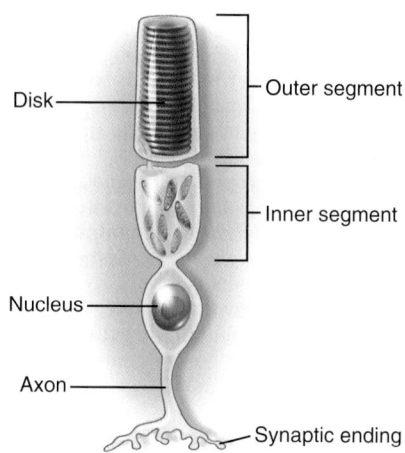

Disk — Outer segment

Inner segment

Nucleus

Axon

Synaptic ending

Rod

rodenticide poisoning /rōden″tisīd/ [L, *rodere,* to gnaw, *caedere,* to kill, *potio,* drink], a toxic condition caused by the ingestion of a substance intended for the control of rodent populations. See also **phosphorus poisoning, thallium poisoning, warfarin poisoning.**

rodent ulcer /rō″dənt/ [L, *rodere,* to gnaw, *ulcus,* ulcer], a slowly developing serpiginous ulceration of a basal cell carcinoma of the skin. See also **basal cell carcinoma.**

rod-monochromat /rod′ monəkrō″mət/, a person who is totally color-blind or who lacks retinal cone function.

rods and cones [AS, *rodd* + Gk, *konos*], the light-sensitive cells of the retina. The rods, under the visual purple pigment epithelium, are mainly located around the periphery of the retina. The cones receive color stimuli.

roentgen (R) /rent″gən, ren″jən/ [Wilhelm K. Roentgen, German physicist, 1845–1923], the conventional unit of x-radiation or gamma radiation that creates 1 electrostatic unit of ions in 1 mL of air at 0° and 760 mm of pressure. In radiotherapy or radiodiagnosis, the roentgen is the unit of the emitted dose. See also **radiation absorbed dose, rem.**

roentgen fetometry, the use of radiographic techniques to measure the fetus in utero.

roentgenologist. See **radiologist.**

roentgenology. See **radiology.**

roentgen ray. See **x-ray,** def. 1.

Roe v. Wade, a 1973 decision of the Supreme Court of the United States in which state laws making it a crime to obtain or attempt an abortion except on medical advice to save the life of the mother were declared unconstitutional.

Roferon-A, a parenteral antineoplastic. Brand name for **interferon alfa-2a.**

Rogers, Martha E. [1914–1994], a nurse theorist who developed the Science of Unitary Human Beings, a nursing theory introduced in 1970. See also **Science of Unitary Human Beings.**

Rohrer's constants, the constants in an empiric equation for airway resistance. It is expressed as $R = K_1 + K_2 V$, where R is resistance, V is instantaneous volumetric flow rate, K_1 is a constant representing gas viscosity and airway geometry, and K_2 is a constant representing gas density and airway geometry.

Rokitansky disease. See **Budd-Chiari syndrome.**

Rolando's fissure /rōlan″dōz/ [Luigi Rolando, Italian anatomist, 1773–1831; L, *fissura,* cleft], the central sulcus of the cerebrum.

Rolando's fracture [Luigi Rolando], a fracture of the base of the first metacarpal.

Rolando's gelatinous substance, the apical part of the posterior horn of the spinal cord's gray matter. It appears gelatinous because of its lack of myelinated nerve fibers. Also called **substantia gelatinosa.**

role [Fr, stage character], a socially expected behavior pattern associated with an individual's function in various social groups. Roles provide a means for social participation and a way to test identities for consensual validation by significant others, for example, roles within the family structure.

role ambiguity, a type of role strain that occurs when the specifications set for an expected role are incomplete or insufficient to tell the involved individual what is desired and how to do it. See **role strain.**

role blurring, the tendency for professional roles to overlap and become indistinct when there is a shared body of knowledge among and between disciplines.

role change, a situation in which status is retained while role expectations change, as when a nurse moves from the role of a primary caregiver to that of an administrator.

role clarification, gaining the knowledge, information, and cues needed to perform a role.

role conflict, the presence of contradictory and often competing role expectations.

role incongruence, role strain that occurs when an individual undergoes role transitions that require a significant modification in attitudes and values. See also **role strain.**

role model [Fr, *role,* stage character; L, *mod us,* small copy], a person who knowingly or unknowingly inspires others to imitate his or her persona. The role model may be a real person, such as a parent, or a symbolic character, such as one depicted in movies or television programs.

role overload, a condition in which there is insufficient time in which to carry out all of the expected role functions.

role overqualification, a type of role strain that occurs when an individual has or is perceived to have education and skill qualifications that exceed job requirements or a role that does not require the full use of a person's resources. See also **role strain.**

role playing, a psychotherapeutic technique in which a person acts out a real or simulated situation as a means of understanding intrapsychic conflicts.

role-playing therapy. See **psychodrama.**

role reversal, the act of assuming the role of another person to appreciate how the person feels, perceives, and behaves in relation to himself or herself and to others.

role strain, stress associated with expected roles or positions experienced as frustration. Kinds include **role ambiguity, role incongruence, role overqualification.**

Rolfing [Ida P. Rolf, 20th-century American biochemist], a form of deep tissue massage. See **structural integration.**

roll [OFr, *rolle*], intrinsic joint movements on an axis parallel to the articulating surface. The axis can remain stationary or move in a plane parallel to the joint surface.

roller bandage, a long, tightly wound strip of material that may vary in width. It is generally applied as a circular bandage wrapped around an extremity or the trunk.

roller clamp, a device, usually made of plastic, equipped with a small roller that may be rolled counterclockwise to close off primary IV tubing or clockwise to open it. The roller clamp may also be manipulated to increase and decrease the flow of the IV solution and is easily moved with the thumb, thus making it a one-handed convenience in the administration of IV therapy. Compare **screw clamp, slide clamp.**

rolling effleurage, a circular rubbing stroke used in massage to promote circulation and muscle relaxation, especially on the shoulder and buttocks. It is performed with the hand flat, the palm and closely held fingers acting as a unit. Compare **effleurage, pétrissage.**

ROM, 1. abbreviation for **range of motion.** 2. abbreviation for **read-only memory.** 3. abbreviation for **rupture of membranes.** 4. abbreviation for *right otitis media.*

Roman chamomile, the dried flowers of *Chamaemelum nobile* (formerly *Anthemis nobilis),* used as a homeopathic preparation and in folk medicine, externally as a counterirritant and internally as a preparation that prevents the expulsion of gas from the gastrointestinal tract.

Romano-Ward syndrome /rō·mä′nō wôrd/ [C. Romano, 20th-century Italian physician; O.C. Ward, 20th-century Irish physician], an autosomal-dominant form of the long QT syndrome, characterized by syncope and sometimes ventricular fibrillation and sudden death. See also **long QT syndrome.**

Romberg sign /rom″bərg/ [Moritz H. Romberg, German physician, 1795–1873; L, *signum,* mark], an indication of loss of the sense of position in which the patient loses balance when standing erect, feet together, and eyes closed. Also called *Romberg test.*

Rondec-DM, a fixed-combination drug containing an antihistamine, an antitussive, and an adrenergic decongestant and bronchodilator. Brand name for **carbinoxamine maleate, dextromethorphan hydrobromide, pseudoephedrine hydrochloride.**

Rood System [Margaret Rood, American physical and occupational therapist], an approach to neurological rehabilitation based on the concept that direct sensory stimulation influences movement.

rongeur forceps /rônzhur′, rôNzhœr″/ [Fr, *ronger,* to gnaw; L, *forceps,* pair of tongs], a kind of biting forceps that is strong and heavy, used for cutting bone. Also called *rongeur.*

R-on-T phenomenon, a cardiac event in which a ventricular stimulus causes premature depolarization of cells that have not completely repolarized. It is noted on the electrocardiogram as a ventricular depolarization falling somewhere within a T wave. The R-on-T phenomenon may result in ventricular tachycardia or ventricular fibrillation.

rooming-in, (in a hospital) a practice that allows mothers and newborn babies to share accommodations, remaining together in the hospital as they would at home, rather than being separated. Also called **living-in unit.**

R

room temperature [AS, *rum* + L, *temperatura*], the air temperature as measured in a specific part of a room.

root /rōot, rŏŏt/ [AS, *rot*], **1.** the lowest part of an organ or a structure by which something is firmly attached, such as the anatomical root of the tooth, which is covered by cementum. Also called **radix. 2.** the part of a plant that anchors it to the surface and provides nourishment. The roots of plants are used in some herbal medicines.

root canal, the inner area of the tooth, consisting of the pulp chamber and pulp canal and ending at the apex. See also **pulp canal.**

root canal file, (in dentistry) a small, round, metal hand instrument or a motor-driven rotary instrument with tightly spiraled blades, used for cleaning and shaping a pulp canal.

root canal filling, a material placed in the pulp canal of a tooth to seal the space previously occupied by the dental pulp and especially the root apex. See also **canal obturation.**

root canal filling spreader, in root canal therapy, a tapered metal instrument used to compress gutta percha and sealer filling material against the sides of the canal to make room for additional gutta percha cones and sealer.

root canal therapy, that aspect of endodontics dealing with the treatment of diseases of the dental pulp, consisting of partial (pulpotomy) or complete (pulpectomy) extirpation of the diseased pulp, cleaning and sterilization of the empty root canal, enlarging and shaping of the canal to receive sealing material, and obturation of the canal with a nonirritating biologically inert hermetic sealing agent. Also called **pulp canal therapy.**

root caries, decay in the dentine and/or the cementum of a tooth.

root curettage, the debridement and planing of the root surface of a tooth with hand instruments and/or ultrasonic scalers to remove accretions and toxins to induce the development of healthy gingival tissues. Usually associated with periodontal disease. Also called **root planing, subgingival curettage.** See also **apical curettage.**

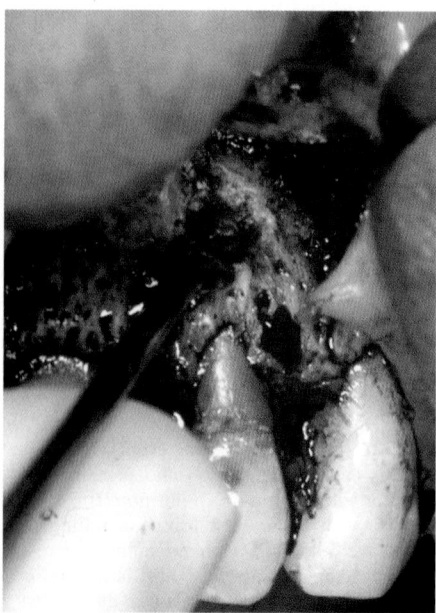

Preparation for root curettage *(Gutman, Dumsha, and Lovdahl, 2006)*

root end cyst. See **radicular cyst.**

root furcation, 1. the anatomical area at which the roots of a multirooted tooth divide. **2.** abnormal intraradicular resorption of bone in multirooted teeth, resulting from periodontal disease.

rooting reflex, a normal response in newborns when the cheek is touched or stroked along the side of the mouth to turn the head toward the stimulated side and begin to suck. The reflex disappears by 3 to 4 months of age but in some infants may persist until 12 months of age.

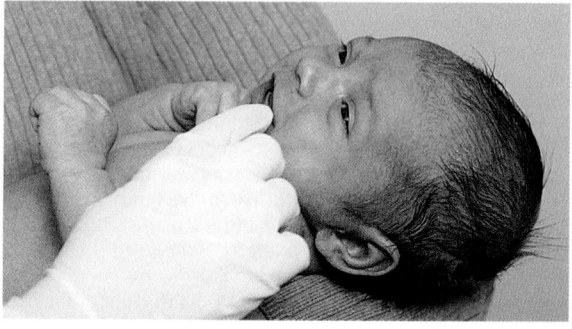

Elicitation of the rooting reflex *(Seidel et al, 2011)*

root of the lung, the structures that pass between the lung and mediastinum and their sleevelike covering of mediastinal pleura. The root joins the medial surface of the lung at the hilum.

root planing. See **root curettage.**

root resection, root-end resection. See **apicoectomy.**

root resorption of teeth [AS, *rot* + L, *resorbere,* to suck back; AS, *toth*], destruction of the cementum or dentin of tooth roots due to osteoclastic activity. If only the apex of the root is affected, the root may become shortened and blunted. If the middle of the root is affected, the pulp canal will generally be penetrated. Root resorption may occur externally or internally within the tooth. See **internal resorption, external resorption.**

root retention, a technique that removes the crown of a root canal-treated tooth and retains enough of the root and gingival attachment to support a prosthesis.

root submersion, a root retention in which the tooth structure is reduced below the level of the alveolar crest and the soft tissue is allowed to heal over it. This technique is used to minimize residual alveolar ridge resorption.

root surface caries, decalcification or cavity formation in or around the junction between the crown and the root and exposed root surfaces. Root surface caries are caused by the neglected daily removal of plaque from the root surface.

ROP, abbreviation for *right occipitoposterior fetal position.*

ropinirole, an antiparkinsonian agent.
- INDICATIONS: It is used to treat parkinsonism.
- CONTRAINDICATIONS: Known hypersensitivity to this drug prohibits its use.
- ADVERSE EFFECTS: Life-threatening effects are hemolytic anemia, leukopenia, and agranulocytosis. Other adverse effects include psychosis, hallucination, dystonia, depression, dizziness, constipation, dyspepsia, flatulence, rash, sweating, tachycardia, hypertension, hypotension, syncope, palpitations, blurred vision, impotence, urinary frequency, pharyngitis, rhinitis, sinusitis, bronchitis, and dyspnea. Common side effects include agitation, insomnia, nausea, vomiting, anorexia, dry mouth, and orthostatic hypotension.

ropivacaine, a local anesthetic.

■ INDICATIONS: It is used to produce peripheral nerve block, caudal anesthesia, central neural block, and vaginal block.

■ CONTRAINDICATIONS: Its use is prohibited in children less than 12 years of age, the elderly, those with severe liver disease, and those with known hypersensitivity to this drug.

■ ADVERSE EFFECTS: Life-threatening effects are convulsions, loss of consciousness, myocardial depression, cardiac arrest, arrhythmias, fetal bradycardia, status asthmaticus, respiratory arrest, and anaphylaxis. Other adverse effects are anxiety, restlessness, drowsiness, disorientation, tremors, shivering, bradycardia, hypotension, hypertension, nausea, vomiting, blurred vision, tinnitus, pupil constriction, rash, urticaria, allergic reactions, edema, burning, skin discoloration at the injection site, and tissue necrosis.

Rorschach test /rôr″shäk, rôr″shokh/ [Hermann Rorschach, Swiss psychiatrist, 1884–1922], a projective personality assessment test developed by Hermann Rorschach. It consists of 10 pictures of inkblots, five in black and white, three in black and red, and two multicolored, to which the subject responds by telling, in as many interpretations as is desired, what images and emotions each design evokes. Replies are evaluated according to whether the response is to the entire or only part of the image; whether color, shading, shape, or location of individual elements is significant; whether movement is seen; and the degree of complexity to which each interpretation is given. Scoring is primarily subjective and is based on both the subject's responses and the general reaction to the circumstances under which the test is administered. The test is designed to assess the degree to which intellectual and emotional factors are integrated in the subject's perception of the environment. See also **Holtzman inkblot technique.**

ROS, abbreviation for **review of systems.**

rosacea /rōzā″shē·ə/ [L, rosaceus, rosy], a chronic inflammatory disease seen in adults of all ages. It has two components: erythema and/or acneiform papules and pustules. It is associated with erythema, pustules, and telangiectasia, especially of the nose, forehead, and cheeks and ocular symptoms of conjunctivitis. See also **rhinophyma.**

rose fever [L, rosa + febris, fever], a common misnomer for seasonal allergic rhinitis caused by pollen (most frequently of grasses) that is airborne at the time roses are in bloom. Because rose pollen is not dispersed by the wind but is carried from flower to flower by insects, roses are not the cause of common spring and summer allergic reactions.

rose hips, an herbal product taken from a plant native to Europe and Asia, now grown widely in North America.

■ INDICATIONS: It is used as a source of vitamin C and as a treatment for colds, fever, and mild infections. Much of vitamin C is, however, reportedly destroyed during the typical drying processes and storage of rose hips, and there are insufficient reliable data regarding efficacy for any of its uses.

■ CONTRAINDICATIONS: It should not be used during pregnancy and lactation or in people with known hypersensitivity to this plant.

Rosenberg-Chutorian syndrome /rō′zən·bergchōō·tor′ē·ən/ [Roger N. Rosenberg, 20th-century American physician; Abe Milton Chutorian, American physician, b. 1929], a rare X-linked hereditary syndrome characterized by optic atrophy, progressive sensorineural hearing loss, and polyneuropathy.

Rosen method, a bodywork technique based on the premise that there is a connection between chronic muscular tension and suppressed emotions or trauma. Using gentle touch and verbal support and guided by careful attention to changes in muscle tension and breathing patterns, the therapist helps the patient to relax the muscular tension and so to bring the underlying repressed memories to the surface and release them.

Rosenmüller's organ. See **epoophoron.**

Rosenthal disease, a deficiency of blood coagulation factor XI resulting in a systemic blood-clotting defect that may resemble classical hemophilia. Also called *Rosenthal syndrome.*

roseo-, prefix meaning "rose-colored," as a roseola rash.

roseola /rōzē″ələ/ [L, roseus], any rose-colored rash. See also **roseola infantum.**

roseola idiopathica, a skin eruption of symmetric reddish patches in a condition not associated with any other well-defined symptoms of disease.

roseola infantum, a benign viral endemic illness of infants and young children, caused by human herpesvirus 6 (of which there are two strains, A and B) and possibly by herpesvirus 7. It is characterized by abrupt, high, sustained or spiking fever, mild pharyngitis, and lymph node enlargement. Febrile seizures may occur. After 4 or 5 days the fever suddenly drops to normal, and a faint, pink, maculopapular rash appears on the neck, trunk, and thighs. The rash may last a few hours to 2 days. Diagnosis is based on high fever and the rash. Sequelae may occur as a result of the seizures. There is no specific therapy or vaccine. Acetaminophen is often used to try to control fever. Also called **exanthema subitum, sixth disease, Zahorsky disease.**

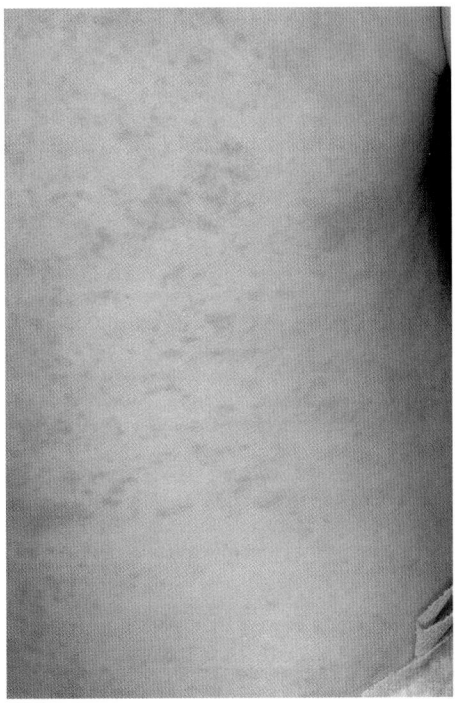

Roseola infantum (Paller and Mancinin, 2006)

roseola symptomatica, a rose-colored eruption that occurs at the onset of a well-defined febrile illness.

Roseolovirus /ro″ze-o′lovi″rus/, a genus of herpesviruses closely related to the genus *Cytomegalovirus* and containing the single species human herpesvirus 6, which is the causal agent of roseola infantum.

rose spots [L, rosa + ME, spotte], small erythematous macules occurring on the upper abdomen and anterior thorax and lasting 2 or 3 days, characteristic of typhoid and paratyphoid fevers.

rosette /rōzet″/, **1.** any structure resembling a rose. **2.** a sporulating body of a malarial parasite.

R

rosette technique, a method of detecting antigens or antibodies on a cell surface using antibody- or antigen-coated particles, which cause erythrocytes to form a rosette pattern.

Rose-Waaler test. See **sheep red cell agglutination test.**

rosiglitazone, an oral antidiabetic drug.

■ INDICATIONS: It is used to treat stable type 2 diabetes mellitus.

■ CONTRAINDICATIONS: Lactation, diabetic ketoacidosis, and known hypersensitivity to thiazolidinediones prohibit its use. It is also contraindicated in children.

■ ADVERSE EFFECTS: Adverse effects include upper respiratory infection, sinusitis, anemia, back pain, diarrhea, edema, fatigue, headache, and hyperglycemia or hypoglycemia.

rosin /roz″in/, a solid oleo resin produced by steam distillation of balsam from various species of pine trees. After extraction of turpentine in the process, the rosin remains as an amber mass. It is used in plasters, ointments, and pharmaceutical coatings.

rost-, rostr-, combining form meaning "a beak": *rostellum, rostral, rostrum.*

rostellum /rostel″əm/ [L, *rostrum*, beak], **1.** the anterior of a tapeworm scolex, commonly featuring hooklike jaws. **2.** tubular mouth parts of some insects.

rostral /ros″trəl/, beak-shaped. **–rostrum,** *n.*

rostrum /ros″trəm/ [L, beak], a beaklike projection, as the rostrum of the sphenoid bone.

rosuvastatin, an antilipemic.

■ INDICATIONS: This drug is used as an adjunct in primary hypercholesterolemia (types IIa and IIb), mixed dyslipidemia, elevated serum triglycerides, and homozygous low-density lipoprotein receptor disorder.

■ CONTRAINDICATIONS: Pregnancy, lactation, active liver disease, and known hypersensitivity to this drug prohibit its use.

■ ADVERSE EFFECTS: Adverse effects of this drug include vomiting; leg, shoulder, or localized pain; insomnia; paresthesia; photosensitivity; rhinitis; sinusitis; bronchitis; and increased cough. Life-threatening side effects include liver dysfunction, myositis, rhabdomyolysis, thrombocytopenia, hemolytic anemia, and leukopenia. Common side effects include nausea, constipation, abdominal pain, flatus, diarrhea, dyspepsia, heartburn, asthenia, muscle cramps, arthritis, arthralgia, myalgia, headache, dizziness, rash, pruritus, and pharyngitis.

rot [AS, *rotian*], **1.** *v.,* to decay. **2.** *n.,* decomposition.

ROT, abbreviation for *right occipitotransverse fetal position.*

rot-, combining form meaning "turned" or "to turn": *rotator, rotating, rotary.*

rotameter. See **flowmeter.**

rotary nystagmus /rō″tərē/ [L, *rotare,* to rotate; Gk, *nystagmos,* nodding], a form of nystagmus in which the eyeball makes rotary motions around an axis.

RotaTeq, a vaccine used to prevent rotavirus infection in children. Brand name for **rotavirus vaccine live oral.**

rotating tourniquet /rō″tāting/ [L, *rotare,* to rotate; Fr, *tourniquet,* garrote], one of four constricting devices used in a rotating order to pool blood in the extremities. The purpose is to relieve congestion in the lungs in the treatment of acute pulmonary edema. Use of the rotating tourniquet has declined with the development of vasodilating drugs and diuretics.

rotation /rōtā″shən/ [L, *rotare*], **1.** the gyration of a bone around its central axis, one of the four basic movements allowed by the various joints of the skeleton. The central axis may lie in a separate bone, as in the pivot formed by the dens of the axis around which the atlas turns. Some bones, such as the humerus, rotate around their own longitudinal axis. Alternatively, the axis of rotation may not be quite parallel to the long axis of the rotating bone, as in movement of the radius on the ulna during pronation and supination of the hand. Compare **angular movement, circumduction, gliding. 2.** a turning around an axis. **3.** the turning of the fetal head to descend through the pelvis during birth. **4.** a clinical experience in hospitals and clinics for students in the health professions, designed as an integral component of the curriculum.

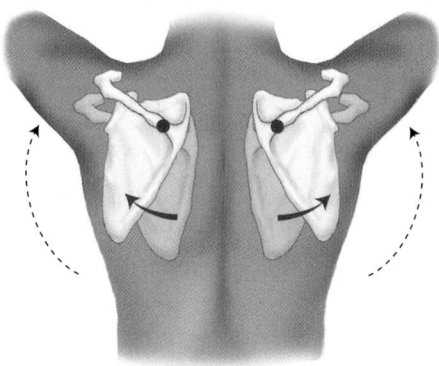

Upward rotation *(Muscolino, 2011)*

rotator /rō″tātər/ [L, *rotare,* to rotate], a muscle that rotates a structure around its axis, as the cervical, thoracic, and lumbar musculi rotatores, which function to extend and rotate the vertebral column toward the opposite side.

rotator cuff, a musculotendinous structure about the capsule of the shoulder joint, formed by the inserting fibers of the supraspinatus, infraspinatus, teres minor, and subscapularis muscles, which blend with the capsule and provide mobility, stability, and strength to the shoulder joint.

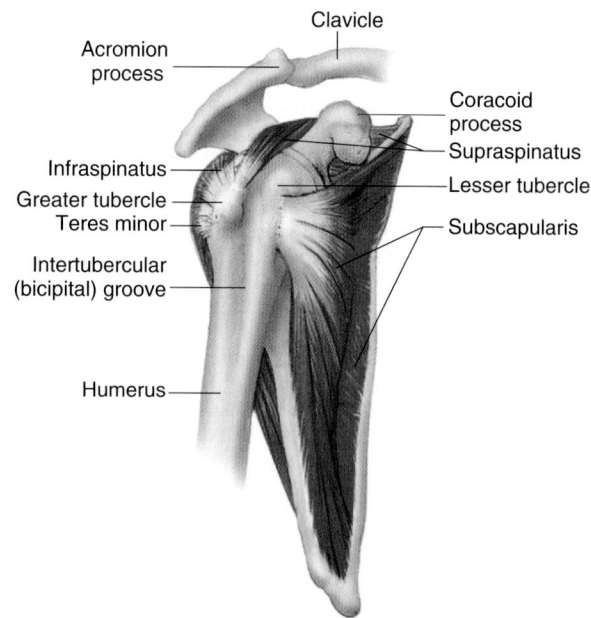

Rotator cuff *(Patton and Thibodeau, 2010)*

rotatores muscles, the deepest muscles of the transversospinales group. These small muscles are present throughout the length of the vertebral column but are best developed in the thoracic region. See also **multifidus, semispinalis muscles.**

rotavirus /rō′təvī″rəs/, a double-stranded ribonucleic acid virus that appears as a tiny wheel, with a clearly defined outer layer, or rim, and an inner layer of spokes. The virus replicates in the epithelial cells of the intestine and is a cause of acute gastroenteritis with diarrhea, particularly in infants. Rotavirus is the most common cause worldwide of severe diarrheal illness in children, with fecal-oral transmission. Various strains also infect domestic and wild animals. In the United States, infections tend to peak during the winter months. Rotavirus vaccines are available.

rotavirus diarrhea, diarrhea caused by a rotavirus, usually seen in children.

rotavirus gastroenteritis, viral gastroenteritis caused by a rotavirus infection, one of the most common causes of diarrhea in the United States. The virus is usually ingested in contaminated food or water. Young children are particularly susceptible and can suffer severe dehydration or even death. The availability of a vaccine has dramaticlly reduced the incidence of diarrhea associated with rotovirus infection.

rotavirus vaccine live oral, a live, oral vaccine that protects against rotavirus serotypes G1, G2, G3, G4, and P1.

■ INDICATIONS: This drug is used to prevent rotavirus gastroenteritis in infants.

■ CONTRAINDICATIONS: Bone marrow and lymphatic disorders, immunodeficiency, administration of blood products within 6 weeks, and known hypersensitivity to this drug prohibit its use. Infants with a history of intussusception should not receive the vaccine.

■ ADVERSE EFFECTS: Adverse effects of this drug include runny nose, sore throat, ear infection, diarrhea, vomiting, wheezing, and coughing. Life-threatening side effects include gastroenteritis, urinary tract infection, pneumonia, and pyrexia.

Rothmund-Thomson syndrome /rot′mo͞ond tom′son/ [August von Rothmund, Jr., German physician, 1830–1906; Mathew Sidney Thomson, English dermatologist, 1894–1969], an autosomal-recessive syndrome, occurring principally in females and characterized by the presence of reticulated, atrophic, hyperpigmented, telangiectatic cutaneous plaques and often accompanied by juvenile cataracts; saddle nose; congenital bone defects; disturbances in the growth of hair, nails, and teeth; and hypogonadism. Also called **poikiloderma congenitale.**

Roth spots /roth, rōt/ [Moritz Roth, Swiss physician and pathologist, 1839–1914], pale-centered oval hemorrhages on the retina, observed in several disorders but classically seen in bacterial endocarditis.

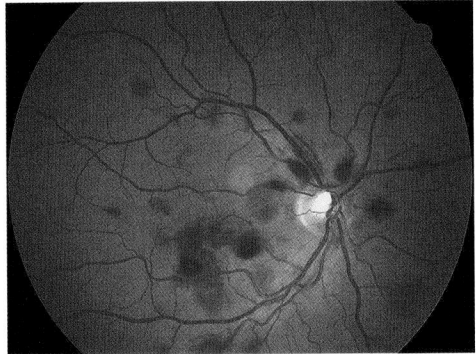

Roth spots *(Swartz, 2009)*

rotigotine, an antiparkinson agent.

■ INDICATIONS: This drug is used to treat idiopathic Parkinson disease.

■ CONTRAINDICATIONS: Defibrillation, MRI, and known hypersensitivity to this drug prohibit its use.

■ ADVERSE EFFECTS: Adverse effects of this drug include drowsiness, hallucinations, headache, malaise, paresthesia, vertigo, confusion, dizziness, dyskinesia, fatigue, fever, insomnia, sudden sleep onset, edema, hypertension, sinus tachycardia, orthostatic hypotension, dyspepsia, anorexia, constipation, vomiting, xerostomia, weight gain, urinary incontinence, dermatitis, erythema, rash, pruritus, purpura, arthralgia, and back pain. A life-threatening side effect is anaphylaxis. A common side effect is nausea.

Rotokinetic treatment table /rō′tōkinet″ik/, a special bed equipped with an automatic turning device that completely immobilizes patients while rotating them from 90 to 270 degrees around a horizontal axis. For example, the Roto-Rest, Delta Bed rotates patients up to 124 degrees around a horizontal axis.

Rotor syndrome /rō″tər/, a rare condition of the liver inherited as an autosomal-recessive trait. It is similar to Dubin-Johnson syndrome but can be distinguished by the normal functioning of the gallbladder and lack of liver pigmentation. Jaundice occurs in childhood, caused by impaired biliary excretion. See also **Dubin-Johnson syndrome, hyperbilirubinemia of the newborn.**

rotoscoliosis /rō′təskō′lē·ō″sis/, a condition in which there is both lateral and rotational spinal deviation.

rotula. See **troche.**

roughage. See **dietary fiber.**

rouleaux /ro͞olō″/*sing. rouleau* [Fr, cylinder], red cells in a microscopic roll or "stack-of-coins" formation that may be caused by abnormal proteins, as in multiple myeloma or macroglobulinemia. Compare **hemagglutination.** See also **erythrocyte sedimentation rate.**

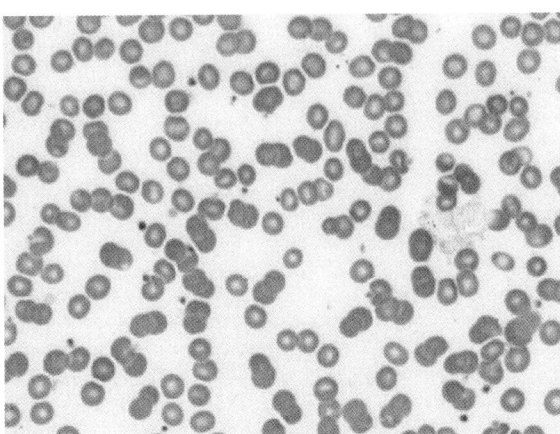

Rouleaux *(Carr and Rodak, 2009)*

round foramen, one of a pair of rounded apertures in the greater wings of the sphenoid bone.

round ligament [L, *rotundus,* round, *ligare,* to bind], **1.** a curved fibrous band that is attached at one end to the fovea of the head of the femur and at the other end to the transverse ligament of the acetabulum. **2.** a fibrous cord extending from the umbilicus to the anterior part of the liver. It is the remnant of the umbilical vein. **3.** in the female, a fibromuscular band that extends from the anterior surface of the uterus through

R

the inguinal canal to the labium majora. The structure is homologous to the spermatic cord in the male.

rounds, *(Informal)* a teaching conference or a meeting in which the clinical problems encountered in the practice of nursing, medicine, or other service are discussed. Kinds include **grand rounds, nursing rounds, teaching rounds, walking rounds, medical rounds.**

round window [L, *rotundus* + ONorse, *vindauga*], a round opening in the medial wall of the middle ear leading into the cochlea and covered by a secondary tympanic membrane. Also called **fenestra cochlea, fenestra rotunda.**

roundworm, any worm of the class Nematoda, including *Ancylostoma duodenale, Ascaris lumbricoides, Enterobius vermicularis,* and *Strongyloides stercoralis.*

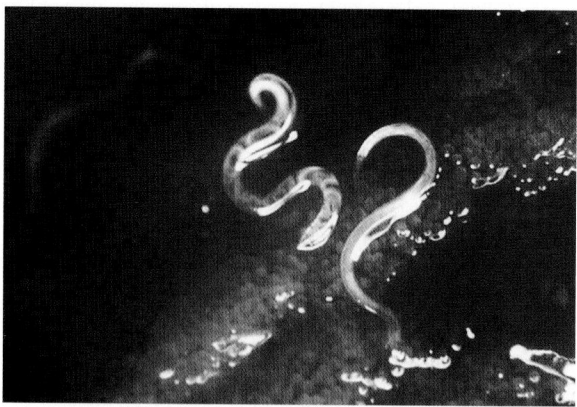

Roundworms attached to the intestinal mucosa
(Courtesy Centers for Disease Control and Prevention)

Roussy-Lévy disease /rōōsē″ lāvē″/ [Gustave Roussy, French pathologist, 1874–1948; Gabrielle Lévy, French neurologist, 1886–1935], an inherited cerebellar ataxia associated with muscle wasting of the extremities, absence of tendon reflexes, and foot deformities.

route of administration /rōōt, rout/ [Fr, *route,* course; L, *administrare,* to serve], (of a drug) any one of the body systems in which a drug may be administered, such as intradermally, intrathecally, intramuscularly, intranasally, intravenously, orally, rectally, subcutaneously, sublingually, topically, or vaginally. Some medications can be given by only one route because absorption or maximum effectiveness occurs by that route only or because the specific substance is toxic or damaging when given by another route.

routine task inventory-expanded (RTI-e), (in occupational therapy) an evidence-based, semistandardized assessment tool developed within the framework of the cognitive disabilities model. The test is comprised of 25 activities of daily living (ADL) and instrumental activities of daily living (IADL). These routine tasks or activities are divided into four subscales: physical scale-ADLs, community scale-IADLs, a communication scale, and a work-readiness scale.

Roux-en-Y /rōō′ en wī′, rōō′änēgrek″/ [César Roux, Swiss surgeon, 1857–1926], a treatment for morbid obesity consisting of surgical division of the small intestine to form two arms; the jejunum is anastomosed to a gastric pouch and the bypassed duodenum connects the pylorus with an end-to-side anastomosis into the lower jejunum.

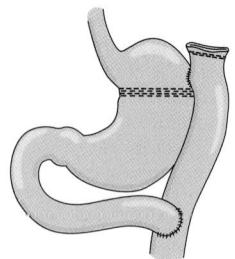

Roux-en-Y *(Phipps et al, 2003)*

Roux-en-Y gastric bypass, a treatment for morbid obesity consisting of surgical division of the small intestine to form two arms. The jejunum is attached to a stoma into a gastric pouch, and the bypassed duodenum connects the pylorus with an end-to-side anastomosis into the lower jejunum.

Rovsing's sign /rov″singz/ [Nils T. Rovsing, Danish surgeon, 1862–1927], an indication of acute appendicitis in which pressure on the left lower quadrant of the abdomen causes pain in the right lower quadrant. See also **appendicitis.**

Royal College of Physicians (R.C.P.), a professional organization of physicians in the United Kingdom.

Royal College of Physicians and Surgeons of Canada (RCPSC), a national Canadian organization that recognizes and confers membership on certain qualified physicians and surgeons.

Royal College of Surgeons (R.C.S.), a professional organization of surgeons in the United Kingdom.

Royal Free disease. See **postviral fatigue syndrome.**

Royer syndrome. See **Prader-Willi syndrome.**

Roy, Sister Callista [b. 1939], a nursing theorist who introduced the adaptation model of nursing in 1970 as a conceptual framework for nursing curricula, practice, and research. In the Roy model the human is viewed as an adaptive system. Changes occur in the system in response to stimuli. If the change promotes the integrity of the individual, it is an adaptive response. Otherwise it is a maladaptive response. The theory provides two mechanisms for coping or adapting. One, a regulator mechanism, is concerned with neural, endocrine, and perception-psychomotor processes. The other, a cognator mechanism, is concerned with perception, learning, judgment, and emotion. Four modes for effecting adaptation of a system are physiological needs, self-concept, role function, and interdependence. The nurse achieves the goal of promoting the patient's adaptation in situations of health and sickness by manipulating stimuli. Nursing intervention is required when the coping mechanism of the patient loses effectiveness in illness.

Rozerem, a sedative medication. Brand name for **ramelteon.**

RPF, abbreviation for **renal plasma flow.**

rpm, a unit of measurement. Abbreviation for *revolutions per minute.*

RPR test, a screening test for syphilis. Abbreviation for **rapid plasma reagin test.**

RQ, abbreviation for **respiratory quotient.**

RRA, abbreviation for **registered record administrator.**

-(r)rhage, combining form meaning "a rupture" or "an excessive fluid discharge": *hemorrhage.*

-(r)rhagia, combining form meaning "a fluid discharge of excessive quantity": *lymphorrhagia, rhinorrhagia, balanorrhagia.*

-(r)rhagic, combining form meaning "a kind or condition of excessive fluid discharge": *hemorrhagic, antihemorrhagic,*

-(r)rhaphy, -(r)rhaphia, combining form meaning "a suturing in place": *angiorrhaphy, nephrorrhaphy, osteorrhaphy.*

-(r)rhea, -(r)rhoea, -(r)rhoeica, combining form meaning "fluid discharge, flow": *diarrhea, leukorrhea, otorrhea.*

-(r)rheic, -(r)rheal, -(r)rhetic, -(r)rhoeic, combining form meaning "fluid discharge": *antiseborrheic.*

-(r)rhexis, suffix meaning "a rupture of a (specified) body part": *karyorrhexis, keratorhexis, myorrhexis.*

-(r)rhine, combining form meaning "having a (specified sort of) nose": *leptorrhine, mesorrhine, platyrrhine.*

-(r)rhinia, combining form meaning "(condition of the) nose": *arrhinia, microrrhinia.*

-(r)rhoea, -(r)rhoeica. See **-(r)rhea, -(r)rhoea, -(r)rhoeica.**

-(r)rhoeic, pertaining to an acid. See **-(r)rheic, -(r)rheal, -(r)rhetic, -(r)rhoeic.**

-(r)rhythmia, combining form meaning "regularly occurring involuntary behavior or actions": *bradyarrhythmia, dysrhythmia, tachyarrhythmia.*

R-R interval, the interval from the peak of one QRS complex to the peak of the next, as shown on an electrocardiogram. It is used to assess the ventricular rate. See also **cardiac cycle.**

rRNA, abbreviation for **ribosomal RNA.**

RRT, abbreviation for **registered respiratory therapist.**

RSD, abbreviation for **reflex sympathetic dystrophy.**

RSNA, abbreviation for **Radiological Society of North America.**

RSV, RS virus, abbreviation for **respiratory syncytial virus.**

RT, **1.** abbreviation for **registered technologist. 2.** abbreviation for **respiratory therapy. 3.** abbreviation for **reverse transcriptase.**

RTA, abbreviation for **renal tubular acidosis.**

r.t.c., chart notation for "return to clinic," usually followed by a date on which a subsequent appointment has been made for the patient.

Ru, symbol for the element **ruthenium.**

RU-486. See **mifepristone.**

rub [ME, *rubben,* to scrape], the movement of one surface moving over another, thereby producing friction, as when pleural membranes produce friction rub.

rub-, rube-, combining form meaning "red": *rubefacient, rubella, rubor.*

rubber. *(Informal)* See **condom.**

rubber-band ligation, a method of treating hemorrhoids by placing a rubber band around the hemorrhoidal part of the blood vessel, causing it to slough off after a period of time. The technique is used in some cases as an alternative to surgery. See also **ligation.**

rubber dam [ME, *rubben,* to scrape; AS, *demman,* to dam up], (in dentistry) a thin sheet of synthetic rubber or natural latex rubber used to isolate one or more teeth during a dental procedure from saliva and bacteria. Also called *dental dam.* See also **dam.**

rubber dam clamps forceps, a type of forceps with beaks designed to engage holes in a rubber dam clamp to facilitate its placement over and around teeth.

rubbing alcohol [ME, *rubben,* to scrape; Ar, *alkohl,* essence], a disinfectant for skin and instruments. It contains 70% isopropyl alcohol by volume, the remainder consisting of water and denaturants, with or without color or perfume. It may cause dryness of the skin. Rubbing alcohol is for external use only and is flammable.

rubefacient /roo′bəfā″shənt/ [L, *ruber,* red, *facere,* to make], **1.** *n.,* a substance or agent that increases the reddish coloration of the skin. **2.** *adj.,* increasing the reddish coloration of the skin.

rubefaction /roo′bəfak″shən/ [L, *ruber,* red, *facer,* to make], a redness of the skin produced by a counterirritant.

rubella /roobel″ə/ [L, *rubellus,* somewhat red], a contagious viral disease that is spread by droplet infection and has an incubation time of 12 to 23 days. It is characterized by fever, symptoms of a mild upper respiratory tract infection, lymph node enlargement, arthralgia, and a diffuse fine red maculopapular rash. Rubella virus is a togavirus belonging to the genus *Rubivirus.* It is most closely related to group A arboviruses. It is an undeveloped RNA virus that does not cross-react with other togaviruses. The virus is spread by droplet infection, and the incubation time is from 12 to 23 days. Also called **German measles, 3-day measles.** Compare **measles, scarlet fever.** Should not be confused with **rubeola.**

■ OBSERVATIONS: The symptoms usually last only 2 or 3 days except for arthralgia, which may persist longer or recur. One attack confers lifelong immunity. If a woman acquires rubella in the first trimester of pregnancy, fetal anomalies may result, including heart defects, cataracts, deafness, and cognitive impairment. An infant exposed to the virus in utero at any time during gestation may shed the virus for up to 12 months after

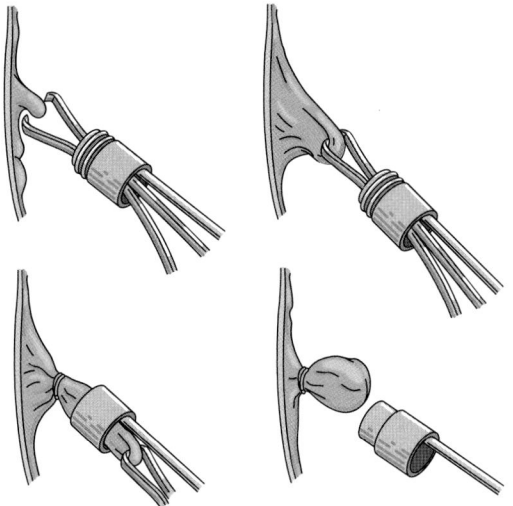

Rubber-band ligation *(Monahan et al, 2007)*

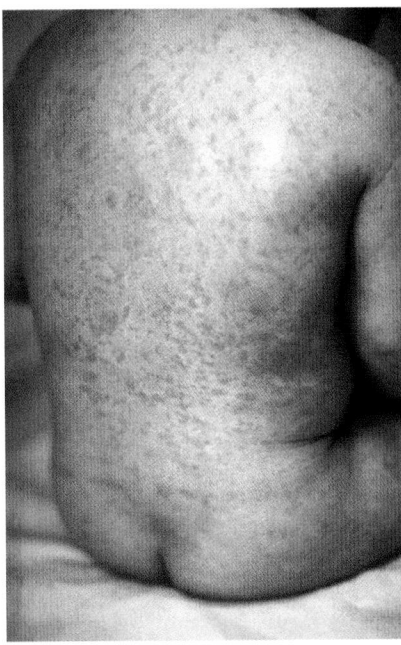

Rubella *(Centers for Disease Control and Prevention Public Health Image Library)*

R

birth. Complications of postnatal rubella are rare. Complications due to rubella infection occur more frequently in adults and include conjunctivitis, testalgia, orchitis, arthralgia or arthritis, encephalitis, and hemorrhagic manifestations.

■ INTERVENTIONS: The illness itself is mild and needs no special treatment. Live attenuated rubella vaccine is advised for all children to reduce chances of an epidemic and thus to protect pregnant women. The vaccine is not given to women already pregnant, and it is recommended that pregnancy be avoided for 3 months after the administration of rubella vaccine. Spread of the virus from a recently vaccinated individual rarely occurs. Immune serum globulin containing rubella antibodies may help prevent fetal infection in exposed susceptible pregnant women, but ordinary gamma globulin will not protect the fetus.

rubella and mumps virus vaccine, a suspension containing live attenuated mumps and rubella viruses.

■ INDICATIONS: It can be prescribed for immunization against rubella, but generally the trivalent mumps-measles-rubella vaccine is administered instead.

■ CONTRAINDICATIONS: Acute infection or known hypersensitivity to avian proteins prohibits its use. It is not given to a patient whose immune function is compromised or to a pregnant woman. It is not given for 3 months after the use of plasma, whole blood, or an immune serum globulin. Pregnancy is avoided for 3 months after immunization.

■ ADVERSE EFFECTS: Among the more serious adverse effects are mild to severe hypersensitivity reactions.

rubella antibody test, a blood test performed to detect immunity to rubella, particularly in pregnant women, and to diagnose rubella in infants.

rubella embryopathy, any congenital abnormality in an infant caused by maternal rubella in the early stages of pregnancy.

rubella panencephalitis. See **panencephalitis.**

rubella titer [L, *rubellus,* somewhat red; Fr, *titre,* standard], a serological test to determine a patient's state of immunity against rubella.

rubella virus, a togavirus that is the causal agent of rubella.

rubella virus vaccine, a suspension containing live attenuated rubella virus.

■ INDICATIONS: It is prescribed for immunization against rubella.

■ CONTRAINDICATIONS: Compromised immune function, fever, acute infection, untreated tuberculosis, or hypersensitivity to proteins of the animal of the vaccine prohibits its use. It is not given to pregnant women, nor is it given for 3 months after the use of plasma, whole blood, or immune serum globulin. Pregnancy should be avoided for 3 months after immunization.

■ ADVERSE EFFECTS: Among the most serious adverse effects are severe hypersensitivity reactions and local pain.

rubeola. See **measles.**

rubeola antibody test, a blood test to measure measles infection in patients who cannot be diagnosed clinically and to establish and document immunity. College students, health care workers, and pregnant women are among those in the commonly tested populations.

rubeosis /roō′bē·ō″sis/, a red discoloration of the skin.

rubeosis iridis, the formation of abnormal blood vessels on the anterior of the iris. It may be associated with diabetes mellitus, retinal ischemia, and neovascular glaucoma.

rubescent /roōbes″ənt/, reddening.

-rubicin, suffix for daunorubicin-type antineoplastic antibiotics.

rubidium (Rb) /roōbid″ē·əm/ [L, *rubidus,* reddish], a soft metallic element of the alkali metals group. Its atomic number is 37; its atomic mass is 85.47. Slightly radioactive, it is used in radioisotope scanning.

Rubinstein-Taybi syndrome /roō′binstīn tā′bē/ [Jack Herbert Rubinstein, American pediatrician, 1925–2006; Hooshang Taybi, American radiologist, 1919–2006], a congenital condition characterized by cognitive impairment and motor delays; broad thumbs and great toes; short stature; characteristic facies, including high-arched palate and straight or beaked nose; various eye abnormalities; pulmonary stenosis; keloid formation in surgical scars; large foramen magnum; and abnormalities of the vertebrae and sternum.

Rubin test [Isador C. Rubin, American gynecologist, 1883–1958], a test performed in the process of evaluating the cause of infertility to assess the patency of the fallopian tubes.

rubivirus /roō′bēvī′rəs/, a member of the togavirus family, which includes the rubella virus.

rubor /roō′bôr/, redness, especially when accompanying inflammation. See also **cardinal signs of inflammation.**

rubratoxin /roō′brətok″sin/, a mycotoxin produced on cereal grains by certain species of *Penicillium* that can cause hepatotoxicity in cattle.

rubricyte /roō′brisīt/ [L, *ruber,* red; Gk, *kytos,* cell], a nucleated red blood cell; the marrow stage in the normal development of an erythrocyte, synonymous with polychromatophilic normoblast.

ructus. See **eructation.**

rudiment /roō″dimənt/ [L, *rudimentum,* beginning], an organ or tissue that is incompletely developed or nonfunctional. **–rudimentary,** *adj.*

rudimentary /roō′dimen″tərē/ [L, *rudimentum,* beginning], pertaining to something either vestigial or embryonic; undeveloped.

Ruffini corpuscles /roofē″nē/ [Angelo Ruffini, Italian anatomist, 1864–1929], a variety of oval-shaped, encapsulated nerve endings in the subcutaneous tissue, located principally at the junction of the dermis and the subcutaneous tissue. Ruffini corpuscles consist of strong connective tissue sheaths, enclosing nerve fibers with many branches that end in small knobs. Compare **Golgi-Mazzoni corpuscles, Krause corpuscles, Pacini corpuscles.**

ruga /roō′gə/ *pl. rugae* [L, ridge], a ridge or fold, such as the rugae of the stomach, which are large folds in the mucous membrane of that organ.

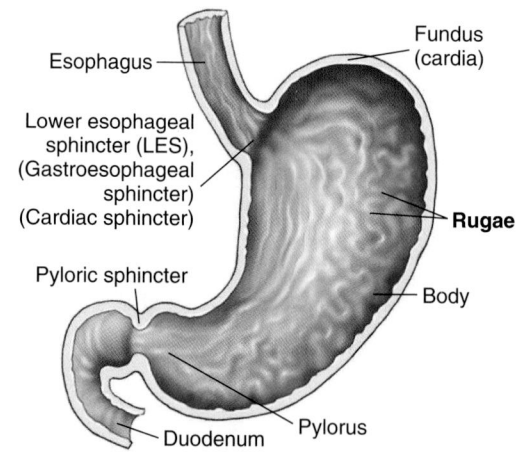

Rugae *(Shiland, 2010)*

rugae of vagina [L, *ruga,* ridge, *vagina,* sheath], the transverse ridges on the mucous membrane lining the vagina. They allow the vagina to stretch during childbirth. Many of the ridges disappear with the atrophy of menopause.

rugitus /roō′jitəs/ [L, roaring], the rumbling sound of flatus in the intestines.

rugose /roo″gōs/, wrinkled or corrugated. Also *rugous*.

RUL, abbreviation for *right upper lobe of lung*.

Ruland, Cornelia M., a nursing theorist who, with Shirley M. Moore, developed the Peaceful End of Life Theory, which asserts that nurses are integral to the creation of peaceful end-of-life care, which includes freedom from suffering, emotional support, closeness to and participation by significant others, and treatment with empathy and respect. The theory was developed from a standard of care created by expert nurses to manage the care of patients with terminal illness.

rule, a guide for conduct or action.

rule of bigeminy [L, *regula,* model, *bis,* double, *geminus,* twin], the tendency of a lengthened ventricular cycle to precipitate a premature ventricular complex.

rule of confidentiality, a principle that personal information about others, particularly patients, should not be revealed to persons not authorized to receive such information. See also **Health Insurance Portability and Accountability Act.**

rule of nines, a formula for estimating the percentage of adult body surface covered by burns by assigning 9% to the head and each arm, twice 9% (18%) to each leg and the anterior and posterior trunk, and 1% to the perineum. This is modified in infants and children because of the proportionately larger head size.

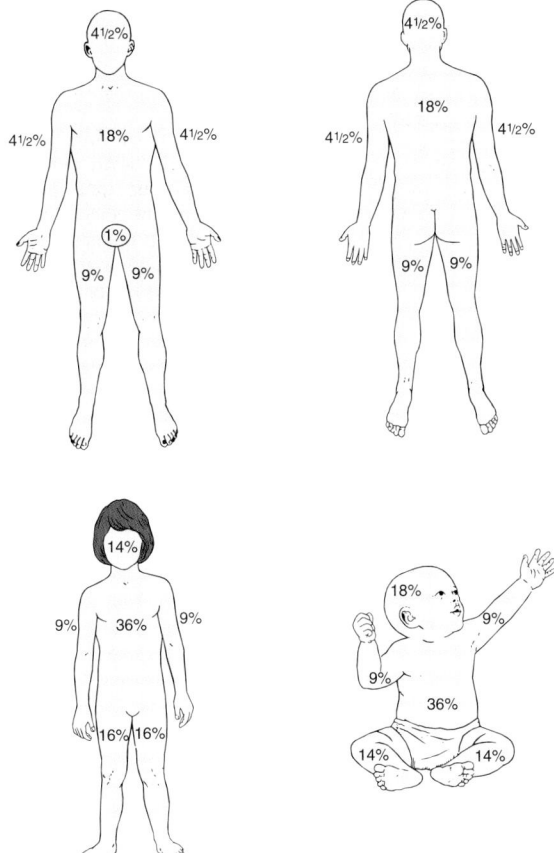

Rule of nines

rule of outlet, an obstetric standard for determining whether the pelvic outlet will allow the passage of a fetus. It is calculated from the sum of the transverse and posterior sagittal diameters of the outlet, which must equal at least 15 cm.

ruminant /roo″minənt/ [L, *ruminare,* to chew again], pertaining to animals that chew their cud and to human infants who may regurgitate and reswallow a meal.

rumination /roo″minā″shən/ [L, *ruminare,* to chew again], **1.** habitual regurgitation of small amounts of undigested food with little force after every feeding, a condition commonly seen in infants. It may be a symptom of overfeeding, of eating too fast, or of swallowing air. It has little or no clinical significance. More copious and forceful regurgitation may indicate a more serious condition such as an allergic intestinal reaction, an infectious disease, an obstruction of the intestinal tract, or a metabolic disorder. Also called **reflux.** See also **vomit. 2.** (in psychology) preoccupation with a thought or idea to a degree that the thinking interferes with activities of daily living or functioning.

runner's high, *(Informal)* a feeling of euphoria experienced by some cross-country runners and joggers as they near the end of a run. The feeling of elation is believed to be associated with the body's production of endorphins during physical stress.

Runyon classification system /run″yən/ [Ernest Runyon, 20th-century American microbiologist], a system of identifying mycobacteria on the basis of pigmentation and growth condition of the organisms. It includes group I, yellow-pigment photochromogens; group II, yellow-to-orange-to-red–pigment scotochromogens; group III, white-to-tan nonphotochromogens; and group IV, rapid-growing saprophytes.

rupia /roo″pē·ə/, a pustular eruption associated with secondary syphilis. It is characterized by encrusted ulcers resembling shells on darkly pigmented skin.

rupture /rup″chər/ [L, *rumpere,* to break], **1.** *n.,* a tear or break in the continuity or configuration of an organ or body tissue, including instances when other tissue protrudes through the opening. See also **hernia. 2.** *v.,* to cause a break or tear.

ruptured hymen, a thin membrane that surrounds or partially covers the external vaginal opening that has been torn as a result of injury, coitus, or surgery.

ruptured intervertebral disk. See **herniated disk.**

rupture of membranes (ROM) [L, *rumpere,* to break, *membrana*], the rupture of the amniotic sac, usually at the start of labor. It may be spontaneous or artificial.

RUQ, abbreviation for *right upper quadrant.*

Rural Clinics Assistance Act /roo″rəl/, an act of the U.S. Congress that permitted the establishment of clinics in certain areas designated rural and underserved and in some inner cities. The clinics are designed to provide primary care through teams of physicians and nurse practitioners. The act is significant for primary care as it is the first federal legislation to allow third-party reimbursement directly to nurses practicing in expanded roles.

rush /rush/, **1.** *(Slang)* a pleasurable feeling experienced by users of recreational drugs following an injection of amphetamine or heroin. An amphetamine rush is described as an abrupt awakening, as distinguished from the drowsy, drifting rush of heroin use. Also called **high.** See also **flash. 2.** (in physiology) a strong wave of contractile activity that travels along the small intestine, usually as a result of irritation or distension.

Rush, Benjamin [1745–1813], American physician, born in Philadelphia and educated at Princeton University and the University of Edinburgh. He was a professor of chemistry while at the same time beginning his practice as a physician. He served as a surgeon in the Continental Army and was the co-founder of the first antislavery society in America. As a member of the Continental Congress, Rush was a signer of the Declaration of Independence, and in 1787 was a member of the Pennsylvania convention that adopted the federal Constitution. Rush protested against improper treatment of the mentally ill and was instrumental in the construction of a facility within Pennsylvania Hospital to provide humane care based on scientific concepts. He is often referred to as "the Father of American Psychiatry."

R

Russell dwarf [Alexander Russell, 20th-century Scottish physician; AS, *dweorge*], a person affected with Russell's syndrome, a congenital disorder in which short stature is associated with various anomalies of the head, face, and skeleton and with varying degrees of cognitive impairment.

Russell bodies [William Russell, Scottish physician, 1852–1940; AS, *bodig,* body], the mucoprotein inclusions found in globular plasma cells in cancer and inflammations. The bodies contain surface gamma globulins, derived from the condensation of internal cellular secretions. Also called **fuchsin bodies,** *cancer bodies.*

Russell's periodontal index [Albert L. Russell, American dentist], a measure of the extent of periodontal disease in an individual that considers the amount of bone loss around the teeth and the degree of gingival inflammation. See also **periodontal index.**

Russell-Silver syndrome [Alexander Russell, 20th-century Scottish physician], a rare congenital disorder in which short stature is associated with asymmetries of the head, face, and limbs with varying degrees of developmental delay. Also called *Silver-Russell syndrome.*

Russell traction [R. Hamilton Russell, Australian surgeon, 1860–1933; L, *trahere,* to pull along], a unilateral or a bilateral orthopedic mechanism that combines suspension and traction to immobilize, position, and align the lower extremities in the treatment of fractured femurs, hip and knee contractures, and disease processes of the hip and knee. Russell traction is applied as adhesive or nonadhesive skin traction and uses a sling to relieve the weight of the lower extremities subjected to traction pull. A jacket restraint is often incorporated to help immobilize the patient. Compare **split Russell traction.**

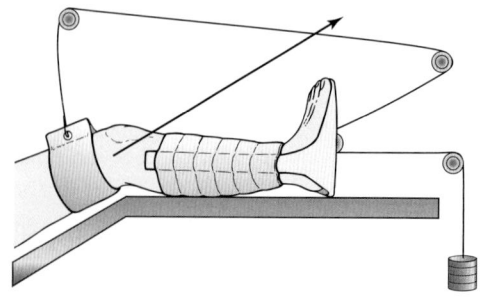

Russell traction *(Lewis, Heitkemper, and Dirksen, 2004)*

Russian bath /rush″ən/, a hot steam bath followed by a plunge into cold water. Also called **sauna bath.**

rusts, microbes that are pathogens of plants, particularly cereal grains. The spores can travel long distances by wind, infecting other plants and causing allergies in humans.

rusty sputum /rus″tē/ [AS, *rust* + L, *sputum,* spittle], *(Informal)* sputum that is reddish, indicative of blood or certain bacteria, such as pneumococcal bacteria, in pneumonia.

ruthenium (Ru) /rōōthē″nē·əm/ [Ruthenia, region of western Ukraine], a hard, brittle, metallic element. Its atomic number is 44, and its atomic mass is 101.07. A compound of ruthenium was used in nuclear testing in the 20th century, increasing the risk of malignancy for those exposed.

rutherfordium (Rf) [Sir Ernest Rutherford, British physicist, 1871-1937], a synthetic transuranic element. Its atomic number is 104, and its atomic mass is 267.

rutin /rōō″tin/, a bioflavonoid obtained from buckwheat thought to have medicinal effects but not approved by the FDA. It is used in a number of supplements primarily for its antioxidant and vasoprotective properties.

Ruvalcaba syndrome /rōō′väl·kä′bä/ [R.H. Ruvalcaba, American physician, b. 1934], abnormal shortness of the metacarpal and metatarsal bones, hypogenitalism, and cognitive impairment of unknown cause present from birth in males. It is characterized by microcephaly, skeletal abnormalities, hypoplastic genitalia, cognitive impairment, and physical disabilities. Also called *osseous dysplasia with mental retardation, Ruvalcaba type.*

RV, abbreviation for **residual volume.**

R wave, the positive component of the QRS complex on an electrocardiogram. See also **QRS complex.**

Ryanodex, a medication used in the management of malignant hyperthermia in conjunction with appropriate supportive measures, as well as prevention in patients at high risk. Brand name for **dantrolene sodium.**

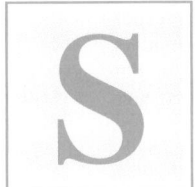

s, 1. (in SI units) abbreviation for *second.* 2. a notation for a Latin word meaning "left." 3. abbreviation for **sinister.** 4. abbreviation for **steady state.**

S, 1. symbol for **sulfur.** 2. symbol for *saturation of hemoglobin.* 3. abbreviation for **siemens.**

s̄, s, a notation for a Latin word meaning "without." Symbol for *sine.*

S₁, the first heart sound in the cardiac cycle, occurring at the outset of ventricular systole. It is associated with closure of the mitral and tricuspid valves and is synchronous with the apical pulse. Auscultated at the apex, it is longer and lower than the second sound (S₂), which follows it. The sound of the mitral valve is loudest at the apex of the heart, and that of the tricuspid valve is loudest at the left sternal border in the fourth intercostal space. See also *lubb.*

S1, S2, ..., symbols for sacral nerves. See also **sacral nerves.**

S₂, the second heart sound in the cardiac cycle. It is associated with closure of the aortic and pulmonic valves at the outset of ventricular diastole. The second sound is louder and shorter than the first. The sound of the aortic valve is loudest on the right sternal border, and that of the pulmonic valve is most distinct on the left sternal border over the second intercostal space.

S₃, the third heart sound in the cardiac cycle. Normally, it is audible only in children and physically active young adults and usually disappears with age. In older people, it is an abnormal finding and usually indicates myocardial failure. It is heard with the bell of a stethoscope placed lightly over the apex of the heart with the patient lying down and facing left. A weak, low-pitched, dull sound, it is thought to be caused by vibrations of the ventricle walls when they are suddenly distended by blood from the atria. Also called **physiological third heart sound, ventricular gallop.**

S₄, the fourth heart sound in the cardiac cycle. It occurs late in diastole on contraction of the atria. Rarely heard in normal subjects, it indicates an abnormally increased resistance to ventricular filling, as in hypertensive cardiovascular disease, coronary artery disease, cardiomyopathy, and aortic stenosis. A left-sided fourth heart sound, it may be heard with the stethoscope's bell at the apex of the heart during expiration. Also called **atrial gallop, physiological fourth heart sound.**

SA, 1. abbreviation for **sinoatrial.** 2. abbreviation for **surface area.** 3. abbreviation for **surgeon's assistant.**

saber-sheath trachea /sā″bər/, an abnormally shaped trachea caused by chronic obstructive pulmonary disease. The diameter of the posterior part of the trachea is increased, and the lateral dimension is decreased.

saber shin, a sharp, anterior bowing of the tibia caused by hereditary syphilis.

Sabin-Feldman dye test /sā″bin feld″mən/ [Albert B. Sabin, American virologist, 1906–1993; H.A. Feldman, American epidemiologist, b. 1914; AS, *deag* + L, *testum,* crucible], a serological test for the diagnosis of toxoplasmosis that depends on the presence of specific antibodies that block the uptake of methylene blue dye by the cytoplasm of the *Toxoplasma* organisms.

Sabin vaccine. See **oral poliovirus vaccine.**

sac /sak/ [Gk, *sakkos,* sack], a pouch or a baglike organ, such as the abdominal sac of the embryo that develops into the abdominal cavity.

saccade /sakād″, sak′ədā″/ [Fr, *saccader,* to jerk], abrupt, rapid, small movements of both eyes.

saccadic eye movement /sakad″ik/, an extremely fast voluntary movement of the eyes, allowing them to accurately refix on an object in the visual field.

sacchari-. See **saccharo-, sacchari-.**

saccharide /sak″ərīd′/, any of a large group of carbohydrates, including all sugars and starches. Almost all carbohydrates are saccharides. See also **carbohydrate, sugar.**

saccharin /sak″ərin/ [Gk, *sakcharon,* sugar], *n.,* a white crystalline synthetic sweetening agent derived from coal tar. Although it is up to 500 times as sweet as sugar, it has no food value.

saccharine /sakxə-rīn/ [Gk, *sakcharon,* sugar], having a sweet taste, especially cloyingly sweet.

saccharo-, sacchari-, prefix meaning "sugar": *saccharometabolism, saccharide, saccharin.*

saccharometabolism /sak′ərōmətab″əliz′əm/, the functioning of sugar within a living body.

Saccharomyces /sak′ərōmī″sēz/ [Gk, *sakcharon* + *mykes,* fungus], a genus of yeast fungi that causes such diseases as bronchitis, moniliasis, and pharyngitis.

saccharomycosis /sak′ərōmīkō″sis/ [Gk, *sakcharon* + *mykes* + *osis,* condition], infection with yeast fungi, such as the genus *Candida* or *Cryptococcus.*

saccular, pertaining to a pouch or shaped like a sac.

saccular aneurysm, a localized dilation of a small area of an artery, forming a saclike swelling or protrusion. It is usually caused by trauma. Also called **ampullary aneurysm, sacculated aneurysm.** Compare **fusiform aneurysm.**

sacculated /sak″yəlā′tid/ [L, *sacculus,* small bag], a condition of small sacs, pouches, or saclike dilations.

sacculated aneurysm. See **saccular aneurysm.**

sacculated pleurisy, inflammation of the pleura with exudate encapsulated in several locations by adhesions.

sacculation /sak′yŏō·lā′shən/ [L, *sacculus*], the quality of being sacculated, or pursed out with little pouches. See also **sacculus.**

saccule /sak″yŏōl/ [L, *sacculus*], a small bag or sac, such as the air saccules of the lungs. See also **sacculus. –saccular,** *adj.*

saccule of larynx. See **laryngocele.**

sacculus /sak″yo͞oləs/ *pl. sacculi,* a little sac or bag, especially the smaller of the two divisions of the membranous labyrinth of the vestibule, which communicates with the cochlear duct through the ductus reuniens in the inner ear. See also **saccule.**

Sachs disease. See **Tay-Sachs disease.**

SA conduction time, the time required for an impulse to travel from the sinus node to the atrial musculature. It is measured from the sinoatrial (SA) deflection in an SA nodal electrocardiogram to the beginning of the P wave in a bipolar record, or to the beginning of the high right atrial electrogram in a unipolar record.

sacral. See **sacrum.**

sacral agenesis. See **caudal regression syndrome.**

sacral bone, a composite bone formed by the fusion during maturation of five sacral vertebrae that were separate at birth. The sacrum forms the back of the pelvis.

sacral canal, an extension of the vertebral canal through the sacrum.

sacral foramen, any one of several openings between the fused segments of the sacral vertebrae in the sacrum through which the sacral nerves pass.

sacral kyphosis, the dorsally convex curve formed by the sacrum when seen from the side.

sacral micturition center, a center in the sacral spinal cord that contributes to control of the bladder and inhibition of tension of the urethral sphincters.

sacral nerves, the five segmental nerves from the sacral part of the spinal cord. The first four emerge through the anterior sacral foramina and the fifth from between the sacral foramen and the coccyx.

sacral node, a node in one of the seven groups of parietal lymph nodes of the abdomen and the pelvis, situated within the sacrum. The sacral nodes are located in relation to the middle and the lateral sacral arteries and receive lymphatics from the rectum and the posterior wall of the pelvis. Compare **lumbar node.** See also **lymph, lymphatic system, lymph node.**

sacral plexus, a network of motor and sensory nerves formed by the lumbosacral trunk from the fourth and fifth lumbar nerves and by the first, second, and third sacral nerves. They converge toward the lower part of the greater sciatic foramen and unite to become a large, flattened band, most of which continues into the thigh as the sciatic nerve. Compare **lumbar plexus.** See also **lumbosacral plexus.**

sacral vertebra, one of the five segments of the vertebral column that fuse in the adult to form the sacrum. The ventral border of the first sacral vertebra projects into the pelvis. The bodies of the other sacral vertebrae are smaller than that of the first and are flattened and curved ventrally, forming the convex, anterior surface of the sacrum. The rudimentary spinous processes of the first several sacral vertebrae surmount the middle sacral crest, and the transverse processes of the sacral vertebrae form the lateral sacral crests. The sacral hiatus at the caudal end of the sacral canal develops from the incomplete growth of the spinous processes of the last two sacral vertebrae. The resultant widened aperture is used by anesthesiologists for the insertion of a needle to administer caudal analgesia. Compare **cervical vertebra, coccygeal vertebra, lumbar vertebra, thoracic vertebra.** See also **sacrum, vertebra.**

sacro-, combining form meaning "sacrum": *sacrococcygeal, sacroiliac, sacrospinalis.*

sacrococcygeal /sā′krōkoksij″ē·əl/ [L, *sacer,* sacred; Gk, *kokkyx,* cuckoo's beak], pertaining to the sacrum and the coccyx.

sacrococcygeal teratoma, a common tumor of newborns, found in the primitive pit. It may represent part of the blastopore of lower vertebrates.

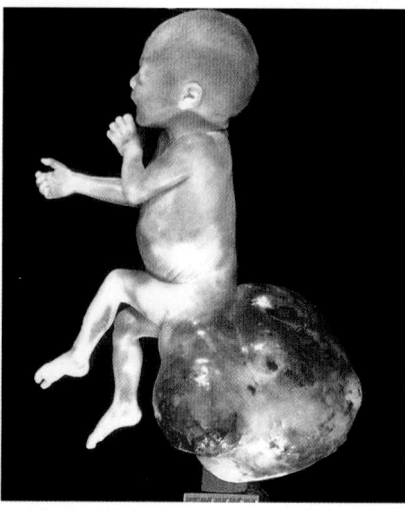

Sacrococcygeal teratoma *(Robbins, Kumar, and Cotran, 2010)*

sacroiliac /sā′krō·il″ē·ak/ [L, *sacer + ilium,* flank], pertaining to the part of the skeletal system that includes the sacrum and the ilium bones of the pelvis.

sacroiliac articulation, an immovable joint in the pelvis formed by the articulation of each side of the sacrum with an iliac bone.

sacroiliac joint, the joint formed by the sacrum and ilium where they meet on either side of the lower back. The tight joint allows little motion and is subject to great stress as the body's weight pushes downward and the legs and pelvis push upward against the joint. The sacroiliac joint must also bear the leverage demands made by the trunk of the body as it turns, twists, pulls, and pushes. When these motions place an excess of stress on the ligaments binding the joint and on the connecting muscles (such as during weightlifting), strain may result.

sacroiliac ligament, one of the three ligaments that stabilizes each sacroiliac joint.

sacroiliitis /sā′krō·il′ē·ī″tis/, an inflammation of the sacroiliac joint.

sacrolumbar. See **lumbosacral.**

sacrosciatic /sā′krōsī·at″ik/, pertaining to the sacrum and ischium.

sacrosidase /sakro′sidās/, an enzyme used as a substitute to replace the sucrase activity lacking in sucrase-isomaltase deficiency. It is administered orally.

sacrospinalis /sak′rōspīnal″is/ [L, *sacer + spina,* backbone], the superficial longitudinal muscle mass on either side of the vertebral column. It is sheathed in the fascia thoracolumbalis and arises in a broad, thick tendon from the sacrum, the ilium, and the lumbar vertebrae. It inserts into the ribs and into certain cervical vertebrae and is innervated by the branches of the dorsal primary divisions of the spinal nerves. It extends and flexes the vertebral column and the head, draws the ribs downward, and bends the trunk to the side. Also called **erector spinae,** *sacrospinal muscle.*

sacrospinous ligament, with the sacrotuberous ligament, an important architectural element of the walls of the true pelvis that links each pelvic bone to the sacrum and coccyx and converts two notches on the pelvic bones into foramina on the lateral pelvic walls.

sacrum /sā″krəm, sak″rəm/ [L, *sacer,* sacred], the large, triangular bone at the dorsal part of the pelvis, inserted like a wedge between the two hip bones. The base of the sacrum articulates with the last lumbar vertebra, and its apex articulates with the coccyx. Various muscles attach to its spinal crest. The sacrum is shorter and wider in women than in men. **−sacral,** *adj.*

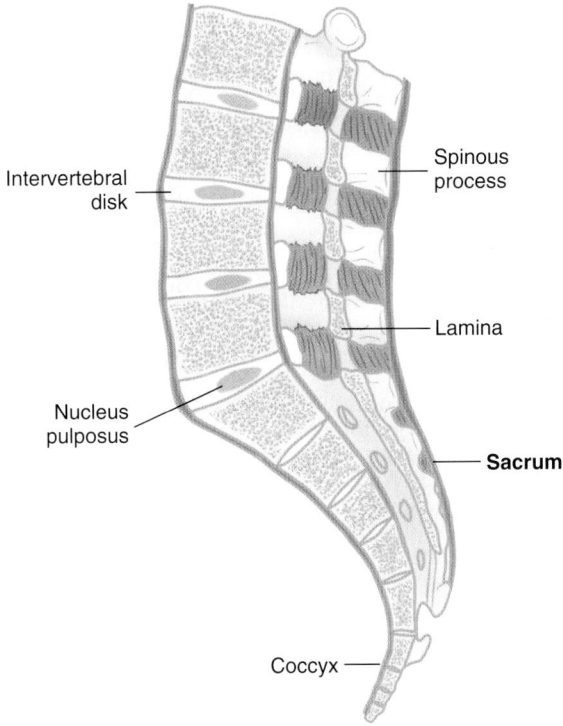

Sacrum *(Seidel et al, 2011)*

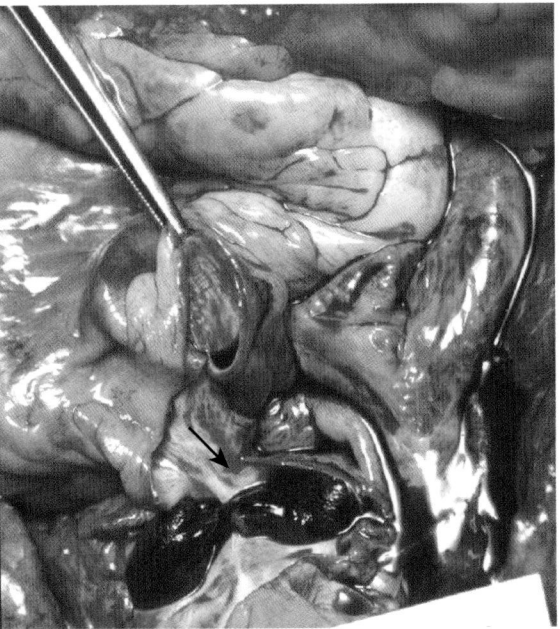

Saddle embolism *(Courtesy Dr. Linda Margraf, Department of Pathology, University of Texas Southwestern Medical School)*

SAD, abbreviation for **seasonal affective disorder.**

saddle /sad′əl/ [AS, *sadol*], **1.** a support whose shape fits the contour of the object resting on it. **2.** a saddle-shaped structure or part. **3.** See **denture base.**

saddleback nose. See **saddle nose.**

saddle block anesthesia [AS, *sadol* + Fr, *bloc* + Gk, *anaisthesia,* lack of feeling], a form of spinal nerve block in which the area of the body that would touch a saddle, were the patient sitting astride one, is anesthetized. It is performed by injecting a local anesthetic into the subarachnoid cerebrospinal fluid space while the patient is in the sitting position. Saddle block anesthesia is utilized in some centers for anesthesia during childbirth; however, epidural analgesia is most commonly given during labor. See also **obstetric anesthesia.**

saddle embolism, a thrombus that straddles a dividing blood vessel. It can block both branches, for example, at the bifurcation of the pulmonary arteries. Also called **straddling embolism.**

saddle joint, a synovial joint in which surfaces of contiguous bones are reciprocally concavoconvex. A saddle joint permits no axial rotation but allows flexion, extension, adduction, and abduction, as in the carpometacarpal joint of the thumb. Also called *articulatio sellaris.* Compare **condyloid joint, pivot joint.**

saddle nose [AS, *sadol* + *nosu*], a sunken nasal bridge caused by injury or disease and resulting in damage to the nasal septum. Also called **saddleback nose.**

sadism /sā″dizəm, sad″izəm/ [Marquis Donatien A.F. de Sade, French writer, 1740–1814], **1.** abnormal pleasure derived from inflicting physical or psychological pain or abuse on others; cruelty. **2.** (in psychiatry) a psychosexual disorder characterized by the infliction of physical or psychological pain or humiliation on another person, either a consenting or a nonconsenting partner, to achieve sexual excitement or gratification. The condition is usually chronic, is seen predominantly in men, may result from conscious or unconscious motivations or desires, and, in severe cases, can lead to rape, torture, and murder. Also called **active algolagnia, sexual sadism.** Compare **masochism.** Kinds include **anal sadism, oral sadism.** See also **algolagnia, sadomasochism.**

sadist /sā″dist/, a person who is afflicted with or practices sadism. Compare **masochist.**

sadomasochism /sā″dōmas″əkiz′əm/ [Marquis de Sade; Leopold von Sacher-Masoch, Austrian author, 1836–1895], a personality disorder characterized by traits of sadism and masochism. See also **algolagnia, masochism, sadism.**

sadomasochist /sā′dōmas″əkist/ [Marquis de Sade; Leopold von Sacher-Masoch], a person who practices sadomasochism.

Saethre-Chotzen syndrome /sā′trə-kot′zən/ [Haakon Saethre, 20th-century Norwegian psychiatrist; F. Chotzen, 20th-century German psychiatrist], an autosomal-dominant disorder characterized by closure of the sutures of the head resulting in an abnormally shaped skull. Intelligence is usually unaffected, but there may be some learning difficulties. Also called **acrocephalosyndactyly, Chotzen syndrome.**

safe period, (*Informal*) the period during the menstrual cycle when conception is considered least likely to occur. It comprises approximately the 10 days after menstruation begins and the 10 days preceding menstruation. See also **contraception.**

safe sex, intimate sexual practices between partners who use condoms or other means to prevent the exchange of body fluids that transmit diseases. Although perfect safety is virtually impossible without abstinence, the known risks of infections by human immunodeficiency virus or other organisms transmitted through sexual contact can be reduced by safe sex practices.

safety director /sāf″tē/ [Fr, *sauver*, to save, *directeur*, manager], a member of a hospital staff whose activities are related to safety functions, such as fire prevention, environmental safety, and disaster planning activities. Also called *safety officer.*

safety glass, a hard, transparent material that resists shattering on impact. It usually is made as a sandwich of two sheets of glass with an intermediate layer of plastic. Safety glass may also be produced as a tempered material that breaks into rounded granules instead of sharp shards. Also called **shatterproof glass.**

safety glasses, impact-resistant lenses that protect the eyes from blows or other kinds of injury. Such lenses are usually made by tempering the glass, substituting plastic for glass, or laminating. Also called **polycarbonate glasses,** *safety lenses.*

safety system /sāf′te sis′tem/, **1.** a system designed to minimize hazards caused by human error. **2.** (in respiratory therapy) a system of connections designed to help prevent accidental interchanging of incorrect equipment or gases.

safflower oil /sef″lou·er/, a liquid fat containing polyunsaturated fatty acids, derived from the seeds of the safflower plant, *Carthamus tinctorius.* It is commonly mixed with other edible vegetable oils.

sagittal /saj″ətəl/ [L, *sagitta*, arrow], (in anatomy) pertaining to a suture or an imaginary line extending from the front to the back in the midline of the body or a part of the body, dividing into right and left parts.

sagittal axis, a hypothetical line through both mandibular condyles that serves as an axis for rotation of the mandible.

sagittal fontanel, a soft area located in the sagittal suture, halfway between the anterior and posterior fontanels. It may be found in some normal newborns and also in some with Down syndrome.

sagittal plane, the anteroposterior plane, or the section parallel to the median plane of the body. Compare **frontal plane, median plane, transverse plane.**

sagittal section, an anteroposterior cross section produced by slicing, laterally or through imaging techniques, a body or body part in a vertical plane parallel to the median plane.

sagittal sinus [L, *sagitta*, arrow, *sinus*, hollow], either of two venous sinuses of the dura mater. The superior venous sinus begins near the crista galli and drains backward to empty into a confluence of sinuses near the occipital area. The inferior venous sinus begins in the lower margin of the cerebral falx and follows the superior venous sinus, emptying into the straight sinus.

sagittal suture, the serrated connection between the two parietal bones of the skull, coursing down the midline from the coronal suture to the upper part of the lambdoidal suture.

sago spleen /sā″gō/, a form of amyloid spleen that mainly affects the malpighian bodies.

SaH, SAH, abbreviation for **subarachnoid hemorrhage.**

Saint John's wort /sānt jonz wort/, any of various species of the genus *Hypericum. H. perforatum* is a medicinal herb that is used as a mild antidepressant, sedative, and anxiolytic; it is also used topically for inflammation of the skin, contusions, myalgia, and first-degree burns. Saint John's wort is one of the most utilized herbal products in the United States. Many brands are now available and sold over the counter as dietary supplements. The patient should be cautioned that this herb interacts with many prescription medications. There is insufficient evidence to support its efficacy in the treatment of depression and anxiety. Also called **St. John's wort.**

Saint's triad [Charles F.M. Saint, 20th-century South African radiologist], a group of three related conditions—cholelithiasis, diverticulosis, and hiatal hernia—occurring together.

Saint Vitus dance /sānt vī″təs/, (*Obsolete*) now called **Sydenham chorea.**

Sakati-Nyhan syndrome /sä′kä·tē·nī′han/ [Nadia Sakati, 20th-century American pediatrician; William Leo Nyhan, American pediatrician, b. 1926], an autosomal-dominant type of acrocephalopolysyndactyly characterized by hypoplastic tibias and deformed, displaced fibulas. Also called *acrocephalopolysyndactyly, type III.* See also **Carpenter syndrome, Goodman syndrome, Noack syndrome.**

SAL, abbreviation for **sterility assurance level.**

sal-, -sal, combining form for salicylic acid derivatives.

salaam convulsion /säläm″/ [L, *convulsio*, cramp], a violent muscle spasm of the sternomastoid muscles marked by head bobbing or bowing. Also called **West syndrome.**

salbutamol. See **albuterol.**

salicylate /səlis″əlāt/ [Gk, *salix*, willow, *hyle*, matter], any of several widely prescribed drugs derived from salicylic acid. Salicylates exert analgesic, antipyretic, and antiinflammatory actions. The most important is acetylsalicylic acid, or aspirin. Sodium salicylate also has been used systemically, and it exerts similar effects. Many of the actions of aspirin appear to result from its ability to inhibit cyclooxygenase, a rate-limiting enzyme in prostaglandin biosynthesis. Aspirin is used in a wide variety of conditions, and, in the usual analgesic dosage, it causes only mild adverse effects. Severe occult GI bleeding or gastric ulcers may occur with frequent use. Large doses taken over a long period can cause significant impairment of hemostasis. Occasionally an asthmalike reaction is produced in hypersensitive individuals. Because of the ready availability of aspirin, accidental and intentional overdosage is common. Symptoms of salicylate intoxication include tinnitus, GI disturbances, abnormal respiration, acid-base imbalance, and central nervous system disturbances. Fatalities have resulted from ingestion of as little as 10 grains of aspirin in adults or as little as 4 mL of methyl salicylate (oil of wintergreen) in children. In addition to aspirin and sodium salicylate, which are used systemically, methyl salicylate is used topically as a counterirritant in ointments and liniments. Methyl salicylate can be absorbed through the skin in amounts capable of causing systemic toxicity. Another salicylate, salicylic acid, is too irritating to be used systemically and is used topically as a keratolytic agent, for example, for removing warts. See also **salicylic acid.**

salicylated /səlis″ilā′tid/ [Gk, *salix*, willow, *hyle*, matter], pertaining to a chemical formed as a salt or ester of salicylic acid.

salicylate poisoning, a toxic condition caused by the ingestion of salicylate, most often in aspirin or oil of wintergreen. Intoxication is characterized by rapid breathing, vomiting, headache, irritability, ketosis, hypoglycemia, and, in severe cases, seizures and respiratory failure.

salicylazosulfapyridine. See **sulfasalazine.**

salicylic acid /sal'isil'ik/, a keratolytic agent.

■ INDICATIONS: It is prescribed in the treatment of hyperkeratotic skin conditions and as an adjunct in fungal infections.

■ CONTRAINDICATIONS: Diabetes, impaired circulation, or known hypersensitivity to this drug prohibits its use.

■ ADVERSE EFFECTS: Among the more serious adverse effects are skin inflammation and salicylism.

salicylism /sal'isil'izəm/ [Gk, *salix,* willow, *hyle,* matter, *ismos,* practice], a syndrome of salicylate toxicity. See also **salicylate poisoning.**

saline /sā''līn/ [L, *sal,* salt], **1.** pertaining to a substance that contains a salt or salts. **2.** pertaining to something that is salty or has the characteristics of common table salt. See also **hypertonic saline, hypotonic saline.**

saline cathartic [L, *sal,* salt; Gk, *katharsis,* cleansing], one of a large group of cathartics administered to achieve prompt, complete evacuation of the bowel. A watery semifluid evacuation usually occurs within 3 to 4 hours. The most common indication for the administration of any of these agents is preparation of the bowel for diagnostic examination. Various preparations, including magnesium sulfate, sodium phosphate, sodium sulfate, and several naturally occurring mineral waters, may be used to achieve catharsis. The palatability of, cost of, and adverse systemic reactions to the saline cathartics depend on the particular agent used and the dose of the agent given.

saline enema [L, *sal,* salt; Gk, *enienai,* to send in], an instillation of a hypertonic solution containing sodium via the rectum to draw water into the lumen of the bowel to stimulate defecation. Overuse of enemas can result in fluid and electrolyte abnormalities, as well as laxative dependence.

saline infusion, the therapeutic introduction of a physiological salt solution into a vein.

saline irrigation, the washing out of a body cavity or wound with a stream of salt solution, usually an isotonic aqueous solution of sodium chloride.

saline solution, a solution containing sodium chloride. Depending on the use, it may be hypotonic, isotonic, or hypertonic with body fluids.

saliva /səlī''və/ [L, spittle], the clear, viscous fluid secreted by the salivary and mucous glands in the mouth. Saliva contains water, mucin, organic salts, and the digestive enzyme ptyalin. It serves to moisten the oral cavity, to initiate the digestion of starches, and to aid in the chewing and swallowing of food. Approximately 1 to 1.5 L is produced per day. –*salivary, adj.*

salivary duct, any one of the ducts through which saliva passes. Kinds include **Bartholin duct, duct of Rivinus, parotid duct, submandibular duct.**

salivary fistula, an abnormal communication from a salivary gland or duct to an opening in the mouth or on the skin of the face or neck.

salivary gland, any one of three pairs of glands secreting into the mouth, thus aiding the digestive process. The salivary glands are the parotid, the submandibular, and the sublingual. They are racemose structures consisting of numerous lobes subdivided into smaller lobules connected by dense areolar tissue, vessels, and ducts. The sublingual gland secretes mucus; the parotid gland, serous fluid; and the submandibular gland, both mucus and serous fluid. The lobules of the salivary glands are richly supplied with

blood vessels and fine plexuses of nerves. The hilum of the submandibular gland contains Langley's ganglion of nerve cells.

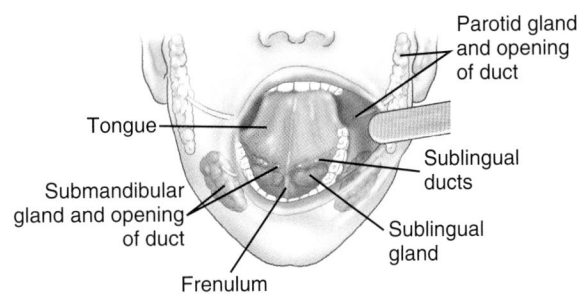

Salivary glands *(Leonard, 2009)*

salivary gland cancer, a malignant neoplastic disease of a salivary gland, occurring most frequently in a parotid gland. About 75% of tumors that develop in the salivary glands are benign, characteristically slow-growing painless mobile masses that are cystic or rubbery in consistency. In contrast, malignant tumors are rapid-growing, hard, lumpy, fixed, and frequently tender. The most common malignant neoplasms are mucoepidermoid, adenoid cystic, solid, and squamous cell carcinomas.

■ OBSERVATIONS: Pain, trismus, and facial palsy may occur, but often there are no symptoms. Diagnostic measures include radiographic studies, with sialographic studies and mandibular and chest films to detect metastases, and cytological studies of saliva from Stensen's duct.

■ INTERVENTIONS: Treatment usually consists of surgical removal of the lobe containing a benign tumor and total parotidectomy with a radical neck dissection if the lesion is advanced. Radiation and chemotherapy may also be employed.

■ PATIENT CARE CONSIDERATIONS: Radiotherapy is administered for residual, recurrent, or inoperable cancers, and chemotherapy may be palliative. It is important to encourage follow-up as the malignancy may recur.

salivary gland nuclear imaging, a nuclear scan of the salivary glands to visualize inflammation, hypofunction, location and character of tumors, and duct obstruction.

saliva substitute. See **artificial saliva.**

salivation /sal'ivā''shən/, the process of saliva secretion by the salivary glands.

salivatory /sal''ivətôr'ē/ [L, *saliva,* spittle], stimulating the production of saliva. Also **sialogenous.**

Salk vaccine. See **poliovirus vaccine.**

sallow /sal''ō/ [ME, *salou,* dirty-gray], yellowish-gray in complexion.

salmeterol, a sympathomimetic, long-acting bronchodilator.

■ INDICATIONS: It is prescribed in the maintenance treatment of reversible bronchospasm associated with asthma (including nocturnal asthma) and chronic obstructive pulmonary disease and to prevent exercise-induced asthma.

■ CONTRAINDICATIONS: It should not be given to patients with allergy to any component of the drug formulation, when patients need a fast-onset inhaled beta$_2$ agonist for bronchodilation, or when patients have used MAO inhibitors within the past 2 weeks. The frequency of salmeterol administration should not be increased. Caution must be used when salmeterol is administered to patients with conditions that have the potential to be exacerbated by sympathomimetic amines, in-

cluding cardiovascular disease, diabetes, prostatic hyperplasia, convulsions, thyrotoxicosis, and narrow-angle glaucoma.
■ ADVERSE EFFECTS: The side effects most often reported include changes in heart rhythm, muscle cramps or stiffness, parkinsonian-like symptoms, pallor, sweating, hives, and tingling of the skin.

salmon calcitonin. See **calcitonin.**

Salmonella /sal′mənel″ə/ [Daniel E. Salmon, American pathologist, 1850–1914], a genus of motile gram-negative rod-shaped bacteria that includes species causing typhoid fever, paratyphoid fever, and some forms of gastroenteritis. *Salmonella* species are widely distributed in animals, frequently producing disease that can be transmitted to humans. The most frequent manifestation of salmonella is food poisoning. See also **salmonellosis.**

Salmonella enteritidis [Daniel E. Salmon; Gk, *enteron,* intestine], a species of *Salmonella* causing food poisoning and gastroenteritis in humans.

Salmonella **enteritis,** bacterial enteritis caused by species of *Salmonella.*

Salmonella **gastroenteritis,** a type of gastroenteritis caused by species of *Salmonella.* Species causing this in humans include *S. choleraesuis* and *S. enteritidis* and usually enter the body in contaminated food. Symptoms include inflammation of the mucosa, nausea, vomiting, abdominal pain, and bloody diarrhea. A more virulent form can occur in immunocompromised patients, sometimes resulting in septicemia.

salmonellosis /sal′mənəlō″sis/ [Daniel E. Salmon; Gk, *osis,* condition], a form of gastroenteritis caused by ingestion of food contaminated with a species of *Salmonella.* It is characterized by an incubation period of 6 to 48 hours followed by sudden colicky abdominal pain; fever; and bloody, watery diarrhea. Nausea and vomiting are common, and abdominal signs may resemble those of acute appendicitis or cholecystitis. Symptoms usually last from 4 to 7 days, but diarrhea and fever may persist for up to 2 weeks. Dehydration may occur. There is no specific treatment. Antibiotics are usually not indicated unless disease has spread beyond the intestine. Adequate cooking, good refrigeration, and careful handwashing may reduce the frequency of outbreaks. See also **food poisoning, typhoid fever.**

salol camphor, a clear, oily mixture of two parts of camphor and three parts of phenyl salicylate, used as a local antiseptic.

Salonica fever. See **trench fever.**

salpingectomy /sal′pinjek″təmē/ [Gk, *salpinx,* tube, *ektomē,* excision], surgical removal of one or both fallopian tubes. It is performed for removal of a cyst or tumor, for excision of an abscess, or, if both tubes are removed, as a sterilization procedure or for tubal pregnancy. Often the operation is done with a hysterectomy or an oophorectomy.

salpingemphraxis /salpinj′emfrak″sis/ [Gk, *salpinx,* tube, *emphraxis,* a stoppage], **1.** an obstruction of the eustachian tube of the ear. **2.** an obstruction of a fallopian tube.

salpinges, salpingian. See **salpinx.**

salpingitis /sal′pinjī″tis/ [Gk, *salpinx* + *itis,* inflammation], **1.** an inflammation or infection of a fallopian tube. See also **pelvic inflammatory disease. 2.** inflammation of the eustachian tube.

salpingo-, prefix meaning "eustachian or fallopian tube": *salpingostomy, salpingraphy, salpingoplasty.*

salpingography /sal″ping·gog″rəfē/, a radiographic examination of the fallopian tube after introduction of a radiopaque contrast medium.

salpingo-oophorectomy /-ō′əfôrek″təmē/, the surgical removal of a fallopian tube and an ovary.

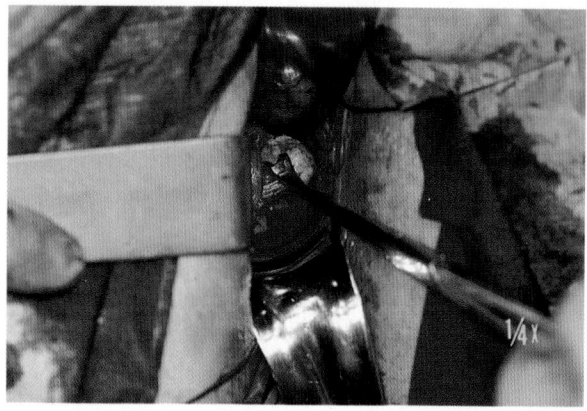

Salpingo-oophorectomy *(Baggish and Karram, 2011)*

salpingo-oophoritis /-ō′əfôrī″tis/ [Gk, *salpinx,* tube, *oophoron,* ovary, *itis,* inflammation], an inflammation of a fallopian tube and associated ovary.

salpingopharyngeal fold, a small vertical fold that descends from the tubal elevation of the nasopharynx and overlies salpingopharyngeus muscle.

salpingoplasty /sal-ping′go-plas″te/, surgical repair of a fallopian tube. Also called **tuboplasty.**

salpingostomy /sal′ping·gos″təmē/ [Gk, *salpinx* + *stoma,* mouth], the formation of an artificial opening in a fallopian tube to restore patency in a tube whose fimbriated opening has been closed by infection or by chronic inflammation or to drain an abscess or a fluid accumulation. A prosthesis may be inserted to maintain the patency of the fallopian tube and to direct the route of the ova to assist fertilization.

salpinx /sal″pingks/ *pl. salpinges* [Gk, *tube*], a tube, such as the fallopian or eustachian tube, the salpinx auditiva, or the salpinx uterina.

salt /sôlt/ [L, *sal*], **1.** a compound formed by the chemical reaction of an acid and a base. Salts are usually composed of a metal cation and a nonmetal anion. **2.** sodium chloride (common table salt). **3.** a substance, such as magnesium sulfate (Epsom salt), used as a purgative.

saltation /saltā″shən/ [L, *saltare,* to dance], a mutation causing a significant difference in appearance between parent and offspring or an abrupt variation in the characteristics of a species. −*saltatory, saltatorial, saltatoric, adj.*

saltatory conduction /sal″tətôr′ē/ [L, *saltere* + *conducere,* to lead together], impulse transmission that skips from node to node, providing rapid transmission.

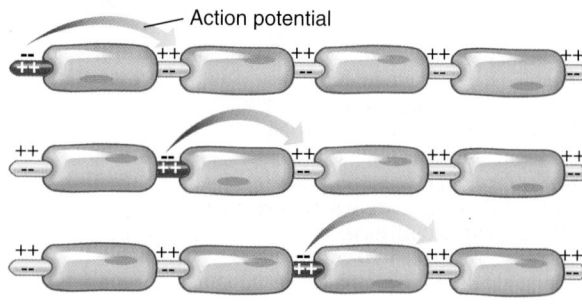

Saltatory conduction

saltatory evolution, the appearance of a sudden change within a species, caused by mutation. The progression of a species by sudden major changes rather than by the gradual accumulation of minor changes. The phenomenon occurs predominantly in plants as a result of polyploidy. See also **emergent evolution.**

salt cake, anhydrous sodium sulfate; a technical grade of sodium sulfate used in detergents, dyes, soaps, and other industrial products. See also **sodium sulfate.**

salt depletion, the loss of salt from the body through excessive elimination of body fluids by perspiration, diarrhea, vomiting, or urination, without corresponding replacement. See also **heat exhaustion, electrolyte imbalance.**

Salter-Harris fracture. See **epiphyseal fracture.**

salt-free diet. See **low-sodium diet.**

salt-losing nephritis, a disorder characterized by abnormal kidney loss of sodium chloride, hyponatremia, azotemia, acidosis, dehydration, and vascular collapse. Causes include kidney tubule damage, endocrine dysfunction, and GI abnormality. Also called **salt-losing syndrome.**

salt-losing nephropathy, intrinsic renal disease causing abnormal urinary sodium loss in persons ingesting normal amounts of sodium chloride, accompanied by vomiting, dehydration, and vascular collapse. Also called **salt-losing nephritis.**

salt-losing syndrome. See **salt-losing nephritis.**

saltpeter /sôlt″pē″tər/ [L, *sal,* salt, *petra,* rock], common name for potassium nitrate, KNO_3, used in gunpowder, pickling substances, and medicines.

salt-poor diet [Gk, *diaita,* way of living], *(Obsolete)* now called **low-salt diet, low-sodium diet.**

salt substitute, a chemical compound for flavoring foods without adding sodium to the diet. Kinds include **potassium chloride, glutamic acid.**

salt wasting, inappropriate sodium excretion in the urine (natriuresis) with hyponatremia and hyperkalemia. See also **salt-losing nephritis.**

Saluron, a thiazide diuretic. Brand name for **hydroflumethiazide.**

salvage therapy /sal″vij/ [Fr, *sauver,* to save; Gk, *therapeia,* treatment], therapy administered after previous therapies have failed and the disease has recurred or failed to respond.

salve. See **ointment.**

samarium (Sm) /səmer″ē·əm/ [Colonel M. von Samarski, 19th-century Russian mine official], a metallic rare earth element. Its atomic number is 62; its atomic mass is 150.35.

samarium Sm 153 lexidronam (Sm 153-EDTMP), samarium 153 complexed with ethylenediaminetetramethylenephosphonic acid, a bone-seeking diphosphonate complex that concentrates in areas of bone turnover. It is administered intravenously in the palliative treatment of patients with osteoblastic metastatic bone lesions.

SAMHSA, abbreviation for **Substance Abuse and Mental Health Services Administration.**

sample [L, *exemplum*], (in research) a group or part of the whole that can be used to demonstrate characteristics of the whole. Kinds include **random sampling, snowball sampling, stratified sample.**

sanatorium. See **sanitarium.**

sanctuary site /sangk′choo-er′ē/ [L, *sanctus,* sacred, *situs,* location], an area of the body that is poorly penetrated by pharmacological agents and therefore is a place in which tumor cells or infectious organisms can escape the effects of drug therapy. For example, because most drugs that are effective against the human immunodeficiency virus (HIV) do not cross the blood-brain barrier, the central nervous system

provides an area in which HIV can avoid the effects of antiviral therapy and from which resistant virus can later emerge.

Sanctura, brand name for **trospium.**

sand bath, **1.** (in health care) the application of warm, dry sand or of damp sand to the body. Also called *ammotherapy.* **2.** (in analytic chemistry) a sealed stainless steel frame or other vessel capable of withstanding high heat filled with sand and placed on a heat source. It is used to facilitate rapid, consistent temperature in a vessel when heat is needed for a chemical reaction.

sand flea. See **chigoe.**

sandfly fever. See **phlebotomus fever.**

Sandhoff disease, a variant of Tay-Sachs disease that includes defects in the enzymes hexosaminidase A and B. It is characterized by a progressively more rapid course and is found in the general population, not a restricted population as is Tay-Sachs disease. Also called **gangliosidosis type II.** See also **Tay-Sachs disease.**

Sandoz Clinical Assessment—Geriatric, an examination of psychological function that is administered to elderly people to assist in the diagnostic process.

sand tumor. See **psammoma.**

sandwich generation, *(Informal)* members of the middle generation who are trying to raise children and help aging parents at the same time.

sandwich technique, a method of identifying antibodies or antibody-synthesizing cells in a tissue preparation. A solution containing a specific antigen is applied to the preparation. If antibodies to the antigen are present in the tissue, they will bind to the antigen. Unbound antigen is washed away, and then a fluorochrome-labeled antibody specific for the antigen is added. The result is a complex of antigen sandwiched between antibodies, which can be detected by fluorescence microscopy. See also **ELISA.**

SANE, abbreviation for **sexual assault nurse examiner.**

Sanfilippo syndrome /san·fi·lip′ō/ [Sylvester J. Sanfilippo, 20th-century American pediatrician], four heterogeneous, biochemically distinct, but clinically indistinguishable, forms of mucopolysaccharidosis characterized biochemically by excretion of the mucopolysaccharide heparan sulfate in the urine and clinically by severe, rapid mental deterioration and relatively mild somatic symptoms. Onset is from 2 to 6 years of age; the head is large, height is normal, Hurler-like features are mild, and hirsutism is generalized; death usually occurs before 20 years of age. The four types are types A through D, each resulting from a different enzymatic defect.

sangui-, prefix meaning "blood": *sanguineous, sanguinopurulent.*

sanguine /sang″gwin/ [L, *sanguis,* blood], pertaining to abundant and active blood circulation, ruddy complexion, and an attitude full of vitality and confidence.

sanguineous /sang·gwin″ē·əs/ [L, *sanguis,* blood], pertaining to blood or containing blood, such as full-blooded. Also spelled **sanguinous.**

sanguinopurulent /sang′gwinōpyoor″ələnt/, containing blood and pus.

sanguinous. See **sanguineous.**

sanies /sā″ni·ēz/, a thin, blood-stained purulent discharge from a wound or ulcer.

sanioserous, containing sanies and serum.

sanious /sā″nē·əs/, pertaining to or resembling sanies.

sanita-, combining form meaning "health": *sanitarium, sanitation, sanitary.*

sanitarian [L, *sanitas,* health], a health professional who is an expert in the science of public health.

sanitarium /san′iter″ē·əm/ [L, *sanitas,* health], a facility for the treatment of patients suffering from chronic mental

S

or physical diseases or for the recuperation of convalescent patients. Also called **sanatorium.**

sanitary landfill /san″iterē/ [L, *sanitas,* health; AS, *land* + *fyllan,* to fill], a disposal site for solid waste. It is usually a swamp area, ravine, or canyon where the waste is compacted by heavy machines and covered with earth.

sanitary napkin, a disposable pad of absorbent material, usually worn to absorb menstrual flow.

sanitation /san′itā″shən/ [L, *sanitas,* health], the science of maintaining a healthful, disease-free, and hazard-free environment.

sanitize /san″itīz/ [L, *sanitas,* health], to take action needed to clean the environment or a part of it, removing or reducing pathogenic microorganisms and their habitats.

San Joaquin fever. See **coccidioidomycosis.**

SA node, abbreviation for **sinoatrial node.** See **sinus node.**

Sanorex, an anorexiant. Brand name for **mazindol.**

Sansert, a vasoconstrictor. Brand name for **methysergide maleate.**

Santyl, an ointment for sterile enzymatic wound debridement. Brand name for **collagenase.**

SaO₂, symbol for *percentage of oxygen saturation of arterial blood.*

saphenous [Gk, *saphenes,* manifest], pertaining to certain anatomical structures in the leg, such as arteries, veins, or nerves.

saphenous nerve /səfē″nəs/ [Gk, *saphenes,* manifest; L, *nervus,* nerve], the largest and longest superficial branch of the femoral nerve, supplying the skin of the medial side of the leg and the skin over the patella. On the lateral side of the knee it joins branches of the lateral femoral cutaneous nerve to form the patellar plexus. One branch of the saphenous nerve below the knee supplies the ankle. Another branch below the knee supplies the medial side of the foot. See also **femoral nerve.**

saphenous vein. See **greater saphenous vein.**

sapo-, combining form meaning "soap": *saponin, saponaceous, saponification.*

saponaceous /sap′ənā″shəs/ [L, *sapo,* soap], pertaining to soap.

saponification /sapon′ifikā″shən/ [L, *sapo,* soap, *facere,* to make], the production of soap.

saponified, pertaining to a substance chemically hydrolyzed into soaps or acid salts and glycerol by heating with an alkali.

saponin /sap″ənin/ [L, *sapo,* soap], a soapy material found in some plants, especially soapwort (bouncing bet) and certain lilies. It is used in demulcent medications to provide a sudsy quality. Saponins can cause cell lysis (e.g., hemolysis). Natural saponins have largely been replaced by synthetic preparations.

sapro-, prefix meaning "decay" or "putrefaction": *saprogen, saprophagus, saprophyte.*

saprogen /sap″rəjən/, a microscopic saprophyte.

saprophagus, an organism that feeds off dead or decaying material.

saprophyte /sap″rəfīt/ [Gk, *sapros,* rotten, *phyton,* plant], an organism that lives on dead organic matter. *−saprophytic, adj.*

SAPS III, a severity score and mortality estimation tool. Abbreviation for *Simplified Acute Physiology Score.*

saquinavir, an antiviral.

■ INDICATIONS: It is used to treat HIV in combination with zidovudine and zalcitabine.

■ CONTRAINDICATIONS: Known hypersensitivity to this drug prohibits its use.

■ ADVERSE EFFECTS: Adverse effects of this drug include buccal mucosa ulceration, headache, musculoskeletal pain, asthenia, and hyperglycemia. Common side effects are diarrhea, abdominal pain, nausea, paresthesia, and rash.

saralasin, a competitive antagonist of angiotensin. It is administered by IV injection to assess the role of the renin-angiotensin system in the maintenance of blood pressure. A decrease in blood pressure is expected in renin-dependent hypertension.

-sarc, combining form meaning "(specified type of) flesh": *angiosarcoma.*

sarco- /sär′kō-/, prefix meaning "flesh": *sarcoadenoma, sarcoidosis, sarcolemma.*

sarcoadenoma /-ad′ənō″mə/ [Gk, *sarx,* flesh, *aden,* gland, *oma,* tumor], a mixed tumor containing both glandular and connective tissue characteristics. Also called **adenosarcoma.**

sarcocarcinoma /-kär′sinō″mə/ [Gk, *sarx,* flesh, *karkinos,* crab, *oma,* tumor], a mixed tumor with characteristics of both sarcomas and carcinomas.

sarcodina. See **protozoan.**

sarcoidosis /sär′koidō″sis/ [Gk, *sarx,* flesh, *eidos,* form, *osis,* condition], a chronic disorder of unknown origin characterized by the formation of tubercles of nonnecrotizing epithelioid tissue. Common sites are the lungs, spleen, liver, skin, mucous membranes, and lacrimal and salivary glands, usually with involvement of the lymph glands. Diminished reactivity to tuberculin frequently accompanies the disorder. The lesions usually disappear over a period of months or years but may progress to widespread granulomatous inflammation and fibrosis. Also called *sarcoid of Boeck.*

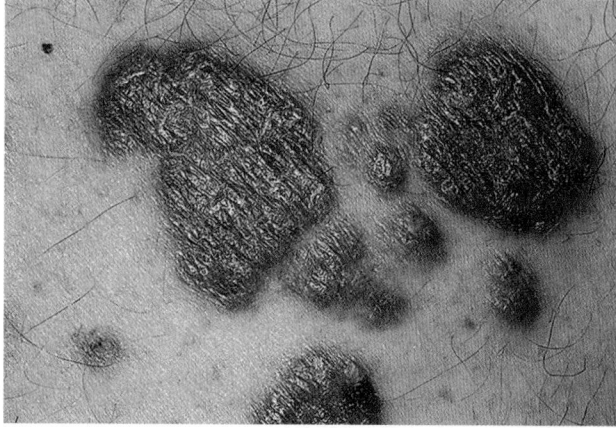

Isolated cutaneous sarcoidosis
(Callen et al, 2000)

sarcoidosis cordis, a form of sarcoidosis in which granulomatous lesions develop in the myocardium. Mild cases with few infiltrates are asymptomatic. In severe cases cardiac failure may result. See also **sarcoidosis.**

sarcolemma /-lem″ə/ [Gk, *sarx,* flesh, *lemma,* sheath], a membrane that covers smooth, striated, and cardiac muscle fibers.

sarcoma /särkō″mə/ *pl. sarcomas, sarcomata* [Gk, *sarx* + *oma,* tumor], a malignant neoplasm of the soft tissues arising in fibrous, fatty, muscular, synovial, vascular, or neural tissue, usually first manifested as a painless swelling. About 40% of sarcomas occur in the lower extremities, 20% in the upper extremities, 20% in the trunk, and the rest in the head, neck, or retroperineum. The tumor is composed of cells in a connective tissue matrix and may be highly invasive. Trauma probably does not play a role in the cause, but sarcomas may arise in burn or radiation scars. Small tumors may be managed by local excision and postoperative radiotherapy, but bulky sarcomas of the extremities may require amputation followed by irradiation for local control and combination chemotherapy to eliminate small foci or neoplastic cells. See *specific sarcomas.* −sarcomatous, *adj.*

-sarcoma,   suffix meaning a "malignant tumor from connective tissue": *angiosarcoma, hemangiosarcoma, lymphosarcoma.*

sarcoma botryoides /bot′rē·oi″dēz/,   a tumor derived from primitive striated muscle cells, occurring most frequently in young children and characterized by a painful edematous polypoid grapelike mass in the vagina or on the uterine cervix or the neck of the urinary bladder. See also **rhabdomyosarcoma.**

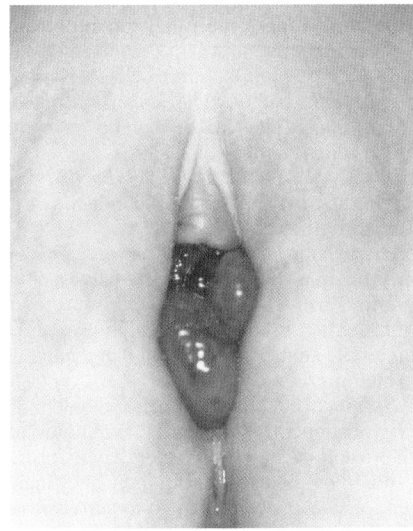

Sarcoma botryoides *(Courtesy Dr. Michael Donovan, Children's Hospital, Boston)*

sarcomagenesis /särkō′məjen″əsis/ [Gk, *sarx* + *oma* + *genesis*, origin],   the process of initiating and promoting the development of a sarcoma. Compare **carcinogenesis, oncogenesis, tumorigenesis.** −sarcomagenetic, *adj.*

sarcomas, sarcomata.   See **sarcoma.**

sarcomere /sär″kōmir/ [Gk, *sarx* + *meros*, part],   the smallest functional, contractile unit of a myofibril. Sarcomeres occur as repeating units, extending from one Z line to the next along the length of the myofibril.

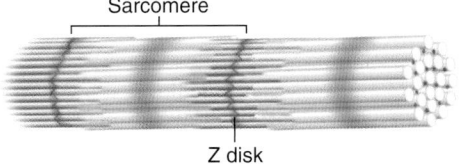

Sarcomere *(Thibodeau and Patton, 2007)*

sarcopenia /-pē″nē·ə/ [Gk, *sarx*, flesh, *penia*, poverty],   a loss of skeletal muscle mass that may accompany aging. Studies indicate that the loss of skeletal muscle for the average normally healthy person amounts to about 20% between

about 30 and 70 years of age. The loss may accelerate as aging progresses. The muscle is replaced by fat, usually in a subtle way that is not noticed by the individual, as areas of muscle loss are padded with extra fat. Muscle-strengthening and muscle-building exercises can prevent or reverse much of this problem.

sarcoplasm /sär″kōplaz′əm/ [Gk, *sarx,* flesh, *plassein,* to mold],   the semifluid cytoplasm of muscle cells.

sarcoplasmic reticulum /-plas″mik/ [Gk, *sarx* + *plassein,* to mold; L, *reticulum,* little net],   a network of tubules and sacs in skeletal muscle fibers that plays an important role in muscle contraction and relaxation by releasing and storing calcium ions. This network is analogous, but not identical, to the endoplasmic reticulum of other cells.

Sarcoptes scabiei /särkop″tēz skā″bē·ī/ [Gk, *sarx* + *koptein,* to cut; L, *scabere,* to scratch],   the genus of itch mite that causes scabies. See also **Norwegian scabies.**

sarcosine /sär′kō·sēn/,   an amino acid occurring as an intermediate in the metabolism of choline in the kidney and liver. It is normally not detectable in human blood or urine.

sarcosinemia,   an inborn error of metabolism caused by a defect of the enzyme that breaks down sarcosine, resulting in elevated levels of sarcosine in the blood. Clinical manifestations include poor feeding in an infant with failure to thrive and developmental delays; however, no consistent clinical syndrome has been reported.

SARS,   abbreviation for **severe acute respiratory syndrome.**

sartorius /särtôr″ē·əs/ [L, *sartor,* tailor],   the longest muscle in the body, extending from the pelvis to the calf of the leg. It is a narrow ribbon-shaped muscle that arises from the anterior superior iliac spine, passes obliquely across the proximal anterior part of the thigh from the lateral to the medial side, and inserts into the tibia. It acts to flex the thigh and rotate it laterally and to flex the leg and rotate it medially. Compare **quadriceps femoris.**

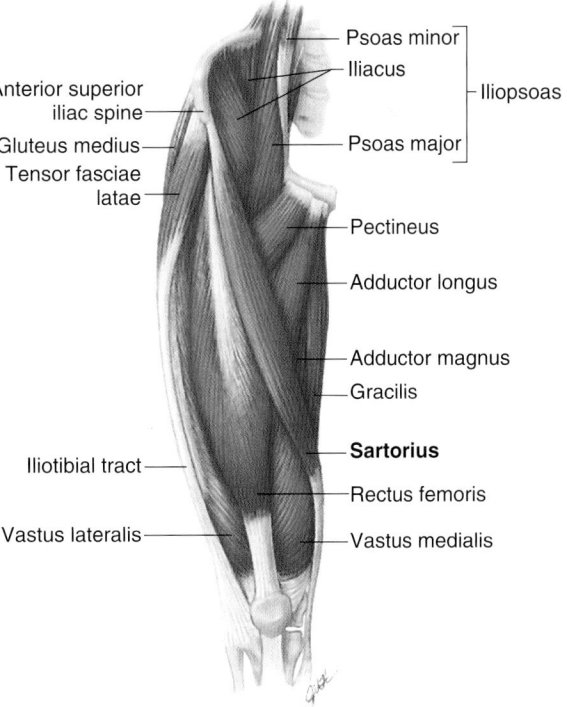

Sartorius *(Patton and Thibodeau, 2010)*

S

satellite cells /sat″əlīt/ [L, *satelles,* attendant, *cella,* storeroom], glial cells (astrocytes) that form around damaged nerve cells and lie close to neuron bodies in the central nervous system.

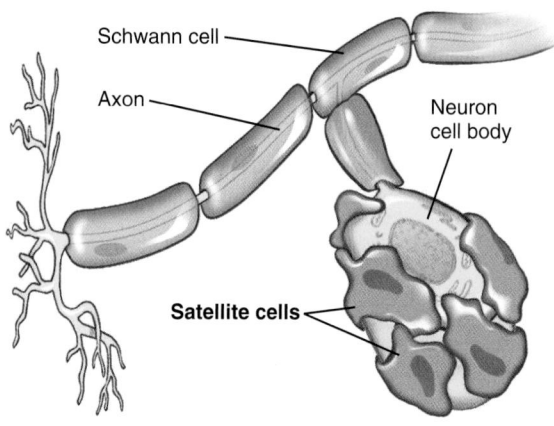

Satellite cells

satellite clinic [L, *satelles,* attendant; Gk, *kline,* bed], a health care facility usually operated under the auspices of a large institution but situated in a location some distance from the larger health center.

satellite virus, a strain of virus unable to replicate except in the presence of a helper virus. The satellite virus is considered to be deficient in coding for capsid formation.

satiety /sətī″ətē/, a state of being satisfied, as in the feeling of being full after eating.

satiety center, a locus of nerve tissue in the ventromedial nucleus of the hypothalamus that controls the appetite.

saturated /sach′ərā′tid/ [L, *saturare,* to fill], **1.** having absorbed or dissolved the maximum amount of a given substance, such as a solution in which no more of the solute can be dissolved. **2.** an organic compound that contains the maximum number of hydrogen atoms so that only single bonds exist in the carbon chain, as in saturated fatty acids. Also called **saturated hydrocarbon.** Compare **unsaturated.**

saturated calomel electrode (SCE), a reference electrode commonly used in polarography and potentiometry.

saturated fatty acid, a fatty acid in which all of the carbon atoms in the hydrocarbon chain are joined by single bonds. They exist mostly as components of fats (triglycerides) or other lipids of animal origin. Foods rich in saturated fatty acids include beef, lamb, pork, veal, whole-milk products, butter, most cheeses, and a few plant products such as cocoa butter, coconut oil, and palm oil. Ordinary oleomargarine and hydrogenated shortenings also contain saturated fatty acids. A diet high in saturated fatty acids may contribute to a high serum cholesterol level and appears to be associated with an increased incidence of coronary heart disease in some populations. Compare **unsaturated fatty acid.**

saturated hydrocarbon. See **saturated.**

saturated solution, a solution in which the solvent contains the maximum amount of solute it can dissolve at a particular temperature. It is often expressed as the number of grams of solute that can dissolve in 100 mL of solution. See also **solute, solvent.**

saturation /sach′ərā″shən/ [L, *saturare,* to fill], **1.** a condition in which a solution contains as much solute as can remain dissolved. **2.** a measure of the degree to which oxygen is bound to hemoglobin, expressed as a percentage of the possible limit. **3.** a chemical compound in which all the valency bonds have been filled.

saturational cuing /sach′ərā″shənəl/, a treatment strategy for visuoconstructive disorders that involves presenting controlled verbal instruction on task analysis and sequence and presenting cues on spatial boundaries.

saturation index of hemoglobin [L, *saturare,* to fill, *index,* pointer], a measure of the amount of hemoglobin in a given amount of blood, compared with normal.

Saturday night palsy [Gk, *paralyein,* to be palsied]. See **radial nerve palsy.**

saturn-, prefix meaning "lead": *saturnine, saturnine tremor.*

saturnine /sat″ərnīn/, pertaining to lead or lead poisoning.

saturnine tremor, a condition of involuntary muscle contractions in the extremities observed in patients with chronic lead poisoning.

satyr ear /sat″ər/, a congenital abnormality in which the helix of the auricle lacks the usual rolled contour and the tubercle is prominent.

satyriasis /sat′irī″əsis/ [Gk, *satyros,* lecherous, *osis,* condition], excessive, pathological, or uncontrollable sexual desire in the male. The cause may be psychological or organic. Also called *satyromania.*

sauna bath /sô″nə/ [Finn, *sauna* + AS, *baeth*], a bath consisting of exposure to dry, hot vapor to induce sweating. Also called **Finnish bath.**

saur-, prefix meaning "lizard" or "reptile."

saw palmetto, an herbal product harvested from the American dwarf palm.

■ INDICATIONS: It is used to treat benign prostatic hypertrophy, and multiple studies have shown that it can improve the urinary symptoms.

■ CONTRAINDICATIONS: Saw palmetto should not be used without verification that the urinary symptoms are caused by benign prostatic hyperplasia rather than by prostate carcinoma. It should not be used during pregnancy and lactation, in children, or in those with known hypersensitivity to this plant.

saxitoxin /sak′sitok″sin/, a powerful neurotoxin found in bivalve mollusks, including mussels, clams, and scallops. It is produced by certain species of dinoflagellates, which are consumed by the mollusks. Saxitoxin may cause a severe food intoxication in humans who eat the contaminated shellfish.

saxophone lung, (*Informal*) an infection related to the inhalation of toxic molds or fungi found in musical instruments, particularly wind instruments such as the saxophone or clarinet. Also called **hypersensitivity pneumonitis.**

Sb, symbol for the element **antimony.**

SBE, 1. abbreviation for **self-breast examination. 2.** abbreviation for **subacute bacterial endocarditis.**

SBT, abbreviation for **Shorted Blessed Test.**

sc, 1. a notation for a Latin phrase meaning "without correction." Abbreviation for *sine correctione.* **2.** abbreviation for *subcutaneously.*

Sc, symbol for the element **scandium.**

SCA, abbreviation for **sudden cardiac arrest.**

scab. See **eschar.**

scabbard trachea /skab′ərd/, a flattening of the trachea caused by lateral compression by swellings or tumors.

scabicide /skab″isīd/ [L, *scabere,* to scratch, *caedere,* to kill], any one of a large group of drugs that destroy the itch mite, *Sarcoptes scabiei.* These drugs are applied topically in a lotion or cream-based preparation. All are potentially toxic and irritating to the skin. They are used with caution in treating children. Kinds include **crotamiton, lindane.**

scabies /skā″bēz/ [L, *scabere,* to scratch], a contagious disease caused by *Sarcoptes scabiei,* the human itch mite, characterized by intense itching of the skin and excoriation from scratching. The mite, transmitted by close contact with infected humans or domestic animals, burrows into outer layers of the skin, where the female lays eggs. From 2 to 4 months after the first infection, sensitization to the mites and their products begins, resulting in a pruritic papular rash most common on the webs of fingers, flexor surfaces of wrists, and thighs. Secondary bacterial infection may occur. Diagnosis may be made by microscopic identification of adult mites, larvae, or eggs in scrapings of the burrows. All contacts are treated simultaneously with topical application of permethrin, crotamiton, or another scabicide. Oral antihistamines and salicylates reduce itching. It is also recommended that clothes and bedding be washed in hot water and dried in a hot dryer. A more severe form of scabies is observed in immunocompromised patients and is characterized by vesicles and thick crusts over the skin. This form is known as Norwegian scabies and is treated with Ivermectin.

scabietic /skā′bē·et″ik/ [L, *scabere,* to scratch], pertaining to scabies.

scabrities unguium /skabrish″i·ēz/, a very pronounced thickening and distortion of the nails, which separate from skin at the base.

scaffolding,   **1.** (in occupational therapy) a technique utilizing a process that begins with the most simple aspects of a skill and builds upon the foundational skills to master more complex skills. The therapist expects errors in the accomplishment of skills, provides feedback, and offers assistance only in aspects of the skill not yet mastered by the client. **2.** (in surgery) the use of a flexible mesh for soft tissue support and repair when weakness or voids exist in anatomical stuctures.

scag,   *(Slang)* heroin.

scala tympani.   See **helicotrema.**

scala vestibuli.   See **helicotrema.**

scald /skôld/ [L, *calidus,* hot], a burn caused by exposure of the skin to a hot liquid or vapor.

scalded skin syndrome.   See **toxic epidermal necrolysis.**

scale [OFr, *escale,* husk], **1.** *n.,* a small, thin flake of keratinized epithelium. **2.** *v.,* to remove encrusted material from the surface of a tooth.

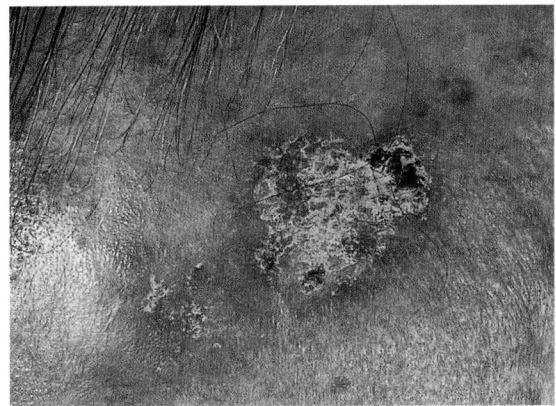

Scale of lupus erythematosus *(du Vivier, 2002)*

scalene /skā′lēn/ [Gk, *skalenos,* uneven], pertaining to one of the scalenus muscles.

scalenus /skālē″nəs/ [Gk, *skalenos*], one of a group of four muscles arising from the cervical vertebrae with insertions on the first or second rib.

scalenus anticus syndrome.   See **Naffziger syndrome.**

scaler /skā′lər/ [OFr, *escale,* husk], a dental hand instrument used to remove calculus from tooth surfaces. See also **scaling.**

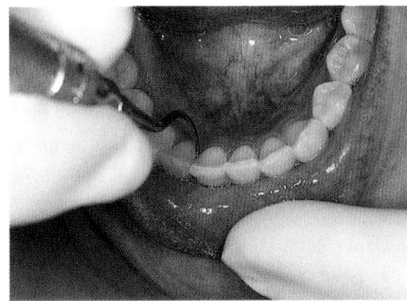

Scaler *(Christensen, 2002)*

scaling /skāl′ing/ [OFr, *escale,* husk], removal of plaque and calculus from the surface of a tooth by means of a scaler.

scalp [ME], the skin covering the head, not including the face and ears.

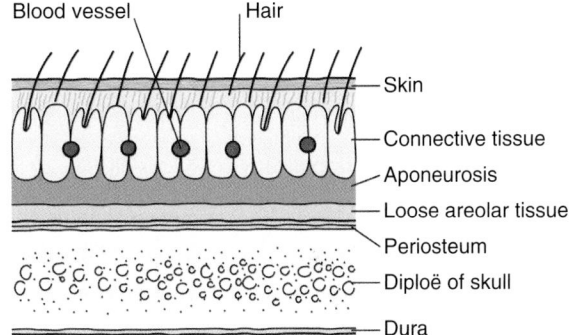

Layers of the scalp *(Drake, Vogl, and Mitchell, 2010)*

scalpel /skal″pəl/ [L, *scalprum,* knife], a small pointed knife with a convex edge. Some scalpels use interchangeable blades for specific surgical procedures, such as operating and amputating. Multiple kinds of scalpels are used; they are identified by number. Number 10 is the most common.

scalp medication,   **1.** a cream, ointment, lotion, or shampoo used to treat dermatological conditions of the scalp. **2.** the application of a medication to the scalp. If a cream, ointment, or lotion is to be applied, a shampoo is usually given first. The hair is dried, combed, and parted in the middle. The medication is most often spread with the fingertips. After treatment the medication may need to be washed off the scalp and hair with an alkaline shampoo. On occasion the affected area may be sharply circumscribed and may not require the scalpwide process.

scalp vein needle,   a thin-gauge needle designed for use in the veins of the scalp or other small veins, especially in infants and children. Also called **butterfly needle.**

scan.   See **scanning.**

scandium (Sc) /skan″dē·əm/ [Scandinavia], a grayish metallic element. Its atomic number is 21; its atomic mass is 44.956.

scanner /skan′ər/ [L, *scandere,* to climb], equipment used for making a digital representation of an original photographic image or printed material. See also **scanning.**

scanning [L, *scandere,* to climb], a technique for carefully studying an area, organ, or system of the body by recording and displaying an image of the area. A concentration of a radioactive substance that has an affinity for a specific tissue may be administered intravenously to enhance the image. The liver, brain, and thyroid can be examined, tumors can be located, and function can be evaluated by various scanning techniques. See also *specific scanning techniques.* **−scan,** *n., v.*

scanning electron microscope (SEM), an instrument similar to an electron microscope in that a beam of electrons is used to scan the surface of a specimen. The beam is moved in a point-to-point manner over the surface of the specimen. These electrons are deflected, collected, accelerated, and directed against a scintillator. The large number of photons thus created are converted into an electric signal that, in turn, modulates the beam scanning the surface of the specimen. The image produced appears to be three-dimensional and lifelike. Compare **electron microscope, transmission scanning electron microscope.**

scanning electron microscopy (SEM), the technique using a scanning electron microscope on a specimen. See also **scanning electron microscope.**

scanning laser ophthalmoscope (SLO), an instrument for retinal imaging in which light from a low-power laser beam that scans the retina is reflected back to a sensor. The light detected by the sensor is used to create a full-color composite digital image.

scanning speech, abnormal speech characterized by a staccato-like articulation in which the words are clipped and broken because the person pauses between syllables. It is most often associated with damage to the cerebellum.

scanography /skanog″rəfē/ [L, *scandere,* to climb; Gk, *graphein,* to record], a method of producing a radiograph of an internal body organ or structure by using a series of parallel beams that eliminate size distortion. The technique is applied most in long-bone radiography. See also **orthoroentgenography.**

scan path, distinct eye movement patterns.

scapegoating /skāp″gōting/ [ME, *escapen,* to escape, *goot*], the projection of blame, hostility, or suspicion onto one member of a group by other members to avoid self-confrontation.

scapho-, combining form meaning "boat-shaped": *scaphocephaly, scaphoid.*

scaphocephaly /skaf′ōsef″əlē/ [Gk, *skaphe,* skiff, *kephale,* head], a congenital malformation of the skull in which premature closure of the sagittal suture results in restricted lateral growth of the head, giving it an abnormally long, narrow appearance with a cephalic index of 75 or less. Also called **dolichocephaly, mecocephaly,** *scaphocephalis, scaphocephalism.* See also **craniostenosis.**

scaphoid /skaf″oid/ [Gk, *skaphe,* skiff, *eidos,* form], boat-shaped, such as the scaphoid bone of the wrist.

scaphoid abdomen, an abdomen with a sunken anterior wall.

scaphoid bone [Gk, *skaphe* + *eidos,* form; AS, *ban*], either of two similar proximal boat-shaped bones of the hand and the foot. The scaphoid bone of the hand is slanted at the radial side of the carpus and articulates with the radius, trapezium, trapezoideum, capitate, and lunate bones. The scaphoid bone of the foot is located at the medial side of the tarsus between the talus and cuneiform bones and articulates with the talus,

the three cuneiform bones, and occasionally the cuboid bone. Also called **navicular bone.**

scaphoid megalourethra. See **urethral diverticulum.**

scapula /skap″yələ/, one of the pair of large, flat triangular bones that forms the dorsal part of the shoulder girdle. It has two surfaces, three borders, three angles, and a prominent dorsal spine. The acromion of the scapula forms the summit of the shoulder. The coracoid process, resembling a raven's beak, accommodates the attachment of various muscles, including the pectoralis minor, and ligaments, including the trapezoid. Also called **shoulder blade.**

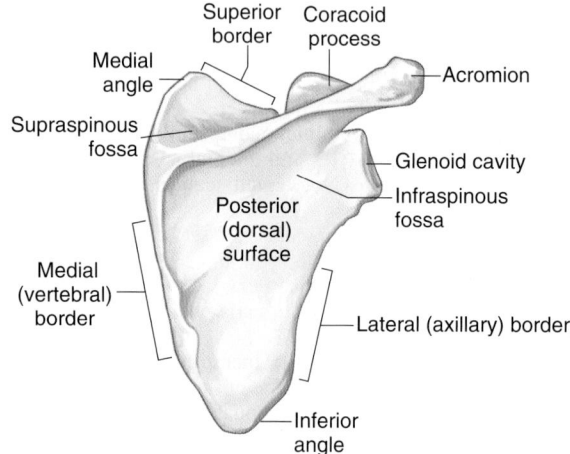

Posterior view of the right scapula *(Patton and Thibodeau, 2010)*

-scapula, suffix meaning "a shoulder blade or a part of it": *subscapularis, suprascapular.*

scapular line /skap″yələr/, an imaginary vertical line drawn through the inferior angle of the scapula.

scapular reflex, a contraction of the rhomboids and approximation of the scapulae when a stimulus is applied to the midline of the back between the scapulae.

scapular winging, a condition in which the vertebral borders of the scapulae move away from the thoracic wall as a result of muscle weakness or nerve damage.

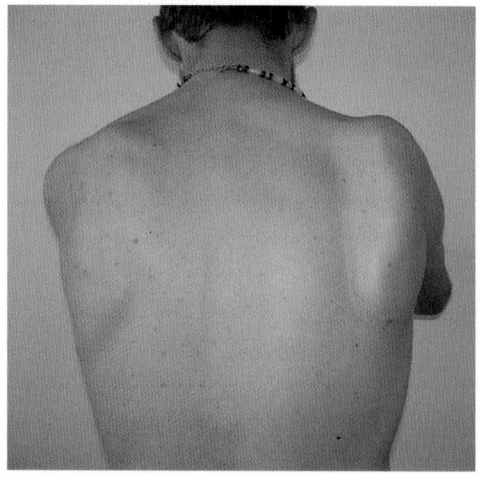

Scapular winging *(Ghosh and Hsich, 2012)*

scapulary /skap″yələr′ē/, a suspender for holding a body bandage in place.

scapulo-, a combining form meaning "scapula or shoulder blade": *scapulohumeral, scapulocostal.*

scapulocostal syndrome /-ōkos″təl/, a condition in which pain radiates from the upper or posterior shoulder area into the neck and back of the head, down the arm, and around the chest. There may also be a tingling in the fingers. The syndrome is associated with a change in the relationship between the shoulder blade and thorax.

scapulohumeral /-ōhyo͞o″mərəl/ [L, *scapula* + *humerus,* shoulder], pertaining to the area around the scapula and humerus.

scapulohumeral muscular dystrophy. See **Erb muscular dystrophy.**

scapulohumeral reflex, a normal response to tapping the vertebral border of the scapula, resulting in adduction of the arm. Absence of the reflex may indicate a lesion in the region of the fifth cervical segment of the spinal cord.

scapus /skā″pəs/ [Gk, *skapos,* rod], a stem or shaft, such as the scapus penis or hair (pili).

scar. See **cicatrix.**

scarf skin, the epidermis, including the cuticle.

scarification /sker′ifikā″shən/ [L, *scarifare,* to scratch open], **1.** multiple superficial scratches or incisions in the skin, such as those made for the introduction of a vaccine. **2.** the process of cutting or burning a design into the skin as a permanent body decoration.

scarify /sker″əfī/ [L, *scarifare*], to make multiple superficial incisions into the skin; to scratch. Vaccination against smallpox was achieved by scarifying the skin under a drop of vaccine. See also **scarification.**

scarlatina. See **scarlet fever.**

scarlatiniform /skär′lətē″nifôrm/ [It, *scarlattina* + L, *forma,* form], resembling the rash of scarlet fever. See also **scarlet fever.**

scarlet fever /skär″lit/ [OFr, *escarlate* + L, *febris,* fever], an acute contagious disease of childhood caused by an erythrotoxin-producing strain of group A hemolytic *Streptococcus.*

■ OBSERVATIONS: Signs and symptoms appear 1 to 3 days after exposure to the agent, starting with an abrupt high fever, chills, tachycardia, nausea, vomiting, headache, abdominal pain, malaise, and a sore throat. The tonsils become enlarged, reddened, and covered with patchy exudate. The pharynx is red and edematous. The tongue is coated and white with red, swollen papillae (white strawberry tongue) until the white coat sloughs off about the fourth day, leaving a red strawberry tongue and red punctate lesions on the palate. A rapidly erupting rash appears 1 to 2 days after the onset of the sore throat. The rash displays as pinhead-size red lesions, which rapidly cover the body except for the face. The rash concentrates in the axial folds, on the neck, and in the groin in bright red lines (Pastia's lines) and lasts 4 to 10 days. The face is flushed on the cheeks with a circumoral pallor. After a week, desquamation and peeling begin on the palms and soles. Diagnosis is made from clinical signs and a rapid strep test or a positive throat culture. Complications include otitis media; sinusitis; peritonsillar abscess; and severe, disseminated toxic or septic disease (fulminating scarlet fever), which may cause septicemia and hepatic damage.

■ INTERVENTIONS: Treatment is aimed at eradicating the streptococcal infection through administration of antibiotics. Antipyretics are given for fever, and analgesics are given for sore throat pain.

■ PATIENT CARE CONSIDERATIONS: Measures are largely supportive and include bed rest during the febrile phase; adequate fluids; gargles, throat lozenges, and throat washes for sore throat; and room humidification for comfort. Respiratory precautions should be instituted until 24 hours after initiation of antibiotics because of the edema in the pharynx and tonsils. Environmentally imposed restraints are used until 24 hours after the initiation of antibiotics to reduce the spread of this communicable disease. Distractive techniques with appropriate developmental activities are used to relieve pain and social isolation. Careful handwashing techniques are used to decrease risk of infection.

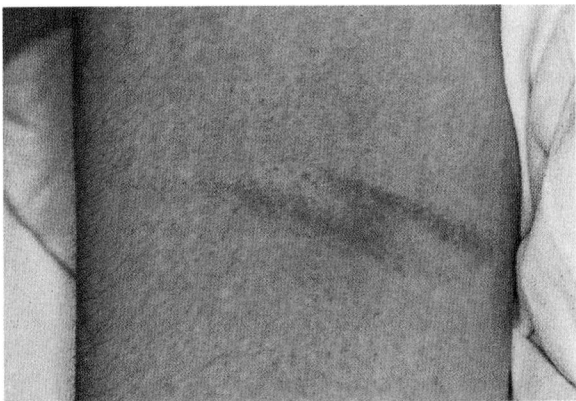

Pastia's lines in scarlet fever (Emond, Wellsby, and Rowland, 2003)

scarlet rash [OFr, *escarlate* + *rasche,* scurf], any scarlatina or rosy skin eruption that accompanies an infection, such as scarlet fever or German measles.

scarlet red, an azo dye that has been used to impart color to pharmaceutic preparations.

Scarpa's fascia, the thin, membranous, deeper layer of fascia in the abdominal wall.

scato-, skato-, prefix meaning "dung" or "fecal matter": *scatology.*

scelotyrbe, an ancient Greek term meaning to walk quickly, used by James Parkinson in his description of the symptoms of Parkinson disease.

scatology /skatol′əjē/ [Gk, *skatos,* dung, *logos,* science], (in biology) the study of feces to obtain information about an individual's diet and health. Also called **coprology.**

scattered radiation /skat″ərd/ [ME, *scateren,* to throw away; L, *radiare,* to emit rays], photons that move in a different direction than the incident photons that produced them, after the interaction of those incident photons. Also called **backscatter radiation.**

scattergram /skat″ərgram′/ [ME, *scateren* + Gk, *gramma,* record], a graph representing the distribution of two variables in a sample population. One variable is plotted on the vertical axis, the second on the horizontal axis. The scores or values of each sample unit are usually represented by dots. A scattergram demonstrates the degree or tendency with which the variables occur in association with each other.

scattering [ME, *scateren*], a change in the direction of photons caused by the interaction between photons and matter. In coherent scattering, an incident photon interacts with matter and excites an atom, causing it to vibrate. The vibration causes the photon to scatter. In unmodified scattering, a small amount of energy changes the direction of the photon path with no net absorption of energy from the original source. In Compton scattering an incident photon interacts with an orbital electron, transferring some of its energy to that electron. The electron is ejected, and the photon is scattered. Also called **Thompson scattering, unmodified scattering.** See also **Compton scatter.**

scavenger cell /skav´ənjər/ [ME, *scavager* + L, *cella,* storeroom], a phagocytic cell that removes tissue debris and some invading pathogens. It may or may not be mobile.

scavenging system. See **gas-scavenging system.**

Sc.D., abbreviation for *Doctor of Science.*

SCE, abbreviation for **saturated calomel electrode.**

scel-, combining form meaning "leg": *scelotyrbe.*

SCFA, abbreviation for **short-chain fatty acids.**

Schamroth window test /sham´rôth/, a test for clubbing of the fingers: the patient holds the fingers back to back against each other. There is normally a diamond-shaped space between the nailbeds and nails of the two fingers. If the space is missing, clubbing is present. See also **clubbing.**

Schedule I, a category of drugs not considered legitimate for medical use. Among the substances so classified by the Drug Enforcement Agency are mescaline, lysergic acid diethylamide, heroin, and marijuana. Special licensing procedures must be followed to use these or other Schedule I substances.

Schedule II, a category of drugs considered to have a strong potential for abuse or addiction but that have legitimate medical use. Among the substances so classified by the Drug Enforcement Agency are morphine, cocaine, pentobarbital, oxycodone, alphaprodine, and methadone.

Schedule III, a category of drugs that have less potential for abuse or addiction than Schedule II or I drugs. Among the substances so classified by the Drug Enforcement Agency are glutethimide and various analgesic compounds containing codeine.

Schedule IV, a category of drugs that have less potential for abuse or addiction than those of Schedules I to III. Among the substances so classified by the Drug Enforcement Agency are chloral hydrate, chlordiazepoxide, meprobamate, and oxazepam.

Schedule V, a category of drugs that have a small potential for abuse or addiction. Among the substances so classified by the Drug Enforcement Agency are many commonly prescribed medications that contain small amounts of codeine or diphenoxylate. The specific drugs in Schedule V vary greatly from state to state.

Schedule for Affective Disorders and Schizophrenia, a semistructured interview administered by a professional and designed to yield diagnostic information about current and lifetime incidences of affective disorders and schizophrenia.

Schedule of Drugs [L, *scheda,* sheet of paper; Fr, *drogue*], a classification system that categorizes drugs by their potential for abuse. The schedule is divided into five groups: Schedules I to V. The assignment of drugs to the categories varies from state to state. Schedule I substances are not approved for medical use. All substances in Schedules II to V require a written prescription signed by a physician. Substances in Schedule V may or may not require a written prescription signed by a physician, depending on state law. Specific regulations for dispensing these substances vary from state to state and from institution to institution. See also **controlled substance, Controlled Substances Act.**

Scheie syndrome /shā/ [Harold Glendon Scheie, American ophthalmologist, 1909–1990], a relatively mild variant of Hurler syndrome, a heritable mucopolysaccharide storage disease, characterized by corneal clouding, claw hand, involvement of the aortic valve, somewhat coarse facies with a broad mouth, genu valgum, and pes cavus. Stature, intelligence, and life span are normal. See also **Hurler syndrome.**

schema /skē´mə/, an innate knowledge structure that allows a child to organize in his or her mind ways to behave in his or her environment.

schematic /skēmat´ik/, pertaining to a schema, model, or diagram representing, without absolute precision, a structure, strategy, or system. An anatomical chart is an example.

schematic eye, 1. a simplified and enlarged illustration of the eye, featuring its anatomical details. **2.** a graphic illustration of the normal eye, with data for curvatures, indices of refraction, and distances between optical elements.

Scheuermann disease /shoi´ərmon/ [Holger W. Scheuermann, Danish surgeon, 1877–1960], an abnormal skeletal condition characterized by a fixed kyphosis that develops at puberty and is caused by wedge-shaped deformities of one or several vertebrae. The cause may be infection, inflammatory processes, aseptic necrosis, disk deterioration, mechanical influences, inadequate circulation during rapid growth, or disturbances of epiphyseal growth caused by protrusion of the intervertebral disk through deficient or defective cartilaginous plates. The most striking pathological feature of Scheuermann disease is the presence of wedge-shaped vertebral bodies, seen on radiographic examination, that create an excessive curvature. Scheuermann disease occurs most frequently in children between 12 and 16 years of age, with the onset at puberty, and the incidence is greater in girls than in boys. The onset is insidious and often associated with a history of unusual physical activity or participation in sports. The most frequent symptom is poor posture, with accompanying symptoms of fatigue and pain in the involved area. Tenderness and stiffness may also affect the area involved or the entire spinal column. In most affected individuals the kyphosis is within the thoracic vertebrae. If the disease is diagnosed at the onset, the associated posture may be corrected. Otherwise, the associated posture becomes fixed within a period of 6 to 9 months. The most effective treatment of Scheuermann disease is immobilization with a cast or Milwaukee brace. The immobilization is continuous for 10 to 12 months, with additional immobilization at night for about the same length of time. Immobilization is usually supplemented with an exercise program that is continued after the immobilization is terminated. In adults persistent pain in the thoracic area may indicate a degenerative alteration secondary to this disease process, and spinal arthrodesis may be required to relieve the symptoms. Also called **adolescent vertebral epiphysitis, juvenile kyphosis.**

Schick test /shik/ [Bela Schick, Austrian-American physician, 1877–1967], a skin test formerly used to determine immunity to diphtheria in which dilute diphtheria toxin was injected intradermally. A positive reaction, indicating susceptibility, was marked by redness and swelling at the site of injection; a negative reaction, indicating immunity, was marked by absence of redness or swelling. This test, along with vaccination, was a major factor in the reduction of diphtheria from epidemic proportions in the 20th century to an extremely rare occurrence.

Schilder disease /shil´dər/ [Paul F. Schilder, Austrian neurologist, 1886–1940], a group of severe progressive neurological diseases beginning in childhood. All are characterized by demyelination of the white matter of the brain, with muscle spasticity, optic neuritis, aphasia, deafness, adrenal insufficiency, and dementia. Many of the signs resemble those of multiple sclerosis. Also called **encephalitis periaxialis diffusa, Flatau-Schilder disease, progressive subcortical encephalopathy,** *Schilder encephalitis.* See also **adrenoleukodystrophy.**

Schiller test /shil´ər/ [Walter Schiller, Austrian pathologist in the United States, 1887–1960], a procedure for indicating areas of abnormal epithelium in the vagina or on the cervix of the uterus as a guide in selecting biopsy sites for cancer detection. A potassium iodide or aqueous iodine solution is painted on the vaginal walls and cervix under direct visualization. Normal epithelium contains glycogen and stains a deep brown; abnormal epithelium, containing no glycogen, will not stain, and nonstaining sites may then be included in tissue biopsy samples. The test is not specific for malignancy, because inflammation, ulceration, and keratotic lesions also may not accept the iodine stain.

Schilling leukemia. See **monocytic leukemia.**

Schilling test /shil″ing/ [Robert F. Schilling, American hematologist, b. 1919], a diagnostic test for pernicious anemia in which vitamin B_{12} tagged with radioactive cobalt is administered orally, and GI absorption is measured by determining the radioactivity of urine samples collected over a 24-hour period. Normal findings show excretion of 8% to 40% of radioactive vitamin B_{12} within 24 hours. In people with pernicious anemia, the ability to absorb vitamin B_{12} from the GI tract is reduced so that excretion of radioactive material in the urine is reduced. This test is rarely used today.

schindylesis /skin′dilē″sis/ [Gk, splintering], an articulation (synarthrosis) of certain bones of the skull in which a thin plate of one bone enters a cleft formed by the separation of two layers of another bone, such as the insertion of the vomer bone into the fissure between the maxillae and the palatine bones.

Schinzel-Giedion syndrome, a rare syndrome, probably of autosomal-recessive inheritance, of hydronephrosis, skeletal abnormalities, flattened midface, hypertrichosis, seizures, and profound growth and developmental delays.

Schiötz tonometer /shē·ets″/ [Hjalmar Schiötz, Norwegian ophthalmologist, 1850–1927; Gk, *tonos,* stretching, *metron,* measure], a tonometer used to measure intraocular pressure by observing the depth of indentation of the cornea made by the weighted plunger on the device after a topical anesthetic is applied.

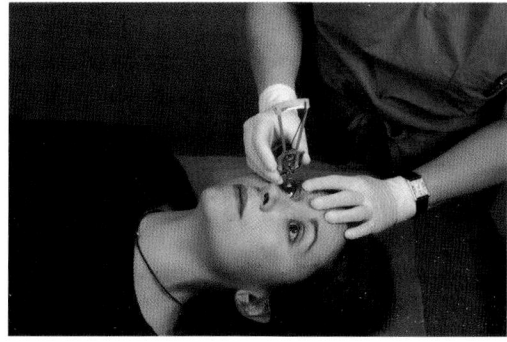

Schiötz tonometer *(Custalow, 2005)*

Schirmer test [Otto W.A. Schirmer, German ophthalmologist, 1864–1917]. See **test for lacrimation.**

schisandra, an herb that is native to China, Russia, and Korea.
- INDICATIONS: It is used for GI disorders, for liver protection, and as a tonic and may have some efficacy.
- CONTRAINDICATIONS: It should not be used during pregnancy and lactation, in children, or in those with known hypersensitivity to this plant.

schisto-, combining form meaning "split" or "cleft": *schistocelia, schistocyte, schistocystis.*

schistocelia /shis′təsē″lyə/, a congenital fissure in the wall of the abdomen.

schistocystis /shis′təsis″tis/ [Gk, *schistos,* cleft, *kystis,* bag], a fissure in the bladder.

schistocyte /shis″təsīt/ [Gk, *schistos,* cleft, *kytos,* cell], an erythrocyte cell fragment characteristic of hemolysis or cell fragmentation associated with severe burns, microangiopathic hemolytic anemias, and intravascular coagulation. Also called **schizocyte.**

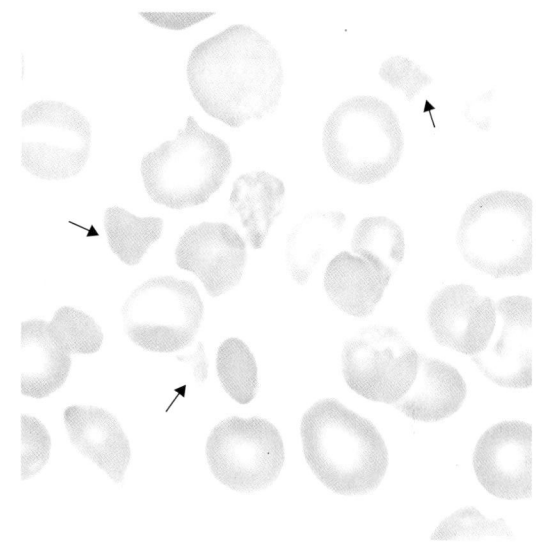

Schistocyte *(Carr and Rodak, 2008)*

Schistosoma /shis′təsō″mə/ [Gk, *schistos,* cleft, *soma,* body], a genus of blood flukes that may cause urinary, GI, or liver disease in humans and that requires fecal contamination of water and freshwater snails as intermediate hosts. *Schistosoma haematobium,* found chiefly in Africa and the Middle East, affects the bladder, ureter, and pelvic organs, causing painful frequent urination and hematuria. *S. japonicum,* found in Japan, the Philippines, and Eastern Asia, causes GI ulcerations and fibrosis of the liver. *S. mansoni,* found in Africa, the Middle East, the Caribbean, and tropical America, causes symptoms similar to those caused by *S. japonicum.*

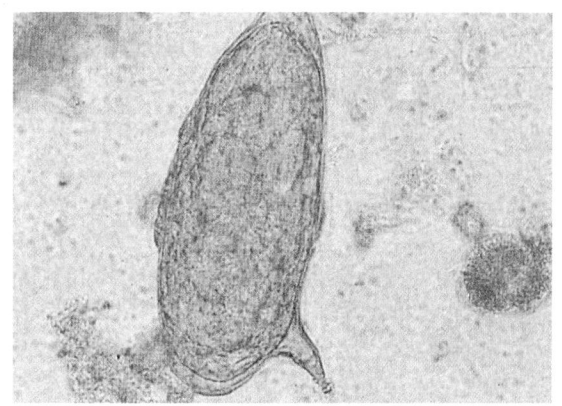

Schistosoma mansoni egg *(Murray, Rosenthal, and Pfaller, 2002)*

schistosome dermatitis. See **swimmer's itch.**

schistosomiasis /shis′təsōmī′əsis/ [Gk, *schistos* + *soma* + *osis,* condition], a parasitic infection caused by a species of fluke of the genus *Schistosoma.* It is transmitted to humans, the definitive host, by contact with water containing the infective stage of the parasite, the cercaria. A single fluke may live in one part of the body, depositing eggs frequently, for up to 20 years. The eggs are irritating to mucous membrane, causing it to thicken and become papillomatous. Symptoms depend on the part of the body infected. *Schistosoma* may be found in the bladder, rectum, liver, lungs, spleen, intestines, and portal venous system. Pain, obstruction, dysfunction of the affected organ, and anemia may result. Diagnosis requires morphological identification of the ova or the parasite. Depending on the species, treatment may be with praziquantel, oxamniquine, or metrifonate. Prevention is more effective. Proper disposal of human urine and feces, chlorination of water, and eradication of the intermediate host, the freshwater snail *Australorbis glabratus,* are totally effective. Second only to malaria in the number of people affected, schistosomiasis is particularly prevalent in the tropics and in Asia. Also called **bilharziasis.** See also **blood fluke,** *Schistosoma.*

schistosomicide /shis′təsō″məsīd/ [Gk, *schistos* + *soma* + L, *caedere,* to kill], a drug destructive to schistosomes, blood flukes transmitted by snails to human hosts in many parts of Africa, Brazil, and Asia. Praziquantel, albendazole, niridazole, metrifonate, oxamniquine hycanthone hydrochloride, and various salts of antimony, including stibophen, are potent antischistosomal agents. −*schistosomicidal, adj.*

schistothorax /-thôr″aks/, a congenital cleft in the wall of the thorax. Also called *schistosternia.*

schizencephaly /skiz′ensef″əlē/, an abnormal cleavage or other division of the brain tissues caused by maldevelopment.

schizo-, combining form meaning "divided" or "related to division": *schizogenesis, schizophrenia.*

schizoaffective disorder /skit′sō·afek″tiv/ [Gk, *schizein,* to split; L, *affectus,* state of mind, *dis,* opposite of, *ordo,* rank], a psychiatric disorder in which either a major depressive or a manic episode develops concurrently with symptoms of schizophrenia, such as hallucinations and delusions.

schizocyte. See **schistocyte.**

schizogenesis /skit′səjen″əsis/ [Gk, *schizein* + *genesis,* origin], reproduction by fission. −*schizogenous, schizogenetic, schizogenic, adj.*

schizogonic, schizogonous, pertaining to a cell that divides by a process of asexual reproduction. See **schizont.**

schizogony, a form of asexual reproduction characteristic of certain protozoa, including sporozoa, in which daughter cells are produced by multiple fission of the nucleus of the parasite (schizont), followed by segmentation of the cytoplasm to form separate masses around each smaller nucleus.

schizogyria /skit′səjī′rē·ə/, the presence of wedge-shaped cracks in the convolutions of the brain.

schizoid /skit″soid, skiz″oid/ [Gk, *schizein,* to split, *eidos,* form], **1.** *adj.,* characteristic of or resembling schizophrenia; schizophrenic. **2.** *n.,* a person, not necessarily a schizophrenic, who exhibits the traits of a schizoid personality.

schizoid personality, a functioning but maladjusted person whose behavior is characterized by extreme shyness, oversensitivity, introversion, seclusiveness, and avoidance of close interpersonal relationships. See also **schizoid personality disorder, schizophrenia.**

schizoid personality disorder, a personality disorder characterized by a defect in the ability to form interpersonal relationships, as shown by emotional coldness and aloofness, withdrawn and seclusive behavior, and indifference to praise, criticism, and the feelings of others. The person is unable to express hostility and ordinary aggressive feelings and reacts to disturbing experiences with apparent detachment. The person neither desires nor enjoys personal relationships, prefers solitary activities, and has no close friends or confidants.

schizont /skitsənt/ [Gk, *schizein* + *genein,* to produce], **1.** reproduction by multiple fission. **2.** the multinucleated cell stage during the asexual reproductive phase in the life cycle of a sporozoon, such as the malarial parasite *Plasmodium.*

schizonticide /skitson″təsīd/ [Gk, *schizein* + *on,* being; L, *caedere,* to kill], a substance that destroys schizonts. −*schizonticidal, adj.*

schizophasia /skit′səfā″zhə, skiz′ə-/ [Gk, *schizein* + *phasis,* speech], the disordered, incomprehensible speech characteristic of some forms of schizophrenia. See also **word salad.**

schizophrenia /skit′səfrē″nē·ə, skiz′ə-/ [Gk, *schizein,* to split, *phren,* mind], any one of a large group of psychotic disorders characterized by gross distortion of reality, disturbances of language and cognitive function, withdrawal from social interaction, disorganization and fragmentation of thought, altered perception, and emotional reaction. The term *schizophrenia* denotes one of the fundamental characteristics of the patients, the splitting off of a part of the psyche. The part that splits off then dominates the psychic life of the patient, even though it may express behavior that is contrary to the original personality of the patient. Apathy and confusion; delusions and hallucinations; rambling or stylized patterns of speech, such as evasiveness, incoherence, and echolalia; withdrawn, regressive, and bizarre behavior; and emotional lability often occur. Most patients have both positive and negative psychotic symptoms. Positive symptoms include hallucinations; negative symptoms include anergia, flatness, and anhedonia. The condition may be mild or require prolonged hospitalization. No single cause of the disorder is known; genetic, biochemical, psychological, interpersonal, and sociocultural factors are usually involved. Although slowly progressive deterioration of the personality may occur, dementia is not an inevitable consequence of the disorder. There may be recovery in some cases, and there may be relapse marked by intermittent episodes that begin after prolonged remission. Formerly called **dementia praecox.**

■ OBSERVATIONS: Characteristics vary in type and severity, and onset may be sudden or insidious. Symptomatic periods may be episodic or continuous. Typical characteristics are divided into prodromal (pre/early), positive (excess/distortion of normal function), and negative (reduction /loss of normal function) symptoms. Prodromal symptoms include withdrawal, social isolation, reduced interest or initiative, elaborate speech, magical thinking, unusual perceptual experiences, and strange behaviors. Positive symptoms include psychosis as evidenced by distortions of thought content (delusions) and/or perceptual distortion (hallucinations) and disorganization evidenced by disorganized speech and behavior. Negative symptoms include restricted emotional expression (flattened affect), poverty of speech (alogia), apathy, decreased ability to experience pleasure (anhedonia), difficulty naming or describing emotions (alexithymia), and a lack of interest in social relationships. These symptoms often resemble depression. The various manifestations greatly impair the ability to function and interfere with work, relationships, and self-care, ultimately leading to social isolation. Deterioration in function is marked in the first 5 years, with a plateau effect later in the disease process. Suicide is the major cause of premature death in schizophrenics. Comorbid substance abuse is a significant problem for about 50% of individuals with schizophrenia and signals the likelihood of a poor outcome. Diagnosis is made primarily through careful clinical history and evaluation. Diagnostic criteria include two or more of the following: delusions, hallucinations, disorganized speech or behavior, catatonia, and negative symptoms for at least a month with evidence of prodromal manifestations or social, occupational, or self-care impairments for at least 6 months. A neurological exam may exhibit soft signs, such as astereognosis, agraphesthesia, dysdiadochokinesia, muscle twitching, increased eye blinks, impaired fine motor movements, or abnormal smooth pursuit eye movements. CT scan or MRI may reveal structural brain abnormalities; medial and superior lobe abnormalities may be seen with positive manifestations; and frontal, cortical, and ventricular system abnormalities may be seen with negative manifestations.

■ INTERVENTIONS: Hospital milieu is helpful for early disease stages to introduce and regulate antipsychotic medications. Crisis care is indicated for high-risk periods for harm (suicide and/or violence). Antipsychotics are used for control of delusions/hallucinations, and sedatives are administered for agitation. Medication compliance is a long-term focus of treatment. Antiparkinsonian agents are used to treat tardive dyskinesia, which may result from use of traditional neuroleptic drugs. Prevention efforts are focused on long-term antipsychotic drug prophylaxis for individuals who have had one schizophrenia episode.

■ PATIENT CARE CONSIDERATIONS: Significant social support is needed for most schizophrenic patients and their families. Support includes supportive psychotherapy, psychosocial skill training, vocational rehabilitation, occupational therapy for activities of daily living, and community support services to promote self-care. Specialized programs and structured, supervised living environments are needed for dual diagnosis patients (schizophrenia and substance abuse). Families may benefit from family therapy and respite care. Individual and family education are needed about the disease process, including psychosis identification, symptoms of relapse, and medication effects and side effects. The importance of long-term medication compliance is stressed. Instruction is needed in coping strategies to increase daily functioning. Information and referral to community support systems can aid individual and family coping (e.g., National Alliance for the Mentally Ill).

schizophrenic /skit′səfren″ik, skiz′ə-/, **1.** *adj.,* pertaining to schizophrenia. **2.** *n.,* a person with schizophrenia.

schizophreniform disorder /-fren″ifôrm/ [Gk, *schizein* + *phren* + L, *forma,* form], a psychiatric disorder exhibiting the same symptoms as schizophrenia but characterized by an acute onset with resolution in 4 weeks to 6 months.

schizophrenogenic /skit′səfren′əjen″ik, skiz′ə-/ [Gk, *schizein* + *phren* + *genein,* to produce], tending to cause or produce schizophrenia.

Schizotrypanum cruzi. See **Chagas disease.**

schizotypal personality disorder /skit′sōtī″pəl/ [Gk, *schizein* + *typos,* mark; L, *personalis,* of a person, *dis,* opposite of, *ordo,* rank], a psychiatric disorder characterized by oddities of thought, perception, speech, and behavior that are not severe enough to meet the clinical criteria for schizophrenia. Symptoms may include magical thinking inconsistent with cultural norms, such as superstitiousness, belief in clairvoyance and telepathy, and bizarre

fantasies; ideas of reference; recurrent illusions, such as sensing the presence of a force or person not actually present; social isolation; peculiar speech patterns, including ideas expressed unclearly or words used deviantly; and exaggerated anxiety or hypersensitivity to real or imagined criticism. See also **schizoid personality disorder, schizophrenia.**

Schlatter-Osgood disease, Schlatter's disease. See **Osgood-Schlatter disease.**

Schlemm's canal. See **canal of Schlemm.**

schlieren optics /shlir″ən/ [Ger, *schlieren,* ulcers, streaks], a system that observes the refractive index gradient in solutions containing macromolecules.

Schmidt syndrome[1] /shmit/ [Adolf Schmidt, German physician, 1865–1918], paralysis on one side affecting the vocal cord, the soft palate, the trapezius muscle, and the sternocleidomastoid muscle, resulting from a lesion in the brain. Also called **vagoaccessory syndrome.**

Schmidt syndrome[2] [Martin Benno Schmidt, German pathologist, 1863–1949], See **polyglandular autoimmune syndromes.**

Schneiderian carcinoma /shnīdir″ē·ən/, an epithelial malignancy of the nasal mucosa and paranasal sinuses.

Schoenhofer, Savina O., a nursing theorist who, with Anne Boykin, wrote *Nursing as Caring: A Model for Transforming Practice,* which postulates that caring is the end, not the means, of nursing.

Schönlein-Henoch purpura. See **Henoch-Schönlein purpura.**

school phobia [AS, *scol* + Gk, *phobos,* fear], an extreme separation anxiety disorder of children, usually in the elementary grades, characterized by a persistent irrational fear of going to school or being in a school-like atmosphere. Such children are usually oversensitive, shy, timid, nervous, and emotionally immature and have pervasive feelings of inadequacy. They typically try to cope with their fears by becoming overdependent on others, especially the parents.

Schüffner's dots [Wilhelm A.P. Schüffner, German pathologist, 1867–1949], coarse pink or red granules seen in the red blood cells of patients with tertiary malaria. They are signs of *Plasmodium vivax* or *P. ovale* and are absent in blood cells of patients infected with other types of malaria.

Schuller method, a technique for positioning a patient's head in a true lateral position to produce a radiographic image of the mastoid and petrous portions of the temporal bone as well as the temporomandibular joint of the side closest to the image receptor. Both temporomandibular joints are imaged with the mouth open and closed.

Schultz-Charlton phenomenon, a reaction that occurs when scarlet fever antitoxin or scarlet fever convalescent serum is injected into an area of the skin showing a bright red rash. A blanching of the skin at the site of the injection occurs. Serum from scarlet fever patients does not produce this reaction.

Schultze's mechanism, the delivery of a placenta with the fetal surfaces presenting.

Schwann cell /shwon/ [Theodor Schwann, German anatomist, 1810–1882], any of the cells of ectodermal origin that make up the neurilemma. They form the myelin sheath around peripheral nerve fibers.

schwannoma /shwonō″mə/ *pl.* schwannomas, schwannomata [Theodor Schwann; Gk, *oma,* tumor], a benign, solitary, encapsulated tumor arising in the neurilemma (Schwann's sheath) of peripheral, cranial, or autonomic nerves. Also called **neurilemmoma,** *Schwann cell tumor.*

S

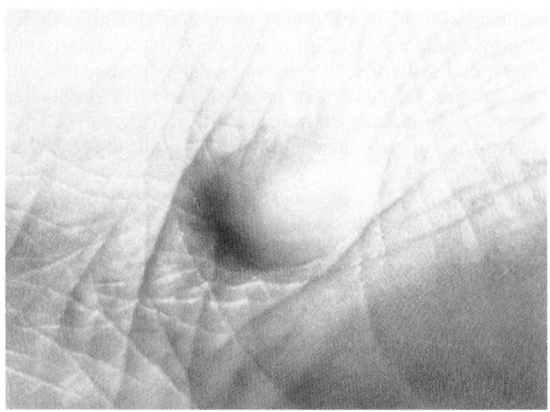

Schwannoma on the sole of the foot (du Vivier, 2002)

schwannosis /shwonō″sis/ [Theodor Schwann; Gk, *osis,* condition], a condition of overgrowth of the neurilemma or sheath of Schwann.

Schwann's sheath. See **neurilemma.**

Schwartz bed. See **hyperextension bed.**

Schwartz-Jampel syndrome /shworts·jam′pəl/ [Oscar Schwartz, American pediatrician, b. 1919; Robert Steven Jampel, American ophthalmologist, b. 1926], an autosomal-recessive disorder characterized by myotonic myopathy, dwarfism, abnormal narrowness of the palpebral fissures in the horizontal direction, joint contractures, and flat facies. Also called **chondrodystrophic myotonia.**

Schwartzman-Sanarelli phenomenon /shvorts′man san′- ərel″ē/ [Gregory Schwartzman, American physician, b. 1896; Giuseppe Sanarelli, Italian bacteriologist, 1864– 1940], a condition induced experimentally in the investigation of the role of coagulation in renal disease. Animals injected twice with a bacterial endotoxin experience massive disseminated intravascular coagulation with blood clots in the vessels of the kidneys. Also called *Schwartzman phenomenon.*

scia-. See **skia-, scia-.**

sciatic /sī·at″ik/ [Gk, *ischiadikos,* hip joint], pertaining to an area near the ischium, such as the sciatic nerve or the sciatic vein.

sciatica /sī·at″ikə/, an inflammation of the sciatic nerve, usually marked by pain and tenderness along the course of the nerve through the thigh and leg. It may result in a wasting of the muscles of the lower leg over time. Also called **sciatic neuritis.**

sciatic dislocation. See **dislocation of the hip.**

sciatic hernia, a protrusion of tissue through the greater sciatic notch.

sciatic nerve, a long nerve originating in the sacral plexus and extending through the muscles of the thigh, leg, and foot, with numerous branches.

sciatic neuritis. See **sciatica.**

sciatic scoliosis, lateral curvature of the spine caused by an asymmetric spasm of the spinal muscles, often resulting in a list to one side.

SCID, abbreviation for **severe combined immunodeficiency disease.**

SCID mouse, (*severe combined immunodeficiency*) a strain of mice lacking in T and B lymphocytes and immunoglobulins, either from inbreeding with an autosomal-recessive trait or from genetic engineering, used as a model for studies of the immune system.

science /sī″əns/ [L, *scientia,* knowledge], a systematic attempt to establish theories to explain observed phenomena and the knowledge obtained through these efforts. Pure science is concerned with the gathering of information solely for the sake of obtaining new knowledge. Applied science is the practical application of scientific theory and laws. See also **hypothesis, law, scientific method, theory.**

Science of Unitary Human Beings, a conceptual model and theory of nursing proposed by Martha Rogers in 1970. Its four basic concepts focus on the nature and direction of "unitary human development": (1) human and environmental energy fields, (2) complete and continuous openness of the energy fields, (3) human energy fields perceived as single waves that give identity to a field, and (4) "pandimensionality," a nonlinear domain without spatial or temporal attributes. See also **Rogers, Martha E.**

scientific method /sī′əntif″ik/, a systematic, ordered approach to the gathering of data and the solving of problems. The basic approach is the statement of the problem followed by the statement of a hypothesis. An experimental method is established to help confirm or negate the hypothesis. The results of the experiment are observed, and conclusions are drawn from observed results. The conclusions may tend to uphold or to refute the hypothesis.

scientific rationale, a reason, based on supporting scientific evidence, that a particular action is chosen.

scimitar sign /sim″ətər/, an arteriographic sign of encroachment on the popliteal or femoral lumen in adventitial cystic disease.

scimitar syndrome, a radiographic sign caused by a congenital disorder in which the right lower pulmonary vein drains into the inferior vena cava. On a chest radiograph, the abnormal vessel configuration produces a scimitar-shaped shadow. Also called *pulmonary venolobar syndrome.*

scintigram /sin″tigram′/ [L, *scintillare,* to sparkle; Gk, *gramma,* record], a recording of the radioactivity emitted by a tracer in an organism or organ system.

scintigraph /sin″tigraf′/, an image showing the distribution and intensity of radioactivity in various tissues and organs after the administration of a radiopharmaceutical.

scintillating scotoma /sin″tilā″ting/ [L, *scintillatio,* sparkling; Gk *skotos* dark, *oma* tumor], an abnormal area of the visual field that is positive and luminous, sometimes becoming hemianopic and appearing in a migraine aura.

scintillation detector /sin″tilā″shən/ [L, *scintillatio,* sparkling], **1.** a device that detects the light emitted by a crystal subjected to ionizing radiation. A photomultiplier tube in the detector converts the light into an electric signal that can be processed further. An array of scintillation detectors is used in a gamma camera. **2.** a device used to measure the amount of radioactivity in an area of the body.

scintillation scanning, the process that results in a scintiscan.

scintiscan /sin″tiscan′/, a visible image display of the distribution of a radiopharmaceutical within the body.

scirrho-, combining form meaning "hard" or "related to a hard cancer or scirrhus": *scirrhous.*

scirrhous carcinoma /skir″əs/ [Gk, *skirrhos,* hard, *karkinos,* crab, *oma,* tumor], a hard, fibrous, particularly invasive tumor in which the malignant cells occur singly or in small clusters or strands in dense connective tissue. Also called **carcinoma fibrosum.** See also **breast cancer.**

scissor gait /siz″ər/ [L, *scindere,* to cut; ONorse, *gata,* way], a manner of walking cross-legged, as observed in spastic paraplegia.

scissor legs [L, *scindere,* to cut; ONorse, *leggr*], legs that are crossed because of a disorder of the adductor muscles of the thigh or a deformity of the hip.

scissors [L, *scindere,* to cut], a sharp instrument composed of two opposing cutting blades held together by a central pin on which the blades pivot. The most common dissecting scissors are the straight Mayo scissors, for cutting sutures; the Snowden-Pencer scissors, for deep, delicate tissue; the long curved Mayo scissors, for deep, heavy, or tough tissue; the short curved Metzenbaum scissors, for superficial, delicate tissue; and the long, blunt curved Metzenbaum scissors, for deep, delicate tissue.

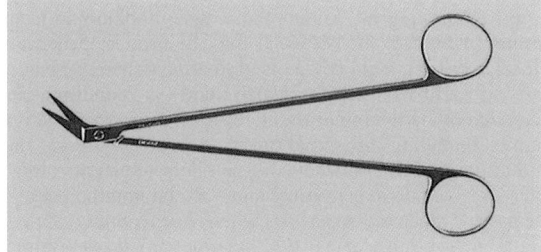

Potts-Smith cardiovascular scissors *(Tighe, 2012)*

SCL, abbreviation for **soft contact lens.**

scler-. See **sclero-, scler-, sklero-.**

sclera /sklir″ə/ [Gk, *skleros,* hard], the tough, inelastic white opaque membrane covering the posterior five sixths of the eyebulb. It maintains the size and form of the bulb and attaches to muscles that move the bulb. Posteriorly it is pierced by the optic nerve and, with the transparent cornea, makes up the outermost of three tunics covering the eyebulb.

scleredema /sklir′ədē″mə/ [Gk, *skleros* + *oidema,* swelling], an idiopathic skin disease characterized by nonpitting induration beginning on the face or neck and spreading downward over the body, sparing the hands and feet. There also may be tongue swelling, restriction of eye movements, and pericardial, pleural, and peritoneal effusions. Resolution occurs after several months, but recurrences are common. The condition often follows a streptococcal infection or an exanthem of childhood. There is no specific treatment. Compare **scleroderma.**

sclerema neonatorum /sklirē″mə/ [Gk, *skleros* + *neos,* new; L, *natus,* birth], a progressive generalized hardening of the skin and subcutaneous tissue of the newborn. It is usually a fatal condition that results from severe cold stress in severely ill premature infants subject to such life-threatening conditions as metabolic acidosis, hypoglycemia, GI or respiratory infection, or gross malformation. Also called *scleredema neonatorum, sclerema adiposum,* **scleroderma neonatorum.**

scleritis /sklirī″tis/ [Gk, *skleros,* hard, *itis,* inflammation], an inflammation of the sclera.

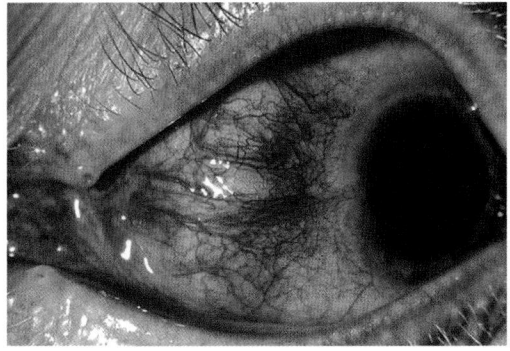

Nodular scleritis *(Courtesy Karen Ann Klima, BA, CRA, COMT, The Johns Hopkins Center for Hereditary Eye Diseases, The Wilmer Eye Institute)*

scleroconjunctival /sklir′ōkon′jungktī″vəl/, pertaining to the sclera and conjunctiva.

sclerocornea /-kôr″nē·ə/, the cornea and sclera of the eye surface considered as a single layer.

sclerodactyly /sklir′ōdak″tilē/ [Gk, *skleros* + *daktylos,* finger], a musculoskeletal deformity affecting the hands of people with scleroderma. The fingers are fixed in a semi-flexed position, with subcutaneous calcification and tightened skin to the wrist. The fingertips may be ulcerated.

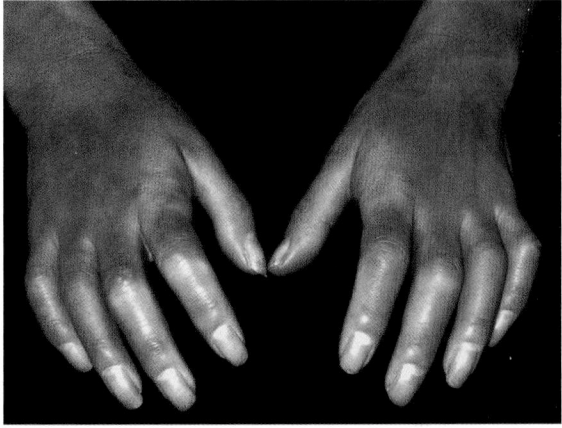

Sclerodactyly *(Firestein and Kelley, 2009)*

scleroderma /sklir′ōdur″mə/ [Gk, *skleros* + *derma,* skin], chronic hardening and thickening of the skin caused by new collagen formation, with atrophy of pilosebaceous follicles. Scleroderma is most common in middle-aged women. It may occur in a localized form (morphea) or as a systemic disease (systemic sclerosis). Progressive systemic sclerosis (PSS) is a relatively rare autoimmune disease affecting the blood vessels and connective tissue. It is characterized by fibrous degeneration of the connective tissue of the skin, lungs, and internal organs, especially the esophagus, digestive tract, and kidneys. See also **morphea, systemic sclerosis.**

■ OBSERVATIONS: The most common initial complaints are changes in the skin of the face and fingers. Raynaud phenomenon occurs with a gradual hardening of the skin and swelling of the distal extremities. In the early stages the disease may be confused with rheumatoid arthritis or Raynaud disease. As the disease progresses, deformity of the joints and pain on movement occur. Skin changes include edema and then pallor; then the skin becomes firm; finally it becomes slightly pigmented and fixed to the underlying tissues. At this stage the skin of the face is taut, shiny, and masklike, and the patient may have difficulty in chewing and swallowing. Patients with mild forms of scleroderma may live to 30 to 50 years of age. Those with cardiac, renal, pulmonary, or intestinal involvement may die at an earlier age. The usual indication that renal disease is present is the abrupt onset of severe arterial hypertension that does not respond to medication. Localized forms of scleroderma may occur; these cases are benign and appear only as small circumscribed patches on the skin. A biopsy of the lesion may be done to diagnose the condition. Radiographic examination of the lungs and GI tract may be diagnostic in the systemic form of the disease. Blood tests may reveal antinuclear antibodies.

■ INTERVENTIONS: There are no drugs to cure scleroderma; however, corticosteroids, immunosuppressants, antacids, and histamine receptor antagonists may be useful in treating the

S

symptoms of the disease, and salicylates and mild analgesics are given to ease pain in the joints. Physical therapy slows the development of muscle contracture and resultant deformity and debility. Nephrectomy or renal transplantation may be performed. ■ PATIENT CARE CONSIDERATIONS: The health care provider advises patients to use mild nonalcoholic astringent soaps; to avoid extreme cold and activities that trigger pain; to wear gloves; to stop smoking; and to eat small, frequent meals. In the advanced stages of scleroderma patients often require help to eat, and care of the mouth and skin is particularly important. As patients deteriorate, there is a need for considerable emotional support.

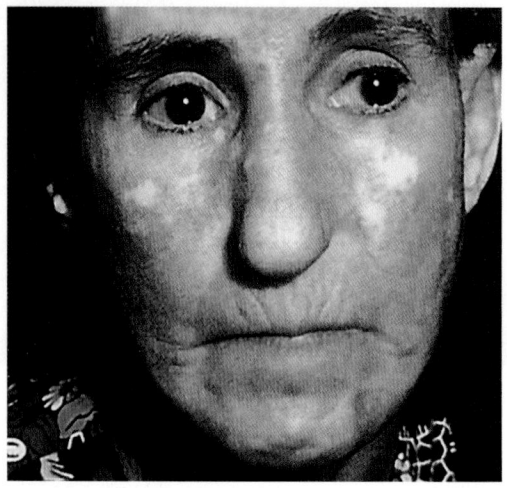

Individual with scleroderma *(Goldman et al, 2008)*

scleroderma heart, a cardiac condition characterized by interstitial myocardial fibrosis and thickening of the small blood vessels in progressive systemic sclerosis.

scleroderma neonatorum. See **sclerema neonatorum.**

sclerodermatitis /-dur′mətī″tis/, an inflammation, thickening, and hardening of the skin.

sclerokeratitis /-ker′ətī″tis/, an inflammation of the sclera and cornea.

-scleroma, suffix meaning "an induration, a hardening of the tissues": *rhinoscleroma.*

scleromalacia perforans /sklir′ōməlā″shə/ [Gk, *skleros* + *malakia,* softening; L, *perforare,* to pierce], a condition of the eyes in which devitalization and sloughing of the sclera occur as a complication of rheumatoid arthritis. The pigmented uvea becomes exposed, and glaucoma, cataract formation, and detachment of the retina may result.

sclero-, scler-, sklero-, combining form meaning "hard," often used to show relationship to the sclera: *scleritis, scleroderma, sclerocornea.*

sclerose /sklərōz″/ [Gk, *skleros*], to harden or to cause hardening. **–sclerotic,** *adj.*

sclerosing /sklirō″zing/ [Gk, *skleros,* hard], pertaining to the tissue changes or other factors involved in the progress of sclerosis.

sclerosing hemangioma [Gk, *skleros* + *haima,* blood, *angeion* vessel, *oma* tumor], a solid cellular tumorlike nodule of the skin or a mass of histiocytes, thought to arise from a hemangioma by the proliferation of endothelial and connective tissue cells.

sclerosing keratitis [Gk, *skleros,* hard, *keras,* horn, *itis,* inflammation], **1.** a form of corneal inflammation in which nodular infiltrates appear near the margin of the cornea in association with a ring of anterior scleritis. **2.** a form of corneal inflammation characterized by an opaque triangle in the deep layers of the cornea, with the base of the triangle near the sclerosing area.

sclerosing phlebitis [Gk, *skleros,* hard, *phleps,* vein, *itis,* inflammation], inflammation of a vein that has become hardened and obstructed.

sclerosing solution [Gk, *skleros* + L, *solvere,* to dissolve], a liquid containing an irritant that causes inflammation and results in fibrosis of tissues. It may be used in cauterizing ulcers, arresting hemorrhage, and treating hemangiomas.

sclerosis /sklirō″sis/ [Gk, *skleros,* hard], a condition characterized by hardening of tissue resulting from any of several causes, including inflammation, the deposit of mineral salts, and infiltration of connective tissue fibers. **–sclerotic,** *adj.*

-sclerosis, combining form meaning "an abnormal hardening of the tissue": *atherosclerosis, arteriosclerosis, dermatosclerosis.*

sclerotherapy /-ther″əpē/ [Gk, *skleros,* hard, *therapeia,* treatment], the use of sclerosing chemicals to treat varicosities such as hemorrhoids or esophageal varices. The agent produces inflammation and later fibrosis and obliteration of the lumen.

sclerotic /sklirot″ik/ [Gk, *skleros,* hard], pertaining to induration or hardening.

sclerotomal pain distribution /-tō″məl/, the referral of pain from pain-sensitive tissues covering the axial skeleton along a sclerotomal segment.

sclerotome /sklir″ətōm/ [Gk, *skleros* + *temnein,* to cut], (in embryology) the part of the segmented mesoderm layer in the early developing embryo that originates from the somites and gives rise to skeletal tissue of the body, specifically the paired segmented masses of mesodermal tissue that lie on each side of the notochord and develop into the vertebrae and ribs. See also **somite.**

sclerotylosis /sklē′rō-tilō″sis/, a rare autosomal-dominant condition of atrophic fibrosis of the skin. Characteristics include hypoplasia of the nails and horny skin covering the palms of the hands and plantar surfaces of the feet. The disorder may be accompanied by cancer of the GI tract. Also called *Huriez syndrome.*

SCMC test, a test for cervical factor infertility. Fresh sperm are put both on a slide with cervical mucus and on a slide without mucus, and motility of the two sperm samples is assessed over time. If the sperm show irregularities of motility through the mucus, there is cervical factor infertility. Also called *Kremer test, sperm–cervical mucus contact test.*

scoleces. See **scolex.**

scoleco-, combining form meaning "worm": *scolecoid.*

scolecoid, resembling a worm; wormlike.

scolex /skō″leks/ *pl.* *scoleces* [Gk, worm], the headlike segment or organ of an adult tapeworm that has hooks, grooves, or suckers by which it attaches itself to the wall of the intestine.

scolio-, combining form meaning "twisted" or "crooked": *scoliokyphosis, scoliometer, scoliosis.*

scoliokyphosis. See **kyphoscoliosis.**

scoliometer /skō′lē·om″ətər/ [Gk, *skoliosis,* curvature], a device for measuring the amount of abnormal curvature in the spine.

scoliosis /skō′lē·ō″sis/ [Gk, *skoliosis,* curvature], lateral curvature of the spine, a common abnormality of childhood, especially in females. Causes include congenital malformations of the spine, poliomyelitis, skeletal dysplasias, spastic paralysis, and unequal leg length. Unequal heights of hips or shoulders may be a sign of this condition. Early recognition and orthopedic treatment may prevent progression of the curvature. Treatment includes braces, casts, exercises, and corrective surgery. See also **congenital scoliosis, idiopathic scoliosis, kyphoscoliosis, kyphosis, lordosis, spinal curvature.**

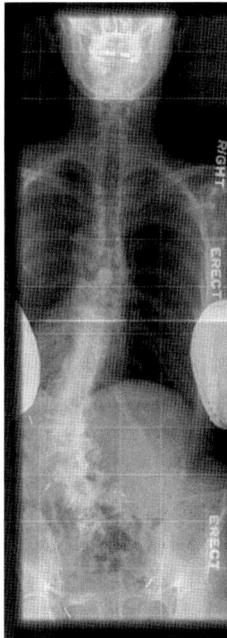

Radiograph of the spine in scoliosis *(Zitelli and Davis, 2007)*

scoliotic pelvis /skō′lē·ot″ik/ [Gk, *skoliosis,* curvature; L, *pelvis,* basin], an effect of scoliosis in which the sacrum bends to one side, distorting the pelvis.

scombroid /skom″broid/ [Gk, *scombros,* mackerel, *eidos,* form], pertaining to fish of the Scombridae and Scomberesocidae families, which include skipjack, mackerel, bonito, and tuna.

scombroid poisoning, toxic effects of eating scombroid fish (such as bonito or tuna) that have begun bacterial decomposition after being caught. Scombroid fish contain large amounts of free histidine in the muscle tissue, which gives rise to toxic levels of histamine under conditions of histidine decarboxylation by any of a dozen species of bacteria. Scombroid poisoning is not limited to consumption of fresh fish; the problem also may affect commercially canned tuna. Symptoms, which usually last no more than 24 hours, include nausea, vomiting, diarrhea, epigastric pain, and urticaria.

scop-, combining form meaning "to examine, observe": *scopophilia.*

-scope, suffix meaning "an instrument for observation" or "a visual examination": *angioscope, episcope, colposcope.*

scopolamine /skōpol″əmēn/ [Giovanni A. Scopoli, Italian naturalist, 1723–1788], an anticholinergic alkaloid obtained from the leaves and seeds of several solanaceous plants. It is a central nervous system depressant. Also called **hyoscine.** See also **transdermal scopolamine.**

■ INDICATIONS: It is prescribed for prevention of motion sickness and as an antiemetic, a sedative in obstetrics, and a cycloplegic and mydriatic.

■ CONTRAINDICATIONS: Narrow-angle glaucoma, asthma, myasthenia gravis, obstruction of the genitourinary or GI tract, severe ulcerative colitis, and known hypersensitivity prohibit its use.

■ ADVERSE EFFECTS: Among the more serious adverse effects are blurred vision, central nervous system effects, tachycardia, dry mouth, decreased sweating, and hypersensitivity reaction.

scopophilia /skō′pəfil″ē·ə, skop″-/ [Gk, *skopein,* to look, *philein,* to love], **1.** sexual pleasure derived from looking at sexually stimulating scenes or at another person's genitals; voyeurism. **2.** a morbid desire to be seen; exhibitionism. Also called **scoptophilia, scoptophilic.** −*scoptophiliac, scopophiliac, scoptophilic, scopophilic, adj., n.*

scopophobia /skō′pə-/ [Gk, *skopein* + *phobos,* fear], an anxiety disorder characterized by a morbid fear of being seen or stared at by others. The condition is commonly seen in schizophrenia. See also **phobia.**

scoptophilia, scoptophilic. See **scopophilia.**

-scopy, combining form meaning "observation" or "a visual examination": *colonoscopy, endoscopy, arthroscopy.*

-scorbic, combining form meaning "prevention or treatment of scurvy": *ascorbic acid.*

-scorbutic, -scorbutical, combining form meaning "scurvy."

scorbutic gingivitis /skôrbyōō″tik/ [NL, *scorbutus,* scurvy; L, *gingiva,* gum; Gk, *itis,* inflammation], an abnormal condition characterized by inflamed or bleeding gums and caused by vitamin C deficiency.

scorbutic pose, the characteristic posture of a child with scurvy, with thighs and legs semiflexed and hips rotated outward. The child usually lies motionless in a state of pseudoparalysis, avoiding voluntary movements of the extremities because of the pain that accompanies any motion. See also **scurvy.**

scorbutus. See **scurvy.**

scorpion sting /skôr″pē·on/ [Gk, *skorpios* + AS, *stingan*], a painful wound produced by a scorpion, an arachnid with a hollow stinger in its tail. The stings of many species are only slightly toxic, but some, including *Centruroides sculpturatus* (bark scorpion) of the southwestern United States, may inflict fatal injury, especially in small children. Initial pain is followed within several hours by numbness, nausea, muscle spasm, dyspnea, and convulsion. Anascorp, an antivenin, is the only approved treatment in the United States and Canada.

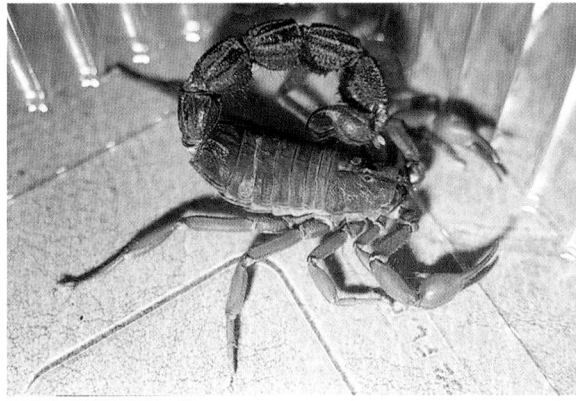

Scorpion *(Courtesy R. David Gaban)*

scoto-, combining form meaning "darkness": *scotoma, scotopic vision.*

scotoma /skōtō″mə/ *pl.* scotomas, scotomata [Gk, *skotos,* darkness, *oma,* tumor], a defect of vision in a defined area of the visual field in one or both eyes. A common prodromal symptom is a shimmering film appearing as an island in the visual field.

scotopic vision /skōtop″ik/ [Gk, *skotos,* darkness; L, *visio,* seeing], the ability of the eye to adjust for vision in darkness or dim light. See also **night vision.**

scrapie /skrā′pē/, the first of the prion diseases to be recognized, occurring in sheep and goats and characterized by severe pruritus, muscular incoordination, and increasing debility ending in death.

scratch test [ME, *scratten* + L, *testum,* crucible], a skin test for identifying an allergen, performed by placing a small quantity of a solution containing a suspected allergen on a lightly scratched area of the skin. The formation of a wheal within 15 minutes indicates an allergy to the substance. Compare **patch test.**

screamer's nodule. See **vocal cord nodule.**

screening [ME, *scren*], **1.** a preliminary procedure, such as a test or examination, to detect the most characteristic sign or signs of a disorder that may require further investigation. **2.** the examination of a large sample of a population to detect a specific disease or disorder, such as hypertension.

screen memory [ME, *scren* + L, *memoria*], a consciously tolerable memory that replaces one that is emotionally painful to recall.

screw /skrōō/ [MFr, *escroue*], a solid cylinder with a helical thread on its exterior surface, used to hold two objects together.

screw artery /skrōō/, a coiled blood vessel in either the uterine mucosa or the retinal macula. Also called **spiral artery.**

screw clamp [OFr, *escroe,* screw; AS, *clam,* fastener], a device, usually made of plastic, equipped with a screw that can be manipulated to close and open the primary IV tubing for regulating the flow of IV solution. Turning the screw clockwise closes the tubing; turning it counterclockwise opens it. Different positions of the screw between the open and the closed positions allow the IV fluid to flow at different rates. Compare **roller clamp, slide clamp.**

scrib-, script-, combining form meaning "write": *prescription.*

Scribner shunt [Belding S. Scribner, American physician, b. 1921], a type of arteriovenous bypass, used in hemodialysis and consisting of a special tube connection outside the body.

scripting /skrip″ting/, a technique of family therapy involving the development of new family transactional patterns.

scrofula /skrof″yələ/ [L, *scrofa,* brood sow], *(Obsolete)* a form of cutaneous tuberculosis with abscess formation, usually of the cervical lymph nodes.

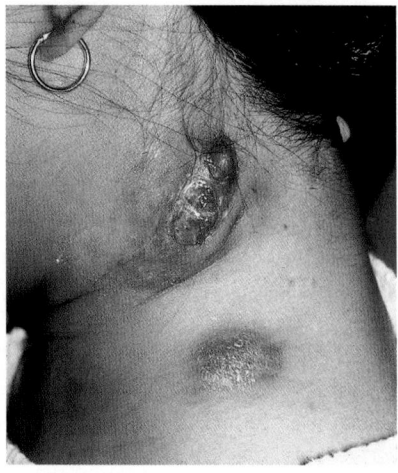

Scrofula *(Stone and Gorbach, 2000)*

scrofulous keratitis, inflammation of the conjunctiva. See **phlyctenular keratoconjunctivitis.**

scroll ear /skrōl/, a distortion of the ear in which the pinna is rolled forward.

scrotal /skrō″təl/, pertaining to the scrotum.

scrotal cancer, an epidermoid malignancy of the scrotum, characterized initially by a small sore that may ulcerate. The lesion occurs most frequently in elderly men who have been exposed to soot, pitch, crude oil, mineral oils, polycyclic hydrocarbons, or arsenic fumes from copper smelting. Treatment involves wide surgical excision of the tumor and resection of inguinal nodes. In the 18th century Sir Percival Pott associated scrotal cancer in chimney sweeps with exposure to soot. It was the first malignancy shown to be caused by an environmental carcinogen. Also called **chimney-sweeps' cancer, soot wart.**

scrotal hernia, an inguinal hernia that has descended into the scrotum.

scrotal nuclear imaging, a nuclear imaging scan, usually done on an emergency basis, that is helpful in diagnosing patients with a sudden onset of unilateral testicular swelling and pain. It can differentiate unilateral testicular torsion from other causes of testicular pain, such as acute epididymitis.

scrotal part of ductus deferens, the initial part of the ductus deferens, which is within the scrotum.

scrotal raphe, a line of union of the two halves of the scrotum. It is generally more highly pigmented than the surrounding tissue.

scrotal septum, an incomplete wall of connective tissue and smooth muscle that divides the scrotum into two compartments, each containing a testis.

scrotal shawl a malformation of the male external genitalia in which the scrotum envelops the penis. It is usually associated with sex chromosome abnormalities or Aarskog syndrome. See also **Aarskog syndrome.**

scrotal swelling, the earliest enlargement of embryonic tissue that will become half of the scrotum.

scrotal tongue, a seldom used term for a nonpathological condition in which the tongue is deeply furrowed and resembles the surface of the scrotum. See **fissured tongue.**

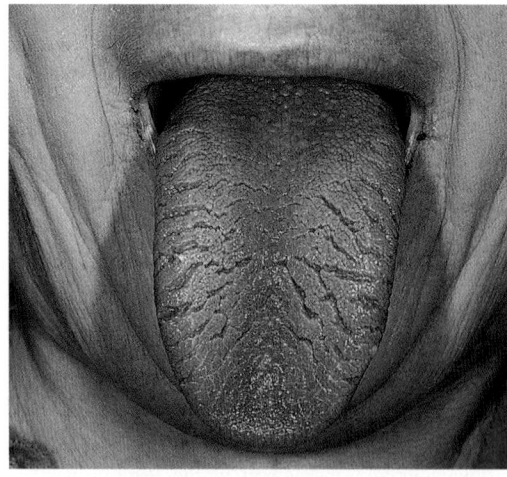

Scrotal tongue *(Callen et al, 2000)*

scrotal ultrasound, an ultrasound test of the scrotum and its contents to diagnose benign and malignant tumors, benign abnormalities such as testicular abscess and orchitis, and extratesticular lesions such as hydrocele, hematocele, and pyocele and to locate cryptorchid testicles.

scrotum /skrō″təm/, the pouch of skin containing the testes and parts of the spermatic cords. It is divided on the surface into two lateral parts by a ridge that continues ventrally to the undersurface of the penis and dorsally along the middle line of the perineum to the anus. In young, robust individuals the scrotum is short and corrugated and closely wraps the testes. In older people and debilitated individuals and in warm environments the scrotum becomes elongated and flaccid. The two layers of the scrotum are the skin and the dartos tunic. The skin is brownish and very thin, is usually wrinkled, and has thinly scattered kinky hairs. The dartos tunic is composed of a thin layer of unstriated muscular fibers around the base of the scrotum. The tunic projects an internal septum that divides the pouch into two cavities for the testes, extending between the scrotal ridge and the root of the penis. The scrotum is highly vascular and contains no fat. See also **testis.** –**scrotal,** *adj.*

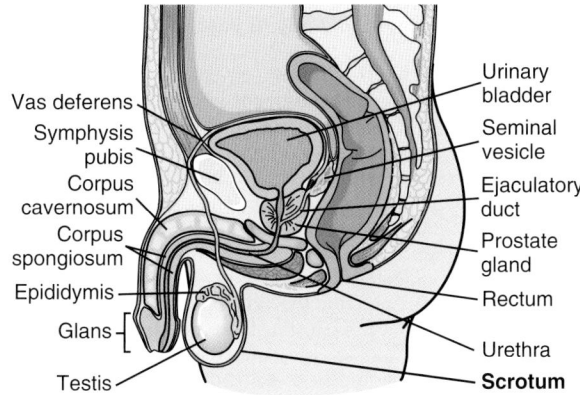

Vas deferens
Symphysis pubis
Corpus cavernosum
Corpus spongiosum
Epididymis
Glans
Testis

Urinary bladder
Seminal vesicle
Ejaculatory duct
Prostate gland
Rectum
Urethra
Scrotum

Scrotum *(Sorrentino, 2008)*

scrub. See **surgical scrub.**

scrubbed team members [ME, *scrobben,* to scrub], the surgeons, physicians, nurses, and technicians who are scrubbed for surgical procedures in a sterile environment.

scrub itch. See ***Leeuwenhoekia australiensis.***

scrub nurse, a registered nurse who assists surgeons during operations.

scrub room, an operative area where surgeons and surgical teams use disposable sterile brushes and bactericidal soaps to wash and scrub their fingernails, hands, and forearms before performing or assisting in surgical operations. Scrub rooms and meticulous washing techniques improve the sterile environment of the operating room and reduce the risk of bacterial infection.

scrub typhus, an acute febrile disease caused by several strains of the species *Orientia tsutsugamushi* (formerly *Rickettsia tsutsugamushi)* and transmitted from infected rodents to humans by mites. It is a serious public health problem in the Asia-Pacific area. The clinical course ranges from mild to severe and is characterized by a necrotic papule or black eschar at the site of the lesion caused by the bite of the small arachnid. Tender enlarged regional lymph nodes, fever, severe headache, eye pain, muscle aches, and a generalized rash usually occur. In severe cases the myocardium and the central nervous system may be involved. The

DNA-PCR and indirect fluorescent antibody tests are useful in diagnosis. Treatment with antibiotics, such as chloramphenicol, doxycycline, or azithromycin, has reduced the mortality rate to nearly zero. Person-to-person transmission is not known to occur. No effective vaccine is available, and second attacks are common because of antigenic differences in various strains of rickettsiae. Prevention includes avoiding mite-infested terrain, reducing the rodent population, destroying scrub vegetation, and using insect repellents. Also called **Japanese flood fever, Japanese river fever, mite typhus, tropical typhus, tsutsugamushi disease.** Compare **Q fever, Rocky Mountain spotted fever, typhus.**

scruple /skrōō″pəl/ [L, *scrupulus,* small stone], a measure of weight in the apothecaries' system equal to 20 grains or 1.296 g. See also **apothecaries' weight, metric system.**

sculpting /skulp″ting/, a technique of family therapy involving construction of a live family portrait that depicts family alliances and conflicts.

Sculptra, brand name for *poly-L-lactic acid.*

Scultetus binder /skəltē″təs/ [Johann Schultes, German surgeon, 1595–1645], a many-tailed binder or bandage with an attached central piece. The tails are overlapped. The last two, tied or pinned, act to secure the others. A Scultetus binder may be opened or removed without moving the bandaged part of the body. Also called *Scultetus bandage, many-tailed bandage.*

scurvy /skur″vē/ [Scand, *scurfa,* scabby], severe ascorbic acid deficiency. It is characterized by weakness; anemia; edema; spongy gums, often with ulceration and loosening of the teeth; a tendency to mucocutaneous hemorrhages; and induration of the muscles of the legs. Treatment and prophylaxis of the disease consist of administration of ascorbic acid and inclusion of fresh vegetables and fruits in the diet. Also called **scorbutus.** See also **ascorbic acid, citric acid, infantile scurvy.**

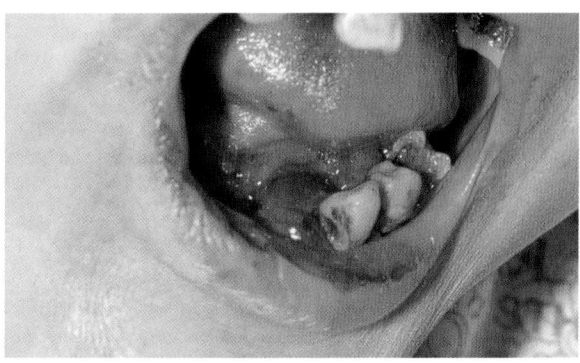

Scurvy *(White and Cox, 2006)*

SD, **1.** abbreviation for **skin dose. 2.** abbreviation for **standard deviation.**

SDAT, abbreviation for **senile dementia–Alzheimer type.**

SDMS, abbreviation for *Society of Diagnostic Medical Sonography.*

Se, symbol for the element **selenium.**

SE, abbreviation for **spin-echo.**

S.E., abbreviation for **standard error.**

sea-blue histiocyte syndrome, a condition of spleen enlargement and mild thrombocytopenia. Histiocytes in the bone marrow contain cytoplasmic granules that stain bright blue.

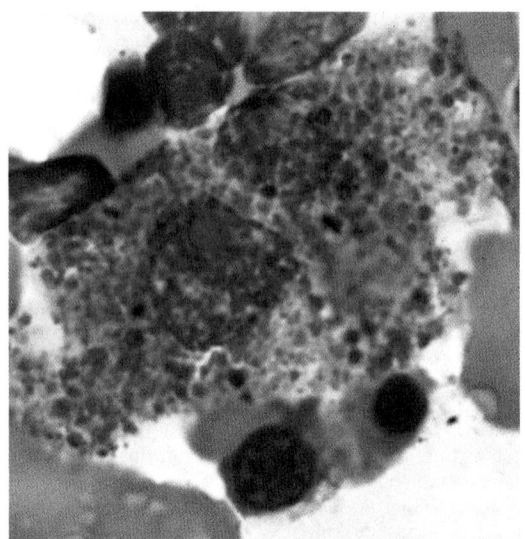

Sea-blue histiocyte syndrome *(Carr and Rodak, 2008)*

seaborgium (Sg) /sēbôr″gē·əm/ [Glenn T. Seaborg, American chemist and educator, 1912–1999],　a synthetic radioactive element with a half-life of 0.9 second. Its atomic number is 106; its atomic mass is 269. It was first synthesized in 1974 by scientists working independently in the United States and Russia.

sealant /sē′lənt/,　an agent that protects against access from the outside or leakage from the inside. See also **dental sealant.**

sealed source [ME, *seel,* mark; Fr, *sourdre,* to spring],　a source of radioactivity that is permanently encased in a container or bonding material to prevent leakage. Sealed sources, such as seeds, needles, and specially designed applicators, are used in the implantation of cesium-137, iodine-125, iridium-192, radium-226, and other radionuclides for the treatment of various malignant tumors.

sealer cement,　a compound used in filling a pulp canal. It is applied as a thick plastic putty that flows and fills depressions in the surface of the canal, solidifies after insertion, and helps close the apex of the root canal.

seal limbs.　See **phocomelia.**

seasickness,　a form of kinesia caused by traveling on an ocean or the sea. Also called **mal de mer.** Compare **air sickness, car sickness.** See also **kinesia.**

seasonal affective disorder (SAD) /sē″zənəl/,　a mood disorder associated with the shorter days and longer nights of autumn and winter. Symptoms include lethargy, depression, social withdrawal, and work difficulties. The patients also consume excess amounts of carbohydrates, gaining weight. The symptoms recede in the spring, when days become longer. The condition is associated with the effect of light on melatonin secretion and is treated with light therapy for 5 to 6 hours per day.

seasonal allergic rhinitis,　hay fever.

Seattle Foot /sē·at″əl/,　a stored-energy foot prosthesis that contains a plastic rod called a keel, which extends from the toe to the heel, where it turns upward toward the ankle. See also **keel, stored-energy foot.**

seatworm.　*(Informal)* See *Enterobius vermicularis.*

sea urchin granuloma,　a type of foreign body granuloma in which nodules of granulation tissue develop in the skin several months after contact with the silicate in the spines of a sea urchin.

sea urchin sting /ur″chin/　[AS, *sae* + *herichon,* hedgehog],　an injury inflicted by any of a variety of sea urchins in which the skin is punctured and, in some species, venom released. A venomous sting is characterized by pain, muscular weakness, numbness around the mouth, and dyspnea. Immediate removal of the spines is necessary and may require the use of a local anesthetic. An antiseptic and a dressing are applied until the wound is healed. In all cases the broken spines cause local pain and irritation. Infection may result. See also **stingray.**

seawater bath [AS, *sae* + *waeter*],　immersion in warm seawater or in saline solution.

seb-,　combining form meaning "sebum": *sebaceous, seborrhea.*

sebaceous /sibā″shəs/　[L, *sebum,* sweat],　pertaining to sebum, the substance secreted by glands of the skin.

sebaceous cyst,　a fluid-filled, noncancerous elevation on the skin, arising from the glands that secrete oily matter lubricating hair and skin. Also called *skin cyst.*

sebaceous epithelioma,　a benign yellowish nodular tumor of sebaceous gland epithelium. It usually appears on the neck or face. It may resemble basal cell carcinoma but is composed mainly of baseloid and sebaceous cells.

sebaceous follicle [L, *sebum,* sweat, *folliculus,* small bag],　a sebaceous gland that opens into a hair follicle.

sebaceous gland,　one of the many small sacculated organs in the dermis. They are located throughout the body in close association with all types of body hair but are especially abundant in the scalp, face, anus, nose, mouth, and external ear. They are rare in the palms of the hands and the soles of the feet. Each gland consists of a single duct that emerges from a cluster of oval alveoli. The ducts from most sebaceous glands open into the hair follicles, but some open onto the skin surface, as in the labia minora and the free margin of the lips. The sebum secreted by the glands oils the hair and the surrounding skin, helps prevent evaporation of sweat, and aids in the retention of body heat. The sebaceous glands in the nose and face are large and lobulated and often swell with accumulated secretion. Compare **sudoriferous gland.**

sebaceous horn,　a solid tissue outgrowth from a sebaceous cyst.

seborrhea /seb′ərē″ə/　[L, *sebum* + Gk, *rhoia,* flow],　any of several common skin conditions in which an overproduction of sebum results in excessive oiliness or scaling. Also spelled **seborrhoea.** See also **seborrheic blepharitis, seborrheic dermatitis.**

seborrhea capitis [L, *sebum,* sweat; Gk, *rhoia,* flow; L, *caput,* the head],　seborrhea of the scalp. See also **cradle cap.**

seborrheic blepharitis,　a form of seborrheic dermatitis in which the eyelids are erythematous and the margins are covered with a granular crust.

seborrheic dermatitis,　a common chronic inflammatory skin disease characterized by greasy scales and yellowish crusts. Common sites are the scalp, eyelids, eyebrows, face, external surfaces of the ears, axillae, central chest, breasts, groin, and gluteal folds. In some people seborrheic dermatitis is associated with paralysis agitans, diabetes mellitus, malabsorption disorders, epilepsy, or an allergic reaction to gold or arsenic. Treatment includes selenium sulfide shampoos, topical and oral corticosteroids, topical antibiotics, proper therapy for any underlying systemic disorder, and avoidance of sweating and external irritants. Kinds include **cradle cap, dandruff, seborrheic blepharitis.**

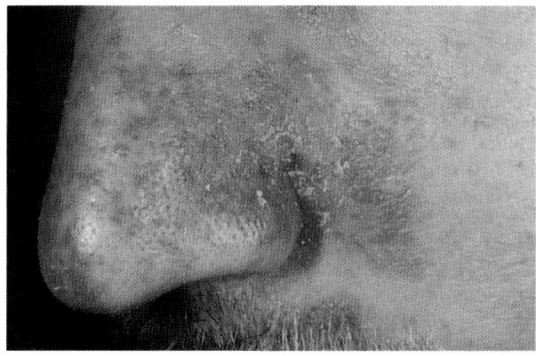

Seborrheic dermatitis *(Courtesy Department of Dermatology, School of Medicine, University of Utah)*

seborrheic keratosis, a benign well-circumscribed, slightly raised, tan to black, warty lesion of the skin of the face, neck, chest, or upper back. The macules are loosely covered with a greasy crust that leaves a raw pulpy base when removed. Itching is common. Treatment includes curettage, electrodesiccation, or cryotherapy. Also called *seborrheic wart,* **acanthoma verrucosa seborrheica.**

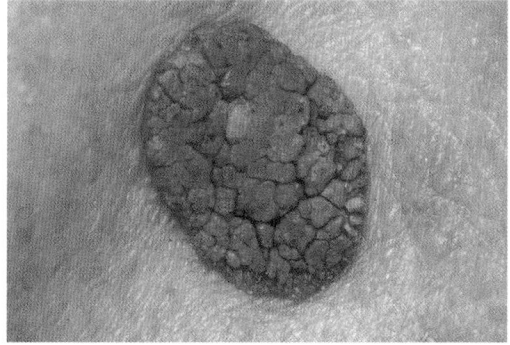

Seborrheic keratosis *(Callen et al, 2000)*

seborrhoea. See **seborrhea.**

sebum /sē″bəm/ [L, grease], the oily secretion of the sebaceous glands of the skin, composed of keratin, fat, and cellular debris. Combined with sweat, sebum forms a moist, oily, acidic film that is mildly antibacterial and antifungal and protects the skin against drying. −**sebaceous,** *adj.*

Seckel syndrome, a congenital disorder characterized by a proportionate short stature; a proportionally small head with jaw hypoplasia, large eyes, and a beaklike protrusion of the nose; cognitive impairment; and various other skeletal, cutaneous, and genital defects. People with the disorder are sometimes referred to as nanocephalic dwarfs.

seclusion /siklōō″zhən/ [L, *secludere,* to isolate], (in psychiatry) the isolation of a patient in a special room to decrease stimuli that might be causing or exacerbating the patient's emotional distress. The room is free from objects that the patient might use to cause self-harm or to harm others.

secobarbital sodium /sek′obär″bital/, a barbiturate sedative-hypnotic.

■ INDICATIONS: It is prescribed in the treatment of insomnia and agitation and as an anticonvulsant and preoperative sedative.

■ CONTRAINDICATIONS: Impaired liver function or known hypersensitivity to this drug or to any barbiturate prohibits its use.

■ ADVERSE EFFECTS: Among the more serious adverse effects are central nervous system and respiratory depression, hypersensitivity reactions, and paradoxical excitement. Kidney damage may result from the polyethylene glycol that is used as a diluent in injectable preparations of the drug.

Seconal, a sedative-hypnotic drug. Brand name for **secobarbital sodium.**

secondary /sek″ənder′ē/ [L, *secundus,* second], second in importance or in occurrence or belonging to the second order of sophistication or development, such as a secondary health care facility or secondary education.

secondary allergen, an agent that induces allergic symptoms in a person through cross-sensitivity with an agent to which the person is hypersensitive.

secondary amenorrhea. See **amenorrhea.**

secondary amputation, amputation performed after suppuration has begun after severe trauma. An area is left open for drainage, and antibiotics are given. Compare **primary amputation.**

secondary amyloidosis. See **amyloidosis.**

secondary analysis, the study of a problem by using previously compiled data.

secondary antibody response, a rapid production of antibodies in response to an antigen in an individual who was exposed previously to the same antigen. Also called **booster response.**

secondary apnea, an abnormal condition in which respiration is absent and will not begin again spontaneously. Resuscitation is initiated immediately with artificial ventilation. Blood gases are analyzed, and oxygen, cardiac massage, and medication specific to the underlying cause may be administered. Secondary apnea may result from any event that severely impedes the absorption of oxygen by the bloodstream. Compare **primary apnea.**

secondary areola, a second ring appearing around the areola of the breast during pregnancy that is more pigmented than the areola before pregnancy.

secondary biliary cirrhosis, an abnormal hepatic condition characterized by obstruction of the bile duct with or without infection. It involves periportal inflammation with progressive fibrosis, destruction of parenchymal cells, and nodular degeneration. Compare **primary biliary cirrhosis.**

secondary bronchial buds, outgrowths of the primary bronchial buds, three on the right side and two on the left, which give rise to the lobes of the lungs and further branch to form the tertiary bronchial buds.

secondary bronchus. See **bronchus.**

secondary care, the provision of a specialized medical service by a physician specialist or a hospital on referral by a primary care physician.

secondary caries. See **dental caries, recurrent caries.**

secondary dementia, dementia resulting from another concurrent form of psychosis. See also **dementia.**

secondary dental caries, dental caries developing in a tooth already affected by the condition. Often a new cavity forms adjacent to or beneath the restorative filling of an old cavity. Compare **primary dental caries.**

secondary dentition, the set of 32 teeth that appears during and after childhood and usually lasts until old age. In each jaw they include four incisors, two canines, four premolars, and six molars. The secondary teeth start to develop

S

in the ninth week of fetal life with the thickening of the epithelium along the line of the future jaw. The permanent first molar in the lower jaw calcifies just after birth, the incisors and the canines approximately 6 months later, the premolars during the second year, the second molar at about the end of the second year, and the third molar at about the twelfth year. The secondary teeth erupt first in the lower jaw, beginning with the first molars in about the sixth year and followed by the two central incisors in about the seventh year, the two lateral incisors in about the eighth year, the first premolars in about the ninth year, the second premolars in about the tenth year, the canines between the eleventh and the twelfth years, the second molars between the twelfth and the thirteenth years, and the third molars between the seventeenth and twenty-fifth years. The eruption of each secondary tooth in the upper jaw lags only slightly behind that of the corresponding tooth in the lower jaw. The third molars in many people are badly oriented or so deeply buried in bone that they must be surgically removed. In some individuals, one or all four of the third molars may not develop completely. Also called **permanent dentition, permanent teeth, secondary teeth.** Compare **primary dentition.** See also **tooth.**

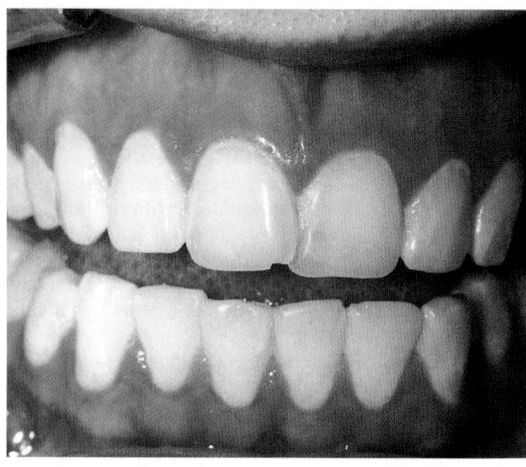

Secondary dentition *(Bird and Robinson, 2012)*

secondary diabetes. See **iatrogenic diabetes mellitus.**

secondary disease, any disorder of bodily functions that follows or results from an earlier injury or medical episode.

secondary distal RTA. See **distal renal tubular acidosis.**

secondary drive. See **drive,** def. 1.

secondary dysmenorrhea. See **inflammatory dysmenorrhea.**

secondary enuresis [L, *secundus,* second; Gk, *enourein,* to urinate], enuresis in an older child who has demonstrated bedtime control for a year or more. It is typically the result of psychological stress but also may be an early sign of an organic disorder, such as diabetes mellitus.

secondary fissure, a fissure between the uvula and the pyramid of the cerebellum.

secondary fracture. See **neoplastic fracture.**

secondary gain, an indirect benefit, usually obtained through an illness or debility. Such gains may include monetary and disability benefits, personal attention, or escape from unpleasant situations and responsibilities. Compare **primary gain.**

secondary gangrene [L, *secundus,* second; Gk, *gagraina*], a form of gangrene in which putrefaction follows

the primary tissue necrosis, generating malodorous, toxic products.

secondary gestation [L, *secundus,* second, *gestare,* to bear], a pregnancy in which the ovum becomes displaced from its original site of implantation but continues development at a different location.

secondary glandular failure, the deficiency of a hormone secreted by a particular gland or gland atrophy caused by absence of a stimulus from another gland, as when a pituitary disorder results in hypogonadism.

secondary health care, an intermediate level of health care that includes diagnosis and treatment, performed in a hospital having specialized equipment and laboratory facilities.

secondary hemorrhage [L, *secundus,* second; Gk, *haima,* blood, *rhegnynai,* to burst forth], a hemorrhage that develops 24 hours or more after the original injury or surgery. It is often caused by an infection.

secondary host. See **intermediate host.**

secondary hydrocephalus [L, *secundus,* second; Gk, *hydor,* water, *kephale,* head], hydrocephalus that develops after an injury, hemorrhage, or infection, such as syphilis or meningitis.

secondary hyperaldosteronism, excessive production of aldosterone caused by an extraadrenal disorder, such as heart failure, kidney disease, cirrhosis, or hypoproteinemia.

secondary hypertension, elevated blood pressure associated with any of several primary diseases, such as renal, pulmonary, endocrine, and vascular diseases. Compare **essential hypertension.** See also **hypertension.**

secondary hypertrophic osteoarthropathy. See **clubbing.**

secondary immunodeficiency, a loss of immunity caused by a disease process or toxic effect of medication rather than by a failure or defect in T or B lymphocytes.

secondary infection, an infection by a microorganism that follows an initial infection by another kind of organism.

secondary infertility, infertility in a patient who has previously conceived.

secondary intention. See **intention.**

secondary iritis [L, *secundus,* second; Gk, *iris,* rainbow, *itis,* inflammation], an inflammation of the iris secondary to another disorder, for example, ankylosing spondylitis or ulcerative colitis.

secondary lymphedema, the swelling of an extremity because of lymph duct obstruction, which may follow surgical removal of lymph channels in mastectomy, obstruction of lymph drainage caused by malignant tumors, or the infestation of lymph vessels with adult filarial parasites. Compare **Milroy disease, Meige disease,** def. 2. See also **lymphedema.**

secondary lymphoid organ, a source of effector lymphocytes, such as the spleen, lymph nodes, or tonsils.

secondary nutrient, a substance that acts as a stimulant to activate the flora of the GI tract to synthesize other nutrients.

secondary occlusal traumatism, occlusal stress that affects previously weakened periodontal structures. The stress may not be excessive for normal tissues but can be damaging to the weakened structures.

secondary oocyte, an oocyte in the period between the first and second maturation division. It is derived from a primary oocyte shortly before ovulation by a division that splits off the first polar body. If fertilized, it divides into an ootid and the second polar body. Otherwise, it perishes. In humans, it is a round cell about 0.1 mm in diameter and consists of protoplasm that contains some yolk enclosed by a thin cell wall, the vitelline membrane. It is surrounded by the zona pellucida and corona radiata.

secondary parkinsonism, a disease of the nervous system caused by degeneration of neurons in the corpus striatum that receive dopaminergic input from the substantia nigra. Unlike idiopathic parkinsonism, the disease does not respond to the administration of levodopa.

secondary peritonitis [L, *secundus,* second; Gk, *peri* + *tenein,* to stretch, *itis,* inflammation], inflammation of the peritoneum caused by the spread of infection from neighboring tissue.

secondary pneumonia [L, *secundus,* second; Gk, *pneumon,* lung], pneumonia that develops during the course of another disease, such as diphtheria or tularemia.

secondary polycythemia [L, *secundus,* second; Gk, *polys,* many, *kytos,* cell, *haima,* blood], a form of polycythemia that develops as a result of oxygen deprivation from a disorder such as a pulmonary or cardiac disease.

secondary port, a control device for regulating the flow of a primary and a secondary IV solution. It consists of a Y-shaped plastic apparatus that attaches to the primary IV tubing and allows the primary and secondary IV solutions to flow separately or to flow simultaneously. Compare **piggyback port.**

secondary prevention, a level of preventive medicine that focuses on early diagnosis, use of referral services, and rapid initiation of treatment to stop the progress of disease processes or a handicapping disability.

secondary proximal renal tubular acidosis. See **proximal renal tubular acidosis.**

secondary radiation, radiation that results from the scattering of primary x-rays. Secondary radiation often accounts for reduced contrast on radiographic images.

secondary relationships, relationships with those who provide or accept services, or with acquaintances and friends, as distinguished from family members and intimate friends.

secondary sensation. See **synesthesia.**

secondary sequestrum, a piece of dead bone that partially separates from sound bone during the process of necrosis but may be pushed back into position. Compare **primary sequestrum.**

secondary sex characteristic, any of the external physical characteristics of sexual maturity secondary to hormonal stimulation that develop in the maturing individual. These characteristics include adult distribution of hair and development of the penis or breasts and the labia.

secondary shock, a state of physical collapse and prostration caused by numerous traumatic and pathological conditions. It develops over time after severe tissue damage and may merge with primary shock, accompanied by various signs, such as weakness, restlessness, low body temperature, low blood pressure, cold sweat, and reduced urinary output. Blood pressure drops progressively in this state, and death may occur within a relatively short time after onset unless appropriate treatment intervenes. Secondary shock is often associated with heat stroke, crushing injuries, myocardial infarction, poisoning, fulminating infections, burns, and other life-threatening conditions. The pathological characteristics of this state reflect changes in the capillaries, which become dilated and engorged with blood. Petechial hemorrhages develop in the serous membranes, edema swells the soft tissues, and the vital organs undergo degenerative changes. Compare **hemorrhagic shock, primary shock.**

secondary symptom. See **symptom.**

secondary syphilis. See **syphilis.**

secondary teeth. See **secondary dentition.**

secondary thrombocytosis. See **thrombocytosis.**

second cranial nerve. See **optic nerve.**

second cuneiform bone. See **intermediate cuneiform bone.**

second-degree burn, a burn that affects the epidermis and the dermis, classified as superficial or deep, according to the depth of injury. The superficial type involves the epidermis and the papillary dermis and is characterized by pain, edema, and the formation of blisters; it heals without scarring. The deep type extends into the reticular dermis, is pale and anesthetic, and results in scarring. See also **burn therapy.**

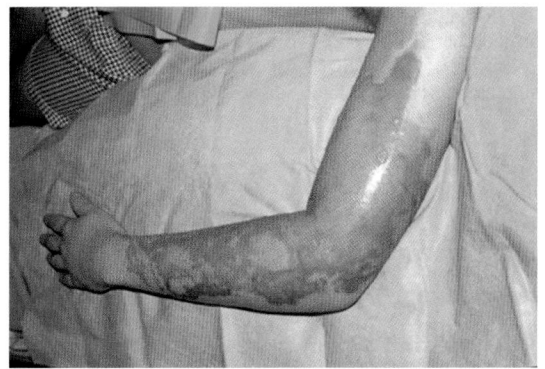

Second-degree burn *(Verbelen et al, 2013)*

second filial generation (F_2), the offspring produced by the mating of two members of the F_1 generation or, broadly, by the crossing of any two heterozygous strains.

secondhand smoke, tobacco smoke from the burning end of a cigarette, cigar, or pipe that is inhaled by nonsmokers. The American Heart Association notes that sidestream smoke (the smoke emanating from the burning end of the cigarette), a major component of secondhand smoke, contains a higher concentration of some toxins than mainstream smoke (inhaled by the smoker directly), making secondhand smoke potentially as dangerous as or even more dangerous than direct smoking. See also **passive smoking.**

second-look operation, a second operation performed within 24 hours of the first to ensure that the first was sufficient and that no further debridement is needed. It is common in cases in which ascertaining whether the bowel is dead or ischemic during the first operation is difficult.

second messenger, a chemical substance inside a cell that carries information farther along the signal pathway from the internal part of a membrane-spanning receptor embedded in the cell membrane. It may be in the form of an enzyme's product or ion fluxes. Ca^{2+}, nitric oxide, and cAMP are common examples.

second opinion [L, *secundus* + *opinari,* to suppose], a patient privilege of requesting an examination and evaluation of a health condition by a second physician to verify or challenge the diagnosis by a first physician. The situation is most likely to arise when an examination by a first physician results in a recommendation for surgery or experimental treatment.

second-order change, a change that alters the system itself.

second-order kinetics, a chemical reaction in which the rate of the reaction is determined by the concentration of two chemical reactants involved or the square of the concentration of one chemical reactant. Also called *second-order reaction.* See also **kinetics.**

second-set rejection, failure of an organ or tissue graft in a host who is already immune to the histocompatibility antigens of the graft because of a previous graft with the same antigens.

second sight, *(Informal)* clairvoyance; precognition.

second stage of labor [L, *secundus,* second; OFr, *estage* + L, *labor,* work], the period of childbirth from full dilation of the cervix to delivery of the fetus.

second-trimester abortion, the termination of a pregnancy approximately 15 to 23 weeks from the first day of the last menstrual period, usually performed for elective reasons, miscarriage management, fetal anomalies, or maternal health conditions. Cervical softening and dilation are performed before the procedure. See also **abortion.**

secretagogue /sikrē″təgog′/, any agent that induces exocrine, endocrine, or paracrine secretion.

secrete. See **secretion.**

secretin /sikrē″tin/ [L, *secernere,* to separate], a digestive hormone that is produced by the S cells lining the duodenum and jejunum when protein of partially digested food enters the intestine from the stomach. It stimulates the pancreas to produce a fluid high in salts but low in enzymes. Secretin has a limited stimulating effect on the production of bile. See also **pancreas.**

secretin-cholecystokinin test, (for pancreatic function) a combination of the secretin test and the cholecystokinin test, measuring pancreatic secretion volume and secretion of bicarbonate, amylase, lipase, and trypsin. Also called *secretin-pancreozymin test.*

secretin test, a test of pancreatic function after stimulation with the hormone secretin. The test measures the volume and bicarbonate concentration of pancreatic secretions. Normal volume findings are 2 to 4 mL/kg body weight HCO_3 (bicarbonate): 90 to 130 mEq/L. A lower-than-normal volume suggests an obstructing malignancy or cystic fibrosis. Reduced bicarbonate and amylase concentration is usually diagnostic of chronic pancreatitis.

secretion /sikrē″shən/ [L, *secernere,* to separate], **1.** the release of chemical substances manufactured by cells of glandular organs. −**secretory,** *adv.* **2.** a substance released or eliminated.

secretoinhibitory /sikrē″tō·inhib″itôr′ē/ [L, *secernere,* to separate, *inhibere,* to restrain], pertaining to a function of inhibiting secretion.

secretor /sikrē″tər/, **1.** a person who releases A, B, or AB blood group antigens into saliva, gastric juice, or other exocrine secretions. **2.** the autosomal-dominant allele that determines this trait.

secretor factor, a substance that triggers the release of ABO blood group antigens into exocrine secretions.

secretory. See **secretion.**

secretory component, a glycopeptide that is attached to immunoglobulin A (IgA). It is necessary for the secretion of IgA into mucosal spaces.

secretory component deficiency, a failure of GI epithelial cells to produce secretory component, a glycopeptide occurring in secretory immunoglobulin A (IgA). It causes a lack of IgA in external secretions, such as tears, saliva, and colostrum, although serum IgA is normal.

secretory cyst. See **retention cyst.**

secretory duct [L, *secernere,* secrete + *ductus,* duct], (of a gland) a small duct that has a secretory function and joins with an excretory duct.

secretory IgA, a dimer of class A immunoglobulins, the principal agents of mucosal immunity. IgA is the only immunoglobulin isotype that can pass through mucosal membranes to reach the lumen of internal organs.

secretory immune system, the part of the immune system that secretes immunoglobulins, primarily immunoglobulin A, onto mucosal surfaces.

secretory phase, the phase of the menstrual cycle after the release of an ovum from a mature ovarian follicle. The corpus luteum, stimulated by luteinizing hormone (LH), develops from the ruptured follicle. It secretes progesterone, which stimulates the development of the glands and arteries of the endometrium, causing it to become thick and spongy. In a negative-feedback response to the increased level of progesterone in the blood, the secretion of LH from the pituitary decreases. In the absence of an embryo and its secretion of chorionic gonadotropin, the secretory phase ends. The corpus luteum involutes, progesterone levels fall, and menstruation occurs. Also called **luteal phase, progestational phase.** Compare **menstrual phase, proliferative phase.**

sect-, -sect, combining form meaning "to cut": *dissect, section, prosector.*

section /sek″shən/ [L, *sectio,* a cutting], **1.** *n.,* a cut surface or slice of tissue. **2.** *v.,* the act of cutting tissue.

sectional arch wire /sek″shənəl/ [L, *sectio,* a cutting, *arcus,* bow; AS, *wir*], a wire attached to only a few teeth, usually on one side of a dental arch or in the anterior segment of the arch, to cause or guide orthodontic tooth movement.

sectional denture. See **partial denture.**

sectional impression [L, *sectio,* a cutting + *imprimere,* to press into], (in dentistry) a molding that captures a desired portion of the total dental arch. The molding, or impression, is created by placing a specially formed tray filled with a gel-like putty material over the area to be captured. The putty material later hardens into a soft, flexible solid.

sector scan /sek″tər/, an ultrasound scan in which the transducer or ultrasound beam is rotated through an angle and the center of rotation is near or behind the surface of the transducer.

Sectral, a beta-adrenergic blocking agent. Brand name for **acebutolol.**

secund-, combining form meaning "second" or "following": *secundigravida, secundines, secundipara.*

secundigravida /səkund′dəgrav″idə/ [L, *secundus,* second, *gravidus,* pregnancy], a woman who is pregnant for the second time. Also called **gravida II** or **2.**

secundines /səkun″dīnz/ [L, *secundus*], the placenta, umbilical cord, and membranes of afterbirth.

secundipara /sek′əndip″ərə/ [L, *secundus* + *parere,* to bear], a woman who has borne two viable children in separate pregnancies.

SED, abbreviation for **skin erythema dose.** See **threshold dose.**

sedation /sidā″shən/ [L, *sedatio,* soothing], an induced state of quiet, calmness, or sleep, as by means of a sedative or hypnotic medication.

sedative /sed″ətiv/ [L, *sedatio,* soothing], **1.** *adj.,* pertaining to a substance, procedure, or measure that has a calming effect. **2.** *n.,* an agent that decreases functional activity, diminishes irritability, and allays excitement. Some sedatives have a general effect on all organs; others principally affect the activities of the heart, stomach, intestines, nerve trunks, respiratory system, or vasomotor system. See also **sedative-hypnotic.**

sedative bath, the immersion of the body in water for a prolonged period as a mechanism to promote relaxation.

sedative filling, a temporary filling material containing agents such as eugenol (also called oil of cloves) to soothe pulpal pain, used to restore missing tooth structure until definitive treatment can be rendered.

sedative-hypnotic, a drug that reversibly depresses the activity of the central nervous system, used chiefly to induce sleep and to allay anxiety. Barbiturates, benzodiazepines, and other sedative-hypnotics have diverse chemical and pharmacological properties that share the ability to depress the activity of all excitable tissue, especially the arousal center in the brainstem. Sedative-hypnotics are used in the treatment of insomnia, acute convulsive conditions, and anxiety states and in facilitation of the induction of anesthesia. Although sedative-hypnotics have a soporific effect, they may interfere with rapid eye movement sleep associated with dreaming and, when administered to patients with fever, may act paradoxically and cause excitement rather than relaxation. Sedative-hypnotics may interfere with temperature regulation, depress oxygen consumption in various tissues, and produce nausea and skin rashes. In elderly patients they may cause dizziness, confusion, and ataxia. Drugs in this group have a high potential for abuse that often results in physical and psychological dependence. Treatment of dependence involves gradual reduction of the dosage because abrupt withdrawal frequently causes serious disorders, including convulsions. Acute reactions to an overdose of a sedative-hypnotic may be treated with an emetic, activated charcoal, gastric lavage, and measures to maintain airway patency. Buspirone, zolpidem, and zaleplon are among the newer nonbarbiturate-nonbenzodiazepine sedative-hypnotic drugs. See also **barbiturate, benzodiazepine derivative.**

sedentary /sed″ənter′ē/ [L, *sedentarius,* sitting], pertaining to a condition of inaction, such as work or recreation that can be performed in the sitting posture.

sedentary living [L, *sedentarius* + AS, *lif*], a pattern of daily living that requires a minimum amount of physical effort.

sediment /sed′imənt/ [L, *sedimentum,* settling], a deposit of relatively insoluble material that settles to the bottom of a container of liquid.

sedimentation /sed′iməntā″shən/ [L, *sedimentum,* settling], the deposition of insoluble materials to the bottom of a liquid. The process may be accelerated by centrifugation.

sedimentation rate (SR) [L, *sedimentum* + *ratum,* rate], the settling rate of red blood cells in a vertical column of anticoagulated whole blood. It is used to monitor inflammatory or malignant disease and to aid in the detection and diagnosis of inflammatory diseases, such as tuberculosis. The test is nonspecific and often unreliable. See also **erythrocyte sedimentation rate.**

sed. rate, *(Informal)* erythrocyte sedimentation rate.

Seeing Eye dog. See **guide dog.**

segment /seg″mənt/ [L, *segmentum,* piece cut off], a component, part, or part of a structure, such as a lobe of the liver or part of the intestine.

segmental bronchus /segmen″təl/ [L, *segmentum,* piece cut off], a secondary bronchus branching from a primary bronchus to a tertiary bronchus.

segmental buds, tertiary bronchial buds.

segmental fracture, a bone break in which several large bone fragments separate from the main body of a fractured bone. The ends of the fragments may pierce the skin, as in an open fracture, or may be contained within the skin, as in a closed fracture.

segmental reflex [L, *segmentum* + *reflectere,* to bend back], a reflex that involves a pathway through only a single segment of the spinal cord.

segmental resection, a surgical procedure in which a part of an organ, gland, or other body part is excised, such as a segmental resection of a part of an ovary performed to

diminish the gland's hormonal secretion by decreasing the amount of secretory tissue in the gland.

segmental spinal artery, feeder arteries that enter the intervertebral foramina at every level. They arise predominantly from the vertebral and deep cervical arteries in the neck, the posterior intercostal arteries in the thorax, and the lumbar arteries in the abdomen. They give rise to anterior and posterior radicular arteries and segmental medullary arteries.

segmentation /seg′məntā″shən/ [L, *segmentum* + *atio,* process], **1.** the division of an animal body into repeating, similar sections, such as somites or metameres. **2.** the division of a zygote into blastomeres; cleavage.

segmentation cavity. See **blastocoele.**

segmentation cell. See **blastomere.**

segmentation method, a technique for filling tooth pulp canals in which a preselected gutta-percha cone is cut into segments. The tip segment is sealed into the apex of a root, and the other segments are usually warmed and condensed against the tip with a plugger. More cone segments are then added until the canal is filled.

segmentation nucleus, the nucleus that results from the fusion of male and female pronuclei in a fertilized ovum. Its formation is the final stage in fertilization and initiates the first cleavage of the zygote. Also called **cleavage nucleus.**

segmented hyalinizing vasculitis /segmen″tid/, a chronic relapsing inflammatory condition of the blood vessels of the lower legs associated with nodular or purpuric skin lesions that may become ulcerated and leave scars. Also called **livedo vasculitis.**

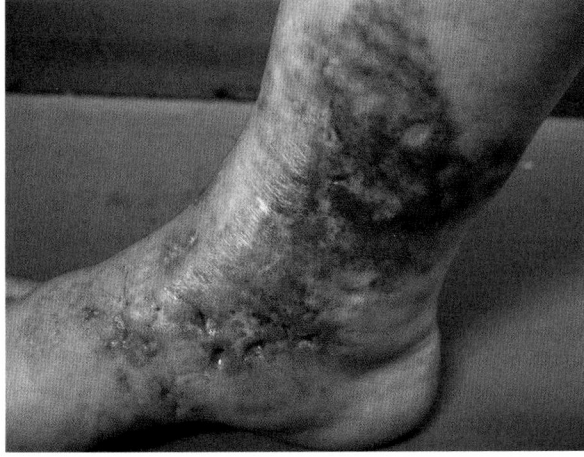

Segmented hyalinizing vasculitis *(Criado et al, 2011)*

segmented neutrophil, a neutrophil with a segmented nucleus. Segments are connected by thin nuclear membrane filaments.

segments of spinal cord. See **spinal cord.**

segregation, the separation of paired alleles during meiosis so that members of each pair of alleles appear in different gametes. See also **Mendel's laws.**

Seitelberger disease. See **infantile neuroaxonal dystrophy.**

seizure /sē″zhər/ [Fr, *saisir,* to seize], a hyperexcitation of neurons in the brain leading to abnormal electric activity that causes a sudden, violent involuntary series of contractions of a group of muscles. It may be paroxysmal and episodic, as in a seizure disorder, or transient and acute, as after a head concussion. A seizure may be clonic or tonic; focal, unilateral, or bilateral; or generalized or partial. Also called **convulsion.**

seizure threshold, the amount of stimulus necessary to produce a convulsive seizure. All humans can have seizures if the provocation is sufficient.

selection /silek″shən/ [L, *seligere,* to choose], **1.** the act or product of choosing. **2.** the process by which various factors or mechanisms determine and modify the reproductive ability of individuals with specific genotypes within a population, thus influencing evolutionary change. Kinds include **artificial selection, natural selection, sexual selection.**

selective absorption. See **differential absorption.**

selective abstraction /silek″tiv/ [L, *seligere,* to choose], a type of cognitive distortion in which focus on one aspect of an event negates all other aspects.

selective angiography, a radiographic procedure that allows selective visualization of the aorta, the major arterial systems, or a particular vessel. It is performed after a few milliliters of a radiopaque contrast medium has been injected through a percutaneous catheter. After the procedure the catheter is withdrawn, and pressure is placed on the puncture site to prevent bleeding.

selective estrogen receptor modulator (SERM), an agent that activates some estrogen receptors but not others, thereby having estrogen-like effects on target tissues without affecting other tissues that have estrogen receptors.

selective grinding, (in dentistry) any modification of the occlusal forms of the teeth to improve occlusion and tooth function, produced by grinding at selected places. See also **occlusal adjustment.**

selective IgA deficiency, a familial or acquired disorder characterized by a lack of serum and secretory immunoglobin A (IgA). The IgA-deficient patient may appear normal or asymptomatic and is diagnosed by demonstration of less than 5 mg/dL of IgA in serum. Patients have an increased risk of respiratory, GI, and urogenital infections.

selective immunoglobulin deficiency, a condition characterized by inadequate levels of one of the major classes of immunoglobulins.

selective inattention, the screening out of unwanted stimuli, particularly the part of a message the listener does not want to hear.

selectively permeable. See **semipermeable.**

selective mutism, a mental disorder of childhood characterized by continuous refusal to speak in social situations by an individual who is able and willing to speak to selected persons.

selective neuronal necrosis, a widespread destruction of neurons caused by hypoxic or ischemic events. Only a fraction of the neurons in a given region are destroyed, selected apparently at random.

selective serotonin reuptake inhibitor (SSRI), an antidepressant drug that blocks reuptake of serotonin without blocking reuptake of other biogenic amines such as norepinephrine and dopamine. Advantages over tricyclic antidepressant drugs include fewer anticholinergic side effects (dry mouth, blurred vision, urinary retention) and fewer antihistaminic side effects (sedation, weight gain).

selectivity /sil′ektiv″itē/ [L, *seligere*], **1.** the ability to discriminate even small differences. **2.** (in chemistry) reactivity of one functional group in the presence of others. **3.** (in biochemistry) the extent to which a given substrate binds two different ligands.

selectivity coefficient, the degree to which an ion-selective electrode responds to a particular ion with respect to a reference ion.

selenious acid /sĕ-le′ne-us/, monohydrated selenium dioxide, a source of elemental selenium. It is administered intravenously.

selenium (Se) /silē″nē·əm/ [Gk, *selene,* moon], a metalloid element of the sulfur group. Its atomic number is 34, and its atomic mass is 78.96. Selenium occurs mainly in iron, copper, lead, and nickel ores in the form of metallic selenides. One of the chief commercial sources is the flue dust produced by the burning of pyrites to make sulfuric acid. Selenium occurs as a trace element in foods, and research continues to determine the most effective daily allowances for different age groups. Dietary experts say that the estimated safe, adequate intake of selenium for infants 6 months of age is 0.04 mg, for adults 0.05 to 0.2 mg. Although selenium deficiency can result in liver problems and degeneration of muscles in some animals, in humans its need has not yet been clearly defined. The bright orange insoluble powder selenium sulfide is used externally in the control of seborrheic dermatitis, dandruff, and other forms of dermatosis. Selenium sulfide, used as a lotion, is used in some therapeutic shampoos as 2.5% of selenium sulfide in a detergent vehicle; it is sold without prescription as a 1% detergent suspension in a scented detergent vehicle. Adverse effects may include conjunctivitis if the preparation enters the eyes, increased oiliness or dryness of the hair, and orange tinting of gray hair. The antidandruff effectiveness of selenium sulfide is thought to stem from its antimitotic activity and its residual adherence to the hair after shampooing. Normal skin absorbs very little of the drug, but inflamed or damaged skin absorbs it readily. Selenium is used in the nuclear medicine compound selenomethionine for diagnosing parathyroid tumors. The element is also used as a photoconductive layer of xeroradiographic plates. Burns and dermatitis venenata may result from prolonged skin contact.

selenium sulfide, an antidandruff and antiseborrheic medication. See also **selenium.**

■ INDICATIONS: It is prescribed for dandruff, for seborrheic dermatitis of the scalp, and for treatment of tinea versicolor.

■ CONTRAINDICATIONS: Acute scalp inflammation or known hypersensitivity to this drug prohibits its use.

■ ADVERSE EFFECTS: Among the more serious adverse effects are dermatitis after prolonged skin contact and keratitis after accidental conjunctival contact.

selenoid cells. See **crescent bodies.**

self selvz/*pl.* selves/ [AS], **1.** the total essence or being of a person; the individual. **2.** those affective, cognitive, and spiritual qualities that distinguish one person from another; individuality. **3.** a person's awareness of his or her own being or identity; consciousness; ego. See also **personality.**

self-acceptance [AS, *self* + L, *accipere,* to take], the recognition and acceptance of one's own qualities and limitations.

self-actualization, (in humanistic psychology) the fundamental tendency toward the maximum realization and fulfillment of one's human potential. In Maslow's hierarchy of needs, self-actualization is the highest need.

self-advocacy, the process of representing oneself, including making one's own decisions about life, developing a network of support, knowing one's rights and responsibilities, reaching out to others when in need of assistance, mastering self-determination, and learning how to obtain information to gain an understanding about issues of personal interest or importance.

self-alien. See **ego-dystonic.**

self-alienation. See **depersonalization.**

self-anesthesia, self-administered inhalation anesthesia in which whiffs of anesthetic gas are inhaled from a handheld breathing device controlled by the patient. This form of anesthesia is most common in England.

self-antigen. See **autoantigen.**

self-breast examination (SBE), a procedure in which a woman examines her breasts and their accessory structures for evidence of change that could indicate a malignant process. The SBE should be performed when the breasts are not swollen or tender. Women may choose not to do SBE or to do SBE occasionally. Women who choose not to do SBE should still be familiar with the usual appearance and feel of their breasts and report any changes immediately to their primary care provider. Also called **breast self-examination.** See also **breast examination.**

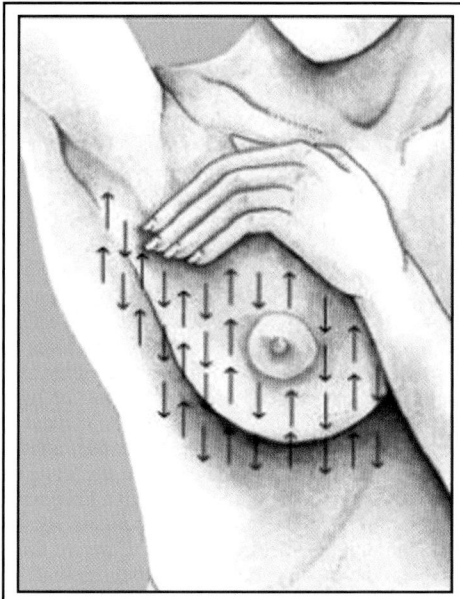

Breast Self-Examination
Examine up to the collarbone,
out to armpit, in to middle of chest,
and down to bottom of rib cage

Self-breast examination *(Seidel et al, 2006)*

self-care, **1.** the personal and medical care performed by the patient, usually in collaboration with and after instruction by a health care professional. The patient's need for assistance and ability to develop a higher level of self-care must be evaluated in forming any nursing care plan. Maximal self-care appropriate to the condition and to the patient is often the ultimate goal of nursing care. Occupational therapy services also help restore, develop, or maintain the skills necessary to permit physically and mentally disabled people to perform the daily living tasks of self-care. **2.** the health care by laypeople of their families, their friends, and themselves, including identification and evaluation of symptoms, medication, and treatment. Self-care is self-limited, voluntary, and wholly outside professional health care systems but may include consultation with a physician or other health care professional as a resource. **3.** personal care accomplished without technical assistance, such as eating, washing, dressing, using the telephone, and attending to one's own elimination, appearance, and hygiene. The goal of rehabilitation medicine is maximal personal self-care.

self-care theory, a model, central to Dorothea Orem's concept of nursing, used to provide a conceptual framework for nursing care directed to self-care by the client to the greatest degree possible. The model requires an assessment of the client's capability for self-care and need for care. The need for care includes biophysical and psychosocial needs and the specific needs that are the result of the illness. See also **Orem, Dorothea E.**

self-catheterization, a procedure performed by a patient to empty the bladder by inserting a catheter into the urethra. The procedure is recommended for patients who cannot empty the bladder completely but can retain urine for 2 to 4 hours at a time and who have mental cognition, some manual dexterity, and the ability to insert a catheter into the urethra. This is generally a clean rather than a sterile procedure.
■ METHOD: Necessary equipment consists of a pan or toilet, two 14 French catheters, a water-soluble lubricant, soap, water, and a clean washcloth and towel; women usually require a magnifying mirror initially to identify the urethral meatus, and men may prefer to perform the procedure sitting on a low stool rather than on a toilet. Women are taught to perform self-catheterization initially in a semi-Fowler's position, using a pan, but later they generally can carry out the procedure sitting on or standing over a toilet. The patient is instructed to clean the urinary meatus and labia or glans penis with soap and water, to grasp the catheter about 2 inches from the tip, and to lubricate the tip before it is gently inserted into the meatus: Women insert about 1½ to 2 inches of the catheter, and men insert 8 inches, or until the urine flows. Urine is allowed to flow into the pan or toilet until the bladder is empty. The catheter is then removed, washed in soap and water, thoroughly rinsed, dried by rolling it in a clean towel, and placed in a clean plastic or paper bag for the next self-catheterization.
■ INTERVENTIONS: The nurse teaches the procedure and ensures that the patient understands its purpose and the need to perform it at designated times, as well as the importance of forcing fluids up to 3000 mL daily unless contraindicated. The nurse makes certain that the patient is able to identify the urinary meatus and perform the procedure.
■ OUTCOME CRITERIA: Regular self-catheterization by the patient who cannot empty the bladder allows the person to work and participate in the normal activities of daily living and to prevent kidney infection and other renal disorders.

self-concept, the composite of ideas, feelings, and attitudes that a person has about his or her own identity, worth, capabilities, and limitations. Such factors as the values and opinions of others, especially in the formative years of early childhood, play an important part in the development of the self-concept.

self-confrontation, a technique for behavior modification that depends on a patient's recognition of and dissatisfaction with inconsistencies in his or her own values, beliefs, and behaviors, or between his or her own personal system and that of a significant other.

self-conscious, **1.** the state of being aware of oneself as an individual entity that experiences, desires, and acts. **2.** a heightened awareness of oneself and one's actions as reflected by the observations and reactions of others; socially ill at ease. −*self-consciousness, n.*

self-curing resin, any plastic resin that can be polymerized by the addition of an activator and a catalyst without the use of external heat. It is used in dental restorations and repairs. Also called **activated resin, autopolymerizing resin, cold-curing resin, quick-cure resin.**

self-defeating personality disorder, a personality characterized by a type of behavior that inhibits the individual from achieving his or her own desires and goals. It is characterized by involvement in situations that continuously lead to failure, rejection, and loss even when other options for involvement are available. Also called **masochistic personality.**

self-destructive behavior, any behavior, direct or indirect, that, if uninterrupted, will ultimately lead to the death of the individual.

self-determination, the abilities or characteristics that enable an individual to develop a greater understanding of self, personal actions, and how those actions support the individual's behavior. Self-determination incorporates goal-setting, the initiative to attain goals, and a belief in the ability to control personal destiny.

self-diagnosis, the diagnosis of one's own health problems, usually without direction or assistance from a physician.

self-differentiation, specialization and diversification of a tissue or body part resulting solely from intrinsic factors.

self-disclosure, the process by which one person lets his or her inner being, thoughts, and emotions be known to another. It is important for psychological growth in individual and group psychotherapy.

self-efficacy, a belief that one has the skills and abilities to accomplish what one wishes to accomplish.

self-esteem, the degree of worth and competence one attributes to oneself.

self-fulfilling prophecy, a principle that states that a belief in or the expectation of a particular resolution is a factor that contributes to its fulfillment.

self-healing squamous epithelioma, an inherited condition of skin tumors that appear on the head and resolve spontaneously after a few months, leaving deep-pitted scars. The tumors resemble squamous carcinoma or keratoacanthoma.

self-help device, an external device that is designed, made, or adapted to assist a person in performing a particular task. Many people with disabilities depend on self-help devices to carry out daily activities and participate actively and productively in community life.

self-help group, a group of people who meet to improve their health through discussion and special activities. Characteristically, self-help groups are not led by a professional. Compare **group therapy.**

self-hypnosis [AS, *self* + Gk, *hypnos,* sleep], the process of putting oneself into a trancelike state by autosuggestion, such as concentration on a single thought or object. Some subjects are more susceptible than others.

self-ideal, a perception of how one should behave based on certain personal standards. The standard may be either a carefully constructed image of the kind of person one would like to be or merely a number of aspirations, goals, or values one would like to achieve. See also **ego ideal.**

self-image, the total concept, idea, or mental image one has of oneself and of one's role in society; the person one believes oneself to be.

self-insurance, a system whereby hospitals or health professionals may, in lieu of commercial insurance, assume financial responsibility for their liability.

self-insured. See **self-insurance.**

self-isolation, the voluntary action of remaining at home, eliminating outside activities, and monitoring one's health following exposure to a communicable disease.

self-limited, (of a disease or condition) tending to end without treatment.

self-limited disease [AS, *self* + L, *limes,* boundary, *dis,* not; Fr, *aise,* ease], a disease restricted in duration by its own pattern of characteristics and not by other influences.

self-management approach, a treatment approach in which patients assume responsibility for their behavior, changing their environment, and planning their future.

self-monitoring of blood glucose (SMBG), the use of a glucose meter to enable a patient to recognize glycemic variations. Most self-monitoring systems use the chemical reaction between glucose oxidase and glucose as a basis for measurement. Some devices depend on hydrogen peroxide, which is a product of the same reaction.

self-other, a concept that characterizes people who believe that the source of power is within the self as opposed to those who believe that it is in others. See also **locus of control.**

self-radiolysis, a process in which a compound is damaged by radioactive decay products originating in an atom within the compound.

self-recognition, the ability of the body's immune system to recognize self-identifying antigens on the body's own cells.

self-regulation, a plan for patients to eliminate health risk behaviors. It includes self-monitoring, self-evaluation, and self-reinforcement.

self-reinforcing adaptation, (in occupational therapy) a therapeutic technique in which each successful stage of adjustment stimulates the next, more complex step.

self-responsibility, a concept of holistic health by which individuals assume responsibility for their own health.

self-retaining catheter, an indwelling urinary catheter that has a double lumen. One channel allows urine to drain from the bladder into a collecting bag; the other has a balloon at the bladder end and a diaphragm at the other end. Several centimeters of air or sterile water is injected through the diaphragm to fill the balloon in the bladder and hold the catheter in place. To remove the catheter, the water or air is withdrawn through the diaphragm. See also **Foley catheter.**

self-stimulation, a system in which patients control their pain by manipulating an electric source of nerve stimulation.

self-system, the organization of experiences that acts as a protective mechanism against anxiety.

self-theory, a personality theory that uses one's self-concept in integrating the function and organization of the personality. See also **humanistic psychology.**

self-threading pin, (in dentistry) a screwlike metal pin placed into a hole whose diameter is slightly smaller in diameter than the pin, used to improve the retention of a restoration.

self-tolerance, the absence of an immune response directed against a person's own tissue antigens.

self-transcendence, the ability to focus attention on doing something for the sake of others, as opposed to self-actualization, in which doing something for oneself is an end goal. See also **altruism.**

Self-Transcendence Theory, the expansion of a person's concept of self through introspection, interaction with other people and the surrounding environment, integration of the past and future, and spirituality. It is based on the belief that to maintain a sense of well-being, older adults must continue their cognitive development during the process of aging. See **Reed, Pamela G.**

sellar diaphragm, a dural partition consisting of a small horizontal shelf of meningeal dura mater that covers the hypophysial fossa in the sella turcica of the sphenoid bone. Also called **diaphragma sellae.**

sella turcica /sel″ə tur″sikə/ [L, *sella,* seat, *turcica,* Turkish], a transverse depression crossing the midline on the superior surface of the body of the sphenoid bone and containing the pituitary gland.

Sellick's maneuver. See **cricoid pressure.**

Selsun, an antidandruff and antiseborrheic medicated shampoo. Brand name for **selenium sulfide.**

Selzentry, an antiviral agent used in the treatment of human immunodeficiency virus. Brand name for **maraviroc.**

SEM, abbreviation for **scanning electron microscope.**

semantics /siman″tiks/ [Gk, *semantikos,* significant], the study of language with special concern for the meanings of words or other symbols.

-seme, suffix meaning "(one) having an orbital (cephalometric) index of less than 84, more than 89, or in between" as specified by the prefix: *megaseme, mesoseme, microseme.*

semeio-, combining form meaning "sign" or "symptom": *semeiotic.*

semeiotic, related to the description of the signs and symptoms of disease.

semen /sē″mən/ [L, seed], the thick, whitish secretion of the male reproductive organs discharged from the urethra during ejaculation. It contains spermatozoa in their nutrient plasma as well as secretions of the prostate, seminal vesicles, and other glands. Also called **seminal fluid, sperm. –seminal,** *adj.*

semen analysis, a fluid analysis that is one of the most important aspects of the fertility workup. This test involves measuring freshly collected semen for volume, counting the sperm, evaluating sperm motility, and studying sperm morphology.

semi- /sem″ē-/, prefix meaning "one half": *semicoma, semicanal, semiconductor.*

semiautomatic external defibrillator /sem″ē-ô′təmat″ik/, a portable apparatus used to restart a heart that has stopped. It is programmed to analyze cardiac rhythms automatically and indicate to a health care professional when to deliver a defibrillating shock.

semicanal /-kənal″/, **1.** a canal with an opening on one side. **2.** a deep groove on the edge of a bone that accommodates part of an adjoining bone.

semicircular canal /-sur′kyələr/ [L, *semi-,* half, *circulare,* to go around, *canalis,* channel], any of three bony fluid-filled loops in the osseous labyrinth of the internal ear, associated with the sense of balance. The posterior, superior, and lateral canals, all about 0.8 mm in diameter and perpendicular to each other, open into the cochlea. The posterior canal is the longest.

semicircular duct, one of three ducts that make up the membranous labyrinth of the inner ear. See also **membranous labyrinth.**

semicoma. See **coma.**

semicomatose /-kō″mətōs/ [L, *semi,* half; Gk, *koma,* deep sleep], pertaining to a condition of stupor from which a patient can be aroused. See also **coma, Glasgow Coma Scale.**

semiconductor /-kənduk″tər/, a solid crystalline substance whose electric conductivity is intermediate between that of a conductor and that of an insulator. An n-type semiconductor has loosely bound electrons that are relatively free to move about inside the material. A p-type semiconductor is one with holes, or positive traps, in which electrons may be bound. The holes may appear to migrate through the material.

semiconscious /-kon″shəs/, pertaining to an impaired state of consciousness, characterized by obtundation, stupor, or hypersomnia, from which a patient can be aroused only by energetic stimulation.

semiflexion /-flek″shən/, a limb position midway between full flexion and full extension.

semi-Fowler position /-fou″lər/ [L, *semi,* half; George R. Fowler, American surgeon, 1848–1906], placement of a patient in an inclined position, with the upper half of the body raised by elevating the head of the bed approximately 30 to 45 degrees.

semihorizontal heart /-hôr′əzon″təl/, an electric "position" of the heart that lies between the horizontal and intermediate positions when the QRS axis is 0 degrees.

semilunar bone. See **lunate bone.**

semilunar fold of the conjunctiva, a fold of membrane that extends laterally from the lacrimal caruncle. It has a concave free border directed to the cornea. In some individuals it contains smooth muscular fibers. Also called **plica semilunaris conjunctivae.**

semilunar hiatus, the deep semilunar groove anterior and inferior to the bulla of the ethmoid bone. The anterior ethmoidal cells, the maxillary sinus, and sometimes the frontonasal duct drain through it via the ethmoid infundibulum.

semilunar valve /-lōō″nər/ [L, *semi* + *luna,* moon, *valva,* folding door], **1.** a valve with half-moon–shaped cusps, such as the aortic valve and the pulmonary valve. **2.** any one of the cusps constituting such a valve. **3.** simple cuplike valves found in the venous and lymphatic vessels. See also **heart valve, mitral valve, tricuspid valve.**

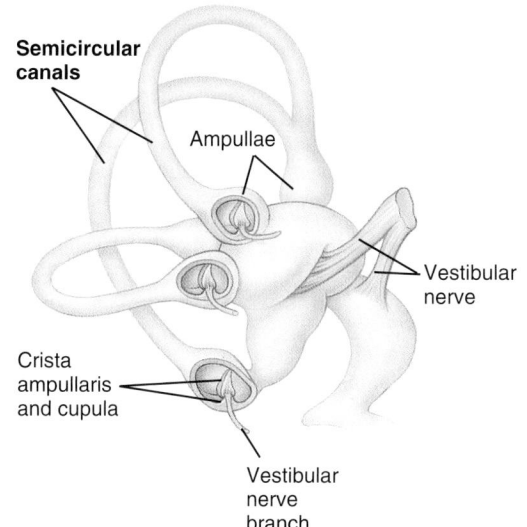

Semicircular canals *(Thibodeau and Patton, 2007)*

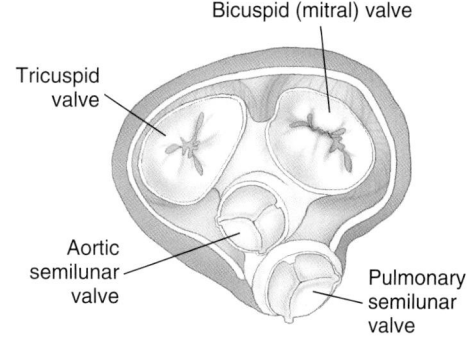

Semilunar valves *(Leonard, 2009)*

semimembranosus /-mem′brənō″səs/ [L, *semi* + *membrana,* membrane], one of three posterior femoral muscles. Situated at the back and medial side of the thigh, it originates in a thick tendon attached to the tuberosity of the ischium and inserts into the horizontal groove on the medial condyle of the tibia. The tendon of insertion passes some fibers laterally and upward to insert on the lateral condyle of the femur and form part of the oblique popliteal ligament behind the knee. The tendon of insertion forms one of the two medial hamstrings. The muscle is innervated by several branches of the tibial part of the sciatic nerve, containing fibers from the fifth lumbar and the first two sacral nerves. The muscle functions to flex the leg, to rotate it medially after flexion, and to extend the thigh. Compare **biceps femoris, hamstring muscle, semitendinosus.**

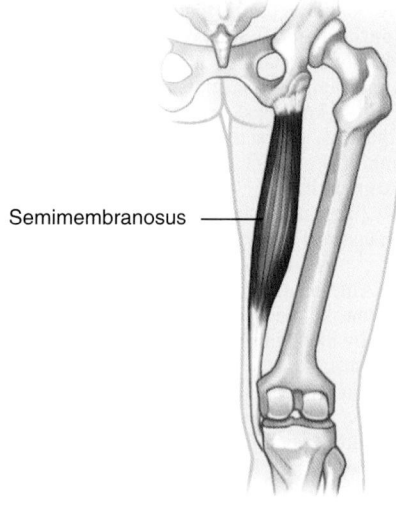

Semimembranosus

semimembranous /-mem″brənəs/ [L, *semi,* half, *membrana*], pertaining to a muscle or other tissue that is partly membrane or fascia, such as the semimembranous hamstring muscle.
seminal. See **semen.**
seminal crest, a prominent portion of the urethral crest on which is the opening of the prostatic utricle and, on either side of it, the orifices of the ejaculatory ducts.
seminal duct /sem′inəl/ [L, *semen,* seed, *ducere,* to lead], any duct through which semen passes, such as the vas deferens or the ejaculatory duct.
seminal emission [L, *semen,* seed, *emittere,* to send out], a discharge of semen.
seminal fluid. See **semen.**
seminal fluid test, any of several tests of semen to detect abnormalities in a male's reproductive system and to determine fertility. Some common factors considered are seminal fluid liquefaction time and spermatic quantity, morphological characteristics, motility, volume, and pH. Normal values in some of these tests are as follows: sperm count, 60 million/mL to 150 million/mL of seminal fluid; pH, higher than 7 (7.7 average); ejaculation volume, 1.5 mL to 5.0 mL; and motility, 60% of sperm.
seminal vesicle, either of the paired saclike glandular structures posterolateral to the urinary bladder in the male and functioning as part of the reproductive system. Each sac is pyramidal in shape and convoluted in appearance and at the anterior extremity becomes constricted into a narrow straight duct that joins the vas deferens to form the ejaculatory duct. The seminal vesicles produce a fluid that is added to the secretion of the testes and other glands to form the semen.
seminal vesicle cyst, a cyst in the wall of a seminal vesicle. It may be congenital and associated with other urinary tract anomalies or acquired, such as a result of obstruction of the vesicle.
seminal vesiculitis, inflammation of a seminal vesicle.

semination /sem′inā″shən/, the introduction of semen into the female genital tract.
seminiferous /sem′inif″ərəs/ [L, *semen* + *ferre,* to bear], transporting or producing semen, such as the tubules of the testis.
seminiferous cords, the primordia of the seminiferous tubules, derived from the gonadal cords of the testis.
seminiferous tubules [L, *semen,* seed, *ferre,* to bear, *tubulus*], long, threadlike tubes packed in areolar tissue in the lobes of the testes.
seminoma /sem′inō″mə/ *pl. seminomas, seminomata* [L, *semen* + *oma,* tumor], a malignant tumor of the testis. It is the most common testicular tumor and is believed to arise from the seminiferous epithelium of the mature or maturing testis. The two types are classic, or typical, and spermatocytic; anaplastic seminoma is a variant of the classic type. Compare **dysgerminoma.**

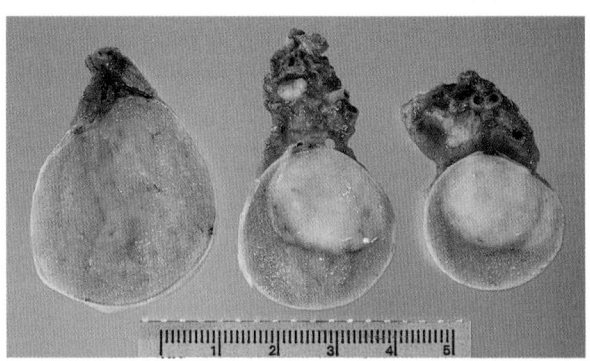

Seminoma *(Kumar, Cotran, and Robbins, 2003)*

semiparametric statistics /sem′ē·par′ə·met′rik/ [L, *semi,* half + Gk, *para,* to, at, or from the side of + *metron,* measure], statistical methodology that combines both parametric and nonparametric elements. It is used for estimating population parameters when a function is unknown (e.g., the distribution function of a random variable that has not been observed).
semipermeable /-pur″mē·əbəl/ [L, *semi,* half, *permeare,* to pass through], pertaining to a membrane that allows the passage of some molecules but prevents the passage of others. Also **selectively permeable.**
semipermeable membrane [L, *semi* + *permeare,* to pass through], a membrane that prevents the passage of some substances but allows the passage of others based on differences in the size, charge, or lipid-solubility of the substances.
semiprone side position, a position in which the patient lies on the side with the knee and thigh drawn upward toward the chest. The chest and abdomen are allowed to fall forward. Left semiprone side position is the position of choice for administering enemas or conducting rectal examinations.

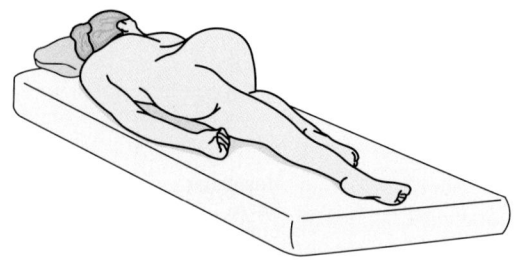

Semiprone side position *(Monahan et al, 2007)*

semirecumbent /-rikum″bənt/, in a reclining position.

semispinalis muscles, the most superficial collection of muscle fibers in the transversospinales group. They are found in the thoracic and cervical regions and attach to the occipital bone at the base of the skull.

semisupine /-səpīn″/, pertaining to a posture that is between a midposition and the supine position.

semisynthetic /-sinthet″ik/ [L, *semi,* half; Gk, *synthesis,* putting together], pertaining to a natural substance that has been partially altered by chemical manipulation.

semitendinosus /sem′iten′dinō″səs/ [L, *semi + tendere,* to stretch], one of three posterior femoral muscles of the thigh, remarkable for the great length of the tendon of insertion. It is a fusiform muscle located in the posterior and medial part of the thigh, arising from the tuberosity of the ischium. It ends just distal to the middle of the thigh in a long round tendon that crosses the semimembranosus and curves around the medial condyle of the tibia and inserts into the medial surface of the tibia. It functions to flex the leg, to rotate it medially after flexion, and to extend the thigh. Compare **biceps femoris, hamstring muscle, semimembranosus.**

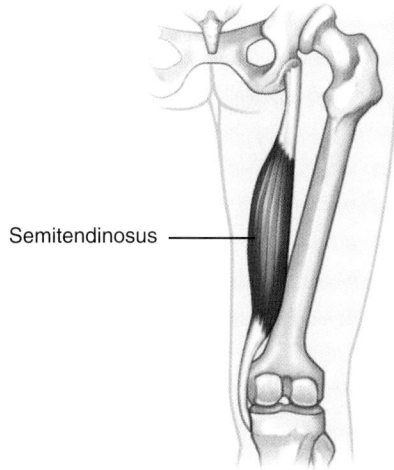

Semitendinosus

semivertical heart /-vur″tikəl/, an electric "position" of the heart that lies between the intermediate and vertical positions when the QRS axis is 60 degrees.

Semmelweis, Ignaz Phillip [Hungarian physician (1818–1865)], born in Buda and educated at the universities of Pest and Vienna. Semmelweis recognized a high rate in puerperal fever and hypothesized that the infection was carried from patient to patient by the physicians. He instituted preventative measures, such as cleansing of the hands with chlorinated lime. He met fierce opposition from his contemporaries and rejection of his theory. He is now considered the pioneer of asepsis in obstetrics.

Semprex-D, a fixed-combination drug containing an antihistamine and a decongestant. Brand name for **acrivastine, pseudoephedrine hydrochloride.**

sender [AS, *sendan,* to send], in communication theory, the person by whom a message is encoded and sent.

seneciosis /senes′ē·ō″sis/, a toxic reaction to the ingestion of plants of the genus *Senecio,* which are used to make bush tea. The poison causes liver damage, particularly in malnourished patients. Common *Senecio* species include ragwort and life root, both used in herbal remedies.

senescence /sənes″əns/ [L, *senescere,* to grow old], the state of being old.

senescent /sənes″ənt/ [L, *senescere,* to grow old], *n.,* pertaining to aging or growing old. See also **senile. –senescence,** *n.*

senescent cell antigen, an antigen that appears on old red blood cells that bind immunoglobulin G autoantibodies. It is also found on lymphocytes, platelets, and neutrophils.

Sengstaken-Blakemore tube [Robert W. Sengstaken, American neurosurgeon, 1923–1978; Arthur H. Blakemore, American surgeon, 1897–1970], a thick catheter having a triple lumen and two balloons, used to produce pressure by balloon tamponade to arrest hemorrhaging from esophageal varices. Attached to a tube, one balloon is inflated in the stomach and exerts pressure against the upper orifice. Similarly attached, another longer and narrower balloon exerts pressure on the walls of the esophagus. The third tube is used for withdrawing gastric contents.

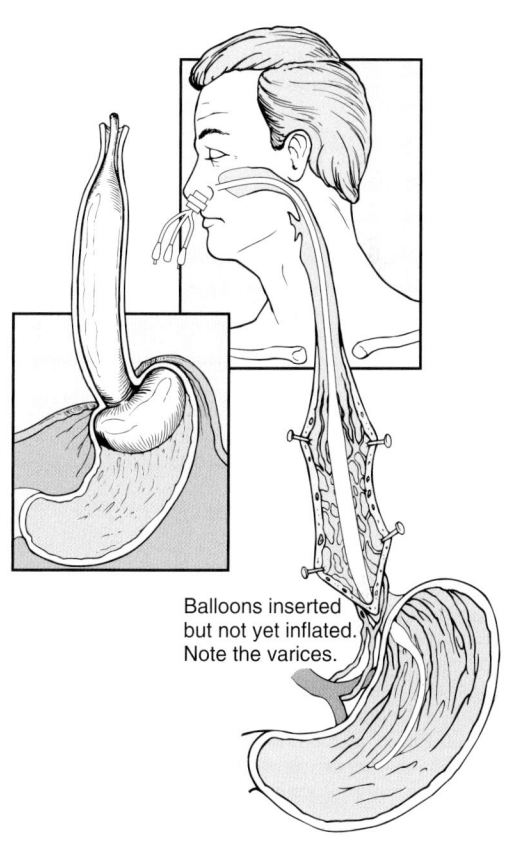

Balloons inserted but not yet inflated. Note the varices.

Sengstaken-Blakemore tube *(Lewis et al, 2007)*

senile /sē″nīl/ [L, *senilis,* aged], pertaining to or characteristic of old age or the process of aging. See also **aging. –senility,** *n.*

senile angioma. See **cherry angioma.**

senile arteriosclerosis, hardening of the arteries associated with aging.

senile cataract, a kind of cataract, associated with aging, in which an opacity forms in the crystalline lens of the eye. See also **cataract.**

senile dementia, dementia occurring in older persons usually over the age of 65. Because most cases are due to Alzheimer disease, the term is sometimes used as a synonym for dementia of the Alzheimer type, late onset.

senile dementia–Alzheimer type (SDAT), **1.** dementia occurring in older persons, usually over the age of

65, resulting from Alzheimer disease. **2.** See **senile dementia.**

senile dental caries, *(Obsolete)* now called **root surface caries.** See also **dental caries.**

senile involution, a pattern of retrograde changes occurring with advancing age and resulting in the progressive shrinking and degeneration of tissues and organs.

senile keratosis. See **actinic keratosis.**

senile lenticular myopia, an early increase in the index of refraction of the lens, resulting in a decrease in hyperopia and an increase in myopia.

senile nanism, dwarfism associated with progeria. See also **progeria.**

senile purpura, bruising associated with advanced age. See **purpura senilis.**

senile tremor [L, *senilis,* aged, *tremor,* shaking], a tremor associated with aging.

senile vaginitis [L, *senilis,* aged, *vagina,* sheath, *itis,* inflammation], a condition of atrophy of the vagina resulting from the postmenopausal loss of estrogen secretion.

senile wart. See **actinic keratosis.**

senility /sinil″itē/ [L, *senilis,* aged], the general state of reduced mental and physical vigor associated with aging.

senior centers /sē″nyər/, community agencies for older adults. The centers offer nutritional, recreational, educational, health, and legal services. Funding is often through the Older Americans Act.

Senior Companion Program, a service that offers personal assistance and peer support to homebound and chronically ill older people.

senior patient, in the United States, a Medicare beneficiary enrolled in a health maintenance organization.

senna, an herbal product taken from several *Cassia* species found across the world.

■ INDICATIONS: It is used as a laxative.

■ CONTRAINDICATIONS: It should not be used during pregnancy and lactation, in children less than 12 years of age (unless prescribed by physician), or in those with known hypersensitivity to this product. Senna is also prohibited in those with intestinal obstruction, ulcerative colitis, GI bleeding, appendicitis, acute surgical abdomen, nausea, vomiting, or congestive heart failure.

Sennetsu fever /sə·net′sōō/, a febrile disease occurring in Japan and Malaysia, caused by the bacterium *Ehrlichia sennetsu.* Symptoms include headache, nausea or vomiting, lymphocytosis, and postauricular and posterior lymphadenopathy. The vector of this disease is unknown; however, infection may occur from ingestion of raw fish.

sens-, combining form meaning "perception" or "feeling": *sensation, sensibility, sensor.*

sensate /sen″sāt/, capable of perceiving sensory stimuli.

sensate focus technique, a therapeutic program for the treatment of erectile dysfunction in males.

sensation /sensā″shən/ [L, *sentire,* to feel], **1.** a feeling, impression, or awareness of a body state or condition that results from the stimulation of a sensory receptor site and transmission of the nerve impulse along an afferent fiber to the brain. Kinds include **delayed sensation, epigastric sensation, primary sensation, referred sensation, subjective sensation. 2.** a feeling or an awareness of a mental or emotional state, which may or may not result in response to an external stimulus.

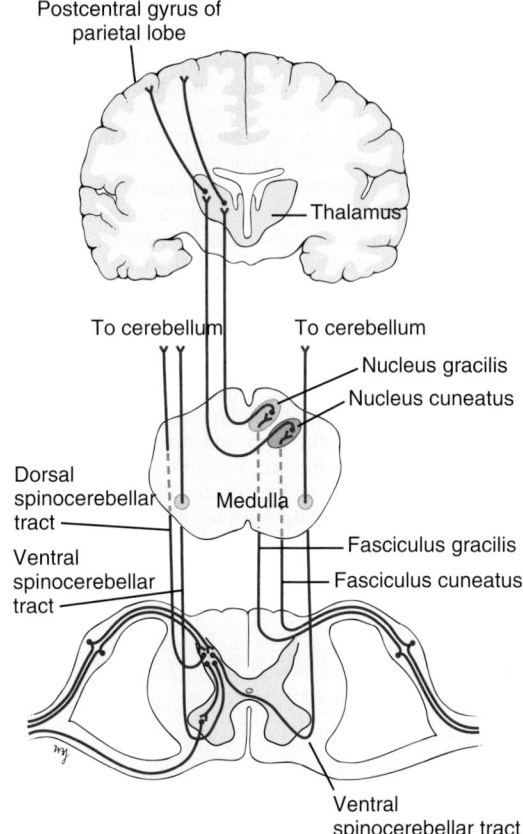

Pathways of sensation *(Swartz, 2009)*

sense [L, *sentire,* to feel], **1.** *n.,* the faculty by which stimuli are perceived and conditions outside and within the body are distinguished and evaluated. The major senses are sight, hearing, smell, taste, touch, and pressure. Other senses include hunger; thirst; pain; temperature; proprioception; and spatial, temporal, and visceral sensations. **2.** *n.,* the ability to feel; a sensation. **3.** *n.,* the capacity to understand; normal mental ability. **4.** *v.,* to perceive through a sense organ. **5.** *adj.,* pertaining to the sense strand of a nucleic acid. Compare **antisense.**

sense strand, the strand of a double-stranded nucleic acid that encodes the product. In DNA it is the strand that encodes the RNA, having thus the same base sequence except changing T for U in the RNA. Also called **coding strand.** Compare **antisense strand.**

sensibility /sen′sibil″itē/, the ability to perceive sensations and impressions, both physical and psychological.

sensible /sen″sibəl/, **1.** capable of sensation. **2.** possessing reason or judgment. **3.** capable of being perceived.

sensible perspiration [L, *sensibilis,* perceptible], loss of body fluid through the secretory activity of the sweat glands in a quantity sufficient to be observed. Compare **insensible perspiration.**

Sensipar, a calcium receptor agonist used in the management of hypercalcemia. Brand name for **cinacalcet.**

sensitive /sen″sitiv/ [L, *sentire,* to feel], **1.** able to perceive and transmit a sensation or stimulus. **2.** affected by low concentrations of antimicrobial drugs, said of microorganisms.

3. abnormally susceptible to a subject, such as a drug or foreign protein.

sensitive volume [L, *sentire* + *volumen,* paper roll], the part of an object from which a magnetic resonance signal is preferentially acquired because of strong magnetic field inhomogeneity elsewhere. This preferential acquisition can be enhanced by the use of a shaped radiofrequency field that is strongest in the sensitive volume.

sensitivity /sen′sitiv″itē/ [L, *sentire*], **1.** capacity to feel, transmit, or react to a stimulus. **2.** susceptibility to a substance, such as a drug or an antigen. See also **allergy, hypersensitivity. 3.** the lowest level of a substance that can be detected by a laboratory test procedure.

sensitivity test, a laboratory method for testing the effectiveness of antibiotics. It is usually done on organisms known to be potentially resistant to antibiotic therapy in vitro. A report of a "resistant" finding means the antibiotic is not effective in inhibiting the growth of a pathogen, whereas use of an effective antibiotic results in a "sensitive" report. See also **antibiotic sensitivity test.**

sensitivity training group, a group that offers members a supportive atmosphere in which to experiment with and alter behavior patterns and interpersonal reactions. Sensitivity training focuses on learning what occurs during group interactions, testing and refining new behavioral responses in light of the reactions they evoke, and applying those responses to situations outside the group setting. Also called **T group.** See also **encounter group, psychotherapy.**

sensitization /sen′sitīzā″shən/ [L, *sentire* + Gk, *izein,* to cause], **1.** reaction in which specific antibodies develop in response to an antigen. Allergic reactions result from excess sensitization to a foreign protein. Sensitization can be induced by immunization, in which a pathogen that has been made noninfectious is introduced into the body. See also **active sensitization. 2.** a photodynamic method of destroying microorganisms through the use of substances, such as fluorescent dyes, that absorb light and emit energy at wavelengths destructive to the organisms. **3.** *(Nontechnical)* anaphylaxis. −*sensitize, v.*

sensitized /sen″sitīzd/, pertaining to tissues that have been made reactive to antigens. See also **allergy.**

sensitized vaccine [L, *sentire,* to feel, *vaccinus,* of a cow], a vaccine that is prepared by suspending microorganisms in their own homologous immune serum.

sensor /sen″sər/, an apparatus designed to react to physical stimuli, such as temperature, light, or movement.

sensoriglandular /sen′sərēglan″dyələr/, pertaining to the reflexive secretion by glands, triggered by sensory stimulation of a nerve.

sensorimotor /sen′sərēmō″tər/ [L, *sentire,* to feel, *moveo,* to move], pertaining to both sensory and motor nerve functions.

sensorimotor phase [L, *sentire* + *moveo,* to move], the developmental phase of childhood, encompassing the period from birth to 2 years of age, according to Piagetian psychology.

sensorimotor therapy, therapy designed to enhance the integration of reflex phenomena and the emergence of voluntary motor behaviors concerned with posture and locomotion.

sensorimuscular /-mus″kyələr/, pertaining to contraction of muscles triggered by sensory stimulation.

sensorineural /sen′sərēnoor″əl/ [L, *sentire,* to feel; Gk, *neuron,* nerve], pertaining to sensory nerves.

sensorineural hearing loss, a form of hearing loss in which sound is conducted normally through the external and middle ear but a defect in the inner ear or auditory nerve results in hearing loss. Sound discrimination may or may not be affected. Amplification of the sound with a hearing aid will help many people with sensorineural hearing loss; if a person demonstrates an intolerance to loud noises, the hearing aid must be adjusted properly to prevent discomfort. Compare **conductive hearing loss.**

sensorium /sensôr″ē·əm/, (in psychology) the part of the consciousness that includes the special sensory perceptive powers and their central correlation and integration in the brain. A clear sensorium conveys the presence of a reasonably accurate memory together with a correct orientation for time, place, and person. Sensorium may be clouded in certain stages of delirium.

sensorivasomotor /-vā′zōmō″tər/, pertaining to the contraction or dilation of a blood vessel in response to a sensory stimulus.

sensory /sen″sərē/ [L, *sentire* to feel], **1.** pertaining to sensation. **2.** pertaining to a part or all of the body's sensory nerve network.

sensory apraxia. See **ideational apraxia.**

sensory area [L, *sentire,* to feel, *area,* space], the regions of the cerebral cortex that receive impulses from sensory nerves, including the thalamic, nucleic, and parietal lobes.

sensory-based language, the use of nonverbal behavior in neurolinguistic communication. Examples include puzzled expressions, scowling, and finger pointing.

sensory deficit, a defect in the function of one or more of the senses.

sensory deprivation [L, *sentire* + ME, *depriven,* to deprive; L, *atio,* process], an involuntary loss of physical awareness caused by detachment from external sensory stimuli. Such deprivation often results in psychological disorders, such as panic, mental confusion, depression, and hallucinations. Sensory deprivation may be associated with various handicaps and conditions, such as blindness, heavy sedation, and prolonged isolation.

sensory desensitization, techniques based on the theory that nerve fibers that carry pain sensation can be positively influenced through the use of pressure, rubbing, vibration, transcutaneous electrical nerve stimulation (TENS), percussion, and active motion.

sensory discrimination, the ability to discern and assign meaning to specific sensory stimuli.

sensory end organ [L, *sentire,* to feel; AS, *ende* + Gk, *organon,* instrument], any of the specialized nerve endings devoted to detection of specific environmental stimuli, such as smell, sight, hearing, temperature, or touch.

sensory integration, the organization of sensory input for use, a perception of the body or environment, an adaptive response, a learning process, or the development of some neural function.

sensory integrative dysfunction, a disorder or irregularity in brain function that makes sensory integration difficult.

sensory integrative therapy, therapy that involves sensory stimulation and adaptive responses to it according to a child's neurological needs. Treatment usually involves full body movements that provide vestibular, proprioceptive, and tactile stimulation. It usually does not include desk activities, speech training, reading lessons, or training in specific perceptual or motor skills. The goal is to improve the brain's ability to process and organize sensations.

sensory modulation, the process of interpreting and filtering sensory information. Sensory modulation originates in the central nervous system as the neurological ability to regulate

S

and process sensory stimuli; this subsequently offers the individual an opportunity to respond behaviorally to the stimulus.

sensory modulation disorder /prə·nən·sē·ā″·shən/ [L, *pro*, unamateurishly, *nuntio*, I declare], impairment in the ability to regulate incoming sensations, or a failure to detect and orient to novel or important sensory information.

sensory nerve, a nerve consisting of afferent fibers that conduct sensory impulses from the periphery of the body to the brain or spinal cord via the dorsal spinal roots.

sensory neuropathy, neuropathy or polyneuropathy of sensory nerves.

sensory nucleus of trigeminal nerve, a collection of nerve cells in the pons that serves as the main nucleus for reception of tactile fibers of the trigeminal area.

sensory overload, a condition in which an individual receives an excessive or intolerable amount of sensory stimuli, as in a busy hospital or clinic or an intensive care unit. The effects of sensory overload are similar to those of sensory deprivation, including confusion and hallucination.

sensory pathway [L, *sentire,* to feel; AS, *paeth* + *weg*], the route followed by a sensory nerve impulse from an end organ to a reflex center in the brain or spinal cord.

sensory-perceptual overload. See **sensory overload.**

sensory processing, means by which the brain receives, detects, and integrates incoming sensory information for use in producing adaptive responses to one's environment.

sensory receptor [L, *sentire,* to feel, *recipere,* to receive], a specialized nerve ending that, when stimulated, initiates an afferent or sensory nerve impulse.

sensory reeducation, a two-part therapeutic intervention strategy employed after a nerve injury to improve functional outcomes. Both protective and discriminative sensory reeducation should begin as soon as possible after a nerve injury to encourage the patient to use the affected extremity before abnormal use patterns can develop.The goal of protective sensory reeducation after a peripheral nerve repair or after a cerebrovascular accident (CVA) that results in sensory loss to a limb is to educate the patient in compensatory techniques that should be used to protect the insensate body part. The goal of discriminative sensory reeducation is the recovery of stereognosis (that is, the ability to recognize the form of an object without using visual or auditory cues). Discriminative sensory reeducation following a peripheral nerve injury incorporates graded training tasks involving localization and discrimination of textures, shapes and objects. A visual-tactile matching process can be used; the patient attempts to correctly identify the stimulus location or modality type, first with eyes closed. If the patient is wrong, then the stimulation is repeated with the eyes open, and the patient concentrates on matching what he feels with what he sees.

sensory root [L, *sentire,* to feel], the proximal end of a dorsal afferent nerve as it is attached to the spinal cord.

sensory seeking, **1.** craving movement, as well as tactile and proprioceptive input, that is associated with a type of sensory-processing disorder. Constant movement and excessive talking are usually prominent. **2.** displaying behavior associated with sensory modulation disorder.

sensory threshold [L, *sentire,* to feel; AS, *therscold*], the point at which increasing stimuli trigger the start of an afferent nerve impulse. Absolute threshold is the lowest point at which response to a stimulus can be perceived.

sensual /sen″shoo·əl/ [L, *sensualis*], pertaining to a great interest in sex, food, or other sense-satisfying topics.

sentient /sen″shənt/ [L, *sentire,* to feel], possessing sensitivity or powers of sensation and perception.

sentinel gland /sen″tinəl/ [Fr, *sentinelle* + L, *glans,* acorn], a node or growth that is associated with the presence of a nearby tumor or ulcer. An example is a supraclavicular node with cancer cells that have metastasized from an undiscovered primary cancer.

sentinel lymph node biopsy (SLNB), a diagnostic procedure to identify metastatic tumor cells from a primary breast tumor or melanoma. See **sentinel node biopsy.**

sentinel node. See **Virchow's node.**

sentinel node biopsy, biopsy of the first lymph node to receive lymphatic drainage from a malignant tumor. Also called **sentinel lymph node biopsy, intraoperative lymphatic mapping.**

■ METHOD: The surgeon injects a radioactive substance and/ or a blue dye near the tumor. Following injection, the agents follow the natural drainage path from the tumor to the first tier of surrounding lymph nodes. The lymph nodes most appropriate for examination then "light up" like sentinels either through the use of a device that monitors the radioactive substance or visualization of their blue stain. The first node is removed by the surgeon and examined by a pathologist.

■ PATIENT CARE CONSIDERATIONS: Sentinel node biopsy assists in the staging of a cancer; it also serves as a mechanism to avoid extensive lymph node surgery.

■ OUTCOME CRITERIA: A negative biopsy eliminates the need for more extensive lymph node surgery, and there is a high probability that other nodes are cancer-free. A positive biopsy assists in developing a plan for the treatment of the malignancy.

Seoul virus /sōl/, a virus of the genus *Hantavirus* that causes mild to moderately severe epidemic hemorrhagic fever in Asia, primarily Korea and Japan. Several species of rats are the natural hosts. See also **epidemic hemorrhagic fever.**

SEP, abbreviation for **somatosensory evoked potential.**

separating spring /sep′ə·rāt·ing/ [L, *separare,* to separate; AS, *springan,* to jump], a spring placed between the teeth to obtain separation.

separating wire, a brass wire threaded between two teeth having tight contact in an effort to wedge them slightly apart before fitting a band in the application of an orthodontic appliance.

separation agent /sep′ərā″shən/, a reagent used to separate bound and free tracers in radioassay.

separation anxiety [L, *separare,* to separate, *atio,* process], fear and apprehension caused by separation from familiar surroundings and significant people. The syndrome occurs commonly in an infant separated from its mother or mothering figure or approached by a stranger. In a separation crisis the child goes through three distinct states. The protest stage is marked by loud cries, which can last for several days and during which the child is inconsolable. In the second phase the child stops crying and becomes depressed as a result of increasing hopelessness, grief, and mourning. The third stage is one of detachment or denial, in which the child outwardly appears to have adjusted.

separation factor. See **selectivity.**

separator /sep′ə·rā·tər/ [L, *separare,* to separate], **1.** a device for separating or moving opposing structures away from each other. **2.** (in dentistry) a device or instrument for wedging teeth apart, especially proximal teeth having tight contact, as for the examination of proximal surfaces, for finishing a restoration, or before banding in orthodontic therapy.

s-EPO, abbreviation for *serum erythropoietin.*

seps-, prefix meaning "decay": *sepsis.*

sepsis /sep″sis/ [Gk, *sepein,* to become putrid], infection; contamination. **−septic,** *adj.* Compare **asepsis.**

-sepsis, combining form meaning "decay caused by a (specified) cause or of a (specified) sort": *antisepsis, asepsis.*

sepsis syndrome, a systemic response to an infection. See also **systemic inflammatory response syndrome.**

sept-, **1.** combining form meaning "nasal septum": *septal, septorhinoplasty.* **2.** combining form meaning "seven": *septuplet.*

septa. See **septum.**

septal /sep″təl/ [L, *saeptum,* enclosure], pertaining to a septum.

septal cartilage. See **nasal cartilage.**

septal defect [L, *saeptum,* fence, *defectus,* failure], a defect in the wall separating the left and right sides of the heart. Depending on the size and the site of the defect, various amounts of oxygenated and deoxygenated blood mix, causing a decrease in the amount of oxygen carried in the blood to the peripheral tissues. The defect is usually congenital. Kinds include **atrial septal defect, ventricular septal defect.**

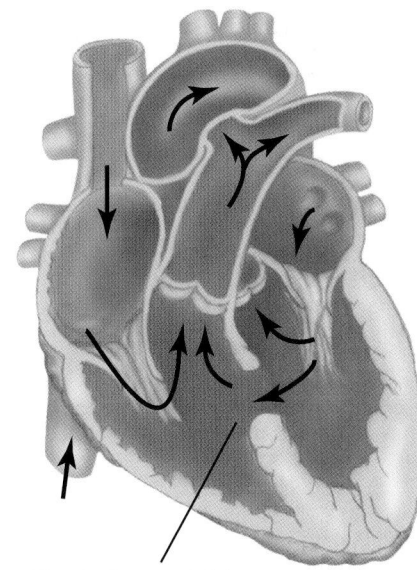

Ventricular septal defect

Ventricular septal defect *(James and Ashwill, 2007)*

septal lines. See **Kerley lines.**

septate /sep″tāt/, pertaining to a structure divided by a septum.

septi-, prefix meaning "seven": *septivalent.*

septic. See **sepsis.**

-septic, combining form meaning "decay or putrefaction": *aseptic, antiseptic.*

septic abortion [Gk, *septikos,* putrid], spontaneous or induced termination of a pregnancy in which the mother's life may be threatened because of the invasion of germs into the endometrium, myometrium, and beyond. The woman requires immediate and intensive care, massive antibiotic therapy, evacuation of the uterus, and often emergency hysterectomy to prevent death from overwhelming infection and septic shock. Compare **infected abortion.** See also **illegal abortion, induced abortion.**

septicaemia. See **septicemia.**

-septicaemia. See **-septicemia, -septicaemia.**

septic arthritis, an acute form of arthritis characterized by bacterial inflammation of a joint caused by the spread of bacteria through the bloodstream from an infection elsewhere in the body or by contamination of a joint during trauma or surgery. The joint is stiff, painful, tender, warm, and swollen. The diagnosis is confirmed by bacteriological identification of an organism in a specimen obtained by aspiration of the joint. Parenteral antibiotics are given to prevent destruction of the joint and are continued for several weeks after inflammation has resolved. Repeated aspiration of the joint or surgical incision and drainage may be performed to relieve pressure on it. Physical therapy as the joint heals is helpful to restore it to full range of motion. Also called **acute bacterial arthritis.**

septicemia /sep″tisē″mē-ə/ [Gk, *septikos* + *haima,* blood], systemic infection in which pathogens are present in the circulating blood, having spread from an infection in any part of the body. It is diagnosed by culture of the blood and is vigorously treated with antibiotics. Characteristically, septicemia causes fever, chill, hypotension, prostration, pain, headache, nausea, or diarrhea. Also called **blood poisoning.** Also spelled **septicaemia.** Compare **bacteremia.** See also **septic shock.** −**septicemic,** *adj.*

-septicemia, -septicaemia, combining form meaning "(condition of the) blood caused by virulent microorganisms": *streptosepticemia, autosepticemia.*

septicemic. See **septicemia.**

septicemic plague /sep″tisē″mik/, a rapidly fatal form of bubonic plague in which septicemia with meningitis occurs before buboes have had time to form. Compare **bubonic plague, pneumonic plague.** See also **plague,** *Yersinia pestis.*

septic fever, an elevation of body temperature associated with infection by pathogenic microorganisms or in response to a toxin secreted by a microorganism.

septic infarct [Gk, *septikos,* putrid; L, *infarcire,* to stuff], an infected segment of dead tissue.

septic shock, a form of shock that occurs in septicemia when endotoxins or exotoxins are released from certain bacteria in the bloodstream, occasionally caused by the presence of fungi or viruses in the blood. These toxins cause vasodilation, resulting in a dramatic fall in blood pressure. Fever, tachycardia, increased respiration rate, and confusion or coma also may occur. Septic shock is usually preceded by signs of severe infection, often of the genitourinary or GI system. The causative bacterium is most frequently gram-negative. Antibiotics, vasopressors, and IV fluids and volume expanders are usually given. In some cases, treatment with monoclonal antibodies may be considered. Compare **hypovolemic shock.** Kinds include **toxic shock syndrome, bacteremic shock.** See also **shock.**

septic sore throat [Gk, *septikos,* putrid; AS, *sar + throte*], a severe throat infection, usually caused by a streptococcus strain, resulting in fever and marked exhaustion.

septivalent. See **heptavalent.**

septooptic dysplasia /sep″tō-op″tik dis·plā″zhə/, a congenital syndrome of hypoplasia of the optic disc with other ocular abnormalities, absence of the septum pellucidum, and hypopituitarism leading to growth deficiency. Also called **de Morsier syndrome.**

septoplasty /sep″tō-plas″tē/ [L, *saeptum,* septum; Gk, *plassein,* to form], surgical reconstruction of the nasal septum.

septorhinoplasty /sep″tōrī″nəplas″tē/ [L, *saeptum,* fence], the surgical correction of defects in the nasal septum.

septostomy /septos″təmē/, the creation of an opening in a septum by surgery.

Septra, an antibacterial agent that is a 1:5 mixture of the antibacterials trimethoprim and sulfamethoxazole. Also called *cotrimoxazole.* Brand name for **trimethoprim and sulfamethoxazole.**

septum /sep″təm/ *pl. septa* [L, *saeptum,* enclosure], a partition or wall, such as the interatrial septum that separates the atria of the heart.

septum pellucidum, a triangular double membrane situated in the median plane and separating the anterior horns of the lateral ventricles of the brain. Also called **transparent septum.**

septuplet /septup″lit/ [L, *septuplum,* group of seven], any one of seven children born of a single pregnancy.

sequela /sikwē″lə/ *pl. sequelae* [L, *sequi,* to follow], any abnormal condition that follows and is the result of a disease, treatment, or injury, such as paralysis after poliomyelitis, deafness after treatment with an ototoxic drug, or scar formation after a laceration.

sequence /sē″kwəns/ [L, *sequi,* to follow], an order of arrangement of objects or events, as the sequence of peptides in a protein molecule.

sequential chemotherapy, chemotherapy in which several agents are administered one at a time rather than concurrently to optimize dosage and increase patient tolerance.

sequential imaging, a diagnostic procedure used to study physiological processes by means of a series of closely timed images of the rapidly changing distribution of a radioactive tracer within the body.

sequential line imaging, the construction of a magnetic resonance image from successive lines through the object.

sequential pacing. See **pacing.**

sequential plane imaging, the construction of a magnetic resonance image from successive planes through the object. The planes may be selected by oscillation of gradient magnetic fields or by selective excitation.

sequential point imaging, the construction of a magnetic resonance image from successive point positions in the object.

sequester /sikwes″tər/ [L, *sequestare,* to lay aside], to detach, separate, or isolate, such as patient sequestration to prevent the spread of an infection.

sequestered antigens hypothesis, a proposed explanation for autoimmunity that stresses the relationship between antigen exposure, immunogenic cells, and body cells. It maintains that immunological tolerance depends on a certain degree of contact between immunological cells and body cells and on a certain degree of antigen exposure. The hypothesis holds that certain sequestered antigens in the brain, the lenses of the eye, and spermatozoa are isolated from the circulation of the blood and the lymph and therefore do not contact the cells of the immune system. When body tissues are damaged, the sequestered antigens are suddenly exposed to the immune system, which treats them as foreign, triggering an autoimmune reaction. Compare **forbidden clone hypothesis.**

sequestered edema, edema localized in the tissues surrounding a newly created surgical wound.

sequestra. See **sequestrum.**

sequestration /sē′kwestrā″shən/ [L, *sequestare,* to lay aside], **1.** the isolation of a patient or group of patients. **2.** a method of controlling hemorrhage of the head or trunk by isolating fluid in the arms and legs from the general circulation. **3.** allowing blood from the systemic circulation to perfuse a nonfunctioning part of a lung.

sequestrum /sikwes″trəm/ *pl. sequestra* [L, a deposit], a fragment of dead bone that is partially or entirely detached from the surrounding or adjacent healthy bone.

sequestrum forceps, a forceps with small, powerful teeth used for extracting necrotic or sharp fragments of bone from surrounding tissue.

sequoiasis /sikwoi″əsis/ [sequoia (tree) + Gk, *osis,* condition], a type of hypersensitivity pneumonitis common among workers in sawmills where redwood is processed. The antigens are the fungus *Pullularia pullulans* and species of the genus *Graphium,* found in moldy redwood sawdust.

Characteristics of the acute disease include chills, fever, cough, dyspnea, anorexia, nausea, and vomiting. Symptoms of the chronic disease include productive cough, dyspnea on exertion, fatigue, and weight loss.

Ser, abbreviation for **serine.**

sera. See **serum.**

Ser-Ap-Es, a fixed-combination antihypertensive drug containing a diuretic (hydrochlorothiazide) and antihypertensives (reserpine and hydralazine hydrochloride). Brand name for **hydrochlorothiazide, reserpine, hydrALAZINE hydrochloride.**

Serax, a benzodiazepine. Brand name for **oxazepam.**

serendipity /ser′əndip″itē/ [Serendip, author Horace Walpole's mythic land of pleasant surprises], the act of accidental discovery. It is one of many factors that lead to new discoveries in health care. For example, the medication sildenafil was originally developed for the treatment of angina pectoris, but during clinical trials it induced penile erections in some patients. Additional research explained the physiological reason for the erections and led to a shift in clinical investigations, resulting in sildenafil being widely used for erectile dysfunction.

Serentil, a phenothiazine antipsychotic drug. Brand name for **mesoridazine.**

Serevent, a long-acting sympathomimetic bronchodilator. Brand name for **salmeterol.**

serial /sir″ē·əl/ [L, *series,* row], pertaining to a succession, arrangement, or order of items.

serial casting, the process of using a sequence of casts to progressively correct a deformity.

serial determination [L, *series,* row, *determinare,* to limit], a laboratory test that is repeated at stated intervals, as in a series of repeated tests for cardiac enzymes in blood samples taken from a patient with suspected myocardial infarction.

serial dilution, a laboratory technique in which a substance, such as blood serum, is decreased in concentration in a series of proportional amounts. In antibody analysis, for example, a serum sample may be distributed in a series of tubes so that each has one half of the amount of the previous tube in the series, resulting in titers of 1:5, 1:10, 1:20, and so on.

serial extraction, a program of selective extraction of primary and sometimes secondary teeth over a period of time, with the objective of relieving crowding and of facilitating the eruption of remaining teeth into improved positions. Close supervision of ensuing eruption is essential because the closing over of spaces is common. Comprehensive orthodontic treatment should almost always be initiated during or after eruption for space management, control of tipping induced by the procedure, and correction of other problems.

serial processing, a specific order of information handled by various computer work centers. Information proceeds sequentially through each of the centers or processes.

serial section [L, *series,* in a row, *sectio*], one of a number of consecutive slices of tissue.

serial speech, overlearned speech involving a series of words, such as counting or reciting the days of the week.

serial static orthosis, a device that immobilizes a joint at its end available range and that is periodically adjusted to provide a sequential progression of end-range stretch to facilitate the development of a greater range of motion.

series /sir″ēs/ *pl. series* [L, in a row], a chain of objects or events arranged in a predictable order, such as the series of stages through which a mature blood cell develops.

serine (Ser) /ser″ēn/, a nonessential amino acid found in many proteins in the body (e.g., casein, vitellin). It is synthesized from glycine or threonin and a precursor of the amino acids purine, cysteine, and others. It can be found in urine. See also **amino acid, protein.**

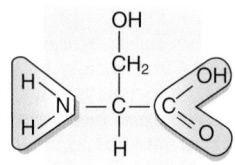

Chemical structure of serine

serine protease inhibitor, serine proteinase inhibitor. See **serpin.**

SERM, abbreviation for **selective estrogen receptor modulator.**

sermorelin /ser″mo-rel′in/, a synthetic peptide corresponding to a portion of growth hormone–releasing hormone, used as the acetate salt in treatment of growth hormone deficiency in prepubertal children. It is administered subcutaneously.

Sernylan, a long-discontinued veterinary anesthetic that is now used illicitly as a euphoric called PCP. Brand name for **phencyclidine hydrochloride.**

sero- /sir″ō-/, combining form meaning "blood serum": *seroconversion, serogroup, seropurulent.*

seroconversion /- kənvur″zhən/ [L, *serum,* whey, *conversio,* turned about], a change in serological test results from negative to positive as antibodies develop in reaction to an infection or vaccine.

serodiagnosis /-dī′əgnō″sis/ [L, *serum,* whey; Gk, *dia,* through, *gnosis,* knowledge], the use of serological tests in the diagnosis of disease.

serofibrinous pericarditis /-fī″brinəs/ [L, *serum,* whey, *fibra,* fibrin; Gk, *peri,* near, *kardia,* heart, *itis,* inflammation], a form of fibrinous pericarditis marked by a serous exudate.

serofibrinous pleurisy, an inflammation of the pleura with a watery effusion and accumulation of fibrin on the pleural membranes.

serogroup /sēr′o-groop/, **1.** a group of bacteria containing a common antigen, sometimes including more than one serotype, species, or genus. This is an unofficial designation, used in the classification of certain genera of bacteria, such as *Leptospira, Salmonella, Shigella,* and *Streptococcus.* **2.** a group of viral species that are closely related antigenically.

seroimmunity /sir′ō-imyoo″nitē/, immunity conferred by administration of an antiserum.

serological /-loj″ik/ [L, *serum,* whey; Gk, *logos,* science], pertaining to the branch of medicine concerned with the study of blood sera.

serological diagnosis /siroloj″ik/ [L, *serum,* whey; Gk, *dia,* through, *gnosis,* knowledge], a diagnosis that is made through laboratory examination of antigen-antibody reactions in the serum. Also called **immunodiagnosis, serum diagnosis.**

serological test [L, *serum,* whey, *testum,* crucible], any diagnostic test made with serum.

serologist /sirol″əjist/ [L, *serum,* + Gk, *logos,* science], a bacteriologist or medical technologist who prepares or supervises the preparation and testing of sera used to diagnose and treat diseases and to immunize people against infectious diseases. Also called **immunologist.**

serology /sirol″əjē/ [L, *serum* + Gk, *logos,* science], the branch of laboratory medicine that studies blood serum for evidence of infection by evaluating antigen-antibody reactions in vitro. Also called **immunology.** −**serologic, serological,** *adj.*

seroma /sirō″mə/, a lump or swelling caused by an accumulation of serum within a tissue or organ.

Seromycin, a tuberculostatic. Brand name for **cycloSERINE.**

seronegative /-neg″ətiv/ [L, *serum,* whey, *negare,* to deny], a serological test with negative results.

seropositive /-pos″itiv/ [L, *serum,* whey, *positivus*], a serological test with positive results.

seroprevalence /-prev″ələns/, the overall occurrence of a disease within a defined population at one time, as measured by blood tests. An example is human immunodeficiency virus seroprevalence.

seroprophylaxis /-prō′filak″sis/, the administration of a serum to prevent disease.

seropurulent /-pyoor″ələnt/, containing serum and pus.

seroreversion /sēr′o-rever″zhun/, spontaneous or induced conversion from a seropositive to a seronegative state.

serosa /sirō″sə/ [L, *serum*], any serous membrane, such as the tunica serosa that lines the walls of body cavities and secretes a watery exudate.

serosanguineous /sir′ōsang·gwin″ē·əs/, **1.** (of a discharge) thin and red. **2.** composed of serum and blood. Also *serosanguinous.*

serotonin /ser′ətō″nin, sir′-/ [L, *serum* + Gk, *tonos,* tone], a naturally occurring derivative of tryptophan found in platelets and in cells of the brain and the intestine. When serotonin is released from platelets on damage to the blood vessel walls, it acts as a potent vasoconstrictor. Serotonin in intestinal tissue stimulates the smooth muscle to contract. In the central nervous system, it acts as a neurotransmitter. It is hypothesized to play a role in appetite, the emotions, and motor, cognitive, and autonomic functions. However, it is not known exactly whether serotonin affects these directly or whether it has an overall role in coordinating the nervous system. It appears to play a key role in maintaining mood balance, as low serotonin levels have been linked to depression. It is a precursor for melatonin, helping to regulate the body's sleep-wake cycles. The normal concentration of serotonin in the urine is 0.05 to 0.2 mcg/mL. Also called **5-hydroxytryptamine.**

serous /sir″əs/ [L, *serum,* whey], pertaining to, resembling, or producing serum.

serous fluid [L, *serum* + *fluere,* to flow], a clear or pale yellow watery fluid.

serous membrane, one of the many thin sheets of tissue that line closed cavities of the body, such as the pleura lining the thoracic cavity, the peritoneum lining the abdominal cavity, and the pericardium lining the sac that encloses the heart. Between the visceral layer of serous membrane covering various organs and the parietal layer lining the cavity containing these organs is a potential space moistened by serous fluid. The fluid reduces the friction of the structures covered by the serous membrane, such as the lungs, which move against the thoracic walls in respiration. Compare **mucous membrane, skin, synovial membrane.**

serovaccination /-vak′sinā″shən/, a technique for producing mixed immunity in which a person is first injected with a serum to establish passive immunity and then vaccinated to produce active immunity.

serpent ulcer /sur″pənt/ [L, *serpens,* snake], an ulceration of the skin that heals in one area while extending to another. Also called *serpiginous ulcer.*

serpin /ser′pin/, any of a superfamily of inhibitors of serine endopeptidase (serine proteinase) found in plasma and tissue. All are similarly structured single-chain glycoproteins, although each one acts specifically on particular endopeptidases. Among their targets are serine proteinases involved in coagulation, complement activation, fibrinolysis,

S

inflammation, and tissue remodeling. The serpins include alpha$_1$-antitrypsin, antithrombin III, alpha$_2$-antiplasmin, C1 inhibitor, and plasminogen activator inhibitor 1. Also called **serine protease inhibitor, serine proteinase inhibitor.**

-serpine, suffix for *Rauwolfia* alkaloid derivatives.

serrate /ser″āt/, having an edge with notches or sawlike teeth. *—serrated, adj.*

serrated suture /ser″ātid/, a suture with sawlike edges, such as most of the sagittal suture.

Serratia /serā″shə/ [L, *serra,* saw teeth], a genus of opportunistic motile, gram-negative bacilli from the family Enterobacteriaceae and the tribe Klebsielleae capable of causing infection in humans, including bacteremia, pneumonia, and UTIs. *Serratia* organisms are frequently acquired in hospitals. See also **nosocomial infection.**

serratus anterior /serā″təs/ [L, *serra,* saw teeth], a thin muscle of the chest wall extending from the ribs under the arm to the scapula. Arising from the outer surface and upper border of the first eight or nine ribs, it inserts into the medial angle, the vertebral border, and the inferior angle of the scapula. It acts to rotate the scapula and to raise the shoulder, as in full flexion and abduction of the arm. Compare **pectoralis major, pectoralis minor, subclavius.**

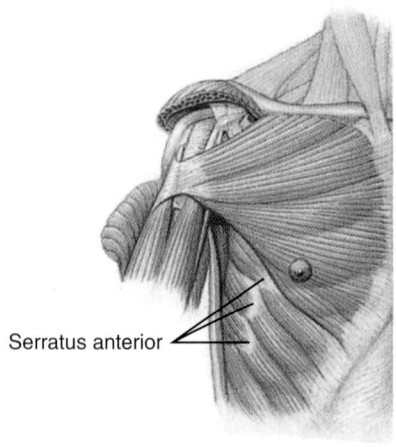

Serratus anterior

Serratus anterior *(Patton and Thibodeau, 2010)*

serratus posterior, muscles in the intermediate group of back muscles that elevate and depress the ribs. They are innervated by segmental branches of anterior rami of intercostal nerves.

Sertoli cell /sertō″lē/ [Enrico Sertoli, Italian histologist, 1842–1910; L, *cella,* storeroom], one of the supporting elongated cells of the seminiferous tubules of the testes. It functions to nourish the developing spermatocytes.

Sertoli-cell–only syndrome [Enrico Sertoli], a form of male sterility in which only Sertoli cells are present in the seminiferous tubules of the testes. Germinal epithelium is absent, resulting in azoospermia.

Sertoli-Leydig cell tumor. See **arrhenoblastoma.**

sertraline /ser′trah-lēn/, a selective serotonin reuptake inhibitor administered orally in the form of hydrochloride salt as an antidepressant and as a treatment for obsessive-compulsive disorder and panic disorder.

serum /sir″əm/ *pl. sera* [L, whey], **1.** the fluid portion of blood that remains subsequent to in vitro clotting. Unlike plasma, serum lacks fibrinogen and several of the coagulation proteins. **2.** any clear watery fluid that has been separated from its more solid elements, such as the exudate from a blister. **3.** a vaccine or toxoid prepared from the serum of a hyperimmune donor for prophylaxis against a particular infection or poison.

serum albumin, a major protein in blood plasma. It is important in maintaining the osmotic pressure of the blood. Normal value is 3.5 to 5.0 g/dL.

serumal calculus. Also called **subgingival calculus.** See **calculus.**

serum bank, a facility for the storage of aliquots of blood serum. The samples are used mainly for medical research.

serum carnosinase deficiency, an autosomal-recessive aminoacidopathy of carnosine metabolism, characterized by urinary excretion of carnosine and accumulation of homocarnosine in the cerebrospinal fluid. This deficiency may cause myoclonic seizures, severe cognitive impairment, and spasticity.

serum C-reactive protein. See **C-reactive protein.**

serum creatinine level, the concentration of creatinine in serum, used as a diagnostic sign of renal impairment.

serum diagnosis. See **serological diagnosis.**

serumfast /sir″əmfast/, **1.** resistant (as bacteria) to the destructive effects of sera. **2.** having (as a serum) little or no change in antibody titer.

serum globulin [L, *serum,* whey, *globulus,* small globe], one of a group of proteins in blood serum with antibody qualities. The various types of serum globulins, designated alpha, beta, and gamma, have different specific properties.

serum glutamic-oxaloacetic transaminase (SGOT). See **aspartate aminotransferase.**

serum glutamic pyruvic transaminase. See **alanine aminotransferase.**

serum hepatitis. See **hepatitis B.**

serum neuritis, a neurological disorder, usually including the cervical nerves or brachial plexus, occurring 2 to 8 days after the injection of a foreign protein.

serum osmolality [L, *serum,* whey; Gk, *ōsmos,* impulse], a measure of the osmotic concentration of blood serum, expressed as the number of osmoles of solute per kilogram of plasma water.

serum protein [L, *serum,* whey; Gk, *proteios,* first rank], any of the proteins in blood serum. See also **serum globulin.**

serum shock, a life-threatening reduction in blood volume and blood pressure caused by the injection of an antitoxic or other foreign serum.

serum sickness, an immunological disorder that may occur 2 to 3 weeks after the administration of an antiserum. It is caused by an antibody reaction to an antigen in the donor serum. The condition is characterized by fever, splenomegaly, swollen lymph nodes, skin rash, and joint pain. Treatment is symptomatic and supportive and may include corticosteroids. See also **angioedema, antigen-antibody reaction, Arthus reaction.**

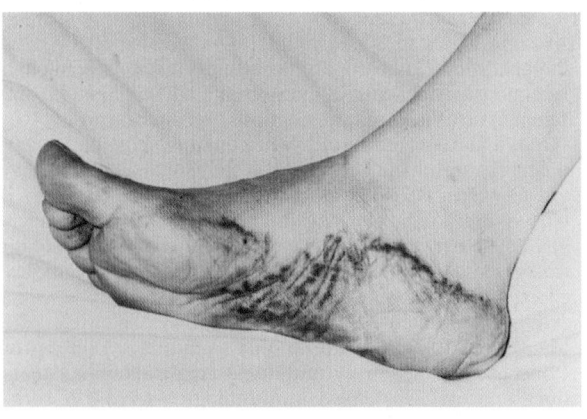

Cutaneous eruptions due to serum sickness
(Hoffman et al, 2009)

serum urea nitrogen. See **blood urea nitrogen.**

service competency, the process of ensuring that two individual practitioners will obtain equivalent results (i.e., replication) when administering a specific assessment or providing intervention.

service dog, a dog trained to aid disabled persons with such tasks as opening or closing doors, picking up dropped items, or pulling a wheelchair.

service of process /sur″vis/ [L, *servus,* a slave, *processus,* going forth], (in law) the delivery of a writ, summons, or complaint to a defendant. Once delivered or left with the party for whom it is intended, it is said to have been served. The original of the document is shown; a copy is served. Service of process gives reasonable notice to allow the person to appear, testify, and be heard in court.

servomechanism /sur″vōmek″əniz′əm/, a control system in which feedback is used to correct errors in another system. A biological example is the mechanism that controls the size of the pupil of the eye as the intensity of light changes.

Serzone, an antidepressant drug. Brand name for **nefazodone hydrochloride.**

sesame oil /ses″əmē/, a liquid fat derived from the seeds of the plant *Sesamum indicum.* The seeds are demulcent and have a laxative effect. Both seeds and oil are used as food flavorings. The oil is also used in skin lotions as an emollient.

sesamoid /ses″əmoid/ [Gk, *sesamon,* sesame, *eidos,* form], nodular objects having the shape and size of sesame seeds. See also **sesamoid bone.**

sesamoid bone [Gk, *sesamon,* sesame, *eidos,* form], any one of numerous small round bony masses embedded in certain tendons that may be subjected to compression and tension. The largest sesamoid bone is the patella, which is embedded in the tendon of the quadriceps femoris at the knee.

sesqui-, prefix meaning "one and one half."

sessile /ses″əl/ [L, *sessilis,* sitting], **1.** (in biology) attached by a base rather than by a stalk or a peduncle, such as a leaf that is attached directly to its stem. **2.** permanently connected. **3.** (in dentistry) a structure or lesion whose base is flattened and spread out over an area of tissue. Compare **pedunculated.**

set, 1. *n.,* a predisposition to behave in a certain way. **2.** *v.,* to reduce a fracture by moving the bones back into a normal position.

set-, combining form meaning "bristle": *setaceous, seton.*

setaceous /sētā″shəs/, having or resembling bristles.

seton /sē″ton/, thread, gauze, or other material passed through subcutaneous tissue or a cyst to create a sinus or fistula to facilitate draining.

settlement [AS, *setlan,* to put in place], (in law) an agreement made between parties to a suit before a judgment is rendered by a court.

setup [AS, *settan,* to set, *up,* on high], **1.** an arrangement of artificial teeth on a trial denture base. **2.** a laboratory procedure in which teeth are removed from a plaster cast and repositioned in wax. It is used as a diagnostic procedure and in creation of a mold for a positioner appliance. **3.** an indication that a plastic material has reached a hardened state after its appropriate setting time has been reached.

sevelamer /sĕvel′ahmer/, a phosphate binder used as the hydrochloride salt to reduce serum phosphorus concentrations in hyperphosphatemia associated with end-stage renal disease. It is administered orally.

7-day fever. See **field fever.**

seventh cranial nerve. See **facial nerve.**

severe acute respiratory syndrome (SARS), an infectious respiratory illness first reported in Asia and characterized by fever over 38° C (100.4° F), dry cough, and breathing difficulties, often accompanied by headache and body aches. It is believed to be caused by a strain of coronavirus, and severity ranges from mild illness to death. The infection appeared to be spread by close contact with infected individuals, by inhalation of droplet nuclei containing the organism, or by contact with infected body fluids. It is now considered eradicated in humans but can still infect animals.

severe combined immunodeficiency disease (SCID) /sivēr″/ [L, *servus,* slave], an abnormal condition characterized by the complete absence or marked deficiency of B cells and T cells, with the consequent lack of humoral and cell-mediated immunity. The disease occurs as an X-linked recessive disorder affecting only males and as an autosomal-recessive disorder affecting both males and females. It results in a pronounced susceptibility to infection and is usually fatal. The precise cause of SCID is not known, but research indicates that the disease may be caused by a cytogenic dysfunction of the embryonic stem cells that normally differentiate into B cells and T cells. The affected individual consequently has a very small thymus and little or no protection against infection.

■ OBSERVATIONS: Pronounced susceptibility to infection usually becomes obvious 3 to 6 months after birth, when maternal immunoglobulin reserves begin to diminish. Diagnosis is difficult because B cell immunity dysfunction is hard to detect in any individual until 5 months after birth, when immunoglobulin levels should reach a low point. Infants with SCID commonly fail to thrive and have a variety of complications, such as sepsis, watery diarrhea, persistent pulmonary infections, and common viral infections that are often fatal. Some infants with SCID have mild infections and low-grade fevers that last for several months while the infant uses maternal immunoglobulin stores. These conditions generally become fatal when maternal antibodies are totally depleted. Some of the more obvious symptoms after the infant has used most of the maternal immunoglobulin stores are cyanosis, rapid respirations, and normal chest sounds with an abnormal chest radiographic picture. Maternal immunoglobulin G (IgG) is persistent, and gram-negative infections usually do not appear until after the sixth month of life. Normal infants less than 5 months of age have very small amounts of IgM and IgA, and normal IgG levels reflect only maternal IgG. The combination of several symptoms may confirm the diagnosis of SCID, including the absence or severe reduction of T cell and B cell immunity; a lymph node biopsy result that shows no lymphocytes, plasma cells, or lymphoid follicles; and no skin reaction to swabbing with dinitrochlorobenzene. Most infants with SCID die from severe infection within 1 year after birth.

■ INTERVENTIONS: Treatment of SCID seeks to develop the immune system and to prevent infection. The only satisfactory treatment available to correct immunodeficiency is histocompatible bone marrow transplantation, but that may cause a graft-versus-host reaction, thus increasing the risk of infection and fatal consequences. Maintained enclosure in a completely sterile environment has prolonged the life of some infants with SCID, but this option is not successful if the infant has already had recurring infections.

■ PATIENT CARE CONSIDERATIONS: Supportive treatment is the primary approach in caring for the SCID patient. The nurse tries to promote an encouraging atmosphere of growth and development while providing the parents with emotional support in the face of the nearly inevitable early death of their child. The infant must remain in strict protective isolation and benefits from diligent nursing attention, frequent parental visits, and gifts of toys, which should be the kind that can be easily sterilized.

S

severe congenital neutropenia, a condition in which there is an absence of neutrophils beginning at birth or early infancy, causing the infant to be more susceptible to infection. It is often associated with decreased bone density and leukemia as the child ages. Formerly called **Kostmann syndrome.**

severe intellectual disability, a category of cognitive impairment in which an individual has a below-average IQ (ranging from 25 to 39) and typically requires extensive support throughout life; generally, individuals with a severe intellectual disability may be able to learn basic self-care skills, although they are unable to live independently as adults.

severity of pitting scale, a common clinical practice in assessment to assign a positive number for the severity of pitting edema in the lower extremities as follows: +1 = a normal foot and leg contour with a barely perceptible pit; +2 = fairly normal lower extremity contours with a moderately deep pit; +3 = obvious foot and leg swelling with a deep pit; +4 = severe foot and leg swelling that distorts the normal contours with a deep pit.

Sever disease. See **calcaneal epiphysitis.**

Sevin, a widely used carbamate insecticide that causes reversible inhibition of cholinesterase. Although less toxic than parathion, carbaryl, when concentrated, may produce skin irritation and systemic poisoning characterized by nausea, vomiting, cramps, diarrhea, diaphoresis, excessive salivation, dyspnea, weakness, loss of coordination, and slurred speech. Large doses may cause coma and death. Carbaryl on the skin is promptly removed by washing with water. Treatment of systemic poisoning includes the immediate IV or intramuscular injection of 1 to 4 mg of atropine sulfate, the administration of artificial respiration and oxygen, gastric lavage, and IV isotonic saline solution to correct dehydration. Brand name for *carbaryl.*

sex [L, *sexus,* sex], **1.** a classification of male or female based on many criteria, among them anatomical and chromosomal characteristics. Compare **gender. 2.** coitus.

sex-, prefix meaning "six": *sexidigitate, sexivalent, sextuplet.*

sex chromatin, a densely staining mass within the nucleus of all nondividing cells of normal mammalian females. It represents the heterochromatin of the inactivated X chromosome. Examination of cells obtained by amniocentesis for the presence of sex chromatin is a technique used for determining the sex of a baby before birth. Sex chromatin is also found as a drumstick-shaped mass attached to one of the nuclear lobes in polymorphonuclear leukocytes in normal females. Also called **Barr body.** See also **Lyon hypothesis.**

sex chromosome, a chromosome that determines the sex of individuals; it carries genes that transmit sex-linked traits and conditions. In humans and other mammals there are two distinct sex chromosomes, designated X and Y, which appear in females as XX and in males as XY. Compare **autosome.**

sex chromosome mosaic, an individual or organism whose cells contain variant chromosomal numbers involving the X or Y chromosomes. Such variations occur in most of the syndromes associated with sex chromosome aberrations, primarily Turner syndrome, and may be caused by nondisjunction of the chromosomes during the second meiotic division of gametogenesis or by some error in chromosome distribution during cell division of the fertilized ovum. Sex chromosome mosaics often have sexual abnormalities, but because of the sex hormones the overall phenotype is uniform and not mosaic in external characteristics, as in certain animals and insects. Also called **sex mosaic.** See also **intersexuality.**

sex-controlled. See **sex-influenced.**

sex determination [L, *sexus,* sex, *determinare*], the process of identifying the sex of an individual on the basis of the presence of the XY chromosome combination in the cells of genetic males or Barr bodies in the cells of genetic females or of secondary sexual characteristics and skeletal variations.

sex deviant, a person whose sexual interests differ markedly from what is accepted as the norm. See also **paraphilia.**

sex factor. See **F factor.**

sex hormone, any of the androgens, estrogens, or related steroid hormones produced mainly by the testes, ovaries, and adrenal cortices.

sex-hormone–binding globulin (SHBG), a protein produced by the liver that binds testosterone and estradiol in the plasma. It has a greater affinity for testosterone. The plasma concentration of SHBG is influenced by liver cirrhosis, hyperthyroidism, obesity (in women), malnutrition, and estrogens.

sexidigitate /sek'sidij″itāt/ [L, *sex,* six], having six digits on one or both hands or feet.

sex-influenced, pertaining to an autosomal genetic trait, such as pattern baldness or gout, that is expressed in both homozygotes and heterozygotes in one sex but only homozygotes in the other sex. Also called **sex-controlled.**

sexism /sek″sizəm/, a belief that one sex is superior to the other and that the superior sex has endowments, rights, prerogatives, and status greater than those of the inferior sex. Sexism results in discrimination in all areas of life and acts as a limiting factor in educational, professional, and psychological development.

sexivalent. See **hexavalent.**

sex-limited, pertaining to an autosomal genetic trait that is expressed in only one sex, although the alleles for it may be carried by both sexes. Such traits are typically influenced by hormonal or environmental conditions.

sex-linked, pertaining to genes carried on the sex chromosomes, particularly the X chromosome, or to the traits they control. See also **sex-linked disorder, X-linked inheritance, Y-linked.** —*sex linkage, n.*

sex-linked disorder, any disease or abnormal condition that is determined by the sex chromosomes or by a defective gene on a sex chromosome. Sex-linked disorders may involve a deviation in the number of either the X or Y chromosomes, as occurs in Turner's syndrome and Klinefelter's syndrome, most occurrences of which are a result of nondisjunction during meiosis. Such aberrations in the number of sex chromosomes do not produce the severe clinical effects that are associated with autosomal aberrations, although they usually cause some degree of mental deficiency. Other sex-linked disorders are transmitted by single-gene defects carried on the X chromosome. X-linked dominant conditions, such as hypophosphatemic vitamin D–resistant rickets, are rare, and males are more seriously affected than females. In inheritance patterns, X-linked dominant conditions are transmitted by affected males to all of their daughters but none of their sons, by affected heterozygous females to one half of their children regardless of sex, and by affected homozygous females to all of their children. More common are X-linked recessive conditions, such as color blindness, ocular albinism, the Xg blood types, hemophilia, Duchenne muscular dystrophy, and inborn errors of metabolism. Such conditions are always transmitted by females. Those predominantly affected are males because they have only one X chromosome, and all of its genes, whether recessive or dominant, are expressed.

Occasionally, females heterozygous for X-linked recessive disorders show varying degrees of expression, but never as severe as those of affected males. There are no known clinically significant traits or conditions associated with the genes on the Y chromosome; their only known function is to trigger the development of male characteristics.

sex-linked ichthyosis, a congenital skin disorder characterized by large, thick dry scales with dark color covering the neck, scalp, ears, face, trunk, and flexor surfaces of the body, such as the folds of the arms and the backs of the knees. It is transmitted by females as an X-linked recessive trait and appears only in males. The condition is managed by topical applications of emollients and the use of keratolytic agents to facilitate removal of the scales. Also called **X-linked ichthyosis.** See also **ichthyosis.**

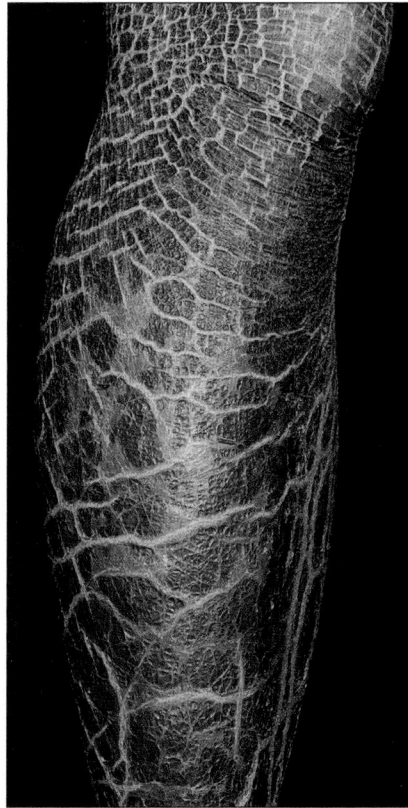

Sex-linked ichthyosis *(James and Berger et al, 2006)*

sex mosaic. See **sex chromosome mosaic.**

sex ratio, the proportion of male-to-female progeny, a relationship that varies with the stage of life. The distribution at birth is usually 106 boys to 100 girls, but the ratio shifts in adulthood, so that, because men have a lower life expectancy, the proportion of females is greater. The ratio may also vary with the effects of a particular disease or trait.

sex role, the expectations held by society regarding what behavior is appropriate or inappropriate for each sex.

sex surrogate [L, *sexus* + *surrogare,* substitute], in sex therapy, a professional substitute trained to help the patient overcome inhibitions. Also called **surrogate partner.**

sextuplet /seks″tup″lit/ [L, *sex,* six], one of six children born of a single pregnancy.

sexual /sek″shoo·əl/, pertaining to sex.

sexual abuse, the sexual mistreatment of another person by fondling, rape, or forced participation in unnatural sex acts or other perverted behavior. Victims tend to experience a traumatic feeling of loss of control of themselves.

sexual asphyxia, accidental strangulation by ligature that occurs in an attempt to induce mild cerebral hypoxia during sexual activity for the purpose of enhancing orgasmic pleasure.

sexual assault, the forcible perpetration of an act of sexual contact on the body of another person, male or female, without his or her consent. Legal criteria vary among different communities.

sexual assault nurse examiner (SANE), a registered nurse with specialized expertise in forensic nursing who has completed educational and clinical programs pertaining to the care of a patient who has experienced sexual assault or abuse.

sexual assault testing, a series of tests performed on sexual assault victims that includes testing of vaginal secretions of women for sperm and of cervical secretions and/or blood for sexually transmitted diseases.

sexual aversion disorder, a persistent or extreme aversion to or avoidance of all or nearly all genital sexual contact with a partner.

sexual deviance. See **paraphilia.**

sexual disorder, 1. any disorder involving sexual functioning, desire, or performance. **2.** any such disorder that is caused at least in part by psychologic factors. Such a disorder characterized by a decrease or other disturbance of sexual desire is called a *sexual dysfunction,* and that characterized by unusual or bizarre sexual fantasies, urges, or practices is called *paraphilia.* Also called **psychosexual disorder, psychosexual dysfunction.**

sexual dwarf, an adult dwarf whose genital organs are normally developed.

sexual dysfunction, a disorder, condition, mental state, or disease that interferes with sexual response in a man, woman, or couple.

sexual fantasy, mental images of an erotic nature that can lead to sexual arousal.

sexual generation. See **sexual reproduction.**

sexual harassment, an aggressive, sexually motivated act of physical or verbal violation of a person over whom the aggressor has some power. Sexual harassment in the workplace is illegal because it represents an abridgment of the victim's right to equal opportunity, privacy, and freedom from assault.

sexual health [L, *sexus* + AS, *haelth*], a condition defined by the World Health Organization as freedom from sexual diseases or disorders and a capacity to enjoy and control sexual behavior without fear, shame, or guilt.

sexual history, in a patient record, the part of the patient's personal history concerned with sexual function and dysfunction. A sexual history is particularly important in gathering data from a patient who has a disease of the reproductive tract, who experiences sexual dysfunction, or who requests contraception, abortion, or sterilization. The extent of the history varies with the patient's age and condition and the reason for securing the history. A short sexual history is recommended as part of every complete physical examination. The therapist needs a detailed sexual history to understand the patient's complaint and to plan treatment. It may include the age at onset of sexual intercourse, the kind and frequency of sexual activity, and the satisfaction derived from it.

S

sexual hormones, chemical substances produced in the body that cause specific regulatory effects on the activity of reproductive organs.

sexual intercourse. See **coitus.**

sexuality /sek′shoo·al″itē/, **1.** the sum of the physical, functional, and psychological attributes that are expressed by one's gender identity and sexual behavior, whether or not related to the sex organs or to procreation. **2.** the genital characteristics that distinguish male from female.

sexually deviant personality /sek″shoo·əlē′/, a sexual behavior that differs significantly from what is considered normal for a society. Either the quality or the object of the sexual drives may be at variance with the accepted cultural norms for adults.

sexually transmitted disease (STD), an infectious disease usually acquired by sexual intercourse or genital contact. These diseases are among the most common communicable diseases, and the incidence has risen in recent years despite improved methods of diagnosis and treatment. Historically, the five venereal diseases were gonorrhea, syphilis, chancroid, granuloma inguinale, and lymphogranuloma venereum. To these have been added scabies, herpes genitalis and anorectal herpes and warts, pediculosis, trichomoniasis, genital candidiasis, molluscum contagiosum, hepatitis B, human papillomavirus infection, nonspecific urethritis, chlamydial infections, cytomegalovirus, and human immunodeficiency virus. Also called **venereal disease.** See also *specific diseases.*

sexually transmitted disease culture, a microscopic examination or blood test used to detect the presence of sexually transmitted diseases, such as gonorrhea, chlamydia, genital herpes, syphilis, hepatitis, and AIDS. Cervical cultures are usually done for women, and urethral cultures for men; rectal and throat cultures are done for people who have engaged in anal and oral intercourse.

sexual mores, socially acceptable sexual behavior, usually based on fixed morally binding customs governing sexual behaviors that are harmful to others or the group, such as rape, incest, and sexual abuse of children.

sexual orientation, the clear, persistent desire of a person for affiliation with one sex rather than the other. Also called *sexual preference.* See also **heterosexual, homosexuality.**

sexual reassignment, a change in the gender identity of a person by legal, surgical, hormonal, or social means.

sexual reflex, in males, a reflex in which tactile or cerebral stimulation results in penile erection, priapism, or ejaculation. Also called **genital reflex.**

sexual reproduction [L, *sexus,* sex, *re + producere,* to produce], replication of an organism by the formation of gametes. Generally this requires the fusion of male spermatozoa and female ova. Parthenogenesis is an exception. Also called **sexual generation, syngenesis.**

sexual response cycle, the four phases of biological sexual response: excitement, plateau, orgasm, and resolution.

sexual sadism. See **sadism.**

sexual selection, the selection of mates on the basis of the attraction of or preference for certain traits, such as coloration or behavior patterns, so that eventually only those particular traits appear in succeeding generations. It explains the wide variety of sexual characteristics among the various species.

sexual tasks, specific skills learned in various phases of development in the life cycle continuum to allow an adult to function normally in the sexual realm.

sexual therapist, a health care professional with specialized knowledge, skill, and competence in assisting individuals who experience sexual difficulties.

sexual therapy, a type of counseling that aids in the resolution of pathological conditions so that a healthy sexuality can be maintained.

Sézary syndrome /sāzärē″/ [A. Sézary, French dermatologist, 1880–1956], a condition of generalized exfoliating erythroderma, lymphadenopathy, and abnormal circulating T cells. The patient experiences pruritus, alopecia, edema, and nail and pigment changes. It is a type of cutaneous T-cell lymphoma.

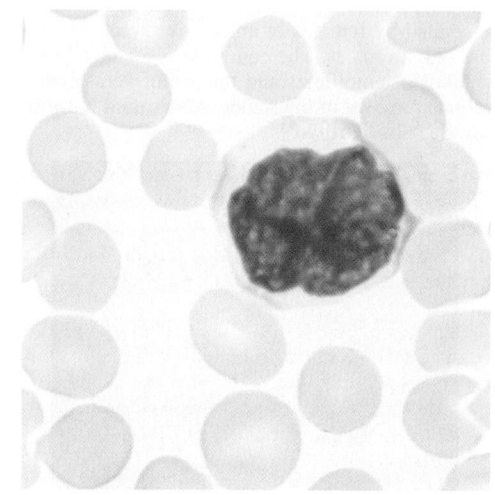

Sézary syndrome *(Carr and Rodak, 2008)*

Sf, abbreviation for *Svedberg flotation unit.*

SFD, abbreviation for *small for dates.* See **small for gestational age (SGA) infant.**

Sg, symbol for the element **seaborgium.**

SGA, abbreviation for *small for gestational age.* See **small for gestational age (SGA) infant.**

SGOT, abbreviation for **serum glutamic-oxaloacetic transaminase.** See **aspartate aminotransferase.**

SGPT, abbreviation for **serum glutamic pyruvic transaminase.** See **alanine aminotransferase.**

shadow /shad″ō/ [AS, *sceadu*], (in psychology) an archetype that represents the unacceptable aspects and components of behavior.

shadowcasting, a technique for enhancing the visualization of a contoured microscopic specimen, in which a chemical film is deposited on it to make it more visible in relief.

shadow cells. See **ghost cells.**

shadowing, 1. *(Informal)* also called **clinical observations. 2.** (in occupational therapy) observing therapists in practice to gain an understanding of the roles and responsibilities of therapists in different settings.

shadow test. See **retinoscopy.**

shaft, an elongated cylindrical object, such as a long bone between the epiphyses.

shaggy chorion. See **villous chorion.**

shaken baby syndrome, a condition of whiplash-type injuries, ranging from bruises on the arms and trunk to retinal hemorrhages, rib fractures, coma, or convulsions, as observed in infants and children who have been violently shaken. This form of child abuse often results in intracranial bleeding from tearing of cerebral blood vessels.

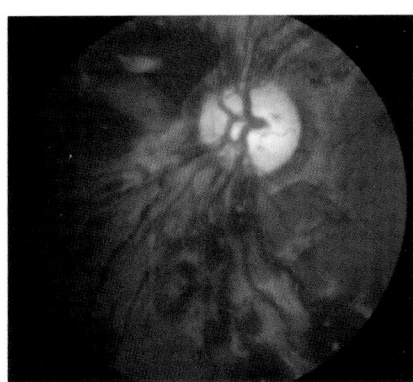

Shaken baby syndrome: retinal hemorrhages *(Courtesy Dr. Daniel Garibaldi, The Johns Hopkins University and Hospital)*

shakes /shāks/, a popular term for the rigor, tremors, or shivering that occurs in intermittent fever or after drug withdrawal.

shake test, a qualitative test for fetal lung maturity. It is more rapid than determination of the lecithin/sphingomyelin ratio. Also called **foam test.**

shaking palsy. *(Informal)* See **parkinsonism.**

shallow breathing /shal′ō/ [ME, *schalowe*, little depth], a respiration pattern marked by slow, shallow, and generally ineffective inspirations and expirations. It is usually caused by drugs and indicates depression of the medullary respiratory center.

shamanism, a form of healing that incorporates personal healing, transformation, and regeneration through access to a "higher power." Sickness, disease, and illness are indicators that the individual is out of balance and in disharmony within the essential nature. Success can be achieved if people are, first, willing to take responsibility for the creation of the disease and, second, open to nonphysical realities of life and willing to engage with their inner spirit and their higher selves. This type of healing has been effective for sexual dysfunction, chronic fatigue syndrome, mental health concerns, and obesity and other eating disorders.

shank, **1.** the tibia. **2.** the part of a device that connects the functional part to a handle.

shaping [AS, *scieppan,* to shape], a procedure used for conditioning a person undergoing behavior therapy to develop new behavioral responses. Initially, any act remotely resembling the desired behavior is reinforced. Gradually, the criterion is made more stringent until the desired response is attained.

shared governance, an organizational framework proposed by Tim Porter-O'Grady that provides for the full use of nursing resources. This system is designed to reflect the professional character of the participants in the nursing organization and to promote certain positive behaviors and practices. The purpose of shared governance is the establishment of a system in which staff participate fully in all activities that have an impact on their work and their ultimate goal of meaningful patient care.

shared paranoid disorder [AS, *scearan,* to shear], a psychopathological condition characterized by identical manifestations of the same mental disorder, usually ideas, in two closely associated or related people. Also called **folie à deux.**

shared services, administrative, clinical, or other service functions that are common to two or more hospitals or other health care facilities and that are used jointly or cooperatively by them.

shark skin. See **dyssebacea.**

Sharpey's fiber [William Sharpey, Scottish anatomist, 1802–1880], any of the many collagenous bundles of fibers of the periodontal ligament that become embedded in the cementum during its formation.

sharps, any needles, scalpels, or other articles that could cause wounds or punctures to personnel handling them. See also **needlestick injuries.**

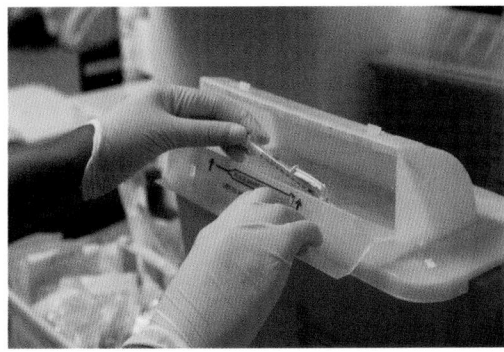

Sharps container *(Perry, Potter, and Elkin, 2012)*

shatterproof glass. See **safety glass.**

shaving stroke [AS, *scafan,* to shave, *strican,* to stroke], a phase of the working stroke of a periodontal curet, used for smoothing or planing a tooth or tooth root surface.

SHBG, abbreviation for **sex-hormone–binding globulin.**

SHCC, abbreviation for **Statewide Health Coordinating Committee.**

SHEA, abbreviation for *Society for Healthcare Epidemiology of America.*

shear /shir/ [AS, *scearan,* to cut], **1.** an applied force or pressure exerted against the surface and layers of the skin as tissues slide in opposite but parallel planes. **2.** a strain in a body structure that causes displacement of the structure.

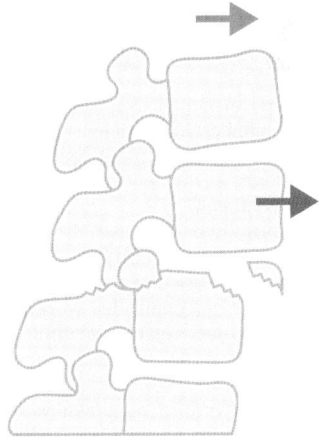

Shear in the vertebral column *(Griffin and Grant, 2013)*

shearling /shir′ling/, a sheepskin placed on a bed to help prevent pressure ulcers.

sheath /shēth/ [AS, *scaeth*], a tubular structure that surrounds an organ or any other part of the body, such as the sheath of the rectus abdominis muscle or the sheath of Schwann, which covers various nerve fibers.

sheath of Schwann [AS, *scaeth*; Theodor Schwann, German anatomist, 1810–1882], a neurilemma sheath of nucleated cells enclosing a nerve fiber.

Sheehan syndrome [Harold L. Sheehan, English pathologist, 1900–1988], a postpartum condition of pituitary necrosis and hypopituitarism after circulatory collapse resulting from uterine hemorrhaging. Lactation may not develop, and loss of pubic and axillary hair may occur.

sheep cell test [AS, *sceap* + L, *cella,* storeroom, *testum,* crucible], a method that mixes human blood cells with the red blood cells of sheep to determine the absence or the deficiency of human T lymphocytes. When mixed with human blood cells, the red blood cells of sheep cluster around the human T lymphocytes and form characteristic rosettes. An electron microscope is used to identify the rosettes. An absence or a decrease in the number of rosettes indicates a deficiency or absence of T cells. The sheep cell test is used to diagnose several diseases, such as DiGeorge's syndrome, that decrease or destroy the cellular immunity provided by T cells.

sheep red cell agglutination test. See **sheep cell test.**

sheet /shēt/ [AS, *scēte*], **1.** a rectangular piece of cotton, linen, or similar cloth for a bed covering. **2.** any structure resembling such a covering.

sheet wadding, stretchable sheets of cotton padding used to cover the skin before a cast is applied. The stretching allows for some extremity edema without the cast becoming too tight.

shelf [AS, *scylf*], a flat, hard anatomical structure that resembles a ridge or platform.

shell [AS, *scell*], **1.** a hard outer protective covering that encloses material. **2.** a principal energy level occupied by an electron in an atom.

shellfish poisoning, an illness caused by toxins or chemicals associated with the ingestion of shellfish (e.g., clams, oysters, mussels, or scallops), causing a variety of symptoms that are dependent on the specific poison.

shell shock [AS, *scell* + Fr, *choc*], any of a number of mental disorders, ranging from extreme fear to dementia, commonly attributed to the noise and concussion of exploding shells or bombs but actually a traumatic reaction to the stress of combat. See also **combat fatigue, posttraumatic stress disorder.**

shell teeth, a type of dental dysplasia in which the teeth have large pulp chambers, insufficient coronal dentin, and, usually, no roots. Both the primary dentition and, more so, the maxillary anterior permanent dentition can be affected. See also **odontodysplasia.**

sheltered workshop [ME, *sheltrun,* body of guards; AS, *werc* + *sceoppa,* stall], a facility or program, either for outpatients or for residents of an institution, that provides vocational experience in a controlled working environment. The workshop also offers related vocational rehabilitation services, such as job interview training, to people with physical or mental disabilities.

Shiatsu, a Japanese form of acupressure involving finger pressure at specific points on the body, mainly for the purpose of balancing energy in the body.

shield [AS, *scild*], a material for preventing or reducing the passage of charged particles or radiation. A shield may be designated by the radiation it is intended to absorb, such as a gamma ray shield, or by the kind of protection it is intended to give, such as a background, biologic, or thermal shield. Lucite and aluminum can be used for beta-radiation shields, but lead is required for gamma ray or x-ray shields.

shift [AS, *sciftan,* to divide], **1.** the particular hours of the day during which a health care professional is scheduled to work. Many innovations in staffing practice currently allow variations on the traditional 5-day, 40-hour workweek. **2.** an abrupt change in an analytic system that continues at the new level.

shift to the left, (in hematology) a predominance of immature leukocytes noted in a differential white blood cell count. It is usually indicative of an infection or inflammation. The term derives from the Arneth classification, a graph of blood components in which immature cell frequencies appear on the left side of the graph.

shift to the right, (in hematology) a preponderance of polymorphonuclear neutrophils having three or more lobes, indicating maturity of the cell. The phenomenon is common in severe liver disease and advanced pernicious anemia. It indicates a relative lack of blood-forming activity.

Shigella /shigel′ə/ [Kiyoshi Shiga, Japanese bacteriologist, 1870–1957], a genus of gram-negative pathogenic bacteria that causes gastroenteritis and bacterial dysentery, such as *Shigella dysenteriae.* It is also associated with hemolytic uremic syndromes. See also **shigellosis.**

Shigella dysenteriae, a species of the bacterial family Enterobacteriaceae that causes a severe form of dysentery in humans. The *dysenteriae* species of *Shigella* is most common in Asia and is particularly virulent. Also called *S. shigae.*

Shigella enteritis, bacterial enteritis caused by the *Shigella* infection of bacillary dysentery.

Shigella gastroenteritis, bacterial gastroenteritis caused by the *Shigella* infection of bacillary dysentery.

shigellosis /shig′əlō″sis/ [Kiyoshi Shiga, Gk, *osis,* condition], an acute, highly contagious bacterial infection of the bowel with a low infectious dose (as few as 180 organisms), characterized by diarrhea, abdominal pain, and fever. It is transmitted by hand-to-mouth contact with the feces of individuals infected with bacteria of a pathogenic species of the genus *Shigella.* Damage is caused by invasion of bacteria (which is dependent on a plasmid-mediated virulence factor) and production of the enterotoxin Shiga toxin. These organisms may be carried in the stools of asymptomatic people for up to several months and may be spread through contact with contaminated objects, food, or flies, especially in poor, crowded areas. The disease occurs in isolated outbreaks in the United States but is endemic in underdeveloped areas of the world. It is especially common and usually most severe in children. Diagnosis is made by isolating and identifying *Shigella* in a specimen of stool. The likelihood of encountering or engendering antibiotic-resistant organisms is very high. Therefore the preferred treatment for shigellosis is supportive, and the major goal is prevention of dehydration. Antimicrobials are given if the disease is severe or if the likelihood of further transmission is great. Antidiarrheal agents should be avoided. Isolation and strict handwashing precautions are instituted. Shigellosis infections must be reported to the public health department. Also called **bacillary dysentery.**

shim, a thin, tapered piece of material used to fill a gap.

shim coils, current-carrying coils that are used in magnetic resonance to improve the magnetic field homogeneity.

shin bone, *(Informal)* See **tibia.**

shingles. See **herpes zoster.**

shin splints [AS, *scinu,* shin; ME, *splinte*], lower-leg pain caused by strain of the long flexor muscle of the toes during strenuous athletic activity, such as running. In many instances, shin splints are the result of inadequate training. Treatment usually involves rest and exercise therapy. Surgery is sometimes necessary.

shipyard eye. See **epidemic keratoconjunctivitis.**

Shirodkar operation /shir′odkär″/ [N.V. Shirodkar, Indian obstetrician, 1900–1971], a surgical procedure called a cerclage in which the cervical canal is closed by a purse-string suture embedded in the uterine cervix encircling the canal. It is performed to correct an incompetent cervix that has failed to retain previous pregnancies. Under spinal block or general anesthesia, a 5-mm–wide band of nonabsorbable material is buried beneath the mucosa of the cervix and pulled in a purse-string manner to close the cervix. The band may be left in place permanently, in which case subsequent deliveries are by cesarean section. Occasionally, a temporary cerclage is done, sewing in the band and leaving the ends exposed in the vagina. The band is then removed before labor and vaginal delivery. Postoperatively, infection or vaginal fistula may occur. If labor begins with the suture in place, the suture is removed promptly or the infant is delivered by cesarean section, before the uterus ruptures.

shivering /shiv″əring/, involuntary contractions of muscles, mainly of the skin, in response to the chilling effect of low temperatures. Shivering may also occur at the onset of a fever when the body's heat balance is disturbed.

shock [Fr, *choc*], an abnormal condition of inadequate blood flow to the body's tissues, with life-threatening cellular dysfunction. The condition is usually associated with inadequate cardiac output, hypotension, oliguria, changes in peripheral blood flow resistance and distribution, and tissue damage. Causal factors include hemorrhage, vomiting, diarrhea, inadequate fluid intake, or excessive fluid loss, resulting in hypovolemia. Kinds include **anaphylactic shock, cardiogenic shock, hypovolemic shock, neurogenic shock, septic shock.**

■ OBSERVATIONS: Hypovolemic shock is the most common kind of shock. There is decreased blood flow with a resulting reduction in the delivery of oxygen, nutrients, hormones, and electrolytes to the body's tissues and a concomitant decreased removal of metabolic wastes. Pulse and respirations are increased. Blood pressure may decline after an initial slight increase. The patient often shows signs of restlessness and anxiety, an effect related to decreased blood flow to the brain. There also may be weakness, lethargy, pallor, and cool, moist skin. As shock progresses, the body temperature falls, respirations become rapid and shallow, and the pulse pressure (the difference between systolic and diastolic blood pressures) narrows as compensatory vasoconstriction causes the diastolic pressure to be elevated or maintained in the face of a falling systolic blood pressure. Urinary output is reduced. Hemorrhage may be apparent or concealed, although other factors, such as vomiting or diarrhea, may account for the deficiency of body fluids.

■ INTERVENTIONS: Fluid volume must be restored quickly so that there can be a rapid return of oxygenated blood to the perfusion-deprived tissues. Supplemental oxygen should be administered. Blood volume is expanded with IV fluids, such as a lactated Ringer's solution or a 5% dextrose in normal saline solution. Packed red blood cells, plasma, and plasma substitutes are also given for shock of hemorrhagic origin. Metabolic acidosis may result from anaerobic metabolism.

■ PATIENT CARE CONSIDERATIONS: After vital functions are restored and diagnosis has been made, the patient in shock must be monitored continuously until recovery is assured. The patient should remain flat in bed, but the lower extremities can be raised to improve venous return (modified Trendelenburg's position). The Trendelenburg position should be avoided because it tends to push the abdominal organs against the diaphragm and increases the work of breathing. Position changes should be made slowly. Vasoactive drugs may be ordered when the blood volume is adequate. The patient's skin color, temperature, vital signs, intake and output, pulse oximetry, and level of consciousness should be monitored closely.

shock liver. See **hepatic ischemia.**

shock lung. See **adult respiratory distress syndrome.**

shock therapy [Fr, *choc* + Gk, *therapeia*], a psychotherapeutic procedure for treating depression and other severe disorders by producing an epileptiform convulsion in the patient. The shock is induced by delivering an electric current through the brain under controlled conditions, using an anesthetic and close monitoring. See also **electroconvulsive therapy.**

shock trousers, a rarely used pneumatic garment designed to produce pressure on the lower part of the body, thereby preventing the pooling of blood in the legs and abdomen. They were also used in emergencies in the treatment of hemorrhagic shock. Shock trousers are contraindicated in patients with pulmonary edema, cardiogenic shock, increased intracranial pressure, or eviscerations.

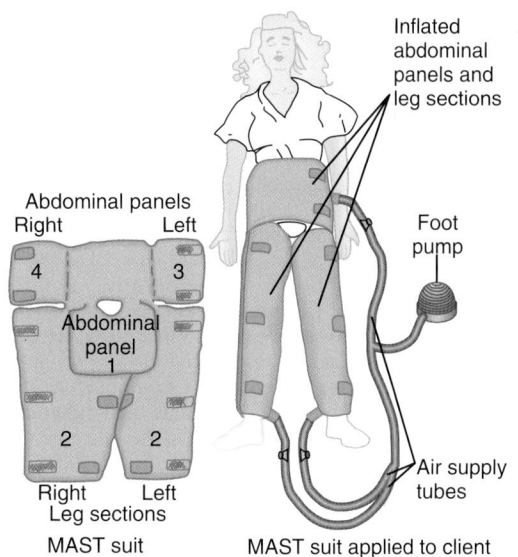

Shock trousers *(Black and Hawks, 2005)*

shock-wave lithotripsy. See **extracorporeal shock-wave lithotripsy.**

shoe cookies. See **navicular pads.**

short-acting [AS, *sceort* + L, *agere,* to do], pertaining to or characterizing a therapeutic agent, usually a drug, with a brief period of effectiveness, generally beginning soon after the substance or measure is administered.

short-acting insulin, a clear preparation of regular (crystalline zinc) insulin with an immediate (15 to 30 minutes) onset of action that reaches a peak of action in 2 to 4 hours. The duration of action is 6 to 8 hours. There is considerable variation in individual patients and with different doses in the same patient. Therefore these data should be considered only as rough guidelines. Also called **rapid-acting insulin.** Compare **intermediate-acting insulin, long-acting insulin.** See also **insulin.**

shortage area /shôr″tij/ [AS, *sceort* + L, *acticum,* process], a geographic area, population group, or area designated by the federal government as being undersupplied with certain kinds of health care services. A shortage area may be eligible for aid under certain federal programs, including the National Health Service Corps or the Rural Clinics Assistance Act.

short-arm cast, an orthopedic cast applied to immobilize the hand or wrist, incorporating the hand below the wrist. The short-arm cast is used in treating fractures, for maintaining postoperative positioning, and for correcting or maintaining the correction of deformities of the hand and the wrist. Compare **long-arm cast.** See also **cast.**

short below-knee (BK) amputation, transtibial amputation in which the division is in the proximal third of the tibia. See also **long below-knee (BK) amputation.**

Short Blessed Test (SBT), a short screening test measuring orientation and memory and designed to assess cognitive impairment. The test can be used to detect early cognitive changes associated with Alzheimer disease or other disorders characterized by dementia.

short bones, bones that occur in clusters and usually permit movement of the extremities, such as the carpals and tarsals.

short-bowel syndrome [AS, *sceort* + OFr, *boel* + Gk, *syn,* together, *dromos,* course], a loss of intestinal surface for absorption of nutrients caused by the surgical removal of a section of bowel. Treatment is with parenteral nutrition in the acute phase.

short central artery, a branch from the precommunical part of the anterior cerebral artery.

short-chain fatty acids (SCFA), those fatty acids having a chain length up to roughly 6 carbon atoms long. They are produced by bacterial anaerobic fermentation, particularly of dietary carbohydrates, in the large intestine. They are readily absorbed and are metabolized in the liver and muscle tissues, producing energy.

short-course tuberculosis chemotherapy, a 6-month treatment regimen for patients with tuberculosis who would otherwise continue to receive medications for at least 18 to 24 months after sputum has a negative finding for tubercle bacilli. The short course requires a combination of four drugs: isoniazid, rifampin, pyrazinamide, and either ethambutol or streptomycin.

short-gut syndrome, **1.** any of the malabsorption conditions resulting from massive resection of the small bowel, the degree and kind of malabsorption depending on the site and extent of the resection. It is characterized by diarrhea, steatorrhea, and malnutrition. **2.** a congenital disorder in which an infant's intestine is too short or underdeveloped to allow normal food digestion. The child is maintained on parenteral nutrition until the intestine grows, develops further, or is replaced by surgical transplantation. A small child who becomes dependent on parenteral feeding may have to be taught chewing and swallowing processes when the short-gut syndrome is eventually corrected.

shorting [AS, *sceort*], the fraudulent practice of dispensing a quantity of drug less than that called for in the prescription and of charging for the quantity specified in the prescription. See also **kiting.**

short-leg cast, an orthopedic cast used for immobilizing fractures in the lower extremities from the toes to the knee. The short-leg cast is also used for treating severe sprains and torn soft tissue of the ankle, for maintaining postoperative positioning and immobilization of the foot and the ankle, and for correcting or maintaining the correction of deformities of the foot or the ankle. Compare **long-leg cast.** See also **cast.**

short-leg cast with walker, an orthopedic cast with rubber walkers on the bottom. It immobilizes the leg from the toes to the knee and allows the patient to walk.

Short Portable Mental Status Questionnaire, a 10-item questionnaire used to screen older adults for cognitive impairment. It tests orientation, remote and recent memory, practical skills, and mathematical ability.

short-PR-normal-QRS syndrome. See **Lown-Ganong-Levine (LGL) syndrome.**

short sight, shortsightedness. See **myopia.**

short stature [AS, *sceort,* short; L, *statura,* man's height], a body height that is less than 70% of the average for a population of the same age, culture, gender, and other peer factors.

short-term memory, memory of recent events, generally the first to be affected in Alzheimer disease.

short-wave diathermy [AS, *sceort* + *wafian* + Gk, *dia* + *therme,* heat], a method of providing heat deep in the body by short-wave electric currents. The high-frequency short-wave uses wavelengths of 3 to 30 meters. It is used to treat chronic arthritis, bursitis, sinusitis, and other conditions.

shotgun therapy [AS, *scot* + ME, *gonne* + Gk, *therapeia,* treatment], *(Informal)* any treatment that has a wide range of effects and that therefore can be expected to correct an abnormal condition even though the particular cause is unknown. Shotgun therapy may cause more than an acceptable rate of side effects and is rarely desirable or necessary.

shoulder [AS, *sculder*], the junction of the clavicle, scapula, and humerus where the arm attaches to the trunk of the body.

shoulder blade. See **scapula.**

shoulder girdle [AS, *sculder* + *gyrdel*], a partial arch at the top of the trunk formed by the scapula and clavicle.

shoulder-hand syndrome, a neuromuscular condition characterized by pain and stiffness in the shoulder and arm, limited joint motion, swelling of the hand, muscle atrophy, and decalcification of the underlying bones. The condition occurs most commonly after myocardial infarction.

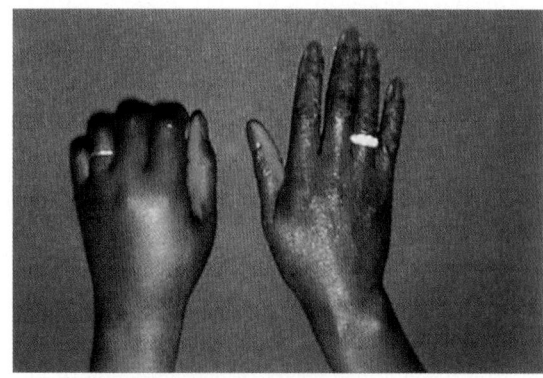

Shoulder-hand syndrome *(Moll, 1997)*

shoulder joint, the ball-and-socket articulation of the humerus with the scapula. The joint includes eight bursae and five ligaments, including the glenoidal labrum that deepens the articular cavity and protects the edges of articulating bones. It is the most mobile joint in the body. Also called **humeral articulation.**

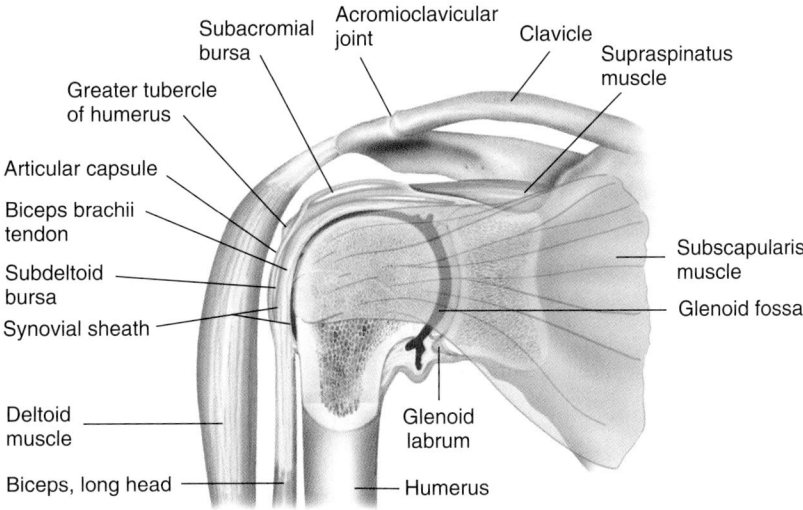

Shoulder joint *(Seidel et al, 2011)*

shoulder presentation [AS, *sculder* + L, *praesentare*, to show], the part of the fetus that occupies the center of the birth canal when the presentation is associated with a transverse or oblique lie.

shoulder spica cast, an orthopedic cast used to immobilize the trunk of the body to the hips, the wrist, and the hand. It incorporates a diagonal shoulder support between the hip and arm parts. The shoulder spica cast is used in the treatment of shoulder dislocations and injuries and in the positioning and immobilization of the shoulder after surgery.

shoulder subluxation, the separation of the humeral head from the glenoid cavity, resulting in strain on the soft tissues surrounding the shoulder joint.

show. See **vaginal bleeding.**

Shprintzen syndrome. See **velocardiofacial syndrome.**

shreds [AS, *screade,* piece cut off], glossy filaments of mucus in the urine, indicating inflammation in the urinary tract. Also called **mucous shreds.**

Shulman syndrome. See **eosinophilic fasciitis.**

shunt [ME, *shunten*], **1.** to redirect the flow of a body fluid from one cavity or vessel to another. **2.** a tube or device implanted in the body to redirect a body fluid from one cavity or vessel to another. See also **left-to-right shunt, right-to-left shunt.**

shu points /shoo/, acupressure points.

Shy-Drager syndrome /shī″ drā″gər/ [G. Milton Shy, American neurologist, 1919–1967; Glenn A. Drager, American physician, b. 1917], a rare progressive neurological disorder of young and middle-aged adults. It is characterized by orthostatic hypotension, bladder and bowel incontinence, atrophy of the iris, anhidrosis, tremor, rigidity, incoordination, ataxia, and muscle wasting. Treatment includes drug therapy to control motor symptoms and to maintain adequate blood pressure. Antigravity stockings may prevent pooling of blood in the lower extremities. See also **orthostatic hypotension.**

Shy-Magee syndrome. See **central core disease.**

Si, symbol for the element **silicon.**

SI, abbreviation for the French name for the International System of Units. Abbreviation for *Système International d'Unités.*

SIADH, abbreviation for **syndrome of inappropriate antidiuretic hormone secretion.**

sial-. See **sialo-, sial-.**

sialadenitis /sī″əlad′ənī′tis/, inflammation of one or more of the salivary glands. Also called **sialoadenitis.**

sialated, a substance that has reacted with sialic acid or its derivatives.

sialemesis /sī′ələmē″sis/, vomiting of saliva, or vomiting associated with excessive salivation.

-sialia, combining form meaning "(condition of the) saliva."

sialic acid /si-al′ik/, any *N*-acyl derivative of neuraminic acid. Various ones are found in polysaccharides, glycoproteins, and glycolipids.

sialidase, an enzyme of the hydrolase class that catalyzes the cleavage of glucosidic linkages between a sialic acid residue and a hexose or hexosamine residue at the nonreducing terminal of oligosaccharides in glycoproteins, glycolipids, and proteoglycans. Deficiency of it is an autosomal-recessive trait and is seen in sialidosis and galactosialidosis. See also **neuraminidase.**

sialidosis /sī″əlidō″sis/, a neuronal storage disease of children caused by a deficiency of the enzyme sialidase (neuraminidase). The condition is characterized by a cherry-red spot on the macula, progressive myoclonus, and seizures. There are two types. Type 1 patients have normal physical features and beta-galactosidase levels. Type 2 patients also have short stature, bony abnormalities, and beta-galactosidase deficiency.

sialo-, sial-, combining form meaning "saliva" or "the salivary glands": *sialoadenitis, sialogogue.*

sialoadenitis. See **sialadenitis.**

sialogenous. See **salivatory.**

sialogogue /sī·al″əgog′/ [Gk, *sialon,* saliva, *agogos,* leading], anything that stimulates, promotes, or produces the secretion of saliva.

sialogram /sī·al″əgram′/ [Gk, *sialon,* saliva, *gramma,* record], a radiographic image of the salivary glands and ducts.

sialography /sī·əlog″rəfē/ [Gk, *sialon* + *graphein,* to record], the radiographic examination of the salivary glands after injection of a radiopaque contrast medium. —*sialographic, adj.*

sialolith /sī·al″əlith/ [Gk, *sialon* + *lithos,* stone], a calculus formed in a salivary gland or duct.

sialolithiasis /-lithī″əsis/, a pathological condition in which one or more calculi, or stones, are formed in a salivary gland or duct.

sialorrhea /sī·al′ərē″ə/ [Gk, *sialon* + *rhoia,* flow], an excessive flow of saliva that may be associated with various conditions, such as acute inflammation of the mouth, cognitive impairment, mercurialism, pregnancy, teething, alcoholism, or malnutrition. Also called **hypersalivation, ptyalism.**

Siamese twins /sī′əmēz/ [Chang and Eng, conjoined twins born in Siam (now Thailand) in 1811], conjoined, equally developed twin fetuses produced from the same ovum. The severity of the condition ranges from superficial fusion, such as of the umbilical vessels, to that in which the heads or complete torsos are united and several internal organs are shared. With modern surgical techniques, most Siamese twins can be successfully separated. See also **conjoined twins.**

sib [AS, *sibb,* kin]. See **sibling.**

Siberian ginseng, an herb harvested from a shrub found throughout the world, primarily in Russia and China. See also **ginseng.**

■ INDICATIONS: It is used to improve appetite; to improve circulation; and to treat memory loss, hypertension, insomnia, rheumatism, heart ailments, diabetes, and headache. It can be efficacious in some instances.

■ CONTRAINDICATIONS: It should not be used during pregnancy and lactation, in children, in those with known hypersensitivity to this product or other ginsengs, or in those with hypertension. Do not use Siberian ginseng for more than 90 days without a rest period.

Siberian tick typhus /sībir″ē·ən/ [Siberia], a mild acute febrile illness seen in north, central, and east Asia, caused by *Rickettsia sibirica,* transmitted by ticks. It is characterized by a diffuse maculopapular rash, headache, conjunctival inflammation, and a small ulcer or eschar at the site of the tick bite. Siberian tick typhus is considered to be a mild form of spotted fever and rarely exhibits further complications. Treatment with chloramphenicol or tetracycline is associated with an excellent prognosis. Also called **North Asian tick typhus.** See also *Rickettsia,* **typhus.**

sibilant /sib″ilənt/ [L, *sibilare,* to hiss], a hissing sound or one in which the predominant sound is /s/. See also **fricative.**

sibilant rhonchus. See **wheeze,** def. 1.

sibling /sib″ling/ [AS, *sibb,* kin], **1.** *n.,* one of two or more children who have both parents in common; a brother or sister. The number, age differences, sex, and birth order of siblings can greatly affect the childhood environment and relationships within a family, which also may include step-siblings and half-siblings. Sibling rivalry and jealousy are common in firstborn children, especially when there is a 2- to 4-year difference in age. In general, sibling relationships help teach the child important social patterns and moral values, such as competitiveness, loyalty, and sharing. Also called **sib. 2.** *adj.,* pertaining to a brother or sister.

sibship /sib″ship/ [AS *sibb,* kin, *scieppan,* to shape], **1.** the state of being related by blood. **2.** a group of people descended from a common ancestor who are used as a basis for genetic studies. **3.** brothers and sisters considered as a group.

sibutramine, an appetite suppressant.

■ INDICATIONS: It is used to treat obesity in conjunction with other treatments.

■ CONTRAINDICATIONS: The following factors prohibit its use: known hypersensitivity to this drug, hypothyroidism, anorexia nervosa, severe hepatic/renal disease, uncontrolled hypertension, cerebrovascular accident, history of coronary artery disease, congestive heart failure, arrhythmias, pregnancy, and lactation.

■ ADVERSE EFFECTS: Tachycardia is a life-threatening effect of this drug. Other adverse effects include headache, insomnia, seizures, stimulation, drowsiness, dizziness, nervousness, emotional lability, hypotension, palpitations, vasodilation, anorexia, constipation, dry mouth, taste aberration, nausea, increased appetite, dysmenorrhea, laryngitis, pharyngitis, rhinitis, sinusitis, rash, and sweating.

sic [L *sic,* thus; *erat,* it was; *scriptum,* written], a notation for a Latin phrase meaning "thus it was written." The term is used to indicate that the materials have been reproduced exactly as they appeared in an original document.

sicc-, combining form meaning "dry": *siccant, sicca complex.*

sicca complex /sik″ə/, abnormal dryness of the mouth, eyes, or other mucous membranes. The condition is seen in patients with Sjögren syndrome, sarcoidosis, amyloidosis, and deficiencies of vitamins A and C.

siccant /sik″ənt/ [L, *siccus,* dry]. See **desiccant.**

sick, experiencing symptoms of physical illness, such as nausea, aches and pains, dizziness, weakness, blurred vision, or malaise.

sick building syndrome, a condition characterized by fatigue, headache, dry eyes, and respiratory complaints affecting workers in certain buildings with limited ventilation. The symptoms seem to be caused by a combination of chemical agents in low concentrations rather than a specific irritant.

sick cell syndrome, a condition characterized by idiopathic hyponatremia in patients with either acute or chronic illness.

sick euthyroid syndrome, a nonthyroidal condition characterized by abnormalities in hormone levels and function test findings related to the thyroid gland. The condition occurs in patients with severe systemic disease.

sickle cell [AS, *sicol,* crescent; L, *cella,* storeroom], an abnormal crescent-shaped red blood cell containing hemoglobin S, characteristic of sickle cell anemia. Also called *drepanocyte.*

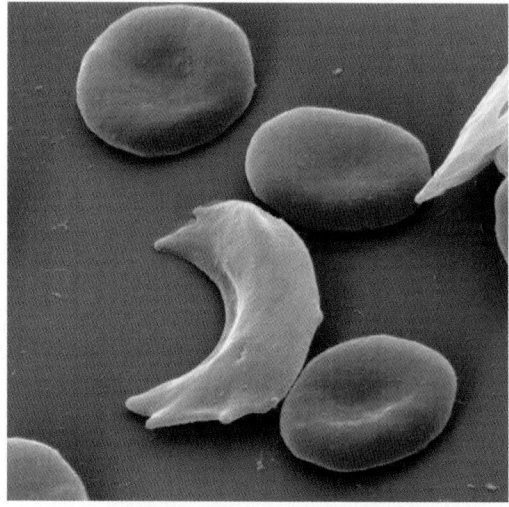

Sickle cell *(Carr and Rodak, 2008)*

sickle cell anemia, a severe, chronic, hemoglobinopathy that occurs in people homozygous for hemoglobin S (Hb S). The abnormal hemoglobin crystallizes and distorts the erythrocytes. Sickle cell anemia is characterized by crises of joint pain, thrombosis, and fever and by chronic anemia, with splenomegaly, lethargy, and weakness. See also **congenital nonspherocytic hemolytic anemia, dactylitis, ellipto-cytosis, hemoglobin S, sickle cell crisis, hemoglobin C disease.**

sickle cell crisis, an acute episodic condition that occurs in children with sickle cell anemia. The crisis may be vasooc-clusive, resulting from the aggregation of misshapen eryth-rocytes, or anemic, resulting from bone marrow aplasia, increased hemolysis, folate deficiency, or splenic seques-tration of erythrocytes. See also **hemoglobin S, sickle cell anemia.**

■ OBSERVATIONS: Painful vasoocclusive crisis is the most common of the sickle cell crises. It is usually preceded by an upper respiratory or GI infection without an exacerbation of anemia. The clumps of sickled erythrocytes obstruct blood vessels, resulting in occlusion, ischemia, and infarction of adjacent tissue. Characteristics of this kind of crisis are leu-kocytosis; acute abdominal pain from visceral hypoxia; pain-ful swelling of the soft tissue of the hands and feet (hand-foot syndrome); and migratory, recurrent, or constant joint pain, often so severe that movement of the joint is limited. Persistent headache, dizziness, convulsions, visual or audi-tory disturbances, facial nerve palsies, coughing, shortness of breath, and tachypnea may occur if the central nervous system or lungs are affected. Other problems associated with vasoocclusion include priapism, hematuria, and retinopathy. Anemic crisis is characterized by a dramatic, rapid drop in hemoglobin levels resulting from various causes. Aplastic crisis resulting in severe anemia occurs because red blood cell production is diminished by acute viral, bacterial, or fun-gal infection. Megaloblastic anemia (another form of anemic crisis) results from folic acid deficiency during periods of accelerated erythropoiesis. Severe anemia between crises is not common unless a generalized state of malnutrition ex-ists. Hyperhemolytic crisis, characterized by anemia, jaun-dice, and reticulocytosis, results from glucose-6-phosphate dehydrogenase deficiency or occurs as a reaction to multiple transfusions. Acute sequestration crisis, which occurs in young children 6 months to 5 years of age, results when large quantities of blood suddenly accumulate in the spleen, caus-ing massive splenic enlargement, severe anemia, shock, and, ultimately, death. Susceptibility to infection is a common problem of young children with sickle cell anemia and may be greatly increased during periods of crisis. Systemic infec-tion and septicemia from pneumococcus or *Haemophilusin-fluenzae* are not uncommon and may be rapidly fatal. In older children, local infection, especially osteomyelitis, rather than generalized septicemia is frequently a complicating factor.

■ INTERVENTIONS: Therapy consists of immediate transfu-sion of packed red blood cells in the acute anemic crisis and alleviation of severe abdominal and joint pain with analgesics or narcotics as needed in vasoocclusive crisis. Short-term oxygen therapy, hydration by oral or IV means, electrolyte replacement to counteract metabolic acidosis re-sulting from hypoxia, and antibiotics to treat any existing infection may be necessary. Pneumococcal and meningo-coccal vaccine is recommended for children between 2 and 5 years of age because they are highly susceptible to infec-tion. Partial exchange transfusions are often mandatory in life-threatening crises, such as when sickling occurs in the vessels of the brain or lungs, and may be used as a preven-tive technique; multiple transfusions, however, increase the risk of hepatitis, hemosiderosis, and transfusion reactions. Oral anticoagulants have been used to relieve the pain of vasoocclusion, but these increase the risk of bleeding. Pria-pism, a painful condition frequently seen in vasoocclusive crisis, may be treated by aspirating the corpora cavernosa.

In children with recurrent splenic sequestration, splenec-tomy may be a lifesaving procedure. The process is not routinely recommended because surgery increases the risk of acidosis and hypoxia from anesthesia, and, in time, the spleen usually atrophies through progressive fibrotic chang-es. Infarction of tissue in any organ is a potential hazard in sickle cell crisis, and special management and treatment are warranted by the specific site of damage. Typical com-plications include uremia (requiring renal transplantation or hemodialysis), chronic functional pulmonary impairment, aseptic necrosis of the hip, and microvascular occlusion that may lead to venous thrombosis.

■ PATIENT CARE CONSIDERATIONS: The primary concern of the nurse during a crisis is to initiate procedures that reduce sickling. Foremost is prevention of tissue deoxygenation and resulting hypoxia by maintaining bed rest to minimize energy expenditure and oxygen use, although some exer-cise is necessary to promote circulation. Hydration and electrolyte balance are essential. A complete record of fluid intake and output is maintained, and adequate therapy is calculated accordingly. Serum sodium level is monitored closely to prevent hyponatremia. Oxygen is given in severe anoxia, although prolonged administration depresses bone marrow activity and thus aggravates anemia. Management of pain in vasoocclusion is often difficult and may require experimentation with various drugs and schedules before the patient receives adequate relief. The application of warmth is often soothing; cold is contraindicated because it enhances vasoconstriction and sickling. The nurse con-stantly monitors the child's condition for splenomegaly, infection, evidence of shock or cerebrovascular accident, hypervolemia, transfusion reaction, or increasing anemia. An important aspect of nursing care is the continued emo-tional support of parents whose child has a chronic illness that is potentially fatal.

sickle cell dactylitis [AS, *sicol* + L, *cella,* storeroom; Gk, *daktylos,* finger, *itis,* inflammation], a painful inflammation of one or more fingers caused by an attack of sickle cell ane-mia. The severe pain affects the bones of the hands, the feet, or both. It is often the first symptom of sickle cell disease in babies.

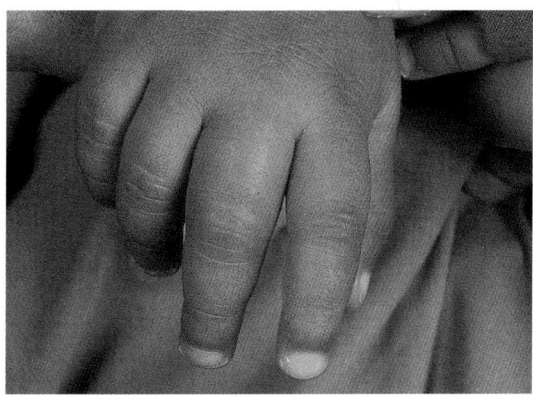

Sickle cell dactylitis *(Hoffbrand et al, 2010)*

sickle cell–hemoglobin C disease. See **hemoglobin SC (Hb SC) disease.**

sickle cell–hemoglobin D disease. See **hemoglobin SD disease.**

sickle cell hepatopathy, the liver damage that accompa-nies sickle cell disease, caused especially by vascular occlu-sion and ischemia, sequestration, and cholestasis.

sickle cell test, a blood screening to detect sickle cell disease and sickle cell trait.

sickle cell thalassemia, a double heterozygous anemia in which the genes for sickle cell and for thalassemia are both inherited. A mild form and a severe form may be identified, depending on the degree of suppression of beta-chain synthesis by the thalassemia gene. In the mild form, synthesis is only partially suppressed, and the red blood cells may contain from 25% to 35% normal hemoglobin A, along with a greater concentration of hemoglobin S. The clinical course is relatively mild. In the severe form, beta-chain synthesis is completely suppressed and only hemoglobin S appears in the red blood cells. The clinical course is generally as severe as in homozygous sickle cell anemia. See also **hemoglobinopathy, hemoglobin S, hemoglobin SC (Hb SC) disease.**

sickle cell trait, the heterozygous form of sickle cell anemia, characterized by the presence of both hemoglobin S and hemoglobin A in the red blood cells. Anemia and the other signs of sickle cell anemia do not occur. People who have the trait are informed of and counseled about the possibility of having an infant with sickle cell disease if both parents have the trait. See also **hemoglobin S.**

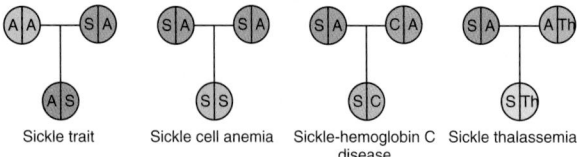

Sickle trait   Sickle cell anemia   Sickle-hemoglobin C disease   Sickle thalassemia

Sickle cell inheritance pattern

sickling, the development of sickle-shaped red blood cells, as in sickle cell anemia.

sick role [AS, *seoc* + Fr, stage character], a behavior pattern in which a person adopts the symptoms of a physical or mental disorder to be cared for, sympathized with, and protected from the demands and stresses of life.

sick sinus syndrome (SSS) [AS, *seoc* + L, *sinus,* hollow], a complex of arrhythmias associated with sinus node dysfunction. The condition may result from a variety of cardiac diseases, ranging from cardiomyopathies to inflammatory myocardial disease. It is most commonly related to either intermittent sinoatrial (SA) block or inadequate SA conduction. SSS is characterized by severe sinus bradycardia, either alone, alternating with tachycardia, or accompanied by atrioventricular block. The most common symptoms are lethargy, weakness, light-headedness, dizziness, and syncope. The severity of symptoms is related to the duration of the asystolic period. Elderly patients with episodes of near-syncope associated with a history of palpitations are most likely to be symptomatic. Accurate diagnosis requires electrocardiography. At present the only treatment is the implantation of a permanent pacemaker.

SICU /sik″yoo̅/, abbreviation for *surgical intensive care unit.*

SID, abbreviation for **source-to-image receptor distance.**

side effect [AS, *side* + L, *effectus*], any reaction to or consequence of a medication or therapy. This can be an effect carried beyond the desired limit, such as hemorrhaging from an anticoagulant, or a reaction unrelated to the primary object of the therapy, such as an anaphylactic reaction to an antibiotic. Usually, although not necessarily, the effect is undesirable and may manifest itself as nausea, dry mouth, dizziness, blood dyscrasias, blurred vision, discolored urine, or tinnitus.

sidero-, combining form meaning "iron": *siderocyte, sideropenia.*

sideroblastic anemia /sid′ərōblas″tik/ [Gk, *sideros,* iron, *blastos,* germ], a heterogeneous group of chronic normocytic or slightly macrocytic anemias characterized by decreased erythropoiesis. The red blood cells contain a perinuclear ring of iron-stained granules. Sideroblastic anemia is an acquired disorder and the cause is not understood. Treatment may include extract of liver, pyridoxine, folic acid, and blood transfusion. Also spelled *sideroblastic anaemia.* Compare **iron-deficiency anemia, siderosis.**

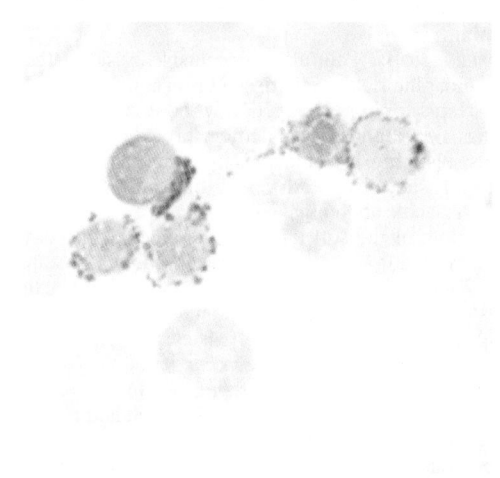

Sideroblastic anemia *(Gilbert-Barness, 2007)*

siderocyte /sid″ərosīt′/ [Gk, *sideros,* iron, *kytos,* cell], an abnormal erythrocyte in which particles of nonhemoglobin iron are visible as siderotic granules, or Pappenheimer bodies.

sideropenia /sid′ərōpē″nē·ə/, an abnormally low level of serum iron.

sideropenic dysphagia. See **Plummer-Vinson syndrome.**

siderosis /sid′ərō″sis/ [Gk, *sideros* + *osis,* condition], **1.** a variety of pneumoconiosis caused by the inhalation of iron dust or particles. **2.** the introduction of color in any tissue caused by the presence of excess iron. **3.** an increase in the amount of iron in the blood. See also **hemochromatosis, hemosiderosis, sideroblastic anemia.**

siderotic granules /sid′ərot″ik/, inclusion bodies seen in the red blood cells of splenectomy patients and in cases of abnormal hemoglobin synthesis, sideroblastic anemia, and hemolytic anemia. The granules contain iron, which takes a Prussian blue stain. Also called **Pappenheimer bodies.**

siderotic splenomegaly, an enlarged spleen associated with fibrosis and an excessive accumulation of iron and calcium. The condition is seen in sickle cell disease and hematochromatosis.

side-to-side anastomosis. See **anastomosis.**

SIDS, abbreviation for **sudden infant death syndrome.**

SIECUS /sē″kəs/, acronym for *Sex Information and Education Council of the United States.*

siemens (S) /sē″mens/ [Ernst Werner von Siemens, German electric inventor, 1816–1892], a unit of electric conductance of a body with a resistance of 1 ohm, allowing 1 ampere of current to flow per volt applied.

sievert (Sv) /sē″vərt/ [R.M. Sievert, 20th-century Swedish physicist], a measure of radiation dose. The sievert has the same units as the gray and is equal to the absorbed dose times the quality factor, which compares the health consequences of that type of radiation with those of x-rays. The rem bears the same relationship to the rad as the sievert does to the gray.

sig, a notation for a Latin word meaning "let it be labeled (according to prescription)." Abbreviation for *signetur.*

sigh. See **periodic deep inspiration.**

sight /sīt/ [AS, *gesiht*], **1.** the special sense that enables the shape, size, position, and color of objects to be perceived; the faculty of vision. It is the principal function of the eye. **2.** that which is seen.

sigma /sig″mə/, Σ, σ, and s, the eighteenth letter of the Greek alphabet.

Sigma Theta Tau International /sig″mə thā″tə tou″/, an international honor society for nurses. Registered nurses and student nurses are invited to join on the basis of academic achievement or contributions to nursing.

sigmoid /sig″moid/ [Gk, *sigma*, the letter S, *eidos*, form], **1.** *adj.,* pertaining to an S shape. **2.** *n.,* the sigmoid colon.

sigmoid-, prefix meaning "sigmoid colon," the section of the colon shaped like the Greek letter *sigma: sigmoidoscope, sigmoidectomy.*

sigmoid colon, the part of the colon that extends from the one descending colon in the pelvis to the juncture of the rectum. Also called **sigmoid flexure.**

sigmoid cystoplasty, augmentation of the bladder using an isolated segment of the sigmoid colon for the graft.

sigmoidectomy /sig″moidek″təmē/ [Gk, *sigma* + *eidos* + *ektomē*, excision], excision of the sigmoid flexure of the colon, most commonly performed to remove a malignant tumor. A large percentage of cancers of the lower bowel occur in the sigmoid colon.

sigmoid flexure. See **sigmoid colon.**

sigmoiditis /sig″moidī″tis/, an inflammation of the sigmoid colon.

sigmoid mesocolon /mez″ōkō″lən/ [Gk, *sigma* + *eidos* + *mesos,* middle, *kolon*], a fold of peritoneum that connects the sigmoid colon with the pelvic wall, forming a curved line of attachment with the apex of the curve located at the division of the left common iliac artery. The fold is continuous with the iliac mesocolon and ends in the median plane over the rectum at the level of the third sacral vertebra. Between the two layers of the fold are the sigmoid and the superior rectal vessels. Compare **mesentery proper, transverse mesocolon.**

sigmoid notch, a concavity on the superior surface of the mandibular ramus between the coronoid and condyloid processes.

sigmoidoscope /sigmoi″dəskōp″/ [Gk, *sigma* + *eidos* + *skopein,* to look], an instrument used to examine the lumen of the sigmoid colon. It consists of a tube and a light, allowing direct visualization of the mucous membrane lining the colon. Compare **proctoscope.**

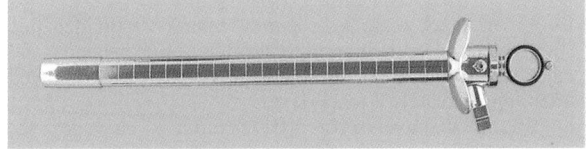

Sigmoidoscope *(Tighe, 2012)*

sigmoidoscopy /sig′moidos″kəpē/, the inspection of the rectum and sigmoid colon by the aid of a flexible lighted tube.

sigmoidostomy /sig′moidos″təmē/, the surgical creation of an anus in the pelvic colon.

sigmoid volvulus, a type of colonic volvulus consisting of twisting of an elongated section of sigmoid colon on its mesenteric axis. It is usually seen in the elderly.

sign /sīn/ [L, *signum,* mark], an objective finding as perceived by an examiner, such as a fever, a rash, the whisper heard over the chest in pleural effusion, or the light band of hair seen in children after recovery from kwashiorkor. Many signs accompany symptoms. For example, erythema and a maculopapular rash are often seen with pruritus. Compare **symptom.**

signal-average electrocardiogram (SAECG), an electrocardiographic study, usually performed on patients with unexplained loss of consciousness or suspected arrhythmias, in which hundreds of QRS complexes are collected, filtered, and analyzed to discover the presence or absence of certain abnormalities in the conducting system of the ventricle.

signal molecule /sig″nəl/ [L, *signum,* mark], a hormone, neurotransmitter, or other agent that transfers information from one cell or organ to another. Examples include steroid hormones, insulin, and growth factors. A photon may have a similar effect on a retinal receptor.

signal node. See **Virchow's node.**

signal symptom. See **symptom.**

signal-to-noise ratio (SNR), the number used to describe the relative contributions to a detected signal of the true signal and random superimposed signals or "noise."

signature /sig″nəchər/ [L, *signare,* (sig) to mark], (in pharmacy) a part of a prescription containing instructions to the patient about dosage and manner and frequency of administration.

signe de journal. See **thumb sign.**

significance /signif″ikəns/ [L, *significare,* to signify], **1.** in research, the statistical probability that a given finding may have occurred by chance alone. The conventional standard for attributing significance is a finding that occurs fewer than 5 times in 100 by chance alone ($p < .05$). **2.** the importance of a study in developing a practice or theory, as in nursing practice.

significance level, the probability of incorrectly rejecting the null hypothesis when such a hypothesis is tested. See also **type I error.**

significant other /signif″ikənt/, a person who is considered by an individual as being special and as having an effect on that individual.

sign language [L, *signum* + *lingua,* tongue], a form of communication often used with and among deaf people, consisting of hand and body movements. Many variations exist, including American Sign Language (ASL). Other forms of manual communication are Signed English and finger spelling. Compare **body language.**

sign-off. See **logoff.**

sign-on. See **login.**

silanization /sil′ənizā″shən/, (in chromatography) the chemical process of converting the SiOH moieties of a stationary form to the ester form.

sildenafil, an erectile agent.

■ INDICATIONS: It is used to treat erectile dysfunction.

■ CONTRAINDICATIONS: Known hypersensitivity to this drug prohibits its use.

■ ADVERSE EFFECTS: Common side effects include headache, flushing, dizziness, dyspepsia, nasal congestion, urinary tract infection, abnormal vision, diarrhea, and rash.

silence, **1.** absence of noise. **2.** a state of producing no detectable signs or symptoms.

silent disease /sī″lənt/ [L, *silens* + *dis* + Fr, *aise,* ease], a disease or other disorder that produces no clinically obvious signs or symptoms. See also **subclinical.**

silent ischemia [L, *silere,* to be silent], an asymptomatic form of myocardial ischemia that may damage the heart muscle. Ischemia is most likely to occur during the first 6 hours after a person awakens in the morning. It is triggered by mental arousal in more than 75% of patients. In contrast, cardiac ischemia accompanied by anginal pains is usually triggered by physical exertion.

silent mutation, an alteration in a DNA sequence that does not result in an amino acid change in a polypeptide.

silent myocardial infarction, an interruption in blood flow to the coronary arteries without the usual signs and symptoms of a heart attack. Such infarctions may be associated with diabetes.

silent peritonitis [L, *silere* + Gk, *peri* + *teinein,* to stretch, *itis,* inflammation], a case of peritonitis that develops without clinical signs or symptoms.

silhouette sign /sil′oo·et′/, a radiographic sign caused by an infiltrate that obscures the demarcating line between lung segments.

silica (SiO₂) /sil′i·kə/ [L, *silex,* flint], silicon dioxide, an inorganic compound occurring in nature as agate, sand, amethyst, flint, quartz, and other stones. It is one of the major constituents of dental porcelain and a common filler in resin composites. In granular form, it serves as a dental abrasive and polishing agent. See also **silicosis.**

silica gel /sil′ikə/, a coagulated form of hydrated silica, used as an absorbent of gases and as a dehydrating agent.

silicic acid /silis′ik/, hydrated silicon dioxide. It is used in thin-layer and column chromatography.

silico-, combining form meaning "silica" or "quartz": *silicosis, silicophosphate cement.*

silicon (Si) /sil′ikon/ [L, *silex,* flint], a nonmetallic element, second to oxygen as the most abundant of the elements in the earth's crust. Its atomic number is 14, and its atomic mass is 28.09. It occurs in nature as silicon dioxide and in silicates. The silicates are used as detergents, corrosion inhibitors, adhesives, and sealants. Elemental silicon is used in metallurgy and in transistors and other electronic components. About 60% of the rocks in the earth's crust contain silicon, and silica dust is associated with many mining operations. Protracted inhalation of silica dust can cause silicosis, which increases the susceptibility to other pulmonary diseases.

silicone /sil′ikōn/ [L, *silex,* flint], any of a large group of inert polymers. Silicones are water-repellent and stable at high temperature. They are useful in medicine as adhesives, lubricants, and sealants. They are used in glass chromatography and in coating of glassware for blood collection because they help reduce platelet loss. They are also used as a substitute for rubber, especially in prosthetic devices. Elastomeric silicone, or silicon rubber, is biologically inert. See also **silicone-gel breast implant.**

silicone-gel breast implant, a type of implant used in reconstructive surgery of the breast and made with synthetic polymers. The implants have been associated with adverse effects on the immune system as well as distorted and painful breasts caused by leakage of the silicone into surrounding tissues. However, a number of statistical studies have not established such a cause-and-effect relationship.

silicone-hydrogel lens, a soft contact lens made of a polymer that contains silicone, which is permeable to oxygen, so that large amounts of oxygen are transmitted to the cornea. Such lenses contain less water than traditional soft lenses and so are more resistant to dehydration and less prone to harbor bacteria and protein deposits. Some are designed to be worn continuously for extended periods, up to 30 days for some types.

silicone oil, any of various fluid silicone polymers. Some are injected into the vitreous of the eye to serve as a vitreous

substitute during or after certain ophthalmological surgical procedures, such as to prevent the recurrence of retinal detachment.

silicone septum, a vascular access device used in IV therapy. It consists of a silicone partition that covers the port chamber housed in the metal or plastic body of an implanted infusion port.

silicophosphate cement /sil′i·kō·fos′fāt/, a mixture of silicate and zinc phosphate cements, formerly used as temporary filling material and for cementation of orthodontic bands, indirect restorations, and porcelain jacket crowns.

silicosis /sil′ikō″sis/, a lung disorder caused by continued long-term inhalation of the dust of an inorganic compound, silicon dioxide, which is found in sands, quartzes, flints, and many other stones. Silicosis is characterized by the development of nodular fibrosis in the lungs. In advanced cases, severe dyspnea may develop. The incidence of silicosis is highest among industrial workers exposed to silica powder in manufacturing processes; in those who work with ceramics, sand, or stone; and in those who mine silica. Also called **grinder's disease, quartz silicosis.** See also **chronic obstructive pulmonary disease, inorganic dust.**

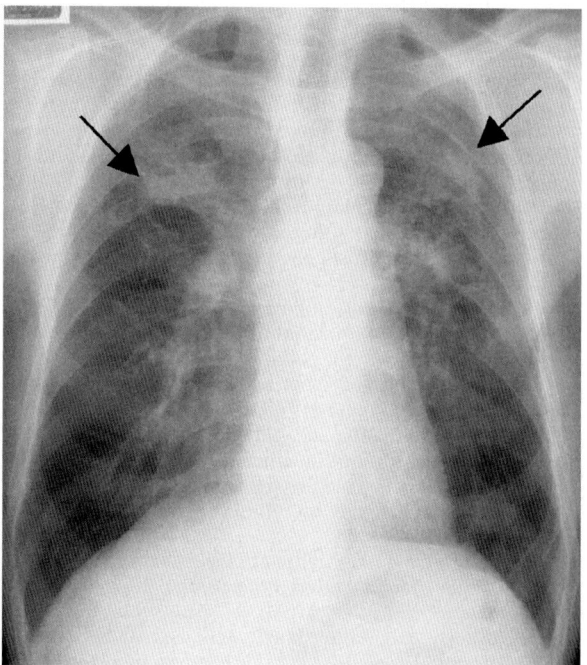

Chest radiograph showing complicated silicosis with bilateral fibrosis in upper lobes (*arrows*) *(Arakawa et al, 2009)*

silk suture [AS, *seolc* + L, *sutura,* seam], a braided fine suture material, usually used to close incisions, wounds, and cuts in the skin. It is not absorbed by the body and is removed after approximately 7 to 21 days.

silo filler's disease /sī′lō/ [Fr, *ensilotage,* ensilage; AS, *fyllan,* to fill], a rare acute respiratory condition seen in agricultural workers who have inhaled nitrogen oxide as they work with fermented fodder in closed, poorly ventilated areas such as silos. Characteristically, symptoms of respiratory distress and pulmonary edema occur several hours after exposure. Loss of consciousness may occur. Observation in the hospital and respiratory assistance often are required. The condition is rarely fatal.

Silvadene, an antibacterial agent. Brand name for **silver sulfadiazine.**

silver (Ag) [AS, *seolfor*], a whitish precious metal occurring mainly as a sulfide. Its atomic number is 47; its atomic mass is 107.88. It is quite soft and is usually alloyed with small amounts of copper to increase its durability. Silver dissolves readily in nitric acid and is used extensively to produce silver halides used in photographic emulsions. It is frequently associated in small amounts with the ores of zinc, copper, and lead and is used extensively as a component of amalgams of dental fillings and in many medications, especially antiseptics and astringents. Some antiseptics containing silver are mild silver protein and strong silver protein, preparations that render silver colloidal in the presence of protein. Mild silver protein contains 19% to 23% silver. Strong silver protein contains 7.5% to 8.5% silver. Both preparations are used externally as antiseptics and do not have irritating properties. Silver nitrate was once widely used externally as an antiseptic and astringent, especially in the prevention of ophthalmia neonatorum. It has been largely replaced with antibiotic eye drops, such as erythromycin. It is also used as a lubricant on the bearings of radiography tubes. Silver picrate, an ionizable salt of silver, is used in the treatment of trichomoniasis and moniliasis of the vagina.

silver amalgam [AS, *seolfor* + Gk, *malagma*], an alloy of silver, tin, copper, mercury, and zinc used in dentistry to fill prepared tooth cavities. See **amalgam.**

silver cone method, a technique for filling tooth pulp canals. It is outdated because the silver corrodes over time, which permits apical fluid leakage and root canal failure. Retreatment of the root canal is necessary. Also called *silver point.*

Silver dwarf [Henry K. Silver, 20th-century American pediatrician], a person who has Silver syndrome, a congenital disorder in which short stature is associated with lateral asymmetry; various anomalies of the head, face, and skeleton; and precocious puberty.

silver-fork fracture. See **Colles fracture.**

Silverman-Anderson score, a system of assessing the degree of respiratory distress.

silver nitrate (AgNO₃), a topical antiseptic.

■ INDICATIONS: A 1% solution was traditionally prescribed for the prevention of gonococcal ophthalmia in newborns, but povidone-iodine is now usually used because it is less expensive and has a broader spectrum of action. Stronger concentrations can also be used on wet dressings for cauterizing wounds, removal of granulation tissue and warts, and prophylaxis following burns.

■ CONTRAINDICATIONS: Known sensitivity to this drug prohibits its use.

■ ADVERSE EFFECTS: Among the more serious adverse effects are severe local inflammation, burns, argyria, and staining.

Silver-Russell syndrome. See **Russell-Silver syndrome.**

silver salts poisoning, a toxic condition caused by the ingestion of silver nitrate, characterized by discoloration of the lips, vomiting, abdominal pain, dizziness, and convulsions.

Silver syndrome, a hereditary spastic paraplegia.

silver sulfadiazine, a topical antibiotic.

■ INDICATIONS: It is prescribed to prevent or treat infection in second- and third-degree burns.

■ CONTRAINDICATIONS: Known hypersensitivity to this drug, to silver, or to sulfonamides prohibits its use. It is not given in the last weeks of pregnancy or to newborn or premature infants.

■ ADVERSE EFFECTS: Among the most serious adverse effects are rash, fungal infection, neutropenia, and kernicterus.

silver-wire arteries, retinal arterioles that appear as white tubes containing a red fluid when viewed through an ophthalmoscope. The condition occurs as replacement fibrosis associated with hypertension continues and the vessel wall obscures the blood column.

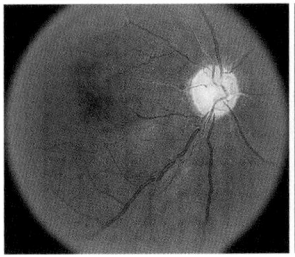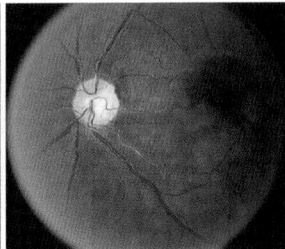

Silver-wire arteries *(Albert et al, 2008)*

simethicone /simeth′ikōn/, an antiflatulent that helps the gases to dissolve in liquid by decreasing the surface tension of gas bubbles.

■ INDICATIONS: It is prescribed to disperse gas pockets in the GI tract.

■ CONTRAINDICATIONS: There are no significant contraindications other than hypersensitivity to the medication.

■ ADVERSE EFFECTS: There are no significant adverse effects.

simian crease /sim″ē·ən/ [L, *simia*, ape; ME, *creste*, crest], a single crease across the palm produced from the fusion of proximal and distal palmar creases, seen in congenital disorders such as Down syndrome. Also called **simian line.**

simian-human immunodeficiency virus, a chimeric, engineered virus with the envelope of human immunodeficiency virus and the cytoplasm and nucleus of simian immunodeficiency virus (SIV). It is used in animal models because it is a better mimic of HIV than SIV is.

simian immunodeficiency virus (SIV), a lentivirus that produces an acquired immunodeficiency syndrome–like disease in nonhuman primates. The cytopathological changes caused by SIV are similar to those caused by the human immunodeficiency virus (HIV). SIV also shares with HIV a group of genes lacking in other retroviruses, and animals infected with either virus experience a similar decrease in the number of CD4⁺ lymphocytes.

simian line. See **simian crease.**

simian virus 40 (SV40), a vacuolating virus isolated from the kidney tissue of rhesus monkeys. SV40 may play a role in the development of malignancies. Exposure to the virus is associated with contaminated polio vaccines administered in the 1960s.

simil-, combining form meaning "like": *Similac, similia similibus curantur.*

Similac preparations, a group of commercial modified milk products that are prepared especially for infant feeding. They are made from a nonfat base of cow's milk supplemented with such substances as lactose, coconut and soy oils, and monosaccharides and disaccharides and are fortified with vitamins and minerals. The ratio of the various nutrients, such as iron or one of the other minerals,

S

is altered in the different preparations to accommodate infants with particular nutritional requirements or nutritional problems, such as nephrogenic diabetes insipidus. The formulas are packaged in both powder and liquid forms.

similia similibus curantur, a homeopathic rule that medication able to produce symptoms in a healthy person will also remove similar symptoms occurring as an expression of disease. See also **homeopathy.**

Simmonds disease. See **panhypopituitarism, postpubertal panhypopituitarism.**

simplate bleeding time test, a blood test for determining how quickly platelets form a plug when an incision is made in the skin. Platelet plug formation is the first step in clotting and, if slower than 8 minutes, indicates platelet deficiency or the effect of a drug, such as aspirin. Also called **template bleeding time test.**

simple, 1. describing something composed of only one or a minimum number of parts or elements. **2.** not involved or complicated.

simple angioma [L, *simplex,* not mixed], a tumor consisting of a network of small vessels or distended capillaries surrounded by connective tissue.

simple astigmatism [L, *simplex,* not mixed; Gk, *a + stigma,* point], **1.** simple myopic astigmatism in which one principal meridian is in focus on the retina and the other in front of it. **2.** simple hyperopic astigmatism in which one meridian is focused on the retina and the other behind it.

simple bone cyst, a benign empty lesion within bone that can result from hemorrhage caused by trauma, inadequate venous drainage of interstitial fluid, disturbance of local bone growth, ischemic bone marrow necrosis, or alteration of bone metabolism resulting in osteolysis. Radiographic or dental imaging of this lesion appears as radiolucent scallops around the roots of teeth. The patient may or may not report a history of trauma to the area. Also called *hemorrhagic bone cyst, idiopathic bone cyst,* **traumatic bone cyst.**

simple cavity, a cavity that involves only one surface of a tooth.

simple diarrhea [L, *simplex,* not mixed; Gk, *dia + rhein,* to flow], a form of diarrhea in which the loose stools contain normal feces.

simple dislocation [L, *simplex,* not mixed, *dis + locare,* to place], displacement of a joint without a penetrating wound or fracture.

simple figure-eight roller arm sling, a sling prepared by placing the patient in a supine or sitting position with the affected arm flexed and adjacent to the chest. The open sling fits under the arm and over the chest. The bandage is fixed with a single turn toward the uninjured side around the arm and chest, crossing the elbow above the external epicondyle. In the next step, the bandage is drawn forward under the tip of the elbow, after making a second turn that overlaps two thirds of the first. Then the bandage is pulled upward along the flexed arm to the base of the neck on the uninjured side. Finally, the bandage is drawn down over the scapula and across the chest and arm, overlapping and continuing in a figure-eight pattern.

simple fission. See **binary fission.**

simple fracture. See **closed fracture.**

simple glaucoma [L, *simplex,* not mixed; Gk, *glaucoma,* cataract], chronic open-angle glaucoma without complications but with visual field loss and optic atrophy.

simple goiter [L, *simplex,* not mixed, *guttur,* sore throat], a goiter not accompanied by signs or symptoms of hyperthyroidism.

simple mastectomy, a surgical procedure in which a breast is completely removed and the underlying muscles and adjacent lymph nodes are left intact, performed to remove small malignant neoplasms of the breast or as a palliative measure to remove an ulcerated carcinoma in advanced breast cancer. It also may be done prophylactically when the patient has severe fibrocystic disease and a strong family history of breast cancer. Compare **modified radical mastectomy, radical mastectomy.** See also **mastectomy.**

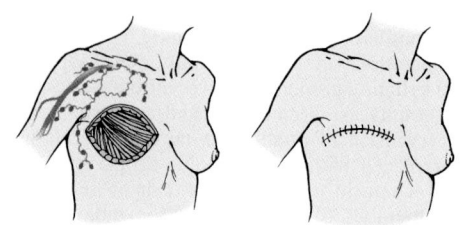

Simple mastectomy *(Ignatavicius and Workman, 2010)*

simple meningitis. See **sterile meningitis.**

simple phobia, an anxiety disorder characterized by a persistent, irrational fear of specific things, such as animals, dirt, light, or darkness. Compare **social phobia.** See also **phobia.**

simple protein, a protein that yields amino acids as the only or chief product of hydrolysis. The class includes albumins, globulins, glutelins, alcohol-soluble proteins, albuminoids, histones, and protamines. See also **complex protein.**

simple reflex [L, *simplex,* not mixed, *reflectere,* to bend back], a reflex with a motor nerve component that involves only one muscle. See also **reflex arc.**

simple stomatitis [L, *simplex* + Gk, *stoma,* mouth, *itis,* inflammation], an inflammation of the mucous membranes of the mouth, with redness, swelling, an excess of mucus, and no accompanying complications. Also called **catarrhal stomatitis.**

simple sugar, a monosaccharide. Kinds include **glucose.**

simple tubular gland, one of the many multicellular glands with only one duct and a tube-shaped part, such as various glands within the epithelium of the intestine.

simple vulvectomy. See **vulvectomy.**

Simplexvirus /sim′pleksvī″rus/, the herpes simplex virus, a genus of herpesviruses that causes herpes simplex. Species pathogenic in humans include human herpesvirus 1 and human herpesvirus 2.

Simpson forceps. See **obstetric forceps.**

simulation /sim′yəlā″shən/ [L, *simulare,* to imitate], **1.** a method of representing the actions of one system by those of another, as a computer program that represents the actions of something in the real world. Computer simulation enables the exploration of situations, such as chemical reactions, that might be too expensive, dangerous, or time-consuming to explore in real life. **2.** a creation of a realistic scenario in a nonclinical setting to facilitate the rehearsal of a situation that a learner might encounter in the clinical setting.

simultanagnosia /sī′multan′agnō″zhə/, a visual disorder in which a person actually perceives only one element of a picture or object at a time and is unable to absorb the whole. See also **Balint syndrome.**

sinus-, combining form meaning "hollow,","cavity,": *sinusitis, sinusoid.*

sinap-, prefix meaning "mustard": *sinapism.*

sinapism. See **mustard plaster.**

sinciput /sin″siput/ [L, half a head], the anterior or upper part of the skull. See also **bregma.**

Sinemet, a fixed-combination drug containing a peripheral dopa decarboxylase inhibitor and an antiparkinsonian that can enter the central nervous system. Brand name for **carbidopa, levodopa.**

Sinequan, a tricyclic antidepressant. Brand name for **doxepin hydrochloride.**

sinew /sin′yōō/ [ME, *sinewe*], the tendon of a muscle, such as the thick, flattened tendon attached to the short head of the biceps brachii. See also **tendon.**

singer's nodule. See **vocal cord nodule.**

single-blind study [L, *singulus,* one by one; AS, *blind* + L, *studere,* to be busy], an experiment in which the person collecting data knows whether the subject is in the control group or the experimental group, but subjects do not. See also **double-blind study.**

single-cell gel electrophoresis, a type of gel electrophoresis used to detect the genotoxic potential of environmental hazards, such as radiation, heavy metals, and toxic chemicals. Such agents may cause breaks in the nuclear DNA of cells. When such a cell is lysed and exposed to electrophoresis that denatures its DNA, the damaged DNA moves toward the electric field, making a formation like the tail of a comet. Also called **comet assay.**

single-chain antigen-binding (SCAB) protein, a polypeptide that joins an antibody's light chain variable region to the antibody heavy chain variable region. SCABs are used as biosensors, in chemical separations, and in the treatment of cancers and heart disease.

single component insulin [L, *singulus* + *componere,* to bring together, *insula,* island], any highly purified insulin with less than 10 ppm of proinsulin. See also **insulin, proinsulin.**

single footling breech. See **footling breech.**

single-locus probe (SLP), a sequence of labeled DNA or RNA that can be used to identify a region of DNA tandem repeats found in the genome only once. It may be used in resolving cases of disputed parentage.

single nucleotide polymorphism (SNP), a genetic polymorphism between two genomes that is based on deletion, insertion, or exchange of a single nucleotide.

single-parent family, a family consisting of only the mother or the father and one or more dependent children.

single-photon emission computed tomography (SPECT), a variation of computed tomography in which the ray sum is defined by the collimator holes on the gamma-ray detector rotating around the patient. SPECT units usually consist of large crystal gamma cameras mounted on a gantry that permits rotation of the camera around the patient. Multiple detectors are used to reduce the imaging time.

single room occupant (SRO), a single person, usually an elderly individual, who lives alone in a single room of a low-cost hotel or apartment building.

single sweep scan, an ultrasonic scan that is completed in a single sweep of the sensing device across the area being examined.

single system ureterocele, a ureterocele involving the ureter of a collecting system that is not double. It is usually orthotopic, intravesical, and seen in adults.

singleton /sing″gəlton/, an offspring born alone.

singlet state /sing″glit/, a state of an atom or molecule in which all electrons have paired spins.

singultus. See **hiccup.**

sinister /sin′istər/ [L], **1.** left, at the left side, at the left hand. **2.** ominous, potentially dangerous; threatening.

sinistral /sinis′trəl/ [L, *sinister,* left], relating to the left side.

sinistrality. See **left-handedness.**

sinistro-, combining form meaning "left" or "related to the left side."

sinoatrial (SA) /sī′nō-ā″trē-əl/ [L *sinus,* hollow, *atrium,* hall], pertaining to the sinus node and atrium. Also called **sinoauricular.**

sinoatrial (SA) block [L, *sinus,* hollow, *atrium,* hall; Fr, *bloc*], a conduction disturbance in the heart during which an impulse formed within the sinus node is blocked or delayed from depolarizing the atria. There are two types of SA block. Type I (SA Wenckebach) is characterized on the electrocardiogram by group beating, shortening of P-P intervals, and pauses that are less than twice the shortest cycle. The P-R intervals are not affected unless there is also an atrioventricular conduction defect. In the case of a 3:2 conduction ratio, a bigeminal sinus rhythm (two sinus-conducted beats and a pause) is noted. Type II SA block is identified on the electrocardiogram by absent P waves without shortening P-P intervals. Causes include excessive vagal stimulation, sinoatrial block acute infections, and atherosclerosis. SA block also may be an adverse reaction to quinidine or digitalis. Treatment for symptomatic SA block includes the use of atropine and isoproterenol; an electronic pacemaker is used if drug therapy is ineffective. See also **atrioventricular block, heart block, intraatrial block, intraventricular block.**

sinoatrial node. See **sinus node.**

sinoatrial valve, the valve at the opening of the sinus venosus into an embryo's right atrium.

sinoauricular. See **sinoatrial.**

sinus /sī′nəs/ [L, hollow], a cavity or channel, such as a cavity within a bone, a dilated channel for venous blood, or one permitting the escape of purulent material.

sinus-. See **sin-, sinus-.**

sinus arrest, a heart disorder in which there is a cessation of activity in the sinus node. The ventricles may continue to contract under the control of pacemakers in the atrioventricular node or the ventricles. Also called **sinus standstill.**

sinus arrhythmia, an irregular cardiac rhythm in which the heart rate usually increases during inspiration and decreases during expiration. It is common in children and young adults and has no clinical significance except in elderly patients.

sinus bradycardia, beating of the sinus node at a rate below 60 beats/min.

sinus dysrhythmia, an irregular heart rhythm characterized by alternate increases and decreases in the heart rate. It is often associated with the vagal effects of respiration, which causes the heart rate to increase on inspiration and decrease on expiration. Nonrespiratory sinus

S

dysrhythmia can be caused by multiple sclerosis, digitalis, myocardial infarction, and increased intracranial pressure. Treatment is not necessary unless the patient is symptomatic with decreased cardiac output; then atropine is given.

sinusitis /sīnəsī″tis/ [L, *sinus* + Gk, *itis,* inflammation], an inflammation of one or more paranasal sinuses. It may be a complication of an upper respiratory infection; dental infection; allergy; or change in atmospheric pressure, as in air travel or underwater swimming; or a structural defect of the nose. See also **sinus surgery.**

■ OBSERVATIONS: With swelling of nasal mucous membranes, the openings from sinuses to the nose may be obstructed, resulting in an accumulation of sinus secretions that cause pressure, pain, headache, fever, and local tenderness.

■ INTERVENTIONS: Treatment includes steam inhalations, nasal decongestants, analgesics, and, if infection is present, antibiotics. Surgery to improve drainage may be performed in the treatment of chronic sinusitis.

■ PATIENT CARE CONSIDERATIONS: Complications include cavernous sinus thrombosis and spread of infection to bone, brain, or meninges.

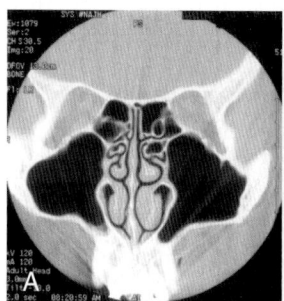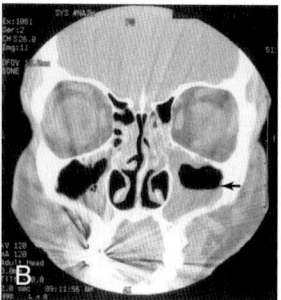

Computed tomography scan of the paranasal sinuses in a patient with normal maxillary sinuses (A) and a patient with bilateral maxillary sinusitis (B) *(Mahon et al, 2015)*

sinus lift, a surgical procedure to add bone to the upper jaw in the area of the molars and premolars by raising the sinus floor and adding bone graft material. Also called *sinus augmentation.*

sinus node, a cluster of hundreds of cells located in the right atrial wall of the heart, near the opening of the superior vena cava. It comprises a knot of modified heart muscle that generates impulses that travel swiftly throughout the muscle fibers of both atria, causing them to contract. Specialized pacemaker cells in the node have an intrinsic rhythm that is independent of any stimulation by nerve impulses from the brain and the spinal cord. Slender fusiform cells making up the sinoatrial node are largely filled with sarcoplasm but contain a few striated fibrillae. The cells are irregularly grouped together and, at the edge of the node, merge with the atrial musculature. The sinoatrial node will normally "fire" at a rhythmic rate of 70 to 75 beats/min. If the node fails to generate an impulse, pacemaker function will shift to another excitable component of the cardiac conduction system, such as the atrioventricular node or Purkinje fibers. Certain hormones and various autonomic impulses can affect the sinoatrial node and cause it to

"fire" faster, such as during strenuous physical activity. During a lifetime of 70 years the node generates about 2 billion impulses. Surgical implantation of an artificial pacemaker is a common procedure for individuals suffering from a defective sinoatrial node. Also called **Keith bundle, Keith-Flack node, pacemaker, sinus pacemaker, sinoatrial node.** Compare **atrioventricular (AV) node, Purkinje network.**

sinus node dysfunction, any disturbance in the normal functioning of the sinus node, such as slow sinus rate or sinoatrial block, that leads to the development of arrhythmias.

sinus of Morgagni. See **aortic sinus.**

sinus of the vena cava, the space in the right atrium posterior to the terminal crest into which empty both vena cava.

sinus of Valsalva. See **aortic sinus.**

sinusoid /sī″nəsoid/ [L, *sinus* + Gk, *eidos,* form], an anastomosing blood vessel that is somewhat larger than a capillary and is lined with reticuloendothelial cells.

sinus pacemaker. See **sinus node.**

sinus rhythm, a cardiac rhythm stimulated by the sinus node. A rate of 60 to 100 beats/min is normal.

sinus standstill. See **sinus arrest.**

sinus surgery, surgery to improve drainage or remove diseased sinus membranes. See also **nasal polyp, sinusitis.**

■ METHOD: Endoscopic surgery is the primary method for treating infected and/or blocked sinuses and has largely replaced other procedures performed with an open approach, such as the Caldwell-Luc procedure. Small polyps, foreign bodies, and infected tissue can be removed, as needed, during sinus surgery.

■ INTERVENTIONS: Surgery for the treatment of chronic sinusitis is most effective when antibiotic therapy is employed first, and then again following surgery to prevent reinfection.

■ OUTCOME CRITERIA: Sinus surgery does not cure sinusitis, and a second procedure may be necessary.

sinus tachycardia [L, *sinus,* hollow; Gk, *tachys,* fast, *kardia,* heart], a rapid heartbeat generated by discharge of the sinus node. The rate is generally 100 to 180 beats/min in the adult, although most clinicians would be suspicious of a rate of 90 beats/min or higher. Sinus tachycardia is also indicated by a heart rate greater than 200 beats/min in an infant and 140 to 200 beats/min in a child. Sinus tachycardia is the body's normal response to exertion, congestive heart failure, cardiogenic shock, acute pulmonary embolism, acute myocardial infarction, and infarct extension.

sinus venosus defect. See **atrial septal defect.**

SiO₂, chemical formula for **silica.**

si op. sit, (in prescriptions) a notation for a Latin phrase meaning "if necessary." Abbreviation for *si opus sit.*

siphonage /sī″fənij/, a process of drawing off fluid from a cavity with a tube using atmospheric pressure.

sireniform fetus. See **sirenomelus.**

sirenomelia /sī″rənəmē″lē·ə/ [Gk, *seiren,* mermaid, *melos,* limb], a congenital anomaly in which there is complete fusion of the lower extremities and no feet. Also called **apodial symmelia.** Compare **dipodial symmelia, monopodial symmelia, tripodial symmelia.** See also **sirenomelus.**

sirenomelus /sī″rənom″ələs/, an infant who has sirenomelia. Also called **sireniform fetus, sympus apus.**

siriasis /sirī″əsis/ [Gk, *sieros,* scorching], sunstroke. See also **heat hyperpyrexia.**

sirolimus, an immunosuppressant.

■ INDICATIONS: It is used after organ transplantation to prevent rejection. Recommended use is in combination with cyclosporine and corticosteroids.

■ CONTRAINDICATIONS: Known hypersensitivity to this drug or any of its components prohibits its use.

■ ADVERSE EFFECTS: Life-threatening effects are anemia, leukopenia, thrombocytopenia, purpura, albuminuria, hematuria, proteinuria, renal failure, pleural effusion, atelectasis, and lymphoma. Other adverse effects include nausea, vomiting, diarrhea, constipation, hypertension, insomnia, chills, fever, urinary tract infections, hyperglycemia, increased creatinine, edema, hypercholesterolemia, hyperlipidemia, hypophosphatemia, weight gain, hyperkalemia, hyperuricemia, hypokalemia, hypomagnesemia, blurred vision, and photophobia. Common side effects include atrial fibrillation, congestive heart failure, hypotension, palpitations, tachycardia, tremors, headache, paresthesia, dyspnea, rash, and acne.

-sis, suffix meaning "an action, process, condition, state, or result of": *centesis, genesis, stasis.*

sister, a term used in the United Kingdom and Commonwealth for a nurse, particularly the head nurse in a hospital, a ward, or an operating room.

Sister Joseph nodule [Sister Mary Joseph Dempsy, U.S. surgical assistant, 1856–1929], a malignant intraabdominal neoplasm of gastric, ovarian, colorectal, or pancreatic origin and metastatic to the umbilicus.

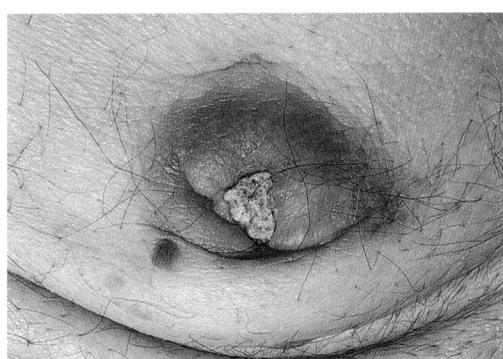

Sister Joseph nodule *(Courtesy Dr. Walter Barkey)*

Sister Kenny's treatment [Elizabeth Kenny, Australian nurse, 1886–1952], poliomyelitis therapy in which the patient's limbs and back are wrapped in warm, moist woolen cloths and, after the pain subsides, the patient is taught to exercise affected muscles, especially by swimming. Equally important is passive movement of affected limbs with simultaneous stimulation at the site of muscle origins, carried out after hot packs.

Sistrurus /sis-troo'rus/, a genus of small rattlesnakes widely distributed throughout the United States, characterized by symmetric plates covering their heads.

sitagliptin, an oral antidiabetic.

■ INDICATIONS: This drug is used alone or in combination with other antidiabetic agents to treat type 2 diabetes mellitus.

■ CONTRAINDICATIONS: Diabetic ketoacidosis and known hypersensitivity to this drug prohibit its use.

■ ADVERSE EFFECTS: Adverse effects of this drug include hypoglycemia and abdominal pain. Common side effects include headache, nausea, and vomiting.

site [L, *situs,* location], **1.** location. See also **situs. 2.** a quantum of space occupied and defined by a cluster of people.

site visit, a visit made by designated officials to gather information about or to evaluate a department or institution. A site visit is a step in the accreditation of an institution and in the funding of many major projects.

siti. See **bejel.**

-sitia, combining form meaning "(condition of) appetite for food": *asitia.*

sito-, sitio-, prefix meaning "food": *sitotherapy.*

sitosterol /sītos″tərôl/ [Gk, *sitos,* food, *stereos,* solid; Ar, *alkohl,* essence], a mixture of sterols derived from plants, such as wheat germ, used for treating hyperbetalipoproteinemia and hypercholesterolemia that are unresponsive to other dietary measures. Its use is controversial, for a dispersing action in the mixture tends to cause loose bowel movements and may lead to diarrhea or interfere with the absorption of concomitantly administered medications. Use in pregnancy is not recommended.

sitotherapy /sī′tōther″əpē/ [Gk, *sitos,* food], a health maintenance system based on food, diet, and nutrition.

sit-to-stand (STS), 1. in the treatment of balance disorders, a movement in which the base of support is transferred from the seat to the feet. The feet begin to accept the weight first by downward pressure through the heels as the pelvis rolls anteriorly. The weight then moves to the front of the feet as the trunk moves forward and the pelvis lifts from the surface. **2.** a transfer activity in which a patient moves from sitting to standing.

situational anxiety /sich′oo·ā″shənəl/ [L, *situs,* location], a state of apprehension, discomfort, and anxiety precipitated by the experience of new or changed situations or events. Situational anxiety is not abnormal and requires no treatment; it usually disappears as the person adjusts to the new experience. See also **anxiety.**

situational characteristics, (in occupational therapy) characteristics that are inconsistent with the way an individual typically behaves when interacting with others. In clinical practice settings, these behaviors are usually linked to stressful circumstances. Situational characteristics are part of the Intentional Relationship Model.

situational crisis, (in psychiatry) an unexpected crisis that arises suddenly in response to an external event or a conflict concerning a specific circumstance. The symptoms are transient, and the episode is usually brief.

situational depression, (in psychiatry) an episode of emotional and psychological depression that occurs in response to a specific set of external conditions or circumstances. See also **mood disorder.**

situational loss, the loss of a person, thing, or quality resulting from alteration of a life situation, including changes related to illness, body image, environment, and death.

situational support, a person who is available and can be depended on to help a patient solve problems.

situational theory, a leadership theory in which the manager chooses a leadership style to match a particular situation.

situational therapy, (in psychiatry) a kind of psychotherapy in which the milieu is part of the treatment program. See also **milieu therapy.**

situation relating /sich′oo·ā″shən/, (in nursing research) a study design used to explain or predict phenomena in nursing practice in which a relationship is thought to exist among certain practices or characteristics of the population being studied.

situation therapy. See **milieu therapy.**

situs /sī″təs/ [L, location], the normal position or location of an organ or part of the body.

situs inversus viscerum.   See **visceral inversion.**

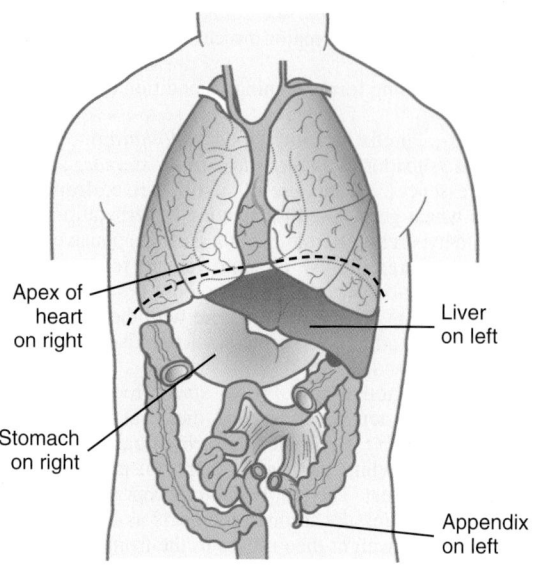

Apex of
heart
on right

Liver
on left

Stomach
on right

Appendix
on left

Complete situs inversus in an adult *(Carlson, 2009)*

sitz bath /sits, zits/   [Ger, *Sitz,* seat; AS, *bjth*],   a therapeutic procedure in which only the rectal and perineal areas are immersed in water or saline solution; used after childbirth and after rectal or perineal surgery to decrease swelling, inflammation, and pain.

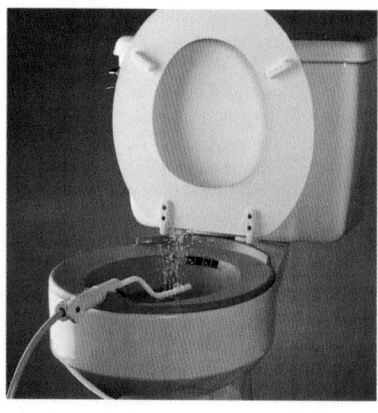

Sitz bath *(Elkin, Perry, and Potter, 2007/Courtesy Andermac, Inc.)*

SI units [Fr, *système international*],   the international units of physical amounts. Examples of these units are the mass of a kilogram, the length of a meter, and the precise amount of time in a second.

SIV,   abbreviation for **simian immunodeficiency virus.**

sixth cranial nerve.   See **abducens nerve.**

sixth disease.   See **roseola infantum.**

Sjögren-Larsson syndrome /shö″gren lär″sən/ [Torsten Sjögren, Swedish pediatrician, 1859–1939; T. Larsson, 20th-century Swedish pediatrician],   a congenital condition inherited as an autosomal-recessive trait, characterized by ichthyosis, cognitive impairment, and spastic paralysis.

Sjögren syndrome [Henrik S.C. Sjögren, Swedish ophthalmologist, 1899–1986],   an immunological disorder characterized by deficient fluid production by the lacrimal, salivary, and other glands, resulting in abnormal dryness of the mouth, eyes, and other mucous membranes. The symptoms primarily affect women over 40 years of age. Atrophy of the lacrimal glands can lead to desiccation of the cornea and conjunctiva with damage to the tissues. Atrophy of the salivary glands results in dental disorders and loss of taste and odor sensations. When the lungs are affected, the dryness increases susceptibility to pneumonia and other respiratory infections. Sjögren syndrome is frequently associated with Raynaud phenomenon, rheumatoid arthritis, Waldenström macroglobulinemia, and lymphoma. Treatment includes applying artificial tears and using soft contact lenses that can be moistened often, sipping fluids frequently to prevent mouth dryness, and avoiding medications that tend to deplete body fluids. See also **dry eye syndrome, keratoconjunctivitis sicca.**

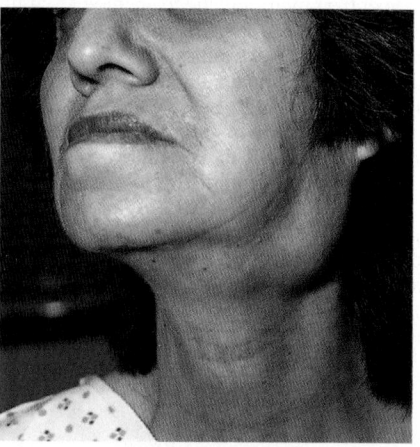

Enlargement of the salivary gland in Sjögren syndrome *(Courtesy Dr. Richard Sontheimer, Department of Dermatology, University of Texas Southwestern Medical School)*

SK,   abbreviation for **streptokinase.**

skato-.   See **scato-, skato-.**

skelalgia [Gk, *skelos,* leg],   pain in the leg.

skeletal.   See **skeleton.**

skeletal fixation /skel′ətəl/ [Gk, *skeletos,* dried up; L, *figere,* to fasten],   any method of holding together the fragments of a fractured bone by attaching wires, screws, plates, or nails. See also **external pin fixation.**

skeletal fluorosis,   skeletal changes caused by long-term ingestion of excessive fluoride, including hyperostosis, osteopetrosis, and osteoporosis.

skeletal muscle.   See **striated muscle.**

skeletal survey,   a radiographic examination of the skeletal system for possible fractures or tumors.

skeletal system,   all of the bones and cartilage of the body that collectively provide the supporting framework for the muscles and organs. See also *Color Atlas of Human Anatomy,* pp. A-2 to A-7.

skeletal traction,   one of the two basic kinds of traction used in orthopedics for the treatment of fractured bones and the correction of orthopedic abnormalities. Skeletal traction is applied to the affected structure by a metal pin or wire inserted into the structure and attached to traction ropes. Skeletal traction is often used when continuous traction is desired to immobilize, position, and align a fractured bone properly during the healing process. Infection of the pin tract is one of the complications that may develop with skeletal traction, and careful scrutiny of pin sites is an important precaution. Some common signs of infection of the pin tracts are erythema, drainage, noxious odor, pin slippage, temperature elevation, and pain. Superficial infection of pin tracts is often treated with antibiotic therapy. Deeper infections usually require pin removal and antibiotic therapy. Compare **skin traction.** See also **Dunlop skeletal traction.**

skeleton /skel′ətən/ [Gk, *skeletos,* dried up], the supporting framework for the body, comprising 206 bones in the adult that protect delicate structures, provide attachments for muscles, allow body movement, serve as major reservoirs of blood, and produce red blood cells, platelets, and most white blood cells. The skeleton is divided into the axial skeleton, which has 74 bones; the appendicular skeleton, with 126 bones; and the 6 auditory ossicles. The four types of bones composing the skeleton are the long bones, including the humerus, the ulna, the femur, the tibia, the fibula, and the phalanges of the fingers and the toes; the short bones, including the carpals and the tarsals; the flat bones, including the frontal bone and the parietal bone of the cranium, the ribs, and the shoulder bones; and the irregular bones, including the vertebrae, the bones of the sacrum, the bones of the coccyx, and certain bones of the skull, such as the sphenoid, the ethmoid, and the mandible. The skeleton changes throughout life as bone formation and bone destruction proceed concurrently. During childhood and adolescence, bone formation proceeds faster than bone destruction. Starting at 35 to 40 years of age, bone destruction proceeds faster than bone formation. In advanced age bone destruction increases, bones become thin and brittle, vertebrae may collapse, and height decreases. See also **bone. −skeletal,** *adj.*

Skene's duct. See **paraurethral duct.**

Skene's glands /skēnz/ [Alexander J.C. Skene, American gynecologist, 1838–1900], the largest of the glands opening into the urethra of women. They contain ducts that open immediately within the urethral orifice.

skew /skyo͞o/ [ME, *skewen,* to escape], a deviation from a line or symmetric pattern, such as data in a research study that do not follow the expected statistical curve of distribution because of the unwitting introduction of another variable.

skia-, scia-, combining form meaning "shadows, especially of internal structures as produced by X- rays": *skiagraph.*

skiagraph, the historical term for the image produced by an x-ray apparatus at the Mayo Clinic in the 1800s.

skill, an observable, goal-directed action that a person uses or demonstrates while performing a task.

skilled nursing facility (SNF) [ME, *skil,* distinction], an institution or part of an institution that meets criteria for accreditation established by the sections of the Social Security Act that determine the basis for Medicaid and Medicare reimbursement for skilled nursing care. Skilled nursing care includes rehabilitation and various medical and nursing procedures. Written policies and protocols are formulated with appropriate professional consultation. Law requires that these policies designate which level of caregiver is responsible for implementation of each policy, that the care of every patient be under the supervision of a physician, that a physician be available on an emergency basis, that records of the condition and care of every patient be maintained, that nursing service be available 24 hours a day, and that at least one full-time registered nurse be employed. Other criteria stipulate that the facility have appropriate facilities for storing and dispensing drugs and biologics, that it maintain a use review plan, that all licensing requirements of the state in which it is located be met, and that an overall budget be maintained.

Skillern fracture /skil″ərn/ [Penn G. Skillern, American surgeon, 1882–1966], an open fracture of the distal radius associated with a greenstick fracture of the distal ulna.

skill play [ME, *skil + plega,* sport], a form of play in which a child persistently repeats an action or activity until it has been mastered, such as throwing or catching a ball.

skills training, the teaching of specific verbal and nonverbal behaviors and the practicing of these behaviors by the patient.

skimmed milk [Dan, *skumme,* scum removal; AS, *meolc*], milk from which the fat has been removed. Most of the vitamin A is removed with the cream, although other nutrients remain. It is available as fluid skimmed milk, fortified skimmed milk, nonfat dry milk, and a form of buttermilk. Also called **nonfat milk,** *skim milk.*

skimming [Dan, *skumme*], a practice, sometimes used by health programs that receive their income on a prepaid or capitation basis, of seeking to enroll only relatively healthy individuals as a means of increasing profit by decreasing costs. See also **skimping.**

skimping [Swed, *skrympa,* to shrink], a practice, sometimes used by health programs that receive their income on a prepaid or capitation basis, of delaying or denying services to enrolled members of the program as a means of increasing profit by decreasing costs. See also **skimming.**

skin [AS, *scinn*], the tough, supple, cutaneous membrane that covers the entire surface of the body. It is composed of a thick layer of connective tissue called the dermis and an epidermis made of five layers of cells. Skin color varies according to the amount of melanin in the epidermis. Genetic differences determine the amount of melanin. The ultraviolet rays of the sun stimulate the production of melanin, which absorbs the rays and simultaneously darkens the skin. Modified skin continues into various parts of the body, such as mucous membrane, as in the lining of the vagina, the bladder, the lungs, the intestines, the nose, and the mouth. Mucous membrane lacks the heavily keratinized layer of the outside skin. The skin helps to cool the body when the temperature rises by radiating the heat of increased blood flow in expanded blood vessels and by providing a surface for the evaporation of sweat. When the temperature drops, the blood vessels constrict and the production of sweat diminishes. Also called **cutaneous membrane, integument.** See also **dermis.**

skin barrier, an artificial layer of skin, usually made of plastic, applied to skin before the application of tape or ostomy drainage bags. It protects the real skin from chronic irritation.

skin button, a plastic and fabric device that covers the drivelines of an artificial heart at their exit point from the skin. Its purpose is to prevent the transmission of pumping pressure to the surrounding tissues.

skin cancer, a cutaneous neoplasm caused by ionizing radiation; certain genetic defects; chemical carcinogens, including arsenics, petroleum, tar products, and fumes from some molten metals; or overexposure to the sun or other sources of ultraviolet light. Skin cancers, the most common and most curable malignancies, are also the most frequent secondary lesions in patients with cancer in other sites. The major risk factor is overexposure to sunlight. Other risk factors include a fair complexion, xeroderma pigmentosa, vitiligo, senile and seborrheic keratitis, Bowen's disease, radiation dermatitis, and hereditary basal cell nevus syndrome. The most common skin cancers are basal cell carcinomas and squamous cell carcinomas. Tumors of the sebaceous glands or sweat glands occur infrequently and are adenocarcinomas. Melanoma is a highly metastatic cancer that has increased in incidence during the past 30 years. Basal cell carcinomas, typically raised hard reddish lesions with a pearly surface, rarely metastasize. Scaly, slightly elevated squamous cell tumors may become growths with extensive ulceration and a nonhealing scab. A definitive diagnosis may be established by incisional biopsy or excisional biopsy, which may be the only treatment required for small lesions. Surgery is usually indicated if the lesion is large, if bone or cartilage is invaded, or if lymph nodes are involved. Radiotherapy may be preferable for some smaller facial lesions and is commonly recommended for the treatment of skin tumors without distinct margins. Because of the possibility of recurrence of cancer, surgery is favored for the treatment of younger patients. Despite the curability of skin cancer, it causes many deaths because people fail to obtain treatment. Lesions caused by actinic rays may be prevented by applying a sunscreen. See also **melanoma.**

skin dose (SD), the amount of radiation absorbed by the skin.

skin erythema dose. See **threshold dose.**

skin flap [AS, *scinn* + ME, *flappe*], a layer of skin usually separated by dissection from deeper layers of tissue.

skinfold calipers, an instrument used to measure the breadth of a fold of skin, usually on the posterior aspect of the upper arm or over the lower ribs of the chest.

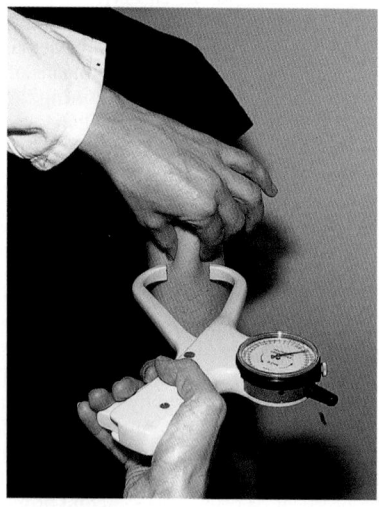

Skinfold calipers (Seidel et al, 2011)

skinfold thickness [AS, *scinn* + *fealden* + *thicce*], a measure of the amount of subcutaneous fat, obtained by inserting a fold of skin into the jaws of a caliper. The skinfolds are usually measured on the upper arm, thigh, or upper abdomen, and the caliper measurements are later compared with precalibrated standard tables to assess an individual's body fat content indirectly.

skin graft, a part of skin implanted to cover areas where skin has been lost through burns or injury or by surgical removal of diseased tissue. To prevent tissue rejection of permanent grafts, the graft is taken from the patient's own body or from the body of an identical twin. Skin from another person or animal can be used as a temporary cover for large burned areas to decrease fluid loss. The area from which the graft is taken is called the donor site; that on which it is placed is called the recipient site. Various techniques are used, including pinch, split-thickness, full-thickness, pedicle, and mesh grafts. In pinch grafting, pieces of skin ¼ inch in diameter are placed as small islands on the recipient site that they will grow to cover. These grafts will grow even in areas of poor blood supply and are resistant to infection. The split-thickness graft consists of sheets of superficial and some deep layers of skin. Grafts of up to 4 inches wide and 10 to 12 inches long are removed from a flat surface—abdomen, thigh, or back—with an instrument called a dermatome. The grafts are sutured into place; compression dressings may be applied for firm contact, or the area may be left exposed to the air. A split-thickness graft cannot be used for weight-bearing parts of the body or for covering those subject to friction, such as the hand or foot. A full-thickness graft contains all skin layers and is more durable and effective for weight-bearing and friction-prone areas. A pedicle graft is one in which a part remains attached to the donor site, whereas the remainder is transferred to the recipient site. Its own blood supply remains intact, and it is not detached until the new blood supply has fully developed. This type is often used on the face, neck, or hand. A successful new graft of any type is well established in about 72 hours and can be expected to survive unless a severe infection or trauma occurs. Before surgery both the donor and the recipient site must be free of infection and the recipient site must have a good blood supply. After surgery, stretching or movement of the recipient site is prevented. Strict sterile technique is used for handling dressings, and antibiotics may be given prophylactically to prevent infection. Good nutrition with a high-protein, high-calorie diet is essential. See also **autograft, graft, xenograft.**

Skinner box [Burrhus F. Skinner, American psychologist, 1904–1990; L, *buxus,* boxwood], a boxlike laboratory apparatus used in operant conditioning of animals, usually containing a lever or other device that when pressed reinforces by either giving a reward, such as food or an escape outlet, or removing a punishment, such as an electric shock. Also called **standard environmental chamber.** See also **operant conditioning.**

skin pigment [AS, *scinn* + L, *pigmentum,* paint], any skin coloring caused by melanin deposits. The coloring may be modified by substances in the blood, such as the several blood pigments, bile, or malarial parasites.

skin prep, a procedure for cleansing the skin with an antiseptic before surgery or venipuncture. Skin preps are performed to kill bacteria and pathological organisms and to reduce the risk of infection. Various skin prep devices are available for this procedure. Such devices are commonly constructed of plastic, filled with a specific antiseptic, and equipped with an applicator. The antiseptic is applied by rubbing the device in a circular motion over the skin. Some of the most common antiseptics contained in skin prep devices are iodine, povidone-iodine, chlorhexidine gluconate, and ethyl alcohol.

skin self-examination (SSE), the practice of studying one's own skin for early signs of premalignant or malignant tumors. A 5-year study by the Sloan-Kettering Cancer Center in New York found that people who examined themselves, looking for moles that change color, shape, or size, were 44% less likely to die of melanoma than those who did not.

skin staple. See **wound clip.**

skin substitute, a material used to cover wounds and burns where extensive areas of skin are missing to promote healing. Effective skin substitutes are bilaminar, with dermal analogue and epidermal analogue layers, and may be synthetic or manufactured from tissue elements.

skin tag. See **cutaneous papilloma.**

skin test, a test to determine the reaction of the body to a substance by observing the results of injecting the substance intradermally or of applying it topically to the skin. Skin tests are used to detect allergens, to determine immunity, and to diagnose disease. Kinds include **patch test, Schick test, tuberculin test.**

skin traction, one of two kinds of traction used for the treatment of fractured bones and the correction of orthopedic abnormalities. Skin traction applies pull to an affected body structure by straps attached to the skin surrounding the structure. Compare **skeletal traction.** Kinds include **adhesive skin traction, nonadhesive skin traction.** See also **Dunlop skin traction.**

skin turgor [AS, *scinn* + L, *turgere,* to swell], the resilience of the normal skin when subjected to physical distortion, such as by pinching or pressing. The relative speed with which the skin resumes its normal appearance after stretching or compression is an indicator of skin hydration. Turgor is slower in older people.

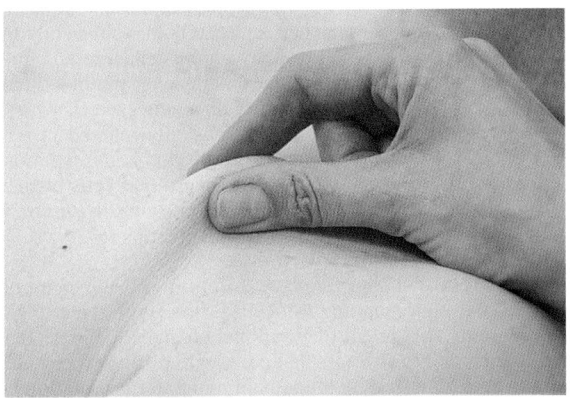

Normal skin turgor (Wilson and Giddens, 2009)

sklero-. See **sclero-, scler-, sklero-.**

skull [ME, *skulle,* shell], the bony structure of the head, consisting of the cranium and the skeleton of the face. The cranium, which contains and protects the brain, consists of 8 bones; the skeleton of the face is composed of 14 bones.

skullcap, an herb that is native to temperate regions of North America.
- INDICATIONS: It has been used as folk medicine to treat convulsions, hysteria, and nervous tension and is a common component of remedies for premenstrual syndrome and other female problems. There is insufficient reliable evidence regarding its effectiveness.
- CONTRAINDICATIONS: Skullcap should not be used during pregnancy and lactation, in children, or in those with known hypersensitivity to this plant.

skull shield, a protective plastic plate worn over a cranial defect.

skull x-ray, radiographic imaging of the bones of the skull, the nasal sinuses, and cerebral calcifications. Skull x-rays have largely been replaced by computed tomography scanning of the brain.

SL, abbreviation for **soda lime.**

slaked lime. See **calcium hydroxide.**

slander [Fr, *esclandre,* scandal], (in law) any words spoken with malice that are untrue and prejudicial to the reputation, professional practice, commercial trade, office, or business of another person. Compare **libel.**

slant of occlusal plane [ME, *slenten,* to slope], the angle between the extended occlusal plane and the axis-orbital plane.

SLE, abbreviation for **systemic lupus erythematosus.**

sleep [AS, *slaepan,* to sleep], a state marked by reduced consciousness, diminished activity of the skeletal muscles, and depressed metabolism. People normally experience sleep in patterns that follow four observable, progressive stages. A device such as an encephalograph is used to record the recurrent pattern of brain waves during the stages. During stage 1 the brain waves are of the theta type, followed in stage 2 by the appearance of distinctive sleep spindles; during stages 3 and 4 the theta waves are replaced by delta waves. These four stages represent three fourths of a period of typical sleep and collectively are called nonrapid eye movement sleep. The remaining time is usually occupied with rapid eye movement (REM) sleep, which can be detected with electrodes placed on the skin around the eyes so that tiny electric discharges from contractions of the eye muscles are transmitted to recording equipment. The REM sleep periods, lasting from a few minutes to half an hour, alternate with the NREM periods. Dreaming occurs during REM time. Individual sleep patterns

normally change throughout life because daily requirements for sleep gradually diminish from as much as 20 hours a day in infancy to as little as 6 hours a day in old age. Infants tend to begin a sleep period with REM sleep, whereas REM activity usually follows the four stages of NREM sleep in adults.

sleep apnea, a sleep disorder characterized by periods in which respiration is absent. The person is momentarily unable to contract respiratory muscles or to maintain airflow through the nose and mouth. See also **apnea, obstructive sleep apnea.**

sleep deprivation [L, *deprivare,* to deprive; ME, *slep* + L, *efficere,* to accomplish], the result of interference with a basic physiological urge to sleep, which appears to be governed by sleep centers in the hypothalamus and reticular activating system. Sleep deprivation can cause significant reductions in performance and alertness. Reducing nighttime sleep by as little as 90 minutes for just one night can affect cognitive processes. Sleep deprivation results in progressive mental aberrations after 30 to 60 continuous hours. After this point, repetitive tasks become intolerable, speech begins to be slurred, and performance becomes increasingly poor. After a week of sleep deprivation, symptoms of psychosis may appear.

sleep epilepsy. See **narcolepsy.**

sleeping pill, **1.** (*Informal*) a prescription sedative taken for insomnia or for postoperative sedation. **2.** an over-the-counter pill classified pharmaceutically as an aid to sleeping. Antihistamines, such as pyrilamine maleate, diphenhydramine, and doxylamine succinate, depend for sedative action on side effects, which may disappear with continued use of such agents. The use of all drugs that depress the central nervous system is contraindicated for pregnant and lactating women and for asthma, glaucoma, or prostatic hypertrophy patients.

sleeping sickness. See **African trypanosomiasis.**

sleep studies, an electrodiagnostic test used to diagnose obstructive sleep apnea. It is performed in a sleep laboratory where the patient is monitored by electrocardiogram, pulse oximetry, electroencephalogram, and electromyography. Also called **polysomnography.**

sleep technologist. See **polysomnographic technologist.**

sleep terror disorder [AS, *slaepan* + L, *terrere,* to frighten], a condition occurring during stage 3 or 4 of nonrapid eye movement sleep. It is characterized by repeated episodes of abrupt awakening, usually with a panicky scream, accompanied by intense anxiety, confusion, agitation, disorientation, unresponsiveness, marked motor movements, and total amnesia concerning the event. The disorder usually occurs in children, is more common in boys than in girls, and is extremely variable in frequency but is more likely to occur if the individual is fatigued or under stress or has been given a tricyclic antidepressant or neuroleptic at bedtime. Compare **nightmare.** See also **pavor nocturnus.**

sleep-wake schedule disorder, a form of dyssomnia caused by a conflict between a person's circadian rhythm and the socioeconomic demands of society, such as work and travel schedules.

sleepwalking. See **somnambulism.**

slice /slīs/ [OFr, *esclice*], (in tomography) a cross-sectional plane of the body selected for imaging.

slice sensitivity profile, a curve showing the effect of broadening the computed tomography slice thickness along the patient axis in helical CT.

slide clamp [AS, *slidan* + *clam,* fastener], a device, usually constructed of plastic, used to regulate the flow of IV solution. The slide clamp has a graduated opening through which the IV tubing passes. Pushing the tube into the narrow end of the opening constricts it and reduces the flow rate of the IV solution. Sliding the wide end of the opening over the tube increases the flow rate. Compare **roller clamp, screw clamp.**

S

slide tracheoplasty, surgical treatment of tracheal stenosis by dividing the stenosis at the midpoint, incising the segments vertically on opposite anterior and posterior surfaces, and sliding the segments together to create an anastomosis with a widened lumen.

sliding esophageal hiatal hernia, a protrusion of the cardioesophageal junction and stomach through the opening in the diaphragm where the esophagus passes from the thoracic to the abdominal cavity.

sliding filaments [AS, *slidan* + L, *filamentum,* thread], interdigitated thick and thin filaments of a sarcomere. In muscle contraction they slide past each other so that the sarcomere becomes shorter although the filament lengths do not change. The action of the sliding filaments contributes to the increased thickness of a muscle in contraction.

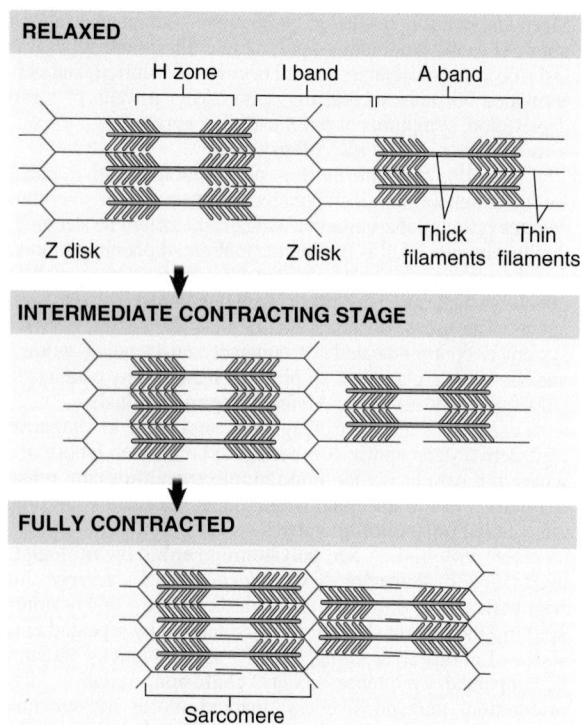

Sliding filaments *(Patton and Thibodeau, 2010)*

sliding inguinal hernia, a protrusion of either the cecum or the sigmoid colon into the parietal peritoneum. Also called **slipped hernia.**

sliding hiatal hernia, a protrusion of the upper stomach and cardioesophageal junction through the diaphragm into the posterior mediastinum.

sliding transfer, the movement of a person in a sitting position from one site to another, such as from a bed to a wheelchair, by sliding him or her along a transfer board.

sling [ME, *slingen,* to hurl], a bandage or device used to support an injured part of the body, especially a forearm. See also **sling restraint.**

sling restraint, a therapeutic device, usually constructed of felt, used to assist in the immobilization of patients, especially orthopedic patients in traction. The sling is placed over the pelvis to reduce pelvic motion with lower extremity traction or over the abdominal area as countertraction with Dunlop traction. With lower extremity traction the sling restraint is attached to both sides of the bedspring frame. Compare

diaper restraint, jacket restraint. See also **Dunlop skeletal traction, Dunlop skin traction.**

slip-on blood pump [ME, *slippen,* slippery, *on*], a plastic mesh device with an attached squeeze bulb, rubber tubing, and pressure gauge, used to help administer large amounts of blood quickly. The plastic mesh slips over the blood bag and exerts pressure on it when the bulb is squeezed. The pressure gauge displays a danger zone, usually marked in red, and indicates pressure limits for safe blood administration. Excessive pressure may damage the red blood cells or may disconnect the primary IV line. *Also called pressure infusion cuff, compression sleeve.*

slipped disk. See **herniated disk.**

slipped femoral epiphysis, a failure of the femoral epiphyseal plate, tending to occur primarily in overweight adolescents as a result of hormonal changes. Clinical features include hip stiffness and pain, with difficulty in walking. There also may be knee pain and external rotation of the affected leg. The condition is treated by orthopedic surgery.

slipped hernia. See **sliding hernia.**

slipping patella [ME, *slippen* + L, *patella,* small dish], a patella that undergoes recurrent dislocation.

slipping rib, a condition in which a loose ligament allows one of the lower five ribs to slip inside or outside an adjacent rib, causing pain or discomfort. The symptoms may mimic those of a disorder of the pancreas, gallbladder, or other upper abdominal organ.

slit diaphragm, a thin membrane that spans the slit pore of the renal glomerulus.

slit lamp [AS, *slitan* + Gk, *lampein,* to shine], an instrument used in ophthalmology for examining the external, surface, and internal segments of the eye, including the eyelid(s), lashes, conjunctiva, cornea, anterior chamber, pupil, iris, vitreous, and retina. A high-intensity beam of light is projected through a narrow slit, and a cross section of the illuminated part of the eye is examined through a magnifying lens. A second, hand-held lens is used to examine the retina.

slit-lamp microscope, a microscope for ophthalmic examination. It permits the viewer to examine the endothelium of the posterior surface of the cornea in a projected band of light that is shaped like a slit.

slit scan radiography, a technique for producing radiographs of body structures without length distortion by scanning a fan-shaped beam of x-rays through a narrow-slit collimator. The beam divergence perpendicular to the scan results in some distortion of width.

slit tongue. See **forked tongue.**

slit-ventricle syndrome, a condition of chronic, positonal headaches affecting individuals with a ventriculoperitoneal (VP) shunt. Radiographic imaging reveals small, slit-shaped ventricles.

SLO, abbreviation for **scanning laser ophthalmoscope.**

Slo-Phyllin, a bronchodilator. Brand name for **theophylline.**

slough /sluf/ [ME, *sluh,* husk], **1.** *v.,* to shed or cast off dead tissue, such as cells of the endometrium, shed during menstruation. **2.** *n.,* the tissue that has been shed.

slow-acting insulin. See **long-acting insulin.**

slow channel, a membrane channel that is slow to become activated. An example is the calcium channel, which allows calcium ions to diffuse across membranes. See also **calcium channel blocker.**

slow diastolic depolarization [AS, *slaw,* dull], the slow loss of membrane polarization that occurs between action potentials in cells of the sinus and atrioventricular nodes.

Slow-K, a slow-release tablet of an electrolyte replacement. Brand name for **potassium chloride.**

slow pain, an unpleasant sensory experience that travels a multisynaptic route to the brain via slow-conducting, non-myelinated nerve fibers.

slow pulse [AS, *slaw,* dull; L, *pulsare,* to beat], a pulse rate of less than 60 beats/min. The rate is common among older people, conditioned athletes, and patients receiving beta-blockers. See also **bradycardia.**

slow-reacting substance of anaphylaxis (SRS-A), a group of active substances, including histamine and leukotrienes, that are released during an anaphylactic reaction. They cause the smooth muscle contraction and vascular dilation that cause the signs and symptoms of anaphylaxis.

slow-response action potential, a cardiac action potential produced by the influx of calcium ions without the typical and much faster influx of sodium ions. Such an action potential has a slow upstroke, low amplitude, and consequent slow conduction.

slow stroking, a therapeutic massage technique of slow continuous movement of the hands over the paravertebral areas along the spine from the cervical through the lumbar region. Usually a lubricant is applied to the skin, and the index and middle fingers are used to stroke both sides of the spinal column simultaneously. Also called **effleurage.**

slow-twitch (ST) fiber, a muscle fiber that develops less tension more slowly than a fast-twitch fiber. The ST fiber is usually fatigue resistant and has adequate oxygen and enzyme activity. Studies indicate that world-class endurance runners apparently have high percentages of ST fibers. It is called red muscle because of the abundance of capillaries serving the fiber muscle. The muscle also contains high amounts of the protein myoglobin that functions to store oxygen inside the muscle cell. See also **fast-twitch (FT) fiber.**

slow virus, a virus, such as lentivirus, that remains dormant in the body after initial infection. Years may elapse before symptoms occur. Several degenerative diseases of the central nervous system are believed to be caused by slow viruses, including subacute sclerosing panencephalitis and kuru.

SLP, **1.** abbreviation for **single-locus probe. 2.** abbreviation for **speech-language pathologist.**

slurred speech /slurd/ [D, *sleuren,* to drag; ME, *speche*], abnormal speech in which words are not enunciated clearly or completely but are run together or partially eliminated. The condition may be caused by weakness of the muscles of articulation, damage to a motor neuron, cerebellar disease, drug use, or carelessness.

slurry /slur″ē/ [ME, *sloor,* mud], a thin suspension of finely divided solids in a liquid.

Sly syndrome /slī/ [William S. Sly, American physician, b. 1932], a mucopolysaccharidosis caused by deficiency of an enzyme important for the degradation of various mucopolysaccharides. It is characterized by excretion of mucopolysaccharides in the urine and by granular inclusions in granulocytes. Onset is between 1 and 2 years of age, with mild to moderate Hurler-like features, including dysostosis multiplex, pigeon breast, organomegaly, cardiac murmurs, short stature, and moderate cognitive impairment. Milder forms exist. Also called **mucopolysaccharidosis.**

Sm, symbol for the element **samarium.**

smack, *(Slang)* heroin.

small bowel follow-through (SBF) test, an x-ray with contrast dye (usually barium) performed to identify abnormalities in the small bowel. X-ray films done at timed intervals follow the progression of the contrast medium through the small intestine. The SBF series is also helpful in identifying and defining the anatomy of small bowel fistulas.

small calorie. See **calorie.**

small cardiac vein [AS, *smael*], one of the five tributaries of the coronary sinus that drain blood from the myocardium. It conveys blood from the back of the right atrium and the right ventricle. Also called **right coronary vein.** Compare **great cardiac vein, middle cardiac vein, posterior vein of left ventricle.**

small cell carcinoma. See **oat cell carcinoma.**

smallest cardiac vein, one of the tiny vessels that drain deoxygenated blood from the myocardium into the atria. A few of these vessels end in the ventricles. Also called **vein of Thebesius.** Compare **anterior cardiac vein.** See also **coronary vein.**

small for gestational age (SGA) infant, a newborn whose weight and size at birth fall below the tenth percentile of appropriate for gestational age infants, whether delivered at term or earlier or later than term. Factors associated with smallness or retardation of intrauterine growth other than genetic influences include any disorder causing short stature, such as dwarfism; malnutrition caused by placental insufficiency; and certain infectious agents, including cytomegalovirus, rubella virus, and *Toxoplasma gondii.* Other factors associated with the smallness of an SGA infant include cigarette smoking by the mother during pregnancy, her addiction to alcohol or heroin, and her having received methadone treatment. Asphyxia may be a significant risk for the SGA infant during labor and delivery if the condition is the result of placental insufficiency. Such an infant has a low Apgar score, becomes acidotic in labor and at birth, and is likely to experience hypoglycemia within the first hours or days of life. Given adequate nutrition and caloric intake, some SGA infants show phenomenal catch-up growth. Also called *small for dates (SFD) infant.* Compare **appropriate for gestational age (AGA) infant, large for gestational age (LGA) infant.** See also **dysmaturity.**

small intestine, the longest part of the digestive tract, extending for about 7 m from the pylorus of the stomach to the iliocecal junction. It is divided into the duodenum, jejunum, and ileum. Decreasing in diameter from beginning to end, it is situated in the central and caudal part of the abdominal cavity and is surrounded by large intestine. It functions in digestion and is the major organ of absorption of prepared food. Compare **large intestine.**

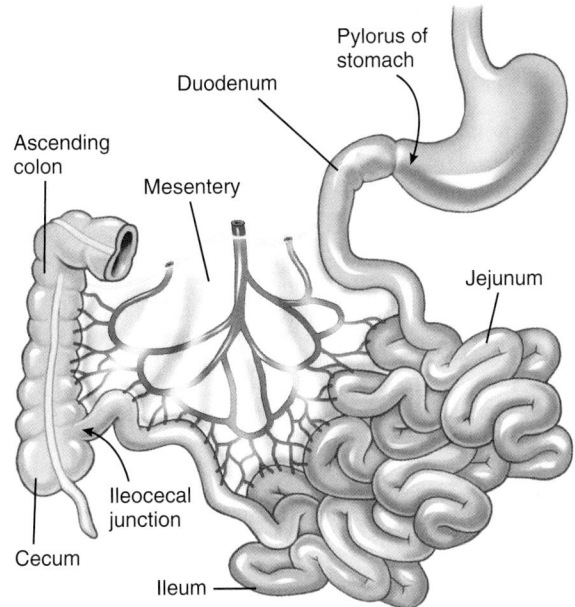

Small intestine

small omentum.   See **lesser omentum.**

smallpox /smôl′poks/   [AS, *smael* + *pocc*],   a highly contagious and sometimes fatal viral disease characterized by fever, prostration, and a vesicular, pustular rash. It is caused by one of two species of poxvirus, variola minor (alastrim) or variola major, the latter being the severe and most common form. Because human beings are the only reservoir for the virus, worldwide vaccination with vaccinia, a related poxvirus, has been effective in eradicating smallpox; the last case of smallpox in the U.S. was in 1949, and the last recorded case in the world was in Somalia in 1977. The only known remaining sources of the virus are stored frozen at the U.S. Centers for Disease Control and Prevention. Smallpox is a potential agent for bioterrorism. Also called **variola, variola major.**

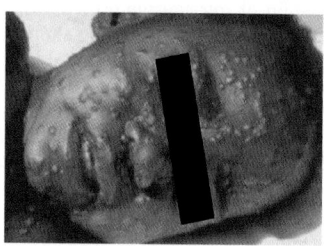

Individual with smallpox *(Courtesy Centers for Disease Control and Prevention/Cheryl Tyron)*

smallpox vaccine,   a vaccine prepared from dried smallpox virus. It is currently indicated only for laboratory workers and certain military personnel who could be exposed to pox viruses, but this recommendation could change with bioterrorism concerns.

smallpox virus,   variola virus.

small saphenous vein,   a large superficial vein embedded in the subcutaneous fascia of the lower limb that passes behind the distal end of the fibula and up the back of the leg to penetrate deep fascia and join the popliteal vein posterior to the knee. The small saphenous veins originate from the lateral side of a dorsal venous arch of the foot.

small sciatic nerve [AS, *smael* + Gk, *ischiadikos,* of the hip joint; L, *nervus*],   the posterior femoral cutaneous nerve, which pierces the fascia and subdivides into filaments, supplying the skin from the level of the greater trochanter to the middle of the thigh.

SMBG,   abbreviation for **self-monitoring of blood glucose.**

smear [AS, *smeoru,* grease],   a laboratory specimen for microscopic examination prepared by spreading a thin film of tissue or fluid on a glass slide. A dye, stain, reagent, diluent, or lysing agent may be applied to the specimen, depending on the purpose of the examination.

smegma /smeg′mə/   [Gk, soap],   a secretion of sebaceous glands, especially the foul-smelling secretion sometimes found under the foreskin of the penis and at the base of the labia minora near the glans clitoris.

smell [ME, *smellen,* to detect odors],   **1.** the special sense that allows perception of odors through the stimulation of the olfactory nerves; olfaction. See also **anosmia. 2.** any odor, pleasant or unpleasant.

smelling salt [ME, *smellen* + AS, *sealt*],   aromatized ammonium carbonate to which ammonia may be added. It is used as a stimulant to arouse a person who has fainted.

Smith fracture [Robert W. Smith, Irish surgeon, 1807–1873],   a fracture of the wrist involving volar displacement and angulation of a distal bone fragment. Also called **reverse Colles fracture.**

Smith-Hodge pessary.   See **pessary.**

Smith-Lemli-Opitz syndrome /ō′pitz/ [John Marius Opitz, German-born pediatrician in United States, b. 1935],   an autosomal-dominant syndrome consisting of hypertelorism and hernias and, in males, hypospadias, cryptorchidism, and bifid scrotum. Cardiac anomalies, laryngotracheal malformations, imperforate anus, renal defects, lung hypoplasia, and downslanted palpebral fissures may also be present. Also called **G syndrome, hypertelorism-hypospadias syndrome.**

Smith-Petersen nail [Marius N. Smith-Petersen, American surgeon, 1886–1953; AS, *naegel,* nail],   a three-flanged, stainless steel nail used in orthopedic surgery to anchor the neck of the femur to its head in the repair of an intertrochanteric fracture. It is introduced below the prominence of the greater trochanter and passed through the fractured part into the head of the femur. See also **nail, pin.**

smog,   a polluting combination of smoke and fog in the atmosphere.

smoke inhalation [AS, *smoca* + L, *in,* within, *halare,* to breathe],   the inhalation of noxious fumes or irritating particulate matter that may cause severe pulmonary damage. Respiratory burns are difficult to distinguish from simple smoke inhalation. Chemical pneumonitis, asphyxiation, and physical trauma to the respiratory passages may occur.

■ OBSERVATIONS: Characteristics include irritation of the upper respiratory tract, singed nasal hairs, dyspnea, hypoxia, dusty gray sputum, rhonchi, rales, restlessness, anxiety, cough, and hoarseness. Pulmonary edema may develop up to 48 hours after exposure.

■ INTERVENTIONS: Airway maintenance and ventilatory assistance are essential. Endotracheal intubation, high-flow oxygen, and mechanical ventilation may be needed. Arterial blood gases are monitored, and corticosteroids may be given.

■ PATIENT CARE CONSIDERATIONS: The characteristics of smoke inhalation and its treatment vary with the nature of the fumes or matter inhaled and the extent of exposure. It is therefore important to know the circumstances, nature, and period of exposure and to know whether the person has a history of chronic respiratory or cardiac disease.

smokeless tobacco [AS, *smoca* + Sp, *tabaco*],   **1.** chewing tobacco or tobacco powder that allows the stimulating components of tobacco to be absorbed through the digestive tract, or through the mucous membrane in the case of snuff. **2.** a transdermal nicotine patch that can be affixed to the upper part of the body to satisfy a person's craving for nicotine.

smooth chorion,   the smooth (nonvillous) and membranous part of the chorion.

smooth muscle [AS, *smoth*],   one of three kinds of muscle, composed of elongated, spindle-shaped cells in muscles not under voluntary control, such as the smooth muscle of the intestines, stomach, and other viscera. The nucleated cells of smooth muscle are arranged parallel to one another and to the long axis of the muscle they form. Smooth muscle fibers are shorter than striated muscle fibers, have only one nucleus per fiber, and are smooth in appearance. Biofeedback devices may help many people gain partial control of contractions of involuntary smooth muscles. Also called **involuntary muscle, unstriated muscle.** Compare **cardiac muscle, striated muscle.**

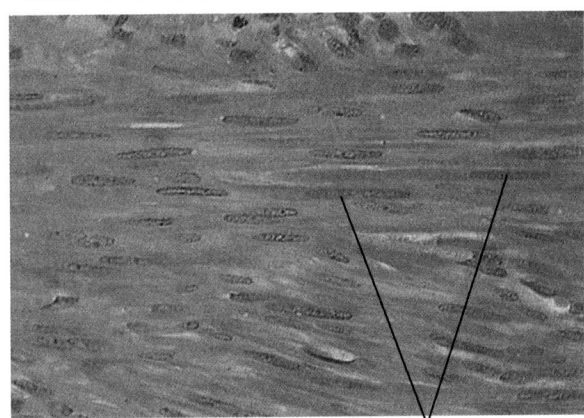

Nuclei of smooth muscle cells

Smooth muscle (© Ed Reschke. Used with permission)

smooth muscle relaxant, an agent that reduces the tone of smooth muscle, such as a bronchodilator or vasodilator.

smooth pursuit eye movement, the tracking by the eyes of a slowly moving object at a steady coordinated velocity, rather than in saccades.

smooth sphincter dyssynergia. See **bladder neck dyssynergia.**

smooth surface cavity, a cavity formed by decay that starts on surfaces of teeth without pits, fissures, or enamel faults.

SMR, abbreviation for **submucous resection.**

smudge cell [ME, *sogen,* to soil], a disrupted lymphocyte, sometimes seen during preparation of blood smears.

Sn, symbol for the element **tin.**

S.N., (in the United States) a notation used by student nurses in signing nursing notes. Abbreviation for *student nurse.*

SNA, **1.** initialism for **State Nurses Association. 2.** initialism for *Student Nurses Association.*

snail [AS, *snagel,* slug], an invertebrate of the order Gastropoda, several species of which are intermediate hosts of the blood flukes that cause angiostrongyliasis in humans.

snakebite [AS, *snacan,* to creep, *bitan*], a wound resulting from penetration of the flesh by the fangs or teeth of a snake. Bites by snakes known to be nonvenomous are treated as puncture wounds; those produced by an unidentified or poisonous snake require immediate attention. The bitten area should be immobilized below heart level, the patient kept still, and prompt transportation arranged to an emergency department. Only polyvalent antivenin is available for bites of all pit vipers, including rattlesnakes, copperheads, and cottonmouths. Pit vipers are responsible for 98% of the poisonous snakebites in the United States. Bites of pit vipers are characterized by pain, redness, and edema followed by weakness, dizziness, profuse perspiration, nausea, vomiting, or weak pulse; subcutaneous hemorrhage; and, in severe cases, shock. Treatment may include the use of antivenin, analgesics, antibiotics, and antitetanus prophylaxis to prevent infections from pathogens found in the mouths of snakes. Patients sensitive to horse serum in antivenin may require antihistamines and steroids for the control of hives, urticaria, and other allergic reactions. Coral snakes rarely bite, but their venom contains a neurotoxin that can cause respiratory paralysis. Antivenin and respiratory support may be indicated.

snake venom [AS, *snacan* + L, *venenum*], a poison produced in glands of certain snakes and injected through fangs into a victim's flesh. The exact composition of snake venoms varies with different species, but generally they are complex mixtures of neurotoxins, proteolytic enzymes, and phosphatases. A venomous snakebite is considered a medical emergency.

snapper /snap′er/, any of various carnivorous marine fish of the family Lutjanidae found in tropical waters; they are often eaten by humans but sometimes contain ciguatoxin and can cause ciguatera.

snapping hip [ME, *snappen* + AS, *hype*], a condition in which a tendon slips over the greater trochanter of the femur when the hip is moved, possibly producing a loud, snapping sound.

snare /sner/ [AS, *sneare,* noose], a device designed for holding a wire noose, used in removing small stalklike growths. The operator tightens the wire around the stalk (peduncle), thus removing the growth.

Sneddon syndrome /sned′ən/ [Ian Bruce Sneddon, English dermatologist, b. 1915], a rare condition in which cerebral arteriopathy and ischemia are accompanied by diffuse noninflammatory livedo reticularis.

sneeze [AS, *snesen,* to sneeze], a sudden forceful involuntary expulsion of air through the nose and mouth occurring as a result of irritation to the mucous membranes of the upper respiratory tract, such as by dust, pollen, or viral inflammation. Also called **sternutation.**

Snellen chart [Hermann Snellen, Dutch ophthalmologist, 1834–1908], one of several charts used in testing visual acuity. Letters, numbers, or symbols are arranged on the chart in decreasing size from top to bottom.

Snellen reflex [Hermann Snellen], unilateral congestion of the ear on stimulation of the distal end of the divided great auricular nerve.

Snellen test [Hermann Snellen], a test of visual acuity using a Snellen chart. The person being tested stands 20 feet from the chart and reads as many of the symbols as possible, reading each line and proceeding downward from the top. A score is assigned in the form of a ratio, comparing the subject's performance to that of a statistically normal subject's performance. For example, a person who can read at 20 feet what the average person can read at this distance has 20/20 vision, whereas a person who can read at 20 feet what the average person can read at 40 feet has 20/40 vision.

SNF, abbreviation for **skilled nursing facility.**

snore /snôr/, a harsh, rough sound of breathing caused by vibration of the uvula and soft palate during sleep.

snout reflex [ME, *snoute,* muzzle], an abnormal sign elicited by tapping the nose, resulting in a marked facial grimace.

snowball sampling, a method of obtaining subjects for a study by soliciting names of potential subjects from those participating in the study.

snow blindness [AS, *snaw* + *blind*], a condition of photophobia, sometimes accompanied by keratitis or conjunctivitis, as a result of overexposure of the eyes to the glare of sun on snow.

Snowden-Pencer scissors, an instrument with an elongated, tapered design for cutting; unique to surgical procedures. See also **scissors.**

SNP, **1.** abbreviation for **sodium nitroprusside. 2.** abbreviation for **single nucleotide polymorphism.**

SNP analysis, analysis of single nucleotide polymorphisms to assess artificially produced genetic modifications or identify different strains of an organism.

SNR, abbreviation for **signal-to-noise ratio.**

snuff, a ground or powdered tobacco that is inhaled through the nostrils.

S

snuff dipping, the practice of extracting juices from moist, fine-cut chewing tobacco placed in the mucobuccal fold of the mouth. The practice has been associated with an increased incidence of leukoplakia, tooth and gum diseases, and oral cancer.

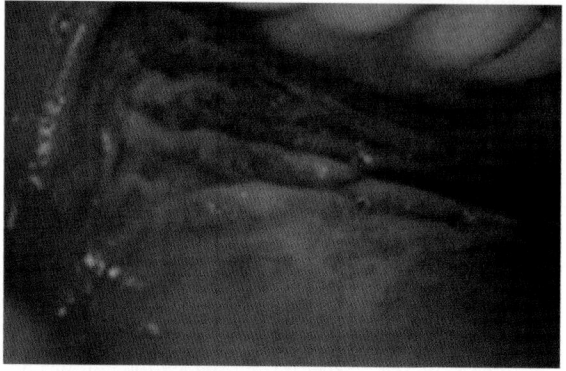

Snuff dipper's pouch (Regezi, Sciubba, and Pogrel, 2000)

snuffles [D, *snuffelen,* to sniff], a nasal discharge in infancy characteristic of congenital syphilis. See also **syphilis.**

soap [L, *sapo*], a salt formed from fatty acids and an alkali. Soap cleanses because molecules of fat are attracted to the fatty part of the anions of soap in a water solution and are pulled off the dirty surface into the water. Compare **detergent.** See also **green soap, surfactant.**

SOAP /sōp′, es″ō′ā′pē″/, (in a problem-oriented medical record) abbreviation for subjective, objective, assessment, and plan, the four parts of a written account of the health problem. In taking and charting the patient history and physical examination, a SOAP statement is made for each syndrome, problem, symptom, or diagnosis. See also **problem-oriented medical record.**

soapsuds enema (SSE) [L, *sapo* + D, *sudse,* marsh water; Gk, *enienai*], an evacuant enema made of 1 ounce of soft soap dissolved in 2 pints of hot water and administered at a temperature of 100° F (38° C). It acts by irritating the colon and stimulating peristalsis.

SOB, abbreviation for *short of breath.*

socia /sō″shē·ə/, an ectopic or displaced part of an organ, such as an accessory parotid gland.

social /so′shal/, **1.** *adj.,* pertaining to societies or groups with a common purpose or identity. **2.** *n.,* an activity undertaken for enjoyment and involving others.

social adjustment rating scale. See **social readjustment rating scale.**

social anxiety disorder. See **social phobia.**

Social Behavior Assessment Scale /sō′shəl/, a semistructured interview guide that elicits information from significant others regarding a patient's functioning.

social breakdown syndrome [L, *socius,* partner; AS, *brecan* + *dune*], deterioration of social and interpersonal skills, work habits, and behavior seen in chronically hospitalized psychiatric patients. Symptoms are a result of long-term hospitalization rather than the primary illness and include excessive passivity, assumption of the chronic sick role, withdrawal, and apathy. Such effects are also seen in long-term inmates of prisons and concentration camps.

social class, a grouping of people with similar values, interests, income, education, and occupations.

social day-care center. See **adult day-care center.**

social determinants of health, economic and social factors in the environment where people live, work, play, worship, and age that impact on health and quality of life. The 5 key determinants include economic stability, education, social and community context, health and health care, and neighborhood and built environment.

social deviance, behavior that violates social standards, engendering anger, resentment, and a desire for punishment in a significant segment of the society or culture.

socialization /sō′shəlīzā″shən/, **1.** the process by which an individual learns to live in accordance with the expectations and standards of a group or society, acquiring its beliefs, habits, values, and accepted modes of behavior primarily through imitation, family interaction, and educational systems; the procedure by which society integrates the individual. **2.** (in psychoanalysis) the process of adjustment that begins in early childhood by which the individual becomes aware of the need to accommodate inner drives to the demands of external reality. See also **internalization.**

socialized medicine /sō′shəlīzd/, a system for the delivery of health care in which the expense of care is borne by a governmental agency supported by taxation rather than being paid directly by the client on a fee-for-service or contract basis. Also called **state medicine.**

social learning theory, a concept that the impulse to behave aggressively is subject to the influence of learning, socialization, and experience. Social learning theorists believe aggression is learned under voluntary control, by observation of aggressive behavior in others, and by direct experience.

social margin, the total of all resources (material, personal, and interpersonal) available to assist an individual in coping with stress.

social medicine, an approach to the prevention and treatment of disease that is based on the study of human heredity, environment, social structures, and cultural values.

social mobility, **1.** the process of moving upward or downward in the social hierarchy. **2.** changes in economic or social status affecting an individual or family over the course of a lifetime or generation(s).

social motivation, an incentive or drive resulting from a sociocultural influence that initiates behavior toward a particular goal. Compare **physiological motivation.**

social network, an interconnected group of cooperating significant others, who may or may not be related, with whom a person interacts.

social network therapy, the gathering together of patient, family, and other social contacts into group sessions for the purpose of problem solving.

social order, the manner in which a society is organized and the rules and standards required to maintain that organization.

social phobia, an anxiety disorder characterized by a compelling desire for the avoidance of and a persistent, irrational fear of situations in which the individual may be exposed to scrutiny by others. Examples of such situations are speaking, eating, or performing in public, or using public lavatories or transportation. Also called **social anxiety disorder.** Compare **simple phobia.** See also **phobia.**

social (pragmatic) speech disorder, difficulties with the use of verbal and nonverbal language for social purposes. Primary difficulties are in social interaction, social cognition, and pragmatics. It may occur with other conditions, including but not limited to intellectual and developmental disabilities.

social psychiatry, a field of psychiatry based on the study of social, cultural, and ecological influences on the development and course of mental illness. In treatment social psychiatry favors the use of milieu or other situational approaches to therapy.

social psychology, the study of the effects of group membership on the behavior, attitudes, and beliefs of the individual.

social readjustment rating scale, a scale of 43 common events associated with some degree of disruption of an individual's life. The scale was developed by the psychologists T.J. Holmes and R. Rahe, who found that a number of serious physical disorders, such as myocardial infarction, peptic ulcer, and infections, and a variety of psychiatric disorders were associated with an accumulation of 200 or more points on the rating scale within a period of 1 year. Most disruptive on one's life, according to the psychologists, was the death of a spouse, which warranted 100 points. The lowest rated event was a minor law violation, rated at 11 points.

social sanctions, the measures used by a society to enforce its rules of acceptable behavior.

Social Security Act, a U.S. federal statute that provides for a national system of old age assistance, survivors' and old age insurance benefits, unemployment insurance and compensation, and other public welfare programs, including Medicare and Medicaid.

social support groups. See **support group.**

social support programs, services both paid and volunteer provided to older persons including visits with older individuals to decrease loneliness and social isolation, telephone contact for older persons for similar purposes, and programs that provide a daily call with emergency procedures that go into effect if the telephone is not answered.

social theories of aging, concepts of social and psychological adjustment in older persons. The theories include activity expressed in adoption of new roles and continuity, which includes retention of physical and social activities from the middle years.

social worker, a person with advanced education in dealing with social, emotional, and environmental problems associated with an illness or disability. A medical social worker usually has completed a master's degree program that includes experience in counseling patients and their families in a hospital setting. A psychiatric social worker may specialize in counseling individuals and families in dealing with social, emotional, or environmental problems pertaining to mental illness.

society /səsīʹətē/, a nation, community, or broad group of people who establish particular aims, beliefs, or standards of living and conduct.

sociobiology /sōʹsē·ō·bīʹol″əjē/ [L, *socius,* companion; Gk, *bios,* life, *logos,* science], the systematic study of biology as a basis for human behavior. Proponents contend that disease, stress, and aggression are natural pressures for maintaining an optimal level of population.

socioeconomic status /sōʹsē·ō·ikʹənom″ik/ [L, *socius,* companion, *oeconomicus,* methodical, *status,* state], the position of an individual on a social-economic scale that measures such factors as education, income, type of occupation, place of residence, and, in some populations, heritage and religion.

sociogenic /-jenʹik/ [L, *socius* + Gk, *genesis,* origin], pertaining to personal or group activities that are motivated by social values and constraints.

sociolinguistics /-ling·gwisʹtiks/, the study of the relationship between language and the social context in which it occurs. *—sociolinguistic, adj.*

sociology /sōʹsē·olʹəjē/ [L, *socius* + Gk, *logos,* science], the study of group behavior within a society.

sociopath, *(Informal)* an individual with antisocial personality disorder.

sociopathic. See **psychopath.**

sociopathic personality. See **antisocial personality.**

sociopathy /sōʹsē·opʹəthē/ [L, *socius,* companion; Gk, *pathos,* disease], a personality disorder characterized by a lack of social responsibility and failure to adapt to ethical and social standards of the community.

sock aid, an adaptive device that enables people who cannot reach their feet to don a pair of socks or stockings. Also called **stocking aid.**

socket, the part of a prosthesis into which the stump of the remaining limb fits. Most modern prosthetic sockets are made of plastic, which is odorless, lighter, and easier to clean than traditional leather sockets. See also **acetabulum, acromion.**

soda [It, *sodo,* solid], a compound of sodium, particularly sodium bicarbonate or sodium carbonate.

soda lime (SL), a mixture of sodium and calcium hydroxides used to absorb exhaled carbon dioxide in an anesthesia rebreathing system. Soda-lime glass beads are used in air-fluidized beds.

sodium (Na) /sōʹdē·əm/ [soda + L, *ium*], a soft grayish metal of the alkaline metals group. Its atomic number is 11; its atomic mass is 22.99. Sodium is one of the most important elements in the body. Sodium ions are involved in acid-base balance, water balance, transmission of nerve impulses, and contraction of muscles. The recommended daily intake of sodium is 250 to 750 mg for infants 6 months to 1 year of age, 900 to 2700 mg for children 11 years of age or older, and 1100 to 3300 mg for adults. Sodium is an important component of more than 8 L of secretions produced by the body every day. These secretions include saliva, gastric and intestinal secretions, bile, and pancreatic fluid. The total daily secretion of sodium into these alimentary tract fluids averages between 1200 and 1400 mEq. A 154-pound adult has a total body pool of 2800 to 3000 mEq. It is also linked to chlorine, which is the most important extracellular anion in the body. Sodium is the chief electrolyte in interstitial fluid, and its interaction with potassium as the main intracellular electrolyte is critical to survival. A decrease in the sodium concentration of the interstitial fluid immediately decreases osmotic pressure, making it hypotonic to intracellular fluid osmotic pressure. The kidney is the chief regulator of sodium levels in body fluids and will excrete sodium-free urine when the body needs to conserve sodium. In high temperatures, such as those associated with fever, the body loses sodium through sweat, and sodium reserves are further diluted with additional water drunk by the affected individual. To prevent serious complications, depleted sodium must be replaced. Sodium salts, such as sodium bicarbonate, are widely used in medications. Sodium bicarbonate has an immediate and rapid antacid action on the stomach, but any excess rapidly enters the intestine so that the substance has a shorter action than that of other antacids. Sodium bicarbonate, which is very effective in rendering the urine alkaline, is an ingredient in many solutions used as douches, mouthwashes, and enemas. Sodium is also important in the transport of sodium and potassium ions through the cytoplasmic membrane.

sodium acid carbonate. See **sodium bicarbonate.**

sodium arsenite poisoning, a toxic condition caused by the ingestion of sodium arsenite, an insecticide and weed killer. The characteristic symptoms of arsenite poisoning are similar to those of arsenic poisoning, as is the treatment. See also **arsenic poisoning.**

S

sodium barbital, the sodium salt of 5,5-diethylbarbituric acid, a hypnotic and sedative drug.

sodium benzoate, an antifungal agent also used in a test of liver function.

sodium bicarbonate, a common salt (baking soda). Sodium is the most important cation in the extracellular fluid, and bicarbonate is the most import buffer in the body. Also called **sodium acid carbonate.**
- INDICATIONS: It is prescribed in the treatment of metabolic acidosis, gastric hyperacidity, and hyperkalemia to alkalinize the urine as part of the treatment for certain poisonings.
- CONTRAINDICATIONS: Alkalosis, hypernatremia, hypocalcemia, severe pulmonary edema, and abdominal pain of unknown cause prohibit its use. It should be administered in cardiac arrest only when there is documented metabolic acidosis of hyperkalemia.
- ADVERSE EFFECTS: Among the more serious adverse effects are tetany, gastric distension, acid rebound, bicarbonate-induced alkalosis, hypernatremia, hypocalcemia, and hypokalemia.

sodium channel blocking agent, any of a class of antiarrhythmic agents that prevent ectopic beats by acting on partially inactivated sodium channels to inhibit abnormal depolarizations. Also called *sodium channel blocker.*

sodium chloride, common table salt used in various concentrations as a fluid and electrolyte replenisher, isotonic vehicle, irrigating solution, and enema.

sodium chloride and dextrose. See **dextrose and sodium chloride injection.**

sodium citrate, a sodium salt of citric acid, used as an anticoagulant for blood or plasma that is to be fractionated or for blood that is to be stored. It is also administered orally as a urinary alkalizer.

sodium etidronate. See **etidronate disodium.**

sodium ferric gluconate, a hematinic used especially in treatment of hemodialysis patients with iron deficiency anemia who are also receiving erythropoietin therapy. It is administered by intravenous injection.

sodium fluoride poisoning, a chronic condition of fluorine poisoning that occurs in some communities where the fluorine concentration in the water supply exceeds 1 ppm. Signs of the condition include mottling of tooth enamel and severe osteosclerosis. Also called **fluorosis.**

sodium glutamate. See **monosodium glutamate.**

sodium hydroxide, NaOH, a strongly alkaline and caustic compound; used as an alkalizing agent in pharmaceuticals.

sodium hypochlorite solution, a 5% aqueous solution of NaOCl (common bleach) used as a disinfectant for utensils and surfaces not harmed by its bleaching action.

sodium iodide, an iodine supplement.
- INDICATIONS: It is prescribed in the treatment of thyrotoxic crisis and neonatal thyrotoxicosis and in the management of hyperthyroidism before thyroidectomy.
- CONTRAINDICATIONS: Hyperkalemia or known hypersensitivity to this drug prohibits its use.
- ADVERSE EFFECTS: Among the more serious adverse effects are salivary gland swelling, metallic taste, rashes, and GI disturbances. Acute poisoning may result in angioedema and pulmonary edema.

sodium lactate injection, an electrolyte replenisher that has been prescribed for metabolic acidosis.

sodium nitrite, an antidote for cyanide poisoning, also used as a preservative in cured meats and other foods.

sodium nitroprusside (SNP), a vasodilator.
- INDICATIONS: It is prescribed primarily in the emergency treatment of hypertensive crises and in heart failure.
- CONTRAINDICATIONS: Certain compensatory forms of hypertension, such as coarctation of the aorta or impaired cerebral circulation, or known hypersensitivity to the drug prohibits its use.
- ADVERSE EFFECTS: Among the most serious adverse effects are a rapid fall in blood pressure or symptoms of cyanide poisoning (cyanide is produced by the metabolism of nitroprusside). Muscle spasms also may occur.

sodium perborate, an oxygen-liberating antiseptic $(NaBO_2 \cdot H_2O_2 \cdot 3H_2O)$ that may be used in treating necrotizing ulcerative gingivitis and other kinds of gingival inflammation and in bleaching pulpless teeth. Prolonged or indiscriminate use of the compound may cause burns of the oral mucosa and blacken the tongue.

sodium phenobarbital. See **phenobarbital.**

sodium phenylbutyrate, an agent used as adjunctive treatment to control the hyperammonemia of pediatric urea cycle enzyme disorders.

sodium phosphate, a saline cathartic.
- INDICATIONS: It is prescribed to achieve prompt, thorough evacuation of the bowel and, in lower dosage, for laxative effect.
- CONTRAINDICATIONS: Congestive heart failure, abdominal pain, edema, megacolon, hypovolemia, salt-restricted diet, or hypersensitivity to this drug prohibits its use. Frequent administration in any dosage is not recommended.
- ADVERSE EFFECTS: Among the more severe adverse effects are dehydration, hypovolemia, abdominal cramping, and electrolyte imbalance.

sodium phosphate P32, an antineoplastic, antipolycythemic radioactive agent.
- INDICATIONS: It is prescribed for treatment of polycythemia vera; for neoplasms, including myelocytic leukemia; and for localizing tumors of the eye.
- CONTRAINDICATIONS: Polycythemia vera with leukopenia or decreased platelet count, chronic myelocytic leukemia with leukopenia or erythrocytopenia, concurrent administration of other alkylating agents, or hypersensitivity to this drug prohibits its use.
- ADVERSE EFFECTS: The most serious adverse effect is radiation sickness.

sodium phosphates, a combination of monobasic and dibasic sodium phosphates used as an electrolyte replenisher.

sodium-potassium pump, a mechanism by which sodium and potassium ions are transferred across a cell membrane by active transport controlled by a specialized plasma membrane protein. See also **calcium pump.**

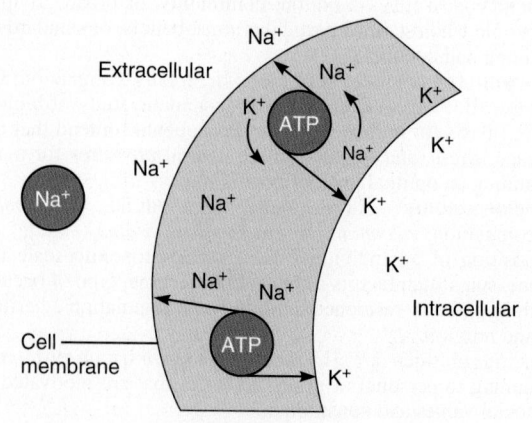

Sodium-potassium pump *(Lewis et al, 2011)*

sodium-restricted diet.   See **low-sodium diet.**

sodium sulfate,   a saline cathartic for chronic constipation caused by peristaltic disorders.

■ INDICATIONS: It is prescribed to achieve prompt, thorough evacuation of the bowel and, in lower dosage, for laxative effect.

■ CONTRAINDICATIONS: Congestive heart failure, hypovolemia, or hypersensitivity to this drug prohibits its use. Frequent administration, in any dosage, is not recommended.

■ ADVERSE EFFECTS: Among the more severe adverse effects are dehydration, hypovolemia, and electrolyte imbalance.

sodium sulfate anhydrous.   See **salt cake.**

sodium sulfide,   the monosulfide salt of sodium, Na_2S, a flammable, highly irritating compound having a variety of industrial uses.

sodoku.   See **rat-bite fever.**

sodomist /sod′əmist/ [Sodom, biblical city in ancient Palestine],   a person who practices sodomy. Also called *sodomite.*

sodomy /sod′əmē/ [Sodom, biblical city in ancient Palestine],   **1.** anal intercourse. **2.** intercourse with an animal. –*sodomize, v.*

soft chancre [AS, *softe* + Fr, *canker*],   a usually painless local genital ulcer that follows an infection by *Haemophilus ducreyi.* It is accompanied by suppuration of the inguinal lymphatic nodes, or inguinal buboes. Complications may include phimosis, urethral stricture or fistula, and marked tissue destruction. Also called **chancroid.**

soft contact lens (SCL) [AS, *softe* + L, *contingere* + *lens,* lentil],   a contact lens made of a flexible plastic material that can be shaped more easily to fit the eyeball than a rigid gas-permeable lens and that typically provides good initial comfort. Among the disadvantages of soft lenses are that they cannot correct all vision problems and that they may not provide vision as sharp as alternative methods. Most contact lens patients are currently being fit into hyperoxygen-permeable silicone-hydrogel soft lenses.

soft data [AS, *softe* + L, *datum,* something given],   health information that is mainly subjective, provided by the patient and the patient's family.

soft diet,   a diet that is soft in texture, low in residue, easily digested, and well tolerated. It provides the essential nutrients in the form of liquids and semisolid foods, such as milk; fruit juices; eggs; cheese; custards; tapioca and puddings; strained soups and vegetables; rice; ground beef and lamb; fowl; fish; mashed, boiled, or baked potatoes; wheat, corn, or rice cereals; and breads. Omitted are raw fruits and vegetables, coarse breads and cereals, rich desserts, strong spices, all fried foods, veal, pork, nuts, and raisins. It is commonly recommended for people who have GI disturbances or acute infections and those unable to tolerate a normal diet.

softening of bones /sô′fəning, sof′əning/ [AS, *softe* + *ban*],   (*Informal*) any disease that results in a loss of the mineral content of the bones. See also **osteomalacia.**

soft fibroma,   a benign tumor composed of fibrous or connective tissue containing many cells. Also called **fibroma molle.**

soft mechanical diet,   a diet containing ground or pureed foods that are easy to chew, often eaten by people who have dental problems or are edentulous. It can contain any foods allowed in a regular diet but in an easy to chew and swallow presentation. It is sometimes inappropriately referred to as a soft diet.

soft neurological sign,   a mild or slight neurological abnormality that is difficult to detect or interpret.

soft palate,   the structure composed of mucous membrane, muscular fibers, and mucous glands suspended from the posterior border of the hard palate forming the roof of the mouth. When the soft palate rises, as in swallowing and in sucking, it separates the nasal cavity and the nasopharynx from the posterior part of the oral cavity and the oral part of the pharynx. The posterior border of the soft palate hangs like a curtain between the mouth and the pharynx. Suspended from it is the conical, pendulous, palatine uvula. Arching laterally from the base of the uvula are the two curved musculomembranous pillars of the fauces. In dentistry, the soft palate serves as the anatomical landmark for construction of a maxillary full denture and establishment of a seal which helps retain the denture in the mouth. Compare **hard palate.** See **posterior palatal seal area.**

soft radiation,   a relatively long wavelength with less penetrating radiation than short wavelength radiation.

soft spot.   See **anterior fontanel.**

soft tissue rheumatism,   a category of disorders producing pain, swelling, or inflammation not caused by arthritis in the tissues and structures around a joint. See also **bursitis, capsulitis, enthesitis, fibromyalgia, myofascial pain, tendinitis,** and **tenosynovitis.**

software,   the programs that control a computer and cause it to perform specific functions. Compare **hardware.** See also **application.**

software bug.   See **bug.**

soft water [AS, *softe* + *waeter*],   water that does not contain salts of calcium or magnesium, which precipitate soap solutions.

sol,   a colloidal state in which a solid is suspended throughout a liquid, such as a soap or starch in water. The fluidity of cytoplasm depends on its sol/gel balance.

sol.,   abbreviation for **solution.**

-sol,   suffix meaning "a colloidal solution": *creosol, nitromersol, ioversol.*

Solanaceae /sō′lənā″si·ē/,   a family of plants that includes the genus *Solanum,* or nightshades, with more than 1800 species, including deadly nightshade (belladonna), henbane, tomatoes, and potatoes.

solanaceous /sō′lənā″shəs/,   pertaining to plants of the Solanaceae family or substances derived from them.

solanine /sō′lə·nēn/,   a steroidal alkaloid found in several species of *Solanum,* such as the nightshades and the green spots on potatoes. It causes hemolysis, central nervous system depression, and often fatal respiratory failure.

Solanum /sō·lā′nəm/ [L, nightshade],   a large genus of plants of the family Solanaceae. It includes the potato, tomato, eggplant, several of the nightshades, and many poisonous and medicinal species.

solar-,   combining form meaning "sun": *solarium.*

solar fever.   See **dengue fever, sunstroke.**

solarium /sōler″ē·əm/ [L, terrace exposed to sun],   a large, sunny room or area serving as a lounge for ambulatory patients in a hospital.

solar keratosis.   See **actinic keratosis.**

solar maculopathy.   See **eclipse scotoma.**

solar plexus /sō′lər/ [L, *sol,* sun, *plexus,* network],   a dense network of nerve fibers and ganglia that surrounds the roots of the celiac and the superior mesenteric arteries at the level of the first lumbar vertebra. It is one of the great autonomic plexuses of the body in which the nerve fibers of the sympathetic system and the parasympathetic system combine. The denser part of the solar plexus lies between the suprarenal glands, on the ventral surface of the crura of the diaphragm and on the abdominal aorta. Also called **celiac plexus.**

solar radiation,   the emission and diffusion of actinic rays from the sun. Overexposure may result in sunburn, keratosis,

S

skin cancer, accelerated aging, or lesions associated with photosensitivity.

solar retinopathy. See **eclipse scotoma.**

solar sneeze reflex [L, *sol,* sun; ME, *snesen* + L, *reflectere,* to bend back], a sneeze that may be caused by exposure to bright sunlight.

solar therapy [L, *sol,* sun; Gk, *therapeia,* treatment], the therapeutic use of sunlight. Also called **heliotherapy.**

solder /sod′ər/ [L, *solidatio,* making solid], **1.** *n.,* a fusible metal or alloy used to unite pieces of metals with higher fusion temperatures. **2.** *v.,* to fasten together pieces of metal through the use of this material.

sole [L, *solea,* sole of foot], the plantar surface of the foot.

soleus /sō″lē·əs/ [L, *solea,* sole of foot], one of three superficial posterior muscles of the leg. It is a broad, flat muscle lying just under the gastrocnemius. The fibers of the soleus merge near the middle of the leg with those of the gastrocnemius to form the tendo calcaneus, which inserts into the calcaneus of the foot. The soleus plantar flexes the foot. Compare **gastrocnemius, plantaris.**

soleus pump. See **calf muscle pump.**

Solganal, a gold salt antirheumatic. Brand name for **aurothioglucose.**

solid /sol′id/ [L, *solidus*], **1.** *n.,* a dense body, figure, structure, or substance that has length, breadth, and thickness, is not a liquid or a gas, contains no significant cavity or hollowness, and has no breaks or openings on its surface. **2.** *adj.,* describing such a body, figure, structure, or substance.

solifenacin, an anticholinergic.

■ INDICATIONS: This drug is used to treat overactive bladder.

■ CONTRAINDICATIONS: Uncontrolled narrow-angle glaucoma, urinary retention, gastric retention, and known hypersensitivity to this drug prohibit its use.

■ ADVERSE EFFECTS: Adverse effects of this drug include anxiety, paresthesia, fatigue, headache, chest pain, hypertension, abdominal pain, dry mouth, dyspepsia, dysuria, urinary retention and frequency, urinary tract infection, rash, pruritus, bronchitis, cough, pharyngitis, and upper respiratory tract infection. Common side effects include dizziness, vision abnormalities, xerophthalmia, nausea, vomiting, anorexia, and constipation.

Soliris, a humanized monoclonal antibody. Brand name for **eculizumab.**

solitary coin lesion /sol″iter′ē/ [L, *solitarius,* standing alone, *cuneus,* wedge, *laesus,* injury], a nodule identified on a chest radiographic image by clear normal lung tissue surrounding it. A coin lesion is often malignant.

solitary play, a form of play among a group of children within the same room or area in which each child engages in an independent activity using toys that are different from the toys of the others, concentrating solely on the particular activity and showing no interest in joining in or interfering with the play of others. Compare **cooperative play.** See also **associative play, parallel play.**

soln, abbreviation for **solution.**

solubility /sol′yəbil″itē/ [L, *solubilis,* able to dissolve], **1.** the maximum amount of a solute that can dissolve in a specific solvent under a given temperature and pressure. **2.** the concentration of a solute in a solvent at its saturation point. −*soluble, adj.*

solubility coefficient. See **coefficient.**

-soluble, combining form meaning "able to be dissolved": *insoluble, liposoluble.*

soluble amyloid beta protein precursor test, a test for a decrease in levels of beta amyloid in cerebrospinal fluid, used in the diagnosis of Alzheimer disease and other forms of senile dementia.

Solu-Cortef, a glucocorticoid. Brand name for **hydrocortisone sodium succinate.**

Solu-Medrol, a glucocorticoid. Brand name for *methylprednisolone sodium succinate.*

solute /sol″yŏŏt, sō″lŏŏt/ [L, *solutus,* dissolved], a substance dissolved in a solvent.

solution (sol., soln) /səlŏŏ′shən/ [L, *solutus*], a mixture of one or more substances dissolved in another substance. The molecules of each of the substances disperse homogenously and do not change chemically. A solution may be a gas, a liquid, or a solid. Compare **colloid, suspension.** See also **solute, solvent.**

-solve, combining form meaning "to loosen": *dissolve.*

solvent /sol′vənt/ [L, *solvere,* to dissolve], **1.** any liquid in which another substance can be dissolved. **2.** *(Informal)* an organic liquid, such as benzene, carbon tetrachloride, and other volatile petroleum distillates, that when inhaled can cause intoxication as well as damage to mucous membranes of the nose and throat and the tissues of the kidney, liver, and brain. Repeated, prolonged exposure can result in addiction, brain damage, blindness, and other serious consequences, some of them fatal. See also **benzene poisoning, carbon tetrachloride, glue sniffing, petroleum distillate poisoning.**

som-, prefix for growth hormone derivatives: *somatotropin.*

soma /sō″mə/ *pl. somas, somata* [Gk, body], **1.** the body, as distinguished from the mind or psyche. **2.** the body, excluding germ cells. **3.** the body of a cell. −*somal,* **somatic,** *adj.*

Soma, a skeletal muscle relaxant. Brand name for **carisoprodol.**

soma-. See **somato-, soma-.**

somal, somas, somata. See **soma.**

-soma, -somus, combining form meaning "a body" or "part of a body": *asoma, hemisomus.*

-somatia, -somatic, combining form meaning "body": *diplosomatia, psychsomatic.*

somatic. See **psychosomatic, soma.**

-somatic. See **-somatia, -somatic.**

somatic cavity. See **coelom.**

somatic cell /sōmat′ik/, any of the cells of body tissue that have the diploid number of chromosomes, as distinguished from germ cells, which contain the haploid number. Compare **germ cell.**

somatic-cell gene therapy. See **gene therapy.**

somatic chromosome, any autosome in a diploid or somatic cell.

somatic delusion, a false notion or belief concerning body image or body function. See also **delusion.**

somatic effects, radiation effects such as cancer that occur in the exposed individual, as opposed to genetic effects, which occur in the individual's offspring.

somatic mutation [Gk, *soma,* body; L, *mutare,* to change], a sudden change in the chromosomal material in somatic cell nuclei affecting derived cells but not offspring.

somatic pain, generally well-localized pain that results from the activation of peripheral nociceptors without injury to the peripheral nerve or central nervous system.

somatic therapy, a form of treatment pertaining to the body that affects one's physiological functioning.

somatist /sō″mətist/, a psychotherapist or other health professional who believes that every neurosis and psychosis has an organic cause.

somatization /sō″mətīzā″shən/ [Gk, *soma,* body], a process whereby a mental event is expressed in a body disorder or physical symptom. Kinds include **peptic ulcer, asthma.** See also **conversion.**

somatization disorder [Gk, *soma* + *izein*, to cause], a psychiatric disorder characterized by recurrent multiple physical complaints and symptoms for which there is no organic cause. The condition typically begins in adolescence or in the early adult years and is less common in men. The symptoms vary according to the individual and the underlying emotional conflict. Some common symptoms are GI dysfunction, paralysis, temporary blindness, cardiopulmonary distress, painful or irregular menstruation, sexual indifference, and pain during intercourse. Hypochondriasis may develop if the condition is untreated. Also called **Briquet syndrome.** See also **conversion disorder.**

somatodyspraxia /-disprak″sē·ə/, inadequate processing of tactile, proprioceptive, and kinesthetic information that causes difficulty in motor planning.

somatoform disorder /sōmat″əfôrm, sō″mətōfôrm′/ [Gk, *soma* + L, *forma,* form], any of a group of disorders characterized by symptoms suggesting physical illness or disease for which there are no demonstrable organic causes or physiological dysfunctions. The symptoms are usually the physical manifestations of some unresolved intrapsychic factor or conflict. Kinds include **conversion disorder, hypochondriasis, psychogenic pain disorder, somatization disorder.**

somatogenesis /sō″matəjen″əsis/ [Gk, *soma* + *genein,* to produce], **1.** in embryology, the development of the body from the germ plasm. **2.** the development of a physical disease or symptoms from an organic pathophysiological cause. Compare **psychogenesis.** −*somatogenic, somatogenetic, adj.*

somatoliberin. See **growth hormone–releasing hormone.**

somatomedin. See **growth hormone.**

somatomedin C. See **insulin-like growth factor.**

somatomedin-C test, a blood test most commonly used to detect levels of somatomedin-C, also called insulin-like growth factor. Screening for somatomedin-C provides an accurate reflection of the mean plasma concentration of growth hormone.

somatomegaly /sō″matōmeg″əlē/ [Gk, *soma* + *megas,* large], a condition in which the body is abnormally large as a result of an excessive secretion of somatotropin or an inadequate secretion of somatostatin.

somatoplasm /sō″mətōplaz″əm/ [Gk, *soma* + *plasma,* something formed], the nonreproductive protoplasmic material of the body cells, as distinguished from the reproductive material of the germ cells. Compare **germ plasm.**

somatopleure /sō″mətōploor′/ [Gk, *soma* + *pleura,* side], the lateral and ventral tissue layer that forms the body wall of the early developing embryo. Consisting of an outer layer of ectoderm lined with somatic mesoderm, it continues as the amnion and chorion external to the embryo. Compare **splanchnopleure.** −*somatopleural, adj.*

somatosensory evoked potential (SEP) /-sen″sərē/ [Gk, *soma* + L, *sentire,* to feel], evoked potential elicited by repeated stimulation of the pain and touch systems. It is the least reliable of the evoked potentials studied as monitors of neurological function during surgery.

somatosensory system, the components of the central and peripheral nervous systems that receive and interpret sensory information from organs in the joints, ligaments, muscles, and skin. This system processes information about the length, degree of stretch, tension, and contraction of muscles; pain; temperature; pressure; and joint position.

somato-, soma-, combining form meaning "body": *somatist, somatization.*

somatosplanchnic /-splangk″nik/ [Gk, *soma* + *splanchna,* viscera], pertaining to the trunk of the body and the viscera.

somatostatin /sō′matōstat″in/, a hormone produced in the hypothalamus that inhibits the release of somatotropin (growth hormone) from the anterior pituitary gland. It also is produced in other parts of the body and inhibits the release of certain other hormones, including thyrotropin, adrenocorticotropic hormone, glucagon, insulin, and cholecystokinin, and of some enzymes, including pepsin, renin, secretin, and gastrin. Also called **growth hormone release inhibiting hormone.**

somatotherapy /-ther′əpē/, the treatment of mental illness using physical modalities (for example, medications or electroconvulsive therapy), as distinguished from psychotherapy.

somatotropic /-trop′ik/ [Gk, *soma,* body, *trope,* a turn], pertaining to an agent that influences the body or body cells.

somatotropic hormone, somatotropin. See **growth hormone.**

somatotropin-releasing hormone. See **growth hormone–releasing hormone.**

somatotype /sō″mətōtīp′/ [Gk, *soma* + *typos,* mark], **1.** body build or physique. **2.** the classification of individuals according to body build on the basis of certain physical characteristics. Kinds include **ectomorph, endomorph, mesomorph.**

somatovisceral reflex /-vis″ərəl/, a reflex in which visceral functions are activated or inhibited by somatic sensory stimulation.

somatrem /sō′mətrem/, a synthetic polypeptide growth hormone produced by recombinant deoxyribonucleic acid technology.

■ INDICATIONS: It is prescribed for growth promotion when patients are not growing because of limited endogenous growth hormone secretion. It is also used to limit cachexia in AIDS patients undergoing antiretroviral treatment and as replacement therapy in adults with documented growth hormone deficiency.

■ CONTRAINDICATIONS: It is contraindicated for pediatric patients with closed epiphyses and for patients with evidence of underlying intracranial lesions, widespread trauma/multiple organ failure, or malignancy. Concurrent use with a glucocorticoid may inhibit the effects of somatrem.

■ ADVERSE EFFECTS: Among reported adverse effects are insulin resistance and hypothyroidism. The adverse effects of somatrem tend to vary with the underlying indication for its use.

Somatuline Depot, a somatostatin analog used in the treatment of acromegaly. Brand name for **lanreotide.**

Somavert, a growth hormone receptor antagonist. Brand name for *pegvisomant.*

-some, combining form meaning "a body" of a specified sort: *chromosome, microsome, neurosome.*

-somia, combining form meaning "(condition of) possessing body": *agenosomia, celosomia, microsomia.*

somite /sō″mīt/ [Gk, *soma,* body], any of the paired segmented masses of mesodermal tissue that form along the length of the neural tube during the early stage of embryonic development in vertebrates. These structures give rise to the vertebrae and differentiate into various tissues of the body, including the voluntary muscle, bones, connective tissue, and dermal layers of the skin. The first somite to appear is in the future occipital region, and the formation of new somites continues in a caudal direction until 36 to 38 have developed.

somite embryo, an embryo in any stage of development between the formation of the first and the last pairs of somites, which in humans occurs in the third and fourth weeks after fertilization of the ovum.

somn-. See **somni-, somn-.**

somnambulism /somnam″byəliz′əm/ [L, *somnus,* sleep, *ambulare,* to walk], **1.** a condition occurring during stage

3 or 4 of nonrapid eye movement sleep that is characterized by complex motor activity, usually culminating in leaving the bed and walking about. The person has no recall of the episode on awakening. The episodes, which usually last from several minutes to half an hour or longer, are seen primarily in children, are more common in boys than in girls, and are more likely to occur if the individual is fatigued or under stress or has taken a sedative or hypnotic medication at bedtime. Seizure disorders, central nervous system infections, and trauma may be predisposing factors, but the condition is more commonly related to anxiety. In adults, the condition is less common and is classified as a dissociative reaction. Also called **noctambulation, sleepwalking,** *somnambulance.* **2.** a hypnotic state in which the person has full possession of the senses but no recollection of the episode. See also **fugue.**

somni-, somn-, prefix meaning "sleep": *somnolent, somnambulism.*

-somnia, suffix meaning "(condition of or like) sleep": *hypersomnia, insomnia.*

somniloquence /somnil″əkwəns/, talking during sleep or under hypnosis.

somnolent /som′nələnt/ [L, *somnolentia,* sleepy], **1.** the condition of being sleepy or drowsy. **2.** tending to cause sleepiness. –*somnolence, n.*

somnolent detachment, (in psychology) a term introduced by H.S. Sullivan for a type of security operation in which a person falls asleep when confronted by a highly threatening, anxiety-producing experience. The mechanism originates in infancy.

Somogyi effect (phenomenon) [Michael Somogyi, American biochemist, 1883–1971; Gk, *phainomenon*], a diabetes mellitus rebound effect in which an overdose of insulin induces hypoglycemia. This releases hormones that stimulate lipolysis, gluconeogenesis, and glycogenolysis, leading to hyperglycemia and ketosis. Treatment involves gradually lowering the insulin dose to achieve an optimal level.

-somus. See **-soma, -somus.**

son-, prefix meaning "sound": *sonorant.*

Sonata /so-nah′tah/, a drug used to treat insomnia. Brand name for **zaleplon.**

sonic scaler, in dentistry, an electromagnetic or compressed air-driven mechanized instrument used to remove calculus, bacterial biofilms, and root surface accretions. Various sized and shaped tips may be placed into the handpiece in order to reach various areas of the tooth and root surface. Compare **ultrasonic scaler.**

sonogram /son′o-gram/, a record, image, or display obtained by ultrasonic scanning. See also **ultrasound.**

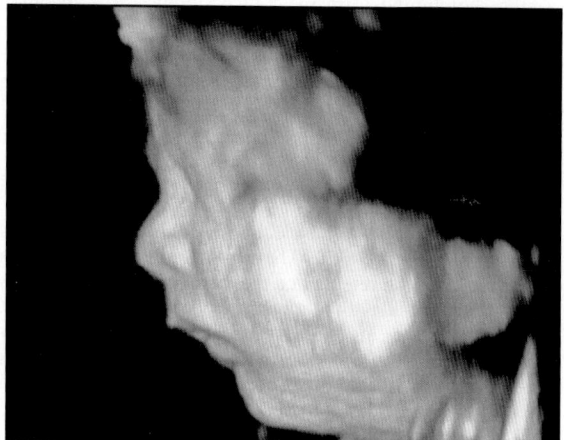

3D sonogram *(Courtesy Dr. Marie O'Toole)*

sonogram imaging, the use of high-frequency sound waves to view structures, tissues, and organs within the body; during pregnancy, the fetus can be viewed using this method. An image is produced when the waves are reflected off the tissues. Also called **ultrasound.**

sonographer /sōnog′rəfər/, an allied health professional with special training in the use of ultrasound equipment for diagnostic and therapeutic purposes. Also called **diagnostic medical sonographer, medical sonographer, ultrasonographer.**

sonography. See **ultrasonography.**

sonorant. See **voiced.**

soot wart. *(Informal)* See **scrotal cancer.**

sopor /sō′pər/ [L, deep sleep], a sleep that is as deep or sound as the state of stupor.

soporiferous /sop′ərif″ərəs/ [L *sopor,* deep sleep, *ferre,* to bear], tending to cause deep sleep, such as an agent that induces deep sleep.

soporific /sop′ərif″ik/ [L, *sopor,* deep sleep, *facere,* to make], **1.** *adj.,* pertaining to a substance, condition, or procedure that causes sleep. **2.** *n.,* a soporific drug. See also **hypnotic, sedative.**

sorafenib, a miscellaneous antineoplastic.

■ INDICATIONS: This drug is used to treat advanced and metastatic murine renal cell carcinoma.

■ CONTRAINDICATIONS: Pregnancy and known hypersensitivity to this drug prohibit its use.

■ ADVERSE EFFECTS: Adverse effects of this drug include fatigue, weight loss, headache, anorexia, mouth ulceration, abdominal pain, constipation, pruritus, erythema, hand-foot rash, acne, flushing, and alopecia. Life-threatening side effects include hypertension, cardiac ischemia, infarction, pancreatitis, hemorrhage, leukopenia, lymphopenia, anemia, neutropenia, thrombocytopenia, and exfoliative dermatitis. Common side effects include nausea, diarrhea, vomiting, dry skin, hypophosphatemia, arthralgia, myalgia, and hoarseness.

sorbent /sôr′bənt/ [L, *sorbere,* to swallow], **1.** *n.,* an agent that attracts and retains substances by absorption or adsorption. **2.** *adj.,* the property of a substance that allows it to interact with another compound, usually to make it bind.

sorbic acid /sôr″bik/, a compound occurring naturally in berries of the mountain ash. Commercial sorbic acid derived from acetaldehyde is used in fungicides, food preservatives, lubricants, and plasticizers.

Sorbitrate, an antianginal. Brand name for **isosorbide dinitrate.**

sordes /sôr″dēz/ *pl. sordes* [L, *sordere,* to be dirty], dirt or debris, especially the crusts consisting of food, microorganisms, and epithelial cells that accumulate on teeth and lips during a febrile illness or one in which the patient takes nothing by mouth. Sordes gastricae is undigested food and mucus in the stomach.

sore /sôr, sōr/ [AS, *sar*], **1.** *n.,* a wound, ulcer, or lesion. **2.** *adj.,* tender or painful.

sore throat [AS, *sar* + *throte*], any inflammation of the larynx, pharynx, or tonsils.

Sorrin operation, a surgical technique for treating a periodontal abscess, used especially when the marginal gingiva appears healthy and provides no access to the abscess. A semilunar incision is made below the abscess area in the attached gingiva, leaving the gingival margin undisturbed. The tissue flap produced by the incision is raised, accessing the abscessed area for curettage, after which the wound is sutured.

s.o.s., a notation for a Latin phrase meaning "if necessary." Abbreviation for *si opus sit.*

sotalol /so'tah-lol/, a noncardioselective beta-adrenergic blocking agent, used as the hydrochloride salt in treatment of life-threatening ventricular arrhythmias.

Soto syndrome. See **cerebral gigantism.**

souffle /soo″fəl/ [Fr, breath], a soft murmur heard through a stethoscope. When detected over the uterus in a pregnant woman, it is usually coincident with the maternal pulse and is caused by blood circulating in the large uterine arteries.

soul food [AS, *sawel* + *foda*], an American cuisine typically associated with African-Americans of the southern United States.

sound [L, *sub,* under, *unde,* wave], an emission detected by an instrument used to locate the opening of a cavity or canal, to test the patency of a canal, to ascertain the depth of a cavity, or to reveal the contents of a canal or cavity. A sound is used to determine the depth of the uterus, to detect stones in the bladder, and, less commonly, to assist in correctly inserting a urinary catheter in the urethra through the urinary meatus.

sounds of Korotkoff. See **blood pressure.**

sound waves, longitudinal waves of mechanical energy that transmit the vibrations interpreted as sound.

Souques sign /sooks/ [Alexandre A. Souques, French neurologist, 1860–1944], in patients with a disease of the corpus striatum, the failure of a seated patient to extend the legs when the chair is pushed backward. The legs normally would be extended to prevent overbalancing. Also called *Souques phenomenon.*

source-to-image-receptor distance (SID) /sôrs, sōrs/ [OFr, *sourse,* origin; L, *imago,* likeness], the distance between the focal spot on the target of an x-ray tube and the image receptor as measured along the beam.

South African genetic porphyria. See **variegate porphyria.**

South American blastomycosis. See **paracoccidioidomycosis.**

South American trypanosomiasis. See **Chagas disease.**

Southern blot test /suth′ərn/, a gene analysis method used in identification of specific deoxyribonucleic acid (DNA) fragments and in diagnosis of cancers and hemoglobinopathies. It involves the placement of a nitrocellulose film on agarose gel surfaces, with dry blotting material on the film. Liquid is then transported from a reservoir beneath the gel through the gel and nitrocellulose layer. The film adsorbs the DNA fragments. The fragments are then analyzed for rearrangements in immunoglobulin or cell receptor genes, chromosomal translocations, oncogene amplifications, and point mutations within oncogenes. Immunoglobulins and T cell receptor genes bear signatures that identify various leukemias and lymphomas. See also **Northern blot test.**

Sp, sp., spp., abbreviation for **species.**

SPA, abbreviation for **sperm penetration assay.**

space [L, *spatium*], an area, region, or segment of the body, such as the complemental spaces in the pleural cavity that are not occupied by lung tissue and the lymph spaces occupied by lymph.

space adaptation syndrome, the ability to accommodate changes in cardiac function, bone mineral changes, and muscle atrophy while in the weightless state of a space traveler.

space maintainer, a fixed or removable appliance for preserving the space created by the premature loss of one or more teeth. It can be unilateral or bilateral. Kinds include *band-loop, crown-loop, lingual arch.*

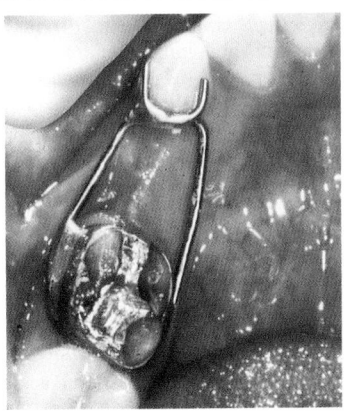

Space maintainer *(Bird and Robinson, 2005)*

space medicine, a branch of medicine concerned with the effects of travel in space, beyond the atmosphere and pull of gravity, including weightlessness, motion sickness, and restricted physical activity.

space obtainer, an appliance for increasing the space between adjoining teeth.

spacer /spās′ər/ [L, *spatium,* space], on a metered dose inhaler, a chamber between the inhaler canister and the patient's mouth where droplets of medication can slow down and evaporate so that there is less direct impact on the oropharynx, with more medication delivered to the lower respiratory tract instead of being lost in the mouth. This is especially helpful for children. See also **metered dose inhaler.**

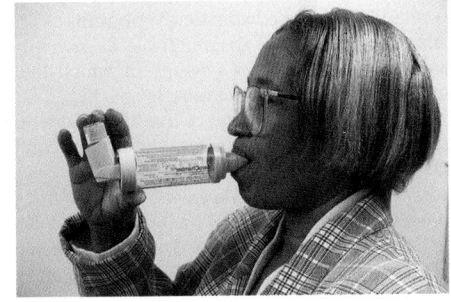

Metered dose inhaler with spacer *(Potter et al, 2011)*

space regainer, a fixed or removable appliance for moving a displaced secondary tooth into its normal position in a dental arch.

space sickness. See **air sickness.**

Spanish fly. See **cantharis.**

spano-, combining form meaning "scanty" or "scarce."

sparfloxacin, an antiinfective.

■ INDICATIONS: It is used to treat community-acquired pneumonia and chronic bronchitis caused by *Klebsiella pneumoniae, Haemophilus influenzae, H. parainfluenzae,* and *Moraxella catarrhalis.*

■ CONTRAINDICATIONS: Known hypersensitivity to quinolones and photosensitivity prohibit its use.

■ ADVERSE EFFECTS: Life-threatening effects are leukopenia and pseudomembranous colitis. Other adverse effects are eosinophilia, anemia, flatulence, diarrhea, QT interval prolongation, vasodilation, rash, pruritus, and photosensitivity.

Common side effects are headache, dizziness, insomnia, nausea, vomiting, and abdominal pain.

sparganosis /spär'gənō"sis/ [Gk, *sparganon,* swaddling clothes, *osis,* condition], a rare infection with larvae of the fish tapeworm of the pseudogenus Sparganum. It is characterized by painful subcutaneous swellings or swelling and destruction of the eye. It is acquired by ingesting larvae in contaminated water or in inadequately cooked infected frog flesh. Treatment includes surgery and local injection of ethyl alcohol to kill the larvae.

Sparine, a phenothiazine antipsychotic and antiemetic. Brand name for *promazine hydrochloride.*

spasm /spaz"əm/ [Gk, *spasmos*], **1.** an involuntary muscle contraction of sudden onset, such as habit spasms, hiccups, stuttering, or a tic. **2.** a convulsion or seizure. **3.** a sudden transient constriction of a blood vessel, bronchus, esophagus, pylorus, ureter, or other hollow organ. Compare **stricture.** See also **bronchospasm, pylorospasm.**

-spasm, suffix meaning "twitching or involuntary contraction" of a specified sort: *blepharospasm, laryngospasm, vasospasm.*

spasmatic croup. See **laryngismus stridulus.**

spasmo-, prefix meaning "spasms": *spasmogen.*

-spasmodic, -spasmodical, combining form meaning "convulsion": *antispasmodic.*

spasmodic asthma /spazmäd'ik/ [Gk, *spasmos + asthma,* panting], an airway obstruction caused by spasms of the bronchioles and inflammation of the bronchial mucosa and characterized by paroxysms of wheezing and coughing.

spasmodic croup. See **laryngismus stridulus.**

spasmodic dysmenorrhea /spazmod"ik/, difficult menstruation accompanied by painful contractions of the uterus.

spasmodic dysphonia [Gk, *spasmodes,* spasms, *dys,* bad, *phone,* voice], a speech disorder in which phonation is intermittently blocked by spasms of the larynx. The cause can be organic. Also called **spastic dysphonia.**

spasmodic stricture [Gk, *spasmodes + L, strictura,* compression], a narrowing of a passage in which there is no organic change but intermittent muscle spasms.

spasmodic tic [Gk, *spasmodes + Fr, tic*], any repetitive movement in which irregular muscle group contractions occur at variable intervals.

spasmodic torticollis [Gk, *spasmodes + L, tortus,* twisted, *collum,* neck], a condition in which the head is inclined to one side as a result of episodes of spasms of the neck muscles. It is often transient, and examination seldom reveals a physical cause. In some cases, it may be brought on by severe stress.

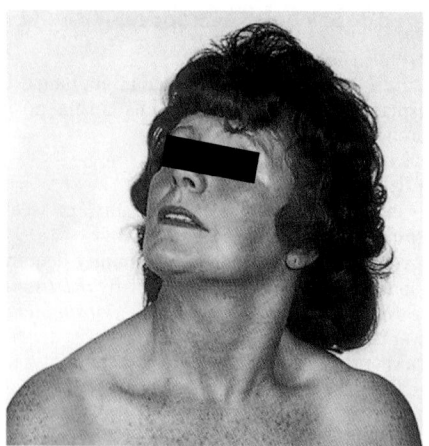

Spasmodic torticollis: characteristic head posture
(Perkin et al, 2011)

spasmogen /spaz"məjən/, any substance that can produce smooth muscle contractions, as in the bronchioles. Kinds include **histamine, bradykinin, serotonin.**

spastic /spas'tik/ [Gk, *spastikos,* drawing in], pertaining to spasms or other uncontrolled contractions of the skeletal muscles. See also **cerebral palsy. –spasticity,** *n.*

spastic aphonia, a condition in which a person is unable to speak because of spasmodic contraction of the abductor muscles of the throat. See also **aphonia.**

spastic bladder, a form of neurogenic bladder caused by conditions affecting sensory and motor neurons in the spinal cord above the voiding reflex center. It is marked by loss of bladder control and bladder sensation; incontinence; and automatic, interrupted, incomplete voiding. Also called **automatic bladder, reflex bladder.** Compare **flaccid bladder.**

spastic colon. See **irritable bowel syndrome.**

spastic constipation [Gk, *spasmos,* spasm; L, *constipare,* to crowd together], a form of constipation associated with neurasthenia and constrictive spasms in part of the intestine. The condition may be a sign of lead poisoning.

spastic diplegia, paralysis of corresponding parts on both sides of the body. See also **cerebral palsy.**

spastic dysarthria, a type of motor speech disorder affecting speech articulation, caused by lesions of the corticobulbar tracts. It affects strength, speed, precision, range of motion, and coordination of speech musculature movements.

spastic dysphonia. See **spasmodic dysphonia.**

spastic dysuria, difficulty in urination caused by involuntary muscular spasms of the bladder.

spastic entropion, entropion that arises from excessive contracture of the orbicularis oculi muscle. See also **entropion.**

spastic gait [Gk, *spasmos,* spasm; ONorse, *gata*], a pattern of walking in which the legs are stiff, the feet are plantarflexed, and movements are made by circumduction. The steps also may be accompanied by toe dragging.

spastic hemiplegia, paralysis of one side of the body with increased tendon reflexes and uncontrolled contraction occurring in the affected muscles.

spastic ileus [Gk, *spasmos,* spasm, *eilein,* to twist], a form of intestinal obstruction caused by sustained, irregular circular musculature contractions in a segment of bowel.

spasticity /spastis'itē/ [Gk, *spastikos,* drawing in], a form of muscular hypertonicity with increased resistance to stretch. It usually involves the flexors of the arms and the extensors of the legs. The hypertonicity is often associated with weakness, increased deep reflexes, and diminished superficial reflexes. Moderate spasticity is characterized by movements that require great effort and lack of normal coordination. Slight spasticity may be marked by gross movements that are coordinated smoothly but combine selective movement patterns that are uncoordinated or impossible.

spastic paralysis, an abnormal condition characterized by the involuntary contraction of one or more muscles with associated loss of muscular function. Compare **flaccid paralysis.**

spastic paraplegia [Gk, *spasmos,* spasm, *para + plege,* stroke], a form of partial paralysis mainly affecting older people. It is accompanied by irritability and spastic contractions of the leg muscles.

spastic primary paraplegia. See **primary lateral sclerosis.**

spastic pseudoparalysis, spastic pseudosclerosis. See **Creutzfeldt-Jakob disease.**

spastic strabismus [Gk, *spasmos + strabismos,* squint], squint caused by spasmodic contractions of ocular muscles.

spatial dance /spā′shəl/ [L, *spatium,* space; ME, *dauncen,* to drag along], the body shifts or movements used by individuals as they try to adjust the distance between themselves and other individuals. See also **spatial zones.**

spatial relationships, **1.** orientation in space; the ability to locate objects in the three-dimensional external world by using visual or tactile recognition and to make a spatial analysis of the observed information. Spatial orientation normally is a function of the right hemisphere of the brain. **2.** the relative locations of staff and equipment in an operating room with particular emphasis on what is sterile, clean, or contaminated. The operating room nurse must maintain an awareness of the arrangement of people and the proximity of sterile to nonsterile areas.

spatial resolution, the ability of an imaging system to discriminate between two adjacent objects.

spatial summation. See **summation,** def. 2.

spatial zones, the areas of personal space in which most people interact. Four basic spatial zones are the intimate zone, in which distance between individuals is less than 18 inches; the personal zone, between 18 inches and 4 feet; the social zone, extending between 4 and 12 feet; and the public zone, beyond 12 feet. See also **proxemics.**

spatula /spach′ə·lə/ [L], **1.** a flat, blunt, usually flexible instrument used for spreading plasters and for mixing ointments, cements, impression materials, and masses. **2.** a structure having a flat, blunt end.

SPCA, factor VII, one of the coagulation factors. Initialism for *serum prothrombin conversion accelerator.*

SPE, abbreviation for **sucrose polyester.**

speaking valve, a one-way valve placed on the end of a cuffless, deflated tracheostomy tube to facilitate normal speech. See **Passy-Muir valve.**

Spearman's rho /spir″mənz rō″/ [Charles E. Spearman, English psychologist, 1863–1945; *rho,* 17th letter in the Greek alphabet], a statistical test for correlation between two rank-ordered scales. It yields a statement of the degree of interdependence of the scores of the two scales.

special care unit /spesh′əl/ [L, *specialis,* individual], a hospital unit with the necessary specialized equipment and personnel for handling critically ill or injured patients, such as a neonatal, burn unit, or cardiac care unit.

special gene system, a plasmid, transposon, or other DNA fragment that is able to transfer genetic information from one cell to another.

specialing /spesh′əling/, **1.** *(Informal)* (in psychiatric nursing) the constant attendance of a professional staff member on a disturbed patient to protect the patient from harming the self or others and to observe the patient's behavior. The patient so cared for is accompanied in all activities by the staff member. **2.** (in nursing) the giving of nursing care to only one person, such as that given by a private-duty nurse or a nurse caring for a patient whose needs are so great that the nurse is required at all times.

specialist /spesh′əlist/, a health care professional who practices a specialty. A specialist usually has advanced clinical training and may have a postgraduate academic degree.

specialist in blood bank technology. See **blood bank technology specialist.**

special sense, the sense of sight, smell, taste, touch, or hearing.

specialty /spesh′əltē/ [L, *specialis*], a branch of health care in which the professional is specially qualified to practice by having attended an advanced program of study, passed an examination given by an organization of the members of the specialty, or gained experience through extensive practice in the specialty.

specialty care, focused health care services provided by a specialist.

species (Sp) /spē″sēz, spē″shēz/ *pl. species (sp., spp.)* [L, form], the category of living things below genus in rank. A species is a genetically distinct group of demes that share a common gene pool and are reproductively isolated from all other such groups. See also **deme, genus.**

species immunity, a form of natural immunity shared by all members of a species. Compare **individual immunity.**

species-specific [L, *specere,* to see, *facere,* to make], **1.** characteristic of a particular species. **2.** having a characteristic effect on, or interaction with, cells, tissues, or membranes of a particular species, said of an antigen, drug, or infective agent.

species-specific antigen, an antigen that is restricted to a single species but occurs in all members of that species.

species specificity. See **specificity.**

specific absorption rate (SAR) /spisif′ik/ [L, *species,* form], (in hyperthermia treatment) the rate of absorption of heat energy (W) per unit mass of tissue in units of watts per kilogram (W/kg).

specific activity, **1.** the radioactivity of a radioisotope per unit mass of the element or compound, expressed in microcuries per millimole or disintegrations per second per milligram. **2.** the relative radioactivity per unit mass, expressed as counts per minute per milligram. For example, the specific activity of potassium in the human body is the same as that in the environment or diet. Because potassium is associated chiefly with muscle tissue, a whole-body count of 40K, after administration of radioactive potassium, can be used to distinguish lean body mass from total body mass.

specific disease, a disorder caused by a special pathogenic organism.

specific granule, a secondary granule in the cytoplasm of polymorphonuclear leukocytes that contains lysozyme, vitamin B_{12}-binding protein, neutral proteases, and lactoferrin.

specific granule deficiency, an immunodeficiency state associated with pyodermas and abscesses in which neutrophils fail to make specific granules. See also **specific granule.**

specific gravity (sp. gr.), the ratio of the density of a substance to the density of another substance accepted as a standard. The usual standard for liquids and solids is water. Thus a liquid or solid with a specific gravity of 4 is four times as dense as water at the same temperature. Hydrogen is the usual standard for gases. See also **density, mass.**

specific immunoglobulin, a preparation obtained from human plasma that is preselected for its high antibody count against a specific pathogen, such as varicella zoster virus.

specificity /spes′əfis″itē/ [L, *species,* form, *facere,* to make], the quality of being distinctive. Kinds include **group specificity, species specificity, type specificity.** See also **diagnostic specificity.**

specificity of association, the uniqueness of a relationship between a causal factor and the occurrence of a disease.

specific mental functions, factors that refer to higher-level cognition, attention, memory, perception, thought, emotion, experience of self and time, and mental functions that regulate the speed, response, quality, and time of motor production.

specific rates, statistical rates in which the events in both the numerator and the denominator are restricted to a specific subgroup of a population.

specific treatment. See **treatment.**

specific ulcer [L, *species + facere,* to make, *ilcus*], ulcer associated with a specific disease, as a syphilitic ulcer.

specific viscosity [L, *species + facere,* to make, *viscosus,* sticky], the internal friction of a fluid, which may be

S

measured by comparing the rate of flow of the fluid through a tube with the rate of a standard liquid under standard conditions.

specimen /spes″imən/ *pl.* **specimens** [L, *specere,* to look], a small sample of something intended to show the nature of the whole, such as a urine specimen.

specimens. See **specimen.**

speckled dystrophy of the cornea /spek″əlt/, a familial condition characterized by irregular mottling of the cornea by spots that vary in shape and size, some with clear centers and sharp margins.

speckled pattern, an immunofluorescence pattern produced when serum from a patient with a particular connective tissue disease is placed in contact with human epithelial cells and stained with fluorochrome-labeled animal antisera. Fine, coarse, or large speckles are observed in disorders such as lupus erythematosus and rheumatoid arthritis.

SPECT, abbreviation for **single-photon emission computed tomography.**

SPECTamine, a lipid-soluble, brain-imaging agent. Brand name for *iofetamine hydrochloride [123]I.*

spectator ions /spek″tātər/, ions that are not involved in a chemical reaction. They may be deleted when writing the net ionic equation.

Spectazole, an antifungal medication. Brand name for *econazole nitrate.*

spectinomycin hydrochloride /spek″tinōmī″sin/, an antibiotic.

■ INDICATIONS: It is prescribed in the treatment of gonorrhea and certain infections in penicillin-allergic patients.

■ CONTRAINDICATIONS: Known hypersensitivity to this drug prohibits its use.

■ ADVERSE EFFECTS: The more serious adverse effects are oliguria, urticaria, chills, fever, dizziness, and nausea.

spectr-, combining form meaning "image": *spectrometer, spectroscope, spectrum.*

spectra. See **spectrum.**

spectro-, prefix meaning "relationship to a spectrum or to an image": *spectrometer.*

Spectrocin, a fixed-combination topical drug containing antibacterials and a local anesthetic (lidocaine). Brand name for **neomycin sulfate, bacitracin, polymyxin B sulfate, lidocaine hydrochloride.**

spectrometer /spektrom″ətər/ [L, *spectrum,* image; Gk, *metron,* measure], an instrument for measuring wavelengths of rays of a spectrum, the deviation of refracted rays, and the angles between faces of a prism. See also **mass spectrometer, Mössbauer spectrometer.**

spectrometry /spektrom″ətrē/, the process of measuring wavelengths of light and other electromagnetic waves. See also **spectrometer.** –*spectrometric, adj.*

spectrophotometer, a measurement device used to capture and evaluate color through the amount of light absorbed or transmitted as it passes through a sample.

spectrophotometry. See **spectrophotometry.**

spectrophotometric analysis. See **quantitative analysis.**

spectrophotometry /spek″trōfətom″ətrē/, the measurement of color in a solution by determining the amount of light absorbed in the ultraviolet, infrared, or visible spectrum, widely used in clinical chemistry to calculate the concentration of substances in solution. –**spectrophotometric,** *adj.*

spectroscope /spek″trə·skōp/ [L, *spectrum,* image; Gk, *skopein,* to examine], an instrument for developing and analyzing bands of color.

spectroscopy /spek·tros″kə·pē/ [L, *spectrum,* image; Gk, *skopein,* to examine], **1.** the propagation and analysis of bands of color. **2.** examination by means of a spectroscope.

spectrum /spek″trəm/ *pl.* **spectra** [L, image], **1.** a range of phenomena or properties occurring in increasing or decreasing magnitude. Radiant or electromagnetic energy is arranged on the basis of wavelength and frequency. Electromagnetic radiation includes spectra of radio waves, infrared waves, visible light, ultraviolet waves, x-rays, and gamma rays. See also **electromagnetic radiation, wave. 2.** the range of effectiveness of an antibiotic. A broad-spectrum antibiotic is effective against a wide range of microorganisms. See also **antibiotic.**

specular reflection, a reflection from a smooth surface, such as a mirror. In ultrasonography, such reflections are from smooth surfaces such as organ walls.

speculum /spek″yələm/ *pl.* **specula** [L, mirror], a retractor used to separate the walls of a cavity to make examination possible, such as an ear speculum, an eye speculum, a nasal speculum, or a vaginal speculum.

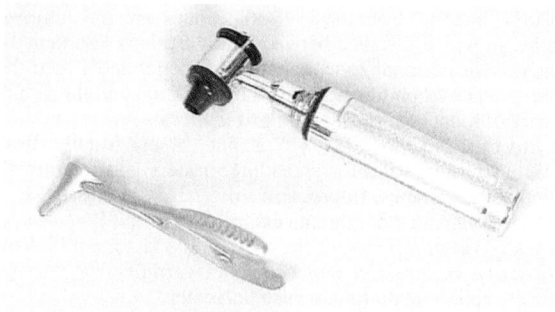

Nasal specula *(Seidel et al, 2011)*

speech [ME, *speche*], **1.** the utterance of articulate vocal sounds that form words of a language to give expression to one's thoughts or ideas. **2.** communication by means of spoken words. **3.** the faculty of language production, which involves the complex coordination of the muscles and nerves of the organs of articulation. Any neurological or muscular injury or defect involving these organs results in various speech impediments or dysfunctions. Kinds include **ataxic speech, explosive speech, scanning speech, slurred speech, staccato speech.**

speech abnormalities, abnormal or difficult function of speech.

speech audiometry. See **audiometry.**

speech banana, the area on an audiogram where sounds of human speech are displayed. See also **audiogram.**

speech centers [AS, *spaec* + Gk, *kentron*], either of two motor areas involved in speech. Broca's motor speech area is a unilateral area in the posterior part of the inferior frontal gyrus and is usually on the dominant hemisphere. Wernicke's second motor speech area is an area comprising the posterior part of the superior temporal gyrus next to the transverse temporal gyri and the supramarginal and temporal gyri, also on the dominant hemisphere. See also **Broca's area, Wernicke center.**

speech dysfunction, any defect or abnormality of the formation of audible and intelligible words, including aphasia, alexia, stammering, stuttering, aphonia, and slurring. Speech problems may result from any of a variety of causes, among them neurological injury to the cerebral cortex; muscular paralysis caused by trauma, disease, or cerebrovascular accident; structural abnormality of the organs of speech; emotional or psychological tension, strain, or depression; hysteria; and severe cognitive impairment. See also **speech.**

speech language disorders, difficulty in communication and related areas, such as oral motor function. Speech and language challenges affect not only communication but also associated abilities that require interactions with others.

speech-language pathologist (SLP), a health professional with graduate education in human communication, its development, and its disorders. An SLP specializes in the measurement and evaluation of language abilities, auditory processes, speech production, and swallowing problems; clinical treatment of speech and language disorders; and research methods in the study of communication problems in children and adults. Also called **speech-language therapist.**

speech-language pathology, **1.** the study of abnormalities of speech and language. **2.** the diagnosis and treatment of abnormalities of speech sounds, language, social communication, voice, fluency, and feeding and swallowing as practiced by a speech pathologist.

speech-language therapist. See **speech-language pathologist.**

speech reading [ME, *reden,* to explain], a method of oral communication in which one uses the visual clues of the speaker's lip and facial movements, along with residual hearing. Gestures and "body language" also are observed. Formerly called **lip reading.** See also **sign language.**

speech reception threshold, the minimum intensity in decibels at which a patient can understand 50% of spoken words; used in tests of speech audiometry. Also called *speech recognition threshold.*

speech synthesizer [AS, *spaec* + Gk, *synthesis,* placing together], an electronic apparatus with a keyboard that produces sounds that imitate the human voice.

speech therapy [AS, *spaec* + Gk, *therapeia,* treatment], the application of treatments and counseling in the prevention or rehabilitation/remediation of speech and language disorders. See also **speech-language pathologist.**

speed [AS, *spedan,* to hasten], **1.** the rate of change of position with time. Compare **velocity. 2.** See **amphetamines. 3.** a reciprocal of the amount of radiation needed to produce an image with various components of an x-ray imaging system, such as screens, film, and image intensifiers. There is often a tradeoff between radiation dose to the patient and the overall image quality. Thus a system using little radiation is "fast," whereas one requiring more radiation is "slow." **4.** the amount of exposure of film to light or x-rays needed to produce a desired image. X-ray film speed usually is indicated as the reciprocal of the exposure in roentgens necessary to produce a density of 1 above the base and fog levels. See also **fogged film fault.**

speed shock, a sudden adverse physiological reaction to IV medications or drugs that are administered too quickly. Some signs of speed shock are a flushed face, headache, a tight feeling in the chest, irregular pulse, loss of consciousness, and cardiac arrest.

sPEEP, abbreviation for **spontaneous PEEP.**

spell of illness [ME, *spel* + *illr,* bad], a period regarded by Medicare rules as the number of days between the admission of an insured patient to a hospital and the day that marks the end of a period during which the insured has not been an inpatient in a hospital or a skilled nursing facility.

sperm. See **semen, spermatozoon.**

-sperm /spurm/, combining form meaning "a seed": *oosperm.*

sperm agglutination test, (for male factor infertility) any of various tests for presence of antisperm antibodies as a cause of infertility, based on the ability of large multivalent isotypes, such as IgM or secretory IgA, to cross-link and agglutinate spermatozoa that have such antibodies. Serum or seminal plasma is mixed with a known concentration of sperm; immunoglobulins in the mixture then begin agglutinating the sperm. After a given period of time at 37° C, the amount of agglutination is assessed.

sperm antibody, a glycoprotein that specifically recognizes the head or tail of a spermatozoon. The antibodies are found often in vasectomized males and infrequently in infertile males.

spermatic cord /spərmat'ik/ [Gk, *sperma,* seed, *chorde,* string], a structure extending from the deep inguinal ring in the abdomen to the testis, descending nearly vertically into the scrotum. The left spermatic cord is usually longer than the right. Consequently, the left testis usually hangs lower than the right. Each cord comprises arteries, veins, lymphatics, nerves, and the vas deferens of the testis.

spermatic duct. See **vas deferens.**

spermatic fistula, an abnormal passage communicating with a testis or a seminal duct.

spermatid /spur'mətid, spərmat'id/ [Gk, *sperma,* seed], a male germ cell that arises from a spermatocyte and becomes a mature spermatozoon in the last phase of spermatogenesis.

spermatocele /spərmat'əsēl', spur'-/ [Gk, *sperma* + *kele,* tumor], a cystic swelling, either of the epididymis or of the rete testis, that contains spermatozoa. It lies above, behind, and separate from the testis. It is usually painless and requires no therapy.

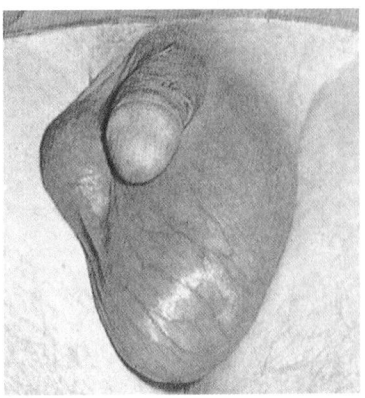

Spermatocele *(Lloyd-Davies et al, 1994)*

spermatocide /spərmat'əsīd, spur'-/ [Gk, *sperma* + L, *caedere,* to kill], a chemical substance that kills spermatozoa by reducing their surface tension, causing the cell wall to break down by a bactericidal effect or by creation of a highly acidic environment. Among many spermatocidal agents used in various contraceptive creams are lactic acid, phenylmercuric acetate, chloramine polyethylene glycol, benzethonium chloride, and certain quinine compounds. Also called **spermicide.**

spermatocyte /spur'mətōsīt'/ [Gk, *sperma* + *kytos,* cell], a male germ cell that arises from a spermatogonium. Each spermatocyte gives rise to two haploid secondary spermatocytes that become spermatids.

spermatogenesis /spərmat'əjen'əsis, spur'-/ [Gk, *sperma* + *genesis,* origin], the process of development of spermatozoa, consisting of two stages. In the first stage, spermatogonia become spermatocytes, which develop into spermatids. In the second stage, called spermiogenesis, the spermatids become spermatozoa. Also called *spermatocytogenesis,* **spermiogenesis.** −*spermatogenic, spermatogenous, adj.*

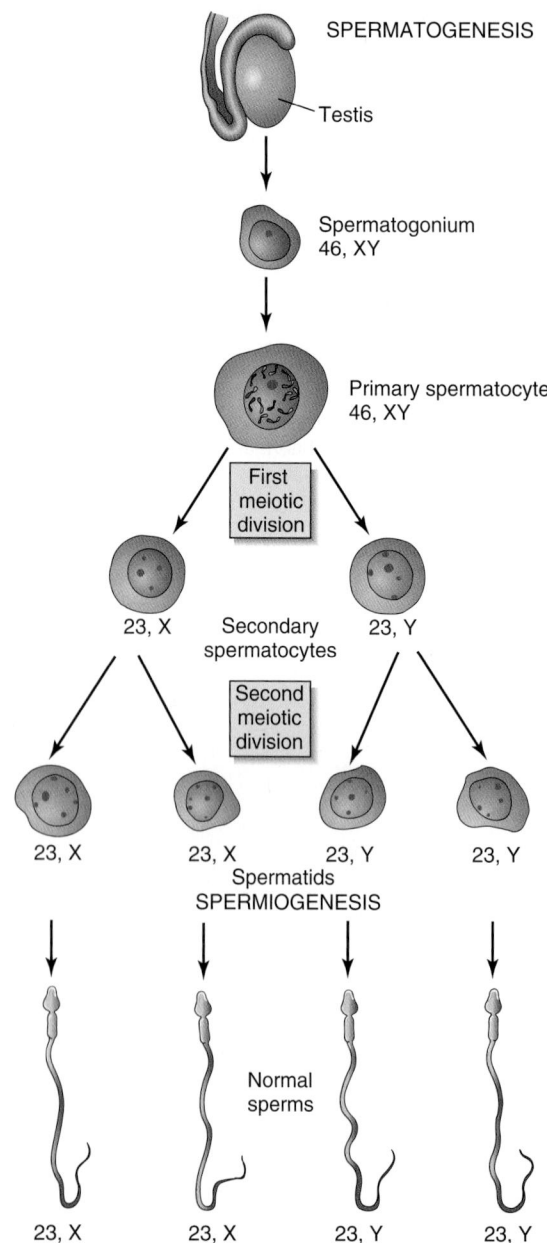

Spermatogenesis *(Moore, Persaud, and Shiota, 2008)*

spermatozoa are the generative component of the semen. See also **spermatogenesis.**

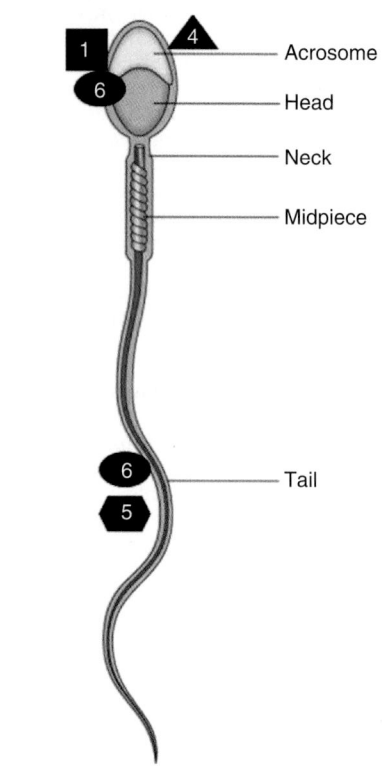

Spermatozoon *(Leonard, 2009)*

spermatogonium /-gō′nē·əm/ [Gk, *sperma* + *gone,* generation], a male germ cell that gives rise to a spermatocyte early in spermatogenesis.

spermatopathia /-path′ē·ə/ [Gk, *sperma,* seed, *pathos,* disease], pertaining to diseased sperm or their associated organs. Also called **spermopathy.**

spermato-, spermo-, combining form meaning "seed, specifically the male generative element": *spermatogenesis.*

spermatozoon /spur′mətəzō″ən, spərmat′-/ *pl. spermatozoa* [Gk, *sperma* + *zoon,* animal], a mature male germ cell that develops in the seminiferous tubules of the testes. Resembling a tadpole, it is about 50 μm ($^1/_{500}$ inch) long and has a head with a nucleus, a neck, and a tail that provides propulsion. Developed in vast numbers after puberty,

sperm bank [Gk, *sperma,* seed; It, *banca,* bench], a facility for storage of semen to be used for artificial insemination.

sperm head, the oval anterior end of a spermatozoon, which contains the male pronucleus and is surrounded by the acrosome.

-spermia, -spermy, combining form meaning "(condition of) possessing or producing seed": *aspermia, bacteriospermia.*

spermicidal /spur′misī″dəl/, destructive to spermatozoa.

spermicide. See **spermatocide.**

sperm immobilization test, (for male factor infertility) a test for antisperm antibodies as a cause of infertility, based on the loss of ability of spermatozoa with such surface antibodies to move when complement is present (as it normally is in the female reproductive tract). Serum from the patient is incubated with motile sperm and complement is added. After 1 hour the mixture is checked to calculate the percentage of formerly motile sperm that can no longer move; a 50% reduction in motility is a positive result for presence of antisperm antibodies. Also called *Isojima test.*

spermiogenesis. See **spermatogenesis.**

spermo-. See **spermato-, spermo-.**

spermopathy. See **spermatopathia.**

sperm penetration assay (SPA), a test for the ability of spermatozoa to penetrate oocytes in vitro. Hamster oocytes that lack the zona pellucida are exposed to the spermatozoa in question. Such zona-free oocytes can undergo heterologous membrane fusion with the membranes of spermatozoa that have undergone the acrosome reaction. An assessment is then made of the proportion of oocytes that have been successfully penetrated.

sperm swim up, the migration of spermatozoa into culture medium.

sperm swim-up technique, any of several methods of checking sperm for motility. A semen sample is centrifuged to form pellets, which are then covered with culture medium. The spermatozoa with greatest motility will swim up into the culture medium and be more suitable for use in in vitro fertilization.

sperm washing, the bathing of fresh sperm with a special solution to remove antibodies and other contaminants so that it can be used for in vitro fertilization or some other technique of artificial insemination. During the sperm washing process sperm is separated from the seminal fluid.

-spermy. See **-spermia, -spermy.**

SPF, abbreviation for **sunscreen protective factor index.**

sp. gr., abbreviation for **specific gravity.**

sphacel-, combining form meaning "gangrene": *sphacelous.*

sphacelous /sfas″ələs/, pertaining to something that is necrotic or gangrenous.

-sphaera, -sphaere. See **sphero-, sphaero-.**

sphaero-. See **sphero-, sphaero-.**

S-phase, the phase of the cell cycle in which DNA is synthesized before mitosis.

spheno-, combining form meaning "sphenoid bone" or "a wedge": *sphenoethmoidal, sphenoiditis, sphenosquamous.*

sphenoethmoidal suture. See **ethmosphenoid suture.**

sphenoethmoid recess /sfē′nō-eth″moid/ [Gk, *sphen,* wedge, *eidos,* form; L, *recedere,* to retreat], a narrow opening in the lateral wall of the nasal cavity bounded above by the cribriform plate of the ethmoid and the body of the sphenoid and below by the superior nasal concha. It opens into the sphenoidal sinus of the skull.

sphenoid /sfē′noid/ [Gk, *sphen,* wedge, *eidos,* form], wedge-shaped. See also **sphenoid bone.**

sphenoidal fissure /sfēnoi′dəl/ [Gk *sphen,* wedge, *eidos* form], a cleft between the great and small wings of the sphenoid bone.

sphenoidal sinus, one of a pair of cavities in the sphenoid bone of the skull, lined with mucous membrane that is continuous with that of the nasal cavity. Compare **ethmoidal air cell, frontal sinus, maxillary sinus.**

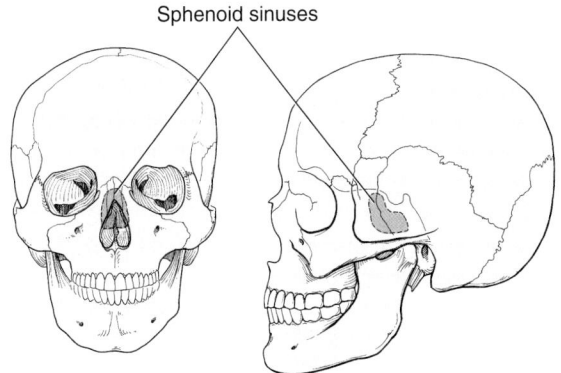

Sphenoidal sinus *(Bontrager, 2005)*

sphenoid bone, the bone at the base of the skull, anterior to the temporal bones and the basilar part of the occipital bone. It resembles a bat with its wings extended. Also called **sphenoid.**

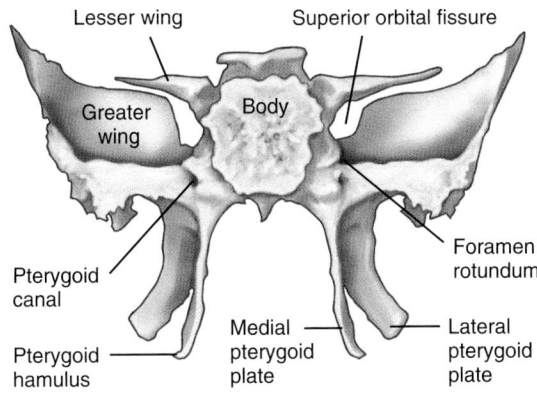

Sphenoid bone

sphenoid fontanel, an anterolateral fontanel that is usually not palpable. See also **fontanel.**

sphenoiditis /sfē′noidī″tis/ [Gk, *sphen,* wedge, *eidos,* form, *itis,* inflammation], an inflammation of the sphenoidal sinus.

sphenomandibular ligament /sfē′nōmandib″yələr/ [Gk, *sphen + eidos +* L, *mandere,* to chew], one of a pair of flat, thin ligaments comprising part of the temporomandibular joint between the mandible of the jaw and the temporal bone of the skull. It is attached to the spine of the sphenoid bone and becomes broader as it descends to the lingula of the mandibular foramen.

sphenopalatine artery, the largest vessel supplying the nasal cavity; the terminal branch of the maxillary artery in the pterygopalatine fossa.

sphenoparietal suture, the articulation of the sphenoid bone with the parietal bone in the calvaria.

sphenosquamous suture, the articulation of the sphenoid bone with the anterior edge of the temporal bone.

sphere /sfir/, a globe-shaped object, theoretically generated by a circle revolving on a diameter as its axis.

-sphere, -sphaera, -sphaere, 1. suffix meaning "a spheric body": *hemisphere.* **2.** suffix meaning "a realm that supports life": *atmosphere.*

sphero-, sphaero-, prefix meaning "round" or "spherical": *spherocyte.*

spherocyte /sfir″əsīt/ [Gk, *sphaira,* sphere, *kytos,* cell], an abnormal spherical red blood cell with a high cytoplasm-to-membrane ration. In Wright-stained peripheral blood films, spherocytes are dense, lack central pallor, and have a reduced diameter. Spherocytes appear most frequently in warm autoimmune hemolytic anemia and hereditary spherocytosis.

spherocytic anemia /sfir′əsit″ik/, autosomal-dominant hemolytic anemia characterized by hemolytic anemia caused by the presence of spherical red blood cells. The cells are fragile and tend to hemolyze in the oxygen-poor peripheral circulatory system. Episodic crises of abdominal pain, fever, jaundice, and splenomegaly occur. Because repeated transfusions are often needed to treat the anemia, hemochromatosis may develop. Splenectomy may then be necessary. Compare **congenital nonspherocytic hemolytic anemia.** See also **elliptocytosis.**

spherocytosis /sfir′ōsītō″sis/, the abnormal presence of spherocytes in the blood. Compare **elliptocytosis.**

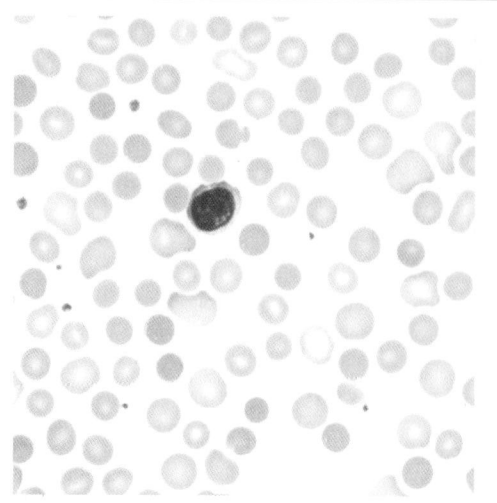

Spherocytosis *(Carr and Rodak, 2009)*

spheroidal /sfir'oidəl/ [Gk, *sphaira*, ball, *eidos*, form], ball-shaped.

spheroidea. See **ball-and-socket joint.**

spherule /sfer'yool/ [Gk, *sphaira*, ball], a small ball.

sphincter /sfingk"tər/ [Gk, *sphingein*, to bind], a circular band of muscle fibers that constricts a passage or closes a natural opening in the body, such as the hepatic sphincter in the muscular coat of the hepatic veins near their union with the superior vena cava, and the external anal sphincter, which closes the anus.

sphincter ani, a double set of circular muscles at the opening of the anus. One, the sphincter ani internus, consists of a thickened inner circular coat of the bowel smooth muscle; the other, the sphincter ani externus, is a flat sheet of striated voluntary muscle surrounding the anal orifice.

sphincter choledochus /kōled'əkəs/, a smooth muscle sphincter that encircles the lower end of the bile duct and is part of the sphincter of Oddi.

sphincter muscle of pancreatic duct, a sphincter that surrounds the pancreatic duct just above the hepatopancreatic ampulla.

sphincter of Oddi [Ruggero Oddi, Italian physician, 1864–1913], a sheath of muscle fibers surrounding the lower end of the common bile and pancreatic ducts as they cross the wall of the duodenum.

sphincter of Oddi dysfunction, abdominal pain or jaundice with failure of the sphincter of Oddi to function properly. It may occur several years after cholecystectomy or as a result of unknown causes. See also **biliary dyskinesia.**

sphincter pupillae, a muscle that contracts the iris, narrowing the diameter of the pupil of the eye. It is composed of circular fibers arranged in a narrow band, about 1 mm wide, surrounding the margin of the pupil toward the posterior surface of the iris. The circular fibers near the free margin of the iris are closely packed; those that are near the periphery of the band are more separated and form incomplete circles. The fibers of the sphincter pupillae blend with the fibers of the dilatator pupillae near the margin of the pupil and are innervated by a motor root of the ciliary ganglion from the oculomotor nerve. Compare **dilator pupillae.**

sphincter spasm, spasm of a sphincter muscle, particularly an anal sphincter.

sphingolipid /sfing'gōlip"id/ [Gk, *sphingein*, to bind, *lipos*, fat], a compound that consists of a lipid and a sphingosine.

It is found in high concentrations in the brain and other tissues of the nervous system, especially membranes.

sphingomyelin /sfing'gōmī"əlin/ [Gk, *sphingein* + *myelos*, marrow], any of a group of sphingolipids containing phosphorus. It occurs primarily in the tissue of the nervous system, generally in membranes, and in the lipids in the blood.

sphingomyelin lipidosis, any of a group of diseases characterized by an abnormality in the ability of the body to store sphingolipids. Kinds include **Gaucher disease, Niemann-Pick disease, Tay-Sachs disease.** See also **angiokeratoma corporis diffusum.**

sphingosine /sfing"gōsēn/, a long-chain, unsaturated amino alcohol, a major constituent of sphingolipids, including sphingomyelins.

sphygm-, sphygmo-, prefix meaning "pulse": *sphygmomanometer.*

-sphygmia, combining form meaning "(condition of the) pulse": *sychnosphygmia.*

sphygmic interval. See **ejection period.**

sphygmo-. See **sphygm-, sphygmo-.**

sphygmogram /sfig"məgram/ [Gk, *sphygmos*, pulse, *gramma*, record], a pulse tracing produced by a sphygmograph. A curve occurs on the tracing with each atrial pulsation. An upward, primary elevation is followed by a sudden drop to a point slightly above the baseline. The curve then gradually descends to the baseline in small decrements of amplitude. Sphygmographic abnormalities of rate, rhythm, and form may be diagnostically useful in an assessment of cardiovascular function.

sphygmograph /sfig"məgraf/, an instrument that records the force of the arterial pulse on a tracing, the sphygmogram. −*sphygmographic, adj.*

sphygmoid /sfig'moid/ [Gk, *sphygmos*, pulse, *eidos*, form], pertaining to or resembling the pulse.

sphygmomanometer /sfig'mōmənom"ətər/ [Gk, *sphygmos* + *manos*, thin, *metron*, measure], an instrument for indirect measurement of blood pressure. It consists of an inflatable cuff that fits around a limb, a bulb for controlling air pressure within the cuff, and an aneroid manometer or a device that uses an electronic pressure sensor within the blood pressure cuff. See also **blood pressure, manometer.**

spica [L, *spica*, spike, or ear of wheat], a figure-eight bandage that, when applied to a joint, resembles the head of a stalk of wheat.

spica bandage /spī"kə/ [L, *spica*, spike of wheat; Fr, *bande*, strip], a figure-eight bandage in which each turn generally overlaps the previous to form a succession of V-like designs. It may be used to give support, to apply pressure, or to hold a dressing in place on the chest, limbs, thighs, or pelvis.

spica cast, 1. an orthopedic cast applied to immobilize part or all of the trunk of the body and part or all of one or more extremities. It is used to treat various fractures, such as of the hip and the femur, and to correct or maintain the correction of hip deformities. Kinds include **bilateral long-leg spica cast, one-and-a-half spica cast, shoulder spica cast, unilateral long-leg spica cast.** See also **cast. 2.** an orthotic device for positioning the thumb. It is commonly used for correcting a thumb-in-palm contracture or a fracture in the thumb or lateral carpal bones.

spicule /spik"yool/ [L, *spiculum*, point], a small sharp body with a needlelike point.

spider angioma [ME, *spithre* + Gk, *angeion*, vessel, *oma*, tumor], a form of telangiectasis characterized by a central elevated red dot the size of a pinhead from which small blood vessels radiate. Spider angiomas are often associated with elevated estrogen levels, such as occur in pregnancy or when the liver is diseased and unable to detoxify estrogens. Also called **spider nevus.** See also **telangiectasia.**

spider antivenin.   See **black widow spider antivenin.**

spider bite [ME, *spithre* + AS, *bitan* + L, *potio,* drink], a puncture wound produced by the bite by any of nearly 60 species of venomous spiders found in North America. Most spiders have fangs that are too short or fragile to penetrate the skin, but some are dangerous to humans. These include the black widow, *Latrodectus mactans*; the brown recluse, *Loxosceles reclusa*; and species of jumping spiders and tarantulas. Spider venom may contain enzymatic proteins, including peptides that may affect neuromuscular transmission or cardiovascular function.

spider mite, either *Tetranychus molestissimus* or *T. telarius.*

spider nevus.   See **spider angioma.**

spider telangiectasia [ME, *spithre* + Gk, *telos,* end, *angeion,* vessel, *ektasis,* dilation], a branched group of dilated capillary blood vessels forming a spiderlike image on the skin. Also called **nevus araneus.**

spike, a sharp peak in an electronic recording, such as an oscillograph.

spikeboard /spīk″bôrd/, a device that enables people with upper extremity disabilities to stabilize foods for meal preparation, typically used by individuals with functional use of only one hand. Also called **paring board.**

spillway [AS, *spillan,* to destroy, *weg,* wagon track], a channel or passageway through which food normally escapes from the occlusal surfaces of the teeth during chewing.

spin [AS, *spinnan,* to draw threads], **1.** the intrinsic angular momentum of an elementary particle or a nucleus of an atom. **2.** intrinsic joint movements about an axis perpendicular to the articular surface.

spina /spī″nə/ *pl. spinae* [L, backbone], **1.** the spinal column. **2.** a spine or a thornlike projection, such as the bony projection on the anterior border of the ilium, forming the anterior end of the iliac crest.

spina bifida /bif″ədə, bī″fədə/, a congenital neural tube defect in which there is a developmental anomaly in the posterior vertebral arch. Spina bifida is relatively common, occurring approximately 10 to 20 times per 1000 births. It may occur with only a small deformed lamina separated by a midline gap, or it may be associated with the complete absence of laminae surrounding a large area. In cases where the separation is wide enough, contents of the spinal canal protrude posteriorly, and a myelomeningocele is evident. Neurological deficits do not usually accompany the anomalies involving only bony deformity. Signs and symptoms are dependent on the size of the defect. Spina bifida that does not involve herniation of the meninges or the contents of the spinal canal (spina bifida occulta) may have no symptoms. Also called **spinal dysrhaphism.** See also **spina bifida occulta.**

spina bifida anterior, incomplete closure along the anterior surface of the vertebral column. The defect is often associated with developmental anomalies of the abdominal and thoracic viscera.

spina bifida cystica, a developmental defect of the central nervous system in which a hernial cyst containing meninges (meningocele), spinal cord (myelocele), or both (myelomeningocele) protrudes through a congenital cleft in the vertebral column. The protruding sac is encased in a layer of skin or a fine membrane that readily ruptures, causing the leakage of cerebrospinal fluid and an increased risk of meningeal infection. The severity of neurological dysfunction and associated defects depends directly on the degree of nerve involvement. The most severe type is lumbosacral myelomeningocele, which is frequently associated with hydrocephalus and the Arnold-Chiari malformation. Compare **spina bifida occulta.** See also **myelomeningocele, neural tube defect.**

spina bifida occulta, defective closure of the laminae of the vertebral column in the lumbosacral region without hernial protrusion of the spinal cord or meninges. The defect, which is quite common, occurs in about 5% of the population. It is identified externally by a skin depression or dimple, dark tufts of hair, telangiectasis, or soft subcutaneous lipomas at the site. Because the neural tube has closed, there are usually no neurological impairments associated with the defect. However, any abnormal adhesion of the spinal cord to the area of the malformation may lead to neuromuscular disturbances, usually problems with gait and foot weakness and with the bowel and bladder sphincters. Compare **spina bifida cystica.**

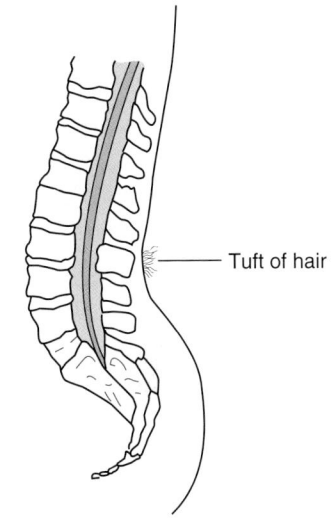

Spina bifida occulta *(Sorrentino, 2008)*

spinae.   See **spina.**

spinal /spī″nəl/ [L, *spina*], **1.** *adj.,* pertaining to a spine, especially the spinal column. **2.** *(Informal) n.,* spinal anesthesia, such as saddle block or caudal anesthesia.

spinal accessory nerve.   See **accessory nerve.**

spinal anesthesia [L, *spina,* backbone; Gk, *anaisthesia,* lack of feeling], a state of lack of sensation in the lower part of the body produced by injection of a local anesthetic drug into the subarachnoid cerebrospinal fluid space. May be combined with narcotics such as preservative-free morphine, and/or Fentanyl for postoperative analgesia. Also called **subarachnoid block anesthesia.** See also **anesthesia, regional anesthesia.**

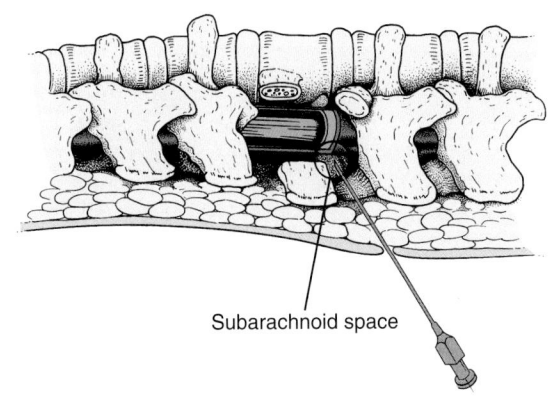

Spinal anesthesia *(Ignatavicius and Workman, 2010)*

spinal aperture,   a large opening formed by the body of a vertebra and its arch.

spinal block [L, *spina,* backbone; OFr, *bloc*],   an obstruction of cerebrospinal fluid circulation. See also **subarachnoid block anesthesia.**

spinal canal,   the cavity within the vertebral column.

spinal caries.   See **tuberculous spondylitis.**

spinal column.   See **vertebral column.**

spinal cord,   a long, nearly cylindric structure lodged in the vertebral canal and extending from the foramen magnum at the base of the skull to the upper part of the lumbar region. A major component of the central nervous system, the adult cord is approximately 1 cm in diameter, with an average length of 42 to 45 cm and a weight of 30 g. The cord is an extension of the medulla oblongata of the brain that extends at the level of the first or second lumbar vertebra. The cord conducts sensory and motor impulses to and from the brain and controls many reflexes. Thirty-one pairs of spinal nerves originate from the cord: 8 cervical, 12 thoracic, 5 lumbar, 5 sacral, and 1 coccygeal. It has an inner core of gray material consisting mainly of nerve cell bodies. The cord is enclosed by three protective membranes (meninges): the dura mater, arachnoid, and pia mater. Also called **chorda spinalis, medulla spinalis.** See also **segments of spinal cord, spinal nerves.**

spinal cord compression,   an abnormal and often serious condition resulting from pressure on the spinal cord. The symptoms range from temporary numbness of an extremity to permanent tetraplegia, depending on the cause, severity, and location of the pressure. Causes include spinal fracture, vertebral dislocation, tumor, hemorrhage, and edema associated with contusion. See also **herniated disk, spondylolisthesis.**

spinal cord injury,   any one of the traumatic disruptions of the spinal cord, often associated with extensive musculoskeletal involvement. Common spinal cord injuries are vertebral fractures and dislocations, such as those commonly suffered by individuals involved in car accidents, airplane crashes, or other violent impacts. Such trauma may cause varying degrees of paraplegia and tetraplegia. Injuries to spinal structures below the first thoracic vertebra may produce paraplegia. Injuries to the spine above the first thoracic vertebra may cause tetraplegia. Injuries that completely transect the spinal cord cause permanent loss of motor and sensory functions activated by neurons below the level of the lesions involved. Spinal cord injuries produce a state of spinal shock, characterized by flaccid paralysis, and complete loss of skin sensation at the time of injury. Within a few weeks the muscles affected may become spastic, and skin sensation may return to a slight degree. The motor and sensory losses that prevail a few weeks after the injury are usually permanent. Musculoskeletal complications are associated with the neurological involvement of spinal cord injuries, and the prevention of pressure ulcers and treatment of any loss of bladder and bowel control are continuing concerns. Treatment of spinal cord injuries varies considerably, depending on the level of injury, and involves numerous approaches by the health care team. See also **hemiplegia, paraplegia, quadriplegia.**

spinal cord tumor,   a neoplasm of the spinal cord of which more than 50% are extramedullary, about 25% are intramedullary, and the rest are extradural. Symptoms depend on the location and rate of growth of the tumor. They usually develop slowly and may progress from unilateral paresthesia and a dull ache to lancinating pain; weakness in one or both legs; abnormal deep tendon reflexes; and, in advanced cases, monoplegia, hemiplegia, or paraplegia. Function of the autonomic nervous system is sometimes disturbed, causing areas of dry, cold, bluish pink skin or profuse sweating of the lower extremities. The diagnosis is made by radiographic and myelographic examination. About 30% of spinal cord tumors are circumscribed, encapsulated meningiomas, and 25% are schwannomas; these two kinds are found chiefly in the thoracic region. Some 20% are gliomas, and the others consist of congenital lipomas, epidermoids, and metastatic lesions. The dura is resistant to invasion, but many extradural tumors are metastatic lesions from primary cancers in the prostate, lung, breast, thyroid, and GI tract. Most extramedullary and nonmetastatic extradural tumors are surgically removed; intermedullary lesions are enucleated, whenever possible; inoperable tumors are treated with radiotherapy and chemotherapy. Tumors of the spinal cord may arise at any age but appear most frequently in the third decade of life and are one fourth as common as brain neoplasms. Care of the patient with a spinal cord tumor involves careful assessment, a coordinated team approach to care, and monitoring of motor and sensory status.

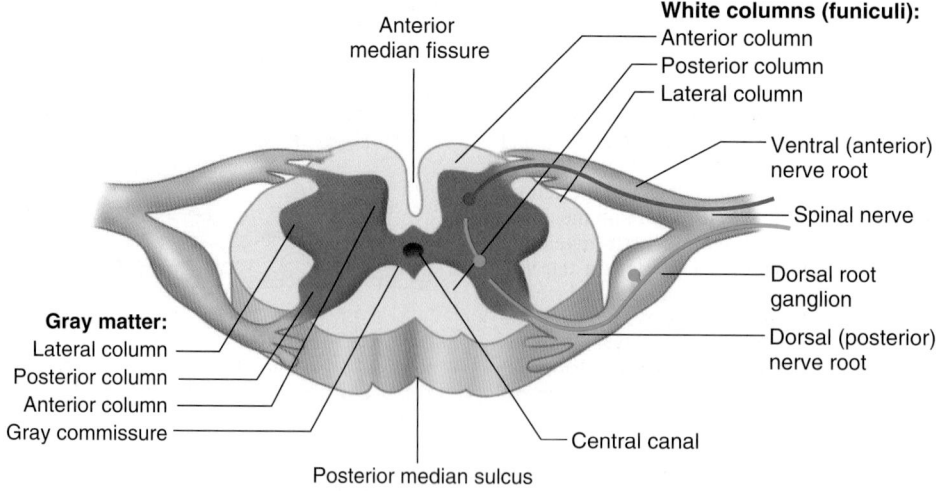

Cross section of the spinal cord *(Patton and Thibodeau, 2010)*

spinal curvature, any persistent, abnormal deviation of the vertebral column from its normal position. Kinds of spinal curvature are kyphoscoliosis, kyphosis, lordosis, and scoliosis. Kinds include **kyphoscoliosis, kyphosis, lordosis, scoliosis.**

spinal dysrhaphism, a term describing congenital anomalies resulting from incomplete or aberrant neural tube fusion. See also **spina bifida.**

spinal fasciculi. See **spinal tract.**

spinal fluid. See **cerebrospinal fluid.**

spinal fusion, the fixation of an unstable segment of the spine. It is sometimes accomplished by skeletal traction or immobilization of the patient in a body cast but most frequently by a surgical procedure. Operative ankylosis may be performed in the treatment of spinal fractures or after diskectomy or laminectomy for the correction of a herniated vertebral disk. Surgical fusion involves the stabilization of a spinal section with a bone graft or synthetic device introduced through a posterior incision in the lumbar region. In the less frequently fused cervical region, the incision may be anterior or posterior. Also called **spondylosyndesis.**

spinal headache, a severe headache occurring after spinal anesthesia, lumbar puncture, or epidural anesthesia, caused by a leak of cerebrospinal fluid from the subarachnoid space. Severe spinal headache may be accompanied by diminished aural and visual acuity. Treatment usually includes keeping the patient flat in bed to relieve the meningeal irritation, promoting increased fluid intake to increase the intravascular volume and increase the production and volume of cerebrospinal fluid, and administering analgesics to reduce pain. If severe headache persists, an autologous blood patch procedure may be performed. Also called **postdural puncture headache.** See also **epidural blood patch.**

spinal manipulation, the forced passive flexion, extension, and rotation of vertebral segments, carrying the elements of articulation beyond the usual range of movement to the limit of anatomical range. Spinal manipulation may be used effectively in physiotherapy for the treatment of vertebral and sacroiliac dislocations, sprains, and adhesions.

spinal meningitis, an inflammation of the membranes of the spinal cord.

spinal motion segment, two adjacent vertebrae and the connecting tissues that bind them together.

spinal muscular atrophy. See **Duchenne disease.**

spinal nerves, the 31 pairs of nerves without special names that are connected to the spinal cord and numbered according to the level of the vertebral column at which they emerge. There are 8 cervical, 12 thoracic, 5 lumbar, 5 sacral, and 1 coccygeal pair. The first cervical pair of nerves emerges from the spinal cord in the space between the first cervical vertebra and the occipital bone. The rest of the cervical pairs and all the thoracic pairs emerge horizontally through the intervertebral foramina of their respective vertebrae, such as the second cervical pair, which emerges through the foramina above the second cervical vertebra. The lumbar, sacral, and coccygeal nerve pairs descend from their points of origin at the lower end of the cord before reaching the intervertebral foramina of their respective vertebrae. Each spinal nerve attaches to the spinal cord by an anterior (or ventral) root and a posterior (or dorsal) root. The nerve impulses enter the cord by way of posterior roots. The posterior roots supply skin and muscles of much of the body with some of the nerve fibers supplying autonomic functions. The posterior roots contain sensory neurons and accompany a distended spinal ganglion within the vertebral foramina. The ventral roots contain motor neuron axons. The sacral plexus in the pelvic cavity comprises certain spinal nerve fibers from the lumbar and sacral regions

and gives rise to the great sciatic nerve in the back of the thigh. See also **spinal cord.**

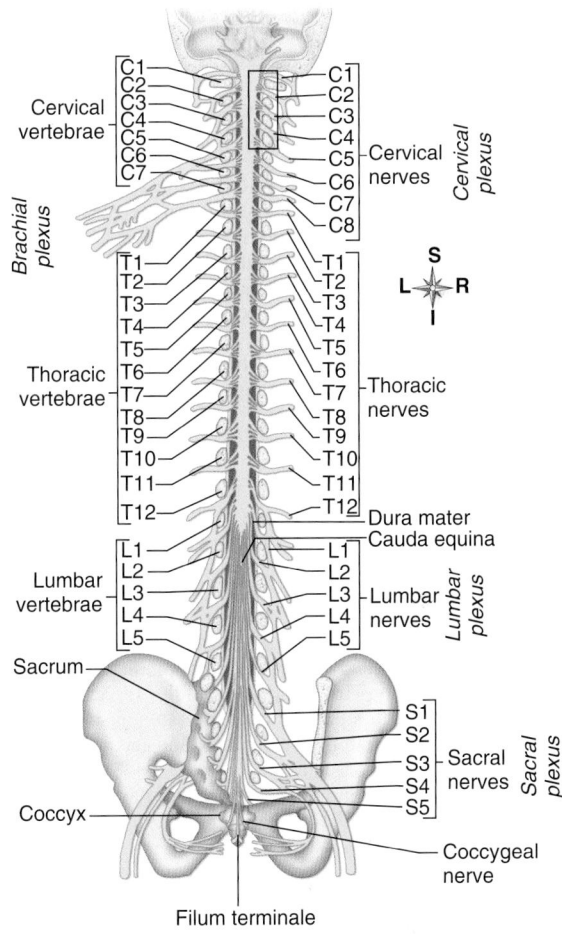

Spinal nerves and spinal column (Drake, Vogl, and Mitchell, 2010)

spinal puncture. See **lumbar puncture.**

spinal reflex [L, *spina* + *reflectere,* to bend back], any reflex with a pathway through the spinal cord but not the brain.

spinal segment, a division of the spinal cord containing a bilateral pair of nerve roots. From the anterior to the posterior, the segments are referred to as cervical (C_1-C_8), thoracic (T_1-T_{12}), lumbar (L_1-L_5), sacral (S_1-S_5), and coccygeal (Co_1-Co_3).

spinal shock, a form of shock associated with acute injury to the spinal cord. Temporary suppression of reflexes is controlled by segments below the level of injury. The period of shock may last from hours to months. See also **shock.**

spinal stenosis, narrowing of the vertebral canal, nerve root canals, or intervertebral foramina of the lumbar spine, caused by encroachment of bone on the space. Symptoms are caused by compression of the cauda equina and include pain, paresthesias, and neurogenic claudication. The condition either may be congenital or may be caused by spinal degeneration. See also **spinal cord compression.**

spinal tract, any one of the ascending (sensory) and descending (motor) pathways for sensory or motor nerve impulses that is found in the white matter of the spinal cord.

Twenty-one different tracts lie within the dorsal, ventral, and lateral funiculi of the white substance. Ascending tracts conduct impulses up the spinal cord to the brain; descending tracts conduct impulses down the cord from the brain. The four major ascending tracts are the lateral spinothalamic, the ventral spinothalamic, the fasciculi gracilis and cuneatus, and the spinocerebellar. The four major descending tracts are the lateral corticospinal, the ventral corticospinal, the lateral reticulospinal, and the medial reticulospinal. Touch, pressure, proprioception, temperature, and pain are sensory stimuli transmitted via the spinal tracts. Reflex and voluntary motor activity is regulated by motor nerve stimulation from the brain and brainstem to the motor neurons of the spinal cord.

spinal x-ray studies, radiographic studies of the spine to diagnose degenerative arthritic changes, traumatic fractures, tumor metastasis, spondylosis, spondylolisthesis, and spinal alignment abnormalities.

spin density, a measure of the hydrogen concentration in magnetic resonance (MR) imaging. It is proportional to the number of hydrogen nuclei precessing at the Larmor frequency and contributing to the MR signal. See also **Larmor frequency.**

spindle [AS, *spinel,* to spin], **1.** the fusiform-shaped body of achromatin in the cell nucleus during the late prophase and the metaphase of mitosis. It consists of tiny fibers radiating out from the centrosomes and connecting them with one another. **2.** a type of brain wave, consisting of a short series of changes in electric potential with a frequency of 14 per second. **3.** any one of the special receptor organs comprising the neurotendinous and neuromuscular spindles distributed throughout the body. These kinds of spindles serve as special receptor organs that detect the degree of stretch in a muscle or at the junction of a muscle with its tendon and are essential in maintaining muscle tone.

spindle cell, any of various cells that are shaped like spindles, being more or less round in the middle with two ends that are pointed.

spindle cell carcinoma, a rapidly growing neoplasm composed of fusiform squamous cells.

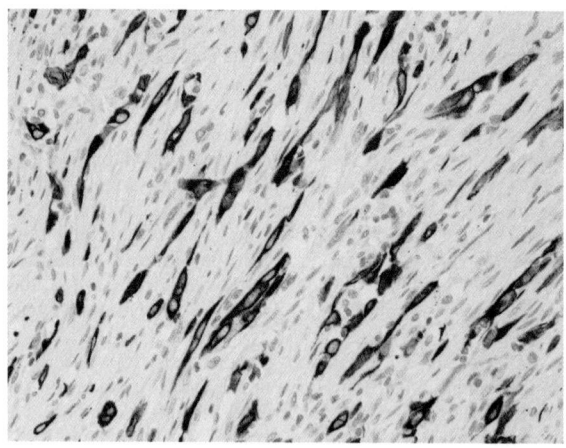

Spindle cell carcinoma *(Fletcher, 2007)*

spindle cell nevus. See **benign juvenile melanoma.**

spine, **1.** the vertebral column, or backbone. **2.** descriptive of a pointed process or prominence, especially on a bone.

spin-echo (SE), a magnetic resonance pulse sequence in which echoes are generated by rephasing spins in the transverse plane using radiofrequency pulses or magnetic field gradients.

spine of scapula [L, *spina,* backbone, *scapulae,* shoulder blades], a sharp-edged plate of bone projecting posteriorly backward from the flattened scapula base.

spin-lattice relaxation time. See **relaxation time.**

spinnbarkeit /spin″bärkīt, shpin″-/ [Ger, threadability], the clear slippery elastic consistency characteristic of cervical mucus during ovulation. The consistency is that of an uncooked egg white, and it is a valuable sign of the peak fertile period in a woman's menstrual cycle. Observation of spinnbarkeit is useful in natural methods of family planning, in the clinical evaluation of infertility, and in discovering the optimal time for artificial insemination. Spinnbarkeit may be evaluated by the length to which a string of mucus can be drawn between the fingers before breaking. See also **ovulation method of family planning.**

spinning top urethra, deformity of the urethra on urination, with narrowing at the urinary meatus and dilation at the proximal end. It is seen sporadically in conditions such as prolonged inflammation of the urethra and detrusor instability. Also called *spinning top deformity.*

spino-, combining form meaning "spine": *spinocerebellar.*

spinocerebellar /spī′nōser′əbel″ər/ [L, *spina + cerebellum,* small brain], pertaining to the spinal cord and the cerebellum.

spinocerebellar disorder, an inherited disorder characterized by a progressive degeneration of the spinal cord and cerebellum, often involving other parts of the nervous system as well. These disorders tend to occur within families and can be inherited as dominant or recessive traits. Onset is usually early, during childhood or adolescence. No effective treatment is known. Kinds include **ataxia-telangiectasia syndrome, Charcot-Marie-Tooth disease, Friedreich ataxia, olivopontocerebellar atrophy, Refsum syndrome.**

spinofallopian tube shunt. See **ventriculofallopian tube shunt.**

spinous /spī″nəs/ [L, *spina,* backbone], pertaining to an object that has the shape of a spine or thorn.

spinous process [L, *spina,* backbone, *processus*], a spinelike projection of bony tissue, such as the spinous process of a vertebra extending posteriorly from a vertebral arch. Also called **spine.**

spin-spin relaxation time. See **relaxation time.**

spinth-, combining form meaning "spark."

spir-, spiro- **1.** combining form meaning "a coil" or "coiled": *spirochete.* **2.** combining form meaning "breath" or "breathing": *spirogram.*

spiral artery. See **screw artery.**

spiral bandage /spī″rəl/ [Gk, *speira,* coil; Fr, *bande,* strip], a roller bandage applied spirally around a limb.

spiral computed tomography. See **helical computed tomography.**

spiral fracture [Gk, *speira,* coil], a bone break that is spiral, oblique, or transverse to the bone's long axis.

spiraling /spī″rəling/, the process by which immunodeficiency allows viral replication, which further depresses the immune system, allowing further viral replication, and so on.

spiral lamina. See **modiolus.**

spiral organ of Corti. See **organ of Corti.**

spiral reverse bandage, a spiral bandage that is turned and folded back on itself as necessary to make it fit the contour of the body more securely.

spirillary rat-bite fever, spirillum fever. See **rat-bite fever.**

spirit /spir″it/ [L, *spiritus,* breath], **1.** any volatile liquid, particularly one that has been distilled. **2.** a volatile substance dissolved in alcohol. See also **volatile.**

spirit of ammonia [L, *spiritus,* breath; *Ammon,* temple in Libya], a solution of 3% ammonium carbonate in alcohol with flavorings added. It is mixed with water for use as a stimulant and carminative.

spirituality, aspects of human thought and behavior that refer to the way individuals and groups seek and express meaning and purpose, particularly in how they relate to religious deities or to sacred or otherworldly matters.

spiritual healing, the use of spiritual practices, such as prayer, for the purpose of effecting a cure of or an improvement in an illness.

spiritual healing and prayer, the offering of prayers to a higher being or authority for the purpose of reducing stress, promoting healing, or arresting disease. Spiritual healing may be practiced by the individual patient, by groups, or by others with or without the patient's knowledge.

spiritual therapy [L, *spiritus,* breath; Gk, *therapeia,* treatment], a form of counseling or psychotherapy that involves moral, spiritual, and religious influences on behavior and physical health; the use of spiritual and religious beliefs and values to strengthen the self.

Spiriva, a bronchodilator. Brand name for **tiotropium.**

Spirochaetales /spī'rō-ke-ta'lēz/, the spirochetes, an order of bacteria in which some species are free-living and some parasitic. It includes the disease-causing genera *Borrelia, Leptospira,* and *Treponema.*

Spirochaeta pallida /spī'rəkē'tə/ [Gk, *speira,* coil, *chaite,* hair; L, *pallidus,* pale], a species of flexible spiral motile microorganisms; the causative agent of human syphilis. Also called *Treponema pallidum.*

spirochete /spī'rəkēt'/ [Gk, *speira,* coil, *chaite,* hair], any bacterium of the genus *Spirochaeta* that is motile and spiral-shaped with flexible filaments. Kinds of spirochetes include the organisms responsible for leptospirosis, relapsing fever, syphilis, and yaws. Also spelled *spirochaete.* Compare ***Bacillus,* coccus, vibrio.**

spirochetemia /spī'rōkətē''mē·ə/ [Gk, *speira,* coil, *chaite* + *haima,* blood], the presence of spirochetal organisms in the blood. See also **spirochete.**

spirogram /spī''rōgram/ [Gk, *speira* + *gramma,* record], a visual record of respiratory movements made by a spirometer, used in the assessment of pulmonary function and capacity.

spirograph /spī'rəgraf/ [Gk, *speira* + *graphein,* to record], a device for recording respiratory movements. See also **spirometer.** −*spirographic, adj.*

spirometer /spīrom''ətər/ [Gk, *speira* + *metron,* measure], an instrument that measures and records the volume of inhaled and exhaled air, used to assess pulmonary function. Volumetric information is recorded on a chart called a spirogram. −*spirometric, adj.*

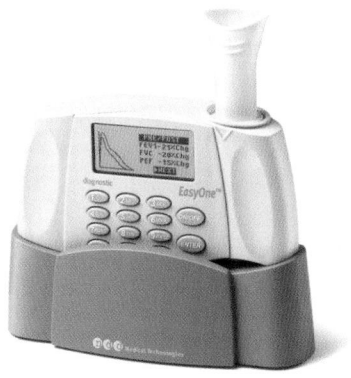

Handheld office spirometer
(Courtesy of Medical Technologies, Inc.)

spirometry /spīrom''ətrē/, laboratory evaluation of the air capacity of the lungs by means of a spirometer. Compare **blood gas determination.** −*spirometric, adj.*

spironolactone /spī'rənəlak''tōn/, a potassium-sparing aldosterone antagonist diuretic.

■ INDICATIONS: It is prescribed in the treatment of primary hyperaldosteronism, edema of congestive heart failure, cirrhosis of the liver accompanied by edema, nephrotic syndrome, essential hypertension, and hypokalemia.

■ CONTRAINDICATIONS: Anuria, acute renal insufficiency, significant impairment of renal function, or hyperkalemia prohibits its use.

■ ADVERSE EFFECTS: Among the most serious adverse effects are hyperkalemia, gynecomastia, mental confusion, ataxia, impotence, amenorrhea, hirsutism, and urticaria.

spittle [AS, *spittan,* spew], saliva.

Spitz nevus. See **benign juvenile melanoma.**

splanchn-. See **splanchno-, splanchn-.**

splanchnic /splangk''nik/. See **visceral.**

-splanchnic, suffix meaning "viscera, entrails": *somatosplanchnic, trisplanchnic.*

splanchnic engorgement, the excessive filling or pooling of blood within the visceral vasculature after the removal of pressure from the abdomen, as in the excision of a large tumor, birth of a child, or drainage of a large quantity of urine from the bladder.

splanchnic nerves [Gk, *splanchna,* viscera, *nervus*], a network of nerves, mainly preganglionic fibers, with filaments innervating the penis and clitoris, as well as the uterus, rectum, and other structures of the abdominal cavity.

splanchno-, splanchn-, prefix meaning "a viscus or splanchnic nerve": *splanchnocele, splanchnopleure.*

splanchnocele /splangk''nōsēl'/ [Gk, *splanchna,* viscera, *kele,* hernia], hernial protrusion of any abdominal viscera. See also **splanchnocoele.**

splanchnocoele /splangk''nōsēl'/ [Gk, *splanchna,* viscera, *koilos,* hollow], a part of the embryonic body cavity, or coelom, that gives rise to the abdominal, pericardial, and pleural cavities. Also called **pleuroperitoneal cavity.**

splanchnopleure /splangk''nōploōr'/ [Gk, *splanchna* + *pleura,* side], a layer of tissue in the early developing embryo, formed by the union of endoderm and splanchnic mesoderm. It gives rise to the embryonic gut and the visceral organs and continues externally to the embryo as the yolk sac and allantois. Compare **somatopleure.** −*splanchnopleural, adj.*

splanchnosomatic reaction. See **viscerosomatic reaction.**

S-plasty /es''plas'tē/, a technique of plastic surgery in which an S-shaped instead of a straight line incision is made to reduce tension and improve healing in areas where the skin is loose.

splay /splā/, **1.** to spread or turn out. **2.** to spread out, as said of the limbs. **3.** to open, as with the end of a tubular structure by making a longitudinal incision. **4.** to dislocate, as said of a bone.

splayfoot [ME, *splaien* + AS, *fot*], a foot that is flat and extremely everted, away from the midline. Also called **talipes valgus.**

spleen [Gk, *splen*], a soft, highly vascular, roughly ovoid organ situated between the stomach and the diaphragm in the left hypochondriac region of the body. It is considered part of the lymphatic system because it contains localized lymphatic nodules. It is dark purple and varies in shape in different individuals and within the same individual at different times. The precise function of the spleen has baffled physiologists for more than 100 years, but research indicates it performs various tasks, such as defense, hemopoiesis, blood storage, and destruction and recycling of red blood cells and platelets. The spleen also produces leukocytes, monocytes, lymphocytes, and plasma cells in response to an infectious agent. It produces red cells before birth and is believed to produce red cells after birth only in extreme and hemolytic anemia. If the body suffers severe hemorrhage, the spleen can contract and increase the blood volume from 350 mL to 550 mL in less than 60 seconds. In the adult the spleen is usually about 12 cm long, 7 cm wide, and 3 cm thick. Its weight increases from 17 g or less in the first year to about 170 g at 20 years of age, then slowly decreases to about 122 g at 75 to 80 years of age. The variation in the weight of adult spleens is 100 to 250 g and, in extreme cases, 50 to 400 g. The size of the spleen increases during and after digestion and often increases during illness. Compare **thymus.** –**splenic,** *adj.*

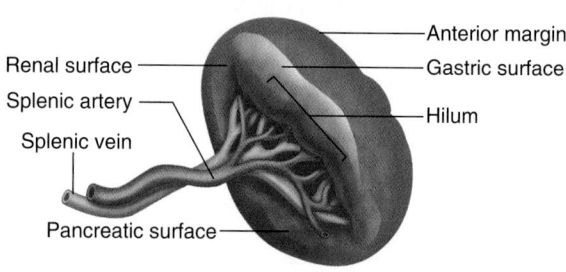

Spleen *(Patton and Thibodeau, 2010)*

spleen scan, a diagnostic scan of the spleen after the injection of radioactive red blood cells, performed to detect a tumor, damage, or other problem.

splen-. See **spleno-, splen-.**

Splendore-Hoeppli phenomenon, the deposition of amorphous, eosinophilic, hyaline material around pathogenic organisms, seen in some fungal and parasitic diseases, as the result of a local antigen-antibody reaction.

splenectomy /splənek″təmē/ [Gk, *splen* + *ektomē,* excision], the surgical removal of the spleen. The spleen is a major phagocytic organ of the reticuloendothelial network and also serves as an important site of antibody production. Infections may follow its removal because the organ plays a vital role in the body's immune system. Splenectomized patients are particularly prone to certain bacterial infections.

-splenia, suffix meaning "condition of the spleen": *asplenia.*

splenic. See **spleen.**

splenic flexure /splen″ik/ [Gk, *splen,* spleen; L, *flectere,* to bend], the left flexure of the colon as it bends at the junction of the transverse and descending segments of the colon, near the spleen.

splenic flexure syndrome [Gk, *splen* + L, *flectere,* to bend], a recurrent pain and abdominal distension in the left upper quadrant of the abdomen caused by a pocket of gas trapped in the large intestine below the spleen, at the flexure of the transverse and descending colon. The symptoms are relieved by defecation or passing of flatus.

splenic gland. See **pancreaticolienal node.**

splenic puncture, a perforation of the parenchyma of the spleen to obtain pressure data or to inject radiopaque material.

splenic vein. See **lienal vein.**

splenius capitis /splē″nē·əs/ [Gk, *splenion,* bandage; L, *caput,* head], one of a pair of deep muscles of the neck and back. Arising from the nuchal ligament, the seventh cervical

vertebra, and the first three or four thoracic vertebrae, it inserts in the occipital bone and the mastoid process of the temporal bone. It acts to rotate, extend, and bend the head.

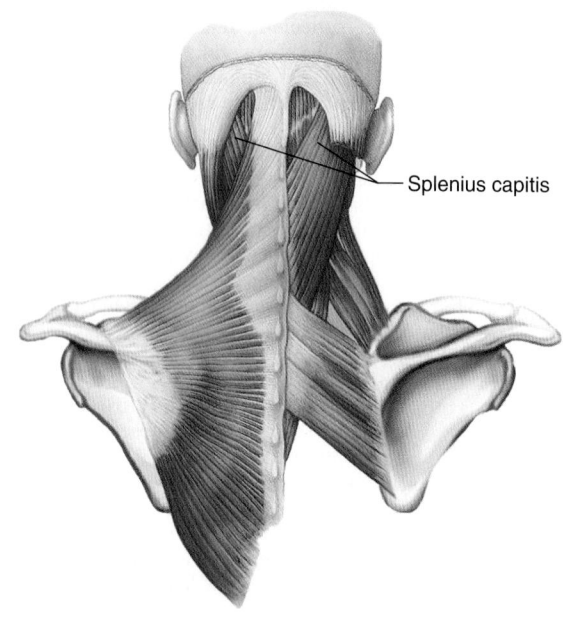

Splenius capitis muscle *(Patton and Thibodeau, 2010)*

splenius cervicis, one of a pair of deep muscles of the neck and back. Arising from a narrow tendinous band from the spinous processes of the third through the sixth thoracic vertebrae, it inserts into the transverse processes of the upper two or three cervical vertebrae. The muscle is innervated by the lateral branches of the dorsal primary divisions of the middle and the lower cervical nerves. The splenius cervicis acts to rotate, bend, and extend the head and neck. Also called *splenius colli.*

spleno-, splen-, combining form meaning "spleen": *splenohepatomegaly, splenomegaly, splenosis.*

splenohepatomegaly /splē′nōhep′ətōmeg″əlē/ [Gk, *splen,* spleen, *hepar,* liver, *megas,* great], an abnormal simultaneous increase in the sizes of the liver and spleen.

splenomedullary leukemia. See **acute myeloid leukemia, chronic myelocytic leukemia.**

splenomegaly /splē′nōmeg″əlē, splen′-/ [Gk, *splen* + *megas,* large], an abnormal enlargement of the spleen, as is associated with portal hypertension, hemolytic anemia, Niemann-Pick disease, or malaria.

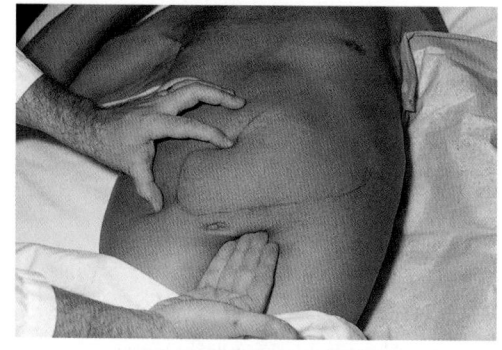

Splenomegaly *(Swartz, 2009)*

splenomyelogenous leukemia. *(Obsolete)* See **acute myeloid leukemia, chronic myelocytic leukemia.**

splenorenal bypass,   a technique of renal revascularization involving creation of a vascular prosthesis from the splenic artery to replace the occluded renal artery.

splenosis /splēnō″sis/,   multiple splenic growths in the peritoneum resulting from splenic rupture or iatrogenic injury.

splint [D, *splinte,* piece of wood],   **1.** *(Obsolete)* (in occupational and physical therapy) now called **orthosis. 2.** (in dentistry) a device, usually made of hard acrylic and wire, for anchoring the teeth or modifying the bite. Compare **brace. 3.** *(Informal)* an external device for immobilization, restraint, or support.

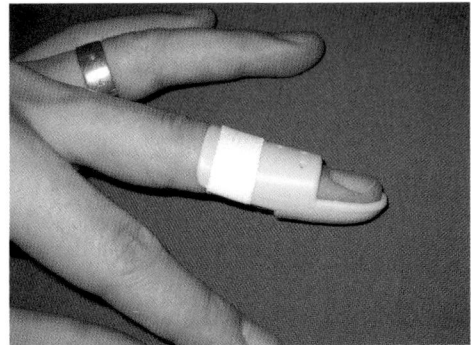

Finger splint *(Miller et al, 2009)*

splinter [D, *splinte*],   a sharp, pointed piece of bone or other substance.

splinter fracture [D, *splinte*],   a comminuted fracture with thin, sharp bone fragments.

splinter hemorrhage,   linear bleeding under a fingernail or toenail, resembling a splinter. It is seen after trauma and in bacterial endocarditis. Also spelled *splinter haemorrhage.*

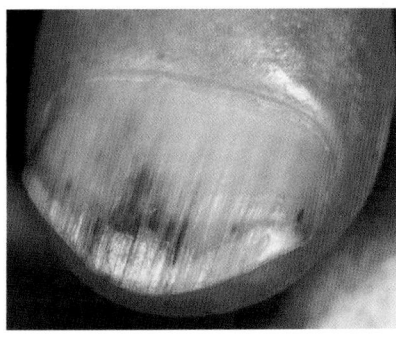

Splinter hemorrhage *(Hordinsky, Sawaya, and Scher, 2000)*

splinter skill,   **1.** (in occupational therapy) the ability to do a specific task that does not generalize to other tasks. **2.** a specific task mastered by a client who lacks the underlying capabilities to perform it; the mastery is usually attained through compensatory methods and practice of the specific task (i.e., walking on a balance board) rather than by remediating the underlying factors.

splinting,   the process of applying a rigid or flexible device (splint or orthosis) to maintain or increase the length of soft tissues, correct biomechanical misalignment, restore muscles to normal resting length, and protect joint integrity. Splinting can be used to position the hand and other body parts to assist in functional activities, promote independence, compensate for weaknesses, and enhance functional positions.

split-brain state,   a condition resulting from the disconnection of the two cerebral hemispheres. It is produced when the corpus callosum is surgically divided completely or partially as a treatment for epilepsy or in congenital absence of corpus callosum. The cognitive effects are identified as a disconnection syndrome.

split gene [D, *splitten,* to split],   a gene whose continuity is interrupted.

split-hand deformity.   See **cleft hand.**

split personality.   See **dissociative identity disorder.**

split Russell traction,   an orthopedic mechanism that combines suspension and traction to immobilize, position, and align the lower extremities in the correction of orthopedic deformities and in the treatment of congenital hip dislocation and hip and knee contractures. Usually applied as adhesive or nonadhesive skin traction, split Russell traction uses a sling to relieve the weight of the lower extremities. The traction weights are suspended from pulley-and-rope systems at the foot and head of the patient's bed. A jacket restraint is often incorporated to help immobilize the patient. Split Russell traction may be applied unilaterally or bilaterally. Compare **Russell traction.**

split-thickness skin graft,   a tissue transplant involving the epidermis and a part of the dermis. This type of graft is the most commonly used method of covering open burn wounds. Also called *split-skin graft.*

split-thickness transplant.   See **deep lamellar endothelial keratoplasty.**

splitting,   a primitive defense mechanism that when overused represents a developmental arrest. It is a failure to synthesize the positive and negative experiences and ideas one has of oneself, other people, situations, and institutions.

spodo-,   combining form meaning "waste materials": *spodogenous.*

spodogenous /spo-doj′ĕ-nus/ [Gk, *spodos,* waste, *gen* producing],   pertaining to an accumulation of waste material in an organ.

spondyl-,   combining form meaning "a physiological condition or change of the vertebrae": *spondylopathy.*

-spondylic /spondil″ik/,   combining form meaning "vertebrae."

spondylitic [Gk, *sphondylos,* vertebra],   pertaining to a person afflicted with spondylitis.

spondylitis /spon′dəlī″tis/ [Gk, *sphondylos,* vertebra, *itis*],   an inflammation of any of the vertebrae, usually characterized by stiffness and pain. The condition may be the result of traumatic injury to the spine, infection, or rheumatoid disease. See also **ankylosing spondylitis. – spondylitic,** *adj.*

spondylitis ankylopoietica.   See **Strümpell-Marie disease.**

spondylo-,   combining form meaning "vertebra" or "the spinal column": *spondylolisthesis, spondylosis, spondylosyndesis.*

spondyloarthropathy /spon′dilō″ärthrop″əthē/,   any of a set of diseases of the joints and spine. Most commonly affected are the lower extremities, sacroiliac joint, and hip. Pain and restricted motion of the hips and lower back are typical complaints. Many patients also experience eye disorders.

spondylolisthesis /spon′dilō′listhē″sis/ [Gk, *sphondylos + olisthanein,* to slip],   the partial forward dislocation of one vertebra over the one below it, most commonly the fifth lumbar vertebra over the first sacral vertebra. Severity of spondylolisthesis is classified by percentage of slip. See also **spinal cord compression.**

S

spondylosis /spon′dilō″sis/ [Gk, *sphondylos* + *osis*], a condition of the spine characterized by fixation or stiffness of a vertebral joint. See also **ankylosing spondylitis, spondylitis.**

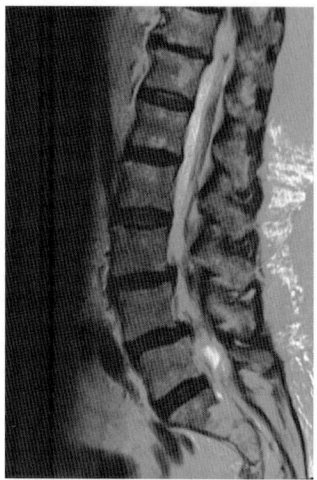

Spondylosis *(Moll, 1997)*

spondylosyndesis. See **spinal fusion.**

spondylothoracic dysplasia. See **Jarcho-Levin syndrome.**

spondylous /spon″diləs/ [Gk, *sphondylos,* vertebra], pertaining to a vertebra.

sponge /spunj/ [Gk, *spongia*], **1.** a resilient absorbent mass used to absorb fluids, to apply medication, or to cleanse. The sponge may be the internal skeleton of a certain marine animal, or it may be manufactured from cellulose, rubber, or synthetic material. **2.** *(Informal)* a folded gauze square used in surgery.

sponge bath, the procedure of washing the patient with a damp washcloth or sponge; it is used when a full bath is unnecessary.

sponge gold. See **mat gold.**

spongio-, combining form meaning "like a sponge" or "related to a sponge": *spongioblastoma, spongiocytoma, spongiositis.*

spongioblastoma /spun′jē-ōblastō″mə/ *pl. spongioblastomas, spongioblastomata* [Gk, *spongia* + *blastos,* germ, *oma,* tumor], a neoplasm composed of spongioblasts, embryonic epithelial cells that develop around the neural tube and transform into cells of the supporting connective tissue of nerve cells or cells of lining membranes of the ventricles and the spinal cord canal. Also called **glioblastoma, gliosarcoma, spongiocytoma.**

spongioblastoma multiforme. See **glioblastoma multiforme.**

spongioblastomas, spongioblastomata. See **spongioblastoma.**

spongioblastoma unipolare, a rare neoplasm composed of parallel spongioblasts. The tumor may occur near the third ventricle, in the pons and brainstem, in basal ganglia, or in the terminal filament of the spinal cord.

spongiocytoma. See **spongioblastoma.**

spongiositis. See **periurethritis.**

spongy /spun″jē/ [Gk, *spoggia*], pertaining to or resembling a sponge.

spongy bone. See **cancellous bone.**

spontaneity, the quality of being natural rather than planned; driven by internal forces.

spontaneous /spontā″nē·əs/ [L, *sponte,* willingly], occurring naturally and without apparent cause, such as spontaneous remission.

spontaneous abortion, a termination of pregnancy before the twentieth week of gestation as a result of abnormalities of the conceptus or maternal environment. Up to 30% of pregnancies may end as spontaneous abortions, many caused by blighted ova that have congenital defects incompatible with life. Also called **miscarriage.** Compare **induced abortion.**

spontaneous delivery, a vaginal birth occurring without the mechanical assistance of obstetric forceps or vacuum aspirator.

spontaneous evolution. See **spontaneous version.**

spontaneous fracture, a fracture that occurs without trauma as a result of bone weakness caused by osteoporosis or by a benign or malignant tumor. Also called **neoplastic fracture, pathological fracture.**

spontaneous generation. See **abiogenesis.**

spontaneous labor, a labor beginning and progressing without mechanical or pharmacological stimulation.

spontaneous PEEP (sPEEP), positive airway pressure applied at the end of the exhalation phase during spontaneous breathing.

spontaneous phagocytosis [L, *sponte,* free will; Gk, *phagein,* to eat, *kytos,* cell, *osis,* condition], ingestion of antigenic particles by phagocytes of the reticuloendothelial system.

spontaneous pneumothorax [L, *sponte,* free will; Gk, *pneuma,* air, *thorax,* chest], the presence of air or gas in the pleural space as a result of a rupture of the lung parenchyma and visceral pleura with no demonstrable cause.

spontaneous remission, 1. the reversal of progress of disease without formal treatment. **2.** the disappearance of symptoms of a mentally ill patient without formal treatment.

spontaneous ventilation, normal, unassisted breathing in which the patient creates the pressure gradient through muscular movements that move air into and out of the lungs.

spontaneous version [L, *sponte,* free will, *vertere,* to turn], a change in the lie of a fetus that occurs without manipulation. Also called **spontaneous evolution.**

spoon nail [AS, *spon* + *naegel*], a nail of the finger or toe that has a thin and concave outer surface.

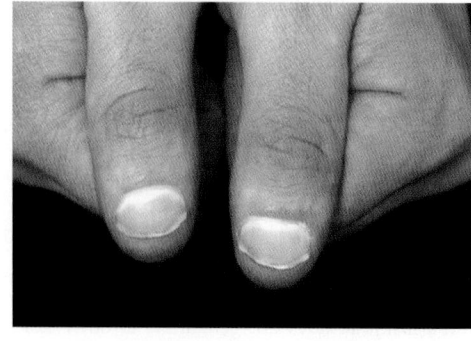

Spoon nails *(Carey, 2010)*

spor-. See **sporo-, spor-.**

sporadic /spôrat″ik/ [Gk, *sporaden,* scattered], (of a number of events) occurring at scattered, intermittent, and apparently random intervals.

-sporangium, combining form meaning "an encasement of spores."

spore [Gk, *sporos,* seed],   **1.** a reproductive unit of some genera of fungi or protozoa. **2.** a form assumed by some bacteria that is resistant to heat, drying, and chemicals. Under proper environmental conditions the spore may revert to the actively multiplying form of the bacterium. Diseases caused by spore-forming bacteria include anthrax, botulism, gas gangrene, and tetanus.

-spore,   combining form meaning "a reproductive element": *azygospore, zygospore.*

sporicidal /spôr´isī´dəl/ [Gk, *sporos,* seed; L, *caedere,* to kill],   spore-killing, as are certain chemicals or other agents.

sporicide /spôr´isīd/ [Gk, *sporos* + L, *caedere,* to kill],   any agent effective in destroying spores, such as compounds of chlorine and formaldehyde and the glutaraldehydes.

sporiferous /spôrif´ərəs/,   producing or bearing spores.

spork,   a spoonlike food utensil with fork tines; it can be used as a spoon or a fork. It is useful for individuals with grip- or strength-related challenges in the upper extremities.

sporo-, spor-,   combining form meaning "spore": *sporocyst, sporogenesis, sporogeny.*

sporoblast /spôr´əblast´/ [Gk, *sporos* + *blastos,* germ],   any cell that gives rise to a sporozoite or spore during the sexual reproductive phase of the life cycle of a sporozoon. It refers specifically to the cells resulting from the multiple fission of the encysted zygote of the malarial parasite *Plasmodium,* from which the sporozoites develop.

sporocyst /spôr´əsist/ [Gk, *sporos* + *kystis,* bag],   **1.** any structure containing spores or reproductive cells. **2.** a saclike structure, or oocyst, secreted by the zygote of certain protists before sporozoite formation. **3.** the second larval stage in the life cycle of parasitic flukes. The saclike organism develops from the miracidium, or first larval stage, in the body of a freshwater snail host and contains germinal cells that give rise either to daughter sporocysts that develop into cercariae or to rediae. See also **fluke.**

sporogenesis /spôr´ōjen´əsis/ [Gk, *sporos* + *genesis,* origin],   **1.** the formation of spores. Also called **sporogeny.** **2.** reproduction by means of spores. −*sporogenic, adj.*

sporogenous /spôroj´ənəs/ [Gk, *sporos* + *genein,* to produce],   describing an animal or plant that produces spores or reproduces by way of spores.

sporogeny.   See **sporogenesis.**

sporogony /spôrog´ənē/ [Gk, *sporos* + *genesis,* origin],   reproduction by means of spores. It refers specifically to the formation of sporozoites during the sexual stage of the life cycle of a sporozoon, primarily the malarial parasite *Plasmodium.* Fusion of the sex cells occurs in the body of the invertebrate host, the female *Anopheles* mosquito in the case of *Plasmodium,* where the encysted zygote undergoes multiple division, giving rise to the sporozoites. Compare **schizogony.**

sporont /spôr´ont/ [Gk, *sporos* + *on,* being],   a mature protozoan parasite in the sexual reproductive stage of its life cycle. It undergoes conjugation to form a zygote, which produces sporozoites by multiple fission. Compare **schizont.** See also **sporogony.**

sporonticide /spôron´tisīd/ [Gk, *sporos* + *on* + L, *caedere,* to kill],   any substance that destroys sporonts, such as chloroquine and other antimalarial drugs. −*sporonticidal, adj.*

sporophore /spôr´əfôr/ [Gk, *sporos* + *pherein,* to bear],   the part of an organism that produces spores.

sporophyte /spôr´əfīt/ [Gk, *sporos* + *phyton,* plant],   the asexual, spore-bearing stage in organisms that reproduce by alternation of generations.

sporotrichosis /spôr´ōtrikō´sis/ [Gk, *sporos* + *thrix,* hair, *osis,* condition],   a common chronic fungal infection caused by the species *Sporothrix schenckii.* It is usually characterized by skin ulcers and subcutaneous nodules along lymphatic channels. It rarely spreads to involve bones, lungs, joints, or muscles. The most severe symptoms are observed in patients with AIDS. The fungus is found in soil and decaying vegetation and usually enters the skin by accidental injury. Outbreaks have occurred in workers at plant nurseries. Treatment may include amphotericin B in severe cases or itraconazole.

Sporotrichum /spôrot´rikəm/ [Gk, *sporos* + *thrix,* hair],   a genus of soil-inhabiting fungi formerly thought to cause sporotrichosis.

Sporozoa /spôr´əzō´ə/ [Gk, *sporos* + *zoon,* animal],   a class of parasite in the phylum Protozoa that is characterized by the absence of any external organs of locomotion. Included in this class are the genera *Toxoplasma* and *Plasmodium.*

sporozoite /spôr´əzō´īt/ [Gk, *sporos* + *zoon,* animal],   any of the cells resulting from the sexual union of spores during the life cycle of a sporozoon. It refers specifically to the elongated nucleated cells produced by the multiple fission of the zygote contained in the oocyst in the female *Anopheles* mosquito during the sexual reproductive stage of the life cycle of the malarial parasite *Plasmodium.* On release from the oocyst, the sporozoites migrate to the salivary glands of the mosquito, where they are transmitted to humans and develop within the parenchymal cells of the liver as merozoites. Also called **falciform body.** See also **malaria,** *Plasmodium.*

sport [ME, *disporten,* to amuse],   **1.** an individual that differs drastically from its parents or others of its type because of genetic mutation; a mutant. **2.** a genetic mutation. **3.** See **lusus naturae.**

sports medicine,   a branch of medicine that specializes in the prevention and treatment of injuries resulting from training for and participation in athletic events. More than 1 million people are treated for sports injuries each year in the United States. Most sports injuries involve muscle sprains, strains, and tears, which frequently result from inadequate preliminary "warm-up" exercises. Among the most common sports injuries are shin splints, runner's knee, pulled hamstring muscles, Achilles tendonitis, ankle sprain, arch sprain, charley horse, tennis elbow, baseball finger, dislocations, muscle cramps, bursitis, myofascitis, costochondritis, hernia, and "Little League elbow."

sporulation /spôr´yəlā´shən/ [Gk, *sporos* + L, *atus,* process],   **1.** a type of reproduction that occurs in fungi, algae, and protozoa and involves the formation of spores by the spontaneous division of a cell into four or more daughter cells, each of which contains a part of the original nucleus. **2.** the formation of a refractile body, or resting spore, within certain bacteria that makes the cell resistant to unfavorable environmental conditions. The cell regains its viability when conditions become favorable. See also **spore.**

spot [ME, *blot*],   (in psychotherapy) a small quantum of space that becomes the territorial object and extension of point behavior.

spot film,   a radiograph made instantly during fluoroscopy. The technique may be used to make a permanent record of a transient effect or to record with definition and detail a small anatomical area.

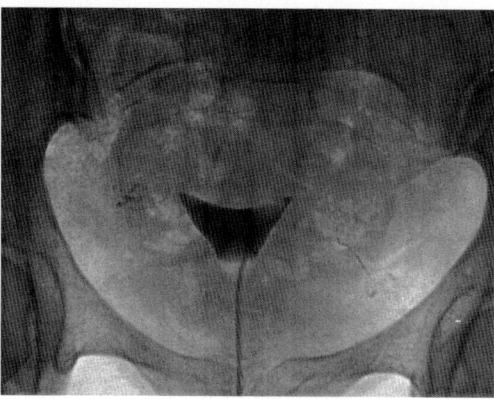

Spot film of contrast media being injected into the uterine cavity *(Bontrager and Lampignano, 2010)*

spotted fever. See **Rocky Mountain spotted fever.**

spotting [ME, *spot,* blot], the appearance of a blood-stained discharge from the vagina between menstrual periods, during pregnancy, or at the beginning of labor.

sprain, a traumatic injury to the tendons, muscles, or ligaments around a joint, characterized by pain, swelling, and discoloration of the skin over the joint. The duration and severity of the symptoms vary with the extent of damage to the tissues. Treatment includes support, rest, and alternating cold and heat. Ultrasound therapy may speed recovery. Radiographic images are often indicated to rule out fractures.

sprain fracture, a fracture that results from the separation of a tendon or ligament at the point of insertion and is associated with the separation of a bone at the same insertion site. Also called **avulsion fracture.**

sprain of ankle or foot [AS, *ancleow* + *fot*], a sudden traction injury to a muscle, ligament, or capsule in the ankle or foot. The injury is not severe enough to cause a rupture of the tissue.

sprain of back [AS, *baec*], a sudden traction injury to muscles and related tissues of the back. The tissues may have undergone traumatic strain without being ruptured.

spreader bar /spred″ər/, a metal bar with curved hoop areas for attaching hooks or pins for traction.

spreadsheet /spred″shēt/, a computer program that simulates a business or scientific worksheet and performs the necessary calculations when data are entered or changed.

Sprengel's deformity /shpreng′gəlz/ [Otto Gerhard Karl Sprengel, German surgeon, 1852–1915], congenital elevation of the scapula resulting from failure of descent of the scapula to its normal thoracic position during fetal life.

spring /spring/ [AS, *springan,* to jump], **1.** a piece of resilient metal, such as a hardened coiled steel wire, that will return to its original shape after bending. **2.** a resilient wire attached to a denture or other appliance.

spring forceps [AS, *springan,* to jump], a kind of forceps that includes a spring mechanism. The forceps are tweezerlike and vary in thickness. With teeth, they can grasp delicate tissue. Without teeth, they can hold thick or slippery tissue. Also called **bulldog forceps.**

spring lancet, a very small knife with a spring-triggered blade. It may be used for collecting small specimens of blood for laboratory tests. See also **lancet.**

sprinter's fracture [Swe, *sprinta,* to spurt; L, *fractura,* to break], a break in the anterior superior or anterior inferior spine of the ilium, caused when the bone is forcibly pulled by a violent muscle spasm.

sprue /sprōō/ [D, *sprouw,* kind of tumor], a chronic degenerative disorder resulting from malabsorption of nutrients from the small intestine and characterized by a broad range of symptoms, including diarrhea; weakness; weight loss; poor appetite; pallor; muscle cramps; bone pain; ulceration of the mucous membrane lining the digestive tract; and a smooth, shiny tongue. It occurs in both tropical and nontropical forms and affects both children and adults. Also called **catarrhal dysentery.** See also **celiac disease, malabsorption syndrome, nontropical sprue, tropical sprue.**

Sprycel, a chemotherapeutic agent. Brand name for **dasatinib.**

SPSS (Statistical Package for the Social Sciences), (in statistics) a computer program often used in research for the analysis of complex data from large samples.

spur [AS, *spura*], a projection of bone from a body structure or of metal from an appliance. See also **exostosis.**

spurious pregnancy. See **pseudocyesis.**

sputum /spyōō″təm/ [L, spittle], material coughed up from the lungs and expectorated through the mouth. It contains mucus, cellular debris, or microorganisms, and it also may contain blood or pus. The amount, color, and constituents of the sputum are important in the diagnosis of many illnesses, including tuberculosis, pneumonia, cancer of the lung, and the pneumoconioses.

sputum collection trap, a plastic trap connected to a suction catheter. Sputum specimens can be contained in the trap and sent for analysis.

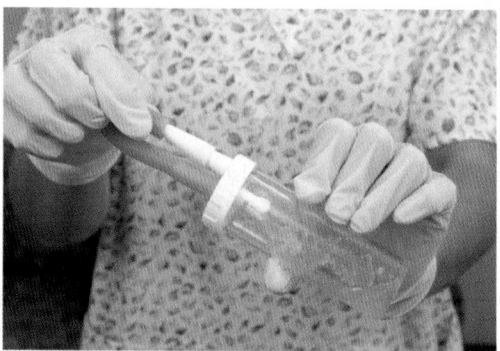

Sputum collection trap *(Perry, Potter, and Elkin, 2012)*

sputum culture and sensitivity test, a test for pathogenic bacteria in the sputum of patients with respiratory infections.

sputum cytology, a sputum test to determine the presence of a pulmonary system malignancy. It is used most frequently in patients who have an abnormal chest x-ray, productive cough, and nothing visible on bronchoscopy. A positive test indicates malignancy, but a negative test means only that, if a tumor exists, it is not shedding cells.

sputum specimen [L, spittle + *specere,* to look], a sample of material expelled from the respiratory passages taken for laboratory analysis to determine the presence of pathogens.

squam-, combining form meaning "scales": *squamous, squamocolumnar junction.*

squama /skwā″mə/ *pl. squamae,* **1.** a flattened scale from the epidermis. **2.** the thin, expanded part of a bone, especially in the cranial wall.

squamocolumnar junction /skwā′mōkəlum″nər/, a region of transition from stratified squamous epithelium to columnar epithelium in the cervical canal. It is a location where cells are obtained for Papanicolaou (Pap) smears.

squamous /skwā″məs/ [L, *squama,* scale], platelike, scaly, or covered with scales.

squamous blepharitis, a kind of nonulcerative blepharitis in which the edge of the eyelid is covered with small white or gray scales.

squamous cell [L, *squama*, scale, *cella*, storeroom], a flat, scalelike epithelial cell.

squamous cell carcinoma, a slow-growing malignant tumor of squamous epithelium, frequently found in the lungs and skin and occurring also in the anus, cervix, larynx, nose, and bladder. The neoplastic cells characteristically resemble prickle cells and form keratin pearls. Although oral cancer is rare (less than 3% of all cancers), 94% of oral malignancies are squamous cell carcinoma. It may appear as a keratotic plaque; a crusted or noncrusted ulcer; a slightly raised lesion with central ulceration and a rolled border; a red, white or red/white combination velvety area; invasive or burrowing into oral tissues; or a verruciform (multilobulated) growth. The most common intraoral site is the tongue, followed in descending frequency by the soft palate, gingiva, buccal mucosa, labial mucosa, and the hard palate. Lesions may metastasize through the lymph nodes. Treatment and prognosis varies according to site, size, and stage of disease progression. Early diagnosis and treatment are essential to increase survival rates. Also called **epidermoid carcinoma.**

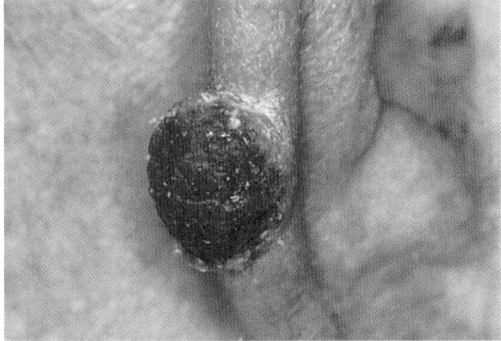

Squamous cell carcinoma *(Courtesy Department of Dermatology, School of Medicine, University of Utah)*

squamous epithelium [L, *squama*, scale; Gk, *epi*, above, *thele*, nipple], a sheet of flattened scalelike cells attached together at the edges. Also called **pavement epithelium.**

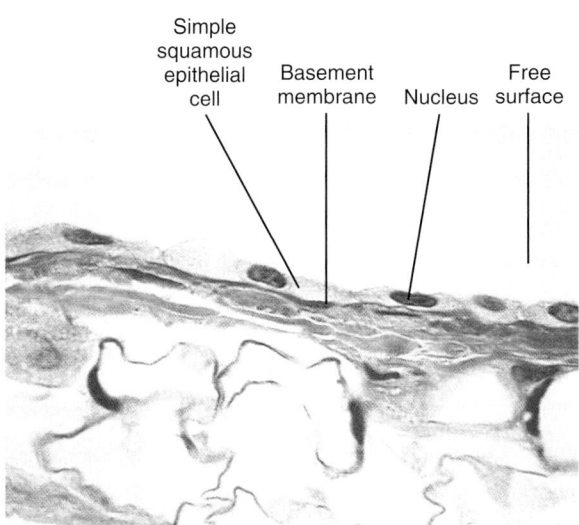

Simple squamous epithelial cell   Basement membrane   Nucleus   Free surface

Simple squamous epithelium *(© Ed Reschke. Used with permission)*

simple squamous epithelium, squamous epithelium having only one layer, such as in endothelium, mesothelium, and pulmonary alveoli. Also called **pavement epithelium.**

squamous epithelium stratified, epithelium, such as that of typical skin, having a basal layer of cuboidal cells and overlying layers of squamous cells.

square centimeter (cm²) /skwer/, a unit of area measurement equivalent to 1 centimeter in length multiplied by 1 centimeter in width, where one centimeter equals 0.3937 inch or 0.03281 foot.

square window [OFr, *esquarre* + ME, *wind*, air, *owe*, eye], an angle of the wrist between the hypothenar prominence and forearm. It is used as a reference point for estimating the gestational age of a newborn.

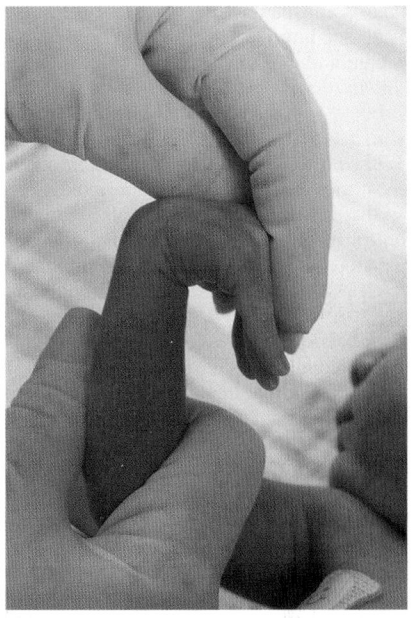

Square window test *(Murray and McKinney, 2006)*

squatting position /skwot″ing/ [Fr, *esquatir*, to press down], a posture in which the knees and hips are flexed and the buttocks are lowered to the level of the heels. It is adopted by children with certain heart diseases as they seek relief from exercise distress.

squeeze dynamometer /skwēz/ [AS, *cwesan*, to press tightly; Gk, *dynamis*, force, *metron*, measure], a device for measuring the muscular strength of the grip of the hand. See also **dynamometer.**

squeeze-film lubrication, the exudation of fluid from the cartilage of joints, forming a film in the transient area of impending contact.

squint. See **strabismus.**

squinting eye /skwin″ting/ [D, *schuinte*, oblique; AS, *eage*], the abnormal eye in a person with strabismus that is not aligned with the fixating eye. See also **strabismus.**

Sr, symbol for the element **strontium.**

SR, abbreviation for **sedimentation rate.**

sRNA, abbreviation for *soluble ribonucleic acid.*

SRO, abbreviation for **single room occupant.**

SRS-A, abbreviation for **slow-reacting substance of anaphylaxis.**

SRY, symbol for a "maleness" gene found on the sex-determining region of the Y chromosome. The gene is believed to function as a master control switch that can turn off or on other genes involved in sexual development.

S

ss, abbreviation for **steady state.**

SSE, 1. abbreviation for **skin self-examination. 2.** abbreviation for **soapsuds enema.**

SSKI, an expectorant. Brand name for **potassium iodide.**

SSRI, abbreviation for **selective serotonin reuptake inhibitor.**

SSS, 1. abbreviation for *sterile saline soak.* **2.** abbreviation for **sick sinus syndrome.**

SSSS, abbreviation for **staphylococcal scalded skin syndrome.**

ST, abbreviation for *slow-twitch.* See **slow-twitch (ST) fiber.**

stab [ME, *stabbe,* piercing wound], a neutrophilic band.

stab culture [ME, *stabbe,* piercing wound; L, *colere,* to cultivate], a culture made by dipping a needle into an inoculum and then into a transparent gelatin or agar medium.

stab form. See **band.**

-stabile, combining form meaning "stable, resistant to change": *tempostabile.*

stabile diabetes. See **type 2 diabetes mellitus.**

stabilization /stab′ilīzā″shən/ [L, *stabilis,* firm, *atus,* process], **1.** the physiological and metabolic process of attaining homeostasis. **2.** the seating of a fixed or removable denture so that it will not tilt or be displaced under pressure. **3.** the control of induced stress loads and the development of measures to counteract such forces so that the movement of the teeth or of a prosthesis does not irritate surrounding tissues.

stabilization exercises, exercises to develop proximal control in symptom (pain)-free positions, such as sitting on a gymnastic ball and extending one knee to maintain balance and control without pain.

stable /stā″bəl/ [L, *stabilis,* firm], remaining unchanged.

stable angina, angina pectoris in which attacks occur with predictable frequency and duration and are precipitated by circumstances such as exercise or emotional stress that increase myocardial oxygen demands. The same circumstances tend to cause the attacks from one episode to another.

stable condition, a state of health or disease from which little if any immediate change is expected.

stable element [L, *stabilis,* firm, *elementum*], a nonradioactive element, one not subject to spontaneous nuclear degeneration. Compare **radioactive element.** Kinds include **calcium, iron, lead, potassium, sodium.** See also **element.**

staccato speech /stəkä″tō/ [It, detached; ME, *speche*], abnormal speech in which the person pauses between words, breaking the rhythm of the phrase or sentence. The condition is sometimes observed in association with multiple sclerosis.

stadium /stā′dē·əm/ *pl. stadia* [Gk, *stadion,* racetrack], a significant stage in a fever or illness, such as the fastigium of a febrile illness or the prodromal stage of a viral infection.

Stadol, an opioid analgesic. Brand name for **butorphanol tartrate.**

staff [AS, *staef*], **1.** the people who work toward a common goal and are employed or supervised by someone of higher rank, such as the nurses in a hospital. **2.** a designation by which a staff nurse is distinguished from a nurse manager or other nurse. **3.** (in nursing service administration) the units of the organization that provide service to the line, or administratively defined hierarchy. For example, the personnel office is staff to the chief nurse executive and the nursing service administration.

staff development, a process that assists individuals in an agency or organization in attaining new skills and knowledge, gaining increasing levels of competence, and growing professionally. Various resources outside the agency employing the individuals may be used. The process may include such programs as orientation, in-service education, and continuing education.

staffing, the process of assigning people to fill the roles designed for an organizational structure through recruitment, selection, and placement.

staffing pattern, (in hospital or nursing administration) the number and types or categories of staff assigned to the particular units and departments of a hospital or other health care facility. Staffing patterns vary with the unit, department, and shift and with the patient acuity levels.

staff of Aesculapius, a staff carried by Aesculapius, the Greek god of medicine. It is used as the traditional symbol of the physician. A single serpent entwines the staff of Aesculapius. It is often confused with the caduceus, a staff with two serpents (which is the staff of Hermes, the Greek god of commerce and travel) symbolizing (because of this misunderstanding) the U.S. Army Medical Corps. See also **Aesculapius.**

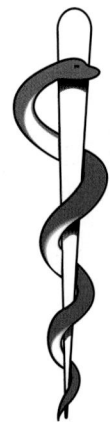

Staff of Aesculapius *(Mosby, 2003)*

stage [OFr, *estage*], **1.** a platform. **2.** a period or phase.

stages of anesthesia, a system for describing the stages and planes of anesthesia based on physical signs observed in the patient. These stages are most applicable to inhalation anesthesia and are difficult to delineate when combination or modern anesthetics are given. Also called **Guedel signs.** See also **anesthesia.**

stages of dying [OFr, *estage,* stage; ME, *dyen,* to lose life], the five emotional and behavioral stages that may occur after a person or family first learns of approaching death. The stages, identified and described by Elisabeth Kübler-Ross, are denial and shock, anger, bargaining, depression, and acceptance. The stages may occur in sequence or they may recur, as the person moves forward and backward—especially among denial, anger, and bargaining. Caring for a dying person requires sensitivity to the signs of each stage. At first, shock may be accompanied by signs of panic. The person may refuse care and deny the diagnosis and prognosis. Denial serves as a defense against the shock. Anger often follows this stage. It is characterized by abusive language, refusal to perform basic self-care responsibilities, negative criticism of anyone who wants to help, and other kinds of angry behavior. The third stage, bargaining, reflects the need of the person for time to accept the situation. A common observation of this period is the patient's attempt to make a bargain, "If I could live until Christmas …" Commonly, the person goes back and forth from anger to bargaining: sometimes silent, sometimes grieving, and sometimes apathetic, depressed, insomniac, and distant. The fourth stage is a time of depression in which the person goes through a period of grieving before death, mourning over past experiences and anticipating impending losses. The final stage, acceptance, is one of inner peace and resolution that death is a certainty. The person may show his or her acceptance by being uninterested in present or future events, being preoccupied with past events, preferring to have few visitors, and wanting quiet and solitude. Nursing care includes administering adequate pain relief, ensuring privacy and dignity, and giving sensitive, honest emotional support to both patient and family. See also **emotional care of the dying patient, hospice.**

staging /stā″jing/, the classification of phases, quantity, or periods of a disease or other pathological process, as in the TMN clinical method of assigning numerical values to various stages of tumor development.

stagnant anoxia /stag″nənt/ [L, *stagnum*, standing water; Gk, *a*, without, *oxys*, sharp, *genein*, to produce], a condition in which there is inadequate blood flow in the capillaries, causing low tissue oxygen tension and reduced oxygen exchange. The condition is associated with shock, cardiac standstill, and thrombosis.

stain [OFr, *desteindre*, to dye], **1.** *n.*, a pigment, dye, or substance used to impart color to microscopic objects or tissues to facilitate their examination and identification. Kinds include **acid-fast stain, Gram stain, Wright stain. 2.** *v.*, to apply pigment to a substance or tissue to examine it under a microscope. **3.** *n.*, an area of discoloration.

stalk /stôk/, an elongated, more or less slender anatomical structure resembling the stem of a plant. See also **peduncle, pedunculus.**

-stalsis, suffix meaning "a contraction in the alimentary canal": *peristalsis, hyperperistalsis.*

stammering [AS, *stamerian*, to stutter], a speech dysfunction characterized by pauses, hesitations, and faltering utterances. The term is not commonly used in clinical practice the United States but is frequently used synonymously with stuttering in Great Britain.

stamp cusp [ME, *stampen* + L, *cuspis*, point], a tooth cusp that works in a fossa, such as any of the maxillary lingual cusps.

stance phase of gait [L, *stare*, to stand; Gk, *phainein*, to show; ME, *gate*, a way], the phase of the normal gait cycle that begins with the strike of the heel on the ground and ends with the lift of the toe at the beginning of the swing phase of gait.

standard [OFr, *estandart*], **1.** *n.*, an evaluation that serves as a basis for comparison for evaluating similar phenomena or substances, such as a standard for the preparation of a pharmaceutic substance or a standard for the practice of a profession. **2.** *n.*, a pharmaceutic preparation or a chemical substance of known quantity, ingredients, and strength that is used to determine the constituents or the strength of another preparation. **3.** *adj.*, of known value, strength, quality, or ingredients. **4.** *n.*, predetermined criteria used to provide guidance in the operation of a health care facility to ensure high-quality performance by the personnel. –*standardize, v.*

standard air chamber, a radiation-measuring device used by national and international calibration laboratories to provide exposure calibrations for ion chambers used in the diagnostic or orthovoltage energy range.

standard bicarbonate, the bicarbonate ion concentration of plasma separated anaerobically from whole blood that has been saturated with oxygen and equilibrated at carbon dioxide pressure of 40 torr at 100° F (38° C). It is a measure of the metabolic disturbance of acid-base balance in a sample of blood after the correction of any respiratory disturbance.

standard curve, a graphic plot of unknown properties versus the known concentration of test substances in a set of standards usually prepared by serial dilution or incremental addition.

standard death certificate, a form for a death certificate that is commonly used throughout the United States. It is the form preferred by the U.S. Census Bureau.

standard deviation (SD), (in statistics) a mathematic statement of the dispersion of a set of values or scores from the mean.

standard environmental chamber. See **Skinner box.**

standard error (S.E.), (in statistics) the variability in scores that can be expected if measurements are made on random samples of the same size from the same universe of populations, phenomena, or observations. The standard error provides a framework within which a determination of the difference between groups may be made. It is an element used in determining statistic significance by means of a wide variety of formulas and methods.

standard error of the mean, (in statistics) an indication of how well the mean of a sample estimates the mean of a population. It is measured by the standard deviation of the means of randomly drawn samples of the same size as the sample in question.

standard gravity (g), the acceleration caused by gravity at mean sea level, 9.80616 m/sec^2.

standard hydrogen electrode, a reference electrode that is assigned a value of 0.00 volt. Also called **normal hydrogen electrode.**

standardization, standardize. See **standard.**

standardized death rate, the number of deaths per 1000 people of a specified population during 1 year. This rate is adjusted to prevent distortion by the age composition of the population. A standard population is used for determining this rate. Also called **adjusted death rate.**

standardized test, any empirically developed examination with established reliability and validity as determined by repeated evaluation of the method and results.

standard of care, a written statement describing the rules, actions, or conditions that direct patient care. Standards of care guide practice and can be used to evaluate performance.

Standard Precautions, guidelines recommended by the Centers for Disease Control and Prevention for reducing the risk of transmission of blood-borne and other pathogens in hospitals. The Standard Precautions synthesize the major features of universal precautions (designed to reduce the risk of transmission of blood-borne pathogens) and body substance isolation (designed to reduce the risk of pathogens from moist body substances) and apply them to all patients receiving care in hospitals regardless of their diagnosis or presumed infection status. Standard Precautions apply to (1) blood; (2) all body fluids, secretions, and excretions except sweat, regardless of whether or not they contain blood; (3) nonintact skin; and (4) mucous membranes. Standard Precautions are designed to reduce the risk of transmission of microorganisms from both recognized and unrecognized sources of infection in hospitals. Compare **Universal Precautions.** See also **Transmission-Based Precautions.**

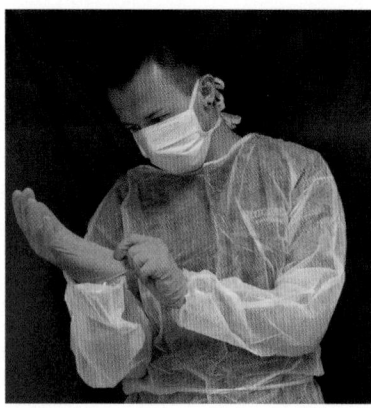

Standard Precautions: personal protective equipment

standard reference gamble, a method of diagnostic testing in which a decision maker is faced with a choice between a certain outcome or intermediate value and a gamble involving a better or worse outcome. The outcomes are assigned arbitrary numeric values of 100 and 0, respectively. All other outcomes can be assigned values relative to the best and worst outcomes.

standards of nursing practice, a set of guidelines for providing high-quality nursing care and criteria for evaluating care. Such guidelines help assure patients that they are receiving high-quality care. The standards are important if a legal dispute arises over the quality of care provided a patient.

standby guardianship, a legal process in the United States that may name an individual to assume specified health care or financial authority for an elderly person who becomes mentally incapacitated.

standing orders [L, *stare,* to stand, *ordo,* rank], a written document containing rules, policies, procedures, regulations, and orders for the conduct of patient care in various stipulated clinical situations. The standing orders are usually formulated collectively by the professional members of a department in a hospital or other health care facility. Standing orders usually name the condition and prescribe the action to be taken in caring for the patient, including the dosage and route of administration for a drug or the schedule for the administration of a therapeutic procedure. Standing orders are commonly used in intensive care units, coronary care units, and emergency departments.

stann-, combining form meaning "tin": *stannous flouride.*

stannous fluoride /stan″əs/ [L, *stannum,* tin, *fluere,* to flow], SnF$_2$, a substance used in prevention of dental caries that is applied topically to the teeth.

stanolone /stan′o-lōn/, a semisynthetic form of dihydrotestosterone, which has been used as an androgenic and anabolic steroid.

stanozolol /stənō″zəlol/, an androgenic anabolic steroid.
■ INDICATIONS: It is prescribed in the treatment of hereditary angioedema.
■ CONTRAINDICATIONS: Cancer of the breast or prostate, nephrosis, pregnancy, or known hypersensitivity to this drug prohibits its use.
■ ADVERSE EFFECTS: Among the most serious adverse effects are various androgenic effects in males and females, hypoestrogenic effects in females, and allergic reactions. GI disturbances may also occur.

St. Anthony's fire. See **ergot poisoning.**

stape-, combining form meaning "stapes": *stapedectomy, stapedius.*

stapedectomy /stā′pədek″təmē/ [L, *stapes,* stirrup; Gk, *ektomē,* excision], the removal of the stapes of the middle ear and insertion of a graft and prosthesis, performed to restore hearing in cases of otosclerosis. The stapes that has become fixed is replaced so that vibrations again transmit sound waves through the oval window to the fluid of the inner ear. Compare **incudectomy.**
■ METHOD: The stapes is removed, and the opening into the inner ear is covered with a graft of body tissue. One end of a small plastic tube or piece of stainless steel wire is attached to the graft. The other end is attached to the two remaining bones of the middle ear, the malleus and the incus.
■ PATIENT CARE CONSIDERATIONS: Headache and dizziness are expected early in the postoperative period. The patient's hearing does not improve until the edema subsides and the packing is removed. Possible complications include infection of the outer, middle, or inner ear; displacement or rejection of the graft or the prosthesis; and leaking of perilymph around the prosthesis into the middle ear, with ringing in the ear and dizziness.

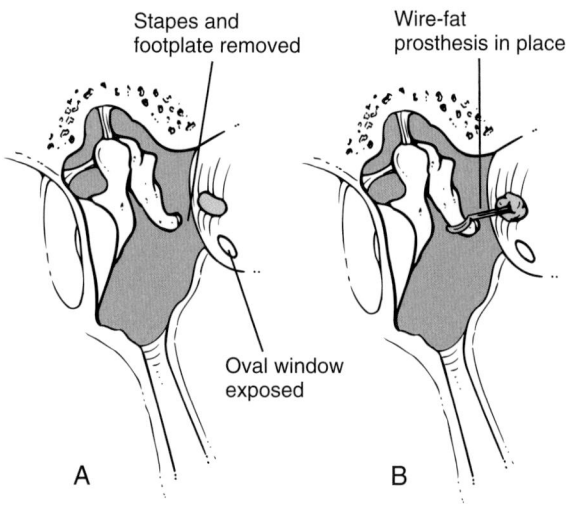

Stapedectomy *(LaFleur, 2011)*

stapedius /stəpē″dē·əs/, a small muscle on the wall of the tympanic cavity of the middle ear. It acts reflexively in response to loud sounds to reduce excessive vibrations that could injure the internal ear by pulling the head of the stapes posteriorly out of the oval window.

stapes /stā″pēz/ [L, stirrup], one of the three ossicles in the middle ear, resembling a tiny stirrup, that fits into the oval window. It transmits sound vibrations from the incus to the internal ear. Compare **incus, malleus.** See also **middle ear.**

Staphcillin, an antibacterial. Brand name for *methicillin sodium.*

staph marginal disease. See **eczematous conjunctivitis.**

staphyl-, staphylo-, 1. combining form meaning "grapelike clusters" or "conditions of the uvula": *staphylopharyngorrhaphy.* 2. combining form meaning "a micrococcal infection": *Staphylococcus.*

staphylococcal. See *Staphylococcus.*

staphylococcal infection [Gk, *staphyle,* bunch of grapes, *kokkos,* berry; L, *inficere,* to taint], an infection caused by any one of several pathogenic species of *Staphylococcus* commonly characterized by the formation of abscesses of the skin or other organs. Staphylococcal infections of the skin include carbuncles, folliculitis, furuncles, and hidradenitis suppurativa. Bacteremia is common and may result in endocarditis, meningitis, or osteomyelitis. Staphylococcal pneumonia often follows influenza or other viral disease and may be associated with chronic or debilitating illness. Acute gastroenteritis may result from an enterotoxin produced by certain species of staphylococci in contaminated food. Treatment usually includes bed rest, analgesics, and an antimicrobial drug that is resistant to penicillinase, an enzyme secreted by many species of *Staphylococcus.* Surgical drainage, especially of deep abscesses, is often necessary.

staphylococcal pneumonia [Gk, *staphyle* + *kokkos* + *pneumon,* lung],   pneumonia caused by a staphylococcus infection.

staphylococcal scalded skin syndrome (SSSS),   an infection or mucous membrane colonization with toxin-producing *Staphylococcus aureus.* It is characterized by epidermal erythema, peeling, and necrosis, which give the skin a scalded appearance. This disorder primarily affects infants 1 to 3 months of age and children, but it may also affect adults. SSSS is more common in the newborn because of undeveloped immunity and renal systems. Treatment of SSSS commonly includes the administration of systemic antibiotics to prevent secondary infections and the replacement of body fluids to maintain fluid and electrolyte balance. Compare **toxic epidermal necrolysis.**

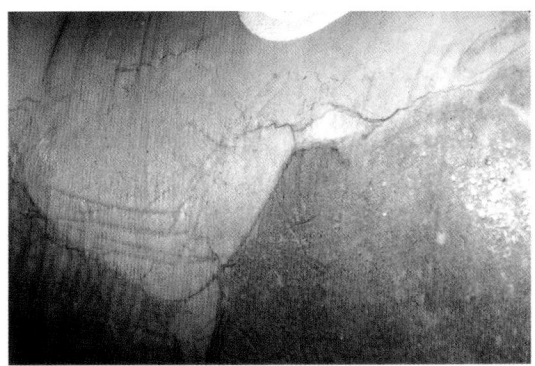

Staphylococcal scalded skin syndrome *(Goldman et al, 2008)*

staphylococcemia /-koksē″mē·ə/,   **1.** the presence of staphylococci in the blood. **2.** septicemia caused by staphylococci.

Staphylococcus /staf′ilōkok″əs/ *pl.* *staphylococci* [Gk, *staphyle* + *kokkos,* berry],   a genus of nonmotile spheric gram-positive bacteria. Some species are normally found on the skin and in the throat. Certain species cause severe purulent infections or produce an enterotoxin, which may cause nausea, vomiting, and diarrhea. Life-threatening staphylococcal infections may arise within hospitals. *Staphylococcus aureus* is a species frequently responsible for abscesses, endocarditis, impetigo, osteomyelitis, pneumonia, and septicemia. *S. epidermidis,* formerly called *S. albus,* occasionally causes endocarditis in the presence of intracardiac prostheses. See also **staphylococcal infection. –staphylococcal,** *adj.*

Staphylococcus aureus [Gk, *staphyle* + *kokkos* + L, *aurum,* gold],   a species of *Staphylococcus* that produces a golden pigment with some color variations and is commonly found on the skin or nose of healthy people. It is also responsible for a number of pyogenic infections, such as boils, carbuncles, and abscesses. *S. aureus* infections have become increasingly more difficult to treat because of the development of resistance to penicillin-related antibiotics. These bacteria are called methicillin-resistant *S. aureus* or MRSAs.

staphylokinase /staf′ilōkī″nās/,   an enzyme produced by certain strains of staphylococci that catalyzes the conversion of plasminogen to plasmin in various animal hosts of the microorganism.

staphyloma /staf′ilō″mə/,   a bulging of eye contents through a thin region of the cornea or sclera.

staphylopharyngorrhaphy.   See **palatopharyngorrhaphy.**

staple /stā″pəl/,   a piece of stainless steel wire used to close certain surgical wounds.

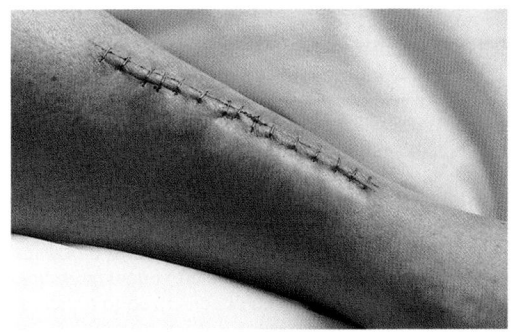

Staples *(Perry, Potter, and Elkin, 2012)*

stapling [ME, *stapel,* stake],   a method of fastening tissues together at the end of surgery by using a U-shaped piece of wire as a suture. The ends of the wire are bent toward the center to close the staple.

starch [AS, *stearc,* strong],   a polysaccharide composed of long chains of glucose subunits. It is the principal molecule used for the storage of energy in plants. See also **carbohydrate, glucose, glycogen.**

Stargardt macular degeneration,   an autosomal-recessive type of eye disorder affecting the retina, usually occurring from 6 to 20 years of age and marked by abnormal pigmentation and other changes in the macular area with rapid loss of visual acuity.

Starling's law of the heart.   See **Frank-Starling relationship.**

Starr-Edwards prosthesis [Albert Starr, American physician, b. 1926; M.L. Edwards, American physician, b. 1906; Gk, *prosthesis,* attachment],   an artificial cardiac valve. It is a caged-ball form of device that obstructs the valve opening and prevents the backward flow of blood. See also **prosthesis.**

start codon.   See **initiation codon.**

start hesitation,   a characteristic of parkinsonism in which the patient has difficulty initiating walking movements, as if the feet were stuck to the floor.

startle reflex /stär″təl/ [ME, *stertlen,* to rush; Gk, *syn,* together, *dromos,* course],   a reflex response to a sudden unexpected stimulus that may be accompanied by physiological effects such as increased heartbeat and respiration, closing of the eyes, and flexion of trunk muscles. The reaction is rapid, pervasive, and uncontrollable, regardless of the unexpected stimulus, which may be as simple as a touch. It is a normal reflex in neonates. However, premature and immature infants may not show the reaction. Also called *startle reaction, startle syndrome.* See also **Moro reflex.**

start point [ME, *sterte* + L, *punctum,* prick],   the initial nucleotide transcribed from a DNA template in the formation of messenger RNA.

starvation /stärvā″shən/ [ME, *sterven,* to die],   **1.** a condition resulting from the lack of essential nutrients over a long period (several days) and characterized by multiple physiological and metabolic dysfunctions. **2.** the act or state of starving or being starved. See also **malnutrition.**

stas-,   combining form meaning "stopped" or "relating to standing or walking": *stasibasiphobia, stasis.*

-stasia, -stasis,   **1.** suffix meaning "a (specified) condition involving the ability to stand": *abasia-astasia, astasia.*

2. suffix meaning "(condition of) stoppage or inhibition": *cholestasis, hemostasis.*

stasibasiphobia /stas′ibas′ifō″bē·ə/, a mental health condition in which a person is convinced that walking or standing is physically impossible. The person may also express a morbid distrust of his or her ability to stand or walk.

stasis /stā″sis, stas″is/ [Gk, standing], **1.** a disorder in which the normal flow of a fluid through a vessel of the body is slowed or halted. **2.** stillness.

-stasis. See **-stasia, -stasis.**

stasis dermatitis, a common result of venous insufficiency of the legs, beginning with ankle edema and progressing to tan pigmentation, patchy erythema, petechiae, and induration. Ultimately, there may be atrophy and fibrosis of the skin and subcutaneous tissue, with ulcerations that are slow to heal. The tan pigment is hemosiderin from blood leaking through capillary walls under elevated venous pressure. The involved skin is easily irritated or sensitized to topical medications. The underlying venous insufficiency must be treated. The dermatitis is often treated by bed rest, antibiotics for infection, and corticosteroids for reduction of inflammation. Also called **venous stasis dermatitis.** See also **stasis ulcer.**

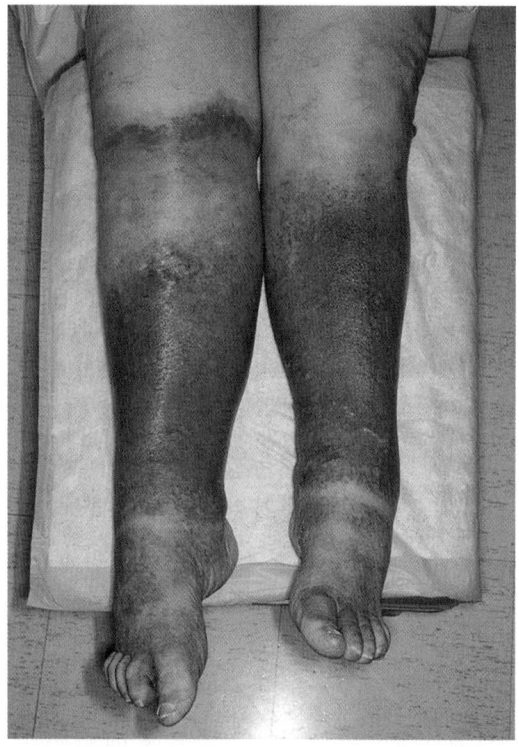

Stasis dermatitis (chronic venous stasis) *(Swartz, 2006)*

stasis syndrome, overgrowth of bacteria in the small intestine resulting from a variety of conditions causing stasis, particularly disturbances to intestinal motility or decreased acid secretion but also structural abnormalities such as diverticula, fistulae between the colon and upper bowel, or chronic obstruction. It is characterized by malabsorption of vitamin B_{12}, steatorrhea, and anemia. Also called **bacterial overgrowth syndrome, blind loop syndrome.**

stasis ulcer, a necrotic craterlike lesion of the skin of the lower leg caused by chronic venous congestion. The ulcer is often associated with stasis dermatitis and varicose veins. Healing is slow, and care to prevent irritation and infection is essential. Bed rest, elevation, and pressure bandages are usually ordered, and antibiotics if needed for infection. Surgery

to improve venous flow may be useful in some cases. Also called **varicose ulcer.** See also **stasis dermatitis.**

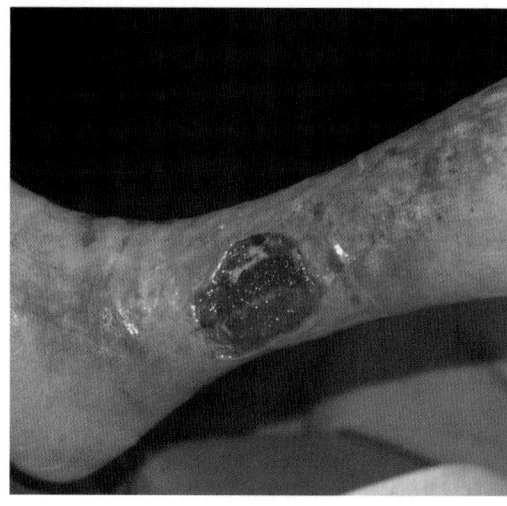

Stasis ulcer *(Black and Hawks, 2009)*

stat, a shortened form of a Latin word meaning "immediately." Abbreviation for *statim.*

-stat, 1. suffix meaning "a device for keeping something stationary": *chemostat.* **2.** suffix meaning an "instrument for the regulation of" something specified: *hemostat, rheostat, thermostat.* **3.** suffix meaning "an agent for stopping the growth of": *bacteriostat.*

state /stāt/ [L, *status,* condition], the circumstances or qualities that characterize a person, thing, or way of being at a particular time.

-state, combining form meaning "the result of a (specified) process": *gestate.*

state medicine. See **socialized medicine.**

State Nurses Association (SNA), an association of nurses at the state level. The various State Nurses Associations are constituent units of the American Nurses Association.

static /stat″ik/ [Gk, *statikos,* causing to stand], without motion; at rest; in equilibrium. Compare **dynamic.**

static cardiac work, the energy transfer that occurs during the development and maintenance of ventricular pressure immediately before the opening of the aortic and pulmonary valves.

static compliance testing, the difference between maximum and minimum compliance of the middle ear, measured with air pressure.

static equilibrium, the ability of an individual to adjust to displacements of his or her center of gravity while maintaining a constant base of support.

static imaging, 1. a diagnostic procedure for visualizing an internal organ or body compartment. A radioactive substance is administered to a patient, and an image or set of images is made of the fixed or slowly changing distribution of the radioactivity. **2.** any diagnostic image that is fixed or frozen in time.

static labyrinth, the vestibule of the inner ear. It contains two communicating chambers, the saccule and the utricle, and elicits tonic reflexes on postural muscles in response to changes in head and body positions.

static pressure [Gk, *statikos,* causing to stand; L, *premere,* to press], a condition of equalized blood pressure throughout the body when the heartbeat is stopped. A nonmoving fluid exerts a uniform pressure in all directions.

static progressive splints, a system of inelastic components that does not allow the person to move the extremity.

It increases range of motion by applying a sustained stretch on the joint.

static reflex [Gk, *statikos,* causing to stand; L, *reflectere,* to bend back], a reflex that helps one maintain normal posture and muscle tone when the body is at rest.

static retinoscopy, a type of retinoscopy in which the patient fixes the gaze on an unmoving target at a long distance to relax accommodation.

static scoliosis [Gk, *statikos,* causing to stand, *skoliosis,* curvature], a form of scoliosis resulting from a difference in the length of the legs.

static symptom. See **passive symptom.**

static tremor, irregular involuntary muscle contractions that occur when a patient makes an effort to hold the trunk or limbs in certain positions.

statin. See **HMG-CoA reductase inhibitor.**

station /stā″shən/ [L, *stare,* to stand], the level of the biparietal plane of the fetal head relative to the level of the ischial spines of the maternal pelvis. An imaginary plane at the level of the spines is designated "zero station." Higher and lower stations are numbered at intervals of 1 cm and labeled as minus above and plus below. For example, "station minus three" is 3 cm above the spines, and "station plus two" is 2 cm below the spines. In breech presentation, the bitrochanteric diameter of the breech is used to determine station. See also **dilation, effacement, labor.**

stationary lingual arch, an orthodontic arch wire that is designed to fit the lingual surface of the teeth and is soldered to the associated anchor bands.

statistic /stetis″tik/ [L, *status,* condition], a number that describes a property of a set of data or other numbers.

statistical model of patient evaluation, a system based on gross quantitative measurements of similar cases used to determine payment for services.

Statistical Package for the Social Sciences. See **SPSS.**

statistical significance [L, *status,* condition, *significare,* to signify], an interpretation of statistical data that indicates that an occurrence was probably the result of a causative factor and not simply a chance result. Statistical significance at the 1% level indicates a 1 in 100 probability that a result can be ascribed to chance.

statistics /stətis″tiks/, a mathematic science concerned with measuring, classifying, and analyzing objective information.

statoconia. See **otoconia.**

statotonic reflex. See **attitudinal reflex.**

status /stā″təs, stat″əs/ [L, condition], **1.** a specified state or condition, such as emotional status. **2.** an unremitting state or condition, such as status asthmaticus.

status asthmaticus, an acute, severe, and prolonged asthma attack. It is caused by critically diminished airway diameter resulting from ongoing bronchospasm, edema, and mucous plugging. Hypoxia, cyanosis, and unconsciousness may follow, and the attack may be fatal. Treatment includes supplemental oxygen given to correct hypoxemia, bronchodilators given intravenously or by aerosol inhalation, corticosteroids, mechanical ventilation, sedation, frequent therapy, and emotional support. See also **allergic asthma, asthma.**

status dysraphicus. See **dysraphia.**

status epilepticus, a medical emergency characterized by continuous seizures lasting more than 30 minutes without interruption. Status epilepticus can be precipitated by the sudden withdrawal of anticonvulsant drugs, inadequate body levels of glucose, a brain tumor, a head injury, a high fever, or poisoning. Therapy includes IV administration of anticonvulsant drugs, nutrients, and electrolytes. An adequate airway is usually maintained with a nasopharyngeal or endotracheal tube.

status lacunaris. See **lacunar state.**

status marmoratus, the presence in full-term infants of basal nucleus lesions resulting from acute total asphyxia.

The lesions have a marbled appearance caused by neuronal loss and an overgrowth of myelin in the putamen, caudate, and thalamus.

statute of limitations /stach″o͞ot/ [L, *statuere,* to set up, *limes,* boundary], (in law) a statute that sets a limit of time during which a suit may be brought or criminal charges may be made. In a malpractice suit, dispute may arise as to whether the time set by the particular statute of limitations begins to run at the time of the injury or at the time of the discovery of the injury.

statutory rape /stach″ətôr′ē/ [L, *statuere,* to place, *rapere,* to seize], (in law) sexual intercourse with a person below the age of consent, which varies from state to state. See also **rape.**

stavudine, a synthetic thymidine nucleoside analog.

■ INDICATIONS: This medication was prescribed in combination with other drugs for the treatment of adults with advanced human immunodeficiency virus (HIV) infection, generally those who are intolerant of other approved therapies, but the World Health Organization advised countries to phase out the use of stavudine due to long-term, irreversible side effects in HIV patients, including wasting and a nerve disorder.

■ CONTRAINDICATIONS: Hypersensitivity to this drug or to any of its components prohibits its use. It is no longer available in the United States.

■ ADVERSE EFFECTS: The side effects most often reported include peripheral neuropathies (occur more commonly than with comparable medications), elevation of hepatic transaminase levels, headache, chills, fever, asthenia, abdominal pain, diarrhea, nausea, and vomiting.

STD, abbreviation for **sexually transmitted disease.**

steady state (s, ss) /sted″ē/ [AS, *stedefast,* firm in its place; L, *status,* condition], a basic physiological concept implying that the various forces and processes of life are in a state of homeostasis. Living organisms are in constant flux, working to balance the internal and external environments in an effort to prevent a deficiency or an excess that might cause illness. Steady state is a complete state of well-being involving total adaptation.

steam sterilization [ME, *steme,* vapor; L, *sterilis,* barren], the destruction of all forms of microbial life on an object by exposing the object to moist heat for 15 minutes at 121° F (49.44° C) under high pressure.

steap-. See **stearo-, steap-, stear-, steato-.**

steapsin, pancreatic enzyme.

stear-, prefix pertaining to fat. See **stearo-, steap-, stear-, steato-.**

-stearic, suffix meaning "(specified) fat or fat derivatives."

stearo-, steap-, stear-, steato-, combining form meaning "fat": *stearrhea.*

stearrhea [Gk, *stear,* fat, *rhoia,* flow], excessive secretion of fat.

stearyl alcohol, a solid substance prepared by the catalytic hydrogenation of stearic acid, used in various ointments.

steato-. See **stearo-, steap-, stear-, steato-.**

steatorrhea /stē′ətərē′ə/ [Gk, *stear,* fat, *rhoia,* flow], greater-than-normal amounts of fat in the feces, characterized by frothy, foul-smelling fecal matter that floats, as in celiac disease, some malabsorption syndromes, and any condition in which fats are poorly absorbed by the small intestine.

steatorrhea simplex. See **seborrhea.**

steatosis, the accumulation of lipids within an organ, most commonly the liver.

Steele-Richardson-Olszewski syndrome [John C. Steele, Canadian neurologist; J. Clifford Richardson, Canadian neurologist, b. 1909; Jerzy Olszewski, Canadian neurologist, 1913–1966]. See **progressive supranuclear palsy.**

steeple head. See **oxycephaly.**

steering wheel injury, a traumatic injury, most commonly to the anterior chest wall, caused by forward propulsion of the body of an automobile driver into the steering wheel during a collision. Injuries include broken ribs and sternum, cardiac and pulmonary damage, and tearing of major blood vessels.

Steinert disease. See **myotonic muscular dystrophy.**

Stein-Leventhal syndrome. See **polycystic ovary syndrome.**

Steinmann pin /stīn″mən/ [Fritz Steinmann, Swiss surgeon, 1872–1932; AS, *pinn*], a wide-diameter pin used for heavy skeletal traction, as in the tibia or femur.

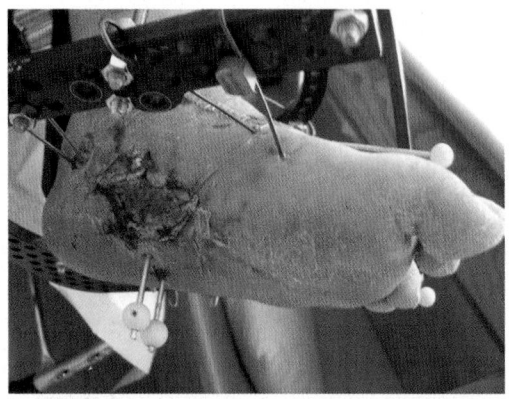

Steinmann pin *(Perry, Potter, and Elkin, 2012)*

Stelazine, a phenothiazine antipsychotic agent. Brand name for **trifluoperazine hydrochloride.**

stell-, combining form meaning "star": *stellate, stellate fracture.*

stellate /stel″it, -āt/ [L, *stella,* star], star-shaped or arranged in the pattern of a star.

stellate fracture, a fracture in which there are numerous fissures radiating from the central point of impact or injury throughout surrounding bone tissue.

stellate ganglion [L, *stella,* star; Gk, *gagglion,* knot], a large irregular ganglion on the lowest part of the cervical sympathetic trunk fused with the first thoracic ganglion. Its branches communicate with the seventh and eighth cervical nerves. Also called **cervicothoracic ganglion.**

stem cell [AS, *stemm,* tree, trunk; L, *cella,* storeroom], a formative cell; a cell whose daughter cells may give rise to other cell types. A pluripotential stem cell is one that has the potential to develop into several different types of mature cells, including lymphocytes, granulocytes, thrombocytes, and erythrocytes. See also **hematopoietic stem cell.**

stem cell leukemia, a neoplasm of blood-forming organs in which the predominant malignant cell is too immature to classify. The acute disease has a rapid, relentless course. Also called **embryonal leukemia, hemoblastic leukemia, hemocytoblastic leukemia, lymphoidocytic leukemia, undifferentiated cell leukemia.**

stem cell lymphoma. See **undifferentiated malignant lymphoma.**

steno-, combining form meaning "short," "contracted," or "narrow": *stenosis.*

stenosis /stinō″sis/ [Gk, *stenos,* narrow, *osis,* condition], an abnormal condition characterized by the constriction or narrowing of an opening or passageway in a body structure. The term is commonly used to describe heart valve and vessel abnormalities, as well as narrowing of joint spaces, as in cervical stenosis. Kinds include **aortic stenosis, pyloric stenosis.**

-stenosis, combining form meaning "narrowed" or "constricted": *arteriostenosis, craniostenosis.*

stenotic [Gk, *stenos,* narrow], pertaining to a structure that is narrowed or strictured.

Stensen's duct. See **parotid duct.**

stent [Charles R. Stent, 19th-century English dentist], **1.** (in dentistry) an acrylic guide, constructed from a model of the patient's mouth, that is inserted over the area where dental implants are to be placed, helping to guide the dental surgeon in the correct angulation and placement of dental implants. The stent contains holes that are predrilled. **2.** a mold or device used in anchoring skin grafts. **3.** a metal rod or mesh device used for supporting tubular structures during surgical anastomosis or for opening or maintaining the patency of coronary arteries during angioplasty.

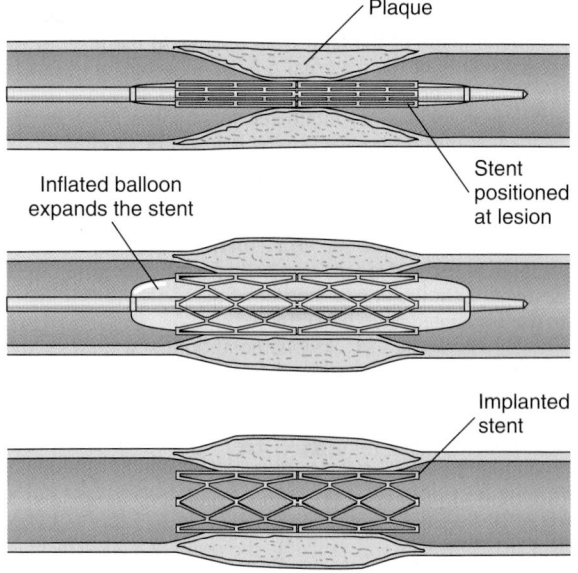

Coronary artery stent *(Lewis et al, 2011)*

step-care therapy, a therapeutic program that begins with a simple, conservative type of treatment but may advance to more complex stages as needed to achieve control of a disease or disorder. An example is step-care therapy of hypertension, in which the first step is limited to nonpharmacological treatments, such as weight control, low-salt diet, and exercise. If the first step fails to produce results, the next step may be the prescription of diuretics, followed by the use of beta-blockers, angiotensin-converting enzyme inhibitors, or other drugs, until an effective form of treatment is found.

steppage gait /step″ij/ [AS, *staepe* + ONorse, *gata,* way], a gait in which the legs are raised abnormally high, as in patients with footdrop.

stepping reflex. See **dance reflex.**

step reflex. See **dance reflex.**

stepwedge /step″wej/, an aluminum device that, when exposed to x-rays, displays a range of exposure intensities on a radiograph. These exposure "steps" are analyzed to determine the speed characteristics of the radiographic film or the dynamic range in digital imaging. Also called **penetrometer.**

Sterapred, a glucocorticoid. Brand name for **predniSONE.**

sterco-, combining form meaning "feces": *stercobilin.*

stereo-, combining form meaning "solid," "three-dimensional," or "firmly established": *stereognosis, stereoisomer, stereopsis.*

stercobilin, the bile pigment responsible for the brown color of feces.

stereognosis /stir′·ē·ŏgnō″sis/ [Gk, *stereos,* solid, *gnosis,* knowledge], **1.** the faculty of perceiving and understanding the form and nature of objects by the sense of touch. **2.** perception by the sense of the solidity of objects. −*stereognostic, adj.*

stereognostic perception /stir′ē·ŏgnos″tik/ [Gk, solid, knowledge], the ability to recognize objects by the sense of touch.

stereoisomer /stir′ē·ō·ī″səmər/ [Gk, *stereos,* solid, *isos,* equal, *meros,* part], one of two or more chemical compounds that contain the same atoms linked in the same way but that are organized differently in space. For example, one may be the nonsuperimposable mirror image of the other.

stereoisomeric specificity /-ī′səmer″ik/ [Gk, *stereos* + *isos,* equal, *meros,* part], specificity of an enzyme for one enantiomer of a racemic mix.

stereoophthalmoscope /stir′·ē·ō′ofthal″məskōp/, an ophthalmoscope fitted with two eyepieces so that the examiner can view the three-dimensional interior of the eye.

stereopsis. See **depth perception.**

stereoradiograph. See **stereoscopic radiograph.**

stereoradiography /-ra′dē·og″rəfē/ [Gk, *stereos* + L, *radiare,* to emit rays; Gk, *graphein,* to record], a technique for producing radiographs that give a three-dimensional view of an internal body structure. The stereoradiographs are produced by combining two separate x-ray images, each made from a slightly different angle without movement of the body part being imaged. The processed images are then viewed through a device that allows the two images to be perceived as one.

stereoscopic microscope /-skop″ik/ [Gk, *stereos* + *skopein,* to look], a microscope that produces three-dimensional images through the use of double eyepieces and double objectives. The three-dimensional image is created because the double optic systems have independent light paths. Also called **Greenough microscope.**

stereoscopic parallax. See **binocular parallax.**

stereoscopic radiograph, *(Obsolete)* a composite of two radiographs made through stereoradiography. Also called **stereoradiograph.** See also **stereoradiography.**

stereotactic mammography, a radiographic procedure using three-dimensional breast imaging to perform a needle breast biopsy and differentiate a benign from a malignant lesion. The three-dimensional imaging assists in locating the lesion and placement of the needle.

stereotactic radiosurgery, surgery utilizing techniques for positioning based on three-dimensional coordinates in which lesions are produced by ionizing radiation. Also called **stereotaxic radiosurgery.** See also **stereotactic surgery.**

stereotactic surgery, any of several techniques for the production of sharply circumscribed lesions in specific tiny areas of pathological tissue in deep-seated structures of the central nervous system. The site to be worked on is localized with three-dimensional coordinates. Methods of producing lesions include heat, cold, x-rays, and ultrasound. Also called **stereotaxic surgery.**

stereotaxic instrument /-tak″sik/, an apparatus that fits on the head and helps locate structures in the brain by means of coordinates.

stereotaxic neuroradiography [Gk, *stereos* + *taxis,* arrangement, *neuron,* nerve; L, *radiare,* to emit rays; Gk, *graphein,* to record], a radiographic procedure commonly performed during neurosurgery to guide the insertion of a needle into a specific area of the brain.

stereotaxic radiosurgery. See **stereotactic radiosurgery.**

stereotaxic surgery. See **stereotactic surgery.**

stereotype /stir″ē·ətīp/ [Gk, *stereos* + *typos,* mark], a generalization about a form of behavior, an individual, or a group.

stereotypical. See **stereotypy.**

stereotypic behavior /stir′ē·ōtip″ik/, a pattern of body movements that has autistic and symbolic meaning for an individual. It may occur in persons with schizophrenia.

stereotypy /ster″ē·ətī″pē/ [Gk, *stereos* + *typos,* mark], the persistent, inappropriate, mechanical repetition of actions, body postures, or speech patterns, usually occurring with a lack of variation in thought processes or ideas. It is often seen in patients with schizophrenia.

sterile /ster″il/ [L, *sterilis,* barren], **1.** free of living microorganisms. **2.** barren; unable to produce children because of a physical abnormality, often the absence of spermatogenesis in a man or blockage of the fallopian tubes in a woman. Compare **impotence.** −**sterility,** *n.* **3.** aseptic.

sterile field, **1.** a specified area, such as within a tray or on a sterile towel, that is considered free of microorganisms. **2.** an area immediately around a patient that has been prepared for a surgical procedure. The sterile field includes the scrubbed team members, who are properly attired, and all furniture and fixtures in the area.

sterile meningitis [L, *sterilis,* barren; Gk, *meninx,* membrane, *itis,* inflammation], a form of nonbacterial meningitis, which usually involves a viral infection but also may be drug-induced, in which there is a primarily lymphocytic response in the cerebrospinal fluid. Also called **benign lymphocytic meningitis, simple meningitis.** See also **aseptic meningitis.**

sterile technique. See **aseptic technique.**

sterile water for inhalation, water for injection that is sterilized and contains no antimicrobial agents, except when used in devices in which it is liable to contamination over a period of time (e.g., humidifiers). It is for inhalation therapy only, not for parenteral administration.

sterile water for irrigation, hypotonic water free from microorganisms and other contaminants; it is intended for use as an irrigation fluid and not for intravenous administration or administration by other parenteral routes.

sterility /stəril″itē/ [L, *sterilis,* barren], a condition of being unable to conceive or reproduce the species.

sterility assurance level (SAL), (in microbiology) the probability that a process makes something sterile. An SAL of 10^{-6} is the recommended probability of survival for organisms on a sterilized device. This level means that there is less than or equal to one chance in a million that an item remains contaminated or nonsterile. See also **sterilization.**

sterilization /ster′ilīzā″shən/ [L, *sterilis* + Gk, *izein,* to cause], **1.** a process or act that renders a person unable to produce children. See also **hysterectomy, tubal ligation, vasectomy. 2.** a technique for destroying microorganisms or inanimate objects using heat, water, chemicals, or gases.

sterilize /ster″ilīz/ [L, *sterilis,* barren], **1.** to make powerless to reproduce (infertile), such as by surgery. **2.** to destroy all living organisms and viruses in a material.

sternal /stur″nəl/ [Gk, *sternon,* chest], pertaining to the sternum.

-sternal, suffix meaning "sternum": *costosternal, presternal, suprasternal.*

sternal node [Gk, *sternon,* chest; L, *nodus,* knot], a node in one of the three groups of thoracic parietal lymph nodes. They are situated at the anterior ends of the intercostal spaces, adjacent to the internal thoracic artery. The afferent vessels of the sternal nodes drain the lymph from the breast, the diaphragmatic surface of the liver, and the deep ventral thoracic wall. Also called **internal mammary node.** Compare **diaphragmatic node, intercostal node.** See also **lymphatic system, lymph node.**

S

sternal puncture [Gk, *sternon,* chest; L, *punctura*], a diagnostic procedure in which a needle is inserted into the marrow of the sternum to remove bone marrow samples for diagnosis.

Sternberg-Reed cell. See **Reed-Sternberg cell.**

Sternheimer-Malbin stain /sturn″hīmər mal″bin/, a crystal violet and safranin stain used in urinalyses to provide additional contrast for certain casts and cells.

-sternia, combining form meaning "(condition of the) sternum."

sterno-, combining form meaning "sternum": *sternocleidal, sternocostal.*

sternoclavicular /stur″nōklavik″yəlar/ [Gk, *sternon,* chest; L, *clavicula,* little key], pertaining to the sternum and clavicle. Also called **sternocleidal.**

sternoclavicular articulation [Gk, *sternon* + L, *clavicula,* little key], the double gliding joint between the sternum and the clavicle. It involves the sternal end of the clavicle, the superior and lateral part of the manubrium, the cartilage of the first rib, and six ligaments.

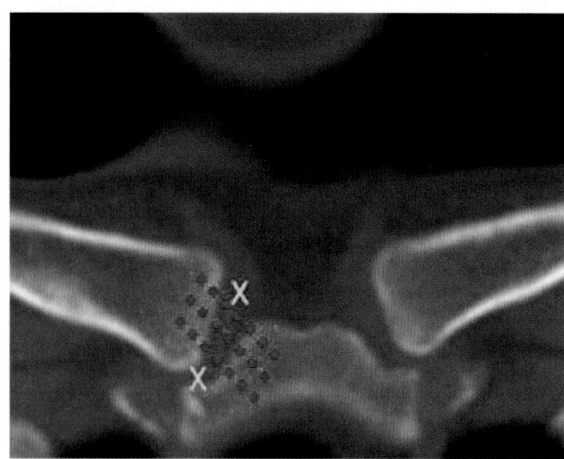

Coronal CT scan of the sternoclavicular joint with superimposed yellow *Xs* on either side of the anterior anteriod ligament, marked with red diamonds
(Imam et al, 2014)

sternocleidal. See **sternoclavicular.**

sternocleidomastoid /-klī′dōmas″toid/ [Gk, *sternon,* chest, *kleis,* key, *mastos,* breast, *eidos,* form], a muscle of the neck that is attached to the mastoid process of the temporal bone and to the superior nuchal line and by separate heads to the sternum and clavicle. They function together to flex the head. Also called **sternomastoid.**

sternocostal articulation /-kos″təl/ [Gk, *sternon* + L, *costa,* rib], the gliding articulation of the cartilage of each true rib and the sternum, except the articulation of the first rib, in which the cartilage is directly united with the sternum to form a synchondrosis. Each sternocostal articulation also involves five ligaments.

sternohyoideus /stur′nōhī·oi″dē·əs/ [Gk, *sternon* + *hyoeides,* upsilon, U-shaped], one of the four infrahyoid muscles. It acts to depress the hyoid bone. Also called *sternohyoid muscle.* Compare **sternothyroideus.**

sternomastoid. See **sternocleidomastoid.**

sternopericardial ligaments, ligaments that attach the fibrous pericardium to the posterior surface of the sternum and help to retain the heart in its position in the thoracic cavity.

sternothyroideus /stur′nōthīroi″de·əs/ [Gk, *sternon* + *thyreos,* shield, *eidos,* form], one of the four infrahyoid

muscles. It acts to depress the thyroid cartilage. Also called *sternothyroid muscle.* Compare **sternohyoideus.**

sternum /stur″nəm/ [Gk, *sternon*], the elongated flattened bone forming the middle part of the thorax. It supports the clavicles; articulates directly with the first seven pairs of ribs; and comprises the manubrium, the gladiolus (body), and the xiphoid process. It is composed of highly vascular tissue covered by a thin layer of bone.

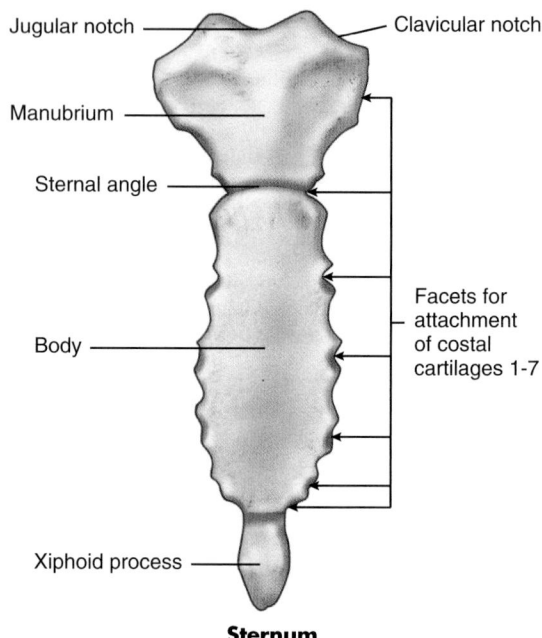

Sternum

sternutation. See **sneeze.**

steroid /stir″oid/ [Gk, *stereos* + *eidos,* form], any of a large number of hormonal substances with a similar basic chemical structure, produced mainly in the adrenal cortex and gonads. Steroids are chemically related to sterols.

steroid acne [Gk, *stereos,* solid; L, *oleum,* oil; Gk, *eidos,* form, *akme,* point], a form of acne caused by the use of corticosteroids.

steroid cell antibody, an immunoglobulin G glycoprotein that interacts with antigens in the cytoplasm of gonadal or adrenal cells that produce steroids.

steroid hormone [Gk, *stereos,* solid; L, *oleum,* oil; Gk, *eidos,* form, *hormaein,* to set in motion], a ductless gland secretion that contains the basic steroid nucleus in its chemical formulae. The natural steroid hormones include androgens, estrogens, and adrenal cortex secretions.

steroid hormone therapy [Gk, *stereos* + L, *oleum,* oil; Gk, *eidos,* form, *hormaein,* to set in motion, *therapeia,* treatment], treatment with any of the steroid hormones, such as the use of estrogen to reduce symptoms of postmenopausal disorders.

steroidogenesis /stiroi′dōjen″əsis/, the biological synthesis of steroid hormones.

sterol /stir″ôl/ [Gk, *stereos* + Ar, *alkohl,* essence], a large subgroup of steroidal compounds which consists of a series of fused carbocyclic rings containing a hydroxyl group at position 3 and a branched aliphatic side chain of eight or more carbon atoms at position 17. Kinds include **cholesterol, ergosterol.**

stertorous /stur″tərəs/ [L, *stertere,* to snore], **1.** pertaining to a respiratory effort that is strenuous or struggling. **2.** having a snoring sound.

stetho-, steth-, combining form meaning "the chest": *stethoscope, stethomimetic.*

stethomimetic /steth′ōmimet″ik/, pertaining to any condition causing or associated with a reduction of chest volume below its normal value. The condition may be congenital, temporary, or permanent.

stethoscope /steth″əskōp/ [Gk, *stethos,* chest, *skopein,* to look], an instrument consisting of two earpieces connected by means of flexible tubing to a diaphragm, which is placed against the skin of the patient's chest or back to hear heart and lung sounds. It is also used to hear bowel sounds.

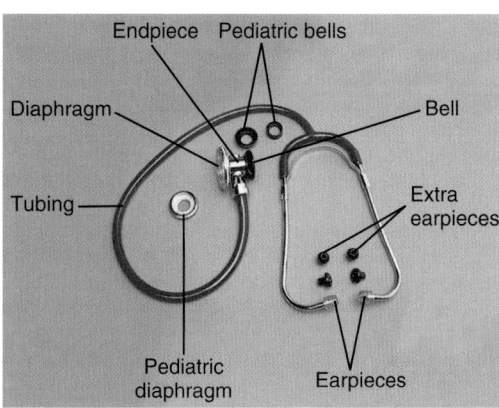

Stethoscope *(Harkreader and Hogan, 2007)*

Stevens-Johnson syndrome [Albert M. Stevens, American pediatrician, 1884–1945; F.C. Johnson, American physician, 1894–1934], a serious, sometimes fatal inflammatory disease affecting children and young adults. It is characterized by the acute onset of fever; bullae on the skin; and ulcers on the mucous membranes of the lips, eyes, mouth, nasal passage, and genitalia. Other complications are pneumonia, pain in the joints, prostration, and perforation of the cornea. It may be an allergic reaction to certain drugs, or it may follow pregnancy, infection by herpesvirus I, or other infection. It is seen rarely in association with malignancy or radiation therapy. Treatment includes bed rest, antibiotics for pneumonia, glucocorticoids, analgesics, mouthwashes, and sedatives. See also **erythema multiforme.**

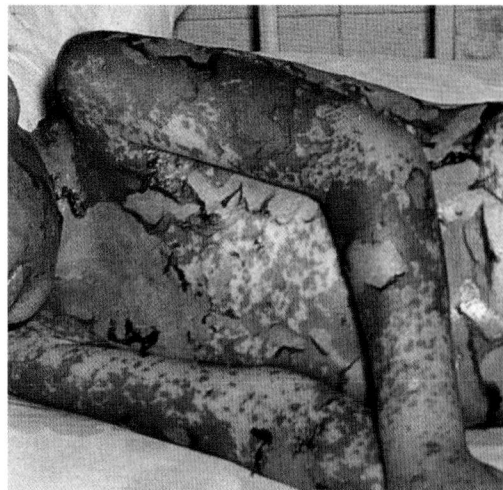

Stevens-Johnson syndrome *(Baren, 2008)*

Stewart, Isabel Maitland [1878–1963], a Canadian-born American nursing educator and writer. The first nurse to receive a master's degree from Columbia University in New York, she succeeded Mary Adelaide Nutting as Professor of Nursing at Teachers College at that university. She was instrumental in upgrading the nursing curriculum and in directing educational policies and became an important figure in international nursing affairs.

STH, abbreviation for *somatotropic hormone.* See **growth hormone.**

sthen-. See **stheno-, sthen-.**

-sthenia, combining form meaning "power" or "strength": *asthenia, myasthenia.*

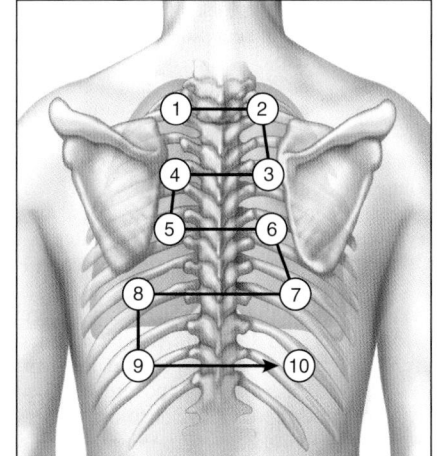

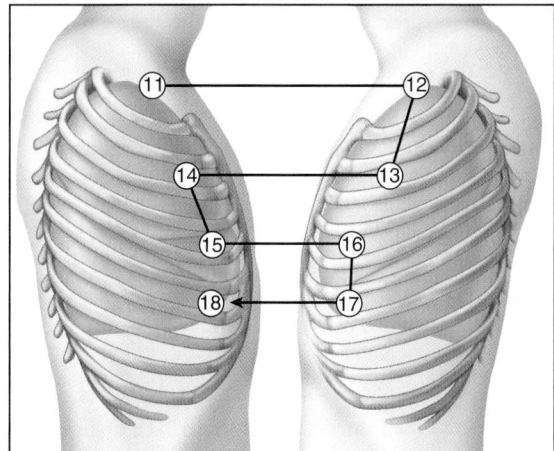

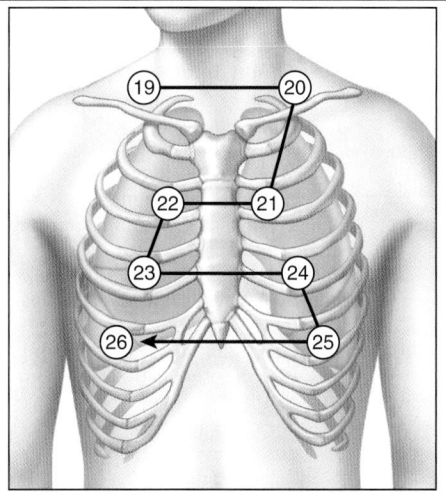

Stethoscope placement for auscultation of breath sounds *(Harkreader and Hogan, 2007)*

sthenic fever /sthen″ik/ [Gk, *sthenos,* power; L, *febris,* fever], high body temperature associated with thirst, dry skin, and often delirium.

stheno-, sthen-, combining form meaning "strength."

-sthenuria, combining form meaning "(condition of) urination or of the specific gravity of urine": *isosthenuria.*

stib-, combining form meaning "antimony": *stibogluconate sodium.*

stibogluconate sodium /stib′ōglōō″kənāt/, an antileishmanial agent. It is a drug of choice for the visceral form of leishmaniasis and has some effect on other forms.

stich-, -stichia, combining form meaning "rows": *polystichia.*

Stickler syndrome /stik′lər/ [Gunnar B. Stickler, 20th-century American physician], an autosomal-dominant disorder consisting of myopia progressing to retinal detachment and blindness and premature degenerative changes in the joints. Sensorineural hearing loss may also occur.

sticky end. See **cohesive terminus.**

Stieda's fracture /stē″dəz/ [Alfred Stieda, German surgeon, 1869–1945], a break in the internal condyle of the femur.

stiff [OE, *stif*], characterized by rigidity or muscular inflexibility.

stiff joint [OE, *stif* + L, *jungere,* to join], a rigid or inflexible joint, as may be caused by tight connective tissue or by arthritis or other rheumatic disorders.

stiff lung. See **adult respiratory distress syndrome.**

stiff-man syndrome, a condition of unknown cause characterized by progressive fluctuating rigidity of axial and limb muscles in the absence of signs of cerebral and spinal cord disease but with continuous electromyographic activity.

stigma /stig″mə/ *pl.* **stigmas, stigmata** [Gk, brand], **1.** a moral or physical blemish. **2.** a mental or physical characteristic that serves to identify a disease or a condition.

stigmatism /stig″mətiz′əm/ [Gk, *stigma,* brand], **1.** normal visual accommodation and refraction whereby light rays fall onto the retina. **2.** a condition of abnormal skin markings.

stilbestrol. See **diethylstilbestrol.**

stilet, stilette. See **stylet.**

stillbirth [AS, *stille* + ME, *burth*], **1.** the birth of a fetus that died before or during delivery. **2.** a fetus, born dead, who weighs more than 500 g and would usually have been expected to live.

stillborn [AS, *stille* + *boren*], **1.** *n.,* an infant who was born dead. **2.** *adj.,* pertaining to an infant who was born dead.

Still disease, *(Obsolete)* now called **juvenile rheumatoid arthritis.**

stimulant /stim″yələnt/ [L, *stimulare,* to incite], any agent that increases the rate of activity of a body system.

stimulant cathartic, a cathartic that acts by promoting the motility of the bowel, especially the longitudinal peristalsis of the colon. Kinds include **cascara sagrada, senna.**

stimulate /stim″yəlāt/ [L, *stimulare,* to incite], to excite, as in the process of increasing a vigorous functional activity.

stimulating bath, submersion in water that contains an aromatic substance, an astringent, or a tonic to enhance physiological or psychological activity.

stimulation /stim′yəlā″shən/ [L, *stimulare,* to incite], the condition of being encouraged to be more active.

stimulus /stim″yələs/ *pl.* **stimuli** [L, *stimulare,* to incite], anything that excites or incites an organism or part to function, become active, or respond. –**stimulate,** *v.*

stimulus control, a strategy for self-modification that depends on manipulating the causes of behavior to increase goals or behaviors desired by a patient while decreasing those that are undesired.

stimulus duration, the length of time a stimulus must be applied for the resulting nerve impulse to produce excitation in the receptor tissue. In general, more intense stimuli require

shorter excitation times to effect cellular response. Any stimulus that acts too briefly to overcome the threshold intensity of the receptor cell will not elicit a response.

stimulus generalization, a type of conditioning in which the reaction to one stimulus is reinforced to allow transfer of the reaction to other occurrences.

sting [AS, *stingan*], an injury caused by a sharp, painful penetration of the skin, often accompanied by exposure to an irritating chemical or the venom of an insect or other animal. In cases of hypersensitivity, a highly venomous sting, or multiple stings, anaphylactic shock may occur. Kinds include **bee sting, jellyfish sting, scorpion sting, sea urchin sting.** See also **stingray, wasp.**

stinging nettle (*Urtica dioica*), a plant that can form large colonies in orchards, farmyards, old pastures, ditches, and waste places. The stinging hairs on the undersides of leaves and the stalk can readily break, allowing chemicals such as acetylcholine, histamine, serotonin, moroidin, and leukotrienes to enter the skin via a painful sting. See also **nettle.**

■ OBSERVATIONS: The sting from the needles is followed by swelling, accompanied by prolonged itching and numbness.

■ INTERVENTIONS: The area exposed to stinging nettle should be irrigated with soap and water but not rubbed as this can release chemicals in needles remaining in the skin. Apply sticky tape to the area of exposure and then pull the tape away from the skin to remove needles.

■ PATIENT CARE CONSIDERATIONS: Although itching can be intense, instruction should be provided not to scratch the area. Cool compresses and topical applications can promote comfort. Although there are medicinal benefits associated with the use of nettle, accidental exposure through the skin can be very uncomfortable.

stingray /sting″rā/ [AS, *stingan* + L, *raia,* ray-fish], a flat, long-tailed fish bearing barbed spines on its back that are connected to sacs of venom. Spasm of the skeletal muscles, severe local pain, seizures, and dyspnea may occur if a person's skin is broken by the spines. See also **sea urchin sting.**

stippling [D, *stippen,* to prick], **1.** the appearance of colored dots in some cells when stained. Red stippling in blood cells stained with eosin hematoxylin is a sign of malaria. Blue stippling in red blood cells stained with Wright's stain can be a sign of lead poisoning. **2.** the appearance of the retina, as if dotted with light and dark points. See also **gingival stippling.**

stitch [ME, *stiche*], **1.** a suture. **2.** a sudden sharp pain.

stitch abscess [ME, *stiche* + L, *abscedere,* to go away], an abscess that develops around a suture.

stitch granuloma, a foreign-body granuloma occurring around a buried nonabsorbable suture.

St. John's wort. See **Saint John's wort.**

St. Louis encephalitis /sānt lōō″is/ [St. Louis, Missouri; Gk, *enkephalon,* brain, *itis,* inflammation], a flavivirus infection of the brain transmitted from birds to humans by the bite of an infected mosquito. It occurs most commonly in the central and southern parts of the United States and is characterized by headache, malaise, fever, stiff neck, delirium, and convulsions. Sequelae may include visual and speech disturbances, difficulty in walking, and personality changes. Convalescence may be prolonged, and death may result. No antivirus agent or vaccine is available. Treatment is supportive. Compare **California encephalitis, equine encephalitis.** See also **encephalitis.**

stochastic effects, effects produced at random without a threshold dose level, the probability of their occurrence being proportional to the dose and their severity being independent of it. In radiation safety, the main stochastic effects are carcinogenesis and genetic mutation.

stocking aid. See **sock aid.**

stock vaccine, an immunizing agent made from a stock microbial strain.

stoker's cramp. See **heat cramp.**

Stokes-Adams syndrome. See **Adams-Stokes syndrome.**

-stole, suffix meaning "contraction, retraction, or dilation of various organs": *asystole, diastole, parasystole.*

stoma /stō″mə/ *pl.* **stomas, stomata** [Gk, mouth], **1.** a pore, orifice, or opening on a surface. **2.** an artificial opening of an internal organ on the surface of the body created surgically, such as for a colostomy, ileostomy, or tracheostomy. **3.** a new opening created surgically between two body structures, such as for a gastroenterostomy, pancreaticogastrostomy, pancreatoduodenostomy, or pyeloureterostomy.

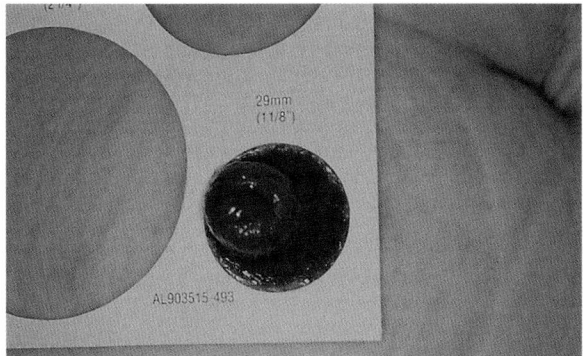

Colostomy stoma *(Courtesy ConvaTec, Bristol-Myers Squibb)*

-stoma, -stome, combining form meaning a "mouth" or "opening": *cystometry, colostomate, ileostomy.*

stomach /stum″ək/ [Gk, *stomakhos,* gullet], the food reservoir and first major site of digestion, located just under the diaphragm and divided into a body and a pylorus. It receives partially processed food and drink funneled from the mouth through the esophagus and gradually feeds liquefied food (chyme) into the small intestine. The stomach lies in the epigastric and left hypogastric regions bounded by the anterior abdominal wall and the diaphragm between the liver and the spleen. The shape of the stomach is modified by the amount of contents, stage of digestion, development of gastric musculature, and condition of the intestines. It is lined with a mucous coat, a submucous coat, a muscular coat, and a serous coat, all richly supplied with blood vessels and nerves, and contains fundic, cardiac, and pyloric gastric glands.

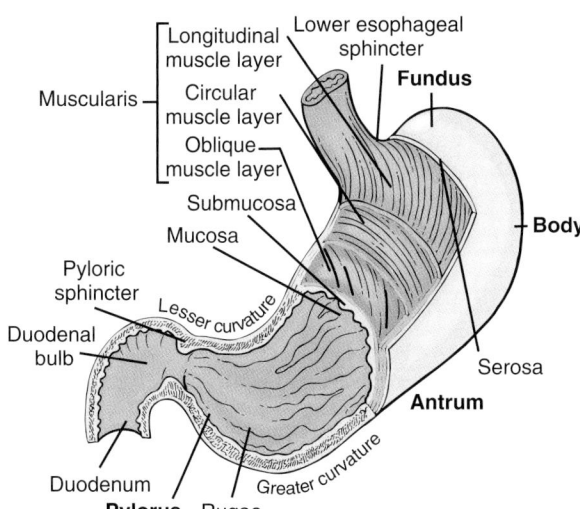

Stomach *(Lewis et al, 2007)*

stomachache [Gk, *stomakhos,* gullet; ME, *aken,* pain], pain in the abdominal area. Also called **gastralgia, gastrodynia.**

stomach cancer. See **gastric cancer.**

stomach drops, a medication that promotes gastric activity.

stomach pump, a pump for withdrawing the contents of the stomach through a tube passed through the mouth or nose into the stomach.

stomach tube. Also called **G tube.** See **gastrostomy tube.**

stomach wall, the layered structure that makes up the stomach, consisting of a serous coat, a muscular coat, a mucous membrane, and other tissue layers in between.

stomadaeal, stomadaeum, stomadeal, stomadeum. See **stomodeum.**

stomal /stō″məl/ [Gk, mouth], pertaining to one or more stomata or mouthlike openings. Also spelled **stomatal.**

stomal peptic ulcer, a marginal peptic ulcer. See also **marginal peptic ulcer, peptic ulcer.**

stomas, stomata. See **stoma.**

stomatal. See **stomal.**

stomatitis /stō″mətī″tis/ [Gk, *stoma* + *itis,* inflammation], any inflammatory condition of the mouth. It may result from infection by bacteria, viruses, or fungi; from exposure to certain chemicals or drugs; from vitamin deficiency; or from a systemic inflammatory disease. Kinds include **aphthous stomatitis, pseudomembranous stomatitis, thrush, Vincent's angina, Vincent's infection.** See also **candidiasis.**

stomatitis parasitica [Gk, *stoma,* mouth, *itis,* inflammation, *parasitos,* guest], an inflammation of the mucous membranes of the mouth by a yeast fungus, *Candida albicans,* typically expressed by a white coating on the tongue. It may affect infants or immunosuppressed people with human immunodeficiency virus or appear as an outgrowth secondary to antibiotic therapy. Also called **thrush.**

stomato-, stomo-, combining form meaning "mouth": *stomatocyte, stomatology, stomodeum.*

stomatocyte /stō′mah-to-sīt/, an abnormal red blood cell in which a slit or mouthlike area replaces the normal central zone of pallor, often due to edema.

stomatocytosis /stō″mah-to-si-to′sis/, the presence of stomatocytes in the blood, as seen in liver disease and Rh-null syndrome, a rare congenital hemolytic anemia. Also called **hydrocytosis.**

stomatognathic system /stō′mətōnath″ik/ [Gk, *stoma* + *gnathos,* jaw, *systema*], the combination of organs, structures, and nerves involved in speech and reception, mastication, and deglutition of food. This system is composed of the teeth, the jaws, the masticatory muscles, the tongue, the lips, the surrounding tissues, and the nerves that control these structures.

stomatology /stō′mətol″əjē/ [Gk, *stoma* + *logos,* science], the study of the morphological characteristics, structure, function, and diseases of the oral cavity.

-stome. See **-stoma, -stome.**

-stomia, combining form meaning "(condition of the) mouth": *xerostomia.*

stomion /stō″mē·on/ [Gk, *stoma*], the median point of the oral slit when the mouth is closed.

stomo-. See **stomato-, stomo-.**

stomodeum /stom′ədē″əm/ *pl.* **stomodeums, stomodea** [Gk, *stoma* + *odaios,* a way], a depression in the ectoderm located in the foregut of the developing embryo that forms the mouth. Also spelled *stomadaeum, stomadeum, stomodaeum.* Compare **proctodeum.** *—stomodeal, stomadeal, stomodaeal, adj.*

-stomy, combining form meaning "surgical opening": *gastrostomy, tracheostomy.*

stone. See **calculus.**

S

-stone, suffix meaning "a calculus in a human organ or duct": *gallstone.*

stone disease, urolithiasis that may have complications when obstructive uropathy or infection develops. See also **urinary calculus.**

stone retrieval basket, a tiny apparatus consisting of several wires that can be advanced through an endoscope into a body cavity or tube, manipulated to trap a calculus or other object, and withdrawn.

stool. See **feces.**

stool culture, a test to determine whether a patient has a bacterial or viral infection of the bowel or parasites.

stool for occult blood test (stool for OB), a stool test performed as part of every routine physical examination to detect the presence of occult blood in the GI tract. Presence of OB in the stool may indicate benign and malignant GI tumors, ulcers, inflammatory bowel disease, arteriovenous malformation, diverticulosis, and hematobilia.

stool softener. See **fecal softener.**

stop [AS, *stoppian,* to stop], a consonantal speech sound produced by closing off the oral cavity and then releasing with a burst of air, such as an initial /p/. Also called **plosive.**

stopcock, a valve or turning plug that controls the flow of fluid from a container through a tube. A three-way stopcock can be used on IV tubing to turn off one solution and turn on another.

stop needle [AS, *stoppian,* to stop, *naedel*], a needle with a shoulder flange that prevents it from penetrating beyond a certain distance.

Stop the Bleed, a national campaign to cultivate grassroots efforts that encourage bystanders to become trained, equipped, and empowered to help in a bleeding emergency before professional help arrives.

storage capacity /stôr″ij/, the amount of data that can be held in computer media, usually expressed in kilobytes (one thousand bytes), megabytes (one million bytes), gigabytes (one billion bytes), or terabytes (one trillion bytes).

storage disease, a metabolic disorder in which certain cells accumulate excessive amounts of lipids, sugars, proteins, or other substances.

storage pool, the area of a platelet organelle, such as a dense body or an alpha granule, where specific chemical constituents are stored.

storage pool disease, inadequate number or contents of platelet delta-granules causing mucocutaneous bleeding. Storage pool disease is usually hereditary and related to oculocutaneous albinism syndromes such as Hermansky-Pudlak syndrome, Chediak-Higashi syndrome, and Wiskott-Aldrich syndrome.

stored-energy foot, a lower-limb prosthesis designed to imitate the springlike action of a natural foot and leg. A device in the prosthesis stores energy when weight is put on the prosthesis. When the weight is shifted to the other leg, the stored energy is released, returning the prosthesis to its original shape.

stork bite. See **telangiectatic nevus.**

storm fermentation [OE, *sturm,* storm; L, *fermentum,* leaven], the rapid gaseous clotting of milk caused by *Clostridium perfringens.*

Stoxil, an antiviral. Brand name for **idoxuridine.**

STP, (Slang) a psychedelic agent, dimethoxy-4-methylamphetamine; the initials stand for serenity, tranquility, and peace.

STPD conditions of a volume of gas, (*s*tandard *t*emperature, standard *p*ressure, *d*ry) the conditions of a volume of gas at 0° C and 760 torr that contains no water vapor (dry). It should contain a calculable number of moles of a particular gas.

Str, abbreviation for ***Streptococcus.***

strab-, combining form meaning "squinting": *strabismus, strabismal.*

strabismal /strabiz″məl/ [Gk, *strabismos,* squint], pertaining to the condition of strabismus.

strabismus /strəbiz″məs/ [Gk, *strabismos,* squint], an abnormal ocular condition in which the visual axes of the eyes are not directed at the same point. There are two kinds of strabismus, paralytic and nonparalytic. Paralytic strabismus results from the inability of the ocular muscles to move the eye because of neurological deficit or muscular dysfunction. The muscle that is dysfunctional may be identified by watching as the patient attempts to move the eyes to each of the cardinal positions of gaze. If the affected eye cannot be directed to a position, the examiner infers that the associated ocular muscle is the dysfunctional one. Because this kind of strabismus may be caused by tumor, infection, or injury to the brain or the eye, an ophthalmologic examination is recommended. Nonparalytic strabismus is a defect in the position of the two eyes in relation to each other. The condition may be inherited. The person cannot use the two eyes together but has to fixate with one or the other. The eye that looks straight at a given time is the fixing eye. Some people have alternating strabismus, using one eye and then the other; some have monocular strabismus, which affects only one eye. Visual acuity diminishes with diminished use of an eye, and suppression amblyopia may develop. Nonparalytic strabismus and suppression amblyopia are treated most successfully in early childhood. The primary treatment to prevent amblyopia consists mainly of covering the fixing eye, forcing the child to use the deviating eye. The earlier it is begun, the more rapid and effective is the treatment. The eyes might be straightened by surgery, but suppression amblyopia will not be corrected. Also called **squint.** See also **anoopsia, esotropia, exotropia.** *—strabismical,* **strabismal,** *strabismic, adj.*

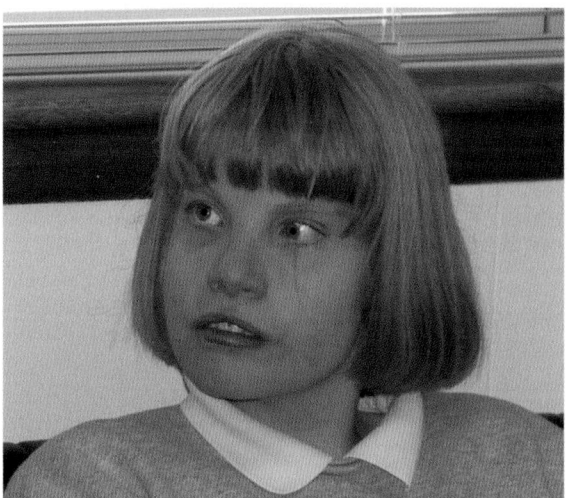

Young child with strabismus *(Wittman, 2009)*

straddle injury, injury to the distal urethra by falling astride a blunt object, such as bicycle handlebars or the top of a fence or railing.

straddling embolism. See **saddle embolism.**

straight catheter, a hollow, flexible instrument passed through body channels for withdrawal or instillation of fluids.

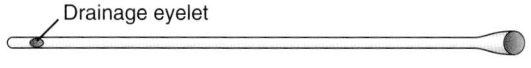

Robinson "straight"

Straight catheter *(Dehn and Asprey, 2013)*

straight chiropractic, the practice of chiropractic in strict accordance with the principles of its founder, D.D. Palmer, without additions made by later practitioners. The original definition of subluxation as a vertebral displacement is adhered to, and chiropractic is considered to be nontherapeutic, its purpose being solely to contribute to health by the correction of vertebral subluxations.

straight-leg-raising (SLR) test, a physical examination technique to determine abnormality of the sciatic nerve or tightness of the hamstrings. The presence of sciatica is confirmed by sciatic nerve pain radiating down the limb when the supine person attempts to raise the straightened limb.

straight line blood set /strāt/ [ME, *streght*], a common device, composed of plastic components, for delivering blood infusions. It includes plastic tubing, a clamp, a drip chamber, and a filter. Some kinds of straight-line blood sets contain filters within drip chambers; others have separate filters. The latter kind can be filled by squeezing the attached drip chamber, but it must not be squeezed itself or it may rupture. The former kind can be filled by squeezing the section of the blood set that contains the filter and the drip chamber. Before infusion, the filter of either kind is tapped with the fingers to dislodge any trapped air bubbles. Compare **component drip set, component syringe set, microaggregate recipient set, Y-set.**

straight sinus [ME, *streght* + L, *sinus*, hollow], one of the six posterior-superior venous channels of the dura mater that drain blood from the brain into the internal jugular vein. It has no valves and is located at the junction of the falx cerebri with the tentorium cerebelli. Compare **inferior sagittal sinus, superior sagittal sinus, transverse sinus.**

straight wire fixed orthodontic appliance, a fixed orthodontic appliance used for correcting and improving malocclusion. It is a variation of the edgewise orthodontic appliance. Its design and placement of arch wire brackets and tubes are intended to limit the need for arch wire adjustments.

strain [ME, *streinen*], **1.** *v.*, to exert physical force in a manner that may result in injury, usually muscular. **2.** *v.*, to separate solids or particles from a liquid with a filter or sieve. **3.** *n.*, damage, usually muscular, that results from excessive physical effort. **4.** *n.*, a taxon that is a subgroup of a species. **5.** *n.*, an emotional state reflecting mental pressure or fatigue.

straitjacket /strāt″jakit/ [OFr, *estreit*, strict, *jaquette*, short coat], a coatlike garment of canvas with long sleeves that can be tied behind the wearer's back to prevent arm movement. It is used for restraining violent or uncontrollable people. Also called **camisole restraint.**

strangle /strang″gəl/ [L, *strangulare*, to choke], to cause an interruption of breathing by compressing or constricting the trachea. Also *strangulate.* —**strangulated,** *adj.*

strangulated /strang″gyəlā′tid/ [L, to choke], pertaining to a constriction or compression of the trachea or other upper airway structure that interrupts the normal flow of air.

strangulated hemorrhoid [L, *strangulare,* to choke; Gk, *haimorrhoise,* vein that discharges blood], a prolapsed hemorrhoid that has become trapped by the anal sphincter, causing the blood supply to become occluded by the sphincter's constricting action.

strangulated hernia [L, *strangulare,* to choke, *hernia,* rupture], a hernia in which the blood vessels have become constricted by the neck of the hernial sac, resulting in ischemia and possible gangrene if blood circulation is not quickly restored.

strangulation /strang′gyəlā″shən/ [L, *strangulare,* to choke], the constriction of a tubular structure of the body, such as the trachea, a segment of bowel, or the blood vessels of a limb, that prevents function or impedes circulation. See also **intestinal strangulation.**

strap [AS, *stropp*], **1.** *n.*, a band, such as that made of adhesive plaster, that is used to hold dressings in place or to attach one thing to another. **2.** *v.*, to bind securely.

strapping, the application of overlapping strips of adhesive tape to an extremity or body area to exert pressure and hold a structure in place, performed in the treatment of strains, sprains, dislocations, and certain fractures.

strata. See **stratum.**

strategic questioning, the use of questions to influence a client's perspective, convey a certain message, or cause a client to reflect on and evaluate personal thinking about a given topic.

strati-, combining form meaning "layer": *stratified, stratiform cartilage.*

stratified /strat″ifīd/ [L, *stratum* + *facere,* to make], arranged in layers.

stratified clot, a semisolid mass of coagulated blood that forms in layers within an aneurysm.

stratified epithelium [L, *stratum* + *facere*; Gk, *epi,* above, *thele,* nipple], closely packed sheets of epithelial cells arranged in layers over the external surface of the body and lining most of the hollow structures. The layers may include stratified squamous, stratified columnar, or stratified columnar ciliated types of cells. There are various subtypes of stratified epithelium, named for the type of cells on the surface (e.g., stratified squamous epithelium, stratified columnar epithelium).

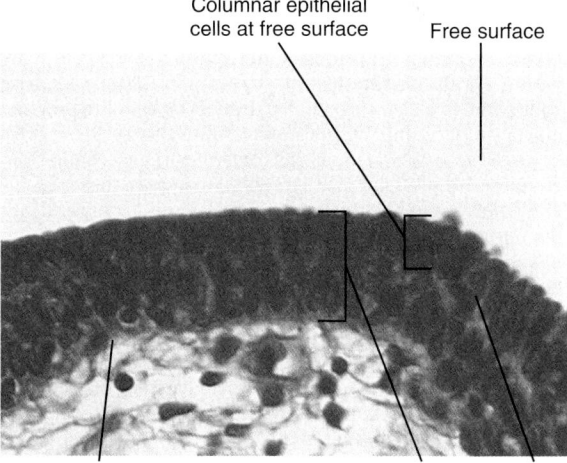

Stratified columnar epithelium *(© Ed Reschke; Used with permission)*

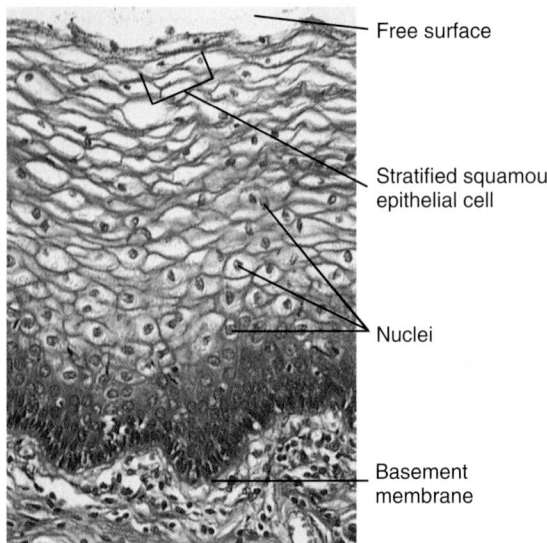

Stratified squamous epithelium (© Ed Reschke; Used with permission)

stratified sample.   See **sample.**

stratiform cartilage.   See **fibrocartilage.**

stratiform fibrocartilage /strat″ifôrm/   [L, *stratum,* layer, *forma,* form, *fibra,* fiber, *cartilago,* cartilage],   a structure made of fibrocartilage that forms a thin coating of osseous grooves through which tendons of certain muscles glide. Small masses of stratified fibrocartilage also develop in the tendons of some muscles that glide over bones, as in the tendons of the peroneus longus and the tibialis posterior. Compare **circumferential fibrocartilage, connecting fibrocartilage, interarticular fibrocartilage.**

stratum /strā″təm, strat″əm/ *pl. strata*   [L, layer],   a uniformly thick sheet or layer, usually associated with other layers, such as the stratum basale of the epidermis.

stratum basale,   **1.** the deepest of the five layers of the epidermis, composed of cuboidal-shaped cells. This layer provides new cells by mitotic cell division. Also called **basal layer, stratum germinativum.** Compare **stratum corneum, stratum granulosum, stratum lucidum, stratum spinosum.** See also **skin. 2.** the deepest layers of the uterine decidua, containing uterine gland terminals.

stratum corneum,   the horny, outermost layer of the skin, composed of dead flat cells converted to keratin that continually flakes away. The thickness of the layer is correlated with the normal wear of the area it covers. The stratum corneum is thick on the palms of the hands and the soles of the feet but relatively thin over most areas. Also called **horny layer.** Compare **stratum basale, stratum granulosum, stratum lucidum, stratum spinosum.** See also **skin.**

stratum germinativum.   See **stratum basale.**

stratum granulosum,   one of the layers of the epidermis, situated just below the stratum corneum except in the thick skin of the palms of the hands and the soles of the feet, where it lies just under the stratum lucidum. The stratum granulosum contains visible granules in the cytoplasm of its cells, which die, become keratinized, move to the surface, and flake away. Compare **stratum basale, stratum corneum, stratum lucidum, stratum spinosum.** See also **skin.**

stratum lucidum,   one of the layers of the epidermis, situated just beneath the stratum corneum and present only in the thick skin of the palms of the hands and the soles of the feet.

It contains translucent eleidin that forms keratin. Also called *clear cell layer.* Compare **stratum basale, stratum corneum, stratum granulosum, stratum spinosum.** See also **skin.**

stratum spinosum,   one of the layers of the epidermis, composed of several layers of polygonal cells. It lies on top of the stratum basale and beneath the stratum granulosum and contains tiny fibrils within its cellular cytoplasm. When the cells of the stratum spinosum are pulled apart, they present minute spines, called desmosomes, at their surfaces. Also called **prickle cell layer.** Compare **stratum basale, stratum corneum, stratum granulosum, stratum lucidum.** See also **skin.**

stratum spongiosum,   one of the three layers of the endometrium of the uterus, containing tortuous, dilated uterine glands and a small amount of interglandular tissue. With the stratum compactum it forms the functional part of the endometrium during pregnancy. Compare **stratum basale.** See also **decidua, placenta.**

strawberry gallbladder /strô″berē/   [AS, *streawberig* + ME, *gal,* gall; AS, *blaedre*],   a tiny yellow gallbladder spotted with deposits on the red mucous membrane, characteristic of cholesterolosis.

strawberry hemangioma, strawberry mark.   See **capillary hemangioma.**

strawberry tongue,   a strawberry-like coloration of inflamed tongue papillae. It is a clinical sign of scarlet fever and is also seen in Kawasaki disease.

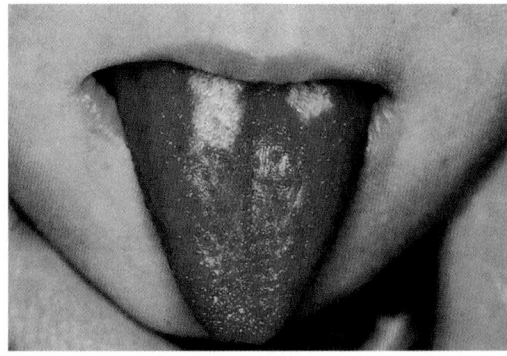

Strawberry tongue (Emond, Wellsby, and Rowland, 2003)

stray light   [OFr, *estraier,* to wander; AS, *leoht,* illumination],   radiant energy that reaches a photodetector and that consists of wavelengths other than those defined by the filter or monochromator.

stray radiation.   See **leakage radiation.**

streak   [AS, *strican,* to stroke],   a line or a stripe, such as the primitive streak at the caudal end of the embryonic disk.

street virus,   a natural infectious agent, such as rabies, that may be transmitted from a domestic animal or may be acquired in the wild, outside the laboratory.

strength   [AS, *strengou*],   the ability of a muscle or a person to produce or resist a physical force.

strength of association,   the degree of relationship between a causal factor and the occurrence of a disease, usually expressed in terms of a relative risk ratio.

strength training,   a method of improving muscular strength by gradually increasing the ability to resist force through the use of free weights, machines, or the person's own body weight. Strength training sessions are designed to impose increasingly greater resistance, which in turn stimulates development of muscle strength to meet the added demand.

streptavidin /strep′təvī″din/,   a biotin-binding protein isolated from *Streptomyces* and used to identify antigens; a widely used reagent for immunoassays.

strep throat [*Streptococcus* + AS, *throte*], *(Informal)* an infection of the oral pharynx and tonsils caused by a hemolytic species of *Streptococcus,* usually belonging to group A. The infection is characterized by sore throat, chills, fever, swollen lymph nodes in the neck, and sometimes nausea and vomiting. The symptoms usually begin abruptly a few days after exposure to the organism in airborne droplets or after direct contact with an infected person. Also called **streptococcal sore throat.**

■ OBSERVATIONS: The throat is diffusely red, and the tonsils often are covered with a yellow or white exudate. Diagnosis is confirmed by bacteriological culture and identification of the streptococcal bacteria in a specimen taken from the throat. Complications of strep throat are otitis media, scarlet fever, and sinusitis; other complications include acute glomerulonephritis and acute rheumatic fever.

■ INTERVENTIONS: Treatment usually includes intramuscular injection of penicillin G benzathine or the administration of penicillin for 10 days. Erythromycin may be given to people allergic to penicillin. For recurrent infections, tonsillectomy may be recommended.

strepticemia. See **streptococcemia.**

strepto-, combining form meaning "twisted": Streptococcus, *streptococcal.*

streptobacillary rat-bite fever. See **Haverhill fever.**

Streptobacillus moniliformis [Gk, *streptos,* curved; L, *bacillum,* small rod, *monile,* necklace, *forma,* form], a species of necklace-shaped nonmotile gram-negative bacteria that can cause rat-bite fever in humans.

streptococcal. See ***Streptococcus.***

streptococcal angina [Gk, *streptos* + *kokkos,* berry; L, *angina,* quinsy], a condition in which feelings of choking, suffocation, and pain result from a streptococcal infection.

streptococcal infection, an infection caused by pathogenic bacteria of one of several species of the genus *Streptococcus* or their toxins. Almost any organ of the body may be involved. The infections occur in many forms, including cellulitis, endocarditis, erysipelas, impetigo, meningitis, pneumonia, scarlet fever, tonsillitis, and urinary tract infection. See also **strep throat.**

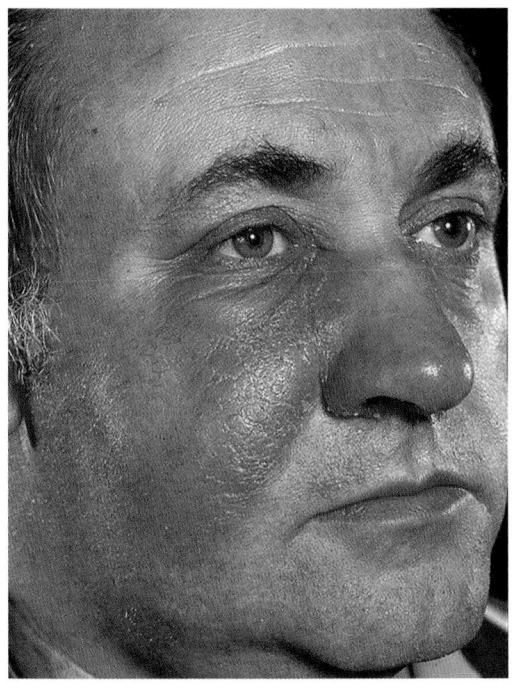

Streptococcal infection *(Weston, 2007)*

streptococcal sore throat. See **strep throat.**

streptococcemia /-koksē″mē·ə/ [Gk, *streptos,* curved, *kokkos,* berry], a condition of the presence of streptococci bacteria in the blood. Also called **streptcemia, streptosepticemia.**

Streptococcus /strep′təkok″əs/ [Gk, *streptos* + *kokkos,* berry], *adj.,* a genus of nonmotile gram-positive cocci classified by serological types (Lancefield groups A through T), by hemolytic action (α, β, γ) when grown on blood agar, and by reaction to bacterial viruses (phage types 1 to 86). The various species occur in pairs, short chains, and chains. Some are facultative aerobes, and some are anaerobic. Some species also are hemolytic, and others are nonhemolytic. Many species cause disease in humans. *Streptococcus faecalis,* a penicillin-resistant group D enterococcus and normal inhabitant of the GI tract, may cause infection of the urinary tract or endocardium. *S. pneumoniae* (formerly *Diplococcus pneumoniae*) causes a majority of the cases of bacterial pneumonia in the United States. *S. pyogenes* belongs to group A and may cause tonsillitis and respiratory, urinary, or skin infections. Some beta-hemolytic strains may lead to rheumatic fever or to glomerulonephritis. *S. viridans,* a member of the normal flora of the mouth, is the most common cause of bacterial endocarditis, especially when introduced into the bloodstream during dental procedures. −**streptococcal,** *adj.*

streptococcus beta-hemolytic, Group A, a strain of streptococcus, group A in the Lancefield classification, that causes necrotizing fasciitis toxic shock syndrome.

streptococcus beta-hemolytic, Group B, a strain of streptococcus that causes human infections such as neonatal sepsis, endocarditis, and septic arthritis.

Streptococcus pneumoniae [Gk, *streptos,* curved, *kokkos,* berry, *pneumon,* lung], any of 70 antigenic types of pneumococcal bacteria that cause pneumonia and other diseases in humans. Bacteria are most commonly community acquired, but there are immunizations for 23 strains.

Streptococcus pyogenes [Gk, *streptos,* curved, *kokkos,* berry, *pyon,* pus, *genein,* to produce], a species of streptococcus with many strains that are pathogenic to humans, including the beta-hemolytics in Lancefield group A. It causes suppurative diseases, such as scarlet fever and strep throat.

Streptococcus viridans [Gk, *streptos,* curved, *kokkos,* berry], a poorly defined species of *Streptococcus* similar to *S. pyogenes* strains. It produces alpha-hemolysis in cultures and is a common cause of subacute bacterial endocarditis and other infections, such as gingivitis, in humans.

streptokinase (SK) /strep′təkī″nās/ [Gk, *streptos* + *kinesis,* motion, (ase) enzyme], a fibrinolytic activator that enhances the conversion of plasminogen to the fibrinolytic enzyme plasmin. It is produced by strains of streptococci. It is used in the treatment of certain cases of pulmonary and coronary embolism.

streptokinase-streptodornase /-strep′tōdôr″nās/, two enzymes derived from a strain of *Streptococcus hemolyticus.*

■ INDICATIONS: It is prescribed for debridement of purulent exudates, clotted blood, radiation necrosis, or fibrinous deposits resulting from trauma or infection.

■ CONTRAINDICATIONS: Active hemorrhage, acute cellulitis, or danger of reopening bronchopleural fistulas prohibits its use.

■ ADVERSE EFFECTS: Among the more serious adverse effects are pyrogenic reactions and irritation.

streptolysin /strepto″līsin/ [Gk, *streptos* + *lysein,* to loosen], a filterable substance, produced by streptococci, that liberates hemoglobin from red blood cells.

streptomycin sulfate /strep′təmī″sin/, an aminoglycoside antibiotic.

■ INDICATIONS: It is prescribed in the treatment of tuberculosis, endocarditis, and certain other infections.

■ CONTRAINDICATIONS: Pregnancy or hypersensitivity to this drug prohibits its use. It must be used with caution in individuals who have vertigo, tinnitus, other manifestations of labyrinthine disease, or impaired renal function and in the elderly.

■ ADVERSE EFFECTS: Among the most serious adverse effects are ototoxicity (generally irreversible), nephrotoxicity (generally reversible), muscle weakness, and allergic reactions.

streptosepticemia. See **streptococcemia.**

streptozocin /strep′təzō″sin/, an antineoplastic used in the treatment of neoplasms, including metastatic islet cell tumors of the pancreas. It is an antibiotic substance from *Streptomyces acromogenes.*

stress [OFr, *estrecier,* to tighten], any emotional, physical, social, economic, or other factor that requires a response or change. Examples include dehydration, which can cause an increase in body temperature, and a separation from parents, which can cause a young child to cry. Stress can be positive or negative. Ongoing chronic stress can result in physical illness. Stress has been theorized as a major contributing factor in many physical diseases, such as asthma. Stress may also be applied therapeutically to promote change, such as implosive therapy for phobic patients, in which the patient is given support while being exposed to the situation that produces anxiety and is thereby gradually desensitized. The nature and degree of stress observed in an individual are frequently evaluated by the health care team. See also **general adaptation syndrome.**

stress-adaptation theory, a concept that stress depletes the reserve capacity of individuals, thereby increasing their vulnerability to health problems.

stress amenorrhea [OFr, *estrecier*; Gk, *a + men,* month, *rhoia,* to flow], a cessation in menstruation caused by a physical change or mental stress.

stress-bearing area, the portion of the natural oral structures that is available to support a denture. Also called **basal seat area, denture-bearing area.**

stress behavior, a change from a person's normal behavior in response to a stressor.

stress echocardiography, echocardiography to assess myocardial function and perfusion that is performed while the patient is under stress, such as during exercise on a treadmill or stationary bike. Medications can be used to increase heart rate when the patient cannot exercise. See also **echocardiogram.**

stress fracture, a fracture, often in one or more of the metatarsal bones, caused by repeated, prolonged, or abnormal stress. It is commonly seen in military recruits, runners, and those who participate in other repetitive movements.

stress incontinence. See **incontinence.**

stress inoculation, a procedure useful in helping patients control anxiety by substituting positive coping statements for statements that bring about anxiety.

stress kinesic, a type of behavioral characteristic of personal conversation, such as the use of body shifts or movements, that marks the flow of speech and generally coincides with linguistic stress patterns.

stress management, methods of controlling factors that require a response or change within a person by identifying the stressors, eliminating negative stressors, and developing effective coping mechanisms to counteract the response constructively. Kinds include **guided imagery, biofeedback, meditation.**

stressor /stres″ər/ [OFr, *estrecier,* to tighten], anything that causes wear and tear on the body's physical or mental resources. See also **general adaptation syndrome.**

stress radiography, the radiographic examination of a body area for soft tissue tears or ruptures. The lesions may appear as abnormal gaps between joint surfaces.

stress reaction, an acute maladaptive emotional response to an actual or perceived stressor.

stress response syndrome. See **posttraumatic stress disorder.**

stress test, a test that measures the function of a system of the body when subjected to carefully controlled amounts of physiological stress, usually exercise but sometimes specific drugs. The data produced allow the examiner to evaluate the condition of the system being tested. Cardiopulmonary function, respiratory function, and intrauterine fetal placental function are tested with stress tests. Also called **thallium stress test, treadmill stress test.** See also **exercise electrocardiogram, oxytocin challenge test.**

stress theory of aging, a stochastic theory of aging that hypothesizes that aging and death result from the effects of environmental stressors that cause wear and tear on cells and disrupt their function. The generation of free radicals during oxidative cell processes is sometimes cited as a specific stressor that disrupts DNA and protein function and so causes aging. See also **theories of aging.**

stress ulcer, a gastric or duodenal ulcer that develops in previously unaffected individuals subjected to severe stress, such as a severe burn. See also **Curling ulcer.**

stretching of contractures [AS, *streccan* + L, *contractura,* drawing together], any of several procedures for release of muscle and other structures that have been shortened because of paralysis, spasm, disuse, or fibrosis. The procedures include stretching exercises, tissue grafts, scar tissue removal, tendon transfer, and incision of a joint capsule.

stretch mark. See **stria.**

stretch pressure, a rehabilitation technique in which the thumb, fingertips, or palm of the hand is used to stretch a target muscle, followed by briefly maintained pressure.

stretch receptor [AS, *streccan* + L, *recipere,* to receive], specialized sensory nerve endings in muscle spindles or tendons that are stimulated by stretching movements.

stretch reflex [AS, *streccan* + L, *reflectere,* to bend back], a reflex muscle contraction after it is stretched as a result of stimulation of proprioceptors in the muscle. Tendon reflexes function in a similar manner. Also called **myostatic reflex.**

stretch release, a rehabilitation technique in which the fingertips are placed over the belly of a large muscle and then spread apart in an effort to stretch the skin and underlying muscle. The stretch is done firmly enough to deform the soft tissue temporarily, stimulating cutaneous and muscle efferents and producing facilitation of the underlying muscle.

stri-, combining form meaning "line," "stripe," or "streak": *striated, myoma striocellulare.*

stria /strī″ə/ *pl.* **striae** [L, furrow], a streak or a linear scar that often results from rapidly developing tension in the skin, such as seen on the abdomen after pregnancy. Purplish striae are among the classic findings in hyperadrenocorticism. Also called **stretch mark.**

stria atrophica, erythematous linear lesions following cleavage lines that are initially red and then fade to white. They are most common in adolescents during growth spurts, in pregnant women in their last trimester, and in individuals with obesity. They are also sometimes noted in individuals with Cushing disease. Also called *striae distensae.*

striae. See **stria.**

stria gravidarum, irregular depressions with red to purple coloration that appear in the skin of the abdomen, thighs, and buttocks of pregnant women.

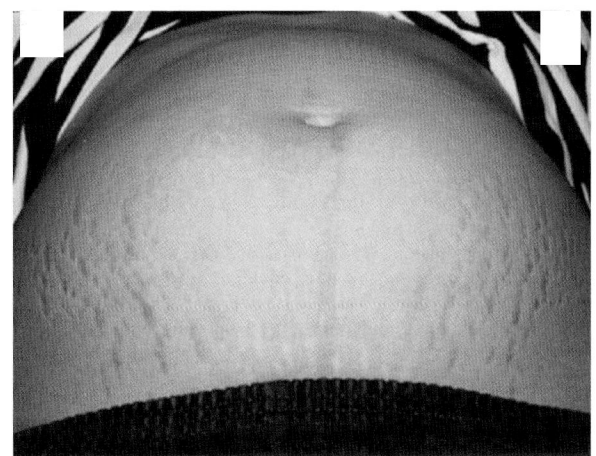

Stria gravidarum *(Courtesy Michael S. Clement)*

striatal /strī·ā″təl, strī″ətəl/ [L, *striatus,* striped], pertaining to the corpus striatum.

striatal toe, hyperextension of the great toe.

striated /strī″āted/ [L, *striatus,* striped], identifying something that is striped, is marked by parallel lines, or has structural lines.

striated muscle /strī″ātid/ [L, *striatus,* striped, *musculus,* muscle], any muscle, including all of the skeletal muscles, in which the fibers are divided by bands of cross-striations (stripes) as a result of overlapping of thick and thin myofilaments. Contractions in such muscles are voluntary. The heart, a striated involuntary muscle, is an exception. Cardiac muscle is often placed in its own category because it has microanatomical and contraction physiological characteristics very different from those of most striated muscle. Also called **skeletal muscle, voluntary muscle.** Compare **cardiac muscle, smooth muscle.**

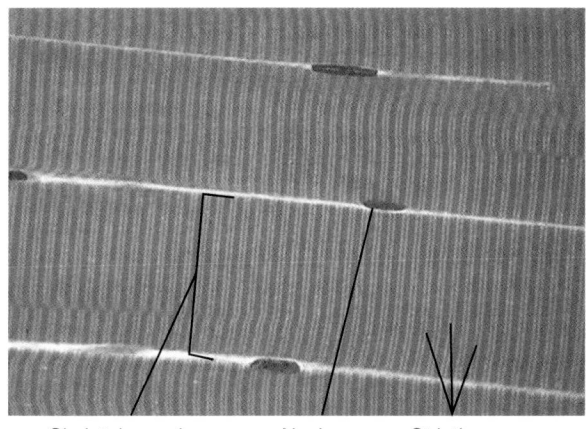

Skeletal muscle   Nucleus   Striations
fiber

Striated muscle *(© Ed Reschke; Used with permission)*

stria terminalis, a slender, compact fiber bundle that functions as a limbic pathway running from the amygdaloid complex to the hypothalamus and septum.

stricture /strik″chər/ [L, *stringere,* to tighten], an abnormal temporary or permanent narrowing of the lumen of a hollow organ, such as the esophagus, pylorus of the stomach, ureter, or urethra. It is caused by inflammation, external

pressure, or scarring. Treatment varies depending on the cause. Compare **spasm.**

strict vegetarian [L, *stringere* + *vegetare,* to grow, *arius,* believer], a vegetarian who consumes no animal products, including meat, fish, poultry, dairy foods, or eggs. All foods consumed are plant-based, including fruits, vegetables, legumes, nuts, seeds, grain, and soy foods. Such diets, unless adequately planned, may be inadequate in many essential nutrients, particularly vitamin B$_{12}$. Also called **vegan.**

stridor /strī″dôr/ [L, harsh sound], an abnormal high-pitched musical sound caused by an obstruction in the trachea or larynx. It is usually heard during inspiration. Stridor may indicate several neoplastic or inflammatory conditions, including glottic edema, asthma, diphtheria, laryngospasm, and papilloma.

strike [AS, *strican,* to advance swiftly], an action taken collectively by the employees of a company or institution in which they stop reporting for work in an effort to cause the employer to accede to certain demands. A strike usually follows unsuccessful negotiations between representatives of the union and management.

string, a cord, usually made of fiber, configured in a long, thin line.

string carcinoma [AS, *strenge,* cord; Gk, *karkinos,* cancer, *oma,* tumor], a malignancy of the large intestine, usually the ascending or transverse colon. On radiological visualization, it causes the intestine to appear to be tied in segments like a string of large beads.

stringiness /string″inəs/, an abnormal tissue texture caused by fine or stringlike myofascial structures.

string sign, a narrow pyloric canal with congenital pyloric stenosis or a narrowed bowel segment with regional ileitis. Use of a radiopaque contrast medium causes the narrowed lumen to appear as a thin string on radiographs.

striocerebellar tremor /strī′ōser′əbel″ər/, a combination of static, active, and intentional voluntary muscle contractions with both striatal and cerebellar components. It is associated with hereditary ataxia and diffuse degeneration of the central nervous system.

strip membranes [Ger, *strippe,* strap; L, *membrana,* thin skin], (in obstetrics) a procedure in which an examiner, with gloved fingers, frees the membranes of the amniotic sac from the wall of the uterus of the lower segment of the uterus in the small area around the cervical os. It is done to stimulate labor.

stripping, 1. *(Nontechnical)* a surgical procedure for the removal of the long and short saphenous veins of the legs. See also **milking, varicose vein. 2.** the mechanical removal of a very small amount of enamel from the mesial or distal surfaces of teeth to alleviate crowding.

stroke. See **cerebrovascular accident.**

stroke prone profile [AS, *strac*], a predictive index using a complex of risk factors that indicate susceptibility of a person to cerebrovascular accident (CVA). The factors include advanced age, hypertension, a history of transient ischemic attacks, cigarette smoking, heart disorders, associated embolism, family history of CVA, use of oral contraceptives, diabetes mellitus, physical inactivity, obesity, hypercholesteremia, and hyperlipidemia.

stroke volume, the amount of blood ejected by a ventricle during contraction.

stroke volume index, stroke volume divided by the body surface area.

stroking /strō″king/, running the entire hand over large parts of the body to relax the muscles reflexively and eliminate muscle spasm, improve circulation, or produce a parasympathetic response. See also **effleurage.**

S

stroma /strō″mə/ *pl.* *stromas, stromata* [Gk, covering], the supporting tissue or the matrix of an organ, as distinguished from its parenchyma. Some kinds of stromata are the vitreous stroma, which encloses the vitreous humor of the eye, and Rollet stroma, which contains the hemoglobin of a red blood cell. −*stromatic, adj.*

stroma-, combining form meaning "connective tissue forming framelike support for an organ": *stromatic.*

-stroma, combining form meaning "supporting tissue of an organ": *myostroma.*

stromas, stromata, stromatic. See **stroma.**

Strongyloides /stron′jiloi″dēz/ [Gk, *strongylos,* round, *eidos,* form], a genus of parasitic intestinal nematode. One species, *S. stercoralis,* causes strongyloidiasis, a potentially life-threatening infection under certain circumstances.

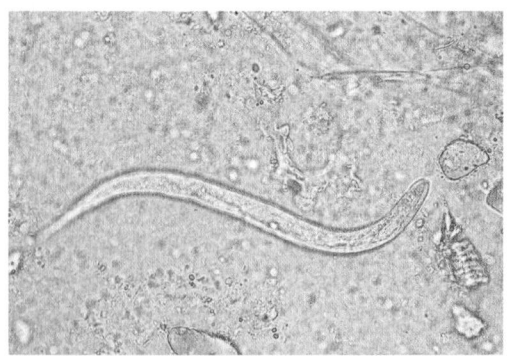

***Strongyloides stercoralis* larvae** *(Murray, Rosenthal, and Pfaller, 2005)*

strongyloidiasis /stron′jəloidī″əsis/, infection of the small intestine by the roundworm *Strongyloides stercoralis.* It is acquired when larvae from the soil penetrate intact skin, incidentally causing a pruritic rash. The larvae pass to the lungs via the bloodstream, sometimes causing pneumonia. They then migrate up the air passages to the pharynx, are swallowed, and develop into adult worms in the small intestine. Bloody diarrhea and intestinal malabsorption may result. Rarely, fatal disseminated strongyloidiasis occurs. Diagnosis depends on finding larvae in freshly passed feces. Treatment of established infections often includes administration of thiabendazole, ivermectin, and albendazole. Early infection is treated with inhaled beta-agonists. Antihelminthic therapy works poorly against the larval stage. Proper sanitary methods for the disposal of excrement can eliminate the disease. Wearing shoes prevents contagion from contaminated soil. Hyperinfection syndrome can arise in immunocompromised patients. Also called **threadworm infection.** See also **Löffler syndrome.**

strontium (Sr) /stron″sh(ē)əm/ [Strontian, Scotland], a metallic element. Its atomic number is 38; its atomic mass is 87.62. Chemically similar to calcium, it is found in bone tissue. Isotopes of strontium are used in radioisotope scanning procedures of bone. Strontium 85 (^{85}Sr) and strontium 87 (^{87}Sr) mimic calcium metabolism and are used in studies of bone physiological characteristics and disorders. These radionuclides can be counted with any standard detector or imaged at a very early stage in bone disease, whereas radiographic films of bone without the use of a radioactive tracer can show decreased density only after approximately 50% of bone is decalcified. Most ^{85}Sr or ^{87}Sr is deposited in bone within 1 hour after injection. Increased deposition of these radionuclides is strongly linked to osteoblastic activity and new bone formation. In addition to four naturally occurring isotopes (^{88}Sr, ^{87}Sr, ^{86}Sr, and ^{84}Sr), 12 artificial strontium isotopes are produced by nuclear reactions. Strontium 90, the

longest-lived, is the most dangerous constituent of fallout from atomic bomb tests. It can replace some of the calcium in food, become concentrated in teeth and bones, and continue to emit electrons that can cause death in the host. Strontium 90 becomes concentrated in cow's milk.

Stroop Color and Word Test (SCWT) [John Ridley Stroop, 1897–1973], a test of cognitive ability that assesses the ability to direct attention to a task. Also called *Stroop test.*

-strophe, strophy, suffix meaning "turning" or "twisting": *algodystrophy, chondrodystrophy, hemidystrophy.*

stropho-, combining form meaning "twisted."

strophulus, a papular eruption on the gingivae of children during teething.

-strophy. See **-strophe, strophy.**

structural /struk″chərəl/ [L, *structura,* arrangement], pertaining to the arrangement or pattern of component parts of an object or organism.

structural chemistry [L, *structura,* arrangement], the science dealing with the molecular structure of chemical substances.

structural gene, a gene that specifies the amino acid sequence of a polypeptide (protein) that has a structural role.

structural integration, a technique of deep massage intended to help in the realignment of the body by altering the length and tone of myofascial tissues. The basis of the practice is the belief that misalignment of myofascial tissues, a result of improper posture and emotional and physical traumas, may have a detrimental effect on a person's energy level, self-image, muscular efficiency, perceptions, and general health. Also called **Rolfing.**

structural model, a model of family therapy that views the family as an open system and identifies subsystems within the family that carry out specific family functions. When faced with demands for change, individual family members, family subsystems, or the family as a whole may respond with growth behaviors or maladaptive behaviors. The goal of family therapy is to help family members learn new scripts or transactional patterns.

structure /struk″chər/ [L, *structura*], a part of the body, such as the heart, a bone, a gland, a cell, or a limb.

structure-activity relationship (SAR), the relationship between the chemical structure of a drug and its activity.

structured learning therapy /struk″chərd/, a rehabilitation technique used with schizophrenic patients.

strum-, combining form meaning "a goiter or scrofula": *struma lymphomatosa.*

struma lymphomatosa. See **Hashimoto disease.**

Strümpell-Marie disease /strim″pəl märē″/ [Ernst A. von Strümpell, German neurologist, 1853–1925; Pierre Marie, French neurologist, 1853–1940; L, *dis;* Fr, *aise,* ease], ankylosing spondylitis. Also called **Marie-Strümpell arthritis, Marie-Strümpell disease, rheumatoid spondylitis, spondylitis ankylopoietica.**

strychnine /strik″nin, strik″nīn/ [Gk, *strychnos,* nightshade], a white crystalline alkaloid obtained from the leaves of the *Strychnos nux-vomica* plant. It is extremely toxic to the central nervous system.

strychnine poisoning [Gk, *strychnos* + L, *potio,* a drink], toxic effects of ingesting strychnine, a central nervous system stimulant. Symptoms include restlessness and hyperacuity of hearing and vision. Minor stimuli may produce convulsions, but there may be complete muscle relaxation between convulsions. One classic sign of strychnine poisoning is an arched back (opisthotonos).

Stryker wedge frame, an orthopedic bed that allows the patient to be rotated as required to either the full supine or full prone position. It is used in the immobilization of patients with unstable spines, in the postoperative management of multilevel spinal fusions, and in the management of severe burn patients. Compare **CircOlectric (COL) bed, Foster bed, hyperextension bed.**

STS,   abbreviation for **sit-to-stand.**

S-T segment,   an isoelectric line after the QRS complex on the electrocardiogram. It represents phase 2 of the cardiac action potential. Elevation or depression of the S-T segment is the hallmark of myocardial ischemia or injury and coronary artery disease.

Stuartnatal Plus,   a fixed-combination oral prenatal drug containing vitamins and minerals.

Stuart-Prower factor.   See **factor X.**

Studer neobladder,   a low pressure type of orthotopic ileal neobladder with ureters attached to the proximal "chimney" of the neobladder.

stump [ME, *stumpe*],   the part of a limb that remains after amputation. Also called **residual limb.**

stump hallucination,   the sensation of the continued presence of an amputated limb. See also **hallucination, phantom limb syndrome.**

stump pain,   pain arising in the stump in a person with an amputated limb. Unlike phantom limb pain, which originates and ends in the brain, it originates from damaged nerves near the site of the amputation.

stunned myocardium,   a condition of impaired myocardial contractile function, cellular biochemical characteristics, and microvasculature function in the absence of gross myocardial necrosis. It can last for minutes to days and is caused by ischemia that is either brief or occurs in the area immediately outside an infarct zone.

stupefacient /st(y)oo′pəfā″shənt/ [L, *stupere,* to stun, *facere,* to make],   an opioid or other agent that has the effect of making a person stuporous.

stupor /st(y)oo″pər/ [L, *stupere,* to stun],   *adj.,* a state of unresponsiveness in which a person seems unaware of the surroundings. The condition occurs in neurological and psychiatric disorders. The person may be totally or almost totally immobile and unresponsive, even to painful stimuli. Kinds include *anergic stupor,* **benign stupor, epileptic stupor.**

Sturge-Weber syndrome /sturj″ web″ər/ [William A. Sturge, English physician, 1850–1919; Frederick P. Weber, English physician, 1863–1962],   a congenital neurocutaneous disease marked by a port-wine–colored capillary hemangioma over a sensory dermatome of a branch of the trigeminal nerve of the face. Radiographic examination of the skull reveals intracranial calcification. The cerebral cortex may atrophy, and generalized or focal seizures, angioma of the choroid, secondary glaucoma, optic atrophy, and new cutaneous hemangiomas may develop. There is no known cure. Treatment is supportive and includes anticonvulsive medication. Also called **encephalotrigeminal angiomatosis.**

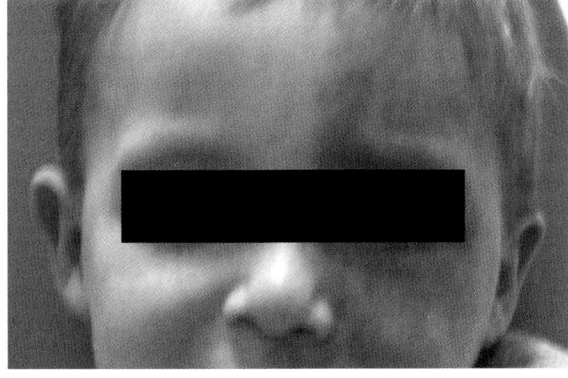

Individual with Sturge-Weber syndrome (Albert, Miller, and Jakobiec, 2008)

stuttering [D, *stotteren*],   a speech disorder usually characterized by excessive abnormal hesitations, blocks, part-word and whole-word repetitions, and audible or silent prolongation of sounds. The cause of stuttering is unknown; it may be hereditary or may result from developmental processes or neurological impairment. Hesitancy and lack of fluency in speech are typical characteristics of normal speech and language development during the preschool years, when a child's physical, psychological, and speech and language development do not match the linguistic demands of talking. The child may become conscious of speaking difficulties associated with acquisition, and a fear of speaking may develop. Early prevention and evaluation are recommended. The health care professional may educate parents by making them aware of the normal dysfluent patterns in a child's speech and by suggesting ways to encourage a child's speech development. If stuttering persists, parents should be encouraged to seek the advice of a speech-language pathologist. Also called **fluency disorder.** See also **stammering.**

sty [ME, *styanye,* eyelid tumor],   a purulent infection of a meibomian or sebaceous gland of the eyelid, often caused by a staphylococcal organism. Also called **hordeolum.** Also spelled *stye.*

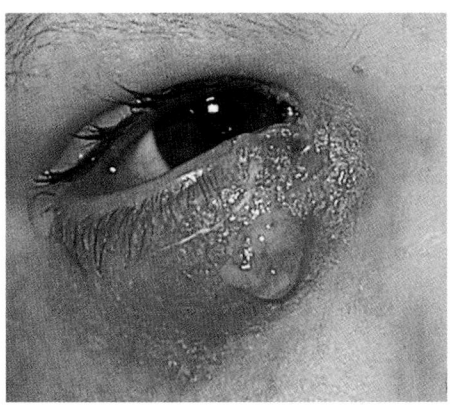

Sty (Kanski and Nischal, 1999)

-style,   combining form meaning "a bone attached to an internal structure."

stylet /stī″lət, stīlet″/ [It, *stiletto,* dagger],   a thin metal probe for inserting into or passing through a needle, tube, or catheter to clean the hollow bore or for inserting into a soft, flexible catheter to make it stiff as the catheter is placed in a vein or passed through an orifice of the body. Also spelled **stilet, stilette.**

stylo-,   combining form meaning "like a pillar, stake, or pole": *styloglossus, stylohyoideus, styloid.*

styloglossus,   a muscle that retracts the tongue and pulls the back of the tongue superiorly. It is innervated by the hypoglossal nerves.

stylohyoideus /stī′lōhī·oi″dē·əs/ [Gk, *stylos,* pillar, *hyoeides,* U-shaped],   one of four suprahyoid muscles, lying anterior and superior to the posterior belly of the digastricus. It is a slender muscle that arises from the styloid process and inserts into the hyoid bone. It serves to draw the hyoid bone up and back. Also called *stylohyoid bone.* Compare **digastricus, geniohyoideus, mylohyoideus.**

stylohyoid ligament /stī′lōhī″oid/,   the ligament attached to the tip of the styloid process of the temporal bone and to the lesser cornu of the hyoid bone. It frequently contains a small cartilage in its center and is often partially ossified.

S

styloid /stī″loid/ [Gk, *stylos,* pillar, *eidos,* form], long and tapered like a pen or stylus.

styloid process [Gk, *stylos* + *eidos* + L, *processus*], any of several projections of bone tissue, particularly a projection on the temporal bone.

stylomandibular ligament /stī″lōmandib″yələr/ [Gk, *stylos* + L, *mandere,* to chew, *ligare,* to bind], one of a pair of specialized bands of cervical fascia forming an accessory part of the temporomandibular joint. It extends from the styloid process of the temporal bone to the ramus of the mandible between the masseter and pterygoideus muscles and separates the parotid gland from the submandibular gland. Compare **sphenomandibular ligament.**

stylus /stī″ləs/, **1.** a fine probe. **2.** a wire inserted into a catheter to stiffen it. **3.** a device that imprints electric activity and wave patterns on electrocardiographic, electroencephalographic, or similar graphic recordings.

styptic /stip″tik/ [Gk, *styptikos,* astringent], **1.** *n.,* a substance used as an astringent, often to control bleeding. A chemical styptic induces coagulation of blood. A cotton pledget used as a compress to control bleeding is a mechanical styptic. **2.** *adj.,* acting as an astringent or agent to control bleeding.

subacromial /sub′əkrō″mē·əl/ [L, *sub,* beneath; Gk, *akron,* extremity, *omos,* shoulder], pertaining to the area below the acromion.

subacromial bursa [L, *sub,* under; Gk, *akron,* extremity, *omos,* shoulder, *byrsa,* wineskin], the bursa separating the acromion and deltoid muscle from the insertion of the supraspinatus muscle and the greater tubercle of the humerus.

subacute /-əkyo͞ot′/ [L, *sub* + *acutus,* sharp], **1.** less than acute. **2.** pertaining to a disease or other abnormal condition present in a person who appears to be clinically well. The condition may be identified or discovered by means of a laboratory test or radiological examination.

subacute bacterial endocarditis (SBE), a chronic bacterial infection of the valves of the heart. It is characterized by a slow, quiet onset with fever, heart murmur, splenomegaly, and development of clumps of abnormal tissue, called vegetations, around an intracardiac prosthesis or on the cusps of a valve. Various species of *Streptococcus* or *Staphylococcus* are commonly the cause of SBE. Dental procedures are associated with infection by *Streptococcus viridans,* surgical procedures with *S. faecalis,* and self-infection (especially by drug abusers) with *Staphylococcus aureus.*
■ OBSERVATIONS: The infected vegetations may separate from the valve or prosthesis and form emboli. Osler nodes, petechiae, Roth spots, and splinter hemorrhages under the fingernails are common manifestations of blood-borne metastases of these emboli. Bacteriological examination of cultures of the blood may allow specific diagnosis and treatment.
■ INTERVENTIONS: Treatment requires prolonged and regular administration of an antibiotic that is known to be effective against the causative organism. If a prosthesis has become infected, it is usually removed. Before surgery or a dental procedure, prophylactic antibiotics are given. During the acute phase of illness the fever is treated with antipyretic medication and bed rest; adequate high-protein diet and fluids are encouraged.
■ PATIENT CARE CONSIDERATIONS: Bed rest and hospitalization may be necessary for several weeks. Emotional and psychological support may help the patient adjust to the necessary inactivity and to understand that SBE is a chronic illness.

subacute care, 1. a level of treatment that is between chronic and acute. **2.** treatment of a disease that is of moderate severity or duration.

subacute combined degeneration of the spinal cord. See **combined system disease.**

subacute glomerulonephritis, an uncommon noninfectious disease of the glomerulus of the kidney characterized by proteinuria, hematuria, decreased production of urine, and edema. Of unknown cause, the disease may progress rapidly, and renal failure may occur. Kidney transplantation and dialysis are the only treatments available. See also **chronic glomerulonephritis, postinfectious glomerulonephritis, uremia.**

subacute infection [L, *sub,* beneath, *acutus,* sharp, *inficere,* to stain], a disease condition that is not chronic and that runs a rapid and severe, but less than acute, course.

subacute inflammation, a reactive sign of inflammation with a gradual onset, later increasing to a chronic or severe type of reaction.

subacute myelooptic neuropathy (SMON), a condition of muscular pain and weakness, usually below the T12 vertebra; painful dysesthesia of the limbs; and, in some cases, optic atrophy. The patient usually experiences a significant alteration of gait.

subacute necrotizing encephalomyelopathy, subacute necrotizing encephalopathy. See **Leigh disease.**

subacute necrotizing lymphadenitis. See **Kikuchi's lymphadenitis.**

subacute sclerosing panencephalitis, a rare, progressive, neurological disorder occurring with primary measles infection in children 2 years of age or younger, with a period of latency for 2 to 10 years. The condition occurs in children and in adolescents who have had measles at a very early age. It is characterized by diffuse inflammation of brain tissue, personality change, seizures, ataxia myoclonus, visual disturbances, dementia, fever, and death. Live measles virus can be cultured from brain tissue. No effective therapy is known; however, some antiviral drugs can slow the progression of the disease. A combination of oral Isoprinosine and interferon alfa injected into ventricles of the brain appears to be the most effective treatment. See also **slow virus.**

subacute spongiform encephalopathy. See **prion disease.**

subacute thyroiditis. See **de Quervain thyroiditis.**

subaortic /-ā·ôr″tik/ [L, *sub* + Gk, *aerein,* to raise], pertaining to the area of the body below the aorta.

subaortic stenosis [L, *sub,* beneath; Gk, *aerein,* to raise, *stenos,* narrow, *osis,* condition], a narrowing of the left ventricle outflow tract below the aortic valve. Also called **aortic valvular stenosis.**

subapical /-ap″ikəl/, below the peak or apex.

subaponeurotic /-ap′ōno͞orot″ik/ [L, *sub,* beneath; Gk, *apo,* from, *neuron,* nerve; L, *tendo*], beneath an aponeurosis.

subarachnoid /sub′ərak″noid/ [L, *sub* + Gk, *arachne,* spider, *eidos,* form], pertaining to the area under the arachnoid membrane and above the pia mater.

subarachnoid block anesthesia. See **spinal anesthesia.**

subarachnoid cistern, any one of many small subarachnoid spaces that serve as reservoirs for cerebrospinal fluid.

subarachnoid hemorrhage (SaH, SAH), an intracranial hemorrhage into the cerebrospinal fluid-filled space between the arachnoid and pial membranes on the surface of the brain. The hemorrhage may extend into the brain if the force of the bleeding from the broken vessel is sudden and severe. The cause may be trauma, rupture of an aneurysm, or an arteriovenous anomaly.
■ OBSERVATIONS: The first symptom of a subarachnoid hemorrhage is a sudden, extremely severe headache that begins in one localized area and then spreads, becoming dull and throbbing. It is frequently described by patients as "the worst headache of my life." The localized pain results from vascular distortion and injury. The generalized ache is the result of meningeal irritation by blood in the subarachnoid space. Other characteristics of subarachnoid hemorrhage can

include dizziness, rigidity of the neck, pupillary inequality, vomiting, seizures, drowsiness, sweating and chills, stupor, and loss of consciousness. A brief period of unconsciousness immediately after the rupture is common; severe hemorrhage may result in continued unconsciousness, coma, and death. Delirium and confusion often persist through the first weeks of recovery, and permanent brain damage is common.

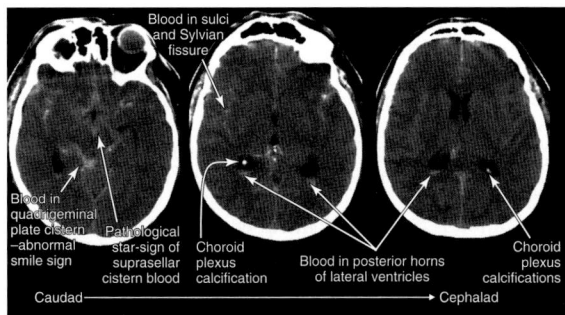

Subarachnoid hemorrhage *(Chabner, 2007)*

subarachnoid space, the space between the arachnoid membranes and pia mater membranes. It contains cerebrospinal fluid.

subatomic /-ətom″ik/ [L, *sub,* beneath; Gk, *atomos,* indivisible], pertaining to the particles and phenomena that are within an atom.

subaxillary /-ak″siler′ē/ [L, *sub,* beneath, *axilla,* wing], pertaining to the area beneath the axilla.

subcapital femoral neck fracture /-kap″itəl/ [L, *sub + caput,* head], a fracture located just below the head of the thigh bone, which pivots in a ball-and-socket joint.

subcapsular /-kap″s(y)ələr/ [L, *sub,* beneath, *capsula,* little box], pertaining to the area below a capsule.

subcapsular cataract [L, *sub + capsula,* little box], a condition marked by opacity or cloudiness beneath the anterior or posterior capsule of the lens of the eye.

subcapsular hematoma, one in the subcapsular space of the kidney. It may be caused by a tumor, trauma, vasculitis, renal infarction, or other disease process.

subcapsular space, the potential space between the renal parenchyma and the renal capsules.

subclavian /-səbklā″vē-ən/ [L, *sub + clavicula,* little key], situated under the clavicle, such as the subclavian vein.

subclavian artery, one of a pair of arteries passing under the clavicle that vary in origin, course, and the height to which they rise in the neck but have six similar main branches supplying the vertebral column, spinal cord, ear, and brain. See also **left subclavian artery, right subclavian artery.**

subclavian catheter, a central venous catheter inserted through the subclavian vein.

subclavian steal syndrome, a vascular syndrome caused by an occlusion in the subclavian artery proximal to the origin of the vertebral artery. It results in a reversal of the normal blood pressure gradient in the vertebral artery and decreased blood flow distal to the occlusion. It is characterized by episodes of flaccid paralysis of the arm, pain in the mastoid and occipital areas, and a diminished or absent radial pulse on the involved side. Markedly different blood pressure measurements obtained from each arm are sometimes indicative of the condition.

subclavian trunk, one of the two lymphatic vessels, right and left, that drain the right upper limb and the superficial regions of the thoracic and upper abdominal wall.

subclavian vein, the continuation of the axillary vein in the upper body, extending from the lateral border of the first rib to the sternal end of the clavicle, where it joins the internal

jugular to form the brachiocephalic vein. It usually contains a pair of valves near its junction with the internal jugular vein. The subclavian vein receives deoxygenated blood from the external jugular vein and, on the left side, at the junction with the internal jugular vein, receives lymph from the thoracic duct. On the right side, at the corresponding junction, it receives lymph from the right lymphatic duct.

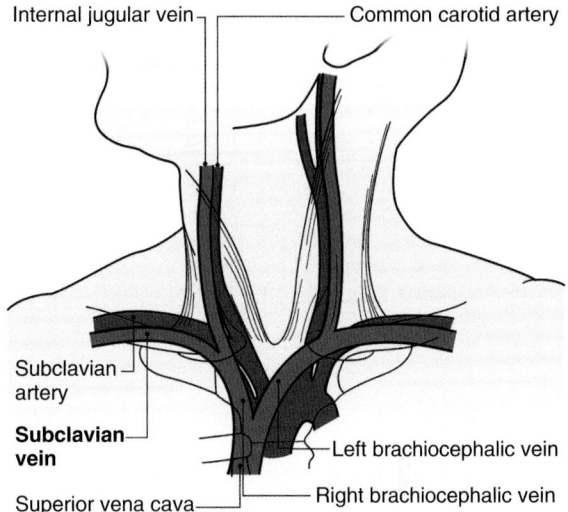

Subclavian vein *(Sanders et al, 2007)*

subclavius /səbklā″vē-əs/ [L, *sub + clavicula*], a short muscle of the chest wall. It is a small cylindric muscle between the clavicle and the first rib and arises in a short thick tendon from the junction of the first rib and its cartilage under the clavicle. It inserts into the groove on the inferior surface of the clavicle between the costoclavicular and conoid ligaments. The subclavius is innervated by a special nerve from the lateral trunk of the brachial plexus, which contains fibers from the fifth and sixth cervical nerves. It acts to draw the shoulder down and forward. Compare **pectoralis major, pectoralis minor, serratus anterior.**

subclinical /-klin″ikəl/ [L, *sub + Gk, kline,* bed], pertaining to a disease or abnormal condition so mild that it produces no symptoms.

subclinical deficiency, (in orthomolecular medicine) deficiency of a nutrient sufficient to affect health but not severe enough to cause classic deficiency symptoms.

subclinical diabetes. See **impaired glucose tolerance.**

subcollateral gyrus /-kəlat″ərəl/ [L, *sub + con + lateralis + Gk, gyros,* turn], a convolution below the collateral fissure or sulcus of the cerebrum.

subconscious /-kon″shəs/ [L, *sub + conscire,* to be aware], a lay or popular term for unconscious or partially conscious. –**subconsciousness,** *n.*

subconscious memory, a thought, sensation, or feeling that is not immediately available for recall to the conscious mind.

subconsciousness. See **subconscious.**

subcostales, muscles that span multiple ribs, extending from the internal surfaces of one rib to the internal surface of the second or third rib below. They are more numerous in the lower regions of the posterior thoracic wall. They parallel the course of the internal intercostal muscles and extend from the angle of the ribs to more medial positions on the ribs below.

subcostal nerve, the spinal nerve T12, which supplies skin and muscle of the abdominal wall.

subcrepitant rale, a fine, moist rale heard over liquid in the smaller tubes. Also called **crackling rale.**

subcrestral periodontal pocket. See **periodontal pocket.**

subculture /sub″kulchər/ [L, *sub + colere,* to cultivate], an ethnic, regional, economic, or social group with characteristic patterns of behavior and ideals that distinguish it from the rest of a culture or society.

subcutaneous /sub′kyo͞otā″nē·əs/ [L, *sub + cutis,* skin], beneath the skin.

subcutaneous adipose tissue [L, *sub,* beneath, *cutis,* skin, *adeps,* fat; OFr, *tissu*], fat deposits beneath the skin.

subcutaneous chronic zygomycosis. See **entomophtho-romycosis basidiobolae.**

subcutaneous emphysema, the presence of air or gas in the subcutaneous tissues. The air or gas may originate in the rupture of an airway or alveolus and migrate through the subpleural spaces to the mediastinum and neck. The face, neck, and chest may appear swollen. Skin tissues can be painful and may produce a crackling or popping sound as air moves under them. The patient may experience dyspnea and appear cyanotic if the air leak is severe. Treatment may require an incision to release the trapped air. Also called *aerodermectasia.*

subcutaneous fascia, a continuous layer of connective tissue over the entire body between the skin and the deep fascial investment of the specialized structures of the body, such as the muscles. It comprises an outer normally fatty layer and an inner thin elastic layer. Between the two layers lie superficial blood vessels, nerves, lymphatics, the mammary glands, most of the facial muscles, and the platysma. Also called **subcutaneous layer.** Compare **deep fascia, subserous fascia.**

subcutaneous fat necrosis. See **adiponecrosis subcutanea neonatorum.**

subcutaneous infusion. See **hypodermoclysis.**

subcutaneous injection, the introduction of a hypodermic needle into the subcutaneous tissue beneath the skin, usually on the upper arm, thigh, or abdomen. A diagram of a plan for the rotation of injection sites helps to prevent overuse of one area of skin.

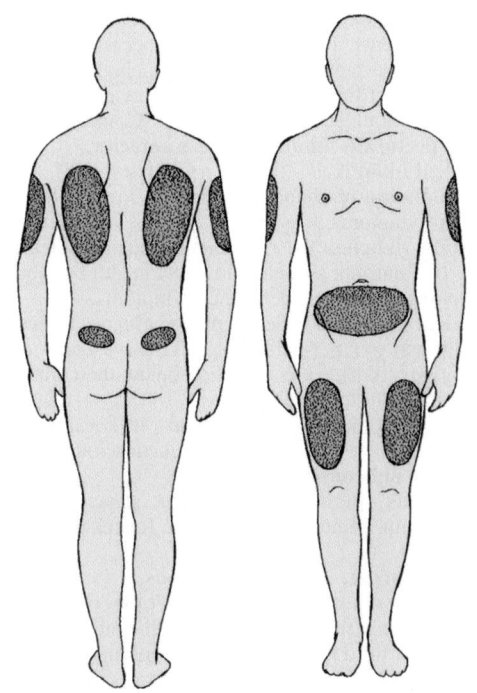

Locations for subcutaneous injections *(Potter et al, 2011)*

subcutaneous layer. See **subcutaneous fascia.**

subcutaneous mastectomy, a surgical procedure in which all of the breast tissue of one or both breasts is removed, leaving the skin, areola, and nipple intact. The adjacent lymph nodes, pectoralis major, and pectoralis minor are not removed. It may be performed on women who are at great risk of development of breast cancer. Reconstruction of the breasts is performed, with the assistance of a plastic surgeon, through the insertion of prostheses to return the normal contour to the breasts.

subcutaneous nodule, a small, solid mass, or node, beneath the skin that can be detected by touch. Subcutaneous nodules consisting chiefly of Aschoff bodies are found in patients with rheumatic fever. Minute subcutaneous nodules formed by the perivascular infiltration of mononuclear cells occur in typhus.

subcutaneous test. See **intradermal test.**

subcutaneous tunnel, a passage under the skin between the exit site of an atrial catheter and the entrance into the vein.

subcutaneous wound [L, *sub,* beneath, *cutis,* skin; AS, *wund*], an injury to internal organs, such as by crushing or another violent force, without a break in the surface of the skin. Also called **internal injury.**

subcuticular suture /-kyo͞otik″yələr/ [L, *sub,* beneath, *cutis,* skin, *sutura*], a continuous suture placed to draw together the tissues immediately beneath the skin. It may be either absorbable or nonabsorbable, requiring later removal.

subdermal /-der″məl/ [L, *sub* + Gk, *derma,* skin], beneath the dermis.

subdural /-d(y)o͞o″rəl/ [L, *sub* + *durus,* hard], pertaining to the area under the dura mater and above the arachnoid membrane.

subdural hematoma, an accumulation of blood in the subdural space, usually caused by an injury or fall. It can be acute with rapid bleeding or subacute with accumulation of blood over a longer period of time. Patients may have a chronic subdural hematoma that slowly occurs over an extended period of time, and some persons may have more than one bleed.

subdural hemorrhage, cerebral hemorrhage into the subdural space, often caused by trauma with resulting damage to the middle meningeal artery. See also **cerebrovascular accident, subdural hematoma.**

subdural hygroma, a collection of fluid between the dura mater and arachnoid layers resulting from a spinal fluid leak through a rupture in the arachnoid tissue.

subdural puncture, a perforation of the space between the dura mater and arachnoid membrane by a needle for the injection of diagnostic or therapeutic medications or for aspiration of blood or other fluid.

subdural space [L, *sub,* beneath, *dura, mater,* hard mother, *spatium*], the potential space between the dura mater and the arachnoid membrane.

subendocardial infarction /-en′dōkär″dē·əl/, a myocardial infarction that involves the innermost layer and, in some cases, parts of the middle layer of the myocardium but does not extend to the epicardium.

subepicardium /sub″ep-ikahr′dē-um/, subepicardial layer.

subepidermal /-ep′idur″məl/ [L, *sub,* beneath; Gk, *epi,* above, *derma,* skin], beneath the epidermis.

subepithelial hematoma of renal pelvis, a hematoma from bleeding in the subepithelial tissue of the renal pelvis, usually the result of a coagulopathy, such as in hemophilia, thrombocytopenia, or anticoagulant therapy. Also called **Antopol-Goldman lesion.**

subfertility /sub″fer-til′-te/, diminished reproductive capacity. Also called **hypofertility.** —*subfertile, adj.*

subgerminal cavity. See **blastocoele.**

subgingival calculus. See **calculus.**

subgingival curettage. See **root curettage.**

subglottic /-glot″ik/, beneath the glottis. Also called **infraglottic.**

subiculum /səbik″yələm/, a part of the hippocampal formation consisting of the transition zone between the parahippocampal gyrus and Ammon's horn.

subintimal /-in″timəl/ [L, *sub* + *intimus,* innermost], pertaining to the area beneath the intima or membrane lining a blood vessel, usually a large artery.

subinvolution, failure of a body part to return to its normal size and condition after enlargement from a functional activity. See **uterine subinvolution.**

subject contrast, the difference in x-ray beam intensities across the beam area after emerging from the part being radiographed.

subjective /-jek″tiv/ [L, *subjectus,* subject], **1.** pertaining to the essential nature of an object as perceived in the mind rather than to a thing in itself. **2.** existing only in the mind. **3.** that which arises within or is perceived by the individual, as contrasted with something that is modified by external circumstances or something that may be evaluated by objective standards. **4.** pertaining to a person who places excessive importance on his own moods, attitudes, or opinions; egocentric.

subjective data collection, the process in which data relating to the patient's problem are elicited from a patient or a patient's family. The data are retrieved from the patient's description of an event rather than from a physical examination, which provides objective data. The interviewer encourages a full description of the onset, the course, and the character of the problem and any factors that aggravate or ameliorate it. Compare **objective data collection.**

Subjective Global Assessment, a method of rating a patient's nutritional status, with subjective observations being given values on an ordinal scale. Factors assessed include weight change, appetite or anorexia, subcutaneous tissue and muscle, and GI symptoms.

subjective sensation, a feeling or impression that is not associated with or does not directly result from any external stimulus. See also **sensation,** def. 1.

subjective symptoms [L, *subjectus,* subject; Gk, *symptoma*], symptoms that are observed only by the patient and that cannot be objectively confirmed.

subjective tinnitus, a variety of sounds (e.g., ringing, buzzing, or humming) heard only by the individual when no external sound is present. The cause may be physical changes in the ear, auditory nerve damage, or intracranial hypertension. Compare **objective tinnitus.**

subjective vertigo, an inappropriate sensation of bodily movement.

subjects /sub″jekts/, participants, people, animals, or events selected for a study to examine a particular variable or condition, such as the effects of a new medication or therapy.

sublethal allele [L, *sub* + *letum,* death; Gk, *genein,* to produce], an allele whose presence causes abnormalities or impairs the functioning of an organism but does not cause its death. Compare **lethal allele.**

sublethal dose /-lē″thəl/ [L, *sub,* beneath, *letum,* death; Gk, *dosis,* giving], a dose of a potentially lethal substance that is not large enough to cause death.

subleukemic leukemia. See **aleukemic leukemia.**

sublimate /sub″limāt/ [L, *sublimare,* to lift up], to refine or divert instinctual impulses and energy from their immediate goal to one that can be expressed in a social, moral, or aesthetic manner acceptable to the person and the society.

sublimation /-limā″shən/ [L, *sublimare*], **1.** an unconscious defense mechanism by which an unacceptable instinctive drive is diverted to and expressed through a personally approved, socially accepted means. **2.** (in psychoanalysis) the process of diverting certain components of the sex drive to a socially acceptable, nonsexual goal. Compare **displacement. 3.** change in a physical state from the solid phase directly to the gas phase.

Sublimaze, an opioid analgesic. Brand name for *fentanyl.*

subliminal /-lim″inəl/ [L, *sub* + *limen,* threshold], taking place below the threshold of sensory perception or outside the range of conscious awareness.

subliminal self [L, *sub,* beneath, *limen,* threshold; AS, *self*], a level of mental activity at which an individual under normal waking conditions may function without consciousness. See also **preconscious, unconscious.**

sublingual /səbling″gwəl/ [L, *sub* + *lingua,* tongue], pertaining to the area beneath the tongue.

sublingual administration of a medication, the administration of a drug, usually in tablet form, by placing it beneath the tongue until the tablet dissolves. Administering drugs such as nitroglycerin by this route rather than by swallowing avoids the extensive first-pass metabolism of nitroglycerin that occurs in the liver.

sublingual caruncle [L, *sub,* beneath, *lingua,* tongue, *caruncula,* small piece of flesh], a small fleshy growth under the tongue.

sublingual duct. See **Bartholin duct, duct of Rivinus.**

sublingual fold, an elongate fold of mucosa raised by the superior margin of the sublingual gland. It extends from the posterolateral aspect of the floor of the oral cavity to the sublingual papilla beside the base of the frenulum of the tongue at the midline anteriorly.

sublingual gland, one of a pair of small salivary glands situated under the mucous membrane of the floor of the mouth, beneath the tongue. It is a narrow, almond-shaped structure and has from 8 to 20 ducts, some of which join to form the sublingual duct. The sublingual gland secretes mucus produced by its alveoli. Compare **parotid gland, submandibular gland.**

subluxation. See **incomplete dislocation.**

subluxation complex /-luksā″shən/, a theoretic chiropractic model of motion-segment dysfunction that incorporates the complex interaction of pathological changes in nervous, muscular, ligamentous, vascular, and connective tissues.

subluxation syndrome, an aggregate of signs and symptoms in chiropractic that relate to pathophysiological characteristics or dysfunction of spinal and pelvic motion segments or to peripheral joints.

submandibular /-məndib″yələr/ [L, *sub* + *mandible*], pertaining to the area beneath the mandible, or lower jaw. Also called **inframandibular.**

submandibular duct [L, *sub* + *mandere,* to chew], a duct through which a submandibular gland secretes saliva. Also called **submaxillary duct of Wharton, Wharton duct.**

submandibular gland, one of a pair of round, walnut-sized salivary glands in the submandibular triangle that open on a small papilla at the side of the frenulum linguae. The gland secretes both mucus and a thinner serous fluid, which aid the digestive process. Compare **parotid gland, sublingual gland.** See also **salivary gland.**

submarginal /sub·mär′ji·nəl/ [L, *sub,* beneath + *margo,* margin], inferior to or beneath a margin.

submaxillary /-mak″siler′ē/ [L, *sub* + *maxilla*], pertaining to the area below the maxilla, or upper jaw.

submaxillary duct of Wharton. See **submandibular duct.**

submeatal /-mē·ā″təl/ [L, *sub,* beneath, *meatus,* passage],   pertaining to tissues beneath a meatus, such as the mastoid air cells under the acoustic meatus or the hard palate beneath the nasal meatus.

submental /-men″təl/   [L, *sub* + *mentum,* chin],   pertaining to the area beneath the chin.

submentovertex /-men′tōvur″teks/   [L, *sub* + *mentum,* chin, *vertex,* peak],   pertaining to a radiographic projection of the skull in which x-rays enter just behind the chin and exit at the top of the head.

submetacentric /sub′metəsen″trik/   [L, *sub* + Gk, *meta,* besides, *kentron,* center],   pertaining to a chromosome in which the centromere is located approximately equidistant between the center and one end so that the arms of the chromosomes are not equal in length. Compare **acrocentric, metacentric, telocentric.**

submucous /-m(y)o͞o″kəs/,   pertaining to a location beneath a mucous membrane. *–submucosal, adj.*

submucous plexus,   one of the two interconnected nerve plexuses of the enteric nervous system. See also **myenteric plexus.**

submucous resection (SMR) [L, *sub* + *mucous* + *re* + *secare,* to cut],   a surgical procedure for correcting a deviated nasal septum, leaving the mucous membrane of the septum intact.

subnormal temperature /-nôr″məl/,   temperature below the normal body level of 98.6° F (37° C).

suboccipital muscles,   a small group of deep muscles in the upper cervical region at the base of the occipital bone that move the head. They include the rectus capitis posterior major, the rectus capitis posterior minor, the obliquus capitis inferior, and the obliquus capitis superior.

suboccipitobregmatic /-aksip′itō′bregmat″ik/   [L, *sub* + *occiput,* back of the head; Gk, *bregma,* front of the head],   pertaining to the smallest anteroposterior diameter of an infant's neck when it is well flexed during labor.

subperiosteal fracture /sub′perē·os″tē·əl/   [L, *sub* + Gk, *peri,* around, *osteon,* bone],   a fracture in a bone beneath the periosteum that does not disrupt the periosteum.

subphrenic /-fren″ik/   [L, *sub* + Gk, *phren,* diaphragm],   pertaining to the area under the diaphragm.

subphrenic abscess [L, *sub,* beneath; Gk, *phren,* diaphragm; L, *abscedere,* to go away],   an abscess that develops on or near the undersurface of the diaphragm, usually as a result of peritonitis or from another visceral site.

subpoena /-pē″nə/   [L, *sub* + *poena,* penalty],   (in law) a document from a court commanding that a person appear at a certain time and place to testify on a specific matter. Subpoenas are governed by federal rules for criminal and civil procedures.

subpoena duces tecum,   (in law) a subpoena commanding a person to take books, papers, records, or other items to the court.

subpopliteal recess,   the smaller of two expansions in the synovial membrane of the knee that lies between the lateral meniscus and the tendon of the popliteus muscle and provides a low-friction surface for the movement of tendons associated with the joint. The larger expansion is the suprapatellar bursa.

subpubic dislocation.   See **dislocation of the hip.**

subscapular artery,   the largest branch of the axillary artery and the major blood supply to the posterior wall of the axilla. It also contributes to the blood supply of the posterior scapular region.

subscapularis /-skap′yəler″is/   [L, *sub,* beneath, *scapulae,* shoulder blades],   the muscle arising from the subscapular fossa with insertion in the humerus. It functions to rotate the arm medially.

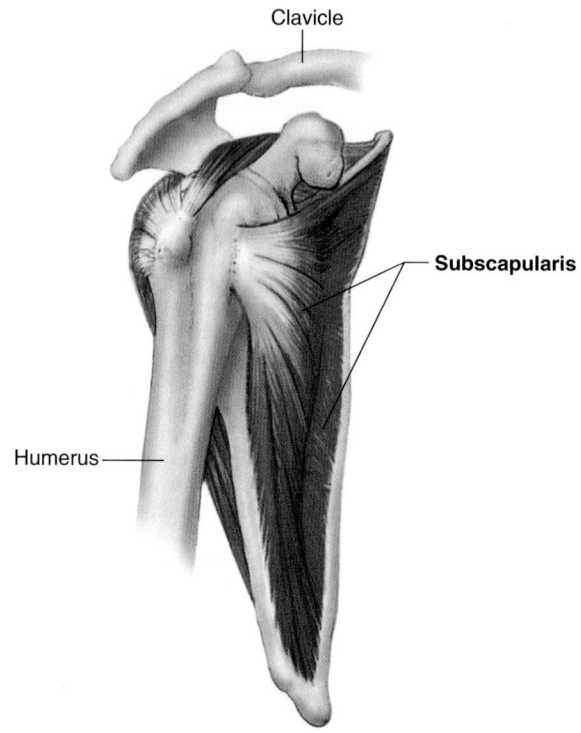

Clavicle

Subscapularis

Humerus

Subscapularis *(Patton and Thibodeau, 2010)*

subscapular nerves,   branches of the brachial plexus that innervate the subscapularis muscle. The inferior subscapular nerve also innervates the teres major muscles.

subscriber,   (in managed care) an individual, agency, or employer that has contracted for services under a health plan.

subserous fascia /-sir″əs/   [L, *sub* + *serum,* whey, *fascia,* band],   one of three kinds of fascia lying between the internal layer of deep fascia and the serous membranes lining the body cavities in much the same manner as the subcutaneous fascia lies between the skin and the deep fascia. It is thin in some areas, such as between the pleura and the chest wall, and thick in other areas, where it forms a pad of adipose tissue. Compare **deep fascia, subcutaneous fascia.**

subsistence /-sis″təns/   [L, *subsistere,* to stand still],   the state of being sustained or remaining alive with a minimum of life essentials.

subspecialty /-spesh″əltē/   [L, *sub* + *specialis,* individual],   a highly specific professional field of practice, such as pediatric oncology, infectious disease, or neonatology. Compare **specialty.**

subspinale /sub′spī·nā′lē/,   the deepest midline point on the maxilla on the concavity between the anterior nasal spine and the prosthion. Also called **point A.**

substance /sub″stəns/   [L, *substantia,* essence],   **1.** any drug, chemical, or biological entity. **2.** any material capable of being self-administered or abused because of its physiological or psychological effects.

substance abuse, the overindulgence in and dependence on a stimulant, depressant, or other chemical substance, leading to effects that are detrimental to the individual's physical or mental health or the welfare of others.

Substance Abuse and Mental Health Services Administration (SAMHSA), an agency of the U.S. Department of Health and Human Services with the function of disseminating accurate and up-to-date information about and providing leadership in the prevention and treatment of addictive and mental disorders.

substance abuse testing, a screening of the urine or blood, or another kind of test, to identify drug use or drug overdose or poisoning from substances such as lead and carbon monoxide.

substance dependence, a maladaptive pattern of substance abuse leading to clinically significant impairment or distress as manifested by three or more episodes within a 12-month period of tolerance, withdrawal, or use of larger amounts or, over a longer period, a persistent desire or unsuccessful effort to control substance abuse or investment of a great deal of time in activities necessary to obtain the substance.

substance P, a polypeptide neurotransmitter that stimulates vasodilation and contraction of intestinal and other smooth muscles. It also plays a part in salivary secretion, diuresis, natriuresis, and pain sensation. It has been isolated from certain cells of the GI and biliary tracts.

substandard /-stan″dərd/ [L, *sub,* beneath; OFr, *estandart*], below the predetermined model or measure.

substantia alba /-stan″shə/ [L, *substantia,* essence, *albus,* white], the part of the central nervous system that is enclosed in myelin sheaths. The myelin contributes a white coloring to otherwise gray nerve tissue.

substantia gelatinosa. See **Rolando's gelatinous substance.**

substantia innominata, nerve tissue immediately inferior to the anterior perforated substance and anterior to the globus pallidus and ansa lenticularis.

substantia nigra [L, *substantia,* essence, *niger,* black], a dark band of gray matter lying between the tegmentum of the midbrain and the crus cerebri.

substantive epidemiology /sub″stəntiv/ [L, *substantia* + Gk, *epi,* upon, *demos,* people, *logos,* science], the body of knowledge derived from epidemiological studies, including, for each disease, the natural history of the disorder, patterns of occurrence, and risk factors for development of the disorder.

substantivity /-stəntiv″itē/, the property of continuing therapeutic action despite removal of the vehicle, such as the action of certain shampoos.

substernal /-stur″nəl/ [L, *sub* + Gk, *sternon,* chest], pertaining to the area beneath the sternum.

substernal goiter [L, *sub* + Gk, *sternon,* chest; L, *guttur,* throat], a nonbacterial inflammation of the lower thyroid isthmus, often preceded by a viral infection causing fever, tenderness, and enlargement of the thyroid gland. Symptoms may last 2 to 4 months and are usually resolved by corticosteroids. See also **thyroiditis.**

substitution /-stit(y)ōō″shən/, a mental defense mechanism, operating unconsciously, by which an unattainable or unacceptable goal, emotion, or object is replaced by one that is more attainable or acceptable.

substitutive therapy /sub″stit(y)ōō″tiv/ [L, *substituere,* to put in place of; Gk, *therapeia,* treatment], a treatment that affects a condition incompatible with or antagonistic to the condition being treated. Also called **allopathy.**

substrate /sub″strāt/ [L, *sub* + *stratum,* layer], a chemical acted on and changed by an enzyme in a chemical reaction.

substrate depletion phase, a period during an enzyme assay when the concentration of substrate is falling and the assay is not following zero-order kinetics.

substratum /-strā″təm/ [L, *sub* + *stratum,* layer], any underlying layer; a foundation.

sub-, suf-, sup-, prefix meaning "under," "below," "down," "near," "almost," or "moderately": *subacute, suffocation.*

subsystem /sub″sistəm/, a smaller component of a large system composed of individuals or dyads, formed by generation, gender, interest, or function.

subtalar joint, the joint between the large posterior calcaneal facet on the inferior surface of the talus and the corresponding posterior talar facet on the superior surface of the calcaneus. It allows gliding and rotation, which are involved in inversion and eversion of the foot.

subtask work, a part of the whole task in a rehabilitation program but distinguished by changes in speed or direction.

subthalamic. See **subthalamus.**

subthalamic nucleus, a biconvex mass of gray matter on the medial side of the junction of the internal capsule and the crus cerebri. Its chief connections are with the globus pallidus.

subthalamus /-thal″əməs/ [L, *sub* + Gk, *thalamos,* chamber], a part of the diencephalon that serves as a correlation center for optic and vestibular impulses relayed to the globus pallidus. It is a transition zone between the thalamus and the tegmentum mesencephali. Compare **epithalamus, hypothalamus, metathalamus, thalamus. –subthalamic,** *adj.*

subtle /sut″əl/ [L, *subtilis*], **1.** having a low intensity. **2.** not severe and having no serious sequelae, such as a mild infection or inflammation.

subtotal /sub″tōtəl/ [L, *sub,* beneath, *totus,* whole], less than complete.

subtotal hysterectomy [L, *sub* + *totus* + Gk, *hystera,* womb, *extome,* excision], the surgical removal of the body of the uterus without removing the cervix. See also **supracervical hysterectomy, supravaginal hysterectomy.**

subtrochanteric osteotomy /-trō′kənter″ik/ [L, *sub* + Gk, *trochanter,* runner, *osteon,* bone, *temnein,* to cut], a surgical procedure that divides the shaft of the femur below the lesser trochanter to correct ankylosis of the hip joint.

subungual /səbung″gwəl/ [L, *sub* + *unguis,* nail], beneath a fingernail or toenail.

subungual hematoma, a collection of blood beneath a nail that usually results from trauma. The pain accompanying this condition may be quickly alleviated by burning or drilling a small hole through the nail to release the blood.

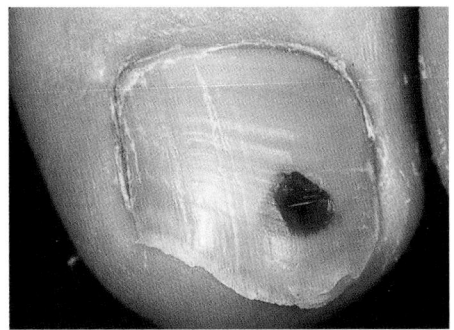

Subungual hematoma *(du Vivier, 2002)*

subunit vaccine /sub″yōōnit/, a viral immunizing agent that has been treated to remove traces of viral nucleic acid so that only protein subunits remain. The subunits have less risk of causing adverse reactions.

subventricular zone /-ventrik″yələr/, an area, located between the ventricular and intermediate zones in the fetal forebrain, in which neurons of the cerebrum are generated.

S

subzonal insemination (SUZI), an older technique of micromanipulation used in cases of male factor infertility. Spermatozoa are inserted into the space between the zona pellucida and the cell membrane surrounding an egg by mechanical or chemical means. Also called *subzonal injection.*

subzygomatic, below the zygomatic bone.

succ-, combining form meaning "juice": *succus, succussion splash.*

succenturiate placenta. See **accessory placenta.**

succi. See **succus.**

succinic acid (HOOC(CH₂)₂COOH) /suksin″ik/, a dicarboxylic acid found in certain hydatid cysts and in lichens, amber, and fossils. Commercial succinic acid, produced by the fermentation of ammonium tartrate, is used in lacquer and dyes. Succinic acid was formerly used in the treatment of diabetic ketoacidosis.

succinylcholine chloride /suk′sinilkō″lēn/, a depolarizing neuromuscular blocker that is a skeletal muscle relaxant.

■ INDICATIONS: It is prescribed to provide an adjunct to anesthesia, to reduce muscle contractions during surgery or mechanical ventilation, and to facilitate endotracheal intubation.

■ CONTRAINDICATIONS: Known hypersensitivity to this drug prohibits its use. Caution is used in administering it to patients with a family history of malignant hyperthermia, those with low pseudocholinesterase levels, and those with myasthenia gravis or renal failure.

■ ADVERSE EFFECTS: Among the more serious adverse effects are cardiac arrhythmia, severe respiratory depression, and (rarely) malignant hyperthermia.

succus /suk″əs/ *pl. succi* [L, juice], a juice or fluid, usually one secreted by an organ, such as succus prostaticus of the prostate.

succussion splash /səkush″ən/ [L, *succutere,* to shake up; ME, *plasche,* puddle], the sound elicited by shaking the body of a person who has free fluid and air or gas in a hollow organ or body cavity. This sound may be present over a normal stomach but also may be heard with hydropneumothorax, large hiatal hernia, or intestinal or pyloric obstruction.

suck [L, *sugere,* to suck], **1.** to draw a liquid or semiliquid into the mouth by creating a partial vacuum through motions of the lips and tongue. **2.** to hold on the tongue and dissolve by the movements of the mouth and action of the saliva. **3.** to draw fluid into the mouth, specifically to draw milk from the breast or nursing bottle.

sucking blisters, the pale soft pads on the upper and lower lips of a baby that look like blisters but are not. They form as soon as the baby begins to suck well at the breast or on a bottle. They seem to augment the seal of the lips around the nipple or breast. Some babies who have sucked on their own fingers, hands, or arms before birth are born with them.

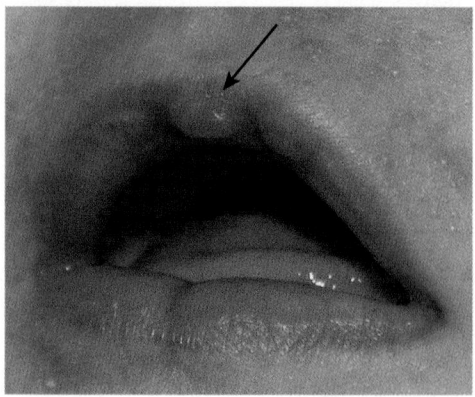

Sucking blisters *(Pride, Yan, and Zaenglein, 2008)*

sucking reflex, involuntary sucking movements of the circumoral area in newborns in response to stimulation. The reflex continues throughout infancy and often occurs without stimulation, such as during sleep. Compare **rooting reflex.**

suckle [L, *sugere*], **1.** to provide nourishment, specifically to breastfeed. **2.** to take in nourishment, especially by feeding from the breast.

suckling, an infant that has not been weaned.

suck-swallow-breathe synchrony, a skill used continuously throughout life that allows an individual to breathe while simultaneously and unconsciously sucking in and swallowing food, drink, and saliva; its disruption can interfere profoundly with development.

suck-swallow reflex, rhythmic sucking and swallowing movements in an infant when a finger or nipple is placed in the mouth.

Sucostrin, a depolarizing neuromuscular-blocker agent. Brand name for **succinylcholine chloride.**

sucrose /soo″krōs/ [Fr, *sucre,* sugar], a disaccharide sugar derived from sugar cane, sugar beets, and sorghum and made up of one molecule of glucose and one of fructose joined together in a glycosidic linkage.

sucrose polyester (SPE), a synthetic nonabsorbable fat that, when added to the diet, reduces plasma cholesterol levels by increasing the excretion of cholesterol in the feces. It is formulated to have the characteristic texture, taste, and consistency of regular margarine or vegetable oil and adds no calories to the diet.

suction /suk″shən/ [L, *sugere,* to suck], the aspiration of a gas or fluid by reducing air pressure over its surface, usually by mechanical means.

suction biopsy [L, *sugere,* to suck; Gk, *bios,* life, *opsis,* view], a procedure for obtaining tissue or fluid samples from lymph nodes or a deep lesion by using suction and a trocar or cannula. Also called **aspiration biopsy.**

suction curettage. See **vacuum aspiration.**

suction drainage. See **drainage.**

suction lipectomy. See **liposuction.**

Sudafed, an adrenergic vasoconstrictor used as a decongestant. Brand name for **pseudoephedrine hydrochloride.**

sudden cardiac arrest (SCA), an abrupt, complete loss of heart function that results in loss of blood circulation within the body. An episode of sudden cardiac arrest may be preceded by arrhythmias, including ventricular tachycardia or fibrillation. It is not caused by the blockage of coronary arteries. Within the United States, as many as 450,000 persons may experience sudden cardiac arrest each year; survivors face a 30% to 50% chance of experiencing a repeat episode. Sudden cardiac arrest is reversible in most patients if it is treated within minutes. Compare **myocardial infarction, acute myocardial infarction.**

sudden death [ME, *sodain,* to come up; AS, *death*], death that occurs unexpectedly and from 1 to 24 hours after the onset of symptoms, with or without known preexisting conditions.

sudden infant death syndrome (SIDS) [ME, *sodain,* to come up; L, *infans,* unable to speak; AS, *death* + Gk, *syn,* together, *dromos,* course], the unexpected and sudden death of an apparently normal and healthy infant that occurs during sleep, with no physical or autopsic evidence of disease. It is the most common cause of death in children under 1 year of age, with an incidence rate of 1 in every 300 to 350 live births. In the last few years, death scene investigations have been helpful in identifying an unsafe sleep environment as a contributing factor in SIDS cases and it is now recognized that many of these infant deaths are due to asphyxiation and suffocation. In 1992 a report by the American Academy of Pediatrics Task Force on Infant Positioning and

SIDS recommended that infants be laid down for sleep in a nonprone position; and in 1994 a "Back to Sleep" campaign was jointly initiated by the American Academy of Pediatrics (AAP) and the National Institute of Child Health and Human Development. Over the next five years, the rate of prone sleep positioning and the rate of SIDS both decreased. Since 2001, the rate has been relatively constant. It is known that the risk of SIDS increases after the first month of life and peaks at 2 to 4 months of age. Infants should be placed for sleep supine as a preventive measure. Nursing considerations consist predominantly of support and counseling, such as assessing how the parents feel about the death to help them through the resolution of grief, learning what they know about the syndrome, supplying them with whatever information and literature they need, and finding out how they are coping with any guilt feelings and how the siblings, if any, are coping with the death. The nurse also can supply information about local groups of parents who have lost a child from SIDS. Also called **cot death, crib death.** See also **parental grief.**

sudo-, combining form meaning "sweat": *sudor, sudiferous, sudorific.*

sudor /soo′dôr/ [L, sweat], perspiration.

sudoriferous duct /soo′dorif″ərəs/ [L, *sudor*, sweat, *facere*, to make], a duct leading from a sweat gland to the surface of the skin. Each sweat duct is the most superficial part of a coiled tube that forms the body of each sweat gland and opens onto the surface through a funnel-shaped opening. The sweat ducts in the armpits and in the groin are larger than in other parts of the body. Also called **sweat duct.**

sudoriferous gland, one of about 2 million tiny structures within the dermis that produce perspiration and secrete it via a sudoriferous duct to the skin's surface. The average quantity of perspiration secreted in 24 hours varies from 700 to 900 g. Each sudoriferous gland consists of a single tube with a deeply coiled body and a superficial duct. The number of glands per square centimeter of skin varies in different parts of the body. The sudoriferous glands are very plentiful on the palms of the hands and on the soles of the feet, least numerous in the neck and the back, and completely absent in the deeper parts of the external auditory meatus, the prepuce, and the glans penis. Most are eccrine glands, producing perspiration that carries away sodium chloride, the waste products urea and lactic acid, and the breakdown products from garlic, spices, and other substances. Apocrine sweat glands associated with the coarse hair of the armpits and the pubic region are larger and secrete fluid that is much thicker than that secreted by the eccrine glands. Also called **sweat gland.** Compare **sebaceous gland.**

sudorific /soo′dərif″ik/ [L, *sudor*, sweat, *facere*, to make], **1.** *adj.,* pertaining to a substance or condition, such as heat or emotional tension, that promotes sweating. **2.** *n.,* a sudorific agent. Sweat glands are stimulated by cholinergic drugs. The alkaloid pilocarpine is a potent sudorific drug, but it is rarely used for that purpose in modern medicine. Also called **diaphoretic.**

suf-. See **sub-, suf-, sup-.**

Sufenta, an opioid analgesic used in balanced anesthesia. Brand name for **sufentanil citrate.**

sufentanil /soo-fen′tah-nil/, an extremely potent opioid analgesic derived from fentanyl; the citrate salt is used as an anesthetic or as an adjunct to anesthesia. It is also used for the treatment of obstetric pain.

sufentanil citrate /sufen″tənil/, an analgesic and anesthetic.
- ■ INDICATIONS: It is administered intravenously as an adjunct to general anesthesia and can be used in higher amounts together with 100% oxygen as a primary anesthetic.

- ■ CONTRAINDICATIONS: Hypersensitivity to sufentanil prohibits its use. It should be used with caution in people with respiratory depression or renal, hepatic, or pulmonary failure.
- ■ ADVERSE EFFECTS: Among the more serious adverse effects are respiratory depression, chest wall rigidity, hypotension, bradycardia, and nausea and vomiting. There must be ready availability of drugs and equipment needed to treat such adverse effects.

suffocation /suf′əkā″shən/ [L, *suffocare*, to choke], an interruption in breathing with oxygen deprivation, usually caused by an obstruction in the airways. The condition may be accidental or intentional or may result from disease or inadequate levels of respirable gases in the atmosphere.

suffocative goiter /suf″əkā′tiv/ [L, *suffocare*, to choke, *guttur*, throat], an enlargement of the thyroid gland that causes a sensation of suffocation when pressed.

sugar /shoog″ər/ [Gk, *sakcharon*], any of several water-soluble simple carbohydrates. The principal categories of sugars are monosaccharides, disaccharides, and polysaccharides. A monosaccharide is a single sugar, such as glucose, fructose, or galactose. A disaccharide is a double sugar, such as sucrose (table sugar) or lactose. A polysaccharide is a sugar made up of repeating units of glucose, such as cellulose, starch, and glycogen. Sugars play an important role in biology by either forming conjugates with other biomolecules (e.g., glycoproteins) or by mediating cell surface recognition events (e.g., bacterial or viral binding to cells). See also **carbohydrate, fructose, galactose, glucose, saccharide, sucrose.**

sugar alcohol, an alcohol produced by the reduction of an aldehyde or ketone of a sugar.

sugar cataract, a visual disorder associated with diabetes in which sorbitol collects within the lens, causing an osmotic gradient of fluid in the lens. This condition leads to a disruption of the lens matrix and loss of transparency.

suggestibility /səjes′tibil″itē/, pertaining to a person's susceptibility to having his or her ideas or actions influenced or altered by others.

suggestion /səjes″chən/ [L, *suggerere*, to propose], **1.** the process by which one thought or idea leads to another, as in the association of ideas. **2.** the use of persuasion, exhortation, or another technique to implant an idea, thought, attitude, or belief in the mind of another as a means of influencing or altering behavior or states of mind. See also **hypnosis. 3.** an idea, belief, or attitude implanted in the mind of another. Compare **autosuggestion.**

suicidal /soo′isī″dəl/ [L, *sui*, of oneself, *caedere*, to kill], of, relating to, or tending toward self-destruction.

suicide /soo″isīd/ [L, *sui*, of oneself, *caedere*, to kill], **1.** the intentional taking of one's own life. **2.** (Informal) the ruin or destruction of one's own interests. **3.** a person who commits or attempts self-destruction. Early signs of suicidal intent include depression; expressions of guilt, tension, and agitation; insomnia; loss of weight and appetite; neglect of personal appearance; giving away of personal or valued possessions; and direct or indirect threats to commit suicide.

suicide gesture, (in psychiatric nursing) an apparent attempt by a patient to cause self-injury without lethal consequences and generally without actual intent to commit suicide. A suicide gesture serves to attract attention to the patient's disturbed emotional status but is not as serious as a suicide attempt, although it may result in suicide, intentional or not.

suicide prevention center, a crisis-intervention facility dealing primarily with people preoccupied with suicidal thoughts. Such facilities are usually operated by professional social workers with special training in counseling possible suicide victims in person or by telephone.

suicidology /so͞o′isīdol″əjē/ [L, *sui* + *caedere* + Gk, *logos*, science], the study of the prevention and causes of suicide. –*suicidologist, n.*

Sular, a calcium channel blocker. Brand name for **nisoldipine.**

sulcate, sulci. See **sulcus.**

sulconazole /sul-kon′ah-zōl/, a broad-spectrum, topical antifungal agent, used as the nitrate salt in treatment of athlete's foot, ringworm, and *Candida* infections.

sulcoplasty. See **vestibuloplasty.**

sulculus /sul′kyələs/ [L, *sulcus*], a small sulcus.

sulcus /sul′kəs/ *pl.* *sulci* [L, furrow], a shallow depression, or furrow on the surface of an organ, such as cerebral sulcus that separates the convolutions of the cerebral hemisphere. A sulcus is usually not as deep as a fissure, but, in the terminology of anatomy, the words *sulcus* and *fissure* are often used interchangeably. –*sulcate, adj.*

sulcus centralis cerebri. See **central sulcus.**

sulcus terminalis cordis. See **terminal sulcus of the right atrium.**

sulfa-, a prefix used for sulfonamide antimicrobials.

sulfacetamide /sul′fəset″əmīd/, a topical antibacterial.
- INDICATIONS: It is most commonly prescribed for the prophylaxis of infection after injury to the cornea and in the treatment of bacterial conjunctivitis and bacterial infections of the skin.
- CONTRAINDICATIONS: Known hypersensitivity to the drug or to other sulfonamides or impaired kidney function prohibits its use.
- ADVERSE EFFECTS: Among known adverse effects are local pain, overgrowth of nonsusceptible pathogens, and hypersensitivity reaction.

Sulfacet-R, a fixed-combination topical antiacne medication containing a keratolytic, an antibacterial, and a physical barrier. Brand name for **sulfur,** *sulfacetamide sodium, zinc oxide.*

sulfADIAZINE /sul′fədī″əzēn/, a sulfonamide antibacterial.
- INDICATIONS: It is prescribed in the treatment of infection, particularly of the urinary tract, and in rheumatic fever prophylaxis.
- CONTRAINDICATIONS: Porphyria, urinary tract obstruction, or known hypersensitivity to sulfonamides prohibits its use.
- ADVERSE EFFECTS: Among the more serious adverse effects are crystalluria, photosensitivity, severe allergic reactions, and blood dyscrasias.

sulfadoxine /sul′fah-dok′sēn/, a long-acting sulfonamide used in combination with pyrimethamine in the prophylaxis and treatment of malaria caused by chloroquine-resistant strains of *Plasmodium falciparum.*

sulfa drugs /sul′fə/, a group of bacteriostatic agents that inhibit the biosynthesis of folic acid.

sulfamethoxazole /sul′fəmethok″səzōl/, a sulfonamide antibacterial.
- INDICATIONS: It is prescribed in the treatment of otitis media, prostatitis, epididymitis, bronchitis, and certain urinary tract infections.
- CONTRAINDICATIONS: It is not given during the last trimester of pregnancy, during lactation, or to children less than 2 months of age. Known hypersensitivity to this drug or to other sulfonamides prohibits its use.
- ADVERSE EFFECTS: Among the more serious adverse effects are crystalluria and rash, fever, and other allergic reactions.

sulfamethoxazole and trimethoprim /trīmeth″əprim/, a fixed-combination antibacterial.

- INDICATIONS: It is prescribed in the treatment of urinary tract infections, otitis media, chronic bronchitis, traveler's diarrhea, and other infections caused by susceptible strains of bacteria and for *Pneumocystisjirovecii* pneumonitis prophylaxis.
- CONTRAINDICATIONS: It is used with caution in patients with impaired renal or hepatic function, possible folate deficiency, or known hypersensitivity either to drug or to sulfonamides. It is not recommended for use in infants less than 2 months of age or in the third trimester of pregnancy.
- ADVERSE EFFECTS: Among the more serious adverse effects are crystalluria and rashes, fever, and other allergic reactions.

Sulfamylon, a topical antiseptic. Brand name for **mafenide acetate.**

sulfanilamide /sul′fah-nil′ah-mīd/, a potent antibacterial compound. Although replaced as a systemic agent by more effective and less toxic derivatives and by antibiotics, it is still used vaginally in the treatment of vulvovaginal candidiasis.

sulfanilic acid /sul′fənil′ik/, a red-tinged white crystalline compound used in the synthesis of sulfonamides and as a reagent in tests for phenol, fecal matter in water, albumin, aldehydes, and glucose. Also called **para-aminobenzenesulfonic acid.**

sulfapyridine /sul′fah-pir′idēn/, a sulfonamide administered orally in the treatment of dermatitis herpetiformis.

sulfasalazine /sul′fəsalaz″ēn/, a sulfonamide and aminosalicylic acid derivative. Also called **salicylazosulfapyridine.**
- INDICATIONS: It is prescribed in the treatment of mild to moderate ulcerative colitis and as adjunctive therapy in severe cases. It is also used to treat juvenile- and adult-onset forms of rheumatoid arthritis and in the treatment of other autoimmune disease, such as ankylosing spondylitis and Crohn's disease.
- CONTRAINDICATIONS: Urinary obstruction, porphyria, or known hypersensitivity to this drug, to other sulfonamide medications, or to salicylates prohibits its use. It is not given during the last trimester of pregnancy.
- ADVERSE EFFECTS: Among the more serious adverse effects are crystalluria, blood dyscrasias, and severe hypersensitivity reactions. GI symptoms and anorexia commonly occur.

sulfatase /sul′fə·tās/, any of a group of enzymes that catalyze the cleavage of inorganic sulfate from sulfate esters to form alcohols.

sulfate (SO$_4$$^{2-}$) /sul′fāt/, an anion of sulfuric acid. A sulfate is usually a combination of a metal with sulfuric acid. Natural sulfate compounds, such as sodium sulfate, calcium sulfate, and potassium sulfate, are plentiful in the body.

sulfatide lipidosis /sul′fətīd/, an inherited lipid metabolism disorder of childhood caused by a deficiency of cerebroside sulfatase enzyme. It results in an accumulation of metachromatic lipids in tissues of the central nervous system, kidney, spleen, and other organs, leading to dementia, paralysis, and death by 10 years of age. Also called **metachromatic leukodystrophy.** See also **lipidosis.**

sulfhemoglobin /sulfhem″əglō′bin/, a trace form of hemoglobin that contains an irreversibly bound sulfur molecule that prevents normal oxygen binding. Also spelled **sulphaemoglobin.**

sulfhemoglobinemia /-ē″mē·ə/, the presence of abnormal sulfur-containing hemoglobin circulating in the blood.

sulfinpyrazone /sul′finpir″əzōn/, a uricosuric drug.
- INDICATIONS: It is prescribed in the treatment of chronic gout and intermittent gouty arthritis.
- CONTRAINDICATIONS: Peptic ulcer, ulcerative colitis, renal dysfunction, or known hypersensitivity to this drug or to phenylbutazone prohibits its use. It is not usually given during an acute attack of gout.

■ ADVERSE EFFECTS: Among the more serious adverse effects are GI ulcers, blood dyscrasias, and dermatitis.

sulfiSOXAZOLE /sul′fisok″səzōl/, a sulfonamide antibiotic.

■ INDICATIONS: It is prescribed in the treatment of conjunctivitis and urinary tract infections, including vaginitis, cystitis, and pyelonephritis.

■ CONTRAINDICATIONS: Porphyria, urinary tract obstruction, or known hypersensitivity to this drug or to sulfonamide medications prohibits its use. It is not given during the last trimester of pregnancy or to children less than 2 months of age.

■ ADVERSE EFFECTS: Among the more serious adverse effects are crystalluria, blood dyscrasias, and severe hypersensitivity reactions.

sulfiting agents /sul″fīting/, food preservatives composed of potassium or sodium bisulfite or potassium metabisulfite. Sulfiting agents are used in the processing of beer, wine, baked goods, soup mixes, and some imported seafood and by restaurants to impart a "fresh" appearance to salad fruits and vegetables. The chemicals can cause a severe allergic reaction in people who are hypersensitive to sulfites. The reactions are marked by flushing, faintness, hives, headache, GI distress, breathing difficulty, and, in extreme cases, loss of consciousness and death.

sulfo- /sul′fō-, sul′fə-/, prefix naming chemical compounds, showing presence of divalent sulfur or of the group SO_2OH: *sulfobromophthalein, sulfonamide.*

sulfobromophthalein /sul′fəbrō′məfthal″ēn, -ē·in/, a substance used in its disodium salt form for evaluating the function of the liver.

sulfobromophthalein test, a liver function test in which the dye sulfobromophthalein sodium is introduced into the circulatory system and a blood sample is withdrawn 30 or 45 minutes later, depending on the dose injected. The parenchymal cells remove almost all of the dye within this time if they are functioning normally. The rate of removal is influenced by the blood flow through the portal circulation, the functioning capacity of the liver cells, and the patency of the biliary tract.

sulfonamide /səlfon″əmīd/, originally one of a large group of synthetic bacteriostatic drugs that are effective in treating infections caused by many gram-negative and gram-positive microorganisms. They are bacteriostatic rather than bactericidal. Some sulfonamides are short-acting, some are intermediate-acting, and some are long-acting, depending on the speed with which they are excreted. They are used in treating many urinary tract infections. A variety of other types of drugs have since been developed that are sulfonamide derivatives, including thiazide diuretics and some of the oral hypoglycemics. Some people are hypersensitive to the sulfonamides. Sulfonamides are given with caution to people who have impaired liver or kidney function, and they are not given in the last trimester of pregnancy or to young infants, because cognitive impairment sometimes can result. Hemolytic anemia; agranulocytosis; thrombocytopenia; or aplastic anemia, drug fever, and jaundice may occur, particularly with long-acting sulfonamides given for more than 10 days. Most sulfonamides are given orally.

sulfonates /sul″fənāts/, a class of anticholinesterase compounds used as insecticides.

sulfonylurea /sul′fənilyo͞or″ē·ə/, an oral antidiabetic agent that stimulates the pancreatic production of insulin. Hypersensitivity to sulfonamides is a contraindication for using such agents, and ethanol consumption is incompatible with all sulfonylureas. These agents cross the placenta, and their use has been associated with a higher incidence of birth defects, making insulin the preferred drug in treating diabetes in pregnancy. Aspirin or other salicylates taken with any sulfonylurea may intensify the hypoglycemic effect.

sulfosalicylic acid /sul′fōsalisil″ik/, a white or faintly pink crystalline substance that is highly water soluble and is used as a reagent in tests for albumin and as an intermediate compound in the manufacture of dyes and surfactants.

Sulfoxyl, a fixed-combination topical antiacne medication containing two keratolytics, benzoyl peroxide and sulfur. Benzoyl peroxide directly inhibits the growth of acne bacteria. Brand name for **benzoyl peroxide, sulfur.**

sulfur (S) /sul″fər/ [L], a nonmetallic, polyvalent, tasteless, odorless chemical element that occurs abundantly in yellow crystalline form or in masses, especially in volcanic areas. Its atomic number is 16, and its atomic mass is 32.07. It is used in the production of sulfuric acid and used in metallurgy, rubber vulcanization, petroleum refining, and many other industrial processes. Sulfur has been used in the treatment of gout, rheumatism, and bronchitis and as a mild laxative. The sulfonamides, or sulfa drugs, are used in the treatment of various bacterial infections. Also spelled **sulphur.**

sulfur dioxide, a colorless nonflammable gas used as an antioxidant in pharmaceutic preparations. It is also an important air pollutant, irritating the eyes and respiratory tract.

-sulfuric /sulf(y)o͞o″rik/, suffix meaning "compounds containing sulfur, especially in its highest valences": hydrosulfuric, persulfuric, thiosulfuric. Also spelled **-sulphuric.**

sulfuric acid (H_2SO_4), a clear, colorless, oily, highly corrosive liquid that generates great heat when mixed with water. An extremely toxic substance, sulfuric acid causes severe skin burns, blindness on contact with the eyes, serious lung damage if the vapors are inhaled, and death if it is ingested. In industry, sulfuric acid is used in the manufacture of fertilizers, dyes, glue, and other acids; in the purifying of petroleum; and in the pickling of metals. Weak solutions of sulfuric acid are used in the treatment of gastric hypoacidity and serous diarrhea. Formerly called **vitriol, oil of.**

sulfurous acid (H_2SO_3) /sul′fərəs/, a weak inorganic acid formed by dissolving sulfur dioxide in water, used as a chemical-reducing and bleaching agent. It has been used in medicine in skin lotions and nasal and throat sprays. Sulfites formed by the acid may be included in antiseptics, antifermentatives, and antizymotics. Sulfurous acid is stable only in aqueous solutions; it decomposes into sulfur dioxide and water on standing. It is a major component of acid rain.

sulindac /sulin″dek/, a nonsteroidal antiinflammatory agent.

■ INDICATIONS: It is prescribed in the treatment of osteoarthritis, rheumatoid arthritis, and ankylosing spondylitis.

■ CONTRAINDICATIONS: Pregnancy (third trimester), lactation, or known hypersensitivity to this drug, aspirin, or nonsteroidal antiinflammatory drugs prohibits its use. It is used with caution in patients who have upper GI tract disease or impaired renal function.

■ ADVERSE EFFECTS: Among the more serious adverse reactions are GI upset, peptic ulcer, dizziness, tinnitus, and skin rash.

sulphaemoglobin. See **sulfhemoglobin.**

sulphur. See **sulfur.**

-sulphuric. See **-sulfuric.**

Sultrin Triple Sulfa, a fixed-combination vaginal drug containing antibacterials. Brand name for *sulfathiazole,* **sulfacetamide,** *sulfabenzamide.*

sumac [Ar, *summaq*], any of a number of species of trees and shrubs in the Anacardiaceae family, including the *Rhus*

S

species, which have poisonous properties. See **poison ivy, poison oak, poison sumac, rhus dermatitis.**

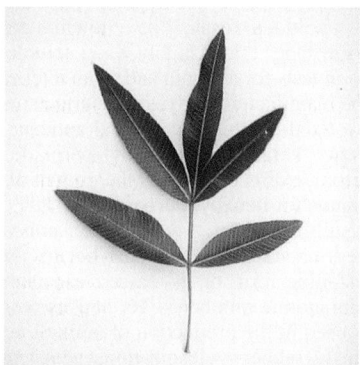

Poison sumac *(Auerbach, 2012)*

summary judgment [L, *summa,* total, *jus,* law, *dicere,* to state], (in law) a judgment requested by any party to a civil action to end the action when it is believed that there is no genuine issue or material fact in dispute. Summary judgment may be directed toward part or all of a claim or defense and may be based on the proceedings in court or on affidavits or other outside materials.

summation [L, *summa,* total], **1.** a cumulative effect or action; a total aggregate; totality. **2.** (in neurology) the concentration of a neurotransmitter at a synapse, either by increasing the frequency of nerve impulses in each fiber (temporal summation) or by increasing the number of fibers stimulated (spatial summation), so that the threshold of the postsynaptic neuron is overcome and an impulse is transmitted. See also **facilitation,** def. 2.

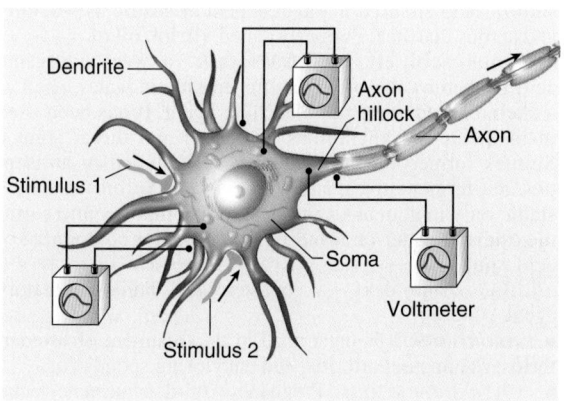

Spatial summation *(Patton and Thibodeau, 2010)*

summation gallop, a gallop rhythm in which the third and fourth heart sounds are superimposed, appearing as one loud sound. It may occur in some patients with tachycardia but is usually associated with cardiac disease. See also **gallop.**

summons /sum″əns/ [OFr, *somondre,* to remind secretly], (in law) a document issued by a clerk of the court on the filing of a complaint. A sheriff, marshal, or other appointed person serves the summons, notifying a person that an action has been begun against him or her. See also **service of process.**

sump drain, a drainage device consisting of two tubes, one to allow fluid to be drained from a cavity and the other to allow air to enter the cavity to replace the fluid. It may be attached to a suction apparatus.

Sumycin, an antibiotic. Brand name for **tetracycline hydrochloride.**

sunburn, a skin injury characterized by redness, tenderness, and possible blistering that results from exposure to actinic radiation from the sun.

sundowning /sun″douning/ [AS, *sunne* + *ofdune,* off the hill], a condition in which persons with cognitive impairment and elderly people tend to become confused or disoriented at the end of the day. Many of them have diminished visual acuity and varying degrees of sensorineural and conduction hearing loss. With less light, they lose visual cues that help them to compensate for their sensory impairments. It may also be a result of decreased sensory stimulation, especially in the evening, when there is less environmental activity and less structure. Sundowning is most common with dementia, Alzheimer type, and is seen with delirium.

sunitinib, a miscellaneous antineoplastic.
■ INDICATIONS: This drug is used to treat advanced renal carcinoma and GI stromal tumors after disease progression or intolerance to imatinib.
■ CONTRAINDICATIONS: Pregnancy, lactation, and known hypersensitivity to this drug prohibit its use.
■ ADVERSE EFFECTS: Adverse effects of this drug include headache, dizziness, insomnia, fatigue, hypertension, altered taste, constipation, stomatitis, mucositis, skin discoloration, depigmentation of hair or skin, alopecia, pain, arthralgia, myalgia, cough, dyspnea, and electrolyte abnormalities. Life-threatening side effects include central nervous system hemorrhage, seizures, left ventricular dysfunction, hepatotoxicity, vomiting, dyspepsia, pancreatitis, neutropenia, thrombocytopenia, and bleeding. Common side effects include nausea, anorexia, abdominal pain, and rash.

sunrise syndrome, a condition of unstable cognitive ability on arising in the morning. Compare **sundowning.**

sunscreen protective factor index (SPF), a system of evaluating the effectiveness of various formulations for protecting the skin from actinic rays of the sun. A sun protective factor of 15 means that the sunscreen provides 15 times the protection of unprotected skin. There are a number of formulations of sunscreen. Some, such as titanium dioxide or zinc oxide, reflect the sun's UVA and UVB rays. Others, such as oxybenzone and octinoxate, are synthetic chemicals absorbed into the skin to filter and absorb UV rays.

sun-setting sign, a characteristic of hydrocephalus in which an infant's eyes appear to look only downward, with the sclera prominent over the iris.

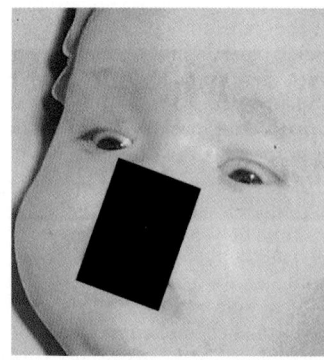

Sun-setting sign *(Kanski and Nischal, 1999)*

sunstroke [AS, *sunne* + *strac*, stroke], a morbid condition caused by overexposure to the sun and characterized by a high temperature and altered level of consciousness. See also **heat hyperpyrexia.**

sup-. See **sub-, suf-, sup-.**

super-, prefix meaning "above," "more than normal," or "implying excess": *supercoat, superficial, supernumerary.*

superantigen, one of a family of related substances, including staphylococcal and streptococcal exotoxins, that can short-circuit the normal sequence of events leading to activation of helper T cells. Superantigens initiate an uncontrolled proliferation of T cells but do not require processing and presentation by macrophages. The result is either an acute and potentially life-threatening disease, such as toxic shock syndrome, or a chronic inflammatory process, such as rheumatic fever.

supercoat, a protective layer of gelatin to provide protection from scratches and pressure damage to radiographic film. Also called *abrasion layer,* **overcoat.**

supercoiling, the underwinding or overwinding of a DNA helix. See also **DNA gyrase.**

supercomputers, high-performance computing equipment capable of handling massive amounts of research and clinical data at speeds more than 1000 times that of most computer equipment. Supercomputer hardware and software may offer a potential of connecting thousands of research facilities and transmitting data at rates up to one billion bits per second. Proposed high-performance computers could quickly analyze archived medical data about worldwide populations, determining, for example, the "normal" human blood pressure on the basis of records of millions of patients.

superego /ē″gō/ [L, *super,* over, *ego,* I], (in psychoanalysis) that part of the psyche, functioning mostly in the unconscious, that develops when the standards of the parents and of society are incorporated into the ego. The superego has two parts, the conscience and the ego ideal. See also **ego, ego ideal, id.**

supereruption. See **overeruption.**

superfecundation /soo̅′pərfekəndā″shən/ [L, *super* + *fecundare,* to be fruitful], the impregnation of two or more ova released during the same ovulation by spermatozoa from successive coital acts.

superfetation /-fētā″shən/ [L, *super* + *fetus,* pregnancy], the fertilization of a second ovum after the onset of pregnancy, resulting in the simultaneous development of two fetuses of different degrees of maturity within the uterus. Also called **superimpregnation.**

superficial /-fish″əl/ [L, *superficies,* surface], **1.** pertaining to the surface. **2.** not grave or dangerous.

superficial abscess [L, *superficialis* + *abscedere,* to go away], an abscess that develops above the fascia layer.

superficial dorsal carpal ligament. See **extensor retinaculum of the hand.**

superficial fading infantile hemangioma, a superficial, temporary, salmon-colored patch in the center of the forehead, face, or occiput of many newborns. It fades during the first 2 years of life, but it may temporarily deepen in color if the child becomes flushed or angry.

superficial fibular nerve, the nerve associated with the lateral compartment of the leg. It originates as one of the two major branches of the common fibular nerve. It innervates fibularis longus and fibularis brevis and then enters the foot where it divides into medial and lateral branches that supply dorsal areas of the foot and toes except for the web space between the great and second toes and the lateral side of the little toe.

superficial inguinal ring, the triangular-shaped opening of the inguinal canal containing the spermatic cord in men or the round ligament in women.

superficial implantation, (in embryology) the partial embedding of the blastocyst within the uterine wall so that it and later the chorionic sac protrude into the uterine cavity. Also called **central implantation, circumferential implantation.**

superficial inguinal node, a node in one of the two groups of inguinal lymph glands in the upper femoral triangle of the thigh. The nodes form a chain distal to the inguinal ligament and receive afferent vessels from the skin of the penis, scrotum, perineum, buttocks, and abdominal wall below the level of the umbilicus. Compare **anterior tibial node, popliteal node.**

superficial nephron, a nephron whose proximal convoluted tubule is in the outer part of the renal cortex and whose loop of Henle goes only a short way into the renal medulla.

superficial penile fascia, subcutaneous tissue of penis. It is the loose external layer of fascial tissue of the penis.

superficial reflex, any neural reflex initiated by stimulation of the skin. Compare **deep tendon reflex.** Kinds include **abdominal reflex, anal reflex, cremasteric reflex.**

superficial sensation, the awareness or perception of feelings in the superficial layers of the skin in response to touch, pressure, temperature, and pain. Such sensations are conveyed to the brain via the spinothalamic system. Compare **deep sensation.**

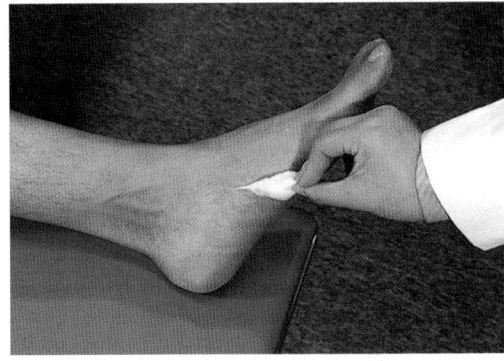

Superficial tactile sensation *(Seidel et al, 2011)*

superficial spreading melanoma, the most common melanoma. It grows outward, spreading over the surface of the affected organ or tissue. It occurs most commonly on the lower legs of women and the torso of men. The lesion is raised and palpable, unevenly pigmented, and irregularly shaped and has an unclear border. See also **lentigo maligna melanoma, nodular melanoma.**

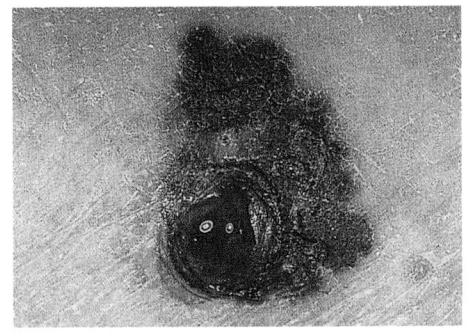

Superficial spreading melanoma *(du Vivier, 2002)*

S

superficial temporal artery, an artery at each side of the head that can be easily felt in front of the ear and is often used for taking the pulse. It is the smaller of the two terminal branches of the external carotid. Compare **deep temporal artery, middle temporal artery.**

superficial transverse perineal muscles, a pair of flat, band-shaped muscles that stabilize the perineal body.

superficial vein, one of the many veins between the subcutaneous fascia just under the skin. Compare **deep vein.**

superimpregnation. See **superfetation.**

superinfection /-infek″shən/ [L, *super* + *inficere,* to stain], an infection occurring during antimicrobial treatment for another infection. It is usually a result of change in the normal tissue flora favoring replication of some organisms by diminishing the vitality and then the number of competing organisms, as yeast microbes flourish during penicillin therapy prescribed to cure a bacterial infection.

superior /səpir″ē·ər/ [L, higher], situated above or oriented toward a higher place, as the head is superior to the torso. Compare **inferior.**

superior aperture of minor pelvis, an opening bounded by the crest and pecten of the pubic bones, the arch-shaped lines of the ilia, and the anterior margin of the base of the sacrum.

superior aperture of thorax, an elliptic opening at the summit of the thorax bounded by the first thoracic vertebra, the first ribs, and the upper margin of the sternum.

superior carotid triangle [L, *superior,* higher; Gk, *karos,* heavy sleep; L, *triangulus*], a triangle bounded by the sternocleidomastoid muscle in front, by the omohyoid muscle below, and by the stylohyoid and digastric muscles above.

superior cervical ganglion, a very large ganglion in the area of the first and second cervical vertebrae that marks the superior extent of the trunk of the sympathetic nervous system.

superior conjunctival fornix, the space in the fold of the conjunctiva created by the reflection of the conjunctiva covering the eyeball and the lining of the upper lid. Compare **inferior conjunctival fornix.**

superior costotransverse ligament, one of five ligaments associated with each costotransverse joint, except that of the first rib. It passes from the neck of each rib to the transverse process of the vertebra immediately above and is associated with the intercostal vessels and the intercostal nerves. The first rib has no superior costotransverse ligament. Compare **posterior costotransverse ligament.**

superior gastric lymph node, a node in one of two sets of gastric lymph glands accompanying the left gastric artery. There are three groups of superior gastric nodes: the upper group of nodes on the stem of the artery, the lower group of nodes accompanying branches of the artery along the cardiac half of the lesser curvature of the stomach, and the paracardial group of nodes around the neck of the stomach. The superior gastric nodes receive their afferent vessels from the stomach and pass their efferent vessels to the celiac group of preaortic nodes. Compare **inferior gastric node.**

superior genial tubercle, superior mental spine. It is the upper part of a small bony projection located on the internal surface of the mandible, near the lower end of the midline and above the anterior end of the mylohyoid line, serving for attachment of the genioglossus muscle.

superior gluteal nerve, a nerve formed by branches of the sacral plexus that supplies muscles in the gluteal region.

superior hemorrhagic polioencephalitis. See **Wernicke encephalopathy.**

superior kidney, superior segment of kidney. It is the renal segment located most superiorly.

superior mediastinum, the upper part of the mediastinum in the middle of the thorax containing the trachea, the esophagus, the aortic arch, and the origins of the sternohyoideus and the sternothyroideus. Compare **anterior mediastinum, middle mediastinum, posterior mediastinum.**

superior mesenteric artery, a visceral branch of the abdominal aorta, arising inferior to the celiac artery, dividing into five branches, and supplying most of the small intestine and parts of the colon. The branches are the inferior pancreaticoduodenal, intestinal, ileocolic, right colic, and middle colic.

superior mesenteric node, a node in one of the three groups of visceral lymph nodes that serve the viscera of the abdomen and the pelvis. The superior mesenteric nodes are associated with branches of the superior mesenteric artery. Compare **gastric node, inferior mesenteric node.** Kinds include **mesenteric node, ileocolic node, mesocolic node.**

superior mesenteric vein, a tributary of the portal vein that drains the blood from the small intestine, the cecum, and the ascending and transverse colons. See also **portal vein.**

superior olivary nucleus [L, *supurus* + *oliva* + *nucleus,* nut kernel], a collection of nerve cells appearing as a clump of gray matter in the pons. The nucleus receives fibers from the cochlear nerve receptors on the same and opposite sides through the trapezoid body. It assists in the localization of sound by comparing the time difference between sounds received by the left and right ears.

superior orbital fissure, an elongated cleft between the small and great wings of the sphenoid bone, which transmits cranial nerves 3, 4, and 6 and the first division of cranial nerve 5 and the ophthalmic vein.

superior profunda artery. See **deep brachial artery.**

superior radioulnar joint. See **proximal radioulnar articulation.**

superior rectal plexus, the submucosal portion of the rectal venous plexus, above the pectinate line.

superior right lateral flexure of rectum, the second bend in the rectum, where it deviates laterally to the right.

superior sagittal sinus, one of the six venous channels in the posterior of the dura mater that drains blood from the brain into the internal jugular vein. It has no valves. The superior sagittal sinus receives the superior cerebral veins, veins from the diploë and near the posterior extremity of the sagittal suture, the anastomosing emissary veins from the pericranium, and the veins from the dura mater. It also anastomoses with veins of the nose, the scalp, and the diploë. Compare **inferior sagittal sinus, straight sinus, transverse sinus.**

superior subscapular nerve /səbskap″yələr/, one of a pair of small nerves on opposite sides of the body that arise from the posterior cord of the brachial plexus. It supplies the superior part of the subscapularis. Compare **inferior subscapular nerve.**

superior tarsal muscle, a collection of smooth muscle fibers in companion with the levator palpebrae superioris passing from the inferior surface of the lavatory to the upper edge of the superior tarsus. Loss of function of either the levator palpebrae superioris or the superior tarsal muscle results in a ptosis of the upper eyelid.

superior temporal gyrus, a rounded elevation on the lateral surface of either temporal lobe of the brain.

superior thoracic artery, a small artery that originates from the anterior surface of the first part of the axillary artery and supplies the upper regions of the medial and anterior axillary walls.

superior thyroid artery, one of a pair of arteries in the neck, usually arising from the external carotid artery, that supplies the thyroid gland and several muscles in the head.

superior ulnar collateral artery,   a long, slender division of the brachial artery, arising just distal to the middle of the arm, descending to the elbow, and anastomosing with the posterior ulnar recurrent and inferior ulnar collateral arteries.

superior vena cava,   the second largest vein of the body, returning deoxygenated blood from the upper half of the body to the right atrium. It is about 2 cm in diameter and 7 cm long. The section of the superior vena cava closest to the heart composes about one-half of the vessel's length and is within the pericardial sac, covered by the serous pericardium. It has no valves. Compare **inferior vena cava.**

superior vena cava syndrome,   a condition of edema and engorgement of the veins of the upper body caused by obstruction of the superior vena cava by thrombi or primary pulmonary tumors. Signs and symptoms include a nonproductive cough, breathing difficulty, cyanosis, central nervous system disorders, and edema of the conjunctiva, trachea, and esophagus.

superior vesical artery,   an artery that originates from the root of the umbilical artery and supplies the superior aspect of the bladder and distal parts of the ureter. In men, it may also give rise to an artery that supplies the ductus deferens.

superlactation.   See **hyperlactation.**

supernatant /-nā″tənt/   [L, *super* + *natare,* to swim],   **1.** *adj.,* situated above or on top of something. **2.** *n.,* the clear upper liquid part of a mixture (a liquid and a solid) after it has been centrifuged.

supernormal excitability /-nôr″məl/,   the ability of the myocardium to respond at the end of phase 3 of the cardiac action potential to a stimulus that would be ineffective at other times.

supernormal period,   a period of supernormal excitability of the myocardium.

supernumerary nipples /-noo″mərer′ē/   [L, *super* + *numerus,* number; ME, *neb,* beak],   an excessive number of nipples, which are usually not associated with underlying glandular tissue. They may vary in size from small pink dots to that of normal nipples.

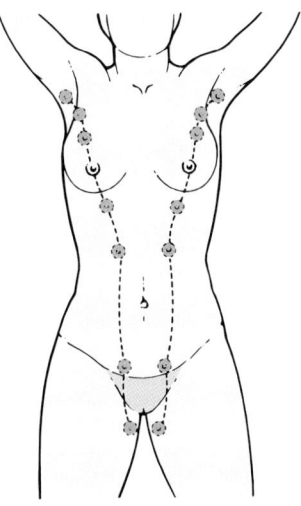

Supernumerary nipples

supernumerary tooth   [L, *super,* above, *numerus,* number; AS, *toth*],   any tooth in addition to the normal 32 teeth in the secondary dentition or the 20 teeth in the primary dentition. See also **hyperdontia, mesiodens.** Compare **peridens.**

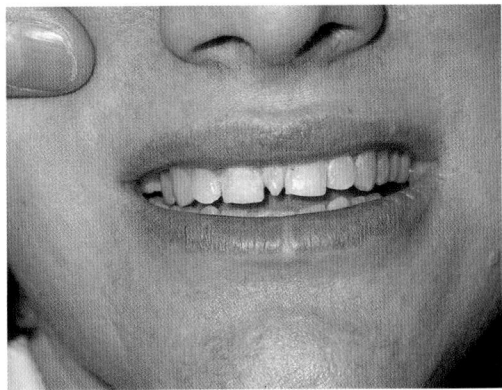

Supernumerary tooth appearing as a conical central incisor *(Van Buggenhout and Bailleul-Forestier)*

superoxide /-ok″sīd/,   a common reactive form of oxygen that is formed when molecular oxygen gains a single electron. Superoxide radicals can attack susceptible biological targets, including lipids, proteins, and nucleic acids.

superoxide dismutase (SOD),   an enzyme composed of metal-containing proteins that converts superoxide radicals into less toxic agents. It is the main enzymatic mechanism for clearing superoxide radicals from the body.

supersaturate /-sach″ərāt/   [L, *super,* above, *saturare,* to fill],   a solution that contains solute at a concentration greater than the solubility at a given temperature. Also called **metastable solution.**

supertwins,   children born from a single pregnancy involving three or more offspring.

superversion.   See **sursumversion.**

supervised fast /soo″pərvīzd/,   a hypoglycemic diagnostic procedure in which glucose levels are measured every 4 to 6 hours in a fasting person until they fall below 50 mg/dL. The fasting person is closely observed, and glucose values are rapidly determined and reported by the laboratory.

supervision /-vizh″ən/,   (in psychology) a process whereby a therapist is helped to become a more effective clinician through the direction of a supervisor who provides theoretic knowledge and therapeutic techniques and supports the working through of transference and countertransference reactions.

supervisor /soo″pərvī′zər/   [L, *super* + *videre,* to see],   **1.** (in hospital or public health nursing) the midlevel management position between the chief nurse executive and nurse managers of a division or of several units. In many hospitals *clinical director* or *director* is the preferred term. The supervisor's responsibilities are primarily administrative, although they may include clinical leadership for the nurses working in a group of units, wards, or divisions. **2.** (in occupational and physical therapy) a therapist responsible for the oversight and coordination of the daily rehabilitation operations and staff, including the monitoring and administration of patient evaluations and quality-of-care initiatives. **3.** (in a health care facility) a professional who oversees and evaluates other members of the professional staff to ensure quality patient care outcomes.

supervitaminosis /-vī′təminō″sis/   [L, *super,* above, *vita* + *amine* + Gk, *osis,* condition],   a condition of ingesting an excessive amount of vitamins in the form of supplements. Signs and symptoms vary with specific vitamin excesses. See also **hypervitaminosis.**

supination /soo″pinā″shən/   [L, *supinus,* lying on the back],   **1.** one of the kinds of rotation allowed by certain skeletal joints, such as the elbow and the wrist joints, which permit the palm of the hand to turn up. **2.** assumption of a supine position, one of lying on the back, face up. Compare **pronation.** –*supinate, v.*

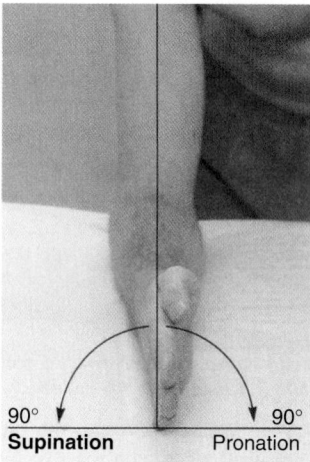

Supination and pronation (Seidel et al, 2011)

supinator jerk reflex. See **supinator longus reflex.**

supinator longus. See **brachioradialis.**

supinator longus reflex /so͞o″pinā′tər/ [L, *reflectere*, to bend back], a contraction of the brachioradialis muscle upon tapping the point of insertion of the supinator longus muscle at the lower end of the radius, causing flexion at the elbow joint. Also called **radial reflex, supinator jerk reflex.**

supine /səpīn′, so͞o″pīn/ [L, *supinus*], **1.** *n.*, position of the arms or body in which the palms of the hands face upward. **2.** *adj.*, lying horizontally on the back. Also called **dorsal decubitus position, dorsal recumbent.** Compare **prone.** See also **body position.**

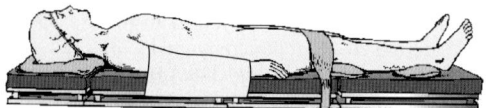

Supine position (Phillips, 2007)

supine hypotension, a fall in blood pressure that occurs when a pregnant woman is lying on her back. It is caused by impaired venous return that results from pressure of the gravid uterus on the vena cava. Also called **vena caval syndrome.**

supine position, the position of a person lying on the back. Also called **dorsal position.**

supplemental air. See **reserve capacity.**

supplemental inheritance /sup′ləmen′təl/ [L, *supplere,* to complete, *in,* in, *hereditare,* hereditary], the acquisition or expression of a genetic trait or condition through the presence of two independent pairs of nonallelic genes that interact in such a way that one gene supplements the action of the other.

supplementary gene /sup′ləmen″tərē/ [L, *supplere* + Gk, *genein,* to produce], one of two pairs of nonallelic genes that interact in such a way that one pair needs the presence of the other to be expressed, whereas the second pair can produce an effect independently of the first.

support /səpôrt″/ [L, *supportare,* to bring up], **1.** *v.,* to sustain, hold up, or maintain in a desired position or condition, as in physically supporting the abdominal muscles with a scultetus binder or emotionally supporting a client under

stress. **2.** *n.,* the assistance given to this end, such as physical support, emotional support, or life support.

support group, **1.** an organization that serves as a link in the network for family caregivers and patients, such as those who are homebound, mentally ill, elderly, or suicidal or who have a specific disorder, such as multiple sclerosis. A support group helps families and patients find a balance of responsibility. The groups are supported by various national and local organizations. **2.** an organization for people who share a common problem. See also **social support groups.**

supporting area [L, *supportare + area,* space], any of the areas of maxillary or mandibular edentulous ridges that are considered best suited to bear the forces of chewing with functioning dentures.

supporting cells, cells that provide support and protection and perhaps contribute to the nutrition of principal or other cells of certain organs. Such cells are found in the labyrinth of the inner ear, organ of Corti, olfactory epithelium, taste buds, and seminiferous tubules. Also called **sustentacular cells.**

supportive psychotherapy /səpôr″tiv/, a form of psychotherapy that concentrates on creating an effective means of communication with an emotionally disturbed person rather than on trying to produce psychological insight into the underlying conflicts. Through such supportive measures as reassurance, reinforcement of the person's defenses, direction, suggestion, and persuasion, the therapist participates directly in the solution of specific problems. Compare **nondirective therapy.**

supportive treatment. See **treatment.**

suppository /səpoz″ətôr′ē/ [L, *sub,* under, *ponere,* to place], an easily melted medicated mass for insertion into the rectum, urethra, or vagina. Theobroma oil, glycerinated gelatin, and high-molecular-weight polyethylene glycols are common vehicles for drugs in suppositories that are cone- or spindle-shaped for insertion into the rectum, globular or egg-shaped for use in the vagina, and pencil-shaped for insertion into the urethra. Drugs administered by rectal suppository are rapidly absorbed systemically, and this route is especially useful in babies, in patients unable to take oral medications, and in cases of vomiting or certain digestive disorders.

suppressant /səpres″ənt/ [L, *supprimere,* to press down], an agent that suppresses or diminishes a physical or mental activity.

suppressed menstruation /səprest″/ [L, *supprimere,* to press down, *menstruare*], a failure of menstruation to occur when expected, as in amenorrhea, or menstruation that is suppressed with the administration of hormones. Also called **suppression of menses.**

suppression /səpresh″ən/ [L, *supprimere*], (in psychoanalysis) the conscious inhibition of or effort to conceal unacceptable or painful thoughts, desires, impulses, feelings, or acts. Compare **repression.**

suppression amblyopia, a partial loss of vision, usually in one eye, caused by cortical suppression of central vision to prevent diplopia. It occurs commonly in strabismus in the eye that deviates and does not fixate. Early recognition of strabismus and amblyopia is essential because occlusive therapy that forces use of the bad eye may dramatically improve the child's vision if begun early. It becomes progressively less effective with increasing age but may improve vision even up to 9 years of age. Without therapy, near-blindness in the affected eye may result, but common acuity loss is 20/40 to 20/400.

suppression of menses. See **suppressed menstruation.**

suppressor gene /səpres″ər/, a gene that is able to reverse the effect of a specific kind of mutation in other genes.

suppressor mutation, a mutation that partially or completely restores a function lost by a primary mutation occurring at a different locus.

suppressor T cell, now called **regulatory CD4 T cell.**

suppurate /sup″yərāt/ [L, *suppurare,* to form pus], to produce purulent matter. −**suppurative,** *adj.,* −**suppuration,** *n.*

suppuration /sup′yərā″shən/ [L, to form pus], the production and exudation of pus.

suppurative /sup′yərā′tiv/ [L, *suppurare,* to form pus], pus-forming.

suppurative arthritis, inflammation of a joint with exudation of pus into the joint fluid.

suppurative fever [L, *suppurare,* to form pus, *febris,* fever], a fever accompanied by pus formation.

suppurative pancreatitis [L, *suppurare,* to form pus; Gk, *pan,* all, *kreas,* flesh, *itis,* inflammation], a form of pancreatic inflammation accompanied by the appearance of small abscesses.

suppurative phlebitis [L, *suppurare,* to form pus; Gk, *phleps,* vein, *itis,* inflammation], a vein inflammation that results from septicemia or a nearby pyogenic infection.

supra-, combining form meaning "above" or "over": *supraclavicular, supraclusion, supracondylar.*

suprabony periodontal pocket. See **periodontal pocket.**

supracallosus gyrus /sōō′prəkəlō″ses/ [L, *supra,* above, *callosus,* hard; Gk, *gyros,* turn], the gray matter covering the corpus callosum of the brain.

supracervical hysterectomy /-sur′vikəl/ [L, *supra,* above, *cervix,* neck; Gk, *hystera,* womb, *ektomē,* excision], a subtotal hysterectomy in which the body of the uterus is removed, leaving the cervix.

supraclavicular /-kləvik″yəl∂r/ [L, *supra,* above, *clavicula,* little key], pertaining to the area above the clavicle, or collarbone.

supraclavicular artery, a branch of the thyrocervical trunk that supplies the muscles on the dorsal surface of the scapula.

supraclavicular nerve, one of a pair of cutaneous branches of the cervical plexus arising from the third and the fourth cervical nerves, mostly from the fourth nerve. The anterior group supplies the skin of the infraclavicular region, the middle group supplies the skin over the pectoralis major and the deltoideus, and the posterior group supplies the skin of the cranial and dorsal parts of the shoulder.

supraclavicular triangle [L, *supra,* above, *clavicula,* little key, *triangulus*], the lower and anterior areas of the neck, bounded by the omohyoid muscle above, the sternocleidomastoid muscle in front, and the clavicle below. The first rib is in the base of the triangle.

supraclusion. See **overeruption.**

supracondylar /-kon′dilər/ [L, *supra,* above; Gk, *kondylos,* knuckle], pertaining to an area above a condyle.

supracondylar fracture [L, *supra* + *kondylos,* knuckle], a fracture involving the area between the condyles of the humerus or the femur.

supracrestal periodontal pocket. See **periodontal pocket.**

supragingival calculus. See **calculus.**

supraglenoid tubercle, the site of attachment on the scapula of the biceps brachii muscle.

suprahyoid muscles, a group of four muscles that attach the hyoid bone to the skull. See also **digastricus, geniohyoideus, mylohyoideus, stylohyoideus.**

suprahyoid pharyngotomy, external pharyngotomy in which the suprahyoid muscles are divided and the epiglottic vallecula is entered by following the hyoepiglottic ligament.

suprainfection /-infek″shən/ [L, *supra* + *inficere,* to stain], a secondary infection usually caused by an opportunistic pathogen, such as a fungal infection after the antibiotic treatment of another infection or pneumonia in a patient debilitated by another illness.

supranasal /sōō′prə·nā′zəl/ [L, *supra,* above + *nasus,* nose], superior to the nose.

supranuclear gaze disturbance /-nōō″klē·∂r/, an inability to direct the eyes to the side contralateral to a lesion in the frontal lobe. If the frontal lobe lesions are bilateral, the patient can maintain fixation and follow visual targets but cannot shift the gaze in any direction in the absence of a target. See also **gaze palsy.**

supraocclusion. See **overeruption.**

supraoptic nucleus /-op″tik/ [L, *supra,* above; Gk, *optikos* + L, *nucleus,* nut kernel], a hypothalamic nucleus that lies above the optic chiasma, with fibers extending to the posterior lobe of the pituitary.

supraorbital /sōō′prə·or′bi·təl/ [L, *supra,* above + *orbita,* wheel track], superior to the orbit.

supraorbital artery, a branch of the ophthalmic artery that supplies the scalp.

suprapatellar /-pətel″ər/ [L, *supra,* above, *patella,* small dish], pertaining to a location above the patella.

suprapatellar bursa, an expansion of the synovial membrane of the knee that is a continuation of the articular cavity superiorly between the distal end of the shaft of the femur and the quadriceps femoris muscle and tendon. It provides a low-friction surface for the movement of knee tendons. See also **subpopliteal recess.**

suprapelvic /sōō′prə·pel′vik/ [L, *supra,* above + *pelvis,* basin], above the pelvis.

suprapubic /-p(y)ōō″bik/ [L, *supra* + *pubes,* signs of maturity], pertaining to a location above the symphysis pubis.

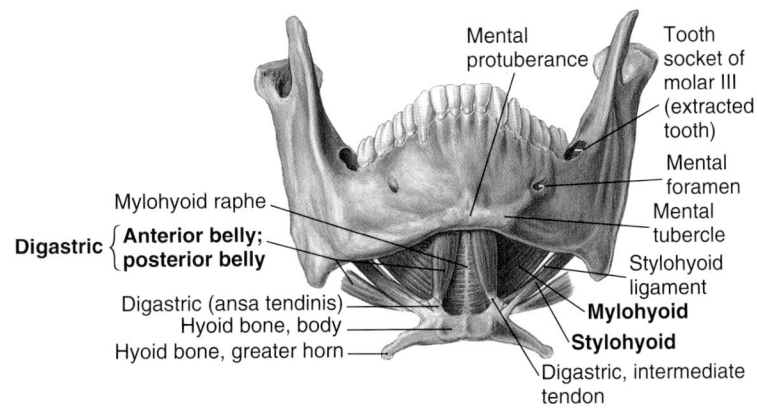

Lower jaw, mandible, and frontal view of the suprahyoid muscles *(Paulsen and Waschke, 2013)*

suprapubic aspiration of urine,　a procedure for draining the bladder by inserting a sterile needle through the skin above the pubic arch and into the bladder. The bladder may also be emptied by inserting a catheter through a suprapubic incision when conditions prohibit use of the conventional insertion. Also called **suprapubic puncture.**

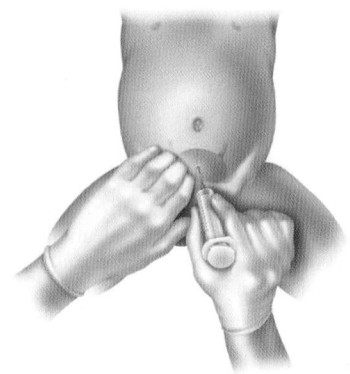

Suprapubic aspiration of urine (Custalow, 2005)

suprapubic catheter [L, *supra* + *pubis* + Gk, *katheter*, a thing lowered into], a urinary bladder catheter inserted through the skin about 1 inch above the symphysis pubis. It is inserted under a general or local anesthetic. It is used for closed drainage and may be left in place for a time, sutured to the abdominal skin. Benefits include a lower incidence of urinary tract infection, ease of voiding naturally when the catheter is clamped, and ease of ambulation. Disadvantages are that they must initially be inserted through the abdominal wall by a physician and the insertion site must be cleaned daily using sterile technique if the patient is in the hospital.

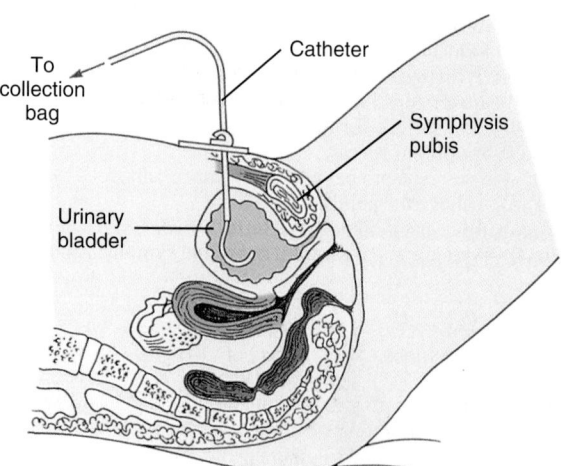

Suprapubic catheter (Elkin, Perry, and Potter, 2007)

suprapubic lithotomy.　See **high lithotomy.**
suprapubic puncture.　See **suprapubic aspiration of urine.**
suprarenal /-rē″nəl/ [L, *supra* + *ren*, kidney], pertaining to a location above the kidney.
suprarenal gland.　See **adrenal gland.**
suprascapular foramen, the route through which structures pass between the base of the neck and the posterior

scapular region. It is formed by the suprascapular notch of the scapula and the superior transverse scapular ligament.
suprascapular ligament /-skap″yələr/ [L, *supra*, above, *scapula*, shoulder blade, *ligare*, to bind], a ligament that extends from the base of the coracoid process to the medial end of the suprascapular notch.
suprascapular nerve [L, *supra* + *scapulae*, shoulder blades], one of a pair of nerve branches from the cords of the brachial plexus. It supplies the shoulder joint, scapula, and associated muscles.
suprasellar /-sel″ər/, above the sella turcica.
suprasellar cyst.　See **craniopharyngioma.**
supraspinal /-spī″nəl/ [L, *supra*, above, *spina*, backbone], pertaining to an area above the spine.
supraspinal ligament [L, *supra* + *spina*, backbone], the ligament that connects the apices of the spinous processes from the seventh cervical vertebra to the sacrum.
supraspinatus /soo͞″prə·spī·nā′tus/ [L, *supra*, above + *spina*, spine], a muscle originating in the supraspinous fossa and inserting in the greater tubercle of the humerus. It functions to abduct the humerus.
supraspinatus syndrome /-spīnā″təs/, pain and tenderness involving the supraspinatus tendon of the arm, restricting abduction of the shoulder.
supraspinous fossa /-spī″nəs/ [L, *supra*, above, *spina*, backbone, *fossa*, ditch], a depressed area on the dorsal surface of the scapula, above the spine.
suprasternal /-stur″nəl/, pertaining to a location above the sternum, adjacent to the neck.
suprasternal notch.　See **jugular notch of the sternum.**
supratentorial /-tentôr″ē·əl/ [L, *supra*, above, *tentorium*, tent], pertaining to a location above a tentorium.
supratrochlear artery, one of the two terminal branches of the ophthalmic nerve, with the dorsal nasal artery.
supravaginal hysterectomy /-vaj″inəl/ [L, *supra*, above, *vagina*, sheath; Gk, *hystera*, womb, *ektomē*, excision], a subtotal hysterectomy in which the body of the uterus is removed but the cervix remains.
supraventricular crest, the muscular ridge on the interior dorsal wall of the right ventricle of the heart. It defines the limit of the arterial cone and extends toward the pulmonary trunk from the ventral cusp of the atrioventricular ring. Compare **moderator band.**
supraventricular tachycardia (SVT) /-ventrik″yələr/ [L, *supra* + *ventriculus,* little belly], any cardiac rhythm with a rate exceeding 100 beats/min that originates above the branching part of the atrioventricular (AV) bundle, that is, in the sinus node, atria, or AV junction.
supraversion /soo͞″prə·ver′zhən/ [L, *supra*, above + *vertere*, to turn], malocclusion in which a tooth or other maxillary or mandibular structure extends farther away from the alveolus than normal, the occluding surfaces of the teeth extending beyond the normal occlusal line.
suprofen /səprō″fən/, an oral nonsteroidal antiinflammatory analgesic.
■ INDICATIONS: It is used in the treatment of mild to moderate pain and primary dysmenorrhea.
■ CONTRAINDICATIONS: It is contraindicated for patients who experience asthma, rhinitis, urticaria, or other allergic reactions from the use of aspirin or other nonsteroidal antiinflammatory drugs. It is not recommended for patients with a history of peptic ulcers or risk of other types of GI bleeding.
■ ADVERSE EFFECTS: Reported side effects include severe flank pain, nausea, vomiting, dyspepsia, abdominal pain, diarrhea, constipation, flatulence, headache, dizziness, sedation, and sleep disturbances.
sural communicating nerve.　See **common fibular nerve.**

sural nerve, a nerve that originates high in the leg between the two heads of the gastrocnemius muscle and supplies skin on the lower posterolateral surface of the leg and the lateral side of the foot and little toe.

sural region /soo͞o″rəl/ [L, *sura,* calf of the leg], the calf of the leg. It is formed by the bellies of the gastrocnemius and soleus muscles.

suramin sodium /soo͞o″rəmin/, an antitrypanosomal and antifilarial available from the U.S. Centers for Disease Control and Prevention. It is used primarily for treatment and prophylaxis of African trypanosomiasis and onchocerciasis.

surcharge, (in the United States) an additional fee charged to health plan enrollees for benefits not provided in the health plan contract.

surface anatomy /sur″fəs/ [L, *superficies,* surface], the study of the structural relationships of the external features of the body to the internal organs and parts. Compare **cross-sectional anatomy.**

surface anesthesia. See **topical anesthesia.**

surface area (SA), the total area exposed to the outside environment. The surface area of an object increases with the square of its linear dimensions. Volume increases as the cube of the object's linear dimensions. Thus the larger of two objects of the same shape will have less surface area per unit volume than the smaller object. Most loss of body heat is from the body surface.

surface biopsy, the removal of living tissue for microscopic examination by scraping the surface of a lesion. It is done primarily to diagnose cancer of the uterine cervix. See also **exfoliative cytology, Papanicolaou (Pap) test.**

surface tension, the tendency of a liquid to minimize the area of its surface by contracting due to intermolecular forces. This property causes liquids to rise in a capillary tube, affects the exchange of gases in the pulmonary alveoli, and alters the ability of various liquids to wet another surface.

surface therapy, a form of radiotherapy administered by placing one or more radioactive sources on or near an area of body surface. The resulting array of sources is called a surface mold, surface applicator, or plaque.

surface thermometer, a device that detects and indicates the surface temperature of any part of the body.

surfactant /sərfak″tənt/ [L, *superficies*], **1.** an agent, such as soap or detergent, dissolved in water to reduce its surface tension or the tension at the interface between the water and another liquid. **2.** one of certain lipoproteins that reduce the surface tension of pulmonary fluids, allowing the exchange of gases in the alveoli of the lungs and contributing to the elasticity of pulmonary tissue. Also called **pulmonary surfactant.** See also **alveolus, atelectasis, surface tension.**

Surfak, a stool softener. Brand name for *docusate calcium.*

surfer's nodules [ME, *suffe,* rush; L, *nodus,* knot], nodules on the skin of the knees, ankles, feet, or toes of a surfer caused by repeated contact of the skin with an abrasive, sandy surfboard. The nodules slowly diminish in size and disappear if surfing is discontinued. When treatment is necessary, injection of corticosteroids is usually effective.

surgeon /sur″jən/, a physician who treats injuries, deformities, and diseases by operative methods.

surgeon general, (in the United States) the chief medical officer of the Army, Navy, Air Force, and Public Health Service. In other countries, the title may indicate any physician with the rank of general.

surgeon's assistant (SA) /sur″jənz/ [Gk, *cheirourgos,* surgeon; L, *assistere,* to cause to stand], a medical professional trained to assist during surgery and in the preoperative and postoperative periods under the supervision of a licensed physician qualified to practice surgery.

surgery /sur″jərē/ [Gk, *cheirourgia*], the branch of medicine concerned with diseases and trauma requiring operative procedures. –**surgical,** *adj.*

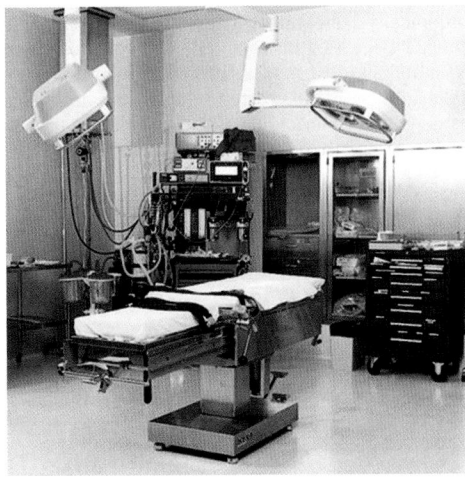

Operating room for surgery *(Courtesy Greg McVicar)*

-surgery, combining form meaning "the treatment of illness or deformity": *chemosurgery, stereotactic radiosurgery.*

surgical /sur″jikəl/ [Gk, *cheirourgia*], pertaining to the treatment of disease by manipulative and operative methods.

surgical abdomen. See **acute abdomen.**

surgical anatomy, (in applied anatomy) the study of the structure and morphological characteristics of the tissues and organs of the body as they relate to surgery.

surgical asepsis. See **asepsis.**

surgical assistant, as defined by the American College of Surgeons (ACS), the surgical assistant, under the direct supervision of the surgeon, provides aid in exposure, hemostasis, and other technical functions that will help the surgeon to perform a safe operation with optimal results for the patient. See also **Certified First Assistant.**

surgical diathermy. See **electrocoagulation.**

surgical fever [Gk, *cheirourgia* + L, *febris*], a fever that develops after surgery.

surgical field. See **operating field.**

surgical gut. See **catgut.**

surgical hospital, a hospital specializing in surgical procedures.

surgical induction of labor. See **induction of labor.**

surgical ligature, **1.** (in dentistry) the exposure of an unerupted tooth by placing a metal tie around its cervix. The free ends of the ligature are fixed to a fine precious-metal chain attached to an orthodontic appliance. These components act together to produce traction on the unerupted tooth and force it through the gingival tissues. **2.** a specialized thread of silk, gut, or wire used to tie off blood vessels to prevent bleeding or to treat abnormalities in other parts of the body that require constriction of tissues during surgical procedures.

surgical menopause [Gk, *cheirourgia* + L, *men,* month; Gk, *pauein,* to cease], the creation of a menopausal state by surgical removal of the ovaries.

surgical microscope. See **operating microscope.**

surgical neck of humerus [Gk, *cheirourgia* + AS, *hnecca* + L, *humerus,* shoulder], the shaft of the humerus distal to the tuberosities. It is a region particularly vulnerable to fracture and surgical correction.

surgical pathology, the study of disease by the analysis of tissue specimens obtained during surgery. The surgical

S

pathologist often examines specimens during surgery to determine how the operation should be modified or completed. The appearance of the specimen is noted. Then, slices of the tissue are prepared by the paraffin or frozen section method and microscopically examined by a physician trained in pathology.

surgical scrub, **1.** a bactericidal soap or solution used by surgeons and surgical nurses before performing or assisting in surgery. **2.** the act of washing the fingernails, hands, and forearms with a bactericidal soap or solution in a prescribed manner for a specific period before a surgical procedure.

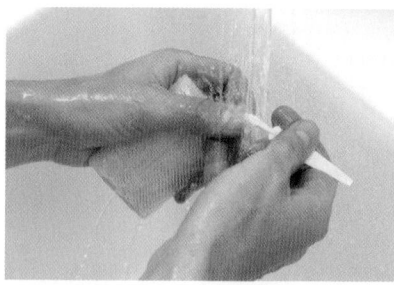
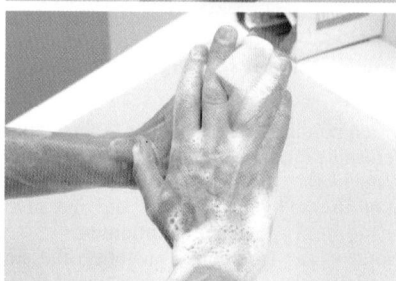
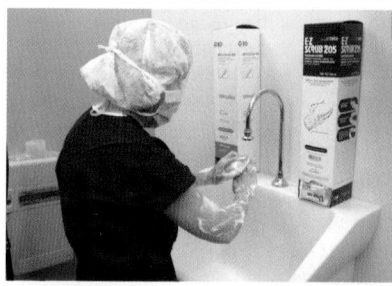
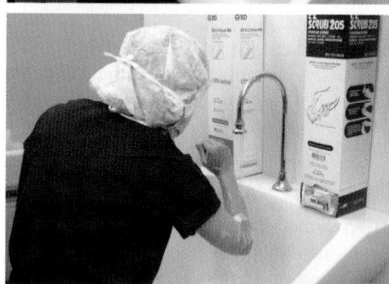
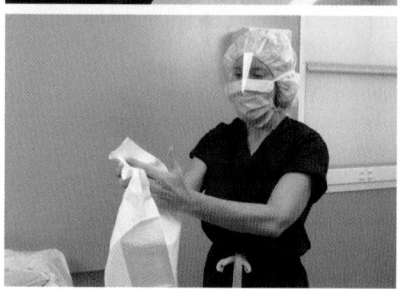

Surgical scrub procedure *(Elkin, Perry, and Potter, 2007)*

surgical sectioning, an oral surgery procedure for dividing a tooth to facilitate its removal. A variety of instruments are used for surgical sectioning, including osteotomes and power-driven burs.

surgical shock [Gk, *cheirourgia* + Fr, *choc*], a condition of shock that may occur during or after surgery, with signs of profound hypotension, decreased urine, increased heart rate, restlessness, and cyanosis of the extremities. Hemoglobin for blood volume may be low, or the patient may be bleeding or have a severe infection.

surgical suite, a group of one or more operating rooms and adjunct facilities, such as a sterile storage area, scrub room, and recovery room.

surgical technology, an allied health profession that focuses on providing an optimal surgical environment for the patient through the performance of sterile and nonsterile roles. See also **Certified Surgical Technologist.**

surgical treatment. See **treatment.**

Surmontil, an antidepressant drug. Brand name for **trimipramine maleate.**

surrogate /sur″əgāt/ [L, *surrogare,* to substitute], **1.** a substitute; a person or thing that replaces another. **2.** a person who represents and acts as a parent, taking the place of the father or mother. **3.** (in psychoanalysis) a substitute parental figure, or a symbolic image or representation of another, as may occur in a dream. The identity of the person represented often remains in the unconscious.

surrogate parenting, a form of artificial insemination in which a fertile woman agrees to be impregnated by a sperm donor and to carry the child to term, at which time the offspring is surrendered to the care of another. The surrogate mother usually receives a fee for bearing the child.

surrogate partner. See **sex surrogate.**

sursum-, combining form meaning "upward": *sursumversion.*

sursumversion /sur′sum·ver′zhən/ [L, *sursum* upward + *vertere,* to turn], binocular conjugate upward rotation of both eyes. Also called **superversion, supraversion.**

surveillance /sərvā″ləns/ [Fr, *surveiller,* to watch over], **1.** supervision or observation of a patient or a health condition. It may include the use of closed-circuit television cameras and monitors to cover unattended locations from a central office. **2.** a detailed examination or investigation for the accurate collection of data to record changes in the character of a population as at a particular time or, in a prospective or longitudinal surveillance, over a period. Retrospective surveillance might study the characteristics of a population in which a previous event occurred. The collection of data may include hospital records, morbidity and mortality statistics, death certificates, records of immunization, age groups, and various ecological and weather factors for the period of investigation, particularly if insect vectors are possible influences.

surveyed height of contour /sərvād″/ [OFr, *surveir,* to survey; AS, *heah,* high; It, *contornare,* to surround], **1.** a line, scribed or marked on a plaster cast of the teeth by the use of a dental surveyor, that designates the greatest convexity relative to a selected path of denture placement and removal, as well as the placement of removable partial denture retention clasps. **2.** See **anatomical height of contour.**

surveyor, a dental instrument composed of a vertical post mounted to a flat metal base and a horizontal arm connected to the vertical post, followed by a vertical stylus that encases a piece of pencil lead. The second portion is a table to which a plaster cast of the teeth is clamped so that a surveyed height of contour can be established.

survival curve /sərvī″vəl/ [Fr, *survivre,* to survive; L, *curvus,* bent], a plot of the number or percentage of organisms surviving for a given period as a function of radiation dose.

survivor guilt /sərvī″vər/ [Fr, *survivre* + ME, *gilt,* sin], feelings of guilt for surviving a tragedy in which others died. In some cases, the person may believe the tragedy occurred because he or she did something bad; in others, the person may feel guilty for not taking proper steps to avert the tragedy. Also called *survival guilt.*

susceptibility /səsep′tibil″itē/ [L, *suscipere,* to undertake], the condition of being vulnerable to a disease or disorder.

susceptible /səsep″tibəl/ [L, *suscipere,* to undertake], being predisposed, liable, or sensitive to the effects of an infectious disease, allergen, or other pathogenic agent; lacking immunity or resistance.

suspension /səspen″shən/ [L, *suspendere,* to hang], **1.** a liquid in which small particles of a solid are dispersed, but not dissolved, and in which the dispersal is maintained by stirring or shaking the mixture. If left standing, the solid particles settle at the bottom of the container. See also **colloid, solution. 2.** a treatment, used primarily in spinal disorders, consisting of suspending the patient by the chin and shoulders. **3.** a temporary cessation of pain or of a vital process.

suspension sling, a sling usually made of muslin or lightweight canvas and used primarily to provide support, such as against the gravitational pull on an injured arm. Kinds include *triangular sling.*

suspensory ligament /səspen″sərē/ [L, *suspendere,* to hang, *ligare,* to bind], any of a number of ligaments that help support an organ or body structure, such as the suspensory ligaments inside the eye that hold the lens in tension.

suspensory ligament of the lens. See **zonule of Zinn.**

sustained release. See **prolonged release.**

sustenance /sus″tənəns/ [L, *sustenare,* to sustain], **1.** the act or process of supporting or maintaining life or health. **2.** the food or nutrients essential for maintaining life.

sustentacular /sus″ten·tak′yo͞o·lər/ [L, *sustentare,* to support], pertaining to a support or serving to support.

sustentacular cells. See **supporting cells.**

sustentaculum tali, a process of the calcaneus that supports the talus.

susto /so͞os″tō/, a culture-bound syndrome found in Central American populations related to stress engendered by a self-perceived failure to fulfill sex-role expectations.

Sutent, a chemotherapeutic agent. Brand name for **sunitinib.**

Sutton disease /sut′ən/ [Richard Lightburn Sutton, American dermatologist, 1878–1952], a recurrent disease of the mucous membranes of unknown cause, generally considered to be a severe form of aphthous stomatitis, characterized by deep crater-like ulcers with inflamed borders that leave scars after healing. It usually involves the mucosa of the lips, cheeks, tongue, palate, and anterior tonsillar pillars, but the pharynx, larynx, and genitalia may also be affected. Also called **Mikulicz aphthae, periadenitis mucosa necrotica recurrens, recurring scarring aphthae.** See also **aphthous stomatitis.**

sutura /so͞ocho͞o″rə/ *pl. suturae* [L, suture], an immovable fibrous joint in which certain bones of the skull are connected by a thin layer of fibrous tissue. Compare **gomphosis, syndesmosis.**

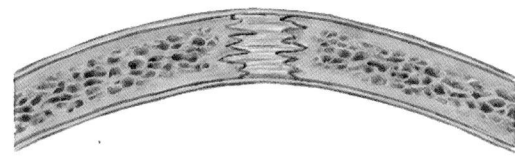

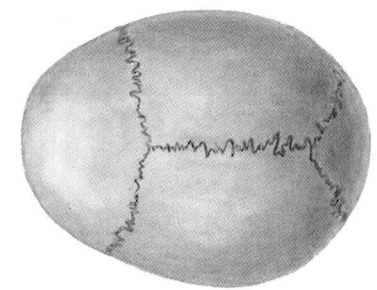

Sutura *(Drake, Vogl, and Mitchell, 2010)*

sutura dentata, an immovable fibrous joint that is one kind of true suture in which toothlike processes interlock along the margins of connecting bones of the skull. Compare **sutura limbosa, sutura serrata.**

suturae, an immovable joint. See **sutura.**

suturae cranii. See **cranial sutures.**

sutura limbosa, an immovable fibrous joint that is one kind of true suture in which beveled and serrated edges of certain connecting bones of the skull, such as the parietal and temporal bones, overlap and interlock. Compare **sutura dentata, sutura serrata.**

sutura plana, a fibrous joint that is one kind of false suture in which rough contiguous edges of certain bones of the skull, such as the maxillae, form a connection. Compare **sutura squamosa.**

sutura serrata, an immovable fibrous joint that is one kind of true suture in which connecting bones interlock along serrated edges that resemble fine-toothed saws. Compare **sutura dentata, sutura limbosa.**

sutura squamosa, an immovable fibrous joint that is one kind of false suture in which overlapping beveled edges unite certain bones of the skull, such as the temporal and the parietal bone. Compare **sutura plana.**

suture /so͞o″chər/ [L, *sutura*], **1.** *n.,* a border or a joint, such as between the bones of the cranium. **2.** *v.,* to stitch together cut or torn edges of tissue with suture material. **3.** *n.,* a surgical stitch taken to repair an incision, tear, or wound. **4.** *n.,* material used for surgical stitches, such as absorbable or nonabsorbable silk, catgut, wire, or synthetic material.

suture forceps. See **needle holder.**

Sv, abbreviation for **sievert.**

SV40, abbreviation for **simian virus 40.**

SV40 papovavirus. See **papovavirus.**

SvO₂, symbol for *percentage of oxygen saturation of mixed venous blood.*

SVR, abbreviation for **systemic vascular resistance.**

SVT, abbreviation for **supraventricular tachycardia.**

swab /swob/ [D, *swabber,* ship's drudge], a stick or clamp holding absorbent gauze or cotton, used for washing,

S

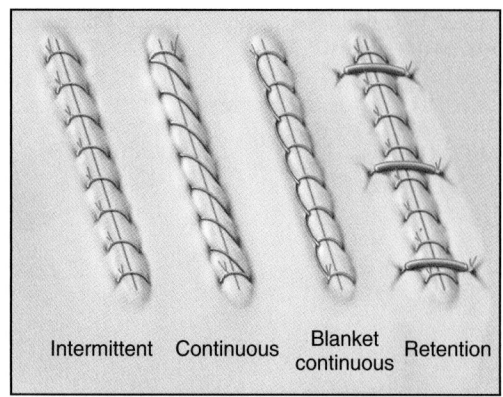

Types of sutures *(Harkreader and Hogan, 2007)*

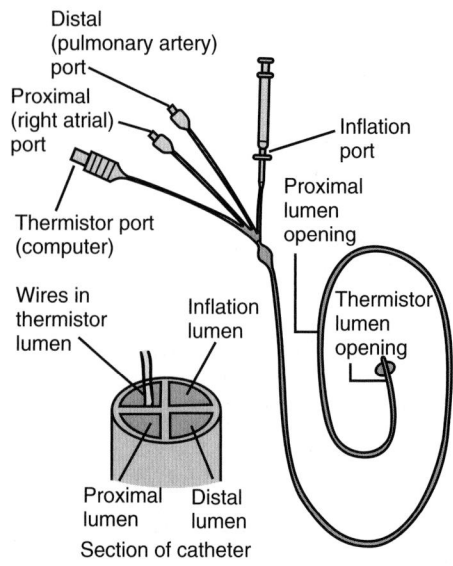

Swan-Ganz catheter *(Black and Hawks, 2009)*

cleansing, or drying a body surface; for collecting a specimen for laboratory examination; or for applying a topical medication.

swaddling /swod″ling/ [OE, *swethel,* swaddling band], **1.** long, narrow bands of cloth once used to wrap a newborn. **2.** a method of wrapping a newborn, especially a premature or at-risk newborn, that provides maximal comfort and containment.

swage /swāj/ [OFr, *souage*], **1.** *v.,* to shape metal by hammering or by adapting it to a die. **2.** *v.,* to fuse suture material to a needle, especially an eyeless needle. **3.** *n.,* a tool or form, often one of a pair, for shaping metal by pressure. Also called *swedge.*

Swain, Mary Ann P. See **Modeling and Role Modeling.**

swallow apnea, absence of respiration during the phase of swallowing when the bolus is passing through the oropharyngeal region.

swallowing /swol″ō·ing/ [AS, *swelgan*], the process that usually involves movement of food from the mouth to the stomach via the esophagus. Coordination of muscles is needed from the tongue to the esophageal sphincter. See also **swallowing reflex.**

swallowing examination, an x-ray with contrast dye (usually barium) that is performed to pinpoint problems that exist in a patient who is unable to swallow. The examination is used to detect tumors; upper esophageal diverticula; inflammation; extrinsic compression of the upper GI tract; problems resulting from surgery to the oropharyngeal tract; motility disorders of the upper GI tract; and neurological disorders such as stroke, Parkinson's disease, and neuropathies.

swallowing reflex [AS, *swelgan* + L, *reflectere,* to bend back], a sequence of reflexes that begins when a bolus of food is manipulated by the tongue and other oral cavity muscles to the palate or the pharynx.

swamp fever. See **leptospirosis, malaria.**

Swan-Ganz catheter /swän″ ganz″/ [Harold J.C. Swan, American physician, b. 1922; William Ganz, American cardiologist, b. 1919; Gk, *katheter,* something lowered], a long, thin cardiac catheter with a tiny balloon at the tip. It is used to determine left ventricular function by measuring pulmonary capillary wedge pressure.

swan neck deformity /swän/ [D, *zwaan* + AS, *hnecca,* neck; L, *deformis,* misshapen], **1.** an abnormal condition of the finger characterized by flexion of the distal interphalangeal joint and hyperextension of the proximal interphalangeal joint. It is caused by a taut profundus tendon in the

presence of a weakened distal interphalangeal joint and may be combined with a volar plate rupture. The condition is seen most often in rheumatoid arthritis. Also called **zig-zag. 2.** a structural abnormality of the kidney tubules associated with rickets. The kidney tubule connecting the glomerulus with the convoluted part of the tubule is narrowed into a configuration referred to as "swan neck." There are also a thinning and atrophy of the distal tubule and a shortening of the convoluted part.

Swanson, Kristen M., a nursing theorist whose Theory of Caring asserts that nursing care is nurturing delivered as a set of interrelated processes that evolve from the nurse's own convictions and knowledge and his or her interaction with the patient. The theory is based on Swanson's Caring Model, which names as the components of caring five basic processes: knowing, being with, doing for, enabling, and maintaining belief (faith in and esteem for the patient). The theory's objective is to help nurses deliver care that promotes the dignity, respect, and empowerment.

Swanson's Caring Model. See **Swanson, Kristen M.**

S wave, the negative component after the R wave in each QRS complex on an electrocardiogram.

sway, to rock, teeter, wobble, or swing back and forth.

sweat. See **perspiration.**

sweat duct. See **sudoriferous duct.**

sweat electrolytes test, a fluid analysis of sweat to indicate whether a patient has cystic fibrosis.

sweat gland. See **sudoriferous gland.**

sweat gland abscess, an abscess in a sweat gland, such as in hidradenitis suppurativa.

sweating. See **diaphoresis.**

sweat test, a method for evaluating sodium and chloride excretion from the sweat glands, often the first test performed in the diagnosis of cystic fibrosis. The sweat glands are stimulated with a drug such as pilocarpine, and the perspiration produced is analyzed. The eccrine glands of patients with cystic fibrosis produce sodium and chloride concentrations that are three to six times normal. Chloride levels above 60 mEq/L and sodium levels above 90 mEq/L are considered diagnostic for the disease. The test is very reliable, and although it may be useful at any age, it is usually performed on infants from 2 weeks to 1 year of age. See also **cystic fibrosis.**

Swedish massage /swē′dish/ [Fr, *masser*], the most commonly used form of classical Western massage, generally performed in the direction of the heart, sometimes with active or passive movement of the joints. It is used especially for relaxation, relief of muscular tension, and improvement of circulation and range of motion.

sweep tapping, a proprioceptive-tactile treatment technique in which the clinician uses a light-touch sweep pattern over the back of the fingers of one of the hands. The stimulus is applied quickly over a dermatomal area, helping the patient to contract the muscle.

Sweet localization method, a radiographic technique for locating a foreign body in the eye by making two radiographic films of the eye while the patient's head is immobilized. A small metal ball and a cone are placed at precise distances from the center of the cornea as register marks while lateral and perpendicular radiographic views of the eye are made. A three-dimensional view of the eye is constructed from the two films, and, guided by the positions of the ball and cone, the location of the foreign body in the eye is plotted from the intersection of lines through the ball and cone.

Sweet syndrome /swēts/ [Robert Douglas Sweet, English dermatologist, 20th century], a condition usually seen on the upper body of middle-aged women, characterized by one or more large, rapidly extending, erythematous, tender or painful plaques and accompanied by fever and dense infiltration of neutrophils in the upper and middle dermis. Also called **acute febrile neutrophilic dermatosis.**

Swift disease. See **acrodynia.**

swimmer's ear [AS, *swimman,* to swim, *eare*], *(Informal)* otitis externa resulting from infection transmitted in the water of a swimming pool. See also **otitis externa.**

swimmer's itch, an allergic dermatitis caused by sensitivity to nonhuman schistosome cercarias that die under the skin, leading to erythema, urticaria, and a papular rash lasting 1 or 2 days. Treatment usually includes oral antihistamines and antipruritic lotions. Also called **schistosome dermatitis.** See also **schistosomiasis.**

swimming reflex, a primitive fetal activity, marked by well-coordinated movements, that is exhibited when the infant's face is placed in water. It normally disappears at 6 months of age.

swineherd's disease, leptospirosis manifested as a benign meningitis and caused by serovariants of *Leptospira interrogans.* It affects people who work with swine or pork or come in contact with the urine of animal or human carriers.

swing phase of gait [AS, *swingan* + Gk, *phasis,* appearance; ME, *gata,* a way], the phase of the normal gait cycle during which the foot is off the ground. The swing phase follows the stance phase and is divided into the initial swing, the midswing, and the terminal swing stages.

switch, **1.** a device used to break or open an electric circuit. **2.** an item that connects, disconnects, or diverts an electric current. **3.** an adaptation used for clients with disabilities to promote successful interaction with computers, battery-operated devices, and powered mobility systems.

switch site, a point on a chromosome where gene segments unite during segment rearrangement, as in the production of immunoglobulins.

swoon [OE, *geswogen,* unconscious], *(Obsolete)* now called **fainting.**

sy-. See **syn-, sy-, syl-, sym-.**

sychnosphygmia, an accelerated heart rate.

sycosis barbae /sikō″sis/ [Gk, *sycon,* fig, *osis,* condition; L, *barba,* beard], an inflammation of hair follicles of skin that has been shaved. Treatment includes light and infrequent shaving, topical and systemic antibiotics, and daily plucking of infected hairs. Also called **barber's itch,** *sycosis vulgaris.*

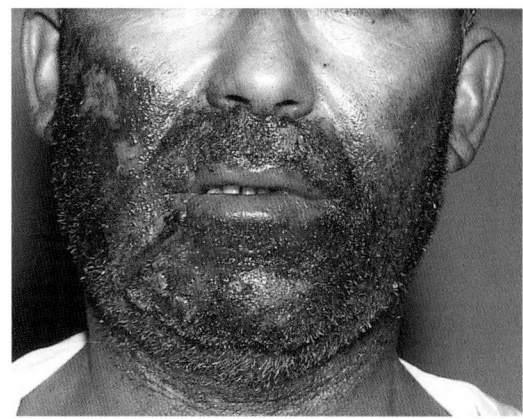

Sycosis barbae (du Vivier, 2002)

Sydenham chorea /sīd″ənham/ [Thomas Sydenham, English physician, 1624–1689; Gk, *choreia,* dance], a form of chorea associated with rheumatic fever, usually occurring during childhood. The cause is unknown but is thought be a streptococcal infection that initiates an autoimmune mechanism. The choreic movements increase over the first 2 weeks, reach a plateau, and then diminish. The child usually recovers within 10 weeks. With undue exertion or emotional strain, the condition may recur. Also called **rheumatic chorea.** Formerly called **Saint Vitus dance, chorea minor.**

syl-. See **syn-, sy-, syl-, sym-.**

sylvatic plague /silvat″ik/ [L, *sylva,* forest, *plaga,* stroke], an endemic disease of wild rodents caused by *Yersinia pestis* and transmitted to humans by the bite of an infected flea. Infection of humans by wild animals is described as a sylvatic stage. It is found on every continent except Australia. See also **bubonic plague.**

sylvian aqueduct /sil″vē·ən/ [Franciscus Sylvius, Dutch anatomist, 1614–1672; L, *aquaductus,* canal], a narrow canal from the third to the fourth ventricle of the midbrain. Also called **aqueduct of Sylvius.**

sylvian fissure [Franciscus Sylvius; L, *fissura,* cleft], the lateral sulcus of the cerebral hemisphere. Also called *sylvian sulcus.*

sym-. See **syn-, sy-, syl-, sym-.**

symbiosis /sim′bē·ō″sis/ [Gk, *syn,* together, *bios,* life], **1.** a mode of living characterized by a close association between organisms of different species. **2.** a state in which two people are emotionally dependent on each other. **3.** a pathologic inability of a child to separate from its mother emotionally and sometimes physically. **–symbiotic,** *adj.*

symbiotic /sim′bē·ot″ik/ [Gk, *syn,* together, *bios,* life], characterized by or concerned with symbiosis or living together.

symbiotic phase, in Mahler's system of preoedipal development, the stage between 1 and 5 months when the infant participates in a "symbiotic orbit" with the mother. All parts of the mother, including voice, gestures, clothing, and space in which she moves, are joined with the infant.

symblepharon, adhesion of the eyelid to the cornea. Also called **corneoblepharon.**

S

symbol /sim″bəl/ [Gk, *symbolon,* sign], **1.** an image, object, action, or other stimulus that represents something else by reason of conscious association, convention, or another relationship, such as a flag or a statue. **2.** an object, mode of behavior, or feeling that disguises a repressed emotional conflict through an unconscious association rather than through an objective relationship, as in dreams and anxiety.

-symbolia, combining form meaning "(condition involving) the ability to interpret symbols": *asymbolia, dyssymbolia.*

symbolism /sim″bəlizəm/, **1.** the representation or evocation of one idea, action, or object by the use of another, as in systems of writing, poetic language, or dream metaphor. **2.** (in psychiatry) an unconscious mental mechanism characteristic of all human thinking in which a mental image stands for but disguises some other object, person, or thought, especially one associated with emotional conflict. The mechanism is a principal factor in the formation of dreams and in various symptoms resulting from such anxious and psychotic conditions as conversion reactions, obsessions, and compulsions. Also called *symbolization.*

symelus. See **symmelus.**

Symlin, a medication used to reduce blood sugar levels in patients with diabetes mellitus. Brand name for **pramlintide.**

symmelia /simē″lyə/ [Gk, *syn,* together, *melos,* limb], a developmental anomaly characterized by apparent fusion of the lower limbs. There may be three feet (tripodial symmelia), two feet (dipodial symmelia), one foot (monopodial symmelia), or no feet (sirenomelia). See also **symmelus, sympus, sirenomelia, monopodial symmelia, dipodial symmelia, tripodial symmelia.**

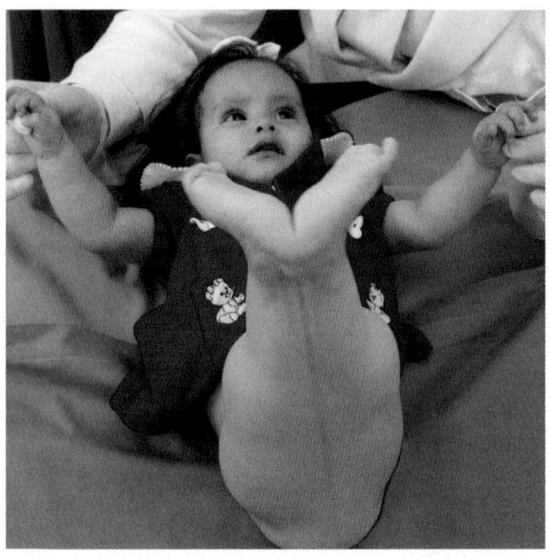

Infant with dipodial symmelia *(Schoenwolf and Bleyl, 2015)*

symmelus /sim″ələs/, a malformed fetus characterized by symmelia. Also spelled **symelus.**

Symmers disease. See **giant follicular lymphoma.**

Symmetrel, an antiviral and antiparkinsonian drug. Brand name for **amantadine hydrochloride.**

symmetric /simet″rik/ [Gk, *syn + metron,* measure], (of the body or parts of the body) pertaining to equality in size or shape. Also *symmetrical.* Compare **asymmetric.**

symmetric lipomatosis. See **nodular circumscribed lipomatosis.**

symmetric orientation, (in neonatal care) midline positioning of the head with similar alignment of the trunk and extremities. The orientation helps promote even development of tone and function in both sides of the body.

symmetric tonic neck reflex, a normal response in infants to assume the crawl position by extending the arms and bending the knees when the head and neck are extended. The reflex disappears when neurological and muscular development allows independent limb movement for actual crawling. Also called **crawling reflex.** See also **tonic neck reflex.**

symmetry /sim″ətrē/ [Gk, *syn,* together, *metron,* measure], (in anatomy) the correspondence of parts on opposite sides of the body, or equality of parts on both sides of a dividing line.

sympathectomize /sim′pəthek″təmiz/ [Gk, *sympathein,* to feel with, *ektomē,* excision], to interrupt the conduction of nerve impulses along part of the sympathetic trunk by surgery or drugs.

sympathectomy /sim′pəthek″təmē/ [Gk, *sympathein,* to feel with, *ektomē,* excision], a surgical interruption of part of the sympathetic nerve pathways to relieve chronic pain or to promote vasodilation in vascular diseases, such as arteriosclerosis, claudication, Buerger disease, and Raynaud phenomenon. The sheath around an artery carries the sympathetic nerve fibers that control constriction of the vessel. Removal of the sheath causes the vessel to relax and expand and allows more blood to pass through it. The operation also may be done with a vascular graft to increase the blood flow through the graft area. Preoperatively the physician may assess the effect of surgery by injecting sympathetic ganglia with a local anesthesia to interrupt temporarily the sympathetic nerve impulses. The nerves lie along the spinal column and are approached through the back or the neck, by using local anesthesia. Postoperatively, the adequacy of circulation and peripheral nervous supply in the affected extremity is monitored. An arteriogram shows a widened pathway.

sympathetic /sim′pəthet″ik/ [Gk, *sympathein,* to feel with], **1.** pertaining to a display of compassion for another's grief. **2.** pertaining to a division of the autonomic nervous system. **3.** See **sympathy.**

sympathetic eye. See **sympathizing eye.**

sympathetic ganglion [Gk, *sympathein,* to feel with, *ganglion,* knot], a collection of multipolar nerve cells along the course of the sympathetic trunk. Nearly two dozen of the ganglia serve as "cell stations" on efferent pathways between the cervical and sacral parts of the sympathetic trunk.

sympathetic imbalance [Gk, *sympathein,* to feel with; L, *in + balance*], pertaining to vagotony, or vagus nerve tension and hyperexcitability of the parasympathetic nervous system, as opposed to the sympathetic nervous system. Also called **vagotonia.**

sympathetic irritation [Gk, *sympathein,* to feel with; L, *irritare,* to tease], inflammation of one organ after inflammation of a related organ, such as when trauma to an eye is followed by similar symptoms in the uninjured eye.

sympathetic nerve [Gk, *sympathein,* to feel with; L, *nervus*], any nerve of the sympathetic branch of the autonomic nervous system.

sympathetic nervous system. See **autonomic nervous system.**

sympathetic ophthalmia, a granulomatous inflammation of the uveal tract of both eyes occurring after an injury to the uveal tract of one eye. Corticosteroids may be helpful in treatment, but surgical enucleation of the originally injured eye may be necessary to preserve vision in the uninjured eye. Also called **metastatic ophthalmia, migratory ophthalmia.**

sympathetic pain, distress that occurs in the hemiplegic shoulder with a loss of joint range as a result of muscle imbalance. It results from loss of active and passive motion, loss of ability to bear weight, and long-standing subluxation without support.

sympathetic stress reaction. See **alarm reaction.**

sympathetic symptom [Gk, *sympathein*, to feel with, *symptoma*, that which occurs], a symptom occurring in one body area when the causative lesion is actually in another area. See also **referred pain.**

sympathetic trunk, one of a pair of chains of ganglia extending along the side of the vertebral column from the base of the skull to the coccyx. Each trunk is part of the sympathetic nervous system and consists of a series of ganglia connected by various types of fibers. Each sympathetic trunk distributes branches with postganglionic fibers to the autonomic plexuses, the cranial nerves, the individual organs, the nerves accompanying arteries, and the spinal nerves.

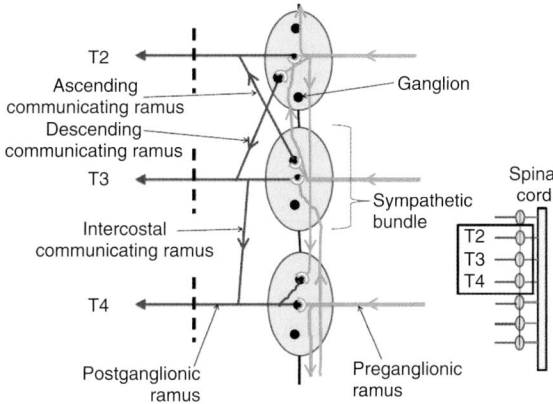

Sympathetic trunk *(Drake, Vogl, and Mitchell, 2010)*

sympathize. See **sympathy.**

sympathizing eye /sim″pəthī′zing/, (in sympathetic ophthalmia) the fellow eye that becomes inflamed by lymphatic or blood-borne metastasis of the causative antigen or microorganism. Also called **sympathetic eye.**

sympatholytic, sympatholytic agent. See **antiadrenergic.**

sympathomimetic /sim′pəthō′mimet″ik/ [Gk, *sympathein* + *mimesis*, imitation], a pharmacological agent that mimics the effects of stimulation of organs and structures by the sympathetic nervous system. It functions by occupying adrenergic receptor sites and acting as an agonist or by increasing the release of the neurotransmitter norepinephrine at postganglionic nerve endings. Various sympathomimetic agents are used as decongestants of nasal and ocular mucosa, such as bronchodilators in the treatment of asthma and vasopressors and cardiac stimulants in the treatment of acute hypotension and shock; they are also used for maintaining normal blood pressure during operations using spinal anesthesia. Drugs in this group include cyclopentamine, DOBUTamine, DOPamine, epHEDrine, isoproterenol, metaproterenol, metaraminol, mephentermine, methoxamine, methoxyphenamine, naphazoline, norepinephrine, phenylephrine, propylhexedrine, protokylol, pseudoephedrine, terbutaline sulfate, tetrahydrozoline, tuaminoheptane, xylometazoline, and epINEPHrine, a synthetic isomer of the hormone secreted by the adrenal medulla. Adverse effects of sympathomimetic drugs may be nervousness, severe headache, anxiety, vertigo, nausea, vomiting, dilated pupils, glycosuria, and dysuria. Also called *adrenergic drug.*

sympathomimetic amine, an amine that mimics the actions of the sympathetic nervous system. The group includes the catecholamines and drugs such as isoprenaline, dobutamine, and dopexamine that mimic their actions. See also **adrenergic.**

sympathomimetic bronchodilator, a medication that reduces bronchial muscle spasm through action that mimics the sympathetic nervous system in producing smooth muscle relaxation. It is commonly a beta₂ receptor agonist agent.

sympathy /sim″pəthē/ [Gk, *sympathein*], **1.** an expressed interest or concern regarding the problems, emotions, or states of mind of another. Compare **empathy. 2.** the relation that exists between the mind and body, causing the one to be affected by the other. **3.** mental contagion or the influence exerted by one individual or group on another and the effects produced, such as the spread of panic, uncontrollable laughter, or yawning. **4.** the physiological or pathological relationship between two organs, systems, or parts of the body.

symphalangia /sim′fəlan″jē·ə/ [Gk, *syn*, together, *phalanx*, finger], **1.** a condition, usually inherited, characterized by ankylosis of the fingers or toes. **2.** a congenital anomaly in which webbing of the fingers or toes occurs in varying degrees, often in conjunction with other defects of the hands or feet. Also called *symphalangism.* See also **syndactyly.**

symphocephalus /sim′fōsef″ələs/ [Gk, *symphes*, growing together, *kephale*, head], twin fetuses joined at the head. The term is often used as a general designation for fetuses with varying degrees of the anomaly. See also **craniopagus, syncephalus.**

Symphonological Bioethical Theory. See **Husted, Gladys L. and James H.**

Symphonological Model for Ethical Decision Making. See **Husted, Gladys L. and James H.**

symphyseal angle /simfiz″ē·əl/ [Gk, *symphysis*, growing together; L, *angulus*, corner], the angle of the chin, which may be classified as protruding, straight, or receding.

symphyses, symphysic. See **symphysis.**

symphysic teratism /simfiz″ik/, a congenital anomaly in which there is a fusion of normally separated parts or organs, such as a horseshoe kidney, or in which parts close prematurely, such as the skull bones in craniostenosis.

symphysis /sim″fəsis/ *pl.* **symphyses** [Gk, growing together], **1.** a line of union, especially a cartilaginous joint in which adjacent bony surfaces are firmly united by fibrocartilage. Also called **fibrocartilaginous joint. 2.** *(Informal)* symphysis pubis. −*symphysic, adj.*

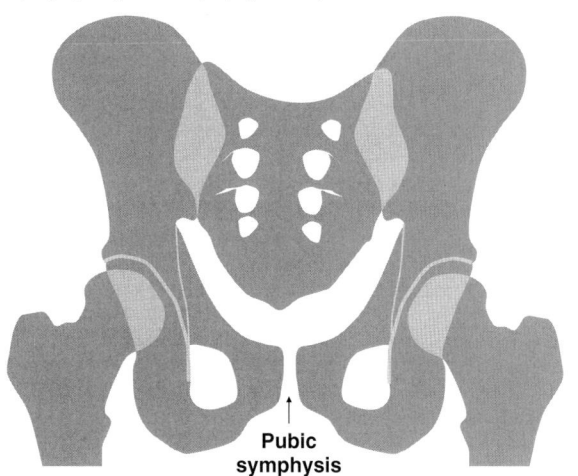

Pubic symphysis

Symphysis *(Drake, Vogl, and Mitchell, 2010)*

S

symphysis menti,   **1.** the junction between the two halves of the mandible. **2.** the prominence of the chin.

symphysis pubis.   See **pubic symphysis.**

sympodia /simpō″dē·ə/ [Gk, *syn,* together, *pous,* foot], a congenital developmental anomaly characterized by fusion of the lower extremities. See also **sirenomelus, sympus.**

symptom /simp″təm/ [Gk, *symptoma,* that which happens], a subjective indication of a disease or a change in condition as perceived by the patient. For example, the halo symptom of glaucoma is seen by the patient as colored rings around a single light source. Many symptoms are accompanied by objective signs, such as pruritus, which is often reported with erythema and a maculopapular eruption on the skin. Some symptoms may be objectively confirmed, such as numbness of a body part, which may be confirmed by absence of response to a pin prick. Primary symptoms are symptoms that are intrinsically associated with a disease. Secondary symptoms are a consequence of illness and disease. Compare **sign.**

symptom focusing, (in occupational therapy) a specific approach to managing an impairment that involves spending a great deal of mental energy, time, and/or physical effort giving in to one's symptoms (or impairment) and spending considerably less time attempting to ignore, implicitly endure, or adjust to symptoms in order to engage in occupations.

symptomatic /simp″təmat″ik/ [Gk, *symptoma,* that which happens], having characteristics of a symptom or indications of a specific disease.

symptomatic esophageal peristalsis, a condition in which peristaltic progression in the body of the esophagus is normal but contractions in the distal esophagus are increased in amplitude and duration. Also called **esophageal peristalsis, nutcracker esophagus.**

symptomatic hyperleukocytosis.   See **leukostasis**.

symptomatic impotence [Gk, *symptoma,* that which happens; L, *in* + *potentia,* power], impotence that is the result of poor health or the use of medications.

symptomatic nanism, dwarfism associated with defects in bone growth, tooth formation, and sexual development.

symptomatic neuralgia [Gk, *symptoma,* that which happens, *neuron,* nerve, *algos,* pain], nerve pain that is secondary to a disease condition.

symptomatic torticollis [Gk, *symptoma* + L, *tortus,* twisted, *collum,* neck], a stiff neck caused by a disease in the neck, such as rheumatoid torticollis or myogenic torticollis.

symptomatic treatment.   See **treatment.**

symptomatology /simp″təmətol″əjē/ [Gk, *symptoma* + *logos,* science], the science of symptoms of disease in general or of the symptoms of a specific disease.

symptom-bearer, (in psychology) a family member frequently perceived as a patient who is functioning poorly because family dynamics interfere with functioning at a higher level. Also called *identified patient.*

symptom complex.   See **syndrome.**

symptomless carrier.   See **passive carrier.**

symptom severity: perimenopause, a nursing outcome from the Nursing Outcomes Classification (NOC) defined as the severity of symptoms caused by declining hormonal levels. See also **Nursing Outcomes Classification.**

symptom severity: premenstrual syndrome (PMS), a nursing outcome from the Nursing Outcomes Classification (NOC) defined as the severity of symptoms caused by cyclic hormonal fluctuations. See also **Nursing Outcomes Classification.**

symptothermal method of family planning /simp″-təthur″məl/ [Gk, *symptoma* + *therme,* heat], a natural method of family planning that incorporates the ovulation and basal body temperature methods of family planning. It is more effective than either method used alone and requires fewer days of abstinence from sexual intercourse because it allows the fertile period of the menstrual cycle to be more precisely identified.

sympus /sim″pəs/ [Gk, *syn,* together, *pous,* foot], a malformed fetus in which the lower extremities are completely fused or rotated and the pelvis and genitalia are defective. Kinds include **sirenomelus, sympus dipus, sympus monopus.** See also **symmelus.**

sympus apus.   See **sirenomelus.**

sympus dipus /dē″pəs/, a malformed fetus in which the lower extremities are fused and both feet are formed.

sympus monopus /mon″əpəs/, a malformed fetus in which the lower extremities are fused and one foot is formed. Also called **monopodial symmelia, uromelus.**

syn-, sy-, syl-, sym-, prefix meaning "union" or "association": *synadelphus, syncephalus, synchronous.*

synactive model of infant behavior /sinak″tiv/, a major theoretic framework for establishing physiological stability as the foundation for the organization of motor, behavioral state, and attentive and interactive behaviors in neonates.

synadelphus /sin″ədel″fəs/ *pl. synadelphi* [Gk, *syn* + *adelphos,* brother], a conjoined twin with a single head and trunk and eight limbs. Also called *cephalothoracoiliopagus,* **syndelphus.**

Synalar, a glucocorticoid. Brand name for **fluocinolone acetonide.**

synapse /sin″aps, sinaps″/ [Gk, *synaptein,* to join], **1.** *n.,* the region surrounding the point of contact between two neurons or between a neuron and an effector organ, across which nerve impulses are transmitted through the action of a neurotransmitter, such as acetylcholine or norepinephrine. When an impulse reaches the terminal point of one neuron, it causes the release of the neurotransmitter. The neurotransmitter diffuses across the gap between the two cells to bind with receptors in the other neuron, muscle, or gland, triggering electric changes that either inhibit or continue the transmission of the impulse. Synapses are polarized so that nerve impulses normally travel in only one direction; they are also subject to fatigue, oxygen deficiency, anesthetics, and other chemical agents. Compare **ephapse.** Kinds include **axoaxonic synapse, axodendritic synapse, axodendrosomatic synapse, axosomatic synapse, dendrodendritic synapse. 2.** *v.,* to form a synapse or connection between neurons. **3.** *v.,* (in genetics) to form a synaptic fusion between homologous chromosomes during meiosis. **−synaptic,** *adj.*

synapsis /sinap″sis/, the pairing of homologous chromosomes during early meiotic prophase in gametogenesis to form double or bivalent chromosomes.

synaptic /sinap″tik/ [Gk, *synaptein,* to join], pertaining to or resembling a synapse.

synaptic cleft, the microscopic extracellular space at the synapse that separates the membrane of the terminal nerve endings of a presynaptic neuron and the membrane of a postsynaptic cell. Nerve impulses are transmitted across this cleft by means of a neurotransmitter. Also called *synaptic gap.* See also **neuromuscular junction.**

synaptic junction, the membranes of both the presynaptic neuron and the postsynaptic receptor cell together with the synaptic cleft. See also **synapse.**

synaptic transmission, the passage of a neural impulse across a synapse from one nerve fiber to another by means of a neurotransmitter. Compare **ephaptic transmission.**

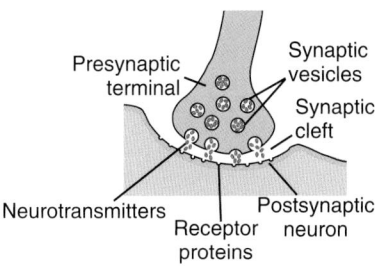

Synaptic transmission *(Black and Hawks, 2009)*

synaptogenesis /sinap'tōjen″əsis/, the formation of synapses between neurons. In humans it begins early in gestation but occurs most rapidly from 2 months before birth to 2 years after birth.

synaptosome /sinap″təsōm'/, a presynaptic nerve terminal that has been separated from the rest of the neuron and isolated from homogenates of brain tissue. It appears as a membrane-bound structure containing synaptic vesicles.

synarthrosis, any of several immovable articulations. See also **fibrous joint.**

syncephalus /sinsef″ələs/ [Gk, *syn + kephale,* head], a conjoined twin having a single head and two bodies. Also called **monocephalus.**

synchilia /singkē″lyə/ [Gk, *syn + cheilos,* lip], a congenital anomaly in which there is complete or partial fusion of the lips; atresia of the mouth. Also spelled *syncheilia.*

synchondrosis /sing'kondrō″sis/ *pl.* **synchondroses** [Gk, *syn + chondros,* cartilage], a cartilaginous joint creating a union between two immovable bones, such as the synchondroses of the cranium, the pubic symphysis, the sternum, and the manubrium.

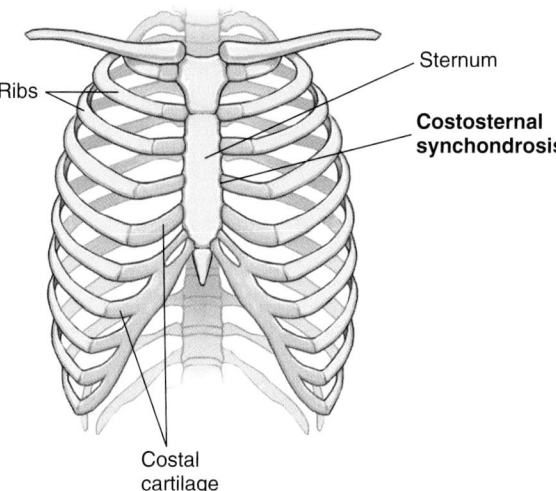

Synchondroses *(Patton and Thibodeau, 2010)*

synchorial /singkôr″ē·əl/ [Gk, *syn + chorion,* skin], pertaining to multiple fetuses that share a common placenta, as in monozygosity.

synchronized intermittent mandatory ventilation (SIMV) /sing″krənīzd/, periodic assisted mechanical ventilation synchronized with the patient's breathing. Spontaneous breathing by the patient occurs between the assisted mechanical breaths, which occur at preset intervals. The ventilator will provide a mechanical breath if the patient fails to do so within the set interval.

synchronous /sing″krənəs/, occurring at the same time.

synclitism /sing″klitiz'əm/ [Gk, *syn + klinein,* to lean], **1.** (in obstetrics) a condition in which the sagittal suture of the fetal head is in line with the transverse diameter of the inlet, equidistant from the maternal symphysis pubis and sacrum. This position is usually found on examination either late in pregnancy or early in labor as the fetal head descends into the pelvic inlet. As labor progresses, posterior asynclitism develops, and, as the head descends farther, anterior asynclitism is evident because of the shape of the true pelvis below the inlet. **2.** (in hematology) the normal condition in which the nucleus and the cytoplasm of the blood cells mature simultaneously and at the same rate.

syncope /sing″kəpē/ [Gk, *synkoptein,* to cut short], a brief lapse in consciousness caused by transient cerebral hypoxia. It is usually preceded by a sensation of light-headedness and often may be prevented by lying down or by sitting with the head between the knees. It may be caused by many different factors, including emotional stress, vagal stimulation, vascular pooling in the legs, diaphoresis, and a sudden change in environmental temperature or body position. Also called **fainting.**

syncretic thinking /singkret″ik/ [Gk, *synkretismos,* combined beliefs; AS, *thencan,* to think], a stage in the development of the cognitive thought processes of the child during which thought is based purely on what is perceived and experienced. The child is incapable of reasoning beyond the observable or of making deductions or generalizations. Through imaginative play, questioning, interaction with others, and the increasing use of language and symbols to represent objects, the child begins to learn to make associations between ideas and to elaborate concepts. In Piaget's classification, this stage occurs between 2 and 7 years of age and is preceded by the sensorimotor stage of development, when the child progresses from reflex activity to repetitive and imitative behavior. Compare **abstract thinking, concrete thinking.**

syncytia. See **syncytium.**

syncytial /sinsish″əl/, pertaining to a syncytium.

syncytial-trophoblast. See **syncytiotrophoblast.**

syncytial virus, a virus that induces the formation of syncytia, particularly in cell cultures.

syncytiotrophoblast /sinsish′ē·ōtrof″əblast'/ [Gk, *syn + kytos,* cell, *trophe,* nutrition, *blastos,* germ], the outer syncytial layer of the trophoblast of an early mammalian embryo. It erodes the uterine wall during implantation and gives rise to the villi of the placenta. Also called **plasmidotrophoblast,** *syncytial trophoblast,* **syntrophoblast.** Compare **cytotrophoblast.** —*syncytiotrophoblastic, adj.*

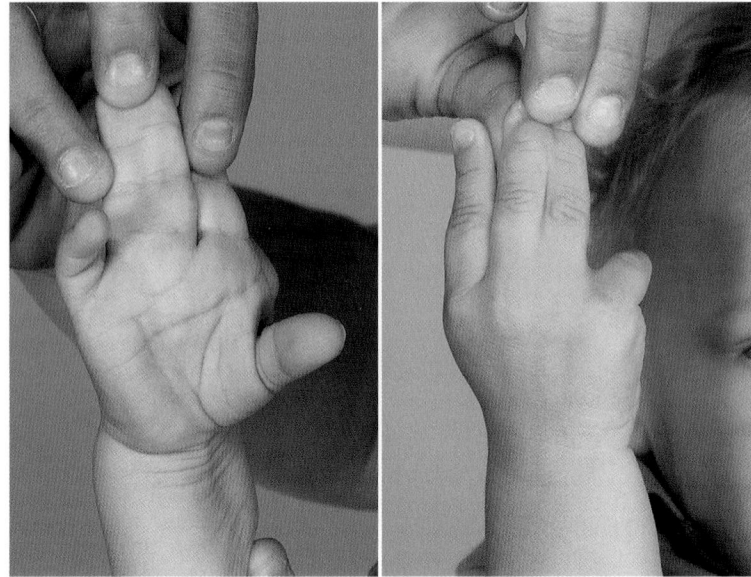

Mild syndactyly of the fingers *(Courtesy Dr. Joseph Imbriglia, Allegheny General Hospital)*

syncytium /sinsit″ē·əm/ [Gk, *syn* + *kytos,* cell], a group of cells in which the cytoplasm of one cell is continuous with that of adjoining cells, resulting in a multinucleate unit. −**syncytial,** *adj.*

syndactyl, syndactylia, syndactylism, syndactylous. See **syndactyly.**

syndactylus /sindak″tiləs/, a person with webbed fingers or toes.

syndactyly /sindak″təlē/ [Gk, *syn* + *daktylos,* finger], a congenital anomaly characterized by the fusion of the fingers or toes. It varies in degree of severity from incomplete webbing of the skin of two digits to complete union of digits and fusion of the bones and nails. Also called *syndactylia, syndactylism.* −*syndactyl, syndactylous, adj.*

syndelphus. See **synadelphus.**

syndesis /sin″dəsis/ [Gk, *syn,* together, *dein,* to bind], surgical fixation of a joint. Also called **arthrodesis.**

syndesmo-, combining form meaning "connective tissue, particularly the ligaments": *syndesmosis, syndesmophyte.*

syndesmophyte /sindez″məfīt/, a bony growth attached to a ligament. It is found between adjacent vertebrae in ankylosing spondylitis.

syndesmosis /sin′desmō″sis/ *pl. syndesmoses* [Gk, *syndesmos,* ligament], a fibrous union in which two bones are connected by interosseous ligaments, such as the anterior and the posterior ligaments in the radioulnar and tibiofibular articulations. Compare **gomphosis, sutura.**

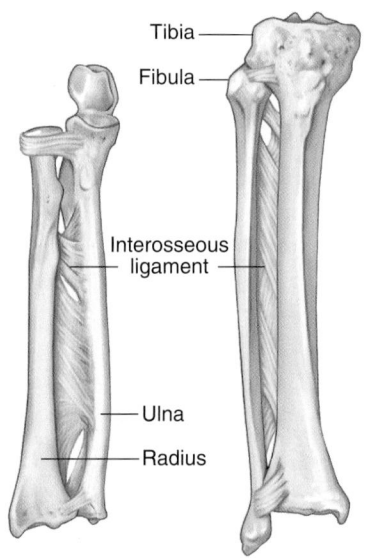

Tibia
Fibula
Interosseous ligament
Ulna
Radius

Syndesmosis *(Patton and Thibodeau, 2010)*

syndrome /sin″drəm/ [Gk, *syn*, together, *dromos*, course], a complex of signs and symptoms resulting from a common cause or appearing, in combination, to present a clinical picture of a disease or inherited abnormality. Also called **symptom complex.** See also *specific syndromes.*

syndrome of inappropriate antidiuretic hormone secretion (SIADH), an abnormal condition characterized by the excessive release of antidiuretic hormone (ADH), which alters the body's fluid and electrolytic balances. It results in various malfunctions, such as the inability to produce and secrete dilute urine, water retention, increased extracellular fluid volume, and hyponatremia. SIADH develops in association with diseases that affect the osmoreceptors of the hypothalamus. Oat cell carcinoma of the lung is the most common cause, affecting about 80% of involved patients. Other causes are disorders that affect the central nervous system, such as brain tumors and lupus erythematosus; pulmonary diseases, such as pneumonia; cancers of the pancreas and the prostate; and pathological reactions to various drugs, such as chlorpropamide, vincristine sulfate, carbamazepine, and clofibrate. Prognosis depends on the underlying disease, promptness of diagnosis and treatment, and the response to treatment.
■ OBSERVATIONS: Common signs and symptoms of SIADH are weight gain despite anorexia, vomiting, nausea, muscle weakness, and irritability. In some patients, SIADH may produce coma and convulsions. Most of the free water associated with this syndrome is intracellular, and associated edema is rare unless excess water volume exceeds 4 mOsm. Confirming diagnosis is based on urine osmolality that exceeds 150 mOsm/kg of water and serum osmolality of less than 280 mOsm/kg of water. Normal urine osmolality is 1.5 times serum osmolality. Other significant results include less-than-normal concentrations of blood urea nitrogen, serum creatinine, and albumin and a concentration of sodium in the urine higher than normal.
■ INTERVENTIONS: Treatment of SIADH commonly includes restriction of water intake and may require administration of normal saline solution to raise the serum sodium level if water intoxication is severe. Furosemide may be administered to block circulatory overload, and drugs, such as demeclocycline hydrochloride and lithium, may be administered to block renal response to ADH. Surgery and chemotherapy are other alternatives to remove or destroy neoplasms that may be the underlying causes of this syndrome.
■ PATIENT CARE CONSIDERATIONS: The SIADH patient is monitored for any signs of hyponatremia, weight change, and fluid imbalance. The patient is carefully advised on the importance of restricted water intake to prevent water intoxication and is closely observed for any indications of restlessness, congestive heart failure, and convulsions.

syndrome X, 1. a condition characterized by hypertension with obesity, type 2 diabetes mellitus, hypertriglyceridemia, increased peripheral insulin resistance, hyperinsulinemia, and elevated catecholamine levels. Formerly called **deadly quartet. 2.** angina pectoris with a normal coronary arteriogram. **3.** an extremely rare condition in which an individual does not age mentally or physically.

synechia /sinek″ē·ə/ *pl. synechiae* [Gk, continuity], an adhesion, especially of the iris to the cornea or lens of the eye. It may develop from glaucoma, cataracts, uveitis, or keratitis or as a complication of surgery or trauma to the eye. Synechiae may prevent or impede flow of aqueous fluid between the anterior and posterior chambers of the eye, resulting in angle-closure glaucoma.

synechiotomy /sinek′ē·ot″əmē/ [Gk, *synechia,* continuity, *temnein,* to cut], the surgical division of an adhesion.

syneresis /siner″əsis/ [Gk, *syn* + *hairein,* to draw], the drawing together or coagulation of particles of a gel with separation from the medium in which the particles were suspended, such as occurs in blood clot retraction.

synergic. See **synergistic.**

synergism. See **synergy.**

synergist /sin″ərjist/ [Gk, *syn* + *ergein,* to work], an organ, agent, or substance that augments the activity of another organ, agent, or substance.

synergistic /sin′ərjis″tik/ [Gk, *syn,* together, *ergein,* to work], pertaining to the acting or working together of a number of components, as when groups of muscles function in a coordinated manner. Also **synergic.**

synergistic agent, a substance that augments or adds to the activity of another substance or agent. See also **synergy,** def. 4.

synergistic muscles, groups of muscles that contract together to accomplish the same body movement.

synergy /sin″ərjē/ [Gk, *syn* + *ergein,* to work], **1.** the process in which two organs, substances, or agents work simultaneously to enhance the function and effect of one another. **2.** the coordinated action of a set of muscles that work together to produce a specific movement, as in a reflex action. **3.** a combined action of different parts of the autonomic nervous system, as in the sympathetic and parasympathetic innervation of secreting cells of the salivary glands, with both systems having a secretory effect. **4.** the interaction of two or more drugs to produce a certain effect, as in the exaggerated response to tyramine in a person who is treated with a monoamine oxidase inhibitor. Also called **synergism.**

synesthesia /sin′esthē″zhə/, a phenomenon in which sensations of two or more modalities accompany one another, as when a visual sensation is experienced when a particular sound is heard. Also called **secondary sensation.**

syngeneic /sin′jənē″ik/ [Gk, *syn* + *genesis,* origin], **1.** denoting an individual or cell that has the same genotype as another individual or cell. **2.** denoting tissues that are antigenically similar. Also called **isogeneic.** Compare **allogenic, xenogeneic.**

syngenesis. See **sexual reproduction.**

synkinesis /sin′kinē″sis/ [Gk, *syn,* together, *kinesis,* movement], an involuntary movement by one part of the body when an intentional movement is made by another part. In imitative synkinesis, movement may be detected in paralyzed muscles when normal muscles are moved, and vice versa.

synophthalmia. See **cyclopia.**

Synophylate GG, a bronchodilator. Brand name for *theophylline sodium glycinate.*

synopsis /sinop″sis/ [Gk, *syn,* together, *opsis,* vision], a brief review, condensation, summary, or abridgment.

synostosis /sin′ostō″sis/ [Gk, *syn,* together, *osteon,* bone], the joining of two bones by the ossification of connecting tissues. It occurs normally in the fusion of cranial bones to form the skull.

synostotic joint /sin′ostot″ik/ [Gk, *syn* + *osteon,* bone], a joint in which bones are connected to bones with no movement between them, as in the bones of the adult sacrum or skull.

synotia /sīnō″shə/ [Gk, *syn* + *ous,* ear], a congenital malformation characterized by the union or approximation of the ears in front of the neck, often accompanied by the absence or defective development of the lower jaw. Compare **agnathia.** See also **otocephaly.**

synotus /sīnō″təs/, a fetus with synotia.

synovectomy /sin′ōvek″təmē/ [Gk, *syn* + L, *ovum,* egg; Gk, *ektomē,* excision], the removal of a synovial membrane of a joint.

synovia /sinō″vē·ə/, a clear, viscous fluid resembling the white of an egg, secreted by synovial membranes and acting as a lubricant for many joints, bursae, and tendons. It contains mucin, albumin, fat, and mineral salts. Also called **synovial fluid.**

synovial /sinō″vē·əl/, pertaining to, consisting of, or secreting synovia, the lubricating fluid of the joints, bursae, and tendon sheaths.

synovial bursa, one of the many closed sacs filled with synovial fluid in the connective tissue between the muscles, the tendons, the ligaments, and the bones. The synovial bursae facilitate the gliding of muscles and tendons over bony and ligamentous prominences. Compare **synovial membrane, synovial tendon sheath.**

synovial chondroma, a rare cartilaginous growth in the connective tissue below the synovial membrane of the joints, tendon sheaths, or bursa. Foci on the surface may develop stalks and then detach, resulting in numerous loose bodies within the joint. Also called *synovial chondromatosis.*

synovial crypt, a pouch in the synovial membrane of a joint.

synovial fluid. See **synovia.**

synovial joint, a freely movable joint in which contiguous bony surfaces are covered by articular cartilage and connected by a fibrous connective tissue capsule lined with synovial membrane. Compare **cartilaginous joint, fibrous joint.** Kinds include **ball-and-socket joint, condyloid joint, gliding joint, hinge joint, pivot joint, saddle joint, uniaxial joint.**

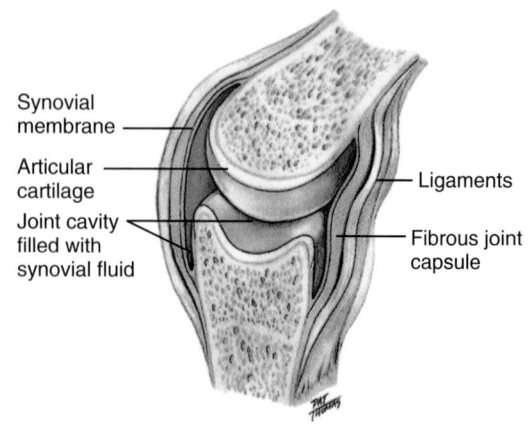

Synovial membrane

Articular cartilage

Joint cavity filled with synovial fluid

Ligaments

Fibrous joint capsule

Synovial joint *(Applegate, 2011)*

synovial membrane, the thin layer of tissue lining the articular capsule surrounding a freely movable joint. The synovial membrane is loosely attached to the external fibrous capsule. It secretes into the joint a thick fluid that normally lubricates the joint but that may accumulate in painful amounts when the joint is injured. Compare **synovial bursa, synovial tendon sheath.**

synovialoma /s-no″ve-ah-lo′mah/, a synovial tumor involving a tendon sheath or joint.

synovial sac, a herniation of a synovial membrane beyond the confines of a joint.

synovial sarcoma, a malignant tumor, composed of synovioblasts, that begins as a soft swelling and often metastasizes through the bloodstream to the lung before it is discovered.

synovial sheath, any one of the membranous sacs enclosing a tendon of a muscle and facilitating the gliding of a tendon through a fibrous or a bony tunnel, such as that under the flexor retinaculum of the wrist.

synovial tendon sheath, one of the many membranous channels or tubes enclosing various tendons that glide through fibrous and bony tunnels in the body, such as those under the flexor retinaculum of the wrist. One layer of the synovial sheath lines the tunnel, and the other covers the tendon. The sheath secretes synovial fluid, which lubricates the tendon. Compare **synovial bursa, synovial membrane.**

synovitis /sin′əvī″tis/, an inflammatory condition of the synovial membrane of a joint as the result of an aseptic wound or a traumatic injury, such as a sprain or severe strain. The knee is most commonly affected. Fluid accumulates around the capsule; the joint is swollen, tender, and painful; and motion is restricted. In most cases, the inflammation subsides and the fluid is resorbed without medical or surgical intervention.

synovium /sinō″vē·əm/, a synovial membrane.

synpolydactyly /sin-pol′e-dak″tile/. See **polysyndactyly.**

syntactic aphasia /sintak″tik/ [Gk, *syn,* together, *taxis,* arrangement, *a, phasis,* not speech], an inability to arrange words in a logical sequence, with the result that what is spoken is not understood.

syntax /sin″taks/ [Gk, *syn* + *taxis,* arrangement], word order; sentence order; a property of language involving structural cues for the arrangement of words as elements in a phrase, clause, or sentence.

syntaxic mode /sintaks″ik/, the ability to perceive whole, logical, coherent pictures as they occur in reality, according to the H.S. Sullivan theory of psychology.

synteny /sin″tənē/ [Gk, *syn* + *taina,* ribbon], (in genetics) the presence on the same chromosome of two or more genes that may or may not be transmitted as a linkage group but that appear to be able to undergo independent assortment during meiosis. The term is used primarily in human genetics, in which linked inheritance patterns are more difficult to determine. See also **linkage.**

synthermal /sinthur″məl/, possessing the same temperature.

synthesis /sin″thəsis/ [Gk, *synthenai,* to put together], a level of cognitive learning in which the individual puts together the elements of previous learning levels to create a unified whole.

-synthesis, combining form meaning "putting together" or "formation of": *psychosynthesis.*

synthesize /sin″thəsīz/ [Gk, *synthesis,* putting together], to form by building, as in the formation of complex chemical compounds such as proteins from simpler units of amino acids.

synthetic /sinthet″ik/, pertaining to a substance that is produced by an artificial rather than a natural process or material.

synthetic chemistry, the science dealing with the formation of more complex chemical compounds from simpler substances.

synthetic human growth hormone, a synthetic form of somatotropin produced by recombinant deoxyribonucleic acid techniques from a strain of *Escherichia coli* bacteria. The polypeptide hormone consists of 191 amino acid residues in a sequence identical to that of natural human growth hormone.

synthetic insulin [Gk, *synthesis,* putting together; L, *insula,* island], a form of insulin synthesized in a non–disease-producing strain of *Escherichia coli* bacteria or in yeast cells that have been genetically altered by the addition of the human gene for insulin production.

synthetic oleovitamin D. See **viosterol.**

synthetic saliva. See **artificial saliva.**

synthetic vaccines, prophylactic immunization substances prepared by artificial techniques, such as by peptide synthesis or cloning of deoxyribonucleic acid.

Synthroid, a thyroid hormone. Brand name for **levothy-roxine sodium.**

Syntocinon, an oxytocic. Brand name for **oxytocin.**

syntrophism /sin″trəfiz′əm/, **1.** mutual dependence for food or other resources. **2.** a condition in which two strains of bacteria can grow together in a mixed culture in a medium that would not support either alone. Each strain produces a nutrient required by the other.

syntrophoblast. See **syncytiotrophoblast.**

syntropy /sin″trəpē/ [Gk, *syn,* together, *trepein,* to turn], a tendency for two diseases to merge into one.

syphilis /sif″ilis/ [from the name of a literary figure (1530) who was thus infected (literally, L, lover of swine)], a sexually transmitted disease caused by the spirochete *Treponema pallidum,* characterized by distinct stages of effects over a period of years. Any organ system may become involved. The spirochete is able to pass through the human placenta, producing congenital syphilis. Also called **lues.** See also **chancre, gumma, Hutchinson teeth, Hutchinson triad, snuffles. −syphilitic,** *adj.*

■ OBSERVATIONS: The first stage (primary syphilis) is marked by the appearance of a small, painless red pustule on the skin or mucous membrane between 10 and 90 days after exposure. The lesion may appear anywhere on the body where contact with a lesion on an infected person has occurred, but it is seen most often in the anogenital region. It quickly erodes, forming a painless, bloodless ulcer, called a *chancre,* exuding a fluid that swarms with spirochetes. The chancre may not be noticed by the patient, and many people may become infected. It heals spontaneously within 10 to 40 days, often creating the mistaken impression that it was not a serious symptom. The second stage (secondary syphilis) occurs about 2 months later, after the spirochetes have increased in number and spread throughout the body. This stage is characterized by general malaise; anorexia; nausea; fever; headache; alopecia; bone and joint pain; and the appearance of a morbilliform rash that does not itch, flat white sores in the mouth and throat, or condylomata lata papules on the moist areas of the skin. The disease remains highly contagious at this stage and can be spread by kissing. The symptoms usually continue from 3 weeks to 3 months but may recur over a period of 2 years. The third stage (tertiary syphilis) may not develop for 3 to 15 or more years. It is characterized by the appearance of soft, rubbery tumors, called *gummas,* that ulcerate and heal by scarring. Gummas may develop anywhere on the surface of the body and in the eye, liver, lungs, stomach, or reproductive organs. Tertiary syphilis may be painless, unnoticed except for gummas, or it may be accompanied by deep, burrowing pain. The ulceration of the gummas may result in punched-out areas of the palate, nasal septum, or larynx. Various tissues and structures of the body, including the central nervous system, myocardium, and valves of the heart, may be damaged or destroyed, leading to mental or physical disability and premature death. Congenital syphilis resulting from prenatal infection may result in the birth of a deformed or blind infant or stillborn child. In some cases, the infant appears to be well until, at several weeks of age, snuffles, sometimes with a blood-stained or mucopurulent discharge, and skin lesions, particularly on the palms and soles or in the genital region, are observed. Such children also may have visual or hearing defects, and progeria and poor health may develop. Diagnosis of syphilis is made by darkfield microscopy of fluid from primary or secondary stage lesions, by bacteriological study of blood samples, and by an examination of cerebrospinal fluid. Because of the slow development of the disease during the early stages, the various serological tests, including the obsolete Wassermann, may not produce accurate findings until months after exposure. Repeated tests and cross-checking with more than one test may be required in some cases. The report by a person that exposure to syphilis has occurred is often the only evidence available to the clinician.

■ INTERVENTIONS: Patients with primary or secondary syphilis are usually given benzathine, penicillin G benzathine, or an equivalent in a single dose of 2.4 million units intramuscularly. The objective is to maintain penicillin in the bloodstream for a number of days because *Treponema pallidum* divides at an average rate of once every 33 hours, and the antibiotic is most effective during the stage of cell division. Larger doses of penicillin, 7.2 million units total, are administered in 3 doses 1 week apart for tertiary syphilis. Infants and small children with congenital syphilis are usually given 50,000 units/kg intramuscularly. Treatment of an infected mother with penicillin during the first 4 months of pregnancy usually prevents the development of congenital syphilis in the fetus. Treating the mother with antibiotics later in the pregnancy usually eliminates the infection but may not protect the fetus. Patients should be reexamined clinically and serologically 3 months and 6 months after treatment. Human immunodeficiency virus–infected patients (also infected with syphilis) should be seen at 1, 2, 3, 6, 9, and 12 months for follow-up observation.

■ PATIENT CARE CONSIDERATIONS: Special care and aseptic precautions are taken while handling the highly contagious fluid from syphilitic lesions used in diagnostic testing because the infection may be acquired through a cut or break in the skin. The nurse discusses with the patient the disease course, its treatment, and ways of preventing future infections. The extremely contagious nature of the infection is explained, and the importance of treatment for all who may have been exposed is emphasized. Tact, patience, and understanding are required to reassure the patient and to secure the patient's cooperation in accepting treatment and in assisting in the identification and location of others needing treatment. Active, serologically documented cases of syphilis must, by law, be reported to local departments of health throughout the United States.

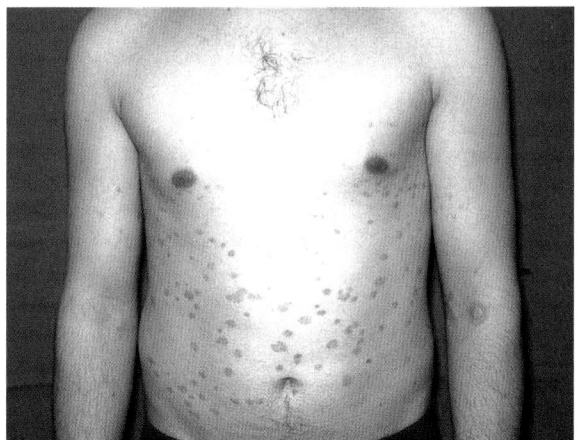

Rash in secondary syphilis *(Sukthankar, 2010)*

syphilitic, pertaining to, resembling, or infected with syphilis. Also **luetic.**

syphilitic aortitis, inflammation of the aorta occurring in tertiary syphilis. It is characterized by diffuse dilation with gray, wheal-like plaques containing calcium on the inside and scars and wrinkles on the outside of the aorta. The middle layer of the aortic wall is usually infiltrated with plasma cells and contains fragments of damaged elastic tissue and many newly formed blood vessels. There may be damage to the cardiac valves, narrowing of the mouths of the coronary arteries, and formation of thrombi. Cerebral embolism may result. Signs of syphilitic aortitis are substernal pain, dyspnea, bounding pulse, and high systolic blood pressure. Penicillin may slow the course of the disease, but it cannot reverse the structural damage to the vessels and the heart. Also called **Döhle-Heller disease, luetic aortitis.**

syphilitic dementia [L, *de* + *mens,* mind], a form of dementia resulting from a syphilis infection. Specific symptoms may vary from memory impairment to personality changes and are severe enough to interfere with social and occupational activities. If untreated, the disease may progress to dementia paralytica, paralysis, and death.

syphilitic endocarditis [L, *endon,* within, *kardia,* heart, *itis,* inflammation], a thickening and stretching of the cusps of the aortic valve, with aortic valve incompetence, caused by a syphilis infection of the aorta.

syphilitic fever [L, *febris*], pyrexia that is caused by a syphilis infection.

syphilitic heart disease. See **cardiovascular disease.**

syphilitic meningoencephalitis. See **general paresis.**

syphilitic periarteritis, an inflammatory condition of the outer coat of one or more arteries occurring in tertiary syphilis and characterized by soft gummatous perivascular lesions infiltrated with lymphocytes and plasma cells. Also called **periarteritis gummosa.** See also **syphilitic aortitis.**

syphilitic retinopathy [L, *rete,* net; Gk, *pathos,* disease], an invasion of the retina and optic nerve by a spreading syphilis infection. Primary retinal lesions are associated with the blood vessels, and the choroid layer is often affected first. There may be occlusion of the retinal vessels.

syphilographer, *n.,* an individual who studies and publishes content related to syphilis.

syr, a notation for a Latin word meaning "syrup." Abbreviation for *syrupus.*

syring-. See **syringo-, syring-.**

syringe /sərinj′, sir″inj/ [Gk, *syrinx,* tube], a device for withdrawing, injecting, or instilling fluids. A syringe for the injection of medication usually consists of a calibrated glass or plastic cylindric barrel with a close-fitting plunger at one end and a small opening at the other to which the head of a hollow-bore needle is fitted. Medication of the desired amount may be pulled up into the barrel by suction as the plunger is withdrawn and injected by pushing the plunger back into the barrel, forcing the liquid out through the needle. A syringe for irrigating a wound or body cavity or for extracting mucus or another body fluid from an orifice or body cavity is usually larger than the kind used for injection. It often has a rubber bulb at one end and a blunt, soft-tipped flexible tube with an opening at the other end. The bulb is squeezed to eject a fluid and is released to withdraw one. Kinds include **Asepto syringe, bulb syringe, hypodermic syringe, Luer-Lok syringe.**

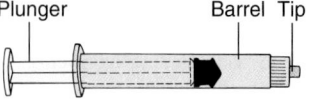
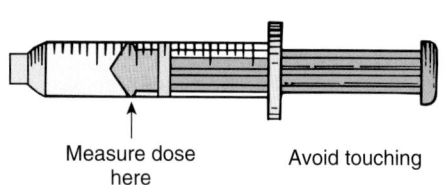

Plunger   Barrel Tip

Measure dose here   Avoid touching

Parts of a syringe *(Potter et al, 2011)*

syringectomy /sir′injek″təmē/ [Gk, *syrinx,* tube, *ektomē,* excision], a surgical procedure for excising the walls of a fistula.

syringo-, syring-, combining form meaning "tube" or "fistula": *syringobulbia, syringoma, syringomyelia.*

syringobulbia /si·ring′gō·bul′bē·ə/ [Gk, *syrinx,* tube; L, *bulbus,* swollen root], syringomyelia in which the cavity extends to involve the medulla oblongata. See also **syringomyelia.**

syringoencephalomyelia /siring′gō·ensef′əlō′mī·ē″lyə/, a progressive disorder characterized by cavitation of the spinal cord. It may occur anywhere from the medulla oblongata to the thoracic segments but usually appears in cervical segments.

syringoma /sir′ing·gō″mə/ *pl.* syringomas, syringomata, a benign tumor derived from an eccrine sweat gland. It appears as a small, smooth papule the color of the underlying skin, often on the upper body of a postpubertal woman. Some are typically multiple, often appearing on the lower eyelids.

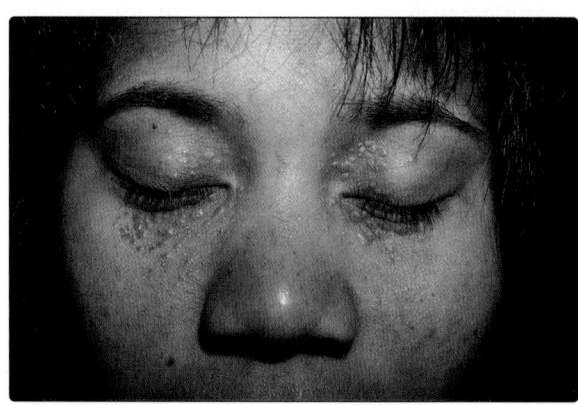

Syringoma *(James and Berger, 2011)*

syringomeningocele /-məning″gōsēl′/ [Gk, *syrinx,* tube, *meninx,* membrane, *kele,* hernia], a meningocele that is connected to the central canal of the spinal cord. See also **spina bifida.**

syringomyelia /-mī·ē″lyə/ [Gk, *syrinx,* tube, *myelos,* marrow], a chronic progressive disease of the spinal cord, marked by elongated central fluid-containing cavities surrounded by gliosis or a proliferation of neurological tissue. Symptoms begin early in adulthood, usually involving the cervical region, with muscular wasting in the upper limbs. The disease is more common in males.

■ OBSERVATIONS: Although present at birth, onset is insidious, and manifestations are often not seen until individuals are in their 20s or 30s. These symptoms are often ambiguous and mimic a host of other diseases. The cervical spine is most commonly affected and manifests as weakness, atrophy, and sensory loss in the shoulders, arms, and hands, including loss of pain and temperature sensation and sweating on the face. Upper extremity reflexes are diminished or absent, whereas weakness, altered gait, spasticity, and hyperreflexia may be noted in the lower extremities. Brainstem involvement may cause dysphagia, ptosis, miosis, or diplopia. GI symptoms include nausea, vomiting, weight loss, and abdominal spasms. Respiratory disturbances may manifest during sleep. Joint arthropathy and trophic skin changes may eventually develop. The course of the disease is variable and may result in slow, long-term incapacitation. Disease progress may slow or stop at any time. Diagnosis is made through MRI. Bony abnormalities at the base of the skull and C1-2 spine and scoliosis may be seen on x-ray.

■ INTERVENTIONS: The primary intervention is a cervical decompression laminectomy at C1-2 spine with repair or removal of bony abnormalities, with possible myelotomy or shunt placement. Although surgical intervention halts disease progression, it seldom leads to significant improvement in current neurological manifestations.

■ PATIENT CARE CONSIDERATIONS: Nursing care after surgery is aimed at careful positioning and turning to maintain proper alignment of the cervical spine and head; control of postoperative pain; surgical wound care; monitoring for CSF leakage and peripheral vital signs; assessment of motor and sensory function in the extremities and bowel and bladder function. Chronic care focuses on rehabilitation for the sequelae from neurological damage that occurred before the surgery. These are varied and may include bowel and bladder programs for management of neurogenic bowel or bladder; protection against injury and breakdown of skin related to decreased sensation; physical therapy to build strength and endurance; occupational therapy to improve or adapt functioning; respiratory therapy to increase vital capacity and tidal volume; and speech therapy if swallowing is affected. Counseling and support services are provided for the individual and family to aid in adaptation.

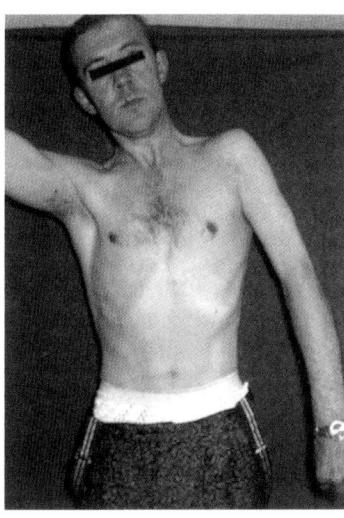

Individual with syringomyelia (Moll, 1997)

syringomyelocele /siring′gōmī″əlōsēl′/ [Gk, *syrinx* + *myelos,* marrow, *kele,* hernia], a hernial protrusion of the spinal cord through a congenital defect in the vertebral column. The cerebrospinal fluid within the central cavities of the cord is greatly increased so that the cord tissue forms a thin-walled sac that lies close to the membrane of the cavity. See also **myelomeningocele, neural tube defect, spina bifida.**

syrup of ipecac /sir″əp/, an emetic preparation of ipecac fluid extract, glycerin, and syrup used to treat certain types of poisonings and drug overdoses. It is no longer routinely used. See also **ipecac.**

system /sis″təm/ [Gk, *systema*], **1.** a collection or assemblage of parts that, unified, make a whole. Physiological systems, such as the cardiovascular or reproductive system, are made up of structures specifically able to engage in processes that are essential for a vital function in the body. **2.** a set of computer programs and hardware that work together for some specific purpose.

systematic /sis′təmat″ik/ [Gk, *systema*], pertaining to a system.

systematic error [Gk, *systema* + L, *errare,* to wander], a nonrandom statistical error that affects the mean of a population of data and defines the bias between the means of two populations.

systematic reviews, a scientific investigation that asks a specific question and uses explicit, rigorous, prespecified methods to identify, critically appraise, select, and summarize findings of similar but separate studies. Systematic reviews are the cornerstone of evidence-based health-care decision making.

systematic tabulation, (in research) mechanical or manual techniques for recording and classifying data for statistical analysis.

system documentation. See **documentation.**

systemic /sistem″ik/ [Gk, *systema*], pertaining to the whole body rather than to a localized area or regional part of the body.

systemic circulation [Gk, *systema* + L, *circulare,* to go around], the general blood circulation of the body, not including the lungs. Also called **greater circulation.**

systemic desensitization, a technique used in behavior therapy for eliminating maladaptive anxiety associated with phobias. The procedure involves the construction by the person of a hierarchy of anxiety-producing stimuli and the general presentation of these stimuli until they no longer elicit the initial response of fear. Also called **desensitization.** Compare **flooding.** See also **reciprocal inhibition.**

systemic hypertension. See **cardiovascular disease.**

systemic immunoblastic proliferation, a condition of immature lymphocyte production resulting in rash, breathing difficulty, enlarged spleen, lymphadenopathy, and increased incidence of immunoblastic lymphoma.

systemic infection [Gk, *systema* + L, *inficere,* to stain], an infection in which the pathogen is distributed throughout the body rather than concentrated in one area.

systemic inflammatory response syndrome (SIRS), the clinical response to infection or trauma that includes two or more of the following symptoms: fever greater than 38° C (100.4° F) or less than 36° C (96.8° F); heart rate >90 beats per minute; respiratory rate >20 breaths per minute or arterial carbon dioxide tension ($PaCO_2$) of less than 32 mm Hg; abnormal white blood cell count (>12,000/μL or <4000/μL or >10% immature [band] forms). Treatment focuses on the underlying cause.

systemic lesion [Gk, *systema* + L, *laesio,* attack], a pathological disturbance that involves a system of tissues with a common function.

systemic lupus erythematosus (SLE), a chronic inflammatory disease affecting many systems of the body. It is an example of an autoimmune connective-tissue disorder. The pathophysiological characteristics of the disease include severe vasculitis, renal involvement, and lesions of the skin and nervous system. The primary cause of the disease has not been determined; viral infection or dysfunction of the immune system has been suggested. Adverse reaction to certain drugs also may cause a lupuslike syndrome. Four times more women than men have SLE. Also called *disseminated lupus erythematosus.* See also **discoid lupus erythematosus.**
■ OBSERVATIONS: The initial manifestation is often arthritis. An erythematous rash ("butterfly rash") over the nose and malar eminences, weakness, fatigue, and weight loss also are frequently seen early in the disease. Photosensitivity, fever, skin lesions on the neck, and alopecia where the skin lesions extend beyond the hairline may occur. The skin lesions may spread to the mucous membranes and other tissues of the body. They do not ulcerate but cause degeneration of the affected tissues. Depending on the organs involved, the patient also may have glomerulonephritis, pleuritis, pericarditis, peritonitis, neuritis, or anemia. Renal failure and severe neurological abnormalities are among the most serious manifestations of the disease. Diagnosis of SLE is made by subjective and objective findings based on physical examination and laboratory findings, including antinuclear antibody in the cerebrospinal fluid and a positive lupus erythematosus cell reaction in a lupus erythematosus preparation. Other laboratory examinations may be useful, depending on the organs, tissues, and systems affected by the disease.
■ INTERVENTIONS: In many cases SLE may be controlled with corticosteroid medication administered systemically. Care and treatment vary with the severity and nature of the disease and the body systems that are affected. Topical steroids may be applied to the rash. Salicylates may be given to alleviate pain and swelling in the joints. Fatigue and stress are prevented, and all body surfaces are protected from direct sunlight. Antimalarial drugs are sometimes given to treat cutaneous lesions, but retinal damage may occur with prolonged use.
■ PATIENT CARE CONSIDERATIONS: The timing, dosage, side effects, and toxic reactions to the medications are explained before discharge. The steroids must be taken exactly as prescribed, and, in the event that the patient cannot take them, the doctor is to be consulted promptly. The patient should carry an identification card bearing his or her diagnosis, a list of all medications and their dosage, and the doctor's name and telephone number. As in any disease marked by chronic remission and exacerbation of many distressing symptoms, the patient may require extensive emotional and psychological support.

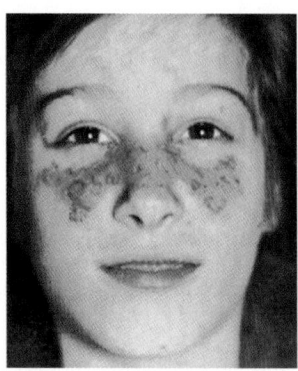

Classic butterfly rash of systemic lupus erythematosus
(Courtesy Department of Dermatology, University of North Carolina at Chapel Hill)

systemic mycosis [Gks, *systema* + *mykes,* fungus, *osis,* condition], a fungal infection that involves more than one body system or area.
systemic oxygen consumption, the amount of oxygen consumed by the body per minute.
systemic remedy, a medicinal substance that is given orally, parenterally, or rectally to be absorbed into the circulation for treatment of a health problem. Many remedies or medications administered locally or regionally are to some degree absorbed systemically. Medication administered systemically may have various local effects, but the intent is to treat the whole body.
systemic sclerosis, a form of scleroderma characterized by formation of thickened collagenous fibrous tissue, thickening of the skin, and adhesion of the skin to underlying tissues. The disease, which may be preceded by Raynaud phenomenon, progresses to involve the tissues of the heart, lungs, muscles, genitourinary tract, and kidneys. See also **scleroderma.**
systemic vascular resistance (SVR), the resistance the left ventricle must overcome to pump blood through the systemic circulation. As peripheral blood vessels constrict, the SVR increases.
systemic vein, one of a number of veins that drain deoxygenated blood from most of the body, as opposed to the pulmonary circulation. Systemic veins arise in tiny plexuses that receive blood from capillaries and converge into trunks that increase in size as they pass toward the heart. They are larger and more numerous than the arteries, have thinner walls, and collapse when they are empty. Groups of systemic veins include the coronary veins, the superior vena cava and its tributaries in the upper body, and the inferior vena cava and its tributaries in the lower body.
systemic venous hypertension, elevation of the venous pressure, usually detected by inspection of the jugular veins and most often caused by disease of the right heart or pericardium.
system of care /sis″təm/, a framework within which health care is provided, comprising health care professionals; recipients, consumers, or patients; energy resources or dynamics; organizational and political contexts or frameworks; and processes or procedures. Current theory recognizes that an analysis of the provision of health care requires knowledge of the systems of care.
system overload, an inability to cope with messages and expectations from a number of sources within a given time limit.
systems integration, the unification of disparate computer hardware and software to achieve usability and transferability of data, such as throughout a managed care or provider network.
systems software, a group of computer utility programs that control the execution of application programs.
systems theory, a holistic medical concept in which the human patient is viewed as an integrated complex of open systems rather than as semiindependent parts. The health care approach in this theory requires the incorporation of family, community, and cultural factors as influences to be considered in the diagnosis and treatment of the patient.
systole /sis″təlē/ [Gk, *systole,* contraction], the contraction of the heart, driving blood into the aorta and pulmonary arteries. The occurrence of systole is indicated by the first heart sound heard on auscultation, by the palpable apex beat, and by the peripheral pulse. −**systolic,** *adj.*

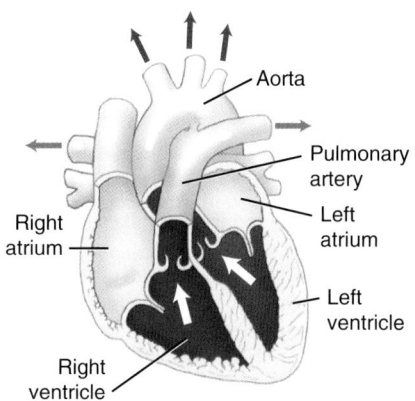

- Aorta
- Pulmonary artery
- Right atrium
- Left atrium
- Left ventricle
- Right ventricle

During systole, the heart contracts and blood is pushed out of the heart *(Leonard, 2008)*

-systole, combining form meaning "types and locations of the higher blood pressure measurement": *extrasystole, hypersystole, parasystole.*

systolic. See **systole.**

systolic click [Gk, *systole,* contraction; Fr, *cliqueter,* to click], a sharp, clicking sound heard in mid- or late systole and believed to originate from the abnormal motion of the mitral valve. The most frequent cause of systolic clicks is prolapse of a mitral valve leaflet, in which case there may be an associated late systolic regurgitant murmur, sometimes called the *click-murmur syndrome.*

systolic click-murmur syndrome. See **Barlow syndrome.**

systolic dysfunction, a loss of cardiac muscle with volume overload and decreased contractility.

systolic ejection period, the amount of time the ventricles spend in systole per minute.

systolic gradient, the difference between the pressure in the left atrium and that in the left ventricle during systole.

systolic murmur, a cardiac murmur occurring during systole. Systolic murmurs include ejection murmurs, often heard in pregnant women or in people with anemia, thyrotoxicosis, or aortic or pulmonary stenosis; pansystolic murmurs, heard in people with incompetence of the mitral or tricuspid valve; and late systolic murmurs, also caused by mitral valve incompetence and, less commonly, by tricuspid regurgitation.

systolic pressure, the blood pressure measured during the period of ventricular contraction (systole). In blood pressure readings, it is the higher of the two measurements.

S

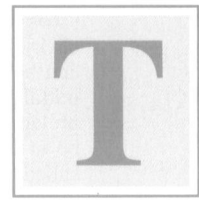

T, abbreviation for **absolute (A) temperature.**

t, symbol for **time.**

T, **1.** symbol for **temperature. 2.** abbreviation for **tumor. 3.** symbol for **occupancy factor.**

T$_{1/2}$, symbol for **radioactive half-life.**

T1, T2, …, symbol for **thoracic nerves.**

T$_1$, T$_2$, See **relaxation time.**

T$_3$, symbol for **triiodothyronine.**

T$_4$, symbol for **thyroxine.**

ta-. See **tono-.**

Ta, symbol for the element **tantalum.**

tabardillo. See **Mexican typhus.**

tabe-, combining form meaning "wasting (away)": *tabes, tabetic crisis, tabes dorsalis.*

tabes /tā′bēz/ [L, *tabes,* wasting], a gradual, progressive wasting of the body in any chronic disease.

tabes dorsalis [L, *tabes,* wasting, *dorsum,* the back], an abnormal condition caused by syphilis. It is characterized by the slow degeneration of all or part of the body and the progressive loss of deep tendon reflexes. This disease involves the posterior columns and posterior roots of the spinal cord and destroys the large joints of affected limbs in some individuals. A wide-base ataxic gait is usually present. It is often accompanied by incontinence and impotence and severe flashing pains in the abdomen and extremities. See also **tabetic gait.**

tabetic crisis /təbet′ik/ [L, *tabes,* wasting; Gk, *krisis,* turning point], an exacerbation of pain in tabes dorsalis because of syphilis.

tabetic gait [L, *tabes,* wasting; ONorse, *gata,* a way], a high-stepping gait caused by degeneration of the spinal cord and sensory nerve trunks, associated with tabes dorsalis. See also **tabes dorsalis.**

tabetic neuritis [L, *tabes,* wasting; Gk, *neuron,* nerve, *itis,* inflammation], a form of neuritis that accompanies a syphilitic infection or tabes dorsalis and involves the dorsal posterior column spinal pathways. See also **syphilis.**

table [L, *tabula*], **1.** any structure with a flat surface. **2.** a chart showing columns of data.

tablet /tab′lit/ [Fr, *tablette,* lozenge], a small, solid dosage form of a medication. It may be compressed or molded in its manufacture, and it may be of almost any size, shape, weight, and color. Most tablets are intended to be swallowed whole.

taboo /təbōō′/, something that is forbidden by a society as unacceptable or improper. Incest is a taboo common to many societies.

taboparesis /tā′bōpərē″sis/ [L, *tabes,* wasting; Gk, *paralyein,* to be palsied], a form of paralysis associated with psychosis in patients with untreated syphilis in the tertiary stage. Also called *taboparalysis.* See also **paresis,** def. 2, **neurosyphilis.**

tabula rasa /tā″bōōlä rä′sä, tab″yəle rä′sə/, a term used to describe a child's mind at birth as a receptive "blank slate."

tache /täsh/ [Fr], a spot, stain, blot, or mark.

tache laiteuse. See **macula albida.**

tache noire /täsh nô·är″/ [Fr, black spot], a local buttonlike ulcer with a black center that marks the point of infection in certain rickettsial diseases such as African tick typhus and scrub typhus.

tachistoscope /təkis″təskōp′/ [Gk, *tachistos,* rapid, *skopein,* to view], a device used to increase the speed of visual perception by displaying visual stimuli only extremely briefly.

tacho-, combining form meaning "swift" or "rapid": *tachometer.*

tachometer /təkom″ətər/, a device for measuring rotational speed.

tachy- /tak′ē-/, combining form meaning "swift" or "rapid": *tachycardia, tachyphagia, tachypnea.*

tachyarrhythmia /tak′ē·ərith″mē·ə/ [Gk, *tachys,* fast, *a + rhythmos,* rhythm], an abnormally rapid heartbeat accompanied by an irregular rhythm.

tachycardia /tak′ēkär′dē·ə/ [Gk, *tachys,* fast, *kardia,* heart], a condition in which the heart contracts at a rate greater than 100 beats/min. It may occur normally in response to fever, exercise, or nervous excitement. Pathological tachycardia accompanies anoxia, such as that caused by anemia; congestive heart failure; hemorrhage; or shock. Tachycardia acts to increase the amount of oxygen delivered to the cells of the body by increasing the rate at which blood circulates through the vessels. Compare **bradycardia.**

tachycardia-bradycardia syndrome. See **bradycardia-tachycardia syndrome.**

tachycardiac /-kär′dē·ak/ [Gk, *tachys,* fast, *kardia,* heart], pertaining to or affected by tachycardia.

tachykinin. See **substance P.**

tachyphagia /-fā″jē·ə/, rapid or hasty eating.

tachyphylaxis /tak′ēfəlak″sis/ [Gk, *tachys + phylax,* guard], **1.** (in pharmacology) a phenomenon in which the repeated administration of some drugs results in a rapidly appearing and marked decrease in effectiveness. **2.** (in immunology) a rapidly developing immunity to a toxin because of previous exposure, such as from previous injection of small amounts of the toxin. Also called **mithridatism.**

tachypnea /tak′ēpnē″ə/ [Gk, *tachys + pnoia,* breathing], an abnormally rapid rate of breathing (more than 20 breaths per minute in adults), such as seen with hyperpyrexia. Also spelled *tachypnoea.*

tack, the degree of stickiness of an adhesive required to affix a therapeutic foreign substance such as a transdermal delivery device to the skin.

tacrolimus, an immunosuppressive drug that modifies biological response.

■ INDICATIONS: This drug is prescribed to suppress the immune system after transplantation of the liver or other organs and can be applied topically for the treatment of dermatitis unresponsive to other medications.

■ CONTRAINDICATIONS: This drug should not be given to patients with allergy to tacrolimus or those receiving potassium-sparing diuretics, cycloSPORINE, or other immunosuppressive agents, with the exception of adrenal corticosteroids.

■ ADVERSE EFFECTS: The side effects most often reported include tremor, headache, diarrhea, hypertension, nausea, renal dysfunction, hyperglycemia, and increased risk of infection.

TAC solution, a solution of tetracaine, epinephrine, and cocaine, used as a local anesthetic in the emergency treatment of uncomplicated lacerations.

tact-, combining form meaning "touch": *tactile, tactile amnesia.*

-tactic, -tactical, -taxic, **1.** combining form meaning "exhibiting agent-controlled orientation or movement": *chemotactic, cytobiotactic, cytobiotaxis.* **2.** combining form meaning "having an arrangement of something": *stereotactic surgery.*

tactile /tak″təl/ [L, *tactus,* touch], pertaining to the sense of touch.

tactile amnesia [L, *tactus* + Gk, *amnesia,* forgetfulness], a loss of the ability to determine the shape of objects through the sense of touch. See also **astereognosis.**

tactile anesthesia, the absence or lack of the sense of touch in the fingers, possibly resulting from injury or disease. This condition can be congenital or psychosomatic and may cause the patient to incur severe burns, serious cuts, contusions, or abrasions. See also **traumatic anesthesia.**

tactile corpuscle. See **Meissner corpuscle.**

tactile defensiveness, a sensory integrative dysfunction characterized by tactile sensations that cause excessive emotional reactions, hyperactivity, or other behavior problems.

tactile discrimination [L, *tactus* + *discrimen,* division], the ability to discriminate among objects by the sense of touch.

tactile fremitus, a tremulous vibration of the chest wall during speaking that is palpable on physical examination. Tactile fremitus may be decreased or absent when vibrations from the larynx to the chest surface are impeded by chronic obstructive pulmonary disease, obstruction, pleural effusion, or pneumothorax. It is increased in pneumonia. Compare **vocal fremitus.**

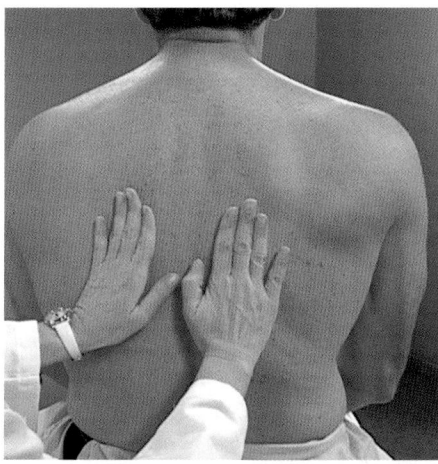
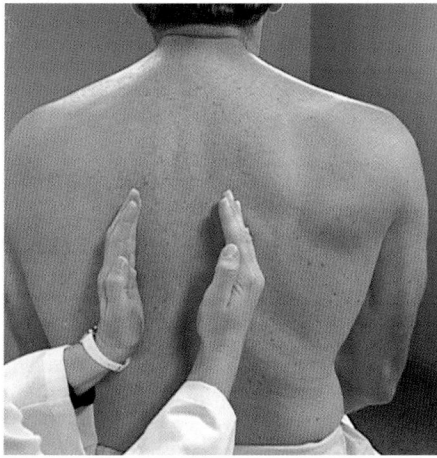

Evaluation of tactile fremitus *(Seidel et al, 2011)*

tactile hair [L, *tactus* + AS, *haer*], a hair shaft that is sensitive to the sensation of touch.

tactile hallucination [L, *tactus* + *alucinare,* to wander in mind], a subjective experience of touch in the absence of tactile stimulation. It is most common in delirium tremens or alcoholic hallucinosis.

tactile hyperesthesia [L, *tactus* + Gk, *hyper,* excessive, *aesthesis,* sensitivity], an abnormal increase in the sense of touch.

tactile image, a mental concept of an object as perceived through the sense of touch. See also **image.**

tactile localization [L, *tactus* + *locus,* place], the ability to identify, without looking, the exact point on the body where a tactile stimulus is applied. The localization test is applied in sensory evaluation tests.

tactile sensation [L, *tactus* + *sentire,* to feel], the sensation of touch.

tactile system [L, *tactus* + Gk, *systema*], the part of the nervous system that is concerned with the sense of touch.

tadalafil, an impotence agent.

■ INDICATIONS: This drug is used in the treatment of erectile dysfunction.

■ CONTRAINDICATIONS: Known hypersensitivity to this drug prohibits its use. Patients who are taking organic nitrates either regularly or intermittently and patients taking any alpha-adrenergic antagonist other than tamsulosin (0.4 mg once daily) should not take this drug.

■ ADVERSE EFFECTS: Adverse effects of this drug include back pain or myalgia, blurred vision, changes in color vision, and pruritus. Life-threatening side effects include myocardial infarction, cardiovascular collapse, and sudden death. Common side effects include headache, flushing, dizziness, dyspepsia, nasal congestion, urinary tract infection, and diarrhea.

Taenia /tē″nē·ə/ [Gk, *tainia,* ribbon], a genus of large parasitic intestinal flatworms of the family Taeniidae, class Cestoda, having an armed scolex and a series of segments in a chain. Taeniae are among the most common parasites infecting humans and include *T. saginata,* the beef tapeworm, and *T. solium,* the pork tapeworm.

taenia-. See **tenia-, taenia-.**

Taenia saginata, a species of tapeworm that inhabits the tissues of cattle during its larval stage and infects the intestine of humans in its adult form. *T. saginata* may grow to a length of between 12 and 25 feet and is the tapeworm species that most often infects humans. Also called **beef tapeworm.** See also **tapeworm, tapeworm infection.**

taeniasis /tēnī″əsis/ [Gk, *tainia* + *osis,* condition], an infection with a tapeworm of the genus *Taenia.* Transmission is through ingestion of undercooked pork containing cysticercus or food contaminated with pig feces containing eggs. See also **tapeworm infection.**

Taenia solium, a species of tapeworm that most commonly inhabits the tissues of pigs during its larval stage and infects the intestine of humans in its adult form. Infrequently humans serve as the intermediate hosts for this tapeworm, and larval infestation of the muscle and brain tissue may occur. Also called **pork tapeworm.** See also **cysticercosis, tapeworm, tapeworm infection.**

TAF, abbreviation for **tumor angiogenesis factor.**

tag, a small piece of epidermal and dermal fibrovascular tissue attached by one margin or a pedicle to a main structure.

Tagamet, a histamine H_2 receptor antagonist medication. Brand name for **cimetidine.**

tai chi, a technique that uses slow, purposeful, motor-physical movements of the body for the purpose of control to increase outer body mass strength and achieve a more

T

balanced physiological and psychological state. Tai chi has positive effects on the respiratory, cardiovascular, and cerebral functions in both children and older adults, including reducing the incidence of falls in older people.

tail, the caudal extremity of an organ or body, such as an axillary tail of a mammary gland.

tail bud. See **end bud.**

tail fold [AS, *taegel* + *fealdan,* to fold], a curved ridge formed at the caudal end of the early developing embryo. It consists of the tail bud, which in lower animals gives rise to the caudal appendage and in humans forms the hindgut.

tail of Spence, the upper outer tail of breast tissue that extends into the axilla.

tail of spermatozoon, the flagellum of a spermatozoon. It has four regions: the neck, middle piece, principal piece, and end piece.

tailor's bunion. See **bunionette.**

Takayasu arteritis /tä′kəyä″soo/ [Mikito Takayasu, Japanese surgeon, 1860–1938], an inflammation of the aorta, its major branches, and the pulmonary artery. It is characterized by progressive occlusion of the innominate, left subclavian, and left common carotid arteries above their origin in the aortic arch. Signs of the disorder are absence of a pulse in both arms and in the carotid arteries, transient paraplegia, transient blindness, and atrophy of facial muscles. Also called **brachiocephalic arteritis, Martorell syndrome, pulseless disease, reversed coarctation.** See **aortic arch syndrome.**

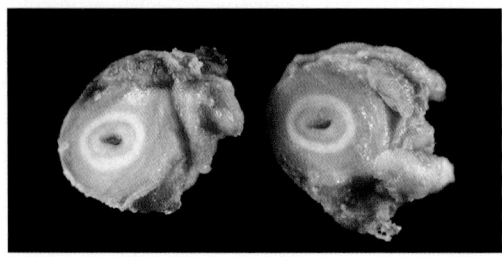

Takayasu arteritis *(Kumar et al, 2007)*

take, a popular term for a satisfactory response, as of a vaccination or tissue graft.

talar dome lesion (injury), a defect in the rounded area of the bone that articulates with the tibia at the ankle, caused by injury to the cartilage and underlying bone. Talar dome injuries are often missed on initial examination of a routine ankle sprain only to be diagnosed weeks after the injury.

talc /talk/ [Ar, *talq*], a native hydrous magnesium silicate, sometimes containing a small proportion of aluminum silicate; used as a dusting powder and adsorbent in clarifying liquids. See also **talcum powder.**

talcosis /talkō″sis/, a silicosis-like respiratory disorder caused by inhalation of magnesium silicate dust.

talcum powder, a fine powder made from talc that is frequently used in cosmetic and baby products. The International Agency for Research in Cancer (IARC) classifies the perineal (genital) use of talc-based body powder as "possibly carcinogenic to humans," based on limited evidence from human studies. See also **talc.**

talip-, combining form meaning "a nontraumatic (usually congenital) twisting defect" or "clubfooted": *talipes, talipes varus.*

talipes /tal″ipēz/ [L, *talus,* ankle, *pes,* foot], a deformity of the foot and ankle, usually congenital, in which the foot is twisted and relatively fixed in an abnormal position. *Talipes* refers to deformities that involve the foot and ankle, whereas *pes* refers only to deformities of the foot. Kinds include

talipes calcaneovalgus, *talipes calcaneovarus,* **talipes equinovarus.** See also **clawfoot, flatfoot.**

talipes calcaneovalgus. See **clubfoot.**

talipes cavus. See **clawfoot.**

talipes equinovarus. See **clubfoot.**

talipes equinus. See **pes equinus.**

talipes valgus. See **splayfoot.**

talipes varus, a deformity of the foot in which the heel is turned inward from the midline of the leg.

talk therapy, 1. *(Informal)* (in psychotherapy) a treatment that focuses on therapeutic communication to assist a client to develop positive ways to improve thoughts and behaviors. **2.** (in occupational therapy) therapeutic groups that use self-disclosure and sharing of experiences and feelings to promote insight and self-understanding. Also called *talk-based therapy.*

tallman lettering, a method of writing medications that are commonly confused. Uppercase lettering is used to draw attention to the differences in the medication names. Kinds include **acetaZOLAMIDE, acetoHEXAMIDE, chlorproPAMIDE, chlorproMAZINE.**

tallow /tal″ō/, **1.** a hard fat obtained from the bodies of ruminant animals such as cattle and sheep and used in soaps and lubricants. **2.** a vegetable fat obtained from plants, such as the wax myrtle.

talo-, combining form meaning "ankle": *talocalcaneonavicular, talofibular, talonavicular.*

talocalcaneonavicular joint, a complex joint in which the head of the talus articulates with the calcaneus and plantar calcaneonavicular ligament below and the navicular in front. It allows gliding and rotation movements, which are involved with inversion and eversion of the foot. It also participates in pronation and supination.

talofibular /tā′lōfib″yələr/, pertaining to the talus and the fibula.

talonavicular /tā′lōnəvik″yələr/ [L, *talon,* bird claw, *naviculus,* scaphoid], pertaining to the talus and the navicular bones.

talus /tā″ləs/ *pl. tali* [L, ankle], the second largest tarsal bone. It supports the tibia, rests on the calcaneus, and articulates with the malleoli and navicular bones. It consists of a body, neck, and head. Also called **ankle bone, astragalus.**

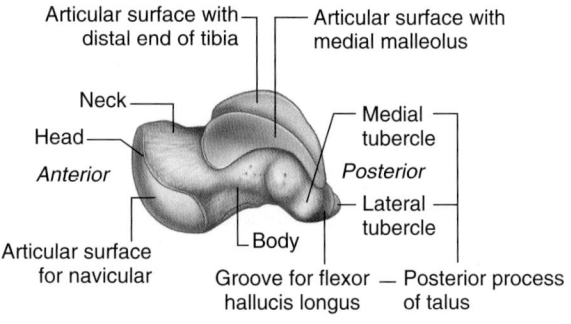

Talus *(Drake, Vogl, and Mitchell, 2010)*

Talwin, a mu antagonist/kappa agonist opioid analgesic. Brand name for **pentazocine hydrochloride.**

Tambocor, an oral antiarrhythmic drug. Brand name for **flecainide acetate.**

tambour /tam″boor/, a cylindric drumlike device connected to an air tube and stylus, used to record sphygmographic or other physiological data.

Tamm-Horsfall protein (THP) [Igor Tamm, American virologist, 1922-1995; Frank L. Horsfall, American virologist, 1906–1971], a mucoprotein found in the matrix of renal tubular casts. THP is secreted in the loop of Henle.

tamoxifen /təmok″səfin/, a nonsteroidal antiestrogen used in the palliative treatment of advanced breast cancer in premenopausal and postmenopausal women whose tumors are estrogen dependent. Tamoxifen has also been used to reduce the incidence of breast cancer in women with a high risk for developing it and for treating gynecomastia, precocious puberty, and other instances of estrogen excess.

tampon /tam′pon/ [Fr, plug], a packed cotton, a sponge, or other material for checking bleeding or absorbing secretions in cavities or canals or for holding displaced organs in position.

tamponade /tam′pənād′/ [Fr, *tamponner,* to plug up], stoppage of the blood flow to an organ or a part of the body by pressure, such as by a tampon or a pressure dressing applied to stop a hemorrhage or by the compression of a part by an accumulation of fluid, such as in cardiac tamponade.

tamsulosin, a selective adrenergic receptor antagonist.
- INDICATIONS: This drug is used to treat symptoms of benign prostatic hyperplasia.
- CONTRAINDICATIONS: Known hypersensitivity to this drug prohibits its use.
- ADVERSE EFFECTS: Adverse effects of this drug include asthenia, insomnia, chest pain, amblyopia, floppy iris syndrome, nausea, diarrhea, dysgeusia, decreased libido, abnormal ejaculation, back pain, rhinitis, pharyngitis, and cough. Common side effects include dizziness and headache.

tandem mass spectrometry (MS/MS), a two-step technique used to analyze a sample for a predetermined set of substances, either by using a separate mass spectroscope for each step or by using the same spectroscope to perform the steps sequentially. In the first stage, a predetermined set of ions is selected for fragmentation; in the second, mass spectra are produced for the fragments. This technique is used in screening newborns for multiple metabolic disorders from a single blood sample.

tandem repeat, appearance of two or more identical segments close to each other within a strand of DNA.

tangentiality /tanjen′chē·al′itē/ [L, *tangere,* to touch], expressions or responses characterized by a tendency to digress from an original topic of conversation, in which a common word connects two unrelated thoughts. It is common in schizophrenia and delirium. Compare **loose associations.**

tangible elements /tan″jibəl/ [L, *tangere + elementum,* first principle], objects that can be seen or touched, as distinguished from emotions, knowledge, or abstractions.

Tangier disease /tanjir″/ [Tangier Island, Virginia], a rare genetic disorder resulting in a deficiency of high-density lipoproteins, characterized by low blood cholesterol and an abnormal orange or yellow discoloration of the tonsils and pharynx. There also may be enlarged lymph nodes, liver, and spleen; muscle atrophy; and peripheral neuropathy. No specific treatment is known.

tangle /tang″gəl/, a dense mass of interlacing of fibers, sometimes appearing as a loose knot. Kinds include *intraneural fibrillary tangle.*

taniae coli, three narrow bands of longitudinal muscles in the walls of the large intestine; the bands are primarily observed in the cecum and colon and less visible in the rectum.

tannic acid /tan′ik/ [Celt, *tann,* oak; L, *acidus,* sour], a substance obtained from the bark and fruit of various trees and shrubs, particularly the nutgalls of oak trees. The acid is used as an astringent and protein precipitant. Also called *tannin.*

tanning [Fr, *tanner,* to tan], a process in which the pigmentation of the skin deepens as a result of exposure to ultraviolet light. Skin cells containing melanin darken immediately. New melanin is formed within 2 to 3 days and moves upward rapidly, allowing the darkening process to continue. Tanning damages skin cells, accelerates the visible signs of aging, and is associated with an increase in the risk for skin cancer.

tantalum (Ta) /tan′tələm/ [Gk, *Tantalus,* mythic king of Phrygia], a silvery metallic element. Its atomic number is 73; its atomic mass (weight) is 180.95. Relatively inert chemically, tantalum is used in prosthetic devices such as skull plates and wire sutures.

tantrum /tan′trəm/, a sudden outburst or violent display of rage, frustration, and bad temper, usually occurring in a maladjusted child and certain emotionally disturbed people. The activity is usually not directed at anyone or anything specific but toward the environment in general and is used primarily as a device for attempting to control others and the surroundings. It most commonly occurs at age 2 to 2½ years. Also called **temper tantrum.**

TAO, an antibacterial medication. Brand name for **troleandomycin.**

tap [ME, *tappen*], **1.** to strike lightly, as in percussion or testing of reflexes. **2.** to draw off fluid through a small opening.

tape [AS, *taeppe*], strips of material, usually with adhesive, used to secure bandages.

tape-compression folliculitis, inflammation of the hair follicles caused by tape dressings placed over foam or cotton-ball pads under a graduated compression stocking. The condition is more likely to occur on patients with hairy legs who may perspire during the summer months.

tapering arch /tā′pəring/ [AS, *tapor,* slender, *arcus,* bow], a dental arch that converges from the molars to the central incisors to such a degree that lines passing through the central grooves of the molars and premolars intersect within 1 inch (2.5 cm) anterior to the central incisors.

tapetoretinopathy /tapē′tōret′inop″əthē/, a hereditary visual disorder characterized by degeneration of the sensory retina and pigmentary epithelium. It occurs in pigmentary retinopathy and other eye diseases.

tapetum, **1.** a carpetlike layer or covering of tissue. **2.** a thin sheet of fibers covering parts of the brain and continuous with the corpus callosum. **3.** the reflective part of the choroid coat of the eye in many mammals.

tapeworm /tāp′wurm/ [AS, *taeppe + wyrm*], a parasitic intestinal worm belonging to the class Cestoda and having a scolex and a ribbon-shaped body composed of segments in a chain. Tapeworms live as larvae in one or more vertebrate intermediate hosts and grow to adulthood in the intestine of humans. In the human alimentary canal the worm develops into an adult with an attaching head, or scolex, and numerous hermaphroditic segments, or proglottids, each of which is capable of producing eggs. Also called **cestode.** Kinds include *Diphyllobothrium latum,* **Taenia saginata, Taenia solium.**

tapeworm infection, an intestinal infection by one of several species of parasitic worms, caused by eating raw or undercooked meat infested with tapeworm, its larvae, or food contaminated with feces containing tapeworm eggs. Symptoms of intestinal infection with adult worms are usually mild or absent, but diarrhea, epigastric pain, and weight loss may occur. Diagnosis is made when eggs or parts of the adult worm are passed in the stool. Treatment is with praziquantel and albendazole. Sanitary disposal of fecal material from affected patients is necessary to prevent the passage of larvae or eggs to other humans or other hosts. Certain species of tapeworm can infect humans during the larval stage, causing a serious, often cystic, condition of larval infestation. Also called **cestode infection, cestodiasis.** See also **cysticercosis, tapeworm.**

T

tapho-, combining form meaning "the grave": *taphophilia, taphophobia.*

taphophilia, a fascination with graves, cemeteries, and other rituals associated with death.

taphophobia, a fear of premature burial.

tapioca /tap′ē-ō″kə/, tiny starchy balls (pearls) or flakes made from the dried paste of grated cassava root, *Janipha manihot.* It is used as a thickener in a variety of easily digested food items, particularly cereals, soups, and puddings.

tapotement /täpôtmäN″/ [Fr, *tapoter,* to pat], a type of massage in which the body is tapped in a rhythmic manner with the tips of the fingers or the sides of the hands, using short, rapid, repetitive movements. The procedure is often used on the chest wall of patients with bronchitis to help loosen the mucus in the air passages. See also **massage.**

Taq polymerase /tak/, an enzyme found in the bacillus *Thermus aquaticus,* which lives in hot springs. It is heat resistant and thus can endure the high temperatures of the polymerase chain reaction.

tar /tär/ [AS, *teoru*], a dark, viscid organic mixture produced by the distillation of coal, wood, or vegetable matter. Some forms of tar are used to treat eczema and other skin disorders.

tarantula /təran″chələ/, a popular name for any of a number of species of large, hairy spiders. Although potentially poisonous, most are relatively harmless to humans. A bite by some species may produce an area of superficial skin destruction and may cause allergic reaction.

Tarceva, a chemotherapeutic agent. Brand name for **erlotinib.**

tardive /tär″div/ [L, *tardus,* late], describing a disease in which a period of time passes between exposure and the first symptoms.

tardive dyskinesia [L, *tardus,* late; Gk, *dys,* difficult, *kinesis,* movement], an abnormal condition characterized by involuntary repetitive movements of the muscles of the face, limbs, and trunk. This disorder most commonly affects older people who have been treated for extended periods with antipsychotics but can be caused by antidopaminergic medication. The involuntary movements associated with the condition may slacken or disappear after weeks or months and have been significantly reduced in some individuals by the administration of cholinergic drugs.

tardy peroneal nerve palsy [L, *tardus* + Gk, *perone,* brooch; L, *nervus* + *paralyein,* to be palsied], a type of mononeuropathy in which the peroneal nerve is excessively compressed where it crosses the head of the fibula. Such compression may occur when an individual falls asleep with the legs crossed.

tardy ulnar nerve palsy, an abnormal condition characterized by atrophy of the first dorsal interosseous muscle and difficulty in performing fine manipulations. It may be caused by injury of the ulnar nerve at the elbow and commonly affects individuals with a shallow ulnar groove or those who persistently rest their weight on their elbows. Signs and symptoms of this disorder may include numbness of the small finger, of the contiguous half of the proximal and middle phalanges of the ring finger, and of the ulnar border of the hand. Treatment concentrates on the prevention of further injury to the ulnar nerve. Therapy may include the use of a doughnut cushion for the elbow to relieve the pressure on the ulnar nerve. Severe cases of this disorder may be corrected by surgical procedures that mobilize and transplant the nerve to a site in front of the medial epicondyle.

target /tär′git/ [OFr, *targuete,* small shield], **1.** any object area subjected to bombardment by radioactive particles or another form of diagnostic or therapeutic radiation. **2.** a device used to contain stable materials and subsequent radioactive materials during bombardment by high-energy nuclei

from a cyclotron or other particle accelerator. **3.** the part of the anode struck by electrons in an x-ray tube.

target cell, **1.** an abnormal red blood cell characterized by a densely stained center surrounded by a pale, unstained ring circled by a dark, irregular band. Target cells occur in the blood after splenectomy, in anemia, in hemoglobin C disease, and in thalassemia. Also called **leptocyte.** Compare **discocyte, spherocyte. 2.** any cell having a specific receptor that reacts with a specific hormone, antigen, antibody, antibiotic, sensitized T cell, or other substance.

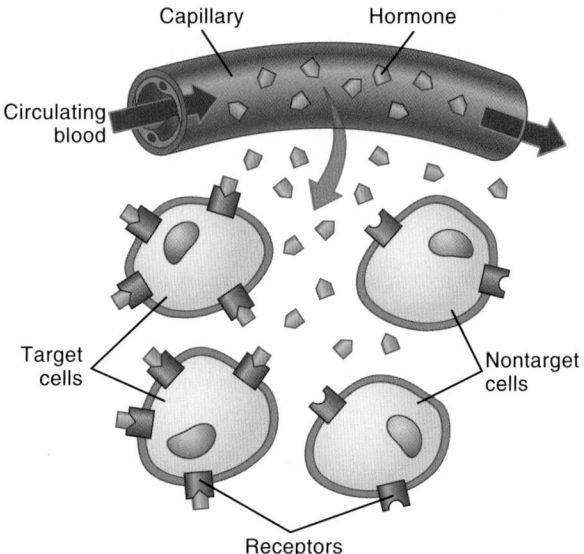

Target cell reaction *(Patton and Thibodeau, 2010)*

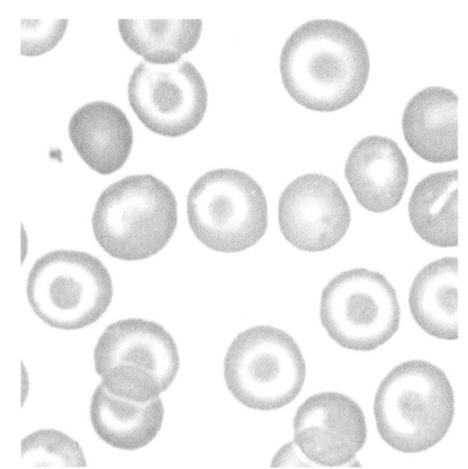

Target cells *(Carr and Rodak, 2008)*

target organ, **1.** an organ intended to receive a therapeutic dose of irradiation, such as the kidney when high-energy x-rays or gamma rays are beamed to the renal area for the treatment of a tumor. **2.** an organ intended to receive the greatest concentration of a diagnostic radioactive tracer, such as the liver, which accumulates Tc-99m sulfur colloid when it is injected intravenously to detect hepatic lesions. **3.** an organ most affected by a specific hormone, such as the thyroid gland, which is the target organ of thyroid stimulating hormone secreted by the anterior pituitary gland.

target symptoms, symptoms of an illness that are most likely to respond to a specific treatment, such as a particular psychopharmacological drug.

targeted therapies, the use of medications and chemotherapeutic agents that attack or block the growth of specific malignant cells and do minimal damage to cells that are growing normally.

tarsal /tär″səl/ [Gk, *tarsos,* flat surface], **1.** pertaining to the tarsus, or ankle bone. **2.** relating to the supporting plate of the eyelid.

tarsal arches [Gk, *tarsos,* flat surface; L, *arcus,* rainbow], the superior and inferior branches of the palpebral artery supplying the eyelid.

tarsal bone, any one of seven bones making up the tarsus of the foot, consisting of the talus, calcaneus, cuboid, navicular, and the three cuneiforms.

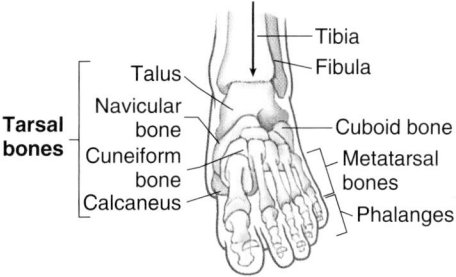

Tarsal bones *(Courtesy Yvonne Wylie Walston)*

tarsal cartilage. See **tarsus.**

tarsalgia /tärsal″jə/, foot pain, usually involving fallen arches. Also called **podalgia.**

tarsal gland, any one of numerous modified sebaceous glands on the inner surfaces of the eyelids. Acute localized bacterial infection of a tarsal gland may cause a sty or a chalazion. Also called **meibomian gland.** Compare **ciliary gland.**

tarsal plate. See **tarsus.**

tarsal tunnel syndrome, an abnormal condition and a kind of mononeuropathy characterized by pain and numbness in the sole of the foot. This disorder may be caused by fractures of the ankle that compress the posterior tibial nerve. It may be corrected by appropriate orthopedic therapy or surgery.

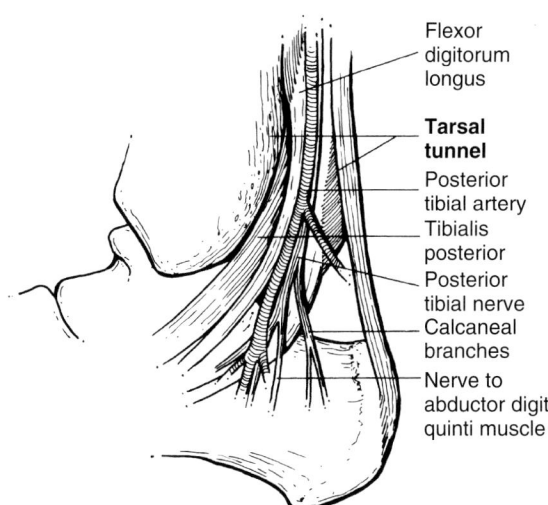

Tarsal tunnel *(DeLee, Drez, and Miller, 2009)*

tarso-, combining form meaning "instep of the foot" or "the edge of the eyelid": *tarsometatarsal, tarsorrhaphy.*

tarsometatarsal /tär′sōmet′ətär″səl/ [Gk, *tarsos,* flat surface, *meta,* beyond, *tarsos*], pertaining to the metatarsal bones and the tarsus of the foot, especially the articulations of the metatarsal bones with the cuneiform and cuboid bones at the instep of the foot.

tarsophalangeal reflex. See **Mendel's reflex.**

tarsorrhaphy /tärsôr″əfē/, a surgical procedure for temporarily or permanently uniting the upper and lower eyelids. It usually is performed in procedures to protect the cornea and may involve only the lateral parts of the eyelids.

tarsus /tär″səs/ *pl.* tarsi [Gk, *tarsos,* flat surface], **1.** the flat area of articulation between the foot and the leg or the edge of the eyelid. **2.** any one of the fibrous plates of cartilage about 2.5 cm long that form the eyelids. One tarsal plate shapes and gives solidity to the edge of each eyelid. Also called **tarsal cartilage, tarsal plate.**

TAR syndrome. See **thrombocytopenia–absent radius syndrome.**

tartar /tär″tär/ [Fr, *tartre*], **1.** *(Informal)* an accumulation of plaque, biofilm, and calculus on the teeth. See **calculus,** def. 2. **2.** any of several compounds containing tartrate, the salt of tartaric acid.

tartaric acid (HOOC(CH₂O)₂COOH) /tärter″ik/, a colorless or white powder found in various plants and prepared commercially from maleic anhydride and hydrogen peroxide. It is used in baking powder, certain beverages, and tartar emetic.

tartrate /tä″trāt/, **1.** a dianion of tartaric acid. **2.** any salt or ester of tartaric acid.

Tarui disease /tah″roo·ē/, a form of glycogen storage disease in which abnormally large amounts of glycogen are deposited in the skeletal muscle. The disorder is characterized by hemolysis and cramping on exercise but no rise in blood lactate. Biopsy of the affected organ reveals the absence of the enzyme phosphofructokinase. Also called **glycogen storage disease, type VII.** See also **glycogen storage disease.**

-tas, a noun-forming suffix: *anxietas, flexibilitas.*

Tasigna, a chemotherapeutic agent. Brand name for **nilotinib.**

task analysis, **1.** (in occupational therapy) a focus on and description of the basic actions required to perform each step of a skill; identification of the cognitive, motor, and social-emotional requirements to accomplish a specific action. **2.** a systematic method of collecting data regarding the knowledge, skills, and attitudes associated with a particular task performed by a member of the health care team.

task functions, behaviors that focus or direct activities toward movements involving work or labor.

task group, **1.** a group in which structured verbal or nonverbal exercises are used to help a person gain emotional, physical, or other personal awareness. **2.** a group of individuals brought together to achieve a certain goal, such as completing a needs assessment, producing a brochure, or recommending changes in work hours or duties.

task-oriented behavior, actions involving a person's cognitive abilities in an attempt to solve problems, resolve conflicts, and gratify the person's needs to reduce or avoid distress.

taste [ME, *tasten*], the sense of perceiving different flavors in soluble substances that contact the tongue and trigger nerve impulses to special taste centers in the cortex and thalamus of the brain. The four basic traditional tastes are sweet, salty, sour, and bitter. The front of the tongue is most sensitive to salty and sweet substances; the sides of the tongue are most sensitive to sour substances; and the back of the tongue is most sensitive to bitter substances. The middle of the tongue produces virtually no taste sensation. Chemoreceptor cells in the taste buds of the tongue detect different substances.

Adults have about 9000 taste buds, most of them situated on the upper surface of the tongue. The sense of taste is intricately linked with the sense of smell, and taste discrimination is very complex. Many experts believe the capacity to perceive different tastes involves a synthesis of chemoreactive nerve impulses and coordinating brain processes that are still not completely understood.

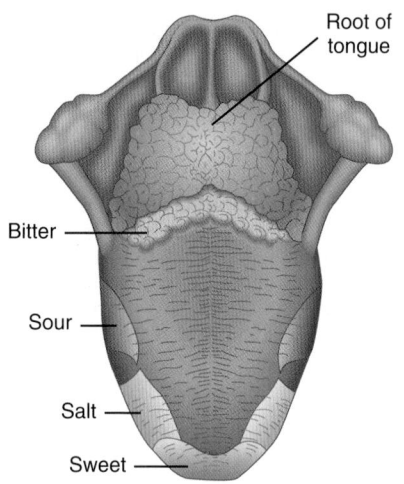

Taste regions of the tongue *(Thibodeau and Patton, 2007)*

taste bud, any one of many peripheral taste organs distributed over the tongue, epiglottis, and the roof of the mouth. The five basic taste sensations registered by chemical stimulation of the taste buds are sweet, sour, bitter, savory, and salty. All other tastes perceived are combinations of these five basic flavors plus the input from olfactory receptors. Each taste bud rests in a spheric pocket, which extends through the epithelium. Gustatory cells and supporting cells form each bud, which has a surface opening and an opening in the basement membrane. Also called **gustatory organ.**

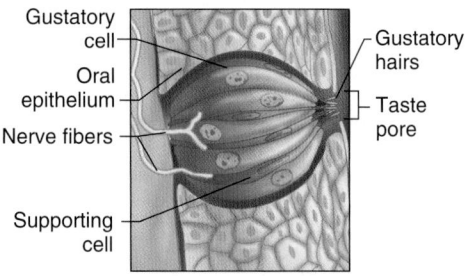

Taste bud *(Patton and Thibodeau, 2010)*

taste papilla [OFr, *taster* + L, *papilla,* nipple], small nipplelike elevations on the tongue. They contain sense organs that are sensitive to the chemicals identified with tastes, which vary with their location on the tongue.

TAT, abbreviation for **tetanus antitoxin.**

tattoo /tatoo′/ [Tahitian, *tatau,* marks], a permanent coloration of the skin by the introduction of foreign pigment. A tattoo may be created deliberately or may accidentally occur when a bit of graphite from a broken pencil point is embedded in the skin. Laser is preferred for removal of tattoos, although small tattoos can be removed by surgical excision. **−tattoo,** *v.*

tau /tou, tō/, T, τ, the nineteenth letter of the Greek alphabet.

tau protein, a microtubule-associated protein that forms insoluble and hyperphosphorylated aggregates in Alzheimer disease.

taurine /tôr″in/, a derivative of the amino acid cysteine. It is present in bile in combination with cholic acid. It is used in the synthesis of bile salts.

taurodontism /tô′rō·don′tiz·əm/ [L, *taurus,* bull; Gk, *odous,* tooth], a variation in tooth form characterized by prism-shaped molars with large pulp spaces and resulting from branching of the root only in the middle (mesotaurodontism) or in the apical third or not at all (hypertaurodontism). See also **mesotaurodontism, hypertaurodontism.**

Taussig-Bing syndrome /tô″sig-bing′/ [Helen B. Taussig, American pediatrician, 1898–1986; Richard J. Bing, American cardiologist, 1909–2010], a developmental anomaly of the heart characterized by transposition of the aorta and pulmonary artery. It is accompanied by a subpulmonary ventricular septal defect and ventricular hypertrophy.

tauto-, combining form meaning "same": *tautology, tautomer.*

tautology, repeating the same statement or idea using different terminology.

tautomer /tôtəmər/, structural isomers that differ only in the position of a hydrogen atom or proton. Because tautomers can be rapidly interconverted by proton transfer in aqueous solutions, they are usually in equilibrium with one another. Kinds include *keto isomer, enol isomer.*

Tavist, an antihistamine medication. Brand name for **clemastine.**

tax-, combining form meaning "order or arrangement": *taxis, taxonomic, taxonomy.*

-taxic. See **-tactic, -tactical, -taxic.**

taxis /tak″sis/, **1.** movement away from or toward a stimulus. **2.** the reduction of a hernia. **3.** a dislocation of a hernia by means of manipulation.

-taxis, -taxia, -taxy, 1. suffix meaning "a (specified) arrangement": *biotaxis.* **2.** suffix meaning "a movement of an organism in response to a stimulus": *chemotaxis, necrotaxis, thermotaxis.*

Taxol, an anticancer medication. Brand name for **paclitaxel.**

taxonomic /tak′sənom″ik/ [Gk, *taxis,* arrangement, *nomos,* law], pertaining to the orderly classification of organisms into appropriate groups, or taxa, on the basis of interrelationships with the use of suitable names.

taxonomy /takson″əmē/ [Gk, *taxis,* arrangement, *nomos,* rule], a system for classifying organisms according to their natural relationships on the basis of such common factors as embryology, structure, or physiological chemistry. The system has seven main levels, or taxa, each more comprehensive than those below it: kingdom, phylum (or division), class, order, family, genus, and species. Humans are members of the species *Homo sapiens* of the genus *Homo,* in the family Hominidae in the order Primates, in the class Mammalia, in the phylum Chordata, in the kingdom Animalia.

-taxy. See **-taxia, -taxis, -taxy, -taxis, -taxia, -taxy.**

Taylor brace [Charles F. Taylor, American surgeon, 1827–1899], a padded steel brace used to support the spine. Also called **Taylor splint.**

Taylor, Effie J. [1874–1970], a Canadian-born American nurse who was graduated from Johns Hopkins School of Nursing. After graduation she continued at Johns Hopkins at the Phipps Psychiatric Institute, served as a nurse in World War I, and went to Yale University School of Nursing in 1923, succeeding Annie Goodrich as dean in 1934. She served as president of the International Council of Nurses during World War II.

Taylor splint. See **Taylor brace.**

Tay-Sachs disease /tā″saks″/ [Warren Tay, English ophthalmologist, 1843–1927; Bernard Sachs, American neurologist, 1858–1944], an inherited, neurodegenerative disorder of lipid metabolism caused by a deficiency of the enzyme hexosaminidase A, which results in the accumulation of sphingolipids in the brain. The condition, which is transmitted as an autosomal-recessive trait, occurs predominantly in families of Eastern European Jewish origin, specifically the Ashkenazic Jews. It is characterized by progressive cognitive impairment and physical delays and early death. Symptoms first appear by 6 months of age, after which no new skills are learned and there is progressive loss of those skills already acquired. Convulsions and atrophy of the optic nerve head occur after 1 year, followed by blindness, with a cherry-red spot on each retina; spasticity; dementia; and paralysis. Most children die between 2 and 4 years of age. There is no specific therapy for the condition, and intervention is purely symptomatic and supportive. The disease can be diagnosed in utero through amniocentesis. Also called *amaurotic familial idiocy,* **gangliosidosis type I, infantile cerebral sphingolipidosis, Sachs disease.** See also **Sandhoff disease.**

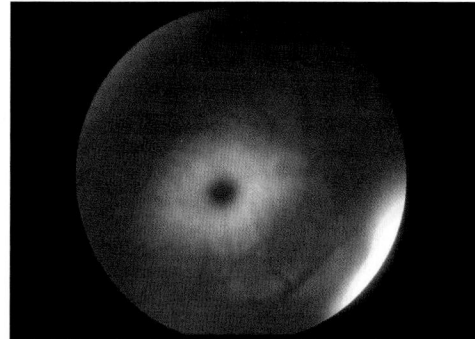

Cherry red spot in Tay-Sachs disease *(Courtesy Dr. Thomas A. Weingeist, Department of Ophthalmology & Visual Science, University of Iowa)*

Tay's spot. See **cherry red spot.**

tazarotene /tah-zar′o-tēn/, a retinoid prodrug used topically in the treatment of acne vulgaris and psoriasis.

Tazicef, a cephalosporin antibiotic medication. Brand name for **ceftazidime.**

tazobactam /taz″o-bak′tam/, a beta-lactamase inhibitor having antibacterial actions and uses similar to those of sulbactam. It is used as the sodium salt.

Tb, symbol for the element **terbium.**

TB, **1.** abbreviation for **tuberculosis. 2.** abbreviation for *tubercle bacillus.*

T bandage, a bandage in the shape of the letter T. It is used for the perineum and sometimes for the head. Also called *crucial bandage.*

TBI, **1.** abbreviation for *total body irradiation.* **2.** abbreviation for *traumatic brain injury.*

T-box, a DNA-binding domain shared by a highly conserved family of genes (Tbx genes) that act as transcription factors involved in the regulation of various developmental processes.

T-box genes, a highly conserved family of transcription factors having a common DNA-binding sequence (the T-box), which are important in the regulation of a wide variety of developmental processes in animals.

Tbs, abbreviation for *tablespoon.*

TBSA, abbreviation for *total body surface area.* See **surface area.**

tbsp, abbreviation for *tablespoon.*

TBT, abbreviation for **tracheobronchial tree.**

TBW, abbreviation for **total body water.**

Tc, symbol for the element **technetium.**

TC, abbreviation for **therapeutic community.**

TCA, abbreviation for **tricyclic antidepressant.**

TCDD, abbreviation for **2,3,7,8-tetrachlorodibenzo-*para*-dioxin.** See **dioxin.**

T cell, a lymphocyte that participates in cellular immunity, including cell-to-cell communication. The major T cell categories are T-helper and T-suppressor cytotoxic cells. Also called **T lymphocyte.** Compare **B cell.** See also **antibody, immune response.**

T cell antigen receptor, a protein present on T cells that combines with antigens to produce discrete immunological components.

T cell lymphomas, a heterogenous group of lymphoid tumors representing malignant transformation of the T lymphocytes. Some types of tumors formerly included in this group have been found to be mixtures of T cells and B cell precursors.

T cell-mediated hypersensitivity reaction, type IV hypersensitivity reaction. See also **hypersensitivity reaction.**

T cell-mediated immunity. See **cellular immunity, immune response, T cell.**

TCV, abbreviation for **total cell volume.**

Td, abbreviation for **tetanus and diphtheria toxoids.**

TD, abbreviation for **toxic dose.**

TD$_{50}$, abbreviation for **median toxic dose.**

TDD, abbreviation for **transdermal drug delivery.**

tDNA, abbreviation for **transfer DNA.**

t.d.s., a notation for a Latin phrase meaning "(to be taken) three times a day." Abbreviation for *ter die sumendum.*

Te, symbol for the element **tellurium.**

tea [Chin, *ch'a*], **1.** a beverage prepared from the leaves and leaf buds of *Thea sinensis,* an evergreen shrub. A member of the camellia family, the plant is grown mainly in Asia. Its pharmacologically active components include caffeine, theobromine, theophylline, and tannin. **2.** maté tea, a caffeine beverage prepared from the leaves of *Ilex paraguayensis,* a shrub grown in South America. **3.** See **cannabis.**

teacher's nodule. *(Informal)* See **vocal cord nodule.**

teaching hospital [AS, *taecan,* to show how], a hospital associated with a university that has accredited programs in various specialties of medical practice.

teaching rounds, informal conferences held regularly, often at the beginning of the day. Various members of the department and staff may attend, including nurses, residents, interns, students, attending physicians, and faculty. Specific problems in the care of current patients, as well as case presentation of patients with specific diseases, are discussed. See also **nursing rounds.**

team nursing [AS, *team,* family; L, *nutrix,* nurse], a decentralized system in which the care of a patient is distributed among the members of a group working in coordinated effort. The charge nurse delegates authority to a team leader, who must be a professional nurse. The team leader assigns tasks, schedules care, and instructs team members in details of care. A conference is held at the beginning and end of each shift to allow team members to exchange information and the team leader to make changes in the nursing care plan for any patient. Compare **primary nursing.**

team practice, professional practice by a group of professionals that may include physicians, nurses, and others, such

T

as a social worker, nutritionist, or physical therapist, who manage the care of a specified number of patients as a coordinated group, usually in an outpatient setting.

tear /ter/ [ME, *teren,* to rend], to rip, rend, or pull apart by force.

teardrop fracture /tir′drop/ [AS, *tear* + *dropa* + L, *fractura,* break], an avulsion fracture of one of the short bones, such as a vertebra, causing a tear-shaped disruption of bone tissue.

tear duct /tir/ [AS, *tear* + L, *ducere,* to lead], any duct that carries tears, including the lacrimal ducts, nasolacrimal ducts, and excretory ducts of the lacrimal glands.

tear gas /tēr/, a gas that produces severe lacrimation by irritating the conjunctivae.

tearing /tir′ing/, watering of the eye usually caused by excessive tear production, resulting from strong emotion, infection, or mechanic irritation by a foreign body. If the normal amount of fluid tears is produced but not drained into the lacrimal punctum at the nasal border of the eye, tear overflow will occur. If the lacrimal punctum, sac, canaliculi, or nasolacrimal duct becomes blocked, tears also will overflow. Also called **epiphora.**

tears /tirz/ [ME, *tere*], a watery saline or alkaline fluid secreted by the lacrimal glands that, along with secretions from the meibomian glands and goblet cells and glands of Zeii, moisten the conjunctiva and cornea. Also called **dacryon.**

tears of the perineum /ters/ [ME, *teren* + Gk, *perineos*], a rending of the tissues between the vulva and anus caused by overstretching of the vagina during child delivery. The degree of damage ranges from a tear of the superficial tissues without injury to the surrounding muscle to a rupture of the perineal skin, vaginal and rectal mucosa, and anal sphincter. The damage is usually repaired by surgery.

teaspoon (tsp), a small spoon that may be used to measure a dose of a liquid medication, equivalent to about 1 fluid dram or 5 mL.

tea tree oil, an herbal product taken from a species of myrtle tree native to coastal Australia.

■ INDICATIONS: This herb is used topically for acne and fungal infections and has proven efficacy. It has also been added to warm bath water and inhaled for treatment of cough and lower respiratory disorders, but there are no reliable data regarding its efficacy in this instance.

■ CONTRAINDICATIONS: This herb should not be used during pregnancy and lactation or in those with known hypersensitivity to this plant. Tea tree oil has been taken orally in the past, but this is not recommended due to safety concerns.

tebutate, a contraction for tertiary butyl acetate.

technetium (Tc) [Gk, *technectos,* artificial], a radioactive, metallic element. Its atomic number is 43, and its atomic mass is 99. The first synthetic element, technetium also occurs in nature. Isotopes of technetium are used in radioisotope scanning procedures of internal organs such as the liver and spleen.

technetium-99m, the radionuclide most commonly used to image the body in nuclear medicine scans. It is preferred because of its short half-life and because the emitted photon has an appropriate energy for normal imaging techniques. The "m" indicates that this radionuclide is metastable. It is generated on site from a molybdenum source.

technic. See **technique.**

-technic, -technics, -technique, -technology, -techny, suffix meaning "skillful way or the mechanics of doing something."

technical [Gk, *technikos,* skillful], pertaining to a procedure or its results that require special techniques, skills, expertise, or knowledge.

technician /teknish′ən/ [Gk, *technikos,* skillful], a person with special training and experience in some form of technical procedures, usually those involving mechanical adjustments, such as maintaining and operating radiological equipment.

-technics. See **-technic, -technics, -technique, -technology, -techny.**

technique /teknēk′/ [Gk, *technikos,* skillful], the method and details followed in performing a procedure, such as those used in conducting a laboratory test, a physical examination, a psychiatric interview, a surgical operation, or any process requiring certain skills or an ordered sequence of actions. Also spelled **technic.**

-technique. See **-technic, -technics, -technique, -technology, -techny.**

techno-, combining form meaning "art", "technical," or "applied technology": *technology.*

technologist /teknol′əjist/ [Gk, *techne,* art, *logos,* science], a person who studies the application of processes for making natural resources beneficial for humans. A medical technologist may work under the supervision of a physician in general clinical laboratory procedures.

-technology. See **-technic, -technics, -technique, -technology, -techny.**

technology /teknol′əjē/ [Gk, *techne,* art, *logos,* study], **1.** the application of science or the scientific method to commercial or industrial objectives. **2.** the knowledge and use of science applied to the conversion of natural resources for the benefit of humans.

-techny. See **-technic, -technics, -technique, -technology, -techny.**

tecto-, combining form meaning "rooflike": *tectorial, tectorium.*

tectonic /tekton′ik/, **1.** pertaining to variations in structure in the cornea or other parts of the eye. **2.** pertaining to plastic surgery or tissue transplants.

tectorial /tektôr′ē-əl/, pertaining to a rooflike structure or cover.

tectorium /tektôr′ē-əm/, a body structure that serves as an overlying structure or roof.

TED, 1. abbreviation for *threshold erythema dose.* See **threshold dose. 2.** abbreviation for *thromboembolic disorder.* See **thromboembolic disorder (TED) hose.**

teenager. See **adolescent.**

teeth. See **tooth.**

teethe. See **teething.**

teether /tē′ther/, an object such as a plastic or rubber teething ring on which an infant can bite or chew during the teething process. Also called **teething ring.**

teething /tē′thing/ [AS, *toth*], the physiological process of the eruption of the primary teeth through the gums. It normally begins around the sixth month of life and occurs periodically until the complete set of 20 teeth has appeared at about 30 to 36 months. Discomfort and inflammation result from the pressure exerted against the periodontal tissue as the crown of the tooth breaks through the membranes. General signs of teething include excessive drooling, biting on hard objects, irritability, difficulty in sleeping, and refusal of food. Low-grade fever or diarrhea often occurs during teething but may be indicative of illness rather than of teething. The pain and inflammation usually may be soothed by cold, such as with a frozen teething ring, cold metal spoon, or ice wrapped in a washcloth. Use of teething powders and procedures such as rubbing or cutting the gums are discouraged because of the possibility of infection or complications from ingestion of the medication. −**teethe,** *v.*

teething ring. See **teether.**

Teflon, a substance (polytetrafluoroethylene) used for the construction of surgical implants in restorative surgery and the coating of surgical blades.

teg-, combining form meaning "a cover": *tegmen, tegmental.*

tegaserod, a 5-HT4 receptor partial agonist used to treat irritable bowel syndrome when the primary bowel symptom is constipation.

tegmen /teg″mən/, a covering, such as the bone that covers the tympanic cavity.

tegmental /tegmen″təl/ [L, *tegmentum,* cover], of or relating to an integument.

Tegretol, an analgesic and anticonvulsant. Brand name for **carbamazepine.**

teicoplanin /ti-ko-pla′nin/, a glycopeptide antibiotic produced by the bacterium *Actinoplanes teichomyceticus,* used as a less toxic alternative to vancomycin in the treatment of moderate to severe infections caused by gram-positive bacteria when other antibiotics cannot be used.

Tekturna, an antihypertensive medication. Brand name for **aliskiren.**

tela-, prefix meaning "a web or weblike structure": *telangiectatic sarcoma.*

-tela, suffix meaning "a weblike membrane."

telangiectasia /təlan′jē·ektā″zhə/ [Gk, *telos,* end, *angeion,* vessel, *ektasis,* swelling], permanent dilation of groups of superficial capillaries and venules. Common causes are actinic damage, atrophy-producing dermatoses, rosacea, elevated estrogen levels, and collagen vascular diseases. See also **Osler-Weber-Rendu syndrome, spider angioma.**

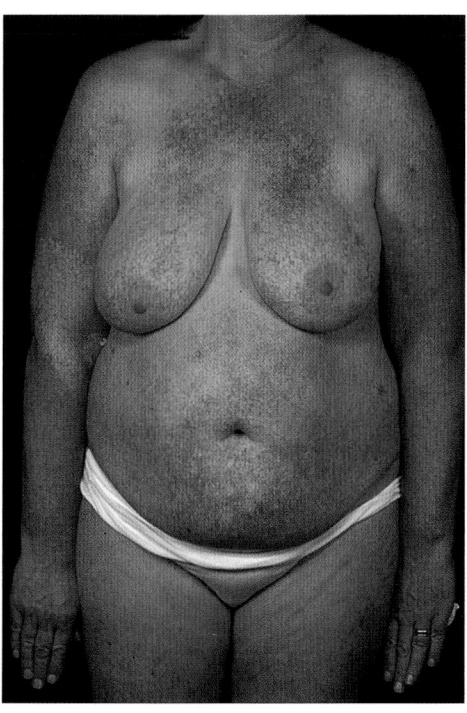

Telangiectasia *(Perez et al, 2010)*

telangiectasia lymphatica [Gk, *telos,* end, *angeion,* vessel, *ektasis,* swelling; L, *lympha,* water], a congenital or acquired condition of obstructed, dilated, lymphatic vessels resulting in lymphangiomas.

telangiectatic angioma /təlan′jē·ektat″ik/, a tumor composed of dilated blood vessels.

telangiectatic epulis, a benign red tumor of the gingiva containing prominent blood vessels. Low-grade or chronic irritation is a risk factor.

telangiectatic fibroma. See **angiofibroma.**

telangiectatic glioma, a tumor composed of glial cells and a network of blood vessels, which give the mass a vivid pink appearance.

telangiectatic granuloma. See **pyogenic granuloma.**

telangiectatic lipoma. See **angiolipoma.**

telangiectatic nevus, a common skin condition of neonates, characterized by flat, deep-pink, localized areas of capillary dilation that occur predominantly on the back of the neck, lower occiput, upper eyelids, upper lip, and bridge of the nose. The areas disappear permanently by about 2 years of age. Also called **capillary flames, stork bite.** Compare **superficial fading infantile hemangioma.**

telangiectatic sarcoma, a malignant tumor of mesodermal cells with an unusually rich vascular network.

telbivudine, an antiretroviral.

■ INDICATIONS: This drug is used in the treatment of hepatitis B.

■ CONTRAINDICATIONS: Lactation and known hypersensitivity to this drug prohibit its use.

■ ADVERSE EFFECTS: Adverse effects of this drug include weakness, taste change, hearing loss, photophobia, abdominal pain, hepatomegaly, lactic acidosis, myalgia, arthralgia, muscle cramps, and cough. Common side effects include fever, headache, malaise, dizziness, insomnia, nausea, vomiting, diarrhea, anorexia, and rash.

tele-, teleo-, prefix meaning "end" or "occurring at a distance": *telekinesis, telehealth.*

telediagnosis /tel′ədī′əgnō″sis/ [Gk, *tele,* far off, *dia,* through, *gnosis,* knowledge], a process whereby a disease diagnosis, or prognosis, is made by the electronic transmission of data between distant medical facilities.

telehealth, the use of telecommunication technologies to provide health care services and access to medical and surgical information for training and educating health care professionals and consumers, to increase awareness and educate the public about health-related issues, and to facilitate medical research across distances.

telekinesis /tel′əkinē″sis/ [Gk, *tele,* far off, *kinesis,* movement], a concept of parapsychology that one can control external events such as the movement of a solid object by the powers of the mind. For example, practitioners of telekinesis may believe it possible, by thought processes alone, to influence the roll of dice. Also called **parakinesis, psychokinesis.**

telemedicine, the use of telecommunication equipment and information technology to provide clinical care to individuals at distant sites and the transmission of medical and surgical information and images needed to provide that care.

telemetry /telem′ətrē/ [Gk, *tele,* far off, *metron,* measure], the electronic transmission of data between distant points, such as the transmission of cardiac monitoring data.

telencephalization /tel′ensef′əlīzā″shən/, a stage in fetal development in which the forebrain begins to assume control over nervous system functions previously directed by more primitive neural centers. Also called **corticalization.**

telencephalon /tel′ensef″əlon/ [Gk, *telos,* end, *egekephalos,* brain], the paired brain vesicles or endbrain from which the cerebral hemispheres are derived.

teleo-. See **tele-, teleo-.**

teleology /tel′ē·ol″əjē/ [Gk, *telos,* end, *logos,* science], **1.** the study of ultimate purpose or design in natural phenomena. **2.** a theory that everything is directed toward some final purpose.

telepathic, the ability or perceived ability to communicate using the mind only. See **telepathy.**

telepathist /təlep″əthist/, **1.** a person who believes in telepathy. **2.** a person who claims to have telepathic powers.

T

telepathy /təlep″əthē/ [Gk, *tele,* far off, *pathos,* feeling], the alleged communication of thought from one person to another by means other than the physical senses. Also called **thought transference.** See also **clairvoyance, extrasensory perception, parapsychology. –telepathic,** *adj.,* –**telepathize,** *v.*

telephone counseling, a strategy system to provide support by telephone for patients or family caregivers who are homebound. The system may offer safety provisions and social contacts for frail older persons or the visually impaired as well as suicide-prevention counseling.

teleradiology /tel′ĕ-ra″de-ol′ah-je/, radiology done through remote transmission and viewing of images.

telereceptive /tel′ərisep″tiv/, pertaining to the exteroceptors of hearing, sight, and smell that detect stimuli distant from the body.

teletherapy /tel′əther″əpē/ [Gk, *tele + therapeia,* treatment], radiation therapy administered by a machine that is positioned at some distance from the patient. Typically a teletherapy unit can rotate around a patient, thus allowing the use of multiple beams that intersect at the tumor and lowering the dose to surrounding normal tissue.

telithromycin, an antiinfective.
- INDICATIONS: This drug is used to treat acute bacterial exacerbation of chronic bronchitis caused by *Streptococcus pneumoniae, Haemophilus influenzae,* and *Moraxella catarrhalis*; acute bacterial sinusitis caused by *S. pneumoniae, H. influenzae, M. catarrhalis,* and *Staphylococcus aureus*; and community-acquired pneumonia.

telluric /teloo″rik/ [L, *tellus,* earth], pertaining to the soil and its possible pathogenic influence.

tellurium (Te) /teloo″rē·əm/ [L, *tellus,* earth], an element exhibiting metallic and nonmetallic chemical properties. Its atomic number is 52; its atomic mass is 127.60. Inhaling vapors of tellurium results in a garlicky breath.

telmisartan, an antihypertensive.
- INDICATIONS: This drug is used to treat hypertension, either alone or in combination with other drugs.
- CONTRAINDICATIONS: Known hypersensitivity to this drug prohibits its use.
- ADVERSE EFFECTS: Adverse effects of telmisartan include dizziness, insomnia, dyspepsia, and cough. Common side effects include anxiety, diarrhea, anorexia, vomiting, myalgia, pain, and upper respiratory infection.

telo-, combining form meaning "end": *telocentric, telomerase, teleology.*

telocentric /tel′əsen″trik/ [Gk, *telos,* end, *kentron,* center], pertaining to a chromosome in which the centromere is located at the end so that the chromosome appears as a straight filament. Compare **acrocentric, metacentric, submetacentric.**

telodendria, the branches of an axon.

telogen, the resting stage of the hair growth cycle. See **hair.**

telogen effluvium (TE), diffuse hair loss due to shedding of hair in the telogen phase, usually developing 3 to 4 months after a stressful event.

telomerase /tə·lō′mər·ās/, a DNA polymerase involved in the formation of telomeres and the maintenance of telomere sequences during replication.

telomere /tel′ō·mēr/, either of the ends of a chromosome. Telomeres possess special properties, among them a polarity that prevents their reunion with any fragment after a chromosome has been broken.

telophase /tel″əfāz/ [Gk, *telos + phasis,* appearance], the final of the four stages of nuclear division in mitosis and in each of the two divisions in meiosis. The newly produced daughter chromosomes from the preceding stage (anaphase) assemble at the poles of the spindle and become long and slender, the nuclear membrane forms around them, the nucleolus reappears, and the cytoplasm begins to divide. See also **anaphase, interphase, meiosis, metaphase, mitosis, prophase.**

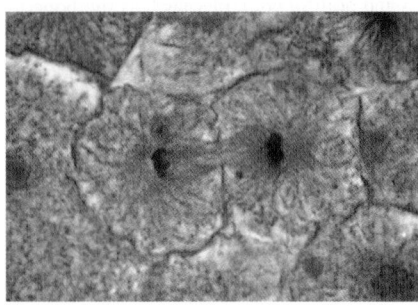

Telophase *(© Ed Reschke; Used with permission)*

temazepam /temaz′əpam/, a benzodiazepine hypnotic agent.
- INDICATIONS: It is prescribed for the relief of transient and intermittent insomnia.
- CONTRAINDICATIONS: Pregnancy or lactation prohibits its use. It is not recommended for patients under 18 years of age. Patients should avoid use of alcohol while also using temazepam.
- ADVERSE EFFECTS: The most serious adverse effects are confusion, euphoria, anorexia, ataxia, palpitations, hallucinations, horizontal nystagmus, and paradoxic reactions.

Temovate, a topical corticosteroid medication. Brand name for **clobetasol propionate.**

temozolomide, a miscellaneous antineoplastic agent.
- INDICATIONS: It is used to treat anaplastic astrocytoma with relapse.
- CONTRAINDICATIONS: Pregnancy, lactation, and known hypersensitivity to this drug or to carbazine prohibit its use.
- ADVERSE EFFECTS: Life-threatening effects are thrombocytopenia, leukopenia, and seizures. Other adverse effects include anemia, urinary incontinence, urinary tract infection, urinary frequency, upper respiratory infection, pharyngitis, sinusitis, cough, headache, fatigue, asthenia, fever, edema, back pain, weight increase, and diplopia. Common side effects include nausea, anorexia, vomiting, hemiparesis, dizziness, poor coordination, amnesia, insomnia, paresthesia, somnolence, paresis, ataxia, anxiety, dysphagia, depression, confusion, rash, and pruritus.

temper [L, *temperare,* to moderate], **1.** *v.,* to moderate or soften the effects. **2.** *n.,* a state of mind regarding calmness or anger.

temperament /temp′(ə)rəmənt/ [L, *temperamentum,* mixture in proper proportions], the features of a persona that reflect an individual's emotional disposition, or the way he or she behaves, feels, and thinks.

temperance /tem″pərəns/, behavior that emphasizes moderation and self-restraint, particularly in the use of alcohol.

temperate phage /tem′pərit/ [L, *temperare,* to moderate; Gk, *phagein,* to eat], a bacteriophage whose genome is incorporated into the host bacterium. It persists through many cell divisions of the bacterium without destroying the host in contrast to a virulent phage, which lyses and kills its host.

temperature (T) /tem′pə(ri)chər/ [L, *temperatura*], **1.** a relative measure of sensible heat or cold. **2.** (in physiology) a measure of sensible heat associated with the metabolism of the human body, normally maintained at a constant level of 98.6° F (37° C) by the thermotaxic nerve mechanism that balances heat gains and heat losses. **3.** *(Informal)* a fever.

temperature of infant [L, *temperatura + infans,* infant], the neonatal temperature, which normally ranges from 97.7° F to 99.5° F (36.5° C to 37.5° C). It is unstable because of immature physiological mechanisms.

temperature scale, a scale for expressing degree of heat, based on absolute zero as a reference point or with a certain value arbitrarily assigned to such temperatures as the freezing point and boiling point of water.

temperature sense. See **thermic sense.**

temper tantrum. See **tantrum.**

template /tem″plit/ [L, *templum,* section], the strand of DNA that acts as a model for the synthesis of messenger RNA. The messenger RNA contains a complementary sequence of nucleotides and travels to the ribosomes, which are located in the cytoplasm, for the synthesis of proteins.

template bleeding time test. See **simplate bleeding time test.**

tempo-, **1.** combining form meaning "time": *tempostabile, temporal, temporary filling.* **2.** combining form meaning "the temples, in the lateral regions of the head": *temporal, temporalis, temporomandibular.*

temporal /tem″pərəl/ [L, *tempus,* time; *tempora,* the temples], **1.** pertaining to a limited time. **2.** pertaining to the temporal bone of the skull.

temporal arteritis [L, *temporalis,* temporary, *arteria,* airpipe, *itis,* inflammation], a progressive inflammatory disorder of cranial blood vessels, principally the temporal artery. It occurs most frequently in women over 70 years of age. Characteristic changes in the involved vessels include granulomatous disruption of the elastic layer and engulfment of fiber fragments by giant cells in the intimal and medial layers. The temporal artery is typically tender, swollen, and pulseless but may be clinically normal. Symptoms are intractable headache, difficulty in chewing, weakness, rheumatic pains, and loss of vision if the central retinal artery becomes occluded. Also called **cranial arteritis, giant cell arteritis, Horton arteritis.**

temporal artery, any one of three arteries on each side of the head: the superficial temporal artery, the middle temporal artery, and the deep temporal artery.

temporal bone, one of a pair of large bones forming part of the lower cranium and containing various cavities and recesses associated with the ear, such as the tympanic cavity and the auditory tube. Each temporal bone consists of four parts: the mastoid, the squama, the petrous, and the tympanic.

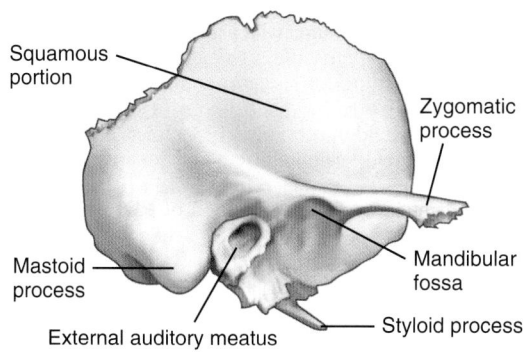

Squamous portion
Zygomatic process
Mandibular fossa
Mastoid process
Styloid process
External auditory meatus

Temporal bone

temporal bone fracture, a break in the temporal bone of the skull, sometimes characterized by bleeding from the ear. Diminished hearing, facial paralysis, or infection of the tympanic cavity leading to meningitis may occur.

temporal context, (in occupational therapy) the experience of time as shaped by engagement in occupations, including the temporal aspects of occupations that contribute to the patterns of daily occupations. The temporal context includes stage of life, time of day or year, duration or rhythm of activity, and history.

temporal fascia, a tough fan-shaped aponeurosis overlying the temporalis muscle and attached by its outer margin to the superior temporal line and by its inferior margin to the zygomatic arch.

temporal fossa, a narrow fan-shaped space that covers the lateral surface of the skull. The major structure in the temporal fossa is the temporalis muscle. Also passing through the fossa are the zygomaticotemporal branches of the maxillary nerve.

temporal gyrus, any of three convolutions, inferior, middle, or superior, on the lateral surface of the temporal lobe of the brain.

temporalis /tem″pəral″is/, one of the four muscles of mastication. It is a broad radiating muscle that acts to close the jaws and retract the mandible. Also called **temporal muscle.** Compare **masseter, internal pterygoid muscle, external pterygoid muscle.**

temporal lobe, the lateral region of the cerebrum, below the lateral fissure. Within the temporal lobe of the brain is the center for smell and some association areas for memory and learning. Compare **frontal lobe, occipital lobe, parietal lobe.**

temporal lobe epilepsy, seizures that arise from the temporal lobe, often associated with mesial sclerosis. Patients may have an aura before these kinds of seizures.

temporal muscle. See **temporalis.**

temporal process, the posterior blunt process of the zygomatic bone that articulates with the zygomatic process of the temporal bone to form the zygomatic arch.

temporal subtraction, the subtraction of two or more digitized x-ray images that were acquired at different times. The subtraction process eliminates information in the image that was static. If contrast material is introduced into the organ during the period between two image acquisitions, the subtracted image will show only the space filled with the contrast material.

temporal summation. See **summation,** def. 2.

temporary absence. See **conditional discharge.**

temporary base. See **baseplate.**

temporary filling, a short-term use material that can restore missing tooth structure until such time as definitive treatment of the tooth is possible. It may incorporate sedative materials for pulpal pain.

temporary pacemaker /tem″pərer″ē/ [L, *temporalis,* temporary, *passus,* step; ME, *maken*], an electronic pacemaker used as an interim treatment when the heart rate is excessively low. It consists of either a pulse generator and battery attached outside the patient's body and connected to a transvenous electrode in the right ventricle or conductive pads placed on the chest and connected to an external pulse generator by cables.

temporary prosthesis. See **preparatory prosthesis.**

temporary removable splint [L, *temporalis,* temporary, *remover* + D, *splint*], any of a variety of dental appliances, including occlusal splints, used when limited stability of the teeth is required. It may be placed on or removed from teeth at will. Kinds include *Haley's orthodontic appliance, Elbrecht's cast metal splint.*

temporary stopping [L, *temporalis* + AS, *stoppian,* to stop up], a mixture of gutta-percha, zinc oxide, white wax, and coloring, used for temporarily sealing dressings in tooth cavities. It softens on heating and rehardens at room temperature but is not hard enough to be used effectively long term in tooth areas under occlusal stress. Compare **sedative filling, temporary filling.**

temporary tooth. See **primary dentition.**

temporomandibular /tem″pərō″mandib″yələr/ [L, *tempora,* the temples, *mandere,* to chew], pertaining to the articulation between the temporal bone and the condyles of the mandible.

T

temporomandibular joint (TMJ) [L, *tempora* + *mandere,* to chew, *jungere,* to join], one of a pair of joints connecting the mandible of the jaw to the temporal bone of the skull. It is a combined hinge and gliding joint formed by the anterior parts of the mandibular fossae of the temporal bone, the articular eminences, the condyles of the mandible, and five ligaments. The TMJ is the only joint in the body in which movement of one joint is always synchronous with movement of the other joint.

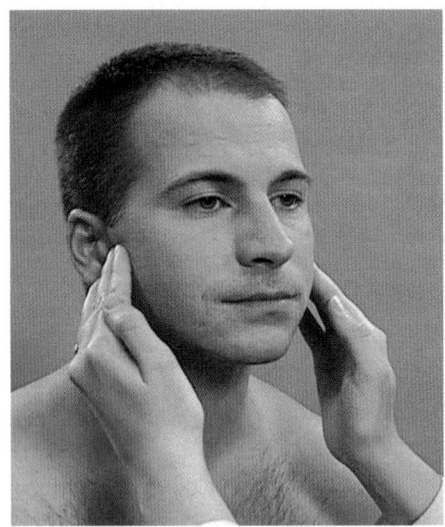

Palpation of the temporomandibular joint *(Seidel et al, 2011)*

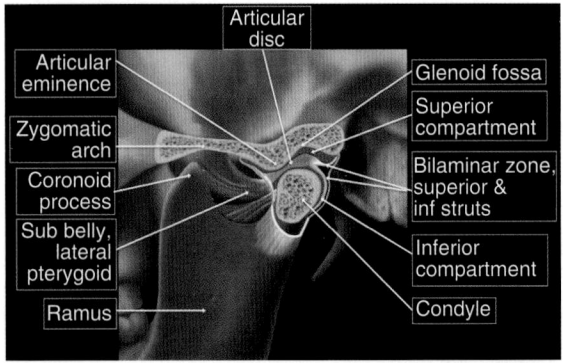

Temporomandibular joint *(Drake, Vogl, and Mitchell, 2010)*

temporomandibular joint capsule, a fibrous protective sheath enclosing the temporomandibular joint of the lower jaw.
temporomandibular joint (TMJ) disorder, dysfunction of the temporomandibular joint, marked by a clicking or grinding sensation in the joint and often by pain in or about the ears, tinnitus, tiredness, slight soreness of the jaw muscles on waking, and stiffness of the jaw or actual trismus. Numerous causes have been proposed, such as mandibular overclosure, stress, and lesions of the joint. Also called **TMJ disorder.**
temporomandibular joint (TMJ) pain dysfunction syndrome, an abnormal condition characterized by facial pain and mandibular dysfunction, apparently caused by a defective or dislocated temporomandibular joint. Some common indications of this syndrome are clicking of the joint when the jaws move, limitation of jaw movement, subluxation, and temporomandibular dislocation.

temporomandibular ligament [L, *temporalis* + *mandere,* to chew, *ligare,* to bind], an oblique band of connective tissue that extends downward and backward from the zygomatic process to the neck of the mandible.
temporomaxillary /-mak″siler′ē/, pertaining to the area of the temporal and maxillary bones.
temporooccipital /tem′pərō·oksip′itəl/, pertaining to the area of the temporal and occipital bones.
temporoparietal. See **parietotemporal.**
temporoparietalis /tem′pərōpərī′ətal″is/ [L, *temporalis* + *paries,* wall], one of a pair of broad, thin muscles of the scalp, which are divided into three parts that fan out over the temporal fascia and insert into the galea aponeurotica. The three parts include an anterior temporal part; a superior parietal part; and, in between, a triangular part. On both sides it acts in combination with the occipitofrontalis to wrinkle the forehead, widen the eyes, and raise the ears. It is innervated by branches of the facial nerve. Compare **occipitofrontalis.**
tempostabile /tem″po-sta′bil/, not subject to change with time.
temsirolimus, a biological response modifier.
- INDICATIONS: This drug is used to treat renal cell carcinoma.
- CONTRAINDICATIONS: Breastfeeding, pregnancy, and known hypersensitivity to this drug, sirolimus, or polysorbate 80 prohibit its use.
- ADVERSE EFFECTS: Adverse effects of this drug include seizures, hypertension, hypertriglyceridemia, hyperlipidemia, hyperglycemia, nausea, vomiting, diarrhea, constipation, pruritus, and metabolic acidosis. Life-threatening side effects include thrombophlebitis, bowel perforation, albuminuria, hematuria, proteinuria, renal failure, anemia, leukopenia, thrombocytopenia, interstitial lung disease, and lymphoma. Common side effects include headache and rash.
TEN, abbreviation for **toxic epidermal necrolysis.**
tenacious /tenā′shəs/ [L, *tenax,* holding fast], pertaining to secretions that are sticky or adhesive or otherwise tend to hold together, such as mucus and sputum.
tenacity /tenas′itē/ [L, *tenax,* holding fast], the ability to be persistent or remain attached.
tenaculum /tənak″yələm/ *pl.* **tenacula** [L, holder], a clip or clamp with long handles used to grasp, immobilize, and hold an organ or a piece of tissue. Kinds of tenacula include the abdominal tenaculum, which has long arms and small hooks; the forceps tenaculum, which has long hooks and is used in gynecological surgery; and the uterine or cervical tenaculum, which has short hooks or open, eye-shaped clamps used to hold the cervix.
tenalgia /tenal″jə/, pain referred to a tendon. Also called **tenodynia.**
tender, responding with a sensation of pain to pressure or touch that would not normally cause discomfort.
tendinitis /ten′dəni″tis/ [L, *tendere,* to stretch; Gk, *itis,* inflammation], inflammation of a tendon, usually resulting from strain. Treatment may include rest, corticosteroid injections, application of ice or heat, and support. Also spelled **tendonitis.**
tendino-. See **teno-, tenonto-, tendo-, tendino-.**
tendinous. See **tendon.**
tendinous arch, a linear thickening in the fascia covering the obturator internus muscle that is part of the attachment of the levator ani muscles to the pelvic wall.
tendinous cords. See **chordae tendineae.**
tendo /ten″dō/, a tendon, such as the tendo calcaneus, the Achilles tendon.
tendo-. See **teno-, tenonto-, tendo-, tendino-.**
tendo calcaneus. See **Achilles tendon.**
tendon /ten′dən/ [Gk, *tenon*], any one of many white, glistening bands of dense fibrous connective tissue that attach muscle to bone. Except at points of attachment, tendons are parallel bundles of collagenous fibers sheathed in delicate

fibroelastic connective tissue. Larger tendons contain a thin internal septum, a few blood vessels, and specialized stereognostic nerves. Tendons are extremely strong, flexible, and inelastic and occur in various lengths and thicknesses. Compare **ligament.** –**tendinous,** *adj.*

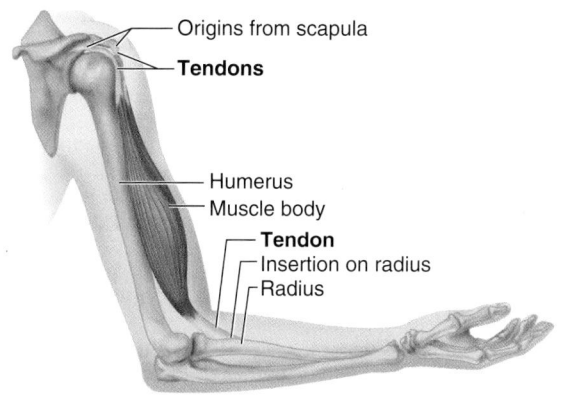

- Origins from scapula
- **Tendons**
- Humerus
- Muscle body
- **Tendon**
- Insertion on radius
- Radius

Tendon *(Patton and Thibodeau, 2010)*

tendon graft, a free graft of tendon used to replace a damaged tendon segment.

tendonitis. See **tendinitis.**

tendon of Achilles. See **Achilles tendon.**

tendon reflex. See **deep tendon reflex.**

tendosynovitis. See **tenosynovitis.**

tenecteplase /tĕ-nek′tĕ-plās/, a modified form of human tissue plasminogen activator produced by recombinant DNA technology; used as a thrombolytic agent in the treatment of myocardial infarction; administered intravenously.

tenesmic /tənez′mik/ [Gk, *tenedere,* to stretch], pertaining to or resembling tenesmus.

tenesmus /tənez″məs/ [Gk, *tendere,* to stretch], persistent, ineffectual spasms of the rectum or bladder, accompanied by the desire to empty the bowel or bladder, or ineffectual straining to evacuate the bowel or bladder. Intestinal tenesmus is a common complaint in inflammatory bowel disease and irritable bowel syndrome. –**tenesmic,** *adj.*

tenia /tē″nē·ə/, **1.** any anatomical bandlike structure, such as a band of muscle fibers. **2.** a bandage or tape.

tenia-, taenia-, combining form meaning "ribbon, band": *taeniasis, teniasis.*

teniasis /tēnī″əsis/, an infection of intestinal tapeworms of the genus *Taenia.*

tenia terminalis. See **terminal crest.**

tennis elbow. See **lateral humeral epicondylitis.**

teno-, tenonto-, tendo-, tendino-, combining form meaning "tendon": *tenodesis, tenodynia, tendinitis.*

tenodesis splint /tənod′əsis, ten′ōdē″sis/, a training device for individuals with no finger strength. The splint stabilizes the thumb with the fingers slightly flexed. When the wrist is extended, an adjustable cord attached to the wrist cuff pulls the long fingers into flexion, creating gross grasp ability and pinch function.

tenodynia. See **tenalgia.**

tenofibril. See **tonofibril.**

tenofovir, an antiretroviral agent.

■ INDICATIONS: This drug is prescribed to treat HIV-1 infection with other antiretrovirals.

■ CONTRAINDICATIONS: Known hypersensitivity to this drug prohibits its use.

■ ADVERSE EFFECTS: Common adverse effects include headache, nausea, vomiting, diarrhea, flatulence, and abdominal pain.

tenofovir disoproxil fumarate, a prodrug of tenofovir, used in the treatment of HIV-1 (human immunodeficiency virus-1) infection.

Tenon's capsule, a thin membranous socket that envelops the eyeball from the optic nerve to the ciliary region sinner surface, is pierced by vessels and nerves, and fuses with the sheath of the optic nerve and with the sclera. The lower part of the membrane thickens into the suspensory ligament, which attaches to the zygomatic arch and the lacrimal bones. Also called **fascia bulbi.**

tenonto-. See **teno-, tenonto-, tendo-, tendino-.**

tenophony /tenof″ənē/, a heart murmur associated with a defect in the chordae tendineae.

Tenormin, a beta-blocker medication. Brand name for **atenolol.**

tenosynovitis /ten′ōsin′əvī″tis/ [Gk, *tenon,* tendon, *syn,* together; L, *ovum,* egg; Gk, *itis*], inflammation of a tendon sheath caused by calcium deposits, repeated strain or trauma, high levels of blood cholesterol, rheumatoid arthritis, gout, or gonorrhea. In some instances, movement causes a crackling noise over the tendon. Most cases not associated with systemic disease respond to rest. Local injections of corticosteroids may provide relief; surgery is indicated if the condition persists. Also called **tendosynovitis.**

tenotomy /tenot″əmē/ [Gk, *tenon,* tendon, *temnein,* to cut], the total or partial severing of a tendon, performed to correct a muscle imbalance, such as in the correction of clubfoot or strabismus of the eye.

TENS, abbreviation for **transcutaneous electrical nerve stimulation (TENS).**

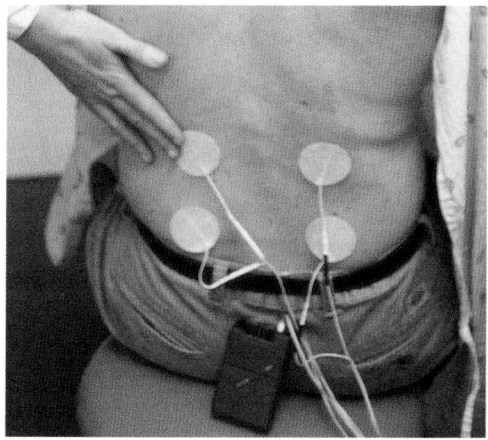

Transcutaneous electrical nerve stimulation (TENS)

Tensilon, an anticholinesterase drug. Brand name for **edrophonium chloride.**

Tensilon test, a diagnostic technique for verifying the signs of myasthenia gravis by testing the power of skeletal muscles before and after injection of edrophonium hydrochloride.

tensiometer /ten′sē·om″ətər/ [L, *tendere,* to stretch; Gk, *metron,* measure], a device for measuring the surface tension of a liquid.

tension /ten′shən/ [L, *tendere,* to stretch], **1.** the act of pulling or straining until taut. **2.** the condition of being taut, tense, or under pressure. **3.** a state or condition resulting from the psychological and physiological reaction to a stressful situation. It is characterized physically by a general increase in muscle tonus, heart rate, respiration rate, and alertness and psychologically by feelings of strain, uneasiness, irritability, and anxiety. See also **stress.**

tension headache, a pain that affects the head as the result of overwork or emotional strain and that involves tension in the muscles of the neck, face, and shoulder.

tension lines, cleavage lines.

tension pneumothorax [L, *tendere,* to stretch; Gk, *pneuma,* air, *thorax*], the presence of air in the pleural space when pleural pressure exceeds alveolar pressure, caused by a rupture through the chest wall or lung parenchyma associated with the valvular opening. Air passes through the valve during coughing but cannot escape on exhalation. Unrelieved pneumothorax can lead to respiratory arrest.

tensor /ten′sər/ [L, *tendere,* to stretch], any one of the muscles of the body that tenses a structure, such as the tensor fasciae latae of the thigh. Compare **abductor, adductor, depressor, sphincter.**

tensor fasciae latae, one of the 10 muscles of the gluteal region arising from the outer lip of the iliac crest, the anterior superior iliac spine, and the deep fascia lata. It lies between the two layers of fascia lata in the proximal third of the thigh and via the iliotibial band inserts onto the lateral tibial condyle (Gerty's tubercle). The tensor fasciae latae functions to flex the thigh and rotate it slightly medially. Also called *tensor fasciae femoris.*

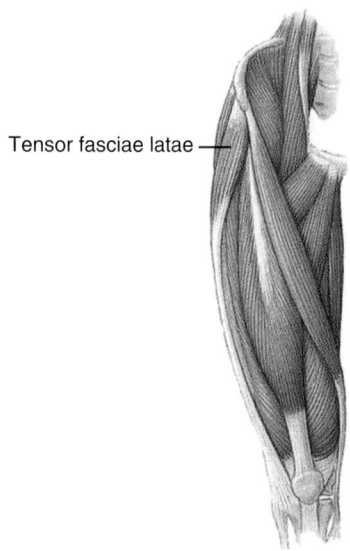

Tensor fasciae latae —

Tensor fasciae latae *(Patton and Thibodeau, 2010)*

tensor tympani /ten′sər tim′pə·nē/, a muscle originating in the cartilaginous portion of the auditory tube and inserting in the manubrium of the malleus. It functions to tense the tympanic membrane during loud noises.

tensor veli palatine, a muscle of the soft palate that is composed of a vertical muscular part and a more horizontal fibrous part that forms the palatine aponeurosis. It tenses the soft palate so that the other muscles attached to the palate can work more effectively, and it opens the pharyngotympanic tube when the palate moves during yawning and swallowing.

tent [ME, *tente*], **1.** a transparent cover, usually of plastic, supported over the upper part of a patient by a frame. Used in the treatment of respiratory conditions, it provides a controlled environment into which steam, oxygen, vaporized

medication, or droplets of cool water may be sprayed, such as an oxygen tent. **2.** a cone made of various materials inserted into a cavity or orifice of the body to dilate its opening, such as a laminaria tent. **3.** a pack placed in a wound to hold it open to ensure that healing progresses from the base of the wound upward to the skin.

tentative /ten′tətiv/ [L, *tentare,* to touch], not final or definite, such as an experimental finding that has not been validated.

tenth cranial nerve. See **vagus nerve.**

tenth-value layer (TVL) [ME, *tenpe* + L, *valere,* to be worth; AS, *lecgan,* to lie], the thickness of material required to attenuate a beam of radiation to one tenth of its original intensity. See also **half-value layer.**

tenting of skin /ten″ting/, a slow return of the skin to its normal position after being pinched, a sign of either dehydration, aging, or both. See also **skin turgor.**

-tention, -tension, combining form meaning "condition of being stretched or strained, or in which pressure is exerted": *attention, distension.*

tentoria, a fold of dura mater. See **tentorium.**

tentorial herniation /tentôr′ē·əl/ [L, *tentorium,* tent, *hernia,* rupture], the protrusion of brain tissue into the tentorial notch, caused by increased intracranial pressure resulting from edema, hemorrhage, or a tumor. Characteristic signs are severe headache, fever, flushing, sweating, abnormal pupillary reflex, drowsiness, hypotension, and loss of consciousness. Also called **transtentorial herniation.**

tentorial notch [L, *tentorium,* tent; OFr, *enochier*], an area occupied by the midbrain and enclosed by the free border of the tentorium cerebelli and the sphenoid bone.

tentorium /tentôr″ē·əm/ *pl. tentoria* [L, tent], any part of the body that resembles a tent, such as the tentorium of the hypophysis that covers the hypophyseal fossa.

tentorium cerebelli. See **cerebellar tentorium.**

Tenuate, an anorexiant medication for the short-term treatment of obesity. Brand name for **diethylpropion hydrochloride.**

tenure /ten′yər/ [L, *tenere,* to hold], **1.** (in a university) a faculty appointment with few limits on the number of years it may be held. **2.** a permanent appointment usually awarded to a person who has advanced to the rank of associate professor and who demonstrates scholarship, community service, and teaching excellence in a specific field of study.

TEP, abbreviation for **tracheoesophageal puncture.**

-tepa, combining form for antineoplastic thiotepa derivatives.

tephr-, combining form meaning "gray" or "ash-colored": *tephra.*

tephra, the material produced by volcanic eruptions.

tepid, moderately warm to the touch.

teprotide /tep″rōtīd/, a bradykinin-potentiating peptide.

tera-, prefix meaning "one trillion": *terabyte, terahertz.*

teramorphous [Gk, *teras,* monster, *morphe,* form], of the nature of or characteristic of a teratic embryo.

teras /ter″əs/ *pl. terata* [Gk, monster], a severely deformed fetus. −*teratic, adj.*

teratic embryo, a fetus that is grossly malformed and usually nonviable. See also **teratism.**

teratism /ter′ətiz′əm/, any congenital or developmental anomaly that is produced by inherited or environmental factors or a combination of the two. Any condition in which a severely malformed fetus is produced. Also called **teratosis.** Kinds include **atresic teratism, ceasmic teratism, ectopic teratism, ectrogenic teratism, hypergenetic teratism, symphysic teratism.**

terato-, combining form meaning "monster": *teratoblastoma, teratogenesis, teratoma.*

teratoblastoma /ter′ətō′blastō″mə/, a teratoma in which not all germ layers are present.

teratogen /ter″ətəjen′/ [Gk, *teras* + *genein,* to produce], any substance, agent, or process that interferes with normal prenatal development, causing the formation of one or more developmental abnormalities in the fetus. Teratogens act directly on the developing organism or indirectly, affecting such supplemental structures as the placenta or some maternal system. The type and extent of the defect are determined by the specific kind of teratogen, its mode of action, the embryonic process affected, genetic predisposition, and the stage of development at the time the exposure occurred. The period of highest vulnerability in the developing embryo is from about the third through the twelfth week of gestation, when differentiation of the major organs and systems occurs. Susceptibility to teratogenic influence decreases rapidly in the later periods of development, which are characterized by growth and elaboration. Among the known teratogens are chemical agents, including such drugs as thalidomide, alkylating agents, and alcohol; infectious agents, especially the rubella virus and cytomegalovirus; ionizing radiation, particularly x-rays; and environmental factors, such as the age and general health of the mother or any intrauterine trauma that may affect the fetus, especially during the later stages of pregnancy. Also called **teratogenic agent.** Compare **mutagen.** –*teratogenic, adj.*

teratogenesis /ter′ətōjen″əsis/, the development of physical defects in the embryo. Also called **teratogeny.** –*teratogenetic, adj.*

teratogenic agent. See **teratogen.**

teratogenous /ter′ətoj″ənəs/ [Gk, *teras,* monster, *genein,* to produce], developed from fetal membranes.

teratogeny. See **teratogenesis.**

teratoid /ter″ətoid/ [Gk, *teras* + *eidos,* form], **1.** pertaining to malformed physical development. **2.** grossly misplaced, misshapen parts.

teratoid tumor. See **dermoid cyst.**

teratologic, teratological, pertaining to abnormalities of the human body. See **teratology.**

teratologist /ter′ətol″əjist/, one who specializes in the causes and effects of congenital anomalies and developmental abnormalities.

teratology /-tol′əgē/ [Gk, *teras* + *logos,* science], the study of the causes and effects of congenital malformations and developmental abnormalities. –*teratological, teratologic, adj.*

teratoma /ter′ətō″mə/, a tumor composed of different kinds of tissue, none of which normally occurs together or at the site of the tumor. Teratomas are most common in the ovaries or testes.

teratosis. See **teratism.**

terazosin /ter′əzō″sin/, a drug approved for the treatment of benign prostatic hypertrophy. It acts by relaxing the smooth muscle fibers of the prostate through its alpha receptor blockage mechanisms. It is also used alone or in combination for the treatment of hypertension.

terbium (Tb) /tur′bē·əm/ [Ytterby, Sweden], a rare earth metallic element. Its atomic number is 65; its atomic mass is 158.294.

terbutaline sulfate /terbyoo′təlēn/, a beta$_2$-adrenergic stimulant.

■ INDICATIONS: It is prescribed as a bronchodilator in the treatment of asthma, bronchitis, and emphysema and as a uterine relaxant to treat premature labor.

■ CONTRAINDICATIONS: Cardiac arrhythmias or known hypersensitivity to this drug prohibits its use. Toxicity is increased by monoamine oxidase inhibitors and tricyclic antidepressants, and beta-adrenergic blocker effects are decreased.

■ ADVERSE EFFECTS: Among the most serious effects are dizziness and palpitations. Nervousness and tremor are common reactions.

teres /tir″ēz, ter′ēz/ *pl. teretes* [L, rounded], a long cylindrical muscle such as the teres minor or the teres major. –**teres,** *adj.*

teres major, a thick, flat muscle of the shoulder. It functions to adduct, extend, and rotate the arm medially. Compare **teres minor.**

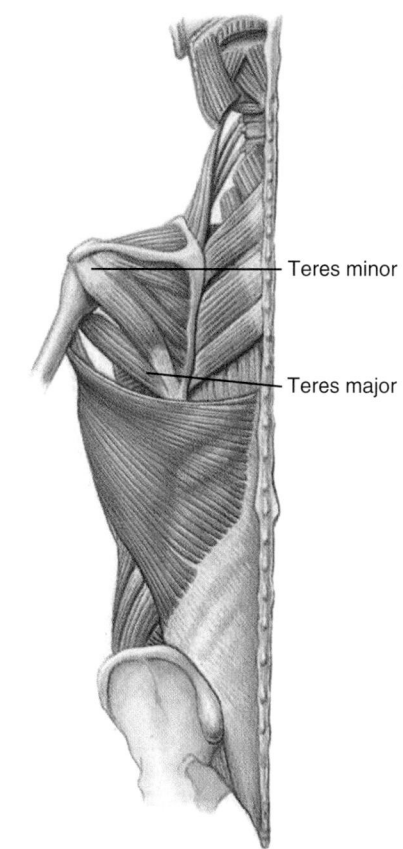

Teres minor

Teres major

Teres major and teres minor *(Patton and Thibodeau, 2010)*

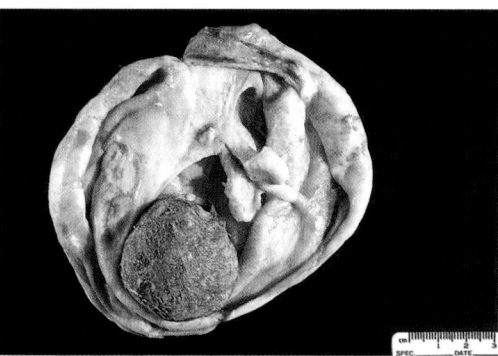

Cystic teratoma of the ovary *(Courtesy Dr. Christopher Crum, Brigham and Women's Hospital)*

teres minor, a cylindric, elongated muscle of the shoulder. It functions to rotate the arm laterally, weakly adduct the arm, and draw the humerus toward the glenoid fossa of the scapula, strengthening the shoulder joint. Compare **teres major.**

teriparatide, a parathyroid hormone used to treat postmenopausal women with osteoporosis and men with primary hypogonadal osteoporosis at high risk for fracture.

term [L, *terminus,* limit], **1.** a specified period of time. **2.** the normal gestation period.

terminal /tur′minəl/ [L, *terminus,* boundary], **1.** (of a structure or process) near or approaching its end, such as a terminal bronchiole or a terminal disease. **2.** an input/output (I/O) device that has two-way communication capability with a computer. A terminal usually has a keyboard and a video display screen, or a text printing facility. −**terminus,** *n.,* −**terminate,** *v.*

terminal arteriole [L, *terminus,* boundary, *arteriola,* little artery], an arteriole that divides into capillaries.

terminal artery. See **end artery.**

terminal bronchiole. See **bronchiole.**

terminal cancer [L, *terminalis* + *cancer,* crab], an advanced stage of a malignant neoplastic disease with death as the inevitable prognosis.

terminal crest, a vertical crest on the interior wall of the right atrium that separates the sinus of the vena cava from the rest of the right atrium. Also called *crista terminalis,* **tenia terminalis.**

terminal drop, a rapid decline in cognitive function and coping ability that occurs 1 to 5 years before death.

terminal illness [L, *terminalis* + ONorse, *illr,* bad], an advanced stage of a disease with an unfavorable prognosis and no known cure.

terminal insomnia, a chronic sleep disturbance occurring at the end of a sleep period. It may be indicative of an underlying depressive disorder and treated with an antidepressant.

terminal nerve, a small nerve originating in the vomeronasal epithelium, projecting to the cerebral hemisphere in the region of the olfactory trigone. It is classified by most anatomists as part of the olfactory, or first cranial, nerve. It courses anteriorly along the olfactory tract and passes through the ethmoid bone. It communicates in the nasal cavity with the ophthalmic division of the trigeminal nerve.

terminal part of ileum, the part just before the ileum meets the cecum at the ileal orifice and ileal papilla. Also called *terminal ileum.*

terminal saccular period, the period or phase of prenatal lung development lasting, in different parts of the lungs, from the twenty-sixth week or later until near term and followed by the alveolar period. Walls of the air spaces become thinner and the spaces divide into alveolar saccules with adjacent capillaries; type I and type II alveolar cells begin functioning, and surfactant is secreted. Also called *terminal saccular phase.*

terminal sacs, thin-walled dilations that develop at the ends of the respiratory bronchioles during fetal development; they develop a close relationship with the capillaries, and their appearance marks the point at which limited respiration becomes possible. Also called *primitive alveoli, primordial alveoli, terminal saccules.*

terminal stance, one of the five stages in the stance phase of a walking gait, directly associated with the continuation of single limb support or the period during which the body moves forward on the supporting foot. Double limb support is initiated during the latter part of terminal stance, which is often a factor in the analysis of many abnormal orthopedic conditions and the diagnosis of weaknesses that may develop in certain muscles used in walking, such as the quadriceps femoris and the gluteus maximus. Compare **initial contact**

stance stage, loading response stance stage, midstance, preswing stance stage. See also **swing phase of gait.**

terminal sulcus of the right atrium, a shallow channel on the external surface of the right atrium between the superior and inferior vena cava. Also called **sulcus terminalis cordis.**

terminal sulcus of the tongue, a V-shaped depression on the oral and pharyngeal surfaces of the tongue that forms the inferior margin of the fauces between the oral and pharyngeal cavities.

terminate. See **terminal.**

termination codon /tur′minā″shən/, a three-nucleotide sequence (UAA, UAG, or UGA) in messenger RNA that specifies the end of the sequence of amino acids in a polypeptide.

termination phase, the last stage of a therapeutic relationship when attained goals are evaluated and outcomes achieved. During this stage practitioners also may help patients establish networks of support, other than the therapist-patient relationship, that may help in coping with future problems.

termination sequence, (in molecular genetics) a deoxyribonucleic acid (DNA) segment at the end of a unit that is transcribed to messenger ribonucleic acid from the DNA template.

term infant [L, *terminus,* limit], any neonate, regardless of birth weight, born after the end of the thirty-seventh and before the beginning of the forty-third week of gestation. Infants delivered at term usually measure from 48 to 53 cm from head to heel and weigh between 2700 and 4000 g.

terminus /tur′minəs/ [L, the end], **1.** a boundary or limit. **2.** See **terminal.**

terpin /tur″pin/, **1.** a diterpene alcohol derived from turpentine oil. **2.** an expectorant ingredient produced through the action of nitric and sulfuric acids on pine oil.

terpin hydrate and codeine elixir /tur″pin/, a preparation of the expectorant terpin hydrate, with sweet orange peel tincture, benzaldehyde, glycerin, alcohol, syrup, water, and the antitussive opiate codeine. Terpin hydrate diminishes secretions and promotes healing of the mucous membrane, and codeine depresses the cough center in the medulla oblongata. Prolonged use may lead to addiction.

Terramycin, an antibiotic medication. Brand name for **oxytetracycline.**

territorial /ter′ətôr″ē·əl/ [L, *territorium,* district], a type of body movement that aids in communication. A territorial will frame an interaction and define an individual's "territory." See also **territoriality.**

territoriality /ter′itôr·ē·al″itē/, an emotional attachment to and defense of certain areas related to one's existence. Humans and animals generally establish a claim to or occupy a defined or undefined area over which they can maintain some degree of control.

terti-, combining form meaning "third": *tertiary, tertian.*

tertian /tur″shən/ [L, *tertius,* third], occurring every 48 hours, including the first day of occurrence, such as vivax or tertian malaria, in which fever occurs every third day. Compare **quartan.** See also **malaria.**

tertian malaria, a form of malaria caused by the protozoan *Plasmodium vivax* or *P. ovale,* characterized by febrile paroxysms that occur every 48 hours. Vivax malaria, caused by *P. vivax,* is the most common form of malaria. Although it is rarely fatal, it is the most difficult form to cure. Relapses are common. Ovale malaria, caused by *P. ovale,* is usually milder and causes only a few short attacks. Both types of tertian malaria are treated with chloroquine. Compare **falciparum malaria, quartan malaria.** See also **malaria.**

tertiary /tur″shē·er·ē, tursh″ərē/ [L, *tertius,* third], **1.** third in frequency or order of use. **2.** belonging to the third level of sophistication of development, such as a tertiary health care facility.

tertiary bronchial buds, outgrowths of the secondary bronchial buds, which become the bronchopulmonary segments of the mature lung.

tertiary bronchus. See **bronchus.**

tertiary health care, a specialized, highly technical level of health care that includes diagnosis and treatment of disease and disability. Specialized intensive care units, advanced diagnostic support services, and highly specialized personnel are usually characteristic of tertiary health care. It offers highly centralized care to the population of a large region and in some cases to the world.

tertiary intention. See **intention.**

tertiary prevention, a level of preventive medicine that deals with the rehabilitation and return of a patient to a status of maximum usefulness with a minimum risk of recurrence of a physical or mental disorder. The scope of tertiary prevention includes the long-term management and treatment of a patient with a terminal disease to maintain the quality of life.

tertiary syphilis [L, *tertius,* third], the most advanced stage of syphilis, resulting in infections of the cardiovascular and neurological systems and marked by destructive lesions involving many tissues and organs. Late-stage syphilis is symptomatic but not contagious.

tervalent. See **trivalent.**

tesla /tes′lə/ [Nikola Tesla, American engineer, 1856–1943], a unit of magnetic flux density, defined by the International System of Units as 1 weber per square meter, the equivalent of 1 volt/second per square meter, or 10,000 gauss.

Teslac, an antineoplastic medication. Brand name for **testolactone.**

Tessalon, a local anesthetic agent. Brand name for **benzonatate.**

test [L, *testum,* crucible], **1.** *n.,* an examination or trial intended to establish a principle or determine a value. **2.** *n.,* a chemical reaction or reagent that has clinical significance. **3.** *v.,* to detect, identify, or conduct a trial. See also **laboratory test.**

test-, combining form meaning "testicle": *testis, testosterone.*

testa /tes′tə/ [L, a shell], **1.** an eggshell. **2.** powdered oyster shells used in antacids. **3.** the outer coat of a seed.

Testacealobosia /tes′təsē′lōbā″zhə/, a subclass of ameboid protozoa in which the cells are enclosed in a chitinous or membranous envelope, vest, or shell. It includes both marine and freshwater forms.

testamentary capacity /tes′təmen″tərē/, a person's competency to make a will, including awareness that a will is being made, awareness of the nature and extent of property covered by the will, and awareness of the identities of beneficiaries.

testcross [L, *testum + crux,* cross], **1.** a cross between a dominant and a recessive phenotype to determine either the degree of genetic linkage or whether the dominant phenotype is a result of a homozygous or a heterozygous genotype. **2.** a subject undergoing such a test. See also **backcross.**

testes, the two male gonads that produce sperm and testosterone.

testes determining factor (TDF) /tes′tēz/, a gene on the Y chromosome that is believed to determine male sexual development. Individuals with the normal female sex chromosome combination (XX) may develop as males if the TDF gene has migrated to one of the X chromosomes. Also, individuals with the normal male sex chromosome pair (XY) may

develop as females if the TDF gene is missing from the Y chromosome.

test for acetone in urine, a part of routine urinalysis. Normal findings are negative because acetone and other ketones are not normally present in urine. Exceptions include such cases as poorly controlled diabetic patients, alcoholics, and people who may be fasting or on special high-protein diets.

test for lacrimation, a test for possible dry eye and/or keratoconjunctivitis sicca conducted by placing a 35-mm long piece of filter paper in the lower fornix of the conjunctiva for 5 minutes. Failure of tears to wet as much as 10 mm of the strip indicates inadequate tear production. Also called **Schirmer test.**

testicle. See **testis.**

testicular /testik″yələr/ [L, *testiculus,* testicle], pertaining to the testicle.

testicular artery, one of a pair of long, slender branches of the abdominal aorta, arising inferior to the renal arteries and supplying the testis.

testicular cancer, a malignant neoplastic disease of the testis occurring most frequently in men between 15 and 35 years of age. An undescended testicle is often involved. In many cases the tumor is detected after an injury, but trauma is not considered a causative factor. Patients with early testicular cancer are often asymptomatic, and metastases may be present in lymph nodes, the lungs, and the liver before the primary lesion is palpable. In the later stages there may be pulmonary symptoms, ureteral obstruction, gynecomastia, and an abdominal mass. Diagnostic measures include transillumination of the scrotum, excretory urography, lymphangiography, and a urine or serum test to evaluate circulating levels of tumor markers. Tumors develop more often in the right than in the left testis. Testis cancers are often curable. Chemotherapeutic agents, used in various combinations, are increasing the survival of patients with testicular cancer. Some of these drugs are actinomycin D, bleomycin, *cis*-platinum, cyclophosphamide, methotrexate, and vincristine. Early detection by testicular self-examination enhances chances of cure.

testicular duct. See **vas deferens.**

testicular feminization. See **feminization.**

testicular hormone, any androgenic steroid hormone secreted by the Leydig cells in the interstitial tissues of the male gonads. Testosterone is the principal hormone secreted by the cells, which also secrete estrogen, the female sex hormone. Testosterone may be converted into estrogen and other steroid hormones, such as dihydrotestosterone, in certain tissues. The secretion of testicular hormones is controlled by luteinizing hormone and follicle-stimulating hormone, both secreted by the anterior pituitary gland.

testicular microlithiasis, the presence of tiny calcifications in the seminiferous tubules. In some cases this precedes development of a tumor.

testicular self-examination (TSE), a procedure for detecting tumors or other abnormalities in the male testes. The TSE is conducted in four simple steps, starting by standing in front of a mirror and looking for any swelling on the skin of the scrotum. One testicle may appear larger than the other, and one may hang lower, which is usually normal. Next, each testicle is examined with both hands, placing the fingers under the testicle while the thumbs are placed on top. The testicle is then rolled gently between the thumbs and fingers. In the next step the epididymis, a normal cordlike structure on the top and back of each testicle, should be found. A small pea-sized lump is felt for on the front or side of a testicle. The lump is usually painless. TSE should

T

be performed once a month, usually after a warm bath or shower because the heat causes scrotal skin to relax, thereby increasing the chances of detecting any tissue abnormality. Testicular cancer almost always occurs in only one testicle. It is highly curable when detected at an early stage.

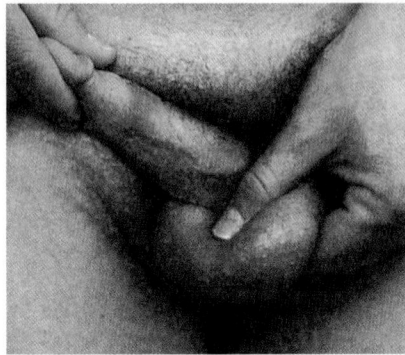

Testicular self-examination *(Seidel et al, 2011)*

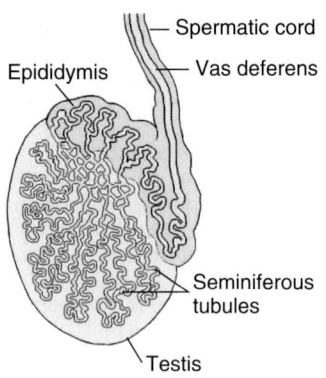

Testis *(Shiland, 2010)*

testicular sperm extraction (TESE), for men with obstructive azoospermia, extraction of spermatozoa directly from the testis through the skin.

testicular vein, one of a pair of veins emerging from convoluted venous plexuses, forming the greater mass of the spermatic cords. The right testicular vein opens into the inferior vena cava, the left testicular vein into the left renal vein. Both testicular veins contain valves. Compare **ovarian vein.**

testimony /tes″timō′nē/ [L, *testimonium,* evidence], the statement of a witness, usually made orally and given under oath, such as at a court trial.

testis /tes″tēz′/ *pl. testes,* one of the pair of male gonads that produces sperm and testosterone. The adult testes are suspended in the scrotum by the spermatic cords; in early fetal life they are contained in the abdominal cavity behind the peritoneum. Before birth they normally descend into the scrotum. The coverings of the testes are the skin and the dartos tunic of the scrotum, the external spermatic fascia, the cremasteric layer, the internal spermatic fascia, and the tunica vaginalis. Each testis is a laterally compressed oval body about 4 cm long and 2.5 cm wide that weighs about 12 g. It is positioned obliquely in the scrotum, with the cranial extremity directed ventrally and slightly laterally and the caudal end directed dorsally and slightly medially. The anterior border, lateral surfaces, and extremities of the organ are convex, free, smooth, and covered by the tunica vaginalis. The convoluted epididymis lying on the posterior border of the testis contains a tightly coiled tube that is about 20 feet long and connects with the vas deferens through which spermatozoa pass during ejaculation. Each testis consists of several hundred conical lobules containing the tiny coiled seminiferous tubules, each about 75 mm long, in which spermatozoa develop. In early life the tubules are pale in color, but in old age they become invested with yellow fatty matter. The tubules converge to form the rete testis, which is drained by the efferent ducts into the head of the epididymis. The testes are supplied with blood by the two internal spermatic arteries that arise from the aorta, are served by the testicular veins that form the pampiniform plexuses constituting the greater part of the spermatic cords, and are innervated by the spermatic plexuses of nerves from the celiac plexuses of the autonomic nervous system. Also called **testicle.** Compare **ovary.** See also **scrotum. –testicular,** *adj.*

test method, a method chosen for experimental testing or study by means of method evaluation.

test of patency of tear duct, a procedure in which drops of a weak sugar solution are placed in the eye. If the patient then detects a sweet taste, the tear duct is assumed open.

testolactone /tes′təlak″tōn/, an antineoplastic androgen analog.

■ INDICATIONS: It is prescribed as palliative treatment of advanced postmenopausal breast cancer and in premenopausal women whose ovarian function has been terminated.

■ CONTRAINDICATIONS: Pregnancy, lactation, or known hypersensitivity to this drug prohibits its use. It is not given to men.

■ ADVERSE EFFECTS: Among the more serious adverse effects are hypercalcemia and peripheral neuropathies with numbness or tingling.

testosterone /testos″tərōn/, a naturally occurring androgenic hormone.

■ INDICATIONS: It is prescribed for androgen deficiency, for female breast cancer, and for stimulation of growth, weight gain, and red blood cell production.

■ CONTRAINDICATIONS: Cancer of the male breast or prostate, liver disease, pregnancy or suspected pregnancy, or known hypersensitivity to this drug prohibits its use.

■ ADVERSE EFFECTS: Among the more serious adverse effects are hepatic dysfunction, fluid retention, masculinization, acne, and erythrocythemia.

testosterone cypionate, a long-acting form of testosterone. Also called *testosterone cyclopentylpropionate.*

testosterone derivative. See **anabolic steroid.**

testosterone enanthate, a long-acting form of testosterone.

testosterone propionate, an androgen given intramuscularly. See also **testosterone.**

testosterone test, a blood test that detects levels of circulating testosterone in men and women. It may be used to evaluate ambiguous sex characteristics, precocious puberty, virilizing syndromes in the female, and infertility in the male. It can also be used as a tumor marker for rare tumors of the ovary and testicle.

test tube, a thin glass container with one open end and one closed end. It is used in many common laboratory procedures. Compare **Veillon tube.** See also **tube.**

test tube baby, *(Informal)* a term for an infant conceived through in vitro fertilization by using an ovum removed from the mother. After fertilization the zygote is transplanted to the mother's uterus to develop normally. See also **in vitro fertilization.**

TET, 1. abbreviation for *treadmill exercise test.* **2.** abbreviation for **tubal embryo transfer.**

-tetanic /tetan'ik/, suffix meaning "tetanus" or "tetany": *posttetanic potentiation.*

tetanic contraction [Gk, *tetanos,* extreme tension; L, *contractio,* drawing together], a condition of continuous contraction in a voluntary muscle caused by a steady stream of efferent nerve impulses. Also called *tetanic convulsion.* See also **physiological tetanus.**

tetanic spasm. See **physiological tetanus.**

tetano-, combining form meaning "tetanus": *tetanolysin.*

tetanolysin, a toxin produced by *Clostridium tetani* bacteria.

tetanus /tet″ənəs/ [Gk, *tetanos,* extreme tension], an acute, potentially fatal infection of the central nervous system caused by the exotoxin tetanospasmin and elaborated by the anaerobic bacillus, *Clostridium tetani.* The toxin is a neurotoxin and one of the most lethal poisons known. *C. tetani* infects only wounds that contain dead tissue. The bacillus is a common resident of the superficial layers of the soil and a normal inhabitant of the intestinal tracts of cows and horses; therefore barnyards and fields fertilized with manure are heavily contaminated.

■ OBSERVATIONS: The bacillus may enter the body through a puncture wound, abrasion, laceration, or burn; via the uterus into the bloodstream in septic abortion or postpartum sepsis; or through the stump of the umbilical cord of the newborn. The dead tissue of the area is low in oxygen. This is the environment essential for the replication of *C. tetani.* The infection occurs in two clinical forms: one with an abrupt onset, high mortality, and a short incubation period (3 to 21 days); the other with less severe symptoms, a lower mortality, and a longer incubation period (4 to 5 weeks). Wounds of the face, head, and neck are the ones most likely to result in fatal infection. The disease is characterized by irritability, headache, fever, and painful spasms of the muscles resulting in lockjaw, risus sardonicus, opisthotonos, and laryngeal spasm; eventually every muscle of the body is in tonic spasm. The motor nerves transmit the impulses from the infected central nervous system to the muscles. There is no lesion; even at autopsy no organic lesion is seen and the cerebrospinal fluid is clear and normal.

■ INTERVENTIONS: Prompt and thorough cleansing and debridement of the wound are essential for prophylaxis. A booster shot of tetanus toxoid is given to previously immunized people; tetanus immune globulin and a series of three injections of tetanus toxoid are given to those not immunized. People who are known to have been adequately immunized within 5 years do not usually require immunization. Treatment of people who have the infection includes maintenance of an airway, administration of an antitoxin as soon as possible, sedation, control of the muscle spasms, and assurance of a normal fluid balance. The room is kept quiet, and benzodiazepines may be given to reduce hypertonicity; penicillin G, metronidazole or doxycycline are antibiotics of choice administered for infection; and a tracheostomy is performed and oxygen given for ventilation.

■ PATIENT CARE CONSIDERATIONS: The health care provider may encourage everyone to be actively immunized against the infection. The vaccine is safe and effective.

tetanus and diphtheria toxoids (Td), an active immunizing agent containing detoxified tetanus and diphtheria toxoids that slowly produce an antigenic response to the diseases.

■ INDICATIONS: This drug is used for prophylaxis when treating wounds and is the preferred method for immunization against tetanus and diphtheria in adults and children over 7 years of age. Younger children should be treated with diphtheria, pertussis, and tetanus trivalent vaccine.

■ CONTRAINDICATIONS: Immunosuppression, concomitant use of corticosteroids, or acute infection prohibits the use of this drug.

■ ADVERSE EFFECTS: Among the most serious adverse effects are allergic reactions and stinging at the site of injection.

tetanus antitoxin (TAT), a tetanus immune serum that neutralizes exotoxins in tetanus infection.

■ INDICATIONS: This drug is prescribed for short-term immunization against tetanus after possible exposure to the organism and in tetanus treatment.

■ CONTRAINDICATIONS: This drug is not given if the more effective tetanus immune globulin is available or if there is a known sensitivity to equine serum.

■ ADVERSE EFFECTS: Among the most serious adverse effects are allergic reactions and pain and inflammation at the site of injection.

tetanus immune globulin (TIG), an injectable solution prepared from the globulin of an immune human. It is effective and much safer than tetanus antitoxin.

■ INDICATIONS: This drug is prescribed for short-term immunization against tetanus after possible exposure to the organism and for tetanus treatment.

■ CONTRAINDICATIONS: Known hypersensitivity to this drug prohibits its use. It should not be substituted for tetanus toxoid.

■ ADVERSE EFFECTS: The most serious adverse effect is anaphylaxis. Fever, pain, and inflammation at the site of injection may occur.

tetanus toxin, the potent exotoxin produced by *Clostridium tetani* and consisting of two components, one a neurotoxin (tetanospasmin) and the other a hemolysin (tetanolysin).

tetanus toxoid, an active immunizing agent prepared from detoxified tetanus toxin that produces an antigenic response in the body, conferring permanent immunity to tetanus infection.

■ INDICATIONS: It is prescribed for primary active immunization against tetanus, generally in combination with diphtheria and pertussis vaccines.

■ CONTRAINDICATIONS: Immunosuppression or immunoglobulin abnormalities, acute infection, or illness prohibits its use.

■ ADVERSE EFFECTS: The most serious adverse effect is hypersensitivity. Pain and inflammation at the site of injection may occur.

tetany /tet′ənē/ [Gk, *tetanos,* extreme tension], a condition characterized by cramps, convulsions, twitching of the muscles, and sharp flexion of the wrist and ankle joints. These symptoms are sometimes accompanied by attacks of stridor. Tetany is a manifestation of an abnormality in calcium metabolism, which can occur in association with vitamin D deficiency, hypoparathyroidism, alkalosis, or the ingestion of alkaline salts. Kinds include **duration tetany, hyperventilation tetany, hypocalcemic tetany.**

tetra- /tet′rə/, combining form meaning "four": *tetrabasic, tetradactyly.*

tetrabasic /tet′rəbā″sik/, **1.** *adj.,* describing a compound that has four acidic hydrogen atoms replaced by metal ions. **2.** *n.,* an alcohol containing four hydroxyl groups.

tetracaine hydrochloride, a local anesthetic used for long-term spinal block and topical anesthesia.

2,3,7,8-tetrachlorodibenzo-*para*-dioxin. See **dioxin.**

tetrachloroethane /-klôr′ō·eth″ān/, a potentially toxic solvent with a sweet, chloroform-like odor. It is used to dissolve fats, waxes, oils, and resins and in the manufacture of paints, varnishes, and rust removers. Symptoms of overexposure include nausea, vomiting, abdominal pain, finger tremors, skin disorders, and liver damage.

tetrachloromethane. See **carbon tetrachloride.**

tetracycline hydrochloride, an antibiotic.

■ INDICATIONS: It is prescribed in the treatment of bacterial infections.

■ CONTRAINDICATIONS: Known hypersensitivity to this drug or to other tetracyclines prohibits its use. Use during pregnancy or in children under 8 years of age may result in discoloration of the child's teeth. It is to be administered with caution with renal or liver impairment.

■ ADVERSE EFFECTS: Among the most serious effects are potentially serious superinfections, allergic reactions, phototoxicity, and GI disturbances.

tetrad /tet″rad/ [Gk, *tetra,* four], a group of four chromatids of a synapsed pair of homologous chromosomes during the first meiotic prophase of gametogenesis. The group is formed in preparation for the two meiotic divisions in the maturation of gametes. −**tetradic,** *adj.*

tetradactyly /-dak′tilē/ [Gk, *tetra* + *dactylos*], the presence of only four fingers on each hand or four toes on each foot (quadridigitate).

tetradic, having four parts. See **tetrad.**

tetraethyl lead /tet′rə·eth″il led/, a potentially toxic gasoline additive. Overexposure can occur in the workplace but is also seen in gas sniffing, a form of substance abuse. Effects of overexposure include insomnia, lassitude, anxiety, nausea, tremor, pallor, hypothermia, anorexia, and psychosis.

tetrahydrobiopterin /tet′rə·hī′drō·bī·op′tər·in/, a compound related to folic acid that functions as a coenzyme in the reactions hydroxylating phenylalanine, tryptophan, and tyrosine by carrying electrons to oxygen. Defects in its biosynthesis or regeneration affect all three hydroxylation reactions, interfere with production of the corresponding neurotransmitter precursors, and result in malignant hyperphenylalaninemia.

tetrahydrocannabinol (THC) /-hi′drōkənab′inol/, the active principle, occurring as two psychotomimetic isomers, in the hemp plant *Cannabis sativa,* used in the preparation of marijuana, hashish, bhang, and ganja. THC increases pulse rate and has variable effects on blood pressure. It causes conjunctival reddening and a feeling of euphoria. The drug affects memory, cognition, and the sensorium; decreases motor coordination; and increases appetite. Nonintoxicating doses of THC are used experimentally in the treatment of glaucoma and to relieve nausea and increase the appetite in patients receiving cancer chemotherapy. See also **cannabis.**

tetrahydrozoline hydrochloride /-hīdroz″əlēn/, an adrenergic vasoconstrictor.

■ INDICATIONS: It is prescribed for the treatment of nasal and nasopharyngeal congestion and as an ophthalmic vasoconstrictor.

■ CONTRAINDICATIONS: Glaucoma or known hypersensitivity to this drug or to other vasoconstrictors prohibits its use. It is used with caution in patients who have cardiovascular disease.

■ ADVERSE EFFECTS: Among the more serious adverse effects are irritation to mucosa, rebound nasal congestion, and effects associated with systemic absorption, including sedation, alterations in cardiovascular function, and hypertension.

tetraiodothyronine. See **thyroxine.**

tetralogy /tetrol′əjē/ [Gk, *tetra,* four, *logos,* word], any group of four writings, symptoms, or other related factors. See also **tetralogy of Fallot.**

tetralogy of Fallot /falō″/ [Gk, *tetra,* four, *logos,* word; Etienne-Louis A. Fallot, French physician, 1850–1911], a congenital cardiac anomaly that consists of four defects: pulmonary stenosis, ventricular septal defect, malposition of the aorta so that it arises from the septal defect or the right ventricle, and right ventricular hypertrophy. The primary symptoms in the infant are cyanosis, hypoxia, difficulty in feeding, failure to gain weight, and poor development. In older children a squatting position and clubbing of the fingers and toes are evident. A pansystolic murmur is usually heard, and the second heart sound is faint or absent. Diagnosis of the condition is primarily based on the patient's history and physical symptoms, although cardiac catheterization is performed to evaluate the severity of the defects. Initial treatment consists mainly of supportive measures and palliative surgical procedures, primarily systemic to pulmonary anastomoses to decrease tissue hypoxia and prevent complications until the child is old enough to tolerate total corrective surgery. The optimal age for surgical repair is approximately 1 year. Also called **Fallot's syndrome.** See also **blue baby, trilogy of Fallot.**

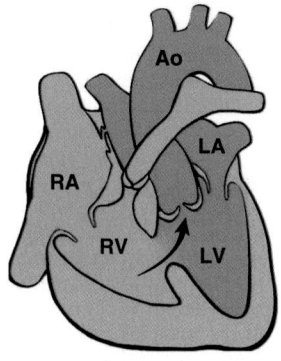

Tetralogy of Fallot *(Courtesy Dr. William D. Edwards, Mayo Clinic)*

tetramer /tet″rəmer/ [Gk, *tetra* + *meros,* part], something that is composed of four parts, such as a protein composed of four polypeptide subunits.

tetraodon poisoning, a reaction caused by a toxin in puffer fish and marine sunfish. It may result in myalgia, paresthesia, and other neuromuscular disorders. Death may result from respiratory paralysis. See also **ciguatera poisoning, fish poisoning, scombroid poisoning.**

tetraparesis /tet′rə·pərē′sis/ [Gk, *tetra,* four + *paresis,* relaxation], muscular weakness affecting all four extremities.

tetrapeptide /-pep″tīd/, a compound formed by four amino acids united by peptide links.

tetraplegia, paralysis of the arms, legs, and trunk of the body below the level of an associated injury to the spinal cord. This disorder is usually caused by spinal cord injury, especially in the area of the fifth to the seventh vertebrae. Automobile accidents and sporting mishaps are common causes. This condition affects about 150,000 Americans, the majority of whom are men between 20 and 40 years of age. Signs and symptoms commonly include flaccidity of the arms and the legs and the loss of power and sensation below the level of the injury. Cardiovascular complications also may develop from any injury that damages the spinal cord above the fifth cervical vertebra because of an associated block of the sympathetic nervous system. A major cause of death from such injury is respiratory failure. Other symptoms may include low body temperature, bradycardia, impaired peristalsis, and autonomic dysreflexia. Diagnosis is based on a complete physical and neurological examination with radiographic pictures of the head, chest, and abdomen to rule out underlying injuries. Spinal x-ray examinations and CT scores and MRI are usually done to evaluate the extent of the injury. Also called **quadriplegia.** Compare **hemiplegia, paraplegia.**

■ INTERVENTIONS: Treatment starts at the accident scene, where the patient's neck and spine are immobilized. Additional immobilization at the hospital commonly includes the use of halo traction. Steroids may be administered to decrease spinal cord edema. Surgery is commonly performed to fuse unstable spinal sections and remove bone fragments.

■ PATIENT CARE CONSIDERATIONS: The care of a patient with a spinal cord injury resulting in quadriplegia is complex—mentally, physically, and socially. The prevention of complications requires a coordinated effort. It is essential that the patient, the patient's family, and an interprofessional rehabilitation team work together to establish short-term and long-term goals.

tetraploid (4n) /tet′rəploid/ [Gk, *tetraploos,* fourfold, *eidos,* form], **1.** an individual, organism, strain, or cell that has four complete sets of chromosomes, quadruple the haploid number characteristic of the species. In humans the tetraploid number is 92; it occurs extremely rarely, in aborted or stillborn fetuses. **2.** *n.,* pertaining to such an individual, organism, strain, or cell. Also *tetraploidic.* Compare **diploid, haploid, triploid.** See also **polyploid, tetraploidy.**

tetraploidy /tet″rəploi′dē/, the state or condition of having four complete sets of chromosomes.

tetrasaccharide /-sak″ərīd/, a sugar containing four molecules of monosaccharide.

tetrascelus /tetras′ēləs/, a fetal anomaly with four legs.

tetravalent /-vā″lənt/, pertaining to a chemical with a valency of four.

tetro-. See **tetra-.**

tetrodotoxism /tet″ro-do-tok′sizm/, the most severe form of fish poisoning, caused by ingestion of inadequately prepared fish that contain tetrodotoxin. After eating such fish, within minutes there are symptoms of malaise, dizziness, and tingling about the mouth, which may be followed by ataxia, convulsions, respiratory paralysis, and death.

Texas catheter. See **condom catheter.**

TF, abbreviation for **transfer factor.**

TFIIE, a general transcription factor involved in complementary DNA encoding. TFIIE consists of two subunits: TFIIE-alpha and TFIIE-beta.

T follicular helper cells, a subset of CD4 helper T cells that regulate the development of antigen-specific effector and memory B cell responses.

T fracture /tē′frakchər/, an intercondylar fracture in which the fracture lines are T-shaped.

TGC, abbreviation for **time gain compensation.**

TGF, abbreviation for **transforming growth factor.**

T group. See **sensitivity training group.**

TGs, abbreviation for **triglycerides test.**

Th, symbol for the element **thorium.**

Th1 cells, a subset of helper T cells that promote cell-mediated immune responses. Th1 cells are induced by cytokines like IL-12 and are essential for the host defense against intracellular pathogens. They secrete the cytokines INFγ, IL-2, and TNFα. See also **helper T cell.**

Th2 cells, a subset of helper T cells that promote humoral immunity. Th2 cells are induced by cytokines like IL-4 and are required for B cell activation. They secrete the cytokines IL-4, IL-5, IL-13. See also **helper T cell, B cell–mediated immunity.**

Th 17 cells, a subset of helper T cells that have a function in the host defense against pathogens by mediating the recruitment of neutrophils and macrophages to sites of infection. They are induced by cytokines like IL-6, TGF-beta and IL-23 and produce the cytokine IL-17.

THA, abbreviation for **total hip arthroplasty.**

thalame. See **thalamus.**

thalamic /thalam′ik/ [Gk, *thalamos,* chamber], pertaining to the thalamus.

thalamic peduncle [Gk, *thalamos,* chamber; L, *pes,* foot], a group of fibers linking the thalamus with the hypothalamus.

thalamic syndrome [Gk, *thalamos* + *syn,* together, *dromos,* course], a vascular disorder involving the ventral and posterolateral nuclei of the thalamus and related nerve fibers. It causes disturbances of sensation and partial or complete paralysis of one side of the body. A major effect is an increased threshold to all stimuli on the opposite side of the body so that any stimuli may cause an exaggerated response. Also called *Dejerine-Roussy syndrome.*

thalamo-, combining form meaning "relating to the thalamus": *thalamotomy.*

thalamotomy /thal′əmot″əmē/, the surgical production of lesions within the nuclei of the thalamus, generally performed to treat diseases of the basal ganglia.

thalamus /thal′əməs/ *pl. thalami* [Gk, *thalamos,* chamber], *adj.,* one of a pair of large oval nervous structures made of gray matter and forming most of the lateral walls of the third ventricle of the brain and part of the diencephalon. It relays sensory information, excluding smell, to the cerebral cortex. It is composed mainly of gray substance and translates impulses from appropriate receptors into crude sensations of pain, temperature, and touch. It also participates in associating sensory impulses with pleasant and unpleasant feelings, in the arousal mechanisms of the body, and in the mechanisms that produce complex reflex movements. Compare **epithalamus, hypothalamus, subthalamus. –thalamic,** *adj.*

thalassemia /thal′əsē″mē·ə/ [Gk, *thalassa,* sea, *a* + *haima,* without blood], production and hemolytic anemia characterized by microcytic, hypochromic red blood cells. Thalassemia is caused by inherited deficiency of alpha- or beta-globin synthesis. See also **hemochromatosis, hemosiderosis.**

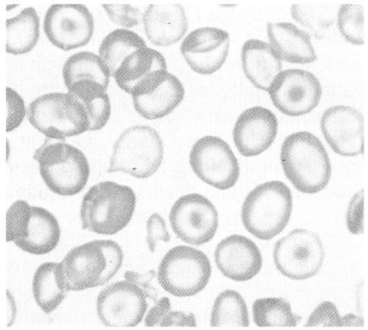

Thalassemia major *(Courtesy Dr. William D. Edwards, Mayo Clinic)*

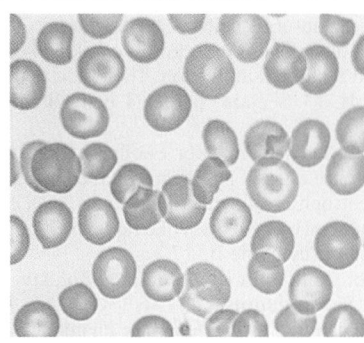

Thalassemia minor *(Damjanov and Linder, 2000)*

thalasso-, combining form meaning "the sea": *thalassophobia, thalassotherapy.*

thalassophobia, a fear of the sea or other deep bodies of water.

thalassotherapy /thalas′ōther″əpē/ [Gk, *tahassa,* seal], a treatment system based on sea bathing and exposure to sea air.

thalidomide /thalid″əmīd/, a sedative-hypnotic sometimes prescribed for the treatment of leprosy. It is never given to women who are or who might become pregnant.

thallium (Tl) /thal′ē·əm/ [Gk, *thallos,* green line], a soft, bluish-white, metallic element that exhibits some nonmetallic chemical properties. Its atomic number is 81; its atomic mass (weight) is 204.38. Many of its compounds are highly toxic. Thallium sulfate is widely used as a rat poison.

thallium poisoning, a toxic condition caused by the ingestion or absorption through the skin of thallium salts, especially thallium sulfate. Characteristic of the condition are abdominal pain, vomiting, bloody diarrhea, tremor, delirium, and alopecia. Thallium has been used in insect and rodent poisons, fireworks, and some cosmetic hair removers, but this extremely toxic and cumulative poison was banned for use in household products in 1965.

thallium stress test. See **stress test.**

thanato-, combining form meaning "death": *thanatology, thanatomania.*

thanatology /than′ətol″əjē/ [Gk, *thanatos,* death, *logos,* science], the study of death and dying. *–thanatologist, n.*

thanatomania /than′ətōmā″nē·ə/ [Gk, *thanatos,* death, *mania,* frenzy], an obsession with death, dying, or suicide.

thanatophidia, *(Obsolete)* a venomous snake.

thanatophoric dwarf /than″ətōfôr″ik/ [Gk, *thanatos* + *phoros,* bearer; AS, *dweorge*], an infant with severe micromelia, the limbs usually extending straight out from the trunk; an extremely narrow chest; and flattened vertebral bodies with wide intervertebral spaces. Death usually occurs from respiratory complications shortly after birth.

Thanatos /than″ətəs/ [Gk, death], a freudian term for the death instinct.

thanotopsy. See **autopsy.**

thaumato-, combining form meaning "marvel" or "miracles."

THC, abbreviation for **tetrahydrocannabinol.**

theater /thē″ətər/, **1.** an operating room or suite of rooms. **2.** a large room used for lectures and demonstrations.

thebesian foramen /thəbē″zē·ən, tābā″zē·ən/ [Adam C. Thebesius, German physician, 1686–1732], any of the openings of the vena cordis minima into the right atrium and ventricles.

thebesian valve, a remnant of the embryonic sinoatrial valves. It is not present in all individuals but, when present, it may interfere with interventional cardiac diagnostic procedures and management involving cannulation of the coronary sinus. Also called **cardiac valve.**

thebesian vein [Adam C. Thebesius], any of the smallest cardiac veins.

thec-, combining form meaning "sheath, such as of a tendon": *thecal, thecodont.*

theca /thē″kə/ *pl. thecae,* a sheath or capsule, such as the theca cordis or pericardium.

theca cells, theca-lutein cells, lutein cells derived from the theca interna.

theca cell tumor [Gk, *theke,* sheath; L, *cella,* storeroom; *tumor,* swelling], an uncommon benign fibroid tumor of the ovary, composed of theca cells and usually containing granulosa (follicular) cells. Characteristically solid masses with yellow fatty streaks, these tumors are frequently associated with excessive estrogen production and tend to develop cystic degeneration. Also called **fibroma thecocellulare xanthomatodes, thecoma.**

thecal /thē″kəl/ [Gk, *theke,* sheath], pertaining to a theca or sheath.

-thecium, combining form meaning "a sack or container": *epithecium.*

thecodont, having teeth that are inserted in sockets in the jawbone.

thecoma, a tumor derived from ovarian mesenchyme, consisting of spindle-shaped cells that may contain fat droplets. It is sometimes associated with excessive estrogen production and precocious sexual development in prepubertal girls.

The Joint Commission (TJC), a private nongovernmental agency that establishes guidelines for the operation of hospitals and other health care facilities, conducts accreditation programs and surveys, and encourages the attainment of high standards of institutional medical care in the United States. Members of The Joint Commission include representatives from the American Medical Association, American College of Physicians, American College of Surgeons, American Dental Association, and American Hospital Association.

thel-, combining form meaning "nipple": *thelarche.*

thelarche /thilär″kē/ [Gk, *thele,* nipple, *archaios,* beginning], the beginning of female pubertal breast development, normally occurring between 9 and 13 years of age. Thelarche occurs before puberty at the beginning of the phase of rapid growth. Premature thelarche is precocious breast development in a female without other evidence of sexual maturation. Compare **menarche.**

-thelia, combining form meaning "(condition of the) nipples": *athelia, macrothelia.*

-thelioma, combining form meaning "a tumor in a cellular tissue": *chondroendothelioma, hemangioendothelioma, reticuloendothelioma.*

-thelium, suffix meaning "a layer of (specified kind of) cellular tissue": *endothelium, mesothelium.*

thely-, *(Obsolete)* prefix meaning "female."

thenar /thē″när/ [Gk, palm of the hand], pertaining to any structure in relation to the ball of the thumb, such as the three thenar muscles.

thenar eminence [Gk, *thenar,* palm of the hand; L, *eminentia,* projection], a raised fleshy area on the palm of the hand near the base of the thumb.

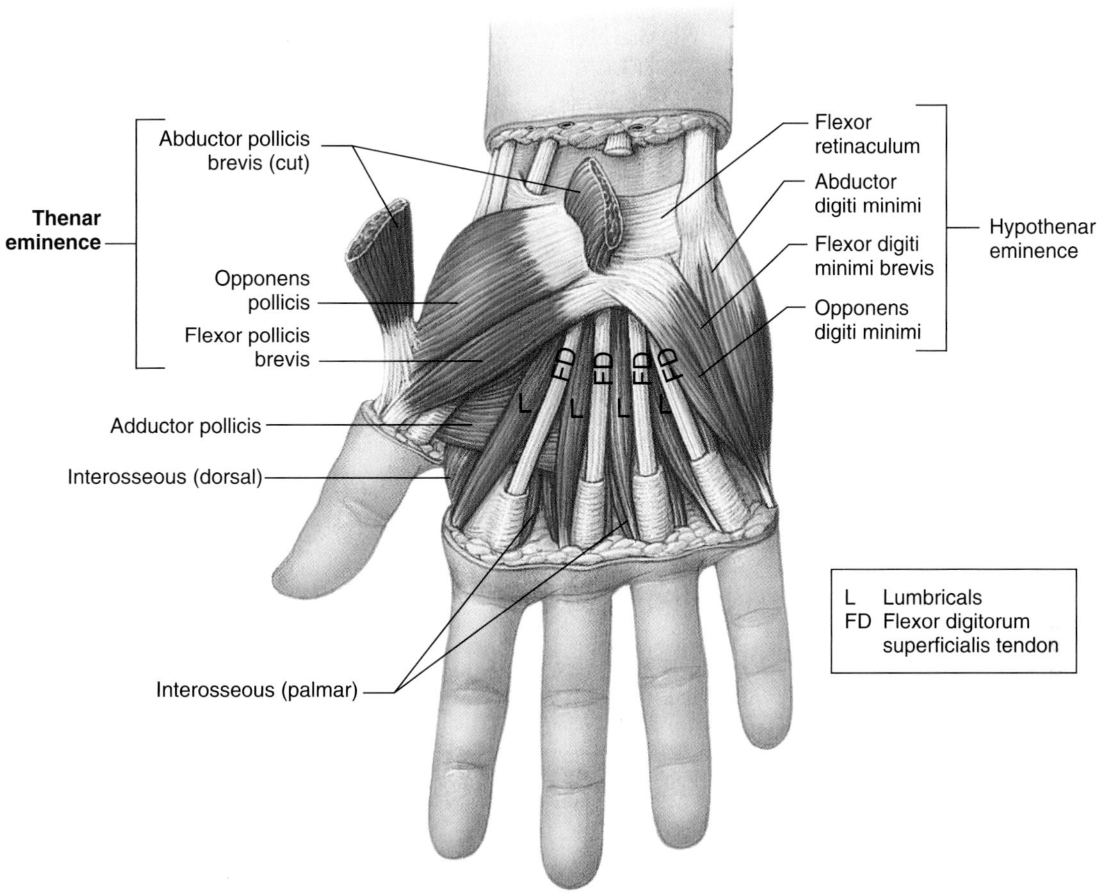
Thenar eminence
Abductor pollicis brevis (cut)
Opponens pollicis
Flexor pollicis brevis
Adductor pollicis
Interosseous (dorsal)
Interosseous (palmar)
Flexor retinaculum
Abductor digiti minimi
Flexor digiti minimi brevis
Opponens digiti minimi
Hypothenar eminence
FD
L
L Lumbricals
FD Flexor digitorum superficialis tendon

Thenar eminence *(Patton and Thibodeau, 2010)*

thenar muscles, the intrinsic muscles at the base of the hand that move the thumb. They include the flexor pollicis brevis, abductor pollicis brevis, and opponens pollicis. **–thenar muscles,** *n.*

theo-, prefix meaning "a god": *theotherapy.*

theobroma oil /thē′ōbrō″mə/, a liquid fat derived from seeds of *Theobroma cacao,* the cocoa plant. It contains a number of fatty acids used in suppositories, ointments, and lubricants.

theobromine /thē′əbrō″min/, a substance (methylxanthine) that is related chemically to caffeine and theophylline but differs from them by the number and distribution of methyl groups. Theobromine occurs naturally in cocoa, cola nuts, and tea. It acts as a diuretic, vasodilator, cardiac stimulant, and smooth muscle relaxant.

Theolair, a bronchodilator medication. Brand name for **theophylline.**

theophylline /thē·əfil″ēn/ [L, *thea,* tea; Gk, *phyllon,* leaf], a bronchodilator.

■ INDICATIONS: It can be prescribed for oral administration to relax the smooth muscle of the bronchial passages in the treatment of bronchospasm in bronchial asthma, bronchitis, and emphysema. Its use has tapered sharply because of the availability of safer and more effective asthma medications that can be administered by inhalation.

■ CONTRAINDICATIONS: Hypertension, cardiac disease, liver disease, renal disease, or concurrent treatment with other xanthines may prohibit its use.

■ ADVERSE EFFECTS: Among the most serious adverse effects are hypersensitivity, GI bleeding, palpitations, and seizures.

theorem /thē′ərəm/ [Gk, *theorein,* to look at], **1.** a proposition to be proved by a chain of reasoning and analysis. **2.** a rule expressed by symbols or formulae.

theoretic effectiveness /thē·əret′ik/ [Gk, *theorein* + L, *efficere,* to do], (of a contraceptive method) the effectiveness of a medication, device, or method in preventing pregnancy if used consistently and exactly as intended without error. Compare **use effectiveness.**

theoretic plate number (N), a number defining the efficiency of a chromatographic column.

theories of aging, theories proposed to explain aging and death of cells and organisms. They are generally divided into two major groupings. The first group consists of programmed causes, with timed functional changes, and is generally based on genetic theories; this group includes programmed senescence of cells, shortening of telomeres, and declines in hormonal or in immunological function. The second group, called stochastic theories, consists of theories based on random events occurring over time and includes free radical generation, gradual wear and tear, mutation over time, and differences in metabolic rate.

theory /thē'ərē/ [Gk, *theorein,* to look at], an abstract statement formulated to predict, explain, or describe the relationships among concepts, constructs, or events. Theory is developed and tested by observation and research supplying factual data.

Theory of Caring.　See **Swanson, Kristen M.**

Theory of Caritative Care.　See **Eriksson, Katie.**

Theory of Chronic Sorrow.　See **Eakes, Georgene Gaskill; Burke, Mary Lermann; Hainsworth, Margaret A.**

Theory of Comfort.　See **Kolcaba, Katharine.**

Theory of Illness Trajectory.　See **Wiener, Carolyn L.; Dodd, Marylin J.**

theotherapy /thē'ōther″əpē/ [Gk, *theos,* god, *therapeia,* treatment], a therapeutic approach to the prevention, diagnosis, and treatment of disease and dysfunction based on religious or spiritual beliefs.

therapeutic /ther'əpyoo″tik/ [Gk, *therapeuein,* to treat], **1.** beneficial. **2.** pertaining to a treatment.

-therapeutic, -therapeutics, suffix meaning "medical treatment by (specified) techniques": *kinetotherapeutic, psychotherapeutics, vaccinotherapeutics.*

therapeutic abortion, **1.** a termination of early pregnancy deemed necessary by a physician. **2.** *(Informal)* any legally induced abortion. Compare **elective abortion.** See also **induced abortion.**

therapeutic communication, a process in which a health care provider consciously influences an individual or helps the individual to a better understanding through verbal or nonverbal communication. Therapeutic communication involves the use of specific strategies that encourage the patient to express feelings and ideas and that convey acceptance and respect.

therapeutic community (TC), (in mental health) a treatment facility in which the entire milieu is part of the treatment. The physical environment, the other clients, the staff, and the policies of the facility influence the function of the individual in the activities of daily living in the community. The concept of a therapeutic community is integral to milieu therapy.

therapeutic dose [Gk, *therapeia,* treatment, *dosis,* giving], the dose that may be required to produce a desired effect.

therapeutic drug monitoring test (TDM), a blood test that entails taking measurements of blood drug levels to determine effective drug dosages and to prevent toxicity. It is also used to identify noncompliant patients.

therapeutic equivalent, a drug that has essentially the same effect in the treatment of a disease or condition as one or more other drugs. A drug that is a therapeutic equivalent may or may not be chemically equivalent, bioequivalent, or generically equivalent. See also **bioequivalent, chemical equivalent, generic equivalent.**

therapeutic exercise, any exercise planned and performed to attain a specific physical benefit, such as maintenance of the range of motion, strengthening of weakened muscles, increased joint flexibility, or improved cardiovascular and respiratory function.

therapeutic gain, the ratio of the biological effect of a therapy on a tumor compared with the effect on surrounding normal tissue. Higher therapeutic gains mean lower complications of therapy.

therapeutic horseback riding, an equine-assisted activity that primarily focuses on providing instruction in riding skills to individuals with disabilities.

therapeutic index (TI), the difference between the minimum therapeutic and minimum toxic concentrations of a drug.

therapeutic media, (in occupational therapy) items used in therapy during the intervention process to address the client's goals and foster participation in desired occupations.

therapeutic plasmapheresis.　See **plasma exchange.**

therapeutic play, a well established therapeutic modality used by psychotherapists, occupational therapists, and other health care providers. Research, both qualitative and quantitative, supports its effectiveness. Sessions may occur with individual children or with groups of children.

therapeutic radiology.　See **radiology.**

therapeutic radiopharmaceutical, a radioactive drug administered to a patient to deliver radiation to body tissues internally. Examples are iodine-131, which is used to ablate thyroid tissue in hyperthyroid patients; cesium-137; iridium-192; radium-226; and strontium-90, which is implanted in a sealed source for the treatment of malignancies.

therapeutic recreation, an allied health treatment service organized by professionals with expertise in organizing and supervising recreational activities designed to accelerate recovery from mental or physical disorders.

therapeutic recreation specialist, a person who assists patients in their recovery or rehabilitation after physical or emotional illness or disability by planning and supervising recreation programs.

therapeutics /ther'əpyoo″tiks/ [Gk, *therapeia,* treatment], a branch of health care that is concerned with the treatment of disease, seeking to relieve symptoms or produce a cure. See also **therapeutic.**

therapeutic touch (TT), a healing method based on the premise that the body possesses an energy field that can be affected by the focused intention of the healer using a consciously directed exchange of energy between practitioner and patient. The practitioner uses the hands as a focus to assess the patient's energy field, to release areas where the free flow of energy is blocked, and to balance the patient's energy by transferring energy from a universal life energy force to the patient.

therapeutic use of self, **1.** the conscious use of one's personality, insights, perceptions, and judgments as part of the therapeutic process. **2.** the art of using oneself to successfully promote engagement in chosen daily activities.

-therapia, -therapy, combining form meaning "a specific type of medical care": *balneotherapy, hypnotherapy, aerotherapy.*

therapist /ther'əpist/, a person with special skills, obtained through education and experience, in one or more areas of health care.

therapy /ther'əpē/ [Gk, *therapeia,* treatment], the treatment of any disease or a pathological condition. An example is inhalation therapy, which administers various medicines for patients suffering from diseases of the respiratory tract.

-therapy.　See **-therapia, -therapy.**

therio-, combining form meaning "beast": *theriotherapy.*

theriotherapy, the care of animals by a veterinarian.

therm-.　See **thermo-, therm-.**

-therm, -thermia, -thermy, combining form meaning "a state of heat": *hypothermia, microthermy, poikilothermic.*

thermal /thur′məl/ [Gk, *thermē*, heat], pertaining to the production, application, or maintenance of heat. Also **thermic.**

thermal biofeedback, the monitoring of skin temperature as an index of blood flow changes because of the dilation and constriction of blood vessels, the feedback being displayed to the patient on a video monitor, accompanied by an audible signal. It is used for stress management and in the treatment of Raynaud disease, hypertension, and migraine.

thermal burn, tissue injury, usually of the skin, caused by exposure to extreme heat. See also **burn.**

thermal dilution. See **thermodilution.**

thermal field size, the area over which therapeutic heating is likely to be produced.

thermalgesia /thur′məljē″zhə/ [Gk, *thermē*, heat, *algos*, pain], pain caused by exposure to high temperatures.

thermalgia /thurmal′jə/, a sensation of intense burning pain sometimes experienced following nerve injuries.

thermal radiation [Gk, *thermē*, heat; L, *radiare*, to shine], the emission of energy in the form of heat.

-thermia. See **-therm, -thermia, -thermy.**

thermic, pertaining to heat. See **thermal.**

thermic fever. See **heat hyperpyrexia.**

thermic sense /thur′mik/ [Gk, *thermē*, heat; L, *sentire*, to feel], the network of sense organs and connecting pathways that allow an appreciation of temperature changes. Also called **temperature sense.**

thermionic emission /ther′mī·on′ik/, the emission of electrons and ions by incandescent bodies.

thermistor /thərmis″tər/ [Gk, *thermē* + L, *resistere*, to withstand], a kind of thermometer for measuring minute changes in temperature. The resistance of a thermistor varies with the ambient temperature, thereby enabling accurate measurements of small temperature changes. See also **temperature, thermometer.**

thermo-, therm-, prefix meaning "heat": *thermochemistry, thermogenesis, thermalgesia.*

thermocautery /thur′mōkô″tərē/ [Gk, *thermē* + *kauterion*, branding iron], the use of a needle or snare heated by direct flame, a heated hydrocarbon vapor, or an electric current in the destruction of tissue.

thermochemistry /-kem′istrē/ [Gk, *thermē*, heat, *chemia*, alchemy], a branch of chemistry that is concerned with the heat changes involved in chemical reactions.

thermocoagulation /-kō·ag′yəlā″shən/ [Gk, *thermē*, heat; L, *coagulare*], the use of high-frequency electric currents to destroy tissue through heat coagulation.

thermocouple /thur″məkup′əl/ [Gk, *thermē* + Fr, *couple*, pair], a temperature-measuring device that relies on the production of a temperature-dependent voltage at the junction of two dissimilar metals.

thermodilution /-dilyoo′zhən/, a method of cardiac output determination. A bolus of solution of known volume and temperature is injected into the right atrium, and the resultant change in blood temperature is detected by a thermistor previously placed in the pulmonary artery with a catheter. Also called **thermal dilution.**

thermodynamics /-dīnam″iks/ [Gk, *thermē*, heat, *dynamis*, power], the science of the interconversion of heat and work.

thermogenesis /thur′mōjen″əsis/ [Gk, *thermē* + *genesis*, origin], production of heat, especially by the cells of the body. –*thermogenetic, adj.*

thermogenic center. See **thermoregulatory center.**

thermograph /thur′məgraf′/ [Gk, *thermē* + *graphein*, to record], **1.** a photographic record of the amount of heat radiated from the surface of the body, revealing "hot spots" of potential tumors or other disorders. **2.** a device consisting of a thermometer, inked stylus, and chart for continuous recording of the ambient temperature.

thermography /thərmog″rəfē/, a technique for sensing and recording on an image hot and cold areas of the body by means of an infrared detector that reacts to blood flow. Disease states that manifest increased or decreased blood flow present thermographic patterns that can be distinguished from those of normal areas. –*thermographic, adj.*

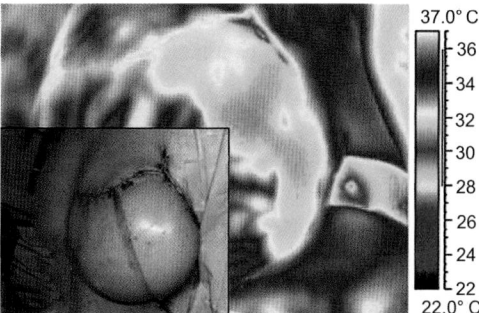

Dynamic infrared thermography (de Weerd, Mercer, and Weum, 2011)

thermoinhibitory center. See **thermoregulatory center.**

thermointegrator /thur′mō·in″təgrā′tər/, an instrument used to create a thermal model of an environment, measuring the warmth and coldness as it might be experienced by a living organism in that environment.

thermokeratoplasty /-ker′ətōplas′tē/, a procedure to correct myopia by applying heat to flatten the cornea. The heat shrinks the collagen in the substantia propria layer of the cornea.

thermolabile /thur′məlā″bəl/ [Gk, *thermē* + L, *labilis*, slipping], easily destroyed or altered by heat. Also called **heat labile.** Compare **thermostable.**

thermoluminescent dosimetry /-loo′mines″ənt/ [Gk, *thermē* + L, *lumen*, light; Gk, *dosis*, something given, *metron*, measure], a method of measuring the ionizing radiation to which a person is exposed by means of a device that contains a radiation-sensitive crystalline material. The material stores the radiation's energy by changing structure. When the material is heated at some later time, it releases the energy as ultraviolet or visible light. The light emitted is detected by a photomultiplier tube that generates an electric signal whose magnitude reflects the amount of ionizing radiation originally received.

thermomassage /-məsäzh″/, a physical therapy technique that combines heat and massage.

thermometer /thermom′ətər/ [Gk, *thermē* + *metron*, measure], an instrument used to measure temperature. The first thermometers consisted of a sealed glass tube, marked in degrees Celsius or Fahrenheit and filled with either mercury or alcohol; the liquid in the tube would rise or fall as it expanded or contracted, based on changes in temperature. There are now many types of thermometers. Kinds include **air thermometer, clinical thermometer, digital thermometer, electronic thermometer, mercury thermometer, rectal thermometer, surface thermometer, tympanic membrane thermometer, wet-and-dry-bulb thermometer.**

thermoneutral environment /-noo′trəl/ [Gk, *thermē* + L, *neutralis*, neutral; ME, *environ*, around], **1.** an environment that keeps body temperature at an optimum point at which the least amount of oxygen is consumed for metabolism.

2. an environment that enables a neonate to maintain a body temperature of 97.7° F (36.5° C) with a minimal requirement of energy and oxygen.

thermonuclear /-nōō′klē·ər/ [Gk, *thermē,* heat; L, *nucleus,* nut kernel], pertaining to a reaction in which isotopes of hydrogen (protium, deuterium, or tritium) can be fused at temperatures of nearly 100,000,000° C into heavier nuclei of helium atoms. The process is the source of energy of the sun and is used in the explosion of thermonuclear weapons.

thermopenetration /-pen′ətrā″shən/ [Gk, *thermē* + L, *penetrale,* passing through], the use of diathermic techniques to produce warmth within the body tissues for therapeutic purposes. Also called **transthermia.**

thermophilic /-fil′ik/ [Gk, *thermē,* heat, *philein,* to love], pertaining to organisms that thrive in very hot environments (e.g., up to 80° C for some bacteria that live in hot springs).

thermophore /thur″məfôr/, a procedure in which heat is applied locally to a body part.

thermoplastic /ther′mō·plas′tik/ [Gk, *thermē,* heat + *plassein,* to mold], a material that softens under heat and becomes capable of being molded into shape with pressure, then hardens on cooling without undergoing chemical change.

thermoradiotherapy /-rā′dē·ō·ther″əpē/, a therapeutic process that applies ionizing radiation to any part of the body in which the temperature has been raised by artificial means. Thermoradiography seeks to increase the radiosensitivity of the body part being treated.

thermoreceptor /-risep′tər/ [Gk, *thermē,* heat; L, *recipere,* to receive], nerve endings that are sensitive to heat or a rise in body temperature.

thermoregulation /-reg′yəlā″shən/ [Gk, *thermē* + L, *regula,* rule], the control of heat production and heat loss, specifically the maintenance of body temperature through physiological mechanisms activated by the hypothalamus.

thermoregulatory center /-reg″yələtôr′ē/ [Gk, *thermē,* heat; L, *regula,* rule; Gk, *kentron,* center], center located in the hypothalamus concerned mainly with the regulation of heat production, heat inhibition, and heat conservation to maintain a normal body temperature. Kinds include **thermoinhibitory center, thermotaxic center, thermogenic center.**

thermoresistance /-risis″təns/, an ability to tolerate heat, as in certain thermophilic bacteria.

thermosetting /ther′mō·set·ing/ [Gk, *thermē,* heat; AS, *settan,* to set], of resins, becoming hard or solid when heat is applied and remaining that way on being cooled. The change is not reversible.

thermostable /-stā′bəl/, unaffected by or resistant to change by an increase in temperature. Compare **thermolabile.**

thermostasis /-stā″sis/, maintenance of a stable body temperature, as in mammals and birds.

thermostat /thur′məstat/ [Gk, *thermē* + *statos,* standing], a device for the automatic control of a heating or cooling system. −*thermostatic, adj.*

thermotaxic center. See **thermoregulatory center.**

thermotaxis /-tak′sis/ [Gk, *thermē* + *taxis,* arrangement], **1.** the normal adjustment and regulation of body temperature. **2.** the movement of an organism in response to heat, either toward the stimulus (positive thermotaxis) or away from the stimulus (negative thermotaxis). Also called **thermotropism.**

thermotherapeutic penetration /-ther′əpyōō″tik/, the depth to which heating to therapeutic temperatures is likely to extend.

thermotherapy /-ther′əpē/ [Gk, *thermē* + *therapeia,* treatment], the treatment of disease by the application of heat. Thermotherapy may be administered as dry heat with heat lamps, diathermy machines, electric pads, or hot water bottles or as moist heat with warm compresses or immersion in warm water. Warm soaks or compresses may be used to treat local infections, relax muscles and relieve pain in patients with motor problems, and promote circulation in peripheral vascular disorders such as thrombophlebitis. −*thermotherapeutic, adj.*

thermotropism, moving toward a source of heat. See also **thermotaxis.**

-thermy. See **-therm, -thermia, -thermy.**

theta /thē″tə, thā″tə/, Θ, θ, the eighth letter of the Greek alphabet.

theta wave [Gk, *theta,* eighth letter of Greek alphabet; AS, *wæfian*], one of the several types of brain waves, characterized by a relatively low frequency of 4 to 7 Hz and a low amplitude of 10 μV. Theta waves are the "drowsy waves" of the temporal lobes of the brain and appear in electroencephalograms when the individual is awake but relaxed and sleepy. Also called *theta rhythm.* Compare **alpha wave, beta wave, delta wave.**

-thetic, -thetical, combining form meaning "to put, place, set": *prosthetics, synthetic.*

thiabendazole /thī′əben″dəzōl/, an anthelmintic with antiinflammatory, antipyretic, and analgesic effects.

■ INDICATIONS: It can be prescribed in the treatment of a range of worm infestations, including hookworms, roundworms, and pinworms, and was the drug of choice for threadworms until recently. Other drugs have fewer adverse effects.

■ CONTRAINDICATIONS: Erythema multiforme, Stevens-Johnson syndrome, or known hypersensitivity to this drug prohibits its use.

■ ADVERSE EFFECTS: Among the more serious adverse effects are anorexia, central nervous system effects, severe GI disturbances, dizziness, and hypotension. Approximately one third of people are incapacitated by this drug for several hours after administration.

thiamin. See **thiamine.**

thiaminase /thī·am″inās/, an enzyme present in raw fish that destroys thiamine. A diet containing a substantial amount of raw fish could result in a thiamine deficiency because of the enzyme. A heat-stable form also exists.

thiamine /thī′əmin/ [Gk, *theion,* containing sulfur, *amine,* ammonia], a water-soluble, crystalline compound of the B vitamin complex, essential for normal metabolism and health of the cardiovascular and nervous systems. Thiamine plays a key role in the metabolic breakdown of glucose to yield energy in body tissues. Rich sources are pork; organ meats; green leafy vegetables; legumes; sweet corn; egg yolk; cornmeal; brown rice; yeast; and the germ and husks of grains, berries, and nuts. It is not stored in the body and must be supplied daily. A deficiency of thiamine chiefly affects the nervous system, the circulation, and the GI tract. Symptoms include irritability, emotional disturbances, loss of appetite, multiple neuritis, increased pulse rate, dyspnea, reduced intestinal motility, and heart irregularities. Severe deficiency causes beriberi. Also called **antiberiberi factor,** *antineuritic vitamin,* **vitamin B₁.** Also spelled **thiamin.**

thiazide diuretics, a group of diuretics in the thiazide family; they decrease reabsorption of sodium by the kidney and thereby increase loss of water and sodium. They also increase urinary secretion of chloride, potassium, and, to some extent, bicarbonate ions. These are the most frequently prescribed diuretics because they are moderately potent and have relatively few side effects. Most act within 1 hour after being taken and are excreted in 3 to 6 hours. Patients who are taking a thiazide diuretic should be monitored for electrolyte imbalances, metabolic acidosis, and, in the case of diabetic patients, hyperglycemia, which may necessitate an increase in insulin dosage. Because GI irritation can occur, it is advisable to take these diuretics at mealtime. See also **diuretic.**

thiazine-eosinate stain,   any of a group of neutral stains used in hematology and histology that combine an eosin dye, usually eosin Y, as the anionic component and one or more thiazine dyes as the cationic component. The prototype is the Romanovsky's stain.

thiemia /thī·ē″mē·ə/   [Gk, *theion,* sulfur, *haima,* blood],   an excess of sulfur in the blood.

thiethylperazine /thī·eth′ilper″əzēn/, a phenothiazine antiemetic.
■ INDICATIONS: It is prescribed to control nausea and vomiting.
■ CONTRAINDICATIONS: Parkinson disease, central nervous system disorders, liver or renal dysfunction, severe hypotension, or known hypersensitivity to phenothiazine medications prohibits its use.
■ ADVERSE EFFECTS: Among the more serious adverse effects are hypotension, liver toxicity, extrapyramidal reactions, blood dyscrasias, and hypersensitivity reactions.

thiethylperazine malate,   the malate salt of thiethylperazine, having the same actions and uses as the base. It is administered intramuscularly.

thiethylperazine maleate,   the maleate salt of thiethylperazine, having the same actions and uses as the base. It is administered orally or rectally.

thigh [AS, *theoh*],   the section of the lower limb between the hip and the knee.

thigh bone.   See **femur.**

thigm-,   combining form meaning "touch": *thigmesthesia.*

thigmesthesia,   sensitivity to pressure.

thinking [AS, *thencan,* to think],   **1.** the cognitive process of forming mental images or concepts. **2.** the process of cognitive problem solving through the sorting, organizing, and classification of facts. Kinds include **abstract thinking, concrete thinking, syncretic thinking.** See also **imagination.**

thin-layer chromatography (TLC),   a method of separating two or more chemical compounds in a solution through their differential migrations across a thin layer of adsorbent spread over a glass or plastic plate.

thio- /thī′ō-/,   combining form designating the presence of sulfur: *thioester, thiobarbituric acid.*

thioamide derivative /thī′ō·am″īd/,   one of a group of antithyroid drugs prescribed in the treatment of hyperthyroidism. Thioamide drugs act by inhibiting the synthesis of thyroid hormone. The principal thioamides are propylthiouracil, methimazole, methylthiouracil, and carbimazole; propylthiouracil and methimazole are the only members of this group still available. Adverse reactions include agranulocytosis, hypersensitivity, and a mild transient pruritus. Because agranulocytosis may occur very rapidly, serial white blood cell counts are not useful in diagnosing that complication of treatment. Instead, the patient is requested to report immediately instances of sore throat and fever, which often herald the onset of agranulocytosis. Prompt discontinuation of the drug before serious depletion of granulocytic white blood cells develops usually results in complete recovery. Use of antithyroid medications in pregnancy may result in fetal hypothyroidism, goiter, and cretinism.

thiobarbituric acid /thī′obahr″bitu′rik/,   a compound that differs from barbituric acid only by the presence of a sulfur atom instead of an oxygen atom at the number 2 carbon. It is the parent compound of a class of drugs, the thiobarbiturates.

thioctic acid /thī·ok″tik/,   a pyruvate oxidation factor found in liver and yeast, used in bacterial culture media.

thioester /thī′ō·es″tər/,   an important group of biological chemicals formed by the hydrosulfides (or mercaptans or thiols) and carboxylic acids and identified by a bond between the acyl carbonyl carbon and the thiol sulfur. Examples include the coenzyme A thioesters.

thioethanolamine   acetyltransferase   /thī′ō·eth′onol′ə min/,   an enzyme that catalyzes the transfer of acetyl groups from acetyl CoA to the sulfur atom of thioethanolamine, producing CoA and *S*-acetylthioethanolamine.

thioflavine T /thī′oflā″vin/,   a yellow dye used as a fluorochrome in histopathology.

thioguanine /thī′ōgwä″nēn/,   a purine analog antagonist, an antineoplastic that acts as an antimetabolite.
■ INDICATIONS: It is prescribed in the treatment of a variety of malignant neoplastic diseases, especially acute and chronic myelogenous leukemias.
■ CONTRAINDICATIONS: Known hypersensitivity or resistance to this drug prohibits its use. It is not given during pregnancy.
■ ADVERSE EFFECTS: Among the most serious adverse effects are bone marrow depression, GI distress, and stomatitis.

thiopental sodium /-pen′təl/,   a potent and short-acting barbiturate formerly widely used as a general anesthetic induction agent. It is administered intravenously in adults. It has no analgesic properties and therefore must be supplemented by analgesics. It has largely been replaced by propofol in the United States and Canada. See also **barbiturate.**

thioridazine hydrochloride /-rid′əzēn/,   a phenothiazine antipsychotic.
■ INDICATIONS: It is prescribed in the treatment of schizophrenia when patients have failed to respond to other therapies and in the management of nonpsychotic behavioral disturbances, senility, alcohol withdrawal, and organic brain disease.
■ CONTRAINDICATIONS: Parkinson disease, concurrent administration of central nervous system depressants, hepatic or renal dysfunction, severe hypotension, or known hypersensitivity to this drug or to other phenothiazine medications prohibits its use.
■ ADVERSE EFFECTS: Among the more serious adverse effects are severe sedation, a potentially life-threatening prolongation of the QT interval, hypotension, hepatotoxicity, extrapyramidal reactions, blood dyscrasias, and hypersensitivity reactions. It should be used with caution in patients with premature ventricular contractions, breast cancer, and respiratory disorders and in patients exposed to extreme heat, cold, and pesticides or insecticides. The herb kava kava may increase the risk and severity of dystonic reactions.

thiotepa /thī′ōtep″ə/,   an antineoplastic alkylating agent.
■ INDICATIONS: It is prescribed in the treatment of malignant neoplastic diseases, including adenocarcinoma of the breast and ovary, and urinary bladder carcinomas.
■ CONTRAINDICATIONS: Bone marrow depression, pregnancy, or known hypersensitivity to this drug prohibits its use. Dosage must be decreased if there is liver or kidney dysfunction.
■ ADVERSE EFFECTS: Among the most serious adverse effects are bone marrow depression, anorexia, nausea, and headache.

thiothixene /-thī′ksēn/,   a thioxanthene antipsychotic.
■ INDICATIONS: It is prescribed in the treatment of acute agitation and mild-to-severe psychotic disorders.
■ CONTRAINDICATIONS: Parkinson disease, concurrent administration of central nervous system depressants, hepatic or renal dysfunction, severe hypotension, or known hypersensitivity to this drug or to phenothiazine medications prohibits its use. It is not recommended for children under 12 years of age.

T

■ ADVERSE EFFECTS: Among the more serious adverse effects are hypotension, hepatotoxicity, extrapyramidal reactions, blood dyscrasias, and hypersensitivity reactions.

thiouracil /thī′ōyŏŏr″əsil/ [Gk, *theion,* sulfur, *ouron,* urine], a chemical compound derived from thiourea that inhibits the formation of thyroxine in the thyroid gland and is used to treat hyperthyroidism.

thioxanthene derivative /thī·oksan″thēn/, any one of a group of antipsychotic drugs, each of which is similar to the phenothiazines in indication, action, and adverse effects.

third cranial nerve. See **oculomotor nerve.**

third cuneiform bone. See **lateral cuneiform bone.**

third-degree AV heart block. See **complete heart block.**

third-degree burn, a burn that destroys both the epidermis and the dermis, often also involving the subcutaneous tissue. Also called *full-thickness burn.*

third-party reimbursement, reimbursement for services rendered to a person in which an entity other than the receiver of the service is responsible for the payment. Third-party reimbursement for the cost of a subscriber's health care is commonly paid in full or in part by a health insurance plan, such as Blue Shield or Blue Cross, Medicare, or Medicaid.

third stage of labor, the expulsion of the placenta, membranes, and a small amount of blood and amniotic fluid, occurring within 5 to 30 minutes after delivery of the fetus.

third ventricle [Gk, *triotus,* below second rank; L, *ventriculus,* little belly], a cavity of the brain bounded on each side by a thalamus and the hypothalamus. It communicates anteriorly with the lateral ventricles and posteriorly with the aqueduct of the midbrain.

third ventriculostomy /ventrik′yəlos″təmē/ [L, *tertius,* three, *ventriculus,* little belly; Gk, *stoma,* mouth], a surgical procedure for draining cerebrospinal fluid into the cisterna chiasmatis of the subarachnoid space in hydrocephalus, usually in the newborn. The procedure is not commonly performed and is used chiefly when the cisterna magna is not available for ventriculocisternostomy. The third ventriculostomy makes an opening on the anterior wall of the floor of the third ventricle into the interpeduncular cistern and is performed to correct an obstructive type of hydrocephalus.

thirst /thurst/ [AS, *Thurst*], a perceived desire for water or other fluid. The sensation of thirst is usually referred to the mouth and throat.

Thiry-Vella fistula /thī″rē vel″ə/ [Ludwig Thiry, Austrian physiologist, 1817–1897; Luis Vella, Italian physiologist, 1825–1886], an artificial passage from the abdominal surface of an experimental animal to an isolated intestinal loop, created surgically for the study of intestinal secretions. The continuity of the animal's gut is restored by anastomosis of the severed sections, and the vascular connections and mesenteric attachment of the isolated loop are preserved. The ends of the isolated segment are attached to two openings in the skin of the abdomen to form a closed internal loop.

thixo-, combining form meaning "touch": *thixotropy.*

thixotropy /thiksot″rəpē/ [Gk, *this,* touch, *terpin,* to turn], a property of certain gels or colloids that become less viscous when shaken or agitated but revert to their original viscosity after standing.

Thomas' splint [Hugh O. Thomas, English surgeon, 1834–1891], **1.** a rigid splint constructed of steel bars that are curved to fit the involved limb and are held in place by a cast or a rigid bandage. It is used in the treatment of chronic joint diseases. **2.** a rigid metal splint that extends from a ring at the hip to beyond the foot. It is used to treat a fractured leg and, in conjunction with various traction and suspension devices, to immobilize and position a fractured femur in a preoperative or postoperative patient. Also called *Thomas' knee splint, Thomas' ring splint.*

Thompson scattering. See **scattering.**

Thomsen disease. See **myotonia congenita.**

thoracentesis /thôr′əsentē″sis/ [Gk, *thorax* + *centesis,* puncture], the surgical perforation of the chest wall and pleural space with a needle to aspirate fluid for diagnostic or therapeutic purposes or to remove a specimen for biopsy. The procedure is usually performed using local anesthesia, with the patient in an upright position. Thoracentesis may be used to aspirate fluid to treat pleural effusion or to collect fluid samples for culture or examination. Also called **thoracocentesis.**

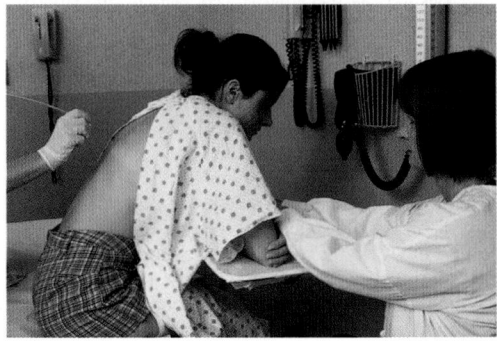

Common position for thoracentesis *(Harkreader and Hogan, 2007)*

thoraces. See **thorax.**

thoracic. See **thorax.**

-thoracic, combining form meaning "the chest": *abdominothoracic arch, cervicothoracic, intrathoracic goiter.*

thoracic actinomycotics. See **actinomycosis.**

thoracic aorta [Gk, *thorax,* chest, *aerein,* to raise], the large upper part of the ascending arch and descending aorta, supplying many parts of the body, such as the heart, ribs, chest muscles, and stomach. Its branches include the coronary brachiocephalic, left common carotid artery, left subclavian, pericardial, bronchial, esophageal, mediastinal, posterior intercostal, subcostal, and superior phrenic. Compare **abdominal aorta.** See also **descending aorta.**

thoracic cage [Gk, *thorax,* chest; L, *cavus,* hollow], the bony framework that surrounds the organs and soft tissues of the chest. It consists of 12 thoracic vertebrae, 12 pairs of ribs, and the sternum.

thoracic cavity [Gk, *thorax,* chest; L, *cavum*], the cavity enclosed by the ribs, the thoracic part of the vertebral column, the sternum, the diaphragm, and associated muscles.

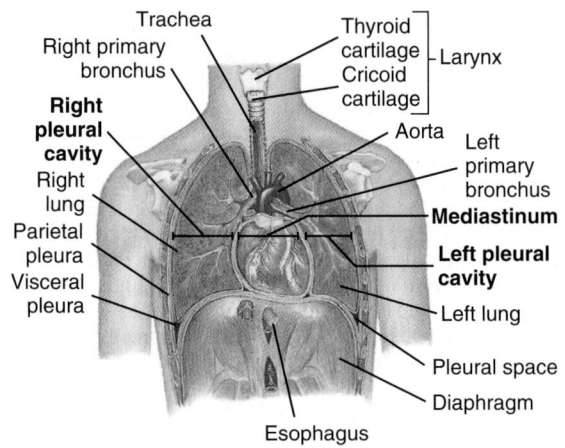

Thoracic cavity *(Thibodeau and Patton, 2003)*

thoracic constriction of esophagus, a narrowing of the thoracic esophagus where it is compressed by the aortic arch and the left main bronchus.

thoracic duct, the common trunk of all the lymphatic vessels in the body, except those on the right and left sides of the head, the neck, and the thorax; the upper abdominal wall; the right and left upper limbs; the right and left lungs; the right side of the heart; and the diaphragmatic surface of the liver. In the adult it is 38 to 45 cm long and 3 to 5 mm in diameter. Also called **alimentary duct.** Compare **right lymphatic duct.** See also **lymphatic system.**

thoracic fistula, an abnormal opening in the chest wall that ends blindly or communicates with the thoracic cavity.

thoracic kyphosis, the dorsally convex curve formed by the thoracic spinal column when seen from the side. Also called *thoracic curvature.*

thoracic medicine, the branch of medicine concerned with the diagnosis and treatment of disorders of the structures and organs of the chest, especially the lungs.

thoracic nerves, the 12 pairs of spinal nerves emerging from the spinal cord at the level of the thorax, including 11 intercostal nerves and one subcostal nerve. They are distributed mainly to the walls of the thorax and the abdomen. The thoracic nerves do not enter a plexus but follow independent courses, making them different from other spinal nerves. The first two intercostal nerves innervate the upper limb and the thorax; the next four supply only the thorax; and the lower five supply the walls of the thorax and the abdomen. Each subcostal thoracic nerve innervates the abdominal wall and the skin of a buttock. See also **autonomic nervous system.**

thoracic outlet syndrome, an abnormal type of mononeuropathy characterized by paresthesia. It may be caused by a nerve root compression by a cervical disk.

thoracic parietal node, one of the lymph glands in the thorax associated with various lymphatic vessels and divided into sternal nodes, intercostal nodes, and diaphragmatic nodes. See also **lymphatic system, lymph node.**

thoracic spine, that part of the spine comprising the thoracic vertebrae.

thoracic surgery [Gk, *thorax,* chest, *cheirourgia,* surgery], the branch of medicine that deals with disease and injuries of the thoracic area by manipulative and operative methods.

thoracic vertebra, one of the 12 bony segments of the spinal column of the upper back designated T1 to T12 or D1 to D12. T1 is just below the seventh cervical vertebra (C7), and T12 is just above the first lumbar vertebra (L1). The thoracic part of the spine is flexible and has a concave ventral curvature. Each vertebra has a broad thick lamina; long, obliquely directed spinous processes; and thick strong articular facets. The thoracic vertebrae are unique in having small lateral facets for articulation with the ribs. The vertebrae are separated from each other by intervertebral disks. The vertebrae become thicker and heavier in descending order from T1 to T12. Compare **cervical vertebra, lumbar vertebra, sacral vertebra.**

thoracic visceral node, a node in the three groups of lymph nodes connected to the part of the lymphatic system that serves certain structures within the thorax, such as the liver, sternum, thymus, pericardium, esophagus, trachea, lungs, diaphragm, and bronchi. Compare **thoracic parietal node.** Kinds include **anterior mediastinal node, posterior mediastinal node,** *tracheobronchial node.* See also **lymph, lymphatic system, lymph node.**

thoracic wall, the musculoskeletal wall of the thorax, consisting of the 12 thoracic vertebrae, the ribs, and the sternum, as well as the intercostals muscles, the subcostales, and the transversus thoracis.

thoraco- /thôr′əkō-/, combining form meaning "the chest": *thoracocentesis, thoracodynia.*

thoracoacromial artery, a short artery originating from the anterior surface of the second part of the axillary artery. It divides into four branches: the pectoral, deltoid, clavicular, and acromial.

thoracocentesis. See **thoracentesis.**

thoracodorsal nerve /thôr′əkōdôr″səl/ [Gk, *thorax* + L, *dorsum,* back], the middle subscapular nerve, a branch of the brachial plexus, usually arising between the upper and lower subscapular nerves. It courses along the posterior wall of the axilla and terminates in branches that supply the latissimus dorsi.

thoracodynia /-din′ē·ə/ [Gk, *thorax,* chest, *odyne,* pain], chest pain.

thoracolumbar fascia /thôr′əkōlum″bər/, a noncontractile structure that functions in a manner similar to a ligament in the lumbar area. It extends from the iliac crest and sacrum to the thoracic cage and envelops the paravertebral musculature. See also **lumbodorsal fascia.**

thoracolumbar junction, the part of the vertebral column from the eleventh thoracic vertebra to the first lumbar vertebra. Here the spinal curvature changes from kyphosis to lordosis and the orientation of the facet joints changes from coronal to sagittal.

thoracolumbosacral orthosis (TLSO) /thôr′əkōlum′bō sā′krəl/ [Gk, *thorax,* chest; L, *lumbus,* loin + *sacrum,* sacred], a spinal orthosis that runs from the thoracic spine caudal to the lumbosacral region and thus limits movement of the thoracic and lumbar spine. Different types vary in rigidity and in the kind of support given to the thorax. See also **body jacket.**

thoracopathy /thôr′əkop″əthē/, any disorder involving the thorax or the organs it contains.

thoracoplasty /thôr″əkoplas′tē/, the surgical reduction in the size of abnormal spaces in the thoracic cavity, such as may result from a collapsed lung.

thoracoscopy, an endoscopic procedure used to directly visualize the pleura, lungs, and mediastinum and to obtain tissue for testing. It is also helpful in staging and dissection of lung cancers.

thoracostomy /thôr′əkos″təmē/ [Gk, *thorax* + *stoma,* mouth], an incision made into the chest wall to provide an opening for the purpose of drainage.

thoracostomy tube, a catheter inserted through the chest wall to drain fluid from the pleural space.

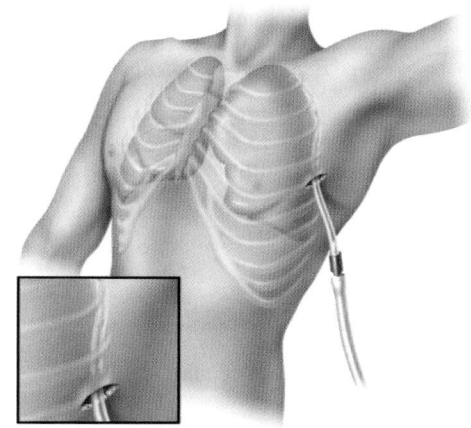

Thoracostomy tube *(Custalow, 2005)*

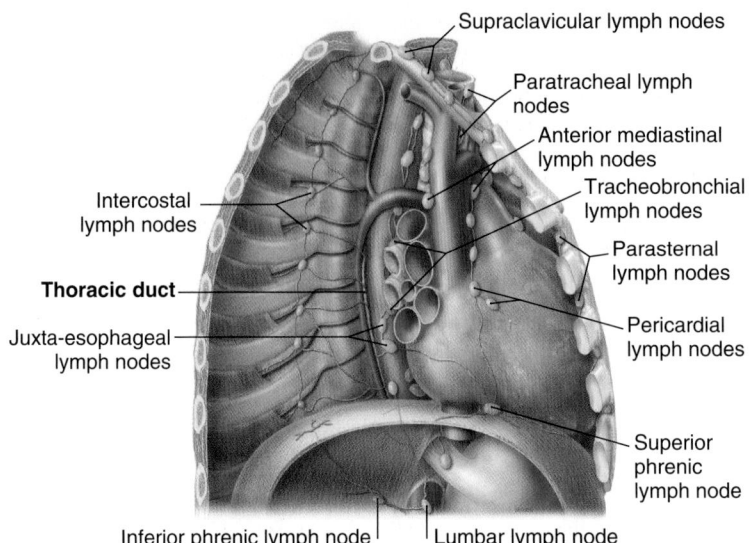

Thorax *(Drake, Vogl, and Mitchell, 2010)*

thoracotomy /thôr′əkot″əmē/ [Gk, *thorax* + *temnein,* to cut], a surgical opening into the thoracic cavity. See also **anterolateral thoracotomy, median sternotomy, posterolateral thoracotomy.**

Thoraeus filters /thôrē′əs/, a combination of metals, usually tin, copper, and aluminum, used to modify the quality of orthovoltage x-ray beams and thus improve their penetrating ability.

Thorazine, a phenothiazine antiemetic and tranquilizer. Brand name for **chlorproMAZINE.**

thorium (Th) /thôr′ē·əm/ [ONorse, *Thor,* god of thunder], a heavy grayish radioactive metallic element. Its atomic number is 90; its atomic mass (weight) is 232.04. Thorium is used in nuclear medicine and in radiation therapy.

thought broadcasting /thôt/ [AS, *thot*], a symptom of psychosis in which the patient believes that his or her thoughts are "broadcast" beyond the head so that other people can hear them.

thought insertion, a belief by some mentally ill patients that thoughts of other people can be inserted into their own minds. See also **schizophrenia.**

thought transference. See **telepathy.**

THP, abbreviation for **Tamm-Horsfall protein.**

Thr, abbreviation for **threonine.**

threadworm. See *Enterobius vermicularis, Acanthocheilonema perstans.*

threadworm infection. See **strongyloidiasis.**

thready pulse /thred′ē/ [AS, *thraed* + L, *pulsare,* to beat], an abnormal pulse that is weak, somewhat difficult to palpate, and often fairly rapid. The artery does not feel full, and the rate may be difficult to count. It is characteristic of hypovolemia, such as occurs with severe hemorrhage.

threatened abortion /thret′ənd/ [AS, *threat,* coercion; L, *ab,* away from, *oriri,* to be born], a condition in pregnancy before the twentieth week of gestation characterized by uterine bleeding and cramping sufficient to suggest that miscarriage may result. A threatened abortion is generally managed with rest and observation. Compare **incomplete abortion, inevitable abortion.**

three-day fever. See **phlebotomus fever.**

3-day measles. See **rubella.**

thorax /thôr′aks/ *pl. thoraxes, thoraces* [Gk, chest], the upper part of the trunk or cage of bone and cartilage containing the principal organs of respiration and circulation and covering part of the abdominal organs. It is formed ventrally by the sternum and costal cartilages and dorsally by the 12 thoracic vertebrae and the dorsal parts of the 12 ribs. The thorax of women has less capacity, a shorter sternum, and more movable upper ribs than that of men. Also called **chest. –thoracic,** *adj.*

3n, abbreviation for **triploid.**

three-point gait [Gk, *treis* + L, *pungere,* to prick; ONorse, *gata,* way], a pattern of crutch-walking in which the crutches and affected leg are advanced together, alternating with the unaffected leg.

three-way irrigation catheter, a hollow, flexible tube with three lumens to faciliate irrigation of a body cavity, especially the urinary bladder. One lumen is for the instillation of fluids; the second is for the evacuation of fluids, clots, and other materials; and the third is to inflate a balloon to hold the catheter in place.

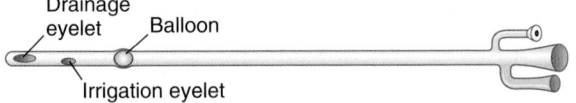

Three-way indwelling irrigation catheter *(Dehn and Asprey, 2013)*

threonine (Thr), an essential amino acid needed for proper growth in infants and maintenance of nitrogen balance in adults. See also **amino acid, protein.**

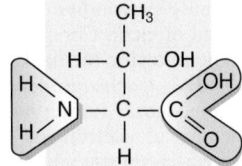

Chemical structure of threonine

threp-, combining form meaning "nutrition": *threptic.*

threptic, related to the care of offspring.

threshold /thresh′ōld/ [AS, *therscold*], the point at which a stimulus is great enough to produce an effect. For example, a pain threshold is the point at which a person becomes aware of pain.

threshold dose [AS, *therscold* + Gk, *dosis,* giving], **1.** a measure of a dose of radiation exposure defined in terms of conditions needed to produce a visible erythema in a given proportion of people exposed. Also called **minimal erythema dose, skin erythema dose,** *threshold erythema dose.* **2.** the minimum dose of a drug needed to produce a measurable response. Administration of drugs at dosages of intervals that do not maintain concentration about the threshold level wastes the medication and, in cases such as antibiotic treatment or cancer chemotherapy, can have additional adverse consequences resulting from the selective growth of cancer cells or microorganisms that are more resistant to the medication.

threshold limit values, the maximum concentration of a chemical to which workers can be exposed for a fixed period, such as 8 hours per day, without developing a physical impairment.

threshold of consciousness [AS, *therscold* + L, *conscire,* to be aware], the lowest limit of perception of a stimulus.

threshold stimulus [AS, *therscold* + L, *stimulare,* to incite], a stimulus that is just sufficient to produce a response. Below that level, no action or response is likely without additional intensity of the stimulus. Also called **limen, liminal stimulus.**

thrill [AS, *thyrlian,* to pierce], a fine vibration, felt by an examiner's hand on a patient's body over the site of an aneurysm or on the precordium, resulting from turmoil in the flow of blood and indicating the presence of an organic murmur of grade 4 or greater intensity. A thrill can also be felt over the carotids if a bruit is present and over an arteriovenous fistula in the patient undergoing hemodialysis. Compare **bruit, murmur.**

thrix /thriks/ [Gk], hair.

throat. See **pharynx.**

throat and nose cultures, a microscopic examination used to isolate and identify pathogens such as streptococci, meningococci, gonococci, *Bordetella pertussis,* and *Corynebacterium diphtheriae.* Identification of streptococci is particularly important in a throat culture because rheumatic heart disease or glomerulonephritis may follow a streptococcal pharyngitis. Nasopharyngeal cultures are often done to screen for infections and carrier states caused by various other organisms such as *Staphylococcus aureus, Haemophilus influenzae, Neisseria meningitidis,* respiratory syncytial virus (RSV), and viruses causing rhinitis.

throb [ME, *throbben,* to beat intensely], a deep, pulsating kind of discomfort or pain. −*throbbing, adj., n.*

thrombapheresis. See **plateletpheresis.**

thrombasthenia /throm′basthē″nē-ə/ [Gk, *thrombos,* lump, *a* + *sthenos,* not strength], decreased platelet function. See **Glanzmann thrombasthenia.**

thrombectomy /thrombek″təmē/ [Gk, *thrombos* + *ektomē,* excision], the removal of a thrombus from a blood vessel, performed as emergency surgery to restore circulation to the affected part. Anticoagulant therapy may begin before surgery. An arteriogram is done to locate the thrombus. During surgery a longitudinal incision is made into the blood vessel, and the clot is removed. After surgery the blood pressure is maintained close to its preoperative level because a decrease would predispose to further clotting. Compare **embolectomy.**

thrombi. See **thrombus.**

thrombin /throm″bin/, the key enzyme produced during coagulation by activation of prothrombin. Thrombin converts fibrinogen to fibrin, activates factors V, VIII, XI, and XIII, and causes platelet aggregation. See also **blood clot, prothrombin.**

thrombo- /throm′bō-/, combining form meaning "clot": *thromboarteritis, thrombocyst, thrombolysis.*

thromboangiitis /throm′bō-an′jē-ī′tis/, an inflammation of the blood vessels associated with thrombosis and accompanied by destruction of the intima.

thromboangiitis obliterans [Gk, *thrombos* + *angeion,* vessel, *itis,* inflammation; L, *obliterare,* to cancel], an occlusive vascular condition, usually of a leg or a foot, in which the small- and medium-sized arteries become inflamed and thrombotic. Early signs of the condition are burning, numbness, and tingling of the foot or leg distal to the lesion. Phlebitis and gangrene may develop as the disease progresses. Pulsation in the limb below the damaged blood vessels is often absent. The goal of therapy is to avoid all factors that decrease the blood supply to the extremity, such as cigarette smoking, and to use all means possible to increase the supply. Amputation may be necessary if the condition progresses to gangrene with chronic infection and extensive tissue destruction. Men are affected more often than women; most affected men smoke and are between 20 and 40 years of age. Also called **Buerger disease.**

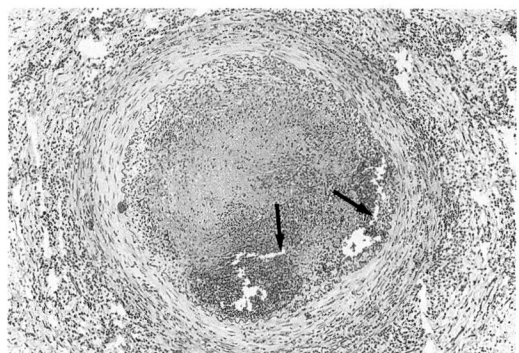

Thromboangiitis obliterans *(Kumar et al, 2007)*

thromboarteritis /throm′bō-är′tərī″tis/, arterial inflammation with thrombus formation.

thrombocyst /throm″bəsist/, a membranous sac enclosing a thrombus.

thrombocyt-, combining form meaning "platelet": *thrombocytopenia, thrombocytosis.*

thrombocyte. See **platelets.**

thrombocythaemia, thrombocythemia. See **thrombocytosis.**

thrombocytopathy /throm′bōsītop″əthē/ [Gk, *thrombos* + *kytos,* cell, *pathos,* disease], any disorder of the blood coagulation mechanism caused by an abnormality or dysfunction of platelets. Kinds include **thrombocytopenia, thrombocytosis.** −*thrombocytopathic, adj.*

thrombocytopenia /throm′bōsī′təpē″nē-ə/ [Gk, *thrombus* + *kytos* + *penia,* poverty], a platelet count below the lower limit of the reference interval, usually 150,000/μL. It may be the consequence of decreased production disorders such as acute leukemia, an idiosyncratic drug response, or increased consumption, such as immune thrombocytopenic purpura. Thrombocytopenia is the most common cause of mucocutaneous (systemic) bleeding. Also called **thrombopenia.**

T

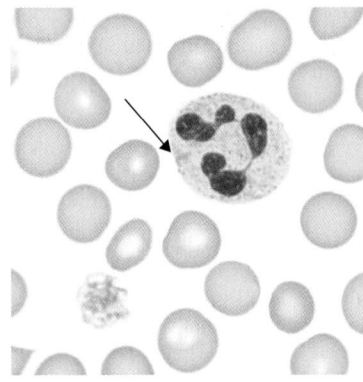

Thrombocytopenia *(Carr and Rodak, 2008)*

thrombocytopenia–absent radius syndrome, an autosomal-recessive syndrome consisting of thrombocytopenia associated with absence or hypoplasia of the radius and sometimes congenital heart disease and renal anomalies. Also called **TAR syndrome.**

thrombocytosis /throm′bōsītō″sis/ [Gk, *thrombos + kytos + osis,* condition], an abnormal increase in the number of platelets in the blood. Benign thrombocytosis, or secondary thrombocytosis, is asymptomatic and usually occurs after splenectomy, inflammatory disease, hemolytic anemia, hemorrhage, or iron deficiency; as a response to exercise; after chemotherapy; in chronic myelogeneous leukemia; or in advanced carcinoma, Hodgkin disease, or other lymphomas. Essential thrombocythemia is characterized by episodes of spontaneous bleeding alternating with thrombotic episodes. The platelets may reach levels exceeding 1,000,000/μL. Compare **thrombocytopenia.** See also **polycythemia.**

thromboembolic disorder (TED) hose. See **antiembolism (AE) hose.**

thromboembolism /-em″bəliz′əm/ [Gk, *thrombos + embolos,* plug], a condition in which a blood vessel is obstructed by a blood clot (thrombus) carried in the bloodstream from its site of formation. The area supplied by an obstructed artery may tingle and become cold, numb, and cyanotic. Treatment includes quiet bed rest, warm wet packs, and anticoagulants to prevent the formation of additional thrombi. Embolectomy may be indicated, especially if the aorta or common iliac artery is obstructed. A thromboembolus in the lungs causes a sudden, sharp thoracic or upper abdominal pain, dyspnea, cough, fever, anxiety, hemoptysis, and associated electrocardiogram changes. Obstruction of the pulmonary artery or one of its main branches may be fatal. Thromboemboli are diagnosed by x-ray films, CT pulmonary angiograms, and other radiological techniques, including lung scans and angiography.

thromboendarterectomy /-en″därtərek′təmē/, removal of thrombus and atherosclerotic inner lining from an obstructed artery.

thrombogenesis /-jen″əsis/, formation of a thrombus or blood clot.

thrombogenic /-jen′ik/ [Gk, *thrombos + genein,* to produce], pertaining to a thrombus or a factor that causes a thrombus.

thromboid /throm″boid/, **1.** clotlike. **2.** resembling a thrombus.

thrombokinase. See **factor X.**

thrombolysis /thrombol″isis/, the dissolution of a thrombus.

thrombolytic /-lit′ik/ [Gk, *thrombos + lysis,* a loosening], pertaining to a drug or another agent that dissolves a thrombus.

thrombolytic therapy (TT), administration of a thrombolytic agent such as tissue plasminogen activator, urokinase, or streptokinase to dissolve an arterial clot, such as a clot in a coronary artery in a patient with an acute myocardial infarction. TT is also used to dissolve clots (thrombi) in venous access devices.

thrombopathy /thrombop″əthē/, a condition in which a clotting ability is deficient for reasons other than thrombocytopenia.

thrombopenia /-pē′nē·ə/ [Gk, *thrombos,* lump, *penia,* poverty]. See **thrombocytopenia.**

thrombopenic purpura. See **hemorrhagic purpura.**

thrombophilia, increased risk of thrombosis secondary to an acquired or inherited thrombotic risk factor.

thrombophlebitis /-fləbī′tis/ [Gk, *thrombos + phleps,* vein, *itis,* inflammation], inflammation of a vein accompanied by the formation of a clot. It occurs most commonly as the result of trauma to the vessel wall; hypercoagulability of the blood; infection; chemical irritation; postoperative venous stasis; prolonged sitting, standing, or immobilization; or a long period of IV catheterization. Also called **phlebitis.**

■ OBSERVATIONS: Thrombophlebitis of a superficial vein is generally evident; the vessel feels hard and thready or cordlike and is extremely sensitive to pressure; the surrounding area may be erythematous and warm to the touch, and the entire limb may be pale, cold, and swollen. Deep vein thrombophlebitis is characterized by aching or cramping pain, especially in the calf, when the patient walks or dorsiflexes the foot (Homans sign).

thrombophlebitis migrans. See **migratory thrombophlebitis.**

thrombophlebitis purulenta, inflammation of a vein associated with the formation of a soft, purulent thrombus that infiltrates the wall of the vessel.

thromboplastic /-plas″tik/, **1.** causing clot formation. **2.** pertaining to the role of thromboplastin in forming a clot.

thromboplastin, a plasma protein that initiates the clotting process by converting prothrombin to thrombin in the presence of calcium ions.

thrombosed /throm″bōst/, **1.** clotted. **2.** pertaining to a blood vessel in which a thrombus has formed.

thrombosis /thrombō″sis/ *pl. thromboses,* an abnormal condition in which a clot (thrombus) develops within a blood vessel. See also **blood clotting.** *–thrombotic, adj.*

thrombosis indicator test, a blood test to support a diagnosis of disseminated intravascular coagulation and to indicate the effectiveness of anticoagulation therapy.

thrombotapheresis. See **plateletpheresis.**

thrombotic microangiopathy, the formation of thrombi in the arterioles and capillaries, as occurs in thrombotic thrombocytopenic purpura and hemolytic uremia syndrome.

thrombotic phlegmasia. See **phlegmasia alba dolens.**

thrombotic thrombocytopenic purpura (TTP) [Gk, *thrombos,* lump, *thrombos + kytos,* cell, *penia,* poverty; L, *purpura,* purple], a disorder characterized by thrombocytopenia, hemolytic anemia, and neurological abnormalities. It is accompanied by a generalized purpura with the deposition of microthrombi within the capillaries and smaller arterioles. It includes a chronic form and an acute fulminating form that may be fatal in weeks. Therapy includes corticosteroids, splenectomy, and therapeutic plasma exchange. Compare **disseminated intravascular coagulation.**

thromboxane, any of several compounds synthesized by platelets and other cells that cause platelet aggregation and vasoconstriction.

thromboxane-A synthase, an enzyme that catalyzes the conversion in platelets of prostaglandin G_2 to thromboxane A_2. A deficiency of the enzyme causes a defect in the release of platelets. See also **thromboxane A_2.**

thromboxane A_2 /thrombok″sān/, biologically active compound derived from prostaglandin H_2 with a 30-second half-life. It increases in concentration after injury to blood vessels and stimulates the primary hemostatic response and irreversible platelet aggregation.

thromboxane B_2, a stable metabolite of thromboxane A_2 that has an effect on polymorphonuclear cells and may possess chemotactic activity. It is released during anaphylaxis in laboratory animals. See also **thromboxane A_2.**

thrombus /throm″bəs/ *pl.* *thrombi* [Gk, *thrombos,* lump], **1.** an aggregation of platelets, fibrin, and red blood cells that attaches to the interior wall of a vein or artery, sometimes occluding the lumen of the vessel. Compare **embolus.** Kinds include **agonal thrombus, hyaline thrombus, laminated thrombus, white thrombus. 2.** a blood clot.

through-and-through drainage /thro͞o/ [ME, *thurgh* + AS, *drachen,* tear drop], a method of irrigating a body organ by inserting two tubes, one to introduce the fluid and another to drain the fluid that accumulates within the organ.

through transmission, a type of ultrasound imaging in which the sound field is transmitted through a specimen and the transmitted energy is picked up on a far surface by a receiving transducer.

thrush [Dan, *troeske,* dryness], candidiasis of the tissues of the mouth. The condition is characterized by the appearance of creamy white patches of exudate on an inflamed tongue or buccal mucosa. It is usually a benign condition in normal children but may be a sign of human immunodeficiency virus infection. See also **candidiasis, stomatitis parasitica.**

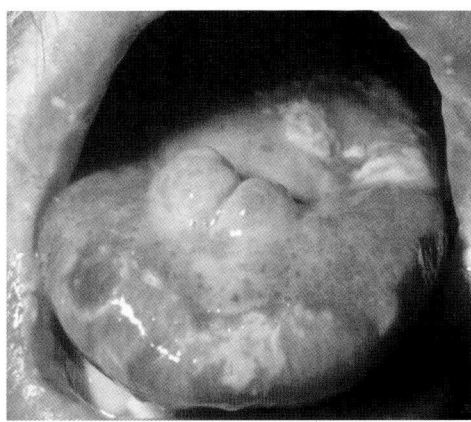

Thrush *(Marks and Miller, 2006)*

thulium (Tm) /tho͞o′lē·əm/ [L, *Thule,* northern island], a rare earth metallic element. Its atomic number is 69; its atomic mass is 168.93. Thulium that has been irradiated in a nuclear reactor gives off gamma radiation.

thumb /thum/ [AS, *thuma*], the first, most lateral digit on the radial side of the hand, classified by most anatomists as one of the fingers because its metacarpal bone ossifies in the same manner as those of the phalanges. Other anatomists classify the thumb separately, noting that it has a much different articulation with the metacarpal bone (a saddle joint) and is composed of one metacarpal bone and only two phalanges. The nerves that innervate the various muscles controlling the thumb include branches of the radial nerve, branches of the median nerve, and the deep palmar branch of the ulnar nerve.

thumb forceps, a surgical instrument used to grasp soft tissue, especially while suturing. Also called **tissue forceps.**

thumb sign [AS, *thuma* + L, *signum*], a swollen, enlarged epiglottis visible on a lateral C-spine x-ray.

thumbsucking, the habit of sucking the thumb for oral gratification. It is normal in infants and young children as a pleasure-seeking or comforting device, especially when the child is hungry or tired. The habit reaches its peak when the child is between 18 and 20 months of age, and it normally disappears as the child develops and matures. Thumbsucking beyond 4 to 6 years of age may lead to malocclusion of the teeth and deformation of the bony tissue of the thumb. Excessive thumbsucking, especially in older children, may be indicative of some emotional problem.

thyme /tīm, thim/ [Gk, *thymon*], the dried leaves and flowering tops of the herb *Thymus vulgaris,* which produces a pungent mintlike aroma. It is the source of a volatile oil, tannin, and gum but is used mainly as a flavoring agent. It also is used in herbal medicine as an infusion for gastrointestinal conditions.

thymectomy /thīmek″təmē/ [Gk, *thymus*], the surgical removal of the thymus.

thymi. See **thymus.**

-thymia, combining form meaning "(condition of the) mind or will": *alexithymia, dysthymia, euthymia.*

thymic /thī″mik/, pertaining to the thymus gland.

thymic hypoplasia, thymic parathyroid aplasia. See **DiGeorge syndrome.**

thymidine (dThd) /thī″mədēn/, one of the four major nucleosides in DNA. It is formed by the condensation of thymine with deoxyribose.

thymidine kinase, an enzyme of the transferase class that catalyzes a phosphorylation reaction of pyrimidine salvage and phosphorylation of drugs, such as acyclovir and ganciclovir, into a form that will be active against viruses.

thymine, a pyrimidine base in animal cells usually occurring condensed with deoxyribose to form the nucleoside deoxythymidine, a component of deoxyribonucleic acid. See also **cytosine, guanine,** *uracil.*

thymo-, 1. combining form meaning "thymus gland": *thymocyte, thymoma.* **2.** combining form meaning "the spirit or mind": *thymogenic.*

thymocyte, the lymphoid cells present in the thymus; heterogeneous population that contains both developing immature T cells and mature naïve T cells.

thymogenic /thī″mō-jen′ik/ [Gk *thymos,* mind, *genesis,* origin], *(Obsolete)* an emotional reaction.

thymol /thī″mol/, a synthetic or natural thyme oil, used as an antibacterial and antifungal, that is an ingredient in some over-the-counter preparations for the treatment of hemorrhoids, acne, and tinea pedis. It is also used as a stabilizer in various pharmaceutic preparations.

T

thymoma /thīmō″mə/ *pl.* **thymomas, thymomata** [Gk, *thymos,* thyme, flowers, *oma,* tumor], a usually benign tumor of the thymus gland that may be associated with myasthenia gravis or an immune deficiency disorder.

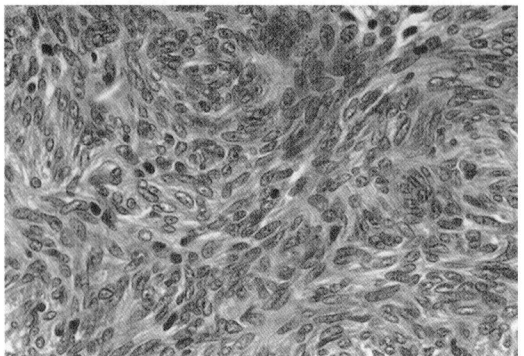

Benign thymoma *(Kumar et al, 2010)*

thymosin /thī″məsin/, **1.** a naturally occurring immunological hormone secreted by the thymus gland. It is present in greatest amounts in young children and decreases in amount throughout life. **2.** an investigational drug derived from bovine thymus extracts and prescribed as an immunomodulator in experimental treatments for certain diseases such as systemic lupus erythematosus or rheumatoid arthritis.

thymus /thī″məs/ *pl.* **thymuses, thymi** [Gk, *thymos,* thyme, flowers], a single unpaired lymphoid organ that is located in the mediastinum, extending superiorly into the neck to the lower edge of the thyroid gland and inferiorly as far as the fourth costal cartilage. The thymus is the primary central gland of the lymphatic system. The endocrine activity of the thymus is believed to depend on the hormone thymosin, which is composed of biologically active peptides critical to the maturation and the development of the immune system. The T cells of the cell-mediated immune response develop in this gland before migrating to the lymph nodes and spleen. The gland consists of two lateral lobes closely bound by connective tissue, which also encloses the entire organ in a capsule. Superficial to the gland is the sternum. Lying deep to the thymus are the great vessels and the cranial part of the pericardium. The two lobes of the gland differ in size, and in many individuals the right lobe overlaps the left lobe. The thymus is about 5 cm long, 4 cm wide, and 6 mm thick. The lobes are composed of numerous lobules, which are separated by delicate connective tissue. Each lobule is composed of a dense cellular cortex and an inner, less dense medulla. The thymus develops in the embryo from the third branchial pouch and increases in size until attaining a weight of 12 to 14 g before birth. The size of the organ relative to the rest of the body is largest when the individual is about 2 years of age. The thymus usually attains its greatest absolute size at puberty, when it weighs about 35 g. After puberty the organ undergoes involution. With aging the gland may change from pinkish-gray to yellow and in the elderly individual may appear as small islands of thymic tissue covered with fat and surrounded by the yellowish capsule. The normal involution of the thymus may be superseded by rapid accidental involution caused by starvation or by acute disease. Compare **spleen.**

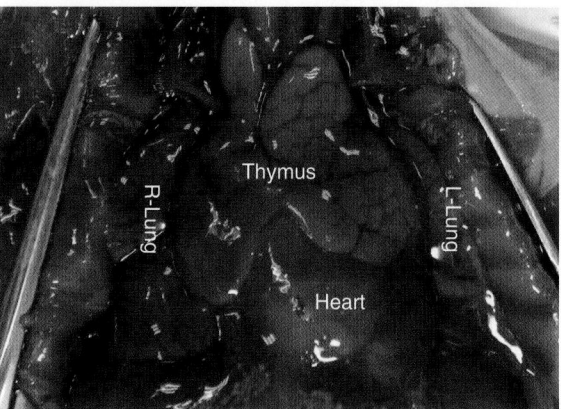

Thymus *(Drake, Vogl, and Mitchell, 2010)*

thymus-dependent antigen, an antigen that requires the interaction between T and B cells to initiate antibody production.

thymus-independent antigen, an antigen that induces antibody (immunoglobulin M) production without direct cooperation from T cells.

Thyrar, a thyroid preparation. Brand name for **thyroid hormone.**

-thyrea, -thyreosis, -thyroidism, combining form meaning "a condition of the thyroid gland": *hyperparathyroidism, hypothyroidism, pseudohyperparathyroidism.*

thyro- /thī′rō-/, **thyroido-, thyreo-,** combining form meaning "a shield" or "pertaining to the thyroid gland": *thyroaplasia, thyroidectomy, thyroiditis.*

thyroaplasia /thī′rō·aplā″zhə/, variations in any of several defects in the thyroid gland and deficiencies of its secretions.

thyroarytenoid muscles, two broad, flat muscles lateral to the fibroelastic membrane of the larynx and the laryngeal entricles and saccules. Each muscle runs from a vertical line of origin on the lower half of the thyroid angle and adjacent external surface of the cricothyroid ligament to the anterolateral surface of the arytenoid cartilage. Some of the fibers may continue into the aryepiglottic fold and reach the margin of the epiglottis. They act as sphincters to the laryngeal vestibule and also narrow the laryngeal inlet. They are innervated by the recurrent laryngeal branches of the vagus nerves.

thyrocalcitonin. See **calcitonin.**

thyrocervical trunk /-sur′vikəl/ [Gk, *thyreos,* shield, *eidos,* form; L, *cervix,* neck, *truncus*], one of a pair of short thick arterial branches arising from the first part of the subclavian arteries close to the medial border of the scalenus anterior and supplying numerous muscles and bones in the head, neck, and back. Each is divided into three branches: the inferior thyroid, the suprascapular, and the transverse cervical.

thyrocricotomy /-krīkot′əmē/ [Gk, *thyreos,* shield, *eidos,* form, *krikos,* ring, *temnein,* to cut], a tracheotomy procedure in which the cricovocal membrane is divided.

thyrogenic /-jen′ik/ [Gk, *thyreos,* shield, *eidos,* form, *genein,* to produce], pertaining to an origin in the thyroid gland. Also *thyrogenous.*

thyroglobulin test, a blood test used primarily to detect well-differentiated thyroid cancers.

thyroglossal /-glos″əl/, pertaining to an embryonic duct connecting the thyroid gland and the tongue. Also **thyrolingual.**

thyrohyoid membrane, a tough fibroelastic ligament that spans between the superior margin of the thyroid cartilage below and hyoid bone above. It is attached to the superior margin of the thyroid laminae and adjacent anterior margins of the superior horns and ascends medial to the greater horns and posterior to the body of the hyoid bone to attach to the superior margins of these structures. An aperture in the lateral part of the membrane on each side allows the passage of the superior laryngeal arteries, nerves, and lymphatics.

thyroid. See **thyroid gland.**

thyroid acropathy /thī′roid/ [Gk, *thyreos,* shield, *eidos,* form, *akron,* extremity, *pathos,* disease], swelling of subcutaneous tissue of the extremities and clubbing of the digits, occurring rarely in patients with thyroid disease and usually associated with pretibial myxedema or exophthalmos.

thyroid cancer, a neoplasm of the thyroid gland, usually characterized by slow growth and a slower and more prolonged clinical course than that of other malignancies. A significant carcinogenic effect of exposure to ionizing radiation is demonstrated by the high rate of thyroid cancer in survivors of exposure to atomic bomb explosions and in individuals who have been treated with radiotherapy for an enlarged thymus in infancy or for acne or other skin disorders in adolescence. Nontoxic colloid goiters and follicular adenomas may be precursors of malignant thyroid tumors. The first sign of cancer may be an increased size of the thyroid gland, a painless palpable nodule, hoarseness, dysphagia, dyspnea, or pain on pressure. Diagnostic measures include x-ray examination, transillumination of the gland, radioisotope scanning, needle biopsy, and ultrasonic examination. More than half of thyroid malignancies are papillary carcinomas, about one third are follicular carcinomas, and the rest consist of rapidly growing invasive anaplastic carcinomas; medullary carcinomas that secrete calcitonin; and metastatic lesions from primary tumors in the breast, kidneys, or lungs. Total or subtotal thyroidectomy with excision of involved lymph nodes is usually recommended. Radioactive iodine may be administered after surgery, and high doses of exogenous thyroid are often used to suppress thyroid-stimulating hormone (TSH) in an effort to cause the regression of residual tumor dependent on TSH. Various chemotherapeutic agents, especially adriamycin, may be effective in patients with metastatic thyroid cancer that is unresponsive to conventional treatment. Thyroid cancer is twice as common in women as in men. Although it is diagnosed most frequently in people between 30 and 50 years of age, it may also occur in children and older individuals.

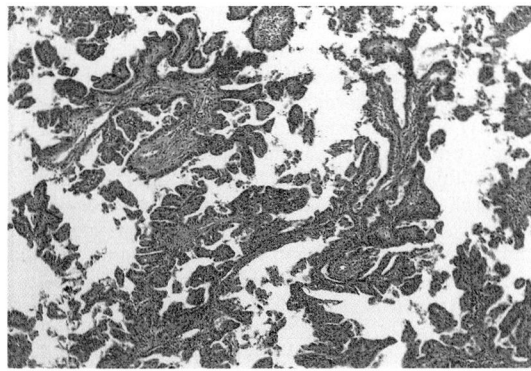

Thyroid cancer: papillary carcinoma *(Belchetz and Hammond, 2003)*

thyroid cartilage, the largest cartilage of the larynx, consisting of two laminae fused together at an acute angle in the midline of the anterior neck to form the Adam's apple. Compare **cricoid.**

thyroid crisis [Gk, *thyreos,* shield, *eidos,* form, *krisis,* turning point], a sudden exacerbation of symptoms of thyrotoxicosis, characterized by fever, sweating, tachycardia, extreme nervous excitability, and pulmonary edema. It usually occurs in a patient whose thyrotoxicosis treatment is inadequate, and the paroxysm is triggered by a stressful infection or injury. If untreated, the crisis is often fatal. Also called **thyroid storm, thyrotoxic crisis.** See also **Graves disease.**

thyroid dermoid cyst, a tumor derived from embryonal tissues that is believed to develop in the thyroid gland or in the thyrolingual duct.

thyroid dermopathy, pretibial myxedema.

thyroidectomized /thī′roidek″təmīzd/ [Gk, *thyreos,* shield, *eidos,* form, *ektomē,* excision], pertaining to a patient or condition in which the thyroid gland has been removed.

thyroidectomy /thī′roidek″təmē/ [Gk, *thyreos* + *eidos,* form, *ektomē,* excision], the surgical removal of the thyroid gland. It is performed for colloid goiter, tumors, or hyperthyroidism that does not respond to iodine therapy and antithyroid drugs. All but 5% to 10% of the gland is removed. Regrowth usually begins shortly after surgery, and thyroid function may return to normal. For cancer of the thyroid, the entire gland is removed, followed by iodine-131 remnant ablation. Before surgery the basal metabolism rate is lowered to normal by giving iodine and antithyroid drugs. If a tumor is present, a frozen section of the affected tissue is examined by a pathologist. If malignant cells are found, all the gland is removed. After surgery the patient is most comfortable in semi-Fowler position with continuous mist inhalation administered to liquefy oral secretions. Oral suctioning may be necessary. A tracheotomy set and oxygen are kept in the room. Calcium gluconate is on hand for use if the patient develops tetany. After surgery the patient is observed for signs of hemorrhage, respiratory difficulty caused by edema of the glottis, and the muscular twitching of tetany from inadvertent removal of a parathyroid gland.

thyroid function test, any of several laboratory tests performed to evaluate the function of the thyroid gland. Thyroid function tests include protein-bound iodine, butanol-extractable iodine, T_3, T_4, free thyroxine index, thyroxin-binding globulin, thyroid-stimulating hormone, long-acting thyroid stimulator, radioactive iodine uptake, and radioactive iodine excretion. Often several of the tests are performed simultaneously.

thyroid gland [Gk, *thyreos,* shield, *eidos,* form], a highly vascular organ at the front of the neck, usually weighing about 30 g and consisting of bilateral lobes connected in the middle by a narrow isthmus. It is slightly heavier in women than in men and enlarges during pregnancy. The majority of the thyroid gland secretes the hormones thyroxin and triiodothyronine, and other clusters of cells produce the hormone calcitonin. These hormones are secreted directly into the blood; thus the thyroid is part of the endocrine system of ductless glands. It is essential to normal body growth in infancy and childhood, and its removal greatly reduces the oxidative processes of the body, producing a lower metabolic rate characteristic of hypothyroidism. The thyroid gland is activated by the pituitary thyrotrophic hormone and requires iodine to elaborate thyroxine. Also called **thyroid.** Compare **parathyroid gland.**

T

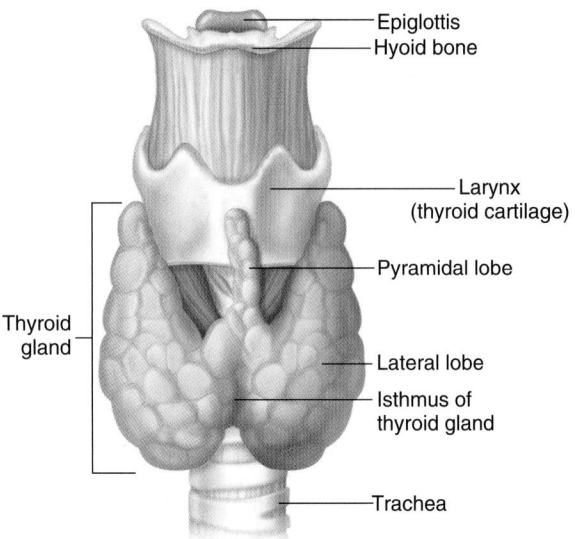

Epiglottis
Hyoid bone

Larynx
(thyroid cartilage)

Pyramidal lobe

Thyroid
gland

Lateral lobe

Isthmus of
thyroid gland

Trachea

Thyroid gland *(Patton and Thibodeau, 2010)*

thyroid hormone, an iodine-containing compound secreted by the thyroid gland, predominantly as thyroxine (T_4) and, in smaller amounts but four times more potent, triiodothyronine (T_3). These hormones increase the rate of metabolism; affect body temperature; regulate protein, fat, and carbohydrate catabolism in all cells; maintain growth hormone secretion, skeletal maturation, and the cardiac rate, force, and output; promote central nervous system development; stimulate the synthesis of many enzymes; and are necessary for muscle tone and vigor. Derivatives of thyronine, T_4 and T_3, are synthesized in the thyroid gland by a complex process involving the uptake, oxidation, and incorporation of iodide and the production of thyroglobulin, the form in which the hormones apparently are stored in thyroid follicular colloid. After the proteolysis of thyroglobulin, T_4 and T_3 are released and transported in the blood in strong, but noncovalent, association with certain plasma proteins; T_4 accounts for approximately 90% of iodine in circulation, and T_3 for 5%. All phases of the production and release of T_4 and T_3 are regulated by the thyroid-stimulating hormone secreted by the anterior pituitary gland. Production of thyroid hormones is excessive in Graves disease and toxic nodular goiter (Plummer's disease), diminished in myxedema, and absent in cretinism. The normal 6- to 7-day half-life of T_4 in blood is reduced to 3 or 4 days in hyperthyroidism and extended to 9 or 10 days in myxedema. T_3 has a normal half-life of 2 days or less and, like T_4, is metabolized most actively in the liver. Pharmaceutic preparations of thyroid hormones extracted from animal glands and the synthetic compounds levothyroxine sodium and liothyronine sodium are used as replacement therapy in patients with hypothyroidism. The dosage is initially low and is gradually increased to the optimal level based on the patient's clinical response and tests of the findings on thyroid function studies. Overdosage or a rapid increase in the dosage may result in signs of hyperthyroidism, such as nervousness, tremor, tachycardia, cardiac arrhythmia, and menstrual irregularity.

-thyroidism. See **-thyrea, -thyreosis, -thyroidism.**

thyroiditis /thī'roidī'tis/, inflammation of the thyroid gland. Acute thyroiditis caused by staphylococcal, streptococcal, or other infections is characterized by suppuration and abscess formation and may progress to subacute diffuse disease of the gland. Subacute thyroiditis is marked by fever, weakness, sore throat, and a painfully enlarged gland containing granulomas composed of colloid masses surrounded by giant cells and mononuclear cells. Chronic lymphocytic thyroiditis (Hashimoto disease), characterized by lymphocyte and plasma cell infiltration of the gland and diffuse enlargement, seems to be transmitted as a dominant trait, may be associated with various autoimmune disorders, and is more common in women. Another chronic form of autoimmune thyroiditis is Riedel's struma, a rare progressive fibrosis, usually of one lobe of the gland but sometimes involving both lobes, the trachea, and surrounding muscles, nerves, and blood vessels. Radiation thyroiditis occasionally occurs 7 to 10 days after the treatment of hyperthyroidism with radioactive iodine 131.

thyroid notch, 1. (superior) a separation above the anterior border of the thyroid cartilage. **2.** (inferior) a depression in the middle of the lower border of the thyroid cartilage.

thyroido-. See **thyro-.**

thyroid-releasing hormone. See **thyrotropin-releasing hormone.**

thyroid scanning, a radionuclear scan that determines the size, shape, position, and physiological function of the thyroid gland. It is useful in patients with neck or substernal masses, thyroid nodules, hyperthyroidism, metastatic tumors without a known primary site, and well-differentiated forms of thyroid cancer. The scan may focus either on the neck area only or on the whole body (done in patients previously treated for thyroid cancer).

thyroid-stimulating hormone (TSH), a substance secreted by the anterior lobe of the pituitary gland that controls the release of thyroid hormone and is necessary for the growth and function of the thyroid gland. The secretion of TSH is regulated by thyrotropin-releasing hormone, elaborated in the median eminence of the hypothalamus and circulating thyroid hormone levels. Normal adult blood levels are 2 to 10 mU/L (SI units). Also called **thyrotropin.** See also **thyroid hormone.**

thyroid-stimulating hormone test (TSH test), a thyroid function test in which thyrotropin (thyroid-stimulating hormone) is administered intramuscularly and the thyroid gland is monitored over time with scintiscanning or radioimmunoassays for a response or areas of decreased responsiveness. It is also used to monitor exogenous thyroid replacement. The test was formerly used for determining whether hypothyroidism was caused by thyroid gland failure or by deficiency in thyrotropin. Also called *thyroid-stimulating hormone assay.*

thyroid-stimulating immunoglobulins test, a blood test to diagnose Graves disease.

thyroid storm, a crisis of uncontrolled thyrotoxicosis caused by the release into the bloodstream of increased amounts of thyroid hormone. Thyroid storm may occur spontaneously or be precipitated by infection, stress, or a thyroidectomy performed on a patient who is inadequately prepared with antithyroid drugs. Characteristic signs are fever that may reach 106° F, a rapid pulse, acute respiratory distress, apprehension, restlessness, irritability, and prostration. The patient may become delirious, lapse into a coma, and die of heart failure. Also called **thyroid crisis.**

thyroid ultrasound, an ultrasound examination of the thyroid gland, used to distinguish cystic from solid thyroid nodules, to determine the efficacy of treatment of a thyroid mass, and to study the thyroid gland of pregnant patients.

Thyrolar, a thyroid preparation. Brand name for **liotrix.**

thyroliberin /thī′rōlib″ərin/, a tripeptide hormone produced by the hypothalamus that stimulates the anterior pituitary gland to release thyrotropin. Also called **thyrotropin-releasing hormone.**

thyrolingual. See **thyroglossal.**

thyromegaly /-meg′əlē/ [Gk, *thyreos,* shield, *eidos,* form, *megas,* large], enlargement of the thyroid gland.

thyrotonine (T₃) triiodothyronine. See **thyroid hormone.**

thyrotoxic crisis. See **thyroid crisis.**

thyrotoxic myopathy /-tok″sik/, a condition in thyrotoxicosis consisting of severe weakness in the limb and trunk muscles, including those used in speech and swallowing.

thyrotoxicosis. See **Graves disease.**

thyrotoxin /-tok″sin/, a theoretic cytotoxin of the thyroid gland, assumed to be a cause of the signs and symptoms of thyrotoxicosis.

thyrotrophic /-trof′ik/ [Gk, *thyreos,* shield, *eidos,* form, *trophe,* nutrition], influencing the thyroid gland, such as the thyroid-stimulating hormone.

thyrotropic hormone. See **thyroid-stimulating hormone.**

thyrotropin. See **thyroid-stimulating hormone.**

thyrotropin alfa, a recombinant form of human thyrotropin. It binds to thyrotropin receptors and stimulates the steps in thyroid hormone synthesis, including iodine uptake and synthesis and secretion of thyroglobulin. It is used as a diagnostic adjunct in serum thyroglobulin testing, with or without radioiodine scanning, in follow-up of patients with well-differentiated thyroid cancer and is administered intramuscularly.

thyrotropin alpha /-trō′pin/, a thyroid-stimulating hormone made with recombinant DNA technology. It increases the uptake of radioactive iodine in the thyroid and the secretion of thyroxine by the thyroid.

■ INDICATIONS: It is prescribed in diagnostic tests and to enhance uptake of ¹³¹I in the treatment of thyroid cancer.

■ CONTRAINDICATIONS: Coronary thrombosis or known hypersensitivity to this drug prohibits its use. It should not be given in untreated Addison disease or after myocardial infarction.

■ ADVERSE EFFECTS: Among the most serious adverse effects are symptoms of hyperthyroidism, allergic reactions, hypotension, and arrhythmias.

thyrotropin-releasing hormone (TRH), a substance produced in the hypothalamus that stimulates the release of thyrotropin (thyroid-stimulating hormone) from the anterior lobe of the pituitary gland. Formerly called *thyrotropin-releasing factor,* **TSH releasing factor.**

thyrotropin-releasing hormone stimulation test, a thyroid function test that assesses release of thyrotropin by the pituitary gland. A bolus of thyrotropin-releasing hormone is administered, and serum concentrations of thyrotropin are assessed at intervals. If serum levels do not increase within 30 to 40 minutes, the pituitary thyrotrophs are dysfunctional. Also called *thyrotropin-releasing hormone test,* **TRH stimulation test, TRH test.**

thyroxine (T₄) /thīrok′sēn/, a hormone of the thyroid gland, derived from tyrosine and deiodinated in the periphery to T₃ (triiodothyronine). Thyroxine stimulates metabolic rate. Also called **tetraiodothyronine.**

thyroxine-binding globulin (TBG), a plasma protein that binds with and transports thyroxine in the blood.

thyroxine-binding globulin test, a blood test used to detect levels of TBG, the major thyroid hormone protein carrier. Elevated TBGs may indicate porphyria or infectious hepatitis, among other conditions, while decreased TBGs may signify various causes of hypoproteinemia (nephrotic syndrome, GI malabsorption, malnutrition).

Ti, symbol for the element **titanium.**

TI, **1.** time to inversion. **2.** the time interval between the initial 180-degree pulse and the subsequent 90-degree radiofrequency pulse in an inversion recovery pulse sequence. **3.** abbreviation for **therapeutic index.**

TIA, abbreviation for **transient ischemic attack.**

tiagabine, an anticonvulsant.

■ INDICATIONS: It is used as an adjunct treatment for partial seizures.

■ CONTRAINDICATIONS: Known hypersensitivity to this prohibits its use.

■ ADVERSE EFFECTS: Adverse effects include dizziness, anxiety, somnolence, ataxia, amnesia, unsteady gait, depression, vasodilation, nausea, vomiting, diarrhea, pruritus, rash, pharyngitis, and coughing. Abrupt discontinuation of this drug can cause sudden onset of seizures. Simultaneous use of the herb ginkgo may decrease anticonvulsant effectiveness.

tibia /tib′ē-ə/ [L, shin bone], the second longest bone of the skeleton, located at the anteromedial side of the leg. It articulates with the fibula laterally, the talus distally, and the femur proximally, forming part of the knee joint. It provides insertion for the quadriceps femoris group of muscles via the patellar ligament and attaches to various muscles, including the popliteus and the flexor digitorum longus. Also called **shin bone.**

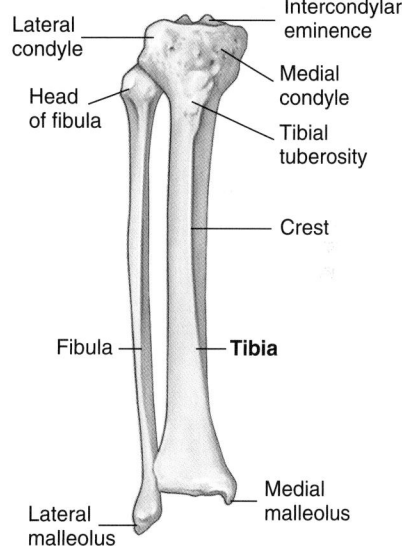

Tibia *(Patton and Thibodeau, 2010)*

tibia-, combining form meaning "the tibia."

tibial /tib′ē-əl/ [L, *tibia,* shin bone], pertaining to the largest long bone of the lower leg.

tibialis anterior /tib′ē-ā″lis/ [L, *tibia* + *anticus,* in front], one of the anterior crural muscles of the leg, situated on the lateral side of the tibia. It is a thick, fleshy muscle proximally and tendinous distally. The muscle dorsiflexes and inverts the foot. Also called *tibialis anticus.* Compare **extensor digitorum longus.**

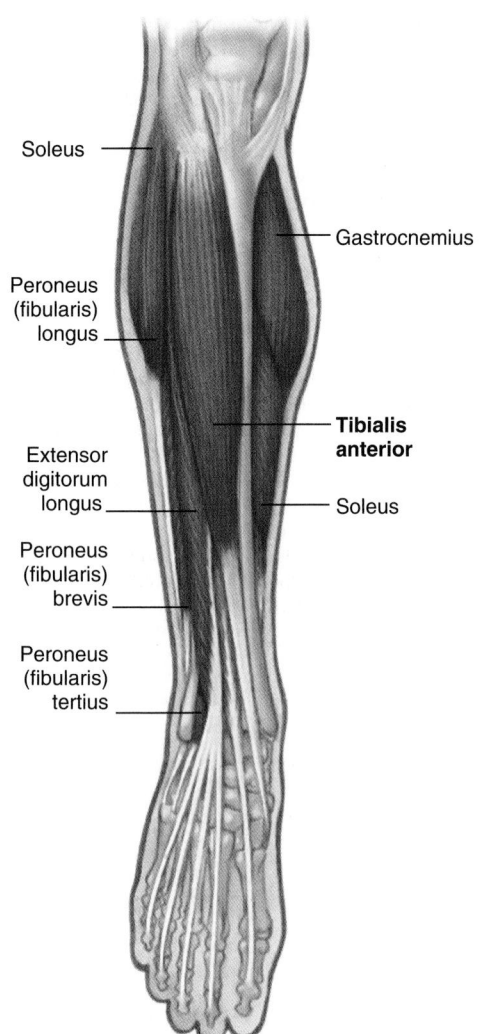

Tibialis anterior *(Patton and Thibodeau, 2010)*

tibial nerve, a major branch of the sciatic nerve that is associated with the posterior compartment of the leg. In the leg it gives rise to branches that supply all the muscles in the posterior compartment of the leg and two cutaneous branches. It enters the foot to supply most of the intrinsic muscles and skin.

tibial torsion [L, *tibia + torquere,* to twist], a lateral or a medial twisting rotation of the tibia on its longitudinal axis. It is similar to pronation of the hand, caused by the contraction of the pronator teres and the pronator quadratus, or supination of the hand caused by the contraction of the supinator muscle. Compare **femoral torsion.**

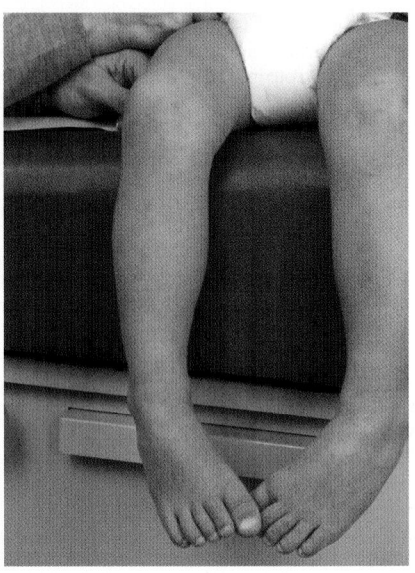

Internal tibial torsion *(Duderstadt, 2006)*

tibia valga [L, *tibia,* shin bone, *valgus,* bowlegged], a bowed tibia with the convex surface toward the outside of the leg.

tic, an involuntary, compulsive, rapid, repetitive, stereotyped movement or vocalization. It can occasionally, but not always, be suppressed and is usually increased by stress. Sleep and engaging activities may reduce occurrence. Kinds include **mimic spasm, coprolalia, echolalia.**

-tic, suffix meaning "pertaining to": *paralytic, therapeutic.*

Ticar, an antibiotic medication. Brand name for **ticarcillin.**

ticarcillin /tik′ärsil″in/, an extended-spectrum penicillin antibiotic.

■ INDICATIONS: It is prescribed in the treatment of bacterial septicemia, as well as skin, soft tissue, and respiratory infections caused by both gram-negative and gram-positive organisms, including some strains of *Pseudomonas.*

■ CONTRAINDICATIONS: A history of allergic reaction to any of the penicillins prohibits its use.

■ ADVERSE EFFECTS: Among the most serious adverse effects are anaphylactic reactions, thrombocytopenia, leukopenia, neutropenia, eosinophilia, vein irritation, and phlebitis.

tic douloureux /tik dōōlōōrœ′/ [Fr, painful spasm], a brief, extremely painful attack of trigeminal neuralgia. It is unilateral and limited to the distribution of the trigeminal (fifth cranial) nerve. An attack is easily and unexpectedly provoked by any stimulus of the facial muscles, from touching to speaking, and may occur repetitively. See also **trigeminal neuralgia.**

tick bite [ME, *tike* + AS, *bitan,* to bite], a puncture wound produced by the toothed beak of a blood-sucking tick, a small, tough-skinned arachnid. Ticks transmit several diseases to humans, and a few species carry a neurotoxin in their saliva that may cause ascending paralysis beginning in the legs. Nervousness, loss of appetite, tingling, and headache, followed by muscle pain and, in extreme cases, respiratory failure may occur. Symptoms often disappear when the attached tick is carefully removed with forceps. See also

Lyme disease, Q fever, relapsing fever, Rocky Mountain spotted fever, tularemia.

tick-borne relapsing fever. See ***Borrelia duttonii.***

tick-borne rickettsiosis [ME, *tike* + *beren* + *Rickettsia* + Gk, *osis,* condition], any disease transmitted by Ixodid ticks carrying the *Rickettsia* pathogens, microorganisms smaller than bacteria but larger than viruses. A common infectious species in North America is *Rickettsia rickettsii,* the cause of Rocky Mountain spotted fever.

tick fever, any of various infectious diseases transmitted by the bite of a tick. The causative parasite may be a *Rickettsia,* as in Rocky Mountain spotted fever; a bacterium, such as *Babesia* or *Borrelia*; or a virus, such as that causing Colorado tick fever.

tickling, a gentle stimulation of the skin surface that produces pleasurable reflexes.

tick paralysis, a rare, progressive, reversible disorder caused by several species of ticks that release a neurotoxin that causes weakness, incoordination, and paralysis. The tick must feed on the host for several days before the symptoms appear, and removal of the tick leads to rapid recovery. Because respiratory or bulbar paralysis can cause death, it is important to search for ticks, frequently hidden in scalp hair, on a patient with these symptoms. This infection is often confused with Guillain-Barré syndrome, botulism, and myasthenia gravis.

ticlopidine /tiklo′pidēn/, a platelet inhibitor used as the hydrochloride salt in the prevention of stroke syndrome.

t.i.d., (in prescriptions) a notation for a Latin phrase meaning "three times a day." Abbreviation for *ter in die.*

tidal /tī′dəl/ [AS, *tid,* time], pertaining to an alternating process, such as a rise-and-fall, ebb-and-flow, or periodic lapse of time.

tidal drainage. See **drainage.**

Tidal Model of Health Recovery, a philosophical approach to the discovery of mental health. This approach emphasizes helping people reclaim the personal story of mental distress by recovering their voices. The use of a person's own language, metaphors, and personal stories is encouraged to faciliate the expression of the meaning of their lives. See **Barker, Phil.**

tidal volume (TV, V$_t$) [AS, *tid,* time; L, *volumen,* paper roll], the amount of air inhaled and exhaled during normal ventilation. Inspiratory reserve volume, expiratory reserve volume, and tidal volume make up vital capacity. See also **pulmonary function test.**

tide [AS, *tid*], a variation, increase, or decrease in the concentration of a particular component of body fluids, such as acid tide or fat tide.

tidemark, a transitional zone, appearing as a wavy line, that marks the junction between calcified and uncalcified cartilage.

Tietze syndrome /tēt″sē/ [Alexander Tietze, German surgeon, 1864–1927], **1.** a disorder characterized by nonsuppurative swellings of one or more costal cartilages that may accompany chronic respiratory infections. It causes pain that may radiate to the neck, shoulder, or arm, mimicking the pain of coronary artery disease. If the pain is severe, infiltration with procaine and hydrocortisone may provide relief. **2.** albinism, except for normal eye pigment, accompanied by deaf mutism and hypoplasia of the eyebrows.

TIG, abbreviation for **tetanus immune globulin.**

Tigan, an antiemetic medication. Brand name for **trimethobenzamide hydrochloride.**

tigecycline, a broad-spectrum antiinfective.

■ INDICATIONS: This drug is used to treat complicated skin and skin structure infections caused by *Escherichia coli, Enterococcus faecalis* (vancomycin-susceptible only), *Staphylococcus aureus, Streptococcus agalactiae, S. anginosus* group, *S. pyogenes, Bacteroides fragilis* and complicated intraabdominal infections caused by *Citrobacter freundii, Enterobacter cloacae, Escherichia coli, Klebsiella oxytoca, K. pneumoniae, E. faecalis* (vancomycin-susceptible only), *S. aureus* (methicillin-susceptible only), *S. anginosus* group, *B. fragilis, B. thetaiotaomicron, B. uniformis, B. vulgatus, Clostridium perfringens,* and *Peptostreptococcus micros.*

■ CONTRAINDICATIONS: Pregnancy, lactation, and known hypersensitivity to this drug prohibit its use. Children under 18 years of age should not use this drug.

■ ADVERSE EFFECTS: Adverse effects of this drug include headache; dizziness; insomnia; hypertension; hypotension; phlebitis; anorexia; constipation; dyspepsia; pruritus; sweating; photosensitivity; increased aspartate aminotransferase, alanine aminotransferase, blood urea nitrogen, lactic acid, alkaline phosphatase, and amylase; hyperglycemia; hypokalemia; hypoproteinemia; bilirubinemia; back pain; fever; abnormal healing; abdominal pain; abscess; asthenia; infection; pain; peripheral edema; and local reactions. Life-threatening side effects include anemia, leukocytosis, and thrombocytopenia. Common side effects include nausea, vomiting, and diarrhea.

tight junction /tīt/ [ME, *thight,* strong; L, *jungere,* to join], the zonula occludens of the junctional complex between cells in which the plasma membranes of adjacent cells are in direct contact and where there is no intercellular space.

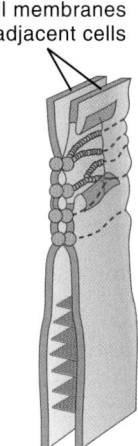

Cell membranes of adjacent cells

Tight junction *(Thibodeau and Patton, 2007)*

tilt table [AS, *tealt,* unsteady; L, *tabula,* board], an examining table that allows a patient to be raised to an approximate 60-degree angle during study of the response of the patient's circulatory system to gravitational forces. A tilt table is also used to assist recovery from orthostatic hypotension after prolonged immobility.

tiludronate, a parathyroid agent (calcium regulator).

■ INDICATIONS: It is used to treat Paget disease.

■ CONTRAINDICATIONS: Factors that prohibit its use include known hypersensitivity to biphosphonates, pathological fractures, colitis, and severe renal disease with creatinine 5 mg/dL. Its use is also contraindicated in children.

■ ADVERSE EFFECTS: Adverse effects include dry mouth, gastritis, vomiting, flatulence, gastric ulcers, rhinitis, rales, sinusitis, upper respiratory infection, headache, somnolence, dizziness, anxiety, vertigo, nervousness, involuntary movements, hyperparathyroidism, rash, epidermal necrosis, pruritus, sweating, nephrotoxicity, decreased mineralization of nonaffected bones, and pathological fractures. Common side effects include nausea, diarrhea, and bone pain.

timbre /tim′bər/ [Fr], **1.** a characteristic sound quality of a voice or musical instrument, as determined by the harmonics of the sound. **2.** a second metallic sound heard in aortic dilation.

time (t) [AS, *tima*], **1.** a measure of duration. **2.** an interval separating two points in a continuum between the past and future.

time agnosia. See **dischronation.**

time constant, a mathematic term of fixed value used in expressing the rate of change of some variable, such as airflow in the airways, as a function of time.

timed collection, the collection of a specimen, such as a urine or stool sample, for a specific period of time.

timed cycling, the delivery of gas under positive pressure during inspiration until an adjustable, preselected time interval has elapsed.

time delay, a period between the application of an input and the beginning of the response.

timed release. See **prolonged release.**

timed vital capacity. See **forced expiratory vital capacity.**

time gain compensation (TGC), increasing amplification of echoes from increasing tissue depths. It is used in ultrasound to correct for increased attenuation of sound with tissue depth.

time-sharing. See **multitasking.**

time trigger, a trigger for initiating assisted ventilation consisting of a mechanism that measures frequency of respirations and starts assisted ventilation when the respiratory frequency is at a given point.

timolol maleate /tim′əlōl/, a beta-adrenergic receptor blocking agent.

■ INDICATIONS: An ophthalmic preparation is used for treating glaucoma, especially chronic open-angle glaucoma. It is administered orally for the treatment of angina and hypertension, to reduce postmyocardial infarction mortality, and as migraine prophylaxis.

■ CONTRAINDICATIONS: Bronchial asthma, chronic obstructive pulmonary disease, sinus bradycardia, cardiogenic shock, pregnancy (second or third trimester), or known hypersensitivity to this drug prohibits its use. It is used with caution in patients (e.g., diabetics) with contraindications to systemic use of beta-adrenergic receptor blocking agents.

■ ADVERSE EFFECTS: The most serious adverse effects of ophthalmic use is blurring of vision. Mild eye irritation also may occur. When it is used systemically, adverse reactions include bronchospasm, cold extremities, decreased sexual ability, drowsiness, and insomnia.

Timoptic, a beta-adrenergic receptor blocking agent. Brand name for **timolol maleate.**

tin (Sn) [AS], a whitish metallic element. Its atomic number is 50; its atomic mass is 118.69. Tin (IV) oxide is used in dentistry as a polishing agent for teeth and in some restorative procedures. See also **stannous fluoride.**

Tinactin, an antifungal medication. Brand name for **tolnaftate.**

tincture, a plant extract made by soaking herbs in a liquid (such as water, alcohol, vinegar, or glycerine) for a specified length of time, then straining and discarding the plant material. The remaining liquid is used therapeutically. Tinctures typically are made at a concentration of 1:5 to 1:10.

tincture (tinct.) /tingk′chər/, a substance in a solution that is dissolved in alcohol.

tincture of iodine [L, *tinctura* + Gk, *ioeides,* violet], *(Obsolete)* a mixture of sodium iodide in an alcohol-water solution; used as a disinfectant.

Tindamax, an antibiotic medication. Brand name for **tinidazole.**

T-independent antigen, an antigen that can trigger B lymphocytes to produce antibodies without the participation of T lymphocytes.

tine, a sharp projecting point, as a prong of a fork.

tinea /tin′ē·ə/ [L, worm], a group of fungal skin diseases caused by dermatophytes of several kinds. The condition is characterized by itching, scaling, and sometimes painful lesions. Tinea is spread by direct contact between humans and even domestic dogs or cats. Diagnosis is made by demonstrating fungus on smear or by culture. Also called **ringworm.** See also **tinea corporis, tinea cruris, tinea pedis, tinea unguium.**

tinea capitis, a superficial fungal infection of the scalp, most common in children. Most infections are caused by species of *Trichophyton.* The infection may lead to hair loss and become secondarily infected with bacteria, causing a severe inflammation. Symptoms include severe itching and scaling of the scalp. Treatment with oral antifungal agents as well as appropriate antibiotics is necessary. Oral steroids may be necessary to prevent scarring hair loss.

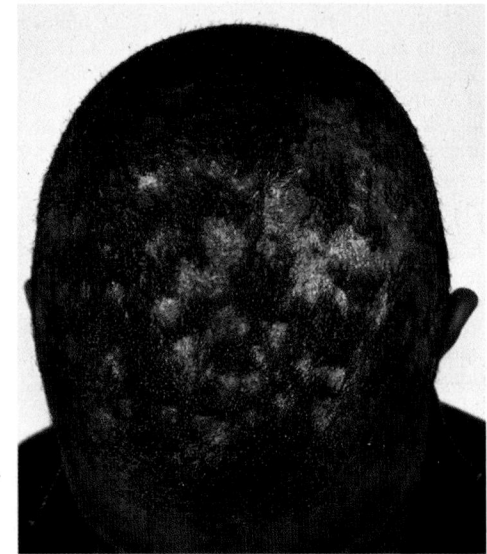

Tinea capitis *(Conlon and Snydman, 2000)*

tinea corporis, a superficial fungal infection of the nonhairy skin of the body, most prevalent in hot, humid climates and usually caused by species of *Trichophyton* or *Microsporum.* Topical fungicides such as miconazole are used for moderate cases; severe infection calls for griseofulvin.

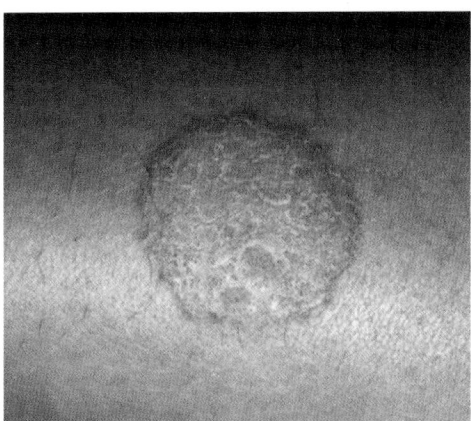

Tinea corporis *(Alter et al, 2018)*

tinea cruris /krōō′ris/, a superficial fungal infection of the groin caused by species of *Trichophyton* or *Epidermophyton floccosum,* the second most common dermatophytosis for clinical presentation. It is most common in the tropics and among males. Topical antifungals such as miconazole and clotrimazole are often prescribed. Griseofulvin is used only for severe resistant cases. Also called **jock itch.**

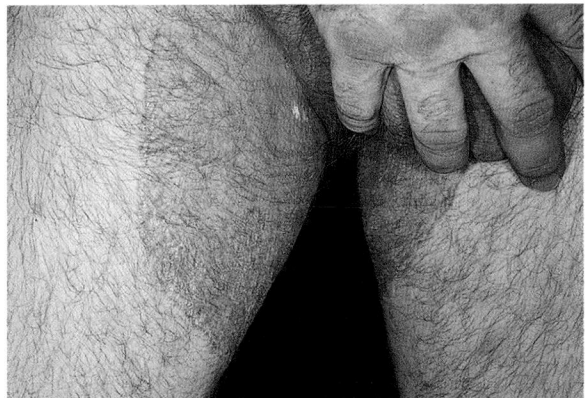

Tinea cruris *(Callen et al, 2000)*

tinea nigra, an uncommon superficial fungal infection caused by *Malassezia furfur* or *werneckii,* formerly classified as *Exophiala werneckii;* it is characterized by dark lesions on the skin of the hands or occasionally other areas. Also called **pityriasis nigra.**

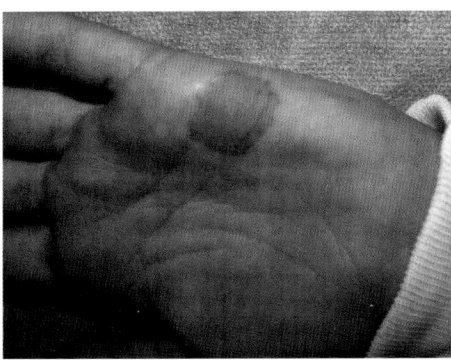

Tinea nigra *(Nazzaro, Poniani, and Cavicchini, 2016)*

tinea pedis, a chronic superficial fungal infection of the foot, especially of the skin between the toes and on the soles. It is common worldwide and is most commonly caused by *Trichophyton rubrum, T. mentagrophytes,* and *Epidermophyton floccosum.* Adults are most susceptible. The wearing of constricting footwear such as sneakers seems to induce the infection. Drying the feet well after bathing and applying powder between the toes help prevent it. Griseofulvin is the most effective treatment, but miconazole and tolnaftate are also used. Recurrence is common. Also called **athlete's foot.**

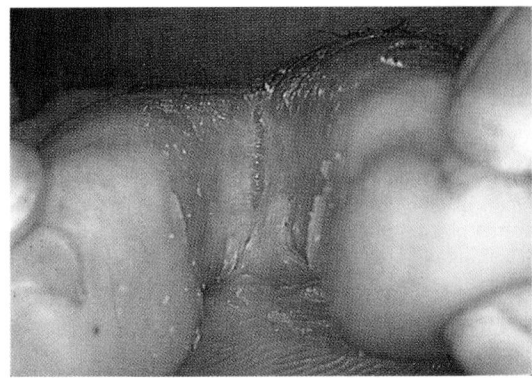

Tinea pedis *(Belchetz and Hammond, 2003)*

tinea unguium /un′gwē·əm/, a superficial fungal infection of the nails caused by various species of *Trichophyton* and occasionally by *Candida albicans.* It is more common on the toes than the fingers and can cause complete crumbling and destruction of the nails. Itraconazole and terbinafine are the drugs of choice, but they must be continued until the nail has regrown completely. See also **onychomycosis.**

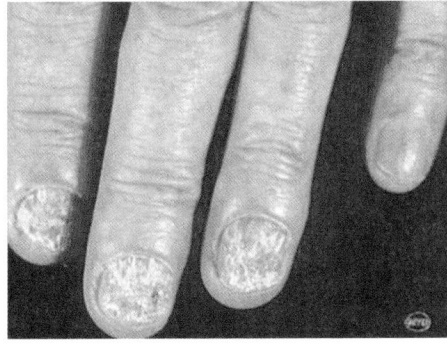

Tinea unguium *(Courtesy American Academy of Dermatology and Institute for Dermatologic Communication and Education)*

tinea versicolor, a fungal infection of the skin caused by *Malassezia furfur* and characterized by finely desquamating, pale tan patches on the upper trunk and upper arms that may itch and do not tan. In dark-skinned people the lesions may be depigmented. The fungus fluoresces under Wood's light and may be easily identified in scrapings viewed under a microscope. Topical and oral antifungal agents may be used, as well as repeated applications of selenium sulfide. The pale patches may persist for up to 1 year after successful treatment, and recurrence is common.

T

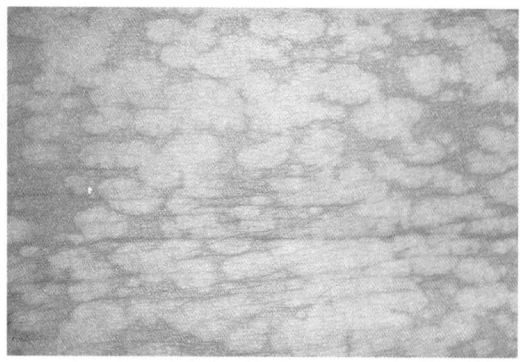

Tinea versicolor *(Goldman et al, 2008)*

Tinel sign /tinel″/ [Jules Tinel, French neurosurgeon, 1879–1952], an indication of irritability of a nerve; a distal tingling sensation on percussion of a damaged nerve. The sign is often present in carpal tunnel syndrome and is produced by tapping over the median nerve on the volar aspect of the wrist.

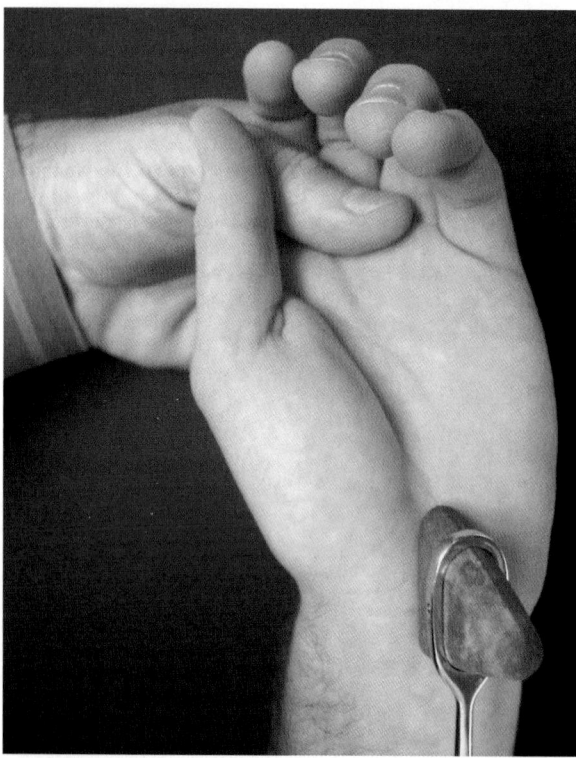

Tinel sign *(Waldman, 2016)*

tine test /tīn/ [ME, *tind*, rake tooth; L, *testum*, crucible], a tuberculin skin test in which a small disposable disk with multiple tines bearing tuberculin antigen is used to puncture the skin. The method is widely used to test for sensitivity to the tuberculin antigen. Induration around the puncture site indicates previous exposure or active disease, requiring further testing. See also **tuberculin test.**

tingling [ME, *tinklen,* to tinkle], a prickly sensation in the skin or a body part, accompanied by diminished sensitivity to stimulation of the sensory nerves.

tinidazole, an antiprotozoal.
■ INDICATIONS: This drug is used to treat amebiasis, giardiasis, and trichomoniasis.
■ CONTRAINDICATIONS: First-trimester pregnancy and known hypersensitivity to nitroimidazole derivative or to this drug prohibit its use.
■ ADVERSE EFFECTS: Adverse effects of this drug include anorexia, increased aspartate aminotransferase and alanine aminotransferase, constipation, abdominal pain, neutropenia, pruritus, urticaria, and oral monilia. Life-threatening side effects include seizures, leukopenia, and angioedema. Common side effects include dizziness, headache, peripheral neuropathy, nausea, vomiting, and rash.

tinnitus /tinī″təs/ [L, *tinnire,* to tinkle], a subjective noise sensation, often described as ringing, heard in one or both ears. It may be a sign of acoustic trauma, aspirin toxicity, multiple sclerosis, Ménière's disease, otosclerosis, presbycusis, or an accumulation of cerumen impinging on the eardrum or occluding the external auditory canal. It occasionally occurs for no apparent reason.

tint, a shade or gradation of a color, usually a pale or less saturated version of the basic shade.

tinted denture base, a denture base that has a color close to that of natural oral tissue.

TINU syndrome, a rare syndrome of tubulointerstitial nephritis and uveitis, often with immunological alterations. Also called *Dobrin syndrome.*

tinzaparin /tin-zap′ah-rin/, a low-molecular-weight heparin obtained by depolymerization of heparin from porcine intestinal mucosa by using a bacterial enzyme. It acts as an anticoagulant and antithrombotic and is used as an adjunct to warfarin in the treatment of deep venous thrombosis with or without pulmonary embolism and is administered subcutaneously.

-tion, suffix meaning "act of, process of, result of": *elongation, dilation.*

tiotropium, an anticholinergic and bronchodilator.
■ INDICATIONS: This drug is used for long-term treatment of chronic obstructive pulmonary disease (COPD) and for once-daily maintenance of bronchospasm associated with COPD, including chronic bronchitis and emphysema.
■ ADVERSE EFFECTS: Adverse effects of this drug include depression, chest pain, increased heart rate, dry mouth, blurred vision, glaucoma, abdominal pain, constipation, dyspepsia, rash, urinary difficulty, urinary retention, sinusitis, upper respiratory tract infection, epistaxis, and pharyngitis. Common side effects include vomiting, cough, and a worsening of symptoms.

tip, **1.** the end of a pointed object. **2.** an attachment fitted to the end of something else. **3.** a point.

tipped uterus /tipt/ [ME, *tipen,* upset; L, *uterus,* womb], a uterus that is displaced from its normal position. See also **uterine anteflexion, uterine anteversion, uterine retroflexion, uterine retroversion.**

tip pinch, a grasp in which the tip of the thumb is pressed against any or each of the tips of the other fingers. Also called **pinch grip.** See also **palmar pinch, pinch.**

tipping, a tooth movement in which the angle of the tooth's long axis is changed.

tipranavir, an antiretroviral.
■ INDICATIONS: This drug is used in combination with other antiretrovirals to treat HIV.
■ CONTRAINDICATIONS: Hepatic disease (Child-Pugh B to C) and known hypersensitivity to this drug prohibit its use.
■ ADVERSE EFFECTS: Adverse effects of this drug include dizziness, somnolence, fatigue, anorexia, dry mouth, nephrolithiasis, rash, pain, asthenia, and hyperlipidemia. Life-

threatening side effects include hepatitis B or C, fatalities when given with ritonavir, insulin-resistant hyperglycemia, and ketoacidosis. Common side effects include headache, insomnia, diarrhea, abdominal pain, nausea, and vomiting.

TIPS,   abbreviation for **transjugular intrahepatic porto-systemic shunt.**

tip seal,   the closure of an ampule accomplished by melting a bead of glass at the neck of the ampule.

tirofiban,   an antiplatelet agent.

■ INDICATIONS: It is used to treat acute coronary syndrome.

■ CONTRAINDICATIONS: The following factors prohibit its use: known hypersensitivity to this drug, active internal bleeding, stroke, major surgery, severe trauma, intracranial neoplasm, aneurysm, and hemorrhage.

■ ADVERSE EFFECTS: Bleeding is a life-threatening effect of tirofiban. Other adverse reactions include bradycardia, dizziness, dissection, coronary artery edema, pain in the legs and/or pelvis, and sweating. Rash is a common side effect.

tisane /tizän″, tizän″/,   a tealike infusion or light drink of a vegetable herb consumed for a claimed medicinal effect.

tissue /tish′o͞o/   [Fr, *tissu,* fabric],   a collection of similar cells in a matrix acting together to perform a particular function.

tissue activator.   See **fibrinokinase.**

tissue bank,   a facility for storing and maintaining a collection of tissues for future use in transplants.

tissue-base relationship,   the interaction between the bottom of a removable dental prosthesis and underlying structures.

tissue committee,   a physician group that evaluates all surgery performed in a hospital or other health care facility. A primary duty is to ensure that unnecessary surgeries have not been performed. See also **tissue review.**

tissue culture   [OFr, *tissu* + L, *colere,* to cultivate],   the maintenance of growth in vitro, under artificial conditions, of tissue or organ specimens.

tissue dextrin.   See **glycogen.**

tissue dose,   the amount of radiation absorbed by tissue in the region of interest, expressed in SI unit gray (or milligray).

tissue factor,   a protein necessary for the initiation of thrombin formation.

tissue fixation,   a process in which a tissue specimen is placed in a fluid that preserves the cells as nearly as is possible in their natural state.

tissue fixative,   a fluid that preserves cells in their natural state so that they may be identified and examined.

tissue forceps.   See **thumb forceps.**

tissue kinase.   See **fibrinokinase.**

tissue macrophage   [OFr, *tissu* + Gk, *makros,* large, *phagein,* to eat],   a large, mobile, highly phagocytic cell derived from monocytes. These cells become mobile when stimulated by inflammation and migrate to the affected area. They are resident in specific tissues (e.g., alveolar macrophages in the lungs).

tissue plasminogen activator (tPA),   a clot-dissolving substance produced naturally by cells in the walls of blood vessels. It is also manufactured synthetically by genetic engineering techniques. tPA activates plasminogen to dissolve clots and has been used therapeutically to open occluded coronary arteries, as well as cerebral arteries.

tissue response,   any reaction or change in living cellular tissue when it is acted on by disease, toxin, or other external stimulus. Kinds include **immune response, inflammation, necrosis.**

tissue review,   a review of the surgery performed in a hospital or other health care facility. The evaluation is usually made on the basis of the extent of agreement of the preoperative, postoperative, and pathological diagnoses and on the relevance and acceptability of the diagnostic procedures. See also **tissue committee.**

tissue typing,   a systematized series of tests to evaluate the intraspecies compatibility of tissues from a donor and a recipient before transplantation. Typing is accomplished by identifying and comparing a large series of human leukocyte antigens in the cells of the body. See also **immune system, transplant, human leukocyte antigen.**

titanium (Ti) /tītā′nē·əm/   [Gk, *Titan,* mythic giant],   a chemical element. Its atomic number is 22; its atomic mass is 47.88. An alloy of titanium is used in the manufacture of orthopedic prostheses and dental implants. Titanium dioxide is the active ingredient in a number of topical ointments and lotions. Titanium dioxide is one of the whitest substances known and is used as a base pigment in many sunscreens.

titer /tī′tər/   [Fr, *titre,* to make a standard,],   **1.** the normality of a solution or substance, determined by titration to find the equivalence of two reactants. **2.** the extent to which an antibody can be diluted before losing its power to react with a specific antigen. **3.** the highest dilution of a serum that causes clumping of bacteria or other visible reaction. Also spelled **titre.**

titillation /tit′ilā″shən/   [L, *titillare,* to tickle],   **1.** tickling. **2.** arousal of the senses.

Title   [L, *titulus,* title],   a section of the Social Security Act that provides for the establishment, funding, and regulation of a service to a specific segment of the population. Examples include Title XIX, which includes medical coverage under Medicaid, and Title X, which awards lump-sum grants for family planning programs.

titration /tītrā″shən/,   a method of estimating the amount of solute in a solution. The solution is added in small, measured quantities to a known volume of a standard solution until a reaction occurs, as indicated by a change in color or pH or the liberation of a chemical product.

titre.   See **titer.**

titubation /tich′əbā″shən/   [L, *titubare,* to stagger],   unsteady posture characterized by a staggering or stumbling gait and a swaying head or trunk while sitting. It may be a manifestation of cerebellar disease. Compare **ataxia.**

TIVA,   abbreviation for **total intravenous anesthesia.**

tizanidine,   a skeletal muscle relaxant and α₂-adrenergic agonist.

■ INDICATIONS: It is used in the acute/intermittent management of increased muscle tone associated with spasticity.

■ CONTRAINDICATIONS: Known hypersensitivity to this drug prohibits its use.

■ ADVERSE EFFECTS: Adverse effects include dry mouth, vomiting, increased ALT, abnormal liver function studies, constipation, somnolence, dizziness, speech disorder, dyskinesia, nervousness, hallucination, psychosis, urinary tract infection, blurred vision, urinary frequency, flulike syndrome, pharyngitis, and rhinitis.

TJC,   abbreviation for **The Joint Commission.**

Tl,   symbol for the element **thallium.**

TLC,   **1.** abbreviation for **total lung capacity. 2.** abbreviation for **thin-layer chromatography. 3.** initialism for *tender loving care.*

TLI,   abbreviation for **total lymphoid irradiation.**

TLR,   abbreviation for **tonic labyrinthine reflex.**

TLSO,   abbreviation for **thoracolumbosacral orthosis.**

T lymphocyte.   See **lymphocyte, T cell.**

Tm,   symbol for the element **thulium.**

TM,   abbreviation for **transcendental meditation.**

TMJ,   abbreviation for **temporomandibular joint.**

T

TMJ disorder. See **temporomandibular joint (TMJ) disorder.**

TMP/SMX, abbreviation for **trimethoprim and sulfamethoxazole.** See also **sulfamethoxazole and trimethoprim.**

TNF, abbreviation for **tumor necrosis factor.**

TNM, a system for staging malignant neoplastic disease. See also **cancer staging.**

TNM staging system, a system maintained by the American Joint Committee on Cancer (AJCC) and the International Union for Cancer Control (UICC) for classification of cancer. Abbreviation for **tumor, node, metastasis.**

t.n.t.c., usually applied to organisms or cells viewed on a slide under a microscope. Abbreviation for *too numerous to count.*

toadstool, popular name for any of various poisonous mushrooms.

toadstool poisoning /tōd'stool/ [AS, *tadige* + *stol* + L, *potio,* drink], a toxic condition caused by ingestion of certain varieties of poisonous mushrooms. See also **mushroom poisoning.**

to-and-fro murmur, a friction sound or murmur heard with both systole and diastole.

tobacco /təbak'ō/ [Sp, *tabaco*], a plant whose leaves are dried and used for smoking and chewing and in snuff. See also **nicotine.**

tobacco withdrawal syndrome, a change in mood or performance associated with the cessation of or reduction in exposure to nicotine. Symptoms may range from lack of concentration to anxiety and temper outbursts. A multitude of physical symptoms can also emerge.

■ OBSERVATIONS: Symptoms associated with tobacco withdrawal can include headache, nausea, gastrointestinal disorders, fatigue, drowsiness, insomnia, and increased hunger.

■ INTERVENTIONS: A combination of drugs and behavior-modification programs can be effective in abstaining from tobacco.

■ PATIENT CARE CONSIDERATIONS: Many activities and events can trigger the urge to smoke. There are numerous evidenced-based strategies that can be individualized to assist a patient in remaining tobacco-free.

TOBEC, abbreviation for **total body electric conductivity.**

tobramycin sulfate /tō'brəmī"sin/, an aminoglycoside antibiotic.

■ INDICATIONS: It is prescribed in the treatment of external ocular infection, septicemia, and lower respiratory tract and central nervous system infections caused by gram-negative bacilli, including *Pseudomonas.*

■ CONTRAINDICATIONS: Kidney dysfunction, use of potent diuretics, or known hypersensitivity to this or other aminoglycosides prohibits its use.

■ ADVERSE EFFECTS: Among the more serious adverse reactions are ototoxicity and nephrotoxicity.

Tobruk plaster /tō'brook/ [Tobruk, Libya], a plaster of paris or soft cast splint with tapes for skin traction coming through openings in the plaster and connected with a Thomas' splint. It covers and immobilizes the leg from foot to groin. Also called *Tobruk splint.* See also **Thomas' splint.**

-tocia, **1.** combining form meaning "condition of labor": *dystocia, oxytocia.* **2.** combining form meaning "the product of parturition."

-tocin, suffix for oxytocin derivatives.

toco-, toko- /tō'kō-/, combining form meaning "childbirth or labor": *tocodynamometer, tocolytic, tocotransducer.*

tocodynamometer /tō'kōdī'nəmom"ətər/ [Gk, *tokos,* birth, *dynamis,* force, *metron,* measure], an electronic device for monitoring and recording uterine contractions in labor. It

consists of a pressure transducer that is applied to the fundus of the uterus by means of a belt, which is connected to a machine that records the duration of the contractions and the interval between them on graph paper. The relative intensity of the contractions is also indicated but cannot be quantified. The tocodynamometer is a component of external monitoring in childbirth. Also spelled **tokodynamometer.** See also **electronic fetal monitor.**

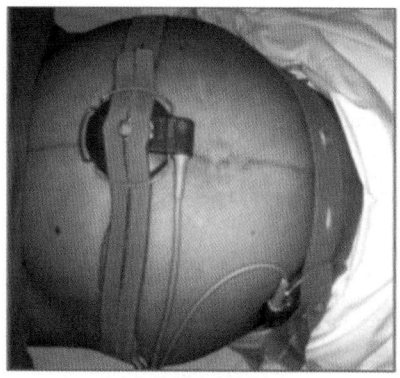

Tocodynamometer *(Ayres-de-Campos and Nogueira-Reis, 2016)*

tocolytic drug /-lit'ik/, any drug used to suppress premature labor.

tocopherol. See **vitamin E.**

tocopherolquinone (TQ) /tōkof'ərōlkwī"nōn/, an oxidized form of tocopherol, or vitamin E.

tocotransducer /-transd(y)oo'sər/ [Gk, *tokos* + L, *trans,* through, *ducer,* to lead], an electronic device used to measure uterine contractions. See also **tocodynamometer.**

toddler [ME, *toteren,* to walk unsteadily], a child between 12 and 36 months of age. During this period of development the child acquires a sense of autonomy and independence through the mastery of various specialized tasks such as control of body functions, refinement of motor and language skills, and acquisition of socially acceptable behavior, especially toleration of delayed gratification and acceptance of separation from the mother or parents. The period is characterized by exploration of the environment and rapid cognitive development as the child strives for self-assertion and personal interaction with others while struggling with parental discipline and sibling rivalry. Of primary importance for the nurse is an understanding of the dynamics of the growth and development of the toddler to help parents deal effectively with appropriate nutrition, toilet training, temper tantrums, prevention of accidental injury (primarily from falls, poisoning, and burns), and childhood fears, especially anxiety as a result of separation from the parents.

toddlerhood /tod'lərhood'/, the state or condition of being a toddler.

Todd paralysis [Robert Bentley Todd, English physician, 1809–1860; Gk, *paralyein,* to be palsied], weakness, usually on one side of the body, after a seizure, usually lasting a few minutes, hours, or, occasionally, several days.

toe, any one of the digits of the feet.

toe clonus [AS, *tá* + Gk, *klonos*], an increased reflex activity in the large toe caused by a sudden extension of the first phalanx.

toe drop [AS, *tá* + *dropa*], a condition in which the toes droop and cannot be lifted because of paralysis of the tibial muscles.

toeing in. See **metatarsus varus.**

toeing out. See **metatarsus valgus.**

toenail [AS, *tá* + *naegel*], one of the heavy ungual structures covering the terminal phalanges of the toes. Also called **unguis.**

Tofranil, a tricyclic antidepressant. Brand name for **imipramine hydrochloride.**

Toga virus. See **hepatitis F.**

toilet training, the process of teaching a child to control the functions of the bladder and bowel. Training programs vary, but all emphasize a positive, consistent, nonpunitive, nonpressured approach. Each program is individualized, depending on the mental and physical age and state of the child, the parent-child relationship, and readiness of the child to learn. Training often begins around 24 months of age, when voluntary control of the anal and urethral sphincters is achieved by most children. When the child has mastered some motor skills, is aware of his or her ability to control the body, and can communicate adequately, training is likely to be easy. Resistance occurs if the parents try to train the child before the child is physiologically and psychologically ready. Bowel training is usually accomplished before bladder training because the urge to evacuate the bowel is stronger than the urge to empty the bladder, and the need is less frequent and more regular. Nighttime bladder control may not be achieved until the child is 4 or 5 years of age or older. Behavior modification, using a system of rewards for each of the various phases of the training, is usually successful. A major function of health care providers working with children is to identify the readiness of the child to learn and to work with the parents, advising them in a nonauthoritarian way of the various techniques.

-toin, suffix for hydantoin derivative antiepileptics.

token economy [AS, *tacen,* to show; Gk, *oikonomia,* household management], a technique of reinforcement used in behavior therapy in the management of a group of people, such as in hospitals, institutions, or classrooms. Individuals are rewarded for specific activities or behavior with tokens that they can exchange for desired objects or privileges.

toko-. See **toco-, toko-.**

tokodynamometer. See **tocodynamometer.**

TOLAZamide /tolaz′əmīd/, an oral sulfonylurea antidiabetic agent.
■ INDICATIONS: It is prescribed in the treatment of stable or type 2 diabetes and for some patients sensitive to other types of sulfonylureas or who have failed to respond to other similar drugs.
■ CONTRAINDICATIONS: Unstable diabetes; serious impairment of renal, hepatic, or thyroid function; pregnancy; or known hypersensitivity to this drug or other sulfonylurea medications prohibits its use.
■ ADVERSE EFFECTS: Among the more serious adverse effects are hypoglycemia and skin reactions. Blood dyscrasias may occur.

tolazoline hydrochloride /tolaz′əlēn/, an alpha-adrenergic receptor blocker.
■ INDICATIONS: It is prescribed in the treatment of persistent pulmonary hypertension of the newborn and in peripheral vascular disease.
■ CONTRAINDICATIONS: Hypersensitivity to this drug prohibits its use.
■ ADVERSE EFFECTS: Among the more serious adverse effects are cardiac arrhythmia, hypotension or hypertension, exacerbation of stress ulcer, hemorrhage, and mitral stenosis.

TOLBUTamide /tolbōō′təmīd/, an oral sulfonylurea antidiabetic.

■ INDICATIONS: It is prescribed in the treatment of stable type 2 diabetes uncontrolled by diet alone and for some patients changing from insulin to oral therapy.
■ CONTRAINDICATIONS: Unstable diabetes, serious impairment of renal, hepatic, or thyroid function, pregnancy, or known hypersensitivity to this drug or to other sulfonylurea medications prohibits its use.
■ ADVERSE EFFECTS: Among the more serious adverse effects are hypoglycemia and skin reactions. Blood dyscrasias may occur.

tolcapone, an antiparkinsonian agent.
■ INDICATIONS: It is used in the treatment of parkinsonism.
■ CONTRAINDICATIONS: Known hypersensitivity to this drug prohibits its use.
■ ADVERSE EFFECTS: Life-threatening effects include hemolytic anemia, leukopenia, and agranulocytosis. Other adverse reactions include dystonia, dyskinesia, dreaming, psychosis, hallucinations, dizziness, chest pain, hypotension, cataract, eye inflammation, diarrhea, constipation, urinary tract infection, urine discoloration, uterine tumor, micturition disorder, sweating, and alopecia. Common side effects include fatigue, headache, confusion, orthostatic hypotension, nausea, vomiting, anorexia, and abdominal distress.

Tolectin, a nonsteroidal antiinflammatory agent. Brand name for **tolmetin sodium.**

tolerance /tol′ərəns/ [L, *tolerare,* to endure], a phenomenon by which the body becomes increasingly resistant to a drug, substance, or activity through continued exposure. Kinds include **work tolerance.**

tolerance dose. See **effective dose equivalent limit.**

tolerance test, 1. an investigation of the ability of the body to metabolize a drug or nutrient, as in a glucose tolerance test. 2. a physical activity drill administered to evaluate the efficiency of blood circulation or of another body system.

Tolinase, an antidiabetic agent. Brand name for **TOLAZamide.**

tolmetin sodium /tol′mətin/, a nonsteroidal antiinflammatory agent.
■ INDICATIONS: It is prescribed primarily in the treatment of rheumatoid arthritis, juvenile rheumatoid arthritis, and osteoarthritis.
■ CONTRAINDICATIONS: Impaired renal function, GI disease, or known hypersensitivity to this drug, to aspirin, or to nonsteroidal antiinflammatory medications prohibits its use. Should not be used during second and third trimesters of pregnancy.
■ ADVERSE EFFECTS: Among the more serious adverse effects are peptic ulcer and GI distress. Dizziness, skin rash, and tinnitus commonly occur. This drug interacts with many other drugs.

tolnaftate /tolnaf′tāt/, an antifungal.
■ INDICATIONS: It is prescribed in the treatment of superficial fungus infections of the skin, including tinea pedis, tinea cruris, tinea corporis, and tinea versicolor.
■ CONTRAINDICATIONS: Known hypersensitivity to this drug prohibits its use. It is also not indicated for nail or scalp infections.
■ ADVERSE EFFECTS: Among the more common adverse effects are hypersensitivity reactions and mild irritation of the skin.

Tolosa-Hunt syndrome /tō·lō′sä·hunt/ [Eduardo S. Tolosa, Spanish neurosurgeon, 1900-1981; William Edward Hunt, American neurosurgeon, 1921-1999], unilateral ophthalmoplegia associated with pain behind the orbit and in the area supplied by the first division of the trigeminal nerve; it is thought to result from nonspecific inflammation and granulation tissue in the superior orbital fissure or cavernous sinus. Compare **cavernous sinus syndrome.**

tolterodine, a muscarinic receptor antagonist.

■ INDICATIONS: It is used to treat overactive bladder (frequency and urgency). It controls bladder incontinence by controlling contractions.

■ CONTRAINDICATIONS: Factors that prohibit its use include known hypersensitivity, uncontrolled narrow-angle glaucoma, urinary retention, and gastric retention.

■ ADVERSE EFFECTS: Adverse effects include paresthesia, fatigue, headache, chest pain, hypertension, vision abnormalities, xerophthalmia, abdominal pain, constipation, dry mouth, dyspepsia, dysuria, urinary retention, urinary frequency, urinary tract infection, rash, pruritus, bronchitis, cough, pharyngitis, and upper respiratory infection. Common side effects include anxiety, dizziness, nausea, vomiting, and anorexia.

toluene ($C_6H_5CH_3$) /tol″yoo·ēn/, an aromatic, colorless, flammable liquid produced from coal tar, petroleum, or Peruvian tolu balsam. It is used in dyes, explosives, gums, and lacquers and in the manufacture of drugs and the extraction of organic chemicals from plants.

-tome, 1. combining form meaning "a cutting instrument": *amniotome, hysterotome, microtome.* 2. combining form meaning "a (specified) segment or region": *dermatome, cytomitome, nephrotome.*

-tomic, -tomical, suffix meaning "incisions or sections of tissue": *anatomical, myotomic.*

tomo-, combining form meaning "preparation of a section or layer": *tomography.*

tomogram /tō″məgram′/ [Gk, *tome,* section, *gramma,* record], a radiograph produced by tomography.

tomograph /tō″məgraf′/ [Gk, *tome,* section, *graphein,* to record], a radiographic apparatus that makes an image of layers of body tissues at various depths.

tomographic DSA /-graf′ik/, the visualization of blood vessels in the body in three dimensions. See also **digital subtraction angiography.**

tomography /təmog″rəfē/ [Gk, *tome* + *graphein,* to record], 1. sectional imaging. 2. a radiographic technique in which the tube and image receptor are moved synchronously during exposure, producing a blurred radiograph in which objects within the focal plane are seen more clearly than objects outside the focal plane. 3. a radiographic technique that produces an image representing a detailed cross section of tissue at a predetermined depth. It is a valuable diagnostic tool for the discovery and identification of space-occupying lesions such as might be found in the brain, liver, pancreas, and gallbladder. See also **computed tomography, positron emission tomography.**

-tomy, combining form meaning "a surgical incision": *cystotomy, lobotomy, phlebotomy.*

tonaphasia. See **amusia.**

tone. See **tonus.**

tone deafness [Gk, *tonos,* stretching; AS, *deaf*], an inability to detect the pitch or changing pitch of a musical note or a voice change.

tongue /tung/ [AS, *tunge*], the principal organ of the sense of taste that also assists in the mastication and deglutition of food. It is located in the floor of the mouth within the curve of the mandible. Its root is connected to the hyoid bone posteriorly. It is also connected to the epiglottis, soft palate, and pharynx. The apex of the tongue rests anteriorly against the lingual surfaces of the lower incisors. The mucous membrane

connecting the tongue to the mandible reflects over the floor of the mouth to the lingual surface of the gingiva and in the midline of the floor is raised into a vertical fold. The dorsum of the tongue is divided into symmetric halves by a median sulcus, which ends posteriorly in the foramen cecum. A shallow sulcus terminalis runs from this foramen laterally and forward on either side to the margin of the organ. From the sulcus the anterior two thirds of the tongue are covered with papillae. The posterior third is smoother and contains numerous mucous glands and lymph follicles. The use of the tongue as an organ of speech is not anatomical but a secondary acquired characteristic. Also called **glossa, lingua.**

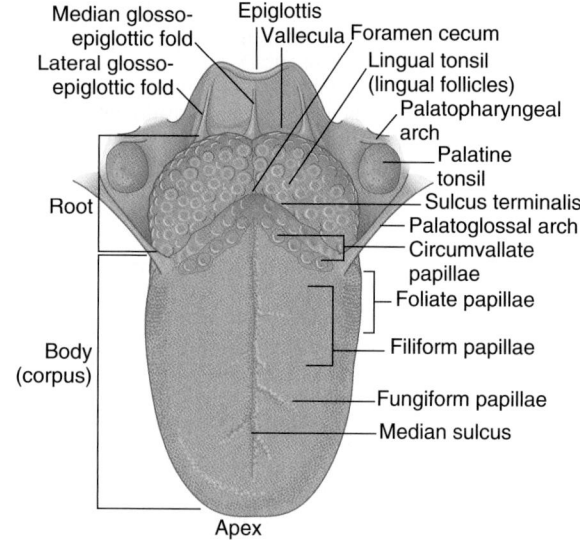

Tongue *(Cohen, 2005)*

tongue deviation. See **deviation of tongue.**

tongue-thrust swallow, an immature form of swallowing in which the tongue is projected forward instead of retracted during the act of swallowing. It may result in forward displacement of the maxilla with consequent malocclusion of the teeth.

tongue-tie. See **ankyloglossia.**

-tonia, -tony, combining form meaning "tone" or "(condition or degree of) muscle tension": *atonia, hemihypertonia, myotonia.*

tonic /ton′ik/, pertaining to a type of afferent or sensory nerve receptor that responds to length changes placed on the noncontractile part of a muscle spindle. It may be triggered by a mechanical external force such as positioning or by an internal stretch caused by intrafusal muscle contraction.

-tonic, 1. combining form meaning "the quality of muscle contraction or tonus": *hypertonic, auxotonic, dystonic.* 2. combining form meaning "a solution with a comparative concentration": *hypertonic, hypotonic, isotonic.*

tonic bite, reflexive, sustained jaw closure, accompanied by increased abnormal tone in the jaw muscles, in response to stimulation of the teeth or gums. It is difficult to release, and its force can damage the teeth or an object placed in the mouth.

tonic convulsion [Gk, *tonos,* stretching; L, *convulsio,* cramp], a prolonged generalized contraction of the skeletal muscles. Also called *tonic contraction.* See also **physiological tetanus.**

tonicity /tōnis″itē/ [Gk, *tonikos,* stretching], the quality of possessing tone, or tonus.

tonic labyrinthine reflex (TLR) [Gk, *tonikos + labyrinthos,* maze; L, *reflectere,* to bend back], a normal postural reflex in animals, abnormally accentuated in decerebrate humans and characterized by extension of all four limbs when the head is positioned in space at an angle above the horizontal in quadripeds or in the neutral erect position in humans. Also called **decerebrate rigidity.**

tonic neck reflex, a normal response in newborns characterized by extension of the arm and the leg on the side of the body to which the head is quickly turned while the infant is supine and to flex the limbs of the opposite side. The reflex, which prevents the infant from rolling over until adequate neurological and motor development occurs, disappears by 3 to 4 months of age, to be replaced by symmetric positioning of both sides of the body. Absence or persistence of the reflex may indicate central nervous system damage. Also called **asymmetric tonic neck reflex.** See also **symmetric tonic neck reflex.**

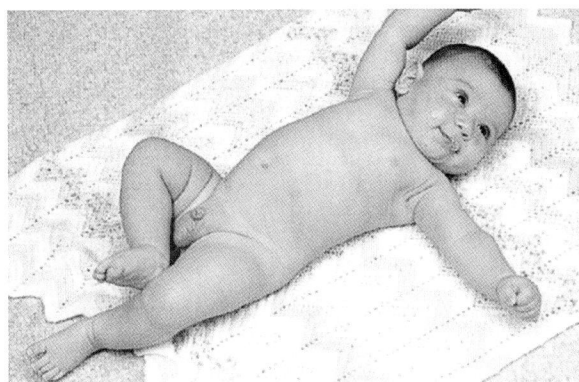

Tonic neck reflex *(Courtesy Marjorie Pyle, RNC, Lifecircle)*

tonic pupil. See **Adie pupil.**

tonic spasm [Gk, *tonos,* stretching, *spasmos*], a sustained contraction of a muscle. See **physiological tetanus.**

tonitrophobia /tonit′rōfō″bē·ə/, an abnormal fear of thunder.

tono-, combining form meaning "tone" or "tension": *tonoclonic, tonofibril, tonoscillograph.*

tonoclonic /ton′əklon″ik/ [Gk, *tonos,* stretching, *klonos,* tumult], pertaining to muscular spasms that are tonic and then clonic.

tonofibril /ton′əfī″bril/ [Gk, *tonos,* stretching, *fibrilla,* small fiber], a bundle of fine filaments found in the cytoplasm of epithelial cells. The individual strands, or tonofilaments, spread throughout the cytoplasm and extend into the intercellular bridge to converge at the desmosome. The system of fibers functions as a supportive element within the cytoskeleton. In keratinizing epithelium the strands are the main precursor of keratin. Also called **epitheliofibril, tenofibril.** See also **keratohyalin, tonofilament.**

tonofilament /ton′ōfil″əmənt/ [Gk, *tonos,* stretching], a proteinaceous fiber found in epithelial cells. Bundles of tonofilaments form a tonofibril, which has a supporting function.

tonograph /ton′əgraf/, an apparatus that makes a record of tension measurements.

tonography /tōnog′rəfē/, **1.** the measurement over time of intraocular pressure with graphic documentation. **2.** the measurement of tension.

tonometer /tōnom″ətər/ [Gk, *tonos + metron,* measure], an instrument used in measuring tension or pressure, especially intraocular pressure.

tonometry /tōnom″ətrē/, the measuring of intraocular pressure by determining the resistance of the eyeball to indentation by an applied force. Several kinds of tonometers are used. The air-puff tonometer, which does not touch the eye, records deflections of the cornea from a puff of pressurized air. The Schiötz impression and the applanation tonometers record the pressure needed to indent or flatten the corneal surface. Applanation tonometry at the slit lamp is considered most accurate. Schiötz tonometry is rarely done today.

tonoscillograph /ton′əsil″əgraf′/, an apparatus that records arterial and capillary pressures with a corresponding pulse tracing.

tonsil /ton′səl/ [L, *tonsilla*], a small rounded mass of tissue, especially lymphoid tissue, such as that composing the palatine tonsils in the oropharynx. Also called **tonsilla.** Compare **intestinal tonsil, lingual tonsil, palatine tonsil, pharyngeal tonsil.**

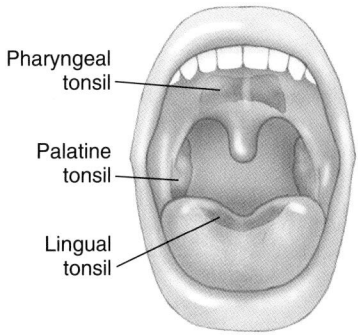

Tonsils *(Leonard, 2009)*

tonsill-, combining form meaning "tonsil": *tonsillectomy, tonsilloliths, tonsillitis.*

tonsilla. See **tonsil.**

tonsillar /ton′silər/ [L, *tonsilla*], pertaining to the palatine tonsil.

tonsillar crypt [L, *tonsilla* + Gk, *kryptos,* hidden], a small slitlike invagination on the surface of a palatine or pharyngeal tonsil.

tonsillar fossa. See **amygdaloid fossa.**

tonsillar herniation [L, *tonsilla + hernia,* rupture], the herniation of tonsils of the cerebellum through the foramen magnum of the skull. It may occur as a result of intracranial pressure from an injury or tumor.

tonsillar ring. See **Waldeyer's throat ring.**

tonsillectomy /ton′silek″təmē/ [L, *tonsilla* + Gk, *ektomē,* excision], the surgical excision of the palatine tonsils, performed to prevent recurrent tonsillitis. Before surgery several laboratory tests, including a bleeding and clotting time, complete blood count, and urinalysis, are done. Tonsillar tissue is dissected and removed, usually with the patient under general anesthesia, and bleeding areas are sutured or cauterized. An increase in pulse rate, falling blood pressure, restlessness, or frequent swallowing warns of possible hemorrhage. When the patient has recovered from anesthesia, ice chips or clear liquids without a drinking straw may be offered. Tonsillectomy is often combined with adenoidectomy. Compare **adenectomy, adenotonsillectomy.**

tonsillitis /-ī′tis/, an infection or inflammation of a tonsil. Acute tonsillitis, frequently caused by *Streptococcus* infection, is characterized by severe sore throat, fever, headache, malaise, difficulty in swallowing, earache, and enlarged tender lymph nodes in the neck. Acute tonsillitis may accompany scarlet fever. Treatment includes systemic antibiotics, analgesics, and warm irrigations of the throat. Soft foods and ample fluids are given. Tonsillectomy is sometimes performed for recurrent tonsillitis or tonsillar abscess. See also **acute tonsillitis, peritonsillar abscess, scarlet fever, strep throat.**

■ OBSERVATIONS: Symptoms include a moderate to severe sore throat, lasting longer than 2 days; difficulty swallowing; pain referred to the ears; enlarged anterior cervical nodes; fever and chills; headache; muscle and joint pain; anorexia; increased secretions from the throat; enlarged, reddened, inflamed tonsils; pus or exudate on the tonsils; halitosis; and edematous or inflamed uvula. Symptoms often last 2 to 3 days after treatment is initiated. Diagnosis is made by direct inspection of the throat and tonsils, and throat cultures are used to identify the causative organism. If not treated, the following can occur: peritonsillar abscess, airway occlusion, rheumatic fever and subsequent cardiovascular disorders, kidney failure, or poststreptococcal glomerulonephritis.

■ INTERVENTIONS: Treatment is directed at the symptoms. Antibiotics are given if the cause is bacterial. Analgesics are used for pain relief. Tonsillectomy is indicated for massive hypertrophy that restricts breathing or obstructs the airway. Adenoidectomy is indicated for hypertrophy of adenoids that obstruct nasal breathing.

■ PATIENT CARE CONSIDERATIONS: Nursing care is focused on provision of comfort and rest. Warm, bland fluids or very cold fluids, saltwater gargles, and throat lozenges may alleviate throat discomfort. A cool mist vaporizer and adequate fluids keep mucous membranes moist. Postsurgical care is aimed at prevention of hemorrhage, prevention of aspiration of drainage, and control of pain. The child is positioned on side until fully alert to facilitate drainage of secretions and prevent aspiration. Suctioning is done with care to prevent trauma to the oropharynx. Frequent assessment for bleeding is done with direct visualization of the surgical site. Continual swallowing by child is an obvious sign of early bleeding. Coughing, clearing of throat, and nose blowing are discouraged and activity is limited to prevent hemorrhage. An ice collar may be applied to help alleviate discomfort from sore throat. Continuous pain control and mild sedation is necessary to prevent crying, which can irritate the operative site and promote hemorrhage. Parents should be educated about signs of hemorrhage and prevention (limiting activity, discouraging coughing, clearing throat, avoiding throat irritants, gargles). Instruction is given to treat any sign of bleeding as a medical emergency.

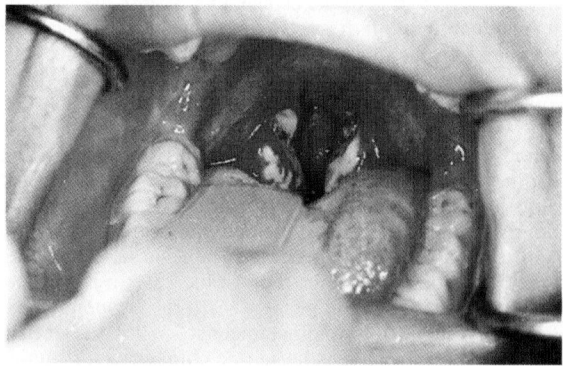

Tonsillitis *(Courtesy Dr. Edward L. Applebaum, Department of Otolaryngology, University of Illinois Medical Center)*

tonsilloadenoidectomy /ton'silō·ad'ɔnoidek″təmē/ [L, *tonsilla* + Gk, *aden,* gland, *eidos,* form, *ektomē,* excision], the surgical removal of tonsil and adenoid tissues.

tonsilloliths, collections of dead bacteria, desquamated epithelium, and food debris within tonsillar crypts, where calcium phosphate, calcium carbonate, and magnesium salts from saliva precipitate to form solid masses that grow by accretion. Also called *tonsil stones.*

tonus /tō″nəs/ [Gk, *tonos,* stretching], **1.** the normal state of balanced tension in the body tissues, especially the muscles. Partial contraction or alternate contraction and relaxation of neighboring fibers of a group of muscles hold the organ or the part of the body in a neutral functional position without fatigue. Tonus is essential for many normal body functions, such as holding the spine erect, the eyes open, and the jaw closed. Also called **muscle tone. 2.** the state of the body tissues being strong and fit. Also called **tone.**

-tony. See -tonia, -tony.

tooth *pl. teeth* [AS, *toth*], any one of numerous dental structures that develop in the jaws. Although derived from modified bone, they are typically classified as part of the digestive system and are used to cut and grind food in the mouth for ingestion. Each tooth consists of a crown, which projects above the gum; two to four roots embedded in the alveolus; and a neck, which stretches between the crown and the root. Each tooth also contains a cavity filled with pulp, richly supplied with blood vessels and nerves that enter the cavity through a small aperture at the base of each root. The solid part of the tooth consists of dentin, enamel, and a thin layer of bone on the surface of the root. The dentin composes the bulk of the tooth. The enamel covers the exposed part of the crown. Two sets of teeth appear at different periods of life: the 20 primary teeth appear during infancy, and the 32 secondary teeth appear during childhood and early adulthood. See also **primary dentition, secondary dentition.**

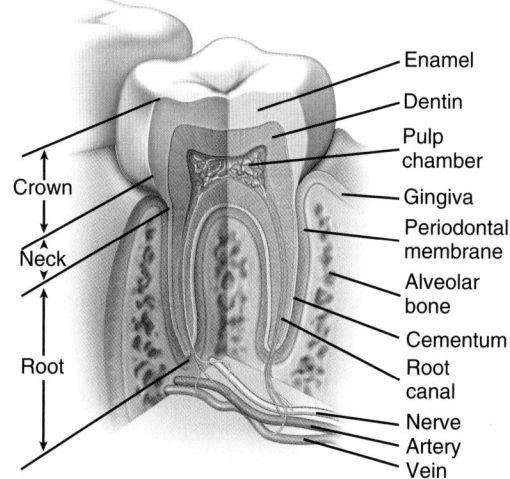

Tooth *(Harkreader and Hogan, 2007)*

tooth abscess [AS, *toth* + L, *abscedere,* to go away], a collection of pus, the body's response to bacterial infection, on a tooth. The abscess is caused either by trauma or by exposure of the pulp to bacterial saliva from caries. The infection is usually close to the root. If untreated, the pressure of the abscess may destroy the alveolar bone and adjoining soft tissues. Treatment includes antibiotics, root canal therapy, or extraction. Also called **dental abscess.** See also **periapical abscess.**

toothache /too″thāk/ [AS, *toth* + *aeca*], pain in a tooth, usually caused by pulpal infection or damage. Also called **dentalgia, odontalgia, odontodynia.** See also **pulpitis.**

tooth alignment, the arrangement of the teeth in relation to their supporting bone or alveolar process, adjacent teeth, and opposing dentition.

tooth bleaching, the process of removing stains or color from teeth by applying chemicals such as hydrogen peroxide or urea peroxide either externally or internally (inside a tooth, performed in conjunction with a root canal).

tooth-borne, describing a dental prosthesis or part of a prosthesis that rests entirely on abutment teeth for support.

tooth-borne base, a denture base restoring an edentulous area that has abutment teeth at each end for support. The residual alveolar ridge tissue that it covers is not used to support the base. See **supporting area.**

toothbrush, an implement of various designs, with bristles, available in a variety of differing amounts of bristle flexibility, fixed to a head at the end of a handle; used for cleaning the teeth and cleaning and massaging the gingival tissues.

tooth eruption, the final stage of odontogenesis, in which a tooth breaks out from its crypt through surrounding tissue into the mouth.

tooth form, the identifying curves, lines, angles, and contours of a tooth that differentiate it from other teeth.

tooth fulcrum, the axis of movement of a tooth subjected to lateral forces. It is considered to be at the middle third of the part of the tooth root embedded in the alveolus.

tooth germ, a primitive cell in the embryo that is the precursor of a tooth.

tooth inclination, the angle of slope of a tooth or teeth from the vertical plane. Inclinations may be mesial, distal, lingual, buccal, or labial.

toothpaste. See **dentifrice.**

tooth rotation [AS, *toth* + L, *rotare,* to rotate], **1.** the turning of a tooth around its longitudinal axis. **2.** the process by which a tooth is turned.

tooth size discrepancy, lack of harmony of size of individual teeth or groups of teeth when related to those within the same arch or the opposing arch.

TOP, abbreviation for *t*emporal, *o*ccipital, and *p*arietal regions of the skull.

top-, topo-, combining form meaning "place" or "location": *topognosis, topology.*

topesthesia. See **topognosis.**

tophaceous /tōfā´shəs/, pertaining to the presence of chalky accumulations of uric acid crystals (tophi). See also **tophus.**

tophaceous gout [L, *tufa,* porous rock], a form of purine metabolism disorder characterized by formation of chalky deposits of sodium biurate under the skin and in the joints. If untreated, the deposits may eventually destroy the involved joints.

tophus /tō´fəs/ *pl.* **tophi** [L, *tufa,* porous rock], *adj.,* a calculus containing sodium urate that develops in fibrous tissue around joints, typically in patients with gout. **–tophaceous,** *adj.*

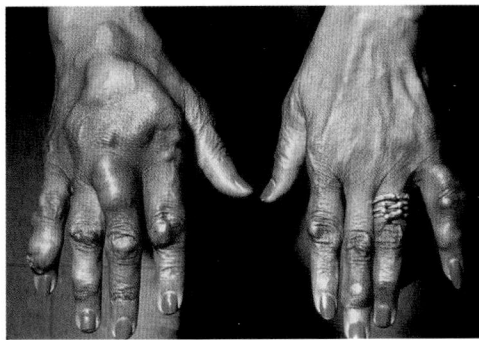

Tophi *(Swartz, 2009)*

-topia, -topy, suffix meaning "(condition of) placement of organs in the body": *heterotopia, cardiectopia, ectopy.*

topical /top´ikəl/ [Gk, *topos,* place], **1.** pertaining to the surface of a part of the body. **2.** pertaining to a drug or treatment applied topically.

topical anesthesia, anesthesia produced by application of a local anesthetic in the form of a solution, gel, or ointment to the skin, mucous membrane, or cornea. The most common agents include benzocaine, lidocaine, and tetracaine. Cocaine may be applied in solution to the mucous membranes of the nasal passages for certain surgical procedures. Also called **surface anesthesia.** Compare **general anesthesia, local anesthesia, regional anesthesia.**

Topicort, a topical glucocorticoid medication. Brand name for **desoximetasone.**

topiramate, a miscellaneous anticonvulsant.

■ INDICATIONS: It is used to treat partial seizures in adults.

■ CONTRAINDICATIONS: Known hypersensitivity to this drug prohibits its use.

■ ADVERSE EFFECTS: Adverse effects include upper respiratory infection, pharyngitis, sinusitis, diplopia, vision abnormality, rash, weight loss, leukopenia, dizziness, fatigue, cognitive disorder, insomnia, anxiety, depression, paresthesia, weight loss, diarrhea, anorexia, nausea, dyspepsia, abdominal pain, constipation, dry mouth, breast pain, dysmenorrhea, and menstrual disorder.

topo-. See **top-, topo-.**

topoanesthesia. See **atopognosia.**

topognosis /top´ognō´sis/ [Gk, *topos* + *gnosis,* recognition], the ability to recognize tactile stimuli. Also called **topesthesia.**

topogometer /top´ōgom´ətər/ [Gk, *topos,* place, *gonia,* angle, *metron,* measure], a movable fixation target attached to an instrument for measuring the radius of curvature of the cornea. It is used in fitting contact lenses of correct curvature.

topographic /top´əgraf´ik/, (in psychiatry) pertaining to a freudian conceptualization of the layers of human consciousness.

topographic anatomy [Gk, *topos,* place, *graphein,* to record, *ana* + *temnein,* to cut], the study of a specific region of a body structure, such as a lower leg, including all of the systems in the part and their relationship to each other. Also called **regional anatomy.**

topographic disorientation, a psychiatric disorder based on Freud's topographic model of the mental apparatus and consisting of conscious, preconscious, and unconscious systems for interpreting perceptions of the outside world and internal perceptions. Under certain conditions, such as frustration or sleep, psychic energy reanimates unconscious memories, resulting in hallucinations in mental disorders.

topography /təpog´refē/ [Gk, *topos,* place, *graphein,* to record], the anatomical description of a body part in terms of the region in which it is located.

topoisomerase /to´po-i´so-mer-ās/, an enzyme involved in mobilization and replication of DNA during cell division.

topoisomerase inhibitors, a class of antineoplastic agents that interfere with the arrangement of DNA in cells.

topology /təpol´əjē/, **1.** orientation of the presenting part of a fetus. **2.** the study of special regions of anatomy. **3.** the science of properties of geometric configuration.

topotecan, an antineoplastic hormone.

■ INDICATIONS: It is used to treat metastatic carcinoma of the ovary after failure of traditional chemotherapy.

■ CONTRAINDICATIONS: Factors that prohibit the use of this drug are known hypersensitivity, lactation, and severe bone marrow depression.

■ ADVERSE EFFECTS: Life-threatening effects are neutropenia, leukopenia, thrombocytopenia, anemia, and sepsis.

T

Other adverse effects are abdominal pain, constipation, diarrhea, obstruction, nausea, stomatitis, vomiting, increased alanine aminotransferase and aspartate aminotransferase, anorexia, arthralgia, asthenia, headache, myalgia, pain, dyspnea, and total alopecia.

TORCH /tôrch/, abbreviation for *t*oxoplasmosis, *o*ther, *r*ubella virus, *c*ytomegalovirus, and *h*erpes simplex viruses, a group of agents that can infect the fetus or the newborn, causing a constellation of morbid effects called TORCH syndrome.

TORCH syndrome, infection of the fetus or newborn by one of the TORCH agents. The outcome of a pregnancy complicated by a TORCH agent may be abortion, stillbirth, intrauterine growth delay, or premature delivery.

■ OBSERVATIONS: At delivery and during the first days after birth an infant infected with any one of the organisms may demonstrate various clinical manifestations, such as fever, lethargy, poor feeding, petechiae on the skin, purpura, pneumonia, hepatosplenomegaly, jaundice, hemolytic and other anemias, encephalitis, microcephaly, hydrocephalus, intracranial calcifications, hearing deficits, chorioretinitis, and microphthalmia. In addition, each of the agents is associated with several other abnormal clinical findings involving abnormal immune response, cataracts, glaucoma, vesicles, ulcers, and congenital cardiac defects.

■ INTERVENTIONS: Before pregnancy, women may be tested for susceptibility to the rubella virus and inoculated against it if not immune. There are currently no vaccines that confer immunity to the other TORCH agents, but the mother may be serologically tested for antibody levels to them. During pregnancy toxoplasmosis is asymptomatic in about 90% of cases, making diagnosis unlikely. If infection is suspected, serial paired serological tests are performed. A high, rising titer indicates recent infection. Transplacental infection occurs in 35% of mothers infected during pregnancy. If the mother contracts infection in the first trimester, before the placenta is fully developed, the infant may not become infected. If the fetus contracts the infection, severe congenital manifestations of the syndrome usually occur. If the fetus is infected after the first trimester, the baby is usually born with asymptomatic or mild disease. The infection may be spread from the baby during the newborn period. Sulfadiazine, pyrimethamine, and folic acid are sometimes given to treat the infection. Primary cytomegalovirus infection during pregnancy is usually asymptomatic. If the infection is suspected, serological testing may be performed to demonstrate primary infection because infants born to mothers infected for the first time during pregnancy are much more likely to develop severe congenital anomalies than if the infection is a reactivation of previous cytomegalovirus infection. There is no specific treatment. The child is considered to be infectious, but contagion among newborns from a congenitally infected infant has not been proven. Transplacental rubella virus infection in pregnancy during the first 8 weeks is likely to cause infection in 50% of fetuses and to result in demonstrable defects in 85% of those infected. The risk becomes less as gestation increases to 24 weeks, after which time infection has not been known to result in defects. Rubella is the only TORCH virus that is usually symptomatic, and therefore it is often recognized. Many mothers infected during the first trimester choose to abort the pregnancy. There is no treatment for the infection, but screening and immunization before pregnancy could prevent virtually all cases of congenital rubella. Herpesvirus infection in pregnancy is rarely transplacentally transmitted to the fetus. Primary infection during pregnancy sometimes results in spontaneous abortion or premature delivery. In the newborn the infection

is usually systemic and life-threatening. The fetus is most apt to become infected by the virus shed from an active genital lesion during vaginal delivery or as the result of vaginal examination or the placement of an intrauterine catheter or a fetal scalp electrode during labor. If the mother has active genital herpesvirus lesions, intrapartal internal monitoring is contraindicated, vaginal examinations are often omitted, regional anesthetic techniques are avoided, and the infant is delivered by cesarean section. The TORCH infections caused by other agents are asymptomatic in pregnancy, revealing themselves by the syndrome after birth. The congenital effects are not amenable to change or to amelioration by any known treatment.

TORCH test, a series of tests (including tests for *t*oxoplasmosis, *o*ther [including syphilis], *r*ubella, *c*ytomegalovirus, and *h*erpes) for diseases that exert recognized detrimental effects on the fetus, such as precipitating abortion or premature labor.

Torecan, a phenothiazine antiemetic medication. Brand name for **thiethylperazine malate.**

toremifene, an antineoplastic.

■ INDICATIONS: It is used to treat advanced breast carcinoma that is not responsive to other therapy in estrogen-receptor–positive patients (usually postmenopausal).

■ CONTRAINDICATIONS: Known hypersensitivity to this drug and pregnancy prohibit its use.

■ ADVERSE EFFECTS: Life-threatening effects are thrombocytopenia and leukopenia. Other adverse effects include altered taste (anorexia), vaginal bleeding, pruritus vulvae, rash, alopecia, chest pain, depression, hypercalcemia, ocular lesions, retinopathy, corneal opacity, and blurred vision (high doses). Common side effects include nausea, vomiting, hot flashes, headache, and light-headedness.

Torisel, a chemotherapeutic agent. Brand name for **temsirolimus.**

Torkildsen procedure. See **ventriculocisternostomy.**

torose /tôr″ōs/ [L, *torosus,* bulging], knoblike, knobby, or bulging.

torpor /tôr″pər/, **1.** a state of mental or physical inactivity. **2.** an absence or slowness of response to a stimulus.

torque /tôrk/ [L, *torquere,* to twist], **1.** a twisting force produced by contraction of the medial femoral muscles that tend to rotate the thigh medially. **2.** (in dentistry) a force applied to a tooth to rotate it on a mesiodistal or buccolingual axis. **3.** a rotary force applied to a denture base. Compare **torsion.**

torr /tôr/ [Evangelista Torricelli, Italian physicist, 1608–1647], a unit of pressure equal to 1333.22 dynes/cm^2, or 1.33322 millibars. One torr is the pressure required to support a column of mercury 1 mm high when the mercury is of standard density and subjected to standard acceleration. These standard conditions are 0° C and 45 degrees latitude, where the acceleration of gravity is 980.6 cm/sec^2. In reading a mercury barometer at other temperatures and latitudes, corrections commonly exceeding 2 torr may be required to compensate for the thermal expansion of the measuring scale used.

tors-, prefix meaning "twisted": *torsiometer, torsades de pointes, torsion.*

torsades de pointes /tôrsäd″ de pô·aNt′, tôr″säd də point″/ [Fr, *torsader,* to twist together, *pointes,* tips], a type of ventricular tachycardia with a spiral-like appearance ("twisting of the points") and complexes that at first look positive and then negative on an electrocardiogram. It is precipitated by a long Q-T interval, which often is induced by drugs (quinidine, procainamide, or disopyramide) but which may be the result of hypokalemia, hypomagnesemia, or profound bradycardia. The first line of treatment is IV magnesium sulfate, as well as defibrillation if the patient is unstable. See also **long QT syndrome.**

torsemide /tor'sĕ-mīd/, a loop diuretic related to sulfonylurea, used in treatment of edema and hypertension. It is administered orally or intravenously.

torsiometer /tôr'sē·om″ətər/, a device for measuring the amount of torsion of an eye around its anteroposterior axis.

torsion /tôr'shən/ [L, *torquere,* to twist], **1.** the process of twisting in a positive (clockwise) or negative (counterclockwise) direction. **2.** the state of being turned. **3.** (in dentistry) the twisting of a tooth on its long axis.

torsion angle, the angle between the axes of any two different portions of long bones, such as between the head and neck of the femur and its long axis.

torsion dystonia. See **dystonia musculorum deformans.**

torsion fracture, a spiral fracture, usually caused by an injury associated with twisting.

torsion of the testis, the axial rotation of the spermatic cord that cuts off the blood supply to the testicle, epididymis, and other structures. Complete ischemia for 6 hours may result in gangrene of the testis. Partial loss of circulation may result in atrophy. Certain testes are anatomically predisposed to torsion because of inadequate connective tissue, but the condition may be caused by trauma with severe swelling. Torsion of the testis occurs more often on the left than on the right side and is most frequent in the first year of life and during puberty. Surgical correction is required in most cases; if performed within 5 hours of the onset of symptoms, the testis can usually be saved.

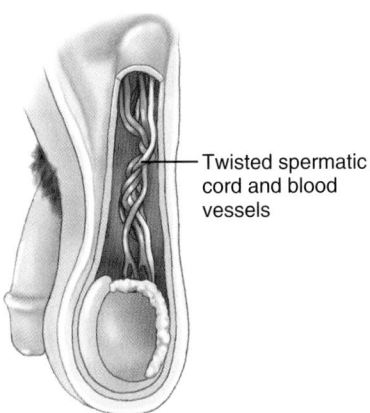

Twisted spermatic cord and blood vessels

Torsion of the testis *(Leonard, 2009)*

torsion spasm. See **dystonia musculorum deformans.**

torso /tôr'sō/ [L, *thyrsus,* stem], the body excluding the head and limbs. Also called **trunk.**

tort [L, *tortus,* twisted], (in law) a civil wrong, other than a breach of contract. Torts include negligence, false imprisonment, assault, and battery. The elements of a tort are a legal duty owed by the defendant to the plaintiff, a breach of duty, and damage from the breach of duty. A tort may be constitutional, in which one person deprives another of a right or immunity guaranteed by the Constitution; personal, in which a person or a person's reputation or feelings are injured; or intentional, in which the wrong is a deliberate act that is unlawful. Many other kinds of torts exist. –**tortious,** *adj.*

torticollis /tôr'tikol″is/ [L, *tortus,* twisted, *collum,* neck], an abnormal condition in which the head is inclined to one side as a result of the contraction of muscles on that side of the neck. It may be congenital or acquired. Treatment may include surgery, heat, support, or immobilization, depending on the cause and severity of the condition. Also called **wryneck.** See also **spasmodic torticollis.**

tortious. See **tort.**

tortipelvis /-pel'vis/ [L, *tortus,* twisted, *pelvis,* basin], a form of muscular dystonia resulting in a distortion of the pelvis or the spine and hips.

tortuous /tôr'choo·əs/ [L, *tortus,* twisted], having or making twists and turns.

Torula histolytica. See *Cryptococcus neoformans.*

Torulopsis, a genus of Fungi Imperfecti of the family Cryptococcaceae; it is closely related to *Candida,* and some authorities have considered it the same genus. Some species are normal inhabitants of the skin, respiratory tract, GI tract, and urogenital region but may also cause opportunistic infections.

Torulopsis glabrata, a species of fungus that is part of the normal flora of the human mouth, gut, and urinary tract but that in weak or immunocompromised patients may cause opportunistic infections such as meningitis, pneumonia, cystitis, and fungemia. Formerly called *Candida glabrata.*

torulopsosis /tôr'yəlopsō″sis, tôr'yoōlop″səsis/ [L, *torulus,* small swelling; Gk, *opsis,* appearance, *osis,* condition], an infection with the yeast *Torulopsis glabrata,* a normal inhabitant of the oropharynx, GI tract, and skin. *T. glabrata* causes disease in severely debilitated patients, in those with impaired immune function, and sometimes in those having prolonged urinary catheterization. Systemic infection is usually treated with amphotericin B.

torulosis. See **cryptococcosis.**

torus fracture. See **lead pipe fracture.**

torus levatorius, a broad fold or elevation in the nasopharynx that appears to emerge from just under the opening of the pharyngotympanic tube, continues medially onto the upper surface of the soft palate, and overlies the levator veli palatini muscle.

torus mandibularis. See **mandibular torus.**

torus palatinus. See **palatine torus.**

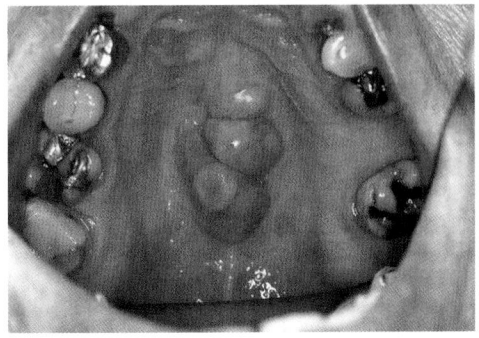

Torus palatinus *(Regezi, Sciubba, and Jordan, 2008)*

torus tubarius, an elevation of the rim of the pharyngotympanic tube where it projects into the nasopharynx. Posterior to the torus tubarius is a deep recess, the pharyngeal recess. Also called **Eustachian cushion, tubal prominence.**

total allergy syndrome, a condition of hypersensitivity to a wide range of substances, including pesticides, insecticides, pharmaceutics, certain metals, and chemicals used in the manufacture of plastics and epoxy resins. Also called **twentieth-century syndrome.**

T

total anomalous venous return [L, *totus,* whole; Gk, *anomalos,* uneven; L, *vena,* vein; ME, *retournen,* to turn back], a rare congenital cardiac anomaly in which the pulmonary veins attach to the right atrium or to various veins draining into the right atrium rather than to the left atrium. These alternate pathways of venous return to the left-sided circulation may be insufficient and cause obstruction, resulting in symptoms. Clinical manifestations include cyanosis, pulmonary congestion, and heart failure. Other cardiac defects also may be present, such as atrial septal defect, which shunts blood from the right atrium to the left atrium and helps decompress the right atrium. Corrective surgery is indicated, usually after 1 year of age, but may be necessary at an earlier age if pulmonary venous obstruction or severe congestive heart failure is present. See also **congenital cardiac anomaly.**

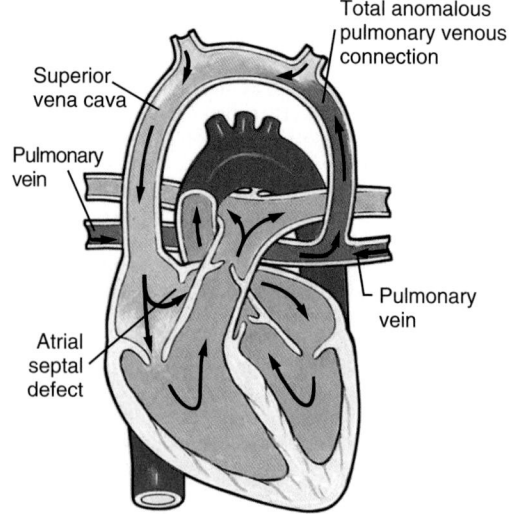

Total anomalous venous return *(Hockenberry and Wilson, 2011)*

total body electric conductivity (TOBEC), a method of measuring body composition by the differences in electric conductivity of fat, bone, and muscle. It is used for monitoring fitness of athletes; in clinical studies of weight control in which physicians want to determine if weight loss is caused by fat, water, or other tissues; and in measurement of fat content of dietary meats. See also **bioelectric impedance analysis.**

total body irradiation, radiation that exposes the entire body and, theoretically, all cells in the body.

total body water (TBW), all the water within the body, including intracellular and extracellular water plus the water in the GI and urinary tracts.

total cell volume (TCV), a measure of the adequacy of urea clearance of a hemodialyzer, calculated as the volume of saline necessary to fill its blood compartment. It declines slightly with each reuse of the dialyzer.

total cleavage, mitotic division of a fertilized ovum into blastomeres. Compare **partial cleavage.**

total color blindness. See **color blindness.**

total communication, the combined use of oral language and manual communication by a person with hearing loss.

total elbow arthroplasty, arthroplasty of both sides of the elbow joint, with humeral and ulnar components.

total filtration, (in radiology) the absorption of lower-energy x-ray photons emitted by the tube and tube housing plus any additional filters before they reach the target.

total hip arthroplasty (THA), arthroplasty of both sides of the hip joint, with acetabular and femoral components. See also **total hip replacement.**

total hip replacement, a surgical procedure to correct a hip joint damaged by degenerative disease, often arthritis. The head of the femur and the acetabulum are replaced with metal components. The acetabulum is plastic-coated to avoid metal-to-metal articulating surfaces. See also **total hip arthroplasty, total joint replacement.**

total hysterectomy. See **hysterectomy.**

total intravenous anesthesia (TIVA), anesthesia using only IV agents without the use of inhalational agents. Drugs used are generally of short duration of action and half-life in order to reduce the risks associated with accumulation. TIVA avoids unwanted effects of inhalational agents.

total iron, the total iron concentration in the blood. The serum reference interval is 50 to 150 mg/dL.

total joint replacement, a surgical procedure for the treatment of severe arthritis and other disorders in which the normal articulating surfaces of a joint are replaced by metal and plastic prostheses. Also called *total joint arthroplasty.*

total lung capacity (TLC), the volume of gas in the lungs at the end of a maximum inspiration. It equals the vital capacity plus the residual capacity.

total lymphoid irradiation (TLI), a method of inducing a strong immunosuppressive effect in patients undergoing bone marrow transplants, treatment of certain lymphomas, or other therapies requiring immunosuppression. TLI involves exposing all lymph nodes, the thymus, and spleen to a total of 2000 rad in 100-rad doses from a linear accelerator before graft implantation.

total macroglobulins, the heavy serum macroglobulins that are elevated in various diseases, such as cancer, and infections. The normal concentrations in serum are 70 to 430 mg/dL.

total parenteral nutrition (TPN), the administration of a nutritionally adequate hypertonic solution consisting of glucose, protein hydrolysates, minerals, and vitamins through an indwelling catheter into the superior vena cava or other main vein. Fat is also provided in a three-in-one solution or "piggy-backed." The high rate of blood flow results in rapid dilution of the solution, and full nutritional requirements can be met indefinitely. The procedure is used in prolonged coma, severe uncontrolled malabsorption, extensive burns, GI fistulas, and other conditions in which feeding by mouth cannot provide adequate amounts of the essential nutrients. In infants and children it is used when feeding via the GI tract is impossible, inadequate, or hazardous, such as in chronic intestinal obstruction from peritoneal sepsis or adhesions, inadequate intestinal length, or chronic nonremitting severe diarrhea. The hyperalimentation solution is infused through conventional tubing with an IV filter attached to remove any contaminates. In adults the catheter is placed directly into the subclavian vein and threaded through the right innominate vein into the superior vena cava. In infants and small children the catheter is usually threaded to the central venous location by way of the jugular vein, which is entered through a subcutaneous tunnel beneath the scalp. Strict asepsis must be maintained because infection is a grave and present danger of this therapy. Also called **hyperalimentation, intravenous alimentation, parenteral hyperalimentation,** *total parenteral alimentation.*

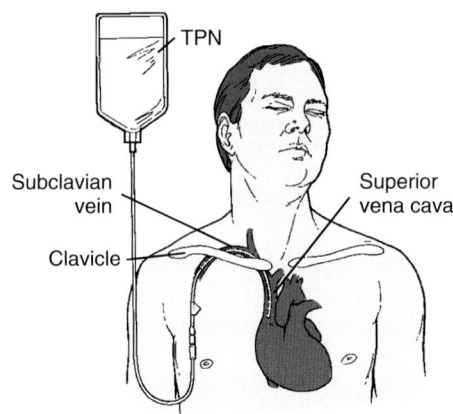

Total parenteral nutrition: adult

total peripheral resistance, the overall resistance to blood flow through the systemic blood vessels, especially in the peripheral arteries and veins.

total quality management (TQM), an approach to the improvement of the provision of services based on the premise that the overwhelming majority of quality failures are the result of flaws in processes and that quality can be improved by controlling these processes. TQM replaces traditional methods of quality management based on the identification and correction of problems as they occur and requires the participation of all members of an organization in improving processes, products, services, and the culture in which they work. TQM involves creation of an organizational structure for identifying and improving processes, the use of data-based statistical analysis to study processes, and the empowerment of employees to take responsibility for their own tasks in a way that encourages both continuous learning and personal responsibility. In a health care setting, this means a shift from an emphasis on tasks to an emphasis on outcomes of care, which provide the data. See also **continuous quality improvement.**

total renal blood flow (TRBF), the total volume of blood that flows into the renal arteries. The average TRBF in a normal adult is 1200 mL per minute. Compare **glomerular filtration rate.**

total thyroxine (T_4) test, a blood test that directly measures the total amount of T_4 present in the patient's blood, with abnormal values indicating either hyperthyroid or hypothyroid states. This test is also used to monitor replacement suppressive therapy.

totem /tō″təm/, an animal, plant, force of nature, or inanimate object that represents a tribal ancestor. It often has spiritual significance to a tribe, clan, family, or individual.

totipotency /tō′tipō″tənsē/, the ability of a cell, particularly a zygote, to differentiate into any of a number of specialized cells and thus form a new organism or regenerate a body part. Also called *totipotence.*

totipotential cell, an embryonic cell that is capable of developing into any variety of body cells. See also **stem cell.**

touch /tuch/ [Fr, *toucher,* to touch], **1.** *n.,* the ability to feel objects and to distinguish their various characteristics; the tactile sense. **2.** *n.,* the ability to perceive pressure when it is exerted on the skin or mucosa of the body. **3.** *v.,* to palpate or examine with the hand.

touch deprivation, a lack of tactile stimulation, especially in early infancy. If continued for a sufficient length of time,

it may lead to serious developmental and emotional disturbances, such as stunted growth, personality disorders, and social regression. See also **hospitalism.**

touch receptors [Fr, *toucher* + L, *recipere,* to receive], specialized sensory nerve endings that are sensitive to tactile stimuli.

Tourette syndrome /too-ret′/. See **Gilles de la Tourette syndrome.**

tourniquet /tur″nikit, toor″-/ [Fr, turnstile], a device used in controlling hemorrhage, consisting of a wide constricting band applied to the limb close to the site of bleeding. The use of a tourniquet is a drastic measure and is to be used only if the hemorrhage is life-threatening and if other safer measures have proved ineffective. A tourniquet is also used routinely to distend veins before venipuncture. See also **hemorrhage.**

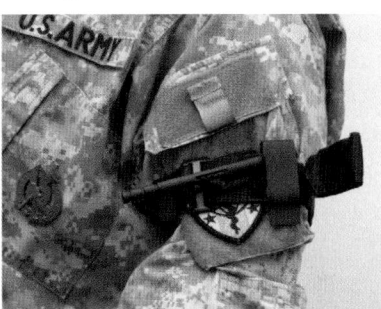

Combat Application Tourniquet *(Welling et al, 2012)*

tourniquet infusion method, a technique of intraarterial regional chemotherapy used in the treatment of osteogenic sarcoma. The technique uses one or two external tourniquets, depending on the location of the tumor, that slow or interrupt the blood flow to a limb temporarily while an anticancer drug, such as adriamycin, is infused into the area. The method increases the concentration of an antineoplastic drug by as much as 100 times compared with an alternative technique of injecting the drug into the circulation without application of a tourniquet, which results in rapid dilution of the drug by the normal blood volume.

tourniquet test, a test of capillary fragility, caused by an abnormality in the capillary wall or thrombocytopenia, in which a blood pressure cuff is applied for 5 minutes to a person's arm and inflated to a pressure halfway between the diastolic and systolic blood pressure. The number of petechiae within a circumscribed area of the skin may be counted, or the results may be reported in a range from negative (no petechiae) to +4 positive (confluent petechiae).

tower head, tower skull. See **oxycephaly.**

Townes method, a technique for producing radiographic images of the occipital bone, foramen magnum, and dorsum sellae. The patient is supine or facing the x-ray tube with the chin depressed so the orbitomeatal line is perpendicular. The x-ray beam is angled 30 degrees toward the patient's feet and enters the frontal bone above the nasal bones and exits the occipital bone. See also **Haas method.**

tox-, toxi-, toxico-, toxo-, prefix meaning "toxins" or "poisons": *toxin, toxicology.*

-toxaemia. See **-toxemia, -toxaemia.**

toxaemia. See **toxemia.**

Toxascaris leonina /toksas″kəris/, a species of nematode found mainly in domestic animals, commonly known as roundworms. It differs from related species in that it spends its entire developmental cycle in the digestive tract, rather than migrating through the lungs.

toxemia /toksē″mē·ə/ [Gk, *toxikon,* poison, *haima,* blood], the presence of bacterial toxins in the bloodstream. Also called **septicemia.** Also spelled **toxaemia.** See also **preeclampsia.** –*toxemic, adj.*

-toxemia, -toxaemia, suffix meaning "a (specified) toxic substance in the blood": *autotoxemia.*

toxemia of pregnancy. See **preeclampsia.**

toxi-. See **tox-, toxi-, toxico-, toxo-.**

toxic /tok′sik/ [Gk, *toxikon*], **1.** pertaining to a poison. **2.** pertaining to a severe and progressive disease or condition.

-toxic, -toxical, suffix meaning "poison": *cardiotoxic, neurotoxic.*

toxic albuminuria [Gk, *toxikon,* poison; L, *albus,* white; Gk, *ouron,* urine], a condition of serum albumin in the urine caused by the presence of toxic substances in the body.

toxic alcohols, poisonous alcohols that can damage the heart, kidneys, and nervous system. Ethylene glycol, commonly used in antifreeze, is a toxic alcohol. Severe poisoning is caused only by ingestion and is marked by progressive stages of central nervous system depression, acidosis, and renal failure. Treatment consists of administration of an antidote, hemodialysis, and supportive care.

toxic allergic syndrome. See **Löffler syndrome, PIE.**

toxic amblyopia, partial loss of vision because of retrooptic bulbar neuritis resulting from poisoning with quinine, lead, wood alcohol, nicotine, arsenic, or certain other poisons.

toxicant /tok″sikənt/, any poisonous agent.

toxic deafness. See **ototoxic hearing loss.**

toxic delirium [Gk, *toxikon,* poison; L, *delirare,* to rave], a symptom of disordered mental status as a result of poisoning.

toxic dementia, dementia resulting from excessive use of or exposure to a poisonous substance. See also **dementia.**

toxic dilation of colon [Gk, *toxikon* + L, *dilatare,* to widen; Gk, *kolon*], a condition of transverse colon dilation as a complication of amebic colitis, ulcerative colitis, or other bowel disease. Symptoms may include cramping, fever, rapid heartbeat, and mental confusion.

toxic dose (TD), (in toxicology) the amount of a substance that may be expected to produce a toxic effect. See also **median toxic dose.**

toxic encephalitis [Gk, *toxikon,* poison, *enkephalos,* brain, *itis,* inflammation], encephalitis caused by heavy metal poisoning. It is characterized by convulsions and cerebral edema.

toxic epidermal necrolysis (TEN), a rare, life-threatening skin disease characterized by epidermal erythema, superficial necrosis, and skin erosions. This condition, which affects mainly adults, makes the skin appear scalded, often leaving scars. It involves more than 30% of body surface area. The cause of TEN is unknown, but it may result from toxic or hypersensitive reactions, an immune response, or severe physiological stress. A similar skin disorder may be the result of a staphylococcal infection. Treatment of TEN commonly involves the administration of IV fluids to replace body fluids and maintain electrolyte balance. Frequent laboratory analyses are necessary to monitor hematocrit and hemoglobin, serum proteins, electrolytes, and blood gases. Also called **scalded skin syndrome.** Compare **staphylococcal scalded skin syndrome.**

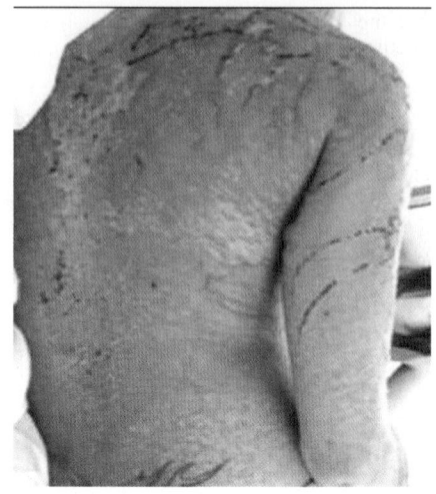

Toxic epidermal necrolysis *(Napolitano et al, 2013)*

toxic erythema [Gk, *toxikon,* poison, *erythema,* redness], an inexact term sometimes applied to reddish skin eruptions of undetermined origin.

toxic erythema of the newborn. See **erythema neonatorum.**

toxic gastritis. See **corrosive gastritis.**

toxic goiter, an enlargement of the thyroid gland associated with exophthalmia and systemic disease. See also **Graves disease, thyroiditis.**

toxic headache, headache caused by systemic poisoning or associated with illness.

toxic hemoglobinuria. See **hemoglobinuria.**

toxic hepatitis, hepatitis produced by a hepatotoxin, such as *Amanita phalloides* toxin, carbon tetrachloride, or any of various drugs.

toxic hepatopathy, liver disease produced by a hepatotoxin such as *Amanita phalloides* toxin, carbon tetrachloride, white phosphorus, or any of various drugs. It can range in severity from subclinical abnormalities to jaundice to fulminant liver failure.

toxicity /toksis″itē/ [Gk, *toxikon*], **1.** the degree to which something is poisonous. **2.** a condition that results from exposure to a toxin or to toxic amounts of a substance that does not cause adverse effects in smaller amounts.

toxic nephropathy, kidney damage caused by the effects of a nephrotoxin. The most common symptoms are dysfunction and then necrosis of the proximal tubules, sometimes progressing to renal failure.

toxic neuritis [Gk, *toxikon,* poison, *neuron,* nerve, *itis,* inflammation], a painful nerve inflammation caused by a metallic, bacterial, or other poison.

toxic nodular goiter, an enlarged thyroid gland characterized by numerous discrete nodules and hypersecretion of thyroid hormones. It occurs most frequently in elderly individuals. Typical signs of thyrotoxicosis such as nervousness, tremor, weakness, fatigue, weight loss, and irritability are usually present, but exophthalmia is rare. Anorexia is more common than hyperphagia, and cardiac arrhythmia or congestive heart failure may be a predominant manifestation. When clinical findings suggest thyrotoxicosis, a therapeutic trial of antithyroid drugs, such as propylthiouracil or methimazol, is indicated, but, after the diagnosis is established, radioactive iodine is considered the treatment of choice, and large doses are usually required.

toxico-.   See **tox-, toxi-, toxico-, toxo-.**

Toxicodendron /tok′sikōden″dron/, a genus of plants that includes poison ivy, poison oak, and poison sumac. The toxic agent in the plants is a nonvolatile oil, toxicodendrol. See also **rhus dermatitis.**

toxicokinetics /tok′sikō′kinet″iks/, the passage through the body of a toxic agent or its metabolites, usually in an action similar to that of pharmacokinetics.

toxicologic, toxicological, pertaining to poisons. See **toxicology.**

toxicologist /tok′sikol″əjist/, a specialist in poisons, their effects, and antidotes.

toxicology /-ol′əjē/, the scientific study of poisons, their detection, their effects, and methods of treatment for conditions they produce. −*toxicological, toxicologic, adj.*

toxicology screening, a blood or urine test that detects the most commonly abused nonprescription drugs. Testing for drug overdose and poisoning is best done on blood, whereas screening for use or abuse of nonprescription drugs is usually done on urine. Toxicology studies are used to implicate drugs as a cause or factor in the death of a person.

toxic or drug-induced hepatitis, hepatitis resulting from a chemical, parasitic, or metabolic poison.

toxicosis /tok′sikō″sis/ [Gk, *toxikon,* poison, *osis,* condition], a disease condition caused by the absorption of metabolic or bacterial poisons.

toxic psychosis, psychosis that results from the poisonous effects of chemicals or drugs, including those produced by the body itself.

toxic shock syndrome (TSS), a severe acute disease caused by infection with strains of *Staphylococcus aureus,* phage group I, that produces a unique toxin, enterotoxin F. It is most common in menstruating women using high-absorbency tampons but has been seen in newborns, children, and men.

■ OBSERVATIONS: The onset of the syndrome is characterized by sudden high fever, headache, sore throat with swelling of the mucous membranes, diarrhea, nausea, and erythroderma. Acute renal failure, abnormal liver function, confusion, and refractory hypotension usually follow, and death may occur. It is probable that mild forms of the syndrome are not reported and therefore are not diagnosed. No seasonal or geographic factor appears involved in the cause of the disease, and there is no evidence of contagion among household members or through sexual contacts of people who have TSS. Bacteremia, or discernible local infection, is absent in most cases. *S. aureus* may be cultured from many sites, including the pharynx, nares, and cervix, but the drastic effects of infection are the result of the toxin released from the organism rather than from the infection itself.

■ INTERVENTIONS: Aggressive volume expansion by the administration of large amounts of IV fluids, assisted ventilation, and administration of vasopressors may be necessary in treating severe TSS. Early recognition and active supportive treatment greatly improve the survival rates and decrease both prolonged morbidity and recurrence.

toxic substance [Gk, *toxikon,* poison; L, *substantia,* essence], any poison.

toxidrome /tok′s-drōm/, a specific syndromelike group of symptoms associated with exposure to a given poison.

toxidromes, signs and symptoms of toxicity consistently associated with classes of medications.

toxin /tok′sin/, a poison, usually one produced by or occurring in a plant or microorganism. See also **endotoxin, exotoxin.**

-toxin, combining form meaning "poison": *biotoxin, histotoxin, zootoxin.*

toxin-antitoxin [Gk, *toxikon,* poison, *anti,* against, *toxikon*], a mixture of toxin and antitoxin. Diph-

theria toxin-antitoxin was formerly used for active immunization.

toxinology /tok′sinol″əjē/, the study of poisons, with particular emphasis on relatively unstable proteinaceous substances. See also **toxicology.**

toxo-.   See **tox-, toxi-, toxico-, toxo-.**

Toxocara /tok′səker″ə/, a genus of ascarid nematodes. *T. canis* affects mainly dogs. *T. mystax* affects cats but may also infect humans, particularly children, causing intestinal and respiratory symptoms and damage to the spleen and liver. See also **toxocariasis.**

toxocariasis /tok′sōkərī″əsis/ [Gk, *toxo,* bow, *kara,* head, *osis,* condition], infection with the larvae of *Toxocara canis,* the common roundworm of dogs, and with *T. cati,* of cats. Human ingestion of viable eggs, commonly found in soil, leads to the spread of tiny larvae throughout the body, resulting in respiratory symptoms, enlarged liver, skin rashes, eosinophilia, and delayed ocular lesions. Children who eat dirt are particularly subject to this disease. Specific drug therapy is not very useful; the outcome is usually good without therapy. Two major forms of the infection exist: ocular larval migrans (OLM), which can cause an eye disease resulting in blindness, occurs when the worm enters the eye. Visceral larval migrans (VLM) is heavy or repeated infection that causes swelling of organs or the central nervous system. Symptoms of this form are caused by movement of the worms and are manifested as fever, asthma, or pneumonia. Severe forms are rare. VLM is treated with antiparasitic drugs and antiinflammatories, whereas OLM is more difficult to treat and usually involves preventing progression of eye damage. Regular worming of pets helps prevent infection. Also called **visceral larva migrans.**

toxoid /tok′soid/ [Gk, *toxikon,* poison, *eidos,* form], a toxin that has been treated with chemicals or heat to decrease its toxic effect but that retains its antigenic power. It is given to produce immunity by stimulating the creation of antibodies. See also **toxin, vaccine.**

toxophore /tok″səfôr′/, the part of a toxic molecule that is responsible for the poisonous effect.

Toxoplasma /tok′sōplaz″mə/ [Gk, *toxikon + plasma,* something formed], a genus of protozoa with only one known species, *T. gondii,* an intracellular parasite of cats and other hosts that causes toxoplasmosis in humans.

toxoplasmosis /tok′sōplazmō″sis/ [Gk, *toxikon + plasma + osis,* condition], a common infection with the protozoan intracellular parasite *Toxoplasma gondii.* The congenital form is characterized by liver and brain involvement with cerebral calcification, convulsions, blindness, microcephaly or hydrocephaly, and cognitive impairment. The acquired form is characterized by rash, lymphadenopathy, fever, malaise, central nervous system disorders, myocarditis, and pneumonitis.

■ OBSERVATIONS: Cats acquire the organism by eating infected birds and mice. Cysts of the organism are transmitted from cat feces to humans or by human ingestion of inadequately cooked meat containing the cysts. Transplacental transmission occurs only during acute infection of the mother, but the disease is very serious in the fetus and in those with human immunodeficiency virus or other immunosuppressive conditions or impaired immune system. Diagnosis is made by demonstrating rising antibody titers or by immunofluorescent antibody tests. Infection confers immunity.

■ INTERVENTIONS: Combinations of sulfonamides with pyrimethamine are recommended as treatment, possibly reducing the severity of the illness in the fetus.

■ PATIENT CARE CONSIDERATIONS: All meat should be heated to at least 140° F (60° C) throughout to kill this parasite. Pregnant women who are not immune are advised not to handle cats, cat feces, or litter boxes.

T

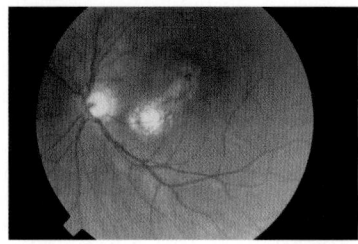

Congenital toxoplasmosis: retinal changes *(Conlon and Snydman, 2000)*

toxoplasmosis antibody titer, a blood test performed on pregnant women to detect toxoplasmosis infection, which is associated with recognized detrimental effects on the fetus. See also **TORCH syndrome.**

Toynbee maneuver /toin′bē/ [Joseph Toynbee, English otologist, 1815–1866], pinching the nostrils and swallowing. If the auditory tube is patent, the tympanic membrane will retract medially.

Toynbee test /toin′bē/ [Joseph Toynbee], performance of the Toynbee maneuver and monitoring of pressure changes in the middle ear. Subsequent middle ear negative pressure or negative pressure followed by ambient pressure usually indicates normal function of the auditory tube.

tPA, abbreviation for **tissue plasminogen activator.**

TPAL. See **parity.**

TPHA, abbreviation for *Treponema pallidum hemagglutination assay.*

TPN, abbreviation for **total parenteral nutrition.**

TPR, abbreviation for *temperature, pulse, respiration.*

TQ, symbol for **tocopherolquinone.**

TQM, abbreviation for **total quality management.**

TR, **1.** abbreviation for **repetition time. 2.** abbreviation for **tricuspid regurgitation.**

trabecula carnea /trəbek″yələ/ *pl. trabeculae carneae* [L, little beam, *carneus,* flesh], any one of the irregular bands and bundles of muscle projecting from the inner surfaces near the apex of the ventricles of the heart. Also called **Rathke bundles.** Compare **chordae tendineae.** See also **left ventricle, right ventricle, heart.**

trabeculae, (in ophthalmology) the part of the eye in front of the canal of Schlemm and within the angle created by the iris and the cornea, responsible for aqueous drainage.

trabecular pattern /trəbek″yələr/ [L, little beam], an irregular meshwork of stress and stress-related struts within a cancellous bone.

trabecula septomarginalis. See **moderator band.**

trabeculated bladder, a noncompliant, hypotonic bladder resulting from hypertrophy of the muscular coat, usually caused by obstruction of the urethra. Increasing postvoid residuals and risk of urinary tract infection may ensue.

trabeculectomy, creation of a fistula between the anterior chamber of the eye and the subconjunctival space by surgical removal of a portion of the trabecular meshwork, performed to facilitate drainage of the aqueous humor in glaucoma.

trabeculoplasty /trabek″yəlōplas′tē/, a plastic surgery procedure used in the treatment of open-angle glaucoma. An argon laser beam is used to blanch the trabecular network of the eye, thereby permitting drainage of the excess fluid that is causing increased pressure within the eyeball.

trabeculotomy /-ot′əmē/, a surgical opening in an orbital trabecula to increase the outflow of aqueous humor.

trace element [L, *trahere,* to draw, *elementum,* first principle], an element essential to nutrition or physiological processes, found in such minute quantities that analysis yields a presence of only trace amounts.

trace gas, any gas that represents an extremely small or insignificant portion of a mixture of gases. See also **gas-scavenging system.**

tracer [L, *trahere,* to draw], **1.** a radioactive isotope that is used in diagnostic x-ray techniques to allow a biological process to be seen. After introduction into the body, the tracer binds with a specific substance and is followed with a scanner or fluoroscope as it passes through various organs or systems. Kinds include **radioactive iodine, radioactive carbon.** See also **radioisotope scan. 2.** a mechanical device that graphically records the outline or movements of an object or part of the body. **3.** a dissecting instrument that is used to isolate vessels and nerves. −*trace, v.*

tracer depot method, a technique used to determine local blood flow through skin or muscle, based on the rate at which a radioactive tracer deposited in a tissue is removed by diffusion into the capillaries and washed out by the local blood supply. If blood flow is diminished or absent, as in dead skin, the deposited tracer does not wash out.

trachea /trā″kē·ə/ [Gk, *tracheia,* rough artery], a nearly cylindric tube in the neck, composed of C-shaped cartilage and membrane and trachealis muscle, that extends from the larynx at the level of the sixth cervical vertebra to the fifth thoracic vertebra, where it divides into two bronchi. The trachea conveys air to the lungs. It is about 11 cm long and 2 cm wide. The ventral surface of the tube is covered in the neck by the isthmus of the thyroid gland and various other structures, such as the sternothyroideus and the sternohyoideus. Dorsally the trachea is in contact with the esophagus. Also called **windpipe.** See also **primary bronchus.**

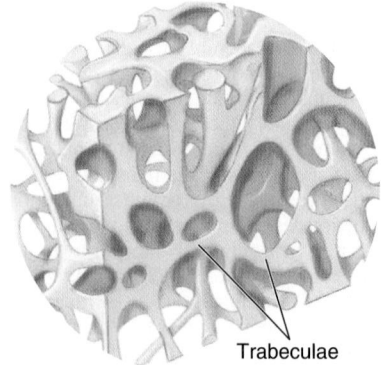

Trabecular pattern *(Patton and Thibodeau, 2010)*

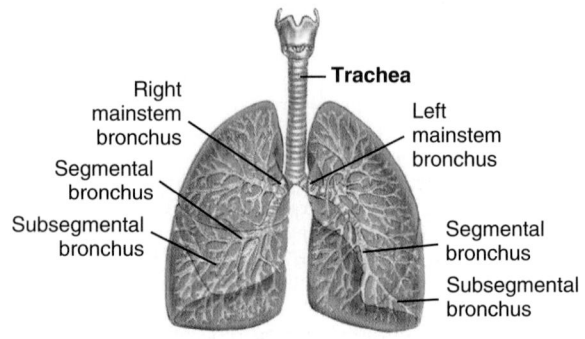

Trachea *(Wilson and Giddens, 2009)*

tracheal /trā′kē·əl/ [Gk, *tracheia,* rough artery], pertaining to the trachea.

tracheal breath sound. See **bronchial breath sound.**

tracheal gas insufflation, continuous insufflation of a low flow of fresh gas to the distal endotracheal tube, believed capable of flushing out the anatomical dead space and thus reducing $PaCO_2$.

tracheal intubation. See **endotracheal intubation.**

tracheal tugging [Gk, *tracheia,* rough artery; ME, *toggen*], an effect of an aortic aneurysm in which the trachea is pulled downward with each heart contraction.

tracheitis /trā′kē·ī′tis/, any inflammatory condition of the trachea. It may be acute or chronic, resulting from infection, allergy, or physical irritation. Also called **trachitis.**

trachelagra, distortion of the muscles of the neck.

trachelo-, combining form meaning "neck" or "necklike structure": *trachelodynia.*

trachelodynia. See **cervicodynia.**

tracheo- /trā′kē·ō-/, combining form meaning "trachea": *tracheobronchial, tracheomalacia, tracheostomy.*

tracheobronchial /trā′kē·ō·brong′kē·əl/, pertaining to the trachea and bronchi. Also called **bronchotracheal.**

tracheobronchial tree (TBT) /-brong′kē·əl/ [Gk, *tracheia + bronchos,* windpipe], an anatomical complex that includes the trachea, bronchi, and bronchial tubes. It conveys air to and from the lungs and is a primary structure in respiration. See also **bronchial tree.**

tracheobronchitis /trā′kē·ōbrongkī′tis/, inflammation of the trachea and bronchi, a common symptom of pulmonary infection.

tracheobronchomegaly /-brong′kōmeg″əlē/, an abnormally large upper airway in which the trachea may be as wide as the spinal column.

tracheoesophageal fistula /trā′kē·ō·ē′səfā′jē·əl/ [Gk, *tracheia + oisophagos,* gullet], a congenital malformation in which there is an abnormal tubelike passage between the trachea and the esophagus. Also spelled **tracheooesophageal fistula.**

tracheoesophageal folds, longitudinal folds in the embryonic respiratory diverticulum that fuse to form the tracheoesophageal septum.

tracheoesophageal puncture (TEP), a one-way synthetic valve placed in a surgically created tracheoesophageal fistula to restore speech after laryngectomy.

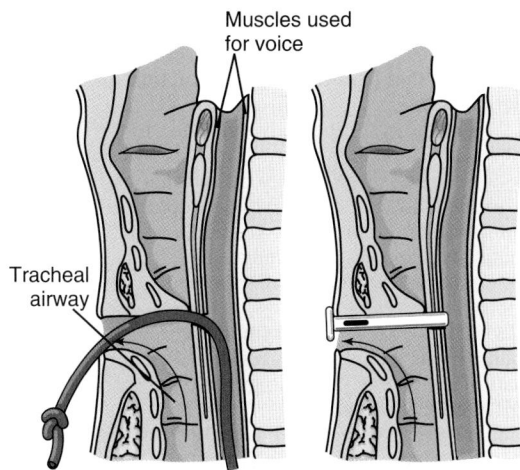

Tracheoesophageal puncture *(Monahan et al, 2007)*

tracheoesophageal shunt, surgical formation of a passageway between the trachea and the esophagus that enables a laryngectomee to speak. The operation results in an ability to produce esophageal speech with normal respiration as a source of air and without the need to belch to produce voice sounds. Also spelled **tracheooesophageal shunt.**

tracheolaryngeal /-lerin″jē·əl/, pertaining to the trachea and larynx.

tracheomalacia /trā′kē·ōmələā″shə/, an eroding of the trachea that is usually caused by excessive pressure from a cuffed endotracheal tube but that can be congenital.

tracheoesophageal fistula. See **tracheoesophageal fistula.**

tracheoesophageal shunt. See **tracheoesophageal shunt.**

tracheopharyngeal /-ferin″jē·əl/, pertaining to the trachea and pharynx.

tracheoplasty /trā″kē·ōplas′tē/, plastic surgery of the trachea.

tracheostenosis /-stənō″sis/, constriction of the lumen of the trachea.

tracheostomy /trā′kē·os′təmē/ [Gk, *tracheia + stoma,* mouth], an opening through the neck into the trachea through which an indwelling tube may be inserted. After tracheostomy the patient's chest is auscultated for breath sounds indicative of bilateral air exchange and pulmonary congestion, mucous membranes and fingertips are observed for cyanosis, oxygenation is monitored with pulse oximeters, and humidified oxygen is given via a trach collar placed over the tracheostomy tube. The patient is reassured that the tube is open and that air can pass through it. The tube is suctioned as needed to keep it free from tracheobronchial secretions by using a suction catheter attached to a Y-connector. The catheter is rotated, and intermittent suction is applied for no longer than 10 seconds. Complications of tracheostomy include pneumothorax, respiratory insufficiency, obstruction of the tracheostomy tube or its displacement from the lumen of the trachea, pulmonary infection, atelectasis, tracheoesophageal fistula, hemorrhage, and mediastinal emphysema. If the procedure was done as an emergency, the tracheostomy is closed after normal breathing is restored. If the tracheostomy is permanent, such as with a laryngectomy, the patient is taught self-care. Compare **tracheotomy.**

tracheostomy care [Gk, *tracheia,* rough artery, *stoma,* mouth], care of the tracheostomy patient consisting of maintenance of a patent airway, adequate humidification, aseptic wound care, and sterile tracheal aspiration. Complications can include injury to the vocal cords, gastric distension and regurgitation, occlusion of the endotracheal tube, and an increased risk of infection.

tracheotomy /trā′kē·ot″əmē/ [Gk, *tracheia + temnein,* to cut], an incision made into the trachea through the neck below the larynx, performed to gain access to the airway below a blockage with a foreign body, tumor, or edema of the glottis. The opening may be made as an emergency measure at an accident site, at a hospitalized patient's bedside, or in the operating room. The patient's neck is hyperextended, and an incision is made through the skin and through the second, third, or fourth tracheal ring. A small hole is made in the fibrous tissue of the trachea, and the opening is then dilated to allow air intake. In an emergency any available instrument may be used as a dilator, even the barrel of a ballpoint pen with the inner part removed. If the blockage persists, a tracheostomy tube is inserted; if not, the incision is closed after normal respirations are established. After surgery the patient is observed for recurrent respiratory difficulty or cyanosis. Compare **tracheostomy.**

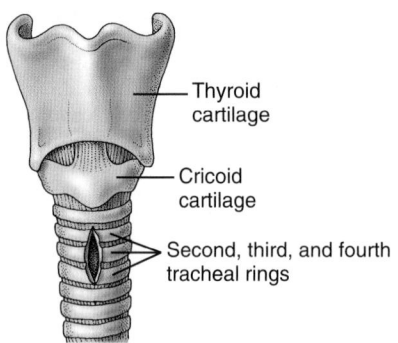

Tracheotomy *(Ignatavicius and Workman, 2010)*

tracheotomy tube [Gk, *tracheia,* rough artery, *temnein,* to cut; L, *tubus*], a curved hollow tube of rubber, metal, or plastic surgically inserted in the trachea to relieve a breathing obstruction.

trachitis. See **tracheitis.**

trachoma /trəkō″mə/ [Gk, roughness], a chronic infectious disease of the eye caused by the bacterium *Chlamydia trachomatis.*

■ OBSERVATIONS: It is characterized initially by inflammation, pain, photophobia, and lacrimation. If untreated, follicles form on the upper eyelids, forming scarring that causes trichiasis and corneal sequelae, eventually causing blindness.

■ INTERVENTIONS: The current recommended treatment is the onetime use of use of oral azithromycin or the topical use of 1% tetracycline ointment. Scarred eyelids may be surgically repaired. Screening communities for the presence of trachoma in children 1 to 9 years of age is an important measure in the eradication of trachoma. When more than 10% of the community has the disease, the entire community is treated with antibiotics.

■ PATIENT CARE CONSIDERATIONS: Trachoma is a significant cause of blindness and is endemic to hot, dry, poverty-ridden areas. In the United States it is found in the Southwest. Teaching an affected population about the spread of trachoma, screening, and having an adequate water supply for washing hands, towels, and handkerchiefs are important factors in eliminating the disease.

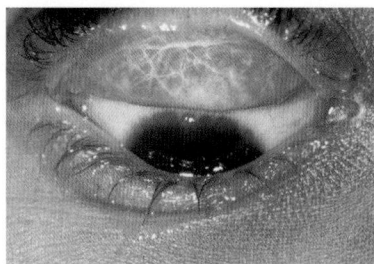

Trachoma *(Conlon and Snydman, 2000)*

tracing [L, *trahere,* to draw], a graphic record of a physical event, such as an electrocardiograph tracing made by pens on a moving sheet of paper while the electric impulses of heart muscle contractions are recorded. Also called **printout.**

trackball, a type of computer peripheral that is larger than a typical mouse. A trackball has one large ball to use to move the cursor and two large buttons for click commands. It is helpful to patients with motor disabilities.

tract [L, *tractus,* trail], **1.** an elongated group of tissues and organs that function together as a pathway, such as the digestive tract or the respiratory tract. **2.** (in neurology) the neuronal axons that are grouped together to form a pathway; a serial arrangement that serves a common function.

traction /trak″shən/ [L, *trahere,* to draw], **1.** (in orthopedics) the process of putting a limb, bone, or group of muscles under tension by means of weights and pulleys to align or immobilize the part to reduce muscle spasm or relieve pressure on it. Kinds include **Bryant's traction, Buck's traction, Russell's traction, skeletal traction, skin traction, split Russell traction.** See also **orthopedic traction. 2.** the process of pulling a part of the body along, through, or out of its socket or cavity, such as axis traction with obstetric forceps in delivering an infant.

traction, 90-90, an orthopedic mechanism, used especially in pediatrics, that combines skeletal traction and suspension with a short-leg cast or a splint to immobilize and position the lower extremity in the treatment of a displaced fractured femur. This type of traction is usually unilateral with the opposite leg in Buck's traction or in split Russell traction for immobilization. The pin used in this kind of skeletal traction is inserted into bone in the knee area and attached to a riser running through a pulley on an overhead traction frame to a pulley and weight system fitted over the foot of the bed. The pulley and weight system at the foot of the bed also accommodates additional attachments to the short-leg cast or splint of the involved lower limb. Application of 90-90 traction may also incorporate a jacket restraint to help immobilize the patient. A variation of this type of traction is often used with adults in the treatment of low back pain.

traction frame, an orthopedic apparatus that supports the pulleys, ropes, and weights by which traction is applied to various parts of the body or by which various parts of the body are suspended. Traction frames are used in the treatment of bone fractures, dislocations, and disease processes of the musculoskeletal system; in the correction of various orthopedic deformities; and in the general immobilization of specific areas of the body. The main components of a traction frame are metal uprights that attach to the bed and support an overhead metal bar. In addition to having traction equipment, traction frames are often rigged with trapeze bars that the patient can grasp to help in changing positions and to exercise the muscles of the arms and the trunk. The components of a traction frame are securely clamped together when in use but can be easily disassembled and reassembled. Compare **Balkan traction frame, claw-type traction frame, IV-type traction frame.**

traction response, the body's reaction to traction applied to the spine. Alterations of certain signs and symptoms of a musculoskeletal disorder may be revealed by traction tests. For example, if traction relieves a symptom, it may indicate impingement of a nerve root. Traction also may be used therapeutically to increase joint range, overcome muscle spasms, shorten soft tissues, or neutralize pressure and relieve pain in various joints.

trademark (™), a word, symbol, or device assigned to a product by its manufacturer, registered or not registered, as a part of its identity. See also **generic name, brand name, registered trademark®.**

tragacanth /trag″əkanth/, a white tasteless vegetable gum derived from the shrub *Astragalus gummifer* and related species. It is used as a suspending agent in pharmaceutic preparations, particularly powders and tinctures.

tragal /trā″gəl/ [Gk, *tragos,* goat], pertaining to the tragus. See also **egophony.**

Trager approach, service mark for a bodywork technique whose purpose is to train patients to develop awareness of movement patterns that relieve pain and promote relaxation. It consists of two components: tablework, in which the practitioner, in a meditative state, uses touch and gentle passive movement to assist the patient in experiencing new movement patterns, and Mentastics, in which the patient is taught a series of movements designed to relieve tension.

tragi, projections external to the ear. See **tragus.**

tragion /traj'ēən/ [Gk, *tragos,* goat], a cephalometric landmark located at the superior margin of the tragus of the ear.

tragophony, voice with a high-pitched or bleating quality. See **egophony.**

tragus /trā″gəs/ *pl.* **tragi** [Gk, *tragos,* goat], a small tonguelike projection of the auricular cartilage of the ear, anterior to the external meatus.

trained reflex. See **conditioned response.**

traineeship /trānē″ship/ [L, *trahere,* to draw; AS, *scieppan,* to shape], a grant of money allocated to an individual for advanced study in a given field. In nursing, many graduate students have been awarded federal traineeships that provide funds for tuition and living expenses.

training effect, a rehabilitation effect in heart patients that can be measured by changes in cardiac function.

training grant, a grant of money or other resources to provide training in a particular field. Many schools of nursing receive federal or state grants to provide specific educational programs. Funds may be allocated for faculty salaries, student aid, or other expenses.

train-of-four, a test for measuring the level of neuromuscular blockade. Four consecutive stimuli are delivered along the path of a nerve, and the response of the muscle is measured to evaluate stimuli that are blocked versus those that are delivered. Four equal muscle contractions will result if there is no neuromuscular blockade, but, if nondepolarizing blockade is present, there will be a loss of twitch height and number, which will indicate the degree of blockade. This test is commonly used in intensive care units.

trait [Fr, trace], **1.** a characteristic mode of behavior or any mannerism or physical feature that distinguishes one individual or culture from another. **2.** any characteristic quality or condition that is genetically determined and inherited as part of a specific phenotype. A trait is inherited as homozygous dominant, homozygous recessive, or heterozygous in the ratio of 1:2:1 among offspring of two heterozygous parents. In medicine the term *trait* is used specifically to denote the heterozygous state of a recessive disorder, such as sickle cell anemia. See also **dominance, gene, Mendel's laws, recessive allele.**

TRALI, abbreviation for **transfusion-related acute lung injury.**

tramadol, a central analgesic.
- INDICATIONS: It is used to manage moderate to severe pain.
- CONTRAINDICATIONS: Factors that prohibit its use are known hypersensitivity to this drug or acute intoxication with any central nervous system depressant.
- ADVERSE EFFECTS: Seizures and GI bleeding are life-threatening effects. Other adverse effects are dizziness, central nervous system stimulation, somnolence, headache, anxiety, confusion, euphoria, hallucination, nausea, constipation, vomiting, dry mouth, diarrhea, abdominal pain, anorexia, flatulence, vasodilation, orthostatic hypotension, tachycardia, hypertension, abnormal electrocardiograms, pruritus, rash, urticaria, vesicles, urinary retention or fre-

quency, menopausal symptoms, dysuria, and menstrual disorders.

TRAM flap, an autogenous myocutaneous flap that uses transverse rectus abdominal muscle (TRAM) to carry lower abdominal skin and fat to the breast for reconstruction. See also **myocutaneous flap.**

trance [L, *transire,* to pass across], **1.** a sleeplike state characterized by the complete or partial suspension of consciousness and loss or diminution of motor activity, as seen in hypnosis, dissociative disorders, and various cataleptic and ecstatic states. **2.** a dazed or bewildered condition; stupor. **3.** a state of detachment from one's immediate surroundings, such as in deep concentration or daydreaming. Kinds include **alcoholic trance,** *death trance,* **hypnotic trance, induced trance.**

Trandate, an antihypertensive drug. Brand name for **labetalol hydrochloride.**

trandolapril, an antihypertensive. Its prototype is enalapril.
- INDICATIONS: It is used to treat hypertension, heart failure, and postmyocardial infarction/left ventricular dysfunction.
- CONTRAINDICATIONS: Factors that prohibit its use include known hypersensitivity, a history of angioedema, and second- or third-trimester pregnancy.
- ADVERSE EFFECTS: Life-threatening effects include myocardial infarction, stroke, agranulocytosis, neutropenia, leukopenia, anemia, proteinuria, and renal failure. Other adverse effects include palpitations, angina, transient ischemic attacks, bradycardia, arrhythmias, paresthesias, headache, fatigue, drowsiness, depression, sleep disturbances, nausea, vomiting, cramps, diarrhea, constipation, ileus, pancreatitis, hepatitis, rash, purpura, dyspnea, hyperkalemia, hyponatremia, and impotence. Common side effects include hypotension, dizziness, dyspepsia, cough, and myalgia.

tranexamic acid /tran″ek-sam′ik/, an agent that combats fibrinolysis by competitively inhibiting activation of plasminogen. It is used in prophylaxis and treatment of hemorrhage associated with excessive fibrinolysis, such as that after oral surgery in patients with hemophilia. It is administered orally or intravenously.

tranquilizer /trang″kwilī′zər/ [L, *tranquillus,* calm], a drug prescribed to calm anxious or agitated people, ideally without decreasing their consciousness. Major tranquilizers are generally used in the treatment of psychoses and are now generally referred to as antipsychotic drugs. Minor tranquilizers are usually prescribed for the treatment of anxiety, irritability, tension, or psychoneurosis and are now generally referred to as antianxiety drugs or sedative-hypnotics. Tranquilizers tend to induce drowsiness and have the potential for causing physical and psychological dependence. Also spelled *tranquillizer.* See also **antipsychotic.**

trans- /trans-, tranz-/, prefix meaning "across, through, over": *transabdominal, transferase, transplacental.*

transabdominal /-abdom′inəl/ [L, *trans,* across, *abdomen,* belly], pertaining to a procedure through the abdominal wall.

transactional analysis (TA) /-ak′shənəl/ [L, *transigere,* to drive through; Gk, *analyein,* to loosen], a form of psychodynamic psychotherapy developed by Eric Berne, based on a role theory that three different coherent organized egos exist throughout life simultaneously in every person, representing the child, the adult, and the parent. Interactions between people are transactions, originating from a person in one of the ego states and received by another person who may be in a complementary or a crossed ego state. Transactions are motivated by a need for recognition and contact called "strokes." Transactions occur in six kinds of "time structure": withdrawal, rituals, pastimes, games, activities, and intimacy. The way in which a person structures time reflects internal conflicts and patterns adopted to cope with those conflicts. The goal of transactional analysis is to enable clients to communicate from the ego state appropriate to the situation and the responses of the individuals, thereby decreasing conflict.

transaminase, now called **aminotransferase.**

transamination /-am′inā″shən/, the reaction between an amino acid and an alpha-keto acid in which the enzyme transaminase induces transfer of the amino group to the alpha-ketoacid.

transaortic /-ā-ôr″tik/ [L, *trans,* across; Gk, *aerein,* to raise], through the aorta.

trans arrangement. See **trans configuration.**

transcellular transport, transport of molecules through the cells of an epithelial cell layer.

transcellular water /-sel″yələr/ [L, *trans* + *cella,* storeroom], the part of extracellular water that is enclosed by an epithelial membrane and whose volume and composition are determined by the cellular activity of that membrane.

transcendence /transen″dəns/ [L, *trans* + *scandere,* to climb], the rising above one's previously perceived limits or restrictions.

transcendental meditation (TM), a psychophysiological exercise designed to lower levels of tension and anxiety and increase tolerance of frustration. TM has been described as a state of consciousness that does not require any physical or mental control. During meditation, the person enters a hypometabolic state in which there is reduced activity of the adrenergic component of the autonomic nervous system.

transcervical femoral neck fracture /transur″vikəl/ [L, *trans,* across; *cervix,* neck, *fractura*], a fracture through the neck of the femur.

transcondylar fracture /transkon″dilər/ [L, *trans* + Gk, *kondylos,* condyle], a fracture that occurs transversely and distally to the epicondyles of any one of the long bones.

trans configuration /-kənfig′yərā″shən/ [L, *trans* + *configurare,* to form from], **1.** an arrangement in which the dominant allele of one pair of genes and the recessive allele of another pair are on the same chromosome. **2.** an arrangement in which at least one mutant gene and one wild-type gene of a pair of pseudoalleles are present on each chromosome of a homologous pair. Also called **trans arrangement, trans position.** Compare **cis configuration,** def. 1. **3.** (in chemistry) a form of geometric isomerism in which two substituent groups occur on opposite sides of a structure such as a ring or a double bond. Also called *E (entgegen) configuration.* Compare **cis configuration,** def. 3.

transcortical /trans·kor′ti·kəl/ [L, *trans,* across + *cortex,* bark], **1.** connecting two different parts of the cerebral cortex. **2.** damage to areas of the cerebral cortex resulting in aphasia. The type of aphasia is related to the specific area of the cortex that is affected.

transcortical apraxia. See **ideomotor apraxia.**

transcortin /-kôr″tin/, a diglobulin protein that binds a majority of cortisol in the plasma. Also called **corticosteroid-binding globulin.**

transcranial Doppler ultrasonography, a form of Doppler ultrasonography in which pulses of ultrasound are directed at vascular formations in the base of the skull, allowing measurements of blood flow velocity in the major basal intracranial arteries on a real-time basis.

transcriptase /transkrip″tās/, an enzyme that induces the formation of RNA from a DNA template during transcription.

transcription /transkrip″shən/ [L, *trans* + *scribere,* to write], the process by which messenger RNA is formed from a DNA template. See also **anticodon, genetic code.**

transcription factor (TF), a protein that binds to DNA to turn specific genes "on" or "off" to facilitate gene expression.

transcultural nursing /-kul″chərəl/ [L, *trans* + *colere,* to cultivate, *nutrix,* nurse], a field of nursing, founded by Madeleine Leininger, in which the nurse transcends ethnocentricity and practices nursing in other cultural environments. Because current nursing process and theory are not culturally bound and the needs of each person are considered individually, transcultural nursing is a part of all nursing practice.

transcutaneous /-k(y)o͞otā″nē·əs/ [L, *trans* + *cutis,* skin], pertaining to a procedure that is performed through the skin.

transcutaneous electrical nerve stimulation (TENS), a method of pain control by the application of electric impulses to the nerve endings. This is done through electrodes that are placed on the skin and attached to a stimulator by flexible wires. The electric impulses generated are similar to those of the body but different enough to block transmission of pain signals to the brain. TENS is noninvasive and nonaddictive, with no known side effects. It is contraindicated in patients with a demand-type cardiac pacemaker. Also called **transcutaneous nerve stimulation.** See also **galvanic electric stimulation.**

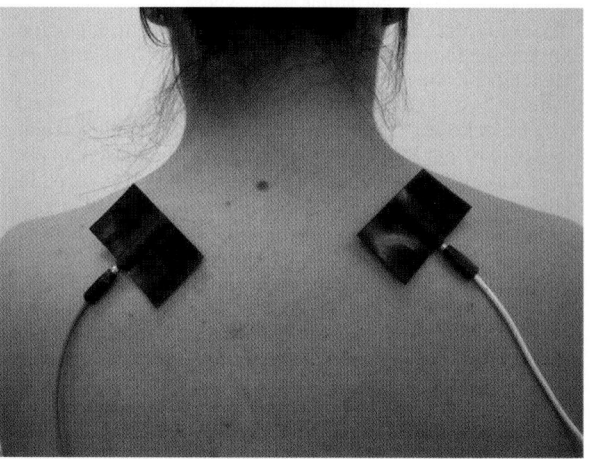

Transcutaneous electrical nerve stimulation (TENS)
(Alves Silverio et al, 2015)

transcutaneous nerve stimulation. See **transcutaneous electrical nerve stimulation (TENS).**

transcutaneous oxygen/carbon dioxide monitoring, a method of measuring the oxygen or carbon dioxide in the blood by attaching electrodes to the skin. Oxygen is commonly measured through an oximeter, which contains heating coils to raise the skin temperature and increase blood flow at the surface. Oxygen content is calculated in terms of light absorption at various wavelengths. Transcutaneous carbon dioxide electrodes are similar to blood gas electrodes, with a Teflon membrane tip that is permeable to gases.

transdermal drug delivery (TDD) /-dur″məl/ [L, *trans* + Gk, *derma,* skin], a method of applying a drug to unbroken skin. The drug is absorbed continuously through the skin and enters the systemic system. It is used particularly for the administration of nicotine, nitroglycerin, scopolamine, testosterone, and contraceptives.

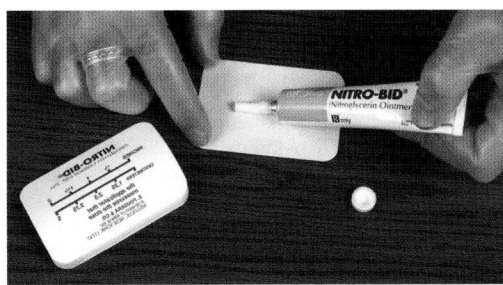

Transdermal drug delivery *(Perry, Potter, and Elkin, 2012)*

transdermal scopolamine, a method of administration of the motion sickness drug scopolamine by application of a skin patch containing the medication.

transducer /-d(y)ōō″sər/ [L, *trans* + *ducere,* to lead], a hand-held device that sends and receives ultrasound signals. It changes electric impulses into soundwaves, receives reflected soundwaves, and converts them back into electric energy.

transductant /-duk″tənt/, a cell that has acquired a new character by the transfer of genetic material.

transduction /-duk″shən/, a method of genetic recombination by which DNA is transferred from one cell to another by a viral vector. Various bacteriophages transfer DNA from one species of bacteria to another.

transect /transekt″/ [L, *trans* + *secare,* to cut], to sever or cut across, as in preparing a cross section of tissue. Also spelled **transsect.** See also **transsection.**

transection. See **transsection.**

transesophageal echocardiography (TEE), an endoscopic/ultrasound test that provides ultrasonic imaging of the heart from a retrocardiac vantage point, thus preventing the interposed subcutaneous tissue, bony thorax, and lungs from interfering with the ultrasound. It is performed to better visualize the mitral valve or atrial septum, to differentiate intracardiac from extracardiac masses and tumors, to diagnose thoracic aortic dissection, to detect valvular vegetation as seen with endocarditis, to determine cardiac sources of arterial embolism, to detect coronary artery disease, and to monitor high-risk patients for ischemia intraoperatively.

***trans*-fatty acids,** stereoisomers of the naturally occurring *cis*-fatty acids, found in margarines and shortenings as artifacts after hydrogenation and in commercially baked cakes, cookies, pies, and crackers. A connection has been found between consumption of large amounts of *trans*-fatty acids and increased low-density lipoprotein levels and, thus, increased risk for coronary heart disease. Also called *trans fats.*

transfection /-fek″shən/ [L, *trans* + *inficere,* to taint], the process by which a bacterial cell is infected with purified DNA or RNA isolated from a virus after a specific pretreatment. Acute transfection is short-term infection. – *transfect, v.*

transfemoral amputation. Also called **above-knee amputation, AK amputation.**

transfer, to move a person or object from one site to another.

transfer agreement /trans″fur/ [L, *transferre,* to carry over, *ad,* toward, *gratus,* pleasure], a written hospital agreement between two health care institutions for the transfer of patients from one to another and the orderly exchange of pertinent clinical information on the patients transferred.

transferase /trans″fərās/ [L, *transferre* + Fr, *diastase,* enzyme], any of a group of enzymes that catalyzes the transfer of a chemical group or radical, such as the phosphate, methyl, amine, or keto groups, from one molecule to another.

transfer belt, a specialized, padded canvas belt 2 to 3 inches in width that is buckled in front over clothing. Compare **walking belt.**

■ METHOD: An assistant grasps the belt from underneath with one hand on either side several inches away from the buckle. The patient leans forward and, on a predetermined count, pushes off a flat surface with feet and hands.

■ OUTCOME CRITERIA: The belt is used as a support and not a device to pull the patient up to a standing position.

transfer DNA (tDNA), DNA transferred from its original source and present in transformed cells.

transference /-fur″əns/ [L, *transferre*], **1.** the shifting of symptoms from one part of the body to another, as occurs in conversion disorder. **2.** (in psychiatry) an unconscious defense mechanism whereby feelings and attitudes originally associated with important people and events in one's early life are attributed to others in current interpersonal situations, including psychotherapy. The phenomenon is used as a tool in understanding the emotional problems of the patient and their origins. See also **countertransference, parataxic distortion.**

transference love, (in psychoanalytic therapy) a projection of libidinal drives expressed by the patient for the psychoanalyst, who has "unconsciously" come to represent a person from the patient's past.

transfer factor (TF), a leukocyte extract that transfers delayed hypersensitivity from one person to another. Transfer factor has been studied for its possible use in the treatment of chronic mucocutaneous candidiasis and Wiskott-Aldrich syndrome and as a means of transferring antitumor immunity to patients with various types of cancer.

transfer factor of lungs. See **diffusing capacity of lungs.**

transferrin /transfer″in/, a plasma protein that is essential in the transport of iron from the intestine into the bloodstream, making it available to the normoblasts in the bone marrow. It also may take part in a slower exchange with ferritin, hemosiderin, and other iron forms in the tissues. See also **hemosiderin, iron transport.**

transferring /-fur″ing/ [L, *trans,* across, *ferre,* to bring], relocating a person in need from one location to another.

transferrin saturation, percentage of iron binding by the major plasma iron transport protein, measured in the blood to detect iron excess or deficiency. The normal transferrin saturation capacity in serum is 20% to 55%. See also **total iron.**

transfer RNA (tRNA), a kind of RNA that carries an anticodon (three nucleotide bases) and a specific amino acid. The identity of the amino acid is determined by the sequence of nucleotides in the anticodon. There are 64 possible anticodons and about two dozen amino acids that are found in proteins. This means that several anticodons may specify to the same amino acid. Each anticodon is complementary to a specific codon in the messenger RNA. The tRNAs (with their amino acids attached) translate the sequence of codons in messenger RNA into a sequence of amino acids in a polypeptide. Also called *adaptor RNA.*

transfixation /-fiksā″shən/, a surgical procedure in which, in an amputation, the soft tissues are cut through from one side to the other, close to the bone. The muscles are then divided from within outward.

transformation /-fôrmā″shən/ [L, *transformare,* to change shape], the integration of exogenous genes into chromosomes in a form that is recognized by the replicative and transcriptional apparatus of the host cell. Transformation occurs rarely in most cell populations.

transformer /-fôr″mər/ [L, *transformare,* to change shape], an electric apparatus that changes alternating current of one voltage into a different voltage of the same frequency.

transforming growth factor (TGF), a group of proteins produced by the cells of a tumor that, when inoculated into a normal cell culture, causes a disorderly increase in the number of cells in the culture.

transforming growth factor-beta, cytokine produced by macrophages and other cells. It controls proliferation, cellular differentiation, and other functions in most cells. It often has an antiinflammatory function during an immune response. It can be up-regulated in some human cancers.

transfusion /-f(y)oo″zhən/ [L, *trans* + *fundere,* to pour], the introduction into the bloodstream of whole blood or blood components, such as plasma, platelets, or packed red blood cells. Whole blood may be infused into the recipient directly from a donor matched for the ABO blood group and antigenic subgroups, but more frequently the donor's blood is collected and stored by a blood bank. See also **blood transfusion.**

transfusion reaction, any adverse event following a blood transfusion, attributed to the transfusion. The most common reactions are allergic, manifested by hives and urticaria, and febrile nonhemolytic, shown by chills and fever. More serious reactions are hemolytic, due to an antibody in the recipient to an antigen on the donor's red cells, anaphylactic, bacterial contamination of the donor unit, transfusion-related acute lung injury (TRALI), and transfusion-associated circulatory overload (TACO). Delayed reactions may include delayed hemolytic, disease transmission, alloimmunization to red cell or HLA antigens, and transfusion-associated graft-versus-host disease. Posttransfusion purpura may occur 5 to 12 days after a transfusion. See also **hemolysis.**

■ OBSERVATIONS: Fever is the most common transfusion reaction; urticaria is a relatively common allergic response. Asthma, vascular collapse, and renal failure occur less commonly. A hemolytic reaction from red blood cell incompatibility is serious and must be diagnosed and treated promptly. Symptoms develop shortly after beginning the transfusion, before 50 mL has been given, and include a throbbing headache, sudden deep severe lumbar pain, precordial pain, dyspnea, and restlessness. Objective signs include ruddy facial flushing followed by cyanosis and distended neck veins; rapid, thready pulse; diaphoresis; and cold, clammy skin. Profound shock may occur within 1 hour.

■ INTERVENTIONS: When a hemolytic reaction is suspected, the transfusion is promptly terminated and the infusion line kept open with a normal solution of IV fluid. The remaining bank blood is saved for a repeat type and crossmatch against a fresh sample of blood from the recipient. Direct and indirect antiglobulin tests are usually ordered to detect hemolytic antibodies, and a sample of urine is examined for free hemoglobin. Immediate treatment may include IV mannitol and a solution of 5% dextrose in water to maintain urine flow of more than 100 mL per hour. In the presence of oliguria, the possibility of acute renal failure is evaluated and the patient managed accordingly. Hypovolemia is corrected with saline or plasma expanders, but the administration of more whole blood is avoided, if possible.

■ PATIENT CARE CONSIDERATIONS: The need for exceptional care to ensure that typed and crossmatched blood conforms to compatibility standards is emphasized. The identifying information on the blood container is always checked against the transfusion records and the patient's identification on the band. Questioning the patient about previous transfusions may elicit warning indications of possible adverse reactions. After the transfusion is started, the patient is watched for objective signs of a transfusion reaction and is questioned for subjective symptoms. Routine temperature checks are done to detect febrile reactions that can be controlled by antipyretic drugs.

transfusion-related acute lung injury (TRALI), a syndrome seen in persons receiving transfusions, characterized by pulmonary edema, dyspnea, hypoxemia, hypotension, and fever; it is thought to be a reaction to antibodies or other components of the donor blood product. The blood transfusion must be immediately stopped. Patients need oxygen support, and in some cases the syndrome can be fatal.

transgender, individuals who do not fit within rigid gender norms and incorporate one or more aspects, traits, social roles, or characteristics of the opposite gender.

transgene /trans″jēn/, a gene that has been transferred from one genome into another. For example, a mouse with a rat hormone gene grows much larger than normal. −*transgenic, adj.*

transient /tran″shənt, tran″zē·ənt/ [L, *transire,* to go through], pertaining to a condition that is temporary, such as transient ischemic attack.

transient global amnesia (TGA) [L, *transire,* to go through, *globus,* ball; Gk, *amnesia,* forgetfulness], a temporary short-term memory loss followed by full recovery. The disorder tends to affect middle-aged adults and may be attributed to cerebral ischemia. It is usually not accompanied by other mental deficiencies.

transhumeral amputation, an amputation of the arm above the elbow. A short amputation results in the loss of shoulder rotation. After a long amputation (just above the elbow), the patient should retain good shoulder function.

transient ischemic attack (TIA), an episode of cerebrovascular insufficiency, usually associated with partial occlusion of a cerebral artery by an atherosclerotic plaque or an embolus. The symptoms vary with the site and degree of occlusion. Disturbance of normal vision in one or both eyes, dizziness, weakness, dysphasia, numbness, or unconsciousness may occur. The attack usually lasts a few minutes. In rare cases symptoms continue for several hours.

transient lower esophageal sphincter relaxation, relaxation of the lower esophageal sphincter in response to gastric distension, lasting for 10 to 30 seconds and resulting in gastroesophageal reflux.

transient monocular blindness, an episode of total or partial loss of vision in one eye, caused by ischemia of the eye and lasting several minutes or longer. The term is sometimes used synonymously with amaurosis fugax and sometimes to designate an episode of longer duration. Also called *transient monocular visual loss.*

transient myeloproliferative disorder, usually transient leukocytosis associated with Down syndrome and generally diagnosed in the first few weeks of life. It is often accompanied by hepatosplenomegaly, pericardial and pleural effusions, hepatic disease, and a pustular rash. Although spontaneous remission occurs in most cases, some affected infants develop a myelodysplastic syndrome or acute leukemia. Also called **congenital leukemoid reaction,** *transient leukemia of infancy.*

transient myopia [L, *transire,* to go through; Gk, *myops,* nearsighted], a temporary change in visual accommodation secondary to trauma, high blood sugar level, sulfanilamide therapy, and other conditions. See also **pseudomyopia.**

transillumination /-iloo′minā″shən/ [L, *trans,* through, *illuminare,* to light up], **1.** the passage of light through a solid or liquid substance. **2.** the passage of light through body tissues for the purpose of examining a structure interposed between the observer and the light source. A diaphanoscope is an instrument introduced into a body cavity to transilluminate tissues.

transient synovitis, an inflammation in the layer of connective tissue in movable joints that is a common cause of joint pain in children. See also **synovitis.**

transition /tranzish″ən/ [L, *transire,* to go through], the last phase of the first stage of labor, sometimes indicated by cervical dilation of 8 to 10 cm.

transitional /tranzish″ənəl/ [L, *transire,* to go through], between a previous and a succeeding state, or in a state of becoming something else.

transitional cell carcinoma, a malignant, usually papillary tumor derived from transitional stratified epithelium, occurring most frequently in the bladder, ureter, urethra, or renal pelvis. The majority of tumors in the collecting system of the kidney are of this kind. They have a better prognosis than squamous cell carcinomas in the same site.

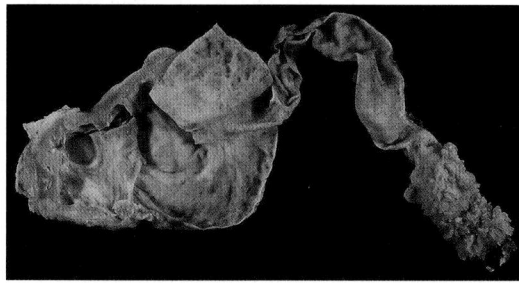

Transitional cell carcinoma of the ureter *(Fletcher, 2007)*

transitional dentition. See **mixed dentition.**

transitional epithelium, a form of stratified epithelium found characteristically in the mucous membrane of ureter and bladder; in the contracted condition it consists of many cell layers, whereas in the stretched condition fewer layers can be distinguished.

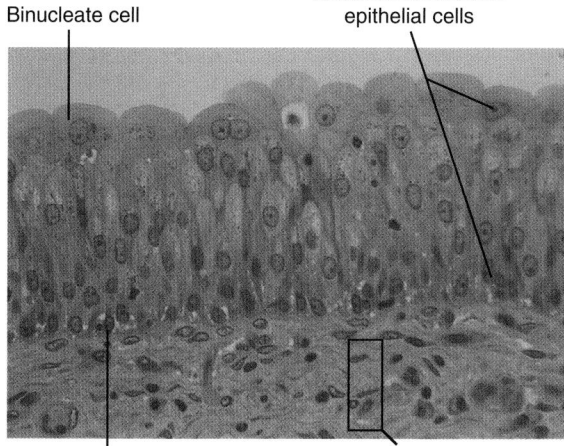

Binucleate cell

Stratified transitional epithelial cells

Basement membrane

Connective tissue

Transitional epithelium *(© Ed Reschke; Used with permission)*

transitional object, an object used by a child to provide comfort and security while he or she is away from a secure base, such as mother or home.

transitory mania /tran″sitôr′ē/ [L, *transire,* to go through; Gk, *mania,* madness], a mood disorder characterized by the sudden onset of manic reactions that are of short duration, usually lasting from 1 hour to a few days. See also **mania.**

transjugular intrahepatic portosystemic shunt (TIPS) /tranz·jug′yoo·lər/, percutaneous creation of a shunt between the hepatic and portal veins within the liver followed by placement of an expandable stent in the tract created, performed by a transjugular route under radiological guidance. It is done for the treatment of bleeding esophageal varices.

translation /-lā″shən/ [L, *translatio,* handing over], the process in which the genetic information carried by nucleotides in messenger RNA directs the amino acid sequence in the synthesis of a specific polypeptide. See also **anticodon, genetic code.**

translocation /-lōkā″shən/ [L, *trans* + *locus,* place], the rearrangement of DNA within a chromosome or the transfer of a segment of one chromosome to a nonhomologous one. In simple translocations, an end segment of one chromosome is transferred onto the end of another, involving a single break in only one of the chromosomes. Translocations in which material from the middle of one chromosome is shifted to the middle of another one are more complex and involve at least three breaks in the participating chromosomes. Such shifting of genetic material can result in serious disorders, such as Down syndrome, which can be caused by a 14/21 translocation, and chronic granulocytic leukemia, in which part of the long arm of chromosome 22 is translocated to the short arm of chromosome 9. Kinds include **balanced translocation, reciprocal translocation, robertsonian translocation.**

translucent /-loo″sənt/ [L, *trans,* across, *lucens,* shining], pertaining to a medium through which light can pass in a diffused manner so that a field is illuminated but objects cannot be seen distinctly. Compare **transparent.**

transmethylation /-meth′ilā″shən/, the transfer of a methyl group from one compound to another.

transmigration /-mīgrā″shən/ [L, *trans* + *migrare,* to migrate], a movement from one side to another, from inside to outside, or from outside to inside.

transmissible /-mis″ibəl/ [L, *transmittere,* to transmit], capable of being passed from one person or place to another, as in the transmission of a disease.

transmissible neurodegenerative disease. See **prion disease.**

transmissible spongiform encephalopathy, a group of fatal neurodegenerative diseases that are unique in having either infectious or genetic causes. A homozygous prion protein genotype predisposes individuals to susceptibility to the diseases. Kinds include **Creutzfeldt-Jakob disease, Gerstmann-Sträussler syndrome.**

transmission /-mish″ən/ [L, *transmittere,* to transmit], the transfer or conveyance of a thing or condition, such as a neural impulse, infectious or genetic disease, or a hereditary trait, from one person or place to another. **—transmissible,** *adj.*

Transmission-Based Precautions, safeguards designed for patients documented or suspected to be infected with highly transmissible or epidemiologically important pathogens for which additional precautions beyond Standard Precautions are needed to interrupt transmission in hospitals. There are three types of transmission-based precautions: Airborne Precautions, Droplet Precautions, and Contact Precautions. They may be combined for diseases that have multiple routes

T

of transmission. They are to be used either singularly or in combination, in addition to Standard Precautions. See also **Airborne Precautions, Contact Precautions, Droplet Precautions, Standard Precautions.**

transmission scanning electron microscope, an instrument that transmits a highly magnified, well-resolved, three-dimensional image on a television screen, thus combining the advantages of the electron and the scanning electron microscopes. Compare **electron microscope, scanning electron microscope.**

transmission scanning electron microscopy (TSEM), a technique using a transmission scanning electron microscope in which the atomic number of the part of the sample being scanned is determined and used to modulate a beam of electrons in a cathode-ray tube and in the beam scanning the sample. The image produced is clear, three-dimensional, and highly magnified. Compare **electron microscopy, scanning electron microscopy.**

transmitted light [L, *transmittere,* to transmit; AS, *leoht*], light that has passed through a transparent medium.

transmitter substance. See **neurotransmitter.**

transmucosal /trans″mu-ko′sal/, entering through, or across, a mucous membrane, as in the administration of a drug via the cavity between the cheek and gum.

transmural /-m(y)$\overline{oo}$″rəl/ [L, *trans* + *murus,* wall], **1.** pertaining to the entire thickness of the wall of an organ, such as a transmural myocardial infarction. **2.** occurring in or completely going through any wall of a hollow structure in the body.

transmural infarction, death of myocardial tissue that extends from the endocardium to the epicardium as a result of a myocardial infarction.

transmutation /-m(y)$\overline{oo}$tā″shən/ [L, *transmutare,* to change], **1.** a mutation that causes a significant species change during evolution. **2.** the conversion of one chemical element into another by radioactive bombardment.

transovarial transmission /-ōver″ē-əl/ [L, *trans* + *ovum,* egg], the transfer of pathogens to succeeding generations through invasion of the ovary and infection of the eggs, such as occurs in arthropods, primarily ticks and mites.

transparent /-per″ənt/ [L, *trans,* across, *parere,* to appear], pertaining to a clear medium that allows for the transmission of light so that objects on the other side are distinguishable. Compare **translucent.**

transparent septum. *(Informal)* See **septum pellucidum.**

transpeptidase /-pep″tidās/, an enzyme that catalyzes the transfer of an amino group from one peptide chain to another.

transpeptidation /-pep′tidā″shən/, the transfer of an amino acid from one peptide chain to another.

transplacental /trans′pləsen″təl/ [L, *trans* + *placenta,* flat cake], across or through the placenta, specifically in reference to the exchange of nutrients, waste products, and other material between the developing fetus and the mother.

transplant /trans″plant, transplant″/ [L, *transplantare*], **1.** *v.,* to transfer an organ or tissue from one person to another or from one body part to another to replace a diseased structure, restore function, or change appearance. Skin and kidneys are the most frequently transplanted structures. Others include cartilage, bone, bone marrow, corneal tissue, parts of blood vessels and tendons, hearts, lungs, and livers. Preferred donors are identical twins or people having the same blood type and immunological characteristics. Success of the transplant depends on overcoming the rejection of the donor tissue by the recipient's immune system. With the patient under local or general anesthesia, the recipient site is prepared, and the donor structure is grafted in place. Its oxygenation and blood supply are preserved during the procedure until the circulation can be restored at the new site. After surgery circulation in the area is observed for signs of impairment. Antirejection drugs are given to suppress the production of antibodies to the foreign tissue proteins. Signs of rejection reaction include fever, pain, and loss of function, usually occurring in the first 4 to 10 days after transplantation. An abscess may form if the reaction is not subdued promptly. The grafted structure may require several weeks to become established. Late rejection may occur several months or even 1 year later. **2.** *n.,* any tissue or organ that is transplanted. **3.** *adj.,* pertaining to a tissue or organ that is transplanted, a recipient of a donated tissue or organ, or a phenomenon associated with the procedure. Also called **graft, transplantation.**

transplantation /-plantā″shən/ [L, *transplantare,* to transplant], the transfer of tissue from one site to another or from one person or organism to another.

transplantation endometriosis [L, *transplantare,* to transplant; Gk, *endon,* within, *metra,* womb, *osis,* condition], endometrial tissue that is accidentally transplanted to the incision wound during pelvic surgery.

transplant list, a list maintained by the United Network for Organ Sharing (UNOS) for the registration of transplant candidates on the national waiting list in the United States. See also **United Network for Organ Sharing.**

transport /trans″pôrt/ [L, *trans,* across, *portare,* carry], the movement or transference of biochemical substances from one site to another. Active transport involves an expenditure of energy, whereas passive transport allows movement down a gradient without an energy expenditure.

transport maximum, the highest rate in milligrams per minute at which the renal tubules can transfer a substance either from the tubular luminal fluid to the interstitial fluid or from the interstitial fluid to the tubular luminal fluid, beyond which it may be excreted in the urine. In kidney function tests, it is expressed as T_m with inferior letters representing the substance used in the test, such as T_{mPAH} (transport maximum for *p*-aminohippuric acid). Also called **tubular maximum.**

transposable element. See **transposon.**

transposase /trans″pəzās/, an enzyme involved in the movement of a DNA fragment from one site in the genome to another.

trans position /-pəsish″ən/ [L, *transponere*], **1.** an abnormality occurring during embryonic development in which a body part normally on the left is found on the right or vice versa. **2.** the shifting of genetic material from one chromosome to another at some point in the reproductive process, often resulting in a congenital anomaly. –*transpose, v.*

transposition of the great vessels, a congenital cardiac anomaly in which the pulmonary artery arises from the left ventricle and the aorta from the right ventricle and there is no communication between the systemic and pulmonary circulations. Life is impossible with this anomaly unless there are associated cardiac defects, such as a septal defect or a patent ductus arteriosus, that enable the mixing of oxygenated and unoxygenated blood. The severity of the condition depends on the type and size of the associated defect. The primary symptoms are cyanosis and hypoxia, especially in infants with small septal defects, although cardiomegaly is usually evident a few weeks after birth. Signs of congestive heart failure develop rapidly, especially in infants with large ventricular septal defects. Definitive diagnosis is based on cardiac catheterization. Surgical correction of the defect is postponed, if possible, until after 6 months of age, when the infant can better tolerate the procedure. Immediate palliative surgical procedures such as the Rashkind procedure may be performed to decrease pulmonary vascular resistance and prevent congestive heart failure. See also **blue baby.**

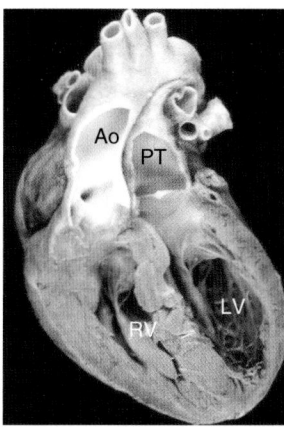

Transposition of the great vessels *(Damjanov and Linder, 2000)*

transposon /transpō″sən/ [L, *transponere* + on], a segment of DNA that can move from one place to another in a cell's genome or between a bacterial cell and a plasmid or virus. Viruses may even carry a transposon from one bacterium to another. Also called **jumping gene, transposable element.**

transpulmonary pressure /-pul″məner′ē/, the difference between intraalveolar and intrapleural pressure, or the pressure acting across the lung from the pleural space to the alveoli.

transsect. See **transect.**

transsection /transek″shən/ [L, *trans*, across, *sectio*], a cross section of a biological specimen or a cut across the long axis. Also spelled **transection.**

transseptal fiber /transep″təl/ [L, *trans* + *saeptum*, wall], any of the many filamentous tissues of the gingival system and periodontal fibers that extend mesially from the supraalveolar cementum of one tooth, through the interdental-attached gingiva above the septum of the alveolar bone, to the distal cementum of an adjacent tooth.

transsexual /transek″choo·əl/, a person whose gender identity is the opposite of his or her biological sex.

transsexualism /-iz′əm/, a condition in which a person has an intense desire to change one's biological sex and live as a member of the opposite sex. It is considered a psychiatric disorder if the condition continues for more than 2 years. Some transsexual individuals cross-dress and seek medical or surgical help to change their physical sex characteristics.

transtentorial herniation /trans′tentôr″ē·əl/ [L, *trans* + *tentorium*, tent, *hernia*, rupture], a bulge of brain tissue out of the cranium through the tentorial notch, caused by increased intracranial pressure. See also **tentorial herniation.**

transthermia. See **thermopenetration.**

transthoracic /trans′thôras″ik/, across or passing through the thorax.

transthoracic impedance, resistance to transmission of electric current represented by the skin, fat, muscle, and lung tissues in a patient's chest.

transthoracic pacemaker /-thôras″ik/ [L, *trans*, across; Gk, *thorax*, chest; L, *passus*, step; ME, *maken*], a permanent pacemaker with the pulse generator located in the abdominal wall and the pacing wires attached directly to the epicardium.

transtibial amputation, an amputation of the lower leg between the ankle and knee. Also called **below-knee (BK) amputation, BK amputation.**

transtracheal oxygen /-trā″kē·əl/ [L, *trans*, across; Gk, *tracheia*, rough artery, *oxys*, sharp, *genein*, to produce], the administration of oxygen via a low-flow catheter inserted directly into the trachea. It is sometimes preferred to the administration of oxygen through a nasal cannula because there is limited loss of oxygen to the environment. Disadvantages include increased risk of infection.

transtrochanteric osteotomy /-trō′kənter″ik/ [L, *trans*, across; Gk, *trochanter*, runner, *osteon* + *temnein*, to cut], a surgical division of the upper end of the femur through the area of the trochanters.

transubstantiation /trans′əbstan′chē·ā″shən/, the replacement or substitution of one kind of tissue for another.

transudate /trans″yədāt/ [L, *trans* + *sudare*, to sweat], a fluid passed through a membrane or squeezed through a tissue or into the space between the cells of a tissue. It is thin and watery and contains few blood cells or other large proteins. See also **edema.**

transudation /-yədā″shən/, **1.** the passage of a substance through a membrane as a result of a difference in hydrostatic pressure. **2.** the passage of a fluid through a membrane with nearly all the solutes of the fluid remaining in solution or suspension.

transudative ascites /transyoo″dətiv/, an abnormal accumulation in the peritoneal cavity of a fluid that characteristically contains scant amounts of protein and cells. Ascitic fluids with protein levels of less than 2.5 g/mL are considered to be transudates. Transudative ascites is indicative of cirrhosis or congestive heart failure rather than infection, inflammation, or a tumor.

transuranic element, any of the elements with atomic numbers above that of uranium (whose atomic number is 92). All are radioactive and have very short half-lives. None, except for neptunium and plutonium in very small amounts, occurs naturally. They are produced artificially in nuclear reactors and particle accelerators. Also called *transuranium element.*

transurethral laser-induced prostatectomy (TULIP), a type of noncontact laser prostatectomy.

transurethral resection (TUR) /trans′yoore″thrəl/ [L, *trans* + Gk, *ourethra*, urethra; L, *re*, again, *secare*, to cut], the surgical removal of a structure performed through the urethra.

transurethral resection of the prostate (TURP), resection of the prostate by means of a cystoscope passed through the urethra.

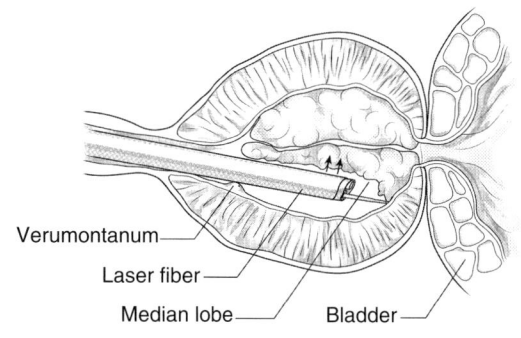

Transurethral resection of the prostate *(Shih et al, 2013)*

transvaginal /trans·vaj′i·nəl/ [L, *trans,* across + *vagina,* sheath], performed through the vagina.

transverse /-vurs″/ [L, *transversus,* oblique], at right angles to the long axis of any common part, such as the planes that cut the long axis of the body into upper and lower parts and are at right angles to the sagittal and frontal planes.

transverse acetabular ligament. See **acetabular labrum.**

transverse cervical nerve, a branch of the cervical plexus arising from the anterior rami of the second and third cervical nerves that provides cutaneous innervation to the neck.

transverse colon, the segment of the colon that extends from the end of the ascending colon at the hepatic flexure on the right side across the midabdomen to the beginning of the descending colon at the splenic flexure on the left side.

transverse colon volvulus, a rare type of colonic volvulus involving the transverse colon.

transverse fissure, a fissure dividing the dorsal surface of the diencephalon and the ventral surface of the cerebral hemisphere. Also called **fissure of Bichat.**

transverse foramen [L, *transversus* + *foramen,* hole], an opening through the transverse process of a cervical vertebra.

transverse fracture, a fracture that occurs at right angles to the longitudinal axis of the bone involved.

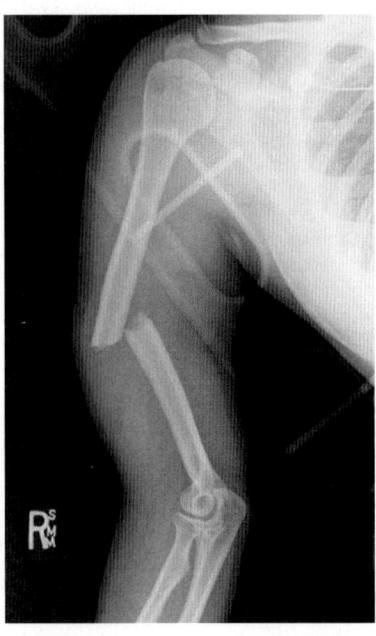

Transverse fracture of the humerus *(Courtesy Ohio State University Medical Center)*

transverse lie, abnormal presentation of a fetus in which the long axis of the baby's body is across the long axis of the mother's body. Unless the baby turns spontaneously or is turned by means of external or internal version, vaginal delivery is impossible.

transverse ligament of the atlas, a thick, strong ligament stretched across the ring of the atlas, holding the dens against the anterior arch. The transverse ligament divides the circular opening of the atlas into posterior and anterior parts. The posterior part transmits the spinal cord and its membranes; the anterior part contains the dens.

transverse magnetization, the magnetization vector oriented in a plane perpendicular to the main external magnetic field in magnetic resonance.

transverse mesocolon /mez″ōkō′lən/, a broad fold of the peritoneum connecting the transverse colon to the dorsal wall of the abdomen. It is continuous with the greater omentum along the ventral surface of the transverse colon and contains between its layers the vessels that supply the transverse colon. Its two layers diverge along the anterior border of the pancreas. Compare **mesentery proper, sigmoid mesocolon.**

transverse myelitis [L, *transversus* + Gk, *myelos,* marrow, *itis,* inflammation], an acute attack of spinal cord inflammation involving both sides of the cord.

transverse palatine suture, the line of junction between the processes of the maxilla and the horizontal parts of the palatine bones that form the hard palate.

transverse pericardial sinus, a passage between the superior and posterior reflections of the serous pericardium. It lies posteriorly to the ascending aorta and the pulmonary trunk, anteriorly to the superior vena cava, and superiorly to the left atrium.

transverse plane, any one of the planes cutting across the body perpendicular to the sagittal and the frontal planes (at right angles to the long axis of the body), dividing the body into superior and inferior parts. Also called **cardinal horizontal plane.** Compare **frontal plane, median plane, sagittal plane.**

transverse presentation [L, *transversus* + *praesentare,* to show], a presentation of the fetal body in an oblique or transverse position across the birth canal.

transverse process, a process of the vertebra that extends posterolaterally from the junction of the pedicle and lamina on each side and is the site for articulation with the ribs in the thoracic region.

transverse rectal folds, semilunar transverse folds in the rectum that support the weight of feces. Also called **Houston's valves.** See also **rectum.**

transverse relaxation time. See **relaxation time.**

transverse septum, a thick plate of mesodermal tissue that occupies the space between the thoracic cavity and yolk stalk in the early embryo, forming a transverse partition partially separating the coelomic cavity into thoracic and abdominal portions. It gives rise to the central tendon of the diaphragm.

transverse sinus, one of a pair of large venous channels in the posterior superior group of sinuses serving the dura mater and draining into the sigmoid sinuses and then into the internal jugular vein. Compare **confluence of the sinuses, inferior sagittal sinus, occipital sinus, straight sinus, superior sagittal sinus.**

transverse tarsal joint, the joint formed by the talocalcaneonavicular and calcaneocuboid joints together.

transversospinales muscles, a group of muscles deep to the erector spinae that consist of the semispinalis, multifidus, and rotatores muscles. When these muscles contract bilaterally, they extend the vertebral column, an action similar to that of the erector spinae group. However, when muscles on only one side contract, they pull the spinous processes toward the transverse processes on that side, causing the trunk to turn or rotate in the opposite direction.

transversus abdominis /-vur″səs/, one of a pair of transverse abdominal muscles that are the anterolateral muscles of the abdomen, lying immediately under the internal abdominal oblique. Arising from the inguinal ligament, the iliac crest, the thoracolumbar fascia, and the last six ribs, it inserts into the linea alba. It serves to constrict the abdomen and, by compressing the contents, to assist in urination, defecation, emesis, parturition, and forced expiration. Also called *transversalis.* Compare **pyramidalis, rectus abdominis.**

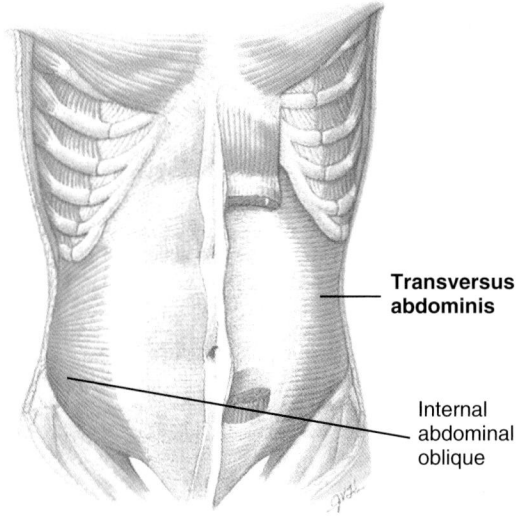

Transversus abdominis *(Thibodeau and Patton, 2003)*

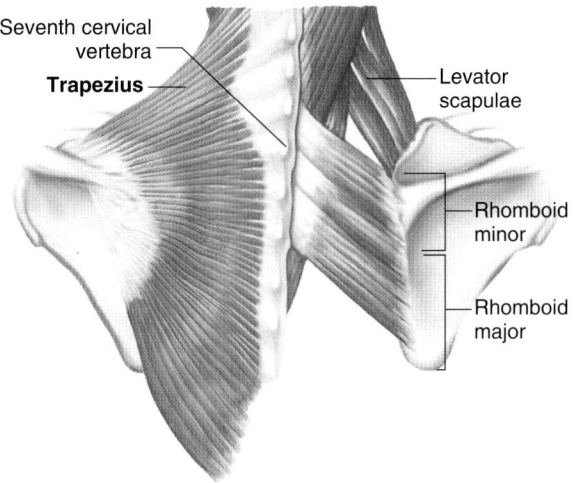

Trapezius *(Patton and Thibodeau, 2010)*

transversus thoracis muscles, muscles found on the deep surface of the anterior thoracic wall that lie deep to the internal thoracic vessels and secure these vessels to the wall.

transvesical prostatectomy, prostatectomy through an incision of the urinary bladder.

transvestism /-ves″tizəm/, a tendency to achieve psychic and sexual relief by dressing in the clothing of the opposite sex.

Tranxene, a benzodiazepine sedative-hypnotic. Brand name for **clorazepate dipotassium.**

tranylcypromine sulfate /tran′əlsip″rəmēn/, a monoamine oxidase inhibitor that acts as an antidepressant.

■ INDICATIONS: It is prescribed in the treatment of severe reactive or endogenous mental depression without melancholia and has an unlabeled use for the treatment of posttraumatic stress disorder.

■ CONTRAINDICATIONS: Cerebrovascular or cardiovascular diseases, paranoid schizophrenia, liver dysfunction, alcoholism, pheochromocytoma, or known hypersensitivity to this drug prohibits its use. It is not given to children under 16 years of age.

■ ADVERSE EFFECTS: Among the most serious adverse effects are severe hypertensive episodes that can be precipitated by ingestion of foods rich in tyramine or by concurrent administration of many sympathomimetic drugs. Common side effects include headache, vertigo, dry mouth, blurred vision, and orthostatic hypotension.

trapeze bar /trapēz″/, a triangular metal apparatus above a bed, used to help the patient move and support weight during transfer or position change.

trapezium /trəpē″zē·əm/ *pl.* *trapezia, trapeziums* [Gk, *trapezion,* small table], a carpal bone in the distal row of carpal bones. The trapezium articulates with the scaphoid proximally, the first metacarpal distally, and the trapezoideum and the second metacarpal medially. Also called **greater multangular, os trapezium.**

trapezius /trəpē″zē·əs/ [Gk, *trapezion,* small table], a large, flat, triangular superficial muscle of the shoulder and upper back. It arises from the occipital bone, the ligamentum nuchae, and the spinous processes of the seventh cervical and all the thoracic vertebrae. It acts to rotate the scapula upward; adduct, raise, or lower the shoulder; and retract the shoulder.

trapezoid /trap″əzoid/ [Gk, *trapezion,* small table, *eidos,* form], having the shape of an irregular four-sided figure with one set of parallel sides.

trapezoidal arch /trap″əzoidəl/ [Gk, *trapezion + eidos,* form; L, *arcus,* bow], a dental arch that has slightly less convergence than that of a tapering arch. The anterior teeth in the arch are somewhat square or abruptly rounded from tip to tip of the canines, which are at the corners of the arch.

trapezoid bone [Gk, *trapezion + eidos + AS, ban*], the carpal bone, located in the distal row of carpal bones between the trapezium and the capitate. It resembles a wedge, with the broad end at the dorsal surface and the narrow end at the palmar surface. Also called **lesser multangular bone, os trapezoideum.**

TRAPS, abbreviation for **tumor necrosis factor receptor–associated periodic syndrome.** Also called **familial periodic fever.**

trastuzumab, a miscellaneous antineoplastic.

■ INDICATIONS: It is used in the treatment of metastatic breast cancer with the overexpression of HER2.

■ CONTRAINDICATIONS: Factors that prohibit its use include known hypersensitivity to this drug or to Chinese hamster ovary cell protein.

■ ADVERSE EFFECTS: Life-threatening effects are tachycardia, congestive heart failure, and leukopenia. Other adverse reactions include depression, insomnia, neuropathy, peripheral neuritis, acne, herpes simplex, nausea, vomiting, anorexia, diarrhea, anemia, arthralgia, bone pain, edema, peripheral edema, cough, dyspnea, pharyngitis, rhinitis, and sinusitis. Common side effects include dizziness, numbness, paresthesias, rash, and flulike syndrome (fever, headache, chills).

trauma /trou″mə, trô″mə/ [Gk, wound], **1.** physical injury caused by violent or disruptive action or by the introduction into the body of a toxic substance. **2.** psychic injury resulting from a severe emotional shock. **–traumatic,** *adj.,* **–traumatize,** *v.*

-trauma, combining form meaning "a wound or injury, psychic or physical": *barotrauma, microtrauma.*

trauma center, a service providing emergency and specialized intensive care to critically ill and injured patients.

trauma-informed interventions, actions by health and social service providers based on psychosocial empowerment principles that recognize the impact of trauma to

T

faciliate both physical and psychosocial healing in a safe, collaborative fashion. See **adverse childhood experiences.**

trauma registry, a repository of data on the incidence, diagnosis, and treatment of acute trauma victims treated by emergency service personnel.

traumatic /trômat″ik/ [Gk, *trauma,* wound], pertaining to an injury, usually a serious and unexpected injury.

traumatic abscess, a pus collection that develops in tissue that has been damaged by a wound or injury.

traumatic anesthesia [Gk, *trauma + anaisthesia,* lack of feeling], a total lack of normal sensation in a part of the body, resulting from injury, destruction of nerves, or interruption of nerve pathways.

traumatic bone cyst. See **simple bone cyst.**

traumatic delirium, delirium after severe head injury, characterized by alertness and consciousness, with disorientation, confabulation, and amnesia apparent. See also **delirium.**

traumatic dislocation [Gk, *trauma,* wound; L, *dis + locare*], a dislocation caused by an injury.

traumatic epilepsy [Gk, *trauma,* wound, *epilepsia,* seizure], a form of motor or sensory seizures caused by a brain injury. Also called **posttraumatic epilepsy.**

traumatic fever, an elevation in body temperature secondary to mechanical trauma, particularly a crushing injury. Such fevers may last 1 or 2 days. The increased body temperature may help provide resistance to subsequent infection, and increased wound temperature may accelerate local healing.

traumatic gangrene [Gk, *trauma,* wound, *gaggraina*], gangrene that follows a severe injury resulting in damage to blood vessels.

traumatic herpes [Gk, *trauma,* wound, *herpein,* to creep], herpes that develops at the site of an injury.

traumatic meningitis [Gk, *trauma,* wound, *meninx,* membrane, *itis,* inflammation], meningitis that develops as a result of injury to the skull or spinal column.

traumatic myelitis [Gk, *trauma,* wound, *myelos,* marrow, *itis,* inflammation], a spinal cord inflammation resulting from an injury.

traumatic myositis, an inflammation of the muscles resulting from a wound or other trauma.

traumatic neuritis [Gk, *trauma,* wound, *neuron,* nerve, *itis,* inflammation], inflammation of a nerve, resulting from an injury.

traumatic neuroma, a mass of nerve elements and fibrous tissue produced by the proliferation of Schwann cells and fibroblasts after severe injury to a nerve. Kinds include **amputation neuroma.**

traumatic occlusion, repeated excessive force in closure of the teeth that injures the teeth, the periodontal tissues, the residual ridge, or other oral structures. The closure extends beyond the reparative ability of the attachment apparatus (cementum, periodontal ligaments, and alveolar bone).

traumatic proctitis, rectal irritation caused by a foreign body in the rectum, such as during a medical procedure or anal intercourse.

traumatic psychosis [Gk, *trauma,* wound, *psyche,* mind, *osis,* condition], a psychiatric disorder that results from injury to the head, with symptoms usually indicating brain trauma. It is differentiated from psychic trauma in which personality damage can be traced to an unpleasant experience, such as sexual assault.

traumatic rhabdomyolysis, skeletal muscle destruction after a crush injury. During reperfusion of the damaged tissue after crushing pressure has been relieved, myoglobin, potassium, and phosphorus are released into the circulation,

causing symptoms of renal failure, hypovolemic shock, and hyperkalemia.

traumatic shock [Gk, *trauma,* wound; Fr, *choc*], the emotional or psychological state after trauma that may produce abnormal behavior. The most common types are hypovolemic shock from blood loss and neurogenic shock caused by a disruption of the integrity of the spinal cord.

traumatic spondylopathy. See **Kümmell disease.**

traumatic thrombosis [Gk, *trauma,* wound, *thrombos,* lump, *osis,* condition], intravascular coagulation of a vein or other blood vessel after injury or irritation. The condition may develop as an adverse effect of an IV injection that damages the wall of a vein. See also **thrombophlebitis.**

traumatize. See **trauma.**

traumato-, combining form meaning "trauma," "injury," "wound": *traumatology, traumatopnea, traumatopathy.*

traumatology /trô′mətol′əjē/ [Gk, *trauma + logos,* science], 1. the study of wounds and injuries. 2. a surgical specialty dealing with the treatment of wounds, injuries, and resulting disabilities. −*traumatological, traumatologic, adj.*

traumatopathy /trô′mətop″əthē/ [Gk, *trauma + pathos,* disease], a pathological condition resulting from a wound or injury. −*traumatopathic, adj.*

traumatophilia /trô′mətōfil″ē·ə/ [Gk, *trauma + philein,* to love], a psychological state in which the individual derives unconscious pleasure from injuries and surgical operations. −*traumatophilic, adj., −traumatophiliac, n.*

traumatopnea /trô′mətop″nē·ə/ [Gk, *trauma + pnein,* to breathe], partial asphyxia with collapse of the patient, caused by a penetrating thoracic wound permitting air to enter the pleural space and compress the lungs. Also called **open pneumothorax.**

traumatopyra /trô′mətōpī″rə/ [Gk, *trauma + pyr,* fire], an elevated temperature resulting from a wound or injury.

traumatotherapy /-ther″əpē/ [Gk, *trauma + therapeia,* treatment], the medical, surgical, and psychological treatment of wounds, injuries, and disabilities resulting from trauma. −*traumatotherapeutic, adj.*

traumatropism /trômat″rəpiz′əm/ [Gk, *trauma + trepein,* to turn], the tendency of damaged tissue to attract microorganisms and promote their growth, frequently causing infections after injuries, especially burns.

travail /trəvāl″/ [OFr, *travaillier,* to work], 1. physical or mental exertion, especially when distressful. 2. in obstetrics, the effort of labor and childbirth.

Travelbee, Joyce [1926–1973], a nursing theorist who developed the Human-to-Human Relationship Model and theory, presented in her book *Interpersonal Aspects of Nursing* (1966, 1971). Travelbee based the assumptions of her theory on the concepts of logotherapy. Logotherapy theory was first proposed by Viktor Frankl, a survivor of Auschwitz, in his book *Man's Search for Meaning* (1963). Travelbee believed nursing is accomplished through human-to-human relationships that begin with the original encounter and then progress through stages of emerging identities, developing feelings of empathy and later feelings of sympathy. The nurse and patient attain a rapport in the final stage. See also **logotherapy.**

traveler's diarrhea [OFr, *travailler,* to work; Gk, *dia,* through, *rhein,* to flow], any of several diarrheal disorders commonly seen in people visiting regions of the world other than their own. Such disorders can be caused by bacterial, viral, or parasitic infections. Some strains of *Escherichia coli,* which produce a powerful exotoxin, are the common cause. Other causative organisms include *Giardia lamblia* and species of *Salmonella* and *Shigella.* Symptoms last for a few days and include abdominal cramps, nausea, vomiting, slight fever, and watery stools. Relapse is rare. Treatment depends on identification of the cause and includes rehydration with beverages containing electrolytes. Preventive measures include using pure or boiled water and beverages for drinking and brushing the teeth and eating only fruits and vegetables with a skin or peel that can be removed and discarded before consumption. Also called *Montezuma's revenge,* **turista.**

travel medicine, the subspecialty of tropical medicine consisting of the diagnosis and treatment or prevention of diseases of travelers. Also called *travelers' medicine.*

traverse /travurs″/, **1.** *v.,* to travel or pass across, over, or through. **2.** *n.,* a single, complete movement of the x-ray tube around the object being scanned in computed tomography.

travoprost /trav′o-prost/, a synthetic prostaglandin analog used in the treatment of elevated intraocular pressure in patients with open-angle glaucoma or ocular hypertension. It is administered topically to the conjunctiva.

tray agglutination test, a type of sperm agglutination test in which small amounts of sperm and serum are mixed on a microscopic tray for examination. Also called *Friberg test.*

trazodone /tra′zo-dōn/, an antidepressant used orally as the hydrochloride salt to treat major depressive episodes with or without prominent anxiety.

TRBF, abbreviation for **total renal blood flow.**

Treacher Collins syndrome [Edward Treacher Collins, English ophthalmologist, 1862–1919], an inherited disorder, characterized by mandibulofacial dysostosis. See also **Pierre Robin syndrome.**

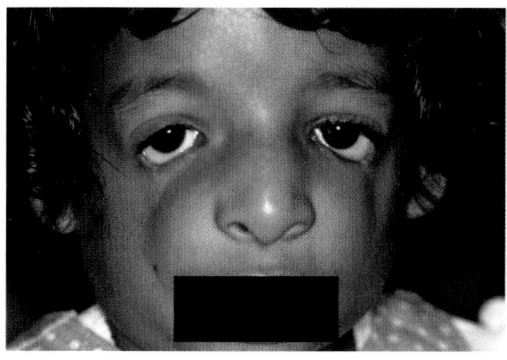

Young girl with Treacher Collins syndrome *(Regezi, Sciubba, and Jordan, 2008)*

treadmill, exercise equipment that allows the individual to walk or run in place on a rotating belt. A treadmill may be flat or inclined.

treadmill stress test. See **stress test.**

treatment [Fr, *traitement*], **1.** the care and management of a patient to combat, ameliorate, or prevent a disease, disorder, or injury. **2.** a method of combating, ameliorating, or preventing a disease, disorder, or injury. Active or curative treatment is designed to cure; palliative treatment is directed to relieve pain and distress; prophylactic treatment is for the prevention of a disease or disorder; causal treatment focuses on the cause of a disorder; conservative treatment avoids radical measures and procedures; empiric treatment uses methods shown to be beneficial by experience; rational treatment is based on a knowledge of a disease process and the action of the measures used. Treatment may be pharmacological, using drugs; surgical, involving operative procedures; or supportive, building the patient's strength. It may be specific for the disorder or symptomatic to relieve symptoms without effecting a cure.

treatment guardian, a person who is appointed by the court for the purpose of consenting to or refusing medical treatment for a patient.

treatment plan [Fr, *traitement* + L, *planta*], (in dentistry) a schedule of procedures and appointments designed to restore, step by step, a patient's oral health. The plan contains the advantages, disadvantages, costs, alternatives, and sequelae of treatment. It must be presented to the patient, as well as to the insurance company, for approval.

treatment room, a room in a patient care unit, usually in a hospital, in which various treatments or procedures requiring special equipment are performed, such as removing sutures, draining a hematoma, packing a wound, or performing an examination.

Trecator-SC, a tuberculostatic drug. Brand name for **ethionamide.**

Trechona /trikōn″ə/, a genus of spiders, family Dipluridae, commonly called funnel web spiders, the bite of which is toxic and irritating to humans.

tree [AS, *treow*], **1.** an anatomical structure with branches that spread out like those of a tree, such as the bronchial tree and the tracheobronchial tree. **2.** a pattern of searching for information in a computer database, following a series of branching options from a general category to reach specific desired items while eliminating unwanted possibilities. MEDLINE and other computer databases are organized in a "logic tree" pattern.

Treg, regulatory T cells. Abbreviation for **regulatory CD4 T cell.**

-trema, 1. suffix meaning "hole," "orifice," or "opening": *helicotrema.* **2.** suffix meaning "creatures possessing an opening": *Eurytrema.*

Trematoda /trem′ətō″də/, a class of flatworms, Platyhelminthes, that includes flukes. The adults are external or internal parasites of vertebrates. Intestinal infections in North America are rare except through flukes in foods imported from Asia or the tropics.

trematode /trem″ətōd/ [Gk, *trematodes,* pierced], any species of flatworm of the class Trematoda, some of which are parasitic to humans, infecting the liver, the lungs, and the intestines. Kinds of trematodes include the organisms causing **clonorchiasis, fascioliasis, paragonimiasis, schistosomiasis.** See also **fluke.**

trematodiasis, infection with trematodes (flukes). Also called *distomiasis.*

trembles /trem″bəls/, a toxic reaction experienced by cattle that have eaten white snakeroot or rayless goldenrod, pasture weeds that contain tremetone, a ketone. The toxic chemical is eliminated in the milk of the cows, causing sickness in humans who drink the milk.

tremor /trem″ər, trē″mər/ [L, shaking], rhythmic, purposeless, quivering movements resulting from the involuntary alternating contraction and relaxation of opposing groups of skeletal muscles, occurring in some elderly individuals, certain families, and patients with various neurodegenerative disorders. Senile tremor is characterized by fine, quick movements, especially of the hands, rhythmic head nodding, and increased trembling during purposeful movements. Familial tremor, which may be hereditary, and the tremor occurring in multiple sclerosis also increase during voluntary movement and may be intensified by anxiety, excitement, and self-consciousness. The tremors of Graves disease, alcoholism, mercury poisoning, and other toxicoses are usually less rhythmic. The tremor in lead poisoning often affects the lips. The fine, quick, continuous tremor present in Parkinson disease sometimes disappears during purposeful movements. Kinds include **resting tremor, intention tremor.**

tremulous /trem″yələs/ [L, *tremulare,* to tremble], pertaining to tremors, or involuntary muscular contractions.

tremulous pulse [L, *tremulare,* to tremble, *pulsare,* to beat], a feeble, fluttering pulse.

trench fever [OFr, *trenchier,* to cut; L, *febris,* fever], a self-limited infection caused by *Bartonella,* a rickettsial organism transmitted by body lice, characterized by weakness, fever, rash, and leg pains. It was common during World War I but is now rare. Also called **5-day fever, quintana fever.**

trench foot [OFr, *trenchier,* to cut; AS, *fot*], a condition of moist gangrene of the foot caused by the freezing of wet skin.

trench mouth. *(Informal)* See **necrotizing ulcerative gingivitis.**

Trendelenburg gait /trendel″ənbərg, tren″d(e) lənboŏrg′/ [Friedrich Trendelenburg, German surgeon, 1844–1924], an abnormal gait associated with a weakness of the gluteus medius. It is characterized by the dropping of the pelvis on the unaffected side of the body at the moment of heelstrike on the affected side. In this deviation the pelvic drop during the walking cycle lasts until heelstrike on the unaffected side and is accompanied by an apparent lateral protrusion of the affected hip. The person with a Trendelenburg gait also shortens the step on the unaffected side and displays a lateral deviation of the entire trunk and the affected side during the stance phase of the affected lower limb. This gait is one of the more common gait deviations. Also called **uncompensated gluteal gait.** Compare **compensated gluteal gait.**

Trendelenburg position [Friedrich Trendelenburg], a position in which the head is low and the body and legs are on an inclined plane. It is sometimes used in pelvic surgery to displace the abdominal organs upward, out of the pelvis.

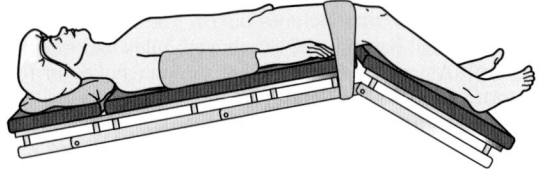

Trendelenburg position *(Phillips, 2007)*

Trendelenburg test [Friedrich Trendelenburg], a simple test for incompetent valves in a person who has varicose veins. The person lies down and elevates the leg to empty the vein, then stands, and the vein is observed as it fills. If the valves are incompetent, the vein fills from above. If the valves are normal, they do not allow backflow of blood, and the vein fills from below.

Trental, an oral hemorrheological drug. Brand name for **pentoxifylline.**

trepan. See **trephine.**

trephination /trif′inā″shən/, the surgical excision of a circular piece of bone or other tissue accomplished with a cylindric saw.

trephine /trifīn′, trifēn″/ [Gk, *trypan,* to bore], a circular sawlike instrument used in removing pieces of bone or tissue, usually from the skull. Also called **trepan.**

trepidation /trep′idā·shən/ [L, *trepidare,* to tremble], a state of anxiety.

Treponema /trep′ənē″mə/ [Gk, *trepein,* to turn, *nema,* thread], a genus of gram-negative spirochetes, including some pathogenic to humans, such as the organisms causing bejel, pinta, syphilis, and yaws.

treponemal antigen test /trep′o-ne″mal/, any of various tests detecting specific antitreponemal antibodies in serum

in the diagnosis of the *Treponema pallidum* infection of syphilis.

Treponema pallidum, an actively motile, slender spirochetal organism that causes syphilis.

treponematosis /trep′ənē′mətō″sis/ *pl.* **treponematoses** [Gk, *trepein* + *nema* + *osis,* condition], any disease caused by spirochetes of the genus *Treponema.* All these infections are effectively treated with penicillin; often one dose given intramuscularly results in cure. Kinds include **bejel, pinta, syphilis, yaws.**

treprostinil, an antiplatelet agent used to treat pulmonary arterial hypertension.

-tresia, suffix meaning "perforation": *atresia.*

tretinoin /tret′inō″in/, a retinoic acid derivative.

■ INDICATIONS: It is prescribed in the topical treatment of acne vulgaris and fine wrinkles and is administered orally for inducing remission in acute promyelocytic leukemia.

■ CONTRAINDICATIONS: Known hypersensitivity to this drug or pregnancy prohibits its use.

■ ADVERSE EFFECTS: Among the more serious adverse effects of topical administration are photosensitivity and red, edematous, blistered, or crusted skin. Almost everybody taking the drug orally experiences some degree of weakness, fatigue, headache, and fever, but adverse effects are seldom reasons for discontinuing use of the drug.

Trevor disease. See **dysplasia epiphysealis hemimelica.**

Trexan, an oral opioid antagonist. Brand name for **naltrexone hydrochloride.**

-trexate, suffix for folic acid analogs used as antimetabolites.

TRF, abbreviation for *thyrotropin-releasing factor.*

TRH, abbreviation for **thyrotropin-releasing hormone.**

TRH stimulation test, TRH test, abbreviation for *thyrotropin-releasing hormone test.* See **thyrotropin-releasing hormone stimulation test.**

tri-, prefix meaning "three" or "thrice": *triad.*

triacetin /trī·as″itin/, an antifungal agent.

■ INDICATIONS: It is prescribed to suppress the growth of superficial fungus infections of the skin, including athlete's foot.

■ CONTRAINDICATIONS: There are no known contraindications.

■ ADVERSE EFFECTS: There are no known serious adverse effects.

triacetyloleandomycin. See **troleandomycin.**

triad /trī″əd/ [Gk, *trias,* three], a combination of three, such as two parents and a child.

triage /trē·äzh″/ [Fr, *trier,* to sort out], **1.** in military medicine, a classification of casualties of war and other disasters according to the gravity of injuries, urgency of treatment, and place for treatment. **2.** a process in which a group of patients is sorted according to their need for care. The kind of illness or injury, the severity of the problem, and the facilities available govern the process, as in a hospital emergency department. **3.** in disaster medicine, a process in which a large group of patients is sorted so that care can be concentrated on those who are likely to survive.

trial /trī″əl/, a process of quality testing.

trial forceps [Fr, *trier,* to sort out], an obstetric operation consisting of an attempt to deliver an infant with obstetric forceps. The forceps are applied to the baby's head, and moderate traction is applied. The delivery is continued only if the trial indicates that delivery can be accomplished safely. The procedure is abandoned if proper application of the forceps or rotation of the baby's head is not possible or if the trial indicates that completion of the delivery with forceps will require inordinately heavy traction likely to be more traumatic to the mother or baby than cesarean section. Trial forceps is usually performed with a double setup so that cesarean section can be carried out immediately if necessary. Compare **failed forceps.** See also **double setup.**

trial of labor [Fr, *trier,* to sort out; L, *labor,* work], childbirth in which there is doubt as to whether the head of the fetus will pass through the pelvic brim. The situation must be monitored and assessed carefully to avoid fetal or maternal distress.

triamcinolone /trī′amsin″əlōn/, a corticosteroid.

■ INDICATIONS: It is prescribed topically as an antiinflammatory agent in the treatment of dermatoses, stomatitis, and lichen planus lesions, is inhaled for the treatment of allergies and asthma, is injected (e.g., into joints) for the treatment of local inflammation, and is taken orally in low doses for treatment of adrenocortical insufficiency and in higher antiinflammatory/immunosuppressive doses for the treatment of systemic diseases such as systemic lupus erythematosus.

■ CONTRAINDICATIONS: Fungal infections or known hypersensitivity to this drug prohibits its systemic use. Viral or fungal infections of the skin, impaired circulation, or known hypersensitivity to this drug prohibits its topical use.

■ ADVERSE EFFECTS: Among the more serious adverse effects to the systemic administration of the drug are GI, endocrine, neurological, fluid, and electrolyte disturbances. Skin reactions may occur from topical administration of this drug.

triamterene /trī·am″tərēn/, a potassium-sparing diuretic.

■ INDICATIONS: It is usually prescribed alone or with another diuretic in the treatment of edema, hypertension, and congestive heart failure.

■ CONTRAINDICATIONS: Anuria, severe liver or kidney dysfunction, hyperkalemia, or known hypersensitivity to this drug prohibits its use.

■ ADVERSE EFFECTS: Among the most serious adverse effects are electrolyte disturbances, particularly hyperkalemia. GI disturbances also may occur.

triangulation [L, *triangulus,* three-cornered], an emotional process that takes place when there is difficulty in a relationship. Triangles represent dysfunctional efforts to reduce fusion or conflict in a relationship. The three corners of a triangle can be composed of three people or of two people and an object, group, or issue.

triangular bandage /trī·ang″gyələr/, a square of cloth folded or cut into the shape of a triangle. It may be used as a sling, a cover, or a thick pad to control bleeding.

triangular bone, the pyramidal carpal bone in the proximal row on the ulnar side of the wrist. Also called **cuneiform bone, os triquetrum.**

triangular dullness. See **Korányi sign.**

triangularis /trī·ang·gyōo·lar′is/ [L], triangular muscle of facial expression.

triangular ligaments, two folds of peritoneum that, with the coronary ligaments, attach the liver to the diaphragm.

Triavil, a central nervous system fixed-combination drug containing a phenothiazine antipsychotic and a tricyclic antidepressant. Brand name for **perphenazine,** *amitriptyline hydrochloride.*

triazolam /tri·az″əlam/, a benzodiazepine hypnotic agent. This drug was withdrawn from the market in the United Kingdom; it continues to be available in the United States. Its prototype is lorazepam.

■ INDICATIONS: It is prescribed in the short-term treatment of insomnia.

■ CONTRAINDICATIONS: Known sensitivity to this drug or to other benzodiazepines or concurrent use of drugs that block CYP3A4 (e.g., ketoconazole) prohibits its use. It is not given to pregnant women, lactating mothers, or patients younger than 18 years.

■ ADVERSE EFFECTS: Among the most serious adverse effects are anterograde amnesia, paradoxical reactions, tachycardia, depression, confusion or memory impairment, and visual disturbances.

triazole /tri′ah-zōl, tri-a′zōl/, **1.** an organic compound in which three atoms of the five that make up the ring are nitrogen atoms. **2.** any of a class of antifungal agents that contain this compound.

tribe [L, *tribus*], a taxonomic division of organisms, subordinate to a family and superior to a genus, or subtribe.

-tribe, combining form meaning "a surgical instrument used to crush a body part."

tribology /tribol″əjē/ [Gk, *tribo,* to rub, *logos,* science], the study of friction, wear, and lubrication of articulating surfaces.

TRIC /trik/, a shortened reference to *Chlamydia trachomatis,* the organism that causes both inclusion conjunctivitis and trachoma. Abbreviation for *trachoma inclusion conjunctivitis agent* (TR, trachoma; IC, inclusion conjunctivitis). See also *Chlamydia.*

tricarboxylic acid cycle. See **citric acid cycle.**

TRICARE, a health care insurance system for military dependents and members of the military services that covers care not available through the usual U.S. military medical service or public health service facilities. CHAMPUS was the first federal third-party reimbursement system to pay for care rendered by nurse-midwives and nurse practitioners. Formerly called **Civilian Health and Medical Programs for Uniformed Services.**

triceps brachii /trī″seps brak″ē-ī/ [L, three-headed, *brachium,* arm], a large muscle that extends the entire length of the posterior surface of the humerus. Proximally it has a long head, a lateral head, and a medial head. The three parts of the muscle converge in a long tendon and insert in the posterior aspect of the olecranon. It functions to extend the forearm and to adduct and extend the arm. Also called *triceps.* Compare **biceps brachii.**

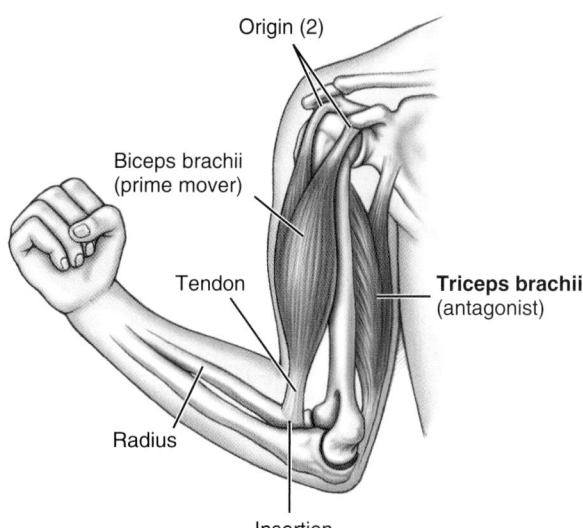

Triceps brachii *(Herlihy, 2011)*

triceps reflex, a deep tendon reflex elicited by tapping sharply the triceps tendon proximal to the elbow with the forearm in a relaxed position. The response is a definite extension movement of the forearm. The reflex is accentuated by lesions of the pyramidal tract above the level of the seventh or eighth vertebra. See also **deep tendon reflex.**

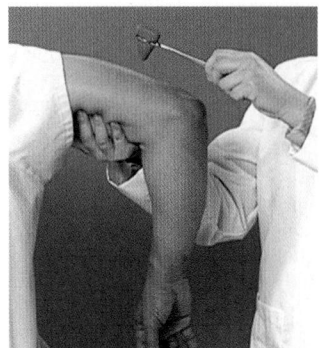

Triceps reflex test *(Seidel et al, 2011)*

triceps skinfold (TSF), the thickness of a fold of skin around the triceps muscle. It is measured primarily to estimate the amount of subcutaneous fat.

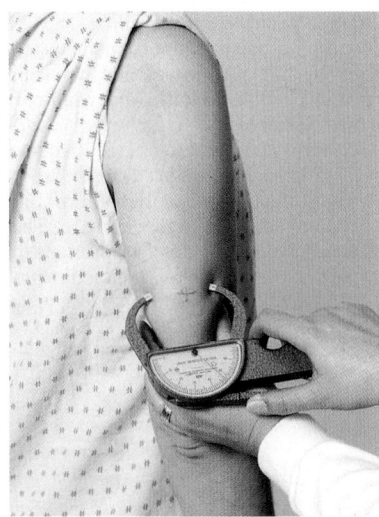

Triceps skinfold measurement *(Seidel et al, 2011)*

triceps surae limp, an abnormal action in the walking or gait cycle, associated with a deficiency in the elevating and propulsive factors on the affected side of the body, especially a deficiency of the triceps surae. Such a deficiency prevents the triceps surae from raising the pelvis and carrying it forward during the walking cycle. The pelvis consequently sags below its normal level and lags behind in the walking movement.

trichi-, tricho-, -trichia, -trichosis, combining forms meaning "hair": *trichiasis, trichophagia, glossotrichia.*

trichiasis /trikī″əsis/ [Gk, *thrix,* hair, *osis,* condition], an abnormal inversion of the eyelashes that irritates the eyeball. It usually follows infection or inflammation. Compare **ectropion.**

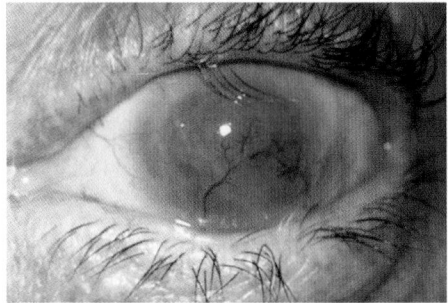

Trichiasis in late trachoma *(Stone and Gorbach, 2000)*

trichinosis /trik′inō″sis/ [Gk, *thrix* + *osis,* condition], infestation with the parasitic roundworm *Trichinella spiralis,* transmitted by eating raw or undercooked meat containing cysts (pork, bear, or other wild game). Early symptoms of infection include abdominal pain, nausea, fever, and diarrhea. Later, muscle pain, tenderness, fatigue, and eosinophilia are observed. Light infections may be asymptomatic. Also called *trichinellosis, trichiniasis.*

trichiuriasis. See **trichuriasis.**

trichlorfon /tri-klor′fon/, an irreversible cholinesterase inhibitor used as an insecticide. Also known as *metrifonate.*

trichlormethiazide /trī′klôrməthī″əzīd/, a thiazide diuretic. The prototype is hydrochlorothiazide.

■ INDICATIONS: It is prescribed in the treatment of hypertension and edema.

■ CONTRAINDICATIONS: Anuria or known hypersensitivity to this drug, to thiazide medications, or to sulfonamide derivatives prohibits its use.

■ ADVERSE EFFECTS: Among the more serious adverse effects are hypokalemia, hyperglycemia, hyperuricemia, and various hypersensitivity reactions.

trichloroethylene /trīklôr′ō-eth″ilēn/, a general anesthetic, administered by mask with N_2O for dentistry, minor surgery, and the first stages of labor. It is too cardiotoxic for deep anesthesia, even in light planes of anesthesia. It is not currently used in clinical anesthesia practice in developed countries.

tricho-. See **trichi-, tricho-, -trichia, -trichosis.**

trichobasalioma hyalinicum. See **cylindroma.**

trichoepithelioma /trik′ō-ep′ithē′lē-ō″mə/ *pl. trichoepitheliomas, trichoepitheliomata* [Gk, *thrix* + *epi,* above, *thele* nipple, *oma,* tumor], a cutaneous tumor derived from the basal cells of the follicles of fine body hair. One form of trichoepithelioma is an inherited condition and usually occurs as multiple growths. Also called **acanthoma adenoides cysticum, epithelioma adenoides cysticum.**

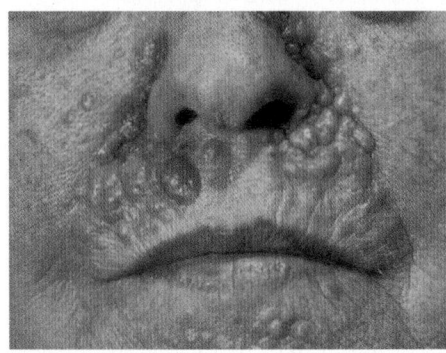

Trichoepithelioma *(Hordinsky, Sawaya, and Scher, 2000)*

trichoid /trik″oid/,   resembling a hair.

trichologia /trik′əlō″jē·ə/   [Gk, *thrix* + *legein,* to pull],   an abnormal condition in which a person pulls out his or her own hair, which may be seen in delirium.

trichology /trikol″əjē/,   the study of the anatomy, development, and diseases of the hair.

trichomania.   See **trichotillomania.**

trichomatous   /trikom″ətəs/ [Gk, *trichoma,* hairy growth],   **1.** pertaining to an introversion of the margin of the eyelid. **2.** pertaining to matted hair or ingrowing hair.

trichomonacide /trik′ōmon″əsīd/   [Gk, *thrix* + *monas,* unit; L, *caedere,* to kill],   an agent destructive to *Trichomonas vaginalis,* a parasitic protozoan flagellate that causes a refractory type of vaginitis, cystitis, and urethritis. Metronidazole, an antimicrobial agent, is used in the treatment of women with trichomoniasis and their asymptomatic partners.

Trichomonas /trik′əmon″əs/,   a genus of flagellate protozoa that includes many species that are parasitic. Some live in the mouth of humans and are found around carious teeth. Other species are found in the vagina and urethra of women. They are a cause of trichomoniasis.

Trichomonas tenax,   a species of protozoa that is found in the human mouth, particularly in cases of pyorrhea.

Trichomonas vaginalis   [Gk, *thrix* + *monas* + L, *vagina,* sheath],   a motile protozoan parasite that causes vaginitis with a copious malodorous discharge and pruritus. See also **trichomoniasis.**

trichomoniasis /trik′əmənī″əsis/   [Gk, *thrix* + *monas* + *osis,* condition],   a vaginal infection caused by the protozoan *Trichomonas vaginalis.* It is characterized by itching; burning; and frothy, pale yellow to green, malodorous vaginal discharge. With chronic infection all symptoms may disappear, although the organisms are still present. In men, infection is usually asymptomatic but may be evidenced by a persistent or recurrent urethritis. Infection is transmitted by sexual intercourse, (rarely) by moist washcloths, or, in newborns, by passage through the birth canal. Diagnosis is by microscopic examination of fresh vaginal secretions. Treatment is by oral metronidazole and tinidazole. Reinfection is common if sexual partners are not treated simultaneously.

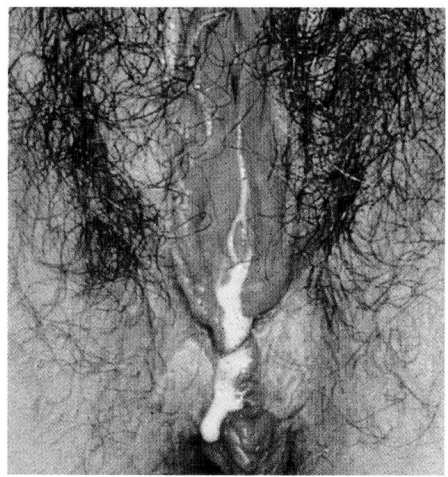

Trichomoniasis *(Courtesy Dr. Ellen Wald, University of Wisconsin Children's Hospital)*

trichopathy /trikop″əthē/   [Gk, *thrix,* hair, *pathos,* disease],   any disease condition involving the hair.

trichophagia /trik″o-fa′jah/,   the habit of eating hair, a form of pica.

trichophytic granuloma.   See **Majocchi granuloma.**

Trichophyton /trikof″iton/   [Gk, *thrix* + *phyton,* plant],   a genus of fungi that infects skin, hair, and nails. See also **dermatomycosis, dermatophyte.**

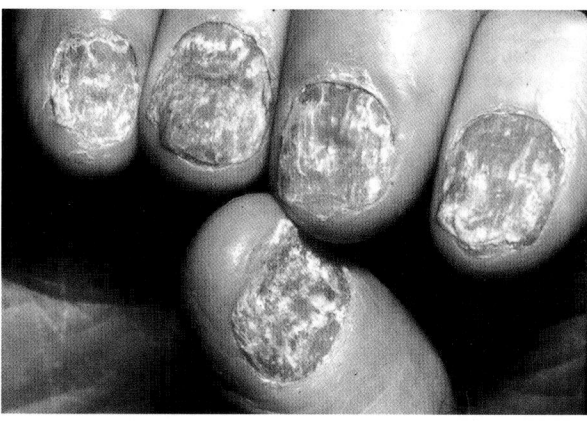

Trichophyton *(Coleman and Fleckman, 2014)*

trichosis /trikō″sis/   [Gk, *thrix,* hair, *osis,* condition],   any abnormal condition of hair growth, including alopecia, excessive female hair growth, or abnormal hair color.

-trichosis.   See **trichi-, tricho-, -trichia, -trichosis.**

trichosporosis   [Gk, *thrix,* hair, *spora,* seed, *osis,* condition],   a fungal disease of the hair shaft, giving the hair a metallic appearance. It is caused by *Trichosporon beigelii.*

trichostrongyliasis   /trik′ōstron′jəlī″əsis/ [Gk, *thrix* + *strongylos,* round, *osis,* condition],   infestation with *Trichostrongylus,* a genus of nematode worm. Also called *trichostrongylosis.* See also **nematode.**

Trichostrongylus /trik′ōstron″jiləs/   [Gk, *thrix* + *strongylos*],   a genus of roundworm, some species of which are parasitic to humans, such as *T. orientalis.*

trichotillomania /trik′ōtil′ōmā″nē·ə/   [Gk, *thrix* + *tillein,* to pull, *mania,* madness],   an impulse disorder characterized by a desire to pull out one's hair, frequently seen in cases of severe cognitive impairment and delirium. Also called **hair pulling, trichomania.** See also **trichologia.** −*trichotillomanic, trichomanic, adj.*

trichromacy /tri-kro′mah-se/,   trichromatic vision.

trichromatic /tri″kro-mat′ik/,   **1.** having or pertaining to three different colors. **2.** able to distinguish the three primary colors. See *trichromatic vision.*

trichromatism /tri-kro′mah-tiz′m/,   trichromatic vision.

trichuriasis /trik′yərī″əsis/   [Gk, *thrix* + *oura,* tail, *osis,* condition],   infestation with the roundworm *Trichuris trichiura.* The condition is usually asymptomatic, but heavy infestation may cause nausea, abdominal pain, diarrhea, and, occasionally, anemia and rectal prolapse. It is common in tropical areas with poor sanitation. Eggs are passed in feces. Contamination of the hands, food, and water results in ingestion of the eggs, which hatch in the intestines where the adult worms embed two thirds of their length in the intestinal mucosa. The worms may live 15 to 20 years. Treatment is with mebendazole; prevention includes proper disposal of feces and good personal hygiene. Also called **trichiuriasis.**

Trichuris /trikyōōr″is/   [Gk, *thrix* + *oura*],   a genus of parasitic roundworms of which the species *T. trichiura* infects the intestinal tract. Adult worms, which are 30 to 50 mm long, resemble a whip, with a threadlike anterior and a thicker posterior. Also called **whipworm.** See also **trichuriasis.**

Trichuris trichiura, a species of whipworms, commonly found in warm, moist regions of the world. Ingestion of whipworm eggs results in infection in humans. The parasites live mainly in the cecum or large intestine. Heavy infections cause abdominal pain and diarrhea. Very heavy infections may result in anemia because of intestinal blood loss.

tricitrates /tri-sit′rāts/, a solution of sodium citrate, potassium citrate, and citric acid. It is used as a systemic or urinary alkalizer and neutralizing buffer and for prevention of kidney stones.

trick knee. *(Informal)* See **locked knee.**

triclosan /tri-klo′san/, an antibacterial effective against gram-positive and most gram-negative organisms and exhibiting slight activity against yeasts and fungi. It is used as a detergent in surgical scrubs, soaps, and deodorants.

tricrotic pulse /trīkrot″ik/, an abnormal pulse that has three peaks of elevation on a sphygmogram, representing the pressure wave from the heart in systole followed by two pressure waves in diastole.

tricuspid /trīkus″pid/ [Gk, *treis,* three; L, *cuspis,* point], **1.** *adj.,* pertaining to three points or cusps. **2.** *adj.,* pertaining to the tricuspid valve of the heart. **3.** *n.,* a tooth with three points or cusps; rare in humans. Also called *tricuspal,* **trident, tridentate.**

tricuspid area [Gk, *treis,* three; L, *cuspis,* point], the region of the chest near the left lower sternum and opposite the fourth and fifth costal cartilages, where sounds of the tricuspid heart valve are best heard by auscultation. Also called **tricuspid-valve area.**

tricuspid atresia, a congenital cardiac anomaly characterized by the absence of the tricuspid valve so that there is no opening between the right atrium and right ventricle. Other cardiac defects, such as atrial and ventricular septal defects, are usually present, allowing some shunting of blood into the lungs. Clinical manifestations include severe cyanosis, dyspnea, anoxia, and signs of right-sided heart failure. Definitive diagnosis is made by cardiac catheterization, although radiographic studies usually reveal a small, underdeveloped right ventricle and large atria, giving the heart a round shape, and decreased pulmonary vascularity. Immediate palliative treatment includes pulmonary artery anastomoses to increase blood flow to the lungs and atrial septostomy if the atrial septal defect is small. Total corrective surgery has been successful in a limited number of older children.

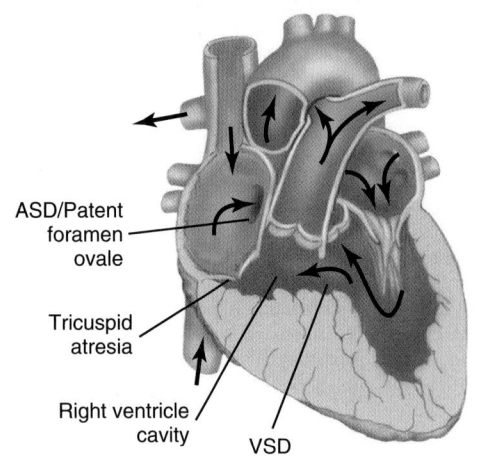

Tricuspid atresia *(James and Ashwill, 2007)*

tricuspid insufficiency, incomplete closure of the tricuspid valve, resulting in tricuspid regurgitation.

tricuspid murmur [Gk, *treis,* three; L, *cuspis,* point, *murmur,* humming], one of the heart murmurs caused by a defective tricuspid valve. The tricuspid diastolic and systolic murmurs resemble mitral valve diastolic and systolic murmurs.

tricuspid oriface. See **right atrioventricular orifice.**

tricuspid regurgitation (TR) [Gk, *treis,* three; L, *cuspis,* point + *re, gurgitare,* again to flow back], the backflow of blood from the right ventricle into the right atrium, resulting from imperfect functioning (insufficiency) of the tricuspid valve.

tricuspid stenosis, narrowing or stricture of the tricuspid valve. It is relatively uncommon and usually associated with lesions, caused by rheumatic fever, of other valves. Clinical characteristics include a diastolic pressure gradient between the right atrium and right ventricle, jugular vein distension, pulmonary congestion, and, in severe cases, hepatic congestion and splenomegaly.

tricuspid valve, a valve with three main cusps situated between the right atrium and right ventricle of the heart. The cusps of the tricuspid valve include the ventral, dorsal, and medial cusps. The cusps are composed of strong fibrous tissue and are anchored to the papillary muscles of the right ventricle by several tendons. As the right and left ventricles relax during the diastolic phase of the heartbeat, the tricuspid valve opens, allowing blood to flow into the ventricle. In the systolic phase of the heartbeat, both blood-filled ventricles contract, pumping out their contents, while the tricuspid and mitral valves close to prevent any backflow. Also called **right atrioventricular valve.** Compare **aortic valve, mitral valve, pulmonary valve, semilunar valve.** See also **atrioventricular (AV) valve, heart valve.**

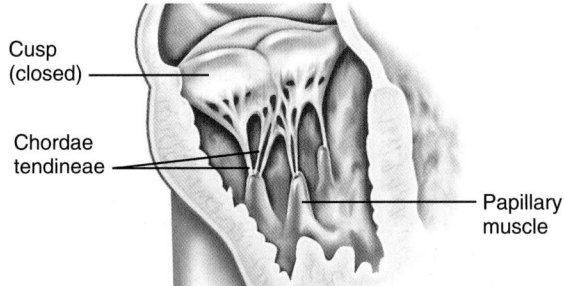

Tricuspid valve

tricuspid-valve area. See **tricuspid area.**

tricyclic antidepressant (TCA), any of a group of antidepressant drugs that contain three fused rings in their chemical structure and that potentiate the action of catecholamines. These drugs rapidly block the reuptake of amine neurotransmitters, but the exact mechanism of their effect is unknown because a period of time is required for the beneficial antidepressant effects to appear. The tricyclic antidepressants include a number of compounds, which may be grouped into four classes on the basis of chemical structure: dibenzazepines, dibenzocycloheptadienes, dibenzoxazepines, and dibenzoxepines. Besides their use to treat depression, various tricyclic antidepressants are used for other conditions, such as obsessive-compulsive disorder, panic disorder, and neurogenic pain.

tricyclic compound /trīsik″lik/ [Gk, *treis + kyklos,* circle; L, *componere,* to put together], a chemical substance containing three rings in the molecular structure, especially a tricyclic antidepressant drug used in the treatment of reactive or endogenous depression. These drugs also have anticonvulsant, antihistaminic, anticholinergic, hypotensive, and sedative effects. See also **antidepressant.**

trident, tridentate. See **tricuspid.**

Tridesilon, a glucocorticoid. Brand name for **desonide.**

Tridione, an anticonvulsant. Brand name for **trimethadione.**

trientene /trī′en-tēn/, a chelating agent used as the hydrochloride salt for chelation of copper in the treatment of Wilson disease; administered orally. See also **chelating agent.**

trientine hydrochloride /trī·en″tēn/, an oral medication for treatment of an inherited defect in copper metabolism (Wilson disease).
- INDICATIONS: It is prescribed for the relief of symptoms of Wilson disease for people who cannot tolerate penicillamine.
- CONTRAINDICATIONS: Known hypersensitivity to this drug prohibits its use.
- ADVERSE EFFECTS: The most serious side effects are possible iron deficiency and hypersensitivity reactions.

triethanolamine polypeptide oleate-condensate /trī-eth″-ənol′əmēn/, a ceruminolytic agent prescribed to reduce excessive earwax, used as a solution in propylene glycol. A possible serious adverse effect is severe contact dermatitis.

trifacial nerve. See **trigeminal nerve.**

trifluoperazine hydrochloride /trī′floo·ō·oper″əzēn/, a phenothiazine antipsychotic.
- INDICATIONS: It is prescribed in the treatment of schizophrenia and other psychoses.
- CONTRAINDICATIONS: Concurrent administration of central nervous system depressants, coma, hepatic or renal dysfunction, severe hypotension, blood dyscrasias, or known hypersensitivity to this drug prohibits its use. It must be used with caution in patients with Parkinson disease.
- ADVERSE EFFECTS: Among the more serious adverse effects are hypotension, hepatotoxicity, extrapyramidal reactions, blood dyscrasias, and hypersensitivity reactions.

trifluorothymidine /trīfloor′ōthī″mədēn/, an antiviral.
- INDICATIONS: It is prescribed in the treatment of keratoconjunctivitis, herpetic keratitis, and other forms of keratitis caused by herpes simplex virus.
- CONTRAINDICATIONS: Known hypersensitivity to this drug prohibits its use. Ocular toxicity may result from continued use beyond 21 days.
- ADVERSE EFFECTS: Among the more serious adverse effects are hypersensitivity reactions, stromal edema, and increased ocular pressure.

trifocal lens /trīfō″kəl/ [Gk, *treis,* three; L, *focus,* hearth, *lens,* lentil], an eyeglass lens ground with three foci to allow correction of near, intermediate, and far vision.

trifurcation /-furkā″shən/ [Gk, *treis,* three; L, *furca,* fork], pertaining to a vessel or other structure with three branches.

trigeminal /trījem″inəl/ [Gk, *treis,* three; L, *geminus,* twins], **1.** pertaining to the three-branch trigeminal (fifth cranial) nerve innervating the face, eyes, nose, mouth, and jaws. **2.** See **trigeminy.**

trigeminal nerve [Gk, *treis + geminus,* twin], either of the largest pair of cranial nerves, essential for the act of chewing and general sensibility of the face. The trigeminal nerves have sensory, motor, and intermediate roots and connect to three areas in the brain. Also called **fifth cranial nerve, nervus trigeminus, trifacial nerve, trigeminus.**

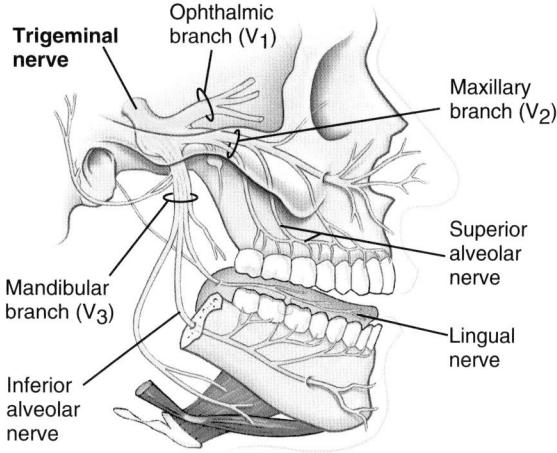

Trigeminal nerve *(Swartz MH: Textbook of physical diagnosis, history and examination, ed 6, Philadelphia, 2009, Saunders.)*

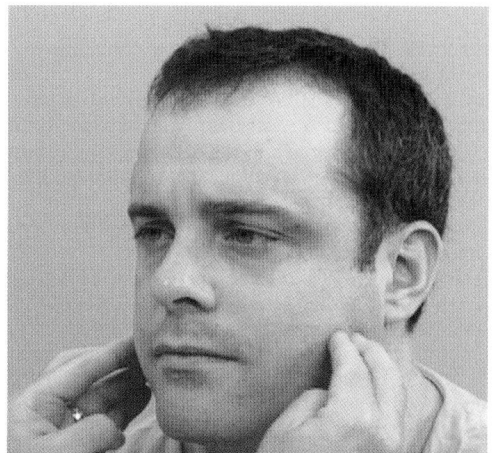

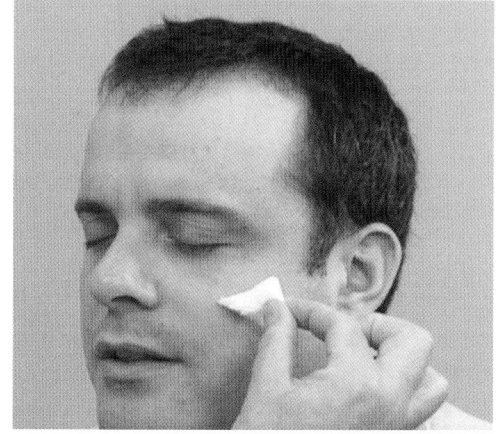

Motor and sensation assessment of trigeminal nerve *(Swartz, 2009)*

trigeminal neuralgia, a neurological condition of the trigeminal facial nerve, characterized by paroxysms of flashing, stablike pain radiating along the course of a branch of the nerve from the angle of the jaw. It is caused by degeneration of the nerve or by pressure on it. Any or all of the three branches of the nerve may be affected. Neuralgia of the first branch results in pain around the eyes and over the forehead; of the second branch, in pain in the upper lip, nose, and cheek; of the third branch, in pain on the side of the tongue and the lower lip. The momentary bursts of pain recur in clusters lasting many seconds. Paroxysmal episodes of the pains may last for hours. Also called **prosopalgia, tic douloureux.**

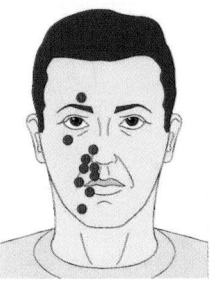

Trigeminal neuralgia: distribution of trigger zones
(Perkin, 2002)

trigeminal pulse, an abnormal pulse in which every third beat is absent. See also **bigeminal pulse, trigeminy.**

trigeminus. See **trigeminal nerve.**

trigeminy /trījem″inē/ [Gk, *treis* + L, *geminus,* twin], **1.** a grouping in threes. **2.** a cardiac arrhythmia characterized by the occurrence of three heartbeats in a repeating pattern: two normal beats coupled to an ectopic beat, or two ectopic beats coupled to a normal beat. **–trigeminal,** *adj.*

trigger [D, that which pulls], a substance, object, or agent that initiates or stimulates an action.

triggered activity [D, *trekker,* that which pulls; L, *activus*], rhythmic cardiac activity that results when a series of afterdepolarizations reach the threshold potential.

trigger finger, a phenomenon in which the movement of a finger is halted momentarily in flexion or extension and then continues with a jerk. Also called **jerk finger.**

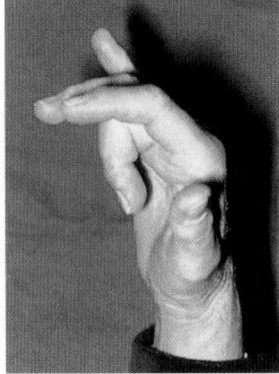

Trigger finger, locked position *(Moll, 1997)*

trigger point, a point on the body that is particularly sensitive to touch and, when stimulated, becomes the site of a painful neuralgia. Also called *trigger zone.*

triglyceride /trīglis″ərīd/, a simple fat compound consisting of three molecules of fatty acid (e.g., oleic, palmitic, or stearic) and glycerol. Triglycerides make up most animal and vegetable fats and are the principal lipids in the blood, where they circulate within lipoproteins. The total amount

of triglyceride and the amount, proportion, and kinds of lipoproteins are important in the diagnosis and treatment of many diseases and conditions, including diabetes, hypertension, and heart disease. Normally the total amount of triglyceride in the blood does not exceed 200 to 300 mg/dL. For improved metabolic health and protection to the heart and blood vessels, the American Heart Association recommends an optimum fasting triglyceride level of 100 mg/dL.

triglycerides test (TGs), a blood test that detects levels of fats existing within the bloodstream that are transported by very low-density lipoproteins (VLDLs) and chylomicrons. It is done as part of a lipid profile, which also evaluates cholesterol and lipoproteins to assess the risk of coronary and vascular disease.

trigonal muscles, a submucous sheet of smooth muscle at the bladder base (trigone), continuous with ureteral muscles above and with those of the proximal urethra below. Its superficial and deep layers are morphologically distinct.

trigone /trī″gōn/ [Gk, *trigonos,* three-cornered], **1.** a triangular space, especially one at the base of the shoulder. **2.** the first three dominant cusps, considered collectively, of an upper molar.

trigonelline /trig′ōnel″ēn/, an alkaloid derived from various kinds of plant products, including coffee beans, fenugreek, and seeds of *Cannabis sativa,* as well as from sea urchins and jellyfish. Trigonelline is used in the manufacture of poultices and other medicinals.

trigone of the bladder /trīgō″n/, a triangular area of the bladder between the opening of the ureters and the orifice of the urethra. Also called **trigonum vesicae.**

trigonitis /trī′gənī″tis/, inflammation of the trigone of the bladder, which often accompanies urethritis.

trigonum vesicae. See **trigone of the bladder.**

trihexyphenidyl hydrochloride /trīhex″ifen″idil/, an anticholinergic agent.

■ INDICATIONS: It is prescribed in the treatment of Parkinson disease and to control drug-induced extrapyramidal reactions.

■ CONTRAINDICATIONS: Narrow-angle glaucoma, asthma, obstruction of the genitourinary or GI tract, severe ulcerative colitis, or known hypersensitivity to this drug prohibits its use.

■ ADVERSE EFFECTS: Among the more serious adverse effects are blurred vision, central nervous system effects, tachycardia, dry mouth, decreased sweating, and hypersensitivity reactions.

trihybrid /trīhī″brid/ [Gk, *treis* + *hybrida,* mixed offspring], **1.** pertaining to an individual, organism, or strain that is heterozygous for three specific traits. **2.** the offspring of parents differing in three specific gene pairs or that is heterozygous for three particular traits or gene loci being followed.

trihybrid cross, the mating of two individuals, organisms, or strains that have different gene pairs that determine three specific traits or in which three particular characteristics or gene loci are being followed.

trihydric alcohol /trīhid″rik/, an alcohol containing three hydroxyl groups. Kinds include **glycerin.**

triiodothyronine (T₃) /trīī·ō′dōthī″rənēn/, a hormone that helps regulate growth and development, helps control metabolism and body temperature, and, by a negative-feedback system, acts to inhibit the secretion of thyrotropin by the pituitary gland. Triiodothyronine is produced mainly from the deiodination of thyroxine in the peripheral tissues but is also synthesized by and stored in the thyroid gland as an amino acid residue of the protein thyroglobulin. Triiodothyronine circulates in the plasma, where it is bound mainly to thyroxine-binding globulin and thyroxine-binding prealbumin, proteins that protect the hormone from metabolism and excretion during its half-life of 2 days or less before it is degraded in the liver. The hormone is the most active thyroid hormone and affects all body processes, including gene expressions. It is a component of various drugs used in the treatment of hypothyroidism and simple goiter, such as liotrix and liothyronine sodium. Normal adult blood levels are 110 to 230 ng/dL. See also **thyroid hormone.**

triiodothyronine resin uptake test, a thyroid function test measuring how many sites on thyroxine-binding globulin are occupied by endogenous triiodothyronine (T_3) and how many sites remain available. An excess of radioactive exogenous T_3 is added to the sample, followed by the addition of a resin that also binds T_3. A portion of the radioactive T_3 binds to sites on TBG not already occupied by endogenous thyroid hormones, and the remainder binds to the resin. The amount of labeled hormones bound to the resin (the T_3 resin uptake) can be subtracted from the total that was added, and the remainder is the amount that was bound to the unoccupied binding sites on the TBG. See also **thyroxine-binding globulin.**

triiodothyronine (T_3) test, a test used to accurately measure thyroid function. Because nonthyroidal diseases can convert thyroxine to T_3 in the liver, and because there is considerable overlap between hypothyroid states and normal thyroid function, T_3 is less useful in indicating hypothyroid states. It is used primarily to determine hyperthyroidism.

trikates /trī′kāts/, a solution of potassium acetate, potassium bicarbonate, and potassium citrate used as a potassium supplement in the treatment and prevention of hypokalemia. It is administered orally.

Trilafon, a phenothiazine antipsychotic. Brand name for **perphenazine.**

trilaminar blastoderm /trīlam″inər/ [Gk, *treis* + L, *lamina,* plate; Gk, *blastos,* germ, *derma,* skin], the stage of embryonic development in which all three of the primary germ layers, the ectoderm, mesoderm, and entoderm, have formed. Compare **bilaminar blastoderm.**

trill [It, *trillare,* to make a ringing sound], a vibratory, quavering, warbling sound, as produced by human voice, birds, insects, or musical instruments.

trilogy of Fallot /tril″əjē, falō′/ [Etienne-Louis A. Fallot, French physician, 1850–1911; Gk, *treis* + *logos,* word], a congenital cardiac anomaly consisting of pulmonary stenosis, interatrial septal defect, and right ventricular hypertrophy. See also **tetralogy of Fallot.**

trimalleolar fracture. See **Cotton fracture.**

trimester /trīmes″tər, trī″-/ [L, *trimestris,* three months], one of the three periods of approximately 3 months into which pregnancy is divided. The first trimester includes the time from the first day of the last menstrual period to the end of 12 weeks of gestation. The second trimester, closer to 4 months in length than 3, extends from the twelfth to the twenty-eighth weeks of gestation. The third trimester begins at the twenty-eighth weeks of gestation and extends to the time of delivery.

trimethadione /trī′methədī″ōn/, an anticonvulsant.
- INDICATIONS: It is prescribed to prevent absence (petit mal) seizures, particularly seizures that are resistant to other therapies.
- CONTRAINDICATIONS: Severe renal or hepatic impairment, blood dyscrasias, or known hypersensitivity to this drug prohibits its use.
- ADVERSE EFFECTS: Among the more serious adverse effects are exfoliative dermatitis, blood dyscrasias, and aplastic anemia. Sedation, diplopia, photophobia and hemeralopia (an inability to see as distinctly in bright light as in dim light) may occur.

trimethobenzamide hydrochloride /trīmeth′ōben″zəmīd/, an anticholinergic and antiemetic.
- INDICATIONS: It is prescribed for the relief of postoperative nausea and vomiting and nausea and vomiting associated with gastroenteritis.
- CONTRAINDICATIONS: Reye syndrome or known hypersensitivity to benzocaine-like local anesthetic or this drug prohibits its use.
- ADVERSE EFFECTS: Among the most serious adverse effects with high doses are drowsiness, allergic reactions, and extrapyramidal reactions. Adverse reactions are rare at usual dosages.

trimethoprim /trīmeth″əprim/, an antibacterial.
- INDICATIONS: It is prescribed in the treatment of infections, particularly of the urinary tract, middle ear, and bronchi.
- CONTRAINDICATIONS: Known hypersensitivity to this drug or megaloblastic anemia resulting from folate deficiency prohibits its use. It should not be used to treat streptococcal pharyngitis.
- ADVERSE EFFECTS: Among the more serious adverse effects are blood dyscrasias and allergic, GI, and central nervous system disorders.

trimethoprim and sulfamethoxazole. See **sulfamethoxazole and trimethoprim.**

trimipramine maleate /trimip″rəmēn/, a tricyclic antidepressant.
- INDICATIONS: It is prescribed in the treatment of depression.
- CONTRAINDICATIONS: Concomitant use of a monoamine oxidase inhibitor within 14 days or known hypersensitivity to this drug prohibits its use. It is not given during recovery from myocardial infarction or to schizophrenic patients. It is not recommended for children.
- ADVERSE EFFECTS: Among the more serious adverse effects are sedation tachycardia, seizures, parkinsonism, blurred vision, hypotension, and aggravation of glaucoma.

Trimox, an antibiotic drug. Brand name for *amoxicillin trihydrate.*

Trimpex, an antibacterial. Brand name for **trimethoprim.**

Trinalin, a fixed-combination medication containing an antihistamine and a decongestant. Brand name for **azatadine maleate,** *pseudoephedrine sulfate.*

trinucleotide. See **codon.**

triolein breath test, a breath test for pancreatic function. The fasting patient is administered triolein labeled with either carbon 13 or carbon 14, and levels of labeled carbon dioxide in the exhaled breath are subsequently measured at regular time intervals; low levels of carbon dioxide indicate inadequate pancreatic lipase, such as with a pancreatic disease or cystic fibrosis.

tripanosomal. See **trypanosome.**

tripelennamine hydrochloride /trī′pelen″əmēn/, an antihistamine.
- INDICATIONS: It is prescribed in the treatment of rhinitis and hypersensitivity reactions of the skin.
- CONTRAINDICATIONS: Asthma, glaucoma, difficulty in emptying the bladder, concomitant administration of a monoamine oxidase inhibitor, or known hypersensitivity to this drug prohibits its use. It is not given to premature infants or newborns or to lactating mothers.
- ADVERSE EFFECTS: Among the more serious adverse effects are sedation, tachycardia, and GI upset.

tripe palms, a condition of thickened velvet or moss-textured palms with pronounced skin ridge pattern. Tripe palms has been associated with certain malignancies, including lung and stomach cancers and pulmonary carcinomas.

triphasic /trīfā″zik/ [Gk, *treis,* three, *phasis,* appearance], having three phases or stages.

triple-dye treatment, a therapy for burns in which three dyes, 6% gentian violet, 1% brilliant green, and 0.1% acriflavine base, are applied.

triplegia /trīplē″jə/ [Gk, *treis,* three, *plege,* stroke], a condition of paralysis on one side of the body plus paralysis of an arm or leg on the opposite side.

triple-lumen catheter [L, *triplus,* triple; L, *lumen,* light; Gk, *katheter,* a thing lowered into], any catheter with three separate passages, each of which is marked with the name of a fluid or medication. Some have infusion plugs and are flushed every 8 hours with a heparin or normal saline solution.

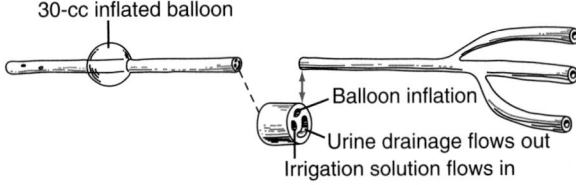

Triple-lumen catheter (cross section) *(Perry, Potter, and Elkin, 2012)*

triple-lumen drain, a drain consisting of three tubes placed one inside another. One passage is for irrigation, one for drainage, and one for inflation of the bulb.

triple point, the combination of temperature and pressure in which a given substance may exist in solid, liquid, and vapor forms, all in equilibrium at the same time. Every substance has a theoretic triple point.

triple response, a triad of phenomena that occur in sequence after an intradermal injection of histamine. First, a red spot develops, spreading outward for a few millimeters, reaching its maximal size within 1 minute and then turning bluish. Next, a brighter red flush of color spreads slowly in an irregular flare around the original red spot. Finally, a wheal filled with fluid forms over the original spot. Also called *triple response of Lewis.*

triple sugar iron reaction, any one of several reactions seen in certain bacterial cultures growing on triple sugar iron agar, a culture medium used to aid in the identification of *Escherichia coli, Proteus, Salmonella, Shigella,* and other pathogenic enteric bacteria.

triple sulfa, a combination of sulfathiazole, sulfacetamide, and sulfabenzamide, administered intravaginally in the treatment of bacterial vaginosis caused by *Gardnerella vaginalis.*

triple sulfonamides. See **trisulfapyrimidines.**

triplet /trip″lit/ [L, *triplus*], **1.** any one of three offspring born over the same gestation period during a single pregnancy. See also **Hellin's law. 2.** (in genetics) the unit of three consecutive bases in one polynucleotide chain of DNA or RNA that codes for a specific amino acid. See also **codon, genetic code.**

triple X syndrome. See **XXX syndrome.**

triploid (*3n*) /trip″loid/ [L, *triplus* + *eidos*], **1.** *n.,* an individual, organism, strain, or cell that has three complete sets of chromosomes, triple the haploid number characteristic of the species. In humans the triploid number is 69. It is found in rare cases of aborted or stillborn fetuses. Of triploid fetuses born alive, all are characterized by gross and multiple malformations; they live for only a few hours. **2.** *adj.,* also pertaining to such an individual, organism, strain, or cell. Also *triploidic.* Compare **diploid, haploid, tetraploid.** See also **polyploid.–triploidy,** *n.*

triploidy /trip″loidē/, the state or condition of having three complete sets of chromosomes.

tripod /trī″pod/ [Gk, *treis,* three, *pous,* foot], any object with three legs or three feet.

tripodial symmelia /trīpō″dē·əl/ [Gk, *treis,* three, *pous,* foot, *syn,* together, *melos,* limb], a fetal anomaly characterized by the fusion of the lower extremities and the presence of three feet. Compare **dipodial symmelia, monopodial symmelia, sirenomelia.**

triprolidine /trī·prol″idēn/, an antihistamine.

■ INDICATIONS: It is prescribed in the treatment of hypersensitivity reactions, including rhinitis, skin rash, and pruritus.

■ CONTRAINDICATIONS: Asthma or known hypersensitivity to this drug prohibits its use. It is not given to newborns or lactating mothers. Adverse reactions may occur in elderly patients.

tripsis /trip″sis/ [Gk, rubbing], **1.** massage. **2.** the process of reducing the particle size of a substance by grinding it with a mortar and pestle. Also called **trituration.**

-tripsis, suffix meaning "to crush, break, or pulverize": *anatripsis.*

-tripsy, suffix meaning "to crush, break, or pulverize": *cholecystolithotripsy, lithotripsy, osteotripsy.*

triptorelin, a gonadotropin-releasing hormone used to treat advanced prostate cancer.

triradiate cartilage, a secondary ossification center of the hip bone, occurring as a Y-shaped strip in the floor of the acetabulum.

trisaccharide /trīsak″ərīd/ [Gk, *treis,* three, *sakcharon,* sugar], a carbohydrate composed of three monosaccharide units linked together.

trisalicylate /trī″sah·lis′ilāt/, a compound containing three salicylate ions.

trismus /triz″məs/ [Gk, *trismos,* gnashing], a prolonged tonic spasm of the muscles of the jaw. Also called **lockjaw.** See also **tetanus.**

trisomy /trī″səmē/ [Gk, *treis* + *soma,* body], a chromosomal aberration characterized by the presence of one more than the normal number of chromosomes in a diploid complement. In humans the trisomic cell contains 47 chromosomes and is designated $2n + 1$. The additional member can join any of the normal homologous pairs, although most human trisomies involve the small chromosomes, such as those in the E or G group or the sex chromosomes. Partial trisomy occurs when only a part of a chromosome attaches to another. In genetic nomenclature, trisomies are indicated by the exact chromosome or karyotypic group in which the addition is made, such as trisomy 13 or trisomy D. Common diseases associated with trisomy include Down syndrome and Patau syndrome. Also called *trisomia.* Compare **monosomy.** See also **aneuploidy, multipolar mitosis, trisomy syndrome.** *–trisomic, adj.*

trisomy 8, a congenital condition associated with the presence of an extra chromosome 8 within the C group. Those with the condition are slender and of normal height and have a large asymmetric head, prominent forehead, deep-set eyes, low-set prominent ears, and thick lips. There are mild to severe cognitive and motor impairments, often with delayed and poorly articulated speech. Skeletal anomalies and joint limitation, especially permanent flexion of one or more fingers, may occur. There are unusually deep palmar and plantar creases, which are diagnostically significant. Most trisomy 8 individuals are mosaic, with no abnormal or only slight clinical manifestations, or they are only partially trisomic, with part of the extra chromosome 8 missing, and show varying degrees of the clinical symptoms. In general, trisomy 8 is a less severe condition than other trisomies, especially trisomy

13 and trisomy 18, so that mortality is low. Also called **trisomy C syndrome.**

trisomy 13, a congenital condition caused by the presence of an extra chromosome in the D group, predominantly chromosome 13, although in rare instances chromosome 14 or 15. It occurs in approximately 1 in 5000 births and is characterized by multiple midline anomalies and central nervous system defects, including holoprosencephaly, microcephaly, myelomeningocele, microphthalmos, and cleft lip and palate. There is also severe cognitive impairment; polydactyly; deafness; convulsions; and abnormalities of the heart, viscera, and genitalia. Most infants with the condition are severely affected and do not survive beyond the first 6 months of life. The symptom combination of cleft lip and palate, polydactylism, and microcephaly is sometimes identified as the triad. Also called **Patau syndrome, trisomy D syndrome,** *trisomy 13-15.*

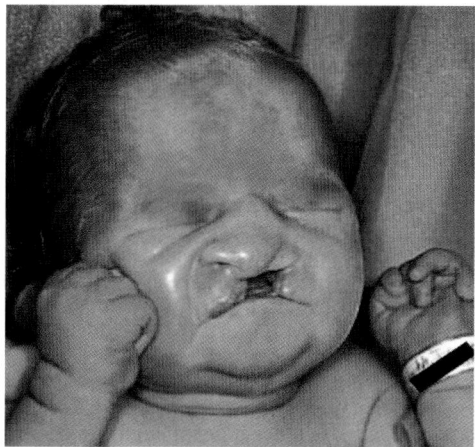

Infant with trisomy 13: midline defect *(Lipson, 2005)*

trisomy 18, a congenital condition caused by the presence of an extra chromosome 18, characterized by severe cognitive impairment and multiple deformities. Among the most common defects are scaphocephaly or other skull abnormalities; micrognathia; abnormal facies with low-set malformed ears and prominent occiput; cleft lip and palate; clenched fists with overlapping fingers, especially the index over the third finger; clubfeet; and syndactyly. Ventricular septal defect, patent ductus arteriosus, atrial septal defect, and renal anomalies are also common. The condition occurs in about 1 in 3000 births and predominantly in females, at a 3:1 sex ratio, and survival for more than a few months is rare. Also called **Edwards' syndrome,** **trisomy E syndrome,** *trisomy 16-18.*

trisomy 21. See **Down syndrome.**

trisomy 22, a congenital condition caused by the presence of an extra chromosome 22 in the G group, characterized by psychomotor delay and various developmental anomalies. Common defects include microcephaly, micrognathia, hypotonia, hypertelorism, abnormal ears with preauricular tags or fistulas, and congenital heart disease. In partial trisomy 22 the extra chromosome is much smaller than the normal pair and causes coloboma of the iris, anal atresia, or both, as well as various other defects. See also **cat-eye syndrome.**

trisomy C syndrome. See **trisomy 8.**

trisomy D syndrome. See **trisomy 13.**

trisomy E syndrome. See **trisomy 18.**

trisomy syndrome, any condition caused by the addition of an extra member to a normal pair of homologous autosomes or to the sex chromosomes or by the translocation of a part of one chromosome to another. Most trisomies occur as a result of complete or partial nondisjunction of the chromosomes during cell division. The more severe conditions are related to trisomies of the autosomes rather than the sex chromosomes. The most common trisomy syndromes with clearly established clinical manifestations are trisomy 8, trisomy 13, trisomy 18, trisomy 21, and trisomy 22. See also **trisomy.**

trisplanchnic /trīsplangk″nik/, pertaining to three visceral body cavities: skull, thorax, and abdomen.

trisulfapyrimidines /trīsul′fəpirim″idīnz/, three antibacterials in combination (sulfadiazine, sulfamerazine, and sulfamethazine), rarely prescribed today. Also called **triple sulfonamides.**

tritium (³H) /trit″ē·əm, trish″əm/ [Gk, *tritos,* third], **1.** the radioactive isotope of the hydrogen atom. See also **deuterium, protium. 2.** a beta emitter and tracer.

trituration, the process of removing impurities from a substance by grinding it under a solvent in which the impurities are much more soluble than the substance itself. See also **tripsis.**

trivalence /trīvā″ləns/ [Gk, *treis* + L, *valere,* to be worth], an ability of an atom or group of atoms to bond with three monovalent elements in a compound.

trivalent /trīvā′lənt/ [Gk, *treis* + L, *valere,* to be worth], **1.** pertaining to an atom or group of atoms with the capability of bonding with or replacing three monovalent elements. **2.** designating a vaccine that can prevent diseases or conditions.

trivial name /triv″ē·əl/, a chemical name that is not derived from a systematic nomenclature system such as the IUPAC nomenclature system. The name may or may not indicate its relationship to molecular structure and to other chemicals. The name may be accepted as an official nonproprietary designation because of common usage.

Tri-Vi-Flor, an oral pediatric fixed-combination drug containing fluoride and vitamins. Brand name for **fluoride, vitamin A, vitamin C, vitamin D.**

tRNA, abbreviation for **transfer RNA.**

Trobicin, an antibacterial. Brand name for **spectinomycin hydrochloride.**

trocar /trō″kär/ [Fr, *trois,* three, *carres,* sides], a sharp, pointed rod that fits inside a tube. It is used to pierce the skin and the wall of a cavity or canal in the body to aspirate fluids, to instill a medication or solution, or to guide the placement of a soft catheter. The trocar is usually removed, and the catheter, tube, or instrument is left in place. See also **cannula.**

trochanter /trōkan″tər/ [Gk, runner], one of the two bony projections on the proximal end of the femur that serves as the point of attachment of various muscles. The two protuberances are the trochanter major and the trochanter minor.

trochanteric fossa, a fossa on the greater trochanter to which the obturator externus muscle is attached.

trochanter major [Gk, *trochanter,* runner; L, *major,* great], a large projection from the proximal end of the shaft of the femur. It is a point of attachment for the gluteus minimus and gluteus medius muscles. Also called **greater trochanter.**

trochanter minor. See **lesser trochanter.**

troche /trō″kē/ [Gk, *trochos,* lozenge], a small, oval, round, or oblong tablet containing a medicinal agent incorporated in a flavored, sweetened mucilage or fruit base that dissolves in the mouth, releasing the drug. Also called **lozenge, rotula,** *trochiscus.*

trochlea /trok″lē·ə/, a pulley-shaped part or structure.

trochlear /trok″lē·ər/ [L, *trochlea*, pulley], **1.** pertaining to a trochlea or something that is pulley shaped. **2.** relating to the trochlear (fourth cranial) nerve.

trochlear nerve [L, *trochlea*, pulley, *nervus*, nerve], either of the smallest pair of cranial nerves, essential for eye movement and eye muscle sensibility. The trochlear nerves branch to supply the superior oblique muscle and communicate with the ophthalmic division of the trigeminal nerve, connecting with two areas in the brain. Also called **fourth cranial nerve, nervus trochlearis.**

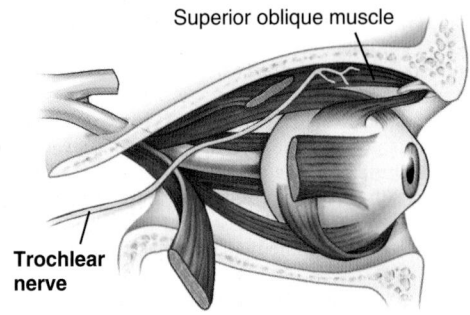

Superior oblique muscle

Trochlear nerve

Trochlear nerve

trochlear notch of ulna, a large depression in the ulna, formed by the olecranon and coronoid processes, that articulates with the trochlea of the humerus.

trochoid joint. See **pivot joint.**

trolamine /trol″əmēn/, a contraction for *triethanolamine.*

troleandomycin /trol′ē·an′dōmī″sin/, a macrolide antibiotic.

■ INDICATIONS: It is prescribed in the treatment of certain infections, including pneumococcal pneumonia and group A streptococcal infections of the upper respiratory tract. It has orphan drug status for the treatment of corticosteroid-dependent asthma due to its steroid-sparing properties.

■ CONTRAINDICATIONS: Known hypersensitivity to this drug or concomitant use of ergot alkaloids prohibits its use.

■ ADVERSE EFFECTS: Among the more serious adverse effects are GI disturbances, mild to severe allergic reactions (including anaphylaxis), and hepatotoxicity.

Trombiculidae /trom′bikyōō″lidē/, a family of mites, including harvest mites, red bugs, and chiggers. The larvae are parasitic and the adults are free-living. The mites are disease vectors of typhus, rickettsiae, scrub itch, tsutsugamushi disease, and other infections.

trombiculosis /trombik′yəlō″sis/ [Gk, *tromein*, to tremble, *osis*, condition], an infestation with mites of the genus *Trombicula*, some species of which carry scrub typhus.

-tron, suffix meaning "a (specified) type of vacuum tube": *betatron, magnetron, cyclotron.*

Tronothane, a local anesthetic agent. Brand name for **pramoxine hydrochloride.**

trop-, -trop, combining form for atropine derivatives.

trop-, tropo-, combining form meaning "turn, turning" or "tendency, affinity": *trophotropism.*

-tropal. See **-tropia, -tropal, -tropic, -tropous.**

-trope, combining form meaning "influencing" or "influenced by": *chromotrope, luteotrope.*

troph-. See **tropho-.**

-troph, **1.** combining form meaning "that which nourishes an embryo": *embryotroph, hemotroph, histotroph.* **2.** combining form meaning "an organism that gets nourishment from a (specified) source": *oligotroph.*

trophectoderm. See **trophoblast.**

trophic /trof″ik/ [Gk, *trophe*, nutrition], pertaining to a nutritive effect on or quality of cellular activity.

-trophic, suffix meaning "a type of nutrition or nutritional requirement": *neurotrophic.*

trophic action [Gk, *trophe*, nutrition; L, *agere*, to do], the stimulation of cell reproduction and enlargement by nurturing and causing growth.

trophic fracture, a fracture resulting from the weakening of bone, caused by nutritional disturbances.

trophic hormones, hormones secreted by the adenohypophysis (anterior lobe of pituitary gland) that stimulate target organs.

trophic ulcer [Gk, *trophe*, nutrition], a pressure ulcer caused by trauma to a part of the body that is in poor condition because of disease, vascular insufficiency, or loss of afferent nerve fibers. Trophic ulcers may be painless or associated with severe causalgia. See also **pressure ulcer.**

trophism /trof″izəm/ [Gk, *trophe*, nutrition], the influence of nourishment.

tropho- /trof″ə-, trō″fə-/, combining form meaning "food" or "nourishment": *trophoblast.*

trophoblast /trof″əblast′/ [Gk, *trophe* + *blastos*, germ], the outermost layer of tissue that forms the wall of the blastocyst of placental mammals in the early stages of embryonic development. It functions in the implantation of the blastocyst in the uterine wall and in supplying nutrients to the embryo. At implantation the cells differentiate into two layers: the inner cytotrophoblast, which forms the chorion, and the syncytiotrophoblast, which develops into the outer layer of the placenta. Also called **trophectoderm.** −*trophoblastic, adj.*

trophoblastic cancer /-blas″tik/, a malignant neoplastic disease of the uterus derived from chorionic epithelium, characterized by the production of high levels of human chorionic gonadotropin (HCG). The tumor may be an invasive hydatid mole (chorioadenoma destruens) formed by grossly enlarged vesicular chorionic villi or a malignant uterine choriocarcinoma that arises from nonvillous chorionic epithelium. One half of the cases of choriocarcinoma follow a molar pregnancy, 25% an abortion, 22.5% a normal pregnancy, and 2.5% an ectopic pregnancy. A hydatid mole invades the myometrium and often forms extrauterine nodules that may spread to distant sites. Choriocarcinoma forms a dark red hemorrhagic nodular tumor on or in the uterine wall and metastasizes early in its course to the lungs, brain, liver, bones, vagina, or vulva. Initial symptoms are vaginal bleeding and a profuse, foul-smelling discharge; a persistent cough or hemoptysis signals pulmonary involvement. As the disease progresses, there may be frequent hemorrhage, weakness, and emaciation. Diagnostic measures include serial assays to determine whether the HCG level in the blood is elevated and histological examination of specimens obtained by curettage. Hysterectomy is indicated in most cases, but surgery does not eliminate the possibility of a recurrence. Chemotherapy is effective in curing a large percentage of patients with trophoblastic tumors. Also called *trophoblastic disease.* See also **choriocarcinoma, hydatid mole.**

trophotropic /trof″ətrop″ik/ [Gk, *trophe* + *trepein*, to turn], pertaining to a combination of parasympathetic nervous system activity, somatic muscle relaxation, and cortical beta rhythm synchronization, such as in a resting or sleep state.

trophotropism /trof′ətrop″izəm/, movement toward or away from nutrient sources.

trophozoite /trof″əzō″īt/ [Gk, *trophe* + *zoon*, animal], an immature ameboid protozoon. Diseases in which trophozoites may be isolated by bacteriological studies include amebic dysentery, malaria, and trichomonas vaginitis. When fully developed, a trophozoite may be identified as a schizont.

-trophy, -trophia, combining form meaning "a condition of nutrition or growth": *dystrophy, embryotrophy, panatrophy.*

-tropia, -tropal, -tropic, -tropous, 1. suffix meaning "a turn or deviation from normal": *esotropia, exotropia.* **2.** suffix meaning "a tendency to have an influence on or to be influenced by": *adrenotropic, pancreatropic, somatotropic.*

tropical acne /trop″ikəl/, a form of acne that is caused or aggravated by high temperature and humidity. It is characterized by large nodules or pustules on the neck, back, upper arms, and buttocks.

tropical medicine [Gk, *tropikos,* of the solstice; L, *medicina*], the branch of medicine concerned with the diagnosis and treatment of diseases commonly occurring in tropical and subtropical regions of the world, generally between 30 degrees north and south of the equator.

tropical sore. See **cutaneous leishmaniasis.**

tropical spastic paraparesis. See **chronic progressive myelopathy.**

tropical sprue, a malabsorption syndrome of unknown cause that is endemic in the tropics and subtropics. It is characterized by abnormalities in the mucosa of the small intestine, resulting in protein malnutrition and multiple nutritional deficiencies, often complicated by severe infection. Symptoms include diarrhea, anorexia, and weight loss. Megaloblastic anemia may result from folic acid and vitamin B_{12} deficiency. Treatment includes administration of antibiotics, particularly tetracycline; folic acid; iron; calcium; and vitamins A, D, K, and B complex; as well as a balanced diet high in protein and normal in fat content. See also **nontropical sprue.**

tropical typhus. See **scrub typhus.**

-tropin, suffix meaning "stimulating effect of a hormone or other substance on a target organ or system": *gonadotropin.*

-tropism. See **-tropy, -tropism.**

-tropo. See **trop-, -trop.**

tropocollagen /trop′əkol″əjən/ [Gk, *trepein,* to turn, *kolla,* glue, *genein,* to produce], fundamental units of collagen fibrils obtained by prolonged extraction of insoluble collagen with dilute acid.

tropomyosin /trop′əmī″əsin/ [Gk, *trepein* + *mys,* muscle], a protein component of sarcomere filaments, which, together with troponin, regulates interactions of actin and myosin in muscle contractions.

troponin /trō″pənin/ [Gk, *trepein,* to turn], a protein in the striated cell ultrastructure that modulates the interaction between actin and myosin molecules. It is believed to be part of the calcium-binding complex of the thin myofilaments. See also **tropomyosin.**

troponins test, blood tests that measure levels of cardiac troponins (T and I), which are the standard biochemical markers for cardiac disease. This test assists in evaluating patients with suspected acute coronary ischemic syndrome. It is particularly useful in differentiating cardiac from noncardiac chest pain, evaluating patients with unstable angina, detecting reperfusion associated with coronary recanalization, estimating myocardial infarction size, and detecting perioperative myocardial infarction.

-tropous. See **-tropia, -tropal, -tropic, -tropous.**

-tropy, -tropism, suffix meaning "influenced by or having an affinity for" something specified: *entropy, monotropy, syntropy.*

trospium, an anticholinergic.

■ INDICATIONS: This drug is used to treat overactive bladder.

■ CONTRAINDICATIONS: Uncontrolled narrow-angle glaucoma, urinary retention, gastric retention, and known hypersensitivity to this drug prohibit its use.

■ ADVERSE EFFECTS: Adverse effects of this drug include fatigue, dizziness, headache, dry eyes, vision abnormalities, flatulence, abdominal pain, and dyspepsia. Common side effects include constipation and dry mouth.

trough /trôf/ [AS, *trog*], **1.** a groove or channel, such as the gingival trough around the neck of a tooth. **2.** (in pharmacology) the time at which a medication is at its lowest concentration in the body. See **peak and trough specimens.**

Trousseau sign /trōōsō′/ [Armand Trousseau, French physician, 1801–1867; L, *signum,* mark], **1.** a test for latent tetany in which carpal spasm is induced by inflating a sphygmomanometer cuff on the upper arm to a pressure exceeding systolic blood pressure for 3 minutes. A positive test may be seen in hypocalcemia and hypomagnesemia. **2.** a reddened streak, the result of drawing a finger across the skin. It is seen with a variety of nervous system disorders.

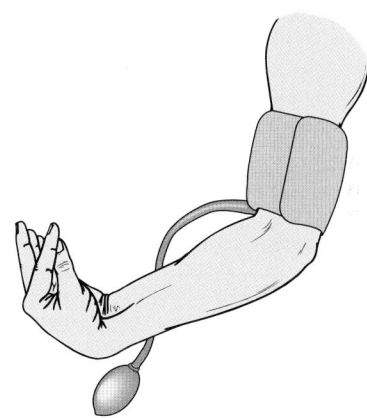

Trousseau sign *(Lewis et al, 2011)*

Trousseau syndrome [Armand Trousseau], superficial migratory thrombophlebitis associated with visceral cancer.

trovafloxacin /tro″vah-flok′sah-sin/, an antibacterial effective against a broad spectrum of gram-positive and gram-negative organisms. It is administered orally as the mesylate salt in the treatment of serious infections.

Trp, abbreviation for **tryptophan.**

true ankylosis, fusion of the bony surfaces of a joint. See also **ankylosis.**

true birth rate [ME, *treue,* faith, *burthe* + L, *reri,* to calculate], the ratio of total births to the total female population of childbearing age, between 15 and 45 years of age. Compare **birth rate, crude birth rate, refined birth rate.**

true chondroma. See **enchondroma.**

true conjugate, a radiographic measurement of the distance from the upper margin of the symphysis pubis to the sacral promontory. It is usually 1.5 to 2 cm less than the diagonal conjugate.

true denticle. See **denticle.**

true diverticulum [ME, *treue,* faith; L, *diverticulare,* to turn aside], diverticulum that includes all the same tissue layers as the organ from which it originates.

true dwarf. See **primordial dwarf.**

true glottis. See **glottis.**

true hermaphroditism [ME, *treue,* faith; Gk, *Hermaphroditos,* son of Hermes and Aphrodite], a condition in which an individual is born with both male and female gonads.

true labor, uterine contractions that result in a change in the cervix and the birth of an infant.

true neuroma, any neoplasm composed of nerve tissue.

true oxygen, the calculated concentration as either a percentage or a fraction that, when multiplied by the expiratory minute volume at STPD, gives oxygen uptake.

true pelvis. See **pelvis.**

true rib. See **rib, vertebrosternal rib.**

true shunt. See **zero V/Q.**

true suture, an immovable fibrous joint of the skull in which the edges of bones interlock along a series of processes and indentations. Compare **false suture.** Kinds include **sutura dentata, sutura limbosa, sutura serrata.**

true twins. See **monozygotic twins.**

true value, (in statistics) a value that is closely approximated by the definitive value and somewhat less closely by the reference value.

true vocal cords [ME, *treue,* faith; L, *vocalis,* of the voice; Gk, *chorde,* string], the vocal folds of the larynx (plicae vocales), as distinguished from the vestibular folds (plicae vestibulares), called false vocal cords. They are located inferior to the false vocal cords. See also **vocal cord.**

truncal /trung″kəl/ [L, *truncus*], pertaining to the trunk of the body or to any arterial or nerve trunk.

truncal ataxia, a loss of coordinated muscle movements for maintaining normal posture of the trunk.

truncal obesity, obesity that preferentially affects or is located in the trunk of the body as opposed to the extremities.

truncated /trung″kātid/, **1.** amputated from the trunk. **2.** cut across at right angles to the long axis.

truncus /trung″kəs/ [L, trunk], the main stem of an anatomical part from which branches may arise, such as the sympathetic nerve chain or jugular lymph trunk.

truncus arteriosus [L, trunk; Gk, *arteria,* airpipe], the embryonic arterial trunk that initially opens from both ventricles of the heart and later divides into the aorta and the pulmonary trunk, the two parts separated by the bulbar septum.

truncus brachiocephalicus, a branch of the aorta that divides into the right common carotid and right subclavian arteries.

trunk [L, *truncus*], **1.** the main stalk of an anatomical structure with many branches, such as an artery or nerve. **2.** the body excluding the head and appendages. Also called **torso.**

trunk balance, the ability to maintain postural control of the trunk, including the shifting and bearing of weight on each side to free an extremity for a particular function such as reaching and grasping. Weight shifting can be anterior, posterior, lateral, or diagonal and involve righting, equilibrium, and protective reactions. Head and neck control allows for dissociation of the shoulder and pelvic girdles from the trunk.

trunk incurvation reflex. See **Galant reflex.**

Trusopt, a carbonic anhydrase inhibitor medication. Brand name for **dorzolamide hydrochloride.**

truss [Fr, *trousser,* to pack up], an apparatus worn to prevent or retard the herniation of the intestines or other organ through an opening in the abdominal wall.

truth [AS, *treowo*], a rule or statement that conforms to fact or reality.

truth serum, a common name for any of several sedatives, such as the short-acting barbiturates, that have been administered intravenously in subjects to elicit information that may have been repressed. It has been used successfully in helping to identify amnesia victims.

trypanocide /tri-pan′o-sīd/, a drug destructive to trypanosomes, especially the species of protozoan parasite transmitted to humans by various insect vectors common in Africa and Central and South America. Various arsenic preparations are used to treat African sleeping sickness, caused by *Trypanosoma gambiense* and *T. rhodesiense,* and Chagas disease, caused by *T. cruzi,* in the Americas. Also called **trypanosomicide.** −*trypanosomicidal, adj.*

Trypanosoma /trip′ənōsō″mə/ [Gk, *trypanon,* borer, *soma,* body], a genus of parasitic organisms, several species of which can cause significant diseases in humans. Most *Trypanosoma* organisms live part of their life cycle in insects and are transmitted to humans by insect bites. See also **trypanosome, trypanosomiasis.**

Trypanosoma brucei gambiense. See **Gambian trypanosomiasis.**

Trypanosoma brucei rhodesiense. See **Rhodesian trypanosomiasis.**

Trypanosoma cruzi. See **Chagas disease.**

trypanosomal infection. See **trypanosomiasis.**

trypanosome /trip″ənōsōm′, tripan″-/, any organism of the genus *Trypanosoma.*

trypanosomiasis /trip′ənō′sōmī″əsis/ [Gk, *trypanon + soma + osis,* condition], an infection by an organism of the *Trypanosoma* genus. Also called **trypanosomal infection.** Kinds include **African trypanosomiasis, Chagas disease.**

trypanosomicide /trip′ənōsō″misīd/ [Gk, *trypanon + soma + L, caedere,* to kill]. See **trypanocide.**

trypsin /trip′sin/ [Gk, *tripsis,* rubbing], a proteolytic digestive enzyme produced by the exocrine pancreas that catalyzes in the small intestine the breakdown of dietary proteins to peptones, peptides, and amino acids.

trypsin, crystallized, a proteolytic enzyme from the pancreas of the ox, *Bos taurus,* that has been used as a debriding agent for open wounds and ulcers.

trypsin inhibitor, one of a group of peptides, present in such varied sources as soybeans, egg white, and human colostrum, that mask or inhibit the active site of the trypsin molecule. Also called **kunitz inhibitor.**

trypsinogen /tripsin″əjən/ [Gk, *tripsis + genein,* to produce], the inactive precursor form of trypsin. Trypsinogen is secreted in pancreatic juice and converted to active trypsin through the action of enterokinase in the intestine. Also called **protrypsin.**

tryptase. See **proteinase.**

tryptophan (Trp) /trip″təfan/, an amino acid essential for normal growth and nitrogen balance. Tryptophan is the precursor of several important biomolecules, including serotonin and niacin. See also **amino acid, protein.**

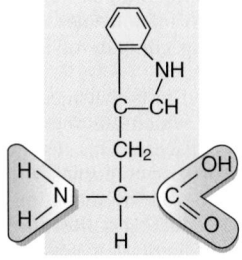

Chemical structure of tryptophan

TSEM, abbreviation for **transmission scanning electron microscopy.**

tsetse fly /tset″sē, tsē″tsē/ [Afr, *tsetse* + AS, *flyge*], a blood-sucking fly found in regions of Africa, mainly south of the Sahara desert. It is an insect of the *Glossina* genus and a secondary host of trypanosomes, which cause African sleeping sickness and other diseases in humans and domestic and wild animals. Also spelled **tzetze fly.** See also **trypanosomiasis.**

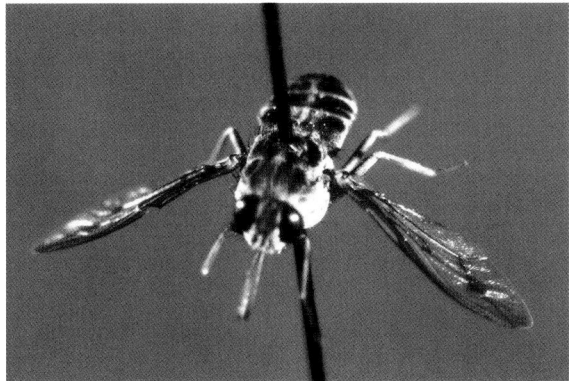

Tsetse fly *(Courtesy Centers for Disease Control and Prevention)*

TSH, abbreviation for **thyroid-stimulating hormone.**

T-shaped fracture, an intercondylar fracture that has both longitudinal and transverse portions in the form of a T.

TSH assay, thyroid-stimulating hormone test.

TSH releasing factor. See **thyrotropin-releasing hormone.**

TSH test, abbreviation for **thyroid-stimulating hormone test.**

tsp, abbreviation for **teaspoon.**

T-spine, thoracic spine.

TSS, abbreviation for **toxic shock syndrome.**

TSA, initialism for **tumor-specific antigen.**

tsutsugamushi disease. See **scrub typhus.**

TT, **1.** abbreviation for **thrombolytic therapy. 2.** abbreviation for **therapeutic touch (TT).**

t test, a statistic test used to determine whether there are differences between two means or between a target value and a calculated mean.

TTP, abbreviation for **thrombotic thrombocytopenic purpura.**

T tube, 1. a tubular device in the shape of a T that is inserted through the skin into a cavity or a wound and used for drainage. **2.** an apparatus used to connect a source of humidified oxygen to the endotracheal tube so that a spirometer can be attached for the evaluation of tidal volume.

T tube cholangiography, a type of biliary tract radiographic examination in which a water-soluble iodinated contrast medium is injected into the bile duct through an indwelling, T-shaped, rubber tube. The tube is inserted in the common bile duct as a routine postoperative procedure to provide drainage.

T tubule system, a system of tubular invaginations along the surface of all striated muscle cell membranes, providing an extension of the membrane into the cells. The system is believed to be part of an extensive endomembrane system involved in storing calcium ions and in the movement of action potentials into the cells. T tubules are likely to be the link between membrane stimulation and the triggering of the release of calcium ions from the sarcoplasmic reticulum.

T.U., 1. abbreviation for *toxin unit.* **2.** abbreviation for *tuberculin unit.*

tubal abortion /t(y)ōō″bəl/ [L, *tubus* + *ab,* away from, *oriri,* to be born], a condition of pregnancy in which an embryo, ectopically implanted, is expelled from the uterine tube into the peritoneal cavity. Tubal abortion is often accompanied by significant internal bleeding, causing acute abdominal and pelvic pain, or it may be asymptomatic, the products of conception being resorbed. Rarely the conceptus reimplants on the peritoneum and continues growing to become an abdominal pregnancy. See also **abdominal pregnancy, ectopic pregnancy, tubal pregnancy.**

tubal air cells, air cells on the floor of the eustachian tube close to the carotid canal.

tubal dermoid cyst, a tumor derived from embryonal tissues that develops in an oviduct.

tubal embryo transfer (TET), 1. a method of artificial reproductive technology consisting of retrieval of oocytes from the ovary, followed by their fertilization and culture in the laboratory with placement of the resulting embryos in the fallopian tubes by laparoscopy more than 24 hours after the original retrieval. **2.** laparoscopic transfer of cryopreserved embryos to the fallopian tubes.

tubal factor infertility, female factor infertility caused by an abnormality of the uterine tubes, such as scarring or obstruction following a urinary tract infection, pelvic inflammation, or sexually transmitted infection.

tubal ligation, one of several sterilization procedures in which both fallopian tubes are blocked to prevent conception from occurring. Through a small abdominal incision, the fallopian tubes are ligated in two places with laser; and the intervening segment is burnt, crushed, or excised. The procedure is less commonly performed vaginally. Complications of the procedure, which are rare but serious, include pulmonary embolism, hemorrhage, infection, and tubal pregnancy. The requirements for informed consent for sterilization procedures vary among states and institutions.

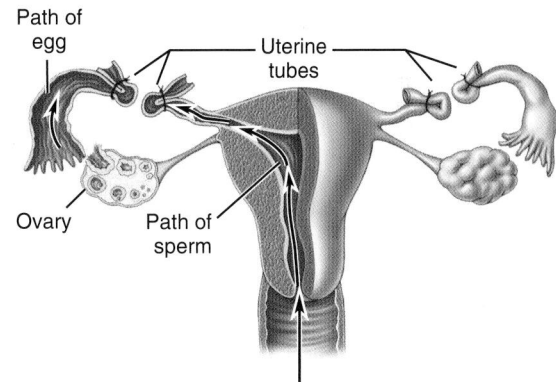

Tubal ligation *(Herlihy, 2011)*

tubal pregnancy, an ectopic pregnancy in which the conceptus implants in the fallopian tube. Approximately 2% of all pregnancies are ectopic; of these, approximately 90% are tubal. Tubal pregnancy seldom occurs in primigravidas. The most important predisposing factor is prior tubal injury. Pelvic infection, scarring and adhesions from surgery, or intrauterine device complications may result in damage that diminishes the motility of the tube. Transport of the ovum through the tube after fertilization is slowed, and implantation takes place before the conceptus reaches the uterine

1832

cavity. Most often the tube, which cannot long contain the growing fetus, ruptures, precipitating an intraperitoneal hemorrhage. If not stopped, the hemorrhaging can lead rapidly to shock and often death. Some conceptuses apparently die and are resorbed in the tube. Diagnosis of tubal pregnancy is often difficult. With rupture of the fallopian tube, women commonly experience sudden sharp pain in one side of the lower abdomen, but signs and symptoms of tubal pregnancy are insidiously variable, and the classic triad of amenorrhea, pelvic pain, and a tender adnexal mass are present only 50% of the time. Recovery of blood from the cul-de-sac by means of culdocentesis is highly suggestive of a ruptured fallopian tube and tubal pregnancy; it requires immediate surgical exploration of the abdomen. Absence of blood on culdocentesis does not rule out the presence of an unruptured tubal pregnancy. Laparotomy may be required, particularly if a woman's pregnancy test is positive, the pelvic findings are suggestive, and sonography of the pelvis cannot demonstrate an intrauterine pregnancy. Because of the lethal potential of an undiagnosed tubal pregnancy, women who report any of the characteristic symptoms early in their pregnancies, particularly during the time before the existence of a normal intrauterine pregnancy can be confirmed, must be considered susceptible. In women who have a history of prior pelvic disease and in those who have symptoms or signs of tubal pregnancy, emergency treatment requires an immediate IV infusion via a large-bore IV catheter, type and crossmatch of blood for blood replacement, and treatment of shock as necessary. In very early ectopic pregnancy, treatment by methotrexate is 90% effective. Otherwise, treatment is surgical and involves laparotomy, removal of the entire products of conception and any intraperitoneal blood present, and the removal or repair of the involved tube. Conditions that predispose to a first tubal pregnancy also predispose to a second; a woman who has had one tubal pregnancy has one chance in five of having another in a subsequent pregnancy. Depending on the location of the developing embryo, the condition is classified as an ampullary, fimbrial, or interstitial tubal pregnancy.

tubal prominence. See **torus tubarius.**

tube /t(y)o͞ob/ [L, *tubus*], a hollow, cylindric piece of equipment or structure of the body.

tube feeding, the administration of nutritionally balanced liquefied foods or nutrients through a tube inserted into the esophagus, stomach, duodenum, or jejunum. Tube feeding may be indicated after mouth or gastric surgery, in cases of severe burns, in paralysis or obstruction of the esophagus, in severe cases of anorexia nervosa, and for unconscious patients or those unable to chew or swallow, among other conditions. Also called *esophageal feeding, gavage feeding,* **jejunostomy feeding, nasogastric feeding.** See also **drip gavage, enteral tube feeding.**

tube gain, the overall electron gain of a photomultiplier tube, calculated as *gn*, where *g* is the dynode gain and *n* is the number of dynodes in the tube. Thus, if *g* is 3 and *n* is 8, the tube gain is 3^8, or 6561. See also **dynode.**

tuber /t(y)o͞o″bər/, a knoblike localized swelling.

tubercle /t(y)o͞o″bərkəl/ [L, *tuber,* swelling], **1.** a nodule or a small eminence, such as that on a bone. **2.** a nodule, especially an elevation of the skin that is larger than a papule, such as Morgagni's tubercles of the areolae of the breasts. **3.** a small rounded nodule produced by infection with *Mycobacterium tuberculosis* and consisting of a gray translucent mass of small spheric cells surrounded by connective cells.

tubercle of sella turcica, the anterior wall of the sella turcica. Also called **tuberculum sellae.**

tubercular /t(y)o͞obur″kyələr/ [L, *tuber,* swelling], pertaining to or resembling tuberculosis.

tuberculid /t(y)o͞obur″kyəlid/, a recurrent skin or mucous membrane lesion in which the tubercle bacillus is absent. It is the result of sensitivity to mycobacterial antigens in patients with tuberculosis.

tuberculin. See **tuberculin test, tuberculosis.**

tuberculin purified protein derivative /to͞obur″kyo͞o lin/, a solution containing a purified protein fraction derived from isolated culture filtrates of strains of *Mycobacterium tuberculosis.* It is used as an aid in the diagnosis of tuberculosis, in the Mantoux test, and, for the same purpose in a dried form, in multiple puncture devices. See also **Mantoux test, tine test.**

tuberculin reaction, hardening or blistering as a delayed reaction at the site of a tuberculin test, a positive result that indicates previous exposure to either the vaccine or the disease.

tuberculin test [L, *tuber + testum,* crucible], a test to determine past or present tuberculosis infection based on a positive skin reaction using one of several methods. A purified protein derivative of tubercle bacilli, called *tuberculin,* is introduced into the skin by scratch, puncture, or intradermal injection. If a raised, red, or hard zone forms surrounding the tuberculin test site, the person is said to be sensitive to tuberculin, and the test is read as positive. A number of factors can affect how the test is interpreted, but an area of induration of 5 mm or less indicates a negative reading. However, a negative tuberculin reaction does not rule out a diagnosis of previous or active tuberculosis. Vaccination with bacille Calmette-Guérin (BCG), a vaccine for tuberculosis, may cause a false-positive reaction to a tuberculin test. Sputum and gastric cultures, acid-fast staining, and x-ray studies often are needed to establish a diagnosis of tuberculosis. Kinds include **Heaf test, Mantoux test, Pirquet test, tine test.**

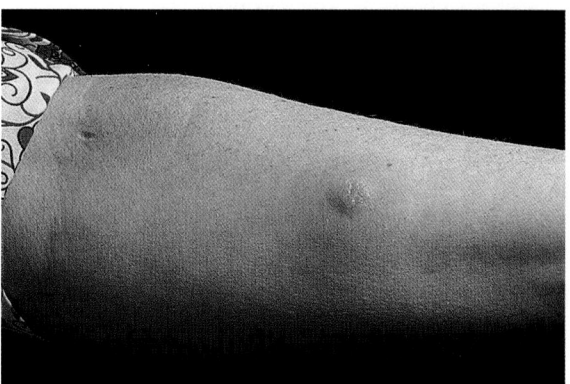

Tuberculin test (positive Mantoux test in a person previously immunized with BCG) *(Cross, 2013)*

tuberculoid leprosy. See **leprosy.**

tuberculoma /t(y)o͞obur′kyəlo̅″mə, to͞obur′kyo͞olo̅″mə/ [L, *tuber* + Gk, *oma,* tumor], a rare tumorlike growth of tuberculous tissue in the central nervous system, characterized by symptoms of an expanding cerebral, cerebellar, or spinal mass. Treatment consists of the administration of antimicrobial drugs to resolve the primary growth and to prevent meningitis.

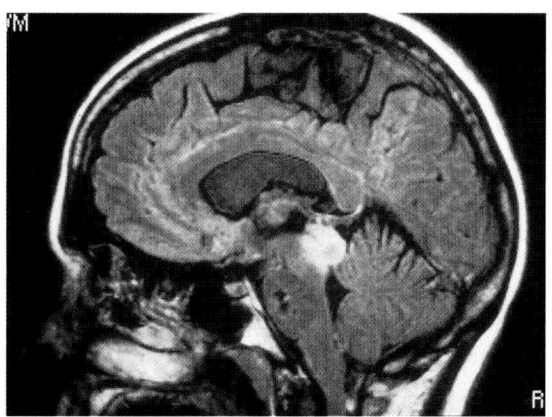

Tuberculoma *(Stone and Gorbach, 2000)*

tuberculosis (TB) /t(y)o͞obur′kyəlō″sis/ [L, *tuber* + Gk, *osis,* condition], a chronic granulomatous infection caused by an acid-fast bacillus, *Mycobacterium tuberculosis.* It is generally transmitted by the inhalation or ingestion of infected droplets and usually affects the lungs, although infection of multiple organ systems occurs. Persons who are immunodeficient, such as those infected with human immunodeficiency virus, may have extrapulmonary tuberculosis. This includes disseminated tuberculosis, which involves multiple organs such as the liver, lung, spleen, bone marrow, and lymph nodes. Diagnosis is through biopsy, stain, sputum and gastric cultures, and x-ray studies. Central nervous system tuberculosis may occur as inflammation of the meninges or a mass lesion (tuberculoma). See also **miliary tuberculosis, tuberculin test.**

■ OBSERVATIONS: Listlessness, vague chest pain, pleurisy, anorexia, fever, and weight loss are early symptoms of pulmonary tuberculosis. Night sweats, pulmonary hemorrhage, expectoration of purulent sputum, and dyspnea develop as the disease progresses. The lung tissues react to the bacillus by producing protective cells that engulf the disease organism, forming tubercles. Untreated, the tubercles enlarge and merge to form larger tubercles that undergo caseation, eventually sloughing off into the cavities of the lungs. Hemoptysis occurs as a result of cavitary spread.

■ INTERVENTIONS: The bacillus is generally sensitive to isoniazid, pyrazinamide, paraaminosalicylic acid, streptomycin, rifampin, ethambutol, dihydrostreptomycin, ultraviolet radiation, and heat. A combination of drugs is prescribed, with regular tests of the function of the kidneys, liver, eyes, and ears to discover early signs of drug toxicity. This is particularly important because drug therapy will usually continue for up to 1 year. The person may be hospitalized for the first weeks of treatment to limit the possible spread of infection, to encourage rest and excellent nutrition, to ensure complete compliance with the prescribed drug regimen, and to observe for adverse drug effects. Samples of sputum are regularly examined. The disease is not infectious after the bacillus is no longer present in the sputum. Care of an outpatient includes continued medication, evaluation for adverse drug effects, sputum analyses, and encouragement to complete the long course of treatment. All contacts are tested periodically with purified protein derivative. People who are at increased risk of infection may be treated empirically, without a positive diagnosis having been made. BCG vaccination has been widely used worldwide but may not be effective at preventing tuberculosis.

■ PATIENT CARE CONSIDERATIONS: Before discharge the patient is taught how to prevent the spread of the disease; the elements of good nutrition; the name, dose, action, and side effects of all medications prescribed; the need to take the drugs regularly; and how and where to get the next supply of drugs. Plans for follow-up care are discussed; they include date, time, and place of the next laboratory tests; referral to community nurses is made. The patient is reminded that a cough, weight loss, fever, night sweats, and hemoptysis are danger signals that are to be reported immediately.

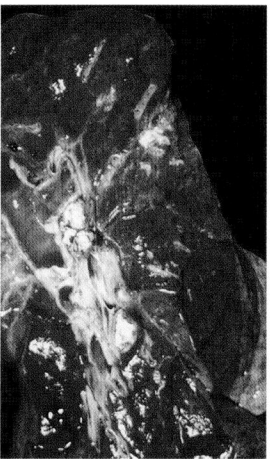

Primary pulmonary tuberculosis *(Kumar et al, 2007)*

tuberculosis culture, a microbiology culture to diagnose tuberculosis. The spread of disease is a possible result of conventional culture techniques, which take 4 to 6 weeks. Newer, more rapid techniques include the BACTEC method, which uses a substrate labeled with radioactive carbon; polymerase chain reaction culture methods, which use genetic DNA probes to detect *Mycobacterium tuberculosis*; and a sputum smear for acid-fast bacillus.

tuberculosis vaccine. See **bacille Calmette-Guérin vaccine.**

tuberculous /t(y)o͞obur″kyələs/ [L, *tuber*], pertaining to tuberculosis.

tuberculous arthritis, a joint inflammation caused by invasion of the joint by tuberculosis bacilli that have migrated from a primary infection, usually in the chest.

tuberculous epididymitis, inflammation and swelling of the epididymis caused by infection with *Mycobacterium tuberculosis,* such as from spread of renal tuberculosis.

tuberculous lymphadenitis [L, *tuber* + *lympha,* water; Gk, *aden,* gland, *itis,* inflammation], an inflammation of the lymph glands caused by the presence of *Mycobacterium tuberculosis.*

tuberculous meningitis. See **meningitis.**

tuberculous peritonitis [L, *tuber* + Gk, *peri* + *teinein,* to stretch, *itis,* inflammation], an inflammation of the peritoneum that is secondary to a tuberculous infection in the viscera.

tuberculous pneumonia [L, *tuber* + Gk, *pneumon,* lung], a complication of tuberculosis in which caseous material is inhaled into the bronchi, leading to bronchopneumonia or lobar pneumonia.

tuberculous prostatitis, a type of granulomatous prostatitis caused by infection with *Mycobacterium tuberculosis.*

tuberculous spondylitis, a rare, grave form of tuberculosis caused by the invasion of *Mycobacterium tuberculosis* into the spinal vertebrae. The intervertebral disks may be destroyed, resulting in the collapse and wedging of affected vertebrae and the shortening and angulation of the spine. Thoracic vertebrae are more frequently involved than the vertebrae of the lumbar, cervical, or sacral segments of the spine. More than one area of the spine may be affected, and normal vertebrae may be evident between affected sections. The infection characteristically dissects vertebrae anterolaterally and produces abscesses. The pressure of the abscess may cause ischemic paralysis in the subjacent spinal cord, and abscesses in the cervical area may displace or obstruct the trachea and the esophagus. Treatment requires an extended regimen of at least three anti-tuberculosis drugs. Also called **Pott's disease, spinal caries.** See also **tuberculosis.**

tuberculum /t(y)oŏbur″kyələm/, a tubercle, nodule, or rounded elevation.

tuberculum sellae. See **tubercle of sella turcica.**

tuberosity /t(y)oŏ′bərosʺitē/ [L, *tuber*], an elevation or protuberance, especially of a bone.

tuberosity of the tibia, a large oblong elevation at the proximal end of the tibia to which the ligament of the patella attaches.

tuberous carcinoma /t(y)oŏʺbərəs/ [L, *tuber* + Gk, *karkinos,* crab, *oma,* tumor], a scirrhous carcinoma of the skin characterized by nodular projections. Also called **carcinoma tuberosum.**

tuberous sclerosis, an autosomal-dominant neurocutaneous disease; it is characterized by epilepsy, mental deterioration, adenoma sebaceum, nodules and sclerotic patches on the cerebral cortex, retinal tumors, depigmented leaf-shaped macules on the skin, tumors of the heart or kidneys, and cerebral calcifications. There is no cure at the present time. Also called **Bourneville disease, epiloia.** See also **adenoma sebaceum.**

tuberous xanthoma, small, firm tumors occurring on the extensor surfaces of the elbows and knees or on the joints of the hands and feet. See **xanthoma tuberosum.**

tube-slide agglutination test, a type of sperm agglutination test in which sperm and serum are mixed in a tube and then transferred to a slide for examination.

tubo- /t(y)oŏ′bō-, t(y)oŏ′bə-/, combining form meaning "tube" or "tubing": *tubular.*

tuboabdominal gestation /-abdom′inəl/ [L, *tubus* + *abdomen,* belly; L, *gestare,* to bear], an ectopic pregnancy in which the embryo develops while partly in the abdominal cavity and partly in the fallopian tube. The condition usually begins as a tubal pregnancy and extends into the abdomen as development continues. Also called *tuboabdominal pregnancy.*

tubocurarine chloride. See **curare.**

tubo-ovarian /t(y)oŏ′bō·ōverʺē·ən/ [L, *tubus* + *ovum,* egg], pertaining to the ovary and fallopian tube. Also *tubo-ovarial.*

tubo-ovarian abscess [L, *tubus* + *ovum* + *abscedere,* to go away], an abscess involving the ovary and fallopian tube. It is commonly associated with salpingitis.

tubo-ovarian cyst [L, *tubus* + *ovum* + Gk, *kystis,* bag], a cyst that forms by adhesion of the ovary at the fimbriated end of the fallopian tube.

tubo-ovarian gestation [L, *tubus* + *ovum* + *gestare,* to bear], an ectopic pregnancy that develops partly in the fallopian tube and partly in the ovary. Also called *tubo-ovarian pregnancy.*

tuboplasty /t(y)oŏʺbōplas′tē/ [L, *tubus,* tube; Gk, *plassein,* to mold], a surgical procedure in which severed or damaged fallopian tubes are repaired in the hope of restoring fertility.

tubular, pertaining to a long, hollow structure.

tubular capillary plexus, a vascular network formed by the capillaries around the renal tubules.

tubular maximum, the highest rate in milligrams per minute at which the renal tubules can transfer a substance. See **transport maximum.**

tubular necrosis [L, *tubulus,* little tube; Gk, *nekros,* dead, *osis,* condition], the death of cells in the small tubules of the kidneys as a result of disease or injury.

tubule /t(y)oŏʺbyoŏl/ [L, *tubulus*], a small tube, such as one of the collecting tubules in the kidneys, the seminiferous tubules of the testes, or Henle's tubules between the distal and proximal convoluted tubules. **−tubular,** *adj.*

tubulin binding agents, a group of medications that bind tubulin and arrest cell mitosis. Abnormal blood vessels in tumors are particularly sensitive to these agents.

tubuloglomerular feedback, a feedback mechanism in the juxtaglomerular apparatus of the kidney so that changes in solute concentration at the macula densa link to control the glomerular filtration rate and help ensure a relatively constant delivery of solutes to the distal tubule.

tuft [Fr, *touffe,* a tuft], an object resembling a tassel, such as a tuft of hair.

tuft fracture [Fr, *touffe,* tuft; L, *fractura,* break], a break in any one of the distal phalanges.

tug [ME, *toggen,* to pull], a dragging or hauling movement or sensation.

tularemia /toŏ′lərē″mē·ə/ [Tulare, California; Gk, *haima,* blood], an infectious disease of animals caused by the bacillus *Francisella (Pasteurella) tularensis,* which may be transmitted by insect vectors or direct contact. It is characterized in humans by fever, headache, and an ulcerated skin lesion with localized lymph node enlargement or by eye infection, GI ulcerations, or pneumonia, depending on the site of entry and the response of the host. This disease can be fatal if not treated with the appropriate antibiotics. Treatment includes streptomycin, chloramphenicol, and tetracycline. Recovery produces lifelong immunity. A vaccine was used in the past to protect laboratory workers but is not currently available; however, a new vaccine is in development. Also called **deerfly fever, rabbit fever.** Also spelled *tularaemia.*

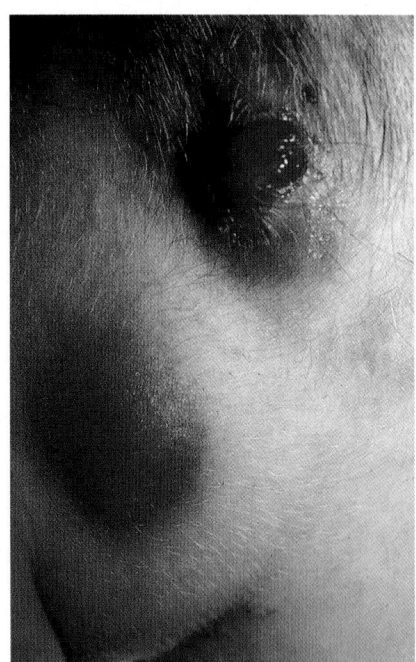

Tularemia *(Stone and Gorbach, 2000)*

TULIP, abbreviation for **transurethral laser-induced prostatectomy.**

tumescence /t(y)oŏmes″əns/ [L, *tumescere,* to begin to swell], a state of swelling or edema.

-tumescence, combining form meaning "a swelling."

tumescent anesthesia, administration of a dilute local infiltration anesthetic (lidocaine) through the use of large volumes of fluid. The technique is applied in liposuction surgery, varicose vein treatment, scalp surgery, dermabrasion, and soft tissue reconstruction.

tummy tuck. *(Informal)* See **abdominoplasty.**

tumor (T) /t(y)o͞o″mər/ [L], **1.** a swelling or enlargement occurring in inflammatory conditions. **2.** a new growth of tissue characterized by progressive, uncontrolled proliferation of cells. The tumor may be localized or invasive, benign or malignant. A tumor may be named for its location, for its cellular makeup, or for the person who first identified it. Also called **neoplasm.**

tumor albus, a white swelling occurring in a tuberculous bone or joint.

tumor angiogenesis factor (TAF), a protein that stimulates the formation of blood vessels in tumors. See also **angiogenin.**

tumoricidal. See **tumoricide.**

tumoricidal agent, an agent that is destructive to cancer cells. See also **antineoplastic.**

tumoricide /t(y)o͞omôr″isīd/, a substance capable of destroying a tumor. **–tumoricidal,** *adj.*

tumorigenesis /t(y)o͞o′mərijen″əsis/, the process of initiating and promoting the development of a tumor. Compare **carcinogenesis, oncogenesis, sarcomagenesis. –tumorigenic,** *adj.*

tumorigenic /-jen″ik/ [L, swelling; Gk, to produce], capable of producing tumors.

tumor-induced osteomalacia (TIO), a rare disorder caused by tumors that secrete fibroblast growth factor 23 (FGF23). It is characterized by bone pain, muscle weakness, and fractures due to bone demineralization. Also called **oncogenous osteomalacia.**

tumor lysis syndrome, an oncological emergency characterized by a decreased calcium level with elevated phosphate, potassium, and uric acid levels occuring after effective induction chemotherapy of rapidly growing malignant neoplasms; thought to be due to release of intracellular products after cell lysis.

tumor marker, a substance in the body that may be associated with the presence of a cancer.

tumor necrosis factor (TNF), a natural body protein, also produced synthetically, with anticancer effects. The body produces it in response to the presence of toxic substances, such as bacterial toxins. Adverse effects are toxic shock and cachexia.

tumor necrosis factor receptor–associated periodic syndrome (TRAPS). See **familial periodic fever.**

tumor registry, a repository of data on the incidence of cancers and personal characteristics, treatment, and treatment outcomes of patients diagnosed with cancer.

tumor-specific antigen (TSA), an antigen produced by a particular type of tumor that does not appear on normal cells of the tissue in which the tumor developed. The marker can be used for diagnostic purposes and, in some cases, holds potential for treatment purposes.

tumor suppressor gene, a gene whose function is to limit cell proliferation and loss of whose function leads to cell transformation and tumor growth. Kinds include the *p53 gene.* Also called **antioncogene.**

tumor viruses [L, *tumor,* swelling, *virus,* poison], viruses that are capable of directly or indirectly inducing tumor formation. Direct tumor formation may result from inoculation of living cells with tumorigenic viruses. Tumor formation may result from the influence of the virus on normal cells that are transformed into tumor cells.

tumor volume, a part of an organ or tissue that includes both the tumor and adjacent areas of invasion.

Tunga penetrans. See **chigoe.**

tungiasis /tung·gī′ə·sis/, infestation of the skin with the chigoe (*Tunga penetrans*).

tungsten (W) /tung″stən/ [SW, *tung,* heavy, *sten,* stone; *wolfram,* the German word for tungsten], a metallic element. Its atomic number is 74; its atomic mass is 183.85. It has the highest melting point of all metals and is used as a target material in x-ray tubes and as filaments in incandescent light bulbs.

tunica /t(y)o͞o″nikə/ [L, tunic], an enveloping coat or covering membrane.

tunica adventitia, the outer layer or coat of an artery or other tubular structure. See also **arterial wall.**

tunica albuginea [L, *tunica + albus,* white], a tissue covering of white collagenous fibers, such as the sclerotic coat of the eyeball and the testes.

tunica dartos. See **dartos fascia.**

tunica intima, the membrane lining an artery. See also **arterial wall.**

tunica media, a muscular middle coat of an artery. See also **arterial wall.**

tunica vaginalis testis, the serous membrane surrounding the testis and epididymis, derived from the peritoneum.

tunica vasculosa bulbi, the uvea of the eye, consisting of the iris, ciliary body, and choroid.

tuning fork /t(y)o͞o″ning/ [Gk, *tonos,* stretching; L, *furca,* fork], a small metal instrument consisting of a stem and two prongs that produces a constant pitch when either prong is struck. It is used by health care providers as a screening test of air and bone conduction.

tunnel [OFr, *tonnel,* fowl trap], a canal or passage, such as the carpal tunnel.

tunneled catheter, a central venous catheter left in place for a long period so that scar tissue forms and anchors it in place.

tunnel vision [OFr, *tonnel,* fowl trap; L, *videre,* to see], a defect in sight in which there is a great reduction in the peripheral field of vision, as if looking through a hollow tube or tunnel. The condition occurs in advanced glaucoma.

tunnel wound [OFr, *tonnel* + AS, *wund*], a break in the surface of the body or an organ in which the entry and exit wounds are the same size.

TUR, abbreviation for **transurethral resection.**

turban tumor /tur″bən/ [Turk, *tulbend,* headdress; L, *tumor,* swelling], a benign neoplasm consisting of pink or maroon nodules that may cover the entire scalp, trunk, and extremities. The growth is familial and often recurs after excision.

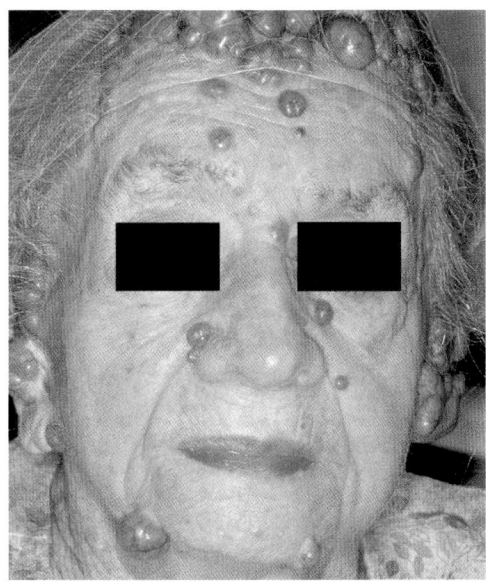

Turban tumor *(du Vivier, 2002/Courtesy Queen Victorial Hospital)*

turbid /tur″bid/ [L, *turbidus,* confused], clouded or obscured, as in solids in suspension in a solution.

turbidimetry /tur″bidim″ətrē/ [L, *turbidus,* confused; Gk, *metron,* measure], measurement of the turbidity (cloudiness) of a solution or suspension in which the amount of transmitted light is quantified with a spectrophotometer or estimated by visual comparison with solutions of known turbidity.

turbidity /tərbid″itē/ [L, *turbidus*], a condition of light scattering in a liquid resulting from the presence of suspended particles. Turbidity increases with the concentration of particles and depends on their shapes and sizes.

turbinate /tur″binit/ [L, *turbinum,* top-shaped], **1.** pertaining to a scroll shape. **2.** pertaining to the concha nasalis.

turgid /tur″jid/ [L, *turgidus*], swollen, hard, and congested, usually as a result of an accumulation of fluid. Compare **flaccid. –turgor,** *n.*

turgor /tur″gər/ [L, *turgere,* to be swollen], the expected resiliency of the skin caused by the outward pressure of the cells and interstitial fluid. Dehydration results in decreased skin turgor, manifested by lax skin that, when grasped and raised between two fingers, slowly returns to a position level with the adjacent tissue. Marked edema or ascites results in increased turgor manifested by smooth, taut, shiny skin that cannot be grasped and raised. The older adult normally has reduced skin turgor because of a lack of skin elasticity, an expected part of aging. An evaluation of the skin turgor is an essential part of physical assessment.

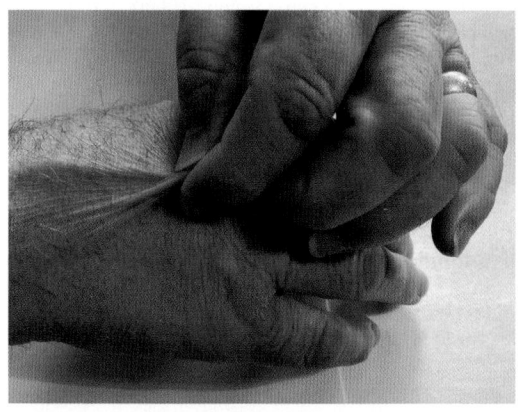

Testing for skin turgor

turista. See **traveler's diarrhea.**

turnbuckle cast [AS, *tyrnan* + ME, *bocle,* small shield; ONorse, *kasta*], an orthopedic device incorporating a hinge with a threaded screw and wingnut; it is used to encase and immobilize an area of the body. An adaptation of the turnbuckle cast is used occasionally as a hyperextension cast for the treatment of kyphosis or kyphoscoliosis. Compare **Risser cast.**

Turner sign, bruising of the flanks. See **Grey Turner sign.**

Turner syndrome [Henry H. Turner, American endocrinologist, 1892–1970], a chromosomal anomaly seen in about 1 in 3000 live female births, characterized by the absence of one X chromosome; congenital ovarian failure; genital hypoplasia; cardiovascular anomalies; dwarfism; short metacarpals; "shield chest"; exostosis of tibia; and underdeveloped breasts, uterus, and vagina. Spatial disorientation and moderate degrees of learning disorders are common. Treatment includes genetic counseling, hormone therapy (estrogens, androgens, pituitary growth hormone), and often surgical correction of cardiovascular anomalies and the webbing of the neck skin. Also called **Bonnevie-Ullrich syndrome, monosomy X.** See also **Noonan syndrome.**

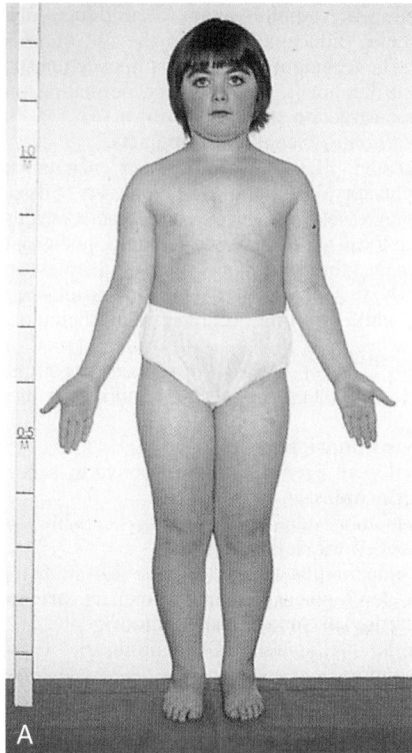
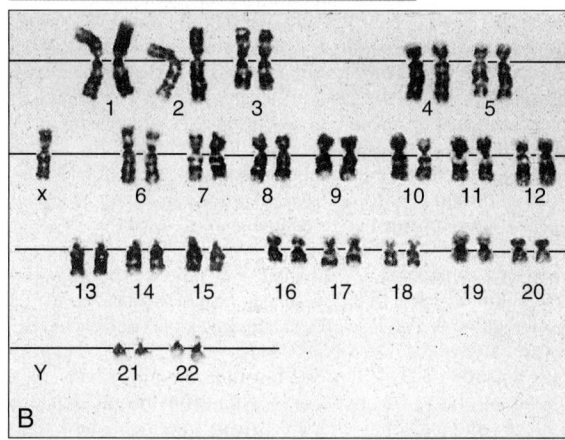

A, Child with Turner syndrome. B, Chromosome map for Turner syndrome *(Patton and Thibodeau, 2010)*

turning sheet. See **drawsheet.**

turnkey /turn″kē/, a term referring to a computer system or installation that is complete on delivery and ready to operate without modification.

TURP, abbreviation for **transurethral resection of the prostate.**

turricephaly. See **oxycephaly.**

TUR syndrome, severe hyponatremia caused by the absorption of fluids used to irrigate the bladder during transurethral resection of the prostate.

-tuse, 1. suffix meaning "dull" or "blunt": *obtuse.* **2.** suffix meaning "to beat or bruise": *contuse.*

Tussionex, a fixed-combination drug containing an antitussive and an antihistamine. Brand name for **hydrocodone bitartrate, phenyltoloxamine citrate.**

tussis /tus″is/ [L, *tussis,* cough], a cough or pertussis.

tussive, pertaining to or due to a cough.

tussive fremitus /tus″iv/ [L, *tussis,* cough, *fremitus,* murmuring], a vibratory cough that can be felt by a hand over the chest of the patient.

tussive headache, pain or discomfort in the head caused by traction on the meninges and cerebral vessels associated with coughing.

tussive syncope, a fainting episode caused by an increase in intrathoracic pressure associated with paroxysms of coughing. Recovery of consciousness and lucidity is rapid.

tutamen, a protective covering or structure, such as the eyelids and eyelashes.

tutorial /t(y)o͞otôr″ē·əl/ [L, *tueri,* to look with care], a form of instruction in which a learner is guided step-by-step through the application of knowledge to a clinical situation or computer application.

TV, the amount of air in milliliters per breath. Abbreviation for **tidal volume.**

TVL, abbreviation for **tenth-value layer.**

T wave, the component of the cardiac cycle shown on an electrocardiogram as a short, inverted, U-shaped curve after the S-T segment. It represents membrane repolarization phase 3 of the cardiac action potential.

Tweed triangle [Charles Tweed, American dentist, 1895–1970; L, *triangulus,* three-cornered], the triangle formed by the mandibular plane, the Frankfort horizontal plane, and the long axis of the lower central incisor. It is used as a diagnostic aid.

Tween 80 /twēn/, a preparation of polysorbate 80, a surfactant.

twelfth cranial nerve. See **hypoglossal nerve.**

twentieth-century syndrome. See **total allergy syndrome.**

24-hour clock system, a method of designating time by using the numeric sequence from 00 to 23 for the hours and the numbers 00 to 59 for the minutes in a daily cycle beginning with 0000 (midnight) and ending with 2359 (1 minute before the next midnight). The system provides a clear distinction between prenoon and afternoon time without requiring the designations AM and PM.

twiddler's syndrome, the nervous habit of slight manipulation of entry portals causing the displacement of inserted wires or catheters.

twilight state [Ger, *Zwielicht,* twilight; L, *status*], an impaired state of consciousness in which the patient may experience visual or auditory hallucinations and responds to them with irrational behavior. The person may be unaware of the surroundings at the time of the experience and have no memory of it later, except perhaps to recall a related dream. It may be induced with certain anesthetics. Also called **deep sedation.**

twin [AS, *twinn,* double], either of two offspring born of the same pregnancy and developed from either a single ovum or from two ova that were released from the ovary simultaneously and fertilized at the same time. The incidence of twin births is approximately 1 in 80 pregnancies. Kinds include **conjoined twins, dizygotic twins, interlocked twins, monozygotic twins, Siamese twins, unequal twins.** See also **Hellin's law.**

twinge /twinj/ [ME, *twengen,* to pinch], a sudden, brief, darting pain.

twinning [AS, *twinn*], **1.** the development of two or more fetuses during the same pregnancy, either spontaneously or through external intervention for experimental purposes in animals. **2.** the duplication of like structures or parts by division.

twin-to-twin transfusion, an intrauterine abnormality of fetal circulation in monozygotic twins in which blood is shunted directly from one twin to the other.

twin-twin transfusion syndrome, a syndrome caused by twin-to-twin transfusion in which the donor twin develops hypovolemia, hypotension, anemia, microcardia, and growth delay while the recipient twin develops hypervolemia, hypertension, polycythemia, cardiomegaly, and congestive heart failure. Hydramnios frequently occurs.

twin-wire orthodontic appliance, a fixed orthodontic appliance that typically uses a pair of 0.01-inch (0.25-mm) wires to form the midsection of the arch wire. It is used to correct the crowding of anterior teeth and to expand the dental arch.

twitch [AS, *twiccian*], **1.** the contraction of small muscle units, manifested as a quick, simple, spasmodic contraction of a muscle. **2.** to jerk convulsively.

twitching [AS, *twiccian*], a series of contractions by small muscle units. Twitching that involves large groups of muscle fibers is identified as fascicular twitching.

two-point discrimination test, a test of the ability of a person to differentiate touch stimuli at two nearby points on the body at the same time. It is used in studies of possible damage to the parietal regions of the brain.

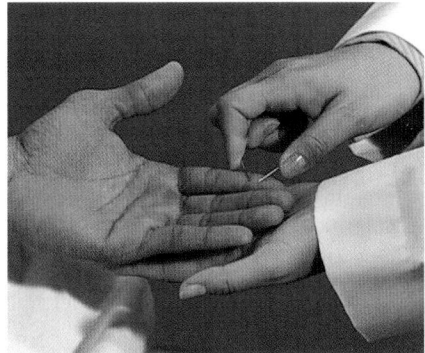

Two-point discrimination test *(Ball et al, 2015)*

two-point gait [OE, *twa* + L, *punctus,* pricked; ONorse, *gata,* way], a pattern of crutch-walking in which the right foot and left crutch advance together, followed by the left foot and right crutch. See also **three-point gait.**

two-way catheter [AS, *twa* + *weg* + Gk, *katheter,* something lowered], a catheter that has a double lumen, one channel for injection of medication or fluids and the other for removal of fluid or specimens.

TXA2, abbreviation for **thromboxane A2.**

TXB2, abbreviation for **thromboxane B2.**

Tygacil, an antibiotic medication. Brand name for **tigecycline.**

tying forceps, a thumb forceps with fine, smooth tips for tying sutures in ophthalmological surgery.

Tykerb, an agent that targets epidermal growth factor receptor (EGFR) and human epidermal growth factor receptor-2 (HER2), both of which are frequently overexpressed in human cancer. Brand name for **lapatinib.**

Tylenol, an analgesic and antipyretic medication. Brand name for **acetaminophen.**

tylosis /tīlō″sis/, a rare autosomal-dominant disease; it is characterized by hyperkeratosis on the palms of the hands and soles of the feet with a high rate of esophageal cancer.

tyloxapol /tīlok″səpôl/, an ocular lubricant used to lubricate, clean, and wet artificial eyes to improve wearing comfort; it also has a detergent action that is used to help break up mucus.

tympan-, combining form meaning "the tympanic membrane": *tympanoplasty, tympanotomy.*

tympana. See **tympanic.**

tympanal. See **tympanic.**

tympanectomy /tim″pənek″təmē/ [Gk, *tympanon,* drum, *ektomē,* excision], the surgical removal of the tympanic membrane.

tympanic /timpan″ik/ [Gk, *tympanon,* drum], *n.,* pertaining to a structure that resonates when struck; drumlike, such as a *tympanic abdomen* that resonates on percussion because the intestines are distended with gas. Also called **tympanal.**

tympanic antrum, a relatively large, irregular cavity in the superior anterior part of the mastoid process of the temporal bone, communicating with the mastoid air cells and lined by the extension of the mucous membrane of the tympanic cavity. The bony tegmen tympani separates the tympanic antrum from the middle fossa of the cranial cavity, and the lateral semicircular canal of the internal ear projects into the antrum. See also **mastoid process.**

tympanic cavity. See **middle ear.**

tympanic cells, tympanic air cells, spaces in the tympanic cavity between the bony projections of the floor or jugular wall that sometimes communicate with the tubal air cells.

tympanic membrane, a thin, semitransparent membrane in the middle ear that transmits sound vibrations to the internal ear by means of the auditory ossicles. It is nearly oval in form, with a vertical diameter of about 10 mm, and separates the tympanic cavity from the bottom of the external acoustic meatus. Also called **eardrum, membrana tympani.**

tympanic membrane thermometer, a device that measures the temperature of the tympanic membrane by detecting infrared radiation from the tissue. Results are obtained within 2 seconds and directly reflect the body's core temperature. *Tympanic thermometer* is the common term. See also **ear thermometry.**

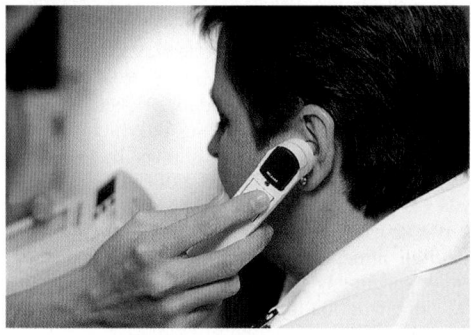

Tympanic membrane thermometer *(Potter et al, 2011)*

tympanic nerve, a branch of the glossopharyngeal nerve that participates in the formation of the tympanic plexus and provides sensory innervation within the middle ear to the mucosa of the cavity, pharyngotympanic tube, and mastoid air cells. It also contributes general visceral efferent fibers, which leave the tympanic plexus in the lesser petrosal nerve.

tympanic reflex, the reflection of a beam of light shining on the eardrum. In a normal ear, a bright, wedge-shaped reflection is seen. Its apex is at the end of the malleus, and its base is at the anterior inferior margin of the eardrum. In disorders of the middle ear or eardrum, this shape may be distorted.

tympanic resonance [Gk, *tympanon* + L, *resonare,* to sound again], a drumlike or hollow sound heard over a large air space of the body such as the pneumothorax.

tympanic sulcus [Gk, *tympanon,* drum; L, *sulcus,* furrow], a narrow circular groove at the medial end of the osseous part of the external acoustic meatus that holds the tympanic membrane.

tympanic temperature, the body temperature as measured electronically at the tympanic membrane. See also **tympanic membrane thermometer.**

tympano-, prefix meaning "eardrum or tympanic membrane": *tympanoplasty, tympanotomy.*

tympanogram /timpan″əgram/, a graphic representation of the acoustic impedance and air pressure of the middle ear and the mobility of the tympanic membrane, measured as part of the audiological test battery. In the normal middle ear, the air pressure is the same as the atmospheric pressure, as shown by a peak in the middle of the tympanogram. Various middle ear pathologies such as otitis media, otosclerosis, or tympanic membrane perforations each yield distinctive tympanograms. See also **acoustic impedance.**

tympanomastoidectomy, mastoidectomy with tympanectomy, done as either closed cavity or open cavity.

tympanometry, a test used to evaluate conditions in the middle ear by evaluating the movement of the tympanic membrane in response to sound and differing air pressures.

tympanoplasty /timpan″əplas′tē/ [Gk, *tympanon* + *plassein,* to mold], any of several operative procedures on the eardrum or ossicles of the middle ear designed to restore or improve hearing in patients with conductive hearing loss. These operations may be used to repair a perforated eardrum, for otosclerosis, or for dislocation or necrosis of one of the small bones of the middle ear. See also **myringoplasty, stapedectomy.**

tympanosclerosis, a condition characterized by the presence of masses of hard, dense connective tissue around the auditory ossicles in the middle ear.

tympanostomy. See **myringotomy.**

tympanotomy. See **myringotomy.**

tympanum, the typanic cavity.

tympany /tim″pənē/ [Gk, *tympanon,* drum], a loud, high-pitched musical sound percussed over the upper gastric area or a pneumothorax.

-type, suffix meaning a "representative form or class": *lysotype, phenotype, somatotype.*

type, the general or prevailing character of any particular case, such as of a disease, person or substance.

type I AV block. See **Mobitz I heart block.**

type 1 diabetes mellitus, an autoimmune disease characterized by inability to metabolize fuels, carbohydrates, protein, and fat because of absolute insulin deficiency. Type 1 diabetes can occur at any age, but its incidence is more common in children. Uncontrolled type 1 diabetes is characterized by excessive thirst, increased urination, increased desire to eat, loss of weight, ketoacidosis, diminished strength, and marked irritability. The clinical onset is usually rapid, but approximately one third of patients have a remission within 3 months (honeymoon phase). This stage may continue for days or months, but type 1 diabetes then progresses quickly to a state of total dependence on insulin. Persons with type 1 diabetes can manage their condition with a carbohydrate-controlled meal plan, exercise, and insulin. Evidence suggests that type 1 diabetes may be triggered by environmental factors, such as a viral infection in genetically susceptible individuals. Compare **type 2 diabetes mellitus.** Formerly called **juvenile diabetes.** See also **diabetes mellitus.**

type 1 antineuronal antibody (ANNA-1).   See **anti-Hu antibody.**

type I error,   **1.** in a test of a statistical hypothesis, the probability of rejecting the null hypothesis when it is true and should be accepted. It occurs when researchers observe a difference when in fact there is none. Also called **alpha error,** *error of the first kind.* **2.** a false negative.

type I hyperlipidemia.   See **hyperlipidemia type I.**

type I hypersensitivity,   hypersensitivity that occurs rapidly, within several minutes, on reexposure to an antigen. Reexposure cross-links the immunoglobulin E present on basophils and mast cells, resulting in degranulation and the secretion of products such as histamine and leukotrienes. Anaphylaxis is a particularly severe type I hypersensitivity reaction. Also called **immediate hypersensitivity reaction.** See **anaphylactic hypersensitivity.**

type 2 antineuronal antibody (ANNA-2).   See **anti-Ri antibody.**

type II AV block.   See **Mobitz II heart block.**

type 2 diabetes mellitus,   a type of diabetes mellitus characterized by insulin resistance, inappropriate hepatic glucose production, and impaired insulin secretion. Onset is usually after 40 years of age but can occur at any age, including during childhood and adolescence. A strong family history of diabetes implies both genetic factors and environmental factors exist. Obesity and a sedentary lifestyle superimposed on genetic susceptibility will hasten the onset of the disease. The majority (>90%) of persons with type 2 diabetes are obese; in these patients glucose tolerance is often improved by modest weight loss and an increase in activity. Persons with type 2 diabetes can manage their disorder with a meal plan; an increase in activity; oral antidiabetes agents such as insulin secretagogues, biguanides, alpha glucosidase inhibitors, and insulin sensitizers; and insulin. Maturity onset diabetes of the young is a rare type 2 diabetes, and an autosomal-dominant inheritance is clearly established. Also called *type II diabetes mellitus.* Formerly called **adult-onset diabetes, ketosis-resistant diabetes, maturity-onset diabetes, non–insulin-dependent diabetes mellitus, stabile diabetes.** See also **diabetes mellitus.**

type II error,   in a test of a statistical hypothesis, the probability of accepting the null hypothesis when it is false and should be rejected. Also called **beta error,** *error of the second kind.*

type II hypersensitivity,   complement-dependent hypersensitivity to foreign cells or to alterations of cell-surface antigens that is mediated by immunoglobulins G (IgG) and M (IgM), causing immediate destruction of cells, as seen in hemolytic disease of the newborn and in severe transfusion reactions. A second type of type II hypersensitivity is called antibody-dependent cell-mediated cytotoxicity (ADCC). Here IgG- or IgM-coated cells are recognized by natural killer cells, and macrophages are subsequently killed. Also called **cytotoxic anaphylaxis.**

type III hypersensitivity,   a local or general inflammatory response caused by the formation of circulating antigen-antibody complexes and their disposition in tissues. Also called *immune complex–mediated hypersensitivity reaction.*

type IV hypersensitivity,   a reaction initiated by antigen-specific T lymphocytes. Unlike hypersensitivity reactions mediated by antibodies, this type takes one or more days to develop, and the hypersensitivity can be transferred by lymphocytes but not by serum. The term is often equated with delayed hypersensitivity reactions that are cytokine-mediated (as contrasted with direct cytolysis). Also called

cell-mediated hypersensitivity, T cell-mediated hypersensitivity reaction.

type A personality [Gk, *typos,* mark],   a parent ego state characterized by a behavior pattern described by Friedman and Rosenman as associated with individuals who are highly competitive and work compulsively to meet deadlines. The behavior also is associated with a higher than usual incidence of coronary heart disease.

type B personality,   a child ego state characterized by a form of behavior associated by Friedman and Rosenman with people who appear free of hostility and aggression and who lack a compulsion to meet deadlines, are not highly competitive at work and play, and have a lower risk of heart attack.

type E personality,   a term introduced by Harriet Braiker to describe professional women who fit neither type A nor type B personality categories but who have a marked sense of insecurity and strive to convince themselves that they are worthwhile. Type E women try to be "all things to all people," according to Braiker, and tend to suffer psychological strain. Also called **adult ego state.**

type specificity.   See **specificity.**

typhlo-,   combining form meaning "cecum": *typhlosole.*

typhlosole,   a fold in the intestinal wall of some invertebrates.

typho-,   prefix meaning "fever" and related to typhus and typhoid fevers.

typhoid /tī″foid/   [Gk, *typhos,* fever, *eidos,* form],   pertaining to or resembling typhus.

-typhoid,   suffix meaning "typhus": *paratyphoid.*

typhoid carrier,   a person without signs or symptoms of typhoid fever who carries the bacteria that cause the disease and sheds the pathogens in body excretions. The typical typhoid carrier has recovered from an attack of the disease.

typhoid fever [Gk, *typhos,* fever, *eidos,* form; L, *febris,* fever],   a bacterial infection usually caused by *Salmonella typhi* and transmitted by contaminated milk, water, or food. It is characterized by headache, delirium, cough, watery diarrhea, rash, and a high fever. The incubation period may be as long as 60 days. Characteristic maculopapular rosy spots are scattered over the skin of the abdomen and chest. Splenomegaly and leukopenia develop first. Complications include intestinal hemorrhage or perforation and thrombophlebitis. The disease is serious and may be fatal. Treatment is with antibiotics. Some people who recover continue to be carriers and excrete the organism, spreading the disease. Two vaccines are available to prevent typhoid fever. Also called **cesspool fever, enteric fever.** Compare **cholera, paratyphoid fever, salmonellosis.**

typhoid nodules [Gk, *typhos,* fever; L, *nodulus,* small knot],   a liver nodule consisting of a cluster of monocytes and lymphocytes surrounding the typhoid fever pathogen, *Salmonella typhi.*

typhoid pellagra,   a form of pellagra in which the symptoms also include continued high temperatures.

typhoid vaccine,   a bacterial vaccine prepared from an inactivated dried strain of *Salmonella typhi.*

■ INDICATIONS: It is prescribed for primary immunization against typhoid fever for adults and children. According to the National Institutes of Health, routine typhoid vaccination is not recommended in the United States. It is only recommended for those who are traveling to areas outside of the United States to areas where typhoid is common.

■ CONTRAINDICATIONS: Acute infection or concomitant use of corticosteroids prohibits its use.

T

■ ADVERSE EFFECTS: Among the more serious adverse effects are anaphylaxis and pain and inflammation at the site of injection.

typhoid vaccine live oral, a preparation of the attenuated strain *Salmonella typhi* Ty21a. It is administered orally.

typhomania /tīfōmā″nē·ə/, a condition characterized by coma and delirium and associated with typhus, typhoid fever, and similar febrile infections.

typhous /tī″fəs/ [Gk, *typhos,* fever], pertaining to typhus fever.

typhus /tī″fəs/ [Gk, *typhos,* fever], any of a group of acute infectious diseases caused by various species of *Rickettsia* and usually transmitted from infected rodents to humans by the bites of lice, fleas, mites, or ticks. Kinds include **epidemic typhus, murine typhus, scrub typhus.** See also **Brill-Zinsser disease, Rocky Mountain spotted fever.**

■ OBSERVATIONS: These diseases are all characterized by headache, chills, fever, malaise, and a maculopapular rash.

■ INTERVENTIONS: Doxycycline and chloramphenicol are the antibiotics of choice for treatment.

■ PATIENT CARE CONSIDERATIONS: A typhus vaccine is available.

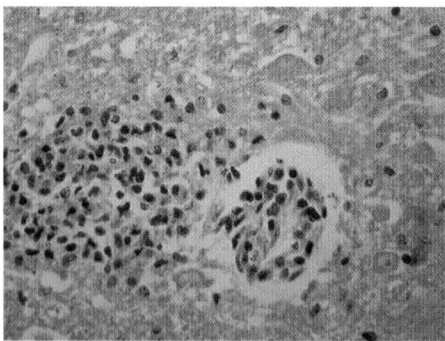

Typhus nodule in the brain *(Kumar et al, 2010)*

typhus vaccine, any one of three vaccines, each of which is prepared for the different rickettsial organisms that cause epidemic typhus, murine typhus, or Brill-Zinsser disease.

■ INDICATIONS: Each is prescribed for immunization against a form of typhus.

■ CONTRAINDICATIONS: Acute infection, debilitating disease, concomitant use of corticosteroids, or hypersensitivity to eggs prohibits its use.

■ ADVERSE EFFECTS: Among the most serious adverse effects are anaphylaxis and various allergic reactions. Pain at the site of injection also may occur.

-typia, suffix meaning "(condition of) conformity to type": *atypia.*

typical /tip″ikəl/ [L, *typicus,* characteristic of a kind], a representative example.

typing [Gk, *typos,* mark], the process of classifying a specimen of blood, tissue, or other substance according to common traits or characteristics. See also **blood typing, tissue typing.**

typo-, combining form meaning "a particular type": *typology.*

typology, a system of classifications.

typoscope, a dark piece of cardboard or plastic with a window cut into it that can be positioned over text to help reduce glare or maintain the place on a page when reading.

Tyr, abbreviation for **tyrosine.**

tyramine /tī″rəmēn/ [Gk, *tyros,* cheese, *amine,* ammonia], an amino acid synthesized in the body from the essential amino acid tyrosine. Tyramine stimulates the release of the catecholamines epinephrine and norepinephrine. People taking monoamine oxidase inhibitors should avoid the ingestion of foods and beverages containing tyramine, particularly aged cheeses and meats, bananas, yeast-containing products, and certain alcoholic beverages, such as red wines. See also **amine, catecholamine, epinephrine, norepinephrine, sympathomimetic, vasoconstriction.**

tyro-, combining form meaning "cheese": *tyroma, tyromatosis.*

tyroma /tīrō″mə/ *pl. tyromas, tyromata* [Gk, *tyros + oma,* tumor], a new growth or nodule with a caseous or cheesy consistency.

tyromatosis /tī″rōmətō″sis/ [Gk, *tyros + oma + osis,* condition], a process in which necrotic tissue is broken down and degenerates to a granular, amorphous, caseous mass.

tyrosine (Tyr) /tī″rəsēn/ [Gk, *tyros*], an amino acid synthesized in the body from the essential amino acid phenylalanine. Tyrosine is found in most proteins and is a precursor of melanin and several hormones, including epinephrine and thyroxine. See also **amino acid, hormone, melanocyte.**

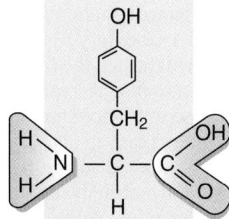

Chemical structure of tyrosine

tyrosinemia /tī″rōsinē″mē·ə/ [Gk, *tyros + haima,* blood], **1.** a benign, transient condition of the newborn, especially premature infants, in which an excessive amount of the amino acid tyrosine is found in the blood and urine. The disorder is caused by an anomaly in amino acid metabolism, usually delayed development of the enzymes necessary to metabolize tyrosine. It is controlled by dietary measures and vitamin C therapy. The metabolic defect disappears with treatment, or it may disappear spontaneously. Also called **neonatal tyrosinemia. 2.** a hereditary disorder involving an inborn error of metabolism of the amino acid tyrosine. The condition, which is transmitted as an autosomal-recessive trait, is caused by an enzyme deficiency and results in liver failure or hepatic cirrhosis, renal tubular defects that can lead to renal rickets and renal glycosuria, generalized aminoaciduria, and cognitive impairment. Treatment consists of a diet low in tyrosine and phenylalanine and high in vitamin C. In severe cases prognosis is extremely poor, and a liver transplantation may be the only lifesaving measure. Also called **hereditary tyrosinemia.**

tyrosinosis /tī″rōsinō″sis/ [Gk, *tyros + osis,* condition], a rare condition resulting from a defect in amino acid metabolism and transmitted as an autosomal-recessive trait. It is characterized by the excretion of an excessive amount of parahydroxyphenylpyruvic acid, an intermediate product of tyrosine, in the urine. There is no known treatment. See also **tyrosinemia.**

tyrosinurea /tī″rōsino͞or″ē·ə/ [Gk, *tyros + ouron,* urine], the presence of tyrosine in the urine.

Tysabri,   a medication indicated for severe cases of multiple sclerosis and Crohn's disease because of its risk for causing a severe brain infection. Brand name for **natalizumab.**

Tyzeka,   an antiviral that is a synthetic analog of the naturally occurring nucleic acid thymine. When substituted into the growing strand of viral DNA, the molecule causes termination of the strand's elongation and decreases viral replication within the cell. Brand name for **telbivudine.**

Tyzine,   an alpha-adrenergic drug. Brand name for **tetrahydrozoline hydrochloride.**

Tzanck test /tsangk/   [Arnault Tzanck, a Russian dermatologist in France, 1886–1954],   a microscopic examination of cellular material from skin lesions to help diagnose certain vesicular diseases. The tissue is scraped from the base of a vesicle, placed on a slide, and stained with Wright or Giemsa stain. Multinucleated giant cells are diagnostic of herpesvirus or varicella. Typical pemphigus and other cells also can be identified.

tzetze fly.   See **tsetse fly.**

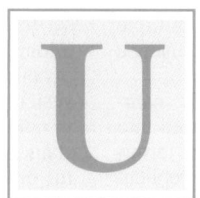

U, 1. abbreviation for **unit. 2.** symbol for the element **uranium.**

UAO, abbreviation for **upper airway obstruction.**

ubiquinone /yoōbik″winōn/, **1.** a naturally occurring organic compound found in the lipid core of mitochondrial membranes. It functions as a carrier in the electron transport chain that produces energy. Formerly called **coenzyme Q. 2.** an herbal supplement used in the treatment of cardiac disease as well as several other chronic and hereditary diseases. The safety and/or effectiveness of this supplement has not been established by the FDA.

ubiquitin /yoōbik″witin/, a small polypeptide that is involved in histone modification and is a marker for intracellular protein transport and breakdown. It is found in all cells of higher organisms.

Uchida technique [Hajime Uchida, Japanese physician, 1921–1996], a method of tubal ligation with injection of saline solution beneath the tubal mucosa to separate it from the underlying tube. A portion of mucosa is removed, and the mucosa-free tube then retracts to form a stump that is closed with sutures.

UGI, abbreviation for **upper GI.**

UICC, abbreviation for **Union for International Cancer Control.**

-ula, combining form meaning "small, little, minute": *macula.*

-ular, 1. combining form meaning "pertaining to" something specified: *appendicular, muscular, papular.* **2.** combining form meaning "resembling" something specified: *circular, granular, tubular.*

ulcer /ul″sər/ [L, *ulcus,* a sore], a circumscribed, crater-like lesion of the skin or mucous membrane resulting from necrosis that accompanies some inflammatory, infectious, or malignant processes. An ulcer may be shallow, involving only the epidermis, as in pemphigus, or deep, as in a rodent ulcer. Kinds include **peptic ulcer, pressure ulcer, serpent ulcer.** *–ulcerative, adj., –ulcerate, v.*

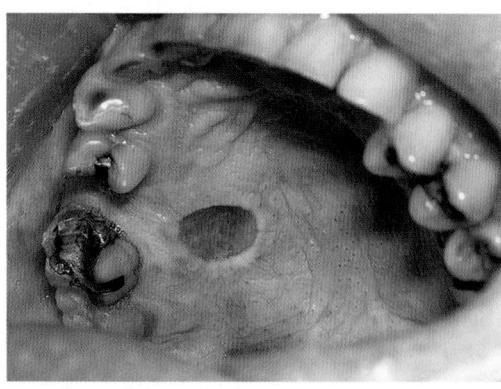

Chronic ulcer of the palate *(Regezi, Sciubba, and Jordan, 2008)*

ulceration /ul′sərā″shən/ [L, *ulcus,* a sore], the process of ulcer formation. *–ulcerate, v.*

ulcerative blepharitis /ul″sərā′tiv, ul″sərətiv′/ [L, *ulcus* + *atus,* relating to; Gk, *blepharon,* eyelid, *itis,* inflammation], an inflammation of the eyelids in which a staphylococcal infection of the follicles of the eyelashes and glands of the eyelids results in sticky crusts forming on the lid margins. If the crusts are pulled off, the skin beneath bleeds. Compare **nonulcerative blepharitis.**

■ OBSERVATIONS: Tiny pustules develop in the follicles of the eyelashes and break down to form shallow ulcers. Other symptoms include burning, itching, swelling, and redness of the eyelids; a loss of eyelashes; irritation of the conjunctiva with tearing; photophobia; and gluing together of the eyelids during sleep by the dried secretions.

■ INTERVENTIONS: Warm compresses may increase comfort. Antibiotics and antibiotic ointments are prescribed for the infection.

■ PATIENT CARE CONSIDERATIONS: Although itching may be intense, the patient should be advised to avoid rubbing the eyes.

ulcerative colitis, a chronic, episodic, inflammatory disease of the large intestine and rectum. It is characterized by profuse watery diarrhea containing varying amounts of blood, mucus, and pus. Some of the many systemic complications of ulcerative colitis include peripheral arthritis, ankylosing spondylitis, kidney and liver disease, and inflammation of the eyes, skin, and mouth. People with severe disease may develop toxic megacolon, a dangerous complication that may lead to perforation of the bowel, septicemia, and death. Also called **inflammatory bowel disease.** See also **Crohn's disease.**

■ OBSERVATIONS: The attacks of diarrhea are accompanied by tenesmus, severe abdominal pain, fever, chills, anemia, and weight loss. Children with the disease may suffer delayed physical growth. The debilitating symptoms often prevent people with ulcerative colitis from carrying on the normal activities of daily living. Diagnosis of the disease is based on clinical signs, the results of barium x-ray films of the colon, and colonoscopy with biopsy. It is often difficult to differentiate between ulcerative colitis and Crohn's disease.

■ INTERVENTIONS: Medical treatment with corticosteroids or other antiinflammatory agents may help control the symptoms in some people. Those with severe disease or life-threatening complications may require surgery. Total proctocolectomy with ileostomy is a permanent cure. Ulcerative colitis carries an increased risk of cancer of the colon, and periodic colonoscopy is performed to rule out this complication.

■ PATIENT CARE CONSIDERATIONS: A person with ulcerative colitis is suffering from a chronic, life-threatening illness and requires frequent evidence of support and understanding during prolonged hospitalization.

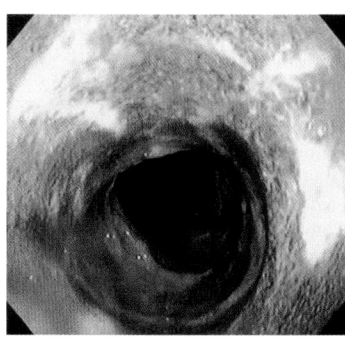

Ulcerative colitis: endoscopic view *(Goldman et al, 2008)*

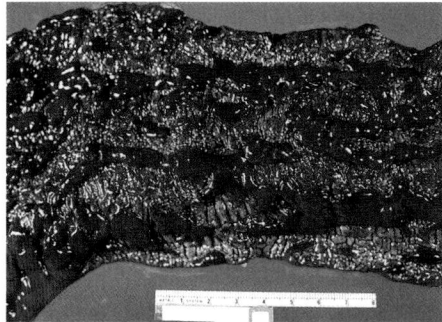

Ulcerative colitis *(Rosai, 2011)*

ulcerative inflammation [L, *ulcus* + *inflammare,* to set afire], the development of an ulcer over an area of inflammation.

ulcerative stomatitis [L, *ulcus* + Gk, *stoma,* mouth, *itis,* inflammation], an infectious disease of the mouth characterized by swollen spongy gums, ulcers, and loose teeth. Also called **trench mouth, ulceromembranous stomatitis, Vincent angina, Vincent infection.**

ulcerogenic drug /ul′sərōjen″ik/, a drug that produces or exacerbates peptic ulcers, such as aspirin, corticosteroids, and nonsteroidal antiinflammatory drugs (NSAIDs).

ulceromembranous /ul′sərōmem″brənəs/, describing an ulcer with a membranous exudation.

ulceromembranous stomatitis. See **ulcerative stomatitis.**

ulcerous /ul″sərəs/, pertaining to ulcers.

ULD, abbreviation for **upper level discriminator.**

ule-. See **ulo-.**

-ule. See **-ulum, -ule, -ulus, -ule.**

ulegyria /yōō′ləjī″rē-ə/, a cerebral cortex abnormality in which the gyri are narrow and distorted by scars.

-ulent, suffix meaning "full of" or "characterized by": *flatulent, pulverulent, seropurulent.*

ulerythema /yōō′lərithē″mə/, a skin eruption characterized by redness and scarring.

ulna /ul″nə/ [L, elbow], the bone on the medial or little finger side of the forearm, lying parallel with the radius. Its proximal end bulges into the olecranon and the coronoid processes and dips into the trochlear and radial notches. The ulna articulates with the humerus and the radius. Also called **elbow bone.** See also **radius.**

ulnar /ul″nər/ [L, *ulna,* elbow], pertaining to the long medial bone of the forearm.

ulnar artery, a large artery branching from the brachial artery, supplying muscles in the forearm, wrist, and hand.

Arising near the elbow, it passes obliquely in a distal direction to become the superficial palmar arch. It has nine branches: four in the forearm, two in the wrist, and three in the hand.

ulnar deviation. See **ulnar drift.**

ulnar drift [L, *ulna,* elbow; AS, *drifan,* to drive], a change in the metacarpophalangeal joints because of rheumatoid arthritis and chronic synovitis. The long axes of the fingers make an angle with the long axis of the wrist so that the fingers are deviated to the ulnar side of the hand. Also called **ulnar deviation.**

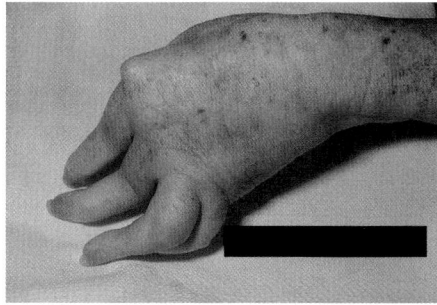

Ulnar drift *(Finkbeiner, Ursell, and Davis, 2009)*

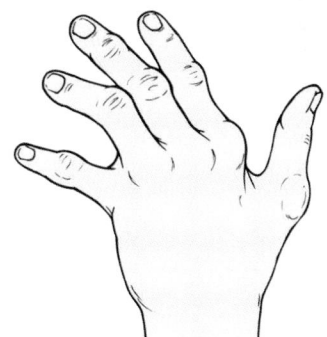

Ulnar drift *(Lewis et al, 2011)*

ulnar nerve, one of the terminal branches of the brachial plexus that arises on each side from the medial cord of the plexus. It receives fibers from both cervical and thoracic nerve roots and supplies the muscles and skin on the ulnar side of the forearm and the hand. It can be easily palpated as the "funny bone" of the elbow as it courses along the groove between the olecranon process and the medial epicondyle of the humerus. Compare **median nerve, musculocutaneous nerve, radial nerve.**

ulnar reflex. See **pronator reflex.**

ulnocarpal /ul′nōkär″pəl/, pertaining to the ulna and carpus or ulnar area of the wrist.

ulnoradial /ul′nōrā″dē·əl/, pertaining to the ulna and radius and the ligaments associated with them.

ulo-, **1.** combining form meaning "scar" or "cicatrix": *ulodermatitis, uloid.* **2.** combining form meaning "gums or gingivae": *ulocarcinoma.*

ulocarcinoma /yōō′lōkär′sinō″mə/ *pl.* *ulocarcinomas, ulocarcinomata* [Gk, *oule,* scar, *karkinos,* crab, *oma,* tumor], any malignant neoplasm of the gums that is classified as a carcinoma.

ulodermatitis /yōō′lōdur′mətī″tis/, dermatitis resulting in the destruction of tissue and scar formation.

uloid /yōō″loid/, resembling scar tissue.

U

ulterior transactions /ultir″ē·ər/, (in transactional analysis), communication that is bilevel. The first level is overt (social), usually of relevant verbal statements. The second level is usually covert (psychological) and nonverbal and has hidden psychological meaning. For example, "Come up to my apartment to see my etchings."

ultimate strain /ul″timit/, the strain at the point of failure.

ultimate stress, the highest load that can be sustained by a material at the point of failure.

ultra- /ul″trə-/, combining form meaning "beyond," "farther," "beyond a certain limit": *ultrafilter, ultrasound, ultraviolet.*

ultrabrachycephalic /-brak′ēsəfal″ik/, describing an extremely short, broad skull.

Ultracef, a cephalosporin antibiotic. Brand name for **cefadroxil monohydrate.**

ultracentrifuge /ul″trəsen″trifyoōj/ [L, *ultra,* beyond; Gk, *kentron,* center; L, *fugere,* to flee], a high-speed centrifuge with a rotation rate fast enough to produce sedimentation of protein and viruses, even in blood plasma. Use of an attached microscope may make it possible to see the sediment.

ultradian /-rā″dē·ən/ [L, *ultra + dies,* day], pertaining to a biorhythm that occurs in cycles of less than 24 hours.

ultrafilter /-fil″tər/, a semipermeable membrane with pores of a known diameter used to separate colloids and large molecules from water and other small molecules.

ultrafiltrate /-fil″trāt/ [L, *ultra* + Fr, *filtre,* filter], a solution that has passed through a semipermeable membrane with very small pores. It usually contains only low-molecular-weight solutes.

ultrafiltration /-filtrā″shən/, a type of filtration, sometimes conducted under pressure, through filters with very small pores, such as those used by an artificial kidney. It can separate large molecules from smaller molecules in body fluids.

ultra–high-speed handpiece, a device for holding rotary cutting instruments, such as burrs, that permits rotational speeds of 100,000 to 450,000 rpm. It is used primarily for the preparation of a tooth or teeth for restorations.

Ultralente, a long-acting form of insulin discontinued in 2005.

ultralente insulin. See **Ultralente.**

ultraligation /-līgā″shən/, tying or closing off a blood vessel beyond the point where it branches.

ultramicroscopy. See **darkfield microscopy.**

ultramicrotome /-mī″krətōm′/, a microtome that cuts very thin slices for examination by electron microscopy.

ultrasonic /ul″trəson″ik/ [L, *ultra,* beyond + *sonus,* sound], pertaining to ultrasound, or sound frequencies so high (greater than 20 kHz) that they cannot be perceived by the human ear.

ultrasonic cardiography. See **echocardiography.**

ultrasonic cleaner, a device that transmits high-energy, high-frequency sound waves into a fluid-filled container, used to remove deposits from instruments and appliances.

ultrasonic cleaning, the use of high-frequency vibrations to dislodge deposits from teeth or other objects.

ultrasonic lithotripsy, lithotripsy in which a rigid probe inserted to the site emits high-frequency sound waves to disintegrate the calculus.

ultrasonic nebulizer, a humidifier in which an electric current is used to produce high-frequency vibrations in a container of fluid. The vibrations break up the fluid into aerosol particles.

ultrasonics /-son″iks/, the science dealing with sound waves having frequencies above the approximately 20-kHz range of human hearing. Ultrasound evolved from the World War II sonar underwater detection apparatus and was first adapted for medical diagnostic purposes in the 1950s. It uses a transducer and generates very short pulses of high-frequency sound that are transmitted into the body. Echoes from interfaces within the body are displayed on a cathode ray tube so that images of normal and abnormal structures can be viewed.

ultrasonic scaler, (in dentistry) a vibrating, crystal-driven, high-frequency (18 to 50 kHz) instrument with a tip for supplying high-frequency vibrations. It produces bubbles that form and collapse, allowing the removal of adherent deposits such as bacteria, biofilm, calculus, and other root surface accretions from the teeth. The water stream washes the gingival pocket and the root surfaces to dilute and remove endotoxins along with bits of inflamed tissue from the walls of the gingival crevice and loose debris. See also **scaler, hand scaling, sonic scaler.**

ultrasonic wave [L, *ultra,* beyond, *sonus,* sound], a sound wave transmitted at a frequency greater than 20,000 Hz/sec, or beyond the normal hearing range of humans. The specific wavelength is equal to the velocity divided by the frequency.

ultrasonographer. See **sonographer.**

ultrasonography /-sənog″rəfē/ [L, *ultra + sonus,* sound; Gk, *graphein,* to record], the process of imaging deep structures of the body by measuring and recording the reflection of pulsed or continuous high-frequency sound waves. It is valuable in many medical situations, including the diagnosis of fetal abnormalities, gallstones, heart defects, and tumors. Also called **sonography.**

ultrasound /ul″trəsound/ [L, *ultra + sonus*], **1.** sound waves at the very high frequency of over 20 kHz (vibrations per second). Ultrasound has many medical applications, including fetal monitoring, imaging of internal organs, and, at an extremely high frequency, the cleaning of dental and surgical instruments. –**ultrasonic,** *adj.* **2.** the image taken by an ultrasound machine.

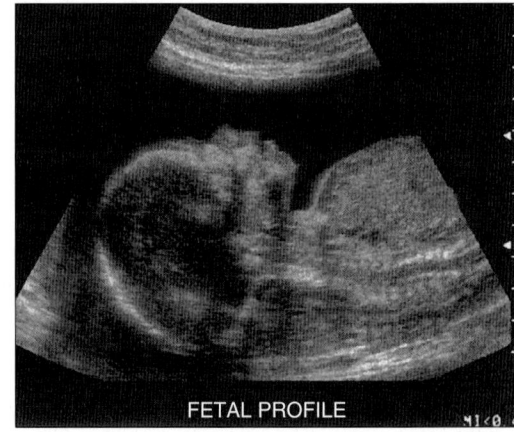

Ultrasound showing fetal profile *(Hagen-Ansert, 2006)*

ultrasound dilution technique, a technique for measuring blood flow and access recirculation in hemodialysis patients. Ultrasound sensors are attached to the venous and arterial catheters in their normal positions and blood flow is checked. Then they are reversed; the ultrafiltration is turned off, and at a known flow rate, a bolus of saline is released into the venous catheter to dilute the blood. The velocity of the dilution as it passes through the access apparatus is measured by ultrasonography.

ultrasound imaging, the use of high-frequency sound (several megahertz or more) to image internal structures by the differing reflection signals produced when a beam of sound waves is projected into the body and bounces back at interfaces between those structures. Ultrasound diagnosis differs from radiological diagnosis in that there is no ionizing radiation involved. Also called *ultrasound diagnosing.* See also **sonogram imaging.**

ultrastructure /-struk″chər/, a structure so small that it can be viewed only with an ultramicroscope or an electron microscope.

ultraviolet (UV) /-vī″ələt/ [L, *ultra* + Fr, *violette*], light beyond the range of human vision at the short end of the spectrum, or that part of the electromagnetic spectrum with wavelengths between about 10 and 400 nm. Equivalently, an ultraviolet photon has an energy between 5 and 500 eV. It occurs naturally in sunlight. It burns and tans the skin and converts precursors in the skin to vitamin D. Ultraviolet lamps are used in the control of infectious airborne bacteria and viruses and in the treatment of psoriasis and other skin conditions. Black light is ultraviolet light used in fluoroscopy. See also **angstrom, light, radiation, spectrum.**

ultraviolet (UV) lamp, a lamp that emits electromagnetic radiation in a range between 4 and 400 nm, or beyond the violet spectrum of visible light. Equipped with a nickel oxide filter, an ultraviolet lamp radiating at wavelengths around 360 nm can be used to examine hairs infected with certain agents. The pathogens reflect the ultraviolet light with a greenish-yellow fluorescence. See also **Wood's light.**

ultraviolet microscopy. See **fluorescent microscopy.**

ultraviolet (UV) radiation, a range of electromagnetic waves extending from the violet, or short-wavelength, end of the visible spectrum to the beginning of the x-ray spectrum. Near-UV radiation covers a range of wavelengths from 400 to 320 nm, middle-UV from 320 to 280 nm, and far-UV from 280 to about 10 nm. About 5% of the energy from the sun consists of UV radiation, but little reaches the earth because much is absorbed by oxygen and ozone in the atmosphere. Window glass also absorbs UV radiation. Artificial sources of UV radiation include the iron arc, the carbon arc, and the mercury vapor arc. For maximum transmission, prisms and lenses used for work in the UV region must be made of quartz, fluorite, or synthetic halides, which are transparent to UV radiation. In medicine, ultraviolet radiation is used in the treatment of rickets and certain skin conditions. Milk and some other foods become activated with vitamin D when exposed to this type of energy. UV radiation also causes certain substances to fluoresce or phosphoresce, a useful characteristic in such diverse applications as lighting and the identification of minerals.

ultraviolet (UV) rays [L, *ultra,* beyond; OFr, *violette* + L, *radius*], electromagnetic radiations found just beyond the violet edge of the visible spectrum, with wavelengths extending to the beginning of x-rays. The wavelengths range from 390 to 290 nm for near-UV rays to 290 to 20 nm for far-UV wavelengths. Ultraviolet radiation in the region of 260 nm can cause photochemical reactions in deoxyribonucleic molecules, causing mutations and destroying microorganisms, including bacteria and viruses.

ultraviolet (UV) therapy [L, *ultra,* beyond; OFr, *violette* + Gk, *therapeia,* treatment], the therapeutic application to the body of electromagnetic radiation in the ultraviolet region of the spectrum. This therapy is useful in the control of infectious airborne bacteria and viruses and in the treatment of psoriasis and other skin conditions.

-ulum, -ule, suffix meaning "small one": *capsule, capitulum, venule.*

-ulus, suffix meaning "small one": *homunculus, loculus, sulculus.*

-um, suffix identifying a noun as singular in number: *cerebellum, datum, jugum.*

umbilical /umbil″ikəl/ [L, *umbilicus,* navel], **1.** See **umbilicus. 2.** pertaining to the umbilical cord.

umbilical artery, the first branch of the anterior trunk of the internal iliac artery and the origin of the superior vesical artery. In the fetus, the umbilical artery is large and carries blood from the fetus to the placenta. After birth, the vessel closes distally to the origin of the superior vesical artery and eventually becomes a solid fibrous cord, the medial umbilical ligament.

umbilical artery catheter [L, *umbilicus,* navel; Gk, *arteria,* airpipe, *katheter,* a thing lowered], a catheter inserted into the umbilical artery of a newborn. See also **umbilical catheterization.**

umbilical catheterization, a procedure in which a radiopaque catheter is passed through an umbilical artery to provide a newborn with parenteral fluid, to obtain blood samples, or both, or through the umbilical vein for an exchange transfusion or the emergency administration of drugs, fluids, or volume expanders.

■ METHOD: Within 1 hour of insertion of the catheter, the position of the tip is validated by x-ray examination. The infant is maintained in a neutral thermal environment as parenteral fluids are delivered by an infusion pump. The rate of flow is checked hourly, and the IV bottle is never allowed to empty. All connections to the umbilical line are checked every 30 to 60 minutes, and only grounded electric equipment is used on or near the infant. At hourly intervals the young patient is repositioned, and the cardiac and respiratory rates are monitored; the axillary temperature is taken every 2 to 3 hours, and the pedal pulses are checked every 2 to 4 hours. The condition of the cord is observed every 2 to 3 hours for signs of infection such as redness, edema, or drainage at the catheter insertion site. The IV tubing is retaped when required, the cord dressing is changed, and antibiotic or antiseptic ointment is applied as ordered. If the umbilical line is displaced, pressure is quickly applied to the cord with a sterile 4 × 4-inch gauze, and an associate is delegated to notify the physician immediately. Fluid intake and output are measured. The infant is observed for oliguria or anuria; signs of vasospasm such as blanching, mottling, or darkening of the legs and absence of peripheral pulses; evidence of sepsis, hemorrhage, or oozing at the catheter insertion site; thromboembolism; and abdominal distension and vomiting, which may indicate necrotizing enterocolitis.

■ INTERVENTIONS: The nurse provides ongoing care, monitoring the catheterized infant for any signs of complications, which are promptly reported. The family is included in the care of the infant as much as possible.

■ OUTCOME CRITERIA: Umbilical catheterization can be an effective method of administering therapeutic fluids and agents or of obtaining diagnostic blood samples from a high-risk newborn, but great care is required in inserting and monitoring the tube.

umbilical cord, a flexible structure connecting the umbilicus with the placenta in the gravid uterus and giving passage to the two umbilical arteries and the umbilical vein. In the newborn it is about 2 feet long and ½ inch in diameter. First formed during the fifth week of pregnancy from the connecting stalk, it contains the yolk sac, stalk, and allantois. Also called **chorda umbilicalis, funiculus umbilicalis.** See also **allantois.**

U

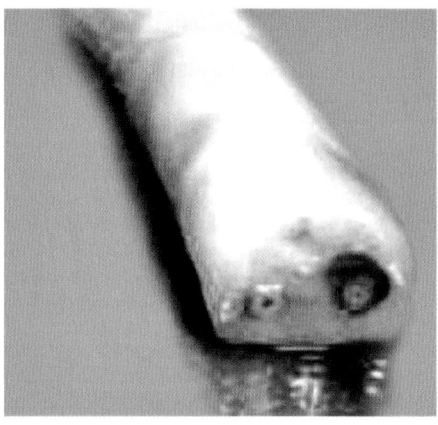

Human umbilical cord *(Moshrefi et al, 2015)*

umbilical duct.   See **vitelline duct.**

umbilical fascia,   a thickening of the fascia transversalis extending along the median umbilical ligament downward from the umbilicus.

umbilical fissure,   a groove on the inferior surface of the liver that holds the round ligament and separates the right and left lobes of the liver.

umbilical fistula,   an abnormal passage from the umbilicus to the intestine or, more frequently, to the remnant of the canal in the median umbilical ligament that connects the fetal bladder with the allantois.

umbilical folds,   folds of peritoneum in the urinary bladder covering the embryological remnants of the urachus and umbilical arteries. The median umbilical fold covers the urachus, and the medial umbilical folds cover the umbilical arteries.

umbilical hernia   a soft, skin-covered protrusion of intestine and omentum through a weakness in the abdominal wall around the umbilicus. It usually closes spontaneously within 1 to 2 years, although large hernias may require surgical closure.

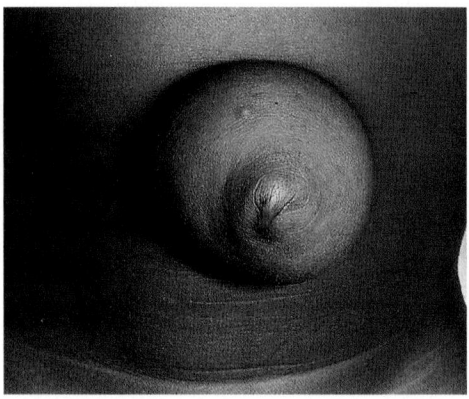

Umbilical hernia *(Salvo, 2014)*

umbilical region,   the part of the abdomen surrounding the umbilicus, in the middle zone between the right and left lateral regions. See also **abdominal regions.**

umbilical vasculitis,   an inflammation of the umbilical cord and its blood vessels.

umbilical vein,   one of three embryonic vessels in the umbilical cord. It functions to return the blood from the placenta and fuses to form a single vein in the umbilical cord.

umbilical vesicle,   a pear-shaped structure formed from the yolk sac at about the fourth week of prenatal development that protrudes into the cavity of the chorion and connects to the developing embryo by the yolk stalk at the region of the future midgut.

umbilication /um′bilikā″shən/ [L, *umbilicus,* navel],   the process of becoming dimpled or pitted or acquiring a depressed area.

umbilicus /umbilī″kəs, umbil″ikəs/ [L, navel],   the point on the abdomen at which the umbilical cord joined the fetal abdomen. In most adults it is marked by a depression; in some, it is marked by a small protrusion of skin. It interrupts the linea alba about halfway between the infrasternal notch and the pubic symphysis. It is located at the level of the interspace of the third and the fourth lumbar vertebrae. Also called **belly button, navel. –umbilical,** *adj.*

umbo [L, knob],   a projection on any rounded surface, such as the inner surface of the tympanic membrane where the malleus is attached.

umbrella filter /umbrəl″ə/,   a small, porous, umbrella-shaped device that can be inserted into the vena cava or other blood vessel to trap blood clots. It is used in patients who have contraindications to anticoagulation or who have failed anticoagulation.

un-,   prefix meaning "not": *unconscious.*

uncal [L, *uncus,* hook],   pertaining to the uncus.

uncal herniation /ung″kəl/ [L, *uncus,* hook, *hernia,* rupture],   a condition in which the medial part of the temporal lobe protrudes over the tentorial edge as a result of increased intracranial pressure. If uncorrected, the progressive disorder causes pressure on the brainstem after first impinging on the third cranial nerve.

■ OBSERVATIONS: The characteristic signs of uncal herniation are an acute loss of consciousness, hemiparesis, and a dilated pupil on the side of the herniation.

■ INTERVENTIONS: A CT or MRI is obtained to determine if there is a need for surgical intervention. The head of the bed should be elevated to 30 degrees or higher to facilitate cerebral venous drainage. Noxious stimuli, such as tracheal suctioning that may elevate intracranial pressure, should be minimized. High-dose corticosteroid therapy is initiated to reduce the pressure.

■ PATIENT CARE CONSIDERATIONS: Uncal herniation is a life-threatening emergency requiring the coordinated efforts of a team focused on monitoring and intervening to prevent further neurological deterioration.

Uncertainty in Illness Theory,   (in nursing) a theory that asserts uncertainty is initially a neutral cognitive state representing the inability of the patient with chronic or life-threatening conditions to interpret the outcome of events related to the illness. Nursing interventions must help patients adapt and cope productively with this uncertainty, integrating it into their lives and improving quality of life. See **Mishel, Merle H.**

unciform bone.   See **hamate bone.**

Uncinaria /un′siner′ē·ə/ [L, *uncinus,* hook],   a genus of nematode that causes hookworm in dogs, cats, and other carnivores, including humans.

uncinate /un″sināt/,   having hooks or barbs.

uncipressure /un'sipresh″ər/, pressure with a hook to control a hemorrhage.

uncompensated care /unkom″pənsā′tid/ [ME, *un,* against, not; L, *compendere,* to be equivalent], services provided by a hospital or other health care professional for which no charge is made and for which no payment is expected.

uncompensated gluteal gait, an uneven pattern of walking because of dysfunction in the muscles of the lower extremities. See **Trendelenburg gait.**

uncompetitive inhibitor /un′kəmpet″itiv/ [ME, *un* + L, *competere,* to compete, *inhibere,* to restrain], an enzymatic inhibitor that appears to bond only to the enzyme-substrate complex and not to free enzyme molecules.

uncomplemented, not united with proteins of the body's immune system and therefore inactive.

unconditioned response /un′kəndish″ənd/ [ME, *un* + L, *conditio,* condition, *respondere,* to reply], a normal, instinctive, unlearned reaction to a stimulus; one that occurs naturally and is not acquired by association and training. Also called **inborn reflex, instinctive reflex,** *unconditioned reflex.* Compare **conditioned response.**

unconjugated, not chemically bound in the serum.

unconjugated bilirubin, the majority of bilirubin in plasma. See **bilirubin.**

unconscious /unkon″shəs/ [ME, *un* + L, *conscire,* to be aware], **1.** unaware of the surrounding environment; insensible; incapable of responding to sensory stimuli. **2.** (in psychiatry) the part of the mental function in which thoughts, ideas, emotions, or memories are beyond awareness and rarely subject to ready recall. It contains data that have never been conscious or that were conscious at one time, usually for a brief period, and later repressed. Compare **preconscious.** See also **collective unconscious, personal unconscious.**

unconsciousness /unkon″shəsnəs/, a state of complete or partial unawareness or lack of response to sensory stimuli as a result of hypoxia caused by respiratory insufficiency or shock; from metabolic or chemical brain depressants such as drugs, poisons, ketones, or electrolyte imbalance; or from a form of pathological brain conditions such as trauma, seizures, cerebrovascular accident, brain tumor, or infection. Various degrees of unconsciousness can occur during stupor, fugue, catalepsy, and dream states. See also **coma.**

unction, the act of anointing an individual with oil, as in a religious rite.

uncus /ung″kəs/ [L, hook], **1.** the hooklike anterior end of the hippocampal gyrus on the temporal lobe of the brain. **2.** a hook-shaped structure.

undecylenic acid /un′desilen″ik/, a topical antifungal agent.

■ INDICATIONS: It is prescribed in the treatment of athlete's foot and ringworm.

■ CONTRAINDICATIONS: Known hypersensitivity to this drug prohibits its use. It is not used in the eyes or on mucous membranes or for fungal infections of the scalp and nails.

■ ADVERSE EFFECTS: Among the more serious adverse effects are skin irritation and hypersensitivity reactions.

underactive bladder, a condition in which bladder contraction is not of sufficient duration or magnitude to empty the bladder completely. Compare **neurogenic bladder.**

undercut, 1. the part of a tooth or artificial crown that lies between the height of contour and the gingivae, only if that part has a smaller diameter than the height of the contour. **2.** the contour of a cross section of a residual ridge that would prevent the placement of a denture or other prosthesis.

3. the contour of flasking stone that interlocks so as to prevent the separation of parts. **4.** the part of a prepared cavity that creates a mechanical lock or area of retention. It may be desirable in a cavity to be filled with gold foil or amalgam but is undesirable in a cavity prepared for a restoration to be cemented.

underdamping /un′dərdam″ping/ [AS, *under,* beneath, *dampen,* to check], the transmission of all frequency components in electrocardiography without a reduction in amplitude.

underlying assumption /un′dərlī′ing/, a set of rules one holds about oneself, others, and the world. These rules are regarded by the individual as unquestionably true.

undernutrition /-noo̅o̅trish″ən/, an inadequate food supply or an inability to use the nutrients in food. Compare **malnutrition.**

underserved /un′dərsurvd″/, individuals, families and/or communities with inadequate access to health care services and resources.

underwater exercise /un″dərwô′tər/ [AS, *under* + *woeter*], any physical activity performed in a pool or large tub, such as a Hubbard tank, where the buoyancy of the water facilitates the movement of weak or injured muscles. Also called **aquatherapy, aquatic exercise.** See also **exercise.**

underwater seal, a seal formed by water allowed to flow over a tube that exits from the chest cavity of a patient. The water acts as a one-way valve and permits the outflow of air but prevents the ingress of air. Also called **water trap.**

underweight /un″dərwāt′/ [AS, *under* + *wiht*], **1.** a body mass index of less than 18.5. See also **body mass index. 2.** less than normal in body weight after adjustment for height, body build, and age.

undescended testis. See **cryptorchidism, monorchism.**

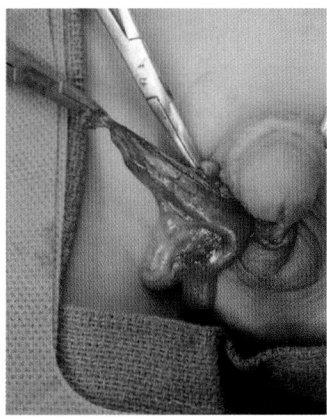

Undescended testis *(Holcomb et al, 2008)*

undifferentiated cell /undif′əren″shē-ā′tid/ [AS, *un,* not; L, *differentia,* difference, *cella,* storeroom], a cell that has not yet expressed signs of its future specific type.

undifferentiated cell leukemia. See **stem cell leukemia.**

undifferentiated family ego mass, (in psychotherapy) a concept introduced by the psychologist Murray Bowen describing an emotional fusion in a family in which all members are similar in emotional expression and know each other's thoughts, feelings, and fantasies.

undifferentiated malignant lymphoma [ME, *un* + L, *differe,* to differ, *atus,* process, *malignus,* evil, *lympha,* water;

Gk, *oma,* tumor], a lymphoid neoplasm containing stem cells that have large nuclei, a small amount of pale cytoplasm, and ill-defined borders. Also called **reticulosarcoma, stem cell lymphoma.**

undifferentiation /un′difərən′shē·ā′shən/, the lack or absence of normal cell differentiation into an identifiable cell type. –*undifferentiated, adj.*

undisplaced fracture /un″displāst, un′displāst″/, a bone break in which cracks in the bone may radiate in several directions but the bone fragments do not separate.

undoing /undoo′ing/ [ME, *un* + AS, *don*], (in psychology) the performance of a specific action that is intended to negate in part a previous action or communication. According to some psychologists, *undoing* is related to the magical thinking of childhood. For example, a spouse brings home flowers and believes this *undoes* a transgression.

undulant /un′dyələnt/ [L, *unda,* wave], wavelike, such as a vibration, fluctuation, or oscillation.

undulant fever. See **brucellosis.**

undulate /un″dyəlit/, to have wavelike fluctuations or oscillations.

undulating pulse /un″dyəlā″ting/, a pulse characterized by a succession of waves without force.

unengaged head /un′engājd″/ [ME, *un* + Fr, *engager,* to involve; AS, *heafod*], the head of a fetus floating freely in the amniotic fluid. See also **ballottement, engagement.**

unequal cleavage /unē″kwəl/ [ME, *un* + L, *aequare,* to make equal; AS, *cleofan,* to split], mitotic division of a fertilized ovum into blastomeres that are larger near the yolky part of the cell (the vegetal pole) and smaller near the nucleus (the animal pole). Compare **equal cleavage.**

unequal pulse [AS, *un,* not; L, *aequare,* to make equal, *pulsare,* to beat], a pulse in which the beats vary in intensity.

unequal twins, two nonjoined fetuses born of the same pregnancy in which only one of the pair is fully formed, with the other showing various degrees of developmental defects.

unfinished business /unfin″isht/, the concerns of a dying patient that require resolution before death can be accepted by the patient. Unfinished business may range from financial matters to personal relationships.

ungual /ung″gwəl/, pertaining to the fingernails.

ungual phalanx. See **distal phalanx.**

unguent. See **ointment.**

unguis. See **nail.**

unheated serum reagin test, a modification of a screening test for syphilis, the VDRL test, using unheated serum; used primarily for screening. Also called **USR test.**

uni- /yoo′nē-/, prefix meaning "one or single": *unicuspid, uniform, unipolar.*

uniaxial joint /yoo′nē·ak″sē·əl/ [L, *unus,* one, *axis,* axle, *jungere,* to join], a synovial joint in which movement is only in one axis, such as a pivot or hinge joint.

unicaliceal kidney, a kidney with a single papilla, calyx, and collecting system.

UNICEF /yoo″nisef′/, abbreviation for **United Nations International Children's Emergency Fund.**

unicellular reproduction. See **parthenogenesis.**

unicentric blastoma. See **blastoma.**

unicuspid, having one leaflet or point. See also **cuspid.**

unidirectional block /-direk″shənəl/ [L, *unus* + *dirigere,* to direct; Fr, *bloc*], a pathological failure of cardiac impulse conduction in one direction while conduction is possible in the opposite direction.

unification model /-kā′shən/ [L, *unus* + *ficare,* to make whole, *atus,* process, *modulus,* small measure], (in academic nursing) an administrative model in which the faculty of the school of nursing hold joint appointments to the school and the hospital, teaching nursing students and providing clinical leadership in nursing service in the hospital. See also **joint appointment.**

uniform /yoo″nifôrm/, **1.** *adj.,* having only one form or shape. **2.** *n.,* distinctive clothing worn by members of a group.

uniform reporting, the reporting of service and financial data by a hospital in conformance with prescribed standard definitions to permit comparisons with other health facilities.

unilaminar /-lam″inər/, composed of only one layer.

unilateral /-lat″ərəl/ [L, *unus,* one, *latus,* side], involving only one side.

unilateral denture. See **partial denture.**

unilateral hypertrophy [L, *unus* + *latus,* side; Gk, *hyper,* above, *trophe,* nourishment], enlargement of one side or a part of one side of the body.

unilateral long-leg spica cast, an orthopedic cast applied to immobilize one leg and the trunk of the body cranially as far as the nipple line. It is used to treat a fractured femur or for the correction or the maintenance of the correction of a hip deformity. Compare **bilateral long-leg spica cast, one-and-a-half spica cast.** See also **cast.**

unilateral neglect, a common behavioral symptom following a cerebrovascular accident in which there is a failure to report or respond to people or objects presented to the side opposite a brain lesion.

unilateral paralysis. See **hemiplegia.**

unilobular /-lob″yələr/, having only one lobe.

unilocular /-lok″yələr/, having only one locus, chamber, or cell.

unimolecular reaction. See **monomolecular elimination reaction.**

uninterrupted suture /unin′tərup″tid/ [AS, *un,* not; L, *interrumpere,* to sever, *sutura*], a continuous suture running forward and backward without interruption.

uniocular diplopia. See **monocular diplopia.**

uniocular squint. See **monocular strabismus.**

uniocular vision. See **monocular vision.**

union /ūn′yən/ [L, *unio*], **1.** the process of healing; the renewal of continuity in a broken bone or between the edges of a wound. See also **healing. 2.** an organized association of employees formed to protect the rights of workers and to advocate for change, fair wages, and other employee concerns.

Union for International Cancer Control, a European nongovernmental association serving as a network for organizations contributing to cancer control on a global scale. Formerly called **International Union Against Cancer.**

uniovular /yoo′nē·ov″yələr/ [L, *unus* + *ovum,* egg], developing from a single ovum, as in monozygotic twins, as contrasted with dizygotic twins. Compare **binovular.**

uniovular twins. See **monozygotic twins.**

Unipen, an antistaphylococcal penicillin medication. Brand name for **nafcillin sodium.**

unipolar /-pō′lər/ [L, *unus,* one, *polus*], pertaining to a nerve cell with only one pole, such as a nerve cell in which the axon and dendrite are fused into a single process a short distance from the cell body.

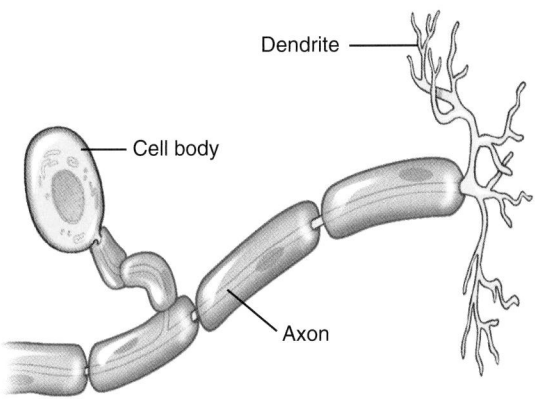

Unipolar neuron

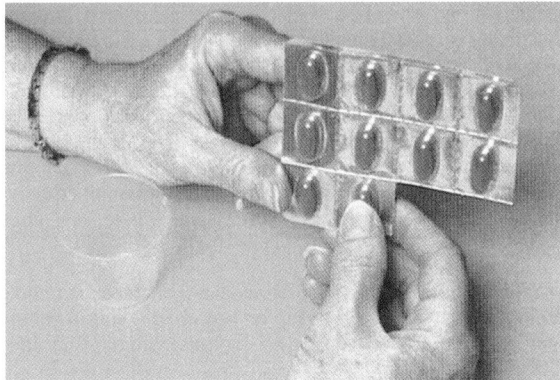

Unit-dose medication *(Potter et al, 2011)*

unipolar depression, a major disorder of mood that is characterized by symptoms of depression only. See also **depression, major depressive disorder.**

unipolar disorder. See **major depressive disorder.**

unipolar electrocautery. See **monopolar electrocautery.**

unipolar lead [L, *unus* + *polus,* pole; AS, *laedan,* to lead], **1.** an electrocardiographic conductor in which the exploring electrode is placed on the precordium or a limb while the indifferent electrode is in the central terminal. **2.** *(Informal)* a tracing produced by such a lead on an electrocardiograph.

unique radiolytic product /yo͞onēk″/, a product such as a food substance that has undergone chemical changes as a result of exposure to ionizing radiation.

uniseptate /-sep″tāt/, having only one septum.

unisex /yo͞o″niseks/ [L, *unus,* one, *sexus,* sex], **1.** concerning only one sex or having reproductive organs of only one sex. **2.** an interchange of sex roles in clothing and hairstyles, work assignments, shared restrooms, and activities, such as encouraging both boys and girls to play with dolls.

unit (U) /yo͞o″nit/ [L, *unus*], **1.** a single item. **2.** a quantity designated as a standard of measurement. **3.** an area of a hospital that is staffed and equipped for treatment of patients with a specific condition or other common characteristics.

unitary human conceptual framework /yo͞o″niter′ē/, a complex theory in nursing introduced by Martha Rogers that emphasizes the importance of holistic health care and an understanding of the human being in relation to the universal environment. See also **Rogers, Martha E.**

unit clerk, a person who performs routine clerical and reception tasks in a hospital inpatient care unit. Certification is available through the National Association of Health Unit Coordinators. Requirements vary by employer. See also **health unit coordinator.**

unit dose, a method of preparing medications in which individual doses of patient medications are prepared by the pharmacy and delivered in individual labeled packets to the patient's unit to be administered by the nurses on an ordered schedule. One intent of unit dose is to decrease administration error.

unit-dose system, a system of drug distribution in which a portable cart containing a drawer for each patient's medications is prepared by a health care facility's pharmacy with a 24-hour supply of the medications.

United Nations International Children's Emergency Fund (UNICEF) /yo͞o″nisef′/, a fund established by the General Assembly of the United Nations in 1946 to aid children in devastated areas of the world. It is funded by contributions from the member nations. It acts to prevent disease, including tuberculosis, whooping cough, and diphtheria, and provides food and clothing to needy children in more than 50 countries. In 1953 UNICEF was made a permanent organization of the United Nations.

United Network for Organ Sharing (UNOS™) /yo͞o′nos/, a national organization for the collection and distribution of body organs that can be used in transplants. Hospitals advise relatives of newly deceased patients about the availability of UNOS service in arranging organ donations. UNOS maintains a computer system that stores information about every person who is waiting for a transplant in the United States. It matches donor organs with transplant candidates 24 hours a day, 365 days a year. See also **transplant list.**

United States Medical Licensing Examination, the standardized three-step examination for medical licensure in the United States sponsored by the Federation of State Medical Boards (FSMB) and the National Board of Medical Examiners®.

United States Pharmacopeia, a compendium recognized officially by the U.S. Federal Food, Drug, and Cosmetic Act that contains descriptions, uses, strengths, and standards of purity for selected drugs and for all of their forms of dosage.

United States Public Health Service (USPHS), an agency of the federal government responsible for the control of the arrival from abroad of any people, goods, or substances that may affect the health of U.S. citizens. The agency sets standards for the domestic handling and processing of food and the manufacture of serums, vaccines, cosmetics, and drugs. It supports and performs research, aids localities in times of disaster and epidemics, and provides medical care for certain groups of Americans.

unit of blood, a standard measure of approximately 450 to 500 mL of whole blood.

unit of service, any individual, family, aggregate, organization, or community given health care. The level at which service is delivered varies with the particular unit entity.

univalent. See **monovalent.**

univalent antiserum. See **antiserum.**

univalent reduction, a phenomenon during intracellular metabolism involving oxygen-reduction reactions in which superoxide radicals are produced because oxygen accepts electrons only one at a time. In the short period between acceptance of the first and second electrons, one electron is unpaired and oxygen is a superoxide radical. The superoxide may then be converted to a second free radical.

Univasc, an angiotensin-converting enzyme inhibitor. Brand name for **moexipril.**

U

universal /yo͞o′nivur″səl/ [L, *universus,* whole world], occurring everywhere and in all things.

universal antidote [L, *universus,* whole world; Gk, *anti,* against, *dotos,* something given], *(Obsolete)* a mixture of 50% activated charcoal, 25% magnesium oxide, and 25% tannic acid, formerly thought to be useful as an antidote for most types of acid, heavy metal, alkaloid, and glycoside poisons. It is now believed that the mixture is no more effective than activated charcoal given with water.

universal choking signal, hands clutched to the throat. See also **Heimlich sign.**

universal cuff, an adaptive device worn on the hand to hold items such as utensils, shaver, or pencil, allowing a patient with a weak or inefficient grasp to participate more in daily activities.

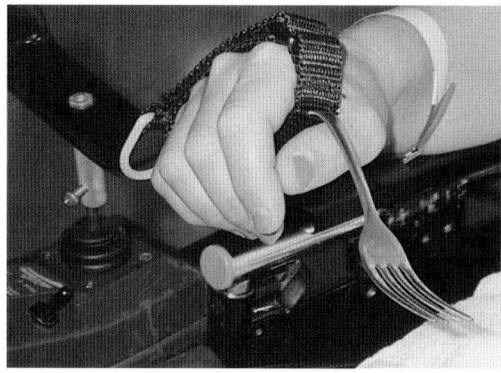

Universal cuff used for feeding. *(Umphred et al, 2013)*

universal design for learning (UDL), a curricular concept that supports flexibility in educational methodologies to reduce barriers for all students; UDL promotes the provision of appropriate supports and challenges so that all students enrolled in primary and secondary public education programs may achieve academic success.

universal donor, type O, Rh negative red blood cells that may be used for emergency transfusion to any ABO type with minimal risk of incompatibility. Group AB plasma can be transfused to all ABO types. See also **blood donor, blood group, transfusion.**

universality, a realization that other members of a group have concerns and feelings similar to oneself and that they may have very similar experiences.

universalizability principle /yo͞o′nivur′səlī′zəbil″itē/, a principle that an act is good if everyone should, in similar circumstances, do the same act without exception.

Universal Precautions, *(Obsolete)* recommendations for the use of gloves, gowns, masks, and protective eyewear when the potential exists for contact with blood or with bodily secretions containing blood. Universal Precautions were initially developed in 1987 by the Centers for Disease Control and Prevention in the United States and in 1989 by the Bureau of Communicable Disease Epidemiology in Canada. It is now recommended that blood and body-fluid precautions should be consistently used for all patients. Compare **Standard Precautions, Transmission-Based Precautions.**

universal qualifiers, in neurolinguistic programming, the use of terms that give general impressions of limitations, such as *all, common, every, only,* and *never.*

universal recipient [L, *universus* + *recipere,* to receive], a person with blood type AB, who can receive a transfusion of any blood type without agglutination or precipitation effects.

universal tooth coding system, (in dentistry) a tooth-numbering system in which the secondary teeth are numbered from 1 (the maxillary right third molar) to 32 (the mandibular right third molar). The primary teeth are similarly numbered from 1 to 20, with the numbers preceded by the letter D (for deciduous). The universal tooth coding system is similar to the American Dental Association (ADA) numbering system, except that the latter uses the letters A (the maxillary deciduous right second molar) to T (the mandibular deciduous right second molar) to identify the deciduous teeth. See also **FDI numbering system, Palmer notation.**

University of Wisconsin solution, a preservation solution used to flush organs before cold storage and before transplantation to prevent cold-induced cell injury.

unlicensed assistive personnel, health care workers in the United States who are not licensed but are prepared to provide certain elements of patient care under the supervision of a registered nurse. Unlicensed assistive personnel include patient care technicians, nurses' aides, and certified nursing assistants. Compare **unregulated care providers.**

unmedullated. See **unmyelinated.**

unmodified scattering. See **scattering.**

unmyelinated /unmī″əlinā′tid/ [AS, *un,* not; Gk, *myelos,* marrow], describing a nerve fiber that is not coated with a myelin sheath. An unmyelinated fiber, lacking the whitish sheath, appears as gray matter in the brain.

Unna paste boot /o͞o″nə/ [Paul G. Unna, German dermatologist, 1850–1929; L, *pasta,* paste; ME, *bote*], a dressing for varicose ulcers formed by applying a layer of a gelatin-glycerin-zinc oxide paste to the leg and then a spiral bandage covered with successive coats of paste to produce a rigid boot. Also called *Unna's boot.*

unoprostone /u″no-pros′tōn/, an antiglaucoma agent that decreases elevated intraocular pressure by increasing the outflow of aqueous humor. It is used as unoprostone isopropyl in the treatment of open-angle glaucoma and ocular hypertension. It is applied topically to the conjunctiva.

UNOS /yo͞o″nos/, abbreviation for **United Network for Organ Sharing.**

unregulated care providers, unlicensed assistants, health care aides (HCAs), long-term care aides (LTCs), and others in Canada providing some services to patients. Compare **unlicensed assistive personnel.**

unresolved grief /un′rizolvd″/, a severe, chronic sorrow reaction in which a person does not complete the resolution stage of the mourning process within a reasonable time.

unresponsive wakefulness syndrome (UWS), a condition associated with brain injury in which the individual is capable of reflexive behaviors such as eye opening and breathing but is unaware of self or the environment.

unroofed coronary sinus, congenital complete or partial absence of the partition dividing the coronary sinus from the left atrium, allowing the shunting of blood from the left atrium through the coronary sinus into the right atrium.

unsaturated /unsach″ərātid/ [ME, *un* + L, *saturare,* to fill], **1.** *adj.,* describing a solution that is capable of dissolving more of the solute; not saturated. **2.** *n.,* an organic compound in which one or more pairs of carbon atoms are united by double or triple bonds, as in unsaturated fatty acids. Also called **unsaturated hydrocarbon.** Compare **saturated.**

unsaturated alcohol, an alcohol derived from an unsaturated hydrocarbon, such as an alkene or olefin. Kinds include *allyl alcohol.*

unsaturated compound [AS, *un,* not; L, *saturare,* to fill, *componere,* to put together], a chemical compound that contains double or triple bonds.

unsaturated fatty acid, a fatty acid in which some of the carbon atoms in the hydrocarbon chain are joined by double or triple bonds. These bonds are easily modified in chemical reactions, either by conversion to other functional groups or for conjugation to other molecules. Monounsaturated fatty acids have only one double or triple bond per molecule and are found as components of fats (triglycerides) in such foods as fowl, almonds, pecans, cashew nuts, peanuts, and olive oil. Polyunsaturated fatty acids have more than one double or triple bond per molecule and are found in fish, corn, walnuts, sunflower seeds, soybeans, cottonseeds, and safflower oil. Diets high in polyunsaturated fatty acids and low in saturated fatty acids have been correlated with low serum cholesterol levels in some study populations. Compare **saturated fatty acid.**

unsaturated hydrocarbon. See **unsaturated.**

unscrubbed team members /unskrubd″/, the members of a surgical team, including the anesthetist and circulating nurse, who wear surgical attire but are not gowned or gloved and do not enter the sterile field.

unsocialized aggressive reaction /unsō″shəlīzd/ [ME, *un* + L, *socialis,* companion, *aggressio,* an attack, *re,* again + *agere,* to act], a behavior disorder of childhood characterized by overt and covert hostility, disobedience, physical and verbal aggression, vengefulness, quarrelsome behavior, and destructiveness, often manifested in acts such as lying, stealing, temper tantrums, vandalism, and physical violence against others.

unstable /unstā″bəl/, **1.** in an excited or active state, such as an atom with a nucleus possessing excess energy. **2.** easily broken down or prone to decomposition. **3.** *(Informal)* (in psychology) unpredictable; labile in mood or behavior.

unstable angina [AS, *un,* not, *stabilis,* firm, *angina,* quinsy], thoracic pain that may mark the onset of acute myocardial infarction. It typically occurs at rest and has a sudden onset, sudden worsening, and stuttering recurrence over days and weeks. It carries a more severe short-term prognosis than stable chronic angina.

unstriated muscle. See **smooth muscle.**

Unverricht disease /un″vərikts, ōōn″ferisht/ [Heinrich Unverricht, German physician, 1853–1912], an inherited condition characterized by progressive degeneration of gray matter, resulting in myoclonic epilepsy. It appears in patients 8 to 13 years of age and is marked by general neurological and intellectual decline. Also called *Unverricht-Lundborg disease.*

unvoiced. See **voiceless.**

upper airway obstruction (UAO), any abnormal condition of the mouth, nose, or larynx that interferes with breathing when the rest of the respiratory system is functioning normally.

upper esophageal sphincter, the upper 3 to 5 cm of the esophagus, including the cricopharyngeus muscle, which prevents the aspiration of air from the pharynx esophagus.

upper extremity suspension, an orthopedic procedure used in the treatment of fractures and in the correction of orthopedic abnormalities of the upper limbs. The procedure uses traction equipment, including metal frames, ropes, and pulleys, to relieve the weight of the involved upper limb rather than to exert traction. Upper extremity suspension is usually unilateral but also may be used bilaterally in postoperative, posttraumatic, or postreduction control of edema. Compare **balanced suspension, lower extremity suspension.**

upper GI (UGI), pertaining to the upper gastrointestinal tract, from the esophagus to and including the duodenum. The term is commonly applied to radiographic or fluoroscopic diagnostic views of the upper gastrointestinal tract after ingestion of a barium sulfate solution. Also called **UGI,** *upper GI series.*

upper GI x-ray study, a series of radiographic images of the upper GI tract, usually with barium sulfate as the contrast medium.

upper level discriminator (ULD), an electronic device used in nuclear medicine to discriminate against all radionuclide pulses whose heights are above a given level.

upper motor neuron paralysis, an injury to or lesion in the brain or spinal cord that causes damage to the cell bodies, axons, or both of the upper motor neurons, which extend from the cerebral centers to the cells in the spinal column. Clinical manifestations include weakness or paralysis; increased muscle tone and spasticity of the muscles involved with little or no atrophy; hyperactive deep tendon reflexes; diminished or absent superficial reflexes; the presence of pathological reflexes, such as Babinski and Hoffmann reflexes; and no local twitching of muscle groups. Compare **lower motor neuron paralysis.**

upper pole of kidney. See **poles of kidney.**

upper pole ureter, the ureter draining the upper pole of a duplex kidney.

upper respiratory tract (URT), one of the two divisions of the respiratory system. The URT consists of the nose, nasal cavity, ethmoidal air cells, frontal sinuses, sphenoidal sinuses, maxillary sinus, larynx, and trachea. The URT conducts air to and from the lungs and filters, moistens, and warms the air during each inspiration. Infection and irritation of the URT are common and often spread to the lower respiratory tract, where they may cause serious complications. Compare **lower respiratory tract.** See also **larynx, nose, trachea.**

upper respiratory tract infection. See **respiratory tract infection.**

UPPP, abbreviation for **uvulopalatopharyngoplasty.** See **palatopharyngoplasty.**

up-regulation /up reg-u-la′shun/, increase in expression of a gene; in the narrowest sense, that in which transcription of a specific mRNA is increased, but also used more broadly to refer to an increase in mRNA levels for a particular gene from any cause, such as increased stability of the specific mRNA. See also **down-regulation.**

upsilon /yōōp″silon, up′-/, Υ, υ, the twentieth letter of the Greek alphabet.

uptake /up″tāk/ [AS, *uptacan*], the drawing up or absorption of a substance.

upward-and-downward squint. See **vertical strabismus.**

ur-. See **uro-.**

UR, abbreviation for **utilization review.**

urachal diverticulum, a usually asymptomatic type of vesical diverticulum resulting from a urachus that has closed at the umbilical end but not at the bladder end. It is seen most often in children, those with prune-belly syndrome, and persons with a bladder outlet obstruction.

urachal sinus, dilation of part of the urachus at the umbilical end, either congenitally or as a result of a urachal cyst that has begun to drain to the surface.

urachus /yōōr″əkəs/ [Gk, *ourachos,* urinary tract], in the fetus, an epithelial tube connecting the apex of the urinary bladder with the umbilicus. It persists throughout life as the median umbilical ligament.

U

uracil, a pyrimidine base found in RNA. Pairs with adenine. See also **thymine.**

-uracil, suffix for uracil derivatives used as thyroid antagonists and as antineoplastics: *fluorouracil.*

uragogue, an agent that increases production of urine.

uraniscus, *(Obsolete)* now called **palate.**

uranium (U) /yo͞orā′nē·əm/ [planet Uranus], a heavy, radioactive metallic element. Its atomic number is 92; its atomic mass is 238.03. Uranium is the heaviest of the natural elements. Isotopes of uranium are used in nuclear power plants to provide neutrons for the nuclear reactions that result in release of energy. The toxicity of uranium varies according to its chemical form and route of exposure.

urano-, combining form meaning "the palate": *uranostaphyloplasty, uranostaphyloschisis, uranoschisis.*

uranoschisis /yo͞o′rənos″kisis/ [Gk, *ouranos,* palate, *schisis,* fissure], *(Obsolete)* now called **cleft palate.**

uranostaphyloplasty /-staf″ilōplas′tē/ [Gk, *ouranos,* palate, *staphyle,* uvula, *plassein,* to mold], the surgical repair of a cleft palate.

uranostaphyloschisis /yo͞o′rənōstaf′ilos″kisis/, a fissure that extends from the hard palate to the soft palate.

urarthritis, inflammation of a joint caused by gout.

urate /yo͞or″āt/, any salt of uric acid, such as sodium urate. Urates are found in urine, blood, and tophi or calcareous deposits in tissues. They also may be deposited as crystals in joints. See also **gout, uric acid.**

uraturia /yo͞or′əto͞or″ē·ə/, the presence of uric acid salts in the urine.

urban typhus. See **murine typhus.**

urceiform /o͞orsē″ifôrm/, pitcher-shaped.

Ur-defenses /o͞or″ dəfen′səs/, (in psychoanalytic therapy) a set of three fundamental beliefs essential for psychological integrity of the individual, as proposed by Jules Masserman. They are a delusion of invulnerability and immortality, faith in a celestial order, and a wishful fantasy that fellow human beings are potential friends available for mutual service.

urea /yo͞or″ē·ə/ [Gk, *ouron,* urine], a normal metabolic waste product from protein metabolism, used as a systemic osmotic diuretic and topical emollient.

■ INDICATIONS: It is prescribed systemically to reduce cerebrospinal and intraocular fluid pressure and is used topically as a keratolytic agent.

■ CONTRAINDICATIONS: Severely impaired kidney function, active intracranial bleeding, marked dehydration, or liver damage prohibits its systemic use.

■ ADVERSE EFFECTS: Among the more serious adverse effects are pain and necrosis at the site of injection, headache, GI disturbances, and dizziness. There are no known severe reactions to topical use.

-urea, suffix meaning "a compound containing urea": *hydroxyurea.*

urea concentration test, a test of renal efficiency based on the fact that urea is absorbed rapidly from the stomach into the blood and is excreted unaltered by the kidneys. 15 g of urea is given with 100 mL of fluid, and the urine collected after 2 hours is tested for urea concentration.

urea cycle, a series of complex enzymatic reactions by which ammonia is detoxified in the liver. In the series of steps for disposing of the ammonia molecule, a waste product of protein metabolism, five enzymatic reactions occur as NH_2 radicals are combined with carbon and oxygen atoms from carbon dioxide to form urea, which is excreted. The amino acid arginine is synthesized during the same process. Also called **Krebs-Henseleit cycle.**

ureagenesis /yo͞or′ē·əjen″əsis/, the process by which urea becomes the final waste product of amino acid metabolism and the detoxification of ammonia from the blood.

urea nitrogen. See **blood urea nitrogen.**

urea nitrogen appearance, the amount of urea in grams produced by a person's body over a specific period of time, closely related to the amount of nitrogen that has not been absorbed by the body. It is calculated as the sum of the urea excreted in the urine plus that found in the blood by calculating blood urea nitrogen. A low figure indicates efficient use of dietary protein. The person's intake of protein must also be known because a low urea nitrogen appearance is also seen with a low protein diet or malnutrition.

urea nitrogen blood (BUN) test, a blood test that detects levels of urea nitrogen in the blood, which serve as an index of liver and kidney function and indicate diseases of these organs as well as other conditions that affect their function. BUN is interpreted in conjunction with the creatinine test in a series known as renal function tests.

Ureaplasma urealyticum /-plaz′mə/, a sexually transmitted microorganism that is a common inhabitant of the urogenital systems of men and women in whom infection is asymptomatic. Neonatal death, prematurity, and perinatal morbidity are statistically associated with colonization of the chorionic surface of the placenta by *Ureaplasma urealyticum.* The mechanisms by which the unfavorable effects on pregnancy occur are not understood. There is no characteristic lesion in the fetus or newborn. Treatment involves oral tetracyclines administered for a period of at least 7 days.

urea rebound, a sudden increase in release of urea into the bloodstream by cells and organs that normally store it, seen in the first 15 minutes to an hour after urea has been removed by dialysis. This is caused by flow-volume dysequilibrium.

urea reduction ratio (URR), the fractional reduction in blood urea nitrogen during a single hemodialysis session, expressed as a percent and measured to assess adequacy of hemodialysis.

urease /yo͞or″ē·ās/, **1.** an enzyme used in the determination of urea in the blood or urine. **2.** an enzyme that catalyzes the hydrolysis of urea to carbon dioxide and ammonia. **3.** an antitumor enzyme.

Urecholine, a cholinergic agonist. Brand name for **bethanechol chloride.**

uremia /yo͞orē″mē·ə/ [Gk, *ouron* + *haima,* blood], the presence of excessive amounts of urea and other nitrogenous waste products in the blood, as occurs in renal failure. Also called **azotemia.** See also **chronic glomerulonephritis, subacute glomerulonephritis.** *−uremic, adj.*

uremic breath, the peculiar odor of the breath in uremic stomatitis.

uremic coma [Gk, *ouron,* urine, *koma,* deep sleep], a stuporous condition resulting from acidosis and the toxic effects of uremia.

uremic convulsion, an episode of involuntary muscle contractions caused by uremia or retention in the blood of substances that would normally be excreted by the kidneys.

uremic frost, a pale frostlike deposit of white crystals on the skin caused by kidney failure and uremia. Urea compounds and other waste products of metabolism that cannot be excreted by the kidneys into the urine are excreted through the small superficial capillaries into the skin, where they collect on the surface.

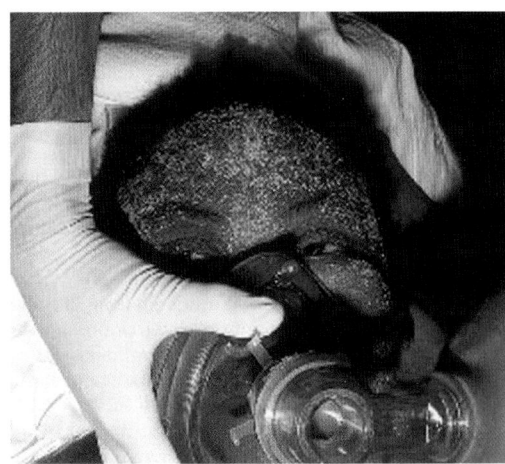

Uremic frost *(Marx et al, 2014)*

uremic gingivitis. See **nephritic gingivitis.**

uremic syndrome, a complication of chronic renal disease. ■ OBSERVATIONS: Symptoms are variable and related to the buildup of urea and other wastes that can not be eliminated by the kidneys. Nausea, weight loss, cardiac symptoms, confusion, and neurological problems such as seizures are often present. ■ INTERVENTIONS: Renal dialysis is necessary unless renal function returns to normal.

-uret, suffix designating a binary compound.

ureter /yo͞or″ətər, yo͞orē″tər/ [Gk, *oureter*], one of a pair of tubes, about 30 cm long, that carries urine from the kidney into the bladder. Each tube is composed of a fibrous, a muscular, and a mucous coat and divides into an abdominal part and a pelvic part. The abdominal part lies behind the peritoneum on the medial side of the psoas major and enters the pelvic cavity by crossing either the termination of the common iliac artery or the commencement of the external iliac artery. In men the pelvic part of the ureter runs caudally along the lateral wall of the pelvic cavity and reaches the lateral angle of the bladder just ventral to the upper tip of the seminal vesicle. In women the pelvic part of the ureter forms the posterior boundary of the ovarian fossa and runs medially and ventrally along the upper part of the vagina. The ureter enters the bladder through a tunnel that functions as a valve to prevent backflow of urine into the ureter when the bladder contracts. Connecting with the kidneys, the ureters expand into funnel-shaped renal pelves that branch into calyces. Urine is pumped through the ureters by peristaltic waves that occur an average of three times a minute. **−ureteral,** *adj.*

ureter-, uretero-, combining form meaning "ureter": *uretercystoscope, ureterocele, ureteroplasty.*

ureteral. See **ureter.**

ureteral duplication, double ureter.

ureteral dysfunction /yo͞orē″terəl/ [Gk, *oureter* + *dys,* bad; L, *functio,* performance], a disturbance of the normal peristaltic flow of urine through a ureter, resulting from dysfunction of ureteral motor nerves. See also **megaloureter.**

ureteral jet, the pattern of fluid seen when dense urine from the ureter is expelled into the more dilute urine in the bladder; it can be studied to assess function and patency of the ureter.

ureteral orifice, the opening of a ureter into the urinary bladder at one corner of the trigone of the bladder. Also called *ureteral meatus.*

ureteral reimplantation, ureteroneocystostomy.

ureteral stent, a stent inserted into the ureter to maintain patency in stenosis or in healing after trauma or surgery.

uretercystoscope /yo͞or″ētər-sis″təskōp′/ [Gk, *oureter,* ureter, *kystis,* bladder, *skopein,* to view], a cystoscope equipped with ureteric catheters that can be inserted into either ureter.

ureteritis /yo͞orē″tərī″tis/ [Gk, *oureter* + *itis*], an inflammatory condition of a ureter caused by infection or by the mechanic irritation of a stone.

uretero-. See **ureter-, uretero-.**

ureteroarterial fistula, a rare, life-threatening fistula that communicates between a ureter and a nearby artery, usually seen as a complication of a surgical procedure of the ureter.

ureterocele /yo͞orē″tərōsēl′/ [Gk, *oureter* + *kele,* hernia], a prolapse of the terminal part of the ureter into the bladder. The condition may lead to obstruction of the flow of urine, hydronephrosis, and loss of renal function. Cystoscopy and pyelography reveal the prolapsed ureter. Surgical correction is performed to prevent permanent damage to the kidney. Compare **cystocele.**

ureterocolonic anastomosis, anastomosis of a ureter to part of the colon, either a detached segment or an in situ segment, so that urine empties into the colon, sometimes as a continent urinary diversion.

ureterography /yo͞orē″tərog′rəfē/ [Gk, *oureter* + *graphein,* to record], the radiological imaging of a ureter, usually conducted as part of an examination of the urinary tract. The examination may involve injection of a radiopaque medium through a urinary catheter with the aid of a ureterocystoscope (the ascending method), or by IV injection of a contrast medium that permits the filtering of the substance through the kidneys (the descending method) to the ureters.

ureterohydronephrosis. See **hydronephrosis.**

ureterolysis, the rupture of a ureter.

ureteroneocystostomy, surgical reimplantation of the ureter into the bladder.

ureteropelvic /u-re″ter-o-pel′vik/, relating to the ureter and renal pelvis.

ureteropelvic junction, the area where the renal pelvis meets the ureter.

ureteroplasty /yo͞orē″tərōplas′tē/ [Gk, *oureter* + *plassein,* to mold], a surgical procedure performed to restructure a ureter, such as when a stricture blocks the normal flow of urine.

ureteropyelonephritis /-pī′əlō′nəfrī″tis/ [Gk, *oureter* + *pyelos,* pelvis, *nephros,* kidney, *itis,* inflammation], an inflammation of the kidney, pelvis, and ureter.

ureterosigmoidostomy /-sig′moidos″təmē/ [Gk, *oureter* + *sigma,* S-shaped, *eidos,* form, *stoma,* mouth], a surgical procedure in which a ureter is implanted in the sigmoid flexure of the intestinal tract. Also called *ureterosigmoid anastomosis.*

ureterostomy /-os″təmē/ [Gk, *oureter* + *stoma,* mouth], the surgical creation of a new opening through which a ureter empties onto the surface of the body or into another outlet.

ureterotomy, an incision into a ureter.

ureterovaginal /-vaj″inəl/, pertaining to the ureters and vagina.

ureterovascular hydronephrosis, hydronephrosis caused by crossed vessels next to the kidney that compress or deform the renal pelvis.

urethra /yo͞orē″thrə/ [Gk, *ourethra*], a small tubular structure that drains urine from the bladder. In women it is

U

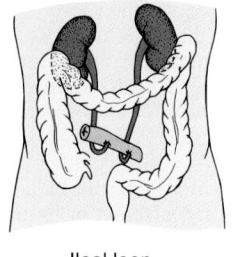

Ileal loop

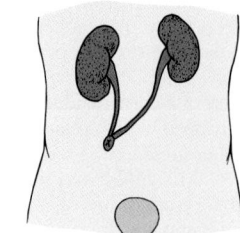

Transureterostomy

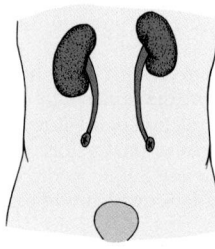

Double ureterostomy

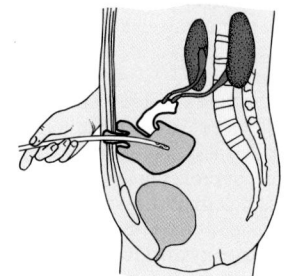

Continent urinary diversion

Ureterostomy *(Potter and Perry, 2007)*

about 3 cm long and lies directly behind the symphysis pubis, anterior to the vagina. In men it is about 20 cm long and begins at the bladder, passes through the center of the prostate gland, goes between two sheets of tissue connecting the pubic bones, and finally passes through the urinary meatus of the penis. In men the urethra is joined by the ejaculatory duct and serves as a passageway for semen during ejaculation, as well as a canal for urine during voiding. See also **ureter.**

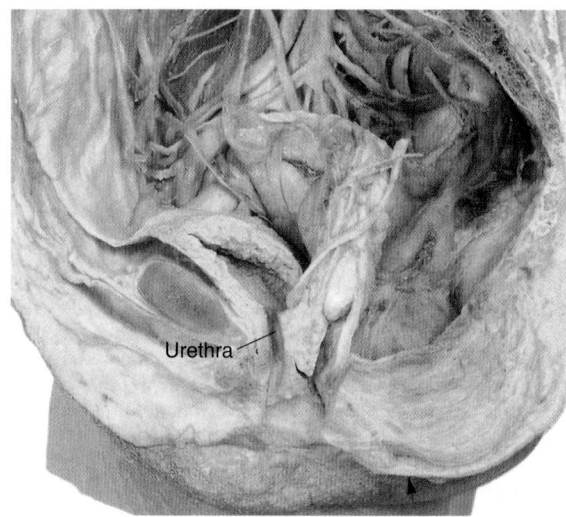

Urethra in sagittal section of female pelvis
(Hagen-Ansert, 2012)

urethral.   See **urethra.**

urethral angle,   the angle at which the urethra exits the bladder neck.

urethral atresia,   imperforation of the urethra.

urethral caruncle [Gk, *ourethra* + L, *caruncula,* small piece of flesh],   a small, painful growth in the mucous membrane of the female urethral meatus. It may be a source of bleeding.

urethral crest,   a longitudinal midline fold of mucosa that marks the lumen of the urethra in men.

urethral diverticula.   See **urethrocele.**

urethral diverticulum,   an outpouching of tissue from the urethra into the potential space surrounding the urethra. It occurs predominantly in women and is associated with chronic urological conditions. The cause is uncertain and symptoms are variable, the most common being frequency, urgency, and dysuria. Formerly called **scaphoid megalourethra.**

urethral duplication,   double urethra.

urethral folds,   a pair of folds derived from the cloacal folds. In male embryos they close over the urethral plate and fuse to form the spongy urethra and ventral aspect of the penis, and in female embryos they fuse only anterior to the anus and form the labia minora.

urethral hematuria [Gk, *ourethra* + *haima,* blood, *ouron,* urine],   blood in the urine as a result of a urethral lesion.

urethral orifice,   **1.** the external opening of the urethra in the glans penis of a male or the vestibule of a female. **2.** internal opening of the urethra at the anterior and inferior angle of the trigone. Also called **meatus,** *urethral meatus.*

urethral papilla.   See **papilla.**

urethral sinus,   the depression on either side of the urethral crest into which empty the ducts of the prostate.

urethral sphincter,   the voluntary muscle at the neck of the bladder that relaxes to allow urination.

urethral swab [Gk, *ourethra* + D, *zwabber*],   an absorbent pad on a slender rod used to treat lesions or to remove secretions.

urethral syndrome,   frequency of urination, urgency, and dysuria with no evidence of infection, obstruction, or other urological abnormality. There may also be suprapubic pain and difficulty in initiating and maintaining the urine stream.

urethritis /yoor´ithrī´tis/,   inflammation of the urethra. The condition is characterized by dysuria and is usually the result of an infection in the bladder or kidneys. An antibiotic, a urinary antiseptic, and an analgesic are usually prescribed after the causative organism is identified by bacteriological culture of a urine specimen. See also **nongonococcal urethritis.**

urethro- /yoorē´thrō-/,   combining form meaning "urethra": *urethrocele, urethrocystitis, urethrospasm.*

urethrocele /yoorē´thrəsēl/   [Gk, *urethra* + *kele,* hernia],   a herniation of the urethra in females. It is characterized by a protrusion of a segment of the urethra and the connective tissue surrounding it into the anterior wall of the vagina. A herniation that is slight and high in the vagina may be palpable only on digital examination when the patient strains downward; one that is large and low in the anterior wall may bulge visibly at the vaginal introitus. A large urethrocele can cause difficulty in voiding, some degree of incontinence, urinary tract infection, and dyspareunia. The condition may be congenital or acquired and may be secondary to obesity, parturition, or poor muscle tone. Surgical repair is the usual treatment. Also called **urethral diverticula.**

urethrocutaneous fistula,   a cutaneous fistula between the urethra and the skin, such as after repair of hypospadias or exstrophy of the bladder.

urethrocystitis /yoorē´thrōsistī´tis/,   inflammation of the urethra and bladder.

urethrocystoscopy /u-re´thro-sis-tos´kah-pe/,   cystourethroscopy.

urethrodynia /-din´ē-ə/,   pain in the urethra.

urethrography /yoor´ethrog´rəfē/,   the radiographic examination of the urethra after the injection of a radiopaque contrast medium into the urethra, usually through a catheter.

The procedure may be performed as a part of a radiographic examination of the lower urinary tract.

urethroplasty /yoorē″thrəplastē′/, a surgical procedure for the repair of a urethra, as in the correction of hypospadias.

urethroscope /-skōp/ [Gk, *ourethra,* urethra, *skopein,* to view], an instrument used to examine the internal surfaces of the urethra.

urethrospasm /-spaz′əm/, a spasm of the musculature of the urethra.

urethrostenosis /-stənō″sis/ [Gk, *ourethra,* urethra, *stenosis,* a narrowing], a stricture of the urethra.

urethrovesical angle, an angle formed by the junction of the bladder wall and the urethra. Analysis of such angles was formerly considered to be a way of gauging the risk for stress incontinence. Also called *vesicourethral angle.*

Urex, a urinary tract antibacterial medication. Brand name for **methenamine.**

urgency /ur″jensē/ [L, *urgere,* to drive on], a feeling of the need to void urine immediately.

-urgy, combining form meaning "the art of working with (specified) tools": *metallurgy.*

URI, abbreviation for **upper respiratory tract infection.**

-uria, 1. combining form meaning "the presence of a substance in the urine": *ammonuria, calciuria, enzymuria.* **2.** combining form meaning "(condition of) possessing urine": *paruria, polyuria, pyuria.*

uric acid /yoor″ik/, a product of the metabolism of protein that is present in the blood and excreted in the urine. Normal adult levels of blood uric acid range from 2.0 to 8.5 mg/dL, with slightly higher values for elderly patients. See also **gout, kidney, liver, purine, urine.**

uricaciduria /yoor′ikas′idoor″ē·ə/ [Gk, *ouron* + L, *acidus,* sour; Gk, *ouron*], an elevated amount of uric acid in the urine, often associated with urinary calculi or gout.

urico-, combining form meaning "uric acid": *uricosuria, uricosuric drugs.*

uricosuria. See **hyperuricosuria.**

uricosuric drugs /yoor′ikōsoor″ik/ [Gk, *ouron* + L, *acidus,* sour; Gk, *ouron* + Fr, *drogue*], drugs administered to increase the elimination of uric acid.

-uridine, suffix for uridine derivatives used as antiviral agents and as antineoplastics.

urinal /yoor″inəl/, an external plastic or metal receptacle for collecting urine.

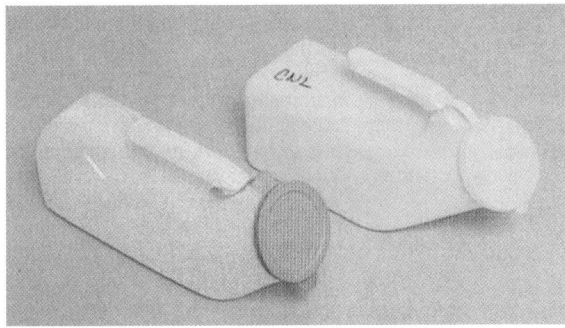

Urinal *(Potter et al, 2011)*

urinalysis /yoor′inal″isis/ [Gk, *ouron* + *analysein,* to loosen], a physical, microscopic, or chemical examination of urine. The specimen is physically examined for color, turbidity, and specific gravity. Then it is spun in a centrifuge to allow collection of a small amount of sediment, which is examined microscopically for blood cells, casts, crystals, pus, and bacteria. Chemical analysis may be performed to measure the pH and to identify and measure the levels of ketones, sugar, protein, blood components, and many other substances.

urinary /yoor″iner′ē/, pertaining to urine or the formation of urine.

urinary albumin [Gk, *ouron,* urine; L, *albus,* white], the presence of albumin, a protein, in the urine. Normally protein is not found in the urine because the spaces in the glomerular membrane of the kidney are too small to allow escape of protein molecules. If the membrane is damaged, however, as in some kidney diseases, albumin molecules can leak through into the urine. The following are normal findings: none or as high as 8 mg/dL; 50 to 80 mg/24 hours at rest; less than 250 mg/24 hours after strenuous exercise. Also called **urine protein.** See also **proteinuria.**

urinary bladder [Gk, *ouron* + AS, *blaedre*], the muscular membranous sac in the pelvis that stores urine for discharge through the urethra. It is connected anteriorly with the two ureters and posteriorly with the urethra.

urinary calculus, a mineral concretion formed in any part of the urinary tract. Calculi may be large enough to obstruct the flow of urine or small enough to be passed with the urine. Calculi can originate in either the kidneys or the bladder. Kinds include **renal calculus, vesical calculus.** See also **calculus.**

urinary casts [Gk, *ouron,* urine; ONorse, *kasta*], cells or particles excreted in the urine having the shape of renal-collecting tubule cells.

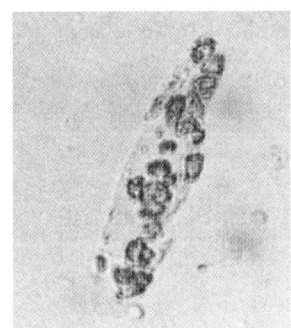

Urinary casts *(Wein et al, 2007)*

urinary diversion, surgical creation of an alternate route of flow for urine to replace an absent or diseased portion of the lower urinary tract to preserve renal function.

urinary flow study. See **uroflowmetry.**

urinary frequency, frequent urination or urgency without an increase in the total daily volume of urine. The condition may result from a bladder or urethral infection, a diminished bladder capacity, or other structural abnormalities. See also **cystitis, cystocele, ureterocele, urethritis, urethrocele.**

urinary hesitancy, a decrease in the force of the stream of urine, often with difficulty in beginning the flow. Hesitancy is usually the result of an obstruction or stricture between the bladder and the external urethral orifice. In men, it may indicate an enlargement of the prostate gland; in women, it may indicate stenosis of the orifice. Cold, stress, dehydration, and various neurogenic and psychogenic factors are common causes of this condition.

urinary incontinence, inability to control urination, caused by acute or chronic factors. Five classes of chronic incontinence are recognized. Functional incontinence is the result of cerebral clouding and/or physical factors that make

U

it difficult to get to bathroom facilities in time. Overflow incontinence occurs when the urinary tract is obstructed or when the detrusor muscle fails to contract as bladder capacity is reached; spinal cord injury or benign prostatic hypertrophy may be the cause. Stress incontinence is precipitated by coughing, sneezing, or straining; it occurs more often in women and is commonly related to anatomic changes. Urge incontinence is the inability to delay voiding after a sensation of bladder fullness is perceived. Reflex incontinence occurs when there is detrusor hyperreflexia and/or urethral relaxation due to neurological causes, such as spinal cord injury. Urinary incontinence can have mixed etiologies. Treatment depends on the underlying cause and may include anticipatory toileting, bladder retraining, exercise of perineal muscles, anticholinergic medications, and surgery. See also **incontinence, retention with overflow.**

urinary infection. See **urinary tract infection.**

urinary meatus, the external opening of the urethra.

urinary output, the total volume of urine excreted daily, normally between 700 and 2000 mL. The smaller number represents the minimum volume needed to excrete waste products. Various metabolic and renal diseases may increase or decrease urinary output. See also **anuria, oliguria, polyuria.**

urinary overflow, a condition that occurs when a patient's bladder is extremely distended with urine and the patient voids or leaks only a small amount of it. It is usually poorly controlled. See also **retention with overflow.**

urinary sediment [Gk, *ouron,* urine; L, *sedimentum,* a settling], solid matter that settles to the bottom of a urine sample that has been allowed to stand for several hours.

urinary space, a narrow chalice-shaped cavity in the renal glomerulus between the visceral layer and the parietal layer of the glomerular capsule, continuous with the lumen of the proximal convoluted tubule.

urinary system. See **urinary tract.**

urinary system assessment, an evaluation of the condition and functioning of the kidneys, ureters, bladder, and urethra and an investigation of concurrent and previous disorders that may be factors in abnormalities in these structures. The assessment aids the urologist in diagnosing the abnormalities.

■ METHOD: In an interview the patient is asked whether painful urination, frequency or burning on urination, dribbling, a decreased urinary stream, nocturia, stress incontinence, headache, back pain, or increased thirst has occurred. The color, odor, and amount of urine voided and obtained via catheter are determined. The patient's vital signs; any bladder distension; skin condition; neurological changes; the location, duration, and character of pain; and the presence of bladder spasms are recorded. It is determined whether the patient has hypertension, diabetes, a venereal disease, vaginal or urethral drainage or discharge, or a history that includes cystitis, pyelonephritis, kidney stones, prostatectomy, renal surgery, a kidney transplant, or a venereal infection. The patient's sexual activity; use of coffee, tea, cola beverages, alcohol, perfumed soaps, feminine hygiene sprays, and prescribed and over-the-counter medication; and habit of bathing in a tub or shower are ascertained. A family history of polycystic kidney disease, hypertension, diabetes, or cancer is noted in the assessment, together with laboratory studies of the specific gravity of the patient's urine, casts, protein, red and white blood cells in the urine, and serum creatinine level. Diagnostic procedures may include cystoscopy, ultrasonic imaging, nuclear imaging, urethroscopy, excretory and IV urography, renal angiography, retrograde studies, and x-ray imaging of the kidneys, ureters, and bladder.

urinary tract, all organs and ducts involved in the secretion and elimination of urine from the body. Also called **urinary system.**

urinary tract infection (UTI), an infection of one or more structures in the urinary system. Most UTIs are caused by gram-negative bacteria, most commonly *Escherichia coli* or species of *Klebsiella, Proteus, Pseudomonas,* or *Enterobacter,* although other strains, such as *Staphylococcus* and *Serratia,* are emerging. Also called **urinary infection.** Kinds include **cystitis, pyelonephritis, urethritis.**

■ OBSERVATIONS: The condition is more common in women than in men. UTIs may be asymptomatic but are usually characterized by urinary frequency, burning pain with voiding, and, if the infection is severe, visible blood and pus in the urine. Fever and back pain often accompany kidney infections. Diagnosis of the cause and location of the infection is made by microscopic examination and bacteriological culture of a urine specimen, physical examination of the patient, and, if necessary, various radiological techniques such as retrograde pyelography or cystoscopy.

■ INTERVENTIONS: Treatment includes antibacterial, analgesic, and urinary antiseptic drugs and increased fluid intake up to 3 L/day unless contraindicated.

■ PATIENT CARE CONSIDERATIONS: Teaching the patient about increased fluid intake, frequent voiding, and good perineal hygiene is also helpful.

urinary urgency, the sudden, almost uncontrollable, need to urinate.

urinate /yo͞or″ĭnāt/ [Gk *ouron* urine], to excrete urine from the bladder.

urination /yo͞or′ĭnā″shən/ [Gk, *ouron* + L, *atus,* process], the act of passing urine. Also called **micturition, voiding.**

urine /yo͞or″ĭn/ [Gk, *ouron*], the fluid secreted by the kidneys, transported by the ureters, stored in the bladder, and voided through the urethra. Normal urine is clear, straw-colored, and slightly acid; has the odor of urea; and has a specific gravity between 1.003 and 1.035. Its normal constituents include water, urea, sodium chloride, potassium chloride, phosphates, uric acid, organic salts, and the pigment urobilin. Abnormal constituents indicative of disease include ketone bodies, protein, bacteria, blood, glucose, pus, and certain crystals. See also **bacteriuria, glycosuria, hematuria, ketoaciduria, proteinuria. –urinary,** *adj.*

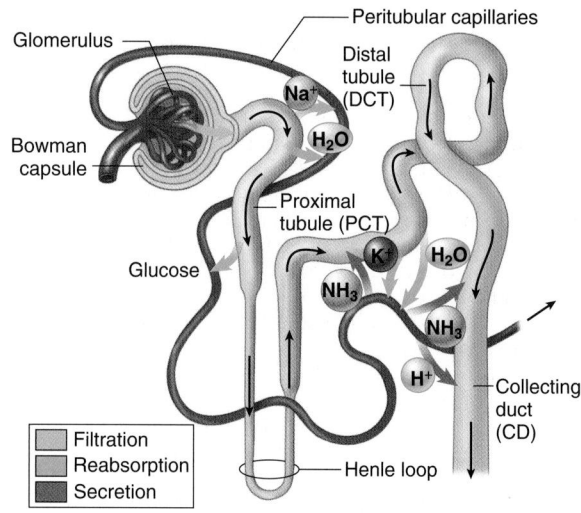

Urine formation *(Patton and Thibodeau, 2010)*

urine culture and sensitivity (C&S), a microscopic study of the urine culture performed to determine the presence of pathogenic bacteria in patients with suspected urinary tract infection.

urine flow studies, a noninvasive, uncomplicated, urodynamic test that measures the volume of urine expelled from the bladder per second. It is indicated to investigate dysfunctional voiding or suspicious outflow tract obstruction and is done before and after any procedure designed to modify the function of the urological outflow tract.

urine glucose test, a qualitative urine test that is usually done as part of a routine urinalysis to screen for the presence of glucose in the urine, which may indicate diabetes mellitus or other causes of glucose intolerance. Other tests are then used to confirm the diagnosis.

urine osmolality, the osmotic pressure of urine, usually greater than the osmolality of serum. The normal values are 500 to 800 mOsm/L after overnight water deprivation. (The term *osmolality* is often used interchangeably with *osmolarity.*)

urine osmolality test, a urine test used in the precise evaluation of the concentrating ability of the kidney. It is also used to monitor fluid and electrolyte imbalance and is valuable in the workup of patients with renal disease, the syndrome of inappropriate antidiuretic hormone secretion, and diabetes insipidus.

urine pH, the hydrogen ion concentration of the urine, or a measure of its acidity or alkalinity. The normal pH value for urine is 4.6 to 8.0.

urine potassium (K⁺) test, a 24-hour urine test that detects the urine concentration of potassium, the major cation within cells. Abnormal findings are associated with chronic and acute renal failure, Cushing syndrome, hyperaldosteronism, alkalosis, diuretic therapy, dehydration, Addison disease, malnutrition, and malabsorption, among other conditions.

urine protein. See **urinary albumin.**

urine sodium test (Na⁺), a 24-hour urine test that evaluates sodium balance in the body by determining the amount of sodium excreted in urine during a 24-hour period. It is useful for evaluating patients with volume depletion, acute renal failure, adrenal disturbances, and acid-base imbalances. It is especially important when the serum sodium concentration is low.

urine specific gravity, a measure of the degree of concentration of a sample of urine. The normal range of urine specific gravity is 1.003 to 1.035, depending on the patient's previous fluid intake, renal perfusion, and renal function.

urinoma /yŏŏr′inō″mə/ *pl. urinoma, urinomata,* a cyst filled with urine.

urinometer /yŏŏr′inom″ətər/ [Gk, *ouron + metron,* measure], any device for determining the specific gravity of urine. Also called **urometer.** See also **hydrometer.**

Urised, a urinary fixed-combination drug used to treat urinary tract infections. Brand name for a combination of antiseptics (**methenamine, methylene blue**, **phenyl salicylate**, **benzoic acid**) and parasympatholytics (**atropine sulfate**, **hyoscyamine**).

Urispas, a smooth muscle relaxant. Brand name for **flavoxate hydrochloride.**

uro- /yŏŏr″ō-/, prefix meaning "urine," "the urinary tract," or "urination": *urodynamics, urogenital, urogram.*

urobilin /yŏŏr′əbī″lin/, a brown pigment formed by the oxidation of urobilinogen, normally found in feces and in small amounts in urine.

urobilinogen /yŏŏr′əbilin″əjən/, a colorless compound formed in the intestine after the breakdown of bilirubin by bacteria. Some of this substance is excreted in feces, and

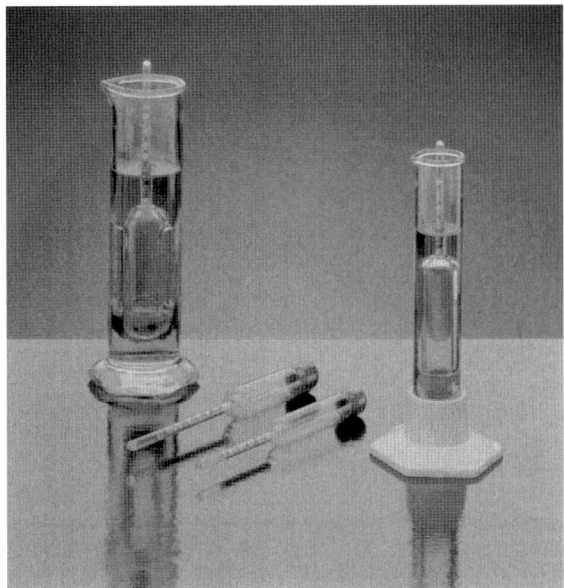

Urinometer *(Zakus, 2001)*

some is resorbed and excreted again in bile or urine. See also **urobilin.**

urobilinuria /yŏŏr′ōbī′linŏŏr″ē·ə/, the presence of excess urobilin in the urine.

urodynamics /-dīnam″iks/ [Gk, *ouron,* urine, *dynamis,* force], the study of the hydrology and mechanics of urinary bladder filling, emptying, and voiding.

uroflowmetry /yŏŏr″ōflō′mətrē/, continuous recording of urine flow by means of a device consisting of a cylinder placed on a transducer that weighs the urine entering the cylinder during voiding and plots the flow rate on a time scale. Also called **flow study.**

urofollitropin /u″rofol′itro″pin/, a preparation of gonadotropins from the urine of postmenopausal women. It contains follicle-stimulating hormone and is used in conjunction with human chorionic gonadotropin to induce ovulation in the treatment of female infertility and to stimulate multiple oocyte development in ovulatory patients using assisted reproductive technologies. Administered by subcutaneous injection.

urogenital /yŏŏr′ōjen″itəl/ [Gk, *ouron* + L, *genitalis,* fruitful], pertaining to the urinary and the reproductive systems. Also called **genitourinary.**

urogenital hiatus, a U-shaped defect in the muscles in the urogenital triangle that allows the passage of the urethra and vagina.

urogenital peritoneum, the peritoneum lining the urogenital structures in the lower pelvis.

urogenital region, the part of the perineal region that surrounds the external genital organs and the urethral orifice.

urogenital sinus, one of the elongated cavities, formed by the division of the cloaca in early embryonic development, into which open the ureter, mesonephric and paramesonephric ducts, and bladder. It also gives rise to the vestibule, urethra, and part of the vagina in the female and part of the urethra in the male.

urogenital system, all of the urinary and genital organs and their associated structures, including the kidneys, ureters, bladder, and urethra; the ovaries, fallopian tubes, uterus, clitoris, and vagina (in women); and the testes, seminal vesicles, seminal ducts, prostate, and penis (in men). Also called

U

genitourinary system. See also *Color Atlas of Human Anatomy,* pp. A-39 to A-41.

urogenital triangle, the triangle in the peritoneum anterior to the imaginary line between the two ischial tuberosities.

urogram /yŏŏr′əgram′/, an x-ray image of the urinary tract obtained by urography. See also **pyelogram.**

urography /yŏŏrog″rəfē/ [Gk, *ouron + graphein,* to record], the radiographic examination of the urinary system. A radiopaque substance is injected intravenously or introduced through a catheter, and radiographs are taken as the substance is passed through or excreted from the part of the system being studied. Kinds include **cystoscopic urography, intravenous pyelography, retrograde pyelography.**

urokinase /yŏŏr′əkī′nās/, an enzyme produced in the kidney and found in urine that is a potent plasminogen activator of the fibrinolytic system. A pharmaceutic preparation of urokinase is administered intravenously in the treatment of pulmonary embolism.

urolagnia /yŏŏr′əlag′nē·ə/, sexual stimulation gained from acts involving urine, such as watching people urinate or being urinated on.

urolithiasis /yŏŏr′ōlithī′əsis/, the presence of calculi in the urinary system.

urological /-loj″ik/ [Gk, *ouron,* urine, *logos,* science], pertaining to the scientific study of the urinary tract.

urologist /yŏŏrol″əjist/, a licensed physician who has completed an approved residency program and who specializes in the practice of urology.

urology /yŏŏrol″əjē/ [Gk, *ouron + logos,* science], the branch of medicine concerned with the study of the anatomy, physiology, disorders, and care of the urinary tract in men and women and of the male genital tract. **–urological,** adj.

uromelus, fusion of the lower limbs. See also **sympus monopus.**

urometer /yŏŏrom″ətər/ [Gk, *ouron,* urine, *metron,* measure], a type of hydrometer used to measure the specific gravity of a urine sample. Also called **urinometer.**

urono-. See **uro-.**

uropathy /yŏŏrop″əthē/ [Gk, *ouron + pathos,* disease], any disease or abnormal condition of any structure of the urinary tract. **–uropathic,** adj.

uroporphyria /yŏŏr′ōpôrfir″ē·ə/ [Gk, *ouron + porphyros,* purple], a rare genetic disease characterized by excessive secretion of uroporphyrin in the urine, blistering dermatitis, photosensitivity, splenomegaly, and hemolytic anemia. Corticosteroid ointments may be helpful for the skin lesions; splenectomy may be necessary to alleviate the hemolytic anemia. Most patients die from hematological complications before they reach middle age. See also **porphyria.**

uroporphyrin /yŏŏr′ōpôr″firin/, a porphyrin normally excreted in the urine in small amounts. See also **uroporphyria.**

uroporphyrinogen-1-synthase test, a blood test used to detect a deficiency of uroporphyrinogen-1-synthase, associated with porphyria.

uroprotective /u″ro-pro-tek′tiv/, providing protection of the urinary tract, especially against urotoxicity.

uroradiology /-rā′dē·ol′əjē/, the radiological study of the urinary tract.

urorectal septum /-rek″təl/ [Gk, *ouron + L, rectus,* straight, *saeptum,* wall], a ridge of mesoderm covered with endoderm that in the early developing embryo divides the endodermal cloaca into the urogenital sinus and the rectum. Also called **cloacal septum.**

uroscopy /yŏŏros″kəpē/ [Gk, *ouron,* urine, *skopein,* to view], diagnostic examination of urine samples.

urostomy /yŏŏros″təmē/, the diversion of urine away from a diseased or defective bladder through a surgically created opening, or stoma, in the skin.

urothelium /yŏŏr″ōthē′lē·əm/, a layer of transitional epithelium in the wall of the bladder, ureter, and renal pelvis.

urotoxicity /yŏŏr′ōtoksis″itē/, the toxic quality or toxic constituents of the urine.

Uroxatral, an alpha₁ blocker used for benign prostatic hypertrophy. Brand name for **alfuzosin.**

ursodeoxycholic acid /ur′sōdē·ok″sikol′ik/, a secondary bile salt. It is used in vivo to dissolve cholesterol gallstones. Also called *ursodiol.* See also **chenodeoxycholic acid.**

urticaria /ur′tiker″ē·ə/ [L, *urtica,* nettle], a pruritic skin eruption caused by capillary dilation in the dermis that results from the release of vasoactive mediators, including histamine, kinin, and the slow reactive substance of anaphylaxis associated with antigen-antibody reaction. Also called **hives.** See also **angioedema, cholinergic urticaria. –urticarial,** adj.

■ OBSERVATIONS: It is characterized by transient wheals of varying shapes and sizes with well-defined erythematous margins and pale centers.

■ INTERVENTIONS: Treatment includes antihistamines and removal of the stimulus or allergen.

■ PATIENT CARE CONSIDERATIONS: It may be a reaction to drugs, food, insect bites, inhalants, emotional stress, exposure to heat or cold, or exercise.

urticaria bullosa [L, *urtica,* nettle, *bulla,* bubble], a skin eruption in which the lesions are capped by blisters. Also called **bullous urticaria.**

urticaria hemorrhagica. See **hemorrhagic urticaria.**

urticarial, pertaining to hives. See **urticaria.**

urticaria maculosa [L, *urtica,* nettle, *macule,* spot], a chronic skin eruption in which red lesions form with little or no edema present.

urticaria medicamentosa [L, *urtica,* nettle, *medicina*], a form of skin eruption that follows the use of certain medications, including those containing quinine.

urticaria papulosa [L, *urtica,* nettle, *papula,* pimple], a form of skin eruption affecting mainly children and characterized by reddish macules on which papules develop.

urticaria pigmentosa, an uncommon form of mastocytosis characterized by pigmented skin lesions that usually begin in infancy and become urticarial on mechanical or chemical irritation. Although duration of the condition is unpredictable, prognosis is good. Treatment is symptomatic and usually includes antihistamines for relief of itching. See also **mastocytosis.**

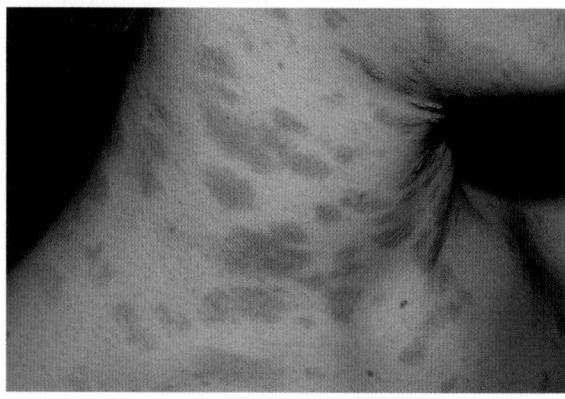

Urticaria pigmentosa *(James, Berger, and Elston, 2006)*

urushiol /ərōō″shē·ôl/, a toxic resin in the sap of certain plants of the genus *Rhus,* such as poison ivy, poison oak, and poison sumac, that produces allergic contact dermatitis in many people.

-us, suffix usually identifying a noun as singular: *thalamus.*

USAN /yōō′san, yōō″es′ā′en′/, an organization that works with pharmaceutical manufacturers to designate names for nonproprietary drugs. A list of USAN-approved drugs is published by U.S. Pharmacopeial Convention, Inc. Abbreviation for *United States Adopted Names.* See also **nonproprietary name.**

use effectiveness [L, *usus,* make use of, *efficere,* to produce], (of a contraceptive method) the actual effectiveness of a medication, device, or method in preventing pregnancy. Inconsistent use and human error usually reduce the theoretic effectiveness of any particular method of contraception. Compare **theoretic effectiveness.**

use factor, (in x-ray shielding design) the fraction of time that an x-ray beam is pointing in any given direction.

useful beam, (in radiology) that part of the primary radiation that is permitted to emerge from the tube head assembly of an x-ray machine, as limited by the aperture or port and accessory collimating devices.

useful radiation, the part of direct radiation that is permitted to pass from an x-ray tube housing through the tube head port, aperture, or collimator. Also called **useful beam.**

user documentation. See **documentation.**

user-friendly, presenting operating information or instructions in a form that is familiar and easy to understand.

user interaction. See **interactive terminal.**

use test, a procedure used to identify offending allergens in foods, cosmetics, or fabrics by the systematic elimination and addition, one at a time, of specific items associated with the lifestyle of the patient involved. Allergic reactions to the use test may be immediate or spread over a considerable period of time. Some patients undergoing the test become frustrated and discouraged, requiring regular encouragement to continue the search for sources of their allergies by this method. See also **allergy testing.**

U-shaped arch, a dental arch in which there is little difference in width between the first premolars and the last molars and in which the curve from canine to canine is abrupt and U-shaped.

Usher syndrome [Charles Usher, Scottish ophthalmologist, 1865–1942], an inherited disorder characterized by retinitis pigmentosa and a sensorineural hearing deficit.

USMLE, abbreviation for **United States Medical Licensing Examination.**

USP, abbreviation for *United States Pharmacopeia.*

USPHS, abbreviation for **United States Public Health Service.**

USP unit, a dose unit as recommended by the *United States Pharmacopeia.* A unit is used in the United States to measure the potency of a vitamin or drug.

USR test. See **unheated serum reagin test.**

uta /yōō′tə/ [Sp, facial ulcers], a mild cutaneous form of American leishmaniasis occurring in the Andes of Peru and Argentina, caused by *Leishmania peruana.* The lesions are small and usually occur on the exposed surfaces of the skin, which ordinarily heal spontaneously within 1 year. The disease has been slowly disappearing because of the increased use of insecticides.

ut dict, a shortened form of a Latin phrase meaning "as directed." Abbreviation for *ut dictum.*

utend, a shortened form of a Latin phrase meaning "to be used." Abbreviation for *utendus.*

uter-, utero-, combining form meaning "relating to the uterus": *uteroplasty, uterotomy.*

uteralgia. See **metralgia.**

uterine /yōō″tərēn/ [L, *uterus,* womb], pertaining to the uterus.

uterine anteflexion [L, *uterus,* womb, *ante,* before, *flectere,* to bend], an abnormal position of the uterus in which the uterine body is bent forward on itself at the juncture of the isthmus of the uterine cervix and the lower uterine segment.

uterine anteversion, a position of the uterus in which the body of the uterus is directed ventrally. Mild degrees of anteversion are of no clinical significance. On speculum examination of the vagina, acute anteversion of the uterus may be deduced from the location of the cervix in the posterior of the vaginal vault. Slight anteversion is the most common uterine position. On speculum examination, the cervix is in the middle of the top of the vagina vault and protrudes directly downward toward the vaginal orifice.

uterine appendages, the ovaries, fallopian tubes, and associated ligaments. Also called **adnexa uteri.**

uterine bleeding [L, *uterus* + ME, *blod*], any loss of blood from the uterus.

uterine bruit, a sound made by the passage of blood through the arteries of the pregnant uterus. The sounds are synchronized with the maternal heart rate. See also **uterine souffle.**

uterine cancer, any malignancy of the uterus, including the cervix or endometrium. See also **cervical cancer, endometrial cancer.**

uterine colic [L, *uterus* + Gk, *kolikos,* pain in the colon], a spasmodic pain originating in the uterus. It is usually caused by dysmenorrhea or extrusion of a fibroid polyp.

uterine fibroid [L, *uterus* + *fibra,* fiber; Gk, *eidos,* form], a growth of fibrous tissue in the uterus, usually a fibroma, fibromyoma, or leiomyofibroma.

uterine fibroma, a benign encapsulated uterine tumor. It affects about 20% of women over the age of 30. The tumor may develop in the wall of the uterus or be attached to a stalk of tissue originating in the wall. Symptoms may include menstrual disorders such as menorrhagia. Symptoms are also likely to be related to the location of the tumor with respect to neighboring organs, as when a uterine fibroma causes pressure on the urinary bladder, producing symptoms of dysuria. Uterine fibromas rarely spread or become life-threatening.

uterine glands, simple tubular glands found throughout the thickness and extent of the endometrium. They become enlarged during the premenstrual period.

uterine hemorrhage, bleeding from the uterus. Types of uterine hemorrhage include fetomaternal hemorrhage, in which fetal blood cells leak into the maternal circulation; postmenopausal bleeding; and dysfunctional uterine bleeding. See also **hemorrhage, intrapartum hemorrhage, postpartum hemorrhage.**

uterine inertia, abnormal relaxation of the uterus during labor, causing a lack of obstetric progress, or after childbirth, causing uterine hemorrhage.

uterine ischemia, a decreasing or ineffective blood supply to the uterus.

uterine peristalsis, rhythmic movements of the myometrium, seen especially during the follicular phase of the menstrual cycle.

uterine prolapse, the falling, sinking, or sliding of the uterus from its normal location in the body.

uterine retroflexion, a position of the uterus in which its body is bent backward on itself at the isthmus of the cervix and the lower uterine segment. This condition has no clinical

U

significance; it does not prevent conception or adversely affect pregnancy. On speculum examination of the vagina, the condition may be deduced by the location of the cervix in the anterior vaginal vault. The fundus of the uterus may also often be felt through the rectal wall upon rectovaginal examination.

uterine retroversion, a position of the uterus in which the body of the uterus is directed away from the midline, toward the back. Mild degrees of retroversion are common and have no clinical significance. Severe retroversion may be accompanied by vague persistent pelvic discomfort and dyspareunia and may prevent the fitting and use of a contraceptive diaphragm. Compare **uterine anteversion.** See also **uterine retroflexion.**

uterine rupture, a rare and life-threatening event in which there is a full-thickness tear or break in the uterus at the site of scarring from a previous cesarean section or other causes, possibly accompanied by displacement of the fetus and amniotic sac into the peritoneal cavity. The mother may experience acute pain because of tissue damage and irritation of the peritoneal tissues. Fetal distress is a classic symptom, usually manifested by fetal bradycardia. Excessive loss of blood may be marked by hypotension, fluid volume deficit, and altered cardiac output in the mother. Surgical intervention as quickly as possible but no longer than 30 minutes after rupture is essential to minimize the risk of maternal complications and permanent perinatal injury to the fetus.

uterine sinus, one of the small irregular vascular channels in the endometrium of the pregnant uterus.

uterine souffle, a soft, blowing sound made by the blood in the arteries of a pregnant uterus. It is synchronized with the maternal pulse.

uterine sound, a long, flexible sound for measuring uterine depth.

uterine subinvolution [L, *uterus* + *sub,* under, *involere,* to roll up], delayed or absent involution of the uterus during the postpartum period. The causes of subinvolution include retained fragments of placenta, uterine fibromyomas, and infection. Regardless of the cause of the condition, it is characterized by longer and heavier bleeding after childbirth and, on pelvic examination, a larger and softer uterus than would be expected at that time. Treatment includes ergonovine given by mouth for 2 or 3 days, and, if an infection is present, an antibiotic. The hemoglobin or hematocrit is also evaluated, and iron is given if necessary. A follow-up examination is performed 2 weeks later. Also called **partial involution.** See also **ergonovine maleate.**

uterine swab [L, *uterus* + D, *zwabber*], an absorbent material on a rod or flattened wire used to obtain specimens or to remove secretions from the uterus.

uterine tenaculum. See **tenaculum.**

uterine tetany, a condition characterized by uterine contractions that are extremely prolonged. This condition may be life threatening to the fetus.

uterine tube. *(Informal)* See **fallopian tube.**

uteritis, inflammation of the walls of uterus. See also **metritis.**

utero-. See **uter-, utero-.**

uteroabdominal pregnancy /yo͞oʹtərō'abdom″inəl/ [L, *uterus* + *abdomen* + *pregnans*], a twin pregnancy in which one fetus develops in the uterus and the other develops in the abdomen.

uteroglobulin. See **blastokinin.**

utero-ovarian varicocele /yo͞oʹtərō″ōverʹē·ən/ [L, *uterus* + *ovum,* egg, *varix,* varicose vein; Gk, *kele,* tumor], a swelling of the ovarian veins of the pampiniform plexus in the female pelvis. Compare **ovarian varicocele.**

uteroplacental apoplexy, *(Obsolete)* now called **Couvelaire uterus.**

uteroplacental sinus /yo͞oʹtərōpləsen″təl/, one of the spaces in the zone of the placenta and the uterine wall where blood is exchanged between the circulations of the fetus and the mother.

uteroplasty. See **metroplasty.**

uterosacral ligament, a ligament that extends from the cervix to the posterior pelvic wall. It is thought to help stabilize the uterus in the pelvic cavity.

uterosalpingography /yo͞oʹtərōsalʹping·gog″rəfē/ [L, *uterus* + Gk, *salpinx,* tube, *graphein,* to record], a radiographic examination of the uterus and fallopian tubes.

uterotomy /yo͞oʹtərot″əmē/ [L, *uterus* + Gk, *temnein,* to cut], a surgical incision into the uterus, such as in a cesarean section.

uterovaginal /yo͞oʹtərovaj″inəl/, pertaining to the uterus and vagina.

uterovesical. See **vesicouterine.**

uterus /yo͞o″tərəs/ [L, womb], the hollow, pear-shaped, internal female organ of reproduction in which the fertilized ovum is implanted and the fetus develops and from which the decidua of menses flows. Its anterior surface lies on the superior surface of the bladder, separated by a fold of peritoneum, the vesicouterine pouch. Its posterior surface, also covered with peritoneum, is adjacent to the sigmoid colon and some of the coils of the small intestine. The uterus is composed of three layers: the *endometrium,* the *myometrium,* and the *parametrium.* The *endometrium* lines the uterus and becomes thicker and more vascular in pregnancy and during the second half of the menstrual cycle under the influence of the hormone progesterone. The *myometrium* is the muscular layer of the organ. Its muscle fibers wrap around the uterus obliquely, laterally, and longitudinally. The muscle fibers contract during childbirth to expel the fetus. After childbirth the meshlike network of fibers contracts again, creating a mass of natural ligatures that stops the flow of blood from the large blood vessels supplying the placenta. The *parametrium* is the outermost layer of the uterus. It is composed of serous connective tissue and extends laterally into the broad ligament. In the adult the organ measures about 7.5 cm long and 5 cm wide at its fundus and weighs approximately 40 g. During pregnancy it is able to grow to many times its usual size, almost entirely by cellular hypertrophy.

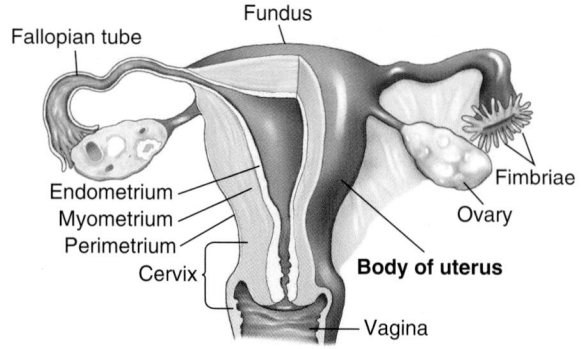

Uterus *(Shiland, 2010)*

uterus bicornis [L, *uterus* + *bis* + *cornu,* horn], a uterus that is divided into two parts, usually separated at the upper end and joined at the lower end. Also called **bicornate uterus.**

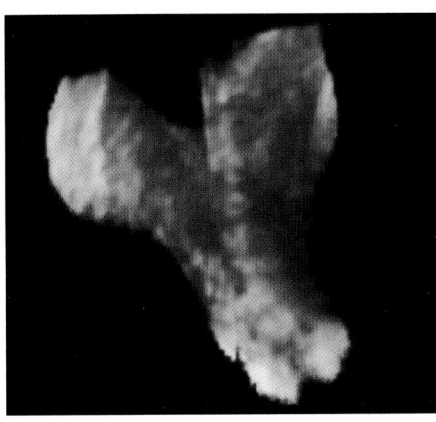

3D surface rendering of uterus bicornis *(Nazzaro et al, 2014)*

uterus masculinus. See **prostatic utricle.**

UTI, abbreviation for **urinary tract infection.**

utilitarianism /yōō′tiliter″ē·əniz′əm/ [L, *utilis,* useful, *isma,* practice], a doctrine of ethics that the purpose of all action should be to bring about the greatest happiness for the greatest number of people and that the value of anything is determined by its utility. The philosophy is often applied in the distribution of health care resources, as in decisions regarding the expenditure of public funds for health services.

utilization review (UR) /yōō′tilīzā″shən/ [L, *utilis + atus,* process], an assessment of the appropriateness and economy of an admission to a health care facility or a continued hospitalization. The length of the hospital stay also is compared with the average length of stay for similar diagnoses.

utricle /yōō′trikəl/ [L, *utriculus,* small bag], **1.** a small sac. **2.** the larger of two membranous pouches in the vestibule of the membranous labyrinth of the inner ear. It is an oblong structure that communicates with the semicircular ducts by five openings and receives utricular filaments of the vestibular branch of the vestibulocochlear nerve. Compare **saccule.**

utriculosaccular duct /yōōtrik′yəlōsak″yələr/ [L, *utriculus + sacculus,* small sack, *ducere,* to lead], a duct connecting the utricle with an endolymphatic duct of the membranous labyrinth.

UV, abbreviation for **ultraviolet.**

uvea /yōō″vē·ə/ [L, *uva,* grape], the vascular, pigmented, middle coat of the eye. Also called **tunica vasculosa bulbi, uveal tract.** *−uveal, adj.*

uveal malignant melanoma /yōō′vē·əl mə·lig′nənt mel′-ə·nō′mə/, the most common type of ocular melanoma, consisting of overgrowth of uveal melanocytes and often preceded by a uveal nevus. See also **ocular melanoma.**

uveal tract, the vascular layer of the eye. See **uvea.**

uveitis /yōō′vē·ī″tis/ [L, *uva* + Gk, *itis*], inflammation of the uveal tract of the eye, including the iris, ciliary body, and choroid. It may be characterized by an irregularly shaped pupil, inflammation around the cornea, pus in the anterior chamber, opaque deposits on the cornea, pain, and lacrimation. Causes include allergy, infection, trauma, diabetes, collagen disease, and skin diseases. A major complication may be glaucoma. See also **chorioretinitis, choroiditis, iritis.**

uvula /yōō″vyələ/ *pl. uvulae* [L, *uva,* grape], the small cone-shaped process suspended in the mouth from the middle of the posterior border of the soft palate, especially the uvula palatina. *−uvular, adj.*

uvular /yōō″vyələr/ [L, *uva,* grape], pertaining to the palatine uvula.

uvulectomy /yōō′vyəlek″təmē/ [L, *uva,* grape; Gk, *ektomē,* excision], the surgical removal of the uvula.

uvulitis /yōō′vyəlī″tis/, an inflammation of the uvula. Common causes are allergy and infection.

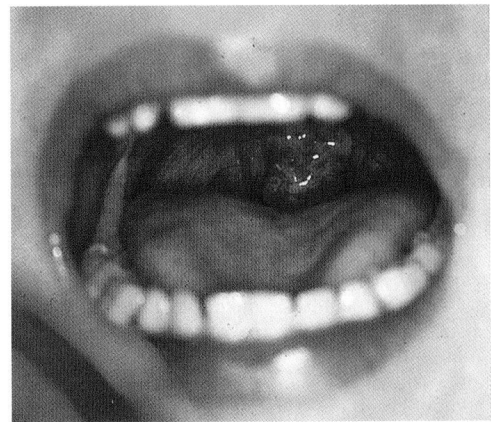

Uvulitis *(Zitelli and Davis, 2007)*

uvulopalatopharyngoplasty. See **palatopharyngoplasty.**

uvulotomy /yōō′vyəlot″əmē/, the surgical removal of all or part of the uvula. See also **uvulectomy.**

U wave, a small, rounded wave that follows the T wave on an electrocardiogram. Normally its polarity is that of the T wave. Its mechanism is unknown. The U wave becomes taller in hypokalemia and inverted in heart disease. It may signify decreased potassium levels in the blood.

U

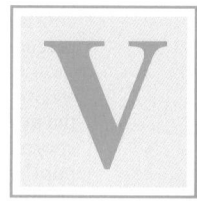

v, **1.** abbreviation for **vein. 2.** abbreviation for **venous blood. 3.** symbol for *speed of a wave.*

V, **1.** symbol for the element **vanadium. 2.** symbol for *ventilation capacity of the lung.* **3.** abbreviation for **volt.**

V̇, symbol for *rate of gas flow.*

V_max, the maximum rate of catalysis.

V_T, abbreviation for **tidal volume.**

VAC, **1.** an anticancer drug combination of vincristine, dactinomycin, and cyclophosphamide. **2.** abbreviation for **Vacuum-Assisted Closure.**

vaccinal /vak″si·nəl/ [L, *vaccinus*], **1.** pertaining to vaccinia, to vaccine, or to vaccination. **2.** having protective qualities when used by way of inoculation.

vaccination (vacc) /vak″sinā″shən/ [L, *vaccinus,* relating to a cow], any injection of attenuated or killed microorganisms, such as bacteria, viruses, or rickettsia, administered to induce immunity or to reduce the effects of associated infectious diseases. Historically, the first vaccinations were administered to immunize against smallpox. Vaccinations are now available to immunize against many diseases, such as flu, diphtheria, measles, varicella, and mumps. –*vaccinate, v.*

vaccine /vaksēn′, vak″sēn, -sin/ [L, *vaccinus*], a suspension of attenuated or killed microorganisms administered intradermally, intramuscularly, orally, or subcutaneously to induce active immunity to infectious disease. Viruses and rickettsia used in some vaccines are grown in avian embryos, rabbit brain tissue, or monkey kidney tissue, and the organisms are usually inactivated by formalin, phenol, or beta-propiolactone. Bacteria for some vaccines may be inactivated by acetone, formalin, heat, or phenol. Vaccines may be used as single agents or in combinations. Compare **antiserum.**

-vaccine, suffix meaning "a preparation containing microorganisms for producing immunity to disease."

vaccinia /vaksin″ē·ə/ [L, *vaccinus*], an infectious disease of cattle caused by a poxvirus that may be transmitted to humans by direct contact or deliberate inoculation as a vaccine against smallpox. A pustule develops at the site of infection, usually followed by malaise and fever that last for several days. After 2 weeks the pustule becomes a crust that eventually drops off, leaving a scar. Satellite lesions may occur, and the virus may be spread to other sites by scratching. Individuals with eczema or other preexisting skin disease may develop generalized vaccinia. Rarely, a severe encephalitis follows vaccinia. Also called **cowpox.** Compare **smallpox.** See also **vaccination.**

vaccinia immune globulin, a hyperimmune gamma globulin developed for the treatment of skin reactions to immunization against the viral disease vaccinia.

vaccinotherapeutics /vak″sinōther″əpyoo″tiks/, a form of therapy that involves injections of bacterial antigens.

VACTERL association, a nonrandom association of congenital anomalies similar to the VATER association but also including cardiac and limb anomalies; the cause is unknown. See also **VATER association.**

vacuole /vak″yoo·ōl/ [L, *vacuus,* empty], **1.** a clear or fluid-filled space or cavity within a cell, such as occurs when a

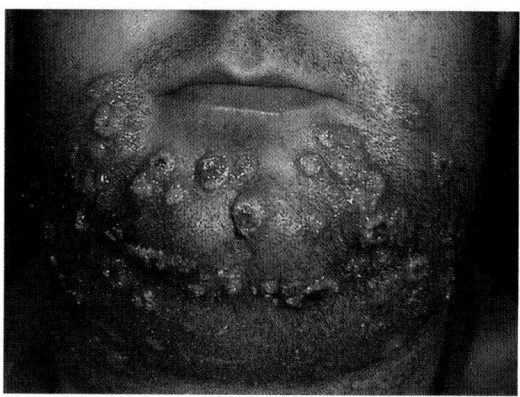

Vaccinia *(du Vivier, 2002)*

droplet of water is ingested by the cytoplasm. **2.** a small space in the body enclosed by a membrane, usually containing fat, secretions, or cellular debris. –*vacuolated, vacuolar, adj.*

Vacutainer tube, a brand of blood-collection tube with a closure that is evacuated to create a vacuum inside the tube facilitating the draw of a predetermined volume of liquid. It is most commonly used to draw blood samples directly from the vein; it is also used in the collection of urine samples. Vacutainer tubes may contain additives designed to stabilize and preserve the specimen prior to analytical testing. Vacutainer is a registered trademark of Becton, Dickinson, and Company.

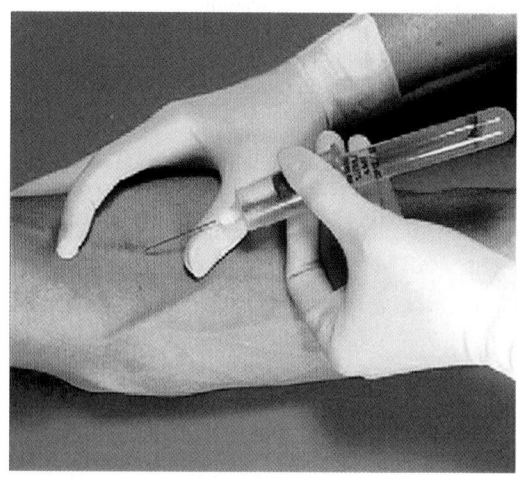

Obtaining a blood sample with a Vacutainer tube
(Sanders et al, 2007)

vacuum aspiration /vak″yoo·əm/ [L, *vacuus,* empty, *aspirare,* to breathe upon], a method of removing tissues from the uterus by suction for diagnostic purposes or to remove elements of conception. With the patient under local or light general anesthesia, the cervix is dilated, and the uterus is emptied with suction. Postoperative care includes the close observation of vital signs for symptoms of blood loss. Also called **suction curettage.** Compare **dilation and curettage.** See also **elective abortion, therapeutic abortion.**

Vacuum-Assisted Closure (VAC), a system that uses the controlled negative pressure of a vacuum to promote healing of certain types of wounds. The edges of the wound are made airtight with foam and a dressing, and a tube is placed in the wound, connecting to a canister that creates a vacuum. Infectious materials and other fluids are then sucked out of the wound.

VAD, abbreviation for **vascular access device.**

vade mecum /vā″dē mē″kəm/ [L, go with me], something carried by a person for constant use—a pocket drug reference, for example.

vagal /vā″gəl/ [L, *vagus,* wandering], pertaining to the vagus nerve.

vagal tone [L, *vagus,* wandering; Gk, *tonos,* stretching], **1.** the level of activity in the parasympathetic nervous system. **2.** the inhibitory control of the vagus nerve over heart rate and atrioventricular conduction.

vagina /vəjī″nə/ [L, sheath], the part of the female genitalia that forms a canal from the orifice through the vestibule to the uterine cervix. It is behind the bladder and urethra and in front of the rectum. In the adult woman the anterior wall of the vagina is about 7 cm long, and the posterior wall is about 9 cm long. The canal is actually a potential space; the walls usually touch. The muscles of the vagina are innervated by the pudendal nerve and perfused by the vaginal artery.

vaginal atrophy /vaj″ənəl/, a postmenopausal condition of gradually declining tissue activity in the female reproductive tract. It is caused by a cessation of follicular inhibin and estrogen secretion. This leads to decreased negative feedback on the release of follicle-stimulating hormone and luteinizing hormone by the anterior pituitary gland. Tissue effects related to estrogen deficiency include atrophy and dystrophy of the vulva and vagina, pruritus vulvae, dyspareunia, cystourethritis, ectropion, and uterovaginal prolapse.

vaginal birth after cesarean section (VBAC), the delivery of a child via the normal passage from the uterus following the previous delivery of a child via an incision directly into the uterus.

■ METHOD: Prenatal assessment will include specific measures to determine whether vaginal delivery is a safe option. A trial of labor with close monitoring is indicated.

■ PATIENT CARE CONSIDERATIONS: Close monitoring is required. Equipment and personnel for an emergency cesarean section should be available.

■ OUTCOME CRITERIA: Complications are rare for most women who receive appropriate prenatal care. Uterine rupture is the most serious complication.

vaginal bleeding, an abnormal condition in which blood is passed from the vagina other than during the menses. It may be caused by abnormalities of the uterus or cervix, an abnormal pregnancy, endocrine abnormalities, abnormalities of one or both ovaries or one or both fallopian tubes, or an abnormality of the vagina. The following terms are commonly used in describing the approximate amount of vaginal bleeding: *heavy vaginal bleeding,* which is greater than heaviest normal menstrual flow; *moderate vaginal bleeding,* which is equal to heaviest normal menstrual flow; *light vaginal bleeding,* which is less than heaviest normal menstrual flow; *vaginal staining,* a very light flow of blood barely requiring the use of a sanitary napkin or tampon; *vaginal*

spotting, the passage vaginally of a few drops of blood; and *bloody show,* an episode of light vaginal bleeding as often occurs in early labor, during labor, and, particularly, at the time of full dilation of the cervix at the end of the first stage of labor because of rupture of the cervical capillaries as dilation occurs.

vaginal cancer, a malignancy of the vagina occurring rarely as a primary neoplasm and more often as a secondary lesion or extension of vulvar, cervical, endometrial, or ovarian cancer. Clear cell adenocarcinoma occurs in young women ages 14 to 30 exposed in utero to diethylstilbestrol, given to their mothers to prevent abortion, but most primary vaginal cancers arise in Caucasian women over 60 years of age. A predisposing factor is cervical carcinoma, HPV infection, and a previous hysterectomy. Vaginal leukoplakia, erythematosus, erosion, or granulation of the mucosa may prove to be carcinoma in situ.

■ OBSERVATIONS: Symptoms of invasive lesions are postmenopausal bleeding, purulent discharge, pain, and dysuria. Diagnostic measures include cervical, endocervical, and vaginal Papanicolaou smears, colposcopy, biopsy, and Schiller iodine test in which malignant cells do not stain dark brown.

■ INTERVENTIONS: Depending on the patient's age and condition and the site and extent of the lesion, treatment may be by irradiation or vaginectomy and radical hysterectomy with lymph node dissection. Cryosurgery, topical 5-fluorouracil, and dinitrochlorobenzene may be used, but chemotherapy is not usually effective.

■ PATIENT CARE CONSIDERATIONS: The majority of vaginal cancers are squamous cell carcinomas; others are clear cell or undifferentiated adenocarcinomas, malignant melanomas, and sarcomas. When diagnosed in the early stages, vaginal cancer can often be cured.

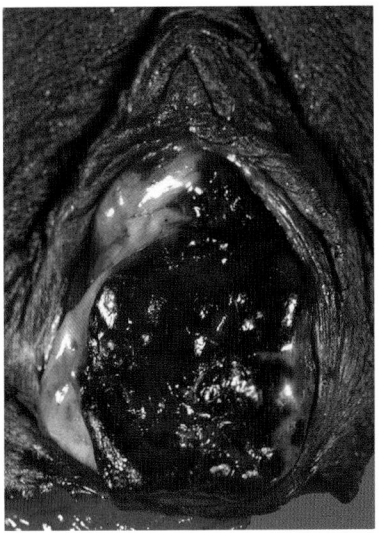

Malignant melanoma involving the vagina *(Kumar, Abbas, and Fausto, 2005)*

vaginal candidiasis. See **vulvovaginal candidiasis.**

vaginal cornification test, a test for the level of estrogen in a urine sample of a female.

vaginal cyst [L, *vagina,* sheath; Gk, *kytis,* bag], an abnormal closed sac or pouch in the vaginal tissues.

vaginal delivery, birth of a fetus through the vagina.

vaginal discharge, any discharge from the vagina. A clear or pearly-white discharge occurs normally. Throughout the

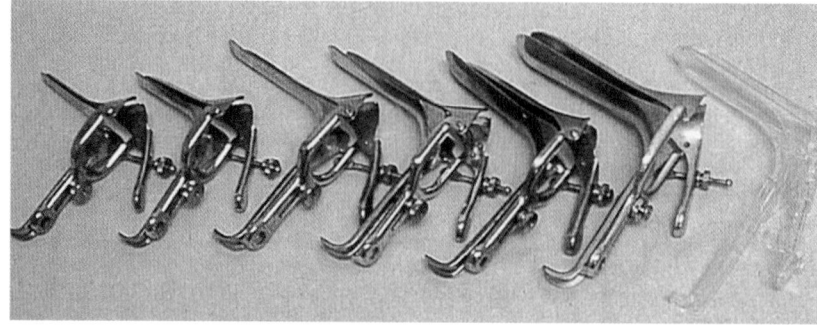

Vaginal specula *(Seidel et al, 2006)*

reproductive years the amount varies greatly from woman to woman, and the amount and character vary in each woman at different times in her menstrual cycle. Before menarche and after menopause, the quantity of discharge is usually less than during the reproductive years. The discharge is largely composed of secretions of the endocervical glands. Inflammatory conditions of the vagina and cervix often cause an increase in the discharge, which may then have a foul odor and cause pruritus of the perineum and external genitalia.

vaginal fornix, a recess in the upper part of the vagina caused by the protrusion of the uterine cervix into the vagina.

vaginal hernia, 1. a hernia into the vagina. **2.** a downward protrusion of the cul-de-sac of Douglas between the posterior vaginal wall and the rectum. Also called **posterior vaginal hernia.**

vaginal hysterectomy [L, *vagina,* sheath; Gk, *hystera,* womb, *ektomē,* excision], the surgical removal of the uterus through the vagina.

vaginal instillation of medication the instillation of a medicated cream, suppository, or gel into the vagina, usually to treat a local infection of the vagina or uterine cervix.

vaginal jelly, a contraceptive product containing a spermicide in a jelly medium. It is usually used in conjunction with a contraceptive diaphragm or cervical cap. Some antimicrobial medications are also supplied in the form of a vaginal jelly.

vaginal lubricant, an ointment or cream used to reduce friction in the vagina.

vaginal mucification test /myoo′sifikā″shən/, a test for the presence of progestins indicated by the stimulation of mucus production in the vaginal epithelium of a laboratory animal. Once used as a test for pregnancy, this test is now used in laboratory studies.

vaginal speculum [L, *vagina,* sheath; L, *speculum,* mirror], a bivalved instrument with two blades used to hold open the vaginal opening for inspection of the vaginal cavity.

vaginal spotting, vaginal staining. See **vaginal bleeding.**

vaginal vault, the enlargement of the internal end of the vagina.

vaginismus /vaj′iniz″məs/ [L, *vagina* + *spasmus,* spasm], a psychophysiological genital reaction of women, characterized by intense contraction of the perineal and paravaginal musculature, tightly closing the vaginal introitus. It occurs in response to fear of painful intercourse before coitus or of pelvic examination. Vaginismus is considered abnormal if it occurs in the absence of genital lesions and if it conflicts with a woman's desire to participate in sexual intercourse or to permit examination, but it may be a normal or physiological response if painful genital conditions exist or if forcible or premature intromission is anticipated. Abnormal vaginismus is uncommon. Sexual adjustment often can be achieved through educative and supportive measures that lead to improved sexual

self-awareness and response. In some cases the condition is a manifestation of serious mental illness and requires formal psychiatric evaluation and treatment. Gender identity conflict, a history of trauma from rape or incest, or an intense suppression of sexuality in childhood and adolescence are factors that often are associated with vaginismus. See also **dyspareunia.**

vaginitis /vaj′inī″tis/, an inflammation of the vaginal tissues, such as trichomonas vaginitis. See also **atrophic vaginitis.**

vagino-, combining form meaning "vagina": *vaginography, vaginolabial, vaginoperineoplasty.*

vaginography /vaj′inog″rəfē/, the radiographic examination of the vagina after the injection of a radiopaque contrast medium. The procedure is performed in the investigation of congenital abnormalities, vaginal fistulae, and other pathological conditions.

vaginolabial hernia /vaj′inōlā″bē-əl/, an inguinal hernia that reaches the tissue of the labium majus.

vaginoperineoplasty /vaj′inōper′inē″əplas″tē/, plastic surgery of the vagina and perineum.

vagoaccessory syndrome. See **Schmidt syndrome.**[1]

vagosympathetic /vā′gōsim″pəthet″ik/ [L, *vagus,* wandering; Gk, *sympathein,* to feel with], pertaining to the vagus nerve and the cervical part of the sympathetic nervous system.

vagotomy /vāgot″əmē/ [L, *vagus,* wandering, *temnein,* to cut], the cutting of certain branches of the vagus nerve, performed with gastric surgery to reduce the amount of gastric acid secreted and lessen the chance of recurrence of a gastric ulcer. With the patient under general anesthesia, a gastrectomy is performed, and the appropriate branches of the vagus nerve are excised. Because peristalsis will be diminished, a pyloroplasty or an anastomosis of the stomach to the jejunum may be done to ensure proper emptying of the stomach. See also **anastomosis, gastrectomy, peptic ulcer, pyloroplasty, vagus nerve.**

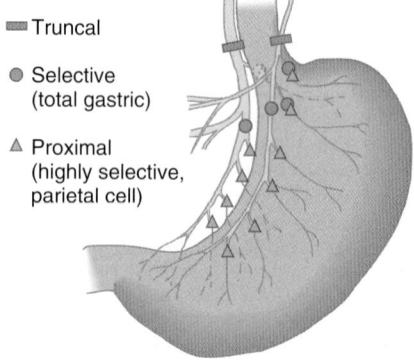

Vagotomy sites *(Black and Hawks, 2009)*

vagotonia.   See **sympathetic imbalance.**

vagotonus /vā′gətō″nəs/ [L, *vagus* + Gk, *tonos,* tension], an abnormal increase in parasympathetic activity caused by stimulation of the vagus nerve, especially bradycardia with decreased cardiac output, faintness, and syncope. Vagotonus may occur in suctioning the oropharynx of a newborn as the syringe, laryngoscope blade, or catheter is inadvertently pressed on the back of the throat, stimulating the nerve. It also occurs in some women after surgical treatment or simple manipulation of the uterine cervix.

vagovagal reflex /vā′gōvā″gəl/ [L, *vagus* + *vagus* + *reflectere,* to bend back], a stimulation of the vagus nerve by reflex in which irritation of the larynx or the trachea results in slowing of the pulse rate.

vagueness /văg″nəs/, a communication pattern involving the use of global pronouns and loose associations that lead to ambiguity and confusion in communication.

vagus nerve /vā″gəs/ [L, *vagus,* wandering, *nervus,* nerve], either of the longest pair of cranial nerves mainly responsible for parasympathetic control over the heart and many other internal organs, including thoracic and abdominal viscera. The vagus nerves communicate through 13 main branches, connecting to four areas in the brain. Also called **nervus vagus, pneumogastric nerve, tenth cranial nerve.**

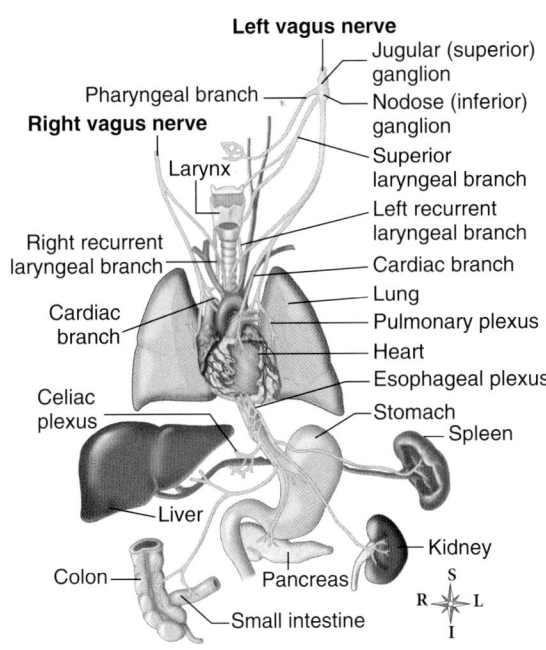

Left vagus nerve
Jugular (superior) ganglion
Pharyngeal branch
Right vagus nerve
Nodose (inferior) ganglion
Larynx
Superior laryngeal branch
Left recurrent laryngeal branch
Right recurrent laryngeal branch
Cardiac branch
Cardiac branch
Lung
Pulmonary plexus
Heart
Esophageal plexus
Celiac plexus
Stomach
Spleen
Liver
Kidney
Colon
Pancreas
Small intestine

Vagus nerve

vagus pulse [L, *vagus,* wandering, *pulsare,* to beat], a slow, regular pulse caused by overactivity of the vagus nerve.

Val, abbreviation for **valine.**

valacyclovir /val″a-si′klo-vir/, a prodrug of acyclovir with improved tolerability. The hydrochloride salt is used as an antiviral agent in the treatment of genital herpes and herpes zoster in patients who are not immunocompromised. It is administered orally.

valdecoxib, a nonsteroidal antiinflammatory drug (NSAID) of the selective cyclooxygenase-2 (COX-2) inhibitors group. It is used to treat acute and chronic rheumatoid arthritis, osteoarthritis, and primary dysmenorrhea. It is no longer manufactured in the United States.

valecular, shallowly grooved. See **vallecula.**

valence /văl″əns/ [L, *valere,* to be strong], **1.** (in chemistry) a numeric expression of the capability of an element to combine chemically with atoms of hydrogen or their equivalent. An element is considered monovalent (or univalent) if each of its atoms can react with only one hydrogen atom or its equivalent, divalent (or bivalent) if each atom can react with two hydrogen or equivalent atoms, trivalent (or tervalent) if each atom can react with three hydrogen atoms, and polyvalent (or multivalent) if each atom can react with many hydrogen atoms. **2.** (in immunology) an expression of the number of antigen-binding sites for one molecule of any given antibody or the number of antibody-binding sites for any given antigen. Most antibody molecules, and those belonging to the IgG, IgA, and IgE immunoglobulin classes, have two antigen-binding sites. Most large antigen molecules are multivalent.

-valence, -valency, a combining form meaning "the combining capacity of an atom compared with that of one hydrogen atom": *electrovalence, trivalence.*

valence electron, any of the electrons in the highest principal energy level of an atom or ion. They are responsible for the bonding of atoms to form crystals, molecules, and compounds.

valency. See **valence.**

-valent, suffix meaning "having a valency of a (specified) magnitude": *divalent, pentavalent, tetravalent.*

valerian, a perennial herb native to Eurasia that is now grown worldwide.

■ INDICATIONS: This herb is used as a sedative; it is generally considered safe and effective for short-term use, but it has not been studied as a drug.

■ CONTRAINDICATIONS: Valerian should not be used during pregnancy and lactation, by those with a known hypersensitivity to it, or by those with hepatic disease. It should be used only with caution in children, as research is lacking. It should be used with caution as efficacy has not been consistently demonstrated.

valeric acid $(CH_3(CH_2)_3COOH)$ /vəler″ik/, an organic acid with a foul odor found in the roots of *Valeriana officinalis.* Commercially prepared, it is used in the production of perfumes, flavors, lubricants, and certain drugs. Also called **pantothenic acid.**

valganciclovir /val″gan-si′klo-vir/, a prodrug of ganciclovir, an antiviral used in the treatment of cytomegalovirus infections in immunocompromised patients; it is administered orally as the hydrochloride salt.

valgus /val″gəs/ [L, bent], describing an abnormal position in which a part of a limb is bent or twisted outward, away from the midline, such as the heel of the foot in talipes valgus (splayfoot). Compare **varus.** See also **hallux valgus.**

validation /val′idā″shən/, the reciprocated communication of respect that conveys that the patient's opinions are acknowledged, respected, and heard regardless of whether the listener actually agrees with the content.

validity /valid″itē/, (in research) the extent to which a test measurement or other device measures what it is intended to measure. A data collection tool should accurately reflect the concept that it is intended to measure. Compare **reliability.** Kinds include **construct validity, content validity, current validity, predictive validity.**

valine (Val) /val″ēn/, an essential amino acid needed for optimal growth in infants and for nitrogen equilibrium in adults. Also called **alpha-aminoisovaleric acid.** See also **amino acid, maple syrup urine disease, protein.**

V

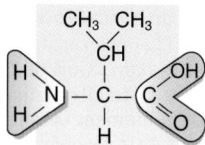

Chemical structure of valine

valinemia. See **hypervalinemia.**

Valisone, a topical glucocorticoid. Brand name for *betamethasone valerate.*

Valium, a benzodiazepine used as an antianxiety agent, anticonvulsant, muscle relaxant, and sedative-hypnotic. Brand name for **diazepam.**

vallecula /vəlek″yələ/ [L, little valley], **1.** any crevice or depression on the surface of an organ or structure. **2.** See **vallecula epiglottica.** *–vallecular, adj.*

vallecula epiglottica, a furrow between the glossoepiglottic folds of each side of the posterior oropharynx. Also called **vallecula.**

vallecular dysphagia /vəlek″yələr/, difficulty or pain on swallowing caused by inflammation of the vallecula epiglottica. Compare **contractile ring dysphagia, dysphagia lusoria.**

valley fever. See **coccidioidomycosis.**

valproate /val-pro′āt/, a salt of valproic acid with anticonvulsant activity similar to that of the acid.

valproic acid /valprō″ik/, an anticonvulsant.
- INDICATIONS: It is prescribed alone or in combination to treat complex partial seizures, absence seizures occurring alone or in combination with other types of seizures, mania associated with bipolar disorder, and migraine prophylaxis.
- CONTRAINDICATIONS: It is not recommended for use during pregnancy or lactation. Hepatic disease or dysfunction, urea cycle disorders, and known hypersensitivity to this drug prohibit its use.
- ADVERSE EFFECTS: Among the more severe adverse effects are decreased platelet function, hepatotoxicity, and pancreatitis. GI disturbances are common. Alopecia, rash, headache, and insomnia also may occur. A sometimes fatal hyperammonemic encephalopathy has occurred in patients with known or suspected urea cycle disorders.

valrubicin, an antibiotic antineoplastic agent.
- INDICATIONS: This drug is used to treat bladder cancer.
- CONTRAINDICATIONS: Factors that prohibit the use of this drug include known hypersensitivity to anthracyclines or Cremophor EL, urinary tract infection, and small bladder size.
- ADVERSE EFFECTS: Life-threatening side effects of this drug include thrombocytopenia and leukopenia. Common side effects include anemia, nausea, vomiting, anorexia, diarrhea, urinary tract infection, urinary retention, hematuria, rash, and chest pain.

Valsalva leak point pressure, the amount of pressure on the bladder by a Valsalva maneuver at which leakage of urine from the urethra occurs. This is a measure of strength of the urethral sphincters.

Valsalva maneuver /valsal″və/ [Antonio M. Valsalva, Italian surgeon, 1666–1723; OFr, *maneuvre,* work done by hand], any forced expiratory effort against a closed airway, such as when an individual holds the breath and tightens the muscles in a concerted, strenuous effort to move a heavy object. Most healthy individuals perform Valsalva maneuvers during normal daily activities without any injurious consequences. However, such efforts are dangerous for many patients with cardiovascular disease, especially if they become dehydrated, increasing the viscosity of their blood and the attendant risk of blood clotting. Constipation increases the risk of cardiovascular trauma in such patients, especially if they perform a Valsalva maneuver in trying to move their bowels. On relaxation after each muscular effort with held breath, the blood of such individuals rushes to the heart, often overloading the cardiac system and causing cardiac arrest. Orthopedic patients often use a Valsalva maneuver in changing their position in bed with the aid of an overhead trapeze bar. Patients who may be endangered by performing a Valsalva maneuver are commonly instructed to exhale instead of holding their breath when they move. Exhalation decreases the risk of cardiovascular trauma. Part of the danger is a bradycardia response.

Valsalva's test [Antonio M. Valsalva; L, *testum,* crucible], a method for testing the patency of the eustachian tubes. With mouth and nose kept tightly closed, the patient makes a forced expiratory effort. If the eustachian tubes are open, air will enter into the middle ear cavities, and the subject will hear a popping sound. See also **Valsalva maneuver.**

valsartan, an angiotensin receptor blocking agent.
- INDICATIONS: It is used to treat hypertension and heart failure, either alone or in combination with other agents.
- CONTRAINDICATIONS: Factors that prohibit its use are known hypersensitivity to valsartan, pregnancy, severe hepatic disease, and bilateral renal artery stenosis.
- ADVERSE EFFECTS: Life-threatening effects are cerebrovascular accident, myocardial infarction, hepatotoxicity, and nephrotoxicity. Major side effects include hypotension, hyperkalemia, dizziness, and acute renal failure.

value /val″yoo/ [L, *valere,* to be strong], a personal belief about the worth of a given idea or behavior.

values clarification, a method whereby a person can discover his or her own values by assessing, exploring, and determining what those personal values are and how they affect personal decision making.

value system, the accepted mode of conduct and the set of norms, goals, and values binding any social group. Such guidelines for determining what is right or wrong, good or bad, and desirable or undesirable serve as a frame of reference for the individual in reaching decisions and in achieving a meaningful life.

valve /valv/ [L, *valva,* folding door], a natural structure or artificial device in a passage or vessel that prevents reflux of the fluid contents passing through it. Valves in veins are membranous folds that prevent backflow of blood. *–valvular, adj.*

-valve, suffix meaning "a thing that regulates the flow of": *bivalve.*

valve of Kerkring. See **circular fold.**

valve of lymphatics, any one of the tiny semilunar structures in the vessels and trunks of the lymphatic system that helps regulate the flow of lymph and prevents venous blood from entering the system. There are no valves in the capillaries of the system, but there are many in the collecting vessels. The valves are attached by their convex edges to the walls of the vessels, leaving their concave edges free and directed along the course of the current of lymph. Usually two valves of equal size are found opposite each other. They are more numerous near the lymph nodes and more prevalent in the lymphatic vessels of the neck and the arms than in the vessels of the legs. The wall of the vessel just above the attachment of each valve bulges with a small sinus that gives the vessel its beaded appearance. See also **lymphatic system.**

valve of vein. See **venous valves.**

valvotomy /valvot″əmē/ [L, *valva* + Gk, *temnein,* to cut], the incision into a valve, especially one in the heart, to correct a defect and allow proper opening and closure. Before surgery a cardiac catheterization is performed. With the patient under general anesthesia, the damaged valve is repaired, if possible, or removed. A prosthetic or biological valve suture is put in its place. Complications peculiar to prosthetic valve surgery are displacement of the valve caused by broken sutures, heart block, leakage and regurgitation from chamber to chamber, infection, and embolus.

valvula, certain small valves in the body and cusps of the heart valves. Also called **valvule.**

valvular, pertaining to a structure that controls the flow of a substance. See **valve.**

valvular endocarditis. See **chronic endocarditis.**

valvular heart disease [L, *valva* + AS, *hoert* + L, *dis,* opposite of; Fr, *aise,* ease], an acquired or congenital disorder of a cardiac valve. It is characterized by stenosis and obstructed blood flow and by valvular degeneration and regurgitation of blood. Diseases of aortic and mitral valves are most common and may be caused by congenital defects, bacterial endocarditis, syphilis, or, most frequently, rheumatic fever. Episodes of rheumatic fever cause the cardiac valves to degenerate and remain open or cause the cusps of the valves to become stiff, calcified, constricted, and fused. Valvular dysfunction results in changes in intracardiac pressure and pulmonary and peripheral circulation. It may lead to cardiac arrhythmia, heart failure, and cardiogenic shock. Cardiotonics, diuretics, analgesics, sodium restriction, and antibiotics, if indicated, are used in the conservative treatment of valvular heart disease. Surgery is usually performed when the symptoms are incapacitating. A diseased valve may be repaired by removing the calcium deposits and opening the fused commissures or by removing a cusp and reconstructing the valve, or it may be replaced with a porcine or artificial valve. Kinds include **aortic regurgitation, aortic stenosis, mitral regurgitation, mitral valve stenosis, pulmonary stenosis, tricuspid stenosis.**

valvular regurgitation [L, *valva,* folding door, *re* + *gurgitare,* to flow], a backflow of blood that occurs when the heart contracts but a heart valve fails to close properly.

valvular stenosis, a narrowing or stricture of any of the heart valves. The condition may result from a congenital defect or may be caused by disease. See also **aortic stenosis, congenital cardiac anomaly, mitral valve stenosis, pulmonary stenosis.**

valvule. See **valvula.**

valvulitis /val′vyəlī′tis/, an inflammation of a valve, especially a cardiac valve. Inflammatory changes in the aortic, mitral, and tricuspid valves of the heart are caused most commonly by rheumatic fever and less frequently by bacterial endocarditis and syphilis. Infected valves degenerate, or their cusps become stiff and calcified, resulting in stenosis and obstructed blood flow.

valvuloplasty /val′vyəlōplas′tē/ [L, *valva,* folding door; Gk, *plassein,* to shape], the use of a balloon-tipped catheter to dilate a cardiac valve.

VAMP /vamp/, abbreviation for a combination drug regimen, used in the treatment of cancer and containing three antineoplastics (vinCRIStine sulfate, methotrexate, and mercaptopurine) and a glucocorticoid (predniSONE).

vanadium (V) /vənā″dē-əm/ [ONorse, *Vanadis,* Freya, goddess of fertility], a grayish metallic element. Its atomic number is 23; its atomic mass is 50.942. Absorption of vanadium compounds results in a condition called *vanadiumism,* characterized by anemia, conjunctivitis, pneumonitis, and irritation of the respiratory tract.

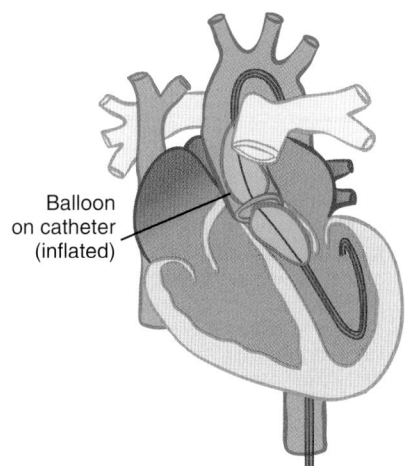

Balloon on catheter (inflated)

Valvuloplasty (Black and Hawks, 2009)

van Bogaert's disease /van bō″gərts/ [Ludo van Bogaert, Belgian neurophysiologist, b. 1897], a rare familial disorder of lipid metabolism in which the substance cholestanol is deposited in the nervous system, blood, and connective tissue. Individuals with the disease develop progressive ataxia and dementia, premature atherosclerosis, cataracts, and xanthomas of the tendons. No effective treatment has been found. Also called **cerebrotendinous xanthomatosis.**

Van Buchem's syndrome. See **endosteal hyperostosis.**

Vanceril, an inhaled glucocorticoid. Brand name for **beclomethasone dipropionate.**

Vancocin Hydrochloride, a glycopeptide antibiotic. Brand name for *vancomycin hydrochloride.*

vancomycin /van′kōmī″sin/, a glycopeptide antibiotic.

■ INDICATIONS: It is prescribed in the treatment of infections, particularly staphylococcal infections resistant to other antibiotics and antibiotic-associated pseudomembranous colitis caused by *Clostridium difficile.*

■ CONTRAINDICATIONS: Concomitant administration of neurotoxic, nephrotoxic, or ototoxic drugs or known hypersensitivity to this drug prohibits its use.

■ ADVERSE EFFECTS: Among the more serious adverse effects are anaphylaxis, dizziness, and tinnitus. The most common adverse effect is red neck syndrome, an infusion reaction that may develop with the first administration of vancomycin. Other side effects include ototoxicity (tinnitus, vertigo, loss of hearing) and nephrotoxicity (change in urine output, elevated serum creatinine and blood urea nitrogen).

Van Deemter's equation /van dēm″tərz/, an expression of a gas chromatography relationship between the height equivalent to the theoretic plate and the linear velocity of the carrier gas.

Van de Graaff generator /van′ də gräf″/ [Robert J. Van de Graaff, American physicist, 1901–1967], a device in which electrically charged particles are sprayed on a moving belt and carried by it to an insulated terminal, where they cause a large electrostatic charge to build up. The charged particles are then accelerated along a discharge path through a vacuum tube by the potential difference between the insulated terminal and the opposite end of the device. The generator often is used to inject charged particles into a larger accelerator.

van den Bergh's test /van″ dən burgs′/ [Albert A.H. van den Bergh, Dutch physician, 1869–1943], a test for the presence of bilirubin in the blood serum. Blood is obtained from a patient, and the diluted serum is added to diazo

V

reagent. A blue or violet color indicates the presence of bilirubin. The rate and magnitude of the color change are noted. See also **bilirubin.**

van der Waals forces /van′ der wäls′, fän-/ [Johannes D. van der Waals, Dutch physicist and Nobel laureate, 1837–1923], weak attractive forces between neutral atoms and molecules. They occur because a fluctuating dipole moment in one molecule induces a dipole moment in another and the two dipole moments interact in an attractive manner. The activity accounts for some deviation from Boyle's law at very low temperatures or very high pressures. Also called **dispersion forces.**

van der Woude's syndrome /van·der·wō′dəz/, an autosomal-dominant syndrome consisting of cleft lip with or without cleft palate, with cysts of the lower lip.

vanillylmandelic acid (VMA) /vənil′ilməndel″ik/, a urinary metabolite of epinephrine and norepinephrine. It may be measured in the urine to determine the levels of these catecholamines. A greater-than-normal amount of VMA is characteristic of a pheochromocytoma or neuroblastoma. Increased concentrations of this acid may raise the blood pressure and indicate the presence of tumors of the adrenal glands or nervous system, muscular dystrophy, and myasthenia gravis; they may be caused by stress, exercise, or certain drugs or foods. Normal amounts in the urine of adults after 24-hour collection are 1.5 to 7.5 mg; in the urine of infants, it is 83 mg/kg of body weight. Also called **3-methoxy-4-hydroxymandelic acid.**

vanillylmandelic acid and catecholamines test, a 24-hour urine test that is performed primarily to diagnose hypertension secondary to pheochromocytoma. It is also used to detect the presence of neuroblastomas and rare adrenal tumors.

vanishing testis, a testis that was originally present in the fetus but atrophied in utero because of torsion.

vanishing twin /van″ishing/, a twin embryo or fetus that is aborted during pregnancy.

vanity surgery /van″itē/, plastic surgery performed primarily to make the patient appear more youthful.

Vanoxide, a topical fixed-combination drug containing an antibacterial keratolytic and an antiinflammatory corticosteroid. Brand name for **benzoyl peroxide, hydrocortisone.**

vape /ˈvāpə/ [L, vapor, steam], |v.,| to inhale and exhale the contents of an e-cigarette or similar apparatus.

Vaponefrin, an adrenergic agonist, sympathomimetic. Brand name for *epINEPHrine hydrochloride.*

vapor /vā′pər/ *pl. vapors* [L], **1.** an atmospheric dispersion of the gaseous form of a substance that in its normal state is a liquid or solid. **2.** steam, gas, or an exhalation.

vapor bath /vā″pər/, the exposure of the body to vapor, such as steam.

vaporization /vā′pərīzā″shən/ [L, *vapor,* steam], the changing of a liquid or solid (such as dry ice) to a gaseous state.

vaporizer, **1.** a device for reducing medicated liquids to a vapor, useful for inhalation or application to accessible mucous membranes. **2.** a device for converting potent liquid anesthetic agents to a vapor useful for inhalation.

vapor pressure depression, a phenomenon in which the addition of a solute molecule to a solvent will decrease the vapor pressure of the solvent in equilibrium with the liquid phase.

vapor therapy, the therapeutic use of vapors or sprays. See also **vaporizer.**

Vaprisol, a nonpeptide inhibitor of antidiuretic hormone. Brand name for **conivaptan.**

Vaquez's disease. See **polycythemia rubra vera.**

vardenafil, an agent used to treat impotence.
- INDICATIONS: This drug is used to treat erectile dysfunction.
- CONTRAINDICATIONS: Known hypersensitivity to this drug prohibits its use. Alpha-blockers or nitrates should not be co-administered with this drug.
- ADVERSE EFFECTS: Common side effects include headache, flushing, and hypotension. Other adverse effects of this drug include conjunctivitis, tinnitus, photophobia, diminished vision, glaucoma, abnormal ejaculation, priapism, myalgia, arthralgia, neck pain, rhinitis, sinusitis, dyspnea, pharyngitis, epistaxis, rash, gastroesophageal reflux disease, and increased gamma glutamyl transpeptidase. Life-threatening side effects include myocardial infarction and cardiovascular collapse.

varenicline, a smoking-cessation agent.
- INDICATIONS: This drug is used as a smoking deterrent.
- CONTRAINDICATIONS: Eating disorders or known hypersensitivity to this drug prohibits its use.
- ADVERSE EFFECTS: Common side effects include blurred vision, nausea, vomiting, dry mouth, and constipation. Adverse effects of this drug include headache, agitation, dizziness, insomnia, abnormal dreams, fatigue, malaise, arrhythmias, changes in blood pressure, palpitations, tachycardia, angina, tinnitus, anorexia, increased or decreased appetite, flatulence, gastroesophageal reflux disease, erectile dysfunction, urinary frequency, menstrual irregularities, rash, pruritus, weight loss or gain, dyspnea, and rhinorrhea. A life-threatening side effect is myocardial infarction.

variability /ver′ē·əbil″itē/ [L, *variare,* to diversify], the degree of divergence or ability of an object to vary from a given standard or average.

variable /ver″ē·əbəl/, **1.** a factor in an experiment or scientific test that tends to vary, or take on different values, while other elements or conditions remain constant. See also **categoric variable, dependent variable, independent variable. 2.** an attribute of a person that is measurable and that varies (heart rate, age).

variable behavior [L, *variare,* to diversify; AS, *bihabban,* to behave], a response, activity, or action that may be modified by individual experience. Compare **invariable behavior.**

variable interval (VI) reinforcement, reinforcement that is offered after varying lapses of time.

variable number of tandem repeats (VNTR), different numbers of tandemly repeated oligonucleotide sequences in the alleles of a gene.

variable-performance oxygen delivery system. See **low-flow oxygen delivery system.**

variable ratio (VR) reinforcement, reinforcement that requires variable numbers of responses.

variable region, the part of an immunoglobulin in which the amino acid sequence can differ among molecules of that class of immunoglobulin. The variable region includes the antigen-binding site. Compare **constant region.**

variance /ver″ē·əns/ [L, *variare*], **1.** (in statistics) a numeric representation of the dispersion of data around the mean in a given sample. It is represented by the square of the standard deviation and is used principally in performing an analysis of variance. **2.** *(Nontechnical)* the general range of a group of findings.

variant /ver″ē·ənt/ [L, *variare,* to diversify], an individual or subpopulation that differs from other individuals or subpopulations of its species.

variant angina. See **Prinzmetal angina.**

varicella. See **chickenpox.**

varicella gangrenosa /ver′isel″ə/, a potentially fatal form of varicella characterized by gangrenous lesions. A fulminating subvariety of the skin disorder may become fatal within a few hours if complicated by hemolytic streptococcus.

varicella virus vaccine live, a preparation of live, attenuated human herpesvirus 3 (varicella zoster virus) administered subcutaneously for production of immunity to varicella and herpes zoster.

varicella-zoster immune globulin (VZIG) /zos″tər/ [L, *varius,* diverse; Gk, *zoster,* girdle; L, *immunis,* free from, *globulus,* small globe], extracted and purified immune globulin made from the blood of people who have high titers of varicella zoster virus antibodies. The immune globulin can be administered to people exposed to chickenpox to prevent or modify symptoms of the infection. See also **immunoglobulin, zoster immune plasma.**

varicella zoster virus (VZV) [L, *varius,* diverse; Gk, *zoster,* girdle; L, *virus,* poison], a member of the herpesvirus family, which causes the diseases varicella (chickenpox) with primary infection and herpes zoster (shingles) of the virus reactivator. The virus has been isolated from vesicle fluid in chickenpox, is highly contagious, and may be spread by direct contact or droplets. Dried crusts of skin lesions do not contain active virus particles. Herpes zoster is produced by reactivation of latent varicella virus, usually several years after the initial infection. There is no simple test for measuring antibodies to this virus. However, zoster immune globulin (ZIG) obtained from convalescing zoster patients will prevent varicella in susceptible children if injected within 3 days of their exposure. The temporary nature of this protection and the relative scarcity of ZIG warrant reservation of its use to children receiving immunosuppressive therapy or suffering from immune deficiency diseases. Herpes zoster should be treated promptly with acyclovir, desciclovir, valaciclovir, or penciclovir to speed healing. (Famciclovir is used for postherpetic neuralgia.) A licensed vaccine is available and highly effective. See also **chickenpox, herpes zoster.**

varicelliform /ver′isel″ifôrm/, resembling the rash of chickenpox.

varices. See **varix.**

varicocele /ver′əkōsēl′/ [L, *varix,* varicose vein; Gk, *kele,* tumor], a dilation of the pampiniform venous complex of the spermatic cord. The varicocele forms a soft, elastic swelling that can cause pain. It is usually more pronounced and painful when the patient is standing. Varicoceles are most common in men between 15 and 25 years of age and affect the left spermatic cord more often than the right. Compare **ovarian varicocele.**

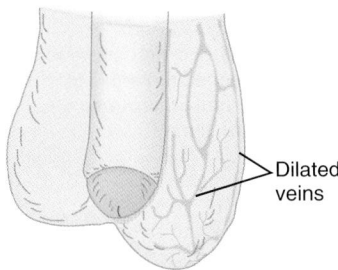

Varicocele *(Black and Hawks, 2009)*

varicose /ver″əkōs/ [L, *varix*], abnormally swollen or dilated.

varicose aneurysm, a blood-filled, saclike projection that connects an artery and one or several veins and that is formed from a localized dilation of the adjoining vessels.

varicose ulcer. See **stasis ulcer.**

varicose vein, a tortuous, dilated vein with incompetent valves. Causes include congenitally defective valves, thrombophlebitis, pregnancy, and obesity. Varicose veins are common, especially in women, and are usually painless. The saphenous veins of the legs are most often affected. Elevation of the legs and use of elastic stockings are frequently sufficient therapy for uncomplicated cases. Ligation of the vein above the varicosity and removal of the distal part of the vessel may be indicated for more severe cases if deeper vessels can maintain the return of venous blood. Injection of sclerosing solutions helps prevent or treat postphlebitic syndrome.
- OBSERVATIONS: Initially the vein may be palpated but invisible, and the individual may have a feeling of heaviness in the legs that gets worse at night and in hot weather. A dull aching, burning, and cramping also occur after prolonged standing or walking, during menses, when fatigued, and at night. Over time the veins can be seen as dilated, purplish, and ropelike. Venous insufficiency and venous stasis ulcers are the two most common complications. Initial diagnosis is made by inspection and palpation and is checked by a manual compression test that reveals a palpable impulse. A Trendelenburg test can help pinpoint the location of incompetent valves. Plethysmography and duplex ultrasound scans can be used to detect venous backflow.
- INTERVENTIONS: Conservative treatment involves elevation and rest of affected extremity, application of lightweight compression hosiery, and avoidance of prolonged standing. Sclerotherapy may be used for removal of unsightly superficial varicosities. Stripping and ligation may be indicated for chronic venous insufficiency, recurrent thrombophlebitis, and persistent varicosities that are painful or ulcerated and are not responsive to conservative treatment.
- PATIENT CARE CONSIDERATIONS: Long-term management of varicosities is directed at improving circulation and preventing stasis, relieving discomfort, and preventing complications. Instruction is given to avoid prolonged standing and sitting and to make frequent position changes. Restrictive and/or occlusive clothing should be avoided, and lower extremities should be periodically elevated above the heart. Compression stockings should be applied while lying down and before rising in the morning. A regular exercise aerobic program should be instituted to promote circulation, and weight reduction is advocated if obesity is a problem.

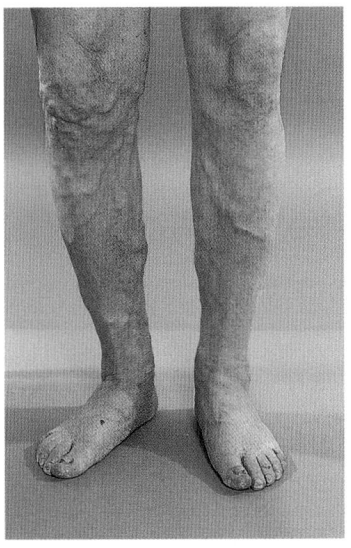

Varicose veins *(Forbes and Jackson, 2003)*

V

varicosis /ver″ikō″sis/ [L, *varix* + Gk, *osis,* condition], a common condition characterized by one or more tortuous, abnormally dilated vessels, usually in the legs or the lower trunk. It most often occurs in persons between 30 and 60 years of age. Varicosis may be caused by congenital defects of the valves or walls of the veins or by congestion and increased intraluminal pressure resulting from prolonged standing, poor posture, pregnancy, abdominal tumor, or chronic systemic disease. Symptoms include pain and muscle cramps with a feeling of fullness and heaviness in the legs. Dilation of superficial veins is often evident before the condition produces discomfort.

varicosity /ver″ikos″itē/, **1.** an abnormal condition, usually of a vein, characterized by swelling and tortuosity. **2.** a vein in this condition.

variegate /ver″ē·əgāt″/ [L, *varius,* diverse], having characteristics that vary, especially as to color.

variegate porphyria (VP), an uncommon form of hepatic porphyria, characterized by skin lesions and photosensitivity. The condition may be congenital or acquired. The congenital form is more serious, resulting in crises of acute abdominal pain and certain neurological complications. See also **porphyria.**

variola minor. See **alastrim.**

variola, variola major. See **smallpox.**

varioliform gastritis. See **erosive gastritis.**

varioloid /ver″ē·əloid″/ [L, *varius* + Gk, *eidos,* form], **1.** *adj.,* resembling smallpox. **2.** *n.,* a mild form of smallpox in a vaccinated person or one who has previously had the disease.

varix /ver″iks/ *pl. varices* [L, varicose vein], a tortuous, dilated vein, artery, or lymphatic vessel.

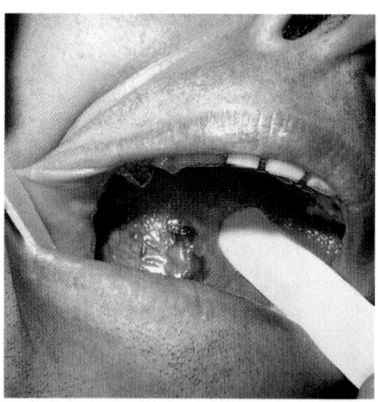

Varix *(Swartz, 2009)*

varnish /vär″nish/, (in dentistry) a solution of natural resins and gums or concentrated fluoride used as a protective coating over the surfaces of a dental cavity preparation before restorative material is applied or over a tooth surface after sealing and root planing. Fluoride varnish is a protective coating that occludes dentinal tubules and applies fluoride to calcified dental tissues, resulting in caries prevention and reduced dental hypersensitivity.

varus /ver″əs/ [L, bent], describing an abnormal position in which a part of a limb is turned inward toward the midline, such as the great toe in hallux varus. Compare **valgus.** See also **hallux varus.**

vas /vas/ *pl. vasa* [L, vessel], any one of the many vessels of the body, especially those that convey blood, lymph, or spermatozoa.

vas afferens, a small arteriole that supplies blood to a renal glomerulus. Also called **afferent glomerular arteriole.**

vasa previa, a rare condition in which blood vessels within the placenta or the umbilical cord obstruct the internal os of the uterus. There is no risk to the fetus until delivery; at that time the fetal vessels are at risk for rupture. A caesarean birth is warranted.

vasa vasorum [L, *vas,* vessel], small blood vessels that supply the walls of the arteries and veins.

vascular /vas″kyələr/ [L, *vasculum,* little vessel], pertaining to a blood vessel.

vascular access device (VAD), an indwelling catheter, cannula, or other instrument used to obtain venous or arterial access.

vascular death, a death caused by vascular pathological conditions.

vascular endothelial growth factor (VEGF), a peptide factor that stimulates the proliferation of cells of the endothelium of blood vessels. It promotes tissue vascularization and is important in blood vessel formation in tumors. It exists in four forms with different lengths (121, 165, 189, and 206 amino acids). Levels are elevated in hypoxia. Also called **vascular permeability factor.**

vascular endothelium, the endothelium that lines the blood vessels.

vascular fasciculus, a fasciculus in the zona externa of the renal medulla.

vascular headache, a classification for certain types of headaches based on a proposed cause involving abnormal functioning of the blood vessels or vascular system of the brain; included are migraine, cluster headache, toxic headache, and headache caused by elevated blood pressure.

vascular insufficiency, inadequate peripheral blood flow. Causes include occlusion of vessels by atherosclerotic plaques, thrombi, or emboli; damaged, diseased, or intrinsically weak vascular walls; arteriovenous fistulas; hematological hypercoagulability; and heavy smoking. Signs of vascular insufficiency include pale, cyanotic, or mottled skin over the affected area; swelling of an extremity; absent or reduced tactile sensation; tingling; diminished sense of temperature; muscle pain, such as intermittent claudication in the calf; and, in advanced disease, ulcers and atrophy of muscles in the involved extremity. Diagnosis may be made by comparing peripheral pulses in contralateral extremities or by angiography, plethysmography, ultrasonography, and skin temperature tests. Treatment of vascular insufficiency may include a diet low in saturated fats, moderate exercise, sleeping on a firm mattress, avoidance of tobacco products, proper standing or sitting posture, elevation of the involved extremity, use of a vasodilating drug, and, if indicated, repair of an arteriovenous fistula or aneurysm or bypass surgery. See also **arterial insufficiency.**

vascularity /vas″kyələr″itē/ [L, *vasculum,* little vessel], the state of blood vessel development and functioning in an organ or tissue.

vascularization /vas″kyələr·īzā″shən/, the process by which body tissue develops proliferating capillaries. It may be natural or induced by surgical techniques. −*vascularize, v.*

vascularized graft, a graft in which the blood supply to the grafted tissue is maintained, as with a pedicle flap.

vascular leiomyoma, a neoplasm that has developed from smooth muscle fibers of a blood vessel.

vascular permeability factor. See **vascular endothelial growth factor.**

vascular pole of renal corpuscle, the end of the corpuscle and glomerulus where afferent arterioles enter and efferent arterioles exit.

vascular sclerosis [L, *vasculum* + Gk, *skerosis,* harden-ing], a condition of hyaline degeneration of the blood ves-sels with hypertrophy of the tunica media and subintimal fibrosis. There also may be a weakening and loss of elasticity in the artery walls.

vascular spider. See **spider angioma.**

vascular tumor, lesions that are the result of pathological development of new blood vessels. See **aneurysm.**

vascular ultrasound studies, ultrasound studies of the extremities, used to identify vein or artery occlusion.

vasculature /vas″kyəlā′chər/ [L, *vasculum*], the blood vessels in an organ or tissue.

vasculitis /vas′kyəlī′tis/, inflammation of the blood vessels. It may be caused by a systemic disease or an allergic reac-tion. Kinds include **allergic vasculitis, necrotizing vascu-litis, segmented hyalinizing vasculitis.** See also **angiitis.**

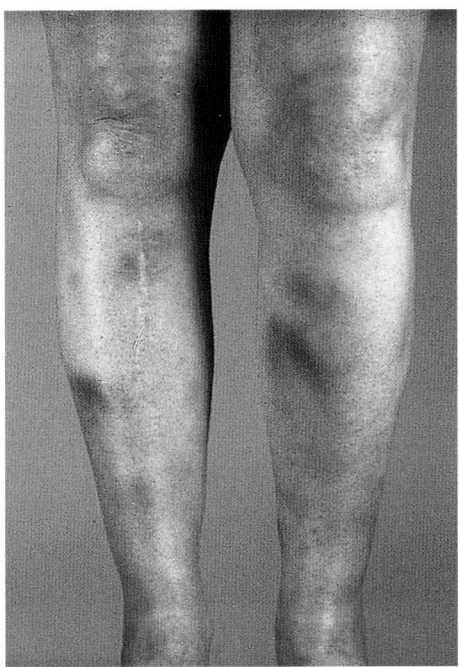

Nodular vasculitis *(du Vivier, 2002)*

vasculogenic impotence /vas′kyəlōjen′ik/ [L, *vascu-lum,* little vessel; Gk, *genein,* to produce; L, *in + potentia,* power], impotence resulting from an inadequate supply of arterial blood to the penis or venous leakage.

vasculomotor. See **vasomotor.**

vas deferens /def″ərənz/ *pl. vasa deferentia* [L, *vas + def-erens,* carrying away], the extension of the epididymis of the testis that ascends from the scrotum into the abdominal cavity and joins the seminal vesicle to form the ejaculatory duct. It is enclosed by fibrous connective tissue with blood vessels, nerves, and lymphatics and passes through the ingui-nal canal as part of the spermatic cord. Also called **deferent duct, ductus deferens, spermatic duct, testicular duct.** See also **testis.**

vasectomy /vasek″təmē/ [L, *vas* + Gk, *ektomē,* exci-sion], a procedure for male sterilization involving the bilat-eral surgical removal of a part of the vas deferens. Vasectomy is most commonly performed at an outpatient surgery cen-ter with local anesthesia. The procedure is also performed routinely before removal of the prostate gland to prevent inflammation of the testes and epididymides. Potency is not affected.

vasectomy reversal. See **vasovasostomy.**

vaso- /vas″ō-, vā″sō/, prefix meaning "vessel or duct": *vaso-constrictor, vasodilation, vasoganglion.*

vasoactive /vā′zō·ak″tiv/ [L, *vas + activus,* active], (of a drug) affecting blood vessels by either constriction or dilation.

vasoactive intestinal polypeptide (VIP), a glucagon-secretin hormone found in the pancreas, intestine, and cen-tral nervous system. The hormone stimulates insulin and glucagon release. Gastric secretion, gastric motility, and peripheral vasodilation, as well as hyperglycemia by hepatic glycogenolysis, are inhibited. See also **VIPoma.**

vasoconstriction [L, *vas + constrigere,* to tighten], a decrease in the diameter of a blood vessel. It plays an important role in the control of blood pressure and the dis-tribution of blood throughout the body. Vasoconstriction is triggered by stimulation of the vasomotor constriction center in the medulla. Impulses from this center travel along sym-pathetic nerve fibers and cause contraction of the smooth muscle layers of arteries, arterioles, and, to a lesser extent, venules, and veins, bringing about constriction of these ves-sels. Vasoconstriction is also induced by vasomotor pressure reflexes, chemical reflexes, the medullary ischemic reflex, and impulses from the cerebral cortex and the hypothalamus. Compare **vasodilation. −vasoconstrictive,** *adj.*

vasoconstrictive /-kənstrik″tiv/ [L, *vas,* vessel, *constring-ere,* to draw tight], able to cause a constriction of blood vessels.

vasoconstrictor /-kənstrik″tər/ [L, *vas + constrigere*], **1.** *adj.,* pertaining to a process, condition, or substance that causes the constriction of blood vessels. **2.** *n.,* an agent that promotes vasoconstriction. Cold, fear, stress, and nicotine are common exogenous vasoconstrictors. Internally secreted epinephrine and norepinephrine cause blood vessels to con-tract by stimulating alpha-adrenergic receptors on the vas-cular smooth muscle. Other endogenous vasoconstrictors are angiotensin, which is formed in the blood through the action of renin, and antidiuretic hormone, which is secreted by the pituitary. Alpha-adrenergic sympathomimetic drugs also cause vasoconstriction, and several of these agents are used for this action in maintaining blood pressure during anesthesia and in treating pronounced hypotension result-ing from hemorrhage, myocardial infarction, septicemia, sympathectomy, or drug reactions. Also called **vasopressor.** Kinds include **phenylephrine hydrochloride, metarami-nol bitartrate, norepinephrine.**

vasodepressor syncope. See **vasovagal syncope.**

vasodilation /-dīlā″shən/ [L, *vas + dilatare*], an increase in the diameter of a blood vessel. It is caused by a relaxation of the smooth muscles in the vessel wall. Also called *vasodi-latation.* Compare **vasoconstriction.**

vasodilator /vā′zōdī″lātər/ [L, *vas + dilatare*], a nerve or agent that causes dilation of blood vessels by promoting the relaxation of vascular smooth muscle. Chemical vasodilators include hydralazine, nitroglycerin, nitroprusside, nesiritide, and trimethaphan. They have been useful in the treatment of acute heart failure in myocardial infarction, in cases associ-ated with severe mitral regurgitation, in hypertensive emer-gencies, and in failure resulting from myocardial disease.

vasoganglion /-gang″glē·on/, a spherical mass of small blood vessels.

vasogenic shock /-jen″ik/ [L, *vas + genein,* to produce; Fr, *choc*], shock resulting from peripheral vascular dilation pro-duced by factors such as toxins that directly affect the blood vessels. Kinds include **anaphylactic shock, septic shock.**

V

vasohypertonic /-hī'pərton″ik/, causing constriction of blood vessels.

vasoinhibitor /vas'ō·inhib″itər/, an agent that opposes the action of vasomotor nerves, thereby causing arterial dilation and reduced blood pressure.

vasoinhibitory /vas'ō·inhib″itôr′ē/, inhibiting the activity of vasomotor nerves.

vasomotor /-mō″tər/ [L, *vas + movere,* to move], pertaining to the nerves and muscles that control the diameter of the blood vessels. Circularly arranged smooth muscle fibers of arteries and arterioles can contract, causing vasoconstriction, or they can relax, causing vasodilation. Also called **vasculomotor.**

vasomotor center, a collection of cell bodies in the medulla oblongata of the brain that regulates or modulates blood pressure and cardiac function, primarily via the autonomic nervous system.

vasomotor epilepsy, a form of epilepsy characterized by episodes of autonomic dysfunction and extreme contractions of the arteries. Also called **autonomic epilepsy.**

vasomotor paralysis, hypotonia of blood vessels caused by blockage of activity in nerves that stimulate vascular constriction. Also called **vasoparalysis.** See also **vasoparesis.**

vasomotor reflex [L, *vas,* vessel, *movere,* to move, *reflectere,* to bend back], any reflex response of the circulatory system caused by stimulation of vasodilator or vasoconstrictive nerves.

vasomotor rhinitis, chronic rhinitis and nasal obstruction, without allergy or infection, characterized by sneezing, rhinorrhea, nasal obstruction, and vascular engorgement of the mucous membranes of the nose. A vaporizer or humidifier and systemic vasoconstrictive agents are used to alleviate discomfort. Nose drops and nasal sprays should be avoided because continued use may cause further vasodilation of the mucous membrane and aggravation of the condition. Topical vasoconstrictors should also be avoided because the nasal mucous membrane loses sensitivity to stimuli. Vasomotor rhinitis is common in pregnancy.

vasomotor spasm. See **angiospasm.**

vasomotor system, the part of the nervous system that controls the constriction and dilation of the blood vessels. See also **vasoconstriction, vasodilation.**

vasoparalysis. See **vasomotor paralysis.**

vasoparesis, a mild form of vasomotor paralysis.

vasopressin. See **antidiuretic hormone.**

vasopressor. See **vasoconstrictor.**

vasospasm. See **angiospasm.**

vasospastic /-spas″tik/, **1.** *adj.,* relating to a spasmodic constriction of a blood vessel. **2.** *n.,* any agent that produces spasms of the blood vessels.

vasospastic angina, chest pain caused by spasms of the coronary arteries. It has features that differ from those of angina pectoris. See also **Prinzmetal angina.**

vasostimulation /-stim′yəlā″shən/ [L, *vas,* vessel, *stimulare,* to incite], the promotion of vasomotor activity.

Vasotec, an angiotensin-converting enzyme inhibitor. Brand name for **enalapril maleate.**

vasovagal reflex, a stimulation of the vagus nerve by reflex in which irritation of the larynx or the trachea results in slowing of the pulse rate.

vasovagal syncope, a sudden loss of consciousness resulting from cerebral ischemia, secondary to decreased cardiac output, peripheral vasodilation, and bradycardia and associated with vagal activity. The condition may be triggered by pain, fright, or trauma and is accompanied by symptoms of nausea, pallor, and perspiration. Also called **vasodepressor syncope.**

vasovasostomy /vas'ōvəsos″təmē/ [L, *vas* + *vas* + Gk, *stoma,* mouth], a surgical procedure in which the function of the vas deferens on each side of the testes is restored, having been cut and ligated in a preceding vasectomy. The procedure is performed if a man wants to regain his fertility. In most cases the patency of the canals is achieved, but, in many cases, fertility does not result, probably because of circulating autoantibodies that disrupt normal sperm activity. The antibodies apparently develop after vasectomy because the developing sperm cannot be excreted through the urogenital tract. Also called **vasectomy reversal.**

vastus intermedius /vas″təs/ [L, *vastus,* enormous, *inter,* between, *mediare,* to divide], one of the four muscles of the quadriceps femoris group, situated in the center of the thigh under the rectus femoris. It arises from the front and lateral surfaces of the femur and the medial and lateral intermuscular septa. Its fibers end in a superficial aponeurosis that forms the deep part of the quadriceps femoris tendon, inserted under the patella and onto the tibial tuberosity. It functions with the other three muscles of the quadriceps to extend the leg. Its deepest fibers are called articularis genus. Also called **crureus.** Compare **rectus femoris, vastus lateralis, vastus medialis.** See also **quadriceps femoris.**

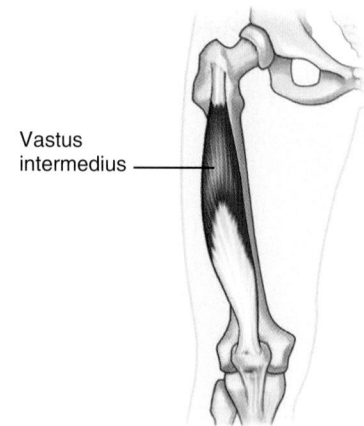

Vastus intermedius

Vastus intermedius

vastus internus. See **vastus medialis.**

vastus lateralis, the largest of the four muscles of the quadriceps femoris group, situated on the lateral side of the thigh. It is a large, dense mass originating in a broad aponeurosis that is attached to the intertrochanteric line of the femur, the greater trochanter, the lateral lip of the gluteal tuberosity, and the lateral lip of the linea aspera. The fibers of the muscle are gathered to form a strong aponeurosis that converges to become a flat tendon before inserting under the patella and onto the lateral condyle of the tibia. The muscle functions to help extend the leg. Compare **rectus femoris, vastus intermedius, vastus medialis.** See also **quadriceps femoris.**

vastus medialis, one of the four muscles of the quadriceps femoris group, situated in the medial part of the thigh. It originates from the intertrochanteric line of the femur, the linea aspera, the medial supracondylar line, the tendons of the adductor longus and the adductor magnus, and the medial intermuscular septum. The vastus medialis extends to the lower anterior aspect of the thigh and inserts by an aponeurosis under the patella as part of the quadriceps femoris tendon and onto the medial condyle of the femur. An expansion of the aponeurosis passes to the capsule of the knee joint. The muscle functions in combination with other parts of

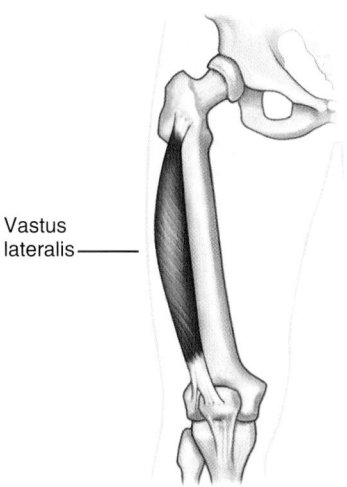

Vastus lateralis

the quadriceps femoris to extend the leg. Also called **vastus internus.** Compare **rectus femoris, vastus intermedius, vastus lateralis.** See also **quadriceps femoris.**

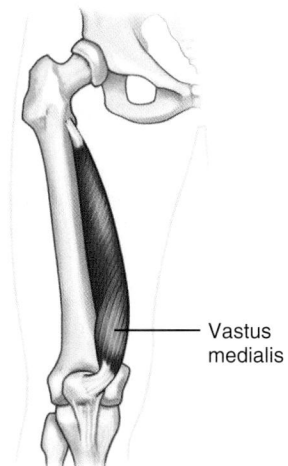

Vastus medialis

VATER association. See **VATER complex.**

VATER complex, a nonrandom association of congenital anomalies consisting of *v*ertebral defects, imperforate *a*nus, *t*racheo*e*sophageal fistula, and *r*adial and *r*enal dysplasia. Also called **VATER association.**

Vater-Pacini corpuscles /fä″tər päsē″nē/ [Abraham Vater, German anatomist, 1684–1751; Filippo Pacini, Italian anatomist, 1812–1883], kinesioceptors located in joint capsules and ligaments. They may transmit nerve impulses at an increasing rate as a joint approaches its maximal range of motion and are believed to have a protective function of signaling the cerebral cortex when a joint has reached the end position of its range. They are the most complicated of the nerve endings.

Vater's ampulla. See **hepatopancreatic ampulla.**

VBP, an anticancer drug combination of vinBLAStine, bleomycin, and cisplatin. Also called **PVB.**

VC, abbreviation for **vital capacity.**

VCO₂, symbol for *carbon dioxide output per unit of time.*

VCU, abbreviation for **voiding cystourethrography.**

VD, abbreviation for **venereal disease.** See **sexually transmitted disease.**

V deflection /diflek″shən/, a deflection on the His bundle electrogram that represents ventricular activation.

VDRL, abbreviation for *Venereal Disease Research Laboratory.*

VDRL test, a serological flocculation test for syphilis. It is also positive in other treponemal diseases such as yaws. False-positive and false-negative results may occur. A positive test must be confirmed by further, more definitive testing. Abbreviation for *Venereal Disease Research Laboratory test.*

V-drugs, vaporized medications that are inhaled.

VDT, abbreviation for **video display terminal.**

V̇e, symbol for *expired volume.*

V̇E, symbol for *volume expired in 1 minute.* See also **minute ventilation.**

Vectibix, a chemotherapeutic agent. Brand name for **panitumumab.**

vector /vek″tər/ [L, carrier], **1.** a quantity having direction and magnitude, usually depicted by a straight arrow. The length of the arrow represents magnitude, and the head represents direction. **2.** a carrier, especially one that transmits disease. A biological vector is usually an arthropod in which the infecting organism completes part of its life cycle. A mechanical vector transmits the infecting organism from one host to another but is not essential to the life cycle of the parasite. Kinds of vectors include dogs, which carry rabies; mosquitoes, which transmit malaria; and ticks, which carry Rocky Mountain spotted fever. **3.** a retrovirus that has been modified by alteration of its genetic component. Through recombinant deoxyribonucleic acid techniques, genes that cause harmful effects such as cancer are removed and genes that mediate synthesis of essential enzymes are added. The vector then can be injected into a patient who suffers from an enzyme deficiency, such as Lesch-Nyhan syndrome. −**vectorial,** *adj.,* −**vector,** *v.*

vectorcardiogram /-kär″dē·əgram′/ [L, *vector,* carrier; Gk, *cardia,* heart, *gramma,* record], a tracing of the direction and magnitude of the heart's electrical activity during a cardiac cycle. It is produced by an oscilloscope, which simultaneously records three standard leads.

vectorcardiography /-kär′dē·og″rəfē/ [L, *vector,* carrier; Gk, *kardia,* heart, *graphein,* to record], a method of recording the direction and magnitude of the heart's electrical activity.

vectorial. See **vector.**

vecuronium bromide /vek′yərō″nē·əm/, a neuromuscular blocking drug.

■ INDICATIONS: This drug is used as an adjunct to general anesthesia to facilitate endotracheal intubation and to relax skeletal muscles during surgery or mechanical ventilation.

■ CONTRAINDICATIONS: This drug should be used cautiously in patients with myasthenia gravis or other neuromuscular disorders and in patients who have been given drugs that produce or increase neuromuscular block. Effects of vecuronium may be prolonged in patients with liver disease.

■ ADVERSE EFFECTS: Adverse effects include muscle weakness, difficulty in breathing, and irregular heartbeat.

VEE, abbreviation for **Venezuelan equine encephalitis.** See **equine encephalitis.**

Veetids, an oral penicillin antibacterial drug. Brand name for *penicillin V potassium.*

vegan. See **strict vegetarian.**

veganism /vej″əniz′əm/ [L, *vegetare,* to grow, *ismus,* practice], the adherence to a strict vegetarian diet, with the exclusion of all protein of animal origin.

V

vegetable albumin /vej″(i)təbəl/, albumin protein produced in plants.

vegetal pole /vej′ətəl/ [L, *vegetare* + *polus,* pole], the relatively inactive part of an ovum where the yolk is situated, usually opposite the animal pole. Also called **antigerminal pole, vegetative pole.** Compare **animal pole.**

vegetarian /vej′əter″ē·ən/ [L, *vegetare*], a person who eats only foods of plant origin, including fruits, grains, and nuts. Many vegetarians eat eggs and milk products but avoid all animal flesh. Kinds include **lacto-ovo-vegetarian, ovo-vegetarian, strict vegetarian.**

vegetarianism /vej′əter′ē·əniz″əm/, the theory or practice of eating only foods of plant origin, including fruits, grains, and nuts.

vegetate, to behave or grow in the manner of a plant. See **vegetative.**

vegetation /vej′ətā″shən/, an abnormal growth of tissue around a valve, composed of fibrin, platelets, and bacteria.

vegetative /vej′ətā′tiv, vej′ətətiv′/ [L, *vegetare*], **1.** pertaining to nutrition and growth. **2.** pertaining to the plant kingdom. **3.** denoting involuntary function, as produced by the parasympathetic nervous system. **4.** resting, not active; denoting the stage of the cell cycle in which the cell is not replicating. **5.** leading a secluded, dull existence without social or intellectual activity; sluggish; lacking animation. **6.** (in psychiatry) emotionally withdrawn and passive, as may occur in schizophrenia and depression or in unipolar depression in severe cases.

vegetative endocarditis [L, *vegetare,* to grow; Gk, *endon,* within, *kardia,* heart, *itis,* inflammation], a subacute form of bacterial endocarditis characterized by vegetation on the heart valves. The vegetation may cause ulceration and perforation of the heart valve cusps.

vegetative pole. See **vegetal pole.**

vegetative state a clinical condition after a brain injury that is characterized by a patient's lack of awareness and responsiveness to usual environmental stimuli although reflexes may be present. The term is considered by some to be pejorative. See **unresponsive wakefulness syndrome.**

VEGF, abbreviation for **vascular endothelial growth factor.**

vehicle /vē′ikəl/ [L, *vehiculum,* conveyance], **1.** an inert substance with which a medication is mixed to facilitate measurement and administration or application. **2.** any fluid or structure in the body that passively conveys a stimulus. **3.** any substance, such as food or water, that can serve as a mode of transmission for infectious agents.

veiling glare, loss of contrast because of light scattering within a lens system, as in a fluoroscopic image intensifier.

Veillonella /vā′yənel′ə/ [Adrien Veillon, French bacteriologist, 1864–1931], a genus of gram-negative anaerobic bacteria. The species *Veillonella parvula* is normally present in the alimentary tract, especially in the mouth. This infection is often mistaken for more serious gonococcal infection.

Veillon tube /vāyōn″/, a transparent tube, the ends of which are closed with removable stoppers, one cotton and one rubber. It is used for the laboratory growth of bacteriological cultures.

vein (v) /vān/ [L, *vena*], any one of the many vessels that convey blood from the capillaries as part of the pulmonary venous system, the systemic venous network, or the portal venous complex. Most of the veins of the body are systemic veins that convey blood from the whole body (except the lungs) to the right atrium of the heart. Each vein is a macroscopic structure enclosed in three layers of different kinds of tissue homologous with the layers of the heart. The outer tunica adventitia of each vein is homologous with the epicardium, the tunica media with the myocardium, and the tunica intima with the endocardium. Deep veins course through the more internal parts of the body, and superficial veins lie near the surface, where many of them are visible through the skin. Veins have thinner coatings and are less elastic than arteries and collapse when cut. They also contain semilunar valves at various intervals to control the direction of the blood flow back to the heart. Compare **artery.** See also **portal vein, pulmonary vein, systemic vein.** –**venous,** *adj.*

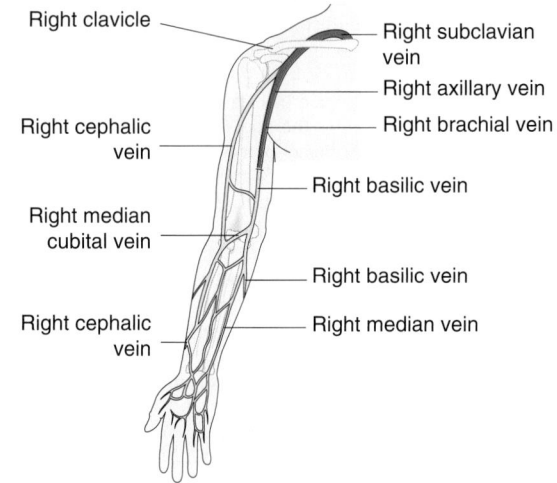

Right clavicle
Right subclavian vein
Right axillary vein
Right cephalic vein
Right brachial vein
Right basilic vein
Right median cubital vein
Right basilic vein
Right cephalic vein
Right median vein

Veins in the arm *(Shade et al, 2007)*

vein ligation and stripping, a surgical procedure consisting of the ligation of the saphenous vein and its removal from groin to ankle. It is performed for the treatment of recurrent thrombophlebitis or severe varicosities or for obtaining a blood vessel to graft in another site, such as in a coronary bypass operation.

vein lumen, the central opening through which blood flows in a vein.

vein of Thebesius. See **smallest cardiac vein.**

veins of the vertebral column, the veins that drain the blood from the vertebral column, adjacent muscles, and meninges of the spinal cord. Along the entire vertebral column these veins form plexuses that are divided into internal and external groups according to their locations inside or outside the vertebral canal. The plexuses and veins of the vertebral network are the external plexus, internal plexus, basivertebral veins, intervertebral veins, and spinal cord veins.

vein wrapping, the wrapping of an injured nerve with an autologous vein (usually saphenous vein) graft to provide insulation and cushioning following decompression in treatment of entrapment neuropathy.

Velban, an antineoplastic. Brand name for **vinBLAStine sulfate.**

Velcade, a chemotherapeutic agent. Brand name for **bortezomib.**

Velcro, a type of fastening device with a surface of tiny hooks that adhere to the opposite side, used mainly on fabric products.

vellus hair, the fine, soft hair covering all parts of the body except the palms, soles, and areas where other types of hair are normally found.

velocardiofacial syndrome /vel′ō·kär′dē·ō·fā′shəl/, an autosomal-dominant syndrome of cardiac defects and characteristic craniofacial abnormalities, including cleft palate, jaw abnormalities, and prominent nose. It is often associated with abnormalities of chromosome 22. Learning disabilities occur often; short stature, slender hyperextensible hands and digits, scoliosis, cognitive impairment, inguinal hernia, auricular abnormalities, and microcephaly occur less frequently. Also called **Shprintzen syndrome.**

velocity /vəlos″itē/ [L, *velox,* quick], the rate of change in the position of a body moving in a particular direction. Velocity along a straight line is linear velocity. Angular velocity is that of a body in circular motion. Compare **speed.**

velocity of growth, the rate of growth or change in growth measurements over a period of time.

velocity of ultrasound, the speed of ultrasound waves in a particular medium. The velocity varies from 331 meters per second (m/sec) in air to 1450 m/sec in fat, 1570 m/sec in blood, and 4080 m/sec in the skull.

velocity spectrum rehabilitation, a rehabilitation program that uses strength training at multiple speeds of movement from slow to fast.

velopharyngeal closure, closure of the nasal airway by the elevation of the soft palate and contraction of the posterior and lateral pharyngeal wall. It is needed for vowels and for all consonants except /n/, /m/, and /ng/.

velopharyngeal insufficiency, an abnormal condition resulting from a congenital defect in the structure of the velopharyngeal sphincter. Closure of the oral cavity beneath the nasal passages is not complete, as seen in cleft palate. Food may be regurgitated through the nose, and speech is impaired. Surgical correction is usually successful.

Velosef, a cephalosporin antibiotic. Brand name for **cephradine.**

Velpeau's bandage /velpōz″/ [Alfred A.L.M. Velpeau, French surgeon, 1795–1867], a roller bandage that immobilizes the elbow and shoulder by holding the brachium against the side and the flexed forearm on the chest. The palm of the hand rests on the clavicle on the opposite side.

ventricular phonation, a disorder of speech usually caused by muscular dysfunction and/or folds that vibrate with the vocal cords. It is characterized by a deep tone and strained sound.

vena cava /vē″nə kā″və/ *pl.* venae cavae [L, *vena,* vein, *cavum,* cavity], one of two large veins returning blood from the peripheral circulation to the right atrium of the heart. See also **inferior vena cava, superior vena cava.** –vena caval, *adj.*

vena caval foramen, an opening in the diaphragm through which the inferior vena cava and vagus nerve pass.

vena caval syndrome. See **supine hypotension.**

vena comitans *pl.* venae comites, one of the deep, paired veins that accompany the smaller arteries on each side of the artery. The three vessels are wrapped together in one sheath. Some of the arteries accompanied by such venous pairs are the brachial, the ulnar, and the tibial.

vena cordis magna. See **great cardiac vein.**

veneer /vənir″/ [Fr, *fournir,* to furnish], **1.** a layer of tooth-colored material, usually porcelain or acrylic, attached to the surface of a crown or artificial tooth by direct fusion; a porcelain prosthesis used to change the shape, size, and color of a tooth or teeth. The prosthesis is directly cemented to the crown of the tooth or teeth. **2.** a thin layer of calculus usually not visible until dried with air. See **calculus.**

venepuncture. See **venipuncture.**

venereal /vənir″ē·əl/ [L, *Venus,* goddess of love], pertaining to or caused by sexual intercourse or genital contact.

venereal bubo [L, *Venus,* goddess of love; Gk, *boubon,* groin], a swollen, inflamed lymph gland or node, usually in the groin and sometimes purulent. It is associated with a sexually transmitted disease.

venereal disease. See **sexually transmitted disease.**

venereal sore. *(Informal)* See **chancre.**

venereal ulcer. See **chancroid.**

venereal urethritis, an inflammation of the male urethra caused by sexually transmitted microorganisms. See also **gonococcal urethritis.**

venereal wart. See **genital wart.**

venereologic, venereological, pertaining to sexually transmitted diseases. See **venereology.**

venereologist /vənir′ē·ol″əjist/ [L, *Venus,* goddess of love; Gk, *logos,* science], a health professional who specializes in the study of the causes and treatments of venereal diseases.

venereology /-ol″əjē/, the study of the causes and treatments of venereal diseases. –venereological, venereologic, *adj.,* –venereologist, *n.*

venerupin poisoning /ven′əroo″pin/, a potentially fatal form of shellfish poisoning that results from ingestion of oysters or clams contaminated with venerupin, a toxin that causes impaired liver functioning, GI distress, and leukocytosis. The shellfish toxin occurs in waters around Japan. About one third of the cases are fatal. See also **shellfish poisoning.**

venesection. See **phlebotomy.**

Venezuelan equine encephalitis. See **equine encephalitis.**

Venezuelan hemorrhagic fever, a hemorrhagic fever caused by an arenavirus transmitted to humans by contact with or inhalation of aerosolized excreta of infected rodents. The disease occurs in west central Venezuela, primarily in settlers moving into areas of cleared forest. Initially it is characterized by the gradual onset of fever, malaise, myalgia, and anorexia, followed by prostration, dizziness, headache, back pain, and GI disturbances. Bleeding of the gums is a typical finding, and there may be petechiae on the palate and axillae. Neurological manifestations, such as tremor of tongue and hands, diminished deep tendon reflexes, lethargy, and hyperesthesia, often occur. Most patients begin to improve after 1 or 2 weeks, but the disease takes a more serious course in about a third; some patients develop a hemorrhagic diathesis; some develop severe neurological deterioration marked by delirium, coma, and convulsions; and still others develop a mixed hemorrhagic-neurological syndrome with shock. Treatment is supportive, with careful attention to fluid and electrolyte balance. If untreated, the case fatality rate may reach 30% or more. With aggressive treatment, the usual prognosis is complete recovery.

veni- [L, *vein*], prefix meaning "vein": *venipuncture.*

venipuncture /ven′əpungk″chər/ [L, *vena + pungere,* to prick], the transcutaneous puncture of a vein by a sharp rigid stylet or cannula carrying a flexible plastic catheter or by a steel needle attached to a syringe or catheter. It is done to withdraw a specimen of blood, perform a phlebotomy, instill a medication, start an IV infusion, or inject a radiopaque substance for radiological examination of a part or system of the body.

veno-, combining form meaning "vein": *venoatrial, venospasm, venostasis.*

venoatrial /vē′nō-ā″trē·əl/, pertaining to the right atrium and either vena cava.

venogenic impotence, vasculogenic impotence caused by a disorder in the veins draining the penis, such as a failure to maintain venous occlusion.

venogram. See **phlebogram.**

venography. See **phlebography.**

venom /ven″əm/ [L, *venenum,* poison], a toxic fluid substance secreted by some snakes, arthropods, and other animals and transmitted by their stings or bites.

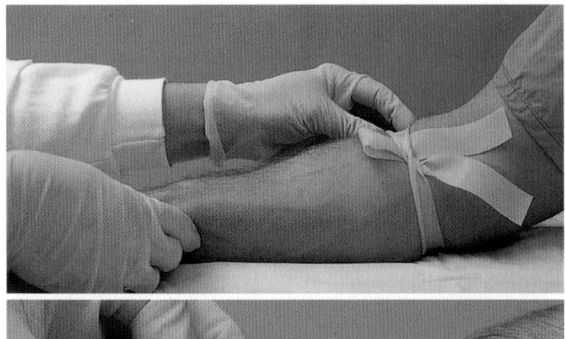

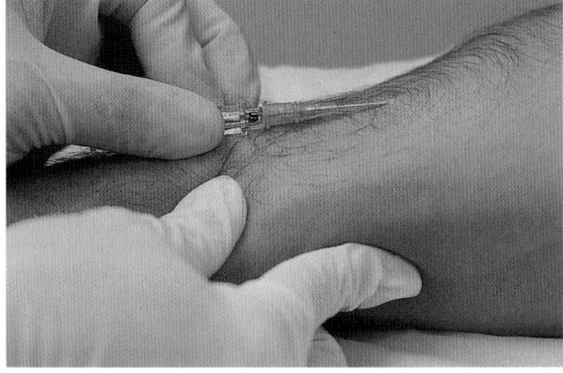

Venipuncture *(Potter and Perry, 2005)*

venom extract therapy, the administration of antivenin as prophylaxis against the toxic effects of the bite of a specific poisonous snake or spider or other venomous animal.

venom immunotherapy, the reduction of sensitivity to a specific venom by the administration of gradually increasing amounts of that venom. See also **immunotherapy.**

venomous snake /ven″əməs/, a snake that secretes a poison. See also **adder, coral snake, pit viper, snakebite, snake venom.**

venospasm /vēn″əspaz′əm/ [L, *vena*, vein; Gk, *spasmos*, spasm], a spasmodic constriction of a vein.

venostasis, sluggish blood flow in the venous system. See **phlebostasis.**

venothrombotic /vē′nəthrombot″ik/, producing a venous thrombus.

venotomy /vēnot″əmē/, the surgical opening of a vein.

venous. See **vein.**

-venous, suffix meaning "veins": *intravenous, arteriovenous.*

venous access device, a catheter designed for continuous access to the venous system. Such devices may be required for long-term parenteral feeding or the administration of IV fluids or medications for a period of several days.

venous access device (VAD) maintenance, a nursing intervention from the Nursing Interventions Classification (NIC) defined as management of the patient with prolonged venous access via tunneled and nontunneled (percutaneous) catheters and implanted ports. See also **Nursing Interventions Classification.**

venous blood (v) [L, *vena*, vein; AS, *blod*], dark red deoxygenated blood that has passed from the left ventricle through the systemic circulation en route to the right atrium.

venous blood gas [L, *venosus*, full of veins; AS, *blod* + Gk, *chaos*, gas], the oxygen and carbon dioxide levels in venous blood. Venous blood gas is measured by various methods to assess the adequacy of oxygenation and ventilation and to determine the acid-base status. The oxygen tension of venous blood normally averages 40 mm Hg; the dissolved oxygen content, 0.1% by volume; the total oxygen content, 15.2%; and the oxygen saturation of venous hemoglobin, 75%. The carbon dioxide tension normally averages 46 mm Hg; the

dissolved carbon dioxide content, 2.9% by volume; and the total carbon dioxide content, 50%. The normal average pH of venous plasma is 7.37. Venous blood gas in an extremity pertains chiefly to that limb. A sample from a central venous catheter is usually an incomplete mix of venous blood from various parts of the body; a sample of completely mixed venous blood may be obtained from the pulmonary artery for an accurate determination of venous blood gas.

venous capillaries [L, *vena*, vein, *capillaris*, hairlike], capillaries that terminate in venules.

venous circulation [L, *vena,* vein, *circulare,* to go around], the movement of blood from the venules, which drain deoxygenated blood from the capillaries, through the veins to the vena cava, and from there through the right atrium and ventricle to the pulmonary circulation of the lungs, where the blood is oxygenated for return to the systemic circulation.

venous cutdown, a small surgical incision made in a vein of a patient who has suffered vascular collapse to permit the introduction of IV fluids or drugs. A cutdown also may be performed for the insertion of a cannula for the withdrawal of blood.

venous foramen, an aperture in the greater wing of the sphenoid bone through which a small vein passes from the cavernous sinus. Also called **foramen of Vesalius.**

venous hemorrhage, excessive bleeding from a vein.

venous hum, a continuous murmur heard on auscultation over the major veins at the base of the neck and around the umbilicus. It is most audible in the neck when the patient is anemic, upright, and looking to the contralateral side. It is also heard in some healthy, young individuals.

venous insufficiency, an abnormal circulatory condition characterized by decreased return of venous blood from the legs to the trunk of the body. Edema is usually the first sign of the condition. Pain, varicosities, and ulceration may follow. Treatment usually consists of elevation of the legs, use of elastic hose, and correction of the underlying condition.

venous lake a small benign blue-purple sessile, compressible papule, or bleb; seen most often on the lips, ears, and faces of elderly persons. Histologically, venous lakes represent dilated capillaries filled with red blood cells and lined with flattened endothelial cells.

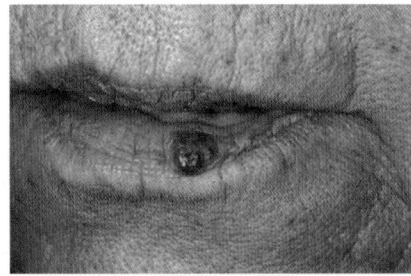

Venous lake *(Habif et al, 2018)*

venous ligation, the ligation of varicose veins whose valves are ineffective, performed to remove weakened parts of tissues in which thrombi might lodge. During surgery the saphenous vein is ligated at the groin, where it joins the femoral vein. A wire device, called a stripper, is threaded through the lumen of the vein from groin to ankle. The wire and the vein are then pulled from the groin incision. Incisions may be made at several sites along the leg. Bleeding is minimal. After surgery a pressure bandage is applied from foot to thigh, and the foot of the bed is elevated 6 to 9 inches, raising the legs above heart level. The patient is encouraged to walk but discouraged from standing or sitting. Cyanosis of the toes indicates possible constriction by the dressings. Elastic bandages remain in place until the seventh day after surgery, when the sutures are usually removed. Possible complications include hemorrhage, infection, nerve damage, and thrombosis.

venous occlusion, the blocking of venous return. It occurs naturally in the penis during an erection or it may be induced artificially in a part, such as in the arm, during venous occlusion plethysmography.

venous plethysmography, a manometric test that measures changes in the volume of an extremity. It is usually performed on a leg to exclude deep vein thrombosis.

venous pressure, the blood pressure in the veins. It is elevated in congestive heart failure, acute or chronic constrictive pericarditis, and venous obstruction caused by a clot or external pressure against a vein. Indications of increased venous pressure are continued distension of veins on the back of the hand when it is raised above the sternal notch and distension of the neck veins when the individual is sitting with the head elevated 30 to 45 degrees.

venous pulmonary thromboembolism (VTE) a blood clot that forms in a vein. There are two types of VTE—deep vein thrombosis and pulmonary embolism. See also **deep vein thrombosis, pulmonary embolism.**

venous pulse, the pulse of a vein usually palpated over the internal or external jugular veins in the neck. The pulse in the jugular vein is taken to evaluate the pressure of the pulse and the form of the pressure wave, especially in a person with a cardiac conduction defect or cardiac arrhythmia.

venous return, the return of blood to the heart via the superior and inferior vena cavae and the coronary sinus.

venous sinus, any one of many sinuses that collect blood from the dura mater and drain it into the internal jugular vein. Each sinus is formed by the separation of the two layers of the dura mater, the outer coat of the sinus consisting of fibrous tissue and the inner coat consisting of endothelium continuous with that of the veins.

venous stasis, a disorder in which the normal flow of blood through a vein is slowed or halted.

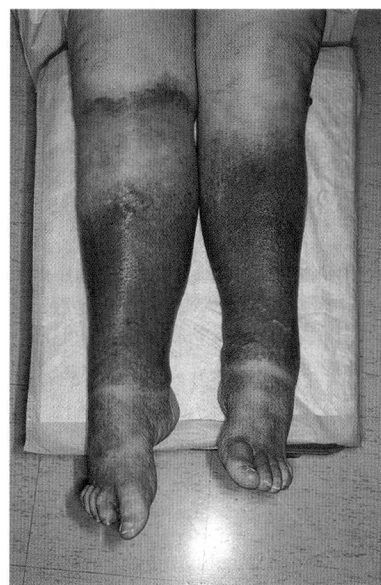

Venous stasis *(Swartz, 2009)*

venous stasis dermatitis. See **stasis dermatitis.**
venous thrombosis. See **phlebothrombosis.**
venous valves, any of the small cusps or folds found in the tunica intima of many veins, serving to prevent backflow of blood.

ventilate /ven″tilāt/ [L, *ventilare*, to fan], **1.** to provide with fresh air. **2.** to provide the alveoli of the lungs with air from the atmosphere and to aerate or oxygenate blood in the pulmonary capillaries. **3.** to open discussion of something, such as one's feelings. −**ventilatory,** *adj.*

ventilation. See **respiration,** def. 2.

ventilation lung scan, a radiographic examination of the lungs to detect nonfunctional or impaired lung areas or other abnormalities, performed while the patient inhales a radioactive gas as a contrast medium.

ventilation-perfusion defect, a disorder in which one or more areas of the lungs receive air but no blood flow or receive blood flow but no air.

ventilation/perfusion (V/Q) ratio, the ratio of pulmonary alveolar ventilation to pulmonary capillary perfusion, both quantities expressed in the same units.

ventilator /ven″tilā″tər/, any of several devices used in respiratory therapy to provide assisted respiration and intensive positive-pressure breathing. Kinds include **pressure ventilator, volume ventilator.** See also **IPPB unit.**

ventilator-associated pneumonia, the most common type of nosocomial pneumonia, a frequently fatal type seen in patients breathing with a ventilator. It is usually caused by aspiration of contaminated secretions or stomach contents and may be bacterial, viral, or fungal.

ventilatory. See **ventilate.**

ventilatory compliance /ven″tilātôr″ē/, the sum of the dynamic compliance of the lung and the compliance of the thoracic cage.

ventilatory rate [L, *ventilare*, to fan, *ratum,* to calculate], the volume of air passing into and out of the lungs per minute. Compare **respiration rate.**

ventilatory standstill [L, *ventilare*, to fan; AS, *standan* + *stille*], the complete cessation of breathing activity. Compare **apnea.**

Ventolin, a sympathomimetic bronchodilator. Brand name for **albuterol.**

ventral /ven″trəl/ [L, *venter,* belly], pertaining to a position toward the anterior surface of the body; frontward. Compare **dorsal.**

-ventral, suffix meaning "of the stomach or abdominal region": *dorsoventral.*

ventral column. See **anterior horn.**

ventral corticospinal tract. See **anterior corticospinal tract.**

ventral hernia. See **abdominal hernia.**

ventral horn. See **anterior horn.**

ventral recumbent. See **prone.**

ventral root [L, *venter,* belly; AS, *rot*], the anterior or motor division of each spinal nerve.

ventri-. See **ventro-, ventri-.**

ventricle /ven″trikəl/ [L, *ventriculus,* little belly], a small cavity, such as the right and the left ventricles of the heart or one of the cavities filled with cerebrospinal fluid in the brain.

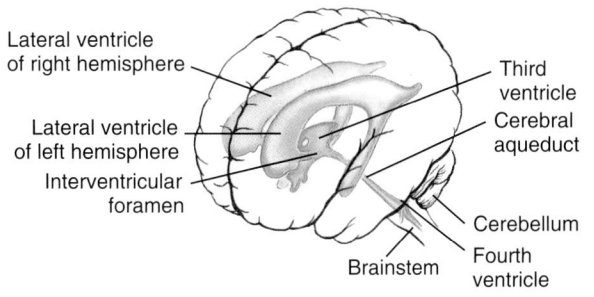

Ventricles of the brain *(Applegate, 2011)*

ventricles of the brain, the cavities within the brain that are filled with cerebrospinal fluid, including the two lateral, the third, and (linked by the aqueduct) the fourth ventricles. They are lined by ependyma, which, in certain regions, is invaginated by vascular fringes of pia mater to form the choroid plexuses.

ventricular /ventrik″yələr/ [L, *ventriculus*, little belly], pertaining to a ventricle.

ventricular aberration. See **aberrant ventricular conduction.**

ventricular aneurysm, a localized dilation or saccular protrusion in the wall of a ventricle, occurring most often after a myocardial infarction. Scar tissue is formed in response to the inflammatory changes of the infarction. This tissue weakens the myocardium, allowing its walls to bulge outward when the ventricle contracts. A typical sign of the lesion is a recurrent ventricular arrhythmia that does not respond to treatment with conventional antiarrhythmic drugs. Diagnostic measures are echocardiography and cardiac catheterization. Treatment may involve surgical removal of the scar tissue. Also called **cardiac aneurysm.**

ventricular assist device (VAD), a circulatory support device that augments function of the left ventricle, the right ventricle, or both. It consists of one or two implanted or extracorporeal pumps with afferent and efferent conduits attached to provide mechanically assisted blood flow.

ventricular bigeminy [L, *ventriculus* + *bis* + *geminus*, twin], a cardiac arrhythmia in which every other beat consists of a premature ventricular beat.

ventricular block [L, *ventriculus* + OFr, *bloc*], an obstruction of the flow of cerebrospinal fluid. Causes usually are closure of the foramina of Magendie or Luschka. The condition results in a distension of the brain ventricles because of an increased accumulation of cerebrospinal fluid. See also **hydrocephalus.**

ventricular compliance, a property of a heart ventricle in its resting state that determines the relation between the filling of the ventricle and its diastolic pressure.

ventricular dysfunction, an abnormality in the contraction of the ventricles or the motion of the cells.

ventricular ejection [L, *ventriculus* + *ejicere*, to cast out], the forceful expulsion of blood from the ventricles into the aorta and the pulmonary arteries.

ventricular escape [L, *ventriculus* + OFr, *escaper*], the discharge of a normal ventricular pacemaker cell when the sinus or junctional rate of discharge falls below that of the ventricular pacemaker cells.

ventricular extrasystole, a premature beat arising from a ventricle.

ventricular fibrillation (VF), a cardiac arrhythmia marked by rapid depolarizations of the ventricular myocardium. The condition is characterized by a complete lack of organized electric activity and of ventricular ejection. Blood pressure falls to zero, resulting in unconsciousness. Death may occur within 4 minutes. Cardiopulmonary resuscitation must be initiated immediately, with defibrillation and resuscitative medications given according to advanced cardiac life support protocol.

ventricular flutter, a condition of very rapid contractions of the ventricles of the heart. Electrocardiograms show poorly defined QRS complexes occurring at a rate of 250 beats/min or higher. Cardiac output is severely compromised or absent. The condition is fatal if untreated. Compare **ventricular fibrillation.**

ventricular gallop. See **S₃.**

ventricular gradient, the sum of the areas within the QRS complex and the T wave on the electrocardiogram.

ventricular hypertrophy [L, *ventriculus* + Gk, *hyper*, excessive, *trophe*, nourishment], abnormal enlargement of the heart caused by enlargement of the myocardium. It is often caused by hypertension, a valvular disease, or heart failure.

ventricular pacing. See **pacing.**

ventricular remodeling, progressive myocardial ventricular dilation, eccentric ventricular hypertrophy, and distortion of left ventricular geometry that persist in the noninfarcted myocardium after a myocardial infarction has healed. It is associated with impaired functional capacity, congestive heart failure, and premature death. Angiotensin-converting enzyme inhibitors can limit the ventricular dilation.

ventricular rhythm [L, *ventriculus* + Gk, *rhythmos*], the recurrent beating of the ventricles, normal or abnormal.

ventricular septal defect (VSD), the most common congenital cardiac anomaly, characterized by one or more abnormal openings in the septum separating the ventricles. The openings, which may range in size from 1 to 2 mm to several centimeters, permit oxygenated blood to flow from the left to the right ventricle and to recirculate through the pulmonary artery and lungs. Small defects may close spontaneously, and children with such defects are usually asymptomatic. Large defects may lead to bacterial endocarditis, lower respiratory tract infections, pulmonary vascular obstructive disease, aortic regurgitation, or congestive heart failure. Children with large defects may show rapid breathing, poor weight gain, restlessness, and irritability. Diagnosis is established by echocardiography and cardiac catheterization. Treatment consists of surgical repair of the defect, preferably in early childhood. In certain cases, the defect may be closed via a percutaneous approach.

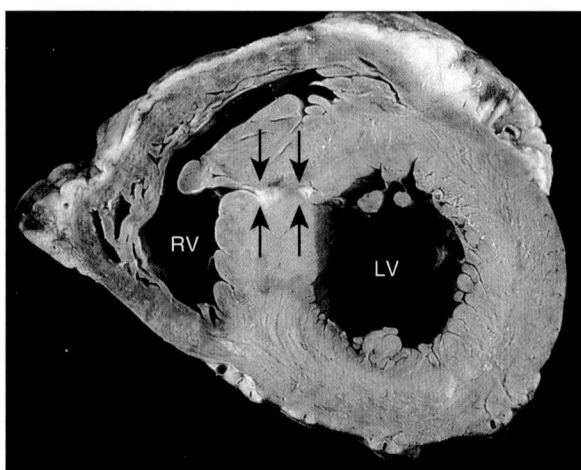

Ventricular septal defect that has undergone spontaneous closure *(Damjanov and Linder, 2000)*

ventricular septum. See **interventricular septum.**

ventricular standstill, a complete cessation of electric and mechanical activity in the ventricles of the heart.

ventricular systole [L, *ventriculus* + Gk, *systole*, contraction], the contraction of the heart ventricles. It begins with the first heart sound.

ventricular tachycardia, tachycardia of at least three consecutive ventricular complexes with a rate greater than 100 beats/min. It usually originates in a focus distal to the branching of the atrioventricular bundle.

ventriculo- /ventrik″yəlō-/, combining form meaning "ventricle of the heart or brain": *ventriculocisternostomy, ventriculogram, ventriculography.*

ventriculoatrial shunt /ventrik′yəlō-ā″trē-əl/ [L, *ventriculus* + *atrium*, hall; ME, *shunten*], a surgically created passageway consisting of plastic tubing and one-way valves, implanted between a cerebral ventricle and the right atrium of the heart to drain excess cerebrospinal fluid from the brain in hydrocephalus.

ventriculoatriostomy. See **auriculoventriculostomy.**

ventriculocisternostomy /-sis′tərnos″təmē/ [L, *ventriculus* + *cisterna,* vessel; Gk, *stoma,* mouth], a surgical procedure performed to treat hydrocephalus. An opening is created that allows cerebrospinal fluid to drain through a shunt from the ventricles of the brain into the cisterna magna. Also called **Torkildsen procedure, ventriculostomy.**

ventriculofallopian tube shunt /-fəlō″pē·ən/, a surgical procedure with limited effectiveness for diverting cerebrospinal fluid into the peritoneal cavity. A polyethylene tube is passed from the lateral ventricle or from the spinal subarachnoid space into a ligated fallopian tube and finally into the peritoneal cavity, where the shunted cerebrospinal fluid is absorbed. This procedure is used to correct both the obstructive and the communicating types of hydrocephalus. Also called **spinofallopian tube shunt.**

ventriculogram /ventrik″yəlōgram′/, a radiograph of the cerebral ventricles or the ventricles of the heart.

ventriculography /ventrik′yəlog″rəfē/ [L, *ventriculus* + *graphein,* to record], **1.** the radiographic examination of a ventricle of the heart after injection of a radiopaque contrast medium. **2.** the radiographic examination of the head following cerebrospinal fluid removal from the cerebral ventricles and its replacement by a contrast medium, usually air.

ventriculoperitoneal shunt /-per′itənē″əl/ [L, *ventriculus* + Gk, *peri,* around, *teinein,* to stretch; ME, *shunten*], a surgically created passageway consisting of plastic tubing and one-way valves between a cerebral ventricle and the peritoneum for the draining of excess cerebrospinal fluid from the brain in hydrocephalus.

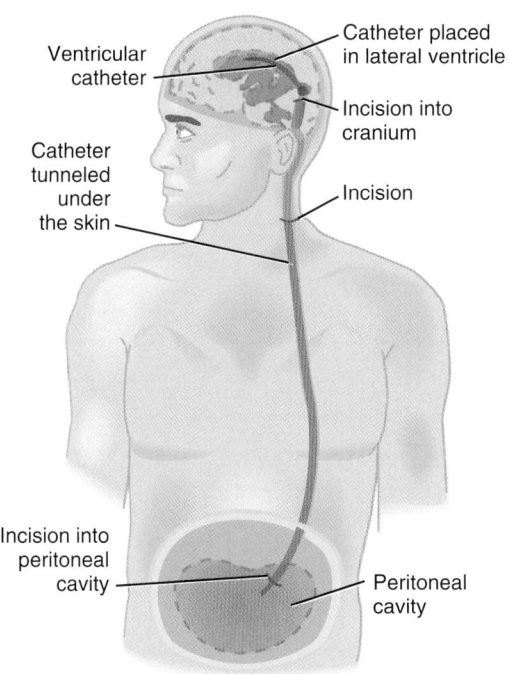

Ventriculoperitoneal shunt *(Black and Hawks, 2009)*

ventriculoperitoneostomy /ventrik′yəlōper′itō′nē·os″təmē/ [L, *ventriculus* + Gk, *peri,* around, *teinein,* to stretch, *stoma,* mouth], a surgical procedure for temporarily diverting cerebrospinal fluid in hydrocephalus, usually in the newborn. In this procedure, which spares the kidney but is less efficient than a ventriculoureterostomy, a polyethylene tube is passed from the lateral ventricle subcutaneously down the dorsal spine and is reinserted into the peritoneal cavity, where the diverted fluid is absorbed. This procedure is used

to correct both the communicating and the obstructive types of hydrocephalus.

ventriculopleural shunt /-ploor″əl/ [L, *ventriculus* + Gk, *pleura,* rib; ME, *shunten*], a surgical procedure for diverting cerebrospinal fluid from engorged ventricles in hydrocephalus, usually in the newborn. In this procedure, cerebrospinal fluid is diverted from the lateral ventricle into the pleural cavity. It is used to correct both the obstructive and the communicating types of hydrocephalus.

ventriculostomy. See **ventriculocisternostomy.**

ventriculoureterostomy /ventrik′yəlō′yoorē′təros″təmē / [L, *ventriculus* + Gk, *oureter,* ureter, *stoma,* mouth], a surgical procedure for directing cerebrospinal fluid into the general circulation. It is performed in the treatment of hydrocephalus, usually in the newborn. In this procedure a polyethylene tube is passed from the lateral ventricle down the dorsal spine subcutaneously to the twelfth rib; the tube is inserted through the paraspinal muscles into a ureter. Rarely used, the method is an alternative to auriculoventriculostomy, especially if the obstruction to cerebrospinal fluid includes the basilar and cerebral subarachnoid spaces, the posterior fossa, and the spinal subarachnoid spaces. The procedure is performed to correct an obstructive type of hydrocephalus.

ventriculovenous shunt, a surgically created communication between a cerebral ventricle and the internal jugular vein by a plastic tube with an in-line pressure-flow regulator; used to permit drainage of cerebrospinal fluid for relief of hydrocephalus.

ventro-, ventri-, combining form meaning "belly" or "to the front of the body": *ventrolateral, ventromedial.*

ventrolateral /ven′trōlat″ərəl/, pertaining to the part of the body opposite the back and away from the midline.

ventromedial /ven′trōmē″dē·əl/, pertaining to the part of the body opposite the back and near the midline.

Venturi effect /ventoo′rē/ [Giovanni B. Venturi, Italian physicist, 1746–1822], a modification of Bernoulli's principle, which states that the pressure of a gas is reduced just beyond an obstruction or restriction in the vessel through which the gas is flowing. The pressure drop can be nearly eliminated if dilation of the vessel does not exceed 15 degrees. The effect is a factor in the design of respiratory therapy equipment for mixing medical gases.

Venturi mask, a respiratory therapy face mask designed to allow inspired air to mix with oxygen, which is supplied through a jet at a fixed concentration.

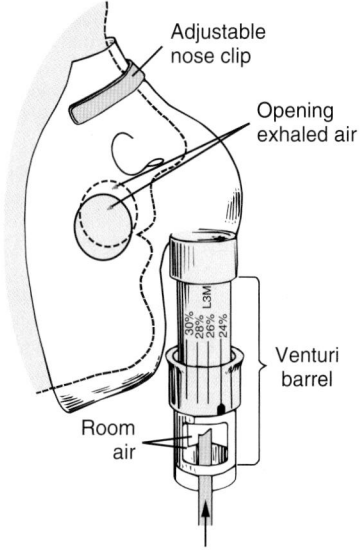

Venturi mask *(Perry, Potter, and Elkin, 2012)*

venul-, combining form meaning "venule."

venule /ven″yōōl/ [L, *venula,* small vein], any one of the small blood vessels that gather blood from the capillary plexuses and anastomose to form the veins. *–venular, adj.*

VEP, abbreviation for **visual-evoked potential.**

VePesid (VP-16), an antineoplastic agent. Brand name for **etoposide.**

verapamil /verap″əmil/, a calcium channel blocker.

- INDICATIONS: It is prescribed for the treatment of vasospastic and exertional angina, supraventricular tachycardia, atrial fibrillation, and atrial flutter. It is also prescribed for hypertension.
- CONTRAINDICATIONS: Severe left ventricular dysfunction, hypotension, cardiogenic shock, sick sinus syndrome, or second- or third-degree atrioventricular (AV) block prohibits its use.
- ADVERSE EFFECTS: Among the more serious adverse effects are hypotension, peripheral edema, AV block, bradycardia, congestive heart failure, pulmonary edema, constipation, and dizziness.

Veratrum /vərā′trəm/ [L, hellebore], a genus of poisonous herbs of the lily family. The dried rhizomes of the British and American hellebore provide alkaloids that may be used with great caution in herbalism.

verbal aphasia. See **motor aphasia.**

verbal language /vur″bəl/ [L, *verbum,* a word, *lingua,* tongue], a culturally organized system of vocal sounds that communicates meaning between individuals.

Verdeso, a corticosteroid indicated for the topical treatment of mild to moderate atopic dermatitis. Brand name for **desonide.**

Veregen, an herbal treatment for warts. Brand name for **kunecatechins.**

vergence /vur″jəns/, movement of the eyes in opposite directions (convergence and divergence).

vergence ability. See **amplitude of convergence.**

-verine, suffix for spasmolytics having a papaverine-like action.

vermes. See **vermis.**

vermicide /vur″misīd/ [L, *vermis,* worm, *caedere,* to kill], an agent that kills worms, particularly those in the intestine. Compare **anthelmintic, vermifuge.**

vermicular /vərmik″yələr/ [L, *vermis,* worm], resembling a worm.

vermicular pulse, a small, rapid pulse that feels like a writhing worm when palpated.

vermiform /vur″mifôrm/ [L, *vermis,* worm, *forma,* form], resembling a worm. Also **lumbrical.**

vermiform appendix [L, *vermis + forma,* form, *appendix,* appendage], a wormlike blunt process extending from the cecum. Its length varies from 7 to 15 cm, and its diameter is about 1 cm. Also called **appendix vermiformis, cecal appendix, mesoappendix.** See also **appendicitis.**

vermifuge /vərmifyōōj″/ [L, *vermis+fugare,* to chase away], an agent that causes the evacuation of intestinal parasitic worms.

vermilion border /vərmil″yən/ [L, *vermillium,* bright red; OFr, *bordure,* frame], the external pinkish-to-red area of the upper and lower lips. It extends from the junction of the lips with the surrounding facial skin on the exterior to the labial mucosa within the mouth.

vermin /vur″min/ [L, *vermis,* worm], any parasitic insect or small animal, such as a louse, bedbug, mouse, or rat, regarded as a destructive or disease-carrying pest.

vermis /vur″mis/ *pl. vermes* [L], **1.** a worm. **2.** a structure resembling a worm, such as the median lobe of the cerebellum. *–vermiform, adj.*

vermis cerebelli /vər″mis ser′ə·bel′ī/ [L, worm of cerebellum], the narrow median part of the cerebellum between the two lateral hemispheres. The cranial or superior portion extends from the lingula to the folium vermis, and the inferior or caudal portion extends from the tuber vermis to the nodulus. Also called *vermis of cerebellum.*

Vermox, an anthelmintic. Brand name for **mebendazole.**

vernal conjunctivitis /vur″nəl/ [L, *vernare,* spring-like, *conjunctivus,* connecting; Gk, *itis,* inflammation], a chronic, bilateral inflammation of the conjunctiva, thought to be allergic in origin, that occurs most frequently in men under 20 years of age during the spring and summer. The most common symptoms include intense itching and a crusting discharge. Topical corticosteroids may be applied, and desensitization to pollen may be helpful. Compare **allergic conjunctivitis.**

vernal keratoconjunctivitis, an ocular inflammatory disease caused by allergic reaction, often occurring in the spring but sometimes year-round. It is characterized by the presence of cobblestonelike bumps on the upper eyelid. There may also be swelling and thickening of the conjunctiva, a mucous discharge, itching, and sensitivity to light.

Verner-Morrison syndrome, a rare syndrome of profuse watery diarrhea, hypokalemia, and achlorhydria, usually associated with excess levels of vasoactive intestinal polypeptide resulting from a tumor (VIPoma) in the pancreas. Also called **pancreatic diarrhea.**

Vernet syndrome /vernā″/ [Maurice Vernet, French neurologist, 1887–1974], a neurological disorder caused by injury to the 9th, 10th, and 11th cranial nerves as they pass through the jugular foramen when leaving the skull. The syndrome is often associated with vascular neoplasms or carotid dissections or aneurysms. Symptoms include unilateral flaccid paralysis of the palatal, pharyngeal, and intrinsic laryngeal muscles and the sternocleidomastoid and trapezius muscles. The patient also experiences dysphagia, a nasal and hoarse voice, and occasionally some loss of taste sensations. Also called **jugular foramen syndrome.**

Verneuil neuroma. See **plexiform neuroma.**

vernix caseosa /vur″niks kas′ē·ō″sə/ [Gk, resin; L, *caseus,* cheese], a grayish-white cheeselike substance, consisting of sebaceous gland secretions, lanugo, and desquamated epithelial cells, that covers the skin of the fetus and newborn. It acts as a protective agent during intrauterine life and is thought to have an insulating effect against heat loss.

verocytotoxin /ver′ō-sī′tō-tok′sin/, either of two toxins found in certain strains of *Shigella dysenteriae* and *Escherichia coli,* causing a type of hemolytic uremic syndrome. Humans are infected by ingesting undercooked meat, unpasteurized milk, and foods contaminated with cattle feces.

verruca /vərōō″kə/ *pl. verrucae* [L, wart], a benign, viral, warty skin lesion with a rough, papillomatous surface. It is caused by a common contagious papovavirus. Methods of treatment include salicylic acid, cantharidin, electrodesiccation, curette excision, laser excision, and liquid nitrogen. Also called **verruca vulgaris, wart.** *–verrucous, verrucose, adj.*

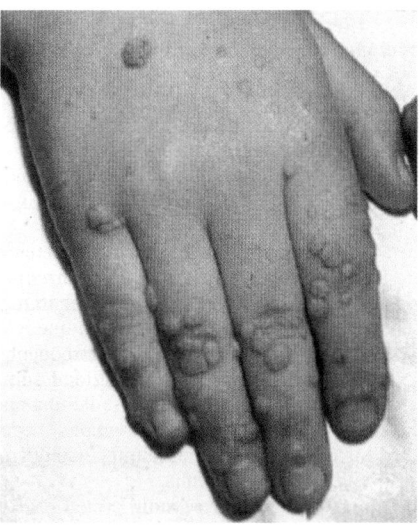

Verrucae *(Courtesy American Academy of Dermatology and Institute for Dermatologic Communication and Education)*

verruca acuminata. See **genital wart.**

verruca plana, a small, slightly elevated, smooth, tan or flesh-colored wart, sometimes occurring in large numbers on the face, neck, back of the hands, wrists, and knees, especially in children. Also called **flat wart.**

verruca senilis. See **basal cell papilloma.**

verruca vulgaris, a common wart. See **verruca.**

verrucose, verrucous, the presence of warts. See **verruca.**

verrucous carcinoma /vəroo″kəs/, a well-differentiated squamous cell neoplasm of soft tissue of the oral cavity, larynx, or genitalia. A slow-growing tumor with displacement of surrounding tissue, rather than invasion or metastasis, occurs.

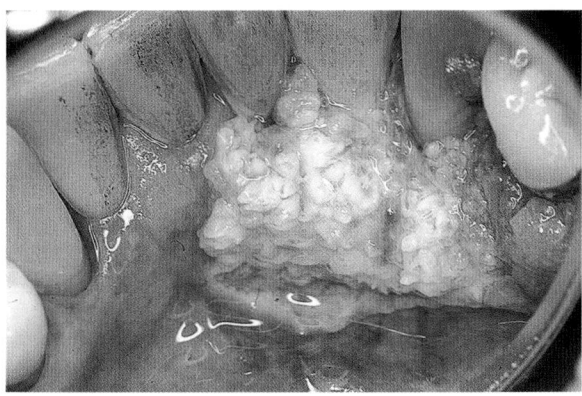

Verrucous carcinoma *(Regezi, Sciubba, and Pogrel, 2000)*

verrucous dermatitis, any skin rash with wartlike lesions.

verrucous endocarditis [L, *verruca,* wart; Gk, *endon,* within, *kardia,* heart, *itis,* inflammation], a form of heart inflammation characterized by the development of wartlike growths on the heart valves.

verruga peruana. See **bartonellosis.**

-verse, 1. suffix meaning "to turn": *reverse curve, transverse.* **2.** suffix meaning "turned," "changed": *adverse reaction.*

Versed, a parenteral benzodiazepine that acts as a central nervous system depressant. Brand name for **midazolam hydrochloride.**

version /vur″zhən/ [L, *vertere,* to turn], the changing of the fetal position in the uterus, usually done to facilitate delivery. Version may occur spontaneously as a result of uterine contractions or be performed by internal or external manipulation by the physician.

version and extraction, an obstetric operation in which a fetus presenting head first is turned and delivered feet first. It is performed by reaching deeply into the uterus, grasping the feet and pulling them down, and extracting the infant. The procedure is considered outmoded and hazardous and has been replaced by cesarean section, although it still may be done to deliver a second twin. Also called **internal podalic version and total breech extraction.** Compare **external version.** See also **breech birth.**

-vert, suffix meaning "a person who has turned (metaphorically)" in a specified direction: *extrovert, introvert.*

vertebra /vur″təbrə/ *pl.* **vertebrae** [L, joint], any one of the 33 bones (26 in the adult) of the spinal column, comprising the 7 cervical, 12 thoracic, 5 lumbar, 5 sacral (1 in adult), and 4 coccygeal vertebrae (1 in adult). The vertebrae, with the exception of the first and second cervical vertebrae, are much alike and are composed of a body, an arch, a spinous process for muscle attachment, and pairs of pedicles and processes. The first cervical vertebra is called the atlas and has no vertebral body. The second cervical vertebra is called the axis and forms the pivot on which the atlas rotates, permitting the head to turn. The body of the axis also extends into a strong, bony process (the dens).

vertebral /vur″təbrəl/ [L, *vertebra,* joint], pertaining to one or more vertebrae.

-vertebral, combining form meaning "spinal column": *costovertebral, paravertebral, intervertebral.*

vertebral angiography [L, *vertebra* + Gk, *angeion* + *graphein,* to record], the radiographic examination of blood circulation in the spinal area after the injection of radiopaque contrast medium. See **angiography.**

vertebral arch [L, *vertebra,* joint, *arcus,* bow], the arch formed on the back of the vertebral body by the pedicles and laminae.

vertebral artery, one of a pair of arteries branching from the subclavian arteries, arising deep in the neck from the cranial and dorsal subclavian surfaces. Each vertebral artery divides into two cervical and five cranial branches, supplying deep neck muscles, the spinal cord and spinal membranes, and the cerebellum.

vertebral-basilar system, an arterial complex in which two vertebral arteries join at the base of the skull to form the basilar artery.

vertebral body, the weight-supporting, solid, central part of a vertebra. The pedicles of the arch project from its dorsolateral surfaces.

vertebral canal [L, *vertebra,* joint, *canalis*], the passage formed anterior to the vertebral arches and posterior to the vertebral bodies and occupied by the spinal cord. The vertebral canal courses within the vertebral column and contains the spinal cord. The canal is formed by the posterior arches of the vertebrae and is large and triangular in the cervical and lumbar sections of the column, the most flexible parts. The canal is small and rounded in the thoracic region, where motion is more restricted.

vertebral column, the flexible structure that forms the longitudinal axis of the skeleton. In the adult it includes 26 vertebrae arranged in a straight line from the base of the skull to the coccyx. The vertebrae are separated by intervertebral disks. They provide attachment for various muscles such as the iliocostalis thoracis and the longissimus thoracis that give the column strength and flexibility.

V

In the adult the five sacral and four coccygeal vertebrae fuse to form the sacrum and the coccyx. The average length of the vertebral column in men is about 71 cm. The cervical part measures about 12.5 cm, the thoracic part about 28 cm, the lumbar part about 18 cm, and the sacrum and the coccyx about 12.5 cm. The vertebral column in women measures approximately 61 cm. Several curves in the column increase its strength, such as the cervical, thoracic, lumbar, and pelvic curves. The cervical curve is convex ventrally from the apex of the dens to the middle of the second thoracic vertebra and is the least marked of all the curves. The thoracic curve, concave ventrally, starts at the middle of the second and ends at the middle of the 12th thoracic vertebra. The lumbar curve, more pronounced in women than in men, begins at the middle of the last thoracic vertebra and ends at the sacrovertebral angle. The pelvic curve starts at the sacrovertebral articulation and ends at the point of the coccyx. The thoracic and the sacral curves constitute primary curves, present during fetal life; the cervical and lumbar curves constitute secondary curves, which develop after birth. Also called **spinal column, spine.** See also **vertebra, vertebral canal.**

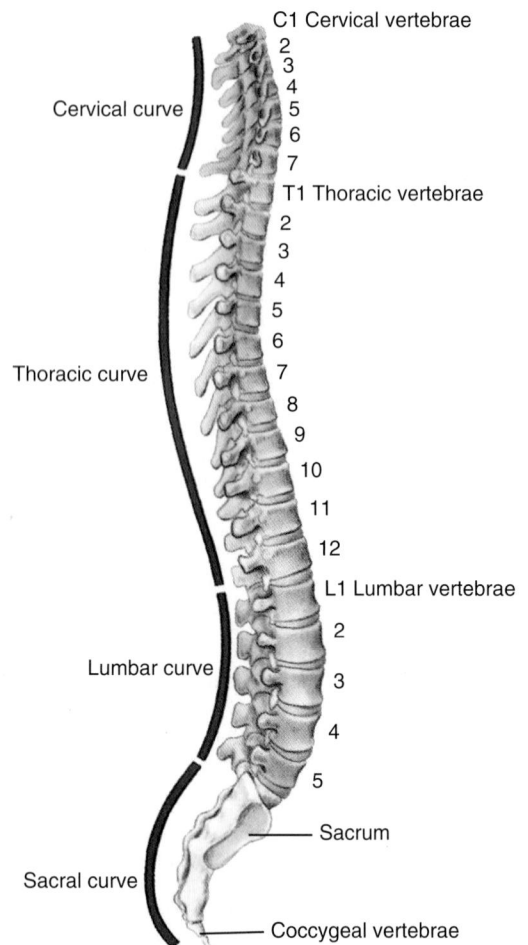

Vertebral column: right lateral view (Applegate, 2011)

vertebral foramen [L, *vertebra,* joint, *foramen,* a hole], the opening between the neural arch and the body of a vertebra through which the spinal cord passes.

vertebral groove [L, *vertebra,* joint; D, *groeve*], a shallow depression on each side of the spinous processes of the vertebrae, occupied by the deep back muscles.

vertebral notch [L, *vertebra,* joint; OFr, *enochier,* notch], either of the concavities on the lower or upper border of a vertebral pedicle.

vertebral rib, one of two lower ribs on either side that are not attached anteriorly. Also called **floating ribs.** See also **rib.**

vertebral subluxation complex, (in chiropractic) malfunction of organs or tissue caused by impairment of nerve function that results from restriction of normal motion or from abnormal position of spinal segments.

vertebral-venous system, a group of four interconnected venous networks surrounding the vertebral column.

vertebrate [L, *vertebra,* joint], any animal that possesses a backbone and thus is a member of the subphylum Vertebrata of the phylum Chordata. Vertebrates include fish, amphibians, birds, reptiles, and mammals.

vertebro-, combining form meaning "vertebral column" or "vertebra": *vertebrocostal, vertebrochondral.*

vertebrochondral /vur'təbrōkon"drəl/, pertaining to a vertebra and a costal cartilage.

vertebrocostal /-kos"təl/, pertaining to a vertebra and a rib or to a vertebra and a costal cartilage.

vertebrocostal rib, one of the 8th, 9th, and 10th ribs on either side that articulate posteriorly with the vertebrae and have their costal cartilages connected anteriorly by capsular ligaments. Also called **false rib.** See also **rib.**

vertebrosternal rib /-stur"nəl/, one of the seven upper ribs on either side that have cartilage articulating directly with the sternum. Also called **true rib.** See also **rib.**

verteporfin /ver"tĕ-por'fin/, a photosensitizing agent that accumulates preferentially in neovasculature, including that in the choroid, such as occurs in age-related macular degeneration, ocular histoplasmosis, or pathological myopia. The agent is then activated by light of a specific wavelength in the presence of oxygen and causes local damage to the neovascular endothelium followed by vessel occlusion. It is administered intravenously before irradiation of the lesion with light from a compatible laser.

vertex /vur"teks/ [L, summit], **1.** the top of the head; crown. **2.** the apex or highest point of any structure.

vertex presentation, (in obstetrics) a fetal presentation in which the vertex of the fetus is the part nearest to the cervical os and can be expected to be born first. Compare **breech presentation.**

vertical /vur"tikəl/ [L, *vertex,* summit], perpendicular or at a right angle to the plane of the horizon.

vertical angulation [L, *vertex + angulus,* corner], the angle within the vertical plane, relative to a reference in the horizontal or occlusal plane, at which the central x-ray beam is directed during radiography or dental imaging of oral structures. Compare **horizontal angulation.**

vertical coordination, a system of community health nurses who serve as links between their level in the organization and those above and below their level. They also serve as links between the agency and the patient.

vertical diplopia [L, *vertex* + Gk, *diploos,* double, *opsis,* vision], a form of double vision in which one image is displaced vertically above the other.

vertically integrated health care, a health delivery system in which the complete spectrum of care, including financial services, is provided within a single organization, such as a health maintenance organization.

vertical nystagmus, a visual abnormality in which the eyes involuntarily move up and down.

vertical plane. See **cardinal frontal plane.**

vertical resorption, a pattern of bone loss in which the alveolar bone adjacent to an affected tooth is destroyed without simultaneous crestal loss. See also **resorption.**

vertical squint. See **vertical strabismus.**

vertical strabismus [L, *vertex* + Gk, *strabismos,* squint], a deviation of one eye in a vertical direction from a point of fixation. A common cause is overaction by the inferior oblique muscles or a weakness of the superior oblique muscle, resulting in a quick vertical movement of the eyeball on adduction. Also called **upward-and-downward squint, vertical squint.**

vertical transmission, the transfer of a disease, condition, or trait from one generation to the next either genetically or congenitally, such as the spread of an infection through breast milk or through the placenta.

vertical vertigo, a sense of instability caused by looking up or down.

verticosubmental /vur′tikō′submen″təl/ [L, *vertex* + *sub,* below, *mentum,* chin], pertaining to a radiographic projection of the head in which the central ray passes from the vertex of the skull through its base.

vertigo /vur″tigō, vurtī″gō/, a sensation of instability, giddiness, loss of equilibrium, or rotation, caused by a disturbance in the semicircular canal of the inner ear or the vestibular nuclei of the brainstem. The sensation that one's body is rotating in space is called subjective vertigo, whereas the sensation that objects are spinning around the body is termed objective vertigo. See also **dizziness, positional vertigo, vestibular neuronitis.**

very low–density lipoprotein (VLDL), a plasma lipoprotein that is composed chiefly of triglycerides, with small amounts of cholesterol, phospholipid, fat-soluble vitamins, and protein. It transports triglycerides primarily from the liver to peripheral sites in the tissues for use or storage. The triglycerides are quickly converted to smaller, more soluble intermediate lipoproteins and eventually to low-density lipoproteins. Elevations in VLDL are associated with increased risk of atherosclerosis. See also **high-density lipoprotein, low-density lipoprotein.**

vesical /ves″ikəl/ [L, *vesica,* bladder], pertaining to a fluid-filled sac, usually the urinary bladder.

vesical calculus, a small hardened mass found in the urinary bladder. Also called **bladder calculus,** *bladder stone,* **cystolith.**

vesical fistula [L, *vesica,* bladder, *fistula,* pipe], an abnormal passage communicating with the urinary bladder. Vesical fistulae may communicate with the skin, vagina, uterus, or rectum.

vesical glands, mucous glands sometimes found in the wall of the urinary bladder, especially in the area of the trigone.

vesical hematuria [L, *vesica,* bladder; Gk, *haima,* blood + *ouron,* urine], the presence of blood in the urine caused by bleeding in the bladder. The urine is bright red.

vesical lithotomy. See **cystolithotomy.**

vesical reflex, the sensation of a need to urinate when the bladder is moderately distended. See also **micturition reflex.**

vesical sphincter, a circular muscle surrounding the opening of the urinary bladder. It is normally contracted to prevent leakage from the bladder.

vesicant /ves″ikənt/, a drug capable of causing tissue necrosis when extravasated.

vesicants. See **blister agents/vesicants.**

VESIcare, an antimuscarinic agent used to treat overactive bladder. Brand name for **solifenacin.**

vesicle /ves″ikəl/ [L, *vesicula*], a small bladder or blister containing clear fluid. Compare **bulla.** **–vesicular,** *adj.*

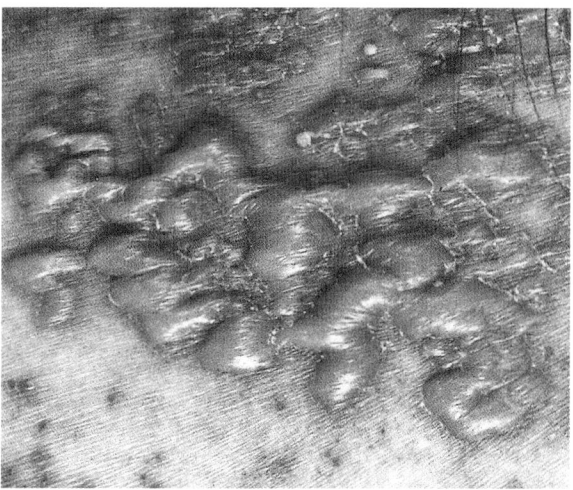

Vesicles *(du Vivier, 2002)*

vesico-, combining form meaning "bladder" or "blister": *vesicoabdominal, vesicocele, vesicovaginal.*

vesicoabdominal /ves′ikō·abdom″inəl/, pertaining to the urinary bladder and abdominal wall.

vesicocele. See **cystocele.**

vesicocolonic fistula, a passageway connecting the colon and the urinary bladder. See **colovesical fistula.**

vesicoenteric fistula, enterovesical fistula. Also called *vesicointestinal fistula.*

vesicosphincter dyssynergia. See **detrusor-sphincter dyssynergia.**

vesicoureteral reflux /ves′ikōyŏŏrē″tərəl/ [L, *vesica* + Gk, *oureter,* ureter; L, *refluxus,* backflow], an abnormal backflow of urine from the bladder to the ureter resulting from a congenital defect, obstruction of the outlet of the bladder, or edema or scarring secondary to infection of the lower urinary tract. Reflux increases the hydrostatic pressure in the ureters and kidneys and may cause permanent damage. The condition is characterized by abdominal or flank pain, enuresis, pyuria, hematuria, proteinuria, and bacteriuria accompanied by persistent or recurrent urinary tract infections. Diagnosis is made by cystoscopy and voiding cystourethrography. Obstruction of the ureter or defective implantation of the ureter in the bladder may be surgically corrected. Antibacterial medication, urinary tract antiseptics, and analgesia are usually prescribed for any infection that causes or results from this condition.

vesicouterine /ves′ikōyŏŏ″tərin, -ēn/ [L, *vesica* + *uterus,* womb], pertaining to the bladder and uterus. Also called **uterovesical.**

vesicouterine pouch, a shallow pouch that occurs anteriorly between the bladder and uterus.

vesicovaginal /ves′ikōvaj″inəl/, pertaining to the urinary bladder and vagina.

vesicovaginal fistula, a fistula between the bladder and the vagina.

vesicula /vəsik″yələ/ [L], a vesicle or small bladder.

vesicular /vesik″yələr/, pertaining to a blisterlike condition.

vesicular appendix, a cystic structure on the fimbriated end of each of the fallopian tubes. It represents a remnant of the mesonephric ducts.

vesicular breath sound (V.S.), a normal sound of rustling or swishing heard with a stethoscope over the lung periphery. It characteristically has a higher pitch during inspiration and fades rapidly during expiration. Compare **bronchial breath sound.**

V

vesicular emphysema.   See **panacinar emphysema.**

vesicular mole.   *(Obsolete)* See **hydatid mole.**

vesicular ovarian follicle,   graafian follicle.

vesiculitis /vəsik′yəlī″tis/,   an inflammation of any vesicle, particularly a seminal vesicle. Clinical manifestations of this condition are minimal; it is usually associated with prostatitis.

vesiculography /vəsik′yəlog″rəfē/,   the radiological examination of the seminal vesicles and adjacent structures, usually after injection of a radiopaque contrast medium into the deferent ducts or, by catheterization, into the ejaculatory ducts. The technique is used to examine the seminal vesicles, vas deferens, and ejaculatory duct for possible tumors, cysts, or other disorders.

vesiculotympanitic,   both vesicular and tympanitic; said of auscultatory sounds.

vespid,   a wasp. See **bee sting.**

vessel /ves″əl/   [L, *vascellum,* small vase],   any one of the many tubules throughout the body conveying fluids, such as blood and lymph. Kinds include **artery, vein, lymphatic vessels.**

vestibular /vestib″yələr/   [L, *vestibulum,* courtyard],   pertaining to a vestibule, such as the vestibular part of the mouth, which lies between the cheeks and the teeth.

vestibular apparatus,   the inner ear structures that are associated with balance and position sense. Kinds include **vestibule, semicircular canal.**

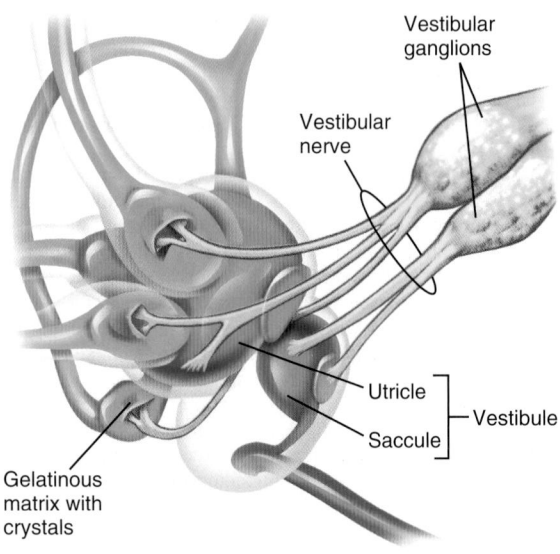

Vestibular apparatus

vestibular caecum of cochlear duct,   a small blind outpouching at the vestibular end of the cochlear duct.

vestibular extension,   oral surgery. See **vestibuloplasty.**

vestibular fold.   See **false vocal cord.**

vestibular fossa,   the vaginal vestibule between the vaginal orifice and the fourchette (frenulum of pudendal labia). Also called **fossa of vestibule of vagina,** *navicular fossa.*

vestibular function,   the sense of balance.

vestibular gland,   any one of four small glands, two on each side of the vaginal orifice. One pair of the small structures constitutes the greater vestibular glands; the other pair constitutes the lesser vestibular glands. The vestibular glands secrete a lubricating substance. Compare **Cowper's gland.** See also **Bartholin gland.**

vestibular nerve   [L, *vestibulum,* courtyard, *nervus*],   a branch of the eighth cranial nerve associated with the sense of equilibrium. It arises in the vestibular ganglion (Scarpa's ganglion) of the ear.

vestibular neuronitis,   a sudden, severe attack of vertigo without symptoms of deafness or tinnitus. It usually affects young or middle-aged adults, is temporary, and follows an upper respiratory infection.

vestibular surface,   the surface of a tooth that is directed outward toward the vestibule of the mouth, including the buccal and labial surfaces, and opposite the lingual (or oral) surface.

vestibular toxicity,   toxic effects (commonly of drugs) on the vestibule of the ear, resulting in dizziness, vertigo, and loss of balance.

vestibular window.   See **oval window.**

vestibule /ves″tibyool/   [L, *vestibulum,* courtyard],   a space or a cavity that serves as the entrance to a passageway, such as the vestibule of the vagina or the vestibule of the ear.

vestibule of the aorta,   Anatomy and Physiology Cardiovascular a space within the left ventricle of the heart at the root of the aorta.

vestibule of the ear,   the central part of the inner ear, within the osseous labyrinth, involved with the sensation of position and movement.

vestibule of the mouth,   the portion of the oral cavity bounded on one side by the teeth and gingivae, or the residual alveolar ridges, and on the other side by the lips (labial vestibule) and cheeks (buccal vestibule).

vestibulocochlear nerve,   either of a pair of cranial nerves composed of fibers from the cochlear nerve and the vestibular nerve in the inner ear, conveying impulses of both the sense of hearing and the sense of balance. Also called **acoustic nerve, eighth cranial nerve.**

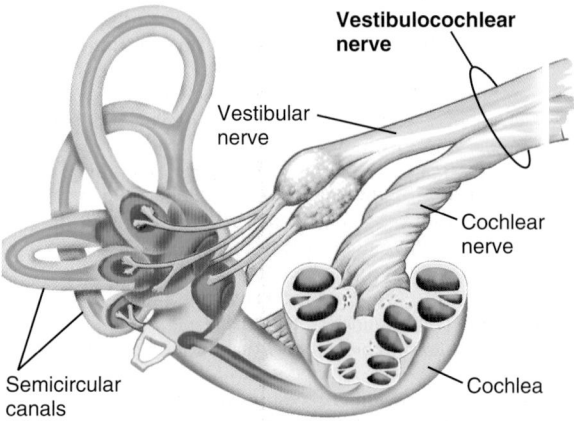

Vestibulocochlear nerve

vestibulo-ocular reflex /vestib″yəlō·ok′yələr/,   a normal reflex in which eye position compensates for movement of the head. It is induced by excitation of the vestibular apparatus.

vestibuloplasty /vestib″yəlōplas′tē/   [L, *vestibulum,* courtyard; Gk, *plassein,* to shape],   plastic surgery of the oral vestibule, particularly modification of the gingival and mucosal tissues to create a deeper or better-shaped vestibule, usually to aid in the creation of a supporting area for a full denture or partial denture base. Also called **sulcoplasty, vestibular extension.** See also **supporting area, stress-bearing area.**

vestige /ves″tij/   [L, *vestigium,* trace],   an imperfectly developed, relatively useless organ or other structure of the body that had a vital function at an earlier stage of life or in a more primitive form of life. The vermiform appendix is a vestigial organ. −*vestigial, adj.*

veterinarian /vet″əriner″ē·ən/ [L, *veterinarius,* beast of burden], a health professional who specializes in the causes and treatment of diseases and disorders of domestic and wild animals.

veterinary medicine /vet″əriner′ē/, the field of medicine concerned with the health and diseases of animals other than humans.

VF, **1.** abbreviation for **ventricular fibrillation. 2.** abbreviation for **visual field. 3.** abbreviation for **vocal fremitus.**

VH, abbreviation for **viral hepatitis.**

VI, abbreviation for *variable interval.* See **variable interval (VI) reinforcement.**

via /vī″ə, vē″ä/ [L, a way], any passage or course, such as the esophagus or trachea.

viability /vī′əbil″itē/ [L, *vita,* life], the ability to continue living.

viable /vī″əbəl/ [Fr, likely to live], capable of developing, growing, and otherwise sustaining life, such as a normal human fetus at 24 weeks of gestation. −**viability,** *n.*

viable infant, an infant who at birth weighs at least 500 g or is 24 weeks or more of gestational age.

Viagra /vi-ag′rah/, a phosphodiesterase inhibitor used for treatment of erectile dysfunction. Brand name for **sildenafil.**

vial /vī″əl/, a glass container with a metal-enclosed rubber seal.

Vibramycin Monohydrate, a tetracycline antibiotic. Brand name for **doxycycline.**

vibrating. See **cupping and vibrating.**

vibration /vībrā″shən/ [L, *vibrare,* to vibrate], a type of massage administered by quickly tapping with the fingertips or alternating the fingers in a rhythmic manner or by a mechanical device. See also **massage.**

vibratory /vī″brətôr′ē/ [L, *vibrare,* to vibrate], causing vibrations or a state of vibration.

vibratory massage, the manipulation of body surfaces with an instrument that produces a rapid tapping sensation. Also called **vibrotherapeutics.**

vibratory sense [L, *vibrare,* to vibrate, *sentire,* to feel], the ability to perceive vibratory sensations. Vibration receptors in the body are found in a variety of locations, from the skin surface to the membranes covering bones. Some respond only to certain vibration frequencies.

vibrio /vib″rē·ō/ [L, *vibrare*], any bacterium that is curved and motile, such as those belonging to the genus *Vibrio.* Cholera and several other epidemic forms of gastroenteritis are caused by members of the genus.

Vibrio cholerae, the species of comma-shaped, motile bacillus that is the cause of cholera.

Vibrio fetus. See *Campylobacter.*

vibrio gastroenteritis, an infectious disease caused by *Vibrio parahaemolyticus* acquired from contaminated seafood. It is characterized by nausea, vomiting, abdominal pain, and diarrhea. Headache, mild fever, and bloody stools also may be present. Spontaneous recovery usually occurs in 2 to 5 days. Compare **salmonellosis, shigellosis.**

Vibrio parahaemolyticus /per″əhē′mōlit′ikəs/, a species of halophic (salt-tolerant) microorganisms of the genus *Vibrio,* found in brackish water. It is the causative agent in food poisoning associated with the ingestion of raw or undercooked shellfish, especially crabs and shrimp. This microorganism is a common cause of gastroenteritis in Japan, aboard cruise ships, and in the eastern and southeastern coastal areas of the United States. Thorough cooking of seafood prevents the infection associated with *Vibrio parahaemolyticus,* which

causes watery diarrhea, abdominal cramps, vomiting, headache, chills, and fever. This microorganism has an incubation period of 2 to 48 hours, after which the symptoms of infection appear. The food poisoning from this agent usually subsides spontaneously within 2 days but may be more severe, even fatal, in debilitated and elderly people. This organism can also cause infection of the skin when an open wound is exposed to seawater. Confirming diagnosis must rule out other causes of food poisoning and acute GI disorders and requires bacteriological examination of the vomitus, stool, and blood. Treatment usually includes bed rest and the oral replacement of fluids. IV replacement of fluids is seldom required.

Vibrio vulnificus, a halophilic (salt-tolerant) species of microorganism whose strains are similar to *V. parahaemolyticus* but differ in that they can ferment lactose. Infection by eating raw seafood causes septicemia, gastroenteritis, and cellulitis and may be especially severe or even fatal in those with preexisting hepatic disease. Wound infection may occur following exposure to seawater or from injury when handling crabs.

vibrotherapeutics. See **vibratory massage.**

vicarious menstruation /vīker″ē·əs/ [L, *vicarius,* substituted, *menstruare,* to menstruate], discharge of blood from a site other than the uterus at the time when the menstrual flow is normally expected. Such bleeding is usually caused by the increased capillary permeability that occurs during menstruation.

vidarabine /vider″əbēn/, an antiviral agent. Also called **adenine arabinoside.**

■ INDICATIONS: This drug is an ophthalmic ointment prescribed to treat keratoconjunctivitis and nearby epithelial or superficial keratitis caused by herpes simplex virus type 1 or type 2.

■ CONTRAINDICATIONS: Known hypersensitivity to this drug prohibits its use, and it should not be used for ophthalmic ulcers that are sterile.

■ ADVERSE EFFECTS: Local irritation, photophobia, and corneal edema may occur in topical ophthalmic applications.

Vidaza, a chemotherapeutic agent. Brand name for **azacitidine.**

videoconference /vid″e-o-con′fer-ens/, a meeting between persons in different locations by means of computerized audiovisual displays.

video display terminal (VDT) [L, *videre,* to see, *displicare,* to scatter, *terminus,* end], a device with a surface similar to a television screen, used in word processors, computer terminals, and similar equipment to display information.

videoendoscopy /vid″e-o-en-dos′kah-pe/, endoscopy performed under the guidance of a video camera in the tip of the endoscope.

videolaparoscopy /vid″e-o-lap″ah-ros′kah-pe/, laparoscopic surgery performed under the guidance of a video camera in the tip of the laparoscope.

videostroboscopy, an endoscopic examination of the larynx while speaking.

Videx, a nucleoside analog reverse transcriptase inhibitor for HIV. Also called **ddI.** Brand name for **dideoxyinosine.**

view /vu/, (in radiology) a projection related to the position of the body and the direction of an x-ray beam.

vigilambulism /vij′ilam″byəliz′əm/, a condition in which walking or other motor acts are performed in an unconscious but waking state.

vigilance /vij″iləns/ [L, *vigil,* awake], a state of being attentive or alert.

vigil coma /vij″əl/ [L, *vigil* + Gk, *koma,* deep sleep], a semiconscious state of delirium in which the patient may appear awake, with eyes open and staring, and may make verbal sounds.

vignetting, the peripheral reduction of light intensity in fluoroscopic image intensifiers.

villi. See **villus.**

villoma /vilō″mə/ *pl.* **villomas, villomata** [L, *villus,* hair; Gk, *oma,* tumor], a villous neoplasm or papilloma occurring in the bladder or rectum. Also called *villioma.*

villous. See **villus.**

villous adenoma /vil″əs/ [L, *villus,* hair], a slow-growing, soft, spongy, potentially malignant papillary growth of the mucosa of the large intestine.

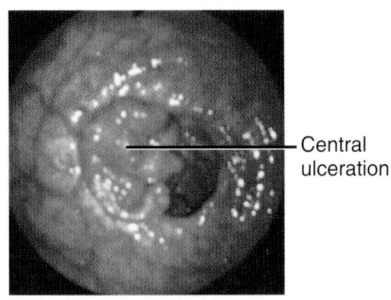

— Central ulceration

Villous adenoma: endoscopic view *(Skarin, 2010)*

villous carcinoma, an epithelial tumor with many long, velvety, papillary outgrowths. Also called **carcinoma villosum.**

villous chorion, the region of the chorion that bears villi. Also called **shaggy chorion.**

villous papilloma, a benign tumor with long, slender processes, usually occurring in the bladder, breast, or a cerebral ventricle.

villus /vil″əs/ *pl.* **villi** [L, shaggy, hair], one of the many tiny projections, barely visible to the naked eye, clustered over the entire mucous surface of the small intestine. Villi are covered with epithelium that diffuses and transports fluids and nutrients. They are larger in some parts of the intestine than in others and flatten out when the intestine distends. Each villus has a core of delicate areolar and reticular connective tissue supporting the epithelium, various capillaries, and often a single lymphatic lacteal that fills with milky white chyle during the digestion of a fatty meal. —**villous,** *adj.*

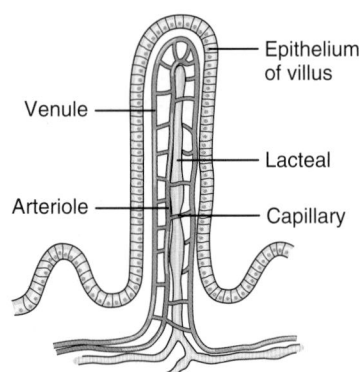

Epithelium of villus

Venule

Lacteal

Arteriole

Capillary

Villus *(Phipps et al, 2003)*

vin-, -vin, combining form for antiviral substances.

vinBLAStine sulfate /vinblas″tēn, -tin/, an antimitotic antineoplastic agent.

■ INDICATIONS: It is prescribed in the treatment of many neoplastic diseases, such as choriocarcinoma, testicular carcinoma, lung cancer, breast cancer, renal cancer, Hodgkin disease, and non-Hodgkin lymphoma.

■ CONTRAINDICATIONS: Leukopenia, bacterial infection, or known hypersensitivity to this drug prohibits its use. It is not prescribed in pregnancy and should not be administered intrathecally.

■ ADVERSE EFFECTS: Among the typical adverse effects are leukopenia (dose-limiting toxicity), nausea, diarrhea, stomatitis, and alopecia. Neurotoxicity seldom occurs at usual clinical doses but can become significant at higher doses. Vinblastine is a vesicant, so prompt attention is required if extravasation occurs.

Vincent angina, Vincent infection. See **necrotizing ulcerative gingivitis.**

Vincent's stomatitis [Henri Vincent, French physician, 1862–1950; Gk, *stoma,* mouth, *itis,* inflammation], a painful bacterial infection of the mouth and gums causing ulceration (gingivitis). See **necrotizing ulcerative gingivitis.**

vinCRIStine sulfate /vinkris″tēn, -tin/, an antimitotic antineoplastic agent.

■ INDICATIONS: It is prescribed in the treatment of many neoplastic diseases, such as leukemia, neuroblastoma, lymphomas, and sarcomas. It is often used in combination therapy because its dose-limiting toxicity is different from that of most other cancer chemotherapy drugs.

■ CONTRAINDICATIONS: Pregnancy, leukopenia, preexisting neuromuscular disease, or known hypersensitivity to this drug prohibits its use. Intrathecal administration of vincristine has caused deaths and is therefore also contraindicated.

■ ADVERSE EFFECTS: Neurotoxicity is the dose-limiting toxicity. Constipation, abdominal pain, and alopecia also may occur. Vincristine is a vesicant, so prompt attention is required if extravasation occurs. Leukopenia seldom occurs at usual clinical doses but can become significant at higher doses.

Vineberg operation /vīn″bərg/ [Arthur M. Vineberg, Canadian thoracic surgeon, 1903–1988], *(Obsolete)* a technique in which the internal mammary artery is implanted into the myocardium to improve blood flow to the heart. Common in the 1950s, the procedure has been replaced by others, such as saphenous vein grafting.

vinegar acid. See **acetic acid.**

vinorelbine tartrate, an anticancer mitotic inhibitor.

■ INDICATIONS: It is prescribed in the treatment of non–small cell lung cancer.

■ CONTRAINDICATIONS: It should not be given to patients with low blood counts or those who may have an allergy or sensitivity to vinorelbine. It should be used with caution in patients with comprised bone marrow; bronchospasm; or kidney, liver, or lung disease.

■ ADVERSE EFFECTS: The side effects most often reported include granulocytopenia, leukopenia, or anemia.

Viokase, an enzyme mixture of amylase, lipase, and protease derived from hog pancreas. Brand name for *pancrelipase.*

violence /vi′o-lens/, great force, either physical or emotional, usually exerted to damage or otherwise abuse something or someone.

viosterol /vī·os″tərôl/, synthetic vitamin D_2 in an oil base. Also called **synthetic oleovitamin D.** See also **calciferol, ergosterol.**

VIP, **1.** abbreviation for **vasoactive intestinal polypeptide.** **2.** *(Informal)* a term used to refer to someone famous or influential. A VIP suite in a hospital is one reserved for such people. Abbreviation for *very important person.*

viperid /vi′perid/. See **viperine.**

viperine,   **1.** *adj.,* pertaining to the true vipers. **2.** *n.,* true viper. Also called **viperid.**

VIPoma /vipō″mə/,   a type of pancreatic tumor that causes changes in secretion of vasoactive intestinal polypeptide (VIP). VIP causes dilation of blood vessels throughout the body and secretion of fluid and salt in the intestinal tract, resulting in diarrhea. The VIP effects mimic the symptoms of cholera (severe diarrhea, hypokalemia, and hypochlorhydria) and can result in death from dehydration and subsequent kidney failure if treatment is not begun early. See also **vasoactive intestinal polypeptide.**

vir-, -vir,   combining form for antiviral substances.

Vira-A,   an antiviral drug. Brand name for **vidarabine.**

viraemia.   See **viremia.**

viral cultures,   cultures of the blood, urine, stool, throat, and skin to definitively diagnose viral disease.

viral cystitis,   cystitis caused by a viral infection, most often seen in immunocompromised persons infected with BK virus.

viral disease.   See **viral infection.**

viral dysentery /vī″rəl/ [L, *virus,* poison; Gk, *dys,* bad, *enteron,* intestine],   a form of dysentery caused by a virus and usually characterized by an acute watery diarrhea.

viral gastroenteritis,   an inflammation of the intestine caused by a virus. The symptoms usually include abdominal cramps, diarrhea, nausea, and vomiting.

viral hepatitis (VH),   a viral inflammatory disease of the liver caused by one of the hepatitis viruses: A, B, C, delta, E, F, G, or H. All have chronic forms except hepatitis A. The disease is transmitted sexually and through blood transfusions and is common among people with behavior risks or human immunodeficiency virus infection. Speed of onset and probable course of the illness vary with the kind and strain of virus, but the characteristics of the disease and its treatment are the same. See also **hepatitis A, hepatitis B, hepatitis C, hepatitis D.**

■ OBSERVATIONS: Diagnosis is made through antibody (A + C) or antigen (B + D). Characteristic of viral hepatitis are anorexia, malaise, headache, pain over the liver, fever, jaundice, clay-colored stools, dark urine, nausea and vomiting, and diarrhea. Laboratory analyses reveal increased amounts of aspartate aminotransferase (AST) and bilirubin and an abnormal coagulation of the blood. Severe infection, especially with hepatitis B virus, may be prolonged and result in tissue destruction, cirrhosis, and chronic hepatitis or in hepatic coma and death.

■ INTERVENTIONS: Treatment is with alpha-interferon. Depending on the specific type of hepatitis, treatment with alpha-interferon is effective in 40% of patients with chronic hepatitis B virus infection. Improvement in liver function has been noted in 50% of the patients infected. Treatment is also largely supportive. It includes bed rest; isolation, if necessary; fluids; a low-fat, high-protein, high-calorie diet; special skin care if pruritus is present; emotional support; vitamins B_{12}, K, and C; and monitoring of liver and kidney function. Sedatives, analgesics, antiemetics, and steroids may be ordered. However, the patient is carefully observed for adverse reaction to medication because the liver may not be able to break down and detoxify the drugs. Decrease in the amount or frequency of administration or change of the medication may be necessary.

■ PATIENT CARE CONSIDERATIONS: The person is taught the importance of rest and avoiding fatigue, washing the hands carefully after urinating or defecating to avoid spreading the virus, eating well, following written dietary instructions after discharge, and avoiding alcohol, usually for at least 1 year. The patient is encouraged to have certain blood tests performed periodically, including AST and serum bilirubin,

to report any symptoms of recurrence immediately, and to avoid contact with people having infections. The person is told not to donate blood and not to take over-the-counter drugs without medical consultation.

viral hemorrhagic fever,   any of a group of severe multisystem syndromes caused by a virus. Typically the illness is characterized by bleeding, which is usually not life threatening. However, viral hemorrhagic fever can cause a range of other symptoms from mild to life-threatening in severity, depending on the virus.

viral infection,   any of the diseases caused by one of approximately 200 viruses pathogenic to humans. Some are the most communicable and dangerous diseases known; some cause mild and transient conditions that pass virtually unnoticed. If cells are damaged by the viral attack, disease exists. The signs of the infection reflect the anatomic location of the damaged cells. Viruses are introduced into the body through nonintact skin or mucous membranes or through a transfusion into the bloodstream or transplantation, by droplet infection through the respiratory tract, or by ingestion through the digestive tract into the GI system. The pathogenicity of the particular virus depends on the rapidity of replication, the enzymes released, the part of the body infected, and the particular action of the virus. After it enters the body, the virus attaches to and enters a cell. The virus directs the cell to produce new virions, using chemical building blocks and energy available in the parasitized cell. The virus has now taken over the cell. After a variable period of time, masses of fully grown viruses appear, each able to survive outside the cell until more susceptible cells are found. In poliovirus infection, one parasitized cell may produce more than 100,000 poliovirus particles in a few hours. Techniques used in viral identification and immunization are based on the essential fact that viruses can multiply only inside living cells. Inoculation of susceptible animals, tissue culture media, and chick embryos allows cultivation of viruses for study and identification and for the preparation of vaccine. Other techniques can also be used in the diagnosis of the cause of viral infection, including serological tests, fluorescent antibody microscopic examination, microscopic examination, and skin tests. In many viral diseases, including mumps, smallpox, and measles, one attack confers permanent immunity. In others, immunity is short-lived. The incubation period for viral infection is usually short, the viruses do not circulate in the bloodstream, antibodies do not form, and most often immunity does not develop. Exposure to a few viruses results in immunity to that virus and to other closely related viruses. Some vectors are able to spread several viruses, but only one at a time. Mechanisms of natural resistance to viral infection are poorly understood, but susceptibility to a particular virus is somehow species-specific; for example, chickenpox, caused by the varicella zoster virus, is seen only in humans. A protective substance, interferon, is elaborated naturally in small amounts in the body. It is cell-specific and species-specific but not virus-specific. Interferon may act as a broad-spectrum antiviral agent, protecting the body from the effects of many viral infections and stopping the synthesis of viral nucleic acid within the parasitized cell. Also called **viral disease.** See also *specific viral infections.*

viral keratoconjunctivitis [L, *virus,* poison; Gk, *keras,* horn; L, *conjunctivus,* connecting; Gk, *itis,* inflammation],   a combination of inflammation of the cornea and conjunctiva caused by a viral infection.

viral load,   measurement of the amount of human immunodeficiency virus in the blood expressed as copies per milliliter. Plasma viremia is used to guide treatment decisions and monitor response to treatment. See also **viremia.**

viral meningitis,   meningitis caused by various viruses, such as the coxsackieviruses, mumps virus, and the virus of lymphocytic choriomeningitis, characterized by malaise, fever, headache, nausea, cerebrospinal fluid pleocytosis (principally lymphocytic), abdominal pain, stiffness of the neck and back, and a short uncomplicated course. See also **aseptic meningitis.**

viral myocarditis, inflammation of the myocardium caused by coxsackievirus.

viral pneumonia, pulmonary infection caused by a virus.

viral therapy, Immunology (Autoimmune)Procedures the use of genetically altered viruses to deliver genes to specific sites.

Viramune, a nonnucleoside reverse transcriptase inhibitor for HIV. Brand name for **nevirapine.**

Virazole, an aerosol antiviral drug. Brand name for **ribavirin.**

Virchow-Robin spaces. See **perivascular spaces.**

Virchow's node /fir″shōz/ [Rudolf L.K. Virchow, German pathologist, 1821–1902], a firm supraclavicular lymph node, particularly on the left side, that is so enlarged that it is palpable. Also called **sentinel node, signal node.**

Virchow's spaces. See **perivascular spaces.**

Viread, a nucleoside analog reverse transcriptase inhibitor. Brand name for **tenofovir.**

viremia /vīrē″mē·ə/ [L, *virus* + Gk, *haima,* blood], the presence of viruses in the blood. Also spelled **viraemia.** Compare **bacteremia, fungemia, parasitemia.**

virgin /vur″jən/, **1.** a person who has never had sexual intercourse. **2.** uncontaminated.

virginity /vurjin″itē/, the state of being a virgin.

virile /vir″əl/ [L, *virilis,* masculine], **1.** pertaining to or characteristic of an adult male; masculine; manly. **2.** possessing or exhibiting masculine strength, vigor, force, or energy. **3.** pertaining to the male sexual functions; capable of procreation. Compare **virilism. –virility,** *n.*

virilism /vir″əliz′əm/ [L, *virilis* + *ismus,* practice], **1.** a syndrome in which excessive adrenal androgens cause virilization. See **virilization. 2.** pseudohermaphroditism in a female. **3.** premature development of masculine characteristics in the male. Kinds include **adrenal virilism, prosopopilary virilism.**

virility. See **virile.**

virilization /vir′əlīzā″shən/ [L, *virilis* + *atus,* process], a process in which secondary male sexual characteristics are acquired by a female, usually as the result of adrenal dysfunction or hormonal medication. Also called **masculinization, virilism.** See also **adrenal virilism.**

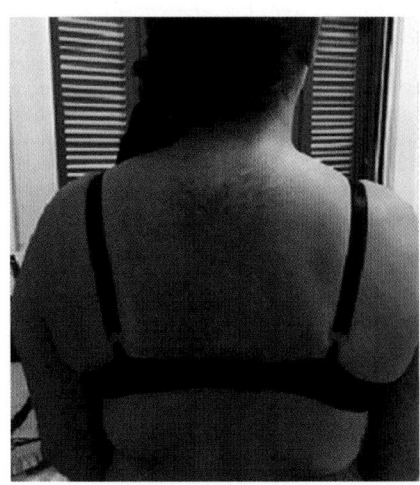

Virilization *(Dotto et al, 2019)*

virion /vir″ē·on, vī″rē·on/ [L, *virus,* poison], a single virus particle with a central nucleoid surrounded by a protein coat or capsid. The complete nucleocapsid with a nucleic acid core may constitute a complete virus, such as the adenoviruses and the picornaviruses, or it may be surrounded by an envelope, as in the herpesviruses and the myxoviruses. Such an envelope is a membrane that contains lipids, proteins, and carbohydrates and projects spikelike structures from its surface. See also **capsid.**

virocytes /vī″rəsīts/ [L, *virus* + Gk, *kytos,* cell], lymphocytes altered in appearance and in staining that are seen in blood smears from patients with viral diseases.

viroid /vī″roid/, a small infective segment of nucleic acid, usually ribonucleic acid (RNA). It is not translated and is replicated by host cell enzymes. Viroids include segments that are complementary to introns and may bind to intron RNA. Viroids are responsible for several plant diseases. Although they have not been associated with animal diseases, viroid-like DNA has been found in cancer cells, and some authorities believe that viroids can evolve into infectious animal viruses. See also **intron, plasmid, transposon.**

virologic, virological. See **virology.**

virologist /vīrol″əjist, vir-/, a specialist who studies viruses and diseases caused by viruses.

virology /-l″əjē/ [L, *virus* + Gk, *logos,* science], the study of viruses and viral diseases. –*virological, virologic, adj.*

Viroptic, an ophthalmic antiviral drug. Brand name for *trifluridine.*

virtual colonoscopy, an imaging technique, used for examination of the colon, in which cross-sectional images acquired by computed tomography or magnetic resonance imaging are processed by computer to reconstruct a three-dimensional display of the colonic lumen.

virtual endoscopy, an imaging technique in which cross-sectional images acquired by computed tomography or magnetic resonance imaging are processed by computer to reconstruct a three-dimensional display similar to that seen through an endoscope.

virtual reality /vur″cho͞o·əl/, a system of computer-generated, three-dimensional, imaginary environments with which a person can subjectively interact. Examples include medical research to monitor brain activity in the hippocampus of subjects trying to solve maze problems. It is also used for simulations and gaming.

virucidal /vī″rəsī″dəl/, pertaining to the destruction of viruses.

virucide /vī″rəsīd/ [L, *virus* + *caedere,* to kill], any agent that destroys or inactivates a virus.

virulence /vir″yələns/ [L, *virulentus,* poisonous], the power of a microorganism to produce disease.

virulent /vir′yələnt/ [L, *virulentus*], pertaining to a very pathogenic or rapidly progressive condition.

virus /vī″rəs/ [L, poison], **1.** a minute parasitic microorganism much smaller than a bacterium that, having no independent metabolic activity, may replicate only within a cell of a living plant or animal host. A virus consists of a core of nucleic acid (deoxyribonucleic acid or ribonucleic acid) surrounded by a coat of antigenic protein, sometimes surrounded by an envelope of lipoprotein. The virus provides the genetic code for replication, and the host cell provides the necessary energy and raw materials. More than 200 viruses have been identified as capable of causing disease in humans. Kinds include **adenovirus,** *Arenavirus, Enterovirus,* **herpesvirus, rhinovirus.** See also **viral infection. 2.** (in computer technology) a type of malicious computer code that is designed to spread from computer to computer, or from computer system to computer system, for the purpose of interfering with normal operations.

virus shedding, the movement by any route of a virus from an infected host.

virustatic /vī′rəstat″ik/, pertaining to the inhibition of the growth and development of viruses, as distinguished from their destruction.

vis /vis, vēs/ [L, force], energy or power.

Visagraph /ve′zah-graf/, a device that records and measures eye movements while the patient is reading.

viscera /vis″ərə/*sing. viscus* [L, *viscus,* internal organs], the internal organs enclosed within a body cavity, including the abdominal, thoracic, pelvic, and endocrine organs.

visceral /vis″ərəl/ [L, *viscus,* internal organs], pertaining to the viscera, or internal organs in the abdominal cavity. Also **splanchnic.**

visceral abdominal fascia, the fascia that invests the abdominal viscera.

visceral afferent fibers, the nerve fibers of the visceral nervous system that receive stimuli, carry impulses toward the central nervous system, and share the sensory ganglia of the cerebrospinal nerves with the somatic sensory fibers. Peripheral distribution of the visceral afferent fibers constitutes the main difference between them and the somatic afferents. The visceral afferent fibers produce sensations different from those of the somatic afferent fibers. The visceral efferent fibers connect with both the somatic and visceral afferent fibers. The number and extent of the visceral afferent fibers is not clearly established. Their peripheral processes reach the ganglia by various routes. Most of the visceral afferent fibers accompany blood vessels for part of their course, and various afferent fibers run in the cerebrospinal nerves. Some of the parts of the body with visceral afferent fibers are the face, scalp, nose, mouth, descending colon, lungs, abdomen, and rectum. See also **autonomic nervous system.**

visceral cavity [L, *viscus,* internal organs, *cavum*], **1.** the abdominal cavity containing the viscera. **2.** the cavity of any viscus, such as the stomach.

visceral efferent system [L, *viscus,* internal organs, *effere,* to bear out; Gk, *systema*], the part of the autonomic nervous system that supplies efferent nerve fibers from the central nervous system to the visceral organs.

visceral inversion, the transposition of the abdominal and thoracic organs to opposite sides of the body. Also called **situs inversus viscerum, situs inversus viscerum, situs inversus viscerum.**

visceral larva migrans, infestation with parasitic larvae, *Toxocara,* or, occasionally, *Ascaris, Strongyloides,* or other nematodes. See also **toxocariasis.**

visceral layer of glomerular capsule, the layer of the glomerular capsule overlying the capillaries and composed of podocytes. It is separated from the parietal layer by the urinary space.

visceral leishmaniasis. See **kala-azar.**

visceral lymph node, a small oval nodular gland that filters lymph circulating in the lymphatic vessels of the thoracic, abdominal, and pelvic viscera. The visceral lymph nodes of the thorax include the anterior mediastinal nodes, posterior mediastinal nodes, and tracheobronchial nodes. The visceral lymph nodes of the abdomen and pelvis include those that follow the course of the celiac artery, superior mesenteric artery, and inferior mesenteric artery. Compare **parietal lymph node.** See also **lymph, lymphatic system, lymph node.**

visceral nervous system, the visceral part of the peripheral nervous system that comprises the whole complex of nerves, fibers, ganglia, and plexuses by which impulses travel from the central nervous system to the viscera and from the viscera to the central nervous system. It contains the usual afferent fibers that receive stimuli and carry impulses toward the central nervous system and efferent fibers that carry impulses from the appropriate centers to the active effector organs, such as the nonstriated muscle, cardiac muscle, and glands of the body. Also called **involuntary nervous system.** See also **autonomic nervous system, visceral afferent fibers.**

visceral obesity, android obesity; so-called from the theory that deep intraabdominal (visceral) fat plays a large role in the associated morbidity and mortality.

visceral pain, pain that results from the activation of nociceptors of the thoracic, pelvic, or abdominal viscera. It is felt as a poorly localized aching or cramping sensation and is often referred to cutaneous sites.

visceral pericardium [L, *viscus* + Gk, *peri,* around, *kardia,* heart], the surface of the pericardial membrane that is in direct contact with the heart. Also called **epicardium.**

visceral peritoneum, a continuation of the parietal peritoneum reflected at various places over the viscera, forming a complete covering for the stomach, spleen, liver, intestines from the distal duodenum to the upper end of the rectum, uterus, and ovaries; it also partially covers some other abdominal organs. It holds the viscera in position by its folds, including the mesenteries; the omenta; and the ligaments of the liver, spleen, stomach, kidneys, bladder, and uterus. The potential space between the visceral and the parietal peritoneum is the peritoneal cavity. The general cavity communicates by the omental foramen with the bursa omentalis (or lesser peritoneal cavity).

visceral pleura. See **pulmonary pleura.**

visceral protein status, the amount of protein that is contained in the internal organs.

visceral reflex. See **viscerosomatic reaction.**

visceral skeleton [L, *viscus* + Gk, *skeletos,* dried up], the part of the skeleton, including sternum, ribs, pelvis, and vertebrae, that encloses the viscera.

visceral swallow, an immature swallowing pattern of an infant, resembling wavelike contractions of peristalsis.

viscero-, combining form meaning "organs of the body": *viscerocranium, visceromotor, viscerosomatic.*

viscerocranium, the facial skeleton.

visceromotor /vis′ərōmō″tər/, **1.** pertaining to nerve impulses that control visceral smooth muscle. **2.** pertaining to movement of the viscera.

viscerosomatic reaction /vis′ərō′sōmat″ik/ [L, *viscus* + Gk, *soma,* body; L, *re* + *agere,* to act], a muscular response to stimulation of a nerve-receptor organ in a visceral organ. Also called **splanchnosomatic reaction, visceral reflex.**

viscoelasticity /vis′kō-ē′lastis″itē/, the quality or condition of being both viscous and elastic.

viscosity /viskos″itē/ [L, *viscosus,* sticky], *adj.,* the ability or inability of a fluid solution to flow easily. A solution that has high viscosity is relatively thick and flows slowly because of the adhesive effect of adjacent molecules. −*viscous, adj.*

viscous fermentation [L, *viscosus*], the formation of viscous material in milk, urine, or wine by the action of various bacilli.

viscus. See **viscera.**

visibility /vis′əbil″itē/ [L, *visibilitas,* being seen], a condition of being visible under the circumstances of light, distance, and other factors.

visible /viz″ibəl/ [L, *visibilis,* visible], perceptible to the eye.

visible light [L, *visus,* sight; AS, *leoht*], the radiant energy in the electromagnetic spectrum that is visible to the human eye. See also **visible spectrum.**

visible radiation [L, *visibilis,* vision, *radiare,* to shine], electromagnetic radiation in the wavelengths between infrared and ultraviolet that can be perceived by most normal humans.

visible spectrum [L, *visibilis,* vision, *spectrum,* image], the colors of the spectrum that can be observed by most people, from violet at about 4000 angstrom units (400 nm) through blue, green, yellow, and orange, to red, at about 6500 angstrom units (650 nm).

vision /vizh″ən/ [L, *visus,* vision], the capacity for sight.

vision therapy technician, an allied health professional who evaluates clients and plans and implements vision therapy programs under the supervision of an optometrist.

visit /viz′it/ [L, *visitare,* to see often], **1.** *n.,* a meeting between a practitioner and a client or patient. In the hospital and the home, the practitioner makes a visit to the patient; in the clinic or office the patient makes a visit to the practitioner. **2.** *v.,* (of a patient) to meet a practitioner to obtain professional services or (of a practitioner) to see a patient or client to render a professional service.

visiting nurse, a nurse who is responsible for a group of patients in a home setting, usually in a defined geographic area. The nurse makes visits to provide skilled nursing care as prescribed by a physician, particularly for persons unable to leave home for professional care, and to educate patients in matters of self-care. See also **home health nurse.**

Vistaril, an antianxiety/antihistamine drug. Brand name for *hydroxyzine pamoate.*

visual /vizh″oo·əl/ [L, *visus,* vision], pertaining to the sense of sight.

visual accommodation, a process by which the eye adjusts and is able to focus, producing a sharp image at various, changing distances from the object seen. The convexity of the anterior surface of the lens may be increased or decreased by contraction or relaxation of the ciliary muscle. With increasing age the lens becomes harder and less flexible, resulting in a loss of accommodation and usually of the ability to focus on nearby objects. Compare **presbyopia.**

visual acuity [L, *visus,* vision, *acuitas,* sharpness], **1.** a measure of the resolving power of the eye, particularly with its ability to distinguish letters and numbers at a given distance. **2.** the sharpness or clearness of vision.

visual agnosia. See **object blindness.**

visual amnesia [L, *visus,* vision; Gk, *amnesia,* forgetfulness], an inability to recognize objects, including written words, previously seen.

visual angle [L, *visus,* vision, *angulus*], the angle between two lines passing from the extremities of an object looked at, through the nodal point of the eye. Also called **optic angle.**

visual aphasia [L, *visus,* vision; Gk, *a + phasis,* not speech], the inability to understand written language caused by a lesion in the left visual cortex and the connections between the right visual cortex and the left hemisphere.

visual center, the center of the brain concerned with vision.

visual center of the cornea, the point of intersection of the line of sight with the cornea.

visual-evoked potential (VEP), an evoked potential elicited by a repeatedly flashing light or a pattern stimulus. It may be used to confirm optic nerve or visual pathway damage.

visual field (VF), the area of physical space visible to an eye in a given position. The average VF is 65 degrees upward, 75 degrees downward, 60 degrees nasally, and 90 degrees temporally.

visual field defect, one or more spots or defects in the vision that remain constant in position, unlike a floater. This fixed defect is usually caused by damage to the retina or visual pathways, such as by retinal detachments, chorioretinitis, traumatic injury, macular degeneration, glaucoma, or a vascular occlusion of the eye or the brain. Sudden loss of a noticeable part of the visual field warrants ophthalmological examination. An Amsler grid detects defects only in the central 30 degrees—not the entire visual field.

visual hallucinations [L, *visus,* vision, *alucinari*], a subjective visual experience in the absence of objective evidence of a corresponding stimulus. Such hallucinations are most likely to be associated with acute organic disorders such as toxic confusional psychoses, delirium, and focal brain diseases and may occur with any stage of schizophrenia.

visualization /vizh′oo·əlīzā″shən/, an effective means of deepening relaxation and desensitizing a real-life situation that is generally met with stress and tension. The imagery combines positive experiences with actual or perceived negative events or situations in an effort to desensitize the person to the trauma. Also called **guided imagery,** *visual imagery.*

visual memory, the ability to create an eidetic image of past visual experiences. Also called **eye memory.**

visual-motor coordination, the ability to coordinate vision with the movements of the body or parts of the body.

visual-motor function, the ability to draw or copy forms or to perform constructive tasks.

visual pathway, a pathway over which a visual sensation is transmitted from the retina to the brain. A pathway consists of an optic nerve, the fibers of an optic nerve traveling through the optic chiasm to the lateral geniculate body of the thalamus, and optic radiations terminating in an occipital lobe. Each optic nerve contains fibers from only one retina. The optic chiasm contains fibers from the nasal parts of the retinas of both eyes; these fibers cross to the opposite side of the brain at the optic chiasm. The fibers from the temporal part of each eye do not cross at the optic chiasm, pass through the lateral geniculate body on the same side of the brain, and continue back to the occipital lobe. Thus the optic tracts, occipital lobe, lateral geniculate bodies of the thalamus, and optic chiasm each contain nerve fibers from both eyes. If the right optic tract were destroyed, a person would lose partial vision in both eyes—the right nasal and the left temporal fields of vision.

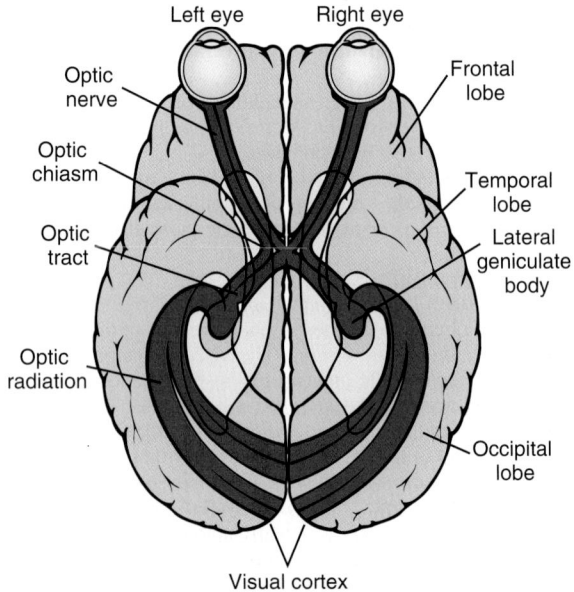

Visual pathway (Lewis et al, 2007)

visual plane, the plane in which the two optic axes lie.

visual purple. See **rhodopsin.**

visual rehabilitation services, professional services provided to individuals who have lost vision or have low vision. Services are designed to facilitate full participation and independence in activities of daily living.

visual response audiometry (VRA), a technique for testing the hearing of older infants and children between the ages of 12 and 30 months. Sounds such as speech and tones are presented through loudspeakers. When the child looks toward the source of the sound, he or she is rewarded by seeing a toy on top of the speaker move or light up. See also **conditioned orientation reflex.**

visual-spatial agnosia, an inability to analyze spatial relationships or to perform simple constructional tasks under visual control.

visuospatial /vizh′oo·ōspā″shəl/, pertaining to the ability to comprehend visual representations and their spatial relationships.

vita-, combining form meaning "life": *vital, vitamin.*

vital /vī″təl/ [L, *vita,* life], pertaining to or contributing to life forces.

vital capacity (VC) [L, *vita,* life, *capacitas,* capacity], the maximum volume of air that can be expelled at the normal rate of exhalation after a maximum inspiration, representing the greatest possible breathing capacity. The VC equals the inspiratory reserve volume plus the tidal volume plus the expiratory reserve volume. The average normal value of 4 to 5 L is affected by age, the physical dimensions of the chest cage, physical fitness, posture, and gender. The VC may be reduced by a decrease in the amount of functioning lung tissue resulting from atelectasis, edema, fibrosis, pneumonia, pulmonary resection, or tumors; by limited chest expansion resulting from ascites, chest deformity, neuromuscular disease, pneumothorax, or pregnancy; or by airway obstruction. Compare **forced expiratory volume, forced expiratory vital capacity, residual volume.**

vitality test /vītal″itē/, a group of thermal, transillumination, and electric tests used to evaluate the health of dental pulp. Also called **pulp test.**

vital signs, the measurements of pulse rate, respiration rate, and body temperature. Although not strictly a vital sign, blood pressure is also customarily included. Abnormalities of vital signs are often clues to diseases, and alterations in vital signs are used to evaluate a patient's progress. See also **blood pressure, pulse, respiration, temperature.**

vital stain [L, *vita,* life; OFr, *desteindre,* to dye], any dye used to impart color to tissues or cells of living organisms.

vital statistics, data relating to births or natality, deaths or mortality, marriages, health, and disease or morbidity.

vital ultraviolet (UV), the ultraviolet wavelengths between 320.0 and 290.0 nm, which are believed to be necessary or helpful for normal growth and health. Ultraviolet radiation at this wavelength converts vitamin D to its first active form.

vitamin /vī″təmin/ [L, *vita* + *amine,* ammonia], an organic compound essential in small quantities for normal physiological and metabolic functioning of the body. With few exceptions, vitamins cannot be synthesized by the body and must be obtained from the diet or dietary supplements. No one food contains all the vitamins. Vitamin deficiency diseases produce specific symptoms, usually alleviated by the administration of the appropriate vitamin. Vitamins are classified according to their fat or water solubility, their physiological effects, or their chemical structures. They are designated by alphabetic letters and chemical or other specific names. The fat-soluble vitamins are A, D, E, and K. The B complex and C vitamins are water soluble. See also **avitaminosis, hypervitaminosis, oleovitamin, provitamin.**

vitamin A, a fat-soluble, solid terpene alcohol essential for skeletal growth, maintenance of normal mucosal epithelium, reproduction, and visual acuity. It is derived from various carotenoids, mainly beta-carotene, and is present in leafy green vegetables and yellow fruits and vegetables as a precursor and is found preformed in fish-liver oils, liver, milk, cheese, butter, and egg yolk. Deficiency leads to atrophy of epithelial tissue resulting in keratomalacia, xerophthalmia, night blindness, and lessened resistance to infection of mucous membranes. Symptoms of hypervitaminosis A are irritability, fatigue, lethargy, abdominal discomfort, painful joints, severe throbbing headache, increased intracranial pressure, insomnia and restlessness, night sweats, loss of body hair, and brittle nails. Also called *antiinfection vitamin,* **antixerophthalmic vitamin.**

vitamin A₁, one of the two forms of vitamin A that occur in nature. It is a fat-soluble unsaturated alcohol formed by hydrolysis of beta-carotene, one molecule of which yields two molecules of vitamin A_1. Natural sources include fish-liver oils, butterfat, and egg yolk. The vitamin is needed for healthy vision and skin epithelium. Also called **retinol.**

vitamin A₂, an alternative form of vitamin A found in the tissues of freshwater fish but not in mammals or saltwater fish. Differences in ultraviolet light absorption spectra are used to distinguish the vitamin A forms.

vitamin B₁. See **thiamine.**

vitamin B₂. See **riboflavin.**

vitamin B₆. See **pyridoxine.**

vitamin B₉. See **folic acid.**

vitamin B₁₂. See **cyanocobalamin.**

vitamin B₁₂ test (cyanocobalamin), a blood test that measures levels of vitamin B_{12}, which is necessary for conversion of the inactive form of folate to the active form, a process that is crucial in the formation and function of red blood cells. Abnormal levels may indicate leukemia, severe liver dysfunction, myeloproliferative disease, pernicious anemia, malabsorption syndromes, inflammatory bowel disease, and Zollinger-Ellison syndrome, among other conditions.

vitamin B₁₇. See **Laetrile.**

vitamin B complex, a group of water-soluble vitamins (such as pyridoxine, or vitamin B_6, and cyanocobalamin, or vitamin B_{12}), differing from one another structurally and in their biological effect. All of the B vitamins are found in large quantities in liver and yeast, and they are present separately or in combination in many foods. Heat and prolonged cooking, especially cooking with water, can destroy B vitamins. See also **folic acid, B complex vitamins.**

vitamin C. See **ascorbic acid.**

vitamin D, a fat-soluble vitamin chemically related to the steroids and essential for the normal formation of bones and teeth and for the absorption of calcium and phosphorus from the GI tract. The vitamin is present in natural foods in small amounts, and requirements are usually met by artificial enrichment of various foods, especially milk and other dairy products, and exposure to sunlight. Ultraviolet rays activate a form of cholesterol in an oil of the skin that is converted to a form of the vitamin in the kidney. The natural foods containing vitamin D are of animal origin and include saltwater fish, especially salmon, sardines, and herring; organ meats; fish-liver oils; and egg yolk. Deficiency of the vitamin results in rickets in children, osteomalacia, osteoporosis, and osteodystrophy. Hypervitaminosis D produces a toxicity syndrome characterized by anorexia, vomiting, headache, drowsiness, diarrhea, and calcification of the soft tissues of the heart, blood vessels, renal tubules, and lungs. Treatment

V

consists of discontinuing the vitamin dosage and initiating a low-calcium diet until symptoms resolve. See also **calciferol, vitamin D₃**.

vitamin D₂. See **calciferol**.

vitamin D₃, an antirachitic, white, odorless, crystalline, unsaturated alcohol that is the predominant form of vitamin D of animal origin. It is found in most fish-liver oils, butter, brain, and egg yolk and is formed in the skin, fur, and feathers of animals and birds exposed to sunlight or ultraviolet rays. Also called **activated 7-dehydrocholesterol, cholecalciferol**.

vitamin deficiency, a state or condition resulting from the lack of or inability to use one or more vitamins. The symptoms and manifestations of each deficiency vary, depending on the specific function of the vitamin in promoting growth and development and maintaining body health.

vitamin D–resistant rickets, a genetic disease clinically similar to rickets but resistant to treatment with large doses of vitamin D. It is caused by a congenital defect in renal tubular resorption of phosphate and usually occurs in men. See also **rickets**.

vitamin E, any or all of the group of fat-soluble vitamins that consist of the tocopherols and are essential for normal reproduction, muscle development, resistance of erythrocytes to hemolysis, and various other biochemical functions. It is a fat-soluble antioxidant and acts in maintaining the stability of polyunsaturated fatty acids and other fatlike substances, including vitamin A and hormones of the pituitary, adrenal, and sex glands. Deficiency is rare and may take from months to years to occur but results in muscle degeneration, vascular system abnormalities, megaloblastic anemia, hemolytic anemia, infertility, creatinuria, and liver and kidney damage and is associated with the aging process. The richest dietary sources are wheat germ; soybean, cotton seed, peanut, and corn oils; margarine; whole raw seeds and nuts; soybeans; eggs; butter; liver; sweet potatoes; and the leaves of many vegetables, such as turnip greens. It is stored in the body for long periods of time so that any deficiency is rare. It is considered nontoxic except in hypertensive patients and those with chronic rheumatic heart disease. Alpha-tocopherol is the most physiologically active form of the group. Toxicity is also rare. Also called **alpha-tocopherol, tocopherol**.

vitamin H. See **biotin**.

vitamin K, a group of fat-soluble vitamins known as quinones that are essential for the synthesis of prothrombin in the liver and of several related proteins involved in the clotting of blood. The vitamin is widely distributed in foods, especially leafy green vegetables, pork liver, yogurt, egg yolk, kelp, alfalfa, fish-liver oils, and blackstrap molasses, and is synthesized by the bacterial flora of the GI tract. It is also produced synthetically. Deficiency results in hypoprothrombinemia, characterized by poor coagulation of the blood and hemorrhage, and usually occurs from inadequate absorption of the vitamin from the GI tract or the inability to use it in the liver. It is used to reduce the clotting time in patients with obstructive jaundice and in hemorrhagic states associated with intestinal diseases and diseases of the liver; it is given prophylactically to infants to prevent hemorrhagic disease of the newborn. Natural vitamin K is stored in the body and produces no toxicity. Excessive doses of synthetic vitamin K may cause anemia in newborns and hemolysis in people with glucose-6-phosphate deficiency. See also **vitamin K₁, vitamin K₂, menadione**.

vitamin K₁, a yellow, viscous, oil-soluble vitamin occurring naturally, especially in alfalfa, and produced synthetically. It is used as a prothrombinogenic agent. Vitamin K is a cofactor in the clotting process. Also called **phylloquinone, phytonadione**.

vitamin K₂, a pale yellow fat-soluble crystalline vitamin of the vitamin K group that is more unsaturated than vitamin K₁ and slightly less active biologically. It is isolated from putrefied fish meal and synthesized by various bacteria in the GI tract. See also **vitamin K**.

vitamin K₃. See **menadione**.

vitamin loss [L, *vita,* life, *amine*], reduction in vitamin content of food resulting from the handling and preparation of fresh foods during harvesting, heating, pickling, salting, milling, canning, and other food-processing techniques. Further vitamin losses can occur because of digestive disorders that prevent nutrient absorption and the use of drugs such as isoniazid that are vitamin antagonists.

vitaminology /vī'təminol″əjē/ [L, *vita* + *amine* + Gk, *logos,* science], the study of vitamins, including their structures, modes of action, and function in maintaining body health.

vitamin P. See **bioflavonoid**.

vitamin supplements, any vitamins or provitamins consumed in addition to nutrients in the food eaten.

vitellin /vitel″in/ [L, *vitellus,* yolk], a lipoprotein containing lecithin, found in the yolk of eggs. Also called **ovovitellin.** *–vitelline, adj.*

vitelline artery /vitel″in, -ēn/ [L, *vitellus* + Gk, *arteria,* airpipe], any of the embryonic arteries that circulate blood from the primitive aorta of the early developing embryo to the yolk sac. Also called **omphalomesenteric artery**.

vitelline circulation, the circulation of blood and nutrients between the developing embryo and the yolk sac by way of the vitelline arteries and veins. Also called **omphalomesenteric circulation.** See also **fetal circulation**.

vitelline duct, (in embryology) the narrow channel connecting the yolk sac with the intestine. Also called **umbilical duct**.

vitelline membrane, the delicate cytoplasmic membrane surrounding the ovum. Also called **yolk membrane.** See also **zona pellucida**.

vitelline sac. See **yolk sac**.

vitelline sphere. See **morula**.

vitelline vein, any of the embryonic veins that return blood from the yolk sac to the primitive heart of the early developing embryo. Also called **omphalomesenteric vein**.

vitellogenesis /vitel″ōjen″əsis/ [L, *vitellus* + Gk, *genein,* to produce], the formation or production of yolk. *–vitellogenetic, adj.*

vitellus. See **yolk**.

vitiligo /vit'ilē″gō, -ī″gō/ [L, *vitium,* blemish], a benign acquired skin disease of unknown cause, consisting of irregular patches of various sizes totally lacking in pigment and often having hyperpigmented borders. The hypopigmented area is caused by loss of melanocytes. Exposed areas of skin are most often affected. Treatment using 8-methoxypsoralen requires extreme care and carefully regulated sun exposure. Some success has been achieved with the use of narrowband ultraviolet light and topical application of protopic. Waterproof, sun-protective cosmetics are often used to cover the patches. Compare **albinism, piebald.** *–vitiliginous, adj.*

vitrectomy /vitrek″təmē/ [L, *vitreus,* glassy; Gk, *ektomē,* excision], a surgical procedure for removing the contents of the vitreous chamber of the eye, which are then replaced by oil, air, or a vitreous substitute.

vitreous /vit″rē·əs/ [L, *vitreus,* glassy], pertaining to the vitreous body of the eye located in the posterior chamber of the eye.

vitreous body. See **vitreous humor**.

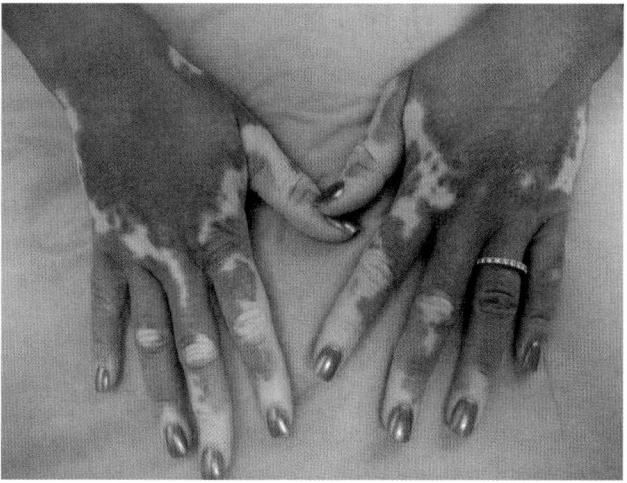

Vitiligo *(Lebwohl et al, 2018)*

vitreous cavity [L, *vitreus,* glassy, *cavum,* cavity], the cavity in the eye posterior to the lens that contains the vitreous body and vitreous membrane and is transected by the vestigial remnants of the hyaloid canal.

vitreous degeneration [L, *vitreus,* glassy, *degenerare,* to deviate from kind], a form of hyaline degeneration; the formation of glassy material in the connective tissue of blood vessels and other tissues.

vitreous hemorrhage, a hemorrhage into the vitreous humor of the eye.

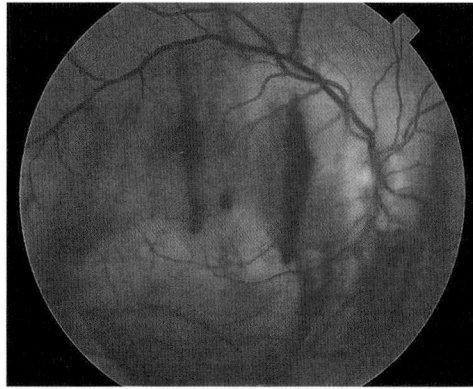

Vitreous hemorrhage *(Albert, Miller, and Jakkobiec, 2008)*

vitreous humor, a transparent, semigelatinous substance contained in a thin hyoid membrane and filling the cavity behind the crystalline lens of the eye. Some indications of the hyaloid canal may persist in the vitreous humor, which is not penetrated by any blood vessels and is nourished at its periphery by vessels of the retina and the ciliary processes. The vitreous humor is concave anteriorly to accommodate the crystalline lens and is closely applied to the retina around the wall of the eyeball. Also called **corpus vitreum, vitreous body.**

vitreous membrane, a membrane that lines the posterior cavity of the eye and surrounds the vitreous body.

vitrification /vit′rifikā″shən/, the conversion of a silicate material by heat and fusion to a glassy substance. Heat converts the material into a viscous liquid, which hardens on cooling.

vitriol, oil of. See **sulfuric acid.**

vitronectin /vit″ro-nek′tin/, a multifunctional adhesive glycoprotein found in serum and various tissues. Its functions include regulation of the coagulation, fibrinolytic, and complement cascades, and it plays a role in hemostasis, wound healing, tissue remodeling, and cancer. It mediates the inflammatory and repair reactions at sites of tissue injury and promotes adhesion, spreading, and migration of cells. It has been shown to be identical to S protein, which was identified as an inhibitor of complement activation, binding the membrane attack complex and preventing its insertion into the membrane.

Vivactil, a tricyclic antidepressant. Brand name for **protriptyline hydrochloride.**

vivax malaria. See **tertian malaria.**

vivi-, prefix meaning "being alive": *vivisection, viviparous.*

viviparous /vivip″ərəs/ [L, *vivus,* alive, *parere,* to bear], bearing living offspring, such as most mammals and some fishes and reptiles, rather than laying eggs. Compare **oviparous, ovoviviparous.**

vivisection /viv″əsek′shən/ [L, *vivus,* alive, *secare,* to cut], the performance of surgical operations on living animals, particularly experimental surgery for the purpose of research.

Vivitrol, an extended-release injectable suspension used to treat alcohol dependence after drinking has been stopped or to prevent relapse to opioid dependence after opioid detoxification. Brand name for *naltrexone.* See also **naltrexone hydrochloride.**

Vivonex, a nutritional supplement containing protein, carbohydrate, and fat.

VLDL, abbreviation for **very low–density lipoprotein.**

VMA, abbreviation for **vanillylmandelic acid.**

VNA, abbreviation for *Visiting Nurses Association.*

VNTR, abbreviation for **variable number of tandem repeats.**

VO₂, symbol for **oxygen uptake.**

vocal apparatus /vō′kəl/ [L, *vocalis,* voice, *ad + parare,* to prepare], the larynx, pharynx, and oral and nasal cavities involved in the production of sound.

V

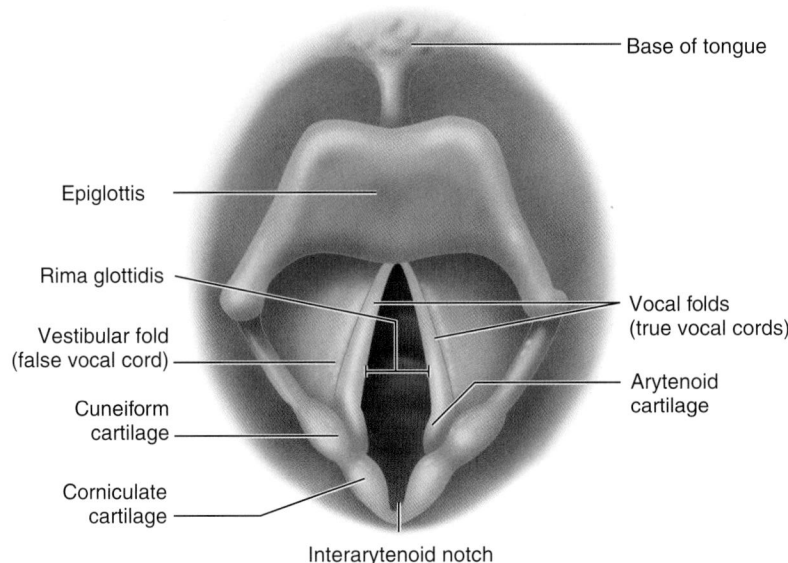

Base of tongue

Epiglottis

Rima glottidis

Vestibular fold
(false vocal cord)

Cuneiform
cartilage

Corniculate
cartilage

Vocal folds
(true vocal cords)

Arytenoid
cartilage

Interarytenoid notch

Vocal cords *(Patton and Thibodeau, 2010)*

vocal cord [L, *vocalis,* voice; Gk, *chorde,* string], one of a pair of strong bands of yellow elastic tissue in the larynx enclosed by membranes called vocal folds and attached ventrally to the angle of the thyroid cartilage and dorsally to the vocal process of the arytenoid cartilage. Also called **true vocal cords, vocal ligament.** Compare **false vocal cord.**

vocal cord dysfunction, a disorder with asthmalike symptoms caused by abnormal closure of the vocal cords.

vocal cord nodule, a small inflammatory or fibrous growth that develops on the vocal cords of people who constantly strain their voices. Also called **screamer's nodule, singer's nodule, teacher's nodule.** See also **chorditis.**

vocal cues, a category of nonverbal communication that includes all the noises and sounds that are extra-speech sounds and convey meaning.

vocal folds [L, *vocalis* + AS, *fealdan*], the true vocal cords.

vocal fremitus (VF), the vibration of the chest wall as a person speaks or sings that allows the person's voice to be heard by auscultation of the chest with a stethoscope. Vocal fremitus is decreased in emphysema, pleural effusion, pulmonary edema, and bronchial obstruction and is increased in consolidation, as in pneumonia. The classic physical examination technique is to ask the patient to say the letter "e"; if there is consolidation, the examiner will hear the letter "a" through the stethoscope.

vocal ligament. See **vocal cord.**

vocal paralysis, the inability of one or both of the vocal cords to move.

vocal register, any of the perceptually distinct regions of vocal quality, each with a characteristic range of pitches, pattern of vocal cord vibration, and tone quality. Also called **register.**

vocal resonance [L, *vocalis* + *resonare,* to sound again], **1.** auscultation. **2.** modification of the laryngeal tone as it passes through the pharynx and oral cavity to produce an increase in the intensity and quality of the sound.

vocal tract, the passages from the glottis through the nose and throat that influence the quality of the voice.

Vogt-Koyanagi-Harada syndrome /fōkt kō ·yah·nah′ge hah-rah′dah/, a syndrome of uveomeningitis associated with retinochoroidal detachment; temporary or permanent deafness and blindness; and, sometimes (usually not permanent), alopecia, vitiligo, and poliosis. The cause is unknown, but it may be an inflammatory autoimmune condition. Also called *Harada syndrome.*

Vogt-Spielmeyer disease /fōkt shpēl′mī·er/, the juvenile form of neuronal ceroid-lipofuscinosis, with onset between 5 and 10 years of age. It is characterized by rapid cerebroretinal degeneration, massive loss of brain substance, and excessive neuronal storage of lipofuscin. The prognosis is poor.

voice, the acoustic component of speech that is normally produced by vibration of the vocal folds of the larynx.

voice box. See **larynx.**

voiced /voist/ [L, *vox,* voice], said of speech sounds produced with vibration of the vocal cords, such as /b/, /d/, or /z/. Also **sonorant.**

voiceless /vois′ləs/ [L, *vox,* voice + AS, *laes,* less], said of speech sounds produced without vibration of the vocal cords, such as /p/, /t/, or /s/. Also **unvoiced.**

voiceprint /vois″print/, a graphic representation of a person's speech pattern as electronically recorded. Like a fingerprint, the speech pattern for any individual is distinctive.

voice sounds, auscultatory sounds heard over the lungs or airways when the patient speaks. Increased resonance indicates consolidation or an airless lung underlying an effusion. Kinds include **bronchophony, egophony, pectoriloquy.**

void /void/ [ME, *voide,* empty], to empty or evacuate, such as urine from the bladder.

voiding. See **urination.**

voiding cystourethrography (VCU) [ME *voide,* empty; Gk, *kystis,* bag + *ourethra,* urethra + *graphein,* to record], cystourethrography in which radiographs are made before, during, and after voiding. See also **cystourethrography.**

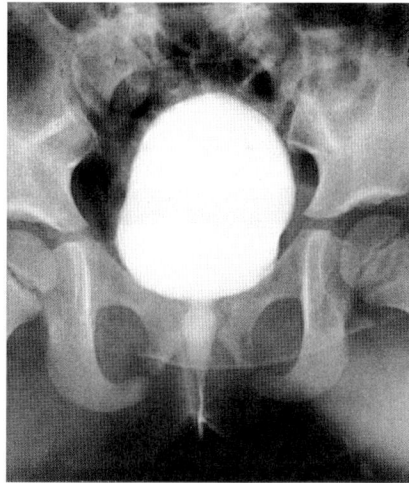

Voiding cystourethrography *(Frank et al, 2007)*

voiding urethrography [ME, *voide,* empty; Gk, *ourethra* + *graphein,* to record], radiography of the urethra during micturition after the introduction of a radiopaque fluid into the bladder.

vol., abbreviation for **volume.**

vol.%, abbreviation for *volume percent.*

volar /vō″lər/ [L, *vola,* palm, sole], pertaining to the palm of the hand.

volar wrist brace, an orthotic device worn on the volar aspect of the distal forearm, wrist, and hand for the treatment of wrist sprains, contusions, and carpal tunnel syndrome. It may also be used for buckle fractures of the radius. Also called **wrist hand orthotic.** Formerly called **cockup splint.**

volatile /vol″ətəl/ [L, *volatilis,* flying], (of a liquid) easily vaporized.

volatile solvent, an easily vaporized solvent.

-volemia, suffix meaning "(condition of the) volume of plasma in the body": *hypervolemia, hypovolemia.*

volition /vōlish″ən/ [L, *voluntas,* inclination], **1.** the act, power, or state of willing or choosing. **2.** the conscious impulse to perform or to abstain from an act.

volition. See **will.**

volitional /vōlish′ənəl/ [L, *velle,* to wish], pertaining to the use of one's own will in performing or abstaining from an action.

volitional tremor [L, *velle,* to wish, *tremor,* shaking], a trembling that begins during voluntary effort, sometimes spreading throughout the body. It may occur in multiple sclerosis and cerebellar disorders. Also called **intention tremor.**

Volkmann's canal /fōlk″munz/ [Alfred W. Volkmann, German physiologist, 1800–1877], any one of the small blood vessel canals connecting haversian canals in bone tissue. Compare **haversian canaliculus.** See also **haversian system.**

Volkmann contracture [Richard von Volkmann, German surgeon, 1830–1889], a serious persistent flexion contraction of forearm and hand caused by ischemia. A pressure or crushing injury in the region of the elbow usually precedes this condition, and pressure from a cast or tight bandage about the elbow is a common cause. Permanent fibrosis, muscle degeneration, and a clawlike hand may result. Health care providers must watch for swelling, pallor, coldness, cyanosis, or pain distal to the injury site so that prompt loosening of constriction can restore circulation. Also called **ischemic contracture, Volkmann paralysis.**

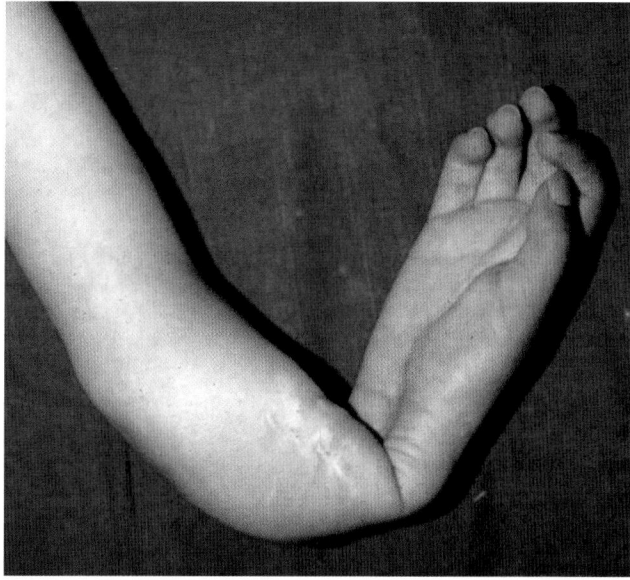

Volkmann ischemic contracture *(Stevanovic and Sharpe, 2006)*

V

Volkmann paralysis. See **Volkmann contracture.**

Volkmann splint [Richard von Volkmann; AS, *splinte*, thin board], a splint that supports and immobilizes the lower leg. A foot-piece extends from the foot to the knee on both sides of the splint, allowing ambulation.

volsella forceps /volsel″ə/ [L, *vosella*, tweezers, *forceps*, tongs], a kind of forceps having a small, sharp-pointed hook at the end of each blade. Also called *volsella, volsellum forceps*, **vulsella forceps.**

volt (V) /vōlt/ [Alessandro Volta, Italian physicist, 1745–1827], the unit of electric potential. In an electric circuit a volt is the force required to send 1 ampere of current through 1 ohm of resistance, or the difference in potential between two points on a conductor carrying a charge of 1 ampere when there is a dissipation of 1 watt between them. See also **ampere, circuit, current, ohm, watt.**

voltage /vō″tij/ [Alessandro Volta], an expression of electromotive force in terms of volts.

voltage ripple. See **waveform ripple.**

voltammetry /voltam″ətərē/, the measurement of an electric current as a function of potential.

voltmeter /vōlt″mētər/, an instrument such as a galvanometer that measures in volts the differences in potential between different points of an electric circuit.

volume (vol.) /vol″yəm, -yo͞om/ [L, *volumen*, paper roll], the amount of space occupied by a body, expressed in units of cubic distance.

volume ATPS, abbreviation for ambient temperature, ambient pressure, saturated with water vapor conditions of a volume of gas. The conditions exist in a water-sealed spirograph or gasometer when the water temperature equals ambient temperature.

volume BTPS, abbreviation for body temperature, ambient pressure, saturated with water vapor. These conditions of a volume of gas are used in respiratory physiology to assess lung volume and flow. For humans, the normal respiratory tract temperature is measured at 37° C, ambient pressure, and the partial pressure of water vapor at 37° C at 47 mm Hg.

volume control fluid chamber, any one of several types of transparent plastic reservoirs with graduated volumetric markings, used to regulate the flow of IV solutions. These devices are components of IV volume control sets and accommodate the injection and mixing of medications by means of special built-in ports. The volume control fluid chamber contains a filter that must be primed to function.

volume cycling, the delivery of gas under positive pressure during inspiration until an adjustable, preselected volume has been delivered.

volume dose. See **integral dose.**

volume expander, intravenous fluids administered to increase the oncotic pressure in the intravascular space.

volume imaging, magnetic resonance (MR) imaging techniques in which MR signals are gathered at once from the whole object volume to be imaged. Many sequential plane imaging techniques can be categorized as volume imaging, at least in principle. Advantages include potential improvement in the signal-to-noise ratio as a result of the inclusion of signals from the whole volume. Disadvantages include a bigger computational task for image reconstruction and longer image acquisition times, although the entire volume can be imaged from one set of data.

volumetric analysis. See **quantitative analysis.**

volumetric flow rate (Q) /vol″yəmet″rik/, the rate at which a volume of fluid flows past a designated point, usually measured in liters per second.

volumetric glassware, (in chemistry) glassware designed and marked to contain or to deliver specific volumes of liquid solutions.

volume unit (VU), a unit of a logarithmic scale for expressing the power level of a complex audiofrequency electrical signal such as that transmitting sound.

volume ventilator, a ventilator that delivers a predetermined volume of gas with each cycle.

voluntary /vol″ənter″ē/ [L, *voluntas*, inclination], referring to an action or thought originated, undertaken, controlled, or accomplished as a result of a person's free will or choice.

voluntary abortion. See **elective abortion.**

voluntary agency, a service agency legally controlled by individuals who serve without reimbursement rather than by owners or a paid staff.

voluntary hospital system, a nationwide complex of autonomous, self-established, and self-supported private not-for-profit and investor-owned hospitals in the United States.

voluntary muscle. See **striated muscle.**

volunteer /vol″əntir″/ [Fr, *volontaire*], an individual who performs a task through personal choice and usually without pay.

-voluted, suffix meaning "to roll or turn around": *convoluted.*

volutrauma /vol″u-traw″mah/, damage to the lung caused by overdistension by a mechanical ventilator set for an excessively high tidal volume. It results in a syndrome similar to adult respiratory distress syndrome.

volvulus /vol″vyələs/ [L, *volvere*, to turn], a twisting of the bowel on itself, causing intestinal obstruction. The condition is frequently the result of a prolapsed segment of mesentery and occurs most often in the ileum, the cecum, or the sigmoid parts of the bowel. If it is not corrected, the obstructed bowel becomes necrotic, peritonitis and rupture of the bowel occur, and death may ensue. Severe gripping pain, nausea and vomiting, an absence of bowel sounds, and a tense distended abdomen suggest the diagnosis, which is confirmed by x-ray examination. Compare **intussusception.**

volvulus neonatorum, an intestinal obstruction in a newborn resulting from a twisting of the bowel caused by malrotation or nonfixation of the colon. Typical symptoms include abdominal distension; persistent regurgitation, often accompanied by fecal vomiting; and nonpassage of stools. Characteristic barium enema x-ray studies confirm the diagnosis. The condition requires immediate surgical correction to prevent necrosis and gangrene of the affected segment of bowel.

vomer /vō″mər/ [L, plowshare], the plow-shaped bone forming the posterior and inferior part of the nasal septum and having two surfaces and four borders.

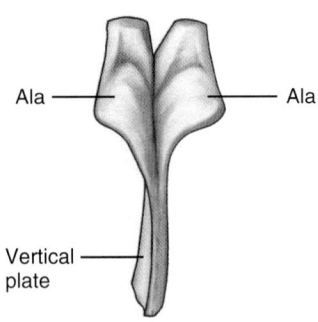

Vomer

vomeronasal organ, a structure on each side of the nasal septum believed to be a chemical sensory center for detection of pheromones.

vomit /vom″it/ [L, *vomere,* to vomit], **1.** *v.,* to expel the contents of the stomach through the esophagus and out of the mouth. **2.** *n.,* the material expelled from the stomach through the mouth. Also called **emesis, vomitus.**

vomiting [L, *vomere,* to vomit], the forcible voluntary or involuntary emptying of the stomach contents through the mouth.

vomiting agents, chemicals that induce nausea and vomiting. Vomiting agents include adamsite, diphenylchlorarsine, and diphenylcyanoarsine. They are used as aerosols, and exposure is primarily by inhalation but also by ingestion and by skin and eye contact. They initially act like tear gas, and their effects progress to difficulty in breathing, nausea, and vomiting. Effects are self-limited, generally disappearing within 2 hours. Death may occur with exposure to high concentrations in confined spaces.

vomiting of pregnancy, vomiting that occurs during the early months of pregnancy. Factors contributing to the condition include delayed stomach emptying during pregnancy, relaxation of the esophageal sphincter at the opening into the stomach, and relaxation of the diaphragmatic hiatus, all of which increase the risk of gastric reflux. Also called **morning sickness.** See also **hyperemesis gravidarum.**

vomiting reflex. See **reflex emesis.**

vomitus /vom″itəs/ [L, *vomere,* to vomit], pertaining to the material expelled from the stomach during vomiting. Vomitus is sometimes classified by color or other appearances as an indicator of the cause of illness, such as a "coffee-ground" vomitus being a clinical sign of gastric bleeding.

VON abbreviation for **Victorian Order of Nurses for Canada.**

von Economo encephalitis. See **epidemic encephalitis.**

von Gierke disease /fôn gir″kə/ [Edgar von Gierke, German pathologist, 1877–1945], a form of glycogen storage disease in which abnormally large amounts of glycogen are deposited in the liver and kidneys. The disorder is characterized by hypoglycemia, metabolic acidosis, dyslipidemia, and hepatomegaly. Biopsy of the affected organs reveals the absence of glucose-6-phosphatase, an enzyme necessary for glycogen metabolism. There is no effective treatment for the disorder. Medical efforts are directed at preventing hypoglycemia and acidosis. Also called **glycogen storage disease, type Ia.** See also **glycogen storage disease.**

von Hippel–Lindau disease [Eugen von Hippel, German ophthalmologist, 1867–1939; Arvid Lindau, Swedish pathologist, 1892–1958], a hereditary disease characterized by congenital tumorlike vascular nodules in the retina and hemangioblastomas of the cerebellar hemispheres. Similar spinal cord lesions; cysts of the pancreas, kidneys, and other viscera; seizures; and cognitive impairment may be present. Also called **cerebroretinal angiomatosis, Lindau-von Hippel disease, retinocerebral angiomatosis.**

von Pirquet test. See **Pirquet test.**

von Recklinghausen canal. See **Recklinghausen canal.**

von Recklinghausen disease. See **neurofibromatosis.**

von Recklinghausen tumor. See **Recklinghausen tumor.**

von Willebrand disease [Erick A. von Willebrand, Finnish physician, 1870–1949], a congenital, autosomal-dominant, mucocutaneous bleeding disorder caused by von Willebrand factor deficiency and subsequent impairment of platelet adhesion to the damaged blood vessel wall.

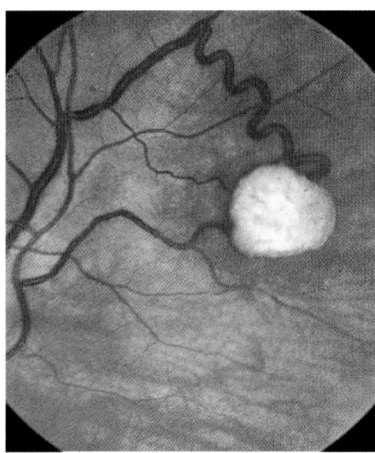

von Hippel–Lindau disease *(Spalton, Hitchings, and Hunter, 2005)*

Also called *vascular hemophilia.* See also **hemophilia, thrombasthenia.**

voracious [L, *vorax*], greedy or gluttonous, with an insatiable appetite.

voriconazole, an azole antifungal agent used to treat invasive aspergillosis and serious fungal infections.

-vorous, suffix meaning "feeding on something": *omnivorous, panivorous.*

vortex *pl.* **vortexes, vortices** [L, whirl], a whirlpool effect produced by the whirling of a more or less cylindric mass of fluid (liquid or gas). The velocity of the motion increases as the radius of the circle described by the motion decreases; the velocity decreases as the radius increases. Tornadoes and whirlpools are examples of free vortexes.

vorticose veins, four large veins involved in the venous drainage of the eyeball. They exit through the sclera from each of the posterior quadrants of the eyeball and enter the superior and inferior ophthalmic veins.

voxel /vok″səl/, abbreviation for *vo*lume element, the three-dimensional version of a pi*xel.*

voyeur /voiyur″, vô·äyœr″/ [Fr, *voir,* to see], one whose sexual desire is gratified by the practice of voyeurism. The female counterpart is a voyeuse. Also called **Peeping Tom.**

voyeurism /voi″yəriz′əm, voiyur″izəm/ [Fr, *voyeur* + L, *ismus,* practice], a psychosexual disorder in which a person derives sexual excitement and gratification from looking at naked bodies and genital organs or from observing the sexual acts of others, especially from a secret vantage point. See also **compulsion.**

VP, abbreviation for **variegate porphyria.**

VPF, abbreviation for **vascular permeability factor.** See **vascular endothelial growth factor.**

V/Q, abbreviation for *ventilation/perfusion.* See **ventilation/perfusion (V/Q) ratio.**

VR, abbreviation for *variable ratio.* See **variable ratio (VR) reinforcement.**

VRA, abbreviation for **visual response audiometry.**

VRE, abbreviation for *vancomycin-resistant enterococci.*

V.S., 1. abbreviation for **vesicular breath sound. 2.** abbreviation for *veterinary surgeon.* **3.** abbreviation for *volumetric solution.* **4.** abbreviation for **vital signs.**

VSD, abbreviation for **ventricular septal defect.**

VU, abbreviation for **volume unit.**

vulgaris /vulger″is/ [L, *vulgus,* common people], common or ordinary.

vulnerable /vul″nərəbəl/ [L, *vulnus,* wound], being in a dangerous position or condition and thereby susceptible to being infected or injured.

vulnerable period, a short period in the cardiac cycle during which activation may result in an ectopic beat. The ventricular vulnerable period corresponds to the apex of the T wave toward its ascending side.

vulnerable population, groups at risk because of difficulties meeting basic needs and/or access to needed resources and services. See **population at risk.**

vulsella forceps. See **volsella forceps.**

vulva. See **pudendum.**

vulvar /vul″vər/, pertaining to the vulva.

vulvar dystrophy, a disorder characterized by skin eruptions of white atrophic pustules, squamous cell hyperplasia, and lichen sclerosis et atrophicus.

vulvectomy /vulvek″təmē/ [L, *vulva,* wrapper; Gk, *ektomē,* excision], the surgical removal of part or all of the tissues of the vulva, performed most frequently in the treatment of malignant or premalignant neoplastic disease. Simple vulvectomy includes the removal of the skin of the labia minora, labia majora, and clitoris. Radical vulvectomy involves excision of the labia majora, labia minora, clitoris, surrounding tissues, and pelvic lymph nodes.

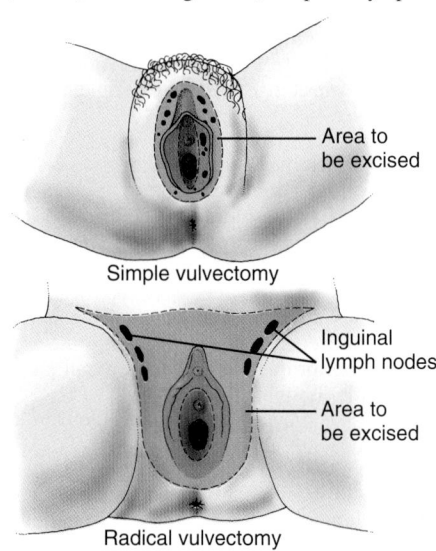

Area to be excised

Simple vulvectomy

Inguinal lymph nodes

Area to be excised

Radical vulvectomy

Vulvectomy *(Ignatavicius and Workman, 2010)*

vulvitis /vulvī″tis/ [L, *vulva,* wrapper; Gk, *itis,* inflammation], an inflammation of the vulva.

vulvo-, combining form meaning "relating to the vulva": *vulvectomy, vulvovaginal.*

vulvocrural /vul′vōkroo″rəl/ [L, *vulva* + *crus,* leg], pertaining to the vulva and the thigh.

vulvodynia /vul′vōdin″ē·ə/, chronic pain and discomfort in the female external genitals.

vulvovaginal /vul′vōvaj″inəl/ [L, *vulva* + *vagina,* sheath], pertaining to the vulva and the vagina.

vulvovaginal candidiasis, candidal infection of the vagina, and usually also the vulva, commonly characterized by pruritus, creamy white discharge, vulvar erythema and swelling, and dyspareunia. Also called ***Candida* vaginitis, *Candida* vulvovaginitis, vaginal candidiasis.**

vulvovaginitis /vul′vōvaj″inī″tis/, an inflammation of the vulva and vagina or of the vulvovaginal glands.

vv, abbreviation for *veins.*

v/v, **1.** symbol for *volume of dissolved substance per volume of solvent.* **2.** symbol for *volume per volume.*

VVI pacing, a specific type of electrical heart pacemaker mode. The letters indicate *v*entricular pacing, *v*entricular activity sensing, and *i*nhibition of ventricular pacing by a sensed QRS complex. Compare **DDD pacing.**

v/w, symbol for *volume of substance per unit of weight of another component.*

vWF, abbreviation for *von Willebrand factor.*

VY plasty /vē″wī″ plas′tē/, a surgical incision made in a V shape and sutured in a Y shape to lengthen the tissue area. In a variation of the procedure, the incision is made in a Y shape and sutured in a V shape to shorten the tissue area. Also called Y-**plasty.** See also **flap.**

Vyvanse, a central nervous system stimulant. Brand name for **lisdexamfetamine.**

VZIG, abbreviation for **varicella-zoster immune globulin.**

VZV, abbreviation for **varicella zoster virus.**

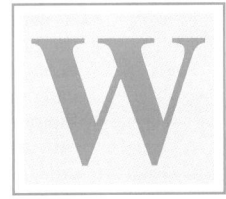

w, the amount of energy required to ionize a molecule of air, as expressed by w = 33.85 eV/ion pair. This is an important quantity for radiation dosimetry because it allows the extraction of dose from ionization measurements.

W, 1. abbreviation for **watt. 2.** symbol for the element **tungsten.**

Waardenburg syndrome /vär′den·bərg/ [Petrus Johannes Waardenburg, Dutch ophthalmologist, 1886–1979], a group of conditions related to an autosomal-dominant disorder. The syndrome is characterized by wide bridge of the nose resulting from lateral displacement of the inner canthi and puncta; pigmentary disturbances, including white forelock; different colors in the iris of the eye; white eyelashes; localized loss of pigmentation of the skin; and sometimes cochlear deafness. There are four known types.

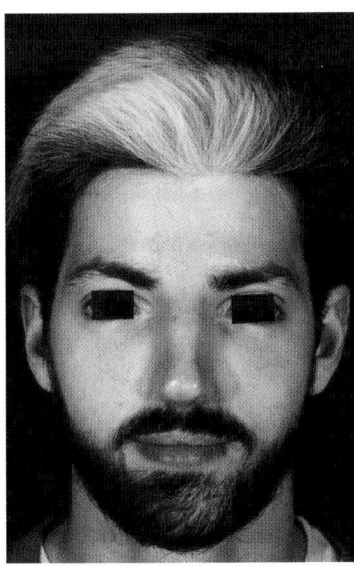

Individual with characteristics of Waardenburg syndrome *(Hordinsky, Sawaya, and Scher, 2000)*

waddling gait /wod′ling/ [ME, *waden,* to wade; ONorse, *gata,* way], a gait characterized by exaggerated lateral trunk movements and hip elevations. It is observed in pregnancy and in patients with osteoarthritis of the hip or progressive muscular dystrophy.

WAGR syndrome, a syndrome of Wilms tumor, absence of the iris, genitourinary abnormalities or gonadoblastoma, and intellectual disability resulting from a small interstitial deletion on chromosome 11. WAGR is the acronym for *W*ilms tumor, *a*niridia, *g*enitourinary abnormalities, and *r*etardation.

Wagstaffe fracture /wag′staf/ [William Wagstaffe, English surgeon, 1834–1910; L, *fractura,* break], a fracture characterized by separation of the medial malleolus of the tibia.

waiting list, a roll of persons waiting to fill a vacancy. Kinds include **transplant list.**

waiver, 1. a legally binding statement or document indicating the relinquishment of a right, entitlement, or privilege. **2.** a mechanism used by Medicaid and the Children's Health Insurance Program to encourage the development of novel ways to improve and finance health care through a formal request documenting the efficacy of other types of services or reimbursement.

wakefulness /wāk′fulnəs/, **1.** an alert state of mind. **2.** sleeplessness or insomnia.

waking imagined analgesia (WIA) [AS, *wacian,* to awaken; L, *imaginari,* to picture oneself; Gk, *a + algos,* without pain], the pain relief experienced by a patient who uses the psychological technique of concentrating on previous pleasant personal experiences that produced tranquility, such as lying on a summer beach beside cooling ocean water or drifting down a quiet river in a canoe. The patient using the WIA technique is encouraged to verbalize such experiences, thereby reinforcing recollection with attendant soothing biological responses. This technique is often effective in reducing mild to moderate pain, especially when used with a mild nonnarcotic analgesic and the compassionate interaction of an attending health care professional. See also **pain assessment, pain intervention.**

waking paralysis, paralysis experienced momentarily upon awakening, usually improving within seconds.

waking ptosis. See **morning ptosis.**

Waldenström macroglobulinemia. See **macroglobulinemia.**

Waldeyer's throat ring /wäl′dī·ərz/ [Heinrich W.G. von Waldeyer, German anatomist, 1836–1921; AS, *hring*], the palatine, pharyngeal, and lingual tonsils that encircle the pharynx. Also called **lymphoid ring, tonsillar ring.**

Wald, Lillian [1887–1940], an American public health nurse, settlement leader, and social reformer. She founded the Henry Street Settlement in New York to bring nursing care into the homes of the poor. This led to the development of the Visiting Nurse Service of New York. She was also instrumental in establishing the school nursing system, the federal government's Children's Bureau, and the Nursing Service Division of the Metropolitan Life Insurance Company. She was the first nurse to be elected into the Hall of Fame for Great Americans.

walker /wô′kər/ [AS, *wealcan,* to roam], **1.** an assistive device made of metal tubing, used to aid a patient in walking. It has four widely placed, sturdy legs. The patient holds onto the walker and takes a step with each leg and then moves the walker forward and takes another step with each leg. Wheeled walkers may have wheels on the front or rear two legs or on all four legs. A walker can be used by an individual with a lower extremity that is full, partial, or non–weight-bearing. It should be used only on flat, level surfaces. The walker is considered the most stable of the ambulatory assistive devices. Compare **crutch. 2.** A small, rubber or plastic heel attached to the bottom of a walking cast to prevent the cast from slipping on hard surfaces. Also called **walking heel.**

W

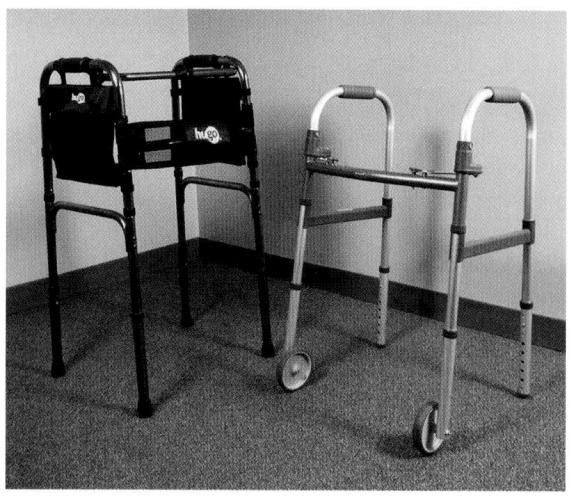

Two types of walkers *(Bonewit-West, 2012)*

Walker-Warburg syndrome /waw′kər·vär′boŏrg/ [Arthur Earl Walker, American surgeon, 1907–1995; Mette Warburg, Danish ophthalmologist, 1926–2015], a congenital syndrome, usually fatal before the age of 1 year, consisting of hydrocephalus; agyria; various ocular anomalies such as retinal dysplasia, corneal opacity, or microphthalmia; and sometimes encephalocele. Also called **HARDE syndrome,** *Walker lissencephaly,* **Warburg syndrome.**

walking belt, a leather or nylon device with handles that fastens around the patient's waist and assists the health care provider with the patient's ambulation. Also called **gait belt.** Compare **transfer belt.**

walking cast [AS, *wealcan,* to roam; ONorse, *kasta*], a cast that immobilizes the movement of the ankle, foot, and calf, allowing ambulation. See also **long-leg cast with walker, short-leg cast with walker.**

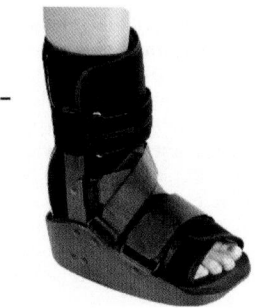

Short walking cast *(Rizzone and Gregory, 2013)*

walking heel. See **walker,** def. 2.

walking pneumonia. *(Informal)* See **mycoplasma pneumonia.**

walking program, an aerobic exercise regimen of walking, usually 30 to 45 minutes a day 5 or 6 days a week. It may be part of a program to maintain health, lose weight, condition the heart, or lower blood pressure.

walking reflex, a series of steplike motions of an infant's legs when the infant is held under the arms and with the feet in contact with a surface. The reflex disappears at approximately 4 to 8 weeks of age.

walking rounds [AS, *wealcan* + Fr, *rond*], interactions at the point of care in which a clinician leads a group of students, less experienced clinicians, colleagues responsible for care, or an interdisciplinary team to interact with patients for the purpose of improving patient care.

walking typhoid [AS, *wealcan,* to roam; Gk, *typhos,* fever, *eidos,* form], an ambulatory subclinical case of typhoid fever. The person may be infected with typhoid but have mild symptoms that do not interfere with the activities of daily living.

walking wounded [AS, *wealcan,* to roam, *wund*], a triage term for an injured person who is ambulatory and has minor injuries.

wall [L, *vallum,* palisade], a limiting structure within the body, such as the wall of the abdominal, thoracic, or pelvic cavities or the wall of a cell.

Wallenberg syndrome /väl′en·berg/ [Adolf Wallenberg, German physician, 1862–1949], a syndrome resulting usually from occlusion of the vertebral artery and less often from occlusion of its branch, the posterior inferior cerebellar artery; it is marked by loss of temperature and pain sensations of the face on the same side as the lesion, contralateral loss of these sensations in the trunk and extremities, and a variety of other neurological and ocular symptoms, including Horner syndrome. Also called **lateral medullary syndrome, posterior inferior cerebellar artery syndrome.**

wallerian degeneration /waler″ē·ən/ [Augustus V. Waller, English physician, 1816–1870; L, *degenerare,* to degenerate], the fatty degeneration of a nerve fiber after it has been severed from its cell body.

wall stress, the tension within the wall of the left ventricle. It is determined by the pressure in the ventricle, the internal radius of the ventricle, and the thickness of the wall. Also called *wall tension.*

wander /won″dər/ [AS, *wandrian*], **1.** to move about purposelessly. **2.** to cause to move back and forth in an exploratory manner; for example, in inserting an intrauterine catheter, the tip of the inserter usually must be wandered around the fetal head in the cervix to find a space through which the catheter may be passed upward into the uterus. **3.** to be cognitively unfocused.

wandering abscess [AS, *wandrian* + L, *abscedere,* to go away], an abscess that moves through tissue openings to a point some distance from its origin.

wandering atrial pacemaker [AS, *wandrian* + L, *passus* + ME, *maken*], a sinus arrhythmia with an atrial or junctional escape rhythm during the slow phase of the sinus rhythm. Frequently there are atrial fusion beats when impulse from the two pacing sources collide within the atrium. An accelerated junctional rhythm that competes with the sinus rhythm is often mislabeled "wandering pacemaker."

wandering goiter. See **diving goiter.**

wandering rash. See **geographic tongue.**

wandering spleen. See **floating spleen.**

Wangensteen apparatus /wang″ənstēn/ [Owen H. Wangensteen, American surgeon, 1898–1981; L, *ad* + *parare,* to prepare], a nasogastroduodenal catheter and suction apparatus used for constant gentle drainage and decompression of the stomach or duodenum. It may be used to relieve abdominal distension that often occurs after surgery or that may complicate a GI disorder, especially an intestinal obstruction. See also **Wangensteen tube.**

Wangensteen tube [Owen H. Wangensteen], the catheter component of a Wangensteen apparatus.

Warburg syndrome. See **Walker-Warburg syndrome.**

ward /wôrd/ [AS, *weard,* guard], **1.** a large room in a hospital for the accommodation of several patients. **2.** a division within a hospital for the care of numerous patients having the same condition (e.g., a maternity ward). See also *specialty units.*

warfarin poisoning /wôr″fərin/ [Wisconsin Alumni Research Foundation + coumarin], a toxic condition caused by the ingestion of warfarin accidentally in the form of a rodenticide or by overdose with the substance in its pharmacologic anticoagulant form. The poison accumulates in the body and results in nosebleed, bruising, hematuria, melena, and internal hemorrhage. Vitamin K is the antidote to warfarin.

warfarin sodium, an oral anticoagulant.
- INDICATIONS: It is prescribed for the prophylaxis and treatment of thrombosis, atrial fibrillation, and embolism.
- CONTRAINDICATIONS: Pregnancy, severe renal or hepatic disease, uncontrolled hypertension, hemorrhage, hemorrhagic tendencies (e.g., due to hemophilia), leukemia, and known hypersensitivity to this drug are among the things that prohibit its use.
- ADVERSE EFFECTS: The most serious adverse effect is hemorrhage. Many other drugs interact with this drug to increase or decrease its effects.

warm-blooded [AS, *wearm* + *blod*], having a relatively high and constant body temperature, such as the temperatures maintained by humans, other mammals, and birds, despite changes in environmental temperatures. Heat is produced in the warm-blooded human body by the catabolism of foods in proportion to the amount of work performed by the tissues in the body. Heat is lost from the body by evaporation, radiation, conduction, and convection. About 80% of the body heat that is dissipated in humans is lost through the skin. The rest is lost through the mucous membranes of the respiratory, the digestive, and the urinary systems. The average temperature of the healthy human is 98.6° F (37° C). Also called **homoiothermal, homothermal.** Compare **cold-blooded.**

warmup, light calisthenics and stretching exercises intended to increase flexibility, minimize risk of musculoskeletal complications, and gradually increase heart rate before the start of strenuous athletic activity.

war neurosis. *(Obsolete)* Compare **posttraumatic stress disorder.** Now called **combat fatigue.**

wart. See **verruca.**

Warthin tumor [Aldred Scott Warthin, American pathologist, 1866–1931], a benign tumor of the salivary gland. See **papillary adenocystoma lymphomatosum.**

washout /wosh″out/ [AS, *wascan,* to wash; ME, *oute*], the elimination or expulsion of a gas such as nitrous oxide or volatile anesthetic agent from the lung alveoli by the administration or flushing out by a carrier gas such as oxygen.

wasp /wosp/ [L, *vespa*], a thin, narrow-waisted hymenopteran insect with two pairs of membranous wings that are folded lengthwise when at rest, like parts of a fan. Many species of wasps can give painful stings that produce severe effects in hypersensitive individuals. Unlike bees, a wasp can sting more than once. Treatment is as for bee stings. See also **bee sting, yellow jacket venom.**

Wassermann blood test /was″ərmən, vos″ərmun/ [August P. von Wassermann, German bacteriologist, 1866–1925], *(Obsolete)* the first standard diagnostic blood test (no longer used) for syphilis based on the complement fixation reaction.

wasted ventilation, the volume of air that ventilates the physiological dead space in the respiratory system.

waste products [L, *vastare,* to destroy, *producere,* to produce], the products of metabolic activity after oxygen and nutrients have been supplied to a cell. These include mainly

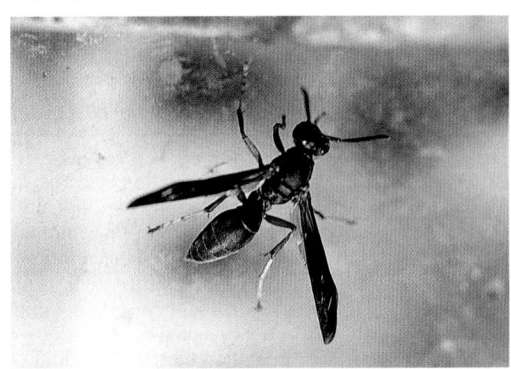

Paper wasp *(Auerbach, 2007)*

carbon dioxide and water along with sodium chloride and soluble nitrogenous salts and are excreted in feces, urine, and exhaled air.

wasting [L, *vastare,* to destroy], a process of deterioration marked by weight loss and decreased physical vigor, appetite, and mental activity. See also **wasting syndrome.**

wasting syndrome, a condition characterized by weight loss associated with chronic fever and diarrhea. Over a period of 1 month, the patient may lose 10% of baseline body weight. In cases of human immunodeficiency virus infection, the malnutrition of wasting exacerbates the condition.

watchfulness /woch″fəlnes/, continuous supervision, either open or unobtrusive, as the situation indicates.

water (H_2O) /wô″tər/ [AS, *waeter*], a chemical compound, one molecule of which contains one atom of oxygen and two atoms of hydrogen. Almost three quarters of the earth's surface is covered by water. Essential to life as it exists on this planet, water makes up more than 70% of living things. Pure water freezes at 32° F (0° C) and boils at 212° F (100° C) at 760 mm Hg.

waterbed, a closed rubber bag filled with water and used as a mattress to prevent or treat pressure ulcers by equalizing the patient's weight against the support. Also called **water mattress.** Compare **fluidized air bed.**

water birth, *(Informal)* an alternate birthing practice in which the mother lies partially submerged in a pool of water heated to 97° to 100° F during the first stage of labor and, if desired, the second stage. It is usually recommended that this alternate birth practice be limited to normal, unassisted labor in the vertex presentation in an uncomplicated, normal-term, singleton pregnancy. Also called *immersion in water during labor and delivery.* See also **birthing pool.**
- METHOD: Protocols must be in place to assure that the water is not contaminated, that there are appropriate maternal and fetal evaluations during labor, and for rapid removal of the mother from immersion to a facility where assisted vaginal birth and cesarean section, as well as neonatal resuscitation, are immediately available if complications arise. Water immersion also requires protocols for rapid, careful extraction to avoid aspiration of water by the infant.
- PATIENT CARE CONSIDERATIONS: Proponents cite easier and faster labor, a greater sense of maternal well-being and control, a decreased risk of perineal trauma (i.e., fewer vulvar and vaginal tears), and less need for analgesia. Other health professionals dispute these claims, noting a relative dearth of controlled, peer-reviewed literature supportive of immersion in water during labor and delivery.
- OUTCOME CRITERIA: Water birth is promoted by some practitioners as a method to facilitate a more comfortable and gentle first stage, allowing the mother greater and easier

W

movement, buoyed in water rather than recumbent on a bed or seated in a birthing chair. Because of risk, many recommend that if water birth is used in the second stage of labor, it be considered an experimental birthing procedure.

water-borne, carried by water, such as a water-borne epidemic of typhoid fever.

water brash, heartburn with regurgitation into the mouth of fluid that may be sour or almost tasteless.

water for hemodialysis, water for use in hemodialysis, produced by subjecting water that meets the requirements of drinking water regulations to further treatment to reduce chemical and microbiological components. It contains no added antimicrobials and is not intended for injection.

water-hammer pulse, a pulse that is bounding and has great force then collapses. See also **collapsing pulse, Corrigan pulse.**

Waterhouse-Friderichsen syndrome /wô″tərhous′ frid″ərik′sən/ [Rupert Waterhouse, English physician, 1873–1958; Carl Friderichsen, Danish physician, 1886–1979], the most severe form of cerebrospinal meningitis, most often caused by meningococcal infection, characterized by the sudden onset of fever, cyanosis, petechiae, and collapse from massive bilateral adrenal hemorrhage. It requires immediate emergency treatment, hospitalization, and intensive care. Emergency treatment includes vasopressor drugs, IV fluids, plasma, and oxygen. No sedatives or narcotics are given. Specific treatment is intensive antibiotic therapy given parenterally and continued for several days after symptoms subside. Care includes close observation and adequate provision of fluids and nutrients.

water hemlock, (*Cicuta douglasii*) a highly poisonous plant commonly found in wet meadows and pastures and along the banks of streams.

watering can perineum (WCP), (*Informal*) a perineum with numerous fistulas leaking urine as a result of abscesses or sometimes strictures of the urethra.

water-in-oil emulsion, a mixture in which water or aqueous solution is the dispersed phase and oil or an oily substance is the continuous phase, resulting in water droplets dispersed in oil.

water intoxication, an increase in the volume of free water in the body, resulting in dilutional hyponatremia. Common causes are excessive ingestion of water, increased infusions of hypotonic IV solutions, or excess secretions of antidiuretic hormone. Clinical manifestations are abdominal cramps, nausea, vomiting, lethargy, and dizziness. It can potentially lead to convulsions and coma. See also **syndrome of inappropriate antidiuretic hormone secretion.**

water mattress. See **waterbed.**

water moccasin, a snake. See **cottonmouth.**

water pollution, the contamination of lakes, rivers, and streams by industrial or community sources of substances. The contamination may result in unsafe and/or unsanitary water supplies.

waters. (*Nontechnical*) See **amniotic fluid.**

watershed infarct /wô″tərshed/, an area of necrosis in the brain caused by an insufficiency of blood where the distributions of cerebral arteries overlap. The condition resembles that of an agricultural field irrigation system, in which the most distant sections may not be irrigated if there is a fall in water pressure.

water-soluble contrast medium, an iodinated contrast medium that is absorbed by the blood and excreted by the kidneys. Among the advantages of a water-soluble contrast medium are that it does not need to be removed after a procedure and that it may reduce the length of the procedure.

water trap. See **underwater seal.**

Watson-Crick helix /wôt″sən krik″/ [John Dewey Watson, American geneticist, b. 1928; Francis H. Crick, British biochemist, 1916–2004; Gk, *helix,* coil], a model of the deoxyribonucleic acid (DNA) molecule proposed by Watson and Crick as two right-handed polynucleotide chains coiled around the same axis as a double helix. The purine and pyrimidine bases of each strand are on the inside of the double helix and paired according to a Watson-Crick hydrogen-bonding base-pairing rule. Variations in the sequences of the bases determine the genetic information transmitted by the DNA molecule. Watson and Crick received the Nobel Prize in 1962.

Watson, Jean, a nursing theorist who proposed a philosophy and science of caring in 1979 in an effort to reduce the dichotomy between theory and practice. Her theory of human caring reflects an existential phenomenologist's view of psychology and humanities. Caring is a universal social phenomenon that is only effectively practiced interpersonally. Watson identified 10 caring factors: (1) the formation of a humanistic-altruistic system of values; (2) the instillation of faith-hope; (3) the cultivation of sensitivity to self and others; (4) the development of a helping-trust relationship; (5) the promotion and acceptance of the expression of positive and negative feelings; (6) the systematic use of the scientific problem-solving method for decision making; (7) the promotion of interpersonal teaching-learning; (8) the provision for a supportive, protective, and corrective mental, physical, sociocultural, and spiritual environment; (9) assistance with the gratification of human needs; and (10) the allowance for existential-phenomenological forces. According to Watson, caring is a nursing term, and nursing concerns itself with health promotion, restoration, and prevention of illness as opposed to curing. Clients require holistic care that promotes humanism, health, and quality of living.

watt (W) /wot/ [James Watt, Scottish engineer, 1736–1819], the unit of electric power or work in the meter/kilogram/second system of notation. The watt is the product of the voltage and the amperage. One watt of power is dissipated when a current of 1 ampere flows across a difference in potential of 1 volt. See also **ampere, current, ohm, volt.**

watt per square centimeter (W/cm²), a unit of power density or intensity used in ultrasonography.

wave [AS, *wafian,* to fluctuate], a periodic disturbance in which energy moves through a medium without permanently altering the constituents of the medium. Electromagnetic waves, such as light, x-rays, and radio waves, can travel through a vacuum. Sound waves can be transmitted only through matter. See also **electromagnetic radiation, light, sound, x-ray.**

waveform, **1.** the graphic representation of a wave, derived by plotting a characteristic wave against time. **2.** the form of an arterial pressure pulse or displacement wave. **3.** the representation of a neuromuscular electric stimulation unit, which is usually a symmetric or asymmetric biphasic pulse with two phases in each pulse. The two phases continually alternate or reverse in direction between positive and negative polarity.

waveform ripple, a temporal variation in the voltage across the x-ray tube. Also called **voltage ripple.**

wavelength, the distance between a given point on one wave cycle and the corresponding point on the next successive wave cycle. A pure color is produced by light of a specific wavelength. Electromagnetic waves of different wavelengths account for many of the transmission characteristics of radio and television.

wax, a low-melting, high-molecular-weight, organic mixture or compound similar to fats and oils but lacking glycerides. See also **cerumen.**

wax bath. See **paraffin bath.**

waxy flexibility. See **cerea flexibilitas.**

Wb, abbreviation for **weber.**

WBC, abbreviation for **white blood cell.** See **leukocyte.**

wc, abbreviation for **wheelchair.**

W chromosome, the sex chromosomes of certain insects, birds, and fish. Females of such animals are heterogametic and have one W and one Z chromosome, whereas males are homogametic and have two Z chromosomes. The ZZ-ZW nomenclature was chosen to differentiate this system from the XX-XY system, which occurs in humans and various other animals and in which the female is homogametic and the male is heterogametic.

W/cm², abbreviation for **watt per square centimeter.**

W/D, abbreviation for **withdrawal.**

weakness /wēk″nəs/, a condition of being feeble, fragile, frail, or decrepit or lacking physical strength, energy, or vigor. Causes of weakness include muscle disuse and nerve injury. Partially denervated muscle shows some degree of weakness, whereas completely denervated muscle becomes flaccid. Concomitant with partial denervation is a patient's complaint of rapid fatigue and diminished capacity to perform activities of daily living. Deep tendon reflexes are diminished or absent, and electromyographic readings are abnormal.

wean [AS, *wenian,* to accustom], **1.** to induce a child to give up breastfeeding and accept other food in place of breast milk. Many children are ready for weaning during the second half of the first year; some wean themselves. **2.** to withdraw a person from something on which he or she is dependent. **3.** to remove a patient gradually from dependency on mechanical ventilation.

weanling, a child who has recently been weaned.

weapons of mass destruction (WMD), weapons, such as nuclear or chemical weapons, whose purpose is to kill large numbers of people indiscriminately.

wear-and-tear theory /wer/, one theory of biological aging in which structural and functional changes occur during the aging process (e.g., osteoarthritis). Damage accumulates when the body fails to repair itself.

weaver's bottom [AS, *wefan,* to weave, *botm,* undersurface], a form of bursitis affecting the ischial bursae in people whose work requires prolonged sitting in one position. See also **bursitis.**

web, a network of fibers and cells forming a tissue or a membrane.

webbed neck /webd/, a congenital thick fold of skin and fascia that stretches from the mastoid process to the clavicle on the lateral aspect of the neck. It occurs in such genetic conditions as Noonan syndrome and Turner syndrome. Also called **pterygium colli.**

webbed penis, a penis enclosed by the skin of the scrotum.

webbed toes [AS, *wefan,* to weave], an abnormality in which the digits of the feet are connected by a thin, flexible sheet of skin.

webbing, skinfolds connecting adjacent structures such as fingers or toes or the neck from the acromion to the mastoid, associated with genetic anomalies.

weber (Wb) /web″ər/ [Wilhelm Edward Weber, German physicist, 1804–1891], a unit of magnetic flux equal to 1 m²kg/s²A.

Weber sign /web″ərz/ [Hermann D. Weber, English physician, 1823–1918], ipsilateral oculomotor nerve paresis and contralateral paralysis of the face, tongue, and extremities caused by a midbrain lesion. Also called *Weber paralysis.*

Weber tuning fork test, a method of screening auditory acuity. It is especially useful in determining whether a hearing loss in one ear is a conductive or a sensorineural loss. The test is performed by placing the stem of a vibrating tuning fork in the center of the person's forehead, or the midline vertex. The loudness of the sound is equal in both ears if hearing is normal or if there is a symmetric hearing loss. If the person has a sensorineural loss in one ear, the unaffected ear perceives the sound as louder. When conductive hearing loss is present in one ear, the sound is perceived as louder in that ear because it does not hear ordinary background noise conducted through the air and receives only vibrations by bone conduction.

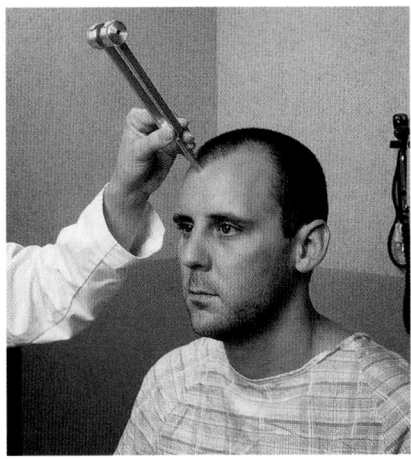

Weber tuning fork test *(Harkreader and Hogan, 2007)*

web of causation, an interrelationship of multiple factors that contribute to the occurrence of a disease.

Webril, a stretchable cotton material applied over the skin to protect it from plaster irritation.

Wechsler intelligence scales /weks″lər/ [David Wechsler, American psychologist, b. 1896], a series of standardized tests designed to measure the intelligence at several age levels, from preschool through adult, by means of questions that examine general information, arrangement of pictures and objects, vocabulary, memory, reasoning, and other abilities.

wedge /wej/ [AS *wecg*], **1.** a piece of material thick at one end and tapering to a thin edge at the other end. **2.** to force something into a space of limited size. See also **wedge pressure.**

wedge fracture /wej/ [AS, *wecg,* peg; L, *fractura,* break], a fracture of the vertebral body with anterior compression.

wedge pressure, the blood pressure in the left atrium, determined with a cardiac catheter wedged in the most distal segment of the pulmonary artery. See also **pulmonary wedge pressure.**

wedge resection, the surgical excision of part of an organ, such as part of an ovary containing a cyst. The segment excised may be wedge-shaped.

WEE, abbreviation for **western equine encephalitis.** See **equine encephalitis.**

weed. *(Informal)* See **cannabis.**

weeping [AS, *wepan,* to cry], **1.** crying, lacrimating. **2.** oozing or exuding fluid, such as a sore or rash.

weeping lubrication, a form of hydrostatic lubrication in which the interstitial fluid of hydrated articular cartilage flows onto its surface when a load is applied.

W

Wegener granulomatosis /wā″gənər/ [Friedrich Wegener, German pathologist, 1907–1990; L, *granulum,* little grain; Gk, *oma,* tumor, *osis,* condition], now called **granulomatosis with polyangiitis (GPA)**.

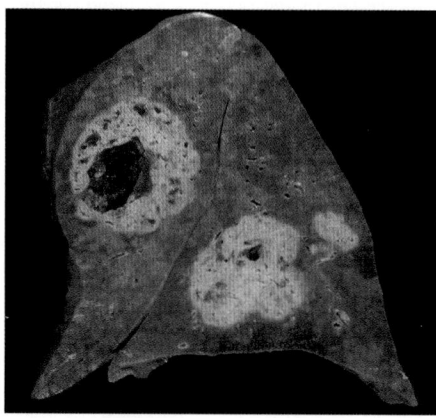

Wegener granulomatosis *(Courtesy Dr. Sidney Murphree, Department of Pathology, University of Texas Southwestern Medical School)*

Weigert-Meyer rule, in cases of double ureter, the ureter from the upper pole of the kidney usually opens below and medial to the one from the lower pole. Also called *Weigert-Meyer law.*

weight (wt) /wāt/ [AS, *gewiht*], the force exerted on a body by gravitational attraction. As a body moves away from the earth, the weight of the body decreases, but the mass remains constant. In empty space a body has mass but no weight. Weight is sometimes measured in units of force such as newtons or poundals, but it is usually expressed in pounds or kilograms, as is mass. See also **mass.**

weight holder, a metal, T-shaped bar that holds weights for traction.

weightlessness [AS, *gewiht* + ME, *les*], a state of absence of apparent weight, as in being beyond the effects of gravitational force in space travel. See also **space medicine.**

weightlifter's headache, a type of headache sometimes experienced by weightlifters and others engaged in resistance forms of exercise. The headache is commonly occipital or upper cervical and comes on suddenly while straining, perhaps as a result of cervical ligament damage. The pain may be severe, steady, burning, or boring and may last for days.

weightlifting, a resistance form of exercise that involves the lifting of maximum heavy weights in a prescribed manner.

weight loss, a reduction in body weight. The loss may be the result of a change in diet or lifestyle or a febrile disease. To lose 1 pound a week a person must consume 500 fewer calories daily and/or expend 500 more calories daily through physical activity. See also **wasting.**

weight per volume (w/v) solution, the relationship of a solute to a solvent expressed as grams of solute per milliliter of the total solution. An example is 50 g of glucose in 1 L of solution, considered a 5% w/v solution.

weight per weight, a unit of concentration used for concentrated solutions, typically acids and bases, expressed as a percentage.

weight-reduction diet, a diet used to decrease body weight. It must supply fewer calories than the individual expends each day while supplying all the essential nutrients for maintaining health.

weights and measures, a system of establishing units or parts of quantities of substances, including standards of mass or volume.

weight traction [AS, *gewiht* + L, *trahere,* to draw], traction applied to a limb or part of a limb by means of a suspended weight.

weight training, a type of resistance-training exercise using barbells, dumbbells, or machines to increase muscle strength. See also **strength training.**

Weill-Marchesani syndrome /vīl mär·kə·sä′nē/ [Georges Weill, French ophthalmologist, 1866–1952; Oswald Marchesani, German ophthalmologist, 1900–1952], a congenital disorder of connective tissue, autosomal dominant or recessive, characterized by brachycephaly, shortened digits, short stature with broad chest and heavy musculature, reduced joint mobility, and a variety of ocular defects. Also called **Marchesani syndrome.**

Weil disease. See **leptospirosis.**

Weiss' sign. See **Chvostek sign, Chvostek-Weiss sign.**

well baby care [AS, *wyllan,* to wish; ME, *babe* + L, *garrire,* to chatter], periodic health supervision for infants and children to promote optimal physical, emotional, and intellectual growth and development. Such health care measures include routine immunizations to prevent disease, screening procedures for early detection and treatment of illness, and parental guidance and instruction in proper nutrition, accident prevention, and specific care and rearing of the child at various stages of development. The recommended preventive health care schedule for children who are developing normally is at months 1, 2, 4, 6, 9, 12, 15, 18, and 24 and at years 3, 4, 5, 8, 10, 12, 14, 16, and 18. Well baby care may be provided in a clinic, a convenient local meeting place, a private doctor's office, the office of a community health nursing service, or a school. Nurses or nurse practitioners frequently provide the care.

well baby clinic, a clinic that specializes in medical supervision and services for healthy infants.

well-being [AS, *wyllan* + *beon,* to be], achievement of a good and satisfactory existence as defined by the individual.

well-differentiated lymphocytic malignant lymphoma /-dif′ərən″shē·ā′tid/, a lymphoid neoplasm characterized by the predominance of mature lymphocytes. Also called **lymphocytic lymphoma, lymphocytic lymphosarcoma, lymphocytoma.**

Wellens syndrome, the electrocardiographic signs of critical proximal left anterior descending coronary artery stenosis in patients with unstable angina. The signs are: normal or minimally elevated enzyme; little or no S-T segment elevation; no loss of precordial R waves; and progressive, deep, symmetric inversion of the T waves in leads V2 and V3 and sometimes in other leads. The signs are seen when the patient is without pain and represent reperfusion following transient occlusion.

wellness, a dynamic state of health in which an individual progresses toward a higher level of functioning, achieving an optimum balance between internal and external environments.

Wells syndrome /welz/ [G.C. Wells, 20th-century British dermatologist], cellulitis with erythema, edema, and often blistering of the skin accompanied by eosinophilia, flame figures, and a mild fever. A single episode lasts 2 to 6 weeks, and recurrences or exacerbations are common. Also called **eosinophilic cellulitis.**

welt [OE, *wealtan,* to roll], a raised ridge on the skin, usually caused by a blow or occurring in dermatographism.

wen. See **pilar cyst.**

Wenckebach heart block. See **Mobitz I heart block.**

Werdnig-Hoffmann disease /verd″nig hôf″mun/ [Guido Werdnig, Austrian neurologist, 1844–1919; Johann Hoffmann,

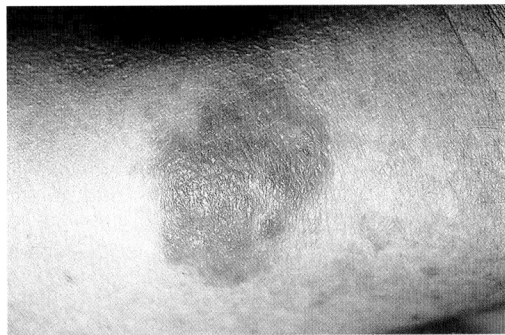

Wells syndrome *(Callen et al, 2000)*

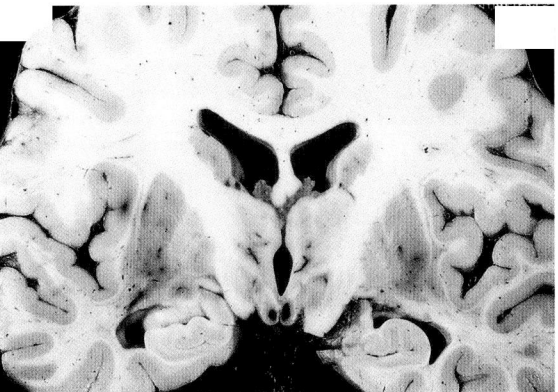

Wernicke encephalopathy *(Kumar, Cotran, and Robbins, 2003)*

German neurologist, 1857–1919], a genetic disorder beginning in infancy or young childhood, characterized by progressive atrophy of the skeletal muscle resulting from degeneration of the cells in the anterior horn of the spinal cord and the motor nuclei in the brainstem. Onset occurs within the first year of life, with the condition usually apparent at birth. Symptoms include congenital hypotonia; absence of stretch reflexes; flaccid paralysis, especially of the trunk and limbs; lack of sucking ability; fasciculations of the tongue and sometimes of other muscles; and often, dysphagia. Treatment is symptomatic, and death generally occurs in early childhood, often from respiratory complications. The condition is transmitted as an autosomal-recessive trait and occurs more frequently in siblings than in successive generations. Also called **familial spinal muscular atrophy, Hoffmann disease, infantile spinal muscular atrophy, progressive spinal muscular atrophy of infants,** *Werdnig-Hoffmann paralysis.*

Werlhof disease, now called **immune thrombocytopenic purpura.**

Werner syndrome /wur″nər, wer″nər/, an inherited condition of progeria with scleroderma, juvenile cataracts, diabetes mellitus, and hypogonadism.

Wernicke-Korsakoff syndrome, the coexistence of Wernicke encephalopathy and Korsakoff syndrome.

Wernicke aphasia /ver″nikē/ [Karl Wernicke, German neurologist, 1848–1905], a form of aphasia affecting comprehension of written and spoken words, possibly caused by a lesion in the Wernicke center. The patient may articulate normally, but speech is incoherent, with malformed or substitute words and grammatical errors. Compare **Broca aphasia.**

Wernicke center [Karl Wernicke, German physician; Gk, *kentron,* center], a sensory speech center located in the posterior temporal gyrus and adjacent angular gyrus in the dominant hemisphere. Wernicke observed in 1874 that patients with brain damage in that area also suffered a loss of speech comprehension. Also called **Wernicke field, Wernicke zone.** See also **speech centers.**

Wernicke encephalopathy [Karl Wernicke], an inflammatory, hemorrhagic degenerative condition of the brain. It is characterized by lesions in several parts of the brain, including the hypothalamus, mammillary bodies, and tissues surrounding the ventricles and aqueducts, double vision, ophthalmoplegia, involuntary and rapid movements of the eyes, lack of muscular coordination, and decreased mental function, which may be mild or severe. Wernicke encephalopathy is caused by a thiamine deficiency and is seen in association with chronic alcoholism. It also occurs as a complication of GI tract disease and hyperemesis gravidarum associated with malabsorption and malnutrition. Also called **Wernicke syndrome.**

Wernicke field. See **Wernicke center.**

Wernicke syndrome. See **Wernicke encephalopathy.**

Wernicke zone. See **Wernicke center.**

West African sleeping sickness. See **Gambian trypanosomiasis.**

Westcort, a topical glucocorticoid. Brand name for *hydrocortisone valerate.*

Westermark's sign [Neil Westermark, German radiologist, b. 1904], on a radiograph of the lung, the absence of blood vessel markings beyond the location of a pulmonary embolism.

Western blot test, a laboratory blood test to detect the presence of antibodies to specific antigens. It is regarded as more precise than the enzyme-linked immunosorbent assay (ELISA) and is sometimes used to check the validity of ELISA tests.

western equine encephalitis. See **equine encephalitis.**

West Indian smallpox. See **alastrim.**

West Nile encephalitis /west nīl/ [West Nile River valley and region in northern Uganda, where the disease was first observed in 1937], a mild, febrile, sporadic disease caused by the West Nile virus, transmitted by *Culex* mosquitoes and occurring chiefly in the summer; infection often does not lead to encephalitis. It may be of sudden onset, and symptoms may include drowsiness, severe frontal headache, maculopapular rash, abdominal pain, loss of appetite, nausea, and generalized lymphadenopathy. Most people infected with West Nile encephalitis are asymptomatic or experience flulike symptoms. Care is supportive. Many recover quickly but may experience prolonged malaise. Also called *West Nile fever.*

West Nile fever. See **West Nile encephalitis.**

West Nile virus /west nīl/, a virus of the genus *Flavivirus* that causes West Nile encephalitis. It is transmitted by *Culex* mosquitoes, with wild birds serving as the reservoir, and occurs widely in Africa, Europe, the Middle East, and Asia; since 1999 it has been present in the United States and Canada.

West Nile virus testing, a test of the blood or cerebrospinal fluid to identify the West Nile antibody.

West nomogram, a graph used in estimating the body surface area. See also **nomogram.**

West syndrome, an infantile encephalopathy characterized by spasms, arrest of psychomotor development, and an electroencephalogram abnormality of random high-voltage slow waves and spikes from multiple loci.

wet-and-dry-bulb thermometer, an instrument used to measure the relative humidity of the atmosphere. It consists of a thermometer with a bulb that is wet or moist and one that is kept dry. The relative humidity is calculated from the

W

difference in readings of the thermometers when water evaporates from the wet bulb, decreasing its temperature.

wet cough. *(Slang)* See **productive cough.**

wet dream. *(Slang)* See **nocturnal emission.**

wet wrap dressing [AS, *waet* + Ofr, *dresser,* to arrange], a moist dressing usually consisting of a cream or ointment applied to the skin with a double layer of cotton bandages (a moist first layer and a dry outer layer). It is used to relieve the symptoms of some skin diseases.

wet lung. See **adult respiratory distress syndrome.**

wet nurse, a woman who cares for and breastfeeds another's infant.

wet pleurisy [AS, *waet* + Gk, *pleuritis*], pleurisy in which the inflammation has progressed to a true exudate (also termed an effusive state). The escaped fluid has a high specific gravity because of the presence of blood clots and fibrin. See **pleurisy.**

wet tap, accidental puncture of the dura mater during injection of epidural anesthesia, so-called from the leakage of cerebrospinal fluid from the needle hub.

wetting agent, **1.** a substance that lowers the surface tension of water to promote wetting. **2.** a detergent such as tyloxapol used as a mucolytic in respiratory therapy.

wet-to-dry dressing, *(Obsolete)* a wet dressing that is allowed to dry and then is removed. It was once thought that in removal the wound would be lightly debrided. It is now known that wet-to-dry dressings allow the wound base to dry and that healing cells are removed when the dressing is removed.

Wharton duct. See **submandibular duct.**

Wharton jelly /wôr″tən/ [Thomas Wharton, English anatomist, 1614–1673; L, *gelare,* to congeal], a gelatinous mesenchymal tissue that remains when the embryonic body stalk blends with the yolk sac within the umbilical cord.

wheal /wēl/ [AS, *walu,* pimple], smooth, slightly elevated area on the skin that is redder or paler than the surrounding skin. A wheal usually itches and can change size or shape or disappear within hours. It is the typical lesion of urticaria. Subdermal or intradermal injections can also create a wheal.

wheal-and-flare reaction [AS, *walu* + *flare* + ME, *fleare,* to blaze up; L, *re,* again, *agere,* to act], a skin eruption that may follow injury or injection of an antigen. It is characterized by swelling and redness caused by a release of histamine. The reaction usually occurs in three stages, beginning with the appearance of an erythematous area at the site of injury, followed by development of a flare surrounding the site; finally a wheal forms at the site as fluid leaks under the skin from surrounding capillaries.

wheat weevil disease, a hypersensitivity pneumonitis caused by allergy to weevil particles found in wheat flour.

wheel, **1.** a rigid circular frame designed to revolve about an axis in the center of the disk. **2.** a round cutting or polishing dental instrument.

wheelchair (wc), a mobile chair equipped with large wheels and brakes. If long-term use of the chair is expected, a physical therapist may prescribe certain personalized requirements, such as size, left- or right-hand propulsion, type of brakes, height of armrests, and special seat pads.

wheelie /wē″lē/, a wheelchair mobility skill in which the front casters are raised and balance is maintained over the large rear wheels. It is used for negotiating steep ramps, steps, curbs, and other rough terrain.

wheeze [AS, *hwesan,* to hiss], **1.** a form of rhonchus, characterized by a high-pitched or low-pitched musical quality. It is caused by a high-velocity flow of air through a narrowed airway and is heard during both inspiration and expiration. It may be caused by bronchospasm, inflammation, or obstruction of the airway by a tumor or foreign body. Wheezes are associated with asthma and chronic bronchitis. Unilateral wheezes are characteristic of bronchogenic carcinoma, foreign bodies, and inflammatory lesions. In asthma, expiratory wheezing is more common, although inspiratory and expiratory wheezes are heard. **2.** to breathe with a wheeze. Compare **crackle, rhonchus.**

whiplash injury [ME, *whippen* + *lasshe* + L, *ijuria*], an injury to the cervical vertebrae or their supporting ligaments and muscles marked by pain and stiffness. It usually results from sudden acceleration or deceleration, such as in a rear-end car collision that causes violent back-and-forth movement of the head and neck.

Whipple procedure /hwip′əl/ [Allen O. Whipple, American surgeon, 1881–1963], radical pancreaticoduodenectomy with removal of the distal third of the stomach, the entire duodenum, and the head of the pancreas, a portion of the jejunum, and the lower half of the common bile duct, with gastrojejunostomy, choledochojejunostomy, and pancreaticojejunostomy. See also **pancreaticoduodenectomy.**

Whipple disease [George Hoyt Whipple, American pathologist, 1878–1976], a rare intestinal disease characterized by severe intestinal malabsorption, steatorrhea, anemia, weight loss, arthritis, and arthralgia. People with the disease are severely malnourished and have abdominal pain, chest pain, and a chronic nonproductive cough. The diagnosis is made by jejunal biopsy. Penicillin and tetracycline may alleviate the symptoms. See also **malabsorption syndrome.**

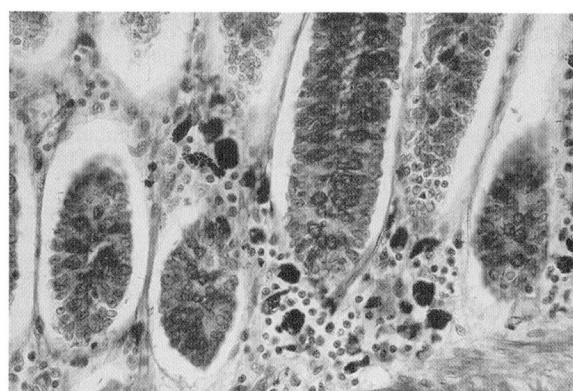

Whipple disease *(Kumar, Abbas, and Fausto, 2005)*

whipworm. See *Trichuris.*

whirlpool bath /(h)wurl/, the immersion of the body or a part of the body in a tank of warm water agitated by a jet of equally hot water and air, often used to clean infected wounds.

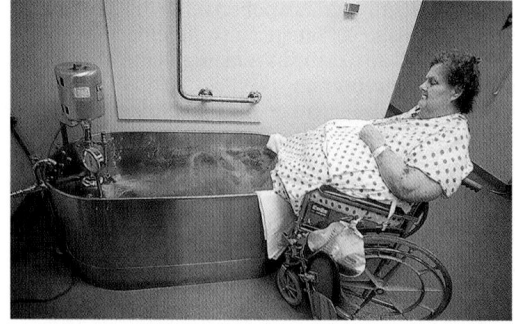

Whirlpool bath *(Elkin, Perry, and Potter, 2007)*

whistling face syndrome, whistling face-windmill vane hand syndrome. See **Freeman-Sheldon syndrome.**

white blood cell. See **leukocyte.**

white blood cell cast, a hyaline cast that contains white blood cells, such as in tubulointerstitial nephritis, pyelonephritis, or glomerulonephritis. Also called *leukocyte cast.*

white blood cell (WBC) count and differential count, a two-component blood test that first counts the total number of WBCs (leukocytes) in 1 cubic millimeter of peripheral venous blood and then measures the percentage of each type of leukocyte present in the same specimen (the differential count). The WBC and differential count are routinely measured as part of a complete blood count and, when done serially, have both diagnostic and prognostic value.

white blood cell scan, a nuclear scan to identify and localize an area of inflammation or infection. The scan is performed 4 to 24 hours after the white blood cells are separated from blood drawn from the patient, labeled with technetium or indium, and reinjected.

white cell, *(Informal)* white blood cell. See also **leukocyte.**

white corpuscle. See **leukocyte.**

white damp. See **damp.**

white fibrocartilage [AS, *hwit* + L, *fibra,* fiber, *cartilago*], a mixture of tough, white fibrous tissue and flexible cartilaginous tissue. It is divided into four types: interarticular fibrocartilage, connecting fibrocartilage, circumferential fibrocartilage, and stratiform fibrocartilage. Compare **hyaline cartilage, yellow cartilage.**

white gold, a gold alloy with a high content of palladium or platinum used in dental restorations, such as prepared tooth cavities and gold crowns. It has a higher fusion range, lower ductility, and greater hardness than a yellow gold alloy.

whitehead. *(Informal)* See **comedo.**

white infarct. See **pale infarct.**

white leg. See **phlegmasia alba dolens.**

white line. See **linea alba.**

white matter, the tissue of the central nervous system and much of the part of the cerebrum, consisting mainly of myelinated nerve fibers, but with some unmyelinated nerve fibers, embedded in a spongy network of neuroglia. It is subdivided in each half of the spinal cord into three funiculi: the anterior, the posterior, and the lateral white column. Each column subdivides into tracts that are closely associated in function. The anterior column divides into two ascending tracts and five descending tracts. The posterior column divides into two large ascending tracts, one small descending tract, and one intersegmental tract. The lateral column divides into six ascending tracts and four descending tracts. Also called **white substance.** Compare **gray matter.** See also **cerebrum, spinal cord, spinal tract.**

white noise, a sound in which the intensity is the same at all frequencies within a designated band.

white piedra. See **trichosporosis.**

whitepox. See **alastrim.**

white radiation, a form of radiation that results from the rapid deceleration of high-speed electrons striking a target, as occurs when the electron beam of a tungsten cathode strikes the tungsten or molybdenum target of the anode in an x-ray tube. Most of the x-rays emitted from a diagnostic or therapeutic x-ray unit represent white radiation. Also called **bremsstrahlung radiation.**

white ramus communicans, the communicating nerve branch between sympathetic ganglions and spinal nerves that is largely myelinated and located mainly in the thoracic and upper lumbar region.

white spot disease. See **lichen sclerosis et atrophicus.**

white substance. See **white matter.**

white thrombus, a clot composed of some combination of blood platelets, fibrin, clotting factors, and white blood cells but containing few or no erythrocytes.

white willow bark, a preparation of the bark of various *Salix* species native to central and southern Europe and collectively known as white willow, containing salicin, a precursor of salicylic acid, to which it is converted metabolically. It is used as an antiinflammatory and antipyretic.

whitlow /(h)witˮlō/ [Scand, *whick,* nail, *flaw,* crack], an inflammation of the end of a finger or toe that results in suppuration. See also **felon.**

WHO, abbreviation for **World Health Organization.**

WHO classification of lymphoid neoplasms, a classification of lymphomas, descended from the REAL classification, that divides them into three main categories (B-cell neoplasms, T-cell neoplasms, and Hodgkin lymphoma) based on morphology, immunophenotype, and genetic abnormalities.

whole blood /hōl/ [AS, *hal* + *blod*], donor blood that is unmodified except for the presence of an anticoagulant. Whole blood is rarely used for transfusion because it is typically separated into red cells, plasma, or other components after collection.

whole body dose, a measure of radiation exposure equal to the total amount of ionizing radiation absorbed by the body divided by the body's mass. It is meaningful only for fairly uniform irradiation over the entire body. See also **effective dose.**

whole-body irradiation, ionizing radiation exposure that affects the entire body. Short-term whole-body irradiation can cause injury or death in humans, mainly from damage to the GI tract and the bone marrow. However, such injury occurs only with doses far beyond the diagnostic range, such as with exposure to nuclear weapons. The effective dose equivalent limit for whole-body occupational exposure is 20 mSv per year. The nonoccupational effective dose equivalent limit is 1 mSv per year. Also called **total body irradiation.**

whole bowel irrigation, a method of treating poisoned patients by flushing large volumes of fluid through the GI tract.

whole milk, cow's milk from which no constituent such as fat has been removed. To be called whole milk it must contain 3.5% fat, 8.5% nonfat milk solids, and 88% water.

wholism, consideration of all aspects of an individual-mind, body, and spirit. Compare **holistic.**

whoop /hoop, (h)woop/, a noisy spasm of inspiration that terminates a coughing paroxysm in cases of pertussis. It is caused by a sudden sharp increase in tension on the vocal cords.

whooping cough. See **pertussis.**

whorl /(h)wurl/ [ME, *hwarwy*], a spiral turn, such as one of the turns of the cochlea or of the dermal ridges that form fingerprints.

WIA, abbreviation for **waking imagined analgesia.**

wick humidifier, a respiratory care device in which a piece of paper, sponge, or similar material that absorbs water by capillary action is inserted in the path of the airflow. With the addition of heat, high levels of humidity can be achieved over a wide range of flows and temperatures.

Widal test /vēdälsˮ/ [Georges F. I. Widal, French physician, 1862–1929], an agglutination test used to aid in the diagnosis of *Salmonella* infections such as typhoid fever. This test measures the level of cold or febrile agglutinins in the blood that causes red blood cells to stick together at low or high temperatures. A fourfold increase in titer of agglutinins to O or H antigens is highly suggestive of active infection. A high titer may persist for years after the disease or after immunization against typhoid fever.

wide-angle glaucoma. See **glaucoma.**

wide area network (WAN), a computer network that uses long-distance communications methods, such as telephone

W

lines, satellite links, or microwave transmission, to cover a geographic area larger than that which can be covered by a local area network (LAN).

Wiedenbach, Ernestine /wē″dənbak/, a German-born American nursing educator and writer. She taught maternal and newborn health nursing at Yale School of Nursing, was a leader in family-centered maternity nursing, and developed the full range of the art and science of obstetric nursing.

Wiener, Carolyn L., a nursing theorist who, with Marylin J. Dodd, developed the Theory of Illness Trajectory, which involves not only the patient but the family and caregivers. The theory helps elucidate how patients and families tolerate the states of uncertainty caused by the illness and manage the illness.

Wigraine, a vasoconstrictor containing an ergotamine and caffeine combination for the treatment of migraine. Brand name for **ergotamine tartrate.**

wild-type allele [AS, *wilde,* untamed; Gk, *typos,* mark, *genein,* to produce], a normal or standard form of a gene, as contrasted with a mutant form.

will [AS, *wyllan*], **1.** the mental faculty that enables one to consciously choose or decide on a course of action. **2.** the act or process of exercising the power of choice. **3.** a wish, desire, or deliberate intention. **4.** a disposition or attitude toward another or others. **5.** determination or purpose; willfulness. **6.** (in law) an expression or declaration of a person's wishes as to the disposition of property to be performed or take effect after death. Also called **volition.**

Williams syndrome /wil′yəmz/ [J.C.P. Williams, 20th-century New Zealand cardiologist], a condition characterized by supravalvular aortic stenosis, cognitive impairment, elfin facies, and transient hypercalcemia in infancy. Also called **elfin facies syndrome.**

Willis circle.   See **circle of Willis.**

willow fracture.   See **greenstick fracture.**

Wilms tumor /vilms/ [Max Wilms, German surgeon, 1867–1918], a malignant neoplasm of the kidney occurring in young children before the fifth year in 75% of the cases. It is slightly more common among females than males and among African-American children than Caucasian children. The most frequent early signs are hypertension, a palpable mass, pain, and hematuria. Diagnosis can be established by an excretory urogram with tomography. The tumor, an embryonal adenomyosarcoma, is well encapsulated in the early stage, but it may extend into lymph nodes, the renal vein, or the vena cava and metastasize to the lungs or other sites. Removal of resectable tumors by transperitoneal nephrectomy is recommended. Radiotherapy is used before or after surgery or palliatively in inoperable cases. Chemotherapy combined with surgery and irradiation is proving highly effective. Also called **adenomyosarcoma, nephroblastoma.** See also **kidney cancer.**

Wilson disease [Samuel A.K. Wilson, English neurologist, 1878–1937], a rare inherited disorder whereby a decrease in ceruloplasmin causes copper to accumulate slowly in the liver, to then be released, and to be taken up in other parts of the body. Hemolysis and hemolytic anemia occur as the copper accumulates in the red blood cells. Accumulation in the brain destroys certain tissue and may cause tremors, muscle rigidity, poorly articulated speech, and dementia. Kidney function is diminished. The liver becomes cirrhotic. Treatment of Wilson disease includes a reduction of copper in the diet and the prescription of copper-binding agents and penicillamine. Also called **hepatolenticular degeneration.**

Winckel disease [Franz Von Winckel, German gynecologist, 1837-1911], a fatal disease of the newborn caused by colon bacilli entering the stump of the umbilical cord.

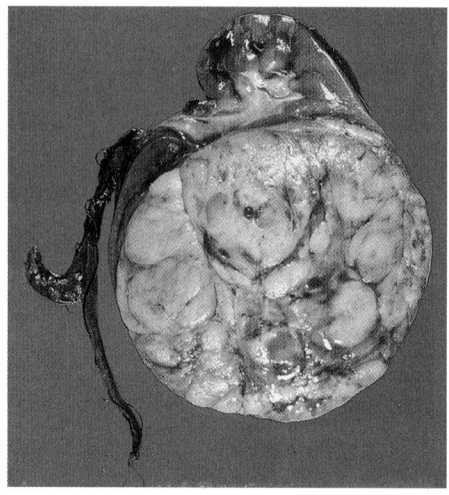

Wilms tumor *(Kumar et al, 2007)*

Characterized by hematuria, jaundice, enlarged spleen, collapse, and convulsions. See also **hemoglobinuria.**

windburn /wind″burn/ [AS, *wind,* air, *baernan*], a skin disorder caused by exposure to wind.

windchill /win′chil/, the loss of heat from the body when it is exposed to wind of a given speed at a given temperature and humidity.

windchill factor [AS, *wind,* air, *cele,* cold], the amount of chilling of the body, beyond that resulting from a cold ambient temperature, because of exposure to cool air currents. The windchill factor is expressed in degrees Celsius or Fahrenheit as the effective temperature felt by a person exposed to the weather. Because windchill factors are based on exposure of dry skin to cool air currents, air blowing at the same speed over a wet skin surface would cause additional loss of body heat and a greater windchill.

windchill index, a chart that compares temperatures of the atmosphere with various wind speeds, enabling one to calculate the windchill factor. The comparison is expressed in kilocalories per hour per square meter of skin surface.

winding sheet /wīn″ding/, a shroud for wrapping a dead body.

window [AS, *wind,* air, *owe,* eye], **1.** a surgically created opening in the surface of a structure or an anatomically occurring opening in the surface or between the chambers of a structure. **2.** a specific time period during which a phenomenon can be observed, a reaction monitored, or a procedure initiated.

windowed /win″dōd/, referring to an orthopedic cast that has an opening designed to relieve pressure that may irritate and inflame the skin or to provide access to an incision or a wound.

windpipe.   See **trachea.**

winegrower's lung /wīn″grō·ərs/, a type of hypersensitivity pneumonitis caused by contact with mold on grapes.

winged scapula /wingd/ [ONorse, *vaengr* + L, *scapulae,* shoulderblades], an abnormal prominence of the scapula caused either by projection of posterior angles of the ribs in a flat chest or by paralysis of the serratus anterior muscle.

wink reflex, an automatic closure of the eyelids in response to an appropriate stimulus. Also called **eye-closure reflex.**

Winstrol, an androgen used as an anabolic agent. Brand name for **stanozolol.**

winter cough [AS, *winter* + *cohhetan*], *(Nontechnical)* a chronic condition characterized by a persistent cough occasioned by cold weather. See also **cough.**

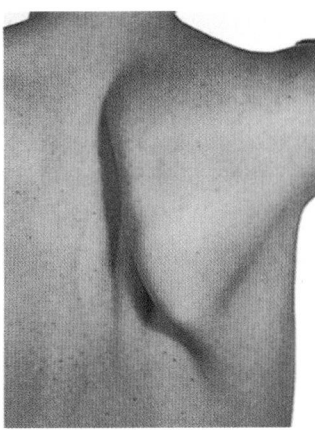

Winged scapula *(Perkin et al, 2011)*

wintergreen oil, a volatile oil with a characteristic odor and taste; used as a counterirritant in ointments or liniments for muscle pain and also as a flavoring agent. Also called **methyl salicylate.**

winter itch, *(Informal)* pruritus occurring in cold weather in people who have dry skin, particularly in those who have atopic dermatitis. Warmer temperature, an increase in humidity, and topical antipruritic emollients may offer relief. Also called **pruritus hiemalis.**

wire /wīr/, **1.** *n.,* a long, slender, flexible structure of metal, used in surgery and dentistry. **2.** *v.,* to insert such metal strands into a body structure, as into a broken bone to immobilize fragments.

wire suture [AS, *wir* + L, *sutura*], a stainless steel or silver wire used for uniting bone fracture fragments or in dentistry.

wiry pulse /wī″(ə)re/ [AS, *wir* + L, *pulsare,* to beat], an abnormal pulse that is strong but small.

wisdom tooth [AS, *wisdom* + *toth*], a third molar; the last tooth to erupt on each side of the upper and lower jaws, numbered 1, 16, 17, and 32. Wisdom teeth usually erupt between 17 and 25 years of age, often causing considerable pain, dental problems, and the need for extraction. Formerly called **dens serotinus.** See also **molar.**

wish fulfillment [AS, *wiscan,* to wish, *fullfyllan,* to fulfill], **1.** the gratification of a desire. **2.** (in psychology) the satisfaction of a desire or the release of emotional tension through such processes as dreams, daydreams, and neurotic symptoms. **3.** (in psychoanalysis) one of the primary motivations for dreams in which an unconscious desire or urge, unacceptable to the ego and superego because of sociocultural restrictions or feelings of personal guilt, is given expression.

wishful thinking [AS, *wiscan* + *thencan,* to think], the interpretation of facts or situations according to one's desires or wishes rather than as they exist in reality, usually used as an unconscious device to avoid painful or unpleasant feelings.

Wiskott-Aldrich syndrome /wis″ko tôl″drich/ [Alfred Wiskott, German pediatrician, 1898–1978; Robert Anderson Aldrich, American pediatrician, b. 1917], an immunodeficiency disorder inherited as a recessive X-linked trait, characterized by thrombocytopenia, eczema, inadequate T and B cell function, and an increased susceptibility to viral, bacterial, and fungal infections and to cancer. Treatment includes the prescription of appropriate antibiotics for specific infectious organisms and the administration of transfer factor from activated lymphocytes to increase the resistance to infection and to clear the eczema. See also **transfer factor.**

witch doctor, a shamanistic healer whose primary function is to cure the sick members of the community.

witch hazel [AS, *wican,* to bend; Ger, *hasel*], **1.** the common name for the shrub *Hamamelis virginiana,* indigenous to North America, from which an astringent extract is derived. **2.** a solution comprising the extract, alcohol, and water, used as an astringent. Also called **hamamelis water.**

witch's milk, a milklike substance secreted from the breast of the newborn, caused by circulating maternal lactating hormone. Also called **hexenmilch.**

withdrawal /withdrô″əl/ [ME, *with* + *drawen,* to take away], a common response to physical danger or severe stress characterized by a state of apathy, lethargy, depression, retreat into oneself and, in grave cases, catatonia and stupor. It is pathological if it interferes with a person's perception of reality and ability to function in society, such as in various forms of schizophrenia. See also **schizophrenia.**

withdrawal behavior, the physical or psychological removal of oneself from a stressor.

withdrawal bleeding, the passage of blood from the uterus, associated with the shedding of endometrium that has been stimulated and maintained by hormonal medication. It occurs when the medication is discontinued. In the endocrine evaluation of a woman with amenorrhea, withdrawal bleeding constitutes evidence that the woman's endometrium is responsive to hormonal stimulation and that the cause of her amenorrhea is probably not uterine.

withdrawal method, a contraceptive technique in coitus wherein the penis is withdrawn from the vagina before ejaculation. It is not reliable because small amounts of seminal fluid carrying millions of spermatozoa may be emitted without sensation before full ejaculation. Also called **coitus interruptus.**

withdrawal reflex. See **flexor withdrawal reflex.**

withdrawal symptoms, the unpleasant, sometimes life-threatening physiological changes that occur when some drugs are withdrawn after prolonged, regular use. The effects may occur after use of an opioid, antipsychotic, stimulant, sedative-hypnotic, alcohol, corticosteroid, or other substance to which the person has become physiologically or psychologically dependent. Other drug therapy may be used to relieve symptoms of withdrawal, such as methadone for heroin withdrawal, buprenorphine for opioid withdrawal, or chlordiazepoxide or clonazepam for alcohol withdrawal. Withdrawal symptoms can also be managed by gradually reducing the drug dose over time, as with the tapering of corticosteroids.

withdrawal syndrome [ME, *with* + *drawen,* to take away; Gk, *syn,* together, *dromos,* course], a physical and mental response after cessation or severe reduction in intake of a substance such as alcohol or opiates that has been used regularly to induce euphoria, intoxication, or relief from pain or distress. The body tissues become dependent on the regular reinforcing effect of the chemical so that interruption of the dosage induces an organic mental state characterized by anxiety, restlessness, insomnia, irritability, impaired attention, and often physical illness. Also called **abstinence syndrome.**

withdrawn behavior, a condition in which there is a blunting of the emotions and a lack of social responsiveness.

witness, a person who is present and can testify that he or she has personally observed an event, such as the signing of a will or consent form.

Wittmaack-Ekbom syndrome. See **restless legs syndrome.**

WMD, abbreviation for **weapons of mass destruction.**

WOB, abbreviation for **work of breathing.**

W

wobble /wob″əl/, an eccentric rotation that permits increased resolution of tomographic imaging devices composed of discrete detector systems. Typical eccentric excursions are 1 to 2 cm.

WOCN, abbreviation for *wound, ostomy, and continence nurses.* See **Wound, Ostomy and Continence Nurses (WOCN) Society.**

Wohlfart-Kugelberg-Welander disease. See **juvenile spinal muscular atrophy.**

Wolbachia /wol-bak′e-ah/, a genus of bacteria that infect a wide variety of invertebrates, including insects, spiders, crustaceans, and nematodes.

Wolff-Chaikoff effect /woolf″ chī″kəf/, the decreased formation and release of thyroid hormone in the presence of an excess of iodine.

wolffian body. See **mesonephros.**

wolffian cyst /wôl″fē·ən/ [Kaspar F. Wolff, German anatomist, 1733–1794; Gk, *kystis,* bag], **1.** a cyst of the wolffian duct. **2.** a cyst of a broad ligament of the uterus.

wolffian duct. See **mesonephric duct.**

Wolff-Parkinson-White syndrome /woolf″ pär″kinsən-(h) wīt″/ [Louis Wolff, American physician, 1898–1972; John Parkinson, English cardiologist, 1885–1976; Paul Dudley White, American cardiologist, 1886–1973], a disorder of atrioventricular (AV) conduction involving an accessory pathway. This syndrome is often identified by a characteristic delta wave seen on an electrocardiogram at the beginning of the QRS complex. It is amenable to radiofrequency ablation. See also **Lown-Ganong-Levine (LGL) syndrome.**

Wolff's law /wôlfs/ [Julius Wolff, German anatomist, 1836–1902], the principle that changes in the form and function of a bone are followed by changes in its internal structure.

Wolf-Herschorn syndrome, a genetic disorder of infants characterized by psychomotor and growth retardation, hypertonicity, seizures, and microcephaly. Other features include craniofacial anomalies, ocular malformations, cleft lip or palate, heart malformations, and scoliosis.

wolfram. See **tungsten.**

Wolfram syndrome /wool′frəm/ [D.J. Wolfram, 20th-century American physician], an autosomal-recessive syndrome, first evident in childhood, consisting of diabetes mellitus, diabetes insipidus, optic atrophy, and neural deafness. Also called **DIDMOAD syndrome.**

Wolman disease. See **cholesteryl ester storage disease.**

woman, an adult female human.

woman-year [AS, *wifman* + *year*], (in statistics) 1 year in the reproductive life of a sexually active woman; a unit that represents 12 months of exposure to the risk of pregnancy. Woman-years are used in calculating a pregnancy rate in the assessment of the effectiveness of the various methods of family planning and of the adverse effect on the birthrate of various environmental factors.

womb. See **uterus.**

wood alcohol. See **methanol.**

wood creosote, a substance obtained by distilling wood tar, mainly beech *(Fagus sylvatica).* It is a colorless to yellowish, oily, refractive liquid composed mainly of the phenol derivatives guaiacol and creosol. It was formerly used as an expectorant and external antiseptic but is now rarely used in the United States.

Wood lamp [Robert W. Wood, American physicist, 1868–1955; AS, *glaes*], an illuminating device with a nickel oxide filter that holds back all light except for a few violet rays of the visible spectrum and ultraviolet wavelengths of about 365 nm. It is used extensively to help diagnose fungal infections of the scalp and erythrasma. The light causes hairs infected with a fungus such as *Tinea capitis* to become brilliantly fluorescent. Also called **black light.**

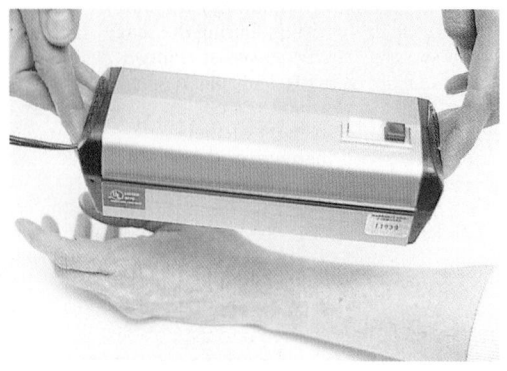

Wood lamp *(Wilson and Giddens, 2009)*

Wood's light. See **ultraviolet (UV) lamp.**

wood tick [AS, *wudu* + ME, *tike*], a hardshelled tick of the Ixodidae family and a natural reservoir of *Rickettsia rickettsii.* One species of wood tick, *Dermacentor andersoni,* is the principal vector in western North America of Rocky Mountain spotted fever, transmitted by *R. rickettsii.*

wool fat, a fatty substance obtained from sheep's wool and of which lanolin is a common chemical component. It consists primarily of lanosterol and cholesterol and its esters.

woolsorter's disease [AS, *wull* + Fr, *sorte* + L, *dis,* opposite of; Fr, *aise,* ease], the pulmonary form of anthrax, so named because it is an occupational hazard to those who handle sheep's wool. Early symptoms mimic those of influenza, but the patient soon develops high fever, respiratory distress, and cyanosis. If the disease is not treated at this stage, it is often fatal. Also called **pulmonary anthrax.** See also **anthrax.**

word association. See **controlled association.**

word association test. See **association test.**

word blindness [AS, *word* + *blind*], an inability to understand written language. A form of receptive aphasia caused by lesions in the parietal or parietal-occipital areas of the brain. The condition may be congenital or acquired as a result of disease or injury. Also called **alexia.** Compare **dyslexia.**

word deafness. See **auditory amnesia.**

word processor, a computer software application designed for the keyboarding, formatting, correcting, and storing of text, including correspondence, reports, manuscripts, and books or other publications.

word salad, a jumble of words and phrases that lacks logical coherence and meaning, often characteristic of disoriented individuals and persons with schizophrenia.

work conditioning, a physical exercise program designed to restore specific strength, flexibility, and endurance for return to work following injury, disease, or medically imposed rest; it may be part of a complete work hardening program when other aspects of functional restoration are required. Compare **work hardening.**

work hardening, a highly structured, goal-oriented individualized treatment program designed to maximize a person's ability to return to work. Work hardening uses work (real or simulated) as a treatment modality. Compare **work conditioning.**

working diagnosis, the identification of an illness based on subjective criteria and clinical judgment before confirmation by definitive diagnostic studies.

working occlusion [AS, *weorc* + L, *occludere,* to shut], the biting (occlusal) contacts of teeth on the side of the jaw toward which the mandible is moved.

working phase, (in psychology) the second stage of the therapist-client relationship. During this stage clients explore their experiences. Therapists assist clients in this process by helping them to describe and clarify their experiences, to plan courses of action and try out the plans, and to begin to evaluate the effectiveness of their new behavior. Should new behavior prove ineffective, therapists can assist clients in revising their courses of action.

working pressure, the recommended pressure, usually about 34 Pa (50 p.s.i.), for oxygen or compressed air leaving a cylinder. It is reduced by a pressure regulator for clinical use in respiratory therapy.

working through, a process by which repressed feelings are released and reintegrated into the personality.

workload, an amount of work to be performed within a specific time period.

work of breathing (WOB), the effort required to inspire air into the lungs. WOB accounts for 5% of total body oxygen consumption in a normal resting state but can increase dramatically during acute illness.

work of worrying, a coping strategy in which inner preparation through worrying increases the level of tolerance for subsequent threats.

workout, **1.** a test of ability and endurance. **2.** a physical exercise session.

work simplification, the use of special equipment, ergonomics, functional planning, and behavior modification to reduce the physical and psychological stresses of home maintenance for disabled people or their family members.

workstation, **1.** an area, as in an office, equipped with a computer or computer terminal. **2.** an electronic monitor, such as a computer or television screen, with controls for manipulating images.

work therapy [AS, *weorc* + Gk, *therapeia,* treatment], (in occupational therapy) a therapeutic approach in which the client sets objectives that can be addressed through activities, performs useful activities, learns valuable life skills (cognitive, psychosocial, emotional, and physical), or learns an occupation.

work tolerance, the kind and amount of work that a physically or mentally ill person can or should perform.

workup, the process of performing a complete patient evaluation, including history, physical examination, laboratory tests, and x-ray or other diagnostic procedures, to acquire an accurate database on which a diagnosis and treatment plan may be established.

World Health Organization (WHO), an intergovernmental organization within the United Nations system whose purpose is to aid in the attainment of the highest possible level of health by all people. Programs include education for current health issues, proper food supply and nutrition, safe water and sanitation, maternal and child health, immunization against major infectious diseases, and prevention and control of diseases. WHO is coordinating global strategies to control and prevent acquired immunodeficiency syndrome. Its functions include furnishing technical assistance, stimulating and advancing epidemiological investigation of diseases, recommending health regulations, promoting cooperation among scientific and professional health groups, and providing information and counsel relating to health matters. The headquarters for WHO is in Geneva, Switzerland.

worm /wurm/ [AS, *wyrm*], any of the soft-bodied, elongated invertebrates of the phyla Annelida, Nemathelminthes, or Platyhelminthes. Some worms are parasitic for humans. Kinds include **hookworm, pinworm, tapeworm.** See also **fluke, roundworm.**

wormian bone /vôr″mē-ən/ [Olaus Worm, Danish anatomist, 1588–1654; AS, *ban*], any of several tiny smooth bones, usually found at the serrated borders of the sutures between the cranial bones.

worthlessness /wurth″ləsnəs/, a component of low self-esteem, characterized by feelings of uselessness and inability to contribute meaningfully to the well-being of others or to one's environment.

wound /wo͞ond/ [AS, *wund*], **1.** any physical injury involving a break in the skin, usually caused by an act or accident rather than by a disease, such as a chest wound, gunshot wound, or puncture wound. **2.** to cause an injury, especially one that breaks the skin.

wound clip, a heavy metal clip used to approximate the edges of a skin incision. Also called **skin staple.**

wound culture and sensitivity (C&S), a microscopic examination done to determine the presence of pathogens in patients with suspected wound infections, which are most often caused by pus-forming organisms. Most organisms require approximately 24 hours to grow in the laboratory, but when antibiotic therapy needs to be instituted before lab results are available, Gram stain of the specimen smeared on a slide can be reported in less than 10 minutes to help determine the organism's possible identity and decide on an appropriate antibiotic treatment.

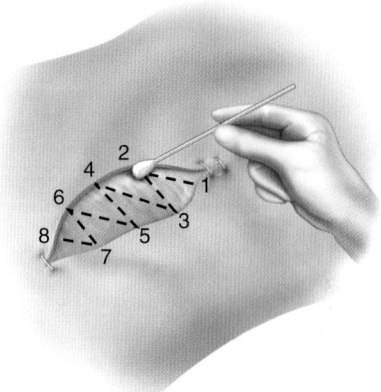

Wound culture and sensitivity: swabbing the wound bed *(Harkreader and Hogan, 2007)*

wound healing, a process to restore to a state of soundness any injury that results in an interruption in the continuity of external surfaces of the body. Also called **wound repair.** See also **healing, intention.**

wound irrigation, the rinsing of a wound or the cavity formed by a wound using a medicated solution, water, saline, or an antimicrobial liquid preparation.

Wound, Ostomy and Continence Nurses (WOCN) Society, an organization of nurses who manage conditions such as stomas, draining wounds, fistulas, vascular ulcers, pressure ulcers, neuropathic wounds, urinary incontinence, fecal incontinence, and functional disorders of the bowel and bladder. See also **enterostomal therapist.**

wound repair. See **wound healing.**

Wright-Giemsa stain, a modified stain using a combination of Wright stain and Giemsa stain in order to detect

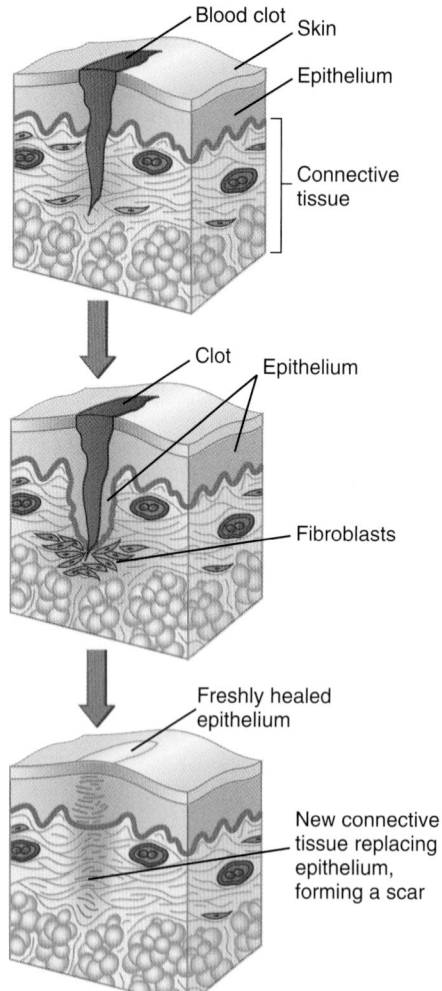

Stages of wound healing *(Patton and Thibodeau, 2010)*

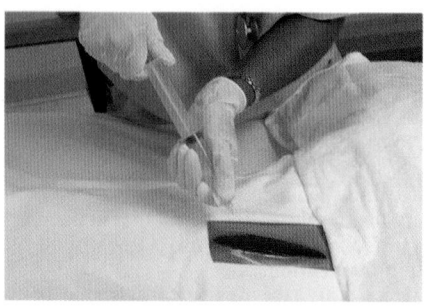

Wound irrigation *(Harkreader and Hogan, 2007)*

parasites, fungi, viral inclusion bodies, and other organisms in blood smears. See also **Giemsa stain, Wright stain.**

Wright stain /rīt/ [James H. Wright, American pathologist, 1869–1928; Fr, *teindre,* to dye], a stain containing methylene blue and eosin that is used to color blood specimens for microscopic examination, such as for complete blood count and particularly for malarial parasites.

wrinkle test /ring″kəl/ [AS, *gewrinclian,* to wind; L, *testum,* crucible], a test for nerve function in the hand by observing the presence of skin wrinkles after the hand has been placed in warm water for 20 to 30 minutes. Denervated skin does not wrinkle.

wrist. See **carpal bones.**

wrist clonus reflex /rist/, a sustained clonic muscle spasm caused by the sudden hyperextension of the wrist joint.

wristdrop [AS, *wrist + dropa*], a condition caused by paralysis of the extensor muscles of the hand and fingers or by injury of the radial nerve, resulting in inability to flex the wrist. An orthotic device can be used to provide support. Surgery is sometimes required if there is nerve impingement.

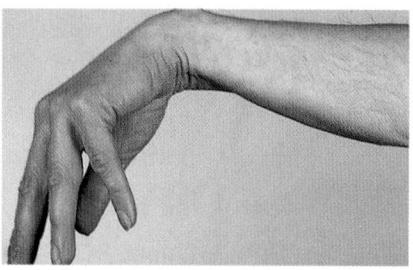

Wristdrop *(Perkin, 2002)*

wristdrop orthosis, an orthotic device the holds the hand in extension to support a weak or flaccid wrist. Modifications can be made so that it assists with daily activities such as writing or eating.

wrist ganglion, a cystic enlargement of a tendon sheath on the back of the wrist.

wrist-hand orthotic (WHO), a device used to immobilize the wrist and leave the fingers free. Formerly called **cockup splint.**

wrist joint. See **radiocarpal articulation.**

writer's cramp [AS, *writan,* to write, *crammian,* to fill], a painful, involuntary contraction of the muscles of the hand in a person attempting to write. It often occurs after long periods of writing. Also called **chirospasm, graphospasm.**

wrongful birth /rông″fəl/ [OE, *wrang,* twisted; ME, *burth*], a belief that a birth could have been avoided if the parents had been properly advised by a physician or health care provider that a pregnancy could occur or that a fetus would be deformed.

wrongful death statute [AS, *wrang + death +* L, *statuere,* to place], (in law) a statute existing in all states that provides that the death of a person can give rise to a cause of legal action brought by the person's beneficiaries in a civil suit against the person whose willful or negligent acts caused the death. Before the existence of these statutes, a suit could be brought only if the injured person survived the injury.

wrongful life [OE, *wrang,* twisted; AS, *lif*]. See **wrongful birth.**

wrongful life action, (in law) a civil suit usually brought against a physician or health facility on the basis of negligence that resulted in the wrongful birth or life of an infant. The parents of the unwanted child seek to obtain payment from the defendant for the medical expenses of pregnancy and delivery, for pain and suffering, and for the education and upbringing of the child. Wrongful life actions have been brought and won in several situations, including malpracticed tubal ligations, vasectomies, and abortions. Failure to diagnose pregnancy in time for abortion and incorrect medical advice leading to the birth of a defective child also have led to malpractice suits for a wrongful life.

wryneck. See **torticollis.**

wt, abbreviation for **weight.**

Wuchereria /vōō′kərē″rē·ə/ [Otto Wucherer, German physician, 1820–1873], a genus of filarial worms found in warm, humid climates. *Wucheria bancrofti,* transmitted by mosquitoes, is the cause of elephantiasis. See also **filariasis.**

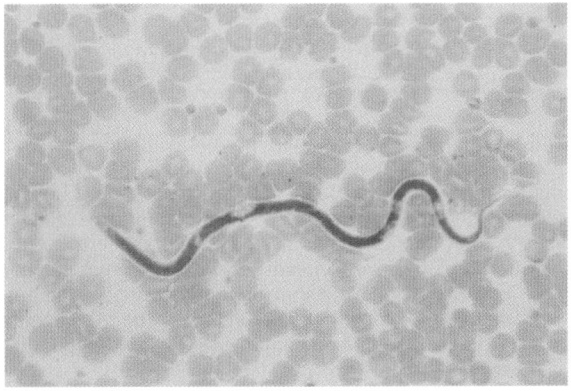

***Wuchereria bancrofti* microfilaria** *(Mahon, Lehman, and Manuselis, 2011)*

w/v, abbreviation for *weight per volume.* See **weight per volume (w/v) solution.**

w/w, abbreviation for **weight per weight.**

Wyburn-Mason's syndrome /wī′bərn·mā′sənz/ [Roger Wyburn-Mason, 20th-century British physician], a rare, nonhereditary condition characterized by arteriovenous aneurysms on one or both sides of the brain, with ocular anomalies, especially in the retina, facial nevi, and sometimes cognitive impairment.

Wycillin, a penicillin antibiotic agent. Brand name for **penicillin.**

Wydase, a medication injected to enhance the absorption of other medications. It also is used to treat extravasation and to aid in hypodermoclysis and in helping contrast dyes be more visible in subcutaneous urography. Brand name for **hyaluronidase.**

Wymox, a penicllin antibiotic medication. Brand name for **amoxicillin.**

Wytensin, a centrally acting alpha$_2$ agonist used to treat hypertension. Brand name for **guanabenz acetate.**

W

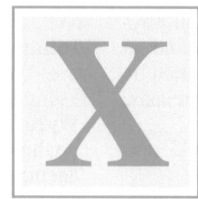

X

Xanax, an antianxiety, anticonvulsant muscle relaxant and sedative-hypnotic. Brand name for **alprazolam.**

-xanox, combining form for antiallergic respiratory tract drugs of the xanoxic acid group.

xanthan gum solution, a solution of xanthan gum, methylparaben, and propylparaben in purified water. It is used as a suspending, stabilizing, emulsifying, and thickening agent.

xanthelasma /zan'thəlaz'mə/ [Gk, *xanthos,* yellow + Gk, *elasma,* plate], a planar xanthoma involving the eyelid(s). Also called **xanthoma palpebrarum.** See also **xanthoma.**

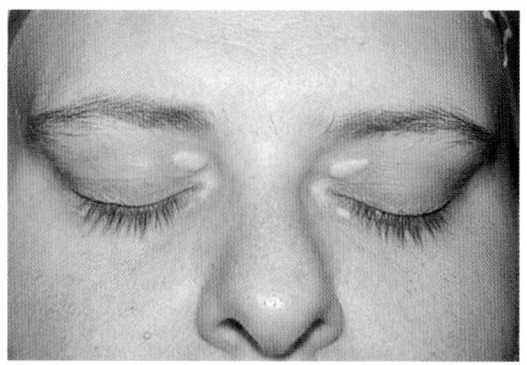

Xanthelasma *(Courtesy Dr. John W. Payne, The Wilmer Ophthalmological Institute, The Johns Hopkins University and Hospital)*

xanthelasmatosis /zan'thilaz'mətō'sis/ [Gk, *xanthos,* yellow, *elasma,* plate, *osis,* condition], a disseminated, generalized form of planar xanthoma frequently associated with reticuloendothelial disorders, especially multiple myeloma.

xanthene /zan'thēn/ [Gk, *xanthos,* yellow], a crystalline organic compound in which two benzene rings are fused to a central pyran ring. The pyran oxygen bridges the two benzene rings. It is a parent chemical structure of many medicinal elements.

xanthine /zan'thīn/ [Gk, *xanthos,* yellow], a nitrogenous by-product of the metabolism of nucleoproteins. It is normally found in the muscles, liver, spleen, pancreas, and urine. −*xanthic, adj.*

xanthine base [Gk, *xanthos,* yellow], a purine compound occurring in plants and animals as a metabolite of adenine and guanine. It is the parent structure of the methylxanthine alkaloids, which include caffeine in coffee, theophylline in tea, and theobromine in cocoa.

xanthine derivative, any one of the closely related alkaloids caffeine, theobromine, and theophylline. They are found in plants widely distributed geographically and are variously ingested as components in beverages such as coffee, tea, cocoa, and cola drinks. The xanthine derivatives or methylxanthines have pharmacological properties that stimulate the central nervous system, produce diuresis, and relax smooth muscles. Theobromine has low potency

and is seldom used as a pharmaceutic. Caffeine produces greater central nervous system stimulation than theophylline or theobromine and is a vasoconstrictor. Caffeine and theophylline affect the circulatory system, tending to dilate the systemic blood vessels but increasing cerebrovascular resistance with an associated decrease in cerebral blood flow and the oxygen tension of the brain. The xanthine derivatives are used as bronchodilators in the treatment of airway diseases such as asthma and COPD. Theophylline is most effective in such treatment and markedly increases vital capacity. The methylxanthines reinforce the release of certain secretions of various endocrine and exocrine tissues, except for mast cells and, possibly, certain other mediators of inflammation. Excess consumption of xanthine beverages may cause various problems, including seizures, restlessness and inability to sleep, GI irritation, and excessive myocardial stimulation characterized by premature systole and tachycardia. See also **caffeine, theobromine, theophylline.**

xanthinuria /zan'thinyŏŏr'ē·ə/ [Gk, *xanthos* + *ouron,* urine], **1.** the presence of excessive quantities of xanthine in the urine. **2.** a rare disorder of purine metabolism, resulting in the excretion of large amounts of xanthine in the urine because of the absence of an enzyme, xanthine oxidase, that is necessary in xanthine metabolism. This inherited deficiency may cause the development of kidney stones made of xanthine precipitate.

xanthism /zan'thizəm/, a genetic pigment anomaly characterized by yellow or yellowish-red hair, coppered skin, and reddish-brown irises.

xantho-, combining form meaning "yellow": *xanthochromia, xanthomatosis, xanthomasarcoma.*

xanthochromia /zan'thəkrō'mē·ə/, a pale yellow or straw-colored discoloration of cerebrospinal fluid. It is caused by the presence of hemoglobin breakdown products, indicating that the cerebrospinal fluid has contained blood in the recent past.

xanthochromic /zan'thəkrō'mik/ [Gk, *xanthos* + *chroma,* color], having a yellowish color, such as cerebrospinal fluid that contains blood or bile. Also called *xanthochromatic.*

xanthoderma /zan'thədur'mə/, skin that has a yellow coloration, as in jaundice.

xanthogranuloma /zan'thəgran'yəlō'mə/ *pl. xanthogranulomas, xanthogranulomata* [Gk, *xanthos* + L, *granulum,* little grain; Gk, *oma,* tumor], a tumor or nodule of granulation tissue containing lipid deposits. Kinds include **juvenile xanthogranuloma.**

xanthogranulomatous cholecystitis, a type of chronic cholecystitis characterized by proliferative fibrosis and infiltration by lipid-laden macrophages. It is often accompanied by obstruction from gallstones or calculi.

xanthoma /zanthō'mə/ *pl. xanthomas, xanthomata* [Gk, *xanthos* + *oma,* tumor], a benign, fatty, fibrous, yellowish plaque, nodule, or tumor that develops in the subcutaneous layer of skin, often around tendons. The lesion is characterized by the intracellular accumulation of cholesterol and cholesterol esters. It is associated with high cholesterol and/or triglycerides.

xanthoma disseminatum, a benign chronic condition in which small orange or brown papules and nodules develop on many body surfaces, especially on the mucous membrane of the oropharynx, larynx, and bronchi and in skinfolds and fissures. Also called **xanthoma multiplex.**

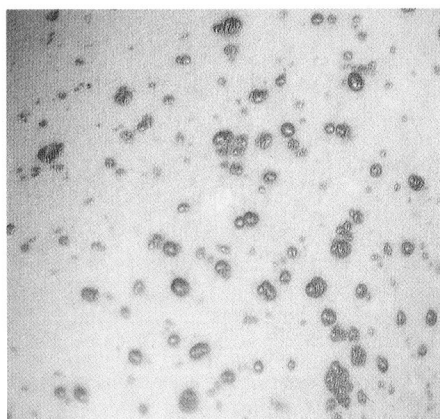

Xanthoma disseminatum (Callen et al, 2000)

xanthoma eruptivum. See **eruptive xanthoma.**
xanthoma multiplex. See **xanthoma disseminatum.**
xanthoma palpebrarum. See **xanthelasma.**
xanthoma planum. See **planar xanthoma.**
xanthomasarcoma /zan′thōməsärkō′mə/ *pl. xanthomasarcomas, xanthomasarcomata* [Gk, *xanthos + oma + sarx,* flesh, *oma,* tumor], a giant cell sarcoma of the tendon sheaths and aponeuroses that contains xanthoma cells.
xanthoma striatum palmare, a yellow or orange flat plaque or slightly raised nodule occurring in groups on the palms of the hands.
xanthoma tendinosum, a yellow or orange, elevated or flat, round papule or nodule occurring in clusters on tendons, especially the extensor tendons of the hands and feet, of individuals with hereditary lipid storage disease.

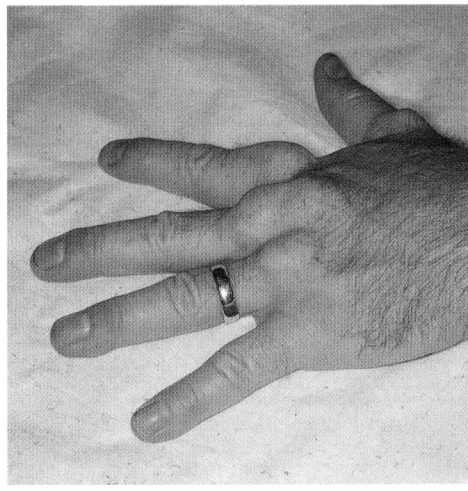

Xanthoma tendinosum (Swartz, 2009)

xanthomatosis /zan′thōmətō′sis/ [Gk, *xanthos + oma + osis,* condition], an abnormal condition in which there are deposits of yellowish fatty material in the skin, internal organs, and reticuloendothelial system. It may be associated with hyperlipoproteinemia, paraproteinemia, lipoid storage diseases, and other disorders of adipose tissue. Also called **xanthosis.** See also **lipemia, xanthoma, xanthoma palpebrarum.**
xanthomatosis bulbi, a fatty degeneration of the cornea.
xanthoma tuberosum, a round, flat or elevated, yellow or orange papule occurring in clusters on the skin of joints, especially the elbows and knees, usually in people who have a hereditary lipid storage disease such as hyperlipoproteinemia. The xanthomatous papules also may be associated with biliary cirrhosis and myxedema. Also called **tuberous xanthoma,** *xanthoma tuberosum multiplex.*

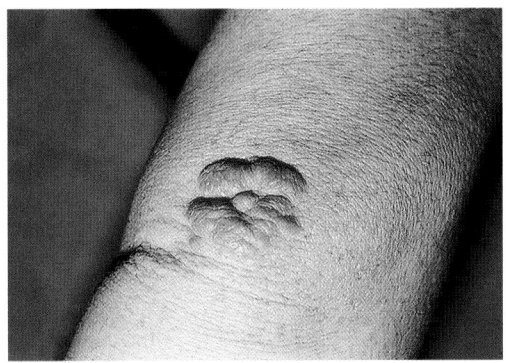

Xanthoma tuberosum (Callen et al, 2000)

Xanthomonas /zan′thəmon′əs/, a genus of gram-negative, rod-shaped aerobic bacteria of the family Pseudomonadaceae that produces a yellow pigment.
Xanthomonas maltophilia, a species of *Xanthomonas* bacteria commonly found in water, milk, and frozen food and in the upper respiratory tract, blood, and urine of humans. It is an opportunistic cause of infections in hospitalized and immunocompromised patients. This organism has been reclassified as *Stenotrophomonas maltophilia.*
xanthopsia /zanthop′sē·ə/ [Gk, *xanthos + opsis,* sight], an abnormal visual condition in which everything appears to have a yellow hue. It is sometimes associated with jaundice or digitalis toxicity.
xanthosis /zanthō′sis/ [Gk, *xanthos + osis,* condition], **1.** a yellowish discoloration sometimes seen in degenerating tissues of malignant diseases. **2.** See **xanthomatosis. 3.** See **carotenemia.**
xanthosis of retina, a generalized yellow discoloration of the retina between the macula and the optic disk, sometimes found in diabetic retinopathy.
xanthurenic acid /zan′thoore̅′nik/, a metabolite of tryptophan that occurs in normal urine and in elevated levels in patients with vitamin B_6 deficiency.
xanthurenic aciduria, a genetic disorder of tryptophan metabolism characterized by a deficiency of the kynureninase liver enzyme. It is also seen in vitamin B deficiency.
X chromosome, a sex chromosome that in humans and many other animals is present in both sexes, appearing singly in the cells of normal males and in duplicate in

X

the cells of normal females. The chromosome is present in all of the female gametes and in half of the male gametes, is much larger than the Y chromosome, and has many sex-linked genes associated with clinically significant disorders, such as hemophilia, Duchenne muscular dystrophy, and Hunter syndrome. Compare **Y chromosome.**

Xe, symbol for the element **xenon.**

xen(o), word element [Gk.], meaning *strange, foreign.*

xeno- /zē′ne-, zen′ō-/, combining form meaning "strange" or "pertaining to foreign matter": *xenodiagnosis, xenogenesis, xenology.*

xenoantibody, an antibody produced in one species to an antigen derived from a different species.

xenoantigen /zē′nō·an′təjən/, an antigen that occurs in organisms of more than one species.

xenobiotic /-bī·ot′ik/ [Gk, *xenos,* strange, *bios,* life], an exogenous chemical compound foreign to a given biological system. With respect to animals and humans, xenobiotics include drugs, drug metabolites, and environmental compounds, such as pollutants that are not produced by the body. In the environment, xenobiotics include synthetic pesticides, herbicides, and industrial pollutants that would not be found in nature.

xenodiagnosis /-dī·agnō′sis/, a method of diagnosing a vector-transmitted infection, for example Chagas disease, in which a laboratory-reared, pathogen-free insect is allowed to suck blood from a patient. The insect is then examined for the presence of the pathogen.

xenogeneic /-jənē′ik/ [Gk, *xenos + genein,* to produce], **1.** denoting individuals or cell types of different species and different genotypes. **2.** denoting tissues from different species that are therefore antigenically dissimilar. Also called **heterologous.** Compare **allogenic, syngeneic.**

xenogenesis /zen′əjen′əsis/, **1.** alternation of traits in successive generations; heterogenesis. **2.** the theoretic production of offspring that are totally different from both of the parents. −*xenogenetic, xenogenic, adj.*

xenograft /zen′əgraft′/ [Gk, *xenos + graphion,* stylus], tissue from another species used as a temporary graft in certain cases, as in treating a severely burned patient when sufficient tissue from the patient or from a tissue bank is not available. It is quickly rejected but provides a cover for the burn for the first few days, reducing fluid loss from the open wound. Also called **heterograft.** Compare **allograft, autograft, isograft.** See also **graft.**

xenology /zēnol′əjē/ [Gk, *xenos,* stranger, *logos,* science], the study of parasites.

xenoma /zēnō′mə/, a tumor that develops on tissue infected with certain parasites. Xenomas are most often noted in fish.

xenon (Xe) /zen′on, zē′non/ [Gk, *xenos,* strange], a gaseous nonmetallic element. Its atomic number is 54, and its atomic mass is 131.30. It has some anesthetic properties.

xenon-133 [Gk, *xenos,* strange], a radioactive isotope of xenon gas, used in radiographic studies of the lung.

xenoparasite /-per′əsīt/, an ectoparasite that has become pathogenic as a result of weakened resistance of the host.

xenophobia /-fō′bē·ə/ [Gk, *xenos + phobos,* fear], an anxiety disorder characterized by a pervasive, irrational fear or uneasiness in the presence of strangers, especially foreigners, or in new surroundings.

Xenopsylla /zen′ōsil′ə/, a genus of parasitic fleas responsible for the transmission of bubonic plague, murine typhus, and other infections. Many of more than 30 species of *Xenopsylla* are vectors of pathogens, including *X. cheopis,* a rat flea found worldwide. It is a vector of *Yersinia pestis,* the bacterial source of murine typhus, as well as of the plague.

xenotransplant. See **cross-species transplant.**

xenotype /zen′ətīp/, molecular variation based on differences in structure and antigenic specificity, such as immunoglobulin from different species.

xero- /zir′ō-/, combining form meaning "dryness": *xerostomia, xeroderma, xerophthalmia.*

xeroderma /zir′ədur′mə/ [Gk, *xeros,* dry, *derma* skin]. See **ichthyosis.**

xeroderma pigmentosum (XP), a rare inherited skin disease resulting from faulty DNA repair, characterized by extreme sensitivity to ultraviolet light, exposure to which results in freckles, telangiectases, keratoses, papillomas, carcinoma, and, possibly, melanoma. Keratitis and tumors developing on the eyelids and cornea may result in blindness. Exposure to sunlight must be avoided. Also called **Kaposi disease.**

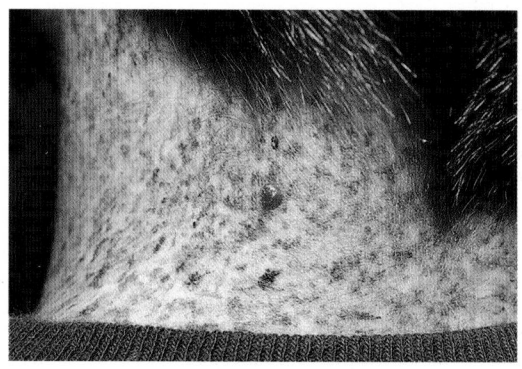

Xeroderma pigmentosum *(Callen et al, 2000)*

xerogram /zir′əgram′/ [Gk, *xeros + gramma,* record], *(Obsolete)* an x-ray image produced by xeroradiography.

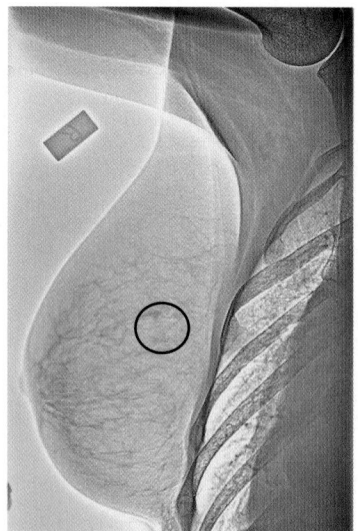

Xerogram *(Frank, Long, and Smith, 2012)*

xeromammography /-mamog′rəfē/, *(Obsolete)* the use of xerographic methods to produce radiographic images of the breasts.

xerophthalmia /zir′ofthal′mē·ə/ [Gk, *xeros + ophthalmos,* eye], a condition of dry and lusterless corneas and conjunctival areas, usually the result of vitamin A deficiency and associated with night blindness.

xeroradiography /-rā′dē·og′rəfē/ [Gk, *xeros +* L, *radiare,* to emit rays; Gk, *graphein,* to record], *(Obsolete)* a diagnostic x-ray technique in which images were produced electrically rather than chemically. The latent image was made visible with a powder toner similar to that used in a copying machine. The powder image was transferred and heat-fused to a sheet of paper. Also called *xerography.*

xerosis. See **dry skin.**

xerostomia /zir′əstō′mē·ə/ [Gk, *xeros + stoma,* mouth], dryness of the mouth caused by cessation of normal salivary secretion. The condition is a symptom of various diseases such as diabetes, acute infections, hysteria, and Sjögren syndrome and can be caused by paralysis of facial nerves. It may also result from radiation treatments for cancers of the face, head, or neck. It is also caused by an adverse reaction to drugs.

xerotic eczema /zi·rot′ik ek′zə·mə/. See **asteatosis.**

xerotic keratitis /zirot′ik/ [Gk, *xeros,* dry, *keras,* horn, *itis,* inflammation], an inflammation of the cornea resulting from dryness of the conjunctiva. Underlying causes may be malnutrition, a deficiency of vitamin A, or autoimmune diseases.

xi /zī, sī/, Ξ, ξ, the 14th letter of the Greek alphabet.

Xifaxan, an antibiotic medication. Brand name for **rifaximin.**

X-inactivation. See **Lyon hypothesis.**

xiphi-. See **xipho-, xiphi-.**

xiphisternal articulation /zif′istur′nəl/ [Gk, *xiphos,* sword, *sternon,* chest; L, *articulare,* to divide into joints], the cartilaginous connection between the xiphoid process and the body of the sternum. This joint usually ossifies at puberty. Compare **manubriosternal articulation.**

xipho-, xiphi-, combining form meaning "sword" or "xiphoid process": *xiphodynia, xiphoid, xiphopagus.*

xiphodynia /zī′fōdin′ē·ə/, a pain in the xiphoid process.

xiphoid /zif′oid/ [Gk, *xiphos,* sword, *eidos,* form], **1.** shaped like a sword. **2.** the pointed section of cartilage at the lower end of the sternum. See **xiphoid process.**

xiphoid process /zif′oid/ [Gk, *xiphos + eidos,* form; L, *processus,* going forth], the smallest of three parts of the sternum, articulating with the inferior end of the body of the sternum above and laterally with the seventh rib. Several muscles of the abdominal wall are attached to the xiphoid process, including the rectus abdominis. Also called **ensiform cartilage, ensiform process,** *xiphisternum,* **xiphoid,** *xiphoid appendix.* Compare **manubrium.**

xiphopagus /zīfop′əgəs/, conjoined twins united at the xiphoid process of the sternum.

X-linked /eks′ lingkt/, pertaining to genes or to the characteristics or conditions they transmit that are carried on the X chromosome. Compare **Y-linked.** See also **sex-linked disorder.** *–X linkage, n.*

X-linked bulbospinal neuropathy, a hereditary disorder of the spinal cord and medulla oblongata in males, with associated endocrine features that include azoospermia, gynecomastia, glucose intolerance, and feminized skin changes.

X-linked disorder, disease or disorder associated with genetic abnormalities on the X chromosomes. Kinds include **muscular dystrophy, hemophilia.**

X-linked–dominant inheritance, a pattern of inheritance in which the transmission of a dominant allele on the X chromosome causes a characteristic to be manifested. Hypophosphatemic vitamin D-resistant rickets is an example of such inheritance. X-linked–dominant inheritance closely resembles autosomal-dominant inheritance. Compare **X-linked–recessive inheritance.** See also **sex-linked disorder.**

X-linked gene, a gene carried on the X chromosome; the corresponding trait, whether dominant or recessive, is always expressed in males, who have only one X chromosome. The term "X-linked" is sometimes used synonymously with "sex-linked," because no genetic disorders have as yet been associated with genes on the Y chromosome.

X-linked ichthyosis. See **sex-linked ichthyosis.**

X-linked inheritance, a pattern of inheritance in which the transmission of traits varies according to the sex of the person, because the genes on the X chromosome have no counterparts on the Y chromosome. The inheritance pattern may be recessive or dominant. The trait determined by a gene on the X chromosome is always expressed in males. Transmission from father to son does not occur. Compare **autosomal inheritance.** Kinds include **X-linked–dominant inheritance, X-linked–recessive inheritance.** See also **sex-linked.**

X-linked lymphoproliferative syndrome, a rare X-linked immunodeficiency in which there is a normal response to childhood infection but infection with Epstein-Barr produces a fatal lymphoproliferative disorder. Most patients die of acute infection. Others develop hypogammaglobulinemia, B-cell lymphoma, aplastic anemia, or agranulocytosis. See also **Epstein-Barr virus.**

X-linked mucopolysaccharidosis. See **Hunter syndrome.**

X-linked–recessive inheritance, a pattern of inheritance in which the transmission of a recessive allele on the X chromosome results in a carrier state in females and characteristics of an abnormal condition in males. Affected people have unaffected parents (except for the rare situation in which the father is affected and the mother is a carrier). One half of the female siblings of an affected male carry the trait. Unaffected male siblings do not carry the trait. Sons of affected males are unaffected, and daughters of affected males are carriers. Unaffected male children of a carrier female do not carry the trait. Compare **X-linked–dominant inheritance.**

XO, the designation of a cell in an individual in whom only one sex chromosome is present. Either the other X or the Y chromosome is missing so that each cell is monosomic and contains a total of 45 chromosomes. All XO individuals are females with Turner syndrome. Individuals with only a Y chromosome do not survive. See also **Turner syndrome.**

Xolair, a monoclonal antibody used to treat more severe cases of asthma not responding to standard options. Brand name for **omalizumab.**

XP, abbreviation for **xeroderma pigmentosum.**

x-ray, 1. electromagnetic radiation with wavelengths between about 0.005 and 10 nm. X-rays are produced when electrons traveling at high speed strike certain materials, particularly heavy metals such as tungsten. They can penetrate most substances and are used to investigate the integrity of

X

certain structures, to therapeutically destroy diseased tissue, and to make radiographic images for diagnostic purposes, as in radiography and fluoroscopy. *Discrete x-rays* are those with precisely fixed energies that are characteristic of differences between electron binding energies of a particular element. Tungsten, for example, has 15 different effective energies and no more, representing emissions from 5 different electron shells. Also called **roentgen ray,** *x radiation.* **2.** an image made by projecting x-rays through organs or structures of the body onto an image receptor. Structures that are relatively radiopaque (allow few x-rays to pass through), such as bones and cavities filled with a radiopaque contrast medium, cast a shadow on the image receptor. **3.** to make a radiograph. See also **contrast medium, electron, fluoroscopy, radiopaque.**

x-ray dermatitis, a skin inflammation caused by exposure to x-rays. Excessive exposure to x-rays can lead to skin cancer. Also called **radiation dermatitis.**

x-ray film, a radiograph made by projecting x-rays through organs or structures of the body onto a photographic film. The latent image is made manifest and permanent through chemical processing of the film. It is not widely used in current practice. Compare **radiographic image.**

x-ray fluoroscopy, real-time imaging using an x-ray source that projects through the patient onto an image intensifier or an electronic signal that is converted to a digital image.

x-ray image, a record or representation of an area exposed to x-rays or similar radiation. It is used in the assessment of health and illness. Also called **radiograph.**

x-ray microscope, a microscope that produces images using x-rays and records them or projects them as enlargements. Images produced by x-ray microscopes may be examined at large magnifications with a light microscope.

x-ray pelvimetry, a radiographic examination used to determine the dimensions of the bony pelvis of a pregnant woman and, if possible, the biparietal diameter of her baby's head. It is performed when doubt exists as to whether the head can pass safely through the pelvis in labor. Because minor degrees of cephalopelvic disproportion are often overcome safely in labor by molding of the fetal skull and because major disproportions may be detected by clinical pelvimetry without x-rays, the value of x-ray pelvimetry is frequently judged to be insufficient to warrant the risk of radiation exposure. Other diagnostic tools, among them ultrasonography, often provide the necessary information with less apparent risk. Compare **clinical pelvimetry.** See also **cephalopelvic disproportion, contraction, dystocia.**

x-ray technologist, now called *radiologic technologist.* See also **radiologic technologist.**

x-ray tube, a large vacuum tube containing a tungsten filament cathode and an anode that often is a tungsten disk. When heated to incandescence, the cathode emits a cloud of electrons that produce x-rays when they strike the surface of the anode at high speed. The anode is designed to deflect the x-rays toward an object to be radiographed. X-ray tubes are produced in a variety of designs for different purposes. Low-kilovoltage x-ray tubes may contain anodes made of molybdenum rather than tungsten. Some anodes are stationary and others rotate at high speed. Because of the intense heat generated by x-ray production, the specific design usually includes devices to help dissipate the heat.

XX /ekseks′/, the designation for the normal sex chromosome complement in the human female. See also **X chromosome.**

XXX syndrome /trip′əleks′/, a human sex chromosomal aberration characterized by the presence of three X chromosomes and two Barr bodies instead of the normal XX complement, so that somatic cells contain a total of 47 chromosomes; trisomy X. The condition occurs approximately once in every 1000 live female births and is confirmed diagnostically by the presence of the extra Barr body in the cells. Individuals with the anomaly show no significant clinical manifestations, although there is usually some degree of intellectual disability. Because selective migration of the X chromosome occurs during meiosis, half of the offspring of a trisomy X female will be both chromosomally and phenotypically normal. Also called **triple X syndrome.**

XXX, XXXX, XXXXX /fôreks′, fīveks′/, the designations for abnormal sex chromosome complements in the human female in which there are, respectively, three, four, or five instead of the normal two X chromosomes so that each somatic cell contains a total of 47, 48, or 49 chromosomes. Although there is no consistent phenotype associated with such aberrations, the risk of congenital anomalies and intellectual disability in the affected individual increases significantly as the number of X chromosomes increases.

XXXY, XXXXY, XXYY /thrē′ekswī, fôr′ekswī, dob′əleks′-dob′əlwī′/, the designations for abnormal sex chromosome complements in the human male in which there are more than the normal one X and one Y chromosome, resulting in a total of 48, 49, or more chromosomes in each somatic cell. The aberration is a variant of Klinefelter syndrome. In general, the more X chromosomes there are, the greater the number of congenital defects and the severity of intellectual disability in the affected individual. See also **Klinefelter syndrome.**

XXY syndrome. See **Klinefelter syndrome.**

XY /ekswī′/, the designation for the normal sex chromosome complement in the human male. See also **X chromosome, Y chromosome.**

xylitol /zī′litôl/, a five-carbon sugar alcohol derived from xylose and as sweet as sucrose. Used as a noncariogenic sweetener and also as a sugar substitute in diabetic diets.

xylo-, combining form meaning "wood": *xylose.*

Xylocaine, a local anesthetic agent. Brand name for **lidocaine hydrochloride.**

xylometazoline hydrochloride /zī′lōmetaz′əlēn/, a topical alpha-adrenergic vasoconstrictor.

■ INDICATIONS: It is prescribed as an intranasal medication spray for the treatment of congestion due to colds, hay fever, sinusitis, and other upper respiratory allergies.

■ CONTRAINDICATIONS: Glaucoma or known hypersensitivity to this drug or to sympathomimetic medications prohibits its use. It should be used with caution in patients with cardiovascular disease. The topical application should not exceed 3 to 5 days of use.

■ ADVERSE EFFECTS: The most common adverse effects associated with topical application are local irritation and rebound congestion. Serious adverse effects associated with systemic absorption include sedation, restlessness, and alterations in cardiovascular function.

xylose /zī′lōs/, an aldopentose sugar produced by hydrolyzing straw and corn cobs. It is incompletely absorbed when taken by mouth and is used in diagnostic studies of the digestive tract.

xylose absorption test, a laboratory test for intestinal absorption of the monosaccharide D-xylose. Absorption of

D-xylose occurs readily in the normal intestine but is diminished in patients experiencing malabsorption.

xysma /zis′mə/, membranous shreds sometimes found in the feces of patients with diarrhea.

XYY syndrome /eks′dob′əlwī′/, the phenotypic manifestation of an extra Y chromosome, which tends to have a positive effect on height and may have a negative effect on mental and psychological development. However, the anomaly also occurs in normal males. See also **trisomy.**

Xyzal, a second-generation antihistamine medication. Brand name for **levocetirizine.**

X

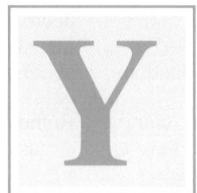

Y, symbol for the element **yttrium**.

-y, suffix meaning "a condition or process having the nature or quality of": *myopathy*.

YAC, abbreviation for **yeast artificial chromosome**.

YAG, a crystal used in some types of lasers. Abbreviation for *yttrium aluminum garnet*.

Yallow, Rosalyn Sussman [U.S. scientist, 1921–2011], a medical physicist whose research involved the discovery and development of a process for recognizing and verifying minute particles of biological active substances.

yang, a polarized aspect of ch'i that is active or positive energy. Compare **yin**. See also **ch'i, yin/yang principle**.

Yangtze edema /yang'sē/, a localized pruritic and erythematous subcutaneous induration caused by *Gnathostoma spinigerum* larvae in gnathostomiasis. Also called **gnathostomiasis**.

Yankauer suction catheter [S. Yankauer, American otolaryngologist, 1872–1932], a rigid hollow tube made of metal or disposable plastic with a curve at the distal end to facilitate the removal of thick pharyngeal secretions during oral pharyngeal suctioning.

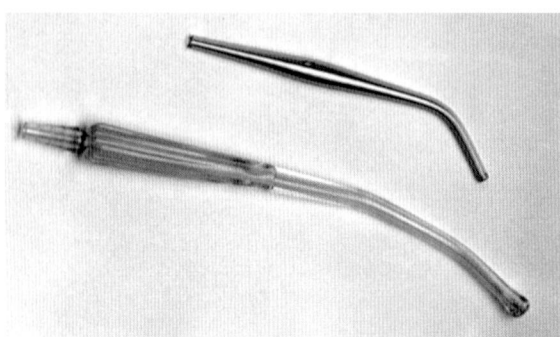

Yankauer suction catheters. Pediatric *(top)* and adult *(bottom)* *(Aitkenhead et al, 2013)*

yarrow, an herb native to Europe and Asia, now grown in North America.

■ INDICATIONS: This herb may help heal cuts and bruises and may treat other bleeding disorders of the GI tract. Chemical analysis supports the possibility of beneficial effects, but there are insufficient reliable data from human studies to assess its efficacy.

■ CONTRAINDICATIONS: Yarrow should not be used during pregnancy and lactation. It is also contraindicated in those with known hypersensitivity to this plant or other members of the Compositae family, such as *Chamomilla recutita*, *Tanacetum parthenium*, or *T. vulgare*.

yaw /yô/ [Carib, *VaVa*], a lesion of the syphilis-like tropical disease of yaws. The initial lesion or primary sore is identified as the mother yaw.

yawn /yôn/ [AS, *geonian*], an involuntary act of opening the mouth wide and taking a deep breath. It tends to occur when a person is bored, drowsy, or depressed and may be

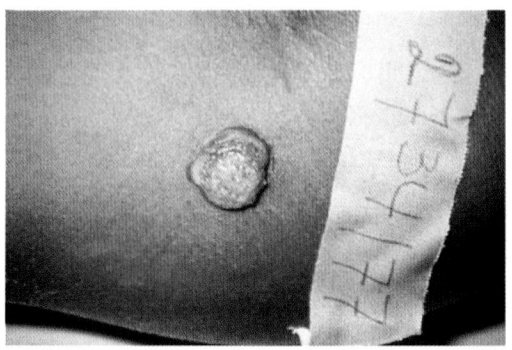

Mother yaw on thigh *(Bennett et al, 2015)*

accompanied by upper body movements or the act of stretching to aid chest expansion. There is a contagious aspect of yawning; the etiology of this phenomenon is unknown.

yaws /yôs/ [Afr, *yaw*, raspberry,], a chronic bacterial infectious disease caused by *Treponema pallidum* subspecies *pertenue*. The World Health Organization identifies two stages of the disease: early (infectious) and late (noninfectious). Also called **bouba, buba, frambesia, framboesia, parangi, patek, pian**. Compare **bejel, pinta, syphilis**.

■ OBSERVATIONS: Yaws is characterized by chronic ulcerating sores anywhere on the body but usually on the legs. The initial lesion, the mother yaw, occurs at the point of entry for the bacteria. The sores associated with yaws are yellowish or reddish in shape and appearance often resemble currants, strawberries, or raspberries. In the late stage, bone, joint, and soft tissue deformities may occur. Lesions are not contagious at this point. Serologic tests confirm the diagnosis of yaws.

■ INTERVENTIONS: A single oral dose of the antibiotic azithromycin can completely cure yaws. An intramuscular injection of penicillin G can also be used in treatment.

■ PATIENT CARE CONSIDERATIONS: Without treatment, infection can lead to chronic disfigurement and disability. Eradication efforts in countries where yaws remains an endemic disease are ongoing. Overcrowding, poor hygiene, and socioeconomic factors contribute to the persistence of this disease.

Yb, symbol for the element **ytterbium**.

Y-cartilage, a Y-shaped band of connective tissue that extends through the acetabulum to join the ilium, ischium, and pubis.

Y chromosome, a sex chromosome that in humans and many other animals is present only in the male, appearing singly in the normal male. It is present in one half of the male gametes and none of the female gametes, is much smaller than the X chromosome, and has genes associated with triggering the development and differentiation of male characteristics. Compare **X chromosome**.

years of potential life lost (YPLL), an evaluation of the economic, social, and other consequences of a premature

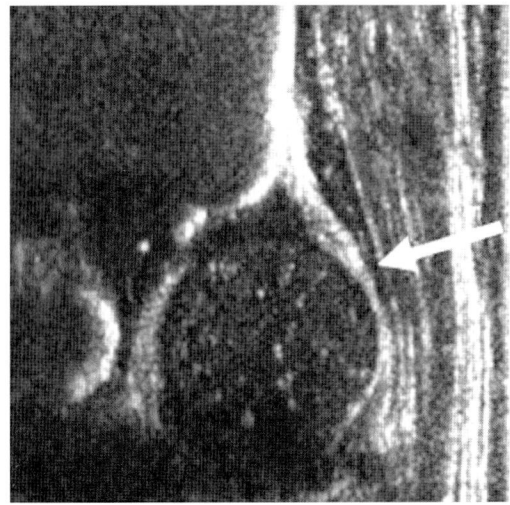

Y-cartilage sonogram *(Zitelli et al, 2012)*

death from injury or disease; such evaluations take into consideration the potential productivity of deceased individuals if they had lived normal life spans.

yeast /yēst/ [AS, *gist*], any unicellular, usually oval, nucleated fungus that reproduces by budding. *Candida albicans* is a kind of pathogenic yeast.

yeast artificial chromosome (YAC), a yeast chromosome used in recombinant DNA procedures. It can carry large segments of foreign DNA.

yellow cartilage. See **elastic cartilage.**

yellow fever, an acute arbovirus infection transmitted by mosquitoes. It is characterized by headache, fever, jaundice, vomiting, and bleeding. There is no specific treatment, and mortality is about 5%. Recovery is followed by lifelong immunity. Immunization for travelers to endemic areas is advised. The vaccine against yellow fever is highly effective, producing a greater-than-10-year immunity to the disease. Nonhuman primates are a reservoir of infection.

yellow fever vaccine, a vaccine produced from live, attenuated yellow fever virus grown in chick embryos.
■ INDICATIONS: It is prescribed for immunization against yellow fever. It is recommended for people who are traveling to or living in areas at risk for yellow fever virus in Africa and South America,
■ CONTRAINDICATIONS: Immunosuppression, pregnancy, or known hypersensitivity to chicken or egg protein prohibits its use.
■ ADVERSE EFFECTS: Among the more serious adverse effects are fever, malaise, and hypersensitivity reactions.

yellow hepatization. See **hepatization.**

yellow jacket venom, a toxin injected by the stings of wasps and hornets. It can induce potentially fatal anaphylactic shock.

yellow marrow, bone marrow in which the fat cells predominate in the meshes of the reticular network. See also **bone marrow.**

yellow nail syndrome, a rare condition in which there is complete or almost complete cessation of nail growth and loss of cuticle because of lymph in the soft layers of tissue under the skin. Nails become thickened, convex, opaque, and pale yellow to yellowish green. The condition is associated with pulmonary disorders and lymphedema.

yerba maté, an herbal product taken from an evergreen tree belonging to the holly family that is native to parts of South America.

■ INDICATIONS: This herb is used as a diuretic and depurative. It is also used in chronic fatigue syndrome.
■ CONTRAINDICATIONS: Yerba maté should not be used during pregnancy and lactation, in children, or in those with anxiety disorders, hypertension, or known hypersensitivity to this plant.

Yersinia /yersin″ē·ə/ [Alexandre E.J. Yersin, French bacteriologist, 1862–1943], a genus of nonmotile ovoid or rod-shaped gram-negative bacteria of the Enterobacteriaceae family.

Yersinia **arthritis** [Alexandre E.J. Yersin], a polyarticular inflammation occurring a few days to 1 month after the onset of infection caused by *Yersinia enterocolitica* or *Y. pseudotuberculosis* and usually persisting longer than 1 month. Knees, ankles, toes, fingers, and wrists are most often affected. Cultures of synovial fluid yield no infectious organism. The clinical presentation may mimic juvenile rheumatoid arthritis, rheumatic fever, or Reiter syndrome and may be associated with erythema nodosum or erythema multiforme. Treatment is with antibiotics.

Yersinia enterocolitica, a ubiquitous species isolated from mammals, birds, and frogs, and from material contaminated by feces; it is transmitted by infected food and water and by person-to-person contact and causes yersiniosis in humans. Some strains produce a heat-stable enterotoxin.

Yersinia pestis [Alexandre E.J. Yersin; L, *pestis,* plague], a species of small gram-negative bacteria that causes plague. The primary host is the rat, but other small rodents also harbor the organism. A person without symptoms may be a carrier, but this happens rarely. *Yersinia pestis* is hardy, living for long periods in infected carcasses, the soil of the host's habitat, or sputum. Also called *Pasteurella pestis.* See also **plague, bubonic plague, pneumonic plague, septicemic plague.**
■ OBSERVATIONS: Symptoms of infection are dependent on the method of exposure; however, fever and weakness are common.
■ INTERVENTIONS: Antibiotics should be administered as soon as the infection is recognized. Circulatory and other supportive care based on symptoms is necessary.
■ PATIENT CARE CONSIDERATIONS: When treatment is not provided, serious illness and death can occur. Infection can occur anywhere but is more common in Africa and Asia.

Yersinia pseudotuberculosis, a species found in the intestinal tract of birds, rodents, and other animals. It causes mesenteric adenitis and pseudotuberculosis in humans who have contact with infected food or animals.

yersiniosis /yər·sin′·ē·ō′sis/, infection with bacteria of the genus *Yersinia,* especially *Y. enterocolitica.*
■ OBSERVATIONS: Symptoms of infection include acute gastroenteritis and mesenteric adenitis in children and arthritis, septicemia, and erythema nodosum in adults.
■ INTERVENTIONS: Uncomplicated cases of diarrhea due to *Y. enterocolitica* usually resolve on their own without antibiotic treatment. However, in more severe or complicated infections, antibiotics are required.
■ PATIENT CARE CONSIDERATIONS: Careful hand washing and caution in the preparation and storage of food play a major role in the prevention of the disease.

Y fracture, a Y-shaped fracture of the tissue between condyles.

yield, 1. an amount or quantity produced in return for an effort or investment. **2.** the energy released by a nuclear reaction.

yin, a polarized aspect of ch'i that is passive or negative energy. See also **ch'i, yang, yin/yang.**

yin/yang, a Chinese philosophy that each entity is one but contains two equal and opposite forces. The forces of yang

Y

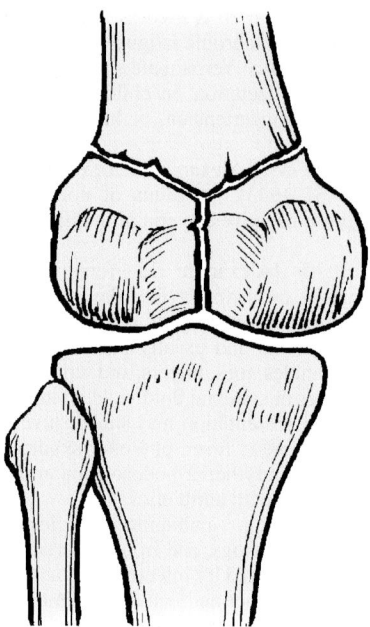

Y fractures of the femoral condyles
(Dandy and Edwards, 2009)

include maleness, the sun, and heat. The forces of yin include femaleness, darkness, and cold. Many holistic care practices are rooted in the belief that there must be a balance between yin and yang forces for health and that illness is the result of imbalance. See also **ch'i, yin/yang principle.**

yin/yang principle, in Chinese philosophy, the concept of polar complements existing in dynamic equilibrium and always present simultaneously. In traditional Chinese medicine, a disturbance of the proper balance of yin and yang causes disease, and the goal is to maintain or to restore this balance.

-yl, suffix used in naming radicals: *alkyl, methyl, hydroxyl.*

-ylene, suffix for chemical terms relating to a bivalent hydrocarbon radical.

Y-linked /wī″lingkt/, pertaining to genes or to the characteristics or conditions they transmit that are carried on the Y chromosome. Excess hair on the pinna of the ear may be Y-linked. Compare **X-linked.** See also **sex-linked.** *–Y linkage, n.*

Yodoxin, an antiamebic agent. Brand name for **diiodohydroxyquin, iodoquinol.**

yoga, a discipline that focuses on the body's musculature, posture, breathing mechanisms, and consciousness. The goal of yoga is attainment of physical and mental well-being through mastery of the body, achieved through exercise, holding of postures, proper breathing, and meditation.

yogurt /yō″gərt/ [Turk, *yoghurt*], a slightly acid, semisolid, curdled milk preparation made from either whole or skimmed cow's milk and milk solids by fermentation with organisms from the genus *Lactobacillus.* It is rich in B complex vitamins and a good source of protein. It also provides a medium in the GI tract that retards the growth of harmful bacteria and aids in mineral absorption. Also spelled *yoghurt.*

yohimbe, an herbal product taken from the bark of a tree that is native to areas of West Africa.

■ INDICATIONS: This herb is used to treat male sexual dysfunction.

■ CONTRAINDICATIONS: Yohimbe can be dangerous. It interacts with many medications, and it should not be used without medical supervision. Prolonged use is contraindicated,

as is the use of this herb in persons with renal or hepatic disease, hypertension, angina pectoris, gastric or duodenal ulcers, bipolar disorder, anxiety disorder, schizophrenia, suicidal tendencies, and prostatitis.

yohimbe bark, a preparation of the bark of *Pausinystalia yohimbe,* used for the same indications as yohimbe; it has also been used traditionally as an aphrodisiac and for skin diseases and obesity.

yoke /yōk/ [L, *jungere,* to join], a connector used to link small cylinders of medical gases, such as portable oxygen tanks, to respiratory equipment.

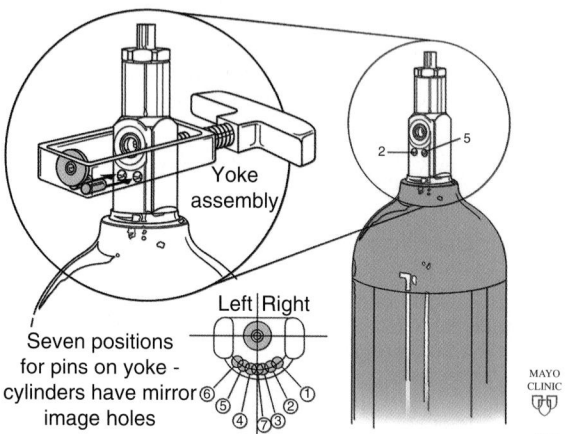

Yoke connector for medical gases *(Murray et al, 2015)*

yolk /yōk, yelk/ [AS, *geolca*], a material rich in fats and proteins that is contained in an ovum and that supplies nourishment to the developing embryo. The amount and distribution of the yolk within the ovum depend on the species of animal and the type of reproduction and development of offspring. In humans and most other mammals, yolk is absent or greatly diffused through the ovum. Mammalian embryos absorb nutrients directly from the mother through the placenta. Also called **vitellus.** Compare **deutoplasm.**

yolk membrane. See **vitelline membrane.**

yolk sac, a structure that develops in the inner cell mass of the embryo and expands into a vesicle with a thick part that becomes the primitive gut and a thin part that grows into the cavity of the chorion. The cells of the extraembryonic mesoderm differentiate to develop endothelium, primitive blood plasma, and hemoglobin. The yolk sac usually disappears during the seventh week of pregnancy. See also **allantois, Meckel diverticulum.**

yolk sphere. See **morula.**

yolk stalk, the narrow duct connecting the yolk sac with the midgut of the embryo during the early stages of prenatal development. It connects at the region of the future ileum and usually undergoes complete obliteration but occasionally may appear as a diverticulum. Also called **omphalomesenteric duct, umbilical duct, vitelline duct.** See also **Meckel diverticulum.**

young and middle adult, the stages of life from 22 to 65 years of age.

Young-Helmholtz theory of color vision [Thomas Young, English physician, 1773–1829; Hermann L.F. von Helmholtz, German physician, physicist, and physiologist, 1821–1894], the concept that all color sensations are mediated by three types of retinal receptors, which correspond to three primary colors: red, green, and blue-violet. By their individual and combined activities, the receptors produce the perception of all visible hues.

young offender, a child or adolescent who has committed a crime.

young-old, a term used to denote a person who is between 55 and 75 years of age.

Young prostatic retractor [Hugh Young, American urologist, 1870–1945], a short, straight surgical instrument with blades operated by a knob, for use in open perineal prostatectomy. The device can be inserted through the prostatic urethra and by direct traction used to draw down the prostate gland into the operative field.

Young's operation [Hugh Young], **1.** the surgical construction of a new urethra to repair a structural defect of the penis. **2.** perineal prostatectomy.

Y-plasty /wī″plas′tē/, a method of surgical revision of a scar, using a Y-shaped incision to reduce scar contractures. Also called **VY plasty.** Compare **Z-plasty.**

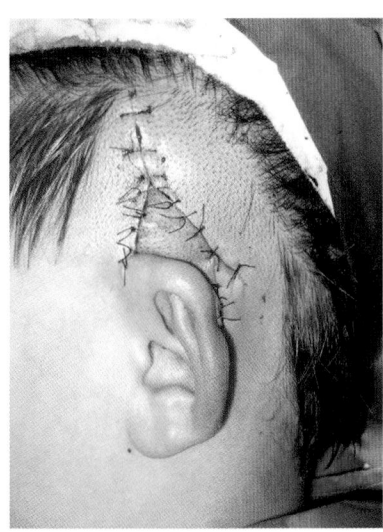

Y-plasty *(Jung et al, 2009)*

YPLL, abbreviation for **years of potential life lost.**

Y-set, a device composed of plastic components, used for delivering IV fluids through a primary IV line connected to a combination drip chamber filter section from which two separate plastic tubes lead to fluid sources. The Y-set also includes three clamps, one for the primary IV line and one for each of the two separate tubes. It is often used to transfuse blood cells for any type of blood administration that must be diluted with saline solution to decrease their viscosity. In such a transfusion one of the tubes is connected to the container of blood cells. The other tube is connected to the container of saline solution. Also called *Y-tubing.* Compare **component drip set, component syringe set, microaggregate recipient set, straight line blood set.**

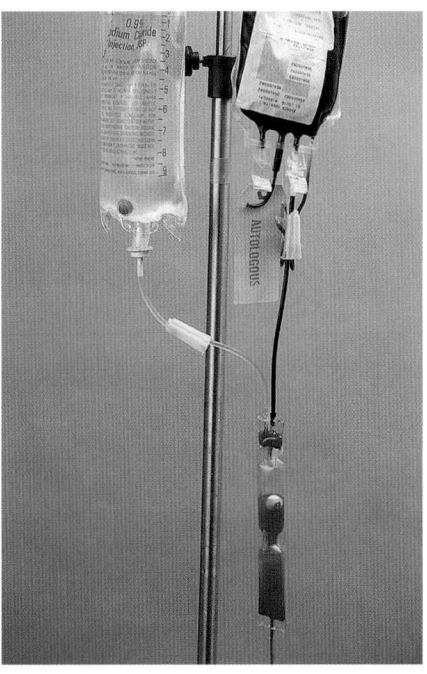

Y-set *(Perry, Potter, and Elkin, 2012)*

ytterbium (Yb) /itur″bē·əm/ [Ytterby, Sweden], a rare earth metallic element. Its atomic number is 70, and its atomic mass (weight) is 173.04. It has been used as a radiation source in portable x-ray machines and is also used in lasers.

yttrium (Y) /it″rē·əm/ [Ytterby, Sweden], a scaly, grayish metallic element. Its atomic number is 39, and its atomic mass (weight) is 88.905. Radioactive isotopes of yttrium have been used in cancer therapy.

yttrium 90 Y ibritumomab tiuxetan, a monoclonal antibody used in refractory non-Hodgkin lymphoma.

Y

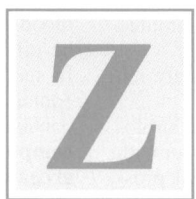

zafirlukast, a leukotriene receptor antagonist interfering with substances that cause swelling and tightening of the airway.

- INDICATIONS: This drug is used for prophylaxis and chronic treatment of asthma in children and adults.
- CONTRAINDICATIONS: Known hypersensitivity to this drug prohibits its use. It should not be used in patients with active liver disease or cirrhosis.
- ADVERSE EFFECTS: Adverse effects of this drug include headache, dizziness, nausea, diarrhea, abdominal pain, vomiting, infections, pain, asthenia, myalgia, fever, dyspepsia, and increased ALT. Adverse effects also include a change in behavior and suicidal thoughts.

Zahorsky disease [J. Zahorsky, American pediatrician, 1871–1963], *(Obsolete)* now called **roseola infantum.**

Zakrzewski, Marie /zakshef″skē/ [1829–1902], a Polish-German-American midwife who studied medicine in Berlin before emigrating to the United States. In New York she met Elizabeth Blackwell, who encouraged her to continue her medical studies. After receiving her medical degree in Cleveland, she worked at Blackwell's New York Infirmary before going to Boston. In 1872 she organized the first successful American school of nursing at the New England Hospital for Women and Children.

zalcitabine, a nucleoside analog reverse transcriptase inhibitor. It was prescribed in combination with other drugs for the treatment of human immunodeficiency virus infections. The sale and distribution of this medication was discontinued in the United States in 2006. Also called **ddC, dideoxycytidine, Hivid.**

zaleplon, a sedative-hypnotic agent.

- INDICATIONS: This drug is used to treat insomnia.
- CONTRAINDICATIONS: Known hypersensitivity to this drug prohibits its use.
- ADVERSE EFFECTS: Adverse effects of this drug include dizziness, confusion, anxiety, amnesia, depersonalization, hallucinations, hypesthesia, paresthesia, somnolence, tremor, vertigo, nausea, abdominal pain, constipation, anorexia, colitis, dyspepsia, dry mouth, vision changes, ear/eye pain, oversensitivity to sound, problems with smell detection, lethargy, fever, headache, muscle aches, and dysmenorrhea. Common side effects include lethargy, drowsiness, and daytime sedation. It should not be used longer than 2 to 3 weeks or with alcohol. Its effectiveness is decreased when taken with a high-fat meal. Insomnia medications, including zaleplon, can cause various complex sleep behaviors that may lead to rare but serious injuries or death. These complex sleep behaviors may include sleepwalking, sleep driving, or engaging in other activities while not fully awake. It is recommended that the agent be taken immediately before sleep is intended.

zanamivir, an antiviral neuraminidase inhibitor administered by oral inhalation.

- INDICATIONS: Zanamivir is used in the treatment and prophylaxis of type A and B influenza in patients who have had symptoms for no more than 2 days.

- CONTRAINDICATIONS: Known hypersensitivity to this drug prohibits its use.
- ADVERSE EFFECTS: Adverse reactions to this drug include fatigue, ear-nose-throat infections, diarrhea, nasal symptoms, cough, sinusitis, and bronchitis. Common side effects include headache, dizziness, nausea, and vomiting.

Zarontin, an anticonvulsant. Brand name for **ethosuximide.**

Zaroxolyn, a diuretic and antihypertensive. Brand name for **metolazone.**

zar syndrome, a belief by an individual that he or she is possessed by an evil spirit. Some cultural groups believe that winds can be evil and cause symptoms of disease or mental illness.

Zavesca, a treatment for Gaucher disease. Brand name for **miglustat.**

Z band. See **Z line.**

Z chromosome, a sex chromosome of certain insects, birds, and fish. See **W chromosome.**

Z disk, the smallest functional unit in striated muscle. Also called **Z line.**

ZDV, abbreviation for **zidovudine.**

Zeeman effect /sē″man, tsā″mon/ [Pieter Zeeman, Dutch physicist and Nobel laureate, 1865–1945], a splitting of lines in an emission spectrum into three or more symmetrically placed lines when the radiation source is in a magnetic field. An important application in health care is magnetic resonance imaging.

ZEEP, abbreviation for **zero-end expiratory pressure.**

zeitgeist /tsīt″gīst/ [Ger], literally, the spirit of the time, a climate of opinion, a convention of thought, or implicit assumptions.

Zellweger syndrome [Hans Ulrich Zellweger, American pediatrician, 1909–1990]. See **cerebrohepatorenal syndrome.**

Zemuron, a nondepolarizing neuromuscular blocking agent. Brand name for **rocuronium bromide.**

Zenapax /ze″nah-paks/, a monoclonal antibody used after transplantation and in the treatment of multiple sclerosis. Brand name for **daclizumab.**

Zenker diverticulum /tseng″ker/ [Friedrich A. Zenker, German pathologist, 1825–1898; L, *diverticulare,* to turn aside], a saclike outpouching of the mucosa and submucosa of the pharynx as it joins the esophagus, just proximal to the cricopharyngeus muscle. It is the most common type of diverticulum of the esophagus. Food may become trapped in the diverticulum and can be aspirated. Diagnosis is confirmed by x-ray studies. In most cases the herniation is small, causes no dysfunction, is not diagnosed, and requires no treatment. Larger diverticula are usually symptomatic and managed with endoscopic procedures.

zeolites, hydrated silicates of aluminum used in ion exchange water softeners. Synthetic zeolites are used as porous molecular containers for reagents and drugs.

Zephiran Chloride, a disinfectant. Brand name for **benzalkonium chloride.**

zeranol /zer″ənol/, a nonsteroidal estrogenic substance used to enhance growth in livestock in the United States and beef cattle in Canada.

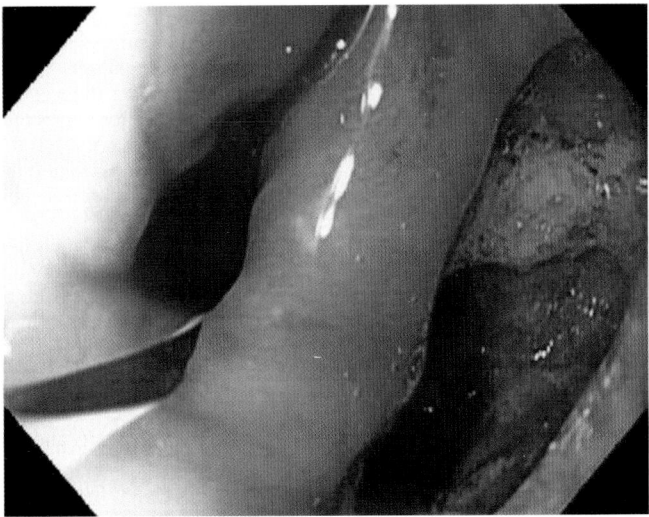

Zenker diverticulum (endoscopic view of hypopharynx) *(Ginsberg et al, 2012)*

Zerit, a nucleoside analog reverse transcriptase inhibitor active against the human immunodeficiency virus. Discontinued in 2020. Brand name for **stavudine.**

zero /zir″ō/ [Ar, *sifr,* cipher], **1.** nothing. **2.** the point on most scales from which measurements begin. **3.** absolute zero (0° K) on the Kelvin scale, the temperature at which there is no molecular movement, corresponding to −273.15° C or −459.67° F.

zero dose, **1.** (in pharmacology) the administration of a vaccine that does not count as a part of the series. **2.** (in biochemistry) the absence of added ligand.

zero-end expiratory pressure (ZEEP) [Ar, *zefiro* + ME, *ende*], pressure in the airways that has returned to ambient or atmospheric pressure at the end of exhalation.

zero fluid balance, a state in which the amount of fluid intake is equal to the amount of fluid output.

zero gravity, a physical state of weightlessness in space or during flight.

zero order kinetics, (in chemistry) a state at which the rate of an enzyme reaction is independent of the concentration of the substrate.

zero population growth (ZPG), a situation in which there is no population increase during a given year because the total of live births is equal to the total of deaths.

zero station, (in labor) when the biparietal diameter of the fetal head passes the diameter of the pelvic inlet; measured from the sacral promontory and the anterior aspect of the symphysis pubis.

zero-to-three early intervention groups, groups that facilitate the provision of therapeutic services for children from birth to 3 years of age, an age group not yet eligible for public school placement.

zero V/Q, an intrapulmonary shunt that allows blood to pass through the lungs without entering alveolar capillaries, causing hypoxemia. Also called **true shunt.**

Zestril, an angiotensin-converting enzyme (ACE) used for various cardiovascular indications, including hypertension and heart failure. Brand name for **lisinopril.**

zeta /zē″tə, zā″tə/, Z, ζ, the sixth letter of the Greek alphabet.

zetacrit /za′tah-krit/, the packed-cell volume produced by the zeta sedimentation ratio procedure. It is a sensitive indicator of the erythrocyte sedimentation rate (ESR) because it is not affected by anemia.

Zetafuge /za′tah-fūj/, a specially designed centrifuge used in determination of the zeta sedimentation ratio.

zeta potential [Gk, *zeta,* sixth letter of Greek alphabet; L, *potentia,* power], the potential produced by the effective charge of a macromolecule, usually measured at the boundary between what is moving in a solution with the macromolecule and the rest of the solution.

Zetar, a topical antieczematic or keratoplastic agent. Brand name for **coal tar.**

zeugmatography /zoog′mətog″rəfē/ [Gk, *zeugnynai,* to join, *graphein,* to record], *(Obsolete)* the joining of a magnetic field and a radiofrequency field to generate a two-dimensional display of anatomic structures. Now called **magnetic resonance imaging.**

zidovudine (ZDV) /zīdov″ədēn/, a pyrimidine nucleoside analog active against human immunodeficiency virus. Also called **azidothymidine, AZT.**

■ INDICATIONS: Its function is to inhibit the reverse transcriptase enzyme of the human immunodeficiency virus (HIV). It is used in combination with other antiretroviral medications in the management of patients with HIV infection who have some evidence of impaired immunity. It also may be used for prophylaxis after exposure to HIV and to prevent perinatal transmission of HIV from mother to fetus.

■ CONTRAINDICATIONS: It must be used cautiously in patients with impaired renal or hepatic function. It must also be used cautiously in patients with preexisting bone marrow suppression.

■ ADVERSE EFFECTS: Headache, GI disturbances, insomnia, flulike symptoms, rash, fatigue, myalgia, and central nervous system symptoms may occur during the first weeks of therapy. The drug may cause granulocytopenia and macrocytic anemia, particularly in patients with advanced HIV disease.

Ziehl-Neelsen test /zēl″ nēl″sən/ [Franz Ziehl, German bacteriologist, 1857–1926; Friedrich K.A. Neelsen, German pathologist, 1854–1894], one of the most widely used methods of acid-fast staining, commonly used in the microscopic examination of a smear of sputum suspected of containing *Mycobacterium tuberculosis.*

Ziehl stain [Franz Ziehl, German bacteriologist, 1859–1926], a bacteriologic process using a chemical wash to color acid-fast organisms, mainly mycobacteria, so that they can be viewed in a specimen. Also called **acid-fast stain.** See also **carbol-fuchsin stain.**

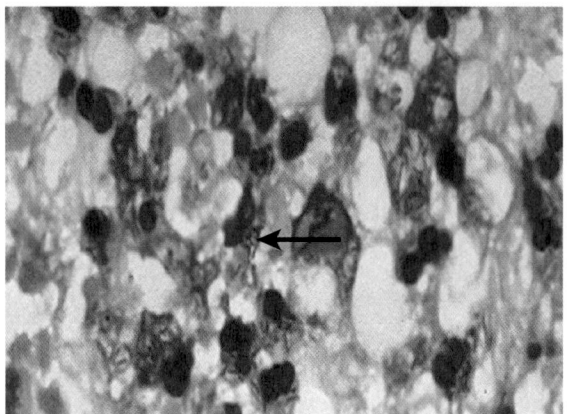

Mycobacteria retain the red carbol-fuchsin stain
(Walker et al, 2014)

Zieve syndrome [Leslie Zieve, American physician, 1915–2000], an acute hemolytic anemia with transient jaundice and hyperlipidemia found in patients with acute alcoholism and liver cirrhosis.

ZIFT, abbreviation for **zygote intrafallopian transfer.**

ZIG, abbreviation for **zoster immune globulin.**

zig-zag deformity, hyperextension of the interphalangeal joint of the thumb with flexion of the metacarpophalangeal joint. See also **swan neck deformity.**

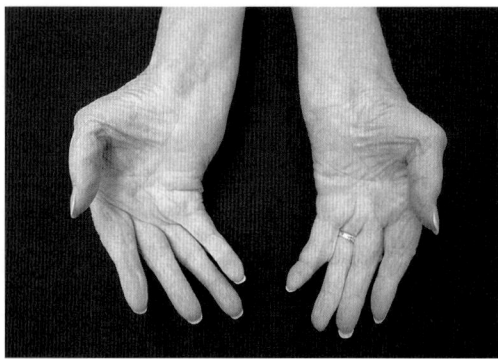

Classic zig-zag deformity *(Rizzo and Cooney, 2011)*

zika virus /zē″ kə/, a small, spherical, single-stranded, enveloped RNA virus belonging to family Flaviviridae, genus *Flavivirus.*

Zika virus disease, a flulike infection caused by the Zika virus. Its primary vector is the mosquito (*Aedes aegypti* and *Aedes albopictus*). It can also be sexually transmitted.

■ OBSERVATIONS: One of the most common symptoms is a rash that begins on the face and usually lasts a week or more. Other symptoms include conjunctivitis, mild fever, chills, and joint and muscle aches. Fatigue, malaise, abdominal pain, and vomiting may also be present.

■ INTERVENTIONS: The disease is usually self-limiting, and there is no specific treatment.

■ PATIENT CARE CONSIDERATIONS: The World Health Organization (WHO) and the U.S. Centers for Disease Control and Prevention (CDC) have issued warnings to those living in or traveling to areas of Zika transmission to practice ab-

stinence and/or avoid unprotected sexual contact for up to 6 months after infection with this virus. Any woman who is pregnant and suspects infection should consult with her health care provider to receive serologic testing for the virus and an evaluation for microcephaly, which is associated with the viral infection. A referral to experts in maternal-child health and infectious disease management is recommended.

zileuton, a 5-lipoxygenase inhibitor, preventing leukotriene formation.

■ INDICATIONS: This drug is used to treat allergic rhinitis and to prevent and control the symptoms of asthma.

■ CONTRAINDICATIONS: Factors that prohibit the use of this drug are hepatic disease, liver function test results three times higher than upper limits, and known hypersensitivity to zileuton.

■ ADVERSE EFFECTS: Adverse effects of this drug include dizziness, insomnia, fatigue, paresthesias, headache, nausea, abdominal pain, dyspepsia, diarrhea, liver function test abnormalities, hives, myalgia, and asthenia.

Zimmermann reaction /zim″ərman, tsim″ərmon/ [Wilhelm Zimmermann, German physician, b. 1910], a chromogen reaction used for detecting androgens with the 17-keto configuration. It involves a reaction between an alkaline solution of meta-dinitrobenzene and an active methylene group.

Zinacef, a cephalosporin antibiotic. Brand name for **cefuroxime sodium.**

zinc (Zn) /zingk/ [Ger, *Zink*], a bluish-white crystalline metal commonly associated with lead ores. Its atomic number is 30; its atomic mass is 65.38. It is ductile in its pure form and occurs abundantly in minerals such as sphalerite, zincite, and franklinite. It has many commercial uses, such as a protective coating for steel and in printing plates. It is an essential nutrient in the body and is used in numerous pharmaceutics, such as zinc acetate, zinc oxide, zinc permanganate, and zinc stearate.

zinc chill. See **metal fume fever.**

zinc deficiency a condition resulting from insufficient amounts of zinc in the diet. It is characterized by abnormal fatigue, decreased alertness, a decrease in taste and odor sensitivity, poor appetite, oral inflammation, sores at the corners of the mouth, white spots on the nails, retarded growth, delayed sexual maturity, prolonged healing of wounds, and susceptibility to infection, injury, and myocardial infarction. Other conditions that may precipitate the deficiency include ulcers and alcoholic cirrhosis and other liver diseases. Prophylaxis and treatment consist of a diet of foods high in protein that are also rich in zinc, including meats, eggs, liver, seafood, legumes, nuts, peanut butter, milk, and whole-grain cereals.

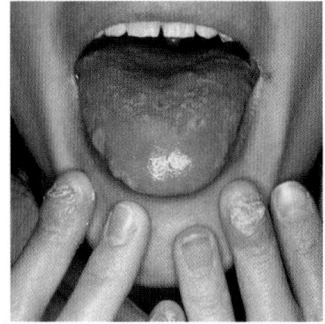

Oral inflammation related to zinc deficiency *(Ferri, 2019)*

zinc finger, a loop of a transcription factor that is stabilized by a zinc ion coordinated with histidine nitrogen atoms or cysteine sulfur atoms at critical junctures in a protein. It is an important step in the cloning and sequencing of human general transcription factors because individual proteins appear to be involved in the regulation of transcription and in RNA transport. See also **transcription factor.**

zinc gelatin, a topical protectant for varicosities and other lesions of the lower limbs. It is available as a smooth jelly containing zinc oxide (10%), gelatin (15%), glycerin (40%), and purified water (35%). It is also available impregnated in gauze.

zinc ointment [Ger, *Zink* + OFr, *oignement*], a preparation of 20% zinc oxide in mineral oil or a white petrolatum semisolid base. It is used as a local surface treatment for various skin disorders, minor skin irritations, and the prevention of diaper rash. Some preparations also may contain salicylic acid.

zinc oxide, a mineral used topically in a wide variety of balms, cosmetics products, and sunscreens. It is also used as an ingredient in rectal suppositories to relieve itching associated with hemorrhoids.

zinc oxide and eugenol (ZOE), a sedative dental cement composed primarily of zinc salts, eugenol (oil of cloves), and rosin, used chiefly in temporary tooth fillings. It has low relative strength and low abrasion resistance, but its nearly neutral pH causes minimal irritation to dental pulp. It is intended as a sedative dressing until pain subsides, a more permanent filling can be inserted, or until it can be determined whether other treatment, such as a root canal or extraction, is needed. See **temporary filling.**

zinc phosphate dental cement, a material for coating or attaching dental inlays, crowns, bridges, and orthodontic appliances and for some temporary restorations of teeth. It is prepared by mixing a powder composed of zinc and magnesium oxides and a liquid composed of phosphoric acid, water, and buffering agents.

zinc protoporphyrin, a compound present in red blood cells when low iron or high lead levels are present.

zinc salt poisoning, a toxic condition caused by the ingestion or inhalation of a zinc salt, which can be present in industrial dyes and paints. Symptoms of ingestion include a burning sensation of the mouth and throat, vomiting, diarrhea, abdominal and chest pain, and in severe cases shock and coma. Inhalation of zinc salts may cause metal fume fever; skin contact may produce blisters. A poison control center should be contacted if zinc poisoning is suspected.

zinc sulfate, an astringent given in the form of a nasal spray for nasal congestion or as eye drops to reduce redness and irritation of the eyes. It is applied topically in deodorants and given orally in tablets as a supplement to decrease the duration of cold symptoms.

Zinecard, a cardioprotective agent. Brand name for **dexrazoxane.**

ZIO patch, a small, water-resistant, single-lead, single-use device used for continuous cardiac monitoring.

ZIP, abbreviation for **zoster immune plasma.** See **chickenpox.**

ziprasidone /zipra'sidōn/, an atypical antipsychotic medication, administered orally as the hydrochloride salt.

■ INDICATIONS: The drug is used in the treatment of schizophrenia and bipolar disorders.

■ CONTRAINDICATIONS: Elderly patients with dementia-related psychosis treated with antipsychotic drugs are at an increased risk of death.

■ ADVERSE EFFECTS: Common side effects include drowsiness, extrapyramidal symptoms, headache, dizziness, and nausea. The drug can also increase levels of prolactin. Serious adverse effects include fainting, tachycardia, fever, stiff muscles, confusion, and diaphoresis.

zirconium (Zr), a chemical element with the atomic number 40. Its primary use is in the production of nuclear power.

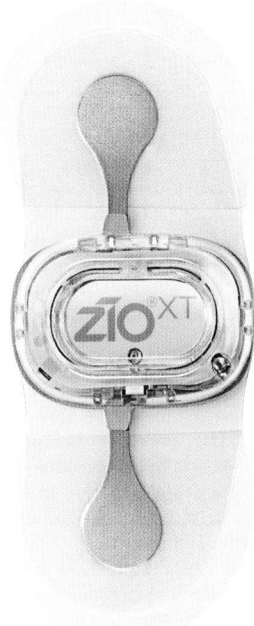

ZIO patch *(Courtesy iRhythm Technologies, Inc.)*

zirconium granuloma, an inflammatory lesion, usually occurring in the axilla as a reaction to zirconium salts in antiperspirants.

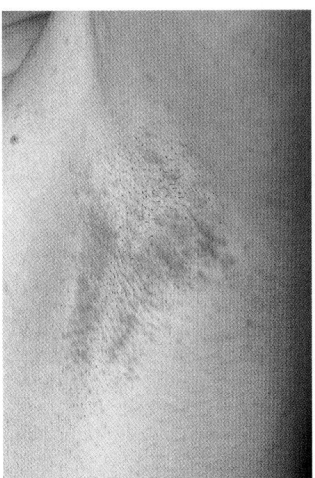

Zirconium granuloma secondary to antiperspirant use
(James et al, 2016)

Zithromax, a macrolide antibiotic. Brand name for **azithromycin.**

Z line, 1. a narrow, darkly staining cross-striation that bisects the I band of skeletal muscles. The distance between Z lines is the length of the sarcomere. Also called **intermediate disk, Z band, Z disk.** See also **I band, sarcomere. 2.** a demarcation of the anatomic junction between squamous epithelium in the esophagus and columnar epithelium in the stomach.

Zn, symbol for the element **zinc.**

zoacanthosis /zō'akanthō"sis/, a dermatitis caused by retention in the skin of foreign bodies such as insect stingers, animal hairs, or bristles.

zoanthropy /zō·an″thrəpē/ [Gk, *zoon,* animal, *anthropos,* human], the delusion that one has assumed the form and characteristics of an animal. –*zoanthropic, adj.*

ZOE, a cement that is used in dentistry. Abbreviation for **zinc oxide and eugenol.**

-zoite, combining form meaning a "simple organism" of a specified sort: *merozoite, sporozoite.*

zoledronic acid /zo′lĕ-dron″ik/, a bisphosphonate that inhibits bone resorption; it is used intravenously in the treatment and prevention of osteoporosis and hypercalcemia of malignancy.

Zollinger-Ellison syndrome /zol″injər el″isən/ [Robert M. Zollinger, American surgeon, 1903–1992; Edwin H. Ellison, American physician, 1918–1970], a condition in which tumors in the pancreas produce excessive amounts of gastrin, which in turn increases the production of gastric acid, leading to gastric ulcers. See also **peptic ulcer.**

■ OBSERVATIONS: The condition is characterized by severe peptic ulceration, gastric hypersecretion, elevated serum gastrin, and gastrinoma of the pancreas or the duodenum. Severe abdominal pain, bloating, gastrointestinal bleeding, and anemia are common symptoms.

■ INTERVENTIONS: The administration of proton pump inhibitors is usually effective in reducing excess gastric secretions. Surgery may be required if complications occur related to the peptic ulcers. The tumors producing gastrin are often difficult to remove, or they may be so numerous that this procedure is ineffective. However, removal or ablation may be considered.

■ PATIENT CARE CONSIDERATIONS: The syndrome is uncommon and may occur in early childhood but is seen more frequently in people between 20 and 50 years of age. Two thirds of the tumors are malignant. Careful monitoring and follow-up are essential.

zolmitriptan, a selective serotonin receptor-1 agonist used in the treatment of migraine headaches.

■ INDICATIONS: Acute treatment of migraine with or without aura.

■ CONTRAINDICATIONS: Factors that prohibit the use of this drug include angina pectoris, a history of myocardial infarction, documented silent ischemia, ischemic heart disease, concurrent use of ergotamine-containing preparations, uncontrolled hypertension, known hypersensitivity to this drug, and basilar or hemiplegic migraine.

■ ADVERSE EFFECTS: Adverse effects of this drug include palpitations, abdominal discomfort, myalgia, and chest tightness and pressure. Common side effects include weakness, neck stiffness, tingling, hot sensation, burning, a feeling of pressure and tightness in the head, numbness, dizziness, and sedation.

Zoloft /zo′loft/, a selective serotonin reuptake inhibitor used to treat depression and anxiety along with other mental health disorders. Brand name for **sertraline.**

zolpidem /zōl-pi′dem/, a nonbenzodiazepine sedative and hypnotic used orally as the tartrate salt.

■ INDICATIONS: This drug is used in the short-term treatment of insomnia. Patients taking zolpidem should be in the bedroom ready for sleep when the dose is taken.

■ CONTRAINDICATIONS: Known hypersensitivity to zolpidem prohibits its use. This medication should not be combined with alcohol, opioids, or other central nervous system depressants.

■ ADVERSE EFFECTS: The most common adverse effects are drowsiness, dizziness, and light-headedness. The medication has been associated with sleep-related activities, such as sleep-driving or sleepwalking, that the patient cannot recall after waking up.

zona /zō″nə/ *pl. zonae* [Gk, *zone,* belt], a zone, or a girdle-like segment of a rounded or spheric structure. See also **zone.**

zona ciliaris. See **ciliary zone.**

zona fasciculata, the middle part of the adrenal cortex, which is the site of production of glucocorticoids and sex hormones.

zona glomerulosa, the outer part of the adrenal cortex, where mineralocorticoids are produced.

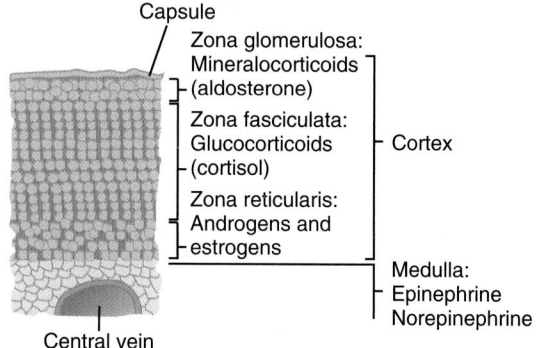

Adrenal gland: cross section showing zona glomerulosa, zona fasciculata, and zona reticularis
(Black and Hawks, 2009)

zona pellucida /pəloo″sidə/, the thick, transparent, noncellular membrane that encloses a mammalian ovum. It is secreted by the maturing oocyte during its development in the ovary and is retained until near the time of implantation. Also called **oolemma.** See also **vitelline membrane.**

zona radiata, a zona pellucida that has a striated appearance caused by radiating canals within the membrane. Also called **zona striata.**

zona reticularis, the innermost part of the adrenal cortex, which borders on the adrenal medulla part of the gland. It acts in consort with the zona fasciculata in producing various sex hormones and glucocorticoids.

zona striata. See **zona radiata.**

zonate /zō″nāt/, having ringed layers with differing colors or textures.

zone [Gk, belt], an area with specific boundaries and characteristics, such as the epigastric, mesogastric, and hypogastric zones of the abdomen. See also **zona.**

zone of equivalence, a region of an antibody-antigen reaction in which concentrations of both reactants are equal.

zone therapy, a complementary therapy in which there is treatment of a disorder by mechanical stimulation and counterirritation of a body area in the same longitudinal zone as the affected organ or region.

zonifugal /zōnif″yəgəl/ [Gk, *zone,* belt; L, *fugere,* to flee], moving from within a zone or area outward.

zonisamide /zo-nis′ah-mīd″/, a sulfonamide that acts as an anticonvulsant, used as an adjunct in the treatment of partial seizures in adults. It is administered orally.

zonography /zōnog″rəfē/ [Gk, *zone* + *graphein,* to record], *(Obsolete)* an x-ray imaging technique used to produce sectional images of the body similar to those made by tomography.

zonula /zōn″yələ/ *pl. zonulae* [Gk, *zone,* belt], a small zone or band. Also called *zonule.*

zonula adherens [L, *zone,* belt, *adhaerere,* to stick], a continuous zone running around the outer surface of a cell in which there is an intercellular space of about 15 to 20 nm wide. A component of the junctional complex between cells, the zone contains dense filamentous material.

zonula ciliaris. See **zonule of Zinn.**

zonulae, zonule. See **zonula.**

zonula occludens [L, *zona,* belt, *occludere,* to close up], a component of the junctional complex between cells in which there is no intercellular space and the plasma membranes of adjacent cells are in direct contact.

zonule of Zinn, a ligament composed of straight fibrils radiating from the ciliary body of the eye to the crystalline lens, holding the lens in place and relaxing by the contraction of the ciliary muscle. Relaxation of the ligament allows the lens to become more convex. Also called **zonula ciliaris.** See also **ciliary zone.**

zoo-, zo- /zō'ə-/, combining form meaning "animal": *zoonosis.*

zoobiology /-bī·ol″əjē/ [Gk, *zoon,* animal, *bios,* life, *logos,* science], the biology of animals.

zoochemistry /-kem″istrē/ [Gk, *zoon,* animal, *chemeia,* alchemy], the biochemistry of animals.

zooerastia. See **bestiality.**

zoogenous /zō·oj'ənəs/ [Gk, *zoon,* animal, *genein,* to produce], acquired from or originating in animals. See also **zoonosis.**

zooglea, (*Obsolete*) a mass of bacteria bound by gelatinous material.

zoograft /zō″əgraft/ [Gk, *zoon + graphion,* stylus], tissue of an animal transplanted to a human, such as a heart valve from a pig to replace a damaged heart valve in a human.

zoologist /zō·ol'əjist/ [Gk, *zoon,* animal, *logos,* science], a person concerned with the scientific study of animals.

zoology /zō·ol'əjē/, the study of animal life.

zoom /zo͞om/, **1.** a feature of a camera that allows an object to remain in focus when the camera approaches or recedes or when the object is viewed close-up or at a distance. **2.** a feature of digital imaging in which an image can be enlarged or magnified for improved visualization.

zoomania /zō·əmā″nē·ə/ [Gk, *zoon + mania,* madness], a psychopathological state characterized by an excessive fondness for and preoccupation with animals. −*zoomaniac, n.*

-zoon, combining form meaning "a living being": *spermatozoon.*

Zoon balanitis [J. J. Zoon, Dutch dermatologist, 1902–1958], a benign erythroplasia of the inner surface of the prepuce or the glans penis, characterized histologically by plasma cell infiltration of the dermis and clinically by a moist, erythematous lesion. Plasma cell vulvitis is a corresponding condition in females. Also called **balanitis circumscripta plasmacellularis.**

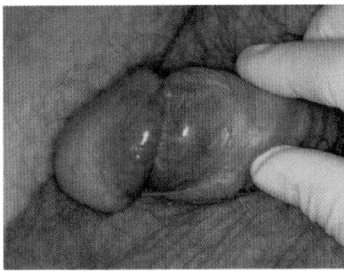

Zoon balanitis *(Teichman et al, 2010)*

zoonosis /zō·on″əsis, zō'ənō″sis/ [Gk, *zoon + nosis,* disease], a disease of animals that is transmissible to humans from its primary animal host. Kinds include **equine encephalitis, leptospirosis, rabies, yellow fever.**

zoonotic filariasis. See **dirofilariasis.**

zooparasite /zō·əper″əsīt/ [Gk, *zoon + parasitos,* guest], any parasitic animal organism. Also called **pinworm.** Kinds include **arthropod-borne virus, protozoal infection.** −*zooparasitic, adj.*

zoopathology /-pəthol″əjē/, the study of the diseases of animals.

zoophilia /zō·əfil″ē·ə/ [Gk, *zoon + philein,* to love], (in psychiatry) a psychosexual disorder in which sexual excitement and gratification are derived from the fondling of animals or from the fantasy or act of engaging in sexual activity with animals. Also called *zoophilism.* See also **paraphilia.**

zoophobia /-fō″bē·ə/ [Gk, *zoon + phobos,* fear], an anxiety disorder characterized by a persistent, irrational fear of animals, particularly dogs, snakes, insects, and mice. The condition is seen more often in women than in men, nearly always begins in childhood, and can typically be traced to some frightening or unpleasant experience involving an animal. Treatment consists of psychotherapy to uncover the cause of the phobic reaction followed by behavioral therapy, specifically the techniques of systemic desensitization and flooding.

zoopsia /zō·op″sē·ə/ [Gk, *zoon + opsis,* vision], a visual hallucination of animals or insects, often occurring in delirium tremens.

zootoxin /zō″ətok″sin/ [Gk, *zoon + toxikon,* poison], a poisonous substance from an animal, such as the venom of snakes, spiders, and scorpions. −*zootoxic, adj.*

zoster. See **herpes zoster.**

zoster auricularis /zos″tər/, an acute earache with herpetic blebs on the eardrum and external auditory meatus caused by the herpes zoster virus and often associated with shingles. Also called **Ramsay Hunt syndrome.**

zosteriform /zoster″ifôrm/ [Gk, *zoster,* girdle; L, *forma,* form], resembling the pocks seen in herpes zoster infection.

zoster immune globulin (ZIG) [Gk, *zoster + L, immunis,* freedom, *globulus,* small sphere], a passive immunizing agent for postexposure prevention of varicella in individuals who are at high risk of herpes zoster virus infection.

zoster immune plasma (ZIP), human plasma containing high levels of varicella zoster virus antibodies. See also **immunoglobulin G.**

zoster ophthalmicus [Gk, *zoster,* girdle, *ophthalmos,* eye], a herpes infection of the eye and the first division of the trigeminal nerve.

■ OBSERVATIONS: The infection frequently involves the cornea. There may be lid edema, ciliary and conjunctival involvement, and pain. Keratitis may be severe. Scarring and glaucoma are common sequelae.

■ INTERVENTIONS: The administration of oral acyclovir or valacyclovir is used to treat the herpes virus. Cool compresses can be applied as a comfort measure. Concurrent infection is treated with broad-spectrum antibiotics. Topical steroids may also be of use. The pain associated with this condition can be significant. Analgesia is frequently required.

■ PATIENT CARE CONSIDERATIONS: The herpes zoster vaccine can reduce significantly the burden of herpes zoster among older people. Health care providers should discuss and encourage vaccination.

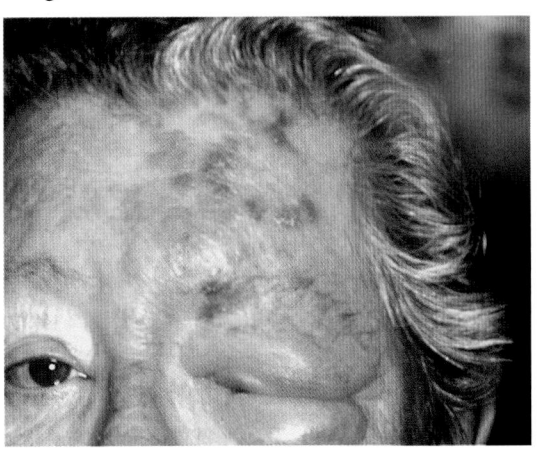

Zoster ophthalmicus *(Yanoff and Duker, 2014)*

Z

Zovirax, a purine nucleoside analog in the antiviral drug class. Brand name for **acyclovir.**

ZPG, abbreviation for **zero population growth.**

Z-plasty /zē″plas′tē/, a method of surgical revision of a scar or closure of a wound using a Z-shaped incision to reduce contractures of the adjacent skin. See also **Y-plasty.**

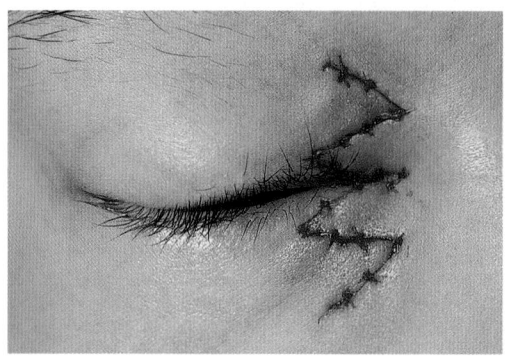

Z-plasty *(Tyers and Collin, 2008)*

Zr, symbol for the element *zirconium.*

z-score, a measurement of the number of standard deviations above or below the mean. See also **z-value.**

z-test, a statistical test using normalized data (*z*-values) to determine if differences in proportions between sets of data or between individual members of different sets of data are large enough to be statistically significant.

Z-track, a technique for injecting irritating preparations into muscle without tracking residual medication through sensitive tissues. The tissue to be injected is pulled downward and in the direction of the body's midline. It is held in this position until the drug is injected. When the tissue is released, the usually straight needle track will become a broken line similar to the letter Z. This allows the medication to remain deep in the muscle and prevents upward seepage through the tissue along the needle track. The area is not massaged after injection. A separate needle is used after the medication is withdrawn from the vial. This eliminates depositing the drug along the needle track while it is piercing the skin.

Zuckerkandl fascia, the posterior part of the renal fascia.

Zung Self-Rating Depression Scale, a "self-report test" of 20 descriptors of depression on which clients rate themselves on a four-point scale ranging from "a little of the time" to "most of the time." The scale is useful in determining the depth or intensity of a client's depression.

z-value, (in statistics) a normalized value created from a member of a set of data in units of standard deviation. Also called **z-score.**

zwieback /zwī″bak, zwē″-/ [Ger, *zwie,* twice, *backen,* to bake], a sweetened bread that is enriched with eggs and baked, then sliced and toasted until dry and crisp. It is used as a snack food for children, especially teething infants.

zwitterion /tsvit″ərī′ən/, a molecule that has regions of both negative and positive charge. Amino acids such as glycine are almost always present as zwitterions when in neutral solutions. Also called **dipolar ion.**

zyg-, zygo- /zī″gō-/, combining form meaning "union or fusion, yoked or joined, a junction or a pair": *zygomatic, zygogenesis, zygote.*

zygapophyseal joint. See **facet joint.**

zygocyte. See **zygote.**

zygogenesis /zī′gōjen″əsis/ [Gk, *zygon,* yoke, *genesis,* origin], 1. the formation of a zygote. 2. reproduction by the union of gametes. −*zygogenetic, zygogenic, adj.*

zygoma /zīgō″mə, zig-/ [Gk, *zygon,* yoke], 1. a long slender zygomatic process of the temporal bone, arising from the lower part of the squamous part of the temporal bone, passing forward to join the zygomatic bone, and forming part of the zygomatic arch. 2. the zygomatic bone that forms the prominence of the cheek.

zygomatic /-mat″ik/ [Gk, *zygon,* yoke], pertaining to the zygoma, or malar bone of the face.

zygomatic arch [Gk, *zygon* + L, *arcus,* bow], an arch formed by the temporal process of the zygomatic bone with the zygomatic process of the temporal bone. The tendon of the temporal muscle passes beneath it.

zygomatic bone [Gk, *zygon* + AS, *ban*], one of the pair of bones that forms the prominence of the cheek, the lower part of the orbit of the eye, and parts of the temporal and infratemporal fossae.

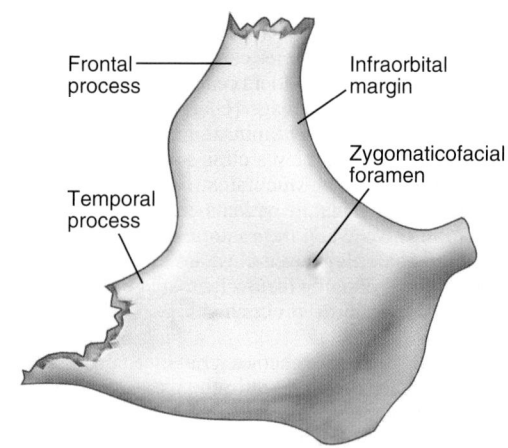

Zygomatic bone

zygomatic head. See **zygomaticus minor.**

zygomatic nerve, a nerve originating from the maxillary nerve that divides into two branches that supply skin over the temple and skin adjacent to the zygomatic bone.

zygomaticofacial /zī′gōmat′ikōfā″shəl/, pertaining to the facial surface of the zygomatic bone.

zygomatic process [Gk, *zygon* + L, *processus*], 1. a projection of the frontal bone forming the lateral boundary of the superciliary arch. 2. a process of the maxilla. 3. a process of the temporal bone.

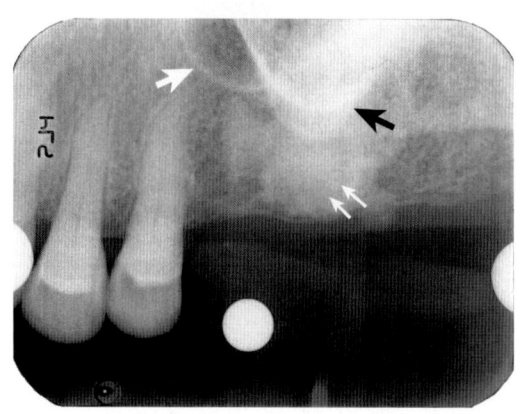

Zygomatic process *(Newman et al, 2015)*

zygomatic reflex [Gk, *zygon* + L, *reflectere,* to bend back], movement of the lower jaw toward the percussed side when the zygoma is tapped lightly but sharply.

zygomaticus major /zī′gōmat″ikəs/, one of the 12 muscles of the mouth. Arising from the zygomatic bone and inserting into the corner of the mouth, it acts to draw the angle of the mouth up and back to smile or laugh. Also called *zygomaticus.* Compare **zygomaticus minor.**

zygomaticus minor, one of the 12 muscles of the mouth. Arising from the malar surface of the zygomatic bone and inserting into the upper lip, it acts to deepen the nasolabial furrow in a sad facial expression. Also called **zygomatic head.** Compare **zygomaticus major.** Formerly called **quadratus labii superioris.**

zygomaxillare. See **key ridge.**

Zygomycetes /zi″go-mi-se′tēz/, a class of saprobic and parasitic fungi of the phylum Zygomycota; important pathogenic organisms are in the orders Entomophthorales and Mucorales. The fungi live in soil or on decaying plant or animal material. Some species can be used in the production of lipases and proteases; others can cause infection.

zygomycosis /zi′gōmīkō″sis/ [Gk, *zygon* + *mykes,* fungus], an acute, often fulminant, and sometimes fatal fungal infections caused by a class of phycomycetal water molds in the orders Mucorales or Entomophthorales. They occur primarily in patients with chronic debilitating diseases, especially uncontrolled diabetes mellitus. The fungus may enter blood vessels and spread to the brain and other organs. Transmission is usually by inhalation. Kinds include **mucormycosis, phycomycosis, basidiobolomycosis.**

■ OBSERVATIONS: The infection characteristically begins with fever, pain, and discharge in the nose and paranasal sinuses that progresses to invade the eye and lower respiratory tract. The diagnosis is confirmed by biopsy and pathological examination of sputum.

■ INTERVENTIONS: Treatment includes improved control of diabetes mellitus, extensive debridement of craniofacial lesions, and amphotericin B, administered intravenously.

■ PATIENT CARE CONSIDERATIONS: The disorder is also associated with natural disasters, when it is difficult to cleanse open wounds that are contaminated with soil or vegetative matter contaminated with a fungus.

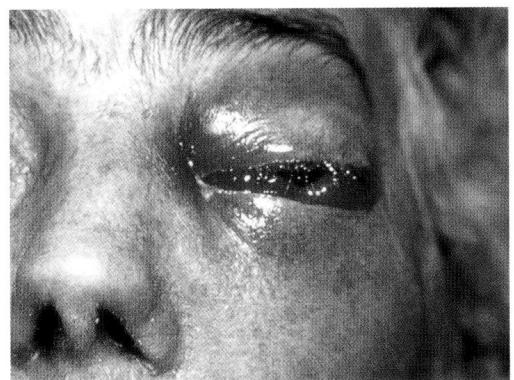

Acute zygomycosis of the orbit *(Procop and Pritt, 2015)*

zygonema /zī′gənē″mə/ [Gk, *zygon* + *nema,* thread], the synaptic chromosome formation that occurs in the zygotene stage of the first meiotic prophase of gametogenesis. −*zygonematic, adj.*

zygopodium /zī′gōpō″dē·əm/, the part of an embryonic limb consisting of the radius and ulna or the tibia and fibula.

zygopophysial joints, the synovial joints between superior and inferior articular processes on adjacent vertebrae. A thin articular capsule attached to the margins of the articular facets encloses each joint.

zygosis /zīgō″sis/, a form of sexual reproduction in unicellular organisms, consisting of the union of the two cells and fusion of their nuclei. −*zygotic, adj.*

zygosity /zīgos″itē/, the characteristics or conditions of a zygote. The form occurs primarily as a suffix denoting genetic makeup, referring specifically to whether the paired alleles determining a particular trait are identical (homozygosity) or different (heterozygosity) or to the condition in twins of having developed from the fertilization of one ovum (monozygosity) or two (dizygosity).

zygospore /zī″gōspôr′/ [Gk, *zygon* + *sporos,* seed], the spore resulting from the conjugation of two isogametes, as in certain fungi and algae. Also called *zygosperm.*

zygote /zī″gōt/ [Gk, *zygon,* yoke], the combined cell produced by the union of a sperm pronucleus and an egg pronucleus at the completion of fertilization until the first cleavage. Also called **zygocyte.**

zygote intrafallopian transfer (ZIFT), retrieval of oocytes from the ovary, followed by their fertilization and culture in the laboratory and placement of the resulting zygotes in the fallopian tubes by laparoscopy 24 hours after oocyte retrieval. Used as a means of establishing pregnancy in treatment of infertility.

zygotene /zī″gətēn/ [Gk, *zygon* + *tainia,* band], the second stage in the first meiotic prophase of gametogenesis, in which synapsis of homologous chromosomes occurs. See also **diakinesis, diplotene, leptotene, pachytene.**

Zyloprim, a xanthine oxidase inhibitor. Brand name for **allopurinol.**

-zyme, zymo-, combining form meaning a "ferment" or "enzyme": *lysozyme.*

zymogen, an inactive precursor that is converted into an active enzyme by action of an acid, another enzyme, or other means.

zymogen granules /zī″məjən/ [Gk, *zyme,* ferment, *genein,* to produce; L, *granulum,* little grain], granules found in some secretory exocrine cells. They contain the precursors of enzymes that become active after the granules leave the cell.

zymogenic cell. See **chief cell.**

zymoprotein /-prō″tēn/ [Gk, *zyme,* ferment, *proteios,* first rank], **1.** a yeast protein. **2.** any protein that functions as an enzyme.

zymorphic /zīmôr″fik/ [Gk, *zyme,* ferment, *morphe,* form], pertaining to fermentation properties.

Z.Z.:Z.", symbol for *increasing strength or intensity of contraction.*

Z

ILLUSTRATION CREDITS

AACN (Carlson): *AACN advanced critical care nursing*, Philadelphia, 2008, Saunders.

Abajian M, Schoepke N, Altrichter S, Zuberbier T, Maurer M: Physical urticarias and cholinergic urticaria, *Immunol Allerg Clin North Am* 1(34):73–88, 2014.

Adam A, Dixon AK, Grainger RG, Allison DJ: *Grainger and Allison's diagnostic radiology*, ed 5, New York, 2008, Churchill Livingstone.

Adams J: *Emergency medicine*, Philadelphia, 2008, Saunders.

Aehlert B: *ACLS study guide*, ed 4, St Louis, 2012, Mosby.

Ahn JE, Ko MS, Park SH, Lee MG: Neuroendocrine carcinoma of the gallbladder causing hyperinsulinaemic hypoglycaemia, *Clin Radiol* 62(4):391–394, 2006.

Aitkenhead AR, Moppett IK, Thompson JP: *Smith and Aitkenhead's textbook of anesthesia*, ed 6, Oxford, 2013, Elsevier Ltd.

Akram H, Sewell MD, Cheng LH: Pseudoxanthoma elasticum, *Br J Oral Maxillofac Surg* 46(3):237–238, 2007.

Albert DM, Miller JW, Azar DT, Blodi BA: *Albert & Jakobiec's principles and practice of ophthlamology*, ed 3, Philadelphia, 2008, Saunders.

Al-Shaikh B, Stacey S: *Essentials of anaesthetic equipment*, ed 4, Oxford, 2013, Elsevier Ltd.

Alter SJ, McDonald MB, Schloemer J, Simon R, Trevino J: Common child and adolescent cutaneous infestations and fungal infections, *Curr Prob Pediatr Adolesc Health Care* 48(1):3–25, 2018.

Alves Silverio KC, Brasolotto AG, Siqueria LTD, Carneiro CG, Fukushiro AP, de Jesus Guirro RR: Effect of application of transcutaneous electrical nerve stimulation and laryngeal manual therapy in disphonic women: clinical trial, *J Voice* 29(2):200–208, 2015.

Alwattar BJ, Bharam S: Hip arthroscopy portals, *Oper Techn Sports Med* 19(2):74–80, 2011.

Amielh D, Seblini M, Desloover F, Chambon JP, Pruvot FR, Zerbib P: Severe erosive ischemic gastritis healed after surgical revascularization, *Eur J Vasc Endovasc Surg Extra* 18(3):35–37, 2009.

Amplatz S, Piazzi L, Felder M, Comberlato M, Benvenuti S, et al.: Extracorporeal shock wave lithotripsy for clearance of refractory bile duct Gs, *Diges Liver Dis* 39(3):267–272, 2006.

Anderson VL: Uncovering a pediatric immunodeficiency part 2, *J Nurse Pract* 2(4):237–246, 2006.

Andreoli TE: *Andreoli and Carpenter's cecil essentials of medicine*, ed 8, Philadelphia, 2010, Saunders.

Andrews G: *Women's sexual health*, Edinburgh, New York, 2005, Elsevier.

Andrews JR, Harrelson GL, Wilk KE: *Physical rehabilitation of the injured athlete*, ed 4, Philadelphia, 2012, Saunders.

Aouthmany M, Weinstein M, Zirwas MJ, Brodell RT: The natural history of halo nevi: a retrospective case series, *J Ame Acad Derm* 67(4):582–586, 2011.

Apaydin N, Kaya B, Loukas M, Tubbs RS: The topographic anatomy of the masseteric nerve: a cadaveric study with an emphasis on the effective zone of botulinum toxin a injections in masseter, *J Plas Recons Aesth Surg* 67(12):1663–1668.

Applegate E: *The anatomy and physiology learning system*, ed 4, St Louis, 2011, Saunders.

Arakawa H, Shida H, Saito Y, Johkoh T, Tomiyama N, Tsubamoto M, et al.: Pulmonary malignancy in silicosis: factors associated with radiographic detection, *Eur J Radiol* 69(1):80–86, 2009.

Aster JC, Poznyakova O, Kutok JL: *Hematopathology: a volume in the high yield pathology series*, Philadelphia, 2013, Saunders.

Atrice: *Umphred's neurological rehabilitation*, ed 6, St. Louis, 2012, Mosby.

Auerbach PS: *Wilderness medicine*, ed 5, St Louis, 2007, Mosby.

Auerbach PS: *Wilderness medicine*, ed 6, Philadelphia, 2012, Mosby.

Ayres-de-Campos D, Nogueira-Reis Z: Technical characteristics of current cardiotocographic monitors, *Best Pract Res Clin Obstetrics Gynaecol* 30:22–32, 2016.

Baggish M, Karram M: *Atlas of pelvic anatomy and gynecologic surgery*, ed 3, St Louis, 2011, Saunders.

Bailey RH, et al.: *Colorectal surgery*, Philadelphia, 2013, Saunders.

Ball JW, Dains JE, Flynn JA, Solomon BS, Stewart RW: *Seidel's guide to physical examination*, ed 8, St Louis, 2015, Mosby.

Baren JM: *Pediatric emergency medicine*, Philadelphia, 2008, Saunders.

Barkauskas VH, Baumann L, Darling-Fisher C: *Health and physical assessment*, ed 3, St Louis, 2002, Mosby.

Bath-Balogh M, Fehrenbach M: *Illustrated dental embryology, histology, and anatomy*, ed 3, St Louis, 2011, Saunders.

Baynes J, Dominiczak M: *Medical biochemistry*, ed 4, Philadelphia, 2015, Saunders.

Beare PG, Myers JL: *Adult health nursing*, ed 3, St Louis, 1998, Mosby.

Beigel R, Cercek B, Luo H, Siegel R: Noninvasive evaluation of right atrial pressure, *J Am Soc Echocard* 26(9):1033–1042, 2013.

Beischer NA, Mackey EV, Coblitz PB: *Obstetrics and the newborn*, ed 3, Philadelphia, 1997, Saunders.

Beksinska M, Smit J, Joanis C, Usher-Patel M, Potter W: Female condom technology: new products and regulatory issues, *Contracep* 84(4):316–321, 2011.

Belchetz PE, Hammond P: *Mosby's color atlas and text of diabetes and endocrinology*, London, 2003, Mosby Ltd.

Belder: *Essential interventional cardiology*, ed 2, St. Louis, 2008, Elsevier Health Sciences.

Bennett JE, Dolin R, Blaser MJ: *Mandell, Douglas, and Bennett's principles and practice of infectious diseases*, ed 8, St. Louis, 2015, Elsevier/Saunders.

Bertolini J, Pelucio M: The red eye, *Emerg Clin North Am* 13(3):561–579, 1995.

Beth-Jones J: Psoriasis, *Med* 6(41):334–340, 2013.

Bieber EJ, Horowitz IR, Sanfilippo JS: *Clinical gynecology*, St. Louis, 2006, Churchill Livingstone.

Bindels RJM, Hoenderop JGJ, Biber J: Transport of calcium, magnesium, and phosphate. In Taal MW, editor: *Brenner and Rector's the kidney*, ed 9, Philadelphia, 2012, Saunders.

Bird DL, Robinson DS: *Torres and Ehrlich modern dental assisting*, ed 8, Philadelphia, 2005, Saunders.

Bird DL, Robinson DS: *Torres and Ehrlich modern dental assisting*, ed 10, St Louis, 2012, Saunders.

Bird DL, Robinson DS: *Torres and Ehrlich modern dental assisting*, ed 11, St Louis, 2015, Saunders.

Bischoff: *Pediatric gastrointestinal and liver disease*, ed 5, St. Louis, 2015, Elsevier.

Biswas D, Saha S, Bera SP: Relative distribution of the tumours of ear, nose and throat in the paediatric patients, *Int J Ped Otorhinolaryngol* 71(5):801–805, 2007.

Black JM, Hawks JH: *Medical-surgical nursing: clinical management for positive outcomes*, ed 7, Philadelphia, 2005, Saunders.

Black JM, Hawks JH: *Medical-surgical nursing: clinical management for positive outcomes*, ed 8, St Louis, 2009, Saunders.

Black MM, Ambros-Rudolph C, Edwards L, Lynch PJ: *Obstetric and gynecologic dermatology*, ed 3, 2008, Elsevier Ltd.

Blake EA, Cheng G, Post MD, Guntupalli S: Cotyledonoid dissecting leiomyoma with adipocytic differentiation: a case report, *Gynecol Oncol Rep* 11:7–9, 2014.

Blaustein M, Kao J, Matteson D: *Cellular physiology and neurophysiology*, ed 2, St Louis, 2012, Mosby.

Block MS: *Color atlas of dental implant surgery*, ed 4, St Louis, 2015, Saunders.

Bloom A, Ireland J: *Color atlas of diabetes*, ed 2, London, 1992, Mosby-Wolfe.

Bolognia JL, Jorizzo JL, Schaffer JV: *Dermatology*, ed 3, Philadelphia, 2012, Mosby.

Bolognia JL, Schaffer JV, Duncan KO, Ko CJ: *Dermatology essentials*, St Louis, 2014, Saunders.

Bonewit-West K: *Clinical procedures for medical assistants*, ed 8, St Louis, 2012, Saunders.

Bonewit-West K: *Clinical procedures for medical assistants*, ed 9, St Louis, 2015, Saunders.

Bonewit-West K, Hunt S, Applegate E: *Today's medical assistant: clinical and administrative procedures*, ed 2, St Louis, 2013, Saunders.

Bontrager KL, Lampignano JP: *Textbook of radiographic positioning and related anatomy*, ed 6, St Louis, 2005, Mosby.

Bontrager KL, Lampignano JP: *Textbook of radiographic positioning and related anatomy*, ed 7, St Louis, 2010, Mosby.

Bork K, Brauninger W: *Skin diseases in clinical practice*, ed 2, Philadelphia, 1999, Saunders.

Boron W, Boulpaep E: *Medical physiology (updated)*, ed 2, St Louis, 2012, Saunders.

Bos EM, Kuijper CF, Chrzan RJ, Dik P, Klijn AJ, et al.: Epispadias in boys with an intact prepuce, *J Pediatr Urol* 10(1):67–73, 2013.

Boyd: *Diagnostic gynecologic and obstetric pathology*, ed 3, St Louis, 2018, Elsevier.

Brandt ML: Pediatric hernias, *Surg Clin North Am* 88(1):27–43, 2008.

Braunstein: *Dermatological signs of systemic disease*, ed 5, St Louis, 2017, Elsevier.

Brazitikos PD, Tsinopoulos IT, Papadopoulos NT, Fotiadis K, Stangos NT: Ultrasonographic classification and phacoemulsification of white senile cataracts, *Ophthalmol Times* 106(11):2178–2183, 1999.

Brightbill FS: *Corneal surgery*, ed 4, St Louis, 2009, Mosby.

Brinster NK, Liu V, Diwan AH, McKee PH: *Dermatopathology: high-yield pathology*, Philadelphia, 2011, Saunders.

Bristow R, Armstrong D: *Early diagnosis and treatment of cancer: ovarian cancer*, Philadelphia, 2010, Saunders.

Broaddus V, Mason RJ, Ernst JD, King TE, Lazarus SC, et al.: *Murray and Nadel's textbook of respiratory medicine*, ed 6, Philadelphia, 2016, Saunders.

Brown M, Mulholland JL: *Drug calculations*, ed 8, St Louis, 2008, Mosby.

Browner BD, Fuller RP: *Musculoskeletal emergencies*, Philadelphia, 2013, Saunders.

Brucato MP, Patel K, Mgbako O: Diagnosis of gas gangrene: does a discrepancy exist between the published data and practice, *J Foot Ankle Surg* 53(2):137–140, 2014.

Bryant R, Nix D: *Acute and chronic wounds: current management concepts*, ed 4, St Louis, 2011, Mosby.

Buck CJ: *STEP-BY-STEP medical coding, 2015 edition*, St Louis, 2015(a), Mosby.

Buck CJ: *2015 ICD9CM, volumes 1 & 2, professional edition*, St Louis, 2015(b), Mosby.

Burt AD, Portmann BC, Ferrell LD: *MacSween's pathology of the liver*, Edinburgh, 2011, Churchill Livingstone.

Butcher GP: *Gastroenterology: an illustrated colour text*, London, 2004, Churchill Livingstone.

Callen JP, Greer KE, Paller AS, Swinyer LJ: *Color atlas of dermatology*, ed 2, Philadelphia, 2000, Saunders.

Calonje JE, Brenn T, Lazar AJ, McKee PH: *McKee's pathology of the skin*, ed 4, Philadelphia, 2012, Saunders.

Cameron JL: *Current surgical therapy*, ed 11, Philadelphia, 2014, Saunders.

Cameron JL: *Current surgical therapy*, ed 13, St. Louis, 2020, Elsevier.

Cameron MH, Monroe LG: *Physical rehabilitation for the physical therapist assistant*, Philadelphia, 2011, Saunders.

Campbell MF, Walsh PC, Retik AB: *Campbell's urology*, Philadelphia, 2002, Saunders.

Canale ST, Beaty JH: *Campbell's operative orthopaedics*, ed 11, Philadelphia, 2008, Mosby.

Canale ST, Beaty JH: *Campbell's operative orthopaedics*, ed 12, Philadelphia, 2013, Mosby.

Canard JM, Létard JC, Palazzo L, Penman I, Lennon E, Lennon AM: *Gastrointestinal endoscopy in practice*, Oxford, 2011, Elsevier Ltd.

Cañueto J, Santos-Briz Á, Yuste-Chaves M, Nieto G, Unamuno P: Turret exostosis or acquired osteochondroma. Dermatology, *Actas Dermo-Sifiliográficas* 102(6):474–475, 2010, English Edition.

Carey WD: *Cleveland clinic: current clinical medicine*, ed 2, Philadelphia, 2010, Mosby.

Carlson BM: *Human embryology and developmental biology*, ed 4, Philadelphia, 2009, Mosby.

Carpentier A, Adams DH, Filsoufi F: *Carpentier's reconstructive valve surgery: from valve analysis to valve reconstruction*, Philadelphia, 2010, Saunders.

Carr JH, Rodak BF: *Clinical hematology atlas*, ed 3, St Louis, 2009, Saunders.

Carr JH, Rodak BF: *Clinical hematology atlas*, ed 4, St Louis, 2013, Saunders.

Carty H, McCullough P, Aluwihare N, Matey P: Breast conserving surgery for breast cancer involving the nipple, *Breast* 17(1):107–110, 2007.

Cattermole GN, Leung PYM, Mak PSK, Graham CA, Ranier TH: Mid-arm circumference can be used to estimate children's weights, *Resuscitation* 81(9):1105–1110, 2010.

Cevasco: *Current clinical medicine*, ed 2, St. Louis, 2010, Saunders Elsevier.

Chabner D: *The language of medicine*, St Louis, 2007, Mosby.

Chan SK, Burrows NP: Atopic dermatitis, *Med* 37(5):242–245, 2009.

Chandrashekhar Y, Westaby S, Narula J: Mitral stenosis, *Lancet* 374(9697):1271–1283, 2009.

Chandrasekhara V, Elmunzer BJ, Khashab M, Muthusamy VR: *Clinical gastrointestinal endoscopy*, ed 3, Philadelphia, 2019, Elsevier.

Chang P: Diagnosis using the proximal and lateral nail folds, *Dermatol Clin* 33(2):207–241, 2015.

Chang Y: Fetoscopic guide laser therapy for twin–twin transfusion syndrome, *Gynecol Minim Invasive Ther* 2(1):8–12, 2012.

Chaudhry B, Harvey D: *Mosby's color atlas and text of pediatrics and child health*, St Louis, 2001, Mosby.

Chen W, Li S, Li Y, Wang Y: Medial epicanthoplasty using the palpebral margin incision method, *J Plast Reconstr Aesthet Surg* 62(12):1621–1626, 2009.

Chen WG, Dai MS, Ho CL, Huang TC: Isolated hypoglossal nerve paralysis, *Am J Med* 127(10):926–927, 2014.

Chen Z, Zhang X, Deng X: A new design of the retrievable vena cava filter, *Med Hypotheses* 79(5):635–636, 2012.

Cheng YP, Chiu HY, Hsiao CH, Lin CC, Liao YH: Scalp melanoma in a woman with LEOPARD syndrome: possible implication of PTPN11 signaling in melanoma pathogenesis, *J Am Acad Dermatol* 69(4):e186–e187, 2013.

Chester GA: *Modern medical assisting*, Philadelphia, 1999, WB Saunders.

Chhabra AB, Browne JA: *Orthopaedic surgical approaches*, Philadelphia, 2008, Saunders.

Chhabra L, Spodick DH: Himalayan osborn waves, *Canadian J Cardiol* 29(12):1743.e7–1743.e8, 2013.

Chiang YC, Lin TS, Yeh MC: Povidone-iodine-related burn under the tourniquet of a child – a case report and literature review, *J Plast Reconstr Aesthet Surg* 64(3):412–415, 2011.

Choo EK, McElroy S: Spontaneous Bowel Evisceration in a patient with Alcoholic Cirrhosis and an Umbilical Hernia, *J Emerg Med* 34(1):41–43, 2008.

Chopita N, Landoni N, Ross A, Villaverde A: Malignant gastroenteric obstruction: therapeutic options, *Gastrointest Endosc Clin N Am* 17(3):533–544, 2007.

Christensen B, Kockrow E: *Foundations and adult health nursing*, ed 6, Mosby, 2011.

Christensen BL, Kockrow E: *Adult health nursing*, ed 6, St Louis, 2010, Mosby.

Christensen GJ: *A consumer's guide to dentistry*, ed 2, St Louis, 2002, Mosby.

Chung KC: *Hand and upper extremity reconstruction*, New York, 2009, Saunders.

Cibas ES, Ducatman BS: *Cytology*, ed 4, Philadelphia, 2014, Saunders.

Ciocca L, Corinaldesi G, Marchetti C, Scotti R: Gingival hyperplasia around implants in the maxilla and jaw reconstructed by fibula free flap, *Int J Oral Maxillofac Surg* 37(5):478–480, 2007.

Cioffi WG, Asensio JA, Adams CA, Connolly MD, Biffl WL, et al.: *Atlas of trauma/emergency surgical techniques*, Philadelphia, 2014, Saunders.

Clark DA, Thompson JE, Barkemeyer BM: *Atlas of neonatology*, Philadelphia, 2000, Saunders.

Clayton BD, Willihnganz M: *Basic pharmacology for nurses*, ed 16, St Louis, 2013, Mosby.

Coad J, Dunstall M: *Anatomy and physiology for midwives*, ed 3, St Louis, 2011, Elsevier.

Cochard LR, Goodhartz LA, Harmath CB, Major NM, Mukundan S: *Netter's introduction to imaging*, Philadelphia, 2012, Saunders.

Cohen BA: *Pediatric dermatology*, ed 3, London, 2005, Mosby.

Cohen BA: *Pediatric dermatology*, ed 4, Philadelphia, 2013, Saunders.

Cohen BA, Davis HW, Mallory SB, Zitelli JA: *Pediatric dermatology: slide atlas of pediatric physical diagnosis*, Philadelphia, 1993, Saunders.

Cohen J, Opal SM, Powderly WG: *Infectious diseases*, ed 3, Oxford, 2010, Elsevier Ltd.

Cohen J, Powderly WG: *Infectious diseases*, ed 2, London, 2004, Mosby.

Cohen Jr MM, Lemire RJ: Syndromes with cephaloceles, *Teratology* 25:161–172, 1982.

Coleman NW, Fleckman P, Huang JI: Fungal nail infections, *J Hand Surg Am* 39(5):985–988, 2014.

Colledge N, Walker BR, Ralston SH: *Davidson's principles and practice of medicine*, ed 21, London, 2010, Churchill Livingstone.

Conlon CP, Snydman DR: *Mosby's color atlas and text of infectious diseases*, London, 2000, Mosby Ltd.

Connolly AJ, Finkbeiner WE, Ursell PC, Davis RL: *Autopsy pathology*, ed 3, Philadelphia, 2016, Elsevier.

Constantinescu R, Leonard C, Kurlan R: Assistive devices for gait in Parkinson's disease, *Parkinsonism Relat Disord* 13(3):133–138, 2006.

Cooper K, Gosnell K: *Foundations of nursing*, ed 7, St Louis, 2015, Mosby.

Copstead-Kirkhorn LE, Banasik JL: *Pathophysiology*, ed 5, Philadelphia, 2014, Saunders.

Coran, et al.: *Pediatric surgery*, ed 7, Philadelphia, 2012, Elsevier.

Cordoro KM, Ganz JE: Training room management of medical conditions: sports dermatology, *Clin Sports Med* 24(3):565–598, 2005.

Corradi D, Contini G, Gherli T, Nicolini F: A left atrial mixomalike rhabdomyosarcoma, *J Thorac Cardiovasc Surg* 144(1):e7–e10, 2012.

Costamagna: *Clinical gastrointestinal endoscopy*, ed 2, St. Louis, 2012, Saunders.

Coughlin MJ, Saltzman CL, Anderson RB: *Mann's surgery of the foot and ankle*, ed 9, Philadelphia, 2014, Saunders.

Cowan GM, Lockey RF: Oral manifestations of allergic, infectious, and immune-mediated disease, *J Allergy Clin Immunol Pract* 2(6):686–696, 2014.

Criado P, Rivitti E, Sotto M, de Carvalho J: Livedoid vasculopathy as a coagulation disorder, *Autoimmun Rev* 10(6):353–360, 2011.

Cronenwett JL, Johnston KW: *Rutherford's vascular surgery*, ed 8, Philadelphia, 2014, Saunders.

Cross S: *Underwood's pathology: a clinical approach*, ed 6, St Louis, 2013, Elsevier.

Crossman AR, Neary D: *Neuroanatomy: an illustrated colour text*, London, 2010, Churchill Livingstone.

Crum CP, Lee K, Nucci M, Granter S, Howitt B, Parast M, et al: *Diagnostic gynecology and obstetric pathology*, ed 3, Philadelphia, 2018, Elsevier.

Cummings NH, Stanley-Green S, Higgs P: *Perspectives in athletic training*, St Louis, 2009, Mosby.

Custalow C: *Color atlas of emergency department procedures*, Philadelphia, 2005, Saunders.

Dallaudière B, Salut C, Hummel V, Pouquet M, River P, et al.: MRI atlas of ectopic endometriosis, *Diagn Interv Imag* 94(3):263–280, 2013.

Damjanov I: *Pathology for the health professions*, ed 3, St Louis, 2006, Saunders.

Damjanov I: *Pathology for the health professions*, ed 4, St Louis, 2012, Saunders.

Damjanov I: *Pathophysiology*, Philadelphia, 2008, Saunders.

Damjanov I, Linder J: *Pathology: a color atlas*, St Louis, 2000, Mosby.

Daniel SJ, Harfst SA, Wilder RS: *Mosby's dental hygiene: concepts, cases and competencies*, ed 2, St Louis, 2008, Mosby.

Danzer E, Johnson MP: Fetal surgery for neural tube defects, *Semin Fetal Neonatal Med* 19(1):2–8, 2014.

Darlymple NC, Leyendecker J, Oliphant M: *Problem solving in abdominal imaging*, St. Louis, 2009, Elsevier.

Dasouki M, Jawdet O, Almadhoun O, Pasnoor M, McVey AL, et al.: Pompe disease, *Neurol Clin* 32(3):751–776, 2014.

Davey AJ, Diba A: *Ward's anaesthetic equipment*, ed 6, Oxford, 2012, Elsevier.

David T, Hoyt CS: *Pediatric ophthalmology and strabismus*, London/New York, 2005, Saunders.

Dayton P, Feilmeier M, Hensley NL: Technique for minimally invasive reduction of calcaneal fractures using small bilateral external fixation, *J Foot Ankle Surg* 3(53):376–382, 2014.

De Berker D: Nail anatomy, *Clin Dermatol* 5(31):509–515, 2013.

Dean J, McDonald R, Avery D: *McDonald and Avery dentistry for the child and adolescent*, ed 9, St Louis, 2011, Mosby.

de Graaf DC, Aerts M, Danneels E, Devreese B: Bee, wasp and ant venomics pave the way for a component-resolved diagnosis of sting allergy, *J Proteomics* 72(2):145–154, 2009.

Dehn RW, Asprey DP: *Essential clinical procedures*, ed 3, Philadelphia, 2013, Saunders.

DeLee JC, Drez D, Miller MD: *DeLee and Drez's orthopaedic sports medicine: principles and practice*, ed 3, Philadelphia, 2009, Saunders.

Demetracopoulos C, Sponseller P: Spinal deformities in Marfan syndrome, *Orthop Clin North Am* 4(38):563–572, 2007, 4.

de Weerd L, Mercer JB, Weum S: Dynamic infrared thermography, *Clin Plast Surg* 38(2):277–292, 2011.

deWit SC, O'Neill P: *Fundamental concepts and skills for nursing*, ed 4, St Louis, 2014, Saunders.

Dias FM, Marçal F, Oliveira J, Póvoas M, Mouzinho A, Marques JG: Exuberant varicella-zoster exanthema and pneumonia as clinical clue for HIV infection, *J Pediatr* 166(1):199, 2015.

Dim CC, Umeh UA, Ezeqwui HU, Ikeme AC: Uterine procidentia in an African adolescent: an uncommon gynecological challenge, *J Pediatr Adolesc Gynecol* 21(1):37–39, 2008.

Dotto RS, Marx G, Bastos M, Machado JL, Glufke V, De Oliveira Freitas DM: A rare case of virilizing adult ectopic adrenal tumor, *Urol Case Rep* 27(100907), 2019.

Doty D, Doty J: *Cardiac surgery: operative technique*, ed 2, Philadelphia, 2012, Saunders.

Douglas G, Nicol F, Robertson C: *Macleod's clinical examination*, ed 13, Oxford, 2013, Elsevier Ltd.

Drake RL, Vogl AW, Mitchell AWM: *Gray's anatomy for students*, Philadelphia, 2005, Churchill Livingstone.

Drake RL, Vogl AW, Mitchell AWM: *Gray's anatomy for students*, ed 2, Philadelphia, 2010, Churchill Livingstone.

Drake RL, Vogl AW, Mitchell AWM: *Gray's anatomy for students*, ed 3, Philadelphia, 2015, Churchill Livingstone.

du Vivier A: *Atlas of clinical dermatology*, ed 2, London, 1993, Gower Medical Publishing.

du Viver A: *Atlas of clinical dermatology*, ed 3, London, 2002, Gower Medical Publishing.

du Vivier A: *Atlas of clinical dermatology*, ed 4, London, 2013, Saunders.

Duderstadt K: *Pediatric physical examination: an illustrated handbook*, St Louis, 2006, Mosby.

Dujardin M, Luypaert R, Vandenbrouke F, Van der Niepen P, Sourbron S, et al.: Combined T1-based perfusion MRI and MR angiography in kidney: first experience in normals and pathology, *Eur J Radiol* 69(3):542–549, 2007.

Edmond RT, Welsby PD, Rowland HA: *Color atlas of infectious diseases*, ed 4, St. Louis, 2003, Mosby.

Ehrlich RA: *Patient care in radiography: with an introduction to medical imaging*, ed 8, St Louis, 2013, Mosby.

Eichenfield L, Frieden I, Mathes E, Zaenglein A: *Neonatal and infant dermatology*, ed 3, St Louis, 2015, Elsevier.

Eisen D, Lynch DP: *The mouth: diagnosis and treatment*, St Louis, 1998, Mosby.

Eisenberg R, Johnson N: *Comprehensive radiographic pathology*, ed 5, St Louis, 2012, Elsevier.

Elkin MK, Perry AG, Potter PA: *Nursing interventions and clinical skills*, ed 4, St Louis, 2007, Mosby.

Ellison D, Love S, Chimelli L, Harding B, Lowe JS, et al.: *Neuropathology*, ed 3, Oxford, 2013, Elsevier Ltd.

Elsevier: *Clinical skills: essentials collection: fundamentals and health assessment*, St Louis, 2016, Mosby.

Elsharawy MA: Outcome of midfoot amputations in diabetic gangrene, *Ann Vasc Surg* 25(6):778–782, 2011.

Emre A, Akbulut S, Yilmaz M, Kanlioz M, Aydin BE: Double Meckel's diverticulum presenting as acute appendicitis: a case report and literature review, *J Emerg Med* 4(44):e321–e324, 2013.

ENA: *Sheehy's emergency nursing: principles and practice*, ed 6, St Louis, 2010, Mosby.

Epstein O, Perkin D, Cookson J: *Clinical examination*, ed 3, St Louis, 2003, Mosby.

Errico TJ, Lonner BS, Moulton AW: *Surgical management of spinal deformities*, Philadelphia, 2009, Saunders.

Evans RC: *Illustrated orthopedic physical assessment*, ed 3, St Louis, 2009, Mosby.

Everett T, Kell C: *Human movement: an introductory text*, ed 6, St Louis, 2010, Elsevier.

Falcone T, Hurd WW: *Clinical reproductive medicine and surgery*, Philadelphia, 2007, Mosby.

Farrar J, Hotez P, Junghanss T, Kang G, Lalloo D, White NJ: *Manson's tropical diseases*, ed 23, Oxford, 2014, Elsevier Ltd.

Farrar WE: *Atlas of infections of the nervous system*, London, 1992, Mosby-Wolfe.

Fatemi MJ, Jalilimanesh M, Dini MT: Evaluation of moving and static two point discriminations of volar forearm skin before and after transfer as a sensate radial forearm island flap in reconstruction of degloving injury of the thumb, *J Plast Reconstr Aesthet Surg* 60(4):356–359, 2007.

Fehrenbach M, Herring S: *Illustrated anatomy of the head and neck*, ed 4, Philadelphia, 2012, Saunders.

Fehrenbach MJ, Popowics T: *Illustrated dental embryology, histology, and anatomy*, Philadelphia, 2016, Saunders.

Feldman M, Friedman LS, Brandt LJ: *Sleisenger and Fordtran's gastrointestinal and liver disease*, ed 8, Philadelphia, 2006, Saunders.

Feldman M, Friedman LS, Brandt LJ: *Sleisenger and Fordtran's gastrointestinal and liver disease*, ed 9, Philadelphia, 2010, Saunders.

Feldman M, Friedman LS, Brandt LJ: *Sleisenger and Fordtran's gastrointestinal and liver disease*, ed 10, Philadelphia, 2016, Saunders.

Ferri FF: *Ferri's clinical advisor 2016*, Philadelphia, 2016, Elsevier.

Ferri FF: *Ferri's clinical advisor 2018*, Philadelphia, 2018, Elsevier.

Ferri FF: *Ferri's color atlas and text of clinical medicine*, Philadelphia, 2009, Saunders.

Ferri FF: *Ferri's fast facts in dermatology*, ed 2, Philadelphia, 2019, Elsevier.

Fewkes JL, Cheney ML, Pollack SV: *Illustrated atlas of cutaneous surgery*, London, 1992, Gower Medical Publishing.

Fielding JR, Brown DL, Thurmond AS: *Gynecologic imaging: expert radiology series*, Philadelphia, 2011, Saunders.

Finkbeiner WE, Ursell PC, Davis RL: *Autopsy pathology: a manual and atlas*, ed 2, Philadelphia, 2009, Saunders.

Firestein GS, Kelley WN: *Kelly's textbook of rheumatology*, Philadelphia, 2009, Saunders.

FitzGerald MJT, Gruener G, Mtui E: *Clinical neuroanatomy & neuroscience*, ed 6, Oxford, 2012, Elsevier Ltd.

Fitzpatrick JE, High WA: *Urgent care dermatology: Symptom-based diagnosis,* St Louis, 2018, Elsevier.

Fleshman JW, Birnbaum EH, Hunt SR, Mutch MG, Kodner IJ, Safar B, et al.: *Atlas of surgical techniques for colon, rectum and anus*, Philadelphia, 2013, Saunders.

Fletcher DM: *Diagnostic histopathology of tumors*, ed 3, Edinburgh, 2007, Churchill Livingston/Elsevier Ltd.

Flint PW, Haughey BH, Lund VJ, Niparko JK, Robbins KT, et al.: *Cummings otolaryngology head & neck surgery*, ed 6, St Louis, 2015, Mosby.

Flint PW, Richardson MA, Haughey BH, Lund VJ, Niparko JK, et al.: *Cummings otolaryngology head & neck surgery*, ed 5, St Louis, 2010, Mosby.

Flynn J, Garner M, D'Italia J, Davidson RS, Ganley TJ, et al.: The treatment of low-energy femoral shaft fractures: a prospective study comparing the "walking spica" with the traditional spica, *J Bone Joint Surg* 93(23):2196–2202, 2011.

Fogo AB, Kashgarian M: *Diagnostic atlas of renal pathology: a companion to Brenner & Rector's the Kidney*, ed 2, Philadelphia, 2012, Saunders.

Folpe AL, Inwards CY: *Bone and soft tissue pathology*, Philadelphia, 2010, Saunders.

Fons ME, Stein DJ, Patel A, Ferrer MS, Ammon H, et al.: Extracolonic gastrointestinal tract morphologic findings in a case of pseudomembranous collagenous colitis, *Ann Diagnos Pathol* 17(3):291–294, 2013.

Forbes B, Sahm D, Weissfeld A: *Bailey & Scott's diagnostic microbiology*, ed 12, St Louis, 2007, Mosby.

Forbes CD, Jackson WF: *Color atlas and text of clinical medicine*, ed 3, London, 2003, Mosby Ltd.

Fortinash K, Holoday-Worret P: *Psychiatric mental health nursing*, ed 4, St Louis, 2008, Mosby.

Frank ED, Long BW, Smith BJ: *Merrill's atlas of radiographic positioning and procedures*, ed 11, St Louis, 2007, Mosby.

Frank ED, Long BW, Smith BJ: *Merrill's atlas of radiographic positioning and procedures*, ed 12, St Louis, 2012, Mosby.

Frantzides CT, Carlson MA: *Video atlas of advanced minimally invasive surgery*, Philadelphia, 2013, Saunders.

Frazier M: *Essentials of human diseases and conditions*, ed 5, Philadelphia, 2013, Saunders.

Frazier MS, Drzymkowski JW: *Essentials of human diseases and conditions*, ed 3, Philadelphia, 2004, Saunders.

Frazier MS, Drzymkowski JW: *Essentials of human diseases and conditions*, ed 4, Philadelphia, 2009, Saunders.

Freund KB, et al: *The retinal atlas*, ed 2, 2017, St Louis.

Friedman-Kien AE, Cockerell CJ: *Color atlas of AIDS*, ed 2, Philadelphia, 1996, Saunders.

Froberg B, Ibrahim D, Furbee RB: Plant poisoning, *Emerg Med Clin North Am* 25(2):375–433, 2007.

Frownfelter D, Dean E: *Cardiovascular and pulmonary physical therapy*, ed 4, St Louis, 2006, Mosby.

Fugate JE, Lyons JL, Thakur KT, Smith BR, Hedley-Whyte ET, Mateen FJ: Infectious causes of stroke, *Lancet Infect Dis* 14(9):869–880, 2014.

Fuhrman BP, Zimmerman JJ: *Pediatric critical care*, ed 4, St Louis, 2011, Mosby.

Fujimori K, Shiroto T, Kuretake S, Gunji H, Sato A: An omphalopagus parasitic twin after intracytoplasmic sperm injection, *Fertil Steril* 82(5):1430–1432, 2004.

Gabbe SG, Niebyl JR, Simpson JL, Landon MB, Galan HL, Jauniaux ERM, et al.: *Obstetrics: normal and problem pregnancies*, ed 6, Philadelphia, 2012, Saunders.

App

Garden OJ, Bradbury AW, Forsythe JLR, Parks RW: *Principles and practice of surgery*, ed 6, London, 2012, Churchill Livingstone.

Garfin SR, et al.: *Rothman-Simeone and Herkowitz's the spine*, ed 7, St. Louis, 2018, Elsevier.

Garrels M, Oatis CS: *Laboratory testing for ambulatory settings: a guide for health professionals*, ed 2, St Louis, 2011, Saunders.

Garrels M, Oatis CS: *Laboratory and diagnostic testing in ambulatory care: a guide for health care professionals*, ed 3, Philadelphia, 2015, Saunders.

Gartner LP, Hiatt JL: *Color textbook of histology*, ed 3, Philadelphia, 2007, Saunders.

Gattuso P, Reddy VB, David O, Spitz DJ, Haber MH: *Differential diagnosis in surgical pathology*, ed 3, Philadelphia, 2015, Saunders.

Gaw A, Murphy M: *Clinical biochemistry: an illustrated colour text*, ed 5, Oxford, 2013, Churchill Livingstone.

Gawkrodger DJ: *Dermatology: an illustrated colour text*, ed 6, Oxford, 2017, Elsevier Ltd.

Gawkrodger DJ, Ardern-Jones MR: *Dermatology: an illustrated colour text*, ed 5, Oxford, 2012, Elsevier Ltd.

Gazendam MGJ, Hof AL: Averaged EMG profiles in jogging and running at different speeds, *Gait Posture* 25(4):604–614, 2006.

Gearhart JG, Rink RC: *Pediatric urology*, Philadelphia, 2010, Saunders.

Ghander C, Tenenbaum F, Tissier F, Silvera S, Lelej D, Dousset B, et al.: When adrenal Cushing's and phaeochromocytoma meet, *Lancet* 380(9854):1683–1683, 2012.

Gilbert-Barness E: *Potter's pathology of the fetus, infant, and child*, ed 2, Philadelphia, 2007, Mosby.

Ginsberg GG, et al.: *Clinical gastrointestinal endoscopy*, ed 2, St. Louis, 2012, Elsevier.

Giulio I, et al.: Lung ultrasound findings undetectable by chest radiography in children with community-acquired pneumonia, *Ultrasound Med Biol* 44(8):1687–1693, 2018.

Gleason C, Juul S: *Avery's diseases of the newborn*, ed 10, St Louis, 2018, Elsevier.

Glynn M, Drake W: *Hutchinson's clinical methods: an integrated approach to clinical practice*, ed 23, London, 2012, Saunders/Elsevier Ltd.

Goetz CG: *Textbook of clinical neurology*, ed 3, Philadelphia, 2007, Saunders.

Goldbloom RB: *Pediatric clinical skills*, ed 4, Philadelphia, 2011, Saunders.

Goldblum, JR, et al: *Enzinger and Weiss's soft tissue tumors*, ed 6, Philadelphia, 2014, Elsevier.

Goldman L, Ausiello DA, Arend W, Armitage JO, Clemmons D, et al.: *Cecil textbook of medicine*, ed 23, Philadelphia, 2008, Saunders.

Goldman L, Ausiello DA, Arend W, Armitage JO, Drazen JM, et al.: *Cecil textbook of medicine*, ed 22, Philadelphia, 2004, Saunders.

Goldman L, Schafer AI: *Goldman's Cecil medicine*, ed 24, Philadelphia, 2012, Saunders.

Goldman L, Schafer AI: *Goldman-Cecil medicine*, ed 25, Philadelphia, 2016, Saunders.

Goldstein BJ, Goldstein AO: *Practical dermatology*, ed 2, St Louis, 1997, Mosby.

Goljan EF: *Rapid review pathology*, ed 4, Philadelphia, 2013, Saunders.

Gómez G, Lopez N, Gómez G, Méndez M: Linear scleroderma en coup de sabre and epilepsy: presentation of a case in a child, *Neurol* 27(7):449–451, 2012.

Gonzalez AL, Cates JMM: Osteosarcoma: differential diagnostic considerations, *Surg Pathol Clin* 5(1):117–146, 2012.

González R, Farias J, Seguel E, Alarcón E: Azygous lobe, *J Am Coll Surg* 209(5):673, 2009.

Gore RM, Levine MS: *Textbook of gastrointestinal radiology*, ed 4, Philadelphia, 2015, Saunders.

Gosling JA, Harris PF, Humpherson JR, Whitmore I, Willan PLT: *Human anatomy: color atlas and textbook*, ed 5, Oxford, 2008, Elsevier Ltd.

Gould B, Dyer R: *Pathophysiology for the health professions*, ed 4, Philadelphia, 2011, Saunders.

Gould KC, Hubert RJ: *Gould's pathophysiology for the health professions*, ed 5, St Louis, 2014, Saunders.

Graham JM, Smith DV: *Smith's recognizable patterns of human deformation*, ed 3, Philadelphia, 2007, Saunders.

Graham-Brown R, Bourke J: *Mosby's color atlas and text of dermatology*, ed 2, London, 2007, Mosby.

Gravante G, Filingeri V, Delogu D, Santeusanio G, Palmieri MB, Esposito G, et al.: Apoptotic cell death in deep partial thickness burns by coexpression analysis of TUNEL and Fas, *Surgery* 139(6):854–855, 2006.

Greig JD, Garden OJ: *Color atlas of surgical diagnosis,* 1996, Times Mirror International.

Griffin N, Grant L: *Grainger & Allison's diagnostic radiology essentials*, London, 2013, Churchill Livingstone.

Gruber G, Hansch A: *Kompaktatlas Blickdiagnosen in der Inneren Medizin*, Munchen, 2007, Urban & Fischer.

Gudson S, de Macêdo MP: Effects of a dynamic orthosis in an individual with claw deformity, *J Hand Ther* 28(4):425–428, 2015.

Gurley L, Callaway WJ: *Introduction to radiologic technology*, ed 7, St Louis, 2011, Mosby.

Gutmann JL, Dumsha TC, Lovdahl PE: *Problem solving in endodontics: prevention, identification, and management*, ed 4, St Louis, 2006, Mosby.

Guyuron B, Eriksson E: *Plastic surgery: indications and practice*, Philadelphia, 2009, Saunders.

Haack J, Papel ID: Caudal septal deviation, *Otolaryngol Clin North Am* 42(3):427–436, 2009.

Haarmann S, Budihardja AS, Hölzle F, Wolff KD: Subcutaneous temporal abscess as a clinical manifestation of pulmonary arteriovenous malformations in a patient with hereditary haemorrhagic telangiectasia (Rendu-Osler-Weber disease), *Int J Oral Maxillofac Surg* 36(12):1211–1214, 2007.

Habif T: *Clinical dermatology*, ed 6, Oxford, 2016, Elsevier.

Habif TP: *Clinical dermatology: a color guide to diagnosis and therapy*, ed 3, St Louis, 1996, Mosby.

Habif TP: *Clinical dermatology: a color guide to diagnosis and therapy*, ed 4, St Louis, 2004, Mosby.

Habif TP: *Clinical dermatology: a color guide to diagnosis and therapy*, ed 5, St Louis, 2010, Mosby.

Habif TP, Campbell Jr JL, Chapman MS, Dinulos JGH, Zug KA: *Skin disease diagnosis and treatment*, ed 3, St Louis, 2011, Saunders.

Habif TP, et al.: *Skin disease: diagnosis and treatment*, ed 4, Elsevier, 2018.

Hadj I, Meziane M, Mikou O, Inani K, Harmouch T, Mernissi FZ: Tuberculous gummas with sporotrichoid pattern in a 57-year-old female: a case report and review of the literature, *Int J Mycobacteriol* 3(1):66–70, 2013.

Hagberg CA: *Benumof and Hagberg's airway management*, ed 3, Philadelphia, 2013, Saunders.

Hagen-Ansert SL: *Textbook of diagnostic ultrasonography*, ed 6, St Louis, 2006, Mosby.

Hagen-Ansert SL: *Textbook of diagnostic ultrasonography*, ed 7, St Louis, 2012, Mosby.

Halberg M: Nummular eczema, *J Emerg Med* 43(5):e327–e328, 2012.

Hall JE, Guyton AC: *Guyton and Hall textbook of medical physiology*, ed 12, Philadelphia, 2011, Saunders.

Hammond DC: *Atlas of aesthetic breast surgery*, Philadelphia, 2009, Saunders.

Han JC, Lawlor DA, Kimm SY: Childhood obesity, *Lancet* 375(9727):1737–1748, 2010.

Hansell DM: *Imaging of diseases of the chest*, ed 5, St. Louis, 2009, Elsevier Health Sciences.

Hansen 3rd RT, Zhang HT: Senescent-induced dysregulation of cAMP/CREB signaling and correlations with cognitive decline, *Brain Res* 1516:93–109, 2013.

Harkreader H, Hogan MA, Thobaben M: *Fundamentals of nursing*, ed 3, Philadelphia, 2007, Saunders.

Hegde V, Mitrut I, Singh J: Episcleritis: an association with IgA nephropathy, *Cont Lens Ant Eye* 32(3):141–142, 2009.

Henry MC, Stapleton ER: *EMT prehospital care*, ed 3, Philadelphia, 2004, Saunders.

Herendael BHV, Dreessen P, Jeurissen A: Fishy business: the value of the QuantiFERON-TB Test in the diagnosis of Mycobacterium marinum skin lesions, *Clin Microbiol Newsl* 34(12):98–100, 2012.

Herlihy B: *The human body in health and illness*, ed 4, St Louis, 2011, Saunders.

Herlihy B: *The human body in health and illness*, ed 5, Philadelphia, 2014, Saunders.

Hernandez A: *Sabiston textbook of surgery*, ed 20, St Louis, 2017, Elsevier.

Herring JA: *Tachdjian's pediatric orthopaedics*, Philadelphia, 2008, Saunders.

Herring JA: *Tachdjian's pediatric orthopaedics*, ed 5, Philadelphia, 2014, Saunders.

Herzig DO, Lu KC: Anal fissure, *Surg Clin North Am* 90(1):33–34, 2010.

Heymann HO, Swift EJ: *Sturdevant's art and science of operative dentistry*, ed 5, St Louis, 2006, Mosby.

Hisi ED: *Hematopathology*, ed 2, Philadelphia, 2012, Saunders.

Hochberg MC, Silman AJ, Smolen J, Weinblatt ME: *Rheumatology*, ed 6, St Louis, 2015, Mosby.

Hockenberry MJ, Wilson D: *Wong's nursing care of infants and children*, ed 8, St Louis, 2007, Mosby.

Hockenberry MJ, Wilson D: *Wong's nursing care of infants and children*, ed 9, St Louis, 2011, Mosby.

Hockenberry MJ, Wilson D: *Wong's nursing care of infants and children*, ed 10, St Louis, 2015, Mosby.

Hoff NP, Gerber PA: Herpetic whitlow, *Can Med Assoc J* 184(17):E924-E924, 2012.

Hoffbrand AV, Pettit JE, Vyas P: *Color atlas of clinical hematology*, ed 4, Philadelphia, 2010, Mosby Elsevier.

Hoffman R, Benz EJ, Silberstein LE, Heslop H, Furie B, et al.: *Hematology: basic principles and practice*, ed 5, Philadelphia, 2009, Churchill Livingstone.

Hoffman R, Benz EJ, Silberstein LE, Heslop H, Weitz JI, Anastasi J, et al.: *Basic principles and practice*, ed 6, Philadelphia, 2013, Saunders.

Ho-Fung VM, Zapala MA, Lee EY: Musculoskeletal traumatic injuries in children: characteristic imaging findings and mimickers, *Radiol Clin North Am* 55(4):785–802, 2017.

Holcomb GW, et al.: *Atlas of pediatric laparoscopy and thoracoscopy*, Philadelphia, 2008, Saunders.

Hordinsky MK, Sawaya ME, Scher RK: *Atlas of hair and nails*, Philadelphia, 2000, Churchill Livingstone.

Howard MR, Hamilton PJ, Haematology: *An illustrated colour text*, ed 4, Oxford, 2013, Elsevier Ltd.

Hoyt CS, Taylor D: *Pediatric ophthalmology and strabismus*, ed 4, Philadelphia, 2013, Saunders.

Huang H, Wu Y, Hsieh Y: Dendritic cell neurofibroma with pseudorosettes: one case report and literature review, *Dermatol Sin* 30(2):75–77, 2012.

Huether SE, McCance KL: *Understanding pathophysiology*, ed 4, St Louis, 2008, Mosby.

Huether SE, McCance KL: *Understanding pathophysiology*, ed 5, St Louis, 2012, Mosby.

Hunt RB: *Text and atlas of female infertility and surgery*, ed 3, St Louis, 1999, Mosby.

Hurwitz S: *Clinical pediatric dermatology*, ed 2, Philadelphia, 1993, Saunders.

Husain AN: *High-yield thoracic pathology*, Philadelphia, 2012, Saunders.

Ibsen OAC, Phelan JA: *Oral pathology for the dental hygienist*, ed 5, St Louis, 2009, Saunders.

Ibsen OAC, Phelan JA: *Oral pathology for the dental hygienist*, ed 6, St Louis, 2014, Saunders.

Igai H, Yamamoto Y, Chang SS, Yamamoto M, Tabata Y, et al.: Tracheal cartilage regeneration by slow release of basic fibroblast growth factor from a gelatin sponge, *J Thor Cardiovasc Surg* 134(1):170–175, 2007.

Ignatavicius DD, Workman ML: *Medical-surgical nursing: critical thinking for collaborative care*, ed 4, Philadelphia, 2002, Saunders.

Ignatavicius DD, Workman ML: *Medical-surgical nursing: critical thinking for collaborative care*, ed 5, Philadelphia, 2006, Saunders.

Ignatavicius DD, Workman ML: *Medical-surgical nursing: patient-centered collaborative care*, ed 6, St Louis, 2010, Saunders.

Ignatavicius DD, Workman ML: *Medical-surgical nursing: patient-centered collaborative care*, ed 7, St Louis, 2016, Saunders.

Irwin S, Tecklin JS: *Cardiopulmonary physical therapy: a guide to practice*, ed 4, St Louis, 2004, Mosby.

Izadpanah A, Hogeling M, Buka RL, Eichenfield LF, Bird LM: Digitocutaneous dysplasia, *J Am Acad Dermatol* 56(Suppl 2):S6–9, 2007.

Jacob JJ, Paul TV, Mathews SS, Thomas N: Perrault syndrome with marfanoid habitus in two siblings, *J Ped Adol Gynecol* 20(5):305–308, 2007.

Jaffe ES, Harris NL, Vardiman JW, Campo E, Arber DA: *Hematopathology*, Philadelphia, 2011, Saunders.

Jaffe NS: *Atlas of ophthalmic surgery*, ed 2, London, 1996, Times Mirror International.

James SR, Ashwill JW: *Nursing care of children: principles and practice*, ed 3, St Louis, 2007, Saunders.

James SR, Ashwill JW: *Nursing care of children: principles and practice*, ed 4, St Louis, 2013, Saunders.

James WD, Berger TG, Elston DM: *Andrews' diseases of the skin: clinical dermatology*, ed 10, Philadelphia, 2006, Saunders.

James WD, Berger TG, Elston DM: *Andrews' diseases of the skin: clinical dermatology*, ed 11, Philadelphia, 2011, Saunders.

James WD, Berger TG, Eston DM: *Andrews' diseases of the skin: clinical dermatology*, ed 12, Philadelphia, 2016, Elsevier.

John Hopkins Hospital: *Harriet lane handbook*, ed 20, Philadelphia, 2015, Saunders, as seen in Cohen BA. Dermatology image atlas. Available at, 2001. http://www.dermatlas.org/.

Johnson RJ, Feehally J, Floege J: *Comprehensive clinical nephrology*, ed 5, Philadelphia, 2015, Saunders.

Jorde LB, Carey JC, Bamshad MJ, White RL: *Medical genetics, updated edition for 2006-2007*, ed 3, St Louis, 2006, Mosby.

Juan PA, José IV, Carolina M, Marco A: Black hairy tongue during interferon therapy for hepatitis C, *Ann Hepatol* 14(3), 2015.

Jung SN, Park SH, Hwang DY, Kwon H, Yim YM, V-Y-Z: Plasty for correcting cryptotia, *Br J Oral Maxillofac Surg* 47(7):562–563, 2008.

Kaban LB, Seldin EB, Kikinis R, Yeshwant K, Padwa BL: Clinical application of curvilinear distraction osteogenesis for correction of mandibular deformities, *J Oral Maxillofac Surg* 67(5):996–1008, 2009.

Kalu PU, Williams G: Scalding as an unusual cause of *Pyoderma gangrenosum*, *Burns* 33(1):105–108, 2007.

Kanski JJ: *Clinical diagnosis in ophthalmology*, London, 2006, Mosby.

Kanski JJ: *Clinical ophthalmology: a systematic approach*, ed 6, London, 2007, Butterworth Heinemann.

Kanski JJ: *Clinical ophthalmology: a test yourself atlas*, ed 2, New York, 2002, Butterworth-Heinemann.

Kanski JJ, Bowling B: *Clinical ophthalmology: a systematic approach*, ed 7, London, 2011, Saunders.

Kanski JJ, Nischal KK: *Ophthalmology: clinical signs and differential diagnosis*, London, 1999, Mosby International.

Kanski JJ, Thomas DJ: *The eye in systemic disease*, ed 2, St Louis, 2014, Elsevier.

Kassolik K, Andrzejewski W, Wilk I, Brzozowski M, Voyce K, et al.: The effectiveness of massage based on the tensegrity principle compared with classical abdominal massage performed on patients with constipation, *Arch Geronto Geriatr* 61(2):202–211, 2015.

Kaufman DM: *Clinical neurology for psychiatrists*, ed 6, Philadelphia, 2007, Saunders.

Kelly Jr RE: Pectus excavatum: historical background, clinical picture, preoperative evaluation and criteria for operation, *Semin Pediatr Surg* 17(3):181–193, 2008.

Kerr D, Partridge H: Deus ex machina: the use of technology in type 1 diabetes, *Prim Care Diabetes* 5(3):159–165, 2011.

Kim D, Chang U, Kim S, Bilksy MH: *Tumors of the spine*, Philadelphia, 2008, Saunders.

App

Kim M, Oh Y, Hong SP, Jeon S, Lee W: Does segmental lipodystrophy represent mosaicism of inherited lipodystrophy? *J Am Acad Dermatol* 60(3):519–521, 2008.

Kim S, Chung DH: Pediatric solic malignancies: neuroplastoma and Wilms' tumor, *Surg Clin North Am* 86(2):469–487, 2006.

King TE, Zamora AC: Neurofibromatosis. In Laurent GJ, Shapiro SD, editors: *Encyclopedia of respiratory medicine*, Academic Press, 2006.

Kinney M: *Andreoli's comprehensive cardiac care*, ed 8, St Louis, 1996, Mosby.

Kiss A, Polovitzer M, Merksz M, Kardos A, Schaffer P, et al.: Treatment of posttraumatic high-flow priapism in 8-year-old boy with percutaneous ultrasound-guided thrombin injection, *Urol Times* 69(4):779, 2007.

Kittur MA, Padget J, Drake D: Management of macroglossia in Beckwith–Wiedemann syndrome, *Br J Oral Maxillofac Surg* 51(1):e6–e8, 2012.

Klatt EC: *Robbins and Cotran atlas of pathology*, ed 2, Philadelphia, 2010, Saunders.

Klatt EC: *Robbins and Cotran atlas of pathology*, ed 3, Philadelphia, 2015, Saunders.

Klein E: *Urology*, St Louis, 2010, Elsevier, pp 791–793.

Kliegman RM, Stanton St BMD, Geme J, Schor NF: *Nelson textbook of pediatrics*, ed 20, Philadelphia, 2016, Saunders.

Kliegman RM, Stanton St BMD, Geme J, Schor NF, Behrman RE: *Nelson textbook of pediatrics*, ed 19, Philadelphia, 2011, Saunders.

Ko CJ, Elston DM: Pediculosis, *J Am Acad Dermatol* 50:1–12, 2004.

Kobayashi S: Fournier's gangrene, *Am J Surg* 195(2):257–258, 2008.

Koeppen B, Stanton B: *Berne & Levy physiology (updated)*, ed 6, St Louis, 2010, Mosby.

Komotar RJ, Mocco J, Kaiser MG: Surgical management of cervical myelopathy: indications and techniques for laminectomy and fusion, *Spine J* 6:259S, 2006.

Koo YJ, Kim DY, Kim KR, Kim JH, Kim YM, Kim YT, et al.: Small cell neuroendocrine carcinoma of the endometrium: a clinicopathologic study of six cases, *Taiwan J Obstet Gynecol* 53(3):355–359, 2014.

Kost GJ, et al.: Point-of-care testing for disasters: needs assessment, strategic planning, and future design, *Clin Lab Med* 29(3):583–605, 2009, Elsevier.

Kouba DJ, Moy RL: Complications and pitfalls of skin cancer Surgery/Mohs micrographic surgery. In Nouri K, editor: *Comp Dermatol Surg*, St Louis, 2008, Mosby.

Kouchoukos NT: *Kirklin/barratt-boyes cardiac surgery*, ed 4, Philadelphia, 2013, Saunders.

Kowalczyk N, Mace J: *Radiographic pathology for technologists*, ed 6, St Louis, 2013, Mosby.

Kowalczyk N, Mace J: *Radiographic pathology for technologists*, ed 5, St Louis, 2009, Mosby.

Krachmer JH: *Cornea atlas*, ed 3, St Louis, 2013, Elsevier.

Kradin RL: *Diagnostic pathology of infectious disease*, Philadelphia, 2010, Saunders.

Kumar P, Nyirjesy S, Robinson WA, Vaccaro AR, Harrod CC: Surgical treatment of odontoid fractures: posterior approach, *Semin Spine Surg* 26(3):192–202, 2014.

Kumar V, Abbas AK, Aster JC, Fausto N: *Robbins and Cotran pathologic basis of disease*, ed 8, Philadelphia, 2010, Saunders.

Kumar V, Abbas AK, Aster JC: *Robbins basic pathology*, ed 9, Philadelphia, 2013, Saunders.

Kumar V, Abbas AK, Fausto N, Mitchell R: *Robbins basic pathology*, ed 8, Philadelphia, 2007, Saunders.

Kumar V, Cotran RS, Robbins SL: *Basic pathology*, ed 7, Philadelphia, 2003, Saunders.

LaFleur Brooks M, LaFleur Brooks D: *Exploring medical language*, ed 8, St Louis, 2012, Mosby.

LaFleur Brooks M, LaFleur Brooks D: *Exploring medical language*, ed 9, St Louis, 2014, Mosby.

Lambert S, Lyons C: *Taylor and Hoyt's pediatric ophthalmology and strabismus*, ed 5, St Louis, 2017, Elsevier.

Lang R: *Dynamic echocardiography*, Philadelphia, 2011, Saunders.

Lanza GA: The electrocardiogram as a prognostic tool for predicting major cardiac events, *Prog Cardiovasc Dis* 50(2):87–111, 2007.

Larcher L, Plötzeneder I, Riml S, Kompatscher P: Management of complications following aesthetic procedures can lead to significant additional cost, *J Plast Reconstr Aesthet Surg* 64(8):1096–1099, 2011.

LaTrenta G: *Atlas of aesthetic face and neck surgery*, Philadelphia, 2004, Saunders.

Lawrence CM, Cox NH: *Physical signs in dermatology*, ed 2, London, 2002, Mosby Ltd.

Lebwohl MG, Heymann WR, Berth-Jones J, Coulson I: *Treatment of skin disease: comprehensive therapeutic strategies*, ed 4, Philadelphia, 2014, Saunders.

Lebwohl MG, Heymann WR, Berth-Jones J, Coulson I: *Treatment of skin disease: comprehensive therapeutic strategies*, ed 5, Philadelphia, 2018, Saunders.

Lee: *Ashcraft's pediatric surgery*, ed 6, St. Louis, 2014, Saunders.

Lehmeyer L, Stumpfe F: *BASICS Anamnese und Untersuchung*, Munchen, 2009, Urban & Fischer.

Leifer G: *Introduction to maternity & pediatric nursing*, ed 6, St Louis, 2011, Elsevier.

Lemmi FO, Lemmi CAE: *Physical assessment findings CD-ROM*, Philadelphia, 2000, Saunders.

Leonard PC: *Building a medical vocabulary: with Spanish translations*, ed 7, St Louis, 2009, Saunders.

Leonard PC: *Building a medical vocabulary: with Spanish translations*, ed 8, St Louis, 2012, Saunders.

Leonard PC: *Building a medical vocabulary: with Spanish translations*, ed 9, St Louis, 2015, Mosby.

Leonard PC: *Quick & easy medical terminology*, ed 6, St Louis, 2011, Saunders.

Leonard PC: *Quick & easy medical terminology*, ed 7, St Louis, 2014, Saunders.

Lester F, Stenson A, Meyer C, Morris J, Vargas J, Miller S: Impact of the Non-pneumatic Antishock Garment on pelvic blood flow in healthy postpartum women, *Am J Obstet Gynecol* 204(5):409.e1–409.e5, 2011.

Lester JD, Watson JN, Hutchinson MR: Physical examination of the patellofemoral joint, *Clin Sports Med* 33(3):403–412, 2014, 1918.

Levine SM, Levine E, Taub PJ, Weinberg H: Electrosurgical excision technique for the treatment of multiple cutaneous lesions in neurofibromatosis type I, *J Plast Reconstr Aesthet Surg* 8(61):958–962, 2007.

Levy M, Koeppen B, Stanton B: *Berne & Levy principles of physiology*, ed 4, St Louis, 2006, Mosby.

Lewis SL, Dirksen SR, Heitkemper MM, Bucher L, Camera I: *Medical-surgical nursing: assessment and management of clinical problems*, ed 8, St Louis, 2011, Mosby.

Lewis SL, Heitkemper MM, Dirksen SR: *Medical-surgical nursing: assessment and management of clinical problems*, ed 6, St Louis, 2004, Mosby.

Lewis SL, et al.: *Medical-surgical nursing: assessment and management of clinical problems*, ed 7, St Louis, 2007, Mosby.

Likens GE: *Encyclopedia of inland waters*, New York, 2009, Academic Press.

Lilley LL, Collins SR: *Pharmacology and the nursing process*, ed 6, St Louis, 2011, Mosby.

Lilley LL, Collins SR, Snyder JS: *Pharmacology and the nursing process*, ed 7, St Louis, 2014, Mosby.

Lim EKS: *Medicine & surgery: an integrated textbook*, Oxford, 2007, Elsevier Ltd.

Limsuwan T, Demoly P: Acute symptoms of drug hypersensitivity (urticaria, angioedema, anaphylaxis, anaphylactic shock), *Med Clin North Am* 94(4):691–710, 2010.

Lipson MH: Common neonatal syndromes: common neonatal syndromes, *Semin Fetal Neonatal Med* 10(3):221–231, 2005.

Lissauer T, Clayden G, Craft A: *Illustrated textbook of paediatrics*, ed 4, Oxford, 2012, Elsevier Ltd.

Little JW, Miller C: *Dental management of the medically compromised patient*, ed 8, St Louis, 2013, Mosby.

Liu GT, Volpe NJ, Galetta SL: *Neuro-ophthalmology: diagnosis and management*, ed 2, Philadelphia, 2010, Saunders.

Lloyd-Davies RW, Llyod-Davies W: *Color atlas of urology*, ed 2, London, 1994, Mosby.

Lo S, Hallam MJ, Smith S, Cubison T: The tertiary management of pretibial lacerations, *J Plast Reconstr Aesthet Surg* 65(9):1143–1150, 2012.

Long SS, Prober CG, Fischer M: *Principles and practice of pediatric infectious diseases*, ed 5, St Louis, 2018, Elsevier.

Long CJ, Srinivasan AK: Percutaneous nephrolithotomy and ureteroscopy in children, *Urol Clin North Am* 1(42):1–17, 2015.

Lovaasen KR, Schwerdtfeger J: *ICD-9-CM coding: theory and practice with ICD-10*, 2015 ed, St Louis, 2015, Saunders.

Lowdermilk DL, Alden KR, Cashion MC, Perry SE: *Maternity and women's health care*, ed 10, St Louis, 2012, Mosby.

Lowdermilk DL, Perry SE: *Maternity and women's health care*, ed 8, St Louis, 2004, Mosby.

Lowdermilk DL, Perry SE, Cashion KC, Alden KR: *Maternity and women's health care*, ed 11, St Louis, 2016, Mosby.

Lowe JS: *Stevens & Lowe's human histology*, ed 4, St. Louis, 2014, Elsevier Health Sciences.

Lusardi MM, Jorge M, Neilson CC: *Orthotics and prosthetics in rehabilitation*, ed 3, Philadelphia, 2013, Saunders.

Lynch VA, Duval JB: *Forensic nursing science*, ed 2, St Louis, 2011, Mosby.

Lyons K, Cassady C, Jones J, et al.: Current role of fetal magnetic resonance imaging in neurologic anomalies, *Semin Ultrasound CT MR* 36(4):298–309, 2015.

Magee D: *Orthopedic physical assessment*, ed 6, Philadelphia, 2014, Saunders.

Magill AJ, Ryan ET, Hill D, Solomon T: *Hunter's tropical medicine and emerging infectious disease*, ed 9, Philadelphia, 2013, Saunders.

Magione S: *Physical diagnosis secrets*, ed 2, Philadelphia, 2008, Mosby.

Maglinte DDT: Fluoroscopic and CT enteroclysis, *Radiol Clin North Am* 51(1):149–176, 2013.

Maguiness SM, Liang MG: Management of capillary malformations, *Clin Plast Surg* 38(1):65–73, 2011.

Mahon CR, Lehman DC, Manuselis G: *Textbook of diagnostic microbiology*, ed 3, Philadelphia, 2007, Saunders.

Mahon CR, Lehman DC, Manuselis G: *Textbook of diagnostic microbiology*, ed 4, St Louis, 2011, Saunders.

Mahon CR, Lehman DC, Manuselis G: *Textbook of diagnostic microbiology*, ed 5, St Louis, 2015, Saunders.

Malamed SF: *Sedation: a guide to patient management*, ed 5, St Louis, 2010, Mosby.

Mangold AR, Torgerson RR, Rogers RS: Diseases of the tongue, *Clin Dermatol* 34(4):458–469, 2016.

Mann DL, Zipes DP, Libby P, Bonow RO: *Braunwald's heart disease: a textbook of cardiovascular medicine*, ed 10, Philadelphia, 2015, Saunders.

Mansel RE, Webster D, Hughes: *Mansel & Webster's benign disorders and diseases of the breast*, ed 3, Edinburgh, 2009, Saunders.

Mansour JC, Niederhuber JE: *Abeloff's clinical oncology*, ed 5, Oxford, 2014, Churchill Livingstone.

Marcdante K, Kliegman R: *Nelson essentials of pediatrics*, ed 7, Philadelphia, 2015, Saunders.

Marks Jr JG, Miller JJ: *Lookingbill & Marks' principles of dermatology*, ed 4, London, 2006, Saunders.

Marks Jr JG, Miller JJ: *Lookingbill and Marks' principles of dermatology*, ed 5, St Louis, 2013, Saunders.

Maroñas-Jiménez L, Krakowski AC: Pediatric acne: clinical patterns and pearls, *Dermatol Clin* 34(2):195–202, 2016.

Marsh GB: *Miller-Keane encyclopedia & dictionary of medicine, nursing & allied health*, ed 7, Philadelphia, 2003, Saunders.

Marx JA: *Rosen's emergency medicine*, ed 7, Philadelphia, 2010, Mosby.

Marx JA, Hockenberger R, Walls R: *Rosen's emergency medicine*, ed 8, Philadelphia, 2014, Mosby.

Maximilian BL: *Netter's illustrated human pathology*, ed 2, Philadelphia, 2014, Saunders.

McCance KL, Huether SE: *Pathophysiology: the biologic basis for disease in adults and children*, ed 6, St Louis, 2010, Mosby.

McCance KL, Huether SE: *Pathophysiology: the biologic basis for disease in adults and children*, ed 7, St Louis, 2014, Mosby.

McIntosh N, Helms PJ, Smyth S, Logan S: *Forfar and Arneil's textbook of paediatrics*, ed 7, St. Louis, 2008, Elsevier.

McKee GT: *Cytopathology*, London, 1997, Mosby-Wolfe.

McKee PH, Calonje E, Granter SR, editors: *Pathology of the skin with clinical correlations*, ed 3, St Louis, 2005, Mosby.

McKenry LM, Salerno E: *Mosby's pharmacology in nursing*, ed 21, St Louis, 2001, Mosby.

McKinney ES, James S, Murray S, Nelson K, Ashwill J: *Maternal-child nursing*, ed 4, St Louis, 2013, Saunders.

McLaren DS: *Colour atlas and text of diet-related disorders*, London, 1992, Mosby-Wolfe.

McPherson RA, Pincus MR: *Henry's clinical diagnosis and management by laboratory methods*, ed 22, Philadelphia, 2011, Saunders.

Mettler F: *Essentials of radiology*, ed 3, Philadelphia, 2014, Saunders.

Mettler Jr FA, Guiberteau MJ: *Essentials of nuclear medicine imaging*, ed 6, Philadelphia, 2012, Saunders.

Mikuła T, Wasilewski R, Stańczak W, Wiercińska-Drapało A: Porphyria cutanea tarda (PCT) after 16 years of HIV/HCV coinfection—case report, *HIV AIDS Rev* 11(3):73–75, 2012.

Milford C, Rowlands A: *Shared care for ENT, Isis medical media, Ltd.,* Martin Dunitz Publishers, UK, 1999, Taylor and Francis Books.

Miller M, Hart J, MacKnight J: *Essential orthopaedics*, Philadelphia, 2010, Saunders.

Miller M, et al.: *Essential orthopaedics*, Philadelphia, 2009, Saunders.

Miller-Keane, O'Toole M: *Miller-Keane encyclopedia & dictionary of medicine, nursing & allied health*, Philadelphia, 1998, Saunders.

Miller-Keane, O'Toole M: *Miller-Keane encyclopedia & dictionary of medicine, nursing & allied health: revised reprint*, ed 7, Philadelphia, 2005, Saunders.

Millett D, Welbury RR: *Orthodontics and paediatric dentistry*, London, 2000, Churchill Livingstone.

Mir MA: *Atlas of clinical diagnosis*, ed 2, Edinburgh, 2003, Saunders.

Misra DP, Lawrence A, Agarwal V: Gangrene in Takayasu's arteritis, *Ind J Rheumatol* 8(3):137–138, 2013.

Mohankumar TS, Kanchan J, Pinakini KS, et al.: Gas geyser: a cause of fatal domestic carbon monoxide poisoning, *J Forens Legal Med* 19(8):490–493, 2012.

Moll JMH: *Rheumatology*, ed 2, London, 1997, Churchill Livingstone.

Monahan FD, Neighbors M: *Medical-surgical nursing: foundations for clinical practice*, ed 2, Philadelphia, 1998, Saunders.

Monahan FD, Sands JK, Neighbors M, Marek JF, Green CJ: *Phipps' medical-surgical nursing: health and illness perspectives*, ed 8, St Louis, 2007, Mosby.

Moore KL, Persaud TVN: *The developing human: clinically oriented embryology*, ed 8, Philadelphia, 2008, Saunders.

Moore KL, Persaud TVN, Shiota K: *Color atlas of clinical embryology*, ed 2, Philadelphia, 2000, Saunders.

Moore KL, Persaud TVN, Torchia MG: *The developing human: clinically oriented embryology*, ed 10, Philadelphia, 2016, Saunders.

Morgan SL, Weinsier RL: *Fundamentals of clinical nutrition*, ed 2, St Louis, 1998, Mosby.

Mori M, Yoshimatsu K, Shinohara S, Tanaka F: Chest wall stabilization with intercostal Z-suture and mesh for rib fractures, *Trauma Case Rep* 28:100311, 2020, https://doi.org/10.1016/j.tcr.2020.100311, Published 2020 May 22.

Moriuchi R, Akiyama M, Onozuka T, Shimizu H: A novel ATP2A2 missense mutation p.Asp254Gly in Darier disease restricted to the extremities, *J Am Acad Dermatol* 5(58):S116–S118, 2008, Supplement 1.

Morse SA, Holmes KK, Ballard RC: *Atlas of sexually transmitted diseases and AIDS*, ed 4, London, 2010, Saunders.

Mosby: *Mosby's dental dictionary*, ed 2, St Louis, 2008, Mosby.

Mosca NG, Hathorn R: HIV-positive patients: dental management considerations, *Dental Clin North Am* 50(4):635–657, 2006.

Mottram C: *Ruppel's manual of pulmonary function testing*, ed 10, St Louis, 2013, Mosby.

Mounsey AL, Halladay J, Sadiq TS: Hemorrhoids, *Am Fam Physician* 84(2):204–210, 2011.

Mourad LA: *Orthopedic disorders*, St Louis, 1991, Mosby Yearbook.

Muller NL, Silva CIS: *Imaging of the chest*, Philadelphia, 2008, Saunders-Elsevier.

Murphy C, Allen L, Jamieson MA: Ambiguous genitalia in the newborn: an overview and teaching tool, *J Pediatr Adolesc Gynecol* 24(5):236–250, 2011.

Murray MJ, Harrison BA, Mueller JT, Rose SH, Wass CT, Wedel DJ: *Faust's anesthesiology review*, ed 4, Philadelphia, 2015, Saunders.

Murray PR: *Medical microbiology*, ed 8, St. Louis, 2015, Elsevier.

Murray PR, Rosenthal KS, Pfaller MA: *Medical microbiology*, ed 4, St Louis, 2002, Mosby.

Murray PR, Rosenthal KS, Pfaller MA: *Medical microbiology*, ed 5, St Louis, 2005, Mosby.

Murray PR, Rosenthal KS, Pfaller MA: *Medical microbiology*, ed 7, St Louis, 2013, Mosby.

Murray SS, McKinney ES: *Foundations of maternal-newborn nursing*, ed 4, St Louis, 2006, Saunders.

Muscolino JE: *Kinesiology: the skeletal system and muscle function*, ed 2, St Louis, 2011, Mosby.

Myers EN, Carrau RL: *Operative otolaryngology: head and neck surgery*, ed 2, Philadelphia, 2008, Saunders.

Naeye RL: *Disorders of the placenta, fetus, and neonate*, St Louis, 1992, Mosby.

Naidich TP, Castillo M, Cha S, Smirniotopoulos JG: *Imaging of the brain*, Philadelphia, 2013, Saunders.

Naish J, Court DS: *Medical sciences*, ed 2, Philadelphia, 2015, Saunders.

Nanci A: *Ten Cate's oral histology*, ed 8, St Louis, 2013, Mosby.

Nanda R: *Biomechanics and esthetic strategies in clinical orthodontics*, Philadelphia, 2005, Saunders.

Nanda VS: Common dermatoses: part II, *Am J Obstet Gynecol* 174(4):1273–1278, 1996.

Napolitano M, Giampetruzzi AR, Didona D, Papi M, Didona B: Toxic epidermal necrolysis-like acute cutaneous lupus erythematosus successfully treated with a single dose of etanercept: report of three cases, *J Am Acad Dermatol* 69(6):e303–e305, 2013.

Naveen KN, Pai VV, Bagalkot P, Kulkarni V, Rashme P, et al.: Pellagra in a child–A rare entity, *Nutrition* 29(11):1426–1428, 2013.

Nazzaro G, Ponziani A, Cavicchini S: Tinea nigra: a diagnostic pitfall, *J Am Acad Dermatol* 75(6):e219–e220, 2016.

Nazzaro G, Locci M, Marilena M, Salzano E, Palmier T, et al.: Differentiating between septate and bicornuate uterus: Bi-dimensional and 3-dimensional power Doppler findings, *J Min Invas Gynecol* 21(5):870–876, 2014.

Nelson PC: *Plastic surgery*, ed 3, Philadelphia, 2013, Saunders.

Neuman TS, Thom SR: *Physiology and medicine of hyperbaric oxygen therapy*, Philadelphia, 2008, Saunders.

Neville BW, Damm DD, Allen CM, Chi AC: *Oral and maxillofacial pathology*, ed 4, St Louis, 2015, Elsevier.

Newman MG, Takei HH, Klokkevold PR, Carranza FA: *Carranza's clinical periodontology*, ed 12, Philadelphia, 2015, Saunders.

Newton RW: *Color atlas of pediatric neurology*, London, 1995, Times Mirror International.

Nguyen TT, Maartens NF: Complication of subacute bacterial endocarditis, *J Clin Neurosci* 11(8):872, 2004.

Niamtu J: *Cosmetic facial surgery*, St Louis, 2011, Mosby.

Nicol M, Bavin C, Cronin P, Rawlings-Anderson K, Cole E, Hunter J: *Essential nursing skills*, ed 4, St Louis, 2012, Mosby.

Nikolaidis P, Gabriel H, Khong K, Brusco M, Hammond N, et al.: Computed tomography and magnetic resonance imaging features of lesions of the renal medulla and sinus, *Curr Prob Diag Radiol* 37(6):262–278, 2008.

Nisa L, Giger R: Black hairy tongue, *Am J Med* 124(9):816–817, 2011.

Nix S: *Williams' basic nutrition and diet therapy*, ed 13, St Louis, 2009, Mosby.

Nix S: *Williams' basic nutrition & diet therapy*, ed 14, St Louis, 2013, Mosby.

Nolte J, Angevine JB: *The human brain in photographs and diagrams*, ed 3, Philadelphia, 2007, Mosby.

Norell M, Perrins J, Meier B, Lincoff A: *Essential interventional cardiology*, ed 2, Philadelphia, 2008, Elsevier.

Nouri K: *Complications in dermatologic surgery*, St Louis, 2008, Mosby.

Numajiri T, Nishino K, Fujiwara T, Takeda K, Sowa Y: Juvenile xanthogranuloma presenting rapid progression after curettage: a case report with clinicopathological findings, *J Plast Reconstr Aesthet Surg* 60(11):1248–1251, 2006.

Nymberg SM, Crawford AH: *Video-assisted thoracoscopic releases of scoliotic anterior spines*, AORN, Inc., 1996.

O'Doherty N: *Neonataology: micro atlas of the newborn*, Nutley, New Jersey, 1986, Hoffman-LaRoche.

Odze RD, Goldblum JR: *Surgical pathology of the GI tract, liver, biliary tract, and pancreas*, ed 2, Philadelphia, 2009, Saunders.

Ogawa R: Keloid and hypertrophic scarring may result from a mechanoreceptor or mechanosensitive nociceptor disorder, *Med Hypotheses* 71(4):493–500, 2008.

Olivier P, Simoneau-Roy J, Francoeur D, Sartelet H, Parma J, et al.: Leydig cell tumors in children: contrasting clinical, hormonal, anatomical, and molecular characteristics in boys and girls, *J Pediatr* 161(6):1147–1152, 2012.

Onda S, Ogura R, Sano T, Imoto A, Masuda D, et al.: Successful removal of intrahepatic bile duct stone using a novel basket catheter, *Gastrointest Endosc* 81(5):1267, 2015.

Orkin SH, Fisher DE, Ginsburg D, Look AT, Lux SE, et al.: *Nathan and Oski's hematology and oncology of infancy and childhood*, ed 8, Philadelphia, 2015, Saunders.

O'Ryan F: Mandibular asymmetry: condylar elongation/hypertrophy. In Bagheri SC, editor: *Current therapy in oral and maxillofacial surgery*, St Louis, 2012, Saunders.

Oshimo T, et al.: *J Dermatol Sci* 52(1):58–66, 2008.

Osiecka BJ, Nockowski P, Jurczyszyn K, Ziólkowski P: Photodynamic therapy of vulvar lichen sclerosus et atrophicus in a woman with hypothyreosis: case report, *Photodiag Photodynam Ther* 9(2):186–188, 2012.

Pagana KD, Pagana TJ: *Mosby's manual of diagnostic and laboratory tests*, ed 3, St Louis, 2006, Mosby.

Palay DA, Krachmer JH: *Primary care ophthalmology*, Philadelphia, 2005, Mosby.

Paller AS, Mancini AJ, editors: *Hurwitz clinical pediatric dermatology*, ed 3, Philadelphia, 2006, Saunders.

Paller AS, Mancini AJ, editors: *Hurwitz clinical pediatric dermatology*, ed 4, Philadelphia, 2011, Saunders.

Palmason S, Marty FM, Treister NS: How do we manage oral infections in allogeneic stem cell transplantation and other severely immunocompromised patients? *Oral Maxillofac Surg Clin North Am* 23(4):579–599, 2011.

Panigrahi I, Bhushan M, Yadav M, Khandelwal N, Singhi P: Macrocephaly-capillary malformation syndrome: three new cases, *J Neurol Sci* 313(12):178–181, 2012.

Pannier S, Legeaui-Mallet L: Hereditary multiple exostoses and enchondromatosis, *Best Pract Res Clin Rheumatol* 22(1):45–54, 2008.

Papathanassiou D, Liehn JC: The growing development of multimodality imaging in oncology, *Crit Rev Oncol Hematol* 68(1):60–65, 2008.

Parillo JE, Dellinger RP: *Critical care medicine: principles of diagnosis and management in the adult*, ed 4, Philadelphia, 2014, Saunders.

Passarini B, Balestri R, D'Errico A, Pinna A, Infusino SD: Lack of recurrence of malignant atrophic papulosis of Degos in multivisceral transplant: insights into possible pathogenesis? *J Am Acad Dermatol* 2(65):e49–e50, 2010.

Patel NA, Jerry JM, Jimenez XF, Hantus ST: New-onset refractory status epilepticus associated with the use of synthetic cannabinoids, *Psychosomatics* 58(2):180–186, 2017.

Patel KB, Taghinia AH, Proctor MR, Warf BC, Greene AK: Extradural myelomeningocele reconstruction using local turnover fascial flaps and midline linear skin closure, *J Plast Reconstr Aesthet Surg* 65(11):1569–1572, 2012.

Patel M, Pilcher J, Travers J, Perrin K, Shaw D, et al.: Use of metered-dose inhaler electronic monitoring in a real-world asthma randomized controlled trial, *J Allergy Clin Immunol Pract* 1(1):83–91, 2012.

Patton KT, Thibodeau GA: *Anatomy and physiology*, ed 7, St Louis, 2010, Mosby.

Patton KT, Thibodeau GA: *Anatomy & physiology*, ed 8, St Louis, 2013, Mosby.

Patton KT, Thibodeau GA: *Anatomy and physiology*, ed 9, St Louis, 2016, Mosby.

Patton KT, Thibodeau GA: *The human body in health & disease*, ed 6, St Louis, 2014, Elsevier.

Paulson F, München: *Sobotta atlas of human anatomy*, ed 15, vol. 3. Elsevier, 2013.

Peng H, Huang K, Chueh H, Adlan AS, Chang SD, Lee CL: Term delivery of a complete hydatidiform mole with a coexisting living fetus followed by successful treatment of maternal metastatic gestational trophoblastic disease, *Taiwan J Obstet Gynecol* 53(3):397–400, 2014.

Perez A, Wain ME, Robson A, Groves RW, Stefanato CM: Cutaneous collagenous vasculopathy with generalized telangiectasia in two female patients, *J Am Acad Dermatol* 63(5):882–885, 2010.

Perkin GD: *Mosby's color atlas and text of neurology*, ed 2, London, 2002, Mosby Ltd.

Perry AG, Potter PA: *Mosby's pocket guide to nursing skills & procedures*, ed 7, St Louis, 2011, Mosby.

Perry AG, Potter PA, Elkin MK: *Nursing interventions and clinical skills*, ed 5, St Louis, 2012, Mosby.

Perry AG, Potter PA, Ostendorf WR: *Nursing interventions and clinical skills*, ed 6, St Louis, 2016, Elsevier Inc.

Petiti-Martin GH, Villar-Buill M, de la Hera LF, Burgues-Calderon M, Rivera-Diaz R, et al. Deep vein thrombosis in a patient with lepromatous leprosy receiving thalidomide to treat leprosy reaction. *Dermatol (Actas Dermo-Sifiliográficas, English Edition),* 104(1):67-70, 2011 Elsevier España.

Pfenninger J: *Pfenninger and Fowler's procedures for primary care*, ed 3, Philadelphia, 2011, Saunders.

Pfenninger JL, Zainea GG: Common anorectal conditions, *Obstet Gynecol* 98(6):1130–1139, 2001.

Phalen T, Aehlert A: *The 12-Lead ECG in acute coronary syndromes*, ed 3, St Louis, 2012, Elsevier.

Phillips N: *Berry & Kohn's operating room technique*, ed 11, St Louis, 2007, Mosby.

Phillips N: *Berry & Kohn's operating room technique*, ed 12, St Louis, 2013, Mosby.

Pincus LB: Mycosis fungoides, *Surg Pathol Clin* 7(2):143–167, 2014.

Plotkin SA, Orenstein WA, Offit PA: *Vaccines*, ed 5, Philadelphia, 2008, Saunders.

Podesta M, Urcullo J: Perineal mobilization of the common urogenital sinus for surgical correction of high urethrovaginal confluence in patients with intersex disorders, *J Pediatr Urol* 4(5):352–358, 2008.

Pollard TD, Earnshaw W: *Cell biology*, ed 2, Philadelphia, 2007, Saunders.

Potter PA, Perry AG: *Basic nursing: essentials for practice*, ed 5, St Louis, 2003, Mosby.

Potter PA, Perry AG: *Basic nursing: essentials for practice*, ed 6, St Louis, 2007, Mosby.

Potter PA, Perry AG: *Fundamentals of nursing*, ed 6, St Louis, 2005, Mosby.

Potter PA, Perry AG, Stockert P, Hall A: *Basic nursing: essentials for practice*, ed 7, St Louis, 2011, Mosby.

Potter PA, Perry AG, Stockert P, Hall A: *Fundamentals of nursing*, ed 8, St Louis, 2013, Mosby.

Pretorius ES, Solomon JA: *Radiology secrets plus*, ed 3, St Louis, 2011, Mosby.

Price SA: *Pathophysiology: clinical concepts of disease processes*, ed 6, St Louis, 2003, Mosby.

Pride HB, Yan AC, Zaenglein AL: *Pediatric dermatology*, Oxford, 2008, Elsevier Ltd.

Proctor D, Adams A: *Kinn's the medical assistant: an applied learning approach*, ed 12, Philadelphia, 2014, Saunders.

Proffit WR, Fields HW, Sarver D: *Contemporary orthodontics*, ed 5, St Louis, 2013, Mosby.

Purrucker JC, Capper D, Behrens L, Veltkamp R: Secondary hematoma expansion in intracerebral hemorrhage during rivaroxaban therapy, *Am J Emerg Med* 32(8):947, 2014.

Quick CRG: *Essential surgery: problems, diagnosis and management*, ed 20, St Louis, 2014, Elsevier.

Qureshi SM: Measurement of respiratory function: gas exchange, *Anaesthes Intens Care Med* 9(11):487–491, 2008.

Raftery AT, Lim E, Östör AJK: *Churchill's pocketbook of differential diagnosis*, ed 4, Oxford, 2014, Elsevier Ltd.

Rakel RE, Rakel D: *Textbook of family medicine*, ed 8, Philadelphia, 2011, Saunders.

Rakel RE, Rakel D: *Textbook of family medicine*, ed 9, Philadelphia, 2016, Saunders.

Ramé A, Thérond S: *Anatomie et physiologie*, ed 2, Issy-les-Moulineaux, 2011, Elsevier Masson.

Regezi JA: *Oral pathology*, ed 7, St. Louis, 2016, Saunders.

Regezi JA, Sciubba JJ, Jordan R: *Oral pathology: clinical pathologic correlations*, ed 6, St Louis, 2012, Saunders.

Regezi JA, Sciubba JJ, Jordan RCK: *Oral pathology: clinical pathologic correlations*, ed 5, Philadelphia, 2008, Saunders.

Regezi JA, Sciubba JJ, Pogrel MA: *Atlas of oral and maxillofacial pathology*, Philadelphia, 2000, Saunders.

Rennie JM: *Rennie and Roberton's textbook of neonatology*, ed 5, Oxford, 2012, Churchill Livingstone.

Riascos: *CT and MRI of the whole body*, ed 6, St Louis, 2017, Elsevier.

Rich RR, Fleisher TA, Shearer WT, Schroeder H, Frew AJ, Weyand CM: *Clinical immunology: principles and practice*, ed 4, London, 2013, Elsevier Ltd.

Richards: *Tachdjian's pediatric orthopaedics*, ed 5, St Louis, 2014, Elsevier.

Richert B, Caucanas M, André J: Diagnosis using nail matrix, *Dermatol Clin* 2(33):243–255, 2015.

Rimoin DL: *Emery and Rimoin's principles and practice of medical genetics*, ed 6, Edinburgh, 2013, Churchill Livingstone.

Roberson JK, Hanke W, Siegel DM, Fratila A, Bhatia AC, Rohrer TE: *Surgery of the skin*, ed 3, Philadelphia, 2015, Saunders.

Roberts JR: *Roberts and Hedges' clinical procedures in emergency medicine*, ed 6, Philadelphia, 2014, Saunders.

Roberts JR, Hedges JR: *Clinical procedures in emergency medicine*, Philadelphia, 2010, Saunders.

Robinson C, Clegg G: The critically ill. In Douglas G, Nicol F, Robertson C, editors: *Macleod's clinical examination*, Oxford, 2013, Churchill Livingstone.

Robinson JK, Hanke CW, Siegel DM, Fratila A: *Surgery of the skin: procedural dermatology*, London, 2010, Mosby.

Rodak BF, Carr JH: *Clinical hematology atlas*, ed 4, St Louis, 2013, Saunders.

Rodríguez-Pazos L, Ginarte M, Vega A, Toribio J: Autosomal recessive congenital ichthyosis, *Actas Dermosifiliogr* 104(4):270–284, 2011.

Rosai J: *Rosai and Ackerman's surgical pathology*, ed 10, Philadelphia, 2011, Mosby.

Roselli EE, Sepulveda E, Pujara AC, Idrees J, Nowicki E: Distal landing zone open fenestration facilitates endovascular elephant trunk completion and false lumen thrombosis, *Ann Thorac Surg* 92(6):2078–2084, 2011.

Rothrock JC: *Alexander's care of the patient in surgery*, St Louis, 1992, Mosby.

Rothrock J: *Alexander's care of the patient in surgery*, ed 13, St Louis, 2007, Mosby.

Rothrock JC: *Alexander's care of the patient in surgery*, ed 14, St Louis, 2011, Mosby.

Rothrock J: *Alexander's care of the patient in surgery*, ed 15, St Louis, 2015, Mosby.

App

Roy FH, Fraunfelder FW, Fraunfelder FT: *Roy and Fraunfelder's current ocular therapy*, Philadelphia, 2008, Saunders.

Rudnicka L, Rakowska A, Olszewska M: Trichoscopy: how it may help the clinician, *Dermatol Clin* 31(1):29–41, 2013.

Ruppel G: *Manual of pulmonary function testing*, ed 9, St Louis, 2009, Mosby.

Russ R: *Crash course: cardiovascular system*, St Louis, 2006, Mosby.

Russi EG, Corvò R, Merlotti A, Alterio D, Franco P, et al.: Swallowing dysfunction in head and neck cancer patients treated by radiotherapy: review and recommendations of the supportive task group of the Italian Association of Radiation Oncology, *Cancer Treat Rev* 8(38):1033–1049, 2012.

Saadeh R, Lisi EC, Batista DA, McIntosh I, Hoover-Fong JE: Albinism and developmental delay: the need to test for 15q11-q13 deletion, *Pediatr Neurol* 37(4):299–302, 2007.

Saadi A, Borck G, Boddaert N, Chekkour MC, Imessaoudene B, et al.: Compound heterozygous ASPM mutations associated with microcephaly and simplified cortical gyration in a consanguineous Algerian family, *Eur J Med Genet* 52(4):180–184, 2009.

Salamon P, Shoham NG, Puxeddu I, Paitan Y, Levi-Schaffer F, Mekori YA: Human mast cells release oncostatin M on contact with activated T cells: possible biologic relevance, *J Allerg Clin Immunol* 2(121):448–455.e5, 2008.

Salvo SG: *Massage therapy: principles and practice*, ed 4, St Louis, 2012, Elsevier.

Salvo SG: *Mosby's pathology for massage therapists*, ed 2, St Louis, 2009, Elsevier.

Salvo SG: *Mosby's pathology for massage therapists*, ed 3, St Louis, 2014, Elsevier, 1921.

Sanders MJ, McKenna KD: *Mosby's paramedic textbook*, ed 3, St Louis, 2007, Mosby JEMS.

Sapp JP: *Contemporary oral and maxillofacial pathology*, ed 2, St Louis, 2004, C.V. Mosby.

Sasseville D: Clinical patterns of phytodermatitis, *Dermatol Clin* 27(3):299–308, 2009.

Savage SA, Atler BP: Dyskeratosis congenita, *Hematol Oncol Clin North Am* 23(2):215–231, 2009.

Saxena R: *Practical hepatic pathology: a diagnostic approach*, Philadelphia, 2011, Saunders.

Schaaf H, Santo G, Gräf M, Howaldt H: En bloc resection of the lateral orbital rim to reduce exophthalmos in patients with Graves' disease, *J Cranio-Maxillofacial Surg* 38(3):204–210, 2009.

Schachner LA, Hansen RC: *Pediatric dermatology*, ed 4, St Louis, 2011, Mosby.

Schipper P, Schoolfield M: Minimally invasive staging of N2 disease: endobronchial ultrasound/transesophageal endoscopic ultrasound, mediastinoscopy, and thoracoscopy, *Thorac Surg Clin* 4(18):363–379, 2008.

Schlenker E, Gilbert JA: *Williams' essentials of nutrition & diet therapy*, ed 11, St Louis, 2015, Mosby.

Schoenwolf GC, Bleyl SB, Brauer PR, Francis-West PH: *Larsen's human embryology*, ed 5, Oxford, 2015, Churchill Livingstone.

Scott WN: *Insall & Scott surgery of the knee*, ed 5, Oxford, 2012, Churchill Livingstone.

Scully C: *Scully's medical problems in dentistry*, ed 7, London, 2014, Elsevier Ltd.

Seidel HM, Ball JW, Dains JE, Benedict GW: *Mosby's guide to physical examination*, ed 5, St Louis, 2003, Mosby.

Seidel HM, Ball J, Dains J, Benedict GW: *Mosby's guide to physical examination*, ed 6, St Louis, 2006, Mosby.

Seidel HM, et al.: *Mosby's guide to physical examination*, ed 7, St Louis, 2011, Mosby JEMS.

Shade BR, Collins Jr TE, Wertz E, Jones SA, Rothenberg MA: *Mosby's EMT-intermediate textbook for 1999 national standard curriculum*, ed 3, Mosby, 2007.

Shah BR, Laude TA: *Atlas of pediatric clinical diagnosis*, Philadelphia, 2000, Saunders.

Shah J, Patel S, Singh B: *Jatin Shah's head and neck surgery and oncology*, ed 4, St Louis, 2012, Mosby.

Shah PV: Flexible bronchoscopy, *Med* 36(3):151–154, 2007.

Sharma H, Bell I, Schofield J, Bird G: Primary peritoneal mesothelioma: case series and literature review, *Clin Res Hepatol Gastroenterol* 35(1):55–59, 2011.

Shaw RW, Luesley D, Monga A: *Gynaecology*, Edinburgh, 2011, Churchill Livingstone.

Shepherd RK, et al.: Visual prostheses for the blind, *Trend Biotechnol* 31(10):562–571, 2013.

Shih H-J, Chen J-T, Chen Y-L, Chiang H-C: Laser-assisted bipolar transurethral resection of the prostate with the oyster procedure for patient with prostate glands larger than 80 mL, *Urology* 81(6):1315–1319, 2013.

Shiland B: *Mastering healthcare terminology*, ed 3, St Louis, 2010, Mosby.

Shiland B: *Mastering healthcare terminology*, ed 5, St Louis, 2016, Mosby.

Shin JS, Seo YS, Kim JH, Park KH: Nomogram of fetal renal growth expressed in length and parenchymal area derived from ultrasound images, *J Urol* 5(178):2150–2154, 2007.

Silverberg SG, et al.: *Silverberg's principles and practice of surgical pathology and cytopathology*, ed 4, London, 2006, Churchill Livingstone.

Shoukry NH, Pelletier S, Chang KM: A view to natural killer cells in hepatitis C, *Gastroenterology* 141(4):1144–1148, 2011.

Silvestri L: *Saunders comprehensive review for the NCLEX-RN examination*, ed 5, St Louis, 2011, Saunders.

Simonetto DA, Shah VH, Kamath PS: Primary prophylaxis of variceal bleeding, *Clin Liver Dis* 18(2):335–345, 2014.

Skarin AT: *Atlas of diagnostic oncology*, ed 3, London, 2003, Mosby Ltd.

Skarin AT: *Atlas of diagnostic oncology*, ed 4, Philadelphia, 2010, Mosby.

Skidmore-Roth L: *Mosby's 2016 nursing drug reference*, St Louis, 2016, Mosby.

Sole ML, Klein D, Moseley M: *Introduction to critical care nursing*, ed 6, Philadelphia, 2013, Saunders.

Solomon EP: *Introduction to human anatomy and physiology*, ed 3, Philadelphia, 2009, Saunders.

Sorrentino SA: *Mosby's textbook for nursing assistants*, ed 7, St Louis, 2008, Mosby.

Sorrentino SA, Remmert L: *Mosby's textbook for nursing assistants*, ed 8, St Louis, 2012, Mosby.

Sorrentino SA, Remmert L: *Mosby's textbook for nursing assistants*, ed 9, St Louis, 2016, Mosby.

Spalton DJ, Hitchings RA, Hunter PA: *Atlas of clinical ophthalmology*, ed 3, London, 2005, Mosby.

Squire LR: *Encyclopedia of neuroscience*, vol. 1. Academic Press, 2009.

Standring S: *Gray's Anatomy: the anatomical basis of clinical practice*, ed 40, Oxford, 2008, Elsevier Ltd.

Stein HA, Stein RM, Freeman MI: *The ophthalmic assistant*, ed 9, Philadelphia, 2013, Saunders.

Stephenac SJ, Nesbit SP: *Diagnosis and treatment planning in dentistry*, ed 3, St. Louis, 2017, Elsevier.

Stevanovic M, Sharpe F: Management of established Volkmann's contracture of the forearm in children, *Hand Clin* 22(1):99–111, 2006.

Stevens A, Lowe J, Scott I: *Core pathology*, ed 3, Oxford, 2009, Elsevier Ltd.

Stone DR, Gorbach SL: *Atlas of infectious diseases*, Philadelphia, 2000, Saunders.

Stoopler ET, Thoppay JR, Sollectio TP: Psychological parameters associated with geographic tongue: a clinical observation, *Oral Surg Oral Med Oral Pathol Oral Radiol* 119(1):122–123, 2015.

Stuart GW: *Principles and practice of psychiatric nursing*, ed 10, St Louis, 2013, Mosby.

Suda S, Ueda M, Sakurazawa M, Nishiyama Y, Komaba Y, et al.: Clinical and neuroradiological progression in diffuse neurofibrillary tangles with calcification, *J Clin Neurosci* 8(16):1112–1114, 2009.

Sueki D, Brechter J: Orthopedic rehabilitation clinical advisor, St Louis, 2010, Mosby. In Magee D, editor: *Orthopedic physical assessment*, ed 5, St Louis, 2008, Saunders.

Sugano K: Gastric cancer: pathogenesis, screening, and treatment, *Gastrointest Endosc Clin North Am* 18(3):513–522, 2008.

Sukthankar A: Syphilis, *Medicine* 38(5):263–266, 2010.

Sun Z, Guan X, Li N, Liu X, Chen X: Chemoprevention of oral cancer in animal models, and effect on leukoplakias in human patients with ZengShengPing, a mixture of medicinal herbs, *Oral Oncol* 46(2):105–110, 2009.

Suresh SS: Periostitis of the metatarsal caused by a date palm thorn in a child: a case report, *J Foot Ankle Surg* 50(2):227–229, 2011.

Suzuki A, Kimura Y, Sasaki E, Narita A, Takagi M, Ishibashi Y: Recurrent patellar dislocation with spontaneous valgus knee deformity treated by distal femoral osteotomy alone: a report of two cases, *J Orthop Sci* 25(2):359–363, 2020.

Swartz MH: *Textbook of physical diagnosis, history and examination*, ed 5, Philadelphia, 2006, Saunders.

Swartz MH: *Textbook of physical diagnosis, history and examination*, ed 6, Philadelphia, 2009, Saunders.

Swartz MH: *Textbook of physical diagnosis: history and examination*, ed 7, Philadelphia, 2014, Saunders.

Symonds E, McPherson M: *Color atlas of obstetrics and gynecology*, London, 1994, Mosby-Wolfe.

Talab SS, Preston MA, Elmi A, Tabatabaei S: Prostate cancer imaging, *Radiol Clin North Am* 50(6):1015–1041, 2012.

Tang JB, Amadio PC, Guimberteau JC, Chang J: *Tendon surgery of the hand*, Philadelphia, 2012, Saunders.

Tanner N, Diaper R, King M, Metcalfe SA: Case study: a case of debilitating gout in the 1st metatarsophalangeal joint, *Foot* 25(1):45–50, 2014.

Taussig LM, Landau LI: *Pediatric respiratory medicine*, ed 2, Philadelphia, 2008, Saunders.

Taylor D, Hoyt CS: *Pediatric ophthalmology and strabismus*, New York, 2005, Saunders.

Taylor D, Pappo E, Aronson IK: Polymorphic eruption of pregnancy, *Clin Dermatol* 34(3):383–391, 2016.

Teichman J, Sea J, Thompson AM, Elston D: Noninfectious penile lesions, *Am Fam Phys* 81(2):167–174, 2010.

Tempkin B: *Sonography scanning: principles and protocols*, ed 4, St Louis, 2015, Saunders.

Thaha KA, Varma RL, Nair MG, Sam Joseph VG, Krishnan U: Interaction between octenidine-based solution and sodium hypochlorite: a mass spectroscopy, proton nuclear magnetic resonance, and scanning electron microscopy-based observational study, *J Endod* 43(1):135–140, 2017.

Thibodeau GA, Patton KT: *Anatomy and physiology*, ed 5, St Louis, 2003, Mosby.

Thibodeau GA, Patton KT: *Anatomy and physiology*, ed 6, St Louis, 2007, Mosby.

Thibodeau GA, Patton KT: *The human body in health and disease*, ed 5, St Louis, 2010, Mosby.

Thiers BH, Tosti A, Iorizzo M, Peraccini BM, Starace M: The nail in systemic diseases, *Dermatol Clin* 24(3):341–347, 2006.

Thurnher D, Moukarbel RV, Novak PT, Gullane PJ: The glottis and subglottis: an otolaryngologist's perspective, *Thorac Surg Clin* 17(4):549–560, 2007, 1922.

Tiodorovic-Zivkovic D, Argenziano G, Lallas A, et al.: Age, gender, and topography influence the clinical and dermoscopic appearance of lentigo maligna, *J Am Acad Dermatol* 72(5):801–808, 2015.

Tighe SM: *Instrumentation for the operating room: a photographic manual*, ed 8, St Louis, 2012, Mosby.

Tighe SM: *Instrumentation for the operating room: a photographic manual*, ed 9, St Louis, 2016, Mosby.

Tille PM: *Bailey & Scott's diagnostic microbiology*, ed 13, St Louis, 2014, Mosby.

Townsend CM, Beauchamp RD, Evers BM, Mattox KL: *Sabiston textbook of surgery: the biological basis of modern surgical practice*, ed 18, Philadelphia, 2008, Saunders.

Townsend CM, Beauchamp RD, Evers BM, Mattox KL: *Sabiston textbook of surgery: the biological basis of modern surgical practice*, ed 19, Philadelphia, 2012, Saunders.

Trelease R: *Netter's surgical anatomy review P.R.N.*, Philadelphia, 2011, Saunders.

Tummawanit S, Shrestha B, Thaworanunta S, Srithavaj T: Late effects of orbital enucleation and radiation on maxillofacial prosthetic rehabilitation: a clinical report, *J Prosthet Dent* 109(5):291–295, 2013.

Tyers AG, Collin JR: *Colour atlas of ophthalmic plastic surgery*, ed 3, London, 2008, Butterworth Heinemann.

Ulbricht C: *Natural standard herbal pharmacotherapy: an evidence-based approach*, St Louis, 2010, Mosby.

Umphred DA, Burton GU, Lazaro RT, Roller ML: *Umphred's neurological rehabilitation*, ed 6, St Louis, 2013, Mosby.

Urden LD, Stacy KM, Lough ME: *Priorities in critical care nursing*, ed 5, St Louis, 2008, Mosby.

Valentine J: *Diagnosis and treatment planning in dentistry*, ed 3, St Louis, 2017, Elsevier.

Velez NF, Jellinek NJ: Simple onycholysis: a diagnosis of exclusion, *J Am Acad Dermatol* 70(4):793–794, 2014.

Verbelen J, et al.: Aquacel® Ag dressing versus Acticoat™ dressing in partial thickness burns: a prospective, randomized, controlled study in 100 patients. part 1: burn wound healing, *Burns* 40(3):416–427, 2013.

Vetrugno L, Muzzi R, Giordano F: Pectoral muscle hematoma after axillary artery catheterization in a patient undergoing minimally invasive mitral valve surgery, *J Cardiothorac Vasc Anesthes* 21(1):96–98, 2007.

Vincent JL, Abraham E, Moore FA, Kochanek PM, Fink MP: *Textbook of critical care*, ed 6, Philadelphia, 2011, Saunders.

Vindas-Cordero JP, Sands M, Sanchez W: Austrian's triad complicated by suppurative pericarditis and cardiac tamponade: a case report and review of the literature, *Int J Infect Dis* 13(1):e23–e25, 2008.

Waldman SD: *Pain management*, ed 2, St. Louis, 2012, Saunders.

Waldman SD: *Physical diagnosis of pain*, ed 3, Philadelphia, 2016, Elsevier.

Waldman SD: *Physical diagnosis of pain: an atlas of signs and symptoms*, ed 2, Philadelphia, 2010, Saunders.

Walker BR, Colledge N, Ralston SH, Penman I: *Davidson's principles and practice of medicine*, ed 22, London, 2014, Churchill Livingstone.

Walker C, Chung J: *Muller's imaging of the chest*, ed 2, Philadelphia, 2019, Elsevier.

Walker G, deValois B, Davies R, Young T, Maher J: Alternative medicine: acupuncture for acute pain, *Comp Ther Clin Pract* 13(4):250–257, 2007.

Walsh D, Caraceni AT, Fainsinger R, Foley KM, Glare P: *Palliative medicine*, Philadelphia, 2009, Saunders.

Wang: *Andreoli and Carpenter's Cecil essentials of medicine*, ed 9, Saunders, 2016.

Waugh A, Grant A: *Ross and Wilson anatomy and physiology in health and illness*, ed 12, London, 2014, Churchill Livingstone.

Wei J, O'Brien D, Vilgelm MB, Piazuelo PC, Washington MK, El-Rifai W, et al.: Interaction of Helicobacter pylori with gastric epithelial cells is mediated by the p53 protein family, *Gastroenterol* 134(5):1412–1423, 2008.

Wein AJ, Kavoussi LR, Novick AC, Partin AW, Peters CA: *Campbell-Walsh urology*, ed 9, Philadelphia, 2007, Saunders.

Wein AJ, Kavoussi LR, Novick AC, Partin AQ, Peters CA: *Campbell-Walsh urology*, ed 10, Philadelphia, 2012, Saunders.

Weinberger S, Cockrill B, Mandel J: *Principles of pulmonary medicine*, ed 6, Philadelphia, 2014, Saunders.

Welling D, McKay PL, et al.: A brief history of the tourniquet, *J Vasc Surg* 55(1):286–290, 2012.

Wesley K: *Huszar's basic dysrhythmias and acute coronary syndromes: interpretation and management*, ed 4, St Louis, 2012, Mosby.

Weston WL, Lane AT, Morelli JG: *Color textbook of pediatric dermatology*, ed 4, St Louis, 2007, Mosby.

White JA: Lymphogranuloma venereum (LGV), *Medicine* 42(7):39–402, 2014.

White GM, Cox NH: *Diseases of the skin: a color atlas and text*, ed 2, St Louis, 2006, Mosby.

William JD: *Andrews' diseases of the skin*, St Louis, 2018, Clinical Atlas.

Williams MV, et al.: *Comprehensive hospital medicine*, Philadelphia, 2007, Saunders.

Willis A: How to perform a neurological examination, *Med* 26:515–519, 2008.

Wilson SF, Giddens JF: *Health assessment for nursing practice*, ed 2, St Louis, 2001, Mosby.

Wilson SF, Giddens JF: *Health assessment for nursing practice*, ed 4, St Louis, 2009, Mosby.

Wilson SF, Giddens JF: *Health assessment for nursing practice*, ed 5, St Louis, 2013, Mosby.

Winn HR: *Youmans neurological surgery*, ed 6, Philadelphia, 2011, Saunders.

Wittman RA, Vallone SA: Inclusion of chiropractic care in multidisciplinary management of a child with Prader-Willi syndrome: a case report, *J Chiropr Med* 8(4):193–199, 2009.

Wodajo FM, Gannon FH, Murphey MD: *Visual guide to musculoskeletal tumors: a clinical-radiologic-histologic approach*, Philadelphia, 2010, Saunders.

Woo JY, et al.: A case of acute compression in block vertebra, *Spine J* 9430(15):01521-1, 2015.

Wu CW, Kao YH, Chen CM, Hsu HJ, Chen CM, Huang IY: Mucoceles of the oral cavity in pediatric patients, *Kaohsiung J Med Sci* 27(7):276–279, 2011.

Wyllie R, Hyams J, Kay M: *Pediatric gastrointestinal and liver disease*, ed 5, St. Louis, 2016, Elsevier.

Yanoff M, Duker JD: *Ophthalmology*, ed 4, Philadelphia, 2014, Elsevier.

Yanoff M, Fine BS, editors: *Ocular pathology*, ed 4, London, 1996, Mosby.

Yanoff M, Sassani JW: *Ocular pathology*, ed 6, St Louis, 2008, Mosby.

Yao Y, Hong W, Chen H, et al.: Cervical spinal epidural abscess following acupuncture and wet-cupping therapy: a case report, *Complement Ther Med* 108(10), 2016.

Yarom N, Epstein J, Levi H, Porat D, Kaufman E, Gorsky M: Oral manifestations of habitual khat chewing: a case-control study, *Oral Surg Oral Med Oral Pathol Oral Radiol Endod* 109(6):e60–e66, 2010.

Young B, O'Dowd G, Woodford P: *Wheater's functional histology*, ed 6, Oxford, 2014, Churchill Livingstone.

Young-Adams AP, Proctor DB: *Kinn's the medical assistant: an applied learning approach*, ed 11, St Louis, 2011, Saunders.

Zakus SM: *Mosby's clinical skills for medical assistants*, ed 4, St Louis, 2001, Mosby.

Zhou M, Netto GJ, Epstein JI: *High-yield uropathology*, Philadelphia, 2012, Saunders.

Zitelli BJ, Davis HW: *Atlas of pediatric physical diagnosis*, ed 2, St Louis, 1992, Mosby.

Zitelli BJ, Davis HW: *Atlas of pediatric physical diagnosis*, ed 4, St Louis, 2002, Mosby.

Zitelli BJ, Davis HW: *Atlas of pediatric physical diagnosis*, ed 5, St Louis, 2007, Mosby.

Zitelli BJ, Davis HW: *Atlas of pediatric physical diagnosis*, ed 6, St Louis, 2012, Mosby.

APPENDIXES

NURSING INTERVENTIONS CLASSIFICATION (NIC) DEFINITIONS[a]

A

Abuse Protection Support: identification of high-risk dependent relationships and actions to prevent further infliction of physical or emotional harm

Abuse Protection Support: Child: identification of high-risk, dependent child relationships and actions to prevent possible or further infliction of physical, sexual, or emotional harm or neglect of basic necessities of life

Abuse Protection Support: Domestic Partner: identification of high-risk, dependent domestic relationships and actions to prevent possible or further infliction of physical, sexual, or emotional harm or exploitation of a domestic partner

Abuse Protection Support: Elder: identification of high-risk, dependent elder relationships and actions to prevent possible or further infliction of physical, sexual, or emotional harm; neglect of basic necessities of life; or exploitation

Abuse Protection Support: Religious: identification of high-risk, controlling religious relationships and actions to prevent infliction of physical, sexual, or emotional harm and/or exploitation

Acid-Base Management: promotion of acid-base balance and prevention of complications resulting from acid-base imbalance

Acid-Base Management: Metabolic Acidosis: promotion of acid-base balance and prevention of complications resulting from serum HCO_3 levels lower than desired or serum hydrogen ion levels higher than desired

Acid-Base Management: Metabolic Alkalosis: promotion of acid-base balance and prevention of complications resulting from serum HCO_3 levels higher than desired

Acid-Base Management: Respiratory Acidosis: promotion of acid-base balance and prevention of complications resulting from serum $PaCO_2$ levels higher than desired

Acid-Base Management: Respiratory Alkalosis: promotion of acid-base balance and prevention of complications resulting from serum $PaCO_2$ levels lower than desired

Acid-Base Monitoring: collection and analysis of patient data to regulate acid-base balance

Active Listening: attending closely to and attaching significance to a person's verbal and nonverbal messages

Activity Therapy: prescription of and assistance with specific physical, social, and spiritual activities to increase the range, frequency, or duration of an individual's or group's activity

Acupressure: application of firm, sustained pressure to special points on the body for therapeutic effect

Admission Care: facilitating entry of a patient into a health care facility

Airway Insertion and Stabilization: insertion or assistance with insertion and stabilization of an artificial airway

Airway Management: facilitation of patency of air passages

Airway Suctioning: removal of secretions by inserting a suction catheter into the patient's oral, nasopharyngeal or tracheal airway

Allergy Management: identification, treatment, and prevention of allergic responses to food, medications, insect bites, contrast material, blood, and other substances

Amnioinfusion: infusion of fluid into the uterus during labor to relieve umbilical cord compression or to dilute meconium-stained fluid

Amputation Care: promotion of physical and psychological healing before and after amputation of a body part

Analgesic Administration: use of pharmacologic agents to reduce or eliminate pain

Analgesic Administration: Intraspinal: administration of pharmacologic agents into the epidural or intrathecal space to reduce or eliminate pain

Anaphylaxis Management: promotion of adequate ventilation and tissue perfusion for an individual with a severe allergic (antigen-antibody) reaction

Anesthesia Administration: preparation for and administration of anesthetic agents and monitoring of patient responsiveness during administration

Anger Control Assistance: facilitation of the expression of anger in an adaptive, nonviolent manner

Animal-Assisted Therapy: purposeful use of animals to provide affection, attention, diversion, and relaxation

Anticipatory Guidance: preparation of patient for an anticipated developmental or situational crisis

Anxiety Reduction: minimizing apprehension, dread, foreboding, or uneasiness related to an unidentified source of anticipated danger

Area Restriction: use of least restrictive limitation of patient mobility to a specified area for purposes of safety or behavior management

Aromatherapy: administration of essential oils through massage, topical ointments or lotions, baths, inhalation, douches, or compresses (hot or cold) to calm and soothe, provide pain relief, and enhance relaxation and comfort

Art Therapy: facilitation of communication through drawings or other art forms

Artificial Airway Management: maintenance of endotracheal and tracheostomy tubes and prevention of complications associated with their use

Aspiration Precautions: prevention or minimization of risk factors in the patient at risk for aspiration

Assertiveness Training: assistance with the effective expression of feelings, needs, and ideas while respecting the rights of others

Asthma Management: identification, treatment, and prevention of reactions to inflammation/constriction in the airway passages

Attachment Promotion: facilitating the development of an affective, enduring relationship between infant and parent

Autogenic Training: assisting with self-suggestions about feelings of heaviness and warmth for the purpose of inducing relaxation

Autotransfusion: collecting and reinfusing blood that has been lost intraoperatively or postoperatively from clean wounds

B

Bathing: cleaning of the body for the purposes of relaxation, cleanliness, and healing

Bed Rest Care: promotion of comfort and safety and prevention of complications for a patient unable to get out of bed

Bedside Laboratory Testing: performance of laboratory tests at the bedside or point of care

Behavior Management: helping a patient to manage negative behavior

Behavior Management: Overactivity/Inattention: provision of a therapeutic milieu that safely accommodates the patient's attention deficit and/or overactivity while promoting optimal function

Behavior Management: Self-Harm: assisting the patient to decrease or eliminate self-mutilating or self-abusive behaviors

Behavior Management: Sexual: defined as delineation and prevention of socially unacceptable sexual behaviors

Behavior Modification: promotion of a behavior change

[a]Data from Bulechek GM, et al: *Nursing Interventions Classification (NIC),* ed 6, St Louis, 2013, Mosby.

Behavior Modification: Social Skills: assisting the patient to develop or improve interpersonal social skills

Bibliotherapy: therapeutic use of literature to enhance expression of feelings, active problem solving, coping, or insight

Biofeedback: assisting the patient to gain voluntary control over physiological responses using feedback from electronic equipment that monitor physiological processes

Bioterrorism Preparedness: preparing for an effective response to bioterrorism events or disaster

Birthing: delivery of a baby

Bladder Irrigation: instillation of a solution into the bladder to provide cleansing or medication

Bleeding Precautions: reduction of stimuli that may induce bleeding or hemorrhage in at-risk patients

Bleeding Reduction: limitation of the loss of blood volume during an episode of bleeding

Bleeding Reduction: Antepartum Uterus: limitation of the amount of blood loss from the pregnant uterus during the third trimester of pregnancy

Bleeding Reduction: Gastrointestinal: limitation of the amount of blood loss from the upper and lower gastrointestinal tract and related complications

Bleeding Reduction: Nasal: limitation of the amount of blood loss from the nasal cavity

Bleeding Reduction: Postpartum Uterus: limitation of the amount of blood loss from the postpartum uterus

Bleeding Reduction: Wound: limitation of the blood loss from a wound that may be a result of trauma, incisions, or placement of a tube or catheter

Blood Products Administration: administration of blood or blood products and monitoring of patient's response

Body Image Enhancement: defined as improving a patient's conscious and unconscious perceptions and attitudes toward his/her body

Body Mechanics Promotion: facilitating the use of posture and movement in daily activities to prevent fatigue and musculoskeletal strain or injury

Bottle Feeding: preparation and administration of fluids to an infant via a bottle

Bowel Incontinence Care: promotion of bowel continence and maintenance of perianal skin integrity

Bowel Incontinence Care: Encopresis: promotion of bowel continence in children

Bowel Management: establishment and maintenance of a regular pattern of bowel elimination

Bowel Training: assisting the patient to train the bowel to evacuate at specific intervals

Breast Examination: inspection and palpation of the breasts and related areas

C

Calming Technique: reducing anxiety in a patient experiencing acute distress

Capillary Blood Sample: obtaining an arteriovenous sample from a peripheral body site, such as the heel, finger, or other transcutaneous site

Cardiac Care: limitation of complications resulting from an imbalance between myocardial oxygen supply and demand for a patient with symptoms of impaired cardiac function

Cardiac Care: Acute: limitation of complications for a patient recently experiencing an episode of an imbalance between myocardial oxygen supply and demand resulting in impaired cardiac function

Cardiac Care: Rehabilitative: promotion of maximum functional activity level for a patient who has experienced an episode of impaired cardiac function that resulted from an imbalance between myocardial oxygen supply and demand

Cardiac Risk Management: prevention of an acute episode of impaired cardiac function by minimizing contributing events and risk behaviors

Caregiver Support: provision of the necessary information, advocacy, and support to facilitate primary patient care by someone other than a health care professional

Case Management: coordinating care and advocating for specified individuals and patient populations across settings to reduce cost, reduce resource use, improve quality of health care, and achieve desired outcomes

Cast Care: Maintenance: care of a cast after the drying period

Cast Care: Wet: care of a new cast during the drying period

Central Venous Access Device Management: care of the patient with prolonged venous access through the use of a device inserted into the central circulation

Cerebral Edema Management: limitation of secondary cerebral injury resulting from swelling of brain tissue

Cerebral Perfusion Promotion: promotion of adequate perfusion and limitation of complications for a patient experiencing or at risk for inadequate cerebral perfusion

Cesarean Birth Care: provision of care to a patient delivering a baby through an abdominal incision into the uterus

Chemical Restraint: administration, monitoring, and discontinuation of psychotropic agents used to control an individual's extreme behavior

Chemotherapy Management: assisting the patient and family to understand the action and minimize side effects of antineoplastic agents

Chest Physiotherapy: assisting the patient to mobilize airway secretions via percussion, vibration, and postural drainage

Childbirth Preparation: providing information and support to facilitate childbirth and to enhance the ability of an individual to develop and perform the parental role

Circulatory Care: Arterial Insufficiency: promotion of arterial circulation

Circulatory Care: Mechanical Assist Device: temporary support of the circulation through the use of mechanical devices or pumps

Circulatory Care: Venous Insufficiency: defined as promotion of venous circulation

Circulatory Precautions: protection of a localized area with limited perfusion

Circumcision Care: preprocedural and postprocedural support to males undergoing circumcision

Code Management: coordination of emergency measures to sustain life

Cognitive Restructuring: challenging a patient to alter distorted thought patterns and view self and the world more realistically

Cognitive Stimulation: promotion of awareness and comprehension of surroundings by utilization of planned stimuli

Commendation: offering statements of praise and admiration to identify and emphasize the strengths and capabilities evident in the individual, family, or community

Communicable Disease Management: working with a community to decrease and manage the incidence and prevalence of contagious diseases in a specific population

Communication Enhancement: Hearing Deficit: use of strategies augmenting communication capabilities for a person with diminished hearing

Communication Enhancement: Speech Deficit: use of strategies augmenting communication capabilities for a person with impaired speech

Communication Enhancement: Visual Deficit: use of strategies augmenting communication capabilities for a person with diminished vision

Community Disaster Preparedness: preparing for an effective response to a large-scale disaster

Community Health Development: assisting members of a community to identify a community's health concerns, mobilize resources, and implement solutions

Complex Relationship Building: establishing a therapeutic relationship with a patient to promote insight and behavioral change

Conflict Mediation: facilitation of constructive dialogue between opposing parties with a goal of resolving disputes in a mutually acceptable manner

Constipation/Impaction Management: prevention and alleviation of constipation/impaction

Consultation: using expert knowledge to work with those who seek help in problem solving to enable individuals, families, groups, or agencies to achieve identified goals

Contact Lens Care: assisting patients in the proper use of contact lenses

Controlled Substance Checking: promoting appropriate use and maintaining security of controlled substances

Coping Enhancement: facilitation of cognitive and behavioral efforts to manage perceived stressors, changes, or threats that interfere with meeting life demands and roles

Cost Containment: management and facilitation of efficient and effective use of resources

Cough Enhancement: promotion of deep inhalation by the patient with subsequent generation of high intrathoracic pressures and compression of underlying lung parenchyma for the forceful expulsion of air

Counseling: use of an interactive helping process focusing on the needs, problems, or feelings of the patient and significant others to enhance or support coping, problem-solving, and interpersonal relationships

Crisis Intervention: use of short-term counseling to help the patient cope with a crisis and resume a state of functioning comparable to or better than the precrisis state

Critical Path Development: constructing and using a timed sequence of patient care activities to enhance desired patient outcomes in a cost-efficient manner

Cultural Brokerage: the deliberate use of culturally competent strategies to bridge or mediate between the patient's culture and the biomedical health care system

Cup Feeding: Newborn: preparation and administration of fluid to a newborn using a cup

Cutaneous Stimulation: stimulation of the skin and underlying tissues for the purpose of decreasing undesirable signs and symptoms such as pain, muscle spasm, inflammation, or nausea

D

Decision-Making Support: providing information and support for a patient who is making a decision regarding health care

Defibrillator Management: External: care of the patient receiving defibrillation for termination of life-threatening cardiac rhythm disturbances

Defibrillator Management: Internal: care of the patient receiving permanent detection and termination of life-threatening cardiac rhythm disturbances through the insertion and use of an internal cardiac defibrillator

Delegation: transfer of responsibility for the performance of patient care while retaining accountability for the outcome

Delirium Management: provision of a safe and therapeutic environment for the patient who is experiencing an acute confusional state

Delusion Management: promoting the comfort, safety, and reality orientation of a patient experiencing false, fixed beliefs that have little or no basis in reality

Dementia Management: provision of a modified environment for the patient who is experiencing a chronic confusional state

Dementia Management: Bathing: reduction of aggressive behavior during cleaning of the body

Dementia Management: Wandering: provision of care for a patient experiencing pacing patterns, elopement attempts, or getting lost unless accompanied

Deposition/Testimony: provision of recorded sworn testimony for legal proceedings based upon knowledge of the case

Developmental Enhancement: Adolescent: facilitating optimal physical, cognitive, social, and emotional growth of individuals during the transition from childhood to adulthood

Developmental Enhancement: Child: facilitating or teaching parents/caregivers to facilitate the optimal gross motor, fine motor, language, cognitive, social, and emotional growth of preschool and school-aged children

Developmental Enhancement: Infant: Facilitating optimal physical, cognitive, social, and emotional growth of child under 1 year of age

Dialysis Access Maintenance: preservation of vascular (arterial-venous) access sites

Diarrhea Management: management and alleviation of diarrhea

Diet Staging: instituting required diet restrictions with subsequent progression of diet as tolerated

Diet Staging: Weight Loss Surgery: instituting required diet changes in progressive phases following bariatric surgery

Discharge Planning: preparation for moving a patient from one level of care to another within or outside the current health care agency

Distraction: purposeful diverting of attention or temporarily suppressing negative emotions and thoughts away from undesirable sensations

Documentation: recording of pertinent patient data in a clinical record

Dressing: choosing, putting on, and removing clothes for a person who cannot do this for self

Dry Eye Prevention: prevention and early detection of dry eye in an individual at risk

Dying Care: promotion of physical comfort and psychological peace in the final phase of life

Dysreflexia Management: prevention and elimination of stimuli which cause hyperactive reflexes and inappropriate autonomic responses in a patient with a cervical or high thoracic cord lesion

Dysrhythmia Management: preventing, recognizing, and facilitating treatment of abnormal cardiac rhythms

E

Ear Care: prevention or minimization of threats to ear or hearing

Eating Disorders Management: prevention and treatment of severe diet restriction and overexercising or binging and purging of food and fluids

Electroconvulsive Therapy (ECT) Management: assisting with the safe and efficient provision of electroconvulsive (ECT) therapy in the treatment of psychiatric illness

Electrolyte Management: promotion of electrolyte balance and prevention of complications resulting from abnormal or undesired serum electrolyte levels

Electrolyte Management: Hypercalcemia: promotion of calcium balance and prevention of complications resulting from serum calcium levels higher than desired

Electrolyte Management: Hyperkalemia: promotion of potassium balance and prevention of complications resulting from serum potassium levels higher than desired

Electrolyte Management: Hypermagnesemia: promotion of magnesium balance and prevention of complications resulting from serum magnesium levels higher than desired

Electrolyte Management: Hypernatremia: promotion of sodium balance and prevention of complications resulting from serum sodium levels higher than desired

Electrolyte Management: Hyperphosphatemia: promotion of phosphate balance and prevention of complications resulting from serum phosphate levels higher than desired

Electrolyte Management: Hypocalcemia: promotion of calcium balance and prevention of complications resulting from serum calcium levels lower than desired

Electrolyte Management: Hypokalemia: promotion of potassium balance and prevention of complications resulting from serum potassium levels lower than desired

Electrolyte Management: Hypomagnesemia: promotion of magnesium balance and prevention of complications resulting from serum magnesium levels lower than desired

Electrolyte Management: Hyponatremia: promotion of sodium balance and prevention of complications resulting from serum sodium levels lower than desired

Electrolyte Management: Hypophosphatemia: promotion of phosphate balance and prevention of complications resulting from serum phosphate levels lower than desired

Electrolyte Monitoring: collection and analysis of patient data to regulate electrolyte balance

Electronic Fetal Monitoring: Antepartum: electronic evaluation of fetal heart rate response to movement, external stimuli, or uterine contractions during antepartal testing

Electronic Fetal Monitoring: Intrapartum: electronic evaluation of fetal heart rate response to uterine contractions during intrapartal care

Elopement Precautions: minimizing the risk of a patient leaving a treatment setting without authorization when departure presents a threat to the safety of patient or others

Embolus Care: Peripheral: management of a patient experiencing occlusion of peripheral circulation

Embolus Care: Pulmonary: management of a patient experiencing occlusion of pulmonary circulation

Embolus Precautions: reduction of the risk of an embolus in a patient with thrombi or at risk for thrombus formation

Emergency Care: providing evaluation and treatment measures in urgent situations

Emergency Cart Checking: systematic review and maintenance of the contents of an emergency cart at established time intervals

Emotional Support: provision of reassurance, acceptance, and encouragement during times of stress

Endotracheal Extubation: purposeful removal of the endotracheal tube from the nasopharyngeal or oropharyngeal airway

Enema Administration: instillation of a solution into the lower gastrointestinal tract

Energy Management: regulating energy use to treat or prevent fatigue and optimize function

Enteral Tube Feeding: delivering nutrients and water through a gastrointestinal tube

Environmental Management: manipulation of the patient's surroundings for therapeutic benefit, sensory appeal, and psychological well-being

Environmental Management: Comfort: manipulation of the patient's surroundings for promotion of optimal comfort

Environmental Management: Community: monitoring and influencing of the physical, social, cultural, economic, and political conditions that affect the health of groups and communities

Environmental Management: Home Preparation: preparing the home for safe and effective delivery of care

Environmental Management: Safety: monitoring and manipulation of the physical environment to promote safety

Environmental Management: Violence Prevention: monitoring and manipulation of the physical environment to decrease the potential for violent behavior directed toward self, others, or environment

Environmental Management: Worker Safety: monitoring and manipulation of the worksite environment to promote safety and health of workers

Environmental Risk Protection: preventing and detecting disease and injury in populations at risk from environmental hazards

Examination Assistance: providing assistance to the patient and another health care provider during a procedure or exam

Exercise Promotion: facilitation of regular physical activity to maintain or advance to a higher level of fitness and health

Exercise Promotion: Strength Training: facilitating regular resistive muscle training to maintain or increase muscle strength

Exercise Promotion: Stretching: facilitation of systematic slow-stretch-hold muscle exercises to induce relaxation, to prepare muscles/joints for more vigorous exercise, or to increase or maintain body flexibility

Exercise Therapy: Ambulation: promotion and assistance with walking to maintain or restore autonomic and voluntary body functions during treatment and recovery from illness or injury

Exercise Therapy: Balance: use of specific activities, postures, and movements to maintain, enhance, or restore balance

Exercise Therapy: Joint Mobility: use of active or passive body movement to maintain or restore joint flexibility

Exercise Therapy: Muscle Control: use of specific activity or exercise protocols to enhance or restore controlled body movement

Eye Care: prevention or minimization of threats to eye or visual integrity

F

Fall Prevention: instituting special precautions with patients at risk for injury from falling

Family Integrity Promotion: promotion of family cohesion and unity

Family Integrity Promotion: Childbearing Family: facilitation of the growth of individuals or families who are adding an infant to the family unit

Family Involvement Promotion: facilitating participation of family members in the emotional and physical care of the patient

Family Mobilization: utilization of family strengths to influence patient's health in a positive direction

Family Planning: Contraception: assisting patient in determining and providing method of pregnancy prevention

Family Planning: Infertility: management, education, and support of the patient and significant other undergoing evaluation and treatment for infertility

Family Planning: Unplanned Pregnancy: facilitation of decision-making regarding pregnancy outcome

Family Presence Facilitation: facilitation of the family's presence in support of an individual undergoing resuscitation and/or invasive procedures

Family Process Maintenance: minimization of family process disruption effects

Family Support: promotion of family values, interests, and goals

Family Therapy: assisting family members to move their family toward a more productive way of living

Feeding: providing nutritional intake for patient who is unable to feed self

Fertility Preservation: providing information, counseling, and treatment that facilitate reproductive health and the ability to conceive

Fever Treatment: management of symptoms and related conditions associated with an increase in body temperature mediated by endogenous pyrogens

Financial Resource Assistance: assisting an individual/family to secure and manage finances to meet health care needs

Fire-Setting Precautions: prevention of fire-setting behaviors

First Aid: providing immediate care for minor burns, injuries, poisoning, bites, and stings

Fiscal Resource Management: procuring and directing the use of financial resources to assure the development and continuation of programs and services

Flatulence Reduction: prevention of flatus formation and facilitation of passage of excessive gas

Fluid/Electrolyte Management: regulation and prevention of complications from altered fluid and/or electrolyte levels

Fluid Management: promotion of fluid balance and prevention of complications resulting from abnormal or undesired fluid levels

Fluid Monitoring: collection and analysis of patient data to regulate fluid balance

Fluid Resuscitation: administering prescribed intravenous fluids rapidly

Foot Care: cleansing and inspecting the feet for the purposes of relaxation, cleanliness, and healthy skin

Forensic Data Collection: collection and recording of pertinent patient data for a forensic report

Forgiveness Facilitation: assisting an individual's willingness to replace feelings of anger and resentment toward another, self, or higher power, with beneficence, empathy, and humility

App

G

Gastrointestinal Intubation: insertion of a tube into the gastrointestinal tract

Genetic Counseling: use of an interactive helping process focusing on assisting an individual, family, or group, manifesting or at risk for developing or transmitting a birth defect or genetic condition, to cope

Grief Work Facilitation: assistance with the resolution of a significant loss

Grief Work Facilitation: Perinatal Death: assistance with the resolution of a perinatal loss

Guided Imagery: purposeful use of imagination to achieve a particular state, outcome, or action or to direct attention away from undesirable sensations

Guilt Work Facilitation: helping another to cope with painful feelings of actual or perceived responsibility

H

Hair and Scalp Care: promotion of healthy, clean, and attractive hair and scalp

Hallucination Management: promoting the safety, comfort, and reality orientation of a patient experiencing hallucinations

Healing Touch: providing a noninvasive, biofield therapy using touch and compassionate intentionality to influence the energy system of a person, affecting their physical, emotional, mental, and spiritual health and healing

Health Care Information Exchange: providing patient care information to other health professionals

Health Education: developing and providing instruction and learning experiences to facilitate voluntary adaptation of behavior conducive to health in individuals, families, groups, or communities

Health Literacy Enhancement: assisting individuals with limited ability to obtain, process, and understand information related to health and illness

Health Policy Monitoring: surveillance and influence of government and organization regulations, rules, and standards that affect nursing systems and practices to ensure quality care of patients

Health Screening: detecting health risks or problems by means of history, examination, and other procedures

Health System Guidance: facilitating a patient's location and use of appropriate health services

Heat/Cold Application: stimulation of the skin and underlying tissues with heat or cold for the purpose of decreasing pain, muscle spasms, or inflammation

Hemodialysis Therapy: management of extracorporeal passage of the patient's blood through a dialyzer

Hemodynamic Regulation: optimization of heart rate, preload, afterload, and contractility

Hemofiltration Therapy: cleansing of acutely ill patient's blood via a hemofilter controlled by the patient's hydrostatic pressure

High-Risk Pregnancy Care: identification and management of a high-risk pregnancy to promote healthy outcomes for mother and baby

Home Maintenance Assistance: helping the patient/family to maintain the home as a clean, safe, and pleasant place to live

Hope Inspiration: enhancing the belief in one's capacity to initiate and sustain actions

Hormone Replacement Therapy: facilitation of safe and effective use of hormone replacement therapy

Humor: facilitating the patient to perceive, appreciate, and express what is funny, amusing, or ludicrous in order to establish relationships, relieve tension, release anger, facilitate learning, or cope with painful feelings

Hyperglycemia Management: preventing and treating above-normal blood glucose levels

Hyperthermia Treatment: management of symptoms and related conditions associated with an increase in body temperature resulting from thermoregulation dysfunction

Hypervolemia Management: reduction in extracellular and/or intracellular fluid volume and prevention of complications in a patient who is fluid overloaded

Hypnosis: assisting a patient to achieve a state of attentive, focused concentration with suspension of some peripheral awareness to create changes in sensation, thoughts, or behavior

Hypoglycemia Management: preventing and treating low blood glucose levels

Hypothermia Induction Therapy: attaining and maintaining core body temperature below 35° C and monitoring for side effects and/or prevention of complications

Hypothermia Treatment: heat loss prevention, rewarming, and surveillance of a patient whose core body temperature is abnormally low as a result of noninduced circumstances

Hypovolemia Management: expansion of intravascular fluid volume in a patient who is volume depleted

I

Immunization/Vaccination Management: monitoring immunization status, facilitating access to immunizations, and providing immunizations to prevent communicable disease

Impulse Control Training: assisting the patient to mediate impulsive behavior through application of problem-solving strategies to social and interpersonal situations

Incident Reporting: written and verbal reporting of any event in the process of patient care that is inconsistent with desired patient outcomes or routine operations of the health care facility

Incision Site Care: cleansing, monitoring, and promotion of healing in a wound that is closed with sutures, clips, or staples

Infant Care: provision of developmentally-appropriate, family-centered care to the child under 1 year of age

Infant Care: Newborn: provision of care to the infant during the transition from birth to extrauterine life and subsequent period of stabilization

Infant Care: Preterm: aligning caretaking practices with the preterm infant's individual developmental and physiological needs to support growth and development

Infection Control: minimizing the acquisition and transmission of infectious agents

Infection Control: Intraoperative: preventing nosocomial infection in the operating room

Infection Protection: prevention and early detection of infection in a patient at risk

Insurance Authorization: assisting the patient and provider to secure payment for health services or equipment from a third party

Intracranial Pressure (ICP) Monitoring: measurement and interpretation of patient data to regulate intracranial pressure

Intrapartal Care: monitoring and management of stages one and two of the birth process

Intrapartal Care: High-Risk Delivery: assisting with vaginal delivery of multiple or malpositioned fetuses

Intravenous (IV) Insertion: insertion of a cannulated needle into a peripheral vein for the purpose of administering fluids, blood, or medications

Intravenous (IV) Therapy: administration and monitoring of intravenous fluids and medications

Invasive Hemodynamic Monitoring: measurement and interpretation of invasive hemodynamic parameters to determine cardiovascular function and regulate therapy as appropriate

J

Journaling: promotion of writing as a means to provide opportunities to reflect upon and analyze past events, experiences, thoughts, and feelings

K

Kangaroo Care: facilitation of skin-to-skin contact between parent or other caregiver and physiologically-stable preterm infant

L

Labor Induction: initiation or augmentation of labor by mechanical or pharmacological methods

Labor Suppression: controlling uterine contractions prior to 37 weeks of gestation to prevent preterm birth

Laboratory Data Interpretation: critical analysis of patient laboratory data in order to assist with clinical decision-making

Lactation Counseling: assisting in the establishment and maintenance of successful breastfeeding

Lactation Suppression: facilitating the cessation of milk production while minimizing painful engorgement

Laser Precautions: limiting the risk of laser-related injury to the patient

Latex Precautions: reducing the risk of a systemic reaction to latex

Learning Facilitation: promoting the ability to process and comprehend information

Learning Readiness Enhancement: improving the ability and willingness to receive information

Leech Therapy: application of medicinal leeches to help drain replanted or transplanted tissue engorged with venous blood

Life Skills Enhancement: developing an individual's ability to independently and effectively deal with the demands and challenges of everyday life

Limit Setting: establishing the parameters of desirable and acceptable patient behavior

Listening Visits: empathic listening to genuinely understand an individual's situation and work collaboratively over a number of home visits to identify and generate solutions to reduce depressive symptoms

Lower Extremity Monitoring: collection, analysis, and use of patient data to categorize risk and prevent injury to the lower extremities

M

Malignant Hyperthermia Precautions: prevention or reduction of hypermetabolic response to pharmacological agents used during surgery

Massage: stimulation of the skin and underlying tissues with varying degrees of hand pressure to decrease pain, produce relaxation, and/or improve circulation

Mechanical Ventilation Management: Invasive: assisting the patient receiving artificial breathing support through a device inserted into the trachea

Mechanical Ventilation Management: Noninvasive: assisting a patient receiving artificial breathing support that does not necessitate a device inserted into the trachea

Mechanical Ventilation Management: Pneumonia Prevention: care of a patient at risk for developing ventilator-associated pneumonia

Mechanical Ventilatory Weaning: assisting the patient to breathe without the aid of a mechanical ventilator

Medication Administration: preparing, giving, and evaluating the effectiveness of prescription and nonprescription drugs

Medication Administration: Ear: preparing and instilling otic medications

Medication Administration: Enteral: delivering medications through a tube inserted into the gastrointestinal system

Medication Administration: Eye: preparing and instilling ophthalmic medications

Medication Administration: Inhalation: preparing and administering inhaled medications

Medication Administration: Interpleural: administration of medication through a catheter for diffusion within the pleural cavity

Medication Administration: Intradermal: preparing and giving medications via the intradermal route

Medication Administration: Intramuscular (IM): preparing and giving medications via the intramuscular route

Medication Administration: Intraosseous: insertion of a needle through the bone cortex into the medullary cavity for the purpose of short-term, emergency administration of fluid, blood, or medication

Medication Administration: Intraspinal: administration and monitoring of medication via an established epidural or intrathecal route

Medication Administration: Intravenous (IV): preparing and giving medications via the intravenous route

Medication Administration: Nasal: preparing and giving medications via nasal passages

Medication Administration: Oral: preparing and giving medications by mouth

Medication Administration: Rectal: preparing and inserting rectal suppositories

Medication Administration: Skin: preparing and applying medications to the skin

Medication Administration: Subcutaneous: preparing and giving medications via the subcutaneous route

Medication Administration: Vaginal: preparing and inserting vaginal medications

Medication Administration: Ventricular Reservoir: administration and monitoring of medication through an indwelling catheter into the lateral ventricle of the brain

Medication Management: facilitation of safe and effective use of prescription and over-the-counter drugs

Medication Prescribing: prescribing medication for a health problem

Medication Reconciliation: comparison of the patient's home medications with the admission, transfer, and/or discharge orders to ensure accuracy and patient safety

Medication Facilitation: facilitating a person to alter his/her level of awareness by focusing specifically on an image or thought

Memory Training: facilitation of memory

Milieu Therapy: use of people, resources, and events in the patient's immediate environment to promote optimal psychosocial functioning

Mood Management: providing for safety, stabilization, recovery, and maintenance of a patient who is experiencing dysfunctionally depressed or elevated mood

Multidisciplinary Care Conference: planning and evaluating patient care with health professionals from other disciplines

Music Therapy: using music to help achieve a specific change in behavior, feeling, or physiology

Mutual Goal Setting: collaborating with patient to identify and prioritize care goals, then developing a plan for achieving those goals

N

Nail Care: promotion of clean, neat, attractive nails and prevention of skin lesions related to improper care of nails

Nasal Irrigation: enhancing nasal mucosa functioning using saline lavage

Nausea Management: prevention and alleviation of nausea

Neurologic Monitoring: collection and analysis of patient data to prevent or minimize neurologic complications

Nonnutritive Sucking: provision of sucking opportunities for the infant

Normalization Promotion: assisting parents and other family members of children with chronic illnesses or disabilities in providing normal life experiences for their children and families

Nutrition Management: providing and promoting a balanced intake of nutrients

Nutrition Therapy: administration of food and fluids to support metabolic processes of a patient who is malnourished or at high risk for becoming malnourished

Nutritional Counseling: use of an interactive helping process focusing on the need for diet modification

Nutritional Monitoring: collection and analysis of patient data pertaining to nutrient intake

O

Oral Health Maintenance: maintenance and promotion of oral hygiene and dental health for the patient at risk for developing oral or dental lesions

Oral Health Promotion: promotion of oral hygiene and dental care for a patient with normal oral and dental health

Oral Health Restoration: promotion of healing for a patient who has an oral mucosa or dental lesion

Order Transcription: transferring information from order sheets to the nursing patient care planning and documentation system

Organ Procurement: guiding families through the donation process to ensure timely retrieval of vital organs and tissue for transplant

Ostomy Care: maintenance of elimination through a stoma and care of surrounding tissue

Oxygen Therapy: administration of oxygen and monitoring of its effectiveness

P

Pacemaker Management: Permanent: care of the patient receiving permanent support of cardiac pumping through the insertion and use of a pacemaker

Pacemaker Management: Temporary: temporary support of cardiac pumping though the insertion and use of a temporary pacemaker

Pain Management: alleviation of pain or a reduction in pain to a level of comfort that is acceptable to the patient

Parent Education: Adolescent: assisting parents to understand and help their adolescent children

Parent Education: Childrearing Family: assisting parents to understand and promote the physical, psychological, and social growth and development of their toddler, preschool, or school-aged child

Parent Education: Infant: instruction on nurturing and physical care needed during the first year of life

Parenting Promotion: providing parenting information, support, and coordination of comprehensive services to high-risk families

Pass Facilitation: arranging a leave for a patient from a health care facility

Patient Contracting: negotiating an agreement with an individual that reinforces a specific behavior change

Patient-Controlled Analgesia (PCA) Assistance: facilitating patient control of analgesic administration and regulation

Patient Identification: positive verification of a patient's identity

Patient Rights Protection: protection of health care rights of a patient, especially a minor, incapacitated, or incompetent patient unable to make decisions

Peer Review: systematic evaluation of a peer's performance compared with professional standards of practice

Pelvic Muscle Exercise: strengthening and training the levator ani and urogenital muscles through voluntary, repetitive contraction to decrease stress, urge, or mixed types of urinary incontinence

Perineal Care: maintenance of perineal skin integrity and relief of perineal discomfort

Peripheral Sensation Management: prevention or minimization of injury or discomfort in the patient with altered sensation

Peripherally Inserted Central Catheter (PICC) Care: insertion and maintenance of a peripherally inserted catheter for access into the central circulation

Peritoneal Dialysis Therapy: administration and monitoring of dialysis solution into and out of the peritoneal cavity

Pessary Management: placement and monitoring of a vaginal device for treating stress urinary incontinence, uterine retroversion, genital prolapse, or incompetent cervix

Phlebotomy: Arterial Blood Sample: obtaining a blood sample from an uncannulated artery to assess oxygen and carbon dioxide levels and acid-base balance

Phlebotomy: Blood Unit Acquisition: procuring blood and blood products from donors

Phlebotomy: Cannulated Vessel: aspirating a blood sample through an indwelling vascular catheter for laboratory tests

Phlebotomy: Venous Blood Sample: removal of a sample of venous blood from an uncannulated vein

Phototherapy: Mood/Sleep Regulation: administration of doses of bright light in order to elevate mood and/or normalize the body's internal clock

Phototherapy: Neonate: use of light therapy to reduce bilirubin levels in newborn infants

Physical Restraint: application, monitoring, and removal of mechanical restraining devices or manual restraints used to limit physical mobility of patient

Physician Support: collaborating with physicians to provide quality patient care

Pneumatic Tourniquet Precautions: applying a pneumatic tourniquet, while minimizing the potential for patient injury from use of the device

Positioning: deliberative placement of the patient or a body part to promote physiological and/or psychological well-being

Positioning: Intraoperative: moving the patient or body part to promote surgical exposure while reducing the risk of discomfort and complications

Positioning: Neurologic: achievement of optimal, appropriate body alignment for the patient experiencing, or at risk for, spinal cord injury or vertebral irritability

Positioning: Wheelchair: placement of a patient in a properly selected wheelchair to enhance comfort, promote skin integrity, and foster independence

Postanesthesia Care: monitoring and management of the patient who has recently undergone general or regional anesthesia

Postmortem Care: provision of care to the deceased patient and family

Postpartal Care: providing care to a woman during the 6-week time period beginning immediately after childbirth

Preceptor: Employee: assisting and supporting a new or transferred employee through a planned orientation to a specific clinical area

Preceptor: Student: assisting and supporting learning experiences for a student

Preconception Counseling: screening and providing information and support to individuals of childbearing age before pregnancy to promote health and reduce risks

Pregnancy Termination Care: management of the physical and psychological needs of the woman undergoing a spontaneous or elective abortion

Premenstrual Syndrome (PMS) Management: alleviation/attenuation of physical and/or behavioral symptoms occurring during the luteal phase of the menstrual cycle

Prenatal Care: provision of health care during the course of pregnancy

Preoperative Coordination: facilitating preadmission diagnostic testing and preparation of the surgical patient

Preparatory Sensory Information: describing in concrete and objective terms the typical sensory experiences and events associated with an upcoming stressful health care procedure/treatment

Prescribing: Diagnostic Testing: ordering a diagnostic test to identify or monitor a health problem

Prescribing: Nonpharmacologic Treatment: ordering nonpharmacologic treatment for a health problem

Presence: being with another, both physically and psychologically, during times of need

Pressure Management: minimizing pressure to body parts

Pressure Ulcer Care: facilitation of healing in pressure ulcers

Pressure Ulcer Prevention: prevention of pressure ulcers for an individual at high risk for developing them

Product Evaluation: determining the effectiveness of new products or equipment

Program Development: planning, implementing, and evaluating a coordinated set of activities designed to enhance wellness, or to prevent, reduce, or eliminate one or more health problems for a group or community

Progressive Muscle Relaxation: facilitating the tensing and releasing of successive muscle groups while attending to the resulting differences in sensation

Prompted Voiding: promotion of urinary continence through the use of timed verbal toileting reminders and positive social feedback for successful toileting

Pruritus Management: preventing and treating itching

Q

Quality Monitoring: systematic collection and analysis of an organization's quality indicators for the purpose of improving patient care

R

Radiation Therapy Management: assisting the patient to understand and minimize the side effects of radiation treatments

Rape-Trauma Treatment: provision of emotional and physical support immediately following a reported rape

Reality Orientation: promotion of patient's awareness of personal identity, time, and environment

Recreation Therapy: purposeful use of recreation to promote relaxation and enhancement of social skills

Rectal Prolapse Management: prevention and/or manual reduction of rectal prolapse

Referral: arrangement for services by another care provider or agency

Reiki: using a specific sequence of hand positions and symbols to channel the universal life force for recharging, realigning, and rebalancing the human energy field

Relaxation Therapy: use of techniques to encourage and elicit relaxation for the purpose of decreasing undesirable signs and symptoms such as pain, muscle tension, or anxiety

Religious Addiction Prevention: prevention of a self-imposed controlling religious lifestyle

Religious Ritual Enhancement: facilitating participation in religious practices

Relocation Stress Reduction: assisting the individual to prepare for and cope with movement from one environment to another

Reminiscence Therapy: using the recall of past events, feelings, and thoughts to facilitate pleasure, quality of life, or adaptation to present circumstances

Reproductive Technology Management: assisting a patient through the steps of complex infertility treatment

Research Data Collection: collecting research data

Resiliency Promotion: assisting individuals, families, and communities in development, use, and strengthening of protective factors to be used in coping with environmental and societal stressors

Respiratory Monitoring: collection and analysis of patient data to ensure airway patency and adequate gas exchange

Respite Care: provision of short-term care to provide relief for family caregiver

Resuscitation: administering emergency measures to sustain life

Resuscitation: Fetus: administering emergency measures to improve placental perfusion or correct fetal acid-base status

Resuscitation: Neonate: administering emergency measures to support newborn adaptation to extrauterine life

Risk Identification: analysis of potential risk factors, determination of health risks, and prioritization of risk reduction strategies for an individual or group

Risk Identification: Childbearing Family: identification of an individual or family likely to experience difficulties in parenting, and prioritization of strategies to prevent parenting problems

Risk Identification: Genetic: identification and analysis of potential genetic risk factors in an individual, family, or group

Role Enhancement: assisting a patient, significant other, and/or family to improve relationships by clarifying and supplementing specific role behaviors

S

Seclusion: solitary containment in a fully protective environment with close surveillance by nursing staff for purposes of safety or behavior management

Security Enhancement: intensifying a patient's sense of physical and psychological safety

Sedation Management: administration of sedatives, monitoring of the patient's response, and provision of necessary physiological support during a diagnostic or therapeutic procedure

Seizure Management: care of a patient during a seizure and the postictal state

Seizure Precautions: prevention or minimization of potential injuries sustained by a patient with a known seizure disorder

Self-Awareness Enhancement: assisting a patient to explore and understand his/her thoughts, feelings, motivations, and behaviors

Self-Care Assistance: assisting another to perform activities of daily living

Self-Care Assistance: Bathing/Hygiene: assisting patient to perform personal hygiene

Self-Care Assistance: Dressing/Grooming: assisting patient with clothes and appearance

Self-Care Assistance: Feeding: assisting a person to eat

Self-Care Assistance: IADL: assisting and instructing a person to perform instrumental activities of daily living (IADL) needed to function in the home or community

Self-Care Assistance: Toileting: assisting another with elimination

Self-Care Assistance: Transfer: assisting a patient with limitation of independent movement to learn to change body location

Self-Efficacy Enhancement: strengthening an individual's confidence in his/her ability to perform a health behavior

Self-Esteem Enhancement: assisting a patient to increase his or her personal judgment of self-worth

Self-Hypnosis Facilitation: teaching and monitoring the use of a self-initiated hypnotic state for therapeutic benefit

Self-Modification Assistance: reinforcement of self-directed change initiated by the patient to achieve personally important goals

Self-Responsibility Facilitation: encouraging a patient to assume more responsibility for own behavior

Sexual Counseling: use of an interactive process focusing on the need to make adjustments in sexual practice or to enhance coping with a sexual event or disorder

Shift Report: exchanging essential patient care information with other nursing staff at change of shift

Shock Management: facilitation of the delivery of oxygen and nutrients to systemic tissue with removal of cellular waste products in a patient with severely altered tissue perfusion

Shock Management: Cardiac: promotion of adequate tissue perfusion for a patient with severely compromised pumping function of the heart

Shock Management: Vasogenic: promotion of adequate tissue perfusion for a patient with severe loss of vascular tone

Shock Management: Volume: promotion of adequate tissue perfusion for a patient with severely compromised intravascular volume

Shock Prevention: detecting and treating a patient at risk for impending shock

Sibling Support: assisting a sibling to cope with a brother or sister's illness/chronic condition/disability

Skin Care: Donor Site: prevention of wound complications and promotion of healing at the donor site

Skin Care: Graft Site: prevention of wound complications and promotion of graft site healing

Skin Care: Topical Treatments: application of topical substances or manipulation of devices to promote skin integrity and minimize skin breakdown

Skin Surveillance: collection and analysis of patient data to maintain skin and mucous membrane integrity

Sleep Enhancement: facilitation of regular sleep/wake cycles

Smoking Cessation Assistance: helping another to stop smoking

Social Marketing: use of marketing principles to influence the health beliefs, attitudes, and behaviors to benefit a target population

Socialization Enhancement: facilitation of another person's ability to interact with others

Specimen Management: obtaining, preparing, and preserving a specimen for a laboratory test

Spiritual Growth Facilitation: facilitation of growth in patient's capacity to identify, connect with, and call upon the source of meaning, purpose, comfort, strength, and hope in their lives

Spiritual Support: assisting the patient to feel balance and connection with a greater power

Splinting: stabilization, immobilization, and protection of an injured body part with a supportive appliance

Sports-Injury Prevention: Youth: reduce the risk of sports-related injury in young athletes

Staff Development: developing, maintaining, and monitoring competence of staff

Staff Supervision: facilitating the delivery of high-quality patient care by others

Stem Cell Infusion: infusion of hematopoietic stem cells and monitoring of the patient's response

Subarachnoid Hemorrhage Precautions: reduction of internal and external stimuli or stressors to minimize risk of rebleeding prior to surgery or endovascular procedure to secure ruptured aneurysm

Substance Use Prevention: prevention of an alcoholic or drug use lifestyle

Substance Use Treatment: care of patient and family members demonstrating dysfunction as a result of substance abuse or dependence

Substance Use Treatment: Alcohol Withdrawal: care of the patient experiencing sudden cessation of alcohol consumption

Substance Use Treatment: Drug Withdrawal: care of patient experiencing drug detoxification

Substance Use Treatment: Overdose: care of a patient demonstrating toxic effects as a result of consuming one or more drugs

Suicide Prevention: reducing the risk for self-inflicted harm with intent to end life

Supply Management: ensuring acquisition and maintenance of appropriate items for providing patient care

Support Group: use of a group environment to provide emotional support and health-related information for members

Support System Enhancement: facilitation of support to patient by family, friends, and community

Surgical Assistance: assisting the surgeon or dentist with operative procedures and care of the surgical patient

Surgical Instrumentation Management: managing the requirements for materials, instruments, equipment, and sterility of the surgical field

Surgical Precautions: minimizing the potential for iatrogenic injury to the patient related to a surgical procedure

Surgical Preparation: providing care to a patient immediately prior to surgery and verifying required procedures/tests and documentation in the clinical record

Surveillance: purposeful and ongoing acquisition, interpretation, and synthesis of patient data for clinical decision-making

Surveillance: Community: purposeful and ongoing acquisition, interpretation, and synthesis of data for decision-making in the community

Surveillance: Late Pregnancy: purposeful and ongoing acquisition, interpretation, and synthesis of maternal-fetal data for treatment, observation, or admission

Surveillance: Remote Electronic: purposeful and ongoing acquisition of patient data via electronic modalities (telephone, video, conferencing, e-mail) from distant locations, as well as interpretation and synthesis of patient data for clinical decision-making with individuals or populations

Sustenance Support: helping an individual/family in need to locate food, clothing, or shelter

Suturing: approximating edges of a wound using sterile suture material and a needle

Swallowing Therapy: facilitating swallowing and preventing complications of impaired swallowing

T

Teaching: Disease Process: assisting the patient to understand information related to a specific disease process

Teaching: Foot Care: preparing a patient at risk and/or significant other to provide preventive foot care

Teaching: Group: development, implementation, and evaluation of a patient teaching program for a group of individuals experiencing the same health condition

Teaching: Individual: planning, implementation, and evaluation of a teaching program designed to address a patient's particular needs

Teaching: Infant Nutrition 0-3 Months: instruction on nutrition and feeding practices through the first three months of life

Teaching: Infant Nutrition 4-6 Months: instruction on nutrition and feeding practices from the fourth month through the sixth month of life

Teaching: Infant Nutrition 7-9 Months: instruction on nutrition and feeding practices from the seventh month through the ninth month of life

Teaching: Infant Nutrition 10-12 Months: instruction on nutrition and feeding practices from the tenth month through the twelfth month of life

Teaching: Infant Safety 0-3 Months: instruction on safety through the first three months of life

Teaching: Infant Safety 4-6 Months: instruction on safety from the fourth month through the sixth month of life

Teaching: Infant Safety 7-9 Months: instruction on safety from the seventh month through the ninth month of life

Teaching: Infant Safety 10-12 Months: instruction on safety from the tenth month through the twelfth month of life

Teaching: Infant Stimulation 0-4 Months: teaching parents and caregivers to provide developmentally appropriate sensory activities to promote development and movement through the first four months of life

Teaching: Infant Stimulation 5-8 Months: teaching parents and caregivers to provide developmentally appropriate sensory activities to promote development and movement from the fifth month through the eighth month of life

Teaching: Infant Stimulation 9-12 Months: teaching parents and caregivers to provide developmentally appropriate sensory activities to promote development and movement from the ninth month through the twelfth month of life

Teaching: Preoperative: assisting a patient to understand and mentally prepare for surgery and the postoperative recovery period

Teaching: Prescribed Diet: preparing a patient to correctly follow a prescribed diet

Teaching: Prescribed Exercise: preparing a patient to achieve or maintain a prescribed level of exercise

Teaching: Prescribed Medication: preparing a patient to safely take prescribed medications and monitor for their effects

Teaching: Procedure/Treatment: preparing a patient to understand and mentally prepare for a prescribed procedure or treatment

Teaching: Psychomotor Skill: preparing a patient to perform a psychomotor skill

Teaching: Safe Sex: providing instruction concerning protection during sexual activity

Teaching: Sexuality: assisting individuals to understand physical and psychosocial dimensions of sexual growth and development

Teaching: Toddler Nutrition 13-18 Months: instruction on nutrition and feeding practices from the thirteenth month through the eighteenth month of life

Teaching: Toddler Nutrition 19-24 Months: instruction on nutrition and feeding practices from the nineteenth month through the twenty-fourth month of life

Teaching: Toddler Nutrition 25-36 Months: instruction on nutrition and feeding practices from the twenty-fifth month through the thirty-sixth month of life

Teaching: Toddler Safety 13-18 Months: instruction on safety from the thirteenth month through the eighteenth month of life

Teaching: Toddler Safety 19-24 Months: instruction on safety from the nineteenth month through the twenty-fourth month of life

Teaching: Toddler Safety 25-36 Months: instruction on safety from the twenty-fifth month through the thirty-sixth month of life

Teaching: Toilet Training: instruction on determining the child's readiness and strategies to assist the child to learn independent toileting skills

Technology Management: use of technical equipment and devices to monitor patient condition or sustain life

Telephone Consultation: eliciting patient's concerns, listening, and providing support, information, or teaching in response to patient's stated concerns, over the telephone

Telephone Follow-Up: providing results of testing or evaluating patient's response and determining potential for problems as a result of previous treatment, examination, or testing, over the telephone

Temperature Regulation: attaining or maintaining body temperature within a normal range

Temperature Regulation: Perioperative: attaining and maintaining desired body temperature throughout the surgical event

Therapeutic Play: purposeful and directive use of toys or other materials to assist children in communicating their perception and knowledge of their world and to help in gaining mastery of their environment

Therapeutic Touch: attuning to the universal energy field by seeking to act as a healing influence using the natural sensitivity of hands and passing them over the body to gently focus, direct, and modulate the human energy field

Therapy Group: application of psychotherapeutic techniques to a group, including the utilization of interactions between members of the group

Thrombolytic Therapy Management: collection and analysis of patient data to expedite safe, appropriate provision of an agent that dissolves a thrombus

Total Parenteral Nutrition (TPN) Administration: delivery of nutrients intravenously and monitoring of patient response

Touch: providing comfort and communication through purposeful tactile contact

Traction/Immobilization Care: management of a patient who has traction and/or a stabilizing device to immobilize and stabilize a body part

Transcutaneous Electrical Nerve Stimulation (TENS): stimulation of skin and underlying tissue with controlled, low-voltage electrical pulses

Transfer: moving a patient with limitation of independent movement

Transport: Interfacility: moving a patient from one facility to another

Transport: Intrafacility: moving a patient from one area of a facility to another

Trauma Therapy: Child: use of an interactive helping process to resolve a trauma experienced by a child

Triage: Disaster: establishing priorities of patient care for urgent treatment while allocating scarce resources

Triage: Emergency Center: establishing priorities and initiating treatment for patients in an emergency center

Triage: Telephone: determining the nature and urgency of a problem(s) and providing directions for the level of care required, over the telephone

Truth Telling: use of whole truth, partial truth, or decision delay to promote the patient's self-determination and well-being

Tube Care: management of a patient with an external drainage device exiting the body

Tube Care: Chest: management of a patient with an external device exiting the chest cavity

Tube Care: Gastrointestinal: management of a patient with a gastrointestinal tube

Tube Care: Umbilical Line: management of a newborn with an umbilical catheter

Tube Care: Urinary: management of a patient with urinary drainage equipment

Tube Care: Ventriculostomy/Lumbar Drain: management of a patient with an external cerebrospinal fluid drainage system

U

Ultrasonography: Limited Obstetric: performance of ultrasound exams to determine ovarian, uterine, or fetal status

Unilateral Neglect Management: protecting and safely reintegrating the affected part of the body while helping the patient adapt to disturbed perceptual abilities

Urinary Bladder Training: improving bladder function for those with urge incontinence by increasing the bladder's ability to hold urine and the patient's ability to suppress urination

Urinary Catheterization: insertion of a catheter into the bladder for temporary or permanent drainage of urine

Urinary Catheterization: Intermittent: regular periodic use of a catheter to empty the bladder

Urinary Elimination Management: maintenance of an optimum urinary elimination pattern

Urinary Habit Training: establishing a predictable pattern of bladder emptying to prevent incontinence for persons with limited cognitive ability who have urge, stress, or functional incontinence

Urinary Incontinence Care: assistance in promoting continence and maintaining perineal skin integrity

Urinary Incontinence Care: Enuresis: promotion of urinary continence in children

Urinary Retention Care: assistance in relieving bladder distention

V

Validation Therapy: use of a method of therapeutic communication with elderly persons with dementia that focuses on emotional rather than factual content

Values Clarification: assisting another to clarify her/his own values in order to facilitate effective decision-making

Vehicle Safety Promotion: assisting individuals, families, and communities to increase awareness of measures to reduce unintentional injuries in motorized and nonmotorized vehicles

Ventilation Assistance: promotion of an optimal spontaneous breathing pattern that maximizes oxygen and carbon dioxide exchange in the lungs

Visitation Facilitation: promoting beneficial visits by family and friends

Vital Signs Monitoring: collection and analysis of cardiovascular, respiratory, and body temperature data to determine and prevent complications

Vomiting Management: prevention and alleviation of vomiting

W

Weight Gain Assistance: facilitating gain of body weight

Weight Management: facilitating maintenance of optimal body weight and percent body fat

Weight Reduction Assistance: facilitating loss of weight and/or body fat

Wound Care: prevention of wound complications and promotion of wound healing

Wound Care: Burns: prevention of wound complications due to burns and facilitation of wound healing

Wound Care: Closed Drainage: maintenance of a pressure drainage system at the wound site

Wound Care: Nonhealing: palliative care and prevention of complications of a malignant or other wound that is not expected to heal

Wound Irrigation: rinsing or washing out wound with solution

App

APPENDIX 2

NURSING OUTCOMES CLASSIFICATION (NOC) DEFINITIONS[a]

A

Abstract Thinking: ability to recognize multiple meanings and patterns of concepts and generalize to new meanings, ideas, or contexts

Abuse Cessation: evidence that the victim is no longer hurt or exploited

Abuse Protection: protection of self and/or dependent others from abuse

Abuse Recovery: extent of healing following physical or psychological abuse that may include sexual or financial exploitation

Abuse Recovery: Emotional: extent of healing of psychological injuries due to abuse

Abuse Recovery: Financial: extent of control of monetary and legal matters following financial exploitation

Abuse Recovery: Physical: extent of healing of physical injuries due to abuse

Abuse Recovery: Sexual: extent of healing of physical and psychological injuries due to sexual abuse or exploitation

Abusive Behavior Self-Restraint: personal actions to refrain from abusive and neglectful behaviors toward others

Acceptance: Health Status: personal actions to reconcile significant changes in health circumstances

Activity Tolerance: physiologic response to energy-consuming movements with daily activities

Acute Respiratory Acidosis Severity: severity of signs and symptoms of decreased pH and increased partial arterial carbon dioxide pressure due to hypoventilation and retention of carbon dioxide

Acute Respiratory Alkalosis Severity: severity of signs and symptoms of increased blood pH and decreased partial arterial carbon dioxide pressure due to hyperventilation and increased elimination of carbon dioxide

Adaptation to Physical Disability: personal action to adapt to a significant functional challenge due to a physical disability

Adherence Behavior: self-initiated actions to promote optimal wellness, recovery, and rehabilitation

Adherence Behavior: Healthy Diet: self-initiated actions to monitor and optimize a balanced nutritional dietary regimen

Aggression Self-Restraint: personal actions to refrain from assaultive, combative, or destructive behaviors toward others

Agitation Level: Severity of disruptive physiologic and behavioral manifestations of stress or biochemical triggers

Alcohol Abuse Cessation Behavior: personal actions to eliminate alcohol use that poses a threat to health

Allergic Response: Localized: severity of localized hypersensitive immune response to a specific environmental (exogenous) antigen

Allergic Response: Systemic: severity of systemic hypersensitive immune response to a specific environmental (exogenous) antigen

Ambulation: personal actions to walk from place to place independently with or without assistive device

Ambulation: Wheelchair: personal actions to move from place to place in a wheelchair

Anger Self-Restraint: personal action to eliminate or reduce intense hostile thoughts, feelings, and behaviors

Anxiety Level: severity of manifested apprehension, tension, or uneasiness arising from an unidentifiable source

Anxiety Self-Control: personal actions to eliminate or reduce feelings of apprehension, tension, or uneasiness from an unidentifiable source

Appetite: desire to eat

Aspiration Prevention: personal actions to prevent the passage of fluid and solid particles into the lung

B

Balance: ability to maintain body equilibrium

Blood Coagulation: extent to which blood clots within a normal period of time

Blood Glucose Level: extent to which glucose levels in plasma and urine are maintained in normal range

Blood Loss Severity: severity of signs and symptoms of internal or external bleeding

Blood Transfusion Reaction: severity of complications with blood transfusion reaction

Body Image: perception of own appearance and body functions

Body Mechanics Performance: personal actions to maintain proper body alignment and to prevent muscular skeletal strain

Body Positioning: Self-Initiated: personal actions to change own body position independently with or without assistive device

Bone Healing: the extent of regeneration of cells and tissues following bone injury

Bottle Feeding Establishment: Infant: establishment of bottle feeding for hydration and nourishment of an infant

Bottle Feeding Performance: caregiver actions to provide fluids to an infant using a bottle

Bowel Continence: control of passage of stool from the bowel

Bowel Elimination: formation and evacuation of stool

Breastfeeding Establishment: Infant: infant attachment to and sucking from the mother's breast for nourishment during the first 3 weeks of breastfeeding

Breastfeeding Establishment: Maternal: maternal establishment of proper attachment of an infant to and sucking from the breast for nourishment during the first 3 weeks of breastfeeding

Breastfeeding Maintenance: continuation of breastfeeding from establishment to weaning for nourishment of an infant/toddler

Breastfeeding Weaning: progressive discontinuation of breastfeeding of an infant/toddler

Burn Healing: extent of healing of a burn site

Burn Recovery: extent of overall physical and psychological healing following major burn injury

C

Cardiac Pump Effectiveness: adequacy of blood volume ejected from the left ventricle to support systemic perfusion pressure

Cardiopulmonary Status: adequacy of blood volume ejected from the ventricles and exchange of carbon dioxide and oxygen at the alveolar level

Caregiver Adaptation to Patient Institutionalization: defined as adaptive response of family caregiver when the care recipient is moved to an institution

Caregiver Emotional Health: emotional well-being of a family care provider while caring for a family member

Caregiver Home Care Readiness: preparedness of a caregiver to assume responsibility for the health care of a family member in the home

Caregiver Lifestyle Disruption: severity of disturbances in the lifestyle of a family member due to caregiving

Caregiver-Patient Relationship: positive interactions and connections between the caregiver and care recipient

Caregiver Performance: Direct Care: provision by family care provider of appropriate personal and health care for a family member

Caregiver Performance: Indirect Care: arrangement and oversight by family care provider of appropriate care for a family member

[a]Data from Moorhead et al: *Nursing Outcomes Classification (NOC)*, ed 5, St Louis, 2013, Mosby.

Caregiver Physical Health: physical well-being of a family care provider while caring for a family member

Caregiver Role Endurance: factors that promote family care provider's capacity to sustain caregiving over an extended period of time

Caregiver Stressors: severity of biopsychosocial pressure on a family care provider caring for another over an extended period of time

Caregiver Well-Being: extent of positive perception of primary care provider's health status

Child Adaptation to Hospitalization: the adaptive response of a child from 3 years through 17 years of age to hospitalization

Child Development: 1 Month: milestones of physical, cognitive, and psychosocial progression by 1 month of age

Child Development: 2 Months: milestones of physical, cognitive, and psychosocial progression by 2 months of age

Child Development: 4 Months: milestones of physical, cognitive, and psychosocial progression by 4 months of age

Child Development: 6 Months: milestones of physical, cognitive, and psychosocial progression by 6 months of age

Child Development: 12 Months: milestones of physical, cognitive, and psychosocial progression by 12 months of age

Child Development: 2 Years: milestones of physical, cognitive, and psychosocial progression by 2 years of age

Child Development: 3 Years: milestones of physical, cognitive, and psychosocial progression by 3 years of age

Child Development: 4 Years: milestones of physical, cognitive, and psychosocial progression by 4 years of age

Child Development: 5 Years: milestones of physical, cognitive, and psychosocial progression by 5 years of age

Child Development: Middle Childhood: milestones of physical, cognitive, and psychosocial progression from 6 years through 11 years of age

Child Development: Adolescence: milestones of physical, cognitive, and psychosocial progression from 12 years through 17 years of age

Circulation Status: unobstructed, unidirectional blood flow at an appropriate pressure through large vessels of the systemic and pulmonary circuits

Client Satisfaction: extent of positive perception of care provided by nursing staff

Client Satisfaction: Access to Care Resources: extent of positive perception of access to nursing staff, supplies, and equipment needed for care

Client Satisfaction: Caring: extent of positive perception of nursing staff's concern for the client

Client Satisfaction: Case Management: extent of positive perception of case management services

Client Satisfaction: Communication: extent of positive perception of information exchanged between client and nursing staff

Client Satisfaction: Continuity of Care: extent of positive perception of coordination of care as the client moves from one care setting to another

Client Satisfaction: Cultural Needs Fulfillment: extent of positive perception of integration of cultural beliefs, values, and social structures into nursing care

Client Satisfaction: Functional Assistance: extent of positive perception of nursing assistance to achieve mobility and self-care

Client Satisfaction: Pain Management: extent of positive perception of nursing care to relieve pain

Client Satisfaction: Physical Care: extent of positive perception of nursing care to maintain body functions and cleanliness

Client Satisfaction: Physical Environment: extent of positive perception of living environment, treatment environment, and equipment and supplies in acute or long-term care settings

Client Satisfaction: Protection of Rights: extent of positive perception of protection of a client's legal and moral rights provided by nursing staff

Client Satisfaction: Psychological Care: extent of positive perception of nursing assistance to cope with emotional issues and perform mental activities

Client Satisfaction: Safety: extent of perception of procedures, information, and nursing care to prevent harm or injury

Client Satisfaction: Symptom Control: extent of positive perception of nursing care to relieve symptoms of illness

Client Satisfaction: Teaching: extent of positive perception of instruction provided by nursing staff to improve knowledge, understanding, and participation in care

Client Satisfaction: Technical Aspects of Care: extent of positive perception of nursing staff's knowledge and expertise used in providing care

Cognition: ability to execute complex mental processes

Cognitive Orientation: ability to identify person, place, and time accurately

Comfort Status: overall physical, psychospiritual, sociocultural, and environmental ease and safety of an individual

Comfort Status: Environment: environmental ease, comfort, and safety of surroundings

Comfort Status: Physical: physical ease related to bodily sensations and homeostatic mechanisms

Comfort Status: Psychospiritual: psychospiritual ease related to self-concept, emotional well-being, source of inspiration, and meaning and purpose in one's life

Comfort Status: Sociocultural: social ease related to interpersonal, family, and societal relationships within a cultural context

Comfortable Death: physical, psychospiritual, sociocultural, and environmental ease with the impending end of life

Communication: reception, interpretation, and expression of spoken, written, and non-verbal messages

Communication: Expressive: expression of meaningful verbal and/or non-verbal messages

Communication: Receptive: reception and interpretation of verbal and/or non-verbal messages

Community Competence: capacity of a community to collectively problem solve to achieve community goals

Community Disaster Readiness: community preparedness to respond to a natural or man-made calamitous event

Community Disaster Response: community response following a natural or man-made calamitous event

Community Grief Response: community response to members' grief that involves loss of life or property

Community Health Screening Effectiveness: quality of community actions to screen members for potential health risks or presymptomatic conditions

Community Health Status: general state of well-being of a community or population

Community Immune Status: resistance of community members to the invasion and spread of an infectious agent that could threaten public health

Community Program Effectiveness: quality of coordinated program activities that promote health and prevent, reduce, or eliminate health problems for an aggregate or population

Community Resiliency: community actions to collectively adapt and function in response to adverse socioeconomic, geopolitical, and physical environmental challenges

Community Risk Control: Chronic Disease: community actions to eliminate or reduce the incidence of chronic diseases and related complications

Community Risk Control: Communicable Disease: community actions to eliminate or reduce the spread of infectious agents that threaten public health

Community Risk Control: Lead Exposure: community actions to reduce lead exposure and poisoning

Community Risk Control: Obesity: community actions to reduce obesity and related chronic diseases

Community Risk Control: Unhealthy Cultural Traditions: community actions to promote customs, beliefs, values, and laws that support members' health and lifestyle modifications within the culture

Community Risk Control: Violence: community actions to eliminate or reduce intentional violent acts resulting in serious physical or psychological harm

Community Violence Level: incidence of violent acts compared with local, state, or national values

App

Compliance Behavior: personal actions to follow recommendations from a health professional for a specific health condition

Compliance Behavior: Prescribed Activity: personal actions to follow daily physical activities recommended by a health professional for a specific health condition

Compliance Behavior: Prescribed Diet: personal actions to follow food and fluid intake recommended by a health professional for a specific health condition

Compliance Behavior: Prescribed Medication: personal actions to administer medication safely to meet therapeutic effects for a specific condition as recommended by a health professional

Concentration: ability to focus on a specific stimulus

Coordinated Movement: ability of muscles to work together voluntarily for purposeful movement

Coping: personal actions to manage stressors that tax an individual's resources

Cup Feeding Establishment: Infant: establishment of cup feeding for hydration and nourishment of an infant

Cup Feeding Performance: caregiver actions to provide fluids to an infant using a cup

D

Decision-Making: ability to make judgments and choose between two or more alternatives

Delirium Level: severity of disturbance in consciousness and cognition that develops over a short period of time and is reversible

Dementia Level: severity of irreversible disturbances in consciousness and cognition that leads to mental, physical, and social functional losses over an extended period of time

Depression Level: severity of melancholic mood and loss of interest in life events

Depression Self-Control: personal actions to minimize melancholy and maintain interest in life events

Development: Late Adulthood: cognitive, psychosocial, and moral progression from 65 years of age and older

Development: Middle Adulthood: cognitive, psychosocial, and moral progression from 40 through 64 years of age

Development: Young Adulthood: cognitive, psychosocial, and moral progression from 18 through 39 years of age

Dignified Life Closure: personal actions to maintain control when approaching end of life

Discharge Readiness: Independent Living: readiness of a patient to relocate from a health care institution to living independently

Discharge Readiness: Supported Living: readiness of a patient to relocate from a health care institution to a lower level of supported living

Discomfort Level: severity of observed or reported mental or physical discomfort

Distorted Thought Self-Control: self-restraint of disruptions in perception, thought processes, and thought content

Drug Abuse Cessation Behavior: personal actions to eliminate drug use that poses a threat to health

Dry Eye Severity: severity of signs and symptoms of insufficient tears

E

Eating Disorder Self-Control: personal actions to eliminate maladaptive behaviors and to adopt and maintain healthy eating patterns and optimum body weight

Electrolyte & Acid/Base Balance: balance of electrolytes and non-electrolytes in the intracellular and extracellular compartments of the body

Electrolyte Balance: concentration of serum ions necessary to maintain equilibrium among electrolytes

Elopement Occurrence: number of times that an individual with a cognitive impairment escapes a secure area

Elopement Propensity Risk: the propensity of an individual with cognitive impairment to escape a secure area

Endurance: capacity to sustain activity

Energy Conservation: personal actions to manage energy for initiating and sustaining activity

Exercise Participation: personal actions to perform a self-planned, structured, and repetitive regimen to maintain or advance the level of fitness and health

F

Fall Prevention Behavior: personal or family caregiver actions to minimize risk factors that might precipitate falls in the personal environment

Falls Occurrence: number of times an individual falls

Family Coping: capacity of the family to manage stressors that tax family resources

Family Functioning: capacity of a family to meet the needs of its members during developmental transitions

Family Health Status: overall health and social competence of a family

Family Integrity: capacity of family members to maintain cohesion and emotional bonding

Family Normalization: capacity of a family to develop strategies for optimal functioning when a member has a chronic illness or disability

Family Participation in Professional Care: capacity of a family to be involved in decision-making, care delivery, and evaluation of care provided by health care personnel

Family Resiliency: capacity of a family to positively adapt and function following a significant adversity or crisis

Family Risk Control: Obesity: capacity of a family to understand, prevent, or eliminate obesity among members

Family Social Climate: capacity of a family to provide a supportive milieu as characterized by family member relationships and goals

Family Support During Treatment: capacity of a family to be present and to provide emotional support for an individual undergoing treatment

Fatigue: Disruptive Effects: severity of observed or reported disruptive effects of chronic fatigue on daily functioning

Fatigue Level: severity of observed or reported prolonged generalized fatigue

Fear Level: severity of manifested apprehension, tension, or uneasiness arising from an identifiable source

Fear Level: Child: severity of manifested apprehension, tension, or uneasiness arising from an identifiable source in a child from 1 year through 17 years of age

Fear Self-Control: personal actions to eliminate or reduce disabling feelings of apprehension, tension, or uneasiness from an identifiable source

Fetal Status: Antepartum: extent to which fetal signs are within normal limits from conception to the onset of labor

Fetal Status: Intrapartum: extent to which fetal signs are within normal limits from onset of labor to delivery

Fluid Balance: water balance in the intracellular and extracellular compartments of the body

Fluid Overload Severity: severity of signs and symptoms of excess intracellular and extracellular fluids

G

Gait: ability to walk with correct body alignment, with smooth gait cycle, and at a steady pace

Gastrointestinal Function: ability of the gastrointestinal tract to ingest and digest food products, absorb nutrients, and eliminate waste

Grief Resolution: personal actions to adjust thoughts, feelings, and behaviors to actual or impending loss

Growth: normal increase in bone size and body weight during growth years

Guilt Resolution: personal actions to adjust intense and frequent thoughts, feelings, and behaviors due to actual or perceived self-blame

H

Health Beliefs: personal convictions that influence health behaviors

Health Beliefs: Perceived Ability to Perform: personal conviction that one can carry out a given health behavior

Health Beliefs: Perceived Control: personal conviction that one can influence a health outcome

Health Beliefs: Perceived Resources: personal conviction that one has adequate means to carry out a health behavior

Health Beliefs: Perceived Threat: personal conviction that a threatening health problem is serious and has potential negative consequences for lifestyle

Health Orientation: personal commitment to health behaviors as lifestyle priorities

Health Promoting Behavior: personal actions to sustain or increase wellness

Health Seeking Behavior: personal actions to promote optimal wellness, recovery, and rehabilitation

Hearing Compensation Behavior: personal actions to identify, monitor, and compensate for hearing loss

Heedfulness of Affected Side: personal actions to acknowledge, protect, and cognitively integrate affected body part(s) into self

Hemodialysis Access: functionality of a dialysis access site and health of surrounding tissues

Hope: optimism that is personally satisfying and life-supporting

Hydration: adequate water in the intracellular and extracellular compartments of the body

Hyperactivity Level: severity of patterns of inattention or impulsivity in a child from 1 year through 17 years of age

Hypercalcemia Severity: severity of signs and symptoms of increased serum calcium

Hyperchloremia Severity: severity of signs and symptoms of increased serum chloride

Hyperglycemia Severity: severity of signs and symptoms of elevated blood glucose levels

Hyperkalemia Severity: severity of signs and symptoms of increased serum potassium

Hypermagnesemia Severity: severity of signs and symptoms of increased serum magnesium

Hypernatremia Severity: severity of signs and symptoms of increased serum sodium

Hyperphosphatemia Severity: severity of signs and symptoms of increased serum phosphorus

Hypertension Severity: severity of signs and symptoms of chronic elevated blood pressure

Hypocalcemia Severity: severity of signs and symptoms of decreased serum calcium

Hypochloremia Severity: severity of signs and symptoms of decreased serum chloride

Hypoglycemia Severity: severity of signs and symptoms of decreased blood glucose levels

Hypokalemia Severity: severity of signs and symptoms of decreased serum potassium

Hypomagnesemia Severity: severity of signs and symptoms of decreased serum magnesium

Hyponatremia Severity: severity of signs and symptoms of decreased serum sodium

Hypophosphatemia Severity: severity of signs and symptoms of decreased serum phosphorus

Hypotension Severity: severity of signs and symptoms of episodic low blood pressure

I

Identity: distinguishes between self and non-self and characterizes one's essence

Immobility Consequences: Physiological: severity of compromise in physiological functioning due to impaired physical mobility

Immobility Consequences: Psycho-Cognitive: severity of compromise in psycho-cognitive functioning due to impaired physical mobility

Immune Hypersensitivity Response: severity of inappropriate immune responses

Immune Status: natural and acquired appropriately targeted resistance to internal and external antigens

Immunization Behavior: personal actions to obtain immunization to prevent a communicable disease

Impulse Self-Control: self-restraint of compulsive or impulsive behaviors

Infant Nutritional Status: amount of nutrients ingested and absorbed to meet metabolic needs and foster growth of an infant

Infection Severity: severity of signs and symptoms of infection

Infection Severity: Newborn: severity of signs and symptoms of infection during the first 28 days of life

Information Processing: ability to acquire, organize, and use information

J

Joint Movement: active range of motion of all joints with self-initiated movement

Joint Movement: Ankle: active range of motion of the ankle with self-initiated movement

Joint Movement: Elbow: active range of motion of the elbow with self-initiated movement

Joint Movement: Fingers: active range of motion of the fingers with self-initiated movement

Joint Movement: Hip: active range of motion of the hip with self-initiated movement

Joint Movement: Knee: active range of motion of the knee with self-initiated movement

Joint Movement: Neck: active range of motion of the neck with self-initiated movement

Joint Movement: Passive: joint movement with assistance

Joint Movement: Shoulder: active range of motion of the shoulder with self-initiated movement

Joint Movement: Spine: active range of motion of the spine with self-initiated movement

Joint Movement: Wrist: active range of motion of the wrist with self-initiated movement

K

Kidney Function: ability of the kidneys to regulate body fluids, filter blood, and eliminate waste products through the formation of urine

Knowledge: Acute Illness Management: extent of understanding conveyed about a reversible illness, its treatment, and the prevention of complications

Knowledge: Anticoagulation Therapy Management: extent of understanding conveyed about the therapeutic purposes, actions, and risks of chemical agents that lengthen blood clotting time

Knowledge: Arthritis Management: extent of understanding conveyed about arthritis, its treatment, and the prevention of disease progression and complications

Knowledge: Asthma Management: extent of understanding conveyed about asthma, its treatment, and the prevention of complications

Knowledge: Body Mechanics: extent of understanding conveyed about proper body alignment, balance, and coordinated movement

Knowledge: Bottle Feeding: extent of understanding conveyed about providing fluids to an infant using a bottle

Knowledge: Breastfeeding: extent of understanding conveyed about lactation and nourishment of an infant through breastfeeding

Knowledge: Cancer Management: extent of understanding conveyed about cancer, its treatment, and the prevention of disease progression and complications

Knowledge: Cancer Threat Reduction: extent of understanding conveyed about causes, prevention and early detection of cancer

Knowledge: Cardiac Disease Management: extent of understanding conveyed about heart disease, its treatment, and the prevention of disease progression and complications

Knowledge: Child Physical Safety: extent of understanding conveyed about safely caring for a child from 1 year through 17 years of age

Knowledge: Chronic Disease Management: extent of understanding conveyed about a specific chronic disease, its treatment, and the prevention of disease progression and complications

Knowledge: Chronic Obstructive Pulmonary Disease Management: extent of understanding conveyed about chronic obstructive pulmonary disease, its treatment, and the prevention of disease progression and complications

Knowledge: Conception Prevention: extent of understanding conveyed about prevention of unintended pregnancy

Knowledge: Coronary Artery Disease Management: extent of understanding conveyed about coronary heart disease, its treatment, and the prevention of disease progression and complications

Knowledge: Cup Feeding: extent of understanding conveyed about providing fluids to an infant using a small cup

Knowledge: Dementia Management: extent of understanding conveyed about progressive dementia, its course over an extended period of time, and plan for supportive care as the disease progresses

Knowledge: Depression Management: extent of understanding conveyed about depression and interrelationships among causes, effects and treatments

Knowledge: Diabetes Management: extent of understanding conveyed about diabetes, its treatment, and the prevention of complications

Knowledge: Disease Process: extent of understanding conveyed about a specific disease process and potential complications

Knowledge: Dysrhythmia Management: extent of understanding conveyed about cardiac conduction irregularity, its treatment, and the prevention of disease progression and complications

Knowledge: Eating Disorder Management: extent of understanding conveyed about an eating disorder, its treatment, and the prevention of disease progression and complications

Knowledge: Energy Conservation: extent of understanding conveyed about energy conservation techniques

Knowledge: Fall Prevention: extent of understanding conveyed about prevention of falls

Knowledge: Fertility Promotion: extent of understanding conveyed about fertility testing and the conditions that affect conception

Knowledge: Health Behavior: extent of understanding conveyed about the promotion and protection of health

Knowledge: Health Promotion: extent of understanding conveyed about information needed to obtain and maintain optimal health

Knowledge: Health Resources: extent of understanding conveyed about relevant health care resources

Knowledge: Healthy Diet: extent of understanding conveyed about a balanced nutritious diet

Knowledge: Healthy Lifestyle: extent of understanding conveyed about a healthy, balanced lifestyle consistent with one's values, strengths, and interests

Knowledge: Heart Failure Management: extent of understanding conveyed about heart failure, its treatment, and the prevention of disease progression and complications

Knowledge: Hypertension Management: extent of understanding conveyed about high blood pressure, its treatment, and the prevention of complications

Knowledge: Infant Care: extent of understanding conveyed about caring for a baby from birth to first birthday

Knowledge: Infection Management: extent of understanding conveyed about infection, its treatment, and the prevention of disease progression and complications

Knowledge: Inflammatory Bowel Disease Management: extent of understanding conveyed about the inflammatory bowel disease process, its treatment and the prevention of relapses or complications

Knowledge: Kidney Disease Management: extent of understanding conveyed about kidney disease, its treatment, and the prevention of disease progression and complications

Knowledge: Labor & Delivery: extent of understanding conveyed about labor and vaginal delivery

Knowledge: Lipid Disorder Management: extent of understanding conveyed about hyperlipidemia, its treatment, and the prevention of complications

Knowledge: Medication: extent of understanding conveyed about the safe use of medication

Knowledge: Multiple Sclerosis Management: extent of understanding conveyed about multiple sclerosis, its treatment and the prevention of relapses or complications

Knowledge: Osteoporosis Management: extent of understanding conveyed about osteoporosis, its treatment, and the prevention of disease progression and complications

Knowledge: Ostomy Care: extent of understanding conveyed about maintenance of an ostomy for elimination

Knowledge: Pain Management: extent of understanding conveyed about causes, symptoms, and treatment of pain

Knowledge: Parenting: extent of understanding conveyed about provision of a nurturing and constructive environment for a child from 1 year through 17 years of age

Knowledge: Peripheral Artery Disease Management: extent of understanding conveyed about peripheral artery disease, its treatment and the prevention of disease progression and complications

Knowledge: Personal Safety: extent of understanding conveyed about risk reduction and prevention of unintentional injuries to self

Knowledge: Pneumonia Management: extent of understanding conveyed about pneumonia, its treatment, and the prevention of complications

Knowledge: Postpartum Maternal Health: extent of understanding conveyed about maternal health in the period following birth of infant

Knowledge: Preconception Maternal Health: extent of understanding conveyed about maternal health prior to conception to ensure a healthy pregnancy

Knowledge: Pregnancy: extent of understanding conveyed about promotion of a healthy pregnancy and prevention of complications

Knowledge: Pregnancy & Postpartum Sexual Functioning: extent of understanding conveyed about sexual function during pregnancy and postpartum

Knowledge: Prescribed Activity: extent of understanding conveyed about physical activity recommended by a health professional for a specific condition

Knowledge: Prescribed Diet: extent of understanding conveyed about a diet recommended by a health professional for a specific health condition

Knowledge: Preterm Infant Care: extent of understanding conveyed about the care of a premature infant born 24 to 37 weeks (term) gestation

Knowledge: Sexual Functioning: extent of understanding conveyed about sexual development and responsible sexual practices

Knowledge: Stress Management: extent of understanding conveyed about the stress process and strategies to reduce or cope with stress

Knowledge: Stroke Management: extent of understanding conveyed about stroke, its treatment, and the prevention of disease progression and complications

Knowledge: Stroke Prevention: extent of understanding conveyed about the causes and the prevention of stroke

Knowledge: Substance Use Control: extent of understanding conveyed about controlling the use of addictive drugs, toxic chemicals, tobacco, or alcohol

Knowledge: Thrombus Prevention: extent of understanding conveyed about causes, prevention, and early detection of blood clots within the circulatory system

Knowledge: Time Management: extent of understanding conveyed about strategies to complete commitments within an expected timeframe with minimum stress

Knowledge: Treatment Procedure: extent of understanding conveyed about a procedure required as part of a treatment regimen

Knowledge: Treatment Regimen: extent of understanding conveyed about a specific treatment regimen

Knowledge: Weight Management: extent of understanding conveyed about the promotion and maintenance of optimal body weight and fat percentage congruent with height, frame, gender, and age

L

Leisure Participation: use of relaxing, interesting, and enjoyable activities to promote well-being

Lifestyle Balance: personal actions to live a healthy, balanced lifestyle consistent with one's values, strengths, and interests through conscious adherence to daily health habits and efforts to reduce or minimize stress

Liver Function: ability of the liver to manufacture, store, alter, and secrete substances essential for metabolism and other body functions

Loneliness Severity: severity of emotional, social, or existential signs and symptoms of isolation

M

Maternal Status: Antepartum: extent to which maternal well-being is within normal limits from conception to the onset of labor

Maternal Status: Intrapartum: extent to which maternal well-being is within normal limits from onset of labor to delivery

Maternal Status: Postpartum: extent to which maternal well-being is within normal limits from delivery of placenta to completion of involution

Mechanical Ventilation Response: Adult: alveolar exchange and tissue perfusion are effectively supported by mechanical ventilation

Mechanical Ventilation Weaning Response: Adult: respiratory and psychological adjustment to progressive removal of mechanical ventilation

Medication Response: therapeutic and adverse effects of prescribed medication

Memory: ability to cognitively retrieve and report previously stored information

Metabolic Acidosis Severity: severity of signs and symptoms of decreased blood pH due to decreased bicarbonate and increased hydrogen ions

Metabolic Alkalosis Severity: severity of signs and symptoms of increased blood pH and bicarbonate due to conditions that cause excessive acid loss or increased bicarbonate retention

Mobility: ability to move purposefully in own environment independently with or without assistive device

Mood Equilibrium: appropriate adjustment of prevailing emotional tone in response to circumstances

Motivation: inner urge that moves or prompts an individual to positive action(s)

Mutilation Self-Restraint: personal actions to refrain from intentional self-inflicted injury (non-lethal)

N

Nausea & Vomiting Control: personal actions to control nausea, retching, and vomiting symptoms

Nausea & Vomiting: Disruptive Effects: severity of observed or reported disruptive effects of chronic nausea, retching, and vomiting on daily functioning

Nausea & Vomiting Severity: severity of signs and symptoms of nausea, retching, and vomiting

Neglect Cessation: evidence that the victim is no longer receiving substandard care

Neglect Recovery: extent of physical, emotional, and spiritual healing following the cessation of substandard care

Neurological Status: ability of the peripheral and central nervous systems to receive, process, and respond to internal and external stimuli

Neurological Status: Autonomic: ability of the autonomic nervous system to coordinate visceral and homeostatic functions

Neurological Status: Central Motor Control: ability of the central nervous system to coordinate skeletal muscle activity for body movement

Neurological Status: Consciousness: arousal, orientation, and attention to the environment

Neurological Status: Cranial Sensory/Motor Function: ability of the cranial nerves to convey sensory and motor impulses

Neurological Status: Peripheral: ability of the peripheral nervous system to transmit impulses to and from the central nervous system

Neurological Status: Spinal Sensory/Motor Function: ability of the spinal nerves to convey sensory and motor impulses

Newborn Adaptation: adaptive response to the extrauterine environment by a physiologically mature newborn during the first 28 days

Nutritional Status: extent to which nutrients are ingested and absorbed to meet metabolic needs

Nutritional Status: Biochemical Measures: body fluid components and chemical indices of nutritional status

Nutritional Status: Energy: extent to which nutrients provide cellular energy

Nutritional Status: Food & Fluid Intake: amount of food and fluid taken into the body over a 24-hour period

Nutritional Status: Nutrient Intake: nutrient intake to meet metabolic needs

O

Oral Health: condition of the mouth, teeth, gums, and tongue

Ostomy Self-Care: personal actions to maintain ostomy for elimination

P

Pain: Adverse Psychological Response: severity of observed or reported adverse cognitive and emotional responses to physical pain

Pain Control: personal actions to control pain

Pain: Disruptive Effects: severity of observed or reported disruptive effects of chronic pain on daily functioning

Pain Level: severity of observed or reported pain

Parent-Infant Attachment: parent and infant behaviors that demonstrate an enduring affectionate bond

Parenting Performance: parental actions to provide a child a nurturing and constructive physical, emotional, and social environment

Parenting Performance: Adolescent: parental actions to provide an adolescent with a safe, nurturing and positive physical, emotional, spiritual, and social environment from 12 years through 17 years

Parenting Performance: Adolescent Physical Safety: parental actions to prevent physical injury in an adolescent from 12 years through 17 years of age

Parenting Performance: Early/Middle Childhood Physical Safety: parental actions to avoid physical injury of a child from 3 years through 11 years of age

Parenting Performance: Infant: parental actions to provide an infant a safe, nurturing and positive physical, emotional, spiritual and social environment from 28 days to first birthday

Parenting Performance: Infant/Toddler Physical Safety: parental actions to prevent physical injury of a child from birth through 2 years of age

Parenting Performance: Middle Childhood: parental actions to provide a child with a safe, nurturing and positive physical, emotional, social, and spiritual environment from 6 years through 11 years

Parenting Performance: Preschooler: parental actions to provide a preschooler with a safe, nurturing and positive physical, emotional, spiritual, and social environment from 3 through 5 years

Parenting Performance: Psychosocial Safety: parental actions to protect a child from social contacts that might cause harm or injury

Parenting Performance: Toddler: parental actions to provide a child with a safe, nurturing and positive physical, emotional, spiritual, and social environment from 1 year through 2 years

Participation in Health Care Decisions: personal involvement in selecting and evaluating health care options to achieve desired outcome

Perimenopause Symptom Severity: severity of reported adverse physical and emotional responses due to declining hormonal levels

Peripheral Artery Disease Severity: severity of signs and symptoms of reduced peripheral blood flow due to atherosclerotic arteries in the extremities

Personal Autonomy: personal actions of a competent individual to exercise governance in life decisions

Personal Health Screening Behavior: personal actions to obtain recommended screening for early detection of a communicable or undetected disease

Personal Health Status: overall physical, psychological, social, and spiritual functioning of an adult 18 years or older

Personal Resiliency: positive adaptation and function of an individual following significant adversity or crisis

Personal Safety Behavior: personal actions to prevent unintentional physical injury to self

Personal Time Management: personal actions to complete commitments within an expected timeframe with minimum stress

Personal Well-Being: extent of positive perception of one's current health status

Physical Aging: normal physiological changes that occur with the natural aging process

Physical Fitness: performance of physical activities with vigor

Physical Injury Severity: severity of signs and symptoms of bodily injuries

Physical Maturation: Female: normal physical changes in the female that occur with the transition from childhood to adulthood

Physical Maturation: Male: normal physical changes in the male that occur with the transition from childhood to adulthood

Play Participation: use of activities by a child from 1 year through 11 years of age to promote enjoyment, entertainment, and development

Postpartum Maternal Health Behavior: personal actions to promote health of a mother in the period following birth of infant

Post-Procedure Recovery: extent to which an individual returns to baseline function following a procedure or minor surgery requiring anesthesia or sedation

Premenstrual Syndrome (PMS) Severity: severity of reported and adverse physical and emotional responses due to cyclic hormonal fluctuations

Prenatal Health Behavior: personal actions to promote a healthy pregnancy and a healthy newborn

Pre-Procedure Readiness: readiness of a patient to safely undergo a procedure requiring anesthesia or sedation

Preterm Infant Organization: extrauterine integration of physiologic and behavioral function by the infant born 24 to 37 (term) weeks gestation

Psychomotor Energy: personal drive and energy to maintain activities of daily living, nutrition, and personal safety

Psychosocial Adjustment: Life Change: adaptive psychosocial response of an individual to a significant life change

Q

Quality of Life: extent of positive perception of current life circumstances

R

Relocation Adaptation: adaptive emotional and behavioral response of a cognitively intact individual to a required change in living environment

Respiratory Status: movement of air in and out of the lungs and exchange of carbon dioxide and oxygen at the alveolar level

Respiratory Status: Airway Patency: open, clear tracheobronchial passages for air exchange

Respiratory Status: Gas Exchange: alveolar exchange of carbon dioxide and oxygen to maintain arterial blood gas concentrations

Respiratory Status: Ventilation: movement of air in and out of the lungs

Rest: quantity and pattern of diminished activity for mental and physical rejuvenation

Risk Control: personal actions to understand, prevent, eliminate, or reduce modifiable health threats

Risk Control: Alcohol Use: personal actions to understand, prevent, eliminate, or reduce the threats to health associated with alcohol use

Risk Control: Cancer: personal actions to understand, prevent, eliminate, or reduce the threat of cancer

Risk Control: Cardiovascular Disease: personal actions to understand, prevent, eliminate, or reduce the threat of cardiovascular disease

Risk Control: Drug Use: personal actions to understand, prevent, eliminate, or reduce the threats to health associated with drug use

Risk Control: Dry Eye: personal actions to understand, prevent, eliminate, or reduce the threat of dry eye

Risk Control: Hearing Impairment: personal actions to understand, prevent, eliminate, or reduce threats to hearing function

Risk Control: Hypertension: personal actions to understand, prevent, eliminate, or reduce the threat of high blood pressure

Risk Control: Hyperthermia: personal actions to understand, prevent, eliminate, or reduce the threat of high body temperature

Risk Control: Hypotension: personal actions to understand, prevent, eliminate, or reduce the threat of low blood pressure

Risk Control: Hypothermia: personal actions to understand, prevent, eliminate, or reduce the threat of low body temperature

Risk Control: Infectious Process: personal actions to understand, prevent, eliminate, or reduce the threat of acquiring an infection

Risk Control: Lipid Disorder: personal actions to understand, prevent, eliminate, or reduce the threat of hyperlipidemia

Risk Control: Osteoporosis: personal actions to understand, prevent, eliminate, or reduce the threat of osteoporosis

Risk Control: Sexually Transmitted Diseases (STD): personal actions to understand, prevent, eliminate, or reduce the threat of acquiring a sexually transmitted disease

Risk Control: Stroke: personal actions to understand, prevent, eliminate, or reduce the threat of a cerebral vascular accident

Risk Control: Sun Exposure: personal actions to understand, prevent, or reduce threats to skin and eyes from sun exposure

Risk Control: Thrombus: personal actions to understand, prevent, eliminate, or reduce the threat of thrombus formation or embolus

Risk Control: Tobacco Use: personal actions to understand, prevent, eliminate, or reduce the threats to health associated with tobacco use

Risk Control: Unintended Pregnancy: personal actions to understand, prevent, or reduce the possibility of unintended pregnancy

Risk Control: Visual Impairment: personal actions to understand, prevent, eliminate, or reduce threats to visual function

Risk Detection: personal actions to identify personal health threats

Role Performance: congruence of an individual's role behavior with role expectations

S

Safe Health Care Environment: physical and system arrangements to minimize factors that might cause physical harm or injury in the health care facility

Safe Home Environment: physical arrangements to minimize environmental factors that might cause physical injury in the home

Safe Wandering: safe, socially acceptable moving about without apparent purpose in an individual with cognitive impairment

Seizure Self-Control: personal actions to reduce or minimize the occurrence of seizure episodes

Self-Awareness: acknowledges one's strengths, limitations, values, feelings, attitudes, thoughts, and behaviors in relationship to the environment and others

Self-Care Status: personal actions to perform basic personal care activities and instrumental activities of daily living

Self-Care: Activities of Daily Living (ADL): personal actions to perform the most basic physical tasks and personal care activities independently with or without assistive device

Self-Care: Bathing: personal actions to cleanse own body independently with or without assistive device

Self-Care: Dressing: personal actions to dress self independently with or without assistive device

Self-Care: Eating: personal actions to prepare and ingest food and fluid independently with or without assistive device

Self-Care: Hygiene: personal actions to maintain own personal cleanliness and kempt appearance independently with or without assistive device

Self-Care: Instrumental Activities of Daily Living (IADL): personal actions to perform activities needed to function in the home or community independently with or without assistive device

Self-Care: Non-Parenteral Medication: personal actions to administer oral and topical medications to meet therapeutic goals independently with or without assistive device

Self-Care: Oral Hygiene: personal actions to care for own mouth and teeth independently with or without assistive device

Self-Care: Parenteral Medication: personal actions to administer parenteral medications to meet therapeutic goals independently with or without assistive device

Self-Care: Toileting: personal actions to toilet self independently with or without assistive device

Self-Direction of Care: care recipient actions taken to direct others who assist with or perform physical tasks and personal health care

Self-Esteem: personal judgment of self-worth

Self-Management: Acute Illness: personal actions to manage a reversible illness, its treatment, and to prevent complications

Self-Management: Anticoagulation Therapy: personal actions to manage therapy to maintain blood clotting time within a prescribed range and prevent complications

Self-Management: Asthma: personal actions to manage asthma, its treatment, and to prevent complications

Self-Management: Cardiac Disease: personal actions to manage heart disease, its treatment, and to prevent disease progression and complications

Self-Management: Chronic Disease: personal actions to manage a chronic disease, its treatment, and to prevent disease progression and complications

Self-Management: Chronic Obstructive Pulmonary Disease: personal actions to manage chronic obstructive pulmonary disease, its treatment, and to prevent disease progression and complications

Self-Management: Coronary Artery Disease: personal actions to manage coronary artery disease, its treatment, and to prevent disease progression and complications

Self-Management: Diabetes: personal actions to manage diabetes, its treatment, and to prevent complications

Self-Management: Dysrhythmia: personal actions to manage cardiac dysrhythmia, its treatment, and to prevent disease progression and complications

Self-Management: Heart Failure: personal actions to manage heart failure, its treatment, and to prevent disease progression and complications

Self-Management: Hypertension: personal actions to manage high blood pressure, its treatment, and to prevent complications

Self-Management: Kidney Disease: personal actions to manage kidney disease, its treatment, and to prevent disease progression and complications

Self-Management: Lipid Disorder: personal actions to manage hyperlipidemia, its treatment, and to prevent complications

Self-Management: Multiple Sclerosis: personal actions to manage multiple sclerosis and to prevent relapses and complications

Self-Management: Osteoporosis: personal actions to manage osteoporosis, its treatment, and to prevent disease progression and complications

Self-Management: Peripheral Artery Disease: personal actions to manage peripheral artery disease, its treatment, and to prevent disease progression

Sensory Function: ability to correctly sense skin stimulation, sounds, proprioception, taste and smell, and visual images

Sensory Function: Hearing: ability to correctly sense sounds

Sensory Function: Proprioception: ability to correctly sense position and movement of the head and body

Sensory Function: Tactile: ability to correctly sense stimulation of the skin

Sensory Function: Taste & Smell: ability to correctly sense chemicals that are inhaled or dissolved in saliva

Sensory Function: Vision: ability to correctly sense visual images

Sexual Functioning: integration of physical, socioemotional, and intellectual aspects of sexual expression and performance

Sexual Identity: acknowledgment and acceptance of own sexual identity

Shock Severity: Anaphylactic: severity of signs and symptoms of blood flow inadequate to perfuse tissues due to vasodilation and capillary permeability with a rapid-onset systemic hypersensitivity reaction

Shock Severity: Cardiogenic: severity of signs and symptoms of blood flow inadequate to perfuse tissues due to the heart's inability to contract and pump blood

Shock Severity: Hypovolemic: severity of signs and symptoms of blood flow inadequate to perfuse tissues due to a severe decrease in intravascular fluid volume

Shock Severity: Neurogenic: severity of signs and symptoms of blood flow inadequate to perfuse tissues due to sustained vasodilation resulting from a parasympathetic-sympathetic system imbalance

Shock Severity: Septic: severity of signs and symptoms of blood flow inadequate to perfuse tissues due to vasodilation resulting from the release of endotoxins with widespread infection

Skeletal Function: ability of the bones to support the body and facilitate movement

Sleep: natural periodic suspension of consciousness during which the body is restored

Smoking Cessation Behavior: personal actions to eliminate tobacco use

Social Anxiety Level: severity of irrational avoidance, apprehension, and distress in anticipation of or during social situations

Social Interaction Skills: personal behaviors that promote effective relationships

Social Involvement: social interactions with persons, groups, or organizations

Social Support: reliable assistance from others

Spiritual Health: connectedness with self, others, higher power, all life, nature, and the universe that transcends and empowers the self

Stress Level: severity of manifested physical or mental tension resulting from factors that alter an existing equilibrium

Student Health Status: overall physical, psychological, and social functioning of a school-age child

App

Substance Addiction Consequences: severity of change in health status and social functioning due to substance addiction

Substance Withdrawal Severity: severity of signs and symptoms of withdrawal from addictive drugs, tobacco, or alcohol

Suffering Severity: severity of signs and symptoms of long-term anguish due to a distressing event, injury, or loss

Suicide Self-Restraint: personal actions to refrain from gestures and attempts at killing self

Surgical Recovery: Convalescence: extent of physiologic, psychological, and role function following discharge from postanesthesia care to the final post-operative clinic visit

Surgical Recovery: Immediate Post-Operative: extent to which an individual achieves physiological baseline function following major surgery requiring anesthesia

Swallowing Status: safe passage of fluids and/or solids from the mouth to the stomach

Swallowing Status: Esophageal Phase: safe passage of fluids and/or solids from the pharynx to the stomach

Swallowing Status: Oral Phase: preparation, containment and posterior movement of fluids and/or solids in the mouth

Swallowing Status: Pharyngeal Phase: safe passage of fluids and/or solids from the mouth to the esophagus

Symptom Control: personal actions to minimize perceived adverse changes in physical and emotional functioning

Symptom Severity: severity of adverse physical, emotional, and social responses

Systemic Toxin Clearance: Dialysis: clearance of toxins from the body with peritoneal dialysis or hemodialysis

T

Thermoregulation: balance among heat production, heat gain, and heat loss

Thermoregulation: Newborn: balance among heat production, heat gain, and heat loss during the first 28 days of life

Tissue Integrity: Skin & Mucous Membranes: structural intactness and normal physiological function of skin and mucous membranes

Tissue Perfusion: adequacy of the blood flow through body organs to function at the cellular level

Tissue Perfusion: Abdominal Organs: adequacy of blood flow through the small vessels of the abdominal viscera to maintain organ function

Tissue Perfusion: Cardiac: adequacy of blood flow through the coronary vasculature to maintain heart function

Tissue Perfusion: Cellular: adequacy of blood flow through the vasculature to maintain function at the cellular level

Tissue Perfusion: Cerebral: adequacy of blood flow through the cerebral vasculature to maintain brain function

Tissue Perfusion: Peripheral: adequacy of blood flow through the small vessels of the extremities to maintain tissue function

Tissue Perfusion: Pulmonary: adequacy of blood flow through pulmonary vasculature to perfuse alveoli/capillary unit

Transfer Performance: ability to change body location independently with or without assistive device

U

Urinary Continence: control of elimination of urine from the bladder

Urinary Elimination: collection and discharge of urine

V

Vision Compensation Behavior: personal actions to compensate for visual impairment

Vital Signs: extent to which temperature, pulse, respiration, and blood pressure are within normal range

W

Weight: Body Mass: extent to which body weight, muscle, and fat are congruent to height, frame, gender, and age

Weight Gain Behavior: personal actions to gain weight following voluntary or involuntary significant weight loss

Weight Loss Behavior: personal actions to lose weight through diet, exercise, and behavior modification

Weight Maintenance Behavior: personal actions to maintain optimum body weight

Will to Live: desire, determination, and effort to survive

Wound Healing: Primary Intention: extent of regeneration of cells and tissues following intentional closure

Wound Healing: Secondary Intention: extent of regeneration of cells and tissues in an open wound

COMMONLY USED ABBREVIATIONS

NOTE: Abbreviations in common use can vary widely from place to place. Each institution's list of acceptable abbreviations is the best authority for its records.

ACLS	Advanced cardiac life support
ADD	Attention deficit disorder
ADL	Activities of daily living
AIDS	Acquired immunodeficiency syndrome
ALS	Advanced life support; amyotrophic lateral sclerosis
AM	Morning
AMI	Acute myocardial infarction
ASD	Atrial septal defect
AST	Aspartate aminotransferase (formerly SGOT)
A-V; AV; A/V	Arteriovenous; atrioventricular
BCLS	Basic cardiac life support
BE	Barium enema
bid; b.i.d.	Twice a day (bis in die)
BM	Bowel movement
BMR	Basal metabolic rate
BP	Blood pressure
BPH	Benign prostatic hypertrophy
bpm	Beats per minute
BSA	Body surface area
BSE	Breast self-examination
BUN	Blood urea nitrogen
Bx	Biopsy
c̄	With
CABG	Coronary artery bypass graft
CAD	Coronary artery disease
CAT	Computerized (axial) tomography scan
CBC; cbc	Complete blood count
CCU	Coronary care unit; critical care unit
CF	Cystic fibrosis
CHD	Congenital heart disease; coronary heart disease
CHF	Congestive heart failure
CK	Creatinine kinase
CMV	Cytomegalovirus
CNS	Central nervous system
c/o	Complaints of
CO	Carbon monoxide; cardiac output
CO_2	Carbon dioxide
COPD	Chronic obstructive pulmonary disease
COX	Cyclooxygenase
CP	Cerebral palsy; cleft palate
CPAP	Continuous positive airway pressure

CPK	Creatine phosphokinase
CPR	Cardiopulmonary resuscitation
CSF	Cerebrospinal fluid
CT	Computed tomography
CVA	Cerebrovascular accident; costovertebral angle
CVP	Central venous pressure
D & C	Dilation (dilatation) and curettage
dc; DC; D/C	Discontinue
DIC	Disseminated intravascular coagulation
diff	Differential blood count
DKA	Diabetic ketoacidosis
DM	Diabetes mellitus; diastolic murmur
DNA	Deoxyribonucleic acid
DNR	Do not resuscitate
DOA	Dead on arrival
DOB	Date of birth
DPT	Diphtheria-pertussis-tetanus
DRG	Diagnosis-related group
DSM-V	*Diagnostic and Statistical Manual of Mental Disorders*
DT	Delirium tremens
D_5W	Dextrose 5% in water
Dx	Diagnosis
EBV	Epstein-Barr virus
ECG	Electrocardiogram; electrocardiograph
ECHO	Echocardiography
ECT	Electroconvulsive therapy
ED	Emergency department
EDD	Estimated date of delivery
EEG	Electroencephalogram; electroencephalograph
EENT	Eye, ear, nose, and throat
ELISA	Enzyme-linked immunosorbent assay
EMG	Electromyogram
EMS	Emergency medical service
EMT	Emergency medical technician
ENT	Ear, nose, and throat
ER	Emergency room (hospital)
ERV	Expiratory reserve volume
ESR	Erythrocyte sedimentation rate
ESRD	End-stage renal disease
FBS	Fasting blood sugar
FEV	Forced expiratory volume
FH; Fhx	Family history
FHR	Fetal heart rate
FTT	Failure to thrive
fx	Fracture
GB	Gallbladder

GC	Gonococcus; gonorrheal
GI	Gastrointestinal
Grav I, II, etc.	Pregnancy one, two, three, etc. (Gravida)
GSW	Gunshot wound
gtt	Drops (guttae)
GU	Genitourinary
Gyn	Gynecology
H & P	History and physical
HAV	Hepatitis A virus
Hb	Hemoglobin
HBV	Hepatitis B virus
HCG	Human chorionic gonadotropin
HCT	Hematocrit
HDL	High-density lipoprotein
HEENT	Head, eye, ear, nose, and throat
HIV	Human immunodeficiency virus
h/o	History of
H_2O_2	Hydrogen peroxide
HR	Heart rate
HSV	Herpes simplex virus
HT; HTN	Hypertension
hx; Hx	History
I & O	Intake and output
IBW	Ideal body weight
ICP	Intracranial pressure
ICU	Intensive care unit
Ig	Immunoglobulin
IM	Intramuscular
IUD	Intrauterine device
IV	Intravenous
IVP	Intravenous pyelogram; intravenous push
KCl	Potassium chloride
KUB	Kidney, ureter, and bladder
L	Liter
lab	Laboratory
L & D	Labor and delivery
LDL	Low-density lipoprotein
LE	Lower extremity; lupus erythematosus
LMP	Last menstrual period
LOC	Level/loss of consciousness
LP	Lumbar puncture
LR	Lactated Ringer's
LVH	Left ventricular hypertrophy
MAP	Mean arterial pressure
MD	Muscular dystrophy
MDI	Medium dose inhalant; metered-dose inhaler
mEq	Milliequivalent
MI	Myocardial infarction
mm Hg	Millimeters of mercury

MMR	Maternal mortality rate; measles-mumps-rubella	PKU	Phenylketonuria	SIDS	Sudden infant death syndrome
MRI	Magnetic resonance imaging	PM	Evening	SLE	Systemic lupus erythematosus
MVA	Motor vehicle accident	PMH	Past medical history	SOB	Shortness of breath
N/A	Not applicable	PMI	Point of maximal impulse	s/s	Signs and symptoms
NaCl	Sodium chloride	PMN	Polymorphonuclear neutrophil leukocytes (polys)	Staph	Staphylococcus
NANDA	North American Nursing Diagnosis Association	PMS	Premenstrual syndrome	stat	Immediately (statim)
N & V; N/V	Nausea and vomiting	PO; p.o.	Orally (per os)	STD	Sexually transmitted disease
NG; ng	Nasogastric	PRN; p.r.n.	As required (pro re nata)	Strep	Streptococcus
NICU	Neonatal intensive care unit	pro time	Prothrombin time	Sx	Symptoms
NKA	No known allergies	pt	Pint	T	Temperature; thoracic
NPO; n.p.o.	Nothing by mouth (nil per os)	PT	Prothrombin time; physical therapy	T & A	Tonsillectomy and adenoidectomy
NSAID	Nonsteroidal antiinflammatory drug	PTT	Partial thromboplastin time	TB	Tuberculosis
NSR	Normal sinus rhythm	PVC	Premature ventricular contraction	TENS	Transcutaneous electrical nerve stimulation
O_2	Oxygen	R	Respiration; right; Rickettsia; roentgen	TIA	Transient ischemic attack
OB	Obstetrics	RBC; rbc	Red blood cell; red blood count	TMJ	Temporomandibular joint
OBS	Organic brain syndrome			TPN	Total parenteral nutrition
OR	Operating room	RDA	Recommended daily/dietary allowance	TPR	Temperature, pulse, and respiration
OTC	Over-the-counter	RDS	Respiratory distress syndrome	TSE	Testicular self-examination
PALS	Pediatric advanced life support	Rh	Symbol of rhesus factor	TSH	Thyroid-stimulating hormone
PACU	Postanesthesia care unit	RNA	Ribonucleic acid	Tx	Treatment
PCA	Patient-controlled analgesia	ROM	Range of motion	UA	Urinalysis
PE	Physical examination	ROS	Review of systems	URI	Upper respiratory infection
PEEP	Positive end-expiratory pressure	RR	Recovery room; respiratory rate	UTI	Urinary tract infection
PERRLA	Pupils equal, regular, reactive to light and accommodation	R/T	Related to	VC	Vital capacity
		$\bar{s}$	Without	vol	Volume
PET	Positron emission tomography	SGOT	Serum glutamic oxaloacetic transaminase	VS; v.s.	Vital signs
				VSD	Ventricular septal defect
PICC	Percutaneously inserted central catheter	SGPT	Serum glutamic pyruvic transaminase	WBC; wbc	White blood cell; white blood count
PID	Pelvic inflammatory disease	SI	Système International		